Brief Contents *Continued*

Medical-Surgical Nursing

CLINICAL MANAGEMENT for POSITIVE OUTCOMES

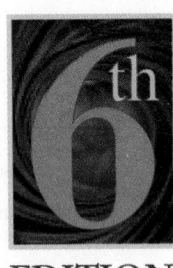

EDITION

Joyce M. Black, PhD, RN, CPSN, CCCN, CWCN
Assistant Professor
College of Nursing
University of Nebraska Medical Center
Omaha, Nebraska

Jane Hokanson Hawks, DNSc, MSN, RN, C
Associate Professor of Nursing
Midland Lutheran College
Fremont, Nebraska

Annabelle M. Keene, MSN, RN, C
Bellevue Public Schools
Bellevue, Nebraska
Formerly, Associate Professor
College of Saint Mary
Omaha, Nebraska

W.B. SAUNDERS COMPANY
An Imprint of Elsevier Science
Philadelphia London New York St. Louis Sydney Toronto

W.B. SAUNDERS COMPANY
An Imprint of Elsevier Science

The Curtis Center
Independence Square West
Philadelphia, Pennsylvania 19106

NOTICE

Nursing is an ever-changing field. Standard safety precautions must be followed, but as new research and clinical experience broaden our knowledge, changes in treatment and drug therapy may become necessary or appropriate. Readers are advised to check the most current product information provided by the manufacturer of each drug to be administered to verify the recommended dose, the method and duration of administration, and contraindications. It is the responsibility of the treating physician, relying on experience and knowledge of the patient, to determine dosages and the best treatment for each individual patient. Neither the Publisher nor the editor assumes any liability for any injury and/or damage to persons or property arising from this publication.

The Publisher

Library of Congress Cataloging-in-Publication Data

Medical-surgical nursing: clinical management for positive outcomes / edited by Joyce M. Black, Jane Hokanson Hawks, Annabelle Keene.—6th ed.

p.; cm.

Includes bibliographical references and index.

ISBN 0–7216–8198–0 (single volume)

ISBN 0–7216–8197–2 (2 vol set)

1. Nursing. 2. Surgical nursing. 3. Psychophysiology. I. Black, Joyce M. II. Hawks, Jane Hokanson. III. Keene, Annabelle.
[DNLM: 1. Nursing Care. 2. Perioperative Nursing. WY 150 M489365 2001]

RT41.L87 2001
610.73—dc21

99–089356

Vice-President and Nursing Editorial Director: Sally Schrefer
Executive Editor: Thomas Eoyang
Production Managers: Linda Garber, Natalie Ware
Developmental Editor: Victoria Legnini
Manuscript Editor: Carol J. Robins
Illustration Coordinator: Rita Martello
Design Coordinator: Karen O'Keefe Owens

MEDICAL-SURGICAL NURSING: Clinical Management for Positive Outcomes

Single volume 0–7216–8198–0
Two-volume set: 0–7216–8197–2

Printed in the United States of America.

Last digit is the print number: 9 8 7 6 5 4 3

There are several people at the University of Nebraska who seemingly never tire of my questions on how to explain or teach something more clearly. Thank you, Drs. Janet Cuddigan, Louise LaFramboise, and Barbara Manz. I also appreciate the countless students and patients who taught me the value of caring and teaching. I appreciate the expertise of the contributors to this text. And I thank my family for their ongoing understanding of the considerable strain on my time and energy.

J. M. B.

I want to thank my family, parents, and nursing friends from my doctoral and master's programs; my colleagues at Midland Lutheran College, Fremont, Nebraska; and my peers from the Iowa Nurses' Association and Society of Urologic Nurses and Associates (SUNA) who helped me with words of encouragement and support.

J. H. H.

To Chuck, Alice, and Clair. Words cannot express my thanks for your support of my projects, including this book. May you have similar support to pursue your dreams.

A. M. K.

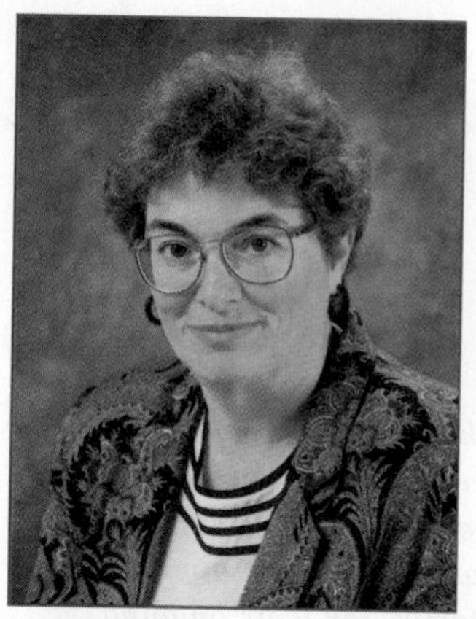

At the time of publication of the fifth edition, **Joyce M. Black, PhD, RN, CPSN, CCCN, CWCN,** was a Nursing Specialist with the Adult Health and Illness Department of the University of Nebraska Medical Center (UNMC). In December 1999 she received her Doctorate from the University of Nebraska College of Nursing. Her dissertation research focused on patient, wound, treatment, and health care system risk factors affecting the rate of pressure ulcer healing. Since graduation, she has returned to her position as Assistant Professor at UNMC, where she teaches medical-surgical nursing. She received her Master's degree from UNMC and her undergraduate degrees from Winona State University in Winona, Minnesota, and Rochester Community College in Rochester, Minnesota.

Dr. Black has also had several years of experience as a medical-surgical nurse at Saint Mary's Hospital, which is affiliated with the Mayo Clinic in Rochester, Minnesota. Her practice has included critical care, burns, respiratory disorders, orthopedics, and plastic surgery. She is certified by the American Society of Plastic and Reconstructive Surgical Nurses and Wound, Ostomy, and Continence Nurses, and she serves as editor of *Plastic Surgical Nursing*. Her area of research concerns pressure ulcers.

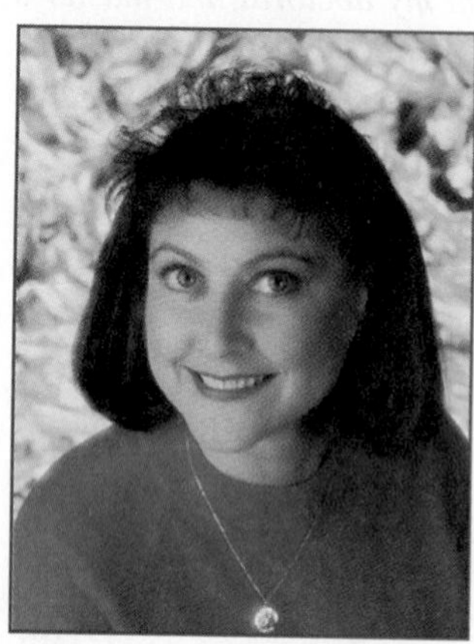

Jane Hokanson Hawks, DNSc, RN, C, is an Associate Professor of Nursing at Midland Lutheran College, Fremont, Nebraska. She teaches sophomore students in medical-surgical nursing and senior students in advanced medical-surgical nursing and nursing management. Dr. Hawks received her Doctorate of Nursing Science in collegiate nursing education from Widener University in Chester, Pennsylvania; her Master of Science degree in Nursing in medical-surgical nursing and nursing administration from UNMC in Omaha, Nebraska; and her Bachelor of Science degree in Nursing from St. Olaf College in Northfield, Minnesota.

Dr. Hawks has worked in and taught medical-surgical nursing for more than 22 years. She has practiced in a variety of areas, including critical care, renal transplantation, orthopedics, general surgery, and urology. She serves as the editor of *Urologic Nursing*. Her areas of research include empowerment and alcoholism. She and her colleagues developed the NANDA nursing diagnosis Altered Family Process: Alcoholism.

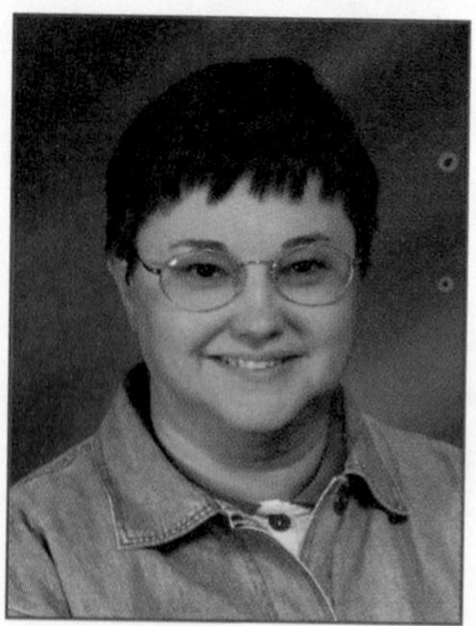

Annabelle M. Keene, MSN, RN, C, is a School Nurse with Bellevue Public Schools in Bellevue, Nebraska. She directs the health offices of several school buildings (approximately 2000 students and staff) and is certified by the State of Nebraska as a school nurse for grades K through 12. She also is a data analysis consultant for nursing graduate students who are studying nurses' perceptions of ethical problems across various specialty areas. Ms. Keene received her Master's degree from UNMC and her B.S.N. from Cornell University–New York Hospital School of Nursing, New York, New York.

Anne Keene has worked in and taught medical-surgical nursing for more than 25 years. She has been a staff nurse, a head nurse, a staff development instructor, and a nursing instructor in a multitude of clinical areas. She has been Assistant Professor at the University of Nebraska College of Nursing, teaching health assessment and medical-surgical nursing to undergraduate students. Anne also has been Associate Professor at the College of Saint Mary, Omaha, Nebraska, teaching in the undergraduate program. Ms. Keene is certified in medical-surgical nursing by the American Nurses Credentialing Center.

Contributors

Mary A. Allen, MS, RN
Clinical Trials Specialist, National Institute of Allergy and Infectious Diseases, National Institutes of Health, Bethesda, Maryland

Chris Stewart Amidei, MSN, RN, CNRN, CCRN
Clinical Nurse Specialist, University of Chicago, Chicago, Illinois

Helen Andrews, RN, BSN
Care Manager, Alegent Health Bergan Mercy Medical Center, Omaha, Nebraska

Jane Allen Austgen, RN, BSN, CRNH
Hospice Nurse Care Manager, Alegent Health Home Care & Hospice, Omaha, Nebraska

Susan Baker, DNS, RN
Instructor, Indiana University School of Nursing, Indianapolis, Indiana

Patricia McCallig Bates, BSN, CURN
Clinical Urology Nurse, Urology Department, Kaiser-Permanente, Portland, Oregon

Deborah L. Bayliss, MS, RN
Community Nurse Care Manager, Poudre Valley Health System, Fort Collins, Colorado

Francie Bernier, BSN, RN, C
Clinical Consultant for Continence Care, Independent Urologic/Urogynecologic Clinical Consultant, Specialist in Continence Care, Leesburg, Virginia

Deborah S. Bjerstedt, MSN, RN, CS, FNP
Family Nurse Practitioner, Allina Medical Group, Shoreview, St. Paul, Minnesota

Hilary S. Blackwood, MSN, RN
Clinician III, Surgical Nutrition Support Services, University of Virginia Health System, Charlottesville, Virginia

Meg Blair, BA, BSN, MSN
Assistant Professor, Nebraska Methodist College of Nursing and Allied Health; Staff Nurse, Emergency Department, St. Joseph's Hospital, Omaha, Nebraska

R. B. Boley, PhD
Professor (Ret.), Biology Department, University of Texas at Arlington, Arlington, Texas

Cynthia A. Bolin, RN
Program Coordinator, Congestive Heart Failure Management Center, St. Luke's Hospital, St. Louis, Missouri

Shawnda Braun, RN
Case Manager, Allied Health Alternatives, Inc., Faribault, Minnesota

Sarah Jo Brown, PhD, RN
Principal and Consultant, Practice-Research Integrations, Norwich, Vermont

Terri Sellin Brown, BSN, RN
School Nurse, Omaha Public Schools, Omaha, Nebraska

Mary Vorder Bruegge
Clinician IV, Nerancy Neuro ICU, University of Virginia Health System, Charlottesville, Virginia

Candace Cantwell, RD
Clinical Dietitian, Clinical Nutrition Support Services, University of Pennsylvania Health System, Philadelphia, Pennsylvania

Robert G. Carroll, PhD
Professor of Physiology, Brody School of Medicine, East Carolina University, Greenville, North Carolina

Bernice B. Christopher, BSN, RN
Keystone Mercy Health Plan, Philadelphia, Pennsylvania

Linda K. Clarke, MS, RN, CORLN
Head and Neck Nurse Specialist, Greater Baltimore Medical Center, Towson, Maryland

Marsha E. Cloud, BSN, RN
Clinician II, Surgical Services, University of Virginia Health System, Charlottesville, Virginia

Linda Carman Copel, PhD, RN, CS, DAPA, ACFE, CGP, CFLE
Associate Professor, Villanova University, Villanova, Pennsylvania; Psychotherapist, Private Practice, Ardmore, Pennsylvania

Pamela Cornwell, MA, RN
Manager, Intensive and Intermediate Care Units, Shriners Hospitals for Children, Northern California, Sacramento, California

Sherill Nones Cronin, PhD, RN, C
Professor of Nursing, Bellarmine College; Nurse Researcher, Jewish Hospital, Louisville, Kentucky

Janice Z. Cuzzell, MA, RN
Vice President, Island Home Care, Inc., Savannah, Georgia

Jean Elizabeth DeMartinis, PhD, APRN, FNP-C
Assistant Professor and Director of the Masters in Cardiac Health and Rehabilitation CNS/ANP Program, Creighton University School of Nursing, Omaha, Nebraska

Kaye M. Dietrich, MS, RN, C
Consultant, Kiel, Wisconsin

Peggy Doheny, PhD, MSN, RN
Associate Professor, Kent State University College of Nursing, Kent, Ohio

Rebecca M. Dudley, RN
Staff Nurse, Fairview Lakes HomeCaring & Hospice, Chisago City, Minnesota

Kimberly Elgin, BSN, RN
Clinician III, Clinical Manager, Surgical Services, University of Virginia Health System, Charlottesville, Virginia

Charlotte Eliopoulos, PhD, MPH, RN, C
President, Health Education Network, Glen Arm, Maryland

James A. Fain, PhD, RN, FAAN
Associate Professor and Director, PhD Nursing Program, University of Massachusetts Graduate School of Nursing, Worcester, Massachusetts

Kathryn Fiandt, DNS, ARNP
Associate Professor, University of Nebraska College of Nursing; Coordinator, Family Nurse Practitioner Program, University of Nebraska Medical Center; Clinical Director, Family Health Care Center, Omaha, Nebraska

Mary L. Fisher, PhD, RN, CNAA
Associate Professor, Nursing Administration, Indiana University School of Nursing, Indianapolis, Indiana

Susan Flannigan, MPH, RN, ANP
Adult Nurse Practitioner, Fairview Lakes Medical Center, Chisago City, Minnesota

Ann K. Frantz, BSN, RN
Independent Health Care Consultant, Pontiac, Michigan

Anne Marie Johnson Fredrichs, MSN, RN, CPNP
Research Coordinator, Nebraska Foundation for Spinal Research, Omaha, Nebraska

Peggy Gerard, DNSc, RN
Professor, School of Nursing, Purdue University, Calumet, Hammond, Indiana

Nancy Girard, PhD, MSN, RN
Associate Professor and Chair, Acute Nursing Care Department, University of Texas Medical School at San Antonio, School of Nursing, San Antonio, Texas

Elizabeth W. Good, MSN, RN, C
Clinician III, Urology Care Coordinator, Surgical Services, University of Virginia Health System, Charlottesville, Virginia

Michelle Goodman, MS, RN, OCN
Assistant Professor of Nursing, Rush University College of Nursing; Oncology Clinical Nurse Specialist, Section of Medical Oncology, Rush Cancer Institute, Rush Presbyterian–St. Luke's Medical Center, Chicago, Illinois

Lisa A. Gorski, MS, RN
Clinical Nurse Specialist, Covenant Home Health and Hospice, Milwaukee, Wisconsin

Maribeth Guzzo, MSN, RN, CRNP
Nurse Practitioner, Division of Cardiology, the Hospital of the University of Pennsylvania, Philadelphia, Pennsylvania

Sheila A. Haas, PhD, RN
Dean and Professor, Loyola University of Chicago Marcella Niehoff School of Nursing, Chicago, Illinois

Diana P. Hackbarth, PhD, RN
Professor, Department of Community, Mental Health, and Administrative Nursing, Loyola University of Chicago Marcella Niehoff School of Nursing, Chicago, Illinois

Linda R. Haddick, MSN, RN
Clinical Nurse Specialist, Alegent Health Home Care & Hospice, Omaha, Nebraska

Margie Hansen, PhD, RN
Clinical Associate Professor, Family Nurse Practitioner Program, University of North Dakota College of Nursing, Grand Forks, North Dakota

Karen A. Hanson, MS, RN, CNP
Urology Nurse Practitioner, Mayo Clinic, Rochester, Minnesota

Tammi G. Hardiman, BSN, RN
Nurse Consultant, Community Services Quality Assurance, Department of Social and Health Services, State of Washington, Arlington, Washington

Jeannine Mueller Harmon, MSN, RN, FNP, CS
Family Nurse Practitioner, Metropolitan State University, St. Paul, Minnesota

Debra E. Heidrich, MSN, RN, AOCN, CHPN
Nursing Consultant, West Chester, Ohio

Esther A. Hellman, PhD, RN
Assistant Professor, Creighton University School of Nursing, Omaha, Nebraska

Beverley E. Holland, PhD, MSN, ARNP
Associate Professor, Lansing School of Nursing, Bellarmine College, Louisville, Kentucky

Rhonda Holloway, BSN, RN, MBA, NP
Women's Wellness Center, Lone Tree, Colorado

Roberta Jorgensen, BSN
Gastrointestinal Nurse Coordinator, Mayo Clinic, Rochester, Minnesota

Juanita Fogel Keck, DNS, BSN
Associate Professor, Indiana University School of Nursing, Indianapolis, Indiana

Catherine A. Kernich, MSN, RN
Clinical Faculty, Frances Payne Bolton School of Nursing, Case Western Reserve University; Director, Ambulatory Practice, Department of Medicine; University Faculty Services, University Hospitals Health Systems, Cleveland, Ohio

Helene J. Krouse, PhD, ARNP, CORLN
Associate Professor of Nursing, University of Florida College of Nursing, Gainesville, Florida

Kim K. Kuebler, MN, RN, ANP-CS
Adjunct Faculty, College of Nursing and Health Sciences, Saginaw Valley State University, University Center, Michigan; Adult Nurse Practitioner, Oncology/Palliative Care, Private Practice, Adjuvant Therapies, Inc., Lake, Michigan

Joanie J. Kush, MS, RN
Director of Hospice, Visiting Nurse Association of Omaha, Omaha, Nebraska

Louise Nelson LaFramboise, PhD, RN
Assistant Professor, University of Nebraska College of Nursing, Omaha, Nebraska

Joan Lappe, PhD, RN
Associate Professor, Creighton University Schools of Nursing and Medicine, Omaha, Nebraska

Anne Larson, PhD, MS, BA, RN, C
Associate Professor of Nursing, Midland Lutheran College, Fremont, Nebraska

Joyce Larson-Presswalla, PhD, RN
President, "Culture Counts," Marketing Coordinator, James A. Haley Veterans Hospital, Tampa, Florida

Cindi Leo-Gofta, BSN, RN
Operations Director, Resource and Referral/Business Development, Alegent Health Home Care & Hospice, Omaha, Nebraska

James Higgy Lerner, RN, LAc
Private practice of acupuncture, traditional Oriental medicine, and biofeedback, Chico, California

Cindy Ludwig, MS, RN
Nurse Manager, Providence Saint Joseph Medical Center, Burbank, California

Cyndy Hunt Luzinski, MS, RN
Community Nurse Case Manager, Poudre Valley Health System, Fort Collins, Colorado

Donna W. Markey, MSN, RN, ACNP-CS
Clinician IV, Surgical Services, University of Virginia Health System, Charlottesville, Virginia

Karen S. Martin, MSN, RN, FAAN
Health Care Consultant, Martin Associates, Omaha, Nebraska

Cynthia McCurren, PhD, MSN
Associate Professor, University of Louisville School of Nursing; Nurse Researcher, University of Louisville Hospital, Louisville, Kentucky

James McLean, BSN, RN, WOCN
Enterostomal Therapist, Fort Worth, Texas

Norma D. McNair, MSN, RN, CCRN, CNRN, CS
Assistant Clinical Professor, University of California, Los Angeles, School of Nursing; Clinical Nurse III, Liver Transplant and Surgical Subspecialties, Intensive Care Unit, UCLA Medical Center, Los Angeles, California

Mary E. McQuinn, RPT
Physical Therapist, Visiting Nurse Association of Omaha, Omaha, Nebraska

Colette H. McVaney, BSN, RN
Lead Nurse, Geriatric Clinic, Nebraska Health System, Omaha, Nebraska

Patricia Meier, MA, BSN, RN, AOCN
Nurse Manager, Shady Grove Adventist Hospital, Rockville, Maryland

Stephanie Mellon-Reppen, MSN, RN, ACNP, OCN
Acute Care Nurse Practitioner and Oncology Certified Nurse, Section of Bone Marrow Transplant and Cell Therapy, Rush Presbyterian–St. Luke's Medical Center, Chicago, Illinois

Melanie Minton, BSN, RN, MBA, CNRN
Lead Adjunct Faculty, Le Tourneau University; Nurse Specialist, Nursing Support and Patient Education, The Methodist Hospital, Houston, Texas

Kim Miracle, MSN, RN, C
Clinical Nurse Specialist, Outcomes Manager, Jewish Hospital, Louisville, Kentucky

Anita E. Molzahn, PhD, MN
Professor, School of Nursing, and Dean, Faculty of Human and Social Development, University of Victoria, Victoria, British Columbia, Canada

Bernadette K. Mruz, RN
Clinical Manager, Visiting Nurse Association of Omaha, Omaha, Nebraska

Elizabeth A. Murphy-Blake, MSEd, MS, RN, ARNP
Assistant Professor of Nursing, Midland Lutheran College, Fremont, Nebraska

Pamela J. Nelson, MS, RN
Assistant Professor of Nursing, Bethel College, St. Paul, Minnesota

Noreen Heer Nicol, MS, RN, FNP
Clinical Senior Instructor, University of Colorado School of Nursing; Director of Nursing, Dermatology Clinical Specialist and Nurse Practitioner, National Jewish Medical and Research Center, Denver, Colorado

Cheryl Noetscher, MS, RN
Director of Case Management, Crouse Hospital and Community–General Hospital, Syracuse, New York

Janice D. Nunnelee, PhD, RN, CS/ANP, CRN
Clinical Associate Professor of Nursing, University of Missouri–St. Louis. Adult Nurse Practitioner, Vascular Nurse Practitioner, Unity Medical Group, St. Louis, Missouri

Barbara B. Ott, PhD, RN, CCRN
Associate Professor, Villanova University College of Nursing, Villanova, Pennsylvania

Arlene L. Polaski, MEd, MSN, RN
Program Director (Ret.), York Technical College/University of South Carolina Lancaster Cooperative Program in Associate Degree Nursing, Rock Hill, South Carolina

Kathleen Popelka, DNSc, CFNP
Family Nurse Practitioner, Women's Veterans Coordinator, Veterans Administration Medical Center, Omaha, Nebraska

David Porta, PhD
Associate Professor, Bellarmine University; Adjunct Faculty, University of Louisville School of Medicine, Louisville, Kentucky

Kathleen Rea, BSN, RN
Clinician III, Clinical Manager, Surgical Services, University of Virginia Health System, Charlottesville, Virginia

Marlene Reimer, PhD, RN, CNN(C)
Associate Dean, Research and Graduate Programs, University of Calgary Faculty of Nursing, Calgary, Canada

Roxanne Rivard, BSN, RN, CWOCN
Enterostomal Therapy Nurse, Fairview Lakes, HomeCaring & Hospice, Chisago City, Minnesota

Dottie Roberts, MSN, MACI, RN, C, ONC, CNS
Medical-Surgical Clinical Nurse Specialist, Penrose–St. Francis Health Services, Colorado Springs, Colorado

Helen Murdock Rogers, BS, MS, DNSc
Associate Professor, Adult Health, Research, and Physical Assessment, Department of Nursing, Worcester State College; Community Nurse, University of Massachusetts, Memorial Home Health, Worcester, Massachusetts

Amy Perrin Ross, MSN, RN, CNRN
Neuroscience Program Coordinator, Loyola University Medical Center, Maywood, Illinois

Vicki M. Ross, MSN, RN
Nurse Clinician, Nutritional Support Services, Truman Medical Center, Kansas City, Missouri

Pamela K. Schaid, MA, RN
Administrator, Seasons Hospice, Rochester, Minnesota

Nancy J. Scheet, MSN, RN
Compliance Officer, Visiting Nurse Association of Omaha, Omaha, Nebraska

Linda Ludy Scott, MS, CFNP
Nurse Practitioner, National Institute of Allergy and Infectious Diseases, Laboratory of Allergic Diseases, National Institutes of Health, Bethesda, Maryland

Carol Sedlak, PhD, MSN, RN
Assistant Professor, Kent State University College of Nursing, Kent, Ohio

Judy Selfridge-Thomas, MSN, RN, CEN, FNP
Nurse Practitioner, Department of Emergency Medicine, St. Mary Medical Center, Long Beach, California; General Partner, Selfridge, Sparger, Shea and Associates, Ventura and Orange Counties, California

Carol Sharkey, MSN, PhD
Associate Professor, Department of Nursing, Regis University, Denver, Colorado

Sandra Sharma, PhD, ARNP, CS
James A. Haley Veterans Hospital, Tampa, Florida

Suzanne Shaw, BSN, RN
Director, Walls Regional Hospital Home Health, Cleburne, Texas

Nancy Shoemaker, MS, RN, CS-P
Nursing Program Consultant, State of Maryland, Department of Public Safety and Correctional Services, Jessup, Maryland

Mary Sieggreen, MSN, RN, CS, NP, CUN
Assistant Professor, Wayne State University; Clinical Nurse Specialist/Nurse Practitioner, Vascular Surgery, Harper Hospital, Detroit Medical Center, Detroit, Michigan

Pamela Singh, CS, MSN, RN, FNP
Family Nurse Practitioner, San Diego, California

Dianne Smolen, PhD, MSN, RN, C
Associate Professor and Director of Continuing Nursing Education, Medical College of Ohio School of Nursing, Toledo, Ohio

Debra A. Solomon, MSN, RN, FNP-C
Clinical Coordinator, Fairview Lakes HomeCaring & Hospice, Chisago City, Minnesota

Kimberly Stallo, BSN, RN, CETN
Wound, Ostomy, and Continence Nurse, Fort Worth, Texas

Mary M. Stasiak, MA, BSN, RN, PHN
Case Manager, Allied Health Alternatives, Inc., Rochester, Minnesota

Eleanor M. Stockbridge, MS, CRRN, FNP
Community Nurse Case Manager, Poudre Valley Health System, Fort Collins, Colorado

Nancy Evans Stoner, MSN, RN, CNSN
Education Manager, Clinical Nutrition Support Services, University of Pennsylvania Health System, Philadelphia, Pennsylvania

Linda J. Svatora, OTR/L, MBA
Occupational Therapist, Visiting Nurse Association of Omaha, Omaha, Nebraska

Janice Tazbir, MS
Assistant Professor, Purdue University Calumet, Hammond, Indiana

Jill E. Timm, BAN, RN, PHN
Public Health Nurse II, Washington County Department of Public Health and Environment, Stillwater, Minnesota

Peter J. Ungvarski, MS, RN, FAAN, ACRN
Clinical Associate Professor, City University of New York, Hunter College–Bellevue School of Nursing; Clinical Nurse Specialist, HIV/AIDS, and Clinical Director, AIDS Services, The Visiting Nurse Service of New York, New York, New York

Linda A. Vader, BS, RN, CRNO
Head Nurse, W. K. Kellogg Eye Center, University of Michigan, Ann Arbor, Michigan

Amy Verst, MSN, RN, CPNP, ATC
Assistant Professor, Bellarmine College; Pediatric Nurse Practitioner, Jefferson County Health Department, Louisville, Kentucky

Bernadette White, MSN, RN
Assistant Professor, Creighton University School of Nursing, Omaha, Nebraska

Connie White-Williams, MSN, RN, FNP
Affiliate Faculty and Cardiothoracic Transplant Coordinator, University of Alabama, Birmingham, Alabama

Gail F. Wilkerson, MSN, RN, CS
Disease Management Specialist, Heart Failure, Group Health Plan, St. Louis, Missouri

Linda Yoder, MSN, MBA, PhD
Colonel, United States Army Nurse Corps, McDonald Army Community Hospital, Fort Eustis, Virginia

Nancy York, MSN, RN
Assistant Professor of Nursing, Bellarmine College, Lansing School of Nursing, Louisville, Kentucky

Bridget A. Young, BSN, RN, MBA
Vice President of Clinical Services, Visiting Nurse Association of Omaha, Omaha, Nebraska

Reviewers

Jan Anderson, MSN, RN, CNS
Assistant Director, ADN Program, Santa Barbara City College, Santa Barbara, California

Linda J. Becker, MSN, RN, C
Department Chair, St. Clair County Community College, Port Huron, Michigan

Barbara J. Benz, MS
Roswell Park Cancer Institute, Buffalo, New York

Veronica K. Casey, MA, RN, C
Assistant Professor, Norwalk Community-Technical College, Norwalk, Connecticut

Joy Churchill, MSN, RN
Northern Kentucky University, Highland Heights, Kentucky

Betty R. Ferrell, PhD, RN, FAAN
City of Hope National Medical Center, Duarte, California

Kay Fitterer, MA, RN
Central Lakes College, Brainerd, Minnesota

Gloria J. Green, PhD, MSN, RN
Southeast Missouri State University, Cape Girardeau, Missouri

Angie B. Greer, MSN, RN, CS
Henderson State University, Arkadelphia, Arkansas

Joyce Harris, MA, RN
Director, Butler County Program of Practical Nursing Education, Hamilton, Ohio

JoAnn Romanzi Herne, MS, RNC, FNP-CS
Student Health Supervisor, Crouse Hospital School of Nursing, Syracuse, New York

Robin Higley, MSN
Fairview Hospital, Cleveland, Ohio

Sheilagh Helen Hunt, BA, RN
Certificate in Palliative Care and Thanatology; Professor, Fanshawe College, London, Ontario, Canada

Mary Jane Jones, MN, RN
Associate Professor, Henderson Community College, Henderson, Kentucky

Elizabeth A. Kassel, MSN, RN
Assistant Professor, Syracuse University, Crouse Hospital School of Nursing, University Hospital, Syracuse, New York

Anne Larson, PhD, RN, C
Associate Professor, Midland Lutheran College, Fremont, Nebraska

Suzanne K. Marnocha, MSN, RN, CCRN
Assistant Professor, University of Wisconsin, Oshkosh, Oshkosh, Wisconsin

Jeanette A. McNeill, DrPH, RN, AOCN
Associate Professor/Department Chair, School of Nursing, University of Texas, Houston, Houston, Texas

Captain John J. Melvin, BSN, RN, CCRN
Brooke Army Medical Center, Fort Sam Houston, Texas

Christine C. Mihal, MS, RN, CS
Lecturer, Fairleigh Dickinson University, Teaneck, New Jersey

Carla Mueller, MS, RN
Associate Professor, Department of Nursing, University of Saint Francis, Fort Wayne, Indiana

Elizabeth A. O'Connor, MSN, RNCS, FWP, CCRN
Montana State University at Bozeman, College of Nursing, Great Falls, Montana

Netha O'Meara, MS, RN, CNS
Former Director of Associate Degree Nursing, Wharton County Junior College, Wharton, Texas

Kay B. O'Neal, MSN, RN
El Centro Community College, Dallas, Texas

Molly R. Parker, MHR, BSed, RN
Practical Nursing Program Director, Green Country Area Vocational-Technical School, Okmulgee, Oklahoma

Diana Reding, MS, RN
El Centro College, Parkland Hospital, Dallas, Texas

Lisa Anderson Shaw, DrPH, MSN, MA, RN, CS
Clinical Instructor, Medical/Surgical Nursing, University of Illinois at Chicago College of Nursing; Clinical Ethics Consultant, University of Illinois at Chicago Medical Center, Chicago, Illinois

Beth Ann Stevenson, MSN, RN, CS
School Nurse, Columbus Public Schools; Nurse Clinician, Ohio Department of Health, Columbus, Ohio

Martha Summers, MSN, C-FNP
West Virginia University, Morgantown, West Virginia

Janice M. Thompson, PhD, MSN, RN, C
Associate Professor, Quinnipiac College, Hamden, Connecticut

Lieutenant Michael Welker, BSN, RN, AN
Brooke Army Medical Center, Fort Sam Houston, Texas

Charlene A. Winters, DNSc, RNCS
Montana State University, Missoula, Montana

Preface

It is our conviction that a book is not a static document. Certainly, a book—bound and printed—portrays health care at a given moment in time. The sixth edition of *Medical-Surgical Nursing* is our best attempt to provide instructors and students with a guide to delivering safe and appropriate nursing care. To that end, we see this book as a "work in progress." Future editions will continue to improve, and we appreciate your comments, questions, and corrections to guide our ongoing work. We can improve only with your input. We also realize that educators and students must share in the task of bringing the book to life.

PHILOSOPHY AND APPROACH

This text grows out of the belief that nurses and physicians do not compete with each other but instead collaborate to reach certain outcomes in cooperation with the client and family. Nonetheless, nursing and medicine are separate disciplines. Consequently, in this text nursing and medical content are not intermingled. However, because nursing and medicine are collaborative efforts, it is often difficult for nursing students to understand one without having an understanding of the other. We therefore present thorough coverage of both nursing management and medical management.

With the increased emphasis on outcomes in health care, we have organized client care under the heading of Outcome Management. Several headings appear under this heading, including: Medical Management, Nursing Management of the Medical Client, Surgical Management, and Nursing Management of the Surgical Client, as appropriate.

In this text, we use the nursing process to describe nursing management but we do not apply the nursing process to every disorder. Instead, we have designated the nursing process for major or prototypical disorders. Within the presentation of the nursing process for those disorders, we have developed nursing diagnoses and collaborative problems, as appropriate, with their own outcomes and interventions. Collaborative problems define those client problems that are not resolvable through independent nursing actions; they are potential complications that may develop because of a disorder, a surgical procedure, or a nonsurgical treatment. Collaborative problems complete the picture of nursing care and eliminate the need to force-fit every client problem into the framework of nursing diagnosis. We have written Outcomes and Intervention sections for *each* identified nursing diagnosis and collaborative problem because we have found, from our teaching experience, that students cannot easily pull apart lists of diagnoses, followed by lists of outcomes and interventions, and rebuild them into care plans.

ORGANIZATION

This edition is organized from simple to complex and from common to uncommon disorders. The early portion of the text focuses on care of clients usually assigned to beginning students. The book then progresses to address care of clients with more complex disorders, which are more commonly taught in upper division classes.

Another change in organization is the use of separate chapters for complex disorders, such as renal failure, the need for transplantation, AIDS/HIV, respiratory failure, myocardial infarction, and central nervous system trauma. These disorders are complex and more commonly addressed in upper division course work. We also separate some other material on fluids and electrolytes, stroke, immune disorders, and nutrition to provide adequate coverage and to differentiate major concepts for these disorders.

The sixth edition is divided into 17 units. The first three units are devoted to content that is applicable to all medical-surgical clients. The material in this first portion of the book will guide the student in learning to provide comprehensive care regardless of the specific diagnosis or problem. Concepts that span medical-surgical practice, such as health promotion, care delivery settings, pain, perioperative care, and oncology, are found in this portion of the book. The remainder of the text is divided into common responses to health disorders. Most of these units begin with a review of anatomy and physiology, followed by a chapter on health and diagnostic assessment; thereafter, one or more "Nursing Care" chapters present the nursing care of clients with specific disorders.

Unit 2 presents an overview of nursing and health care today. Chapter 4 describes the "stakeholders" in health care delivery, because medical-surgical nurses (not just managers) in all areas of practice must be increasingly aware of how health care is financed. Because the practice of medical-surgical nursing is not confined to certain areas, more material has been added to this edition on nursing care and philosophy in various care settings. Chapters 5 through 8 address nursing care in ambulatory, acute, home health, and long-term care settings.

Unit 3 covers health assessment, physical examination, and diagnostic testing. The format for health assessment and physical examination that is introduced in Chapters 9 and 10 is carried through in the Assessment chapters for each body system. This structure helps the student to become familiar with one form of thorough assessment and then to apply it in a focused way for clients with specific disorders.

Unit 4 looks at concepts that are common to many medical-surgical clients. Fluid and electrolyte disorders have been separated into two chapters. Other chapters address acid-base disorders, the surgical experience, wound healing, infectious disorders, cancer, psychosocial and mental health concerns, and sleep and sensory disorders, including new material on fatigue and pain. New to this edition is a chapter on end-of-life concerns (Chapter 22). Material on substance abuse has been moved forward into the introductory material because of the increasing numbers of people with substance abuse problems. Chapter 24 discusses the effects of substance abuse on major body systems. It also identifies populations at risk for substance abuse and presents strategies for care.

Units 5 through 16 focus on management of clients with specific disorders. Each unit begins with a structure and function overview of the pertinent body systems as well as a nursing assessment chapter. The structure and function overview has been shortened and redesigned, with more artwork added for each body system.

Discussion of specific disorders generally includes headings for Etiology, Pathophysiology, Clinical Manifestations, and Outcome Management. Because more and more nursing care is being directed toward health promotion, in this edition we have added content focusing on health promotion, health maintenance, and health restoration to the Risk Factors and Etiology topics in chapters on disorders. To emphasize the importance of understanding pathophysiology and its relationship to treatment of a disorder, we have incorporated headings in the management sections that will help the student see the relationship between the pathophysiologic changes and specific strategies to promote positive outcomes in nursing management. The term "clinical manifestations" has been selected to encompass signs and symptoms along with diagnostic findings. The term "manifestations" replaces "signs and symptoms" in all chapters except one; in Chapter 22, "end-of-life symptom management" is the preferred term.

The major content areas for Units 5 through 16 are mobility disorders (Unit 5); nutritional disorders, including ingestive and digestive disorders as well as a new chapter on malnutrition (Unit 6); elimination disorders, including urinary and intestinal problems (Unit 7); sexuality and reproductive disorders (Unit 8); metabolic disorders (Unit 9); integumentary disorders (Unit 10); circulatory disorders (Unit 11); cardiac disorders (Unit 12); oxygenation disorders (Unit 13); sensory disorders (Unit 14); cognitive and perceptual disorders (Unit 15); and protective disorders (Unit 16).

Unit 17 presents care of clients with multisystem disorders. A new chapter, Chapter 79, covers care of the client with HIV infection and AIDS. Chapter 80, also new, looks at organ donation issues, the transplantation process, quality of life issues, and specific interventions for clients requiring organ transplantation. Shock and multisystem disorders are discussed in Chapter 81. Chapter 82 examines the basic concepts of triage, ethical issues, and maintaining the chain of custody of medicolegal evidence. The chapter organizes emergency conditions by various nursing diagnoses identified and treated.

SPECIAL FEATURES

Bridging the gap between classroom instruction and clinical nursing care is difficult. We find that students often think, "I learned that for a test last year," and question how the material is relevant to the clinical situations that they face today. To address those questions, Joyce Black has devised a method of clinical teaching in which the pathophysiology of a disorder is presented graphically and is then overlaid with corresponding clinical manifestations and treatments. The overlays allow students to visualize how changes in pathophysiology lead to certain manifestations and how a particular treatment is designed to block the progression of the pathophysiologic changes into the development of clinical manifestations. Underlying this teaching method is the assumption that it is easier to "transfer" material if you can visualize the links among pathophysiology, clinical manifestations, and interventions. The fifth edition incorporated this teaching method in special features called **Pathophysiology/Treatment Algorithms (PTAs).** These features are presented on such topics as "Understanding Asthma and Its Treatment." A new PTA on Cushing's disease has been added because of the positive response to the PTAs from the fifth edition.

As another way to help students, particularly at the upper level, to integrate material that they have learned in many courses over the span of a number of years, we have retained all six **Case Studies** from the fifth edition and have added four new ones. The Case Studies, some of which are illustrated, present complex client scenarios that are typical of the situations that students will encounter in clinical practice. Following each scenario is a series of questions for students to consider. The discussions for these questions are included on the CD-ROM packaged with the text.

More and more, students are recognizing the importance of providing quality nursing care to clients with backgrounds different from their own. To help them, this edition includes **Diversity in Health Care** boxes about such topics as "Cultural Perspectives on Pain," "Cultural Aspects of Death and Dying," and "Cultural Influences on Nutrition."

The increased use of alternative and complementary therapies by clients affects their health care management. A new feature, **Alternative Therapies,** has been added to help the student understand what complementary therapies may be used by their clients and the impact that these treatments might have on prescribed therapy ordered by the health care provider. Although many of the alternative therapies are not scientifically supported, they are widely endorsed and should be considered as part of the nursing assessment.

Client Education Guides are presented throughout the text. This important feature helps nurses teach clients how to collaborate in their own care and are worded in client-centered language.

Unlicensed assistive personnel continue to provide direct client care in hospitals. We also recognize that few nursing students have had the opportunity to learn how to delegate care safely. In this edition, we have added 10 additional **Management and Delegation** features, for a total of 19. These discuss assessments and interventions that can, under certain circumstances, be delegated to assistive personnel. They also provide guidance about how to decide whether a particular aspect of care is safe to delegate, and they emphasize that in all cases the responsibility for client care, analysis of client data, and the safety of the client rests squarely on the nurse.

Case management is another area of ongoing change in hospital nursing, and one of the hallmarks of case management is the use of clinical pathways. Two features in this revision highlight the importance of this content area. The first is Case Management. This feature, written by a practicing case manager, presents key coordination and anticipatory issues under consistent headings of "Assess," "Advocate," and "Prevent Readmission," thus linking nursing care with patient-focused case management. Many textbooks now incorporate clinical pathways. In this book we have gone a step further by including a group of **Clinical Pathway Guides** (or CareMap) that have been carefully selected by two experts in case management as among the best in use today. We have included portions of the clinical pathway and a guide to orient the student to the value and important components of each pathway.

The growing use of standardized language in nursing has been addressed by including a list of appropriate **Nursing Outcomes Classification (NOC)** labels at the start of each nursing management chapter. The outcomes chosen include those that may apply to clients with any of the conditions presented within the chapter.

Critical Monitoring features highlight for the student those clinical manifestations that must be reported to the physician without delay. **Care Plans** summarize the nursing diagnoses, outcomes, interventions and rationales, and evaluation criteria for selected disorders.

We have found that students often struggle with how to record normal assessment findings. This edition again includes **Physical Assessment Findings in the Healthy Adult** features, which serve both to remind students of the relevant normal findings for each body system and to demonstrate how to chart those findings with clinical precision.

Bridging the distance from the theoretical to the practical, and from the hospital to the home, is essential in nursing today. To that end, we have asked practicing home care nurses to write new **Bridge to Home Health Care** features for this edition. These features provide practical suggestions on the ever more critical skill of adapting medical-surgical care to the home.

Nursing research is providing evidence to guide practice decisions for all nurses. No longer can just one study be summarized and included in a chapter. We have examined nursing research findings and have incorporated them into the discussion of nursing care. A new feature has been designed to help the student gain a sense of the "state of the science" in selected areas of practice. The **Bridge to Evidence-Based Practice** features examine an integrative review of research evidence for a specific topic by identifying the research questions, studies examined, findings of the studies, limitations, and application to practice. These features appear at the end of units in which the content is related.

Another feature, the **Bridge to Critical Care,** highlights common treatment modalities and assessments performed in critical care. Rather than attempt to discuss all of critical care nursing in these features, we have tried to impart through them a basic understanding of hospital-based critical care treatments as they are used in inpatient care. Some examples are the use of pulmonary pressure monitors, ventilators, and arterial lines.

The prevalence of many diseases in older adults and the special needs of older adults prompted retention of sections called **Modifications for Elderly Clients** for many disorders. Because it is often difficult to differentiate normal manifestations of aging from pathologic conditions in the elderly, we have also included content on normal aging for each body system.

Because of the growing importance of being able to "think critically" as a nurse, we have concluded each nursing care chapter in the book with a series of **Thinking Critically** exercises. Each of these exercises presents a typical client scenario and poses several questions about what actions to take. To give the student clues about how to think through these clinical problems, each exercise includes one or more *Factors to Consider.* On the enclosed CD-ROM, we provide a brief discussion of each of these exercises. Because there is no one right answer to a *Thinking Critically* question, these are *discussions* rather than hard-and-fast *answers.*

SUPPLEMENT PACKAGE

Student Study CD-ROM

Packaged with each copy of the text, this new feature provides students with a wealth of study materials. All of the Case Studies from the text, plus two *bonus* Case Studies, are presented with the corresponding questions and a discussion for each question. Each Case Study also provides 7 to 10 multiple choice questions for further review and presents a nursing care plan in summary. The Thinking Critically questions, with discussions written by the authors, are also included. Students will also benefit from the more than 700 NCLEX-style test questions included for study and review. Icons throughout the text provide reminders for students to refer to the CD-ROM.

Study Guide

The *Study Guide* is designed to improve understanding of each chapter of the textbook. Learning objectives are provided to help the student focus on critical content in each chapter. In addition, *Study Guide* chapters include the following sections, as appropriate:

- Learning the Language
- Critical Thinking: Understanding Rationales
- Thinking Clinically: Knowing What to Do and Why
- Client Education: Knowing What to Teach and Why
- Putting It All Together
- Diagnostic Tests: Knowing Why You Do What You Do
- At-a-Glance Worksheets

Instructor's Electronic Resource

The *Instructor's Electronic Resource* (IER) is designed to help faculty develop lectures, assignments, and clinical assignments based on the content of the textbook and is free to textbook adopters. The IER is a CD-ROM composed of four components:

- A 2000 multiple-choice question test bank in the ExaMaster format
- Image Collection of approximately 200 illustrations from the text
- NEW! LectureView composed of more than 1000 Powerpoint slides
- Instructor's Manual

ExaMaster, a computer test bank, provides approximately 2000 NCLEX-style questions from which instructors can automatically or manually generate examinations. Provided for each question is the correct answer, the rationale for the correct answer, the cognitive level according to Bloom's taxonomy, and the corresponding learning objective in the *Study Guide* and *Instructor's Manual.* These questions are also available to textbook adopters in printed form.

Approximately 300 color illustrations from the text are available through the **Image Collection** and provide exciting visual aids to help the instructor with classroom presentations.

LectureView presents more than 1000 Powerpoint slides organized by each unit of the text. These slides provide instructors with ready-made lectures and are an effective teaching tool.

The **Instructor's Manual** repeats the Learning Objectives from the Student Study Guide and includes Facilitating Student Learning ideas and Critical Points to Emphasize summaries.

SIMON WEB SITE

The SIMON Web site provides instructors and students who are using this textbook with several tools to enhance teaching and learning. It acts as an "Internet"-based ancillary that includes Web links that connect the content of each chapter to numerous Web sites. These linkages are updated during the life of the book so that the content is always current. The Web site also provides content updates, ethics challenges, and other relevant and helpful material.

(http://www.wbsaunders.com/SIMON/Black/medsurg/)

ACKNOWLEDGMENTS

We have been asked several times, "Isn't a revision a lot less work than a new book?" You would think so, but it's amazing—a revision is no less work than a new book.

A project of this size certainly could not be accomplished without the collaboration of many people. First and foremost, we recognize the importance of the clinical expertise of our many contributing authors, which enables us to present a new edition that continues to be the "gold standard" for textbooks of medical-surgical nursing. We would also like to thank the special feature contributors and to acknowledge Anne Larson for her contribution of the Case Studies.

There are also many people at W. B. Saunders Company who have made this monumental task a "do-able" task. Thank you, Thomas Eoyang, former Editorial Manager, Nursing Books, for your ongoing encouragement, help, and support. Thank you, Terri Ward, former Developmental Editor, and Victoria Legnini, Developmental Editor; without your help and day-to-day management, we would still be behind on the deadlines. Your organization made this project move well. Thank you, Ceil Roberts and Rita Martello, for your meticulous coordination of a massive art program. Thank you, Observatory Group, for your stunning new full-color illustrations. Thank you, Karen O'Keefe Owens, Designer, for your fresh, appealing, full-color design. Thank you, Carol J. Robins, Manuscript Editor, for finding just the right words when we could not, for coordinating the work of other copy editors, and for fielding countless changes, additions, and deletions with unfailing grace. Thank you, Linda Garber and Natalie Ware, Production Managers, for keeping the book on schedule against overwhelming odds. Thank you, Fran Murphy, for coordinating the peer reviews of the book, and Adrienne Simon for handling the countless administrative tasks associated with the publication of the book. Thank you, Barbara Nelson Cullen, Executive Editor, for developing and producing the book's supplement package.

Finally, we want to thank *you*—educators and students—for allowing us to join you in the teaching and learning of medical-surgical nursing. We trust that you will find the sixth edition of *Medical-Surgical Nursing: Clinical Management for Positive Outcomes* a valuable asset.

JOYCE M. BLACK
JANE HOKANSON HAWKS
ANNABELLE M. KEENE

Contents

UNIT 3

UNIT 11

UNIT 12

UNIT 13

Special Features

Alternative Therapies

Bridges to Critical Care

Bridges to Evidence-Based Practice

Bridges to Home Health Care

Care Plans

Case Management

Case Studies

Client Education Guides

Clinical Pathway Guides

Critical Monitoring

Diversity in Health Care

Management and Delegation

Physical Assessment Findings in the Healthy Adult

Pathophysiology/Treatment Algorithms

UNIT 1

Promotion of Self-Care

CHAPTER 1

Theories of Health Promotion and Illness Management

Esther A. Hellman

As a result of the growing prevalence of chronic conditions and related cost burden, health promotion and illness prevention will be increasingly important. This chapter describes epidemiologic concepts and health promotion theories and shows how these concepts and theories are used in managing chronic conditions, which can occur across the life span. Health promotion concepts in two groups of the adult population are described in Chapters 2 and 3.

HISTORY OF HEALTH CARE

Disease and illness have plagued humans since the beginning of time. Familiarity with dominant ideas about the health care and diseases of each era is useful in understanding the antecedents of the current health care system. Through the ages, people have wondered why some individuals become sick while others remain healthy. When the populace of early civilizations had little knowledge of disease processes, magic and superstition were the mainstays in treating illness. As medical knowledge increased, treatment became more science-based. Table 1–1 presents an overview of health care history from prehistoric times to the 19th century.

During prehistoric times, diseases were thought to be caused by the stars, angry spirits, or demons. Sorcerers and priests treated disease by exorcism or by placating the evil spirits. As medical knowledge progressed, Asians in India and China and Greeks believed that a body fluid imbalance caused illness. Early forms of immunizations, medications, and surgeries were developed during this period. During the Dark Ages, physicians could not stop smallpox, cholera, or bubonic plague from killing millions of people. People believed that they had no control over disease and illness. During the Dark Ages, minimal progress was made toward understanding health or illness; medical care consisted of magic and superstitious practices. During the Renaissance, interest in science revived and medical knowledge advanced through direct observation during autopsies and analyses of urine and blood. It was not until the late 19th century that scientists began to discover causes of infectious diseases.

■ THEORIES OF DISEASE CAUSATION

Scientific concepts about the causes of disease and illness are relatively new ideas. Table 1–2 describes some theories of disease causation. One of the earliest theories, Pasteur's *germ theory,* described microorganisms, such as viruses and bacteria, as the causative factor in infectious disease. Although the germ theory helped to increase medical knowledge and to reduce deaths from infection, it did not explain the causes of all diseases.

The *biomedical model* described disease as malfunctioning cells or organs with consistent signs and symptoms. This model focused on cause-and-effect relationships while ignoring psychosocial components of disease.

Multicausal theories, such as Bernard and Cannon's Theory of Homeostasis and Selye's Theory of the General Adaptation Syndrome, explained the influence of lifestyle, genetic background, diet, and stress response on disease and illness.

Psychosocial theories integrate physiologic, psychological, and sociologic factors to better explain disease development. Examples of psychosocial theories are Mason's Theory of Specificity of the Stress Response; Lazarus' Theories of Stress Response; Wolff's Theory of Stress, Organ Maladaptation, and Disease; and Holmes and Rahe's Theory of Life Change and the Onset of Illness.

Multicausal and psychosocial theories of disease causation more closely approximate reality and increase the likelihood of discovering factors susceptible to intervention.

■ CONCEPT OF HEALTH

The word "health," as it is used today, did not appear in writing until about 1000 A.D. Until the 19th century, being healthy was the norm and sick people were ostracized. The dawn of the 19th century scientific era led to new discoveries and better understanding of human physi-

TABLE 1–1 THE HISTORY OF HEALTH CARE

Time Period	Theories of Disease Development	Health Care Practices
Prehistoric	Illnesses are sent from the angry spirits of dead animals or people	Sorcerers claimed to be able to placate evil spirits with herbs or potions. They practiced trephining (perforation of the skull). The skull holes supposedly enabled evil spirits to leave the body
Early civilizations Sumerians (Mesopotamia) Egyptians	Medicine is based on astronomy A person's destiny is told in the stars Demons, infesting the earth, produced diseases	Priests treated disease by exorcism. A wide range of drugs, obtained from plants, fruits, animals, and minerals, were also used
Asian civilizations India	Illness is described as an imbalance Belief that imbalance occurs between three physical humors: spirit, bile, and phlegm	Physicians specialized in plastic surgery, especially rhinoplasty (reshaping of the nose)
China	Imbalance occurs between *Yin* (negative, passive, feminine) and *Yang* (positive, active, masculine)	Chinese physicians were the first to vaccinate against smallpox and to prescribe iron for anemia; developed acupuncture
Israelite civilization	Illness represents a visible sign of God's wrath on sinful people who have broken rules of faith related to food preparation and hygiene. Dietary and other religious practices promote health	Faith brought health. Priests treated disease (e.g., leprosy treated with isolation and cleansing); then the recovered person was reintroduced into the community
Greek civilization Hippocrates, the "Father of Medicine," author of the Hippocratic Oath Aristotle described body's organs in elaborate detail	Nature has power to heal. Health and illness are due to balance or imbalance between blood, phlegm, yellow bile, and black bile. Human suffering and disease can be reduced through good hygiene, not magic. Proven cures for diseases are used, not relying on religious and demonic explanations	The body had the means to cure itself. Fevers, inflammation, boils, and diarrhea were seen as the body's way of purging itself
Roman civilization Galen wrote 22 massive volumes on health, illness, and health care	Superstition and magic are central to health care	Various gods were called on to help people through specific troubles (Opigena called on to help women in childbirth) Animal liver was used to cure various ailments Public health improvements were introduced (sewers, aqueducts)
Dark Ages	Superstitions prevail	Plagues killed millions of people. Physicians powerlessness to help. Society moved away from reason and back to superstition. The common practice of bloodletting allowed the body to get rid of bad "humors"
The Renaissance Leonardo da Vinci described muscles and arteries Vesalius described human anatomy Paré developed principles of surgery Harvey discovered how blood circulates	Culture is revived, and science begins again. Direct observation of the natural world leads to knowledge	Diagnosis of illness made by analyses of urine and bloodletting; physicians, educated in universities
18th and 19th centuries Florence Nightingale established the profession of nursing	Germ theory is developed Believed that controlling the environment promotes health and healing and prevents disease	Basic means to inhibit spread of disease by hand-washing and disinfection began
Semmelweis thought puerperal fever was contagious	Ordered hand-washing and disinfection practices	
Lister and Pasteur	Introduced disinfection techniques into hospitals and operating rooms	

TABLE 1–2 THEORIES OF DISEASE CAUSATION

Theory	Description	Components
Germ theory	Pasteur proposed that a specific microorganism was capable of causing infectious disease	Antibiotics, vaccinations, and other treatments were developed as a result of this theory. *Weakness of theory:* Does not explain causes of all diseases (i.e., most diseases today are not infectious).
Biomedical model	Disease is a result of malfunctioning organs or cells	Diseases are observable and quantifiable, in that most findings are objective (called "signs") and symptoms are subjective reports of disease. *Weakness of model:* Does not account for many other factors specific to each individual (lifestyle, diet, genetic background, stress response) that may also contribute to disease.
Multicausal theories (factors specific to each client must be examined; an individual's lifestyle and genetic background play an underlying role in development of disease)	1. Bernard and Cannon's *Theory of Homeostasis* a. Bernard hypothesized that if an organism is to live, it must have the capacity to maintain its internal environment b. Canon developed the concept of *feedback mechanisms* to explain Bernard's theory of regulation of the internal environment	 a. Illness occurs as the result of an imbalance in the body's internal environment, and disease is an adaptive effort by the body to restore its balance. b. Homeostasis is a dynamic equilibrium, flexible and ongoing, that maintains certain factors within a given range, e.g., body temperature, blood pressure, fluid and electrolyte balances. The fight-or-flight response prepares the body to react in an emergency and to move quickly away from danger.
	2. Selye's *Theory of the General Adaptation Syndrome:* A framework to describe how people respond to stress; involves generalized changes that affect several body systems *Local Adaptation Syndrome* takes place in a single organ or specific section of the body (e.g., inflammation)	2. Both syndromes develop in three distinct stages: (a) alarm reaction, or fight-or-flight response, (b) resistance, and (c) exhaustion. The most important regulators are the central and autonomic nervous systems and pituitary and adrenal glands. Disease occurs when the adaptive capacity of the body is exceeded.
Psychosocial theories (integrate physiologic, psychological, and sociologic factors that explain disease development)	1. Mason's *Theory of Specificity of the Stress Response:* The stress response is dependent on psychological factors (e.g., a person's perception of the stressor rather than the stressor itself)	1. Cortisol hormonal responses to stress increase when (a) we first experience a new stimulus, (b) we learn to avoid noxious stimuli, and (c) we receive punishment. We can modify the cortisol response by coping effectively with a stressor.
	2. Lazarus' *Theories of the Stress Response:* The degree of resistance to infection depends on how well a person copes with stress and general life experiences	2. The brain, through one's perception of the stressor, appears to be the mediating influence on how the body responds to stress. Daily hassles are irritating, frustrating, minor life events that everyone experiences, such as losing things and being delayed in traffic. Daily uplifts are buffers to daily hassles. People who cope poorly with stress have significantly impaired immune responses, as shown by diminished leukocyte activity levels.

Table continued on following page

TABLE 1–2 THEORIES OF DISEASE CAUSATION *Continued*

Theory	Description	Components
	3. Wolff's *Theory of Stress, Organ Maladaptation, and Disease:* It is hypothesized that disease often results from adaptive attempts to restore homeostasis that were appropriate in kind but incorrect in magnitude. Inappropriate adaptation attempts occur because: a. Humans can symbolize, recall the past, and project themselves into the future; therefore, threats of possible danger and symbols of danger are just as important a cause of disease as noxious chemicals, microbes, and mechanical forces b. People depend on others for much of their satisfaction in life	3. Stressors are created by the need to be successful at work and with other people. Some individuals consistently respond to frustrating situations through a response by a particular body system or organ, perhaps the stomach, back muscles, colon, or nasal mucous membranes. Pathologic changes that occur regularly and that are combined with other chemical, biologic, or physical stressors can eventually lead to tissue damage.
	4. Roy's *Adaptation Model:* Health is a state of being and a process of becoming an integrated whole	4. Human behavior is a result of adaptation to internal and external stimuli. The model provides a framework to help understand human adaptive responses and interventions that can be used to foster adaptation and minimize stress. The four modes of adaptation are (a) physiologic responses, (b) self-concept responses, (c) role function, and (d) interdependent relations.
	5. Holmes and Rahe's *Theory of Life Change and the Onset of Illness:* Life changes (both positive and negative) are a form of stress to which people must learn to adapt, both psychologically and physically	5. If we must adapt to too many significant changes over a short period of time, we expend too much energy trying to adapt, which may result in illness. Minor ailments, serious disease, depression, and suicide attempts typically follow a cluster of both positive and negative life changes.
Biopsychosociospiritual theories	A person's body, mind, and environment all function together to determine whether illness develops	
	1. Wolf's *Concept of Disease as a Way of Life:* The brain has a role in regulating bodily processes and in causing disease when it defines situations that can evoke chemical and nervous system reactions	1. The body needs high levels of epinephrine, blood glucose, and other hormones during times of physical threat when a person must literally fight or flee. When these responses occur inappropriately or chronically, the excess hormones can cause harm, including disease. Disease can arise from evoked reaction patterns that are meant to be protective when a person is physically threatened but that are destructive when used inappropriately to fight symbolic battles.
	2. Schwartz's *Model of the Brain as an Adaptive Regulator:* The brain is an adaptive system for regulation of the body through a feedback system with the peripheral organs	2. The brain is central to any change in health because it is the mediator between the external and internal environments. Through the brain's interpretation, a person can (a) change an environment, (b) leave it, (c) engage in it, or (d) rest, exercise, or diet. People have the ability to regulate themselves and move toward health on the health care continuum.

TABLE 1–2 THEORIES OF DISEASE CAUSATION *Continued*

Theory	Description	Components
Mediators of the stress response: 1. Internal variables (personality, personal resources, temperament, history, genes)	1. Behavior Patterns a. Friedman and Rosenman described two behavior types: (1) *Type A* personality is characterized by constant mobilization of inner resources to combat real or imagined stresses	(1) People with a type A personality are described as aggressive, often hostile, hard-driving, and deadline-ridden, with a chronic sense of urgency. Between ages 35 and 60 years, they are almost three times more likely to have coronary artery disease than type B people.
	(2) *Type B* personality characteristically takes life with all its stresses in stride	(2) Although often intelligent and ambitious, type B people do not allow activity to become self-destructive. They can relax without feeling guilty and can work without a sense of time urgency.
	b. Kobasa's *Model of Hardiness:* A personality component that moderates or buffers the response to stress. Hardy clients can remain healthy under stressful situations and can view the stressor as an opportunity to practice mastery and undergo personal growth	Concepts of hardiness have been associated with health maintenance in the following areas: (1) *Control:* The sense of mastery or self-confidence needed to appraise and interpret health stressors appropriately (2) *Commitment:* Presence of active involvement in efforts to maintain or improve health (3) *Challenge:* Presence of flexibility and persistence in coping with health stressors
2. Environment (social supports, physical setting, organizational factors)	2. Social support: More socially isolated or less socially integrated people are less healthy psychologically and physically and are more likely to die than more socially oriented people	2. Physiologic studies show a link between the amygdala and the hypothalamus in the brain and positive social relationships. Social contact decreases hormones such as cortisol, epinephrine, and norepinephrine.

ology and disease origins. At the same time, society began to treat illness with less disgust and defined health simply as the absence of disease.

In 1947, the World Health Organization (WHO) definition of health emphasized several holistic qualities: "Health is a state of complete physical, mental, and social well-being and not merely the absence of disease or infirmity."[44] Since 1947, alternate definitions of health have been proposed. Some definitions portray health and illness on an interactive continuum, with multiple configurations ranging from depletion of health (death) to high-level wellness.[29] High-level wellness is further conceptualized as self-actualization and maximization of an individual's potential. Other definitions describe health as a unidirectional developmental process consisting of a unitary patterning of person and environment. When each person is viewed as being part of a complex, interconnected social, biologic, and environmental system, health can be better understood. Table 1–3 lists various definitions of health.

In general, today's definitions of health reflect a multidimensional, holistic, and subjective view. Individual definitions and perceptions of health are taken into account. The meaning of health can be viewed in many contexts, such as historical, social, personal, scientific, philosophical, and spiritual. These meanings will always exist in the various contexts of individual human experience, are sometimes contradictory, and often overlap. Cultural ideologies and tradition also influence one's image of health.

Support client participation in the process of actualizing a defined image of health, and do not negate the ability of clients to form their own image of health. Include clients' perceptions when assessing their health to fully understand the priority of their values and perceptions of these very complex interactions.

■ CONCEPT OF WELLNESS

Dunn was the first to define and describe wellness, a term and an ideal that was the precursor to the health promotion movement.[10] His now-classic definition of what he termed *high-level wellness* is "an integrated method of functioning which is oriented toward maximizing the potential of which the individual is capable within the environment where he is functioning." Dunn stressed that wellness is an ongoing process directed toward higher potential, not a static goal; and that high-level wellness is a feeling of being "alive to the tips of the fingers, with energy to burn, tingling with vitality."[10] He postulated

TABLE 1–3 DEFINITIONS OF HEALTH

Nursing Model	Definition
King's goal attainment theory	Health is a dynamic life experience. "Dynamic" implies a continuous adjustment to stressors in internal and external environments and the use of one's resources to achieve maximum potential.
Leininger's transcultural model	Health refers to "beliefs, values, and action patterns that are culturally known and used to preserve and maintain personal or group well-being, and to perform daily role activities."[23a]
Levine's conservation principles	Health is defined in terms of an Anglo-Saxon word meaning "whole." Patterns of wholeness change with growth and development. Health and disease patterns reflect adaptive change.
Neuman's systems model	Health is a condition in which the parts and subparts of the whole person are in harmony.
Orem's self-care model	Health is a state of wholeness, including a person's parts and modes of functioning.
Pender's health promotion model	"Health is a manifestation of evolving patterns of person-environment interaction throughout the life span."[31]
Rogers' unitary person model	Health and illness are seen as expressions of the interaction of a person and the environment in the process of unfolding consciousness.
Roy's adaptation model	Health is a process or state of being and a process of becoming an integrated whole.
Watson's model of human caring	Health is more than the absence of disease. It is a harmony within the mind, body, and soul.
World Health Organization	Health is a "state of complete physical, mental, and social well-being and not merely the absence of disease or infirmity."[44]

that health professionals tend to focus on disease rather than on wellness because their training is disease-focused rather than wellness-oriented or prevention-oriented. It is easier to fight against disease than to fight for a condition of greater wellness.

Travis popularized the theoretical concept of wellness through development and teaching of the wellness model (Fig. 1–1). The effect of this model resulted in the recognition that wellness requires attention; it does not happen automatically. The left side of the figure represents the biomedical model. The client exhibits manifestations of a disease, is treated, and is brought back to a neutral point where disease manifestations have been alleviated. In the case of chronic illness, disease manifestations are controlled and minimized. The right side represents the wellness model and the potential for high-level health and wellness. The nurse can use the wellness model at any point by directing clients beyond the neutral point and encouraging them to move as far toward high-level wellness as possible. The biomedical and wellness models can work in harmony. For example, if clients are ill, treatment is important, but clients should not stop there. After recovery, clients should practice healthy behaviors (such as regular exercise and eating a low-fat, balanced diet) to minimize future illnesses.

Wellness is the quality or condition of being well, even among people with chronic illness, especially of being robust, healthy, and fit. Wellness is not simply the absence of clinical manifestations; it incorporates positive mental, physical, and spiritual well-being. High-level wellness is a method of functioning oriented toward maximizing individual potential within the environment. High-level wellness involves (1) progression toward a higher level of functioning, (2) integration of the whole being, and (3) an open-ended future with the challenge of fuller potential.

■ RELATIONSHIP BETWEEN DISEASE, ILLNESS, HEALTH, AND WELLNESS

In the biomedical model, disease is a biomedical term, identified by clinical manifestations. A person who has a disease has a medically defined condition similar to that suffered by others (e.g., diabetes mellitus or hepatitis).[8] From a multicausal perspective, disease may be defined as "the failure of a person's adaptive mechanisms to adequately counteract stimuli and stresses, resulting in functional or structural disturbances."[12] As mentioned earlier, multicausal and psychosocial theories of disease causation more closely approximate reality and increase the chances of discovering factors that are amenable to intervention.

In contrast to the concept of disease, illness has a broader meaning and includes the perception and the response of clients and those around them. Illness is a state of being with social and psychological as well as biomedical components. Illness is a disenabling response, a mismatch between a person's needs and the resources available to meet those needs; it signals that the present balance is not working.[12] A person can have a disease without feeling ill. A seemingly healthy person may have an early form of disease without clinical manifestations. For example, young people in their 20s may already have heart disease, such as atherosclerosis (or "hardening of the arteries"), without evidence of disease. Although such people appear healthy, if they continue unhealthy habits such as smoking, eating a high-fat diet, and not exercising, the heart disease will progress until clinical manifestations appear. Similarly, injury changes the balance on the wellness continuum (see Fig. 1–1). Injuries usually require treatment; after recovery or rehabilitation, people can achieve higher levels of wellness by practicing healthy behaviors.

In summary, disease, illness, health, and wellness are related concepts. Disease and health must be considered together because without disease, there is no need to discuss health.[12] Disease is a state of disequilibrium, whereas health is a state of equilibrium, or balance.[14]

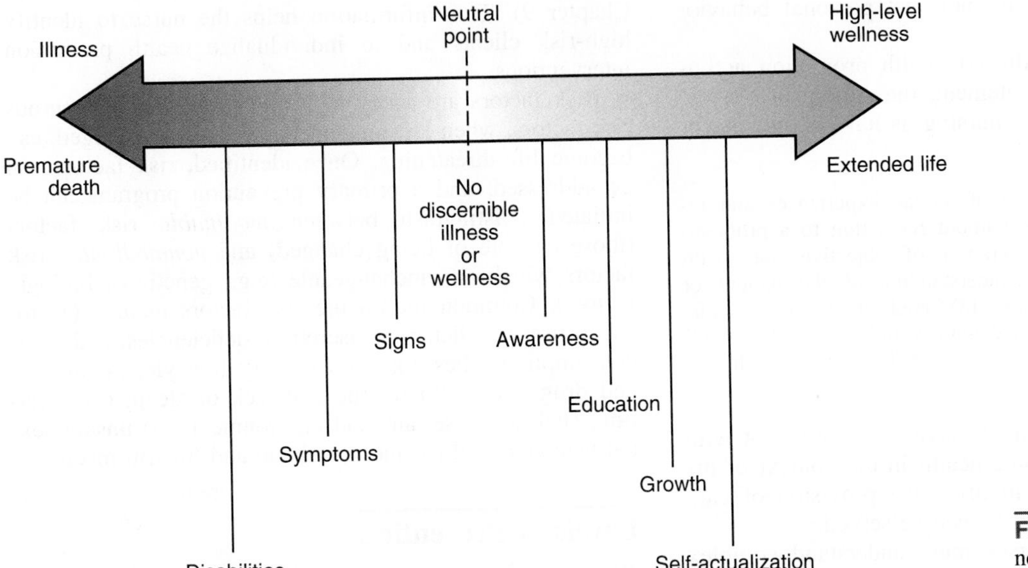

FIGURE 1–1 Travis' wellness model.

Health and illness are dynamic patterns that change with time and social circumstances; they are not mutually exclusive. There are degrees of health and illness; clients with cancer and others with chronic diseases can achieve personal levels of wellness. Health is a resource for everyday living. High-level wellness maximizes one's potential capacity and is a component of the highest level of health.

Concept of Health Promotion

Health promotion is the process of fostering awareness, influencing attitudes, and identifying alternatives so that people can make informed choices and change behavior to achieve an optimal level of physical and mental health and improve their physical and social environments. According to WHO, health promotion includes activities that encourage healthy lifestyles, create supportive environments for health, strengthen community action, reorient health service, and build healthy public policy. Health promotion has to do with acquiring mental, physical, and spiritual assets to protect and buffer people from disease as well as to move them along a continuum toward high-level wellness.

Health promotion programs are designed to improve the health and well-being of individuals and communities through empowerment. Clients are empowered through the provision of information, skills, services, and support needed to undertake and maintain positive lifestyle changes. Health promotion activities are geared toward individuals, families, and communities. WHO defines *community* as a social group determined by geographical boundaries or common values and interests. Community members know and interact with one another. The community within a particular social structure creates norms, values, and social institutions.

Health is affected by the extent of control or mastery people have over their lives or by the amount of power or powerlessness felt. Health promotion involves empowering the client. *Empowerment* gives the client power by transferring from the nurse knowledge, skills, resources, access, and language. The nurse can empower the client by teaching about self-care.

■ EVOLUTION OF THE CONCEPT OF HEALTH PROMOTION

During the 1970s and 1980s, the field of health promotion grew alongside the emerging ideology and practice of wellness. Initially, it found expression in Canada with the Lalonde Report[21] and in the United States in the Surgeon General's Report, *Healthy People.*[38] Both documents discussed the significance of environmental factors in influencing health and were not limited to mention of individual lifestyle or personal behavior issues, which are hallmarks of the wellness movement. The Lalonde Report made recommendations in four equally weighted areas: (1) human biology, (2) environment, (3) lifestyle, and (4) health care organization. The Surgeon General's Report noted that lifestyle influenced health more than the other categories did. The Surgeon General's Report argued that Americans are killing themselves, not only by careless habits but also by polluting the environment and permitting harmful social conditions to exist. For the first time, attention was directed toward environmental issues such as control of toxic agents and occupational health and safety.

In 1991, *Healthy People 2000* was published.[39] This report introduced a set of clearly articulated, measurable goals for improving the health of the nation by the year 2000. Three broad goals were identified: (1) increasing the span of healthy life for Americans, (2) reducing health disparities among Americans, and (3) achieving access to preventive services for all Americans. Specific goals, objectives, and strategies were delineated for achieving 22 priorities in health promotion, health protection, and preventive services. More recently, *Healthy People 2000: Review 1997*[41] was published and work on objectives for the next decade is under way. These reports prompted agencies to focus on prevention and promotion through institutional change strategies, legislation, and public policy, and not just personal behavior change.

Nurses have long conducted health promotion activities. In its social policy statement, the American Nurses' Association (ANA) defined nursing as having four essential features[2]:

> (1) attention to the full range of human experiences and responses to health and illness without restriction to a problem-focused orientation; (2) integration of objective data with knowledge gained from an understanding of the patient or group's subjective experience; (3) application of scientific knowledge to the processes of diagnosis and treatment; and (4) provision of a caring relationship that facilitates health and healing.

Therefore, a focus on health behaviors is consistent with nursing's focus on a person's health in the context of his or her total life. Nursing involves the provision of care that promotes well-being in the people served.[2]

To promote health, nurses must understand complex social, political, and economic forces that shape clients' lives. A nurse who is active socially and politically models the ANA social policy statement that delineates involvement in social reform as being a part of nursing practice. The policy states, among other concerns, the "provision for the public health through use of preventive and environmental measures and increased assumption of responsibility by individuals, families, and other groups."[2] Labonte, a health educator, believed that the ultimate challenge is to create social and health conditions that allow all of the world's citizens to achieve a state of good health.

EPIDEMIOLOGIC CONCEPTS

Epidemiology is the study of patterns of health, disease, disability, death, and other problems in a population. Epidemiology focuses on how diseases originate and spread.[24] A major epidemiologic goal is identifying aggregates, or subpopulations, at high risk for acquiring a disease and then modifying or reducing those risks. For example, smokers have a three-fold higher risk for development of cardiac disease compared with nonsmokers. Nurses can modify or reduce a smoker's risk of cardiac disease by counseling about how to accomplish smoking cessation. Risk factors and levels of prevention are epidemiologic concepts.

Risk Factors

Risk factors are factors whose presence is associated with increased probability of the occurrence of an illness or disease. Health risk factors can be categorized:

- *Genetic* or *biologic* (age, race, family history)
- *Behavioral* (health habits, such as eating a high-fat diet, not exercising, smoking)
- *Environmental* (living in an area with frequent smog warnings)

The risk level for disease or illness is assessed through health risk appraisal. Health risk appraisal identifies potential health threats prior to illness or disease development and provides clients with a way to evaluate their vulnerability to identified potential health threats (see Chapter 9). This information helps the nurse to identify high-risk clients and to individualize health promotion interventions.

Risk factors are a key to health promotion. Numerous risk factors, when left unattended or unacknowledged, can become life-threatening. Once identified, risk factors can be addressed, and a primary prevention program can be initiated. Distinguish between *modifiable* risk factors (those capable of being changed) and *nonmodifiable* risk factors which are unchangeable (e.g., genetic or biologic factors). Common modifiable risk factors include (1) tobacco use; (2) dietary indiscretion, deficiencies, and overconsumption (obesity); (3) sedentary lifestyle; (4) alcohol and drug abuse; (5) fatigue and lack of sleep; (6) pollution, such as noise, air, and environment; (7) unsafe sexual behavior; and (8) motor vehicle and firearm misuse.

Levels of Prevention

"Prevention" means averting the development and progression of disease.[23] Preventive health care is more dynamic than health maintenance. Prevention deals with health enhancement and promotion, whereas health maintenance is concerned with maintaining the status quo. Thinking about the levels of prevention implies a commitment to wellness and a conscious desire to prevent illness and disease. The levels of prevention are primary, secondary, and tertiary. Table 1–4 identifies selected behaviors associated with these levels.

PRIMARY PREVENTION

Primary prevention involves health promotion activities that provide protection against the occurrence of a specific illness or disease.[23] Primary prevention does not include therapeutic treatment or identification of symptoms. It does include health promotion (e.g., teaching clients about healthy lifestyle behaviors) and specific protection interventions (e.g., immunizations) to decrease vulnerability to illness or dysfunction. A health promotion program or enhancement activities can be developed to increase immunity and strengthen the body and mind. Everyday behavior can be examined in order to guide primary prevention. The objective is to achieve maximum functioning in each health potential.

For example, impaired mobility is usually preventable. If a client is at risk for impaired mobility, nursing intervention can prevent impairment. For the client who has arthritis and currently does not have mobility problems but is at risk for impaired mobility, for example, encouraging the client to eat a well-balanced diet and to engage in specific exercises may help delay the development of mobility problems.

SECONDARY PREVENTION

Secondary prevention refers to health behavior that promotes the early detection (case-finding or screenings) and treatment of disease, and limitation of disability[23] (also known as "health maintenance"). Screening primarily identifies cases in an early stage of disease, when treatment is more effective.

When working with a client:

1. Identify risk factors that cannot be modified but that leave the client vulnerable to disease.

TABLE 1-4 BEHAVIORS ASSOCIATED WITH EACH LEVEL OF PREVENTION

Level of Prevention	Type of Behavior*
PRIMARY	Stop smoking, or do not start smoking Avoid overexposure to the sun Support antipollution legislation Practice safe sex, monogamy, or abstinence Obtain genetic counseling for family-linked disorders Design and follow a regular exercise plan Maintain ideal body weight Maintain a low-cholesterol, low-fat, high-fiber nutritious diet Wear a seat belt and helmet Identify and eliminate stressors Limit alcohol intake, and never drink and drive Have regular dental care
SECONDARY	Obtain genetic counseling for family-linked disorders Undergo screening for tuberculosis Obtain tonometry yearly after age 40 for glaucoma screening Have yearly Papanicolaou smears and mammograms per recommended guidelines Have eye examinations every 2 years Practice monthly self-breast, self-testicular, self-skin, and self-oral examinations Undergo a physical examination yearly after age 40 Self-monitor blood pressure for hypertension
TERTIARY	Have a complete blood count before chemotherapy Have speech therapy after a stroke Participate in cardiac rehabilitation Have breast reconstruction Participate in stroke or coma rehabilitation

*Preventive behaviors identified are representative and not intended to be inclusive.

2. Using secondary prevention, analyze assessment data in order to derive nursing diagnoses and to identify problems common to target populations that exhibit nonmodifiable risk factors.
3. Rank intervention priorities, identify nursing management approaches within the secondary prevention mode, and evaluate outcomes.
4. Obtain assessment data by interview, observation, and physical examination.
5. Proceed to work with the client to develop a means of early detection, such as screening for the disease.

Using the immobility example to examine secondary prevention, consider subconcepts that emerge if immobility is thought of as the prescribed or unavoidable restriction of movement in any area. Immobility can be (1) physical, (2) emotional or psychological, (3) intellectual, or (4) social.

Causes of physical immobility may be (1) decreased energy from ischemia, hypoxia, malnutrition, and electrolyte imbalance; (2) lack of innervation, as in central nervous system or peripheral nerve impairment; (3) decreased musculoskeletal strength, as in endocrine diseases, disuse syndrome, and scar tissue formation; and (4) pain, which inhibits movement and the desire to move.

When looking at problems of immobility, consider individual norms. Although complications may not always be preventable, manifestations can be detected early and thus some complications can be avoided. Nursing interventions, such as applying heat, balancing exercise and rest, and administering prescribed anti-inflammatory drugs, can help prevent a serious mobility problem.

Tertiary Prevention

Tertiary prevention is directed toward rehabilitation after a disease or condition already exists to minimize disability and help the client learn to live productively with limitations. Tertiary prevention is used when disability is permanent and irreversible. It minimizes effects of disease and disability by surveillance and maintenance aimed at preventing complications and deterioration. Incorporate creative problem-solving approaches in the design, implementation, and evaluation of nursing intervention to support the client's achievement of successful adaptation to known risks, optimal reconstitution, or establishment of high-level wellness.

Continuing the immobility example, muscle and joint degeneration and metabolic and circulatory disturbances occur when a client is immobile for any length of time. Identifying immobility as an actual diagnosis permits development of a rehabilitation plan and restoration to high-level wellness. The plan would implement (1) active exercise, (2) passive mobilization, and (3) frequent position changes. Tertiary preventive outcome goals are optimal rehabilitation within parameters that the client can achieve.

■ MODELS OF HEALTH PROMOTION

Social scientists have worked on models of health-related behavior change or health promotion behavior. The models look at factors that affect individual readiness to take health action. Nurses use health promotion models to motivate clients to make health behavior changes.

Social Cognitive Theory

Bandura developed the Social Cognitive Theory to explain human behavior. The model is based on the premise that human behavior is influenced by "reciprocal determinism" between cognition, behavior, and environment.[4] According to this theory, both efficacy and outcome expectations are crucial for behavioral change. The central concept is self-efficacy. Perceived self-efficacy or efficacy expectation is a judgment of one's ability to execute a specific behavior.

People with high self-efficacy are more confident of their abilities to maintain behavioral change (e.g., exercise adherence, smoking cessation, or achievement of ideal weight). They will attempt to execute the behavior more readily, with greater intensity, and with greater perseverance in response to initial failure than people with comparatively weaker self-efficacy. Interventions to increase self-efficacy include (1) *performance attainment*—having clients successfully execute the behavior; (2) *vicarious experiences*—watching others successfully enact the behavior; (3) *verbal persuasion*—convincing clients of their capability to execute the behavior; and (4) *physiologic states*—helping clients to expect and interpret various physiologic states (e.g., stress, anxiety, fatigue, pain) that may occur when the behavior is executed.

Interventions to increase perceived self-efficacy may be beneficial when the nurse is encouraging health-protecting and health-promoting behaviors. Social Cognitive Theory affects behavior change through phases:

1. Promoting and motivating clients to change a target behavior
2. Providing skills training so that clients can acquire the specific behavioral change skills
3. Developing support networks to help maintain the new behavior
4. Maintaining the behavior through reinforcement
5. Generalizing to other levels of interaction, from the family to the community

Health Belief Model

The Health Belief Model attempts to explain why some people who are illness-free take actions to avoid illness, whereas others do not. This model is based on the idea that people want to avoid negatively valued outcomes or personal threats, such as illness, disability, nonproductivity, discomfort, and death. The Health Belief Model includes five factors, identified and illustrated in Box 1–1. Cognitive and emotional beliefs identify an individual's readiness to change behavior.[36] Before people take action to change a behavior, they must decide that the selected behavior (whether it is smoking, not being immunized, or engaging in unprotected sexual activity) creates a serious health harm and that moderating or stopping the behavior will be beneficial.[14]

BOX 1–1 The Health Belief Model: Client Characteristics and Starting an Exercise Program

1. *Perceived susceptibility to a problem.* Negative effects of not exercising (identified as threatening) include difficulty managing weight, lack of energy, and increased risk of coronary artery disease.
2. *Perceived seriousness of a problem.* The client feels that the identified negative effects of not exercising are serious problems.
3. *Perceived benefits and barriers to taking action.* If an exercise program is started, the benefits (weight loss and maintenance, more energy, better health) will be greater than any barriers (lack of time, cost of equipment, lack of an exercise partner).
4. *Cues to action.* The client has been exposed to action cues. An exercise room is available to employees at work, and the company's nurse practitioner has advised the client to begin an exercise program.
5. *Self-efficacy* (the behavior is doable). The client is confident that he or she will be able to begin and continue a regular exercise program.

Health Promotion Model

Pender's Health Promotion Model emphasizes developing individual resources to enhance well-being.[31] This model demonstrates complex biopsychosocial processes that motivate people to engage in behaviors directed toward health enhancement.[14] The model links individual characteristics and experiences, and behavior-specific cognitions and affects (including benefits of and barriers to action and interpersonal and situational influences), to a commitment to a health-promoting behavior. The final behavioral outcome is also influenced by the immediate competing demands and preferences, which can derail an intended health-promoting action (e.g., selecting a meal with a high-fat rather than a low-fat content because of taste preferences).

Transtheoretical Model

The Transtheoretical Model, developed by Prochaska and DiClemente,[33] identifies stages of change: The individual moves from (1) not thinking about change in the near future *(precontemplation),* (2) to seriously thinking about making a change *(contemplation),* (3) to actively planning and starting a behavior change *(preparation),* (4) to overtly making changes *(action),* and (5) to taking steps to maintain changes and avoid relapse *(maintenance).* This model stages the client's readiness to change and incorporates (1) pros and cons of a behavior change, (2) self-efficacy, and (3) change processes. For example, a client who states no intention of beginning an exercise program would be in the precontemplation stage for exercise. The model is a guide for assessing a client's readiness to change and for developing stage-specific health interventions.

■ TEACHING AND MOTIVATING CLIENTS

Nurses encounter clients during times of major health changes and are in key positions to help them make decisions and adopt behaviors that greatly alter health. To effectively assist others in making healthy decisions and changes, nurses must teach about healthy behaviors, function as role models, and understand the concepts of motivation. The previously described health promotion models can be used as client teaching guides to identify potential areas for assessment and crucial teaching content to facilitate desired behavioral changes. An example of health behavior client teaching, using the Transtheoretical Model, follows.[33] This example can be applied to any health behavior change, such as quitting smoking, starting a regular exercise program, or eating a low-fat, balanced diet.

According to the Transtheoretical Model, assessment of the client's readiness to change must be done before any health behavior change instruction is initiated. First determine the stage of change and by assessing the client's willingness to modify or reduce health risk by making the desired healthy behavior change and by assessing the client's progress toward making the change. Then use an intervention that is appropriate for the client's stage of change. Both practice and research have demonstrated that giving information to clients does not in itself bring about healthy behaviors. Nurses frequently give up trying to teach because of a lack of client motivation. When this occurs, the client may be labeled as "noncompliant" or "difficult." Instead, it may be that the client cannot relate to the intervention because it is not directed at the client's specific stage of behavioral change, situation, or cultural perspective. Ask clients about their perceived benefits of changing the behavior as well as about barriers to changing the behavior.

Motivating others to change health behaviors involves the following:

- Clients must believe that the problem is solvable.
- Clients must view the solution as something they want to do.
- Clients must feel competent to successfully carry out the behavior.
- Clients must feel able to overcome barriers to change.
- Clients must experience positive feedback and consequences.

The nurse's role is to use multiple skills to empower clients to engage in healthy behaviors. Approaches include helping clients to identify their values and to explore feelings about themselves, with emphasis on identifying strengths. Helping clients set goals (developing intrinsic motivation) greatly enhances the likelihood of achieving the desired behavioral changes. Nurses assist clients in differentiating perceived from actual barriers and in promoting behaviors to overcome the actual barriers. Whenever possible, nurses should act as models of health with a joyful zest for living, thus providing a living example.

CHRONIC CONDITIONS OR ILLNESSES

Since the 1920s, chronic conditions have become an increasingly larger challenge to health care providers and health care delivery systems.[16] In the ensuing 80 years, chronic conditions replaced infectious diseases as the dominant health care challenge. The number of people who have chronic conditions is increasing with the ever-growing number of older people and the increasing number of people who survive major illness. In 1995, it was estimated that 99 million people in the United States had chronic conditions.[16] Of these, 41 million were limited in their daily activities, and 12 million were unable to go to school or work or to live independently. By the year 2030, it is estimated that nearly 150 million Americans will have a chronic condition; 42 million of these will be limited in their ability to go to school or work or to live independently. In addition, the lives of family members and others are affected by the related caregiving responsibilities.

A *chronic illness* or *condition* has been defined as a long-term health problem caused by an irreversible disorder (e.g., a severe spinal cord injury), an accumulation of disorders (e.g., neuropathy and retinopathy as complications of diabetes), or a latent disease (e.g., development of lung cancer after years of exposure to asbestos). A *chronic condition* is a general term that includes both chronic illnesses and impairments, such as developmental disabilities or impairments caused by injuries. From this broad definition, it is apparent that chronic conditions are prevalent. Whether in an acute care, an ambulatory, or a long-term care setting or in the community, nursing care is provided to clients who have chronic conditions. A "chronic condition" is consistent with the concept of health as multidimensional, so that some dimensions of health exist until death. Health promotion, illness prevention, and health maintenance interventions are extremely important for people who have a chronic condition.

In 1995, chronic conditions cost the economy $470 billion (in 1990 dollars)[18] in direct medical costs and more than $230 billion in lost productivity.[16] These estimated costs would be even higher if they were expressed in the current year's dollars as a result of inflation. The cost of chronic conditions increases daily and affects the health care system. The health care system is undergoing a paradigm shift involving changes in philosophies about health, chronic illness, disability, and the roles of health care professionals, clients, and families in the management of chronic conditions. Increased emphasis is being given to prevention of chronic conditions and finding ways to help people live with and shape the course of such conditions.

■ MULTIFACTORIAL ASPECTS OF CHRONIC DISEASE

As mentioned earlier, a century ago our ancestors fought infectious and communicable diseases. Although serious infectious diseases are still a public health threat, most life-threatening diseases today are those that become chronic as a result of metabolic abnormalities induced by health risk factors such as genetic or biologic (aging), behavioral (nutrition), and environmental influences. Figure 1–2 shows the association between multiple risk factors and chronic diseases. Health risk factors reflect a multicausal disease causation theory. The relationships among health risk factors and disease are examined in the following text.

Genetic or Biologic Health Risk Factors

HEREDITY AND DISEASE

Genetic aspects of disease have been recognized for many years. Recent technology has allowed researchers to identify the actual gene that is faulty in some disorders. Most recently, therapy has been developed to treat altered gene structures and to clone a new being.

More than one fifth of the human genes differ in form from one person to another. This remarkable degree of genetic variation among normal people is what accounts for natural variations in attributes such as height, hair color, intelligence, personality, and blood pressure. These genetic differences also affect each person's ability to handle environmental challenges, including those that produce disease. In every disease, there is some degree of genetic interaction with the environment. For example, lung cancer may develop in many smokers, but not in all. In 1990, medical researchers identified a single gene linked to lung cancer risk. Perhaps a person's genetic makeup allows the body to kill early cancer cells.

More than 5000 diseases are known to have a genetic

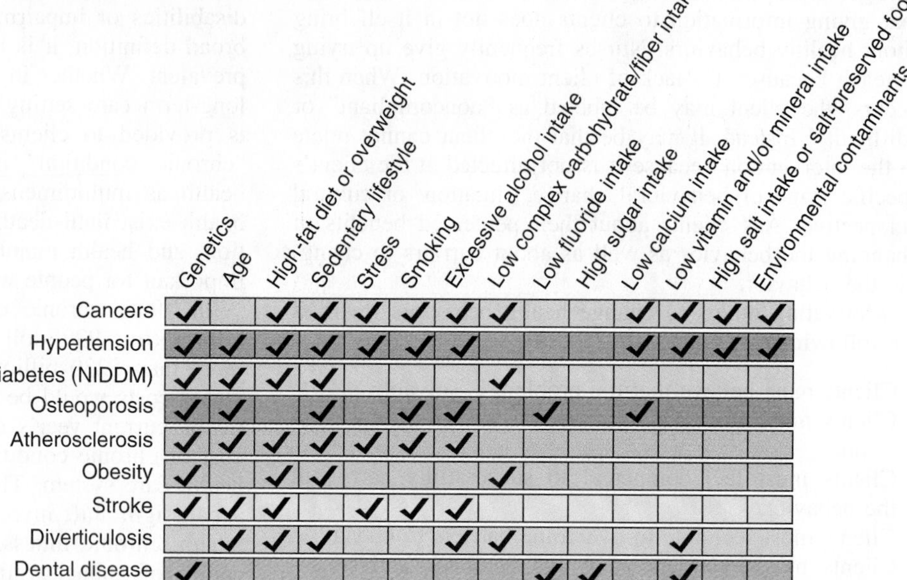

	Genetics	Age	High-fat diet or overweight	Sedentary lifestyle	Stress	Smoking	Excessive alcohol intake	Low complex carbohydrate/fiber intake	Low fluoride intake	High sugar intake	Low calcium intake	Low vitamin and/or mineral intake	High salt intake or salt-preserved foods	Environmental contaminants
Cancers	✓		✓	✓	✓	✓	✓	✓			✓	✓	✓	✓
Hypertension	✓	✓	✓	✓	✓	✓	✓				✓	✓	✓	✓
Diabetes (NIDDM)	✓	✓	✓	✓				✓						
Osteoporosis	✓	✓		✓		✓	✓		✓		✓			
Atherosclerosis	✓	✓	✓	✓	✓	✓	✓							
Obesity	✓		✓	✓				✓						
Stroke	✓	✓	✓		✓	✓	✓							
Diverticulosis		✓	✓	✓			✓	✓				✓		
Dental disease	✓								✓	✓		✓		

FIGURE 1–2 Multiple risk factors have been linked to most of the chronic diseases. NIDDM, non–insulin-dependent diabetes mellitus. (From Whitney, E. N., & Rolfes, S. R. [1993]. *Understanding nutrition* [6th ed., p. 93]. Belmont, CA: West Publishing Company. Reprinted by permission of Wadsworth Publishing Co.)

component. In certain diseases, however, the genetic component is so overwhelming that the disease occurs in a predictable manner. Such diseases are termed *genetic disorders;* an example is Huntington's chorea, which is a progressive neurologic disease.

New approaches to the treatment of genetic disease include gene therapy. *Gene therapy* involves the injection of deoxyribonucleic acid (DNA) fragments into cells. The fragments find their way to the nucleus and repair enzymes to restore normal function to the cell. Today research is being conducted on the use of gene therapy in the treatment of Alzheimer's disease, muscular dystrophy, cystic fibrosis, and some forms of primary and secondary epilepsy. Gene therapy is a rapidly evolving form of treatment, and other new approaches include the promotion of new blood vessel growth *(angiogenesis)* for clients who have impaired circulation.

AGING AND DISEASE

There is an increased risk for all diseases with aging, especially cancer. Older clients tend to attribute aches and pains to aging itself and often are less likely to have routine preventive screenings. Older clients are more prone to injury, acute infections (especially respiratory), and other acute illnesses than younger clients. Contributing to this are the increased occurrence of chronic illness, decreased reserves of energy, and decreased ability to respond physiologically to stress. It is common to see an older client who is mentally competent become confused during the stress of acute illness often resulting from renal and hepatic changes. Recovery from acute illness takes longer than in a younger client, and it is possible that the previous level of functioning will not be regained.

Common problems in the care of the older client include promotion of physical safety, prevention of alterations in skin integrity, promotion of social interactions, and promotion of adequate nutrition. Do not presume that all elderly clients are weak and debilitated. The older client and the nurse's role are described in Chapter 3.

Behavioral Health Risk Factors

NUTRITION AND DISEASE

Heart disease, cancer, stroke, and liver disease are associated with nutritional factors. These disorders are four of the 10 leading causes of death in the United States (Box 1–2). The role of nutrition in these diseases is discussed, and more information is presented later.

LIPIDS. There are three types of lipids, or fats: (1) triglycerides and their component fatty acids, (2) phospholipids, and (3) sterols. Triglycerides are an energy source, and stored fat is used as body insulation. Triglycerides contain one molecule of glycerol and three fatty acid molecules. The fatty acids can be saturated, monounsaturated, or polyunsaturated. The polyunsaturated and monounsaturated fats lead to a lower blood cholesterol level. Fatty acids are used as starting points for the manufacture of hormonal regulators. Phospholipids and sterols build cell membranes and manufacture hormones, vitamin D, and bile.

LIPOPROTEINS. As fats are digested, they must be "packaged" for transport in the blood because they are not soluble in water. Fats cluster together with special proteins, forming lipoproteins. There are four types: chy-

BOX 1–2 Ten Leading Causes of Death

1. Heart disease
2. Cancer
3. Stroke
4. Unintentional injuries
5. Chronic obstructive lung disease
6. Pneumonia and influenza
7. Diabetes mellitus
8. Suicide
9. Chronic liver disease and cirrhosis
10. Homicide

lomicrons, very-low-density lipoproteins (VLDLs), low-density lipoproteins (LDLs), and high-density lipoproteins (HDLs). High HDL levels and low LDL levels are associated with reduced risk of heart disease. Laboratory values for VLDLs and LDLs are found in Appendix C. Lipoproteins are explained in Chapter 56.

CHOLESTEROL. Cholesterol is carried in several lipoproteins, primarily in LDLs. A high level of cholesterol carried in LDL is directly correlated with atherosclerosis. A *direct correlation* means that as one factor rises, so does the other; in this case, the higher the cholesterol and LDL, the higher the incidence of heart disease from atherosclerosis. High blood cholesterol in HDL correlates *inversely* with risk of heart disease. Appendix C describes the range of normal laboratory values for cholesterol. The pathophysiology of atherosclerosis and heart disease is discussed in Chapter 56.

ALCOHOL. Alcohol intake plays several roles in health. Research indicates that moderate alcohol intake (one glass of red wine per day) raises HDL levels and reduces the risk of heart disease.[43] A high intake of alcohol, however, is associated with hypertension, stroke, liver disease, and several types of cancer, including some found in the head, neck, and reproductive system.

OBESITY. Obesity has been associated with increased risk of heart disease, stroke, hypertension, and diabetes (see Chapters 28 and 29). The pathophysiology of these disorders is discussed in Chapters 45 (diabetes), 52 (hypertension, 56 (heart disease), and 70 (stroke).

NUTRITION AND CANCER

Cancer is a disease of multiple origins, such as heredity, smoking, and environmental exposure. Some cancers have dietary links. Many people fear that food additives are *carcinogens* (cancer-causing substances). In fact, food additives have little to do with cancer. Contaminants of food, entities that get into foods by accident, may be powerful carcinogens, such as pesticides and bacteria. Fat has been implicated in cancer. Fat does not cause cancer; however, animals that have been exposed to a carcinogen and given a high-fat diet appear to have greater numbers of tumors than animals given a low-fat diet. Thus, fat appears to be a cancer promoter, perhaps by (1) causing the body to secrete more hormones, such as estrogen; (2) promoting the secretion of bile into the intestine, where organisms can convert the bile into compounds that cause cancer; or (3) incorporating into cell membranes and changing them so they offer less resistance to carcinogenic invaders. It is thought that fiber and vegetables might help reduce the risk of some forms of cancer by speeding excretion of bile from the body, decreasing transit time of food through the colon, and reducing exposure.

Beta-carotene (vitamin A) regulates cellular differentiation, a process that goes awry in cancer. Some people think that if they take vitamin A supplements, their risk of cancer will be reduced. This area is still being studied, but it appears that the fiber in foods containing vitamin A is more important than the vitamin itself. Other antipromoters of cancer include vitamin B_6, folate, pantothenic acid, vitamin B_{12}, iron, zinc, selenium, and antioxidants, such as vitamins C and E. Some non-nutrient compounds are found in foods from the cabbage family. These foods produce chemicals that activate enzymes that destroy carcinogens. The research base for the synthetic form of antioxidants and other cancer-preventing vitamin supplements is less conclusive. Dietitians recommend eating vegetables and consuming various foods to dilute the effects of harmful cancer promoters but may or may not recommend taking vitamin supplements.

OXYGEN FREE RADICALS AND DISEASE

Oxygen free radicals, or superoxide radicals, are by-products of energy production. Superoxide radicals are atoms or molecules with one or more pairs of unpaired, free electrons that are reactive. The radicals commonly bind to oxygen for stabilization. The oxygen then binds to hydrogen for stabilization. The product of this reaction is hydrogen peroxide, which is toxic to cells. The most unbalanced form of free radicals is free hydroxy radicals. The free hydroxy radicals bind to polyunsaturated fatty acids, which are commonly found in cell membranes and membranes of organelles within the cell. If the free radical binds to the lysosome, the cell is destroyed.

The body is equipped to handle some of these radicals with antioxidants for the conversion of the radical back to usable oxygen. The antioxidants include vitamins C and E and beta-carotene (vitamin A). Vitamin E and selenium in cell membranes are oxidized by the free radicals, much as fatty acid is. Vitamin E neutralizes the free radical and prevents it from attaching to a fatty acid. In the process, vitamin E is damaged. The damaged vitamin E is restored by vitamin C. The role of beta-carotene is not clear in free radical antioxidation. Vitamins A and E are carried by the LDLs.

Environmental Health Risk Factors

Studies in cancer causation have revealed that chemicals in the workplace are responsible for specific cancers. Such discoveries have left the impression that most human cancers are associated with environmental chemical contamination. This opinion has led to public pressure on government to control chemical contamination as a key means of cancer prevention. In most of today's industrialized world, however, work-related cancer is rare and should remain infrequent if regulations are followed. A careful analysis of the causative elements in each type of cancer has shown that prevailing lifestyles in a given population (especially tobacco use, nutritional variations, and physical activity) account for the incidence of cancer.

Sun exposure increases the risk of skin cancers. The populations most sensitive to the sun's effects are those with fair skin, such as people of Celtic descent. The chief cause of skin cancer is damage to DNA from ultraviolet light. An allegedly "healthy" look (tanned skin) can have unhealthy consequences. The belief that sun exposure is needed for vitamin D absorption is obsolete in most countries, because milk is supplemented with vitamin D. Children who have no sun exposure and do not drink milk can be at risk for rickets from low vitamin D levels. Adults who do not consume adequate vitamin D develop osteomalacia. Arabic women constitute a high-risk group because they shield their skin from the sun and do not drink milk.

Air and water pollution can lead to disease. Water pollution has caused endemic infections with various microorganisms throughout the world. Air pollution increases the risk of asthma and lung cancer.

Interrelationship of Health Risk Factors

A person's body, mind, and environment all function together to determine whether illness develops. The brain helps maintain an internal milieu and assists the body in adapting to the external environment. The response can affect the body's functioning. The way the brain defines a situation can evoke chemical and nervous system reactions. When people habitually respond to every frustration, disappointment, or loss as if it is a matter of life and death, the endocrine, musculoskeletal, and autonomic nervous systems respond. If people view life as requiring constant domination of things and people, they can have excessive production of cholesterol, triglycerides, norepinephrine, adrenocorticotropic hormone (ACTH), and insulin. This attitude may contribute to deficient levels of pituitary growth hormone.

The function and balance of neurotransmitters (chemical messengers, such as enkephalins and endorphins) can be influenced by drugs, viruses, bacteria, poor nutrition, defective genes, aging, or the perception of stress. Tissue damage can result from normal bodily processes that go awry or are disrupted; these processes include (1) neurotransmitter activity in the brain, (2) the stress hormones of the adrenal glands and nervous system, and (3) the helper and suppressor cells of the immune system. For example, excessive stress hormones (corticosteroids, catecholamines) can lead to artery damage or may suppress the action of antibodies and natural killer cells, which protect the body from foreign invaders and tumor development. Deficient suppressor cells may permit overaction of the immune system to the point at which the body starts attacking itself, such as in rheumatoid arthritis. Autoimmune disorders are discussed in Chapter 77.

The brain is central to any change in health because it is the mediator between the external and internal environments. Through the brain's interpretation, we can change an environment, leave it, or engage in it, or we can decide to rest, exercise, or diet. Ultimately, illness involves a combination of mind-body factors. These factors interact to produce symptoms. It is not uncommon to experience depression with physical illness or to have physical manifestations of mental or emotional illness.

Increasingly, scientific study is directed toward the mind-body interactions. The increase in chronic conditions and the disillusion with medical care have led to increased use of alternative, or complementary, practices which are often based on mind-body connection theory, are wellness-oriented, are less intrusive, and have fewer side effects. The Office of Alternative Medicine within the National Institutes of Health (NIH) funds research to evaluate the effectiveness of alternative medical treatment. This research provides support for the interactive nature of systems (the mind-body connection) and presents evidence other than the biomedical model.

MANAGEMENT OF CHRONIC CONDITIONS AND ILLNESS

Nursing management can strengthen the client's and family's ability to live with, and can shape the course of, chronic conditions. For effective management of chronic conditions it is essential to know (1) the time pattern of chronic conditions; (2) commonalities in physical, psychological, and social adaptation to different chronic conditions; (3) health promotion and illness prevention nursing interventions in the care of people with chronic conditions; and (4) patterns of health care delivery for people with chronic conditions. This chapter addresses these aspects.

Stages of a Chronic Condition

In general, chronic conditions evolve in a typical pattern. Various terms are used to describe this process; it can be called the *course of illness,* the *trajectory,*[4] or *time phases.*[44] Awareness of the effect of time on chronic disease creates an appreciation for the challenges experienced by clients and their families living with chronic conditions. Awareness of the pattern also promotes an appreciation that management of chronic conditions is accomplished largely by clients and families in the home. Knowledge of the time pattern of chronic conditions helps broaden the focus of health care to include all levels of prevention and to increase the percentage of health care dollars allocated to prevention.

The three stages of the pattern in all chronic conditions are (1) *prediagnostic,* (2) *diagnostic,* and (3) *chronic.* Some chronic conditions also have a *terminal stage.*

PREDIAGNOSTIC STAGE

In the prediagnostic stage, manifestations of chronic conditions are vague or absent. Risk factors common to one or more chronic conditions may be present. This chapter presents an overview, and several other chapters are devoted to specific chronic conditions.

Some risk factors are modifiable, and others are not. Modifying behavioral and environmental risk factors can prevent the development or may extend the prediagnostic phase of some chronic conditions. For example, not smoking or stopping smoking is a controllable behavior that decreases the risk for development of a chronic condition in the respiratory, cardiovascular, or other systems. These chronic conditions include asthma, emphysema, bronchiectasis, coronary artery disease, angina, myocardial infarction, hypertension, and cancer. A low-fat diet appears to decrease the risk of obesity, coronary disease, diabetes, hypertension, stroke, and cancer. Seat belts protect against injury in vehicular accidents. Reducing high stress levels may help lower the risk of cardiovascular disease, peptic ulcers, asthma, ulcerative colitis, multiple sclerosis, cancer, and accidental trauma. Specific immunizations can prevent the development of certain diseases.

DIAGNOSTIC STAGE

In the diagnostic stage, the client recognizes that something is wrong and seeks medical attention, and a disorder is diagnosed. In some cases, chronic conditions are sequelae to acute illness, trauma, or treatment. In these instances, the health care provider may simply inform the client that he or she has a given disorder. This stage occurs in all cases because chronic disorders affect all ages.

Clinical manifestations range from vague to severe or even life-threatening. Manifestations differ because the client may have ignored early warning signs or may have been able to cope with early clinical manifestations, or the condition's course may be variable. Hypertension, for example, is called a "silent killer" because most people have no clinical manifestations. Thus, hypertension may be diagnosed incidentally when a client has a routine physical examination, receives treatment for another problem, or has suffered a stroke from untreated hypertension.

CHRONIC STAGE

The chronic stage has been referred to as the "long haul" because the client must live with the condition for a prolonged time. In fact, this stage may last for the rest of the client's life.

Clinical manifestations may be controlled or out of control. Changes in function may be stable or may be marked by remissions and exacerbations, or function may progressively decline. If the onset has been acute (i.e., stroke, spinal cord injury, myocardial infarction), the greatest return of function frequently occurs within the first 6 months. Remissions and exacerbations may be frequent or infrequent. Progressive decline may be rapid or slow. Changes in function and the rate of change are more predictable for some chronic conditions than for others. Acute episodes of illness during this stage frequently relate to exacerbations, sudden decline in body system function, or side effects or complications of treatment. With medical and surgical advances (i.e., liver and heart transplants, chemotherapy), life spans have been extended but new health problems may develop. Some acute episodes can be managed at home; others must be managed in the hospital. When death occurs at this stage, it is sudden and unexpected.

TERMINAL STAGE

Transition to the terminal stage occurs (1) when changes in body systems become irreversible and the loss of these functions is incompatible with life and (2) when death is expected within 6 months.

For many chronic conditions (e.g., arthritis), there is no terminal stage. Death for these clients is due to other causes. Technological advances have eliminated the terminal stage for other chronic conditions. For example, organ transplants in clients with organ failure may reverse this stage to the chronic stage. Recent cure for some types of childhood cancers has changed the time pattern from terminal to an "at-risk" stage.

Process of Adaptation

Adaptation to chronic conditions is complex and continuous and involves physiologic, psychological, social, technological, and time factors. Knowledge related to adaptation factors has been generated by many disciplines. Adaptation is pivotal for the client with a chronic condition. In this chapter, *adaptation* refers to the body's or mind's response to a chronic condition. However, some adaptations are not positive and can worsen the condition. The nurse's role is to monitor and prevent adaptations that are not beneficial and to assist the client and family to adapt their lifestyles to the condition.

PHYSIOLOGIC ADAPTATION

Chronic conditions can interfere with physiologic functions. The body's intake, digestion, and expenditure of physical energy for cellular metabolism and protein synthesis can be altered. When physical energy demands exceed the intake and processing of physical energy, general resistance to physiologic stressors is impaired. Neuroendocrine responses to psychological distress have been implicated in adaptation to (1) anorexia, pain, fatigue, shortness of breath, and decreased immune response; (2) progressive decline or exacerbations of chronic conditions; and (3) delayed recovery from acute episodes of illness during the chronic stage. It is thought that adaptive energy from neuroendocrine sources becomes exhausted over time.

Another physiologic adaptation is the loss of coordinated function of various body systems. Clients whose levels of mobility become limited because of self-imposed inactivity, progression of chronic health problems, surgery, trauma, or acute episodes of medical treatment are at high risk for experiencing changes in body system functions. Collectively, these adaptive responses are commonly referred to as "hazards of immobility" or the "disuse syndrome." Clearly, these adaptive responses increase levels of disability.

PSYCHOLOGICAL ADAPTATION

Psychological adaptation to a chronic condition is difficult and demanding. This adaptation process is ongoing and overlaps other biologic and psychosocial processes associated with gains, losses, and challenges throughout the remaining life span. Box 1–3 identifies common concerns, fears, and events of personal change associated with a chronic condition.

As with other ongoing processes, psychological adaptation to a chronic condition is characterized by periods of changing demands and transitions. Some of these are predictable; others are not. Predictable periods of changing demands and transitions include onset and diagnosis, hospitalizations for treatment, exacerbation of illness, treatment failures, and loss of self-care abilities. These times can be expected to be especially stressful. Some periods are marked by depression when clients realize they may not get better and may get worse. The client and family must redefine their roles, expectations, and life goals. Clients in the terminal stage must adapt to a shortened life span and to the process of dying.

Although chronic diseases, such as acquired immunodeficiency syndrome (AIDS), cancer, diabetes mellitus, and multiple sclerosis, may differ in their impact on each client, psychological adaptation to various chronic conditions, over varying lengths of time, has many similar characteristics. Therefore, some general statements can be made. The incidence of clinical depression in persons living with chronic conditions ranges from "no difference from" to "higher than" that of community-dwelling adults without chronic health problems. Risk factors for depression have been identified as (1) biologic changes, (2) medications (e.g., digoxin, droperidol, ethanol), and (3) psychological vulnerability. Some cases of depression may be resolved with medical treatment or by a change in medication. If these interventions are not effective, the client should receive psychiatric evaluation and treatment.[1]

Different clients adapt to the same diagnosis and stage of illness in different ways. During the diagnostic stage, one client may appear overwhelmed and may assume a

BOX 1–3 Common Concerns, Fears, and Events of Personal Change Associated with Chronic Conditions

Concerns and Fears

Loss of sense of self
Loss of control and predictability
Heightened sense of mortality
Loss of productivity
Loss of valued roles
Loss of relationships
Loss of opportunity or ability for sexual expression or reproduction
Uncertainty about the future
Loss of purpose and meaning in life
Fear of procedures
Fear of death

Events of Personal Change

Life plans and goals
Established roles and patterns of interacting within family and outside the home
Relationships with others
Work (job) or school roles, relationships, and patterns of interaction
Daily routines
Loss of gratifying behaviors
Changes in health maintenance and management behaviors
Activity and sleep patterns
Financial resources
Appearance

lower level of physical, psychological, or social functioning than the physical condition warrants. Another client may evidence minimal distress and may regain or maintain a high level of physical, psychological, and social functioning.

General Pattern of Adaptation. A general pattern of psychological adaptation to personal change perceived as a loss or threat of loss has been described by sociologists, psychologists, physicians, and nurses. Phases of this pattern have been labeled in various ways by different authors. The pattern has been referred to as the *grief process* and the *mourning process.*

Disbelief. The first phase is commonly referred to as disbelief or *resistance.* Denial (unconscious refusal to acknowledge painful realities) of the changes or the need for personal change is characteristic. This phase is similar to the "fight-or-flight" response and is believed to protect the client from being psychologically overwhelmed.

Developing Awareness. The second phase, commonly referred to as the *anger* phase, is developing awareness. It is characterized by withdrawal, preoccupation with self, crying, depression, expression of anger toward others, and feelings of guilt for having brought the disease on oneself, being different, and being alone. In this phase, the client experiences acute awareness of what has been lost and grieves for it.

Integration. The third phase is characterized by rational acceptance that a physical or psychological change has occurred and by attempts to keep emotional distress within manageable limits. Other cognitive behaviors associated with this phase are reestablishing a sense of self, meaning, and purpose; revising life goals; learning to live with uncertainty; and acquiring new strategies for coping with one's environment.

Some people describe experiencing intermittent chronic sorrow.[11] Triggers of sadness include the anniversary date of the condition's onset, special events, birthdays, and losses in physical function. Knowledge that feelings of sorrow are commonly felt may help mitigate the distress associated with the experience.

Coping Behaviors. Clients with the same medical diagnosis and in the same phase of chronic illness use a variety of physical, cognitive, and verbal behaviors to manage distress. The type of behaviors used and their effectiveness are highly individual. Some coping behaviors are passive; others are active. *Emotion-focused (affective)* behaviors have been defined as thoughts or actions that make a person feel better but do not alter the distressing situation. *Problem-focused* behaviors are efforts taken to change or resolve distressing situations. A number of behaviors fall into both categories. The prevailing assumption is that problem-focused behaviors are more efficacious, but some research suggests that a combination of both behaviors may be most efficacious, especially when the problem cannot be resolved and must be managed.

Interestingly, some clients report that talking about their illness helps them cope.[22] Others report that *not* talking about their illness helps them cope. Strategies reported as being effective in managing distressful situations include avoiding, ignoring, accepting, thinking out, and changing the situation. Shopping, driving, going out to eat, and exercising are types of activities that some people find helpful in relieving stress. Other reported helpful strategies include taking naps; seeking information and advice; changing values, attitudes, and goals; hope; prayer; putting the problem in God's hands; humor; positive thinking; positive self-talk; trying to maintain some control over the situation; trying to look at the problem objectively; and drawing on past experiences.[27] Although many strategies are constructive, others can be destructive, such as imagining the worst, taking anger out on others, blaming others, taking illegal drugs, overeating, smoking, and abusing alcohol.

Social Adaptation

The roles of clients with chronic conditions overlap social roles related to age, sex, family, work, and recreation. The impact of health and illness roles on social roles ranges from minimal to severe, with health and illness roles being dominant. The degree to which clients adapt socially is influenced by (1) changes in physical appearance, (2) ability to communicate, (3) ability to navigate the physical environment, (4) social resources (e.g., people, money, and community services), and (5) societal values and attitudes. Society responds more favorably to clients who have less apparent chronic conditions than to those with more visible signs of illness. Beliefs and values influence social acceptance related to attractiveness,

DIVERSITY IN HEALTH CARE

Health and Illness Beliefs and Practices

Whether we consider ourselves well or ill is primarily a matter of cultural definition. Kleinman and colleagues[3] describe illness as culturally shaped, in that it is individually perceived. What is important is how one explains one's illness, such as:

- How it was caused
- How long it will last
- What type of treatment should be received
- What type of practitioner should deliver the treatment

Illness includes the subjective experiences of the person who is ill and how the illness is perceived and experienced by the social group also.

In many cultures, illnesses are defined as "natural" or "unnatural."[2] In the folk health tradition, *natural* illnesses are those that occur because of some known external factors in the environment, such as bad air, night air, bad food, bad water, or infestations. An example of a folk illness or culture-bound syndrome that is considered to be the result of natural factors is *Empacho,* an illness recognized by Hispanics in which pain and cramping in the abdomen are believed to be due to food forming into a ball and clinging to the stomach or intestines.[1] Another example of a natural illness is "high blood," believed among some African Americans and Haitians to be the result of eating too many rich foods or red meat.[1] Treatment may involve consuming an astringent substance to promote "sweating out" the excess blood nutrients.

Unnatural illnesses are believed to be caused by supernatural forces, such as punishment from God or a hex or curse by a witch, a root doctor, or other practitioner. An unnatural illness that shows up in many cultures around the world is the Evil Eye, known as *Mal Ojo* in Spanish or as other names in other languages. The Evil Eye is usually considered to be a disorder in which a child falls ill as a result of a stranger's attention or admiration. In *Mal Ojo,* the practice of touching a child by one who is admiring him or her is believed to prevent the disorder.[2] *Susto,* or magical fright, is another unnatural illness and is believed to result from the loss of the spirit from the body. Treatment at times includes the use of ceremonies along with herbs.[4]

The concept of "balance" is also important in many cultures in understanding and maintaining health and treating illnesses. For health, a balance must exist among a person's psychological, physical, social and spiritual realms. If imbalance is present, illness results. The "hot-cold" theory related to the balance needed for health exists in many cultures and is a classification in which illnesses, treatments, and foods are identified as to their hot and cold qualities; these qualities are not related to temperature.[6] If an illness is considered "cold," a "hot" treatment, such as particular herbal tea, food (e.g.,meat), or a medication is given to help restore balance. The opposite is done with a "hot" illness. Whether or not a particular illness or substance is considered hot or cold varies across cultures.

In Asian cultures following Taoist philosophy, the concepts of the opposing forces in nature of *Yin* and *Yang* are the bases for determining balance.[1] *Yin* is considered to be all that is female, dark, cold, quiet, empty, and negative; *Yang* is all that is male, light, warm, and positive. What is especially important to nurses and other caregivers about these belief systems is that clients may not want to follow a treatment regimen if they consider that the wrong treatment is being given for the illness and thus that balance will not be achieved. If a client identifies the illness as hot, such as in an infection, and the medication is also considered hot, such as an antibiotic, the client may throw away the medication in favor of a cold treatment. If a nurse elicits the client's belief system, the nurse can then help to make the treatment more acceptable, such as by adding a substance (e.g., herbal tea) that is considered cold to a regimen that includes a hot treatment.

In relation to her theory of culture care, Leininger emphasizes the need for the nurse to understand the client's view of illness in order to provide culturally congruent care. One of the theory-based modes of nursing action identified by Leininger is that of cultural care *repatterning,* which refers to the supportive and facilitative professional actions and decisions that help clients reorder or modifiy their health care patterns in a more health-promoting direction while respecting their cultural values and beliefs.[5] By understanding the client's view of illness and providing care that respects and incorporates the beliefs of the client, the nurse can improve the probability that the client will achieve the most positive health outcomes possible.

References

1. Andrews, M. M., & Boyle, J. S. (1999). *Transcultural concepts in nursing care* (3rd ed.). Philadelphia: Lippincott–Williams & Wilkins.
2. Giger, J. N., & Davidhizar, R. E. (1999). *Transcultural nursing: Assessment and intervention* (3rd ed.). St. Louis: Mosby.
3. Kleinman, A., Eisenberg, L., & Good, B. (1978). Clinical lessons from anthropologic and cross-cultural research. *Annals of Internal Medicine, 88,* 251–258.
4. Purnell, L. D., & Paulanka, B. J. (1998). *Transcultural health care: A culturally competent approach.* Philadelphia: F. A. Davis.
5. Reynolds, C. L., & Leininger, M. (1993). *Madeleine Leininger: Cultural care diversity and universality theory.* Newbury Park, CA: Sage.
6. Spector, R. E. (1996). *Cultural diversity in health and illness* (4th ed.). Stamford, CT: Appleton & Lange.

Sandra Sharma, PhD, ARNP, CS, *James A. Haley Veterans Hospital, Tampa, Florida*

productivity, independence, self-reliance, normality, individual rights, and health and illness. These beliefs and values also influence the availability of social resources and health services as well as job, recreational, and housing opportunities.

Social Beliefs. Social beliefs and expectations about behavior appropriate for people experiencing physical illness have changed since the 1950s when Parsons described the "sick role" in our society.[30] Parsons stated that people are not responsible for their illness. This pattern of thinking has shifted to an idea that a client may have a role in the development of some illnesses. Parsons also stated that society believed that all clients should be released from the usual role responsibilities. The belief today is shifting to one in which clients try to maintain responsibility for personal, family, and social activities that they are capable of doing or learning. The expectation that clients should view illness as undesirable and try to get well is shifting to one in which cure is not possible for all illnesses and that clients should maintain an active role in managing incurable health problems. The expectation persists that clients should seek medically competent help; however, clients are more actively involved in decision-making related to care options and management of health problems than they were 50 years ago. Differences in beliefs and expectations about clients who have chronic conditions and how they respond to their sick role are a frequent source of conflict among caregivers, clients, and families. See Diversity in Health Care.

SOCIAL CHANGE EVENTS. Events of social change commonly associated with a chronic condition relate to roles and interaction patterns, mobility patterns, employment, living arrangements, recreation, finances, time and place for vacations, and health insurance.

FAMILY ADAPTATION

Because of the long-term nature of chronic conditions and the role of the family in maintaining the health of its members, a chronic condition is also a family condition. Families must cope with unusual ongoing adaptive challenges related to the presence of a chronic condition. Some families are more effective than others in meeting adaptive challenges. Types of physical impairments, family resources, family perception, the developmental stage of family members and the family unit, behaviors of the client, the health care environment, and society's expectation are interrelated factors that affect family adaptation. Some family units become stronger, whereas others disintegrate.

Challenges to family adjustment vary with different stages of the condition. Adaptive challenges during the *diagnostic* stage are the same as those related to acute illness, such as (1) pulling together, (2) learning to cope with the acute care environment and treatment, and (3) establishing relationships with caregivers. Other challenges include (1) identifying the meanings of health and illness, (2) assessing potential changes in the family, (3) moving toward integration of temporary and permanent changes while maintaining a sense of continuity between past and present, and (4) developing an attitude of flexibility toward future personal and family goals.

Adaptive challenges during the *chronic* stage include (1) maintaining a sense of normality, (2) adjusting to changing expectations of each family member, (3) striving to balance family resources, and (4) maintaining autonomy of all family members despite the pull toward mutual dependency, caretaking, or focus on the family member who has the chronic condition. Some demands during the chronic stage result from treatment, for example, changing work schedules to accommodate treatment, or loss of strength related to treatment side effects. Similarly, the client's roles may have to be assumed by other family members or friends. If the client is the primary wage earner, the tasks of earning a living may have to be undertaken by another. Initially, the condition may generate a lot of support from extended family members and friends; after several months, support may decline.

When a family has a member with a long-term disabling condition and limited financial resources, complex issues must be managed. Some couples divorce so that they can qualify for funding to care for a family member. If the family member has impaired judgment or reduced ability to conduct personal business, another family member may need to obtain power of attorney. If the chronic condition is terminal, families must also manage issues related to the family member's death and to resuming a normal family life after the death.

Health Care and Chronic Conditions

Health care management after the diagnostic stage occurs in various settings, such as (1) rehabilitation centers, units, and programs; (2) home health care agencies; (3) long-term health care facilities; (4) nurse-managed clinics; (5) case management; (6) hospice care; and (7) community service agencies. During the other phases of chronic conditions, care may be provided in acute care hospitals, rehabilitation units, nursing homes, or the client's home.

Chronic care is different from *acute* care.[18] The goal of acute care is to restore a person to the previous level of functioning. The goal of chronic care is to maintain independent living, facilitate successful personal and social adjustment, and minimize further deterioration of physical and mental health. The aim of chronic care is not to "fix" or "cure." Chronic care requires interdisciplinary collaboration and multidisciplinary approaches. Medical management varies with the type and stage of the chronic condition and the technology available. Management and management outcomes are better defined for some conditions than others. Medical management includes prevention, diagnosis, treatment of acute episodes, and helping clients manage and shape the course of their chronic condition. Multidisciplinary approaches are employed in promoting maximal use of the client's functional abilities and adaptation to deficits. Increasingly, goals for management are established in conjunction with other health team members, the client, and family.

In the United States, chronic conditions are the leading cause of illness, disability, and death.[18] Today's health care system is not very effective in treating chronic conditions, because available care is often fragmented, inappropriate, and difficult to obtain. New health problems may result when clients who have chronic conditions face barriers in accessing services such as preventive care, durable medical equipment, medications, or home nursing care. These secondary health problems might have been prevented through better coordination of health care services and more preventive care. Managed care or the case management approach has the potential to provide the range of integrated services required by people with chronic conditions.

FUNDING ISSUES

Chronic conditions cost $470 billion (in 1990 dollars) in direct medical costs.[18] This cost has the potential to be reduced. Table 1–5 demonstrates how more health promotion and illness prevention interventions might be cost-effective in chronic care.

TABLE 1–5 THE OPPORTUNITY COSTS OF CHRONIC CARE

America's lack of investment in an adequate system of chronic care carries an *opportunity cost;* that is, when money is spent on "X"—usually acute care services—it is not available to spend on "Y"—early, up-front prevention and treatment of chronic conditions, or coordinated systems of supportive services.

Examples:

More money spent on	*May mean less money spent on*
1. Screening, nutrition, and education to prevent heart attacks	1. Emergency department treatment and subsequent care for a heart attack victim
2. Relatively inexpensive preventive care for a client with diabetes	2. Complications leading to amputation and lifelong disability
3. Breast cancer screening for early detection, when treatment is less expensive and more effective than later detection	3. Chemotherapy, radiation, or surgery for breast cancer
4. Modest cost of installing a handrail to prevent falls	4. Hip replacement surgery
5. Adult day care	5. Nursing home care

From The Institute for Health and Aging, University of California, San Francisco.

One example of the current chronic care system's fragmentation is the lack of distribution of assistive technology (e.g., wheelchair, walker, hearing aid, brace, or artificial limb) among those in need. The 1990 National Health Interview survey showed that more than 2.5 million people reported a need for assistive technology but did not receive it.[18] Of these, nearly half were adults of working age (25 to 64 years old), and more than half reported that they could not afford a device. Clients with physical disabilities benefit from assistive devices and techniques that compensate or substitute for lost function. Acquiring skills in using these devices improves functional levels. Unfortunately, many clients and families who would benefit are not referred because some health care professionals lack knowledge about rehabilitation services, or third-party payers may not reimburse clients for these services.

Outcome Management in Chronic Conditions

The focus of the health history varies with the stage of the chronic condition. In the *prediagnostic* phase, emphasis is on obtaining the history, determining the client's current health status, and identifying risk factors. In the *diagnostic* phase, the emphasis is on manifestations and the client's related experiences, for example:

- When did they start?
- What makes them better or worse?
- To what degree are they interfering with sleep and the activities and demands of daily living?

In the *chronic* phase, assessment focuses on several aspects of the major manifestations: (1) change or stability, (2) frequency and severity, (3) triggers, and (4) means of relief. Manifestations common to a number of chronic conditions are anorexia, fatigue, pain, shortness of breath, and sleep and sexual disturbances.

Ask about (1) facilitators and barriers encountered in carrying out prescribed health care regimens in the home, (2) recreational and work environments, (3) general energy level, (4) sleep pattern, (5) activity level and amount of assistance needed in conducting activities, and (6) demands of daily living. Levels of mobility and self-care are on a continuum ranging from complete or modified independence to modified or complete dependence.

Assess the client for treatment-related, environmental, and psychological factors as well as illness-related factors that may be contributing to physical symptoms and immobility. Self-reported symptoms are better predictors of functioning than objective measurements of physical function. Assessing the client's strengths is beneficial and provides a positive starting point for health promotion interventions. Assessment is described in Chapters 9 and 10.

■ IDENTIFYING CLIENT STRENGTHS

Everyone has both strengths and weaknesses. Help the client to recognize this fact, and encourage the client to take the necessary time to identify them. Consider questions such as the following:

- What do I like best about myself?
- What are my personal strengths?
- What goals do I set for myself?
- Am I able to complete goals I set for myself?
- How do I perceive my personal strengths as a way of understanding these patterns?

Evaluating one's strengths can help build an individual's belief system. Gaining knowledge of strengths and weaknesses fosters a sense of personal worth, which may be severely tested or destroyed during periods of stress or crisis. Our thoughts affect our life patterns. Working on acknowledging one's strengths allows them to be called into consciousness during stressful periods. Positive cognitive thoughts connect with all the human potentials so that the body responds positively. When activating and acting from one's strengths, a person is more likely to develop positive attitudes. Developing positive attitudes enhances one's ability to cope effectively with stress during the inevitable everyday life struggles that confront us all. Active interventions, such as recognizing strengths, enable individuals to call up inner resources to combat stress on the journey toward becoming healthy.

■ NURSING DIAGNOSIS

A number of interrelated physiologic, psychological, and sociologic nursing diagnoses are associated with chronic conditions (Box 1–4). Etiologic factors for the diagnoses

BOX 1–4 Physiologic, Psychological, and Social Nursing Diagnoses Commonly Associated with Chronic Conditions

Physiologic Diagnoses

Activity intolerance
Constipation
Disuse syndrome, risk for
Fatigue
Fluid volume deficit
Fluid volume excess
Health maintenance, altered
Impaired physical mobility
Incontinence, bowel
Infection, risk for
Injury, risk for
Nutrition: less than body requirements, altered
Nutrition: more than body requirements, altered
Pain
Pain, chronic
Self care deficit (bathing/hygiene, dressing/grooming, feeding, toileting)
Urinary elimination, altered

Psychological Diagnoses

Anxiety
Body image disturbance
Decisional conflict (specify)
Fear
Grieving, anticipatory
Grieving, dysfunctional
Growth and development, altered
Hopelessness
Knowledge deficit (specify)
Powerlessness
Self-esteem disturbance
Spiritual distress

Social Diagnoses

Communication, impaired verbal
Diversional activity deficit
Family processes, altered
Parenting, altered
Role performance, altered
Sexuality patterns, altered
Social interaction, impaired
Social isolation

differ according to individual characteristics, stage of chronic condition, changes in physiologic structure or function, treatment, and environment.

■ EXPECTED OUTCOMES

The expected outcomes for the client with a chronic condition are directly related to the specific diagnosis, physiologic changes, treatment, and adaptive energy. In general, a cure is not expected and some outcomes are more predictable than others. *Long-term* outcomes are usually written with months allowed for achievement. *Short-term* outcomes that are achievable and measurable provide positive feedback to clients, families, and caregivers. This feedback is believed to decrease the potential for caregiver burnout. The client, family, and other health team members should be involved in determining long-term and short-term outcomes.

When clients and families identify seemingly unrealistic goals, tell them that they may not achieve them and that most people with similar problems have not done so. Then identify incremental goals that can be achieved. For example, for the client with a spinal cord injury who has a goal of walking, the work would be on maintaining range of motion, which is necessary for walking. As clients and families work toward more modest goals, they will, with time, readjust their goals. In some cases, clients and families have achieved goals that were perceived as unrealistic by others.

■ EVALUATION

Expected outcomes for clients living with chronic conditions are achieved over time. Evaluation examines outcome achievement and movement to another level of care. For example, a client in acute care may become physiologically stable and may be discharged to the home for home care, to a skilled or long-term care facility, or to an acute rehabilitation center.

When gains in physical function stabilize with or without assistive devices, the client can be moved to less skilled care areas or discharged to the home. Of course, the original goals may not have been met. In these instances, determine the cause, keeping in mind that the condition may have worsened and that the expected outcome and interventions may require revision.

■ INTERVENTIONS

Nursing interventions should strengthen the client's and family's ability to live with and shape the course of the chronic condition. General strategies used in the care of clients with chronic conditions include providing direct care, teaching, counseling, working things out, making arrangements, and advocating. Interventions must be specific to the client and the setting. Use the health promotion theories presented earlier as a guide to motivate health behavior change.

Providing Client Education

Most chronic illnesses exist in a balance between control and crisis. Client education includes teaching how to determine when an illness is becoming uncontrolled, how to treat it, and when to contact the health care provider; for example:

1. Teach diabetic clients to recognize the clinical manifestations of hyperglycemia and hypoglycemia,

how to begin treatment, and when to notify the health care provider.
2. Instruct diabetic clients to carry a blood glucose testing device, a fast-acting carbohydrate, and insulin at all times.
3. Advise asthmatic clients to carry a rescue bronchodilator and angina clients to carry nitroglycerin.

Preventive actions (e.g., annual influenza vaccinations) and healthy behaviors (e.g., regular exercise) will help the client with chronic illness achieve the highest possible level of wellness.

Most chronic illnesses require some degree of daily treatment. These treatments can range from taking medication to receiving multiple injections to running a home dialysis unit. Assess the client's and the family's ability to follow the treatment guidelines, and ask whether they have experienced problems in carrying out the treatment regimen. When formulating your questions, consider these characteristics:

- *Degree of difficulty in learning the regimen.* Are there several steps involved? What complications might result from using equipment or giving medications incorrectly? Does the client or family member have the dexterity required to complete the regimen successfully? Does the client or a family member have limitations that can interfere with performing tasks?
- *Amount of time required to implement the regimen.* How much time does the treatment regimen require? How many times each day must the regimen be performed?
- *The monetary cost.* Can the client afford this regimen? Are there alternatives?
- *Amount of discomfort and exertion associated with the regimen.* How painful or inconvenient is the treatment? Do you believe the client will comply or that a family member will be persuasive enough to ensure compliance?
- *Visibility of the regimen to other people, and its social acceptance.* Will the client need to take equipment everywhere, as with oxygen? Does the client have a disfiguring condition, such as a tracheostomy or a fistula?
- *Effectiveness and speed of the regimen in controlling the condition or its manifestations.* Will the client or family members have to wait a long time for results of the regimen? What complications might occur because of the regimen (e.g., drug side effects)?

On the basis of these and other questions, develop a comprehensive teaching plan to help the client implement the treatment regimen successfully.

Controlling Clinical Manifestations

In addition to implementing a treatment regimen properly, the client and family may need to learn ways to control the chronic condition's influence on their lives. Some clients must plan ahead so that needed items will be available. For example, they may need to buy adequate supplies before leaving on a trip. The client may need to hand-carry supplies when traveling or may need adaptive equipment. Clients with arthritis, for example, may benefit from using fastening tape (Velcro) closures rather than zippers or buttons.

Restructuring Time

Assess the client's time requirements. A client who is unemployed because of a chronic condition may have too much free time; a client who spends hours each day undergoing a medical regimen may have little time to enjoy life.

Focus the teaching plan on helping the client maintain enough free time to enjoy a high-quality life. Examine areas of the client's life that include wasted time. Encourage a hobby or a support group, which may help to build a support system and to cultivate interests. Consult a recreational therapist at a local physical rehabilitation center about recreational activities in the home or community.

Adjusting to Changes

The teaching plan can provide invaluable assistance in helping clients cope with the course of a chronic disorder. With some disorders, the course is stable; for others, it is unpredictable. For example, the course of chronic ulcerative colitis usually is stable, whereas that of multiple sclerosis can be erratic.

Inform the client and the family about predictable flare-ups. For example, depression is common 4 to 6 months after a cerebrovascular accident or a myocardial infarction. Educate the client and family ahead of time, so that they can watch for signs of depression and can consult a health care provider if necessary. Support groups exist for many chronic conditions and should be included in the teaching plan along with instruction on how to access a local group.

Promoting Physiologic Adaptation

Physical adaptation to a chronic condition can be improved by a change in medication, dosages, or schedules or diet and activity patterns. Identifying environmental or behavioral factors that trigger manifestations, improve sleep, increase energy levels, or substitute for lost function can increase feelings of wellness. Early detection of complications, knowledge about the condition and its management, and how to substitute and compensate for changes in physical function facilitate physiologic adaptation.

Promoting Psychological Adaptation

Interventions to enhance psychological adaptation during the diagnostic stage include (1) encouraging the client's active involvement in the diagnostic process and treatment decisions, (2) facilitating the client's expressions of feelings, and (3) helping a client to seek appropriate information.

Some clients may perceive hospitalization during the *chronic* stage as a crisis episode; other clients may view hospitalization during this stage as a reprieve from day-to-day hassles and concerns or as a period of hope because new treatments may be available. In the *terminal* stage, one client may fear death whereas another may view death as a preferable alternative to suffering and disability. Personal factors that may contribute to the individual nature of psychological adaptation include hope, commitment, confidence, appraisal of changes, perception of the effectiveness of management, coping strategies, and personal, spiritual, and social resources. Appraisals of change are based on an individual's beliefs, knowledge, skills, previous losses, and threat of loss. Each client's ability to manage loss, the threat of loss, and challenges also differs. Spiritual adaptation can positively affect the mental and physical health of clients during this time of adjustment to the chronic illness. Relaxation, meditation, distraction, social support, spiritual guidance, and cognitive therapies are interventions that may promote psychological adaptation.

Promoting Sociologic Adaptation

Interventions that promote sociologic adaptation include teaching and counseling related to management of the chronic condition in home, work, and recreational environments and assisting the client and family in locating professional and community resources to lower barriers to social integration. Vocational rehabilitation and job skills training may help a client gain employment. Interventions that foster and support role changes include (1) *role-playing* in anticipated situations; (2) imaginative *role-taking,* in which the client imagines how another person would respond to behaviors; and (3) *role-modeling,* in which the individual is introduced to another person who has the same chronic condition and has adapted positively to enforced changes. Role-modeling may help the client gain practical tips about hunting for a job, finding accessible housing, and meeting new friends.

Role clarification is a strategy in which the client is given information about behaviors necessary to play a particular role. Reference group interaction brings together people with similar problems and concerns. These groups are helpful for exchanging ideas for solving problems and relieving feelings of isolation and helplessness.

Encourage clients to normalize their lives and to resume social activities. Some visible deformities can be disguised with clothing, such as scarves, or make-up to reduce self-consciousness. Similarly, clients with dyspnea, by looking in a store window, can disguise the fact that they are stopping to catch their breath. If a condition cannot be disguised, prepare the client to sometimes be the object of rude stares and comments. Encourage the client to educate others. Eventually, the client will learn to ignore the stares and comments.

Health Promotion and Illness Prevention Interventions

Health promotion and illness prevention interventions are essential for everyone, including people who have chronic conditions. Chronic conditions account for approximately 80% of all medical expenses.[13] Chronic conditions usually cannot be cured, but health promotion and illness prevention interventions can improve the quality of life for those with chronic conditions and have the potential to reduce medical expenses. A health risk appraisal should be done, with risk reduction interventions tailored to each individual's need. A general discussion of health promotion follows. Health promotion for young and middle-aged adults is described in Chapter 2; for older clients, see Chapter 3.

■ MODIFYING BEHAVIORAL HEALTH RISK FACTORS

Nutrition and exercise are addressed together because they work synergistically to promote high-level wellness. Sedentary living and the lack of sound nutrition contribute to major risk factors, such as hypercholesterolemia, obesity, and muscular atrophy. When people begin to modify one of these two areas, the other area often receives attention at the same time.

Nutrition

Nutrition has moved into the forefront as a prominent component of health promotion and disease prevention. A correlation exists between what we eat and how we feel; the potential for development of disease is also correlated with nutritional status and habits. Cardiovascular disease, cancer, and osteoporosis are three common afflictions that are directly related to nutrition to some degree. Scores of other conditions related to poor nutrition may be less crippling, but they clearly affect how we feel (e.g., dental caries, constipation, and acne). The U.S. Department of Agriculture (USDA) has revised its dietary recommendations and has created the "food pyramid" (see Chapter 2), which includes food groupings and provides suggested servings from each group.

Nutritional Deficits

Deficits in nutritional intake can result in stunted growth, reduced metabolic function, delayed or premature cessation of reproductive function, and increased risk for less serious illnesses. Mechanisms of homeostasis protect the body from temporary deficits, but chronic nutritional deprivation creates a susceptible host for the diseases of malnutrition. Three classic deficiency diseases are scurvy (vitamin C deficiency), beriberi (thiamin deficiency), and pellagra (niacin deficiency). Malnutrition also increases susceptibility to infection (see Chapter 17) and decreases wound-healing ability (see Chapter 16).

Nutritional Excesses

Overeating or eating too many of the wrong foods can also cause illness and disease. Many people, especially those in the lowest socioeconomic group, eat foods that are high in fat, sugar, protein, simple carbohydrates, caffeine, and alcohol. Over time, diseases of overconsumption or malconsumption appear. Obesity, atherosclerosis, alcoholism, constipation, hypertension, cardiorespiratory disorders, and some cancers are, to some extent, thought to be related to nutritional imbalance (see Chapter 2).

Balanced Nutrition

Healthy nutrition is defined as a balance of nutrients, fiber, fluids, vitamins, and minerals. Whenever possible, foods should be free of chemicals, additives, preservatives, and toxins. Clients should eat fresh foods, fruits, vegetables, legumes, and lean meats and should avoid high-fat, overprocessed, and fried foods. The U.S. government recommends a diet with less fat and more complex carbohydrates (see Chapter 2). Clients can use a food diary (see Chapter 28) to assess their food intake.

Exercise

Until recently, physical fitness was directed primarily toward building muscle groups for the purpose of preparing for competition. A new way of thinking about fitness is depicted in Chapter 2. Exercise, like nutrition, should be balanced and performed on a regular basis; it cannot be effective if it is performed sporadically. Exercise tones and strengthens internal organs and the circulatory, respiratory, and musculoskeletal systems. It is more than calisthenics. The components of fitness are multiple, and all aspects should be part of a routine.

Exercise does not reverse pathophysiologic changes but is believed to condition muscles to work more efficiently and to use less oxygen. Exercise also stimulates the production of endorphins (which promote the feelings of well-being), increases production of high-density lipoproteins (HDLs), assists in weight control, decreases risk of some cancers, and increases activity tolerance.

A physical exercise program coupled with a balanced nutritional diet is the most effective way to actualize promotion of physical health. Eating and exercising wisely develop strength and endurance, a more youthful appearance, increased vitality, straight posture, and general physical stamina (see Chapters 2 and 3).

Empowerment

Empowerment involves helping clients assume control and mastery over all aspects of their lives. This involves health care as well as social and political environments. Accept clients as the experts in their own experience and definition of health. At the basic level, empowerment means a transfer of skills, resources, access, and language, so that the client with a chronic condition can be as independent as possible. Empowerment can occur only in a supportive environment. Learn how to establish and maintain an empowering environment in which the client sees the potential and value in seizing power and being independent.

In the United States, changing social beliefs about individual rights and normality have influenced state and federal laws. This legislation has contributed to a decrease in attitudinal and architectural barriers to social integration as well as to increased availability of health care, housing, employment, recreation, and transportation for ill people. Nurses can encourage clients to be politically active and can also be active themselves in advocating for the health care rights of those with chronic conditions.

Developing Human Potential

Current definitions of health refer to the achievement of maximum potential, or *self-actualization* (see Table 1–3). In the domain of health promotion, people develop and maintain life potentials, becoming the best and healthiest that they can. The more time and energy devoted to developing strengths, the less likely problems are to develop. The physical potentials of nutrition and exercise have been discussed earlier.

Figure 1–3 represents the circle of human potentials, each of which needs to be developed to maximize health. Each physical body is unique. Through the senses of sight, hearing, touch, taste, and smell, we gather experience of the world. When the body is nurtured, it increases in strength, vitality, energy, sexuality, and the capacity to communicate and connect with other potentials.

Our picture of the world is created uniquely from mental stimuli. It is through logical processes that we learn to fully understand, enjoy, and appreciate many of life's greatest pleasures. Growth is possible when we are receptive to information, suggestions, and help.

Emotions are feelings, the inner and outer responses to the events encountered in life. One of the greatest challenges is to acknowledge, own, express, and understand one's emotions. Increasing attention to the development and balancing of this potential allows spontaneity and positive zest for living to emerge.

Spirit comes from one's roots and inner core of being. It is related to the universal need to understand the human experience of life on Earth. Where did we come from? Where are we going? What is our purpose? Why do good and evil exist? What occurs after death? Who or what put this life form together? Development of the spiritual potential allows for the transcendence of the experience of oneness, peace, harmony, and connection with the universe.

We cannot live purposeful lives without meaningful relationships. We may not share a house with anyone, but many of us live in neighborhoods and all of us are part

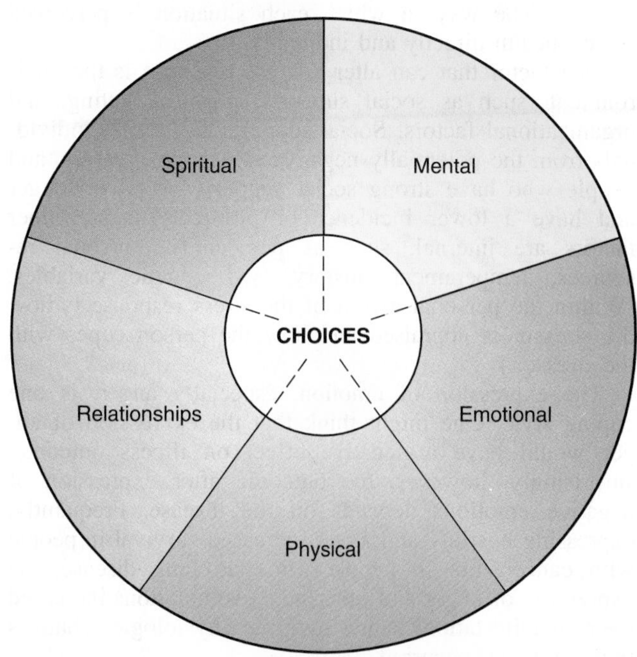

FIGURE 1–3 The circle of human potentials.

of communities, cities, and states. Our relationships extend to our nation and to the whole of planet Earth. The challenge in relationships is to extend ourselves and to learn how to exchange feelings of honesty, trust, intimacy, compassion, openness, and harmony. When we share our feelings and experiences, true interchange occurs. It is through our attitude and orientation that we affect the outcome of all of our encounters.

People have enormous capacity for making choices either consciously or unconsciously. Health and balance occur when we use the skill of effective choice-making. Each of us is responsible for assessing our values and desires. No one else can make decisions for us.

Milio[26] contends that the focus on choice is paramount in shaping the overall health for the person as well as for the society as a whole. Our range of choices is affected by personal resources, which include awareness, knowledge, our own beliefs, and our family's beliefs. Time, money, support of family and friends, and the urgency of other priorities influence what choices are made. Milio notes that "most human beings, professional or nonprofessional, provider or consumer, make the easiest choices available to them most of the time."[26] Try to recognize this tendency when working with clients. Lifestyle behavioral patterns are not isolated choices unrelated to social, personal, or economic circumstances.

Stress Management

All of us have experienced stress, but each of us has different perceptions and thoughts about it. What are your perceptions? Think of a recent stressful event at home or at work that involved you and someone else. How did you react? How did the other person react? Was there a different reaction to the same event? Stress is an individual matter. No two people respond in completely the same manner. In a given situation, one person may perceive a challenge whereas the other perceives a serious stressor. The way in which each situation is perceived affects health directly and indirectly.

One factor that can alter a stress response is the environment, such as social supports, physical setting, and organizational factors. Social supports can buffer individuals from the potentially negative effects of stressors, and people who have strong social supports may live longer and have a lower incidence of physical illness. Other factors are internal, such as personality, personal resources, temperament, history, and genetic variables. (Within the personal aspect of the stress response is how the stressor is appraised and how the person copes with the stressor.)

The expression of emotion, especially anger, is one coping style. One might think that the expression of anger would have a negative effect on illness outcome; surprisingly, however, the outcome after expression of negative emotions depends on the disease. Frequently, expressing hostility and anger increased survival in people with cancer, but in people who had lung disease, the expression of anger and other negative emotions increased their manifestations and adverse physiologic changes (e.g., hypoxia) occurred.

Social Support

Scientists have long noted a link between social relationships and health. Socially isolated people are less healthy, psychologically and physically, and are more likely to die than people who are more socially integrated; however, the actual cause and effect are not clear. Are unhealthy people less likely to have and maintain social relationships, or does the lack of social relationships cause people to become ill and die? Do people in a social network provide a basis of health?

As we learn more about chronic illnesses, the role of social support seems even stronger. Physiologic studies have shown a link between the amygdala and the hypothalamus in the brain and positive social relationships. Social contact decreases levels of hormones such as cortisol, epinephrine, and norepinephrine. From a psychological standpoint, social relationships provide a sense of meaning or coherence that promotes a healthy lifestyle. Social support may help a client adhere to medical treatment and seek of medical care. Marriage, a widely studied area of social support, may be simultaneously a source of stress and support, but regardless of the quality of the interaction, marriage is a form of support. Frequently, a quick deterioration in the health of a survivor is seen after the death of a spouse. Health care providers must make use of a client's social support network, including the network in the treatment regimen and assessing the impact of illness on the partner.

Self-Help Groups

Self-help groups are growing in industrialized nations. It is estimated that there are at least 500,000 to 750,000 self-help groups in the United States, with at least 10 to 15 million members. Some groups are approved by various organizations. Reach for Recovery, an organization for women who have had a mastectomy, is approved by the American Cancer Society. Informal groups also exist, such as people caring for older, infirm parents in their homes, who meet to discuss common problems. Self-help groups are recognized and accepted as a form of assistance to meet people's needs. The largest groups help people with mental illnesses, and the second largest groups help people with AIDS.

There are two types of self-help groups. One is the Twelve-Step program, of which Alcoholics Anonymous is the prototype. The other is a group whose members share common experiences. Characteristics of both types of groups include (1) helping with cognitive restructuring of an event or experience, (2) instructing in adaptive skills, and (3) fostering emotional support, personal disclosure, socialization, taking actions together, empowerment, self-reliance, and self-esteem.

Developing Coping Skills

Many practical methods exist to cope with stress. Planning is one effective way to reduce adverse effects. For example, we prepare for predictable life changes, such as marriage, job change, or retirement. We plan by establishing goals. Through planning, we develop a belief system that allows us to dictate our life and our experience. Setting goals facilitates this belief system because it serves as a reminder that we have the power to create new experiences in our lives. Goals should include areas such as meaning and purpose, fun and play, exercise, nutrition, work, and relaxation.

The most widely practiced and possibly the most effective exercise for immediate stress reduction is to evoke the relaxation response:

1. When first learning to do this, remove yourself from the source of stress, assume a relaxed posture, and begin taking deep breaths through your nose.
2. Consciously and progressively relax all of your muscles.
3. Begin thinking of your strengths and imagining a successful outcome.
4. Realize that, in the great scheme of things, this event, whatever its nature, is only a minor event. Evoking the relaxation response induces a decrease in sympathetic nervous system activity and produces an altered, quieted state of consciousness.
5. As you begin to appreciate the effects of the simple progressive relaxation technique, you may want to explore and develop more long-term stress management techniques, such as biofeedback training, yoga, *Tai Chi,* meditation, and guided imagery.

Mind-Body Views and Alternative Therapies

Various mind-body therapies have been introduced to Western medicine. Biofeedback, autogenic training, therapeutic touch, guided imagery, and focused thought are examples. Mind-body therapies can influence the immune system, help manage pain, and reduce stress and anxiety. An example of the positive influences of a mind-body therapy is teaching a client to slow down, simplify, and fully relax, so that the client might experience enhanced life satisfaction and beneficial immune system changes.

Alternative medicine (complementary medicine) refers to a wide range of treatments that include mind-body therapies, homeopathy, and herbal medicine. In 1992, Congress established the Office of Alternative Medicine within the National Institutes of Health to evaluate alternative medicine therapies. Table 1–6 lists seven fields of alternative and complementary medicine.

About 40% of Americans surveyed in 1997 reported using some form of alternative health care. There is a growing demand for these therapies, but more needs to be

TABLE 1–6 CATEGORIES OF COMPLEMENTARY AND ALTERNATIVE MEDICINE

1. *Alternative systems of medical practice.* Seventy per cent to 90% of world health care ranges from self-care based on folk principles to organized health care that is based on an alternative tradition or practice
   a. *Popular* (informal practices in the home, such as using herbal teas for a cold)
   b. *Community-based* (care that reflects the natural environment, health needs, and health beliefs of those who use it, such as nonprofessional practices occurring in many urban and rural communities)
   c. *Professionalized* (a health care delivery system based on theories of health and disease, including traditional oriental medicine, acupuncture, Ayurvedic medicine, homeopathy, anthroposophically extended medicine, naturopathy, and environmental medicine)
2. *Mind-body interventions.* Therapies that make use of the interconnectedness of the mind and body and of the power of each to affect the other
   a. Psychotherapy
   b. Meditation
   c. Hypnotherapy
   d. Yoga
   e. Prayer and mental efforts
   f. Support groups
   g. Guided imagery and relaxation
   h. Dance, music, and art therapy
   i. Biofeedback
   j. Humor
3. *Manual healing methods.* Therapy that includes touch and manipulation of soft tissues or realignment of body parts to correct a dysfunction that affects the function of other body parts
   a. Osteopathic medicine
   b. Massage and other physical healing methods
   c. Chiropractic
   d. Biofield therapeutics (laying on of hands)
   e. Acupuncture
   f. Reflexology
   g. Rolfing
4. *Bioelectromagnetic applications.* Based on the ways living organisms interact with electromagnetic fields
   a. *Nonthermal non-ionizing radiation* (includes bone repair, nerve stimulation, wound healing, osteoarthritis treatment, electroacupuncture, tissue regeneration, and immune system stimulation)
   b. *Thermal non-ionizing radiation* (includes radiofrequency [RF], hyperthermia, laser and RF surgery, RF diathermy)
5. *Herbal medicine.* The use of plants and plant products as remedies, often self-administered and purchased through herbalists, health food stores, and certain practitioners. In the United States, these products are marketed as food supplements without specific health claims because of the lack of Food and Drug Administration (FDA) approval related to insufficient standards for safety and efficacy of herbal remedies
6. *Pharmacologic and biologic treatments.* The use of drugs, vaccines, and other agents (including antioxidants, oxidizing agents, chelation treatments, cell treatment, and metabolic therapy) not yet accepted by conventional medicine; clinical safety and effectiveness trials to meet FDA approval have not been fully investigated because of lack of sponsors and funding
7. *Diet, nutrition, and lifestyle changes.* Therapy that uses foods to affect biochemical and physiologic processes in the body. This field includes orthomolecular medicine (high-dose vitamins, a Macrobiotic diet, nutritional supplements, and dietary and other lifestyle changes in the treatment of chronic diseases such as AIDS; bronchial asthma; cancer; cardiovascular diseases, heart attacks, and stroke; lymphedema; and mental and neurologic disorders)

Modified from U.S. Office of Alternative Medicine. (1994). *Alternative medicine: Expanding medical horizons* (pp. 3–206). Washington, DC: National Institutes of Health.

AIDS, acquired immunodeficiency syndrome.

known about their effectiveness. Recently, there has been a call for higher standards in the evaluation of alternative medicine, especially in regard to herbal medicine.[3] Herbs are considered to be dietary supplements that are exempt from U.S. Food and Drug Administration (FDA) guidelines for prescribed medications. Some authorities claim that alternative therapies should be subjected to the same scientific testing as conventional treatments.[3]

The Office of Alternative Medicine recently reviewed the use of acupuncture for treatment of chronic conditions. Acupuncture was found to be effective for addictions and psychiatric disorders; allergy and immunology; general pain; headaches; and nausea, vomiting, and postoperative problems.[28] Another effective therapy was the integration of behavioral and relaxation approaches into the treatment of chronic pain and insomnia (see also Chapters 21 and 23).[28]

■ MODIFYING ENVIRONMENTAL HEALTH RISK FACTORS

Environment is one of the four primary determinants of health. It is not enough to think solely in terms of self or of our immediate surroundings when we think of health promotion. We are not just members of families, communities, states, or regions; we are intertwined with one another and linked as a global family. What affects one of us now has a ripple effect and affects us all. Because of the population explosion and congested urban living conditions, it is easy to affect another person's living environment. For example, it is possible to pollute the air by driving a car with a defective exhaust pipe, to impinge on auditory air space by playing loud music, or to create an eyesore by littering. Collectively, we can pollute the environment to such a great degree that life itself is threatened.

Health promotion, because it addresses the whole self and the whole human family, must also address protection of the environment. It is not within the scope of this chapter to delineate ways to do this; its purpose is to stimulate an awareness that each of us can play a role in cleaning, maintaining, and striving to improve environmental conditions to the best of our ability.

CONCLUSIONS

Health promotion is a key watch phrase for the 21st century. Nurses are encouraged to develop a consciousness that includes attention to the social, political, and economic aspects of the environment. Once we recognize that establishing health-promoting behaviors can alter the presence or absence of good health, specific interventions must be delineated and disseminated to the subsets of the population that can benefit. Clients with chronic conditions are a subset of the population that has potential to achieve improvements in quality of life and health care savings with interventions of health promotion and illness prevention. Appraisal of health risk can reveal which risk reduction interventions would be helpful. Models of health promotion serve as a guide for motivating clients to make health behavioral changes. A broad understanding of chronic conditions will widen the nurse's role and will assist the nurse in providing holistic nursing care to facilitate client and family adaptation and ameliorate the course of a chronic condition.

BIBLIOGRAPHY

1. Agency for Health Care Policy and Research. (1993). *Clinical practice guideline No. 5: Depression in primary care.* Rockville, MD: U.S. Department of Health and Human Services.
2. American Nurses' Association. (1995). *Nursing's social policy statement.* Washington, DC: Author.
3. Angell, M., & Kassirer, J. (1998). Alternative medicine: The risks of untested and unregulated remedies. *New England Journal of Medicine, 339*(12), 839–841.
4. Bandura, A. (1986). *Social foundations of thought and action: A social cognitive theory* (p. 22). Englewood Cliffs, NJ: Prentice-Hall.
5. Cassileth, B. R. (1998). *The alternative medicine handbook: The complete reference guide to alternative and complementary therapies.* New York: W. W. Norton.
6. Clark, C. (1996). *Wellness practitioner: Concepts, research, and strategies* (2nd ed.). New York: Springer.
7. Dossey, B. (1998). Holistic modalities and healing moments. *American Journal of Nursing, 98*(6), 44–47.
8. Downie, R., Tannahill, C., & Tannahill, A. (1996). *Health promotion models and values* (2nd ed.). New York: Oxford University Press.
9. Duke, J. A. (1997). *The green pharmacy.* Emmaus, PA: Rodale Press.
10. Dunn, H. (1961). *High-level wellness.* Arlington, VA: R. W. Beatty.
11. Eakes, G., Burke, M., & Hainsworth, M. (1998). Middle-range of chronic sorrow. *Image: Journal of Nursing Scholarship, 30,* 179–184.
12. Edelman, C., & Mandle, C. (Eds.). (1997). *Health promotion throughout the life span* (4th ed.). St. Louis: Mosby–Year Book.
13. Fox, P., & Fama, T. (1996). *Managed care and chronic illness: Challenges and opportunities.* Gaithersburg, MD: Aspen.
14. Gochman, D. (Ed.). (1997). *Handbook of health behavior research: I: Personal and social determinants.* New York: Plenum Press.
15. Gorin, S., & Arnold, J. (1998). *Health promotion handbook.* St. Louis: Mosby–Year Book.
16. Hoffman, C., Rice, D., & Sung, H. (1996). Persons with chronic conditions: Their prevalence and costs. *Journal of the American Medical Association, 276,* 1473–1479.
17. Hover-Kramer, D. (1996). *Healing touch: A resource for health care professionals.* Albany, NY: Delmar.
18. Institute for Health and Aging, University of California–San Francisco. (1996). *Chronic care in America: A 21st century challenge.* Princeton, NJ: The Robert Wood Johnson Foundation.
19. Kobasa, S., Maddi, S., & Zola, M. (1983). Type A and hardiness. *Journal of Behavioral Medicine, 6,* 41–51.
20. Labonte, R. (1994). Health promotion and empowerment: Reflections on professional practice. *Health Education Quarterly, 21*(2), 253–268.
21. Lalonde, M. (1974). *A new perspective on the health of Canadians.* Ottawa: Government of Canada.
22. Lazarus, R., & Folkman, S. (1984). *Stress, appraisal, and coping.* New York: Springer.
23. Leavell, H., & Clark, E. (1965). *Preventative medicine for the doctor in his community: An epidemiologic approach.* New York: McGraw-Hill.

23a. Leininger, M. (1978). *Transcultural nursing: Concepts, theories and practices.* New York: John Wiley and Sons.

24. Lilienfeld, A. (1976). *Foundations of epidemiology.* New York: Oxford University Press.
25. Micozzi, M. S. (Ed.). (1996). *Fundamentals of complementary and alternative medicine.* New York: Churchill Livingstone.
26. Milio, N. (1976). A framework for prevention: Changing health damaging to health-generating life patterns. *American Journal of Public Health, 66,* 435–439.
27. Morse, J., & Doberneck, B. (1995). The concept of hope. *Image, 27,* 227–286.
28. National Institutes of Health, Office of Alternative Medicine. Grant award and research data. Bethesda, MD: Office of Alternative Medicine. Available: *http://altmed.od.nih.gov.*
29. Newman, M. (1987). Health conceptualizations: Nursing emergency paradigm: The diagnosis of pattern. In McLean (Ed.), *Class of*

nursing diagnosis. St. Louis: Proceedings of the Seventh Conference.

30. Parsons, T. (1951). *The social system.* New York: Free Press.
31. Pender, N. (1996). *Health promotion in nursing practice* (3rd ed.). Stamford, CT: Appleton & Lange.
32. Portnoy, B., et al. (1989). Application of diffusion theory to health promotion research. *Family Community Health, 12,* 63–71.
33. Prochaska, J., Redding, C, & Evers, K. (1996). The Transtheoretical Model and stages of change. In K. Glanz, F. Lewis, & B. Rimer (Eds.), *Health behavior and health education: Theory, research, and practice* (2nd ed., pp. 60–84). San Francisco: Jossey-Bass.
34. Randall, J., & Lazar, J. (1997). Complementary and alternative therapies in primary care. *Primary Care: Clinics in Office Practice, 24*(4).
35. Roy, C., & Andrews, H. (1998). *The Roy adaptation model* (2nd ed.). Englewood Cliffs, NJ: Prentice-Hall.
36. Strecher, V., & Rosenstock, I. (1996). The Health Belief Model. In K. Glanz, F. Lewis, & B. Rimer (Eds.), *Health behavior and health education: Theory, research, and practice* (2nd ed., pp. 41–59). San Francisco: Jossey-Bass.
37. Turner, J. (1986). World Health Organization: Charter for health promotion. *Lancet, 2,* 1407.
38. U.S. Department of Health and Human Services. (1979). *Healthy people: The Surgeon General's report on health promotion and disease prevention.* Washington, DC: U.S. Government Printing Office.
39. U.S. Department of Health and Human Services. (1991). *Healthy people 2000: National health promotion and disease prevention objectives.* (PHS No. 91-50213.) Washington, DC: U.S. Government Printing Office.
40. U.S. Department of Health and Human Services. (1996). *Physical activity and health: A report of the Surgeon General.* Atlanta: National Center for Chronic Disease Prevention and Health Promotion.
41. U.S. Department of Health and Human Services. (1997). *Healthy people 2000: Review 1997.* (DHHS No. 98-1256.) Hyattsville, MD: U.S. Government Printing Office.
42. U.S. Office of Alternative Medicine. (1994). *Alternative medicine: Expanding medical horizons.* Washington, DC: National Institutes of Health.
43. Wannamethee, S., & Shaper, A. (1999). Type of alcoholic drink and risk of major coronary heart disease events and all-cause mortality. *American Journal of Public Health, 89,* 685–690.
44. World Health Organization. (1947). Constitution of the World Health Organization. *Chronicle of the World Health Organization, 1*(1–2), 29–43.

CHAPTER 2

Health Promotion in Young and Middle-Aged Adults

Kathryn Fiandt

It is essential that nurses be knowledgeable regarding health promotion and disease prevention. When providing holistic care, think beyond current health problems to the client's general well-being and future risk for illness or injury. This can be particularly important when you are working with young and middle-aged adults who rarely visit health care providers except for family planning, child-bearing needs, acute illness, or injury episodes. It is not uncommon for young and middle-aged adults to go 10 years between health care visits. Because of the rarity of contacts with this population, take every opportunity to address health risks and risk management in these age groups.

HEALTH RISKS

The leading causes of death in young adults are motor vehicle and other unintentional injuries, homicide, suicide, malignant neoplasms, and heart disease. In middle-aged adults, the risk of premature death from cancer or heart disease increases.[47] In both age groups, death from human immunodeficiency virus (HIV) infection has increased; of the more than 1 million people with acquired immunodeficiency syndrome (AIDS) in the United States, the majority are 20 to 40 years old.[12]

Healthy People 2000, the federal population-based health objectives (1995 revisions), identified health-related goals that apply to young and middle-aged adults (Table 2–1). Nurses can assist in achieving these goals by assessing the client's lifestyle and risk status and by intervening to modify poor habits and to reduce risk. This chapter describes the components of a healthy lifestyle, including health promotion (primary prevention), risk assessment, and risk management, specifically disease prevention (*primary* prevention) and early detection (*secondary* prevention) in the young and middle-aged populations.

HEALTH PROMOTION

Health promotion involves activities that promote general well-being. These activities are categorized as patterns of healthy eating, healthy activity, and effective coping with stress. The concept of health promotion is described in Chapter 1. The following topics describe specific health promotion activities.

HEALTHY EATING

Healthy eating is a cornerstone of a healthy lifestyle. The U.S. Department of Agriculture (USDA) and the U.S. Department of Health and Human Services (USDHHS) developed the *Dietary Guidelines for Americans* (Table 2–2). Be familiar with these guidelines as the foundation for healthy eating. A useful tool for explaining these guidelines to clients is the *Food Guide Pyramid,* a pictorial representation of the principles described in the dietary guidelines (Fig. 2–1).

To use the guidelines effectively for achieving healthy eating patterns, clients must be able to identify a serving size and to read nutrition labels. The food labeling system mandated by the U.S. Food and Drug Administration (FDA) is designed to assist consumers in making informed decisions regarding the foods they purchase. The Nutrition Facts label (Fig. 2–2) is a tool to identify both serving size and the nutritional components of the food item.

Nurses who are knowledgeable regarding the Dietary Guidelines for Americans, the Food Guide Pyramid, and the Nutrition Facts label can assist clients to adopt healthy eating patterns. Young and middle-aged adults are often in excellent health but may have poor eating patterns that lay the foundation for future health problems. In addition, these clients may already have health problems as a result of poor eating patterns. Health patterns of concern include obesity, cancer risk, osteoporosis, and cardiovascular disease. Obesity and cancer risk are discussed here. Chapter 26 covers osteoporosis; Chapters 55 and 58 cover heart disease; and Chapter 52 covers hypertension.

Obesity

Although the *Healthy People 2000* goals include reducing the number of overweight Americans to 20%, the per-

TABLE 2-1 *HEALTHY PEOPLE 2000* GOALS FOR YOUNG AND MIDDLE-AGED ADULTS

1. Decrease motor vehicle deaths to no more than 14.2/100,000
2. Reduce motor vehicle deaths caused by alcohol to no more than 5.5/100,000
3. Reduce prevalence of overweight to no more than 20%
4. Reduce coronary heart disease deaths to no more than 100/100,000
5. Reduce cancer deaths to no more than 130/100,000
6. Reduce diabetes to a prevalence of 25/1,000
7. Confine the prevalence of HIV infection to no more than 400/100,000
8. Reduce the incidence of vaccine-preventable disease
9. Reduce suicide deaths to no more than 10.5/100,000
10. Increase to 30% the proportion of people who exercise regularly
11. Reduce cigarette smoking to no more than 15% of people 18+ years old
12. Reduce alcohol consumption to an annual average of no more than 2 gallons/person
13. Reduce unplanned pregnancies to no more than 30% of all pregnancies
14. Increase to at least 20% the proportion of people who seek help in coping with personal and emotional problems
15. Increase the number of people who meet U.S. Preventive Services Task Force guidelines for screening, vaccinations, and counseling services
16. Reduce deaths caused by unintentional injuries to 29.3/100,000

HIV, human immunodeficiency virus.

Modified from U.S. Department of Health and Human Services. (1996). *Healthy People 2000: Midcourse review and 1995 revisions.* Sudbury, MA: Jones & Bartlett.

TABLE 2-2 DIETARY GUIDELINES FOR AMERICANS

1. Eat a variety of foods
2. Maintain a healthy weight
3. Choose a diet low in fat, saturated fat, and cholesterol:
   a. 30% or less of calories from fat
   b. Less than 10% of calories from saturated fat
4. Choose a diet with plenty of vegetables, fruit, and grain products:
   a. 3 or more daily servings of various vegetables
   b. 2 or more daily servings of fruit
   c. 6 or more servings of grain products per day
5. Use sugar only in moderation
6. Use salt and sodium only in moderation
7. If you drink alcohol, do so in moderation:
   a. 1 drink per day for women
   b. 2 drinks per day for men

Modified from U.S. Department of Health and Human Services. (1994). *Clinician's handbook of preventive services.* Washington, DC: U.S. Government Printing Office.

centage of overweight people has actually increased from 26% (1976–1980 data) to 34% (1988–1991 data).[45] Obesity poses serious health risks. Obese people have an increased risk for heart disease, hypertension, type 2 diabetes, degenerative joint disease, sleep apnea, and gallbladder disease. When obesity is associated with a high-fat diet, the risk of breast, colon, rectum, and prostate cancer increases. Take every opportunity to measure height and weight, and calculate body mass index (BMI) (see Chapter 28). Obesity is defined as a BMI of 30 or greater. Advise clients when they fall outside the range of healthy weight.

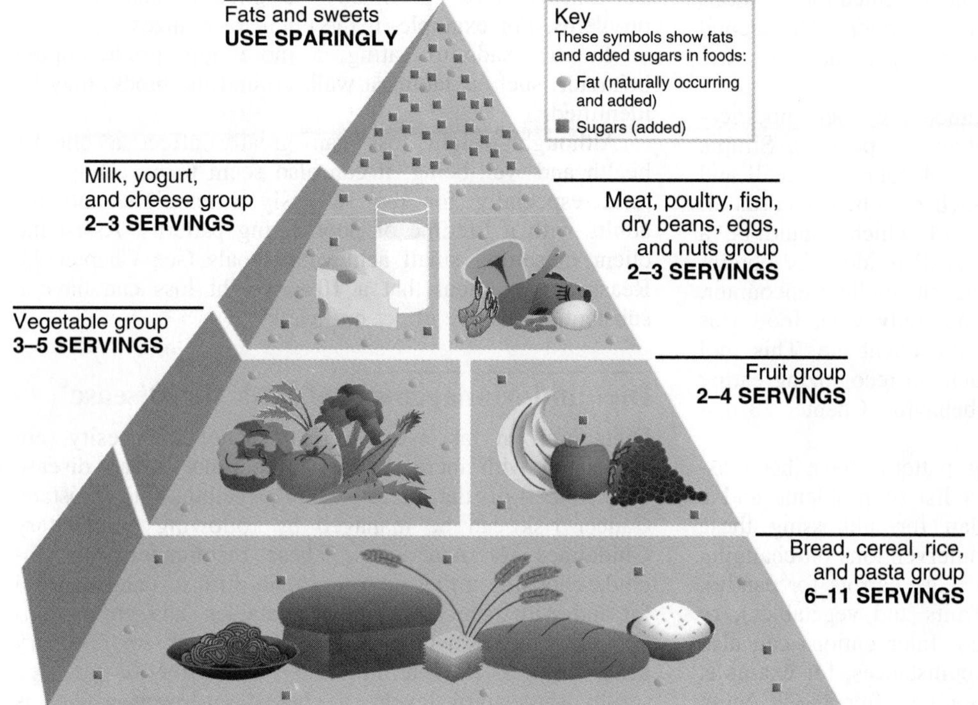

FIGURE 2–1 The USDA Food Guide Pyramid. (From U.S. Department of Agriculture and U.S. Department of Health and Human Services, Washington, DC.)

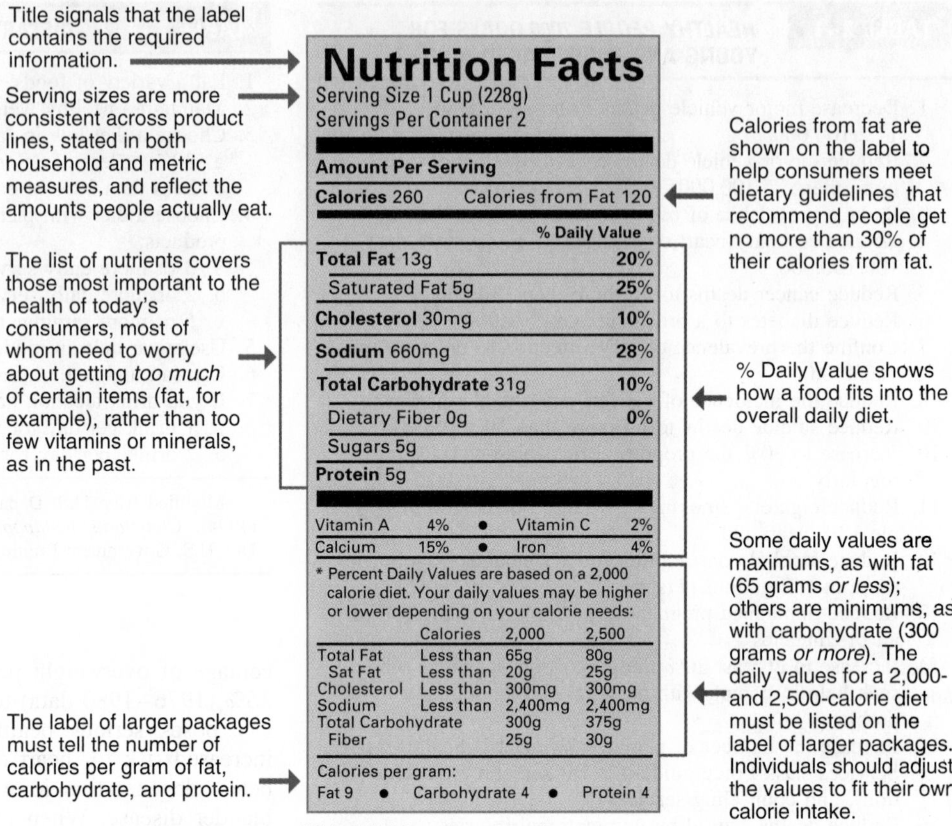

Title signals that the label contains the required information.
Serving sizes are more consistent across product lines, stated in both household and metric measures, and reflect the amounts people actually eat.
The list of nutrients covers those most important to the health of today's consumers, most of whom need to worry about getting *too much* of certain items (fat, for example), rather than too few vitamins or minerals, as in the past.
The label of larger packages must tell the number of calories per gram of fat, carbohydrate, and protein.
Nutrition Facts
Serving Size 1 Cup (228g)
Servings Per Container 2
Amount Per Serving
Calories 260 Calories from Fat 120
% Daily Value *
Total Fat 13g 20%
Saturated Fat 5g 25%
Cholesterol 30mg 10%
Sodium 660mg 28%
Total Carbohydrate 31g 10%
Dietary Fiber 0g 0%
Sugars 5g
Protein 5g
Vitamin A 4% • Vitamin C 2%
Calcium 15% • Iron 4%
* Percent Daily Values are based on a 2,000 calorie diet. Your daily values may be higher or lower depending on your calorie needs:
Calories 2,000 2,500
Total Fat Less than 65g 80g
Sat Fat Less than 20g 25g
Cholesterol Less than 300mg 300mg
Sodium Less than 2,400mg 2,400mg
Total Carbohydrate 300g 375g
Fiber 25g 30g
Calories per gram:
Fat 9 • Carbohydrate 4 • Protein 4
This label is only a sample.
Calories from fat are shown on the label to help consumers meet dietary guidelines that recommend people get no more than 30% of their calories from fat.
% Daily Value shows how a food fits into the overall daily diet.
Some daily values are maximums, as with fat (65 grams *or less*); others are minimums, as with carbohydrate (300 grams *or more*). The daily values for a 2,000- and 2,500-calorie diet must be listed on the label of larger packages. Individuals should adjust the values to fit their own calorie intake.

FIGURE 2–2 Guide to using a food label. (Modified from U.S. Food and Drug Administration. [December 10, 1992]. The new food label. *FDA Backgrounder,* 1–9.)

MANAGEMENT OF THE OBESE CLIENT

The basic therapeutic approach to obesity is to modify eating patterns through improving the *quality* (versus *quantity*) of foods eaten. The focus is on making positive changes in eating patterns. Specific modifications include (1) decreasing portion size, (2) modifying the composition of the diet through substitution and modification of foods consumed, and (3) changing eating behaviors. The second therapeutic component of obesity management is improving activity patterns (see later).

ASSESSMENT. Before recommending diet modifications, assess the client's current eating patterns. Simple dietary assessment tools include a 24-hour diet recall and use of a 3-day dietary log in which the client records all food and drink for 3 days, one of which should be a weekend day. The 24-hour diet recall is ideal for obtaining information at the time of the nurse-client encounter. The 3-day dietary log includes not only what food was eaten but when, why, and how the client ate. This tool assists both the nurse and the client in recognizing eating patterns and problematic eating behavior. Chapter 28 discusses nutritional assessment.

INTERVENTION. Once eating patterns have been assessed, collaboratively develop a list of problems and a mutually agreed-on, realistic plan for addressing these problems with the client. Focus interventions on changing foods eaten through substitution (e.g., carrots for candy), increasing certain foods (e.g., fruits and vegetables), or decreasing other foods (e.g., fats). Interventions can also include modifying the eating circumstances, for example, adding a breakfast meal, not eating after the evening meal, setting the eating utensil down between bites, and eating only at the table.

Eating behavior has a strong emotional component. Poor eating patterns are used to cope with emotional discomfort such as depression or anger. Understanding circumstances under which the client eats helps to identify interventions specifically designed to address these problems. For example, if the client recognizes that anger or fatigue leads to eating, a more appropriate coping behavior, such as taking a walk around the block, may be identified.

Although weight loss can greatly affect a client's health and well-being, it can also seem to be a hopeless task, especially for the seriously overweight and for adults with a lifetime of poor eating patterns. Assist the client in setting small achievable goals (see Chapter 1). Reassure the client that a 10% weight loss can have a substantial positive effect on health.[15]

Diet and Management of Risk for Disease

Diets high in fat, even in the absence of obesity, are associated with increased risk of coronary heart disease and cancer of the breast, colon, rectum, and prostate. Cancer risk can be managed by following the Dietary Guidelines for Americans. These recommendations include choosing a diet with less than 30% of calories from fat and with plenty of fruits, vegetables, and grain products. For clients who are at increased risk for coronary heart disease, as determined by borderline or elevated serum cholesterol levels, a cholesterol-lowering diet is recommended by the National Cholesterol Education Panel (NCEP).[30] The NCEP Step I diet includes decreasing dietary cholesterol to less than 300 mg/day and decreasing total dietary calories from saturated fat to between 8% and 10%. Step II includes a reduction of dietary cholesterol to below 200 mg/day and an intake of less than 7% of total daily calories from saturated fat. Referral to a dietitian is recommended for clients needing a Step II cholesterol-lowering diet.

■ HEALTHY ACTIVITY

Another cornerstone of a healthy lifestyle is healthy activity. People who are active throughout life live longer and are healthier than their less active counterparts.[33] However, more than 60% of adults do not achieve the recommended level of regular physical activity and 25% of adults get no activity. Physical inactivity increases with age, and women are more inactive than men.[46] Physical inactivity is a serious, nationwide problem resulting in a significant burden of unnecessary illness and premature death. It is associated with increased risk for coronary heart disease, type 2 diabetes, hypertension, and obesity.

Benefits of physical activity include (1) weight maintenance, (2) lower blood pressure, (3) improved mood, (4) relief from depression, (5) improved sense of well-being, (6) decreased risk of type 2 diabetes, (7) reduced mortality from coronary heart disease, and (8) increased levels of peak bone mass. In people with chronic, disabling conditions, activity improves stamina, muscle strength, and quality of life[17] (see Chapter 1). Given these benefits, take every opportunity to assess clients' activity patterns and work with them to improve activity levels.

MANAGEMENT OF THE INACTIVE CLIENT

Current activity recommendations are that every adult in the United States should accumulate "30 minutes or more of moderate-intensity physical activity on most, preferably, all days of the week."[34] Activity can be accumulated, but it should occur in blocks of at least 8 minutes and should be perceived as moderate or difficult in intensity.[4, 21] Simple walking is an excellent initial activity that requires no special equipment and can be done anywhere. Although this is a minimum standard, important benefits can be obtained through modest amounts of daily physical activity.[34]

Most research indicates that counseling individuals to increase their physical activity is rarely effective in initiating behavioral change. However, a trial of the effect of brief counseling suggests that highly structured and specific programs might, with minimal expense or time, be effective in promoting healthy patterns of physical activity in clients (see Chapter 1).[5]

ASSESSMENT. Intervention to improve activity patterns begins with assessment of the client's current activity pattern. Two effective tools are the 24-hour recall and a 3-day activity log. In the 24-hour recall, help the client identify all forms of activity during that day. Focus on activity that was sustained for at least 8 minutes and perceived as moderate to heavy exertion. Encourage the client to be thorough by giving examples, such as time spent doing housework. Then sum the total number of minutes spent in moderate or heavy activity per day.[4] During assessment, begin developing ideas for new activity opportunities. This information will be useful later for developing an intervention plan.

Benefits outweigh the risks with the current recommendation for moderate physical activity. Before beginning an activity program, however, all clients should be screened for risks that contraindicate unsupervised activity. People with known health problems, especially those involving cardiac risk including hypertension, elevated serum cholesterol, cigarette smoking, diabetes, and a family history of early heart disease, should be evaluated by their health care provider before increasing physical activity levels.[44]

INTERVENTION. Once the activity pattern has been assessed and there are no evident risks requiring further evaluation, work with the client to identify problem areas and develop a plan to increase physical activity. The *Activity Pyramid* is an excellent tool for beginning instruction (Fig. 2–3). Like the Food Guide Pyramid, the Activity Pyramid is a pictorial representation of the principles of healthy activity and can be used during nurse-client encounters to provide basic information.

Another tool for counseling clients regarding physical activity is the Project PACE (Physician-Based Assessment and Counseling for Exercise).[25, 35] Project PACE, a system of materials initially developed for physicians, is designed to assess a client's readiness to modify physical activity, to screen for activity contraindications, and to develop and implement an individualized activity program. Whichever tools are used, the intervention program should include a personalized exercise prescription and a plan for identifying and overcoming probable barriers to implementation and maintenance of the plan (see Chapter 1).

The Exercise Prescription. A written exercise prescription specifies recommended activity. The exercise prescription has four major components:

- *Mode,* or the type of activity engaged in
- *Intensity* with which the activity is performed
- *Duration* of time
- *Frequency*

As noted earlier, the minimum goal for an exercise program is a moderate-intensity (intensity) physical activity performed for a total of at least 30 minutes (duration) most days of the week (frequency). Many activities (Table 2–3) that are a part of most people's daily routine can serve as the mode of a physical activity program, including walking, housework, child care, and gardening.

Intensity is an essential component of an activity. Instruct clients how to assess exertion level. One simple means of measuring perceived exertion is the *talk test;* clients should be able to talk but only a few words at a time when engaged in the activity. If they can carry on a normal conversation they are not working hard enough; if they cannot talk at all, they are working too hard. Another measure of intensity is the *Borg rating* of perceived exertion (Fig. 2–4).

Overcoming Barriers. Research indicates that people who successfully incorporate physical activity into their daily lives are confident in their ability to perform the activity, find it pleasurable, and have social support.[2, 4] Activities should also be convenient and realistic.

Simple strategies can increase the likelihood of success in implementing an activity program. On the basis of the

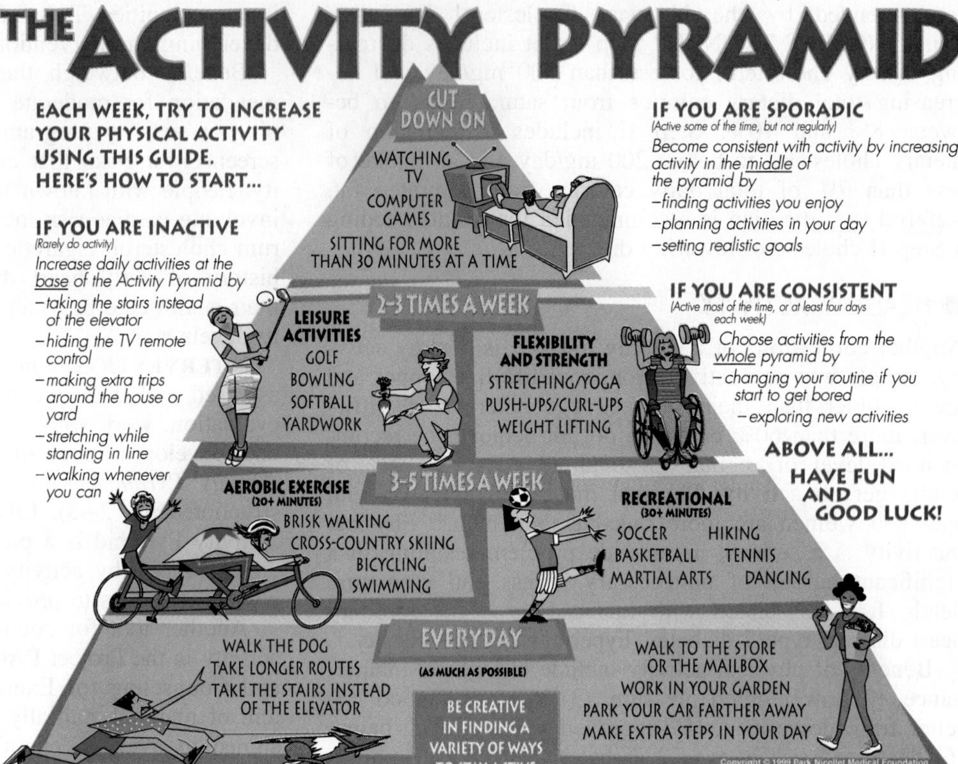

EACH WEEK, TRY TO INCREASE YOUR PHYSICAL ACTIVITY USING THIS GUIDE. HERE'S HOW TO START...
IF YOU ARE INACTIVE
(Rarely do activity)
Increase daily activities at the base of the Activity Pyramid by
–taking the stairs instead of the elevator
–hiding the TV remote control
–making extra trips around the house or yard
–stretching while standing in line
–walking whenever you can
CUT DOWN ON
WATCHING TV
COMPUTER GAMES
SITTING FOR MORE THAN 30 MINUTES AT A TIME
IF YOU ARE SPORADIC
(Active some of the time, but not regularly)
Become consistent with activity by increasing activity in the middle of the pyramid by
–finding activities you enjoy
–planning activities in your day
–setting realistic goals
2-3 TIMES A WEEK

EVERYDAY
(AS MUCH AS POSSIBLE)
WALK THE DOG
TAKE LONGER ROUTES
TAKE THE STAIRS INSTEAD OF THE ELEVATOR
BE CREATIVE IN FINDING A VARIETY OF WAYS TO STAY ACTIVE
WALK TO THE STORE OR THE MAILBOX
WORK IN YOUR GARDEN
PARK YOUR CAR FARTHER AWAY
MAKE EXTRA STEPS IN YOUR DAY
Copyright © 1999 Park Nicollet Medical Foundation

FIGURE 2–3 The activity pyramid. (Copyright © 1999, Park Nicollet *HealthSource* ® Institute for Research and Education.)

assessment of the client's activity level, (1) advise the client to increase time spent in current moderate-intensity activities, (2) help the client identify pleasurable activities to incorporate into the current routine, and (3) encourage the client to identify friends or family members who can serve as a support system and, ideally, who can join in the planned activity.

Activity plans should include a monitoring method, such as a log, and a reward system. Help clients identify potential barriers and assist them in developing a plan to overcome them (Table 2–4). Although the primary goal of a regular activity plan is to improve physical health, many benefits relate to feelings of well-being. When working with a client to improve activity patterns, use interventions that increase self-efficacy by choosing realistic activities and goals.

TABLE 2–3 EXAMPLES OF MODERATE LEVELS OF ACTIVITY

AROUND THE HOUSE

- Washing windows or floors
- Washing and waxing the car
- Walking and running with children
- Climbing stairs
- Pushing a stroller
- Raking leaves
- Shoveling snow
- Digging and weeding in the garden

SPORTS AND LEISURE ACTIVITIES

- Volleyball or basketball
- Bicycling
- Social dancing (fast)
- Walking (briskly)
- Skiing
- Swimming

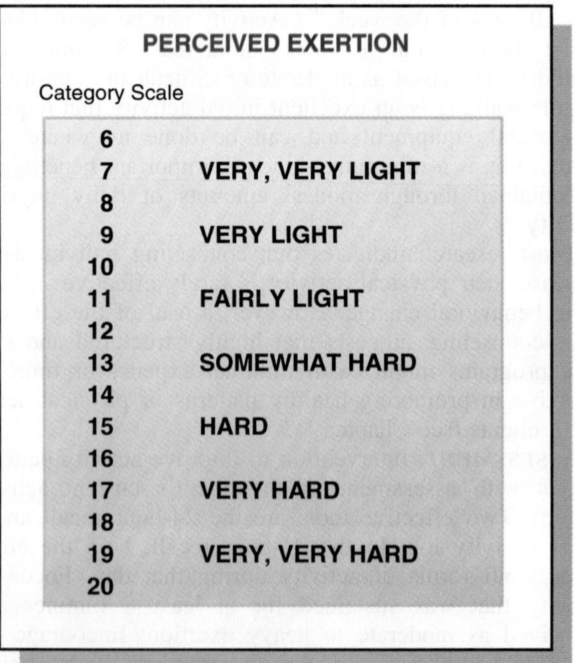

PERCEIVED EXERTION
Category Scale
6
7 VERY, VERY LIGHT
8
9 VERY LIGHT
10
11 FAIRLY LIGHT
12
13 SOMEWHAT HARD
14
15 HARD
16
17 VERY HARD
18
19 VERY, VERY HARD
20

GOLF
BOWLING
SOFTBALL
YARDWORK
FLEXIBILITY AND STRENGTH
STRETCHING/YOGA
PUSH-UPS/CURL-UPS
WEIGHT LIFTING
IF YOU ARE CONSISTENT
(Active most of the time, or at least four days each week)
Choose activities from the whole pyramid by
–changing your routine if you start to get bored
–exploring new activities
ABOVE ALL... HAVE FUN AND GOOD LUCK!
3-5 TIMES A WEEK
AEROBIC EXERCISE
(20+ MINUTES)
BRISK WALKING
CROSS-COUNTRY SKIING

RECREATIONAL
(30+ MINUTES)
SOCCER
HIKING

TENNIS
MARTIAL ARTS

FIGURE 2–4 The Borg perceived exertion scale. (From Strauss, R.H. [Ed.]. [1991]. *Sports medicine* [2nd ed.]. Philadelphia: W. B. Saunders.)

TABLE 2–4 OVERCOMING BARRIERS TO EXERCISE

Barrier	Suggested Response
Exercise is hard work.	Pick an activity that you enjoy and that is easy for you.
I do not have the time.	We are talking about only three 20-minute sessions per week. Could you do without three television shows each week?
I am usually too tired for exercise.	Tell yourself, "This activity will give me more energy." See if it happens.
I hate to fail, so I will not start.	Physical activity is not a test. You will not fail if you choose an activity you like and start off slowly.
I do not have anyone to work out with.	Maybe you have not asked. A neighbor or coworker may be a willing partner, or you can choose an activity that you enjoy doing by yourself.
There is not a convenient place.	Pick an activity you can do at a convenient place. Walk around your neighborhood or do exercises with a television show or a videotape at home.
I am afraid of being injured.	Walking is a safe and excellent exercise. Choose a safe and well-lit area.
The weather is too bad.	There are many activities that you can do in your home, in any weather.
Exercise is boring.	Listening to music during your activity keeps your mind occupied. Walking, biking, or running can take you past lots of interesting things.
I am too overweight.	You can benefit regardless of your weight. Pick an activity that you are comfortable with, such as walking.
I am too old.	It is never too late to start. People of any age, including older people, can benefit from physical exercise.

Modified from Project PACE. (1991). *Physician-based assessment and counseling for exercise.* San Diego, CA: San Diego State University. Project PACE material is available from San Diego State University, Student Health Services, 550 Campanile Dr., San Diego, CA, 92182 (619-594-5949).

One successful strategy for increasing physical activity is to increase social support within the community as well as within the client's social circle. Use every opportunity to support community projects that promote physical activity, such as developing hiking, walking, and biking trails or opening schools for community recreation. If security is a concern, support efforts to organize a community watch unit or to develop a walking club to take advantage of safety in numbers. Occupational health nurses can encourage employers to develop on-site programs to support employee health. Nurses who regularly work with clients to develop activity programs can maintain a comprehensive listing of community resources available to support activity plans. Community nursing organizations can develop a volunteer pool to work with walking clubs in area malls, perform blood pressure screenings, and provide health education classes.

■ STRESS MANAGEMENT

Stress, the body's response to demands, seems to be increasing in today's world. Physical demands for adaptation are compounded by the adaptive responses required by the volume of information and decisions required for existence in today's society. Stress is usually the result of an imbalance between the demands placed on a person and one's ability to adapt. Stress management, the final cornerstone of a healthy lifestyle, is the ability to cope with these adaptive demands effectively.

Dysfunction in one's ability to adapt and manage stress has a negative effect on health[6]:

1. *Behavioral* responses to stress include decreased ability to think clearly and function, increased tobacco and alcohol use, overeating, and disrupted sleep patterns.
2. *Emotional* responses include depression, anger, decreased self-esteem, apathy, and impatience.
3. *Physical* responses to stress can include tight, sore neck and shoulder muscles, increased blood pressure and heart rate, palpitations, chest discomfort, headaches, gastrointestinal upset, and fatigue.

Management of Stress

Assessment. Today it seems that people are always "stressed," often blaming stress for their physical and mental problems. As a result, clients may request help in coping with stress. Assessment of the problem is the first step in intervention. Include a thorough history of the cognitive, emotional, and physical manifestations that lead clients to conclude that they are stressed. Assess the problems or situations that seem to precipitate stress and the behavioral and emotional response (i.e., how clients feel and act when the problem is present). Also evaluate how clients currently cope with the problem (see discussion of coping in Chapters 1 and 20). Help the person recognize ineffective coping and develop a plan to cope effectively with the stress.

Intervention. Stress management has three components: stress resistance, cognitive reappraisal, and effective coping skills.

Stress Resistance. Stress resistance involves decreasing the body's response to stress, healthy eating and activity, and relaxation techniques. Physical activity can be a *positive* stressor; that is, activity requires an adaptive response, and when performed properly, it results in physical changes that counter the normally negative effects of stress. Physical activity improves mental function, decreases depression, and increases physical endurance.

Healthy eating can increase resistance to stress, and unhealthy eating adds to stress. Healthy eating, based on the Dietary Guidelines for Americans, aids stress resistance; however, some foods are associated with effective or ineffective coping. Complex carbohydrates (e.g., breads, beans, grains) provide a sustained source of energy and have a relaxing effect, whereas fruits, vegetables, and protein provide energy and increased physiologic ability to cope. Intake of simple carbohydrates (e.g., sugar) can temporarily increase energy, but this rise is then quickly followed by weakness and lethargy as the blood glucose level drops. Overeating, an ineffective means of coping, can result in decreased energy and lowered self-esteem. The stimulant caffeine induces the fight-or-flight biologic response and can exacerbate the physical damage that results from stress when it is consumed in excess.

Sleep and rest are natural forms of relaxation that are essential for healing and repairing the physiologic consequences to stress. Inadequate rest worsens stress, especially through impaired mental functioning. Chapter 21 discusses promoting positive outcomes in clients with sleep and rest disorders. In addition to sleep and rest, people can practice techniques to facilitate physical and mental relaxation. *Progressive relaxation* is a technique of slowly focusing on each muscle group, tensing the muscles for 5 to 7 seconds, and then relaxing them. This process promotes learning how to relax the entire body and particularly benefits people with muscle tension or spasm, insomnia, and neck or back pain. Many forms of relaxation involve *breathing techniques,* such as breath awareness, deep breathing, and the purifying breath.[9]

Meditation, once considered an alternative practice, is an established form of relaxation therapy. Research has shown that physiologic changes, such as lowering blood pressure and decreasing heart disease risk, occur as a result of meditation. There are several active or passive forms of meditation, including focusing on breath awareness or a *mantra,* meditative movement such as *yoga* or *Tai Chi,* mindfulness, and prayer.

Cognitive Reappraisal. The goal of cognitive reappraisals or restructuring is to change the perception or interpretation of events as stressors. Cognitive reappraisal is based on the assumption that a major factor in stress is the individual's perception of the event or experience as a stressor.[26] Three common techniques are presented.

Thought stopping is an ideal intervention for "worriers" (i.e., people who obsessively maintain ongoing inner dialogues of "what if". . . or "I can't"). Clients identify the obsessive thought and allow the self to imagine a situation involving the thought. As the obsessive dialogue begins, the person interrupts the dialogue with a loud "STOP!" and substitutes a positive thought. The goal of this process is to learn to automatically disrupt obsessive and nonproductive thoughts with a positive message.

Refuting irrational ideas, like thought stopping, involves interventions designed to disrupt obsessive, nonproductive thoughts. The intervention derives from Rational Emotive Therapy. It is based on the belief that much stress is related to common irrational beliefs such as "I must be perfect in everything I do" and "It's absolutely necessary that I have love and approval from my peers and family at all times." To overcome these stressful beliefs, the client first identifies the irrational idea and then identifies the facts, such as "no one is perfect all the time." Clients also need to explore their emotional response to stressful thoughts. The client then substitutes rational self-talk for the previous irrational self-talk. This particular intervention is very effective for self-directed, empowered people.

Guided imagery, a form of relaxation, is an excellent method of cognitive reappraisal. Guided imagery is usually practiced under the direction of a trained therapist. The therapist assists the client to visualize a stressful event, become worried, and then to switch to a relaxing event or to rework the situation so that it is less stressful. Alternatively, the therapist may help the client into a guided dialogue with his or her inner self or may act as a guide to help with problem-solving.

Effective Coping. Effective coping involves recognition of the problem causing stress and, through problem-solving skills, development and implementation of an effective strategy to cope with or solve the problem. Effective coping skills include time management, assertiveness, solution-oriented therapy, and development of a support system.[9, 26] Often clients use ineffective coping strategies, usually designed to avoid the problem, resulting in repression of associated unpleasant emotions. Addictive behaviors, such as alcohol abuse and overeating, often begin as ineffective coping strategies.

Effective coping starts with identifying the problem. Help the client to differentiate the problem from the emotional response to the problem. Once the problem is identified, several issues must be addressed before one can work on problem-solving skills.

First, does the problem really exist, or is it imagined? People often worry about imagined problems. Help the client assess validity of the problem before working on a solution.

Second, is the problem really important or just a nuisance? If the problem is not important, use cognitive reappraisal techniques to put the problem in perspective.

Third, does the problem have feasible solutions? Some problems (an untimely death or catastrophic illness) are beyond control. In these cases, the goal is not problem resolution but acceptance. The individual will need support to learn from the problem and to develop an ongoing support system for assistance through the crisis.

Important, controllable problems are amenable to intervention or action responses using standard problem-solving, assertiveness, and time management skills. Nurses often assist people in distress. Mastering effective coping skills can be an asset in clinical practice. However, nurses often work with people experiencing crises in which basic coping strategies are not enough. Develop a network of counseling and support resources to which clients can be referred.

PREVENTION OF INJURY AND ILLNESS

The greatest causes of injury and premature death in young and middle-aged adults include accidents, particularly motor vehicle accidents, and violence, particularly suicide and homicide.[47] Risk identification and risk management counseling can prevent illness and injury in these populations. Place particular emphasis on preventable causes of accidents, specifically the use of drugs and alcohol, and preventable causes of cancer, specifically smoking. In addition, always be aware of the risk for domestic or spouse abuse.

■ ACCIDENTS

Because motor vehicle accidents are the leading cause of death in young adults, focus prevention counseling on regular use of lap and shoulder belts and refraining from drug or alcohol use while driving. Because of the significant impact drugs, alcohol, and tobacco have on health, most prevention measures are devoted to screening and intervening in alcohol, drug, and tobacco abuse. The following discussion focuses on screening and primary prevention measures. Chapter 24 describes secondary intervention for clients who have abuse problems.

■ ALCOHOL ABUSE

Alcohol abuse results in specific health problems, including withdrawal syndrome; hepatitis, cirrhosis, and pancreatitis; and cancers of the liver, oropharynx (especially in smokers), and esophagus as well as an increased risk of breast cancer. In addition to diseases clearly associated with alcohol abuse, "problem drinkers" have increased mortality from all causes, beginning with four drinks per day for men and two drinks per day for women. Alcohol is associated with more than 50% of all injuries (44% of all traffic accidents), fires, drownings, homicides, and suicides.[47]

Problem drinkers are more likely to be seen in primary care clinics and hospitals. They often do not present with manifestations of dependence that would immediately result in identification of the problem. All clients, not just those with obvious problems, should be screened for problem drinking. Nurses are in a position to identify problem drinking because their role includes obtaining a comprehensive psychosocial history (see Chapter 9).

A variety of tools are available to screen for problem drinking. The mnemonic CAGE is a useful popular 4-item tool[47]:

- *C* = Have you ever felt you ought to *Cut* down on drinking?
- *A* = Have people *Annoyed* you by criticizing your drinking?
- *G* = Have you ever felt bad or *Guilty* about your drinking?
- *E* = Have you ever had a drink first thing in the morning to steady your nerves or get rid of a hangover *(Eye-opener)*?

If problem drinking is suspected or if the client answers "yes" to any item, the Alcohol Use Disorders Identification Test (AUDIT) may be administered. The AUDIT is a 10-item tool developed by a six-nation team in conjunction with the World Health Organization (WHO). The AUDIT is highly sensitive and specific[22, 40] and can easily be included in a social history format. Score the AUDIT tool (Table 2–5) by summing the total points for all answers. Drinking is considered problematic if the score is 8 points or more.

Do not hesitate to screen for problem drinking. If you suspect that a client has a drinking problem (based on screening), briefly state so to the client. Be sure to have an established support and referral network of clinical specialists to assist the client and family with acceptance and management of problem drinking.[47] Chapter 24 details interventions for clients who have substance abuse problems.

■ DRUG ABUSE

Unfortunately since 1992, after years of decline in drug use, abuse of illicit and legal drugs has been on the increase. More than 5.5 million Americans are affected by drug abuse, and 50% of these people are in the criminal justice system. Drug abuse is more common among men, the unemployed, and people without a high school education. Although drug abuse is more prevalent in urban communities, rural communities are not immune. Drug abusers are at increased risk for HIV infection and other communicable diseases. Drug abuse is a significant factor in homicides, suicides, and motor vehicle accidents.[47]

Be aware of the hazards of drug abuse and of the possibility of drug abuse in clients. Several standardized tools can be used to screen for drug abuse, but none has well-established validity or reliability.[47] Take every opportunity to assess for drug abuse. Ask the client about drug use as a routine part of lifestyle assessment, following questions regarding tobacco and alcohol use (see Chapter 9). State questions directly ("Do you currently use any other drugs such as marijuana ['pot,' 'weed'] or cocaine ['crack']?"). If the answer is "no," follow with "Have you ever used any other drugs?" If the client indicates current or past use of illicit drugs, further explore the patterns of use.

Advise abusing and high-risk clients (adolescents, males, people exposed to users of drugs) of the hazards of substance abuse. Advise users to stop or cut down, and offer help through referral. See Chapter 24 for interventions for substance abuse problems.

■ SMOKING CESSATION

More than 25% of Americans smoke, and thousands of children begin smoking every day.[32] Smoking is directly linked to many forms of cancer, heart disease, and hypertension. It is a risk factor in health problems as diverse as osteoporosis, ulcer disease, and low birth weight in babies. Smoking accounts for one of every five deaths in the United States.[47] All nurses should have the skills necessary to help people who are ready to stop smoking and to help motivate people who are not at a point where they can stop. The Agency for Health Care Policy and Research (AHCPR) has published guidelines for smoking cessation intervention (Table 2–6).[1]

INTERVENTION. Smoking cessation intervention can be seen as a stepped process. First, ask all clients if they smoke or are exposed to secondary smoke. When a person who smokes or is regularly exposed to smoke is identified, advise him or her to stop or to avoid exposure. Personalize the need to stop smoking. For example, remind parents of young children of the increased risk for ear infections and asthma the child may have or of the type of role model the parent is presenting. Remind women that smoking increases the risk of osteoporosis and premature aging of the skin. Remind asymptomatic men of the increased risk for emphysema, heart disease, and lung cancer.

Once the client is identified as a smoker and is advised

TABLE 2–5 THE ALCOHOL USE DISORDERS IDENTIFICATION TEST (AUDIT) STRUCTURED INTERVIEW

Question	Score*				
	0	*1*	*2*	*3*	*4*
How often do you have a drink containing alcohol?	Never	Monthly or less	2–4 times/mo	2–3 times/wk	4 or more times/wk
How many drinks do you have on a typical day when you are drinking?	None	1 or 2	3 or 4	5 or 6	7–9†
How often do you have 6 or more drinks on one occasion?	Never	Less than monthly	Monthly	Weekly	Daily or almost daily
How often during the last year have you found that you were unable to stop drinking once you had started?	Never	Less than monthly	Monthly	Weekly	Daily or almost daily
How often last year have you failed to do what was normally expected from you because of drinking?	Never	Less than monthly	Monthly	Weekly	Daily or almost daily
How often during the last year have you needed a first drink in the morning to get yourself going after a heavy drinking session?	Never	Less than monthly	Monthly	Weekly	Daily or almost daily
How often during the last year have you had a feeling of guilt or remorse after drinking?	Never	Less than monthly	Monthly	Weekly	Daily or almost daily
How often during the last year have you been unable to remember what happened the night before because you had been drinking?	Never	Less than monthly	Monthly	Weekly	Daily or almost daily
Have you or has someone else been injured as a result of your drinking?	Never	Yes, but not in last year (2 points)		Yes, during the last year (4 points)	
Has a relative, doctor, or other health worker been concerned about your drinking or suggested you cut down?	Never	Yes, but not in last year (2 points)		Yes, during the last year (4 points)	

*Score of greater than 8 (out of 41) suggests problem drinking and indicates need for more in-depth assessment. Cut-off of 10 points recommended by some to provide greater specificity.

†Five points if response is 10 or more drinks on a typical day.

From U.S. Preventive Services Task Force. (1996). *Guide to clinical preventive services* (2nd ed.). Baltimore: Williams & Wilkins.

TABLE 2–6 RECOMMENDATIONS FOR SUCCESSFUL SMOKING CESSATION TREATMENT

1. Every person who smokes should be offered smoking cessation treatment at every office visit.
2. Clinicians should ask and record tobacco-use status of every client.
3. Cessation treatments even as brief as 3 minutes per visit are effective.
4. More intense treatment is more effective in producing long-term abstinence from tobacco.
5. Nicotine replacement therapy (patches or gum or nasal spray), clinician-delivered social support, and skills training are the three most effective components of treatment.
6. Health care systems should make institutional changes that result in the systematic identification of, and intervention with, all tobacco users at every visit.

From Agency for Health Care Policy and Research. (1996). *Smoking cessation: Information for specialists.* Washington, DC: U.S. Government Printing Office, AHCPR Pub. No. 96-0694.

of the need to stop smoking, assess motivation to change (see Chapter 1). If a client expresses any interest in changing the smoking behavior, from cutting down to stopping, ask what can be done to help. Success is more likely if people spend thoughtful time planning the behavior change in preparation to quit. Help the client evaluate his or her smoking patterns to personalize the plan. Suggestions include (1) cleaning the house to rid tobacco odor just prior to stopping; (2) getting rid of all cigarettes; and (3) setting up a support network. Advise the client to inform friends who smoke that he or she is trying to quit and that they should respect this by not smoking around the client or not offering cigarettes. If the client's history indicates a high degree of nicotine addiction, offer advice about or referral for nicotine replacement.

Finally, address how the client will manage "triggers" to smoking (e.g., alcohol or anxiety-producing situations) and alternatives to smoking. When the urge to smoke strikes, advise the client to walk and learn deep breathing

TABLE 2–7 THINGS TO DO INSTEAD OF SMOKING

Take a slow deep breath of fresh air.
Take a walk.
Chew on a piece of gum or a carrot or hard candy.
Drink a glass of water.
Think about your children.
Brush your teeth.
Play with worry beads.
Pray or meditate.
Think about the money you are saving.
Smile.

to work through the urge. Table 2–7 lists suggested activities to substitute instead of smoking.

In addition to explaining smoking cessation, be aware of community resources to which clients can be referred for assistance. Provide a variety of motivational literature to clients, such as the excellent materials by the American Cancer Society and the American Lung Association. Support community-based smoking cessation interventions. These include a smoke-free work environment and participation in such community programs as the National Smoke-Off day. Whatever the practice environment, seek out ways to support smoking cessation.

Passive Smoking

Passive smoking, or exposure to second-hand smoke, also places people at increased risk for heart disease and cancer. The Atherosclerosis Risk in the Community (ARIC) study in 1994 indicated that non-smokers who are regularly exposed to environmental tobacco smoke have a 20% increase in progression of atherosclerosis compared with non-smokers who are not exposed to tobacco smoke.[22] Identify people who are exposed to environmental tobacco smoke, and help them devise ways to modify their risk. Ideally, risk modification involves smoking cessation on the part of a family member. However, people are often exposed to tobacco smoke in their work environment (e.g., bars, casinos), and the client may have to make difficult decisions regarding risk management versus livelihood and family.

■ DOMESTIC ABUSE

The Surgeon General's report in the mid-1980s identified domestic violence as a public health issue. Estimates range from 1 million[47] to 4 million[18] women as victims of assault, robbery, or rape by a spouse, ex-spouse, or intimate partner each year. Too often, this violence escalates to murder; 50% of murders are committed by an intimate partner.[18] It is estimated that 35% of women are seen in emergency departments for abuse and that 30% of women seen in primary care are abuse victims.[39] One study of inpatient female psychiatric clients found that 64% reported abuse as adults.[39] Although men are not immune from domestic abuse, most victims are women; therefore, this discussion focuses on abuse of women.

Nurses in all clinical settings see women who are abused; they must, therefore, be aware of the risk of violence and must be comfortable addressing abuse risk issues in client encounters. The American Nurses' Association position paper, *Physical Violence Against Women,*[7] supports the need to (1) increase nurses' awareness of and sensitivity to the problem of physical violence against women; (2) work to reduce injuries, psychological trauma, and cost that are a result of such violence; and (3) increase nurses' awareness of their role in assessing, intervening for, and preventing physical violence against women.[39]

ASSESSMENT. Although nurses often work with women who are victims of abuse, this text emphasizes (1) identification of risk for abuse and (2) interventions to prevent abuse before it starts. Identification begins with recognizing characteristics common to abused women. Characteristics of women at increased risk for violence include living in households with high degrees of stress, being abused as a child, and marrying young.[39, 47] Abused women often display low self-esteem and experience helplessness.[18, 39] In addition, certain characteristics in the woman's partner can increase her risk, such as having been abused or observed abuse as a child, abusing drugs or alcohol, having controlling behaviors, and pathologic jealousy. In addition, men who repetitively abuse women verbally often escalate to physical violence over time, during periods of high stress, or when a woman is pregnant.[39] Remember, any woman can be a victim of abuse, and any man can be an abuser. Routine screening for a history of abuse or current abuse in all women is an appropriate component of a psychosocial history (see Chapter 9).

The Partner Violence Screen (PVS)[13] is brief, easy to use, and accurate in identifying abuse. The tool consists of three questions:

1. Have you been hit, kicked, punched, or otherwise hurt by someone within the past year? If so, by whom?
2. Do you feel safe in your current relationship?
3. Does a partner from a previous relationship make you feel unsafe now?

INTERVENTION. Once a woman is identified as being at risk for violence either through having established risk factors or having been abused in the past, work with her to develop an individualized plan designed to prevent future violence. The plan may include assertiveness training, participation in a woman's empowerment or support group, self-esteem work, and social services assistance to improve her educational and economic status.[19, 27] Additional prevention strategies include community health nurse visits to high-risk families and community-wide media campaigns to enhance public awareness of the problem.[39] Explain stress management strategies, especially effective coping (see earlier), to help the client to avoid violence.

If a woman is identified as being in a currently violent relationship, focus intervention on safety. This woman is at high risk for sustaining significant injury or death. Therefore, nurses who screen for domestic violence must have a clearly established protocol for ensuring that every effort has been made to protect the woman. This protocol should be developed in collaboration with local law enforcement agencies and women's safety groups (e.g., YWCAs or other agencies).[10]

INFECTIOUS DISEASES

With the exception of HIV disease, infectious diseases are not a major cause of illness or premature death in young and middle-aged adults. However, these groups are not immune to problems related to infectious diseases. Two activities are essential for protection from infectious diseases in these populations: maintaining up-to-date immunizations and practicing safe sex.

Immunization

The U.S. Preventive Services Task Force (USPSTF)[47] recommends that all young and middle-aged adults have a tetanus-diphtheria booster vaccination every 10 years and that women of child-bearing age who do not have proven immunity to rubella have a rubella vaccination. In addition, people at risk for hepatitis B (Table 2–8) should receive the hepatitis B vaccination series.

Safe Sex

There are dozens of infectious sexually transmitted diseases (STDs). Of these, HIV infection and hepatitis B and C can result in significant morbidity and premature death; others result in permanent infection (e.g., herpes simplex) or infertility (e.g., gonorrhea). Risk factors for contracting a STD include:

1. Having a high number of sex partners.
2. Having sex with a person who engages in high-risk behavior (e.g., multiple partners).
3. Having sex for money.
4. Having sex with an intravenous (IV) drug user.

People who abuse drugs and alcohol are at increased risk, even if they do not abuse IV drugs, because they are more likely to engage in high-risk sexual behaviors while in an impaired state.

Do not hesitate to screen for high-risk sexual behavior, and advise clients about the risks and behaviors to protect from infection. Safe sex behavior includes:

1. Abstaining from sex
2. Maintaining a mutually monogamous relationship with a non-infected partner
3. Avoiding sexual contact with casual or high-risk partners
4. Using male or female condoms consistently and appropriately.

TABLE 2–8 PEOPLE AT HIGH RISK FOR HEPATITIS B

1. Recipients of blood products (including hemodialysis clients)
2. People with frequent occupational exposure to blood or blood products
3. Men who have sex with men
4. Injection drug users and their sex partners
5. People with multiple sexual partners
6. People with a history of sexually transmitted diseases
7. Travelers to countries where hepatitis B is endemic

From U.S. Preventive Services Task Force. (1996). *Guide to clinical preventive services* (2nd ed.). Baltimore: Williams & Wilkins.

Present information regarding referral sources in the community to assist clients with free or low-cost screening and treatment for STDs and information regarding sources of low-cost condoms. If you work in an ambulatory clinic or a community-based practice, consider finding a source of low-cost condoms and making them available at little or no cost to people at high risk.[47] Chapters 41 and 79 cover working with clients who have STDs, including AIDS.

SCREENING FOR DISEASE

Secondary prevention includes early detection of illness. Early identification is key to preventing premature death from many catastrophic illnesses, including coronary heart disease, cancer, and type 2 diabetes mellitus. Be aware of the risks for diseases and the current recommendations regarding screening, and take every opportunity to advise clients of the need for regular screening (see Chapter 9). Facilitating early detection of disease saves lives.

RECOMMENDATIONS FOR SCREENING

The Preventive Services Task Force issued its landmark report regarding the effectiveness of preventive services in 1989 and updated its recommendations in 1996. These recommendations are the "gold standard" regarding screening services, and you should be familiar with them. In addition to screening, the Task Force recommends the counseling, immunization, and chemoprophylaxis measures discussed earlier in this chapter. The recommendations are specific to age groups (except for pregnant women) and differentiate screenings recommended for all people in the group from screenings recommended for those with high-risk characteristics.

Screening recommendations are based on several factors that apply to populations rather than to individuals. The screening test must be reasonably priced, sensitive, and specific to the problem. In addition, there is generally no value to screening for diseases for which there is no treatment or when treatment does not improve either the quality of life or longevity. As a result, many tests do not meet requirements for an effective screening program.

Screenings recommended for the general population between the ages of 11 and 24 years are listed in Table 2–9. Screenings recommended for the general population between the ages of 25 and 64 years are listed in Table 2–10.

Many other organizations, particularly the American Cancer Society and the American Academy of Family Physicians, publish additional screening guidelines that have been addressed by the Task Force but that do not meet its criteria for recommendation. The American Cancer Society recommends that all women over age 20 perform breast self-examination (BSE) on a monthly basis.[42, 47] Although the American Cancer Society does not formally recommend that men practice regular testicular self-examination (TSE), its literature does support the practice.[43] Nurses can teach individuals how to do these self-examinations.

TABLE 2–9 RECOMMENDED SCREENINGS FOR THE GENERAL POPULATION AGES 11 TO 24 YEARS

Screening	Frequency	For
Height and weight	Periodic*	Obesity
Blood pressure	Periodic*	Hypertension
Papanicolaou (Pap) test (females)	At least every 3 years	Cervical cancer
Chlamydia screen (females)	With Pap test	*Chlamydia trachomatis*
Rubella serology (females)†	Once	Non-immune status
Assess for problem drinking	Periodic	Problem drinking

*Clinician discretion.

†In women with childbearing potential with incomplete vaccination history.

Modified from U.S. Preventive Services Task Force. (1996). *Guide to clinical preventive services* (2nd ed.). Baltimore: Williams & Wilkins.

■ BREAST SELF-EXAMINATION

BSE is a technique that women can use to assess their breasts. When women perform BSE properly and regularly, they can note early changes in their breasts and seek further evaluation. A major barrier to BSE is lack of confidence. Take time when working with the woman to ensure that she is confident of her skill and has had all her questions addressed. The BSE technique is described in Figure 2–5.

When teaching, emphasize that the examination should be done every month and at the end of menses in all menstruating women. Advise nonmenstruating women to pick one day a month (e.g., the first day of the month) to do BSE. Inform women that most breast lumps are benign but it is essential that they seek professional evaluation if they find anything that concerns them. Chapter 37 discusses physical assessment of the breast, including the clinical breast examination.

■ TESTICULAR SELF-EXAMINATION

TSE is a simple technique that men can use to assess for changes in their testicles that may signal testicular cancer. The risk is highest in adolescents and in men under age 35 years. As with BSE, the man should become familiar with the normal appearance and feel of his genitals to feel confident of his ability to perform TSE. Advise the man to schedule a regular time each month to assess his genitals. The best time is after bathing, because the warm water causes the scrotum to relax and makes the testicles easier to examine.

Teach the client to perform TSE as follows (Fig. 2–6):

1. Hold the scrotum in the palms of your hands, and examine each testicle with the thumbs and fingers of both hands. The index and middle fingers should be on the underside of each testicle with the thumbs on the top.
2. The testicle is rolled between your thumb and fingers. A normal testicle is shaped like an egg and is about 4 cm (1⅗ inches) long. It feels firm but not hard (like an ear lobe) and should be smooth without lumps.
3. After examining the testicles, examine the epididymides (behind the testicles); they should be soft and may feel sponge-like.
4. Examine the spermatic cords, which ascend from the epididymides up into the body. They are normally firm, smooth tubular structures.

■ PROSTATE CANCER

Nearly 40,000 men die annually of prostate cancer. Men at increased risk include those who have a first-degree relative (e.g., father, brother, son) with prostate cancer and African Americans. Despite the prevalence of the disease, both the Task Force and the American Academy of Family Physicians do not recommend screening for prostate cancer because early screening and treatment have not proved beneficial. However, the American Cancer Society and American Urological Association recommend screening for prostate cancer using a prostate-specific antigen (PSA) test and a digital rectal examination for all men over age 50 (over age 40 for African American men) (see Chapter 37).

When advising men about screening, keep in mind the man's prostate cancer risk factors, his general health, and his desires. Generally, prostate cancer screening should not be done in men over 70 years or who have significant underlying illness that would result in a life expectancy of less than 10 years.[29]

TABLE 2–10 RECOMMENDED SCREENINGS FOR THE GENERAL POPULATION AGES 25 TO 64 YEARS

Screening	Frequency	For
Blood pressure	Periodic*	Hypertension
Height and weight	Periodic*	Obesity
Total blood cholesterol†	Every 5 years	Coronary heart disease risk
Papanicolaou (Pap) test (females)	At least every 3 years	Cervical cancer
Fecal occult blood test‡	Annually	Colorectal cancer
Mammogram and clinical breast exam§	Annually	Breast cancer
Rubella serologic testing (females)ǁ	Once	Non-immune status
Assessment for problem drinking	Periodic*	Problem drinking

*Clinician discretion.

†Males age 35–64; females age 45–64.

‡Over age 50, or sigmoidoscopy less often.

§Females ≥ 50 years.

ǁIn women of childbearing age with an inaccurate vaccination history.

From U.S. Preventive Services Task Force. (1996). *Guide to clinical preventive services* (2nd ed.). Baltimore: Williams & Wilkins.

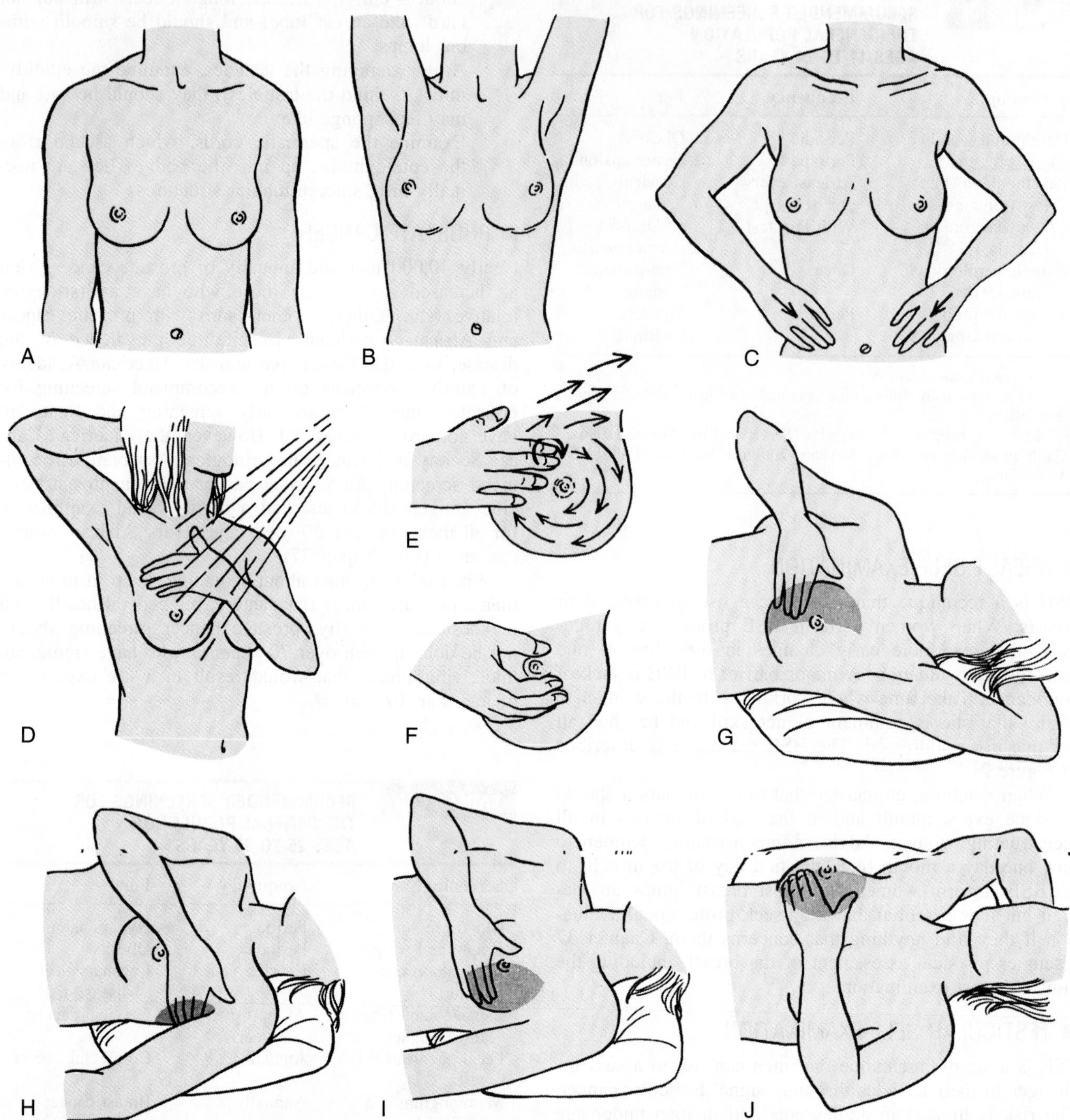

FIGURE 2–5 Self-examination of female breasts and axillae. Accomplished by observation and palpation. The client assumes various positions for observation while standing in front of a mirror. *A*, Arms relaxed at sides. Next, lean forward. *B*, Raise arms high overhead. Press arms behind head. *C*, Rest palms on hips, and firmly press inward to flex chest muscles. *D*, In shower, examine breast contours. *E*, Method of palpating breast. With fingers flat, gently press with small circular motions around an imaginary clock face; begin at 12 o'clock. Move an inch at a time toward the nipple. *F*, As a final step, squeeze the nipple gently between the thumb and index finger. Palpation of the breast is accomplished while lying down. *G*, Position to examine inner breast. *H*, Position to examine axilla. *I*, Position to examine outer breast. *J*, Repeat entire process for opposite breast and axilla. (See text and Chapter 37 for discussion of technique and observations.)

■ COLORECTAL CANCER

Colorectal cancer is the second most common form of cancer in the United States and accounts for more than 55,000 deaths per year. If the disease is found while still localized, survival rates are at 91%. If the disease is found when it has spread, the survival rate is much lower.[47] Therefore, early detection of the disease is essential. Risk factors include uncommon hereditary familial polyposis syndromes and ulcerative colitis of greater than 10 years' duration. More common risk factors include a

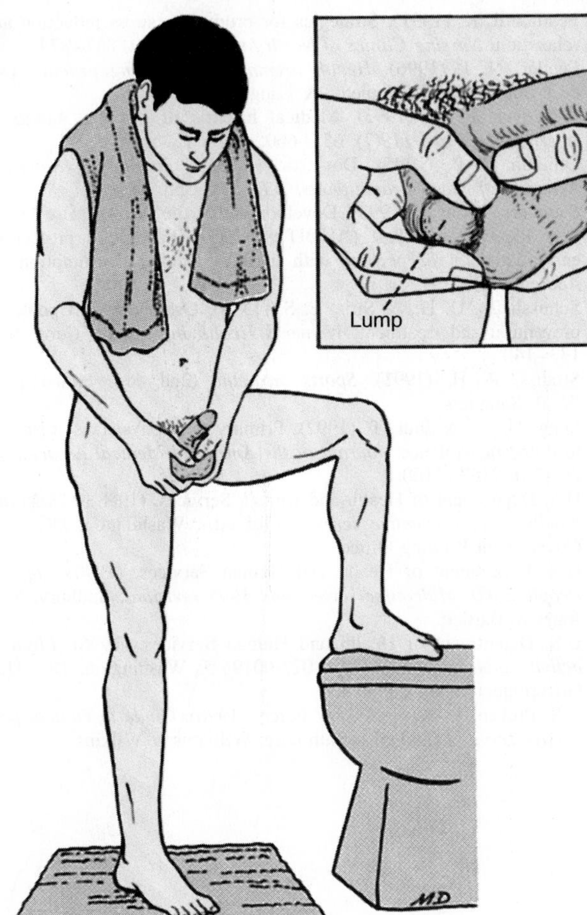

FIGURE 2–6 Testicular self-examination.

family history of colorectal cancer, especially in young and middle-aged adults, and possibly high-fat and low-fiber diets.[47]

Current recommendations are for annual screening using fecal occult blood testing (FOBT) for adults over 50 years of age.[47] People who are at increased risk would benefit from beginning screening at age 40. Fecal occult blood testing is easily done at home, but the client should be instructed on dietary restrictions, specifically, no raw meat; no aspirin or nonsteroidal anti-inflammatory agents (NSAIDs), and no vitamin C in doses over 250 mg for 48 hours prior to and during specimen collection. Specimens should be kept away from heat and should be tested within 2 weeks of collection. Advise clients at increased risk to discuss the benefits of regular sigmoidoscopy screening with a health care provider. Current Task Force recommendations include consideration of a sigmoidoscopy at age 50.

CONCLUSIONS

Health promotion and disease prevention activities are at the core of health care for young and middle-aged adults. Be familiar with current recommendations regarding healthy eating and activity patterns and with strategies for coping with daily stressors. Take every opportunity to work with clients to assist them to implement healthy lifestyles. Include risk assessment, risk management, and appropriate screening for diseases when working with these populations. Based on assessment results, provide education and appropriate referral.

BIBLIOGRAPHY

1. Agency for Health Care Policy and Research. (1996). *Smoking cessation: Information for specialists.* Washington, DC: U.S. Government Printing Office, AHCPR Pub. No. 96-0694.
2. Bonheur, B., & Young, S. (1991). Exercise as a health-promoting life-style choice. *Applied Nursing Research, 4*(1), 2–6.
3. Burns, C. M. (1993). Assessment and screening for substance abuse: Guidelines for the primary care nurse practitioner. *Nurse Practitioner Forum, 4*(4), 199–206.
4. Burns, K. (1996). A new recommendation for physical activity as a means of health promotion. *Nurse Practitioner, 21*(9), 18, 21–22, 26, 27.
5. Calfas, K., et al. (1996). A controlled trial of physician counseling to promote the adoption of physical activity. *Preventive Medicine, 25,* 225–233.
6. Chrousos, G., & Gold, P. (1992). The concepts of stress and stress system disorders. *Journal of the American Medical Association, 267*(9), 1244–1252.
7. Council of Community Health Nurses. (1991). *Physical violence against women: ANA position statement.* Kansas City, MO: American Nurses' Association.
8. Daughton, D., et al. (1994, September). Confronting cigarette addiction: A guide to efficient clinical intervention. *Internal Medicine,* 68–70, 73–77.
9. Davis, M., Eshelman, E., & McKay, M. (1995). *The relaxation and stress reduction workbook* (4th ed.). Oakland, CA: New Harbinger Publications.
10. Domestic violence: Ending the cycle of abuse. (1998). *Clinician Reviews, 8*(1), 55–57, 61–62, 67–68, 71.
11. Edmunds, M. (1991). Strategies for promoting physical fitness. *Nursing Clinics of North America, 26*(4), 855–866.
12. Ferri, R. (1998, June 25). Treating HIV infection. *The Clinical Advisor,* 30–36.
13. Feldhaus, K., et al. (1997). Accuracy of three brief questions for detecting partner violence in the emergency department. *Journal of the American Medical Association, 277,* 1357–1361.
14. Franklin, B., Buchal, M., & Hollingsworth, V. (1991). Exercise prescription. In R. Strauss (Ed), *Sports medicine* (2nd ed.). Philadelphia: W. B. Saunders.
15. Goldstein, D. J. (1992). Beneficial effects of modest weight loss. *International Journal of Obesity, 16,* 397–415.
16. Gorin, S. S. (1998). Smoking cessation. In S. S. Gorin & J. Arnold (Eds.), *Health promotion handbook.* St. Louis: Mosby–Year Book.
17. Grubbs, L. (1993). The critical role of exercise in weight control. *Nurse Practitioner, 18*(4), 20, 22, 25–26, 29.
18. Hoff, L. A. (1992). Battered women: Understanding, identification, and assessment. *Journal of the American Academy of Nurse Practitioners, 4*(4), 148–155.
19. Hoff, L. A. (1993). Battered women: Intervention and prevention. *Journal of the American Academy of Nurse Practitioners, 5*(1), 34–39.
20. Howard, G., et al. (1998). Cigarette smoking and progression of atherosclerosis: The Atherosclerosis Risk in Communities (ARIC) study. *Journal of the American Medical Association, 279*(2), 119–124.
21. Jones, K. D., & Jones, J. M. (1997). Physical activity and exercise. *Clinician Reviews, 7*(3), 81–83, 86–88, 93–94, 97–98, 101–102, 104.
22. Isaacson, J., Butler, R., & Zackarek, M. (1994). Screening with the Alcohol Use Disorders Identification Test (AUDIT) in an inner-city population. *Journal of General Internal Medicine, 9,* 550–553.
23. Krawiec, J. V., & Pohl, J. M. (1998). Smoking cessation and nicotine replacement therapy: A guide for primary care providers. *American Journal of Nurse Practitioners, 2*(1), 15–16, 19–22, 27–33.

24. Kushner, R., & Hopson, S. (1998). Obesity therapy: What works—what doesn't? *Consultant, 38*(3), 511–518.
25. Long, B. J., et al. (1996). A multisite field test of the acceptability of physical counseling in primary care: Project PACE. *American Journal of Preventive Medicine, 12*(2), 73–81.
26. McCloskey, J. C., & Bulechek, G. M. (1996). *Nursing intervention classification* (2nd ed.). St. Louis: Mosby–Year Book.
27. McWhirter, E. H. (1994). *Counseling for empowerment.* Alexandria, VA: American Counseling Association.
28. Melkus, G. D. (1994). Obesity: Assessment and intervention in primary care practice. *Nurse Practitioner Forum, 5*(1), 28–33.
29. Naitoh, J., Zeiner, R. L., & Dekernion, J. B. (1998). Diagnosis and treatment of prostate cancer. *American Family Physician, 57*(7), 1531–1539.
30. National Cholesterol Program. (1993). *Second report of the National Cholesterol Education Expert Panel on detection, evaluation, and treatment of high blood cholesterol in adults (Adult Treatment Panel II),* NIH Pub. No. 93-3085. Bethesda: National Institutes of Health, National Heart, Lung, and Blood Institute.
31. National Institutes of Health Consensus Panel on Optimal Calcium Intake. (1992). Optimal calcium intake. *Journal of the American Medical Association, 272*(24), 1942–1948.
32. Novak, J. C. (1998). Effective smoking cessation strategies. *Clinical Letter for Nurse Practitioners, 2*(1), 1–6.
33. Paffenbarger, R. S., et al. (1986). Physical activity, all-cause mortality, and longevity in college alumni. *New England Journal of Medicine, 314*(10), 605–613.
34. Pate, R. R., et al. (1995). Physical activity and public health. *Journal of the American Medical Association, 273*(5), 402–407.
35. Patrick, K., et al. (1994). A new tool for encouraging activity. *The Physician and Sportsmedicine, 22*(11), 45–55.
36. Peddicord, K. (1991). Strategies for promoting stress reduction and relaxation. *Nursing Clinics of North America, 26*(4), 867–874.
37. Pender, N. J. (1996). *Health promotion in nursing practice* (3rd ed.). Stamford, CT: Appleton & Lange.
38. Pi-Sunyer, F. X. (1993). Medical hazards of obesity. *Annals of Internal Medicine, 119*(7), 655–660.
39. Quillian, J. P. (1995). Domestic violence. *Journal of American Academy of Nurse Practitioners, 7*(7), 351–358.
40. Saunders, J., et al. (1993). Development of the Alcohol Use Disorders Identification Test (AUDIT): WHO collaboration project on early detection of persons with harmful alcohol consumption. II. *Addiction, 88,* 791.
41. Schussheim, D. H., & Siris, E. S. (1998). Osteoporosis: Update on prevention and treatment. *Women's Health in Primary Care, 1*(2), 133–140.
42. Strauss, R. H. (1991). *Sports medicine* (2nd ed.). Philadelphia: W. B. Saunders.
43. Sugg, N. K., & Inui, T. (1992). Primary care physicians' response to domestic violence. *Journal of the American Medical Association, 267*(23), 3157–3160.
44. U.S. Department of Health and Human Services. (1998). *Clinician's handbook of preventive services* (3rd ed.). Washington, DC: U.S. Government Printing Office.
45. U.S. Department of Health and Human Services. (1996). *Healthy People 2000: Midcourse review and 1995 revisions.* Sudbury, MA: Jones & Bartlett.
46. U.S. Department of Health and Human Services. (1996). *Physical activity and health,* S/N 017-023-00196-5. Washington, DC: U.S. Government Printing Office.
47. U.S. Preventive Services Task Force. (1996). *Guide to clinical preventive services* (2nd ed.). Baltimore: Williams & Wilkins.

CHAPTER 3

Health Promotion in Older Adults

Beverley E. Holland
Cynthia McCurren

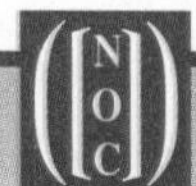

NURSING OUTCOMES CLASSIFICATION (NOC)
for Nursing Diagnoses—Clients at Risk for Relocation Stress Syndrome

Relocation Stress Syndrome
Anxiety Control
Caregiver Adaptation to Patient Institutionalization
Coping
Depression Control
Depression Level
Grief Resolution
Loneliness
Mood Equilibrium
Psychosocial Adjustment: Life Change
Quality of Life
Sleep
Social Support

As a result of the phenomenon of the aging of the United States population and related issues, health promotion in older adults merits special attention. According to the American Association of Retired Persons,[28] almost 34 million Americans were age 65 years or older in 1996. This figure represents 12.8% of the population, about one in every eight Americans. The older population will continue to grow (Fig. 3–1). The most rapid increase is expected between the years 2010 and 2030, when the "baby boom" generation (those born between 1946 and 1964) reach age 65. By 2030, there will be about 70 million elderly, more than twice the number in 1996; they will represent 20% of the population. The elderly population is currently the fastest-growing segment in the nation. Concern for rapidly increasing aging populations is an international dilemma.

The aging of America has profound implications for nursing practice across all settings, including acute care, the community, and long-term care. Among all hospital admissions in the United States, nearly 60% involve clients over age 65.[10] Nurse experts on aging agree that nurses need information to provide appropriate care to older people. Nurses who care for older clients must be aware of the unique physical, psychosocial, legal, ethical, and economic issues surrounding the aging process. Knowing what resources, services, and options are available at the federal, state, and local levels is essential.

Nurses must understand the normal aging process and must be prepared to care for clients who have chronic disorders and complex acute conditions. Normal aging changes the structure and function of various organ systems. Pathologic processes often present and progress differently in the elderly, necessitating adaptation of interventions. Selected effects of aging as they relate to assessment, disease presentation, and nursing intervention appear throughout this book in discussions of the different body systems and their disorders.

This chapter examines late adulthood and the implications for nursing practice from a holistic perspective. The focus is on issues associated with health promotion and disease prevention in older adults.

NURSING AND THE STUDY OF AGING

Two terms are used in the study of aging[8]:

1. *Geriatrics,* from Greek *geras* (old age) and *iatrike* (medicine), is the branch of medicine concerned with medical problems and care of older people. Geriatrics pertains to all health care disciplines, and

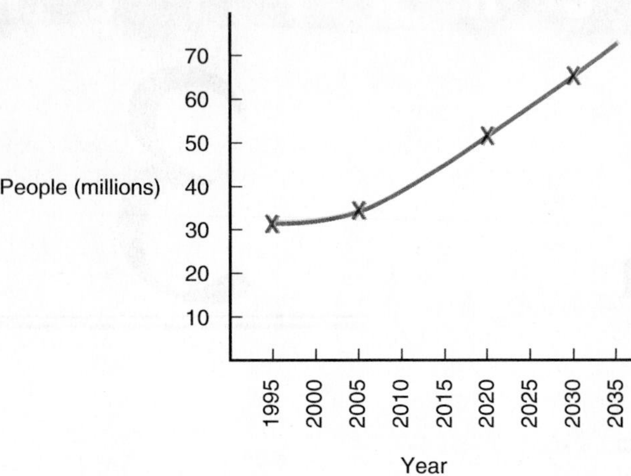

FIGURE 3–1 Projected rise in America's 65-and-older population.

professionals who care for these clients should be familiar with the illnesses that affect them.

2. *Gerontology* takes a broader perspective. It is the scientific study of the process and problems of aging and focuses on the biologic, sociologic, and psychological aspects of normal aging.

Ebersole and Hess studied aging within the discipline of nursing.[10] They assert that *geriatric nursing* occurs primarily with the ill elderly in a medical setting. These authors use the term *ærontic nursing,* defined as the specialized nursing care of older adults that occurs in any setting in which nurses use knowledge, expertise, and caring abilities to promote optimal functioning. Herontic nursing includes a comprehensive understanding of aging within a holistic perspective. It is more than the medical or scientific approach and encompasses nursing's concept of the spiritual biopsychosocial person.

The American Nurses' Association (ANA) identifies standards of *gerontological nursing* practice.[1] "Gerontological nursing" is the ANA's term for nursing specializing in the care of older adults. These standards include practice guidelines for health promotion, health maintenance, disease prevention, and self-care, with a goal of restoring and maintaining optimal physical, psychological, and social functioning. Organizational standards for nursing service, research, ethics, and professional development are also included. *Standards of Gerontological Nursing Practice* defines what gerontological nurses can do and outlines their unique contributions by describing and prescribing professional nursing practice related to care of older adults.

The ANA provides three levels of gerontological nursing certification:

- Gerontological nurse
- Gerontological clinical nurse specialist (GCNS)
- Gerontological nurse practitioner (GNP)

Advanced-practice nurses (GNPs and GCNSs) have diverse opportunities for practice. They can manage many health problems that occur among residents in skilled nursing facilities, retirement communities, day care settings, ambulatory care settings, hospitals, and private practice. Gerontological nurse specialists can also assume roles in education, counseling, case management, and long-term care administration.

THE OLDER POPULATION

■ TRENDS AMONG THE ELDERLY

Aging trends have profound implications for nursing practice and the delivery of health care. The Pew Health Professions Commission report, *Healthy America: Practitioners for 2005,*[31] summarized the aging population growth trends. The 65-and-older group was expected to increase between 1995 and 2005. After 2010, there will be rapid growth to the year 2030 as baby boomers age. Figure 3–1 depicts this rapid rise. Not only is the total U.S. population aging; the elderly population is aging too. In 1987, 9.6% of the elderly population was older than 85 years; by 2010, this percentage will increase to 15.5%. There are now 36,000 centenarians in the United States. If present trends continue, there may be 266,000 centenarians by the year 2020.

Ethnicity

In 1997, 15.3% of persons 65 years and older in the United States were minorities. By 2030, this percentage is expected to increase to 25%.[28] It is projected that Hispanics will represent 13%; blacks, 17%; Asians and Pacific Islanders, 12%; and Native Americans, Eskimos, and Aleuts, 11% of the older population. Whites will make up 47% of the total elder population.[28] Caregivers who work with diverse older Americans must consider ethnic origin in relation to health and illness issues, family and social support, and interaction within the health care system.

Aging, Sex, and Marital Status

Of the 33.9 million Americans over age 65 years, nearly 20 million are women and 13.9 million are men.[28] Life expectancy for men is 80 years, and 84 years for women. Among people 65 years and older, 76% of men live with their spouses, compared with only 43% of women.[10] The implications for nursing practice are evident. Most older women living alone are an at-risk population, frequently encountering problems accessing and obtaining quality health care. Traditionally, women assumed dependent roles, letting others make their decisions, including treatment choices. In general, these women are vulnerable; nurses need to ensure that they receive their share of medical resources and quality health care.

Economic Forces

The largest single income source for an older adult is the Social Security benefit, about 40%. Other contributing sources include earnings, property income, pensions, and public assistance. In 1997, the median yearly income for older men was $17,768; for older women, it was $10,062.[28] The poverty and near-poverty rate was 16.9% among all elderly in 1997.[28] Among minority ethnic groups, poverty levels are even higher. Approximately 26% of elderly black Americans currently fall below the federal poverty line, compared with 9% of elderly white Americans and nearly 51% of elderly Native Americans.

Although most older adults receive Medicare benefits, Medicare does not provide comprehensive coverage of health care expenses. Medicare does not cover most preventive care, including vision, hearing, or dental examinations. For a person living at or near poverty level, supplemental health insurance is not an option. Medicare reimburses only for limited home health care services and does not cover a large part of nursing home costs.

Educational Issues

In 1987, fewer than half of the elderly population were high school graduates.[11] Current trends indicate that by the year 2000, 66% of all elders will have completed high school and more older adults will have advanced degrees.[8] There is great disparity in educational levels among various ethnic groups. Many blacks older than 65 years of age have not had a formal education. Hispanic elderly people have the least amount of formal education, whereas Asians are the most educated minority.

■ CULTURAL ASPECTS OF AGING

Diverse Definitions of "Elderly"

The United States has many ethnocultural groups interacting within one society. Culture defines who is old, establishes rituals for identifying the elderly, sets socially acceptable roles and expectations for behavior of older adults, and influences attitudes toward aged members.

The definitions of functional and chronological aging indicate that there are no arbitrary or widely accepted markers for old age. The prevailing definition of old age in the United States is considered to be age 65; there are diverse perceptions of old age in various cultures. People may be recognized as elders as early as age 40 among Southeast Asian and Native American groups. Social changes, such as becoming grandparents and retirement, or changes in functional status rather than chronological age, mark entrance into old age in different cultures. Clients may be chronologically old but, in functional terms, are active and productive.

When working with older people, use a holistic approach. Holistic care encompasses understanding the interaction of culture, socioeconomic background, and spirituality as well as the physiological and psychological processes of the person. Chapter 9 discusses psychosocial and cultural assessment. A holistic approach takes into account the complexities of the interactions and delivers individualized care to meet each client's needs.[24]

Family Support

Nurses who care for older clients and families from different cultural backgrounds notice that family relationships vary within a cultural context. The availability of physical and personal support from family members can facilitate the older person's ability to maintain independence, cope effectively with acute and chronic illnesses, remain functional and productive despite disability, and experience a peaceful death.

Since decision-making in the Hispanic culture usually includes the family, the following guidelines apply:

1. Involve the relatives in the plan of care and consult with them.
2. In the inpatient setting, do not be surprised to see a room full of guests visiting the client. Be sensitive to this, and know that Hispanic elders value close family contact.
3. Encourage this if it is not contraindicated by the current therapy, and view it as a necessary integral part of the client's recovery.[24]

Some older adults from culturally diverse backgrounds who have given material and social support to children and grandchildren may expect reciprocity during their aging years. In many Hispanic, Native American, Asian American, Amish, Arab American, and first-generation immigrant ethnic groups, the cultural norm is to care for aging parents, grandparents, and extended family members.

The importance of family support is compounded for older refugees. In instances of forced migration, the traditional family structure may have been altered or destroyed in the country of origin, sometimes in extremely violent ways. When older refugees arrive in the new host country, they may be isolated. Older refugees may have limited or no English language skills and have lost their social status, their country, and their home. The psychological stress related to cultural change is more intense. The older refugee is more likely to rely on younger family members for economic and social support, housing, and access to health services.[24]

Older adults from cultures that highly value independence and self-reliance may refuse offers of assistance from their children, grandchildren, and extended family members. Depending on personal finances, these individuals may have planned carefully for their aging in ways that rely on personal resources. They may seek assistance on a fee-for-service basis from organizations that provide services and homes for the elderly but may refuse help from relatives.

A national sample of older Hispanics revealed that 30% reported providing child care to younger family members, 50% reported assisting in family decisions, and 12% provided financial assistance to family members. This compares with a national average of 19% of older Americans providing child care regularly, and 15% occasionally caring for their grandchildren. More grandparents in Japan and France (51%) provide regular care than grandparents in Great Britain (19%).[24] In black American households, the grandmother often takes a direct role in childrearing. More than twice as many young blacks live in households headed by elderly family members compared with whites.

Cultural Influences on Caregiving

Historically, a higher proportion of older adults among minority ethnic groups have been cared for in home environments than older white Americans have. Research indicates that family care of the elderly in other cultures is supportive for several reasons: as a substitute for formal services, as a more affordable alternative, as a caring option that is consistent with cultural values and preferences, and as an effective strategy for overcoming language barriers. In large extended families, more relatives are likely to be available to provide partial services and care for an older family member.[24]

In Hispanic families, the elder has a position of respect and is usually cared for at home by the family. Should institutionalization occur, a Hispanic elder may suffer feelings of isolation, anguish, and perhaps betrayal by loved ones. The Hispanic male in a traditional authority role may be greatly affected by the transition to a dependent, passive role.[24]

Economic Issues

The work histories of cultural groups, including long careers in agricultural and domestic labor, often preclude coverage within the Social Security or Medicare system. For this reason, many elderly members from diverse cultural backgrounds face out-of-pocket health care expenses on limited incomes and have difficulty paying health care costs. Nurses who work with aged clients in their homes often find them also unable to afford these costs. In many cases, family members of culturally diverse older adults bear the burden of such expenses.[24]

Older adults who have made major lifestyle adjustments from their homelands to the United States and from rural to urban settings may be unaware of health care alternatives (e.g., preventive programs, benefits, and screening programs) for which they are eligible. The nurse can help clients in evaluating their social networks, seeking assistance for health care needs, activating social contacts for support, and developing culturally competent care plans.

HEALTH PROMOTION, MAINTENANCE, AND RESTORATION IN OLDER CLIENTS

Older adults are more likely to suffer from multiple chronic and disabling illnesses than younger adults (see Chapter 2). Approximately 80% of elderly people in the United States have one or more chronic diseases.[28] Chronic conditions result in limitations in *activities of daily living* (ADL) for 50%, major limitations in activities for 18%, and home confinement for 5%. Heart disease, cancer, and strokes account for 80% of deaths in people older than age 65. Clients with hypertension, arthritis, pulmonary disorders, diabetes, visual and hearing problems, dementia, and depression require ongoing care and rehabilitation.[10]

A traditional definition of *health* as the absence of disease or disability is clearly not applicable to most older people. A more appropriate focus is on health as a state of mind and on the ability to live and function effectively in society. Health encompasses an interaction of physical, functional, and psychosocial factors. Health promotion goals, therefore, must include individual and group efforts related to spiritual, emotional, psychosocial, and physical concerns (see Chapter 1). Desired outcomes of health promotion programs should include:

1. Maximizing functional independence, thereby reducing dependency.
2. Decreasing mortality.
3. Decreasing morbidity, including impairment.
4. Maintaining or improving quality of life.
5. Promoting behavioral change when necessary.
6. Increasing productivity.

Elders can make efforts to control aspects of their health and move toward wellness (Table 3–1). Nursing

TABLE 3–1 HEALTH PROMOTION, MAINTENANCE, AND RESTORATION ACTIVITIES FOR OLDER ADULTS

Promotion*	Maintenance†	Restoration‡
Primary Prevention (prevents occurrence of specific disease and provides specific protection)	*Secondary Prevention* (early detection and treatment and limitation of disability)	*Tertiary Prevention* (rehabilitation after disease)
Smoking cessation programs Diet low in fat, high in fiber Regular weight-bearing exercise Weight control Limiting alcohol ingestion Testicular self-examination Breast self-examination Education in osteoporosis: calcium and vitamin D intake Use of seat belt Vaccinations Tetanus-diphtheria toxoid Pneumococcus Influenza	**Complete physical examination** Blood pressure Electrocardiogram Total cholesterol with high-density lipoprotein Clinical breast examination Mammography Digital rectal examination Fecal occult blood testing Thyroid-stimulating hormone test Pelvic examination with Papanicolaou smear Prostate examination Sigmoidoscopy **Counseling** Sexuality Urinary incontinence Depression/life satisfaction **Counseling and referral** Hearing examination Visual examination with glaucoma test Dental examination and cleaning	Post-stroke rehabilitation Cardiac rehabilitation Pulmonary rehabilitation Orthopedic rehabilitation

*Health promotion activities for older adults are similar to recommendations for all adults.

†Recommendations on frequency of examinations vary, depending on the recommending organization (American College of Physicians, American Cancer Society, U.S. Preventive Services Task Force, and American Geriatrics Society) and the risk factors and presenting manifestations of the individual.

‡Rehabilitation programs are interdisciplinary and developed to meet the specific needs and deficits of the person.

has a prominent role in helping elders practice health promotion, including self-care, physical activity, nutritional awareness, and stress management.

Self-Care and Self-Responsibility

As older adults become better informed and increasingly aware of the self-help movement, health care expectations also rise. There is an increasing desire to be in control of one's body, mind, and spirit and to assume responsibility for one's own wellness. This does not mean that traditional health care providers are ignored. Instead, strategies are taught that enable people to respond to their body signals and to take action accordingly. You can help the aging person understand this shared role (between the individual and health care professionals) for maintaining wellness, counsel elders about factors that can alter wellness, and provide information about available alternatives (see Chapter 1). Given adequate information, elders can practice effective self-care through a process of examining choices and making informed, meaningful decisions.

Most older people want to have as much control as possible over their body, mind, and spirit. Assessment should include an evaluation of self-care, with an emphasis on abilities rather than disabilities. Suggested preventive practices are discussed in Chapters 1, 2, and 9. Physical activity, nutrition, and stress management are also factors in geriatric wellness.

Physical Activity

Exercise and activity are essential for health promotion and maintenance and for achieving an optimal level of functioning (see Chapters 1 and 2). Approximately half of the physical deterioration in the elderly population is caused by disuse rather than by the aging process or disease. Positive effects of exercise on health include (1) increased energy, (2) improved eating and sleeping, (3) decreased discomfort and stress, and (4) decreased smoking and alcohol use.[10]

Physiologically, benefits to the cardiopulmonary, vascular, and musculoskeletal systems result in (1) improved oxygen transport, (2) decreased blood pressure and pulse rate, (3) increased vital lung capacity, (4) decreased body fat and increased lean body mass, (5) reduced osteoporosis, and (6) increased muscle strength and joint flexibility. Positive psychological changes occur as well, including improved cognitive functioning and a heightened sense of well-being.

Before beginning an exercise program, older clients should have a physical examination, which may include an exercise stress test. One of the best exercises for an older adult is walking, with progression to 30-minute sessions three to five times each week (Fig. 3–2). Swimming and dancing are also beneficial. Age alone does not preclude older people from pursuing a range of physical activities; the issue is simply one of physical tolerance. Elders confined to a chair or with limited mobility can perform adapted exercises. At many senior centers, wellness programs, and fitness clubs, consultants, instructors, or physical therapists can help the client establish an individualized exercise program (Fig. 3–3).

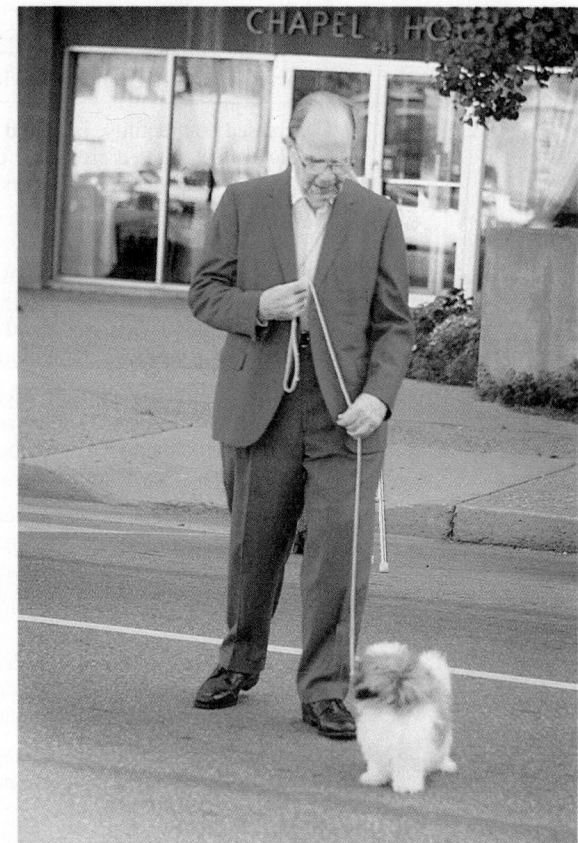

FIGURE 3–2 Walking provides a multitude of physiologic benefits for the older person.

Nutrition

Nutritional status is important to an older person's ability to remain healthy, to maintain structural integrity, think clearly, and to possess the necessary energy to engage in social and fitness activities. Several physiologic changes related to aging can affect nutritional status (Table 3–2).

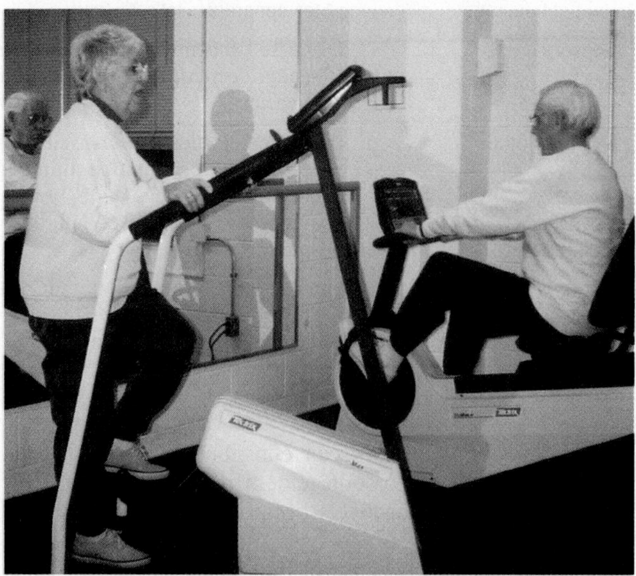

FIGURE 3–3 Today's older adult is interested in maintaining strength and endurance.

TABLE 3–2 **STRUCTURAL AND FUNCTIONAL CHANGES AND COMMON HEALTH PROBLEMS IN OLDER ADULTS**

System	Normal Changes Associated with Aging	Common Health Problems
Cardiovascular	Decreased contractility, impaired coronary artery blood flow, altered preload and afterload, increased atherosclerotic plaques	Hypertension, ischemic heart disease, heart failure, cardiac dysrhythmia, valvular heart disease, peripheral vascular disease, varicose veins, dehydration, stroke/transient ischemic attack
Neurologic/behavioral	Decreased speed of neural conduction, decreased number of brain cells, decreased neurotransmitters, decreased rapid eye movement sleep, decreased cerebral circulation	Parkinsonism, essential tremor, Alzheimer's disease or dementia, depression, anxiety, psychosis or paranoid state, sleep disturbance, subdural hematoma, trigeminal neuralgia
Respiratory	Increased rigidity of thoracic cage, decreased elasticity, decreased vital capacity, increased residual volume, decreased cough efficiency, decreased ciliary action	Pneumonia, chronic obstructive pulmonary disease, dyspnea
Gastrointestinal	Decreased secretion of gastric acid, delayed gastric emptying, decreased gastrointestinal motility, altered nutrient digestion, altered bowel function, weakening of lower esophageal sphincter	Diverticula or diverticulitis, constipation, diarrhea, gastroesophageal reflux or hiatus hernia, fecal incontinence, colorectal cancer, rectal prolapse, dysphagia, anorexia, gallbladder disease
Genitourinary	Decreased bladder capacity, decreased concentrating and diluting abilities, decreased creatinine clearance, increased prostate size	Renal insufficiency, urinary incontinence, urinary tract infection, enlarged prostate or prostate cancer, sexual dysfunction
Endocrine/metabolic	Decreased basal metabolism, altered pancreatic function, decreased testosterone, estrogen, progesterone	Diabetes mellitus, hyperthyroidism or hypothyroidism, thyroid cancer, hypercalcemia or hypocalcemia, hyperlipidemia, hypokalemia, hyponatremia, gout
Musculoskeletal	Decreased bone density, decreased muscle size and strength, degenerated joint cartilage	Paget's disease, osteoporosis, osteomalacia, rheumatoid arthritis, osteoarthritis, polymyalgia rheumatica, spondylosis, fractures, foot pathology, gait disturbance, falls
Autonomic nervous system	Decreased reaction time and coordination, decreased temperature regulation, decreased sensitivity of baroreceptors	Falls, accidental injuries, orthostatic hypotension, impaired body temperature regulation
Hematologic and immune	Decreased erythropoietin production, decreased intrinsic factor, decreased functioning T and B cells and monocytes	Iron deficiency anemia, pernicious anemia, anemia of chronic disease, cancer, autoimmune disorders
Oral	Decreased salivary secretion, decreased oral motor apparatus, loss of teeth	Periodontal disease; problems with speech, chewing, and swallowing
Sensory	Decreased accommodation, decreased visual acuity, decreased hearing of high-pitched frequencies	Visual impairment, hearing impairment, diminished smell or taste
Dermatologic	Decreased elasticity, decreased secretion of natural oil and perspiration, thinning of skin, decreased heat regulation, decreased epidermal renewal, decreased inflammatory response	Pressure sores, basal cell and squamous carcinoma, herpes zoster, seborrheic and actinic keratosis, stasis dermatitis, pruritus, hypothermia or hyperthermia
Reproductive	Female: vaginal mucosa thinning, atrophy, decreased breast tissue, sexual dysfunction Male: decreased sexual desire	Female: cervical cancer, breast cancer Male: prostate cancer, impotence

Socioeconomic factors can contribute to malnutrition. With reduced income, some elders may restrict food intake to near-starvation levels because they may choose to pay rent and buy medicine over spending for food. Diets may be unbalanced because of the expense of fresh fruits, vegetables, and meats. Lack of transportation and the inability to carry heavy quantities of groceries can prohibit some people from obtaining food. Living alone can also be associated with poor nutrition, since many older adults may lose the motivation to prepare a balanced diet for just themselves.

Psychologically, depression and stress can affect nutritional status. Both conditions can lead to overeating or undereating. Medications can influence nutrition, producing side effects of increased or decreased appetite, constipation, nausea, or decreased absorption. Additionally, drugs such as diuretics can affect fluid and electrolyte balance, leading to problems with dehydration and constipation.

Physiologically, energy requirements lessen with age because of a decline in basal metabolic rate and often a reduction in physical activity. There is an increased need for vitamin D, vitamin B_6, and calcium to protect against osteoporosis. Increased fiber intake is recommended to reduce the apparent risk of some forms of cancer and to promote bowel function. Unexplained weight loss of more than 5% in 1 month or more than 10% in 6 months is cause for concern. Clients at risk for nutritional problems should be identified (Box 3–1; see also Chapter 28). When no physical cause can be identified, elders with altered nutrition should be referred to community resources for assessment and assistance related to food, finances, and dental care.

Stress Management

Any real or perceived threat to one's physical, emotional, and social well-being can create stress (see Chapters 1 and 2). Life's later years can include changes such as acute or chronic illness, retirement, death of significant others, financial hardship, or relocation resulting in stress that can be overwhelming. Although the sources of stress may vary, the physiologic outcomes are similar. Stimulation of the sympathetic nervous system results in the release of epinephrine, norepinephrine, and adrenal glucocorticoids. Prolonged stress can result in serious consequences, including heart disease, hypertension, cerebrovascular accident, cancer, gastric ulcers, skin problems, complications of underlying disorders, and numerous social and emotional problems.

The way in which an older person adapts to change and stress is influenced by personality traits, past coping strategies, and spirituality. Spirituality extends beyond religion to include contemplation, experiential learning, recognition through growth, discovery and acceptance, new connections, and letting go. Growth, self-discovery, and connecting with others support older people in times of stress, reinforce a sense of self-worth, and provide confidence to overcome obstacles.

Encourage the client to respond to stress in a healthy manner. Balancing nutrition, rest, and exercise, remaining connected with others, and having a sense of inner peace help with stress management. Explain methods of relaxation, including biofeedback, meditation, progressive relaxation, breathing control exercises, physical activity, and involvement in pastimes that provide respite from stressful demands should also be emphasized (see Chapters 1 and 2).

Teaching

Encouraging health promotion and disease prevention among elders requires effective teaching. Teaching elders is similar to teaching members of any age group, in that individual characteristics and learning needs must be considered. General guidelines for teaching older adults are listed in Box 3–2.

BOX 3–1 Risk Factors for Malnutrition in the Elderly Population

*D*isease
*E*ating poorly
*T*ooth decay or oral pain
*E*conomic hardship
*R*educed social contact
*M*ultiple medications
*I*nvoluntary weight loss or gain
*N*eeds assistance with self-care
*E*lder older than 80 years

From the Nutrition Screening Initiative in conjunction with the American Academy of Family Physicians, the American Dietetic Association, and the National Council on the Aging.

BOX 3–2 Guidelines for Effectively Teaching Older Adults

Vision

1. Provide large, easy-to-read typeface
2. Emphasize contrasting colors: black and white
3. Avoid blues and greens
4. Use nonglare paper
5. Write short, simple paragraphs
6. Make sure eyeglasses are in place and clean

Hearing

1. Speak slowly
2. Enunciate clearly
3. Lower the pitch of your voice
4. Eliminate background noise
5. Face the learner
6. Use nonverbal cues
7. Make sure client's hearing aid is in place and working properly

Energy Level/Attention

1. Use short teaching sessions
2. Offer liquid refreshment and bathroom breaks
3. Promote comfort

Information Processing and Memory

1. Present most important information first
2. Clarify information with use of examples that the client can relate to
3. Motor skills: Teach one step at a time, demonstrate, allow for return demonstration
4. Encourage association between items
5. Be concrete and specific
6. Eliminate distractions
7. Encourage verbal interactions
8. Correct wrong answers and reinforce correct answers
9. Offer praise and encouragement

Normal Aging and Commonly Occurring Pathologic Processes

Aging has been defined as a universal, internally predictable biologic process following maturity. It is characterized by changes accumulated over time that increase susceptibility to disease and ultimately lead to death. Physiologically, aging in the absence of disease involves a steady decline in the functional reserve of organ systems and homeostatic controls, especially when a person is under stress. In addition to disease, nutritional status and other extrinsic factors (i.e., environment, activity, medication, depression) are superimposed on the basic process of aging and create individual differences in how one experiences aging.

Presentation of Illness

With advanced age, the body does not respond as vigorously to illness or disease because of diminished physiologic reserve. People often attribute discomforts to "old age" and accept the changes as inevitable, thus failing or refusing to seek help for potentially treatable conditions. A frequent complicating factor in identifying and treating disease in older people is the presence of multiple ailments. The number of pathologic conditions that a person has at one time is strongly correlated with age.[14] The presenting picture may be further complicated by atypical or altered presentation of disease (i.e., weakness, weight loss, confusion, or failure to thrive). Each of these factors presents a challenge; conduct careful and thorough assessments and analyses of manifestations to promote appropriate treatment.

Atypical or altered presentation of disease can be displayed in various ways. For example, an older adult with pneumonia may exhibit confusion, have an increased respiratory rate, and generalized weakness instead of the classic symptoms of productive cough, fever, and chest pain. Frequently, manifestations in one organ system may cause abnormality in another system. This results in manifestations unrelated to the actual problem, such as confusion accompanying a urinary tract infection. Chronic conditions can mask the presence of acute illness. This can be seen in new-onset heart failure, when orthopnea might be hidden if a person regularly uses multiple pillows because of gastroesophageal reflux, arthritis, or obesity.

Finally, expected manifestations may not be present at all, as in the case of a myocardial infarction unaccompanied by chest pain. Table 3–2 summarizes common structural and functional changes associated with normal aging and presents common diseases, disorders, and injuries frequently seen in older adults. Risk factors for many chronic diseases in old age are manifested in early-to-middle adulthood (see Chapters 45, 52, 61, and 70). Increasing age and chronic disease, functional disabilities, and hospitalization intensify the demand and need for health care services. This has implications in any health care setting.

Functional Status

Assessment of functional status of the older adult is important when one is considering the client's level of independence within the environment. Assess basic and instrumental activities of daily living, balance and mobility, cognitive abilities, vision and hearing, bowel and bladder function, nutritional status, and environmental factors. Research has found that functional impairments (both physical and psychosocial) are reliable early indicators of active illness in older people.[5, 10]

Basic activities of daily living (BADL) are the essential activities and tasks performed to get through the day. BADL can be remembered by the mnemonic DEATH: *d*ressing, *e*ating, *a*mbulating, *t*oileting, and *h*ygiene. BADL assessment helps to determine the need for daily personal care and to plan long-term care. There is a corresponding rise in functional dependency related to BADL with increasing age (Fig. 3–4).[28]

Instrumental activities of daily living (IADL) are more complex and are essential to community living situations. IADL include all the daily activities of BADL and SHAFT (*s*hopping, *h*ousework, *a*ccounting (managing money), *f*ood preparation, and *t*ransportation. Evaluation of IADL is used to decide what type of assistance is needed by people in independent or semi-independent settings. The ability to perform IADL is less important in institutional settings than in community settings, although the assessment can prove important for discharge planning when the client is returning to the home environment.

Upon completion of a functional assessment, the individual's problems can be categorized as "functional," "medical," or "support" issues, and a management plan

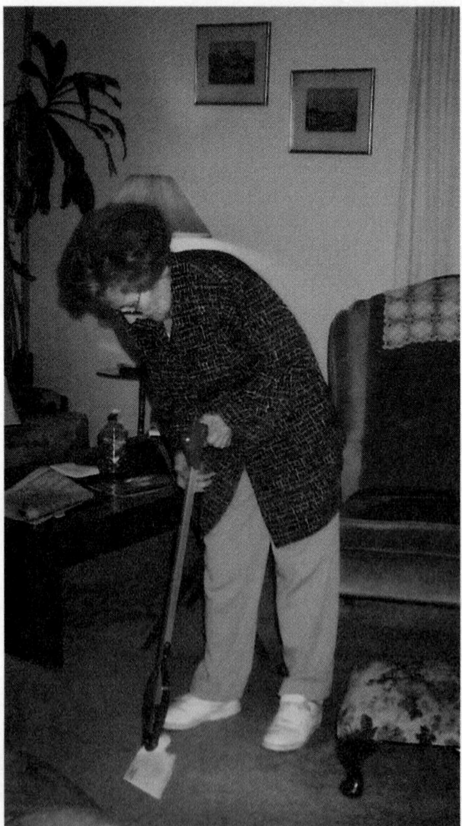

FIGURE 3–4 Use of a grabber to retrieve a dropped object from the floor.

can be developed. This plan may include coordination of environmental changes, facilitation for the use of assistive devices (Figs. 3–5 and 3–6), and arrangements for community referrals (Table 3–3) for services that would allow the person to remain in the chosen environment.

Functional assessment instruments generally include scales for measuring BADL and IADL. The Barthel,[21] Katz,[17] and Older Americans Resources and Services (OARS) indexes[16] are commonly used. Observation, interview, mental status screening,[12] and a screen for depression can assess psychosocial functioning. These provide information about cognitive functioning, perceptual-motor skills, insight, reasoning, and contact with reality. Chapters 9 and 67 describe mental status assessment.

■ PHYSIOLOGIC FACTORS THAT INFLUENCE FUNCTIONAL STATUS

Sleep

Older adults fall asleep with more difficulty, awaken more readily and more frequently, spend more time in the drowsiness stage, and spend less time in deep sleep than do younger adults.[34] Functionally, these changes have little impact on the daily life of the older adult. However, adverse reactions can occur when these changes coincide with illness, stress, daily demands, or certain medications, such as hypnotic, antidepressant, diuretic, and some antihypertensive medications. Sleep disorders and their treatment are discussed in Chapter 21.

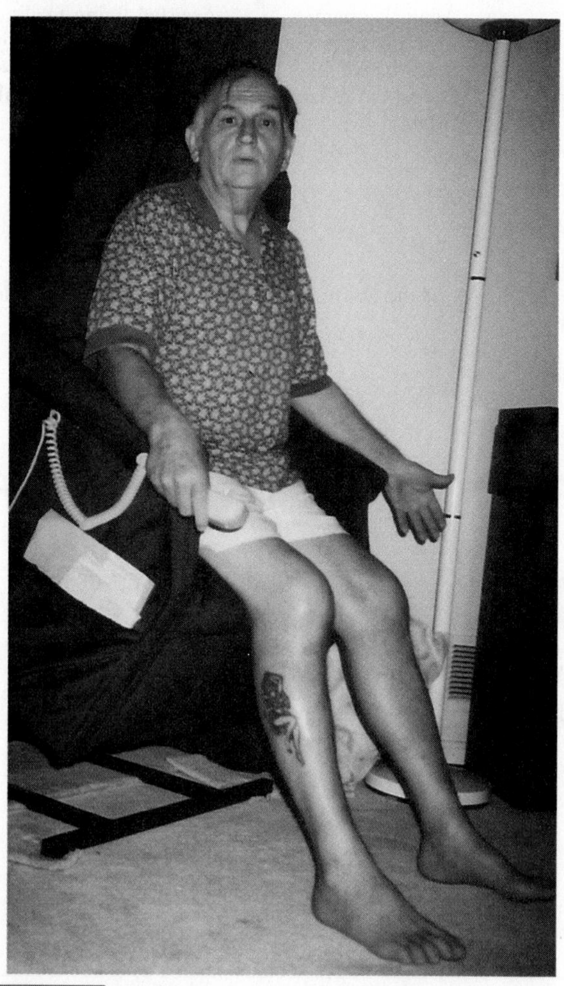

FIGURE 3–5 An electric recliner lifts a person from a sitting to standing position or assists in lowering a person from a standing to sitting position.

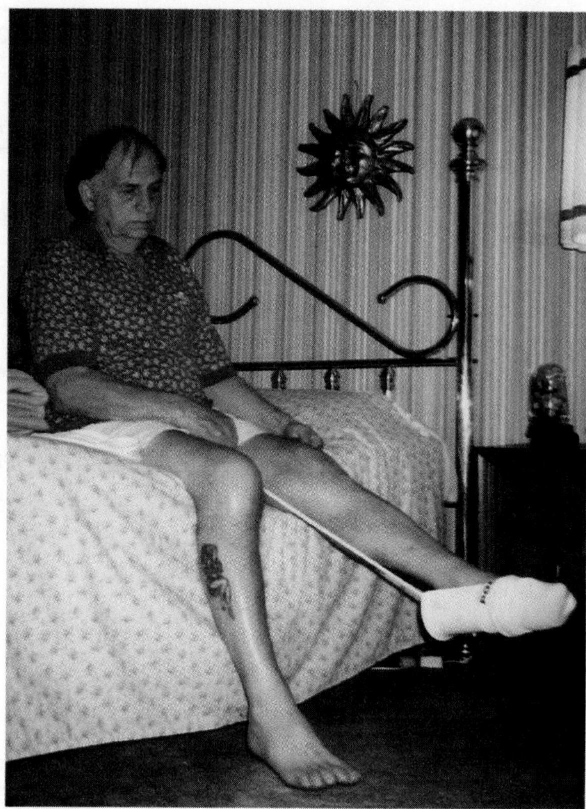

FIGURE 3–6 A sock slide allows a person to put on socks independently.

Sensory Impairments

Normal aging results in some sensory impairment (see Table 3–2). Vision and hearing are senses that individuals rely on to communicate and to function in the environment. Sensory impairments can affect safety, communication with others, performance of daily activities, and quality of life. Assessment suggests that limitations in ADL are more likely to occur in older people with sensory impairments than in those without sensory loss. Vision changes can affect the performance of a variety of daily activities: driving a vehicle; shopping for groceries; negotiating stairs; maneuvering safely in dark or unfamiliar environments; seeing markings on clocks, radios, thermostats, appliances, and televisions; and reading newspapers, signs, directories, and labels on food items and medication containers. Besides influencing daily activities, impaired vision increases the risk of falling. Impairments and treatment for vision and hearing disorders are discussed in Chapters 65 and 66.

Mobility and Balance

Mobility is essential for maintaining independence. Serious consequences occur when mobility declines. Older

TABLE 3–3 CONTINUUM OF CARE: COMMUNITY RESOURCES, SERVICES, AND HOUSING OPTIONS*

Functional Level of Care	Nursing Functions	Services Needed: In the Home	Services Needed: In the Community	Living and Housing Options
Older adults of all functional levels	Support individual in achieving highest level of autonomy possible in situation. Provide health surveillance. Identify health, social, spiritual, and economic need. Make clients and families aware of options and resources		Support groups (e.g., for illness or bereavement). Advocacy services. Outpatient nurse-run clinics. Mental health clinics. Private physicians	
Older adults who are functionally independent	Assist client and family to modify patterns detrimental to health. Evaluate deviations from normal and advise clients of appropriate action. Identify existing or impending illness. Educate clients regarding self-responsibility for health	Gatekeepers	All of the above, *plus:* Senior centers Meal sites	Own home Retirement community House-sharing
Older adults who need some help with IADL	Teach clients and families. Consult and collaborate with agencies and multiprofessional representatives. Provide appropriate information to clients and families about treatment plan, medications, and diagnosis in collaboration with physician	Chore services Housekeeping Escort Transportation Emergency response system Home modifications Home-delivered meals Friendly visitors Telephone reassurance Gatekeepers	All of the above, *plus:* Adult day care Case management Respite care Outpatient rehabilitation	Retirement community Assisted-living facilities Congregate or shared housing Sheltered living Family care homes
Older adults who need help with IADL and BADL	Promote health through clinic and home contact. Provide appropriate resources. Counsel clients and family members	All of the above, *plus:* Personal care services Home health aides Public health nurse Respite care at home	All of the above	Assisted-living facilities Sheltered living
Older adults who need help with most IADL and BADL	Give treatments, medications, and rehabilitative exercises. Observe and evaluate response to treatment and medication	All of the above	All of the above, *plus:* Adult day care Case management	Nursing homes
Older adults who are acutely ill, need rehabilitation, or are dying	Keep physician aware of changes in client's conditions. Ensure adequate medical, dental, and podiatric care. Maintain hydration, nutrition, aeration, and pain management. Provide emotional support	All of the above, *plus:* Visiting nurse Visiting rehabilitation therapist Hospice care at home	Case management	Hospitals Rehabilitation facilities Nursing homes

*Availability of resources and services varies from community to community.
IADL, instrumental activities of daily living; BADL, basic activities of daily living.

people use mobility and balance to assess whether they are in relatively good or poor health. At least half of older adults have some limitation in function that prevents them from being fully independent.

Mobility depends on the ability to maintain balance and strength. Decreased functioning of various body systems can affect balance and strength and may place the person at risk. Decreases in functional status can be caused by impaired sensory ability (vision and hearing), cardiopulmonary disorders (dysrhythmia, postural hypotension, chronic obstructive pulmonary disease), neurologic disorders (parkinsonism and problems that affect gait, balance, sway, and reaction time), and depression. Side effects from medications also increase risk. The side effects of hypovolemia, postural hypotension, excessive sedation, decreased cognitive functioning, and loss of postural control can negatively affect mobility and balance.[35] Chronic disorders that increase with age and affect functional ability include osteoporosis, osteoarthritis, and rheumatoid arthritis (see Chapters 26 and 77).

Unstable balance is of concern because the risk of falling increases with age. Falls occur in 32% of 65- to 74-year-olds, 35% of 75- to 84-year-olds and 51% of those aged 85 years and older.[35] In hospitals, falls make up the largest category of reported incidents.

The effect of falls in the elderly is far-reaching. Falls contribute to significant morbidity and mortality.[35] Consequences of falls consume a large portion of health care dollars in the United States, and fear of subsequent falls contributes to restricted activity and mobility and to reduced independence. This self-restriction contributes to functional decreases and social isolation, thus setting up a spiral of downward decline. Up to 40% of all nursing home admissions are related to falls and instability.[35]

■ PSYCHOSOCIAL FACTORS THAT INFLUENCE FUNCTIONAL STATUS

Although physiologic changes and chronic illnesses associated with aging may affect functional abilities, psychosocial changes are often the most challenging and demanding. Some challenges arise from physical changes, but many are caused by changes in roles, relationships, and living environments. These changes tax coping abilities and energies.

Ageism

"Ageism" refers to the prejudices and stereotypes applied to older people purely because of their age. Ageism, like racism and sexism, is a way of labeling a group of people and not allowing them to be individuals with unique ways of living. Prejudice toward the elderly is often an attempt by younger generations to shield themselves from their own eventual aging and death. Such stereotyping allows younger individuals to see older people as different from themselves, and they ultimately cease to identify with older people as human beings. An awakening comes when these younger people age and find themselves the victims of the same stereotypes and attitudes.

The significance of ageism is considerable. Ageism can affect a person's self-confidence, disempower by limiting potential, and cause early or excessive dependency. It can also affect well-being by influencing the attitudes of health care providers and political powers. Typically, diagnosis and treatment of disease in the elderly are less aggressive; programs are generally underfunded; and the ability of older people to remain a contributing force, as perceived by society, is reduced simply because of chronological age.[10]

Negativism can have a devastating effect and cause the elder to adopt modes of dependency, helplessness, and a negative self-image. This can lead to increased vulnerability to biopsychosocial stressors.[32] Images of older persons as being dependent, deteriorating beyond rehabilitative efforts, and being physically and mentally unappealing can lead to reluctance among professionals to care for them. This can result in carelessness about the quality of care delivered. However, each elderly person has potential for rehabilitation, treatment, self-actualization, or improvement in quality of life and well-being, regardless of how small that potential may be.

Multiple Losses

Many losses inevitably occur in later life. Assessing the impact of the losses and supporting the elder are major goals. Aging persons experience personal, social, and economic losses. Among the most devastating are "people" losses—parents, friends, spouse, or children (Fig. 3–7). Other typical losses may include loss of one's home, possessions, pets, employment, social position, or financial security. An "overload" state can result when losses become multiple; the emotional upheaval becomes a catalyst, and the result is mental confusion, withdrawal, helplessness, and depression.

King and coworkers[18] examined the loss of one's traditional dwelling and the effect of relocation. Central to the reaction and adjustment to relocation was whether the move was voluntary or involuntary. Individuals at high risk for poor relocation adjustment have low self-esteem, no friends or support, many worries, high levels of alienation, poor self-perception of health, and depression. Interventions to help with relocation include assessing for risk factors, empathizing with the difficulties of the move,

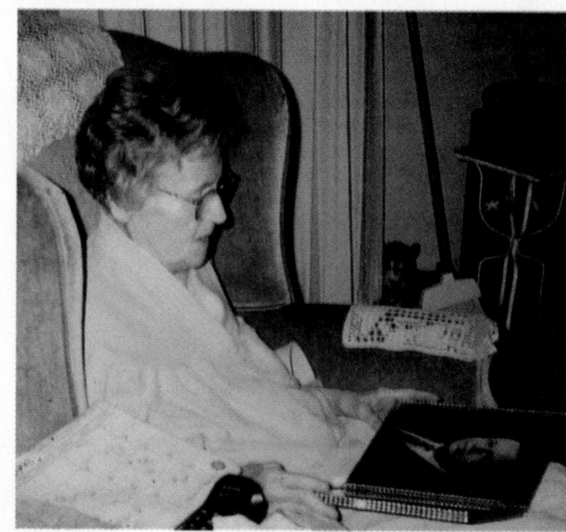

FIGURE 3–7 Loss of loved ones may result in an emotional burden accompanied by mental and physical effects.

C A R E   P L A N

THE OLDER CLIENT AT RISK FOR RELOCATION STRESS SYNDROME

Nursing Diagnosis. Risk for Relocation Stress Syndrome related to changes associated with health care facility transfer or admission to long-term care facility as evidenced by anxiety, insecurity, and changes in health status.

Outcomes. (1) Resident will verbalize feelings, expectations, and disappointments with staff and/or family. (2) Resident will react in a positive manner to staff efforts to assist in adjustment to new facility. (3) Resident will socialize with staff and/or other residents. (4) Resident will maintain stable preadmission weight, appetite, and sleep patterns.

Interventions	Rationales
1. Assess for low self-esteem, anxiety, feeling of insecurity, and disorientation related to move.	1. These are risk factors associated with poor adjustment to relocation.
2. Assess resident's current health status, medications, and needs for additional health services after move.	2. Provides a current baseline of health status and opportunity to review medication, chronic health conditions, and need for additional services.
3. Encourage resident to express emotions associated with the relocation.	3. Allowing resident to express emotions provides an opportunity to correct misconceptions, answer questions, and reduce anxiety.
4. Assist resident and family to prepare for the move by providing information, arranging a visit to the new facility, and introducing them to the new staff if possible.	4. Allows the resident and family to become familiar with the new environment and reduce the stress of relocation.
5. Educate family members about relocation stress syndrome and its potential effects.	5. Family needs to know that family member may exhibit anxiety and other stress-related symptoms and that visiting and providing emotional support during transition period are helpful.
6. Communicate all aspects of the resident's care plan to appropriate staff members at the new location.	6. Communication with staff allows for continuity of care and reduces stress for the resident.

Evaluation. Accomplishment of expected outcomes may require considerable time. Reassessment and revision of plan are important.

and suggesting positive resources to effectively cope. The accompanying Care Plan offers additional information. Adjustment to loss is a challenge at any age. For older adults, resolution of grief loss may not always be achieved but can be integrated into their lives without causing dysfunction.

Neglect and Abuse

Neglect and abuse are complex, serious issues affecting older adults. Research suggests that *elder abuse* is widespread. It occurs among all subgroups of the population and affects up to two million older people a year. Elder abuse encompasses physical, psychological, and financial abuse or neglect by oneself or by a caregiver. It is not uncommon for adults to experience several types of abuse simultaneously. Without intervention, abuse tends to escalate. See Bridge to Home Health Care: Detecting Elder Abuse.

The typical abuse victim is a woman of advanced age with few social contacts, who has a history of mental illness, cognitive impairment, and poor health. These factors often limit her ability to perform BADL. In addition, she frequently lives alone or with the abuser and depends on the abuser for care.[2, 38]

Elder abuse has emerged as a significant aspect of family violence for several reasons. One is the increased number of older adults. As more people live to an advanced age, more adult children are assuming the caregiver role. If the adult child is unprepared for this responsibility, abuse and neglect may occur. Because an older person's dependency needs increase with time, the stress and burden of caregiving also increase, thus raising the risk of abuse. It is the responsibility of the health care provider, both ethically and legally, to be aware of the obvious and subtle signs of abuse and neglect. As a client advocate, encourage and coordinate assistance for victims and abusers. The passage of elder abuse and adult protective services laws has led to increased reporting of mistreatment and self-neglect. This has resulted in greater recognition of the problem.

MENTAL HEALTH DISORDERS IN THE ELDERLY

■ DEMENTIA, DELIRIUM, AND DEPRESSION

Dementia (specifically Alzheimer's disease) and delirium (also known as "confusion") are discussed in Chapter 72 along with their pathophysiology, clinical manifestations, assessment, and management. The focus here is on three important conditions in the elderly: dementia, delirium, and depression. Clinically, the presenting manifestations of these conditions in older clients can be very similar. A differential diagnosis is essential.

Disorders associated with cognitive decline are among the most common and frightening problems faced by the elderly. A common myth is that older adults inevitably experience cognitive decline as a consequence of aging. Serious difficulties with thinking clearly and remembering are abnormal consequences at any age and are manifestations of medical illness or altered psychosocial well-being.[29]

The stereotypical view that cognitive decline is a normal part of aging prevails. For this reason, an acute deterioration in cognition is frequently overlooked; undetected cases of cognitive disorders have ranged from 16% to 72%.[13] Because many older adults believe that cognitive decline is part of aging, they do not seek medical attention when they notice changes in processing stimuli

BRIDGE TO HOME HEALTH CARE

Detecting Elder Abuse

In the home care setting, factors beyond the physical condition of the client—such as the environment of care, relationships, and support systems—are crucial to the achievement of positive outcomes. This is especially true when abuse of a client is suspected. When you suspect abuse, you must incorporate the client, family, and caregiver into your total assessment and care plan.

When providing home care, listen carefully to the client and observe overt and covert behaviors. In addition to completing a history and physical assessment related to the client's current condition, confirm the caregiver's report of the client's condition. For example, if the caregiver attributes bruises to a fall, determine whether gait instability is consistent with the client's condition.

It may be difficult for a client to admit that a caregiver is abusive. Many times, abusive caregivers provide assistance with activities of daily living (ADL), financial assistance, or emotional support, which allows the client to continue to live in the community.

Situations can appear to indicate abuse when, in reality, a caregiver is simply uninformed about providing care. Inform the client and family about nutrition, transfers, ambulation, and positioning so that caregivers can adequately meet the needs of clients. In addition, the frustration of providing care can contribute to abuse. Encourage caregivers to arrange for regular absences from care.

When you suspect abuse, a multidisciplinary plan of care is essential. Inform the physician of the situation and of any clinical manifestations. A social worker can coordinate family counseling, make referrals to community resources, and facilitate day care. Homemakers and home health aides can help to relieve the burden of care. Volunteers can provide respite for the caregiver. In most states, reporting abuse is mandatory for health care professionals; contact the local Adult Protection Service department for investigation of suspected abusive situations.

Do not be reluctant to confront suspicious situations for fear of jeopardizing rapport with the client and family. Although maintaining a relationship is important, client safety and advocacy are your first priorities.

Bridget A. Young, RN, BSN, MBA, *Vice President of Clinical Services, Visiting Nurse Association of Omaha, Omaha, Nebraska*

or in responding to stressful life events. Family members may react to acute cognitive changes as the "beginning of the end" and may prematurely plan for alternative living arrangements and entertain other actions and thoughts that may be unnecessary.[3]

Dementia

Dementia is a clinical syndrome characterized by severe intellectual deterioration that interferes with one's ability to cope with daily life. It is gradually progressive and *irreversible.* Deficits occur in memory, language, perception, praxis, learning, problem-solving, abstract thinking, and judgment. Approximately 3% of people 65 to 74 years of age have dementia; the prevalence increases to 47.2% for those older than 85 years.[32] Dementia can be *primary,* as with Alzheimer's disease, multi-infarct dementia, alcoholism, and Pick's disease, or *secondary* to other causes, as with Parkinson's disease and trauma. Causes of dementia can vary, but the clinical presentation is similar regardless of cause. Therefore, the descriptive term *dementia of Alzheimer's type* (DAT) is generally used.

Before a diagnosis of dementia is made, all potential physical and psychosocial causes of cognitive decline should be ruled out. The onset and progressive nature of the cognitive decline should be documented, and serial neuropsychological testing should be performed. The diagnosis can be complicated when delirium, depression, or both are superimposed on dementia.

Delirium

Delirium is a syndrome characterized by global cognitive impairment of abrupt onset that is *reversible.* This condition becomes irreversible only if underlying causes are undetected or treated unsuccessfully. Delirium is also known as acute confusion, reversible dementia, pseudosenility, acute brain failure, and clouded state. Attention deficits are the most salient feature of delirium. Other diagnostic criteria include disorganized thinking, reduced level of consciousness, perceptual disturbances, disturbances of the sleep-wake cycle, increased or decreased psychomotor activity, disorientation, and memory impairment.

Delirium is one of the most prevalent cognitive disorders among hospitalized older clients. It is associated with higher mortality, prolonged hospital stays, a greater nursing time than necessary for the admitting diagnosis, and a higher rate of nursing home placement.[6, 23] Delirium is often the presenting manifestation of physical illness in an older person, exceeding the indicators of fever, pain, and tachycardia. It has been associated with a variety of conditions, especially adverse drug reactions, metabolic disorders (e.g., electrolyte disorders, renal failure, respiratory failure, and endocrinopathies), cardiac failure, cerebrovascular disorders, infection (especially pulmonary, renal, or neurologic), anemia, and surgery. Psychosocial factors can also cause or contribute to a delirious state; these include bereavement, relocation, and sensory deprivation or overstimulation.

The key to differentiating delirium from dementia is the assessment of the onset of the cognitive manifestations. Onset of delirium is rapid, occurring within hours to days; dementia onset is slower and more gradual. It is imperative that reversible delirium not be classified as dementia. A comprehensive investigation of all possible physical and psychosocial factors that might cause altered cognition must be conducted.

Depression

Research suggests that significant manifestations of depression occur in approximately 10% to 15% of all community-dwelling elders over 65 years; among institutionalized elders, the prevalence rate increases to 50% to 75%.[32] Depression is a complex syndrome that manifests itself in a variety of ways in older people. The most common manifestations are *vegetative,* which include insomnia, fatigue, weight loss, constipation, preoccupation with physical health, and thoughts of death. Elders suffering from depression may also exhibit sadness, crying, anxiety, irritability, or paranoia.

Depression can also lead to cognitive impairment. It is estimated that depression-associated cognitive disorders occur in 10% to 29% of depressed elderly clients.[29] Therefore, differentiation between depression-related cognitive alteration and dementia may be difficult. Depressed clients often look and act demented, and they perform poorly on mental status tests; however, the vegetative signs of depression are not usually seen in demented people. Features supporting a diagnosis of depression versus dementia include recent onset of depressive symptoms and inconsistencies with actual functional performance and cognitive testing. Table 3–4 contrasts the primary clinical features of delirium, dementia, and depression.

Treatment Strategies

Several strategies are used to help older clients who have dementia, delirium, or depression. Four strategies are commonly used by gerontological nurses: (1) reality orientation, (2) validation therapy, (3) remotivation therapy, and (4) reminiscence therapy. Treatment modalities and their specific application are described in gerontological nursing and psychiatric literature.[10]

■ SUBSTANCE USE DISORDERS

Substance use disorders refer to ingestion of any compound in quantities that may be harmful to health or well-being. This includes overindulgence in legal drugs, alcohol, nicotine, caffeine, nonprescription over-the-counter (OTC) drugs and preparations, prescription drugs, controlled drugs (e.g., meperidine or codeine), and illegal drugs (see Chapter 24). Dependence on alcohol, nicotine, and prescription and OTC drugs is far more common among the elderly population than is generally thought. The addictive experience includes alterations in mood and sensation, immediate gratification, and enhanced sense of control and power. These are elements that may be missing in the lives of some elders.

As many as 15% of community-dwelling elders and 18% to 44% of hospitalized elders have serious problems

TABLE 3–4 COMMON MENTAL HEALTH DISORDERS IN THE ELDERLY: CLINICAL FEATURES

	Delirium	Dementia	Depression
DESCRIPTION	A reversible, acute confusional state	A gradually progressive, irreversible cognitive decline	A reversible affective feeling associated with sadness, which may vary from mild downheartedness or a feeling of indifference to a feeling of great despair beyond hope
ONSET	Rapid, acute, often at night	Slow, gradual	Gradual or sudden
DURATION	Days to weeks, but usually less than 1 month	Continuous, ongoing, months to years	Varies from weeks to years
DISORIENTATION	Present, especially for time; tendency to mistake unfamiliar for familiar persons, place	May be absent in mild states of dementia	May seem disoriented to place or time
THINKING	Slow or accelerated; may be dream-like, impoverished	Impoverished; poor abstracting ability	Slowed thinking, indecisiveness
MEMORY	Short-term memory impaired; long-term memory intact	Short-term memory impaired; long-term memory may be affected	May seem impaired for recent and remote events
ATTENTION	Consistently impaired; easily distracted; fluctuates	Typically intact	Complaints or evidence of diminished ability to concentrate
ALERTNESS	Reduced or increased, but awareness always affected	Typically normal; may be reduced	Psychomotor agitation or retardation
PERCEPTION	Invariably affected, especially at night; often have hallucinations	May be intact; usually no hallucinations	May have auditory hallucinations
SLEEP	Sleep-wake cycle altered	Usually normal for age	Insomnia or hypersomnia
COURSE	Typically fluctuates with lucid intervals and exacerbations	Relatively stable over course of a day	Usually rapid progression
AFFECT	Intermittent fear, perplexity, bewilderment	Flat or indifferent	Sad, worried, anxious, hopeless; may show agitation or apathy
CAUSE	Multiple potential causes (e.g., surgery, infection, drugs)	Unknown, possible environmental, hereditary, chemical	Secondary to other mental illness; related to loss, physical illness, medications, loneliness

Data from American Psychiatric Association. (1994). *Diagnostic and statistical manual of mental disorders* (4th ed.). Washington, DC: Author.

related to alcohol use.[40] Alcohol abusers can be divided into two types: (1) long-term and (2) recent-onset. Long-term drinkers who live to old age can be called survivors. They may be at risk for serious medical problems and generally have alienated their families and social support systems.

Drinkers who have a relatively recent onset of problems with alcohol may be reacting to some event, such as loss of a loved one, or they may have general negative feelings, such as helplessness or depression stemming from role losses in later life.[40] The recent-onset alcohol abuser is more successful in substance abuse treatment than the long-term abuser. Learning new coping skills and increasing socialization often help the recent-onset drinker to overcome problems.

Older individuals who drink are at risk for developing medical, relationship, and social problems. Medical problems include:

- Liver and pancreatic disease
- Gastrointestinal problems (gastritis, ulcers and hemorrhage, malnutrition, nausea and vomiting, electrolyte disturbance, dehydration, hypoglycemia)
- Central nervous system damage
- Cognitive changes of impairment and confusion
- Cardiac problems (cardiomyopathy, dysrhythmia, systolic hypertension, peripheral edema)
- Injuries and accidents because of decreased tolerance to alcohol and the normal changes in dexterity, balance, and proprioception associated with aging

Psychosocially, these people may have alienated family and friends, exhausted their funds, and estranged themselves from health care and social service providers.[40]

It is difficult to determine the extent of prescription drug abuse by older people. Researchers contend that thousands of older Americans are "hooked" on their prescription drugs in an "inadvertent addiction."[27] The cycle of addiction usually begins benignly with a medication or a drink for pain or anxiety. Physicians often are unaware of the problem, and they may also be unaware of the number of medications that a client may be taking because the prescriptions may be issued by several different physicians.

Medication Use in the Elderly

In the United States, adults age 65 years and over consume 30% of all prescription medications and 40% to 50% of all OTC medications.[10, 33] Elders who live in long-term care facilities typically take four to seven different medications,[32] or approximately 4.5 medications at any one time. Among Medicare beneficiaries who rate their health as poor, an average of 31 prescriptions per year is reported. Of community-dwelling elders, 90% took an average of three OTC and five prescription drugs daily (Fig. 3–8). See Bridge to Home Health Care: Managing Multiple Medications.

The most commonly prescribed and used drugs are cardiovascular, anti-infective, antipsychotic, antidepressant, and diuretic agents.[9, 33] Analgesics, laxatives, and antacids are the most frequently used OTC drugs. The trend of multiple drug use will continue as more sophisticated drug therapies are developed. When used properly, drugs can be beneficial; when used inappropriately, they threaten one's functional abilities and health.

■ PHARMACOKINETICS

Age-related changes affect a medication's pharmacokinetics, or how the body handles the drug. The term includes (1) absorption of the medication into the systemic circulation, (2) distribution of the drug to the tissues, (3) metabolism (breakdown) of the medication, and (4) elimination (removal) of the drug from the body.

Absorption refers to the movement of a drug from the site of administration into the circulation. Absorption is not greatly affected by age, but the rate of absorption is. Age-related changes in stomach emptying, changes in gastric pH, gastrointestinal motility, and nutritional status may influence absorption rate.

Distribution is the movement of the drug throughout the body. This activity depends on the adequacy of the circulatory system and the ability of the drug to exit the circulation and enter the cell. Altered cardiac output and sluggish circulation can delay the arrival of medication at the target receptors. Age-related changes in body composition influence drug distribution. Total body water decreases with age and adipose tissue or fat content increases; the result can be higher than usual blood levels of water-soluble drugs and storage of lipid-soluble drugs in the fatty tissue. This can result in higher concentration of drug levels (toxicity), with less drug reaching the site

BRIDGE TO HOME HEALTH CARE

Managing Multiple Medications

Clients who take several medications often need help to understand the best procedures and follow instructions as closely as possible. Failure to take the right drug at the right time and in the proper way often results in relapses, rehospitalizations, or nursing home placement.

Nurses play a crucial role when they foster client independence and assess and facilitate the client's ability to follow a prescribed medication regimen. Review all prescription and nonprescription medications, and carefully explain the administration schedule to the client and family members. Tailoring the schedule to the client's lifestyle increases the likelihood that the instructions will be followed. For example, if the client goes to bed at 7:00 P.M., be sure that the last dose is scheduled at that hour.

Some people need minimal help with organizing their drugs and dosages. They may benefit from any number of compliance aids that can be purchased at pharmacies, such as containers with separate compartments for each day of the week. The challenge is greater when the client has a complex medication program; reduced strength and dexterity; or a visual, hearing, cognitive, or other impairment in functional status. These clients may need to purchase an automated medication dispenser that emits visual cues, such as flashing strobe lights, or audible cues, such as beeps. Dispensers that beep are ideal for people with visual impairments, whereas dispensers that flash a strobe light are good for people with hearing impairments.

Although units vary, an automated dispenser must be simple to use. One such dispenser can be programmed easily to provide a reminder at the right time for up to four times a day for a week. This dispenser helps the client manage complex schedules, is tamper-proof, and dispenses only the pills needed from a supply cassette in a removable drawer. Other automated dispensers have light-emitting diode (LED) screens on which preprogrammed messages, such as "Take with food" or "Take 30 minutes before food," serve as additional reminders.

Determine how and when the client will obtain refills. If the client has no transportation, a pharmacy may have a delivery service or a family member can obtain them. A social service referral is needed if the client cannot pay for prescriptions.

Monitor the client for side effects. Many people stop taking essential medications because of unpleasant side effects. Sometimes the client can manage this problem effectively by changing the times of doses or by taking the medication with food.

Instruct the client on drug storage. Some drugs are sensitive to light; others must be secured to decrease the risk of overdoses. All medications must be safely kept away from any children who visit or live in the household.

Simplicity is the key to successful medication management. Regularly evaluate the client's regimen and household routines, and discuss any changes that would make things easier with the client, family members, and physician.

Kaye M. Dietrich, RN,C, MS, *Consultant, Kiel, Wisconsin*

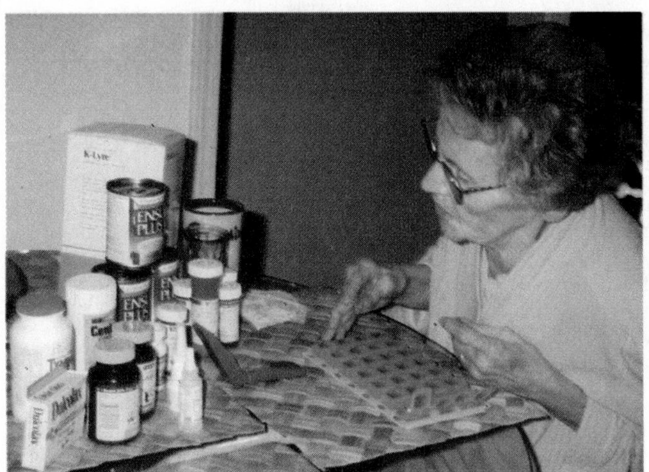

FIGURE 3–8 Use of a medication planner assists older people in managing multiple medications.

of action because of storage in the adipose tissue, thereby reducing the drug's effect.

Metabolism occurs primarily in the liver. There is an age-related decrease in liver size and blood flow, contributing to decreased hepatic clearance. As a result of this slowed metabolism, the drug remains in the body longer, with prolonged responses.

Elimination of the drug from the body occurs primarily through the renal system but also through bile, feces, sweat, and saliva. Age-related changes in renal function include reductions in renal blood flow, glomerular filtration rate, and tubular secretion. These changes affect both the duration and intensity of the drug responses in the body.

■ PHARMACODYNAMICS

Pharmacodynamics, or drug activity, refers to the actual effects of the drug in the body. An altered pharmacodynamic response is considered an adverse effect. An interaction occurs when drugs with similar actions or similar adverse effects are administered together. Drug interactions increase with age and the number of drugs taken. The interactive effect may be (1) additive, (2) synergistic, (3) antagonistic, or (4) potentiated. These effects can be beneficial or harmful. Nearly one third of elderly clients report adverse reactions to medications, accounting for as many as 10% of their hospitalizations.[10]

An *additive* effect occurs when two drugs with same or similar adverse effects are combined, resulting in a summative effect from the doses taken. The additive effects for an older person taking a diuretic (e.g., furosemide) for a cardiovascular disorder and an aminoglycoside antibiotic (e.g., tobramycin) for an infection can be adverse, resulting in increased damage to the organs of hearing and balance *(ototoxicity)* and to the kidneys *(nephrotoxicity)*.

A *synergistic* effect occurs when two drugs with or without the same effects are combined for an outcome that is greater than the sum of the individual drugs. The effect is greater than that seen in additive effects. Positive synergistic interaction is experienced when hypertension is treated with a diuretic (e.g., hydrochlorothiazide) and a beta-adrenergic blocker (e.g., atenolol). This combination lowers blood pressure better than either drug alone.

An *antagonistic* reaction occurs when the combined effect of two drugs is less than that of either active drug alone (the opposite of a synergistic effect). Often the addition of a second drug diminishes or eliminates the effect of the first. Protamine sulfate (an anticoagulant antagonist) is given as an antidote when a person is bleeding as a result of the anticoagulant action of heparin. The protamine binds with the heparin to form a stable compound with no anticoagulant effect. A thiazide diuretic can counter the hypoglycemic action of an antidiabetic medication.

Potentiation describes a synergistic effect in which the effect of only one of the two drugs is made greater by the presence of the second drug. When acetaminophen is given with codeine, the result is increased analgesia.

■ POLYPHARMACY

Polypharmacy, the use of large quantities of different drugs to relieve symptoms of illness or symptoms resulting from drug therapy, has become one of the major causes of *iatrogenic* (treatment-acquired) illness and complications in the elderly. The use of generic drugs or the substitution of OTC drugs compounds it. Polypharmacy occurs because of the multiple medications prescribed by different specialists for treating concurrent conditions, the beliefs and practices of older clients, and the use of multiple pharmacies for prescription filling.[34] Table 3–5 presents suggestions for helping elders to manage medication regimens.

HEALTH CARE FOR THE ELDERLY CLIENT

In the United States, older people historically did not use as many health care services as they do today. Before Medicare and Medicaid, only a small proportion of the federal budget went toward health care for older people, and government agencies paid little attention to their health and medical needs. Today, older people constitute the largest group of health care consumers, and it is projected that by the year 2040, they will account for 45% of health care expenditures.[39]

In this current period of health care reform, the political climate is one of change. Legislatures are looking for ways to reduce government spending. Government health insurance (Medicare) and government health assistance (Medicaid) programs will change, and these changes will have ramifications for all Americans.

■ RESOURCES, SERVICES, AND OPTIONS FOR OLDER PEOPLE

An outgrowth of gerontology has been development of programs and services designed to address the unique needs of older adults. These programs and services recognize that these adults have varied individual needs and health conditions that call for different service options at different stages of aging as the clients move along the health-illness continuum.

The continuum of care refers to services designed to provide diagnostic, preventive, therapeutic, rehabilitative, supportive, and maintenance care. These services can be

TABLE 3–5 HELPING OLDER CLIENTS TO MANAGE MEDICATION REGIMENS

Potential Problem	Strategy
Motivation	▪ Assess the client's understanding of need for medication and desire to take medication. Provide information as needed to promote informed decision-making
Knowledge deficit related to drug regimen	▪ Assess vision, hearing, comprehension, and best learning style ▪ Teach the client about medication's purpose, correct dosage, and administration instructions ▪ Identify common side effects for each drug. If side effects occur, advise what to do, what changes in administration to make, and when to notify the physician ▪ Reinforce information with written instructions when appropriate ▪ Include family members and other support persons in teaching sessions
Safety	▪ Assess for any over-the-counter drugs being used to avoid possible interaction effects; advise the client to avoid any over-the-counter drugs unless approved by the physician ▪ Basic rules to teach the client: ▪ Take only the amount of drug prescribed by the physician ▪ Never take medication prescribed for someone else ▪ Do not share medication with others ▪ Dispose of outdated medications in a sink or toilet, never in the trash within reach of children ▪ Keep drugs in the original, labeled container
Physiologic limitations	
▪ Swallowing	▪ Assess need for liquids versus pills or thickened liquids for administration of drugs ▪ Discuss which drugs cannot be chewed or crushed
▪ Vision	▪ Larger label for medication bottles ▪ Color coding (e.g., red heart for heart medication) ▪ Braille labels where appropriate
▪ Memory impairment	▪ Memory aids include calendars; day, week, month pill containers; timers or voice mail reminders
▪ Fine motor coordination deficit	▪ Teach about availability and use of non-childproof caps and organization containers or any automated medication dispenser
Economic limitations	▪ Assess for transportation or monetary problems ▪ Use social services to identify community resources for financial assistance with pharmaceutical needs and transportation and delivery of medications
Information overload	▪ Keep the number of medications to a minimum, and keep instructions clear, concise, and simple

provided in a variety of institutional, non-institutional, and community health care settings. The continuum also includes an expanded variety of living arrangements. The goal behind the concept of continuum of care services is to ensure that clients have control over their environment by offering services that are supportive, preserve health, and counteract dependency. Table 3–3 presents a variety of available services to help people maintain independence and live in their chosen environment as long as possible.

The changing economy promotes structural changes in health care institutions that affect the continuum of care. Many institutions, facilities, and services are merging into integrated systems. An *integrated* system provides a seamless delivery of services and encompasses the entire range of health, community-based, and in-home services. Advantages of an integrated system include a single point of access and entry, assessment and coordination of appropriate care services, and assured quality of care in a cost-effective, time-efficient system.

In the United States, approximately 32 million people over age 65 years have a current or potential need for more assistance and support in their living environment.[10] These individuals frequently choose alternative living arrangements. The continuum of housing, or alternative living arrangements, offers choices to meet a variety of needs. Options include:

1. Retirement communities for the older person who is fully independent but wants socialization, security, emergency medical services, and some supplemental services without homeowner responsibilities.
2. Sheltered living environments (rest homes, family care homes, shared congregate housing), which provide minimal assistance with BADL in a family setting environment.
3. Nursing facilities (nursing homes, intermediate care, skilled care) for the person who needs long-term sheltered care and cannot function independently.

Intermediate care facilities (ICFs) do not provide round-the-clock professional nursing care but do provide medication and BADL assistance and safety supervision. *Skilled care facilities* (SNFs) provide care for a person requiring 24-hour observation and highly technical care of unstable medical conditions; this may include rehabilitative services. Nursing home facilities rarely have only intermediate or skilled care; there is usually a mixture of both types of services (see Table 3–3). Not all programs, services, and housing options are available in every community. Area agencies on aging or the American Association of Homes and Services for the Aging can provide information about what is available in individual communities (Box 3–3).

■ MANAGED CARE

The way in which health care is delivered is changing. Among the major shifts taking place is the rapid growth

BOX 3–3 Aging Resources

Administration on Aging
330 Independence Ave., SW
Cohen Building, Room 4760
Washington, DC 20201
(202) 619-0556
http://www.aoa.dhhs.gov

Aging Network
http://www.mfaaa.org/agingnet.html

Alzheimer's Association
919 N. Michigan Ave.
Suite 1000
Chicago, IL 60657-1676
(312) 335-8870 or 1/800-272-3900
http://www.alz.org

American Association of Homes and Services for the Aging
901 E St. NW
Suite 500
Washington, DC 20004
(202) 783-2242
http://www.aahsa.org

American Association of Retired Persons
601 E Street NW
Washington, DC 20049
(202) 434-2277
http://www.aarp.org

American Geriatrics Society
770 Lexington Ave.
Suite 400
New York, NY 10021
(212) 308-1414
http://www.americangeriatrics.org

American Society on Aging
833 Market St.
Suite 511
San Francisco, CA 94103-1824
(415) 882-2910

Area Agencies on Aging
http://www.mfaaa.org/aging_aaa.html

Family Caregiver Alliance
425 Bush St.
Suite 500
San Francisco, CA 94108
(415) 434-3508
http://www.caregiver.org

Gerontological Society of America
1275 K St. NW
Suite 350
Washington, DC 20005-4006
(202) 842-1275
http://www.gsa.iog.wayne.edu

Gray Panthers
1424 16th St. NW
Suite 602
Washington, DC 20036
(202) 387-1111

Internet and e-mail Resources on Aging
http://www.aoa.dhhs.gov/aoa/pages/jpost1st.html

National Association of State Units on Aging
2033 K St. NW
Suite 304
Washington, DC 20006
(202) 785-0707
http://www.mfaaa.org/aging_state.html

National Citizen's Coalition for Nursing Home Reform
1424 16th St. NW
Suite 202
Washington, DC 20036
(202) 332-2275
http://www.aoa.dhhs.gov/aoa/dir/144.html

National Council on Aging
409 3rd St. SW
Suite 200
Washington, DC 20027
(202) 479-1200

National Council of Senior Citizens
1311 F St. NW
Suite 200
Washington, DC 20004-1174
(202) 347-8800
http://www.ncscinc.org

National Institute on Aging/National Institutes of Health
Federal Bldg. 31-C, Room 5C27
9000 Rockville Pike
Bethesda, MD 20892
http://www.senior.com/npolnia.html

National Senior Citizens Law Center
1815 H St. NW
Suite 700
Washington, DC 20006
(202) 887-5280

Older Women's League (OWL)
666 11th St. NW
Suite 700
Washington, DC 20001
(202) 783-6686
http://www.scn.org

of managed care. This transition represents a fundamental change. Managed care is a system that provides generalized structure and focus for overseeing the use, cost, quality, and effectiveness of health care services. The basic concept revolves around accountability and standardization of care for a given disorder or for a specific population. The increasing number of frail older persons with chronic disorders has resulted in pressure to move Medicare into a managed care system. The thrust of services will be to coordinate and integrate health services and resources in order to improve quality, to provide service flexibility, to contain cost, and to help the older person maintain function and independence as long as possible.

■ ACUTE CARE

Most nurses who care for older adults provide care in an inpatient hospital setting. This setting can be for an emergency or acute illness, such as a stroke or hip fracture (see Chapter 6). These facilities are driven by diagnosis-related group (DRG) assessment. DRGs determine the length of stay (LOS) according to the diagnosis. Medicare generally pays for most necessary and appropriate treatments, tests, and equipment after a deductible is met. Medicare provides for 150 days of hospitalization.

Hospitals are developing new ways of delivering care to older adults in order to improve both quality and efficiency. Some hospitals are establishing geriatric units with specially trained staff who work together as an interdisciplinary team. The team typically includes nurses, a geriatrician, a pharmacist, a social worker, various rehabilitation therapists (e.g., speech, physical, and occupational), and mental health professionals (e.g., psychologists or psychiatrists). These programs focus on helping older adults with complex problems to remain at their highest possible level of functioning. Geropsychiatric and geriatric rehabilitation programs are other models of hospital-based geriatric care that are evolving to address the unique needs of older people.

■ LONG-TERM CARE

Long-term care refers to a continuum of care that ranges from informal assistance provided by family and friends, to formal medical and supportive services provided in the home, to specialty facilities for rehabilitation, to care in a nursing home (see Chapter 8). Long-term care services assist those with chronic disabilities and decreasing health status to maintain their physical, social, and psychologic functioning. Traditionally, nursing home care has been synonymous with long-term care, but this is misleading. Many older persons with disabilities are as likely to receive long-term care at home as in a nursing home. Long-term care accounts for 25% of all health care expenditures for older persons.[10]

Specialty Facility

Rehabilitation centers are specialty facilities that provide intensive inpatient care to rehabilitate functional disabilities. The older individual must be able to tolerate 3 to 5 hours of intensive rehabilitation daily. The usual length of stay is 2 to 4 weeks, depending on evaluations. Medicare pays 80% of the costs.

Nursing Home Care

The close association between nursing home and long-term care arises from the late 1970s, when nursing homes were the primary (and usually the only) resource for people who needed long-term care. Nursing homes are licensed by the state, and most are certified for Medicare or Medicaid reimbursement. Round-the-clock care averages $38,000 annually for basic nursing home care. About 5% of the population 65 years and older are in nursing homes at any given time.[28]

People in this age group have a 50% chance of being in a nursing home at some point in their lives.[22] Typical nursing home populations are as follows[27, 37]:

- Average age is 82 years
- There is no living spouse
- Women outnumber men by a ratio of 3:1
- More than half have a progressive dementia or arthritis, cardiovascular disorder, or both
- One third have impaired vision or impaired hearing
- Most require assistance in several or all ADL
- Twenty per cent return home, and 70% stay for longer than 1 year

Two levels of care are provided in nursing homes, with many facilities offering both. Residents needing highly *skilled* nursing care may have feeding tubes, tracheotomies, extensive wounds, or infections or may need medications that require round-the-clock supervision and treatment by a registered nurse under the direction of a physician. The length of stay is variable. Medicare Part A generally pays 100% for the first 20 days, then 80% after a co-payment. After 100 days, Part A pays nothing. Medicare Part B pays a portion of the cost after 100 days.

Intermediate care is suitable for clients who need supervision and moderate assistance with ADL and medications. Generally, nurse's aides give primary care. The average length of stay varies. Medicare does not pay for this type of care.

Subacute Care

Many hospitals and nursing homes have added subacute care units to their facilities. The typical subacute unit looks much like a medical-surgical hospital unit; however, in contrast to a hospital, it is more family-focused and flexible, with a relaxed and adaptable atmosphere.[10] Medicare Part A pays for subacute care in a manner similar to that for skilled nursing home care.

Clients in subacute units typically have short-term stays. They frequently need skilled nursing care, rehabilitation, and other services, but they may no longer meet the criteria for hospitalization. Often because of their age and frailty, they cannot tolerate the daily amount of rehabilitation mandated in inpatient rehabilitation facilities; thus, they transfer to a subacute unit to complete rehabilitation before returning home.

The goal of subacute care is to discharge the client back to home or to an appropriate living environment.

The picture of the "typical" nursing home resident mentioned earlier would accurately depict a long-term resident, but it does not apply to the many who are in nursing homes for subacute, short-term care.

Home Care

Home health care is skilled care consisting of rehabilitation services that can be received in the home if the person is homebound, has a physician's referral, needs intermittent skilled care, is making progress, and receives rehabilitation three to five times a week. The average length of stay is six weeks. Medicare Part A pays the full, approved cost for five visits a week. Home health care can provide a wide variety of services, such as social services, nutritional counseling, provision of some medical supplies and equipment, and personal care assistance (see Chapter 7). Medicare may cover some of these services for a limited time for clients who meet specific criteria.

Outpatient Rehabilitation

Outpatient rehabilitation is for the older client who has a physician's prescription for therapy. The client is responsible for a deductible and noncovered amounts. Medicare pays 80% of the fee up to a specified limit but does not pay for services by independent speech pathologists.

Hospice

Hospice is a program of care for the terminally ill, either on an inpatient basis or at home. The emphasis is on alleviation of pain, terminal care, and support for the individual and family (see Chapter 22). Physicians must certify that the client has less than 6 months to live. Medicare covers hospice care, and there is no deductible. Medicare also covers nursing, physicians, drugs, rehabilitation, homemaker, social services, short-term care, counseling, and *respite care* (short-term relief for family members who care for an older person at home).

Respite Care

The elderly client may receive respite care at home or at such locations as day care centers and health care facilities. Trained individuals care for the older person while the family member is away. Medicare generally does not pay for respite care unless the client is in a hospice program.

Adult Day Care

Day care refers to daily supervised programmed activities for moderately to minimally impaired elders. Community-based adult day care centers focus on maintaining or improving the functional abilities of the impaired older person. Typically, participants need safety supervision or assistance in several areas of functioning. Centers usually emphasize either rehabilitation or social activities and provide a variety of services ranging from health care to social programs. Most participants cannot be left at home alone during the day when family members are at work or are unavailable. This arrangement allows the family caregiver to work outside the home. Medicare does not cover the cost of day care.

Case Management

Nursing case management provides comprehensive, individualized, and economic care for older clients with complex chronic health needs. The goal is to meet client and support caregiver needs while coordinating access to cost-effective services. The nurse case manager functions as the primary care representative and coordinates with others to form a team of acute, long-term, and community care services as needed. The nurse case manager serves as a client advocate, has a holistic view of the situation, and can help solve problems as they arise in a cost-efficient, high-quality manner. Nursing case management can become involved through a health provider referral, social service intervention, or family contact with independent case management services.

Legislation Affecting the Elderly Population

Federal and state laws govern legal issues that affect the elderly and the services provided. Table 3–6 lists the major laws that affect the older population. Three of the most significant acts are Title XVIII–Medicare of 1965, the Older Americans Act of 1965, and the Omnibus Budget Reconciliation Act (OBRA) of 1987.

The Nursing Home Reform Act, part of OBRA 1987, mandated the most comprehensive legislative requirements ever to affect nursing homes and the delivery of long-term care. The intent was to improve quality of care by establishing a set of conditions for certification and regulations for resident care, rights, behaviors, quality of life, interdisciplinary evaluation, staffing requirements, and facility practices. Important changes resulted from this act. These changes include the Minimum Data Set (MDS), a standardized resident assessment that provides a nationwide research data base; (2) improved resident rights with emphasis on resident-driven rather than provider-driven care; (3) a more "humane" environment with a focus on quality of life rather than custodial care; and (4) movement toward a restraint-free environment that has reduced the use of physical and chemical restraints.

Ethical Issues That Affect the Elderly

Whatever the setting, there are daily challenges to be advocated for the older client. An advocate represents the interests of others by acting in their behalf or influencing policies that affect them.[10] Issues of autonomy and self-determination arise frequently. Know the issues in order to serve as a client advocate and to ensure that both the client and family are informed.

■ AUTONOMY

Autonomy is the personal freedom and independence to direct one's own life and make decisions for and about

TABLE 3–6 LEGISLATION AND EVENTS AFFECTING THE ELDERLY

Legislation	Content and Concerns
1935, Social Security Act (SSA)	Provides income after retirement, based on individual's average earnings paid into social security over a defined period of years before retirement
1961, First White House Conference on Aging (WHCOA) 1971, 1981, 1995 subsequent WHCOA	Each conference focused on different concerns of the aging. Outcomes included establishment of Senate Special Committee on Aging (1961), Cabinet-level Domestic Council Committee on Aging (1971), revision of mandatory retirement laws (1981), and preservation of Medicare, Medicaid, and Older Americans Act (1995)
1965, Amendment to SSA: Title XVIII—Medicare	Provides health insurance for all eligible individuals over age 65 and some younger disabled individuals. Part A: Hospital insurance, covers important hospital care, skilled nursing home care, and some home health care. Part B: Supplemental medical insurance, covers physician services; in some outpatient services, there is an additional monthly charge
1965, Amendment to SSA: Title XIX—Medicaid	Health assistance program for low-income individuals (<21 years and >64 years of age), frequent source of long-term care payment for elderly
1965, Older Americans Act; amended 1975, 1976, 1992	Provides federal funds to states for services, training, and research to help older persons. Amended objectives focus on health care, housing, residential repair, in-home services, transportation, senior centers, nutrition and ombudsman program, legal services, crime prevention, job counseling, and case management
1973, Area Agencies on Aging (AAA)	Coordinates plans for comprehensive Aging Service delivery at the local level
1974, Amendments to SSA: Title XV—Supplemental Security Income (SSI)	Income maintenance program for low-income people who are aged, blind, or disabled; guarantees a minimum income level
1976 Tax Reform Act	Provides income tax break on post-retirement income, sale of residence, and estate and gifts
1981 Omnibus Budget Reconciliation Act; amended 1987, 1990	Standardized assessment and process of care planning and provision in all long-term care facilities receiving federal funds; includes right to self-determination, freedom from restraints, and ombudsman advocacy
1983, Diagnosis-Related Groups (DRGs)	Instituted by Health Care Financing Administration in attempts to limit and control Medicare health costs
1990 Patient Self-Determination Act	Requires all health care facilities to provide written information concerning right to make health care decisions
1996, Managed care and Medicare	Medicare changes move most older clients into managed care systems

oneself. Autonomous people are capable of rational thought and problem-solving. They can identify problems, understand the situation, search for alternatives, and select solutions that allow continued personal freedom.

Loss of autonomy, and therefore independence, is a real fear among the elderly. No autonomous adult wishes to give up the right to decide when to get up, when to go to bed, what to eat, or what interests and activities to pursue. In many institutional settings, autonomy becomes scarce when schedules must be met and the older person moves slowly, when decreases in hearing and processing slow decision-making, and when the person's decision does not coincide with the health care provider's ideas.

Encourage the older person's autonomy in any way possible, supervise and educate staff to listen and allow the person time to make choices, and discuss with family members what is occurring and how they can enhance the older person's autonomy.

■ COMPETENCE

The term competence is used to describe a person's decision-making abilities. Competence is the ability to adequately fulfill one's role and handle one's affairs.[27] Increasingly, nurses encounter clients who are confused or mentally impaired. Are these individuals competent to give consent for tests and procedures? Can they decide whether to proceed with, stop, or refuse treatment? Can they make end-of-life decisions?

Competence usually describes a status—the ability to make all or no decisions for oneself. Competence is a legal determination made by a judge. Adults are presumed to be legally competent unless there is evidence of an inability to care for oneself or to manage affairs or both. The court generally appoints a guardian for the individual judged to be incompetent.

In recent years, the notion of capacity to make health care decisions has become an alternative to the traditional concept of competence. Determining capacity is a criteria-based judgment similar to that made by an informed lay person.[26] The criteria include that the client (1) understand there is the right to make a choice; (2) understand the medical situation, prognosis, and risks, benefits, and consequences of treatment; (3) have the ability to communicate the decision; and (4) make a decision that is stable and consistent over time. Capacity is not absolute; it recognizes that a person may be able to make some decisions and not others or may have decisional capacity only at certain times and that some decisions require a higher level of capacity than others. Health care professionals must be sensitive to the fact that some residents are lucid during certain hours of the day and disoriented or confused at others. At the appropriate time, discuss treatment options and matters that require a decision.

■ SELF-DETERMINATION

The Patient Self-Determination Act (PSDA) reaffirmed the common law right of self-determination as guaranteed by the Fourteenth Amendment.[20] This act requires all health care facilities receiving Medicare and Medicaid reimbursement to recognize *advance directives.* Self-determination encourages individuals to be active partners in guiding their medical treatment and to claim their rights in treatment decisions. Self-determination, competency, and autonomy are closely related in decision-making associated with future treatment and end-of-life decisions.

Advance Directives

"Advance directive" is an umbrella term for any document used to protect the individual's wishes for and interests in decisions about life-sustaining measures. If used, advance directives can minimize potential conflict within the family once the person loses decision-making capacity and alleviate the burden of guilt that family members may feel about decisions to withdraw or withhold treatment. These documents include the *living will* and the *durable power of attorney* for health care or health care *proxy*.

Advance directives are valuable planning tools for all adults. However, the documents have special relevance for older people because a significant percentage of them will lose decision-making capacity at some time before death.[32] Discussion of advance directives does not come easily. Many clients want to talk about advance directives with their physician but are reluctant to initiate discussion because of a belief that it is the physician's role. Only about 15% of elderly patients have advance directives.[30] Studies have shown that most older people expect and anticipate that "someone" will know what to do when the time comes,[20, 25, 32] and they prefer family members, rather than health care providers, to be surrogate decision makers.

Many factors influence a person's decisions about advance directives including religion, education, knowledge of these instruments, and cultural and ethnic values.[24] Blacks rarely execute advance directives, Hispanics use them 25% of the time, and about half of older whites and Asians have them. Elders older than 80 years of age are more likely to have recorded health care wishes. Cultural importance of family ties, religion, and death may explain some of these differences.

Living Will

A living will affirms a person's right and desire to refuse a life-prolonging intervention and becomes effective when the person is determined to be terminally ill or near death. A living will, sometimes called a *treatment directive,* is typically a series of instructions regarding the withholding, withdrawing, or implementing of life-sustaining medical care in the event of terminal illness. It is limited to the instructions in the document. A living will can be used only for terminal illness or when death is imminent.[27] It is often less flexible, covers fewer medical decisions, and can lead to disagreement about whether a condition is terminal or not. Such disagreement affects implementation of the living will. Relatives who disagree with the stated terms have been known to override the individual's wishes and not honor the living will. In most states, a living will is in effect until the writer revokes it, creates a new one, or destroys the document.

Durable Power of Attorney for Health Care or Health Care Proxy

Durable power of attorney for health care is assigned to a trusted person, often called the proxy, designated to make decisions regarding medical care for the older person in the event of future mental incapacity rather than in situations of terminal illness. A health care proxy can make all treatment decisions, not just decisions about life-sustaining measures. The proxy can guide the overall course of the elder's treatment by consenting to treatment as well as by refusing care. The proxy can clarify a living will or make decisions independently according to the client's values in situations that a living will might not address. Use of a proxy is a recommended procedure for clients with dementia and other disorders in which capacity is anticipated to decline. Older people generally name a spouse or an adult child as proxy. The proxy designee must be able to seek and understand medical information, communicate with health care professionals, and advocate effectively on the elder's behalf. The proxy must be faithful to the elder's wishes and well-being and must be willing to assume the burden of difficult decisions to honor the client's wishes.

An advance directive, although a legal document, can be disregarded or overridden. Situations in which advance directives have been disregarded include (1) family opposition; (2) caregiver disregard for, or lack of knowledge about an advance directive; and (3) state laws that mandate responding Emergency Medical Technicians (EMTs) and paramedics to resuscitate before transporting to a hospital. To guard against these occurrences, families should discuss end-of-life decisions before their occurrence, especially if the condition is one of terminal illness. All parties should understand the decisions that are made.

To educate the public about advance directives, nurses must know the different types and must have a sensitivity to individual cultural and ethnic values. Once an advance directive is available and placed on the client's chart, all caregivers should be made aware of its existence and every effort should be made to honor the individual's wishes (see Chapter 22).

Prehospital Advance Directive for Emergency Medical Services

Depending on state or local law, an advance directive may or may not be honored when an emergency medical service (EMS) system (9-1-1) is activated. California, Texas, and New Jersey have legislation that requires special forms to be prepared in order that EMTs not resuscitate a person. It is important to let families know the laws that EMTs must uphold when advance directives are involved.

CONCLUSIONS

Opportunities to care for elders exist in all settings. The number of elderly people requiring health care is considerable. The proportion of all hospital patient days accounted for by people over 65 years of age was 38% in 1980 and is expected to rise to 58% by 2000.[39] Many of these hospitalized clients will be discharged to their homes with continued care needs. The role of the nurse in acute care and community settings—to act as an advocate and to promote the physical and mental well-being of older people—will be extremely important.

Given that the elderly are the fastest growing segment of the population in the United States, every nurse involved with adult health care will undoubtedly at some point be challenged to meet the unique needs of these clients. A holistic perspective is necessary, and the physiologic, psychological, sociologic, and spiritual needs of older people must be considered.

BIBLIOGRAPHY

1. American Nurses' Association. (1995). *Scope and standards of gerontological nursing practice.* Washington, DC: Author.

1a. American Psychiatric Association. (1994). *Diagnostic and statistical manual of mental disorders* (4th ed.). Washington, DC: Author.

2. Anetzberger, G. J. (1990). Abuse, neglect and self-neglect: Issues of vulnerability. In Z. Hanel, P. Ehrlich, & R. Hubbard (Eds.), *The vulnerable aged: People, services, and policies* (pp. 140–148). New York: Springer.

3. Batt, L. (1989). Managing delirium; Implications for geropsychiatric nurses. *Journal of Psychosocial Nursing and Mental Health Services, 27*(5), 22–25.

4. Beare, P. G., & Graveley, E. (1995). Health teaching and compliance. In M. Stanley & P. Beare (Eds.), *Gerontological nursing* (pp. 63–96). Philadelphia: F. A. Davis.

5. Besdine, R. W. (1983). The educational utility of comprehensive functional assessment in the elderly. *Journal of the American Geriatrics Society, 31,* 651–656.

6. Binder, E., & Robins, L. (1990). Cognitive impairment and length of hospital stay in older persons. *Journal of the American Geriatrics Society, 38,* 759–766.

7. Burnside, I. (1988). *Nursing and the aged.* New York: McGraw-Hill.

8. Carnaveli, D., & Patrick, H. (Eds.). (1993). *Nursing management for the elderly* (3rd ed.). Philadelphia: J. B. Lippincott.

9. Darnell, J. C., et al. (1986). Medication use by ambulatory elderly: An in-home survey. *Journal of the American Geriatrics Society, 34*(1), 1–4.

9a. Davies, H. (1999). Delirium and dementia. In J. K. Stone, et al. (Eds.), *Clinical Gerontological Nursing* (2nd ed., pp. 413–443). Philadelphia: W. B. Saunders.

10. Ebersole, P., & Hess, P. (Eds.). (1998). *Toward healthy aging* (5th ed., pp. 1–29). St. Louis: Mosby–Year Book.

11. Eliopoulos, C. (1987). *Gerontological nursing.* Philadelphia: J. B. Lippincott.

12. Folstein, M. F., Folstein, S., & McHugh, P. R. (1975). Mini mental state: A practical method for grading the cognitive states of patients for the clinician. *Journal of Psychiatric Research, 12,* 189–198.

13. Foreman, M. (1989). Confusion in the hospitalized elderly: Incidence, onset, and associated factors. *Research in Nursing and Health, 12,* 21.

14. Hogstel, M. O. (Ed.). (1992). *Clinical manual of gerontological nursing.* St. Louis: Mosby–Year Book.

15. Johnson, J., Sullivan, E., & Gottlieb, G. (1987). Delirium in elderly patients on internal medicine services. *Journal of the American Geriatrics Society, 35,* 972.

16. Kane, R. A., & Kane, R. (1981). *Assessing the elderly* (pp. 59–64). Lexington, MA: Lexington Books.

17. Katz, S., et al. (1963). Studies of illness in the aged. The index of ADL: A standardized measure of biological and psychosocial functions. *Journal of the American Medical Association, 185,* 915–919.

18. King, K., Diamond, M., & McCanie, K. (1987). Coping with relocation. *Geriatric Nursing, 8*(5), 258–261.

19. Levkoff, S., Besdine, R., & Wetle, T. (1986). Acute confusional states (delirium) in the hospitalized elderly. In C. Eisdorfer (Ed.), *Annual review of gerontology and geriatrics* (Vol. 6, pp. 1–26). New York: Springer.

19a. Lipowski, A. (1983). Transient cognitive disorders (delirium, acute confusional states) in the elderly. *American Journal of Psychiatry, 140,* 1426–1436.

20. Madson, S. K. (1993). Patient self-determination act: Implications for long-term care. *Journal of Gerontological Nursing, 19*(2), 15–18.

21. Mahoney, F. I., & Barthel, D. W. (1965). Functional evaluation: The Barthel index. *Maryland State Medical Journal, 14,* 61–65.

22. McConnel, C. E. (1984). A note on the lifetime risk of nursing home residency. *The Gerontologist, 24,* 193–198.

23. McCurren, C. (1991). *Hospitalized elders: Attention deficits and confusion.* Doctoral dissertation. Lexington KY: University of Kentucky.

24. McKenna, W. A. (1995). Transcultural perspectives in nursing care of the elderly. In M. M. Andrews & J. S. Bole (Eds.), *Transcultural concepts in nursing care* (pp. 203–234). Philadelphia: J. B. Lippincott.

25. Meyer, C. (1993). "End-of-life" care: Patients' choices, nurses' challenges. *American Journal of Nursing, 93*(2), 40–47.

26. Mikulencak, M. (1993). The "graying of America": Changing what nurses need to know. *The American Nurse, 25*(7), 1, 12.

27. Miller, C. A. (1995). *Nursing care of older adults: Theory and practice* (2nd ed.). Philadelphia: J. B. Lippincott.

28. Program Resource Development, American Association of Retired Persons. (1998). *A profile of older Americans (1997)* [brochure]. Washington, DC: Author.

29. Ramsdell, J., et al. (1990). Evaluation of cognitive impairment in the elderly. *Journal of General Internal Medicine, 5,* 55–64.

30. Shawler, E., et al. (1992). Clinical considerations: Surrogate decision making for hospitalized elders. *Journal of Gerontological Nursing, 18*(6), 5–11.

31. Shugars, D. A., O'Neil, E. H., & Bader, J. D. (Eds.). (1994). *Healthy America: Practitioners for 2005.* Durham, NC: The Pew Health Professions Commission.

32. Stanley, M., & Bare, P. (Eds.). (1995). *Gerontological nursing.* Philadelphia: F. A. Davis.

33. Stewart, R. B., et al. (1991). Changing patterns of therapeutic agents in the elderly: A ten-year overview. *Age and Aging, 20*(3), 182–188.

34. Stone, J. K., Wyman, J. F., & Salisbury, S. A. (1999). *Clinical gerontological nursing: A guide to advanced practice* (2nd ed.). Philadelphia: W. B. Saunders.

35. Tideiksaar, R. (1997). *Falling in old age* (2nd ed.). New York: Springer.

36. U.S. Bureau of the Census. (1991). *Statistical abstracts of the U.S.* (111th ed.). Washington, DC: U.S. Government Printing Office.

37. U.S. House Select Committee on Aging. (1986). *The rights of America's institutionalized aged: Lost in confinement* (Committee Publication No. 99-543). Washington, DC: U.S. Government Printing Office.

38. U.S. House Select Committee on Aging. (1990). *Elder abuse: A decade of shame and inaction.* Washington, DC: U.S. Government Printing Office.

39. U.S. Senate Special Committee on Aging. (1989). *Developments in aging: 1988* (Committee Publication No. 101-4). Washington, DC: U.S. Government Printing Office.

40. Valanis, R., Yeaworth, R., & Mullis, M. (1987). Alcohol use among bereaved and nonbereaved older persons. *Journal of Gerontological Nursing, 13*(5), 26–32.

The Trait and Process of Resilience

QUESTIONS
What is meant by resilience?
How does it affect responses to illness and adversity?

CITATION
Jacelon, C. S. (1997). The trait and process of resilience. *Journal of Advanced Nursing, 25,* 123–129.

STUDIES

The author of this review selected studies to demonstrate the breadth and diversity of ideas about resilience and diversity in the behavioral science and clinical literature. Other than these goals, the method of locating and choosing the studies for inclusion was not described. The studies were conducted by researchers from social, psychological, and health care disciplines. Studies about adults are emphasized in this synopsis.

Summary of Findings

"Resilience as a Trait" (p. 123)

Resilience can be defined either as a personal trait or as a process by which people "spring back" from adversity and continue with their lives.[5] *Vulnerability* may be an opposite trait, referring to how people are easily "beaten down" by adversity and succumb to dysfunction in their lives.[9]

Resilience is manifested differently in children and adults. Studies of children in poverty,[5] of children who have parents with major affective disorders,[2] of children whose parents are divorced,[7] and of children with attention deficit disorder[6] suggest a constellation of characteristics that constitute resilience. Important contributors include:

- Personal disposition to high activity levels, self-understanding, intelligence, and positive responsiveness to others
- The presence of a caring adult or a warm cohesive family
- Strong community support and role models[5]

Adult homosexual men who are long-term survivors of acquired immunodeficiency syndrome (AIDS) were also found to have extraordinary personal resources: intelligence, education, wide-ranging interests, a positive outlook, and goals.[8] Most of them also had a confidant, access to community resources, and adequate housing.

The personality traits and responses of adults with cancer have also been studied. A correlational study examined the relationship between personality traits and the degree of atypical neoplastic growth on the cervix of 75 women who had abnormal Papanicolaou (Pap) smears.[1] An interview was conducted and a health inventory questionnaire was administered before the examination results were reported to the women. Several associations were revealed between personality variables and the degree of neoplastic growth. Women with cancer had significantly higher scores in pessimism, future despair, life-threat reactivity, and somatic anxiety than women with a very low level of or no neoplastic growth. Thus, we might infer that a positive life outlook affords resistance to development of cancer.

As part of a qualitative study, in-depth interviews were conducted with 24 older women who had adjusted well after a major loss. The themes that emerged from the interview data were:[10]

- A balanced perspective of their life experiences
- Persistence in the face of adversity
- A belief in their own abilities
- The realization that life has purpose and that one can always make a contribution
- A belief that each person's life path is unique

An experimental instrument to measure the trait of resilience has been tested on 810 older adults.[11] Resilience was found to be positively correlated with life satisfaction, morale, and physical health and negatively correlated with depression. The instrument was found to measure two main factors: personal competence and acceptance of life and self.

"Resilience as a Process" (p. 126)

The process of resilience has been described as the complex interaction of intrapsychic and social responses with demands and stresses that occur over time.[4,9] Two stages have been delineated: (1) the *disruption* phase, "during which energy is directed at minimizing the impact of the stress or stressor"; and (2) the *reorganization* phase, "during which a new reality is accepted in part or in whole."[3] The literature suggests that resilience as a process can be learned at any point in life.[3]

Overall, studies of resilience as a *process* are fewer than studies of resilience as a personal *trait.* One investigator working with the physically disabled concluded that personal perceptions and responses to major life events are "crucial elements of survival, recovery, and rehabilitation."[3]

Limitations/Reservations. We as health care workers seem to be intrigued by the ability of children, adolescents, adults, couples, and families to bounce back from adversity and persevere. We understand the personal traits that serve as protective factors to the hurts, losses, and difficulties of adverse experiences, but we do not know why some people have these resources while other people lack them. We also do not understand how people acquire resilience and remain resilient over a long time.

The concept of resilience has been defined in various ways and is not well differentiated from other similar concepts such as hardiness, thriving, self-efficacy, and coping. Perhaps most lacking from a nursing perspective is that it is not clear whether or not interventions can promote and support resilience during difficult times.

Continued on following page

The Trait and Process of Resilience *Continued*

Research-Based Practice

Resilient people have a constellation of traits, including (1) the ability to form and maintain meaningful relationships with others, (2) a balanced perspective of life's joys and difficulties, and (3) a belief that we can determine our own future. The review author envisions that if an instrument for measuring resilience existed, "Nurses in practice could then better focus resources by capitalizing on the resilient person's strengths and by providing assistance to people who are not inherently resilient" (p. 128). This is an intriguing idea, but further development is needed to specify what should be done differently for the two groups of people; the proposed interventions would need to be tested to ensure that they work and to specify the people with whom they work. Another issue to be addressed would be how one helps people whose trait score is in the mid-range.

Attempts have been made to teach coping and problem-solving skills to clients with chronic health problems, but the extent to which the learning of these skills results in resilience has not been examined. Similarly, conducting personal resource inventories with clients who face chronic illness may help them realize what protective resources they do have and then tap into them.

Promoting support groups is another intervention that may foster resiliency. Support groups seem to benefit people who already have resiliency traits in place. It is not known whether people with tentative resiliency traits are bolstered by support groups. For older adults and clients with life-threatening illness, a life review may build resilience by helping them realize how strong they have been over their lifetime and by helping them place the current adversity into perspective.

In summary, some of the interventions already used to "support" people during difficult times may succeed by bolstering, tapping into, or bringing into conscious awareness a client's resiliency traits that were developed earlier in life.

Cited References

1. Antoni, M. H., & Goodkin, K. (1988). Host moderator variable in the promotion of cervical neoplasia. I. Personal facets. *Journal of Psychosomatic Research, 32,* 327–338.
2. Beardslee, W. R., & Poderefsky, D. (1988). Resilient adolescents whose parents have serious affective and other psychiatric disorders: Importance of self-understanding and relationships. *American Journal of Psychiatry, 145,* 63–69.
3. Fine, S. B. (1991). Resilience and human adaptability: Who rises above adversity? *American Journal of Occupational Therapy, 45,* 493–503.
4. Fonagy, P., et al. (1993). The Emanuel Miller memorial lecture 1992: The theory and practice of resilience. *Journal of Child Psychology and Psychiatry, 35,* 231–257.
5. Garmezy, N. (1993). Children in poverty: Resilience despite risk. *Psychiatry, 56,* 127–136.
6. Hechtman, L. (1991). Resilience and vulnerability in long term outcome of attention deficit hyperactive disorder. *Canadian Journal of Psychiatry, 36,* 415–421.
7. Mulholland, D. J., et al. (1991). Academic performance in children of divorce: Psychological resilience and vulnerability. *Psychiatry, 54,* 268–280.
8. Rabkin, J. G., et al. (1993). Resilience in adversity among long-term survivors of AIDS. *Hospital and Community Psychiatry, 44,* 162–167.
9. Rutter, M. (1985). Psychosocial resilience and protective mechanisms. *American Journal of Orthopsychiatry, 57,* 316–331.
10. Wagnild, G., & Young, H. M. (1990). Resilience among older women. *Image: Journal of Nursing Scholarship, 22,* 252–255.
11. Wagnild, G., & Young, H. M. (1993). Development and psychometric evaluation of the resilience scale. *Journal of Nursing Measurement, 1,* 165–178.

Sarah Jo Brown, PhD, RN, *Principal and Consultant, Practice-Research Integrations, Norwich, Vermont*

UNIT

2

Health Care Delivery Systems

CHAPTER 4

Overview of Health Care Delivery

Mary L. Fisher

Nurses in the United States practice within a diverse and complex health care system. During the 1980s and 1990s, the system experienced a dramatic growth in scientific knowledge, coupled with an explosion of technology. This also was a period of increased competition and regulation. Additionally, the financing of health care was revolutionized in 1983, when prospective payment was introduced, and later, as managed care began to dominate the market. These events have had a profound impact on the practice of nursing. Understanding who the major stakeholders are within the field of health care and understanding recent health care history are crucial to the practice of professional nurses. This chapter strives to inform beginning practitioners of these changes and trends to prepare them for active roles in shaping the health care system for the new millennium.

MAJOR STAKEHOLDERS IN THE HEALTH CARE SYSTEM

■ GOVERNMENT

The role of government in the administration of health care in the United States cannot be overestimated. Health care expenditures accounted for 20% of the federal government's budget in 1995; by 1997, expenditures amounted to $485 billion.[16, 20] In 1997, 46.4% of health care dollars spent were funded by government programs, especially Medicare (a federal program funded at $214 billion for 1997) and Medicaid (a joint federal-state initiative funded at $160 billion for 1997).[14, 16] Other important sources of federal government funding are the Department of Veterans Affairs (VA), funded at $16.6 billion for 1997, which oversees the VA health care system, and the Department of Defense, funded at 13.4 billion for 1997, which funds health care for members of the armed forces and their dependents.[14] Workers' compensation, a joint federal and state program, was funded at $14.1 billion for 1997.[14] In addition, state and local governments support local indigent care through various mechanisms.

As the major payer, the federal government has been active in regulating the health care industry. Approximately 40% of hospital beds are occupied on any given day by Medicare recipients. Therefore, hospitals have great incentive to comply with regulations promulgated by the federal government, because they can be fined or "decertified" as a provider of care to Medicare clients if they do not. Noncompliance can result in the loss of millions of dollars of income for the hospital.

Government regulation is frequently opposed by the health care industry because it often affects the health care practitioner's autonomy. In 1991, for example, the U.S. Supreme Court upheld the right of the federal government to restrict health care providers in family planning clinics that receive federal funds from informing pregnant women about abortion options (*Rust v. Sullivan*). Since the Supreme Court ruling, health care workers in the clinics had to alter their practice or be subject to penalty. Strong condemnation of this restriction was voiced by the American Nurses' Association (ANA) and the American Medical Association (AMA), among others. Legislation to modify the regulation was eventually passed.

The federal government is the biggest source of funding for biomedical research. The Agency for Health Care Policy and Research (AHCPR), established in 1989, conducts research on costs, quality, and medical effectiveness of health care. It received $171 billion in 1999, two thirds of which was awarded in grants and contracts.[2] The National Institutes of Health (NIH), the principal biomedical research agency of the government through its 17 institutes, received $15.6 billion for fiscal year 1999, 82% of which supports research and training.[21] The House of Representatives passed $17.9 billion for fiscal year 2000.[8] The government also directs public health programs through the Centers for Disease Control and Prevention (CDC), which received $3.1 billion for fiscal year 2000.[9] The growth of scientific knowledge related to health care is highly dependent on government funding. Nurse researchers are recipients of research grants through various government agencies, most notably the National Institute for Nursing Research at NIH. Its budget for 1999 was $70 million.[22] Research funds are an important source of revenue for major medical centers and university-affiliated hospitals.

This chapter includes material from the fifth edition written by Bonita Ann Pilon.

DIVERSITY IN HEALTH CARE

Health Care Practitioners

Americans have been socialized to believe that the United States has the best health care system in the world. This ethnocentric attitude interferes with nurses' recognition and acceptance of the value and use of traditional healers. Terms used for traditional healers include folk practitioners, indigenous healers, native healers, primitive healers, and witch doctors. Whatever the terms, they generally are given a negative connotation, and it is implied that they are not as good as Western practitioners. Health care needs to reflect an understanding of the values of diverse populations.[2]

The table identifies culture and folk practitioners, their preparation, and scope of practice.

Culture/Folk Practitioners

Practitioner	Preparation	Scope of Practice
Hispanic		
Family member	Possesses knowledge of folk medicine.	Common illnesses of a mild nature that may or may not be recognized by modern medicine.
Curandero	May receive training in an apprenticeship. May receive a "gift from God" that enables her or him to cure. Knowledgeable in use of herbs, diet, massage, and rituals.	Some may not treat illness caused by witchcraft for fear of being accused of possessing evil powers. Usually admired by community. Treats almost all of the traditional illnesses.
Espiritualista or spiritualist	Born with the special gifts of being able to analyze dreams and fortell future events. May serve apprenticeship with an older practitioner.	Emphasizes prevention of illness or bewitchment through use of medals, prayers, and amulets. May also be sought for cure of existing illnesses.
Yerbero	No formal training. Knowledgeable in growing and prescribing herbs.	Consulted for preventive and curative use of herbs for traditional and Western illnesses.
Sabador	Knowledgeable in massage and manipulation of bones and muscles.	Treats many traditional illnesses, particularly those affecting the musculoskeletal system. May also treat nontraditional illnesses.
Black		
"Old Lady"	Usually an older woman who has successfully raised her own family. Knowledgeable in child care and folk remedies.	Consulted about common ailments and advice for child care.
Spiritualist	Called by God to help others. No formal training. Usually associated with a fundamentalist Christian church.	Assists with financial, personal, spiritual, or physical problems. Predominantly found in urban communities.
Voodoo priest or priestess or *Hougan*	May be trained by another priest or priestess. In the United States, the oldest son of a priest becomes a priest. A daughter of a priest or priestess becomes a priestess if she is born with a veil (amniotic sac) over her face.	Knowledgeable about properties of herbs and interpretation of signs and omens. Can cure illness caused by voodoo. Uses communication to establish a therapeutic milieu (like a psychiatrist). Treats African Americans, Mexican Americans, and Native Americans.
Chinese		
Herbalist	Knowledgeable in diagnosis of illness and herbal remedies.	Both diagnostic and therapeutic. Diagnostic techniques include interviewing, inspection, auscultation, and assessment of pulses.
Acupuncturist	3½ to 4½ years (1500 to 1800 hours) of courses on acupuncture, Western anatomy and physiology, and Chinese herbs. Usually requires a period of apprenticeship under someone who is licensed or certified. Licensure required in North America.	Diagnosis and treatment of *Yin* and *Yang* disorders by inserting needles into meridians (pathways through which life energy flows). Heat may be applied to the acupuncture needle (moxibustion). May combine acupuncture with herbal remedies and/or dietary recommendations. Acupuncture is sometimes used as an anesthetic in surgery.

DIVERSITY IN HEALTH CARE *Continued*

Amish		
Braucher or *baruch-doktor*	Apprenticeship.	Men or women use a combination of modalities, including physical manipulation, massage, herbs, teas, reflexology, and *brauche,* folk-healing art with origins in 18th and 19th century Europe. Especially effective in the treatment of bed-wetting.
Lay midwives	Apprenticeship.	Cares for women before, during, and after delivery.
Greek		
Magissa "magician"	Apprenticeship.	Woman who cures *matiasma* (evil eye). May be referred to as a doctor.
Bone setters	Apprenticeship.	Specializes in treating uncomplicated fractures.
Priest (Orthodox)	Ordained clergy. Formal theological study.	May be called on for advice, blessings, exorcisms, or direct healing.
Native American		
Shaman	Spiritually chosen. Apprenticeship.	Uses incantations, prayers, and herbs to cure physical, psychological, and spiritual illnesses.
Crystal gazer, hand trembler (Navajo)		Diviner diagnostician who can identify the cause of a problem by using crystals or by placing a hand over the sick person. Does not implement treatment.

Traditional healers existed long before modern nursing or medicine. It is only recently that health care professionals are becoming aware of their value. Ideally, traditional healers will soon be an integral part of the health care team.[1]

References

1. Leininger, M. (1997). Founders focus alternative to what? Generic vs. professional caring, treatments and healing modes. *Journal of Transcultural Nursing, 9*(1), 37.
2. Purnell, L., & Paulanka, B. (1998). *Transcultural health care: A culturally competent approach.* Philadelphia: F. A. Davis.

Modified from Andrews, M., & Herberg, P. (1999). Transcultural nursing care. In M. Andrews & J. Boyle (Eds.), *Transcultural concepts in nursing care* (pp. 42–43). Philadelphia: J. B. Lippincott.

Joyce Larson-Presswalla, PhD, RN, *President, "Culture Counts," Marketing Coordinator, James A. Haley Veterans Hospital, Tampa, Florida*

■ PHYSICIANS

The role of physicians in the health care system in the United States is an important one. Physicians provide direct medical services to clients in a variety of settings, including offices, clinics, hospitals, and freestanding centers. In addition, physicians control 60% to 80% of hospital costs through their decisions about the use of resources. As gatekeepers to inpatient care, physicians decide which clients to admit, where to admit clients, the length of stay, the quantity of ancillary services, whether to perform surgery, when to initiate and to discontinue treatment regimens, and which medications to prescribe.

Because physicians strongly influence health care use, health care agencies and clients are often dependent on physicians. Agencies such as hospitals rely on their medical staffs to admit clients who generate income for the hospital. Therefore, physicians are customers of the hospital, just as clients are. As a result, physicians and their lobby groups, such as the AMA, usually have strong political influence within hospital organizations, the health care system, legislatures, and government-regulating agencies.

Many physicians perceived a decline in their dominance and control of health care during the 1980s and 1990s. These perceived and real losses have created anxiety and defensive tactics among some members of the profession toward a restructured health care system. The traditions that define medical practice, such as autonomy, professional control, solo medical practice, and fee-for-service entrepreneurialism, are being questioned and reformed. Some contend that physicians will enjoy less control in a restructured health care environment than they did before. In keeping with this trend toward the loss of physician power, the AMA took the unprecedented step in 1999 of forming a collective bargaining arm to assist physicians in seeking input into practice changes.

While Western practitioners are the main group sanctioned by American society to treat disease, traditional cultural and folk practitioners are a presence in ethnic segments of our society. Providers must recognize the place of traditional healers for an ethnically diverse population (see Diversity in Health Care).

HOSPITAL ADMINISTRATORS AND GOVERNING BOARDS

The chief executive, chief financial officer, chief nursing officer, and governing boards of hospitals strongly influence health care delivery in their institutions. In addition, most hospitals are members of the American Hospital Association (AHA), which represents the industry's efforts to influence legislation, regulation, judicial decisions, and health policy. The AHA filed a suit in the early 1990s to stop the National Labor Relations Board from implementing new collective bargaining rules. The suit went to the Supreme Court, where the rules were upheld, but they have had little impact in fostering collective bargaining, as the AHA has feared.[7] The AHA also worked to block regulations from the Health Care Financing Administration (HCFA), which effectively decreased reimbursement for capital costs to hospitals from Medicare.[30]

BUSINESS AND INDUSTRY

By the year 2000, health care costs were projected to represent 19% of the gross national product (GNP), or $1.6 trillion.[17, 26] These costs are the highest of any industrialized nation, making American products less competitive in the world economy. For example, health care costs for automobile workers add $1100 to the cost of every car made in America.[13] This continuing trend is best illustrated by comparing the cost of prescription drugs in the United States with that of other wealthy nations: Great Britain's cost is 33% less; Canada's, 37% less; and France's and Italy's, 47% less.[1]

One can understand why American industries have a big stake in controlling these costs. As health care costs rose in the mid-1990s (~5% per year),[15] the influence of business and industry increased as well. Health insurance programs, such as Blue Cross/Blue Shield and commercial insurance, are purchased mainly through employee benefit programs. As the cost of health care rises, insurance costs rise as well, forcing businesses to assume greater financial burdens to insure employees and their dependents. Costs for products increase accordingly.

One major reason for the increase is the health care industry's practice of cost shifting by increasing charges to individuals and small payers to offset underpayment by Medicare, Medicaid, and other contracted payers. The result is that the private sector, insured clients, and employers pay more for care. During the past decade, business and industry leaders protested the increased costs and began to take collective action to drive costs down. Some strategies have included:

- Increased deductibles
- Larger and more frequent co-payments
- Reduced benefits and services
- Initiation of managed care programs
- Mandatory second opinions
- Precertification of admission
- Increased contracting of care to health maintenance organizations (HMOs) and preferred provider organizations (PPOs)

By 1997, 85% of the enrolled work force was in some type of managed care plan.[14]

In some areas of the United States, industry leaders have formed coalition groups that lobby their state government for laws to restrict health care spending, limit malpractice liability, and provide major reform for the health care system. Increasingly, large businesses have contracted for health care services directly with hospitals and physician groups, demanding—and receiving—significant discounts for care. The influence of large employers is expected to remain strong within the health care industry.

THE PUBLIC

Despite decades of public policy designed to reduce health costs, U.S. health care spending is estimated to exceed $1.6 trillion or $5700 per capita annually by 2000.[13] The American public has a stake in health care from several perspectives. First, as consumers of health care services, the public is concerned with the quality, cost, and access to care. Many Americans believe that health care is a right and should be universally available to all citizens ragardless of the cost. Paradoxically, however, most do not want to pay these costs in the form of increased taxes.

People who are uninsured (approx. 44 million, 86% of whom are employed workers and their families) or underinsured (Medicare recipients have no prescription medication coverage) do not have equal access to health care services that income and insurance provide.[13] This uninsured figure represents 16% of the non-elderly population.[15] Women and children are among those who suffer the most, since 25% of the uninsured are children.[15] Because people have not agreed on the model for health care reform or the role of government, several ideas are being explored by various interest groups.

The public also is composed of voters who can elect representatives to enact laws protecting their health care interests. Often, citizens band together to influence the passage of health-related legislation. In 1990, activist groups concerned about acquired immunodeficiency syndrome (AIDS) strongly lobbied Congress to ensure passage of the Ryan White bill (Public Law 101-381), which provided funds for AIDS education, service, and research. The American Association of Retired Persons (AARP) is another prominent group that actively supports health care legislation targeted to older people. Although many other consumer groups are concerned with health care issues, AIDS and breast cancer activist groups and the AARP represent some of the larger and more vocal constituencies that currently influence the health care industry.

Overall, public values regarding health care are changing. People are interested in receiving quality health care at a reasonable cost. In addition, the public has a more positive view of health promotion and illness prevention than in the past. Health care resources remain focused on illness, however, with only 1% of health care expenditures going to public health.[30]

NURSES

Nurses outnumber physicians, dentists, pharmacists, and every other single group of health care providers in the United States. As of 1996, there were 2.6 million Licensed Professional Nurses (LPNs), 1.93 million of whom were employed in nursing.[19] Among those 1.93 million

Registered Nurses (RNs), slightly fewer than two thirds worked in hospitals—a distribution that has remained constant since the mid-1980s. The supply of RNs has increased by 40% since 1980. During that time, the percentage employed in hospitals had been stable at 67% through the mid 1990s. The percentage dipped to 60% in 1996, reflecting trends toward community and outpatient care and nurses' growing concern with health maintenance, health promotion, and health education.[11, 19]

The average age of nurses has risen steadily since the 1980s. The median age for RNs neared 40 in 1996.[19] Racial and ethnic minorities except Asians are underrepresented.[23] The U.S. Bureau of Census in 1996 estimated that 72% of Americans were white, in contrast to 90% of nurses being white.[29]

Although the influence of such a large group of health care providers should be noticed, the greatest impact—and the most frequently discussed aspect of nursing—has been the recurring shortage of RNs. The voice of nursing has been heard lately, as thousands protest downsizing of hospitals, replacement of RNs by less skilled workers, and layoffs. However, the collective expertise and leadership of nurses has not yet been fully utilized to shape the reform era. Nursing's response to rapid market changes has been largely reactionary.

In 1991, the ANA, in collaboration with the National League for Nursing, the American Organization of Nurse Executives, the American Association of Colleges of Nursing, and other organized nursing groups, introduced *Nursing's Agenda for Health Care Reform.* The authors[3] stated that

> Nurses provide a unique perspective on the health care system. Our constant presence in a variety of settings places us in contact with individuals who reap the benefits of the system's most sophisticated services, as well as those individuals seriously compromised by the system's inefficiencies. . . . America's health care system is . . . very costly, its quality inconsistent, and its benefits unequally distributed. . . . In short, health care is neither fairly nor equitably delivered to all segments of the population.

Nursing's health care reform proposal attempted to address the cost, quality, and access dilemmas facing the nation. This endeavor was a proactive attempt by the nursing profession to significantly alter existing health policy. A 1999 publication by ANA, *Legislative and Regulatory Initiatives for the 106th Congress* proposed mobilizing nurses politically to enact continuing influence on health care policy.[4]

FINANCING OF HEALTH CARE SERVICES

FUNDING MECHANISMS

Health care is paid for in various ways. The major funding programs are defined in Box 4–1.

The health care industry has evolved through significant phases since the 1920s with regard to quality, cost, and access. To understand current issues, it is useful for nurses to understand the past, which was characterized by two major periods: (1) the *period of expansion* and (2) the *period of regulation and cost containment.* The current climate is known as the *period of reform.*

PERIOD OF EXPANSION

During the late 1920s, a congressional committee studied various facets of health care organization and financing. It was found that the cost of health care per illness had substantially increased with the emergence of hospitalization as the appropriate method of treating illness.[24] These rising costs, coupled with the financial problems created by the Depression of 1929, led to financial difficulties for community general hospitals. Consequently, the need to spread financial risk across the community was recognized. Prepayment plans for hospital care spread slowly during the 1930s and evolved into the Blue Cross system.

PRIVATE HEALTH INSURANCE

Blue Cross plans had two goals: (1) to provide a stronger financial base for community hospitals and (2) to move the risk of economic loss caused by hospitalization away from single individuals to larger groups of people. Because these objectives were considered socially desirable, Blue Cross, and later Blue Shield organizations, benefited from favorable legislation exempting them from some of the more stringent requirements for commercial insurance companies.

The evolution of Blue Cross/Blue Shield plans and their availability to the average worker signaled the beginning of an era in which the actual cost of health care became separated from the person who purchased the care (the insurance effect). Such a separation causes the cost of health care to appear artificially low to the client, who in turn, can afford to buy more services.

Demand for health care services, as a result of insurance, grew rapidly in the 1940s and 1950s. Because of economic wage and price controls during and after World War II, salary increases to workers were limited. Fringe benefits came into vogue as a means of attracting and retaining workers. Unions began bargaining for fringe benefits in lieu of unobtainable salary increases. As a consequence, health insurance became widely available to American workers and their families. The consumption of health care services, in turn, increased.

Another important event was the passage of the Social Security Act of 1935. This legislation established as social policy the right of older people to financial security. Although health care was not affected by this law at the time of its passage, the Social Security Act would later become the vehicle through which health care needs of older people and the poor would be addressed.

HILL-BURTON ACT

After World War II, it was apparent that the nation's hospitals were obsolete and poorly distributed to meet the population's needs. There had been great shifts from rural to urban areas during the War. Immediately after the War, the baby boom began. The private sector had difficulty meeting the need for improved health care facilities.[6] Congress responded by passing the Hospital Survey and Construction Act of 1946 (the Hill-Burton Act).

The overt purpose of the Hill-Burton Act was to eliminate shortages of hospitals, especially in rural and economically depressed areas. Ratios of beds-to-population were used to measure shortage. Funds generated by the Act were dispersed over 28 years (1946 to 1974). The Act was amended during that time to include not only

BOX 4–1 Major Health Care Funding Programs in the United States

Medicare

A federally funded and administered national health insurance program for citizens age 65 years and older and for certain other clients, such as those with end-stage renal disease, regardless of age. Medicare began in 1966 and is paid for through payroll taxes of all workers (a portion of Social Security deductions) and through monthly premiums paid by recipients. The program covers both hospitalization and physician costs, but deductibles and restrictions apply. Medicare determines the maximum allowable fee for service. Health care providers receive 80% of this fee from Medicare and can bill only for the balance of the allowable fee. The maximum allowable fee is often much less than the true value of the service.

In 1983, the federal government instituted major changes in the way hospitals were reimbursed for Medicare clients. Previously, hospitals had been reimbursed costs plus an additional amount. Since 1983, hospitals have received compensation on a *prospective* basis. Hospitals are paid one predetermined sum for a given diagnosis. Similar types of diagnoses and conditions are grouped together, weighted for severity or intensity of illness, and assigned a dollar value for compensation; these are called diagnosis-related groups (DRGs). If the client's care (e.g., acute myocardial infarction) costs the hospital *more* than Medicare's payment, the hospital *loses* money. If the costs are less than the reimbursement amount, the hospital keeps the profit. This system has caused dramatic changes as hospitals struggle to survive financially. Congress is now debating whether Medicare should fund prescription coverage for recipients.

Medicaid

A joint federal and state program administered by the state governments. This insurance program provides limited funding for hospital and medical care costs of low-income citizens. Each state sets the income levels that determine eligibility. As a result, some states provide more services than others can afford. The state must budget money from its own revenues for the program matched by the government. The federal portion is always larger than the state portion.

Blue Cross and Blue Shield

Private not-for-profit health insurance companies set up through special legislation in the 1930s. The "blues" are the largest single insurer outside the federal government from which businesses and industry can purchase health insurance for employees. Both hospital and medical care insurance are available.

Commercial Insurance Companies

For-profit businesses (e.g., Traveler's, Metropolitan Life). These agencies usually sell a host of insurance packages. Businesses or individuals may buy health insurance from a commercial carrier.

Self-Insurance

Businesses that develop their own insurance programs for employees. More companies are setting aside funds (which can be millions of dollars) to cover the risk of their self-insurance program. The company may hire Blue Cross and Blue Shield or a commercial insurer to administer the program, including receiving, reviewing, and paying claims.

HMO

A health maintenance organization representing a system of bundled services. Clients pay a monthly premium to the HMO, which entitles them to checkups and preventive care, medical care, prescriptions, and hospitalization if needed. The HMO employs its own physicians and other health care providers and may own or manage its own hospitals. Some HMOs charge the clients a co-payment for some services, such as prescriptions and office visits. Clients are restricted to using only HMO facilities and physicians. If clients go outside the system, they must pay for past or all of their expenses (except in emergencies or during travel).

PPO

A preferred provider organization is a group consisting of physicians, usually at least one hospital, as well as ancillary providers that coalesces to form a system of care. This system is marketed and sold, contractually, to employers. The physicians, hospital, and others remain independent agents who agree to treat certain clients (those who join the PPO) at discounted prices.

Workers' Compensation

A federally mandated, state-funded and state-administered insurance program available to workers injured on the job. Each employer is assessed a payroll tax, which funds the plan. Clients file claims through the employer to secure funds for treatment.

Private Pay

A term used to describe clients who have no insurance and who must pay the entire health care bill.

Uncompensated Care

Health care delivered that is not paid for by an insurance program or by clients themselves. Many private pay clients contribute to the amount of uncompensated care when they cannot pay the high costs of health care. Other sources of uncompensated care include the differences between what the care costs and what Medicare or Medicaid pays the provider. By law, providers cannot bill anyone for the difference and must absorb the loss of revenue.

Capitation

A form of payment between the purchaser of health care and the provider. Capitation is often used when a large organization contracts for health services from a provider, such as a hospital or home health agency. The provider is paid in one of two ways: (1) a flat fee is paid per incident of care (no care, no payment) or (2) the provider receives a flat fee per person enrolled in the health plan for a defined level of care whether or not the enrollee seeks care. If few enrollees use the service, the provider does well financially. If not, the provider must care for every enrollee who seeks care regardless of whether the total money received covers the cost of the care provided.

construction of new facilities but also modernization of existing facilities and, later, construction of emergency departments and neighborhood health centers.[6]

Implicit within this legislation was the social policy of ensuring access to health care for all. The solution to the social problem of inadequate access was to construct more health care facilities. To ensure that people with limited ability to pay were actually served by the agencies receiving Hill-Burton Act money, the legislation stipulated a unique payback scheme. Each facility had to provide care to indigent clients, on an annual basis, that was equal in dollar value to the amount of money received by the hospital, prorated over a specified time period, usually 20 years. Much like a mortgage payment, the hospital provided free care each year equal to its annual repayment amount. These health services were provided, in lieu of payment, to people with limited access because of poverty.

The Hill-Burton Act's approach to indigent care was a noble one but did not succeed in providing access for all indigent clients. During the long payback period, the cost of health care increased dramatically as a result of new technology and inflation. Many hospitals began meeting their obligations for free care in a few weeks' time each year. After those obligations were met, hospitals were not legally bound to treat indigent clients. By the early 1970s, the bed shortage addressed by Hill-Burton legislation had reversed itself and an oversupply appeared to exist. In 1974, the Act was allowed to expire.

MEDICARE/MEDICAID ENACTED

The early 1950s featured continued wage and price controls, growth of health insurance coverage among workers, and increased discussion of a national health insurance program. National health insurance was viewed as a means of insuring every American citizen against economic loss caused by the high cost of illness, regardless of employment status, age, or health status. This concern repeatedly asserted itself during President Truman's administration. The medical and hospital lobby successfully fought such legislation as late as 1952.[25]

By the middle of the 1960s, a new social problem was identified as the nation's priority: poverty. The War on Poverty during the Johnson Administration (1963 to 1968) provided the impetus for passage of the first national health insurance plans, for which the federal government was both the insurance carrier and the payer of a large portion of the premium. These insurance programs, known as Medicare and Medicaid, were passed as amendments to the Social Security Act in 1965. The social problem of poverty was translated more specifically into limited access to health care services by the elderly and the non-elderly poor as the result of inability to pay. The social policy expressed by both pieces of legislation implied that access to health care for all citizens was a right. Government had an obligation to ensure that right.

Funding for the Medicare hospitalization plan (Part A) is provided by a payroll tax collected from every worker who pays Social Security taxes. The medical payment component (Part B) for physician care is paid by the enrollee through monthly premiums. The Medicare program is administered by the federal government through the Department of Health and Human Services (DHHS) Health Care Financing Administration.

Administration of Medicaid is delegated to the states, which must provide certain core services but are free to tailor other services to meet specific population needs. The states also determine eligibility requirements, which vary considerably from state to state. Funding for Medicaid is provided by a matching formula specific to each state. The federal funds are always the greatest portion of each Medicaid dollar spent. States receive differing amounts of federal money—and thus, provide different ranges of care—because some states can match more federal dollars than others through larger state tax revenues.

Implementation of Medicare and Medicaid substantially increased the federal government's (and, to a lesser extent, the state governments') role in the health care market. The federal government became the single largest purchaser of health care services. Subsequently, it played a growing role in regulating the health care industry in both cost and quality.

■ PERIOD OF REGULATION AND COST CONTAINMENT

In 1974, Congress passed the National Health Planning and Resources Act (Public Law 93-641), which required states to develop a statewide health plan for the use of resources. States were also required to review providers' requests to initiate or expand health services.[18] This review process, known as *certificate of need* (CON) review, required providers to demonstrate sufficient need for the service before the request was approved. This legislation represented the first federal government effort to combine health planning and regulation in one program. It was also the first significant attempt to control health care costs through the elimination of duplicate services and facilities. It was designed to curb the oversupply and increasing technology of facilities that arose during the period of expansion.

Because the CON regulation did nothing to change incentives to hospitals in the competitive health care market, it could not control costs and by the late 1970s was curtailed as a federal effort.[18] Results of CON studies support this evaluation. Steinwald and Sloan[27] suggested that "certificate-of-need controls, initiated by the states and mandated by PL 93-641, may be regarded as a classic example of regulatory failure."

During the 1970s, some state governments undertook their own regulatory programs. Rate controls were in place in at least eight states by the end of the decade. According to Steinwald and Sloan,[27] such programs "all respond to the evils of cost-based reimbursement—they seek to counteract the unrestrained nature of hospital reimbursement by superimposing constraints that the market cannot provide."

States with mandatory rate-setting programs represented the most stringent group of prospective reimbursement programs operating during the late 1970s. The rates of increase in total hospital expenses in the eight mandatory states were 9.7% and 8.6% for the years of 1976 to 1977 and 1977 to 1978, respectively, versus 15.8% and 14% for the other states and the District of Columbia.[27]

These data and other studies clearly indicated that prospective rate-setting was more effective in controlling health care costs than the CON controls were. Reimbursement for Medicaid patients also had moved to a prospective system in many states, whether or not the state had mandatory rate-setting.

Federal Prospective Payment Systems

The federal government, very aware of the rising cost of health care and continuing as the nation's largest purchaser of care, began to look at methods of prospective reimbursement that could be used by the Medicare program. Research studies were under way at Yale University and other centers to develop a system of prospective payment. These studies were closely followed and sometimes funded by DHHS, previously called the Department of Health, Education, and Welfare (DHEW).

The hospital industry adopted its own form of regulation in December 1977. Known as the Voluntary Effort (VE), it consisted of "joint activities at the state level by the American Hospital Association, the American Medical Association, and the Federation of American Hospitals (the for-profit hospitals' trade organization) to control the rate of growth of hospital costs."[27] Results of the Voluntary Effort were mixed. A study by the Congressional Budget Office indicated a small, nonsignificant negative effect on hospital expenditures. A second study found a significant negative effect on the cost per admission and cost per patient day. However, the second study indicated that the cost savings were not passed on to the consumers because hospital profits increased during the same period (1978 to 1980).[27]

The inability of various regulatory programs to control the rising cost of health care (from 9% of the gross national product in 1978 to 13% by 1992) became a primary issue with Congress. The nation was trying to recover from economic recession, and inflation in all sectors of the economy was of grave concern. In addition, the population was aging and the ratio of workers (who paid Medicare taxes for hospitalization insurance) to older people (who spent the dollars paid in by using hospital services) was shrinking. Projections that the Medicare Trust Fund would be bankrupt began in the mid-1980s and continue to this day, with Congress taking only intermediate steps to bail out the program instead of overhauling the entire health care system.

For example, the Tax Equity and Fiscal Responsibility Act (TEFRA), passed by Congress in July 1982, contained temporary limits on Medicare payments and directed the Secretary of DHHS to develop a *prospective payment system* (PPS) for Medicare. The Secretary was instructed to report back to Congress by December 1982 on the status of such a system.

In December 1982, Secretary Richard Schweiker recommended to Congress that a PPS based on *diagnosis-related groups* (DRGs), developed by researchers at Yale University, be used for all Medicare patients. In March 1983, Congress passed amendments to the Social Security Act authorizing such a system. This system was to replace the *cost-based retrospective payment system* used to determine Medicare payments to hospitals. All hospitals serving Medicare clients were to switch to PPS except for certain sole community providers, specialty hospitals, and some psychiatric units within general hospitals.

The program became operational on October 1, 1983. Hospitals were phased into the system over the next 11 months, when their fiscal year began. A formula was calculated for each hospital to determine its initial reimbursement rate under DRGs. Data were gathered from the hospital's own cost history (using a base year) and from a cost history by geographical region; a national rate was also established. These rates were weighted and blended to determine the exact rate of reimbursement per DRG. Since the PPS was initiated, several adjustments have been made in blending. The goal is still to move all hospitals toward one national rate.

Private Sector Response

Government was not the only entity involved with rising health care costs during the early 1980s; business and industry were also concerned because they paid the majority of the health insurance premium costs for employees. Local and regional business leaders come together to discuss and try to remedy the worsening situation. With the implementation of PPS for Medicare clients, these business coalitions were joined by Blue Cross organizations and other commercial insurers. These new groups held a common fear: that hospitals would shift uncompensated costs generated by Medicare clients to clients who were still reimbursed retrospectively on a cost-plus basis. As a result of that fear, Blue Cross and other insurers have begun to restructure their payment systems to protect themselves from potential or actual cost shifting. These fears were warranted, because cost shifting became and remains a reality.

PPS has yielded other results as well. Hospitals and other health care providers increasingly compete for non-Medicare clients who are more favorably reimbursed. Hospitals also compete for certain Medicare clients whose DRG rate has been profitable for the hospital. Much traditional inpatient care has been shifted to the outpatient system or to the client's home, where the cost of care is less. Insurers and providers have teamed up in creative arrangements designed to hold down costs and yet remain competitive. Such arrangements have created alternative delivery systems based on greater efficiency and decreased costs. Among these are HMOs, PPOs, and independent practice associations (IPAs). The number of outpatient surgical centers (freestanding and hospital-based) and freestanding emergency clinics has increased rapidly.

Providers have been marketing health services to businesses and the public. HMOs and PPOs, for example, seek to contract with employers to be the sole insurer for employee groups. *Capitation* has emerged as a popular form of PPS within these arrangements. Capitation is a per-member per-month fee paid in advance for a specified set of health care services. This money is given to providers up front, whether or not clients use services. The health care provider must provide care even if all of the up front fees have been used.

Medicare also is interested in capitation as a means of payment for its enrollees. In some regions, Medicare enrollees already receive care through an HMO that receives capitation payments from the federal government. The American Hospital Association projected that most Medicare clients would be covered by capitation by the early 1990s.[12] This prediction has yet to become a reality, with many HMO providers threatening to pull out of the Medicare sector because of reimbursement concerns.

Complex *oversight systems* within managed care limited the rate of cost growth through the 1990s, but this restraint did not come without costs. The public grew wary of roadblocks to receiving needed services and applied growing pressure on Congress to control HMO gatekeeping abuses. Perhaps heralding a new trend, United Health Care, (UHC) the nation's second largest health insurer, began dismantling the costly oversight structure in late 1999.[5] Physicians in UHC plans no longer need permission for client tests and admissions. Citing studies indicating the oversight cost more than it saved and disrupted coordination of care, the insurer led the way for the next phase of managed care reform.[5]

■ PERIOD OF REFORM

By 1992, the United States began to reform its health care financing system. With the election of President Clinton, a Democrat, and with continued control of Congress by the same party, passage of national health care reform legislation seemed inevitable. President Clinton introduced the Health Security Act in early 1994, after almost a year of deliberation by economists, business people, and health care providers. First Lady Hillary Rodham Clinton chaired the panel, which attempted to examine the current system's problems (access, cost, quality) to identify the national priorities, including a new emphasis on illness prevention.[23] Much controversy surrounded this ad hoc group. No representation was allowed from organized medicine or other provider organizations. Testimony was sought from these groups, but the actual crafting of the reform plan and ensuing legislation was carried out by the task force. The plan that emerged was so complex that it contained more than 100 pages in published form. The legislation that was sent to Congress was more than 1000 pages.

President Clinton's plan met opposition from within his own party as well as from outside. Everyone publicly agreed that the system needed to be reformed, but no one could agree about how much reform was needed or could be afforded. At one point in 1994, at least six different pieces of health care reform legislation were being considered by Congress. The main points of contention centered on (1) universal access and how to pay for it and (2) employer mandates, which require all employees to be covered by insurance provided by the employer. As a result of these issues and of a general lack of political support by Congress for the President, federal health care reform initiatives did not pass. In fact, no bill was moved out of committee for a vote.

The support for reform, however, did not die in Washington. A number of states passed legislation and policy directives to halt the escalation of costs and to provide increased access to services for citizens regardless of ability to pay. Tennessee led the way in 1994, when it moved all Medicaid recipients into a managed care plan, with capitation paid to managed care companies, which in turn provided a full range of health care services to recipients. Today, Tennessee is still in the forefront of state managed care reform, with 1.3 million Medicaid eligible and uninsured and uninsurable people covered.[28]

By 1996, more than one third of all Medicaid recipients nationwide were enrolled in some form of managed care. The Balanced Budget Act (BBA) of 1997 enabled states to convert to managed care without the need for a federal Medicaid waiver.[10] The law established minimum standards for Medicaid managed care contracts, added qualifying conditions for companies to participate in the program, and ensured better access and coverage for recipients.[10]

Reform also is being driven by the health care industry itself. During 1994, Columbia Health Care System, based in Dallas, acquired Hospital Corporation of America and Health Trust (HCA), both based in Nashville, to form the largest for-profit health care delivery system in the world. In addition to owning 220 hospitals, this corporation aggressively acquired primary care practices of physicians in both rural and urban areas. Using such a strategy, Columbia is creating a network of integrated delivery systems that focuses on primary care as the most desirable and least costly level of care, with secondary and tertiary care available when needed. With such a network in place in numerous markets across the United States, Columbia actively seeks managed care contracts from large employers, generally paid on a capitation basis, although discounted reimbursement mechanisms are still mixed with fee-for-service in most markets.

The response by the not-for-profit sector has varied. In some competitive markets, the not-for-profit hospitals have banded together to form their own integrated delivery systems to compete for managed care contracts. In other areas, some not-for-profits have entered into joint venture arrangements with the for-profit sector or have been purchased by large for-profit systems. This consolidation trend continued throughout the 1990s.

Since the early 1980s, the health care system has undergone rapid change. The system is still evolving, however, and the end product is difficult to foresee. Scarcity of and competition for human and financial resources are the dominant forces operating. This situation creates a dilemma with regard to social values of the past: health care as a right versus scarcity. Nurses must recognize and grapple with these forces and the dilemmas involved in shaping the nation's future health care system.

CONCLUSIONS

Our health care system is large and complex, with many stakeholders. It is also a system under considerable pressure to change as a direct result of rising costs and lower accessibility to basic care for many citizens. This is the environment in which nursing practice takes place. Nurses are in the mainstream of service to both advantaged and disadvantaged clients. Nurses play a crucial role in delivering health care. Many believe that nurses may be the key to revamping the health care system to one that provides access to basic primary care for all citizens. The contribution of the nursing profession to the nation's health has never been more important as we move into the 21st century.

BIBLIOGRAPHY

1. Abundis, J., & Rechin, K. (1999, November 18). Drug prices cheaper abroad. *USA Today*, p. 1.

2. Agency for Health Care Policy and Research. (1999). *AHCPR at a glance.* Agency for Health Care Policy and Research, U.S. Department of Health and Human Services [On-line]. Available: *http://www.ahcpr.gov/news/glance/htm.*
3. American Nurses' Association. (1991). *Agenda for health care reform.* Kansas City, MO: Author.
4. American Nurses' Association. (1999). *Legislative and regulatory initiatives for the 106th Congress.* Kansas City, MO: Author.
5. Appleby, J. (1999, November 9). Health plan eases doctor oversight. *USA Today,* p. 1.
6. Bice, T. W. (1980). Health services planning and regulation. In S. J. Williams & P. R. Torrens (Eds.), *Introduction to health services* (pp. 267–321). New York: John Wiley.
7. Blouin, A. S., & Brent, N. J. (1994). Revisiting collective bargaining. *Journal of Nursing Administration, 24*(9), 9–10, 36.
8. Campbell, P. W., & Healy, P. (1999 November, 5). House approves 15% budget increase for the NIH—but with a hitch. *Chronicle of Higher Education,* A36, 38.
9. Centers for Disease Control and Prevention. (1999). *2000 budget.* Centers for Disease Control and Prevention, U.S. Department of Health and Human Services [On-line]. Available: *http://www.cdc.gov/2000bdg/cdcbud.pdf*
10. Center for Health Policy Research. (1999). *A nationwide study of Medicaid managed care contracts* (2nd ed.). The George Washington University Medical Center [On-line]. Available: *http://www.chcs.org/oview.htm*
11. Clemen-Stone, S., Eigsti, D. G., & McGuire, S. L. (1998). Clients with long-term care needs: Home health, hospice, and other services. In S. Clemon-Stone (Ed.), *Comprehensive community health nursing* (5th ed., pp. 630–663). St. Louis: Mosby–Year Book.
12. Clemen-Stone, S., Eigsti, D. G., & McGuire, S. L. (1998). Occupational health nursing. In S. Clemon-Stone (Ed.), *Comprehensive community health nursing* (5th ed., pp. 537–566). St. Louis: Mosby–Year Book.
13. Clemen-Stone, S., Eigsti, D. G., & McGuire, S. L. (1998). U.S. health and welfare legislation and services. In S. Clemon-Stone (Ed.), *Comprehensive community health nursing* (5th ed., pp. 67–98). St. Louis: Mosby–Year Book.
14. Health Care Financing Administration. (1999). *Expenditures for health services and supplies under public programs by type of expenditure and program: Calendar year 1997.* Health Care Financing Administration, U.S. Department of Health and Human Services [On-line]. Available: *http://www.hcfa.gov/stats/nhe-oact/tables/t18.htm*
15. Health Care Financing Administration. (1999). *Highlights of the national health expenditure projections: 1997–2007.* Health Care Financing Administration, U.S. Department of Health and Human Services [On-line]. Available: *http://www.hcfa.gov/stats/nheproj/hilites/htm*
16. Health Care Financing Administration. (1999) *Highlights: National health expenditures, 1997.* Health Care Financing Administration, U.S. Department of Health and Human Services [On-line]. Available:*http://www.hcfa.gov/stats/nhe-oact/hilites/htm*
17. Huber, D. (1996). *Leadership and nursing care management.* Philadelphia: W. B. Saunders.
18. Jacobs, P. (1995). Economics of healthcare. In G. L. Deloughery (Ed.), *Issues and Trends in Nursing* (pp. 97–128). St. Louis: Mosby–Year Book.
19. Moses, E. B. (1997). *The registered nurse population: Findings from the national sample survey of RNs.* Rockville, MD: Division of Nursing, Bureau of Health Professions, Health Resources and Services Administration, Public Health Service, U.S. Department of Health and Human Services.
20. National Center for Health Statistics. (1995). *Health, United States, 1994.* Hyattsville, MD: Public Health Service, U.S. Department of Health and Human Services.
21. National Institutes of Health. (1999). *Welcome.* National Institutes of Health, U.S. Department of Health and Human Services. [On-line]. Available: *http://www.nih.gov/welcome/nihnew.htm*
22. National Institute for Nursing Research (1999). National Institute for Nursing Research, U.S. Department of Health and Human Services. [On-line]. Available: *http.//www.nih.gov/ninr/openingstatement99.htm*
23. O'Neil, E., & Coffman, J. (Eds.). (1998). *Strategies for the future of nursing.* San Francisco: Jossey-Bass.
24. Pilon, B. A., & Davis, S. (1988). Healthcare delivery cost containment practices: History, current status, future directions. In N. Sanders (Director), *Cost management education for nurses* (Contact No. 240-86-0064) Washington, DC: Division of Nursing, Bureau of Health Professions, Health Resources and Services Administration, U.S. Department of Health and Human Services.
25. Poen, M. (1979). Politics, then health: The medicare compromise. In *Harry S. Truman versus the medical lobby* (pp. 174–209). Columbia, MO: University of Missouri Press.
26. Shortell, S. M., & Kaluzny, A. D. (1997). *Essentials of health care management.* Albany, NY: Delmar.
27. Steinwald, B., & Sloan, F. (1981). Regulatory approaches to hospital cost containment: A synthesis of the empirical evidence. In M. Olsen (Ed.), *A new approach to the economics of health care* (pp. 272–307). Washington, DC: American Enterprise Institute.
28. TennCare. (1999). *TennCare fact sheet* [On-line]. Available: *http// www.state.tn.us/health/tenncare/*
29. U.S. Bureau of Health Professions. (1996). *National sample survey of registered nurses.* Washington, DC: Government Printing Office.
30. Williams, C. A. (1996). Community-based population-focused practice: The foundation of public health nursing. In M. Stanhope & J. Lancaster (Eds.), *Community health nursing: Process and practice for promoting health* (4th ed., pp. 21–33). St. Louis: Mosby–Year Book.

CHAPTER 5

Ambulatory Health Care

Sheila A. Haas
Diana P. Hackbarth

In any given year, most Americans are not hospitalized, but the average person makes 3.6 visits to ambulatory care per year.[23] This makes ambulatory settings the major site for health care delivery in the United States. Ambulatory care visits have increased for several reasons:

1. The number of hours or days people stay in hospitals for illness, surgery, or complex treatments has decreased. More clients are seen in ambulatory settings for post-hospital visits and follow-up care.
2. New technology has made ambulatory settings the site for people to undergo many surgical and complex procedures that previously required hospitalization.
3. Advances in the treatment of chronic health problems have made it possible to treat and monitor a client's progress in ambulatory care settings and to avoid costly hospitalization. As a result, both the numbers and the acuity of people cared for in ambulatory settings have increased.

There are numerous advantages to providing health care in ambulatory settings. Clients often feel less stress because they are not separated from their family, significant others, and community. Care in the community decreases exposure to nosocomial infections and other hazards of hospitalization. Ambulatory care is often less costly than hospitalization, saving money for clients, insurance companies, employers, and the government.

Socioeconomic factors have also encouraged the growth of ambulatory care. The growth of managed care organizations has increased the demand for primary care services and ambulatory facilities. Clients who are insured through a managed care plan often must see a primary care provider before obtaining referrals to specialty or hospital care. The variety of care modalities offered in ambulatory care has escalated, and the demand for professional nurses to work in ambulatory care has never been greater. The opportunities for professional nurses to work in ambulatory care settings are expected to increase in the years to come.

■ DEFINITION AND CHARACTERISTICS OF AMBULATORY CARE NURSING

Nurses have worked in ambulatory care settings for many years. Ambulatory care nurses take care of people in all age groups and with all diagnoses, both those who are healthy and those with acute, chronic, or life-threatening health problems. The definition of ambulatory nursing was developed by a panel of expert ambulatory care nurses who participated in focus groups of ambulatory care nurses across the United States.[3] The following themes arose consistently in discussions about the unique characteristics of ambulatory care nursing[3]:

- Nursing autonomy
- Client advocacy
- Skillful, rapid assessment
- Holistic nursing care
- Client teaching
- Wellness and health promotion
- Coordination and continuity of care
- Long-term relationships with clients and families
- Telephone triage, instruction, and advice
- Client and family control as major caregivers, users of the health care system, and decision-makers regarding compliance with care regimen
- Collaboration with other health care providers
- Case management

Based on these themes, the American Academy of Ambulatory Care Nursing (AAACN)[1, 3] defined ambulatory care nursing as follows:

> Professional ambulatory care nursing includes those clinical, management, educational, and research activities provided by registered nurses for and with individuals who seek care for health-related problems or concerns or seek assistance with health maintenance and/or health promotion. These individuals engage predominantly in self-care and self-managed health activities or receive care from family and significant others outside an institutional setting.
>
> Ambulatory care nursing services are episodic, less than 24 hours in duration, and occur as a single encounter or a series of encounters over days, weeks, months, or years. Ambulatory nurse-patient encounters take place in health care facilities as well as in community-based settings, including schools, workplaces, or homes.
>
> They occur as personal visits or as encounters using the telephone and other communication devices. Ambulatory care nursing services focus on cost-effective ways to maximize wellness; prevent illness, disability, and disease; minimize symptoms of acute minor aliments; and support patients in the management of chronic disease to affect more positive health states throughout the life span up to and including a peaceful death.

Challenges are an inherent characteristic of ambulatory care nursing:

1. *Visit encounters are short,* the number of client visits per day is great, and the assessment time is compressed. In contrast to the hospital nurse, who can return to a client confined to bed to retrieve data that may have been missed, the ambulatory care nurse who misses collecting data may not be able to obtain it until the next visit. Because visits are short, the ambulatory care nurse cannot do an extensive assessment on every client but must do a focused assessment. This aspect is often a difficult transition for nurses who have worked in hospital settings.
2. Control of care and treatment modalities is in the hands of the *client and family,* not the *health care provider.* In the hospital, the nurse administers medications, administers the treatments, or supervises others providing care to the client. In ambulatory care, however, the client chooses to schedule a visit, keep an appointment, take prescribed medications, or undergo treatments as he or she sees fit. The nurse must become a teacher, coach, and advocate as well as a treatment provider because clients and families must follow through with the treatment plan on their own between visits.
3. In ambulatory care, many members of the health care team work together, and their roles always do not have clear boundaries. Nurses must be strong communicators and collaborators, often functioning as a team leader or team facilitator.
4. In ambulatory care, contacts with the nurse are often maintained through *communication devices* such as the telephone and computer. Ambulatory care nurses need highly developed assessment and communication skills, as well as critical thinking and judgment, in order to interpret data and to refer the client for appropriate follow-up.

Finally, there is *constant pressure* to increase efficiency and effectiveness of care. Nurses are working to standardize care so that health promotion, disease prevention, and early detection and treatment of health problems will be integral to the ambulatory care client encounter.[3]

Conceptual Models That Influence Ambulatory Care Nursing Practice

■ THE CLINICAL MODEL

The organization of ambulatory care services in the United States is based on a complex mix of historical, philosophical, political, and economic factors. The way in which policy-makers, health care providers, and ordinary citizens conceptualize health and disease has a profound effect on how health care is delivered.

Most health policy experts agree that our current health care system is based on the clinical or medical model.[6, 22, 24] In this model, health is conceptualized as the absence of the signs or symptoms of disease.[25] It is assumed that the body is a machine and that modern medical technology can employ physical and chemical interventions to "fix the machine" whenever it is broken.[22] This has led to great emphasis on expensive, acute care with high-technology treatments and relatively little attention to prevention, public health, environmental measures, or personal responsibility for health.

Most ambulatory care services, except for certain public health programs in the community, are outgrowths of this clinical model. Services were traditionally organized around physicians' delivery of reimbursable clinical model care to people who sought care only when they were ill. The traditional nursing role in ambulatory care supported physician control and the clinical model of care delivery. Although the clinical model has led to great advances in scientific medicine and technology, the focus on body parts rather than the whole and the lack of emphasis on prevention have been problematic.

Many nurse theorists, primary care providers, and public health advocates look at health in a *holistic* way. Nurses are educated to (1) consider the whole person, family, and environment; (2) to address both actual and potential health problems; and (3) to emphasize health teaching, prevention, and self-care as well as care of the sick. Newer, more holistic conceptual models are becoming increasingly important in ambulatory care. These models have been delineated by health care scholars, national and international health advocacy organizations, and ambulatory care nurses themselves.

■ LEVELS OF PREVENTION MODEL

The Levels of Prevention Model, advocated by Leavell and Clark in 1965,[20] has influenced both public health practice and ambulatory care delivery worldwide. This model suggests that the natural history of any disease exists on a continuum, with health at one end and advanced disease at the other. The model delineates three levels of the application of preventive measures that can be used to arrest the disease process at different points along the continuum.[20] The goal is to maintain a healthy state and to prevent disease or injury.

People experiencing acute or chronic disease, as well as healthy populations, are all candidates for primary prevention measures. The Levels of Prevention Model is appropriate in all health care settings and in any population group. The *Healthy People 2010 Objectives for the Nation* includes objectives at all three levels of prevention.[29] Most of these objectives can be implemented in ambulatory settings.

Primary Prevention. Primary prevention encompasses both health promotion and specific protection.[20] Health promotion includes interventions such as health education, information on growth and development, nutrition, and exercise as well as the provision of adequate housing, safe working conditions, and other services. For example, an ambulatory care nurse might provide telephone consultation and teaching to a new mother concerned about well baby care.

Specific protection interventions are targeted at specific health risks, injuries, or diseases. For example, immunizations protect against particular infectious diseases; seat belts reduce injuries in auto crashes; smoking cessation reduces the risk of cancers and heart disease; reducing air pollution prevents exacerbations of asthma and bronchitis; encouraging a high-calcium diet with over-the-counter calcium supplements and weight-bearing exercise helps menopausal women prevent osteoporosis. Primary prevention interventions may be targeted at individual clients, families, groups, communities or populations.

SECONDARY PREVENTION. Secondary preventive measures include early diagnosis and prompt treatment as well as disability limitation.[20] Case finding, screening, and treatment of disease by medical or surgical interventions to arrest the disease process and prevent further complications are all part of secondary prevention. An ambulatory care nurse carrying out a multiphasic health screening for hypertension, diabetes, and hypercholesterolemia would be practicing secondary prevention. Other examples are administering chemotherapy to a client with cancer and positioning a client in the recovery room after outpatient surgery to ensure proper alignment of the extremities.

TERTIARY PREVENTION. Tertiary prevention is the provision of measures to rehabilitate a person or groups so they can maximize their remaining capacities.[20] Cardiac rehabilitation nurses, physical and occupational therapists, and many home care nurses focus on tertiary prevention. An example in the ambulatory surgery recovery room would be teaching crutch walking to a client after foot surgery.

■ PRIMARY HEALTH CARE, PRIMARY CARE, AND MANAGED CARE MODELS

Primary health care focuses on the universal right to basic health care. *Primary care* focuses on integrated care coordinated by one primary provider. *Managed care* approaches the use of health care services from a cost-containment perspective. *Primary prevention* is often confused with the concepts of primary health care and primary care.[14] In addition, many managed care organizations use primary care providers, such as family practice physicians and nurse practitioners, in a "gatekeeper" function, causing further confusion. Box 5–1 compares and contrasts these conceptual models. They, as well as the clinical model and the ambulatory care nursing conceptual framework, have influenced the organization of practice in ambulatory care settings.

AMBULATORY CARE NURSING CONCEPTUAL FRAMEWORK

The Ambulatory Care Nursing Conceptual Framework was developed by a think tank of experts who are also members of the AAACN.[7] The AAACN member experts

BOX 5–1 Prevention and Health Care Models

Primary Prevention

- Includes health promotion and specific protection
- May be directed at individuals, groups, or populations
- May be targeted at well or ill populations
- Goal: to prevent disease or injury and to reduce risk factors
- Includes individual lifestyle changes as well as healthy environments and positive social change
  - Education
  - Legislation
  - Regulation
  - Taxation
  - Health policy
  - Risk reduction and lifestyle change
- *Healthy People 2010* goals: primary prevention

Primary Care

- IOM definition (1994)[17]: "provision of integrated accessible health care services by clinicians who are accountable for addressing a large majority of personal health care needs, developing a sustained partnership with patients, and practicing in the context of family and community.
- IOM definition (1978)[18]: personal health care services that are accessible, comprehensive, coordinated, and continuous. Care delivered by accountable providers of personal health services.
- Starfield definition (1992)[26]:
  - First contact—source of care available in a timely manner
  - Longitudinal—not episodic, focused on person not episode of disease; client sees provider as regular source of care
  - Comprehensive—includes services for common problems
  - Coordinated—provider coordinates care when client is sent elsewhere for referrals, procedures, and therapies

Primary Health Care

- WHO definition (1978)[31]: "essential health care—made universally accessible to individuals and families in the community through their full participation and at a cost the community and country can afford"
  - Assumes community involvement
  - Includes both personal health care services and population-based public health services
  - Aimed at prevention as well as treatment of disease
  - Aimed at improving health status of the population or community

Managed Care

- Enthoven definition (1993)[5]:
  - Integrated financing and delivery systems with per capita prepayment and with providers placed at risk for cost and quality of care
  - First contact—ensure access to basic services; restrict access to specialized services through "gatekeeper" function of primary provider
- Starfield definition (1992)[26]:
  - Longitudinal—not addressed
  - Comprehensive—not addressed
  - Coordinated—gatekeeper as coordinator; goal is to eliminate unnecessary and inappropriate care; may also restrict access to appropriate care
  - Reduction in cost; cost containment
  - Health status of population—not addressed; in HMO organizations, goal is to keep enrolled population healthy in order to reduce utilization cost

IOM, Institute of Medicine; WHO, World Health Organization.

work in ambulatory care settings, perform research, and write about ambulatory care nursing. A conceptual framework is a diagram that:

- Specifies major concepts, skills, and responsibilities in an area of practice
- Reflects values and beliefs as well as the experiential knowledge of a practice discipline
- Delineates the relationships between major concepts and skills
- Acts as a model to help organize practice, guide the development of educational materials, create test items for certification examinations, and develop orientation programs
- Forms the basis of performance appraisal instruments for ambulatory care

The conceptual framework shown in Figure 5–1 delineates three roles for ambulatory care nurses: (1) the Clinical Nursing Role, (2) the Organizational/Systems Role, and (3) the Professional Role.[7] Each role has several dimensions that vary, depending on the size of the ambulatory care setting. For example, staff nurses working in larger settings, where there are multiple nurses and nurse managers, do not need to do many of the more managerial dimensions under the Organizational/Systems Role. In smaller settings, they would likely practice in all three roles. The Ambulatory Care Nursing Conceptual Framework was used to structure the Ambulatory Care Nursing Core Curriculum written for nurses to use in preparation for certification in ambulatory care.

As seen in Figure 5–1, client populations may be healthy, acutely ill, chronically ill, or terminally ill. Role dimensions highly valued by nurses are all included in this conceptual framework:

- Primary, secondary, and tertiary prevention
- Teaching and client advocacy
- Care management, a feature of primary care
- Evidence-based practice

AMBULATORY CARE PRACTICE SETTINGS

Historically, health services in the United States were delivered to people in their homes by itinerant physicians,

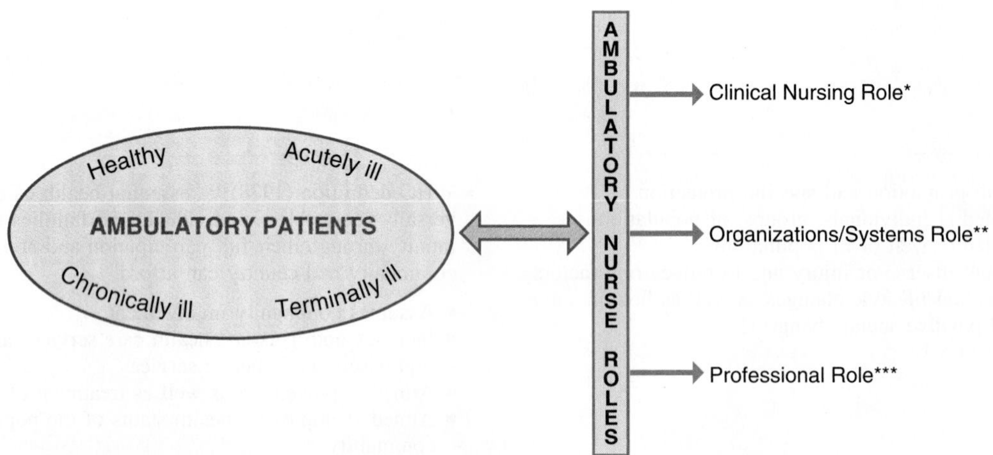

***Clinical Nursing Role**
Patient Education
Advocacy (compassion, caring, emotional support)
Care Management
Assessment, Screening, Triage
Telephone Practice
Collaboration/Resource Identification and Referral
Clinical Procedures, Independent/Interdependent/Dependent
Primary, Secondary, and Tertiary Prevention
Communication/Documentation
Outcome Management
Protocol Development/Usage

****Organizations/Systems Role**
Practice/Office Support
Healthcare Fiscal Management (reimbursement and coding)
Collaboration/Conflict Management
Informatics
Context of Care Delivery/Models
Care of the Caregiver
Priority Management/Delegation/Supervision
Ambulatory Culture/Cross Cultural Competencies
Ongoing Political/Entrepreneurial Skills
Structuring Customer-focused Systems
Workplace Regulatory Compliance (EEOC, OSHA)
Advocacy Inter-organizational and in Community
Legal Issues

*****Professional Role**
Evidence-based Practice
Leadership Inquiry and Research Utilization
Clinical Quality improvement
Staff Development
Regulatory Compliance (risk management)
Provider Self-Care

FIGURE 5–1 Ambulatory Care Nursing Conceptual Framework. (Modified from Haas, S. [1998]. Ambulatory care nursing conceptual framework. *AAACN Viewpoint, 20*[3], 16–17.) Reprinted with permission of publisher.

midwives, barbers, nurses, and "medicine men," who learned their trade through an unregulated apprentice system. In some urban areas, freestanding dispensaries were established as charity for the poor and a place for would-be physicians to learn their trade.[27] These dispensaries dissolved into outpatient departments once a system of voluntary hospitals was developed and nursing and medical education was upgraded and standardized in the beginning of the 20th century.[27]

For the purposes of data collection, the National Center for Health Statistics classifies ambulatory care settings into three main groups: physician offices, hospital outpatient departments, and hospital emergency departments.[23] Each of these may sponsor many types of ambulatory care programs, both on-site and geographically dispersed in communities. With the advent of managed care insurance plans, health maintenance organizations (HMOs) and preferred provider organizations (PPOs) have grown in importance as both sites and financiers of ambulatory care delivery.

Physician Group Practices. Almost 82% of all ambulatory care visits occur in physicians' offices.[23] Physician group practices arose out of the perceived need to enhance services offered to clients and to provide for more equal distribution of work among physicians. Increasingly, physicians are abandoning solo practice and aligning themselves in group practices in order to consolidate resources to meet the challenges of managed care contracting. In the past, many group practices consisted of groups of specialists, such as cardiologists or oncologists; today, larger group practices now seek to add primary care physicians.

Physician group practices usually operate on a for-profit basis and seek fee-for-service payment. In a *fee-for-service* system, providers generate more revenue the more services they provide. *Integrated* delivery systems have been developed in which hospitals align with several physician group practices to increase the hospital referral rate and provide increased coordination of care. Many physician group practices also contract with HMOs and PPOs and offer either reduced rate fee-for-service or *capitated* (prepaid at a fixed rate) services along with their traditional fee-for-service practices.

The predominant way of viewing health and disease in most physician group practices is the *clinical model.* However, family practice physicians may adhere to the *primary care model.* In the past, nurses in physician offices often served a clerical as well as an assistive function. The role of the ambulatory care nurse in physician group practices is evolving to meet the need for increasingly skilled technical services, especially in specialty practices such as oncology, freestanding birthing centers, and surgical centers.

Community Hospital Outpatient Departments. Community hospital clinic services began in the latter part of the 19th century and took over the functions of the freestanding dispensaries.[27] Clinic services were consistent with the mission of the religious and ethnic groups that organized voluntary community hospitals. This mission included both a charitable function for the community and a place for local physicians to practice.[6] Physicians were often assigned to staff hospital clinics as a duty, in return for the privilege of hospitalizing their clients.[19, 24] Nurses trained in diploma schools staffed both the hospital and clinics.

Today, nonprofit community hospitals still provide varying amounts of uncompensated care in their outpatient departments as part of their obligation to provide "community benefits" as not-for-profit corporations. However, their goal is to maximize revenues by attracting individuals or employee groups who have insurance coverage. Thus, outpatient services constitute a key source of revenue for hospitals.

Both primary care and specialized care in a clinical model may be offered. Ambulatory services may be housed adjacent to the hospital or be freestanding in the community. Services may include outpatient surgery, emergency centers, cardiac rehabilitation centers, drug and alcohol treatment programs, mobile vans, women's health or breast centers, work site health promotion, oncology centers, home care, hospice, and community health promotion.[24] Many integrated health care systems have freestanding satellite ambulatory care sites that offer primary care services for managed care enrollees. Specialized clinics and health promotion programs staffed by nurses also exist in community hospital outpatient settings. Some of these programs are organized around the ambulatory care nursing conceptual framework.

Teaching Hospital Outpatient Departments. Outpatient departments of teaching hospitals were developed to fulfill the mission of academic health centers: to provide medical and other health professional education, biomedical research, and client care services.[4] University hospital outpatient departments and most large hospitals run by local governments provide learning experiences for medical, nursing, and other health science students as well as opportunities for clinical research on populations of patients with highly specialized needs. Veterans Administration ambulatory care departments serve a similar function.

Clinical services are often organized around medical specialty areas for the convenience of providers. Some are regional referral centers, whereas others, especially those that are tax-supported, may provide a full range of services, including primary care for the poor.[24] Most teaching hospitals maintain a nonprofit status and provide care for those with public or private insurance as well as uncompensated care for uninsured clients (whose diseases may provide good learning experiences). Many hospitals have satellite ambulatory care centers. With the growth of managed care, increased competition, and decreased reimbursement from Medicaid and Medicare, teaching hospitals are increasingly concerned with maximizing revenue from insured clients and ensuring a flow of paying clients to make up for empty inpatient beds.

University hospital outpatient departments have traditionally espoused the clinical model and have been driven and controlled by physicians. There are, however, some nurse-managed hospital clinics that deal with specific client populations, such as clients with chronic leg ulcers or those who need monitoring of warfarin (Coumadin) therapy. Nurses play a major role in patient and family teaching and as case managers for clients with catastrophic and chronic illnesses. For example, nurses case manage the care of heart transplant clients, trauma victims, oncology clients, and high-risk mothers and infants.

Health Maintenance Organizations. HMOs began more than 50 years ago and proliferated during the 1990s in response to both federal enabling legislation and market forces. HMOs provide a defined population with a stated range of services through the prepayment of an annual or monthly capitation fee. With *capitation,* providers receive the same amount of money per patient per month, no matter how many or how few services a client uses that month or year. Thus, there is no incentive to provide expensive tests or treatments that the client may not need. HMOs are systems of care that integrate the insurance and payment mechanisms and the actual delivery of health care services.

HMOs began as nonprofit organizations but increasingly have been purchased by the for-profit sector. Philosophically, the concept of an HMO differs from traditional ambulatory services, in that value is placed on prevention and maintaining health in order to avoid more costly specialist or inpatient services. Care is coordinated by a primary care provider who acts as a gatekeeper. The goal is to lower costs through the provision of primary care, coordination of services, utilization management, and elimination of the "incentives" of the fee-for-service payment system.

Many HMOs employ nurse practitioners, nurse-midwives, and physician assistants as primary care providers. In addition to the clinical model, HMOs espouse wellness, health maintenance, and primary care. Nursing, with its more holistic approach to client care, can play an influential role in managed care settings.

Emergency Departments. Almost 10% of ambulatory care visits are provided in emergency departments (EDs).[23] Although some of these visits are for true emergency conditions, more than half of ED visits in the United States are for non-urgent care.[21] Uninsured people and those on Medicare and Medicaid use disproportionately more ED services for non-urgent care than those who have private insurance.[23] In the United States, there are 45 million uninsured and underinsured people who lack access to appropriate primary care services in their communities.[24] Because EDs are organized according to the clinical model and are set up to meet acute care needs, they are far from the ideal place to provide primary care services.

Other Ambulatory Care Settings. Many other settings provide a wide array of ambulatory care services. One unique type of ambulatory care organization is a Nurse-Managed Center or Nursing Center. These nurse-staffed community centers may provide primary health care services, home care, hospice, college health services, work site health promotion, school nursing, or wellness services. Many Nursing Centers were developed by schools of nursing as faculty practice sites and clinical sites for undergraduate and graduate students. Others were federally funded demonstration projects. Most Nurse-Managed Centers employ Advanced Practice Nurses (APNs) and are organized around a nursing or primary health care model.

Other settings in which ambulatory care nurses practice include government-funded public health clinics, migrant and community health centers, homeless shelters, school-based health centers, Native American Health Service clinics, and other community-based organizations that serve special population groups. These are either tax-supported or private nonprofit organizations and are organized around a primary health care or public health model. Most include population-based preventive services as well as personal health care.

CHARACTERISTICS OF AMBULATORY CARE CLIENT POPULATION

Each year in the United States, people make more than 960 million ambulatory visits. Women make more visits than men, and older adults make an average 7.5 visits a year, compared with about three visits a year for children.[23] The overall visit rate for whites is not significantly different than that for African Americans.[23] Figure 5–2 shows the distribution of ambulatory care visits, categorized by clients' expressed reasons for the visit. Figure 5–3 depicts the distribution of ambulatory care visits by primary diagnosis in the United States in 1997. Difficulty breathing, a manifestation of many problems including lung, heart, and allergic conditions, is a common reason for visits.

Ambulatory clients are often classified by their *health status.* A client may be essentially healthy but acutely ill at the time of the visit, such as a client with otitis media or appendicitis. The client can be expected to return to wellness once the acute problem is cured. Another client may be chronically ill but managing the chronic illness well. A young asthmatic person with peak flow readings within normal limits is an example. A client may be chronically ill and have an acute episode, such as an elderly diabetic client with influenza. Finally, a client may be terminally ill with end-stage renal disease or liver failure and require supportive care.

Ambulatory clients may also be classified by a major *illness,* body system, and typical *treatment* needed. For example, teaching hospital outpatient settings often have specific clinics for people with diabetes or heart failure; some have ear, nose, and throat (ENT) clinics or urology clinics for people with maladies of certain body systems; and others have programs such as a "Coumadin clinic" and "cast clinic," which classify clients according to the type of treatment to be administered.

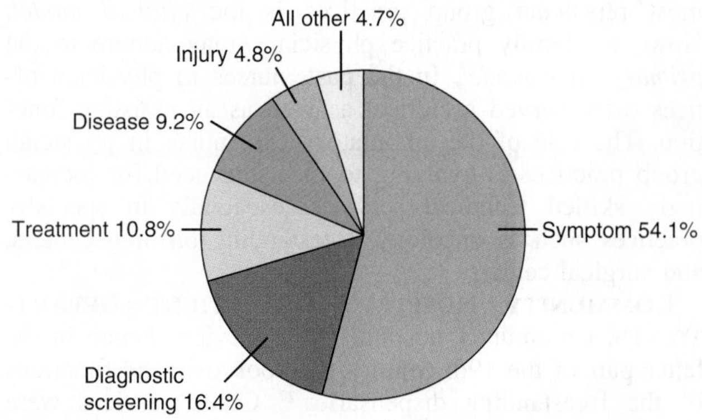

FIGURE 5–2 Per cent distribution of ambulatory care visits by patients' expressed reason for visit: United States, 1997. (From National Center for Health Statistics. [1999]. *Ambulatory care statistics: United States, 1997.* Hyattsville, MD: Centers for Disease Control and Prevention, National Center for Health Statistics.)

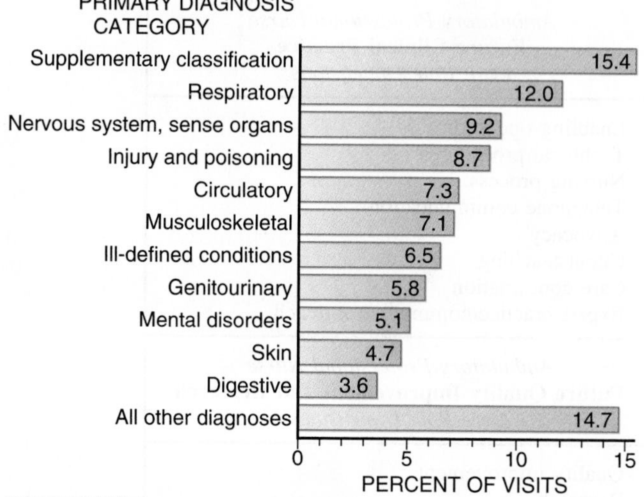

FIGURE 5–3 Per cent distribution of ambulatory care visits by primary diagnosis category: United States, 1997. The category "supplementary classification" is used for diagnoses not related to illness or injury, such as general medical examinations and normal prenatal care. (From National Center for Health Statistics. [1999]. *Ambulatory care statistics: United States, 1997.* Hyattsville, MD: Centers for Disease Control and Prevention, National Center for Health Statistics.)

Ambulatory clients may also be classified in terms of *age,* such as pediatric, adolescent, and geriatric.

Another means of categorizing clients is by the type or source of *reimbursement* for the care provided; (e.g., private insurance, Medicare, Medicaid, worker's compensation, or self-pay). Ambulatory care clients also may be defined by the type of *service,* such as primary care, which includes pediatrics, obstetrics and gynecology, family practice, and internal medicine.

As mentioned previously, in ambulatory care it is the client, client's family, or significant other who initiates an encounter or visit, travels to and from the ambulatory care setting, and chooses to collaborate with the ambulatory interdisciplinary team regarding wellness behaviors and the treatment regimen. Thus, the ambulatory care team must know, understand, and respect the client's culture, traditions, and perspective on health and illness. Cultural competence is essential, because the client, family, or significant other manages and provides health care during visits and during the interval between visits and the client controls health care decisions. Respectful communication facilitates the long-term relationships that clients often have with ambulatory care nurses and other providers.

RESEARCH IN AMBULATORY CARE NURSING

Although nurses have been working in ambulatory settings for many years, little research on the work and role of ambulatory care nurses has been done. Such research is needed for many reasons[15]:

- To help develop new models of nursing care delivery
- To delineate position descriptions for nurses working in ambulatory care
- To develop standards of client care and professional nursing practice
- To create both performance improvement programs and nursing intensity systems to determine the number and types of nursing personnel needed.[15]

One of the earliest studies, done by Hooks and colleagues in 1980,[16] delineated barriers to ambulatory nursing practice. Verran, in 1981,[30] developed seven areas of nursing responsibility in ambulatory care using a Delphi method and the opinion of expert ambulatory care nurses. Tighe and associates,[28] in 1985, further refined Verran's areas of responsibility by adding planning. In 1995, Hackbarth and co-workers[15] and Haas and colleagues[10–13] conducted a national survey of ambulatory care nurses working in many types of ambulatory care settings. An analysis of these data provided insight into the dimensions of the current staff nurse role and the dimensions of the future staff nurse role in ambulatory care.

In current practice, Hackbarth and co-workers[15] found that ambulatory care nurses spent much of their time performing activities in dimensions named Enabling Operations and Technical Procedures. These activities include locating records, ordering supplies, taking vital signs, setting up rooms, assisting with procedures, and administering oral or intramuscular (IM) medications. Some of these activities could have been done by clerks or nursing assistants. Relatively less of the staff nurses' time was spent on more professional activities in the dimensions named Telephone Communication, Advocacy, Teaching, and Care Coordination.

When nurses surveyed by Haas and Hackbarth[12] were asked what they would like to be doing in the future, they indicated that they would prefer to accomplish more activities in higher-level professional dimensions such as Teaching, Care Coordination, and Expert Practice. They even foresaw another dimension, labeled High Tech Procedures (Fig. 5–4). The implications of this research are clear. Nurses in many ambulatory settings need to have sufficient numbers of competent assistive personnel to whom they can delegate Enabling and Technical procedures if they are to have sufficient time to perform activities in higher-level dimensions such as Teaching, Advocacy, Care Coordination, High Tech Procedures, and Expert Practice.

DIMENSIONS UNIQUE TO NURSING PRACTICE IN AMBULATORY CARE

TELEPHONE NURSING PRACTICE. One dimension of the professional nurse's role that is unique in ambulatory care settings is Telephone Communication, or Telephone Nursing Practice. Telephone Nursing Practice is defined as "nursing practice using the nursing process to provide care for individual patients or defined patient populations over the telephone."[2] Defined criteria include:

- Using protocols, algorithms, or guidelines to assess and address client needs systematically
- Prioritizing the urgency of client needs
- Developing a collaborative plan of care with clients and their support systems, including wellness promotion, prevention education, advice, care counseling, disease state management, and care coordination
- Evaluating outcomes of practice and care

Ambulatory Professional Nurse **Current Clinical Practice** *Core Role Dimensions*	*Ambulatory Professional Nurse* **Future Clinical Practice** *Core Role Dimensions*
Enabling operations Technical procedures Nursing process Telephone communication Advocacy Teaching Care coordination Expert practice within setting	Enabling operations Technical procedures Nursing process Telephone communication Advocacy Client teaching Care coordination Expert practice/community outreach
Ambulatory Professional Nurse **Current Quality Improvement and Research** *Core Role Dimensions*	*Ambulatory Professional Nurse* **Future Quality Improvement and Research** *Core Role Dimensions*
Quality improvement Research Continuing education	Quality improvement Research Continuing education

FIGURE 5–4 Current and future ambulatory professional nurse role dimensions. (Data from Haas, S. A., & Hackbarth, D. P. [1995]. *Nursing Economics, 13*[4], 230–241; and Hackbarth, D. P., et al. [1995]. *Nursing Economics, 13*[2], 89–98.)

Telephone Nursing Practice is not new and has been described in the literature since the 1960s. Communication by telephone for health guidance is common in pediatric practices, obstetrics and gynecology practices, primary care, and the ED. Clients often call ambulatory care settings to report symptoms of illness and to seek advice. A 1997 document published by the AAACN identifies standards that define the responsibilities of both clinical nurses and managers when providing care via the telephone.[3]

The *Nursing Intervention Classification* (NIC) lists four telephone nursing practices:

- Telephone consultation
- Telephone follow-up
- Telephone triage
- Telephone surveillance

Each of these interventions was proposed by Haas and Androwich in 1999.[8]

1. *Telephone consultation.* The nurse assesses the client's need and readiness to learn, teaches clients, and provides advice based on protocols approved for use with telephone nursing practice. Assessing a client by telephone is far more difficult for the nurse than a face-to-face meeting with a client. The nurse must have expert communication skills to elicit information when no visual or physical assessment cues are available. The nurse must listen for nuances in the client's communication, such as inflection, pitch, volume, and rate of speech. The telephone encounter time is very limited. There is no time to reflect or have second thoughts. Although telephone assessment has some pitfalls, there are some benefits too (see later).
2. *Telephone follow-up* is used for clients who have had ambulatory surgery or complex treatments. The nurse calls the client within a specified period to assess how well the client is recovering and to provide guidance for any problems. Especially when the nurse is calling the client, the nurse must protect the confidentiality of the client and should speak with family members or significant others only if the client has given permission. Many clients appreciate telephone follow-up. It connotes caring and concern on the part of the nurse and the ambulatory care organization, and it gives the client ready access to a health professional.
3. With *telephone triage,* clients are sorted by telephone encounter based on the immediacy of the need and the type of problem. In ambulatory care, a nurse talks with a client calling from home and assesses the type of problem, how the problem should be resolved, how soon, whether the client should be seen in person, and who should resolve the problem.
4. Nurses use *telephone surveillance* to work with data coming into a central ambulatory site from monitoring equipment used by clients at home. For example, cardiac monitoring or high-risk obstetric monitoring can be accomplished by connecting the monitoring equipment to a computer or telephone in the client's home.

Telephone triage and telephone consultation by nurses has increased with the growth of managed care health insurance plans. Nurses use commercially available protocols or protocols that have been developed by physicians and nurses in their own ambulatory care organization to assess the client over the telephone and to recommend approved interventions. Nurse telephone consultation and telephone triage have some advantages. They make nurses and expert health advice readily available; they may save a trip to the ambulatory care site; and for many clients, they provide a knowledgeable and caring person to ask about a problem.

Professional nurses have stated strongly that Telephone Nursing Practice should be part of the professional nurse role.[3] It should not be done by Licensed Practical Nurses (LPNs) or assistive personnel such as receptionists or schedulers. It requires critical thinking and judgment as well as assessment and evaluation skills. Nurses need to attend educational programs designed to help them develop the knowledge and skills needed to practice these techniques effectively. Every telephone encounter should be documented on the client's medical record, including assessment data, analysis, recommendations made to the client, and the client's level of understanding of instructions, (e.g., when to come in or to call back).

Expert Practice Within the Setting. Another unique dimension of the current clinical nurse role in ambulatory care is Expert Practice Within the Setting. Ambulatory care nurses who develop expertise with specific client populations often are in charge of nurse-run clinics such as incontinence clinics, Coumadin clinics, or wound care clinics. In a nurse-run clinic, a nurse with at least a Bachelor's Degree in Nursing, plus experience and continuing education, works with physicians to develop protocols. Nurses monitor clients during ambulatory visits and suggest interventions for common problems that clients experience.

Nurses and clients express high levels of satisfaction with nurse-run ambulatory programs. Clients have a nurse they can call who knows them and their problems and who has insight into what works for them. The nurse often acts as their advocate in the health care system. Nurses find this type of work rewarding because they have long-term relationships with clients and families and can see the results of their teaching, advocacy, and nursing interventions.

■ AMBULATORY CARE INTERDISCIPLINARY TEAM

Nurses working in ambulatory settings are members of an interdisciplinary team. They work collaboratively with physicians; midlevel providers, such as Nurse-Practitioners (NPs), nurse-midwives, or Physician Assistants (PAs); LPNs or Licensed Vocational Nurses (LVNs); medical assistants (MAs); Nurse Assistants (NAs); and clerks, receptionists, and schedulers.

The challenges in working with a large team are numerous. Roles often are blurred, especially when people have worked together in the same clinic for many years. Sometimes team members may be asked to perform beyond their legal scope of practice; at other times, nurses may do assistive or clerical work. Both situations can prevent clients from receiving care from the best prepared provider. Nurses must continually negotiate and advocate for clients within and beyond the team.

Nurses must also delegate appropriately to assistive workers. Nurses must be aware of the specifications of their state Nurse Practice Act and delegate to LPNs or LVNs only what is legally within their scope of practice. For example, MAs in some states may administer immunizations when they have the requisite training and when they are supervised by licensed professional nurses or physicians; in other states, this might be illegal. Supervision in ambulatory care is challenging.[9] State Nurse Practice Acts often legally define both the delegation and the supervision to be done by professional nurses.

Professional and Legal Considerations

Standards of Care

Standards are written authoritative statements developed and disseminated by a professional organizational or governmental or regulatory agency by which the quality of practice, services, research, or education can be judged.[1] In 1987, the AAACN developed Ambulatory Care Nursing Administration and Practice Standards. These have been revised and updated periodically, most recently in 2000.[1] There are nine standards: Structure and Organization of Ambulatory Care Nursing, Staffing in Ambulatory Care, Competency, Ambulatory Nursing Practice, Continuity of Care, Ethics and Patient's Rights, Environment, Research, and Quality Management. AAACN also developed and published the Telephone Nursing Practice Administration and Practice Standards in 1997.[2]

Ambulatory care nurses are also guided by other sets of standards. To provide services, an ambulatory care setting must be in compliance with each state's Department of Health rules and regulations and must operate in compliance with Occupational Safety and Health Administration (OSHA) standards. Evidence-based practice standards are available through the Agency for Health Care Research and Quality (AHRQ), which has standards for many common health problems such as chronic pain, incontinence care, depression, and sickle cell anemia. These are available on the World Wide Web at *http://www.ahcpr.gov*. Professional nursing organizations, such as the American Nurses' Association (ANA) and Oncology Nurses Society (ONS), also have specific patient population standards.

Competence

Competence is the "demonstrated knowledge, skills, and ability to effectively carry out the requirements of a given role. Nurse competence is circumscribed by the individual nurse's education, knowledge, certification, experience and abilities."[3] Ambulatory care nurses demonstrate competence in core clinical practice dimensions, such as client teaching. They also have competencies that reflect the unique clinical dimensions of ambulatory care nursing, such as telephone nursing, and that correspond to the needs of the particular client populations served and the nursing interventions commonly required by such populations. For example, ambulatory oncology clients are a specific population for whom competence with chemotherapy administration is a requisite nursing intervention competence. Ambulatory care nurses who work in smaller ambulatory settings may also be required to exhibit competencies in dimensions within the leadership role, such as regulatory compliance and risk management. Any nurse who works with assistive personnel must be competent in delegation and supervision.

Certification

Holding certification in a specialty practice area such as ambulatory care nursing is a way of demonstrating competence to consumers and colleagues. To obtain certification, practicing nurses prepare for and take an examination that is developed by a panel of experts and administered by a recognized certification agency. With increasing numbers of nurses practicing in ambulatory care and the evolution of the Ambulatory Care Nursing Conceptual Framework,[7] the AAACN and the American Nurses Credentialing Center (ANCC) service have developed a certification examination for nurses working in staff nursing positions in ambulatory care. The examination was administered for the first time in the fall of 1999.

To qualify for the examination, ambulatory care nurses must have a Baccalaureate degree in nursing and meet the requirement for hours of experience in ambulatory care nursing. To maintain certification, ambulatory nurses must continue to practice in the clinical area for the specified number of hours per year and attend a specified number of hours of sanctioned continuing education. Ambulatory care nurses are often certified in more than one area of specialty nursing practice. A nurse working with oncology clients might be certified in oncology nursing as well as ambulatory care nursing. AAACN has led the development of the Ambulatory Care Nursing Conceptual Framework, core curriculum, and ambulatory certification. AAACN Web site address is *http://www.inurse.com* and the e-mail address is *aaacn@ajj.com.*

REGULATORY COMPLIANCE

Ambulatory settings must be licensed in the state in which they are located; they may earn and maintain credentials, such as accreditation by a national association like the Joint Commission on Accreditation of Healthcare Organizations (JCAHO). Accreditation offers the opportunity for an organization to be evaluated by an external group that assesses the quality of care provided. Accreditation demonstrates compliance with a uniform set of standards; it allows comparisons with other organizations and enhances the organization's competitive edge.

Three accreditation agencies publish standards and offer external validation of quality of care for ambulatory care organizations:

1. JCAHO serves hospital-affiliated ambulatory care organizations as well as freestanding ambulatory care settings.
2. The National Committee for Quality Assurance (NCQA) serves managed care organizations and uses the Health Plan Employer Data and Information Set (HEDIS) Report Cards.
3. The Accreditation Association for Ambulatory Health Care (AAAHC) serves freestanding ambulatory surgery centers, medical group practices, student health centers, and office-based surgeons' practices.

All accreditation organizations use standards developed by the accreditation organization and on-site surveys done by teams of experts.

MULTI-STATE LICENSURE

Multi-state licensure is an issue that has emerged because (1) there are increasing numbers of national health care systems, (2) telephone nursing practice is more common, and (3) people are more mobile in seeking care. The legal authority for practice is a concern for any professional nurse who provides care for people located in a state in which the nurse is not licensed. Examples of nurses who must be concerned about multi-state licensure are (1) nurses working in integrated delivery systems and regional referral health care systems in which people come in for care from other states; (2) flight nurses; and (3) telephone practice nurses. If a nurse cares for a client by telephone, computer, or monitoring device and the client is located in a state where the nurse is not licensed, the nurse faces the risk of being cited for practicing without a license in the client's home state.

The *Mutual Recognition Model,* implemented through an *Interstate Compact,* has been recognized as the preferred model of nurse licensure. The National Council of State Boards of Nursing (NCSBN) has been working to educate nurses about the Interstate Compact. Information is available on their Web site at *http://www.ncsbn.org.* The Interstate Compact is a legal document that must be adopted by each state legislature. After adoption, nurses would obtain a license in their home state but would be able to communicate with clients in other states without violating the Nurse Practice Act in the client's home state if that state has also passed Compact legislation. The advantages of the Interstate Compact or "the one license concept" are reduced barriers to interstate practice, improved tracking for disciplinary purposes, cost-effectiveness, unduplicated counts of nurses, maintenance of a state-based system of licensure, and expanded consumer access to qualified nurses. Only a few states have adopted the Interstate Compact thus far. It will take several years for all states to sign on. Until all states have adopted the Interstate Compact, nurses need to be aware of the implications of practicing across state lines.

TRENDS AND DIRECTIONS FOR THE FUTURE

Demographic and socioeconomic trends in the United States are expected to continue to challenge ambulatory care nurses. Among these are (1) rapid changes in technology; (2) increased emphasis on demonstrated outcomes; (3) aging of the population; (4) reduced revenue to health care organizations from managed care contracts; and (5) the large number of uninsured people. A unified system ensuring access to health care for all Americans does not seem imminent. In addition, a nursing shortage is on the horizon.

Many believe, however, that the nation is experiencing a fundamental shift in emphasis on the concept of health itself, with the focus changing from the old clinical model to a wellness orientation. According to Shi and Singh,[24] health care is changing (1) from an *illness* orientation to a *wellness* orientation; (2) from an *acute* care emphasis to *primary* care; (3) from *inpatient* to *outpatient* services; (4) from *individual* health to *community* well-being; (5) from *fragmented* care to *managed* care; (6) from *independent* institutions to *integrated* systems; and (7) from service *duplication* to a *continuum* of services. If these predictions are correct, the well-educated ambulatory care nurse will be at the forefront of the health care delivery system in the new millennium.

CONCLUSIONS

Ambulatory care nursing is one of the fastest-growing areas of nursing specialty practice. Ambulatory care nurses are not only expert clinicians but also expert communicators. They play key roles in facilitating clients' successful progress through our integrated delivery systems. Ambulatory nurses make quality health care accessible for clients calling and coming into our health care delivery systems.

BIBLIOGRAPHY

1. American Academy of Ambulatory Care Nursing. (2000). *Ambulatory care nursing administration and practice standards.* Pitman, NJ: Anthony J. Jannetti, Inc.
2. American Academy of Ambulatory Care Nursing. (1997). *Telephone nursing practice administration and practice standards.* Pitman, NJ: Anthony J. Jannetti, Inc.
3. American Academy of Ambulatory Care Nursing and American Nurses Association. (1997). *Nursing in ambulatory care: The future is here.* Washington, DC: American Nurses Publishing.
4. Bentley, J., et al. (1991). Faculty practice plans: The organization and characteristics of academic medical practice. *Academic Medicine, 66*(8), 433–439.
5. Enthoven, A. (1993). The history and principles of managed competition. *Health Affairs* (suppl.), 24–28.
6. Ginzberg, E. (1994). *The road to reform.* New York: The Free Press.
7. Haas, S. (1998). Ambulatory care nursing conceptual framework. *AAACN Viewpoint, 20*(3), 16–17.
8. Haas, S., & Androwich, I. (1999). Telephone consultation. In G. Bulecheck & J. McCloskey (Eds.), *Nursing interventions: Effective nursing treatments.* Philadelphia: W. B. Saunders.
9. Haas, S., & Gold, C. (1997). Perspectives in ambulatory care: Supervision of unlicensed assistive workers in ambulatory settings. *Nursing Economics, 15*(1), 57–59.
10. Haas, S. A., & Hackbarth, D. P. (1995). Dimensions of the staff nurse role in ambulatory care: Part IV: Developing nursing intensity measures, standards, clinical ladders, and QI programs. *Nursing Economics, 13*(5), 285–294.
11. Haas, S. A., & Hackbarth, D. P. (1997). The role of the nurse manager in ambulatory care: Results of a national survey. *Nursing Economics, 15*(4), 191–203.
12. Haas, S. A., & Hackbarth, D. P. (1995). Dimensions of the staff nurse role in ambulatory care: Part III: Using research data to design new models of nursing care delivery. *Nursing Economics, 13*(4), 230–241.
13. Haas, S. A., et al. (1995). Dimensions of the staff nurse role in ambulatory care: Part II: Comparison of role dimensions in four ambulatory settings. *Nursing Economics, 13*(3), 152–165.
14. Hackbarth, D. (1995). Institute of Medicine revised definition of ambulatory care. *Viewpoint, 17*(4), 1–4.
15. Hackbarth, D. P., et al. (1995). Dimensions of the staff nurse role in ambulatory care: Part I: Methodology and analysis of data on current staff nurse practice. *Nursing Economics, 13*(2), 89–98.
16. Hooks, M., Dewitz-Arnold, D., & Westbrook, L. (1980). The role of the professional nurse in the ambulatory care setting. *Nursing Administration Quarterly, 4*(4), 12–17.
17. Institute of Medicine. (1994). *Defining primary care: An interim report.* Committee on the future of primary care. Washington, DC: National Academy Press.
18. Institute of Medicine. (1978). Primary care medicine: A definition. In *A manpower policy for primary health care: Report of a study.* Washington, DC: National Academy Press.
19. Kovner, A. (1996). *Health care delivery in the United States* (6th ed.). New York: Springer.
20. Leavell, H. R, & Clark, E. (1965). *Preventive medicine for the doctor in his community: An epidemiologic approach.* New York: McGraw-Hill.
21. McCaig, L. F. (1994). *National hospital ambulatory medical care survey: 1992 emergency department summary.* Atlanta: Centers for Disease Control and Prevention, National Center for Health Statistics.
22. McKeown, T. (1978). Determinants of health. *Human Nature, 1*(4), 60–67.
23. National Center for Health Statistics. (1999). *Ambulatory care statistics: United States, 1997.* Hyattsville, MD: Centers for Disease Control and Prevention, National Center for Health Statistics.
24. Shi, L., & Singh, D. (1998). *Delivering health care in America.* Gaithersburg, MD: Aspen.
25. Smith, J. (1983). *The idea of health: Implications for the nursing professional.* New York: Teachers College Press.
26. Starfield, B. (1992). *Primary care: Concept, evaluation and policy.* New York: Oxford University Press.
27. Starr, P. (1982). *The social transformation of American medicine.* Cambridge, MA: Basic Books.
28. Tighe, M. G., et al. (1985). A study of the oncology nurse role in ambulatory care. *Oncology Nursing Forum, 12*(6), 23–27.
29. U.S. Department of Health and Human Services, Office of Public Health and Science (1998). *Healthy people 2010 objectives: Draft for public review and comment.* Hyattsville, MD: Author.
30. Verran, J. A. (1981). Delineation of ambulatory care nursing practice. *Journal of Ambulatory Care Management, 4*(2), 1–13.
31. World Health Organization. (1978). *Primary health care: Report of the international conference on primary health care. Alma-Ata, USSR.* Geneva: Author.

CHAPTER 6

Acute Health Care

Cindy Ludwig

If you talk to a nurse who has worked in a hospital setting for the past 15 to 20 years, you are likely to hear about how much hospitals have changed. It is true. Today's hospitalized clients are sicker than they were years ago, in part because of advances in health care technology that have enabled them to survive disease and serious medical conditions longer. In the past, some of the nurse's case load included clients who were nearly well. Today, clients who are not acutely ill are discharged from the hospital and are treated in outpatient settings and by their families or significant others at home. Therefore, the case load for hospital nurses today consists of very ill clients. Chapter 4 discusses the many reasons for this change. This chapter addresses what it is like to work in a hospital today.

History of Hospital Nursing

Professional nursing in the United States is only about 100 years old. Although nursing is a young profession, it is an indispensable one. The need for nursing care is the major reason for hospitalization.

At the beginning of the 20th century, most nurses were employed by affluent clients in the client's home. Nurses worked on a fee-for-service basis and were paid by the client or the client's family. A nurse worked with only one client all day long. This early form of nursing care was called *private duty nursing*. Private duty nurses became well versed in the total care of a person because they provided physical, psychological, and social care. When care of the ill moved into the hospitals, many nurses moved into a hospital setting.

During the Great Depression, many nurses could no longer find employment in the client's home. They were forced to work in hospitals, and in many instances they worked for room and board rather than for a salary. The Blue Cross plan, developed in 1929, offered a form of prepayment of insurance to help people pay their hospital bills. During the 1930s and 1940s, more and more people purchased such insurance to protect themselves against hospital costs. The fact that hospitals could be more assured of payment put them on a sounder financial footing, and the demand for hospital-based nurses rose dramatically. Private duty nurses also moved into the hospital and provided one-to-one care for the hospitalized client at the client's request. Home-based private duty nursing care dwindled.

Today, private duty nurses can still be employed by hospitalized clients, but they are commonly employed elsewhere and are usually hired on a short-term basis. Hospitals contract with agencies, which provide a list (called a *registry*) of nurses who will work as private duty nurses.

In the 1970s and 1980s, the demand for hospital nurses continued to soar. Many schools of nursing met the demand by increasing the number of students they enrolled and graduated. History reveals cycles of nursing shortages. Nursing programs and hospitals must develop strong alliances to match the demand. There has been, and continues to be a nursing shortage. Hospital-based nurses are in shortest supply. Those who formerly chose nursing as a profession have broader career options available to them today, in home health care and other settings.

As health care costs have risen, third-party payers have begun to try to control hospital costs and soaring debts. Early discharge and the use of outpatient treatments now place clients back home quickly, even though they are still very ill. Not surprisingly, home health care nursing is increasing. Nurses still work in hospitals, but a rising percentage of nurses are caring for people in their homes.

Acute Care Hospitals

The American Hospital Association defines a hospital as an institution with the primary function of providing diagnostic and therapeutic patient services for a variety of medical conditions, both surgical and nonsurgical. Hospitals are of three types: government-owned, voluntary, and for-profit.

Government-Owned Hospitals. Government-owned hospitals are official agencies designed to provide care for people who receive local, state, or federal government support. Their services are often provided at no cost or at a reduced cost to the client. Many of the clients have no health care benefits. The clients may be employed, but the employer does not provide health care insurance programs.

Government-owned hospitals can be federally, state, or locally funded. Examples include the Army, Navy, Veterans Affairs, Public Health Service, and Department of Justice prison hospitals. State-supported facilities include psychiatric hospitals, state university hospitals, and state prison hospitals. Locally supported institutions include county and city hospitals.

VOLUNTARY HEALTH AGENCIES. Voluntary health agencies are nonprofit, tax-exempt organizations designed to meet the health care needs of the general public. Despite their name, nonprofit organizations still need to be concerned with their financial status. Although no stockholders are interested in profit, the hospital must have adequate resources to meet its expenses, plan for expansion, and be sustainable during economic depressions. Examples include church-affiliated, community, union, and Kaiser-Permanente hospitals. This category also includes hospitals owned by special interest groups, such as the Shriners, and hospitals for treatment of cancer or other chronic disorders.

FOR-PROFIT HOSPITALS. For-profit (*proprietary*) hospitals have the same goal as businesses: to generate profit. Like voluntary hospitals, they serve the general public. The hospitals are privately owned by large corporations, are parts of chains of hospitals, or are owned by single owners. These hospitals have stockholders. An advantage to the larger chains of hospitals is that they can purchase medical supplies in greater volume and, therefore, at less cost. They also have a slight advantage when contracting for third-party payment because of their ability to reduce costs.

Magnet hospitals are medium-sized to large urban medical for-profit centers that have a reputation for providing excellent nursing care and for having good medical outcomes. These hospitals often provide medical services for complex problems that require a team of health care providers who would be too expensive to replicate in multiple sites. For example, clients who require organ transplantation or care after a serious injury are commonly cared for in these institutions. The hospitals have a high retention rate of their staff because of their high morale and good payment systems. Most magnet hospitals employ very competent, experienced nurses who need little direct supervision.

Client Admissions

Clients in acute care hospitals include those who are acutely ill, are victims of trauma, have a potentially critical condition, need intensive monitoring, need complex diagnostic studies, need surgery or complex treatments, or have an exacerbation of a chronic disorder.

Clients can be admitted to a hospital in several ways (Box 6–1). Once the client is admitted, a primary physician (also called the *attending physician*) oversees the client's care. Consultants may be used to diagnose problems outside the physician's speciality. *Acute care* is a costly service that relies on technology and the expertise of the health care team to arrive at a diagnosis, begin treatment, stabilize the condition, and prepare for a transition to a less costly level of health care. Many people are involved in a client's care (Box 6–2).

BOX 6–1 How Clients Are Admitted to a Hospital

Direct

A client is seen in a physician's office, and it is determined that the client needs nursing care and specialized monitoring.

Emergency

A client is seen in the emergency department, and it is determined that the client needs surgery, nursing care, and/or specialized monitoring. The disease that has been diagnosed or is considered likely cannot be managed on an outpatient or self-care basis.

Scheduled

A client has elected to undergo surgery or special diagnostic testing that requires specialized monitoring or nursing care during recovery.

Efficiency Measures

Hospitals continuously assess their outcomes and financial health by reviewing cost-benefit and clinical analysis data from their service lines. *Service lines* can be defined as care given to groups of clients with similar problems. For example, care of clients with heart disease or heart surgery would make up one service line. Many communities with two or more hospitals collaborate and then delineate service lines for each institution. For example, one hospital might provide all psychiatric services, another might provide acute service, and another might provide rehabilitation service. This is a cost-effective and a resource-effective method of providing care because duplication of effort is eliminated. Clinical outcomes are generally improved when the volume of cases increases because the staff become familiar with typical responses of clients and can detect complications earlier. In addition, equipment used to provide care can be purchased at lower costs when purchased in larger quantities.

During the late 1990s, many hospitals merged with others in efforts to reduce cost, combine services, and attract third-party payment contracts. Some of the mergers are collaborative, in which both parties are served by the merger. Some mergers are done to rescue ailing hospitals; other mergers are contested or surprise mergers. The environment of the hospital during a merger can be very volatile. Many employees realize that jobs might be lost in an effort to redesign the work environment and delivery systems, and morale often falls. Nurses should keep client care foremost in their minds and continue to provide high-quality care during the turmoil.

Subacute Care

Subacute care is designed to fill the gap between acute care hospitals and long-term care. Clients may follow a continuum from acute care to a transitional care unit (usually located within the acute care hospital but defined as a separate area) and a skilled nursing facility. If the client can provide his or her own care at home, discharge to home is appropriate. If some nursing care is still required, home health care may be used to assist the client.

Subacute care is more intensive than traditional nursing home care and less acute than acute care hospitals. For example, a client may have many complex conditions that require a lower level of care than would be given in an acute care setting but higher than could be pro-

BOX 6–2 Personnel and Departments in a Hospital

Professional Services

Medical staff. Consists of private practice or group practice physicians who have their own offices and use the hospital services for care of specific problems. Also made up of physicians who may work for the hospital in such departments as surgery, laboratory, radiology, and emergency.

Nursing Service. Largest group of client care providers in the hospital. Nurses are employed by the nursing service department and provide client care on one unit or ward in the hospital; in areas where no direct client care is given (such as administration and hospital-based education programs); and by the "patient care" department.

Pharmacy. Consists of pharmacists and assistants who dispense medications prescribed by physicians. Pharmacy staff also monitor the use of regulated medications, such as narcotics. Many pharmacists also teach clients about their medications.

Rehabilitation Services. Physical therapists treat diseases and injuries by restoring, improving, or maintaining the client's functional ability or status to increase musculoskeletal strength to prevent further problems. Occupational therapists teach clients ways to overcome or reduce the problems in activities of daily living resulting from their disabilities.

Support Services

Administration. Hospital staff who are accountable for the operation of the entire hospital or institution. May include the hospital president, vice-presidents, and nurse-managers who supervise client care on a given nursing unit.

Biomedical Engineering Department. Maintains the elaborate equipment in the hospital to ensure safe and proper functioning and adherence to government regulations.

Business Departments. Several departments manage the business of the hospital based on both client income and outgoing expenses (salaries, purchasing, operation of the building). The admitting office collects information on insurance and assigns a room to the client. The business office lists all client charges, prepares the hospital bill, submits it to insurance companies, and records payments received. Payroll departments monitor hours worked, disperse salaries to the employees, and keep records. Purchasing departments disperse money for purchase of new supplies.

Central Service/Material Management Department. Maintains supplies needed for client care. Provides stock supplies of routinely used items on the nursing units. Cleans and resterilizes reusable supplies.

Dietary. Prepares food for client and staff daily. Dietitians assess and manage nutritional needs of hospitalized clients.

Environmental Services. Clean the hospital, including client rooms.

Foundation. Volunteers and professional staff who often raise funds for various hospital projects (e.g., building projects). May be combined with the marketing department.

Information Technology. Computer support staff is growing in most hospitals because of the increasing use of computers. Staff members focus on design and support mechanisms for electronic data retrieval and storage.

Laboratory. Conducts diagnostic tests to help identify illness. Technicians commonly work in radiology and the various laboratories. Laboratory technicians usually collect blood samples from clients; nurses often collect all other specimens and may collect blood.

Laundry. Launders, sorts, and presses several hundred pounds of linen each day. New linen is delivered to each nursing unit daily. These services may be contracted out ("outsourced") to local providers.

Medical Records. Stores medical records for all clients. If a client is rehospitalized, former medical records are often important in diagnosis of new problems. Also compiles data for retrieval for reimbursement, service trending, and outcomes research.

Personnel/Human Resources Department. Hires new employees and concentrates on employee relations. Human resources departments may serve in public relations roles to inform the hospital staff, clients, media, and the public about the hospital and its operations. Public relations services may also be provided by the marketing department.

Volunteer Services. Operates coffee shops and gift shops, delivers mail to clients, and often raises funds for various hospital projects.

vided by nurses in a traditional transitional care unit in a skilled nursing facility. The requirements as outlined by the Department of Health Services are shown in Box 6–3.

Several factors have made subacute care facilities one of the fastest-growing segments of health care through the mid-1990s. Subacute care provides health care for clients with complex problems at a fraction of the cost, or at about 30% of the cost of the acute care general hospital. At one time, reimbursement was more lucrative for these care settings, and many hospitals augmented their physical structure to add subacute care units. This financial incentive changed when legislation was enacted to slow down early discharge from acute to subacute care. In some hospitals today, nursing units or beds on a given unit or actual beds can serve a dual purpose. These *swing beds* can be used either for acute care or for subacute care, depending on the circumstances.

Subacute care areas are designed for clients who are out of the fragile phase of their illness and need routine monitoring and rehabilitation. Typical candidates are clients with diagnoses of stroke, cancer, acquired immunodeficiency syndrome (AIDS), head injury, total hip replacement, vascular diseases, chronic obstructive pulmonary disease, renal failure, and wounds needing care. These clients do not need surgery or other invasive procedures, but they do require frequent assessment and longer stays. Subacute care provides coordinated services to clients by a team of nurses, nursing assistants, physicians, specialized therapists, social workers, and dietitians. Outcomes after subacute care stays are the same as, or better than, those after hospital stays.

Subacute care areas have attracted nurses from the hospital setting, because nurses feel they have more time, less pressure, and a more interdisciplinary approach to client care. Another attractive feature of most subacute

BOX 6–3 Nursing Hours per Day in Various Levels of Care

- *Skilled nursing:* LPN or RN + CNA = 2.5 hours/day
- *Transitional care unit:* LPN or RN + CNA = 4.9 hours/day
- *Subacute care* (distinct portion of acute care hospital) = LPN or RN + CNA = 6.0 hours/day
- Subacute care (freestanding) = LPN or RN + CNA = 5.8 hours/day

CNA, Certified Nursing Assistant; LPN, Licensed Practical Nurse; RN, Registered Nurse.

units is that the environment seems more like home to the client and family.

The four categories of subacute care units are (1) transitional, (2) general, (3) chronic, and (4) long-term transitional.

TRANSITIONAL. Transitional subacute care provides for short stays (10 days) with high levels of nursing care. It serves as a hospital step-down unit, an alternative to continued hospitalization in an acute care setting. Typical clients in transitional subacute care include those recovering from myocardial infarction (heart attack) or open heart surgery; those who must be weaned from a ventilator; those who need wound management after burn injury or for multiple pressure ulcers; those who require more rehabilitation after stroke or orthopedic surgery; or those who have complex medical conditions such as diabetes or digestive or renal problems.

GENERAL. General subacute units have some overlap with transitional units; the key difference is the *acuity level* (severity of illness) of the clients. Many clients in these units are Medicare beneficiaries, whose younger counterparts with the same level of disability would receive home care. General subacute units are used for clients who require about 3.5 hours of nursing care and 1 to 3 hours of therapy daily. Typical clients are the same as those in transitional units, although the stay is longer (10 to 40 days). The goal of care is to send clients home or to a less expensive level of care, such as to long-term care or assisted-living centers.

CHRONIC. Chronic subacute units manage clients with little hope of ultimate recovery and functional independence. Typical clients include those who cannot be successfully weaned from a ventilator, are in a long-term comatose state, or have progressive neurologic disorders. Nursing intensity is similar to that in general subacute care units. The goal of care is to stabilize the client's condition so that he or she can be transferred to home or to a long-term care center. The average length of stay is 60 to 90 days.

LONG-TERM. Long-term transitional subacute facilities provide care for clients with medically complex problems or those who are ventilator-dependent. The average length of stay is about 25 days, but it can be more. The units are staffed primarily by Registered Nurses (RNs), and each client requires about 6 to 9 hours of care per day.

ROLES OF NURSES IN HOSPITALS

Nursing is a service provided both to individual clients and to aggregates of people (e.g., families, groups, communities, populations). To fulfill nursing's commitment to contribute to the health care of people, professional nurses assume multiple roles and responsibilities. Although these roles tend to overlap, they are important to distinguish. Nurses are providers of direct care, educators, and managers.

Provider of Direct Care

Most people are familiar with nurses as providers of *direct care.* Nurses assess, care for, educate, and comfort clients. Nurses provide direct care in all settings and along all dimensions of the health-illness continuum, from health promotion to critical care and death.

Indirect care consists of processes that go on in support of the actual bedside nursing care given. Sometimes this level of care is labeled *interdependent.* The nurse interprets physicians' orders, administers medication, and provides treatment for the client when performing interdependent care.

Educator

Professional nurses provide formal and informal education to their clients, individually and in groups. Informal education goes on almost continually, as clients are taught about medications while the medications are being administered, about the importance of eating a balanced diet when they choose their menu selections, and so on. The importance of informal education should not be underestimated.

Formal education is usually provided to groups of clients and their families. The nurse may use a classroom or bring videotapes or audio tapes into the client's room. Advantages to formal education are that the client is usually prepared for learning, significant others are included, and the material presented is consistent from client to client. Many hospitals have formal educators on their staff for clients with complex learning needs. Certified diabetes educators, certified lactation specialists, oncology nurse specialists, and enterostomal therapists are examples of nurses who teach clients in the hospital and often follow up with clients when they are back in the community.

Finally, some nurses specialize in education and rehabilitation. These nurses often work in cardiac and pulmonary rehabilitation and may have a subspecialty in physical therapy or exercise physiology. Their role is to assist in the rehabilitation of clients after myocardial infarction, heart failure, or chronic obstructive pulmonary disease.

Manager

The term *manager* in this discussion means the person who coordinates human and material resources in providing care to clients. *Human resources* include (1) the client, (2) the nurse, (3) the family or significant others, (4) professional colleagues, (5) support groups (e.g., the American Cancer Society), and (6) resource groups (e.g., Vocational Rehabilitation). *Material resources* include equipment and supplies. Time is also an important resource. Finally, outcome is an important consideration in health care management. Outcomes are detailed in the next section.

The first episode of client management that you encounter as a nurse is your provision of timely care to one client. Effective time management of only one client is difficult at first because of interruptions and lack of familiarity with equipment and procedures. Even while you are caring for only one client, stay on time with assessments, medications, and treatments. Most of these aspects of nursing care are scheduled more than once every 24 hours; if you are late, the next treatment or medication may have to be delayed. As you gain experience, care of one client becomes efficient. When caring for more than one client, time management becomes even more important.

NURSING CARE DELIVERY SYSTEMS

How client care is delivered on any nursing unit is very important. Several techniques are in use today, and each has its advantages and disadvantages.

Total Care Nursing

Total care nursing is the oldest of the care delivery systems. One nurse is assigned to one client and provides all care. The one-to-one pattern is common in critical care, with student nurses, and with private duty nurses. The advantage is that the client needs to work with only one nurse and that one nurse can focus on meeting all the biopsychosocial needs of the client and family. The disadvantage is that any given nurse must be proficient in all nursing tasks and problem-solving areas.

Functional Nursing

Functional nursing is a system of care borrowed from industry, which concentrates on duties. It can be seen as an "assembly line" of care. Functional nursing began during World War II, when the demand for patient care outstripped the supply of nurses. The RN would coordinate care for an entire unit or team. Other nurses might be assigned to pass medications and perform treatments. Personnel with less training would be assigned to provide more basic care (e.g., giving baths, making beds).

An advantage of this system is that care can be provided at a lower cost. Disadvantages are that the client interacts with several people, psychosocial needs are seldom met, and the RN seldom cares for the client and must rely on other people's assessments of the client's problems. Each member of the working group is highly dependent on the other members, and the nurse is in an autocratic position. Functional nursing is still commonly used in skilled nursing and long-term care facilities.

Team Nursing

In team nursing, the RN leads a group of health care personnel in providing care for 10 to 20 clients. Team nursing was developed in the 1950s because of social and technological changes. World War II had drawn many nurses from hospitals, causing gaps in the nursing population. In addition, several technological advances required specialized knowledge. Team nursing was felt to be one approach to using people's skills more effectively.

Advantages are that an experienced RN is head of the team and generally knows the clients. In addition, the team leader can provide guidance to new or inexperienced nurses. As in functional nursing, the talents and abilities of each member of the health care team are used. Disadvantages are that (1) it is fairly expensive (because care is fragmented), (2) a lack of delegation skills by RNs may reduce efficiency, and (3) some redundancy may occur if each team leader must perform several managerial tasks, such as making assignments.

Primary Nursing

Primary nursing is a model of care delivery and a model of organizing care to achieve high-quality care outcomes. This style of care delivery emerged during the 1980s to meet the increasingly complex needs of clients. The goal is for each client's care to be comprehensive and coordinated, from admission to discharge. Each client is assigned an RN as the primary nurse, and that nurse always provides care for that client when he or she is working. In addition, associate nurses provide care when the primary nurse is absent.

Advantages are obvious: (1) the client has the same nurse, (2) the client's psychosocial needs can be met, (3) communication with the physician is improved, and (4) the nurse feels autonomous. Disadvantages are (1) the increased cost in hiring a large RN staff, (2) possible role confusion between primary and associate nurses, and (3) many calls to physicians from one nursing unit. (When a charge nurse system is used, the charge nurse makes telephone calls and often handles several issues in one telephone call.)

Case Management

The nurse can serve a pivotal role in coordinating all of the events required for a timely recovery. Many hospitals have developed sophisticated guides, called *care pathways* or case management plans, to direct client care and recovery from predictable problems. Case management is a care delivery mode that incorporates concepts of continuity and efficiency in addressing long-term physical, psychological, and social needs of clients. The primary goals of case management are promoting self-care, upgrading the quality of life, and using resources efficiently. Case managers are nurses who coordinate care of a group of clients, monitor the implementation of interdisciplinary care plans, and maintain communication with third-party payers and referral sources.

A key distinction in the nurse's role in the case management system is that it transcends nursing unit and physician service (e.g, cardiology) boundaries. The nurse follows the client through the entire stay in the health care system and back into the community. Case managers must have a thorough knowledge of third-party reimbursement patterns and rules, community resources, and discharge planning techniques. Several care pathways are presented in this book with a discussion of how to use them.

MANAGEMENT AND DELEGATION

Today, in an effort to control costs, almost all hospitals have hired *unlicensed assistive personnel* to provide care. Other than on-the-job training, these personnel receive little formal training. The use of less trained and educated personnel to perform nursing duties is changing the face of nurse staffing in hospitals. The use of unlicensed assistive personnel is increasing despite the inconclusive amount of research demonstrating their effectiveness on client outcomes.

Different terms are used for "nurse extenders" (which may include unlicensed assistive personnel), such as *unit assistants, primary practice partners,* and *unit hostesses.* Nurse extenders with more advanced skills might be called *clinical technicians.* Assistive personnel may help with clinical duties, nonclinical duties, or both. Some of the duties that may be delegated include giving baths, taking vital signs, serving food and collecting trays, performing unit-based laboratory tests (e.g., finger sticks for blood glucose assessment), 12-lead electrocardiograms (ECGs), and skin care.

Nurses need to learn when to delegate. For example, the nurse may delegate a bed bath and linen change for a client who is stable and may give the bath herself to an unstable or new client. This book offers many examples of appropriate delegation to unlicensed assistive personnel (see, for example, the Management and Delegation features in Chapters 27 and 46).

In planning the use of nurse extenders, nurse managers and their staff must consider many key questions (Box 6–4). Two issues that demand particular attention are the functions that only an RN can perform and the minimum level of RN staffing required to provide safe client care. Nurses may have been taught that only RNs can or should perform certain clinical duties, and they may therefore have difficulty delegating them to less qualified personnel. As the pressure mounts to delegate tasks to lower-paid workers, nurses will need to develop managerial skills, especially those of leadership, delegation, and supervision. Nurses will remain professionally accountable for client outcomes whether or not the specific tasks that contribute to those outcomes have been performed by nurses or by nurse extenders. Each nurse must clearly understand what the agency defines as the role and duties of the RN, the Licensed Practical Nurse or Vocational Nurse, and the various nurse extenders.

BOX 6–4 Critical Considerations for Delegating Care to Unlicensed Assistive Personnel

- What are the appropriate core duties of a Registered Nurse?
- Who should perform which tasks?
- What can be delegated?
- What is an appropriate and cost-effective staff mix?
- What is the risk management and liability at each level of caregiver?
- Who can substitute for whom?
- Who is the least expensive worker to do each task?
- How much management or supervision is needed?
- What is the philosophical commitment to the provision of total patient care by the RN here?
- Will lowering the qualification of staff add further stress and frustration to our staff?
- How will this affect recruitment?
- What is the impact on collective bargaining?

From Gardner, D. L. (1991). Issues related to the use of nurse extenders. *Journal of Nursing Administration, 21*(10), 40–45.

ENSURING QUALITY HEALTH CARE DELIVERY

Amid the fast-paced changes occurring in health care delivery, health care professionals remain responsible for ensuring quality client care. Quality client care is the outcome of the integrated health care team approach that involves the corporate and hospital or agency administration, medical staff, board of trustees, employees, community, and client. Contract services, community resources, transfer agreements, and expertise of social workers or case managers enable client transitions to alternate levels of care to occur in a continuous, coordinated, and almost seamless fashion.

Through work-redesign and skill-mix reallocation, institutions are focusing goals on achieving efficient client outcomes. *Work-redesign* involves studying a job over a fixed period to discover if and how a certain job function might be made more efficient. *Skill-mix* is determined by studying the ratio of RNs to Licensed Practical Nurses or Vocational Nurses and nursing assistants on a unit. The best skill-mix delivers quality care while also controlling costs.

The "one-level-of-care" philosophy ensures that clients receive optimal care in all areas of an institution. For example, the same monitoring pertains when intravenous (IV) conscious sedation is administered in the endoscopy unit as when general anesthesia is administered in the operating room or emergency department.

The Client's Rights to Quality Care

Clients have an increased awareness of the quality-of-care issue. They are demanding and receiving more information before the initiation of treatments. Increasingly, clients' requests for information about costs, risks, benefits, and alternatives to suggested therapies are being honored. No longer automatically submissive to the suggested care, the client is becoming a participant and partner in health care, with the expectation of receiving quality care from all health care professionals.

Client rights have also reached a new level of importance for the health care consumer. Regulating agencies, insurance carriers, third-party payers, and providers are responding to ensure that these fundamental rights are maintained and that clients receive quality services.

Providing Quality Client Care

Any plan for providing client care involves the following aspects:

- Budgeting process, to assist the institution in studying, spending, and using the information to reduce costs or maintain them at the present rate
- Strategic planning, to serve as a guideline for the continued or expanded services provided by the health care agency
- Performance improvement plan, to show the steps taken to improve performance based on monitoring and evaluation of staff performance
- Risk management input, to identify and eliminate potential injuries to staff and clients
- Utilization review data, to explore items such as acuity levels (a degree of severity of illness that affects the amount and complexity of care the client requires), outcomes, and costs, and to discover what is and is not effective care
- Client satisfaction survey results, which gather data from clients at various stages of their stay in the agency (e.g., preprocedure, admission procedure, discharge)
- Physician input, to incorporate professional input into client care planning
- Census data, to plot current and future trends of health care in the organization
- Acuity levels, as designated by the health care organization, to plan an appropriate skill-mix for staffing

Changes in client population, diagnoses, programs, or staffing that would necessitate changes in the type, level, or amount of care are reviewed on an ongoing basis. Other factors contributing to quality care include (1) the adherence to, monitoring of, and evaluation of care given according to professional standards; (2) Joint Commission on the Accreditation of Healthcare Organizations (JCAHO) and Department of Health criteria; and (3) input from other regulatory agencies. In addition, clinical pathways, clinical practice guidelines, standards of practice and care, and competence standards serve as models for professional delivery of client care.

Staffing for Quality Care

Health care institutions use a combination of methods to ensure a staff of caregivers who can deliver quality care to clients. Two methods include (1) daily collection of census data (a count of the number of clients occupying beds on any given day); and (2) determination of acuity levels.

Staff are assigned or reassigned to units that have the greatest need for their expertise and experience. Staffing adjustments caused by the fluctuation of census data and acuity levels are accomplished by using per diem (daily) staff and other creative measures to ensure safe client care.

Although staffing adjustment decisions in the past were typically made at higher levels of administration, today service line leaders and empowered directors and managers are instrumental in adjusting strategies based on the many shifting variables that affect client care. These personnel are closer to the actual care setting (clients and staff) and can use their expertise to make informed decisions about staffing for quality care.

Input from the employees who actually provide care is helpful in redesigning and improving the quality of care. Because caregivers are directly involved with client care, they can contribute in important ways by reporting problems that can be addressed in a timely fashion. Such input, especially when acted on by management, helps staff members feel valued.

Unfortunately, adequate staffing is not always ensured. In 1995, nurses marched on Washington, D.C., to protest clinical staffing shortages that had already endangered and might further endanger client care. Today, RNs are still in short supply.

In an attempt to make the most effective use of available nursing staff, *cross-training* has evolved in hospitals. Whereas in the past nurses were typically assigned to one unit where they could become familiar with the other personnel and the unit routine, today's hospital nurses may be cross-trained to work effectively in two or more units (e.g., a surgical unit and a cardiac intensive care unit). Nurses are assigned to the unit where they are most needed and may arrive for work not knowing in advance the work assignment for that day. Nurses may also be assigned to similar areas (e.g., orthopedics) but at different hospitals within the larger system as a result of mergers and acquisitions. This new scenario is often stressful for nurses and other staff members.

Nursing Intensity Classification

To ensure that staffing is adequate, one must understand how ill any given group of clients is and how much nursing care they will require. Hospitalized clients are classified according to several systems in an attempt to determine *nursing intensity,* a combination of the amount of care and the skill level at which care is provided. Usually, physical care and psychosocial or teaching skills are included. For example, a stable comatose client might require a large amount of low-complexity care that could be provided by unlicensed assistive personnel. In contrast, a newly diagnosed diabetic teenager with several personal and family problems may require less time for care, but the care should be provided by an RN.

Any patient classification system has several purposes, such as:

1. *Providing staffing.* The system will establish a unit of measure for nursing time. The unit of measure will be used to determine the number and kinds of health care providers needed for any given shift.
2. *Reducing cost.* The system can be used to determine the cost of nursing care. Profits and losses can then be calculated.
3. *Tracking changes.* The acuity of care needed may change as the case mix changes or during certain times of the year.

Two methods are generally used to determine acuity.

1. *Factor evaluation method.* Each client is rated on independent elements of care; each element is scored (weighted); scores are summarized, and the client is placed in a category based on the total numerical value obtained.

2. *Prototype evaluation method.* Each client is categorized according to a broad description of care requirements. The prototypes usually have four categories that describe (a) the client's ability to perform activities of daily living (ADL), (b) general health, (c) emotional support, and (d) treatment modalities (Table 6–1).

■ MONITORING HEALTH CARE OUTCOMES

New ideas are coming into play about health care outcomes. The shift in health care originally focused on cost reduction. Fortunately, it has become recognized that cost reduction may equate to losses in quality of care. New ideas are addressing the *value* of health care (cost of care for procedure or health problem as well as outcome of care). This is a needed change in the direction of quality health care. Third-party payers in the future will probably consider the value of health care provided at various institutions before signing contracts. Some of the ways health care outcomes are monitored in an effort to track outcomes and value are now presented.

Patient Satisfaction Surveys

As in business, health care providers have learned that it is easier to keep customers than to find new ones. Patient satisfaction surveys are commonly given to the client on discharge or sent to the client's home shortly after discharge. The basic question is, "Would you return to our institution for health care in the future?" Clients are often asked about their perception of medical care, nursing care, ancillary care, the environment, and follow-up care.

Sometimes patient satisfaction surveys are discounted because of the fact that the patient has limited knowledge of what would constitute "reasonable" care. To overcome this feeling of helplessness by the client, some hospitals inform clients of the services they can reasonably expect while hospitalized. For example, clients are told that they can reasonably expect adequate pain relief. Then clients are asked to evaluate whether the outcome was met during the stay. This excellent change reminds all health care providers that the client's opinion should always be one indicator of quality of care.

Measurement of Functional Status

Functional status is a composite measurement of many components of physical health and psychosocial well-being. Because it is a composite, several instruments can be used to measure functional status; these include:

- General perception of health
- Limitations in physical ability because of health problems
- Ability to engage in social activities (including work)
- General mental health
- Pain
- Energy
- Fatigue
- Depression

Some hospitals are using these measures to monitor how interventions affect functional status. For example, it is expected that functional status will improve after coronary bypass surgery. Valid data to show improvement in a group of clients served by the hospital provides excellent evidence of health care value.

Accessibility

Because people are mobile, the location of the hospital and access to the agency are important factors. Hospitals are concerned about convenience, location, wait time, and lead time needed to find a primary care provider, to arrange an outpatient procedure, or to schedule a diagnostic procedure.

■ REGULATORY REQUIREMENTS AND ISSUES

Regulatory agencies have the primary goal of enhancing the public's ability to secure adequate health care. Health care agencies are surveyed periodically to ensure that they comply with specific rules and regulations. A survey is an in-depth study of a health care institution (e.g., a hospital or a long-term care facility) according to specific criteria set forth by the regulating agencies involved. All aspects of the institution's services are inspected. Important performance areas include client assessment, medication administration, use of restraints, client and family education, staff training, information management, and organizational performance. After the survey is completed, a report of findings is compiled and the institution is notified of its status. If a criterion is not met satisfactorily, the institution is notified, given time to correct the deficiency, and reevaluated at a later date. Sometimes the reevaluation is unannounced.

Public disclosure of survey findings has begun. Hospital surveys completed after 1994 are made available to the public, media sources, insurance companies, third-party payers, clients, and competing institutions. Other health care delivery services function under the same disclosure rules for compliance with regulations of the inspecting agencies.

Regulatory Agencies and Statutes

Several regulatory agencies have statutes that must be met by hospitals. These laws govern hiring and employment, quality controls, and conditions of the work site to reduce hazards. A full description of these laws is beyond the scope of this book; we will only look at a few of them. Employment laws include the equal employment opportunity laws that ensure equal rights in the workplace for racial and ethnic minorities, women, the elderly, and the handicapped. Contemporary changes in workplace rights for everyone would probably be incomprehensible to a worker from the 1920s.

The *Civil Rights Act* of 1964 laid the foundation for equal employment in the United States. The thrust of Title VII of the Civil Rights Act is two-fold: (1) it prohibits discrimination based on factors unrelated to job qualifications, and (2) it promotes employment based on ability and merit. The areas of discrimination specifically mentioned are race, color, religion, sex, and national origin. The Equal Employment Opportunity Commission (EEOC) is responsible for enforcing Title VII of the Civil

TABLE 6–1 PATIENT CARE CLASSIFICATION USING FOUR LEVELS OF NURSING CARE INTENSITY

Area of Care	Category 1	Category 2	Category 3	Category 4
Eating	Feeds self or needs little food	Needs some help in preparing; may need encouragement	Cannot feed self but is able to chew and swallow	Cannot feed self and may have difficulty swallowing
Grooming	Almost entirely self-sufficient	Needs some help in bathing, oral hygiene, hair combing, and so forth	Unable to do much for self	Completely dependent
Excretion	Up and to bathroom alone or almost alone	Needs some help in getting up to bathroom or using urinal	In bed, needs bedpan or urinal placed; may be able to partially turn or lift self	Completely dependent
Comfort	Self-sufficient	Needs some help with adjusting position or bed (e.g., tubes, IV lines)	Cannot turn without help, get drink, adjust position of extremities, and so forth	Completely dependent
General health	Good—in for diagnostic procedure, simple treatment, or surgical procedure (D & C, biopsy, minor fracture)	Mild symptoms—more than one mild illness, mild debility, mild emotional reaction, mild incontinence (not more than once per shift)	Acute symptoms—severe emotional reaction to illness or surgery, more than one acute illness, medical or surgical problem, severe or frequent incontinence	Critically ill—may have severe emotional reaction
Treatments	Simple—supervised ambulation, dangle, simple dressing, test procedure preparation not requiring medication, reinforcement of surgical dressing, change pad, vital signs once per shift	Any category 1 treatment more than once per shift, Foley catheter, care, I & O, bladder irrigations, sitz bath, compresses, test procedures requiring medications or follow-ups, simple enema for evacuation, vital signs every 4 hr	Any treatment more than twice per shift, medicated IV lines, complicated dressings, sterile procedures, care of tracheotomy, Harris flush, suctioning, tube feeding, vital signs more than every 4 hr	Any elaborate or delicate procedure requiring two nurses, vital signs more often than every 2 hr
Medications	Simple, routine, not needing preevaluation or postevaluation; medications no more than once per shift	Diabetic, cardiac, hypotensive, hypertensive, diuretic, anticoagulant medications, prn medications, more than once per shift, medications needing preevaluation or postevaluation	Unusual amount of category 2 medications; control of refractory diabetics (need to be monitored more than every 4 hr)	More intensive category 3 medications; IV lines with frequent, close observation and regulation
Teaching and emotional support	Routine follow-up teaching; clients with no unusual or adverse emotional reactions	Initial teaching of care of ostomies, new diabetics, tubes that will be in place for periods of time; conditions requiring major change in eating, living, or excretory practices; clients with mild adverse reactions to their illness (e.g., depression, being overly demanding)	More intensive category 2 items; teaching of apprehensive or mildly resistive clients; care of moderately upset or apprehensive clients; confused or disoriented clients	Teaching of resistive clients, care and support of clients with severe emotional reaction

D & C, dilatation and curettage; I & O, input and output; IV, intravenous.

Modified from Marquis, B. L., & Huston, C. J. (1996). *Leadership roles and management functions in nursing* (p. 266). Philadelphia: J. B. Lippincott.

Rights Act. When a charge of discrimination is proven, the agency attempts to mediate the problem through persuasion and conciliation.

In 1967, Congress enacted the *Age Discrimination and Employment Act* (ADEA). Its purpose was to promote employment of older people based on their ability rather than their age. In early 1978, the ADEA was amended to increase the protected age to 70 years. Although people feared that this act would have serious consequences for labor-intensive occupations, such as nursing, many people are opting for earlier retirement and problems have not been reported.

The *Rehabilitation Act* of 1973 required all employers with government contracts of more than $25,000 to take affirmative action to recruit, hire, and advance handicapped people who are qualified. In 1990, Congress passed the *Americans with Disabilities Act* to eliminate discrimination against Americans with physical or mental disabilities in the workplace and in social life. Disability is defined as "any physical or mental impairment that limits any major life activity." This includes not only all individuals with obvious physical disabilities, but also individuals with cancer, diabetes, human immunodeficiency virus (HIV) infection, AIDS, and recovering alcoholics and drug users. The act not only prohibits discrimination but also delineates clear, enforceable standards.

The *Occupational Safety and Health Act* (OSHA) is broadly written legislation that requires a place of employment to be free from recognized hazards and to develop environmental safety laws for the safety of the employees. The Department of Labor enforces this act. Since the inception of OSHA, many companies have vehemently criticized the act, specifically its administration. Companies have charged that the costs of meeting OSHA standards have excessively burdened American business. However, unions have asserted that the federal government has never adequately staffed or funded the Occupational and Health Administration. They have charged that OSHA has been negligent in setting standards for toxic substances, carcinogens, and other disease-producing agents.

Finally, quality assurance standards must be met by several areas of the hospital. Laboratories must test control solutions of known substances routinely to ensure that test results are accurate. Equipment used for sterilization of instruments and other supplies must be tested daily. These precautions are critical to safe care.

Ethical Issues

Ethical issues in acute care commonly occur when the nurse is caught in the middle between clients, physicians, administrators, and other nurses and feels powerless to change the situation. Ethical distress can lead to negative consequences for everyone involved. Nurses are often called on to assist families in making informed decisions about client care, and they must be familiar with ethical, legal, economic, and emotional factors that affect the family's decision.

Legal Issues

Nurses have more responsibility today than in the past. These expanded roles open the doors to greater legal risk. The nurse's employer is obligated to carry malpractice insurance for its employees. You should know what is covered in the policy. In addition, you should carry individual malpractice insurance.

Proper documentation is crucial to serve as evidence of the quality of nursing care provided. The court still assumes that if something was not noted in a chart, it was not done. Be specific, and document nursing actions taken and the client's response (e.g., pain relief). If unusual events occur, complete an incident report. The benefit of incident reports is that they allow the analysis of adverse client events. They should not be treated as a punitive activity but rather as a method of promoting quality care and risk management. Errors are examined to determine whether the error was due to a system problem (e.g., a faulty electrical outlet that leads to a fire or an improperly mounted side rail that allows a client to fall). If a lawsuit is filed, incident reports are usually not revealed; instead, the court system relies on the information in the medical record.

Cultural Issues

Nurses who practice in the 21st century will be interacting with an increasingly multicultural American society. It is projected that most of the American population will include groups of minorities from other cultures. Areas of the United States that seldom had immigrants now see people from all over the world. This diverse population requires that nurses be able to recognize differences and be sensitive to those differences in perceptions of health and illness, in communication styles, and in nontraditional approaches to health care. Culturally competent care in its broadest sense is knowing, explaining, interpreting, and predicting nursing care within the knowledge of the client's cultural and ethnic beliefs and practices, whether the client is well or sick.[14]

■ PERFORMANCE IMPROVEMENT AND GOALS

Hospitals and other health care organizations have been challenged by their goal of attaining a planned, systematic, multidisciplinary, nationwide approach to designing, measuring, assessing, and improving performance. These institutions generally seek to enhance their measurement activities as they relate to institutional quality indicators (Box 6–5). These indicators generally include:

- Results of basic clinical indicators
- Continuous quality improvement
- Access to care issues
- Consumer satisfaction and judgment input
- JCAHO indicators
- Human resource management
- Organization performance

Health care organizations are in the midst of a transition to performance improvement from traditional quality assurance. Relevant goals include:

- Enhancing clinical leaders' abilities to set expectations, develop plans, and manage processes to assess, improve, and maintain the quality of the organization's clinical and support activities
- Enhancing health care outcomes and the perception of these outcomes and expectations by all consumers

BOX 6–5 Clinical Indicators with a Focus on High-Volume, High-Risk, and Problem-Prone Issues

The community/clinic focus includes the following:

- Communicable diseases (e.g., TB, HIV)
- Low birth weight as a percentage of live births
- Births to mothers 10 to 17 years of age as a percentage of all live births
- Percentage of women receiving prenatal care during the first trimester
- Breast cancer rates and mammography statistics
- Immunization rates
- Return visits to the same level of care or visit within 72 hours to a higher level of care
- Accessibility, availability, and acceptability of care
- Appropriateness and relevance of care (e.g., based on diagnostic laboratory work, symptomatology)
- Appropriateness of treatment frequency
- Intake system
- Provision for information on an emergency or after-hours basis
- Client education
- Consultation
- Documentation including, for example, transfers and advance directives
- Availability of emergency carts/equipment
- Use of leasing for expensive/alternative resources
- Client record
- Client rights, including advance directives, informed consent, and special concern for abuse victims and for those with cultural diversity

From Polaski, A., & Tatro, S. (1996). *Luckmann's core principles and practice of medical-surgical nursing.* Philadelphia: W. B. Saunders.

- Measuring outcomes to determine priorities for improvement
- Systematically improving performance of important functions and maintaining stability of these functions
- Implementing quality improvement activities that optimally affect client outcomes and cost of services and then measuring the ongoing effect of these changes on the services provided
- Instituting a flexible performance improvement plan so that new or changed services and clinical practices serve as triggers for new indicator development
- Enhancing reporting and communication mechanisms of performance improvement results so that the greatest benefit is realized
- Strengthening the client education component as a result of quality assurance and improvement of information
- Supporting performance by improving existing processes
- Designing improvement activities for new processes
- Supporting client advocacy and customer response functions by responding to complaints at the closest level of client care
- Using available resources to produce all-inclusive information and to minimize data collection by staff
- Exploring automated methods of improving clinical information systems

Qualities that enhance the important dimensions of performance are listed in Box 6–6.

RISK MANAGEMENT

Risk management follows the current trend of adapting business strategies to health care systems. Risk management is a planned program of loss prevention and liability control. Its purpose is to identify, analyze, and evaluate risks followed by a plan of reducing the frequency of accidents and injuries. The program requires a team of people from all departments in the institution. The risk manager or safety committee administers the program and serves as the liaison between the hospital administration, the risk management committee, and others as well as between insurance representatives, institution attorneys, and others. Risk managers have no typical profile and can be nurses, administrators, lawyers, or former insurance representatives.

Nursing personnel are crucial to a successful risk management program. The five areas of highest risk in the hospital are (1) medication errors, (2) complications from diagnostic or treatment procedures, (3) falls, (4) client or family dissatisfaction, and (5) refusal of treatment or refusal to sign consent for treatment. Most medication errors are omissions or transcription errors, not dosage calculation errors. Medical records and incident reports serve as documents of accountability. Incident reports are used to analyze problems within the five categories and to plan for corrective actions.

BOX 6–6 Qualities That Enhance Performance of Services

- Efficacy: the degree to which the care and intervention for the client have been shown to accomplish the desired or projected outcomes
- Appropriateness: the degree to which the care and intervention provided are relevant to the client's clinical needs, given the current state of knowledge
- Availability: the degree to which appropriate care and intervention are available to meet the needs of the client
- Timeliness: the degree to which the care and intervention are provided to the client at the most beneficial or necessary time
- Effectiveness: the degree to which the care and intervention are provided in the correct manner, given the current state of knowledge, to achieve the desired or projected outcome for the client
- Continuity: the degree to which the care and intervention for the client are coordinated among practitioners, among organizations, and over time
- Safety: the degree to which the risk of an intervention and the risk in the care environment are reduced for the client and others, including health care providers
- Efficiency: the relationship between the outcomes and the resources used to deliver client care
- Respect and caring: the degree to which the client or a designee is involved in his or her own care decisions and to which those providing services do so with sensitivity and respect for the client's needs, expectations, and individual differences

From Polaski, A., & Tatro, S. (1996). *Luckmann's core principles and practice of medical-surgical nursing.* Philadelphia: W. B. Saunders.

The Future of Acute Care Hospital Nursing

Acute care nursing is changing, but a bright future exists. Major changes will continue in health care delivery, and it will be essential that nurses take a primary position to help ensure that client care remains a priority. With health care costs continuing to rise, cost containment will also remain a major concern. As a result of cost containment, goals for acute care health providers are to:

- Increase the efficiency of care to speed transfer to a less costly level of care
- Streamline care to ease movement into capitated services or managed care contracts
- Monitor clinical pathways for variances and then implement quality improvement strategies to correct the variances
- Enhance client understanding of the disease and its management through education and early discharge planning
- Target high-risk, problem-prone, high-volume client care activities for quality improvement endeavors
- Act on client satisfaction concerns to promote client advocacy
- Extract applicable client, physician, and employee satisfaction data to allow a realistic focus on pertinent issues
- Support institutional quality indicators and quality improvement team endeavors to increase the value of health care
- Enhance the dimensions of performance through the use of appropriateness, availability, timeliness, effectiveness, continuity, safety, efficiency, respect, and caring

CONCLUSIONS

Acute care hospital-based nursing has changed. Years ago, clients could stay in the hospital until they felt well enough to go home. Cost-containment issues have demanded that clients today spend as little time as possible in acute care and quickly move to less expensive areas for care. Professional nurses have become more pivotal providing high-quality care during these shortened stays. All health care providers are trying to maintain excellence in health care during these changing times.

BIBLIOGRAPHY

1. Alfred, C. A., et al. (1995). A cost-effectiveness analysis of acute care case management outcomes. *Nursing Economics, 13*(3), 129–136.
2. Badovinac, C. C., Wilson, S., & Woodhouse, S. (1999). The use of unlicensed assistive personnel and selected outcome indications. *Nursing Economics, 17*(4), 194–200.
3. Brazino, J. (1997). Reinventing nurse extenders: The emergence of UAP. *Nursing Spectrum, 6*(4), 4–5.
4. Buchan, J. (1999). Still attractive after all these years? Magnet hospitals in a changing health care environment. *Journal of Advanced Nursing, 30*(1), 100–108.
5. Doswell, W., & Erlen, J. (1998). Multicultural issues and ethical concerns in the delivery of nursing care interventions. *Nursing Clinics of North America, 33*(2), 353–361.
6. Douglas, L. M. (1996). *The effective nurse: Leader and manager* (5th ed.). St. Louis: Mosby–Year Book.
7. Fletcher, C. (1997). Failure mode and effects analysis: An interdisciplinary way to analyze and reduce medication errors. *Journal of Nursing Administration, 27*(12), 19–26.
8. Gardner, D. L. (1991). Issues related to the use of nurse extenders. *Journal of Nursing Administration, 21*(10), 40–45.
9. Huber, D. (1996). *Leadership and nursing care management.* Philadelphia: W. B. Saunders.
10. Huggins, D., & Lehman, K. (1997). Reducing costs through case management. *Nursing Management, 28*(12), 34–37.
11. Joint Commission on Accreditation of Healthcare Organizations. (1995). *Accreditation manual for hospitals* (Vol. I). Oak Brook Terrace, IL: Author.
12. Johnson, K. (1994). A practical approach to patient classification. *Nursing Management, 25,* 50–55.
13. Krapohl, G. L., & Larson, E. (1996). The impact of unlicensed assistive personnel on nursing care delivery. *Nursing Economics, 14*(2), 99–108, 122.
14. Leninger, M. (1996). Cultural care: Theory, research and practice. *Nursing Science Quarterly, 9*(2), 71–78.
15. Lipson, J., & Steiger, N. (1996). *Self-care nursing in a multicultural context.* Thousand Oaks, CA: Sage Publications.
16. Marquis, B. L., & Huston, C. J. (1996). *Leadership roles and management functions in nursing* (2nd ed.). Philadelphia: J. B. Lippincott.
17. Moore, B. W., et al. (1996). Patient care leadership within an emerging integrated delivery network. *Nursing Administration Quarterly, 20*(2), 54–64.
18. Nolan, M., et al. (1998). Preparing nurses for the acute care case manager role: Educational needs identified by existing case managers. *Journal of Continuing Education in Nursing, 29*(3), 130–134.
19. Prescott, P. A., et al. (1991). The patient intensity for nursing index: A validity assessment. *Research in Nursing and Health, 14*(3), 213–221.
20. Schaefer, J. A., & Moos, R. H. (1996). Effects of work stressors and work climate on long-term care staff's job morale and functioning. *Research in Nursing and Health, 19*(1), 63–73.
21. Sowell, R. L., & Meadows, T. M. (1994). An integrated case management model: Developing standards, evaluation and outcome criteria. *Nursing Administration Quarterly, 18*(2), 53–64.
23. Swansburg, R. C. (1996). *Management and leadership for nurse managers* (2nd ed.). Sudbury, MA: Jones & Bartlett.
24. Wagner, N., & Ronen, I. (1996). Ethical dilemmas experienced by hospital and community nurses: An Israeli survey. *Nursing Ethics, 3,* 294–302.
25. Wyld, D. C. (1996). The capitation revolution in health care: Implications for the field of nursing. *Nursing Administration Quarterly, 20*(2), 1–12.

CHAPTER 7

Home Health Care

Karen S. Martin

This chapter is intended to serve as a bridge for nurses making the transition from inpatient or long-term care facilities to home health care and community-focused service settings. Including a summary of the trends, general philosophy, risks, and practice of home health care, it is designed for the student or clinician whose primary or recent clinical experience has been in hospital, assisted living, nursing home, or other long-term care facilities. *Community health nursing* is defined as a synthesis of nursing and public health practice that is comprehensive and is intended to promote and preserve the health of populations.[27] In this chapter, community health nursing is used as an umbrella term to cover all the diverse types of home health care and community-focused services, settings, and providers. Community health settings in which nurses commonly practice include hospital-based home health care agencies, visiting nurse associations, tax-supported home health agencies, and privately or corporately owned agencies. Other community health settings include tax-supported public health agencies, nursing centers, schools, wellness and occupational health programs, parish nursing programs, clinics for the homeless, case management programs, and other programs that offer related nursing services.

Scattered throughout this book are features called Bridge to Home Health Care, written by nurses and other community-focused professionals to describe their practice. These features address environmental, psychosocial, physiologic, and health-related behavior concerns experienced by clients and their families. For example, in "Living with Failing Vision" in Chapter 65, Bernadette Mruz shares ideas that you might use with clients with vision problems who are leaving your facility to return to the challenges of living at home. The Bridge to Home Health Care features help you gain insight into the roles and responsibilities of the nurse in home health care as it is practiced with clients and families every day. You can use this information as you consider and make referrals for follow-up care.

The Bibliography in this chapter provides more extensive information about home care, public health, and related topics. After reading the chapter, you may discuss what community-focused opportunities you will have as a nursing student. If you are a staff nurse, you may consider making an appointment to accompany a colleague who practices in a home care, public health, clinic, or school setting to learn more about the specialty. Together, this chapter and the Bridge to Home Health Care features provide a review of or introduction to the world of home health care and community-focused practice.

Trends

The need for home health care and community-focused services has grown explosively as a result of consumer demand, the advent of Medicare reimbursement for home health services, the aging of the population, federal legislation that encouraged the expansion of home care, escalating health care costs, and the rise of managed care.[19, 20, 31] By 1996, more than 20,000 Medicare-certified and non-certified home health agencies were operating in the United States, a 1000% increase over 20 years.[31] Between 1967 and 1998, Medicare home health expenditures grew from $50 million to $42 billion.[6, 31]

These trends reflect a shift in the delivery of health care services from the hospital to the community. Ideally, this shift will decrease fragmentation and produce an improved health care system in which providers work together in the interest of their clients. The shift also has the potential to increase provider accountability and result in a more systematic delivery model that is driven by outcome data. A "seamless health care system" is the term being used to describe that new model, a system that includes a wide array of services and providers who collaborate as team members.

Although the recipients of home health care have diverse needs, circulatory disease is the primary medical diagnosis for more than half of home health clients admitted. Diabetes and cancer are the next most frequent diagnoses.[31] In general, the clients who receive home health care tend to be in the elderly population; this trend is likely to continue. Consider these projections[30, 40]:

- Since 1900, the percentage of people older than age 65 has tripled.
- More than 35 million people will be older than age 65 by the year 2000.
- People older than age 65 account for one third of health care consumption; they may represent half of the total health care dollars spent by the year 2040.
- Nearly half of all hospital admissions nationally involve older people.
- Up to 60% of older adults do not take their medications properly.

- The 4 million men and women older than age 85 constitute the fastest-growing subset of older adults, with a growth rate nearly three times that of the overall elderly population.

Because the growth of home health care promises to continue, community health nurses face challenges unlike any they have faced before. The number of clients and complexity of their needs are increasing dramatically, as are the numbers and types of community health staff members and agency programs. At the same time, demands from consumers and payers for comprehensive, economical services are increasing, the availability of staff and reimbursement is decreasing, and regulatory demands are increasing.

For example, during 1997, dramatic legislative and regulatory events occurred that cut home care reimbursement and reflected a growing federal opposition to the rate of home health care expansion. The *Interim Payment System,* scheduled to become the *Prospective Payment System* in 2000, required that all Medicare- and Medicaid-certified agencies, home health staff nurses, and physical therapists complete a 95-item start-of-care Outcome and Assessment Information Set (OASIS).[6, 7] Versions of the data set were to be completed soon after adult clients were admitted to service, at interim periods, and at client dismissal.[10, 22] Home health agencies throughout the United States oriented their staff to OASIS, developed new policies and procedures for collection and transmission of data, and purchased new paper forms or computer equipment. Two months after agencies implemented the federal regulation, it was announced that the regulation was delayed and agencies would not be required to collect OASIS data until further notice. Partly as a result of these changing demands, more than 3000 home health agencies closed because of financial losses, more than 500 agencies in Texas alone.[32]

Although some home care requirements are still in flux, some are not. Reimbursement is a challenge and responsibility that frequently confronts the staff nurse who practices in home health or community settings (see Bridge to Home Health Care: Finding Financial Help). A staff nurse in a hospital, nursing home, or other long-term care facility may not know the cost of service or supplies and may not need to discuss charges with clients and their families. In home health care agencies, however, it is usually nurses who collect financial data, either at intake or when providing the initial services. Data include:

- The source of payment
- Verification of eligibility for Medicare, Medicaid, or other programs providing payment
- Preauthorization approval from a managed care or other third-party payer
- Other concerns

Home health agencies bill third-party payers for most services; Medicare and managed care are the most common. Some clients pay for services themselves (private pay) or receive services that are paid for by taxes, United Way, foundations, or grants. Often, reimbursement regulations are complex and require extensive paperwork for both nurses and clients.[6, 22] Clients may ask their nurses for assistance as they try to deal with those regulations. The Bridge to Home Health Care: Medicare and Medicaid Coverage of Home Health Services feature summarizes eligibility, requirement, and coverage information that home health nurses must know.

BRIDGE TO HOME HEALTH CARE

Finding Financial Help

Finding financial help and support services for a chronically ill client requires patience and perseverance. As clients, families, and informal caregivers assume more responsibility for providing home health care, it is essential that the multidisciplinary health care team help in locating and obtaining needed services.

This process must start early. Waiting periods for federal, state, county, and local services—such as Medicare, Medicaid, Social Security Disability, and county assistance—make early referral not only helpful but necessary. Applications to these agencies can be started while the client is still hospitalized. Make a complete assessment of the client's present and future needs. Your assessment should address financial, environmental, and emotional concerns in addition to physical ones. Your evaluation should focus on the client's, family's, and community's ability to provide for the needs and to mobilize available resources. The health care team should be sensitive to the client's ethnic, cultural, privacy, and value diversities by affirming the client's choices and goals.

A stopgap approach may provide temporary relief for the client's problem, but a more permanent or long-term solution is preferable and avoids having to address the problem repeatedly. Consider, for example, a client who has no money to purchase medications. Finding a resource to help the client obtain medications for a few days may require only a phone call to a local community help group. A long-term solution will require additional time and creative problem-solving. Many managed care and Medicare supplement plans include prescription benefits that allow clients to purchase medications at a set fee. Selecting such a prescription program may be the best alternative for a client who has high monthly medication bills—even if the plan has relatively few additional services and benefits.

To provide the best service to your client, all team members must keep their resource materials updated. Include all team members when attempting to find a solution to a client's financial problem. They may know of appropriate resources, and they may know the staff members or volunteers who serve as gatekeepers for those resources. Local churches, human service agencies, clubs, community action groups, and health service organizations can provide numerous resources for supportive care.

Cindi Leo-Gofta, RN, BSN, *Operations Director, Resource and Referral/Business Development, Alegent Health Home Care & Hospice, Omaha, Nebraska*

BRIDGE TO HOME HEALTH CARE

Medicare and Medicaid Coverage of Home Health Services

Program	Eligibility	Requirement	Coverage
Medicare	Age 65 years or older and established entitlement to Social Security or Railroad Retirement benefits End-stage renal disease (waiting period applies) Younger than age 65 years and established eligibility for Social Security or Railroad Retirement disability benefits (waiting period applies)	Physician-prescribed plan of care Services "medically necessary" Intermittent skilled nursing, physical therapy, or speech-language pathology service Homebound	Skilled nursing, physical therapy, and speech-language pathology services Skilled occupational therapy service if initiated in conjunction with coverable skilled nursing, physical therapy, or speech-language pathology service Medical social and home health aide services if provided in conjunction with skilled service Medical supplies and equipment
Medicaid	Recipients of Aid to Families with Dependent Children (AFDC) Recipients of Aid to Aged, Blind, and Disabled (AABD) who meet specific income guidelines Others who meet federal or state income and categorical guidelines	Physician-prescribed plan of care Services "medically necessary" Homebound; requirements vary by category Additional requirements may be established by each state and may include case management and prior authorization for services	*Required* Intermittent nursing service Home health aide service Medical supplies and equipment *Optional* Physical therapy service Speech-language pathology service Occupational therapy service Private duty nursing service Personal care or housekeeping service Registered dietitian service

Nancy J. Scheet, RN, MSN, *Compliance Officer, Visiting Nurse Association of Omaha, Omaha, Nebraska*

PERSPECTIVES

The specialty of home health care and community-focused nursing has a long and distinguished history in the United States, even though it received little attention from the public or the nursing profession until the 1990s. In 1877, Francis Root was employed in New York City as the first home visit nurse. In 1893, Lillian Wald and Mary Brewster established the Henry Street Settlement in the same city. Their goal was to offer public health nursing and community programs to people of all ages who were at high risk of developing health problems and to those with acute and chronic health problems. Lillian Wald had the vision to:

- Initiate programs and group activities at the settlement to meet the community's health-related, educational, social, and employment needs
- Send nurses from the settlement to make home visits and provide care to new mothers, infants, and the sick
- Forge alliances with business and political leaders to obtain support for her programs

This comprehensive approach to health can be called *community health nursing* and represents a true blend of public health and home care practice. Collaboration between the Henry Street staff and the New York City Mission home visit staff followed and led to the formation of the Visiting Nurse Service of New York, the largest single provider of home health care services in the United States. Soon, organized home visit programs were established in populated areas along the East Coast. Lillian Wald's vision of preventive, curative, and social services for the entire community spread throughout New York City and the rest of the nation. By 1912, 2500 nurses were employed by 900 independent visiting nurse associations.[11]

By 1963, there were 1100 home health and home care aide organizations and hospices in the United States that employed professional registered nurses. The enactment of national Medicare legislation in 1965 accelerated the rate of agency growth. More than 20,000 Medicare and non-Medicare certified home care agencies now offer services to 8 million clients.[31] About 200,000 community health nurses are employed by home care and public health agencies, school systems, and industry. That number is expected to escalate dramatically in the next 10 years.

Agencies that provide Medicare- and Medicaid-certified services must meet minimum national standards; state standards also exist. Agencies voluntarily participate in national accreditation programs such as those sponsored by the National League for Nursing and the Joint Commission on Accreditation of Healthcare Organizations. Nurses and other professional staff are required to meet licensure requirements but not consistent competence standards. Accreditation and competence are becoming important concerns to administrators, clinicians, and the public because of the increased use of technology and high-risk procedures and medications in the home. To be competent, clinicians need adequate orientation, equipment, and supervision; they also need to repeat high-risk procedures with sufficient frequency that they maintain their skills.

Collaboration and communication among members of all disciplines are necessary in home health care and community-focused settings. Nurses make up the largest group of clinicians, although most home health agencies also employ or contract with home health aides and other paraprofessionals as well as other professionals. Physical therapists, occupational therapists, social workers, and speech pathologists are usually on staff. Registered dietitians, pharmacists, dentists, physicians, and clergy may be part of the team as well. Agency staff members also need to coordinate referrals and communicate about client services with various community providers.

Historically, Lillian Wald at Henry Street and other community-focused nurses demonstrated collaboration and communication skills as part of their practice. During the 1990s, a new role, that of case manager, has developed. Nurse case managers are employed by home health agencies, hospice programs, health maintenance organizations, physician group practices, private insurance companies, public health departments, school systems, and managed care organizations. Although their responsibilities vary, they attempt to coordinate the delivery and payment of services that target clients' needs.

COMMUNITY-FOCUSED PHILOSOPHY

The client who receives services may be an individual, a family, a group, or a community.[1, 27, 37, 38] As home health care and community-focused clinicians have had the opportunity to work with clients over time, they have espoused a number of core values that influence their practice. Multidisciplinary collaboration and a seamless health care environment have already been mentioned. In addition, community health nurses have frequently conducted prevention and health promotion programs involving immunizations, smoking cessation, breast self-examination, and similar concerns.[34, 37]

Nurses in home health care and community-focused settings refer to those they serve as clients, patients, consumers, or customers. Regardless of the term they use or whether they use the terms interchangeably, they tend to base their practice on beliefs related to the consumer movement. Included are beliefs that people have both rights and responsibilities and that they must be knowledgeable about their own health care and actively involved in decisions. These beliefs are linked to issues of access, cost, and quality as well as the concepts of primary health care applicable at a national and an international level. For international use, the World Health Organization[42] defined *health* as a state of complete physical, mental, and social well-being and not merely the absence of disease or infirmity; the definition further states that health is a fundamental human right and that attainment of the highest possible level of health is an important worldwide social goal.

The power of the client is an important core value for home health care and community-focused providers.[35, 37] When a clinician enters a client's home, it is the client, not the clinician, who is in charge. In the hospital or nursing home, the nurse gives the client medications and changes dressings. In the home, nurses assist clients in providing their own care or assist family members or informal caregivers in providing that care.[23, 35] The family and other informal caregivers are critical members of the health care team. Their beliefs about health care practice and treatment, the extent of their skills, and their availability influence or even determine whether a client can remain at home and the outcome of the client's care.

Hospice programs provide some of the most dramatic examples of the power of clients. The agency's hospice team usually consists of nurses, home health aides, social workers, pharmacists, registered dietitians, chaplains, and volunteers. Team members also work with the client's physician and other social service agencies. The role of the team is to support end-of-life decisions made by clients and their families as described in the Bridge to Home Health Care: Providing End-of-Life Care in Chapter 22.

Staff members who provide services to clients, their families, and other informal caregivers in their homes are human bridges to home health care. This is true whether the staff member is a nurse, another professional, or a paraprofessional. To maximize outcomes of care, all members of the home health and community-focused team should follow some basic principles as they practice their specialty:

- Remember that you are a guest in your client's home and neighborhood. Your behavior and your manners must convey that you recognize this role.
- Respect the client's cultural, religious, and ethnic heritage. Hesitate before contradicting that heritage. Clients are more likely to follow their heritage than your advice.
- It is possible that the client will not respect *your* cultural, religious, and ethnic heritage. If you are a male nurse, the client may expect, and even request, a female nurse. Develop interpersonal skills—and a tough skin.
- Almost every home health client has family members or significant others who will offer advice and will serve as your advocate or foe. Try to enlist them as your advocates.
- The client "owns" the health-related problem that initiated your services. That problem is just one portion of the client's past, present, and future. Thus, it is the client who experiences, learns to understand, and ultimately solves the problem. It is your goal to help clients and their families become independent as quickly as possible. Talk to your peers and supervisors if you sense that you may be losing that perspective.
- Enjoy the unique autonomy and challenges of providing highly complex care in the home and community setting. Home health practice requires integration of high-technology skills, teaching, case management, and monitoring. Remember the need for communication with other members of the health care team. The nurse is usually responsible for judging whether or not the client can safely remain at home, and other team members

need to share the information the nurse has through oral and written means.
- Maintain your sense of humor. You will need it!

■ RISKS

Home health care staff and students should consistently practice the Boy Scout motto, "Be prepared." Preparedness is essential regardless of your responsibilities, the size of your agency or organization, or its geographical location. If you work in a hospital or nursing home, colleagues, technology, supplies, and references are nearby. When you visit a home, school, clinic, or other community site, you are usually on your own. Help and information may be available via extra supplies in the trunk of your car, the telephone, a computer, a pager, or a Fax machine, but help may not be available immediately.

You must always consider your safety and that of your client. Plan carefully to minimize the risks of accidents or violence; make sure you know your agency's disaster plan.[18] If an accident or violence occurs, you must know how to intervene immediately and appropriately. For example, when selecting individuals, families, or groups for a student assignment, it is necessary to evaluate the client's needs, the student's educational and life experiences, the faculty member's skills and availability, where the clients are located, the timing of the visit, the availability of other sources of help, and the student's method of transportation to and familiarity with the neighborhood.

It is also important to establish an excellent working relationship among the students, faculty, and staff of the agency or institution to enhance safety and the quality of the experience for all. To improve communication and safety for both clients and students, strategies such as shared home visits, student learning centers, nursing centers, and homeless clinics are being used.[8, 15, 24, 39] The Nightingale Tracker, a computerized communication system, and other tools and techniques are additional strategies to link faculty and students (see later in this chapter).

■ RESOURCES

The home health care student and staff nurse have valuable resources that contribute to their ability to provide high-quality care: education, experience, and common sense. Use these resources consistently when making home visits.

Education

Regardless of the stage of your education or the length of time since graduation, faculty and materials provide valuable professional information. Formal and informal education beyond the professional program is important for practicing community health nurses; many educators are increasingly interested in partnerships with practitioners and agencies.[36] Consider courses in first aid; cardiopulmonary resuscitation; computers; the Internet; cultural awareness; community resources; current affairs; and political, legal, financial, and ethical issues. Read relevant publications, and attend relevant conferences. Remember what you learned, and keep updating your knowledge.

Experience

Your professional and life experiences contribute to your technical and interpersonal skills. Know where you are, and take action in the areas in which you need to improve.[2] Discuss your career goals and opportunities with a trusted friend. Take every opportunity to observe a colleague providing care or completing other responsibilities, such as documentation. Learn how to organize your practice and avail yourself of excellent practice pointers, such as the Bridge to Home Health Care features in this book.

Common Sense

Practice in community-focused settings is not the same as practice in the acute care setting. Develop and use your intuition, and listen to it.[18, 27] Expert home health care clinicians are known for their caring, flexibility, persistence, and ability to improvise. They use sound judgment to alter everything from their schedule to their interventions according to their circumstances and the available resources. Expert clinicians have more than a plan A as they begin to work with a client; they can move to a plan B or plan C at a moment's notice.

PROVIDING CARE

The concepts and principles involved in home health care and other community-focused practice settings are closely related to those of nursing practice in the hospital, outpatient departments, and long-term care. The assessment, problem identification (diagnosis), planning, intervention, and evaluation steps of the nursing process provide an important foundation for that practice. Specific systems that you may use in home health or community-focused care include the Omaha System and the Nightingale Tracker.

■ THE OMAHA SYSTEM

The Omaha System was developed and refined during three Visiting Nurse Association (VNA) of Omaha research projects funded by the Division of Nursing, U.S. Department of Health and Human Services, between 1975 and 1986. Research on reliability, validity, and usability was also completed.[25, 27, 28]

The Omaha System is designed to facilitate nursing practice, documentation, and information management. It is a series of cues or feedback loops that help remind the user about possible client problems and intervention options and about ways to evaluate the effect of the care provided. Structured language and codes enhance the precision of recording and ease of communication. Users can communicate their conclusions orally, through printed paper forms, or electronically.

The Omaha System provides a clinical data framework for agencies or programs that use manual or automated versions of client records. Establishing a clinical database that is reliable and valid enables a user to generate reports that contribute to program evaluation, long-range planning, complying with regulations required by accreditation organizations and third-party payers, and outcome statistics required as part of managed care contracts.

Many home health and community-focused agencies are making progress in their efforts to improve their client records and to develop integrated clinical and financial management information systems. The time and costs required for development of such information systems, however, are significant constraints.

Initial users of the Omaha System were community-focused home care, public health, and school practice professionals in the United States. Both the number and type of Omaha System users are expanding dramatically to include nursing center staff, hospital-based and managed care case managers, nursing educators and students, acute care staff, researchers, and the international community. Such expansion reflects the trends already described in this chapter and the trend among all types of health care providers to automate the handling of clinical data.[3, 4, 9, 12, 21, 29, 41] The Omaha System includes one of the vocabularies recognized and disseminated by the American Nurses Association.[16, 17]

Figure 7–1 illustrates the concepts of the nursing process as they relate to the Omaha System. The circular model shown depicts the dynamic, interactive nature of the nursing process; the nurse-client relationship; and related theories of diagnostic reasoning and clinical judgment, sometimes referred to as *analytic reasoning* or *expert knowledge.* The Omaha System is a research-based nursing diagnosis, intervention, and outcome measurement classification or taxonomy developed by practicing nurses.[21, 26, 27] The Problem Classification Scheme, the Intervention Scheme, and the Problem Rating Scale for Outcomes are components of the system. The relationships among the nursing process, the Omaha System, and home health care practice are described next.

A community health nurse begins service to a client after an intake or referral process. During a nurse's initial visit and all other visits, the vital importance of establishing and maintaining a positive nurse-client relationship must be recognized. Freeman and Heinrich[14] emphasized that a positive relationship is developed, not discovered. Such a relationship promotes quantity and quality of data and enhances the potential for success and client progress in relation to all components of the nursing process.

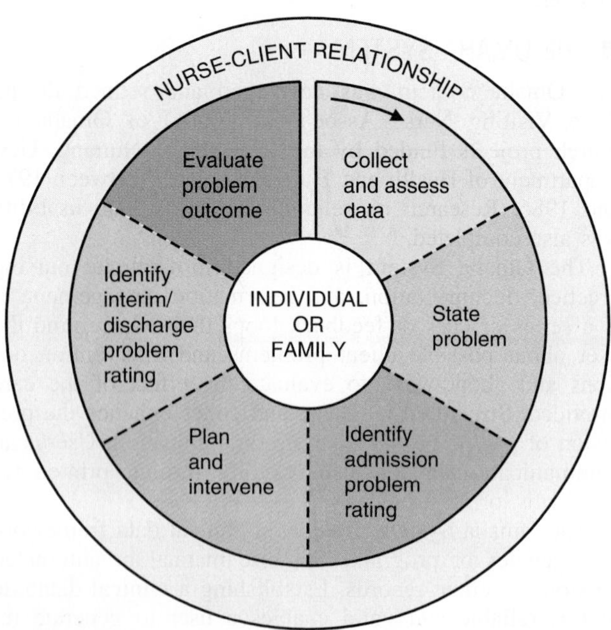

FIGURE 7–1 Steps of the nursing process as they relate to the Omaha System. (From Martin, K. S., & Scheet, N. J. [1992]. *The Omaha System: Applications for community health nursing* [p. 34]. Philadelphia: W. B. Saunders.)

A nurse's initial activities include data collection, assessment, and analysis (i.e., Problem Classification Scheme). This process involves gathering, clustering, combining, summarizing, and validating diverse subjective and objective information about each family member, the family as an interacting unit, and the sociocultural and physical environment. A community health nurse uses principles of epidemiology to enhance systematic data collection and assessment and to identify patterns within client data. . . . The conclusion and logical end product of the data collection and assessment process is problem identification or diagnosis, which involves interpretation of the acquired data.

Planning and intervening are two of the most important concepts of the model to both a client and a nurse (i.e., Intervention Scheme). Campbell[5] described a broad interpretation of planning and intervention involving nurse and family collaboration to:

- Set priorities
- Identify client status and expected outcome(s) criteria or goals relative to specific nursing problems and time frames
- Delineate alternative courses of action
- Choose and take action

Identification of admission, interim, and discharge ratings quantifies the evaluation process (i.e., Problem Rating Scale for Outcomes). Each rating provides a baseline for contrast with later ratings during the period of client service. The evaluation component of the Omaha System allows a nurse to compare a client's health status at different points in time to determine the degree of nursing effectiveness. The nurse uses data from the evaluation process to revise and modify plans and interventions with an individual, family, or group. Thus, evaluation is both ongoing and terminal.[27]

The Problem Classification Scheme, the Intervention Scheme, and the Problem Rating Scale for Outcomes follow principles of taxonomy and consist of terms and codes arranged from general to specific. Terms are intended to be simple, clear, and concise.

The Problem Classification Scheme

The Problem Classification Scheme is a taxonomy of client problems or nursing diagnoses that has been developed from actual client data (Box 7–1). It consists of four levels[26, 27]:

Domains are four general areas that represent community health practice and provide organizational groupings for client problems: Environmental, Psychosocial, Physiological, and Health-Related Behaviors.

Problems are 40 nursing diagnoses that represent matters of difficulty and concern that adversely affect any aspect of the client's well-being. Examples include Caretaking/parenting, Integument, and Nutrition.

BOX 7–1 Domains and Problems of the Problem Classification Scheme

Domain I. Environmental

The material resources, physical surroundings, and substances both internal and external to the client, home, neighborhood, and broader community.

1. Income
2. Sanitation
3. Residence
4. Neighborhood/workplace safety
5. Other

Domain II. Psychosocial

Patterns of behavior, communication, relationships, and development.

6. Communication with community resources
7. Social contact
8. Role change
9. Interpersonal relationship
10. Spirituality
11. Grief
12. Emotional stability
13. Human sexuality
14. Caretaking/parenting
15. Neglected child/adult
16. Abused child/adult
17. Growth and development
18. Other

Domain III. Physiological

Functional status of processes that maintain life.

19. Hearing
20. Vision
21. Speech and language
22. Dentition
23. Cognition
24. Pain
25. Consciousness
26. Integument
27. Neuromusculoskeletal function
28. Respiration
29. Circulation
30. Digestion-hydration
31. Bowel function
32. Genitourinary function
33. Antepartum/postpartum
34. Other

Domain IV. Health-Related Behaviors

Activities that maintain or promote wellness, promote recovery, or maximize rehabilitation potential.

35. Nutrition
36. Sleep and rest patterns
37. Physical activity
38. Personal hygiene
39. Substance use
40. Family planning
41. Health care supervision
42. Prescribed medication regimen
43. Technical procedure
44. Other

Data from Martin, K. S., & Scheet, N. J. (1992). *The Omaha System: A pocket guide for community health nursing*. Philadelphia: W. B. Saunders.

Modifiers are the two sets of terms used to identify ownership of the problem and degree of severity in relation to client interest, risk factors, and signs/symptoms.

Signs and symptoms are the objective and subjective evidence of a client's problem.

The Problem Classification Scheme offers a view of the wide range of client concerns that the home health or community-focused provider addresses. These include physical, emotional, social, spiritual, and economic concerns. Thus, this tool is used as a framework for assessment during a home or clinic visit and for documentation of the service provided. In that way, it constantly reminds the provider that the client needs to be viewed holistically and not as a "colostomy case" or a drug user, for example. The OASIS data set was not designed to be an assessment framework, but OASIS items can be integrated into the agency's assessment form, such as a form based on the Problem Classification Scheme.[41]

Caretaking/parenting, a problem from the Psychosocial domain, appears in Box 7–2. It has nine signs/symptoms, including difficulty providing physical care/safety and expectations incongruent with stage of growth and development. For example, you visit a 14-year-old mother and her newborn to provide information about infant growth, development, and care. You may record:

1. The problem, Caretaking/parenting.
2. Signs/symptoms, difficulty providing physical care/safety and expectations incongruent with stage of growth and development.
3. More specific descriptive and quantitative clinical data on the client's manual or automated record.

Integument, a problem from the Physiological domain, also appears in Box 7–2. Integument has 10 signs/symptoms, including lesion and drainage. If you care for a client whose infected wound requires cleaning and a dressing change, you may record[26]:

1. The problem, Integument.
2. Signs/symptoms, lesion and drainage.
3. More specific descriptive and quantitative clinical data on the client's form or automated record.

Table 7–1 illustrates these two examples of assessment and nursing diagnosis documentation as well as terms and codes from the other two Omaha System schemes. Note that it depicts only part of the documenta-

BOX 7–2 Problems, Modifiers, and Signs/Symptoms from the Problem Classification Scheme

14. Caretaking/parenting:
    Health promotion
    Potential impairment
    Impairment
    01. difficulty providing physical care/safety
    02. difficulty providing emotional nurturance
    03. difficulty providing cognitive learning experiences and activities
    04. difficulty providing preventive and therapeutic health care
    05. expectations incongruent with stage of growth and development
    06. dissatisfaction/difficulty with responsibilities
    07. neglectful
    08. abusive
    09. other
26. Integument:
    Health promotion
    Potential impairment
    Impairment
    01. lesion
    02. rash
    03. excessively dry
    04. excessively oily
    05. inflammation
    06. pruritus
    07. drainage
    08. ecchymosis
    09. hypertrophy of nails
    10. other

Data from Martin, K. S., & Scheet, N. J. (1992). *The Omaha System: A pocket guide for community health nursing.* Philadelphia: W. B. Saunders.

tion for two nurse-client visits, not complete record entries.

The Intervention Scheme

The Intervention Scheme is a systematic arrangement of nursing actions or activities designed to help users identify and document plans and interventions in relation to specific client problems and other concepts of the nursing process (Box 7–3). It represents a research-based effort to link the effectiveness of interventions with diagnoses.[26]

The first level consists of four categories:

- Health Teaching, Guidance, and Counseling
- Treatments and Procedures
- Case Management
- Surveillance

Categories are broad areas that provide a structure for describing actions or activities. One or more categories are used to develop a plan or document an intervention specific to a client problem.

The second level is an alphabetical listing of 62 targets. *Targets* are objects of nursing intervention or nursing activities that further describe problem-specific intervention categories. For the problem Integument and the category Treatments and Procedures, useful targets include dressing change/wound care and signs/symptoms—physical. For Caretaking/parenting and the category Health Teaching, Guidance, and Counseling, possible targets are anatomy/physiology, bonding, and growth/development.

The third level is designed for client-specific information. Users generate pertinent, concise words or phrases as they develop plans or document care provided to a specific client. Although it was not part of the research

TABLE 7–1 APPLICATION OF OMAHA SYSTEM

Client Data	Problems and Signs/Symptoms	Problem Rating Scale for Outcomes	Intervention Categories	Intervention Targets
PSYCHOSOCIAL DOMAIN				
Jane Doe: 14-year-old new mother with 2-day-old infant boy. Says she is "scared." Has not cared for infants; asking how to hold and feed. Wants son to sleep at least 6 hr. No family in area.	14. Caretaking/parenting: actual/family 01. difficulty providing physical care/safety 05. expectations incongruent with stage of growth and development	Knowledge = 2 Behavior = 3 Status = 2	I. Health teaching, Guidance, and Counseling III. Case Management	01. Anatomy/physiology 04. Bonding 08. Caretaking/parenting skills 59. Support group
PHYSIOLOGICAL DOMAIN				
John Brown: 82-year-old just discharged after hemicolectomy. Has infected incision. Recalls some of discharge instructions.	26. Integument: actual/individual 01. lesion 07. drainage	Knowledge = 4 Behavior = 3 Status = 3	I. Health teaching, Guidance, and Counseling II. Treatments and Procedures	14. Dressing change/wound care 50. Signs/symptoms—physical 14. Dressing change/wound care 50. Signs/symptoms—physical

BOX 7–3 Intervention Scheme

Categories

I Health Teaching, Guidance, and Counseling

Health teaching, guidance, and counseling are nursing activities that range from giving information, anticipating client problems, encouraging client action and responsibility for self-care and coping, to assisting with decision-making and problem-solving. The overlapping concepts occur on a continuum with the variation due to the client's self-direction capabilities.

II Treatments and Procedures

Treatments and procedures are technical nursing activities directed toward preventing signs and symptoms, identifying risk factors and early signs and symptoms, and decreasing or alleviating signs and symptoms.

III Case Management

Case management includes nursing activities of coordination, advocacy, and referral. These activities involve facilitating service delivery on behalf of the client, communicating with health and human services providers, promoting assertive client communication, and guiding the client toward use of appropriate community resources.

IV Surveillance

Surveillance includes nursing activities of detection, measurement, critical analysis, and monitoring to indicate client status in relation to a given condition or phenomenon.

Targets

1. Anatomy/physiology
2. Behavior modification
3. Bladder care
4. Bonding
5. Bowel care
6. Bronchial hygiene
7. Cardiac care
8. Caretaking/parenting skills
9. Cast care
10. Communication
11. Coping skills
12. Day care/respite care
13. Discipline
14. Dressing change/wound care
15. Durable medical equipment
16. Education
17. Employment
18. Environment
19. Exercises
20. Family planning
21. Feeding procedures
22. Finances
23. Food
24. Gait training
25. Growth/development
26. Homemaking
27. Housing
28. Interaction
29. Laboratory findings
30. Legal system
31. Medical/dental care
32. Medication action/side effects
33. Medication administration
34. Medication set-up
35. Mobility/transfers
36. Nursing care, supplementary
37. Nutrition
38. Nutritionist
39. Ostomy care
40. Other community resource
41. Personal care
42. Positioning
43. Rehabilitation
44. Relaxation/breathing techniques
45. Rest/sleep
46. Safety
47. Screening
48. Sickness/injury care
49. Signs/symptoms—mental/emotional
50. Signs/symptoms—physical
51. Skin care
52. Social work/counseling
53. Specimen collection
54. Spiritual care
55. Stimulation/nurturance
56. Stress management
57. Substance use
58. Supplies
59. Support group
60. Support system
61. Transportation
62. Wellness
63. Other

Data from Martin, K. S., & Scheet, N. J. (1992). *The Omaha System: A pocket guide for community health nursing.* Philadelphia: W. B. Saunders.

projects, VNA of Omaha staff organized their suggestions into care planning guides.[26]

Table 7–1 presents the use of intervention categories, targets, and client-specific information to describe and document a plan or intervention category specific to a client problem such as Integument or Caretaking/parenting. Again, note the definitions and diversity of community-focused interventions. Nurses and other providers who practice in the community must be generalists and must develop competence in providing "hands-on" bedside care and technical skills as well as educational, referral, monitoring, and motivational skills. Recall the previous comments about the client's owning the health-related problem and being the only one who ultimately solves the problem.

Problem Rating Scale for Outcomes

The Problem Rating Scale for Outcomes is a framework for measuring a client's problem-specific Knowledge, Behavior, and Status. The scale is intended to measure the client's progress and provide both a guide for practice and a method of documentation. The scale was designed for use throughout the time of client service. When establishing the initial ratings for client problems, the user creates an independent data baseline, capturing the condition and circumstances of the client at a given point in time. This admission baseline is used to compare and contrast the client's condition and circumstances with those at the ratings completed at later intervals and at client discharge. The comparison or change in ratings over time can be used to identify the client's progress in relation to interventions and the effectiveness of the plan of care.[25–27]

The Problem Rating Scale for Outcomes is a five-point, ordinal scale comprising three subscales, or concepts (Table 7–2). *Concepts* are three major areas that represent the basic client issues of knowing (Knowledge), doing (Behavior), and being (Status):

TABLE 7–2 **PROBLEM RATING SCALE FOR OUTCOMES**

Concept	1	2	3	4	5
Knowledge: the ability of the client to remember and interpret information	No knowledge	Minimal knowledge	Basic knowledge	Adequate knowledge	Superior knowledge
Behavior: the observable responses, actions, or activities of the client fitting the occasion or purpose	Not appropriate	Rarely appropriate	Inconsistently appropriate	Usually appropriate	Consistently appropriate
Status: the condition of the client in relation to objective and subjective defining characteristics	Extreme signs/symptoms	Severe signs/symptoms	Moderate signs/symptoms	Minimal signs/symptoms	No signs/symptoms

Data from Martin, K. S., & Scheet, N. J. (1992). The *Omaha System: A pocket guide for community health nursing.* Philadelphia: W. B. Saunders.

Knowledge refers to the ability of the client to remember and interpret information.

Behavior consists of the observable responses, actions, or activities of the client fitting the occasion or purpose.

Status is the condition of the client in relation to objective and subjective defining characteristics.

The scale for each of the concepts has five categories or degrees for response. For example, for the problems Integument and Caretaking/parenting, the nurse would identify baseline Knowledge, Behavior, and Status ratings during the first home or clinic visit.

■ AUTOMATION AND THE NIGHTINGALE TRACKER

The Omaha System has been described as a model for practice, documentation, and information management. The critical need to generate, store, analyze, and distribute clinical data with the help of automated information systems exists in all health care settings. For a few years early in the 1980s, the VNA developed and sold computer software. Soon other groups and agencies developed their own Omaha System software. Early in the 1990s, software companies started to develop commercially available software for home health agencies, public health departments, nursing centers, and colleges and schools of nursing.[12, 13, 21, 33, 41]

The presence of faculty and nursing students in service settings, especially students who are just beginning their nursing education, introduces additional challenges related to practice, documentation, and information management. Unlike hospital practice, community health practice may involve faculty remaining at the college or service setting while their eight or more students make independent visits and see clients at homes, clinics, schools, or other sites. These faculty and students, especially students in their early semesters of education, need to maintain communication while traveling and providing client care. Students may need to communicate with faculty quickly and often for the safety of both clients and students. These needs can be met by using reliable and efficient automated point-of-care information systems.

To help nursing students and faculty, the Helene Fuld Trust provided a 3-year (1994 to 1997) research and development grant to FITNE (formerly the Fuld Institute for Technology in Nursing Education). Staff members at FITNE developed the Nightingale Tracker, a computerized communication system using portable hand-held computers. Students use the Nightingale Tracker to document the services they provide, send and receive Fax and e-mail messages, and browse the Internet. They can also use it as a speaker phone.[12, 13]

The Omaha System terminology was selected as the clinical vocabulary for the Nightingale Tracker and is used by students as they complete clinical assignment activities. Such activities include assignment generation, preplanning, postclinical documentation, and evaluation follow-up. When the Nightingale Tracker was released in 1998, the first users were students and faculty in seven colleges and schools of nursing. These schools were selected for diversity in geographical location, size, and educational programs and included associate degree, baccalaureate degree, registered nurse completion, and graduate nurse programs.[9, 12, 33] Since 1998, the number and types of students who use the Nightingale Tracker and the Omaha System have increased to include schools and colleges that base their curriculum on the Omaha System.[29]

CONCLUSIONS

Home health care and community-focused service settings are experiencing both unprecedented growth and financial constraints. Decreased agency revenue can lead to layoffs, decreased salary and benefits, increased workloads, and a sense of insecurity. Increases in client caseloads and services, staff, and budget can be exciting. At the same time, when the internal systems of agencies experience extra pressure and become overloaded, employees are more likely to become frustrated and stressed and to make errors. Teamwork and development and improvement of systems are critical. Clinicians, administrators, students, and faculty need to use a variety of methods to communicate efficiently and work together to provide effective, high-quality services.

BIBLIOGRAPHY

1. Anderson, E. T., & McFarlane, J. M. (1996). *The community as partner* (2nd ed.). Philadelphia: J. B. Lippincott.
2. Benner, P. (1984). *From novice to expert.* Menlo Park, CA: Addison-Wesley.
3. Bowles, K. H. (1999). The Omaha System: Bridging hospital and home care. *On-line Journal of Nursing Informatics* [On-line], *3*(1). Available: *http://cac.psu.edu/~dxml2/ojni.html.*
4. Button, P., et al. (1998). Challenges and issues related to implementation of nursing vocabularies in computer-based systems. *Journal of the American Medical Informatics Association, 5*(4), 332–334.
5. Campbell, C. (1984). *Nursing diagnosis and intervention in nursing practice* (2nd ed.). New York: John Wiley & Sons.
6. *Caring.* (1998). XVII(2).
7. *Caring.* (1998). XVII(10).
8. Coenen, A., Marek, K. D., & Lundeen, S. P. (1996). Using nursing diagnoses to explain utilization in a community nursing center. *Research in Nursing and Health, 19*(5), 441–445.
9. Connolly, P. M., Huynh, M. T., & Gorney-Moreno, M. J. (1999). Cutting edge or over the edge? Implementing the Nightingale Tracker. *On-line Journal of Nursing Informatics* [On-line], *3*(1). Available: *http://cac.psu.edu/~dxm12/ojni.html.*
10. Crisler, K. S., Campbell, B. M., & Shaughnessy, P. W. (1997). *OASIS basics: Beginning to use the Outcome and Assessment Information Set.* Denver: Center for Health Services and Policy Research.
11. Dolan, J. A., Fitzpatrick, M. L., & Herrmann, E. K. (1983). *Nursing in society: A historical perspective* (15th ed.). Philadelphia: W. B. Saunders.
12. Elfrink, V. L. (1999). The Omaha System: Bridging nursing education and information technology. *On-line Journal of Nursing Informatics* [On-line], *3*(1). Available: *http://cac:psu.edu/~dxm12/ojni.html.*
13. Elfrink, V. L., & Martin, K. S. (1996). Educating for community nursing practice: Point of care technology. *Healthcare Information Management, 10*(2), 81–89.
14. Freeman, R., & Heinrich, J. (1981). *Community health nursing practice* (2nd ed.). Philadelphia: W. B. Saunders.
15. Frenn, M., et al. (1996). Symposium on nursing centers: Past, present, and future. *Journal of Nursing Education, 35*(2), 54–62.
16. Helmlinger, C. (1998). New classification system recognized. *American Journal of Nursing, 98*(12), 63.
17. Lang, N. M. (Ed.). (1995). *Nursing data systems: The emerging framework.* Washington, DC: American Nurses Publishing.
18. Leahy, L. (1997). Decrease violence—increase safety. *Home Health FOCUS, 4*(1), 1, 4.
19. Martin, K. S. (1998). Economics, home health style. *Home Health FOCUS, 4*(11), 82.
20. Martin, K. S. (1998). Economics: Wishes, magic wands, and reality. *Home Health FOCUS, 4*(12), 90.
21. Martin, K. S. (1999). The Omaha System: Past, present, and future. *On-line Journal of Nursing Informatics* [On-line], *3*(1). Available: *http://cac.psu.edu/~dxm12/ojni.html.*
22. Martin, K. S. (2000). Home health care, outcomes management, and the Land of Oz. *Outcomes Management for Nursing Practice, 4*(1), 7–12.
23. Martin, K. S., & Gorski, L. A. (1998). Managed care: Effects on home health providers and stroke survivors. *Topics in Stroke Rehabilitation, 5*(3), 11–24.
24. Martin, K. S., & Norris, J. (1996). The Omaha System: A model for describing practice. *Holistic Nursing Practice, 11*(1), 75–83.
25. Martin, K. S., Norris, J., & Leak, G. K. (1999). Psychometric analysis of the Problem Rating Scale for Outcomes. *Outcomes Management for Nursing Practice, 3*(1), 20–25.
26. Martin, K. S., & Scheet, N. J. (1992). *The Omaha System: A pocket guide for community health nursing.* Philadelphia: W. B. Saunders.
27. Martin, K. S., & Scheet, N. J. (1992). *The Omaha System: Applications for community health nursing.* Philadelphia: W. B. Saunders.
28. Martin, K. S., Scheet, N. J., & Stegman, M. R. (1993). Home health clients: Characteristics, outcomes of care, and nursing interventions. *American Journal of Public Health, 83*(12), 1730–1734.
29. Merrill, A. S., et al. (1998). Curriculum restructuring using the practice-based Omaha System. *Nurse Educator, 23*(3), 41–44.
30. Mikulencak, M. (1993, July–August). Facts you should know. *American Nurse, 25*(7), 13.
31. National Association for Home Care. (1999). *Basic statistics about home care 1999.* Washington, DC: Author.
32. National Association for Home Care. (1999, March 19). *Home health agency closures rise* (NAHC Report. No. 802:1). Washington, DC: Author.
33. Nightingale Tracker Field Test Nurse Team. (1999). Designing an information technology application for use in community-focused nursing curriculum. *Computers in Nursing, 17*(2), 73–81.
34. Pender, N. J. (1996). *Health promotion in nursing practice* (3rd ed.). Norwalk, CT: Appleton & Lange.
35. Reif, L. J., & Martin, K. S. (1996). *Nurses and consumers: Partners in assuring quality in the home.* Washington, DC: American Nurses Publishing.
36. Rothert, M. L., Talarczyk, G. L., & Awbrey, S. M. (1997). Distance learning: An integral part of transforming the university and nursing education. In J. C. McCloskey & H. K. Grace (Eds.), *Current issues in nursing* (5th ed., pp. 180–184). St. Louis: Mosby–Year Book.
37. Stanhope, M., & Lancaster, J. (Eds.). (2000). *Community and public health nursing: Promoting health of aggregates, families, and individuals* (5th ed.). St. Louis: Mosby.
38. Swanson, J. M., & Neis, M. (1997). *Community health nursing: Promoting the health of aggregates* (2nd ed.). Philadelphia: W. B. Saunders.
39. Tully, M., & Bennett, K. (1992, March). Extending community health nursing services: The student learning center. *Journal of Nursing Administration, 22*, 38–42.
40. U.S. Bureau of the Census. (1996 & 1998). Resident population of the United States: Estimates and projections. Available: *http://www.census.gov/population.* Accessed: April 1, 1999.
41. Westra, B. L., & Solomon, D. A. (1999). The Omaha System: Bridging home care and technology. *On-line Journal of Nursing Informatics* [On-line], *3*(1). Available: *http://cac.psu.edu/~dxm12/ojni.html.*
42. World Health Organization/UNICEF. (1978). *Primary health care: Alma-Ata Conference.* Geneva: Author.

CHAPTER 8

Long-Term Care

Charlotte Eliopoulos

Of all the types of health care settings, long-term care facilities (LTCFs) are perhaps the most misunderstood and criticized. The media give prime coverage to the small minority of facilities that have substandard conditions while ignoring the majority that provide compassionate, competent care on a daily basis. Some professionals who have never worked in an LTCF believe that this setting is a simple, nonchallenging environment in which to work. Many families assume that nursing home staff are untrustworthy, uncaring, and lazy.

In reality, residents of LTCFs receive proper care and enjoy a good quality of life. Despite significantly fewer resources available to them, compared with those found in hospitals and other care settings, LTCFs provide adequate care for highly dependent residents. The wide range of physical and mental conditions of residents, combined with their advanced age, make them a complex population for whom to care. Because physicians typically are not on the premises at all times, nurses must be highly competent in assessing residents, recognizing changes in status, and communicating needs to physicians. It is not unusual to find very special relationships between residents and their caregivers, who often assume a family surrogate role. Why is there such a discrepancy between the reality and perception of the LTCF? Much of this is the result of the manner in which these facilities have developed. A brief review of the growth of LTCF may offer some insight into the current challenges confronting this care setting.

GROWTH OF LONG-TERM CARE FACILITIES

By the end of the 17th century, most European countries had created institutions to care for the mentally ill, aged, developmentally disabled, orphaned, poor, criminals, and people with contagious diseases. It was not unusual for a single institution to house all of these various types of people together. The interest was not to provide highly specialized and individualized care but to segregate these people from the rest of society. Not surprisingly, low public interest and limited funds caused conditions to become severe in these institutions.

Until the 19th century, the United States had few institutions. People who were sick, old, or disabled were expected to receive care at home, from private help or family. As the population grew, however, so did the number of people without the financial or family resources to provide care, and hospitals and other forms of inpatient care were needed. Hospitals, staffed by physicians who at that time were from society's elite, were less than enthusiastic about having poor people with long-term care needs remaining in their beds for extended periods. Pressure grew to create facilities that could house and care for persons over the long term. In response, communities developed institutions that were given names such as almshouse hospital, asylum, homes for the incurable, and chronic disease hospital. Most often, these institutions were located on the outskirts of town so that the average citizen would not have to have contact with the residents.

Because these early facilities relied on charities and meager public funds for their existence, needless to say, conditions were quite poor. A physician from that era, writing about those early institutions, described conditions such as grossly inadequate supplies, food so insufficient that many residents experienced recurrent incidents of scurvy, and residents forced to sleep on the floor because of overcrowding, rampant theft, open drunkenness, and sex between residents and their caregivers.[7] Residents were expected to work for their keep, and recovered residents who had no family or home in the community, remained in the institution and cooked, cleaned, or cared for other residents in exchange for room, board, and a small salary. In this environment, high quality of life, rehabilitation, residents' rights, and individuality were foreign concepts. With these conditions, most people did not view institutions that provided long-term care as highly desirable options.

The enactment of Social Security in 1935 afforded older adults the means to purchase care privately and not rely on charitable or public institutions. An informal long-term care system began to grow as people rented rooms of their homes to elders who needed room, board, and perhaps some basic personal care assistance. Many of these homes were operated by nurses, or women who called themselves nurses, thus, the term *nursing home* began to be more widely used. Small nursing homes began to appear, often developed by religious or public agencies (e.g., Jewish homes for the aged, county rest homes) and sometimes by private individuals. At this time, the government had little involvement in nursing home operations; there were no government regulations pertaining to nursing home care and no government reimbursement for long-term care services.

In 1946, the federal government took a noticeable step in promoting nursing home growth through the Hill-Burton Hospital Survey and Construction Act. This Act provided funds for hospital construction, but other institutions, such as nursing homes, could obtain funds if they met the conditions required by the Act. Since the construction requirements were developed from hospitals, the nursing homes who obtained these funds constructed facilities that were very similar to hospitals. Rather than an environment designed for the unique needs of chronically ill individuals who would reside in the setting for an extended period of time, nursing homes resembled acute hospitals in appearance and style of operation (e.g., white uniforms, rigid schedules, limited visitation schedules, subservient role of residents).

By the 1960s, the graying of the population was being realized. As the numbers of elders grew, so did their need for health services. During the Kennedy-Johnson era, federal programs proliferated to assist the disabled, the aged, and other special groups. In 1965, Medicare and Medicaid were developed to ensure a minimum level of health care for the aged and poor. There was considerable interest in the existing health care system in providing nursing home reimbursement through Medicare and Medicaid. The American Medical Association lobbied to have reimbursement for extended care facilities to ease the problems acute hospitals were experiencing in having people who no longer needed acute care services remaining in their beds because of the lack of means to pay for nursing home care. The owners of LTCFs also lobbied Congress to provide government funding for care in their facilities. Congress responded by including provisions for reimbursement for nursing home care in Medicare and Medicaid.

Along with funding came regulations—the standards or conditions that facilities had to meet in order to qualify for funds. Initially, the regulations included requirements for 24-hour licensed nursing coverage, individualized care plans, provisions for special diets, and other good standards of practice. Unfortunately, only a small minority of the existing LTCFs could meet the standards at the time and protested that it would not be possible for them to participate in the Medicare and Medicaid programs. Again, with strong lobbying efforts, these conditions were waived, and facilities were able to take advantage of government reimbursement for long-term care without having to meet what were good, basic standards. (It is interesting that there was no noticeable voice from nurses, even though these facilities were called *nursing* homes.)

With eased standards and an influx of government reimbursement, the number of nursing homes grew (Table 8–1). This rapid and unregulated growth led to problems, some of which made front page headlines. Short staffing, substandard care, and abuse were among the conditions that the media exposed and that helped to generate the negative image of LTCFs that continues to shadow this care setting. The public was outraged and demanded action. In response, the Department of Health and Human Services (DHHS) commissioned the Institute of Medicine (IOM) to study these facilities and recommend changes. The IOM study confirmed the widespread poor quality of care that existed in LTCFs and emphasized the need to develop stricter regulations.[5] In response, highly stringent regulations were enacted under legislation called the *Omnibus Budget Reconciliation Act of 1987* (OBRA) which produced profound reforms in nursing home care. Some of the conditions that LTCFs must meet are described in Box 8–1. Both the conditions and enforcement provisions are more stringent. Facilities that do not meet the conditions described in regulations can receive sanctions that include termination of Medicare and Medicaid reimbursement. As a result of the new regulations and strict enforcement of them, conditions in LTCFs have improved.

TABLE 8–1 GROWTH OF NURSING HOMES AND NURSING HOME RESIDENTS IN THE 20TH CENTURY

Year	No. of Nursing Homes	Residents (in Thousands)
1940	1,200	25
1960	9,582	290
1970	22,004	1,076
1980	30,111	1,396
1990	14,744	1,558
1996	16,800	1,700

From U.S. Department of Commerce, Table 204: Nursing and Related Care Facilities. *Statistical Abstract of the United States: 1996* (116th ed., p. 136). Washington, DC: Bureau of the Census.

This history can help you to understand some of the reasons for the persistent negative image of LTCFs. Further, it demonstrates that the importance of an active role for nursing in developing new services and defining nursing services that contribute to high-quality care. Nursing leadership was sorely lacking as nursing homes grew and as non-nurses determined nursing's function, role, and staffing requirements, and the results speak for themselves.

RESIDENTS OF LONG-TERM CARE FACILITIES

Residents of LTCFs can be of any age, although most are old. The risk of being in an LTCF increases with each decade of life; the average age of residents is 82 years. Women outnumber men by a ratio of 3 to 1, and 90% are single or widowed.

Most residents have conditions that impair their self-care capacity or require interventions that they cannot perform independently. About one half have a progressive cognitive impairment, such as Alzheimer's disease, arthritis, cardiovascular disease, or a combination. One third have impaired vision, and another third have impaired hearing. Most residents need assistance with at least several activities of daily living (ADL). Although most residents will spend the remainder of their lives in the facility, an increasing number will recover, have restored function, and return to the community. In the past, some who might have remained in the hospital during recovery are now convalescing in nursing homes as a result of changes in reimbursement policies. The quality and quantity of caregiver support available, rather than the medical diagnosis, determine one's risk of being admitted to an LTCF. For every resident in a nursing home, at least two

BOX 8–1 Protections Afforded to Residents of Long-Term Care Facilities as Described in Regulations*

Resident Rights

- to have rights as citizen and resident protected
- to be informed of rights, rules, regulations and responsibilities
- to inspect and obtain copies of records
- to be informed of health status
- to refuse treatment or participation in research
- to be informed of charges
- to be informed of eligibility for Medicaid
- to be informed of process for filing a complaint with the state agency
- to choose and know physician and method of contacting physician
- to be informed of changes in status, room, roommate, or rights
- to proper management of personal funds
- to have privacy respected
- to voice grievances
- to examine survey results
- to perform or refuse to perform services for the facility, and to be compensated for services performed
- to send and receive mail
- to have access to stationery, postage, and writing implements
- to receive visitors
- to use telephone privately
- to retain and use personal possessions
- to share a room with a spouse
- to self-administer drugs unless determined to be unsafe

Admission, Transfer, Discharge

- to have legitimate reason for discharge
- to be free from solicitation of gifts or money as condition for admission
- to have written policies regarding services provided by facility

Resident Behavior and Facility Practices

- to be free from restraints used for purpose of discipline or staff convenience
- to be free from verbal, physical, or mental abuse, punishment or seclusion
- to have alleged and known abuse incidents investigated and reported according to state law

Quality of Life

- to have dignity maintained and promoted
- to choose activities and care
- to organize and participate in resident groups
- to participate in social, religious, and community activities
- to have program of activities directed by qualified personnel
- to have social services provided by qualified personnel
- to have clean, safe, home-like environment
- to have private closet space, adequate lighting, and comfortable room temperatures

Resident Assessment

- to have a comprehensive assessment conducted within the first 14 days of admission and at least annually thereafter
- to be reassessed whenever there is a change in status
- to have a comprehensive care plan developed within 7 days after completion of assessment
- to have a discharge plan and summary as needed

Quality of Care

- to receive necessary services and treatments to maintain or improve condition
- to be free from developing pressure ulcers, incontinence, contractures, or dehydration unnecessarily
- to be adequately nourished and hydrated
- to not receive unnecessary drugs
- to be free from significant medication errors

Nursing Services

- to have nursing personnel provided consistent with level of care and needs of residents

Dietary Services

- to have at least 3 well balanced meals provided daily, including special diets
- to have department employ qualified personnel and follow standards for safe food procurement, preparation, and storage

Physician Services

- to be under the care of a physician
- to have the physician adhere to standards of practice

Specialized Rehabilitative Services

- to have physical therapy, occupational therapy, or speech-language therapy arranged for or provided as needed

Dental Services

- to be assisted in obtaining dental services

Pharmacy Services

- to have the facility adhere to standards for prescribing, pouring, administering, and monitoring medications

Infection Control

- to have the facility establish and maintain an infection control program

Physical Environment

- to have the facility follow standards of Life Safety Code

Administration

- to have facility be licensed by state
- to have qualified administrator
- to have nursing assistants complete training program and competency evaluation
- to have a designated medical director
- to provide or arrange for laboratory and diagnostic services
- to have clinical records safeguarded and maintained as required by state law
- to have facility emergency and disaster plans
- to have facility make transfer agreements with hospitals
- to have a utilization review committee in effect
- to have facility maintain a quality assessment and assurance committee that meets at least quarterly and develops and implements corrective actions for deficiencies

*This represents a brief outline of regulations included in the Omnibus Budget Reconciliation Act (OBRA). Please consult the full set of OBRA and state regulations for a complete description of regulatory requirements.

equally disabled people are living in the community, receiving care from family or paid caregivers.[6] Often it is a change in status of the caregiver that precipitates the dependent person's admission to an LTCF. This reinforces the importance of assessing the family and assisting these caregivers in using interventions and resources that will promote and maintain their health and well-being.

Staff of Long-Term Care Facilities

Of the more than 1.3 million people who work in nursing and personal care facilities in the United States, about 1 million are nursing employees. Most of these are unlicensed personnel.[13] Regulatory standards are basic, and the only specific staffing requirements in federal regulations are that (1) a Registered Nurse must be on duty at least 8 consecutive hours per day, 7 days a week and (2) a full-time director of nursing must be on staff if the facility has more than 60 beds. The proportion of other nursing staff is not stated, although it is required that "the facility provide 24-hour nursing services which are sufficient to meet total nursing care needs."[4] The fact that most direct nursing care is provided by nursing assistants presents special challenges to nurses who must supervise these caregivers.

Nursing Responsibilities

■ ASSESSMENT

The facility is required to assess residents within the first 14 days of admission and at least annually thereafter; residents are to be reassessed whenever there is a change in their status. The Minimum Data Set (MDS) is the tool on which the assessment is to be documented, and a Registered Nurse coordinates its completion (Fig. 8–1). Problems in need of care planning are generated from the information on the MDS.

As numerous as the items are on the MDS, it is not a *comprehensive* assessment; it a *minimum* assessment. Important pieces of information are not captured, such as the client's self-concept, spirituality, sense of power, knowledge of health condition and self-care practices, sexuality, patterns of solitude, sense of purpose, immunity, stress management, use of alternative therapies, and attitudes regarding health status and death. Since these are important areas for consideration in the long-term care of residents, you may want to supplement the MDS with these additional assessment data. Although the MDS assessment tool may be formally completed periodically, high-quality care relies on the nurse's assessment of residents with every nurse-resident contact. For example, when administering a medication, you can observe the resident's coloring and respirations, note any change in mood, and ask about the status of a previous manifestation. Often residents do not have the ability to identify and report changes in their own health status, and astute nursing assessment is thus crucial. The need to be alert to changes in status is reinforced by the reality that physicians typically do not see residents on a daily basis and must rely on nurses to detect and report manifestations.

The advanced age of the residents can create challenges in assessment. Age-related changes can cause atypical manifestations in older adults. For example, clinical manifestations of pneumonia in elders, instead of high fever and coughing, may include confusion, loss of appetite, and fatigue with activities that caused no difficulties in the past. This challenges nurses to know the norms for individual residents and to identify subtle clues of illnesses so that problems can be identified early. Timely recognition and communication of manifestations to the physician can help prevent complications.

■ CARE PLANNING

Regulations require that a care plan be written for each resident within 7 days after completion of the assessment. The care plan is an *interdisciplinary* one; nurses coordinate the input offered by each discipline and ensure that the plan is written in a correct, timely manner (Box 8–2). To the extent possible, the resident and the family should actively participate in the development of the care plan.

A care plan is not merely a paperwork requirement but a working tool to guide nursing actions; it is a blueprint for nursing actions. Goals and actions that are no longer relevant need to be revised. All members of the team, particularly nursing assistants who will perform most direct care activities, must be familiar with the care plan.

■ CAREGIVING

The direct caregiving role of nurses varies from facility to facility. In some LTCFs, nurses perform selected roles, such as administering medications and treatments; in others, they may be involved in total care activities. During the pre-employment interview, nurses should review the job descriptions for their specific positions to ensure that they have a realistic view of their role.

In addition to caregiving activities that might be performed in any setting (e.g., medication administration, treatments), special nursing support is required by residents and their families as they adjust to the LTCF. Few individuals have had experiences that prepared them for living in or having a loved one in a nursing home. Residents face many adjustments.

Environment

Many people have lived in the same home for several decades before admission and could probably locate ob-

BOX 8–2 Characteristics of an Effective Care Plan

- Is based on needs as identified in the Minimum Data Set assessment tool
- Contains goals and actions to address current needs and to prevent new problems
- States goals that are realistic, clear, specific, and measurable
- Lists actions that are related to each goal that include discipline responsible for implementation and specific directions
- Is accessible and utilized by all caregivers
- Is evaluated at least quarterly and revised as necessary

Resident ____________ Numeric Identifier ____________

MINIMUM DATA SET (MDS) — *VERSION 2.0*
FOR NURSING HOME RESIDENT ASSESSMENT AND CARE SCREENING
FULL ASSESSMENT FORM
(Status in last 7 days, unless other time frame indicated)

SECTION A. IDENTIFICATION AND BACKGROUND INFORMATION

1.	RESIDENT NAME	a. (First) b. (Middle Initial) c. (Last) d. (Jr./Sr.)
2.	ROOM NUMBER	
3.	ASSESSMENT REFERENCE DATE	a. *Last day of MDS observation period* — Month – Day – Year b. Original (0) or corrected copy of form (enter number of correction)
4a.	DATE OF REENTRY	Date of reentry from most recent temporary discharge to a hospital in last 90 days (or since last assessment or admission if less than 90 days) Month – Day – Year
5.	MARITAL STATUS	1. Never married 3. Widowed 5. Divorced 2. Married 4. Separated
6.	MEDICAL RECORD NO.	
7.	CURRENT PAYMENT SOURCES FOR N.H. STAY	*(Billing Office to indicate; **check all that apply in last 30 days**)* Medicaid per diem a. Medicare per diem b. Medicare ancillary part A c. Medicare ancillary part B d. CHAMPUS per diem e. VA per diem f. Self or family pays for full per diem g. Medicaid resident liability or Medicare co-payment h. Private insurance per diem (including co-payment) i. Other per diem j.
8.	REASONS FOR ASSESSMENT *[Note—If this is a discharge or reentry assessment, only a limited subset of MDS items need be completed]*	a. Primary reason for assessment 1. Admission assessment (required by day 14) 2. Annual assessment 3. Significant change in status assessment 4. Significant correction of prior full assessment 5. Quarterly review assessment 6. Discharged—return not anticipated 7. Discharged—return anticipated 8. Discharged prior to completing initial assessment 9. Reentry 10. Significant correction of prior quarterly assessment 0. NONE OF ABOVE b. *Codes for assessments required for Medicare PPS or the State* 1. Medicare 5 day assessment 2. Medicare 30 day assessment 3. Medicare 60 day assessment 4. Medicare 90 day assessment 5. Medicare readmission/return assessment 6. Other state required assessment 7. Medicare 14 day assessment 8. Other Medicare required assessment
9.	RESPONSIBILITY/ LEGAL GUARDIAN	*(Check all that apply)* Legal guardian a. Other legal oversight b. Durable power of attorney/health care c. Durable power of attorney/ financial d. Family member responsible e. Patient responsible for self f. NONE OF ABOVE g.
10.	ADVANCED DIRECTIVES	*(For those items with supporting documentation in the medical record, **check all that apply**)* Living will a. Do not resuscitate b. Do not hospitalize c. Organ donation d. Autopsy request e. Feeding restrictions f. Medication restrictions g. Other treatment restrictions h. NONE OF ABOVE i.

SECTION B. COGNITIVE PATTERNS

1.	COMATOSE	*(Persistent vegetative state/no discernible consciousness)* 0. No 1. Yes ***(If yes, skip to Section G)***
2.	MEMORY	*(Recall of what was learned or known)* a. Short-term memory OK—seems/appears to recall after 5 minutes 0. Memory OK 1. Memory problem **2** b. Long-term memory OK—seems/appears to recall long past 0. Memory OK 1. Memory problem **2**
3.	MEMORY/ RECALL ABILITY	*(**Check all** that resident was **normally able to recall during last 7 days**)* Current season a. Location of own room b. Staff names/faces c. That he/she is in a nursing home d. NONE OF ABOVE are recalled e.
4.	COGNITIVE SKILLS FOR DAILY DECISION-MAKING	*(Made decisions regarding tasks of daily life)* 0. *INDEPENDENT*—decisions consistent/reasonable 1. *MODIFIED INDEPENDENCE*—some difficulty in new situations only **2** 2. *MODERATELY IMPAIRED*—decisions poor; cues/ supervision required **2** 3. *SEVERELY IMPAIRED*—never/rarely made decisions **2, 5B**
5.	INDICATORS OF DELIRIUM—PERIODIC DISORDERED THINKING/ AWARENESS	*(Code for behavior in the **last 7 days**.)* **[Note: Accurate assessment requires conversations with staff and family who have direct knowledge of resident's behavior over this time.]** 0. Behavior not present 1. Behavior present, not of recent onset 2. Behavior present, over last 7 days appears different from resident's usual functioning (e.g., new onset or worsening) a. EASILY DISTRACTED—(e.g., difficulty paying attention; gets sidetracked) 2 = **1, 17*** b. PERIODS OF ALTERED PERCEPTION OR AWARENESS OF SURROUNDINGS—(e.g., moves lips or talks to someone not present; believes he/she is somewhere else; confuses night and day) 2 = **1, 17*** c. EPISODES OF DISORGANIZED SPEECH—(e.g., speech is incoherent, nonsensical, irrelevant, or rambling from subject to subject; loses train of thought) 2 = **1, 17*** d. PERIODS OF RESTLESSNESS—(e.g., fidgeting or picking at skin, clothing, napkins, etc.; frequent position changes; repetitive physical movements or calling out) 2 = **1, 17*** e. PERIODS OF LETHARGY—(e.g., sluggishness; staring into space; difficult to arouse; little body movement) 2 = **1, 17*** f. MENTAL FUNCTION VARIES OVER THE COURSE OF THE DAY—(e.g., sometimes better, sometimes worse; behaviors sometimes present, sometimes not) 2 = **1, 17***
6.	CHANGE IN COGNITIVE STATUS	Resident's cognitive status, skills, or abilities have changed as compared to status of **90 days ago** (or since assessment if less than 90 days) 0. No change 1. Improved 2. Deteriorated **1, 17***

SECTION C. COMMUNICATION/HEARING PATTERNS

1.	HEARING	*(With hearing appliance, if used)* 0. *HEARS ADEQUATELY*—normal talk, TV, phone 1. *MINIMAL DIFFICULTY* when not in quiet setting **4** 2. *HEARS IN SPECIAL SITUATIONS ONLY*—speaker has to adjust tonal quality and speak distinctly **4** 3. *HIGHLY IMPAIRED*/absence of useful hearing **4**
2.	COMMUNICATION DEVICES/ TECHNIQUES	*(**Check all that apply** during last 7 days)* Hearing aid, present and used a. Hearing aid, present and not used regularly b. Other receptive comm. techniques used (e.g., lip reading) c. *NONE OF ABOVE* d.
3.	MODES OF EXPRESSION	*(**Check all used by** resident to make needs known)* Speech a. Writing messages to express or clarify needs b. American sign language or Braille c. Signs/gestures/sounds d. Communication board e. Other f. *NONE OF ABOVE* g.
4.	MAKING SELF UNDERSTOOD	*(Expressing information content—however able)* 0. *UNDERSTOOD* 1. *USUALLY UNDERSTOOD*—difficulty finding words or finishing thoughts **4** 2. *SOMETIMES UNDERSTOOD*—ability is limited to making concrete requests **4** 3. *RARELY/NEVER UNDERSTOOD* **4**
5.	SPEECH CLARITY	*(Code for speech in the **last 7 days**)* 0. *CLEAR SPEECH*—distinct, intelligible words 1. *UNCLEAR SPEECH*—slurred, mumbled words 2. *NO SPEECH*—absence of spoken words
6.	ABILITY TO UNDERSTAND OTHERS	*(Understanding verbal information content—however able)* 0. *UNDERSTANDS* 1. *USUALLY UNDERSTANDS*—may miss some part/ intent of message **2, 4** 2. *SOMETIMES UNDERSTANDS*—responds adequately to simple, direct communication **2, 4** 3. *RARELY/NEVER UNDERSTANDS* **2, 4**
7.	CHANGE IN COMMUNICATION/ HEARING	Resident's ability to express, understand, or hear information has changed as compared to status of ***90 days ago*** *(or since last assessment if less than 90 days)* 0. No change 1. Improved 2. Deteriorated **17***

[shaded box] = When box blank, must enter number or letter.

[a.] = When letter in box, check if condition applies

Code "—" if information unavailable or unknown

TRIGGER LEGEND
1 - Delirium
2 - Cognitive Loss/Dementia
4 - Communication
5B - ADL Maintenance
17* - Psychotropic Drugs
(For this to trigger, O4a, b, or c must = 1-7)

Form 1728RHH

3 of 9

MDS 2.0 1/30/98

FIGURE 8–1 Sample section of the Minimum Data Set (MDS) assessment tool for nursing home resident assessment and care screening. Other sections would include Vision Patterns, Mood and Behavior Patterns, Psychosocial Well-Being, Physical Functioning and Structural Problems, and Continence in Last 14 Days. (© 1997, Briggs Corporation, West Des Moines, IA.)

jects in their homes blindfolded. Now they are faced with adapting to the layout of a new setting, paging systems, new odors, and sounds, and other new components of their environment. They no longer have ready access to their own refrigerator if they are hungry or a spare bedroom where a grandchild can spend the night. Their personal space has shrunk to a bed, a few chairs, a closet, and several drawers. People can enter their space and invade their privacy at any hour of the day or night.

Routines

New residents soon learn that they must adjust to routines and schedules. They may now have to take a morning shower, although they may have taken a bedtime bath for more than 70 years. They may have a full breakfast placed before them at 8 AM when they seldom ate a bite of food before noon. After decades of staying awake and listening to the radio until 2 AM, they now are told that "lights out" is 9 PM.

People

After years of being on a first-name basis with neighbors, store clerks, the mail carrier, and auto repairman, residents must learn a cast of new players. In addition to other residents, they will meet at least three nurses and three nursing assistants who will care for them over a 24-hour period, the facility's medical director, administrator, social worker, housekeeper, dietitian, activities therapist, clergy, and several therapists. They must learn not only the names but also the roles of these people and how to communicate with them.

Independence

Despite a staff's best efforts to afford residents the right to make decisions, there is a loss of independence when people become residents of a nursing home. They cannot scramble an egg in the middle of the night, have a friend stay over for a few days, or paint the walls the color of their choice. They must report their whereabouts and needs to staff, and depend on others for the basics of bringing them food and taking them to the toilet.

These adjustments also affect family members at the same time that they are facing their own changing roles and responsibilities in regard to their relationship with the resident. Both residents and their families can experience such reactions as anxiety, depression, anger, helplessness, withdrawal, grief, and inattention to self-care practices. You can protect the health of residents and their families and facilitate a positive adjustment to the LTCF by taking some of the actions described in Box 8–3.

During caregiving activities, make sure that *holistic care* is provided; such care implies that every aspect—body, mind, spirit—is being addressed. This integration of body, mind, and spirit results in more powerful and meaningful care than if each aspect were addressed separately. Some ways in which holistic nursing is demonstrated are offered in Box 8–4.

■ COMMUNICATION

As mentioned earlier, the LTCF nurse carries significant responsibility for identifying and obtaining timely treatment of complications and new health problems. Because of their regular and close contact with residents, nursing assistants may be the first and only caregivers to detect changes in health status (e.g., a developing pressure ulcer or a change in eating pattern); therefore, effective channels of communication are crucial in reporting these findings. Conducting rounds, reading what has been documented, and asking specific questions are among the measures you can use to learn about a resident's condition.

You also must make sure that physicians learn of changes in a resident's condition in a timely manner. Documenting in a resident's record is not necessarily sufficient, particularly since most attending physicians do not visit LTCF residents on a daily basis. You must promptly communicate any changes and relevant information (e.g., abnormal laboratory results, family complaints) to physicians.

In between their scheduled visits to the facility, physicians may generate new orders, and most of the time these are communicated by telephone. Facilities may differ in regard to the personnel who can accept telephone orders; therefore, it is best to check with the individual facility's policy. To promote safety in telephone orders:

1. Provide the physician with complete information that can aid in medical decision-making (e.g., clinical manifestations, current and usual vital signs, prescribed medications, unusual incidents, and other relevant facts).
2. Avoid making a medical diagnosis.
3. Take the order directly from the prescribing physician, not office staff.
4. Repeat the order; if possible, have the physician fax a copy of the written order.
5. Have the order signed within 24 hours.

■ MANAGEMENT

Nurses hold a variety of administrative and managerial positions in LTCFs, such as director of nursing, assistant director of nursing, supervisor, unit manager or head nurse, charge nurse, and staffing coordinator. Even if they do not hold these formal titles, most LTCF nurses must perform some management functions, such as:

- Delegating assignments
- Supervising other staff
- Evaluating performance
- Implementing disciplinary actions
- Completing reports
- Reviewing and auditing records
- Communicating needs to other departments
- Investigating, reporting, and recording incidents and accidents
- Handling complaints
- Ordering supplies
- Communicating with insurers, regulatory agencies, and other parties

To manage effectively, your knowledge and skills must exceed those used in clinical nursing activities. You must be knowledgeable of regulations, reimbursement programs, and legal aspects of nursing practice and employee-employer relations. You must also be skillful in

BOX 8–3 Helping New Residents and Families

1. *Learn about the unique characteristics of each resident.*
   a. Find out not only about the health conditions residents have but also who they are as people and the lives they have lived.
   b. Engage residents and families in conversations about residents' histories.
   c. Complete a *Profile Poster* similar to the one shown below to help staff and other residents learn about the unique backgrounds of residents and who they are as individuals.

Profile Poster

Name: *Mary Auchmeyer Luggi*
Recent home: *New York City*
Childhood home: *Frankfurt, Germany*
Schools attended: *New York City College*
Spouse's name: *Gus Luggi (deceased)*
Occupation: *High school home economics teacher*
Children: *Son: Gus Luggi Jr, Daughter: Emily Smythe*
Grandchildren: *Tom 21, Amelia 19, Gus 15, Ginny 14, Sammie 13*
Hobbies, interests: *Quilting, baseball, singing*
Other tidbits: *Travelled on several missionary trips to India, speaks German, Italian, and French*

Photos of resident and family can be added

2. *Identify residents' needs, preferences, and level of physical and mental function.*
   a. Assess how well residents can meet their activities of daily living and the assistance they need.
   b. Ask about their preferences in regard to food likes and dislikes, sleep and nap habits, bathing, and other activities.
   c. Incorporate findings into their plan of care.
3. *Explain and educate.*
   a. Orient residents and families to the layout of the facility, staff, routines, and activities.
   b. Explain procedures before doing them.
   c. Be available to discuss residents' and families' concerns and to answer questions.
4. *Promote maximum independence.*
   a. Encourage residents to do as much for themselves as possible.
   b. Explain to residents and families the value of residents being independent.
   c. Give residents opportunities to make decisions regarding their care and activities.
5. *Make residents and families feel comfortable.*
   a. Be courteous and patient; understand that the stress associated with admission can cause residents and family members to make demands, complain, ask many questions, and forget what has been told to them.
   b. Provide privacy during visitation.
   c. Inform families of the location of visitor lounges, cafeteria, and vending machines.
6. *Be holistic.*
   a. Being holistic means that we are concerned with the whole person: body, mind, and spirit.
   b. Try to help residents meet physical, emotional, social, and spiritual needs to promote their physical, emotional, social, and spiritual health.

From Eliopoulos, C. (1997). Helping new residents and families. *Long-Term Care Educator, 8*(12), 6.

BOX 8–4 Holistic Nursing in Long-Term Care Facilities

Nurses can promote holistic care in long-term care facilities by:

- Assisting residents to achieve a higher potential of functioning
- Supporting residents in their efforts to promote health and prevent complications
- Learning about the unique life stories of residents
- Ensuring that residents receive care that is consistent with their values and beliefs and respecting cultural differences
- Aiding residents and families in discovering meaning in health status and in life and death
- Strengthening residents' abilities to live in harmony with their health condition
- Assisting residents in maintaining their connections with family, friends, and the community within and outside the facility
- Helping residents boost their natural healing abilities
- Facilitating hope and a sense of purpose in residents' lives
- Supporting residents as they respond to their spiritual identity or relate to a higher power
- Providing a nurturing, healing caregiving environment
- Offering opportunities for residents to experience joy and satisfaction
- Protecting residents from threats to their health or well-being, and promoting highest quality of life
- Adhering to accepted standards of nursing practice

From Eliopoulos, C. (1999). *Nursing administration of long-term care facilities* (3rd ed). Glen Arm, MD: Health Education Network.

assertiveness, coaching, counseling, accurate documentation, organization, time management, and communication.

Other Forms of Long-Term Care

So far this chapter has focused on the role of nurses in the LTCF. However, the LTCF is only one part of the long-term care system, and other forms of long-term care are available. Box 8–5 presents additional resources.

1. *Subacute or transitional care.* For people who require ongoing care or recovery for an acute condition but do not need to receive the services on an acute hospital unit. The subacute care unit can be separate parts of a hospital or nursing home, or it can be an entire facility dedicated to this purpose.
2. *Assisted living facility.* A form of housing that provides 24-hour staffing, meals, supervision of medications, and personal care assistance.
3. *Adult day care.* A daytime program for people who typically have the same level of impairments as nursing home residents but who receive care in the community, usually by family members. The client is transported to the center and receives structured activities, meals, personal care assistance, and health care supervision.
4. *Home care.* For community-based people who are homebound and who need caregiving assistance or special treatments.
5. *Hospice.* For people who are terminally ill and in need of care. This care can be provided in the home or in a day hospital setting.

Each of these types of care have unique regulations and conditions for reimbursement.

Conclusions

The roles and responsibilities of nurses in LTCFs are varied and complex. Residents possess a wide range of physical and mental conditions that require expert assessment, interventions, and monitoring. The inability of many residents to accurately express their needs and age-related alterations in the presentation of clinical manifestations presents special challenges in detecting changes in status. The absence of physicians in the facility on a daily basis places a greater burden on nurses to identify and seek treatment of residents' problems. The high proportion of unlicensed staff demands that nurses be effective managers. An abundance of regulatory and reimbursement requirements demand that nurses be knowledgeable of these topics.

The reality that most residents will not only receive

BOX 8–5 Resources to Learn More About Long-Term Care

Adult Day Care

National Institute on Adult Day Care
600 Maryland Ave., S.W.
Washington, DC 20024
(202) 479-1200

Home Health and Community Services

American Public Health Association
Section on Gerontological Health
1015 18th St., N.W.
Washington, DC 20036

International Senior Citizens Association, Inc.
11753 Wilshire Blvd.
Los Angeles, CA 90025

National Association of Home Care
205 C St., N.E.
Washington, DC 20002

National Association of Home Health Agencies
426 C St., N.E., Suite 200
Washington, DC 20002
(202) 547-1717

National Home Caring Council
235 Park Ave. South
New York, NY 10003

Visiting Nurse Associations of America
3801 E. Florida Ave., Suite 900
Denver, CO 80210
(800) 426-2547

Long-Term Care Facilities

American Association of Homes for the Aging
901 E St., N.W., Suite 500
Washington, DC 20036
(202) 783-2242

American Health Care Association
1200 15th St., N.W.
Washington, DC 20005
(202) 833-2050

American Nurses Association, Inc.
Council on Nursing Home Nurses
600 Maryland, Ave., S.W., Suite 100 West
Washington, DC 20024
(800) 274-4262
www.nursingworld.org

National Association of Directors of Nursing Administration in Long Term Care
10999 Reed Hartman Hwy, Suite 234
Cincinnati, OH 45242
(800) 222-0539

National Citizens Coalition for Nursing Home Reform
1424 16th St., N.W.
Washington, DC 20036
(202) 332-2275

National Gerontological Nursing Association
7250 Parkway Drive, Suite 510
Hanover, MD 21076
(800) 723-0560
www.nursingcenter.com/people/nrsorgs/ngna

care, but will *live* in the facility for the remainder of their lives causes nurses often to serve as surrogate family. Very few practice settings offer nurses the opportunity to fill such a wide and varied range of roles. Rather than a simple, nonchallenging practice setting, LTCFs challenge nurses to use a wide range of knowledge and skills as they establish meaningful long-term relationships with residents and their families. To fill the roles and responsibilities competently, LTCF nurses must be among their profession's best.

BIBLIOGRAPHY

1. Eliopoulos, C. (1998). *Transforming nursing homes into healing centers: A holistic model for long-term care* (p. 48). Glen Arm, MD: Health Education Network.
2. Eliopoulos, C. (1999). *Integrating alternative and conventional therapies: Holistic care for chronic conditions.* St. Louis: Mosby.
3. Eliopoulos, C. (1999). *Nursing administration of long-term care facilities* (3rd ed.). Glen Arm, MD: Health Education Network.
4. *Federal Register.* (1989). Rules and Regulations (Vol. 54, No. 21). Section 483.26(c), February 2, 1989.
5. Institute of Medicine, Committee on Implications of For-Profit Enterprise in Health Care. (1986). Profits and health care: An introduction to the issues. In B. H. Gray (Ed.), *For-profit enterprise in health care* (pp. 3–18). Washington, DC: National Academy Press.
6. Kane, R. L., & Kane, R. A. (1997). Long-term care. In C. K. Cassel, et al. (Eds.), *Geriatric medicine* (3rd ed., pp. 81–96). New York: Springer.
7. Lawrence, C. (1905). *History of the Philadelphia almshouses and hospitals* (pp. 52, 123). Privately printed.
8. Muder, R. R., Brennen C., & Swenson, D. L. (1996). Pneumonia in the long-term care facility. *Archives of Internal Medicine, 156,* 2365–2370.
9. National Committee to Preserve Social Security and Medicare. (1997). *Nurse staffing in nursing homes: Viewpoint.* Legislative Agenda for the 105th Congress, April 1997.
10. Rice, V. H. (1997). Ethical issues relative to autonomy and personal control in independent and cognitively impaired elders. *Nursing Outlook, 45,* 27–34.
11. Rosenberg, C. E. (1987). *The care of strangers: The rise of America's hospital system.* New York: Basic Books.
12. Thomas, W. H. (1996). *Life worth living. How someone you love can still enjoy life in a nursing home.* The Eden Alternative in action. Acton, MA: VanderWyk & Burnham.
13. U.S. Department of Commerce. (1996). Table 654: Nonfarm industries: Employees and earnings. *Statistical Abstract of the United States: 1996* (116th ed., p. 421). Washington, DC: Bureau of the Census.

UNIT 3

Health Assessment

CHAPTER 9

Health History

Annabelle M. Keene

The nursing process hinges on assessment of the client to provide baseline data. Assessment enhances identification of physical and psychosocial needs. The amount, depth, and level of assessment skills vary with the nurse's knowledge and expertise. Some assessment skills are basic, such as taking a temperature. Advanced assessment skills are learned and practiced in order to provide interventions and to evaluate health maintenance and promotion practices.

Familiarity with the parameters of human behavior and physiology is necessary in order to recognize abnormal situations. Normal ranges for psychosocial behavior may vary, whereas many physiologic manifestations have narrowly defined limits. For example, cell death occurs if body temperature is either too high or too low; the defined parameters are a matter of a few degrees. In contrast, depression in survivors following the death of a loved one is expected, but prolonged depression may signal mental illness. Skillful assessment requires careful observation along with the ability to decide whether an observation is normal. Consider the client's unique circumstances when comparing assessment findings to standardized norms.

Evaluate the client's reaction to the assessment process as well as the possible implications of the findings. Nursing diagnoses common to clients experiencing health assessment include *Anxiety, Fear, Knowledge Deficit, Pain, Powerlessness,* and *Situational Low Self Esteem.* Each nursing diagnosis is followed by a related factor identifying the specific cause leading to the problem. For example, a woman having a breast examination may be anxious because she never has had such an examination before or she may fear that a lump will be found.

Assessment requires skill and judgment. Chapters 9 and 10 provide information to begin developing expertise in health assessment. Proficiency requires extensive practice. Seek guidance from a skilled, competent practitioner. A broad knowledge base, repeated practice, and access to a mentor foster the ability to discriminate between findings.

Health assessment focuses on the client and is divided into two portions. The health history contains subjective information, whereas the physical examination is objective information about a client's health status. The client is a unique person with complex physical and psychosocial interactions. Keep the health history interview free from bias, prejudice, and stereotyping. For example, an elderly client with several chronic health problems may or may not have immediate health care needs, yet the potential for complex health problems exists. Conversely, a young adult may appear "healthy" when in fact he or she may have overwhelming psychosocial problems or needs affecting both current and future health status. An individualized approach to health assessment provides a valid database for nursing care.

The Health History

■ ACCURACY

Assess the accuracy and completeness of the data throughout the health history interview. Validation allows formulation of accurate nursing diagnoses. Determine whether the client is a reliable historian, able and willing to provide information. The client may be (1) unconscious or disoriented and, therefore, may be unable to cooperate; (2) willing to cooperate but hindered by circumstances, such as a language barrier, or anxiety; (3) unwilling and mistrustful about cooperating because of anger or depression.

If the client cannot provide information, seek secondary sources, such as significant others or an interpreter. Information content and accuracy may be influenced by the perceptions and biases of the secondary sources as well as by their knowledge of the problem and recall ability.

Stereotyping jeopardizes collection of accurate data. False assumptions and generalizations may lead to questions that alienate the client and that interfere with development of trust. A mistrustful client is reluctant to divulge sensitive information, perhaps fearing rejection or ridicule, resulting in inaccurate or missed nursing diagnoses.

Similarities among people result in their being grouped according to age, sex, ethnic background, common occupation, recreational activity, health risk behavior, or type of health problem. Each person is also unique. Reliable research findings concerning group characteristics or similarities may be applied to a specific client who belongs to that group. For example, the incidence of hypertension is higher in blacks than in whites, and regular blood pressure screening should be included at every health care visit. Generalizations, particularly those grounded in assumptions or prejudice or based on limited experience, are potentially harmful.

Physical appearance or presenting manifestations may bias one's perception of a client. Similar manifestations may have different origins. For example, a client with an uneven, lurching gait and garbled speech may appear to be intoxicated or under influence of a controlled substance. In fact, the client might have residual neurologic deficits from a head injury. Initial inaccurate judgment may be costly in wasted time and effort and may result in a strained nurse-client relationship. Box 9–1 includes guidelines that may reduce stereotyping during health assessment.

Computerized health history assessment is available in clinical settings, particularly ambulatory care. Computer programs for history taking result in accurate, legible databases when data are entered correctly. Either the client or the nurse, using interactive programs, records the data directly. Data also may be entered from a client-completed questionnaire, which is reviewed and validated by a nurse skilled in health assessment. Computerized health histories tend to be complete because pertinent assessment areas are included in the programs. Branching programs direct collection of additional data when the client responds with significant information.

■ DEPTH

Many factors influence the level of assessment. Ideally, data are collected at one time and in sufficient depth to allow problem identification; however, this may not always be practical. The interview setting may be less than ideal (e.g., the scene of a motor vehicle accident). The client's reason for seeking health care may preclude in-depth interviewing (e.g., if the client has a ruptured appendix). The client's attention span, energy, and comfort level may affect ability to participate (e.g., if pain is present).

In an acute situation:

1. Collect data pertinent to the immediate problem, and assess the client's present health status.
2. Tailor the health history interview to include pertinent data while striving to be thorough.
3. Update and enlarge the database as indicated by the client's condition.

In clinical practice, many agencies provide specific health history formats. These formats are designed to meet agency purposes and may vary considerably in depth and level. Tailor the health history interview to the needs of the client and the agency. For example, you might arrange to meet several brief times with clients who have limited abilities or special needs (e.g., impaired hearing or limited intellectual capacity), or an interpreter may be required when a language barrier exists.

Long Format

The health history model presented in this chapter is an *exhaustive,* or long format (Box 9–2). This holistic approach, although time-consuming, elicits a wealth of data and allows thorough assessment of how the client functions within multiple aspects. The exhaustive approach may be impractical in an acute care setting, especially in one sitting. However, to make accurate nursing diagnoses and to identify etiology, you must know each component of the history and should learn how to collect a complete database, over time if necessary. Students often learn history-taking skills in a laboratory setting using the exhaustive model. They must also learn to modify the technique to an actual setting and to a client's ability.

Short Format

An *episodic* health history assessment often suffices when a client presents with an uncomplicated, short-term health problem, such as an earache. Use a systematic approach to collect data significant to the problem (Box 9–3). Proficiency in all areas of health history assessment, which are discussed in this chapter, is necessary to conduct an accurate episodic assessment.

BOX 9–1 Guidelines That May Reduce Stereotyping During Health Assessment

- Do not manipulate a client's information to make it congruent with a cultural image.
- Do not assume that all of a client's reported symptoms stem from the identified medical diagnosis.
- Do not classify a client on the basis of appearance or behavior.
- Do not ignore any aspect of the client's presentation.

GUIDELINES FOR THE HEALTH HISTORY INTERVIEW

External (environmental and interpersonal) and *internal* (intrapersonal and physiologic) factors affect the health history interview. Data quality and quantity are enhanced by sensitivity to the client and by one's skill level with the interview process.

■ PREPARATION OF THE ENVIRONMENT

The following guidelines apply:

1. When possible, conduct the interview in a comfortable setting. A quiet room with a closed door decreases interruptions. If the client cannot leave a setting (e.g., a multibed room or an emergency department cubicle), screen the area by drawing the privacy drapes.
2. Reduce or eliminate distractions (e.g., turn off the television) and inform colleagues to avoid interruptions.
3. Use facing comfortable chairs to help establish rapport. Adjust their distance to the client's preference and sense of personal space.
4. Ensure a moderate room temperature to promote comfort.
5. Provide indirect lighting to prevent glare and strong shadows that may distort observation of nonverbal cues.

■ PREPARATION OF THE CLIENT

The following guidelines apply:

1. After introductions, explain the nature and purpose of the health history interview.

Text continued on page 135

BOX 9–2 An Exhaustive Health History Format

Interview date (included as a baseline for later reference)

Biographical and Demographic Data

Full name (include aliases, if applicable)
Age
Sex
Race
Nationality or ethnic background
Primary language
Date and place of birth
Significant others and relationship to client
Home address (and alternate contact address, if applicable)
Phone number(s)
Occupation (usual and current)
Social Security number
Religion
Emergency contact or next of kin
Legal guardian (if necessary)
Source of information and reliability as a historian (note use of an interpreter, if needed)
Source of referral to agency and/or usual primary health care provider
Health insurance information
Advance directive information

Current Health

Reason for seeking health care, or chief complaint (recorded in client's own words)
Symptom analysis (in-depth analysis of manifestations):

- Last time client was well (discriminate between onset of symptom and when client became concerned about it)
- Date and time of onset, including time period during which symptom evolved (slow? abrupt?)
- Setting (what was client doing and where was the client when symptom began?)
- How was client feeling before problem's onset?
- Duration or how long symptom lasts (minutes? hours? days? intermittent? constant? goes away completely?)
- Frequency or how often symptom occurs (daily? weekly? monthly?)
- Location (localized? diffuse? radiating?)
- Quality (description) of symptom's characteristics (burning? piercing? stabbing? dull? aching? throbbing?)
- Quantity or severity rated by client using an analog scale such as 1 to 10, with 1 being the least and 10 being the most or worst)
- Does symptom interfere with client's usual daily activities? Do interferences cause problems for the client? What types of problems? (sleeping? eating? activity tolerance?)
- Factors that seem to precipitate (bring on) the symptom
- Factors that seem to worsen (aggravate) the symptom (activity? weather? eating? medication? position? fatigue? time of year or day?)
- Factors that relieve symptom (rest? sleep? medication [name, strength, amount taken, and frequency]? heat? cold?)
- Associated factors or symptoms in other body systems that seem concurrent—review the associated body system at this time instead of later

Past Health History

Developmental (may not be appropriate for all adults)

- Any known problems with growth and development including prenatal or birth history (e.g., premature delivery or low birth weight) or delay in language, speech, motor skills, and so forth

Immunizations

- Record childhood immunizations and whether kept up to date (tetanus, diphtheria, pertussis, measles, mumps, rubella, chickenpox, polio, *Haemophilus influenzae* b conjugate, hepatitis B)
- Note last dates of tetanus booster and influenza vaccination
- Note whether client has received pneumococcal vaccination if age 65 or over or if there is a history of chronic illness

Past illnesses (childhood and adulthood)

- Ask about measles (rubeola), mumps, rubella, chickenpox (collectively called "usual childhood diseases"), whooping cough (pertussis), scarlet fever, strep throat, rheumatic fever, poliomyelitis, asthma, tuberculosis, pneumonia, and any sequelae or residual effects

Serious or chronic illnesses

- Note the presence of diabetes mellitus, heart disease, hypertension, kidney problems, ulcers, thyroid problems, migraine headaches, seizure disorders, stroke (cerebral vascular accident), arthritis, Lyme disease, cancer, anemia, sickle cell anemia, bleeding tendencies, or human immunodeficiency virus (HIV) infection

Hospitalizations

- Date and reason for each admission
- Summary of treatment, length of hospitalization
- Name of primary care physician
- Reaction to these events and their outcomes

Surgeries

- Date and type of procedures performed
- Name of surgeon
- Note whether procedure was performed on inpatient or outpatient basis
- Client's reaction to each procedure and its outcome

Serious injuries or accidents

- Date and type of injury or accident
- Ask specifically about head injuries, fractures, burns, or other trauma
- Note client's reaction to each and their outcomes

Obstetric history (if applicable)

- For completed pregnancies: number; course of each pregnancy, labor, delivery, and postpartum period; delivery date; birth weight, sex, and health of infant
- For incomplete pregnancies: number; duration of pregnancy; date and circumstances of termination (spontaneous or induced abortion, stillbirth)
- Complications (describe)

Last visit to health care provider

- Record most recent dates for dental, physical, vision, and hearing examinations. Identify provider if different from primary care provider
- Date and results of screening or diagnostic tests performed such as electrocardiogram (ECG), radiology studies, laboratory tests, Papanicolaou (Pap) smear, purified protein derivative (PPD) test, or tuberculosis tine test

Allergies

- Describe allergens and reactions (rash, urticaria, pruritus, watery or itching eyes, nasal congestion, running nose, breathing difficulty including asthma, pulse irregularity, convulsions, collapse)

Box continued on following page

BOX 9–2 An Exhaustive Health History Format *Continued*

- Include medications (true allergic reactions only and not side effects), food, contact agents (fabric, nickel), and environmental agents (dust, dander, pollens, cigarette smoke)

Medications currently taken, including prescriptive, nonprescriptive over-the-counter, and recreational (street) drug use

- Ask about common over-the-counter medications by name (such as aspirin, vitamins, herbals, antacids, birth control pills, cold and allergy preparations, topical creams and lotions—many people do not think of these as medications)
- For all medications, ask for: name; dose; route; frequency and time of day taken; reason for taking; any problems with drug regimen; who prescribed each drug and when

Family Health History

- Include ages, cause of death, and age at death of family members
- Ask specifically about heart disease, hypertension (high blood pressure), cerebrovascular accidents (stroke), epilepsy (seizures), migraines or headaches, mental illness, Alzheimer's disease, Huntington's chorea, alcoholism, tuberculosis, asthma, allergies, diabetes mellitus, thyroid problems, eating disorders (overeating, undereating, self-induced vomiting), obesity, kidney disease, arthritis, cancer (type), sickle cell anemia, anemia, hemophilia, HIV infection, developmental delay
- Data may be displayed in a diagram of the family tree (see Fig. 9–1)

Psychosocial History

Explore history of psychosocial problems

- Personal history
- Family history

Assess psychologic components

- General appearance

  Dress
  Hygiene and grooming
  Posture
  Motor activity
  Facial expression

- Behavior

  Verbal
  Nonverbal
  Reaction to interview

- Recent level of stress

  Current perceived level of stress
  Adjustment to past stressors
  Signs of response to stress
  Usual coping pattern

- Mental status and level of understanding

  Level of consciousness
  Orientation
  Mood and affect
  Speech and communication (language)
  Thought process and content
  Attention span
  Memory
  General fund of knowledge
  Calculation ability
  Ability to reason and think abstractly
  Perception
  Judgment
  Insight

- Personality style
- Motivation
- Personal strengths
- Values and beliefs

  Self-concept, self-esteem
  Body image
  Locus of control

- Spirituality
- Psychosocial risk factors (including coping ability, suicidal ideation)

Assess sociologic components

- Psychosocial level of development
- Social network and support systems (including pets)
- Socioeconomic status
- Lifestyle (including habits, recent travel within and outside of country)
- Sexuality

Assess cultural components (see Table 9–1)

Review of Systems

General

Do the following symptoms occur: fever, chills, sweats, night sweats, weakness, weight loss or gain (in past 6 months), fatigue, malaise, nausea or vomiting, headaches, mood changes?

Nutrition

Describe the kinds of food usually eaten, including likes and dislikes. Describe everything eaten during the last 24 hours. How much of each food was eaten? Is the client on a special type of diet, such as avoiding salt, sugar, fats, or caffeine? Does the client take vitamin or mineral pills, or anything else believed necessary in the diet? Does the client have an appetite? Has it changed recently (describe)? Has the client ever had an eating problem or disorder such as anorexia or bulimia nervosa (describe)? What is the client's usual weight? Does the weight vary (ask client to describe maximum and minimum weights)? Has the client gained or lost weight recently? (How much? Over how long a time period did this happen?) Who does the food shopping in the household? Who usually prepares meals? Does the client usually have someone to share meals with? Does the person who plans and prepares food use a system such as the Food Guide Pyramid? Does food have a special meaning for the client? Are there foods that the client looks forward to eating on special occasions (such as a religious holiday)? Are there any foods that cannot be eaten because of allergies or for other reasons? Are there any problems with following a special diet (describe)? Are there any problems with being able to swallow or chew food (describe)?

Integument

- Skin

Inquire about past skin problems (e.g., scars; birthmarks; moles; burns). Ask if the following problems occur: dryness; pruritus (itching); rashes or other skin eruptions; odor; a change in skin color, texture, or temperature; a change in any skin lesion; growths; easy bruising; psoriasis; eczema. Has the client had any skin lesions removed (describe)? Does the client have any tattoos or pierced body parts? Ask the client to describe skin care habits (e.g., use of soap, lotions, skin oils, etc.) that may affect skin texture and moisture. How much sun exposure has the client had (e.g., sunbathing, tanning salon, severe sunburns)?

BOX 9–2 An Exhaustive Health History Format *Continued*

- Hair

Are there any problems with alopecia (hair loss), dryness, brittleness, or dandruff? Does the client use hair dyes or have a permanent wave? Ask the client to describe hair care habits (e.g., frequency of shampooing, use of conditioner, combing versus brushing) that may affect hair texture.

- Nails

Are there any problems with brittleness, cracking, or splitting? Has there been a change in nail texture? Does the client bite his or her nails? Does the client wear nail polish? Have artificial nails?

Hematopoietic

Are there any problems with fatigue, unusual bleeding, easy bruising, ecchymoses (bruises), anemia, or leukemia? Has the client ever been exposed to radiation or toxic agents (describe)? Has the client ever had a transfusion of blood or a blood product (were there any problems?)? Does the client know his or her blood type (if a female is Rh-negative and has been pregnant, does she recall receiving Rho-GAM)? Does the client know if he or she has any unusual type of antibodies (describe)?

Endocrine

Have there been past problems with diabetes, goiter or thyroid, or growth and development? Has the client ever been treated with hormones (describe)? Has the client ever had neck surgery (describe)? Are there problems with polydipsia, polyuria, or polyphagia (increased thirst, urination, or hunger); heat or cold intolerance; weakness; tremors; nervousness; dry skin or hair; excessive sweating; change in hair distribution or hirsutism (excess hair growth in unusual places); impotence or a change in sexual activity or libido?

Head

Has the client ever had a blow, trauma, or injury to the head? Ask about problems with headaches (unusual or severe), dizziness or lightheadedness, syncope (fainting or loss of consciousness), vertigo, seizures.

Eyes

Has the client had past problems with eye infections (conjunctivitis or pink eye), chalazion (eyelid cyst), hordeolum (stye), glaucoma, cataracts, amblyopia (lazy eye), detached retina, or strabismus? Has the client ever received a blow to the eye? Has the client ever had eye surgery (describe)? Does the client wear an eye prosthesis (ask the client to describe how he or she cares for it)? Are there problems with a change in vision (either in general or in part of the visual field, or in night vision), failing vision or blindness, blurred vision, diplopia (double vision), spots or floaters, redness, pain, itching, lacrimation (excess tearing), dryness, discharge or drainage, swelling around the eyes, unusual sensations or twitching, photophobia (light sensitivity)? Is there difficulty reading or seeing distant objects? Do vision problems interfere with daily activities? Does the client wear eyeglasses or contact lenses (when was the last prescription change)? When was the last eye examination (results)? Last glaucoma check (results)?

Ears

Inquire about past problems with ear infections or earaches; diminution of or loss of hearing. Are there problems with difficulty hearing; deafness; increased sensitivity to sound; tinnitus (ringing), crackling, buzzing, or other sounds in the ears; feeling of fullness in the ear; ear pain; discharge or drainage (describe); vertigo? Does the client have problems with excess cerumen (ear wax)? Ask how the client cleans his or her ears (is a cotton-tipped swab, hairpin, or other sharp, foreign object used that may damage the ear canal or tympanic membrane?). Does the client wear a hearing aid? When was the last ear and hearing examination performed (results)?

Nose and Sinuses

Ask if there is a history of frequent colds, sinus infections, nasal stuffiness, allergies, hay fever, or nasal trauma or fracture. Are there current problems with sneezing, postnasal drip, rhinitis (runny nose), difficulty breathing through the nose, pain over the sinuses, or epistaxis (nosebleed)? Has there been a change in the sense of smell? Does the client use a nasal spray or other cold, allergy, or sinus medication (type, amount, frequency)?

Mouth and Pharynx

Does the client have a history of sore throats or oral infection such as strep throat, herpes (cold sores), or *Candida* (thrush)? Are there problems with mouth or tongue lesions (sore, abscess, ulcer); bleeding gums; increased saliva or dry mouth; mouth pain; sore throat; hoarseness or voice change; difficulty chewing or swallowing (dysphagia); change in taste; halitosis? Does the client use tobacco products (describe type, amount, frequency, and current use patterns)? Does the client have any dentures or bridges? Do they fit well? Are they worn most of the time?) Ask the client to describe dental hygiene practices (brushing, flossing, use of fluoride dentifrice). Has the client ever had oral or dental surgery (describe)? When was the last dental examination and the results (if known)? Were x-ray films obtained at that time?

Neck

Have there been past problems with neck injury, goiter, pain, limited movement, or swollen glands? Does the client currently have stiffness, tenderness, pain, swelling, or lumps in the neck?

Breasts and Axillae

Ask the client about a history of fibrocystic breast disease and cancer of the breast (is there a family history of breast cancer?). If the client is a woman with children, ask if she breast-fed her infants. Are there current problems with breast pain, tenderness, or swelling; gynecomastia (enlargement); pruritus (itching); nipple discharge; breast lumps; dimpling or change in breast skin texture or color; change in appearance of the nipples? Does the client perform breast self-examination (if so, ask for a description of when it is done and the technique used)? If the client is a woman, has she had mammograms? When? Results, if known? How often done? Does the client take any estrogen (e.g., birth control) or corticosteroid medications (describe)? Is there a history of breast surgery (describe)?

Lungs

Inquire about a history of breathing problems, such as asthma, emphysema, wheezing, pleurisy, pneumonia, or bronchitis. Has the client ever had tuberculosis (describe any treatment

Box continued on following page

BOX 9–2 An Exhaustive Health History Format *Continued*

received) or whooping cough? Has the client smoked or used tobacco products (describe type, amount, length of time used, attempts to stop)? If the client is a former smoker, ask how long it has been since quitting. Current problems might include chronic cough, sputum production (describe), hemoptysis (blood in sputum), night sweats, dyspnea (shortness of breath) with or without exertion, inability to tolerate exercise or activities of daily living without becoming short of breath, orthopnea (difficulty breathing without elevating the head when supine), pain with breathing, and cyanosis (blue-tinged nail beds or lips). Has the client ever had a chest x-ray (results)? Has the client ever had a skin test for tuberculosis (results)?

Heart

Ask the client about a history of rheumatic fever, congenital heart problems, heart murmur, myocardial infarction, coronary artery disease, cardiac surgery, hypertension, or thyroid problems. Is there a family history of hypertension or myocardial infarction before age 50? Are there current problems with chest discomfort or pain, syncope, vertigo, palpitations, paroxysmal nocturnal dyspnea (sudden awakening at night with difficulty breathing), dyspnea on exertion, orthopnea, sudden weight gain, edema of hands or feet, hyperlipidemia, or hypercholesteremia? Has the client ever had any cardiac tests, such as an electrocardiogram (ECG), stress ECG, coronary angiograms, echocardiogram, or electrophysiologic studies (results)?

Peripheral Vascular

Has the client had previous problems with varicose veins, diabetes, hypertension, pain in the extremities, injury to an extremity (describe), or edema of the hands or feet? Are there problems with lymph node swelling or tenderness, claudication (pain in legs with walking relieved by resting), numbness or coldness of an extremity, discoloration or ulceration on extremities (especially feet and ankles), hair loss over an extremity; nail changes? Has the client ever had any vascular tests, such as Doppler studies (results)? Ask what type of hose the client wears (e.g., support hose). Does the client use garters or other means of securing the hose? Does the client spend prolonged periods of time standing?

Gastrointestinal

Inquire about a history of ulcers, indigestion, heartburn, hernia, liver disease, hepatitis (type if known), gallbladder disease, pancreatic disease, appendicitis, and use of alcohol. Is there a family history of alcohol abuse or cancer of the stomach, liver, pancreas, intestines, or colorectal area? Ask the client to describe the usual bowel pattern and characteristics. Are there problems with weight loss or gain, a change in appetite or taste, food intolerance, belching, nausea or vomiting, hematemesis (blood in emesis), pain or indigestion with eating, difficulty swallowing, diarrhea or constipation, bowel incontinence, flatulence (excess gas), changes in bowel habits or stool characteristics (e.g., clay-colored or blood in stool, ribbon-like stools), hemorrhoids (is there any pain or bleeding especially with defecation), rectal pain or itching, pain in the abdomen, ascites (swelling of the abdomen) or jaundice? Does the client use digestive aids, laxatives, enemas, or suppositories (describe)? Has the client had tests of the gastrointestinal (GI) system, such as a barium swallow, upper GI series, barium enema, sigmoidoscopy or colonoscopy, Hemoccult test, gallbladder x-rays or ultrasound, or liver scan (results)?

Urinary

Does the client have a history of bladder infection, kidney problems, urinary tract stones, or sexually transmitted disease (STD)? Is there a family history of renal disease? Are there current problems with a change in the urinary patterns, hesitancy, frequency, dysuria (pain), pyuria (pus in the urine), urgency, weak stream, dribbling or incontinence, stress incontinence, nocturia, polyuria or oliguria (increased or decreased amount of urine), flank or low back pain, a change in the color of the urine, foam in the urine (proteinuria), or discharge from the urethra. Has the client ever had tests of the urinary system such as urinalysis, cystoscopy, or intravenous pyelogram (results)?

Genitoreproductive

- General

Is there a history of genital lesions, sores, or ulcers; urethral discharge; odor; pain, burning, or pruritus; STDs (identify); infertility; problems with sexual performance? Has the client ever had surgery involving the genitoreproductive system (describe)? Does the client use a contraceptive (type)? Is the client satisfied with the type used or is a change desired? Is the client knowledgeable about STD preventive practices or is information wanted?

- Female

Ask about a history of pelvic inflammatory disease, endometriosis, or abnormal Pap test results. Is there a personal or family history of reproductive cancer (e.g., cervix, uterus, ovary, breast)? Review the menstrual cycle history for age at menarche and menopause (if applicable), duration and amount of menstrual flow, and last menstrual period. Are there problems with premenstrual bloating, weight gain, fatigue, or mood changes; irregular menstrual periods; menorrhagia (excessive menses); dysmenorrhea (painful menses); amenorrhea (absence of menses); metrorrhagia (bleeding other than with menses); dyspareunia (painful intercourse); postcoital pain or bleeding? Ask when the woman's last pelvic examination and Pap test were done (results).

- Male

Inquire about a history of inguinal hernia, prostate problems, or impotence. Is there a family history of reproductive cancer (e.g., penis, testis, prostate)? Does the man have current problems with testicular pain or mass, or blood in the ejaculate? Ask when the man's last examination was, including checking the prostate and for hernia (results). Does the man know how to perform testicular self-examination (How often?) Has the man had a prostate-specific antigen (PSA) test (results)?

Musculoskeletal

Ask about past problems with sprains, strains, fractures, dislocations, arthritis, gout, backache, bursitis, osteomyelitis, scoliosis, or flat feet. Is there a family history of arthritis, gout, or muscular dystrophy? Are there current problems with muscle twitches, cramps, spasms, involuntary movements, pain, or weakness; muscle atrophy; joint pain, stiffness, swelling, redness, deformity, or limited movement; crepitation (noise or grating with joint movement); backache; spinal deformity; limitation in walking, gait, running, sports activities, or activities of daily living? Has the client ever had tests involving the musculoskeletal system such as skeletal x-rays or electromyography (results)?

BOX 9–2 An Exhaustive Health History Format *Continued*

Neurologic

Is there a history of loss of consciousness, fainting, seizures, paralysis, paresthesia (numbness or tingling), trauma to the nervous system, cerebrovascular accident (CVA)? Is there a family history of CVA, seizures, or neurologic disease such as Huntington's chorea? Are there current problems with vertigo, syncope, paresthesia, paralysis, headache, loss of balance, seizures, uncoordinated or involuntary movements (e.g., tics, tremors, spasms, clumsiness), speech problems, memory problems (short or long term)? Are there interferences with the activities of daily living from neurologic problems (describe)? Has the client ever had neurologic tests, such as electroencephalography, lumbar puncture, or computed tomography of the head (results)?

Psychiatric

Ask about a history of depression, bipolar disease, schizophrenia, obsessive-compulsive tendency (does it interfere with the client's activities of daily living?); sleeping problems; eating disorders (e.g., anorexia or bulimia nervosa); memory problems; or anxiety attacks. Is there a family history of mental health problems, such as depression, bipolar disease, or schizophrenia? Has the client ever been treated for mental or emotional health problems or taken psychotropic substances (describe)? Is there a history of suicide attempts? Does the client currently have problems with mood swings; sleeping problems, such as insomnia; anxiety, especially that interferes with activities of daily living; nervousness; increased or decreased appetite; memory lapses; inability to concentrate; change in energy level or inability to complete tasks; phobias; delusions; hallucinations? Has there been a change in relationships with significant others recently (describe)? Has there been a change in living arrangements or housing recently (describe)? Has there been a change in jobs recently (describe)?

2. Speak in a moderate tone of voice, calmly and patiently.
3. Ask nonprobing, client-centered questions, which help put the client at ease. As the interview progresses, focused questions and therapeutic communication techniques help identify problem areas.
4. Alternate between open-ended and closed questions, depending on the data being elicited.
5. Throughout the interview, observe nonverbal communication for signs of discomfort with topics under discussion. These areas may need gentle, further exploration (with client permission), either during the interview or at a later time.
6. Respect the client's wish to decline discussing a topic.
7. Be aware of your interview style and skills. Nonverbal behavior can either facilitate or inhibit client responses and affect the quality of the historical data.

■ PREPARATION OF THE INTERVIEWER

The following guidelines apply:

1. Reduce repetitious questioning, and proceed in a structured yet flexible manner. Until you are comfortable with the format, use a pocket-sized outline of the health history as an aid.
2. Take *brief* notes, and inform the client in advance that you will be taking notes so as not to disrupt the flow of the interview. Avoid extensive note taking, because it suggests that you are not listening attentively.
3. Compile the written history after the interview.
4. Terminate the interview by summarizing highlights and allowing the client to add or clarify information.
5. Inform the client about how the physical examination will proceed.

BOX 9–3 An Episodic Health History Format

Include these elements in an episodic (short) health history:

- Client's statement of the problem (i.e., chief complaint)
- Symptom analysis
- Review of the body system to which the symptom belongs
- Exploration of the symptom's relationship to other body systems (including a review of the associated body systems)
- Investigation of the current problem's relationship to the client's past health and health maintenance and promotion practices

COMPONENTS OF THE HEALTH HISTORY

The health history includes subjective data regarding:

- Biographical and demographic information
- The health history including review of systems (ROS)
- Family health history
- Psychosocial assessment
- Appraisal of the client's health maintenance and health promotion behaviors to assess health risks

Health history assessment may be organized according to a nursing theory (e.g., Orem's theory of self-care) or by health behavior patterns (e.g., Gordon's functional health patterns). A *format* is a tool for collecting comprehensive data. In this chapter, the health history format is an extended health database model (see Box 9–2). A health history format that integrates the assessment of functional health patterns is found in Appendix B.

If data are available in other forms, compile them, thereby enhancing and expediting the interview. A single complete database is preferable for reference and retrieval of information.

■ BIOGRAPHICAL AND DEMOGRAPHIC INFORMATION

The extent and type of biographical and demographic information vary, depending on agency protocol (see Box 9–2). The date of the interview is important because the information gathered constitutes the baseline assessment. Should the client's health status change, the health history and physical examination will reflect the extent of the change over time.

ALTERNATIVE THERAPY

Alternative and Complementary Modalities Used by Clients

A landmark study by Eisenberg and coworkers[1] found that an estimated 60 million Americans were using some form of alternative or complementary therapy. This therapy ranged from the taking of vitamins and herbs to visits to massage therapists and acupuncturists along with a number of other modalities. Visits to alternative practitioners were estimated to exceed those to primary care physicians, with more than $13 billion spent annually on alternative care and products, and perhaps most important for physicians and nurses, more than 70% of clients using alternative therapies did not inform their medical caregivers of such use.

In a follow-up study, Eisenberg and coworkers[3] reported an increase in use of at least one of 16 identified therapies in from 33.8% to 42.1% of the respondents. Again, of particular concern, the follow-up study found that nearly 20% of clients taking prescription medications were concurrent users of herbs or high-dose vitamins.

It is being increasingly recognized that this information, or the lack thereof, about clients' use of alternative methods is of great importance to health care providers. There is much of promise in many alternative therapies, and the power of many of them, especially those involving the ingestion of herbs, vitamins, and other substances, is such that they can cause problems when combined with medications. Sometimes this is true of substances that are quite commonplace and thought to be innocuous because of their common usage. For example, several herbs may interfere with warfarin anticoagulant treatment, including celery, chamomile, fenugreek, garlic, ginger, and some Chinese medicinal herbs.[4]

The chief author of the studies cited, David Eisenberg, M.D., strongly believes in the need to explore with clients their use of alternative therapies. "Undoubtedly, talking with patients about alternative therapies requires additional skills and time. Yet, is this responsibility significantly different from exploring patients' use of alcohol or drugs, exposure to abuse, or preferences for cardiopulmonary resuscitation?"[2]

The key to this process is to be nonjudgmental about what the client is using. People use alternative and complementary therapies in an effort to become healthier, and this attempt deserves respect. Many clients believe that what they are doing is helping to achieve their goals of better health. Our task is to increase both their and our understanding of what clients are using and whether there is any potential danger in such use, either intrinsically or in combination with medical treatment. If a client is taking herbs that might have an anticoagulant effect, for example, this might be a problem if surgery is scheduled.

If clients perceive disdain or ridicule from physicians and nurses about their use of these modalities, they will continue to keep knowledge of such use from their caregivers. Many practitioners of both mainstream and alternative medicine are looking toward an "integrated" approach to medicine and health care, including the proper use and appropriate combination of all therapies relevant to a client's individual needs. A forthright and open-minded approach is the best way to communicate with clients about their use of alternative and complementary methods.

As Eisenberg has written: "We as a profession must address the challenge of discussing alternative therapies with our patients and put an end to the 'don't ask, don't tell' approach that characterizes communication in this area." Such a discussion can be a fruitful learning experience for all involved.

References

1. Eisenberg, D. M., et al. (1993). Unconventional medicine in the United States: Prevalence, costs, and patterns of use. *New England Journal of Medicine, 328:*246–252.
2. Eisenberg, D. M. (1997). Advising patients who seek alternative medical therapies. *Annals of Internal Medicine, 127:*61–69.
3. Eisenberg, D. M., et al. (1998). Trends in alternative medicine use in the United States, 1990–1997: Results of a follow-up national survey. *JAMA, 280:*1569–1575.
4. Miller, L. G. (1998). Herbal medicinals, selected clinical considerations focusing on known or potential drug-herb interactions. *Archives of Internal Medicine, 158:*2200–2211.

James Higgy Lerner, RN, LAc, *Private practice of acupuncture, traditional Oriental medicine, and biofeedback*

Biographical and demographic data provide clues about personal health risk. For example, some health risk may be ascribed to age, sex, family history, and location of residence. Various health screening procedures or recommendations are made based on age, sex, or other background data. Examples of recommended procedures include periodic pelvic examinations and monthly breast self-examinations for women, periodic prostate examinations and monthly testicular self-examinations for men, and regular screening of visual acuity and testing for glaucoma as a person ages.

■ CURRENT HEALTH

Current health status describes the reason for the health care visit.

Chief Complaint

Begin with the client's subjective statement of the reason for seeking health care (the *chief complaint*). The response may indicate concerns or anxiety on the part of the client or significant others and reveals the client's perception of the health problem. The client may talk about what the problem means and how he or she is coping. Allowing the client to elaborate can assist in avoiding generalizations. When the client reports a past or current health problem, proceed with a *symptom analysis* (see Box 9–2).

Symptom Analysis

Symptom analysis is a detailed description of the health problem. In this book, the term "manifestations" is used synonymously with "symptoms." In addition to assessing the following characteristics, ask the client to provide an opinion about the cause of the symptom or problem. Clients often have insight as to the nature and the cause of their problems and sometimes express fears and concerns while discussing them. Explore fears and concerns to identify and treat client responses to health problems.

TIMING

Timing includes onset, duration, and frequency. *Onset* refers to when a symptom was first noticed (e.g., hours, days, months). *Duration* is how long the symptom lasts (e.g., minutes, hours, days, weeks). The symptom may occur continuously, intermittently, regularly, or irregularly. *Frequency* is how often a symptom occurs (e.g., daily, weekly, monthly).

QUALITY

Ask the client to discriminate symptom quality with adjectives such as sharp, stabbing, dull, aching, cramping, cold, searing, burning, numb, tingling, loose, solid, soft, hard, tight, or crushing.

QUANTITY

Assist the client in describing the size, amount, number, or extent of symptoms as well as the severity or intensity. Quantify pain severity by asking the client to rate it on a scale (e.g., 1 to 10). Assess the symptom's effect by asking how usual daily activities have been affected, for example, "Describe how the pain has interfered with what you usually do. Does it keep you awake at night? Has it affected your appetite?"

LOCATION

Ask where a symptom, such as pain, is located on the body and whether it moves or is stationary, for example, "Does the pain stay in one place, or does it move around?" Asking the client to point helps define the location.

PRECIPITATING FACTORS

Ask what the client was doing at the time the symptom was first noticed. Does the client know what may have led to the symptom's occurrence?

AGGRAVATING AND RELIEVING FACTORS

Ask the client to recall whether any factors alleviate the symptom or make it worse, for example, "Is there anything that makes the symptom go away or become less uncomfortable?" "Is there anything that makes the symptom become worse?"

ASSOCIATED MANIFESTATIONS

Inquire whether the client has noticed anything in conjunction with the symptom. For example, "Does the symptom ever occur at other times or only when ________?"

When a symptom is reported, assess all associated physiologic areas; for example, for reported epigastric pain, review gastrointestinal, endocrine, and psychological systems. The epigastric pain may be related to problems in any of these body systems. If the reported symptom is urinary incontinence, include the following:

1. Timing
2. Quality (e.g., are incontinent episodes accompanied by dysuria?)
3. Quantity (e.g., amount of urine leakage per occurrence, effect of episodes on daily activities)
4. Precipitating factors (e.g., obesity, pregnancy, vaginal delivery)
5. Aggravating factors (e.g., coughing, sneezing, straining, lifting, caffeine intake)
6. Relieving factors (e.g., frequent toileting, medication, pelvic muscle toning exercises)
7. Associated manifestations (e.g., urgency, urinary retention, constipation).

Location does not apply in this example.

The review of body systems (described later in this chapter) should include the urinary (renal), reproductive, and gastrointestinal systems as well as a careful diet history.

■ PAST HEALTH HISTORY

The past health history may be important for determining both current and future health risk status. For example, the client who has not had chickenpox may be at risk when a community outbreak occurs or when exposed to herpes zoster (shingles). Further assess risk status, and provide information about the varicella vaccination. Box 9–2 lists the data to assess for the past health history. Throughout this part of the health history interview, note areas to explore, such as use of alternative or complementary therapies (see Alternative Therapies feature).

■ FAMILY HEALTH HISTORY

The family health history helps to identify family-linked (familial) diseases that affect health status and risk for potential health problems. The nurse should:

1. Inquire about relationships of family members to the client, their ages (if living), the age at which they died, the cause of death (if known), and the presence of significant illness or health problems.
2. Diagram the data (Fig. 9–1) as a visual display to help track the client's health risk status.
3. Include a statement summarizing health problems in the family.

Box 9–2 lists important health problems in the family health history.

■ PSYCHOSOCIAL HISTORY

Psychosocial assessment is an important part of the health history. A complete psychosocial assessment, although lengthy, is essential to a client-centered approach. Integrate psychosocial assessment throughout the history interview. If in-depth assessment is indicated, do this after the physical health history assessment, once you have established rapport. Psychosocial assessment also may come earlier (see Box 9–2), after the family health history.

Psychological status affects multiple areas of human development and behavior, such as intellectual development and capability, motivation, perception and insight, decision-making, speech and communication, motor ability, sleep and rest patterns, and nutrition and elimination patterns. It is impossible to separate a human being into discrete components. Multiple dimensions (psychological, sociologic, physiologic) interact and affect each person's behavior and responses to the environment. Interrelationships among the dimensions are neither static nor always predictable. Physiologic responses to health problems are more predictable and objectively observed, whereas two people who are faced with identical problems may not react the same way emotionally. For this reason, psychosocial assessment may be less reliable than objective assessment of physical findings. However, one may be able to develop skill and expertise in psychosocial assessment by collecting both subjective and objective data.

Psychosocial assessment assists the nurse in understanding a client's response to circumstances and events, which in turn influences the client's ability to function.

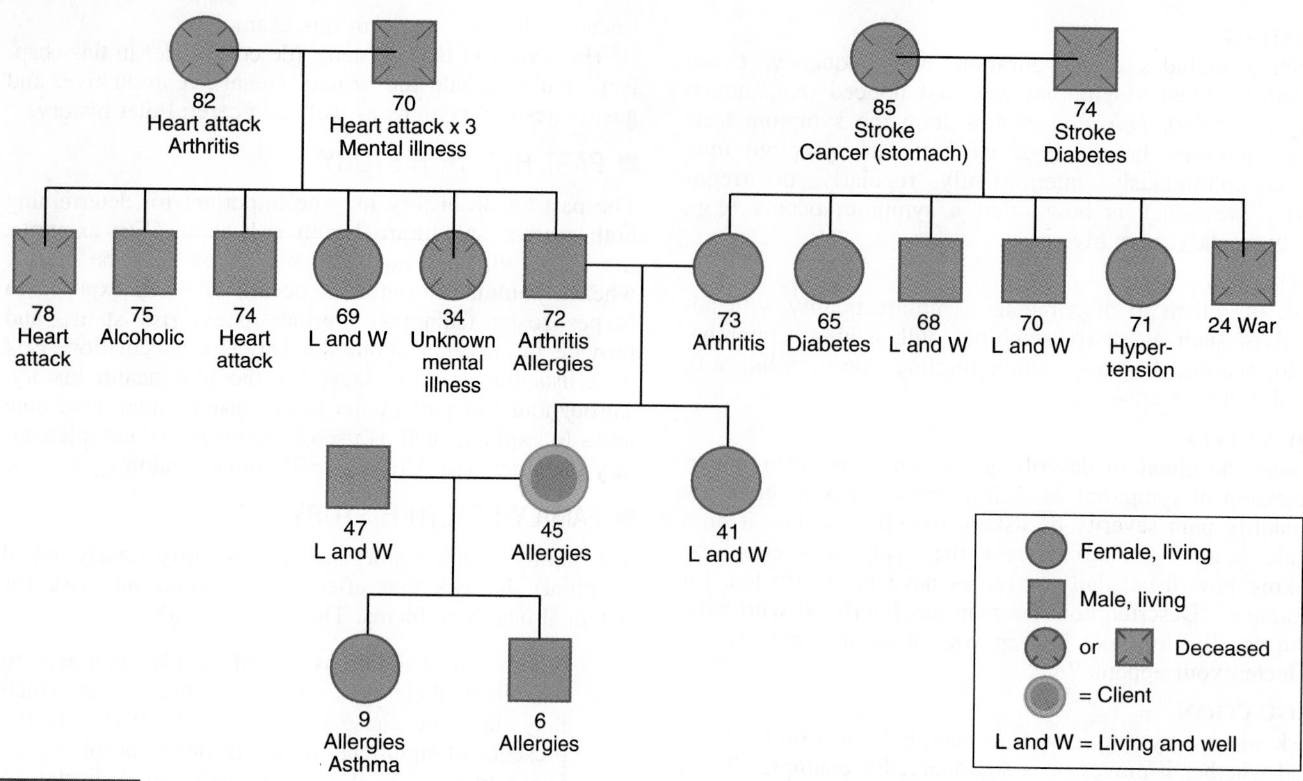

FIGURE 9–1 Family history diagram. A diagram such as this one assists in determining a client's risk for various disorders. In this case, the diagram indicates a woman with an increased inherited risk of cardiovascular disease (heart attack and stroke) and arthritis.

This understanding enables comprehensive care based on accurate nursing diagnoses. Approximately two thirds of the disorders that nurses independently identify and treat are psychosocial. Accurate assessment of responses to health problems enables the client to return to optimal levels of both physiologic and psychological functioning.

Performing the psychosocial assessment requires sensitivity and interpersonal skills. Ability to establish a therapeutic relationship directly affects the quality of the data. Because many topics are highly personal, it is imperative to be tactful and nonjudgmental and to handle confidential information professionally. An atmosphere of trust encourages the client to divulge sensitive information. Convey interest by listening attentively, making eye contact, and using skillful interview techniques. Your personal value system may influence or bias perception of a client's behavior and experiences. Self-awareness helps one to remain nonjudgmental. Free from bias, a trusting relationship promotes sharing of relevant information. Making accurate observations and sharing them allow the client opportunity to validate the nurse's perceptions and inferences.

Nature of the Psychosocial Assessment

Psychosocial assessment encompasses gathering information about *psychological patterns* (nonphysical components, such as thoughts, feelings, motivations, mental status, personal strengths, and weaknesses) and *social experiences* (parts of life that are affected by or dependent on others). The term *psychosocial* denotes the melding of the two dimensions; it is impossible to separate the effects of psychological factors from those of social factors. Similarly, the psychosocial dimension intertwines with the physiologic dimension. All dimensions interact to produce a unique individual.

Psychosocial Risk Factors

During the health history interview, assess for factors indicating risk for or an actual psychosocial problem. Box 9–4 lists guidelines for identifying psychosocial risk factors. If risk factors are present, proceed with a detailed assessment. Table 9–1 is an interview guide for in-depth assessment of selected areas of psychosocial status, including questions that may be asked during a cultural assessment.

Psychological Assessment

The psychological dimension includes perceptions about mood, thoughts, feelings, motivations, stressors, personal strengths and weaknesses, values and beliefs, and spirituality. Responses and interpretations are reflected in thought processes and in what is said and done. Observe the client's appearance and behavior throughout the interview. Observations, when validated, assist in understanding psychological status. Subjective data are recorded in the health history, and objective data are recorded in the physical examination report.

General Appearance

Appearance and behavior reflect the client's mental status and comfort level with the interview. Observe the client's

BOX 9-4 Guidelines for Identifying Psychosocial Risk Factors

Social History

Social history includes information about the client's family members, social network, and lifestyle. Ask if others are available to provide emotional support to the client during stressful times. This support system may include pets.

Personal and Family History

A personal or family history of psychosocial problems increases a client's risk of having problems. A client may fear recurrence of an emotional or mental health problem or worry that he or she has inherited a family-linked illness, such as schizophrenia.

Level of Stress

Change and loss are two major influences that produce stress in individuals. Clients who have experienced stressful events within the past year are at risk for development of health problems. Assess the client's present stress level compared to the response to previous stressful events.

Usual Coping Pattern

The usual coping pattern refers to how the client copes with a serious problem or manages high levels of stress. Ask the client to describe a particularly stressful situation and how it was managed. Assess whether the client's usual coping style is adequate and appropriate for the current situation. Other coping strategies may be necessary. Psychosocial reactions to health problems are highly individual and usually occur as the client and significant others cope with the effects of illness.

Changes in Neurophysiologic Function

Neurophysiologic changes include physical manifestations of psychological stress. The stress response, regardless of its cause, results in altered levels of neurotransmitters, such as norepinephrine and serotonin, which then affect the sympathetic and parasympathetic nervous systems. The client's usual body functions, such as sleep and rest patterns, appetite, energy level, sexual function, and elimination patterns, can be affected.

Level of Understanding about Health Problem

Explore the client's level of understanding. The client may not comprehend what has happened or could happen as a result of a health problem. The client may have unrealistic expectations of the health care team. Determine how threatening a particular health problem is and whether the client has been able to prepare psychologically for its effects.

Mental Status

Mental status refers to the client's current emotional, intellectual, and perceptual functioning. If a dysfunction is evidenced, describe the problem.

Personality Style

Personality style is the way a client usually interacts with others. Examples include dependent, independent, controlled, relaxed, dramatic, suspicious, accepting, self-sacrificing, superior, inferior, uninvolved, involved, mixed (a combination of two predominant styles), or no predominant style.

Major Psychosocial Reactions

Reactions include disruption in the ability to trust, maintain self-esteem, retain feelings of control, cope with loss and guilt, and maintain intimacy.

posture, nonverbal behavior, facial expression, manner of dress with regard to the climate and occasion, grooming and hygiene, and attitude toward the assessment interview (e.g., cooperative, hostile, withdrawn). For example, "The client is dressed neatly, sits back in the chair, and answers questions without hesitation."

MOTOR ACTIVITY

Note motor ability, gait, coordination, reaction time, and unusual body movements (e.g., gestures, tics, tremors, foot tapping, hand wringing, grimacing, or other repetitive movements). For example, "The client drummed his fingers on the table before answering."

BEHAVIOR

Activities observed by others constitute behavior. *Verbal* behavior is what is said and includes voice tone; *nonverbal* behavior is everything done that may be observed, such as posture, movement, and facial expression. Observe and record both verbal and nonverbal behaviors.

Behavior is central to psychological assessment. Accurate assessment dictates that observed behavior be *described* rather than *interpreted.* "The client is crying" is an observed behavior, whereas "The client is depressed" is a judgmental statement. Without further assessment, the nurse does not know why the client is crying. If the client states, "I feel depressed," the recorded statement reads, "States she feels depressed."

MENTAL STATUS

Mental status assessment consists of evaluating behavior (verbal and nonverbal) and asking a series of questions. The purpose is to discover problems that may require further assessment and intervention. The level and depth of questioning vary, depending on individual circumstances. Assess a client who is alert and cooperative by listening and observing carefully during the interview. The client's responses provide information about orientation, mood, memory, attention span, general knowledge, language abilities, thought processes, judgment, and insight.

If a client demonstrates impaired cognitive function, perform a Mini-Mental State Examination (see Chapter 67). Disturbances in mood or thought processes (such as suicidality) warrant a complete, detailed mental status examination. Even though mental status data are collected during the health history, record this information with the physical examination data. The following areas are included.

LEVEL OF CONSCIOUSNESS. Level of consciousness (LOC) is the state of awareness. The client must be alert, not just awake, for a mental status assessment (see Chapter 67). The nurse should cue the client that the questions may seem "silly" but are to be answered anyway.

TABLE 9–1 INTERVIEW GUIDE FOR ASSESSMENT OF SELECTED AREAS OF A CLIENT'S PSYCHOSOCIAL STATUS

Assessment Area	Key Questions or Issues to Include*
Values and beliefs	What things in your life are important to you and help you want to live each day (e.g., health; respect for others; happiness; loving relationships with significant others; time to spend with your loved ones; friendships; religious beliefs; financial security; having a job or work to do)? How important is your health to you? to your family or significant others? (Ask person to rate importance on a scale of 1 to 10, with 10 being of most importance and 1 being of least.) What do you hope to accomplish in your lifetime (e.g., rear children successfully; become rich or famous; have a satisfying job or career)? Have you accomplished what you set out to do in your life? Are you satisfied/dissatisfied? If you were to come into a lot of money (win a lottery, receive an inheritance), what would you do with it? Do specific factors influence you when you have to make important decisions (e.g., being fair/honest; getting a fair deal; examining all sides of the issue)? Have any of your beliefs or values been challenged recently? Are you uncomfortable that this has happened? Have you changed any of your values or beliefs recently? Has this change put a strain on your relationship with significant others? Are you comfortable with the change?
Self-concept, self-esteem, body image	Describe yourself as you believe others see you and as you see yourself (e.g., emotional health; usual mood and what affects it; ability to cope with daily stressors; physical appearance; stamina; intelligence). Describe your major strengths and areas that you would like to improve. What do you like about yourself? What do you wish you could change about yourself? Has anything happened recently to change your feelings about yourself (e.g., change in health status or physical agility; a loss of some kind; a role change)? Do you feel more positive or negative about yourself because of this change? Describe how you feel when you become ill or in some way incapacitated and are unable to carry on your daily activities.
Locus of control	Do you feel that you can control or manage factors that affect your state of health or illness (e.g., whether or not you smoke or exercise; what you do/do not eat; getting regular checkups)? Do you feel that you can control or manage factors that affect your life (e.g., your job; where you live; who your friends are)? Is there anything or anybody that you believe is responsible for what happens to you in your life (e.g., a supreme being; fate; luck; people who are more powerful than you)?
Spirituality	Do you have a preferred religion or religious beliefs? Is your religion an important influence in your life? Does it give you guidance in your daily life? Are there other things besides religion that are important to you as you go about your daily life? How often do you attend worship services? Does it bother you if you are ill or unable to attend worship services? What do you do if you cannot attend services? Is there someone you consider to be your spiritual advisor? Do you need to talk to this person regularly? Is there anything special that you do when you feel a need for spiritual support? Do you need help to practice your beliefs at this time? Do you have any religious or spiritual beliefs about health and illness (e.g., illness as a punishment; certain foods to eat or avoid, or practices that should be done or avoided) that the health care team should be aware of? Can the health care team be of spiritual help to you?
Social network and support system	Describe your family: Who are its members and what are their relationships to you? What roles do you and your family members have (e.g., parent, child, spouse, sibling, other relative, teacher, provider, role model, best friend, authority figure, peacemaker)? Who in your family do you feel closest to? Are there other people not related to you whom you consider important (i.e., significant others)? Do you and your family members (or significant others) get along with one another? Are there any problems within your family or with significant others that have strained your relationships with one another (e.g., change in living space; marital problems; arguments)? Are friendships important to you? Are you satisfied with the friendships that you have now? Whom would you identify as your best friend? Are your friends accepted by your family and significant others? Describe your relationships with your friends and coworkers. What types of groups, clubs, or organizations do you belong to? If you had a problem or were in a crisis, whom would you turn to for help? Is this person available? Is there someone at work whom you confide in? Are there other things that help you when you need support during stressful times (e.g., a pet or inanimate object)?

TABLE 9–1 INTERVIEW GUIDE FOR ASSESSMENT OF SELECTED AREAS OF A CLIENT'S PSYCHOSOCIAL STATUS *Continued*

Assessment Area	Key Questions or Issues to Include*
	Do you have a pet or animals that are important to you? Is there someone who will take care of them for you if you are unable to do so?
Sexuality	Are you satisfied with being a man (or a woman)? Have you ever wished you were of the opposite sex?
	Are you satisfied in your sexual relationships with your spouse, significant other, or other sexual partners (e.g., frequency and quality of interactions)? Has there been a change in your sexual function? If so, describe what is different and how long it has been this way. Is this change for the better or worse?
	Have you experienced any problems with sexual activity (e.g., impotence, pain, premature ejaculation, bleeding, lack of privacy, infertility, other)? Do you feel that this may be related to a health problem or some other cause? If so, have these problems affected your relationship with your sexual partner?
	How long have you been sexually active?
	How long have you been in your current relationship?
	Can you recall whether you used protection against venereal diseases with past sexual partners?
	Do you use contraceptives? If not, are you interested in information about this? Do you have any questions about the method you are using now?
	Do you use any type of protection against venereal diseases (e.g., condoms)? Have you ever been treated for a venereal disease?
	Do you have reason to believe that you have been exposed to a venereal disease such as syphilis, gonorrhea, or human immunodeficiency virus?
Cultural components	***Identification with a cultural group***
	How do you identify yourself to others when you are asked to what nationality or what ethnic group you belong?
	Describe how strongly you feel about your ethnic roots. Do you see yourself as a member of your ethnic group first, or do you think of yourself as a/an ________ (American, Canadian, or other) first?
	How do you identify yourself when you are asked about your racial background (e.g., black, white, Native American, Hispanic, Asian)?
	Where were you born? Where were your parents born?
	What countries (or regions of this country) have you lived in and when?
	Communication
	What language do you speak at home? Do you speak or read other languages? Do you prefer to speak in a language other than English? Is there someone (e.g., friend, relative) whom you want to act as an interpreter for you? Do you want a professional interpreter? Is there anyone (e.g., someone of the opposite sex; a person who is older/younger than you; a person you see as a rival or enemy) who should not act as an interpreter?
	Whom do you prefer to take care of you when you need health care (e.g., a person of the same cultural background/same sex/same age as you)?
	Values, beliefs, and attitudes
	Can you identify any special beliefs or practices of yours that are influenced by your ethnic or cultural background? For example, are there things that you or your significant others do when a baby is born? When someone dies? When you or your family members are ill?
	Is there anything special that you or your family do to stay healthy (e.g., eat or avoid certain foods; use herbs; call in someone who has special powers or gifts to help you stay well or get well)?
	Is leisure time important to you? Do you take time to relax and have fun? Describe what you do when you want to relax.
	Cultural sanctions and restrictions
	Is there anything the health care team should know about when taking care of you? For example, do you need to keep parts of your body covered to prevent others from seeing them?
	Are there certain types of procedures that are forbidden for you to have done (e.g., hysterectomy, vasectomy)?
	If you were to have a serious operation in which part of your body had to be removed (amputation) or cut out (excision), how should this body part be handled (e.g., preserved, buried, cremated, no special treatment)?
	Are there any topics or subjects that you do not wish to talk about because it is not allowed by your beliefs (e.g., discussing people who have died)?

Table continued on following page

TABLE 9–1 INTERVIEW GUIDE FOR ASSESSMENT OF SELECTED AREAS OF A CLIENT'S PSYCHOSOCIAL STATUS *Continued*

Assessment Area	Key Questions or Issues to Include*
	Health-related beliefs and practices
	Is there anything in your beliefs that you feel helps you to be (or to stay) healthy? For example, do you believe certain foods, herbs, or beverages (potions) are good for you?
	Is there anything special that you do or wear to help you stay healthy or bring you luck (e.g., an amulet; prayers to ancestors; praying to a saint, supreme being, or other being; certain rituals)?
	Is there anything that you believe is not good for your health or that causes illness or sickness (e.g., illness is a punishment for doing something "wrong"; you are under a spell or curse; your body is not in harmony or balance with nature; there is an imbalance between good/bad [positive/negative] forces within your body such as *Yin/Yang* or hot/cold)?
	Is there anything in your religious beliefs that influences what you believe about health and illness? Describe.
	Do you believe in or use other types of people to help you get better or heal when you are sick (e.g., curandero; shaman; minister, priest, or other spiritual adviser)? How do you know when to contact this person?
	Are there any types of healing practices or beliefs that you have or feel you need (e.g., use of herbal remedies or potions; massage or other type of special touch; wearing a special charm or talisman to ward off evil spirits; special prayers or incantations; specific healing practices or ceremonies)?
	When you are ill or sick, does your family and significant others expect you to act in a certain way (e.g., to play a particular "sick role")?
	Who decides when you are sick or when you are no longer sick?
	Who usually helps take care of you when you are sick?
	Nutritional beliefs and practices
	Do you have any special beliefs that certain foods are better for you and help keep you healthy? Are there specific foods that you believe should be eaten if you have a certain kind of illness?
	Identify foods that you believe are healthy for you to eat and foods that you believe you should avoid because they are unhealthy.
	Describe how food is prepared in your home (e.g., frying; steaming; use of cooking oils [type]; how long foods are cooked; what types of seasonings are used or avoided; what foods may/may not be served together at the same meal; use of special cookware or dishes to serve food).
	Do you have certain religious beliefs that control the type of foods you eat/should not eat (e.g., kosher diet) or how food is prepared? (Also see previous question.)
	Do you fast or abstain from specific foods at certain times during the week or year because of religious beliefs?
	If you believe in "fasting" for religious reasons, describe what this means to you. Do you avoid certain foods or beverages? Do you eat only at specified times during the day?
	Are you ever allowed to break your religious rules of diet or fasting if you are ill? Who makes this decision and who would tell you that it is acceptable to break a dietary rule?
	Socioeconomic issues
	Is there anyone in your circle of family, friends, significant others, or spiritual advisers (i.e., social network) who you feel influences your health or illness status?
	Are there special things that the members of your social network and support system do to help you when you are sick or to help you get better? Describe how these people would help take care of you if you were ill (e.g., stay by your side continuously; do things for you or your family; help your family).
	Describe the roles that your family members play when one of the members is ill.
	Do you expect your family members to help take care of you when you are sick? Describe what types of activities they might do (e.g., give you a bath; prepare your food; help to feed you; be with you).
	Will your illness put a financial strain on your family? Who is the main wage earner in the family? Does anyone else help contribute to the family's income? Are there other sources for the family for financial income?
	Educational background
	Can you read and write in English, or do you feel more comfortable with another language?
	How much education have you had in schools?
	When you learn about new things, is there a special way that you prefer to learn? For example, do you like to read information first, or do you like to watch someone do a new skill and then try to repeat it? Does it help for you to talk to someone and ask questions?

TABLE 9–1 INTERVIEW GUIDE FOR ASSESSMENT OF SELECTED AREAS OF A CLIENT'S PSYCHOSOCIAL STATUS *Continued*

Assessment Area	Key Questions or Issues to Include*
	Religious beliefs and practices Do your religious beliefs or practices influence you in how you feel or act when you are sick or when you are well? Are there special practices or healing rituals that you believe help to keep you well or to get better faster when you are ill? Is there someone special who performs healing rituals for you (e.g., shaman, priest)? Is it important to you to have a special religious person with you when you are sick or who comes to visit you (a priest or elder; imam; monk)? If so, describe how this person helps you feel better.

* The items in this guide are representative of but not inclusive for each assessment area.

ORIENTATION TO PERSON, PLACE, TIME, AND CIRCUMSTANCES. Ask the client to explain the reason for seeking health care. If the reply is unclear or if the client digresses, ask the client to state his or her name, to identify the present location, and to specify the date and time.

MOOD AND AFFECT. *Mood* is the subjective description of a personal emotion that is pervasive and sustained. Record whether the described mood matches the present situation. For example, "The client stated she was 'happy and going to celebrate' when informed that the results of her tests were normal."

Affect is the observable, outward demeanor that depicts the current emotional state, such as fear, anger, resentment, depression, anxiety, or elation. A *flat* affect is a lack of any facial expression or emotional response and is accompanied by a monotonous voice. A *blunted* affect is greatly reduced in intensity but still appropriate to the situation. Note whether the observed affect matches the immediate circumstances. For example, "When informed that discharge from the hospital was postponed because of an infection, the client first cried, then shouted at the nurse to leave the room." This indicates the client first was upset and then became angry that the discharge was delayed because of a complication. Both reactions are understandable, given the situation.

SPEECH AND COMMUNICATION (LANGUAGE). Evaluate the physical ability to speak and communicate by focusing on *how* the client talks, not the topic of speech. Observe tone of voice, pitch, rate of speech, articulation, length of responses, pauses, and pauses before the client replies to questions (latency).

THOUGHT PROCESSES AND CONTENT. Assess whether speech progresses logically and whether the stream of thought is spontaneous, natural, organized, logical, relevant, coherent, and goal-directed. What the client says should be consistent.

ATTENTION SPAN. Assess the client's ability to focus or concentrate on a task or activity over time, such as completing history forms or answering questions. If results are uncertain, further evaluate the attention span using the following tests:

1. *Digit span,* a test in which a series of five to seven numbers forward and up to five numbers backward is repeated that have been identified by the nurse.
2. *Serial 7s* and *3s,* which test attention span as well as calculation ability. Ask the client to subtract 7 (or 3) from 100 and continue to subtract by 7 (or 3) until the client cannot go any further.

MEMORY: IMMEDIATE, RECENT, AND REMOTE. Assessment of memory usually begins with recall of the past health history. Ask the client to recall information: (1) within seconds (e.g., repeat a series of numbers); (2) within several minutes to hours (e.g., recall specific words later during the interview or recall what was eaten yesterday); and (3) within hours, months, or years (e.g., identify where the client grew up). Be able to verify the client's answers.

GENERAL FUND OF KNOWLEDGE. Ask the client to identify commonly known places, events, and people. This can be done casually during conversation.

CALCULATIONS. Ask the client to perform simple arithmetic functions (addition, subtraction, multiplication, division) without using pencil or paper (see Serial 7s).

ABSTRACT REASONING AND THINKING. Answers to general questions (e.g., explaining the reason a course of action was taken for a health problem) are usually sufficient to assess abstract reasoning. If reasoning is impaired, ask the client to think beyond the concrete dimension by explaining a common proverb or by explaining similarities or differences between selected concepts. For example, "A bird in the hand is worth two in the bush." "What is the difference between a tree and a bush?"

PERCEPTUAL DISTORTION. The client should be able to discriminate reality from misperceptions. Ask the client to describe any illusions or hallucinations by asking about each of the senses. For example, "Do you ever feel that you are hearing sounds that other people do not?"

JUDGMENT. Judgment (decision-making ability) may be assessed within the context of the health history interview as the client discusses actions and decisions made in daily living. To assess further, ask about a realistic rather than a hypothetical situation. For example, "What would you do when a prescribed medication has run out?"

INSIGHT. Assess the client's insight throughout the interview as the client explains the nature of the current health problem and his or her expectations of the health care team. Evaluate whether the client demonstrates ability to perceive the self realistically and accurately.

When assessing mental status, individualize questions to the client's circumstances. Variables affecting one's ability to respond to specific questions include:

- Level of education
- Cultural background
- Degree of exposure to knowledge and information
- Familiarity with the language and vocabulary
- The client's perceived acceptance by the nurse

For example, it may be revealing to ask a teenager the name of a current popular singer but inappropriate to ask the same question of an older person. A client who has not progressed beyond a third grade level of education may be incapable of performing complicated arithmetic calculations. A proverb widely known in one culture may be meaningless to someone from a different cultural background. Finally, you must have access to correct answers for the questions asked, particularly those relating to personal circumstances, such as the location of the client's home, date and place of birth, and names of family members.

OTHER PSYCHOLOGICAL FACTORS

Assess additional psychological factors, such as personality style (see Box 9–3), motivation, and personal strengths, while interacting with the client and significant others. Although nurses do not usually participate in formal psychological testing, data from formal testing can be used to supplement psychosocial data collected in nurse-client interactions and in the health history.

MOTIVATION. Motivation is highly individual and is influenced by personal needs and desires, goals, hopes, and aspirations. Attempt to determine motivation for seeking health care. If the client is ill, ascertain the motivation for returning to an optimal level of wellness.

PERSONAL STRENGTHS. When planning care, use the client's strengths. *Resources* are personal elements that determine an individual's capability to adapt to challenges and threatening stressors. *Internal* resources are *physiologic* (e.g., immune system, nutritional state, physiologic defense systems, genetic predisposition to health, current state of each body system) and *psychological* (e.g., defense mechanisms, interpersonal style, usual coping ability, current coping ability, and spiritual state, such as the will to live). *External* resources include the social environment (e.g., usual coping style of the family, availability of social support, and the assessment skills of the health care providers) and the physical, economic, and cultural environments.

VALUES AND BELIEFS. The value system and beliefs determine whether or not the client views health care as worthwhile. The client's values and beliefs may differ from yours. Accept them as valid because they help provide insight into behavior.

SPIRITUALITY. Spiritual beliefs have implications for well-being, such as sustaining hope or assisting with coping during periods of stress. Include spirituality assessment as part of the health history, and explain the purpose for asking about it. This portion of the history is usually addressed at the end of the interview after a trusting nurse-client relationship is established. Because spirituality is very personal, respect a client's wishes not to discuss this topic. Ask whether the client prefers to consult someone else when spiritual support is needed.

Sociologic Assessment

The *sociologic dimension* includes information about social roles and functions. Assess psychosocial development, social network, socioeconomic status, lifestyle, and sexuality. View the client both as an individual and as a member of a social network.

PSYCHOSOCIAL DEVELOPMENT

Psychosocial development refers to a person's level of growth and development, including the life developmental processes and phases of growth and maturation. Psychosocial development occurs across the life span and includes physical, emotional, psychological, social, and cognitive components. These components are not distinct from one another, nor is progress through life's stages and phases always predictable or inflexible. An understanding of human growth and development provides a foundation from which to assess the client.

SOCIAL NETWORK

A *social network* is the group of people that surrounds, interacts with, and sustains a person with intimacy, social integration, nurturing, reassurance, and assistance. The nurse becomes part of a client's social network when the client enters the health care system; however, the client continues to receive support from the established social network.

Collect social network data by observing the client during interactions with family and visitors; ask questions about interpersonal relationships, and determine whether there are certain individuals with whom the client prefers to maintain contact. Do not assume that only family members are the most important people. When planning care, include the significant others who may be experiencing stress along with the client.

SOCIOECONOMIC STATUS

An individual's economic position within society is referred to as *socioeconomic status.* Ask about factors that affect financial and social well-being because they have implications for planning individualized health care, such as (1) occupation, (2) current employment status, (3) work-related concerns, (4) financial concerns, (5) effect of the client's health status on the ability to work and on finances, (6) perceived effect that the client's socioeconomic status has on access to the health care system, (7) educational background, and (8) hopes and goals for the future.

LIFESTYLE

Usual daily patterns of living are referred to as *lifestyle.* Lifestyle is closely associated with socioeconomic status but also includes relationships with others. Assess the following as they apply to the client's health:

- Usual roles and functions
- Work and study habits
- Leisure and relaxation activities
- Type and location of residence
- Living arrangements

- Usual manner of transportation
- Proximity of close friends
- Importance and influence of cultural beliefs on diet and health-seeking behavior or treatment
- Health habits (e.g., use of alcohol, medications, nicotine, recreational drugs)
- Stress level
- Coping methods used to relieve stress and their effectiveness
- Usual sleep pattern
- Degree of satisfaction with current status

SEXUALITY

Sexuality is the behavioral expression of one's sexual identity. It involves sexual relationships between people as well as the perception of one's maleness or femaleness (gender identification). Many aspects of sexuality affect health status and have significance in relation to nursing care and client outcomes. Aspects include (1) physical health problems that affect sexual behavior (e.g., mastectomy, colostomy, skin lesions, venereal diseases, paralysis, physical deformities), (2) concerns with sexual performance (e.g., impotence, premature ejaculation, inability to achieve orgasm, infertility), (3) issues of sex role function (e.g., homosexuality, bisexuality, sexual ambiguity, transsexual surgery), and (4) effects of environmental restrictions on sexual performance (e.g., residency in a long-term care facility).

Sexuality and sexual behavior are sensitive topics to discuss. Clients may want to talk about sexuality issues and may look for permission and encouragement to do so. Become comfortable with sexuality issues, and do not allow personal beliefs and values to interfere with professional care. Accept and interact with clients without judging them or their behavior.

Cultural Assessment

Cultural assessment is a systematic examination of the cultural beliefs, values, and practices as they apply to determining health care needs. These needs, and any culture-based interventions, must be viewed from the client's cultural context. Cultural assessment tends to be broad because it seeks information about group values, beliefs, and behaviors. The nurse also assesses what the larger group's tenets mean to the individual. Table 9–1 includes guidelines for assessing cultural components as part of the psychosocial assessment. Also see the Diversity in Health Care features.

A GUIDE TO PSYCHOSOCIAL ASSESSMENT

Although discussed separately, psychological and sociologic assessments are often combined (see Box 9–2). You may collect psychosocial data that indicate a psychiatric disorder. If this situation occurs, consult with other health care professionals, such as a psychiatric clinical nurse specialist and the client's physician.

■ REVIEW OF SYSTEMS

The review of systems (ROS) is a head-to-toe review of the physical health history for each body system. This review provides a focus for the physical examination. Box 9–2 presents the information assessed. These data often are collected by having the client complete a checklist form that is then reviewed, and expanded as necessary, by a health care professional. In an episodic (short-format) health history, focus on those systems pertinent to the problem.

HEALTH PROMOTION AND HEALTH RISK APPRAISAL

Health risk appraisal examines factors that affect potential for developing a particular health problem. Risk factors are (1) *genetic* or *biologic* (e.g., race, family history, personal history), (2) *behavioral* (e.g., health habits such as smoking), or (3) *environmental* (e.g., living in a locale with smog). Determining health risk status identifies high-risk clients who may benefit from timely intervention. Explain the difference between being *at increased risk for development of* a health problem and the inevitability of *actual development of* a health problem. In health risk appraisal, assess the client's willingness and motivation to modify or reduce risk factors. For example, a client who smokes is at higher risk for pulmonary disease than a nonsmoker. You may believe that the client *should* stop smoking; however, if there is no desire to stop, your teaching will be ineffective. This client may be labeled "noncompliant" by the health care team when the client is only following a personal decision to keep smoking. Conversely, a female client at risk for osteoporosis tells you that she is concerned and desires to reduce her risk. This client is receptive to teaching about increasing dietary calcium intake and engaging in regular weight-bearing activity.

Health risk factors are categorized for assessment purposes. Some risk factors are potentially hazardous for many people (e.g., ground water pollution in a community that depends on wells for the water supply). Other risk factors may adversely affect a limited group of individuals (e.g., particle inhalation in workers who install insulation materials). Still other risk factors are significant for a family group (e.g., genetic diseases, such as Huntington's chorea). Risk categories include:

- Race and genetic or family-related factors
- Age-related factors
- Biologic factors
- Personal habits
- Lifestyle
- Environmental and occupational factors
- Socioeconomic factors

Table 9–2 summarizes examples of health risk factors, their commonly associated health problems, and suggested health promotion behaviors or screening procedures that may reduce potential risk or facilitate early detection. Awareness of health risk factors may motivate a client to seek screening procedures and to practice health promotion behaviors, particularly for health problems that are treatable or manageable through timely intervention. Environmental and occupational risk factors are linked with specific health problems and may be sus-

DIVERSITY IN HEALTH CARE

Introduction to Cultural Aspects of Health Care

Cultural knowledge is an important ingredient in health care because both health caregivers and clients interpret actions in light of their own belief systems. If clients do not respond as the nurse expects, the nurse may interpret this as unconcern or resistance. The nurse then can become anxious and frustrated. In order to incorporate cultural knowledge in care, it is important to understand some definitions and cultural components that are important in health care. Some pertinent definitions are the following:

1. *Culture:* "The learned and shared beliefs, values, and lifeways of a designated or particular group which are generally transmitted intergenerationally and influence one's thinking and action modes."[3]
2. *Ethnicity:* A characteristic of groups in which a shared social and cultural heritage is passed on to each successive generation and in which there is a sense of identity.[1]
3. *Ethnocentrism:* "The belief that one's own beliefs and ways of doing things are the best."[3]

Before we can truly appreciate and respect the belief systems of others, we must be able to recognize our own belief systems for what they are, where they originated, and how they influence perception of what others believe and do. Shaking up our own ethnocentrism is a necessary step in delivering culturally relevant care.

Another important part of delivering culturally relevant care is the use of information about the culture of the ethnic group to which the client belongs as well as the client's particular beliefs and practices. To understand the information, it is helpful to consider components of a cultural system that are pertinent to health caregivers, which are described as follows[4]:

1. *Religion:* May affect practice of health care in all phases. Religious rituals mark stages in the life cycle, influence dietary and health habits, and affect beliefs about cause of illness and effectiveness of treatment and caregiver. Religion may also influence interpreting illness as punishment from God or viewing the health professional as an instrument of God. The beliefs of some religious groups (Christian Science, Jehovah's Witnesses) have a direct influence on what is acceptable in the provision of health care (see Appendix A). Religion can also provide solace in times of stress and illness to client and family.
2. *Value Orientations*[2]
   a. *Time:* past, present, or future. All societies deal in all three but differ in their emphasis. The *past* focuses on ancestors and tradition. The *present* focuses on now; caregivers should focus on the present value of information. The *future* is concerned with progress and change and is not concerned with present. Caregivers should focus on the long-term importance of information. All societies must deal in all three orientations.
   b. *Activity:* "doing" versus "being" versus "being-in-becoming" (self-contained; inner-controlled). *Doing* encompasses one's being valued for accomplishments. In a *being-oriented* culture, one is valued for one's existence. *Being-in-becoming* involves the value of one's striving for growth of self.
   c. *Relational:* "Collateral" versus "lineal" versus "individualistic." *Collateral* refers to the emphasis on the laterally extended group (siblings or same-age group); group goals are the primary focus. *Lineal* emphasizes kinship and continuity through time. *Individualistic* emphasizes personal autonomy and independence; individual goals dominate.
   d. *Individual-to-Nature:* "subjugated to nature" versus "dominating nature" versus "in harmony with nature." *Subjugated to nature* encompasses a fatalistic view that whatever nature causes will happen. *Dominating nature* is a major theme in the Western medical system. *In harmony with nature* concerns beliefs that balance is necessary to health.
3. *Health and illness beliefs and practices:* Involve beliefs as to causation of illness, defining of illness, toleration of pain and suffering, when to seek help, and choice of treatments and practitioners.
4. *Communication:* Differences in language or dialect, meaning, norms of social gestures, etiquette, touch, eye contact, distance zones (intimate, personal, social, public), and communication of emotions.
5. *Family and lifestyle patterns:* Includes organization and roles and relationships of family, nuclear versus extended family, gender roles, clothing, and diet.

Gathering information, both generally about the ethnic group to which the client belongs and individually about the client's beliefs and practices pertinent to these cultural components, greatly enhances nursing care and client outcomes.

References

1. Giger, J. N., & Davidhizar, R. E. (1999). *Transcultural nursing: Assessment and intervention.* (3rd ed.). St. Louis: Mosby.
2. Kluckhohn, F. (1979). Dominant and variant value orientations. In P. J. Brink (Ed.), *Transcultural nursing: A book of readings* (pp. 63–81). Englewood Cliffs, NJ: Prentice Hall.
3. Leininger, M. (1995). *Transcultural nursing: Concepts, theories, research and practices.* New York: McGraw-Hill.
4. Sharma, S. (1988). *Bridging the gap: Anthropological brokerage in nursing care.* Unpublished doctoral dissertation, University of South Florida, Tampa.

Sandra Sharma, PhD, ARNP, CS, *James A. Haley Veterans Hospital, Tampa, Florida*

ceptible to change. Socioeconomic risk factors are less easily eliminated; however, their effects may be modified through skillful case finding and risk management.

Assess the client's risk profile throughout the health history interview. A client with multiple risk factors linked to specific health problems is at greater risk for development of those problems than the client with fewer or no risk factors. People in hazardous occupations include firefighters, police, miners, heavy equipment operators, lumber and construction workers, factory and textile workers, musicians, and workers who use chemicals or pesticides, such as farmers, landscapers, gardeners, painters, and artists. Risk for *accidental injury* or *trauma* has been linked to multiple stressors, inadequate coping abil-

DIVERSITY IN HEALTH CARE

Communicating with Culturally Diverse Clients

Nurses increasingly find themselves caring for clients from diverse cultures. In such a situation, it can be expected that the client's first language will not always be English. Most clients experience illness with some degree of anxiety. Certainly clients' anxiety is increased when language barriers do not allow them to communicate with their caregivers. The communication component of Purnell and Paulanka's Model for Culture Competence[2] describes essential variables that the nurse must assess when identifying the complexities of communication that exist when interacting with culturally diverse clients. Communication is essential to providing culturally competent care.

Certification of medical interpreters would help to ensure communication with clients who are not fluent in English.[1] Until medical interpreters are consistently available, techniques that facilitate communication can still be used.

Upon first contact with the culturally diverse client, it is essential to identify the dominant language of the client and to obtain someone who can help interpret the meaning.[2] Guidelines for communicating with clients who are not fluent in English are provided next.

Guidelines for Communicating with Clients Not Fluent in English[2]

1. Assess the client's fluency in English. Remember, clients often understand more than they can express, and they need time to think in their own language. Stress interferes with the client's ability to think and speak in English.
2. Determine whether there is a dialect that interferes with communication.
3. Given the difficulty of knowing the precise meaning of words in a language, it is best to obtain someone who can interpret the meaning and message, not just translate the individual words.
4. If there *is* an interpreter available:
   a. Use dialect-specific interpreters, not translators.
   b. Avoid using children and relatives as interpreters.
   c. Select same-age and same-gender interpreters.
   d. Give the client and interpreter time alone together.
   e. Address your questions to the client, not the interpreter.
   f. Build in time for translation and interpretation.
5. If there *is not* an interpreter available:
   a. Determine whether a third language is common to you and the client. If not, use a translator.
   b. Use pantomime for simple words and actions.
   c. Use pictures when possible (a picture is worth a thousand words).
   d. Use and also give the client paper and pencil.
   e. Avoid using technical terms.

Nonverbal Cultural Communication Patterns

Nonverbal communication is as important as verbal communication. Be attentive to both your own and the client's nonverbal messages. Nonverbal cultural communication patterns may vary from one client to another. Consequently, it is important to[2]:

1. Explore the willingness of clients to share their thoughts, feelings, and ideas.
2. Explore the practice and meaning of touch in their society: within the family, between friends, with strangers, with members of the same sex, with members of the opposite sex, and with health care providers.
3. Identify personal spatial and distancing characteristics when communicating on a one-to-one basis. Explore how distancing changes with friends versus strangers.
4. Explore the use of eye contact within this group. Does avoidance of eye contact have special meanings? How does eye contact vary among family, friends, and strangers? Does eye contact change among socioeconomic groups?
5. Explore the meaning of various facial expressions. Do specific facial expressions have special meanings? Do people tend to smile a lot? How are emotions displayed or not displayed in facial expressions?
6. Determine whether there are acceptable ways of standing.

The Challenge

It would be very convenient if there were a universal language; in reality, there is none. Cultural diversity with its accompanying many languages *is* reality. The United States has an emerging population composed of peoples from all over the world. Nurses are confronted with the challenge of communicating with and caring for these clients.

References

1. Lester, N. (1998). Cultural competence: A nursing dialogue, 1. *American Journal of Nursing, 98*(8), 26–34.
2. Purnell, L., & Paulanka, M. (1998). *Transcultural health care: A culturally competent approach.* Philadelphia: F. A. Davis.

Joyce Larson-Presswalla, PhD, RN, *President, "Culture Counts," Marketing Coordinator, James A. Haley Veterans Hospital, Tampa, Florida*

ity, mental and physical fatigue, decreased reaction time, and substance abuse. Stressors include strained interpersonal relationships, physical or psychological abuse, inadequate financial resources, a recent change in lifestyle, sensory stimulation overload, nutritional deficits, and hazardous environments. Lifestyle and personal habits greatly affect health status, and many are modifiable.

After assessing the risk profile, evaluate the client's health risk status. Examine each identified risk factor with the client to determine whether its effects can be modified. If the client is interested in reducing health risks (e.g., stopping smoking or wearing seat belts), intervene either directly or indirectly. Discuss approaches to behavior changes. *Direct* interventions include teaching sessions to provide information and counseling to reinforce behavior. *Indirect* interventions include referral to an appropriate community resource or other health care professional (e.g., nutritionist, smoking-cessation program, counselor, support group for substance abusers, dieters' support programs).

The goals for the client are (1) to take responsibility for modifying factors that can affect health and (2) to

Text continued on page 155

TABLE 9–2 HEALTH PROMOTION AND RISK MANAGEMENT

Risk Factor	Potential Health Problem	Screening and Preventive Measures: *Self-Care*	Screening and Preventive Measures: *Professional Level*
RACE			
Black	Hypertension	Self-monitor BP Avoid salt in diet Maintain ideal body weight Seek professional care if systolic BP > 140 or diastolic BP > 90	Monitor if BP is elevated or client is taking antihypertensive medications
White (fair skin tones)	Skin cancer	Limit exposure to sun Wear protective clothing Use sunscreen with SPF 15 or above Perform monthly head-to-toe skin inspection Seek professional care if change noted in any moles or birthmarks, or new growths or patches do not heal	Monitor skin lesions Skin biopsy or excision and follow-up treatment
	Osteoporosis	See self-care and professional level measures listed under "Personal Habits—Inadequate calcium intake"	
Japanese	Stomach cancer	Know suspicious GI symptoms: pain, hematemesis, melena, weight loss, nausea, and so on*	Follow-up for laboratory tests and special diagnostic procedures
Hispanic	Diabetes mellitus	Regular exercise and weight control Consume balanced diet of no more than 30% fats with complex carbohydrates Know symptoms of hyperglycemia: polydipsia, polyuria, polyphagia, and delayed wound healing*	Diet counseling Follow-up for laboratory tests, diagnostic procedures, and blood glucose monitoring and control
Native American	Alcohol abuse and related diseases	Abstinence Limit alcohol intake to 1 oz/day or less if personal tendency (e.g., 1 to 2 mixed drinks or cans of beer) Know symptoms of alcoholism* Join self-help support group such as Alcoholics Anonymous (AA)	Assessment of history and physical condition Referral to a detoxification program Counseling for client and family
GENETIC OR FAMILY-RELATED			
Overweight	Obesity-related disease	Monitor weight once per week Perform regular, sustained exercise Consume balanced diet (no more than 30% fats, and calories should not exceed metabolic needs) Join self-help group such as Weight Watchers	Diet counseling Follow-up for moribund obesity (>100% of ideal body weight)
Diabetes mellitus	Diabetes mellitus or glucose intolerance	Regular exercise and weight control Consume balanced diet Know symptoms of hyperglycemia: polydipsia, polyuria, polyphagia, and delayed wound healing*	Follow-up for laboratory tests, special diagnostic procedures, and blood glucose monitoring and control
Hypertension	Cardiovascular disease Renal disease Retinopathy Cerebrovascular accident	Regular, sustained exercise Consume balanced diet Avoid excess salt intake Maintain ideal body weight Regular BP checks (self or professional) Take BP medication daily	Regular follow-up for diagnostic studies and laboratory work Monitor compliance
Heart disease (onset before age 50)	Cardiovascular disease	See "Hypertension" Know symptoms of heart disease: chest pain, dyspnea, cyanosis*	Annual physical examination, including ECG and laboratory tests

TABLE 9–2 HEALTH PROMOTION AND RISK MANAGEMENT *Continued*

Risk Factor	Potential Health Problem	Screening and Preventive Measures: *Self-Care*	Screening and Preventive Measures: *Professional Level*
		Stop smoking Monitor resting pulse rate Low saturated fat diet Regular exercise	Refer to smoking cessation clinics Diet counseling
Breast cancer (in mother or sister)	Breast cancer	Learn to perform BSE Perform BSE monthly	Regular professional breast examination as indicated for age and personal history Regular mammography as indicated for age
AGE-RELATED			
Vision changes	Strabismus	Monitor for difficulty focusing, especially on near objects See ophthalmologist if symptoms occur Schedule regular eye examinations as indicated for age	Follow-up for complete eye examination and possible neurologic examination
	Visual acuity changes, cataracts, glaucoma, or macular degeneration	Monitor visual acuity See ophthalmologist if vision is "fuzzy," or seeing halos around lights Schedule regular eye examinations	Complete eye examination to screen for cataracts, glaucoma, and macular degeneration as indicated for age
	Injury or trauma	Wear protective eye gear when engaging in activity likely to result in projectiles or blunt trauma See ophthalmologist if injury should occur	Provide prompt diagnosis and treatment if injury occurs
Falls	Injury or trauma	Keep environment illuminated Remove loose scatter rugs Use a night-light Install handrails and grab bars Wipe up spills immediately	Provide prompt diagnosis and treatment if injury occurs
Self-medication errors	Overmedicating or undermedicating	Request and use prepackaged unit dose medications Prepare medicines in a well-lit area Wear corrective lenses when preparing medicines	Careful assessment of medication history; monitor for toxic response
Hearing problem	Presbycusis	Avoid exposure to loud noises Wear ear plugs when exposed to loud noise levels and limit lengths of exposure	Complete audiometric screening as appropriate for age and personal history
	Injury or trauma	Avoid putting sharp objects into ear canals Know symptoms of ear infections: pain, discharge from ear canal, vertigo, and fever*	Follow-up for prompt diagnosis and treatment if injury or infection occurs
Inadequate dental hygiene	Dental caries Periodontal disease Premature loss of teeth	Brush teeth regularly after meals and at bedtime Floss teeth daily Have damaged teeth repaired or replaced promptly Follow recommendations for fluoride treatments; use fluoridated toothpaste Schedule regular dental checkups	Provide complete dental checkups, with yearly follow-up Fluoride treatments as indicated for age and locale
Impaired immune system integrity	Community-acquired infections	Keep immunizations current as recommended for age Receive vaccinations for influenza yearly and pneumococcal infection as indicated Seek professional care if symptoms of infection occur	Provide prompt diagnosis and treatment if a contagious disease or infection is suspected

Table continued on following page

TABLE 9–2 HEALTH PROMOTION AND RISK MANAGEMENT *Continued*

Risk Factor	Potential Health Problem	Screening and Preventive Measures: *Self-Care*	Screening and Preventive Measures: *Professional Level*
Impaired mobility	Falls	See self-care measures listed for falls related to vision changes under Age-Related Use mobility-assistance devices (e.g., cane or walker) Avoid hazardous surfaces, such as wet floors and icy pavements	Provide prompt diagnosis and treatment if injury occurs
BIOLOGIC			
Hyperlipidemia, hypercholesteremia	Cardiovascular disease	Consume balanced diet low in saturated fats Exercise regularly Avoid or stop smoking Have blood lipid and cholesterol levels monitored periodically as recommended	Regular follow-up for monitoring serum levels
Hyperglycemia	Diabetes mellitus	Consume diet low in fats and simple carbohydrates Include complex carbohydrates Exercise regularly Have blood glucose levels monitored periodically as recommended Self-monitor blood glucose levels if diabetic and following a prescribed medical regimen	Regular follow-up for monitoring control of blood glucose levels Adjustment of medical treatment as indicated by laboratory results
Hypersensitivity reactions	Allergic reactions, including rhinitis, bronchospasm, asthma, eczema, and atopic dermatitis	Avoid known allergens Seek prompt medical treatment if self-care measures are ineffective Discuss with physician whether allergen sensitivity testing and treatment for desensitization is indicated Wear a Medic-Alert tag Learn to use and carry an emergency kit (e.g., epinephrine [Adrenalin] if indicated)	Provide prompt diagnosis and treatment if severe reactions or complications occur Initiation of desensitization therapy if indicated
PERSONAL HABITS			
Inadequate rest and sleep	Fatigue Lowered resistance to illness	Obtain sufficient sleep to feel rested on awakening (amount varies with individual need) (see Chapter 21) Avoid sedatives, caffeine, alcohol Seek professional care if chronic fatigue interferes with activities of daily living	Complete history and physical examination Evaluation in a sleep laboratory
Irregular diet habits	Obesity, diabetes, hypertension, cardiovascular disease, irritability, depression, and hyperactivity or hypoactivity	Consume meals at regular times each day Eat three balanced meals per day Limit intake of salt, caffeine, refined sugar, and fats Perform regular exercise Monitor weight weekly See self-care measures listed under obesity, diabetes, hypertension, and cardiovascular disease	Regular follow-up to monitor existing health problems Provide prompt diagnosis and treatment if a health problem arises
Inadequate calcium intake	Osteoporosis	Consume elemental calcium in recommended amount per day for age and sex. Recommended amounts range from 1000 to 1500 mg/day	Follow-up for periodic physical examination Possible estrogen hormone replacement therapy, when indicated

TABLE 9–2 HEALTH PROMOTION AND RISK MANAGEMENT *Continued*

Risk Factor	Potential Health Problem	Screening and Preventive Measures: *Self-Care*	Screening and Preventive Measures: *Professional Level*
		Limit milk products as source of calcium; include other sources of dietary calcium, such as broccoli, carrots, green beans, spinach, collard greens, and rhubarb Consume 400–800 IU/day of vitamin D Engage in daily weight-bearing activity such as walking	Diet counseling
Excess fat intake	Colon cancer Possible breast cancer	Consume diet low in saturated fats, such as that found in beef. Substitute with fish, poultry, and beans Limit milk products and eggs Include fiber in diet such as from grains and cereals Know symptoms of colon cancer (blood in stool, change in bowel habits) and breast cancer (lump, discharge, pain)* Have stool specimen tested for occult blood Perform BSE monthly	Follow-up for laboratory tests and possible diagnostic procedures Diet counseling
Low fiber intake	Colon cancer	Consume diet high in fiber, including cereals and grains, especially bran Know symptoms of colon cancer (see earlier)* Have stool specimen tested for occult blood	Follow-up for laboratory tests and diagnostic procedures Supplemental fiber to include in diet
Alcohol abuse	Alcoholism Cancer of mouth, throat, esophagus, larynx, and liver Accidents, including those that result in death Cirrhosis Esophageal varices Pancreatitis Dementia	Abstinence, if high risk for alcoholism Limit alcohol intake to 1 oz or less per day if no personal tendency (e.g., 1 to 2 mixed drinks or cans of beer) Know the symptoms of alcoholism* Join self-help support group, such as Alcoholics Anonymous, if alcohol consumption interferes with performance of job or interpersonal relationships	Careful assessment of history and physical condition Referral to a detoxification program, if indicated Provide counseling Family counseling and support are often necessary (e.g., Al-Anon, Ala-Teen)
Drug abuse	Harmful side effects Drug interactions Allergic reactions Hepatitis HIV	Use prescribed medications only as directed Discard outdated medications Limit use of over-the-counter drugs to only those necessary Avoid recreational drug use Know symptoms of substance abuse* If using intravenous drugs, do not share needles or syringes	Careful assessment of history and physical condition Referral to a detoxification program, if indicated Provide counseling Family counseling and support are often necessary Screening for HIV infection
Tobacco use	Cancer of mouth or lung Cardiovascular disease Respiratory disease	Avoid tobacco use in any form Limit use, if unable to quit Know symptoms of tobacco-related health problems: persistent cough, oral sore that does not heal, hoarseness that persists, blood in sputum* Have regular health checkups Avoid exposing others to sidestream smoke Attend support group to help stop smoking, such as Smokers Anonymous	Follow-up for laboratory tests and special diagnostic procedures Counseling for help to stop smoking Referral of family members (if indicated) for health assessment if exposed to sidestream smoke
Safety	Unintentional injury or death	Use safety equipment as indicated (seat belts, helmet, eye shield, life vest)	Thorough teaching about medications and their side effects

Table continued on following page

TABLE 9–2 HEALTH PROMOTION AND RISK MANAGEMENT *Continued*

Risk Factor	Potential Health Problem	Screening and Preventive Measures: *Self-Care*	Screening and Preventive Measures: *Professional Level*
		Learn how to swim Never drink and drive. Appoint a designated driver Do not operate equipment or engage in hazardous activity if taking medication that causes drowsiness Develop safety awareness; e.g., learn to identify unsafe situations and avoid them or take corrective action	Provide prompt diagnosis and treatment if an injury occurs
Sun exposure	Sunburn Skin cancer	See self-care measures listed under skin cancer related to race	See measures listed under skin cancer related to race
LIFESTYLE			
Lack of regular exercise	Obesity Cardiovascular disease	Engage in regular aerobic exercise (brisk walking, biking, jogging, swimming) at least 3 times/week for 30 to 40 minutes each Warm up prior to exercising to increase flexibility and reduce chance of injury Do not begin an exercise program until evaluated by health care professional for a baseline health assessment Follow professional advice regarding type of exercise program and intensity of training Wear appropriate gear for activity as protection Consume a balanced diet Know warning signals of when to stop exercising (e.g., dizziness, chest pain)*	Baseline health assessment prior to beginning exercise program Provide prompt diagnosis and treatment if complications or injury occurs Periodic assessment of cardiovascular status and endurance
Stress and coping ability	Many health problems are related to high stress levels and inadequate coping	Decrease level of stress whenever possible Develop a variety of coping skills Practice relaxation techniques (e.g., biofeedback, imagery, meditation, self-hypnosis) Recognize effects of stress on self Develop a support network* Modify lifestyle to reduce stress	Provide counseling for stress management Refer to appropriate support system as indicated by the individual circumstances Teach regarding relaxation techniques Carefully assess and treat if psychosomatic health problems develop
Lack of self-care activities to promote health	Cancer of breast, testis, or prostate	Monthly practice of BSE or TSE Regular professional examination as indicated for age	Periodic, regular examination
	Cancer of the cervix	Obtain regular pelvic examination and Papanicolaou (Pap) test as indicated for age and sexual activity status	Periodic, regular examination with follow-up as necessary
	Vision and hearing problems	See self-care measures under age-related health problems	See measures listed under age-related health problems for vision and hearing
	Dental and gum disease	See self-care measures under age-related health problems	See measures listed under age-related health problems for dental hygiene
	Tetanus Influenza Pneumonia	Keep immunizations current*	Provide prompt diagnosis and treatment if an infectious disease occurs

TABLE 9–2 HEALTH PROMOTION AND RISK MANAGEMENT *Continued*

Risk Factor	Potential Health Problem	Screening and Preventive Measures	
		Self-Care	*Professional Level*
	Cancer	Know the seven warning signs: change in bowel or bladder habits, a nonhealing sore, unusual bleeding or discharge, lump or thickening in breast or other area, difficulty swallowing or indigestion, change in mole or wart, and persistent cough or hoarseness* Know and follow current recommendations for prevention and early entry into the health care system	Follow-up for laboratory tests and special diagnostic procedures Provide prompt diagnosis and treatment
High-risk sexual activity	Unplanned pregnancy	Use contraceptive method acceptable to self and partner Prenatal care	Provide counseling regarding options for contraceptives Provide counseling regarding pregnancy outcome options
	Cervical cancer	Abstain from early, frequent sexual activity Limit number of sexual partners Limit number of childbirths Schedule regular Pap test as recommended for age	Regular professional pelvic examinations and Pap tests as indicated by health behavior profile
	STDs, such as HIV infection and herpes	Limit number of sexual partners Avoid anal intercourse Use condoms Avoid oral-genital intercourse Avoid oral contact with body fluids (semen, blood, feces, urine) Seek professional care for regular, periodic assessment if engaging in high-risk sexual activity Know symptoms of STDs, e.g., sore on genitals or mucous membranes, discharge from penis or vagina, abnormal bleeding, dyspareunia Refrain from sexual activity if symptoms of STDs develop	Follow-up for prompt diagnosis and treatment should STD be suspected Provide counseling regarding safe sex practices Refer to public health for contact and follow-up of possible infected partners
Travel	Diseases prevalent in locale	Obtain necessary vaccinations before departure Seek prompt treatment if illness develops while traveling or after return	Provide prompt diagnosis and treatment if illness occurs
ENVIRONMENTAL AND OCCUPATIONAL			
Sports	Fractures, sprains, and strains	Have a baseline health assessment prior to beginning a sport Wear protective gear to avoid injury (e.g., eye shield, helmet, padding)* Follow recommendations for warm-up and cool-down exercises Limit mobility of injured body part until rehabilitation begins	Provide prompt diagnosis and treatment of injuries Rehabilitation
Outdoor activity	Sunburn Skin cancer Frostbite Hypothermia or hyperthermia	Wear protective gear appropriate for the weather Use sunscreen with an SPF of 15 or above Limit exposure to extremes of heat or cold Learn survival tactics relative to activity Know early signs of hypothermia (disorientation) and hyperthermia (dry, hot skin)	Provide prompt diagnosis and treatment if a problem occurs See measures listed under skin cancer related to race

Table continued on following page

TABLE 9–2 HEALTH PROMOTION AND RISK MANAGEMENT *Continued*

Risk Factor	Potential Health Problem	Screening and Preventive Measures: *Self-Care*	Screening and Preventive Measures: *Professional Level*
		Attempt to seek medical treatment as soon as possible if a problem arises Avoid future exposure to extremes of heat or cold because of increased vulnerability	
Loud noise	Hearing loss	Limit exposure to loud music and machinery Wear protective ear plugs Have regular screening of hearing and seek professional care if hearing loss is evident	Regular, complete audiometric screening, as appropriate
Chemical fumes, airborne particle exposure	Respiratory diseases Cancer	Provide adequate ventilation Wear protective gear (goggles, respirators) Limit exposure when possible (chemicals, dry cleaning fluid, film processing, mining, asbestos exposure, household cleaners) Evaluate occupational risks Reduce exposure by changing jobs, if necessary Know symptoms of possible disease, such as hoarseness, persistent cough, hemoptysis, chronic dyspnea* Avoid smoking	Prompt diagnosis and treatment if disease should occur
Stress-provoking activity	Many stress-related health problems may occur	See "Stress and coping ability" under Lifestyle	Provide counseling regarding stress management
High-accident-risk activity (also see "Safety" under Personal Habits)	Unintentional injury or death	Avoid high-accident-risk activities Learn safety measures Practice safety measures so they become habitual Use safety equipment such as goggles, helmets Get sufficient rest Avoid alcohol, drugs, or medications known to cause drowsiness when engaging in high-risk activity Obtain treatment if injury occurs	Provide prompt diagnosis and treatment if an accidental injury occurs
Low-level electromagnetic radiation exposure	Cancer of brain or eye Leukemia Sarcoma Possible birth defects	Limit exposure Monitor immediate environment for radiation levels Promptly seek health assessment and treatment for possible problems	Provide prompt diagnosis and treatment if a health problem occurs
SOCIOECONOMIC			
Recent immigration	Diseases common to locale of origin or where traveled	Obtain necessary immunizations before departure Seek professional care if symptoms of disease occur, especially during or after recent travel	Careful assessment of history and physical examination Provide prompt diagnosis and treatment if a health problem occurs
Lack of adequate health insurance coverage	Delayed or postponed treatment of health problems Undetected health problems	Use free walk-in health care facilities	Refer client to social services or welfare agency for assistance with applying for available health care, such as Medicaid or Medicare

*Seek professional care if symptoms are present.

BP, blood pressure; BSE, breast self-examination; ECG, electrocardiogram; GI, gastrointestinal; HIV, human immunodeficiency virus; IU, international units; SPF, sun protection factor; STDs, sexually transmitted diseases; TSE, testicular self-examination.

BOX 9–5 Example of Integrating Health Risk Appraisal into the History Interview

Biographical and Demographic Data

S. W. is a 28-year-old, single, white, female, self-employed clothing designer. Self-insured. Admitted to nursing unit after surgical repair of the right knee.

Health Maintenance Activities

Annual examinations for teeth, vision, Pap smear. No breast self-examination. Last physical examination 18 months ago.

Personal Habits

Denies smoking. Consumes one to two alcoholic drinks or glasses of wine most days. Uses own automobile frequently, wears seat belts "when [she] remembers to put them on." Uses tanning room at health spa twice a week for 30 minutes.

Diet

No restrictions, likes most foods. Prefers to limit sugar and salt intake. Typical 24-hour diet includes Food Guide Pyramid groups. Usually eats breakfast and dinner; lunch consumed "on the run." Dines out often with clients at restaurants.

Exercise

Jogs once per week for 2 to 3 miles and performs step aerobics once per week at health spa. Tripped and fell while jogging 3 weeks ago; twisted right knee.

Stress Management

Feels "moderate" pressure to succeed in business. Life becomes "hectic" when new fashion lines shown. Uses imagery for relaxation (usually effective). Denies current problems with stress management.

Sleep and Rest

Gets approximately 6 to 7 hours' sleep per night and feels rested.

Sexuality

Sexually active since age 18. Reports five or six partners in past 10 years, with one partner for past 2 years. Prescribed oral contraceptive for 6 years. Partner does not use condoms.

Past Health History

No previous illness, injury, or surgery. No allergies.

Family Health History

Mother had breast cancer at age 42; treated with surgery and is currently healthy. No other known family-linked health problems.

Health Risk Appraisal

S. W. is at risk for (1) breast cancer, (2) possible skin cancer, (3) automobile-related injury or death, (4) possible sexually transmitted diseases, including human immunodeficiency virus infection, and (5) recurrent injury to the right knee. She also is at risk for health problems related to alcohol consumption, inadequate nutrition, inadequate exercise patterns, and a stress-producing lifestyle. There may be concerns about financial security that can be explored with S. W. during further questioning.

strive for optimal health. Box 9–5 provides an example of how to integrate health risk appraisal into the history interview.

■ HEALTH PROMOTION ACROSS THE LIFE SPAN

Health promotion needs change with age and sex. For example, the risk for development of cancer of the bowel or breast is higher in people over age 50 years than in younger people.

Specific screening procedures are performed during health assessment to determine potential and actual health problems. For example, after age 40, glaucoma screening is recommended every 2 years. For health maintenance and prevention, specific health management behaviors are recommended based on age. For example, routine childhood vaccinations for immunization against contagious diseases are administered according to a schedule that correlates with the development of the immune system as well as with periods when exposure is most likely to occur. Adults may be deficient in routine vaccinations or may not have had previous exposure to childhood contagious diseases. These clients should have screening antibody assays and immunizations if indicated.

Recommendations for common screening procedures and health management behaviors across the life span are listed in Table 9–3. Recommendations change periodically as research and epidemiologic studies reveal information about occurrence and as newer, more easily applied or sensitive screening methods are developed. Become familiar with the most current recommendations.

Chapter 18 discusses risk factors for the common types of cancer as well as primary risk factors and secondary type of cancer prevention. The American Cancer Society Guidelines are given for early detection in asymptomatic populations.

■ SCREENING TESTS AND PROCEDURES

Screening tests and procedures are used to assess for a health problem (e.g., a skin test for tuberculosis) or for risk of future health problems (e.g., serum cholesterol screening for the risk of atherosclerosis). When inquiring whether the client has had a specific screening test or procedure, such as an eye examination or mammogram, ask when the test was last performed and what the results were. Use this information to assess health risk status and to recommend further follow-up or screening procedures.

Text continued on page 160

TABLE 9-3 RECOMMENDATIONS FOR COMMON SCREENING PROCEDURES AND HEALTH MANAGEMENT BEHAVIORS ACROSS THE LIFE SPAN*

Potential Health Problem	Recommended Preventive/ Screening Examination†	Birth to 18 Months	2 to 6 Years	7 to 12 Years	13 to 18 Years	19 to 39 Years	40 to 64 Years	65 Years and over
Growth and developmental concerns	History—re: developmental disorders	Parent/family dysfunction. Physical, mental, emotional, and social growth. Behavioral and learning disorders				Relationships with significant others. Parenting behaviors. Job satisfaction.		Retirement planning; declining mental acuity
			Discipline, school readiness		Sexual practices			
	Nutrition history	Breastfeeding, iron intake	Sweets, between-meal snacks, fats (saturated), cholesterol, sodium, iron, calcium			Fats (saturated), cholesterol, complex carbohydrates, fiber, sodium, calcium		
						Iron for women until menopause		
			Caloric balance and selection of exercise program					
	Complete physical examination	Birth, 2–4 weeks, and 2, 4, 6, 9, 12, 15, and 18 months	Every year until age 5	Every 2 years	Every 2 years	Every 5 years	Every 2 years ages 40 to 50, then yearly	Every year
Vision problems	Strabismus check, amblyopia	Every visit						
	Assessment of visual acuity		Every year beginning at age 3	One time	One time	Every 2 to 4 years	Every 1 to 2 years to include glaucoma screening	
Hearing problems	Audiometry	18 months	Every year	One time	One time		Every 3 years	Every year
Dental problems	Assessment of teeth/cleaning	Every visit (baby bottle tooth decay)	Every 6 months beginning at age 3		Every 6 months to 1 year			
	Fluoride	+	+	+	+			
	Brushing and flossing		+	+	+	+	+	+

Infectious diseases	Routine immunizations	DTP, OPV/IPV, MMR, Hib, HBV, VZV per protocol	DTP, OPV/IPV, MMR per protocol	MMR at age 11 to 12 if not given at 4 to 6 years				
	PPD or tine test	At age 1	One time	One time	One time	One time	One time	One time
	Tetanus-diphtheria booster		One time between 4 and 6 years		One time between 14 and 16 years	Every 10 years		
	Influenza vaccine			Every year if high risk under age 65				Every year
	Pneumococcal vaccine			Every 6 to 10 years if in high-risk category (e.g., asthma, cystic fibrosis, chronic pulmonary disease)				
Accidents and injuries	Automobile restraints	Car seats	Car seats until age 4; seat belts	+	+	+	+	+
	History—re: risk factors	Burns, falls, choking, poisoning, drowning	Poisoning, drowning, burns, bicycle accidents, choking	Bicycle accidents, burns, poisoning, firearms, drowning	Bicycle accidents, burns, firearms, drinking while driving, suicide	Drinking while driving, firearms, back injury, burns, suicide	Drinking while driving, burns, back injury, falls	Falls
Substance abuse	History—re: use of tobacco, drugs, alcohol			+	+	+	+	+
Birth defects	Rubella titer				Unimmunized/unexposed female			
	Amniocentesis					Over age 35		
Unplanned pregnancy	Sex education			+	+	+	+	
	Contraceptive information				+	+	+	
Anemia	Hemoglobin and hematocrit	One time, early infancy	Age 3 and 5 years	Ages 8, 10, and 12	Ages 15 and 18	One time	Every 3 years	Every year
Bacteriuria	Urinalysis		One time at age 3	One time	One time	Every 1 to 3 years		Every year

Table continued on following page

TABLE 9–3 RECOMMENDATIONS FOR COMMON SCREENING PROCEDURES AND HEALTH MANAGEMENT BEHAVIORS ACROSS THE LIFE SPAN *Continued*

Potential Health Problem	Recommended Preventive/ Screening Examination†	Birth to 18 Months	2 to 6 Years	7 to 12 Years	13 to 18 Years	19 to 39 Years	40 to 64 Years	65 Years and over
Bowel cancer	Rectal examination					Every year from ages 30 to 40	Every year	
	Stool examination for occult blood						Every year beginning at age 40	
	Sigmoidoscopy						Every 3 to 5 years after two negative test results 1 year apart, beginning at age 40	
Breast cancer	Breast self-examination (BSE)					Every month		
	Professional examination					Every 3 years	Every year	
	Mammogram					One time between ages 35 and 39 if high risk	Every 1 to 2 years until age 50; then every year until age 75	
Cervical cancer/ gynecologic problems	Papanicolaou (Pap) smear				Every 1 to 3 years if sexually active	Every year until 3 examination results in a row are negative; then decrease frequency		
	Pelvic examination					Every 1 to 3 years	Every year	
Heart disease	History—re: exercise program or physical activity		Every visit					
	Electrocardiogram					Every 5 years after age 35; every 2 years after age 50		
Hypertension	Blood pressure		Every year beginning at age 3	Every 1 to 2 years				Every year
Hyperlipidemia	Blood cholesterol level		Age 3 if family history			Every 5 years if below 200 mg/dl		Every 3 to 5 years
Obesity	Height and weight	Every visit	+	+	+	+	+	+
Oral cancer	Professional examination					Annually	Annually	Annually

Scoliosis	Back examination			Every year beginning at age 8	Every visit			
Sexually transmitted diseases (STDs)	VDRL/RPR				One time if sexually active	One time	One time	One time
	Chlamydial testing Gonorrhea culture HIV counseling and testing				+ + +	+ + +	+ + +	+ + +
Testicular/ prostate problems	Testicular self-examination (TSE)					Every month	Every month	Every month
	Professional examination					Every 5 years	Every 2 to 3 years between ages 40 and 50, then every year	Every year
Prostate cancer	Prostate-specific antigen (PSA)						Every year between ages 50 and 70 years	

*Recommendations are subject to change, based on the most current information available. Recommendations in this table are based on guidelines from the American Academy of Family Physicians, the American Academy of Ophthalmology, the American Academy of Pediatrics, the American Cancer Society, the American College of Obstetricians and Gynecologists, the American College of Physicians, the National Cancer Institute, the National Heart, Lung, and Blood Institute, Centers for Disease Control and Prevention, and the U.S. Preventive Services Task Force.

† The list of preventive/screening services is not exhaustive, nor are all services listed indicated for every client at every visit. Type and frequency of visits and services is determined by individual and family health history and personal habits.

DTP, diphtheria and tetanus toxoids combined with pertussis vaccine; HBV, hepatitis B vaccine; Hib (or HbCV [*Haemophilus* b conjugate vaccine]); HIV, human immunodeficiency virus; IPV, injectable polio virus; MMR, measles-mumps-rubella vaccine; OPV, oral polio vaccine; PPD, purified protein derivative; RPR, rapid plasma reagin test (for syphilis); VDRL, Venereal Disease Research Laboratory test (for syphilis); VZV, varicella-zoster virus vaccine; +, ongoing preventive behavior (these items should be assessed during each contact with the client).

Organizing the Health History Interview

Organize the data collected during the health history interview by topical areas. Use a comprehensive, flexible approach while allowing for in-depth focus assessment in areas of concern. Include a head-to-toe assessment. Various formats are helpful for conducting a health history interview. Gordon's functional health patterns (FHPs) are an example.

Functional health patterns may be used to collect health history data (Box 9–6). This approach assists in identifying health patterns, deviations from these patterns, and actual or potential nursing diagnoses. Each of the 11 patterns has its own assessment criteria (see Appendix B).

Recording the Health History Interview

Record interview data in the health record according to agency protocol. The format is organized and may be a narrative, an outline, or a checklist with written supplementary comments. Record all pertinent data (both positive and negative findings). Data are clear, concise, comprehensive, and consistent, with no gaps or areas of ambiguity. Use approved agency abbreviations and terminology, whenever possible, to promote communication among health care team members.

Applying the Nursing Process to Health Assessment

In health assessment, seek to gather as much data about the client as possible, both subjective and objective. Analyze the data to determine the client's needs and responses to potential and actual health problems. Consider the client's preferences when formulating nursing diagnoses that are amenable to intervention. Establishing realistic goals and outcome criteria and planning interventions follow in logical order (Box 9–7).

CONCLUSIONS

The health history is the first component of health assessment. The history constitutes the subjective data and guides thorough assessment of specific concerns or areas identified through health risk appraisal. The history can be recorded in many ways, such as through computerized database assessments or on paper. Although a thorough history may seem time-consuming, the data provided are crucial to fully understanding the client's special needs.

BOX 9–6 Gordon's Functional Health Patterns

Health Perception and Health Management

The client's perception and understanding of the health status; this includes lifestyle and behaviors to promote, maintain, and restore health and well-being.

Nutritional-Metabolic

Food and fluid consumption in relation to the body's metabolic needs, including adequacy of nutrient supply to local tissues. Multiple factors influence behavior, such as physiologic (e.g., dehydration), pathophysiologic (e.g., peptic ulcer), psychosocial (e.g., the emotional significance of food), and socioeconomic (e.g., financial ability to purchase food).

Elimination

Patterns of excretory function, including bowel, bladder, and skin. Habits of excretory regularity and perceived difficulties are assessed.

Activity-Exercise

Activities of daily living requiring energy expenditure; these include self-care measures, physical exercise, stamina, and leisure and recreational activities.

Sleep-Rest

The usual habits of sleep, rest, relaxation, and energy level. Patterns are assessed for a 24-hour period so that circadian rhythmicity can be considered.

Cognitive-Perceptual

The ability to perceive, comprehend, and use information. The sensory functions are also involved. Pain is included in this pattern.

Self-Perception and Self-Concept

View of self, including attitudes, identity, body image, sense of self-worth, and self-esteem.

Role Relationship

The client's roles in society and interpersonal relationships.

Sexuality-Reproductive

Satisfaction or dissatisfaction with sexuality and reproductive functions; these include sex role behavior and identification, physiologic and biologic functions, and sociocultural aspects of sexual behavior.

Coping–Stress Tolerance

General coping strategies and effectiveness in managing stress, including the perception of stressors and their effect on the client.

Value-Belief

Values, beliefs (including spiritual), and goals that guide the choices and decisions, particularly in health care. Sources of strength and meaning are identified.

BOX 9–7 Applying the Nursing Process to Health Assessment: Case Example

Introduction

Mrs. L. is a 58-year-old, healthy-looking woman who visits a glaucoma screening booth at a health fair. The nurse integrates health assessment data and nursing process while talking to Mrs. L. and testing her visual acuity.

Biographical Data

Married. Works full time as a legal secretary. Has one married child who lives out of state.

Physical Health History

History negative for significant health problems. Postmenopausal. Reports seeing rings around lights and decreased side vision most noticeable when reading.

Health Risk Appraisal

Mother had cataracts. Family history positive for hypertension. Nearsighted since age 10 and wears corrective lenses. Last eye examination 5 years ago. Has smoked one pack of cigarettes per day for 40 years.

Physical Examination

Snellen chart results (with corrective lenses) are O.D. (right eye) = 20/40, O.S. (left eye) = 20/30, O.U. (both eyes) = 20/30. Visual fields to confrontation reveal superior fields less than those of the examiner. Pupils react sluggishly to accommodation. Further physical examination limited because of setting.

Nursing Diagnosis

High risk for altered health maintenance related to visual changes (decreased visual acuity and peripheral vision), family history of hypertension, and smoking history.

Expected Outcomes

Long Term

Mrs. L. will maintain present visual acuity and prevent further loss of vision.

Short Term

1. Mrs. L. will verbalize understanding of the need for an immediate, complete ophthalmologic examination.
2. Mrs. L. will identify an ophthalmologist whom she will contact no later than tomorrow for an appointment.

Interventions

1. Discuss results of visual screening with Mrs. L. and their significance.
2. Explain risk factors for glaucoma and Mrs. L.'s risk profile.
3. Assist Mrs. L. in choosing an ophthalmologist.
4. Provide Mrs. L. with pamphlets about glaucoma from the National Society to Prevent Blindness.
5. Give Mrs. L. a self-addressed, stamped postcard that is to be returned by the ophthalmologist after the first visit.

Evaluation

Long Term

Ask Mrs. L. to restate her understanding of the need to have regular visual check-ups by an ophthalmologist and to follow the recommended medical regimen for eye care.

Short Term

Ask Mrs. L. whom she plans to contact for an eye appointment and when she intends to do this.

BIBLIOGRAPHY

1. Ainslie, G., et al. (1998). Psychosocial history by automated self-report. *Federal Practitioner, 15*(3), 33–40.
2. Alfaro-LeFevere, R. (1998). *Applying nursing process: A step-by-step guide* (4th ed.). Philadelphia: J. B. Lippincott.
3. American Academy of Family Physicians (AAFP). (1996). *Summary of policy recommendations for periodic health examination.* (AAFP No. 962, reprint No. 510.) Kansas City, KS: Author.
4. American Academy of Pediatrics. (1988). *Guidelines for health supervision II* (2nd ed.). Elk Grove Village, IL: Author.
5. American Academy of Pediatrics, Committee on Infectious Diseases. (1999). Recommended childhood immunization schedule—United States, January–December 1999. *Pediatrics, 103,* 182–185.
6. Andresen, G. P. (1992). How to assess the older mind. RN, *55*(6), 34.
7. Andrews, M. M., & Boyle, J. S. (Eds.). (1995). *Transcultural concepts in nursing care* (2nd ed.). Philadelphia: J. B. Lippincott.
8. Barry, P. D. (1996). *Psychosocial nursing: Care of physically ill patients and their families.* Philadelphia: J. B. Lippincott.
9. Bozzo, J. (1999). Databases and nursing outcomes. *American Journal of Nursing, 99*(4), 22.
10. Braverman, B. G. (1990). Eliciting assessment data from the patient who is difficult to interview. *Nursing Clinics of North America, 25,* 743–750.
11. Brennan, P. F., & Romano, C. A. (1987). Computers and nursing diagnoses: Issues in implementation. *Nursing Clinics of North America, 22,* 935–941.
12. Brink, P. (1984). Value orientations as an assessment tool in cultural diversity. *Nursing Research, 35,* 198.
13. Brink, P. J. (1987). Cultural aspects of sexuality. *Holistic Nursing Practice, 1,* 12–20.
14. Buckley, G. E. (1995). Traveling healthy: A guide for counseling the international traveler. *Nurse Practitioner, 20*(10), 38–50.
15. Burnard, P. (1988). Discussing spiritual issues with clients. *Health Vision, 61*(12), 371–372.
16. Cameron, C. T., & McNeil, E. L. (1976). The importance of history. *Journal of Emergency Nursing, 2*(3), 21–22.
17. Carpenito, L. J. (1997). *Nursing diagnosis: Application to clinical practice* (8th ed.). Philadelphia: J. B. Lippincott.
18. Carson, V. B. (1999). *Spiritual dimensions of nursing practice* (2nd ed.). Philadelphia: W. B. Saunders.
19. Centers for Disease Control and Prevention. (1999). Recommended childhood immunization schedule—United States, 1999. *Morbidity and Mortality Weekly Report, 48,* 12–6.
20. Chilton, B. A. (1998). Recognizing spirituality. *Image, Journal of Nursing Scholarship, 30*(4), 400–401.
21. Clark, C. C. (1996). *Wellness practitioner: Concepts, research, and strategies* (2nd ed.). New York: Springer.
22. Diaz-Duque, O. F. (1982). Advice from an interpreter. *American Journal of Nursing, 82*(9), 1380–1382.
23. Dirckx, J. H. (1985). Talking with patients, the art of history taking. *Clinical Nurse Practitioner, 3,* 13–14.
24. Edelman, C., & Mandle, C. (Eds.). (1997). *Health promotion throughout the life span.* (4th ed.). St. Louis: Mosby–Year Book.
25. Geissler, E. M. (1994). *Pocket guide to cultural assessment.* St. Louis: C. V. Mosby.
26. Giger, J., & Davidhizar, R. (Eds.). (1995). *Transcultural nursing: Assessment and intervention* (2nd ed.). St. Louis: Mosby–Year Book.

27. Gordon, M. (1994). *Nursing diagnosis: Process and application* (3rd ed.). New York: McGraw-Hill.
28. Grasska, M. A., & McFarland, T. (1982). Overcoming the language barrier: Problems and solutions. *American Journal of Nursing, 82*(9), 1376–1379.
29. Grimes, J., & Burns, E. (1996). *Health assessment in nursing practice* (4th ed.). Boston: Little, Brown.
30. Grossman, D. (1994). Enhancing your "cultural competence." *American Journal of Nursing, 94*(7), 58–62.
31. Halloran, E. J. (1988). Computerized nurse assessments. *Nursing and Health Care, 9,* 497–499.
32. Helman, C. (1994). *Culture, health and illness* (3rd ed.). Boston: Wright.
33. Hogstel, M. O. (1996). *Practical guide to health assessment through the lifespan* (2nd ed.). Philadelphia: F. A. Davis.
34. Huff, R. M., & Kline, M. V. (Eds.). (1998). *Promoting health in multicultural populations: A handbook for practitioners.* Thousand Oaks, CA: Sage.
35. Iyer, P. W., Taptich, B. J., & Bernocchi-Losey, D. (1995). *Nursing process and nursing diagnosis* (3rd ed.). Philadelphia: W. B. Saunders.
36. Jarvis, C. (2000). *Physical examination and health assessment.* (3rd ed.). Philadelphia: W. B. Saunders.
37. Landis, B. J., & Brykczynski, K. A. (1997). Employing prevention in practice. *American Journal of Nursing, 97*(8), 40–46.
38. Lester, N. (1998). Cultural competence: A nursing dialogue. Part One. *American Journal of Nursing, 98*(8), 26–33.
39. Lester, N. (1998). Cultural competence: A nursing dialogue. Part Two. *American Journal of Nursing, 98*(9), 36–42.
40. Lipson, J. G., Dibble, S. L., & Minarik, P. A. (1996). *Culture and nursing care: A pocket guide.* San Francisco: University of California, San Francisco, Nursing Press.
41. Longo, D. C., & Williams, R. A. (1986). *Clinical practice in psychosocial nursing: Assessment and intervention* (2nd ed.). Norwalk, CT: Appleton-Century-Crofts.
42. McConnell, E. A. (1998). Communicating with a hearing-impaired patient. *Nursing, 28*(1), 32.
43. Miya, P. A., & Megel, M. E. (1997). Confidentiality and electronic medical records. *MEDSURG Nursing, 6*(4), 222–224, 212.
44. Murray, R. B., & Zentner, J. P. (1993). *Nursing assessment and health promotion: Strategies through the life span* (5th ed.). Norwalk, CT: Appleton & Lange.
45. North American Nursing Diagnosis Association (NANDA). (1999). *NANDA definitions and classification, 1999–2000.* Philadelphia: Author.
46. Pender, N. J. (1996). *Health promotion in nursing practice* (3rd ed.). Norwalk, CT: Appleton & Lange.
47. Poss, J. E., & Rangel, R. (1995). Working effectively with interpreters in the primary setting. *Nurse Practitioner, 20*(12), 43–47.
48. Purnell, L., & Paulanka, B. (1998). *Transcultural health care: A culturally competent approach.* Philadelphia: F. A. Davis.
49. *Quick reference to cultural assessment.* (1994). St. Louis: Mosby–Year Book.
50. Rahe, R. H. (1975). Life changes and near-future illness reports. In L. Levi (Ed.), *Emotions: Their parameters and measurement.* New York: Raven Press.
51. Risen, C. B. (1995). A guide to taking a sexual history. *Psychiatric Clinics of North America, 18*(1), 39–53.
52. Schneiderman, H. (1982, June). The review of systems, an important part of comprehensive examination. *Postgraduate Medicine, 71,* 151–158.
53. Spillane, R. K. (1987). Getting the patient's point of view: Early. *Nursing Manager, 18*(5), 20–28.
54. Strub, R. L., & Black, F. W. (1995). *The mental status examination in neurology* (3rd ed.). Philadelphia: F. A. Davis.
55. Tom, C. K. (1976). Nursing assessment of biological rhythms. *Nursing Clinics of North America, 11,* 621–630.
56. U.S. Department of Health and Human Services. (1998). *Clinician's handbook of preventive services* (3rd ed.). Washington, D.C.: U.S. Government Printing Office.
57. U.S. Preventive Services Task Force. (1996). *Guide to clinical preventive services* (2nd ed.). Baltimore: Williams & Wilkins.
58. VanDongen, C. J. (1998). Environmental health risks. *American Journal of Nursing, 98*(9), 16B–16F.
59. Warner, P. H., Rowe, T., & Whipple, B. (1999). Shedding light on the sexual history. *American Journal of Nursing, 99*(6), 34–40.
60. Wenger, A. F. Z. (1993). Cultural meaning of symptoms. *Holistic Nursing Practice, 7*(2), 22–35.
61. Woolf, S. H., Jonas, S., & Lawrence, R. S. (Eds.). (1996). *Health promotion and disease prevention in clinical practice.* Baltimore: Williams & Wilkins.

CHAPTER 10

Physical Examination

Annabelle M. Keene

The physical examination is performed after the health history interview. Physical examination skills require use of the ears, eyes, and senses of touch and smell. Repeated practice reinforces integration of these skills. Learn the techniques and correct use of equipment as well as how to discriminate "normal" from "abnormal" findings.

Collect objective data systematically during the examination to supplement and validate subjective data. Evaluate both types of data to enhance holistic perception of the client. Ask the client questions about abnormal physical findings. For example, if a mass is found during palpation, ask whether the area is tender to touch. Record the client's reply in the physical examination portion of the database (e.g., "nontender") even though the data are subjective. If you are palpating a lump or mass that the client did not report initially during the history interview, ask the client whether he or she is aware of the mass's existence. If the client knows that the mass is present or reports related symptoms, proceed with a symptom analysis (see Chapter 9). Record these subjective data in the health history.

Physical examination is used in many settings. Health fairs, screening clinics, physicians' offices, independent practice clinics, home health care, and hospitals are some examples. Client health needs determine the extent and depth of examination. For example, a home health nurse visits a client who has had total hip replacement surgery. During the initial visit, the nurse performs a baseline assessment. During subsequent visits, the initial assessment findings guide evaluation of the client's progress (e.g., increased mobility and strength in the operative leg). Similarly, a coronary care nurse conducts periodic examinations of a client after a myocardial infarction to assess for life-threatening complications.

Purpose of the Examination

The purpose of physical examination is to differentiate normal from abnormal physical findings. A foundation of basic anatomy (structure) and physiology (function) is key to developing skill, expertise, and an appreciation for the wide range of findings that are considered normal. In addition to collecting baseline data, use assessment skills to make clinical judgments about health status and to evaluate the effectiveness of health care interventions. The home health care and coronary care scenarios are examples.

Levels of Physical Examination

Several levels of physical examination are available, depending on client needs.

1. A *screening* physical examination is an organized, superficial check of major body systems for detecting abnormalities or possible problems.
2. If a problem is detected, the examination focuses on a *regional* or *branching* examination, which is an in-depth assessment of a specific body system. This chapter describes the screening adult physical examination. Table 10–1 shows regional examination assessments (see following unit assessment chapters for specific body systems).
3. A *complete* physical examination, which includes ancillary procedures such as x-ray studies and clinical laboratory tests, is beyond the scope of this text.

In the clinical setting, *periodic head-to-toe assessment* updates baseline data and assesses changes in health status. Individualize the depth of body system examinations according to client needs. For example, assess a client with a neurologic problem using the Glasgow Coma Scale in addition to the rest of the head-to-toe evaluation (see Chapter 68). A client with intact neurologic function would not require this depth of assessment. An example of a head-to-toe periodic assessment guide appears in Box 10–1.

Accuracy of Physical Examination

The physical examination helps to validate data collected during the health history interview. As with the health history, strive to collect accurate, thorough data. If you encounter difficulty with an assessment technique or question the accuracy of a finding, consult with colleagues. A second opinion or evaluation may be needed.

Physical Examination and the Nursing Process

An accurate database is essential for formulating individualized nursing diagnoses. It may be misleading to diagnose a problem on the basis of one assessment finding. *Significant* findings (i.e., data that are either abnormal or indicate a potential risk) cue the nurse to collect addi-

Text continued on page 174

TABLE 10–1 ASSESSMENTS PERFORMED DURING REGIONAL EXAMINATIONS

Assessment Area	Client Position or Activity*	Technique†	Equipment	What to Observe
1. General survey	▪ Standing and walking during entrance (a, c) ▪ Sitting during health history interview (a, c) ▪ Changing into examining gown (a, c, f) ▪ Walking to examining table (a, b, c, d, f) ▪ Sitting on edge of examining table (a, c, e, f)	▪ Inspection (a, b, c, d, e, f) ▪ Olfaction (a)		a. General appearance and behavior; apparent age; sex; race; general state of health; signs of distress; body build; posture; gait; obvious deformity; movements and gross ROM; skin color and texture of exposed areas; dress, hygiene, and grooming; body or breath odor; mental status (expression, affect, speech, memory, eye contact); level of consciousness; level of cooperation
			b. Balance scale with height measure	b. Height and weight measurements
				c. Balance, coordination (Romberg's test, arm drift)
			d. Snellen chart	d. Visual acuity (CN II)
			e. Thermometer; watch with second hand; sphygmomanometer; stethoscope	e. Vital signs: temperature; pulse; respirations; blood pressure, including check for auscultatory gap
			f. Tape measure; skinfold calipers	f. Nutritional status: body frame (wrist circumference); MAC; TSF; MAMC; IBW
2. Head and neck	▪ Sitting on edge of examining table (a, b, c, d, e, f, g)	▪ Inspection (a, b, c, d, e, f, g) ▪ Palpation (a, b, c, d, e, f, g) ▪ Percussion (e) ▪ Auscultation (a, f, g) ▪ Olfaction (a, f)		a. *Head*
			(1) Tape measure	(1) Inspect and palpate: skull size, shape, symmetry, contour, tenderness, lesions; measure circumference if abnormal size
				(2) Inspect hair and scalp: color, integrity; hair distribution and texture; presence of nits or lice; hygiene
			(3) Stethoscope	(3) Palpate temporal arteries: thickening, tenderness; auscultate for bruits if abnormality noted; rate amplitude
				b. *Face*
				(1) Inspect symmetry, skin color, hair distribution; facial movements (CN V and VII): clenched jaws, puffed cheeks, raised eyebrows, frown, eyelid strength
				(2) Palpate TMJ; temporal and masseter muscles (CN V); nodules
			(3) Cotton wisp; sterile safety pin	(3) Test facial sensation for light touch, pressure and pain (CN V) over forehead, cheeks, and jaw
				c. *Eyes*
			(1) Snellen chart; eye cover	(1) Visual acuity, if not performed earlier (CN II)
			(2) Eye cover; penlight or pen	(2) Visual fields (peripheral vision) by confrontation method (CN II)
			(3) Penlight or pen	(3) EOMs through six cardinal positions of gaze (CN III, IV, VI, VIII)
			(4) Penlight or pen	(4) Convergence and accommodation (CN III, IV, VI)

	(5) Eye cover	(5) Cover/uncover test (CN III, IV, VI) for movement
	(6) Penlight	(6) Corneal light reflex (CN III, IV, VI) for alignment (Hirschberg's test)
	(7) Penlight; cotton wisp; cotton applicator	(7) Inspect and palpate external eye structures: (a) Eyebrow symmetry, alignment (b) Eyelash symmetry, hair distribution, direction of growth (c) Eyelid position, skin characteristics, blinking (d) Lacrimal apparatus function (e) Eyeball symmetry, firmness (f) Conjunctiva and sclera color, texture, lesions, foreign bodies (g) Cornea texture, transparency; corneal reflex (CN V); omit corneal reflex testing if blinking intact (h) Anterior chamber transparency, depth (i) Iris and pupil symmetry, color, size, reaction to light and accommodation (CN III, IV, VI)
	(8) Ophthalmoscope	(8) Inspect internal eye structures: red reflex, retina, retinal vessels, optic disc, macula, fovea
		d. *Ears*
	(1) Otoscope	(1) Inspect and palpate external ear structures: (a) Auricle symmetry, placement, skin integrity, color, mobility, tenderness over tragus (b) Ear canal skin integrity, cerumen, obstruction, foreign body, discharge (c) Tympanic membrane symmetry, color, light reflection, landmarks, scars, fluid
	(2) Tuning fork (512 Hz)	(2) Hearing acuity: response to normal conversation, whisper test, Weber's test for sound lateralization, Rinne's test for air and bone conduction of sound (CN VIII)
		e. *Nose and sinuses*
		(1) Inspect and palpate external nose alignment, symmetry; skin color, lesions, tenderness, discharge, nasal flaring, patency
	(2) Penlight	(2) Inspect vestibule color, mucous membrane, septum alignment
	(3) Nasal speculum and penlight; or otoscope head with nasal speculum	(3) Inspect nasal mucosa for color, moisture; septum for alignment, masses, perforation; turbinates for color, exudate, inflammation
		(4) Palpate and percuss frontal and maxillary sinuses for swelling and tenderness
	(5) Penlight or transilluminator	(5) Transilluminate frontal and maxillary sinuses if client reports a problem
	(6) Various substances to smell (coffee grounds, cinnamon, cloves, peppermint)	(6) Sense of smell (CN I) not usually tested, but if done, test with coffee grounds, cinnamon, cloves, peppermint

Table continued on following page

TABLE 10–1 ASSESSMENTS PERFORMED DURING REGIONAL EXAMINATIONS *Continued*

Assessment Area	Client Position or Activity*	Technique†	Equipment	What to Observe
			f. Gloves; tongue blade; penlight	f. *Mouth and pharynx*
				(1) Inspect and palpate lips and oral mucosa for color, symmetry, texture, hydration, lesions, Stensen's ducts
				(2) Inspect teeth and gums and palpate gums for state of repair, hygiene, teeth alignment, missing teeth, gum bleeding, gum integrity
				(3) Inspect and palpate tongue and floor of mouth for symmetry, color, tongue position and size, texture, mobility, lesions, presence of papillae
				(4) Tongue mobility and strength (CN IX, XII)
				(5) Inspect Wharton's duct under tongue, floor of mouth, and base of tongue for lesions
				(6) Inspect roof of mouth, palates, and uvula for color, symmetry, texture, bone deformity
				(7) Test rise of uvula and soft palate with phonation (CN X)
				(8) Inspect tonsils and pillars for color, size, shape
				(9) Inspect pharynx for color, discharge on posterior wall
				(10) Test gag reflex (CN IX, X) if swallowing impairment reported or noted
				(11) Note characteristics of voice, ability to swallow (CN IX, X)
				(12) Note presence of breath odor
			(13) Various substances to taste (sugar, salt, lemon juice, bitters)	(13) Test sense of taste (CN VII, IX) only if abnormality reported with sugar, salt, lemon juice, bitters
				g. *Neck*
				(1) Inspect neck muscle symmetry, ROM, strength (CN XI); shoulder shrug
				(2) Palpate and inspect over parotid and submandibular salivary glands for swelling, tenderness
				(3) Palpate all cervical lymph nodes
				(4) Inspect and palpate trachea for symmetry and alignment
			(5) Stethoscope	(5) Inspect and palpate thyroid gland for symmetry, masses; auscultate for bruits if enlarged
			(6) Stethoscope	(6) Inspect and palpate carotid arteries; rate amplitude; auscultate for bruits
				(7) Inspect jugular venous distention

3. Upper extremities and spine	▪ Sitting on edge of examining table (a, b)	▪ Inspection (a, b) ▪ Palpation (a) ▪ Percussion (b)		a. *Upper extremities*
				(1) Inspect skin for lesions and palpate turgor
				(2) Inspect limbs for alignment and symmetry
				(3) Inspect fingernails and blanch to test capillary refill; inspect for clubbing
				(4) Palpate peripheral pulses: brachial, radial, ulnar; rate amplitude
				(5) Palpate epitrochlear lymph nodes
			(6) Tape measure	(6) Inspect and palpate muscle groups for size, symmetry, tone; measure if they appear unequal
				(7) Evaluate and rate muscle strength: upper arms, forearms, wrists, fingers
				(8) Inspect and palpate joints for swelling and tenderness, crepitus
			(9) Goniometer	(9) Assess ROM: shoulders, elbows, wrists, fingers; measure ROM if limitation noted
				b. *Spine*
			(1) Reflex hammer	(1) Test DTRs and rate response: biceps, triceps, brachioradialis; test lower extremity DTRs: patellar, Achilles, and plantar cutaneous reflexes
				(2) Assess cerebellar functions: finger-to-finger touch; hand supination and pronation; finger-to-thumb opposition
4. Posterior thorax	▪ Sitting on edge of examining table; nurse stands behind client (a, b, c)	▪ Inspection (a, b) ▪ Palpation (a, b) ▪ Percussion (a, b, c) ▪ Auscultation (b)		a. *Spine, ribs, muscles*
				(1) Inspect spine for alignment; palpate spine processes for tenderness; inspect skin integrity
				(2) Inspect rib cage for symmetry, shape, movement with respiration
				(3) Measure anteroposterior-to-lateral diameter
				(4) Inspect and lightly palpate paravertebral muscles for tenderness, spasm
				(5) Assess thoracic expansion (respiratory excursion)
				b. *Lungs*
				(1) Observe respiratory pattern
				(2) Palpate tactile fremitus and respiratory excursion
				(3) Percuss posterior and lateral thorax and diaphragmatic excursion
			(4) Ruler and pen	(4) Measure diaphragmatic excursion
			(5) Stethoscope	(5) Auscultate breath sounds, posterior and lateral thorax
			(6) Stethoscope	(6) Auscultate voice sounds if fremitus abnormal (bronchophony, egophony, whispered pectoriloquy)
				c. *Kidneys*
				Percuss over CVAs for kidney tenderness

Table continued on following page

TABLE 10–1 ASSESSMENTS PERFORMED DURING REGIONAL EXAMINATIONS *Continued*

Assessment Area	Client Position or Activity*	Technique†	Equipment	What to Observe
5. Anterior thorax	▪ Sitting on edge of examining table; nurse stands on right side of client (a, b, c, d, e) ▪ Sitting up and leaning forward (b, e) ▪ Sitting with arms at sides; with hands on hips; with arms raised over head (e) ▪ Supine, arm behind head (e) ▪ Supine, head elevated 30 degrees (f, g) ▪ Left lateral recumbent (f)	▪ Inspection (a, b, c, d, e, f, g) ▪ Palpation (a, b, e, f) ▪ Percussion (a) ▪ Auscultation (a, b, c, f)		a. *Lungs and thorax* (1) Inspect skin integrity (2) Observe respiratory pattern (3) Inspect rib cage for symmetry, movement with respiration, shape, use of accessory muscles (4) Palpate respiratory excursion (5) Palpate tactile fremitus (6) Percuss anterior thorax
			(7) Stethoscope	(7) Auscultate breath sounds and voice sounds (if fremitus abnormal)
				b. *Heart* (1) Inspect precordium for lifts, heaves, apical impulse (2) Inspect epigastrium for aortic pulsations (3) Palpate precordium for thrills, apical impulse, lift, heaves
			(4) Stethoscope	(4) Auscultate heart sounds with client sitting up, then leaning forward
			(5) Stethoscope	(5) Assess heart rate and rhythm
				c. *Carotid vessels*
			(1) Stethoscope	(1) Auscultate for bruits (2) Rate amplitude if not done during neck examination
				d. *Jugular veins* Inspect for distention
				e. *Breasts and axillae* (1) Inspect breasts in 3 positions for size, shape, symmetry, contour, skin characteristics, lesions (2) Inspect areolae and nipples for size, shape, color, contour, symmetry, lesions (3) Inspect axillae for rashes, masses, lesions, pigmentation (4) Palpate axillae for lymph nodes (5) Palpate breasts for lumps, masses, consistency ▪ **Assist client to supine position** (6) Palpate breasts, areolae, and nipples with client supine and arm behind head
				f. *Heart* (1) Inspect precordium for lifts, heaves, apical impulse (2) Inspect epigastrium for aortic pulsations (3) Palpate precordium for thrills, lifts, heaves, apical impulse
			(4) Stethoscope	(4) Auscultate heart sounds with client supine, then in left lateral recumbent position

				g. *Jugular veins* (1) Inspect for level of venous distention with client's head elevated 30 to 45 degrees; measure level of distention between angle of Louis and angle of jaw (2) Assess for hepatojugular reflux if right ventricular failure suspected
6. Abdomen	▪ Supine with arms relaxed at sides or crossed over chest; may have knees flexed slightly (a, b, c, d, e, f, i) ▪ Turned to right lateral recumbent (g, h)	▪ Inspection (a, i, j) ▪ Auscultation (a) ▪ Percussion (a, b, c, h, j) ▪ Palpation (a, b, d, e, f, g, h)		a. *Abdomen (general)* (1) Inspect skin integrity and characteristics: striae, venous pattern, hair distribution
			(2) Tape measure	(2) Inspect contour, symmetry, umbilicus, pulsations, peristalsis, rectus muscles with straining; measure girth if distention noted
			(3) Stethoscope	(3) Auscultate all quadrants for bowel sounds
			(4) Stethoscope	(4) Auscultate major vessels for bruits: abdominal aorta; renal, iliac, and femoral arteries
			(5) Stethoscope	(5) Auscultate over epigastrium for venous hum
			(6) Stethoscope	(6) Auscultate over liver and spleen for peritoneal friction rub
				(7) Percuss all quadrants for masses, tenderness, gastric bubble; over bladder and spleen (8) Blunt percussion over anterior right (liver) and left (spleen) lower rib margins for tenderness (9) Lightly palpate all quadrants for masses, tenderness (10) Deep palpation for masses and tenderness, all quadrants (11) Assess rebound tenderness over RLQ and LLQ b. *Liver*
			(1) Pen	(1) Percuss liver size at RMCL and MSL and mark borders
			(2) Ruler	(2) Measure liver span at RMCL and MSL
				c. *Spleen* (1) Percuss spleen size (2) Percuss for splenic enlargement if indicated d. *Aorta* Palpate for area of pulsation in epigastrium e. *Inguinal areas* (1) Palpate femoral arteries and rate amplitude (2) Palpate inguinal lymph nodes; note characteristics f. *Liver* Palpate for size, masses, nodules g. *Spleen* Palpate for size if enlargement suspected h. *Kidneys* (1) Palpate right and left kidneys for enlargement (2) Blunt percussion over CVAs (posterior thorax) for tenderness if not done earlier

Table continued on following page

TABLE 10–1 ASSESSMENTS PERFORMED DURING REGIONAL EXAMINATIONS *Continued*

Assessment Area	Client Position or Activity*	Technique†	Equipment	What to Observe
			i. Tongue blade	i. *Abdominal reflexes* Assess each quadrant for presence of reflex j. Test for ascites if indicated
7. Lower extremities and spine	▪ Supine with arms relaxed (a, b) ▪ Prone if needed to assess popliteal lymph nodes (a)	▪ Inspection (a, b) ▪ Palpation (a) ▪ Percussion (b)	(7) Tape measure (9) Tape measure (12) Goniometer	a. *Lower extremities* (1) Inspect skin for lesions, hair distribution (2) Inspect limbs for alignment and symmetry (3) Inspect toenails and blanch to test capillary refill (4) Palpate peripheral pulses: popliteal, posterior tibial, dorsalis pedis; rate amplitude (5) Palpate popliteal lymph nodes (6) Inspect for edema and palpate for pitting if present (7) Palpate for phlebitis, varicosities; measure circumference of calves or thighs if phlebitis present (8) Assess for presence of Homans' sign (9) Inspect and palpate muscle groups for size, symmetry, tone; measure if appear unequal (10) Evaluate and rate muscle strength: hips, hamstrings, quadriceps, ankles, toes, feet (11) Inspect and palpate joints for swelling, tenderness, crepitus (12) Assess ROM: hips, knees, ankles, feet, toes; measure ROM if limitation noted b. *Spine* (1) Test DTRs if not done before at time of upper extremity evaluation; test patellar, Achilles, and plantar cutaneous reflexes (2) Assess cerebellar functions: ability to slide heel down opposite shin; foot tapping
8. General neurologic and spine	▪ Supine with arms at sides, eyes closed (a) ▪ Walking heel to toe (b) ▪ Walking on toes, then heels (b) ▪ Hopping on each foot (b) ▪ Knee bends (b) ▪ Standing with arms relaxed at sides (c)	▪ Inspection (a, b, c)	(1) Cotton wisp (2) Sterile safety pin or needle (3) Tuning fork (128 Hz) (5) Key, coins, safety pin, paper clip (6) Closed pen (7) Two sterile safety pins (8) Test tubes filled with hot water and cold water	a. *Sensory function* (1) Test perception of light touch over symmetric dermatomes distally, then proximally; trunk, face, neck (2) Test perception of pain vs. pressure over symmetric dermatomes distally, then proximally; trunk, face, neck (3) Test perception of vibration distally on toes and fingers; progress proximally if abnormal (4) Test position sense, fingers and toes (5) Test object identification, both hands (stereognosis) (6) Test graphism, both hands (7) Test two-point discrimination, both index fingers (8) Test temperature perception only if pain perception is impaired: distally, then proximally; trunk, face, neck

			(9) Finger touch	(9) Test point localization and tactile localization (double simultaneous stimulation) only if light touch perception is impaired ▪ **Help client to a standing position** b. *Gross motor and balance* (1) Inspect gait and balance while client walks heel to toe, then on toes, then on heels (2) Observe balance while client stands on one foot, then the other (3) Observe balance and lower extremity strength while client hops on one foot, then the other (4) Observe balance and strength while client performs shallow knee bends c. *Spine* (1) Inspect spine from anterior, lateral, and posterior views for kyphosis, lordosis, or scoliosis (2) Assess spine ROM
9A. Genitalia (male)	▪ Standing facing nurse (a, b, c, d, e, f, g, h, i) ▪ Standing and performing Valsalva's maneuver (g, h, i)	▪ Inspection (a, b, d, f, g) ▪ Palpation (c, e, h, i)	A. Gloves worn throughout b. Culture medium f. Transilluminator or flashlight	A. *Male genitalia* a. Inspect pubic hair and skin for hair distribution, rashes, lesions, parasites b. Inspect penis: shaft, prepuce, glans, urethral meatus; culture discharge if present c. Palpate penile shaft for nodules, tenderness d. Inspect scrotum for size, symmetry, shape, swelling e. Palpate scrotum for presence of testes, epididymis, vas deferens f. Transilluminate scrotum if swelling or mass palpated g. Inspect inguinal areas for hernia, first with client standing quietly, then during Valsalva's maneuver h. Palpate for direct inguinal hernia with client at rest and performing Valsalva's maneuver i. Palpate for indirect inguinal hernia with client at rest and performing Valsalva's maneuver
9B. Anus and rectum (male)	▪ Standing and bending over examining table (a, c, f, g) ▪ Standing and bending over examining table, performing Valsalva's maneuver (b, d, e)	▪ Inspection (a, b, g) ▪ Palpation (c, d, e, f)	B. Gloves worn throughout c. Lubricant	B. *Anus and rectum (male)* a. Inspect perianal skin for integrity, color, excoriation, rash, lesions, fissures, ulcers, hemorrhoids b. Inspect anal area for rectal prolapse, fissures, fistulas, inflammation, hemorrhoids, polyps with client performing Valsalva's maneuver c. Palpate anus, anal canal, sphincter tone, anorectal junction, rectal walls, coccyx with client at rest d. Palpate anal sphincter tone during Valsalva's maneuver e. Palpate for a descending rectal mass with client performing Valsalva's maneuver f. Palpate prostate gland: median sulcus, two lateral lobes

Table continued on following page

TABLE 10–1 ASSESSMENTS PERFORMED DURING REGIONAL EXAMINATIONS *Continued*

Assessment Area	Client Position or Activity*	Technique†	Equipment	What to Observe
			g. Hemoccult test; culture medium	g. Inspect gloved finger as it is withdrawn for stool and test stool for occult blood; obtain rectal culture if indicated ▪ **Female client is assisted to assume lithotomy or dorsal recumbent position**
10A. Genitalia (female)	▪ Lithotomy position if both external and internal genitalia examined (a, b, c, d, e, f, g, h, i, j, k, l, m, n) ▪ Dorsal recumbent if only external genitalia examined (a, b, c, d, e, f, g, h, i)	▪ Inspection (a, b, c, d, e, g, j, k) ▪ Palpation (f, h, i, l, m, n)	A. Gloves worn throughout	A. *Female genitalia* a. Inspect mons pubis for pubic hair distribution and texture; perineal skin for color, lesions, irritation, parasites b. Inspect labia majora for edema, symmetry c. Inspect labia for minora symmetry d. Inspect clitoris for color, presence of lesions e. Inspect introitus and hymen f. Palpate Bartholin's glands if inflamed or enlarged for size, tenderness g. Inspect urethral meatus for discharge, inflammation, swelling
			h. Culture medium; change gloves if discharge present	h. Palpate Skene's glands for discharge and obtain specimen for culture if present i. Assess integrity of pelvic floor muscles: strength, presence of cystocele or rectocele, discharge of urine
			j. Vaginal speculum; light source; wooden spatula; cotton-tipped applicator; glass slides; fixative; culture medium	j. Insert vaginal speculum and inspect cervix; adjust light as needed; note shape, position, color, lesions, discharge; obtain cervical specimens if indicated: cervical scraping, endocervical swab, vaginal pool scraping k. Inspect vagina as speculum is removed: color, rugae, mucosa
			l. Lubricant	l. Palpate vagina and cervix for nodules, masses; cervix position, mobility, consistency, tenderness m. Bimanually palpate pelvic structures (1) Uterus (anterior wall and fundus) for masses, tenderness, position (2) Ovary and adnexa for ovary size, masses, tenderness
			n. Change gloves if vaginal examination performed; lubricant	n. Rectovaginal palpation of uterus for masses, position, tenderness

10B. Anus and rectum (female)	▪ Lithotomy position if done at same time as internal genitalia examination (a, b, c, d, e, g) ▪ Dorsal recumbent if done after external genitalia examination (a, b, c, d, e, f, g) ▪ Performing Valsalva's maneuver (b, d, e)	▪ Inspection (a, b, g) ▪ Palpation (c, d, e, f)	B. Gloves worn throughout c. Lubricant g. Hemoccult; culture medium	B. *Anus and rectum (female)* a. Inspect perianal skin for integrity, color, excoriation, rash, lesions, fissures, ulcers, hemorrhoids b. Inspect anal area for rectal prolapse, fissures, fistulas, inflammation, hemorrhoids, polyps with client performing Valsalva's maneuver c. Palpate anus, anal canal, sphincter tone, anorectal junction, rectal walls, coccyx with client at rest d. Palpate anal sphincter tone during Valsalva's maneuver e. Palpate for a descending rectal mass with client performing Valsalva's maneuver f. Palpate cervix through anterior rectal wall for shape, position, mobility, tenderness g. Inspect gloved finger as it is withdrawn for stool and test stool for occult blood; obtain rectal culture if indicated
11. Examination complete	▪ Sitting			After removal of finger, assist client in cleaning the perineum and in sitting comfortably before leaving to allow client to dress

*Letters in parentheses after the client position or activity denote what the nurse observes.

†Letters in parentheses after technique denote the examination portions during which the nurse uses these skills to assist observations.

CN, cranial nerve; CVAs, costovertebral angles; DTRs, deep tendon reflexes; EOMs, extraocular movements; IBW, ideal body weight; LLQ, left lower quadrant; MAC, midarm circumference; MAMC, midarm muscle circumference; MSL, midsternal line; RLQ, right lower quadrant; RMCL, right midclavicular line; ROM, range of motion; TMJ, temporomandibular joint; TSF, triceps skinfold thickness.

BOX 10–1 Head-to-Toe Periodic Assessment Guide

1. *Vital signs:* Temperature, pulse, respirations, blood pressure
2. *Pain:* Location, type, quality, intensity
3. *Neurologic:* Orientation (person, place, time, situation), level of consciousness, gait, extremity color/movement/sensation (CMS), pupillary responses to light
4. *Pulmonary:* Respiratory pattern and effort; breath sounds; cough quality; sputum production, color, and quantity
5. *Cardiovascular:* Heart sounds and rhythm, pulses (radial, dorsalis pedis, and right and left posterior tibial), capillary refill, edema (location and amount), skin color and temperature
6. *Gastrointestinal:* Oral assessment, abdominal appearance, bowel sounds, bowel elimination pattern
7. *Genitourinary:* Bladder distention, voiding pattern
8. *Integument:* Skin integrity, wounds, dressings, drainage
9. *Psychosocial:* Sociability, affect, anxiety, attitude

Note: Perform additional assessments according to the client's specific health status and needs.

tional information. A complete assessment is necessary before data can be grouped and a cause determined. The initial physical assessment is the baseline for the client's functional ability. Physical assessment is also used as intervention (e.g., monitoring lung sounds) to evaluate changes in the client's physical condition and to determine whether expected outcomes have been achieved.

TECHNIQUES OF PHYSICAL EXAMINATION

Four primary techniques are used in physical assessment: *inspection, palpation, percussion,* and *auscultation.* These techniques enhance the data collected by observation of the ears, eyes, and senses of touch and smell and are used as indicated during the examination of each body region (Fig. 10–1).

■ INSPECTION

Inspection is the systematic, deliberate visual examination of the entire client or a region. Inspection yields information about size, shape, color, texture, symmetry, position, and deformities. It is the first technique of examination and begins at the outset of the client-nurse interaction. For example, inspect facial skin while collecting the history. Complete this inspection before progressing to the hands-on techniques of palpation, percussion, and auscultation.

Conduct inspection in a well-lighted setting. Uncover the body region or part sufficiently to permit complete visualization while draping the rest of the body to preserve modesty and comfort. During inspection, compare observations with the known parameters of normal findings in clients of similar age, sex, race, and ethnicity.

Inspection is enhanced with special instruments such as a penlight, oto-ophthalmoscope, and various specula (e.g., nasal and vaginal) that permit visual access to body cavities and orifices (Fig. 10–2). Other equipment includes tongue blades, a marking pen, a ruler, a tape measure, skinfold calipers, a goniometer, and eye charts.

■ PALPATION

Palpation, generally the second physical assessment technique, is the use of touch. During palpation, exert varying amounts of pressure to determine information about masses, pulsation, organ size, tenderness or pain, swelling, tissue firmness and elasticity, vibration, crepitation, temperature, texture variation, and moisture. In addition, use palpation to assess masses for position, size, shape, consistency, and mobility.

TECHNIQUE

Use the most sensitive parts of your hands and fingers to palpate specific characteristics. For example, the *fingertips* or *pads* are the most sensitive for fine touch and are used to palpate pulses, lymph nodes, and breast tissue. The *dorsum,* or back of the hand and fingers, is used to discriminate changes in skin temperature (see Fig. 48–3). Use the *palmar surface* of the hand over the metacarpophalangeal joints and the *ulnar aspect* to assess vibration of the lung with vocalization (tactile fremitus). Assess position, consistency, mobility, size, shape, and skin turgor by lightly grasping tissue between the *thumb* and *index finger.*

Facilitate palpation by positioning the client comfortably. This minimizes muscle tension and lessens the possibility of mistaking such tension for muscle rigidity. Improve client relaxation by having warm hands and short fingernails and by using a gentle approach. Encourage the client to take slow, deep breaths. Apply tactile pressure, and increase pressure gradually. Prolonged pressure decreases sensitivity in the palpating hand.

Before palpating, ask the client to indicate tender areas. Palpate tender areas last while you observe for nonverbal signs of discomfort or pain. Examine these areas, but note that this may result in client discomfort and reluctance to continue with examination.

LEVELS OF PALPATION

Palpation proceeds from light to deep (Fig. 10–3).

For *light* palpation, depress the underlying tissue approximately 1 to 2 cm (½ to ¾ inch). After light palpation, use deep palpation to determine the size and condition of underlying structures, such as abdominal organs.

For *deep* palpation, depress the underlying tissue approximately 4 to 5 cm (1½ to 2 inches), proceeding cautiously, because prolonged pressure can potentially injure internal organs. Use one or both hands (i.e., bimanual palpation).

For *bimanual* palpation, place one hand lightly on the client's skin (the sensing hand). Place the other hand (active hand) over the sensing hand to apply pressure. The sensing hand does not apply direct pressure and remains sensitive to underlying organ characteristics.

In one *variation* of bimanual palpation, one hand positions or stabilizes an organ while the other hand palpates (e.g., liver, spleen, kidney, or breast, or uterus and adnexae during gynecologic examination). Another variation involves trapping structures that move between the two hands, such as the kidney with respiration. (See also gynecologic assessment, Chapter 37.)

PRECAUTIONS

Take precautions during palpation. For example, palpate an artery so that blood flow is not obstructed. Do not

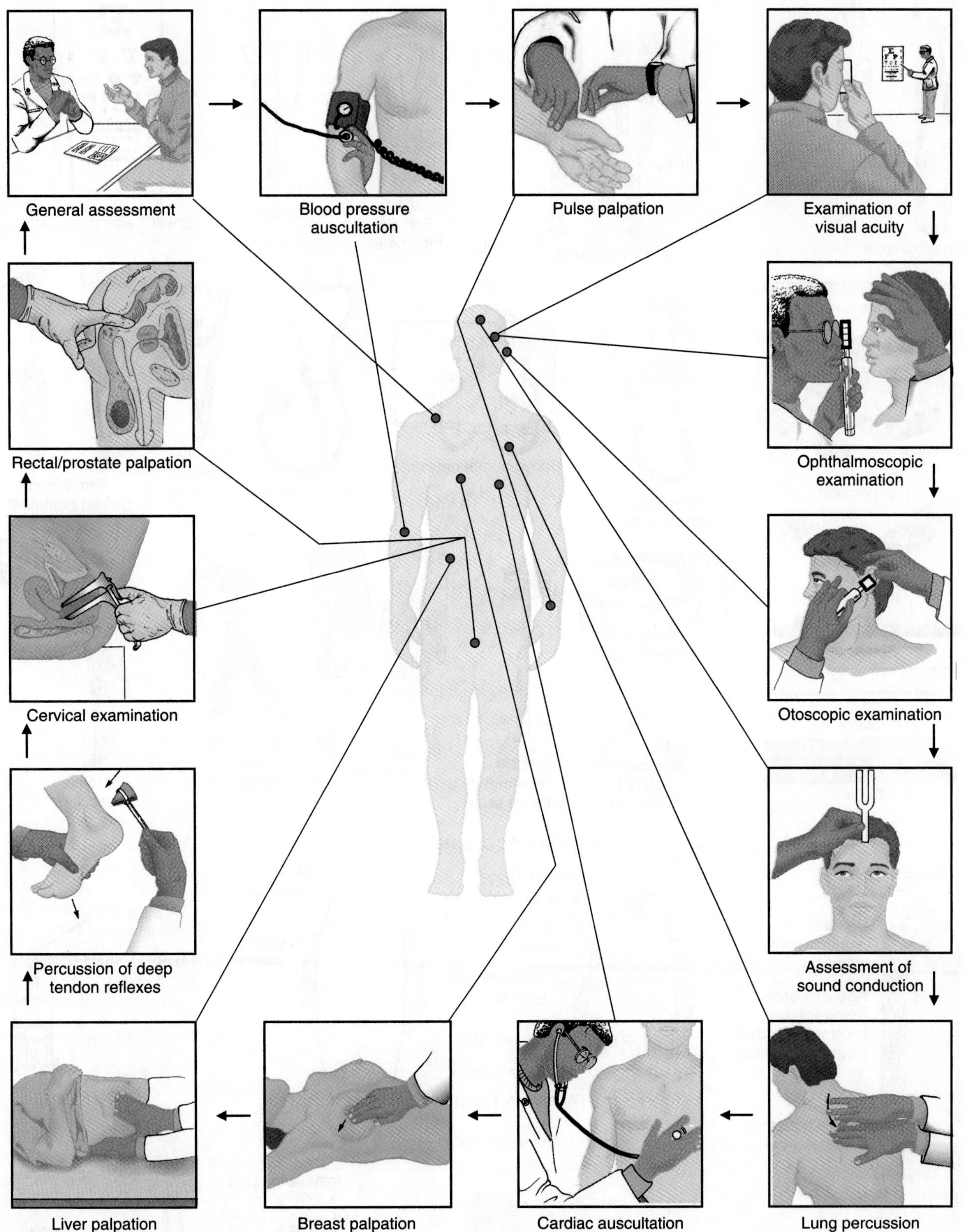

FIGURE 10–1 Common techniques of physical assessment used in a head-to-toe screening examination. The examiner wears gloves for the pelvic, rectal, and prostate examinations.

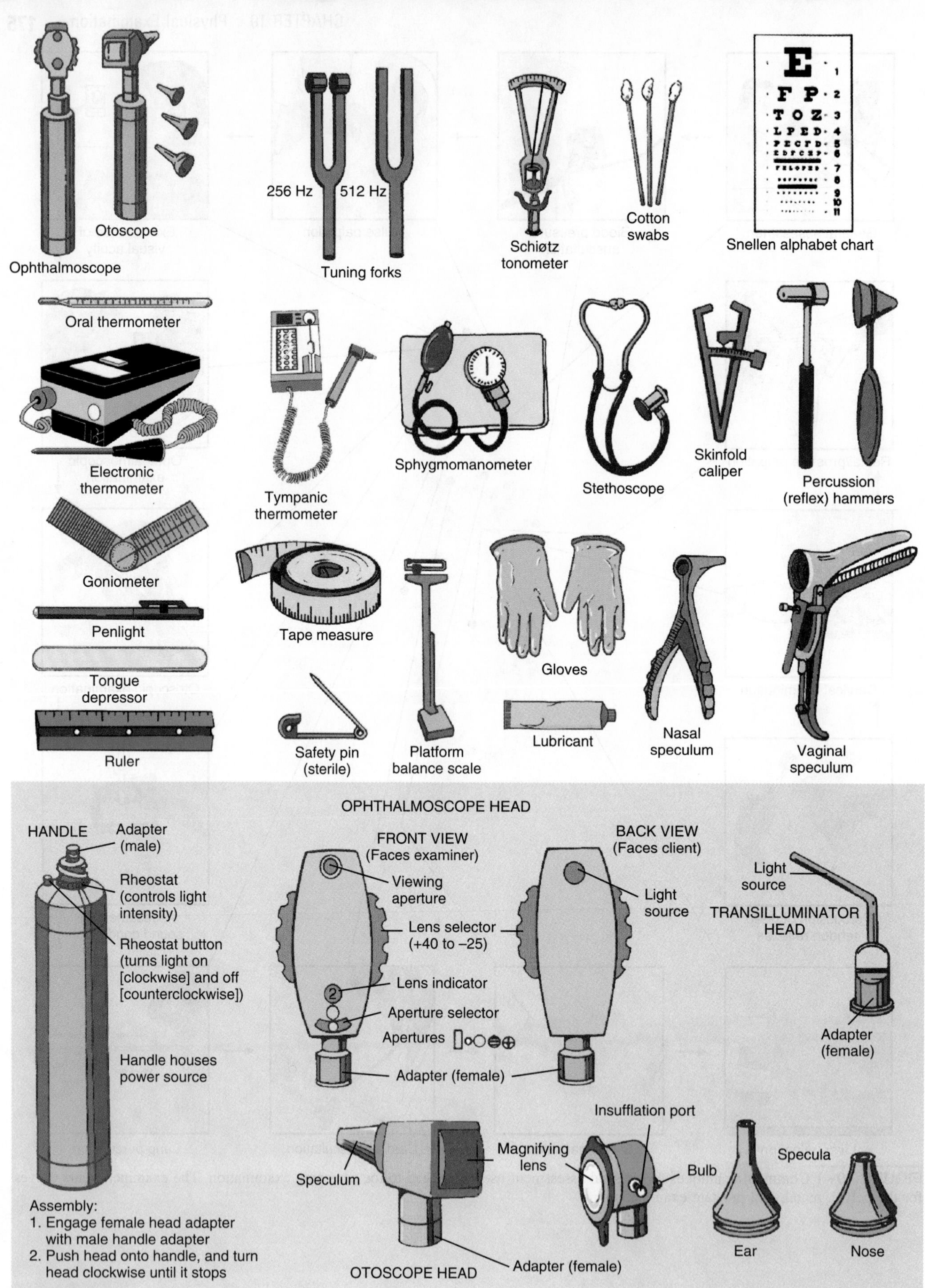

FIGURE 10–2 Instruments used in a physical examination.

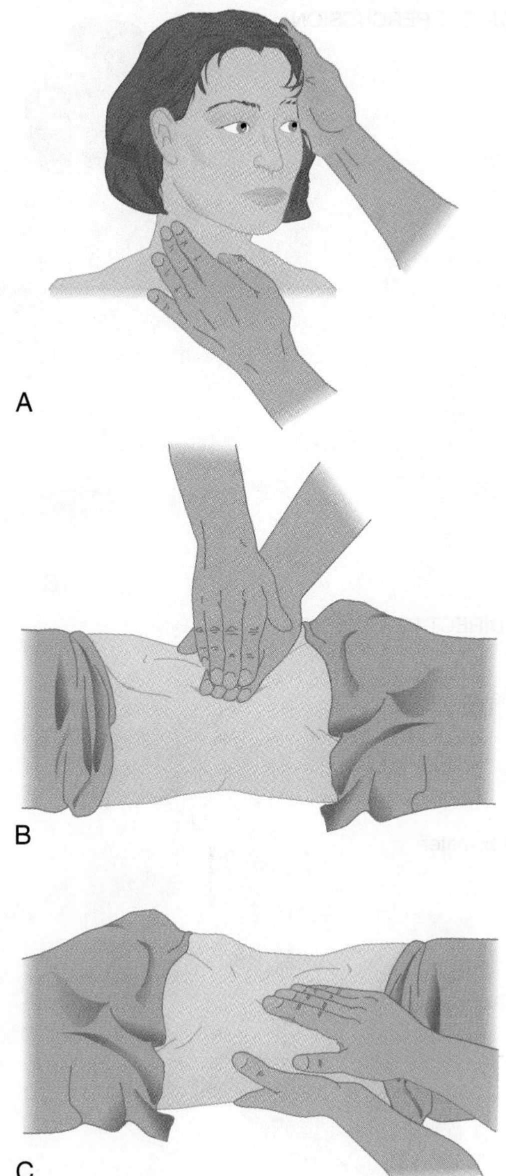

FIGURE 10–3 Palpation techniques. *A,* Light palpation employs the lightest possible pressure to assess structures under the surface of the skin, such as lymph nodes. *B,* Deep palpation is used to assess the condition of underlying organs, such as in the abdomen, using one or both hands. *C,* Bimanual palpation is used to trap and assess hard-to-palpate organs, such as the kidneys, or to stabilize an organ with one hand while the other hand palpates, as in liver palpation.

palpate the carotid arteries simultaneously because of the possibility of restricting blood flow to the brain.

■ PERCUSSION

Percussion is a technique to assess tissue density by sound produced from striking the skin. With this step, which is usually the third technique in physical assessment, 3 to 5 cm of tissue depth can be examined. Evaluate the sounds and tissue vibrations that result from percussion in relation to the underlying body structures. Percussion of body structures containing air, fluid, and solids produces various sounds, depending on their densities. Percussion helps to confirm suspected abnormal findings from palpation and auscultation, such as a mass or consolidation in the lungs.

There are two primary methods of percussion: direct and indirect (Fig. 10–4).

Direct Percussion

Direct percussion involves striking the body surface with either one or two fingers or the fist (i.e., *blunt* percussion). Use it primarily to assess the sinuses and over the thin chest wall of a small adult or a child. Perform *blunt* percussion to elicit tenderness from an underlying structure, such as the liver or kidney, not to produce a sound. Use of a reflex hammer is another example of blunt percussion.

Indirect Percussion

TECHNIQUE

Indirect percussion involves striking an intermediary finger or hand that is placed firmly on the body's surface. Dexterity and practice are required to attain proficiency in this technique. Place the distal phalanx of the middle finger (*pleximeter*) (see Fig. 10–4) firmly on the skin surface over soft tissue. Hyperextend the remaining fingers so that only the single digit is in contact with the skin. The *plexor* must strike the pleximeter sharply and quickly; do this by relaxing the wrist, keeping the forearm stationary, and striking with the fingertip (not the pad). Errors in technique diminish (damp) the sound produced. Common errors include (1) placing the pleximeter over bone, (2) resting the palm or other fingers of the nondominant hand on the body surface, (3) losing contact between pleximeter and skin surface, (4) delivering a weak blow with the plexor, and (5) striking the pleximeter at a point other than the distal joint.

For an accurate comparison of sounds, deliver the same amount of force with each blow. A light, quick blow produces the clearest sound. The blows may be repeated rapidly two or three times to assess the sound.

TYPES OF SOUNDS

Indirect percussion results in five characteristic sounds:

1. *Flatness,* a soft, high-pitched, short sound produced by very dense tissue such as muscle. Percussion of the thigh reproduces a characteristic flat sound.
2. *Dullness,* a soft to moderately loud sound of moderate pitch and duration. It is produced by less dense, mostly fluid-filled tissue, such as the liver and spleen, and has a thudding quality.
3. *Resonance,* a moderate to loud sound of low pitch and long duration. It results from the air-filled tissue of the normal lung and has a hollow quality.
4. *Hyperresonance,* a very loud, low-pitched sound lasting longer than resonance. It is produced by the overinflated, air-filled lungs of a person with pulmonary emphysema, or it may be heard in a child's lung because of a thin chest wall. Hyperresonance has a booming quality.
5. *Tympany,* a loud, high-pitched, moderately long sound with a drum-like, musical quality. It results from enclosed, air-containing structures, such as the

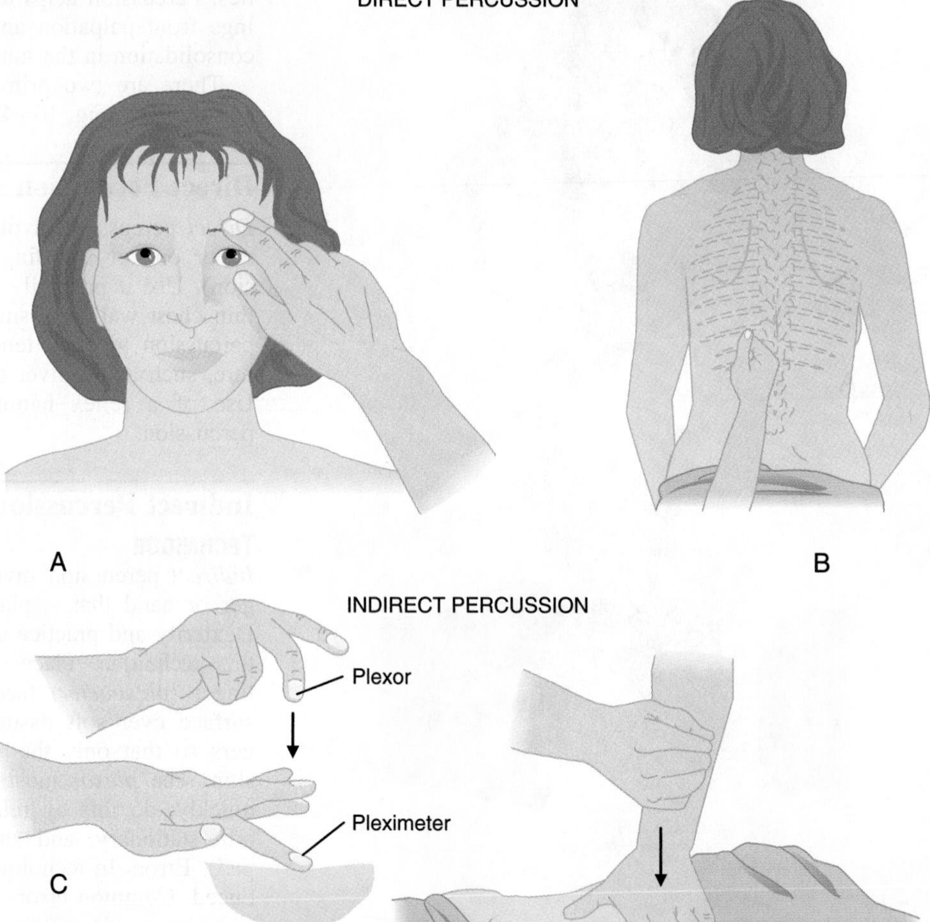

FIGURE 10–4 Techniques for the two primary types of percussion, direct and indirect. *A* and *B, Direct percussion. A,* Use one or two fingers to percuss directly against a body surface, such as over the sinuses, to elicit tenderness. *B,* Use the ulnar surface of your fist to gently strike the surface of the client's body over an underlying organ, such as at the costovertebral junction to assess for kidney tenderness. *C–E, Indirect percussion. C,* Place the distal phalanx of the middle finger of your nondominant hand (the pleximeter) on the client's skin over soft tissue. Bend the middle finger of your dominant hand at its distal interphalangeal joint to create a "hammer" (or plexor). *D,* Pivot the plexor down quickly in an arc to strike the pleximeter. *E,* Place the palm of your left hand over the area to be percussed. Gently strike the left hand with the ulnar surface of your right fist.

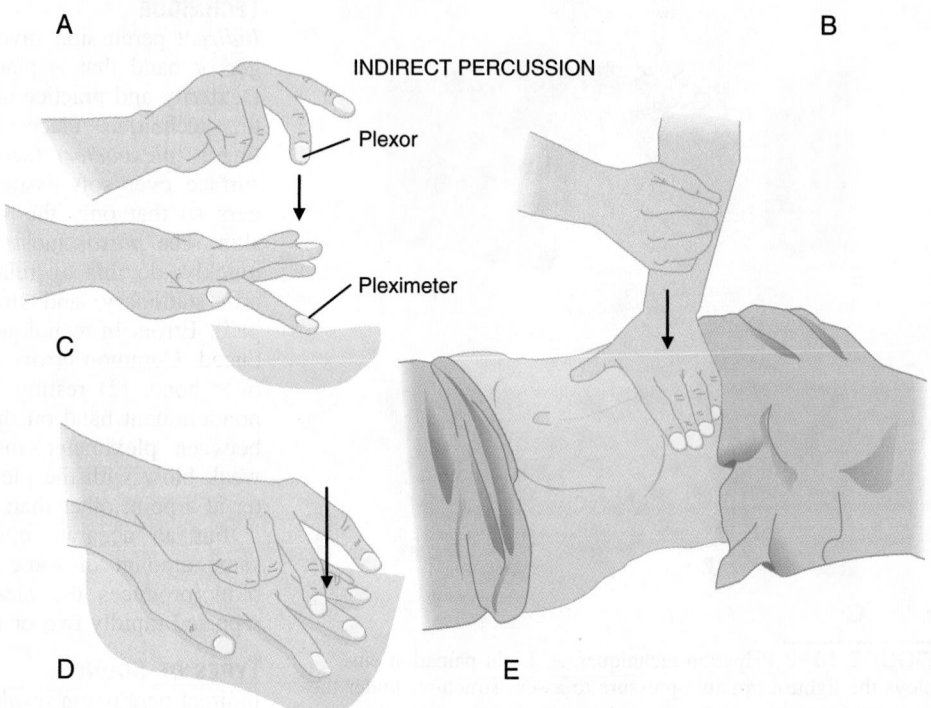

stomach (gastric bubble) and bowel. It can be reproduced by percussion over a puffed cheek.

■ AUSCULTATION

Auscultation is listening to internal body sounds to assess normal sounds and detect abnormal sounds. It is the final step in the physical examination. Use a stethoscope to enhance sounds. The sounds commonly assessed by auscultation include those produced by the heart, lungs, abdomen, and vascular system. Become proficient at auscultation by knowing which sounds are produced by each body structure and the location at which they are most readily heard. Recognizing abnormal sounds is easier once the normal sounds have been mastered.

Acute hearing ability, a reliable stethoscope, and knowing how to use the stethoscope are essential. Stethoscopes that amplify sounds are available for those who have difficulty hearing. The basic stethoscope (Fig. 10–5) has a chestpiece with a bell and diaphragm and single or double tubing connected to double ear tubes (i.e., binaurals). A tension bar between the binaurals holds the ear pieces firmly in place and reduces kinking of the tubing.

TECHNIQUE

Hold the *diaphragm* between the index and middle fingers firmly against the skin surface; use it to hear *high-pitched* sounds, such as lung sounds, heart sounds, and blood pressure. Place the *bell* lightly in contact with the skin to hear *low-pitched* sounds, such as murmurs and bruits. Place the *chestpiece* on the skin so that it is between bones and not over them, because bone does not transmit sound. Clothing and excessive chest hair interfere with sound transmission and may introduce artifacts. Snug-fitting *earpieces* occlude the external ear canal to

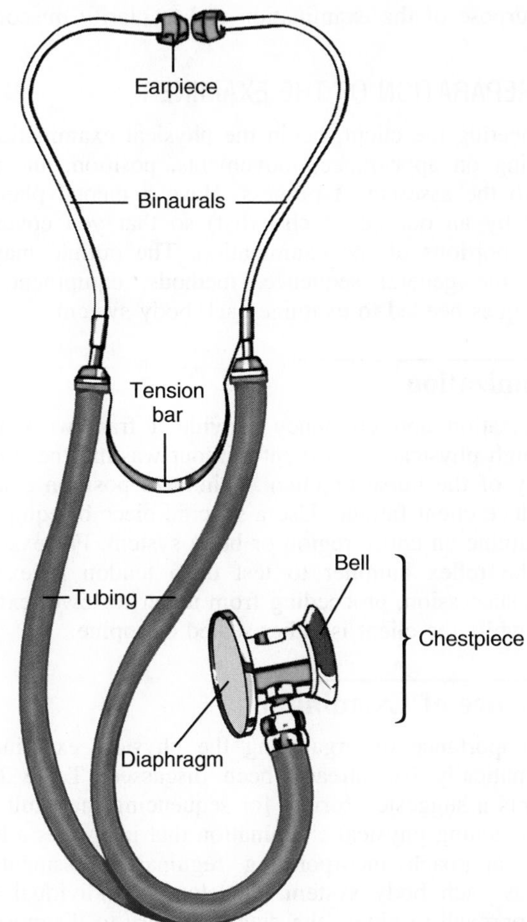

FIGURE 10–5 Components of a stethoscope. The *bell* is used to listen for low-pitched sounds, such as bruits. The *diaphragm* is used to assess high-pitched sounds, such as lung sounds and sounds heard in the assessment of blood pressure.

enhance sound transmission from the chestpiece. Keep the *tubing,* no longer than 12 to 15 inches for the best sound transmission, free of contact with all surfaces to prevent extraneous noises.

A quiet environment is essential for auscultation. Close the door, and draw the cubicle curtains. If necessary, turn down the television or radio volume after informing the client about the importance of decreasing external sounds. Concentrate on the part being auscultated to determine what is causing the sounds that are heard. Once you understand the source and characteristics of normal body sounds, it is easier to recognize abnormal sounds and their origin.

TYPES OF SOUNDS

There are four characteristic auscultation sounds:

1. *Pitch,* the number or frequency of sound wave cycles per second. By varying the frequency, one may alter the pitch. For example, a high frequency results in a high-pitched sound, whereas a low frequency produces a low-pitched sound. Heart murmurs can be either high-pitched or low-pitched, depending on the structural cause. Pitch is a diagnostic clue.
2. *Intensity,* the amplitude of a sound wave. The greater the amplitude, the louder the sound; the lower the amplitude, the softer the sound.
3. *Duration,* the length of time a sound endures; it may be long, medium, or short.
4. *Quality,* a description of a sound's character, such as "gurgling," "blowing," "whistling," or "snapping."

■ OLFACTION

Olfaction is the use of the sense of smell to detect body odors. The sense of smell helps detect abnormalities not readily recognized by other means, such as inspection. For example, the smell of ammonia in urine suggests a urinary tract infection; a strong, musty odor from a casted body part suggests a wound infection under the cast; a strong, fruity breath odor indicates enhanced production of ketone by-products. Consider olfactory findings with other assessments to determine the nature of the client's health problem.

GUIDELINES FOR PHYSICAL EXAMINATION

Physical examination proceeds in a logical, orderly fashion. The approach commonly used follows a head-to-toe organization so that findings are complete. This is not an absolute rule, and the nurse who is beginning to use physical assessment skills must practice and develop a system that is comfortable to use. Once a system is developed, use it routinely to avoid inadvertently omitting portions of the examination. For a successful physical assessment, you must know both the techniques and the parameters of normal findings. Consult the following guidelines to plan and conduct a physical examination.

■ PREPARATION OF THE ENVIRONMENT

To prepare for physical examination, ensure that the environment is private, quiet, comfortable (neither too warm or too cool), and well lighted. An examination may be conducted in a special room in an office or clinic; in a client's bedroom in the home; or in the area enclosed by drawn curtains around a client's bed in a hospital room. Eliminate or control extraneous noises to enhance concentration and to encourage the client to feel free to discuss problems or concerns.

■ PREPARATION OF EQUIPMENT

Assemble all necessary equipment before beginning. Arrange equipment in order of use to facilitate examination. Practice picking up equipment, holding it in the position of use, making adjustments, assembling, and disassembling. Check equipment for adequate functioning. It is embarrassing as well as time-consuming to hunt for a replacement bulb for the oto-ophthalmoscope or to discover that the battery needs recharging in the middle of an examination.

Equipment commonly used in physical examination is shown in Figure 10–2. Additional equipment may include cotton balls, gauze sponges, a watch with a second hand, supplies for specimens, and substances to test the senses of taste and smell.

■ PREPARATION OF THE CLIENT

Prepare the client physically and psychologically for the physical examination. Before beginning, instruct the client to empty the bladder. If a urine specimen is needed, instruct the client in the technique for collection at this time. An empty bladder facilitates examination of the abdomen, genitalia, and rectum.

Draping

Physical preparation also includes instructing the client to dress according to the type and extent of examination to be conducted. A gown and drapes provide privacy (Fig. 10–6).

Positioning

During the examination, assist the client in assuming different positions to facilitate assessment. Figure 10–6 illustrates common positions for examination and the areas of the body that are assessed. Consider any limitations of the client that may prevent optimal positioning, such as arthritis, back injury, joint deformities, or weakness. Alternative positions may have to be assumed to complete the examination. The client may find some positions uncomfortable or embarrassing. Keep the client in these positions only as long as required and drape to prevent unnecessary exposure. Table 10–1 shows a sequence that minimizes position changes during the examination.

Psychological Preparation

Approach the client professionally and calmly. An organized, efficient approach and a relaxed tone of voice and facial expression put the client at ease and promote trust. The client may be anxious about the examination and about the possibility of finding something abnormal. Some agencies require the presence of a second staff person of the same sex as the client for examination of breasts and genitalia when the examiner is of the opposite sex. Explain what will be done before proceeding so that the client knows what to expect and cooperates to the fullest extent possible.

Explain the examination in general terms, and then provide a detailed explanation as you examine each body system. Simple terms are less confusing and less threatening than complicated explanations. Encourage the client to verbalize discomfort as the examination proceeds.

Be sensitive to the client who is uncomfortable with exposing body parts to anyone other than those who are culturally sanctioned. For example, in some cultures, a woman is restricted from revealing most of her body to a male other than her husband or immediate family. In other cultures, women are restricted from touching men other than their immediate male relatives.

Watch facial expressions and body language throughout the examination. Nonverbal communication may convey anxiety, fear, or concern. For example, the client may pull the drape closely around the body, or muscles may be tight and tense. In extreme instances, the client may wish to stop the examination and you should comply. Never coerce the client to continue. Attempt to explain the purpose of the examination and to clarify misconceptions.

■ PREPARATION OF THE EXAMINER

On meeting the client, begin the physical examination by focusing on appearance, movements, position, and reaction to the assessment process. Have a mental plan (assisted by an outline or checklist) so that you cover the major portions of the examination. The outline may include the general sequence, methods, equipment, and techniques needed to examine each body system.

Organization

Organization and efficiency provide a framework for a thorough physical assessment without wasting the time or energy of the nurse or client. Minimize position changes to reduce client fatigue. Use a specific piece of equipment to examine an entire region or body system. For example, use the reflex hammer to test deep tendon reflexes in quick succession, proceeding from upper to lower extremities, while the client is either seated or supine.

Sequence of Examination

The importance of organizing the physical examination systematically has already been discussed. Table 10–1 presents a suggested format for sequencing the adult general screening physical examination that integrates a head-to-toe approach incorporating regional assessments as well as each body system. Develop an individual style and approach to obtain the data necessary to diagnose the client's responses to physical problems, yet be flexible enough to accommodate individual needs.

Knowledge of Structure and Function

Anatomic landmarks are reference points for locating areas to examine and for use in recording findings. Reference to an anatomy book is recommended for the beginning practitioner in physical examination. Descriptive terms and anatomic reference points are discussed further with the examination of the respective body systems.

ADULT GENERAL SCREENING PHYSICAL EXAMINATION

■ GENERAL SURVEY

The general survey begins the physical examination and includes observing the overall appearance and behavior, taking vital signs, and measuring height and weight.

General Appearance and Behavior

Evaluate observations regarding general appearance and behavior in relation to the client's background (i.e., culture, educational level, socioeconomic status, current health, and illness status). Signs of problems or abnormalities direct attention to specific body areas as the examination proceeds. For example, the client who is unkempt and has obvious body odor needs thorough examination of the hair, skin, and nails for assessment of hygiene.

POSITION	AREAS EXAMINED	RATIONALE	CONTRAINDICATIONS
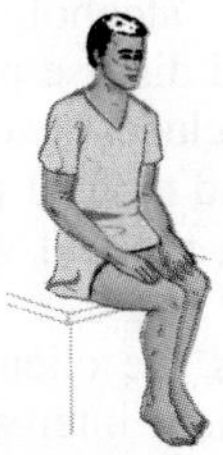 Sitting	Vital signs, head and neck, back, posterior and anterior thorax and lungs, breasts, axillae, heart, upper and lower extremities, reflexes	Sitting upright allows for full lung expansion and better visualization of upper body symmetry.	Elderly and weak clients may be unable to sit without support. An alternate position is supine with the head of the bed elevated.
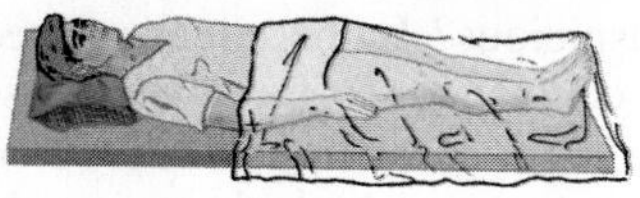 Supine	Vital signs, head and neck, anterior thorax and lungs, breasts, axillae, heart, abdomen, extremities, peripheral pulses	This is a relaxed position for most clients. It provides access to pulse sites and prevents contracture of abdominal muscles, especially if a small pillow is placed under the knees.	Clients with cardiovascular and respiratory problems may be unable to lie flat without becoming short of breath. An alternate position is to raise the head of the bed. Clients with lower back pain may be unable to lie flat without flexing the knees.
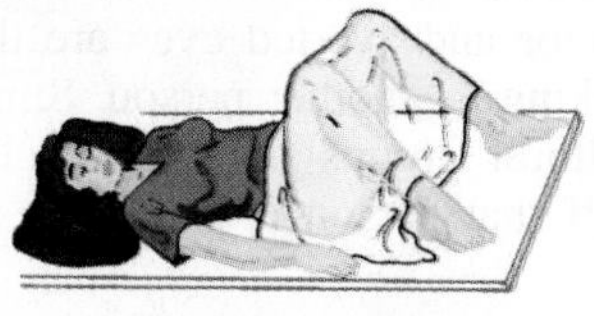 Dorsal recumbent	Abdomen and external genitalia	Flexed knees reduce tension on lower back and abdominal muscles and increase client comfort.	Same as for supine. The client should not raise the arms over the head or clasp the hands behind the head because this increases contraction of the abdominal muscles.
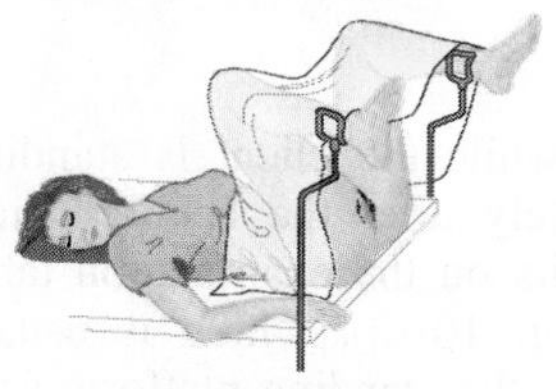 Lithotomy	Female genitalia, reproductive tract, and rectum	This position maximally exposes the genitalia and facilitates the insertion of a vaginal speculum.	This position is assumed immediately before it is needed because it is embarrassing and uncomfortable. The client is kept draped. Clients with arthritis or joint deformity may be unable to assume this position. Alternate positions are dorsal recumbent and Sims'.
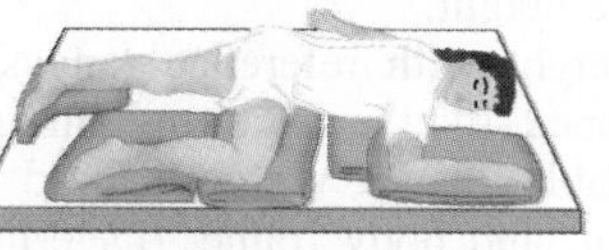 Sims' (posterior view)	Rectum, vagina	Flexion of the upper hip and knee improves exposure of the rectal area.	Clients with deformities of the hip or knee may be unable to assume this position. Elderly and obese clients may be uncomfortable.
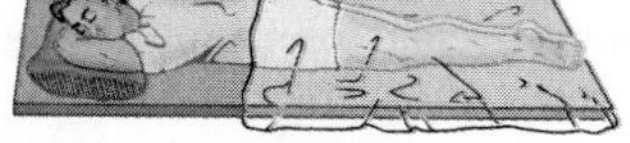 Prone	Posterior thorax, hip movement, popliteal pulses	This position is used to assess hip extension. Sometimes popliteal pulse palpation is facilitated in this position.	This position is not well tolerated by the elderly or clients with cardiovascular or respiratory problems.
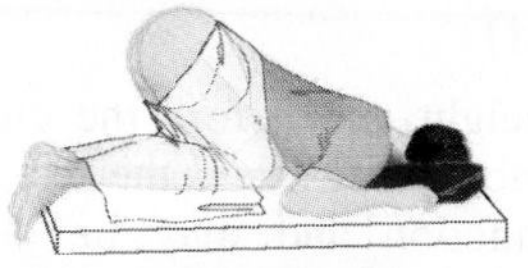 Knee-chest	Rectum, prostate	This position provides maximal exposure of the anal and rectal areas and facilitates insertion of instruments into the rectum.	Poorly tolerated by clients with cardiovascular or respiratory problems. Clients with difficulty flexing hips or knees may be unable to assume this position.
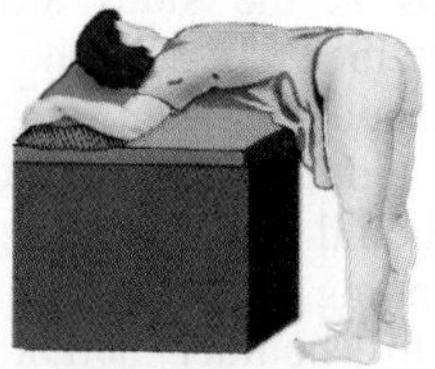 Standing, bent over examining table	Rectum, prostate	This is a more comfortable position than knee-chest and allows for palpation of the prostate gland.	This position is assumed immediately before it is needed because it is embarrassing. Clients with back problems may need assistance.

FIGURE 10–6 Draping and positioning the client to facilitate assessment and protect privacy.

General appearance and behavior assessments include the following.

APPARENT AGE, SEX, AND RACE. Because a client's appearance may or may not match chronologic age, direct assessment to each body system for potential problems related to aging. Other assessments are sex-specific and affect the type of procedures performed. Interpret data, and make recommendations for health teaching and further screening based on the client's health risk profile (see Chapter 9).

APPARENT STATE OF HEALTH. Assess whether the client looks "healthy," frail, or ill. Note deformities or absent body parts.

SIGNS OF DISTRESS OR DISCOMFORT. The client may display obvious signs of pain (wincing), anxiety (eyes darting around room), difficulty breathing (gasping), or other problems. Adapt the examination by including only the necessary assessments. The ideal situation is one in which the client is comfortable and in no acute distress.

BODY BUILD, HEIGHT, AND WEIGHT. Assess the client's body build for proportionate distribution of weight for height. Body build may be thin, obese, trim, or muscular, and it reflects the level of wellness, age, and lifestyle.

POSTURE. Posture may reflect mood or the presence of a physical problem. Observe the client's posture throughout the assessment process. Normal findings are an erect posture while the client is standing, with the shoulders and hips aligned over the knees and ankles. Sitting posture is with a straight back and slight rounding of the shoulders. Deviations from normal include stooping, slouching, and a curved posture. An ethnic variation may include an increased forward lumbar spine curvature (i.e., lordosis) accompanied by a forward tilt of the pelvis and abdominal protrusion.

GAIT. Observe gait as the client enters the examination room or ambulates. The gait should be smooth and coordinated as arms swing freely at the sides, in a direction opposite that of leg movement. The head and face should orient in the direction of movement. Shuffling steps and hesitancy are abnormal findings. Note devices to assist ambulation.

MOVEMENTS. Observe body movements as the examination proceeds. They are usually purposeful and controlled without tremors, tics, muscle fasciculations, signs of spasticity, or decreased muscle tone. Note immobile body parts.

DRESS. The client's manner of dress should be appropriate to the time of year, temperature, age, socioeconomic status, and current circumstances. A depressed client may wear clothing that is dull, unkempt, or mismatched. A client with a thyroid disorder may be dressed more warmly than others (hypothyroid) or may wear lightweight clothing despite a cool or cold environment (hyperthyroid).

HYGIENE AND GROOMING. Note the cleanliness of hair, nails, skin, and clothes. Does the client present a pleasant image? Consider what activity the client engaged in before the examination and whether it affects appearance.

BODY AND BREATH ODOR. Note these in relationship to activity level, such as strenuous exercise. Deficient hygiene may result in body and breath odors that are considered unpleasant or offensive. Odors include cigarette smoke, perfume, perspiration, alcohol, acetone, blood, decaying tissue, or an associated disease process.

MENTAL STATUS. Mental status includes level of consciousness, orientation, affect, speech, and thought processes. If abnormalities are noted in these areas, proceed with a full mental status assessment (see Chapters 9 and 67).

LEVEL OF COOPERATION. Assess the client's cooperation with the examination. Is the client interested, concerned, and willing to discuss information, or silent, withdrawn, hostile, angry, or suspicious? Is the client relaxed and able to engage in eye contact, or is the client tense and avoiding eye contact? Also consider cultural influences when assessing eye contact and body language. In some cultures, direct eye contact is perceived as being hostile or as dominant behavior and averted eyes are the norm when one person is talking to another person. Similarly, members of some cultural groups do not directly face a person while talking if that person is perceived as an authority figure.

Height and Weight

Measure height and weight while the client is standing. This often is done immediately after the health history interview, before the client sits on the examination table. Use a balance scale (see Fig. 10–2), which is usually very accurate. (Alternatives to the standing platform scale include bed and chair scales.) The standing scale has a telescoping ruler to measure height.

Compare height and weight with reference ranges in tables such as that developed by the Metropolitan Life Insurance Company (see Table 28–7). Weight should fall within range for sex, height, and body frame. (Determining body frame and ideal body weight is discussed in Chapter 28.) Adjust weight for clients who are missing all or part of an extremity (e.g., amputation) to account for the absent body mass using a chart or table for segmental weights.

Balance (Romberg's Test)

After measuring height and weight and before the client sits down, assess balance. Romberg's test and the test for pronation assess cerebellar function and may be done later, during the neurologic examination. Instruct the client to stand quietly with hands at the sides and feet together. Once equilibrium is attained, instruct the client to close the eyes. The client should be able to stand upright with minimal swaying and no loss of balance. Stand close by and intervene should the client begin to lose balance and fall. While standing, the client is asked to raise and extend the arms to shoulder height, then close the eyes. The client should be able to maintain the arms in extension with no downward drifting or pronation (pronation sign). (See other cerebellar assessments in Chapter 67.)

Once Romberg's test is completed, you may assess visual acuity if the eye chart is located at the correct distance from the examination table. Otherwise, test visual acuity when the eyes are examined. Instruct the cli-

MANAGEMENT AND DELEGATION

Measuring and Recording Vital Signs and Other Client Data

The measurement and recording of routine vital signs may be delegated to unlicensed assistive personnel. Delegate collection of data only when you are caring for a stable client. Emphasize the following when delegating these tasks to assistive personnel.

1. *Blood pressure.* Place the blood pressure cuff 1 to 2 inches above the antecubital fossa, with the cuff bladder overlying the brachial artery. For the leg, place the blood pressure cuff 1 to 2 inches above the popliteal space, with the cuff bladder overlying the popliteal artery. The size of the cuff should accommodate the circumference of the client's arm or leg. If the client has contraindications to blood pressure measurement on the arm or leg, inform the assistive personnel.
2. *Pulse.* Count the radial pulse for 30 seconds and multiply by 2. If the pulse seems irregular, count it for a full minute.
3. *Respiratory rate.* Count the rate of respiration without the client's being aware that it is being done. This prevents the client from consciously controlling the respiratory rate. If the respiratory rate is regular, count the rate for 30 seconds and multiply by 2. If the respiratory rate is irregular, count the rate for a full minute.
4. *Temperature.* Designate the route by which the temperature should be taken. Delay taking oral temperatures for 15 minutes if the patient has just eaten, smoked, or consumed a hot or cold liquid. If the client has dry mucous membranes and cannot hold the thermometer under the tongue with the lips closed, use the axillary, rectal, or tympanic route. If the client has contraindications to rectal temperature measurement, inform the assistive personnel.
5. *Oxygen saturation.* Designate the type of pulse oximeter sensor to be used. If a finger or toe sensor is used, you may need to remove nail polish or artificial nails. The skin at the sensor site should be clean, dry, and intact.

Findings that are immediately reportable to you, the R.N., should be described for the assistive personnel. These findings may include a blood pressure outside the range of 95/60 to 140/90 mm Hg or may be defined by the client's baseline blood pressure. For example, in a client with known controlled hypertension, a systolic reading of 140 to 170 mm Hg may be acceptable. Pulse rates less than 60 or greater than 110 beats per minute as well as any irregular pulse or inability to locate a pulse should be reported. Adult respiratory rates less than 10 or greater than 20 should be reported to you, as should any irregular respiratory rate. Temperatures outside the normal range of 97.6° to 99.4° F should be reported. An oxygen saturation level below 96% should be brought to your attention.

Even though you have delegated the collection of this information, you remain responsible for the review and interpretation of the data as well as for the full health assessment of the client. Assess cardiovascular and respiratory status daily and more frequently as the client's clinical condition warrants.

Verify the competence of the assistive personnel in performing each of these tasks during orientation and annually thereafter. Include the proper recording of the vital signs and any other client data delegated for collection.

Donna W. Markey, MSN, RN, ACNP-CS, *Clinician IV, Surgical Services, University of Virginia Health System, Charlottesville, Virginia*

ent to sit on the edge of the examination table for assessment of vital signs (see Table 10–1).

Vital Signs

Once the client is comfortably seated, measure vital signs after a brief stabilization period. Measure body temperature and blood pressure during the general survey. You may measure specific vital signs during examination of the upper extremities or heart (peripheral pulse) and thorax (respirations). A nursing fundamentals textbook would describe the techniques of vital signs measurement and equipment selection. (See Management and Delegation.)

TEMPERATURE. Oral body temperature ranges from 96.8° to 99.5° F (36° to 37.5° C), with an average of 98.6° F (37° C). Body temperatures above the normal range are *hyperthermic;* those below are *hypothermic.*

PULSE. Resting pulse rate ranges from 60 to 100 beats per minute (BPM). A rate above 100 BPM is *tachycardia;* a rate below 60 BPM is *bradycardia.* Note general characteristics of the pulse, such as rhythm (regular or irregular), amplitude (weak or bounding), and pattern. Rhythm is regular, with pulsations occurring at equal intervals, and are of similar amplitude. A slight variation in rhythm occurs with respiration and is normal. Describe *pulse amplitude* (Box 10–2) and any irregular patterns. See also Chapter 51.

RESPIRATION. Respirations range from 12 to 20 per minute. They have a regular, smooth pattern and are of consistent depth. They are quiet and effortless, without abnormal sounds such as wheezing. Respiratory depth reflects *tidal volume* (i.e., the amount of air taken in with each breath). Use the rise and fall of the chest to estimate whether respirations are shallow, moderate, or deep. Note

BOX 10–2 Pulse Amplitude

The following terms are commonly used to describe and record pulse amplitude:

Absent. The pulse is indiscernible to palpation.
Weak, thready. The pulse is difficult to palpate and easily obliterated by slight pressure.
Normal. The pulse is easily palpable and can be obliterated only with strong pressure.
Bounding. The pulse is easily palpable, forceful, and not easily obliterated by pressure.

RESPIRATORY PATTERN	DESCRIPTION
A. Eupnea (Normal) 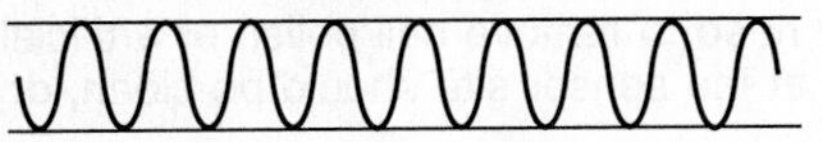	Rate = 12 to 20 breaths per minute Depth = Average tidal volume 350-500 mL (adults) Rhythm = Regular, occasional sigh breath deeper than baseline tidal volume I:E Ratio* = 1:2
B. Hyperventilation 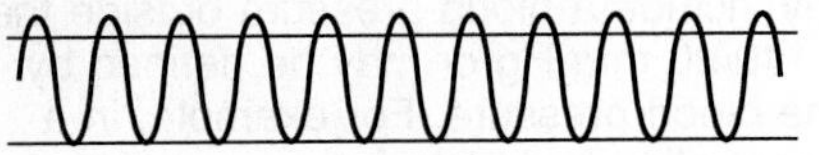	Rate = May increase Depth = Deep—large tidal volumes Rhythm = Usually regular I:E Ratio = Approaches 1:1 Comment = May be associated with CO_2 loss (respiratory alkalosis)
C. Tachypnea 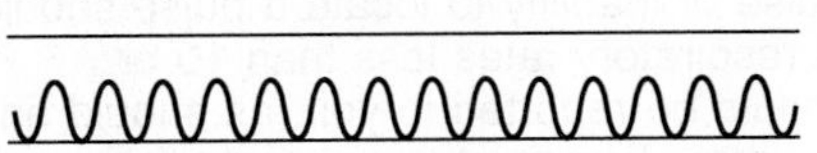	Rate = Rapid Depth = Shallow—small tidal volume with each breath Rhythm = Regular I:E Ratio = Approaches 1:1 Comment = May be associated with CO_2 retention (respiratory acidosis)
D. Bradypnea 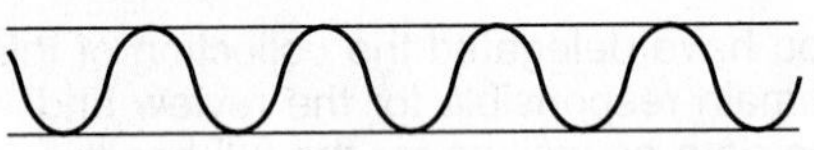	Rate = Slow Depth = Tidal volumes vary depending on the cause Rhythm = Regular I:E Ratio = 1:2
E. Apnea 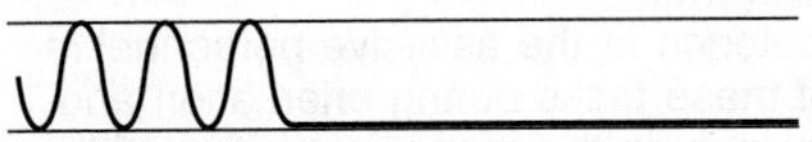	Complete absence of breathing Comment = May be temporary
F. Cheyne-Stokes 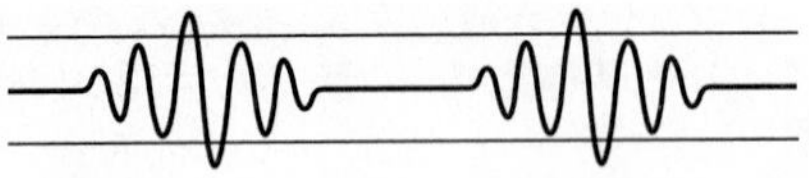	Rate = Variable Depth = Depth of each breath varies in a cyclical pattern: Shallow before and after apnea, deep with hyperventilation Rhythm = Apneic periods alternate with hyperventilation Comment = Regular-irregular—crescendo-decrescendo pattern
G. Biot's 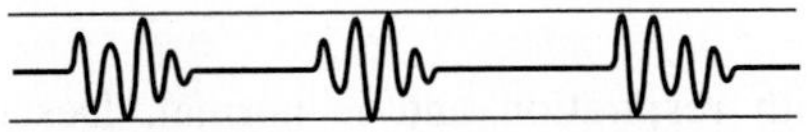	Rate = Variable Depth = Depth variable—predominantly shallow Rhythm = Unpredictable irregularity Comment = Long periods of apnea alternate with breathing periods
H. Kussmaul's 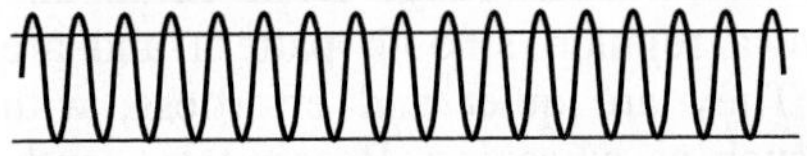	Rate = Rapid Depth = Deep without pauses Rhythm = Regular Comment = Associated with diabetic ketoacidosis
I. Apneustic 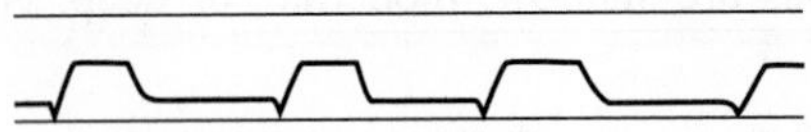	Rate = Rapid Depth = Shallow Comment = Prolonged inspiration followed by short, ineffective expiration

* Inspiration to Expiration (I:E) ratio

FIGURE 10–7 Assessing respiratory patterns.

the respiratory pattern, and record its characteristics (Fig. 10–7). See also Chapters 59 and 67.

Blood Pressure. Blood pressure varies greatly among individuals. Normal systolic pressure ranges from 100 to 140 mm Hg, and diastolic pressure ranges from 60 to 90 mm Hg. It is more accurate to evaluate consecutive blood pressure readings over time rather than make an isolated measurement for determining blood pressure abnormalities. *Hypotension* is a systolic pressure below 95 mm Hg or diastolic pressure below 60 mm Hg. *Hyper-*

tension is a systolic pressure above 140 mm Hg or diastolic pressure above 90 mm Hg. Note the difference between the systolic and diastolic pressure readings (i.e., *pulse pressure*). Report a difference of more than 40 mm Hg, which is abnormal. A slightly elevated blood pressure may be considered a normal finding in older people.

Assess blood pressure by using the bell of the stethoscope initially. Assess both arms, and compare the two readings. A pressure difference of 5 to 10 mm Hg between the two arms is insignificant. Report larger differences. Assess for an *auscultatory gap* the first time a client's blood pressure is measured. This phenomenon occurs as a period of silence between two levels of systolic pressures that may range as much as 40 mm Hg. See also Chapter 51.

Skin Color

Assess overall skin color during the health history interview, but conduct a more thorough assessment during the remainder of the examination. Observe the face and visible skin surfaces for color tones that should be congruent with the client's stated race. Abnormal findings include pallor (paleness), flushing or a ruddy complexion, cyanosis (blue cast), jaundice (yellow cast), and areas of irregular pigmentation. See also Chapter 48.

PROCESSING THE DATA

COMPARISON OF FINDINGS

Use the client as a "control," or self-standard, for comparison during the physical examination. Compare findings from one side of the body with those from the opposite side (*bilateral comparison*). Even though both sides of the human body are not exactly identical (i.e., symmetrical), similarities in structure and appearance are individualized and unique. Comparisons are useful and valid for findings such as a joint deformity or an extremity swelling. If a part of a limb is missing (such as from an amputation), a bilateral comparison is impractical; compare findings with a known standard.

COMPARISON WITH KNOWN STANDARDS

Compare physical examination findings with known parameters of "normal" for age, sex, and racial background. For example, decreased skin elasticity and loss of subcutaneous adipose tissue are expected findings for an older client but not for a 30-year-old.

SUSPECTED PROBLEM AREAS

Examine known or suspected problem areas carefully. Include areas identified during the health history interview as well as those predicted to be at risk based on the client's history and reactions to the physical examination. For example, thoroughly assess mouth and neck structures of the client who reports difficulty swallowing (see Chapters 28 and 42). To allay client anxiety, explain why a particular portion of the examination is more thorough.

HEALTH TEACHING

The physical examination process lends itself to health teaching and opportunities for providing accurate information and correcting misconceptions. Examples include reinforcing techniques for self-examination and having the client perform a return demonstration.

TERMINATING THE HEALTH ASSESSMENT

After completing the examination, close the client's gown or allow the client to dress (assist if needed) and to assume a comfortable position. Summarize findings in understandable terms. If a serious abnormality is found, consult with the client's health care provider or refer the client to another health care professional for further assessment after explaining the general nature of the abnormality and the need for further examination.

Discard disposable, used equipment and supplies according to agency protocol. Clean or restock nondisposable equipment for future use.

RECORDING THE FINDINGS

Document physical examination findings using accurate, descriptive terms. Avoid vague, subjective terminology, such as "normal," "slight," "moderate," "healthy," or "poor," because they are easily misinterpreted. Strive to be objective, concise, clear, and thorough in the recording. However, it is better to err on the side of verbosity than to describe a significant finding vaguely or inadequately. A detailed recording is helpful as a baseline for comparison with future physical findings.

During the examination, briefly note abnormal assessment findings for later retrieval and detailed documentation. This avoids interrupting the flow of the examination to record detailed observations. After the examination, combine normal and abnormal findings in the final document.

HEALTH ASSESSMENT, NURSING DIAGNOSIS, AND NURSING PROCESS

After the collection of baseline data, which include both the health history and the physical examination results, summarize the client's health problems. Assess the client's areas of strength and health risk profile. Formalize and prioritize nursing diagnoses. Reexamine and validate the tentative diagnoses formulated after the health history interview in light of the physical examination findings.

Determine which health problems are nursing diagnoses and which are collaborative problems. Make referrals when indicated so that the client receives continuity of care and either resolution or effective management of the health problems.

CONCLUSIONS

The physical examination is the second portion of physical assessment, following the health history, in which objective data are collected through inspection, palpation, percussion, and auscultation. Once all data are collected, compare the findings with known standards and make appropriate referrals, intervene, or provide health teaching.

BIBLIOGRAPHY

1. Alfaro-LeFevre, R. (1995). *Critical thinking in nursing: A practical approach.* Philadelphia: W. B. Saunders.
2. Andrews, M. M., & Boyle, J. S. (Eds.) (1995). *Transcultural concepts in nursing care* (2nd ed.). Philadelphia: J. B. Lippincott.
3. Bates, B. (1995). *A guide to physical examination* (6th ed.). Philadelphia: J. B. Lippincott.
4. Braunwald, E. (1997). *Heart disease* (5th ed.). Philadelphia: W. B. Saunders.
5. ——— (1997). *Expert 10-minute physical examinations.* St. Louis: Mosby–Year Book.
6. Geissler, E. M. (1994). *Pocket guide to cultural assessment.* St. Louis: Mosby–Year Book.
7. Giger, J. N., & Davidhizar, R. E. (Eds.). (1995). *Transcultural nursing: Assessment and intervention* (2nd ed.). St. Louis: Mosby–Year Book.
8. Grimes, J., & Burns, E. (1996). *Health assessment in nursing practice* (4th ed.). Boston: Little, Brown.
9. Hogstel, M. O. (1996). *Practical guide to health assessment through the lifespan* (2nd ed.). Philadelphia: F. A. Davis.
10. Hurst, J. W., et al. (Eds.). (1990). *The heart* (7th ed.). New York: McGraw-Hill.
11. Iyer, P. W., Taptich, B. J., & Bernocchi-Losey, D. (1995). *Nursing process and nursing diagnosis* (3rd ed.). Philadelphia: W. B. Saunders.
12. Jacobson, N., Gift, A., & Jacox, A. (1990). Advances in physical assessment. *Nursing Clinics of North America, 25*(4), 743–833.
13. Jarvis, C. (2000). *Physical examination and health assessment* (3rd ed.). Philadelphia: W. B. Saunders.
14. Joint National Committee on Detection, Evaluation, and Treatment of High Blood Pressure. (1993). The fifth report of the Joint National Committee on detection, evaluation, and treatment of high blood pressure. *Archives of Internal Medicine, 153,* 154–188.
15. Leasia, M. S., & Monahan, F. D. (1997). *A practical guide to health assessment.* Philadelphia: W. B. Saunders.
16. Morton, P. (1994). *Quick reference to cultural assessment.* St. Louis: Mosby–Year Book.
17. Purnell, L., & Paulanka, B. (1998). *Transcultural health care: A culturally competent approach.* Philadelphia: F. A. Davis.
18. Seidel, H. M., et al. (1995). *Mosby's guide to physical examination* (3rd ed.). St. Louis: Mosby–Year Book.
19. Society of Actuaries and Association of Life Insurance Medical Directors of America. (1983). *Metropolitan Life Insurance Co. build study.* New York: Author.
20. Solomon, E. P. (1992). *Introduction to human anatomy and physiology.* Philadelphia: W. B. Saunders.
21. Strub, R. L., & Black, F. W. (1993). *The mental status examination in neurology* (3rd ed.). Philadelphia: F. A. Davis.
22. Swartz, M. H. (1997). *Textbook of physical diagnosis* (3rd ed.). Philadelphia: W. B. Saunders.
23. Thomas, C. L. (1998). *Taber's cyclopedic medical dictionary* (18th ed.). Philadelphia: F. A. Davis.
24. Weber, J. (1997). *Nurses' handbook of health assessment* (3rd ed.). Philadelphia: J. B. Lippincott.

CHAPTER 11

Diagnostic Assessment

Annabelle M. Keene

Diagnostic assessment refers to the various tests used to detect disease and to evaluate the nature and extent of a disease, if present. During diagnostic assessment, you may have many responsibilities, ranging from preparing a client to interpreting test results to determining whether a client requires immediate medical intervention. This chapter discusses the general nursing management of clients undergoing a variety of common laboratory, imaging, endoscopic, and cytologic diagnostic tests. Specific information about individual tests is also found throughout the book.

GENERAL NURSING MANAGEMENT

■ ASSESSMENT

If your client is scheduled for a diagnostic test, you will need to assess his or her ability to participate in the test. Limitations in the client's physical condition, sensory ability, psychological condition, and functional status can all affect the successful performance of a diagnostic test. For instance, disorders of the cardiovascular or respiratory system may severely limit the client's tolerance for required position changes. Sensory limitations (such as impaired hearing or speech) or mental impairment may interfere with the client's ability to understand or carry out his or her role in accomplishing the test.

Assessment of the client's self-care ability, mobility, and nutritional status can also help you determine the client's ability to participate in diagnostic testing. Clients with impaired mobility, restricted self-care ability, or nutritional deficits may require interventions to help prepare for testing; they may need extra assistance during testing as well. If clients are agitated or unable to lie still, for instance, they may need a sedative before undergoing a lengthy imaging test. Many imaging tests require the client to lie motionless for 30 minutes or more. Similarly, for many tests, the client must have fasted for 6 to 8 hours; if the client does not follow the directions for fasting time, the test will probably need to be postponed.

■ NURSING INTERVENTIONS

Independent nursing interventions commonly needed by clients undergoing diagnostic tests include (1) preparation of the client (based in part on your assessment of the client's ability to participate), (2) collection of data, (3) collection and transport of clients and specimens, (4) monitoring of clients during diagnostic testing, and (5) supportive teaching. Naturally, it is crucial that you obtain adequate specimens (Box 11–1).

Interdependent nursing interventions commonly include (1) transcribing orders, (2) consulting with laboratory and radiology technicians, (3) sedating the client, and (4) interpreting test results to determine whether immediate action is required. Consider the underlying pathophysiologic status, current medical treatment, and laboratory result when assessing the need for immediate attention from a physician. For example, if a client's serum potassium level rises from 2.5 to 2.8 mEq/L, he has no dysrhythmias, and 80 mEq of potassium is being infused in 1 liter (L) of intravenous (IV) fluid, you may notify the physician about the potassium level during usual rounds. In contrast, if the potassium level drops from 2.5 to 2.0 mEq/L and the client has a flattened T wave and ventricular dysrhythmia, immediately notify the physician about the change in the client's status.

SPECIFICITY AND SENSITIVITY OF DIAGNOSTIC TESTS

It would be ideal if all diagnostic (or screening) tests were 100% accurate. They are not. False-positive and false-negative results occur. The concepts used to evaluate the effectiveness of a test are its specificity and its sensitivity.

Specificity is the ability of a test to correctly identify a person who is disease free. It equals the number of *true negative* results divided by the sum of true negative and false-positive results. A *false-positive* result indicates that a client has the disease or disorder being tested for when, in fact, he does not have that disease or disorder.

Sensitivity is the ability of a test to correctly identify a disease. Sensitivity equals the number of true-positive results divided by the sum of true-positive and false-negative results. A *false-negative* result indicates that a client does not have the disease or disorder being tested for when, in fact, he does have that disease or disorder.

No test is 100% specific and 100% sensitive because of (1) limitations inherent in the test and (2) various factors that can affect all tests. For example, the antinu-

This chapter incorporates material written by Cynthia Hromek from the fifth edition.

BOX 11–1 Obtaining Adequate Specimens

- Ensure confidentiality and privacy for the client.
- If a culture is required, obtain it prior to initiating antibiotics, if possible.
- Avoid contamination of the specimen with secretions or excretions from uninvolved areas.
- Collect the correct amount of fluid or tissue for the sample.
- Use the proper instruments and collection tubes or bottles.
- To avoid contamination, do not open the collection bottle until you have the specimen.
- Label all containers accurately. Include the name of the client, source of the specimen, and date and time collected.
- Deliver the specimen to the laboratory immediately or keep it at the recommended temperature.

clear antibody (ANA) test is highly sensitive for detecting systemic lupus erythematosus but is not specific because clients with rheumatoid arthritis may also have positive ANA results. The closer a test is to 100% on both counts, the more reliable its results.

MEASUREMENTS USED TO REPORT LABORATORY TEST RESULTS

REFERENCE VALUES

The term *reference value* (rather than "normal value") is used for reporting laboratory studies because different laboratories may produce different values. In addition, some tests (e.g., serum calcium level) have more than one accepted reference value.

Laboratory results may be influenced by several factors. The time of day, temperature, altitude, stress felt by the client, medications taken, and underlying disorder may all affect the test. When analyzing a client's laboratory test results, consider all of these influencing variables.

INTERNATIONAL SYSTEM OF UNITS

A comprehensive modern form of the metric system is the *International System of Units,* commonly called the *SI system* (from its French name, Système Internationale d' Unités). The SI system provides a common international language for units of measurement. The meter and kilogram are used for length and weight. Moles are used to express amounts per volume. A *mole* is the quantity of a substance in grams that is equal to its molecular weight.

Most Americans are more familiar with mass concentration units (such as milligrams) than with moles, and the United States has been slow to adopt the SI system. The rationale for changing to SI units is that biologic components react in vivo on a molar basis. Thus, moles offer a better understanding of the relative amounts of components of body fluids and of biologic processes and their interrelationships.

LABORATORY DIAGNOSTIC TESTING

Many diagnostic tests in all practice settings are performed by nurses. Some can even be delegated to assistive personnel, as discussed in the Management and Delegation feature. No matter who performs a test, its accurate outcome depends on collecting the proper specimen, in the proper manner, in the proper container, at the proper time. Anyone performing a test should:

1. Carefully follow the instructions on diagnostic test kits, and maintain the integrity of all test materials.
2. When necessary, protect the test materials from light and moisture.
3. Always check the expiration dates.

In addition to performing tests, you may be responsible for the ongoing care of portable testing equipment. Equipment requires routine maintenance, quality assur-

MANAGEMENT AND DELEGATION

Performing Specimen Collection and Testing

Collection of the following specimens may be delegated to unlicensed assistive personnel:

Specimen	Procedure
Sputum	Culture and sensitivity testing
Urine	Routine urinalysis Urine electrolyte measurements 24-hour urine collection Culture and sensitivity testing for clean-catch and indwelling catheter specimens
Stool	Culture and sensitivity testing

Testing of the following specimens may be delegated to unlicensed assistive personnel:

Specimen	Procedure
Blood	Bedside blood glucose monitoring
Urine	Test-strip (dipstick) analysis Specific gravity determination
Stool	Occult blood test

Delegation of the tasks listed above requires that you give instructions on the following topics:

- Type of specimen to be collected and collection container in which it should be placed
- Client label with the appropriate information required by your laboratory
- Specimen request form to accompany the specimen
- Proper method of recording blood glucose, urine test-strip analysis, specific gravity, and stool occult blood results

After initial orientation, the assistive personnel should demonstrate competence in the performance of these tasks. Describe any findings that assistive personnel should report immediately to you, such as blood glucose levels outside the range of 70 to 180 mg/dl, urine that looks cloudy or seems to contain sediment, and obvious evidence of blood in urine, sputum, or stool. Inability to obtain the specimen should also be reported immediately.

Note: Delegating the collection of blood specimens may be permitted in some institutions, in states whose practice acts permit this. This very specialized skill requires venipuncture training and competence beyond the scope of most unlicensed assistive personnel.

Donna W. Markey, MSN, RN, ACNP-CS, *Clinician IV, Surgical Services, University of Virginia Health System, Charlottesville, Virginia*

ance checks, and recalibration, just as in a full-scale diagnostic laboratory. Standardized specimens should be analyzed on a routine schedule according to the agency's quality control standards and those mandated by the American Society of Pathologists and the Joint Commission on the Accreditation of Healthcare Organizations (JCAHO). The reliability of test results depends on the accuracy of procedures and equipment and the integrity of test materials.

■ MICROBIOLOGY STUDIES

Many microbiology studies can be used to identify infection-causing organisms—such as bacteria, viruses, fungi, and protozoa—and to guide treatment. Several tests can be performed to identify a specific microorganism:

1. A *smear* is a specimen that has been spread across a glass slide. It is examined under a microscope, usually after being stained.
2. A *stain* is the application of dye or a combination of dyes to help identify microorganisms. Gram's stain is a quick, commonly used method to identify general strains of bacteria by their color. Gram-positive organisms stain purple-black. Gram-negative organisms stain pink. Knowing whether a bacterium is gram-positive or gram-negative can assist in choosing an initial treatment until the specific bacterium is identified by culture.
3. A *culture* is the placement of microorganisms on culture plates to facilitate their growth. Afterward, the microorganisms can be isolated and identified. The culture process may take a few hours to several weeks, depending on the organism.

Sensitivity studies determine the type of antibiotic that will impede the growth of the organism. Small discs saturated with antibiotics are placed on the culture plate. In time, the culture is examined again. If the antibiotic stopped the growth of the microorganism, the microorganism is said to be *sensitive* to the antibiotic. If the antibiotic does not halt the growth of the microorganism, the organism is said to be *resistant* to it. Sensitivity reports typically list several antibiotics to which an organism is susceptible. The physician then chooses an appropriate treatment on the basis of cost, adverse drug effects, and so on.

Culture and sensitivity tests are commonly performed together to both identify an infecting microorganism and to determine appropriate drugs for treating it. On a physician's order, you may see these tests abbreviated as *C & S.*

Specimen collection and handling are common procedures that can raise the risk of disease transmission if they are done incorrectly. To help prevent disease transmission, wash your hands thoroughly and frequently, and wear appropriate personal protective equipment—especially gloves—whenever you could be exposed to a client's body fluids. Properly label specimens, and place in plastic containers to reduce the risk of transmission to other personnel.

Blood Cultures

Normally, blood is sterile. If bacteria enter the bloodstream, they can cause severe infections. *Bacteremia* is the term used to describe bacteria in the bloodstream. *Septicemia* is systemic disease caused by bacteria and their toxins in the blood. Blood cultures are commonly obtained for clients who have unexplained fever, a high risk of sepsis, or the appearance of being in septic shock.

To collect blood for culture, thoroughly clean the client's skin at the selected puncture site. Draw samples at specific intervals (30 minutes apart, for example) or draw a second specimen from the client's other arm. Blood samples may be examined for anaerobic or aerobic microorganisms. Ideally, blood culture specimens should be collected before antibiotic therapy begins or other blood samples are collected (if ordered at the same time).

If the client has already received an antibiotic, certain enzymes can be added to the growth medium by laboratory personnel to eliminate the activity of the antibiotic. Note on the laboratory request slip that the client is receiving an antibiotic. Once the specimen is obtained, the client should receive any prescribed antibiotics and antipyretics.

Wound Cultures

Healing is delayed in wounds that are infected. Therefore, material from inside the wound may be obtained for culture to detect and identify microorganisms in the wound. Ideally, the specimen should be collected before the client receives an antibiotic. Aseptic technique is used. Additional precautions, such as the wearing of mask, gown, and gloves, may be needed to collect specimens from draining wounds.

Culturettes (sterile, cotton-tipped applicators in special containers) are commonly used for collecting specimens for a wound culture; they should be used as follows:

1. Place the cotton tip deep into the wound without touching the surrounding skin.
2. Swab the wound where the purulent drainage is most profuse.
3. Return the applicator to the holder, and break the bottom of it to release the culture medium.

A syringe and needle can also be used to aspirate infectious material from the wound.

Note on the request slip any antibiotics the client is taking and the specific site from which the specimen was obtained. After collecting the specimen, administer any antibiotics prescribed.

Urine Cultures

Normally, urine is sterile. However, urinary tract infection (UTI) is a common disorder. Women are susceptible to UTIs because of their short urethras. In addition, nosocomial UTI is a common sequela (consequence) of indwelling catheterization. The culture test used most often to detect bacteria in the urine uses a clean-catch (or midstream) specimen. The goal of clean-catch collection is to minimize contamination of the specimen by organisms on the perineal skin. To obtain the specimen correctly, the client (1) cleans the perineum, (2) starts voiding, (3) stops voiding, (4) resumes voiding, then (5) catches the specimen in a sterile container.

As an alternative, you may need to collect a specimen

from an indwelling catheter. Urine standing in the collection bag undergoes chemical changes, may be contaminated with bacteria, and does not reflect the client's current urinary status; as a result, it should never be used as a urine specimen. Instead, obtain a specimen from the catheter or drainage tubing. Avoid opening the drainage system to air, which might introduce microorganisms. Most urinary drainage systems have a self-sealing, rubber-covered specimen collection port built into the top of the drainage tubing. Clean this area, and then aspirate the urine specimen with a sterile needle and syringe. You may need to clamp the tubing below the port for 15 to 20 minutes to allow enough urine to accumulate.

If there is no collection port and the catheter is not rubber-like silicone (Silastic), use a small 25-gauge needle and syringe to aspirate urine from the catheter itself. Using aseptic technique, insert the needle into the catheter distal to the sleeve leading to the balloon, slant the needle toward the drainage tubing, and make sure it does not enter the balloon lumen. Puncture the catheter at an angle to allow it to reseal after you withdraw the needle. This procedure cannot be performed with a Silastic catheter because it will not reseal after being punctured.

Sometimes you may need to perform a straight catheterization to obtain a urine specimen for culture. To do so, use a straight catheter of the smallest size. Insert it into the bladder under aseptic conditions, allowing urine to flow directly from the end of the catheter into the sterile specimen container. Some agencies provide special kits that include a catheter attached to a test tube. Only rarely will you obtain urine specimens by catheterization because the catheter may introduce organisms into the client's urinary tract.

■ BLOOD STUDIES

Types of blood collection methods are venipuncture, microcapillary collection, serial port sampling, and arterial blood sampling. Check your facility's laboratory procedure manual to review collection procedures, available equipment, biohazard disposal procedures, and standard precautions.

Venipuncture

The procedure for venipuncture is described in Box 11–2. Table 11–1 shows the various tubes, called Vacutainer tubes, used for drawing blood. The tubes are vacuums and fill automatically with blood. Before drawing a specimen, make sure that (1) you have the proper tube and (2) specimens from one type of tube are not mixed with those from another tube. Remember, when cells are damaged, potassium leaks and platelets migrate. A concern is that multiple venipuncture attempts or contamination with EDTA (ethylenediaminetetraacetic acid, an anticoagulant) may distort serum potassium test results. Therefore, draw specimens for potassium measurements early and consider that abnormal serum potassium readings may result from multiple punctures or contamination.

BOX 11–2 Procedure for Venipuncture

1. Check physician's request to verify test and time requested, client's name, and client's identification number.
2. Select materials needed: alcohol swabs, cotton or gauze swab, adhesive bandage, gloves, labels, needle, sharps container, tube holders, tourniquets, and Vacutainer tube or syringe (if using a butterfly needle).
3. Label Vacutainer tube with client's name and identification number, collection date and time, specimen source, and test.
4. Greet client, check test requested and client's name and identification number, and determine client's preparation for test. Wash your hands.
5. Place the client's arm in a position comfortable for the client and convenient for you. Support it on a firm surface. The client should be sitting or lying down.
6. Assemble the needle, needle holder, Vacutainer tube, alcohol swabs, cotton or gauze swab, and bandage. Take care not to engage the Vacutainer tube. Place any additional Vacutainer tubes in a convenient location. Use a 20- or 21-gauge, 1- to 1½-inch needle for antecubital veins.
7. Apply the tourniquet tightly enough to distend the veins but not so tightly that it cuts off circulation. Tell the client to open and close his fist several times and to keep it closed while you locate a vein. If it is difficult to locate a vein, wrap the arm in a warm compress to promote venous distention. Instead, you may use a blood pressure cuff to distend the veins; obtain a pressure between the client's systolic and diastolic readings. Remember that a tourniquet or blood pressure cuff should never remain on the client's arm for more than 1 to 2 minutes.
8. Choose the site. Try to locate the median cubital vein. Other acceptable veins are the cephalic and basilic veins. If hand veins are selected, use a 23- or 25-gauge needle.
9. Put on gloves. Clean the venipuncture site with 70% isopropyl alcohol by making outward concentric circles. Allow the site to air-dry or wipe with sterile gauze.
10. Anchor the vein by stretching the skin below the site with your thumb. Reassure the client that any discomfort will be brief. Insert the needle bevel-up into the vein, and engage the Vacutainer tube. The needle should be at about a 15-degree angle to the client's arm and directly in line with the vein. If multiple samples are needed, remove the tube as soon as the blood flow stops and insert the next tube into the needle holder. Once good blood flow is established and before the final tube is filled, release the tourniquet.
11. Remove the last Vacutainer tube from the needle holder. Remove the needle with a swift motion, and quickly apply clean cotton or gauze over the puncture site. Apply pressure, or ask the client to apply pressure to the puncture site. Properly dispose of the needle in the sharps container. (Do not lay down or recap the needle.) Immediately label the specimen. Remove your gloves, and wash your hands. Record the client's name, the test performed, disposition of the specimen, and any condition not meeting specimen collection criteria.

Specimens for vacuum collection tubes without additives should be drawn first to prevent contamination by samples for additive-containing vacuum tubes.

A suggested sequence for blood specimen collection to prevent specimen contamination is as follows:

1. Microbiology culture specimen tubes.
2. Tubes without additives (red, speckled, or gold top).
3. Citrate-containing tubes (blue top).
4. Heparin-containing tubes (green or dark blue top).
5. EDTA-containing tubes (lavender top).
6. Oxalate/fluoride-containing tubes (gray top).

When you need to obtain blood from a superficial hand vein, use a butterfly needle (Fig. 11–1). Insert the needle and, after blood flashback is noted in the tubing, use a syringe or Vacutainer tube to withdraw blood from the vein.

Microcapillary Collection

Microcapillary blood collections may be used for a variety of purposes, including peripheral testing in clinics, for very young or very old clients, and for clients with skin disorders. The procedure for microcapillary collection is similar to that for venipuncture. The site of the skin puncture is usually the finger tip. (An ear lobe may be used for clients with edema.) No tourniquet is used.

Use the following procedure for microcapillary blood collection:

1. Hold the finger firmly.
2. Clean the area with povidone-iodine or 70% alcohol.
3. Using a microlance instead of a needle and Vacutainer tube, make a puncture perpendicular to the fingerprint lines and off the center of the finger.
4. Wipe away the first drop of blood with sterile gauze because it contains plasma, which may affect the accuracy of results.
5. Place the hand in a dependent position, and allow the next drops to flow without squeezing. A microtube or pipette may be used to collect the blood specimen.
6. After blood collection, you or the client must maintain pressure on the puncture site until the bleeding has stopped.

Serial Port Sampling

Serial port sampling refers to collection of blood specimens from an indwelling venous catheter. The advantage of this method is that it reduces client discomfort caused by multiple venipunctures. The preparation for serial port sampling is similar to that for venipuncture:

1. Stop the intravenous fluid flow.
2. After opening the stopcock or choosing the lumen, use a 10-ml syringe to aspirate 10 ml of blood from the indwelling catheter.
3. Discard the first sample.
4. Use another 10-ml syringe (or 20-ml syringe, depending on the number of tests needed) to aspirate the blood specimen needed for the study.
5. Flush the indwelling line with saline and heparin according to agency protocol.
6. Return the stopcock to the original position and adjust the intravenous fluid rate as needed.

Arterial Blood Sampling

A sample of blood is collected from an artery for blood gas analysis and, rarely, for other studies. The technique of arterial blood sampling is discussed in Chapter 59. Because this method raises a risk of bleeding and nerve injury, arterial blood sampling is performed only by staff with special training. Blood gas analysis is discussed in Chapter 14.

■ URINE STUDIES

Urinalysis

Urinalysis is one of the oldest and most common laboratory tests. It is noninvasive, the specimen is easily obtained, results are available quickly, and it is economical. It yields a large amount of information about possible disorders of the kidney and lower urinary tract as well as about systemic disorders that alter the composition of urine. Normal urinalysis results can be used to exclude a number of alternative diagnoses (Table 11–2).

Data from a urinalysis include color, specific gravity, pH, and the presence of protein, red blood cells (RBCs), white blood cells (WBCs), bacteria, leukocyte esterase, bilirubin, urobilirubin, glucose, ketones, casts, and crystals. Normal urine does not contain protein, bilirubin, urobilirubin, glucose, ketones, bacteria, or leukocyte esterase. A few RBCs, WBCs, casts, and crystals are normal (see Chapter 32).

A random-specimen urinalysis can be collected at any time. In general, an early-morning specimen gives more definitive results because the urine is concentrated and is not influenced by diet. Generally, no specific client preparation is needed. The urine should be collected in a clean container. This type of specimen cannot be used for culture and sensitivity tests because neither the container nor the collection technique is sterile.

12- or 24-Hour Urine Collection

A timed collection of urine allows for quantitative analysis of specific substances and, because the specimen is collected over time, is more accurate than a random one-time specimen. A 12- or 24-hour specimen is usually collected in one large container. The procedure may require a chemical preservative in the container and refrigeration during the collection process. If appropriate refrigeration is not available, the specimen container may be placed in ice or in insulated ice packs; in this case, make sure the cooling agent is replaced frequently to maintain the specimen at the necessary temperature. Furthermore, if the client has an indwelling catheter, the bag can be placed on ice to collect a 24-hour specimen.

TABLE 11–1 TUBES USED FOR VENIPUNCTURE

Stopper Color	Principal Anticoagulant/Additive	Mode of Action	Commonly Used for
Red	None Clot activator and gel separator	None Enhances clot formation	Cell/blood typing Serum blood group antibody testing Alkaline phosphatase Amylase Blood urea nitrogen (BUN) Creatine phosphokinase (CPK) Calcium Cholesterol
Speckled			Compatibility testing Drug monitoring Glucose High-density lipoprotein (HDL) Human immunodeficiency virus (HIV) Iron profile Low-density lipoprotein (LDL)
Gold (Hemoguard)			Liver enzymes Potassium Protein Rapid plasma reagin (RPR) Sodium Triglycerides
Lavender	Ethylenediaminetetraacetic acid (EDTA)	Binds calcium	Complete blood count (CBC) Erythrocyte sedimentation rate (ESR) Hemoglobin electrophoresis Platelet count Reticulocyte count Sickle cell screen White blood cell differential

When specimen collection begins, the client voids (or the urine collection bag is emptied) and this specimen is discarded. All urine voided over the next 12 or 24 hours, as appropriate, is placed in the container. After 12 or 24 hours from the time of the first voiding, instruct the client to void again (or empty the urine collection bag) and add this urine to the specimen. One of the major requirements during this collection process is careful communication among all persons involved. If any single urine specimen is inadvertently discarded, the entire procedure must begin anew. The client should also be instructed to moderately limit the amount of fluids consumed and to avoid alcohol. Other specific instructions may be needed, such as avoiding certain foods or medications.

DIAGNOSTIC IMAGING

Imaging refers to representations produced by radiography (x-rays), nuclear magnetic resonance, tomograms, ultrasound, radioisotopes, and so forth. Methods range from simple x-ray studies to very complex and expensive imaging using magnetic fields and radiowaves. Review the protocol to be followed at your facility, especially the guidelines for preparation and follow-up care. You may need to consult with the imaging (radiology) department to obtain written guidelines for preparation and postimaging care, or to coordinate studies. For example, barium studies may make visualization for other abdominal tests impossible for up to 2 days.

Explain the procedure to the client and family and answer their questions. Many procedures may take up to an hour (follow-up x-rays are sometimes taken 30 minutes after an injection). Suggest that the client void before the procedure, unless the bladder must be full for the procedure.

■ X-RAY STUDIES

PROCEDURE

Radiography is the most widely used diagnostic procedure for the study of soft tissues and bones. A radiograph, commonly called an "x-ray," is an image of a negative on photographic film made by exposing the film to x-rays that have passed through the body. The energy of the x-rays is adjusted by varying the voltage in the x-ray tube. Because each part of the body absorbs some of the x-rays, variable amounts of exposure are needed for optimal results, depending on the body part being examined.

TABLE 11–1 TUBES USED FOR VENIPUNCTURE *Continued*

Stopper Color	Principal Anticoagulant/Additive	Mode of Action	Commonly Used for
Blue 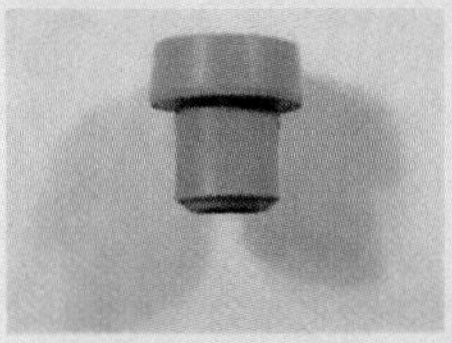	Sodium citrate	Binds calcium	Activated partial thromboplastin time (aPTT) Individual coagulation factor studies Fibrin degradation products (FDPs) Fibrinogen Prothrombin time (PT)
Green 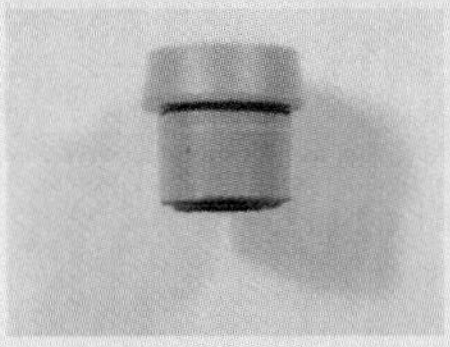	Heparin	Inactivates thrombin and thromboplastin	Ammonia Chromosome screening Lupus erythematosus cell, preparation HLA typing
Gray 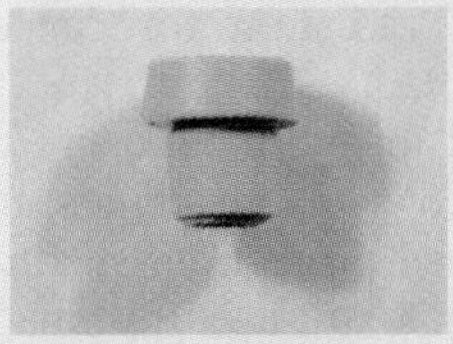	Potassium oxalate/sodium fluoride	Binds calcium Inhibits glycolysis	Glucose
Dark or royal blue 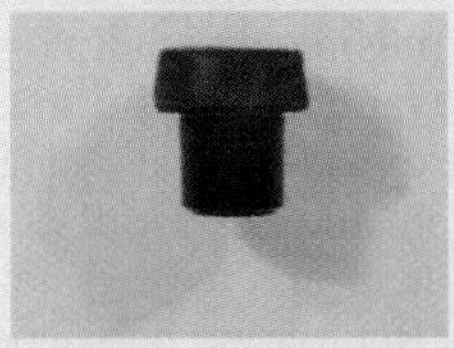	Heparin	Inactivates thrombin and thromboplastin	Trace metals (e.g., lead)

From Flynn, J. C., Jr. (1994). *Procedures in phlebotomy.* Philadelphia: W. B. Saunders.

Tissue is called *radiopaque* when transmission of x-rays is partially blocked, such as by bone. Bone appears white on x-ray film. Tissues are said to be *radiolucent* when they allow x-rays to penetrate. Lung is translucent and therefore appears dark on x-ray film. The images on x-ray films are two-dimensional, so that multiple views are often needed, such as anteroposterior (AP, front to back), posteroanterior (PA, back to front), lateral (LAT, from the side), or oblique (OBL, at an angle). It is impor-

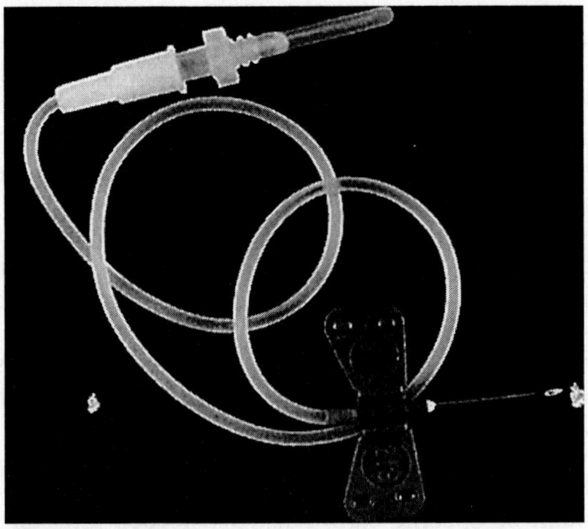

FIGURE 11–1 A butterfly needle used for venipuncture. (From Flynn, J. C., Jr. [1994]. *Procedures in phlebotomy.* Philadelphia: W. B. Saunders.)

TABLE 11–2 NORMAL FINDINGS IN A ROUTINE URINALYSIS

Component	Normal Values
Color	Pale yellow to deep amber
Opacity	Clear
Specific gravity	1.002–1.035
Osmolality	275–295 mOsm/L
pH	4.5–8.0
Glucose	Negative
Ketones	Negative
Protein	Negative
Bilirubin	Negative
Red blood cells	None to 3
White blood cells	None to 4
Bacteria	None
Casts	None
Crystals	None

tant to note the position of the view of an x-ray for proper interpretation; this information is usually recorded by the x-ray technician.

X-ray examinations are important to (1) establish the presence of a mobility or structural problem, (2) follow its progress, and (3) evaluate the effectiveness of treatment. Features shown by an x-ray can help diagnose a suspected problem; for example:

- A radiopaque (rather than radiolucent) area in the lung, which may mean pulmonary edema, pneumonia, or a tumor (Fig. 11–2)
- Alterations in normal contour or density of bones, as in fractures or osteoporosis (Fig. 11–3)
- Changes in fat lines around soft tissues (e.g., with tumor or inflammation present, fat tissue is replaced by soft tissues)
- Enlargement in shadows produced by organs (e.g., an enlarged heart shadow possibly meaning an enlarged heart from heart failure or athletic activity)

Two potential risks from repeated exposure to radiation are genetic and somatic. The *genetic risk* involves changes in the chromosomes. If a developing (first-trimester) fetus is exposed to radiation, the chromosomes can mutate and the baby can be born with deformities; the eggs and sperm can be damaged by radiation, which may lead to deformities in future offspring.

Somatic changes occur in body tissues that receive excessive or repeated doses of radiation. The risks from radiation exposure are cumulative and therefore are potentially more dangerous to health care personnel than to clients. Side effects of the use of radiation for cancer treatment are discussed in Chapter 19.

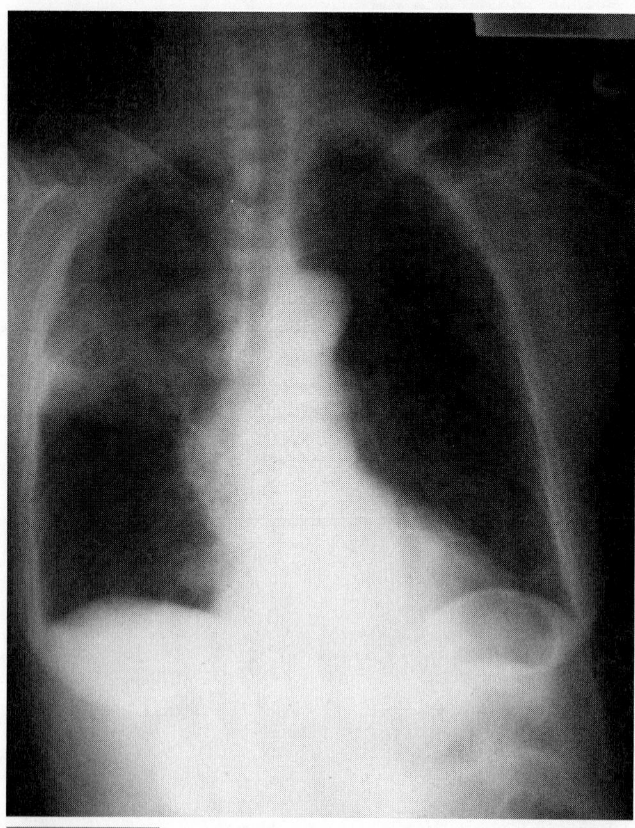

FIGURE 11–2 A chest x-ray showing right middle lobe pneumonia. The consolidation of lung tissue makes the area appear radiopaque.

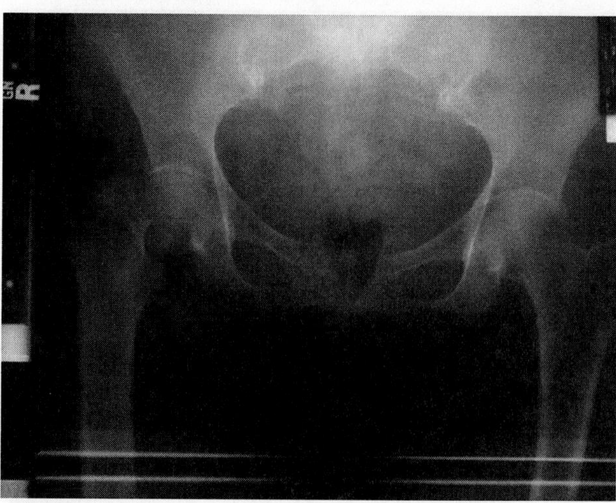

FIGURE 11–3 An x-ray showing a hip fracture.

Several safety measures are used to avoid exposure to x-rays. The walls in rooms in which x-ray machines are located are lined with lead. Lead-lined protection, such as aprons, eyeglasses, and thyroid shields, are used by imaging personnel. Maintaining adequate distance is also important, and x-ray rooms have a protective divider for the technician. When x-rays are taken outside the radiology department, less protection may be available. If you must remain with a client during x-ray exposure, wear a lead apron. Other personnel should step outside the room during the exposure. Clients are given lead aprons to shield their reproductive organs (gonads). Radiology personnel also wear a film badge to monitor accidental exposure.

Preprocedure Care

Before the x-ray procedure, ask the client to remove any radiopaque objects (such as jewelry, belts, or metal buttons) and to wear a gown. Additional preparation depends on the type of study. The client may be asked to move into various positions, if possible, so that x-ray films can be taken from the most useful angles.

Because various positions may be difficult or painful and x-ray tables are hard, the client may need analgesia and other pain-relieving interventions before and after the x-ray study. Nursing care for the client having diagnostic imaging studies focuses on client preparation and follow-up care.

Occasionally, you may be asked to monitor an unstable client during an imaging procedure. You will need an oximetry monitor, sphygmomanometer to measure blood pressure, stethoscope, extra intravenous fluids, and an emergency cart. Note pertinent findings—such as the presence of a pacemaker or an artificial joint—on the x-ray request.

Postprocedure Care

Although no specific care is usually needed after an x-ray procedure, in some instances specific postprocedure care is needed. See headings corresponding to the specific x-ray procedures.

Chest X-rays

Chest x-rays may be taken to detect pulmonary disease and the status of respiratory problems or trauma and to confirm the placement of an endotracheal or tracheostomy tube. Complete details are presented in Chapter 59. There is no specific follow-up care.

Plain Abdominal Films

A plain abdominal film—known as a *flat plate* or a KUB, which stands for *k*idney, *u*reter, *b*ladder—can reveal such abnormalities as tumors, obstructions, abnormal gas collections, and strictures. No follow-up care is needed for this study.

Skeletal X-rays

When fractures are suspected, x-rays are ordered for the bones in question. Generally, the procedure is not painful unless the extremity has to be moved for positioning. Examples of some x-ray projections are:

- Waters' projection, which is a posteroanterior view of the skull to show the orbits and maxillary sinuses. If the client may have a cervical spine fracture, the physician will order a lateral cervical spine x-ray instead.
- Towne's projection, which is an anteroposterior view to demonstrate the occipital bone and facial structures, such as the zygomatic arch.
- Panoramic (sometimes called Panorex, from the name of a machine used to take panoramic x-rays), a 180-degree view of the teeth and jaw.

Fluoroscopy

Fluoroscopy is a radiographic technique that permits direct observation of the body. The body part under examination is positioned between an x-ray tube and a fluorescent screen. X-rays pass through the body and project the targeted organs or bones onto the fluoroscopic screen as visual images. The benefit of fluoroscopy is that joint actions, organs, and entire body systems can be observed directly and dynamically (as they move). Radiopaque and radiolucent media enhance visualization.

Fluoroscopy can be used to monitor the progress of other diagnostic studies. For example, the progress of a radiopaque catheter can be observed as it is threaded through an artery or vein; or the progress of radiopaque barium can be seen as it is swallowed and moves through the gastrointestinal (GI) tract.

Tomography

Tomography is a radiographic technique that produces images of body tissues in a single plane or slice. Sequential images are obtained by moving the x-ray tube as it projects views at varying levels of tissue depth. Tomograms can be static body-section radiographs or can be combined with reconstruction tomography, as in computed tomography (CT) and positron emission tomography (PET), which are discussed later in this chapter.

Contrast X-rays

Contrast studies use radiopaque media to enhance visualization of an organ system or tissue under study. Contrast media include barium (a radiopaque contrast medium) and various dyes.

Upper Gastrointestinal Series

An upper GI series, also known as a *barium swallow,* permits radiologic visualization of the esophagus, stomach, and duodenum using fluoroscopy. It can aid in the detection of strictures, ulcers, tumors, polyps, hiatal hernias, and motility problems. A detailed discussion of the upper GI series and related client care is found in Chapter 28.

Lower Gastrointestinal Series

A lower GI series, which requires a barium enema, is performed to visualize the position, movements, and filling of the colon. Barium is instilled rectally, and x-rays are taken with or without fluoroscopy. This test can aid in detecting tumors, diverticula, stenoses, obstructions, inflammation, ulcerative colitis, and polyps. See Chapter 32 for a detailed discussion of this procedure and related client care.

Computed Tomography

Procedure

Computed tomography scans highlight differences in bone and soft tissue. The images are generated by computerized synthesis of x-ray data obtained in many different directions in a cross-sectional plane or slice. The computed data are assembled as three-dimensional images. CT is used to identify space-occupying lesions (masses) and shifts of structures caused by neoplasms, cysts, focal inflammatory lesions, and abscesses of the head, chest, abdomen, pelvis, and extremities (Fig. 11–4). To distinguish normal tissue from abnormal masses, a contrast

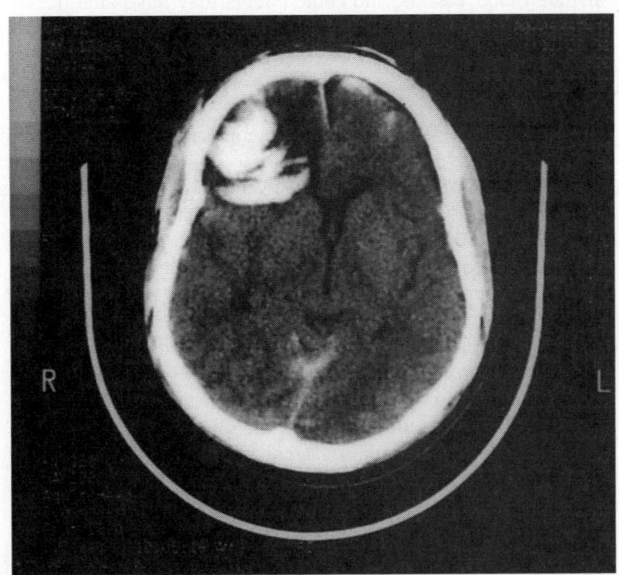

FIGURE 11–4 A computed tomography scan of the head. The brain tissue is gray, and the skull is white. The mass in the left frontal lobe is blood from a head injury.

medium (dye) may be administered. The CT scan can be performed quickly, within 20 minutes, not including analysis.

PREPROCEDURE CARE

Before a CT scan, make sure that the client has given informed consent and answer any questions the client and family may have about the procedure. Explain that fasting usually is not required for a CT scan of the head, but ask whether or not the client becomes nauseated easily; if so, adjust food and fluid intake accordingly. For example, some clients prefer a light breakfast to reduce nausea and others prefer an empty stomach. Fasting is usually required for a CT scan of the abdomen. Explain that a contrast agent is commonly given. Because the contrast material is iodine-based, ask whether the client has allergies to iodine or contrast dyes (Box 11–3).

If the CT scan will be of the client's head, remove any objects from the hair (wigs, barrettes, earrings, hair pins) before the test begins. The client's hair should be combed smooth.

Explain the client's role during the scan. The client is positioned supine, and the body part to be scanned is placed into the doughnut-shaped ring of the scanner. The technician moves the table from a control room during the scan to direct the study to different areas. The client should expect to hear mechanical noises coming from the scanner. Some clients may feel claustrophobic during the test, but assure them that it is possible to communicate with the technician during the scan.

Emphasize that the client must remain still during the scan. If the client is unable to comply, sedation or even general anesthesia may be required. If sedation is needed, tell the client to (1) avoid alcohol and caffeine on the day of the scan, (2) avoid eating for 2 hours before the scan, (3) arrange for someone to drive him home after the scan, and (4) avoid driving for at least 12 hours.

POSTPROCEDURE CARE

After the test, assess the client for reactions to the contrast agent, for hematoma at the injection site, and for the quality of pulses in the limb used for injection of the contrast agent. The client may resume normal activities unless additional diagnostic tests are planned. Tell the client to expect to experience diuresis from the dye. Encourage the client to drink plenty of fluids to flush the dye and prevent nephrotoxic injury.

■ MAGNETIC RESONANCE IMAGING

PROCEDURE

Magnetic resonance imaging (MRI) is a noninvasive imaging test that uses powerful magnetic fields and radiofrequency pulses to produce the image; therefore, the client is not exposed to ionizing radiation. The magnet in the scanner is 30,000 times more powerful than the earth's magnetic field. Consequently, this test cannot be performed if clients have pacemakers, metal implants, some types of ventilators, or embedded metal fragments, such as shrapnel. The powerful magnet may move these objects inside the client's body or may interfere with their

BOX 11–3 Use of Contrast Agents

Certain disorders, such as tumors, are better visualized with the use of a contrast agent. Other disorders, such as bleeding and edema, can be seen better without a contrast agent. The use of contrast agents is potentially dangerous. They may irritate blood vessels, and some clients may have allergic reactions to them that, if untreated, may develop into anaphylactic shock.

Preprocedure Care

Before a test involving a contrast agent, ask the client whether he has ever had an allergic reaction to contrast dye or iodine. Note the type of allergic response on the record; for example, "Client states that he developed hives when a dye was injected for another test." Some clients report allergies, but when asked to explain the reaction, they state that they "feel warm" when given the dye. This is a normal reaction, not an allergic one.

Some clients are given contrast agents even though they report contrast allergy. To reduce the severity of the reaction, these clients are pretreated with an antihistamine or corticosteroids. Therefore, do not assure the client with a reported allergy to dye that a contrast agent will not be given. Even if the client says that he has no history of allergy, watch for symptoms of an allergic reaction after injection of contrast agent. Some anaphylactic reactions have occurred with the first dose of dye. Tell the client that it is normal to feel a hot, flushed sensation and metallic taste in the mouth when the dye is injected. Tell the client to report any difficulty breathing or itching to staff in the radiology department.

Postprocedure Care

After the procedure, the client can usually resume normal activities. Diuresis will occur shortly after the use of a contrast agent. If the client is able to do so, encourage drinking at least one glass of water or other liquid an hour after the procedure. Replacement fluid may be needed, and the client should be assessed for fluid balance. The fluid balance in clients with renal or cardiac disease should be assessed carefully after a series of tests requiring intravenous contrast agents.

Complications

Complications rarely occur with the use of contrast agents but include local and systemic allergic reactions, spasm, occlusion of the vessel by a clot, and bleeding at the injection site. Assess the affected limb for color, warmth, pulses distal to the injection site, bleeding or hematoma formation, and mobility.

Assess the client for clinical manifestations of an allergic reaction, which include pallor, tachycardia, restlessness, sneezing, coughing, erythema, tachypnea, respiratory distress, facial flushing, urticaria, pruritus, hypotension, nausea, vomiting, headache, convulsions, flank pain, hematuria, and oliguria. Assess for these reactions after the dye is injected, because clients have experienced respiratory or cardiac arrest while undergoing x-ray study. Emergency equipment should always be available.

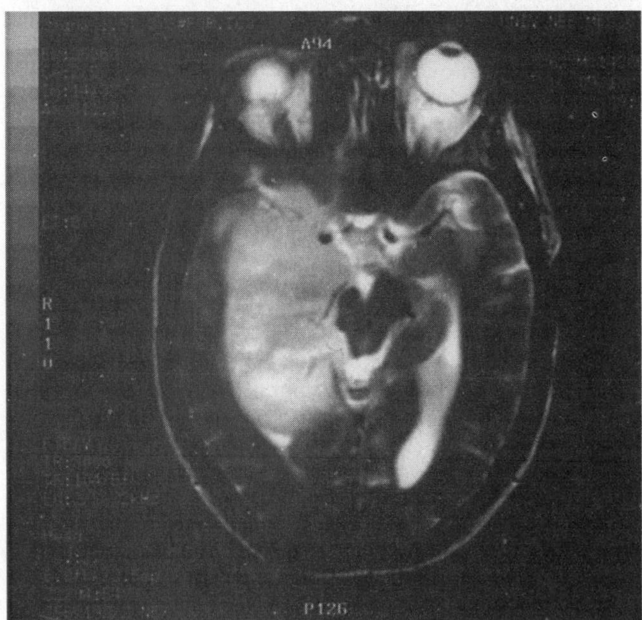

FIGURE 11–5 Magnetic resonance imaging of the head. The eyes are evident at the top of the image. The client has a brain tumor.

function. MRIs also are not performed for pregnant clients.

When looking at an MRI, remember that the image is opposite to that of a CT scan: Bone appears black on an MRI and white on a CT scan (Fig. 11–5). A contrast agent may be used to augment the images.

Preprocedure Care

Explain to the client and family the purpose of the MRI, the sounds and sensations that the client will hear and feel during the examination, and the client's role during the test. Obtain an informed consent.

Before the test, the client should remove all metal-containing objects (brassiere, jewelry, watch, and so on). Note the presence of any internal metal objects, such as a prosthesis or pacemaker, for the physician. Intravenous fluid pumps need to be removed during the test. Special MRI-compatible monitoring devices, such as pulse oximeters and electrocardiogram (ECG) leads, can be used.

The client can eat normally and take any prescribed medication before an MRI of the head. When the scan involves the GI system, the client must fast for 6 hours before the procedure. Explain that he must lie still during the procedure, which can take from 60 to 90 minutes. Clients who are agitated or unable to remain motionless may require sedation before the scan (see instructions for CT). If the use of a contrast agent is planned, ask whether the client tends to become nauseated easily, and adjust the intake of food and fluids accordingly.

The client lies supine on a narrow padded table. Because the scanner makes loud clanging noises, the client should wear earplugs or headphones. Some clients may feel claustrophobic during the test; assure them it is possible to communicate with the technician during the scan.

Postprocedure Care

After the test, the client may resume previous activities and diet. Tell the client to expect to experience diuresis if a contrast agent was used for the MRI (see instructions for CT).

■ POSITRON EMISSION TOMOGRAPHY

Procedure

Positron emission tomography (PET) scanning produces images of metabolic and physiologic function. PET scans have diagnostic value because the function of diseased tissue commonly differs from that of normal tissues. The client is given doses of strong radioactive tracers (*radionuclides*), which emit signals to show the uptake and distribution of the traces. The images are formed by computer analysis of photons detected by annihilation of positrons emitted by the radionuclides (Fig. 11–6). PET has three primary uses:

- To determine the amount of blood flowing into specific body tissues
- To reveal how adequately tissues use blood receptors, such as medications and neurotransmitters
- To measure blood flow, glucose metabolism, and oxygen extraction

PET is used in the diagnosis of stroke, brain tumors, and epilepsy and to chart the progress of Alzheimer's disease, Parkinson's disease, head injury, schizophrenia, bipolar disorder, and cardiac hypoxemia.

Preprocedure Care

Explain to the client and family the purpose of the test, the sounds and sensations that the client will hear and feel during the examination, and the client's role during the test. Obtain an informed consent. In contrast to CT and MRI machines, the PET scanner is quiet. The client should fast for 4 hours before the scan. If the client is diabetic, it is preferred that the blood glucose be below 150 g/dl. The client must remain motionless for about 45

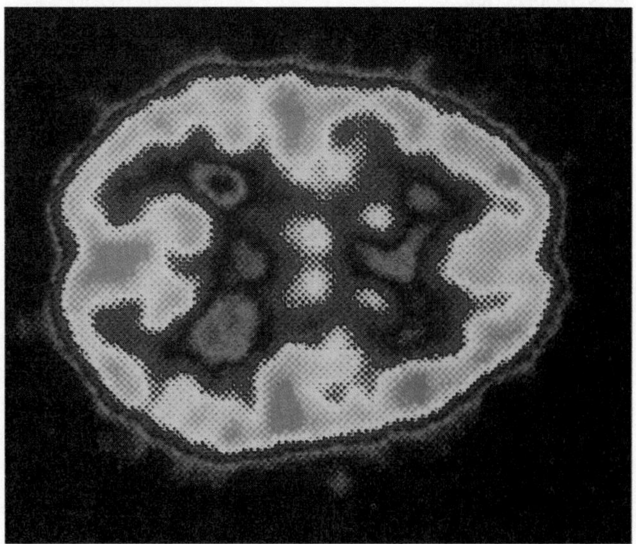

FIGURE 11–6 A positron emission tomographic scan showing decreased metabolic activity after a seizure (noted as green areas on the scan).

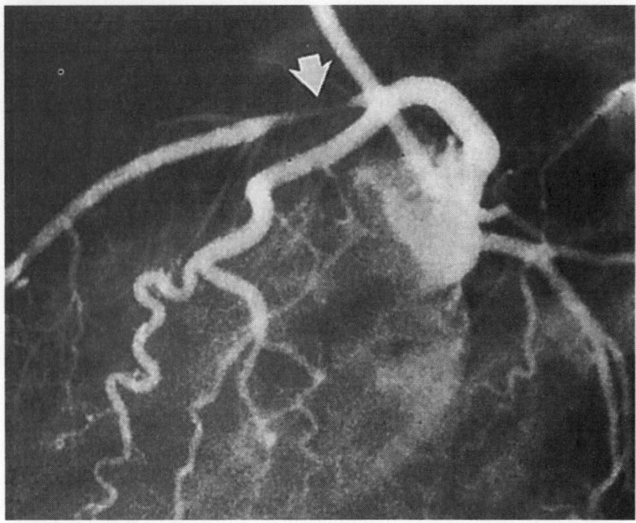

FIGURE 11–7 Coronary angiography shows stenosis, or narrowing (*arrow*), of the left anterior descending coronary artery. (From Braunwald, E. [1992]. *Heart disease: A textbook of cardiovascular medicine* [4th ed.]. Philadelphia: W. B. Saunders.)

minutes. An agitated client may require sedation. (See instructions for sedation under CT Preprocedure Care earlier.)

Postprocedure Care

No special care is required after a PET procedure.

■ ANGIOGRAPHY

Procedure

Angiography is a radiographic technique that uses a contrast agent to assess blood vessels and the blood flowing through them. A common form of angiography is coronary angiography, which is performed to determine the degree of obstruction in the myocardial circulation (Fig. 11–7). Angiography can also be used to outline veins (*venography*) or lymphatic vessels (*lymphography*). The terms *angiogram* and *arteriogram* are used interchangeably in practice.

Preprocedure Care

Before angiography, make sure the client understands the planned procedure and has given informed consent. Note any known allergies to contrast agents or iodine. Collect baseline assessment data: vital signs, quality and symmetry of pulses in the limbs, level of consciousness, speech patterns, and estimates of limb strength. The same assessments are made after the procedure. *A detailed baseline is crucial to accurate assessment of postprocedure changes.*

In most facilities, the client is given nothing by mouth for 6 to 8 hours before angiography. Some facilities allow fluids to reduce the risk of dehydration and clotting. Follow your facility's protocol. The planned puncture site may be shaved.

Postprocedure Care

Decreased perfusion of the distal limb from hemorrhage or hematoma at the puncture site and an allergic reaction to the contrast agent are the two major complications that can develop after angiography. Assessment is crucial to their early detection. Follow your facility's protocol for postprocedure care. Usually, it consists of the following steps:

1. If the femoral approach was used, keep the leg immobile; tell the client not to flex the hip or leg for 12 hours. If the brachial approach was used, release the pressure dressing and apply an elastic bandage to the client's arm; the arm must remain straight. Movement of the limb can dislodge the clot at the puncture site and result in bleeding.
2. Monitor the client's vital signs every 15 minutes for 2 hours, then hourly until stable. Review the signs of an allergic reaction (see Box 11–3).
3. Keep a sandbag on a femoral puncture site to maintain pressure on the site. Check puncture sites every 15 minutes for 2 hours, then hourly.
4. Monitor distal pulses every 15 minutes for 2 hours, then hourly until stable. Assess the quality of the pulses and note capillary filling time. Notify the physician if the quality of the pulse changes.
5. Expect diuresis, provide ample fluids, and keep a urinal or bedpan nearby.
6. Resume medications, if prescribed, and the client's usual diet.

■ ULTRASONOGRAPHY

Procedure

Ultrasonography (also called *ultrasound* or *echography*) uses high-frequency sound waves to depict soft tissues. Ultrasonography works on the same principle as sonar and radar. When the ultrasound waves are directed into the body, they spread through the tissues. Because tissues differ in density, the sound waves are reflected (bounced back) in various ways in different tissues. The reflected waves are processed, shown as an image, and then recorded.

Ultrasound can be used to assess many structures in the body, including the heart, great vessels, liver, gallbladder, pancreas, breast, uterus and ovaries, scrotum, kidney, and thyroid gland (Fig. 11–8). It is commonly

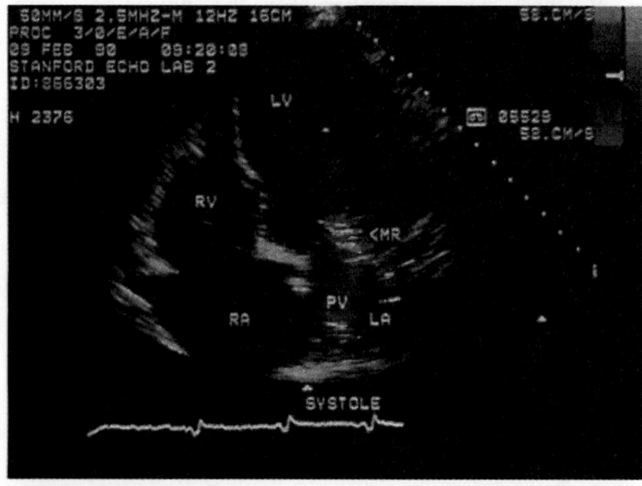

FIGURE 11–8 An ultrasound image of the heart, also known as an echocardiogram. (From Bennett, J. C., & Plum, F. [1996]. *Cecil textbook of medicine* [20th ed.]. Philadelphia: W. B. Saunders.)

used in obstetrics to determine gestational age. There is no exposure to ionizing radiation during this test, and it is noninvasive.

Preprocedure Care

No special care is required before ultrasonography. Tell the client the purpose of the test and what to expect. A gel is applied to the skin, and a transducer (a device that changes reflected high-frequency sound to electrical energy) is moved on the skin surface above the organ. The procedure is painless and fairly quick.

Sometimes a bowel preparation with laxatives is used for viewing the abdominal organs. The bladder must be very full for the uterus to be viewed. Sometimes the lighting must be dimmed for the oscilloscope to be seen.

Postprocedure Care

No special care is required after an ultrasound study.

■ RADIONUCLIDE IMAGING

Procedure

Radionuclides are radioisotopes (radioactive forms of some elements) or tracers that are used to visualize organs or regions that cannot be seen on plain films. Radioisotopes are treated the same as normal elements by living cells. Their radiation can be detected by suitable counters. Radionuclide studies may be used to diagnose disorders of the heart, thyroid, liver, brain, bone, kidney, spleen, pancreas, lung, and gallbladder.

Various isotopes are used because they concentrate in one organ or body fluid. For example, thallium concentrates in the heart, whereas iodine concentrates in the thyroid. An artificial radioactive element (technetium) is used extensively. Technetium emits gamma radiation only and therefore is safer than other isotopes that emit more damaging radiation. When combined with pyrophosphate given intravenously, technetium is taken up by bone and the entire skeleton can be surveyed. This technique is helpful in detecting bone tumors (Fig. 11–9). When combined with albumin, technetium concentrates in the lung and can be used to estimate pulmonary blood flow. It can also be used to investigate lesions in other organs and has largely replaced radioactive iodine for thyroid assessment.

Depending on the intended diagnostic purpose, a blocking agent may be administered before the radionuclide to prevent uptake by certain tissues. The blocking agent is not radioactive. For example, iodine is normally concentrated in the thyroid gland. When iodine-tagged radionuclides are used other than in thyroid studies, Lugol's solution is given to block the uptake of iodine-tagged radionuclides by the thyroid.

The radionuclide is administered orally or intravenously about 1 to 3 hours before the test to allow time for distribution. During this time, have the client drink extra fluids to clear the portion not taken up by the tissues. After the waiting period, the client is placed on a table and an imaging device records the activity of the emitted radiation.

Radioactivity may be increased or decreased in comparison with normal activity in the organ. Areas of decreased activity, called *cold-spot imaging,* usually indicate tissues that are functioning improperly. This is common when normal tissues have been replaced by tumor. Increased activity, called *hot-spot imaging,* may occur in tissues that are metabolically more active. For example, a diseased thyroid gland or bone infection may be detected by hot-spot imaging.

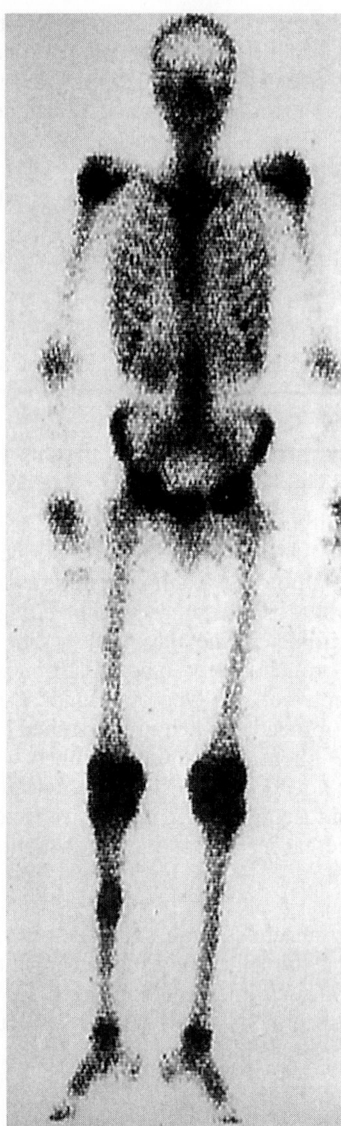

FIGURE 11–9 A technetium scan of the skeleton shows an area of increased radionuclide density on the right tibia that is a bone tumor. (From Walter, J. B. [1992]. *An introduction to the principles of disease* [3rd ed.]. Philadelphia: W. B. Saunders.)

Preprocedure Care

Tell the client that the radionuclide contains very little radioactivity. If an abdominal scan is scheduled, the client may need an enema first. Make sure that the radionuclide test is scheduled before any tests that use iodinated contrast agents or barium. These substances block the exit of protons from radionuclides. This is especially important with radioactive iodine thyroid scans. The use of contrast agents for other studies can block uptake of radioactive iodine for months. Obtain an informed consent.

Obtain the following information from the client:

- Age, weight, and height to calculate the amount of radioactive substance to be used

- Menstrual history to rule out pregnancy (pregnancy is a contraindication to many radionuclide studies)
- Whether the client is breast-feeding (breast-feeding is a contraindication to many radionuclide studies)
- A history of allergy
- Recent exposure to radionuclides
- Presence of internal prostheses that could block the view of the organ
- Current treatments, such as the need for oxygen, telemetry, or timed specimen collections

POSTPROCEDURE CARE
Tell the client to drink extra fluids; otherwise, no special care is required.

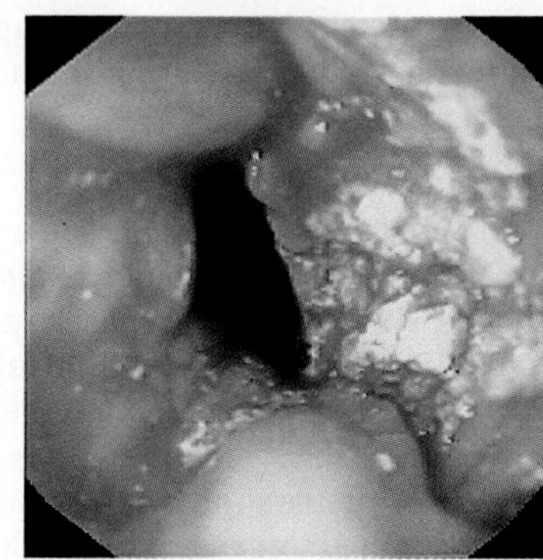

FIGURE 11–10 An endoscopic view of the esophagus showing an esophageal ulcer.

ENDOSCOPY

Endoscopy is direct visualization of a body system or part by means of a lighted, flexible tube. This method is more accurate than radiologic examination because the physician can directly observe sources of bleeding and surface lesions and can determine the status of healing tissues. Arthroscopy, bronchoscopy, and gastrointestinal endoscopy are examples of this type of diagnostic technique.

Endoscopic procedures require a signed consent. Provide complete client education to enhance cooperation. Tell the client not to drive a motor vehicle for at least 12 hours after endoscopy if sedation was used during the procedure. (See earlier instructions for sedation.)

■ ARTHROSCOPY

Arthroscopy is an endoscopic examination of a joint. An arthroscope is a thin fiberoptic instrument that allows examination of various joints without need for a large incision. Biopsy specimens can be taken, articular cartilage abnormalities assessed, loose bodies removed, and cartilage trimmed. Further discussion of arthroscopy is found in Chapter 25.

■ BRONCHOSCOPY

Bronchoscopy is the passage of a lighted bronchoscope, either rigid or flexible, into the bronchial tree for diagnostic or therapeutic purposes. This procedure is covered in Chapter 59.

■ ENDOSCOPY OF THE GASTROINTESTINAL TRACT

Endoscopy of the upper GI tract consists of esophagoscopy and esophagogastroduodenoscopy (Fig. 11–10). These procedures are useful for assessing acute or chronic GI bleeding, pernicious anemia, esophageal injury, dysphagia, substernal pain, and epigastric discomfort (see Chapter 28). Endoscopy of the lower GI tract consists of proctosigmoidoscopy and colonoscopy (see Chapter 32).

CYTOLOGIC STUDIES

Cytology is the study of the anatomy, physiology, pathology, and chemistry of the cell. One of the most common cytologic studies is a staining technique developed by George Papanicolaou—the *Pap test,* which is used to detect malignant cells. Usually, this test is used to study vaginal or cervical cells. Sometimes it may be used for other tissues obtained easily by smearing or scraping, such as the mouth, genital tract, or anus.

Tissues not available for scraping must be obtained by *biopsy,* which is the removal of tissue for diagnostic study. The tissue removed must be (1) representative of the tissue in question, (2) large enough to be examined, and (3) kept intact until studied. Many times a fixative or refrigeration is used to prevent tissue decomposition. Some tissues are not placed in fixative, such as breast tissue to be analyzed for hormones.

Biopsy procedures are either closed or open.

■ CLOSED BIOPSY

In a closed biopsy, no surgical incision is used. Examples include:

- *Needle aspiration biopsy.* A trocar or needle is inserted into the tissue. The aspirated cells are then examined. This technique is common for the biopsy of breast masses.
- *Stereotactic needle aspiration biopsy.* A three-dimensional view of the abnormal tissue is created. On the basis of the imaging results, a needle is inserted into the mass. The client must be able to remain motionless for 20 to 60 minutes while the coordinates are determined. This technique is used for biopsy of certain lung lesions.
- *Core needle biopsy.* A special needle cuts a specimen from tissues not in view. This technique is common for biopsy of the kidney, prostate, liver, lung, and thyroid gland.
- *Punch biopsy.* A small specimen is removed by means of a special instrument that pierces the organ directly or through the skin. This technique is commonly used for biopsy of the skin or the cervix.
- *Brush biopsy.* Cells and tissue fragments are removed by a stiff bristle brush. The brush is advanced into the target area through an endoscope. Areas sampled in this way are the renal pelvis and bronchus.
- *Shave biopsy.* Skin lesions are shaved from the skin surface with a surgical blade or razor blade.

■ OPEN BIOPSY

A surgical incision is needed for an open biopsy. There are two types:

- *Excisional biopsy.* The entire lesion and a margin of surrounding normal tissue are removed. This is the procedure of choice in most cases.
- *Incisional biopsy.* A selected part of the lesion is removed. This form of biopsy is commonly completed during endoscopic examination.

■ SECTIONS

Two methods are used to assess for malignant cells from tissue samples:

1. *Frozen sections* are used for rapid microscopic diagnosis. A thin slice of tissue is cut from the frozen specimen and examined. The procedure requires about 10 to 15 minutes. The pathologist can determine whether malignancy is present and whether the entire tumor has been removed by looking for a margin of tumor-free tissue.
2. *Permanent sections* require about 48 hours. The tissue is placed in a fixative and then examined. It can be stained to facilitate pathologic study.

Preprocedure Care

Before a biopsy, tell the client about the purpose of the procedure and obtain informed consent. The client may express concern or anxiety about the possible results of the biopsy; be empathetic with the client and family. Some clients sign a permit that allows surgical excision of the mass if it is found to be malignant on frozen section. In these situations, perform a complete baseline assessment for postoperative comparison. Certain types of biopsy require the client's cooperation. For example, to reduce the risk of liver laceration during biopsy of the liver, the client is instructed to hold his breath.

Postprocedure Care

Postprocedure care varies with the type of biopsy done. If organs such as the liver, lung, or kidney are sampled, the client has a risk of bleeding, peritonitis, and pneumothorax. Tailor the specific interventions to match the client's needs. Guidelines for care are offered in assessment chapters throughout this book.

CONCLUSIONS

Diagnostic testing is common in both hospital and ambulatory care settings. In all likelihood, a growing number of tests will be performed, processed, or both at the point of care rather than in a laboratory. Become familiar with the various tests on urine, blood, and other body fluids. In many settings, nurses are now required to be prepared to collect these specimens. Understanding how to collect the specimen and knowing the care needed by the client before and after the procedure are important aspects of nursing management. Diagnostic assessment of organs mandates an understanding of the test and the proper scheduling of multiple tests to avoid losing time. In addition, most laboratories call or fax results to the nurse, who is then responsible for determining whether the results warrant notification of the physician.

BIBLIOGRAPHY

1. Brunzel, N. A. (1994). *Fundamentals of urine and body fluid analysis.* Philadelphia: W. B. Saunders.
2. Chernecky, C. C., & Berger, B. J. (1997). *Laboratory tests and diagnostic procedures* (2nd ed.). Philadelphia: W. B. Saunders.
3. Cook, L. (1999). The value of lab values. *American Journal of Nursing, 99*(5), 66–75.
4. Corbett, J. (1996). *Laboratory tests and diagnostic procedures with nursing diagnosis* (4th ed.). Norwalk, CT: Appleton & Lange.
5. Edelman, R. R., & Warach, S. (1993). Magnetic resonance imaging: Part I. *New England Journal of Medicine, 328*(10), 708–716.
6. Edelman, R. R., & Warach, S. (1993). Magnetic resonance imaging: Part II. *New England Journal of Medicine, 328*(11), 785–791.
7. Fishbach, F. T. (1996). *A manual of laboratory & diagnostic tests* (5th ed.). Philadelphia: Lippincott-Raven.
8. Flynn, J. C., Jr. (1994). *Procedures in phlebotomy.* Philadelphia: W. B. Saunders.
9. Frizzell, J. (1998). Avoiding lab test pitfalls. *American Journal of Nursing, 98*(2), 34–37.
10. Greenberg, J. (1993). Physiologic imaging. *Neuroimaging, 7,* 166–174.
11. Malarky, L. M., & McMorrow, L. M. (1996). *Nurse's manual of laboratory tests and diagnostic procedures.* Philadelphia: W. B. Saunders.
12. McFarland, M. (1994). *Nursing implications of laboratory tests.* Albany, NY: Delmar.
13. Mettler, F. A. (1996). *Essentials of radiology.* Philadelphia: W. B. Saunders.
14. O'Toole, M. T. (Ed.). (1997). *Miller-Keane encyclopedia and dictionary of medicine, nursing, and allied health* (6th ed.). Philadelphia: W. B. Saunders.
15. Pagana, K. D., & Pagana, T. J. (1997). *Mosby's diagnostic and laboratory test reference* (3rd ed.). St. Louis: Mosby–Year Book.
16. Putnam, C., & Ravin, C. (1994). *Textbook of diagnostic imaging.* Philadelphia: W. B. Saunders.
17. Scheffer, K. J., & Tobin, R. S. (1997). *Better x-ray interpretation.* Springhouse, PA: Springhouse.

BRIDGE TO EVIDENCE-BASED PRACTICE

Patient-Centered Communication

QUESTIONS:
What is patient-centered communication?
Does patient-centered communication affect patient outcomes?
How is patient-centered communication used in clinical problem-solving?

CITATION:
Brown, S. J. (1999). Patient-centered communication. *Annual Review of Nursing Research, 17,* 85–104.

The definition of patient-centered communication (PCC) used for the review was an orientation to patient-provider discourse by which patient and provider co-produce mutual understandings and decisions.

STUDIES

The term "patient-centered communication" is used in the clinical literature quite aften, yet a comprehensive search of *CINAHL* and *MEDLINE* (1984–1998) produced only five relevant research studies. Unfortunately, the definition of PCC used in these studies was not consistent with the term's usage in the North American clinical literature. However, many studies did examine a communication behavior and then related the behavior to PCC in the conclusion. As a result, the body of studies included in the review focus more on the behavioral components of PCC than on PCC as a comprehensive health care communication style. Findings from 63 nursing and medicine studies and reviews were included.* Most studies were conducted in office settings.

Summary of Findings

What Is Patient-Centered Communication?

The following behaviors were associated with PCC:

- Allowing clients to give their accounts in their own language[9]
- A conversational style of interview[4, 13]
- Eliciting the client's thoughts, perspectives, expectations, values, and goals
- Inquiring about the client's home, work, and social lives[4]
- Responding to the client's indirect and nonverbal clues regarding emotions and problems[5]
- Providing clients with information for self-care and participation in health care decisions[7, 13]
- Creating shared understandings with clients[9]
- Collaboratively developing health care plans with clients[7]
- Expressing concern for the client's well-being[4, 13]
- Creating social connectedness with clients by humor, touch, and modest personal sharing[4, 13]

Does PCC Affect Patient Outcomes?

Contrary to what some providers think, when the behaviors of PCC are used, more accurate and more useful information about the client's illness or health status is obtained than when the provider asks a series of specific questions.[11, 14] Other outcomes associated with the behaviors of PCC include

- Increased client compliance and resolution of client concerns[6]
- Greater client satisfaction[2]
- Better physiologic outcomes[8]
- Higher overall health ratings[8]
- Increased trust in the health care provider[16]

How Is Patient-Centered Communication Used in Clinical Problem-Solving?

Three different strategies are used for incorporating PCC into clinical problem-solving discourse:

1. Some providers open the interview with a client-centered phase in which the clients take the lead and present their health problems and issues. Then the provider takes control and asks specific questions about these health problems.[10, 15]
2. Some providers allow the client's story to structure the entire interview. Interestingly, it has been found that when clients were given an uninterrupted opportunity to present their concerns, they on average took only 38 seconds to do so and never more than 2½ minutes.[1] Providers using this strategy ask questions that arise out of what the client has just said and keep the story intact as a life experience rooted in events, sequence, places, and relationships. They also avoid use of medical language and specific disease-centered questions.[4, 7, 12, 13] These providers then offer their thoughts on the underlying illness meanings of the client's experiences, carefully linking these interpretations to the client's statements.
3. In the *windows-of-opportunity approach,*[3] the provider asks an initial open-ended question, followed by specific questions that help pinpoint the health problem or diagnosis. However, the provider remains sensitive to the client's desires to talk about personal, emotional, or family issues. The provider responds to these comments by asking about them, thus allowing the client to introduce concerns and psychosocial issues into the interview.

There is no one best strategy; each has its benefits and is employed in different situations. The *integrated approach* (i.e., with the entire interview structured around the client's story) may work best when there are few health or illness problems, whereas the *phased approach* may work best when the client has an immediate concern to be addressed. The issue of when to use one strategy or another still needs to be studied.

Limitations/Reservations: We know a lot about the separate interpersonal processes that compose PCC but very little about it as a multiprocess, integrated health care communication strategy. We do not know whether or how integrated PCC affects the client's clinical outcome. In addition, most of the studies in this review focus on physicians because relatively few studies of nurses' communication processes have been conducted. The studies on communication have been performed mainly in office settings because appointments are scheduled and take place in a room, a setting that lends itself to audiotap-

*Not all studies for each behavior are cited.

Patient-Centered Communication *Continued*

ing or videotaping. In contrast, communication between nurses and clients in hospital is typically not scheduled and takes place as a series of short contacts, not one longer contact as in offices. Hence, we know little about how nurses and clients communicate over time (e.g. a shift or consecutive days) in hospitals.

Research-Based Practice

A wide range of communication behaviors and styles is used by health care providers in their conversations with clients. Some of the behaviors associated with PCC may help the client feel at ease (e.g., humor, touch, brief social chit-chat). Others actually help clients tell their stories (e.g., asking about home life, responding to indirect and nonverbal clues regarding emotions and psychosocial issues).

Skilled clinicians let clients tell their whole stories before asking questions. They build on what clients have said and ask focused-but-open question (not questions with yes or no answers). Then they ask a few specific questions to complete their understanding of the situation. Clients who feel that they are appreciated as unique persons and whose providers allow them to tell their stories in the sequence and manner that makes sense to them may be socially more comfortable in the health care interview. As a result, they may disclose more personal information than they would in a more traditional health care interview.

More controlling communication behaviors force clients to tell their stories in ways that impose medical or nursing language and sequences on what clients say. For example, a client may say he "gets winded." A PCC nurse might continue to listen to the rest of a story about when this happens, or might say, "Tell me more about when you get winded." In contrast, a nurse who is disease-centered may say, "Do you get this shortness of breath when you climb a short set of stairs?" This response, which changes what clients call their problem and moves it away from how clients are thinking about it, subtly "medicalizes" the description of what clients are experiencing. More relevant information will be provided by clients if nurses do not introduce specific questions at this point.

All nurses should listen to themselves and note to what extent they interrupt clients, change the language clients use to describe problems, or otherwise control the conversation. The nurse should be committed to getting in touch with the client's view of the situation and the meanings it holds for them. Each nurse should attempt to become a partner with the client, a partner who works with the client to create a true conversation. When true conversation takes place, a mutual understanding of the client's problems and mutually agreed upon ways of addressing them become possible. The plans that PCC nurses and clients make together are more likely to be realistic, to address all the important aspects of a situation, and to produce good clinical outcomes.

Cited References

1. Beckman, H. B., & Frankel, R. M. (1984). The effect of physician behavior on the collection of data. *Annals of Internal Medicine, 91,* 692–696.
2. Bertakis, K. D., Roter, D., & Putnam, S. M. (1991). The relationship of physician medical interview style to patient satisfaction. *Journal of Family Practice, 32,* 175–181.
3. Branch, W. T., & Malik, T. K. (1993). Using "windows of opportunities" in brief interviews to understand patients' concerns. *Journal of American Medical Association, 269,* 1667–1668.
4. Brown, S. J. (1994). Communication strategies used by an expert nurse. *Clinical Nursing Research, 3,* 43–56.
5. Brykcznski, K. A. (1989). An interpretive study describing the clinical judgment of nurse practitioners. *Scholarly Inquiry for Nursing Practice: An International Journal, 3,* 75–104.
6. Henbest, R. J., & Stewart, M. A. (1990). Patient-centredness in the consultation: Does it really make a difference? *Family Practice, 6,* 249–253.
7. Johnson, R. (1993). Nurse practitioner-patient discourse: Uncovering the voice of nursing in primary care practice. *Scholarly Inquiry for Nursing Practice: An International Journal, 7,* 143–157.
8. Kaplan, S. H., Greenfield, S., & Ware, J. E. (1989). Assessing the effects of physician-patient interaction on the outcomes of chronic disease. *Medical Care, 33,* 1176–1187.
9. Kristjanson, L., & Chalmers, K. (1990). Nurse-client interactions in community-based practice: Creating common ground. *Public Health Nursing, 7,* 215–223.
10. Levenstein, J. H., et al. (1986). The patient-centred clinical method. 1. A model for doctor-patient interaction in family medicine. *Family Practice, 3,* 24–30.
11. Marshall, R. S. (1988). Interpretation in doctor-patient interviews: A sociolinguistic analysis. *Culture, Medicine, and Psychiatry, 12,* 201–218.
12. Mishler, E. G. (1984). *The discourse of medicine: Dialectics of medical interviews.* Norwood, NJ: Ablex.
13. Morten, A., et al. (1991). Certified nurse midwifery care of the postpartum client: A descriptive study. *Journal of Nurse-Midwifery, 36,* 276–288.
14. Roter, D. L., & Hall, J. A. (1987). Physicians' interviewing styles and medical information obtained from patients. *Journal of General Internal Medicine, 2,* 325–329.
15. Smith, R. C. (1996). *The patient's story: Integrated patient-doctor interviewing.* Boston: Little, Brown.
16. Thom, D. H., & Campbell, B. (1997). Patient-physician trust: An exploratory study. *Journal of Family Practice, 44,* 169–176.

Sarah Jo Brown, PhD, RN, *Principal and Consultant, Practice-Research Integrations, Norwich, Vermont*

UNIT 4

Foundations of Medical-Surgical Nursing

Anatomy and Physiology Review

The Cell

R. B. Boley
Arlene L. Polaski
David Porta

The cell is the basic unit of structure and function in biologic systems. Two fundamental types of cells are recognized on the basis of composition and organization: *prokaryotic* and *eukaryotic.* Cells found in the human body and in higher plants and animals are eukaryotic; a bacterial cell is prokaryotic. All life systems use one of these two patterns except for viruses, which are acellular and are placed in a separate kingdom: the Akaryotae.

NORMAL CELL STRUCTURE AND FUNCTION

All cells, regardless of type, have the same basic structural pattern: a cytoplasmic matrix surrounded by a plasma membrane (Fig. U4–1). Numerous *organelles* (membrane-limited structures with a complex infrastructure and unique functions) are scattered within the cytoplasm of eukaryotic cells. Their compartmentalization allows multistage metabolic and physiologic events to occur simultaneously while keeping one function separate from another. In contrast, prokaryotic cells do not have organelles and have minimal infrastructural organization. The differences between these two cell types allow clinicians to attack a prokaryotic pathogen selectively in vivo and to use drugs that do not damage eukaryotic cells.

Despite some marked differences in structure and composition, both cell types perform the same basic functions. All cells transfer energy, take up and assimilate materials from outside the cell, synthesize macromolecules, maintain a homeostatic environment, and reproduce themselves as required (Table U4–1).

Most of a cell's mass is water (60% to 95%), which aids in thermal regulation and serves as a solvent for (1) electrolytes, (2) organic molecules, and (3) chemical reactions. *Electrolytes* in the cytoplasm help maintain stable electrical and pH environments and assist with various metabolic and physiologic activities. The most common intracellular electrolytes are calcium, magnesium, phos-

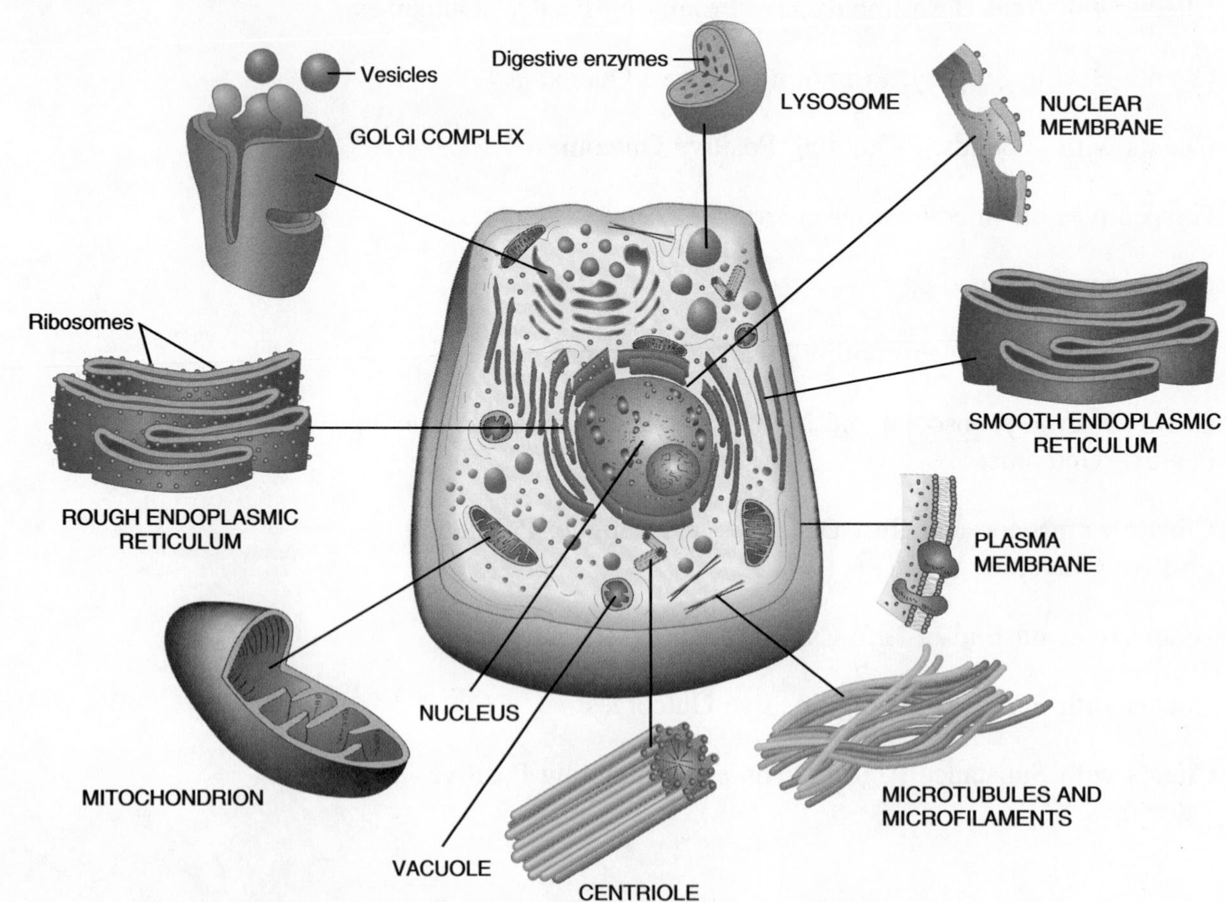

FIGURE U4–1 A "typical" cell showing the internal organelles in the cytoplasm and the nucleus.

TABLE U4–1 CELL STRUCTURES AND THEIR FUNCTIONS

Structure	Description	Function
Cell Nucleus		
Nucleus	Large structure surrounded by double membrane, contains nucleolus and chromosomes	DNA is transcribed using RNA to make proteins
Nucleolus	Granular body, consists of RNA and protein	Ribosomal RNA synthesis; ribosome subunit assembly
Chromosomes	Complexes of DNA and protein known as chromatin become visible as rodlike structures when cell divides	Contain genes that transmit hereditary information and govern cell structure and activity
Cytoplasmic Organelles		
Cell membrane	Boundary of cell	Encloses cell contents; regulates movement of materials in and out of the cell; maintains cell structure; communicates with other cells
Endoplasmic reticulum (ER)	Network of internal membranes extending throughout the cytoplasm. Two types: smooth and rough. Smooth lacks ribosomes on the outer surface; rough has ribosomes on the outer surface	Site of membrane lipids and proteins; origin of intracellular transport vesicles carrying proteins to be secreted. Smooth ER is used for lipid biosynthesis and drug detoxification; rough ER is site of protein manufacturing
Ribosomes	Granules composed of RNA and protein, some attached to ER, some free in cytoplasm	Synthesize polypeptides
Golgi complex	Stacks of flattened membrane sacs	Modifies proteins; packages secreted proteins; sorts other proteins to vacuoles and other organelles
Lysosomes	Membranous sacs	Contain enzymes to break down ingested materials, secretions, and waste
Vacuoles	Membranous sacs	Transport and store materials, waste, and water
Mitochondria	Sacs consisting of two membranes; inner membrane is folded to form cristae and encloses matrix	Site of most reactions of cellular respiration; transformation of energy originating from glucose or lipids into ATP
Microbodies (e.g., peroxisomes)	Membranous sacs containing a variety of enzymes	Sites of many diverse metabolic reactions
Cytoskeleton		
Microtubules	Hollow tubes made of tubulin protein	Provide structural support; provide for cell movement and cell division
Microfilaments	Solid, rodlike structures consisting of actin protein	Provide structural support; provide for cell movement and cell division
Centrioles	Pairs of hollow cylinders located near center of the cell	Spindles form between centrioles during mitosis; may anchor or organize microtubule formation
Cilia	Short projections extending from the surface of the cell, covered by plasma membrane	Regulate movement of material on surface of cell and some tissues
Flagella	Long projections made of microtubules, extend from surface of the cell, covered with plasma membrane	Provide for cellular locomotion by sperm cells

ATP, adenosine triphosphate; DNA, deoxyribonucleic acid; RNA, ribonucleic acid.

phate, bicarbonate, and potassium (the most abundant intracellular cation). *Molecules* within the cell consist mostly of sugars, fatty acids, amino acids, and nucleotides. These are metabolized for energy or used to synthesize macromolecules (lipids, proteins, nucleic acids, and their conjugates).

CELL DEVELOPMENT

Human life begins as an undifferentiated single cell, derived from the fusion of a male gamete (sperm) with a female gamete (ovum). By about the 7th day after fertilization, the original cell (or zygote) has already undergone several cycles of proliferation. The progeny cells begin to develop into distinctive tissues. In the embryo and fetus, these fully differentiated cells can be distinguished on the basis of both form and function.

When tissues in the developing organism reach genetically programmed size limits, the rate of cell reproduction begins to slow and finally stops or attains a steady-state replacement level. This form of growth regulation (called *contact* or *density-dependent inhibition*) is initiated by physical (contact) and chemical (nutrient and cytokine) levels. Cell replication is described later in this review.

■ CELL MEMBRANE

The cell membrane is a fluid phospholipid bilayer with a variety of proteins and conjugated proteins attached to or embedded within it (Fig. U4–2). Proteins that are weakly bound to the inner surface are called *peripheral* proteins. Those that span the lipid bilayer are called *integral;* they function as junctions or channels for the selective transport of ions and other water-soluble molecules or as receptors for various signaling molecules, including transmitters, hormones, and drugs.

The cell selectively regulates entry and exit of materials across the membrane by mechanisms that permit transport either down the concentration gradient (from high to low concentration) or up the gradient (from low to high). In general, a mechanism is termed *passive* or *active* according to the use of energy from the hydrolysis of adenosine triphosphate (ATP). The basic transport mechanisms are summarized in Table U4–2 and are illustrated in Figure U4–3.

The fate of material after uptake in vesicles is controlled by the presence of signal sequences on molecules within the cell and by other, as yet undetermined, factors. Some substances are degraded by enzymes, and the fragments are metabolically assimilated. Viruses may be uncoated, releasing their nucleic acid component into the cytoplasm. Bacterial toxin molecules may be split and the active portion released to combine with a cytoplasmic or nuclear receptor. Other materials may be exocytosed on another side (e.g., transcytosis of substances across mucosal epithelia in the gut).

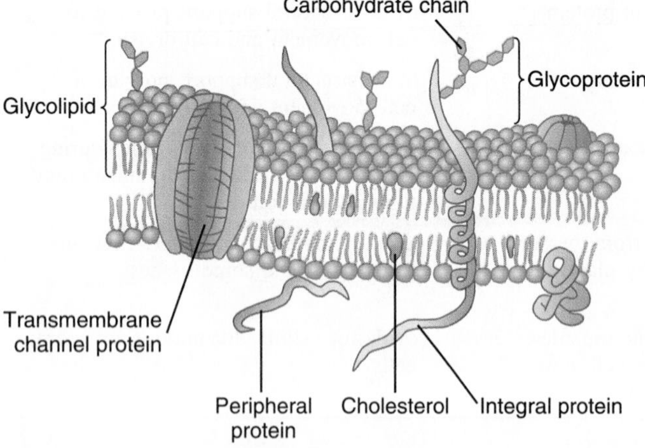

FIGURE U4–2 The cell membrane is composed of a bimolecular layer of lipids, primarily phospholipid and cholesterol. Proteins can be attached or embedded in the membrane. Peripheral proteins are attached to the surface; integral proteins are embedded in the cell membrane.

Membrane Channels

Proteins in the cell membrane provide channels into the cell. Some of the channels leak continuously, and some are gated (opened by stimuli). A *ligand-gated* channel

TABLE U4–2 MECHANISMS OF MEMBRANE TRANSPORT

Mechanism	Common Examples
Passive (High to Low, No ATP)	
Osmosis	Movement of water through a lipid portion of the membrane
Diffusion	Movement of gasses and small hydrophilic molecules (oxygen, carbon dioxide, nitrogen, glycerol, urea) through the lipid portion of a membrane
Facilitated diffusion	Movement of glucose, some ions, and amino acids via specific carrier proteins
Active (Low to High, Uses ATP)	
Pumps	Hydrogen, sodium, and potassium ions moved by protein pumps
Endocytosis	Intake of substance by creating a vesicle
Pinocytosis	Random uptake of small amounts of extracellular fluid and solutes
Phagocytosis	Large-scale uptake of particles and cells, especially important in defense
Receptor-mediated	Specific uptake of molecules after binding to a ligand
Exocytosis	Secretion of products and wastes via secretory vesicles

ATP, adenosine triphosphate.

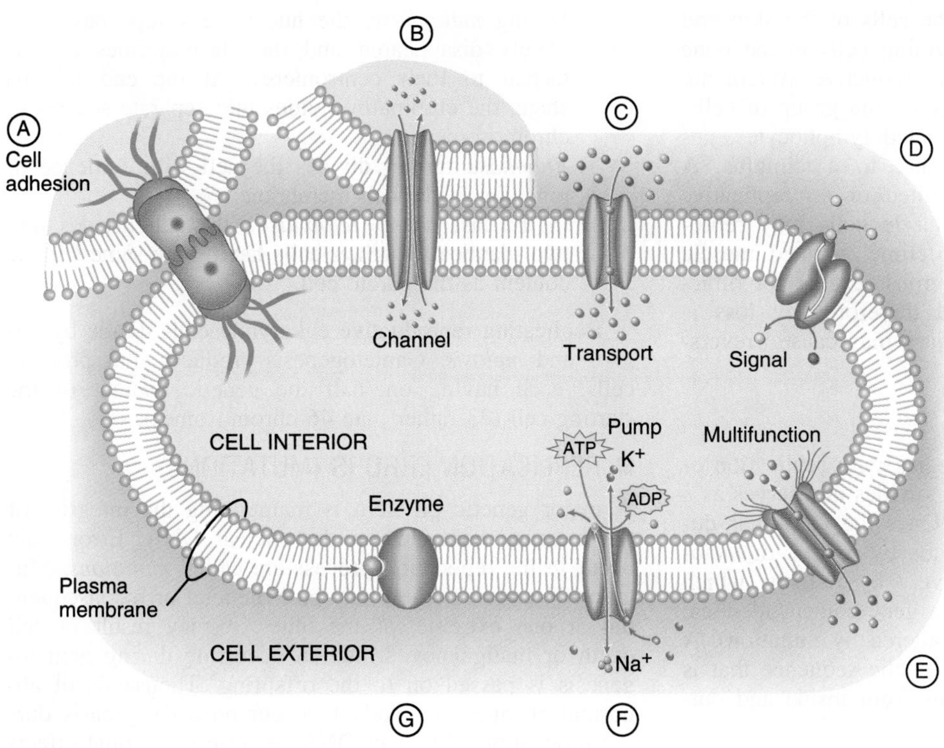

FIGURE U4–3 The cell membrane is responsible for adhesion to adjacent cells (A) and movement of substances in and out of the cell. Several mechanisms are required: gap junctions allow communication between neighboring cells by transfer of small molecules (B); passive transport of molecules (C); signal receptor proteins that bind to surface signal molecules and transfer a message to the cell interior (D); use of integral proteins to transport specific molecules (E); ATP-driven pumps to actively transport ions from one compartment to another (F); and use of membrane bound enzymes, which have active sites on either side of the cell membrane (G). ADP, adenosine diphosphate; ATP, adenosine triphosphate.

changes shape when a protein binds to it, then opens and closes. These channels are seen in cells that respond to hormones, drugs, or neurotransmitters. A *voltage-gated* channel opens or closes when there are changes in the electrical voltage across the membrane. These channels are seen in all three types of muscle cells: skeletal, smooth and cardiac.

A *mechanically gated* channel opens in response to deforming forces, such as pressure or friction. These channels are found in blood vessels, skin, and sensory nerves. Channels that leak are important in the cardiac, nervous, and muscle tissue for the rapid transmission of electrical pacemaker messages.

Intercellular Communication

Special sites on cell membranes play a role in communication and interaction between cells, both nearby and at a distance. Membrane proteins mediate this communication, serving as ligand-binding receptors and as transducers that initiate enzymatic function in the cell. Hormones as well as an extensive group of molecules called *cytokines* are involved in intercellular signaling.

Some cell surface molecules serve as mammalian blood group isoantigens (e.g., ABO, Rh). Others act as histocompatibility antigens, which detect self and non-self in immune function and in tissue and organ transplants.

■ NUCLEUS

The nucleus is the most prominent organelle in the eukaryotic cell. It is surrounded by a porous double membrane (the *nuclear envelope*). Within the nucleus are one or more nucleoli, visible among a mass of chromosomes. The nucleus contains the genetic material of the cell in the form of chromatin threads composed of deoxyribonucleic acid (DNA). Each cell, except the reproductive cells, contains a person's full genetic complement of DNA (46 chromosomes).

The DNA contains the recipes for all the proteins in the body. The DNA in the nucleus is unable to pass through the nuclear envelope into the cytoplasm; yet it is in the cytoplasm that polypeptides and proteins are synthesized. These proteins are used for structure or control of all metabolic and physiologic activities of the cell. Therefore, DNA must transfer its instructions for synthesizing proteins to molecules that can carry the information from the nucleus to the cytoplasm. It does this through a two-step process: transcription and translation.

TRANSCRIPTION. DNA serves as a template for the assembly of molecules of ribonucleic acid (RNA). The two linked chains of DNA separate from one another, exposing part of the base sequence. RNA links to the DNA template and then serves as the messenger (mRNA) and moves from the nucleus to the cytoplasm for protein synthesis.

TRANSLATION. At the ribosome, mRNA is used to assemble proteins in specific order. This step (translation) requires that the mRNA bind to the ribosome and that the ribosome "read" the RNA. Transfer RNA (tRNA) transports the amino acids in the cytoplasm to the ribosome, and the protein is assembled. In a human body, roughly 100,000 genes produce about 60,000 essential proteins. A single cell can synthesize about 20,000 different proteins (an awesome achievement).

CELL REPLICATION

Besides producing proteins, most body cells also must reproduce themselves. In the healthy adult body, somatic cells replicate at varying rates. The cells of the skin and mucous membranes, the blood-forming cells in the bone marrow, and some cells in the reproductive system are replaced at a high constant rate. A second group of cells, such as hepatocytes and differentiated lymphocytes, undergoes replication only in response to a stimulus. A third group of cells has very limited or no replicative capabilities. Individual smooth muscle cells may reproduce only once or twice in a lifetime; striated muscle cells (heart and skeleton) and neurons (except for olfactory cells) do not replicate, and therefore any loss is permanent. Thus, a spinal cord injury may cause irreversible paralysis.

■ STAGES OF REPLICATION

The process of cell replication begins with replication of the genetic information. The DNA divides and serves as a template for its own duplication. Once the DNA has duplicated, eukaryotic cells may divide by *mitosis* or *meiosis.* Somatic cells divide exclusively by mitosis, which produces two daughter cells with a gene content identical to that of the parent cell (unless altered by mutation). A cell undergoing mitosis follows a cyclic sequence that is driven by a combination of signals from inside and outside the cell (Fig. U4–4).

Mitosis involves several steps:

1. In *prophase,* two centrioles move toward opposite poles of the cell, fibers become visible, and the nucleolus disappears. The chromatin threads of DNA become visible as structures called *chromosomes.*

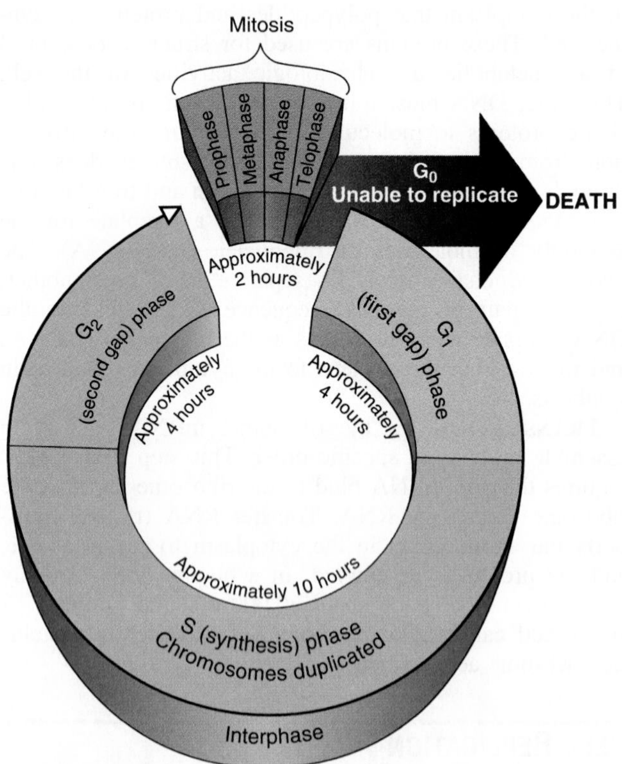

FIGURE U4–4 Phases in the life cycle of a cell. Actual times vary, depending on the type of cell.

2. During *metaphase,* the nuclear envelope has completely disappeared and the chromosomes are attached to their centromeres. At the end of this stage, the chromatin divides into separate strands of chromosomes.
3. *Anaphase* further divides the cell with evidence of pinching of the cell membrane.
4. In the last phase *(telophase),* the cell divides into two identical daughter cells having the same genetic content as the parent cell.

Replicating reproductive eukaryotic cells divide by *mitosis* and *meiosis.* Gametogenesis produces four progeny cells, each having one-half the genetic content of the starting cell (23 rather than 46 chromosomes).

■ REPLICATION ERRORS (MUTATIONS)

A major genetic problem is maintaining the integrity of the message contained in the nuclear DNA. Errors that occur in the replication process are called *mutations.* Mutation in a somatic cell may be beneficial or inconsequential at one extreme; at the other, it may result in cell death or malignancy. Mutation occurring during gametogenesis is passed on to the offspring. Thousands of abnormal changes are likely to occur on a daily basis during replication of human DNA because of thermal effects and inappropriate metabolic events. In nearly all cases, however, the DNA is restored to normal configurations by a variety of repair mechanisms. Abnormal genes that escape repair may result in diseases such as phenylketonuria or sickle cell disease.

Biotechnologists are applying recent advances in genetic engineering to the prevention and therapy of diseases. Using restriction *endonuclease* (which hydrolyzes or cuts DNA at specific sequences) and *DNA ligase* (which recombines the cut ends of DNA fragments), biotechnologists can cut selected genes out of sections of human DNA molecules, insert them into bacterial *plasmids* (extrachromosomal genetic elements in bacteria that can incorporate segments of human DNA), and produce large quantities of the gene product. Many benefits are being realized and anticipated from the use of this technology:

- Increased yields and improved antimicrobial action of antibiotics
- More effective and safer virus vaccines (prepared from gene components)
- Ability to produce mammalian proteins, including clotting factors, insulin, human growth hormone, and interferons
- Development of "magic bullets" for treating many conditions, including tumors, through precise modification of reactive sites in antibodies
- Development of transgenic plants and animals for increasing and improving nutritional sources for humans.

CELLS IN TISSUES AND ORGANS

Cells working together as a unit are called *tissues.* Tissues unite to form individual *organs.* The four major specialized types of cells that unite into larger tissue units are the following:

1. *Epithelial cells* are arranged in sheets. They cover the outside of the body (epidermis) and form the absorptive linings of the body's cavities and tubular structures (such as mucosa and glands).
2. *Nerve cells* form the highly specialized, irritable, and conductive nerve tissue. Destroyed nerve cells cannot be replaced.
3. *Muscle cells* allow mobility of body parts as well as mobility of substances (such as air, blood, and waste) within the body by contracting and relaxing.
4. *Connective tissue cells* support other cells and tissues. They include blood cells and structural cells found in bones, tendons, and ligaments. Blood cells carry oxygen to the tissues and carbon dioxide and wastes from the tissues. They also defend the body against foreign substances. Structural cells build the bony scaffolding and form the critical intercellular proteins that bind together the cells of the body. Collagen is an important extracellular connective tissue protein.

ALTERATIONS IN CELL STRUCTURE AND FUNCTION

The major causes of cellular alterations include changes in gene structure and function (either newly acquired or hereditary) and degeneration of normal tissue due to aging, excessive use, or infiltration by foreign substances (including fat, water, glycogen, and proteins).

ATROPHY

Atrophy is the wasting or decrease in size of a normally developed organ. This condition results from a decrease either in the number of cells or in the size of the cells composing it. Atrophy may follow disuse of an organ. For example, muscle atrophy may develop following denervation or prolonged immobilization. Muscular atrophy caused by aging can be greatly minimized by physical activity. Because the adrenal glands normally secrete corticosteroids, atrophy of these glands can occur when large doses of corticosteroids are administered over a prolonged period. Atrophy also accompanies the normal physiologic aging process. The thymus gland increases in size during childhood and very gradually starts to atrophy during adolescence. The ovaries atrophy after menopause.

HYPERTROPHY

Hypertrophy is an increase in the size of an organ or tissue resulting from an increase in the size of the cells. Hypertrophy sometimes represents the response of an organ to a greater workload. For example, when the heart is subjected to great strain, the left ventricle of the heart enlarges (hypertrophies) in order to handle the additional stress. Another example is the increased size of the biceps muscle in people engaged in strenuous physical activity.

PRECANCEROUS CHANGES

Hyperplasia is an increase in the number of cells. Hyperplasia can be an expected cellular response, such as increased cell regeneration in the formation of calluses. Pathologic hyperplasia can become cancerous.

Dysplasia is deranged cellular growth or a form of hyperplasia. It results from persistent severe injury or irritation.

Metaplasia is the transformation of one mature cell type or tissue into another. Usually, the new cell does not perform the functions of the cell it replaced. Metaplastic cells can transform into malignant cancer cells.

NEOPLASTIC (CANCEROUS) CHANGES

Neoplastic change is characterized by disturbances in cell differentiation and growth. When normal cells undergo transformation into cancerous cells, they fail to respond to normal regulatory forces and instead show unrestrained growth. These unregulated replicating cells *(neoplasms)* may then invade contiguous healthy tissues or become detached from the primary tumor and spread *(metastasize)* to other parts of the body where they continue to divide. This alteration in normal cell reproduction is discussed in greater detail in Chapter 18.

AGING

In a young healthy person, cells are biochemically active, have a high turnover rate (in some tissues), and have a high rate of metabolic and physiologic efficiency. In older adults, cells are less active, have a slower turnover rate, and begin to decline in efficiency. Aging cells shrink in size, protein synthesis slows, the Golgi apparatus shows signs of disintegration, and the mitochondria may undergo fragmentation. Aging affects every system of the body (Table U4–3).

Numerous theories exist regarding the aging process, but little is certain about how age-related changes occur. The age range of a cell is great. In the mature adult, an epithelial cell lining the intestinal tract lives only about 1½ days; a red blood cell can survive for 120 days. At the other extreme, nerve cells have a potential life expectancy of 100 years or more. In the immune system, immunocompetent cells appear to remain constant in numbers as people age but lose some of their interactive and regulatory properties. The resulting alteration in immune function is responsible for the increased incidence of autoimmune disease, the appearance of tumors, and the greater susceptibility to infection seen in the elderly population.

One theory of aging is that unrepaired mutations accumulate on DNA, causing changes that lead to aging. For example, highly specialized cells (such as nerve cells) do not reproduce. When these cells die from injury or disease and are not replaced, the remaining cells must assume their functions. The greater workload may stress these cells, cause them to age faster, and hasten their dying.

Another hypothesis is that each of us is born with a genetic clock that governs our life span. This theory is based on the observation that each cell type has a finite number of divisions. This concept is supported in part by similarities in life spans seen in various family groups.

TABLE U4–3 PHYSIOLOGIC CHANGES OF AGING: AN OVERVIEW

System	Physiologic Changes
Cardiovascular	Decreased vessel elasticity due to calcification and connective tissue (increased pulmonary vascular resistance) Decreased number of heart muscle fibers, with increased size of individual fibers (hypertrophy) Decreased filling capacity Decreased stroke volume Decreased sensitivity of baroreceptors Degeneration of vein valves
Respiratory	Decreased chest wall compliance due to calcification of the costal cartilage Decreased alveolar ventilation Decreased respiratory muscle strength Air trapping and decreased ventilation due to degeneration of lung tissue (decreased elasticity)
Renal and urinary	Decreased glomerular filtration rate due to nephron degeneration (decreased 33%–50% by age 70) Decreased ability to concentrate urine Decreased ability to regulate hydrogen (H^+)
Gastrointestinal	Decreased muscular contraction Decreased esophageal emptying Decreased bowel motility Decreased production of hydrochloric acid (HCl), enzymes, and intrinsic factor Decreased hepatic enzyme production and metabolic capacity Thinning of stomach mucosa
Neurologic and sensory	Degeneration and atrophy of nerve cells Decrease of 25% to 45% in neurons Decrease in neurotransmitters Decreased rate of conduction of nerve impulses Loss of taste buds Loss of auditory hair cells and sclerosis of the eardrum
Musculoskeletal	Decreased muscle mass Bone demineralization Joint degeneration, erosion, and calcification
Immune	Decreased inflammatory response Decrease in T-cell function due to involution of the thymus gland
Integumentary	Decreased subcutaneous fat Decreased elastin Atrophy of the sweat glands Atrophy of the epidermal arterioles, causing altered temperature regulation

From Copstead, L. C., & Banasik, J. (2000). *Pathophysiology.* Philadelphia: W. B. Saunders.

MECHANISMS OF CELL DAMAGE

When cells are injured, injured organelles no longer carry out their specific functions (e.g., mitochondria stop producing ATP). The extent of the damage depends on (1) the nature, intensity, and duration of the stressor; (2) whether the blood supply to the cells is affected; and (3) the state of differentiation or metabolic activity of the cells. Indeed, two clients exposed to the same injurious substance may not sustain the same degree of injury because of the influence of modifying factors. For example, a person's nutritional and emotional state can have a profound impact on the extent and consequences of a slight to moderate level of injury. However, there is a point after which cell death inevitably occurs. The mechanisms responsible for the transition from reversible to irreversible cellular damage are not completely understood.

■ HYPOXIA

Hypoxia (inadequate tissue oxygenation) is a leading cause of cell injury and death. Hypoxia can occur as a result of:

- Vascular disease or injury, which impedes blood flow to tissues
- Insufficient oxygenation of blood caused by conditions such as carbon monoxide poisoning

Depending on the severity of the hypoxic state, cells compensate and recover or are killed. (For example, if the femoral artery becomes stenotic, the skeletal muscles of the legs will eventually atrophy as a result of the inadequate blood flow and the consequent reduced oxygen supply. Severe or chronic hypoxia will result in cell injury or death.)

The most common cause of hypoxia is *ischemia,* or reduced blood supply. Progressive hypoxia caused by gradual narrowing of arteries *(atherosclerosis)* is better tolerated than sudden anoxia caused by an obstruction in the blood supply.

■ TEMPERATURE EXTREMES

Extreme heat damages cells by coagulating cytoplasmic protein. Even mild heat results in permanent cellular damage if it is applied over a prolonged period to people with impaired circulation, as seen in peripheral vascular disease. Heat in these cases increases the metabolic needs of cells and tissues and leads to insufficient oxygen levels. Coupled with a reduced capacity to dispose of waste products, this process accelerates the damage to the affected tissue.

Cold constricts the smaller blood vessels, thereby decreasing the circulation of blood and oxygen to tissues. Freezing temperatures may cause the intracellular water to crystallize, which destroys the cell's structure. Cold injury can result in frostbite, permanently injuring the tissues involved. Very low temperatures cause stasis of blood, clot formation, arterial occlusion, ischemia, and ultimately cell death and necrosis.

■ IONIZING RADIATION

Exposure to radiation causes mutations, inactivates enzymes, and interrupts cell division. The fact that radiation inhibits mitosis makes this therapy important in the treatment of cancer, a disease involving pathologic cell reproduction. Radiation affects virtually all cells, but certain cells are more susceptible than others. Reproductive cells, cells in the lymph nodes and gastrointestinal tract, and bone marrow cells are highly sensitive to damage by radiation exposure, whereas cells of cartilage, muscle, brain, and endocrine glands are relatively insensitive. People who work with radioactive materials or nuclear fission reactors or who are giving or receiving radiotherapy are most at risk for cellular trauma from radiation.

■ ELECTRICAL INJURY

Electrical energy generates heat when it passes through the body and may thus produce burns. It also interferes with neural conduction and often causes death from cardiac dysrhythmias. The extent of damage from electrical energy depends on its voltage and amperage, tissue resistance, and the pathway of the current as it passes through the body. Users of electrical equipment should be aware that exposure to 100 milliamperes (mA) can be lethal to humans. Electrical burns are discussed in Chapter 50.

■ CHEMICAL INJURY

Chemicals harm cells by destroying or altering their structure and by disrupting their metabolism. The capacity of a chemical to injure a cell depends on the strength and toxicity of the chemical as well as on the susceptibility of the cell. Many chemicals can injure cells. Highly toxic substances are called *poisons.* Minute amounts of poisonous substances, such as cyanide and arsenic, can cause death. Some of the most toxic substances known are bacterial exotoxins, such as diphtheria toxin and botulinum toxin.

Environmental chemicals, such as herbicides, pesticides, and air pollutants, are potential causes of cellular injury. Lead-based paint, which tastes sweet, is often eaten by children. Lead-based paint on walls and window blinds comes off in dust particles and can be inhaled. Dangerous amounts of lead may also be found in water pipes and drinking water in older homes. Ingested or inhaled lead destroys cells in the nervous system (which may lead to mental retardation in young children), affects blood cell production, and damages the kidneys.

Workers around machinery and home owners with gas appliances must guard against carbon monoxide poisoning. Carbon monoxide binds tightly and 210 times more rapidly than oxygen to hemoglobin, preventing normal exchange of oxygen and carbon dioxide.

■ BACTERIAL INJURY

Microorganisms such as bacteria injure host cells by direct attack or by the toxins they produce. Bacterial toxins are classified as (1) endotoxins or (2) exotoxins.

Endotoxins may act directly with macrophages and T lymphocytes, causing the release of cytokines. Endotoxins acting on macrophages stimulate the production of interleukin-1 (IL-1) and tumor necrosis factor (TNF), two cytokines that in large quantities cause bacterial septic shock, a condition that is often fatal. Endotoxins may also activate the complement cascade, producing disseminated intravascular coagulation (DIC), another potentially fatal condition. Successful intervention in endotoxemia is difficult and often impossible to achieve.

Exotoxins are proteins and have specific toxic effects. For example, *Clostridium tetani,* the organism that causes tetanus, produces a neurotoxin that blocks processes that inhibit neural transmission in the central nervous system (CNS). Preventive immunization is possible with a few exotoxins (such as *C. tetani*), and in some cases an exotoxemia can be successfully treated with antitoxins (e.g., diphtheria).

■ VIRAL INJURY

Viruses have been described as mobile genetic elements protected by outer layers of protein and lipoprotein. Viruses attach to specific receptors on host cell surfaces and are taken up by endocytosis. The nucleic acid core of the virus passes through the vesicular membrane into the interior of the host cell. The viral genome then subverts the host cell metabolic machinery and begins to make viral components. While inside the host cell, the virus is protected from the host's reactive cells and solutes. The assembled *virions* may then exit the cell either by lysing the cell remnant or by permitting the host cell to remain viable while continuously secreting virions across the cell membrane. Viruses damage host cells by killing them, depriving them of nutrients, or causing cells to transform into a tumor state.

■ MECHANICAL INJURY

Cells can be damaged by physical impact or irritation. Examples of this type of injury include blisters from tight shoes, abrasions, lacerations, and contusions (bruises). Cells can be injured in other ways as well. Light can damage cells of the cornea. Noise can damage the eardrum (tympanic membrane), the ossicle in the middle ear, and the organ of Corti in the inner ear. Prolonged contact with vibrating objects can alter muscle and bone structure as well as nerve conduction. Clients at risk for these injuries are those who work with power tools.

■ NUTRITIONAL IMBALANCE

Inadequate protein intake decreases the function of the intestinal mucosa and pancreas, which in turn reduces nutrient absorption. Plasma proteins, especially albumin, help retain fluid in blood vessels. When levels of plasma proteins decline, fluid tends to move into interstitial spaces, causing edema. Antibodies or immunoglobulins are protein; therefore, the lack of proteins adversely affects immune system function and increases the risk of infection.

Inadequate carbohydrate intake forces the body to use fats for energy. The liver becomes overwhelmed and ketone bodies are formed that accumulate in the blood, a condition known as *ketosis.* Ketosis develops because of the rapid breakdown of fatty acids stored in adipose tissue. Fatty acids are used for energy when the daily intake of carbohydrates is less than 50 g. Clients at high risk for ketosis include those with diabetes, those on starvation diets, and those on low-carbohydrate diets.

Increased fat intake often causes fat deposition in heart, liver, and muscle and may lead to obesity, coronary heart disease, stroke, or breast and colon cancer.

Growth factors include amino acids, purines and pyrimidines, and vitamins. These nutrients are required but cannot be synthesized. Insufficient quantities of these substances can seriously impair the ability of the cell to take up and metabolize nutrients or to synthesize macromolecules for structural building and reproduction.

■ CELL DEATH

Cells die as a result of being traumatized, through alteration by disease, from failure caused by genetic alterations, or through a programmed process called *apoptosis.* Apoptosis usually does not disturb the steady-state nature of the tissue and thus gives no sign of its occurrence.

CONCLUSIONS

Cells are the basic units of life, and they serve many functions. The integrity and existence of the organism is dependent on the individual and collective ability of body cells to digest and assimilate substances, protect themselves by reacting to stimuli, replicate, metabolize, and produce energy. When cells lose their ability to function normally because of injury or attack by pathogens, the organism will show signs of distress and disease will develop.

Recent advances in molecular biology are providing the means for great improvements in the diagnosis and treatment of many human diseases. Only those professionals who keep current in the field will be able to comprehend the nature and consequences of the pathologic changes associated with disease processes and will know how to make and evaluate therapeutic decisions.

BIBLIOGRAPHY

1. Alberts, B. D., et al. (1994). *Molecular biology of the cell* (3rd ed.). New York: Garland.
2. Barnes, D. E., Lindahl, T., & Sedgwick, B. (1993). DNA repair. *Current Opinion in Cell Biology, 5,* 424.
3. Becker, W. M., Reece, J. B., & Poenie, M. F. (1995). *The world of the cell* (3rd ed.). New York: Benjamin/Cummings.
4. Berridge, M. J. (1994). The biology and medicine of calcium signalling. *Molecular and Cellular Endocrinology, 98,* 119.
5. Hartwell, L. H., & Kastan, M. B. (1994). Cell cycle control and cancer. *Science, 266,* 1821.
6. Mulligan, R. C. (1993). The basic science of gene therapy. *Science, 260,* 926.
7. Welch, W. J. (1993). How cells respond to stress. *Scientific American, 268,* 56.
8. Yeh, E. (1998, August 15). Life and death of the cell. *Hospital Practice,* 85–92.

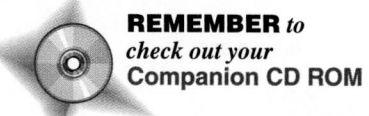

CHAPTER 12

Clients with Fluid Imbalances: Promoting Positive Outcomes

Bernadette White

Dehydration is the most common fluid and electrolyte imbalance in the United States. The Health Care Financing Administration has identified dehydration as one of the most frequent diagnoses upon hospital admission, present in more than 1 million admissions per year. Dehydration is especially common among older adults and therefore is expected to increase as our population ages. Dehydration carries a 17% to 45% morbidity and mortality rate.[36] The cost to society includes not only the cost of admission, diagnosis, and treatment of the dehydration and secondary complications but also the financial and psychological loss to the family and society of a productive contributor.

This chapter provides the basic knowledge necessary to promote positive health outcomes for clients at risk for fluid and electrolyte imbalances. Positive health outcomes are achieved through health promotion, health maintenance, and health restoration strategies. Clearly, water is not only responsible for the body's structure and function; it is also necessary for the maintenance of equilibrium and of life itself.

OVERVIEW

Fluids exist in two compartments in the body: (1) the *intracellular* fluid (ICF) compartment, inside the cells, and (2) the *extracellular* fluid (ECF) compartment, outside the cells. Two thirds of body fluid is intracellular. Although water is the predominant component in each of these compartments, the word *fluid* is used to indicate that other substances (glucose, sodium, waste products) are also found in these compartments and that they influence the water balance in and between compartments.

The ECF compartment is further divided into the *intravascular* (e.g., plasma) and *interstitial* (between cells) compartments. Cerebrospinal, lymphatic, synovial, and eye fluids are also part of the ECF compartment. Interstitial fluid compartments are also known as *tissue spaces* or *third spaces.*

Fluids move between the intracellular, intravascular, and interstitial compartments to maintain fluid balance. Fluid in the cells is the most stable; cells are fairly resistant to major fluid shifts. Fluids in the bloodstream are the most changeable, quickly lost or gained by intake of fluids or by loss of fluids through sweat, urination, diarrhea, and so on. Fluids in the interstitial spaces are the reserve fluids, replacing fluid in the cells or the blood.

About 60% of the body's total weight is water, although this percentage varies with stature and lean body mass. Among short and obese people, 50% of body mass is water. In athletes and lean people, water comprises 70% of total body weight.

■ FLUID MOVEMENT FROM PRESSURE CHANGES

Fluids move between compartments to maintain homeostasis. Changes in pressure promote fluid movement. Most fluid movement, (i.e., water and dissolved particles in the water) takes place across the capillary wall. Forces that move fluids are constantly at work and allow the fluid taken in orally to maintain blood pressure and hydrate cells and eventually to be excreted as urine.

Figure 12–1 demonstrates *hydrostatic* and *oncotic pressures* within the capillary. Blood moves through the vascular system from areas of high pressure (arteries) to areas of low pressure (capillaries and veins) via hydrostatic pressure. *Hydrostatic pressure* is the pressure exerted against the wall of the blood vessel by the blood inside it. *Oncotic* (sometimes called *osmotic*) *pressure* results from the presence of "nondiffusible" (too large, opposing ionic charge) proteins. These proteins create a pressure that draws fluid to it. Oncotic pressures pull fluids back into the vessel on the venous end of the capillary.

As arterial blood enters the capillary, it is at higher pressure than the surrounding tissues. Fluids are pushed into the interstitial spaces from the arterial end. This passive form of fluid movement is known as *filtration.* As blood continues to flow through the capillary, the volume of blood is reduced, thereby reducing the pressure. By the time blood reaches the venous end of the capillary, pressure is higher in the interstitial space and fluid returns to

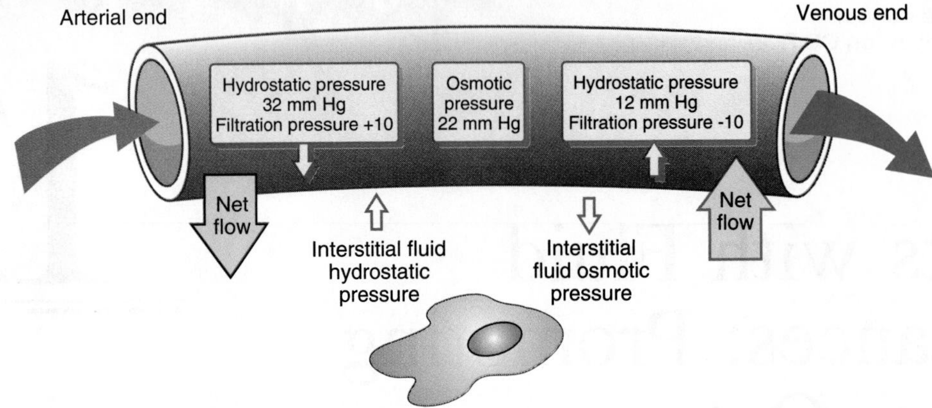

FIGURE 12–1 Pressure differences inside the capillary are responsible for movement of fluids. Fluid moves out of the capillary at the arterial end because hydrostatic pressure in the vessel exceeds pressure in the tissues. Fluids return to the vessel at the venous end because proteins (colloids) in the vessel exert a pulling pressure on them. Under normal conditions, movement of fluids is almost equal, and neither dehydration nor edema results. Fluid that remains in the interstitium is transported via the lymphatics to the vascular system. Abnormal conditions occur with the presence of too much fluid, too few proteins, changes in the capillary wall, or lymphatic obstruction.

the capillary. This form of fluid movement is known as *reabsorption.* The terms “reabsorption,” “absorption,” and “resorption” are clarified in Box 12–1. The movement of fluids is based on the presence of proper amounts of pressure on both sides of the capillary wall.

Proteins in the interstitial spaces and in the capillary pull fluids toward themselves. Therefore, proteins promote fluid movement both ways: into the interstitial space and into the capillary. Because these forces are due to protein, this process is often called *colloid (protein) osmotic pressure.* The most common protein in plasma is *albumin,* which is responsible for most of the fluid movement at the capillary level. Albumin comprises 50% of the plasma proteins but contributes to 80% of the osmotic force inside the capillary. The proper movement of fluids is also based on adequate amounts of protein on both sides of the capillary wall.

As blood moves through the capillary, not all of the fluid that passed into the interstitial spaces is recaptured. The remainder is returned to the central circulation by the lymphatic system. As interstitial and tissue fluid pressures increase, one-way valves in the terminal lymphatic capillaries open and fluid enters. Pressure or skeletal muscle movement from outside of the lymphatics propels the fluid forward into larger lymphatic vessels and eventually to the thoracic duct or the right lymph duct and then into the left subclavian vein. Valves inside the lymphatic vessels prevent back flow of fluid. The lymphatics also return small proteins that have leaked into the tissues.

BOX 12–1 Concepts: Absorption, Reabsorption, and Resorption

In addition to many other concepts, three often confusing concepts are discussed in this chapter: absorption, reabsorption, and resorption.

- *Absorption* usually refers to the initial movement of substances, such as the end products of digestion or medications, into the vascular spaces from an organ, such as the gastrointestinal tract, muscle, subcutaneous or dermal tissue, or buccal or pharyngeal tissues.
- *Reabsorption* refers to the movement of water, electrolytes, vitamins, amino acids, glucose, lactate, or other essential substances from one compartment, such as the interstitium or renal tubules, back into capillaries.
- *Resorption* refers to the process of calcium salts leaving the bone and moving into the blood in an ionized form.

FLUID MOVEMENT BY DIFFUSION AND OSMOLALITY

Diffusion is the most important means by which substances such as nutrients and waste products move between blood and the interstitial spaces. It is the movement of fluids or substances across a membrane because of differences in concentration. Substances diffuse across the membrane to equal the concentration on each side of the membrane.

Osmolality and a related concept, *osmolarity,* refer to the concentration of solutes (electrolytes, glucose, urea, protein) in 1 liter (L) of solution. The more solute present, the higher the osmolality. Fluids of high osmolality tend to pull water across a membrane to reduce the osmolality by reducing the ratio of solute to solvent.

Osmolality is measured by the number of dissolved particles per kilogram of water. Because 1 L of water is equal to 1 kg of weight, the terms osmolality and osmolarity are frequently used interchangeably. Electrolytes, especially sodium and protein, contribute the largest number of particles to the osmolality. Urea and glucose also contribute to osmolality.

Sodium is the most abundant and easily accessible electrolyte in plasma. The concentration of sodium is used to measure osmolality. Normal plasma osmolality is 275 to 295 mOsm/kg of water. This is an *iso-osmolar* state because the fluid contains particles (*solutes*) and water (*solvent*) in approximately equal proportions. When there are *more than* 295 mOsm/kg of water, a *hyperosmolar* (*hypertonic*) state results. In contrast, fluid with *less than* 275 mOsm/kg of water is *hyposmolar* (*hypo-*

tonic) fluid because it has fewer particles than water. Thirst is regulated in the hypothalamus, and changes in the osmolality of circulating blood produce thirst.

■ HORMONAL REGULATION OF FLUID BALANCE

The hypothalamus regulates osmolality by producing *antidiuretic hormone* (ADH), also called vasopressin. The term *diuresis* means to produce and excrete urine; therefore, this hormone slows the production of dilute urine, thereby retaining body fluids.

ADH is stored in the posterior pituitary gland. Increasing serum osmolarity is sensed by the hypothalamus, and it signals the posterior pituitary gland to release ADH into circulation. ADH reduces urinary output by enlarging the size of the pores in the distal and collecting tubules in the nephron, returning fluids to the body rather than excreting them. ADH allows the kidneys to produce a range of urine volumes and concentrations. When body fluid levels are dangerously low, ADH also constricts arterioles to shunt blood from the peripheral areas and promote perfusion of the major organs.

ADH is released continuously in response to many conditions, not just during emergencies. These conditions include a lack of water intake (as from nothing by mouth [NPO] status), uncontrolled water loss (as from watery diarrhea), consumption of concentrated food or fluids, pain, and use of certain medications, such as narcotics, barbiturates, and anesthetics. Emotional or physiologic stress can also trigger ADH release, during surgery, trauma, severe anxiety, or prolonged exercise.

Factors that suppress ADH include hyposmolality of the ECF, increased blood volume, exposure to cold, acute alcohol ingestion, carbon dioxide inhalation, and administration of some diuretics, lithium, and some antipsychotic medications. Disorders of the pituitary gland can also lead to failure to release ADH. These situations lead to increased urine output (diuresis). Sometimes diuresis is desirable, but other times it is dangerous. Can you see potential problems with uncontrollable diuresis or with diuresis in clients who are unable to respond to thirst?

Aldosterone, another hormone that controls fluid balance, is secreted by the adrenal cortex and conserves body sodium by promoting potassium excretion from the kidneys. Sodium retains fluid, and under the action of aldosterone fluid is thus also retained.

Aldosterone secretion is a four-step process:

1. When arterial blood flow is decreased to the kidneys, renin is released by the juxtaglomerular apparatus of the kidney.
2. In the blood, renin converts angiotensinogen to angiotensin I.
3. Angiotensin I is further converted to angiotensin II by a converting enzyme from the lungs.
4. The presence of angiotensin II stimulates secretion of aldosterone from the adrenal cortex.

This process is called the *renin-angiotensin system.* Adrenocorticotropic hormone (ACTH) from the anterior pituitary is necessary for aldosterone secretion, but its effect is limited. When ACTH levels are low, the kidney is less able to respond to sodium depletion. Figure 12–2 illustrates how the kidneys interact with hormones and the thirst mechanism to maintain fluid balance.

The two most powerful stimulants for aldosterone release are (1) decreased arterial blood flow in the kidney and (2) increased plasma potassium. Conditions such as hemorrhage, dehydration, and an upright posture reduce renal blood flow. An increased plasma sodium level slightly decreases aldosterone secretion.

Atrial natriuretic peptides, prostaglandins, and *kinins* also contribute to the regulation of sodium balance. Because their major action is on sodium, and secondarily on water, they are discussed in Chapter 13.

EXTRACELLULAR FLUID VOLUME DEFICIT

Extracellular fluid volume deficit (ECFVD), commonly called *dehydration,* is a decrease in intravascular and interstitial fluids. ECFVD is a common and serious fluid imbalance that results in vascular fluid volume loss (*hypovolemia*). With *mild* ECFVD, 1 to 2 L of water or 2% of body weight is lost; with *moderate* ECFVD, 3 to 5 L of water or 5% body weight is lost; and with *severe* ECFVD, 5 to 10 L of water or 8% of body weight is lost.

Etiology

Fluid balance is maintained in the body because the intake of fluids equals the excretion of fluids. This simple concept can be used to explain common causes of fluid imbalances. A lack of fluid intake, excessive fluid output, or both can lead to dehydration. Conversely, excessive fluid intake and a lack of fluid excretion can lead to overhydration. Further, alteration in any of the regulators of fluid balance—thirst, hormones, lymphatic system, and kidneys—increases the risk for or can cause an actual fluid imbalance.

LACK OF FLUID INTAKE

Average daily fluid intake for adults is about 1500 to 2000 ml. In addition, about 800 ml of fluid is consumed through solid foods; however, cognitive and physical impairments can quickly reduce water intake. For example, clients who are hospitalized, chairbound, or bedbound may not be able to reach their glass of water or may be too confused to recognize thirst. People with dysphagia or at risk for aspiration may not be able to swallow fluids safely. Tube-fed people who are not given adequate free water, or are fed hypertonic formulas, are also at risk. Community-dwelling older adults may have decreased access to fluids because of financial or transportation barriers or debilitation. For many of these reasons, nursing home residents older than 85 years of age appear to be at greatest risk for dehydration.

Impaired thirst mechanisms can also decrease fluid intake. Thirst usually develops from low blood pressure or fluid volume depletion as small as 0.5%. Low blood pressure can be seen in people who are losing fluids because of diuresis, diarrhea, bleeding, or drainage tubes. Excessive urination can be due to the use of diuretics (e.g., furosemide), intake of hypertonic fluids (e.g., hypertonic intravenous solutions), excretion of large volumes of glucose (e.g., ketoacidosis with diabetes mellitus), or, less commonly, neurologic problems (e.g., a lack of ADH production from diabetes insipidus). The sensation of a

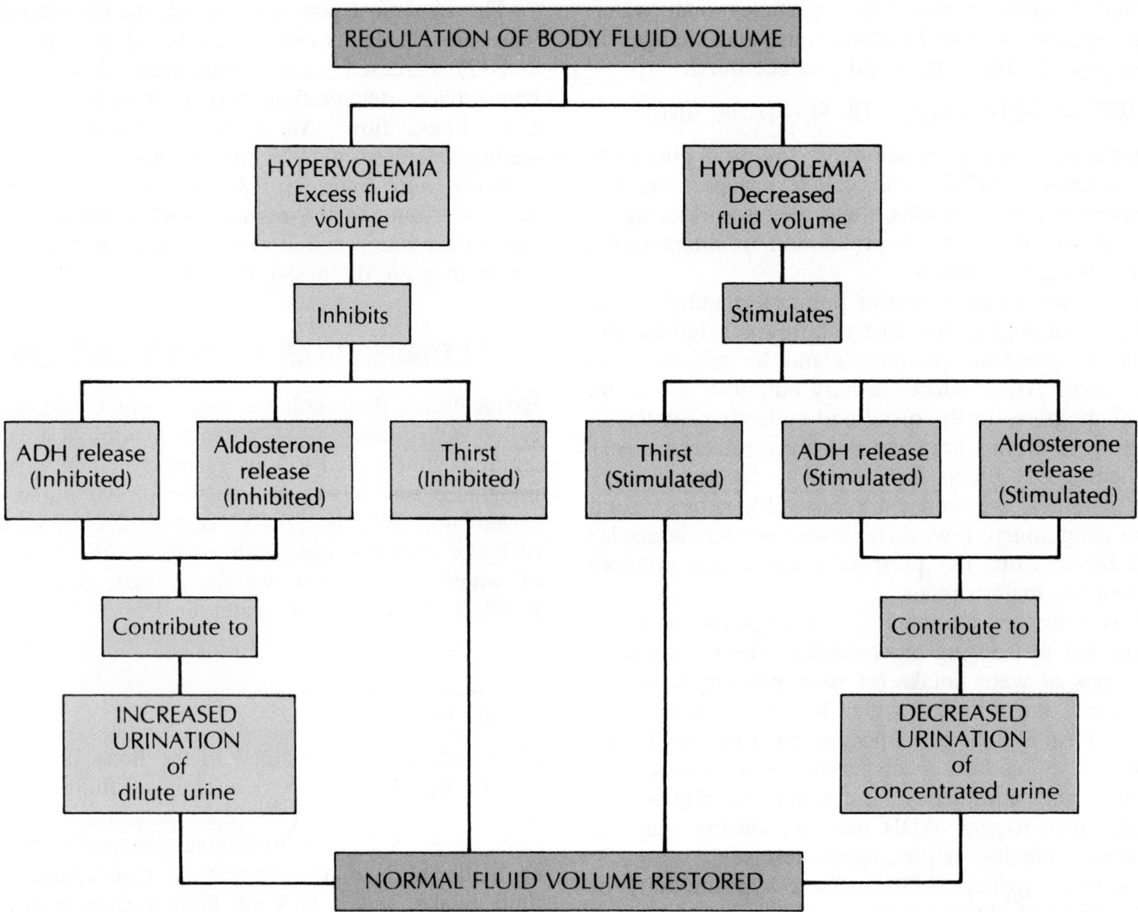

FIGURE 12–2 Regulation of body fluid volume depends on antidiuretic hormone (ADH), aldosterone, and thirst and fluid dynamics. (From White, B. [1994]. Maintaining fluid and electrolyte balance. In V. B. Bolander, [Ed.], *Sorensen and Luckmann's basic nursing: A psychophysiologic approach* [3rd ed.]. Philadelphia: W. B. Saunders.)

dry mouth also stimulates thirst. Clients may experience dry mouth from salivary gland dysfunction, head or neck radiation, smoking, mouth breathing, oxygen therapy, hyperventilation, and anticholinergic medications (such as atropine).

Most healthy people respond to decreased fluid levels by drinking fluids and thus maintain balance. However, the thirst mechanism is depressed in people with debilitating illnesses and in older adults, even the healthy elderly.[36] Several disorders also lead to inappropriate thirst mechanisms. People with excess fluids in the interstitial space, but depleted fluids in the vascular space, are commonly thirsty. Thirst is due to an increased renin-angiotensin-aldosterone response. Clients with congestive heart failure commonly experience this problem.

Osmolarity also influences thirst. Hyposmolarity inhibits the thirst response. Conversely, hyperosmolarity leads to thirst. It is common to find comatose and confused people with high plasma osmolarity, but they are unable to recognize the urge to drink.

Excess Fluid Losses

Severe vomiting and diarrhea are common causes of dehydration. These conditions are commonly associated with other clinical manifestations as well, such as changes in electrolytes. Potential causes of fluid loss include fever, diaphoresis, hyperglycemia, gastrointestinal suction, ileostomy, fistulae, burns, blood loss, hyperventilation, hyperthyroidism, decreased ADH secretion, diabetes insipidus (nephrogenic and neurogenic),[31] Addison's disease or adrenal crisis, diuretic phase of acute renal failure, and the use of diuretics.

Again, the elderly population is at risk for excessive fluid losses for several reasons: (1) decreased renal concentration of urine, (2) an altered ADH response, and (3) an increase in body fat and thus a decrease in total quantity of body water in proportion to body weight.[14, 36] Increased drug-drug interactions and multiple chronic diseases potentiate the risk for fluid imbalances.

Third-space fluid shifts (shifting of fluid from the vascular space to interstitial space where fluid cannot be easily exchanged) can result in a fluid deficit in the vascular compartment. Spaces that are prone to third-spacing include the peritoneal, pericardial, pleural, and joint cavities. Abdominal third-spacing is called ascites.

Pathophysiology

When fluids are lost from the ECF, fluids move in from the interstitial spaces to restore vascular volume and dilute the hypernatremic state. ADH and aldosterone are secreted to retain fluids by decreasing urine output. Fluids are also recruited from fecal matter in the colon. Decreased blood volume is sensed by *baroreceptors,* which send messages to the sympathetic nervous system to increase peripheral vasoconstriction and the heart rate in an attempt to move fluids from the periphery into circulation. Low blood volume is also sensed by the osmoreceptors in the hypothalamus, which signals the thirst mechanism. These compensatory processes occur over and over again in normal healthy people. When fluid loss continues or when the compensation fails to restore blood volume, the person becomes dehydrated.

If the dehydration is not corrected, fluid is shifted from the cells because the ECF is hypertonic in relation to the ICF. The salivary glands become less active. There is less cerebrospinal fluid (CSF) and less fluid in the fat pads around the eyes. Less fluid is available for temperature regulation via sweating, and a lowered blood volume decreases the body's ability to transport core heat to the periphery for conductive loss. If cerebral cells become dehydrated, the vessels may bleed or go into spasm, and thought processes may be impaired. If sodium is lost, the muscle and nerve functions that depend on this electrolyte are slowed. A full discussion of sodium imbalances is provided in Chapter 13.

Clinical Manifestations

There are three types of extracellular fluid (ECF) volume deficits:

- *Hyperosmolar* fluid volume deficit: water loss is greater than electrolyte (sodium) loss
- *Iso-osmolar* fluid volume deficit: water and electrolyte (sodium) losses are equal
- *Hypotonic* fluid volume deficit: electrolyte loss is greater than fluid loss (rare)

Loss of Body Weight

Because water is a major portion of body weight, fairly rapid weight loss is an early and common result of fluid loss. A mild ECFVD exists when weight loss equals 2% of body weight. For example, in a client who weighs 150 pounds (68 kg), a 2% loss equals 1.4 L of water. Severe fluid loss exceeds 6% of body weight. In mild forms of dehydration, weight loss may not occur because it is masked by trapped fluids in the third space.

Changes in Intake and Output

Intake and output (I & O) measurements provide another means of assessing fluid balance. These data provide insight into the cause of the imbalance (such as decreased fluid intake or increased fluid loss). I & O measurements are not as accurate as body weight, however, because of relative risk of errors in recording.

Thirst is an early clinical manifestation of ECFVD in a conscious person. Clients often request plain, cold water rather than carbonated or caffeinated beverages. This is advantageous because caffeine is a diuretic and sweet fluids may not quench thirst.

Urine output usually decreases with ECFVD because of the effects of ADH and aldosterone. Urine is usually concentrated, with specific gravity above 1.030 and urine osmolarity above 1000 mOsm/kg. For many years, it had been thought that the kidneys had to excrete at least 30 ml of urine per hour as a mechanism for waste removal. Today, a urine output of 400 to 500 ml/day (16–20 ml/hr) is considered *oliguria* and indicates a marked compromise in kidney function. In most people (perhaps not the critically ill), urine output varies throughout the day. Normally, urine output is low and concentration is higher during the night. Thus, the view that urine should flow constantly at 30 to 40 ml/hr appears to lack justification.

Two groups of clients can become dehydrated because they do not have the ability to concentrate urine: (1) those with diabetes insipidus who do not produce ADH, and (2) those with kidney failure that prevents urine concentration.

Changes in Vital Signs

Inadequate fluid volume also leads to a decrease in systolic blood pressure, a weak pulse, and a decrease in central venous pressure (CVP) and pulmonary capillary wedge pressure (PCWP). For every liter of fluid lost, the cardiac output decreases by 1 L/min, the heart rate increases eight beats per minute (BPM), and the core temperature increases by 0.3° C (0.6° F).[15] Postural hypotension is a classic sign of decreased fluid volume. It is defined as a drop in systolic blood pressure of more than 25 mm Hg, a drop in diastolic pressure of more than 20 mm Hg, and a pulse increase of 30 BPM or more when the client stands up.

Sympathetic nervous system stimulation leads to vasoconstriction and increases the heart rate in an attempt to compensate for the altered tissue perfusion. Without restoring fluids, the vasoconstrictive and tachycardic (rate > 100 BPM) responses provide only a minimal and temporary solution. If these responses continue, tissue perfusion is further compromised. Serious fluid loss can lead to systolic blood pressures below 70 mm Hg. Low systolic pressure impairs tissue perfusion to vital organs that have high metabolic demands, such as cerebral, cardiac, and kidney tissues.

Flat jugular veins in a supine position and a prolonged peripheral venous filling time of more than 5 seconds are also noted. Because of the inability to cool the body core, an elevated temperature is common and can reach 105° F.

Manifestations of Cellular Dehydration

The mucous membranes of the mouth and eyes become dry even though fluid is recruited from the interstitial spaces. The lips can crack, and furrows may be seen on the tongue. Swallowing can become difficult.

Tenting of the skin (decreased turgor) occurs when the skin tissues tend to stick together because of the decreased interstitial fluid. Tenting is not diagnostic of fluid deficit in older adults because tenting commonly results from loss of elastin in the skin in this population. Soft and sunken eyes may be noted. Muscle weakness from an imbalance of sodium and potassium occurs early and becomes worse as the deficit progresses. Feces become hard and decreased in number because the colon is trying to restore fluid balance.

Cerebral signs are always considered serious because it means that ICF compartmental shifting has occurred. Early signs include apprehension, restlessness, and headache. As the deficit progresses, hallucinations, maniacal behavior, and confusion occur, followed by coma.

DIAGNOSTIC FINDINGS

In hyposmolar fluid loss, more solvent is lost than solutes, which creates hemoconcentration. Plasma sodium concentration is also increased (*hypernatremia*). The following elevations are typical findings secondary to a hemoconcentrated state:

- Osmolality above 295 mOsm/kg
- Plasma sodium level above 145 mEq/L
- Blood urea nitrogen (BUN) above 25 mg/dl
- Plasma glucose above 120 mg/dl
- Hematocrit above 55%
- Urine specific gravity above 1.030

Specific gravity is a numeric value of urine concentration using solute-solvent relationships. Very concentrated urine has a high specific gravity. High specific gravity readings indicate dehydration or increased ADH. Glucose, protein, and dyes falsely elevate specific gravity. You can measure urine specific gravity by using a urinometer or by sending a urine sample to the laboratory for testing.

Hypernatremia usually indicates hyperosmolality, and hyponatremia usually indicates hyposmolality. Box 12–2 shows how to calculate plasma osmolality. Urine specific gravity may also be used as an indirect measurement of osmolality.

Outcome Management

The seriousness of a client's manifestations and the aggressiveness of treatment are related to both the *amount* and *acuteness* of the fluid loss and the client's state of health at the time of loss. Sudden loss of fluid does not give the compensatory mechanisms time to adapt; severe loss is often beyond the potential of compensatory mechanisms to adapt, resulting in vascular collapse or shock. A thorough history and physical examination, including collection of such demographic variables as age, gender, culture, presence of chronic diseases, and socioeconomic status, are critical to identifying realistic and measurable outcomes.

Medical treatment of fluid volume deficit depends on the acuteness and severity of the fluid deficit. The goals of treatment of ECFVD are to replace fluids and electrolytes (sodium primarily) that have been lost and to correct the underlying problem (such as vomiting or diarrhea).

BOX 12–2 How to Calculate Plasma Osmolality

To calculate plasma osmolality, you must know the plasma sodium (Na) level. Additionally, you should know the glucose level and blood urea nitrogen (BUN). The first formula may be used as a rough estimate of the plasma osmolality; the second formula gives a more exact plasma osmolality value.

$$2 \times \text{plasma Na} = \text{plasma osmolality}$$

$$2 \times \text{plasma Na} + (\text{BUN}/3) + (\text{glucose}/18) = \text{plasma osmolality}$$

FLUID RESTORATION

ORAL REHYDRATION. If the fluid loss is mild, the thirst mechanism is intact, and the client can drink fluid, fluids can be replaced orally. Oral glucose replacement solutions are palatable, inexpensive, and a good source of fluid, glucose, and electrolytes (Table 12–1). These solutions are quickly absorbed even if the client has diarrhea or is vomiting. Avoid cola drinks because they do not contain adequate electrolyte replacement; the sugar content also may lead to osmotic diuresis, and the caffeine may lead to diuresis.

INTRAVENOUS REHYDRATION. Whenever possible, use the oral route for replacement therapy. When the fluid loss is severe or life-threatening, intravenous (IV) fluids are used for replacement. The volume of fluid is calculated on the basis of the client's weight and the presence of any cardiac, renal, or pulmonary disorders. The type of solution used is based on the type of fluid lost from the body. Generally, isotonic ECFVD is treated with isotonic solutions, hypertonic ECFVD is treated with hypotonic solutions, and hypotonic ECFVD is treated with hypertonic solutions. Common IV fluids are listed in Table 12–2. Remember, a client with a terminal illness may have specific wishes about fluid maintenance.

MONITOR FOR COMPLICATIONS OF FLUID RESTORATION. Fluid needs must be assessed within the context of the client's overall condition. A client with severe ECFVD accompanied by severe heart, liver, or kidney disease cannot tolerate large volumes of fluid or sodium

TABLE 12–1 CONTENTS OF ORAL REHYDRATION SOLUTIONS

Brand Name	Calories per Liter*	Sodium (mEq/L)	Potassium (mEq/L)	Chloride (mEq/L)	Citrate (mEq/L)
Gastrolyte	75	60	20	60	10
Lytren	84	50	25	45	30
Naturalyte	100	45	20	35	48
Oralyte	100	45	20	25	48
Pedialyte	100	45	20	35	30
Rapolyte	84	90	20	80	30
Rehydralyte	100	75	20	65	30
Resol	84	50	20	50	34
Ricelyte	126†	50	25	45	34

* From dextrose.
† From rice syrup.

TABLE 12–2 **INTRAVENOUS WATER AND ELECTROLYTE SOLUTIONS**

Solution (Abbreviation)	Contents	Uses	Comments
HYPOTONIC			
5% dextrose in water (D_5W)	50 g dextrose No electrolytes	Replace deficits of total body water Not used alone to expand ECF volume because dilution of electrolytes can occur	Supplies 170 kcal/L and free water Distilled water cannot be given IV because it would cause hemolysis of RBCs Dextrose is metabolized on first pass through the liver, leaving a solution of water but without the hemolytic problems
ISOTONIC			
0.9% NaCl (normal saline solution, NS, 0.9% NS)	154 mEq/L of Na and Cl	ECF deficits in patients with low serum levels of Na or Cl and metabolic alkalosis Before and after the infusion of blood products	Not used for routine administration of IV fluids because it contains more sodium than ECF (140 mEq of NaCl and 103 mEq of Cl) Expands plasma and interstitial volume and does not enter cells
Lactated Ringer's solution (LR)	130 mEq/L Na 4 mEq/L K 3 mEq/L Ca 109 mEq/L Cl 28 mEq/L lactate	ECF deficits, such as fluid loss with burns and bleeding and dehydration from loss of bile or diarrhea	Solution is roughly isotonic to plasma but does not contain magnesium or phosphate Lactate is equivalent to bicarbonate, and solution can be used to treat many forms of acidosis Cannot be used in people with alkalosis; solutions of acetate Ringer's are better for these clients
HYPERTONIC			
Lactated Ringer's solution with 5% dextrose (D_5/LR)	50 g dextrose 130 mEq/L Na 4 mEq/L K 3 mEq/L Ca 109 mEq/L Cl 28 mEq/L lactate	ECF deficits, such as fluid loss with burns and bleeding and dehydration from loss of bile or diarrhea Provides modest calories (170 kcal)	This solution is hypertonic because it is the combination of two solutions (D_5W and LR) See other comments on individual solutions
5% dextrose and normal saline (D_5/0.9 NS)	50 g dextrose 154 mEq/L Na and Cl	ECF deficits in patients with low serum levels of Na or Cl and metabolic alkalosis Before and after the infusion of blood products Provides modest calories (170 kcal)	This solution is hypertonic because it is the combination of two solutions (D_5W and NS) See other comments on individual solutions
5% dextrose and 0.45% normal saline (D_5/0.45 NS; D_5/½ NS)	50 g dextrose 77 mEq/L Na and Cl	Can be used as an initial fluid for hydration because it provides more water than sodium Provides modest calories (170 kcal)	Commonly used as a maintenance fluid
5% dextrose and 0.225% normal saline (D_5/0.2 NS; D_5/¼ NS)	50 g dextrose 34 mEq/L Na and Cl	Can be used as an initial fluid for hydration because it provides more water than sodium Provides modest calories (170 kcal)	Commonly used as a maintenance fluid

Na, sodium; Cl, chloride; K, potassium; Ca, calcium; ECF, extracellular fluid; NS, normal saline; RBC, red blood cells; IV, intravenously; kcal, kilocalories.

without the risk for development of heart failure. For unstable clients, monitors to detect increasing pressures from fluids are used (e.g., measurement of CVP and pulmonary artery pressure). If the deficit has existed for more than 24 hours, it is dangerous to correct this deficit too rapidly. Sodium solutions should be infused at a rate of 0.5 to 1 mEq/L/hr. If fluid is given too rapidly, cerebral edema may result.[7]

Urine output, body weight, and laboratory values of sodium, osmolarity, BUN, and potassium are monitored closely.

CORRECTION OF UNDERLYING PROBLEM. Antiemetic and antidiarrheal drugs may be prescribed to correct problems with nausea and vomiting or diarrhea. Antibiotics may be used in clients with infectious diarrhea. Antipyretic agents may be used to reduce body temperature.

Nursing Management of the Medical Client

ASSESSMENT

Obtain the client's history of fluid losses. Consider whether the cause is infectious and whether isolation is warranted to reduce the spread of organisms.

Assess the client's vital signs every 2 to 4 hours, depending on the severity of the fluid loss; compare them with baseline vital signs and report marked differences. Assess for postural (orthostatic) blood pressure and pulse changes by taking blood pressure and pulse with the client lying down. Then have the client stand up; repeat the blood pressure and pulse measurements after 1 minute. Report a drop in standing systolic blood pressure of 25 mm Hg or more from the supine blood pressure; report pulse increases of more than 30 BPM. Autonomic neuropathy seen in diabetes, dysrhythmias, and some medications (e.g., antihypertensive agents) can also cause postural hypotension.

Assess the peripheral vein filling time daily. Veins with normal fluid volume should fill in 3 to 5 seconds when the arm is lowered below the level of the heart.

Monitor intake, output, and daily weights accurately in high-risk clients. Comparison of I & O data necessitates that all sources of intake (including liquids with meals and between meals, with medications, in IV lines, in tube-feedings, and in IV or tube flushes) and all sources of output (including urine, diarrhea, diaphoresis, and hyperventilation) be recorded accurately. If the ECFVD is mild, assess urine output every 8 hours and compare daily outputs. Absence of adequate renal perfusion for several hours may result in permanent renal damage. Whenever the output drops below 30 ml/hr for 2 consecutive hours, urinary output must be assessed hourly.

Teach unlicensed assistive personnel to report urine outputs of less than 30 ml/hr for 2 consecutive hours or less than 240 ml for an 8-hour period. Provide other instructions as well (see the Management and Delegation feature). Instruct the client to report fluids consumed in addition to the fluids on food trays and urine output not measured.

Monitor plasma sodium, BUN, glucose, and hematocrit levels to determine plasma osmolality. Assess the client for confusion, which is an early manifestation of ICF involvement.

MANAGEMENT AND DELEGATION

Care of Clients with Fluid Volume Deficit

When working with unlicensed assistive personnel in the care of clients with fluid volume deficit, remind them to:

- Keep fresh water or other fluids in an easily accessible location. Remind older clients to drink fluids hourly because their thirst mechanism is diminished.
- Try to provide fluids of choice every 1 to 2 hours.
- Encourage family members to assist with fluid intake.
- Provide oral care every 2 hours to help decrease discomfort from dry mucous membranes.
- Record intake accurately. Remember, a cup of ice chips provides one-half cup of water.
- Assist clients as necessary to the bathroom, commode, or bedpan every 2 hours. If the client is wearing disposable briefs, assess for incontinence and the need for perineal care at least every 2 hours.
- Record all output accurately. Include the amount of urine, the number of episodes of incontinence, and the measured amount of any diarrhea.
- Report diarrhea, excessive sweating, or rapid breathing to the nurse.
- Report urine that is dark, produced at less than 30 ml/h over 2 consecutive hours, or produced at more than 150 ml/hr to the nurse.
- Report weight changes of 2 pounds or more from the previous day.

Donna W. Markey, MSN, RN, ACNP-CS, *Clinician IV, Surgical Services, University of Virginia Health System, Charlottesville, Virginia*

Determine a history of chronic illnesses that may impair the ability to tolerate fluids at rapid speeds. Lung, renal, and heart disease reduce the body's ability to move fluids through the vascular system. Note the client's lung sounds on admission to serve as a baseline for later comparison.

Assess the client's weight and height. Do not rely on the client's stated weight because it may have decreased with fluid loss. Weigh the client daily. To increase accuracy of the measurement, weigh on the same scale, at the same time of day, with the client wearing clothing of similar weight. Help the client onto the scale; orthostatic hypotension may be present. Analyze changes in daily weights. A loss of 2.2 pounds is equivalent to 1 L of fluid. Therefore, an 8-pound weight loss equals about 3.5 L of fluid, or a moderate fluid volume deficit.

Assess the oral cavity between the gums and cheek for dryness of the mucous membranes and the tongue for dryness and longitudinal furrows.[17] A reliable method of testing for dryness of the mouth is to place your finger on the mucous membranes where the gums and cheek meet. When ECFVD is present, your finger will not glide easily because of dryness. Note any speech and swallowing difficulty. Assess closely for dried and adherent mucus on the soft palate.

Check skin turgor by gently pinching and lifting the skin (Fig. 12–3). Usually, skin returns to a normal position within 1 or 2 seconds in people younger than 60 years of age. A slower response may indicate loss of

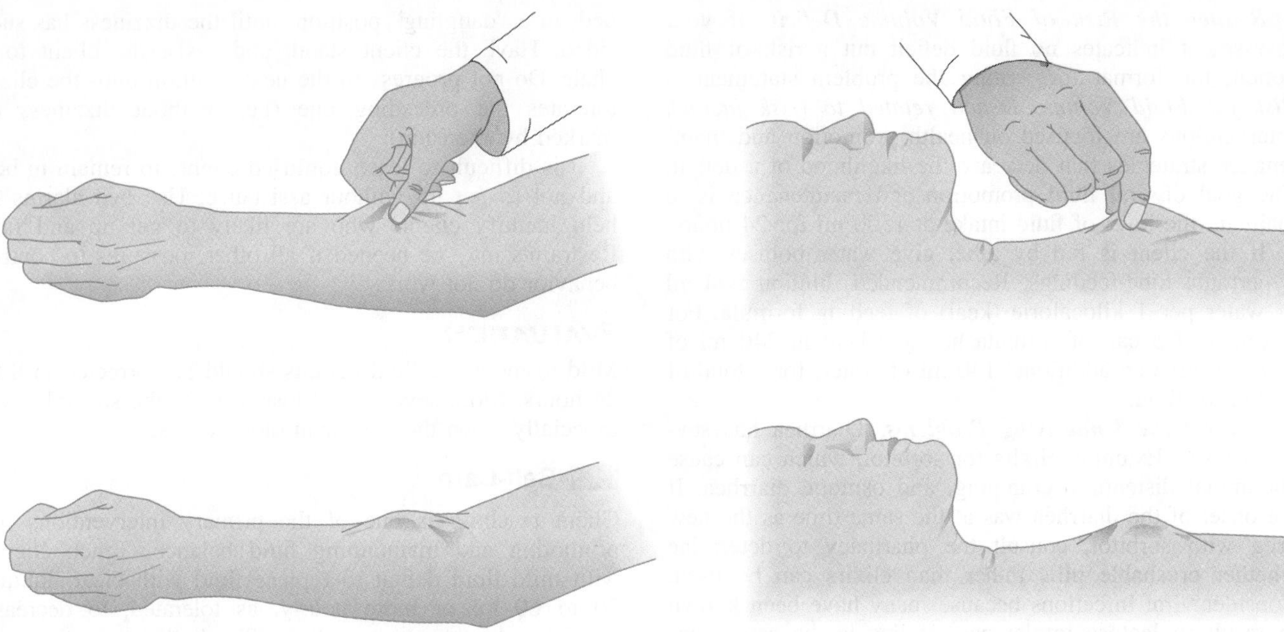

A Assessment of skin turgor on the forearm
B Assessment of skin turgor on the sternum

FIGURE 12–3 Skin turgor assessment. This assessment can be done on the forearm (*A*) of a young to middle-aged adult. For older adults, skin turgor should be assessed over the sternum (*B*) because using a forearm yields inaccurate results because of natural loss of subcutaneous tissue.

interstitial fluids. Generalized weakness may develop because of changes in sodium levels.

DIAGNOSIS, OUTCOMES, INTERVENTIONS

Fluid Volume Deficit. Fluid volume deficit (FVD) is the state in which a person has vascular, interstitial, or intracellular dehydration. The diagnosis is *Fluid Volume Deficit related to insufficient fluid intake, vomiting, diarrhea, hemorrhage, or third-space fluid loss such as ascites or burns.*

Outcomes. The desired outcome is return of normal levels of body fluids. Indicators of adequate fluid volumes include:

- Oral intake between 1500 and 2500 ml or more in 24 hours
- Urine output greater than 600 ml in 24 hours
- Stable blood pressure and pulse in the supine and standing positions
- Increasing body weight of about 0.5 to 1.0 pound per day
- Absence of crackles (fluid in alveoli), an indicator of fluid overload from overcompensation
- Moist tongue and mucous membranes
- BUN plasma sodium hematocrit and osmolality levels approaching normal ranges over the first 48 to 72 hours

Interventions

Restore Oral Fluid Intake. Give small amounts of fluids "of choice" hourly to elderly, confused, or debilitated clients and to those who require restraints. Keep fluids fresh and within reach. Use orthotic devices as appropriate for those who can assist in their own fluid intake. Use antiemetics as needed to control nausea before drinking. When appropriate, begin with clear liquids, such as oral replacement fluids, broth, or gelatin. Progress to full liquids and then solid foods, if tolerated without vomiting or aspiration. Encourage family members to participate in feeding.

If dysphagia (difficulty in swallowing) is present, consult the physician for swallowing studies. Once the problem has been identified, a speech pathologist can provide exercises to help the client. Reinforce the speech therapist's prescription during each feeding. You may need to give thickened fluids, elevate the headrest to 90 degrees before meals and for 1 hour after feeding, and flex the client's head slightly forward at the start of a swallow. Decrease the risk of aspiration by placing small amounts of food on the side of the mouth that has the best sensation and muscle strength. Teaching the client to chew slowly and to swallow two or three times with each mouthful and inspecting the mouth for food pocketing can also decrease the risk of aspiration. Assessing the fit of dentures is also important.

Restore Fluids by Intravenous Routes. Administer IV fluids cautiously to clients with ECFVD. Ideally, a large IV gauge (e.g., 18- to 20-gauge) should be used; however, most clients have venous collapse, and it is difficult to find a vein. A small IV site may be used initially; once fluids are reestablished, a larger needle can be inserted if fluids or an IV access is still needed. Use an IV pump or a mini-drop infusion set to regulate IV infusion and to decrease the risk of too rapid an infusion. Monitor IV solutions, IV sites, and client outcomes hourly.

Rapid fluid replacement often results in overflow diuresis without cellular replacement. Diuresis compounds dehydration and may result in hypernatremia. In elderly people or those with renal or cardiac disease, rapid fluid administration may also result in pulmonary overload.

Reduce the Risk of Fluid Volume Deficit. If your assessment indicates no fluid deficit but a risk of fluid deficit, the format for writing the problem statement is *Risk for Fluid Volume Deficit related to (risk factor).* Interventions are focused on health promotion and maintenance strategies that decrease the likelihood of a deficit. The goal of oral fluid promotion and maintenance is to maintain the level of fluid intake at 1500 ml for 24 hours.

If the client is fed by tube, give water boluses with hypertonic tube-feedings. Recommended dilution is 1 ml of water per 1 kilocalorie (kcal) of feeding formula. For example, if a can of formula has 380 kcal in 240 ml of formula, give an additional 140 ml of water, for a total of 380 ml of fluid.

Control the Underlying Problems. Diarrhea has several causes. Examine elixirs for sorbitol, which can cause abdominal distention, cramping, and osmotic diarrhea. If the onset of the diarrhea was at the same time as the new drug with sorbitol, consult the pharmacy to determine whether crushable pills rather than elixirs can be used. Consider viral infections because many have been known to result in lactose intolerance. If this is the cause, encourage the client to avoid milk-based products. Avoiding fatty or fried foods also decreases diarrhea and enhances digestion.

Give prescribed antiemetics for nausea, antipyretics for fever, and antibiotics for infection.

Monitor for Complications. When fluid balance is compromised, a person is at risk for tissue breakdown. Apply a moisturizer or skin barrier to protect the skin from the irritants, enzymes, and microorganisms found in urine and feces. Continue to assess lung sounds for manifestations of fluid overload (crackles) from overcorrection.

Altered Oral Mucous Membranes. The nursing diagnosis of *Altered Mucous Membranes related to lack of oral intake, or other causes* is a common problem in clients with dehydration.

Outcomes. The desired outcome is that the client's mouth, gums, and teeth remain clean and free of accumulations of dried mucus.

Interventions. Give oral care with a regular toothbrush or a foam toothbrush every 2 to 4 hours, and apply lip moisturizer. Rinse the client's mouth every 1 to 2 hours. Examine the client's mouth with a penlight to make sure that it remains free of debris. Avoid mouthwashes with an alcohol base, which can dry the mucous membranes. The frequency of oral care may need to be increased to hourly if evaluation of the skin and oral assessment findings indicate lack of improvement. Artificial saliva can also be used for the client with a very dry and fissured mouth.

Risk for Injury. If orthostatic hypotension is present, *Risk for Injury* is another problem that needs to be addressed.

Outcomes. The desired outcome is that the client will remain free of injury, as evidenced by no manifestations of falls (bruises, bumps, abrasions) or reported episodes of falls.

Interventions. Provide safety through step-progression position changes. Step-progression gives the client's body time to adapt to changes in position. First, raise the head of the bed. Next, assist the client to sit at the edge of the bed, in a "dangling" position, until the dizziness has subsided. Have the client stand, and assist the client to a chair. Do not progress to the next position until the client tolerates the preceding one (i.e., without dizziness or marked hypotension).

It is difficult to teach confused clients to remain in bed and not to get up without assistance. Use bed alarms to help identify clients who are likely to get up and fall. Restraints may be needed if all other measures to control behavior do not work.

EVALUATION

Mild to moderate fluid deficits should be corrected in 8 to 24 hours. More severe fluid losses may take several days, especially when they occur in older adults.

Self-Care

Client teaching is one of the primary interventions for promoting and maintaining fluid balance. Teach clients with mild fluid deficit to replace fluid with clear liquids, 30 to 60 ml or more hourly, as tolerated, to decrease nausea and replace electrolytes. Teach the importance of consulting a physician if an illness lasts longer than 24 hours or if the person is older or has a chronic illness, such as diabetes mellitus or liver, kidney, or heart disease.

Health promotion teaching is critical for those who actively exercise.[15] Teach people who exercise to:

- Understand the importance of exercise and heat acclimatization
- Avoid exercise during high heat and humidity
- Wear appropriate clothing (excess clothing decreases evaporation)
- Use more caution to prevent heat exhaustion if they are obese, because obesity impairs the sweating mechanism
- Drink cool water before exercise, 150 to 200 ml every 15 minutes during exercise, and after finishing exercise, and add 500 to 700 kcal of carbohydrates (for energy and sodium), if exercise is prolonged
- Avoid rapid fluid replacement, since this fluid only overflows to the kidneys
- Use caution when taking medications that interfere with thermoregulation, such as thyroid replacement, amphetamines, beta-blockers, haloperidol, antihistamines, anticholinergic drugs, and phenothiazines

Encourage diabetic clients who exercise to wear or carry Medic-Alert identification, to increase their protein intake, to decrease refined sugar intake, and to reduce insulin to half the usual dosage or to an amount recommended by the physician.[23] Teach people taking cortisone the importance of not missing doses, of carrying Medic-Alert identification, and of consulting a physician about increased dosage during physical or emotional stress to prevent Addison's crisis.

Reducing fluid intake as a way of decreasing urinary incontinence in older adults is inappropriate. Limited fluid intake increases bladder irritability, leading to uninhibited contractions, and alters the neurologic stimulus that controls normal bladder emptying. Emphasizing the importance of drinking even in the absence of thirst, teaching pelvic muscle exercises, and instituting a toilet schedule may help an older person overcome the problem of incontinence.

INTRACELLULAR FLUID VOLUME DEFICIT

Dehydration can become so severe that the cells become dehydrated. This condition is relatively rare in a healthy adult, but it occurs quite often in older clients and in clients with conditions that result in acute water loss. Compensatory attempts to combat the fluid deficit have the same physiologic basis as in ECFVD. Thirst and oliguria are the most common compensatory signs. Cellular manifestations are due to the dysfunction in the cerebral cells and include fever and central nervous system (CNS) changes, such as confusion, coma, and cerebral hemorrhage.

The desired outcome is restoration of fluid volume, which is initially addressed through IV replacement. Once the client becomes stable, the focus of medical management is correction or control of the underlying cause. The focus of nursing management is on prevention or early detection of complications secondary to the pathology or the treatment. Interdisciplinary communication is critical to the achievement of positive outcomes.

EXTRACELLULAR FLUID VOLUME EXCESS

ECF volume excess (ECFVE) is fluid overload or overhydration. Excess fluids can be found in the vascular system, a problem called *hypervolemia,* or in the interstitial spaces, a problem usually called *third-spacing* (see later). The water and sodium retained is in the same proportions as it exists in other ECF, and therefore is referred to as *isosmolar fluid volume excess.*

Etiology

ECF volume excess can develop from two processes: (1) simple overloading with fluids and (2) failure to excrete fluids. ECFVE often results from an increase in the total body sodium. Causes of ECFVE are shown in Table 12–3.

TABLE 12–3 ETIOLOGY OF EXTRACELLULAR FLUID VOLUME EXCESS

Etiologic Factor	Examples
Compromised regulation of fluid movement and excretion	Cirrhosis of the liver Decreased plasma protein Heart failure Hypothyroidism Lymphatic or venous obstruction Renal disorders
Excessive ingestion of fluids or foods containing sodium	Excessive amounts of saline intravenous fluids Ingestion of high-sodium foods Excessive use of enemas with sodium (e.g., Fleet's) or medications with sodium (e.g., Alka-Seltzer)
Increased antidiuretic hormone (ADH) and aldosterone	Certain barbiturates and narcotics (e.g., morphine) Cushing's syndrome General anesthesia Glucocorticoid use Hyperaldosteronism Syndrome of inappropriate secretion of ADH

Pathophysiology

With a fluid volume excess, the hydrostatic pressure of the fluid is higher than usual at the arterial end of the capillary. Excess amounts are moved out into the interstitial spaces because of the pressure. The fluid is not reabsorbed at the venous end because pressure remains high in the arteriole and resists flow from the tissues. Peripheral and pulmonary edema may result (Fig. 12–4*A*).

As the fluid pressure increases in the interstitial area and tissues, it creates a resistance to forward blood flow and increases resistance throughout the circulatory system. A resistance to arterial flow occurs, which leads to increased pressure in the left ventricle and then in the left atrium. From the atrium, fluid is unable to be propelled forward and it backs up across the alveolocapillary membrane of the lungs, resulting in pulmonary edema. Because the lungs are low-pressure organs, they also offer little resistance to fluid accumulation. Pulmonary edema develops quickly in clients with distention of the left side of the heart muscle, and the heart cannot pump adequately. If the right side of the heart fails, peripheral edema occurs through the same retrograde process. Left-sided heart failure leads to right-sided failure and vice versa, and both pulmonary and peripheral edema may thus exist simultaneously.

When fluid overload results from renal disorders, sodium and water excretion are decreased. As fluid volume rises, the heart compensates through tachycardia and hypertrophy. When compensatory mechanisms fail, heart failure results. Uncontrolled heart failure can lead to multiple organ failure and death from massive water retention, also known as *anasarca.*

In severe liver disease, renal disease, burns, or protein malnutrition, the plasma protein and albumin levels are decreased. Therefore, oncotic pressure is decreased in the vascular fluids, resulting in less fluid reabsorption from the tissue spaces at the venous end. Peripheral edema and ascites result (see Fig. 12–4*B*).

When lymphatic channels are obstructed, tissue oncotic pressure rises and leads to edema (see Fig. 12–4*C*). Chapter 53 discusses lymphedema. Edema can also develop from conditions that increase capillary permeability, such as tissue trauma (see Fig. 12–4*D*). This form of edema is discussed in Chapter 27.

Clinical Manifestations

Fluid volume excess leads to respiratory and cardiovascular manifestations. The respiratory manifestations are from increasing hydrostatic pressure in the pulmonary capillaries, which results in shifting of fluid to the alveolar sacs. Fluid congestion in the alveoli manifests as coughing, dyspnea, and crackles that can be auscultated over the involved lung area. The alveolar fluid accumulation

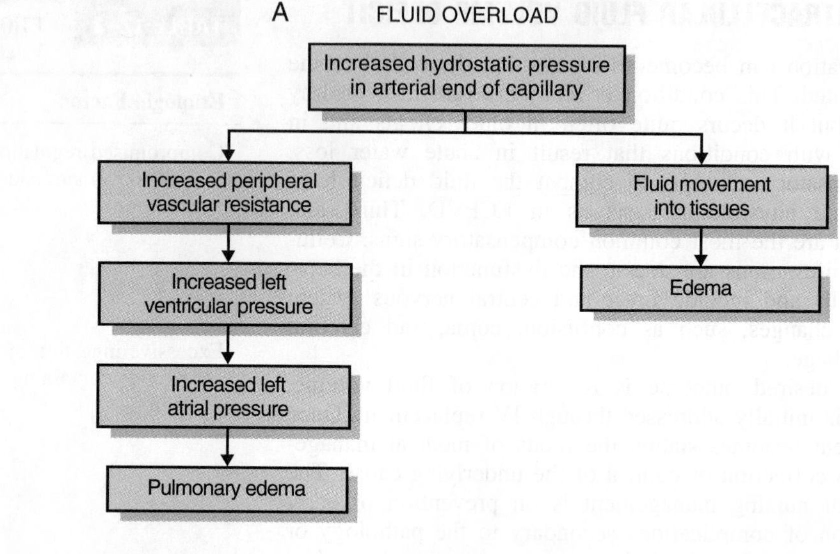

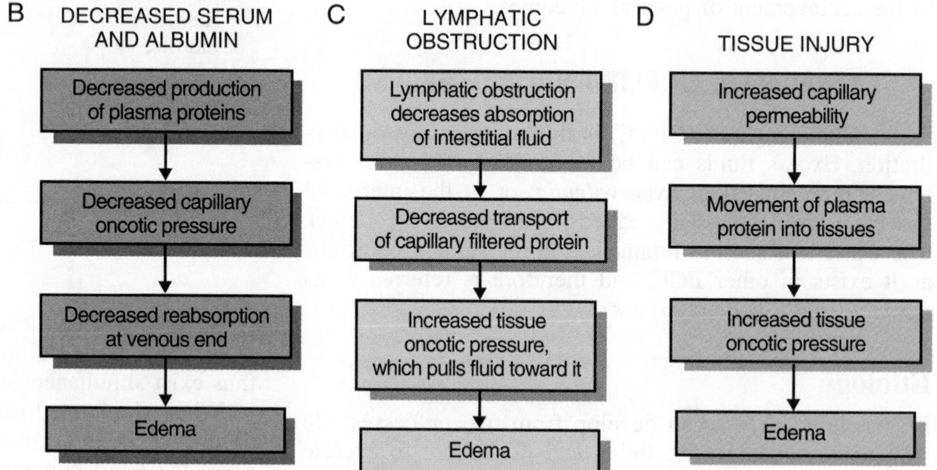

FIGURE 12–4 Mechanisms of edema formation. *A,* Fluid overload. *B,* Decreased plasma and albumin. *C,* Lymphatic obstruction. *D,* Tissue injury.

also leads to impaired oxygen (O_2) and carbon dioxide (CO_2) transport between the capillaries and alveoli, resulting in pallor, cyanosis, decreased tissue perfusion (measured by pulse oximetry) and increased CO_2 blood gas abnormalities. If hydrostatic pressure continues to rise, fluid shifts into the pleural spaces as well; this is known as *pleural effusion.*

Cardiovascular manifestations are numerous. Delayed emptying and filling of the right ventricle leads to systemic venous engorgement, including signs of jugular venous distention, peripheral vein filling time above 5 seconds, a bounding pulse and elevated blood pressure, and increased CVP and pulmonary capillary wedge pressure (PCWP). If the delayed ventricular filling overdistends the ventricles, an extra heart sound, called S_3, can often be auscultated.

Fluid accumulates in the interstitial compartments, especially in the gravity-dependent tissues of the legs and sacrum. Edema may develop in the feet in ambulatory people and in the sacrum of bedridden clients. The continued increase in fluid pressure also causes fluid shifting into the visceral tissues. Thus, the client may exhibit signs of organ dysfunction specific to the tissues involved (e.g., anorexia and bloating from stomach involvement). Rapid weight gain is a classic sign of fluid overload regardless of the system responsible for the overload.

If any early changes in cerebral function develop, such as confusion and headache, suspect ICF shifting. As the fluid excess increases in the cerebral cells, lethargy occurs, followed by seizures and then coma.

With fluid overload, the concentration of solutes is decreased by the excess fluid volume. Typical findings include:

- Plasma osmolality less than 275 mOsm/kg
- Plasma sodium less than 135 mEq/L, depending on the type of fluid excess
- Hematocrit less than 45%
- Specific gravity less than 1.010
- BUN less than 8 mg/dl

Remember, these results must be evaluated in the context of the client's manifestations and the possibility of other pathologic processes. For example, blood loss would also cause a decreased hematocrit; a decreased protein intake would result in a decreased BUN. Chapters 56 and 63 describe heart failure and acute pulmonary edema. The plasma sodium level may appear to be within the normal range because of excess water retention, even though the actual sodium level is increased.

Outcome Management

A thorough clinical history of contributing and causative factors, medication history, manifestations of fluid overload, and laboratory findings are essential to identifying appropriate interventions. Reduction of dietary sodium, restriction of fluids, and pharmacologic interventions are the major treatments of ECFVE.

RESTRICTION OF SODIUM AND FLUIDS. According to the usual definitions, a *mildly* restricted sodium diet contains 4 to 5 g of sodium, a *moderately* restricted diet contains 2 g of sodium, and a *severely* restricted diet contains 0.5 g of sodium[1] (see Chapter 13, Box 13–2, for a list of high- and low-sodium foods). To convert milligrams of sodium to milliequivalents, divide the number of milligrams by 23 (the atomic weight of sodium). For example, 1000 mg sodium is equivalent to 43 mEq of sodium.

PROMOTING URINE OUTPUT. Mild diuretics and digitalis promote fluid loss and improve myocardial contractility. Many diuretics cause potassium and magnesium to be excreted along with the sodium and water. To counteract this, a combination of potassium-wasting and potassium-sparing diuretics may be prescribed.

Several studies have found improved myocardial contractility and decreased morbidity and mortality in clients with heart failure who, in addition to digitalis, have received angiotensin-converting enzyme (ACE) inhibitors and low-dose beta-blockers. Many of these clients showed such an improvement in their overall cardiac function that they did not need diuretics. When ACE inhibitors are used, clients should be monitored for hyperkalemia because of the potassium-sparing effect of the ACE inhibitor.[24]

Nursing Management of the Medical Client

ASSESSMENT

Monitor the client's vital signs for a bounding pulse, elevated blood pressure, or both every 4 to 8 hours. Assess the apical pulse if the radial pulse is irregular or if the client is taking cardiac medication. Assess breath sounds every 4 to 8 hours for crackles, rhonchi (abnormal lung sounds indicating retention of secretions), or wheezes, noting changes in location or severity. Assess for changes in respiratory effort with activity or rest.

Each morning, palpate the sacrum and legs for pitting edema and observe the client for hand and bilateral neck vein engorgement. Jugular vein distention at or above a 45-degree headrest suggests ECFVE. Hand veins that do not flatten within 3 to 5 seconds when the hand is raised above the heart level suggest fluid overload. Assess the condition of skin on the legs. Edematous skin is very fragile and can tear easily.

Compare I & O every 4 to 8 hours. Weigh the client daily; do not rely on stated weights. Determine whether the client has had expected weight loss or unexpected weight gain. Edema does not usually occur until 3 L or more of excess fluid has accumulated. Measure extremities if edema seems pronounced.

Monitor plasma osmolality, sodium level, hematocrit, and urine specific gravity. Observe for changes in level of consciousness, which may indicate the more serious complication of ICF shifting.

DIAGNOSIS, OUTCOMES, INTERVENTIONS

Fluid Volume Excess. The diagnostic statement is written *Fluid Volume Excess* related to (specific cause, such as heart, renal, or liver failure). Be certain to specify the cause in your client's case. If your client has heart failure, also consider using the diagnosis *Decreased Cardiac Output.*

Outcomes. The desired outcome is return of normal levels of body fluids. Indicators of adequate fluid volumes include:

- Stable blood pressure and pulse
- Decreasing body weight of about 0.5 to 1.0 pound per day
- Absence of manifestations of ICFVE such as confusion
- Absence of manifestations of ECFVE such as coughing, crackles, dyspnea, jugular venous distention, peripheral edema, S_3 gallop rhythm
- BUN, plasma sodium, hematocrit, and osmolality approaching normal levels in 48 to 72 hours
- Absence of manifestations of overcorrection, such as hypotension, dry mucous membranes

Interventions

Reduce Sodium and Fluid Intake. Fluid management becomes extremely important in clients with ECFVE. Strict I & O may be crucial. Include fluids on meal trays and those given with medications as part of the total fluid intake. Collaborate with the dietitian in planning fluid restrictions. Schedule oral medications at meal times, if possible, to limit fluid intake. Use minimal amounts of water (5 to 10 ml) to dissolve crushed medications that need to be given by feeding tube. Flushing the tube with cola may decrease the need for large amounts of water and may keep the tube patent. Cold fluids decrease the sensation of thirst more than warm or hot fluids do. Give the client ice chips, if allowed, and provide frequent oral care to decrease the thirst sensation (1 cup of ice equals ½ cup of water). Instruct the client about the rationale for fluid and sodium restrictions.

Use IV pumps and/or mini-drop tubing to control IV fluid intake. Use only isotonic saline for bladder and nasogastric tube irrigations. For clients on continuous bladder irrigation, consult the physician about changing hypotonic bladder irrigations to normal saline during the postoperative period.

Sodium is a common ingredient in foods, and to many clients the low-sodium diet is bland. Suggest alternatives for seasoning to enhance the taste of foods and increase dietary compliance. Salt substitutes are available; they use potassium as the cation but taste bitter to many people. Clients who take ACE inhibitors cannot use potassium salt substitutes.

Mobilize Fluid. Instruct the client who has dependent leg edema to avoid long periods of standing and to sit with legs elevated. Bed rest alone promotes diuresis, particularly in clients with heart failure. Mobilization of edema in the supine position is probably due to diminished pooling of venous blood, a resultant increase in effective circulating blood volume and thus renal perfusion.

Reduce Complications. Elevate the head of the bed 30 to 45 degrees to decrease venous return to the heart, which decreases cardiac workload and allows for improved diaphragmatic excursion, both of which improve oxygenation. This position also promotes jugular venous drainage, which improves cerebral perfusion. If dyspnea or orthopnea is present, position the client in semi-Fowler's or Fowler's position. Give oxygen to keep oxygen saturation above 90%, according to the provider's orders.

If the client is taking diuretics and digitalis, monitor plasma electrolytes and anticipate digitalis toxic effects secondary to hypokalemia. Report the levels of plasma electrolytes, especially potassium levels.

When peripheral tissue perfusion is altered because of edema or vascular disease, provide frequent skin care, turn the client often, control moisture, and prevent friction and shear. The heel is especially at risk for decreased capillary blood flow. Therefore, it is important to keep the client's heels elevated off the mattress and to remove elastic stockings when redness is noted.

Modifications for Elderly Clients

In general, the interventions for each of these outcomes are the same for the older client; however, response time is usually slower and the risk for side effects is higher because of poorer renal and liver function and problems with drug interactions.[32] For instance, digitalis toxicity is much more common in the elderly. Some diagnostic studies may not be as accurate in this population. For example, a person with protein malnutrition, which is more common in the elderly, may have renal insufficiency but may have a normal BUN because of the lack of protein.

EVALUATION

Correcting ECFVE is a slow process, especially when it results from an organ disorder. Most clients are discharged without complete resolution of peripheral edema but with improvement in pulmonary edema and breathing. Self-care instructions are critical.

Self-Care

If the client is going home on a low-sodium diet, review allowed and restricted foods with the client and the person who prepares the meals. Canned foods should be avoided; fresh and frozen foods are usually lower in sodium. Buying these items in season and freezing them for later use save money and provide more nutrients. Encourage the food purchaser to read food labels and to avoid products with high levels of sodium or salt and food whose labels contain the word "sodium" or the symbol "Na" as a prefix. Avoid drinking or cooking with softened water, which is high in sodium. Water may need to be obtained from another source, or a water distiller may be needed.

Suggest alternatives for seasoning to enhance the taste of foods and to increase dietary compliance. Adding fresh lemon to vegetables and main dishes, condiments that come in powder form (such as garlic), or other low-sodium seasonings that can be found at health food stores can increase satiety. Remember, people taking ACE inhibitors cannot use potassium salt substitutes.

If the client is going home with fluid restriction, help the client and family plan for how fluids can be spaced. Recognize the cultural variations in fluid consumption. In Western society, offering a guest something to drink is a common practice and may influence total fluid consumption.

Instruct the client and family to notify the physician about a weight gain of more than 3 pounds per week, a marked reduction in urine output, increased shortness of breath with exertion or especially at rest, new-onset headaches, confusion, seizures, or a deterioration in level of consciousness.

INTRACELLULAR FLUID VOLUME EXCESS: WATER INTOXICATION

Although the cells are usually quite resistant to fluid shifts, certain conditions can lead to an intracellular fluid volume excess (ICFVE). Conditions that cause acute or severe fluid volume excesses have a higher incidence of ICF overload. This is because the adaptive mechanisms may be unable to compensate for large or sudden fluid excesses.

ICFVE results from either water excess or solute deficit, primarily from sodium loss. In water excess, the number of solutes is normal but they are diluted by excessive water. In solute deficit, the amount of water is normal but there are too few particles per liter of water.

The most common cause of ICFVE is the administration of excessive amounts of hyposmolar IV fluids, such as 0.45% (half-normal) saline solution or 5% dextrose in water (D_5W). ICFVE may occur in clients who receive continuous IV D_5W or in older clients who consume excessive amounts of tap water without adequate nutrient intake. Syndrome of inappropriate antidiuretic hormone (SIADH) also leads to ICFVE regardless of whether the SIADH is caused by CNS trauma, the stress of surgery, pain, or narcotic use.

People with certain psychiatric disorders, such as schizophrenia, often have compulsive water consumption behaviors. Studies have found that as many as 80% of people admitted to a hospital with a diagnosis of schizophrenia have water intoxication. You must monitor for compulsive water consumption in people with a history or current manifestations of an organic psychiatric illness.[12, 13, 35]

Hyposmolar fluids in the vessels move by osmosis to the region of higher concentration of sodium in the cells in an attempt to maintain equilibrium. Unfortunately, too much fluid accumulates in the cells, causing cellular edema. Cerebral cells absorb hyposmolar fluid more quickly than do other cells. Thus, these cell changes often present the earliest warning signs of intracellular shifting.

All neurologic manifestations are secondary to the increasing intracranial pressure (ICP). Most ICP syndromes progress cephalocaudally. Thus, the early signs are cortical and, as pressure increases, pupillary. The vital signs then change. A complete discussion of the changes caused by increasing ICP is presented in Chapter 73.

Because ICF excess is often associated with ECF excess, it is common to see a plasma sodium level of less than 125 mEq/L and a decreased hematocrit. However, there is no plasma test to reflect the cell fluid volume. Diagnostic tests, such as computed tomography (CT) and magnetic resonance imaging (MRI), are more helpful in identifying causes underlying the syndrome of ICFVE.

Neurologic cells are very vulnerable to fluid excess or deficit. The first priority is to reduce ICP with steroids and osmotic diuretics. Equally as important is identifying and addressing the cause of the fluid volume excess. Immediate surgical intervention may be critical. The interventions specific to varying causes are discussed in Chapters 68, 69, 70, and 73.

If SIADH is an impending risk, early administration of IV fluids containing some sodium chloride (NaCl) may prevent it. Saline solutions, such as D_5/0.45% NaCl, increase the osmolality of vascular fluid and prevent or help correct hyposmolality.

Because brain tissue has a very narrow margin in which life is sustained, frequent monitoring and early intervention are critical. Perform neurologic checks, including level of consciousness, vital signs, reflexes, and pupillary responses, every hour if cranial changes are present. Cerebral perfusion is altered if systolic blood pressure drops too low or rises too high. Notify the provider if the client's sensorium changes from the baseline assessment, if systolic blood pressure is less than 100 mm Hg or greater than 150 mm Hg, or if other signs persist or worsen.

Monitor IV fluids and I & O hourly, and monitor weight daily. Polyuria is a good sign and indicates that fluid has shifted to the vascular space and to the renal tubules, where it can be excreted. Administer antiemetics prophylactically, as appropriate, to promote food and fluid ingestion and retention and to decrease the risk of vomiting, which worsens the increased ICP.

Provide safety measures when the client displays behavioral changes, such as confusion or disorientation. Keep the bed in a low position with bedside rails raised. Keep suction equipment at the bedside in anticipation of seizures. If a client has a seizure, turn the client to one side to displace the tongue. Remain at the bedside until the client is safe, and document all phases of the seizure. See Chapter 69 for care of the client during a seizure.

If the manifestations of increased ICP are improving, then the client is at less risk for complications. Remember, time equals brain cell survival. The longer the manifestations of increased ICP persist and the more serious they are, the graver the prognosis.

EXTRACELLULAR FLUID VOLUME SHIFT: THIRD-SPACING

A fluid volume shift is basically a change in the location of ECF between the intravascular and the interstitial spaces. Fluid shifts are of two types: (1) *vascular* fluid shifts to interstitial spaces and (2) *interstitial* fluid shifts to vascular spaces. Fluid that shifts into the interstitial spaces and remains there is referred to as *third-space fluid.* This abnormal fluid accumulation not only results from pathologic conditions but also reflects an inability of the lymphatic system to compensate. Common sites of third-spacing include the pleural cavity, peritoneal cavity, and pericardial sac. Third-space fluid is physiologically useless because it does not circulate to provide nutrients for cells.

Etiology

Fluids can move into interstitial spaces because of increased capillary permeability, decreased serum protein levels, obstruction of the venous portion of the capillary, or nonfunctional lymphatic drainage systems.

Any pathologic process that increases capillary permeability can cause third-spacing. Any tissue injury can lead to fluid shifting. Massive fluid shifts from the vascular to the interstitial spaces can be seen in crush injuries, major tissue trauma, major surgery, extensive burns, acid-base imbalance, bowel obstruction, and sepsis. Capillary permeability can also be altered by ischemia.

Decreased protein intake, production, or storage, as seen in protein-calorie malnutrition, leads to hypoalbuminemia. Bowel disorders that reduce protein absorption can reduce serum levels. Conditions that cause a loss of protein, such as kidney and liver disease or large draining wounds or burns, also deplete protein stores. Increased protein anabolism can occur in the healing phase of fractures or wounds; increased protein catabolism can occur with fever, infection or sepsis, and malignancy.

Lymphatic obstruction and venous thrombosis slow fluid returning through the venous system.

Pathophysiology

Tissue injury causes the release of histamine and bradykinin, resulting in increased capillary permeability, which allows more fluid, protein, and other solutes to move into the interstitial spaces than normal. This form of fluid shift is time-limited. Once the early stages of inflammation pass in about 24 to 48 hours, the capillary closes and fluid returns to the venous system.

Protein malnutrition leads to fluid shifts because protein is not present to pull fluid back into the capillary at the venous end. This form of fluid shifting is usually long term and can be seen in children who are malnourished and have large protruding abdomens and pencil-thin legs.

Two phases of fluid shift are associated with tissue injury:

1. Fluid shift from vascular to interstitial spaces, which leads to a fluid volume deficit (*hypovolemia*) (see Fig. 12–4*D*). Severe hypovolemia may lead to vascular collapse and death. If cellular damage is severe, a toxic response may occur from intracellular ions, such as potassium, which leak into the vascular spaces.
2. Fluid shift back from the interstitial to the vascular space, which leads to a fluid volume excess (*hypervolemia*). If the hypervolemia is severe, it may lead to heart failure. Intracellular potassium ions shift back into the cell during this phase, which increases the risk for hypokalemia.

Clinical Manifestations

Clinical manifestations of a fluid shift from the vascular to the interstitial spaces are similar to the manifestations of hypovolemic shock because the fluid is not in the vascular system. Typical clinical manifestations include pallor, cold limbs, weak and rapid pulse, hypotension, oliguria, increased skin turgor, and decreased levels of consciousness. Body weight does not change because fluid has not been lost; it has been redistributed.

If fluid collects and obstructs an organ, nerve, or vessel, other clinical manifestations may arise. For example, bowel sounds may change throughout the abdomen. Extremities may become pale, cool, and pulseless if fluid obstructs blood vessels or nerves. Laboratory results may indicate an elevated hematocrit and an elevated BUN. Urine has an elevated specific gravity.

When fluid returns to the blood vessels, the clinical manifestations are similar to those of fluid overload. Signs may include a bounding pulse, crackles, engorgement of peripheral and jugular veins, and an increase in blood pressure. Laboratory results may indicate a decrease in hematocrit and BUN. Other abnormal findings depend on the area of the body affected.

Outcome Management

As with fluid volume deficit and fluid volume excess, third-spacing is only a manifestation. It is crucial that the underlying cause be identified through a thorough history and physical examination so that interventions can be targeted to the desired outcomes.

Medical treatment begins with determining the cause of the fluid volume shift. If the third-spacing of fluid has occurred as a result of pericarditis, pericardiocentesis may have to be done to preserve organ function. If third-spacing is from a bowel obstruction, paracentesis (removal of peritoneal fluid via a large-bore needle) is the procedure of choice (see Chapters 30 and 62).

Replace Fluids

When hypovolemia results from tissue injury, such as burns or crush injuries, a large volume of isosmolar IV fluid administration is required to replace intravascular volume. When there is evidence of capillary sealing, as when urine output increases without additional fluids, albumin may be given to replace the protein lost from the trauma and to promote restoration of capillary oncotic pressures. Because third-spacing is a common occurrence after major surgery, maintaining IV fluid intake is essential to maintaining kidney perfusion. The amount of fluid infusion may be three times greater than urine output. Generally, fluids are titrated to maintain an adequate blood pressure, PCWP or PAWP, and urine output. If replacement is too aggressive, a fluid overload can occur, in part because of increased ADH.

When the capillary walls regain integrity, fluid shifts from the tissue spaces back into the vessels. If fluid replacement is too aggressive during this phase, a fluid overload can also occur.

Stabilize Other Problems

The diagnosis of sepsis is confirmed by culture, and treatment is with antibiotics. Vasoactive medications may be needed to maintain blood pressure. Bowel obstructions are decompressed and surgically repaired. Inflammatory disorders are treated with massive doses of steroids to stabilize the mast cell membrane.

Nursing Management of the Medical Client

Assess vital signs often according to the client's condition. The frequency can vary from every 1 to 8 hours. If shock-like symptoms are present, assess vital signs every hour during the shock-like state. If fluid loss is a result of ascites or peripheral edema, the fluid shift is slower and changes in vital signs are usually subtle.

Monitor IV fluid replacement needs. If fluids are administered too rapidly, fluid overload or hypervolemia may occur. Assess for early signs of fluid overload, such as pulmonary crackles, difficulty in breathing, and neck vein engorgement. Notify the provider if these signs are present. Anticipate a reduction in IV fluid needs as the third-space fluid shifts back into the plasma during the capillary repair stage.

If the third-spacing is in the abdomen, as with ascites, measure the client's abdominal girth every 8 hours. If a limb is involved, measure the circumference of the limb and assess peripheral pulses every 8 hours. Use preventive measures to prevent skin breakdown of edematous areas.

Monitor urine output every hour, and report an output of less than 30 ml/hr if it persists for more than 2 hours. The client may need more fluids, not diuretics. Urine output is usually reduced after tissue injury because of decreased renal circulation and a fluid shift into the injured tissue spaces. One to 3 days after tissue injury, fluid returns to the circulation and excess fluid is excreted by the kidneys unless renal function is impaired. Monitor plasma levels of BUN and creatinine.

CONCLUSIONS

Fluid imbalances are common problems, especially in high-risk populations, such as older adults and clients with acute illnesses or multiple pathologic processes. Many health care disciplines work collaboratively toward maintaining or retoring fluid balance. The role of nursing in this collaborative effort is focused on health promotion activities, including teaching positive health behaviors, health maintenance activities (including early detection and consultation with other disciplines), and prevention and early detection of complications from the underlying diseases, coexisting conditions, or treatment. Through these interventions, you play a critical role in assisting clients and their families achieve positive health outcomes in a cost-effective manner.

THINKING CRITICALLY

1. The admitting receptionist has just called your floor to secure a room for a 69-year-old woman with a history of 2 days of vomiting and diarrhea and a fever of 103° F secondary to suspected influenza virus. The client has a history of hypertension and heart failure. Home prescriptions include digoxin, 0.125 mg/day; furo-

semide (Lasix), 40 mg bid; and potassium chloride, 40 mEq/day. The client has also been advised to consume a low-sodium diet. An IV line of D_5/NS with 30 mEq of potassium chloride was started.

Factors to Consider. What is the priority risk or problem in this scenario? What are the desired outcomes? What are the critical assessments? What medical management and nursing strategies do you anticipate?

2. **A middle-aged client is admitted to your unit with shock-like symptoms from a massive burn wound. He has pale skin, cold limbs, hypotension, and a weak, rapid pulse. Urine output via the indwelling catheter is decreased. His level of consciousness varies from an adequate response to little or no response to external stimuli.**

Factors to Consider. What is the priority risk or problem in this scenario? What are the desired outcomes? What are the critical assessments? What medical management and nursing strategies do you anticipate during this phase of fluid shifting from the vascular spaces to the interstitial spaces? How will they change when the fluid shifts back into the vascular spaces?

BIBLIOGRAPHY

1. Abraham, W., & Schrier, R. (1994). Body fluid volume regulation in health and disease. *Advances in Internal Medicine, 39,* 23–43.
2. Andrews, M., et al. (1993). Dehydration in terminally ill patients. *Postgraduate Medicine, 93*(1), 201–208.
3. Arief, I. (1999). Fatal postoperative pulmonary edema: Pathogenesis and literature review. *Chest, 115*(5), 1371–1377.
4. Banasik, J. (1995). Alterations in cardiac function. In L. Copstead (Ed.), *Perspectives on pathophysiology* (pp. 346–374). Philadelphia: W. B. Saunders.
5. Batcheller, J. (1994). Syndrome of inappropriate antidiuretic hormone secretion. *Critical Care Nursing Clinics of North America, 6*(4), 687–692.
6. Bergeron, M., Armstrong, L., & Maresh, C. (1995). Fluid and electrolyte losses during tennis in the heat. *Clinics in Sports Medicine, 14*(1), 23–32.
7. Brown, R. (1993). Disorders of water and sodium balance. *Postgraduate Medicine, 93*(4), 227–246.
8. Burge, F. (1993). Dehydration symptoms of palliative care cancer patients. *Journal of Pain and Symptom Management, 8*(7), 454–464.
9. Casa, D. J. (1999). Exercise in heat: I. Fundamentals of thermal physiology, performance implications, and dehydration. *Journal of Athletic Training, 34*(3), 246–252.
10. Carrougher, G. J. (1997). Management of fluid and electrolyte balance in thermal injuries: Implications for perioperative nursing practice. *Seminars in Perioperative Nursing, 6*(4), 201–209.
11. Corbett, J. V. (1996). *Laboratory tests and diagnostic procedures with nursing diagnoses* (4th ed.). Stamford, CT: Appleton & Lange.
12. Cosgray, R., et al. (1993). A program for water-intoxicated patients at a state hospital. *Clinical Nurse Specialist, 7*(2), 55–61.
13. Davidhizar, R., & Kriesl, R. (1993). Water intoxication: One nursing staff's response and intervention. *Journal of Advanced Nursing, 18,* 1975–1980.
14. Faull, C., Holmes, C., & Baylis, P. (1993). Water balance in elderly people: Is there a deficiency of vasopressin? *Age and Ageing, 22,* 114–120.
15. Galloway, S. D. (1999). Dehydration, rehydration, and exercise in the heat: Rehydration strategies for the athletic competition. *Canadian Journal of Applied Physiology, 24*(2), 188–200.
16. Gisolfi, C. (1996). Fluid balance for optimal performance. *Nutrition Reviews, 54*(4), S159–S166.
17. Gross, C., et al. (1992). Clinical indicators of dehydration severity in elderly patients. *Journal of Emergency Medicine, 10*(3), 267–274.
18. Hall, J. (1994). Caring for corpses or killing patients? *Nursing Management, 25*(10), 81–89.
19. Held, J. (1995). Cancer care: Correcting fluid and electrolyte imbalances. *Nursing, 95*(4), 24–28.
20. Hoot-Martin, J., & Larsen, P. (1994). Dehydration in the elderly surgical patient. *AORN Journal, 60*(4), 666–671.
21. Iggulden, H. (1999). Dehydration and electrolyte disturbance. *Elderly Care, 11*(3), 17–23.
22. Kaufmann, M. (1996). Preventing dehydration in the elderly. *Provider, 9,* 65–66.
23. Koivisto, V., et al. (1992). Fuel and fluid homeostasis during long-term exercise in healthy subjects and type I diabetic patients. *Diabetes Care, 15*(4), 1736–1742.
24. Krueger, S., et al. (1994). Treatment of heart failure: Update 1994. *Nebraska Medical Journal, 8,* 292–297.
25. Maughan, R. J. (1999). Exercise in the heat: Limitations to performance and the impact of fluid replacement strategies. *Canadian Journal of Applied Physiology, 24*(2), 149–151.
26. May D. L. (1998). The relationship between self-induced water intoxication and severity of psychiatric symptoms. *Archives of Psychiatric Nursing, 12*(6), 335–343.
27. McClousky, J., & Bulechek, G. (1996). *Nursing interventions classification (NIC): Iowa intervention project* (2nd ed.). St. Louis: Mosby–Year Book.
28. McConnell, E. (1995). What's wrong with this patient? Assessing altered level of consciousness. *Nursing, 95*(6), 66–67.
29. Miller, C. (1995). *Nursing care of older adults: Theory and practice* (2nd ed.). Philadelphia: Lippincott-Raven.
30. Miller, K. (1996). Diabetes insipidus. *Journal, 23*(3), 285–292.
31. Moseley, M. J. (1997). Perioperative problems: Nutrition and electrolytes in the elderly. *Seminars in Perioperative Nursing, 6*(1), 21–30.
32. O'Donnell, M. (1995). Assessing fluid and electrolyte balance in elders. *American Journal of Nursing, 95*(11), 41–45.
33. Oster, J., & Materson, B. (1992). Renal and electrolyte complications of congestive heart failure and effects of therapy with angiotensin-converting enzyme inhibitors. *Archives of Internal Medicine, 152,* 704–710.
34. Rehrer, N. (1994). The maintenance of fluid balance during exercise. *International Journal of Sports Medicine, 15,* 122–125.
35. Ribbe, D., & Thelander, B. (1994). Patients with disordered water balance. *Journal of Psychosocial Nursing, 32*(10), 35–42.
36. Sansevero, A. (1997). Dehydration in the elderly: Strategies for prevention and management. *Nurse Practitioner, 22*(4), 41–70.
37. Smith, S. (1995). Patient-induced dehydration: Can it ever be therapeutic? *Oncology Nursing Forum, 22*(10), 1487–1497.
38. Smith, S. (1997). Controversies in hydrating the terminally ill patient. *Journal of Intravenous Nursing, 20*(4), 193–199.
39. Spangler, A. A. (1998). Age, dependency and other factors influencing fluid intake by long term care residents. *Journal of Nutrition for the Elderly, 18*(2), 21–35.
40. Steiner, N. & Bruera, E. (1998). Methods of hydration in palliative care patients. *Journal of Palliative Care, 14*(2), 6–13.
41. Sutcliffe, J., & Holmes, S. (1994). Dehydration: Burden or benefit to the dying patient? *Journal of Advanced Nursing, 19,* 71–76.
42. Theston-Aurand, J., Olmsted R., Allen-Bridson, K., & Craig, C. (1997). Impact of dressing materials on central venous catheter infection rates. *Journal of Intravenous Nursing, 20*(4), 201–204.
43. Vonfolio, L. (1995). Back to basics: Would you hang these IV solutions? *AJN, 95*(6), 37–39.
44. Zerwekh, J. (1997). Do dying patients really need IV fluids? *AJN, 97*(3), 26–30.

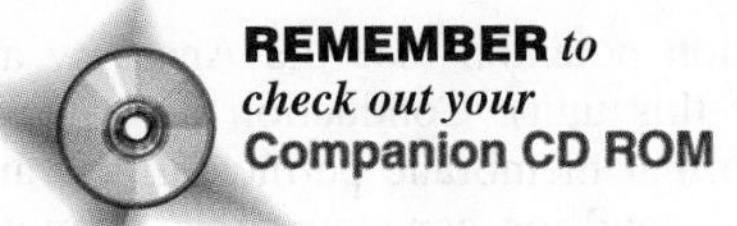

CHAPTER 13

Clients with Electrolyte Imbalances: Promoting Positive Outcomes

Bernadette White

Electrolytes are substances found in extracellular and intracellular fluid that dissociate into electrically charged particles known as ions. Ions that carry a positive charge are called *cations;* those that carry a negative charge are called *anions.* Sodium, potassium, calcium, magnesium, and hydrogen are the major cations in the body. Major anions are chloride, phosphate, bicarbonate, and protein. The principal cation in the intracellular fluid (ICF) is potassium. The principal cation in the extracellular fluid (ECF) is sodium (Fig. 13–1). Chapter 14 discusses the role of hydrogen and bicarbonate in maintaining acid-base balance. The concentrations of electrolytes in various body fluids are given in Table 13–1.

Electrolytes have several functions in the body. They regulate fluid balance and osmolality. Because of the abundance of sodium in the ECF, this ion has a major effect on fluid balance. Problems related to fluid balance are discussed in Chapter 12. The continual fluctuation of anions and cations also allows for transmission of nerve impulses and stimulation of muscle activity.[29]

ELECTROLYTE BALANCE

■ DIETARY INTAKE

Under normal circumstances, humans ingest far more electrolytes than are needed each day. Food sources for some important electrolytes are listed later in the chapter (see Boxes 13–2 to 13–5). Only when food intake is restricted does the intake of electrolytes become a concern.

■ REGULATED OUTPUT

Several hormones govern the output of electrolytes. Sodium, potassium, and chloride are closely regulated by aldosterone, antidiuretic hormone (ADH), and atrial natriuretic peptide (ANP). Calcium and phosphorus are regulated by vitamin D and calcitonin. Insulin and epinephrine promote the uptake of potassium by cells. Hormones such as gastrin, cholecystokinin, and secretin affect some degree of electrolyte absorption in the intestines. Finally, weight-bearing and stress on bones promote calcium uptake by the bone.

ELECTROLYTE IMBALANCES

An electrolyte imbalance is present whenever there is an excess or deficit in the plasma level of a specific ion. Terms used to describe the imbalance contain the prefix *hyper-* for increased or *hypo-* for decreased, followed by the name of the electrolyte (in its Latin form for sodium and potassium) and then the suffix *-emia* to indicate presence in the blood—as measured in the plasma. For example, *hyponatremia* means low plasma sodium, and *hyperkalemia* means elevated plasma potassium. *Hypercalcemia* and *hypermagnesemia* indicate elevated calcium and magnesium levels, respectively.

Although electrolyte imbalances are very common, the literature is scant on the topic. One study found that 94% of clients coming into the emergency department with certain presenting characteristics had significant electrolyte imbalances. These variables included poor oral intake, history of vomiting or muscle weakness, use of diuretics, signs of abnormal mental status, and history of chronic hypertension, alcoholism, recent seizure or electrolyte imbalance, and age 65 years or older.

As with fluid imbalance, a client's response to electrolyte imbalance is related to several variables. The relationship of fluid status to the electrolyte level, age, health status, potential for adaptive mechanisms, and the severity and acuteness of the imbalance all influence the client's response.

To help clients achieve the most positive health outcomes, you must understand the underlying causative disorders and conditions as well as the risk factors for electrolyte imbalance and become an active participant in health promotion, health maintenance, and health restoration interventions. By increasing the emphasis on health promotion and maintenance from a community perspective, you can also decrease the need for acute care intervention, which decreases the cost of health care in addition to improving health outcomes.

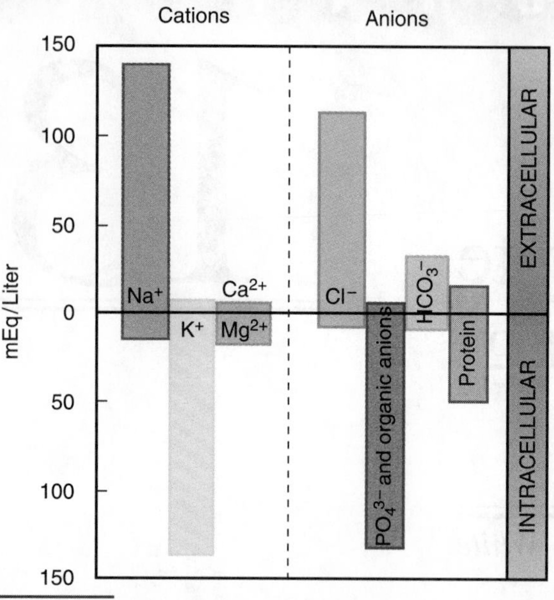

FIGURE 13–1 A comparison of electrolyte composition of the extracellular and intracellular fluid compartments. (From Guyton, A. C., & Hall, J. E. [1996]. *Textbook of medical physiology* [9th ed., p. 300]. Philadelphia: W. B. Saunders.)

Etiology and Risk Factors

Anyone who has decreased intake, decreased availability, or increased loss of electrolytes is at risk for electrolyte deficit. When body fluids are lost, the electrolytes in them are also lost. For example, the loss of gastric juice through vomiting may lead to the loss of several electrolytes. Conversely, increased intake or increased retention of an electrolyte or decreased ability to excrete certain electrolytes may increase the risk for electrolyte excess. For example, ingestion of excess sodium bicarbonate for indigestion can alter both sodium level and acid base balance.

Pathophysiology

Before you can fully understand the pathophysiology of electrolyte imbalances, you need to first understand the physiology of the action potential (see the Anatomy and Physiology section of this unit). Conduction of electrical current depends on normal membrane permeability, transportation of electrolytes, and ion concentrations. Common problems that alter the conduction of electrical current include problems with membrane permeability, ionic gradients, and concentrations.

Cells are quickly damaged by lack of blood flow or oxygen. Cardiac, nerve, and muscle cells can be damaged by lack of blood flow (as during periods of ischemia), altered by toxins (as from various medications), or directly injured (as in crush or stab injuries). Such damage typically increases the permeability of the cell membrane and increases its tendency to "fire." This phenomenon can be seen in cardiac cells after ischemia. Cells that normally do not generate action potentials begin to do so, causing abnormal heart rhythms. This same phenomenon can be the cause of seizures following brain injury.

Potassium levels can significantly influence the resting membrane potential (Fig. 13–2). When potassium levels are lower than normal, the resting membrane potential becomes more positive. It requires less stimulus to make it "fire." Cells so affected are called *hypopolarized* and respond to a weaker stimulus. Conversely, when potassium levels are higher, the resting membrane potential falls and the cell is less excitable. Such cells are called *hyperpolarized* and require a stronger-than-normal stimulus to reach threshold potential and to generate an action potential. Sodium and calcium also alter resting membrane potential.

Diagnosis

A wide range of clinical manifestations should raise suspicion about a possible electrolyte imbalance, as suggested in the Critical Monitoring feature. The diagnosis of electrolyte imbalance is made through clinical assessment and measurement of plasma levels in laboratory studies. Currently, measurement of intracellular levels of electrolytes is too costly; thus, plasma levels are used for diagnostic evaluation (Box 13–1). Plasma electrolyte studies are relatively inexpensive.

Plasma values for electrolytes can be expressed as milliequivalents per liter (mEq/L), or milligrams per deciliter

TABLE 13–1 CONCENTRATION OF ELECTROLYTES IN VARIOUS BODY FLUIDS*

Fluid	Concentration (mEq/L)				
	Na^+	*K^+*	*Cl^-*	*HCO_3^-*	*H^-*
Plasma	135–145	3.5–5.0	98–106	25–29	7.35–7.45
Gastric juice	55–100	10–15	120	5–10	90
Pancreatic juice	145–160	5	65–90	50–80	—
Bile	130–145	5–9	75–100	10–45	—
Ileum	125	10–80	55	60	—
Sweat					
Insensible	8	10	15	—	—
Sensible	10–80	6	5–85	—	—

*Levels may vary according to the physiologic state of the body.
Na^+, sodium; K^+, potassium; Cl^-, chloride; HCO_3^-, bicarbonate; H^+, hydrogen.
From White, B. (1994). Maintaining fluid and electrolyte balance. In V. B. Bolander (Ed.), *Sorenson and Luckmann's basic nursing: A psychophysiologic approach* (3rd ed.). Philadelphia: W. B. Saunders.

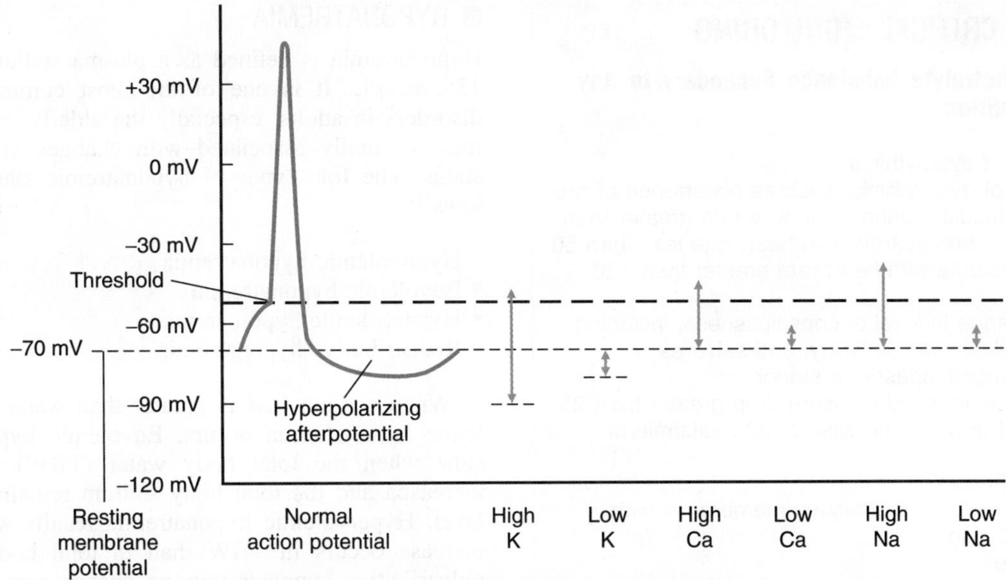

FIGURE 13–2 Effects of electrolyte imbalances on the membrane potential. Conductile tissue rests at negative millivolts, called a *resting membrane potential.* When the nerve is stimulated, ion channels for sodium, potassium, and calcium open to change the firing potential. Potassium tends to lower the potential by decreasing the millivolts to more negative levels. Sodium does the opposite: It raises the action potential to more positive values (above zero). Calcium also raises the resting membrane potential to a more positive value. The closer the resting membrane potential to threshold, the more rapid the nerve firing.

(mg/dl). Values reported as mEq/L can be converted to mg/dl by multiplying by 1.2.

Using a "Collaborative Problem" Format

Currently there are no NANDA diagnoses for electrolyte imbalances. The Iowa Interventions Project approached these disorders as collaborative problems and developed a research-based list of critical and supporting activities for management of 15 fluid and electrolyte disorders. Because the nursing role primarily involves collaborating with the physician, the goal statements are also phrased differently. Note that each expected outcome is preceded by the phrase "The nurse will monitor the client for. . . ."[20] Nursing diagnoses that may apply to clients with electrolyte imbalances include *Risk for Injury, Risk for Activity Intolerance, Risk for Decreased Cardiac Output, Altered Mucous Membranes,* and *Risk for Impaired Skin Integrity.* Or you may use the appropriate collaborative problem taxonomy to identify the problem—*hyponatremia* or *hypernatremia, hypokalemia* or *hyperkalemia, hypocalcemia* or *hypercalcemia, hypomagnesemia* or *hypermagnesemia* and *hypophosphatemia* or *hyperphosphatemia.*

BOX 13–1 Plasma Ranges for Electrolytes*

Sodium	135–145 mEq/L
Chloride	98–106 mEq/L
Potassium	3.5–5.0 mEq/L
Calcium	4.5–5.5 mEq/L
Ionized calcium	1.18–1.30 mEq/L
Phosphorus	1.2–3.0 mEq/L
Magnesium	1.5–2.5 mEq/L

*Ranges may vary somewhat between laboratories.

SODIUM IMBALANCES

A sodium imbalance occurs when sodium concentration in plasma either decreases or increases. A sodium deficit is known as *hyponatremia.* Sodium excess is known as *hypernatremia.* Chloride is the anion that usually accompanies sodium; therefore, levels of chloride fall or rise along with levels of sodium. Manifestations of chloride imbalance are usually associated with the cation imbalance.

Sodium balance is regulated by the interaction among neural, hormonal, and vascular mechanisms. Sensing mechanisms in the atria, aorta, carotid sinus, liver, pulmonary tissue, and juxtaglomerular apparatus (JGA) in the kidneys detect changes in sodium intake and ECF volume by sensing an increase or decrease in blood pressure. Central nervous system (CNS) receptors also respond to changes in the sodium concentration in the cerebrospinal fluid (CSF).

One example of a neural-hormonal interaction is the JGA sensory mechanism in the nephron, which promotes a stimulation response of the renin-angiotensin-aldosterone hormonal system. Renin, excreted in response to hypotension, results in increased aldosterone secretion, which stimulates sodium reabsorption across the renal tubule. Prostaglandins, kallikrein, and atrial natriuretic peptide also control sodium homeostasis. Prostaglandins secreted by the kidney stimulate the production of renin to maintain renal blood flow during periods of reduced blood volume. Kallikreins are high-molecular-weight pro-

CRITICAL MONITORING

Fluid and Electrolyte Imbalance Secondary to Any Disorder/Condition

- New onset of dysrhythmia
- Worsening of dysrhythmia, such as occurrence of premature ventricular contractions at a rate greater than 6 per minute, bradycardia with heart rate less than 50 BPM, tachycardia with heart rate greater than 120 BPM
- Sudden change in level of consciousness, including sudden restlessness, lethargy, and seizures
- Tetany, laryngeal spasm, or stridor
- Postural systolic blood pressure drop greater than 25 mm Hg, with a pulse increase of 30 beats/min or more
- Rapid weight loss
- Severe dryness of oral mucous membranes with tongue furrowing
- Hemorrhage
- Urinary output less than 30 ml/hr for 2 consecutive hours
- Rapid weight gain, especially with pulmonary signs of sudden onset such as crackles, dyspnea, S_3 gallop

teins produced by the distal convoluted tubule that secrete kinin. Kinin is a potent renal vasodilator that increases renal excretion of sodium. Atrial natriuretic peptide (ANP) balances the effects of ADH by promoting urinary sodium excretion (natriuresis), vasodilatation, and increased urinary output.[13] See the Nervous System review in Unit 11 and Chapter 52 for review of the influence of the baroreceptors.

The phenomenon of glomerular capillary filtration is an example of how vascular dynamics influence sodium homeostasis. The renal glomerulus filters 1000 mEq of sodium every hour, and about 99% of this is reabsorbed. Reabsorption is influenced by the pressure of the blood entering the glomeruli. Increased blood pressure promotes filtration of water and sodium and other electrolytes across the glomerular membrane. Sodium is reabsorbed in the loop of Henle, and reabsorption of the rest of the electrolytes occurs in the proximal tubule.

HYPONATREMIA

Hyponatremia is defined as a plasma sodium level below 135 mEq/L. It is one of the most common electrolyte disorders in adults, especially the elderly.[21, 30] Hyponatremia is usually associated with changes in fluid volume status. The four types of hyponatremic states are as follows[21]:

- Hypovolemic hyponatremia
- Euvolemic hyponatremia
- Hypervolemic hyponatremia
- Redistributive hyponatremia

When sodium loss is greater than water loss, hypovolemic hyponatremia occurs. Euvolemic hyponatremia results when the total body water (TBW) is moderately increased and the total body sodium remains at a normal level. Hypervolemic hyponatremia results when a greater increase occurs in TBW than in total body sodium. In redistributive hyponatremia, no change occurs in TBW or total body sodium; water merely shifts between the intracellular and extracellular compartments relative to the sodium concentration.

Etiology and Risk Factors

Table 13–2 lists the most common pathophysiologic causes of hyponatremia. Hyponatremia can also occur in persons who are considered healthy. For example, athletes[3, 12] and outdoor laborers are at risk for hyponatremia from excessive perspiration. Any person with an altered thirst mechanism or without access to fluids, or one who attempts to rehydrate too rapidly after excessive fluid loss, is at risk for hyponatremia. Older adults are at increased risk because of their relatively lower percentage of TBW. The preoperative use of laxatives, multiple pathologic conditions, spinal anesthesia, and noninfectious postoperative complications increase risk factors for death from hyponatremia in elderly people after surgery.

With cardiac, renal, and liver disease, the total body sodium is usually high, although the plasma sodium level may appear normal or low because of dilution from water retention. In such instances, the increase in TBW is generally greater than the sodium indicates. Renal causes of hyponatremia stem from the inability to excrete suffi-

TABLE 13–2 CLINICAL CONDITIONS AND DISORDERS THAT MAY CAUSE HYPONATREMIA

Type of Hyponatremia	Clinical Conditions and Disorders
Hypovolemic hyponatremia	Renal loss of sodium from diuretic use, diabetic glycosuria, aldosterone deficiency, intrinsic renal disease Extrarenal loss of sodium from vomiting, diarrhea, increased sweating, burns, high-volume ileostomy
Euvolemic hyponatremia	Sodium deficit resulting from SIADH or the continuous secretion of ADH due to pain, emotion, medications; many cancers; CNS disorders
Hypervolemic hyponatremia	Edematous disorders resulting in sodium deficits; congestive heart failure, cirrhosis of the liver, nephrotic syndrome, acute and chronic renal failure
Redistributive hyponatremia	Pseudohyponatremia, hyperglycemia, hyperlipidemia

ADH, antidiuretic hormone; CNS, central nervous system; SIADH, syndrome of inappropriate (secretion of) antidiuretic hormone.

ciently dilute urine.[25] Normally, when hyponatremia and hyposmolality occur, diuresis follows to promote the return of sodium and water reabsorption.

Pathophysiology

Most pathophysiologic changes caused by hyponatremia result from the decreased excitability of the membranes from a loss of sodium and changes in water volume. Recall that most sodium is outside the cell. Less sodium is available to move across the excitable membrane, resulting in delayed membrane depolarization. Excitable tissues vary in their response to decreased sodium. The cells most sensitive to change are the CNS cells.

As the concentration of sodium decreases in the ECF, the difference in gradient between the ECF and ICF compartments also decreases. When the extracellular sodium level falls, the ECF becomes hypo-osmolar. This osmotic shift can lead to intracellular edema. Water moves into the cell to the area of greater concentration to rebalance the water concentration. An increase in brain cell volume as small as 5% can cause brain herniation.[27] Brain cells attempt to compensate by reducing cerebral blood flow, shifting CSF, and decreasing the brain's intracellular osmolality. Intracellular osmolality is reduced through decreasing the amount of intracellular ions, such as sodium and potassium, and amino acids.[21, 27]

Clinical Manifestations and Diagnostic Findings

Clinical manifestations of hyponatremia vary with the cause, type, and rate of onset of sodium or fluid imbalance. A plasma sodium level of 120 mEq/L that developed slowly may be asymptomatic. The same plasma sodium level resulting from an acute loss may be life-threatening.[10]

When plasma sodium concentration is greater than 125 mEq/L, clinical manifestations may not be apparent.[10, 30] Early neurologic manifestations of headache and apprehension are from increased fluid shift into the cerebral cells. As intracranial pressure rises and plasma sodium level drops to 115 mEq/L, severe neurologic changes such as confusion, hallucinations, behavioral changes, and seizures occur. Continued shifting of water into the intracellular compartment leads to brain herniation, resulting in coma and death.[21, 27, 30]

Cardiovascular manifestations—such as a decrease in systolic and diastolic blood pressures, orthostatic hypotension, and a weak, thready pulse—are due to a decrease in vascular volume secondary to sodium and water loss. Tachycardia is a compensatory response that is the direct result of triggering of the release of sympathetic catecholamines by the baroreceptor reflex (see Unit 12 review). Chemoreceptors in the aortic arch and carotid bodies also trigger sympathetic responses if the oxygen, carbon dioxide, or hydrogen levels become affected. In severe hypovolemic hyponatremia, a shock-like state occurs, with blood pressures of 60 mm Hg and below. An exception is hypervolemic hyponatremia, in which the excess volume causes elevated blood pressure and a full, rapid pulse.

Crackles in the lungs are from fluid shifting into the pulmonary alveoli secondary to increasing fluid pressures in the pulmonary capillaries. The increasing left ventricular fluid pressure leads to a retrograde increase in pressure in the left atrium and pulmonary vasculature. The changes in respiratory rate and difficulty breathing—such as tachypnea, dyspnea, orthopnea, and feeling short of breath—are from presence of fluid in the alveoli, which alters oxygen and carbon dioxide levels. Alterations in respiratory pattern, such as with Cheyne-Stokes respirations, neurogenic hyperventilation, apneustic breathing, or ataxic breathing, are from increasing intracranial pressure.

Hyponatremia causes gastrointestinal (GI) manifestations, such as nausea, vomiting, hyperactive bowel sounds, abdominal cramping, and diarrhea, because sodium is a crucial component of normal neuromuscular activity of smooth muscle. A decrease in sodium causes increased excitability of the neurons that innervate the smooth muscle.

Although not life-threatening, the dryness of the skin, tongue, and mucous membranes that results from the decreased interstitial volume caused by a sodium deficit has other, more serious implications. There is a higher risk for altered integrity of the skin and oral mucous membranes, which increases the risk of infection and results in increased health care needs and costs.

A laboratory finding of a plasma sodium level below 135 mEq/L is diagnostic of hyponatremia. However, as noted previously, most clients are not symptomatic until levels reach 125 mEq/L or less. Because chloride is the main anion associated with sodium, a chloride level below 98 mEq/L is a very common finding. A decreased concentration of sodium is also reflected in a plasma osmolality of less than 275 mOsm/kg. The kidney attempts to compensate for the body's loss of sodium by decreasing urinary losses; thus, a typical urine sodium level is below 40 mEq/L.[36]

If the hyponatremic state and body fluid volume disorders are not corrected, potassium, calcium, chloride, and bicarbonate electrolyte imbalances may also occur.

Outcome Management

Medical Management

Medical management is determined by the cause of the hyponatremia, the type of hyponatremia, and the severity of the clinical manifestations. The more serious the manifestations, the more aggressive the treatment. The goal of medical intervention is correction of the body water osmolality, with restoration of cell volume, by raising the ratio of sodium to water in the ECF. The increased ECF osmolality draws water from the cells, thereby decreasing cellular edema.

Restoring Sodium Levels

If the client has hyponatremia from fluid volume excess, fluids are restricted to allow the sodium to regain balance. Intake of balanced diet is usually adequate therapy for mild hyponatremia, with sodium levels of 126 to 135 mEq/L. Fluids may be restricted to a range of 1000 to 1500 ml/day.

If the plasma sodium level declines below 125 mEq/L, sodium replacement is needed. For sodium levels of 125 mEq/L or less, intravenous (IV) therapy is the treatment of choice. Dietary supplementation may still be appropriate for a client who can ingest oral fluids or food. Foods high in sodium are listed in Box 13–2. For moderate hyponatremia, with sodium levels of 125 mEq/L, IV normal saline solution (0.9% NaCl) or lactated Ringer's solution may be ordered if the client is symptomatic. When the plasma sodium level is 115 mEq/L or less, a concentrated saline solution such as 3% NaCl may be indicated until the plasma sodium reaches 125 mEq/L. A diuretic such as furosemide (Lasix) is often given intravenously to prevent fluid overload. Demeclocycline (a tetracycline), an agent that antagonizes ADH, is the preferred agent for treatment of hyponatremia secondary to syndrome of inappropriate antidiuretic hormone (SIADH).[10, 28, 33, 77]

Rapid elevation of plasma sodium concentrations to more than 125 mEq/L increases intravascular fluid volume and may result in hypernatremia and CNS damage. Recommendations for IV replacement therapy include an infusion rate of 0.5 mEq/L/hr if the loss is chronic, not to exceed a total of 12 mEq of sodium in 48 hours, or of 1.0 mEq/L/hr if the loss is acute, not to exceed 25 mEq in 48 hours.[5] To prevent fluid shifts and exacerbation of vasospasm in persons with subarachnoid hemorrhage, normal saline is usually the IV solution of choice.[21, 37]

Nursing Management of the Medical Client

ASSESSMENT

Take a complete history of risk factors and presenting manifestations. Emphasize diet and medication history, including over-the-counter medications. Older adults are especially prone to drug-drug interactions that may alter sodium balance. The client and family members should be asked about behavioral changes, headaches, increased weakness or sleepiness, dizziness, and palpitations.

Measure the client's body weight, because the stated weight may not be accurate. Calculate ideal body weight by using height, weight, and body frame; then compare measurements. Assess intake and output, peripheral vein filling time, and vital signs every 4 to 8 hours. Also, monitor plasma sodium levels and estimate the plasma osmolality. It is important to remember that in hyponatremic conditions, such as hypervolemic hyponatremia, plasma sodium levels may appear to be normal to low.

DIAGNOSIS, OUTCOMES, INTERVENTIONS

Risk of Hyponatremia. There is no specific diagnosis for hyponatremia; therefore, the collaborative problem of *Risk for Hyponatremia* can be used to label this client problem. State the problem as *Risk for Hyponatremia related to unreplaced fluid loss or limited oral intake.*

When actual hyponatremia is present, the collaborative problem is stated as *Hyponatremia related to* (e.g., *vomiting, diarrhea, gastric suctioning, burns, SIADH, surgery, or fluid overload*). The cause needs to be clear because it relates directly to the interventions.

Outcomes. The nurse will have a high index of suspicion for high-risk clients and will monitor clients who have had fluid losses or limited fluid intake for manifestations of hyponatremia. When your assessment indicates an actual sodium deficit, restoration is the primary goal. An outcome may be as follows: The nurse will monitor laboratory sodium and chloride levels and will continue to monitor for clinical manifestations of hyponatremia.

BOX 13–2 High- and Low-Sodium Foods

High-Sodium Foods (~250 mg per serving)

Breads/Cereals

Cold cereal, 1 oz
Corn chips, 14 chips
Instant hot cereal, ½ cup
Potato chips, 14 chips

Cheeses

Natural cheese, 1 oz
Processed cheese, 1 oz
Creamed cheese, ½ cup

Meats

Sausage, 1 oz
Luncheon meats, 1 oz
Frankfurters, 1 oz
Cooked bacon, 2 slices
Ham, 1 oz

Convenience Foods

Pizza, 2 to 3 slices
Pot pies, 8 oz
Ravioli, canned, 8 oz
Soups (canned/dehydrated), 1 cup

Low-Sodium Foods (<50 mg per serving)

Fruits/Vegetables

Fresh or canned, ½ cup
Fresh, frozen, ½ cup

Breads/Cereals

Unsalted pastas, ½ cup
Oatmeal, cooked, 1 cup
Popcorn (unsalted), 1 oz
Puffed rice, 1 cup
Shredded wheat, 1 biscuit

Meats

Fresh meat, 1 oz
Fresh chicken, 1 oz
Fresh fish, 1 oz

Data from Laquarta, I., & Gerlach, M. (1990). *Nutrition in clinical nursing.* Albany, NY: Delmar; and Burtis, G., et al. (1988). *Applied nutrition and diet therapy.* Philadelphia: W. B. Saunders.

Interventions

Reduce Sodium Loss in High-Risk Clients. If plasma sodium levels are above 125 mEq/L, encourage intake of 30 to 60 ml of clear liquids or more per hour as tolerated. If the client is on a low-sodium diet, do not be concerned about sodium restriction until the vomiting or diarrhea subsides and the client is taking whole foods.

To prevent sodium loss, irrigate nasogastric tubes and wounds with isotonic saline and give only minimal ice chips, even if ordered, when a nasogastric tube is connected to suction. Never give more than three tap water enemas in succession without consulting the physician about converting the enema fluid to normal saline. Treat nausea with prophylactic antiemetics. If hyponatremia is from hypervolemia, consult the dietitian for assistance in total fluid restriction. Consult the physician if (1) the sodium level is less than 125 mEq/L or sooner if client is symptomatic or (2) the client is receiving nothing by mouth (NPO status) and has no intake of electrolytes or has an increased loss of electrolytes.

Restore Sodium Balance. Encourage the intake of a well-balanced diet. Give nutrient-dense supplements between meals. If the client is receiving nutrition only through tube feedings, it is sometimes necessary to add extra salt to the feeding to achieve the desired sodium level.[29] If the hyponatremia is secondary to hypervolemia, consult with the physician and dietitian to coordinate therapeutic fluid restriction. Strict behavioral modification or psychiatric consultation may be necessary for a client who drinks water compulsively.

To decrease the thirst that accompanies fluid restriction, offer ice chips, cold fluids, and frequent oral care. Some clients feel less thirsty if they hold the fluids in their mouth first to fully moisten the oral mucous membranes before swallowing. Restricting fluids is contraindicated in persons with subarachnoid hemorrhage because it increases the risk of cerebral vasospasm and cell death.[10]

When plasma sodium levels are 125 mEq/L or less and the client is symptomatic, notify the physician immediately. Administration of hypertonic IV saline (3% saline) is the most commonly prescribed therapy. *Caution:* Hypertonic saline must be given very slowly by IV piggyback infusion in a large vein to decrease the risk of hypernatremia, pulmonary congestion, and phlebitis. If the client is confused or agitated, also initiate safety and seizure precautions.

EVALUATION

Mild to moderate deficits are usually corrected in 8 to 24 hours. More severe deficits may take several days, especially in older adults. Evaluate the client's and family members' understanding of positive health behaviors that prevent further occurrences of sodium deficit.

Self-Care

Teach the client to consult the physician if vomiting or diarrhea persists for more than 48 hours, or sooner if extreme weakness, dizziness, palpitations, irregular pulse of new onset, cough or dyspnea, or CNS changes (such as headache, confusion, or seizures) develop. Anyone who has a chronic disease—such as renal, liver, or heart disease or diabetes mellitus—should consult a physician if any signs or symptoms persist for more than 24 hours.

Teach clients to consult a physician before taking over-the-counter medications. Review the exercise precautions discussed in Chapter 12. Refer people with eating disorders to counseling and community support groups.

HYPERNATREMIA

Hypernatremia is defined as a plasma sodium level above 145 mEq/L. It occurs in about 1% of hospitalized clients and carries a high mortality rate, whether it has an acute or a chronic onset. Hypernatremia is usually associated with water loss or sodium gain. It can occur with increased, decreased, or normal total body sodium levels and decreased or increased TBW levels. The underlying cause of hypernatremia is a TBW deficit relative to the total body sodium content, which results in hyperosmolality.

Etiology and Risk Factors

Body fluid loss resulting in hypernatremia may be from renal or extrarenal causes, such as GI or skin problems. Hypernatremia can be classified as one of three types:

- Hypovolemic hypernatremia, in which TBW is greatly decreased relative to sodium (loss of hypotonic fluid)
- Euvolemic hypernatremia, in which TBW is decreased relative to the normal total body sodium
- Hypervolemic hypernatremia, in which TBW is increased but the sodium gain exceeds the water gain

Hypervolemic hypernatremia is the least common type of hypernatremia. Table 13–3 presents clinical conditions and disorders that may contribute to the development of hypernatremia.[24] Elderly and debilitated people are at highest risk for developing hypernatremia. Major risk factors include inadequate water intake in conjunction with decreased thirst (hypodipsia), lack of access to drinkable water, physical or chemical restraint, mental confusion, and NPO status. Excessive water loss and insufficient fluid replacement associated with fever, vomiting, diarrhea, excess drainage, polyuria, tube-feeding, or prolonged hyperventilation are also major risk factors.

Other factors that increase the risk for hypernatremia include increased sodium intake, such as with IV administration of hypertonic saline or hypertonic tube feedings. Retention of sodium occurs in heart, renal, or liver disease; Cushing's syndrome; hyperaldosteronism with corticosteroid therapy; and uncontrolled diabetes mellitus or insipidus. Uncontrolled diabetes mellitus results in polyuria, leading to dehydration and secondary hypernatremia. Fortunately, hypernatremia from untreated diabetes insipidus tends to be mild. Although the ADH mechanism is

TABLE 13–3 CLINICAL CONDITIONS AND DISORDERS THAT MAY CONTRIBUTE TO HYPERNATREMIA

Type of Hypernatremia	Clinical Conditions and Disorders
Hypovolemic hypernatremia	Renal losses; osmotic diuresis, diuretics, severe hyperglycemia Extrarenal losses: profuse diaphoresis, decreased thirst, diarrhea occurring with inadequate volume replacement or fluid replacement with hyperosmolar solutions, burns
Euvolemic hypernatremia	Excess fluid losses from the skin and lungs Hypodipsia in the elderly and infants Diabetes insipidus
Hypervolemic hypernatremia	Administration of concentrated saline solutions; hypertonic feedings, excess mineralocorticoids Accidental or intentional salt ingestion; commercially prepared soups and canned vegetables

altered, the thirst mechanism is intact and stimulates the client to drink water and fluids, which helps balance water losses and hypernatremia. See Chapter 44 for a more in-depth discussion of diabetes insipidus.

Pathophysiology

When sodium levels rise, water moves to maintain balance. However, the osmotic shift of water from the cells to the ECF in an attempt to dilute the hyperosmolar state only creates another problem: cellular dehydration. If the hypernatremia evolves slowly or is chronic, the brain develops its own osmotic particles, called *idiogenic osmoles,* to prevent fluid shifts into and out of the brain cells.[30]

The heart is sensitive to the increasing sodium levels. Calcium must move through the calcium channels for cardiac muscle contraction to occur. However, in hypernatremia, sodium molecules compete with calcium in the slow calcium channels of the heart, resulting in decreased myocardial contractility. Myocardial depolarization, however, occurs more easily with the increased sodium levels.

Generally, the body responds to increased sodium levels by suppressing the effects of aldosterone and ADH. These two substances normally act to increase renal blood flow and cause excretion of sodium and water. In hypernatremia, the magnitude of the problem overwhelms the ability of these adaptive mechanisms to compensate.

Clinical Manifestations and Diagnostic Findings

In the early stages of hypernatremia, clinical manifestations are nonspecific because two thirds of body water is intracellular; primary water losses tend to cause only modest effects on circulating blood volume. Early manifestations include polyuria followed by oliguria, anorexia, nausea, vomiting, weakness, and restlessness. The anorexia, nausea, and vomiting are related to increased fluid retention in the gastric cells. Early neurologic manifestations of restlessness, agitation, irritability, and muscle weakness are related to the sensitivity of brain cells to fluid shifting.

The response of the kidneys varies with the type of hypernatremia. In a hypervolemic state, the kidneys excrete some of the excess water. In a hypovolemic state, oliguria is the method of renal compensation. As fluid levels decrease in the interstitial compartments, the skin becomes dry and flushed, the mucous membranes become dry and sticky, and tongue furrows develop. The person experiences increasing thirst and fever. Temperature elevation is from the decreasing amount of fluid available for dissipating heat.

Cardiovascular manifestations are related to the type of hypernatremia. In hypovolemic hypernatremia, orthostatic hypotension with compensatory tachycardia (rapid heart beat) occurs. In hypervolemic hypernatremia, signs of hypertension, jugular venous distention, prolonged peripheral vein emptying, an extra heart sound (S_3 gallop), and generalized weight gain and edema are often present.

Dysrhythmia can result from the competition of sodium ions with calcium ions in the slow channels of the heart cells. Pulmonary manifestations, such as crackles, dyspnea, and pleural effusion, are also due to the increasing hydrostatic pressure seen in hypervolemic hypernatremia.

When sodium levels reach 155 mEq/L or more, cells (especially brain cells) shrink because of the increased ECF osmolality. More severe neurologic changes occur, manifested as confusion, seizures, or coma, in some cases with irreversible brain damage. Altered neuromuscular contractility and irritability lead to muscle twitching, tremor, hyperreflexia, and seizures. The development of rigid paralysis is a grave sign.

The diagnosis of hypernatremia is validated through increased plasma sodium concentration and osmolality. A plasma sodium level above 145 mEq/L and plasma osmolality above 295 mOsm/kg are diagnostic for hypernatremia. Because chloride is the major ECF ion that balances sodium, it is common to find a plasma chloride level above 106 mEq/L. Unless the sodium elevation is an acute change, many clients will not be symptomatic until plasma sodium reaches 155 mEq/L or more.

Outcome Management

Again, a thorough history and physical examination, as well as the aforementioned plasma studies, are necessary for accurate diagnosis of hypernatremia. Awareness of demographic variables is essential for choosing the appropriate interventions for restoring sodium balance.

Medical Management

Medical management is determined by the type of hypernatremia. The goal of medical intervention is correction of the body water osmolality, with restoration of cell volume, by decreasing the ratio of sodium to water in the ECF.

For a client experiencing minor manifestations from hypovolemia or euvolemic hypernatremia, the focus is on correcting the underlying disorder and giving oral fluid replacement. However, clients with cardiovascular, pulmonary, or neurologic manifestations from severe hypernatremia usually require hospitalization and the more aggressive approach of IV hypotonic saline.

To decrease total body sodium and replace fluid loss, either a hyposmolar electrolyte solution (0.2% or 0.45% NaCl) or 5% dextrose in water (D_5W) is administered. These solutions do not cause a considerable dilution of body sodium; instead, the plasma sodium level gradually decreases as excess sodium is excreted. When administered continuously, D_5W is considered to be a hypoosmolar solution because the dextrose is metabolized quickly and only water remains. If the plasma sodium level is lowered too rapidly, fluid shifts from the vascular fluid into the cerebral cells, causing cerebral edema. Slow administration of IV fluids with a goal of reducing plasma sodium levels, at a rate of not more than 2 mEq/L/hr for the first 48 hours, decreases this risks.[5, 10]

Hypernatremia due to sodium excess may be treated with administration of D_5W and a diuretic, such as furosemide (Lasix).[31, 32] When hypernatremia results from diabetes insipidus, desmopressin acetate, in the form of a nasal spray, is commonly ordered to slow the rate of diuresis. It has a 20-hour duration of action compared with the 4- to 6-hour duration of vasopressin oil nasal spray.[10]

Although dietary sodium restriction is useful in preventing hypernatremia in high-risk clients, it cannot bring a high sodium level down to normal. People with renal disease may need sodium intake restricted to 500 to 2000 mg/day (see Box 13–2). In hypervolemic hypernatremia, fluids must also be restricted. Clients with diabetes insipidus who are receiving antidiuretic medications must be taught to avoid excessive water intake. Drinking excess water defeats the purpose of the medication.

Nursing Management of the Medical Client

ASSESSMENT

Assess for the usual clinical manifestations, especially in head-injured and other high-risk clients. Obtain a thorough diet and medication history, including the use of corticosteroids and over-the-counter medications, such as cough medicine, and food flavorings and spices (salt).

Depending on the client's condition, assess vital signs and peripheral vein filling time every 4 to 8 hours, measure intake and output every 8 hours, and monitor body weight daily. Use oral membrane and skin assessment tools to guide your interventions. Monitor for changes in plasma sodium and plasma osmolality (by estimated values). Report early signs of altered mental status, such as agitation, irritability, or confusion, to prevent the progression of hypernatremia and to detect lack of response to therapy or signs of overcorrection (resulting in hyponatremia). Monitor lung sounds every 2 to 4 hours, and notify the physician of increasing pulmonary overload.

DIAGNOSIS, OUTCOMES, INTERVENTIONS

Risk of Hypernatremia. The format for writing the collaborative problem is as follows: *Hypernatremia related to* (e.g., *decreased thirst, excessive administration of salt solutions,* or *impaired excretion of sodium and water*). The cause needs to be identified specifically, as it guides the choice of interventions.

Outcomes. The nurse will maintain a high index of suspicion for high-risk clients and will monitor plasma sodium and chloride levels and clinical manifestations of hypernatremia.

Interventions. Monitor the client for response to IV fluid replacement of hyposmolar electrolyte solutions, absence of clinical manifestations of hypernatremia, and return to normal sodium levels. Prevent osmotic diuresis from D_5W by maintaining the prescribed rate. Use IV pumps in high-risk clients. Initiate safety and seizure precautions if the client manifests weakness or cerebral changes.

Offer water and fluids hourly to clients with hypovolemic or euvolemic hypernatremia. Consult with the dietitian and the physician concerning the need for fluid and sodium restriction in those with hypervolemic hypernatremia. Teach the client and family members the food items that should be restricted as well as the rationale for these restrictions.

Give 1 ml of fluid per kilocalorie (kcal) of hypertonic feeding solution. Initiate new gastric feedings slowly. Increase the rate if the client tolerates the feeding, as evidenced by no diarrhea, with residuals less than half the amount of the feeding per hour, or up to 100 ml.

Consult the physician for signs that indicate worsening of the hypernatremia or fluid overload, such as increasing weight gain or pulmonary, cardiovascular, or neurologic manifestations.

Altered Oral Mucous Membranes. The problem statement *Altered Oral Mucous Membranes related to lack of body water secondary to hypernatremia* can be used.

Outcomes. There are several options for outcome statements, depending upon the condition of the mouth initially. If the oral membranes are simply dry, but not open or cracked, an outcome of maintaining moist oral mucous membranes is appropriate. If the oral mucous membranes are cracked or open, the outcome should state that no further deterioration will occur and that the mouth will be moist. Additional nursing diagnoses for pain from oral ulcerations or inadequate nutrition related to mouth pain should be considered.

Interventions. Provide oral care every 2 hours with a nonalcoholic mouthwash. Avoid lemon-glycerin swabs because they dry the membranes and may cause pain. Dilute saline and non-alcoholic rinses have been found to be effective. Use a soft toothbrush to prevent injury to the mucosa. Moisten the client's lips every 1 to 2 hours. Offer cool, nonacidic fluids such as apple juice. Low-acid juices provide fluid while decreasing pain and irritation. Limited ice chips may also decrease the discomfort from dry mucous membranes.

Caregivers often feel uncomfortable about giving oral care, and often the client's mouth is simply rinsed or lightly "brushed" with foam toothbrushes. This "light touch" oral care is appropriate when clients are in pain from mouth ulcers. However, lack of thorough oral care also leads to mouth ulcers, dental decay, and malnutrition. Mucus can accumulate on the roof of the mouth and impair swallowing or even breathing. Assess the mouth before and after mouth care, and be aggressive in cleaning the mouth.

EVALUATION

Even if the desired outcome of sodium maintenance has been met, continue to monitor clients at high risk. The key to evaluating health promotion strategies is evaluating not only whether the client and family members understand the health promotion activities but, more important, asking whether they have incorporated the necessary changes into their lifestyle. If change has not occurred, investigate the barriers and recommend alternatives or resources.

If the desired outcome of sodium restoration has been met or partially met, the manifestations of excess should be absent or at least lessened. Mild to moderate excesses are usually corrected in 8 to 24 hours. If the excesses are more severe or occur in very young or older clients, intervention must be more cautious, necessitating 48 hours or more before positive outcomes are noticeable. Evaluate the client with altered oral mucous membranes every nursing shift. If improvement is not seen within a few hours, increase the frequency of oral care.

Self-Care

Teach clients the importance of taking hourly fluids—30 to 60 ml of clear liquids or more as tolerated—and avoiding excessive caffeinated beverages (because they lead to diuresis). Impress upon family members the importance of keeping fresh foods and a variety of fluids on hand, especially for the client who lives alone. Encourage the use of community resources, such as Meals on Wheels. Instruct on reading labels and avoiding foods with high "Na" (sodium) content and over-the-counter medications unless physician-approved.

Teach the client to consult the physician if vomiting or diarrhea persists for more than 48 hours or sooner if extreme weakness, dizziness, palpitations, change in mental state, new onset of cough, or increasing restlessness occurs. Persons with a concurrent chronic disease (such as diabetes mellitus or disease of the liver, heart, or kidneys) should consult a physician if any of these manifestations persist for longer than 24 hours. Explain the importance of reporting weight gains of more than 3 pounds in 1 week.

Some clients are managed at home with IV fluids. Home health care nurses see their clients often (see Bridge to Home Health Care).

POTASSIUM IMBALANCES

Potassium helps regulate intracellular osmolality and promotes the transmission and conduction of nerve impulses and the contraction of skeletal, cardiac, and smooth muscle. It promotes enzyme action for cellular metabolism and glycogen storage in the liver. Potassium also fosters acid-base balance through cellular exchange with hydrogen.

Potassium is plentiful in cells. About 96% (150 mEq/L) of potassium is in ICF, and 4% (5 mEq/L) is in intravascular fluid. Potassium is also plentiful in the GI tract secretions. Because the greatest amount of potassium is intracellular, the plasma range is very narrow. Normal values of plasma potassium range from 3.5 to 5.0 mEq/L. Life-threatening changes occur when the plasma potassium concentration is altered; levels less than 2.5 mEq/L or greater than 7.0 mEq/L can result in cardiac arrest.

Requirements for a person with no active loss of potassium are 40 to 60 mEq/day. Because potassium is

BRIDGE TO HOME HEALTH CARE

Managing Intravenous Therapy

Intravenous (IV) therapy is commonly administered in the home setting. Some recognized advantages include increased comfort, increased client participation in care, reduced cost of services, and a reduced risk of infection compared with the hospital. However, home therapy has associated risks, including those related to the presence of an invasive device (i.e., the IV catheter) and potential adverse reactions to certain medications or with specific modalities. Thus, it is important to provide home IV therapy with a primary goal of ensuring client safety.

Clearly delineated policies and procedures and careful client selection are essential. Client selection criteria to consider in planning home IV therapy include client (1) willingness and motivation, (2) ability to learn and remember procedures, (3) visual acuity, and (4) manual dexterity.

Some degree of self-care is usually the goal of home IV therapy. Depending on the type of therapy, clients or their caregivers may assume all or part of the responsibility for administering IV therapy. This includes taking care of the IV catheter site, flushing the catheter with heparin or normal saline to maintain patency, and administering IV medications. Home IV therapies usually taught to a client or caregiver include antibiotic treatment, simple hydration, continuous chemotherapy with selected drugs, and parenteral nutrition. However, nurses administer blood transfusions and complicated chemotherapy drug regimens.

Prescribed IV medications and all necessary IV supplies (e.g., syringes, catheter valves, site dressings, IV pole) are provided and usually delivered to the client's home by the designated pharmacy. Improvisation with IV supplies is rarely needed or appropriate, although a coat hanger suspended from a curtain rod can serve as an IV pole. Home as well as inpatient-based IV therapy demands strict adherence to aseptic technique, storage of medications and IV fluids at proper temperatures, and maintenance of IV supplies and use within expiration dates.

Various methods are used to administer IV therapy in the home setting. The simple *gravity drip method* and *IV push* are cost-effective and appropriate ways to administer most antibiotics. Infusion pumps are used when rate control is necessary. Typically, home infusion pumps have computers that can be programmed, are battery-powered, and are small—about the size of a portable radio. The pump is placed in a small nylon pouch with the IV fluid container. The pouch is often worn with an over-the-shoulder strap or sometimes as a "fanny pack." IV tubing is threaded through the client's clothing to the IV catheter. The client can then ambulate while the pump is infusing the IV fluid.

Electronic home infusion pumps include complete alarm systems; the alarm sounds if a battery is low or if IV tubing is occluded. Most home infusion pumps also have "lock-out" capabilities to reduce the risk of tampering or of accidentally changing the program. The latest in home infusion pump technology allows infusion pumps to be programmed or alarms to be cleared via "telehealth" technology; a special modem can be placed in the client's home and attached to the telephone. The home care pharmacist or nurse can view the pump screen from the pharmacy and make necessary program changes without going to the client's home.

Specific client education to be addressed when an infusion pump is used includes teaching the client how to safely maneuver while the pump is in use. Client education should address bathing, dressing, checking pump function, and troubleshooting alarms.

The Intravenous Nursing Society (617-441-3008; *www.INS1.org*) is a national nursing organization devoted to the education of nurses practicing the specialty of IV nursing. This professional group is an excellent resource for home IV therapy; specific benefits include a professional journal, ongoing educational conferences, and local chapter meetings.

Lisa A. Gorski, RN, MS, *Clinical Nurse Specialist, Covenant Home Health and Hospice, Milwaukee, Wisconsin*

poorly stored in the body, *daily* potassium intake is necessary. A standard diet contains 50 to 100 mEq/day. Foods rich in potassium include vegetables, fruits (especially if dried), nuts, and meats.

Eighty per cent to 90% of potassium is excreted through the kidneys, and the remainder is excreted in feces. Renal excretion of potassium is influenced by plasma potassium concentration, blood flow into the kidney, acid-base status, and various hormones. An increased sodium intake promotes potassium loss.

Plasma and cellular levels of potassium are affected by acid-base imbalances. Alkalosis can cause hypokalemia. In an alkalotic state, hydrogen moves out of the cells to correct the alkalosis, and potassium moves into the cells, thus lowering the plasma potassium level. In acidosis, the reverse is true: Potassium leaves the cell, and extracellular levels rise.

Several substances can alter potassium levels. *Insulin* promotes potassium uptake by the cells by stimulating the sodium-potassium pump. Insulin-deficient clients often have hyperkalemia. *Glucagon* increases plasma levels of potassium by stimulating potassium release from the liver, and it may promote potassium movement from muscle cells. *Adrenocortical hormones,* such as cortisol and aldosterone, promote potassium excretion and sodium retention via the kidneys. During stress, cortisol and aldosterone levels are increased. Thus, hypokalemia is a risk factor in stress. *Catecholamines* and *beta-adrenergic agonists* promote cellular uptake of potassium. In response, hepatic stores of potassium are released and muscle storage is altered. Conversely, *alpha-adrenergic* agonists increase plasma potassium concentration. *Epinephrine,* which has both alpha- and beta-adrenergic properties, causes an initial transient rise in potassium. The beta-adrenergic properties subsequently become dominant, and the major effect is a reduced plasma potassium level.

HYPOKALEMIA

Hypokalemia is defined as a plasma potassium level of less than 3.5 mEq/L. It is a common electrolyte disorder, especially in the elderly population.

Etiology and Risk Factors

The body does not conserve potassium; thus, potassium deficit commonly results from inadequate potassium intake. Fortunately, potassium is found in most foods and fluids. People at high risk for hypokalemia include those who are debilitated, confused, restrained, or lacking access to dietary sources for financial or other reasons, or who are malnourished, anorexic, or bulimic.[7] Clients on potassium-restricted diets or some weight reduction diets or those receiving potassium-free IV solutions compounded by lack of dietary potassium are also at risk. Older adults are at especially high risk.

Potassium levels can also fall when the excretion or loss of potassium exceeds intake. People at high risk for loss include those with vomiting or diarrhea, nasogastric suctioning, intestinal fistulae, or ileostomy. Potassium is also lost with the osmotic diuresis that occurs with diabetic ketoacidosis. Surgical clients often develop hypokalemia secondary to the increased cortisol levels during the stress adaptation period and to the effects of general or spinal anesthesia. Some studies suggest that hypokalemia in alcoholic clients, as well as hypocalcemia, hypophosphatemia, and hypomagnesemia, is secondary to alcohol-induced nephrotoxicity. After several weeks of alcohol abstinence, electrolyte levels returned to normal.[8]

Medications that commonly cause hypokalemia include the potassium-wasting diuretics (thiazide, loop, and osmotic diuretics), cathartics, steroids, aminoglycosides, amphotericin B, digitalis preparations, beta-adrenergic drugs, cisplatin, and bicarbonate. People who ingest large amounts of natural licorice may develop hypokalemia secondary to an aldosterone-like effect.

Several conditions cause redistribution of potassium. Increased levels of insulin promote the movement of not only glucose but also potassium into the cell. In alkalosis, potassium exchanges with hydrogen across the cell wall, thus increasing the level of hydrogen but decreasing the level of potassium in the plasma. Clients who are in the healing phase after a severe tissue injury or burn also experience hypokalemia secondary to the shifting of potassium into the cell.[34]

Other factors associated with an increased risk of hypokalemia include Cushing's syndrome, the diuretic phase of renal failure, hyperaldosteronism, liver disease, cancer, wounds, and Bartter's syndrome, a chronic electrolyte-wasting syndrome.

Pathophysiology

When plasma potassium levels decrease, a decrease in potassium gradient occurs between the ICF and the plasma. The decreased gradient causes the resting membrane potential to increase, thus increasing excitability. Therefore, cell membranes are more responsive to stimuli (see Fig. 13–2). Almost all of the manifestations that occur with hypokalemia are secondary to the changes in neuronal excitability and its consequent effect on muscle function.

Clinical Manifestations and Diagnostic Findings

The clinical manifestations of hypokalemia include abnormal findings on the electrocardiogram (ECG) and GI, cardiac, renal, respiratory, and neurologic disturbances. Abnormalities may not be apparent with mild hypokalemia (3.3 to 3.4 mEq/L), especially if the decrease in the potassium concentration is gradual. Slowed smooth muscle contraction leads to early GI manifestations, which include anorexia, abdominal distention, and constipation. Slowed skeletal muscle contraction results in muscle weakness and flabbiness and leg cramps. Increased conduction of nerve impulses leads to the neurologic manifestations of fatigue, paresthesias, hyporeflexia, and irritability.

With severe hypokalemia, ECG changes (Fig. 13–3) may occur. The depressed and prolonged ST segment, depressed and inverted T wave, and prominent U wave are due to the prolongation of myocardial repolarization. Dysrhythmias are common because of increased cellular excitability. Ventricular fibrillation and cardiac arrest are the most serious consequences of impaired cellular action potentials. Hypokalemia also leads to a decrease in myo-

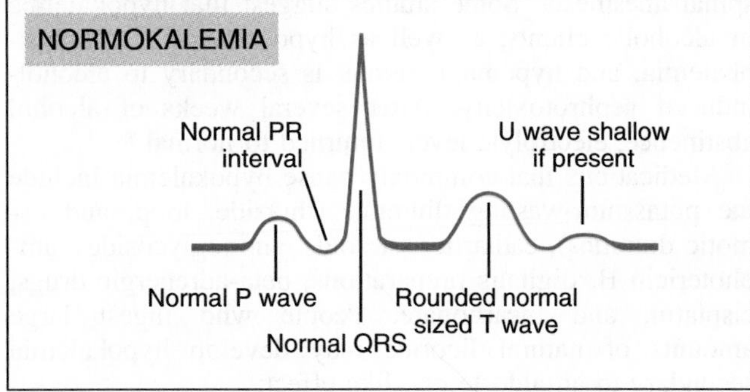

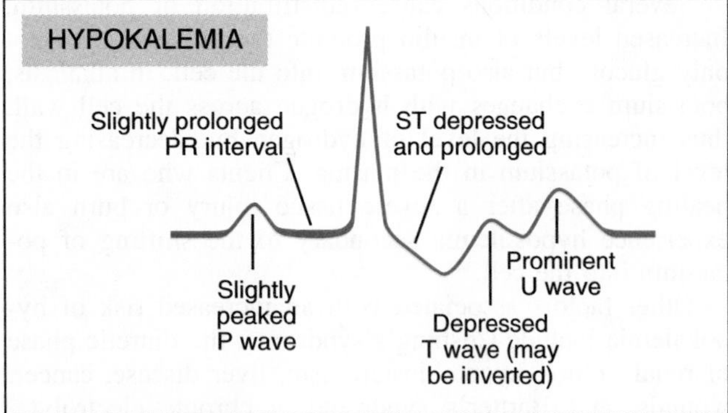

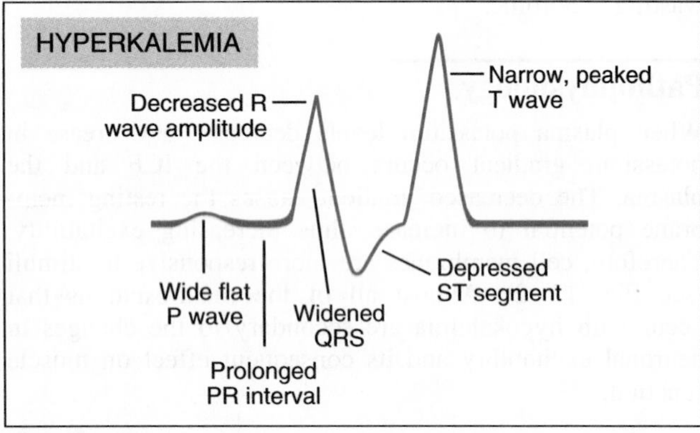

FIGURE 13–3 Electrocardiographic changes seen in potassium imbalances. (From McCance, K. L., & Huether, S. E. [1994]. *Pathophysiology: The biologic basis for disease in adults and children* [2nd ed.]. St. Louis: Mosby–Year Book.)

cardial contraction, which is manifested as hypotension and a slow, weakened pulse. Pulmonary manifestations of shallow respirations, shortness of breath, and apnea, culminating in respiratory arrest, are also from progressive deterioration of respiratory muscular contraction.

The progressive neurologic consequences of altered nerve conduction are manifested as dysphasia, confusion, depression, convulsions, areflexia, and coma. Extreme smooth muscle slowing leads to vomiting and an ileus as well as urinary retention. Skeletal muscle weakness may progress to paralysis. Hypokalemia also inhibits the kidney's ability to concentrate urine, which leads to polyuria, nocturia, and a decreased plasma osmolality.

Although plasma potassium levels below 3.5 mEq/L are diagnostic for hypokalemia, the ECG is the most reliable tool for identifying abnormalities in intracellular potassium level.

Outcome Management

A thorough history and physical examination with appropriate diagnostic studies are essential in accurate diagnosis and management of hypokalemia.

Medical Management

Medical management is focused on identifying and correcting the cause of the imbalance. The aggressiveness of the therapy is determined by the potassium level and the clinical manifestations. Extreme hypokalemia necessitates cardiac monitoring.

RESTORE POTASSIUM LEVELS

Maintenance doses for clients not taking any source of potassium are 40 to 60 mEq/day in the IV solution. Larger amounts are needed with coexisting potassium losses.

For clients with minor potassium deficits or for those who have potassium-wasting conditions, administering foods high in potassium helps correct the deficit and offsets losses. The adult recommended allowance for potassium is 1875 to 5625 mg/day. Box 13–3 includes examples of foods that are high and low in potassium.

Mild to moderate hypokalemia is treated by correcting or controlling the cause of the loss or by supplementing potassium intake through the diet and/or with medication. Oral potassium replacement therapy is usually prescribed for mild hypokalemia (plasma potassium, 3.3 to 3.5 mEq/L) or for potassium-wasting conditions. Oral potassium (chloride or gluconate) is extremely irritating to the gastric mucosa, therefore, it must be taken with a glass of water or juice or with meals.

Severe hypokalemia requires IV intervention. A client with a plasma potassium level between 3.0 and 3.4 mEq/L needs approximately 100 to 200 mEq of IV potassium for the potassium level to rise 1 mEq/L. If the plasma potassium level is less than 3.0 mEq/L, it takes approximately 200 to 400 mEq of IV potassium to raise the level 1 mEq/L.[34] Potassium given intravenously *must always be diluted in IV fluids.* The usual concentration of IV potassium is 20 to 40 mEq/L. Potassium is *not* given intramuscularly and is *never* given as a bolus (IV push) injection. Giving potassium by IV push creates sudden, severe hyperkalemia, which may result in cardiac arrest.

For severe potassium deficits, 10 to 20 mEq of potassium can be given every hour if *diluted* in IV fluids; a cardiac monitor must be used to ensure safety. Use of saline as a dilutent is recommended; avoid dextrose as a diluent, because it increases intracellular potassium shifting. Because potassium is irritating to the veins, concentrations higher than 20 to 40 mEq/L increase the risk of phlebitis, and large veins should be used for administration.

If hypokalemia is refractory to the usual treatments, assess for manifestations of hypomagnesemia. Many clients who are hypokalemic are also hypomagnesemic. Hypokalemia that does not respond to treatment is frequently associated with hypomagnesemia. Magnesium is necessary for the kidney to conserve potassium.[1]

Nursing Management of the Medical Client

ASSESSMENT

Assessment focuses on identifying risk factors for hypokalemia through history-taking and a thorough physical

BOX 13–3 High- and Low-Potassium Foods

High-Potassium Foods (average: 7 mEq per serving)

Vegetables (½ cup cooked or 1 cup raw)

Artichokes
Broccoli
Brussels sprouts
Cabbage
Carrots
Celery
Collards
Cucumber
Mushrooms
Potatoes with skins
Spinach
Tomatoes

Fruits

Apricots, fresh, 4 medium
Apricots, canned, 4 halves
Apricots, dried, 7 halves
Banana, 7 inches
Cantaloupe, ¼ small
Guava, 1 medium
Honeydew melon, ⅛ medium
Nectarine, ½
Orange, 1 small
Prunes, 3 medium
Strawberries, 1¼ cups
Tangerine, 2 medium
Watermelon, 1¼ cups

Beverages

Brewed coffee
Tomato juice
Vegetable juice cocktail, unsalted

Low-Potassium Foods (average: 3 mEq per serving)

Vegetables

Corn, ⅓ cup
Sweet potato, yams, ¼ cup
Lima beans, ⅓ cup
French fried potatoes, 10 pieces

Fruit

Apple, 1 small
Apple juice, ½ cup
Applesauce, ½ cup
Blueberries, ¾ cup
Cranberries, 1¼ cups

Beverages

Coffee, instant
Cola
Cranberry juice cocktail, ⅓ cup
Ginger ale
Noncarbonated drinks
Root beer
Lemon-lime soda

Data from Mahan, K. L., & Arlin, M. (1992). *Food, nutrition & diet therapy* (8th ed.). Philadelphia: W. B. Saunders.

examination. Obtaining a diet history that focuses on intake, conditions promoting loss, and drugs such as diuretics, cortisone, and over-the-counter medications is very important. Review laboratory reports of potassium levels. Report even borderline plasma potassium levels to the physician, especially in high-risk clients, particularly those about to undergo surgery. General anesthesia not only promotes potassium loss but, in combination with lower plasma potassium levels, synergistically increases the risk of cardiac dysrhythmia. Consult the physician about the need for potassium supplementation in anyone who has been on NPO status or who has an obvious cause of potassium loss or marked decrease in potassium intake.

Ongoing assessments of the client with hypokalemia include all the body systems, because the effect of low potassium is widespread. Assess cardiac function, including apical pulses, and renal function every hour in the client with severe hypokalemia, and progress to every 8 hours as the client's condition improves. Assess neuromuscular and bowel function every 4 to 8 hours. A urine output of 30 ml/hr is necessary to prevent rebound hyperkalemia. Hypokalemia increases the risk of digitalis toxicity because low potassium levels increase the sensitivity of the myocardium to digitalis-induced dysrhythmia.[48] If the client receives digitalis, monitor for anorexia, nausea, vomiting, diarrhea, headache, weakness, blurring or visual halos, or marked change in cardiac rate or rhythm.

If the apical pulse is irregular, assess for pulse deficits. Because this procedure is impractical for self-monitoring, at least ensure that the client or a family member is able to assess a radial pulse accurately for 1 minute and is aware of the need to notify the physician if the pulse is below 60 BPM (beats/minute).

DIAGNOSIS, OUTCOMES, INTERVENTIONS

Hypokalemia. Because there is no nursing diagnosis for hypokalemia, a collaborative problem format is used. It is commonly written as *Hypokalemia related to* (specific etiology). Causative factors often include vomiting, diarrhea, Cushing's disease, prolonged or intensive diuretic use, cortisone therapy, decreased intake, and NPO status.

Outcomes. The client's potassium level will be 3.5 to 5.0 mEq/L. Because the nurse cannot treat the problem independently, the outcome can also be written: "The nurse will monitor potassium levels."

Interventions. Give oral or IV potassium as prescribed, ensuring that it is *diluted in IV fluids; it cannot be given as an IV push.* Always *agitate* IV bags before hanging them up in order to prevent giving a loading dose, which can cause cardiac arrest.[34] Monitor IV sites hourly for phlebitis, infiltration, and rate of infusion. Change IV sites every 72 hours or sooner if the vein becomes tender to palpation. Tenderness indicates damage to the intima of the vein; this is an early sign of phlebitis.

Use the smallest IV catheter possible to allow maximum plasma flow around the site at which the potassium enters the vein. This promotes dilution of the potassium, thereby decreasing the risk of phlebitis. If an IV solution containing potassium infiltrates surrounding tissue, consult the physician for advice. Potassium can cause tissue sloughing. Give IV fluids with potassium chloride by a controlled infusion pump to ensure the correct flow rate.

Notify the physician if signs of hypokalemia persist or worsen, such as dysrhythmia of increasing severity, or if signs of overcorrection occur, such as manifestations of hyperkalemia. During the administration of IV potassium, consult the physician if the client's urinary output is less than 30 ml/hr for 2 consecutive hours, if the pulse deficit is greater than 20 BPM, or if signs of impaired peripheral tissue perfusion are present. Anticipate the need for additional potassium with increased IV glucose, such as in total parenteral nutrition (TPN) resulting from the increased shift of potassium into the cell caused by the increased insulin levels.

Risk of Injury. Because potassium is needed for normal nerve conduction and muscle function, low plasma potassium levels often lead to weakness and can lead to seizures. The nursing diagnosis is stated as *Risk for Injury related to muscle weakness and hypotension or seizures secondary to hypokalemia.*

Outcomes. The client will sustain no injury, as evidenced by an absence of falls, bruises, and contusions.

Interventions. Employ safety and seizure precautions to reduce the risk of injury. Keep the bed in a low position with side rails up. Before the client walks, clear the path of obstacles and place non-slippery shoes and a gait belt on the client. Use restraints only after all other alternatives to prevent inadvertent harm to self or others have been tried. It is imperative that health care providers comply with the client's rights and follow the defined protocols for use of restraints. Refer to your agency's policy and procedure manuals for explicit guidelines for action and documentation.

Altered Nutrition: Less Than Body Requirements. If the main cause of the client's hypokalemia is inadequate consumption of foods rich in potassium, then use the nursing diagnosis *Altered Nutrition: Less than Body Requirements related to insufficient intake of foods rich in potassium.* However, this diagnosis can be used *only* if the client can eat and drink.

Outcomes. The client will demonstrate improved nutrition, as evidenced by consumption of adequate amounts of food and fluid to maintain a normal potassium level.

Interventions. Instruct the client to choose and consume foods rich in potassium, such as fruits, fruit juices, dried fruits, and vegetables, including potato skins. Fish (but not shellfish), whole grains, and nuts, such as peanuts, almonds, and walnuts, are also good sources of potassium. Some fruits have a relatively higher potassium content; bananas, cantaloupe, and honeydew melons have twice as much potassium as that in oranges. Meat and milk have moderate amounts of potassium. Instruct the client to take liquid or tablet potassium supplements with a glass or more of water or juice and food.

EVALUATION

If the desired outcome of potassium maintenance has been met, continue to monitor high-risk clients for evidence of deficit. Continue to reinforce strategies for prevention. If the outcome of potassium restoration has been met or partially met, the manifestations of deficit should be absent or at least lessened in severity. Mild to moderate deficits are usually corrected in 8 to 24 hours. Correction of more severe deficits may take several days, especially in the older adult. Continue to evaluate the client's and family members' understanding of positive health behaviors, and assess for barriers to achieving those behaviors.

Self-Care

Teaching is essential to the promotion and maintenance of potassium balance. Provide a copy of the list of food groups, and emphasize the importance of eating a well-balanced diet. Review alternative cooking methods, reinforcing that prolonged cooking of vegetables may result in potassium and vitamin wasting. Suggest steaming, microwaving, and, if possible, eating raw vegetables as methods to increase nutrient retention.

Teach the basic principles of sick care. These principles include ingestion of 30 to 60 ml hourly of fluids with electrolytes; for example, cola contains potassium and reduces nausea. Sick care also involves teaching clients when to consult a physician. People with chronic diseases, such as heart, liver, or kidney disease or diabetes mellitus, should consult a physician for any illness that interferes with food ingestion or causes loss of nutrients and persists for more than 24 hours. Anyone who becomes symptomatic—who develops weakness of sudden onset, irregular heartbeat, or change in mental status—should consult a physician.

Teach the importance of not taking over-the-counter medicine, especially laxatives, without physician approval. Encourage clients who are lactose-intolerant to avoid milk products or to take lactase. Reinforce the label instruction that potassium products should be taken with food to avoid GI irritation.

Encourage use of support services—first, the family or extended family and then the religious community as well as respite services, Meals on Wheels, food stamps, Alcoholics Anonymous, or other community services.

HYPERKALEMIA

Hyperkalemia is defined as an elevation of the potassium level above 5.0 mEq/L. Hyperkalemia is rare in clients with normal kidney function but affects more than half of people with acute renal failure.

Etiology and Risk Factors

The three major causes of hyperkalemia are as follows:

- Retention of potassium by the body because of decreased or inadequate urine output
- Excessive release of potassium from the cells during the first 24 to 72 hours after traumatic injury or burns, or from cell lysis or acidosis
- Excessive infusion of IV solutions that contain potassium or excessive oral intake, especially in a person who has renal disease

All three potential causes of hyperkalemia limit the ability of the kidneys to excrete the excess potassium. Because the kidneys are responsible for 80% to 90% of potassium excretion, the underlying cause of hyperkalemia is often related to decreased kidney function. People with as little as 5% glomerular function can maintain normal plasma potassium levels if urine output is at least 1 L/day. Shock compounds the problem because of a low volume of circulating vascular fluids and diminished kidney function. Other routes of excretion are less effective to rid the body of potassium. The GI tract and skin cannot excrete enough potassium to compensate for an acute state of hyperkalemia.

Recall that most potassium is inside the cell. Therefore, conditions that destroy cells release potassium into the circulation. People with fast-growing cancers, such as non-Hodgkin's lymphoma, acute leukemia, small cell carcinomas, and some metastatic cancers, are at risk for *tumor lysis syndrome* (TLS). TLS is the consequence of rapid destruction of tumor cells secondary to chemotherapy and/or irradiation, which results in hyperkalemia, hyperphosphatemia, hypocalcemia, and hyperuricemia. Hyperkalemia can also result from burns, crush injuries, or severe infections involving extensive cell destruction. Potassium levels can also rise after the use of stored blood, and after open-heart surgery or other surgical procedures in which a perfusion pump is used.

Therapy with potassium-sparing diuretics or concurrent use of potassium supplements and angiotensin-converting enzyme (ACE) inhibitors may also cause hyperkalemia. Disorders that decrease or inhibit secretion of aldosterone, such as adrenal insufficiency, may also cause hyperkalemia. Acidosis also increases hyperkalemia owing to the compensatory shifting of potassium out of the cell in exchange for hydrogen; the exception to this mechanism is in diabetic acidosis (see Chapter 45). See earlier discussion of hypokalemia.

Pathophysiology

Hyperkalemia increases the cell membrane's excitation threshold, causing the cell to become less excitable. Decreased irritability (excitability) of nerve and muscle results. As hyperkalemia becomes more severe, muscles become weak, flaccid, and paralyzed.

Clinical Manifestations and Diagnostic Findings

Clinical manifestations are related to the plasma potassium level and the mode of onset of the imbalance. Acute hyperkalemia may cause manifestations when the plasma level is only moderately elevated, to 6.0 mEq/L. However, if the condition developed slowly, manifestations may not be present until the plasma level reaches 7.0 mEq/L. Clinical manifestations can involve many body systems, including GI, cardiac, renal, and neurologic systems. Mild to moderate hyperkalemia (a plasma level near 6.0 mEq/L) causes nerve and muscle irritability, resulting in paresthesia (numbness, tingling), tachycardia, and intestinal colic and diarrhea.

As the plasma potassium level approaches 7.0 mEq/L, sodium channels become progressively inactivated, which causes disturbances in nerve and muscle function: impaired cardiac conduction, ventricular contraction, hypotension, cardiac arrest, convulsions, and severe neuromuscular weakness progressing to flaccid paralysis and respiratory muscle paralysis. The acidosis that occurs with hyperkalemia has a synergistic effect on the progressive impairment of depolarization. The renal abnormalities oliguria and anuria are commonly precursors to hyperkalemia rather than consequences of the imbalance.

As noted previously, the key to the level of severity is the amount of time the body has had to adapt to the imbalance. Although a plasma potassium level above 5.0 mEq/L is diagnostic for hyperkalemia, the ECG is the most reliable tool for identifying an imbalance (see Fig. 13–3). Blood studies may yield false-positive results when hemolysis of blood specimens has occurred, when tourniquets are applied too tightly, when multiple attempts are made to obtain a sample from the same site, or when excess force is used to transfer blood into tubes or to aspirate blood into a syringe. Under these conditions, the cell ruptures and releases potassium into the sample of blood.

Other useful laboratory studies include determination of blood urea nitrogen (BUN), serum creatinine, and carbon dioxide levels. Elevated BUN and serum creatinine levels, which reflect decreased renal function, are important laboratory indicators for determining the risk of hyperkalemia. If the total carbon dioxide levels in the venous blood are low, an arterial blood gas study should be done to rule out metabolic or respiratory acidosis as a possible cause of hyperkalemia.

Outcome Management

Medical Management

The goals of medical management are to correct the potassium level as quickly as possible to prevent life-threatening consequences. Although a thorough history and physical examination are desirable, if the client's state is critical, intervention may preempt a thorough assessment.

Restore Potassium Balance

If the plasma potassium level is less than 5.5 mEq/L, dietary restriction of potassium may be all that is needed (see Box 13–3).

If the level is higher or if the client is symptomatic, pharmacologic intervention is usually necessary. The onset of symptoms and the need for aggressive intervention are usually related to the suddenness of the development of hyperkalemia. Improving urine output by forcing fluids, giving IV saline, or giving potassium-wasting diuretics usually corrects mild hyperkalemia.

When hyperkalemia is severe, immediate action is needed to avoid lethal cardiac disturbances. Temporary corrective measures may include the following: infusion of IV calcium gluconate to decrease the antagonistic effect of the potassium excess on the myocardium; infusion of insulin and glucose or sodium bicarbonate to promote potassium uptake into the cells (useful in metabolic acidosis); and use of the beta-agonist albuterol (0.5 mg IV), which results in a decrease in plasma potassium level within 30 minutes, lasting for 6 hours.[30] These are only temporary methods for decreasing plasma potassium; repeating these methods may not be effective.[9]

As hyperkalemia persists or increases, a cation-exchange resin such as sodium polystyrene sulfonate (Kayexalate) may be given orally or rectally as a retention enema. When this medication is given, the potassium ion is exchanged for the sodium ion in the intestinal tract; the potassium ion is then excreted in the stool. To prevent the constipating effect of this drug, it is usually combined with sorbitol, and diarrhea often results. In marked renal failure, peritoneal dialysis or hemodialysis may be needed.[9]

Prevention is central to the management of TLS. Adequate hydration is the key: 3000 ml of IV fluid is given 24 hours before therapy, during therapy, and for 48 hours after therapy. Diuretics, to decrease the risk of pulmonary overload, and a uric acid blocker such as allopurinol, to increase the excretion of uric acid, are also given to prevent renal failure.

If hyperkalemia is secondary to respiratory acidosis, enhancing pulmonary function is the primary focus. If it is from metabolic acidosis, the immediate risks associated with the acidosis and hyperkalemia are addressed first, and then interventions are targeted at the system in which the acidosis originated.

Nursing Management of the Medical Client

Assessment

Assessment focuses on identifying risk factors for hyperkalemia through history-taking and a thorough physical examination. Obtain a history of medical conditions associated with potassium elevations. Review laboratory reports of potassium levels. Report even borderline plasma potassium levels to the physician, especially in high-risk clients, such as those who have cancer or are undergoing chemotherapy.

Ongoing assessments include checking vital signs, bowel function, urine output, lung sounds (crackles), and peripheral edema every 4 to 8 hours. Monitor plasma levels of potassium and creatinine and BUN. In severe hyperkalemia, perform hourly checks of vital signs, including apical pulses. ECG changes should be monitored continuously. In the absence of ECG monitoring, apical pulses constitute the next most valuable indicator of abnormality in intracellular potassium concentration. Monitor urine output hourly if severe hyperkalemia or a history of renal insufficiency exists or if the urine output drops to less than 30 ml/hr for 2 consecutive hours.

Monitor not only for a therapeutic response to treatment (improvement) but also for signs of overcorrection. Rapid correction places a client at risk for hypokalemia and metabolic alkalosis. In a client taking digitalis, the occurrence of hypokalemia is associated with a digitalis toxic response.

Diagnosis, Outcomes, Interventions

There is no nursing diagnosis for hyperkalemia. The problem can be written using the following collaborative problem statement: *Hyperkalemia related* to (specify etiology). Consider the contribution of renal dysfunction, shock from traumatic injuries, or burns (tissue destruction).

Outcomes. The client will have and maintain a potassium level of 3.5 to 5.0 mEq/L. Because you cannot treat the problem independently, the outcome can also specify: "The nurse will monitor potassium levels."

Interventions. Administer fluids as ordered to promote renal excretion of potassium. Report manifestations indicating the development of hypokalemia and urine outputs of less than 30 ml/hr for 2 consecutive hours, or less than 720 ml/day.

If the client is to receive a blood transfusion and is at risk for hyperkalemia, notify the blood bank so that "old" blood (more than 2 weeks old) is not supplied. Use a 19-gauge needle or 20-gauge catheter to deliver the packed cells, to prevent red blood cell (RBC) rupture with release of intracellular potassium. When obtaining blood specimens, use vacuum tubes when possible to avoid false-positive results on tests for hyperkalemia.

High potassium levels have the potential to induce life-threatening dysrhythmias. Treat them according to protocol, and report ECG changes that indicate worsening hyperkalemia or overcorrection resulting in hypokalemia.[13] Set cardiac monitor alarms with narrow limits to ensure early detection of lethal dysrhythmias. *Remember, a machine cannot replace your bedside assessment.* Cardiopulmonary resuscitation may be required, but it is seldom successful in cases of severe hyperkalemia because the heart muscle cannot respond to medications or countershock. Consult the physician for any serious change, including progression of altered tissue perfusion, especially in the heart, lungs, brain, or kidneys.

Evaluation

Evaluate the client's responses to therapy every hour if severe hyperkalemia is present or every 8 hours if mild hyperkalemia exists. Hyperkalemia must be corrected quickly because of the risk of dysrhythmia.

Self-Care

Teaching still remains one of the primary interventions to promote and maintain normal potassium balance for those at high risk for hyperkalemia. Explain the significance of potassium restriction. Crucial elements of teaching include dietary potassium sources and the importance of reading labels, avoiding salt substitutes, which are usually made from a potassium salt, and avoiding over-the-counter medication not approved by a physician. Clients must also understand the importance of consulting a physician if renal function worsens or if an acute illness lasts more than 24 hours. Occasionally, a person with renal insufficiency is in a state of hypokalemia secondary to an acute loss. To ensure safe administration of potassium to any client with renal insufficiency, see that a cardiac monitor is used.

Calcium Imbalances

Calcium, an extracellular and intracellular cation, has a normal plasma range of 4.5 to 5.5 mEq/L, or 9 to 11 mg/dl. About 99% of the body's calcium is in the bones and teeth. The other 1% is in the tissues and intravascular fluid. About half of the portion of calcium in the blood is bound to protein, mostly albumin, and the remaining half is free (ionized calcium). Therefore, the total plasma calcium level does not indicate the exact amount of free, active calcium in the body.

Calcium has many functions in the body:

- Acts as a catalyst in the transmission and conduction of nerve impulses

- Stimulates the contraction of skeletal, smooth, and cardiac muscle
- Maintains normal cellular permeability; increased plasma calcium levels decrease cellular permeability, and decreased plasma calcium levels increase cellular permeability
- Promotes coagulation of blood in all phases but mostly in the prothrombin to thrombin phase
- Promotes absorption and utilization of vitamin B_{12}. Promotes strong and durable bones and teeth; vitamin D is needed to absorb calcium from the GI tract

Parathyroid hormone (PTH) regulates plasma levels of calcium and phosphorus (see later discussion on phosphorus [phosphate]) by increasing resorption from bone, and reabsorption from the renal tubule or the GI tract. Thus, increased PTH increases plasma ionized calcium levels and decreases plasma phosphorus levels. Calcitonin from the thyroid gland also promotes calcium balance by opposing the action of PTH; it inhibits bone resorption.

When the level of plasma calcium falls even slightly, PTH secretion increases. Within minutes, calcium is reabsorbed from the kidney tubules; within hours, bone resorption occurs; and within days, increased absorption from the GI tract occurs (Fig. 13–4). Notice in Figure 13–4*B* and *C* how calcium and phosphate intake and output remain in balance.

■ HYPOCALCEMIA

Hypocalcemia is defined as a plasma calcium level below 4.5 mEq/L, or 8.5 mg/dl. Calcium levels are often reciprocal with phosphorus levels. Phosphate imbalances are discussed separately later on the chapter, however.

Low calcium levels are common in older adults because of inadequate intake. Hypocalcemia can also develop from an inadequate intake of vitamin D due to intentional changes in the diet or to diseases that impair absorption. Diets can be deficient in vitamin D in people with lactose intolerance, GI disease, liver disease, alcoholism, anorexia, and bulimia.[7] Decreased intake for several days, such as with NPO status, or for longer periods, as in high-protein and other weight-reduction diets, has also been linked to hypocalcemia.

Parathyroid disease decreases serum calcium levels. A deficiency of PTH results in a drop in plasma calcium levels secondary to decreased bone resorption and GI absorption and increased urinary excretion of calcium. Inadvertent (unplanned) removal of the parathyroid can occur when the thyroid is removed.

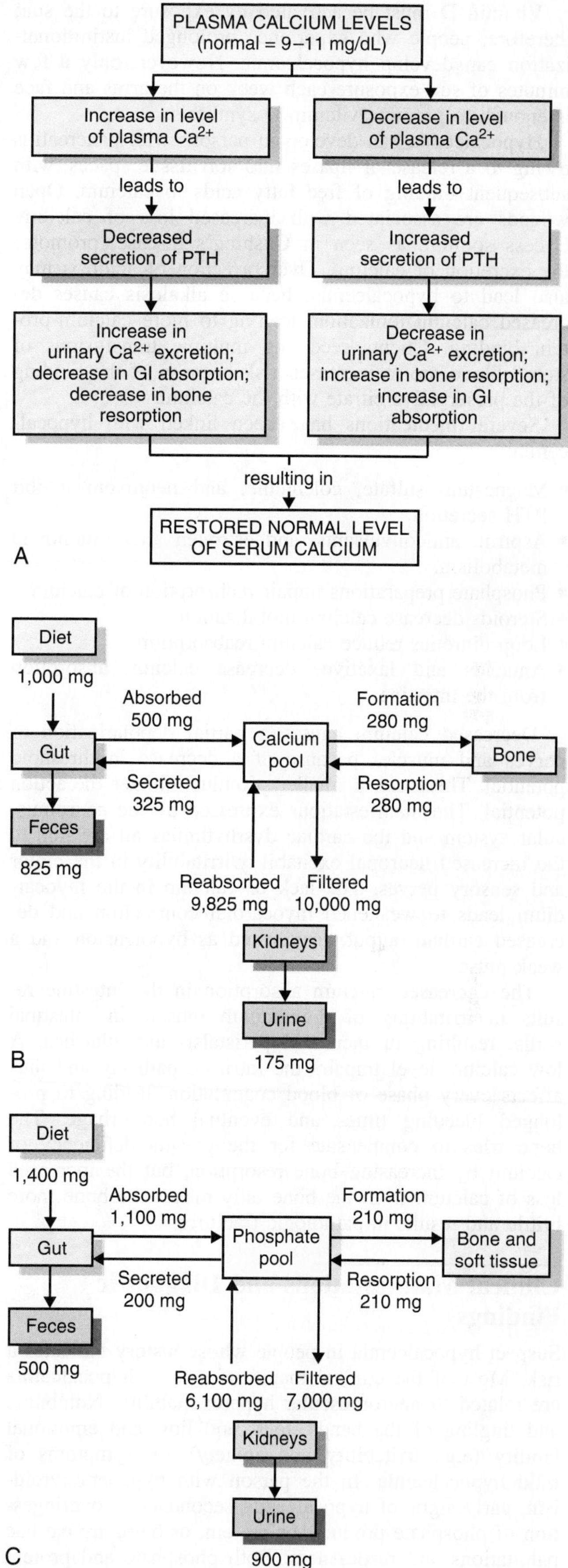

FIGURE 13–4 *A,* Parathyroid hormone (PTH) regulation of plasma calcium level. GI, gastrointestinal. *B,* Calcium homeostasis. A pool of calcium exists in the body and remains in balance by dietary intake, bowel and kidney excretion, and bone formation and resorption. *C,* Phosphate homeostasis. A pool of phosphate exists in the body and remains in balance by dietary intake, urine and bowel excretion, and bone and soft tissue formation and resorption.

Vitamin D must be activated by exposure to the sun; therefore, people who experience prolonged institutionalization can develop hypocalcemia. However, only a few minutes of sun exposure each week on the arms and face is enough to promote vitamin D synthesis.

Hypocalcemia can develop in persons with pancreatitis owing to a release of lipases into soft tissue spaces, with subsequent binding of free fatty acids to calcium. Open wounds are associated with increased loss of calcium. Excess sodium, as seen in Cushing's disease, promotes the excretion of calcium. Overcorrection of acidosis may also lead to hypocalcemia, because alkalosis causes decreased calcium ionization, leading to more calcium-protein binding. Clients receiving multiple transfusions of stored blood are at increased risk because of the binding of the preservative citrate with the calcium.

Several medications have been linked with hypocalcemia:

- Magnesium sulfate, colchicine, and neomycin inhibit PTH secretion.
- Aspirin, anticonvulsants, and estrogen alter vitamin D metabolism.
- Phosphate preparations impair reabsorption of calcium.
- Steroids decrease calcium mobilization.
- Loop diuretics reduce calcium reabsorption.
- Antacids and laxatives decrease calcium absorption from the intestine.

Decreased calcium causes a partial depolarization of nerves and muscles because of a decrease in threshold potential. Therefore, a smaller stimulus initiates the action potential. The manifestations expressed by the neuromuscular system and the cardiac dysrhythmias all are due to the increased neuronal excitability/irritability in the motor and sensory nerves. The lack of calcium in the myocardium leads to weakened myocardial contraction and decreased cardiac output, manifested as hypotension and a weak pulse.

The decreased calcium absorption in the intestine results in irritability of the smooth muscle in intestinal walls, resulting in increased peristalsis and diarrhea. A low calcium level impairs the intrinsic pathway and thus affects every phase of blood coagulation, leading to prolonged bleeding times and eventual hemorrhage. The bone tries to compensate for the plasma deficiency of calcium by increasing bone resorption, but the increased loss of calcium from the bone only makes the bone more brittle and results in pathologic fractures.

Clinical Manifestations and Diagnostic Findings

Suspect hypocalcemia in people whose history indicates a risk. Most of the clinical manifestations of hypocalcemia are related to neuromuscular hyperexcitability. Numbness and tingling of the hands, toes, and lips; and emotional lability (e.g., irritability and anxiety) are symptoms of mild hypocalcemia. In the person with hypoparathyroidism, early signs of hypocalcemia secondary to overingestion of phosphate products or protein, or both, are cardiac palpitations and restlessness. Both phosphate and protein increase calcium binding. Findings in severe hypocalcemia are cardiac insufficiency, hypotension, dysrhythmias, a prolonged QT interval, carpopedal spasm (Trousseau's sign), facial twitching (Chvostek's sign), and prolonged bleeding times; these abnormalities progress to seizures, laryngeal stridor, tetany, hemorrhage, cardiac collapse, and eventual death.[38]

With prolonged hypocalcemia, cataracts may develop because of increased uptake of sodium and water by the lens. Trophic changes, such as dry, sparse hair and rough skin, may also be noted. Spontaneous fractures can occur when the bone is depleted of calcium.

A plasma calcium level below 4.5 mEq/L, or 9 mg/dl, is considered diagnostic for hypocalcemia. This measurement and the clinical manifestations are the validating data used in most situations. However, remember to interpret these findings in the context of the plasma albumin level and pH, and adjust the data if either is abnormal. Also, when clients have manifestations of hypocalcemia but have a normal plasma calcium, an ionized calcium level should be determined, as it is the only value that gives the true level of free calcium. A level below 1.18 mEq/L (<2.36 mg/dl) indicates hypocalcemia.

Also, abnormal plasma albumin and pH levels influence the interpretation of plasma calcium levels. For example, when the albumin level is low, a falsely normal plasma calcium level can be present. Conversely, when plasma albumin is high, the functional ionized calcium level is actually lower than the plasma laboratory level reveals. When albumin levels are abnormal, the total plasma calcium can be adjusted by adding or subtracting 0.8 mg/dl for every 1 g/dl decrease or increase, respectively, in plasma albumin. A basic pH causes an increase in calcium binding. The plasma level may appear normal, but the functional ionized calcium level is actually lower. The opposite is true with an acid pH. Therefore, a plasma ionized calcium (iCa) assay should be done in clients who are critically ill, those with marginal calcium imbalances, or those with an abnormal albumin level or acid-base imbalance. (See Box 13–1 for normal ranges.)

Outcome Management

The goals of medical management are to determine and correct the cause of the hypocalcemia, restore calcium levels to normal values, and determine a method to reduce recurrence.

Medical Management

RESTORE CALCIUM BALANCE

Asymptomatic hypocalcemia is usually corrected with oral calcium gluconate, calcium lactate, or calcium chloride. For increased absorption, the calcium supplement should be given with a glass of milk 30 minutes before meals. The vitamin D in the milk promotes calcium absorption.

Chronic or mild hypocalcemia can be treated in part by having the client consume a diet high in calcium (Box 13–4). If hypocalcemia is secondary to parathyroid deficiency, the client must avoid high-phosphate foods, such as milk products and carbonated beverages, and excess protein. Protein binds with available calcium and only exacerbates the manifestations of hypocalcemia. Maintenance needs are met through calcium and vitamin D supplements.

BOX 13–4 High- and Low-Calcium Foods

High-Calcium Foods (>100 mg per serving)

Dairy Products

Cheese, all types
Ice cream, 1 cup
Milk, 1 cup
Yogurt, low-fat with fruit, 1 cup

Other Foods

Oatmeal, instant, ¾ cup
Rhubarb, cooked, 1 cup
Spinach, frozen, ½ cup
Tofu, regular, ½ cup

Low-Calcium Foods (<25 mg per serving)

Apple, 1 medium
Banana, 1 medium
Chicken breast, baked, 3 oz
Ground beef, lean, 3 oz
Oatmeal, cooked, 1 cup
Pasta, cooked, 1 cup
Vegetable juices

Data from Laquarta, I., & Gerlach, M. (1990). *Nutrition in clinical nursing.* Albany, NY: Delmar; and Burtis, G., et al. (1988). *Applied nutrition and diet therapy.* Philadelphia: W. B. Saunders.

Tetany from acute hypocalcemia needs *immediate* attention. IV calcium chloride or calcium gluconate must be given slowly to avoid hypotension and bradycardia and other dysrhythmias. Use D_5W solutions when dilution is necessary; avoid saline solutions, as they promote calcium loss.

Nursing Management of the Medical Client

A thorough history of the client's current and chronic illnesses, diet intake, and medications, including over-the-counter medications, assists in identifying risks for calcium deficit and guides interventions for health promotion and maintenance. If digitalis and calcium are among the medications identified, assess for digitalis toxicity as well, because hypocalcemia increases the risk of this problem.

Check for Trousseau's and Chvostek's signs in high-risk clients (Fig. 13–5). *Trousseau's sign* is the occurrence of carpopedal spasm, or contraction of the fingers and hand, when a blood pressure cuff is kept inflated on the upper arm for 5 minutes at diastolic pressure. *Chvostek's sign* is occurrence of spasm of the muscles innervated by the facial nerve when the client's face is tapped lightly below the temple. Spasm of the face, lip, or nose is also evidence of tetany. In addition, assess for paresthesias.

Assess the client's cardiac status by monitoring the ECG and vital signs, especially the apical heart rate and rhythm. Frequency of assessment varies from 1 to 4 hours, depending on the client's condition. Assess color, warmth, motion, and sensation (CWMS) and peripheral pulses to provide data for evaluation of the peripheral cardiac output.

Monitor also for bleeding in the gums and petechiae or ecchymosis in the skin. Assess for changes in the clarity of urine, as microscopic bleeding causes clear urine to become cloudy before frank bleeding is apparent. Also,

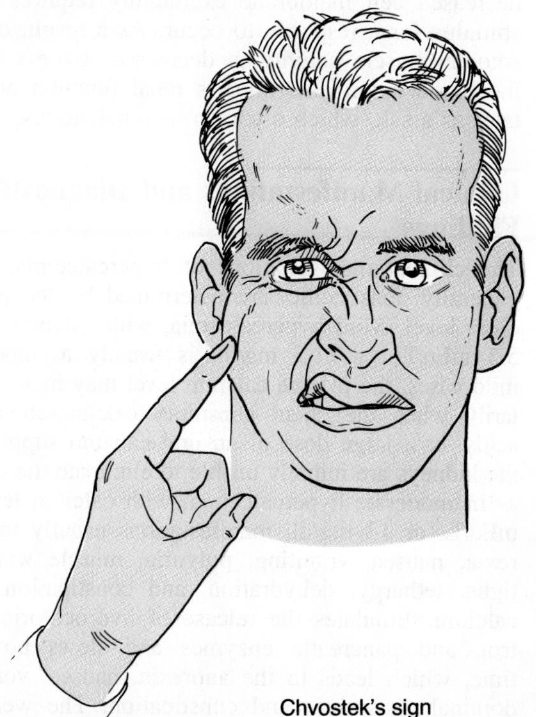

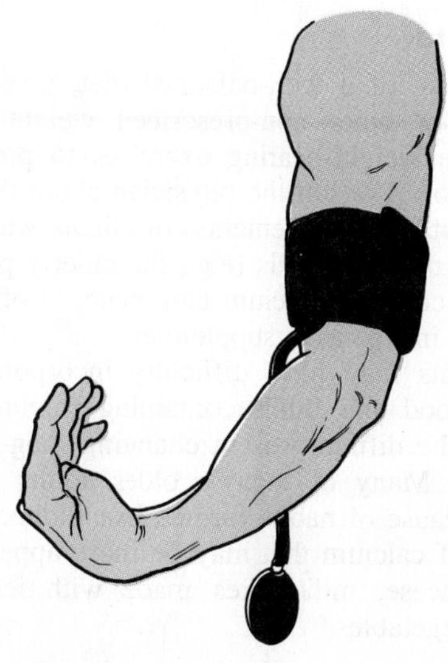

FIGURE 13–5 Chvostek's and Trousseau's signs. A calcium deficit (hypocalcemia) or magnesium deficit (hypomagnesemia) raises the resting potential of nerves. This rise allows nerve stimulation and firing with less stimulus. Touching the facial nerve adjacent to the ear produces twitching of the client's upper lip (Chvostek's sign). The hand and fingers can also go into spasm (Trousseau's sign or carpopedal spasm). These spasms can occur spontaneously or when blood flow is decreased (e.g., during blood pressure cuff inflation).

note black or blood-streaked stool, which may signify occult gastrointestinal bleeding. Be suspicious of an intracerebral hemorrhage when a client reports headaches of new onset. Monitor plasma calcium levels for improvement or worsening.

Monitor IV sites for infiltration or phlebitis when IV calcium is being infused. Calcium chloride is extremely irritating to the subcutaneous tissue. If infiltration occurs, notify the physician immediately, as tissue sloughing may occur. In either situation, change the IV site. Also notify the physician if the client's manifestations do not resolve or if signs of overcorrection (hypercalcemia) occur. When possible, use fresh blood for transfusions. Avoid giving calcium and bicarbonate in the same IV solution, as a precipitate will form. Use filters with TPN solutions.

To prevent pathologic fractures, use caution by obtaining adequate help to turn or move the client. Use gait belts and or extra personnel to walk or transfer the client to and from bed.

Instruct the client about foods that are rich in calcium, such as milk, cheese, yogurt, and green leafy vegetables. Encourage taking calcium supplements before meals and with vitamin D milk for better absorption. *Exception:* For persons with hypocalcemia secondary to hypoparathyroidism, phosphorus intake should be decreased by *omitting* milk, milk products, and other high-phosphorus foods (e.g., carbonated beverages). Calcium and vitamin D supplements are prescribed for this population as well. Several types of vitamin D are available. Therefore, clients with hypoparathyroidism must be advised not to take over-the-counter forms without first consulting with a physician to ensure that the right supplement is taken. These clients should also be advised to ingest protein only in amounts recommended by the American Dietetic Association (ADA). Increased intake of protein leads only to further binding of available calcium. For clients with osteoporosis, see the dietary recommendations in Chapter 26.

Self-Care

Reinforce intake of a well-balanced diet, avoiding high-protein diets or other non-prescribed weight-loss diets, and encourage weight-bearing exercises to prevent bone demineralization. Consult the physician about the need for mineral and vitamin supplements for clients who consume less than half of their meals (e.g., the elderly population). Tums, which contains calcium carbonate, is often recommended as an inexpensive supplement.

Older clients may have difficulty incorporating large amounts of food and fluids containing calcium into the diet. Part of the difficulty is in changing long-established eating habits. Many of today's older adults drink very little milk because of habits formed in childhood. Suggest other forms of calcium that may be more appealing, such as yogurt, cheese, milkshakes made with ice milk, or green leafy vegetables.[6]

HYPERCALCEMIA

Hypercalcemia is defined as a plasma level over 5.5 mEq/L, or 11 mg/dl. Hypercalcemia can occur in any age group. It is a common electrolyte disorder that can have serious physical complications.

Etiology and Risk Factors

The three most common causes of hypercalcemia are (1) metastatic malignancy, (2) hyperparathyroidism, and (3) thiazide diuretic therapy. The most common cancers that cause hypercalcemia are malignancies of the lung, breast, ovary, prostate, bladder, bone (multiple myeloma, leukemia), kidney, head and neck, and lymph tissues. Malignancy-induced hypercalcemia is the result of either bone destruction or an increased secretion of ectopic PTH.

Other causes of hypercalcemia include an excessive intake of calcium supplements with vitamin D or of calcium-containing antacids, prolonged immobilization, metabolic acidosis, and hypophosphatemia. Prolonged immobilization causes resorption of calcium from the bone. Recall that bone density is maintained by weight-bearing stress on bone (see Chapter 26). Metabolic acidosis promotes hypercalcemia by two mechanisms: decreased binding of calcium, which increases the plasma ionized calcium levels, and inhibition of calcium excretion from the kidney. Hypophosphatemia inhibits the kidney's ability to excrete excess calcium.

Pathophysiology

Destruction of bone tissue results in an increased release of calcium into the vascular spaces. See Chapter 19 for more information related to malignancies. Excessive PTH production promotes calcium retention, which leads to hypophosphatemia. Hypophosphatemia compounds the problem by promoting more calcium retention.

When excess calcium is present, the cell membrane threshold potential becomes more positive, which results in membranes that are refractory to depolarization. This decreased cell membrane excitability requires a stronger stimulus for a response to occur. As a result, cardiac and smooth muscle activity is decreased. Excess calcium in the bloodstream also impairs renal function and precipitates as a salt, which often forms renal stones.

Clinical Manifestations and Diagnostic Findings

The clinical manifestations of hypercalcemia, which are generally nonspecific, are determined by the plasma calcium level. Mild hypercalcemia, with calcium levels near 5.5 mEq/L, or 11.5 mg/dl, is usually asymptomatic. In mild cases, the plasma calcium level may increase momentarily when the client consumes calcium-containing antacids, or a large dose of an oral calcium supplement, and the kidneys are initially unable to eliminate the excess.

In moderate hypercalcemia, with calcium levels of 6.2 mEq/L, or 13 mg/dl, manifestations usually include anorexia, nausea, vomiting, polyuria, muscle weakness, fatigue, lethargy, dehydration, and constipation. Increased calcium stimulates the release of hydrochloric acid, gastrin, and pancreatic enzymes and slows bowel transit time, which leads to the anorexia, nausea, vomiting, abdominal distention, and constipation. The weakness, fatigue, depression, and difficulty concentrating are due to neurologic depression. Hypercalcemia also causes osmotic diuresis; the polyuria leads to dehydration and thirst and further exacerbates the constipation.

Calcium precipitates tend to form ureteral or kidney stones, which results in urinary blockage and severe colicky pain. Excess calcium also impairs glomerular blood flow, which in severe cases has led to renal failure. Bone pain is often associated with cancer of the bone and is due to the pressure on nerve endings from the tumor cells. Pathologic fractures are due to the decalcification of the bony matrix and can occur with cancer of the bone or with any condition that causes resorption of calcium.[7, 14, 17]

Progressive neurologic depression from increasing hypercalcemia is manifested as extreme lethargy, a depressed sensorium, confusion, and eventually coma. Severe hypercalcemia may result in hypercalcemic crisis, which carries a 30% to 50% mortality rate. A hypercalcemic crisis occurs when calcium levels reach 7.1 mEq/L, or 15 mg/dl. The resultant increased conduction transmission, shortened repolarization, and severe cardiac depression can cause cardiac dysrhythmias, ECG changes, and cardiac arrest. Hypokalemia may occur as the body eliminates potassium rather than calcium.

A plasma calcium level above 5.5 mEq/L, or 11.5 mg/dl, is considered diagnostic for hypercalcemia. Typical ECG changes include a widened T wave and shortened QT interval.

Outcome Management

Medical Management

The goals of medical management are to determine and correct the cause of the hypercalcemia, restore calcium levels to normal values, and determine a method to reduce recurrence. Prevention and early detection of complications such as renal stones and fractures are also important.

RESTORE CALCIUM BALANCE

Immediate correction of moderate and severe hypercalcemia is essential. IV normal saline, given rapidly with furosemide to prevent fluid overload, promotes urinary calcium excretion. Antitumor antibiotics such as plicamycin inhibit the action of PTH on osteoclasts in bone tissue, which reduces decalcification and the plasma calcium level. However, plicamycin has many dangerous side effects.

Calcitonin decreases the plasma calcium level by inhibiting the effects of PTH on the osteoclasts and increasing urinary calcium excretion. Corticosteroid drugs decrease calcium levels by competing with vitamin D, resulting in decreased intestinal absorption of calcium, and by inhibiting prostaglandins, resulting in decreased bone resorption. IV phosphate decreases plasma calcium; however, it is used as a last resort because it may result in severe calcification of various tissues.

Thiazide diuretics should be changed to furosemide or to another diuretic that does not cause retention of calcium. If the cause of the hypercalcemia is excessive use of calcium or vitamin D supplements or calcium-containing antacids, these agents should be either avoided or used in a reduced dosage. If the client is not nauseated, encourage oral liquids. These actions are designed to lower the calcium level in 36 to 48 hours. Etidronate disodium (Didronel) reduces plasma calcium by inhibiting precursors to calcium mineralization and, secondarily, by reducing bone formation. The client needs to be hydrated with large volumes of normal saline before etidronate administration and must be given loop diuretics to enhance urine output and calcium excretion following drug administration.

Gallium nitrate has been effective in inhibiting bone resorption and in decreasing osteoclastic activity. The drug should be stopped if the urinary output is less than 2 L/day or if the plasma creatinine level is greater than 2.5 mg/dl.[15, 16, 22]

For client teaching, review high-calcium foods that should be restricted (see Box 13–4). Instruct the client that forcing fluids helps to lower plasma levels by flushing excess calcium through the kidney. If manifestations of renal calculi (stones) are present, teach that consumption of foods and fluids that increase urine acidity will help decrease stone formation. These include meat, cheese, eggs, whole grains, cranberry juice, and prune juice.

Nursing Management of the Medical Client

Because plasma calcium levels are not routinely assessed, it is essential that you identify high-risk clients. Screening assessment includes obtaining a thorough history, focusing on risk factors, medications (including over-the-counter calcium supplements or antacids), and diet history. Assess vital signs, apical pulses, and ECG every 1 to 8 hours, depending on the severity of the client's manifestations. Bowel sounds, renal function, and hydration status should be assessed every 8 hours. Also, recall that it is important to monitor for fluid volume depletion secondary to hypercalcemia.

Early treatment may prevent a hypercalcemic crisis. Unless fluids are contraindicated (as in clients with heart failure), increase fluid intake. If flank pain or renal colic is present, strain all urine to capture renal calculi for analysis. Report urine output of less than 30 ml/hr for 2 consecutive hours. Report any manifestations that indicate worsening of the clinical status, such as an increase in severity of dysrhythmias, a decrease in sensorium, or manifestations of overcorrection (hypocalcemia).

Once the crisis is controlled, prevention of complications through teaching and safety interventions becomes the primary focus of health maintenance. Instruct the client to avoid calcium supplements. Sodium intake is increased, unless contraindicated, to promote calcium loss through the kidneys. Consumption of high-fiber foods and fluids should be increased to prevent constipation, and an acid-ash diet may be recommended to decrease the risk of stone formation. The client should also be taught to report clinical manifestations of renal calculi, such as flank pain, hematuria, or cardiac dysfunction (such as an irregular pulse or palpitations).

If the client has confusion, lethargy, or coma, institute safety precautions, including a low bed position with side rails raised. To prevent injury, turn and move the client with extreme caution and with adequate assistance. Gait belts, back braces, tripod canes, and walkers may be used to facilitate safer ambulation. Assist with resistive range of motion and weight-bearing activities to decrease calcium loss from bone. Report clinical manifestations of fractures immediately, such as bone pain or ecchymosis.

Surgical Management

Surgery may be used to remove an ectopic PTH-secreting tumor. Noninvasive or invasive lithotripsy or endoscopic removal of renal or ureteral calculi may be necessary. See Chapters 34 and 35 for more information related to these surgical procedures.

PHOSPHATE IMBALANCES

The normal plasma phosphorus level is 1.2 to 3.0 mEq/L. Less than 1% of phosphorus is contained in the vascular spaces; 85% is contained in the bones, and 14% is contained in the soft tissues. However, rapid shifting between cells and blood can occur, which can create a risk for severe hypophosphatemia or hyperphosphatemia.

Phosphorus promotes strong and durable bones and teeth. Phosphorus is also an integral part of the energy systems in the body—adenosine diphosphate (ADP) and adenosine triphosphate (ATP) and in the phosphate acid-base buffer system. PTH regulates plasma levels of phosphorus by the following mechanisms:

- Increasing resorption of phosphate from the bone
- Inhibiting phosphate reabsorption from the renal tubule
- Increasing phosphate absorption from the GI tract

Thus, increased PTH increases plasma ionized calcium levels and decreases plasma phosphorus levels.

HYPOPHOSPHATEMIA

Hypophosphatemia is defined as plasma phosphorus levels below 1.2 mEq/L. The overall major risk for hypophosphatemia is loss or long-term lack of intake. However, risk factors that are often overlooked include periods of increased growth or tissue repair and recovery from malnourished states. Each of these factors increases the demand for phosphorus.[38] Failure to meet these increased needs results in a state of phosphorus depletion.

Phosphorus depletion can occur as a result of prolonged and excessive intake of antacids. Administration of high levels of glucose via tube feeding or IV line causes phosphorus to enter the cell for glucose phosphorylation. The increased sodium found in Cushing's syndrome, the increased calcium found in hyperparathyroidism, and the decreased arterial partial pressure of carbon dioxide ($PaCO_2$) in chronic respiratory alkalosis also cause phosphorus to move into the cell. Lead poisoning leads to a decreased availability of phosphate. Phosphate loss occurs in burns, and a mild renal loss occurs with metabolic alkalosis.

Pathophysiologic changes that occur with hypophosphatemia can affect every organ system because of the effect of hypophosphatemia on optimal ATP and oxygen supply. Phosphate depletion impairs the conversion of glucose and many other intermediate substances to ATP. The ultimate result is a disruption in the sole mechanism responsible for regeneration of ATP.

Recognition of phosphate deficits is challenging because the plasma level, whether normal or low, does not always reflect the total body phosphate content. Careful review of a client's history, laboratory data, medications, and clinical manifestations, with emphasis on nutritional health in people at high risk, increases the likelihood of identifying phosphate deficiencies. The primary manifestations of hypophosphatemia are decreased cardiac and respiratory function, muscle weakness, fatigue, brittle bones, bone pain, confusion, and seizures.

Mild hypophosphatemia can be treated with diet and dietary supplementation. The major nursing roles are teaching a well-balanced diet and helping the client and family gain access to resources that alleviate barriers to positive health behaviors.

Clients who have a serious phosphate imbalance are often deficient in many other nutrients. TPN is usually the intervention of choice until the plasma levels become stable. Monitoring a client's response to IV TPN is also essential. See Chapter 29 for more information on nursing implications related to TPN.

HYPERPHOSPHATEMIA

Hyperphosphatemia is a rare but serious disorder. It is defined as a plasma phosphate level above 3.0 mEq/L. However, it is the total body phosphate level that determines the seriousness of the imbalance. The most common causes are excessive intake of high-phosphate foods, excess vitamin D (especially with renal insufficiency due to decreased excretion), impaired colonic motility from increased absorption, hypoparathyroidism, and Addison's disease. Clinical manifestations are related to the degree of hyperphosphatemia or to secondary hypocalcemia. Tachycardia, palpitations, and restlessness are among the earliest manifestations. Anorexia, nausea, vomiting, hyperreflexia, tetany, and more serious dysrhythmias may follow if the imbalance worsens.

In certain conditions, an increased intake or decreased excretion of phosphate or an increase in cell lysis results in high levels of phosphorus. In renal failure, the kidney is less able to excrete phosphate; the excess phosphate impairs calcium reabsorption. TLS results in a state of hyperphosphatemia from excess cell rupture. Women are at risk after menopause owing to a slight increase in phosphate secondary to a deficiency of estrogen. Exposure to lead increases the risk of phosphorus imbalances. Hyperphosphatemia leading to death has been associated with administration of Fleet Phospho-Soda enemas in the presence of altered renal or bowel function.[11] Follow manufacturer recommendations when giving Fleet Phospho-Soda enemas.

In mild or asymptomatic hyperphosphatemia, treatment focuses on limiting high-phosphate foods, especially milk, ice cream, cheeses, high amounts of meat and fish, and carbonated beverages, or giving calcium or aluminum products that promote the binding and excretion of phosphate. Dialysis is the primary treatment for renal failure that is refractory to conservative approaches (either peritoneal dialysis or hemodialysis).

For mild or moderate phosphate deficiencies, diet supplementation is usually sufficient. Sources of phosphorus include milk products, eggs, fish, whole grains, vegetables, and carbonated beverages. Hypophosphatemia, if associated with signs of total body phosphate deficit, is usually treated with IV replacement. This is most commonly given in the form of TPN if the client suffers from other electrolyte imbalances.

MAGNESIUM IMBALANCES

Magnesium is the second most abundant intracellular cation. The actions of magnesium in the body and the clinical manifestations of imbalance are similar to those for potassium. Half the body's magnesium is stored in bone, 49% is contained in the ICF, and 1% is contained in the ECF. Of the 1% in the plasma, 30% of the magnesium is bound to protein, 15% is combined with anions, and 55% is in a free, ionized form. Magnesium is absorbed from the small intestine at the same site at which calcium is absorbed. Thus, malabsorption affects both electrolytes. Magnesium is excreted in the urine and in small amounts in feces. Figure 13–6 shows how magnesium balance is maintained.

The functions of magnesium include the transmission and conduction of nerve impulses and the contraction of skeletal, smooth, and cardiac muscle. Magnesium accomplishes this through its effect on more than 300 enzyme systems. It is responsible for the transportation of sodium and potassium across the cell membrane (sodium-potassium pump) and for the synthesis and release of PTH. Therefore, a deficit can lead to hypokalemia and hypocalcemia. Magnesium is necessary for the conversion of ATP to ADP and hence the release of energy. It influences the use of potassium, sodium, calcium, and phosphate, and it activates enzymes that are necessary for the metabolism of carbohydrates, proteins, lipids, and vitamin B_{12}. Finally, magnesium promotes vasodilatation of peripheral arteries and arterioles.

Increased calcium or phosphorus intake can decrease magnesium absorption from the intestines. Conversely, a low calcium level increases magnesium absorption from the intestines.

■ HYPOMAGNESEMIA

Hypomagnesemia is defined as a plasma magnesium level below 1.5 mEq/L, or 1.8 mg/dl. Magnesium deficits are being identified more often as a result of increased knowledge about this ion. Twenty-two per cent to 42% of clients with calcium, phosphate, sodium, and potassium imbalances have been found to have a coexisting magnesium imbalance.[1] However, it is a rare imbalance in people who consume a well-balanced diet. As with other intracellular ions, plasma levels may be normal in the presence of intracellular depletion. Also, hypomagnesemia is often overlooked, because tests for plasma magnesium levels are not routinely ordered until a severe deficit has occurred. Plasma levels may be helpful in severe or acute changes, but a 24-hour urinalysis after an IV magnesium challenge, ion-selective imaging, or nuclear magnetic resonance imaging (MRI) (to determine soft tissue levels) is more predictive of total body magnesium levels, but these studies are rarely done owing to the expense.[2]

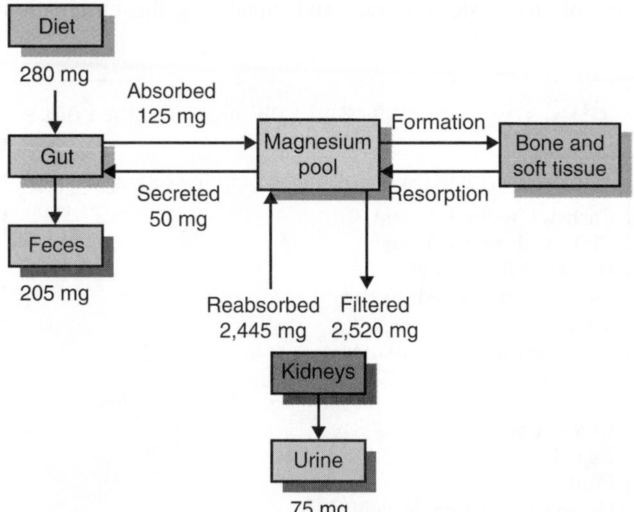

FIGURE 13–6 Magnesium homeostasis. A pool of magnesium exists in the body and is kept in balance by dietary intake, bowel and kidney excretion, and bone and soft tissue formation and resorption.

Hypomagnesemia is becoming recognized as a common cause of refractory (not responsive to treatment) hypokalemia and hypocalcemia.[1] The hypomagnesemic state inhibits potassium reabsorption; the hypomagnesemia therefore needs to be corrected before potassium and calcium imbalances respond to treatment.

Magnesium deficits are often seen in critically ill and alcoholic clients. Alcoholism decreases intestinal absorption secondary to a decrease in enzymes that are normally produced by the liver. Alcoholism also promotes magnesium wasting secondary to nephrotoxicity and leads to malnutrition. Other causes of hypomagnesemia are severe or chronic malnutrition; malabsorption syndromes, such as Crohn's or celiac disease or pancreatitis; and GI losses secondary to vomiting, GI suction, diarrhea, high-volume ileostomies, fistulas, laxative abuse, or radiation enteritis. Mechanisms for renal losses include the diuretic phase of acute renal failure and hyperphosphatemia. Prolonged IV or TPN therapy without magnesium replacement also increases the risk for hypomagnesemia. Excess calcium (as in hyperparathyroidism) and excess sodium (as in Cushing's syndrome or hyperaldosteronism) inhibit magnesium. The hyperglycemia seen in diabetic acidosis causes osmotic diuresis with loss of magnesium. Alkalosis is also associated with hypomagnesemia.

Many medications increase the risk of hypomagnesemia. Excessive amounts of phosphorus in the intestine (as from overuse of antacids) inhibit the uptake of magnesium from the intestinal villi. Some medications interfere with renal handling of magnesium as either a primary action or a side effect. The primary drugs implicated are diuretics and antibiotics. Loop, osmotic, and thiazide diuretics; aminoglycoside antibiotics (gentamicin, tobramycin); carbenicillin; amphotericin B; cisplatin; corticosteroids; and digitalis are the usual offenders. The neurologic trauma associated with cocaine abuse has also been linked to hypomagnesemia.[1]

The myocardial irritability that occurs with hypomagnesemia seems to be a result of changes in the resting membrane potential associated with the altered relationship between potassium and magnesium ions. It is thought to be secondary to the stimulation of $beta_2$-adrenergic cells; more commonly, it is associated with digitalis intake. Magnesium depletion and digitalis both promote potassium loss from myocardial cells. Digitalis uptake also seems to be increased in hypomagnesemia. GI changes from decreased contractility, such as anorexia, nausea, and abdominal distention, can occur. Psychological disorders, such as depression, psychosis, and confusion, may also develop.[35]

Severe hypomagnesemia causes neuromuscular manifestations such as Chvostek's and Trousseau's signs, tetany, convulsions, and vasospasm leading to stroke. Cardiac abnormalities include premature ventricular contractions, atrial or ventricular fibrillation, and ECG changes (prolonged QT intervals, widened QRS complexes, and broadening of T waves). Other ECG changes are related to the concomitant low levels of potassium. Low magnesium levels have been linked with an increased incidence of ventricular dysrhythmias and decreased 1-year survival rates in clients with heart failure as well as with lethal dysrhythmias in clients who have had myocardial infarctions.[2] Studies also suggest a link between estrogen therapy in postmenopausal women and increased coagulation risk; estrogen promotes tissue uptake of magnesium and hence hypomagnesemia.[2]

Management

Treatment of hypomagnesemia includes oral magnesium replacement in the form of magnesium-containing antacids or parenteral magnesium sulfate. Increasing dietary intake of magnesium also helps ensure balance and stability.

IV magnesium reduces the tendency of the small airways to spasm and has been found useful in treating acute asthma that has been refractory to other therapy. The positive inotropic, negative chronotropic, and vasodilatory effects of magnesium have also been found to increase cardiac output and decrease oxygen consumption in people with shock and sepsis. Magnesium has also been successfully used as a mood stabilizer in clients with bipolar disease.[1]

Nursing management includes monitoring vital signs every 4 to 8 hours and reviewing ECG readings hourly. Initiate safety and seizure precautions for clients who are extremely confused or at risk for seizures. Monitor plasma magnesium, potassium, and calcium levels. Also, many experts recommend assessing the client's deep tendon reflexes. Normal reflexes suggest normal magnesium levels.

Consult a physician about the need for magnesium maintenance or replacement if the client has severe malnutrition, is on NPO status for more than 3 days (especially in the presence of coexisting losses), or has manifestations of hypokalemia or hypocalcemia even after treatment. TPN may be necessary to correct coexistent nutrient imbalances, which is common. The presence of hyperglycemia in diabetic clients increases the risk of hypomagnesemia. Therefore, maintaining glucose control in people with diabetes mellitus will decrease the risk of hypomagnesemia.

When administering magnesium intravenously, dilute it according to pharmacy recommendations. Rapid infusion of magnesium sulfate can cause a hot or flushed feeling and phlebitis. Avoid giving magnesium in saline solutions.

Instructing clients and family members about foods rich in magnesium provides information that may be essential to prevent magnesium deficiency or to correct a mild deficit (Box 13–5). Caution clients about taking mineral supplements without the advice of a dietitian or pharmacist. The calcium-to-magnesium ratio should be maintained at 4:1, because a higher ratio can lead to deposition of calcium in the soft tissues and vessels.[2] Taking magnesium without potassium causes shifting of potassium into the cell. In the alcoholic client, magnesium should be given with thiamine to promote nerve regeneration.[1]

HYPERMAGNESEMIA

Hypermagnesemia is defined as a plasma magnesium level greater than 2.5 mEq/L, or 3.0 mg/dl. It is a rare disorder. Hypermagnesemia may occur with renal insufficiency, excessive use of magnesium-containing antacids or laxatives, or administration of potassium-sparing diuretics. Many potassium-sparing diuretics conserve magnesium. Hypermagnesemia is also seen with severe dehydration from ketoacidosis, with decreased synthesis of aldosterone (such as in Addison's disease or after adrenalectomy), and with overuse of IV magnesium sulfate for controlling premature labor or pregnancy-induced hypertension.

Clinical manifestations are related to the blocked release of acetylcholine from the myoneural junction, which results in a decrease in muscle cell activity. With mild hypermagnesemia, peripheral vessels dilate, causing hypotension. ECG changes include prolonged PR and QT intervals. In extreme hypermagnesemia, profound sedative effects on the neuromuscular system lead to severe muscle weakness, lethargy, drowsiness, loss of deep tendon reflexes, respiratory paralysis, and loss of consciousness. Cardiac signs include delayed myocardial conduction manifested on the ECG as wide QRS complexes, elevated T wave, heart block, and premature ventricular contractions.

Management

Management of hypermagnesemia includes decreasing the use of magnesium sulfate and enhancing the elimination

BOX 13–5 High- and Low-Magnesium Foods

High-Magnesium Foods (>75 mg per serving)

Cashews, roasted, ¼ cup
Chili, with beans, 1 cup
Halibut, baked, 3 oz
Swiss chard, cooked, ½ cup
Tofu, ½ cup
Wheat germ, ¼ cup, toasted

Low-Magnesium Foods (<25 mg per serving)

Chicken breast, 3 oz
Egg, 1
Fruits
Green peas, frozen, ½ cup
Ground beef, 3 oz
White bread, 1 slice

Data from Mahan, K. L., & Arlin, M. (1992). *Food, nutrition and diet therapy* (8th ed.). Philadelphia: W. B. Saunders.

of magnesium. A saline infusion with a diuretic increases renal elimination of magnesium. However, a side effect of the treatment is a loss of calcium. Hypocalcemia may intensify the hypermagnesemia. Calcium antagonizes magnesium. Thus, IV calcium salts in solution have been used in the treatment of extreme hypermagnesemia. Albuterol has also been used to reduce magnesium levels. The presence of severe respiratory distress requires ventilatory assistance. If renal failure is present, hemodialysis may be necessary.[35]

Nursing management focuses on monitoring for early signs of hypermagnesemia in high-risk clients. Assessment includes vital signs, respiratory function, ECG recordings, urinary output, and the level of sensorium; these should be checked every 1 to 4 hours, depending on the client's condition. Safety and seizure precautions should be initiated if confusion or seizure risk is present. Changes in deep tendon reflexes should be reported. If the reflexes are normal, body levels of magnesium are normal. Keep IV calcium salts in the code cart for emergency reversal of severe hypermagnesemia.

Teach clients to avoid constant use of laxatives and antacids containing magnesium, especially if urinary output is decreased. Encourage eating foods that contain fiber and drinking adequate fluids to promote fecal elimination.

CONCLUSIONS

Electrolyte imbalances are found in all age groups in every type of health care setting. It is rare for a person to have only one electrolyte imbalance; more commonly multiple electrolyte and fluid imbalances are present, especially in high-risk populations such as the very young, older adults, and people with chronic illnesses.

Nurses play an essential role in health promotion, health maintenance, and health restoration for clients at risk for or experiencing fluid and electrolyte imbalances. Nursing management includes the following pivotal roles:

- *Teaching* clients and their families about positive health behaviors, about the importance of nutrient intake (even during non-acute illnesses), and about manifestations of fluid and electrolyte imbalance that necessitate physician consultation
- *Promoting* nutritional maintenance and replacement in clients who are at high risk for or who are experiencing fluid and/or electrolyte imbalance
- *Assisting* the physician in early detection of imbalances and of poor response to treatment or signs of overcorrection
- *Promoting* balanced nutrition in rehabilitation or extended care settings through family support, early physician referrals for supplements, dietary consultation, or management of imbalances

THINKING CRITICALLY

1. **An elderly, tube-fed resident from a nursing home is admitted with recent changes in level of consciousness. Her skin and mouth are very dry, and her urine is scant and dark yellow. Laboratory assessment reveals sodium, 150 mEq/dl; chloride, 106 mEq/dl; BUN, 52; and creatine, 1.2. Her family calls and wants to know "if she will make it." How would you respond?**

Factors to Consider: What do this assessment findings suggest? What interventions would you expect to be prescribed? What precautions will be needed to prevent further fluid and electrolyte shifts?

2. **A 45-year-old woman was admitted with a rapid heart rate. Her past medical history is negative for cardiac disease. One week ago, she started on a new weight loss program, which included furosemide. Could her heart rate be potentially lethal?**

Factors to Consider: Why would a client take furosemide in a weight-loss program? What side effects may be occurring? What laboratory studies will be ordered? Which electrolytes do you think will be abnormal?

BIBLIOGRAPHY

1. Altura, B., et al. (1994). Magnesium: Growing in clinical importance. *Patient Care, 28*(1), 130–150.
2. Altura, B., et al. (1994). Magnesium therapy: Coming of age. *Patient Care, 28*(2), 79–94.
3. Bergeron, M., Armstrong, L., & Maresh, C. (1995). Fluid and electrolyte losses during tennis in the heat. *Clinics in Sports Medicine, 14*(1), 23–32.
4. Bove, L. (1996). Restoring electrolyte balance: Sodium & chloride. *RN, 96*(1), 25–28.
5. Brown, R. (1993). Disorders of water and sodium balance. *Postgraduate Medicine, 93*(4), 227–246.

5a. Carrougher, G. J. (1997). Management of fluid and electrolyte balance in thermal injuries: Implications for perioperative nursing practice. *Seminars in Perioperative Nursing, 6*(4), 201–209.

6. Constants, T., et al. (1994). Effects of nutrition education on calcium intake in the elderly. *Journal of the American Dietetic Association, 94*(4), 447–448.
7. Crow, S., et al. (1997). Serum electrolytes as markers of vomiting in bulemia nervosa. *International Journal of Eating Disorders, 21*(1), 95–98.
8. DeAngelis, R. (1992). Hypokalemia. *Critical Care Nurse, 12*(7), 71–75.
9. DeAngelis, R., & Lessig, M. (1992). Hyperkalemia. *Critical Care Nurse, 12*(3), 55–59.
10. Diringer, M. (1992). Management of sodium abnormalities in patients with CNS disease. *Clinical Neuropharmacology, 15*(6), 427–444.
11. Fass, R., Son, D., & Hixson, L. (1993). Fatal hyperphosphatemia following Fleet Phospho-Soda in a patient with colonic ileus. *The American Journal of Gastroenterology, 88*(6), 929–932.
12. Gisolfi, C., et al. (1995). Effect of sodium concentration in a carbohydrate-electrolyte solution on intestinal absorption. *Medical Science Sports Exercise, 27*(10), 1414–1420.
13. Guyton, A., & Hall, J. (1996). *Textbook of medical physiology* (9th ed.). Philadelphia: W. B. Saunders.
14. Held, J. (1995). Cancer care: Correcting fluid and electrolyte imbalances. *Nursing, 95*(4), 24–28.

14a. Iggulden, H. (1999). Dehydration and electrolyte disturbance. *Elderly Care, 11*(3), 17–23.

15. Kaplan, M. (1994). Hypercalcemia of malignancy: A review of advances in pathophysiology. *Oncology Nursing Forum, 21*(6), 1039–1046.
16. Kaye, T. (1994). Hypercalcemia. *Postgraduate Medicine, 97*(1), 153–160.
17. King, P. (1995). Oncologic emergencies: Assessment, identification, and interventions in the emergency department. *Journal of Emergency Nursing, 21*(3), 214–217.
18. Klotz, R. (1998). The effects of intravenous solutions on fluid and electrolyte balance. *Journal of Intravenous Therapy, 21*(1), 20–26.

18a. Latzka, W. A., & Montain, S. J. (1999). Water and electrolyte requirements for exercise. *Clinics in Sports Medicine, 18*(3), 513–524.
19. McCance, K., & Huether, S. (1998). *Pathophysiology: The biologic basis for disease in adults and children* (3rd ed.). St. Louis: Mosby–Year Book.
20. McCloskey, J., & Bulechek, G. (1996). *Nursing interventions classification (NIC): Iowa intervention project* (2nd ed.). St. Louis: Mosby–Year Book.
20a. Moseley, M. J. (1997). Perioperative problems: Nutrition and electrolytes in the elderly. *Seminars in Perioperative Nursing, 6*(1), 21–30.
21. Mulloy, A., & Caruana, R. (1995). Hyponatremic emergencies. *Medical Clinics of North America, 79*(1), 155–169.
22. Mundy, G. (1994). Evaluation and treatment of hypercalcemia. *Hospital Practice, 6,* 79–86.
23. O'Donnell, M. (1995). Assessing fluid and electrolyte balance in elders. *American Journal of Nursing, 95*(11), 41–45.
24. Okun, J. (1995). Clinical pathology rounds: Severe hypernatremia. *Laboratory Medicine, 26*(8), 507–509.
25. Radke, K. (1994). The aging kidney: Structure, function, and nursing practice implications. *ANNA Journal, 21*(4), 181–190.
26. Reber, P., & Heath, H. (1995). Hypocalcemic emergencies. *Medical Clinics of North America, 79*(1), 93–107.
27. Rutecki, G. W., & Whittier, F. C. (1994). Hyponatremia: Physiologic clues to a state of disordered tonicity. *Consultant, 34*(5), 688–690, 700–702.
28. Rutecki, G. W., & Whittier, F. C. (1994). Hyponatremia: Cause of hypotonicity directs management. *Consultant, 34*(5), 705–707, 711–712.
29. Seshadri, V., & Meyer-Tettambel, O. (1993). Electrolyte and drug management in nutritional support. *Critical Care Nursing Clinics of North America, 5*(1), 31–36.
30. Sica, D. (1994). Renal disease, electrolyte abnormalities, and acid-base imbalance in the elderly. *Clinics in Geriatric Medicine, 10*(1), 197–211.
31. Simmons-Holcomb, S. (1997). Understanding the ins and outs of diuretic therapy. *RN, 97*(2), 34–40.
32. Stark, J. (1997). Dialysis choices. *RN, 97*(2), 41–46.
33. Sterns, R. (1991). The management of hyponatremic emergencies. *Critical Care Clinics, 7*(1), 127–141.
34. Terry, J. (1994). The major electrolytes: Sodium, potassium, and chloride. *Journal of Intravenous Nursing, 17*(5), 240–247.
35. Toto, K., & Yucha, C. (1994). Magnesium. *Critical Care Nursing Clinics of North America. 6*(4), 767–783.
36. Toto, K., & Yucha, C. (1996). Urine chemistry: Monitoring fluid and electrolytes. *Nursing, 96*(4), 24j, 24l.
37. Vieweg, W. (1994). Treatment strategies in the polydipsia-hyponatremia syndrome. *Journal of Clinical Psychiatry, 55*(4), 154–160.
38. Yucha, C., & Toto, K. (1994). Calcium and phosphorus derangements. *Critical Care Nursing Clinics of North America, 6*(4), 747–766.

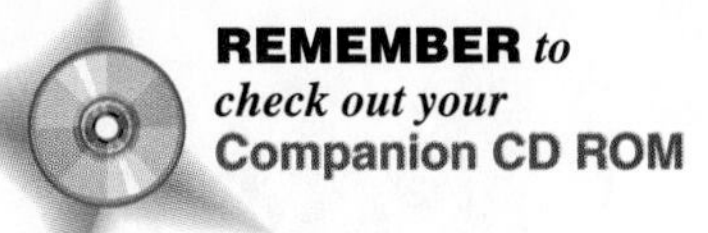

CHAPTER 14

Acid-Base Balance

Margie Hansen

Normal function of body cells depends on regulation of the hydrogen ion (H^+) concentration within very narrow limits. If H^+ levels exceed these normal limits, acid-base imbalances result and are recognized clinically as abnormalities of serum pH. Because acid-base imbalances may be caused by disorders of any body system, their incidence in clinical settings is quite high. Along with other health care professionals, you are responsible for preventing, detecting, and intervening in acid-base imbalances.

Regulation of Acid-Base Balance

The symbol *pH* refers to the negative logarithm of the H^+ concentration. It is used to express the acidity or alkalinity of a solution. A pH of 7.0 is *neutral*, having an equal number of acids and bases. An *acidic* solution has a pH less than 7.0, and an *alkaline* solution has a pH greater than 7.0. Because pH is a *negative* log (indicating a reciprocal relationship), a rise in pH reflects a drop in H^+. Conversely, a decline in pH indicates an increase in H^+.

Normal serum pH is 7.35 to 7.45. The function of cellular proteins is seriously impaired when pH falls to 7.2 or less or rises to 7.55 or more. Rapid rates of change in pH are especially detrimental. A serum pH below 6.8 or above 7.8 typically is fatal.

Three physiologic systems act interdependently to maintain a normal serum pH:

- Buffering of excess acid or base by blood buffer systems
- Excretion of acid by the lungs
- Excretion of acid or regeneration of base by the kidneys

■ MODULATION OF SERUM pH BY BLOOD BUFFER SYSTEMS

A buffer system consists of a weak acid (one that does not readily release H^+ into solution) and a salt of a base. For example, carbonic acid (H_2CO_3), a weak acid, and sodium bicarbonate ($NaHCO_3$), the salt of a base with which H^+ can combine, make up the clinically important bicarbonate buffer in the blood. The organic acids formed during cellular energy metabolism are strong acids; that is, they readily contribute free H^+ to body fluids, potentially producing large alterations in pH. The pH of buffered solutions tends to remain fairly stable despite the addition of strong acids or bases because buffer system components combine with added acids or bases to convert them to weaker forms. Because only free H^+ contributes to pH, changes in pH are minimized. Examples of buffering reactions are presented next.

Strong acid buffered:

$$HCl + (H_2CO_3/NaHCO_3) \rightarrow H_2CO_3 + NaCl$$

where HCl is hydrochloric acid and NaCl is sodium chloride.

Strong base buffered:

$$NaOH + (H_2CO_3/NaHCO_3) \rightarrow NaHCO_3 + H_2O$$

where NaOH is sodium hydroxide.

Several buffer systems are present in the blood, both within red blood cells (RBCs) and in the plasma. The numerous negative charges on proteins permit the binding of large quantities of H^+ cations. Accordingly, proteins such as hemoglobin in RBCs and albumin in the plasma are quantitatively (judged according to amount) the most important buffers.

In clinical settings, however, the bicarbonate buffer is monitored because of its accessibility within the plasma as well as its physiologic importance as an *open* buffer system. In an open buffer system, the end products of acid-buffering reactions are continuously eliminated from the body by the lungs and kidneys, allowing these reactions to continue without being slowed by the accumulation of end products. When bases must be buffered, the carbon dioxide (CO_2) consumed by carbonic acid formation is readily replenished by normal metabolism. Furthermore, the dissociation constant (p*K*a) of this system is ideal for buffering fluids such as plasma, in which the addition of acids is more prevalent than the addition of bases. The *dissociation constant* (p*K*a) of a buffer is the pH at which half its components are in the acid form and half are in the base form. At normal serum pH, the bicarbonate buffer has about 90% of its components in base form.

Since all intracellular and extracellular buffer systems operate interdependently, the status of the bicarbonate buffer is representative of acid-base homeostasis within the body as a whole. Buffer systems act instantly to minimize the impact of adding strong acids or bases to the blood; thus, these systems are the body's first line of defense against acid-base imbalance. Unlike the lungs and kidneys, however, buffers do not actually eliminate acid or base from the body.

■ REGULATION OF VOLATILE ACID BY THE LUNGS

Volatile acids are acids that can be converted to gases. During normal ventilation (breathing), the lungs exhale large quantities of "potential" acid in the form of CO_2 gas. CO_2 is continuously produced by body cells as an end product of complete oxidative metabolism of nutrients for energy. CO_2 diffuses from body cells into the blood, where it may combine with water to form H_2CO_3, which then dissociates, or separates, into its component ions: H^+ and HCO_3^- (bicarbonate). This *hydrolysis reaction*, which is reversible, is shown as

$$H_2O + CO_2 \rightleftarrows H_2CO_3 \rightleftarrows HCO_3^- + H^+$$

It is apparent from this equation that CO_2 and H_2CO_3 are directly related. As serum CO_2 levels rise, H^+ production increases and pH falls, indicating increased acidity. Conversely, lower CO_2 levels are consistent with higher (more alkaline) pH values. The hydrolysis reaction further demonstrates that some of the CO_2 entering the blood forms the base HCO_3^-. Although some hydrolysis occurs in the plasma, most takes place in the cytoplasm of RBCs, where the enzyme carbonic anhydrase (CA) catalyzes the reaction at much more rapid rates than in the plasma. The presence of CA in other cells, notably the renal tubular cells, is also important to acid-base homeostasis (discussed later).

Figure 14–1 demonstrates the hydrolysis reaction at the tissue level. Consistent with the *law of mass action*, the rate and direction of this reaction are determined by (1) the addition of substrate or (2) the removal of end product. In the tissues, the addition of CO_2 to the blood by metabolizing cells drives hydrolysis in the forward direction, forming H^+ and HCO_3^-, mostly in the RBCs. The H^+ formed by hydrolysis is buffered by hemoglobin, thereby minimizing changes in the pH of the RBC cytoplasm. The HCO_3^- formed in RBCs diffuses out into the plasma, while the chloride anion (Cl^-) moves in to maintain electroneutrality. This anion countertransport is known as the *chloride shift*. HCO_3^- formed in this way accounts for the major portion (80%) of CO_2 transported in the blood. Small amounts are transported while dissolved in plasma (8%) or are combined with hemoglobin (as carbaminohemoglobin) or other proteins (12%). The amount of carbonic acid in the blood at any time is negligible (0.0006%).

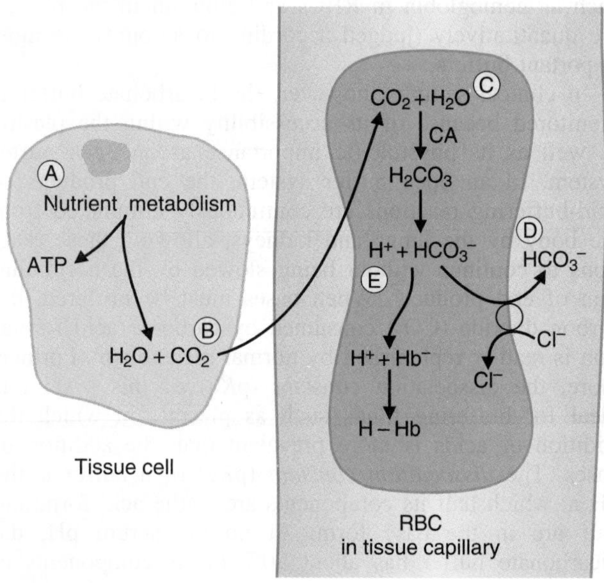

FIGURE 14–1 Tissue level hydrolysis. *A*, Carbon dioxide (CO_2) is formed during cellular energy metabolism. *B*, CO_2 diffuses into plasma, then into red blood cells. *C*, CO_2 enters hydrolysis catalyzed by carbonic anhydrase (CA), yielding hydrogen (H^+) and bicarbonate (HCO_3^-). *D*, HCO_3^- diffuses into plasma in exchange for Cl^- (chloride shift). *E*, H^+ is buffered by hemoglobin (Hb) and other intracellular buffers. RBC, red blood cell; ATP, adenosine triphosphate.

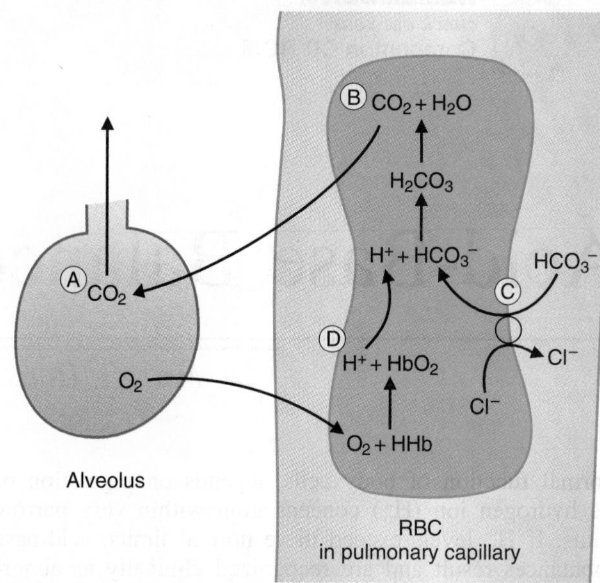

FIGURE 14–2 Reversal of hydrolysis in the lung. *A*, Carbon dioxide (CO_2) is exhaled, creating a gradient for diffusion of CO_2 from the blood to the alveolus. *B*, Removal of CO_2 drives reverse hydrolysis in the red blood cell (RBC). *C*, Bicarbonate (HCO_3^-) reenters the RBC in exchange for Cl^- (reverse chloride shift). *D*, Oxygen binding to hemoglobin (Hb) promotes H^+ release (reverse Haldane effect). HHb, combined hydrogen/hemoglobin.

In the lungs, CO_2 diffuses along its concentration gradient from the plasma to the alveoli, from which it is exhaled. Removal of CO_2 drives the hydrolysis reaction in reverse, as shown in Figure 14–2. In a reversal of the chloride shift, HCO_3^- reenters the RBCs, and Cl^- exits. HCO_3^- combines with H^+, which has been released from its buffers, regenerating CO_2 and H_2O.

■ REGULATION OF FIXED ACIDS AND BICARBONATE BY THE KIDNEYS

Acids that cannot be converted to gases must be eliminated in the urine. These *fixed acids* include:

- Sulfuric, phosphoric, and other acids produced during protein metabolism
- Ketones produced during accelerated lipid metabolism, as in diabetic ketoacidosis

- Lactic acid produced during anaerobic glycolysis, as in shock and hypoxemia
- Occasionally, ingested toxins, such as salicylate (aspirin), drugs, and methanol

The kidneys regulate serum pH by secreting H^+ into the urine and by regenerating HCO_3^- for reabsorption into the blood. At the glomerulus, HCO_3^- is filtered from the blood into the proximal convoluted tubule. Because HCO_3^- is a large, charged particle, it is poorly reabsorbed. Any HCO_3^- filtered in excess of H^+ is excreted in the urine. H^+ is actively secreted into the renal tubules, primarily by proximal tubular cells, but also in the distal tubule and collecting duct. This system operates only until tubular pH falls to about 4.5. At lower pH values, significant amounts of H^+ leak from the tubular lumen back into the blood. Secretion of large amounts of H^+ into the renal tubules would result in a rapid fall in tubular pH and would inhibit further H^+ secretion, if not for the presence of *urinary buffer systems.* These systems permit the tubular fluid to accept large quantities of H^+ while limiting how much the urinary pH decreases.

Urinary Buffer Systems

The three principal buffer systems in renal tubules are the bicarbonate, ammonia, and phosphate (titratable acid) systems.

In the *bicarbonate buffer* (Fig. 14–3), H^+ is secreted into the tubular lumen by tubular cells in countertransport with sodium (Na^+). The combination of H^+ with filtered bicarbonate regenerates CO_2 in a reversal of the hydrolysis reaction. This CO_2 is reabsorbed into tubular cells, where hydrolysis proceeds efficiently because of the presence of CA. The HCO_3^- formed is reabsorbed with sodium into the blood. Thus, for every molecule of H^+ secreted, a molecule of HCO_3^- is returned to the blood to restore components of the plasma bicarbonate buffer system.

The *ammonia buffer* depends on the generation of ammonia (NH_3) from amino acids, such as glutamine, in renal tubular cells (Fig. 14–4). NH_3 diffuses into the tubular lumen, where it may combine with secreted H^+ to form ammonium (NH_4^+), a large, charged particle that cannot be reabsorbed. H^+ in this form is thus trapped in the tubule. NH_4^+ is excreted in the urine in combination with Cl^- from NaCl. Na^+ is actively reabsorbed, along with tubular HCO_3^-.

The *phosphate buffer* operates similarly (Fig. 14–5), resulting in the formation of weak acids that are excreted in the urine. Sodium and bicarbonate are reabsorbed.

Effects of Other Electrolytes

Although H^+ and HCO_3^- are critical determinants of acid-base balance, they are also electrolytes, subject to the *principle of electroneutrality*, which holds that total cations must equal total anions in any fluid compartment. Renal regulation of serum pH is greatly influenced by the concentrations of other electrolytes, particularly potassium (K^+), sodium (Na^+), calcium (Ca^{2+}), chloride (Cl^-), and protein (Pr^-).

When serum potassium is elevated (*hyperkalemia*), renal tubular cells secrete more K^+ but retain H^+ for electroneutrality. The opposite occurs in *hypokalemia*, which promotes renal secretion of H^+. Similarly, H^+ imbalance influences both renal regulation and cellular shifts in potassium. In cases of serum H^+ excess, more H^+ is secreted by renal tubular cells, but K^+ is retained, promoting hyperkalemia. At the tissue level, H^+ moves into cells to be buffered by intracellular proteins, and K^+ moves out into the blood to maintain electroneutrality. This shift does not represent a true K^+ excess but does contribute to clinical manifestations of hyperkalemia, which include potentially lethal cardiac dysrhythmias. Treatment of the H^+ excess causes a shift in the opposite direction, promoting hypokalemia. In response to a deficit in serum H^+, renal cells retain H^+ and secrete more K^+, and cellular proteins release H^+ to the extracellular fluid while K^+ shifts intracellularly.

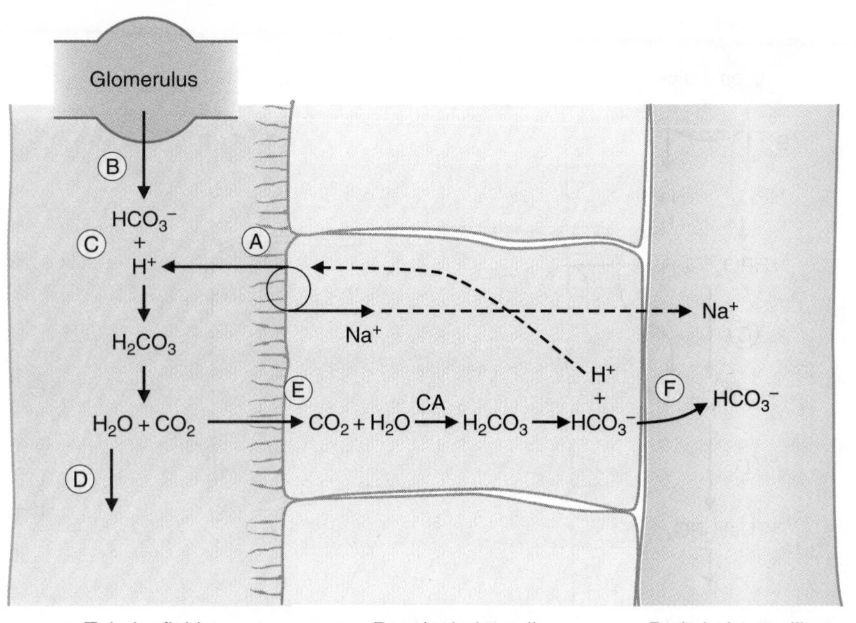

FIGURE 14–3 Function of the urinary bicarbonate (HCO_3^-) buffer. *A*, Hydrogen (H^+) is actively secreted into the tubule in exchange for sodium (Na^+). *B*, HCO_3^- is filtered into the tubule at the glomerulus. *C*, H^+ and $H_2CO_3^-$ enter reverse hydrolysis, yielding water (H_2O) and carbon dioxide (CO_2). *D*, H_2O remains in the tubule as urine unless it is reabsorbed. *E*, CO_2 diffuses into tubular cells and enters hydrolysis, catalyzed by carbonic anhydrase (CA), yielding H^+ and HCO_3^-. *F*, HCO_3^- is reabsorbed, with Na^+, into the blood.

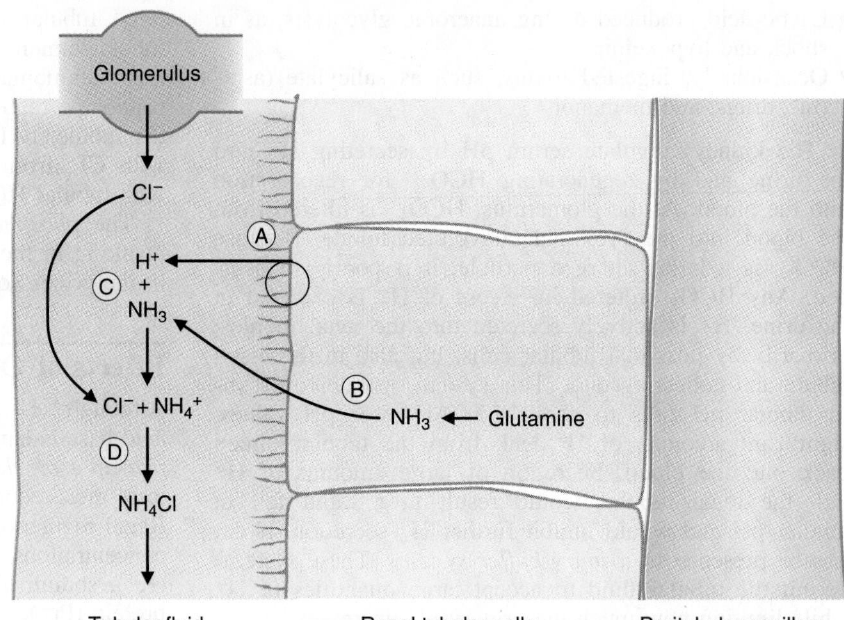

FIGURE 14–4 Function of the ammonia (NH_3) buffer. *A*, Hydrogen (H^+) is actively secreted into the tubular fluid. *B*, NH_3 is formed in the tubular cell and diffuses into the tubular lumen. *C*, Hydrogen (H^+) combines with NH_3 to form ammonium (NH_4^+), which cannot be reabsorbed. *D*, NH_4^+ combines with filtered chloride (Cl^-) for excretion in the urine. NH_4Cl, ammonium chloride.

Na^+ and Cl^- are of particular importance in maintaining fluid balance, and the kidney is the principal site of their regulation. Active reabsorption of Na^+ from the renal tubules creates gradients that drive the reabsorption of anions such as Cl^- and HCO_3^-. The juxtaglomerular cells of the renal glomeruli sense a low extracellular volume, triggering the renin-angiotensin-aldosterone system. Release of the mineralocorticoid hormone aldosterone from the adrenal cortex stimulates renal reabsorption of Na^+ from the distal tubule and proximal collecting duct. Maintenance of electroneutrality requires concurrent increases in the secretion of H^+ and K^+ as well as reabsorption of HCO_3^-. The kidney's priority in such cases is to restore volume balance, but this happens at the cost of worsening pH status. Clinical conditions that cause low serum Na^+ (*hyponatremia*) almost invariably result in low Cl^- (*hypochloremia*) as well. In Cl^- deficit, the kidney reabsorbs more HCO_3^- to maintain electroneutrality. Conversely, in conditions in which excess HCO_3^- is lost in the urine, Cl^- is retained.

Although intracellular proteins are the most important buffers in whole-body acid-base homeostasis, serum proteins such as albumin are also significant. In H^+ excess, for example, serum proteins bind circulating H^+, displacing other cations, such as calcium. The level of free (ionized) Ca^{2+} thus rises, promoting clinical manifestations of hypercalcemia. In H^+ deficit, a greater fraction of serum calcium is bound, decreasing levels of Ca^{2+}. Because H^+ excess creates a need for more urinary buffers, including ammonia (which is derived from protein), in-

FIGURE 14–5 Function of the phosphate buffer. *A*, Hydrogen (H^+) is actively secreted into the tubule. *B*, HPO_4^{2-} (hydrogen phosphate) and Na^+ are filtered into the tubule at the glomerulus. *C*, H^+ and HPO_4^{2-} combine to form dihydrogen phosphate ($H_2PO_4^-$). *D*, $H_2PO_4^-$ combines with filtered Na^+ for excretion in the urine.

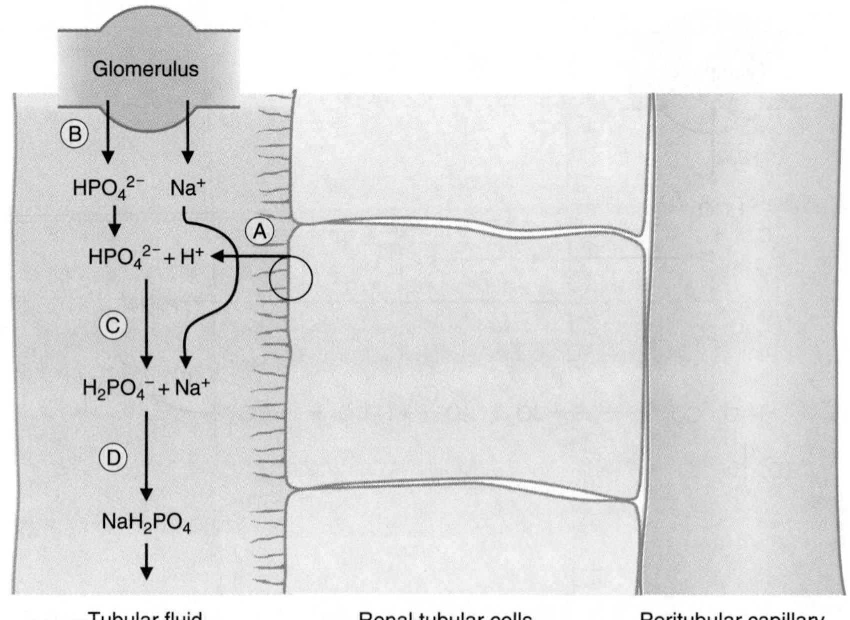

creased buffering of acid promotes depletion of protein. Similarly, deficiency of serum albumin caused by renal disease or other disorders may promote H^+ excess.

INTERACTION OF ACID-BASE REGULATORY SYSTEMS

Clinical evaluation of total acid-base homeostasis is aided by an understanding of the *Henderson-Hasselbalch equation*, which describes the relationships among pH, acid (H_2CO_3), and base (HCO_3^-):

$$pH = pKa + \log([HCO_3^-]/[H_2CO_3])$$

In this equation, p*K*a is a constant value (6.1). The base component is represented by serum HCO_3^- (normal value 24 mEq/L); since carbonic acid levels are negligible, the acid is represented by dissolved CO_2. Dissolved CO_2 is derived from the measurement of Pa_{CO_2}, the partial pressure of CO_2 in arterial blood (normal value 40 mm Hg, multiplied by a unit conversion factor of 0.03 to yield 1.2). When normal values are substituted, the equation becomes

$$7.4 = 6.1 + \log \frac{24}{1.2}$$

This equation reveals that a ratio of 20 parts base to 1 part acid must be present to yield a normal pH. An increase in the numerator (base) promotes an increase in blood pH; a decrease in base lowers pH. An increase in the denominator (acid) lowers pH; a decrease in acid raises pH (Fig. 14–6).

■ ACID-BASE COMPENSATION

When primary disease processes alter either the acid or the base component of the ratio, the lungs or the kidneys (whichever is unaffected by pathologic change) act to restore the 20:1 ratio and normalize pH. This process is known as *acid-base compensation*. When kidney disease impairs excretion of fixed acids, for example, the respiratory system can increase ventilation to "blow off" excess acid as CO_2. In respiratory failure, the kidneys can compensate for retention of acid (CO_2) by secreting H^+ and regenerating HCO_3^-.

As stated, blood buffers act to modulate pH changes but do not eliminate acid or base from the body. The lungs or kidneys alter the actual amounts of acid and base, but regulation by these systems is not as fast. The lungs respond within minutes, but maximal compensation takes up to 24 hours. The kidneys may require up to 72 hours to achieve optimal compensation.

In most cases, compensation does not fully restore normal pH. Respiratory compensation is limited because reducing ventilation to compensate for a renal deficit of H^+ would eventually result in hypoxemia. Because hypoxemia is a respiratory stimulant, ventilation would again increase. Similarly, renal compensation for ventilatory disorders is potentially limited by many factors, including renal blood flow, tubular flow rates, and saturability of tubular transport processes.

■ ACID-BASE CORRECTION

Although compensatory responses for primary acid-base disorders may nearly restore the 20:1 ratio of base to acid, the actual amounts of acid and base remain abnormal. Thus, compensation must be differentiated from *correction*, in which the ratio is restored and the absolute

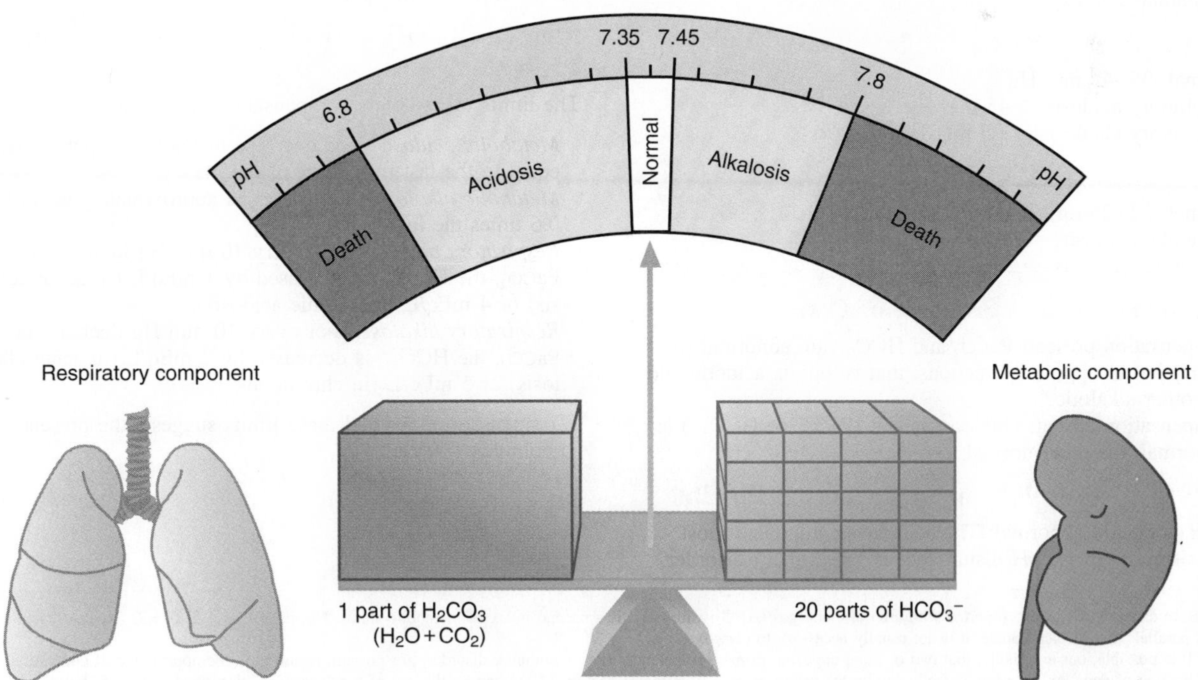

FIGURE 14–6 Regulation of acid-base balance. H_2CO_3, carbonic acid; H_2O, water; CO_2, carbon dioxide; HCO_3^-, bicarbonate.

quantities of dissolved CO_2 (as derived from $PaCO_2$) and HCO_3^- are returned to the normal range. Correction occurs only with resolution of the underlying disorder.

■ ANALYSIS OF ARTERIAL BLOOD GASES

The status of acid-base homeostasis may be monitored clinically through the serial measurement of *arterial blood gases* (ABGs). Among the parameters reported are pH, $PaCO_2$, and HCO_3^-. As illustrated in Box 14–1, these values may be used to (1) determine the presence and type of acid-base imbalance and (2) evaluate the level of compensation.

DISORDERS OF ACID-BASE BALANCE

The four general classes of acid-base imbalance are (1) respiratory acidosis, (2) respiratory alkalosis, (3) metabolic acidosis, and (4) metabolic alkalosis. These disorders are not clinical diagnoses or diseases in themselves; rather, they are clinical syndromes associated with a wide variety of diseases.

Acidosis refers to any pathologic process that causes a relative excess of acid (volatile or fixed) in the body. *Acidemia* is excess acid in the blood. The presence of acidemia does not necessarily confirm an underlying pathologic process; technically, it is merely a laboratory finding.

The same distinction may be made between the terms alkalosis and alkalemia. *Alkalosis* indicates a primary condition resulting in excess base in the body, and *alkalemia* refers more narrowly to elevation of serum pH. Care must be taken not to confuse these terms conceptually, and they must not be used interchangeably in clinical practice.

The incidence of acid-base imbalances in clinical settings is high. A study of 110 consecutive admissions to a general hospital revealed an overall incidence of acid-base imbalances of 56%. The most common disorder was respiratory alkalosis (26 cases), followed by respiratory acidosis (16), metabolic alkalosis (10), and metabolic acidosis (6). Eleven clients had more than one acid-base imbalance concurrently.[11]

■ RESPIRATORY ALKALOSIS

Respiratory alkalosis is a state of relative excess of base in body fluids resulting from increased respiratory elimination of CO_2. *Acute* respiratory alkalosis lasts for 24 hours or less; *chronic* respiratory alkalosis persists for a longer period.

Etiology and Risk Factors

Respiratory alkalosis is caused by alveolar hyperventilation, in which excess CO_2 is eliminated. The most com-

BOX 14–1 Analysis of Arterial Blood Gases

Step 1: Classify the pH

Normal: 7.35–7.45
Acidemia: <7.35
Alkalemia: >7.45

Step 2: Assess $PaCO_2$

Normal: 35–45 mm Hg
Respiratory acidosis: >45 mm Hg
Respiratory alkalosis: <35 mm Hg

Step 3: Assess HCO_3^-*

Normal: 22–26 mEq/L
Metabolic acidosis: <22 mEq/L
Metabolic alkalosis: >26 mEq/L

Step 4: Determine Presence of Compensation

Compensation present: $PaCO_2$ and HCO_3^- are abnormal (or nearly so) in opposite directions; that is, one is acidotic and the other alkalotic.†

Compensation absent: One component ($PaCO_2$ or HCO_3^-) is abnormal, the other normal.

Step 5: Identify Primary Disorder, If Possible

If pH is clearly abnormal: The acid-base component most consistent with the pH disturbance is the primary disorder.

If pH is normal or near-normal: The more deviant component is probably primary.‡ Also, note whether pH is on acidotic or alkalotic side of 7.4. The more deviant component should be consistent with this pH.

Step 6: Classify Degree of Compensation, If Present

The limits of complete compensation are as follows:

- *Metabolic acidosis*: The decrease in $PaCO_2$ is approximately equal to the last two digits of the pH.
- *Metabolic alkalosis*: The $PaCO_2$ is approximately equal to 0.6 times the increase in HCO_3^-.
- *Respiratory acidosis*: For every 10 mm Hg increase in $PaCO_2$, the HCO_3^- is increased by 1 mEq/L (in acute acidosis) or 4 mEq/L (in chronic acidosis).
- *Respiratory alkalosis*: For every 10 mm Hg decrease in $PaCO_2$, the HCO_3^- is decreased by 2 mEq/L (in acute alkalosis) or 5 mEq/L (in chronic alkalosis).

"Compensation" beyond these limits suggests the presence of a complex disorder.

*Base excess (BE) is also reported with arterial blood gas (ABG) values and is a second index of metabolic status. Normal BE is −2 to +2. Because fluctuation in BE parallels that of bicarbonate, it is not usually necessary to classify both.

† It is possible, but less likely, that two or more opposing primary imbalances (i.e., a complex disorder) are present, resulting in the appearance of compensation. The detection of complex disorders is facilitated by the use of an acid-base map (see Fig. 14–1) and by the use of the "formulas" described in Step 6, but a complex disorder cannot always be differentiated from compensation on the basis of laboratory values.

‡ It is unlikely that the more deviant component represents compensation, because except in rare cases the body does not overcompensate for imbalance. When pH approaches the normal range, compensatory mechanisms are no longer triggered.

mon cause of respiratory alkalosis is hypoxemia from such pulmonary disorders as pneumonia, pulmonary embolism, asthma, adult respiratory distress syndrome (ARDS), and pulmonary edema. Transient respiratory alkalosis may also occur secondary to acute anxiety or as a response to respiratory stimulant drugs such as epinephrine and salicylates. Neural disorders, such as stroke and intracranial lesions, may stimulate the central respiratory drive.

The most common causes of mild, chronic respiratory alkalosis are residence in high altitudes and pregnancy. Pulmonary fibrosis and other disorders that limit ventilatory volume result in an increased ventilatory rate, with a possible net excess of CO_2 elimination.

Pathophysiology

A low partial pressure of oxygen in arterial blood (PaO_2) is sensed by peripheral chemoreceptors in the carotid bodies and aortic arch. The rate at which these receptors fire then increases, stimulating the respiratory center in the medulla and increasing the rate and depth of ventilation. Peripheral chemoreceptors are also stimulated in states of low blood flow, such as shock.

Conditions that physically impede expansion of the lungs (such as pulmonary fibrosis) stimulate activation of the respiratory center via the Hering-Breuer, or stretch reflex. The J receptors, located in the alveolar-capillary membrane, are thought to stimulate increased ventilation in disorders such as ARDS, which causes thickening of this membrane.

The central chemoreceptors and respiratory center may be stimulated excessively by chemicals or toxins. In the case of salicylate overdose, it is interesting that adults usually exhibit respiratory alkalosis and that children more often have metabolic acidosis from the acid ingestion. The reason for this difference between children and adults is unknown. In severe alkalemia, changes in the ionization of structural and regulatory proteins result in widespread organ dysfunction. Cellular shifts and increased binding of Ca^{2+} to serum proteins induce electrolyte imbalance.

The buffering response in acute respiratory alkalosis results from (1) shifting of acid from intracellular fluid into the blood and (2) movement of HCO_3^- into cells in exchange for Cl^-. An adaptive increase in lactic acid production occurs secondary to stimulation of glycolysis. Renal compensation in chronic respiratory alkalosis involves decreased H^+ secretion as well as excretion of excess filtered HCO_3^-.

Clinical Manifestations

Signs of respiratory alkalosis in a client's ABG analysis include a high pH and a low $PaCO_2$. HCO_3^- levels fall with compensation in chronic respiratory alkalosis, and serum lactate dehydrogenase levels are often elevated. Hyperventilation, the underlying cause, is clinically apparent.

Central nervous system manifestations of altered blood flow and neurotransmission are usually predominant. They include paresthesias, lightheadedness, and confusion. Musculoskeletal and cardiac manifestations of hypokalemia and hypocalcemia (such as dysrhythmias and muscle weəkness) may be present.

Prognosis

The clinical outcome depends on the severity of the underlying disorder and its response to treatment. Mild alkalosis in pregnancy and at high altitudes is considered to be adaptive. Respiratory alkalosis in a critically ill client is an ominous prognostic sign, with mortality increasing proportionately with the severity of alkalosis.[2] Compensation for severe respiratory alkalosis depletes the bicarbonate buffer, increasing the client's vulnerability to later acidosis.

Outcome Management

Treatment of the Underlying Disorder

Treatment of mild, chronic respiratory alkalosis is usually not warranted because it produces little risk and few symptoms. Aggressive treatment of the underlying causes of hypoxemia is essential in cases of severe respiratory alkalosis. Electrolyte imbalances usually resolve with treatment of the underlying cause.

Respiratory Support

Oxygen therapy may be used to correct underlying hypoxemia. Rebreathing of CO_2 (as from breathing into a paper bag or other closed system) provides prompt but short-term relief in anxiety-related respiratory alkalosis.

■ RESPIRATORY ACIDOSIS

Respiratory acidosis is a state of relative excess of acid in body fluids resulting from retention or excessive production of CO_2. *Acute* respiratory acidosis develops and resolves within 3 days or less; *chronic* respiratory acidosis persists over a longer period.

Etiology and Risk Factors

Respiratory acidosis nearly always results from hypoventilation. Chronic respiratory acidosis is most commonly caused by chronic obstructive pulmonary disease (COPD), also known as "chronic airflow limitation." In end-stage COPD, pathologic changes lead to airway collapse, air trapping, and disturbance of ventilation-perfusion (V/Q) relationships. Acute respiratory acidosis also occurs when respiratory infection or concurrent cardiac disease increases the work of breathing. Hypoventilation with resulting respiratory acidosis is seen in diseases of the neuromuscular junction in which diaphragmatic movement is impaired (such as Guillain-Barré syndrome) and in depression of the medullary respiratory center by drugs or lesions of the central nervous system.

Respiratory acidosis may occur iatrogenically (as a result of treatment) from inadequate mechanical ventilation or from excessive oxygen administration to clients with chronic CO_2 retention (as in COPD). In the latter case, hypoventilation results from:

- Depression of the medullary respiratory center with removal of the hypoxemic stimulus
- Worsening of V/Q relationships secondary to replacement of airway nitrogen (which helps keep airways open) with oxygen

Normally, the most important stimulus for ventilation is an increase in the acidity of cerebrospinal fluid (CSF) resulting from diffusion of CO_2 into the CSF from the blood. However, the higher level of HCO_3^- resulting from renal compensation for chronic respiratory acidosis minimizes the effect of increasing $Paco_2$ in these clients. Oxygen therapy may worsen V/Q relationships because it displaces nitrogen, a much less soluble gas, in alveoli. As oxygen is absorbed, alveoli may collapse, contributing to hypoventilation.

The second, much less common cause of respiratory acidosis is excessive CO_2 production from hypermetabolism, or from excessive metabolism of carbohydrate fuels for energy. Clinical use of enteral feedings or parenteral nutrition formulas that are disproportionately high in carbohydrate may contribute to elevated $Paco_2$ levels, particularly in clients who also have impaired ventilation.

Pathophysiology

CO_2 accumulates in the blood and diffuses readily into all body compartments. This *hypercapnia* drives the hydrolysis reaction forward, generating carbonic acid that dissociates into H^+ and HCO_3^-. Immediate buffering by nonbicarbonate buffers occurs. Renal compensation proceeds over 3 to 5 days, with greater secretion of H^+ and regeneration of bicarbonate. Renal ammonia production increases, enhancing the function of the ammonia urinary buffer but depleting protein stores. As serum HCO_3^- levels rise with compensation, Cl^- is excreted in greater amounts, potentially inducing hypochloremia in chronic respiratory acidosis. Renal retention of K^+ and cellular cation shifts may lead to hyperkalemia. Displacement of Ca^{2+} from albumin may result in hypercalcemia.

In acute respiratory acidosis, the rapid rise in $Paco_2$ results in hypoxemia in clients breathing room air, as retained CO_2 displaces oxygen in alveoli. Hypoxemia poses a more serious threat to life than either acidemia or hypercapnia in severe acute respiratory acidosis. Acidemia alters the ionization of structural and regulatory proteins (enzymes, for example), resulting in widespread manifestations of organ dysfunction.

Clinical Manifestations

An arterial blood sample that has a low pH signifies that the client has acidemia, and a high $Paco_2$ signifies hypercapnia. The client probably has hypoventilation, the usual underlying cause of respiratory acidosis; signs of hypoxemia may be present in severe cases. HCO_3^- levels are normal or, if renal compensation is occurring, elevated. Compensation is present to a greater extent in chronic respiratory acidosis than in acute respiratory acidosis.

Clinical signs of organ system dysfunction from acidemia include hypotension and cardiac dysrhythmias caused by decreased vascular tone, decreased myocardial contractility, and manifestations of electrolyte imbalance. Altered cerebral blood flow and depressed neurotransmission may manifest as tremors, seizures, lethargy, stupor, and, ultimately, coma (hypercapnic encephalopathy).

Prognosis

The clinical outcome in respiratory acidosis depends on the severity and duration of tissue hypoxia as well as on the responsiveness of the underlying disorder to treatment.

Outcome Management

Treatment of the Underlying Disorder

Treatment of respiratory acidosis is primarily focused on resolving the underlying disorder. For example, you may give an antibiotic to treat pneumonia, a narcotic antagonist to treat a drug overdose, or dialysis to clear toxins from the blood. Electrolyte imbalances usually resolve with such treatment; however, life-threatening hyperkalemia may require emergency treatment with dialysis or cation-exchange resins.

Respiratory Support

Mechanical ventilation and supplemental oxygen are often employed in conditions that cause respiratory acidosis. Currently, the trend is to use ventilation at lower tidal volumes than would be required to completely restore $Paco_2$ to the normal range. This *permissive hypercapnia* results in fewer airway injuries but comparable clinical outcomes. However, because the client's own ventilatory drive exceeds that provided by the ventilator, sedation is usually required. Administer oxygen therapy cautiously (at low flow rates or low percentages) to the client with chronic CO_2 retention to minimize the risk of worsening the client's respiratory status via nitrogen washout and blunting of the ventilatory drive.

Administration of Exogenous Alkali

If the client has adequate renal function, administration of base (typically, sodium bicarbonate) to partially correct the pH is not warranted. Such treatment may actually worsen the client's condition because bicarbonate further raises CO_2 levels by driving reverse hydrolysis. An exception may be made if the client has severe bronchospasm, because alkalinization may restore the responsiveness of the airways to beta-agonist drugs.[1]

■ METABOLIC ALKALOSIS

Metabolic alkalosis is a state of relative excess of base (or H^+ deficit) in body fluids resulting from a gain of bicarbonate or a loss of fixed acids.

Etiology and Risk Factors

Metabolic alkalosis develops through a two-phase mechanism. In the *generation phase*, the imbalance is first created by (1) loss of acid (as with HCl loss during vomiting) or gain of base (as with administration of $NaHCO_3$) or (2) loss of intestinal fluids containing more Cl^- than HCO_3^-. Metabolic alkalosis associated with fluid volume loss is referred to as *contraction alkalosis*. Another common type, *posthypercapnic metabolic alkalosis*, results from too-rapid correction of chronic respiratory acidosis, in which case a compensatory increase in HCO_3^- then persists as a primary disorder.

In the *maintenance phase*, alkalosis persists because renal excretion of HCO_3^-, which would otherwise correct the disorder, is impaired. This impairment may result from hypovolemia in contraction alkalosis or, much less commonly, from aldosterone excess. In hypovolemia, greater Na^+ reabsorption by the distal tubule (stimulated by the renin-angiotensin-aldosterone system) results in increases in both H^+ secretion and HCO_3^- regeneration. In primary aldosteronism (or with prolonged corticosteroid administration, in which aldosterone-like effects also arise), the hormone stimulates increased Na^+ reabsorption by the same distal tubular transport mechanism.

Metabolic alkalosis from fluid loss is referred to as "saline-sensitive," because restoration of volume with fluid containing NaCl permits the kidneys to restore acid-base homeostasis. Alkalosis in cases of aldosterone excess is not correctable with administration of a saline solution and so is termed "saline-resistant." Rarely, excessive ingestion of licorice (20 to 40 g) causes metabolic alkalosis because of its structural similarity to aldosterone.

Overcorrection of acidosis with $NaHCO_3$ may cause alkalosis, as can massive transfusion of whole blood. The citrate anticoagulant used for storing blood is metabolized to bicarbonate. Packed RBCs contain much less citrate; thus, their use in multiple transfusion is preferred. Treatment of hypovolemia with lactated Ringer's solution may also contribute, because lactate is metabolized to bicarbonate.

Loss of gastric fluid via nasogastric suction or vomiting further contributes to metabolic alkalosis because of loss of HCl. Additional HCl must be produced by gastric cells via the hydrolysis reaction. H^+ is secreted into the stomach with Cl^-, while the HCO_3^- produced during the reaction is reabsorbed into the blood.

Pathophysiology

Respiratory compensation for metabolic alkalosis is limited by the hypoxemia that quickly develops with hypoventilation. Most buffering occurs in the extracellular fluid, where the buffers are much less effective for base loads than for acid loads. Severe alkalemia leads to widespread organ dysfunction because of altered ionization of body proteins as well as enhanced Ca^{2+} binding to serum proteins. Neurologic and cardiovascular systems are primarily affected. Hypokalemia, which occurs from cellular shifts and renal or intestinal losses, is more prominent in metabolic alkalosis than in respiratory alkalosis.

Clinical Manifestations

Metabolic alkalosis is manifested in ABG values by a high pH and a high HCO_3^-. $PaCO_2$ rises with compensation. Adaptive hypoventilation may be apparent and may induce some hypoxemia. Signs of volume deficit are often present in association with the underlying disorder. Hypokalemia may be manifested as cardiac dysrhythmias. Central nervous system manifestations include lethargy, confusion, and seizures.

Prognosis

The outcome of metabolic alkalosis depends primarily on the severity of the underlying disorder and its responsiveness to treatment. Uncorrected metabolic alkalosis is associated with high mortality from dysrhythmias and poor tissue perfusion.

Outcome Management

Treatment of the Underlying Disorder

Prompt treatment of the underlying disease process is the primary approach. Replacement of lost fluids and electrolytes and support of renal function are often the mainstays of therapy.

Administration of Acetazolamide

Acetazolamide (Diamox) is a diuretic that inhibits carbonic anhydrase and promotes loss of bicarbonate in the urine. Losses of potassium and phosphate are also greater with the use of acetazolamide, however, and may lead to manifestations of electrolyte imbalance.

Administration of Exogenous Acid

In severe alkalemia, the intravenous administration of acid (HCl) or HCl precursors (ammonium chloride or arginine monohydrochloride) may be warranted to enhance physiologic compensation. Risks of acid infusion are substantial, however; they include local tissue injury (sclerosis of veins), hypervolemia, hyperosmolar imbalance (with HCl precursors), increased ammonia levels (with ammonium chloride), and hyperkalemia (with arginine monohydrochloride).

■ METABOLIC ACIDOSIS

Metabolic acidosis is a state of relative acid excess (or base deficit) in body fluids resulting from gain of fixed acids or a loss of bicarbonate.

Etiology and Risk Factors

Metabolic acidosis may be caused by either of two mechanisms: accumulation of fixed acid or loss of base. These mechanisms may be differentiated clinically by the presence or absence of a high *anion gap*. Normally, the anion gap is 6.6 ± 4 mEg/L.[13] It is calculated by subtracting the sum of the serum concentrations of the major anions, bicarbonate and chloride, from the serum concentration of sodium. The difference, or "gap," represents anions in the serum other than HCO_3^- and Cl^-.

When acidosis results from addition of organic acid (as in lactic acidosis), bicarbonate is consumed in buffering but is not lost from the body. Unmeasured anions (primarily proteins) buffer most of the acid load, and the anion gap thus increases. Common causes of *high–anion gap acidosis* are:

- Azotemic renal failure, in which acid end products of protein metabolism cannot be effectively excreted because of impaired glomerular filtration
- Diabetic ketoacidosis, in which ketoacids accumulate because of accelerated lipid metabolism in the absence of insulin
- Lactic acidosis, a consequence of anaerobic carbohydrate metabolism
- Ingestion of toxins with acid metabolites (less common)

Non–anion gap acidosis caused by loss of base is also called *hyperchloremic metabolic acidosis*. In this case, chloride is retained by the kidneys when excess bicarbonate is lost from the body, and the anion gap remains normal. Excess bicarbonate may be lost through either the kidneys or the intestinal tract. In renal tubular acidosis, the renal tubular cells cannot reabsorb bicarbonate, which therefore is lost in the urine. Intestinal secretions, high in bicarbonate, may be lost through enteric drainage tubes (such as an ileostomy tube) or diarrhea. Drugs that inhibit carbonic anhydrase, such as acetazolamide, interfere with bicarbonate regeneration during urinary buffering. In non–anion gap acidosis caused by a gain of mineral acid (such as HCl), chloride is ingested with the acid, and bicarbonate is excreted proportionately.

Pathophysiology

Metabolic acidosis is accompanied by a compensatory increase in ventilation. Severe acidemia induces insulin resistance and depresses glycolytic enzymes, resulting in impairment of energy metabolism. The function of regulatory and structural proteins is impaired by altered ionization, leading to widespread organ dysfunction. Increased protein catabolism also occurs. Hyperkalemia occurs because K^+ shifts out of cells as excess H^+ enters. Insulin deficiency in diabetic ketoacidosis may worsen hyperkalemia because insulin normally promotes cellular uptake of K^+ along with glucose. Uptake of lactic acid by the liver is reduced, whereas hepatic lactate production is increased.

In metabolic acidosis caused by a gain of organic acids, bicarbonate stores are rapidly depleted by buffering. If renal function is not impaired, renal regeneration of HCO_3^- occurs with excretion of H^+. However, this response takes several days.

Clinical Manifestations

Metabolic acidosis is apparent in ABG values as a low pH and a low HCO_3^-. $PaCO_2$ drops as respiratory compensation occurs. Systemic signs of acidemia resulting from altered protein function and electrolyte imbalance are similar to those of respiratory acidosis, except that compensatory hyperventilation is present.

Prognosis

Clinical outcomes of metabolic acidosis depend on the severity of the underlying disorder and its responsiveness to treatment.

Outcome Management

Treatment of the Underlying Disorder

Aggressive intervention aimed at resolving the underlying disorder is the primary form of treatment. Electrolyte imbalance is treated only if life-threatening, because it normally resolves with correction of the underlying disorder.

Administration of Exogenous Alkali

In severe metabolic acidosis, administration of intravenous sodium bicarbonate or other alkalinizing substances may be warranted to minimize the detrimental effects of the acidosis until the underlying disorder is resolved or until physiologic compensation is effective. Such therapy may provide a margin of safety in anticipation of continued acidifying stressors, but it is not without controversy. Fluid overload, hyperosmolar imbalance, and alkalosis due to excessive treatment are risks of this approach. As previously mentioned, administration of bicarbonate results in increased CO_2 levels, which may be detrimental in clients with respiratory disease or advanced cardiac failure. Alternative alkalinizing agents, such as tromethamine (Tham), produce less CO_2 but have not proved more effective than $NaHCO_3$ for the treatment of severe acidemia.[1]

■ COMPLEX ACID-BASE DISORDERS

Mixed acid-base disorders, in which two primary acid-base imbalances coexist, are common. In cardiac arrest, for example, lactic acid quickly accumulates as a result of anaerobic metabolism; the carbonic acid level is elevated because of respiratory arrest. In COPD, underlying respiratory acidosis may be complicated by metabolic alkalosis secondary to diuretic or steroid therapy.

A *triple acid-base disorder* is present when metabolic acidosis and metabolic alkalosis coexist with either respiratory acidosis or respiratory alkalosis. (The two respiratory imbalances cannot coexist because they have opposite effects on ventilation.) As an example of a triple disorder, imbalances due to ingestion of methanol (an exogenous toxin that produces metabolic acidosis), vomiting (which produces metabolic alkalosis), and respiratory arrest from aspiration (which produces respiratory acidosis) may occur simultaneously.

Suspect a complex acid-base disorder when a client's $PaCO_2$ value and HCO_3^- level do not correlate with pH or when ABG evidence of compensation exceeds predicted levels (see Box 14–1). Use of an acid-base map may also facilitate detection (Fig. 14–7). If the plotted ABG values converge at a point outside the usual range for a primary imbalance, a complex disorder is likely.

Nursing Management of the Medical Client

Assessment

You must be alert for signs of acid-base imbalance in clients at risk for these disturbances. There is such a risk in any client who:

- Has a known disease of the pulmonary, cardiovascular, or renal system
- Is in a hypermetabolic state, such as with fever, sepsis, or burns
- Is receiving total parenteral nutrition or enteral tube feedings high in carbohydrate
- Is receiving mechanical ventilation
- Has diabetes
- Has vomiting, diarrhea, or enteric drainage
- Is elderly

Age-related decreases in respiratory and renal function may limit the client's ability to compensate for acid-base disturbances. The normal aging process results in decreased ventilatory capacity as well as loss of alveolar surface area for gas exchange; thus, older adults are susceptible to respiratory acidosis from hypoventilation and to respiratory alkalosis from hypoxemia. Older adults commonly take multiple medications for hypertension or cardiovascular disease; these drugs may contribute to hypokalemia and metabolic alkalosis. Respiratory compensa-

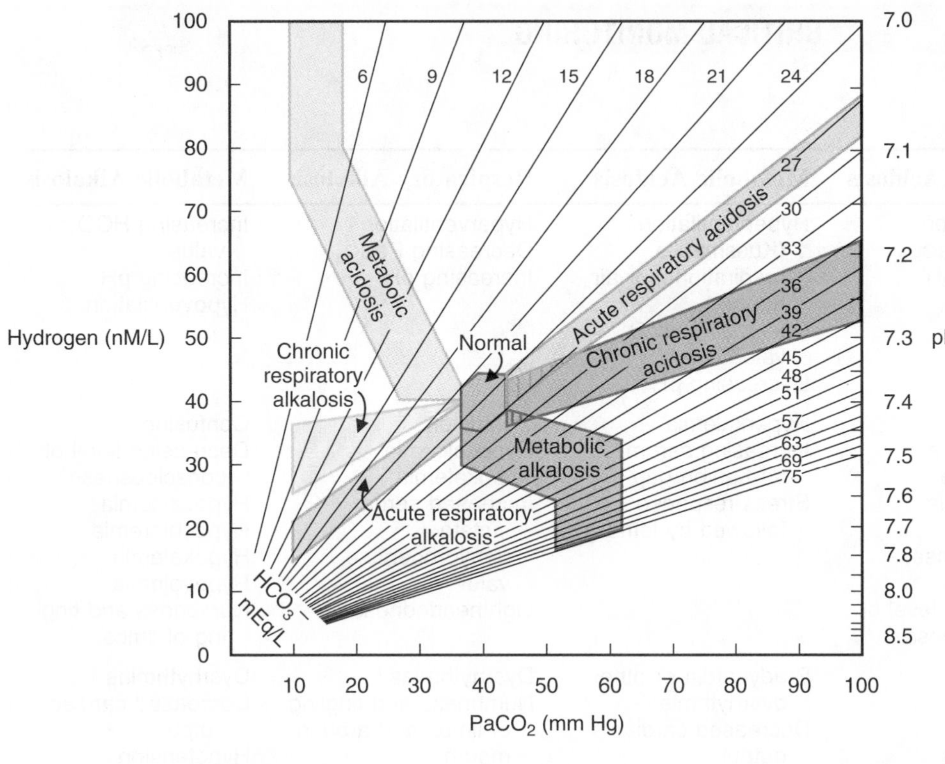

FIGURE 14–7 An acid-base map. To use the acid-base map, plot the pH on the vertical axis and the partial pressure of arterial carbon dioxide ($PaCO_2$) on the horizontal axis. Note the point at which the values intersect. If the result falls outside the normal area or the 95% confidence bands for the major primary disorders, the client probably has a complex acid-base imbalance. However, a point falling within one of the bands does not rule out a complex disorder. HCO_3^-, bicarbonate.

tion in this condition is compromised because of the structural and functional changes mentioned. Decreased cardiac output in the aging person diminishes renal perfusion and glomerular filtration. Aldosterone is less effective in older people, as is ammonia buffering. These changes limit renal compensation for respiratory imbalances and may put an elderly client at higher risk for metabolic imbalance.

To assess for acid-base imbalances, document the findings of a comprehensive physical assessment of ventilatory status, cardiovascular function, and fluid balance, as described in the Critical Monitoring chart. Carefully analyze the trends you see. Consider laboratory values as well, including ABG, electrolyte, blood urea nitrogen, creatinine, and serum lactate dehydrogenase values.

INTERPRET ARTERIAL BLOOD GAS VALUES. Your knowledgeable interpretation of ABG values is critical for timely, appropriate intervention in acid-base disturbances. Often, you are the first to see a client's ABG results. You become the communication link between respiratory therapists and physicians about potential changes in a client's status or treatment. In critical care units, many nurses are using bedside ABG analyzers to obtain these results. Systems for continuous in vivo monitoring of blood gases have recently been developed. Although ABG interpretation is essential to diagnosis and treatment of acid-base imbalance, ABG findings are helpful only when they are considered as part of the total clinical picture.

PROTECT THE CLIENT. Preventing client injury during diagnostic procedures is one of your most important responsibilities. Before a client receives a radial artery puncture for withdrawal of an arterial blood specimen, for example, perform Allen's test to ensure adequate circulation to the hand. Perform this test as follows:

1. Have the client tightly close the intended test hand into a fist.
2. Apply pressure over the pulse points for both radial and ulnar arteries.
3. Ask the client to open the fist; the palm has a blanched look from a lack of blood.
4. Release pressure on the ulnar artery. If the artery has adequate circulation, the client's palm reddens within 10 or 15 seconds; it is safe to use the radial artery to obtain a blood specimen.

Failure to assess collateral circulation may result in severe ischemic injury to the client's hand if the ulnar artery is compromised and the radial artery is injured by the puncture.

Critically ill clients commonly have femoral or radial arterial catheter systems from which blood specimens are drawn. Frequent sampling can result in significant blood loss if an open system is used. Nursing research has demonstrated that a minimal discard specimen of 2 ml is sufficient to clear the arterial line of heparinized solution before blood is aspirated for ABG testing.[15] Closed systems allow reinstillation of initially aspirated heparinized solution and blood. Nursing responsibilities for clients with arterial lines are discussed in Chapter 56.

ENSURE ACCURACY. You are responsible for minimizing errors in ABG analysis caused by faulty specimen collection and handling. Potential sampling errors, their consequences, and nursing implications are summarized in Table 14–1. Despite quality control procedures, erroneous blood gas data are sometimes reported. You should suspect a sampling error or transcription error

CRITICAL MONITORING

Acid-Base Imbalances

	Respiratory Acidosis	Metabolic Acidosis	Respiratory Alkalosis	Metabolic Alkalosis
Defining Signs	Hypoventilation Increasing $PaCO_2$ Decreasing pH	Hyperventilation (Kussmaul's respirations, or air hunger) Decreasing HCO_3^- value Decreasing pH	Hyperventilation Decreasing $PaCO_2$ Increasing pH	Increasing HCO_3^- value Increasing pH Hypoventilation
Commonly Seen	Dyspnea Hypercalcemia Hyperkalemia Hypochloremia Hypoxemia Stress response, followed by decreasing level of consciousness	Hyperkalemia Increasing serum Cl^- and anion gap Stress response followed by lethargy	Confusion Hypocalcemia Hypokalemia Increased serum lactate dehydrogenase value Lightheadedness	Confusion Decreasing level of consciousness Hypocalcemia Hypochloremia Hypokalemia Hypovolemia Numbness and tingling of limbs
Signs of Severe Imbalance	Hypotension Papilledema Seizures Dysrhythmias Muscle tremors	Bradycardia or other dysrhythmia Decreased cardiac output Gastrointestinal distention Hypotension Nausea and vomiting	Dysrhythmias Numbness and tingling of limbs and around mouth Muscle weakness	Dysrhythmias Decreased cardiac output Hypotension Hypoxemia Muscle cramping or tetany Muscle tremors Seizures

TABLE 14–1 SOURCES OF ERROR IN SAMPLING FOR ARTERIAL BLOOD GAS ANALYSIS

Sampling Error	Effect	Nursing Implications
Air bubbles in syringe	↑ PaO_2 ↓ $PaCO_2$ ↑ pH	Expel all air bubbles immediately. Do not agitate syringe. Do not use any sample that appears frothy.
Inadvertent venous sample or venous contamination of arterial sample	↓ PaO_2 ↑ $PaCO_2$ ↓ pH	Avoid use of femoral artery. Use short-beveled needle. Do not overshoot artery and then withdraw to "catch" it. Watch for autofilling of syringe with arterial puncture. Verify questionable results with new sample.
Anticoagulant effects Altered pH	↓ pH	Use lithium heparin, if possible. Use 1:1000 units/ml concentration. Use minimum 2-ml discard sample with arterial line aspiration.
Dilution of sample	↑ pH ↓ all other values	Use syringe with minimal dead space. Use dried heparin if available. Use at least 3-ml sample.
Effects of metabolism of white blood cells in sample	↓ PaO_2 ↑ $PaCO_2$ ↓ pH	Place sample in ice water immediately. Have sample analyzed within 20 min. Cool sample to 5° C if it cannot be analyzed quickly. Have sample analyzed immediately if client has leukocytosis.

$PaCO_2$, partial pressure of carbon dioxide in arterial blood; PaO_2, partial pressure of oxygen in arterial blood; ↑, increase in; ↓, decrease in.
Data from Malley, W. J. (1990). *Clinical blood gases: Application and noninvasive alternatives.* Philadelphia: W. B. Saunders; and Williams, A. J. (1998). ABC of oxygen: Assessing and interpreting arterial blood gases and acid-base balance. *British Medical Journal, 317*(7167), 1213–1216.

when the reported values lack internal consistency or external congruity. *Internal consistency* means that the values make sense when considered as a whole. An alkalotic pH, for example, is inconsistent with excess $PaCO_2$ and deficient HCO_3^-. *External congruity* means that the ABG findings are consistent with other laboratory data and with clinical assessment findings. For example, a client with a pH of 7.10 should appear profoundly ill.

DIAGNOSIS, OUTCOMES, INTERVENTIONS

Nursing Diagnoses. Several nursing diagnoses may apply to the management of underlying causes and clinical manifestations of acid-base disturbances. For example, *Ineffective Breathing Pattern, Altered Tissue Perfusion,* or *Risk of Injury* may be appropriate. Acid-base imbalances are perhaps best conceptualized as collaborative problems, however, because the interventions of several health care professionals, including nurses, respiratory therapists, and physicians, are required for effective treatment.

Outcomes. When acid-base imbalances are approached as collaborative problems, the expected outcomes reflect timely resolution of underlying disorders and minimization of the detrimental effects of acidemia or alkalemia. Your role in promoting these outcomes includes implementing medical management and watching for clinical manifestations of the imbalances and the response to treatment.

Interventions. Corrective interventions address the underlying causes of acid-base imbalances and are the mainstay of treatment in such disorders. Compensatory imbalances are not treated but instead resolve spontaneously as the primary disorder is reversed. You should optimize the client's respiratory and renal function through positioning, pulmonary hygiene, and hydration. Also, help clients cope with the anxiety that often accompanies—and may contribute to—acid-base imbalance. Collaborate in the administration of drug therapy, fluid and electrolyte replacement, oxygen therapy, and mechanical ventilation when indicated.

Provide Respiratory Support. Altered ventilation is a component of all significant acid-base imbalances, whether as a contributing cause or as a result of compensation. You can help to promote optimal ventilation through such measures as repositioning, airway management, hydration, and implementation of oxygen therapy and mechanical ventilation.

Administer Exogenous Acid or Alkali. In extreme circumstances that require intravenous administration of acid or base, you must be knowledgeable about the potential risks of this therapy, and you must carefully monitor administration rates and therapeutic response. For a detailed discussion of appropriate nursing interventions for specific disorders underlying acid-base imbalances, consult the appropriate chapters of this book.

EVALUATION

Acid-base disorders can be acute and corrected quickly, with control of the underlying disorder, or they may be chronic and managed with compensation. Clients with chronic forms of acid-base imbalance must be assessed closely because they decompensate quickly.

CONCLUSIONS

In collaboration with other health care professionals, you may reduce the client's risk for adverse outcomes resulting from acid-base imbalances. Because of the narrow homeostatic range of serum pH, the client at risk must be carefully monitored in order to detect imbalance as early as possible. Nursing interventions that promote optional respiratory and renal function are particularly important in prevention and treatment of acid-base imbalances.

THINKING CRITICALLY

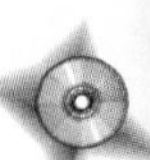

1. **The client is a 65-year-old widow with a long history of type 2 diabetes mellitus. She was a heavy smoker for 40 years but has not smoked in the last 5 years. She is admitted to the general medical unit because of a 1-week history of profuse diarrhea, attributed to food poisoning. She appears to be in respiratory distress. Her admission ABG values are pH, 7.26; $PaCO_2$, 13 mm Hg; HCO_3^-, 5 mEq/L. What acid-base imbalance does she have? Should you encourage her to breathe more slowly? Other than ABGs, what laboratory values should you monitor closely in this case? Why?**

Factors to Consider. What acids or bases are lost through diarrhea? Why might a respiratory change have developed if the client's primary problem is gastrointestinal (e.g., metabolic)?

2. **A 19-year-old college student is brought to the emergency department at 4:30 AM by his friends. While studying for final examinations, he grew increasingly anxious during his "cram session," frequently voicing doubts about passing a particularly difficult course. His breathing became increasingly labored, and he seemed dazed and confused. He says his "face feels numb." His pulse is rapid (165 beats per minute) and he is diaphoretic. The client was seen with bleeding duodenal ulcers 2 years ago. ABG analysis of blood samples drawn in the emergency department reveals pH, 7.58; $PaCO_2$, 21 mm Hg; HCO_3^-, 20 mEq/L. What acid-base imbalance does the client have? What caused it? What bedside assessments should you perform and why? What interventions should you consider that might prevent future episodes?**

Factors to Consider. Can rapid breathing alone alter excretion of components needed for acid-base balance?

3. **A 72-year-old retired college professor has a 55-pack-year history of cigarette smoking and advanced emphysema. He had an acute myocardial infarction 5 years ago, from which he recovered uneventfully. He sees his physician in the clinic, complaining of a "cold" that he "just can't get rid of" and "soreness" in his chest. His blood pressure is 165/90 mm Hg, and he has inspiratory crackles in both lung bases. His ankles are**

edematous. ABG analysis of blood samples drawn during the visit revealed: pH, 7.34; $PaCO_2$, 65 mm Hg; HCO_3^-, 34 mEq/L. What acid-base imbalance does he have? What is the probable cause? What additional information would be helpful in planning his care? What variables should you consider in determining priorities of care?

Factors to Consider. Consider that the client has developed heart failure. When the lungs fill with fluid, what happens to O_2/CO_2 exchange and, thereby, acid-base balance?

BIBLIOGRAPHY

1. Adrogue, H., & Madias, N. (1998). Management of life-threatening acid-base disorders: Part 1. *New England Journal of Medicine, 338*(1), 26–34.
2. Adrogue, H., & Madias, N. (1998). Management of life-threatening acid-base disorders: Part 2. *New England Journal of Medicine, 338*(2), 107–111.
3. Carpenito, L. (1995). *Nursing diagnosis: Application to clinical practice* (6th ed.). Philadelphia: J. B. Lippincott.
4. Dirks, J. (1995). Innovations in technology: Continuous intra-arterial blood gas monitoring. *Critical Care Nurse, 15*(4), 19–20, 22, 24–27.
5. Gilbert, H., & Vender, J. (1995). Arterial blood gas monitoring. *Critical Care Clinics, 11*(1), 233–248.
6. Grogono, A. (1999). *Fundamentals of acid-base balance* [Online]. Available: *http://gasnet.med.yale.edu/gta/acid-base/AB.html.*
7. Hanna, J., Scheinman, J., & Chan, J. (1995). The kidney in acid-base balance. *Pediatric Clinics of North America, 42*(6), 1365–1395.
8. Hansen, M. (1998). *Pathophysiology: Foundations of disease and clinical intervention.* Philadelphia: W. B. Saunders.
9. Laski, M., & Kurtzman, N. (1996). Acid-base disorders in medicine. *Disease-a-Month, 42*(2), 59–125.
10. Malley, W. J. (1990). *Clinical blood gases: Application and noninvasive alternatives.* Philadelphia: W. B. Saunders.
11. Palange, P., Carlone, S., Galassetti, P., et al. (1990). Incidence of acid-base and electrolyte disturbances in a general hospital: A study of 110 consecutive admissions. *Recenti Progressi in Medicina (Roma), 81*(12), 788–791.
12. Preusser, B., Lash, J., Stone, K., et al. (1989). Quantifying the minimum discard sample required for accurate blood gases. *Nursing Research, 38*(5), 276–279.
13. Rutecki, G., & Whittier, F. (1997). Acid-base interpretation: Part 1: Applying five rules in everyday cases. *Consultant, 37*(12), 3067–3070, 3073.
14. Rutecki, G., & Whittier, F. (1998). Acid-base interpretation: Part 2: Applying five rules to simplify complex cases. *Consultant, 38*(1), 131–133, 137–138, 141–142.
15. Rutecki, G., & Whittier, F. (1998). An approach to clinical acid-base problem-solving. *Comprehensive Therapy, 24*(11/12), 553–559.
16. Williams, A. J. (1998). ABC of oxygen: Assessing and interpreting arterial blood gases and acid-base balance. *British Medical Journal, 317*(7167), 1213–1216.
17. Williamson, J. C. (1995). Acid-base disorders: Classification and management strategies. *American Family Physician, 52*(2), 584–590.

REMEMBER *to check out your* **Companion CD ROM**

CHAPTER

15

Clients Having Surgery: Promoting Positive Outcomes

Nancy Girard

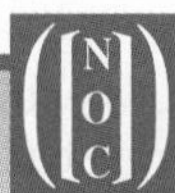

NURSING OUTCOMES CLASSIFICATION (NOC)
for Nursing Diagnoses–Clients Having Surgery

Altered Thought Processes
Cognitive Ability
Cognitive Orientation
Concentration
Decision-Making
Distorted Thought Control
Identity
Information Processing
Neurologic Status: Consciousness
Anxiety
Anxiety Control
Coping
Hypothermia
Thermoregulation
Neurologic Status
Vital Signs Status
Knowledge Deficit
Concentration
Knowledge: Diet
Knowledge: Disease Process
Knowledge: Health Resources
Knowledge: Illness Care
Knowledge: Medication
Knowledge: Prescribed Activity
Knowledge: Treatment Procedure
Knowledge: Treatment Regimen
Information Processing
Pain
Comfort Lever
Pain Control
Pain: Disruptive Effects
Pain Level
Risk for Aspiration
Cognitive Ability
Endurance
Immobility Consequences: Physiologic
Infection Status
Knowledge: Treatment (Procedures)
Neurologic Status
Respiratory Status: Gas Exchange
Respiratory Status: Ventilation
Risk Control
Risk for Injury
Neurologic Status
Risk Control
Safety Behavior: Fall Prevention
Safety Behavior: Home Physical Environment
Safety Status: Physical Injury
Symptom Control

Having surgery is a major event in any person's life. Clients faced with surgery want to know that someone is there with them and will look out for them during a time when they may have no control or any self-protective abilities. The perioperative nurse is the member of the surgical team clients are most likely to look to for advocacy.

Perioperative Nursing

The total surgical episode is called the *perioperative period.* This period in the health care continuum includes the time prior to surgery, or preoperative period; the time spent during the actual surgical procedure, or intraoperative period; and the period after the surgery is completed, or postoperative period. In the broadest definition of perioperative nursing practice, care can range from home, through surgery and recovery, and back to home again. A *perioperative nurse* is a Registered Nurse who uses the nursing process to design, plan, and deliver care to meet the identified needs of a client whose protective reflexes or self-care abilities are potentially compromised because of the operative procedures to be performed. Surgery is performed in a multitude of settings, and the nurse's role as a surgical team member is partially defined by the practice setting. Thus, perioperative nursing is client-centered rather than task-oriented. The perioperative nurse must possess and apply knowledge of anatomy, physiology, psychology, and sociocultural and spiritual beliefs and practices, in addition to knowledge of all aspects of the surgical procedure to be performed. The perioperative nurse must be a good communicator, delegator, and supervisor to ensure that the needs of the patient are being met throughout the surgical experience.

Basic Concepts of Perioperative Nursing

Nursing care of the perioperative patient takes place before, during, and after a surgical procedure. In each of these periods, specific assessments and interventions are performed by nurses acting both as independent clinicians and as members of the health care team. The goals of perioperative nursing practice are to assist clients and their significant others through the surgical episode, to help promote positive outcomes, and to help clients achieve their optimal level of function and wellness after surgery. The management of clients' needs, both unique and predictable, may be through direct or indirect interventions. These interventions are planned to assist the client in meeting the projected outcomes in an efficient and appropriate manner. Perioperative nursing care is implemented by registered nurses who strive to assist the client by functioning in various roles.

PREOPERATIVE PERIOD

Each client responds differently to surgery. Therefore, for each client having surgery, a care plan based on the nursing process is developed. It is vital to identify potential risks and complications that may arise during the perioperative period. In addition, a care plan also identifies the need for supportive services at home or in the hospital after surgery.

■ PREOPERATIVE ASSESSMENT

Assessment is the first step in the nursing process and is designed to provide information that enables the nurse and the client to plan for optimal postoperative outcomes. A complete assessment must be done before surgery whenever possible. Generally, preoperative assessment can take place in many different places, including the physician's office before admission to a health care facility; at home during the days before the operation and on admission; the night before surgery if the client is in the hospital; and on admission on the day of surgery. In the case of emergency surgery, time may not permit complete preoperative assessment, care planning, and teaching. Nevertheless, preparation must be as thorough as possible.

Preoperative assessment includes the medical/health history, the psychosocial history, physical examination, cognitive assessment, and diagnostic testing. When surgery must be performed following a traumatic event (e.g., gunshot wound, stab wound, serious accident, or severe fall), a preoperative assessment must include details of the traumatic event described precisely as possible. If the client was injured in a fall or a motor vehicle accident, information on injury-related factors such as the position in which the injury occurred, or whether the accident appeared to cause the victim to lose consciousness, may help to assess surgical risk or to identify underlying conditions related to the injurious event. Trauma patients are usually admitted to the operating room from an emergency department. Emergency department staff provide a detailed report upon transfer.

MEDICAL/HEALTH HISTORY

Obtaining a health history allows clients to explain their understanding of impending surgery and to establish rapport with the nurse conducting the interview. Reassurance by the nurse through this process may reduce anxiety in the client and family members or significant others. In most instances, the past medical history (PMH) has been previously recorded and is found in the medical record. A complete PMH is critical, and the nurse reviews it to ensure that it is thorough, completing any missing pieces and validating information with the client. The purpose of reviewing the medical history is to determine operative risk.

The past-medical history should include, but is not limited to, the following.

PREVIOUS SURGERY AND EXPERIENCE WITH ANESTHESIA. Any untoward reactions to anesthesia (e.g., high fever, intraoperative death of family members, known malignant hyperthermia, prolonged nausea and vomiting) by the client or anyone in the family must be reported to anesthesia personnel. These problems do not preclude surgery but often require a change in the type of anesthetics used.

SERIOUS ILLNESS OR TRAUMA. This information should cover anything that might influence the surgery and recovery. An ABCDE mnemonic is often used to ascertain information:

- *A*—allergy to medications, chemicals, and other environmental products such as latex. All allergies are reported to anesthesia and surgical personnel before the beginning of surgery. If allergies exist, an allergy band must be placed on the client's arm immediately.
- *B*—bleeding tendencies or the use of medications that deter clotting, such as aspirin or products containing aspirin, heparin, or warfarin sodium. Herbal medications may also increase bleeding times or mask potential blood-related problems.
- *C*—cortisone or steroid use.
- *D*—diabetes mellitus, a condition that not only requires strict control of blood glucose levels but is also known to delay wound healing.
- *E*—emboli; previous embolic events (such as lower leg blood clots) may recur because of prolonged immobility.

Clients whose immune system is suppressed are at a much higher risk for development of a postoperative infection and have a diminished capacity to fight that infection.

ALCOHOL, RECREATIONAL DRUG OR NICOTINE USE. The use of drugs signals potential problem with the administration of anesthesia or analgesia and risk for withdrawal complications. Clients who use alcohol or drugs may experience withdrawal manifestations while the drugs are withdrawn during the postoperative course. In addition, clients addicted to alcohol often have malnutrition or unpredictable reactions to anesthetic agents. As little as two drinks per day can lead to withdrawal manifestations that may require dosage alterations in anesthesia and analgesia.

The abuse of tobacco or inhaled drugs reduces hemoglobin levels, so that less oxygen is available for tissue repair. Smokers may be more susceptible to thrombus (clot) formation because of the hypercoagulability secondary to nicotine use. Smokers are also much more likely to have damage to lung tissue. Clients are instructed to abstain from any nicotine product for at least 1 week prior to surgery. Nicotine is a potent vasoconstrictor, and the flow of blood to surgical sites is an important aspect of healing. The use of nicotine patches and nicotine gum is also inappropriate preoperatively because the body continues to receive nicotine into the bloodstream.

CURRENT DISCOMFORTS. Clients with pre-existing painful conditions may require alternate methods of pain relief while they are receiving nothing by mouth (NPO). Clients who drink a considerable amount of caffeinated beverages such as coffee often develop headaches related to their NPO status, when their caffeine intake ceases abruptly. Without appropriate preoperative assessment, the headache may be misinterpreted as a surgical problem.

CHRONIC ILLNESSES. Arthritis of the neck or back is considered in positioning the client during surgery or in extending the neck during intubation.

ADVANCED AGE. Older clients have specific perioperative needs that should be identified preoperatively and considered in developing and maintaining a plan of care.

MEDICATION HISTORY. Many clients take prescription and over-the-counter (OTC) drugs that may increase operative risks (Table 15–1). Ask if the client is taking any medications and if these have been brought to the hospital. Dosage and administration schedules for all medications should be noted on the chart.

PSYCHOLOGICAL HISTORY

Knowledge of cultural beliefs and practices is a very important component of holistic nursing care. Some cultures practice traditional health care as well as alternative

TABLE 15–1 MEDICATIONS WITH POSSIBLE EFFECTS ON THE SURGICAL CLIENT

Medication	Possible Effects
Antibiotics	
Gentamicin Penicillins	Produces mild respiratory depression; may mask infection and affect metabolism of muscle relaxants
Antiarrhythmic Agents	
Propranolol HCl	Affects tolerance of anesthesia; interacts with epinephrine used in local anesthesia
Quinidine gluconate	Depresses cardiac function
Procainamide HCl	Potentiates anesthetic agents that are neuromuscular blockers
Antihypertensive Agents	
Methyldopa	May alter response to muscle relaxants and narcotics
Captopril	May cause intraoperative or postoperative hypotensive crisis
Corticosteroids	
Dexamethasone Hydrocortisone sodium succinate Prednisone	Delays wound healing Masks infection Increases risk of hemorrhage Increases serum glucose Decreases stress response (replacement needed during surgery)
Anticoagulants	
Heparin sodium Warfarin sodium Aspirin NSAIDs	Increases risk of hemorrhage intraoperatively and postoperatively because of clotting abnormalities
Glaucoma Medications	
Pilocarpine hydrochloride	May cause respiratory or cardiovascular collapse during surgery
Antidiabetic Agents	
Chlorpropamide, glipizide, glyburide, insulin	Insulin needs decrease when client receives nothing by mouth; insulin levels may fluctuate because of physiologic stress Dosage alterations required, with close monitoring of blood glucose
Tricyclic Antidepressants	
Amitriptyline, amoxapine, doxepin	Lowers blood pressure, thus increasing the risk of shock Potentiates the effects of narcotics and barbiturates
Thiazide Diuretics	
Hydrochlorothiazide, Furosemide	Increased risk for dysrhythmias Can deplete potassium and cause electrolyte imbalances
Beta-adrenergic Blockers	
Atenolol, propranolol	Antidysrhythmics and antihypertensives, which can cause adverse effects when combined with anesthetic agents
Street Drugs	
Beer, whiskey, cocaine, heroin	Alcohol and narcotic abuse increase tolerance to narcotics, requiring more anesthesia and analgesia, potential for delirium tremens during surgery or immediately postoperatively; may precipitate a medical crisis

NSAIDs, nonsteroidal anti-inflammatory drugs.

and complementary practices that may include use of candles, rituals, and herbs. Certain rituals are very important to the client and should be respected by all members of the health care team. For example, in some cultures, the family may make decisions regarding health care as a unit. In other cultures, the oldest woman makes all medical decisions. The nurse must be accepting of each individual's beliefs and should play an active advocate role by supporting the client in any manner possible.

ABILITY TO TOLERATE PERIOPERATIVE STRESS

Physiologic stressors in the perioperative client include pain, tissue damage, blood loss, anesthesia, fever, and immobilization. The stressful stimuli imposed by surgery promote the physiologic stress response by combining both psychological factors (such as anxiety and fear of the unknown) and physiologic factors (including blood loss, anesthesia, pain, and immobility). The sympathetic nervous system is activated by any stressor. A person's age, physical condition, and duration of the stress determine the success of the stress response in maintaining homeostatic balance. The ability to tolerate the stress of surgery and anesthesia is decreased significantly in older and debilitated people. All body systems are affected by the stress response; therefore, this assessment is crucial throughout the perioperative experience. The nurse must be able to assess stress and to plan and implement appropriate interventions to effectively reduce or treat complications related to stress.

LIFESTYLE HABITS

Sedentary lifestyles can complicate the surgical course via poor muscle tone, limited cardiac and respiratory reserves, and decreased stress response. On the other hand, an overly active lifestyle may present postoperative compliance problems.

SOCIAL HISTORY

An important component of a social history on a preoperative patient is the support system. Identification of client occupation and physical and mental requirements for job performance also provides important information that may prove useful for care planning.

■ PHYSICAL EXAMINATION

A physical examination is performed on all clients undergoing surgery to identify the present health status and to have baseline information for comparisons during and after surgery. These data are used to determine nursing diagnoses or to identify problems and to develop pertinent outcome goals. Perform a complete physical examination whenever possible. When perioperative time is brief, such as is the case in many trauma cases, you may be required to complete the assessment in minutes. This assessment is of the utmost importance and must be accurate. Report any abnormal findings to the surgical team members immediately, as this information may affect the initiation of the surgery.

Review preoperative laboratory and diagnostic study results, and post them on the client's chart (Table 15–2). Missing laboratory data constitute a common problem in ambulatory surgery settings, especially if the client's tests were ordered days before the scheduled procedure. Missing laboratory reports could lead to cancellation of the surgery.

Examine the part of the body that will be operated on first. Next, complete a general systems assessment. Systems to be assessed include cardiovascular, pulmonary, renal, musculoskeletal, skin, and neurologic. Ask the client whether there are any particularly troublesome manifestations, and include this information in the written assessment for further investigation. Again, document all unusual findings, and communicate them to the surgical team.

The best way to organize a brief assessment in the immediate preoperative period is to develop a personal system for conducting the examination and use it consistently. Although each person will devise a particular method for gathering data, a head-to-toe examination is a common method (see Box 15–1). Assess cognition throughout the examination by noting the client's demeanor and responses to directed questioning. For example, you can assess orientation to time, place, and person in "casual" conversation with the client during the physical assessment. If possible, watch the client walk and move when he or she enters the preparation area. Include this information in the ambulatory status section of the examination.

SPECIFIC BODY SYSTEM ASSESSMENTS

Cardiovascular Assessment

Pathologic cardiac conditions or events that increase operative risk include angina pectoris, the occurrence of a myocardial infarction within the last 6 months, uncontrolled hypertension, heart failure, and peripheral vascular disease. All cardiac conditions can lead to decreased tissue perfusion with impairment of surgical wound healing. In addition to the portion of the cardiovascular assessment completed as part of the head-to-toe assessment, note specific findings that warrant further work-up. Document shortness of breath on minor exertion, hypertension, heart murmurs or S_3 gallops, and chest pain. These manifestations may be present if the client is scheduled for heart or vascular surgery, but they may make the ability to tolerate anesthesia and blood loss questionable. Laboratory studies to measure the function of the cardiovascular system include an electrocardiogram (ECG), especially for those clients over 40 years of age, and determinations of hemoglobin, hematocrit, and serum electrolytes.

Respiratory Assessment

Chronic lung conditions, such as emphysema, asthma, and bronchitis, increase operative risk because these disorders impair gas exchange in the alveoli, predisposing the client to postoperative pulmonary complications. Assessment of pulmonary conditions includes examining for the presence of shortness of breath, wheezing, clubbed fingers, chest pain, cyanosis, and coughing with expectoration of copious or purulent mucus. Question the client carefully about smoking habits. Obtain a complete history of respiratory allergies and infections. If a client demonstrates any respiratory distress at the time of the assessment, notify the surgeon before administration of anesthesia. Abnormal breath sounds may indicate the need for respiratory therapy both before and after surgery. Clients with severe respiratory disease are usually managed preoperatively with aerosol therapy, postural drainage, and antibiotics. Clients who smoke are strongly encouraged to stop smoking as early as possible before surgery. Nicotine patches

TABLE 15-2 COMMON PREOPERATIVE LABORATORY TESTS

Test	Normal Range in Serum	Conditions Often Leading to Abnormal Findings: *Elevated in*	*Decreased in*
Potassium (K^+)	3.5–5.0 mEq/L or mmol/L	Dehydration Renal failure Acidosis Traumatic crush injury Burns Massive hemolysis of test specimen Addison's disease	NPO status when K^+ not replaced through IV fluids Excessive use of non–K^+-sparing diuretics Vomiting Malnutrition Diarrhea Alkalosis Aldosteronism
Sodium (Na^+)	136–146 mEq/L or mmol/L	Dehydration Edema Cardiac failure Renal failure Excessive infusion of sodium-containing fluids Inadequate thirst Diabetic acidosis	GI fluid loss through NG tube drainage, vomiting, diarrhea Excessive use of laxatives or diuretics Excessive infusion of fluids without sodium SIADH
Chloride (Cl^-)	98–107 mEq/L or 98–107 mmol/L	Dehydration Excessive infusion of NaCl-containing fluids Mineralocorticoid deficiency Renal failure Respiratory alkalosis	Diabetic acidosis Excessive GI losses through NG drainage, vomiting, diarrhea Excessive use of diuretics
Calcium (Ca^{2+})	8.6–10 mEq/L or 2.15–2.5 mmol/L	Excessive intake of calcium Excessive intake of vitamin D Renal failure Hyperparathyroidism Bone cancer Immobility Steroid use Adrenal insufficiency	Lack of oral intake Lactose intolerance Inadequate intake of vitamin D End-stage renal disease Low serum protein Alkalosis Acute pancreatitis Damage to parathyroid glands
Glucose (fasting)	60–100 mg/dl or mmol/L	Diabetes mellitus Gluconeogenesis with stress response Steroid use Excessive administration of glucose-containing fluids	Diabetes mellitus Excess insulin
Carbon dioxide	23–31 mEq/L or mmol/L*	Chronic airflow diseases (COPD) Intestinal obstruction Vomiting or NG suction Metabolic alkalosis	Hyperventilation Diabetic ketoacidosis Diarrhea Lactic acidosis Renal failure Salicylate toxicity
Creatinine	0.6–1.2 mg/dl or 53–106 μmol/L†	Acute or chronic renal failure End-stage renal disease Renal disease with destruction of large numbers of nephrons Renal insufficiency Shock Rhabdomyolysis	Atrophy of muscle tissue Hyperthyroidism Muscular dystrophy Paralysis
Blood urea nitrogen (BUN)	8–23 mg/dl or mmol/L*	Dehydration Renal failure Renal insufficiency Excessive dietary protein Liver failure	Overhydration Malnutrition
Albumin	3.5–5.0 g/dl	Dehydration Infection and fever	Acute burns Large open wounds Chronic liver disease Protein-calorie malnutrition

Table continued on following page

TABLE 15–2 COMMON PREOPERATIVE LABORATORY TESTS *Continued*

Test	Normal Range in Serum	Conditions Often Leading to Abnormal Findings: *Elevated in*	Conditions Often Leading to Abnormal Findings: *Decreased in*
Prealbumin	18–40 mg/dl	Protein-calorie malnutrition	Dehydration
Hemoglobin	Females: 11.7–16 g/dl Males*: 13.1–17.2 g/dl	Dehydration Polycythemia Chronic pulmonary diseases Heart failure High altitude	Overhydration
Hematocrit	35%–47%†	Dehydration Polycythemia Chronic pulmonary diseases Heart failure	Blood loss Anemia Renal failure with loss of erythropoietin
White blood cell count	4500–11,000 cells/μl	Acute infection Acute inflammation Stress Lymphoma Leukemia	Bone marrow dyscrasias Use of immunosuppressant medications Systemic lupus erythematosus
Differential count	Segmented neutrophils 56%	Bacterial infection, especially streptococcal or staphylococcal Inflammation with tissue necrosis Malignancy of bone marrow, especially chronic myeloid leukemia	Depletion of available pool of neutrophils during severe infection Bone marrow damage
	Banded neutrophils 3%	Overwhelming infection Early indicator of sepsis	
	Eosinophils 2.7%	Allergy Inflammation of skin Parasitic infection	Bacterial infections
	Basophils 0.3%	Healing phase of wounds Chronic inflammation	Acute infection Hyperthyroidism Stress
	Lymphocytes 34%	Bacterial, viral, or other causes of infection Lymphocytic leukemia	Lymphatic drainage Advanced cancers Bone marrow disease Immune deficiency that decreases T lymphocytes
	Monocytes 4%	Infection (monocytes become macrophages) Granulomatous diseases Collagen disease	Bone marrow failure
Prothrombin time (PT)	11–15 sec	Coagulation defect Liver disease Anticoagulant use	Coagulation (clotting) disorder Extensive cancer
Partial thromboplastin time, activated (aPTT)	35 sec	Coagulation defect Liver disease Anticoagulant use	Coagulation (clotting) disorder Extensive cancer

* Normal values vary slightly by age.
† Normal values vary slightly by age and gender.
COPD, chronic obstructive pulmonary disease; GI, gastrointestinal; IV, intravenous; NaCl, sodium chloride; NG, nasogastric; NPO, nothing by mouth; SIADH, syndrome of inappropriate antidiuretic hormone.

are usually not an appropriate alternative because of vasoconstriction caused by the nicotine.

Laboratory studies performed before surgery to diagnose respiratory conditions include chest radiography and pulse oximetry. Chest radiography (or x-rays) detect abnormalities, if present, in the lungs, such as infections, collapsed alveoli or segments of the lung, tumors, fractures of the ribs, and size of the heart.

The pulse oximeter is used to determine gross levels of tissue oxygenation. Explain the operation and purpose

BOX 15-1 Preoperative Head-to-Toe Assessment

- Assess cognition throughout the examination by noting the client's demeanor and responses to directed questioning. For example, you can check the client's orientation to time, place, and person in the course of eliciting information during the physical assessment.
- Assess muscle strength and coordination, gait, and balance by watching the client walk and move while entering the preparation area. (This may not be possible with all clients.)
- Take a full set of vital sign measurements. Note the ease of respiration.
- Look at the client's eyes and nose, and assess the mobility of the neck.
- Listen to the heart and the lungs. Listen to the rate and rhythm of the heart. Note the character of the lung sounds, listening for any diminution of intensity or the absence of breath sounds. Shortness of breath on minor exertion should also be noted. Dyspnea, wheezing, clubbed fingers, chest pain, cyanosis, and coughing with expectoration of copious or purulent mucus should be reported to anesthesia personnel. Question the client carefully about smoking habits and recent illness with a cold or influenza. Obtain a history of respiratory allergies and infections.
- Assess range of motion of the shoulders and the strength of the arms and hand grip.
- Ask about the ability to urinate and if the client has diabetes.
- Assess the ability to flex the spine (this is important if the client is scheduled to have spinal anesthesia).
- Examine the extremities for edema, coldness to the touch, and cyanosis.
- Assess the range of motion and strength of the legs and feet.
- Assess cognition preoperatively to determine whether any postoperative changes are the effects of surgery. This is particularly important in the older adult. The effects of the operation and of associated medications frequently cause temporary cognitive deficits that can be erroneously identified as a permanent condition by the health care team. Temporary deficits in memory and recall are normal and seen in most clients, but these manifestations can persist in the older adult. Note equal movement of the face and shoulders on both sides of the body if a crude estimate of cranial nerve function is needed. Complete neurologic testing includes assessment of cranial nerve function, reflex response of the upper and lower extremities, and sensory reflexes, as well as cognitive assessment. This level of testing is performed before neurologic surgery.
- During the examination, observe the condition of the skin. Note and document lesions, pressure ulcers, necrotic tissue, skin turgor, erythema or other discoloration of the skin, and the presence of external devices. Record the approximate size, color, and location of any lesions for later comparison.
- Review the chart for results of laboratory and diagnostic tests. Commonly ordered for the client undergoing heart surgery include chest x-ray film, electrocardiogram, hemoglobin, hematocrit, serum electrolytes, and urinalysis.
- During the physical examination, pay attention to the client's verbal and nonverbal communication. Does the client complain of any pain unrelated to the impending surgical procedure?

of the oximeter to the client and why it is important to monitor oxygenation throughout the surgical experience. The definitive laboratory test for blood oxygenation is arterial blood gas (ABG) analysis. Although routine ABG analyses are not ordered preoperatively, a physician may order the test if the client has been determined to be at high risk for surgical complications. Additional pulmonary function tests may be ordered in specific situations (see Chapter 59).

Musculoskeletal Assessment

A history of fractures, contractures, joint injury, or musculoskeletal impairment is an important factor in surgical positioning and postoperative support. The physical examination should reveal any problems with joint mobility or deformities that may interfere with operative positioning as well as with the postoperative course. For example, if the preoperative assessment identifies arthritis of the neck and shoulder, the circulating nurse can incorporate this information into the care plan. Hyperextension of the arthritic neck during general anesthesia can cause postoperative pain and discomfort unrelated to the surgery. The musculoskeletal system can be assessed through passive and active range of motion and a history provided by the client or family member, or the medical record. Documentation of impairment before the surgical procedure assists in the investigation of any impairment postoperatively.

Gastrointestinal Assessment

Gastrointestinal conditions associated with poor surgical outcomes include severe malnutrition and prolonged nausea and vomiting. The client's gastrointestinal system should be assessed if the planned operation is in the abdominal area or if the general physical examination reveals any abnormal data. Because narcotic analgesics increase constipation, obtain information about normal bowel patterns, so that postoperative expectations for return of function are appropriate. A client with a long history of constipation may have more difficulty postoperatively than that experienced by the client with regular bowel function.

Skin Integrity Assessment

Skin integrity must be assessed and documented preoperatively to establish a baseline for comparison postoperatively. Document and report lesions, pressure ulcers, necrotic skin tissue, skin turgor, erythema or discoloration of the skin, and the presence of external devices. Note the size, color, and location of the skin impairment to determine whether the impaired skin remains stable or worsens during and after the surgical procedure. Padding and positioning equipment should be used to maintain skin integrity and to prevent pressure ulcers. Any alterations in skin integrity that can occur intraoperatively and are not related to the actual surgical procedure are preventable by the nurse and other members of the surgical team with adequate padding and repositioning as needed during very long procedures.

Renal Assessment

Adequate renal function is necessary to eliminate protein wastes, to preserve fluid and electrolyte balance, and to remove anesthetic agents. Important renal and related disorders include advanced renal insufficiency, acute nephritis, and benign prostatic hypertrophy (BPH). If renal deficiency exists, the surgical team must be made aware of the problem. To assess renal status, ask about voiding patterns such as frequency and dysuria. Also, observe the appearance of urine if a sample is collected or an indwelling catheter is in place. Document and report abnormal urine characteristics. Monitor fluid balance by recording intake and output throughout the surgical continuum.

The most common preoperative tests to assess renal function are determination of blood urea nitrogen (BUN) and serum creatinine and urinalysis. BUN and serum creatinine levels indicate the ability of the kidney to excrete urea and protein wastes. Elevated levels may reflect dehydration, impaired cardiac output, or renal failure. Elevated creatinine is associated with renal disease. Serious renal disease and urinary infections must be treated, if possible, before surgery. Urinalysis results may indicate urinary infection, diabetes, malnutrition, renal disease, or dehydration.

Liver Function Assessment

Liver disease such as cirrhosis increases a client's surgical risk because an impaired liver cannot detoxify medications and anesthetic agents. The client may also be unable to metabolize carbohydrates, fats, and amino acids. Liver disease may be manifested by decreased albumin levels, leading to decreased immunoglobulin and fibrinogen levels. Low albumin levels predispose the client to fluid shifts, surgical wound infection, and ineffective coagulation. Clients with a history of alcoholism or other substance abuse require a careful assessment of liver function before surgery. If evidence of risk factors for liver disease is uncovered during the immediate preoperative assessment, information must be shared immediately with other members of the surgical team. Because a client with liver disease is often malnourished and debilitated and may have clotting disorders, the surgeon generally orders a high-calorie diet, or hyperalimentation during the preoperative and postoperative periods.

Cognitive and Neurologic Assessment

Serious neurologic conditions, such as uncontrolled epilepsy or severe Parkinson's disease, increase surgical risk. Important preoperative neurologic abnormalities include severe headache, frequent dizziness, light-headedness, ringing in the ears, unsteady gait, unequal pupils, and a history of seizures. Assessment of the client's orientation to time, place, and person can be accomplished by simple questioning. To determine baseline neurologic function, include testing of cranial nerves, reflex responses of the upper and lower extremities, sensory reflexes, and cerebral responses (see Chapter 67).

Assess cognition preoperatively to determine postoperative effects of surgery. This is particularly important in an older adult. The effects of the operation and of associated medications frequently lead to temporary cognitive deficiencies that can be erroneously identified as a permanent condition. Temporary deficits in memory and recall are considered normal and are seen in the majority of clients, but the older adult can experience these symptoms for a longer time.

Endocrine Assessment

Diabetes mellitus is the most common pre-existing endocrine pathophysiologic disorder. In some ethnic groups, especially Hispanic populations, diabetes is rampant. Diabetes mellitus predisposes the affected client to poor wound healing and increased risk of surgical wound infection. Corresponding cardiovascular, peripheral vascular, neurologic, visual, and renal complications may be present as well. These factors can greatly increase the surgical risk for a client with diabetes. A client who has well-controlled diabetes (i.e., blood glucose levels are consistently monitored and kept within a normal range) is less susceptible to infection. Chapter 45 describes the care of clients with diabetes mellitus.

Thyroid functioning may also need to be assessed preoperatively. Thyroid hormone replacement is usually continued throughout the perioperative period. Stopping thyroid medications may precipitate a thyroid storm or crisis, with manifestations of hypertension, tachycardia, and hyperthermia. This event can be devastating if it occurs during surgery or immediately postoperatively. In addition, the presence of hypothyroidism increases the risk of hypotension and cardiac arrest during anesthetic administration.

ADDITIONAL ASSESSMENTS

Other factors that may be considered during the planning of surgical intervention include (1) age, (2) nutrition, (3) fluid and electrolyte balance, (4) infection, and (5) hematologic conditions.

Age

Normal physiologic changes that occur with aging, along with the increased presence of disease, may adversely affect surgical outcomes. Chronic conditions commonly found in the older client that may increase surgical risk include malnutrition, anemia, dehydration, atherosclerosis, chronic obstructive pulmonary disease (COPD), diabetes mellitus, cerebrovascular changes, and peripheral vascular disease. Table 15–3 outlines major physiologic changes that occur in older adults and appropriate perioperative nursing interventions.

Pain

Pain is an important physiologic indicator that must be carefully monitored (see Chapter 23). During the preoperative nursing assessment, ask if the client is experiencing any pain. If pain is present, obtain a full assessment of the pain. Determine whether the pain is chronic and unrelated to the pathologic condition necessitating surgery or is acute and attributable to the surgical procedure. Be aware that although most operations increase pain, older adults who have undergone joint replacement surgery often state that the postoperative pain is minor compared with the chronic pain of a disintegrating joint.

Nutritional Status

Nutritional status (positive nitrogen balance) is directly related to intraoperative success and postoperative recovery. The client who is well nourished preoperatively is better prepared to handle surgical stress and to return to optimal health after surgery. Improving nutrition is usually attended to in a clinic or physician's office weeks before surgery. However, if the operation is performed on an emergency basis or has not been planned, nutritional

TABLE 15-3 INTERVENTIONS FOR PHYSIOLOGIC CHANGES IN OLDER ADULTS UNDERGOING SURGERY

Physiologic Change	Nursing Interventions
Cardiovascular	
Decreased cardiac output Moderate increase in blood pressure Decreased peripheral circulation Dysrhythmias	Know what anesthetic agents are being used. Monitor vital signs carefully. Encourage early ambulation and leg exercises. Assess for hypotension or hypertension or hypothermia. Note changes in baseline ECG; note any changes.
Respiratory	
Decreased vital capacity Reduced oxygenation of blood	Assess for pulmonary aspiration. Monitor respirations carefully. Use vigorous pulmonary hygiene. Postoperatively, auscultate lung sounds. Monitor oxygen saturation using pulse oximeter.
Renal	
Decreased renal blood flow and glomerular filtration rate Decreased ability to excrete waste products	Monitor urine output q 1–2 hr during immediate postoperative period. Evaluate intake and output. Monitor fluid and electrolyte status.
Musculoskeletal	
Decrease in lean body mass Increase in spinal compression Increased incidence of osteoporosis and arthritis	Assess level of mobility. Position the client on operating table with padding to reduce trauma to bones and joints. Assist with early ambulation or exercises in accordance with client's ability. Provide adequate nutrition. Provide effective pain management.
Sensorimotor	
Decreased reaction time Decreased visual acuity Decreased auditory acuity Slowed thermoregulation	Orient client to environment. Plan individual teaching, allowing time to reinforce client learning. Maintain core body temperature.

status may be a risk factor through the perioperative period. In addition, some operations are completed to improve nutrition. For example, a client who is to undergo placement of a permanent feeding tube would be expected to have evidence of malnutrition. Likewise, a client who is to have an intestinal bypass for obesity is also malnourished (in terms of excess intake).

Assessment of nutritional status preoperatively includes obtaining a diet history, observing the general appearance of the client, laboratory diagnostic testing, and comparing current weight with ideal body weight. Laboratory tests that can assist in the assessment of nutritional status include determinations of serum albumin, hemoglobin and hemotocrit, BUN, and creatinine clearance.

Nutritional abnormalities include deficiencies and excesses. Nutritional deficiencies primarily affect clients with chronic illnesses, cancer, gastrointestinal disorders, and advanced age. Malnutrition is directly linked to delayed healing and infection.

Obesity is also associated with poorer surgical outcomes. Adipose (fatty) tissue increases the technical difficulty of surgery. Fatty tissue is less vascular and more prone to postoperative infection, incisional hernias, and wound dehiscence or evisceration. The surgeon may use an alternative closure method for a client with excess adipose tissue at or around the incision.

Obese clients frequently suffer from hypertension, heart failure, and metabolic problems. An obese client is more susceptible to postoperative pulmonary complications. Obesity decreases the efficiency of coughing and deep breathing. The pressure of the abdominal contents on the diaphragm and lungs decreases expansion, which may lead to hypoventilation. An obese client is more prone to postoperative immobility. Immobility increases the risk of venous stasis and deep vein thrombosis or pulmonary embolism. Good preoperative teaching that describes turning, coughing, deep-breathing, and moving after surgery is essential. Most complications related to obesity can be prevented, or the risk of their occurrence reduced, with appropriate interventions.

Fluid and Electrolyte Balance

Fluid volume deficits (dehydration/hypovolemia or fluid volume excess/hypervolemia) predispose a client to complications during and after surgery. Actual or potential fluid imbalance can be assessed by evaluation of skin turgor. A coated tongue can also be a manifestation of fluid volume deficit. A decrease in urine output or an increase in specific gravity is also diagnostic of decreased fluid volume. If dehydration is severe, irritability or confusion can be apparent. Dehydration results from limited fluid intake, prolonged vomiting, diarrhea, or bleeding. Fluids can be administered by the IV route if dehydration is identified.

Electrolyte imbalances also increase operative risk. Preoperative laboratory results should be checked to see whether serum sodium, potassium, calcium, and magnesium concentrations are within the normal range. In-depth assessment and management of fluid and electrolyte imbalances are discussed in Chapters 12 and 13, respectively.

Infection and Immunity

Any pre-existing infection can adversely affect surgical outcomes because bacteria may be released into the bloodstream during surgery. Their release may lead to infection elsewhere in the body. When the surgical site is near a lymph node or lymphatic vessel that is draining infectious material, the likelihood of surgical infection increases. During the preoperative assessment, documentation of any possible exposure to communicable diseases, presence of skin lesions, or manifestations of an infection (such as coughing, sore throat, or elevated body temperature) is vital. An elevated white blood cell (WBC) count also suggests an infection and should be communicated immediately to the surgical team. Because infection greatly increases surgical risk, it may be necessary to reschedule elective surgery.

A low WBC count is also a danger sign and may indicate that the client is at risk for infection. A low WBC count may be a manifestation of immunosuppression. People with diabetes mellitus, those who are undergoing radiation therapy or chemotherapy, and those with chronic medical conditions are at high risk of immunosuppression. Steroid use also decreases the client's ability to fight infection; therefore, the client taking steroids should be assessed and monitored for immunosuppression.

Hematologic Function

Clients with blood coagulation disorders are at risk for hemorrhage and hypovolemic shock during and after surgery. Five factors that should be assessed preoperatively to identify potential hematologic problems are:

- A history of bleeding or a diagnosis of a pathologic condition such as hemophilia or sickle cell anemia
- Manifestations such as easy bruising, excessive bleeding following dental extractions and razor nicks, and severe nosebleeds
- Hepatic or renal disease
- Use of anticoagulants, aspirin, or other nonsteroidal anti-inflammatory drugs (NSAIDs)
- Abnormal bleeding time, prothrombin time, or platelet count.

Remember that many clients take aspirin and other OTC medications that may increase the risk of bleeding. The client may not consider nonprescription medications important and often may not include them in a medication history. Ask specific questions regarding all prescription and nonprescription medications. Specifically ask about the use of herbal preparations. Ginkgo biloba, garlic, ginger, and ginseng may prevent blood clot formation and may lead to excess blood loss in surgery. Two other popular herbs—St. John's wort, an antidepressant, and kava-kava, a relaxant—may prolong the sedative effect of anesthesia. Advise clients to stop taking herbal products at least 2 weeks before elective surgery. Ask how often the client takes the OTC medications and when the last dose of any of those drugs was taken.

For a variety of reasons, blood transfusions are used less frequently than in past years. Many clients fear the transmission of human immunodeficiency virus (HIV) and hepatitis B. If possible, clients are encouraged to donate their own blood for use during or after surgery (autologous transfusion). Blood substitutes or fluid volume expanders can also be used in some cases to replace lost blood until the body can produce new blood cells. Blood transfusions are discussed in Chapter 75.

■ EDUCATIONAL ASSESSMENT

The client's experience with previous surgery and level of anxiety are noted. The client's education level, sensory impairments (e.g., loss of vision), expectations regarding the operation, and availability of support systems are used to guide plans for teaching. In general, clients who have undergone multiple operations need less educational preparation. However, do not assume that such clients need no reinforcement of preoperative and postoperative assessments and interventions.

The client undergoing elective surgery and planning to go home the same day requires some additional planning. See the Case Management feature.

PREOPERATIVE NURSING DIAGNOSES

Common nursing diagnoses during the preoperative period include *Knowledge Deficit related to unfamiliar surgical experience* and *Anxiety related to fear of pain, fear of death, fear of disfigurement,* or *fear of the unknown.* The outcomes for these problems must be achievable in a short preoperative time frame.

ESTIMATING MEDICAL RISK FOR SURGERY

Each surgeon determines the relative risk versus benefit from the operation for the specific client. In addition, the outcomes for many surgical procedures have been researched, and these figures can be presented to the client and family. The natural history of the condition requiring surgery (that is, the outcome if it goes untreated) is also presented. This information can then be considered by the client and family members before consenting to surgery. The surgeon presents a frank but optimistic discussion of risks of the procedure. Well-intentioned friends and family may wish to shield the client from unpleasant facts. Although medical facts may be unpleasant, it is imperative that the client have full and complete information before consenting. Some clients (such as those with malnutrition or anemia) benefit from waiting for surgery.

The type of surgery to be performed also has some inherent risk. The types of operations by category are presented in Table 15–4.

ANESTHESIA AND ANESTHETIC RISK

The anesthesia care provider visits the client before surgery to perform a complete respiratory, cardiovascular, and neurologic examination. The client's general surgical risk (the ability of the client to withstand the surgery) is expressed according to the American Society of Anesthesia (ASA) grading system (see Box 15–2). Generally, the topics discussed with the client during this examination include the type of anesthesia planned and the sensations the client may experience when undergoing anesthesia. Fears the client has concerning anesthesia are also addressed. The client's risk of side effects and complications is assessed at this time.

The pharmacologic preparation for anesthesia is based on many variables, including the client's age and physical and psychological condition, the type of surgery, and the type of anesthesia to be used. The preoperative and anesthetic medications are discussed later in the chapter.

IMMEDIATE PREOPERATIVE CARE

■ PHYSICAL CARE

PREPARE THE SKIN

Explain shower and bathing protocols for the night before a planned surgical procedure. Usually the operative area is cleaned the night before surgery with soap and water to reduce the number of microbes on the skin. Allergies to chemicals (e.g., iodine) necessitate use of other cleansing agents. If the skin assessment has identified fragile and delicate skin in an older client, nursing care must involve a gentle method for cleansing skin and hair and for any needed hair removal. Additional considerations may include use of padding over pressure points and tape that will not irritate or rip the skin, as well as lifting—rather than pulling or sliding—the client from bed to bed, to prevent traumatizing the skin.

CASE MANAGEMENT

The Elective Surgery Client

The elective surgical client presents some unique opportunities. Unlike a client arriving from the emergency department, the client undergoing elective surgery has already agreed to an operation and has had some preoperative assessment and preparation; this client will know what to expect in the perioperative period. This preparation serves as an excellent basis for case management. Case management practices become increasingly important as more procedures are being performed in ambulatory surgery settings or even in offices rather than inpatient areas. Almost all clients present the day of surgery, having undergone outpatient testing and preparation. The length of surgical stays is decreasing, especially as more laparoscopic procedures are developed. The emphasis on one-day surgery and on decreasing inpatient stays requires astute nursing assessment and intervention to prevent surgical complications and readmission.

Assess

Ideally, assessment should be initiated when the client is an outpatient. What do the client and family know about the surgical procedure, the consequences of surgery, and postoperative care needs? What other conditions might affect the client's ability to successfully undergo surgery? For instance, a client with chronic obstructive pulmonary disease having a cholecystectomy may have difficulty performing deep-breathing exercises; a client with diabetes may need to modify the insulin dose. Overlooking these situations can result in unwanted complications and increased length of stay.

How long does the client expect to be hospitalized? What plans are in place for postsurgical care? If short-term rehabilitation is planned, clients can tour facilities and can be helped to make arrangements for care even before the procedure. What is the purpose of surgery—curative, cosmetic, palliative?

Advocate

This is an ideal time to answer questions and to make sure that clients have a health care proxy and advance directives noted on their chart. If a different living situation is planned or required because of the surgery, discuss this situation with the client and family. Even if such planning is temporary, this can be viewed negatively. Be sensitive to the client's feelings about surgery as it relates to body image, especially if it may cause disfigurement or result in changes in normal body function. Many support groups are available for referral.

Prevent Readmission

Helping the client to return to optimal function in activities of daily living is an important outcome. Although simple nursing interventions such as getting the client out of bed, ambulating, and watching for return of bowel function are often dismissed as unimportant, these interventions can help clients return home safely in a shorter time. Consider hospital discharge when (1) the complete blood count and electrolyte levels are within normal range, (2) the client can be hydrated and fed, (3) voiding has occurred, and bowel function returns, and (4) mobility and ambulation are at baseline or improved levels. Especially in short-stay surgical procedures, and with older clients, watch for physical or mental effects of anesthesia. Make sure that clients and families (1) know how to perform wound care or other treatments, (2) recognize manifestations of infection or other complications, and (3) receive clear directions for follow-up.

Help clients to obtain pain medication. Referrals for nursing care, outpatient phlebotomy, physical therapy, or other home services can ensure continued improvement after surgery.

Cheryl Noetscher, RN, MS, *Director of Case Management, Crouse Hospital and Community–General Hospital, Syracuse, New York*

Prepare the Gastrointestinal Tract

The gastrointestinal tract needs special preparation on the evening before surgery to (1) reduce the possibility of vomiting and aspiration, (2) to reduce the risk of possible bowel obstruction, (3) to allow visualization of the intestine during bowel surgery, and (4) to prevent contamination from fecal material in the intestinal tract during bowel or abdominal surgery. Preparation involves restrict-

TABLE 15–4 CATEGORIES OF SURGICAL PROCEDURES

Category	Purpose	Example
Aesthetic	Improvement of physical features that are within the "normal" range	Breast augmentation
Constructive	Repair of a congenitally defective body part	Cleft palate and cleft lip repair
Curative	Removal or repair of damaged or diseased tissue or organs	Hysterectomy
Diagnostic	Discovery or confirmation of a diagnosis	Breast biopsy
Exploratory	Estimation of the extent of disease or confirmation of a diagnosis	Exploratory laparotomy
Emergent	Life-saving	Repair of traumatic punctured lung
Palliative	Relief of symptoms but without cure of underlying disease	Colostomy
Reconstructive	Partial or complete restoration of a body part	Total joint replacement
Urgent	Performed as soon as client is stable and infection is under control	Appendectomy

BOX 15–2 Classification of Physical Status

ASA I

Healthy person with no systemic disease, undergoing elective surgery, and at no extremes of age.

ASA II

Client with one-system, well-controlled disease. Disease does not affect daily activities. Other clients classified in this level include those with mild obesity, alcoholism, and smoking

ASA III

Client with multiple-system disease or well-controlled major system diseases. The disease status limits daily activities. However, there is no immediate danger or death due to any individual system disease.

ASA IV

Client with severe, incapacitating disease. Typically, the disease is poorly controlled, or end-stage disease is present. Danger of death related to organ failure is present.

ASA V

Client is very ill, in imminent danger of death. Operation is deemed to be a last resort attempt at preserving life. The client is not expected to live through the next 24 hours. In some cases, the client had been healthy up to a recent catastrophic event.

Data based on American Society of Anesthesiologists (ASA) classification.

ing food and fluid, administering enemas as needed, and inserting a gastric or intestinal tube when appropriate. Gastrointestinal tubes are usually inserted during surgery for drainage. This procedure is usually performed for clients undergoing major abdominal or intestinal tract surgery.

If a client undergoing surgery is to receive a general anesthetic, foods and fluids are restricted for 8 to 10 hours before the operation. This restriction significantly reduces the possibility of aspiration of gastric contents, which may lead to pneumonia. Because solid food must be withheld for 8 to 10 hours before surgery, clients who are to undergo anesthetic procedures must be instructed not to eat or drink anything after midnight. Therefore, clients are assigned NPO status after midnight the night before surgery is scheduled. If a client scheduled for surgery has eaten or had something to drink after midnight, the surgery may be delayed or postponed. Preoperative care for hospitalized clients also includes the restriction of food and water if anesthesia is to be used.

When a client is on NPO status, perform the following:

- Explain the reason for the fluid and food restriction.
- Remove food and water from the bedside at midnight.
- Place "NPO" signs on the door and on the bed.
- Mark the care plan or Kardex with "NPO."
- Inform the diet and nutrition department about the client's NPO status.
- Inform other caretakers and family members that the client is on NPO status.

If the client has been instructed to take important medications orally, small sips of water are permitted. For example, a client with cardiovascular disease may need to take heart medications such as digoxin on the morning of surgery. However, the client may have heard preoperative instructions not to eat or drink anything. Make sure that the medication is taken with a sip of water and inform the client that this exception is permissible. Record this medication and the amount of fluid taken on the client care record.

Enemas are not routinely ordered during the preoperative period except for surgical procedures involving the gastrointestinal tract, perianal or perineal areas, and the pelvic cavity. The client may perform the enema at home, or the nurse may complete it at the hospital. Some clients may require further bowel cleansing on the morning of surgery. Clients who are to be admitted for same-day surgery are instructed before the surgical date about the need for enemas and whether they will be self-administered. If bowel cleansing is done by the client, ensure that directions are completely understood.

■ NUTRITIONAL CARE

Nursing interventions for clients who are malnourished preoperatively include encouragement of high carbohydrate intake to increase energy, high protein intake to assist in wound healing, and supplementing the diet with vitamins to encourage healing. Vitamin C is beneficial in wound healing, whereas vitamin K will increase blood clotting times. Total parenteral nutrition (TPN) can be used preoperatively to bolster the client's nutritional status.

TPN solutions that contain lipids (fats) supply total nutritional replacement including vitamin and mineral supplements. Tube feeding (enteral nutrition) can be administered via a tube placed in the stomach or small intestine. The tube is placed through the nose or directly into the stomach through a skin incision. Both enteral and parenteral feeding can improve a client's nutritional status; either may be continued postoperatively until satisfactory swallowing or gastrointestinal functioning returns (see Chapter 29).

Treatment of obesity before surgery calls for a reducing diet, mild exercise if possible, and assessing for and controlling conditions such as hypertension and diabetes mellitus. Obese clients are not placed on a weight-reduction diet after surgery while they are healing. Wound healing is delayed when protein intake is inadequate.

■ PREOPERATIVE TEACHING

Preoperative teaching is very important to ensure a positive surgical experience for the client. Numerous research studies have supported the value of preoperative instructions in reducing both the incidence of postoperative complications and the length of stay in the hospital. The client's learning needs, level of anxiety, and fears about surgery are assessed individually so that an individualized teaching plan can be formulated.

The timing of preoperative teaching is highly individualized. Ideally, there would be enough time for the client to be given instructions and time to answer questions. If teaching is done too far in advance, the client may forget important components of the education. On the other hand, a client who is taught immediately before surgery may be too anxious to comprehend what is being taught. In many cases, the client is admitted on the day of surgery. It is imperative that the client has received written or oral instructions before this time, so that the nurse can simply reinforce these instructions and answer individual questions from the client and family members. Many ambulatory surgery or "same-day surgery" centers conduct telephone interviews before admission to educate and allow the client to ask questions.

Being aware of the effects of surgery on cognition, determine learning needs preoperatively and teach both client and family before surgery if at all possible. Only essential activities should be taught in the immediate preoperative period because of the client's total concentration on surviving the surgery. Assess the client's ability to see, hear, and understand verbal communication. Glasses and hearing aids can be worn up until the actual surgical procedure to promote learning of necessary information and to reduce apprehension and fear. As the client moves into surgery, these important items must be carefully stored or given to an accompanying adult. Add careful documentation of the location of items, such as hearing aids and glasses, to the client record to ensure retrieval after surgery. If any items are lost, the institution is responsible for replacing them.

The client should understand what the preoperative, intraoperative, and postoperative course entails. Consult with the physician before speaking to the client about specific or technical details so that you can clarify if needed. Explain all nursing care and any possible discomfort that may result as a consequence of nursing interventions. Tell the client what you will do to minimize any discomfort. If the client is scheduled to go to the surgical intensive care unit (SICU) after the operation, ask what the client and family members already know or have heard about intensive care. Take time to address any misconceptions or incorrect information.

PREOPERATIVE ANXIETY

All people are fearful of surgery. The extent to which a client fears surgery depends on many factors, such as (1) how serious the operation is, (2) individual coping abilities, (3) cultural expectations, and (4) experiences with previous surgery. Well-meaning family members and friends often contribute to the fear level unintentionally. Fear of the unknown is one of the most prevalent causes of preoperative anxiety. During the preoperative phase, clients also fear postoperative pain, the discovery of cancer, the loss of an organ or limb, anesthesia, vulnerability while unconscious, the threat of loss of job or financial security, loss of social and familial roles, disruption of lifestyle, separation from significant others, and death.

Clients respond differently to fear. Some respond by becoming silent and withdrawn, childish, belligerent, evasive, tearful, or clinging. Most clients feel helpless to some extent when admitted to a health care facility. Although surgery may be commonplace for the health care professional, it is a frightening experience for clients and their families. Report extreme anxiety and fear to the anesthesia personnel so that a sedative can be administered. A surgical procedure can be canceled if fear is overwhelming.

Allow the client to take the lead in asking questions concerning surgery and the postoperative period. Provide only as much additional information as the client wants to know. Emphasize that a nurse will be with the client throughout the total surgical experience. Stand close to the client when taking him or her into the operating room. If touch is culturally appropriate, use touch to reassure the client.

If the surgical procedure to be performed has potential long-term effects, support groups may be contacted to offer support preoperatively. Cancer organizations, amputation support groups, and enterostomal therapist associations are examples of large national organizations that offer peer support for surgical and nonsurgical patients.

■ COMPONENTS OF PREOPERATIVE TEACHING

Information provided to the client before surgery should be geared to individual needs. This information can be (1) sensory, (2) psychosocial, or (3) procedural.

Sensory information addresses the sights, sounds, and "feel" of the operating room. Instruct the client that the operating room and skin preparation fluids will be cold but that warm blankets are available. Many surgery suites are now incorporating music into their preoperative and intraoperative areas. Clients may be given headphones and can choose from a variety of music types to help them relax and to reduce external noxious sounds in the operating room environment. If the client wears a hearing aid and music is used, check with the anesthesia personnel to determine whether the hearing aid can remain in place during surgery.

Psychosocial information involves coping abilities and worries about family and similar concerns. Typical questions the client may have are the following: "What if I die?" "Who is going to care for the children?" "What if I become an invalid?" "Who is going to earn enough money to care for my family?" You can provide answers if this information is available, or you can arrange for others, such as a social worker or a member of the clergy, to talk to the client.

Procedural information details activities during the preoperative period and postoperative care. It includes information that the client needs to know and wants to know about what is going to happen. For example, you can state as appropriate: "Your family can be in the presurgical area before you are taken into the operating room," or "There will always be a nurse with you during this time, and I will remain by your side throughout the entire operation." Provide explanations and printed information about the health care facility routines, visiting hours, mealtimes, the location of the chapel and waiting room, and so on. If you find that the client is unclear about what the operation entails, the physician must be notified (see Informed Consent, p. 287). You can elaborate on or clarify information regarding surgery.

The client's role in postoperative care is taught before surgery. The nurse provides instructions on (1) deep breathing, (2) coughing, (3) turning, (4) ambulating, and (5) pain control, and the client's learning of some of these procedures is validated by return demonstration.

DEEP-BREATHING EXERCISES. To help prevent postoperative surgical complications, careful preoperative instructions and practice in deep-breathing and coughing exercises should be completed and reinforced.

Breathing and coughing exercises help to expand collapsed alveoli in the lungs and to prevent postoperative pneumonia and atelectasis. Demonstration of correct deep breathing can be done by inhaling slowly through the nose, distending the abdomen, and exhaling slowly through pursed lips. After demonstrating this method, ask the client to provide a return demonstration to ensure understanding (Fig. 15–1). The client is instructed to use this breathing method as often as possible, preferably 5 to 10 times every hour during the postoperative period of immobilization.

COUGHING EXERCISES. Coughing removes retained secretions from the bronchi and larger airways. Coughing may be painful, and analgesia may be required.

For coughing exercise, the client may remain in a sitting or supine position. Teach the client how to splint the surgical incision, to minimize pressure, and to control pain during coughing. Splinting is accomplished by lacing the fingers and holding them tightly across the incision before coughing. A small pillow or folded towel held over the incision also facilitates splinting. The client is instructed to take three deep breaths, exhaling through the mouth, before coughing from deep in the lungs. Encouragement to perform deep-breathing exercises before coughing is important because the deep breathing assists in stimulating the cough reflex and mobilizing retained secretions. Many clients simply clear their throats when coughing hurts. Encourage true coughing, and use aggressive measures to control pain, with reteaching of the procedure as intended.

Incentive spirometers are often used to promote expansion of the alveoli postoperatively by guiding the client to reach a predetermined level of lung inflation. Use of a spirometer promotes alveolar inflation and strengthens respiratory muscles that were weakened during anesthesia administration. Clients should have the opportunity to practice use of the incentive spirometer before surgery so that they can use it appropriately after surgery. Most

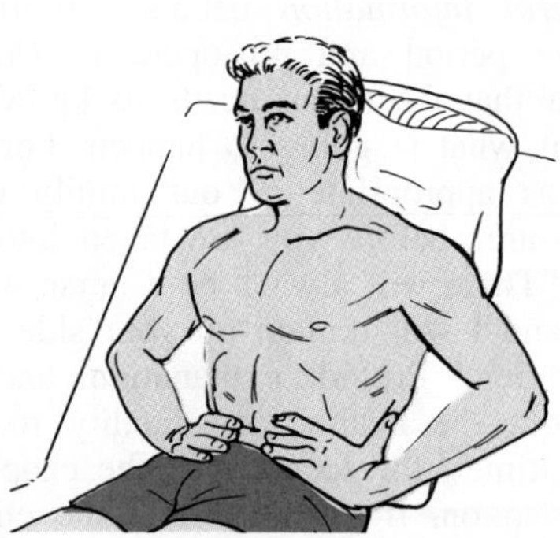

1. Have the client sit upright at the side of the bed or supported in bed in semi-Fowler's position (at right).
2. Instruct the client to place his or her hands on the abdomen to feel whether the chest rises to indicate that the lungs are expanding.
3. Have the client inhale through the nose until the abdomen distends.
4. Instruct the client to exhale through pursed lips while contracting the abdominal muscles.
5. Have the client repeat this exercise every hour during the first postoperative day.

FIGURE 15–1 Deep (diaphragmatic) breathing after surgery.

facilities teach clients to use the incentive spirometer about 10 times an hour after surgery.

TURNING EXERCISES. Preoperative clients also need to practice turning from side to side, using the bedside rails to assist movements. Turning helps to prevent venous stasis, thrombophlebitis, pressure ulcer formation, and respiratory complications. The client should be instructed to turn and reposition in bed every 1 to 2 hours during the postoperative period.

EXTREMITY EXERCISE. Postoperative extremity exercise helps to prevent circulatory problems, such as thrombophlebitis, by facilitating venous return to the heart. The client is taught to flex and extend each joint, particularly the hip, knee, and ankle joints, while lying supine; the lower back is kept flat as the leg is lowered and straightened. The feet can be moved in circular motions while the client is lying down or sitting. The client should be encouraged to practice these exercises before surgery to gain familiarity with the appropriate exercises to be used postoperatively.

Antiembolism stockings may be used on the lower extremities perioperatively. These stockings use a low compression gradient to encourage venous blood flow. Sequential pressure stockings use compression that is applied sequentially up and down the lower extremities to massage the legs rhythmically, for even more effective prevention of clot formation.

AMBULATION. Ambulation should be encouraged whenever appropriate, as it helps to prevent many postoperative complications. Clients are taught an appropriate ambulation schedule preoperatively so that they have an idea of when they are allowed to get out of bed after surgery. Teaching of proper methods of arising from bed to prevent pain and to minimize orthostatic hypotension is important. The client is instructed to sit up slowly and pause before attempting to stand. Teach the client to use the same splinting method for providing support to the incision that is used during coughing and deep-breathing exercises in order to decrease pain on arising and sitting.

PAIN CONTROL. Uncontrolled pain is a common concern among preoperative clients. It is important to reassure clients that their pain will and can be controlled after surgery. Undertreatment of postoperative pain is unacceptable (see Chapter 23). Fears of addiction are unfounded, and clients have suffered needlessly. Preoperatively, explain the type of pain relief that will be used postoperatively. For example, some surgeons inject the surgical site with a long-acting local anesthetic before closing the wound so that the client will not feel any pain in the site until the medication wears off. The ambulatory surgery client probably will be home when the local anesthetic wears off. Because the stress of surgery or side effects of anesthesia can affect memory temporarily, give instructions on taking the postoperative pain medication before surgery to both the client and accompanying family members.

If the client is to be hospitalized after surgery, explain the type of pain medication used. During the immediate postoperative period, clients can receive medications by an IV, intramuscular, or epidural route. Clients on a demand schedule (intramuscular) ask for pain medications when they are beginning to feel uncomfortable. Clients frequently believe that they should be stoic, and they may and hesitate to ask for relief. All clients need to be assured that they will not get addicted to pain medications in the short time for which the pain medication is required. In addition, anticipate pain when the client will be moving for the first time or when the analgesia has worn off. At such times, pain medication should be offered. If the client is to have a patient-controlled analgesia (PCA) pump after surgery, demonstrate how the machine operates, and emphasize that safety features on the equipment prevent overdosing. Without preoperative teaching about these procedures, postoperatively the client will be a groggy, sore client who may not understand how to treat the pain.

Pain can also be controlled through continuous infusion of analgesic agents through an epidural or IV route. Explain the method of planned pain control and how adjustments can be made for comfort.

EQUIPMENT. Whenever possible, explain about the equipment that will be used during the perioperative period. Depending on the type of surgery to be performed, various tubes, drains, and IV lines may be used. Discussion should focus on the purpose of specific pieces of equipment and how their use is related to the surgery.

Tubes. The most common type of tube used during the intraoperative period is an indwelling urinary catheter. Another tube commonly used is a nasogastric (NG) tube, which is used to decompress the stomach and upper bowel or to drain the stomach contents. These tubes are often inserted in the operating room.

Drains. Drains are inserted to promote evacuation of fluid from the dead space (tissue planes created during the operation) in the operative site. Many different types of drains are used. The Penrose drain works by wicking away fluid within the operative site, which then moves through the drain via gravity to an outside dressing or collection container. Drains are frequently attached to mild suction. Hemovac and Jackson-Pratt drains are commonly used suction devices.

Intravenous Infusion Devices. IV infusions are usually started before surgery. The purpose of the infusion is to administer medication, fluids, and nutrition solutions. The surgeon may request IV access for use in case of emergency even if the client is not expected to need IV medications.

■ PREOPERATIVE TEACHING FOR OLDER ADULTS

Older clients usually desire the same basic operative information as that provided for young patients. You must attend to this need in a sensitive and effective way. Preoperative teaching for older clients should include consideration of possible decreased sensory ability. Sit close to the client when teaching. Speak slowly and in a manner that results in a lower tone of voice. High-pitched sounds are frequently hard for an older people to discern. Glare from lights may bother the older client's eyes. Avoid bright lights while preparing the client preoperatively. Because the older client is more prone to hypothermia, apply blankets in the preoperative area and plan an appropriate method of warming for use in the operating room, where temperatures are usually cool.

■ INFORMED CONSENT

Anyone undergoing any invasive procedure must give informed consent for that procedure to be performed. A *consent form* is the legal document that signifies that the client has been told about and understands all aspects of a specific invasive procedure. This document guards the client against unwanted invasive procedures. It also protects the health care facility and health care professionals when a client denies understanding the procedure that was, or is planned to be, performed. Once the operative permit—indicating the client's *informed consent*—is signed, it becomes a permanent part of the client's record. This document accompanies the record to the operating room (Fig. 15–2).

Formal consent is necessary for each invasive procedure. The client or the client's legal surrogate must receive a full explanation of the operation before giving verbal and written consent. Pictures and diagrams may be necessary for a complete understanding of the surgical procedure. Moreover, the client or the surrogate must be told about who will perform the surgery; anesthesia and anesthetic choices; potential risks, complications, and risk of disfigurement or death; and whether organs or body parts may be removed. The client or the surrogate is also informed about alternative treatments. The surgeon must explain the procedure in terms the client or the surrogate readily understands. You are responsible for ensuring that the client or the surrogate receives an honest, accurate, and fair statement of what to expect during and after surgery and that the client understands it before informed consent is given.

The procedure for obtaining an informed consent varies from state to state and according to the individual policy for each health care facility. Generally, the surgeon explains the surgical procedure, the possible risks and complications, and the alternatives. The nurse may obtain and witness the client's signature on the consent form and may help to reinforce what the client has been told by the surgeon. It is not appropriate for the nurse to explain the surgical procedure, risks, complications, and alternatives unless this is done for reinforcement or clarification. The consent must be signed before the client receives any medication that may alter consciousness.

Adults sign their own operative permit unless they are unconscious or mentally incompetent. In such cases a surrogate, such as a relative or a legal guardian, is responsible for consent. If the relative or the guardian is out of state, consent can be secured via the telephone in the presence of one or two witnesses. If no relative or guardian can be found, one can be appointed by court order.

Children under legal age who are not emancipated minors must have consent given by the child's parent or legal guardian. Emancipated minors are considered to be those who are under the legal age of emancipation but because of marriage or other circumstances are independent of the parents. If the child's parent or guardian cannot be present to sign the permit, consent can be obtained from an appropriate person by telephone, Fax, or letter. When a minor's relatives cannot be located, the state in which the surgery is to be performed provides written procedures to follow in order to obtain consent via a court order.

619271 (CH Rev. 7-96)

I, ______________________, hereby consent to the procedures outlined below, to be performed by ______________________, and his/her associates, assistants and appropriate hospital personnel.

The procedure proposed is ______________________

for diagnosis/treatment of ______________________.

This procedure has been explained in terms understandable to me, which include the following:

1. The nature and extent of the procedure to be performed and risks involved, including those which, even though unlikely to occur, involve serious consequences.
2. Alternative procedures and methods of treatment.
3. The dangers and probable consequences of such alternatives (including no procedures or treatment).
4. The estimated period of hospitalization and/or incapacity and the estimated period of convalescence (assuming there are no complications).
5. The expected consequences of the procedure upon my future health.
6. I understand that there are other risks, such as the risks of infection and other serious complications, in the pre-operative and post-operative stages of my care, which can result in serious consequences such as loss of the use of parts of my body and life.
7. I have asked all of the questions which I thought were important in deciding whether or not to undergo treatment or diagnosis. Those questions have been answered to my satisfaction.
8. I understand that no assurance can be given that the procedure will be successful and no guarantee or warranty of success or cure has been given to me.
9. I have been advised that I may have anesthesia, which in rare instances has serious and even fatal complications.
10. I further authorize and request my physician and his/her associates, assistants and appropriate hospital personnel to perform such additional procedures which in their judgement are incidentally necessary or appropriate to carry out my diagnosis/treatment.
11. I have been afforded the opportunity to consult with other physicians to my complete satisfaction before signing this form and I understand that I have the right to refuse any medical and surgical procedures and treatment.
12. I authorize the hospital to dispose of or use for research any tissue or body parts which may be necessary to remove in a manner consistent with state and federal regulations for such disposal.

I certify that I have read and fully understand the above consent statement, that the explanations are understood by me, that all blanks or statements requiring insertion or completion were filled in prior to the time of my signature, that this consent was given freely, voluntarily and without reservation.

Patient's Signature:	Date:	Time:

In the event patient is a minor, unconscious or otherwise not competent to give consent: I, ______________________

the (relationship to patient) ______________, of ______________ hereby give consent on his/her behalf.

Witness to Signature:	Date:	Time:

Clarkson Hospital
4350 Dewey Avenue
Omaha, Nebraska 68105

CONSENT FOR SURGERY OR DIAGNOSTIC/THERAPEUTIC PROCEDURES

FIGURE 15–2 Consent form for blood transfusion. (Courtesy of the Nebraska Health System, Omaha, NE.)

PREPARING THE CLIENT ON THE DAY OF SURGERY

Many clients are admitted into the hospital or surgical center the morning of surgery. These clients can be admitted to the hospital after the procedure if their condition requires specialized observation or nursing care. For so-called ambulatory surgery or same-day surgery, clients come to the hospital or surgery suite the morning of surgery but go home the same day to the care of family members or significant others. The ambulatory surgery approach presents a dilemma in providing preoperative instruction to the client, because time is very limited during the admission period prior to the actual surgical event. Often, the nurse will telephone the night before the procedure to remind the client of any preoperative instructions. Instructions are reinforced about starting NPO status after midnight, wearing washable clothing that is easily removed and put back on, wearing flat shoes, not wearing pantyhose, and securing a ride home after the procedure. Other instructions may be reinforced during this contact with the client. The nurse conducting the telephone educational session should convey a positive attitude about the planned surgical procedure and assist in allaying doubts or fears related to the surgery.

PREOPERATIVE PREPARATION IMMEDIATELY BEFORE SURGERY

Final preoperative preparation begins 1 to 2 hours before surgery for clients in the hospital, and upon admission for clients to have outpatient surgery. The client is asked whether there are any unanswered questions or concerns. Make sure that the client understands the operative procedure to be performed, and continue to assess for manifestations of anxiety. Delays in performing the surgery should be communicated to the client and family.

To prevent omissions in preoperative nursing interventions, most facilities supply nurses with a preoperative checklist. As each intervention on the list is completed, initial it on the form. An example of a preoperative checklist is provided in Box 15–3. Individual surgical centers may include various other actions on this form. You may need to give medications ordered preoperatively to the client before going to the operating room. You must know the approximate time the surgical procedure is scheduled for and must begin the preoperative activities early enough to have them completed when the operating room is ready.

BOX 15–3 Immediate Preoperative Activities

Before the client enters the operating room, check to determine that:

- All known allergies are recorded and allergy wristband is present if indicated.
- Vital signs are checked and recorded. Report marked differences from baseline to the surgeon or anesthesia personnel.
- The identification band is present and correct.
- The consent form is signed and the surgical procedure is listed correctly.
- Skin preparation is completed if ordered preoperatively.
- Any special orders, such as administering enemas or starting an intravenous line, are completed.
- The client has not eaten or had fluids by mouth for the last 8 hours.
- The client has just voided; measure and record the amount of urine (if indicated).
- Oral hygiene or other physical care is completed.
- The presence of dentures, bridgework, or other prostheses is noted, and the anesthesia personnel knows about it.
- Storage is arranged and documented for valuables according to health care facility policy or is given to family members.
- The client has removed jewelry. (Many facilities allow the client to keep the wedding band on as long as it is taped securely.) If jewelry is removed, it should be stored according to policy or given to the family. Assist with the removal of hairpins, wigs, and so on.
- The perioperative nurse is notified about the presence of a hearing aid. Leave it in place so that operating room personnel can communicate with the client.
- The client has a hospital gown and protective cap on. Elastic bandaging or antiembolic hose has been applied, if ordered.
- Colored nail polish has been removed from at least one fingernail for the application of the pulse oximeter (although the device can accurately read oxygen saturation levels through light-colored polish).
- Make-up is removed so that skin color can be observed.

PREOPERATIVE MEDICATIONS

Preoperative medications are given to allay anxiety, to decrease pharyngeal secretions, to reduce side effects of anesthetic agents, and to induce amnesia. Table 15–5 presents an overview of common preoperative medications. Specific drug choices are based on individual client variables, the goals of sedation, and the potential for undesirable side effects. Preoperative medications may be given in the preoperative holding area or on the nursing unit. Before administering preoperative medications, ensure that the operative permit is correctly signed because legal consent cannot be given by a medicated adult. If the preoperative medication is given on the unit, the side rails of the bed must be raised. Once medication is administered, the window shades should be lowered and bright lights turned off to avoid glare. The client is instructed not to get up without assistance because the medications are likely to cause drowsiness or dizziness. Once the client is calm and drowsy, disruptions should take place only when necessary and then be brief. Observe the client for side effects (e.g., hypotension and respiratory distress).

TRANSPORTING THE CLIENT TO SURGERY

When surgical personnel call for the client, the client is gently transferred to a stretcher. Adequate assistance for transfer must be obtained to reduce the possibility of injury to the client and staff. Appropriate covering is provided for the client, and side rails are raised. The medical record accompanies the client to the operating room. The trip to surgery should be as smooth as possible so that the sedated client does not experience nausea and dizziness.

PREPARING THE CLIENT'S ROOM FOR POSTOPERATIVE CARE

The client's room should be prepared so that the initial care of the client on return from surgery can be orderly. Furniture should be arranged so that the stretcher can easily be brought to the bedside. The bed should be placed in high position and made with clean linen in an open position. Bed rails should be down on receiving side, up on other side. An emesis basin should be located close to the bed. Blood pressure monitoring equipment, IV setup, suction, and oxygen should be nearby. All equipment should be tested to ensure it is in working condition before the client returns.

CARING FOR SIGNIFICANT OTHERS

A designated area is usually provided for family members to wait in during surgery. If family members plan on

TABLE 15–5 COMMONLY USED PREOPERATIVE MEDICATIONS

Medication	Desired Effect	Undesired Effect(s)
Tranquilizers		
Diazepam (Valium)	Decreases anxiety	May cause dizziness, clumsiness, or confusion
Droperidol (Inapsine)	Decreases anxiety Produces an antiemetic effect	Anxiety/hypotension during and after surgery
Sedatives		
Midazolam HCl	Induces desired sleepiness Decreases anxiety	Hypotension, undesired respiratory depression
Promethazine HCl (Phenergan)	Same as for droperidol	Hypotension during and after surgery
Secobarbital sodium (Seconal Sodium)	Decreases anxiety Promotes sedation	Disorientation, especially in elderly clients
Pentobarbital sodium (Nembutal Sodium)	Same as for secobarbital sodium	Same as for secobarbital sodium
Analgesics		
Morphine sulfate	Relieves pain Decreases anxiety Sedation	Respiratory depression Hypotension Circulatory depression Decreased gastric motility causing potential for vomiting
Fentanyl citrate (Sublimaze)	Is a short-acting analgesic for minor or outpatient surgery; adjunct to general anesthesia	Same as for morphine sulfate
Meperidine HCl (Demerol)	Same as for morphine sulfate	Same as for morphine sulfate
Anticholinergics		
Atropine sulfate	Controls secretions	Excessive dryness of mouth, tachycardia
Glycopyrrolate (Robinul)	Same as for atropine sulfate	Same as for atropine sulfate
Histamine H_2-Receptor Antagonists		
Cimetidine (Tagamet) (see Table 31–2 for other H_2 antagonists)	Inhibits gastric acid production	Mild dizziness, diarrhea, somnolence, and rash

leaving the facility during the procedure, ensure that there is a way to contact them and supply them with a phone number to the nurses' station and client's room.

When discussing the surgical procedure with the client's significant others, be sure to provide answers congruent with the information that the surgeon has already provided. Family members should also be prepared for any equipment that may accompany the client postoperatively. A preoperative explanation will assist the family in understanding what equipment is attached to their loved one, and why. Significant others need to be informed when surgery is completed or if there are any delays. The surgeon should speak with family members as soon as possible after completion of the procedure.

INTRAOPERATIVE PERIOD

Nursing care during the intraoperative phase focuses on the client's emotional well-being as well as on physical factors such as safety, positioning, maintaining asepsis, and controlling the surgical environment. The preoperative assessment assists the nurse in planning appropriate interventions for this phase of the surgical experience. The nurse remains the client's advocate during this period, anticipating and guarding against potential complications. Whereas the surgeon concentrates on performing the surgical procedure and the anesthesia provider concentrates on the client's breathing and on maintenance of the client's physiologic stability, the circulating nurse is responsible for all other activities that take place in the operating room.

■ MEMBERS OF THE SURGICAL TEAM

The surgical team is a group of highly trained and educated professionals who coordinate their efforts to assure the welfare and safety of the client. Although the specifics of each type of surgical procedure may vary, certain key players must always be present, such as the surgeon, the anesthesiologist, the circulating nurse, and scrub personnel (see Box 15–4).

The surgeon heads the surgical team and makes decisions concerning the surgical procedure. Depending on the surgical procedure to be performed, a second surgeon or a specially trained nurse may serve as an assistant. The anesthesiologist alleviates pain and promotes relaxation with medications. The anesthesia provider maintains the airway, ensures adequate gas exchange, monitors circulation and respiration, estimates blood and fluid loss, in-

BOX 15–4 Roles of the Perioperative Nurse

Many roles are available to the perioperative nurse. The ongoing shift from tertiary care practice to community-focused practice is continuing to create even more new roles. The role these nurses play in the perioperative environment depends on their academic preparation, extended specialty education, experience, career plan, and needs of the employer. The roles of the perioperative nurse include, but are not limited to, the following:

- Circulating nurse
- Scrub nurse
- Registered Nurse First Assistant (RNFA)
- Certified Registered Nurse Anesthetist (CRNA)
- Manager
- Educator
- Case Manager, and Clinical Nurse Specialist (CNS)

Circulating Nurse

The circulating role is a major one for perioperative nurses. A nurse functioning as a circulator should be a Registered Nurse (RN). He or she assesses the client preoperatively, planning for optimal care during the surgical intervention, coordinating all personnel within the operating room, delegating and monitoring unlicensed personnel, and monitoring responsible cost compliance associated with operating room procedures. The circulator does not wear sterile clothing and can go in and out of the operating room. In addition to caring directly for the client, the circulator has very defined activities during surgery. These include:

- Ensuring all equipment is working properly
- Guaranteeing sterility of instruments and supplies
- Assisting with positioning
- Performing surgical skin preparation
- Monitoring the room and team members for breaks in sterile technique
- Assisting anesthesia personnel with induction and physiological monitoring
- Handling specimens
- Coordinating activities with other departments, such as radiology and pathology
- Documenting care provided
- Minimizing conversation and traffic within the operating room suite

Scrub Nurse

An RN or Surgical Technician (ST) can perform the role of scrub person. The duties include gathering all equipment for the procedure, preparing all supplies and instruments using sterile technique, maintaining sterility within the sterile field during surgery, handling instruments and supplies during surgery, and cleaning up after the case. During surgery, the scrub person maintains an accurate count of sponges, sharps, and instruments on the sterile field and counts the same materials with the circulating nurse before and after the surgery.

Registered Nurse First Assistant

The RNFA role is relatively new. In 1980, the American College of Surgeons supported the use of qualified RNs as first assistants in place of second or assisting physicians during surgical procedures. The Association of Operating Room Nurses (AORN) published its official statement on the role of the RNFA in 1984. The RNFA is an experienced perioperative nurse who has had additional specialized education to perform this role. The RNFA works with the primary surgeon during the surgery. This is a role separate from that of the scrub person. Some of the activities of an RNFA include providing exposure of the surgical area, using instruments to hold and cut, retracting and handling tissue, providing hemostasis, and suturing. RNFAs must work with a surgeon and are not independent practitioners.[29]

Certified Registered Nurse Anesthetist

The CRNA is a nurse who has a minimum of 2 years of additional education specializing in the administration of anesthesia. Entry into a CRNA program usually requires a Bachelor of Science degree in nursing or other appropriate field plus one year of acute or intensive care nursing experience. These nurses work under the direction of an anesthesiologist.

Manager

The role of manager of the operating room has extensive experience and has had additional education in management. It can be any Registered Nurse, but hospitals today prefer candidates with a Bachelor of Science in Nursing (BSN). Many large hospitals now require a master's degree, with a major in acute care or management. This nurse has many names, depending on the institution, such as head nurse, clinical nursing director, operating room manager, and others.

Educator

The role of educator can be played by any RN, but usually nurses with a BSN or Master's (MSN) degree who are experienced perioperative nurses are best qualified. They are responsible for staff continuing education, orientation of new staff, and working with staff to learn how to be preceptors to students. These nurses may also fulfill the role of circulator or Clinical Nurse Specialist outside their teaching responsibilities.

Case Manager

The perioperative case manager is also a new role for RNs. The role calls for extensive experience, ability to communicate, and a knowledge of the total surgical episode from home before surgery to home care needs after surgery. These nurses may have different functions within their place of work, depending on the need of the institution or employing agency. As with any role, the role of case manager should be investigated before nurses accept a position of employment.[25]

Clinical Nurse Specialist

The Clinical Nurse Specialist is an Advanced Practice Nurse.[21] These nurses must hold a MSN with a major reflecting their specialty. The major roles (depending on institutional needs) vary but incorporate direct client care; education of staff, clients, family members, people of other disciplines; consultation; and research.[21] A perioperative or surgical Clinical Nurse Specialist may not always be in the operating room but may go on rounds with physicians, interact with clients in homes, clinics, or other sites; and monitor clients in hospital surgical units. These nurses have specialized skills in heart, transplantation, renal, and cancer fields.

Perioperative nursing is performed preoperatively, intraoperatively, and postoperatively. Each of these periods is characterized by specific actions required by nurses, who participate both independently and as part of a health care team.

fuses blood and fluids, administers medications to maintain hemodynamic stability, and alerts the surgeon immediately to any complications. The circulating nurse is a core member of the surgical team and maintains the coordination of all team members while always remaining the client's advocate. Scrub personnel organize the surgical equipment and hand the surgeon appropriate instruments required for the operative procedure. Depending on the specific surgical procedure, the surgical team may include other members—for instance, a pathologist may be called in to identify tissue, an x-ray technician may be needed to perform various radiologic procedures, or a perfusionist may be required when cardiac bypass is necessary. The circulating nurse must control the traffic within the operating suite and know the designated responsibilities of each team member.

ANESTHESIA

Anesthesia is an artificially induced state of partial or total loss of sensation with or without loss of consciousness. Anesthetic agents can produce muscle relaxation, block transmission of pain nerve impulses, and suppress reflexes. It can also temporarily decrease memory retrieval and recall. The depth and effects of anesthesia are monitored by observing changes in respiration, oxygen saturation and end-tidal carbon dioxide (CO_2) levels, heart rate, urine output, and blood pressure.

Most clients are anxious about the anesthesia. Some are concerned about the adequacy of the pain-blocking effects, whereas others are concerned about being "put to sleep" with a drug. Some clients wonder whether they will talk during anesthesia or will experience nausea and vomiting postoperatively. Nurses must respond to these concerns by providing reassurance about the capability of the anesthesiologist, and about the availability of other drugs to reduce any unpleasant side effects of the anesthesia. The client needs frequent reminders to let the nurse or the physician know immediately about any side effects experienced from the anesthesia, and the nurse must remain diligent in assessing for any possible complications. Bring any side effects noted to the immediate attention of the anesthesiologist.

The decision about the type of anesthesia to be used is made by the anesthesia provider in consultation with the surgeon and the client. The choice of anesthetic agent for a surgical procedure depends on many variables. The two major techniques in anesthesia are general and regional.

Agents for *general anesthesia* (general anesthetics) block pain stimulus at the cerebral cortex and induce depression of the central nervous system (CNS) that is reversed either by metabolic change and elimination from the body or by pharmacologic means. General anesthetic agents produce analgesia, amnesia, unconsciousness, and loss of reflexes and muscle tone. The neurologic, respiratory, and cardiovascular systems are affected by these agents. General anesthesia is best suited for surgery on the head, neck, upper torso, and back; for prolonged surgical procedures; or for use in clients who are unable to lie quietly for a long period of time. General anesthetic agents affect all tissues in the body to some degree.

In *regional anesthesia,* drugs are given to block the pain stimulus at its origin, along afferent neurons, or along the spinal cord. Unlike general anesthesia, regional anesthesia produces a loss of painful sensation in only one region of the body and does not result in unconsciousness. In addition to the regional anesthetic agent, the client also may receive sedative agents that produce drowsiness. The client can also receive epidural narcotics, which have a systemic effect and produce some drowsiness.

GENERAL ANESTHESIA

Stages of General Anesthesia

There are four stages of general anesthesia (Table 15–6). Surgery is performed in stage III. These stages were identified many years ago when ether was the most common drug used for anesthesia. The effects of ether allowed these distinct stages to be easily differentiated. The stages were used to guide the surgeon in determining when

TABLE 15–6 THE FOUR STAGES OF ANESTHESIA

Stage	Start-Point	End-Point	Physical Reactions	Nursing Interventions
I: Onset	Anesthetic administration	Loss of consciousness	Client may be drowsy or dizzy Possible auditory or visual hallucinations	Close operating room doors; keep room quiet; stand by to assist client
II: Excitement	Loss of consciousness	Loss of eyelid reflexes	Increase in autonomic activity Irregular breathing Client may struggle	Remain quietly at client's side; assist anesthetist, if needed
III: Surgical anesthesia	Loss of eyelid reflexes	Loss of most reflexes Depression of vital functions	Client is unconscious Muscles are relaxed No blink or gag reflex	Begin preparation (if indicated) only when anesthetist indicates stage III has been reached and client is breathing well, with stable vital signs
IV: Danger (death)	Functions excessively depressed	Respiratory and circulatory failure	Client is not breathing A heartbeat may or may not be present	If arrest occurs, respond immediately to assist in establishing airway; provide cardiac arrest tray, drugs, syringes, long needles; assist surgeon with closed or open cardiac massage

surgery could begin. Ether, which is no longer used because of its explosive nature, has been replaced with greatly improved anesthetic agents that provide rapid induction of anesthesia. With the rapid action of these new drugs, the stages of anesthesia are not readily apparent; however, they still occur. Some signs may be noted if the anesthetic drug is given slowly as the nurse holds the hand of the client during induction. Mild tremors of the hand may be felt as the client moves through stages I and II to stage III.

Because the last sense to be depressed during induction is hearing, remember to maintain a quiet atmosphere during this time. The client can hear and may remember conversations upon awakening. The nurse, always remaining the client's advocate, ensures that all conversation during induction and throughout the case is appropriate. Clients emerge into consciousness backward through all three stages of anesthesia after the anesthetic agents are discontinued. Therefore, hearing is the first sense to return.

Administration of General Anesthesia

General anesthesia can be administered in a variety of ways. The most common method of administering anesthesia is to use a combination of agents based on the client's need with consideration of the type of surgery to be performed. This type of anesthesia is called *neuroleptic* or *balanced anesthesia.* Balanced anesthesia is typically achieved with a combination of an inhalation agent, oxygen, a narcotic, and a neuromuscular blocking agent. Inhalation and the IV route are the most common routes of administration. Table 15–7 describes the most common general anesthetic agents used and the implications for the delivery of nursing care associated with the use of each.

Neuromuscular Blocking Agents. Neuromuscular blocking agents are classified as *depolarizing* and *nondepolarizing.* These agents block the transmission of nerve impulses to the muscle fibers. Neuromuscular blocking agents (Table 15–8) are administered via the IV route and are given mainly to facilitate intubation by easing laryngospasm, and relaxing muscles for controlled ventilation. When general anesthetics are given with neuromuscular blocking agents, the latter can be given in smaller and thus safer doses. Common muscle relaxants are succinylcholine, tubocurarine, pancuronium, and vecuronium.

Types of General Anesthesia

INTRAVENOUS ANESTHESIA. When general anesthesia is administered intravenously the client experiences an extremely rapid induction. Unconsciousness generally occurs about 30 seconds after the medication is administered. This process promotes a rapid transition from the conscious stage to the surgical anesthesia stage. It also prepares the client for a smooth transition to the surgical stage of anesthesia, as the IV anesthetic can act as a calming agent. IV anesthesia is sufficiently potent to be used alone in such minor procedures as dental extractions and pelvic examinations. Examples of IV anesthetics are thiopental sodium and ketamine.

INHALATION ANESTHESIA. For inhalation anesthesia, a mixture of volatile liquids or gas and oxygen is used. These anesthetics are advantageous because of their ease of administration and elimination through the respiratory system. These are usually used to maintain the client in stage III anesthesia following induction. The mixture is given through a mask or through an endotracheal tube (Fig. 15–3), which is inserted once the patient is paralyzed and unconscious. Anesthesia intubation is often more difficult in an obese client because of the typically thickened neck and in the client with arthritis or a neck fracture.

When inhalation anesthetic agents are administered by mask, the gases generally flow into the mask via a finely calibrated vaporizer that is controlled by a machine. When an endotracheal tube is used to give the anesthetic, the gases flow directly into the client's tracheobronchial tree, resulting in a very quick response. Many different liquids and gases are used in inhalation anesthesia. Two commonly employed inhalation anesthetics are halothane and isoflurane. A commonly used gas anesthetic is nitrous oxide.

REGIONAL ANESTHESIA

Regional anesthetics are useful in many clinical situations. Local anesthetic agents, which are used to obtain local anesthesia, can also be administered to function as a central, peripheral, IV, regional, retrobulbar, or transbronchial nerve block. Table 15–10 (see later on) describes agents commonly used for local anesthesia. These anesthetic agents block the conduction of impulses in the nerve fibers without depolarizing the cell membrane.

Epinephrine can be added to many of the local anesthetics in an effort to prolong the anesthetic effect. Epinephrine also causes local blood vessels to constrict, thus delaying absorption of the anesthetic agent. This factor also can reduce bleeding via vasoconstriction. Epinephrine should be used with caution in older adults with cardiovascular or liver disease. Traditionally, epinephrine is not used in hand or foot surgery because of the small blood vessels in the area. Because the effect is vasoconstriction, use of epinephrine could compromise tissue perfusion, leading to adverse outcomes such as poor circulatory response. Recently, the use of epinephrine in hand and foot surgery has been reevaluated.

Types of Regional Anesthesia

Regional anesthesia can be administered in a variety of different ways: spinal, epidural, caudal, topical, local infiltration, field block, peripheral nerve block, and IV regional block.

SPINAL ANESTHESIA. Spinal anesthesia offers many advantages for clients undergoing surgical procedures involving the lower half of the body. It is often the anesthetic technique of choice for older adults because of its overall favorable profile. Benefits of spinal anesthesia include its relative safety, excellent lower body muscle relaxation, and absence of effect on consciousness; furthermore, its use does not require empty stomach. Spinal anesthesia is achieved by injecting local anesthetics into the subarachnoid space (Fig. 15–4). Autonomic nerve fibers are affected first and are also the last to recover. After blockade of the autonomic nervous system, spinal anesthesia blocks the following fibers in this order: (1) touch, (2) pain, (3) motor, (4) pressure, and (5) proprioceptive fibers—these fibers alert the brain of physical orientation. Recovery is in the reverse order.

TABLE 15–7 GENERAL ANESTHETIC AGENTS

Drug	Action	Side Effects	Nursing Implications
Inhalation Agents			
Nitrous oxide	Gas has very low anesthetic potency, so it must be used with other agents; highest analgesic effect of all agents; little or no effect on BP or P; no muscle relaxant properties	Minimal side effects; little or no hypotension or respiratory depression; low incidence of malignant hypothermia	Monitor vital signs, especially BP and P; monitor effects of CNS depressants for 24 hours after administration
Halothane (Fluothane)	Volatile liquid with high anesthetic potency, so it could be used alone; has weak analgesic effect; causes moderate decrease in BP and large decrease in respirations; only a mild muscle relaxant	Hypotension, depression of myocardium with decreased cardiac output, bradycardia, respiratory depression; sensitizes heart to catecholamines; malignant hyperthermia, hepatitis, postoperative mild nausea and vomiting, decreased urine output	Monitor all vital signs closely; monitor body temperature for signs of malignant hyperthermia; keep client warm during recovery, and watch for severe shivering; avoid use of catecholamines (epinephrine or norepinephrine); monitor liver function after surgery; monitor urine output closely
Enflurane (Ethrane)	Volatile liquid with fairly high anesthetic potential; has weak analgesic effect; causes moderate decrease in BP and large decrease in respirations; is a moderate muscle relaxant	Hypotension, respiratory depression; blocks labor; minimal sensitization of heart to catecholamines; seizures with high doses	Do not give to clients with history of seizures; monitor vital signs, especially BP, P, and respirations; not for use during labor
Isoflurane (Forane)	Volatile liquid with high anesthetic potential; has weak analgesic effect; causes moderate decrease in BP and large decrease in respirations; is a moderate muscle relaxant; produces profound vasodilatation	Hypotension related to vasodilating effect; respiratory depression; suppresses uterine contractions	Does not sensitize heart to catecholamines, so it can be used with epinephrine and norepinephrine; monitor vital signs; and avoid rapid position changes because it may lead to hypotension as a result of vasodilatation
Intravenous Drugs			
Thiopental sodium (Pentothal)	Short-acting barbiturate that produces rapid unconsciousness; a weak analgesic and muscle relaxant	Respiratory depression with momentary apnea after injection, retrograde amnesia, myocardial depression, hypotension, headache, and shivering	Monitor for allergic reactions; monitor respiratory function closely, especially during induction; monitor vital signs; cannot be mixed with solutions containing atropine, tubocurarine, or succinylcholine; avoid extravasation
Fentanyl citrate–droperidol (Innovar)	A potent opioid (fentanyl) combined with a neuroleptic (droperidol); produces indifference to surroundings and insensitivity to pain; CNS depressant, which produces calming, analgesia, and reduced motor activity	Emergence delirium with hallucinations, hypotension, vasodilatation, nausea and vomiting, laryngospasm, respiratory depression, shivering, and apnea	Use with caution in clients with head injuries, increased intracranial pressure, COPD, hepatic or renal dysfunction, or bradyarrhythmias, or in elderly clients; monitor vital signs; maintain patent airway; reduce narcotic doses to one fourth or one third for first 24 hr postoperatively; when Innovar is used for induction, fentanyl citrate (Sublimaze) alone is used for maintenance of anesthesia
Ketamine HCl (Ketalar)	Produces state of dissociative anesthesia; causes sedation, immobility, analgesia, amnesia, and unresponsiveness to pain; short-acting (no antagonist)	Delirium, hallucinations, disturbing dreams, tonic and clonic movements, respiratory depression, hypotension or hypertension, decreased or increased pulse, nystagmus, increased salivation, laryngospasms, and mild nausea and vomiting	Contraindicated in clients with history of CVA and severe hypertension; use with caution in clients with alcoholism or elevated CSF; maintain airway; do not give in same syringe as for barbiturates; minimize stimulation as client emerges from anesthesia; use diazepam if hallucinations occur or delusions are severe; excellent for anesthesia in young and elderly; pad side rails of gurney; place client in quiet dark area; do not stimulate client inadvertently; any sudden moves elicit hallucinations

BP, blood pressure; CNS, central nervous system; COPD, chronic obstructive pulmonary disease; CVA, cardiovascular accident; CSF, cerebrospinal fluid; P, pulse.

TABLE 15–8 NEUROMUSCULAR BLOCKING AGENTS

Drug	Action	Side Effects	Nursing Implications
Pancuronium bromide (Pavulon)	Nondepolarizing agent; prevents acetylcholine from binding to receptors on muscle end-plate, blocking depolarization	Tachycardia, hypertension, prolonged dose-related apnea, allergic reaction, and excessive sweating and salivation	Use carefully in older or debilitated clients or in clients with renal, hepatic, or pulmonary disease, myasthenia gravis, or thyroid disease; measure intake and output carefully; have resuscitation equipment available; do not mix in syringe or solution with barbiturates; neostigmine reverses effect
Vecuronium bromide (Norcuron)	Nondepolarizing agent; prevents acetylcholine from binding to receptors on muscle end-plate, blocking depolarization	Transient tachycardia; prolonged dose-related apnea, redness, itching, and induration	Has no effect on cardiovascular system; use with caution in clients with hepatic disease, obesity, or neuromuscular disease; tolerated well in renal disease; reversed with anticholinesterase and neostigmine; have emergency resuscitation equipment available
Succinylcholine chloride (Anectine)	Nondepolarizing agent that prolongs depolarization of muscle end-plate	Increased or decreased pulse rate and blood pressure, dysrhythmias, increased intraocular pressure, prolonged respiratory depression, malignant hyperthermia, postoperative muscle pain, excessive salivation, and hypersensitivity	Monitor vital signs; maintain patent airway; postoperative stiffness is normal; drug of choice for short procedures; keep emergency resuscitation equipment on hand; repeat infusions can prolong apnea; neostigmine reverses effect

Spinal anesthesia can be used for almost any type of major procedure performed below the level of the diaphragm, such as a hysterectomy or appendectomy. Figure 15–5 illustrates proper positioning for injection of drugs for spinal anesthesia. Within minutes of administration the client experiences a loss of sensation and paralysis of the toes, feet, legs, and then abdomen. Most clients exhibit a slight hypotension initially due to the vasodilatation that occurs with administration of the spinal anesthetic. The complications of spinal anesthesia are listed and described in Table 15–9, along with prevention and intervention suggestions for nurses. As with any anesthesia, the client who has undergone spinal anesthesia is at risk for neurologic, respiratory, or cardiovascular complications. However, the risk of spinal anesthesia in general is no higher than with general anesthesia.

EPIDURAL ANESTHESIA. An epidural block is achieved by introduction of an anesthetic agent into the epidural space (see Fig. 15–4). The epidural space is generally entered by a needle at a thoracic, lumbar, sacral, or caudal interspace. The needle is carefully positioned in the epidural space without penetrating the dura and without entering the subarachnoid space. When the needle is properly positioned, the cerebrospinal fluid

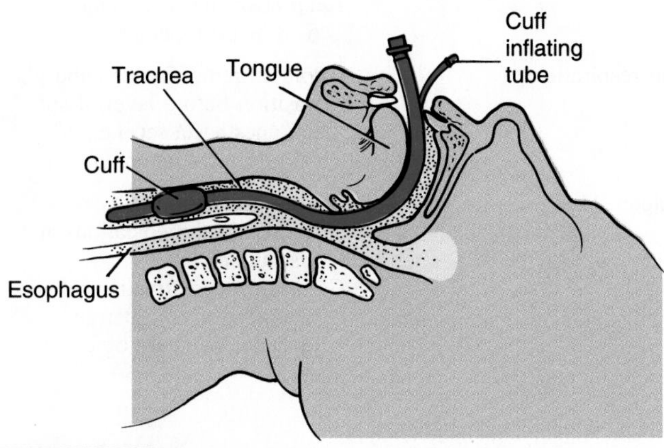

FIGURE 15–3 Correct placement of the endotracheal tube for anesthesia administration.

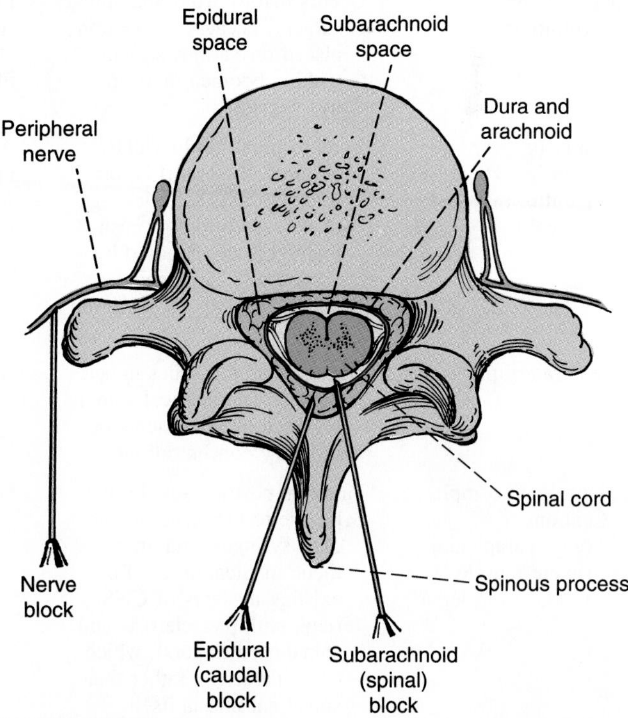

FIGURE 15–4 Cross-section of a lumbar vertebra showing injection sites for anesthesia.

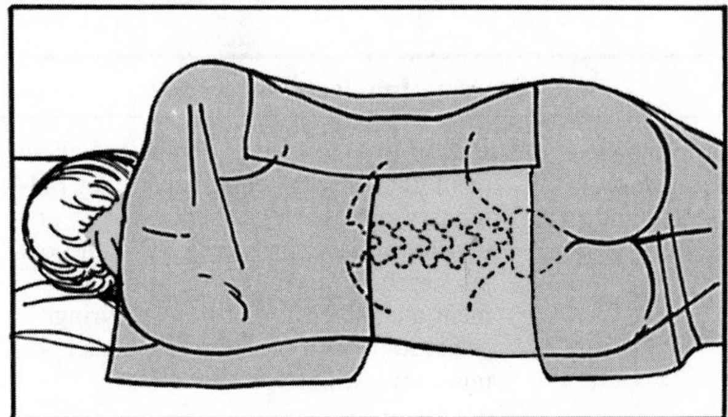
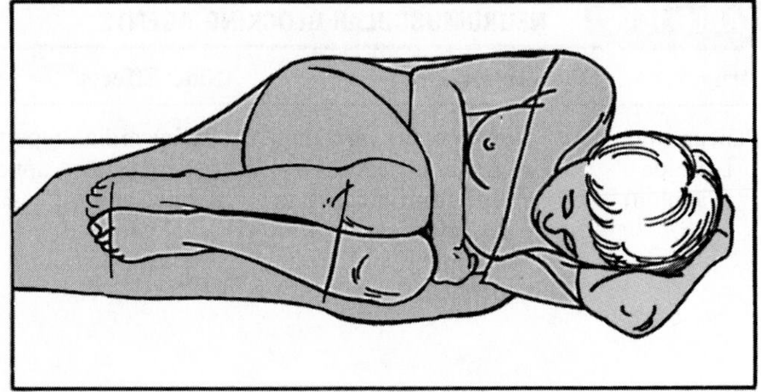

FIGURE 15–5 Proper positioning for spinal anesthesia administration flexes the client's torso to expand the space between the lumbar vertebrae.

(CSF) cannot be aspirated. An epidural block, like spinal anesthesia, produces a blockade of the autonomic nerves and hypotension can result. If the level of the block is too high and the respiratory muscles are affected, then respiratory depression or paralysis may occur.

Caudal Anesthesia. Caudal anesthesia is produced by injection of the local anesthetic into the caudal or sacral canal. Caudal anesthesia is a variation of epidural anesthesia. This method is commonly used with obstetric clients.

TOPICAL ANESTHESIA. Topical anesthetic agents may be directly applied onto the area to be desensitized. The

TABLE 15–9 COMPLICATIONS AND DISCOMFORTS OF SPINAL ANESTHESIA

Complications and Discomforts	Causes	Intervention	Prevention
Hypotension	Paralysis of vasomotor nerves; usually occurs shortly after induction of anesthesia	Administer oxygen by inhalation Vasoactive drugs Trendelenburg's position if level of anesthesia is fixed, 10–20 min after induction	In clients not prone to heart failure, 500–800 ml of IV fluids, administered rapidly before block
Nausea and vomiting	Occurs mainly from abdominal surgery, because of traction placed on various structures within abdomen or from hypotension	Ephedrine Antiemetics Oxygen Fluids	
Headache (can be extremely painful, may last a week)	Cerebrospinal fluid (which cushions the brain) is lost through dural hole; leakage of fluid with loss of cushioning effect increased by (1) use of a large spinal needle or (2) poor hydration	Apply tight abdominal binder Fluids Analgesics In severe cases, inject 10 ml of client's blood to plug hole (blood patch)	Use of very small spinal needle reduces incidence of spinal headache to 0.9% Administer IV and oral fluids before and after induction of spinal anesthesia Keep client flat and quiet 6–8 hr postoperatively
Respiratory paralysis	Occurs if drug reaches upper thoracic and cervical spinal levels in large amounts or in heavy concentrations	Artificial respiration	Avoid extreme Trendelenburg's position before level of spinal anesthesia set, i.e., 10–20 min after induction
Neurologic complications (e.g., paraplegia, severe muscle weakness in legs)	Paralysis postoperatively may be due to (1) unsterile needles, syringes, and anesthetic medications; (2) preexisting diseases of CNS (e.g., multiple sclerosis and spinal cord tumors), which cause paralysis, rather than spinal anesthesia itself	See Chapter 73	Strict sterile technique Heat-sterilized medications and instruments Careful preoperative neurologic examination to ascertain presence of neurologic disease

IV, intravenous; CNS, central nervous system.

TABLE 15–10 LOCAL AND TOPICAL ANESTHETIC AGENTS

Drug	Action	Side Effects	Nursing Implications
Local Agents			
Bupivacaine HCl (Marcaine HCl)	Amide-type local anesthetic that blocks depolarization, preventing generation and conduction of nerve impulses; combined with epinephrine, it has prolonged action	Edema, anaphylaxis; rarely, anxiety, convulsions, respiratory arrest, cardiac arrest, blurred vision, and shivering	Contraindicated in children under 12 years of age, or for spinal or paracervical block or topical anesthesia; use with caution in older clients, or clients with hepatic disease or allergies; onset 4–15 min, duration 3–6 hr; keep resuscitative equipment available
Chloroprocaine HCl (Nesacaine)	Ester-type local anesthetic that blocks depolarization, preventing generation and condition of nerve impulses	Anaphylaxis, edema; rarely, anxiety, convulsions, respiratory arrest, cardiac arrest, blurred vision, and shivering	Contraindicated in clients with allergies to "caines," CNS disease; use cautiously in older adults; check solution for particles or discoloration; keep resuscitative equipment available; do not use solution with preservative for caudal or epidural blocks
Lidocaine HCl (Xylocaine)	Amide-type local anesthetic that blocks depolarization, preventing generation and conduction of nerve impulses; combined with epinephrine, it has prolonged action	Edema, anaphylaxis, dysrhythmias; rarely, anxiety, respiratory arrest, cardiac arrest, and tinnitus	Contraindicated in clients with hypersensitivity, severe hypertension, septicemia, spinal deformities, or neurologic disorders; use cautiously in older clients and those with heart block or general drug allergies or in severe shock; use solutions with epinephrine only in body areas with good blood supply; use preservative-free solution for spinal, epidural, and caudal blocks
Topical Agents			
Benzocaine (Americaine)	Blocks conduction of impulses at sensory nerve endings	Sensitization rash, possible tolerance	Contraindicated in clients with history of hypersensitivity to "caines"; discontinue if rash develops; avoid contact with eyes; avoid inhalation of spray; has short duration of action; do not use over infected area; if used rectally, clean area well first
Ethyl chloride spray	Produces local anesthesia by producing sensation of cold	Frostbite, tissue necrosis from prolonged use, muscle spasms, and increased pain	Do not apply over broken skin; protect adjacent skin; avoid contact with eyes; avoid inhalation; highly flammable, do not use near open flame; very short duration
Tetracaine HCl (Pontocaine HCl)	Blocks conduction of impulses at sensory nerve endings	Local sensitization and rash	Do not use in hypersensitive clients; clean rectal area well before applying; do not use if rash develops
Cocaine	Ester-type topical anesthetic that blocks uptake of norepinephrine by adrenergic neurons	CNS stimulation, euphoria, decreased fatigue, tachycardia, vasoconstriction, and hypertension	For topical use only; produces psychological dependence with prolonged or repeated use; schedule II narcotic; use cautiously in clients with history of severe hypertension or heart disease; combined with epinephrine, it can lead to cardiovascular toxicity; monitor vital signs closely

CNS, central nervous system.

anesthetic may be a solution, an ointment, a gel, a cream, or a powder. This short-acting form of anesthesia can block peripheral nerve endings in the mucous membranes of the vagina, rectum, nasopharynx, and mouth. Topical anesthesia is used in minor procedures such as a rectal examination when painful hemorrhoids are present or before a bronchoscopic examination to desensitize the bronchi. Medications used for local and topical anesthesia are listed in Table 15–10.

One drug commonly used for topical anesthesia is a 4% to 10% solution of cocaine. This agent is for topical use only and is primarily used to anesthetize the eye and the mucous membranes of the nose, mouth, and urethra. Cocaine is highly toxic. If accidentally injected, it may cause severe excitement or seizures, followed by shock, respiratory failure, and cardiac arrest. Emergency resuscitation equipment must be available when cocaine is used. Other agents commonly used for topical anesthesia include tetracaine, procaine, mepivacaine, bupivacaine, and lidocaine. To avoid anaphylactic reactions from previous sensitization to anesthetic agents, check the client's drug allergies before application of any topical anesthetic agent.

LOCAL INFILTRATION ANESTHESIA. Local infiltration anesthesia involves injection of an anesthetic agent such as lidocaine (Xylocaine) into the skin and subcutaneous tissue of the area to be anesthetized. Local anesthesia blocks only the peripheral nerves around the area of the incision. When local anesthetic is administered, the person injecting the drug must aspirate before injection to ensure the needle is not in a blood vessel. If a local anesthetic agent is inadvertently injected into the bloodstream, it becomes systemic, and cardiovascular collapse or convulsions could result.

FIELD BLOCK ANESTHESIA. The area proximal to a planned incision can be injected and infiltrated with local anesthetic agents to produce what is known as a *field block.* This block forms a barrier between the incision and the nervous system. This procedure differs from simple injection of local anesthesia, in which only the area of the incision is injected. A field block actually walls in the area around the incision and prevents transmission of sensory impulses to the brain from that area. The anesthesia provider must take precautions when performing a field block to avoid injection of the agent into a blood vessel.

PERIPHERAL NERVE BLOCK ANESTHESIA. A *nerve block* anesthetizes individual nerves or nerve plexuses rather than all the local nerves anesthetized by a field block. Nerve blocks can be obtained in a finger (digital nerve block), the entire upper arm (brachial plexus nerve block), or the chest or abdominal wall (intercostal nerve block). Nerves most commonly blocked are those within the brachial plexus and the intercostal, sciatic, and femoral nerves. Drugs commonly used as nerve block agents are lidocaine, bupivacaine, and mepivacaine. The anesthesia provider injects the anesthetic along the nerve rather than into the nerve in an effort to decrease the risk of nerve damage. Once the drug has been injected, it takes several minutes for onset of the anesthesia.

Nerve blocks, like local infiltration blocks, can produce severe systemic response if the drug is accidentally injected into a blood vessel. Because epinephrine causes vasoconstriction, particularly in the extremities, anesthetic procedures for surgery performed below the wrist or ankle typically use agents that do not contain epinephrine.

INTRAVENOUS REGIONAL EXTREMITY BLOCK ANESTHESIA (BIER BLOCK). Regional anesthesia of a limb can be achieved with an agent such as lidocaine when it is injected into a vein of the limb to be anesthetized. A pneumatic dual-cuff tourniquet applied to the anesthetized area prevents the lidocaine from circulating beyond the area undergoing the procedure. This type of anesthesia is used most commonly for procedures of the extremities that are of short duration. The tourniquet can be inflated only for 2-hour increments.

MONITORED ANESTHESIA. Monitored anesthesia is used during an operation in which the surgeon infiltrates the surgical site with a local anesthetic and the anesthesia provider supplements the local anesthetic with IV drugs to provide sedation and systemic analgesia. The anesthesia care provider monitors the client's blood pressure, heart rate, and respiration while the local anesthesia and IV support are being provided. *Local standby* and *anesthesia standby* also refer to monitored anesthesia.

Other Methods of Anesthesia and Analgesia

ACUPUNCTURE. Acupuncture is an ancient Chinese pain-killing technique that works by the insertion of long, thin needles into specific acupuncture points located on lines called *meridians* that connect anatomic sites on the body. Practitioners of acupuncture have named and numbered approximately 1000 acupuncture points, each about 0.25 cm in diameter. When performing major surgery, Chinese doctors use acupuncture as a form of anesthesia. Some advantages of acupuncture include (1) decreased anesthesia-related side effects during or after surgery, (2) less blood loss during surgery, and (3) reduced need for postoperative analgesia, because acupuncture's pain-killing effects persist for several hours.

There are several Western hypotheses to explain why acupuncture works. One hypothesis is based on the outdated gate control theory of pain control and contends that the technique stimulates the larger sensory nerve fibers that carry non-pain impulses. Another theory suggests that acupuncture triggers the release of endorphins, endogenous polypeptides with analgesic properties. Some Western physicians remain skeptical about the technique's pain-killing capabilities.

CRYOTHERMIA. Cryothermia is the use of cold to induce anesthesia. Because a very low surface temperature reduces pain, the surgical site is treated with ice preoperatively. Although there are many acceptable alternatives to cryothermia, this technique can be used in extreme conditions that threaten life and when the client cannot tolerate conventional forms of anesthesia.

■ INTRAOPERATIVE NURSING CARE

Intraoperative nursing care is the second component of perioperative nursing. It is often called "operating room nursing." Intraoperative nurses see the client immediately before surgery, either in a holding area or in an admission unit. An initial, brief assessment is completed by the intraoperative nurse. The care plans that were developed and planned preoperatively, along with the findings on the extensive admission examination, are used in this phase. Intraoperative nursing care plans incorporate safety, monitoring of the client, and control of operative resources along with considerations of the individual needs of each client.

MAINTAIN SAFETY AND PREVENT INJURY

Safety is a major consideration in the perioperative nursing. Using data gathered from the preoperative assessment, the nurse implements care individually designed for each client. This care includes positioning, controlling equipment and supplies, maintaining surgical asepsis, monitoring the physiologic status, and monitoring for potential emergencies.

Position the Client

Procedures vary among institutions, but after admission to the operating room the client is identified and then moved to the operating room bed. At this time, the client is anesthetized and positioned, and the skin is prepared and any other procedures that must be completed before draping and creating the sterile field (such as catheterization or shaving) are done. The perioperative nurse understands the various operative positions as well as the physiologic changes that occur when a client is placed in a specific position. Table 15–11 reviews these positions and the changes that may occur. Essential factors to consider in positioning a client on the operating table are (1) the site of the operation, (2) the age and size of the client, (3) the type of anesthetic used, and (4) pain normally experienced by the client on movement, such as that due to arthritis. The position must not hinder respiration or circulation, must not apply excessive pressure to skin surfaces, and must not limit surgical exposure. The following surgical positions are shown in Figure 15–6:

- *Dorsal recumbent (supine).* Commonly used for coronary artery bypass grafting hernia repair, mastectomy, or bowel resection
- *Trendelenburg.* Permits displacement of the intestines into the upper abdomen and is often used during surgery of the lower abdomen or pelvis
- *Lithotomy.* Exposes the perineal and rectal areas and is ideal for vaginal repairs, dilation and curettage, and most types of rectal surgery
- *Lateral.* Used for clients undergoing kidney, chest, or hip surgery

Many other positions can be used, depending on the type of surgery and the visualization of the site required by the surgeon. Laser techniques, endoscopy, or biopsy all may require different client positioning. Interventions may include gathering special supplies that can accommodate an obese client, arranging for an appropriate operating table to withstand excess weight, and providing extra padding to assist in skin integrity maintenance. Additional padding is applied to the operating table for the very thin client or the client with kyphosis.

Whatever the client's position on the operating table, there are general guidelines to promote safety. Most clients feel stiff and sore after a long surgical procedure and may actually complain of the effects of positioning.

Provide Equipment Safety

Almost everything in the operating room can be a source of injury if careful control is not exercised. Every action is designated to prevent accidents. These procedures include counting surgical supplies and equipment that could inadvertently be left inside the surgical incision, such as needles, sponges, and instruments. Counts are performed by two people, usually the circulating nurse and the scrub person, at three different times before the initial incision, during the surgery, and immediately before the incision is closed. A final correct count is announced to the surgeon and charted on the intraoperative chart.

Electrical safety is also controlled during surgery. All plugs and wires are inspected for correct attachment; all equipment is checked to ensure that it is in working order; and measures are taken to prevent electrical burns

TABLE 15–11 GUIDELINES FOR POSITIONING THE CLIENT DURING SURGERY

Nursing Action	Rationale
Explain to the client, in simple, understandable terms, why the positions and restraints are necessary.	Some clients feel that retraining straps are punitive. Some positions can be difficult or embarrassing.
Preserve the client's dignity and avoid undue exposure.	To promote a positive feeling that will encourage healing.
Place restraining straps 2 inches above the knees.	Most secure position on operating bed. Avoids pressure injury from strap on bony prominences.
Nerves, muscles, pressure points and bony prominences are padded.	To prevent nerve and tissue damage; decrease pressure that will impair or slow circulation; prevent pressure sores during long surgical procedures.
Position the client to obtain or maintain adequate respiratory exchange and vascular circulation.	To ensure tissue perfusion, oxygenation, and minimize the pooling of blood. Slow blood flow predisposes to thrombus formation.
Avoid pressure on the chest and on body parts such as the female breast and male genitalia.	Prevent injury and minimize discomfort after surgery.
Do not allow the client's extremities to dangle over the sides of the table.	Hands or feet can be inadvertently compressed against the operating room bed by surgery team personnel as they lean over the client's body. Impairment of circulation or nerve and muscle damage may result.
When using an armboard, do not abduct the upper extremity more than 90 degrees.	Hyperextension can result in permanent nerve damage caused by stretching or crushing the brachial plexus between the first rib and scapula.
Avoid excessive strain on the client's muscles.	Postoperative strain and discomfort may result.
Be certain that the client's ankles are not crossed when in the prone position.	Circulation may be occluded.
Always move both lower extremities at the same time when putting them up in stirrups and when lowering.	Hip joint could be dislocated or the muscles strained when extremities are positioned one at a time.
Monitor the total position throughout surgery.	Remember, the client may remain in one position for hours.

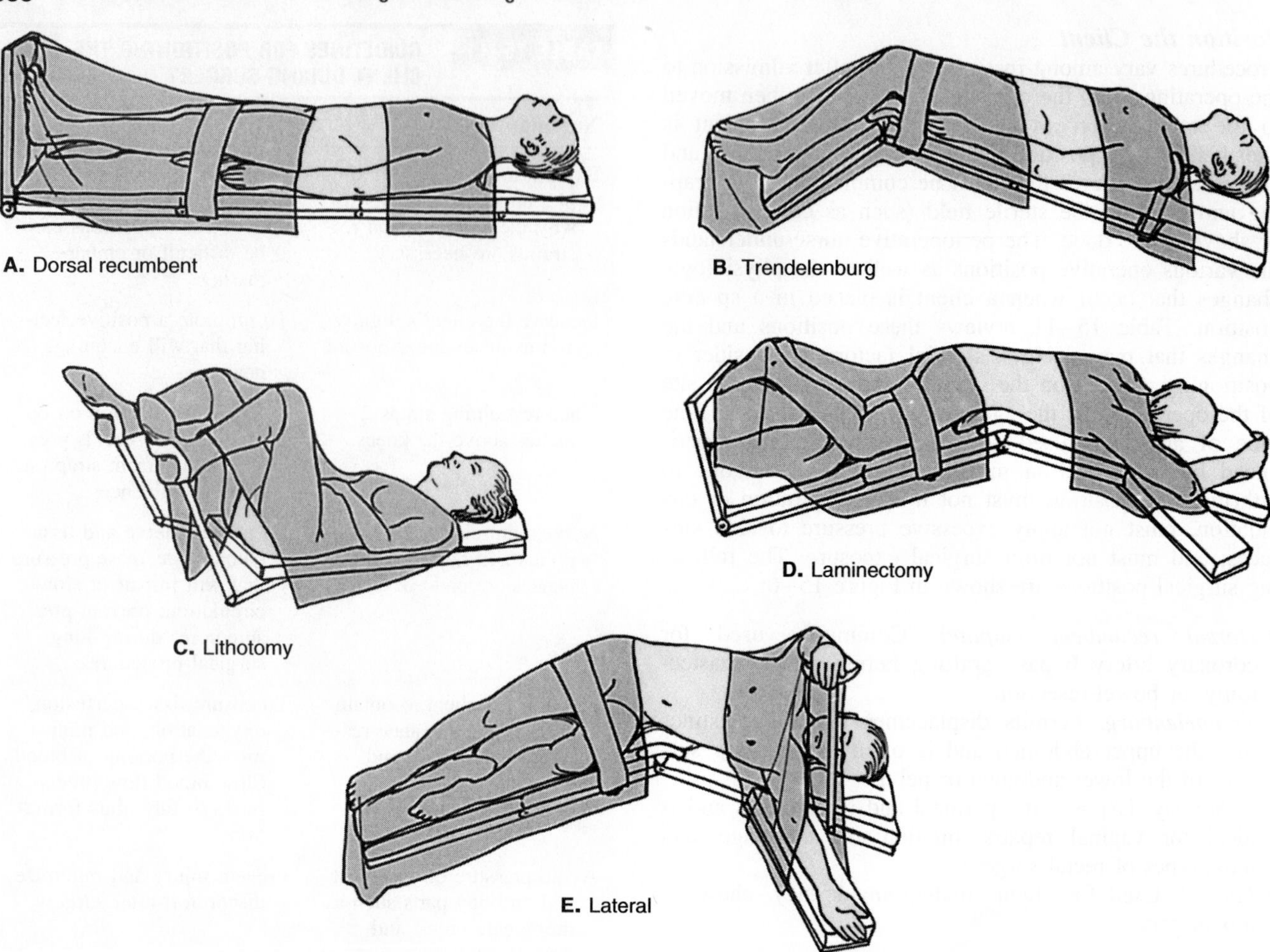

FIGURE 15–6 *A–E,* Five surgical positions.

to the client. An *electrosurgical unit* (ESU) is used to sear the ends of capillaries and blood vessels to control bleeding during surgery. When unipolar cautery is used, place a grounding pad on a large body surface area (thigh or back) to "ground" the client and to prevent sparking and burns. Grounding pads must be placed over intact skin, away from any bony prominences and not over scars or fragile tissue. Many ESUs have a safety feature that does not allow the unit to work if the grounding pad is placed inappropriately. Bipolar cautery does not require a grounding pad.

Maintain Surgical Asepsis

The perioperative nurse ensures the sterility of supplies and equipment. All members of the health care team use sterile technique. If a suspected or actual break in the sterile field occurs, the contaminated instruments and clothing are removed and replaced with new, sterile items. Members of the surgical team who are in the "sterile area" are those actively performing or assisting in the surgical procedure. They include the surgeon and the assistants and the scrub personnel. The circulating nurse is not sterile and monitors the sterile field to maintain sterility of supplies and personnel. Surgical asepsis may be broken but must be immediately rectified. The nurse is the advocate of the client in maintaining a sterile surgical environment.

Assist with Wound Closure

After final counts are completed, the nurse anticipates the type of wound closure needed and obtains the supplies for the surgical team. The surgical wound may be closed with sutures, staples, or other materials or may be left open to heal by secondary intention. Common skin closures are illustrated in Figure 15–7. A drain is placed in a separate small incision parallel to the operative incisions to drain blood or serum from the operative site. The use of a surgical drain promotes wound healing and decreases the potential for infection. There are many types of surgical drains. The drain is chosen by surgeon preference and is based on the size of the wound and the type of drainage expected. Drains may be free-draining, attached to suction apparatus, or self-contained with suction. The intraoperative nurse and the postoperative nurse are responsible for assessing that the drainage is flowing freely through the system. When the client is transferred out of the operative area, the responsible nurse continues to monitor the patency of the drain and the characteristics of the drainage.

MONITORING

Monitor Body Temperature

Hypothermia can occur easily in the operating room. The operating room temperature is maintained at a standard cool level of 60° to 75° F. Humidity is regulated at 50%

to 60%. Temperature control is set to allow optimal performance of the surgical team members, who must wear layers of clothing, and to inhibit bacterial growth. The client can become cold in the operating room if appropriate covering is not provided. Heat is lost from the skin and from the area open for surgery. When tissues that are not covered with skin are exposed to the air, heat loss is greater than normal. The client should be kept as warm as possible to minimize heat loss without causing vasodilatation, which may cause more bleeding. Most operating rooms have a cabinet that warms blankets, and unless the surgical procedure requires cooling, the nurse should offer the client a blanket immediately upon transfer to the operating room bed. Some surgery centers allow the client to wear booties or socks during the operation to provide as much comfort as possible. The intraoperative nurse reports the lowest core body temperature to the postoperative nurse when transferring the client after surgery. Thermia blankets can also be used; these blow warm air over the client's body during the procedure. IV solutions can be warmed to assist in maintaining a warm body temperature during the operative procedure as well.

Certain operations require a hypothermic patient. Cooling of the body reduces the metabolic rate, which protects the brain and other organs during the surgical procedures. Constant monitoring of the core body temperature is needed, and the nurse assists the anesthesia provider in this activity.

At other times a warm operating room is needed. A warm room is preferred for surgery for large body burns, for replantation, or for surgery in infants. Because of immature internal temperature controls, the infant's body temperature quickly equilibrates with the temperature of the room. Thus, room temperatures can be in the 90s. Hyperthermia can be a problem for the surgical team member who has adapted to the cool temperatures over time. If weakness, faintness, or nausea develops, the team member must leave the room at once.

Monitor for Emergencies

The perioperative nurse must be alert for potential emergencies. When these occur, knowledge, instant decision-making, and critical thinking are essential, as is speed in performing needed skills. Although almost any imaginable emergency can occur during an operation, the most common are malignant hyperthermia, cardiac or respiratory arrest, uncontrollable hemorrhage, and drug or allergic reactions.

MALIGNANT HYPERTHERMIA. Malignant hyperthermia is a genetic disorder characterized by uncontrolled skeletal muscle contraction leading to potentially fatal hyperthermia. It occurs in predisposed clients when they

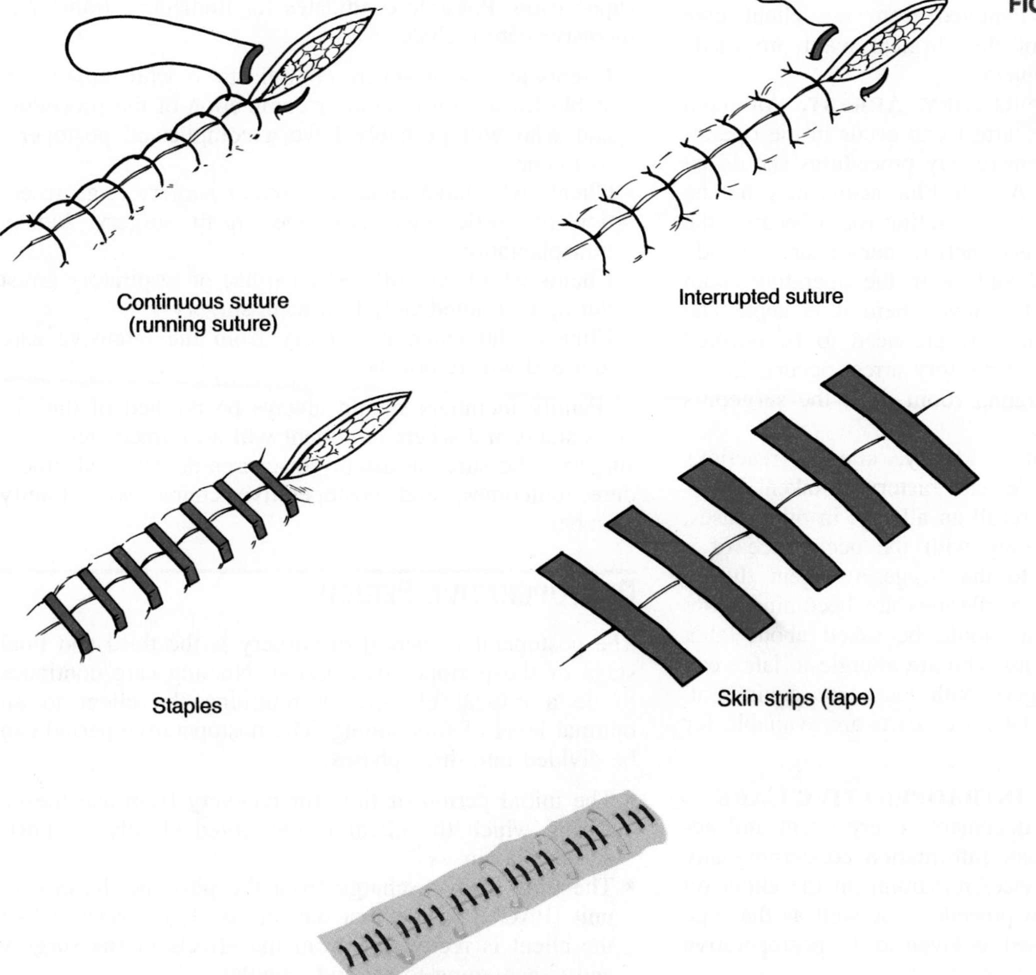

FIGURE 15–7 Skin closures.

receive a combination of succinylcholine and inhalation agents (especially halothane). Unless the triggering event is stopped and the body is cooled, death is the result. This condition can occur within 30 minutes of anesthesia induction or several hours after surgery. The initial manifestation is increased end-tidal carbon dicxide, masseter muscle rigidity, cardiac dysrhythmias, and a hypermetabolic state. The client's fever can rise to as high as 109° F (43° C).

Everyone in the operating room must know the protocol for treatment of malignant hyperthermia. Medications for the emergency treatment of malignant hyperthermia cart should be in the operating room suite. Nurses must know where the cart is and the procedure to follow if this event occurs. Datrolene, a skeletal muscle relaxant, is used to decrease skeletal muscle rigidity. The nurse must know how to reconstitute this drug, supplied as a powder, and must be capable of assisting the surgeon or anesthesia personnel with its administration and with any other treatments needed to save the client's life.

There is a screening test for malignant hyperthermia. A muscle biopsy specimen must be taken from the vastus lateralis or abdominal rectus muscle and sent to a malignant hyperthermia laboratory for testing. This test is very expensive. A diagnosis of malignant hyperthermia can be made if there is any personal or family history of anesthesia problems. High-risk clients or those with a history of malignant hyperthermia can successfully undergo surgery if the condition is known. The triggering drugs and conditions are carefully removed from the client care plan, and all members of the surgical team are made aware of the potential problem.

Cardiac and Respiratory Arrest. Although rare, cardiac or respiratory arrest can occur in the operating room, and the same emergency procedures should be carried out as elsewhere. A code blue status may not be called when a client is in the operating room because the key people (physician, anesthetist, nurse) are already present. The crash cart should be in the operating room suite, and everyone should know where it is kept. The nurse manager and any key people need to be notified immediately if cardiac or respiratory arrest occurs. In the case of death in the operating room, it is the surgeon's duty to talk to the family.

Allergic Reactions. Ideally, allergic reactions should not occur if an adequate history is taken. However, some clients do not recall an allergy; in other cases, the allergy is identified only with the occurrence of a second allergic reaction to the triggering agent during surgery. For example, latex allergies are becoming more frequent, and every client should be asked about latex sensitivity or allergy. Clients who are allergic to latex can successfully undergo surgery with latex-free equipment. In many surgery centers, latex-free carts are available for such situations.

Documentation of Intraoperative Care

The intraoperative nurse documents every event and action in the operating room. Information concerning any drains, tubes, or other devices remaining in the client on completion of the surgical procedure, as well as the type of closure and dressing used, is given to the postoperative care nurse upon transfer.

Moving and Transporting the Client

On completion of the operation, a member of the surgical team wipes off any excess blood, skin preparation, and debris from the client's skin and puts a clean gown and blanket on the client. There should always be enough personnel for moving or transferring a client postoperatively to prevent injuries. Avoid rapid movements when changing the client's position because it can predispose the development of hypotension. In particular, move the client gradually from whatever surgical position was used onto the transportation cart. During emergence (revival) from anesthesia, the client is prone to nausea, confusion, and hypotension. Care must be taken not to catch, kink, or dislodge IV or catheter tubing, drains, or other equipment during the transfer. During transfer to the bed or stretcher, the client's modesty must be maintained. Avoid rough handling, which may damage fragile skin.

After being placed on the stretcher, the client is covered with warm blankets and secured with a safety belt. Make sure that the side rails of the stretcher are up to ensure the client's safety in case the client becomes agitated during transport from the operating room. The anesthesia care provider, as well as another member of the operating room professional staff, and sometimes the surgeon or the assistant accompany the client to the postoperative care unit.

In some hospitals, certain clients are transferred directly from the operating room to the intensive care unit (ICU) for continued specialized care and constant nursing supervision. Possible candidates for immediate transfer to intensive care include:

- Clients at risk of severe complications who remain unstable for a long time after completion of the procedure and who will probably have a complicated postoperative course
- Clients who have undergone major surgery (e.g., resection of aortic aneurysm, open heart surgery, kidney transplantation)
- Clients who have suffered a cardiac or respiratory arrest during or immediately following surgery
- Clients who came to surgery from the intensive care unit and will return there

Family members should always be notified of the client's status and where the client will go immediately after surgery. The surgeon usually discusses the surgical procedure, outcomes, and postoperative course with family members.

Postoperative Period

The postoperative period of surgery is the third and final stage of the perioperative period. Nursing care continues to be a critical element in returning the client to an optimal level of functioning. The postoperative period can be divided into three phases.

- The initial period of time for recovery from anesthesia, during which the client is monitored closely by post-anesthesia nurses
- The time from discharge from the post-anesthesia care unit (PACU) to the first day or so after surgery while the client is recovering from the effects of the surgery and is beginning to eat and ambulate

- The postoperative phase, the time of healing, which may last for weeks, months, or even years after surgery

There is certainly an overlap of these phases, but in the following discussion they are dealt with separately.

POST-ANESTHESIA CARE UNIT NURSING

The goal of post-anesthesia nursing is to assist a noncomplicated return to safe physiologic function after an anesthetic procedure by providing safe, knowledgeable, individualized nursing care for clients and their family members in the immediate post-anesthesia phase. The immediate post-anesthesia period is a critical time for the client. Close and constant observation is essential. The client's vital physiologic functions must be supported until the effects of the anesthetic agents abate. Until then, the client is dependent and drowsy and may be unable to call for assistance. Equipment commonly used in PACU nursing care is listed in Box 15–5.

The client is received in the PACU on a bed or a stretcher, where he or she remains, or is transferred to another bed or to a recovery chair. Proper positioning of a sedated, unconscious, or semiconscious client must ensure airway patency. For an unconscious adult patient, extend the neck and thrust the jaw forward (Fig. 15–8). The position may depend on the surgery performed. The preferred position is the lateral Sims position, because side-lying allows the client's tongue to fall forward and mucus or vomitus to drain from the mouth. Regardless of the position used, carefully monitor the client's respiratory status. Suction equipment must be ready to suction vomit or oral secretions.

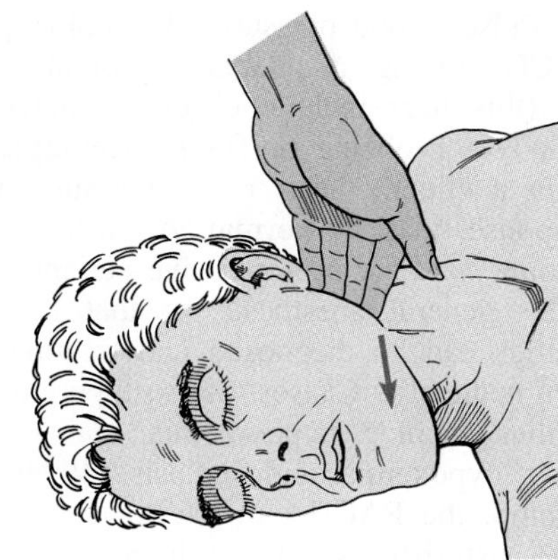

FIGURE 15–8 So that the jaw can be moved forward after anesthesia, the operator's fingers are placed behind the angle of the jaw. As the jaw is moved, the tongue comes forward, opening the airway.

After the client has been positioned safely and has been determined to be stable, the nurse receives a verbal, detailed report of events from members of the operating room team (Box 15–6). The PACU nurse reviews the client's record with the anesthesia provider present, noting specifically (1) the anesthesia record for IV medications and blood received during surgery and (2) the length of time the client was in surgery. Ideally, a preoperative nursing assessment and nursing history are available in the record for comparison with the postoperative assessment.

IMMEDIATE ASSESSMENTS IN THE POST-ANESTHESIA CARE UNIT

After the transfer report from the operating room, the PACU nurse performs an assessment. The ABCs (airway, breathing, and circulation) are critical and must be assessed first. Included in the assessment are the following:

Airway: Patency; presence of tubes and respiratory assistance devices.

Breathing: Respiration rate and depth; presence of bilateral breath sounds, stridor, wheezes, hoarseness, or decreased breath sounds. Stay at the bedside until the client's gag reflex returns.

BOX 15–5 Equipment Used in the Post-Anesthesia Care Unit (PACU)

The PACU nurse prepares and checks the function of the following equipment:

- Sphygmomanometer or automatic blood pressure monitor
- Pulse oximeter—a noninvasive device that measures oxygen saturation of arterial blood and the pulse rate; provides warning of hypoxemia
- Stethoscope—to auscultate breath sounds and blood pressure
- Cardiac monitor and electrodes
- Intravenous equipment (e.g., insertion equipment, fluids, tubing, infusion pumps)
- Suction equipment (e.g., catheters, sterile saline, sterile gloves)
- Supplies to support respiration (e.g., artificial airways, oxygen, tongue depressors, oxygen tubing with masks and cannulas, intubation equipment, and anesthesia machine)
- Medications (e.g., narcotics, narcotic antagonists, hypnotics, antihypertensives, neuromuscular blocking agents)
- Emesis basin, mouth wipes, urinals, bedpans
- Thermometers—oral, rectal, and tympanic membrane types
- Warmed blankets or electric warming units to maintain body temperature
- Emergency cart containing appropriate equipment and medications—drugs including cardiotonics, vasotonics, and respiratory agents; a tracheostomy tray; endotracheal tubes; a defibrillator; a cutdown tray; a ventilator; gastric suction equipment; and chest tube insertion equipment

BOX 15–6 Information Given to the Post-Anesthesia Care Unit Nurse by the Perioperative Team

- Operative procedure performed
- Medical diagnosis, pertinent medical history, and daily medications
- Vital signs
- Blood loss, fluid replacements
- Urine output and presence of bladder catheters
- Anything eventful or complications during surgery
- Anesthetic agents, narcotics, neuromuscular blocking agents, or antibiotics
- Drains inserted and their locations and purpose
- Physician orders to be carried out immediately

Circulation: Pulse, blood pressure, skin color, pulse oximeter, ECG tracing if attached, wound status and dressings (this may include checking underneath the client's body for oozing or frank bleeding). A slight increase in a client's heart rate after surgery, due to stress response, may be normal. A cardiac monitor is also recommended for postoperative patients who have been under general anesthesia so that heart rhythm abnormalities can be diagnosed and treatment can be started immediately. Causes of postoperative cardiac dysrhythmias include hypovolemia, pain, electrolyte imbalances, hypoxemia, and acidosis. When dysrhythmias develop, the PACU nurse follows facility protocols if the disturbances are life-threatening and monitors the client's blood pressure, oxygen saturation, and ventilation.

Other: Level of consciousness, muscle strength, ability to follow commands, IV infusions, dressings, drains, and special equipment, tubes, and drains that must be immediately attached to containers or suction, reddened or bruised areas on skin unrelated to surgery (inspect pressure points and tape and skin preparation sites; look for signs of cautery or thermal burns), temperature (assist client to regain normal core body temperature or anticipate complications).

After receiving the admission report and review of the client's record, the PACU nurse documents all observations. Most PACUs use a flow-type method of charting, which includes a numerical rating scale measuring clients' respirations, level of consciousness, ability to move, body temperature or skin color, and blood pressure (see Fig. 15–9). As the client recovers from the anesthesia, the rating improves to a top score of 10.

NURSING DIAGNOSES

Nursing diagnoses most common during this period of care are *Risk for Injury, Hypothermia, Risk for Aspiration, Pain,* and *Altered Thought Processes.* Most common potential complications are respiratory problems, hypovolemia or hypervolemia, hemorrhage, and cardiac problems.

NURSING CARE IN THE POST-ANESTHESIA CARE UNIT

Protect the Airway

One major complication that occurs in the PACU is airway obstruction or hypoventilation. The primary nursing intervention to protect the airway is positioning the head of a minimally responsive client turned to the side with the chin extended forward to prevent respiratory obstruction. The client who is unable to clear mucus or vomitus from the throat requires suctioning immediately.

An oral or nasal airway may be in place to help maintain patency and control the tongue. The airway is a hollow rubber or plastic tube. It is inserted through the nose or mouth and passes over the base of the tongue to keep the tongue from falling back into the throat and obstructing the anatomic airway (Fig. 15–10). Airways should not be taped in place. When clients awaken and the gag reflex returns, they may spit out the airway. The PACU nurse may also remove the airway for the responsive client who is unable to remove it unassisted. Left in place too long, it can irritate the tissue, stimulate vomiting, or cause laryngospasm.

When the client is extubated, observe for the development of crowing respirations. The client may be experiencing laryngospasm. If this problem develops, the client could progress to respiratory arrest. Immediately try to ventilate the client using a face mask oxygen delivery system, securing a tight fit over the mouth and nose. The use of positive pressure sometimes alleviates the laryngospasm. If the spasm does not abate, succinylcholine is given to temporarily paralyze the voluntary muscles, including the muscles that control respiration. Respiration must be supported by mechanical means (i.e., a ventilator) when muscle relaxants are used. Respiration in clients who have received muscle relaxants must be closely monitored for at least 1 hour after the relaxants appear to have worn off because of the possibility of paralysis reoccurrence. Some clients remain intubated and ventilated, such as those who have undergone open heart surgery. They require close monitoring and intermittent suctioning.

The nurse also consults with the surgeon and the anesthesia provider and administers prescribed medications as needed. Interventions may also include the continued administration of oxygen, positive-pressure airway support, and use of reversal medications. Reversal agents such as naloxone (Narcan) are administered to reverse the respiratory depression from narcotics. Neostigmine with glycopyrrolate (Robinul) is given to reverse the effect of some neuromuscular blocking agents. Most clients receive oxygen. The rate flow of oxygen should be closely checked against physician orders. This may be administered by a respiratory therapist, but the nurse is responsible for assessment and monitoring of treatment. Oxygen levels will vary, depending on the method of delivery, such as nasal canula, simple face masks, or more controlled methods. Flow rates vary from 2 to 15 L/min with a positive pressure mask. Clients with COPD receive no more than 20%/2 L.

Maintain Normal Blood Pressure

Postoperative hypotension can have numerous causes, including inadequate ventilation, side effects of anesthetic agents or preoperative medications, rapid position change, pain, fluid or blood loss, and peripheral pooling of blood after regional anesthesia. A drop in blood pressure slightly below a client's preoperative baseline reading is common after surgery. However, a significant drop in blood pressure, accompanied by an increased heart rate, may indicate hemorrhage, circulatory failure, or fluid shifts. Do not diagnose impending hypovolemic shock on the basis of one low blood pressure reading. If you are concerned about a dropping blood pressure, measure pressure, every 5 minutes for 15 minutes to determine the variability. Decreased blood pressure can also mean that the anesthesia is wearing off or that the client is experiencing severe pain.

In addition to hypotension, manifestations of shock include tachycardia, restlessness and apprehension, and cold, moist, pale or cyanotic skin. When a client appears to be going into shock, the PACU nurse intervenes as follows: (1) administering oxygen or increasing its rate of delivery, (2) raising the client's legs above the level of the heart, (3) increasing the rate of IV fluids (unless contraindicated because of fluid excretion problems), (4) notifying the anesthesia provider and the surgeon, (5)

NHS NEBRASKA HEALTH SYSTEM
CLARKSON HOSPITAL • UNIVERSITY HOSPITAL
A Partner with University of Nebraska Medical Center

Patient Identification (Stamp)

NAME

REG. NO.

LOCATION

DATE

NURSING NOTES:

Nurse Signatures	Nurse Initials

ALDRETESCORE▲	Baseline		Post Recovery
Time			
ACTIVITY Able to move four extremities voluntarily or on command. .... 2 Able to move two extremities voluntarily or on command. .... 1 Unable to move extremities voluntarily or on command. 0			
RESPIRATION Able to deep breathe and cough freely. .... 2 Dyspnea or limited breathing. .... 1 Apneic 0			
CIRCULATION Baseline BP .... ____ Systolic BP +/-20% of preanesthetic level. .... 2 Systolic BP +/-20-49% of preanesthetic level. .... 1 Systolic BP +/-50% of preanesthetic level. 0			
CONSCIOUSNESS Fully awake. .... 2 Arousable on calling. .... 1 Unresponsive. 0			
OXYGENATION Able to maintain O2 saturation > 92% on room air. .... 2 Needs O2 inhalation to maintain saturation > 90%. .... 1 O2 saturation < 90% even with O2 supplement. 0			
TOTAL			

▲Aldrete, J.A. & Kroulik, D.J., *Clinical Anesthesia*, Vol. 7, Feb. 1995 and *Anesthesia & Analgesia*, Vol. 49, No. 6, 1970

Potential alteration in fluid volume and/or urinary elimination
Expected outcome: Maintains fluid levels

INTAKE	
IV	
Oral	
TOTAL:	

OUTPUT	
Urine	
Drain	
TOTAL:	

	On	Off
Sequential Stockings		
Support hose		
Ice		

☐ See extended Outpatient Flowsheet

IV DC'd at ____________

CATHETER TIP INTACT? ☐ YES ☐ NO

Narcotic Waste____ mgs of ______ #1 ______ #2 ______

Potential for Knowledge Deficit: Expected Outcome: Patient or Significant Other will Verbalize Understanding of Instructions.

DISCHARGE CRITERIA	N/A
☐ RX GIVEN AND EXPLAINED.	☐
☐ VITAL SIGNS STABLE ________	☐
☐ NAUSEA, VOMITING, DIZZINESS MINIMAL	☐
☐ POST ANESTHESIA RECOVERY SCORE 9-10	☐
☐ SWALLOW, COUGH AND GAG REFLEX PRESENT	☐
☐ ABSENCE OF RESPIRATORY DISTRESS	☐
☐ DRESSING CHECKED C̄ MINIMAL DRAINAGE	☐
☐ RESPONSIBLE ADULT PRESENT TO ESCORT HOME	☐
☐ ALERT AND ORIENTED	☐
☐ PAIN CONTROLLED	☐

Time discharged ________ per ____________

Accompanied by ____________

Postoperative Phone Call:

Phone Number: ____________ Date: ______ Time: ______

	Yes	No	
			☐ message left
Drsg dry/intact	☐	☐	Unsuccessful Attempts: ______
Nausea/Vomiting	☐	☐	Spoke With: ______
Pain	☐	☐	
Swelling	☐	☐	
Fever	☐	☐	
Voiding easily	☐	☐	☐ Unable to reach, chart returned to MR
Surgeon/Anes. Contacted	☐	☐	

Completed by ____________ RN

NHS-914 (6/99)

OUTPATIENT PACU FLOWSHEET

PROCEDURES TAB

FIGURE 15–9 Post-Anesthesia care unit (PACU) documentation. (Courtesy of Nebraska Health Systems, Omaha, NE.)

providing medications as ordered, and (6) continuing to assess the client and response to interventions.

Hypertension may also develop. Older adults with a history of hypertension may exhibit hypertensive episodes after the stress of surgery. If the blood pressure rises above the baseline, the PACU nurse should consult with the anesthesia provider or the surgeon and administer antihypertensive medication as ordered.

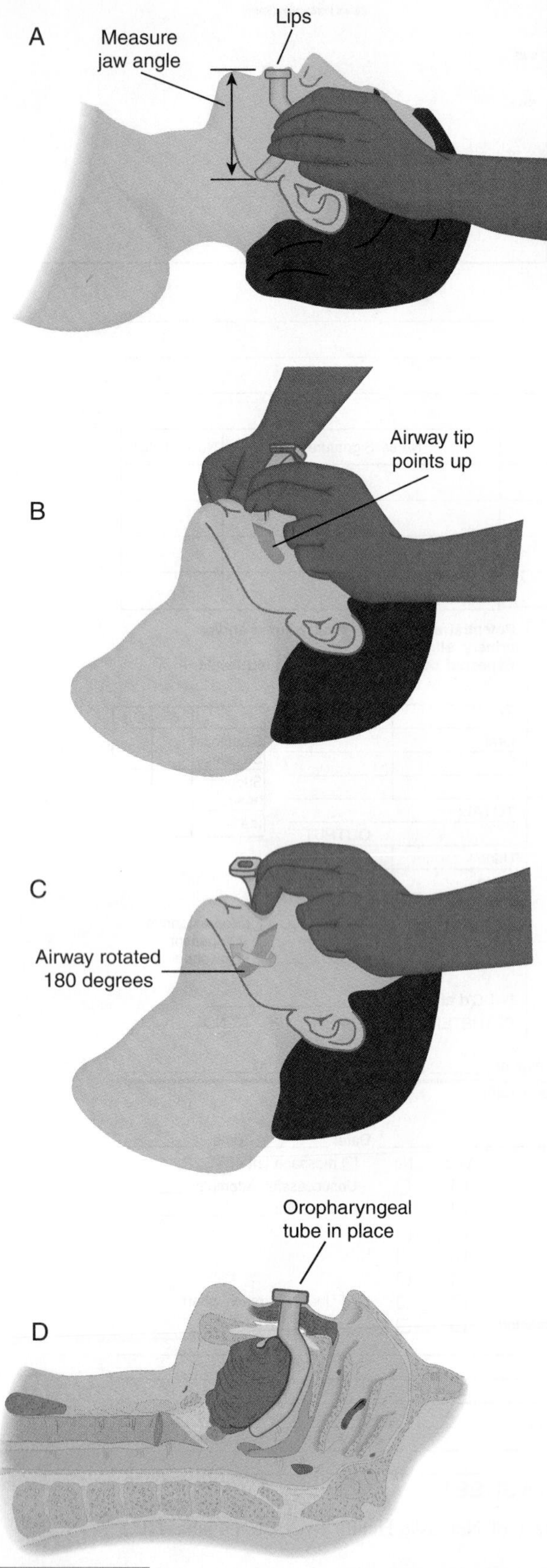

FIGURE 15–10 Artificial airway. The flattened, hollow tube prevents the tongue from falling back and occluding the natural airway.

Monitor for Return of Consciousness

The PACU nurse monitors the level of consciousness. Orientation to person is the first cognitive response to return after anesthesia. Level of orientation is assessed by noting whether the client responds to his or her name. Be certain that a client who normally wears hearing aids has them in place and turned on before you attempt to talk to the client. Orientation to place is also an important indication of postoperative return of cognitive function. Because of confusion from anesthesia and analgesia medications, the client is usually not oriented to time until after the nurse provides this information. Assessment of returning cognitive functioning includes the ability to remember facts after being told. Older adults and clients with liver or kidney impairment may take longer to regain orientation. Postoperative delirium may occur with some procedures, such as open heart surgery; therefore, do not assume that aberrations are due to age-related "senility." Rather, check the present cognitive status against that noted in the preoperative assessment to gain a truer picture of the client's level of consciousness and cognition.

Assess for Return of Sensation and Motion

In the PACU, the client is monitored carefully for return of sensation as the anesthetic agent wears off. Check return of motion to the extremities by asking clients to wiggle their toes. However, the ability to move the toes may not indicate complete recovery if client had spinal anesthesia. In such cases, the toe movement signifies that the motor blockade is wearing off, but blockade of the autonomic nervous system may still be present. Clients who are still experiencing autonomic blockade are prone to hypotension despite the presence of ability to move their toes and extremities.

Assess for Normothermia

The client in the PACU is monitored for temperature and vital signs every 15 minutes until vital signs are stable, or more often if they are unstable. The frequency of monitoring and length of time over which monitoring must be done are dictated by facility PACU policy. Clients are monitored until they are discharged from the PACU. This is usually at least 1 hour. Clients must have a minimum temperature of greater than 96.8° F (36° C) before they are discharged from the PACU. The heat loss that occurs in the operating room can continue in the PACU if the client is not warmed sufficiently. Warming requires the maintenance of temperature without overwarming and causing excessive vasodilatation, which can cause fluid shifts and a decrease in blood pressure. The PACU nurse must also realize that malignant hyperthermia can also occur in the PACU and should repeatedly assess for manifestations of this condition.

Assess Perfusion

Assessment of skin color, warmth, and turgor provides evidence of tissue perfusion. Verify skin color in clients with dark or brown skin with another nurse to avoid making incorrect assumptions. Dusky, pale, cold, moist skin is an important assessment finding that may be a manifestation of shock. Because it is not possible to detect systemic conditions by skin color alone, assessment should include other pertinent data. For example, when impending shock is suspected, check the client's blood pressure, and inspect the lips and nails as well as the skin to detect pallor or cyanosis. Consider these findings in relation to oxygen saturation and hemoglobin before assuming a diagnosis of shock.

Assess the Surgical Site

Check the dressing over the surgical incision frequently. If it is soiled, note the color, type, and amount of drainage. Reinforce the dressing, but do not change it or open it without a physician's order. If seepage is noted, draw an outline of the fluid on the dressing and note the date and time. If oozing continues, the estimation of the amount can be more easily determined by areas outside the previously marked borders. Sometimes bleeding is present but not visible on dressings. If bleeding is suspected, look for blood under the operated leg, or under the back, that may have leaked downward out of sight.

Promote Fluid and Electrolyte Balance

Assess intake and output hourly. Monitor all parenteral fluids to ensure that the proper amount and type of fluids are being infused. Intake can include solutions of IV fluids, medications, blood products, nutritional support, and colloid infusions. Check the amount of solution in the IV bottle on admission of the client to the PACU along with the rate of infusion. All types of delivery systems and lines must be considered: pumps, infusion machines, monitoring machines, IV lines, central venous lines, and arterial lines. Check the insertion sites for redness, soreness, and swelling, as these may be indications of infiltration. Note medications that have been added to solutions, so that when the next dose is ready to be infused a new bag of dilution fluid is present. This procedure ensures that there is no lapse in administration of ordered fluids or medications.

Changes in renal function and fluid and electrolyte balance may develop soon after surgery. The stress response to surgery stimulates the secretion of antidiuretic hormone (ADH) and aldosterone, which cause fluid retention. Until the stress subsides, urine volume decreases regardless of fluid intake. Avoid fluid overload while maintaining the client's blood pressure, cardiac output, and urinary output. If an indwelling bladder catheter is present, document the amount of output and compare it with the amount of input via IV fluids.

Manage Drainage Systems

Drainage tubes, such as a T-tube, gastric tube, urinary catheter, or wound drains, must be constantly monitored. For example, urinary catheters and T-tubes are unclamped and attached to gravity drainage systems. Gastric, chest, and intestinal tubes are attached to wall suction. Wound drainage systems are attached to self-contained suction devices. The PACU nurse must ensure that tubes are patent and draining freely. Check that there are no kinks in the tubes and that they are not occluded. Document the amount and characters of drainage on a regular schedule. Compare the type and amount of drainage with those expected for the surgical procedure.

Promote Comfort

Pain is an expected outcome postoperatively, yet one of the most frequent postoperative problems is inadequate analgesic administration. You must carefully and regularly assess the client's level of pain. Pain may be caused by a factor unrelated to the surgical procedure, such as poor positioning. The discomfort of a full bladder can imitate abdominal pain even when appropriate doses of pain medication have been administered. Provide appropriate pain relief while not overmedicating. If there is any problem in making the postoperative client comfortable, call the anesthesia provider or surgeon to minimize the time the client is in pain.

Maintain Safety

Continue to be the client's advocate, and protect the client from injury that may be caused by equipment, medication, and postoperative risks. Side rails must remain in the up position to protect the client from falling out of the bed. Proper body alignment and frequent repositioning assist in maintaining circulation and relieve skin pressure. Postoperative equipment is checked to ensure that it is working properly before the client is received in the PACU. Place equipment in a safe location and electrical cords or lines out of the way so that they do not present a danger to the client or staff members.

DISCHARGE FROM THE POST-ANESTHESIA CARE UNIT

Common criteria for evaluating the client's readiness for discharge from the PACU are based on a general scoring system. The criteria that are scored include activity, respiration, circulation, consciousness, and skin color. A typical scoring system is shown in Box 15–7.

When the client is considered ready for discharge from the PACU, a report (via telephone or verbal) must be relayed to the receiving unit. The report must include the client's condition along with a summary of details of the operative procedure and events that may affect client care. Thorough documentation of the client's progress in the PACU is included in the client's permanent medical record and is an important source of information for use in providing appropriate care. If for some reason the client is to have an extended stay in the PACU, notify the family immediately, and explain the reasons for the prolonged stay.

"Same-day surgery" clients cannot be discharged until they are able to tolerate fluids by mouth, can ambulate with a steady gait and no orthostatic hypotension, and have voided. A responsible adult must accompany the client being discharged from the ambulatory care center. Taxi cabs are not an appropriate means of transportation after a surgical procedure. Discharge instructions include written and oral information. It is best if this information has been reviewed both preoperatively and postopera-

BOX 15–7 Criteria for Discharge from the Post-Anesthesia Care Unit (PACU)

The vital signs must be stable or at near-preoperative levels.

Each numbered entity is scored from 0 to 3. A score of 9 or 10 usually indicates that the client is ready for transfer out of the PACU.

1. There is only moderate or light drainage from any operative site.
2. All essential postoperative care has been completed.
3. Urine output is at least 30/ml/hr for an adult.

tively. The instructions usually include information about medications, how to care for the surgical wound, the amount and type of activity that is appropriate, when and how to seek help for any problems that may arise, and when and where follow-up appointments are scheduled. The client who has had a same-day procedure is telephoned by a Registered Nurse the day after surgery to ensure that there are no complications or further questions.

■ POSTOPERATIVE NURSING CARE

After the client has been released from the PACU, the nursing assessments and interventions are similar to those performed in the PACU. The most common immediate postoperative complications are those related to spinal anesthesia and those affecting the respiratory, cardiovascular, and renal systems and fluid and electrolyte balance.

ESTABLISHMENT OF POSTOPERATIVE GOALS

At this point, the postoperative care plan is expanded and revised. The plan should include an assessment of the client's needs and goals as well as nursing interventions. Nursing diagnoses are used to specify and define postoperative problems and to guide the plan of nursing care. Findings on the preoperative assessment constitute a very important body of information at this time because the findings can be used as baseline values for comparison with those obtained in postoperative assessments. A general nursing care plan is presented. Specific assessment and care measures are often based upon the surgical procedure performed and the preoperative condition of the client.

ASSESSMENT OF THE POSTOPERATIVE CLIENT

Assess Respiratory Status

Assess for a patent airway. Observe the client and assess the breathing pattern at rest. Listen to sounds; breath respirations should be unlabored and quiet. As a result of effects of general anesthetic agents and narcotics, respiratory drive and depth may be reduced, leading to hypoxia. Clinical manifestations of hypoxia include restlessness, pale skin, pulse oximetry readings below 90%, and cool skin temperature. Although restlessness is an early sign of hypoxia, there may be other causes such as pain. Cyanosis is a very late manifestation of hypoxia.

A major complication following surgery may be decreased lung expansion, atelectasis (collapse of alveolar sacs), or aspiration of retained secretions. Lung assessment should include auscultation in all lobes as well as assessment of rate and rhythm of respirations. For many clients, incentive spirometry (Fig. 15–11) is prescribed to increase respiratory expansion and to open the alveoli. A body temperature of greater than 100° F (37.7 C) in the first 24 hours after surgery is frequently due to atelectasis.

Assess Circulation

Assess vital signs, skin color, and temperature according to facility protocols. Vital signs are assessed frequently (e.g., every 30 minutes). Reassure the client that this pattern of assessment is a matter of routine and does not indicate anything is wrong. Because the client has been immobile during the operation and may have experienced pressure on body parts that diminished circulation, extremities must be evaluated for weakness, circulation, and numbness. Bony prominences should be assessed for stage I pressure ulcers (see Chapter 49). Although all clients must be encouraged to get out of bed and walk as soon as possible after surgery to prevent the formation of thrombus and devastating emboli, early ambulation is especially important after surgery of the abdominal area. The aorta and femoral arteries may have been manipulated during the procedure. In addition, the client may find that the dorsal recumbent position (as in a recliner chair) is most comfortable because it reduces strain on the incision. However, this position slows venous return in the pelvis and can foster thrombus formation.

Thrombus can form in any blood vessel, and you should be especially alert to any complaints of extremity pain, unilateral edema, or warmth in the calf. If the thrombus dislodges and travels via the bloodstream, it can lodge anywhere in the body, producing emergency conditions that need to be treated immediately. It is obvious when a clot suddenly lodges in the lung, heart, or brain, but embolism in other body sites may be less apparent. Walking can nullify much of the threat of thrombus formation. However, most clients do not want to move after surgery. Leg exercises should have been taught preoperatively, and you should emphasize their importance in the prevention of thrombus formation to promote an optimal postsurgical outcome.

Assess Neurologic Status

Assess the client for level of consciousness, orientation, and lingering effects of anesthesia in the first 24 hours. In older adults, cognitive deficits may remain for days or even weeks after surgery. Compare present mental status with preoperative ability to clearly define the client's neurologic status. Medications are slower to clear through aging kidneys, and hypothermia and pain can also affect

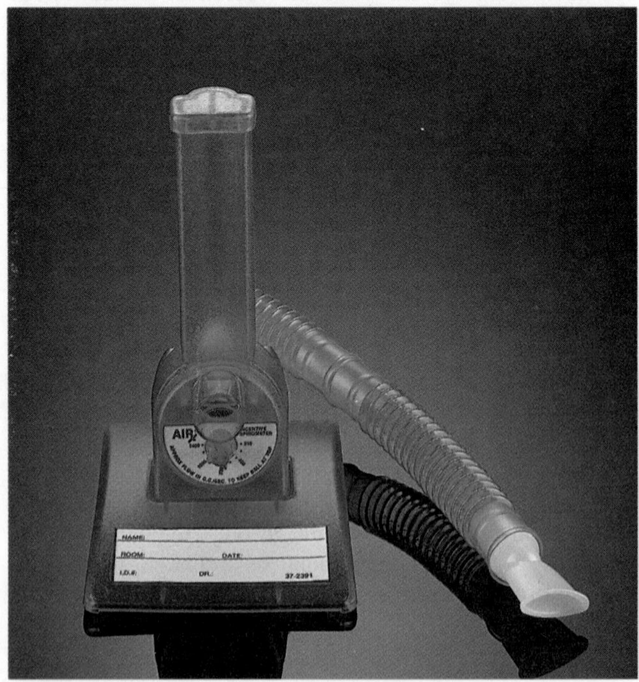

FIGURE 15–11 Use of an incentive deep-breathing exerciser promotes alveolar inflation, restores and maintains lung capacity, and strengthens the respiratory muscles. (Courtesy of Baxter Healthcare Corporation, Roond Lake, IL.)

cognition. Clients need to know that impaired cognition is to be expected—especially older clients, in whom the fear of dementia may be marked. If they are not aware that the condition is temporary, clients may believe that they have had a stroke during surgery from which they will never recover. This in turn can lead to depression with decreased coping ability. Nurses can facilitate recovery by promoting cognitive activity, repeating instructions often if needed, having patience with clients slow in recovery, and fostering hope. Document changes every shift. If a decrease in cognition appears, notify the physician immediately. Most common is the slow steady progress in return to preoperative status.

Obese clients also have a delayed return of consciousness after anesthetic procedures. Greater amounts of anesthetic agents are required for these clients. Anesthetic agents are fat-soluble, and much of the drug dose is deposited from the blood into fatty tissue. In obesity, therefore, excretion of anesthetic agents is slower because of the increased amounts of drug retained before excretion.

Monitor the Wound

Assess the dressing and the amount and character of any drainage that is present. Be alert to the method of care that the surgeon prefers. Most surgeons prefer to do the first dressing change. Some surgeons leave the original surgical dressing intact for 24 to 48 hours. Others request that the dressing be changed as it becomes soiled. If the wound is closed and left to heal by first intention, dressings on the wound may be minimal, and the client may be allowed to shower after 24 hours. If the wound healing is to be by second or third intention, then it is left open to heal from the fascia to the skin, and special wound handling must occur. Measures can include wound packing, dressings, drains, ostomy bags, and so on, depending on wound size, and location and drainage from the wound. Measure and record the amount of drainage for comparison with later assessments to guide future care plan changes (see Chapter 16).

Each client must have an individualized care plan to facilitate the most effective healing. Document the wound's appearance, drainage, and client's reports of discomfort at least every shift. If you are in doubt of how to describe the wound, it is suggested that two nurses compare observations at each change of shift.

Although it is commonplace for nurses to look at wounds, the appearance of the surgical wound is frightening to many clients. It sometimes takes days before a client can even look at the wound. Assess the client's willingness to look at the wound. Do not force the client to look at the wound until he or she is ready. Look for subtle cues—for example, the client may continue to look away from the wound while dressings are being changed. Body image is altered in response to surgery, even surgery on internal organs. Body image reintegration or restoration requires weeks or months to occur. Show acceptance of the client's appearance, and assist the client in verbalizing feelings about the postoperative appearance and the reaction of others.

If wound infection develops, the clinical manifestations appear in the wound 3 to 4 days postoperatively. Clinical manifestations include redness beyond the incision line, edema that remains after the initial swelling, increasing pain, and increased drainage. Sometimes drainage becomes purulent or foul-smelling. The client may also have fever, malaise, anorexia, and leukocytosis (increased WBC count with increased numbers of band WBCs). Notify the surgeon of any suspected wound infection. Wound cultures may be ordered to verify that organisms in the wound are sensitive to the antibiotics taken.

If collagen fibers are not mature enough to hold the incision closed without suture, the wound may open. An opening of a skin wound is called *dehiscence.* Wounds in which dehiscence has occurred are treated as open wounds—that is, they are kept clean, with application of packing or dressings and allowed to heal by secondary or tertiary intention (see Chapter 16).

If abdominal wounds become infected and the abdominal incision opens, the fascia or internal organs may be visible (Fig. 15–12). This condition is called *evisceration* and constitutes an emergency. Return the client to bed. Do not attempt to replace the organs. Cover the wound with sterile dressings moistened with normal saline. Monitor the client's vital signs, keep the client as calm as possible, and notify the surgeon immediately for emergency surgery. In many clients, evisceration is preceded by a gush of serosangineous drainage about 48 hours earlier. Notify the surgeon of this sudden increase in drainage, and plan to put an abdominal binder on the client's body for support.

Clients must learn to care for any dressing before discharge, so education must be a written intervention in the care plan on admission to the nursing unit. Training should proceed daily until the client or a family member feels comfortable with the wound care skills necessary to promote healing.

Routine care of drains and dressings can be delegated to trained unlicensed assistive personnel. See the Management and Delegation feature.

Monitor Intravenous Lines

All IV lines must be checked for patency, type of fluid to be infused, and rate. For any client with an IV line, intake and output monitoring must be completed. This is a nursing decision; although there may be a physician's routine order, none is required to monitor the client. If

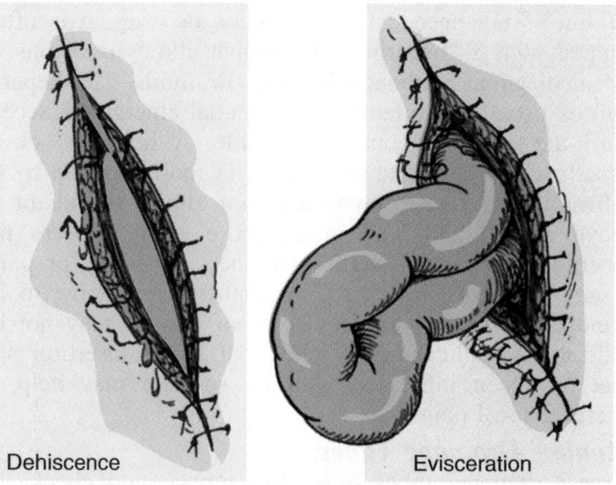

FIGURE 15–12 Clients with wound dehiscence and evisceration after surgery require immediate attention (see text).

MANAGEMENT AND DELEGATION

Postoperative Care: Dressings and Drains

The assessment and care of postoperative wounds, including drain management and dressing changes, are your responsibility. The emptying, measurement, and recording of drainage from a postoperative wound may be delegated to unlicensed assistive personnel who have demonstrated competence in performing this task; the removal and application of some dressings may also be delegated to such personnel with special training competence.

Before delegating the care of postoperative dressings and drains, consider the type of surgical procedure performed, the extent of the wound and dressing care requirements, and the nature of the drainage and type of drain present.

Drains

1. Initially, assess the quality, character, and volume of the drainage expressed via the drain. At this time, note the patency of the drain and any leakage of fluid at the drain insertion site.
2. Ensure that the drain is secured and labeled properly. Your documentation should reflect the appropriate labeling. For example, for a client having two abdominal drains (one a right upper quadrant drain and the second a midline drain) list these as such on the output record. The drains may be labeled by name or location, at the time of placement by the physician.
3. Record the volume of drainage from each drain separately unless otherwise noted by the physician.
4. Perform the irrigation of any drain as ordered.
5. Specify the frequency with which the drain is to be emptied for the assistive personnel. A frequency of every 4 hours or once per shift may be delegated, whereas you may choose to perform more frequent measurement and recording of drainage as appropriate. For example, you might best perform hourly drain emptying with subsequent intravenous (IV) fluid replacement of the volume measured, which requires an hourly adjustment in the IV infusion rate.
6. Perform the assessment for air leak at intervals throughout your shift. Chest tube drainage may be measured and recorded by assistive personnel.

Dressings

1. In many institutions, the physician changes the initial postoperative dressing.
2. Assistive personnel may perform subsequent dressing changes if the wound is closed and does not require special intervention. The physician orders the type and frequency of dressing changes.
3. Delegate the dressing change to assistive personnel after your assessment of the wound. It may also be appropriate to have the assistive personnel remove the dressing in preparation for your assessment and then reapply the dressing after you examine the wound. (*Note:* A Registered Nurse should assess any wound at least once per day, more frequently as guided by the type of wound and required intervention.)
4. Specify the type of dressing (clean or sterile) for assistive personnel.

Describe findings immediately reportable to you for the assistive personnel, including changes in the color, character, and quantity of the drainage from a drain or around a drain site. Additionally, any sign of redness, swelling, tenderness, warmth, pain, bleeding, discharge, or separation of wound edges is reportable. The finding of new drainage or blood on a postoperative dressing is immediately reportable to the Registered Nurse.

In summary, even though you have delegated the completion of these tasks, you remain responsible for assessment and evaluation of the client's postoperative wound and drains. Verify the competency of the assistive personnel in performing each of these tasks during orientation and annually thereafter.

Donna W. Markey, MSN, RN, ACNP-CS, *Clinician IV, Surgical Services, University of Virginia Health System, Charlottesville, Virginia*

there have been no complications during surgery and the IV line is not needed for medication delivery, it is often capped with a "heparin lock," which allows infusions of IV medications without additional IV fluids. The heparin lock is usually maintained for potential emergency access until the client is considered stable. A heparin lock is usually more comfortable than an IV port attached to an infusion line. It also costs less and allows the client to move around and walk much more easily. Assess the insertion site for any signs of redness, swelling, or pain. If any problems are noted, the catheter may have to be removed from the vein; replacement may or may not be indicated. Application of mild heat to an insertion site that has been infiltrated with IV solution may help to decrease local pain.

Monitor Drainage Tubes

Assess drainage tubes (e.g., NG tubes), and check the client's postoperative physician's instructions to determine whether to attach the tubes to suction or to use gravity drainage. Note the amount, color, and consistency of drainage, and document the findings. If the client has a low-suction NG tube, it must remain patent. Irrigate the tube with normal saline according to the surgeon's orders; some tubes cannot be irrigated because of increased risk of injuring internal sutures. Make sure the tube is connected to suction if ordered.

If the tube has a dual lumen and if one side is for air, do not insert medication through the air vent. Medication can easily occlude this port. If the port gurgles, do not plug the port to quiet the system. By plugging up the air vent, the suction system becomes a closed system, thereby increasing the suction on the wall of the stomach, which can cause trauma and bleeding. NG tubes inserted for decompression and removal of intestinal secretions remain in place until peristalsis begins. The removal of an NG tube requires an order by the surgeon. Assess for

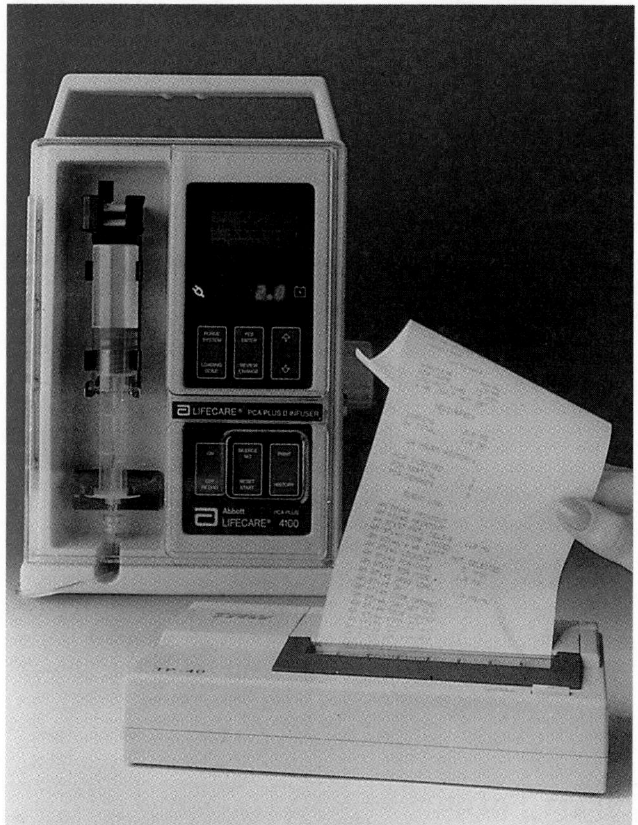

FIGURE 15–13 A patient-controlled anesthesia (PCA) device allows clients to control their own pain relief postoperatively. The printout allows the nurse to assess and record the amount of opioid analgesia. (Courtesy of Abbott Laboratories, Hospital Products Division, North Chicago, IL.)

bowel sounds, passage of flatus, and hunger as signs of peristalsis as long as the tube is in place. When peristalsis returns, the physician will probably order the NG tube to be clamped initially and then removed if the clamping was tolerated without nausea or vomiting.

Promote Comfort

All clients who have just had surgery will experience pain. Pain medication should be given when needed and before the pain becomes severe. When the "demand approach" (prn meds) is used for analgesia, it is crucial to medicate the client at the onset of the pain. When pain becomes too severe, more medication and a longer time are needed for the medication to take effect. Clients may return to the surgical unit with a patient-controlled analgesia (PCA) device for pain medication administration (Fig. 15–13). Repeat instructions on how to use the device, and assure the client that a "lock-out" function prevents inadvertent overdosing.

Document the date and time of the medication, the amount given, and the route of administration. Also include a description of the pain the client is experiencing and the effectiveness of the pain medication in controlling it. Consider the time to onset of medication effect in determining when evaluation of pain control should be assessed. For example, reassess the client 30 minutes after oral pain medication is administered. IV medications should control pain within 5 to 10 minutes. It is usually the nurse who determines whether the client is obtaining a sufficient dose of medication, whether pain is being controlled, or whether it is causing side effects such as nausea and vomiting. Communicating these details to the physician allows for a change to best suit the client's needs, leading to a positive outcome for pain relief. It is vital that pain be managed if the client is to comply with instructions for coughing, deep breathing, and ambulation. Chapter 23 addresses pain and pain management.

Reduce Nausea and Vomiting

Postoperative nausea and vomiting (PONV) do not occur frequently; however, the surgical experience for those clients with PONV will remain uniquely unpleasant. Vomiting is a reflex, and the reflex is stimulated in many ways. Stimuli can arise from gastrointestinal tract distention on irritation, vagal stimulation, centers in the cerebrum, the chemoreceptor trigger zone (CTZ) located in the floor of the fourth ventricle in the brain, rotation or disequilibrium of the vestibular labyrinths of the ear, increased intracranial pressure, pain, or sensory perceptions (such as the sight of blood or an odor or a taste). Several medications stimulate the CTZ, including morphine, meperidine, cardiac glycosides, and amphetamines.

Risk factors are shown in Table 15–12. PONV can be prevented by reducing movement, controlling pain, and early intervention with antiemetics. Several categories of medications are used to control PONV and include (1) anticholinergics and histamine type 1 (H_1) receptor an-

TABLE 15–12 RISK FACTORS FOR POSTOPERATIVE NAUSEA AND VOMITING

Client Factors
Ambulation
Bowel obstruction/ileus
Female gender
History of motion sickness
History of vomiting with previous anesthetic procedure
Hypoglycemia
Hypotension
Obesity
Swallowed blood
Uncontrolled pain
Young age
Type of Surgery
Eye
Intra-abdominal
Intracranial
Laparoscopic
Middle ear
Testicular
Medications
Anticholinesterases
Etomidate
Isoflurane
Nitrous oxide?
Pentothal
Propofol
Regional anesthetics above T5 spinal level

tagonists, which reduce excitability of the labyrinth receptors; (2) antidopaminergic drugs, which depress the CTZ; and (3) gastrointestinal antispasmodics, which promote forward peristaltic movement. PONV has also been controlled with acupuncture.

Discharge Instructions and Care

Regardless of the length of stay in the hospital or surgical center, when the client is ready to go home, ensure that the client and a family member as appropriate have the information and skills needed to continue a successful recovery. Teach skills over a period of days, with ample time for questions and "hands-on" practice. Give all information in writing to the client or family members. Most institutions provide a printed form filled out with specific postoperative information, such as instructions on medications and wound care, an appointment for a postoperative clinic visit, and names and telephone numbers in case there are further questions or an emergency arises. Drug prescriptions are also provided if medications are to be continued at home.

If the client has further health care needs after discharge, collaborate with other health care workers such as those in social services, home nursing (see Bridge to Home Health Care: Recovering from Surgery), or rehabilitation services. Many resources are available in the community for clients, and most institutions have a list for the local area. Determine the resources available in your community for the clients that you care for, what each provides, and how they are contacted. A partial listing of the most common resources follows:

- Child Protection Services
- Emergency social services or hospital social services
- Emergency legal assistance
- Hospice
- Local chapters of organizations offering help (e.g., American Cancer Society, American Heart Association, American Diabetes Association)
- Local mastectomy, laryngectomy, or colostomy support groups
- Local senior citizens assistance program
- Medic Alert Foundation
- Local sexual assault center (by law, suspected sexual abuse of minors must be reported)
- Malignant Hyperthermia Hotline
- Substance abuse treatment programs or groups
- Visiting Nurse Association or home health care services

BRIDGE TO HOME HEALTH CARE

Recovering from Surgery

An 80-year-old man is discharged from 1-day surgery in stable condition after an inguinal hernia repair. Before discharge, he is given postoperative instructions. Because he is elderly and lives alone, his physician orders a home care consultation.

On your initial visit to the client's home, you perform an assessment that includes physical, environmental, and psychosocial status. As you review the client's discharge instructions, you realize that his vision is impaired. He cannot read the instructions without help. Although he was told to take his temperature twice daily, he cannot read the thermometer. The client is on a regular diet but has little food in his house. He tells you that he recently stopped driving because of poor vision and depends on neighbors for transportation, including trips to the grocery store. He was instructed to see his physician in 1 week but is not sure how he will get to the office. The client says the doctor told him to call if there was drainage from his surgical incision; he is not sure what that means.

Before you leave, you review all of the postoperative instructions with the client to be sure that he understands them. You change his dressing and note serosanguineous drainage at the surgical site. You show him the drainage and explain that he should call you if it increases or changes color. You contact a neighbor, who agrees to take his temperature every morning and record it. You also telephone Meals-on-Wheels to have food delivered to the client's home. Most important, you tell the client that you will be back to see him tomorrow and you leave a phone number for him to call if he needs a nurse.

This client's case reflects the variety of issues that can arise during recovery from surgery at home and also illustrates the benefits of home care services in this setting. For the client to qualify for home care, certain guidelines must be followed. Medicare guidelines have required that clients be homebound and require skilled, intermittent care. Payer sources require medical orders for home care; most third-party payers require preauthorization for services.

The primary goals for the home care nurse are:

- To assess and prevent postoperative complications
- To instruct the client or the caregiver
- To assist the client in achieving an optimal level of wellness and functioning

In assessing the postoperative client, ascertain the following:

- Does the client understand the postoperative instructions?
- Does the client need specific equipment, such as a walker or dressings?
- Does the client have prescribed medications and know how to use them?
- If a special diet is ordered, can the client get the food needed for the diet?
- Does the client have needs for skilled care such as wound care or intravenous administration? Can the client or the caregiver be taught to perform this care?
- Does the client understand the prescribed level of activity?

You can help the client learn and cope during the postoperative recovery period.

Deborah L. Bayliss, RN, MS, *Community Nurse Case Manager, Poudre Valley Health System, Fort Collins, Colorado*

CONCLUSIONS

The nurse plays a critical role in the perioperative care of the client. Today, surgery ranges from outpatient procedures to complex inpatient procedures. No matter what type of surgery is performed, however, the client needs expert nursing care. The quality of nursing care can determine whether the client has a successful perioperative experience.

THINKING CRITICALLY

1. A young adult client in the emergency department has acute appendicitis. Surgery is scheduled in 30 minutes. What teaching should be completed before the client has the surgery? What interventions must be completed before the client is taken to the operating area?

Factors to Consider. What important client teaching is completed before any surgery in which general anesthesia is used? Are possible complications discussed at the time? What measures usually appear on a preoperative checklist?

2. An elderly client has undergone major abdominal surgery under general anesthesia. At age 80 years, she is in relatively good health following a cerebrovascular accident about 8 years ago. Her only medication is a 325-mg aspirin tablet taken once a day. What complications are most likely in an 80-year-old client? How can these complications be prevented? How is pain tolerated by the older client?

Factors to Consider. What complications are associated with general anesthesia? How do a thorough history and assessment help you in your plan to prevent complications after surgery? What age-related considerations must be made? Does the use of aspirin increase the risk of any complications?

BIBLIOGRAPHY

1. Acute Pain Management Guideline Panel. (1992). *Acute pain management in adults. Operative procedures.* AHCPR Pub. No. 92-0019. Rockville, MD: Agency for Health Care Policy and Research, Public Health Service, U.S. Department of Health and Human Services.
2. *AORN standards, recommended practices, and guidelines.* (2000). Denver: Association of Perioperative Nurses, Int.
3. Alves, S. L., & Deisering, L. F. (1996). Cardiovascular changes associated with aging: The anesthetic implications. *CRNA: The Clinical Forum for Nurse Anesthetists, 7*(1), 2–8.
4. Badgwell, J. M. (1996). The postanesthesia care unit: A high-risk environment for bloodborne and infectious respiratory pathogens. *Journal of Post Anesthesia Nursing, 11*(2), 66–70.
5. Beerman, C. M. (1997). The nurse's role in bioethics. *AORN Journal, 65*(5), 923–926.
6. Bogart, J. (1998). *Legal nurse consulting: Principles and practice.* American Association of Legal Nursing Consultants. Boca Raton, FL: CRC Press.
7. Britt, B., Joy, N., & Mackay, M. (1998). Anesthesia related trauma caused by patient malpositioning. In N. Gravenstein & R. Kirby, (Eds.), *Complications of anesthesiology* (2nd ed., pp. 3654–3689). Philadelphia, W.B. Saunders,
8. Carpenito, L. J. (1999). *Nursing care plans and documentation: Nursing diagnosis and collaborative problems* (3rd ed.). Philadelphia: Lippincott.
9. Cericola, S. A. (1998). Management. Understanding informed consent. *Plastic Surgical Nursing, 18*(4), 249–251.
10. Chiarella, M. (1998). Legal and ethical issues in perioperative nursing. The nurse's responsibility for the swab and instrument count. *AORN Journal, 11*(1), 39–41.
11. Davila, Y. (1999). Cultural considerations in perioperative nursing. *Seminars in Perioperative Nursing, 8*(3), 128–136.
12. Davidhizar, R., Bechtel, G., & Giger, J. N. (1998). When your client in the surgical suite is Mexican American. *Today's Surgical Nurse, 20*(6), 29–35.
13. Dodd, F. (1996). Under pressure . . . pressure area care in theatre. *British Journal of Theatre Nursing, 6*(9), 33–35.
14. Dunn, D. (1997). Malignant hyperthermia. *AORN Journal, 65*(4), 767–776.
15. Fairchild, S. (1996). *Perioperative nursing: Principles and practice* (2nd ed). Boston: Little, Brown.
16. Fortner, P. (1998). Preoperative patient preparation: Psychological and educational aspects. *Seminars in Perioperative Nursing, 7*(1), 3–9.
17. Girard, N. (2000). Care of the geriatric patient. In M. L. Phippen & M. P. Wells (Eds.), *Patient care during operative and invasive procedures* (pp. 675–695). Philadelphia: W. B. Saunders.
18. Girard, N. (1997). Gerontological nursing in acute care settings. In M. A. Matteson, E. S. McConnell, & A. D. Linton (Eds.), *Gerontological nursing: Concepts and practice* (2nd ed., pp. 855–895). Philadephia: W. B. Saunders.
19. Girard, N. (1997). Preoperative assessment. *Nurse Practitioner Forum, 8*(4), 140–146.
20. Groah, L. K. (1996). *Perioperative nursing* (3rd ed.). Norwalk, CT: Appleton & Lange.
21. Hodson, D. M. (1998). The evolving role of advanced practice nurses in surgery. *AORN Journal, 67*(5), 998–1006, 1008–1009.
22. Ibarra, V., et al. (1997). Clinical pathways in the perioperative setting. *Nursing Case Management, 2*(3), 97–106.
23. Keller, C. (1999). The obese patient as surgical risk. *Seminars in Perioperative Nursing, 8*(3), 109–117.
24. Keller, K. (1997). The role of advanced practice nurses in surgical services. *AORN Journal, 67*(1), 16.
25. Klein, J. N. (1996). Future gazing. Perioperative case management—2001. *Surgical Services Management,* 2(1) 51.
26. McLeskey, S. W., & Korniewicz, D. M. (1998). Understanding latex allergy. *Seminars in Perioperative Nursing, 7*(4), 206–215.
27. Meeker, M. H., & Rothrock, J. C. (1995). *Alexander's care of the client in surgery* (10th ed.). St. Louis: Mosby–Year Book.
28. Murphy, J. M. (1999). Preoperative considerations with herbal medicines. *AORN Journal, 69*(1), 173, 175, 177–178.
29. Poe, D., et al. (1997). Implementation of the RN first assistant role. *AORN Journal, 65*(1), 32–44.
30. Pryor, F. (1997). Practical innovations. Key concepts in informed consent for perioperative nurses. *AORN Journal, 65*(6), 1105–1107, 1109–1110.
31. Ronk, L. (1998). Monitored anesthesia care is not synonymous with low risk. *Seminars in Perioperative Nursing, 7*(1), 54–57.
32. Rothrock, J. C. (1996). *Perioperative nursing care planning* (2nd ed.). St. Louis: Mosby–Year Book.
33. Ruzicka, S. (1997). The impact of normal aging processes and chronic illness on perioperative care of the elderly. *Seminars in Perioperative Nursing, 6*(1) 3–13.
34. Sabiston, D. C. (1997). *Textbook of surgery: The biological basis of modern surgical practice* (15th ed.). Philadelphia: W. B. Saunders.
35. Thompson, H. J. (1999). The management of postoperative nausea and vomiting. *Journal of Advanced Nursing, 29*(5), 1130–1136.
36. Vermette, E. (1998). Emergency! Malignant hyperthermia. *American Journal of Nursing, 98,* 45.
37. Williams, G. D. (1997). Preoperative assessment and health history interview. *Nursing Clinics of North America, 32*(2), 395–416.
38. Williams, H., & Reeves, F. (1998) Anesthetic techniques and positioning: Implications for perioperative nurses. *Seminars in Perioperative Nursing, 7*(1), 14–20.

REMEMBER *to check out your* **Companion CD ROM**

CHAPTER 16

Clients with Wounds: Promoting Positive Outcomes

Joyce M. Black

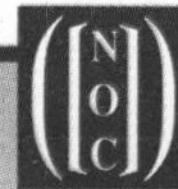

NURSING OUTCOMES CLASSIFICATION (NOC) for Nursing Diagnoses—Clients with Wounds

Impaired Skin Integrity
Tissue Integrity: Skin and Mucous Membranes
Wound Healing: Primary Intention
Wound Healing: Secondary Intention

Healing is a fundamental property of living tissue. If healing did not occur, all species would eventually become extinct. Unfortunately, many health care practices seem to lack respect for this critical attribute of healing and accept the process as passive, inevitable, and unimprovable. Popular literature assumes that if people survive, they heal, and if people are healthy, they heal.

Healing activities have always formed the basis of nursing practice. Florence Nightingale defined the nursing role as preparing the patient for the most favorable conditions for healing. Nurses today still serve as a crucial link in the process of wound healing. Nurses educate clients about disease management and wound care and support them through the physical and psychological processes of healing.

This chapter focuses on tissue injury and repair. Tissue injury is common and is seen in clients who sustain trauma as well as those who have undergone surgery. Because tissue injury is common, the body is well equipped with mechanisms of defense and healing. Defense mechanisms include intact skin and mucous membranes, phagocytes, and the immune and inflammatory responses (see Unit 16 review). In this chapter, the discussion is limited to wound healing in general. Specific information on types of wounds can be found in other chapters: diabetic foot ulcers, in Chapter 45, pressure ulcers, in Chapter 49; and venous stasis ulcers, in Chapter 53.

NORMAL WOUND HEALING

Wound healing has been defined as "a complex and dynamic process that results in the restoration of anatomic continuity and function."[12] Wound healing is a continuous sequence of signals and responses during which several cells come together outside of their usual domains, interact, perform their tasks, and having done so, resume their normal functions. Healing, specifically wound healing, is a process.

Healed wounds constitute a spectrum of repair. An *ideally healed* wound is one that has returned to normal anatomic structure, function, and appearance. In humans, this degree of healing can occur only in epidermal tissue or mucous membrane. Once there is injury through the dermis, normal appearance cannot return because scar tissue replaces missing dermis and epidermis. On the other end of the spectrum, a *minimally healed* wound has anatomic continuity (the wound has closed) but does not have sustained functional result. Hence, the wound may recur. Between these two extremes of healing, an *acceptably healed* wound is characterized by restoration of sustained function and anatomic continuity.[12] The type of wound and the intrinsic and extrinsic environments determine the timeliness of wound healing.

The type of injury has considerable influence on the form of repair. Clean approximated incisions heal with minimal synthesis of new tissue and barely test a client's resources. In sharp contrast, major burn wounds require complete regeneration of tissue and stimulate massive responses from all body systems to sustain life. The location of the wound also influences healing. Perineal wounds are likely to become infected, wounds over joints are subject to motion and therefore increased scarring, and wounds in peripheral areas or those that do not receive adequate blood supply heal slowly.

Wound healing is most apparent on the skin but occurs in all areas of the body. Bones, tendons, organs, and tissues all heal by regenerating cells to restore function. The most favorable outcome of healing is the complete return to normal structure and function. Such an outcome is possible if tissue damage is minor, no complications occur, and the destroyed tissues can regenerate. Body tissues have varying capabilities for regeneration. For example, mucous membrane is completely regenerated. Deep skin injury regenerates with a scar, which restores only a barrier. It has been thought that the central nervous system (CNS) cannot regenerate its damaged cells. Although new information is challenging that belief, today the knowledge does not exist to promote CNS tissue regeneration. It is still assumed that damaged tissues in the CNS are repaired with scar tissue, but they cannot be regenerated to regain their original function.

PHASES OF WOUND HEALING

Regardless of the cause of the wound, healing follows a predictable course. Events can be described in four phases:

- Vascular response
- Inflammation
- Proliferation or resolution
- Maturation, or reconstruction

At the time of injury, many actions occur simultaneously. The course is depicted in Figure 16–1.

VASCULAR RESPONSE PHASE

Within seconds after an injury, regardless of the type, blood vessels constrict to stop bleeding and reduce exposure to bacteria. Smooth muscle in the arterial walls contracts to reduce blood flow. The clotting process begins. Platelets, activated by the injury, aggregate to form a clot and stop bleeding. At the same time, the plasma protein system begins to form a fibrous meshwork. When the platelets come in contact with the fibrin meshwork across the open vessel wall, they become sticky and adhere (aggregate) to the fibers, forming a plug. This meshwork of clotted blood and serum covers the wound while it heals and prevents further loss of blood and plasma. Platelets also release chemicals that promote clotting, such as adenosine diphosphate (ADP), to attract other platelets and a type of prostaglandin that activates other platelets. Platelets also release growth factors to stimulate healing (see later discussion).

Capillaries dilate 10 to 30 minutes after injury and remain dilated for some time because of serotonin released by the platelets. Capillary dilation allows the ingress of plasma. Plasma dilutes toxins secreted by the organisms, brings nutrients necessary for tissue repair, and carries phagocytes into the area. In addition, when the vessels dilate, the flow of blood slows and extra blood and oxygen are brought into the injured area. The capillary dilation causes the classic signs of warmth and redness seen with inflammation.

INFLAMMATION PHASE

Inflammation, the second phase of wound healing, involves a series of physiologic responses to tissue injury induced by trauma or a foreign object. It is nonspecific and occurs after every injury. The inflammatory response is essential for the repair and restoration of the structure and function of damaged tissues. The mustering of the inflammatory response is so necessary to healing that it is commonly said, "no inflammation, no healing."

The inflammatory response occurs *whenever* injury has occurred. Cellular injury can occur from trauma, oxygen or nutrient deprivation, chemical agents, microorganism invasion, temperature extremes, or ionizing radiation. Inflammation also occurs when dead cells are present. Inflammation begins at the moment of injury and may ex-

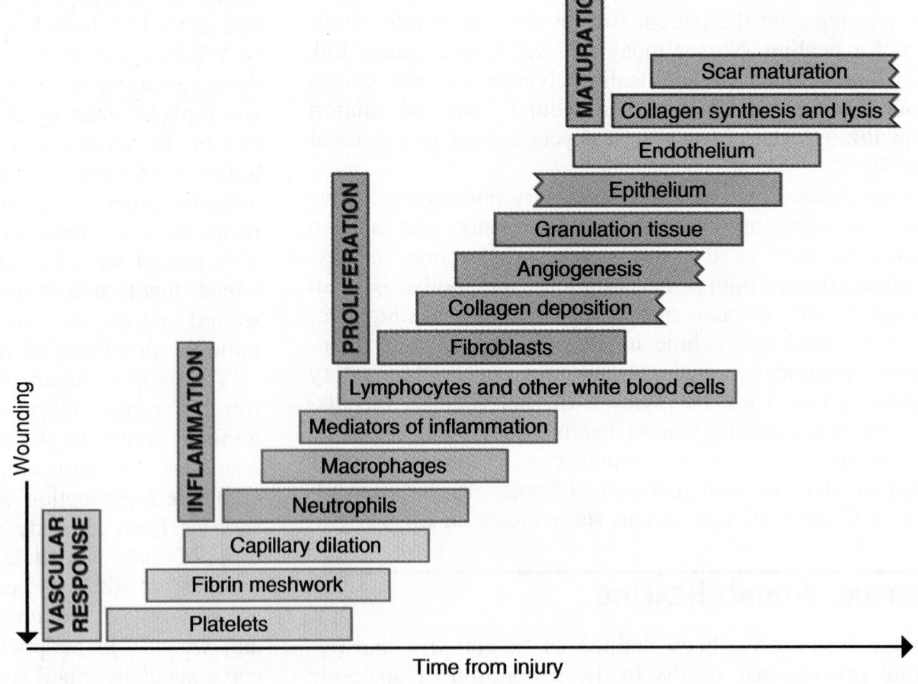

FIGURE 16–1 Normal wound healing. Wound healing proceeds through four phases: (1) the vascular response, (2) inflammation, (3) proliferation of cells to heal the wound, and (4) maturation of the wound. There are many components of each step. The jagged edge depicts an ongoing process. (Adapted from Cohen, I., et al. (Eds.). [1992]. *Wound healing.* Philadelphia: W. B. Saunders.)

tend for 4 to 6 days, depending on the extent of the injury. Inflammation is prolonged in infected wounds or wounds with necrotic tissues.

Thus, inflammation is important for healing. Unfortunately, health care terminology uses the word *inflamed* to describe the wound that is not healing normally. Do not be confused between the normal process of inflammation and the term "inflamed" to mean exaggerated inflammation. Recognize inflammation as an expected response to tissue injury, not necessarily a pathologic process.

Although inflammation can cause additional tissue injury, it is an adaptation to injury. The purpose of inflammation is to limit the effects of harmful bacteria or injury by destroying or neutralizing the organism and by limiting its spread throughout the body. The inflammatory response thereby sets up proper conditions to promote tissue repair. Unlike the *immune response,* which is slow and deliberate, using a system of specific antibodies, the effects of inflammation are immediate.

During the inflammation phase, the white blood cells (WBCs) become active to clean up the wound and initiate further healing processes. We now look closely at these WBCs and the process of phagocytosis (see Understanding Inflammation and Its Treatment).

Role of White Blood Cells

NEUTROPHILS. Neutrophils are vital defense mechanisms because they are both the first and most numerous cell types to arrive at any area of disease or injury. Within 6 hours after release from bone marrow, neutrophils migrate into tissues, where they survive for 4 to 5 days. Their role, along with tissue macrophages, is to

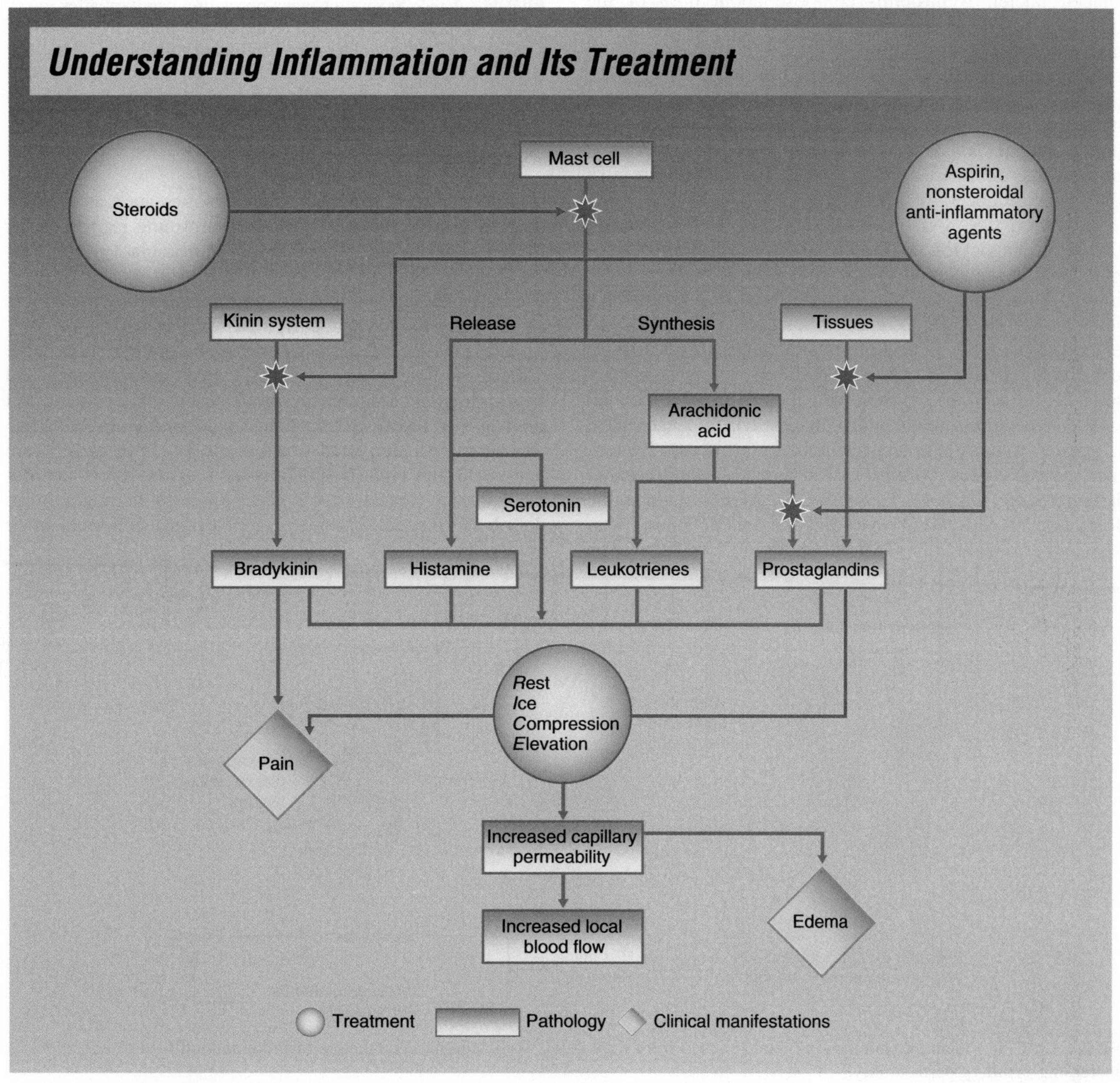

phagocytose (ingest) injurious agents, thereby protecting against bacterial invasion.

Neutrophils are attracted to the injury site by chemotaxis. The slowed flow of blood allows the neutrophil to leave the center of the bloodstream and line the walls of the capillaries, a process called *pavementing,* or *marginating,* because the cells line up like bricks on a sidewalk. Histamine stimulates the cells that line the capillary to constrict, creating spaces in the wall. Neutrophils, which are normally too large to squeeze through the lining, can pass through the capillary wall and enter the site of tissue injury to begin phagocytosis, through a process called *diapedesis* (Figs. 16–2 and 16–3). Neutrophils phagocytose bacteria, dead cells, and cellular debris. These cells are short-lived, but they are effective in clearing a wound of debris if bacteria are not excessive in number (>100,000 per gram of tissue).

Neutrophils are sometimes called *polymorphonuclear neutrophils* (PMNs), or polys, because of their irregularly shaped nuclei. Neutrophils compose about 60% of the circulating WBCs. Mature neutrophils appear segmented and are called "segs." Immature cells are "banded" and called bands. Bands are not effective in phagocytosis. The presence of an increase in segmented WBCs indicates a bacterial invasion. The presence of increased band neutrophils indicates more severe infection because the bone marrow has released immature cells. Leukocytes are also the major producers of interferon.

MONOCYTES AND MACROPHAGES. Monocytes are the next phagocytes on the scene, stimulated by neutrophils and lymphokines. They arrive about 4 days after injury. Monocytes can phagocytose foreign material for a longer time. In addition, a large percentage of monocytes enter the tissues and become macrophages. In the tissue, these cells continue to phagocytose large numbers of bacteria. If the need arises, these cells can reenter the circulation and become mobile macrophages. Macrophages have a greater role in chronic inflammation (discussed later). The macrophage is a critical cell in wound healing because it secretes *angiogenesis factor* (AGF). AGF stimulates the formation of new blood vessels at the end of injured vessels and stimulates fibroblasts to spew forth collagen. The macrophage also secretes other cytokines such as platelet-derived growth factor (PDGF), transforming growth factor (TGF), interleukin-1 (IL-1) and basic fibroblast growth factor (bFGF). This cell has a major role in wound healing. Wounds can heal without leukocytes, but wound healing is significantly impaired without macrophages.

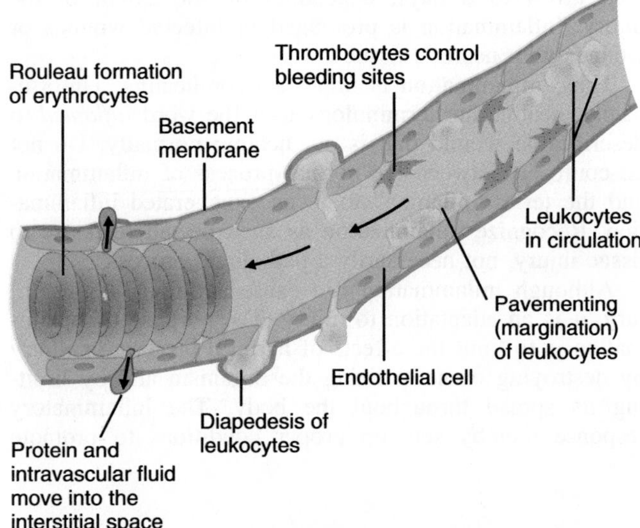

FIGURE 16–2 Several changes occur in a capillary after injury. Neutrophils are attracted to the site of injury by chemotactic factors at the site. The neutrophil leaves the blood vessel by sliding through holes in the vessel wall (diapedesis). The leukocytes also line the vessel wall, and the erythrocytes stack like coins (rouleau formation) to slow blood flow.

The amount of oxygen in the wound influences the effectiveness of phagocytic cells. Both macrophages and neutrophils can function in an anaerobic environment, but their ability to effectively digest bacteria is slowed. Macrophages are inactivated when tissue levels of oxygen are below 30 mm Hg. (Normal tissue oxygen levels are not the same as levels of oxygen bound to hemoglobin or dissolved oxygen. Tissue oxygen levels are normal at or above 30 mm Hg.)

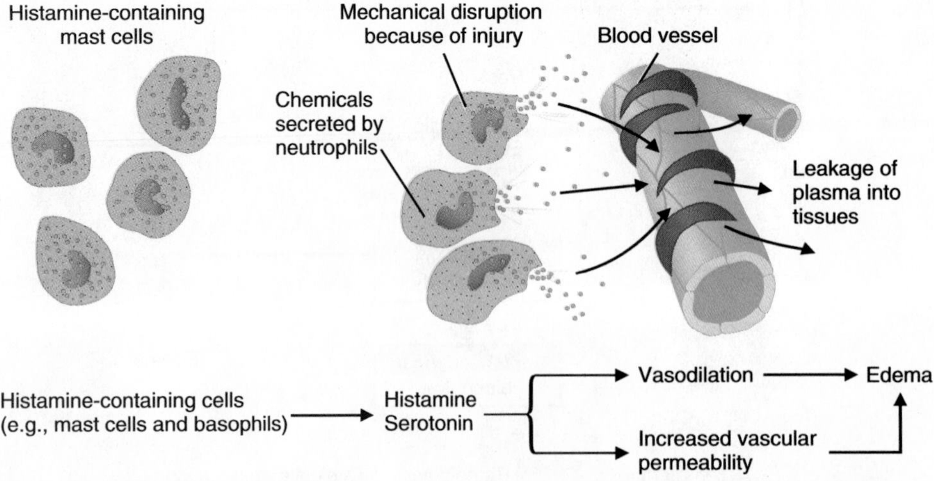

FIGURE 16–3 Histamine and serotonin are released from mast cells. These chemical mediators of inflammation lead to edema by increasing capillary permeability.

LYMPHOCYTES AND OTHER WHITE BLOOD CELLS. Two other forms of WBCs have much less importance in wound healing and are addressed only briefly. The lymphocytes are formed in the lymphoid tissues of the tonsils, intestines, and bone marrow, and they mature in the lymph nodes, thymus, and spleen. Lymphokines are sensitized lymphocytes. Lymphokines help the macrophages to become more effective at the site of local injury through a number of processes. Lymphocytes are controlled by the adrenocortical hormones. Therefore, clients receiving steroid therapy have reduced numbers of lymphocytes. This change places the steroid-dependent client at increased risk for infection and delayed healing.

Eosinophils and basophils may also migrate to the injured area. Eosinophils help control the inflammatory response by secreting antihistamine. Basophils secrete histamine.

"WALLING-OFF" EFFECT. A walling-off effect occurs in the damaged area to prevent the spread of injurious agents to other body tissues. Fibrinogen clots block the lymphatic channels and spaces in the tissues so that fluid barely flows through the area. The process of walling off the area partly depends on the invading agent. For example, staphylococci invade and destroy nearby tissues quickly, and therefore the process of walling off also develops quickly to control the spread. In contrast, streptococci did not cause an intense reaction in the tissues and can digest the walls. This allows the streptococci to multiply and spread. As a result, streptococcal infections have a much greater tendency to invade other organs (such as the heart valves) and are associated with a higher mortality rate.

Mediators of the Inflammation Phase

The specific mediators of inflammation are not shown in Figure 16–1. They are important, and their activity occurs throughout the healing phases. The chemicals that guide inflammation are shown in the feature called Understanding Inflammation and Its Treatment.

MAST CELLS. Several substances mediate (control) inflammation. Mast cells are found in the tissue. Mast cells are filled with histamine and neutrophil chemotactic factors, substances called vasoactive amines. Histamine and serotonin cause capillary dilation (see Fig. 16–2). The mast cell is stimulated by many factors, such as physical injury (wounds, burns, x-ray exposure), chemical injury (toxins, snake and bee venom), or immunologic means (the trigger of hypersensitivity reactions seen in allergies).

Mast cells also synthesize leukotrienes and prostaglandins. These two chemicals cause the same responses as histamine, but the response they generate lasts longer. Prostaglandins also cause pain and tend to appear in the later stages of inflammation. Leukotrienes and prostaglandins are produced from the arachidonic acid released from the mast cell membrane. Aspirin and other nonsteroidal anti-inflammatory drugs (NSAIDs) block the production of prostaglandins and can assist in reducing inflammation and pain (see Understanding Inflammation and Its Treatment). Leukotrienes and prostaglandins increase vascular permeability and enhance the action of neutrophils. The increase in blood flow brings in more nutrients and WBCs. Bradykinin, (see next section) also causes vasodilation, induces pain, and facilitates the action of the leukocyte.

KININ SYSTEM. Kinins are plasma proteins involved in inflammation. Early in injury, kinins increase vascular permeability and allow the leukocytes to enter the tissue. Later in the inflammatory process, kinins act with prostaglandin to cause pain and smooth muscle contraction and to increase leukocyte chemotaxis. Kinins increase vascular permeability, fluid in the wound, and the number of leukocytes available to assist with phagocytosis. The primary kinin is bradykinin.

OXYGEN FREE RADICALS. Free radicals are commonly regarded as the cause of some diseases. During metabolism, an unstable form of oxygen is produced. This is a single oxygen atom, derived from molecular oxygen (O_2), having an unpaired electron. This form of oxygen is called an *oxygen free radical* or a *superoxide radical.* The molecule tries to become stable again by attaching to hydrogen, lipids, or vitamin E. If the molecule attaches to hydrogen, the product is hydrogen peroxide, which is toxic to the cell. If it attaches to lipids, it can enter the cell or organelles and produce damage. When attached to vitamin E, it is stabilized and does not produce damage. Other vitamins support vitamin E; vitamin C restores vitamin E to the cell membrane. Vitamin A (beta-carotene) is present in high-density lipoproteins and is presumed to serve some role as an antioxidant, but that role is not fully understood.

Unrestrained free radicals can injure tissues and induce breaks in both single-stranded and double-stranded deoxyribonucleic acid (DNA), leading to mutations. In wound healing, free radicals serve as mediators of both acute and chronic inflammation, being stimulated by PMNs and the mast cell. They damage vascular endothelium (the inside lining of blood vessels). The exact role of free radicals in wound healing is still under investigation. The use of vitamin E as an antioxidant is becoming popular.

THE COMPLEMENT SYSTEM. The complement system is composed of a group of plasma proteins that normally lie dormant in the blood, interstitial fluid, and mucosal surfaces. Microorganisms (or antigen-antibody complexes) activate the complement system. Complement activation promotes inflammation and induces movement of leukocytes into the area of injury in a process is called *chemotaxis.* The final aspect of complement activation is the coating of microbes to make them vulnerable to phagocytosis. Many bacteria have an outer capsule that resists phagocytosis. (Complement is fully discussed in the Unit 16 review.)

PROLIFERATIVE PHASE

The third phase of wound healing, the proliferative or resolution phase, contains overlapping processes of collagen deposition, angiogenesis (formation of new blood vessels), granulation tissue development, and wound contraction. This phase ends about 2 weeks after injury, but the processes of healing are not complete and continue for 1 to 2 years.

Mediators of the Proliferative Phase

CYTOKINES. Cytokines regulate the mobility, differentiation, and growth of leukocytes. Among the best understood cytokines are interleukins and interferon. *Interleukins* promote the growth and function of several cells. Interleukin can account for many of the clinical manifestations of both acute and chronic inflammation, such as fever, anorexia, cachexia, and movement of PMNs to the site of injury. Interferons augment immunity through several processes, especially the promotion of B-cell maturation and moderating of suppressor T-cell function.

GROWTH FACTORS. Catalysts for wound healing are growth factors released by platelets and macrophages. They can prime other cells to enter a growth phase, or they can move a cell from a growth phase to a DNA production phase. Several types of growth factors have been identified. Only major families of wound healing growth factors are described.

Platelet-derived growth factor (PDGF) is named for the platelet from which it originated. PDGF regulates the synthesis of fibronectin and fibroblasts in the matrix of the wound healing bed. Epidermal growth factor (EGF), named for the target cell, stimulates fibroblasts and endothelial cells. FGF stimulates collagen synthesis and angiogenesis. TGF-α stimulates epithelial cells and macrophages and controls cell growth and synthesis of the components of the matrix. TGF-β increases synthesis of the matrix components. Colony-stimulating factors (CSFs) are secreted by the bone marrow, monocytes, fibroblasts, and keratinocytes. Their major function appears to be enhancing the function of WBCs.

Components of Healing

COLLAGEN. Fibroblasts, normally found in connective tissue, are brought into the wound by various cellular mediators. They are the most important cells in this phase of healing because they synthesize and secrete collagen, elastin, and proteoglycans. These substances reconstruct connective tissue. Initially, collagen is gel-like, but within several weeks to months, it re-forms along lines of mechanical stress, which adds strength to the wound. Several substances are needed for normal collagen deposition, including vitamin C, zinc, oxygen, and iron.

ANGIOGENESIS. Microscopically, the development of new blood vessels (angiogenesis) begins within hours of injury. Over a period of time, the new blood vessels in the wound bed can be identified through clinical assessment. Initially, the skin edges of a wound are bright red and bleed easily. Within hours, the ends of the vessels seal and the wound drainage changes from bright red to dark red.

GRANULATION TISSUE. A matrix of collagen, capillaries, and cells begins to fill the wound space with new connective tissue, forming a scar. This tissue grows from the wound edges and the base of the wound. Granulation tissue is filled with new capillary buds, which give it a red, bumpy, or granular appearance. Fibroblasts and macrophages also surround it. The fibroblasts secrete collagen. The macrophages continue to debride the wound and stimulate fibroblasts and the process of angiogenesis. As granulation tissue is being formed, the process of *epithelialization* begins.

WOUND CONTRACTION. Wound contraction is the mechanism by which the edges of a wound are drawn together as a result of forces within the wound. Contraction is due to the action of myofibroblasts. Myofibroblasts bridge across a wound and then contract to pull the wound closed. The process of wound contraction is crucial for survival. If a wound from an acute injury did not contract, infections would be lethal complications in all acute injuries. Contraction is undesirable in some wounds because of the cosmetic deformities that result from *contracture.*

CONTRACTURE. In large open wounds, such as burns, wound contraction can go on to become the more severe form of contracture. Contracture of the scar can produce profound deformities; contracture of the scar at the neck can pull the chin onto the chest. Wounds over joints can also contract severely. Contracture also occurs in internal organs, such as the intestine, breast, and liver.

EPITHELIALIZATION. Epithelialization is the migration of epithelial cells from surrounding skin. Epithelial buds also line hair follicles in the dermis of shallow wounds or wounds that are healing by secondary intention (discussed later). When epithelium covers a wound, the wound is considered to be closed, or healed. Large wounds or full-thickness wounds may require skin grafting because epidermal migration is normally limited to about 3 cm.

Epithelial buds can be seen in a clean granulating wound. The epithelial cells divide, and eventually the migrating epithelial cells contact similar cells from the other edges and stop migrating. At this point, they begin to differentiate into the various layers of epidermis. Epithelialization can be hastened if a wound is kept moist.

MATURATION PHASE

The final phase of wound healing (maturation or reconstruction) is marked by remodeling of the scar. This phase occurs for a year or more after the wound is closed. Collagen has been deposited, tissue is repaired, and the wound has begun to contract during the proliferative phase. During the maturation phase, the scar is remodeled, capillaries disappear, and the scar tissue regains about two thirds of its original strength. The remodeling is the process of collagen synthesis and lysis. Remodeling provides tensile strength to the wound.

Scar tissue is never as strong or durable as normal tissue. Tensile strength never reaches over 80% in scar tissue. Over the 12 months after injury, the scar becomes mature and appears thin and white instead of the red, raised appearance seen with granulation tissue. Scarring is a normal part of wound healing. Some scars are barely visible, whereas others remain very visible throughout the client's lifetime. Factors that affect scarring are discussed in Chapter 49.

■ WOUND HEALING INTENTION

Wound healing intention refers to the probable process of healing for any wound. Wounds can heal by (1) primary, (2) secondary, or (3) tertiary (delayed primary) intention (Fig. 16–4.)

PRIMARY INTENTION

Primary intention is the use of suture or other wound closures to approximate (place close together) the edges of an incision or clean laceration. Healing is primarily through collagen synthesis, and little scarring or contraction is needed. The risk of infection and tissue defects is minimal. The eventual scar is usually thin and flat.

SECONDARY INTENTION

Wounds healing by secondary intention are left open rather than closed with sutures (stitches) and heal by the generation of connective tissue. Consider open wounds like pressure ulcers or abrasions. Open wounds require

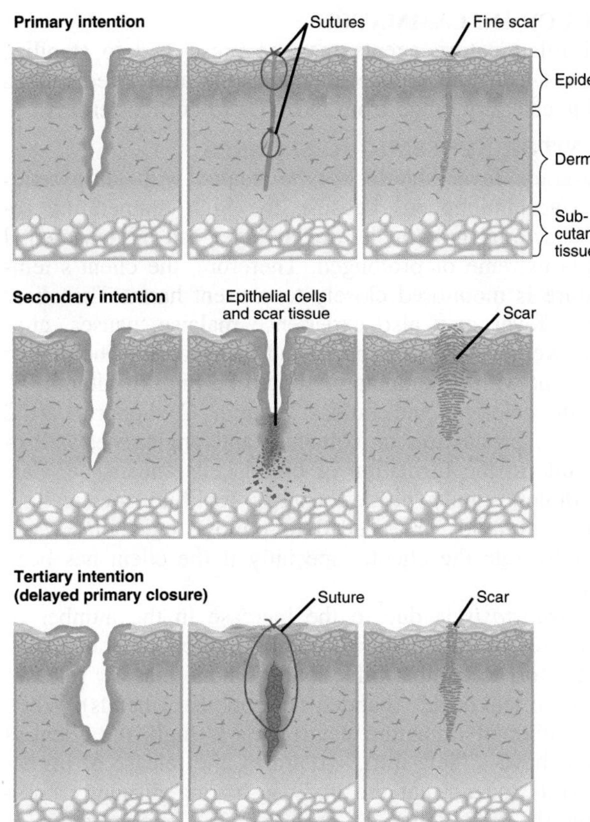

Figure 16–4 Wound healing by primary, secondary, and tertiary intention (delayed primary closure).

the regeneration of much more tissue than does the wound healing by primary intention, and there is also increased risk of infection. Wounds healing by secondary intention have a prolonged phase of inflammation because more time is required for phagocytosis of necrotic tissue. In chronic inflammation, macrophages and lymphocytes are the predominant cells. The ability of epithelial cells to migrate is limited, and epithelialization may not heal the wound. Therefore, the wound is characterized by longer phases of proliferation and maturation, leading to healing by contraction and the formation of scar tissue. Sometimes healing of is hastened by the application of skin grafts or musculocutaneous (myocutaneous) flaps (see Chapter 49).

TERTIARY INTENTION

Certain wounds may be contaminated, and although they can be closed by primary intention (e.g., by suture), they are not. Because of the increased risk of infection, these wounds are closed later, when they are free of debris. This type of wound closure is called healing by tertiary intention, or delayed primary closure.

■ NUTRITION AND WOUND HEALING

Protein and calories are needed for wound healing, and vitamins and minerals are also important components in this process (Table 16–1). Malnutrition leads to impaired collagen synthesis and an increased risk of infection. Protein-calorie malnutrition is an all too common problem in older people, especially those in institutions.

CLIENTS WITH ACUTE INFLAMMATION

Inflammation occurs in all clients who have sustained any form of tissue trauma. The trauma can be due to surgery, injury, changes in oxygen delivery to various tissues, and so on. Therefore, the information herein can be applied to many clinical settings. There are both local and systemic manifestations of inflammation. Because the response to inflammation is the same, regardless of the cause, the manifestations of inflammation are relatively consistent.

There are three systemic reactions to inflammation:

- Fever
- Leukocytosis (a rise in the number of WBCs)
- An increase in the number of plasma proteins.

Fever is caused by a pyrogen (fever-causing chemical) released from leukocytes, macrophages, and tumor necrosis factor (TNF). Prostaglandins also act on the hypothalamus to reset the internal thermostat. Fever is usually adaptive because bacterial reproduction is sensitive to even slight increases in temperature.

Outcome Management

Medical Management

Goals of medical management of a client with acute inflammation include (1) minimizing complications of the edema accompanying inflammation, (2) reducing the inflammatory response, and (3) monitoring systemic responses. Because the inflammatory response is a desired

TABLE 16–1 NUTRITION AND WOUND HEALING

Nutrient	Impairments Related to Nutrient Deficiency
Protein	Decreased collagen production, angiogenesis, and neutrophil and lymphocyte immune response; increased risk of dehiscence and infection
Calories	Too little glucose impairs immune response because energy needs of white blood cells cannot be met
Fats	Impaired inflammation
Vitamin A	Impaired monocyte and macrophage activity; delayed inflammatory response, including macrophage activity; increased risk of infection
Vitamin B complex	Not well understood; lack of B vitamins interferes with enzyme production
Vitamin C	Decreased collagen production, angiogenesis, and contraction; weakness in healed wound; increased risk of infection
Vitamin E	Delayed healing when given in excess
Zinc	Possibly impaired action of vitamin A; phagocytosis; increased risk of infection; decreased protein synthesis
Iron	Impaired oxygenation and secondary healing at very low levels

response to promote wound healing, the client with inflammation often requires only supportive care.

Control the Effects of Edema

*R*est, *I*ce, *C*ompression, and *E*levation (RICE) is a mnemonic that can be used to guide care to reduce the effect of edema. If an extremity is inflamed, it is elevated and wrapped to reduce edema. Most practitioners advocate using ice to control the inflammatory response in the extremities, especially when edema and pain are present. Some physicians order ice for 24 to 72 hours to control inflammation and then apply heat to remove the accumulated waste products. When ice is ordered, be certain that the cold reaches the wound and that it is not rendered ineffective by bulky dressings. Assess for signs of skin damage if ice is applied directly to unprotected skin.

If edema is causing a detrimental alteration of tissue perfusion, anti-inflammatory agents may be required. In certain areas of the body, such as the brain and extremities, the edema that accompanies inflammation can be detrimental to tissue perfusion. These clients may require surgery to release pressure in the area or restore blood flow. Fasciotomy and bur holes are examples of these operations (see Chapters 27 and 73, respectively).

The degree of inflammation is monitored to determine whether it is leading to healing. Analgesics may be required for pain control. Temperature is monitored, and fever is treated with antipyretics when it reaches detrimental levels (e.g., >38.3° C or 101° F). If the inflammation is in response to a probable invasion by organisms, antibiotics may be prescribed.

Reduce Inflammation

Anti-inflammatory agents may be prescribed to stabilize the mast cell and reduce edema in the area. Medications in this category range from NSAIDs to corticosteroids.

Monitor Systemic Responses

Low-grade fever should not be treated with antipyretics (e.g., acetaminophen) because the high temperature retards bacterial growth. However, fever can be detrimental if it is extreme or prolonged. Therefore, the client's temperature is monitored closely to prevent harm. The client with a fever may also experience malaise, nausea, anorexia, weight loss, tachypnea, and tachycardia. The diet of the client with inflammation should be high in vitamin C, protein, calories, and fluids. Vitamin C supports WBC function, production of collagen, and angiogenesis. Protein aids in the formation of blood cells and tissue. Carbohydrates supply needed energy for fuel for healing. Additional fluids are needed to remove metabolic waste and rehydrate the client, especially if the client has been febrile.

Leukocytosis is due to the increase in the number of leukocytes in circulation to combat infection. Sometimes, in an effort to combat infection, the bone marrow releases immature leukocytes (banded neutrophils or bands). When the number of immature neutrophils is high, the client is said to have a "left shift." At times, the release of immature cells means that the body is having difficulty combating the infection with mature cells. Interpretation of the WBC differential is shown in Table 16–2.

The *erythrocyte sedimentation rate* (ESR) also rises

TABLE 16–2 INTERPRETATION OF DIFFERENTIAL COUNTS WITHIN A COMPLETE BLOOD COUNT

Cell Type	Function	Normal Value	Significance of Change
Segmented neutrophils (segs)*	Mature neutrophils act as phagocytes	50%–60%	Elevated with infection; a "left shift" means that many band (immature) cells are present as the body fights infection; "right stuff" is the presence of more mature cells, seen with liver disease and pernicious anemia
Band neutrophils	Immature neutrophils	3%–8%	Elevated in acute stages of infection
Lymphocytes	Produced by lymphoid tissue, participate in humoral response	25%–40%	Elevated in infectious mononucleosis, cytomegalovirus infection, and infectious hepatitis; decreased in acquired immunodeficiency syndrome (AIDS), Cushing's syndrome, chronic uremia, and following trauma (e.g., burn injury)
Monocytes	A second line of defense, increasing in chronic infections	2%–8%	Elevated in chronic bacterial infection, viral disease, Hodgkin's disease, multiple myeloma, and some forms of leukemia
Eosinophils	Phagocytic, destroy antigen-antibody complexes before they can harm the body	1%–4%	Elevated in allergic disorders and parasitic infections; decreased in infectious mononucleosis, congestive heart failure, pernicious anemia, and during the use of steroids, epinephrine, and thyroxine

*To calculate the absolute neutrophil count (also called an absolute granulocyte count):

$$\text{absolute neutrophil count} = \frac{\text{total \% of neutrophils (segs + bands) WBC count (cells/mm}^3\text{)}}{100}$$

When the absolute neutrophil count falls below 1000/mm³, the client is said to be "neutropenic" and precautions must be taken to prevent infection.

with inflammation. The ESR rate ("sed rate") is the rate at which cells settle to the bottom of a glass test tube. Increased levels of fibrinogen cause the red blood cells to stack (like coins) and therefore settle more quickly. Additionally, plasma proteins rise during inflammation (e.g., fibrinogen, C-reactive protein). Most are released by the liver, and they are collectively called *acute phase reactants.* They provide components of coagulation, transportation, and complement production.

Nursing Assessment of the Medical Client

ASSESSMENT

The clinical manifestations of inflammation include redness, swelling, heat, pain, and loss of function. Tissues are red, warm, painful, and swollen and have limited mobility. In addition, an inflammatory exudate is formed. The exudate dilutes the toxins released by bacteria, brings certain nutrients to the wound, and carries phagocytes for defense. Various types of exudate are present, depending on the stage of inflammation and its cause.

Serous exudate is seen in early inflammation and is composed of water with a small amount of colloids, ions, and phagocytic cells. A *blister* is a common example of serous exudate. Hemorrhagic or sanguineous exudate is composed of blood. Drainage is bright red or dark red. Serosanguineous exudate is drainage composed of both serous fluid and blood. It is pink and usually fairly thin. Purulent exudate is filled with more leukocytes (pus) and is common in chronic inflammation from walled-off lesions.

The type of drainage present in the wound is indicative of the phase of healing. For example, a surgical wound initially presents with sanguineous drainage. As hemostasis progresses, the drainage becomes serosanguineous and finally advances to serous drainage (Table 16–3).

Monitor the level of WBCs, differential counts, and fever as indicators of infection. Expect the WBC level to rise in clients with known infections and after acute injury, such as a surgical incision (report elevations in WBC and clinical manifestations of infection to the physician). Monitor also the elderly, who often have infection but not necessarily elevated WBC counts.

DIAGNOSIS, OUTCOMES, INTERVENTIONS

Altered Tissue Perfusion. Edema from the inflammatory response may restrict blood vessels and entrap nerves in the traumatized area. The nursing diagnosis *Altered Tissue Perfusion related to edema* is an important problem.

Outcomes. Tissues will be perfused, as evidenced by the usual skin color, presence of pulses in areas distal to the edema, skin warmth, lack of paresthesias, and lack of escalating pain.

Interventions. Assess clients with visible injury causing inflammation for resolution of bleeding in the area, adequate blood flow, and nerve conduction distal to the affected site. Frequent assessments (every 2 hours) of the edematous area are needed. Measurement of the circumference of the area also enables the examiner to determine whether the area is becoming markedly edematous. To measure the same site, mark the area on the client with a pen to ensure appropriate location of serial measurements.

In addition to assessing the circumference, assess pulses, skin temperature, capillary refill, sensation, and movement in areas distal to the inflammation. Dressings or casts over the affected area can also form a constriction. This response can be called *compartment syndrome.* Clients who have been injured or are undergoing orthopedic surgery are at highest risk for compartment syndrome (see also Chapter 27).

Objects that may become entrapped in edematous tissues, such as rings, should be removed because they can cause serious damage. The inflamed area should be elevated. Application of cold compresses causes vasoconstriction and decreases the amount of edema. Prolonged use of cold compresses may lead to rebound vasodilation and increase the risk of tissue injury. Vasoconstriction can also decrease the inflow of new blood and thereby slow the removal of toxins and waste from the site of injury.

If the extremity is edematous, it should be elevated and assessed for the presence of distal circulation and neurologic response. Factors that impede venous flow should be controlled. For example, rolled stockings that constrict venous return should not be worn. Compression bandages may be used to reduce edema by promoting lymphatic and venous drainage. Explain the appropriate way to apply these bandages and when to rewrap them to maintain compression.

EVALUATION

The outcome of the inflammatory response is usually time-dependent. Most edema subsides over 72 hours with

TABLE 16–3 INFLAMMATORY EXUDATES

Type	Appearance	Significance
Hemorrhagic, sanguineous	Bright red or bloody	Small amounts expected after surgery or trauma; large amounts may indicate hemorrhage; sudden large amounts of dark-red blood may indicate a draining hematoma
Serosanguineous	Blood-tinged yellow or pink	Expected for 48–72 hr after injury or trauma; a sudden increase may precede wound dehiscence
Serous	Thin, clear, yellow	Expected for up to 1 wk after trauma or surgery; a sudden increase may indicate a draining seroma
Purulent	Thin, cloudy, foul-smelling; may be thick if filled with dead cells	Usually indicates infection; may drain suddenly from an abscess (boil)
Catarrhal	Thin, clear mucus	Seen with upper respiratory infection

appropriate RICE measures. If the edema has not subsided in that time frame, consider another cause of the edematous process, such as infection.

Self-Care

Clients capable of caring for a wound or area that is likely to become inflamed need instructions on how to elevate the extremity, how to use heat or ice, how to follow the medication regimen, and how to change dressings. Clinical manifestations of edema and infection must be reported, such as changes in color, pulse, and pain.

CLIENTS WITH CHRONIC INFLAMMATION

Chronic inflammation is differentiated from acute inflammation by its duration and the cells that mediate the response. Acute inflammation is accompanied by altered capillary permeability, release of chemical mediators, and infiltration of leukocytes that engulf and destroy injured tissue and pathogens. If these elements succeed in cleaning the wound, healing begins. If the area is not cleaned, monocytes continue to perpetuate the inflammatory response, but this time the accumulation of inflammatory mediators may actually cause tissue destruction. The lymphocyte and tissue macrophages are the major phagocytes in chronic inflammation.

When the immune system is unable to eliminate the invading organisms during the acute stage of inflammation, it attempts to protect surrounding tissues from further invasion by building a wall around the infected site called a *granuloma.* Some forms of infection, such as fungi, parasites, and perhaps antibody-antigen reactions (autoimmune disease), result in granuloma formation. Tuberculosis is a good example. When tuberculosis develops, a thick wall forms around the mycobacteria. The bacteria continue to live in the walled-off area, and it is soon filled with dead tissue. As the tissue dies, the cellular enzymes are released and the fluid leaves the granuloma. The empty sac remains.

Outcome Management

The chronically inflamed wound has purulent drainage (*suppuration*) and does not heal completely. A common example of chronic inflammation is seen when foreign objects are not removed from tissues (e.g., splinter, glass, and dirt). Chronic inflammation can also occur when certain forms of bacteria cannot be killed by phagocytes. For example, the organisms that cause tuberculosis, syphilis, and leprosy have cell walls with a very high lipid and wax content, which makes them impermeable to the phagocyte.

Care of the client with chronic infection is focused on determining the source of the problem. Wounds may be *debrided* (cleaned and freed of dead tissue), and the client may be given antibiotics or anti-inflammatory agents.

CLIENTS WITH INCISIONS

Outcome Management

Wounds made intentionally with a scalpel and closed with sutures, staples, or strips of tape are called *incisions.* Incisions are the most common example of wounds healing by primary intention. An incision should be assessed every 8 hours. If the incision is not visible, check the dressings or assess for increased girth. The incision normally appears somewhat pink and swollen; small areas of induration around the suture marks are common. However, erythema should not extend beyond a ½ inch from the incision. If the wound was closed primarily, you should be able to palpate the presence of newly synthesized collagen just under an intact suture line. This internal scar is known as a "healing ridge." When this ridge is not present 5 to 7 days after suturing, suspect slowed collagen synthesis. The client may need additional protection of the nonhealing area to prevent infection.

A wound that is healing by primary intention should be protected from further trauma, including external pressure. Keep the wound free of pulling forces that stretch the sutured skin. Keep the wound clean, but do not wash the suture line because water carries microorganisms into the wound along the sutures. Protect it from the external environment and drainage with dressings.

Apply dressings using an aseptic or sterile technique. Sterile gloves are usually not required. Hold the side of the dressing that will not touch the client's incision by the clean or gloved hands and tape it in place. The type of dressing used changes as the wound responds to treatment. Use dressings that best suit the wound. Gauze dressings are used most often on a wound healing by primary intention. Dressings for open wounds are discussed in the following section.

Wound drainage tubes can be placed in the dead space created during exposure of the operative area. Drainage of a wound is indicated when actual or potential fluid accumulation threatens the healing process. The drain facilitates removal of blood and bacteria from the wound. Assess the volume and type of fluid hourly immediately after surgery. If a reservoir is attached to the drain, measure the volume of drainage by markings on the reservoir. If the drainage is emptied from the reservoir, follow universal precautions for its disposal. In addition, if the drainage is caustic (e.g., bile), the skin around the site must be protected with skin barriers.

Teach the client how to care for the incision, the clinical manifestations of wound infection, how to care for and empty the drain reservoir, and when to return for suture removal. Sutures in areas where scarring must be controlled (e.g., on the face) are usually removed in 4 to 7 days; in other areas, sutures are usually removed in 7 to 10 days. Sutures in the hand and foot are removed in 1 to 2 weeks or more.

CLIENTS WITH OPEN WOUNDS

Outcome Management

Medical Management

The goal of medical management of an open wound is to prepare the client and the wound for the quickest and most durable form of healing. The treatment of a wound includes the removal of its cause, the correction of underlying problems that are delaying healing, and the initiation of topical (or systemic) treatments to facilitate healing.

Clients with open wounds often have other problems, such as venous insufficiency or diabetes. These disorders decrease blood flow (and thereby oxygen) into the wound and delay healing. Protein-calorie malnutrition may be present and delays healing because the protein needed to manufacture new cells is not available. If the client is immobile or incontinent, adequate prevention must be given to reduce the incidence of new areas of skin breakdown. If wound healing is delayed because of lack of venous return, the extremity requires elevation. If the cause of the wound is lack of arterial flow, the extremity should be positioned flat. If pressure is a causative or contributing factor, repositioning and proper support surfaces must be considered.

The client's diet should be high in carbohydrates, protein, iron, and vitamins. In addition, the client may remain at risk of further skin breakdown, such as pressure ulcers. Medical management may include antibiotics to reduce infection.

REMOVE DEVITALIZED TISSUE FROM THE WOUND: DEBRIDEMENT

Wound healing is optimized and the risk of infection is reduced when all necrotic (dead) tissue, exudate, and metabolic wastes are removed from the wound. Moist, devitalized tissue supports bacterial growth. Various forms of debridement are used to remove these tissues (see later). Systemic and topical antibiotics seldom stop infection because they cannot penetrate the avascular tissues.

Before a wound can heal, necrotic tissues must be removed. Debridement can be accomplished by means of a variety of techniques: (1) sharp, (2) mechanical, (3) enzymatic, and (4) autolytic (these last three are described later). Timely debridement is necessary to remove the devitalized tissue and reduce the risk of infection and the physical obstacles dead tissue places on the process of granulation. In addition, the true size of the wound cannot be known until the necrotic tissue is removed.

Sharp Debridement

Wounds covered with dead tissue, called *eschar* or *slough,* need to be cleaned to promote healing and reduce infection. *Sharp debridement* is performed by the physician and is the quickest method. The technique allows immediate treatment of the wound bed after the devitalized tissue is removed. The eschar or slough is removed to the level of red, bleeding tissues. The wound must then be protected to begin healing. The wound size, depth of the wound, contamination, and the client's status influence whether the client is in satisfactory condition to tolerate sharp debridement, which may call for general anesthesia or sedation. Pain medications should be used for clients undergoing sharp debridement.

Sharp debridement is carried out under sterile conditions, usually in an operating room, a treatment room, or an outpatient surgical setting. Risks associated with general anesthesia, blood loss, and infection are a major concern. This procedure is used for a large wound, a wound that involves a thick eschar that would not be permeated by any topical agent, and a wound that is acutely infected.

After sharp debridement, the client is monitored for signs of bleeding and bacteremia (sepsis.) Sepsis is suspected if unexplained fever, tachycardia, hypotension, or deterioration in mental status develops. The physician should be notified of these changes. Sepsis can be fatal if it is not recognized early and treated aggressively (see septic shock in Chapter 81.) Other forms of debridement commonly used by nurses are discussed later.

Once the wound is clean, surgery may be used to speed healing and to reduce the risk of infection and contracture. Skin grafts are commonly used to replace the epidermis. The partial-thickness burn wound is the best example of a wound that could heal by secondary intention but is often grafted to speed healing and reduce infection and scarring. Cutaneous or musculocutaneous flaps can also be used to close a large wound (see Chapter 49).

Nursing Management of the Medical Client

ASSESSMENT

The client's history must be taken, including a history of the wound itself. The wound history includes causative and contributing factors, duration of the wound, and current and previous methods of treatment and their corresponding success. Sometimes wound treatments are used that actually impair healing, such as hydrogen peroxide or Dakin's solution, or that do not match the type of wound. This information is important when one is obtaining a complete wound history.

The history obtained by the nurse should include information about the following:

- Medical history
- Previous surgery
- Current and past medications, especially steroids and over the counter (OTC) and herbal preparations
- Nutritional state (type of diet, eats and any supplements)
- Serum glucose level if client is diabetic
- Smoking
- Degree of immobility
- Bowel and bladder continence
- Circulatory status
- Presence of infection

Many factors can lead to impaired wound healing. Assessments should be thorough and should focus on the whole client, not just the wound.

Psychosocial assessment should include the client's age, occupation, living situation, financial status, health care benefits, roles and responsibilities, cultural and spiritual beliefs, body image and self-esteem, and ability to learn self-care and comply with the treatment plan. Also note compliance with treatment of underlying disorders, such as diabetes and collagen diseases.

A complete physical assessment should be performed. Focus the data collection on height and weight; degree of range of motion; muscle wasting and level of activity; circulation, such as peripheral pulses, color, edema, and the temperature of extremities; lung sounds; and level of pain. A complete assessment is needed (Box 16–1). Clearly document data about the wound to allow for an objective evaluation at a later date. Describe the actual size of the ulcer by measuring the length (head to toe) and width (shoulder to shoulder). Describe the depth, color, type of drainage, presence of undermining, and

BOX 16–1 Wound Assessment

When assessing an open wound, obtain the following information:

1. What is the size of the wound? Use objective measures to indicate the length and width (such as centimeters or millimeters). Avoid terms such as "the size of a grape." Use a sterile gloved finger or cotton swab to measure depth. Consider using photographs to provide a baseline and serial evaluations.
2. Where is the wound located anatomically?
3. What is the color of the wound? Estimate the percentage of each color when more than one color is noted.
4. Is there granulation tissue or epithelial tissue? Granulation tissue is red, shiny, and bumpy; epithelial tissue looks like pale skin.
5. Are there sinus tracts, or are the edges undermined? Use a gloved hand or swab to measure the extent. Indicate the location and direction of tunneling.
6. Are there signs of infection in the wound? Look for erythema extending beyond the edges of the wound as well as warmth, edema, odor, and purulent exudate. (Also consider systemic signs.)
7. Is there any drainage? Note the color, odor, consistency, and approximate amount by the number of dressings saturated.
8. What is the condition of the surrounding skin? Is it intact, red, indurated, or macerated?
9. Is the wound painful?

condition of periwound skin in the assessment data for later comparison. A photograph is an excellent means of documentation and determination of the progress in healing. Obtain consent before photographs are taken. Photographs should be taken with a consistent method that includes reproducible distance, color, and grid film.

Examine laboratory values for hemoglobin, hematocrit, albumin, and WBCs, specifically lymphocytes. These values indicate the degree of nutritional impairment that may be contributing to the wound's lack of healing. Generally, the risk of delayed healing correlates with low serum albumin levels. However, albumin levels are a slow-to-change indicator of nutritional state. A pre-albumin level is more indicative of current nutritional status.

DIAGNOSIS, PLANNING, INTERVENTIONS

Impaired Skin Integrity. The nursing diagnosis should be used to indicate an actual loss of skin. The actual statement might be phrased *Impaired Skin Integrity related to delayed wound healing secondary to impaired circulation, to infection, or to malnutrition.*

Outcomes. The client will experience improved skin integrity, as evidenced by a cleaner wound within 1 week and no signs of infection in the wound. A long-term goal might be a smaller wound in 3 weeks.

Interventions. Many agencies have wound care nurses who should be contacted for up-to-date information and for assistance with complex wounds. However, every nurse must properly identify basic concepts of wound assessment and treatment.

Keep the Wound Moist. Wound healing is optimized in a moist environment. When the environment is moist, collagen synthesis and granulation tissue formation are enhanced, cell migration and epithelial resurfacing occur more rapidly, and scab, crust, and eschar cannot form. This moist environment, however, can create a medium conducive to infection, and a clean technique must be used for wound care. Heat lamps or treatments that dry the wound must be avoided.

Wet-to-moist or continuously moist dressings are used in clean and granulating wounds. Insert dressings into the wound or place them on the wound while they are moist, again making certain to protect normal intact skin. Remove the dressings while they are still moist to avoid disrupting the granular bed. Bleeding should not occur when the dressing is removed. If the dressing is too dry to pull off, moisten it with sterile normal saline before attempting to remove it.

Prevent Injury to Healing Tissues. Avoid applying solutions on and in the clean wound that may impair healing. For example, iodine, hydrogen peroxide, and Dakin's solution were once commonly used for wound care; however, these solutions damage the wound. They are toxic to the fibroblast and therefore delay healing. In addition, use of large volumes of iodine in wounds can lead to toxicity from excess iodine absorption.

Normal saline is the only solution for wound care recommended by the Agency for Health Care Policy and Research (AHCPR). Normal saline is physiologic, does not harm tissues, and adequately cleans most wounds. Pressure may be applied to the irrigant for enhanced cleaning. If the wound is covered with adherent material, some solutions contain surfactants that aid in cleaning. Some of these chemicals can harm wound-healing cells (Table 16–4). If used, it is important to limit their use to as short a time as possible.

Protect the Periwound Skin. Moisture on normal, intact skin makes the skin more prone to breakdown. The cardinal rule is to keep the wound bed moist and surrounding skin dry. Figure 16–5 shows wound healing cascade in a dry and moist environment. Note that there is faster migration of epithelial cells on a moist wound bed.

Fill Dead Space. Dead space is empty space within a wound. In an ulcer, it is the space between the base of the ulcer and the underside of the dressing around its perimeter. If this space is closed, empty pockets may develop anaerobic infection. Long-acting normal saline gel and wound packing are good media to fill a clean wound and the pockets of empty space before a topical dressing is applied.

Perform Wound Packing. Deep wounds with channels are at high risk of infection. These wounds can also heal with "false floors," which trap bacteria and lead to further infection. It is important that an open wound heal from the inside out. Deep wounds are often packed with saline or gauze strips soaked in an antibiotic solution to debride the wound or prevent abnormal healing. Strips of gauze must be used to avoid having soiled dressings lost in the wound. The gauze is packed into the wound with enough force to hold the edges of the wound open, but not so much force that the wound is under tension. Wounds packed too tightly compromise blood flow and delay healing. The outer edge of the dressing is covered with dry dressings.

TABLE 16–4 TOPICAL AGENTS USED IN TREATMENT OF OPEN WOUNDS

Agent	Indications	Impact on Wound Healing
ANTISEPTIC SOLUTIONS		
Normal saline	Used to moisten dry eschar; keep a clean wound healing by secondary intention	Speeds healing because solution is iso-osmolar, and it keeps the wound bed moist
Hydrogen peroxide	Used to dissolve clotted blood in a wound	Retards healing; do not use as a dressing on an open wound
Providone-iodine (Betadine)	Used for preparation of intact skin; may be used to clean very contaminated wounds	Retards healing; does not penetrate eschar
Dakin's solution	Used 3 to 2 strength to clean contaminated wounds	Retards wound healing
Acetic acid	Used to treat wounds contaminated with *Pseudomonas*	Retards wound healing slightly
ANTIBIOTIC SOLUTIONS AND OINTMENTS		
Neomycin-bacitracin-polymyxin B (Neosporin)	Used to clean wounds contaminated with gram-negative and gram-positive bacteria	Increases epidermal healing but may sensitize tissues; high incidence of allergy
Polymyxin B-bacitracin (Polysporin)	Treatment of gram-negative organisms	None known
Silver sulfadiazine	Used in wounds with eschar (e.g., burns): effective against gram-negative and gram-positive organisms	Enhances epidermal healing; penetrates eschar
Gentamicin	Most effective against gram-negative organisms, but its use may promote resistance in hospital flora	None known
Bacitracin	Effective against gram-positive and gram-negative organisms	May enhance epidermal healing

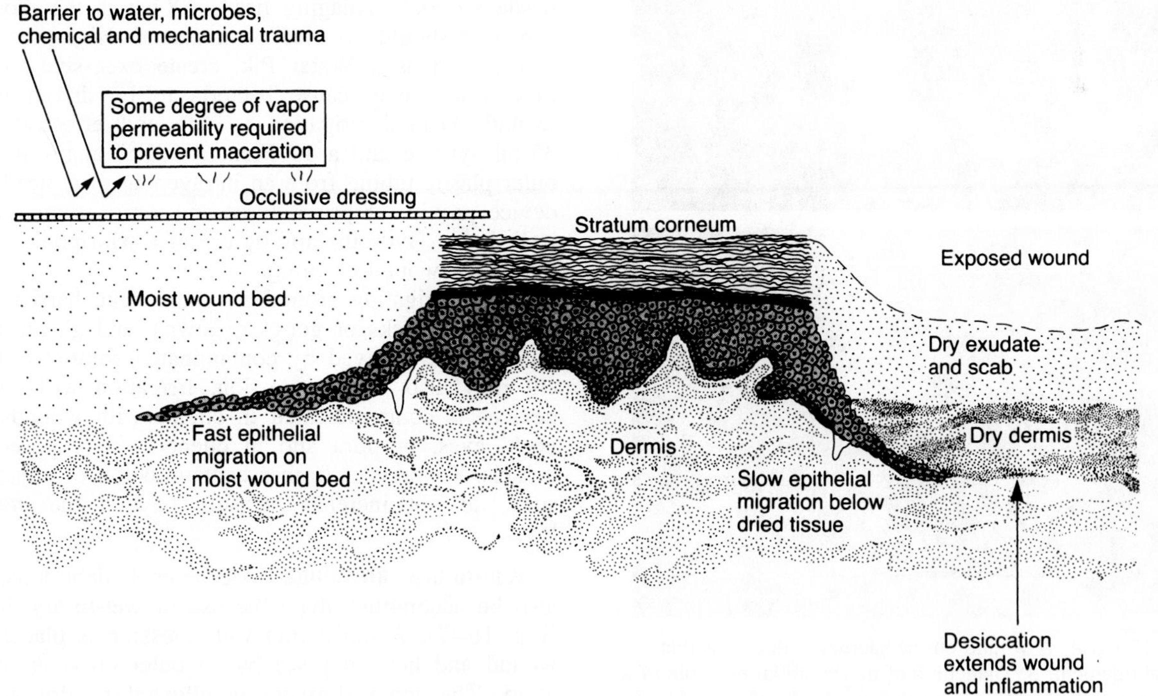

Figure 16–5 Wound healing under an occlusive dressing. (Adapted from Winter, G. D., & Scales, J. T. [1963]. Effect of air drying and dressings on the surface of a wound. *Nature, 197,* 91–92. Copyright 1963 Macmillan Magazines Limited.)

Packing is usually changed every 4 to 6 hours. Some gel packing strips are changed less often. Skin surrounding the wound should be assessed for breakdown from frequent tape removal, and dressings should be secured with other methods if needed (e.g., Montgomery straps).

Select Dressings. Red wound bases need protection to promote healing (Fig. 16–6). Red wounds are filled with granulation tissue and are beginning to heal. These wounds should not be treated with lotions, ointments, or soaps, which generally irritate or infect the area. Topical vasodilators can be used to stimulate capillary flow to the wound, but a physician's order is required. If the wound is shallow, a thin layer of antibiotic ointment and non-adhering dressing (or synthetic dressing) may be used to cover it. If the wound is deep, saline-moistened gauze can be used to pack the wound, but the dressing should not be allowed to dry out before it is changed. When an-

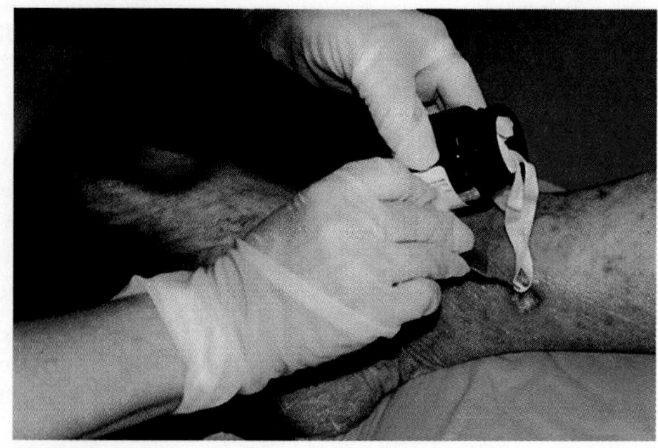

Figure 16–7 Wet-to-dry dressings are placed into a wound with the use of strip gauze.

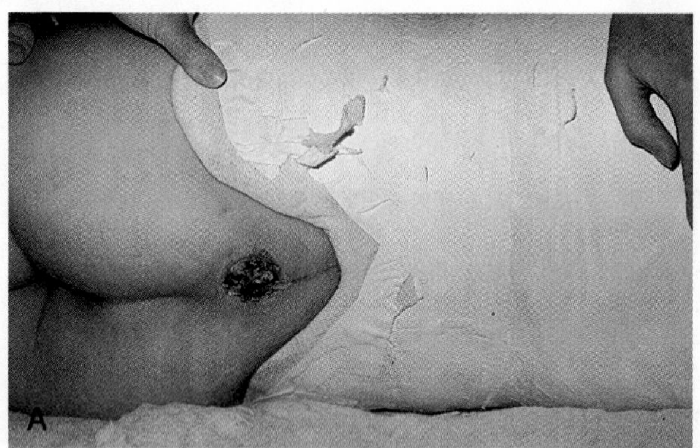

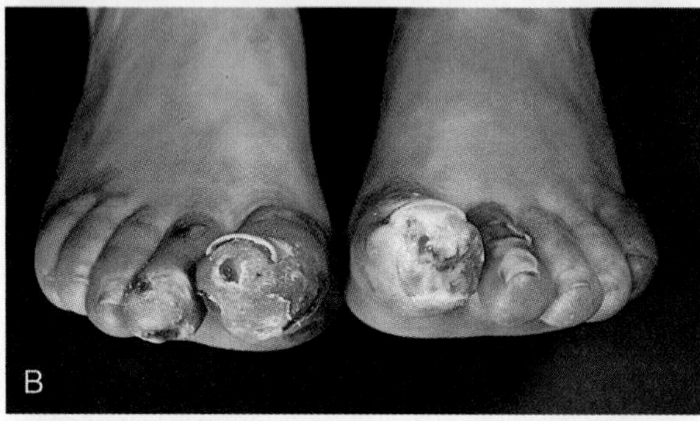

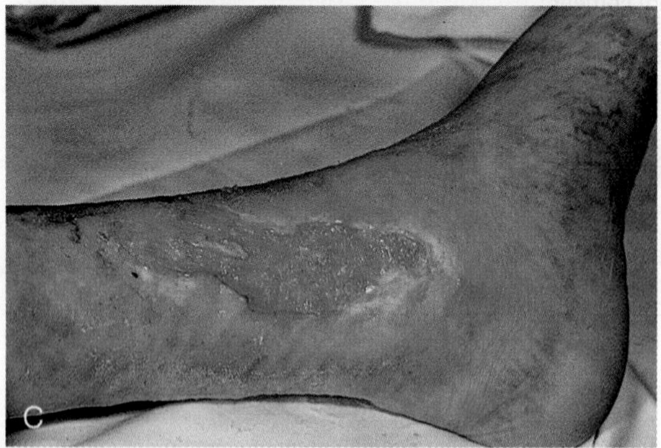

Figure 16–6. *A,* A wound on the sacrum with eschar that needs debridement. *B,* Diabetic foot ulcers are an example of a wound with yellow, soft, slough that needs cleaning. *C,* Healing venous stasis ulcers have a clean wound filled with granulation tissue that needs protection.

adherent dressing is being changed, granulation tissue and new epithelium are also removed. If a wound is healing, the wound should be kept moist to facilitate healing.

A wound that presents with black, leathery material in the wound base is necrotic. This black, nonviable tissue is known as eschar. Yellow material in the wound base is a sloughy, necrotic substance. Black and yellow tissues present in the wound bed can be appropriately classified as devitalized, necrotic, or dead. The risk of infection rises in proportion to the amount of necrotic tissue present. Debridement techniques for removing necrotic tissue include those described in the sections that follow. (Sharp debridement was discussed earlier.)

Perform Mechanical Debridement. Mechanical debridement includes treatments with irrigation and dressings.

Irrigation. Irrigation between 4 and 15 pounds per square inch (psi), removes debris, bacteria, and necrotic tissue without damaging tissues; 8 psi is the most pressure that should be used on a wound. High-pressure devices, such as a Water Pik, create excessive force and trauma and may cause bacteria to be driven into the wound. Wound irrigation is safe and effective with a 35-ml syringe and a 19 French (19Fr.) angiocatheter, or outer plastic tubing from an intravenous (IV) needle. This device provides 8 psi of force and removes most devitalized tissue. Hydrotherapy by use of a whirlpool is also an option for wound cleaning.

When irrigating around a wound, take barrier precautions with masks or goggles, gowns, and gloves because you may be sprayed by contaminated solutions. The client may also need protection. Irrigation with pulsating devices is contraindicated in clients with wounds of the neck, eyes, or dura and in clients with exposed blood vessels. To prevent further contamination of adjacent tissues, do not increase pressure beyond the prescribed level.

Wet-to-dry dressings. Mechanical debridement can also be accomplished by the use of wet-to-dry dressings (Fig. 16–7). A moist (not wet) dressing is placed in the wound and held in place by an outer dressing or gauze wrap. The inner dressing is allowed to dry and then removed. As the dressing dries, debris, necrotic tissue, exudate, and drainage adhere to it. The wound is debrided as the dressing is gently removed. The wet dressing is obtained by saturating an all-gauze dressing with the prescribed solution and wringing the dressing out until it is just moist. The moist dressing should be placed in the wound and left long enough to begin to dry (4 to 6 hours). Use caution so that the dressing does not cause normal (or high-risk) tissues on the edges of the wound to become moist. Topical skin protectants can be used to protect surrounding intact skin. Once the dressing is dry, it is removed along with adherent tissues. The dressings are not remoistened to make removal easier because this practice defeats the purpose of the dressing, which is to debride the wound. The process is often painful, and clients should have adequate analgesia before the dressing is changed. Wet-to-dry dressings are a nonselective form of debridement and can inadvertently remove new granulation tissues as well as necrotic tissue, creating an environment that retards healing. Therefore, they are used only until the wound is clean and granulating.

Perform Enzymatic Debridement. To avoid the risk of damaging new tissue growth, which is often experienced with wet-to-dry dressings, consider chemical agents, such as enzymes, as a nonsurgical option. Enzymatic agents are expensive, requiring diligent care. Some enzymatic agents work by converting denatured proteins to peptides and amino acids. Other enzymatic preparations cause fibrin lysis. These agents cannot be used on wounds communicating with major body cavities, wounds with exposed nerves, or neoplastic ulcers. They must be used with caution around the eyes.

A dry eschar should be *scored* (should have small cuts made into it) before the enzymatic ointment is applied. Scoring enhances penetration. For the agent to work, the wound surface must be kept moist. The ointment is used until the eschar separates from the wound surface. Use of agents necessitates frequent dressing changes, and they should be used only on necrotic tissue. They are usually applied to only about 2 to 4 square inches of necrotic tissue at one time. Medicate clients prior to the use of enzymatic agents, which cause burning. Enzymatic agents should not be placed on viable tissue, as they cause tissue necrosis.

Perform Autolytic Debridement. With this method, a synthetic dressing is placed over the ulcer and the eschar or devitalized tissue is allowed to self-digest through the action of enzymes normally present in the wound fluid. Although not as rapid than other methods, autolytic debridement may be appropriate for clients who cannot tolerate other methods and are not susceptible to infection. Autolytic debridement is contraindicated for most infected wounds.

Select Dressings. Gauze still remains the most commonly used material for a dressing. Gauze is used as a dry cover for surgical wounds or wounds that heal by

TABLE 16–5 WOUND DRESSINGS

Type	Product	Indications for Use	Nursing Implications
Nonadhering, nonimpregnated	Telfa	Shallow, open wounds	Second dressing or tape needed it is nonadhesive
Impregnated	Adaptic gauze, Vaseline gauze, Xeroform	Moist wounds	Nonabsorbent, occlusive, not traumatic to remove
Gauze	Adaptic gauze, Kling gauze, Nu-gauze, Primapore	Wet-to-dry debridement, wound packing	Moderately absorbent; can be used as wound packing for shallow wounds; use long strips of gauze to pack deep wounds; gauze does not provide a bacterial barrier; if allowed to dry on a wound, it may remove viable tissue when removed
Transparent films	Bio-occlusive, Op-Site, Tegaderm	Coverage of shallow wounds, intravenous sites, blisters, abrasions	Adhesive; therefore, no secondary dressing is needed; retain moisture, semipermeable, water-resistant; facilitate autolytic debridement
Hydrocolloids	Comfeel, Duoderm, Intrasite, Restore, Tegasorb, Intact, ulcer dressing	Shallow ulcers, donor sites, second-degree (partial-thickness) burns; do not use on infected wounds	Retain moisture, occlusive or semipermeable, water-resistant, adhesive; require replacement because the dressing melts; reduce pain
Hydrogels	Elastogel, wound gel, Spenco, Vigilon	Pressure ulcers, dermal ulcers, partial-thickness burns, abrasions, blisters	Hydrogels having cooling effect: maintain moist environment, relieve pain, permit autolytic debridement; easily removed unless they dry out
Exudate absorbers	Bard absorption dressing, Envisan	Deep wounds with eschar	Retain moisture, absorbent, promote autolytic debridement
Calcium alginates	Sorbsan, Kaltistat, Algiderm	Clean wounds with profuse drainage	Retain moisture, absorbent, left intact for several days
Foams	Reston, Flexan Lyofoam, Polymen	Full-thickness wounds with moderate to heavy drainage, skin tears	Moisture, absorbent, nonadherent, left intact for several days

primary intention (Table 16–5). Wet-to-dry gauze dressings can be used for nonselective debridement of wounds. More absorbent dressings should be used with exudative wounds. Only mesh gauze dressings should be used in a wound because cotton dressings are likely to leave fibers behind. Use cotton-filled gauze as an outer dressing. If the wound edges are friable or if the wound will be disrupted when the dressing is removed, a nonadherent dressing can be used. The nonadherent dressing can be impregnated or nonimpregnated. This nonadherent dressing is often chosen because when it is removed, disruption of the wound bed is minimal.

Clean granulating wounds do not require daily dressing changes. Apply hydrocolloid dressings for 3 to 5 days. Continue to observe for infection. If purulent drainage develops, do not apply occlusive dressings. Allow the wound to drain by using gauze or alginates.

Excessive exudate can delay healing. If the wound produces exudate, several absorption dressing products can be used. Absorptive dressings, calcium alginates, and hypertonic saline dressings are appropriate choices for moderate or highly exudating wounds. Foams can also be used for absorption and autolytic debridement. Table 16–5 describes the actions, indications, and nursing implications for various categories of wound dressings.

The selection of dressing type changes as the wound responds to treatment. Careful assessment and reassessment will indicate progress, or lack of progress, in wound healing. As the wound changes, variations in the dressing materials are made so that healing is maximized. No single dressing provides the optimal atmosphere required during all healing stages of the wound.

Providing Nutritional Support. In addition to local wound care, the client must be provided with a diet that is high in protein, fat, carbohydrates, vitamins, and minerals to facilitate healing. Regardless of the client's actual body weight (e.g., obesity), this is not the time to begin a weight loss diet. The wound must be healed first. If the client cannot or will not eat, the use of tube feeding or hyperalimentation should be considered.

Reducing Interface Pressure. If the client has pressure ulcers, pressure reduction is key to management and prevention. If venous stasis ulcers or lymphedema is present, use graded pressure wraps. Details on the management of these ulcers may be found in Chapter 53.

EVALUATION

Wound healing should be assessed every 24 hours, especially if the risk of infection remains high. If the wound shows no signs of healing after 2 weeks, the AHCPR suggests a 2-week trial of topical antibiotics. If no healing occurs after another 2 weeks, the AHCPR advises quantitative bacterial cultures to evaluate for infection and a bone scan to assess for osteomyelitis.

Self-Care

The client with open wounds often requires long-term care or community resources for safe self-care. Planning for discharge should begin several days before the client is released so that the home situation can be appraised and the necessary support, supplies, and equipment obtained. Appropriate referral to the home health agency or wound healing clinic should be made before discharge. Social services, home health care, or a discharge planner should be involved in the plan of care. The client's financial status, home environment, and support systems must be evaluated. Third-party reimbursement may cover supplies, equipment, and nursing care.

Several areas of client education are needed. The client or family should demonstrate dressing removal, wound cleaning, and dressing application before discharge. Detailed written instructions on wound care should be provided to the client, family, and home health care nurse. Explain what changes should be expected and what changes should be reported to the health care provider. Fever, a change in drainage, or the development of an odorous drainage should be instructed as a reportable change. If the client has a pressure ulcer, provide the client or caregiver with a copy of *Treatment of Pressure Ulcers*[2] (Pub. No. 95-B0652 from the AHCPR, at 800-358-9295).

The average cost of skilled nursing services for treating wounds in the home is $1600 per healed wound. Some cost-cutting measures for saline and gloves have been designed, and it is now possible to make normal saline for home use on wounds. Use to 1 gal of distilled water or 1 gallon of tap water boiled for 5 minutes; do not use well water or sea water. Add 8 teaspoons of table salt. Mix the solution well and cool to room temperature before use. This solution can be stored for up to 1 week.

In the home, rather than purchasing gloves for dressing changes, soiled dressings can be removed with a plastic sandwich bag (Fig. 16–8). The inside of the bag is used as a glove to remove the dressing, and the dressing is disposed of in the same bag. Methods of obtaining needed wound care supplies should also be discussed with the client and family.

Alert the client to signs of complications, such as infection, and give directions on when and how to contact the health care provider. A balanced diet with frequent high-protein snacks should continue until the wound and contributing factors have been resolved. A vitamin and mineral supplement should be taken as directed. The client is often required to incorporate lifestyle changes into activities of daily living (ADL) in an effort to promote healing.

DISORDERS OF WOUND HEALING

DELAYED WOUND HEALING

Become aware of the factors that affect wound healing in order to maximize the positive factors and to minimize the negative effects of the factors that may delay healing. If the effects of unfavorable conditions in the wound or systemically within the client are compromised, these may delay healing. This not only causes the client distress but also increases the cost of wound care. Consider both the wound surface and the client's general physical condition when assessing the client, the wound, and the environment in which care will be carried out. The factors affecting wound healing are usually *intrinsic* and *extrinsic,* although some factors may fall into both categories.

Awareness of the intrinsic and extrinsic factors that

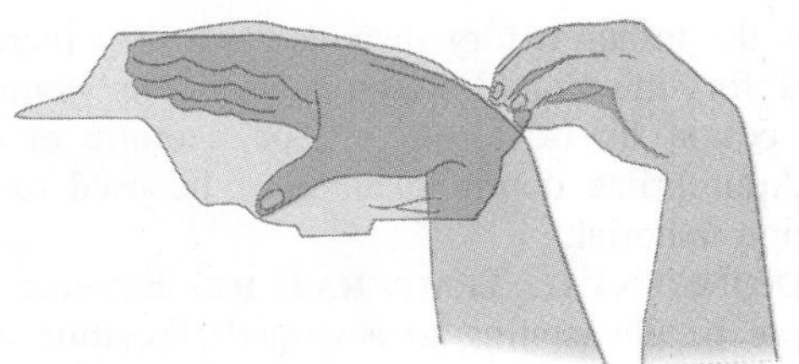

Place a small, clean bag over your hand like a mitten.

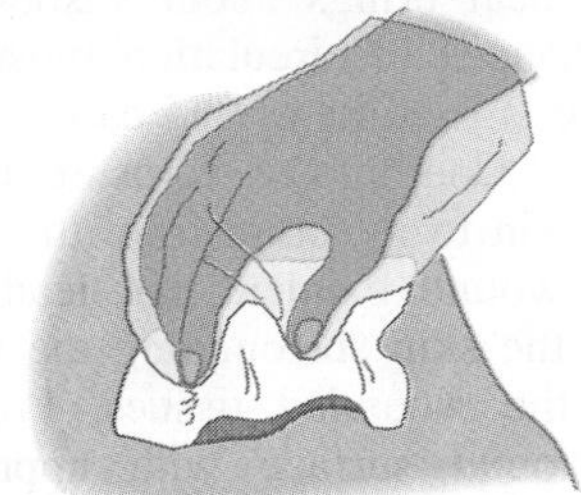

Carefully lift the dressing off the sore.

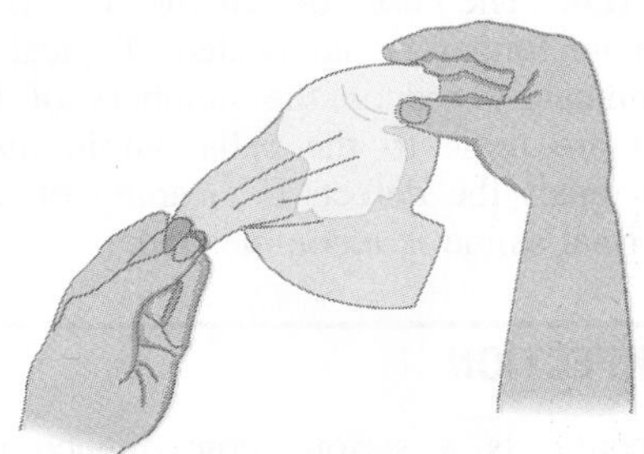

Turn the bag inside out to enclose the dressing.

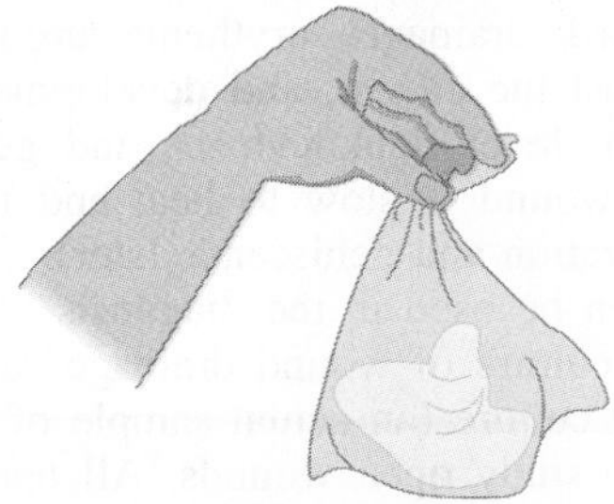

Seal the bag before throwing it away.

Figure 16–8 Plastic bags used as gloves to remove a dressing in the home. (Adapted from Agency for Health Care Policy and Research. (1994). *Treating pressure sores.* Bethesda, MD, U.S. Department of Health and Human Services, AHCPR Publ. No. 95-B0654.)

can affect wound healing is required by staff who are assessing wounds, prescribing wound care products, and evaluating the care. The factors mentioned here are just a small number of conditions that can impede wound healing. As your experience grows, you will become more aware of the intrinsic and extrinsic factors that affect your clients. This knowledge is required to enable the caregiver to enhance the positive factors and to address and reduce the negative effects of intrinsic and extrinsic factors on a wound.

■ INTRINSIC FACTORS

Intrinsic factors can be divided into eight general categories: (1) health status and concurrent systemic illness, (2) age and body build, (3) nutritional status, (4) infection, (5) decreased circulation, (6) diabetes mellitus, (7) smoking, and (8) steroid use.

HEALTH STATUS AND CONCURRENT SYSTEMIC MELLITUS ILLNESS. Any systemic illness (e.g., chronic obstructive pulmonary disease, diabetes mellitus, peripheral vascular disease) may result in a reduced amount of oxygen and nutrients reaching the wound bed. Hypoxia at the tissues reduces collagen synthesis that is required for wound repair. This results in a longer time required for healing. The resulting scar has a reduced tensile strength and may be more vulnerable to reinjury.

AGE AND BODY BUILD. With age, the dermis and epidermis are not as firmly interlocked as before because the junction between them is flattened. The skin also thins and becomes less elastic, muscle tone is lost, and blood flow is reduced. There is slower healing, and the inflammatory response is diminished. Cell migration and division are slower, and all the phases of healing are lengthened. This leads to wounds remaining open for longer periods, which increases the risk of infection and thus further delays wound healing. The elderly population is more likely to have systemic disease, which also takes its toll and has a detrimental effect on wound healing.

Obese clients have increased adipose tissue, which is poorly supplied by the peripheral circulation, and therefore less oxygenated blood and nutrients are delivered to the tissues by the blood. In underweight clients, there may be inadequate storage of suitable energy, which can lead to impaired collagen synthesis and delayed healing. Both obese and underweight clients are at greater risk for pressure sore formation.

NUTRITION. Malnutrition can be present in both obese and underweight clients. Malnutrition results from a diet that is deficient in one or more of the nutrients that are essential for cells to repair damaged tissue and to help prevent damage. An adequate nutritional diet and the body's ability to effectively utilize the energy and deliver the nutrients to the cells are essential for tissue repair and for prevention and elimination of infection. Protein, vitamins, carbohydrates, fats, trace elements, and fluids are necessary and play an essential role in the wound-healing process.

INFECTION. Infection can develop when defense mechanisms are weakened, thus allowing a normal bacterial load to become overwhelming. Alternatively, the bacterial load can be greater than the body's defenses can handle. In healthy clients, the critical number is 100,000 bacteria per gram of tissue. This number is expressed as 10^5 on laboratory cultures of wounds (and other body fluids or tissues). This threshold number for bacteria holds true for all kinds of bacteria except group B streptococci, which can cause infection in lesser quantities. When bacteria are present above 10^5, the body loses control over bacterial proliferation and invasion and infection is present.

The diagnosis of infection is made through quantitative wound biopsy specimen cultures. Results take 24 to 48 hours, and the client receives a broad-spectrum antibiotic while awaiting results. Sometimes, foreign bodies within the wound are a source of infection. Examples include soil, hematoma (accumulations of blood), and bone fragments.

DECREASED CIRCULATION. An adequate blood supply is essential for all aspects of wound healing. The blood supply can be restricted through disorders of the heart, vessels, or lungs. Hypoxia impairs delivery of oxygen and nutrients to the wound and the action of various defensive cells. Neutrophils require oxygen to generate hydrogen peroxide to kill the pathogens. Likewise, fibroblast and collagen proliferation is slowed. The only aspect of wound healing that can proceed in hypoxic states is angiogenesis.

DIABETES MELLITUS. Diabetes predisposes many clients to difficulty in wound healing because of impaired collagen synthesis, angiogenesis, and phagocytosis. Elevated glucose levels interfere with the cellular transport of ascorbic acid into various cells, including fibroblasts and leukocytes. Hyperglycemia also decreases leukocyte chemotaxis. Atherosclerosis, especially of small vessels, is also common in clients with diabetes and impairs tissue oxygen delivery. Diabetic neuropathy further impairs healing by interrupting the neurologic components of healing (e.g., reducing vasodilation and the protective sensation of pain). Control of glucose levels after surgery facilitates normal wound healing.

SMOKING. Smoking causes vasoconstriction and hypoxia because of the carbon monoxide in the smoke. In addition to limiting oxygen supply, smoking increases atherosclerosis and platelet aggregation. These conditions further restrict the amount of oxygen in the wound.

STEROIDS. The use of steroids slows healing by inhibiting collagen synthesis. Clients who are taking steroids have decreased wound strength, inhibited contraction, and impeded epithelialization. Fortunately, vitamin A reverses some of the healing impairments caused by steroids.

■ EXTRINSIC FACTORS

Extrinsic factors are often the initial cause influencing the failure for wounds to respond favorably to local wound management or systemic therapy of chronic disease. Awareness of the extrinsic factors and their effects on the wound is an important component of good, consistent wound care.

Extrinsic factors of delayed wound healing include (1) mechanical stresses, (2) debris, (3) environmental temperature, (4) maceration, and (5) chemical assaults.

MECHANICAL STRESSES. Mechanical stresses that impede wound healing include friction and shear. Friction is the force that occurs when skin is dragged across a coarse surface, such as bed linens. Shearing forces occur when a mechanical force acts on an area of skin in a direction parallel to the body's surface. Shear is affected by the amount of pressure exerted, the coefficient of friction between the materials contacting each other, and the extent to which the body makes contact with the support surface. Shearing force often occurs when clients sit for a long period of time. When sitting, their skin remains stuck to the support surface while the underlying structures slide down because of gravity. This internal pressure can deter wound healing or cause new wounds.

DEBRIS. When foreign material is left in the wound it prolongs the inflammatory response and may increase the potential for infection. Foreign material in wounds may include cotton fibers, loose grit, or necrotic or sloughy tissue. Appropriate debridement must be used to remove the foreign material.

ENVIRONMENTAL TEMPERATURE. Extreme temperatures can be devastating to a wound. Frostbite or burns can delay or prevent healing and cause extensive damage. The caregiver must be cautious when using heat or cold to treat the symptoms of the wound. Cold causes vasoconstriction and heat brings about vasodilation. The effects of these changes in circulation must be considered when temperature is used in wound care.

MACERATION. Continuous exposure of wounds and the surrounding skin to moisture from the outside or poor management of wound exudate can lead to maceration and break down the skin surrounding the wound, causing enlargement of the wounded tissues. Protection of the skin and the wound surface with appropriate wound dressings and care of the skin by careful skin hygiene help to reduce the effects of urine, feces, and sweating or excessive wound exudate.

CHEMICALS. The use of chemical substances on wounds can no longer be advocated. Topical antiseptics do not significantly reduce the numbers of bacteria in wounds and are toxic to the cells within the body attempting to repair the defect. If cleaning of a wound is required, normal saline is recommended.

WOUND INFECTION

Wound infection is a serious consequence and delays wound healing. Infection is often due to lack of blood supply, lack of oxygen, or exposure to environmental pathogens. Clinical manifestations of wound infection include increased drainage, erythema around the entire wound (not just the edges), and development of purulent drainage, pain, fever, leukocytosis, and general malaise. The infected wound is slow to heal and may open (see text on evisceration and dehiscence later).

Cultures can be used in the diagnosis of wound infection. A swab culture of wound drainage can be obtained. A quantitative culture (an actual sample of tissue) is usually needed to study open wounds. All open wounds are colonized, and using a swab culture does not reveal the true offending organisms, only organisms growing on the wound's surface.

Outcome Management

Topical antimicrobial agents can be used as the primary treatment. The ideal antimicrobial is a broad-spectrum agent and preserves the regenerating tissues. All antimicrobials compromise wound healing to some degree by having low efficacy against a particular organism or by interfering with healing. A variety of topical agents can be used to either clean or disinfect the wound (see Table 16–4).

Hydrogen peroxide breaks down into water and oxygen. When hydrogen peroxide is used in a wound, H_2O_2 must be rinsed off the wound bed with normal saline to remove any trapped oxygen before the tissues can absorb it. Povidone-iodine, acetic acid, and sodium hypochlorite are used only in debris-contaminated, infected, and malodorous wounds. These agents are cytotoxic and inhibit granular tissue growth and damage endothelial cells and fibroblasts. Therefore, their use is usually short term.

Medical Management

The goal of medical management of clients with wound infection is to promote healing. The extrinsic and intrinsic factors that lead to nonhealing are examined. Not all of these factors can be eliminated, however. Clients cannot be made younger, and some clients refuse to stop smoking, even though their nonhealing is due to inadequate circulation. At times, bypass surgery may be required to restore adequate blood flow. Cultured epithelial grafts and hyperbaric oxygen are relatively new treatments in the care of nonhealing wounds. Wound healing accelerators, such as topically applied growth factors, electric currents, and negative pressure, are being studied. Most chronic nonhealing wounds are managed by a team of health care providers that may include a wound care physician, vascular or orthopedic surgeons, a wound care nurse, a nutritionist, a physical therapist, hyperbaric medicine specialists, and social workers and psychologists. Even for these teams, chronic nonhealing wounds are a challenge.

Chronic wounds commonly affect several groups of clients. Clients with diabetes, venous or arterial disease of the legs, and collagen diseases (such as scleroderma) often do not heal quickly or completely. Several forms of adjunctive treatment are discussed briefly next.

ADJUNCTIVE WOUND HEALING TREATMENTS

ELECTRIC STIMULATION. Pulsed galvanic stimulation (Diapulse) is a form of electricity applied to the skin's surface. The electric currents stimulate DNA synthesis, increase blood flow, enhance fibroblast proliferation, and promote cell migration across the wound. This modality appears to be effective in promoting healing in wounds that have been refractory to other forms of treatment. Clients who are considering the use of electrotherapy should seek centers that have proper equipment and trained personnel.

HYPERBARIC OXYGEN THERAPY. Hyperbaric oxygen (HBO) is the administration of oxygen at greater than atmospheric pressure. When oxygen is inhaled under pressure, the level of tissue oxygen is greatly increased. The high levels of oxygen promote the action of phagocytes and promote healing of the wound by increasing the action of fibroblasts. HBO is effective in clients with complex wounds, especially clients with osteomyelitis and other types of infection. HBO is becoming more available in the United States. As with electric stimulation, a properly trained staff is critical. Clients who have inner ear problems and claustrophobia require pretreatment care.

TOPICAL APPLICATION OF GROWTH FACTORS. The same growth factors that are found in the wound bed naturally can be grown in a laboratory and applied to the wound bed. Research is ongoing to determine the biologic activity and the potential benefits of topical application of these growth factors. The efficacy of these treatments is still being studied. At the present time, only becaplermin (Regranex), a PDGF for use in diabetic foot ulcers, has gained approval for use by the Food and Drug Administration.

NEGATIVE PRESSURE WOUND THERAPY. The application of controlled negative pressure in a clean wound bed can assist and accelerate wound healing. A black sterile, reticulated foam sponge is placed in the wound bed. A connecting evacuation tube is attached to external suction and removes excess fluid in the wound and peripheral edema. The foam and tube are secured with transparent adhesive dressing. A small electrical unit controls pressure, and drainage is collected in a canister attached to the unit and to the sponge. Negative pressure wound therapy increases healing rates by up to 40%.

Nursing Management of the Medical Client

Your role in the care of the client with a nonhealing wound is to provide ample information for self-care, including how to change dressings, the disease process underlying the wound, and how to return to work or activities without increasing the risk of nonhealing. For example, a woman with venous stasis ulcers may need to return to work but can do so safely only when the ulcer is healed. She also needs to know how to apply bandages, how long to elevate her legs while at work, and how to move her legs while working (e.g., walking rather than standing). You serve a vital role in determining whether these requirements are feasible for the client and employer.

WOUND DISRUPTION

Dehiscence is the interruption of a previously intact suture line (see Chapter 16). A sharp pain in the suture line or a cough and increased serosanguineous drainage from the wound frequently precede dehiscence. *Evisceration* is the opening of a wound with exposure of internal organs. It is obviously more serious than dehiscence. If a client experiences evisceration, cover the exposed organs with sterile wet dressings, notify the physician, and prepare the client for surgery. Also notify the physician about dehiscence, although it is not an emergency.

ALTERED COLLAGEN SYNTHESIS

Hypertrophic scars are scars that are raised above the suture line. They may be painful and itch. In general, hypertrophic scars tend to regress over time. Keloids are scars that extend well beyond the suture line (Fig. 16–9). These scars tend to occur in African Americans and clients of Mediterranean descent. The scars can be excised from a wound but, unfortunately, tend to recur. Newer treatments include the use of topical forms of heat.

CONCLUSIONS

Wound healing is a complex process but often goes on with little effort on the part of the client. Only when the wound does not heal or pressure ulcers develop are the many steps in wound healing evident. Wound care follows some basic principles: debride the wound of nonviable tissues, keep the wound bed moist, protect the surrounding skin, apply the proper dressings, use safe topical agents, and fill dead space.

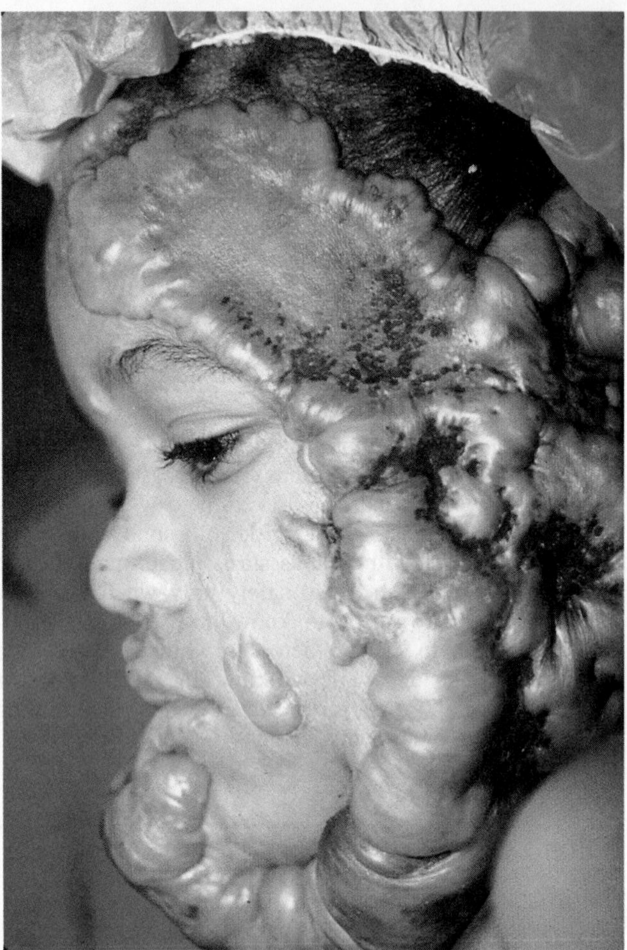

Figure 16–9 Keloid formation. Keloids are overgrowths of scar tissue above and beyond the normal boundaries of the scar. They are fairly resistant to treatment.

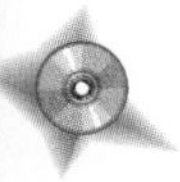

THINKING CRITICALLY

1. You are caring for a man with large venous stasis ulcers on his lower legs. When he was admitted, the ulcers were covered with soft yellow devitalized tissue. He has been treated with wet-to-dry dressings for the past 7 days. Today, you notice that the ulcers are red and wet with a lumpy appearance. What should be done?

Factors to Consider. Is the appearance of red and lumpy tissue in a wound good or bad? What might be happening? What type of dressing is best used on this red and lumpy tissue?

2. You are caring for an older homeless man after emergency abdominal surgery. He has had a nasogastric tube in place for 3 days for ileus and is receiving 1 L of IV fluids of 5% dextrose with 0.45 normal saline with 20 mEq of potassium every 8 hours. Prior to surgery, serum albumin was 3.2 g/dl, hemoglobin was 9.6 g/dl, and WBCs were 17,000/mm^3. His weight was 104 pounds and height 5 feet 5 inches. What are this client's chances of recovery? What interventions should be considered?

Factors to Consider. Does this client have evidence of malnutrition? If so, what effect does malnutrition have on wound healing? What short-term and long-term interventions may need to be initiated? Does this client have a risk of fluid or electrolyte imbalance? If so, which ones, and what can be done (or is being done) to reduce the risk?

BIBLIOGRAPHY

1. Baranoski, S. (1995). Wound assessment and dressing selection. *Ostomy and Wound Management, 41* (suppl. 7A), 7S–12S.
2. Bergstrom, N., et al. (1994). *Treatment of pressure ulcers.* Clinical Practice Guideline, No. 15. Rockville, MD, U.S. Department of Health and Human Services, Public Health Service, Agency for Health Care Policy and Research. AHCPR Pub. No. 95-B0652.
3. Black, S. (1995). Venous stasis ulcers. *Ostomy and Wound Management, 41*(8), 20–32.
4. Brylinsky, C. M. (1995). Nutrition and wound healing: An overview. *Ostomy and Wound Management, 41,* 14–16.
5. Cooper, D. (1995). Indices to include in wound assessment. *Advances in Wound Care, 8*(4), 18–25.
6. Eastman, S. (1997). Negative pressure wound therapy. *Plastic Surgical Nursing, 18*(1), 27–37.

6a. Falanga, V., et al. (1995). Experimental approaches to chronic wounds. *Wound Repair and Regeneration, 3*(2), 132–140.

7. Gentzkow, G. D. (1992). Electrical stimulation for dermal wound healing. *Wounds: A Compendium of Clinical Research and Practice, 4*(6), 227–235.
8. Kerstein, M. (1997). The scientific basis of healing. *Advances in Wound Care, 10*(3), 30–36.
9. Kerstein, M., & Polasky, S. (1995). Wounds associated with decreased sensibility. *Wounds: A Compendium of Clinical Research and Practice, 7*(1), 30–34.
10. Kiy, A. M. (1997). Nutrition and wound healing: A bio-psychosocial perspective. *Nursing Clinics of North America, 32,* 849–862.
11. Ladin, D. A. (1998). Understanding dressings. *Clinics in Plastic Surgery, 25,* 433–441.
12. Lazarus, G., et al. (1994). Definitions and guidelines for assessment of wounds and evaluating healing. *Archives of Dermatology, 130,* 489–493.
13. Netscher, D., & Clamon, J. (1994). Smoking: Adverse effects on outcomes for plastic surgical patients. *Plastic Surgical Nursing, 14*(4), 205–210.
14. Stotts, N., & Hunt, T. (1997). Managing bacterial colonization and infection. *Clinics in Geriatric Medicine, 13*(3), 565–573

CHAPTER 17

Perspectives on Infectious Disorders

Carol Sharkey

For one brief moment in human history (circa 1950 to 1980), management of infectious disease did not dominate health care practice. By the close of that era, sickness and death caused by infectious diseases had plummeted as a result of multifaceted social, public health, and medical control efforts. Environmental sanitation had curbed such killers as yellow fever, cholera, typhus, malaria, typhoid fever, and plague.

International vaccination programs had eradicated smallpox. Organized efforts to vaccinate all children lowered the occurrence of vaccine-preventable diseases, particularly measles, mumps, rubella, diphtheria, tetanus, and poliomyelitis. Improved living conditions and personal hygiene had diminished parasitic diseases and gastrointestinal (GI) infections. The widespread availability of antibiotics quelled the fear of deadly tuberculosis, syphilis, gonorrhea, bacterial meningitis, scarlet fever, and rheumatic fever. Nosocomial (hospital-acquired) infections, which had already responded to medical asepsis, responded further to antibiotics, and medical technology continued to produce anti-infective agents to match the newly developing antibiotic-resistant organisms. As a result, health professionals could focus on prevention and management of chronic disease.

This brief moment in history did not last. The 1980s and 1990s brought new infectious agents, such as *Legionella,* the human immunodeficiency virus (HIV), and the Ebola virus (which actually first appeared in 1976), all reminders of human vulnerability to infectious disease. Hepatitis, tuberculosis, sexually transmitted diseases, and many vaccine-preventable diseases persist, spread, and continue to kill. Nonpathogenic organisms continue to create devastating disease in immunocompromised people and in those with chronic diseases or malnutrition. Antibiotic-resistant organisms have developed with chronic misuse and improper prescription of antibiotics. In addition, many of the major killers of the past, such as cholera and yellow fever, continue to cause death and destruction in parts of the world where poor sanitation, poor hygiene, and poverty are endemic.

All people, particularly health care professionals, must maintain vigilance to infectious diseases—to prevention rather than simply treatment. Prevention requires an understanding of the infectious process and the control measures needed. This chapter describes the process of infection and selected aspects of prevention and control. Other chapters explain the nursing care of clients with specific infectious diseases.

THE PROCESS OF INFECTION

Infection is a process by which an organism establishes a parasitic relationship with its host. The process begins with transmission of an infectious organism. Infection may end in infectious disease, a condition that depends on the response of the host to the invader. The entire process and its outcome hinge on a complex interaction of (1) the *infectious agent,* (2) an *environment* conducive to transmission of the organism, and (3) a susceptible *host.* The agent, the host, and their environmental interaction are prerequisites to infectious disease.

■ AGENT

Humans coexist with many microorganisms in complex, mutually beneficial relationships. Many organisms establish residence on or in the host and usually cause no harm. Other organisms are parasitic, maintaining themselves at the expense of their host. Some parasites arouse a pathologic response in the host and are called *pathogens* or *pathogenic agents.* In one sense, pathogens are ineffective parasites because they stimulate an inflammatory response, leading to a disease that may harm the host and eventually kill the pathogen.

All microorganisms can be distinguished by certain intrinsic properties. These properties provide the basis for identifying and classifying bacteria, viruses, fungi, and helminths. An organism's properties include its shape, size, structure, chemical composition, antigenic make-up, growth requirements, viability under adverse environmental conditions, and ability to produce toxins. Viability is a particularly important property to health care professionals because it determines the pathogen's ability to survive outside its host. Organisms that can survive drying, sunlight, heat, or other adverse environmental conditions require more aggressive tactics to prevent transmission.

■ ENVIRONMENT

Transmission of an infectious agent from a source to a susceptible host occurs within an environment. Organisms live and multiply in a *reservoir,* which can be a person, animal, plant, soil, food, or other organic substance or combination of substances. The reservoir provides what the organism needs for survival at specific stages in its life cycle. Infected people are the reservoirs for most bacteria and viruses that affect humans.

Both human and animal reservoirs may be infected and, therefore, may also be hosts. An infected host may be asymptomatic—a *carrier* of the pathogen. A carrier maintains an environment that promotes growth, multiplication, and shedding of the parasite without exhibiting manifestations of disease.

Organisms can have one or more than one *route of transmission* from the reservoir to a new host. In fact, transmission can occur through five mechanisms:

1. *Contact transmission.* Through *direct* transmission, an organism moves from an infected person (or carrier) to an uninfected person via direct contact between their body surfaces. Through *indirect* transmission, an uninfected person picks up an infectious organism from an intermediate object, such as contaminated gloves, a used needle, or a dirty dressing.
2. *Droplet transmission.* An uninfected person picks up an infectious organism when an infected person coughs, sneezes, or talks. These activities propel droplets a short distance through the air, and they may land on an uninfected person's conjunctivae, nasal mucosa, or oral mucosa. Certain procedures, such as suctioning and bronchoscopy, can generate droplets as well.
3. *Airborne transmission.* Droplets can evaporate into airborne nuclei, or microbes can become attached to floating dust particles. Unlike droplets, dry nuclei and dust particles can float a long way in the air. Relatively few organisms remain viable as airborne nuclei, but those that do can be transmitted in the air and breathed into the lungs.
4. *Common vehicle transmission.* Many uninfected people can pick up an infectious organism from the same contaminated source, such as food, water, a medication, or a device.
5. *Vector transmission,* An infected creature, such as a mosquito, fly, rat, or flea, transmits an infectious organism by biting an uninfected host.

The *portal of exit* is the place whence the parasite escapes the reservoir. Generally, this site corresponds to the *portal of entry* into the next host. For example, the portal of exit for GI parasites is generally the feces and the portal of entry into a new host is the mouth. As is the case with other links in the transmission chain, variability exists. Hookworm eggs, for example, are shed in the feces, but hookworm larvae enter through the skin of a person walking barefoot in soil containing hatched eggs. Common portals of exit include secretions and fluids (respiratory and vaginal secretions, blood, tears, semen, breast milk), excretions (urine and feces), open lesions, and exudates. Some organisms, such as HIV, have more than one portal of exit. Knowledge of the portal of exit is essential for preventing transmission of a pathogen.

A pathogen may enter a new host by ingestion, inhalation, contact with mucous membranes, percutaneously, or transplacentally. Infectious diseases vary as to the number of organisms and the duration of the exposure required to start the infectious process in a new host.

■ HOST

Some humans are more susceptible to infectious disease than others. A susceptible host has characteristics and behaviors that increase the probability of infectious disease. Factors such as age, sex, ethnicity, heredity, altitude, and temperature influence the likelihood of infection. For example, the ethnic custom of eating raw fish may increase the risk of exposure to pathogens. General health and nutritional status, hormonal balance, and the presence of concurrent disease also play a role. Living conditions and personal behaviors—such as drug use, diet, hygiene, and sexual practices—also influence the risk of exposure to pathogens and resistance once exposure has occurred. Susceptibility is also influenced by anatomic and physiologic defenses, sometimes called *lines of defense.* Even though an infectious disease is said to be caused by an etiologic (causal) agent, infection results from interactions among a variety of factors related to agent, host, and environment (Table 17–1).

The host's first-line defenses are external and act to bar invasion by pathogens. These defenses are nonspecific, in that they act against any invading pathogen. First-line defenses include (1) *physical* and *chemical barriers* and (2) the body's own natural flora.

Physical barriers include intact skin and mucous membranes; oil and perspiration on skin; cilia in respiratory passages; gag and cough reflexes; peristalsis in the GI tract; and the flushing action of tears, saliva, and mucus. All act to remove organisms before they have an opportunity to infect. The chemical composition of body secretions such as tears and sweat, together with the pH of saliva, vaginal secretions, urine, and digestive juices, further prevents or inhibits the growth of organisms. Compromise of any of these natural defenses increases host susceptibility to pathogen invasion.

Another important first-line defense is the *normal flora* of microorganisms that inhabit the skin and mucous membranes of the oral cavity, GI tract, and vagina. These microorganisms are indigenous to (occur naturally in) specific tissue. They typically coexist with their host in a mutually beneficial relationship as long as they do not migrate from the specific site. Through a mechanism called *microbial antagonism,* they control the replication of potential pathogens. The importance of this mechanism is evident when the mechanism is disturbed. An example of disturbance is the overgrowth of *Candida albicans* (thrush) that results from extensive antibiotic therapy that destroys normal flora in the GI tract or vagina.

Some normal flora can become pathogenic under specific conditions, such as immunosuppression or displacement of the pathogen to another area of the body. The opportunistic infections experienced by clients with symptomatic HIV infection are an example of immunosuppression. Displacement is seen when *Escherichia coli,* normally found in the GI tract, invades the urogenital tract

TABLE 17–1 AGENTS AND SITES OF SELECTED INFECTIOUS DISEASES

Disease	Infectious Agent	Site of Infection	Reservoir	Mode of Transmission
BACTERIA				
Cholera	*Vibrio cholerae*	Gastrointestinal tract	Humans	Ingestion of water contaminated with feces
Diarrhea	*Escherichia coli*	Gastrointestinal tract	Humans	Ingestion of contaminated food or water
Giardiasis	*Giardia lamblia*	Gastrointestinal tract	Water, humans, wild animals	Ingestion of cysts in fecally contaminated water and food
Gonorrhea	*Neisseria gonorrhoeae*	Genitourinary tract	Humans	Sexual contact
Lyme disease	*Borrelia burgdorferi*	Skin, joints, systemic	Wild rodents and deer	Tick bite
Malaria	*Plasmodium* spp.	Red blood cells, liver	Mosquito	Bite from infected mosquito
Meningitis	*Neisseria meningitidis*	Meninges	Humans	Direct contact with droplets from respiratory passages
Pneumonia	*Streptococcus pyogenes*	Lung	Humans	Inhalation; aspiration of gastric contents
Rocky mountain spotted fever	*Rickettsia rickettsii*	Vascular endothelium	Ticks	Tick bite
Toxoplasmosis	*Toxoplasma gondii*	Eye, lung, brain	Cats	Ingestion of cysts on fecally contaminated fingers or in food; transplacental
Tuberculosis	*Mycobacterium tuberculosis*	Lung	Humans	Inhalation of droplet nuclei
Wound infection	*Staphylococcus aureus*	Connective tissue	Humans	Contaminated hands, surgical instruments
FUNGI				
Candidiasis	*Candida albicans*	Skin, mucous membranes, genital tract	Humans	Overgrowth associated with damaged skin or mucosa or use of antibiotics
Histoplasmosis	*Histoplasma capsulatum*	Lung	Bat or bird feces	Inhalation of spores
HELMINTHS				
Trichinosis	*Trichinella spiralis*	Gastrointestinal tract, muscle	Animals	Ingestion of raw or undercooked meat
VIRUSES				
Acquired immunodeficiency syndrome (AIDS)	Human immunodeficiency virus	Helper T lymphocyte	Humans	Contaminated needles, blood transfusions, sexual contact, transplacental
Hepatitis B	Hepatitis B virus	Liver	Humans	Contaminated needles, blood transfusions, sexual contact, perinatal
Influenza A	Influenza A virus	Respiratory tract	Humans	Direct contact by aerosol droplets; airborne spread
Measles (rubeola)	Paramyxoviridae	Skin, respiratory tract, systemic	Humans	Direct contact with nasal or throat secretions; airborne spread
Rabies	*Lyssavirus*	Systemic	Dogs, wild animals	Animal bite

and becomes pathogenic. Displacement of normal flora is a common cause of nosocomial infections. Invasive procedures increase the risk of displacing these organisms. For this reason, it is essential to maintain meticulous hand-washing and asepsis.

The *second line of defense* (the inflammatory process) and the *third line* (the immune response) share several physiologic components. These include the lymphatic system, leukocytes, and a multitude of proteins and enzymes.

Even after successful transmission of a pathogen, there may be more than one possible outcome. The pathogen may merely contaminate the body surface. The process ends there if the host's first-line defenses, such as intact skin or mucous membranes, block the pathogen from further invasion. Successful invasion with replication of a pathogen that does not lead to clinical manifestations or a detectable immune response is referred to as *colonization.*

When microorganisms in or on the host cause an immune response, an infection is said to be present. The period of time during which the pathogen is replicating but before it is shed from the host is called the *latent period.* During latency, host inflammatory and immune responses may ward off the organism or its by-products, thus preventing tissue damage, or the pathogen or its products may begin to destroy undefended or poorly defended tissue, producing infectious disease. Disease manifestations herald the end of the *incubation period,* which is defined as the time from invasion of the disease to the appearance of manifestations. By definition, *infectious disease* is the pathophysiologic response of a host to the destructive action of the pathogen, to its toxic products, or to the host immune responses to fight the pathogen. This pathophysiologic response is generally symptomatic. An asymptomatic pathologic response is called a *subclinical infection.*

An important point is that an asymptomatic host can still transmit a pathogen. The host may harbor the pathogen in sufficient quantities to shed it at any time after latency and toward the end of the incubation period. The time during which an organism can be shed is called the *period of communicability.* It usually precedes manifestations and coincides with part or all of the clinical disease, sometimes extending to convalescence. The communicable period, like the incubation period, varies with the pathogen and the disease.

TABLE 17–2 THE MOST COMMON CAUSES OF NOSOCOMIAL INFECTION*

Site of Infection	Pathogen
Bloodstream	Coagulase-negative staphylococci *Staphylococcus aureus* *Enterococcus* spp. *Candida albicans* *Enterobacter* spp.
Lung	*Pseudomonas aeruginosa* *Staphylococcus aureus* *Enterobacter* spp. *Klebsiella pneumoniae* *Haemophilus influenzae*
Surgical wound	*Enterococcus* spp. Coagulase-negative staphylococci *Staphylococcus aureus* *Pseudomonas aeruginosa* *Enterobacter* spp.
Urinary tract	*Escherichia coli* *Candida albicans* *Enterococcus* spp. *Pseudomonas aeruginosa* *Klebsiella pneumoniae*

* Organisms are listed by major site and order of importance.
Data from Centers for Disease Control and Prevention. (1997). National Nosocomial Infections Surveillance Report, data summary from October 1986–April 1997, issued May 1997. *American Journal of Infection Control, 25,* 477–487.

RISKS OF HOSPITALIZATION

Nosocomial infections (which arise in a hospital or other health care facility) are a leading cause of death in the United States and are associated with significant morbidity.[18, 27] Infections present or incubating at the time of admission are referred to as *community-acquired.* From 5% to 10% of hospitalized clients acquire a nosocomial infection.[18] Occupationally acquired infections among the staff of a hospital are also considered nosocomial.

The source of nosocomial pathogens in health care facilities varies, but both health care workers and clients are reservoirs in most instances. For example, *Staphylococcus aureus* is often carried on the skin and in the nasopharynx. Respiratory secretions, feces, urine, and blood are reservoirs for some nosocomial organisms. Liquids and inanimate objects in the hospital environment may also serve as sources of nosocomial infections. The most important means of transmission is via the hands of health care workers. Hand-washing, combined with principles of asepsis and proper use of gloves, is the best method of preventing nosocomial infections.

The most common sites of nosocomial infections in clients are the urinary tract, lower respiratory tract, surgical wounds, and the bloodstream.[11] Various pathogens can cause nosocomial infections in multiple sites. For example, *Pseudomonas aeruginosa* is the organism that causes most cases of nosocomial pneumonia, but it also causes urinary tract and surgical site infections. *S. aureus* is a common cause of surgical site infection, pneumonia, and bloodstream infection. Table 17–2 lists common nosocomial pathogens.

■ URINARY TRACT INFECTIONS

Urinary tract infections (UTIs) are the most common nosocomial infections, and about 80% stem from urethral catheterization.[18, 29] Major risk factors for catheter-related UTIs include female sex, increased duration of catheterization, breaks in the closed catheter system, and lack of administration of systemic antimicrobial agents.[27]

In most catheter-related infections in women, bacteria enter the bladder by the periurethral route. Organisms originating primarily from the fecal flora and found at the meatal and perineal areas may be introduced into the bladder during insertion of the catheter or may migrate along the external surface of the catheter into the bladder. In men, catheter-related infections usually result from *cross-infection* (transmission between clients), with bacteria introduced into the collection system at the junction of the catheter and drainage tube or at the outflow spigot; they then migrate to the bladder in 24 to 48 hours. Most nosocomial UTIs are easily managed, but bacteremia develops in 1% to 4% of affected clients. Of these, up to 15% of clients die.[29]

■ PNEUMONIA

Pneumonia is the second most common nosocomial infection and is associated with more deaths than any other nosocomial infection.[29] Most nosocomial pneumonias are caused by gram-negative bacteria. Aspiration of oropharyngeal or stomach organisms is the predominant mechanism by which nosocomial pneumonia develops.[18] Airborne transmission is usually not the cause.

Stasis (stoppage) of respiratory secretions caused by immobility and a decreased cough also contributes to nosocomial pneumonia. Postoperative clients, particularly those who have had thoracic and upper abdominal surgery, and clients who require ventilatory support are at high risk of aspiration. Clients with diminished consciousness, impaired gag reflex, intubation, or tracheostomy are also at increased risk for aspiration of oral secretions. Other risk factors include old age, decreased mobility, and severe disease, such as chronic lung disease, cardiovascular disease, renal insufficiency, and malignancies.

Nosocomial pneumonia is difficult to prevent because in most cases the microorganisms are derived from the client's own flora. Soon after hospitalization, the oropharynx of many clients becomes colonized with gram-negative bacteria that may be aspirated into the lungs. The use of histamine H_2-blockers, antimicrobial therapy, and enteral nutritional therapy have been found to promote colonization of the oropharynx with gram-negative bacteria.[18, 29] Contaminated respiratory therapy equipment can serve as a source of pathogens as well.

■ SURGICAL WOUND INFECTIONS

Surgical wound infections are a major source of hospital morbidity and account for nearly 60% of extra hospital days.[18] These infections usually result from *endogenous* (inside the host) or *exogenous* (outside the host) microorganisms that enter the wound at the time of an operation. The most common source of infecting bacteria is the client's own flora. Although the physical environment of the operating room is an uncommon source of infection, operating room personnel may shed bacteria-laden skin particles that travel through the air to the open wound.

Factors that influence the development of surgical wound infections include (1) number and types of organisms present in the wound, (2) type of operation, (3) surgeon's technique, and (4) duration of the operation. Surgical wound infection rates almost double for each hour of surgery.[18] Old age, obesity, malnutrition, and underlying immunocompromise are client-related factors that increase the risk of postoperative wound infection.

The risk of surgical wound infection also increases with the length of the client's preoperative hospital stay.[18, 29] Shortening the preoperative stay tends to reduce the risk of infection by decreasing the opportunity for colonization with nosocomial bacteria.[18, 29] Proper preparation of the surgical site is also important. Shaving the operative site—once a common practice—is now known to damage the epithelium, impair the skin's defense mechanism, and raise the risk of infection.

■ DEVICE-RELATED INFECTIONS AND BACTEREMIAS

Rates of nosocomial infection of the bloodstream are increasing, particularly in clients admitted to intensive care units.[29] The increase is partly due to the increased use of intravascular devices in this setting. Intravascular devices may include intravenous (IV) lines, intra-arterial infusion lines, and devices used for diagnostic, therapeutic, and hemodynamic monitoring. The risk of infection is influenced by factors related to the device itself, the site of insertion, and the technique used to place the device. Stiff catheters are associated with higher rates of infection than flexible catheters. Partially implantable catheters and totally implanted injection ports are associated with lower infection rates.[18]

Device-related infections and bacteremias are usually caused by microorganisms found on the client's skin that invade disrupted tissue and migrate around the site of insertion and along the device into the intravascular space. The use of semipermeable membrane dressings over the insertion site facilitates the growth of skin flora. Dressing changes following institution-specific protocols must be done at regularly scheduled intervals under aseptic conditions. Colonization of skin flora can also occur around the hub of the device, the tubing-device junction, or other connectors attached to the system. Although liquids given through the device may become contaminated, infusion-related infection is relatively uncommon.

Client factors that contribute to the risk of device-related infections include age, nutritional status, type and severity of underlying illness, skin condition, and immunosuppressive therapy. Bacteremia is especially common in clients with chronic diseases, malnutrition, and cancer.

■ ANTIBIOTIC-RESISTANT MICROORGANISMS

S. aureus is one of the pathogens most frequently reported to cause nosocomial infections because of its remarkable ability to develop resistance to antibiotics. Before the advent of penicillin in the early 1940s, the fatality rate for bacteremia caused by *S. aureus* was about 90%.[22] The use of penicillin dramatically reduced that rate, but within a few years resistant strains of *S. aureus* evolved that produced a penicillin inactivator. New antibiotics, such as methicillin, were effective in the 1960s, but they provided only a temporary solution to the problem. In the 1980s, epidemics of infections with methicillin-resistant *S. aureus* (commonly called MRSA) forced operating rooms and intensive care units to close. Once introduced into a hospital, MRSA is difficult to eliminate.[22] It spreads via nasopharyngeal secretions and via the hands of health care workers and clients.

Prior to the introduction of linezolid (Zyvox) in 2000 and the combination of quinupristin and dalfopristin (Synercid) in 1999, vancomycin was the antimicrobial agent of choice for MRSA[14, 14a]. The action of Zyvox differs from other antibimicrobials in that it blocks bacterial growth by disrupting initiation of the process that microorganisms use to make proteins. Zyvox is administered via intravenous and oral routes and is effective against gram-positive bacteria such as *S. aureus,* streptococci, and enterococci.

Strains of vancomycin-resistant *Enterococcus* (VRE) began to appear in the mid-1980s, and these organisms are now important nosocomial pathogens. Treatment of VRE infections poses a major challenge because these organisms are resistant to a wide variety of antimicrobials. Synercid and Zyvox are the only drugs currently available for treatment of VRE. Environmental cultures in hospital rooms have identified VRE-contaminated client gowns, bed rails, floors, door handles, blood pressure cuffs, stethoscopes, glucose meters, and telephones.

Person-to-person spread, probably by the hands of health care workers, may be a significant mode of transmission.

■ OTHER NOSOCOMIAL INFECTIONS

Effective screening and processing of donated blood and blood products have greatly reduced the risk of HIV transmission to clients in health care settings. The risk of provider-to-client transmission of HIV is remote,[18] although the matter has created much public anxiety. The risk of occupational exposure to HIV in the health care setting has been associated primarily with parenteral exposures to blood from clients infected with HIV. Infection after exposure of mucous membranes to infected blood is much less common.

Nosocomial infection with *hepatitis B virus* (HBV) is another concern in hospitals because the source of a typical nosocomial HBV infection is never identified. Provider-to-client transmission of HBV does not occur with routine client contact. Client-to-provider transmission is a much larger problem and is why health care workers must be vaccinated against HBV.

The resurgence of *tuberculosis* is another major concern in health care facilities. Two factors responsible for this resurgence are (1) poor compliance with therapeutic drug regimens and (2) the emergence of drug-resistant strains of *Mycobacterium tuberculosis.* When clients infected with susceptible strains of the pathogen receive appropriate therapy, sputum smears begin to clear by the third week of treatment. Clients with resistant strains, however, continue to cough up large numbers of viable organisms, exposing many health care workers. Respiratory isolation must be closely followed with high-risk clients until adequate treatment has been given.

Nosocomial infections tend to occur more frequently and with more severity in ill, debilitated, malnourished, immunocompromised, and older clients (Box 17–1). Susceptibility to infection increases when invasive procedures and indwelling devices are used. With the expanding use of invasive devices, more exposure to antimicrobial therapy, and more severely ill hospitalized clients, the risk of nosocomial infections will probably increase. Furthermore, the emergence of resistant organisms is likely to continue, resulting in infections that are more difficult to treat. Although resistance to infection may be enhanced by vaccines and immune globulin, it must be supplemented by manipulation of the physical environment to reduce the risk. This means that nurses must be ever more vigilant in administering care and in supervising those providing care.

PREVENTING AND CONTROLLING INFECTION

To be effective, strategies to prevent and control infection must be based on knowledge of agent-host-environment interactions. The goal in developing and implementing interventions is to prevent the spread of an infectious agent from its reservoir or source to susceptible hosts.

Methods for controlling transmission of infectious disease vary with the characteristics of the organism, its reservoirs, the type of pathologic response it produces, and technology available for control. In general, the aim is to intervene at the point where the greatest number of people can be protected, using the least amount of resources.

BOX 17–1 Infectious Disease in the Elderly

More than any other population, elderly clients are at risk of infection. In fact, studies show that older clients contract about three times as many nosocomial infections as younger clients. Infection frequently leads to hospitalization for nursing home residents, and it is one of the top 10 causes of death in the elderly. Many common infectious diseases, such as pneumonia, urinary tract infection (UTI), sepsis, skin and soft tissue infection, tuberculosis, and herpes zoster, become more common with advancing age.

Elderly clients have an increased risk of infection partly as a normal consequence of growing older. With aging, mechanical barriers—such as skin and mucosa—undergo structural and functional decline. The physiologic reserve capacity of organ systems dwindles, and the immune system falters. When these defense mechanisms are compromised, infection can progress locally and even spread systemically.

Many older adults have chronic diseases that further jeopardize their host defenses. Conditions associated with aging, such as diabetes mellitus and malnutrition, probably exert more influence on immunity than age itself.

Not only do older people contract more infections; they tend to experience more complications of those infections. For example, an older client with pneumonia or a UTI is more likely to develop bacteremia than a younger client with the same infection.

To make matters worse, infection can be more difficult to detect and diagnose in the older client. Older people often do not manifest typical signs and symptoms of infectious diseases. Instead, they may have worsening cognition, an abnormal mental status, lethargy, agitation, loss of appetite, incontinence, or an increased tendency to fall.

Fever—the cardinal sign of infection—may be absent in infected elderly clients, even those who have bacteremia or pneumonia. Many older people have a low baseline temperature. Suspect infection in any elderly client with an oral temperature of 100° F or higher or an increase in baseline temperature of 1.4° F or more. Coexisting diseases may mask the signs of infection even further.

Even drugs used to treat infections are less successful when given to older clients. The drugs produce a weaker response in the older person's body while producing even more adverse reactions. Age-related changes in gastrointestinal, cardiac, and renal function alter the way in which antimicrobial agents are absorbed, distributed, and excreted.

Researchers are looking for better ways to detect and better drugs to treat infections in the elderly. While these agents are being investigated in the elderly population, you can help already infected clients by encouraging individualized dosage regimens and monitoring these clients carefully.

Data from Yoshikawa, T. T., & Normal, D. C. (Eds.). (1994). *Antimicrobial therapy in the elderly client.* New York: Marcel Dekker.

The simplest and most effective way to prevent transmission is meticulous *hand-washing.* Hand-washing is an absolute necessity, even when gloves are worn. Wash your hands before donning gloves and after removing them, before and after each client contact. Teach this procedure to all personnel and continually monitor for compliance. This simple, inexpensive technique, used appropriately, is one of the most potent weapons against the spread of infection. The hygienic hand rub is also effective. This technique involves rubbing 3 to 5 ml of a fast-acting antiseptic preparation onto the hands until dry.[29]

Another method to prevent and control infectious disease involves environmental measures. Some pathogens, such as *S. aureus,* can be controlled by disinfection, sterilization, or anti-infective drugs. Other pathogens can be controlled best by eradicating their non-human reservoirs via environmental sanitation measures, such as water treatment, food safety programs, and control of animals, vectors, sewage, and solid wastes.

Transmission from the portal of exit can often be prevented by detecting and treating clients who are shedding pathogens, such as gonococci. Antimicrobials are among the drugs most frequently prescribed in the United States to treat infections. The use of antibiotics is not without problems, as shown in Box 17–2. Another example of prevention is the use of prophylactic antitubercular medications for clients who are exposed to tuberculosis and whose skin test result is positive.

BOX 17–2 The Problem of Resistance to Antibiotics

Among researchers and health care professionals, there is growing concern over the frequent, widespread use of antimicrobial drugs in hospitals and long-term care facilities. Nursing home studies have revealed frequent orders for antibiotics, often without adequate evidence of underlying infection. Worse, many of these drugs were prescribed for infections not responsive to antibiotic therapy, such as viral respiratory tract infections.

Studies in hospitals have found antimicrobial drugs used routinely as prophylaxis for invasive and even noninvasive surgical procedures.[30] Although prophylaxis may be helpful when applied wisely, more than half the drugs studied were used inappropriately. Sometimes the wrong drug was ordered. Some were prescribed for unjustifiable reasons. Others were administered in the wrong dose or for the wrong duration of therapy.

Misuse of antimicrobial drugs may alter a client's normal flora and encourage resistance of pathogenic organisms. To help avoid growing resistance to antimicrobial drugs, obtain appropriate specimens for culture before starting antibiotic therapy. Also check sensitivity reports to ensure that the client receives an appropriate antibiotic.

Controlling the spread of antimicrobial resistance is difficult and requires appropriate selection and administration of antimicrobials, use of antibiotic combinations, and strict asepsis and infection control efforts. Finally, although infection control practices—such as hand-washing, aseptic techniques, and barrier precautions—do not directly limit the emergence of resistant strains, they do prevent transmission of resistant organisms from one client to another.

■ IMMUNIZATION PROGRAMS

Several infectious diseases have been dramatically reduced by maximizing host defenses through active and passive vaccinations that stimulate the immune system to counteract the infectious agent:

Active vaccination refers to the deliberate administration of a modified infecting agent, called a *vaccine,* or a modified toxin, called a *toxoid,* to stimulate an immune response. Protection is not immediate: a period of time is needed to achieve protective antibody levels. However, induced active immunity usually results in long-lived protection against disease.

Passive vaccination refers to the administration of antibodies to a nonimmune person to provide temporary protection against a pathogenic agent or toxin. Passive immunity provides immediate but short-lived protection that lasts a few weeks.

Vaccination programs in the United States have resulted in a significant reduction in childhood infectious diseases. However, a major resurgence of measles occurred from 1989 to 1991, signaling a major problem with childhood vaccination programs.[15] Baseline data from 1989 indicated that the immunization level of preschool children was approximately 70% to 80%, with some segments of the population having levels below 50%.[28] Urban minority populations, particularly African American and Hispanic American children, had much lower immunization levels than those in the general population.[15] The goal of the Department of Health and Human Services is to vaccinate at least 90% of all children in the United States by age 2 years.[28]

An entire population does not have to be immune for prevention of a disease epidemic. When a large proportion of individual members of a community becomes immune to a disease, the chance of contact between susceptible persons and infected persons decreases. This type of immunity is called *herd immunity.* For example, epidemics of measles are less likely to occur when herd immunity increases and the number of susceptible people in the community decreases.

Vaccination schedules and recommendations are established by the Committee on Infectious Diseases of the American Academy of Pediatrics (AAP) and the Advisory Committee on Immunization Practices (ACIP) of the Centers for Disease Control and Prevention (CDC). The AAP and ACIP recommend that all children be vaccinated against measles, mumps, rubella, diphtheria, pertussis, tetanus, poliomyelitis, *Haemophilus influenzae* type b, HBV, and varicella virus.[8] Hepatitis A (HAV) vaccines are recommended for high-risk children.

Vaccinations are as important for adolescents and adults as they are for children (Table 17–3). Infections seen primarily in children are now occurring in adolescents and adults who never developed active immunity. Adolescents and adults who escaped natural infection or who were not adequately immunized as children are at risk for childhood diseases and their complications. In 1996, the ACIP recommended establishing a routine vaccination visit to a health care provider for adolescents 11 to 12 years old to review their vaccination status and to administer needed vaccines for measles, mumps, rubella,

TABLE 17–3 CDC RECOMMENDATIONS FOR VACCINATION OF OLDER ADOLESCENTS AND ADULTS IN THE UNITED STATES

Disease	Recommendation
Polio	Primary series of oral poliovirus vaccine in childhood is sufficient. If no childhood series, vaccine need not be given except to persons at risk because of health care occupation or foreign travel.
Tetanus, diphtheria	Booster dose of tetanus and diphtheria toxoids (Td) every 10 years after primary series of Td; tetanus toxoid may be repeated in 5 years if a dirty wound is sustained. If no childhood series, initiate series of three doses within 1 year.
Pertussis	Primary series of pertussis vaccine is given in childhood only.
Measles	Documented immunity or two doses of MMR* vaccine at least 1 month apart. People who have received only one dose of vaccine since their first birthday should receive a second dose, particularly on enrolling in college, traveling to a foreign country, or entering a health care field.
Mumps	Documented immunity or two doses of MMR vaccine at least 1 month apart.
Rubella	Documented immunity or two doses of MMR vaccine at least 1 month apart. Vaccine particularly recommended for previously unimmunized women of childbearing age and susceptible health care providers.
Hepatitis A	Two doses of vaccine at least 6 months apart for persons who reside in a community that has a high rate of hepatitis A virus infection, who are at risk because of foreign travel, or who have chronic liver disease.
Hepatitis B	Complete series of three doses within 6 months for high-risk individuals including health care providers, susceptible dialysis clients, people with hemophilia, intravenous drug abusers, sexual and household contacts of hepatitis B virus carriers.
Varicella	Documented immunity or two doses of vaccine separated by 4 to 8 weeks. Recommended for health care providers, teachers of young children, day-care employees, and others at high risk for exposure and for transmitting disease.
Influenza	Annually for people older than 65; residents of nursing homes and other chronic care facilities; people with chronic cardiac or pulmonary disease, diabetes or other metabolic disorders, renal disease, severe anemia, or immunosuppression; health care providers and others in close contact with people in high-risk groups.
Pneumococcal	Single dose of vaccine for people older than 65; those with chronic cardiac or pulmonary disease, cirrhosis, alcoholism, diabetes, Hodgkin's disease, nephrosis, renal failure, cerebrovascular fluid leaks, immunosuppression, sickle cell anemia, and asplenism. Revaccination should be considered after 5 years for people at highest risk.

* MMR, measles-mumps-rubella vaccine.
Data from Centers for Disease Control and Prevention.[2, 5–7, 9, 12, 13]

HAV and HBV infections, tetanus, diphtheria, and varicella.[5]

Adolescents older than 12 years and adults through age 64 should complete a primary series of diphtheria and tetanus toxoids, plus measles-mumps-rubella vaccines if they did not receive them as children.[2] Adults 65 years and older should complete a primary series of diphtheria and tetanus toxoids but are generally considered immune to measles, mumps, and rubella. Most people born before 1957 are likely to have been infected naturally with these diseases. People who have a reliable history of varicella are considered immune; those who do not can be tested to determine their immune status or can be vaccinated without testing.[7] Vaccination for other diseases, such as influenza, pneumococcal pneumonia, HAV and HBV, is recommended for people in certain age, occupational, environmental, and lifestyle groups and for those with special health problems.

The elderly population and people with chronic diseases are at particular risk for infectious diseases because of a decline in their immune system. More than 90% of all deaths from influenza A and B viruses occur in people age 65 years and older.[12] The most effective way to reduce the impact of influenza is to vaccinate people at high risk each year before the influenza season. The ACIP recommends that influenza vaccine be administered annually to adolescents and adults at high risk and to all people age 65 and older. For people living in nursing homes and other chronic care facilities, annual vaccination can reduce the risk of influenza outbreaks by inducing herd immunity. Annual vaccination with the current vaccine is necessary because new variants of influenza continue to occur; vaccination against one strain may not confer immunity to another.

Pneumococcal pneumonia, caused by *Streptococcus pneumoniae,* is an important cause of morbidity and mortality in the very young, the elderly, and others with certain high-risk or chronic conditions. The ACIP recommends that these people receive a single dose of pneumococcal polysaccharide vaccine.

You and other nurses can be instrumental in ensuring that all children, adolescents, and adults are properly immunized. Every visit to a health care provider should be an opportunity to obtain a history of vaccination status and to provide vaccinations as needed. In addition, you and other health care providers should be concerned about improving your own resistance to infectious diseases. One important approach is to maintain your immunization status by being vaccinated against HBV infection, measles, mumps, rubella, polio, tetanus, diphtheria, varicella, and influenza.

HBV infection is a major occupational hazard for all health care providers because of the likelihood of contact with blood and blood-contaminated body fluids from infected clients. The Occupational Safety and Health Administration (OSHA) has developed regulations that require employers to offer at-risk employees the HBV vaccine at the employers' expense. Influenza vaccination is recommended yearly for health care providers in hospital, chronic care, and outpatient settings to reduce the risk of illness and to reduce the possibility of transmitting the virus to clients. The vaccinations you receive protect not only you but your clients as well.

INFECTION CONTROL IN HOSPITALS

Many nosocomial infections can be prevented if health care personnel adhere to infection control practices. The CDC and the Joint Commission on Accreditation of Healthcare Organizations (JCAHO) issue guidelines and establish standards for control of hospital infection. The CDC develops and updates guidelines related to the control and prevention of nosocomial infections, and JCAHO requires hospitals to establish infection control programs that meet accreditation standards. The JCAHO standards require hospital infection control committees to establish surveillance programs, implement infection control policies and procedures, and conduct continuing education for all hospital employees regarding infection control.[21] Most hospitals employ an infection control nurse or infection control practitioner (ICP) who is responsible for the coordination of a hospital-wide infection control program.

Infection control programs in hospitals address two major areas related to nosocomial infection: (1) surveillance and reporting and (2) control and prevention. The purpose of surveillance is to establish and maintain a database to track the rates of nosocomial infections. Surveillance activities include early detection of infections in clients and personnel and reporting of relevant data to designated people for appropriate action. Surveillance systems to detect both organisms and diseases are necessary components of prevention and control strategies. National data on nosocomial infections are obtained from selected hospitals in the United States by the CDC and used to estimate rates and trends.

The focus of infection control strategies is on barrier precautions to reduce infection risk for all clients and personnel and on occupational health practices to protect health care staff from infection.

Barrier Precautions

Barriers are intended to prevent the transfer of an infective organism to a susceptible host. By placing a clean layer of plastic or fabric between a susceptible site and a potential source of pathogenic organisms, we reduce likelihood of transmitting an infection. The prevented transmission can be from client to caregiver or caregiver to client. The risk for a client increases when caregivers have contact with the client's mucous membranes and non-intact skin. The risk for caregivers increases whenever they are in contact with a client's moist body substances. Protective barriers include gloves, gowns, masks, and protective eyewear.

None of the protective barriers are intended to replace hand-washing. *The most important means of preventing the spread of microorganisms is hand-washing.* Hands become soiled during client care, particularly after contact with moist body sites and substances. Soiled hands have played a major role in transferring organisms to new client hosts. Unfortunately, gloves provide a false sense of security because hands can become contaminated even when gloves are used. The use of gloves is not a substitute for hand-washing.

In the past, most barrier precautions were instituted after a client's infection was diagnosed. When an infection was suspected or recognized, a system of barrier precautions, referred to as *isolation procedures,* was instituted to prevent transmission of pathogens among hospitalized clients, health care personnel, and visitors. Depending on the diagnosis, one of several isolation strategies was used. Precautions varied, depending on the methods needed to interrupt transmission of the infection. For the isolation strategy to be effective, the diagnosis of infection had to be made or suspected early. However, most infections are communicable for some period when manifestations are absent and the infection is undetected.

In the early 1980s, unrecognized cases of HBV and HIV infection were identified as important sources of disease. Health care workers could potentially become infected through needle-sticks and body fluids contaminated with clients' blood. In response to this problem, the CDC recommended "universal precautions" as a means of preventing transmission of HIV, HBV, and other blood-borne pathogens.[1] Universal precautions focused on preventing transmission of blood-borne pathogens from infected or potentially infected clients to susceptible caregivers. Universal precautions required the use of protective barriers with all clients regardless of their presumed infection status. These precautions emphasized (1) the use of gloves and gowns to reduce contamination of skin and clothing; (2) the use of masks and goggles to reduce contamination of the mucous membranes of the mouth, nose, and eyes; and (3) prevention of needle-stick injuries. Used needles were not to be recapped by hand, and puncture-resistant containers were to be used for disposal of sharps.

In 1987, the practice of *body substance isolation* (BSI) was proposed as a system to isolate all moist and potentially infectious body substances from all clients, regardless of their presumed infection status.[20] Personnel were to use clean gloves during contact with non-intact skin and mucous membranes and when anticipating contact with blood, feces, urine, sputum, saliva, wound drainage, and other body fluids. BSI was based on the assumption that the blood and body substances of all clients might contain potentially infectious, transmissible organisms.

MANAGEMENT AND DELEGATION

Infection Control

Regulatory agencies have developed specific and complete guidelines for infection control to protect clients and staff from the transmission of infectious diseases. All health care providers must receive training and education on their role in maintaining infection control practices, including Universal Precautions. Your role in providing and delegating care of clients on isolation for known or suspected organisms includes assessment of clients and their environment. Note the level of precaution required according to your institution's system. Ensure that strict attention to isolation techniques is maintained by all who interact with the client. For the newly isolated client, you are responsible for client and family assessment and education regarding infection control measures. Unlicensed assistive personnel may then reinforce your teachings.

Some components of infection control practice may be delegated to unlicensed assistive personnel, such as room setup and maintenance of supplies and equipment. Consider delegating the following tasks:

- Stocking of gloves, gowns, and masks
- Stocking of client-specific equipment, such as thermometers, stethoscopes, and sphygmomanometers
- Cleaning of equipment after use, such as oxygen saturation machines and wheelchairs
- Removal of linen and unused equipment from the client's room

Delegation of direct care provision for clients in isolation to unlicensed assistive personnel should include reinforcement of the outlined precautions. Note: Care of a client in isolation does not change the practice parameters for what unlicensed assistive personnel may provide to the client or what you can delegate. Emphasize the ways in which the isolation status may affect delivery of care. For example, a client isolated because of methicillin-resistant *Staphylococcus aureus* (MRSA) is routinely cared for with gown, gloves, and mask. If that client is actively incontinent, you may need to give unlicensed assistive personnel additional instruction to change gloves between tasks.

Describe findings that are immediately reportable to you for the unlicensed assistive personnel. Such findings may include a disruption of isolation technique or any difficulty the unlicensed assistive personnel experience while providing care.

Kathleen Rea, BSN, RN, *Clinician III, Clinical Manager, Surgical Services, University of Virginia Health System, Charlottesville, Virginia*

In 1996, the Hospital Infection Control Practices Advisory Committee (HICPAC) of the CDC synthesized the various isolation systems into one new set of guidelines.[17] The new guidelines recommend two tiers of isolation strategies: (1) standard precautions and (2) transmission-based precautions (see inside back cover).

Standard precautions are the more important tier and are designed for the care of all clients in hospitals regardless of their diagnosis or presumed infection status. These precautions synthesize the major components of universal precautions and BSI. Standard precautions apply to non-intact skin, mucous membranes, blood, and all body fluids, secretions, and excretions except sweat.

Transmission-based precautions form the second tier and are designed only for the care of clients who have known or suspected infections or have been colonized with transmissible pathogens. These are *additional* precautions needed to interrupt transmission of a nosocomial infection and are used with standard precautions. There are three types of transmission-based precautions, and they may be combined for infections that have more than one route of transmission:

1. *Contact precautions* are designed to reduce direct and indirect contact transmission of microorganisms.
2. *Droplet precautions* are for infections transmitted by large-particle droplets such as those generated during coughing, sneezing, speaking, or suctioning.
3. *Airborne precautions* are designed to reduce the transmission of pathogens on airborne droplet nuclei.

In many cases, the risk of transmitting a nosocomial infection is highest before a diagnosis can be made. Certain clinical syndromes and conditions warrant the addition of transmission-based precautions while the definitive diagnosis is anticipated. For example, contact precautions should be implemented for incontinent or diapered clients who have acute diarrhea with a likely infectious cause such as HAV infection. Clients with infected draining skin lesions or wounds that cannot be covered warrant contact precautions because the wound may be infected with *S. aureus.* Droplet precautions should be implemented for clients with meningitis until infection with *Neisseria meningitidis* is ruled out.

Other examples include clients admitted with rashes or respiratory infections with possible etiologic agents that require additional precautions beyond standard precautions. Additional precautions should also be taken with clients who have a history of infection or colonization with multi-drug–resistant organisms or who had a recent hospital or nursing home stay in a facility where multi-drug–resistant organisms were prevalent.

Control of the spread of nosocomial infections depends on meticulous attention to infection control practices. The CDC has provided excellent institutional infection control guidelines that can be tailored to meet the needs of specific situations or environments. In addition to standard and transmission-based precautions, the CDC has issued special guidelines for preventing nosocomial transmission of tuberculosis,[3] and vancomycin-resistant *S. aureus,*[10] and VRE[4] in health care facilities. See the Management and Delegation feature on infection control.

Occupational Health Practices

The second major component of an infection prevention and control program is to protect health care workers from infection. Occupational health practices include evaluating personnel for existing infections, administering vaccinations, keeping records, managing exposures, educating employees, and developing and enforcing infection control procedures.

When it was recognized that health care workers who had contact with clients' blood were at increased risk for infection by blood-borne pathogens, infection control efforts focused on preventing employee exposure to blood. By 1989, most hospitals had implemented the universal precautions guidelines to protect employees at risk of transmission of HIV and HBV. In addition, efforts focused on HBV vaccination of employees at risk for blood exposure. New employees are screened for susceptibility to tuberculosis, HBV, measles, rubella, and chickenpox. Periodic tuberculin skin testing is recommended for employees at risk for exposure to tuberculosis.

In 1991, OSHA published guidelines—the *blood-borne pathogens standard*—to protect employees exposed to blood and other potentially infectious materials.[24] One of the most important components of the guidelines is the requirement that all health care employees at risk for exposure to blood and body fluids be offered an HBV vaccination free of charge. In addition, OSHA requires all care providers to wear protective attire when they are likely to have contact with blood and other moist body substances that may contain pathogens. Because a third of occupational exposures to HIV result from recapping needles after use, OSHA standards urge the use of needle-less or recessed needle systems. The OSHA blood-borne pathogens standard incorporates most elements of universal precautions plus barrier precautions and needle disposal systems that must be available at the point of use.

Another major area of concern has been the role and selection of respiratory protection equipment to prevent transmission of tuberculosis in hospitals. OSHA has proposed standards for respiratory protection programs to

BRIDGE TO HOME HEALTH CARE

Infection Control

Be alert for signs of high risk in every home situation, focus your teaching on clients' specific needs, and follow infection control guidelines:

1. Use a nursing bag that has a plastic liner or is made from a water-repellent material. Compartments must physically separate clean and dirty items. Store handwashing supplies in an outside pocket.
2. Hang your bag on the back of a sturdy, straight chair or place it on a hard, stable surface, not on the floor, bed, or eating surface. If environmental conditions pose a threat to the bag or its contents, place a barrier beneath the bag. Most agencies recommend clean paper towels or waxed paper and clean plastic bags if moisture is a problem. When the risk of contamination is high because of the environment, pets, children, or infectious agents such as MRSA and VRE, take only the supplies needed for the visit into the home.
3. Wash your hands using your own supplies; do not use the client's bar soap or fabric towels. Wash again after you complete care and remove your gloves. Use a rinse, gel, or foam antimicrobial product if no clean, running water is available. Wash your hands thoroughly as soon as possible after leaving. Teach and remind clients and families to use good technique.
4. Do not carry reusable equipment such as a sphygmomanometer, stethoscope, electronic thermometer, and blood glucose meter in the same compartment as for clean and sterile supplies. For general client use and in low-risk situations, it is not necessary to disinfect these items between use. Do not attempt to disinfect equipment with alcohol or a household disinfectant. If equipment becomes contaminated, follow agency protocols. Leave it in the home or place it in a plastic bag, take it to your office, and follow specific protocols to clean and disinfect it thoroughly under controlled conditions. In high-risk situations, plan to leave a dedicated blood pressure cuff, stethoscope, or other necessary equipment in the home and teach clients and caregivers how to care for it.
5. Use designated containers to dispose of sharps and other biohazardous waste. Make certain that containers are removed from the home when they are full. Agencies should not allow their employees to transport containers because of the risk to employees and numerous regulations; nurses' vehicles are not approved to transport medical waste. Containers should be removed by a service approved to perform waste removal or mailed under strict federal guidelines to an approved waste disposal center. When neither of these plans is used, some agencies require families to make arrangements with local pharmacies or hospitals for disposal.
6. Place wound care supplies in a plastic bag, tie the bag closed, and dispose of it in the family's garbage. Use double bags only if the soiled dressings are heavily saturated or contain blood or if there is a risk that the plastic may rip or tear. Teach families to use safe disposal techniques that are consistent with local regulations.
7. If any area of the home becomes soiled with blood or body fluids, teach the family to use paper towels and then disinfect with a freshly prepared 1:10 solution of household bleach and tap water. For linens and clothing, add a cup of full-strength bleach to the laundry cycle; warn families that bleach, whether or not it is diluted, may discolor fabrics or other surfaces.
8. Encourage families to use a dishwasher with a heated drying cycle; the next best option is to wash dishes with hot soapy water, rinse thoroughly, and store in a secure, dry place.

Suzanne Shaw, RN, BSN, *Director, Walls Regional Hospital Home Health, Cleburne, Texas*

protect hospital personnel from pathogens spread by the airborne route. In particular, surgical masks have not been effective in preventing inhalation of droplet nuclei, and the use of disposable particulate respirators has been recommended instead. Regulations and recommendations are continually being updated by OSHA as health care methods and techniques evolve.[25]

■ INFECTION CONTROL IN LONG-TERM CARE FACILITIES

Nosocomial infections are common among residents of long-term care facilities (LTCFs) and are a major source of morbidity and mortality. UTIs, respiratory infections (influenza, pneumonia), infected pressure ulcers, gastroenteritis, and conjunctivitis are the most common infections found in long-term care facilities.[26] Many long-term care facilities are becoming reservoirs for antimicrobial-resistant organisms, including MRSA and VRE.[23]

Many hospital-oriented infection control guidelines are relevant to long-term care facilities, but they must be adapted, depending on the acuity of residents, facility size, resources, and other factors. The long-term care facility is a home to residents, one in which they usually reside for months or years. Strict barrier approaches used in hospitals can have a negative effect on the residents and the facility's social and rehabilitative goals. Infection control programs must be designed to balance the medical and social needs of long-term care residents. The Association for Practitioners in Infection Control (APIC) has addressed this problem in its guidelines for infection control programs in long-term care facilities.[26]

■ INFECTION CONTROL IN COMMUNITY-BASED SETTINGS

Today, health care is provided to clients in their homes, in physicians' offices, in ambulatory care centers, and in outpatient specialty clinics. Intravenous infusions, hemodialysis, and mechanical ventilation are provided in the home, and nearly half of all surgical procedures are performed in outpatient settings.[29] Venipuncture, wound care, suturing, skin biopsy, bone marrow aspiration and biopsy, plastic and reconstructive surgery, and other minor surgical procedures are commonly performed in physicians' offices. Same-day surgery centers accommodate both minor and major ambulatory surgeries and procedures. Outpatient specialty clinics are available to provide hemodialysis and peritoneal dialysis.

Infections arise during the provision of care in home and outpatient settings, but identifying a break in infection control practices can be difficult. Infection control surveillance programs in community-based settings have been limited, and specific data about infections occurring in homes and outpatient settings are not readily available. Infection control guidelines from the usual resources, such as the CDC, have been written primarily for hospitals. Until setting-specific guidelines are published, commonsense adaptations of hospital infection control practices are recommended.[29] As the shift to managed care continues, it can be expected that infection surveillance and control issues will become more important as a basis for measuring the quality of care and as a requirement for agency certification.

Home care has grown to encompass services provided by family members, partners, and friends as well as health care professionals. Lay caregivers must be given simple guidelines for infection control in the home. Handwashing, use of gloves, and appropriate methods for disposal of contaminated sharps and other waste are examples of infection control practices that must be taught by the home care provider. Clients and their caregivers should be taught about safe food handling, health concerns about pets, and sanitation issues. See Bridge to Home Health Care: Infection Control.

Protecting the health care worker is a critical component of infection control in any health care setting, and the employee health plan should be similar to that used in hospitals. You should not assume that health care workers who work in outpatient settings are at lower risk for infectious diseases than those employed by hospitals. Policies should be developed that meet the requirements of OSHA and other regulating agencies and that acknowledge the unique requirements of the health care setting.

CONCLUSIONS

Infectious diseases have been killers of humans throughout recorded history. For most of this time, conquering infection has been the focus of health care. The nurse's role in preventing, detecting, and treating infectious disease is a vital one. You must be aware of agent-host-environment interactions and take appropriate steps to prevent accidental transmission in all health care settings.

BIBLIOGRAPHY

1. Centers for Disease Control. (1988). Update: Universal precautions for prevention of transmission of human immunodeficiency virus, hepatitis B virus, and other bloodborne pathogens in health-care settings. *Morbidity and Mortality Weekly Report, 37*(24), 377–387.
2. Centers for Disease Control. (1991). Update on adult immunization: Recommendations of the Immunization Practices Advisory Committee (ACIP). *Morbidity and Mortality Weekly Report, 40*(RR-12), 1–94.
3. Centers for Disease Control and Prevention. (1994). Guidelines for preventing the transmission of *Mycobacterium tuberculosis* in health-care facilities. *Morbidity and Mortality Weekly Report, 43*(RR-13), 1–132.
4. Centers for Disease Control and Prevention. (1995). Recommendations for preventing the spread of vancomycin resistance: Recommendations of the Hospital Infection Control Practices Advisory Committee (HICPAC). *Morbidity and Mortality Weekly Report, 44*(RR-12), 1–13.
5. Centers for Disease Control and Prevention. (1996). Immunization of adolescents: Recommendations of the Advisory Committee on Immunization Practices, the American Academy of Pediatrics, the American Academy of Family Physicians, and the American Medical Association. *Morbidity and Mortality Weekly Report, 45*(RR-13), 1–13.
6. Centers for Disease Control and Prevention. (1996). Prevention of hepatitis A through active or passive immunization: Recommendations of the Advisory Committee on Immunization Practices (ACIP). *Morbidity and Mortality Weekly Report, 45*(RR-15), 1–30.
7. Centers for Disease Control and Prevention. (1996). Prevention of varicella: Recommendations of the Advisory Committee on Immunization Practices (ACIP). *Morbidity and Mortality Weekly Report, 45*(RR-11), 1–36.
8. Centers for Disease Control and Prevention. (1999). Notice to readers: Recommended childhood immunization schedule: United States, 1999. *Morbidity and Mortality Weekly Report, 48*(1), 8–16.

9. Centers for Disease Control and Prevention. (1997). Immunization of health-care workers: Recommendations of the Advisory Committee on Immunization Practices (ACIP) and the Hospital Infection Control Practices Advisory Committee (HICPAC). *Morbidity and Mortality Weekly Report, 46*(RR-18), 1–42.
10. Centers for Disease Control and Prevention. (1997). Interim guidelines for prevention and control of staphylococcal infection associated with reduced susceptibility to vancomycin. *Morbidity and Mortality Weekly Report, 46*(27), 626–628, 635.
11. Centers for Disease Control and Prevention. (1997). National Nosocomial Infections Surveillance Report, data summary from October 1986–April 1997, issued May 1997. *American Journal of Infection Control, 25,* 477–487.
12. Centers for Disease Control and Prevention. (1997). Prevention and control of influenza: Recommendations of the Advisory Committee on Immunization Practices (ACIP). *Morbidity and Mortality Weekly Report, 46*(RR-9), 1–25.
13. Centers for Disease Control and Prevention. (1997). Prevention of pneumococcal disease: Recommendations of the Advisory Committee on Immunization Practices (ACIP). *Morbidity and Mortality Weekly Report, 46*(RR-8), 1–24.
14. Centers for Disease Control and Prevention. (1997). Update: *Staphylococcus aureus* with reduced susceptibility to vancomycin: United States, 1997. *Morbidity and Mortality Weekly Report, 46*(35), 813–815.
14a. Centers for Disease Control and Prevention. (2000). *Staphylococcus aureus* with reduced susceptibility to vancomycin—Illinois, 1999. *Morbidity and Mortality Weekly Report, 48*(51), 1165–1167.
15. Cochi, S. L., et al. (1994). Meeting the challenges of vaccine-preventable diseases in child day care. *Pediatrics, 94*(6, Part 2), 1021–1023.
16. Eliopoulos, G. M. (1997). Vancomycin-resistant enterococci: Mechanism and clinical relevance. *Infectious Disease Clinics of North America, 11*(4), 813–849.
17. Garner, J. S., & Hospital Infection Control Practices Advisory Committee. (1996). Guideline for isolation precautions in hospitals. *Infection Control and Hospital Epidemiology, 17,* 54–80.
18. Hoeprich, P. D., Jordan, M. C., & Ronald, A. R. (1994). *Infectious diseases: A treatise of infectious processes* (5th ed.). Philadelphia: J. B. Lippincott.
19. Institute of Medicine. (1992). *Emerging infections: Microbial threats to health in the United States.* Washington, DC: National Academy Press.
20. Jackson, M. M., & Lynch, P. (1991). An attempt to make an issue less murky: A comparison of four systems for infection precautions. *Infection Control and Hospital Epidemiology, 12,* 448–450.
21. Joint Commission on Accreditation of Healthcare Organizations. (1995). *Accreditation manual for hospitals.* Chicago: Author.
22. Maranan, M. C., et al. (1997). Antimicrobial resistance in staphylococci: Epidemiology, molecular mechanisms, and clinical relevance. *Infectious Disease Clinics of North America, 11*(4), 813–849.
23. Nicolle, L. E. (1997). Nursing home dilemmas. *Infection Control and Hospital Epidemiology, 18*(12), 806–808.
24. Occupational Safety and Health Administration. (1991). Occupational exposure to bloodborne pathogens: Final rule. *Federal Register, 56,* 64003–64182.
25. Occupational Safety and Health Administration. (1997). Occupational exposure to tuberculosis: Proposed rule. *Federal Register, 62*(201), 54159–54209.
26. Smith, P. W. & Rusnak, P. G. (1997). SHEA/APIC position paper: Infection prevention and control in the long-term-care facility. *Infection Control and Hospital Epidemiology, 18*(12), 831–849.
27. Soule, B. M., Larson, E. L., & Preston, G. A. (1995). *Infections and nursing practice: Prevention and control.* St. Louis: Mosby–Year Book.
28. U.S. Department of Health and Human Services. (1990). *Healthy people 2000.* Washington, DC: U.S. Government Printing Office.
29. Wenzel, R. P. (Ed.). (1997). *Prevention and control of nosocomial infections* (3rd ed.). Baltimore: Williams & Wilkins.
30. Yoshikawa, T. T., & Normal, D. C. (Eds.). (1994). *Antimicrobial therapy in the elderly client.* New York: Marcel Dekker.

CHAPTER

18

Perspectives in Oncology

Patricia Meier

The face of health care, including scientific knowledge and care delivery systems, is ever changing. Likewise, the experience of cancer is changing for our clients and families. Today, a person confronted with a new diagnosis often knows someone who has survived cancer. Yet, cancer remains a frightening unknown for many. Some clients, especially older ones, still associate the word with death. Cancer nursing requires a clinical knowledge of the disease and its treatment as well as the skills to care for and support clients and their families. The pathophysiology and scientific advances discussed in this chapter provide a foundation for promoting positive outcomes for clients with cancer, discussed in the next chapter.

Approximately 1.2 to 1.3 million new cancers are diagnosed in the United States each year. Survival rates and quality of life for people living with the disease have improved. Yet, each year, approximately 552,000 Americans die of cancer. Cancer remains the second leading cause of death in the United States.[2, 20]

The National Cancer Institute (NCI) estimates that 8.4 million Americans alive today have a history of cancer. This number includes disease-free survivors who may be considered "cured," people living with cancer as a chronic disease, and those currently receiving treatment. Six of 10 clients with cancer diagnosed this year are expected to be alive 5 years after the diagnosis.[2]

TERMINOLOGY

The terms *cancer, neoplasm, malignant neoplasm,* and *tumor* are often used interchangeably by both professionals and the lay public. Strictly speaking, these words are not interchangeable. Although generally used as a synonym for cancer, the word *tumor* simply refers to a lump, mass, or swelling. That swelling can be a neoplastic mass, or it may be only an accumulation of fluid.

The word *neoplasm* (derived from the Greek *neos,* new, and *plasis,* molding) is defined as an abnormal mass of tissue that serves no useful purpose and may harm the host organism. A neoplasm can be either *benign* or *malignant.* A benign neoplasm is *usually* a harmless growth that does not spread or invade other tissues. A benign tumor does occupy space. Consequently, if it is located near a vital tube or organ, it can be fatal, as with a benign brain tumor. A malignant neoplasm is a harmful mass, capable of invasion of other tissues and *metastasis* (spread) to distant organs.

The term *cancer* is used to refer to malignant neoplasms. Cancer is a disease of the cell in which the normal mechanisms of the control of growth and proliferation have been altered. It is invasive, spreading directly to surrounding tissue as well as to new sites in the body.

The term *oncology* refers to the medical specialty that deals with the diagnosis, treatment, and study of cancer. An oncologist is a physician who specializes in cancer therapy. There are surgical, radiation, and medical oncologists. A medical oncologist is a physician with expertise in treating cancer with chemotherapy or biotherapy and in handling general medical problems related to the disease or side effects of cancer treatment. Table 18–1 lists other important terms.

EPIDEMIOLOGY

Epidemiology is the study of the distribution and determinants of diseases and health problems in specified populations. The goal of epidemiologic study is the prevention or control of the health problem. One who uses an epidemiologic approach to cancer evaluates patterns of the disease, identifies possible causes, and infers relationships between patterns of disease and determining factors. Although the causes of many cancers remain unknown, epidemiologic studies have helped to identify factors that underlie theories of causation. Nurses can utilize knowledge of the factors associated with cancer causation in promoting positive outcomes for their clients through nursing assessment and interventions.

The NCI established the Surveillance, Epidemiology, and End Results (SEER) program in 1973 as a way to report population-based data in site-specific incidences of cancer, mortality, and survival rates. This report is based on a sample of 12% of the United States population. It includes four metropolitan areas (Atlanta, Detroit, San Francisco/Oakland, and Seattle/Puget Sound). It also contains data from five states (Connecticut, Hawaii, Iowa, New Mexico, and Utah) and the Commonwealth of Puerto Rico. The SEER reporting areas reasonably represent the subsets of the population. Data are gathered from

TABLE 18–1 CANCER TERMINOLOGY

Terms	Definitions
Adenocarcinoma	Cancer that arises from glandular tissues. Examples include cancers of the breast, lung, thyroid, colon, and pancreas.
Anaplastic	Tumor cells that are completely undifferentiated and bear no resemblance to cells of tissues of their origin.
Aneuploid	Tumor cells that do not have the normal 46 chromosomes in a human cell. Aneuploid tumors often have a worse prognosis.
Antigens	Substances that cause activation of the immune system.
Carcinoma	A form of cancer that is composed of epithelial cells; develops in tissues covering or lining organs of the body such as the skin, uterus, or breast.
Carcinoma in situ	The earliest stage of cancer, in which the tumor is still confined to the local area, before it has grown to a significant size or has spread.
Cytokine	A substance secreted by immune system cells, usually to send messages to other immune cells.
Differentiation	The process of maturation of a cell line of cancer cells. When they are fully differentiated or well differentiated, they more closely resemble the normal cells in the tissue of origin.
Dysplasia	An alteration in the size, shape, and organization of differentiated cells. Cells lose their regularity and show variability in size and shape, usually in response to an irritant. Cells may revert to normal when the irritant is removed but may transform to a neoplasia.
Hyperplasia	An increase in the number of normal cells in a normal arrangement in a tissue or organ; usually leads to an increase in the size of the part and an increase in functional activity.
Metaplasia	The replacement of one type of fully differentiated cell by another fully differentiated cell that is not normal for that part of the body.
Oncogenes	Specific segments of cellular deoxyribonucleic acid (DNA) that, when inappropriately activated, contribute to the transformation of normal cells into malignant cells.
Sarcoma	A cancer of supporting or connective tissue such as cartilage, bone muscle, or fat.
Tumor markers	Chemicals in the blood that are produced by certain cancers.

hospital medical records. Therefore, the accuracy of the data recorded in clients' medical records by physicians, nurses, and others can affect the accuracy of the SEER data. This ongoing project provides a great deal of information about cancer incidence, prevalence, and mortality for different geographical areas and ethnic groups.

INCIDENCE AND PREVALENCE

The *incidence* rate for cancer reflects the number of new cases occurring in a specified population during a year, expressed as the number of cancers per 100,000 people. For the year 2000, about 1,220,100 new diagnoses of cancer were expected (Table 18–2).[20] The incidence gives perspective on the current magnitude of the problem and provides a source for establishing future priorities in cancer control programs. The *prevalence* of cancer is the total number of people alive today, whose cancer has been diagnosed in the current year (incidence) and those whose cancer has been diagnosed previously. The 8.4 million Americans living with a history of cancer (prevalence) include the 1,220,100 people whose cancer has been diagnosed in the current year (incidence).

The reported incidence of cancer appears to have increased since 1900 for several reasons. First, diagnostic methods have become more precise. Utilization of diagnostic tests, such as mammograms for breast cancer and the prostate-specific antigen (PSA) blood test for prostate cancer, has led to earlier detection than previously.

Second, data collection and analysis of cancer statistics have become more sophisticated over the years. Therefore, reported rates of incidence and mortality that are due to cancer are more accurate. Both can result in an increase in the *reported* incidence of cancer but not a true increased incidence of cancer.

Third, Americans are living longer than even a few decades ago. Most cancers take many years to develop. More people are now living long enough for cancer to develop. Therefore, the apparent rise in cancer rates can be somewhat misleading. These factors simply reflect more precise diagnostic and statistical methods combined with the trend toward a longer life span rather than a true increase in the rates of cancer. However, many lifestyle behaviors associated with cancer causation, such as smoking, alcohol intake, and multiple sex partners, are risk factors linked to true changes in cancer rates.

MORTALITY

The mortality rate is the number of deaths caused by cancer that occur in the specified population in a given year, expressed as the number of deaths that are due to cancer per 100,000 persons. Figures 18–1 and 18–2 show changes in the mortality rates for lung cancer for both males and females.[2] A decline in lung cancer deaths for males is a reflection of the decline in smoking by American men. Meanwhile, in the words of a long-running tobacco company advertisement, women have "come a long way baby"—all the way to increased incidence of and mortality from lung cancer. In 1987, for the first time more women died of lung cancer than of breast cancer.[27] It is predicted that neither the incidence of nor the mortality from lung cancer has yet peaked in women. The prevalence of smoking by women has begun to decline, although more recently and more gradually than in men.

TRENDS

In 1992, cancer rates inched down for the first time. The incidence of cancer had increased 1.2% each year between 1973 and 1992. However, from 1992 to 1995 the incidence of cancer fell 0.7% per year. Mortality rates from cancer likewise fell 2.6% (0.5% per year) from

TABLE 18–2 **ESTIMATED NEW CANCER CASES AND DEATHS BY SEX FOR ALL SITES, UNITED STATES, 2000***

	Estimated New Cases			Estimated Deaths		
	Both Sexes	*Male*	*Female*	*Both Sexes*	*Male*	*Female*
All Sites	1,220,100	619,700	600,400	552,200	284,100	268,100
Oral cavity and pharynx	30,200	20,200	10,000	7,800	5,100	2,700
Tongue	6,900	4,500	2,400	1,700	1,100	600
Mouth	10,900	6,500	4,400	2,300	1,300	1,000
Pharynx	8,200	5,900	2,300	2,100	1,500	600
Other oral cavity	4,200	3,300	900	1,700	1,200	500
Digestive system	226,600	117,600	109,000	129,800	69,300	60,500
Esophagus	12,300	9,200	3,100	12,100	9,200	2,900
Stomach	21,500	13,400	8,100	13,000	7,600	5,400
Small intestine	4,700	2,300	2,400	1,200	600	600
Colon	93,800	43,400	50,400	47,700	23,100	24,600
Rectum	36,400	20,200	16,200	8,600	4,700	3,900
Anus, anal canal, and anorectum	3,400	1,400	2,000	500	200	300
Liver and intrahepatic bile duct	15,300	10,000	5,300	13,800	8,500	5,300
Gallbladder and other biliary	6,900	2,900	4,000	3,400	1,200	2,200
Pancreas	28,300	13,700	14,600	28,200	13,700	14,500
Other digestive organs	4,000	1,100	2,900	1,300	500	800
Respiratory system	179,400	101,500	77,900	161,900	93,100	68,800
Larynx	10,100	8,100	2,000	3,900	3,100	800
Lung and bronchus	164,100	89,500	74,600	156,900	89,300	67,600
Other respiratory organs	5,200	3,900	1,300	1,100	700	400
Bones and joints	2,500	1,500	1,000	1,400	800	600
Soft tissue (including heart)	8,100	4,300	3,800	4,600	2,200	2,400
Skin (excluding basal and squamous)	56,900	34,100	22,800	9,600	6,000	3,600
Melanoma-skin	47,700	27,300	20,400	7,700	4,800	2,900
Other non-epithelial skin	9,200	6,800	2,400	1,900	1,200	700
Breast	184,200	1,400	182,800	41,200	400	40,800
Genital system	265,900	188,400	77,500	59,000	32,500	26,500
Uterine cervix	12,800	—	12,800	4,600	—	4,600
Uterine corpus	36,100	—	36,100	6,500	—	6,500
Ovary	23,100	—	23,100	14,000	—	14,000
Vulva	3,400	—	3,400	800	—	800
Vagina and other genital, female	2,100	—	2,100	600	—	600
Prostate	180,400	180,400	—	31,900	31,900	—
Testis	6,900	6,900	—	300	300	—
Penis and other genital, male	1,100	1,100	—	300	300	—
Urinary system	86,700	58,600	28,100	24,600	15,700	8,900
Urinary bladder	53,200	38,300	14,900	12,200	8,100	4,100
Kidney and renal pelvis	31,200	18,800	12,400	11,900	7,300	4,600
Ureter and other urinary organs	2,300	1,500	800	500	300	200
Eye and orbit	2,200	1,200	1,000	200	100	100
Brain and other nervous system	16,500	9,500	7,000	13,000	7,100	5,900
Endocrine system	20,200	5,600	14,600	2,100	1,000	1,100
Thyroid	18,400	4,700	13,700	1,200	500	700
Other endocrine	1,800	900	900	900	500	400
Lymphoma	62,300	35,900	26,400	27,500	14,400	13,100
Hodgkin's disease	7,400	4,200	3,200	1,400	700	700
Non-Hodgkin's lymphoma	54,900	31,700	23,200	26,100	13,700	12,40
Multiple myeloma	13,600	7,300	6,300	11,200	5,800	5,400
Leukemia	30,800	16,900	13,900	21,700	12,100	9,600
Acute lymphocytic leukemia	3,200	1,800	1,400	1,300	700	600
Chronic lymphocytic leukemia	8,100	4,600	3,500	4,800	2,800	2,000
Acute myeloid leukemia	9,700	4,800	4,900	7,100	3,900	3,200
Chronic myeloid leukemia	4,400	2,600	1,800	2,300	1,300	1,000
Other leukemia	5,400	3,100	2,300	6,200	3,400	2,800
Other and unspecified primary sites	34,000	15,700	18,300	36,600	18,500	18,100

*Excludes basal and squamous cell skin cancers and in situ carcinomas except urinary bladder. Carcinoma in situ of the breast accounts for about 42,600 new cases annually, and melanoma carcinoma in situ accounts for about 28,600 new cases annually. Estimates of new cases are based on incidence rates from the National Cancer Institute, Surveillance, Epidemiology, and End Results program 1979–1996.

From American Cancer Society. 2000. *Cancer facts & figures 2000.* Atlanta: Author. Reprinted by permission of the American Cancer Society, Inc.

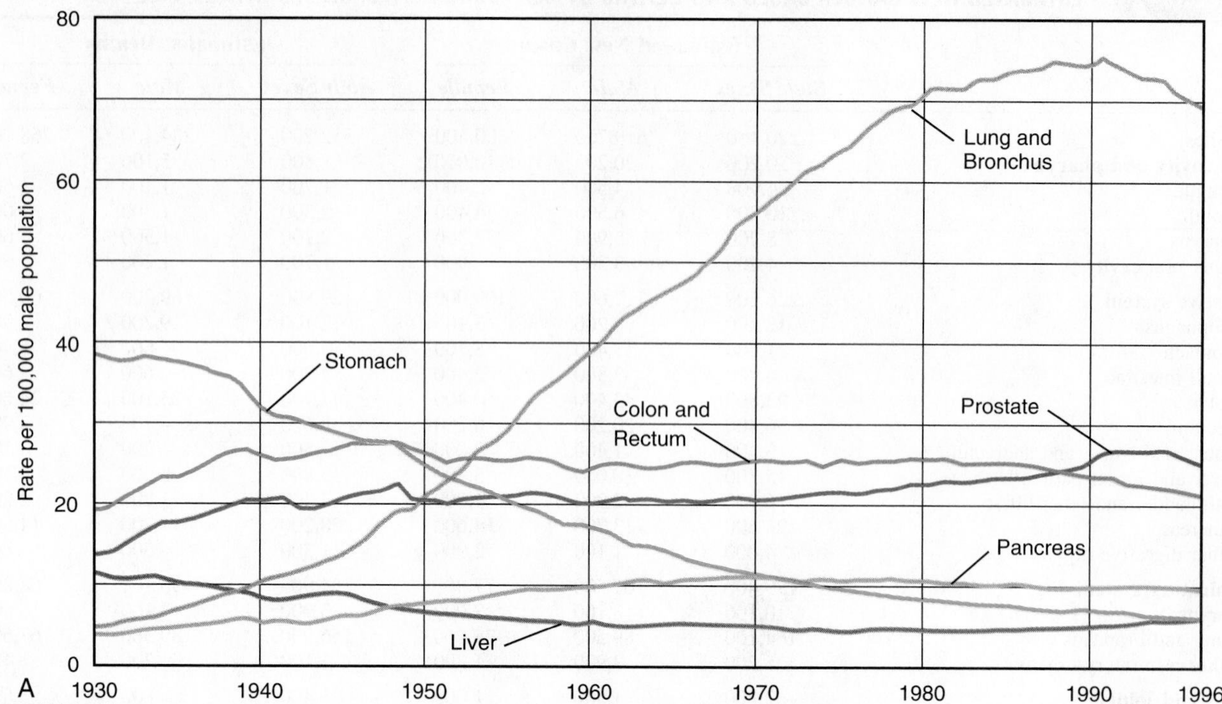

FIGURE 18–1 Cancer death rates by site in males in the United States from 1930 to 1996. Rates are per 100,000 and are age-adjusted to the 1970 U.S. standard population. (From American Cancer Society [2000]. *Cancer facts & figures 2000.* Atlanta: Author. © American Cancer Society, Inc.)

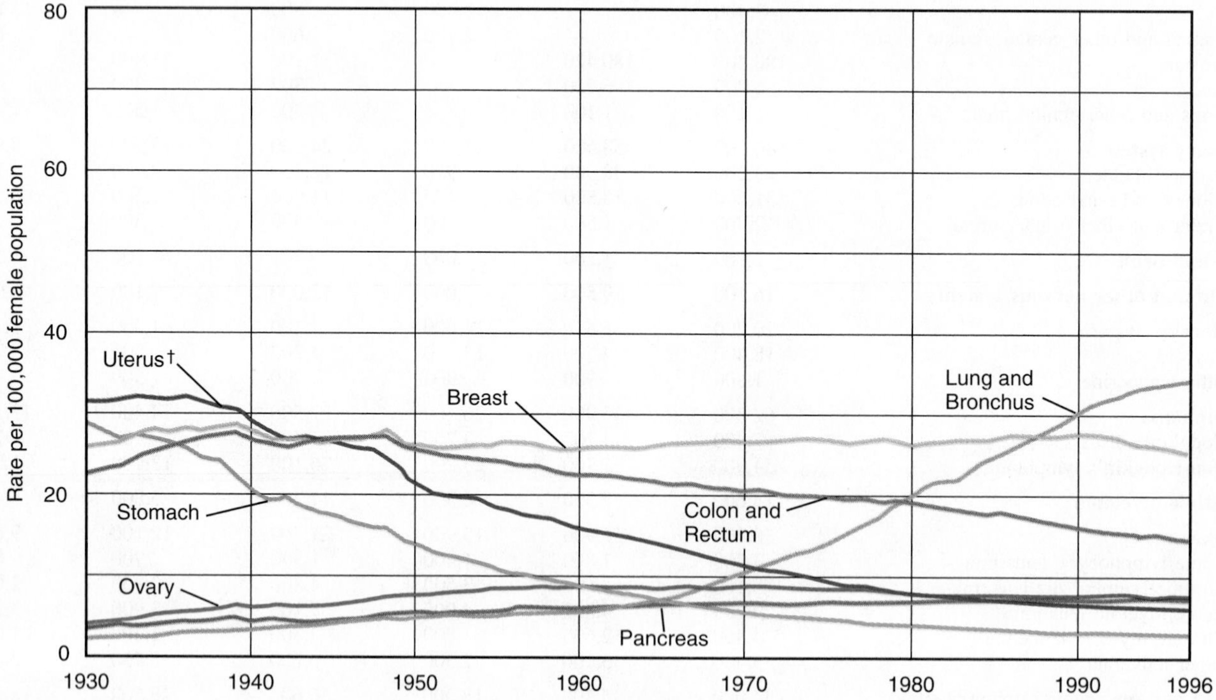

†Uterus cancer death rates are for uterine cervix and uterine corpus combined.

B

FIGURE 18–2 Cancer death rates by site in females in the United States from 1930 to 1996. Rates are per 100,000 and are age-adjusted to the 1970 U.S. standard population. (From American Cancer Society [2000]. *Cancer facts & figures 2000.* Atlanta: Author. © American Cancer Society, Inc.)

1991 to 1995. This represented about 30,000 fewer deaths than had been expected. Factors that may explain this decline include the decrease in tobacco use, better cancer research and treatment, and earlier cancer detection and prevention. Lung cancer incidence dropped 1.1% a year, mostly in men, who began quitting smoking earlier than women. Cancer is not just being treated earlier. Through cancer screening, for example, precancerous colon polyps can be removed before they become cancerous.

Although overall cancer rates inched down, declines were not seen in all areas. The incidence of deadly melanoma from chronic exposure to ultraviolet radiation is actually rising about 4% per year. Incidence rates for non-Hodgkin's lymphoma have increased nearly two-fold since the early 1970s. Although more than 25% of cancers are associated with diet, dietary patterns likely did not have an impact on the decline in overall cancer incidence. Obesity in Americans is actually increasing. Cancer rates also did not improve for some minority populations. Cancer rates increased for black males and remained level for Asian and Pacific Islander females.[2, 20, 26] Figures 18–3*A* and *B* reflect the rates of cancer incidence and mortality by race or ethnicity.[2]

Although the decline in cancer incidence is positive news, the gains are fragile. Lifestyle choices are responsible for most exposure to environmental carcinogens. The recent increase in tobacco use by teenagers may cause a rebound in cancer rates. From 1991 to 1995, the percentage of high school students who smoke frequently increased 3% to 5%. There has also been a resurgence in the use of smokeless tobacco products.[2] Lifestyle choices resulting in severe sunburn from ultraviolet radiation, especially in children, are associated with a greatly increased risk of melanoma in later life. Another concern related to melanoma is the rapid increase in the use of tanning beds. Long-term exposure to ultraviolet radiation is associated with basal cell and squamous cell skin cancers.[14] Prevention, early detection, and treatment of cancer remain significant health care concerns.

PATHOPHYSIOLOGY

Knowledge about the pathophysiology of cancer will help you better understand the significance of clinical observations and plan interventions, including client teaching, for

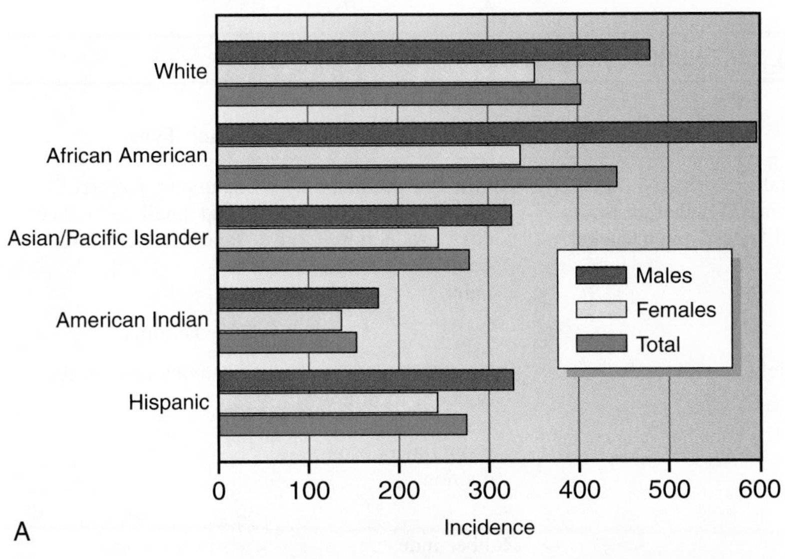

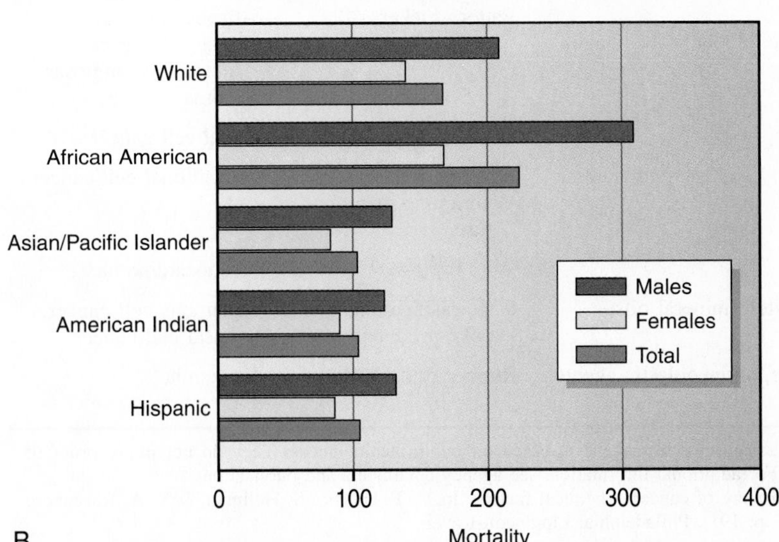

FIGURE 18–3 *A*, Cancer incidence rates (per 100,000) for all sites combined by race, ethnicity, and sex in the United States. *B*, Cancer mortality rates (per 100,000) for all sites combined by race, ethnicity, and sex in the United States. (Data from American Cancer Society. [2000]. *Cancer facts & figures 2000.* Atlanta: Author.)

outcomes management. A common misconception is that cancer is *one* disease. Cancer is many diseases.

Cancers comprise all diseases of cells that are altered or transformed in some way but are able to multiply, grow, and spread. Cancerous cells differ from normal cells in appearance, growth, and function. The change from normal to neoplastic cells is a process, not a single event or a single alteration in cells. The development of a cancer is a series of events that generally occur over many years. Clinical manifestations are only the final stages in the natural history of a cancer.

■ CARCINOGENS

Carcinogens (factors associated with cancer causation) may be (1) radiation, (2) chemicals, (3) viruses, or (4) other physical agents (Table 18–3).[34] In addition, hormones play a significant role in the development of many cancers.[17]

Radiation

More than 80% of exposure to radiation is from natural sources.[6, 14] This includes ionizing radiation from cosmic rays and radioactive minerals, such as radon gas, radium, and uranium. Sunlight and tanning beds are two sources of ultraviolet radiation, a complete carcinogen.

About 15% of radiation exposure comes from diagnostic or therapeutic procedures, including radiographs, radiation therapy, and radioisotopes used in diagnostic imaging. Individual doses vary widely with the numbers and types of procedures done.[14] The levels of radiation emitted by equipment for a given procedure have been falling significantly since the 1980s. Physicians commonly avoid ordering unnecessary procedures for clients. The amount of risk of a second malignancy caused by radiation therapy is still open to debate. At most, about 5% of all secondary cancers are clearly linked to radiation therapy for a previous cancer.[14]

Chemicals

Tobacco, a chemical carcinogen, remains the most important known cause of cancer in the United States, accounting for almost 30% of cancer deaths. It has been linked not only with lung cancer but also with oropharyngeal, bladder, pancreatic, cervical, and kidney cancers. Because there is a clear linear relationship between the amount and number of years of smoking and cancer risk, a nurse

TABLE 18–3 KNOWN OR SUSPECTED CHEMICAL CARCINOGENS IN HUMANS*

Target Organ	Agent	Industry	Tumor Type
Lung	Tobacco smoke, arsenic, asbestos, crystalline silica, benzo[*a*]pyrene, beryllium, bis(chloromethyl)ether, 1,3-butadiene, chromium VI compounds, coal tar and pitch, nickel compounds, soots, mustard gas	Aluminum production, coal gasification, coke production, hematite mining, paint	Squamous, large cell, and small cell cancer and adenocarcinoma
Pleura	Asbestos	—	Mesothelioma
Oral cavity	Tobacco smoke, alcoholic beverages, nickel compounds	Boot and shoe production, furniture manufacturer, isopropyl alcohol production	Squamous cell cancer
Esophagus	Tobacco smoke, alcoholic beverages	—	Squamous cell cancer
Gastric	Smoked, salted, and pickled foods	Rubber industry	Adenocarcinoma
Colon	Heterocyclic amines, asbestos	Pattern makers	Adenocarcinoma
Liver	Aflatoxin, vinyl chloride, tobacco smoke, alcoholic beverages	—	Hepatocellular carcinoma, hemangiosarcoma
Kidney	Tobacco smoke	—	Renal cell cancer
Bladder	Tobacco smoke, 4-aminobiphenyl, benzidine, 2-naphthylamine	Magenta manufacture, auramine manufacture	Transitional cell cancer
Prostate	Cadmium	—	Adenocarcinoma
Skin	Arsenic, benzo[*a*]pyrene, coal tar and pitch, mineral oils, soots	Coal gasification, coke production	Squamous cell cancer, basal cell cancer
Bone marrow	Benzene, tobacco smoke, ethylene oxide, antineoplastic agents	Rubber	Leukemia

*These carcinogen designations are determined by regulatory or review agencies based on public health needs. They do not imply proof of carcinogenicity in individuals. This table is not all-inclusive. For additional information, see agency documents and publications.

Modified from Yuspa, S. H., & Shields, P. G. (1997). Etiology of cancer: Chemical factors. In V. T. DeVita, S. Hellman, & S. A. Rosenberg (Eds.), *Cancer: Principles and practices of oncology* (5th ed., p. 191). Philadelphia: Lippincott-Raven.

can often find in a physician's history the number of pack-years a client has smoked. (A "pack-year" refers to the number of packs of cigarettes smoked per day times the number of years the client has smoked. It provides a measure of the client's cigarette abuse.) Smokeless tobacco (chewing tobacco, snuff) is linked to oral cancers. Long-term users of smokeless tobacco have a nearly 50-fold increased risk of cancer of the cheek and gum.[2]

In addition to lifestyle exposure to the chemicals in tobacco products, people can be exposed to chemicals in the workplace. Occupational exposure causes 2% to 8% of all human cancers. The risk estimates are much higher among the subpopulation of people actually exposed to carcinogens in the workplace. These occupationally occurring cancers are, for the most part, preventable.[31] Health care workers wear radiation badges to ensure that they do not receive unsafe levels of exposure. Before safe handling practices were instituted, the urine of pharmacists and nurses mixing or administering chemotherapy agents was found to show mutagenic changes from cumulative exposure. Today, chemotherapeutic agents are mixed by pharmacists under laminar flow hoods. The hood draws air containing aerosolized drug away and prevents the pharmacist from breathing in the chemicals. Oncology nurses wear gowns and gloves to administer chemotherapy and use special procedures to clean up any spills to prevent absorbing the chemicals through the skin or mucous membranes.

Viruses

Some viruses are strongly associated with cancer. Table 18–4 lists biologic agents, including viruses, judged by the World Health Organization (WHO) to be involved in human cancers.[30] In the 1970s and early 1980s, many lay people thought cancer was contagious and therefore often shunned those with cancer. Occasionally, yet today, a client or family member expresses this fear. Even when there is a viral link, the cancer is not contagious. Rather, a virus at some point infected the cell, causing genetic damage to the cell's deoxyribonucleic acid (DNA), thus leading to the development of cancer.

Age, Sex, Genetics, Ethnicity

Host characteristics influencing cancer susceptibility include age, sex, genetic predisposition, and ethnicity or race. Age is a factor because the person has had more years of potential exposure to carcinogens. Females have a generally lower risk of cancer incidence. Hormonal status is associated with increased risk of neoplasia in tissues that are responsive to hormones, including breast, endometrium, prostate, ovary, thyroid, bone, and testes. In addition to biologic or genetic differences, cultural and socioeconomic factors may put an ethnic or racial group at increased or decreased risk of a specific cancer.[8, 15]

For people who do not smoke, dietary patterns and physical activities become the most important cancer risk factors that they can modify. It is estimated that at least one fourth of cancer deaths in the United States are related to diet. Research into the relationship of diet and cancer is ongoing.[6] A balanced, healthy diet that includes a high proportion of plant foods (fruits, vegetables, grains, and beans), limited intake of high-fat foods, a balance of caloric intake and physical activity, and limited consumption of alcoholic beverages can reduce cancer risks.[2, 30]

TABLE 18–4 BIOLOGIC AGENTS JUDGED BY IARC (WHO) OR OTHERS AS BEING INVOLVED IN HUMAN CARCINOGENESIS

Agent	Site of Cancer
Aflatoxin-producing fungal strains	Liver (hepatocellular)
Hepatitis B virus	Liver (hepatocellular)
Hepatitis C virus	Liver (hepatocellular)
Helicobacter pylori	Stomach
Schistosoma haematobium	Urinary bladder
Opisthorchis viverrini	Liver (cholangiocarcinoma)
HTLV-1	Adult T-cell leukemia or lymphoma
HPV (or other sexually transmitted agent)	Uterine cervix
Epstein-Barr virus	Burkitt's lymphoma, nasopharynx, Hodgkin's disease

HPV, human papillomavirus; HTLV-1, human T-cell lymphotropic virus type I; IARC, International Agency for Research on Cancer; WHO, World Health Organization.

From Trichopoulos, D., et al. (1997). Epidemiology of cancer. In V. T. DeVita, S. Hellman, & S. A. Rosenberg (Eds.), *Cancer: Principles and practices of oncology* (5th ed., pp. 249). Philadelphia: Lippincott-Raven.

■ CARCINOGENESIS: TRANSFORMATION OF NORMAL CELLS INTO CANCER CELLS

The process through which normal cells are transformed into malignant or cancer cells is called carcinogenesis. Figure 18–4 depicts the multistage model of carcinogenesis.[31, 34] There are four broadly identified stages of the process of carcinogenesis:

1. *Initiation* occurs when a carcinogen damages DNA. Carcinogens cause changes in the structure and function of the cell at the genetic or molecular level. This damage may be reversible or may lead to genetic mutations if not repaired; however, the mutations may not lead immediately to cancer.
2. *Promotion* occurs with additional assaults to the cells, resulting in further genetic damage.
3. At some point, these genetic events result in a *malignant conversion.*
4. With *progression,* the cells are increasingly malignant in appearance and behavior and develop into an invasive cancer with metastases to distant body parts.

Clinicians are already using their broad understanding of this process of transformation from normal cells to malignancy. Through health promotion programs, the outcome goal of smoking cessation classes is to decrease lung cancer through prevention. Regular Papanicolaou (Pap) smears are a means of health maintenance through early detection of cervical dysplasia, a precancerous lesion. Likewise, precancerous colon polyps can be removed by colonoscopy before they progress to malig-

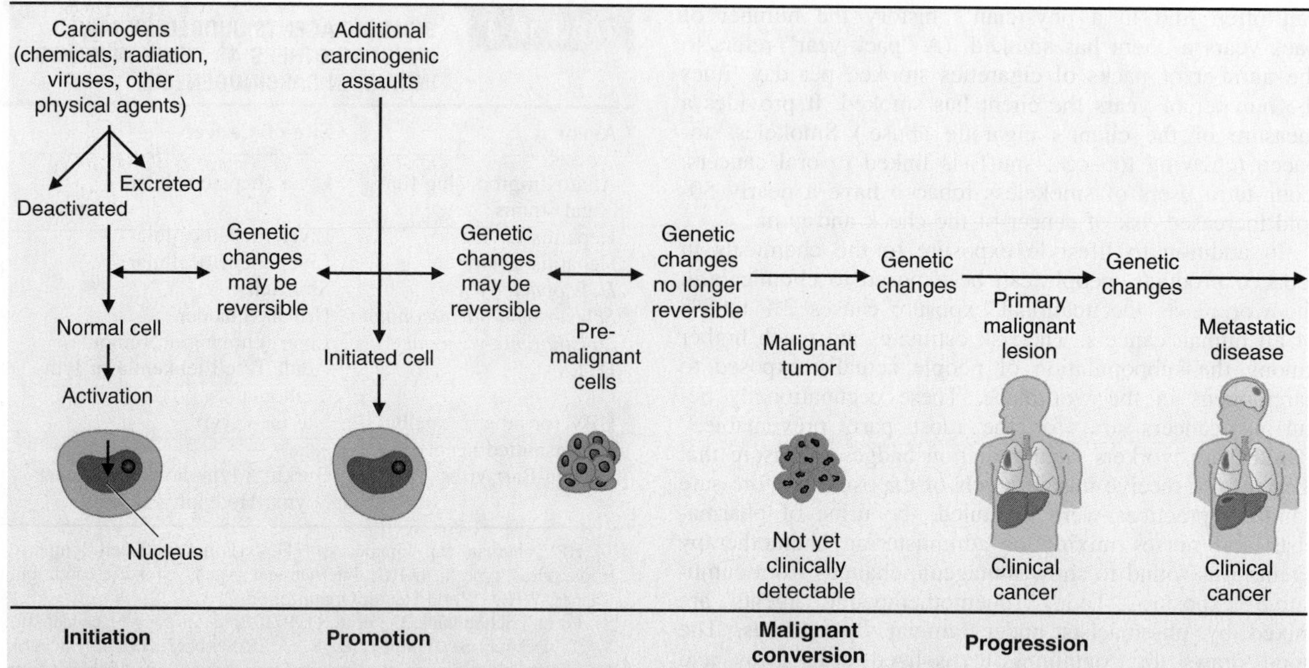

FIGURE 18–4 Multistage model of carcinogeneis. (Adapted from Volker, D. L. [1998]. Carcinogensis. In J. K. Itano & K. N. Taoka [Eds.], *Core curriculum for oncology nursing* [3rd ed., p. 359]. Philadelphia: W. B. Saunders; and Yupsa, S. H., & Shields, G. P. [1997]. Etiology of cancer: Chemical factors. In V. T. DeVita, S. Hellman, & S. A. Rosenberg [Eds.]: *Cancer: Principles and practices of oncology* [5th ed., p. 188]. Philadelphia: Lippincott-Raven.)

nancy. Monitoring moles for early changes can allow a potentially lethal melanoma to be removed while it is still a localized disease.

Increased knowledge of the underlying biology of the process of carcinogenesis is coming quickly. In the 1980s, the identification of oncogenes led to the recognition that cancer is largely a genetic disease. Research shifted from carcinogenesis and mutagens to oncogenes and tumor suppressor genes. In less than a decade, researchers have clarified critically important mechanisms that control cell growth and division, regulate embryologic development, and cause disease.[7] With this knowledge, scientists are developing better treatments. Powerful new chemotherapy drugs and new ways of delivering these drugs are becoming available. *Biotherapy* is now recognized as a fourth treatment modality in addition to surgery, radiation therapy, and chemotherapy. Biotherapy is moving from research to standard treatment.[11, 23]

The process of carcinogenesis transforms normal cells into cancer cells. The Anatomy and Physiology review of the cell (see beginning of Unit 4) explores the characteristics of normal cells. They differ from cancer cells in many key ways (Table 18–5). Specific concepts that help us to understand changes that occur in the neoplastic transformation of cells are (1) the cell cycle, (2) altered differentiation, (3) altered growth characteristics, and (4) metastasis.

The Cell Cycle

The concept of the cell cycle has increased researchers' understanding of how both normal and neoplastic cells replicate (Fig. 18–5). The cell's replication cycle is divided into the following intervals, or steps, with the letter G standing for "gap"—the interval separating cell division, or *mitosis* (M) and *synthesis* (S).

G_0 Phase. This phase is the interval in which the cell is at rest from cell division until a trigger in the immediate environment signals the beginning of the G_1 phase. Some cells do not replicate, or they replicate so infrequently that they are said to always be in a G_0 or resting state.

G_1 Phase. This phase is the interval in which ribonucleic acid (RNA) and protein are synthesized. The period of time the cell is in G_1 varies, depending on the type of cell and the proliferation activity of the tissue. With high activity, the G_1 interval is short. The interval lengthens when activity is low. There is a point in the G_1 phase known as the *restriction point,* after which the cell is committed to progressing into the S phase. One to 3 hours after passing the restriction point, cells initiate DNA synthesis. The acquisition of the ability to begin DNA synthesis marks the termination of the G_1 phase.

S Phase. Synthesis of both DNA and proteins of new chromosomes occurs during the S phase. The interval of time is probably 6 to 8 hours, although it varies in certain cell populations and under different conditions. Cell proliferation can be measured in the laboratory by flow cytometry. In reading a pathology report, you may find a reference to the percentage of cells in S phase. Only a small percentage of cells should be synthesizing DNA. An increase in S phase fraction is a negative predictor of long-term survival.[22]

G_2 Phase. Biochemical processes, including the synthesis of some RNA, occur in preparation for mitosis.

TABLE 18–5 A COMPARISON OF THE CHARACTERISTICS OF NORMAL AND CANCER CELLS

Characteristic	Normal Cells	Cancer Cells
Mitotic cell division	Mitotic division leads to two daughter cells	Mitosis leads to multiple daughter cells that may or may not resemble the parent. Multiple mitotic spindles
Appearance	1. Cells of same type homogeneous in size, shape, and growth 2. Cells cohesive, form regular pattern of expansion 3. Uniform size to nucleus 4. Have characteristic pattern of organization 5. Mixture of stem cells (precursors) and well-differentiated cells	1. Cells larger and grow more rapidly than normal. Pleomorphic, i.e., heterogeneous in size and shape. 2. Cells not as cohesive, irregular patterns of expansion 3. Larger, more prominent nucleus 4. Lack characteristic pattern of organization of host cell 5. Anaplastic, lack of differentiated cell characteristics, specific functions
Growth pattern	1. Do not invade adjacent tissue 2. Proliferate in response to specific stimuli 3. Grow in ideal conditions (e.g., nutrients, oxygen, space, correct biochemical environment) 4. Exhibit contact inhibition 5. Cell birth equals or is less than cell death 6. Stable cell membrane 7. Constant or predictable growth rate 8. Cannot grow outside specific environment (e.g., breast cells grow only in breast)	1. Invade adjacent tissues 2. Proliferation in response to abnormal stimuli 3. Grow in adverse conditions such as lack of nutrients 4. Do not exhibit contact inhibition 5. Cell birth exceeds cell death 6. Loss of cell control a result of cell membrane changes 7. Growth rate erratic 8. Able to break off cells that migrate through bloodstream or lymphatics, or seed to distant sites and grow in other sites
Function	1. Have specific, designated purpose 2. Contribute to the overall well-being of the host 3. Cells function in specific predetermined manners (e.g., cells in the thyroid secrete thyroid hormone)	1. Serve no useful purpose 2. Do not contribute to the well-being of the host; parasitic, actually feed off host without contributing anything 3. If cells function at all, they do not function normally, or they may actually cause damage (e.g., lung cancer cells secrete ACTH and cause excessive stimulation of adrenal cortex)
Other	1. Develop specific antigens, characteristic of the particular cell formed 2. Chromosomes remain constant throughout cell division 3. Complex metabolic and enzyme pattern 4. Cannot invade, erode, or spread 5. Cannot grow in presence of necrosis or inflammation	1. Develop antigens completely different from a normal cell 2. Chromosomal aberrations occur as cell matures 3. Have more primitive and simplified metabolic and enzyme pattern 4. Invade, erode, and spread 5. Grow in presence of necrosis and inflammatory cells such as lymphocytes and macrophages 6. Exhibit periods of latency that vary from tumor to tumor 7. Have own blood supply and supporting stroma

ACTH, adrenocorticotropic hormone.

Little is known about this phase, which lasts only a few hours.

M PHASE. Actual division of the cell (mitosis) occurs during this phase, producing two daughter cells. The M phase usually ranges from less than an hour to a few hours.

In the normal mature organ, cell cycling is carefully controlled so that the organ maintains its function. Cells that die are replaced, but no extra cells are produced. Researchers are investigating the mechanisms of this control, which are not fully understood.

ALTERED CELL DIFFERENTIATION

Cells that were genetically identical in the embryo eventually assume varying structures and functions. One muscle cell looks like all the other muscle cells but not like a kidney or liver cell. In normal growth, cells become more specialized or committed to a particular cell line as they mature. This process of development is called *differentiation.* Most cells contain the entire genome. The growth and function of a particular cell line result from the expression of certain genes and the suppression of others. Transformation of a normal cell to a cancer cell can

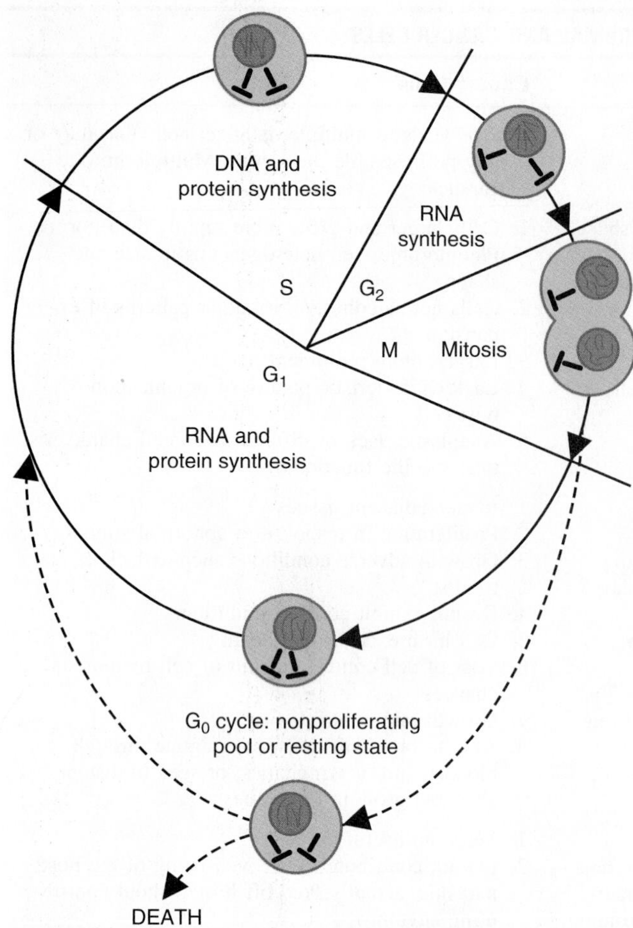

FIGURE 18–5 The cell cycle. Periods of deoxyribonucleic acid (DNA) synthesis (S) and mitosis (M) are divided by gaps (G) in which the cell is in a resting state (G0), producing substances in preparation for DNA synthesis (G1), or producing proteins and some ribonucleic acid (RNA) in preparation for mitosis (G2).

occur at any point in the process of differentiation. Changes in the appearance of the cell, the presence of tumor-specific antigens that are suppressed on the normal cell, and the loss of normal function can result from altered differentiation.

APPEARANCE. An obvious difference from normal cells is in the appearance of cancer cells. Normal cells have well-organized cellular components. Cancer cells have variable sizes and shapes. Nuclei may be disproportionately large, or there may be multiple nuclei. A variety of abnormal mitotic features may be present. There may be an abnormal number of chromosomes (aneuploidy) or an abnormal arrangement of chromosomes.[31] The detection of aneuploidy in a pathology report is an unfavorable prognostic factor.

A pathology report generally describes the grade of the cancer cells. When the cells are well differentiated, or low-grade, they are more mature in appearance and more like the normal cells from which they have arisen than poorly differentiated cancer cells. Anaplastic (undifferentiated) cells appear so disorganized under the microscope that they have no resemblance to the tissue of origin. Poorly differentiated and anaplastic cancers tend to be more aggressive—an unfavorable prognostic factor. During the natural history of many malignant neoplasms, as the cancer cells grow and divide, they often lose more and more of their mature characteristics. As a result, a malignant neoplasm can be heterogeneous with more than one variation of the malignant cell line. This heterogeneity is caused by random mutations during tumor progression.[12]

At times, a neoplasm initially responds to therapy. You may read in a radiology report that the tumor has shrunk back, with a partial remission (PR) or a complete remission (CR) of all radiologic evidence of the neoplasm; then the neoplasm may come back and grow aggressively. A likely explanation is that the treatment successfully eliminated one variant of the cancer cells, causing those cells to die and the overall size of the tumor to shrink. Then other variants of the cancer cells, which were resistant to the treatment, grew and multiplied, so that the tumor increased in size.

Biochemical studies reflect differences resulting from altered cell metabolism. The cell's surface membrane is the interface between the cell and extracellular components. Cell membrane changes may result in the production of enzymes that aid in cancer spread. A loss of glycoproteins results in a loss of cell-to-cell adhesion. Loss of antigens that identify the cell as "self" or production of tumor-specific antigens can alter the immune system's ability to mount a response.[31]

Tumor cell membranes have a greater fluidity than normal cell membranes do. This may be due to changes in the lipid composition of the membrane of tumor cells. Scientists are trying to take advantage of this difference. Some chemotherapy drugs are now being delivered in *liposomes* (spheres with an outer lipid layer and internal core of drug). The tumor cells take in more of the liposomal drug than is taken in by the normal cells. The result is a better treatment effect with fewer harmful effects on the normal cells.

TUMOR-SPECIFIC ANTIGENS. Cell surfaces express antigens. Some tumors express more of an antigen than is expressed by normal cells. These tumor-specific antigens can be used as a diagnostic tool in the detection of cancer or in monitoring the effectiveness of cancer treatment. One example is the PSA test. Normally, a man's blood level of PSA is low (0 to 5 ng/ml). In the presence of prostate cancer, this antigen can be elevated. The PSA blood test is now being utilized as one early detection tool, along with the digital rectal examination, to detect prostate cancer in men who are still asymptomatic.[2] During treatment, a decline in the PSA level is an indicator of the effectiveness of the treatment. During follow-up after treatment ends, a rise in the PSA level can be an early indicator that the cancer has recurred.

FUNCTION. Unlike normal cells, cancer cells typically serve no useful purpose. The result of neoplastic growth is an abnormal tissue mass that does not contribute in any way to the well-being of the host. The mass occupies space and draws nutrition and sustenance from the host. If the cancer cells function at all, they often do not function normally and may even act in a way that causes damage to the host. For example, a functional tumor of the thyroid gland produces excess amounts of thyroid hormone, leading to a hypermetabolic state.

ALTERED GROWTH CHARACTERISTICS

Another obvious difference from normal cells is the uncontrolled growth of cancer cells. Because of changes in their cell surfaces, neoplastic cells differ from normal cells in growth patterns and mobility. Cancer cells lose the contact inhibition of normal cells, can establish metastasis, avoid normal regulation by hormones, and avoid being recognized by the immune system as altered.

CONTACT INHIBITION AND DOUBLING TIME. When normal cells are cultured in the laboratory, they exhibit a behavior known as contact inhibition. This means the cells continue to divide until they cover the bottom of the Petri dish and stop dividing when they touch the edges of the dish. Cancer cells continue to divide, piling up on the other cells. In human tissues, the growth of normal cells is carefully regulated. Cells divide to produce new cells only when needed to replace cells that have died. Cancer cells do not stop dividing and multiplying. They do not necessarily go through the cell cycle at a faster rate than the normal cells of the tissue from which they have arisen. Rather, cancer cells are almost continuously in the process of cell division, spending little time in the G_0 phase.[19]

This continuous growth results in a phenomenon referred to as *doubling time.* The doubling time of a human malignant tumor can vary from weeks to months. As depicted in Figure 18–6, it may take 10 years for a tumor to reach 1 cm in size. In only another year, that same tumor may grow to 8 cm. The smallest clinically detectable mass is about 1 g in weight or 1 cm^3 in size. A *tumor burden* (amount) of 1 kg, which requires only about 10 more doublings, is potentially lethal.[31]

Clients sometimes ask whether exposing the tumor to air during surgery can cause it to grow more rapidly. More likely, if the surgeon did not see evidence of tumor in other areas, it had already spread, but the size of the tumor mass was still too small to be seen or felt. Then in a few more doubling times, without effective treatment, it became evident and proceeded to enlarge.

METASTASIS

Normal cells are adherent to the other normal cells from which they have arisen. Normal breast tissue cells, for example, are never found anywhere in the body except in the breast. Malignant or cancer cells are less adherent and more mobile than normal cells. They have the ability to spread from the original site of the tumor to distant organs. This phenomenon is called *metastasis* (from the Greek *meta,* beyond, and *stasis,* standing).

The capacity of a neoplastic tumor to metastasize to other sites is a major characteristic of malignancy—and the most frequent reason why cancer treatment fails. It is the characteristic that distinguishes malignant from benign growths. Neoplastic cells must overcome multiple barriers to successfully spread to other sites. For the purposes of study, the metastatic cascade is divided into three stages, (Fig. 18–7).

STAGE 1. Neoplastic cells from the primary tumor invade surrounding tissue and penetrate blood or lymph vessels. Increasing tumor size, leading to tissue pressure and mechanical expansion, may cause neoplastic invasion. However, the size of the primary tumor is not the sole predictor of metastasis. Tumors with identical size and histologic cell type can vary markedly in metastatic spread.[28]

Loss of tumor cell cohesiveness with increasing motility is another factor in the metastatic cascade. Tumors, even when very small, shed cells. As many as 10^7 to 10^9 cells per day may be found circulating in the bloodstream of clients with cancer.[28] Although surgery can cure most early breast cancers, some eventually recur because of these shed cells. Adjuvant chemotherapy or hormonal therapy, given when no visible tumor remains, may therefore be considered for early-stage breast cancer clients to decrease the risk of recurrence. Yet, fewer than 1% of circulating cancer cells successfully metastasize.[28] In the future, new scientific knowledge may allow oncologists to identify the clients with early-stage breast cancer who would benefit from adjuvant chemotherapy. This would allow the majority of women for whom surgery alone was curative to avoid the adverse effects of chemotherapy.

Benign neoplasms and cancer in situ do not cause destruction of the host stroma (the supporting tissues of an organ). With progression to invasive disease, the neoplasm penetrates the epithelial basement membrane and invades the interstitial stroma at multiple stages in the metastatic cascade.[28] A client's pathology report often indicates whether there was invasion of the neoplasm into surrounding tissue or into lymphatic, perineural, or vascular tissues. Such invasion may be an indication of occult (as yet undetected) metastatic disease.

Cancer cells that successfully metastasize represent a subpopulation of the primary tumor's cells. Not all cells in the primary mass share the unique genetic and biologic properties necessary for metastasis.[12]

STAGE 2. Cancer cells migrate via the lymph or blood circulation or by direct extension. The lymphatic system

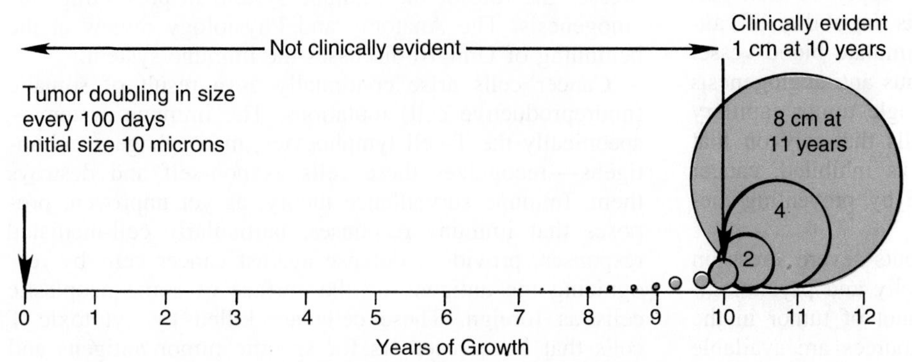

FIGURE 18–6 A depiction of tumor growth, showing doubling time related to tumor size.

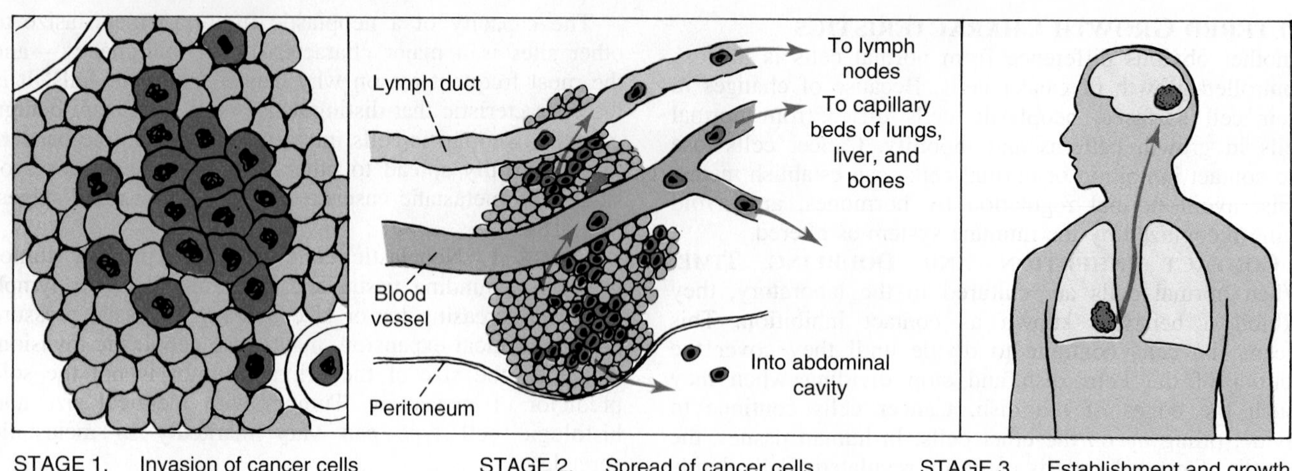

FIGURE 18–7 The three stages of the metastatic process.

provides the most common pathway for the initial spread of malignant cancer cells. There may be spread to the lymph nodes draining the region of the primary tumor site. Lymph node involvement is seen in about 50% of all fatal cancers. The blood vessels (both veins and arteries) carry cancer cells from the primary tumor to the capillary beds of the lungs, liver, and bones. Metastatic spread to distant organs and tissues is almost always the result of cells moving through the bloodstream.

Direct extension of tumors to adjacent tissues also occurs. For example, a breast cancer may spread directly to the chest wall. In body cavities, cells may spread by gravity, resulting in new growths on other serosal surfaces. Cells shed by cancers of the ovary are often found to have fallen onto and "seeded" the entire peritoneal cavity with metastatic sites of the tumor.

STAGE 3. Cancer cells are established and proliferate at the secondary site. Researchers have observed that certain tumor cells have, for unknown reasons, an affinity for certain sites. Although the exact mechanism of metastasis is unclear, the metastatic sites of many cancers are fairly predictable. The predilection of certain malignant neoplasms for particular sites may be due to the ability of the tumor to live within only certain tissues or to some other, unknown factor. The most common site of metastasis is lymphatic tissues; the next most common sites are the liver, lungs, bones, and brain.[28]

ANGIOGENESIS. The metastatic cascade begins and ends with *angiogenesis.* A tumor cannot grow more than a few millimeters without a blood supply to transport nutrients to the tumor. Angiogenesis is the ability of cancer cells to secrete substances that stimulate blood vessel growth.[30] Scientists are studying various anti-angiogenesis strategies.[3, 12] The destruction of a single tumor capillary may be able to kill many cancer cells that rely on that vessel for nutrition. If angiogenesis is inhibited, cancer progression may be halted or slowed by preventing metastasis.[3, 12, 28]

The growth of metastatic tumors puts severe stress on the affected person, both physiologically and psychologically. As the tumor burden (the amount of tumor in the body) increases, fewer metabolic resources are available for normal cells. As mentioned earlier, when the total burden of tumor in the body approaches 1 kg, the shear burden of the tumor is potentially lethal.

When a client's cancer metastasizes to other sites, clients and family members may erroneously believe that the client has multiple cancers; it is one cancer spread to other organs. For example, cells that have spread to the bone from a breast cancer are breast cancer cells, not malignant variants of bone tissue cells; however, a client may have two different cancers at one time. In the process of making a new diagnosis of colon cancer, for example, a clinician may also discover a previously undetected prostate cancer.

Knowing the natural history and the most likely pattern of spread can be very helpful to the clinician. If the cancer is likely to spread to the liver, bone, or brain, the clinician will want to rule out evidence of such spread in making treatment decisions and in monitoring for recurrence following treatment.

■ INABILITY OF IMMUNE SYSTEM TO RECOGNIZE CANCER CELLS

ROLE IN PREVENTING CARCINOGENESIS

The immune system usually defends against bacterial or viral invaders and plays a key role in controlling the growth of cancer cells. There are two critical components of the immune response: (1) the ability to recognize a pathogen as foreign and (2) the ability to mount a response to eliminate the pathogen.[4, 21, 25] This section addresses the role of the immune system in preventing carcinogenesis. The Anatomy and Physiology review at the beginning of Unit 16 discusses the immune system.

Cancer cells arise continually as a result of somatic (nonreproductive cell) mutations. The immune system—specifically the T-cell lymphocytes, macrophages, and antigens—recognizes these cells as non-self and destroys them. Immune surveillance theory, as yet unproven, proposes that immune responses, particularly cell-mediated responses, provide a defense against cancer cells by recognizing the antigens on the surface of some neoplastic cells as foreign. These cells are killed by cytotoxic T cells that have receptors for specific tumor antigens and by interferon-activated natural killer (NK) lymphocytes and macrophages.[4]

Macrophages, the important first line of defense, phagocytize the pathogen and present it as antigen to T and B lymphocytes. T-cell recognition of antigen stimulates proliferation of T and B cells, with B-cell production of antibodies against the pathogen and T-cell secretion of cytokines. Cytokines, hormone-like peptides or glycopeptides, regulate activation of the immune system against cancer cells. Cytokines both enhance and suppress complex immune interactions.

Antigens on cancer cells can take various forms, resulting in T-cell recognition of the cells as abnormal. The cancer cells may express antigens that are not present on normal cells. Cancer cells may have antigens that are "unmasked" and thus visible to the immune system. These same antigens when present on normal cells are masked and thus not recognized by the immune system. Cancer cells may also express antigens that are only present during oncofetal or embryonic development of normal cells. Cytotoxic T cells that have receptors for specific tumor antigens and interferon-activated NK lymphocytes and macrophages can then destroy these cancer cells.

Failure of Immune Defenses

Unfortunately, the immune defenses are not always effective. The immune system may be unable to recognize cancer cells as foreign or to mount an immune response for several reasons.

An immature, old, or weak immune system may contribute to this. People who are malnourished or chronically ill may also be immunocompromised. The tumor burden (number of cancer cells) may be too small to stimulate an immune response. Alternatively, the tumor burden may be so great as to overwhelm the immune system.

Some cancer cells may escape detection because they resemble normal cells. Other cancer cells may produce substances that shield them from recognition. Cancer cells may also escape detection by becoming coated with fibrin. Tumor invasion of the bone marrow can result in decreased production of lymphocytes needed to destroy the tumor mass.

The incidence of malignancy increases with the use of immunosuppressive drugs after organ transplantation to counteract rejection. Chemotherapeutics or radiation used to treat cancer can also induce suppression of the immune response.[4, 25, 31]

■ APOPTOSIS

With the development of molecular biology in the 1980s, scientists began to understand another important step in the process of carcinogenesis: the failure of cells to die.[1, 10, 17] In normal physiology, a damaged cell sacrifices itself for the greater good. There are two pathways to cell death:

1. *Necrosis* is cell death resulting from injury. The dead cells swell, lyse, and release their cellular contents into the intercellular spaces, causing the inflammatory response.
2. In *apoptosis* (from the Greek word for "falling off"), "cellular suicide" results in cells rapidly shrinking with loss of their intercellular contents.[17] They are quickly phagocytized and digested by macrophages and other cells in the vicinity. Inflammation is not triggered. Figure 18–8 depicts this programmed cell suicide. The morphologic changes of apoptosis can be completed in less than an hour.[10]

Most, if not all, cells manufacture a set of proteins that serve as weapons of self-destruction. As long as a cell is useful to the body, it restrains its death machinery. If the cell becomes infected or malignant or otherwise threatens the health of the organism, however, the lethal proteins are unleashed.[10]

Increasingly, scientists view cancer as both a disease of excessive cell growth and a lack of normal cell death. In the process of carcinogenesis, cells accumulate enough damage to genes that control cell growth and survival that the mutation seems irreparable. The affected cell usually kills itself rather than risk becoming deranged and potentially dangerous. If the cell does not die, it or its daughter cells may live long enough to accumulate mutations that make it possible to divide uncontrollably and to metastasize to distant sites.

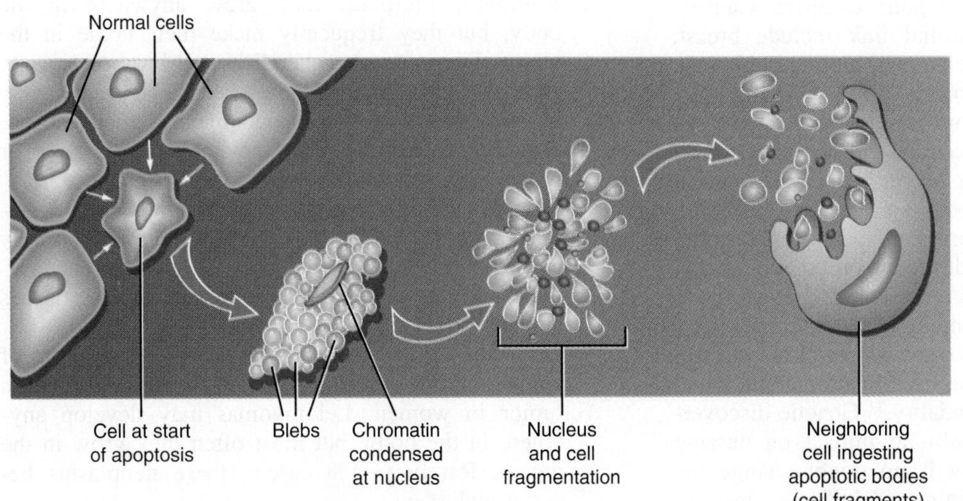

FIGURE 18–8 Programmed cell death resulting from apoptosis (cell "suicide"). The cell shrinks and pulls away from surrounding cells. Blebs appear on the surface of the cell. Chromatin condenses on the edge of the nucleus. The nucleus and then the cell itself breaks up. Cell fragments are ingested by other cells.

Apoptosis may not be induced in response to a cancer cell because there has also been damage to a tumor suppressor gene. In many cancers, genetic damage apparently fails to induce apoptosis because there has been damage to the gene that codes for the p53 protein. The p53 protein is a suppressor gene that can prompt activation of cell suicide. It is estimated that as many as half of solid cancers, including lung, colon, and breast cancers, have damage to the p53 protein.[10]

Still other apoptotic triggers may lead to programmed death of cancerous cells. Normal cells also tend to self-destruct when deprived of their usual growth factors or contact with other like cells. This is probably a built-in defense mechanism against metastasis. Part of the reason some cancers are resistant to the effects of radiation therapy or chemotherapy may be due to the lack of cell death through apoptosis even after cancer treatment. Researchers are investigating genetic therapies that might overcome this resistance to apoptosis.

Genetics and Cancer

As stated earlier, cancers comprise all diseases of cells that have been altered or transformed in some way. Throughout this chapter, genetic damage has been mentioned. The Human Genome Project, a federally funded, multibillion dollar international initiative was begun in 1990, with the goal of locating, mapping, and sequencing the more than 100,000 genes of a human's genetic composition. Approximately 60 genes have been linked to cancer. Many genes are used as molecular biologic markers of tumor prognosis, whereas others are useful markers for the screening and early detection of common cancers, including those of the breast, ovary, and colon. For example, the BRCA1 gene, isolated in 1994, is a mutation that has been linked to the susceptibility to breast, and probably ovarian, cancers in a small percentage of women.[32]

Up to 30% of rare childhood cancers result from genetic predisposition. In adults, approximately 34% of cancers have a *familial* basis; only 5% to 10% of adult cancers are *hereditary*. Some families experience a higher than normal rate of cancer that cannot be explained by environmental exposure or general risk. The cancers may be all of one type or of two or more types. There is no predictable pattern of inheritance because the cancers are probably not linked to a single gene disorder. Cancers that may have a potential familial link include breast, ovarian, colorectal, prostate, melanoma, uterine, leukemia, sarcomas, and primary brain tumors.

Hereditary cancers result from a single inherited gene disorder. Patterns of occurrence are clearly predictable. These cancers usually occur at an early age, in unusual sites, and in paired organs (both breasts, for example). There also may be multiple primary (versus metastatic) sites. Hereditary cancers include some breast, colorectal, melanoma, ovarian, and renal cell cancers as well as retinoblastoma and Wilms' tumor.[33]

Although gene therapy for cancer prevention is still futuristic, there are already some investigational studies of this treatment as a treatment modality.[33] Genetic discoveries are expected to have a profound impact on nursing practice in several areas and will no doubt change the traditional perspective on screening, identifying, preventing, and treating cancer. Precise identification of cancer-causing genetic abnormalities will significantly improve the accuracy of cancer prediction and thus the capacity to target preventive interventions to at-risk populations. As a result, the perspective of nursing will shift from symptomatic clients with cancer to counseling asymptomatic clients. Issues of confidentiality and discrimination, as well as the dilemma of predicting as yet incurable illnesses, may have an enormous negative effect on the client's and family's quality of life and psychological state.

Classification of Neoplasms

■ BENIGN VERSUS MALIGNANT

As stated, neoplastic tumors can be either benign or malignant. The word *benign* comes from the Latin *benigunus,* meaning kind. A benign tumor expands in size as it grows, but it does not infiltrate or metastasize. Because it occupies space, it may be fatal if it is located near a vital tube or organ. As a rule, though, the person with a benign neoplasm has a good prognosis because the tumor can be readily excised. Malignant neoplasms, on the other hand, represent a serious threat to the life and well-being of the host. Table 18–6 compares the characteristics of benign and malignant neoplasms.

■ TISSUE OF ORIGIN

Besides being classified as benign or malignant, neoplasms are also classified according to the tissue from which they arise. Almost all names for neoplasms end in the suffix-*oma,* meaning tumor (Table 18–7). This suffix is usually attached to a term for the parent tissue of the neoplasm. Thus, adenoma comes from the Greek *aden-,* or gland, plus-*oma.* When more than one parent tissue enters into the formation of a neoplasm, the names of the tumors are even more descriptive. For example, an adenomyoma is a benign neoplasm that contains both glandular and muscle (Greek genitive *myos*) cells.

Because epithelial tissues vary greatly, benign tumors of epithelial origin are classified according to either their *microscopic* appearance (e.g., adenoma) or their *macroscopic* appearance (e.g., polyp, from the Greek *polys* for many plus *pous* for foot).

Three of the most common benign neoplasms are:

1. *Fibromas.* Fibromas may grow anywhere in the body, but they frequently make their home in the uterus. Fibromas are generally small but occasionally grow to great size. These encapsulated, relatively harmless neoplasms cause no manifestations unless, because of their location, they press on a bone or nerve. Fibromas are easily removed surgically.
2. *Lipomas.* Lipoma, a very common benign neoplasm, arises in adipose tissue. Lipomas rarely cause manifestations, but they are poorly encapsulated and may exert pressure on surrounding tissues as they expand.
3. *Leiomyomas.* The leiomyoma, a benign neoplasm of smooth muscle origin, is the most common benign tumor in women. Leiomyomas may develop anywhere in the body, but most often they grow in the uterus. Rarely ($\sim$1% cases), these neoplasms become malignant.

TABLE 18–6 COMPARISON OF THE CHARACTERISTICS OF BENIGN AND MALIGNANT NEOPLASMS

Characteristic	Benign Neoplasm	Malignant Neoplasm
Speed of growth	Grows slowly Usually continues to grow throughout life unless surgically removed May have periods of remission	Usually grows rapidly Tends to grow relentlessly throughout life Rarely, neoplasm may regress spontaneously
Mode of growth	Grows by enlarging and expanding Always remains localized; never infiltrates surrounding tissues	Grows by infiltrating surrounding tissues May remain localized (in situ), but usually infiltrates other tissues
Capsule	Almost always contained within a fibrous capsule Capsule does not prevent expansion of neoplasm but does prevent growth by infiltration Capsule advantageous because encapsulated tumor can be removed surgically	Never contained within a capsule Absence of capsule allows neoplastic cells to invade surrounding tissues Surgical removal of tumor difficult
Cell characteristics	Usually well differentiated Mitotic figures absent or scanty Mature cells Anaplastic cells absent Cells function poorly in comparison with normal cells from which they arise If neoplasm arises in glandular tissue, cells may secrete hormones	Usually poorly differentiated Large numbers of normal and abnormal mitotic figures present Cells tend to be anaplastic, i.e., young, embryonic type Cells too abnormal to perform any physiologic functions Occasionally a malignant tumor arising in glandular tissue secretes hormones
Recurrence	Recurrence extremely unusual when surgically removed	Recurrence common following surgery because tumor cells spread into surrounding tissues
Metastasis	Metastases never occur	Metastases very common
Effect of neoplasm	Not harmful to host unless located in area where it compresses tissues or obstructs vital organs Does not produce cachexia (weight loss, debilitation, anemia, weakness, wasting)	Always harmful to host Causes death unless removed surgically or destroyed by radiation or chemotherapy Causes disfigurement, disrupted organ function, nutritional imbalances May result in ulcerations, sepsis, perforations, hemorrhage, tissue slough Almost always produces cachexia, which leaves person prone to pneumonia, anemia, etc.
Prognosis	Very good Tumor generally removed surgically	Depends on cell type and speed of diagnosis Poor prognosis if cells are poorly differentiated and evidence of metastatic spread exists Good prognosis indicated if cells still resemble normal cells and there is no evidence of metastasis

Malignant neoplasms are also categorized by tissue origin. A malignant neoplasm that arises from epithelial tissue is called a *carcinoma;* a malignant neoplasm that arises from mesenchymal origins (i.e., blood vessels, lymphatic tissue, nerve tissue) is called a *sarcoma* (from Greek *sarx,* flesh).

Three representative examples of malignant neoplasms or cancers are:

1. *Carcinoma in situ.* This is a neoplasm of epithelial tissue that remains confined to the site of origin. In situ carcinoma typically affects the cervix, and it may occur in squamous epithelium in other parts of the body. This form of cancer is, by definition, localized and thus can be removed surgically. However, in situ carcinoma can become invasive, eroding into surrounding tissues.
2. *Malignant fibrosarcomas.* These tumors are similar to benign fibromas. Fibrosarcomas tend to grow in the same sites and may originate as benign fibromas, later becoming malignant. These bulky, well-differentiated tumor masses are usually responsive to surgery. Fortunately, they rarely metastasize.
3. *Bronchogenic carcinomas.* These tumors account for 90% of all cases of lung cancer. Bronchogenic carcinomas usually develop in the lower trachea and lower bronchi. Surgical excision of the tumor is the intervention of choice. However, this type of cancer readily gives rise to metastasis; if this occurs, surgery is contraindicated.

CONCLUSIONS

Effective nursing care and client teaching to achieve outcome goals require that you understand the pathophysiol-

TABLE 18–7 CLASSIFICATION OF NEOPLASMS BY TISSUE OF ORIGIN

Tissue of Origin	Benign	Malignant
Connective tissue		Sarcoma
Embryonic fibrous tissue	Myxoma	Myxosarcoma
Fibrous tissue	Fibroma	Fibrosarcoma
Adipose tissue	Lipoma	Liposarcoma
Cartilage	Chondroma	Chondrosarcoma
Bone	Osteoma	Osteogenic sarcoma
Epithelium		Carcinoma
Skin and mucous membrane	Papilloma	Squamous cell carcinoma
Glands		Basal cell carcinoma
		Transitional cell carcinoma
	Adenoma	Adenocarcinoma
	Cystadenoma	Cystadenocarcinoma
Pigmented cells (melanocytes)	Nevus	Malignant melanoma
Endothelium		Endothelioma
Blood vessels	Hemangioma	Hemangioendothelioma
		Hemangiosarcoma
		Kaposi's sarcoma
Lymph vessels	Lymphangioma	Lymphangiosarcoma
		Lymphangioendothelioma
Bone marrow		Multiple myeloma
		Ewing's sarcoma
		Leukemia
Lymphoid tissue		Malignant lymphoma
		Lymphosarcoma
		Reticulum cell sarcoma
Muscle tissue		
Smooth muscle	Leiomyoma	Leiomyosarcoma
Striated muscle	Rhabdomyoma	Rhabdomyosarcoma
Nerve tissue		
Nerve fibers and sheaths	Neuroma	Neurogenic sarcoma
	Neurinoma	
	(Neurilemoma)	
	Neurofibroma	(Neurofibrosarcoma)
Ganglion cells	Ganglioneuroma	Neuroblastoma
Glial cells	Glioma	Glioblastoma
Meninges	Meningioma	Malignant meningioma
Gonads	Dermoid cyst	Embryonal carcinoma
		Embryonal sarcoma
		Teratocarcinoma

ogy of the cancer. You should know the natural history of the disease, such as the normal course of disease progression, likely sites of metastasis, potential for effective treatment, and side effects and complications of both the disease and the treatments. With a basic understanding of cancer, you can build on that knowledge base by listening to the client's history, reviewing the information provided in the medical record, and consulting with colleagues, including nursing peers, nursing leaders, physicians, and oncology nurses, both locally and nationally.

BIBLIOGRAPHY

1. Ameisen, J. C. (1996). The origin of programmed cell death. *Science, 272,* 1278–1279.
2. American Cancer Society. (2000). *Cancer facts & figures—2000.* Atlanta: Author.
3. Baillie, C. T., Winslet, M. C., & Bradley, N. J. (1995). Tumour vasculature—a potential therapeutic target. *British Journal of Cancer, 72,* 257–267.
4. Brophy, L. (1998). Immunology. In J. K. Itano & K. N. Taoka (Eds.), *Core curriculum for oncology nursing* (3rd ed., pp. 383–391). Philadelphia: W. B. Saunders.
5. Calzone, K. A. (1998). Genetics. In J. K. Itano, & K. N. Taoka (Eds.), *Core curriculum for oncology nursing* (3rd ed., pp. 392–403). Philadelphia: W. B. Saunders.
6. Cartmel, B., & Reid, M. (1997). Cancer control and epidemiology. In S. L. Groenwald et al. (Eds.), *Cancer nursing: Principles and practices* (4th ed., pp. 50–74). Boston: Jones & Bartlett.
7. Caudell, K. A., Cuaron, L. J., & Gallucci, B. B. (1996). Cancer biology: Molecular and cellular aspects. In R. McCorkle et al. (Eds.), *Cancer nursing: A comprehensive textbook* (2nd ed., pp. 150–170). Philadelphia: W. B. Saunders.
8. Cortner, J., & Vande Woude, G. F. (1997). Essentials of molecular biology. In V. T. DeVita, S. Hellman, & S. A. Rosenberg (Eds.), *Cancer: Principles and practices of oncology* (5th ed., pp. 3–33). Philadelphia: Lippincott-Raven.

9. DeVita, V. T., Hellman, S., & Rosenberg, S. A. (Eds.). (1997). *Cancer: Principles and practices of oncology* (5th ed.). Philadelphia: Lippincott-Raven.
10. Duke, R. C., Ojcius, D. M., & Young, J. D. (1996). Cell suicide in health and disease. *Scientific American, 275*(6), 80–87.
11. Farrell, M. M. (1996). Biotherapy and the oncology nurse. *Seminars in Oncology Nursing, 12*(2), 82–88.
12. Fidler, I. J. (1997). Molecular biology of cancer: Invasion and metastasis. In V. T. DeVita, S. Hellman, & S. A. Rosenberg (Eds.), *Cancer: Principles and practices of oncology* (5th ed., pp. 135–148). Philadelphia: Lippincott-Raven.
13. Groenwald, S. L., et al. (1997). *Cancer nursing: Principles and practices* (4th ed.). Boston: Jones & Bartlett.
14. Hall, E. J. (1997). Etiology of cancer: Physical factors. In V. T. DeVita, S. Hellman, & S. A. Rosenberg (Eds.), *Cancer: Principles and practices of oncology* (5th ed., pp. 203–218). Philadelphia: Lippincott-Raven.
15. Henderson, B. E., Bernstein, L., & Ross, R. (1997). Etiology of cancer: Hormonal factors. In V. T. DeVita, S. Hellman, & S. A. Rosenberg (Eds.), *Cancer: Principles and practices of oncology* (5th ed., pp. 219–229). Philadelphia: Lippincott-Raven.
16. Hetts, S. W. (1998). To die or not to die. *Journal of the American Medical Association, 279*(4), 300–307.
17. Itano, J. K. & Taoka, K. N. (Eds.). (1998). *Core curriculum for oncology nursing* (3rd ed.). Philadelphia: W. B. Saunders.
18. Johnson, B. E. (1998). Tobacco and lung cancer. *Primary Care, 25*(2), 279–290.
19. Kastan, M. B. (1997). Molecular biology of cancer: The cell cycle. In V. T. DeVita, S. Hellman, & S. A. Rosenberg (Eds.), *Cancer: Principles and practices of oncology* (5th ed., pp. 121–134). Philadelphia: Lippincott-Raven.
20. Landis, S. H., et al. (1998). Cancer statistics. *CA: A Cancer Journal for Clinicians, 48*(1), 6–29.
21. Loescher, L. J. (1998). DNA testing for cancer predisposition. *Oncology Nursing Forum, 25*(8), 1317–1327.
22. Peters, J. A. (1997). Applications of genetic technologies to cancer screening, prevention, diagnosis, prognosis, and treatment. *Seminars in Oncology Nursing, 13*(2), 74–81.
23. Pitler, L. R. (1996). Hematopoietic growth factors in clinical practice. *Seminars in Oncology Nursing, 12*(2), 115–129.
24. Post-White, J. (1996). The immune system. *Seminars in Oncology Nursing, 12*(2), 89–96.
25. Post-White, J. (1996). Principles of immunology. In R. McCorkle et al. (Eds.), *Cancer nursing: A comprehensive textbook* (2nd ed., pp. 171–189). Philadelphia: W. B. Saunders.
26. Ries, L. A., et al. (Eds.). (1998). *SEER cancer statistics review, 1973–1995.* Bethesda, MD: National Cancer Institute.
27. Saenz, R. B., & Phillips, D. M. (1998). *Breast cancer. Primary care, 25*(2), 152–162.
28. Soltis, M., Hubbard, S., & Kohn, E. (1996). The biology of invasion and metastases. In R. McCorkle et al. (Eds.), *Cancer nursing: A comprehensive textbook* (2nd ed., pp. 190–212). Philadelphia: W. B. Saunders.
29. Stellman, J. M., Stellman, S. D. (1996). Cancer and the workplace. *CA: A Cancer Journal for Clinicians, 46*(70), 70–92.
30. Trichopoulos, D., et al. (1997). Epidemiology of cancer. In V. T. DeVita, S. Hellman, & S. A. Rosenberg (Eds.), *Cancer: Principles and practices of oncology* (5th ed., pp. 231–257). Philadelphia: Lippincott-Raven.
31. Volker, D. L. (1998). Carcinogenesis. In J. K. Itano & K. N. Taoka (Eds.), *Core curriculum for oncology nursing* (3rd ed., pp. 357–382). Philadelphia: W. B. Saunders.
32. Williams, J. K. (1997). Principles of genetics and cancer. *Seminars in Oncology Nursing, 13*(2), 68–73.
33. Workman, M. L. (1996). Gene therapy. In R. McCorkle et al. (Eds.), *Cancer nursing: A comprehensive textbook* (2nd ed., pp. 458–469). Philadelphia: W. B. Saunders.
34. Yuspa, S. H., & Shields, P. G. (1997). Etiology of cancer: Chemical factors. In V. T. DeVita, S. Hellman, & S. A. Rosenberg (Eds.), *Cancer: Principles and practices of oncology* (5th ed., pp. 185–202). Philadelphia: Lippincott-Raven.

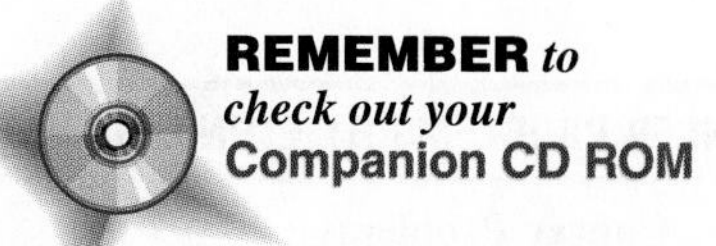

CHAPTER 19

Clients with Cancer: Promoting Positive Outcomes

Patricia Meier

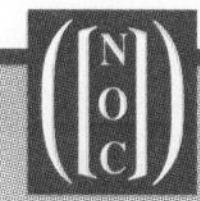

NURSING OUTCOMES CLASSIFICATION (NOC) for Nursing Diagnoses—Clients with Cancer

Altered Nutrition: Less Than Body Requirements
Nutritional Status: Food and Fluid Intake
Fatigue
Activity Tolerance
Endurance
Ineffective Individual Coping
Coping
Decision Making
Role Performance
Social Support
Risk for Infection
Immune Status
Risk Control
Risk Detection
Tissue Integrity: Skin and Mucous Membranes
Risk for Injury
Knowledge: Personal Safety
Neurologic Status
Risk Control
Risk Detection
Symptom Control

The continuum of disease progression begins with precancerous and cellular level changes discussed in the previous chapter on the pathophysiology of malignant neoplasms. The goal of health promotion is to prevent cancer or to detect it early, in its most treatable stage. After a new diagnosis of cancer, the client may experience remission, stable disease, recurrence, progressive disease, end-stage or terminal disease, or long-term survivorship. Treatment modalities depend on the type and extent of the cancer but often include some combination of surgery, radiation therapy (RT), chemotherapy, and biotherapy. Bone marrow transplantation may be part of the treatment plan. Clinical trials offer the hope of new treatments for clients.

Increasingly, complementary approaches are being used in combination with other cancer treatments. The disease process and the effects of treatment on normal tissue present common complications or oncologic emergencies that require effective nursing management to achieve desired outcomes. Cancer care is not just about the disease and treatment; cancer comes in the midst of peoples' lives. Therefore, an important role of the nurse in managing outcomes is to recognize, intervene, and provide support for the human responses to living with cancer.

HEALTH PROMOTION AND MAINTENANCE

■ CANCER PREVENTION AND CONTROL

In the 1980s, the National Cancer Institute (NCI) set a goal to decrease mortality from cancer by 25% to 50% by the year 2000.[53] Cancer prevention and control were major priorities of the NCI's Year 2000 objectives. To achieve this goal, the NCI's objectives included reduction of the smoking rate in the United States to 15% or lower in order to achieve an 8% to 16% reduction in cancer mortality. Another NCI objective was to lower cancer mortality by 8% through dietary modifications. Such modifications involved decreasing fat intake to 30% of total calories and increasing dietary intake of fruits and vegetables to five or more servings daily and of grains to six or more servings daily. Another NCI objective was persuading 60% of the population to limit sun exposure, use sunscreen and protective clothing when exposed to the sun, and avoid artificial sources of ultraviolet light.

Recognizing the role of health professionals in motivating clients to alter lifestyle behaviors, the NCI also set an objective to have at least 75% of primary care providers routinely counsel clients about cessation of tobacco use, modifications of diet and exercise, and guidelines for screening.[53] These goals were difficult to achieve from the outset, given that (1) 20% to 30% of Americans smoke, (2) 90% eat too few fruits, vegetables, and grains while consuming too much fat, and (3) more than half have sedentary lifestyles.

PREVENTION, SCREENING, AND EARLY DETECTION

The three interrelated activities involved in cancer prevention and control are prevention, screening, and early detection. Primary prevention involves measures to avoid or reduce exposure to carcinogens. Screening programs help to identify high-risk populations and individuals. Early detection involves finding a precancerous lesion or a cancer at its earliest, most treatable stage.

Primary prevention activities are aimed at intervention before pathologic change has begun.[37] They can help to reduce cancer risk through alteration of lifestyle behaviors to eliminate or reduce exposure to carcinogens. Many cancers are associated with smoking, dietary habits, and alcohol consumption.[16, 37, 53] All of the cancers caused by combined tobacco and alcohol consumption could be avoided. Adapting a more healthy diet, limiting exposure to sun and other sources of ultraviolet radiation, modifying sexual practices, and decreasing exposure to environmental and occupational carcinogens would lead to further reduction in cancer incidence. Exposure to carcinogens can vary widely among population segments. In lower socioeconomic, medically underserved, and nonwhite segments of the population, the incidence of cancer is increased, and cancer is usually diagnosed at more advanced stages (Table 19–1).[69]

Secondary prevention,[37] also referred to as *early detection*, provides the opportunity to detect precancerous lesions or early-stage cancers before manifestations become readily apparent to the client and to treat them promptly. Screening efforts facilitate early detection. Methods of early detection are (1) inspection, (2) palpation, and (3) the use of tests or procedures. Inspection is useful in identifying lesions of the skin, lip, mouth, larynx, external genitalia, and cervix. Lumps or nodules in the breast, mouth, salivary glands, thyroid, subcutaneous tissue, anus, rectum, prostate, testes, ovaries, and uterus as well as enlarged lymph nodes can be detected through palpation. Mammograms, Papanicolaou (Pap) smear, occult blood testing of feces, endoscopy, and radiologic imaging studies are some of the tests or procedures that can be used. As a result of early detection, (1) premalignant lesions may be arrested, removed, or reversed or (2) cancer treatment can be started earlier, often while the cancer is in a stage more amenable to treatment.

Screening identifies high-risk groups of people more likely to have cancer or precancerous lesions. The current American Cancer Society (ACS) recommendations for screening are listed in Table 19–2. It is estimated that 75% of all cancers in the United States could be cured if all available screening tests and self-examination methods were practiced routinely.[37] Criteria for screening are as follows[30]:

- The population to be screened has a high incidence of the disease.
- The disease is detectable in its presymptomatic stage.
- Prognosis is poor if diagnosis is delayed until manifestations appear.

TABLE 19–1 CANCER PROBLEMS BY ETHNIC GROUPS

Ethnic Group	Cancer Problems
African American	Highest overall cancer incidence rate Highest overall mortality rate Survival 30% lower than for whites High-incidence cancers: prostate, breast, lung, colorectal, cervical, pancreatic, and esophageal
Hispanic	Gallbladder cancer among New Mexico Hispanics of Native American ancestry Liver cancer among Mexican Americans Cervical cancer among women from Central and South America Pancreatic cancer among Mexican Americans Prostate cancer
Asian/Pacific Islander	Nasopharyngeal cancer Stomach cancer
Chinese	Liver cancer Esophageal cancer
Native American	Lowest overall cancer incidence and mortality of all U.S. populations Survival rates uniformly low Important differences in tribal cancer rates

Adapted from Phillips, J., Belcher, A., & O'Neil, J. A. (1997). Special populations. In C. Varricchio et al. (Eds.), *A cancer source book for nurses* (7th ed.). Boston: Jones & Bartlett.

- An effective treatment is available for disease that is diagnosed early.
- There is an effective test for screening.
- The potential benefits of screening outweigh its potential risks and costs.

APPROACHES TO CANCER PREVENTION

Three main approaches to cancer prevention are (1) education, (2) regulation, and (3) host modification.[53] A client's health beliefs can be vital determinants of learning readiness when information is made available.

The beliefs that influence the effectiveness of *education* consist of the client's perception of susceptibility to developing cancer, beliefs about the harmful or beneficial consequences of lifestyle behaviors, and perceptions about the benefits of prevention and early detection.

Methods of *regulation* utilized in this country include prohibiting the sale of tobacco and alcohol to minors, limiting smoking in public places, imposing excise taxes, regulating the use of manufactured carcinogens such as asbestos, and prohibiting carcinogens in foods.

Host modification aims to alter the body's internal environment to decrease the risk of cancer or to reverse a carcinogenic process. Twenty per cent of cancers are associated with viruses (see Chapter 18, Table 18–4). Clinical trials of possible vaccines to immunize against some cancers have begun. Yet another avenue for host modification being studied in clinical trials is chemoprevention. This process is the use of noncytotoxic (non–cell-de-

TABLE 19–2 SUMMARY OF AMERICAN CANCER SOCIETY (ACS) RECOMMENDATIONS FOR THE EARLY DETECTION OF CANCER IN ASYMPTOMATIC PEOPLE

Site	Recommendation
Cancer-related checkup	A cancer-related checkup is recommended every 3 years for people aged 20–40 years and every year for people age 40 and older. This exam should include health counseling and, depending on a person's age, might include examinations for cancers of the thyroid, oral cavity, skin, lymph nodes, testes, and ovaries, as well as for some nonmalignant diseases.
Breast	Women 40 years and older should have an annual mammogram, an annual clinical breast exam (CBE) performed by a health care professional, and should perform monthly breast self-examination (BSE). The CBE should be conducted close to the scheduled mammogram. Women aged 20–39 should have a CBE performed by a health care professional every 3 years and should perform monthly BSE.
Colon and rectum	Men and women aged 50 years or older should follow *one* of the examination schedules below: ▪ A fecal occult blood test every year and a flexible sigmoidoscopy every 5 years. ▪ A colonoscopy every 10 years. ▪ A double-contrast barium enema every 5 to 10 years. ▪ A digital rectal exam should be done at the same time as sigmoidoscopy, colonoscopy, or double-contrast barium enema. People who are at moderate or high risk for colorectal cancer should talk with a doctor about a different testing schedule.
Prostate	The ACS recommends that both the prostate-specific antigen (PSA) blood test and the digital rectal examination be offered annually, beginning at age 50, to men who have a life expectancy of at least 10 years and to younger men who are at high risk. Men in high-risk groups, such as those with a strong familial predisposition (i.e., two or more affected first-degree relatives), or African Americans may begin at a younger age (i.e., 45 years).
Uterus	**Cervix:** All women who are or have been sexually active or who are 18 and older should have an annual Pap test and pelvic examination. After three or more consecutive satisfactory examinations with normal findings, the Pap test may be performed less frequently. Discuss the matter with your physician. **Endometrium:** Women at high risk for cancer of the uterus should have a sample of endometrial tissue examined when menopause begins.

Pap, Papanicolaou.
From American Cancer Society. (2000). *Cancer facts & figures 2000* (p. 34). Atlanta: American Cancer Society. ©American Cancer Society, Inc.

stroying) nutrients, pharmacologic agents, or both to prevent or reverse carcinogenesis.

PREVENTION AND EARLY DETECTION OF COMMON CAUSES

BREAST CANCER. Breast cancer is the most commonly diagnosed cancer, second only to lung cancer for cancer mortality, in American women. Risk factors (early menarche, late menopause, or being either nulliparous or older than 30 years at the birth of a first child) relate to their effect on circulating hormones. Incidence increases with age; more than 77% of women are older than age 50 at diagnosis. Having first-degree relatives with and a previous personal history of breast cancer also are indicators of higher risk. Many women diagnosed with breast cancer have no known risk factors.

One clinical trial has indicated the potential benefit of tamoxifen (Nolvadex), an anti-estrogen hormone, as preventive therapy for high-risk women older than 50 years. Breast cancer mortality could be reduced by 30% through early detection using routine screening mammography alone or together with an annual clinical breast examination by a primary health care provider beginning between ages 40 and 50. The ACS also recommends that women perform monthly breast self-examination (BSE) beginning at 20 years of age. The data are insufficient to determine the role of BSE in decreasing mortality; however, clients who perform BSE generally present with smaller tumors.[3, 30]

LUNG CANCER. Lung cancer is the leading cause of cancer deaths among Americans. More than 80% of lung cancers result from tobacco abuse. Other risk factors are tuberculosis (scar tumor), asbestos, exposure to radiation, and air pollution. To prevent lung cancer, clients should be counseled to not smoke. A healthy diet with at least five servings of fruits and vegetables is an added preventive step. Previous clinical trials have not found chemopreventives effective in preventing lung cancer. There is no reliable, inexpensive early detection method; therefore, screening is not of benefit.[3]

COLORECTAL CANCER. Colorectal cancer has the third highest incidence of all cancers in both men and women; the incidence is greater in men. Risk factors include familial polyposis, familial nonpolyposis syndromes, cancer family syndrome, hereditary site-specific colon cancer, and ulcerative colitis. Incidence of colorectal cancer increased with age after 50 years. A weaker risk factor associated with colorectal cancer may be a high-fat, low-fiber diet. There is no known prevention, although a healthy diet (higher in fiber and low in fat) and physical activity may be of benefit.

Early detection through routine screening is the key to decreasing mortality. The ACS recommends that people with an average risk for colon cancer be screened annually with digital rectal examinations and fecal occult blood tests beginning at age 40 and with sigmoidoscopy every 3 to 5 years beginning at age 50. For people with a high risk for colon cancer, the ACS recommendation is colonoscopy and/or double-contrast screenings beginning at age 40 (see Table 19–2).[3, 30]

PROSTATE CANCER. Age is the greatest risk factor for prostate cancer, 70 years being the median age at diagnosis. The incidence increases with each decade of life beginning at age 50. African-American men have the highest incidence of prostate cancer in the world. Another risk factor is family history; almost 25% of men with prostate cancer have two first-degree relatives with the disease. An occupationally related risk factor is exposure to cadmium. Prevention strategies include limiting exposure of workers handling cadmium batteries and keeping dietary fat intake low.

A clinical trial for prostate cancer prevention is under way with a chemopreventive agent, finasteride (Propecia). The ACS recommends that men at age 50 years and high-risk clients at age 40 years begin receiving a digital rectal examination as part of their annual physical examination as well as a prostate-specific antigen (PSA) blood test. The role of PSA findings in early detection is still unsettled. Early-stage prostate cancer is more amenable to treatment. However, the controversy centers on whether the PSA is leading to the diagnosis and treatment of prostate cancers that would never progress if not detected.[3, 30]

CERVICAL CANCER. Risk factors for cervical cancer are closely linked to sexual behavior and sexually transmitted infections. First intercourse at an early age, multiple sexual partners, or a sexual partner who has had multiple sexual partners put a woman at increased risk. The human papillomavirus and the acquired immunodeficiency syndrome (AIDS) are also risk factors, as are low socioeconomic status and cigarette smoking. Other than changing sexual behavior and avoiding tobacco use, there are no known preventive actions the client can take to avoid cervical cancer.

Routine screening for cervical cancer with the Pap smear should begin with the onset of sexual activity and should be repeated at least as often as every 3 years, annually for clients in nonmonogamous relationships. The Pap smear detects cancer in a premalignant stage, which is very amenable to treatment. With adequate screening, cervical cancer should not exist. However, there remain cultural and social barriers to prevention and early detection of this disease.[3, 30]

HEAD AND NECK CANCER. Men are at greater risk of head and neck cancer than women. A synergistic effect of alcohol and tobacco use increases the risk for cancer of the head and neck. Poor oral hygiene, long-term sun exposure, and occupational exposures (asbestos, tar, nickel, textile, wood or leather work, and machine tool operation) are additional risk factors. Southern Chinese clients are also at greater risk. All clients who smoke or combine smoking with drinking alcohol should be counseled to stop these behaviors. Retinoids have been used as a chemopreventive. The evidence does not support the value of routine screening programs, although early detection by dentists and dental hygienists can identify precancerous lesions.[3]

SKIN CANCER. Approximately 1 million new diagnoses of basal cell and squamous cell skin cancers are made each year. These highly curable cancers are not included in overall cancer statistics. The incidence of the most serious form of skin cancer, melanoma, has been increasing about 4% each year since 1973. Individuals with fair complexion, family history, multiple or atypical nevi (moles), and occupational exposure to coal tar, pitch, creosote, arsenic, or radium are at greater risk. Prevention involves avoiding ultraviolet radiation as well as limiting midday sun exposure, wearing a hat or clothing to protect the skin, using sunscreen with a sun protective factor (SPF) of 15 or higher, and avoiding severe sunburns, especially in childhood.

Early detection, especially for melanomas, is critical. Screening programs should include teaching clients how to inspect their own skin. Moles can be mapped as a baseline for future inspections. Basal and squamous cell skin cancer frequently appears as a pale, wax-like, pearly nodule or a red, scaly patch. Note should be made of any changes, such as new moles or a sore that repeatedly scabs over but fails to heal. Moles that are asymmetrical, that have irregular borders or uneven variations in color, or that change in diameter or height should be checked by a physician. A change in the color, surface appearance, or sensation of a mole should also be reported. Clients should be taught the importance of regular self-inspection and of seeking medical attention.[3]

HEALTH RESTORATION

■ MAINTAINING WELLNESS DURING TREATMENT

For clients with cancer, tertiary prevention[37] consists of limitation of disability and rehabilitation. For any client who must undergo cancer treatment, maintaining optimum wellness is important to both treatment outcome and quality of life in the midst of cancer. The nurse's role in caring for clients undergoing cancer treatment in order to maintain optimum wellness is addressed in the later discussion of outcome management during cancer treatments.

■ REHABILITATION

In addition to disease treatment, rehabilitation therapy is often important to the client's quality of life. Rehabilitation may consist of reconstructive surgery after breast cancer or surgery to reverse a temporary colostomy after colon cancer treatment. An important opportunity for rehabilitation may be an exercise program to help a client counteract chemotherapy-related fatigue.

A client whose treatment resulted in lymphedema is most grateful for the improved quality of life following a rehabilitation referral for lymphedema management. Clinicians often think of lymphedema management as benefiting only clients with breast cancer. However, professionals may overlook the possible secondary effect of lower extremity lymphedema after treatment for prostate cancer or after treatment for other cancers that affects the lymph nodes, such as surgery for melanoma or metastatic colon cancer. Additional rehabilitation strategies, such as speech therapy and prosthetic devices, are described in various chapters of the book, in discussions of specific disorders.

OUTCOME MANAGEMENT

■ DIAGNOSIS OF CANCER

Accurate diagnosis is paramount to effective cancer treatment. The vital first step in the diagnostic process is obtaining a complete history and physical examination. The history and physical assessment, together with diagnostic tests, can be highly predictive of a cancer diagnosis. Further, your careful attention to a client's history and physical status will result in accurate nursing diagnoses and interventions.

OBTAIN HISTORY

Because some cancers are linked with certain genetic and environmental factors, you will be concerned with cancer histories of blood relatives, the client's work history, and the environmental factors that may be associated with cancer causation. (See Chapters 9 and 10 for discussions of health history and physical assessment, respectively.) You should also listen for the client's previous life experiences with cancer—whether of a blood relative, the client's own history, or a friend's experience. This information will be useful in assessing both the client's previous knowledge and perceptions about cancer and the client's readiness for teaching.

ASSESS CLINICAL MANIFESTATIONS

When cancer is in its early stages, there are often few manifestations. Clinical manifestations usually appear once the cancer has grown sufficiently large to cause one or more of the following problems:

- Pressure on surrounding organs or nerves
- Distortion of surrounding tissue
- Obstruction of the lumen of vessels, intestines, ureters, and so on
- Interference with the blood supply of surrounding tissues
- Interference with organ function
- Disturbance of body metabolism
- Parasitic use of the body's nutritional supplies
- Mobilization of the body's defensive response

A localized tumor usually produces manifestations related to increased pressure or obstruction in a single region. Metastatic disease and extensive tumors of major organs may display a variety of local and systemic manifestations.

Common clinical manifestations that may arise secondary to cancer include weight loss, weakness or fatigue, central nervous system (CNS) alterations, pain, and hematologic and metabolic alterations. Close assessment of such manifestations may reveal that they are directly or indirectly related to the cancer.

Anorexia, weight loss, weakness, and fatigue are related to the body's inability to consume and use nutrients appropriately. Mechanical interference by tumors, malabsorption, paraneoplastic endocrine secretions (such as excessive secretion of thyroid hormones), and a tumor's use of nutrients may all contribute to a process that must be interrupted to avoid general physical debility.

The client who has difficulty with vision, speech, coordination, or memory may be experiencing primary or metastatic CNS disease. Increased intracranial pressure caused by tumor growth may cause headache, lethargy, nausea, and vomiting.

Although pain is not a common manifestation of early-stage cancer, it may occur as a result of obstruction or destruction of a vital organ, pressure on sensitive tissues or bone, or involvement of nerves. Pain that is not adequately treated may become constant and progressively severe. Bone cancer is particularly painful because the rigidity of bone allows for little or no expansion as the tumor cells proliferate.[27, 57] The pain worsens when pathologic fractures produce instability and muscle spasms. Even though pain is usually a late manifestation in cancer, it may be the manifestation that brings the client to health care.

COMPLETE DIAGNOSTIC EVALUATION

In addition to the history and physical assessment, laboratory and imaging studies may provide further data to support a cancer diagnosis. Many of the diagnostic laboratory and imaging studies utilized to detect other diseases are used to detect cancer. (See Chapter 11 for a discussion of diagnostic assessment.)

A variety of blood tests can be performed to help diagnose cancer (Table 19–3). Some of the more routine tests, such as the complete blood count (CBC) and differential count, do not test for specific types of cancer but indicate the presence of nonspecific problems. These tests are also vital to monitoring the side effects of treatment. Other blood tests, such as tumor marker measurements and biochemical tests, identify the extent of a particular type of cancer. Tumor markers such as PSA can be indicators of cancer; tumor markers are often even more useful as "barometers" demonstrating the effectiveness of treatment.

Unexplained anemia often indicates a malignancy. Hematologic changes include leukopenia, leukocytosis, and bleeding disorders, which in some diseases may occur before local manifestations. Metabolic manifestations, such as Cushing's syndrome, hypercalcemia, syndrome of inappropriate antidiuretic hormone (SIADH) secretion, and carcinoid syndrome, also signify the possibility of cancer.

■ GRADING AND STAGING OF CANCER

Microscopic evidence of malignant cells from the tumor tissue, generally obtained through a surgical or needle biopsy for cytologic analysis, is the *only* definitive evidence of cancer. Once the diagnosis has been made and the microscopic cell type and grade of the tumor have been determined, the extent of spread (staging) of the tumor also needs to be identified.

Tissue may be obtained through a *biopsy*, the surgical excision of a small piece of tissue and its microscopic examination. After the excision, the pathologist prepares a frozen section or permanent paraffin section of the tissue to examine the specimen. For a frozen (or rapid) section, the tissue is immediately frozen; then the pathologist cuts the tissue into thin sections or slices and examines them

TABLE 19–3 LABORATORY BLOOD TESTS FOR CANCER

Test	Reference Values	Conditions in Which Levels May Be Altered
HEMATOLOGIC (CBC)		
Hemoglobin	M: 14–18 g/dl F: 12–16 g/dl	↓ Anemia; nonspecific; may indicate malignancy
Hematocrit	M: 40–54 ml/dl F: 37–47 ml/dl	↓ Anemia; nonspecific; may indicate malignancy
Leukocytes (WBC count)	4500–11,000/mm^3	↑ Leukemia, lymphomas ↓ Leukemia, metastatic disease to bone marrow
Platelets	150,000–300,000/mm^3	↑ Myeloproliferative disorders, CML, Hodgkin's disease ↓ ALL, AML, multiple myeloma, bone marrow depression
BLOOD OR SERUM		
Acid phosphatase	0.11–0.60 mU/ml	↑ Metastatic prostate cancer
ACTH	10–80 pg/ml (in AM)	↑ Lung cancer
Alkaline phosphatase	20–90 mU/ml	↑ Cancer of bone or bone metastasis, liver cancer, lymphoma, leukemia
Calcitonin	Undetectable	↑ Medullary thyroid cancer if >100 pg/ml
Calcium	9.0–11.0 mg/dl	↑ Bone metastasis, breast cancer, leukemia, lymphoma, multiple myeloma, and lung, kidney, bladder, liver, and parathyroid cancers
Gastrin	<200 pg/ml	↑ Gastric and pancreatic cancers
LDH	100–190 mU/dl	↑ Liver cancer, liver metastasis, lymphoma, acute leukemia
Parathyroid hormone	430–1860 ng/L	↑ Squamous cell lung, kidney, pancreatic, and ovarian cancers
Serotonin	50–200 ng/ml	↑ Carcinoid syndrome
SGPT (AST)	5–35 mU/ml	↑ Metastatic cancer to the liver
SGOT (ALT)	740 mU/ml	↑ Metastatic cancer to the liver
Testosterone	M: 275–875 ng/dl F: 23–75 ng/dl	↑ Adrenal and ovarian cancers
Uric acid	M: 2.5–8.0 mg/dl F: 1.4–7.0 mg/dl	↑ Leukemia, multiple myeloma ↓ Hodgkin's disease, multiple myeloma, lung cancer
TUMOR MARKERS		
AFP	<10 ng/ml	↑ Lung, nonseminomatous testicular, pancreatic, colon, and gastric cancers, choriocarcinoma
CA–125	<35 units	↑ Ovarian and pancreatic cancers
Calcitonin	<100 pg/ml	↑ Medullary thyroid, small cell lung, and breast cancers, carcinoid
CEA	0–2.5 ng/ml nonsmokers <3.0 ng/ml smokers	↑ Colorectal, breast, lung, stomach, pancreatic, and prostate cancers
Estrogen receptors	Positive >10 fmoles/mg	↑ ER + breast cancer
HCG	0–5 IU/L	↑ Choriocarcinoma, germ cell testicular cancer; ectopic production in lung, liver, gastric, pancreatic, and colon cancers
Progesterone receptor assay	Positive >10 fmoles/mg	↑ PR + breast cancer
Prostatic acid phosphatase	0.26–0.83 U/L	↑ Metastatic prostate cancer
PSA	0–4 ng/ml	↑ Prostate cancer
CA-19–9		↑ Pancreatic, colon, and gastric cancers
CA-15–3		↑ Breast cancer

ACTH, adrenocorticotropic hormone; AFP, alpha-fetoprotein; ALL, acute lymphocytic leukemia; ALT, alanine transferase; AML, acute myelogenous leukemia; AST, aspartate transaminase; CBC, complete blood count; CEA, carcinoembryonic antigen; CML, chronic myelogenous leukemia; ER, estrogen receptors; F, female; f, femto-; HCG, human chorionic gonadotropin; LDH, lactic acid dehydrogenase; M, male; mU, milliunits; PSA, prostate-specific antigen; SGOT, serum glutamic-oxalo-acetic transaminase; SGPT, serum glutamate pyruvate transaminase; U, units; WBC, white blood cell; ↑, increase; ↓, decrease.

under the microscope. The main advantage of the frozen section is the speed with which the specimen can be prepared and the diagnosis made. Only minutes are required, enabling the surgeon to receive an initial report during surgery. In contrast, the slower, more classic method of embedding the tissue in paraffin takes about 24 hours. However, the paraffin section demonstrates clearer detail than the frozen section.

The tumor *grade* is an evaluation of the extent to which tumor cells differ from their normal precursors. In low numerical grades, grades I and II, the cells are well-differentiated and deviate minimally from normal cells. High grades, grades III and IV, refer to cells that are poorly differentiated and the most aberrant compared with normal cells. A pathologist determines the grade. Tumor grading involves a histologic and anatomic description of the cancer. The pathologist also evaluates the biopsy specimen for other characteristics that help identify the cell type of the malignancy or provide important indicators of prognosis.

Basic x-rays, computed tomography (CT), magnetic resonance imaging (MRI), ultrasound, and other imaging studies are utilized in the diagnosis of cancer as well as in diagnosis of many other diseases. (See Chapter 11 for more information.) When measurable amounts of tumor remain after surgery, imaging studies such as CT scans are repeated at regular intervals to evaluate the effectiveness of chemotherapy or RT.

When a neoplastic growth is definitely diagnosed, it must be further defined in terms of its extent. This diagnostic process, called *staging*, involves a systematic search for the characteristics of the primary tumor (T), involvement of lymph nodes (N), and evidence of metastasis (M), on the basis of knowledge of the natural history of the disease. The TNM system is the accepted system for cancer staging today (Table 19–4).

According to the TNM classification, cancers may be grouped into one of four stages (I to IV) or indicated as stage 0 for carcinoma in situ (without spread). Higher stages signify more extensive disease, with stage IV consistently representing distant metastasis and the worst prognosis. Grading and staging information guides the physician in choosing the intervention and estimating the client's prognosis.

Other established classifications may be used for particular malignancies, such as Clark's classification for malignant melanomas and Dukes' classification for colorectal cancer. Clark's classification considers the level of invasion of melanomas, and Dukes' system refers to the depth of invasion of colorectal cancer. Hodgkin's disease uses the Ann Arbor classification, which refers to both the distribution of the tumor and the associated manifestations.

IDENTIFYING TREATMENT GOALS

The major objective of cancer therapy is to treat the client effectively with appropriate therapy for a sufficient duration so a cure (or control) of the cancer results with minimal functional and structural impairment. *Cure* is a controversial word because of the chronic nature of most cancers, so many health care providers prefer the term *control*. If a cure is not possible, important alternative goals are:

TABLE 19–4 TNM STAGING SYSTEM

Stage	Characteristics
Primary Tumor (T)	
TX	No primary tumor can be assessed
T0	No evidence of primary tumor
TIS	Carcinoma in situ
T1, T2, T3, T4	Increasing size and extent of the primary tumor
Regional Lymph Nodes (N)	
NX	Cannot be assessed
N0	No regional lymph node involvement
N1, N2, N3	Increasing involvement of regional lymph nodes
Distant Metastasis (M)	
MX	Presence of metastasis cannot be assessed
M0	No distant metastasis
M1	Distant metastasis

From Miaskowski, C., & Buchsel, P. (1999). Oncology nursing assessment and clinical care. St. Louis: Mosby.

- *Control* of the cancer by slowing disease progression
- *Palliation,* or alleviation of manifestations
- *Rehabilitation* to maintain a high quality of life for as long as possible or even when cure results

Decisions made at the time of first diagnosis are crucial, because early aggressive intervention usually offers the best hope of cure. Even when cure is not possible, many clients with cancer have benefited from an extended life span and an improved quality of life as a result of cancer treatment.

DETERMINING TREATMENT MODALITIES

Methods of treating clients with cancer are surgery, RT, chemotherapy, biotherapy, and bone marrow transplantation. The choice of method depends on the type of tumor, the extent of disease, and the client's co-morbid conditions (such as cardiac disease), performance status, and wishes.

Performance status is a way of evaluating a client's overall health status and ability to tolerate treatment. Table 19–5 describes two common performance status scales. In most cases, a client is treated with a combination of methods rather than a single therapy. This approach is called *combined modality* or *multimodal* therapy. Combined modality therapy is used in most cancer treatment regimens because it is more effective in destroying cancerous cells. For example, first surgically debulking (removing as much tumor as possible) an ovarian cancer increases the potential for the chemotherapy to be effective on the remaining tumor volume.

Surgical Management

Surgery plays a major role in the diagnosis, staging, and treatment of cancer. It is also an integral part of the

TABLE 19–5 PERFORMANCE STATUS SCALES

EASTERN COOPERATIVE ONCOLOGY GROUP SCALE	
0	Asymptomatic
1	Symptomatic; fully ambulatory
2	Symptomatic; in bed <50% of day
3	Symptomatic; in bed >50% of day, but not bedridden
4	Bedridden
KARNOFSKY SCALE	
100	Normal; no complaints; no evidence of disease
90	Able to carry on normal activity; minor manifestations of disease
80	Normal activity with effort; some signs or symptoms of disease
70	Can care for self; unable to do normal activity or active work
60	Needs occasional assistance; able to care for most of needs
50	Needs considerable assistance and frequent medical care
40	Disabled; needs special care and assistance
30	Severely disabled; hospitalization and death not imminent
20	Very sick; hospitalization necessary
10	Moribund; fatal processes progressing rapidly
0	Death

Adapted from Powel, L. L. (1996). *Cancer chemotherapy guidelines and recommendations for practice.* Pittsburgh: Oncology Nursing Press; and Ignatavicius, D., Workman, M. L., & Mishler, M. (1999). *Medical-surgical nursing across the health care continuum* (3rd ed.). Philadelphia: W. B. Saunders.

rehabilitation and palliation for clients with cancer. Surgery is used with less frequency as a method of cancer prevention.

Although many aspects of surgical care of the client with cancer are similar to those for all clients undergoing surgery for any reason (see Chapter 15 as well as chapters that address surgery of a specific part of the body), there are some differences. In addition to providing expert physical care, it is important that, preoperatively, you evaluate the client's understanding of the proposed procedure and the changes it involves. The emotional impact of the diagnosis may affect the client's expectations, coping, and ability to learn. Preoperatively, clients with cancer may be nutritionally compromised and may require nutritional therapy before surgery. Those who have undergone adjuvant (treatment after removal of all detected cancer) or palliative (comfort care) chemotherapy or RT may have a low red blood cell (RBC) or white blood cell (WBC) count, which needs correction before surgery. In the client undergoing a palliative surgical procedure, pain must be assessed from the perspective of normal postoperative pain in addition to pain secondary to tumor invasion.

DIAGNOSTIC SURGERY

As mentioned, the diagnosis of cancer is established by microscopic identification of malignant cells from tumor tissue. A variety of methods, most involving a surgical procedure, are used to obtain tissue for diagnostic purposes. The biology of the tumor, its size and location, and the proposed method of treatment determine which biopsy method should be used.

Cytologic specimen collection and needle biopsy are relatively simple procedures. A negative biopsy result does not prove the absence of cancer but rather may be an indication of inadequate or misplaced tissue sampling. Negative needle biopsy results generally must be followed by additional specimen collections to obtain an accurate diagnosis.

CYTOLOGIC SPECIMENS. Cytologic specimens can be obtained from tumors that tend to shed cells from their surface. Tumor cells can often be obtained from cytologic examination of fluids aspirated from effusions or ascitic fluid. The physician may obtain cytologic brushings or tissue biopsy specimens while using an endoscope to examine a questionable area. An endoscopy involves direct visualization of the gastrointestinal (GI) tract, bronchoscopy of the lungs, laryngoscopy of the larynx, colposcopy of the cervix and vagina, cystoscopy of the bladder, laparoscopy of the pelvic or abdominal cavity. During these tests, questionable areas can be examined, tissue samples and aspirates taken for biopsy, the extent of the disease staged, and pathologic processes excised.

NEEDLE BIOPSY. Needle biopsy is a simple method of obtaining tissue samples. In a *fine-needle aspiration*, tumor cells are withdrawn from the tumor with a needle and syringe. A *core-needle biopsy* is essentially the same procedure; however, the needle is larger, and a core or barrel of tissue is obtained. Core-needle biopsy allows the pathologist to examine the cells with their spatial relationships intact, whereas fine-needle aspiration provides individual cells or clumps of cells for review.

Needle biopsy is useful in obtaining samples from tumors in subcutaneous tissue, muscle, breast, pancreas, liver, and lung. Needle (aspiration) biopsy is used mainly to obtain tissue samples for identification from liver, kidney, spleen, lung, or breast. The physician aspirates a core of tissue from a questionable nodule or mass rather than excising it.

EXCISIONAL BIOPSY AND INCISIONAL BIOPSY. The size of the tumor and the purpose of the biopsy are determinants of whether an excisional or incisional biopsy is performed. If the suspected tumor is small, the entire tumor is excised for examination; this is called a *total* or *excisional* type of biopsy. It is used for small tumors (2 to 3 cm) for which the biopsy also may serve as the treatment if the tissue margins contain no tumor cells. If tumor cells remain, a wider excision is required.

If the tumor is large, only a part of the neoplasm is excised. This procedure is termed a *subtotal* or *incisional* type of biopsy. Stereotactic breast biopsy is a radiography-guided method for localizing and sampling small, nonpalpable breast lesions that are discovered on mammography and that suggest malignancy.

SURGERY FOR STAGING

Cancer staging is the process of determining the extent of disease as the basis for treatment decisions. *Clinical staging* is based on evidence acquired before treatment and obtained from physical examination, imaging, endoscopy, biopsy, laboratory tests, surgical exploration, and other diagnostic tests. It is based on all information gathered prior to the first definitive treatment used.

Pathologic staging is based on the microscopic evidence acquired before treatment, which is supplemented or modified by information obtained at surgery and from the pathologic examination of resected specimens, including the primary tumor, regional lymph nodes, and metastatic nodules. For example, the true stage of colon cancer is usually determined after surgery, when the regional lymph nodes are examined for the presence of tumor cells. Staging of ovarian cancer is based on the extent and location of disease found during surgery.

Surgery as Treatment

Surgery is performed in 55% of clients with cancer.[2] Forty per cent of clients who undergo cancer surgery are treated with surgery alone. Cancers that are localized to the organ of origin and the regional lymph nodes are potentially curable by surgery, although multimodal treatment is more likely to be used to control any submicroscopic spread.

Historically, the generally accepted concept of tumor growth was an orderly sequence of growth from the organ of origin to adjacent tissue, regional lymph nodes, and, eventually, distant sites in a systematic fashion. The logical surgical approach to this type of growth was the widest excision possible of the tumor, surrounding tissue, and regional lymph nodes. Thus, radical surgery became the standard for cancer treatment. Analysis of treatment results, however, demonstrated that despite radical excisions, tumors recurred. Current concepts of tumor biology hold that tumors probably shed cells into the systemic circulation throughout their growth and that, therefore, local therapies (surgery and radiation) must be combined with systemic therapies (biotherapy and chemotherapy) to improve client survival.

When surgery is performed with curative intent, the type of tumor determines the extent of the excision. For slow-growing tumors, such as squamous cell carcinoma and adenocarcinoma of the skin, a wide local excision may be sufficient. Tumors of the colon and breast that spread to the regional lymph nodes are removed with an en bloc excision of the tumor and regional lymph nodes. Sentinel node mapping for breast cancer is discussed in Chapter 40 (the procedure is also used for melanoma). Large tumors, such as sarcomas, which tend to spread locally without metastasis, are removed with radical excisions, such as amputations. In all surgical procedures, various operative techniques, such as glove changing, instrument cleaning, and wound irrigation with cytotoxic agents, are used to prevent dissemination of tumor cells into and beyond the operative field.

Surgery for Recurrence and Metastasis

Cancer that recurs locally can be resected, resulting in occasional cure, remission, or both. Local recurrences of sarcomas as well as colon, breast, and skin cancers have been successfully excised. Solitary metastatic lesions that appear in the lungs, liver, or brain can be removed to effect a surgical cure. Excision of metastatic lesions is considered if (1) no other evidence of disease exists and (2) the metastatic lesion has appeared after a relatively long disease-free interval. The metastatic lesion must exhibit some stability and must be refractory (unresponsive) to chemotherapy and RT. Metastatic renal cell carcinomas, sarcomas, melanomas, and colon carcinomas have been removed in selected clients, resulting in cures or prolonged survival times.

Palliative Surgery

Because surgical procedures carry an inherent potential for morbidity, use of surgery in palliative care is carefully considered and is used only if the risk-benefit ratio is favorable. Examples of palliative surgery that can benefit the client with cancer and improve quality of life include procedures that (1) reduce pain by such means as interrupting nerve pathways or implanting pain control pumps, (2) relieve airway obstructions, (3) relieve obstructions in the GI and urinary tracts, (4) relieve pressure on the brain or spinal cord, (5) prevent hemorrhage, (6) remove infected and ulcerating tumors, and (7) drain abscesses.

Reconstructive Surgery

Advances in reconstructive surgery offer a different perspective on rehabilitation to the client who has experienced curative surgery. Restoration of form and function is possible to varying degrees, depending on the site and extent of surgery. Reconstructive surgery may be performed concurrently with the radical procedure or may be delayed. The major goal of reconstructive surgery is to improve the client's quality of life by restoring maximal function and appearance.

Preventive Surgery

The client at unusually high risk for cancer may elect to undergo a preventive (prophylactic) surgical intervention. Certain conditions or diseases increase the risk of cancer occurrence so significantly that removal of the target organ is justified to prevent cancer development. Clients with familial polyposis, for example, have a 50% risk of having colon cancer by age 40 years. By the time they are 70 years old, all clients with this inherited trait have colon cancer. Clients with ulcerative colitis also have a greater risk for colon cancer. Prophylactic subtotal colectomies may be indicated for this group.

Clients with multiple high-risk factors may consider preventive surgery. Prophylactic mastectomy (breast removal) or oophorectomy (ovary removal), although uncommonly indicated, are acceptable forms of preventive therapy in certain high-risk clients.[65]

Nursing Management of the Surgical Client

Cancer operations tend to be more involved than similar procedures for benign conditions. This tendency can lead to the potential for more complications. For the most part, the postoperative care (such as wound care and prevention of infection) of the client with cancer is similar to that of any client having the same surgical procedure for a noncancer diagnosis. The difference lies in what follows. With a benign condition, although there is certainly a period of healing and perhaps rehabilitation, the surgery usually concludes the active treatment.

With cancer surgery, however, the client often has only begun one phase of multimodal treatment. Surgery is not always the first phase of treatment, because many treatment protocols begin with chemotherapy or RT to shrink the tumor mass and decrease the likelihood of micrometastasis. In the midst of the emotional impact of the diagnosis, the client and family are confronted with an often overwhelming amount of information about the diagnosis, necessary tests, treatment alternatives, and decisions to be made. The client will probably be seen or treated in multiple health care settings by many different health professionals. To effectively help the client manage outcomes, the medical-surgical nurse must not only provide excellent care during the hospitalization but also proactively assist the client with continuing care.

Assess Discharge Needs

Questions you can ask as a guide to discharge planning are as follows:

- What does the client need to know, and what does the client need to be able to do?
- Does the client know how to get to the medical oncologist's office or the clinic?
- Will the client need assistance with transportation, such as an ACS Road to Recovery volunteer driver?
- Would the client benefit from initial information about chemotherapy or from talking with someone who has "been there"?
- If the client or family members have questions you cannot answer, is there a social worker, oncology nursing colleague, or chaplain who can provide assistance?

See the Case Management feature.

No one person and no one profession can meet all of the needs of the client with cancer and the family. To effectively manage outcomes requires teamwork involving the client, the family, the nurse, and other health professionals.

CASE MANAGEMENT

The Client with Cancer

A diagnosis of cancer has traditionally evoked fear of pain and death. Many clients believe that there is little to be done. However, newer therapies have made it possible for curative treatment or remission and have led to improved survival rates. As a nurse, you will be working with clients of all ages at various stages in the cancer process.

Case management for these clients involves awareness of the client's emotional, physical, and psychological state; competent clinical care; education about treatment and further options; and helping the client to use preventive measures as possible. As a good example, you should practice preventive measures—no smoking, good nutrition, weight control, screening examinations, and awareness of environmental hazards.

Assess

- Has a definitive diagnosis of cancer been made?
- What do the client and family know about the diagnosis, type of treatment, and prognosis?
- Which treatment modalities will be used—chemotherapy, surgery, radiation, or some combination?
- What does the client anticipate as a result of treatment (e.g., alopecia, nausea, leukopenia)?
- Is pain management adequate?
- Has this diagnosis affected the client's role in the family? The ability to return to work?
- Are there financial or insurance concerns? (Some insurers may not cover all treatments, especially if they are considered investigational. Loss of insurance or inability to obtain insurance or exhaustion of benefits may also be issues.)

Advocate

Clients with cancer may exhibit behavior indicative of stages in the grieving process (e.g., denial, anger). Giving support without taking the client's behavior personally can be a challenge. Always be aware of what the client and family have been told, and make sure that all caregivers are consistent with information given. Sometimes family members will try to shield the client from knowing the extent of the disease. Honesty and knowledge of what to expect are generally more helpful and empower the client to direct treatment choices. Clients may need assistance with advanced directives or in making a will. Be aware of spiritual needs, and elicit support from the pastoral care team as the client desires.

Management of clinical manifestations is another area of advocacy. Certainly, pain management should always be considered, but other physical and psychological problems must be handled as well—nausea and vomiting, diarrhea, stomatitis, skin breakdown, anxiety, withdrawal, and self-image concerns. At some point, you may help the client to decide that palliative care is preferable to aggressive therapy.

Prevent Readmission

There are multiple reasons for readmission, depending on the type of therapy and stage of cancer. Some readmissions may be anticipated, such as a continuing course of chemotherapy or reconstructive breast surgery; others may be unexpected, such as pneumonia or another infection. Before the client leaves the hospital, consider whether the client can return to the previous living arrangement and whether caregiver support is available; also consider respite for the caregiver. Is hospice care appropriate? Many clients will have complicated care regimens, including intravenous lines or ports, total parenteral nutrition and pain medications via pump. Knowledge of treatments, medications, especially for pain and management of manifestations, can assist the client in managing successfully at home. Information and assistance in obtaining wigs, prosthetics, makeup and special clothing, as well as connecting clients with the many cancer support groups, can promote a positive outlook, leading to an improved quality of life.

Cheryl Noetscher, RN, MS, *Director of Case Management, Crouse Hospital and Community–General Hospital, Syracuse, New York*

■ RADIATION THERAPY

More than 50% of all clients with cancer receive RT at some point during the course of their disease. RT may be used as a primary, an adjuvant, or a palliative treatment. When RT is used as a *primary* modality, it is the only treatment used and aims to achieve local cure of the cancer (e.g., early-stage Hodgkin's disease, skin cancer, carcinoma of the cervix). For patients with laryngeal cancer, the potential for cure with RT is equal to the cure rate with surgery—but without the client's loss of the voice box.

As an *adjuvant* treatment, RT can be used either preoperatively or postoperatively to aid in the destruction of cancer cells (e.g., colorectal cancer, early breast cancer). In addition, it can be used in conjunction with chemotherapy to treat disease in sites not readily accessible to systemic chemotherapy, such as the brain. In some situations, chemotherapy is combined with RT and is administered before the RT dose in an attempt to enhance the effects of RT. For example, in rectal cancer, a client may receive the drug 5-fluorouracil (5-FU) by continuous infusion via an ambulatory pump while receiving RT to kill residual cancer cells left behind after the surgery. The 5-FU makes the malignant cells more sensitive to the effects of the RT.

As a *palliative* treatment modality, RT can be used to relieve pain caused by obstruction, pathologic fractures, spinal cord compression, and metastasis.

HOW RADIATION THERAPY WORKS

Radiosensitivity, the relative susceptibility of tissues to radiation, depends on the individual cells and the characteristics of the tissue itself. A highly radiosensitive tumor is greatly affected by radiation because it divides rapidly, is well vascularized, and has high oxygen content.

RT is the use of high-energy ionizing radiation to treat a variety of cancers. Ionizing radiation destroys a cell's ability to reproduce by damaging its DNA. Rapidly dividing cells are more vulnerable to radiation than more slowly dividing cells. Normal cells have a greater ability than cancer cells to repair the DNA damage from radiation. Therefore, the radiation oncologist may deliver a sufficient dose of radiation to kill the cancer cells while sparing normal cells from excessive cell death.

In addition to the DNA effects, a complex chain of chemical reactions occurs in the extracellular fluid, resulting in the formation of free radicals. Well-oxygenated tumors show a much greater response to radiation than poorly oxygenated tumors. Oxygen free radicals formed during ionization interact readily with nearby molecules, causing cellular damage. A well-vascularized tumor may therefore be more responsive to RT than the same type of tumor if it is larger and, as a result, more poorly vascularized.

TYPES OF RADIATION THERAPY

RT can be administered by a variety of methods. The RT may be delivered as external beam therapy or via a radiation source placed close to the surface of the body or inside the body.

EXTERNAL BEAM RADIATION THERAPY. External beam RT, or teletherapy, is the delivery of radiation from a source placed at some distance from the target site. It is administered in the RT department by high-energy x-ray or gamma-ray machines (e.g., linear accelerator, cobalt, betatron, or a machine containing a radioisotope). The major advantage of high-energy radiation is its skin-sparing effect; that is, the maximum effect of radiation occurs at tumor depth in the body and not on the skin surface. Neutron beam therapy delivered from a cyclotron particle accelerator is currently used to treat many types of cancers, including salivary gland tumors, sarcomas, and tumors of the prostate and lung. Therapists do not remain in the room with the client during the treatment but monitor the client via closed-circuit television and remain in voice contact via an intercom.

INTERNAL RADIATION THERAPY. Internal RT involves placement of specially prepared radioisotopes (radioactive isotopes) directly into or near the tumor itself (*brachytherapy*) or into the systemic circulation. The two major types of internal RT are (1) sealed-source RT, in which the radioactive material is enclosed in a sealed container, and (2) unsealed-source RT, in which the radioactive material is administered systemically, such as by injection or orally.

Sealed-Source Radiation Therapy. Sealed-source RT is used for both intracavity and interstitial therapy. In *intracavity* therapy, the radioisotope, usually cesium 137 or radium 226, is put in an applicator, which is then placed in the body cavity for a carefully calculated time, generally 24 to 72 hours. Intracavity RT is used to treat cancers of the uterus and cervix.

In *interstitial* therapy, the radioisotope of choice (e.g., iridium 192, iodine 125, cesium 137, gold 198, or radon 222) is placed in needles, beads, seeds, ribbons, or catheters, which are then implanted directly into the tumor. For example, clients with prostate cancer may receive implanted seeds as therapy. Implants may be left in the tumor either temporarily (when ribbons, needles, or catheters are used) or permanently (when prostatic seeds are used), depending on the half-life of the isotope.

With sealed sources of internal radiation, the radioisotope is completely enclosed by nonradioactive material. Thus, the radioisotope cannot circulate through the client's body nor can it contaminate the client's urine, sweat, blood, or vomitus. Consequently, the client's excretions are not radioactive. However, radiation exposure can result from direct contact with the sealed radioisotope, such as touching the container with bare hands or from lengthy exposure to the sealed radioisotope.

Afterloading devices have been developed in which an empty applicator (the product that holds the radiation source) is placed during an operative procedure, and the radioactive source is not loaded until the client returns to the hospital room or the radiation treatment department. The technique of remote afterloading may be used to deliver frequent, short-term, high doses of radiation directly to a selected tumor. Generally, hollow applicators are surgically placed. The radioactive source is inserted into the applicator and left in place for a specific time afterward. After a treatment, the radioactive source is removed, but the applicator is left in place if more than one treatment is planned. The client is returned to the hospital room until the next treatment. When brachytherapy is used in the hospital room, the radioactive source can be returned to the brachytherapy device while you are in the client's room providing care. Thus, the use of afterloading devices has helped to decrease radiation exposure for staff but lengthens the total time needed to deliver the dose for the client.

Unsealed-Source Radiation Therapy. Unsealed sources of internal radiation are used in systemic therapy. Unsealed sources used for internal RT are colloid suspensions that come into direct contact with body tissues. The radioisotopes may be administered intravenously, orally, or by instillation directly into a body cavity. For example, iodine 131 is given orally in very low doses to treat Graves' disease (see Chapter 43) or in high doses to treat thyroid cancer. Strontium chloride 89 (Metastron) is administered intravenously for relief of painful bony metastases.

With unsealed sources of internal radiation, the radioisotope circulates through the client's body. Therefore, the client's urine, sweat, blood, and vomitus contain the radioactive isotope.

Radiation Safety Standards

Three key principles you should follow to protect yourself and others from excessive radiation exposure are (1) distance, (2) time, and (3) shielding.

The greater the *distance* from the radiation source, the less the exposure dose of ionizing rays. Distance and radiation exposure are inversely related. Thus, the intensity of radiation decreases inversely with the square of the distance from the source. For example, if you stand 4 feet from a source of radiation, you are exposed to approximately one-fourth the amount of radiation you would receive at 2 feet (Fig. 19–1). When providing care to a client with a uterine implant, you will receive less radiation exposure if you stand at the head of the client's bed rather than directly beside the client.

You should aim to minimize the amount of *time* you are exposed to the radiation source, although you must still meet the client's care needs. Your exposure time should generally be limited to 30 minutes of direct care per 8-hour shift.[16] You need to plan your time in the client's room so you can spend it efficiently while providing care to the client. Time required to organize supplies should be spent outside the room. Care for the client should be rotated among available nursing staff to limit exposure for each employee. Pregnant nurses should not be assigned to care for clients receiving RT.

The use of *shielding* devices whenever possible reduces radiation exposure. The dose of x-rays and gamma rays is reduced as the thickness of the lead shield is increased. In practice, nurses have found that lead shielding can be cumbersome to work with. When shielding is not feasible, you should maintain maximum distance from the radioactive source and limit the duration of exposure.

With sealed-source internal radioactive implants, clients require a private room and bath because of the risk of implant dislodgment and consequent exposure of other people to the radiation. Rooms at the ends of halls or stairwells may be designated for use by such clients because their location lessens the chance that others will be exposed to the radiation. Institutions with a high volume of radiation implants may have specially designed rooms with lead-shielded walls. Shields, a lead container called a *pig*, and a pair of long-handled forceps should always be present in the client's room. If the radiation source becomes dislodged, forceps are used to pick it up and place it immediately in the pig. Generally, the radiation therapist and the radiation safety officer are notified *immediately* of the situation.[21] They retrieve and secure the radiation source.

Staff caring for clients with radioactive implants are rotated to limit exposure per employee. Pregnant staff should be assigned to other clients. Staff members must wear their own film badges or dosimeters while in the client's room. Visiting policy is restricted, so the client may experience feelings of isolation. To maintain contact while keeping distance from radiation exposure, talk with the client from the doorway of the room. Encourage family and friends to telephone. Prepare the client ahead of time for limited employee contact. Before the radiation source is inserted, the client should be provided with ways to pass the time, such as reading and handwork. Such clients usually feel well but are isolated and confined to their beds as a safety measure to prevent the appliance from being dislodged when the client is to have radioactive implants inserted in the abdominal cavity. The client has a Foley (indwelling) urinary catheter and should be eating a low-fiber diet after evacuation of the colon prior to insertion of the radioactive implant. The client should not have a bowel movement before the device is removed in 2 to 3 days.

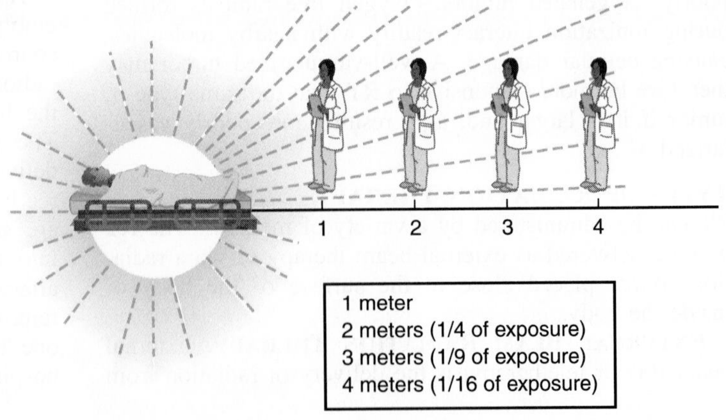

FIGURE 19–1 Inverse relationship of distance and radiation exposure.

The client receiving internal RT with an unsealed source also needs to have a private room and bath. Further precautions must be taken because all body secretions are radioactive. All surfaces, including the floor area the client will be walking on, are covered with Chux, paper, or other protective covering. Foods are served on disposable plates with disposable utensils. Trash and linens are kept in the client's room and are not removed until the client is ready for discharge. To further decrease the risk of radiation exposure of caregivers, bed linens are generally not changed unless they are grossly soiled. Instruct the client to flush the toilet several times after each use.

Visitor and staff contact is limited, as already described for sealed-source RT. Anyone entering the room wears a new pair of booties each time to avoid tracking the radioactive isotope out into the hallway. You must wear gloves to avoid exposure if you are handling body fluids. Any emesis (vomiting), especially that occurring shortly after the client has ingested an oral isotope, should be covered with absorbent pads, and the radiation safety officer should be called immediately. Additional precautions may be necessary, depending on the radioisotope used and the policies and procedures of the individual practice setting.

Prior to discharge, instruct the client about any precautions that should be continued at home. The radiation safety officer will scan the client to be certain that the radiation has decreased to a safe level. All precautions for the room should be continued even after the client has been discharged, until the radiation safety officer has lifted restrictions.

The U.S. Nuclear Regulatory Commission requires that radiation exposure of people be kept as low as reasonably achievable. All institutions using radioactive materials must have written policies concerning radiation protection. In addition, a radiation safety officer licensed by the U.S. Atomic Energy Commission to work with radioactive material must be available at all institutions using radioactive materials.

The law also requires monitoring devices, such as film badges, for health care workers exposed to radiation and the keeping of a record of each worker's exposure. Do not share your film badge with anyone. The film badge provides a measure of whole-body exposure. The general precautions distance, time, and shielding apply for all forms of external and internal RT. Sealed and unsealed sources of internal RT require additional precautionary measures for their safe use.

TREATMENT CONSIDERATIONS FOR RADIATION THERAPY

The goal of RT is to destroy the cancer while keeping dosages within the normal tissue tolerance to avoid harming surrounding normal tissues. Several factors determine the treatment effect and side effects of RT:

1. Tumor location in relation to surrounding normal tissue affects both treatment effect and side effects. Certain normal tissues are more sensitive to radiation and may incur permanent damage as a result of radiation. The spinal cord and the GI, integumentary, and myeloproliferative systems are at greatest risk for damage. If the spinal cord lies in the treatment field, the maximum safe dose of RT is lower than if the RT can be delivered from directions (ports) that avoid the spinal cord. Additionally, customized shielding "blocks" may be created to protect normal tissues from ionizing rays.
2. The size of the treatment field affects the dose of RT. If a small area is treated, the client can tolerate a higher dose of radiation than if a larger area is treated. RT is a regional treatment. Widespread or metastatic disease likely extends beyond the treatment field; in such situations, RT would not be an effective curative treatment modality.
3. The client's overall health or performance status affects the ability to tolerate RT. For example, a client who already has severe chronic obstructive pulmonary disease is less able to tolerate RT to the lung.
4. The therapeutic ratio of the treatment effects on the tumor to the side effects on normal tissue is an important cost-benefit determinant in decision-making about RT.
5. The side effects a client may experience are related to the total dose of radiation. Radiation dose is prescribed in units called *grays* (Gy). This term has replaced the unit of dose known as the *rad* (radiation absorbed dose): 1 Gy equals 100 rad; 1 cGy (centigray) equals 1 rad. The RT dose is higher when the goal is curative eradication of the cancer than when the goal is pain control or palliation. A client receiving 5000 cGy for cure experiences more side effects than a client receiving 2000 cGy to the same body area for palliation.
6. In general, only the area in the treatment field is affected by the radiation. For example, hair loss occurs only in the area being treated with radiation. Therefore, a client receiving RT to the chest experiences hair loss on the chest but usually not on the scalp.
7. Administering the radiation in divided (fractionated) rather than single doses minimizes the side effects by allowing the normal cells time to recover. *Fractionation* refers to dividing the total radiation dose into small, frequent doses. A common dosage schedule for external RT is 150 to 200 cGy, 5 days per week, for a total of 4 to 5 weeks. Fractionation also increases the probability that tumor cells will be in a vulnerable phase of the cell cycle when treated; cells are more sensitive to RT during the late G_2 and early M phases. Fractionation allows normal cells time to repair themselves. At times, an RT dose is *hyperfractionated* (divided into doses given twice daily).

Nursing Management of the Client Receiving Radiation Therapy

The staff of most RT departments includes a nurse to meet the learning and manifestation management needs of the client. Yet nurses in the chemotherapy clinic, inpatient unit, or home care setting may be faced with concerns of or questions from clients and family members about the side effects of RT.

Provide Education

In addition to the emotional impact of the cancer diagnosis, RT can be a source of fear and misunderstanding. Clients may experience fears of being burned or becoming radioactive. Since RT cannot be seen or felt during treatment, the client may also fear that the treatment is not effective. Education can dispel such common fears and misconceptions.

Comparing RT to the effects of the sun can be helpful. One generally does not notice the full effect of the sun immediately after coming indoors. So also, many manifestations of RT do not develop until approximately 10 to 14 days into treatment, and some do not subside until several weeks after treatment. If the cancer was not causing physical manifestations, the client may not have evidence (like seeing a suntan) of the treatment's effect. If, however, the tumor was obstructing air flow, the client may realize a few weeks into the RT that breathing is easier or coughing is diminished—even before imaging studies are performed to verify tumor shrinkage. Likewise, if RT is being delivered for painful bone metastases, the client will probably note a decrease in pain or diminished need for pain medications 1 to 2 weeks into the RT.

Minimize Side Effects

In general, skin reactions and fatigue may occur with RT to any site, whereas other side effects occur only when specific areas are involved in the treatment field. The response of normal skin to RT varies from mild erythema to moist desquamation similar in appearance to a second-degree burn. The term "burn" should not be used to describe these skin reactions, however, because doing so may frighten the client unnecessarily. Because megavoltage and cobalt deliver the maximum dose beneath the skin, skin reactions have become less significant than in years past. The accompanying Client Education Guide offers more teaching information about skin care during RT.

Site-specific manifestations of RT include mucositis, xerostomia (dry mouth), radiation caries, esophagitis, dysphagia (difficulty swallowing), nausea and vomiting, diarrhea, tenesmus (straining at stool or in urination), cystitis, urethritis, alopecia (hair loss), and bone marrow suppression. These may be the result of acute changes associated with inflammation or chronic changes associated with fibrosis. During RT, a CBC is usually performed weekly. The degree of myelosuppression varies with the amount of bone marrow within the treatment field. Areas at greatest risk are the pelvic region, sacrum, skull, lumbar and thoracic spine, ribs, shoulder region, and sternum.

In women of childbearing age, RT may cause prolonged or permanent infertility. In prostate brachytherapy, when radioactive seeds have been permanently implanted, there is a low, weakly penetrating radiation exposure for others. Therefore, the client should use a condom for sexual intercourse in the first weeks after the procedure. Also, the client should avoid close ($<$6 feet) contact with pregnant women and young children (younger than 3 years) for more than 5 minutes a day during the first 2 months following implantation.[1]

Many of the manifestation management strategies for side effects of RT are similar to those for side effects of chemotherapy, described later in this chapter. Information on nursing management of the general side effects of RT is included in the Oncology Nursing Society's *Manual for Radiation Oncology Nursing Practice*.[13] The NCI offers a free client education booklet, *Radiation Therapy and You: A Guide to Self-help*.[62] A nurse or therapist in the RT department is a readily accessible source of information. Furthermore, you can alert the RT staff about the client's concern and thus help the client manage outcomes of the RT side effects.

CLIENT EDUCATION GUIDE

Skin Care Within the Treatment Field

- Keep your skin dry.
- Do not wash the treatment area until you are instructed to do so. When permitted, wash the treated skin gently with mild soap, rinse well, and pat dry. Use warm or cool water, *not* hot water.
- Do not remove the lines or ink marks placed on your skin.
- Avoid using powders, lotions, creams, alcohol, and deodorants on the treated skin.
- Wear loose-fitting clothing to avoid friction over the treatment field.
- Do not apply tape to the treatment site if dressings are applied.
- Shave with an electric razor. Do not use pre-shave or after-shave lotions.
- Protect your skin from exposure to direct sunlight, chlorinated swimming pools, and temperature extremes (e.g., hot water bottles, heating pads, ice packs).
- Consult your radiation therapist or nurse about specific measures for individual skin reactions.

Medical Management

Chemotherapy

As with surgery and RT, the goals of chemotherapy can be cure, control, or palliation of manifestations. Chemotherapy is a systemic intervention and is appropriate when:

- Disease is widespread
- The risk of undetectable disease is high
- The tumor cannot be resected and is resistant to RT

The client who is at high risk for recurrence but shows no evidence of current disease may be a candidate for *adjuvant chemotherapy*; in this type of therapy, after initial treatment with either surgery or RT, chemotherapeutic drugs are used to eliminate any remaining submicroscopic cancer cells that are suspected to be still present. Adjuvant therapy is now well established in the treatment of breast cancer.

Neoadjuvant chemotherapy refers to the preoperative use of chemotherapy to reduce the bulk and lower the stage of a tumor, making it amenable to surgery or possibly even cure with subsequent local therapy.

The objective of chemotherapy is to destroy all malignant tumor cells without excessive destruction of normal cells. Several types of cancer are now considered curable with chemotherapy, even in advanced stages. Unfortunately, these tumors account for only about 10% of all cancers.

HOW CHEMOTHERAPY WORKS. The phases of the cell cycle are common to all cells (see Chapter 18). Normally, cells respond to the body's need for growth, repair, or regeneration in an orderly manner and cease production by entering a resting phase or slowing growth when the need is met. At any given time, normal cells may be found in all phases of growth. Cancer cells reproduce in the same manner as normal cells. However, growth occurs in an uncontrollable manner. In general, cells that are actively dividing are the most sensitive to chemotherapy.

Chemotherapy directly or indirectly disrupts reproduction of cells by altering essential biochemical processes. The desired outcome is control or eradication of all malignant cells. Experiments and clinical experience suggest that most types of chemotherapy do not kill all cancer cells during one exposure. According to the cell kill hypothesis, only a percentage of cancer cells are killed with each course of chemotherapy. Repeated doses—or cycles—of chemotherapy therefore must be used.

The use of drugs in combination, known as *combination chemotherapy*, has consistently been far superior to single-agent therapy. Drugs selected to be used in combination must each be effective against the type of cancer being treated. When combined, chemotherapeutic agents destroy more malignant cells and produce fewer side effects because each drug strikes the cancer cells at a different point in the cell cycle. Combination chemotherapy is now the standard in most situations. The regimens are complex, cyclic, and individualized for the client and the type of cancer. An example of a chemotherapy regimen for Hodgkin's disease is shown in Table 19–6.

CLASSIFICATION OF CHEMOTHERAPEUTIC AGENTS. Chemotherapeutic agents generally are classified according to their pharmacologic actions and effects on the cell generation cycle. However, the method by which cancer cells are inhibited or destroyed is not always known. A classification of common chemotherapeutic agents is shown in Box 19–1.

TABLE 19–6 MOPP REGIMEN FOR HODGKIN'S DISEASE

Drug	Dosage
M = Mechlorethamine HCl (Mustargen)	6.0 mg/m² IV on days 1 and 8
O = Oncovin (vincristine)	1.4 mg/m² IV on days 1 and 8
P = Procarbazine	100 mg/m² PO on days 1–14
P = Prednisone	40 mg/m² PO on days 1–14 during cycles 1 and 4 Repeat cycle every 28 days for at least 6 cycles or at least 2 cycles beyond the attainment of maximum response

IV, intravenously; PO, orally.

Adapted from Greco, F. A. (Ed.). (1996). *Handbook of commonly used chemotherapy regimens.* Chicago: Precept Press.

Nursing Management of the Client Receiving Chemotherapy

Only adequately prepared registered professional nurses who are skilled in the administration of chemotherapeutic agents should assume responsibility for performing it.[76] At a minimum, the nurse should have completed chemotherapy administration classes. Ideally, nurses providing oncology care are also Oncology Certified Nurses (OCNs), who have the specialized knowledge and skills to manage potential outcomes of cancer and its treatment. When the bedside nurse does not have the requisite knowledge, the institutional policies can ensure that a nurse with expertise in cancer care is responsible for supervising care and guiding the bedside nurse in the assessment and administration issues in order to give safe, effective care to the individual client. Recommendations for course content, clinical practicum, and nursing practice can be found in the Oncology Nursing Society's *Cancer Chemotherapy Guidelines.*[76]

ASSESSMENT. A thorough client evaluation is necessary before cytotoxic drugs can be administered. Review the client's medical history to identify potential risk factors for chemotherapy toxicity, such as a history of impaired cardiac, pulmonary, or renal function. Carefully assess the severity and duration of side effects experienced since the previous course of therapy. Abnormal laboratory values may indicate organ-specific toxicities of chemotherapeutic agents. Before a subsequent course of chemotherapy, a CBC with differential count is vital in ensuring adequate bone marrow recovery since the last chemotherapy treatment. The differential count is used to calculate the absolute neutrophil count (ANC) (see later), a means of determining the percentage of mature white cells. Drug doses may have to be modified or delayed on the basis of these results.

The client's chart should contain either a copy of the formal drug protocol or a written summary of the planned chemotherapy regimen. Chemotherapy doses are usually based on body surface area in square meters (m^2), which is determined by the client's height and weight. Clear and complete chemotherapy prescriptions consist of (1) the name of the drug, (2) dose/m^2 and total dose, (3) route of administration, (4) administration rate for intravenous (IV) infusions, and (5) frequency of administration. Plans for antiemetic therapy, hydration, diuresis, and electrolyte supplementation are frequently included as well. It is vital that clients know what side effects to watch for and what to do when side effects arise. See the Care Plan for interventions used to manage the side effects of chemotherapy and related suggestions for client education.

Most serious side effects of the treatment do not occur in the chemotherapy clinic but develop after the client has returned home. Knowing about the expected side effects of cancer treatment and appropriate interventions increases your ability to give prompt, effective care. In a medical-surgical or home care setting, you should be able to recognize variations from normal, perform a complete

BOX 19–1 Classification of Chemotherapeutic Agents

Cell Cycle–Specific Groups

Antimetabolites

Cytarabine (Ara-C, Cytosar)
5-Fluorouracil (5-FU)
Floxuridine (FUDR)
6-Mercaptopurine (6-MP, Purinethol)
Methotrexate (Mexate)
6-Thioguanine (6-TG)
Fludarabine (Fludara)
Pentostatin (Nipent)

Vinca Alkaloids

Vinorelbine (Navelbine)
Vincristine (Oncovin)
Vinblastine (Velban)

Epipodophyllotoxins

Etoposide (VP-16)
Teniposide (VM-26, Vumon)

Taxanes

Paclitaxel (Taxol)

Miscellaneous

L-Asparaginase
Hydroxyurea (Hydrea)

Cell Cycle–Nonspecific Groups

Alkylating Agents

Busulfan (Myleran)
Carboplatin (Paraplatin)
Cisplatin (CDDP, Platinol-AQ)
Cyclophosphamide (Cytoxan)
Ifosfamide (Ifex)
Mechlorethamine HCl (Mustargen)
Thiotepa

Antitumor Antibiotics

Chlorambucil (Leukeran)
Bleomycin (Blenoxane)
Dactinomycin (Cosmegen)
Daunorubicin (Cerubidine)
Doxorubicin (Adriamycin)
Idarubicin (Idamycin)
Mitomycin C (Mitomycin)
Mitoxantrone (Novantrone)
Plicamycin (Mithracin)

Hormonal Therapy

Glucocorticoids

Prednisone (Deltasone)
Methylprednisolone (Solu-Medrol, Medrol)
Dexamethasone (Decadron)

Estrogens

Chlorotrianisene (Tace)
Diethylstilbestrol (DES)
Estradiol (Estrace)

Antiestrogens

Tamoxifen (Nolvadex)

Progestins

Depo-Provera
Megestrol acetate (Megace)
Leuprolide (Lupron)

Nitrosoureas

Carmustine (BCNU)
Lomustine (CCNU)
Streptozocin (Zanosar)

Adapted from Powel, L. L. (1996). *Cancer chemotherapy guidelines and recommendations for practice.* Pittsburgh, PA: Oncology Nursing Press.

assessment of the client's status, and then report that information in a timely manner to the client's oncology caregivers. You can therefore communicate pertinent data to the oncology professional as a basis for a medical or nursing diagnosis. Nurses in all practice settings must work together, sharing information and knowledge, to ensure continuity of care for the client undergoing chemotherapy for cancer.

Administration of Chemotherapy. Before administering antineoplastic agents, consult with the pharmacist and review chemotherapy drug handbooks and investigational drug protocols for detailed information regarding drug actions, dosages, administration guidelines, and potential side effects. A critical step in the administration of chemotherapeutics is the verification of the drug, dose, and schedule.[14, 76] Chemotherapy calculations and drugs should be checked by two nurses against the written orders. Errors in chemotherapy orders may result from such factors as the misplacement of a decimal point or the dispensing of the wrong drug. An overdose of an antineoplastic agent could result in profound toxicity and death.

Educating the client and family about chemotherapy and the identification, prevention, and management of side effects is primarily a nursing function. As already mentioned, the Care Plan in this chapter offers an example of a plan for managing side effects of chemotherapy. The NCI provides an excellent booklet, *Chemotherapy and You*, free of charge for client teaching.[60] Hypersensitivity reaction and extravasation, discussed later in the chapter, can occur during the administration of chemotherapy. Other side effects are most likely to occur after the client is discharged from the outpatient clinic or inpatient unit. Potentially life-threatening side effects, such as infection during neutropenia (see later), are more likely to occur while the client is at home, when no health professionals are available.

Routes of Administration. Two routes are discussed: intravenous and regional.

Intravenous Chemotherapy. Most chemotherapeutic agents are administered intravenously. Extravasation (escape from the vein) of some chemotherapeutic agents can cause significant harm to the surrounding tissue. There-

SIDE EFFECT MANAGEMENT FOR THE CLIENT RECEIVING CHEMOTHERAPY

Nursing Diagnosis. Risk for Injury related to side effects secondary to chemotherapy.

Outcomes. Client will experience minimal side effects of chemotherapy, will demonstrate knowledge of rationale for chemotherapy and treatment plan, and will demonstrate knowledge about potential side effects of drugs and related self-management strategies.

Interventions	Rationales
1. Monitor client during clinic or home visits or when taking phone calls for potential side effects of the drugs—while reinforcing client education of manifestations to report.	1. Some side effects, such as drug extravasation and nausea and vomiting, may occur immediately; others are more likely to occur between treatment cycles.
2. Identify and monitor for known side effects of the drugs utilized in the treatment regimen, including leukopenia, nausea and vomiting, diarrhea or constipation, stomatitis, hair loss, and drug-specific side effects.	2. Early detection and intervention can minimize the morbidity of adverse side effects.
3. Perform more in-depth assessment and additional nursing interventions as indicated for the symptoms identified.	3. See No. 2.

Client Education	Rationales
1. Assess client's learning readiness, including previous life experience related to cancer and expectations related to chemotherapy.	1. A family member's or friend's cancer experience—whether it has any bearing on the client's cancer experience or not—can have a major effect on the client's expectations, anxiety, and even willingness to proceed with treatment.
2. Identify family members and other support persons whom client wished to be included in education; document this information for taking phone calls from support persons.	2. Protects client confidentiality while involving client's support persons.
3. Develop a teaching plan appropriate to the client's individual needs and the specific chemotherapy regimen.	3. Each client's experience will depend on the cancer, the treatment regimen utilized, co-morbid conditions, and ability to cope.
4. Verify client's understanding of the cancer diagnosis, treatment regimen, and informed consent.	4. The information is often overwhelming to hear, the terminology and content are frequently unfamiliar.
5. Provide client and family caregivers with oral and written information regarding: a. Chemotherapy b. Each drug utilized in the treatment regimen. c. Anticipated schedule of administration. d. Rationale for follow-up procedures, including laboratory tests, office visits, and imaging studies. e. Potential side effects—when they may occur, self-care management, and manifestations to report to the physician or nurse.	5. Written information that reinforces teaching is vital. Recall alone is not likely to be efficient. Because most care is provided in outpatient settings, health professionals generally are not present when potentially life-threatening side effects appear.

Nursing Diagnosis. Risk for Infection related to leukopenia secondary to chemotherapy.

Outcomes. Client will remain free of infection, as evidenced by temperature remaining within normal limits. Client demonstrates knowledge related to prevention of infection.

Interventions	Rationales
1. Practice good hand-washing, especially between caring for clients.	1. These interventions will decrease the risk of exposure to a nosocomial infection. Good hand-washing is the most important means of preventing the spread of a nosocomial infection.
2. Keep neutropenic clients separate from others exposed to infections.	2. When neutropenic, a client is at greater risk for infection.
3. Care for neutropenic clients before caring for other clients.	3. This helps prevent nosocomial spread of an infection to client.
4. Use aseptic technique in client care and treatments.	4. See No. 2.
5. Check baseline vital signs.	5. Provides a basis for early detection of manifestations of infection
6. Monitor hematologic laboratory results, especially complete blood count, white blood cell count, differential, and absolute neutrophil count.	6. See No. 5.
7. Monitor for signs of infection, including respiratory, urinary, oral mucosa, and skin.	7. See No. 5.

Care Plan continued on following page

Client Education	Rationales
1. Explain purpose of chemotherapy, how it works, and reason for potential side effects.	1. Because the client is generally home when adverse side effects arise, it is vital that the client be an involved member of the health care team.
2. Explain relationship between effects of treatment on white blood cell (granulocyte) count and potential for infection.	2. See No. 1.
3. Teach measures for preventing infections, including meticulous hand-washing and good oral hygiene.	3. Infection in the neutropenic client is potentially life-threatening.
4. Discuss necessity of avoiding crowds and people who have infection or have recently been vaccinated.	4. See No. 3.
5. If applicable to client, note the need to avoid cleaning cat litter boxes, fish tanks, and canine or human excreta.	5. These are high-risk potential sources of infection.
6. Teach the manifestations that must be reported immediately (e.g., fever, chills, sore throat, burning or pressure with voiding, purulent drainage).	6. When the client is neutropenic, an infection can become rapidly life-threatening.
7. Verify that client has, and is able to read, a thermometer.	7. See No. 6.
8. Verify that client knows how to reach the health professionals after hours.	8. The consequences of not knowing how to reach professionals in an emergency can be both serious and frightening.

Nursing Diagnosis. Altered Nutrition: Less Than Body Requirements related to disease process and treatment.

Outcomes. Client will identify measures to prevent nutritional deficits and will maintain adequate nutritional status, as evidenced by body weight within preset parameters.

Interventions	Rationales
1. Evaluate nutritional status: a. Measure height and weight. b. Compare with prediagnosis weight. c. Assess laboratory values (e.g., serum albumin, complete blood count). d. Obtain anthropometric measurements when indicated.	1. Weight loss over time is an indicator of malnutrition. With significant decrease in weight, chemotherapy dosages must be decreased.
2. Monitor oral cavity for stomatitis, infection, and pain.	2. Client may avoid nutritional intake if it is painful to eat.
3. Arrange for assistance in obtaining and preparing food, if needed.	3. Adequate hydration and a high-protein, high-calorie diet that includes foods high in electrolytes (e.g., Gatorade, fruit juices, salty broths, soups, milk, green leafy vegetables) are vital to recovery of normal cells from the adverse effects of chemotherapy.
4. Refer client to the dietitian if indicators of malnutrition are present.	4. See No. 3.

Client Education	Rationales
1. Discuss relationship of adequate nutrition to disease process and treatment.	1. The client who understands the vital role nutrition plays in the treatment is more likely to make an effort to ensure an adequate intake in spite of the loss of appetite and alterations in the sense of taste.
2. Discuss the elements of a nutritional diet.	2. See No. 1.
3. Help client identify foods that are tolerated and those that cause discomfort or have become distasteful.	3. See No. 1.
4. Discuss strategies for counteracting the loss of appetite or alterations in taste and for ensuring adequate nutritional intake.	4. Suggestions specific to the client's experience (e.g., extra sweetener if foods taste bitter, popsicles for fluid intake) can be very helpful.
5. Emphasize good oral hygiene.	5. Pain and alteration of taste can impair nutritional intake.

Nursing Diagnosis. Fatigue related to cancer treatment.

Outcomes. Client will demonstrate knowledge about methods that may prevent transient tiredness states from progressing to the more intransigent states of acute or chronic fatigue and will be able to engage in a certain percentage of desired activities.

Interventions	Rationales
1. Include evaluation of fatigue in nursing assessment. Obtain data on physical performance status, response to treatments over time, and impact on activities of daily living.	1. The first step in treatment is recognition of the problem. Unfortunately, cancer treatment–related fatigue is often not recognized, and its effect not appreciated, by health professionals.
2. Review laboratory and other clinical data (e.g., oxygen saturation levels) for physiologic manifestations.	2. Fatigue is multidimensional, comprising neuromuscular, attentional, and perceptual factors.
3. Assist client in identifying aggravating and alleviating factors.	3. See No. 2.

4. Administer erythropoietin or blood transfusions as ordered.
   4. Anemia is a common cause of fatigue in clients receiving myelosuppressive therapy.
5. Carry out treatments for dehydration or electrolyte imbalance.
   5. Dehydration and electrolyte imbalance can contribute to fatigue and weakness.
6. Promote sleep and rest.
   6. Clients with cancer report that sleep and rest are helpful but not completely effective in addressing cancer-related fatigue.
7. Assist referrals to community resources that will reduce fatigue (e.g., physical therapy, home health services, transportation services).
   7. This step allows the client to conserve energy for activities that maintain quality of life.

Client Education / **Rationales**

1. Inform client of the relationship of the therapy with fatigue.
   1. Understanding that the fatigue can result from the therapy rather than solely from the disease can alleviate undue anxiety.
2. Prepare client to anticipate periods during chemotherapy treatments when acute fatigue is more likely to be experienced.
   2. Client can plan activities related to anticipated energy levels.
3. Encourage the client to report fatigue and its effect on activities of daily living.
   3. Professionals may be able to offer additional interventions.
4. Help client identify strategies that may prevent transient tiredness from progressing to more intransigent fatigue:
   4. An intervention before fatigue becomes intransigent is more effective.
   a. Vary activities.
      a. A variety of activities prevents boredom.
   b. Use distraction techniques.
      b. Use of distraction helps the client focus on something besides fatigue.
   c. Use relaxation techniques to dissipate the negative effects of stressors.
      c. Relaxation techniques relieve fatigue by reducing effects of stressors.
   d. Maintain good nutritional and fluid intake.
      d. Nutrition provides a source of energy, and hydration promotes excretion of cell destruction end products/toxins.
   e. Schedule activities to balance rest and activity in order to conserve energy.
      e. Results of studies of exercise programs are quite promising, whatever the exercise (bicycle ergometry, walking, or personal).

Nursing Diagnosis. Ineffective Individual Coping related to cancer diagnosis.

Outcomes. Client begins process of adapting to psychoemotional stressors. Client demonstrates functional adaptive behaviors and problem-solving capacity.

Interventions / **Rationales**

1. Develop rapport; utilize active listening skills.
   1. Client will know that you are concerned about his or her well-being as a person. Listening often is the best source of data of the depth of the impact of the cancer experience.
2. Assess coping by directly asking the client how he or she is coping with the cancer and the treatment.
   2. When asked, the client may share fears or concerns. The professional can offer support and suggest related interventions.
3. Provide consistent, empathetic, and positive regard.
   3. See No. 1.
4. Support client's expression of feelings.
   4. See No. 1.
5. Guide the client to community resources such as support groups.
   5. Provides client opportunity to share feelings with and to learn from others who experience cancer.
6. Refer client to appropriate and qualified professional for further intervention as indicated.
   6. For some clients, the emotional impact of the cancer experience—often combined with other life issues—can be overwhelming.

Client Education / **Rationales**

1. Explain relationship between coping and the perception of stressors.
   1. The first step in the problem-solving process is to understand the problem.
2. Help client identify problems, factors over which one has control, and coping methods that have worked for the client during previous life experiences.
   2. Many clients experience a sense of loss of control and feelings of helplessness when confronted with a cancer diagnosis.
3. Teach problem-solving as needed.
   3. The client may not recognize that coping strategies from other life experiences can be utilized in coping with a cancer experience.
4. Teach client about keeping a journal for identification of events, feelings, and strategies utilized for particular problems.
   4. Keeping a journal can help the client identify specific concerns; possible solutions can then be identified.
5. Emphasize the importance of social network and community resources for dealing with concerns.
   5. A social network of support counteracts feelings of isolation.

Data from McNally, J. C., et al. (Eds.). (1991). *Guidelines for oncology nursing practice.* Philadelphia: W. B. Saunders.

fore, you must always know before administering a drug whether it is a vesicant (an agent capable of causing tissue damage).

Great care should be taken in vein selection and in venipuncture technique. Large veins in the fleshy part of the forearm are the preferred peripheral access sites. Avoid areas of impaired lymphatic drainage, phlebitis, invading neoplasm, hematoma, inflammation, sclerosis, impaired venous circulation, the lower extremities, and sites distal to a recent venipuncture site. Also avoid veins that are on the dorsal aspect of the hand or over an area of flexion, such as the wrist or elbow. When administering a vesicant drug, you must be prepared ahead of time to deal with a potential extravasation to limit tissue damage. Preparation includes having immediate availability of an antidote, if there is one.[76]

In the past, vascular access devices (VADs) were placed as a last resort in clients with poor venous access. Today, because chemotherapy regimens are complex and supportive care is extensive, VADs are being used during the initial treatment of clients requiring continuous chemotherapy, multiple access, parenteral fluids, antibiotics, and frequent blood testing.

Implanted and external vascular access catheters are usually inserted into one of the major veins of the upper chest. Centrally implanted VADs are placed by a surgeon, generally during a brief outpatient procedure. The brachial or cephalic vein in the forearm is used for peripherally inserted central catheters (PICCs), which are often placed by specially trained nurses. The distal catheter tip is advanced to the level of the superior vena cava at or above the junction of the right atrium. Proper catheter tip placement of both central and peripheral VADs is confirmed by fluoroscopy or radiography. Various types of VADs are depicted in Figure 19–2.

In addition to VADs, there are arterial, peritoneal, and intraventricular access devices that permit regional delivery of chemotherapy to the liver or peritoneal cavity or into the cerebrospinal fluid of the brain.[2] Each type of device has advantages and disadvantages, including factors such as maintenance requirements, ease of use, cost, ease of insertion, longevity, and effect on body image.

The most commonly reported complications are infection and catheter occlusion.[80] The prevention of VAD infections centers on catheter care, daily assessment for manifestations of infection, and client education. Intraluminal occlusion may occur secondary to a blood clot or precipitate. Prevention strategies include proper flushing, vigilance for drug incompatibilities, and adherence to proper drug dilutions. Other rare complications can also occur with VADs.[41] Procedures for the care and maintenance of VADs vary with each clinical setting and type of device. Nursing management strategies for VADs are extensively described elsewhere.[9, 15, 48, 54]

When the procedure for accessing a VAD is performed according to institutional policy and goes as expected, use of a VAD is relatively easy. Major, even life-threatening, problems can arise, however, if the VAD is not accessed correctly or the nurse does not know how to recognize a problem and the corrective action to take. Nurses who access VADs infrequently should review their institution's procedure before doing so. If the procedure in any way varies from the expected, obtain the advice of a nurse who is more experienced in VADs before proceeding.

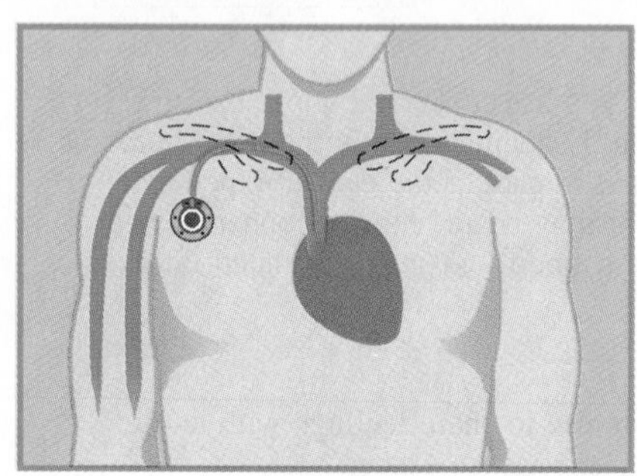

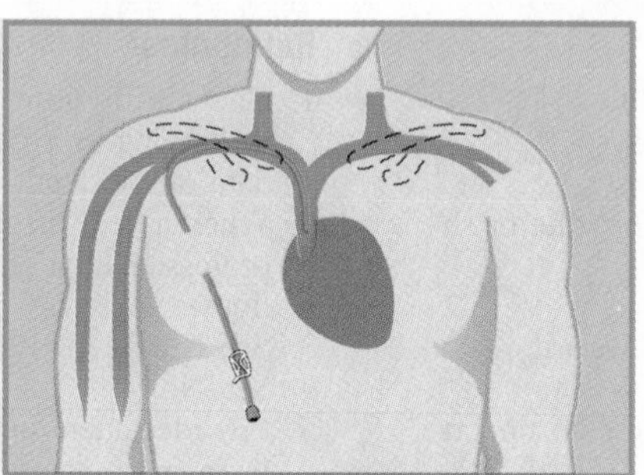

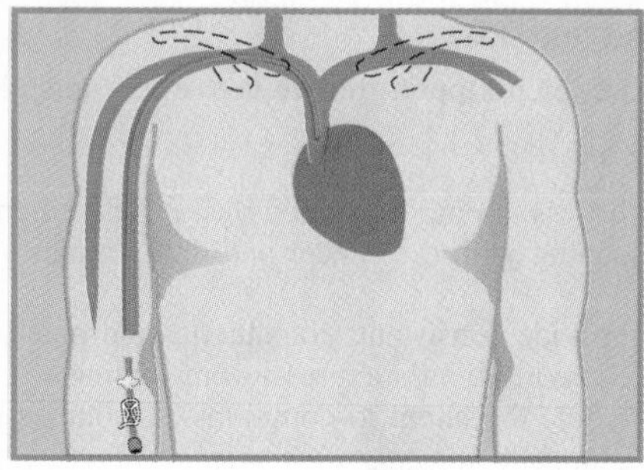

Venous Access Devices

A. Implanted

B. External

C. Peripherally inserted central catheter (PICC)

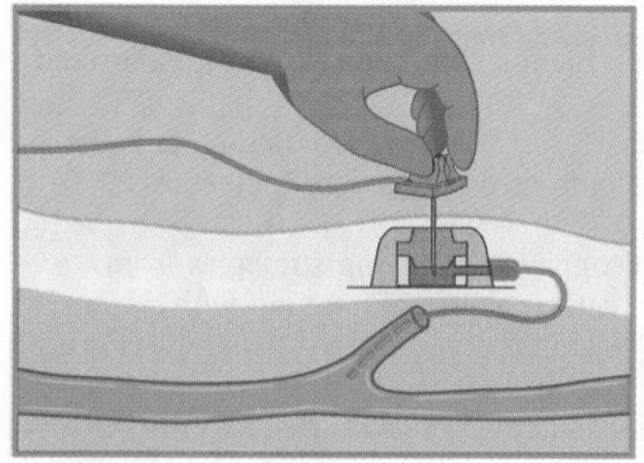

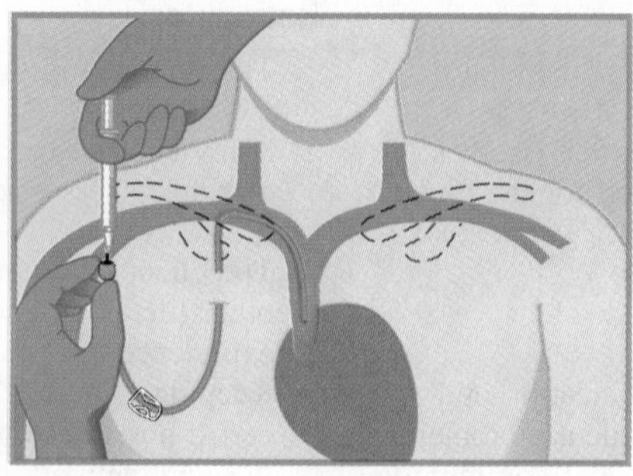

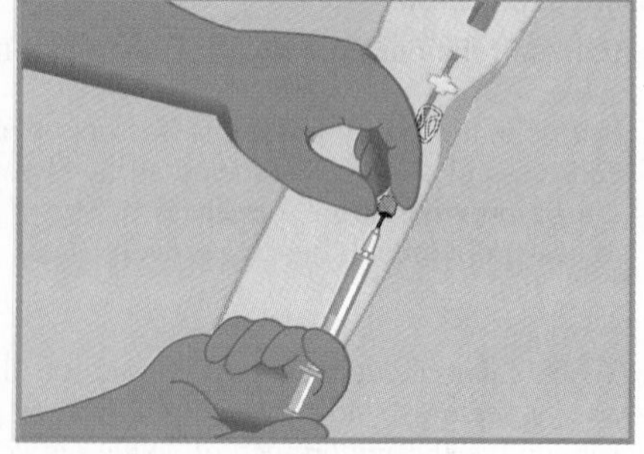

Accessing Venous Access Devices

D. Implanted

E. External

F. Peripherally inserted

FIGURE 19–2*A–F*, Venous access devices.

Regional Chemotherapy. Regional chemotherapy via alternative routes allows high concentrations of drugs to be directed to localized tumors. Methods are (1) topical, (2) intra-arterial, (3) intracavitary, (4) intraperitoneal, and (5) intrathecal.

Topical. Fluorouracil cream may be applied to the skin to treat actinic keratoses (sun keratoses. Squamous cell carcinoma can arise from these precancerous lesions if they are left untreated.

Intra-arterial infusions involve some risk but enable major organs or tumor sites to receive maximal exposure with limited serum levels of medications. As a result, systemic side effects are lessened.

Intracavitary therapy instills the medication directly into an area such as the abdomen, bladder, or pleural space.

Intraperitoneal chemotherapy is an option for cancer involving the intra-abdominal area, such as ovarian cancer. With this method, a high concentration of a chemotherapeutic agent is delivered to the actual tumor site with minimal exposure of healthy tissues, thereby decreasing toxic side effects.

Intrathecal. Most medications given systemically are not effective against central CNS tumors because they cannot cross the blood-brain barrier. The physician may instill chemotherapeutic agents into the CNS through a reservoir placed in the ventricle via an Ommaya reservoir (Fig. 19–3) or via a lumbar puncture. Kosier and Minkler[46] provide an excellent review of the nursing management of clients with an implanted Ommaya reservoir.

ADVERSE REACTIONS. Two potentially serious adverse reactions, the seriousness of which depends on the chemotherapeutic agents, may occur during administration: hypersensitivity reactions and extravasation.

Hypersensitivity Reaction. Hypersensitivity reaction (an exaggerated immune response to a foreign substance) to chemotherapy, although rare, can be serious and life-threatening. The antineoplastic agents most commonly implicated in the development of hypersensitivity reactions are L-asparaginase (Elspar), carboplatin (Paraplatin), cisplatin (Platinol-AQ), paclitaxel (Taxol), bleomycin (Blenoxane), and teniposide (Vumon).[90] When administering a drug with anaphylactic potential (potential to cause a possibly fatal hypersensitivity reaction), take the following precautions to ensure client safety:

- Obtain an allergy history from the client.
- Administer a test dose if ordered by the physician.
- Stay with the client the entire time the drug is being administered.
- Have emergency equipment and drugs readily available.
- Obtain baseline vital signs.
- Establish a free-flowing IV line for the administration of fluids and emergency drugs, in case they are needed.

The manifestations of an immediate hypersensitivity reaction are (1) dyspnea, (2) chest tightness or pain, (3) pruritus (itching), (4) urticaria (wheals), (5) tachycardia, (6) dizziness, (7) anxiety, (8) agitation, (9) inability to speak, (10) abdominal pain, (11) nausea, (12) hypotension, (13) cloudy mental status, (14) flushed appearance, and (15) cyanosis. If an anaphylactic reaction is suspected, take the following actions:

- Immediately stop drug administration.
- Maintain IV access with 0.9% saline.
- Maintain the airway.
- Place the client in a supine position with the feet elevated, unless contraindicated.
- Notify the physician.
- Monitor the client's vital signs every 2 minutes until he or she is stable.
- Administer epinephrine, aminophylline, diphenhydramine (Benadryl), and corticosteroids according to the physician's orders.

Extravasation. Before administering a chemotherapeutic drug, note its vesicant potential—and its antidote, if there is one—in your review of the drug. Careful assessment of the IV site is required during and after the infusion of antineoplastic agents because some agents may cause tissue damage if extravasated (infiltrated).

Nonvesicant agents have no significant soft tissue toxicities. Vesicant chemotherapeutic agents can cause or form a blister and cause tissue destruction. Commonly utilized vesicant drugs are doxorubicin (Adriamycin) and vincristine (Oncovin). Cisplatin (Platinol-AQ) and paclitaxel (Taxol) are also vesicant drugs. Because they are commonly mixed in large volumes of fluid, the extravasation can be detected more easily before serious tissue damage occurs. Irritant drugs can produce venous pain at the site and along the vein, with or without an inflammatory reaction. Pain, erythema, swelling, and lack of a blood return indicate an extravasation.

Procedures for management of extravasation are controversial and unique to each clinical setting. Institutionally approved guidelines for the management of extravasation should be readily available. Guidelines for the management of extravasation are included in the Oncology Nursing Society's *Cancer Chemotherapy Guidelines*.[76] General recommendations are:

- Stop drug administration.
- Leave the needle in place, and attempt to aspirate any residual drug from the tubing, needle, and site.

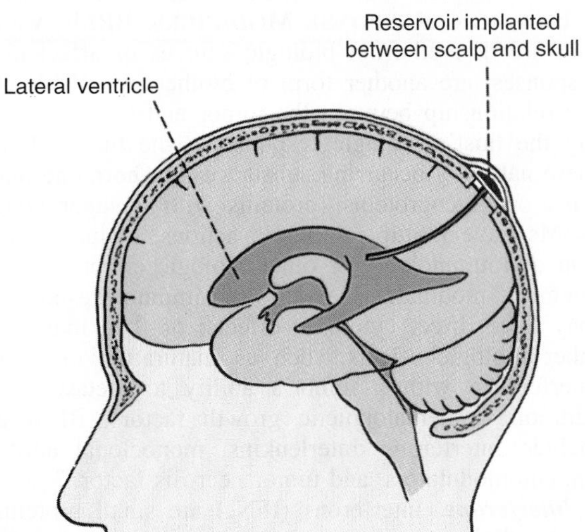

FIGURE 19–3 Ommaya reservoir. An Ommaya reservoir should be accessed only with a small-gauge, non-coring or butterfly needle.

- Administer an antidote, if appropriate, then remove the needle.
- Do not apply direct manual pressure to the site.
- Apply warm (for vinca alkaloid) or cold compresses as indicated.
- Observe the site regularly for pain, erythema, swelling, induration, and necrosis.
- Document the appearance of the site before and after chemotherapy.

Safe Preparation, Handling, and Disposal. The safe administration and disposal of chemotherapeutic agents is controversial. Although evidence suggests that these agents may be carcinogenic, no valid and reliable studies have determined the risks of exposure to the health care provider. Undue exposure to antineoplastic drugs can occur from three major routes:

- Inhalation of aerosols
- Absorption through the skin
- Ingestion of contaminated materials

Several organizations, including the U.S. Occupational Safety and Health Administration (OSHA), the National Study Commission on Cytotoxic Exposure, and the Oncology Nursing Society, have prepared guidelines for the safe preparation, handling, and disposal of antineoplastics.[68, 76] These guidelines call for (1) the wearing of gloves and gowns during preparation and administration and (2) the use of a biologic safety or laminar-flow cabinet for preparation. Antineoplastic agents and their metabolites are found in the excreta and body fluids of clients undergoing chemotherapy. For this reason, you should wear gloves and disposable gowns when handling body secretions, such as blood, vomitus, or excreta, of clients who have received chemotherapy within the previous 48 hours.

Biotherapy

Biotherapy is the use of agents called *biologic response modifiers* (BRMs) to affect a biologic response. The effort to understand and manipulate the human immune system has engaged scientists for decades. The observation of interactions between the immune system and malignant cells, such as spontaneous tumor remissions, continues to fuel the quest to isolate and identify effective biologic agents. Immune response remains at the core of biotherapy. Biotherapy now also includes agents that affect biologic responses in other ways. In the last decade, four major technological advances have assisted scientists in their search[37, 42, 78]:

- A greater understanding of the complex cellular nature of the immune system
- Progress in genetic engineering, enabling the development of recombinant biologic agents
- Advances in molecular biology
- Refined and improved laboratory equipment and computer systems

Hematopoietic Growth Factors. Hematopoietic growth factors are a family of glycosylated proteins that mediate hematopoiesis (formation and development of blood cells). They are used to stimulate bone marrow recovery after courses of chemotherapy. Generally, they are named for the major cell lineage they mediate: GM-CSF (granulocyte and macrophage colony-stimulating factor) affects both the granulocyte and macrophage lineage; G-CSF affects only granulocytes. GM-CSF is approved for myeloid (bone marrow) reconstitution after autologous bone marrow transplantation (BMT) and for use in clients experiencing BMT failure or engraftment delay. G-CSF and GM-CSF are approved for the treatment of chemotherapy-associated neutropenia. GM-CSF is generally well tolerated.

Side effects of these growth factors are (1) mild to moderate flu-like manifestations, such as fever, myalgia (muscular pain), bone pain, fatigue, and headache, (2) rash, (3) a transient increase in liver enzymes, and (4) thrombocytopenia (reduced platelets). The most commonly reported side effect of G-CSF is bone pain. Clients report pain in bone areas that have large marrow reserves, such as the pelvis, sternum, and long bones. This pain may be the result of the marrow expansion that occurs from the rapid increase in the neutrophil pool that G-CSF causes.

Erythropoietin, another hematopoietic growth factor, was approved by the U.S. Food and Drug Administration (FDA) in 1989 for use in treating anemia secondary to end-stage renal failure, and in 1993 to treat anemia associated with cancer chemotherapy (epoetin alfa [Procrit, Epogen]). Clients with serum erythropoietin levels greater than 200 mU/ml are unlikely to show a response to therapy. It is important to maintain adequate levels of iron, folic acid, and vitamin B_{12} because these components are essential for the development of red blood cells. The most commonly reported side effect is transient flu-like manifestations, such as arthralgias (joint pain) and myalgias.

Oprelvekin (Neumega), a hematopoietic growth factor for chemotherapy-induced thrombocytopenia, received FDA approval in November 1997. Its most common side effects are edema, dyspnea, tachycardia, and conjunctival redness. More experience with the use of this treatment is needed before broad generalizations can be made about its usefulness. It is anticipated that oprelvekin will reduce the need for platelet transfusions and allow clients to receive the desired doses of chemotherapy as scheduled.[82]

Biologic Response Modifiers. BRMs, which either are derived from biologic sources or affect biologic responses, are another form of biotherapy. BRMs change the relationship between the tumor and the host by altering the host's biologic response to the tumor. Many of these naturally occurring substances are hormone-like proteins or glycoproteins (proteins with a sugar attached). BRMs have multiple biologic actions, including production of immunologic or other biologic effects. They may augment, modulate, or restore the immune response; they may have direct cytotoxic effects; or they may produce other biologic effects, such as maturation of cells and interference with a tumor's ability to metastasize.[78] In addition to hematopoietic growth factors, BRM agents include interferons, interleukins, monoclonal antibodies, immunomodulators, and tumor necrosis factor.[78]

Interferons. Interferons (IFNs) are small proteins that have cellular activity in three areas: antiviral, immunomodulatory, and antiproliferative. Interferon alpha received FDA approval for use in hairy cell leukemia in 1986. The drug's clinical indications have been broadened to include AIDS-associated Kaposi's sarcoma. Clinical trials are being conducted to investigate its use in other hematologic malignancies, including chronic leukemias, multiple myeloma, cutaneous T-cell lymphoma, and low-grade non-Hodgkin's lymphoma.

Toxicities appear to be dose-related, with lower doses of IFN being associated with few side effects and high doses having side effects that may require therapy to be interrupted or stopped. A flu-like syndrome, a common side effect of IFN therapy, may consist of fever, chills, tachycardia, muscle aches, malaise, fatigue, and headaches. Continued use of IFN produces a tachyphylactic response (rapidly decreasing response after administration of a few doses) such that these manifestations decrease in intensity over time. Premedication with acetaminophen (Tylenol) and diphenhydramine (Benadryl) is helpful in reducing the client's discomfort.

Interleukins. Most interleukins (proteins that serve as regulators of the immune system) are capable of inducing multiple biologic activities. A number of interleukins have been identified. Thus far, only interleukin-2 (IL-2) has received FDA approval. It is derived from T cells, augments various T-cell activities, and enhances the function of natural killer cells. Successes have been seen in renal cell carcinoma and melanoma. Other areas of interest for its use are hematologic malignancies and bone marrow transplantation.

Major toxic responses with IL-2 therapy are due to increased capillary permeability, which may produce hypotension, ascites, pulmonary edema, fatigue, and generalized weight gain. Additionally, integumentary changes occur and may include generalized redness, rash, pruritus, and occasionally skin desquamation. Toxicity resulting from IL-2 varies greatly with the dose of drug administered. Higher doses produce greater toxicity, necessitating astute clinical management.

MONOCLONAL ANTIBODIES. Monoclonal antibodies (MoAbs) are specific antibodies directed against single antigenic determinants on the cell surface.[80] MoAbs provide high specificity lacking in other types of treatment modalities. They can be used either diagnostically or therapeutically. Diagnostic uses of these agents include the early detection of cancer by identification of surface markers on tumor cells and as a delivery agent of radioisotopes to the tumor site to aid in tumor visualization. Therapeutically, MoAbs may be used to deliver immunotoxins, such as ricin, chemotherapeutic agents, and radioisotopes, directly to the tumor site. To date, MoAbs have demonstrated limited success as a therapeutic option, and clinical trials continue for a variety of cancers.

BONE MARROW TRANSPLANTATION

BMT is discussed in Chapter 78. Although it is used as a primary treatment modality in leukemia, BMT may be used to counter the toxic effects of chemotherapy or RT in the treatment of breast cancer, lymphoma, and other cancers. BMT allows the client to receive lethal and potentially more effective doses of chemotherapy and RT without regard to hematopoietic toxicity. With BMT, the damaged bone marrow is replaced by healthy marrow.

The client's own marrow may be harvested prior to the treatment (*autologous* BMT). An *allogeneic* BMT involves the use of marrow from a matching donor. If the client's own marrow was harvested, the marrow may or may not have been chemically treated to destroy any cancer cells. It is then stored (frozen) to be reinfused after the chemotherapy or RT to "rescue" the bone marrow from the lethal effects of the treatment.

■ CLINICAL TRIALS

A *clinical trial* is a study conducted to evaluate a new treatment. New drugs or treatment modalities are first evaluated through basic research studies in the laboratory and with animals. The most promising of these treatment approaches are then further assessed in clinical trials with human subjects. There are four phases of clinical trials[64]:

- *Phase 1:* Only a small number of patients are used as subjects in phase 1 clinical trials. The purpose of the study is to determine the maximum tolerated dose of a drug or treatment. The researchers are also watching carefully for harmful side effects. Although the treatment has been tested in the laboratory and in animals, it is not yet known how humans will respond. No direct benefit in terms of disease remission can be guaranteed. Because phase 1 studies involve significant risk without any promise of benefit, participation is offered only to people with advanced disease and for whom there are no other known treatment options. Safety, comfort, and ethical considerations are primary nursing concerns during this phase of clinical drug trials.
- *Phase 2:* Phase 2 studies are developed from the information gained from the phase 1 studies. The treatment now is offered to people with types of cancer that responded to the treatment in the phase 1 studies. The purpose of a phase 2 study is to determine the effectiveness of the treatment against those cancers while continuing to learn more about the harmful effects of the treatment. As with phase 1 studies, participation in phase 2 studies is offered only to people for whom there are no known treatment alternatives.
- *Phase 3:* In a phase 3 study, a promising new treatment is compared with a standard treatment. On the basis of scientific evidence, the researchers believe that the new treatment is likely to be as good as or better than the current standard treatment. Clients who participate in clinical trials are the first people to benefit from new, more effective treatment modalities.
- *Phase 4:* In phase 4 postmarketing surveillance studies, newly introduced drugs are monitored for adverse effects. Such studies may also compare two standard treatments. For example, surgery and RT may be compared to determine whether the survival rate following RT is similar to that after surgical treatment. Clinical trials are carried out on a nationwide basis, and the pooled results of these investigations are used to determine and validate the effectiveness of treatment regimens.

Nurses have a major role to play in these research trials. Nursing responsibilities associated with caring for a client who is participating in a clinical trial are

- Client education
- Documentation of treatment benefits and side effects
- Anticipation of adverse reactions and early recognition of toxicity
- Management of side effects

Research nurses have even greater responsibilities for monitoring of clients, recruitment of participants, and dissemination of data.

Written informed consents for participation in a clinical trial are often lengthy and can be overwhelming. In most settings, nurses are responsible for reviewing the written consent and the physician's verbal teaching with the client. You can often help by highlighting key information in the consent form, such as the purpose of the study, the treatments being compared, and whom to contact for more information. An NCI pamphlet[64] describes important questions a client should ask when considering participation in a clinical trial.

Self-Care

COMPLEMENTARY APPROACHES

Use by the public of alternative or complementary therapies for chronic conditions, such as back problems, depression, and cancer, is growing. Eisenberg and associates[23] estimated that in 1997, 629 million visits were made to alternative medicine practitioners, exceeding the total number of visits to all U.S. primary care physicians. These researchers found that 42.1% of the population had used at least 1 of 16 alternative therapies in the previous year.

Complementary approaches often combine one or more elements, such as (1) spiritual, psychological, nutritional, physical, pharmacologic, herbal, electromagnetic, or psychic approaches, (2) traditional medicines, (3) unconventional uses of conventional therapies, (4) unconventional instruments, and (5) humane approaches. Of these approaches, Lerner[51] points out that spiritual, psychological, nutritional, and physical approaches represent a "vital quartet of ethical approaches" that have benefited many clients with cancer. In research, prayer has been found to be a coping mechanism that correlates with perceptions of well-being.[10]

Psychological approaches that are widely recognized yet underutilized include support groups, psychotherapy, imagery, biofeedback, and hypnosis. When used with antiemetic drugs, music can be an effective diversional therapy to decrease the frequency of nausea and vomiting.[24] Guided imagery also can help control nausea and vomiting, create a relaxation response, and control pain.[10] Art therapy can be used to help an adult with cancer gain insight into his or her situation.[5]

Although diet is recognized to play a major role in cancer causation, there is no known dietary treatment that slows or cures cancer. Nevertheless, nutritional interventions can enhance a client's ability to tolerate treatment and thereby improve both the quality of life and, potentially, the treatment outcome. Physical therapy approaches, including exercises, massage therapies, and progressive relaxation, are often overlooked by health care providers.

Lerner[51] offers a framework for evaluating unconventional—and conventional—therapies. First, assess the therapy. Is there any significant scientific literature to support the therapy? Second, evaluate the practitioner. What training has the practitioner completed? What do other unconventional practitioners think of the provider? Does the practitioner share data about treatments with other practitioners? Third, assess the usefulness of the service delivery. Do most people who have completed treatment believe that the service was reasonably related to the cost?

To date, Lerner[51] has encountered no decisive and scientifically documented cure for any type of cancer among the complementary therapies. For all their shortcomings, conventional therapies are capable of curing a number of cancers. He finds, however, that some complementary therapies, such as psychosocial support for clients with metastatic breast cancer, appear to extend life and that many complementary therapies enhance the quality of life.

HOME MANAGEMENT OF SIDE EFFECTS

Aggressive, complex, and sophisticated cancer therapies are now being delivered in the ambulatory, office, and home care settings. This shift in care settings presents additional challenges for clients, family members, and health care providers. A high level of commitment is required from the client and family caregivers for the successful management of care in the outpatient setting. Clients and family members require education regarding complex treatment regimens. They must know how to recognize manifestations of side effects or adverse events, how to prevent side effects, and what they can do to treat the manifestations. Most importantly, they must know when to report manifestations and how to reach the physician—especially after office hours. When chemotherapy is administered in the home setting, provisions must be made for the safe handling and disposal of cytotoxic drugs to minimize client, family, and nurse exposure.[76]

FINANCIAL CONCERNS

Cancer care can place a financial burden on the client and family. First are the direct costs of deductibles and co-insurance. Unless the client has a prescription card, some medications, such as the serotonin (5-HT_3 [5-hydroxytryptamine]) antagonist antiemetics, can be more costly than the client can afford.

In addition, cancer and its treatment often involves many hidden costs. Examples are transportation and meals for travel to clinic appointments, new clothing to accommodate weight loss or gain, medical supplies, special foods or nutritional supplements, long-distance telephone calls, and loss of income for the client or family caregiver.[58] Ten per cent, or $104 billion, of the $1 trillion spent on health care annually is utilized for cancer care; of this amount, $35 billion is utilized for direct medical care, $12 billion for lost productivity, and $57 billion for mortality costs.[11]

EVALUATION OF TREATMENT RESPONSE

During and after treatment, the client is monitored for tumor response. Just as with diagnosis, listening carefully to the client's history and the physical examination are fundamental sources of data. If the client's cancer was symptomatic, the client may be able to predict that the treatment is working because the pain has lessened, breathing requires less effort, or other manifestations are subsiding.

When known disease remained after surgical intervention or diagnostic studies, repeating the imaging studies that were performed at the time of the diagnosis can be used to determine treatment effectiveness. Imaging studies are generally repeated after every two to three cycles of chemotherapy. If the tumor was associated with an elevated tumor marker at the time of diagnosis, testing for the marker again can be both a guide to the effectiveness of the chemotherapy and, later, a means of early detection of recurrence of the cancer. With ovarian cancer, a "second-look" surgical procedure may be performed after the completion of the chemotherapy to verify that no detectable disease remains.

After treatment is completed, the client continues to be monitored for manifestations of disease recurrence and for delayed or long-term after-effects of the treatment. Depending on the type of cancer, follow-up appointments may initially be at 3-month intervals, eventually extending to 6-month and then 1-year intervals.

Nursing Management of Oncologic Treatment and Emergencies

Comprehensively and successfully managing cancer-related manifestations—whether they are from the cancer itself or are side effects of treatment—is essential for achieving high-quality outcomes in cancer care. For some clinical manifestations, urgent intervention is required to prevent undue morbidity or even mortality. For example, infection, a potentially life-threatening complication in the client with neutropenia, is an oncologic emergency. When a person has few white cells, infection can quickly progress to septicemia and death unless aggressive intervention is instituted. Failure to recognize, diagnose, and intervene for new-onset back pain can result in paralysis if the pain is secondary to spinal cord compression. Uncontrolled pain, discussed in Chapter 23, is often considered an oncologic emergency in the client with cancer because it so greatly interferes with the client's relationships and activities of daily living.

Both antineoplastic medications and RT can damage and destroy not only cancer cells but also certain normal cells. Box 19–2 summarizes the side effects of antineoplastic drugs. Side effects on normal cells are evaluated or graded according to the degree of severity. Mild to moderate side effects generally do not warrant discontinuation of treatment or a decrease of the dose. More severe

BOX 19–2 Side Effects of Antineoplastic Drugs

Gastrointestinal

Nausea and vomiting
Constipation
Anorexia
Stomatitis
Esophagitis
Alterations in taste
Diarrhea
Weight loss
Pharyngitis

Integumentary

Dermatitis
Alopecia
Perianal ulcers
Vulvar ulcers
Hyperpigmentation
Photosensitivity
Nail changes

Hematopoietic

Anemia
Thrombocytopenia
Neutropenia

Genitourinary

Nephrotoxicity
Urine color change
Hemorrhagic cystitis
Hyperuricemic nephropathy

Hepatic

Hepatotoxicity
Cirrhosis
Hepatic fibrosis
Portal hypertension

Reproductive

Amenorrhea
Sterility
Loss of libido
Impotence
Azoospermia
Gonadal dysfunction
Menopausal manifestations
Irregular menses
Gynecomastia
Oligospermia

Cardiac

Electrocardiogram changes
Dysrhythmias
Cardiomyopathy, chronic heart failure
Tachycardia

Pulmonary

Pneumonitis
Pulmonary fibrosis

Metabolic

Tumor lysis syndrome

Neurologic, Sensory-Perceptual

Ototoxicity
Subacute meningeal irritation
Peripheral neuropathy
Cranial nerve neuropathy
Autonomic neuropathy
Cerebellar toxicity

Data from Hydzik, C. A. (1990). Late effects of chemotherapy: Implications for patient management and rehabilitation. *Nursing Clinics of North America, 25,* 423; and Ruccione, K., & Weinberg, K. (1989). Late effects in multiple body systems. *Seminars in Oncology Nursing, 5,* 4.

or unexpected toxicities require careful evaluation and dose reduction.

The onset of the side effects of chemotherapy may be acute or delayed. *Acute* toxicities (1) tend to occur in tissues composed of rapidly dividing cells (bone marrow, hair, mucosa), (2) are frequently intermittent, and (3) generally resolve with complete recovery. In contrast, *delayed* or *late* effects may produce lifelong problems. Such effects include organ-specific treatment toxicities resulting in cardiac, renal, pulmonary, hepatic, reproductive, and neurologic dysfunction.

Because many of these problems appear when the client has returned home rather than in the clinical setting, the client as well as the health care providers must be aware of, monitor for, and report side effects. When taking a telephone call from a client, you must be prepared to anticipate the potential complications related to the concern that led to the call. Telephone triage is a particularly challenging aspect of ambulatory care because you must depend almost entirely on verbal report to formulate an accurate picture of the client's situation and its urgency.

■ MYELOSUPPRESSION

NEUTROPENIA

Infection and bleeding, often resulting from diminished production of WBCs and platelets (thrombocytopenia) secondary to treatment, are two common causes of death in clients with cancer. The time after chemotherapy administration when the WBC or platelet count is at the lowest point is referred to as the *nadir.* For most chemotherapeutic agents, the nadir occurs within 7 to 14 days after drug administration. Knowledge of blood count nadirs helps the health professional predict when the client is at greatest risk for infection and bleeding. Monitoring the CBC and differential count can identify when the nadir occurs and whether the client has adequate numbers of blood cells and can demonstrate evidence of impending bone marrow recovery.

The etiology of infections associated with cancer is multifactorial. Some cancers cause specific defects in the immune response. Side effects of treatment can result in myelosuppression (decreased RBCs, WBCs, and platelets). An impaired integumentary system can increase vulnerability to infection. Corticosteroids, which are used in many treatment protocols, suppress immune functions. Neutropenia predisposes the client to infection, especially infection by opportunistic endogenous (normally resident in the client's body or surroundings) organisms. More than half of infections in clients with neutropenia are associated with organisms from the local environment. Major sources are food (raw fruits and vegetables), water, inhaled organisms, and organisms passed through direct contact. The client with neutropenia can quickly become septic; the mortality rate with septicemia can range from 30% to 80%.[98] For this reason, a CBC with differential count must be performed before administration of myelosuppressive (most chemotherapeutic) drugs and repeated periodically between treatments.

The two major types of WBCs are granulocytes (which include neutrophils) and agranulocytes. *Neutrophils* are the first and most numerous type of cell to arrive at any area of disease or tissue injury. When the number of neutrophils is substantially reduced, one of the body's prime defenses against infection is impaired. Therefore, it is important to know what proportion of WBCs are neutrophils. The absolute neutrophil count (ANC) is calculated by multiplying the WBC by the percentage of segmented and banded neutrophils in the CBC differential count:

$$\text{ANC} = \text{WBC} \times \text{neutrophils (\%)}$$

On a CBC laboratory report, the neutrophils are often listed as Segs (for segmented neutrophils) and as bands; the percentages of these two cells are added together to obtain the total percentage of neutrophils. For example, if the WBC count is 1200/mm^3 and the percentage of neutrophils (sum of the percentages of segmented and banded neutrophils) is 34%, the ANC is 408 ($1200 \times .34 = 408$).

Neutropenia is commonly defined as an ANC of less than 1000/mm^3. The frequency of infection increases (1) as the ANC decreases below 500/mm^3 and (2) with duration of the neutropenia. In the client with neutropenia, the usual manifestations of infection can be absent because of the lack of neutrophils to produce an adequate inflammatory response to the infection. Therefore, fever is the cardinal, and often the only, manifestation of infection. Three oral temperature readings exceeding 38° C (100.4° F) in 24 hours or one temperature reading exceeding 38.5° C (101.3° F) is considered diagnostic of a fever.

Because infections are associated with greater morbidity and mortality, the development of fever in a client with neutropenia should be treated as an oncologic emergency that mandates prompt assessment, diagnosis, and intervention. Measures to be taken generally consist of (1) cultures, chest x-ray, and physical evaluation to attempt to identify the source, (2) broad-spectrum antibiotic therapy, and (3) monitoring of vital signs. G-CSF or GM-CSF (see earlier) may be prescribed to reduce the duration and severity of neutropenia.

Nursing management of outcomes begins with teaching clients measures to protect against infection and reinforcement of such teachings as WBC counts reach their nadir. These measures are as follows[66]:

- Practice good personal hygiene, especially handwashing.
- Perform oral care daily and frequently rinse the mouth with an alcohol-free mouthwash, such as saline and soda (1 tsp soda to 1 L of normal saline) or even just water four to six times per day.
- Maintain adequate nutrition and fluid intake.
- Do not share eating utensils with anyone.
- Avoid raw or uncooked foods during nadir period.
- Avoid crowds, people with infections, and children who have been recently vaccinated with live or attenuated vaccines.
- Avoid contact with animal excrement (e.g., bird, cat, or dog feces).
- Either avoid having cut flowers in the home, or change the water of fresh flowers daily, with 1 tsp of chlorine bleach added to the new water.
- Get adequate rest and exercise.
- Avoid indiscriminate use of antipyretics (e.g., acetaminophen, aspirin) because they can mask fever.

Clients should also be taught that even with the best precautions, infections cannot always be prevented. The importance of immediately reporting any manifestations of infection must be stressed: (1) temperature reading of more than 38° C (100° F), (2) cough, (3) sore throat, (4) chills or sweating, and (5) frequent or painful urination.

THROMBOCYTOPENIA

Thrombocytopenia due to chemotherapy may cause subtle to life-threatening bleeding. A high risk of hemorrhage exists when the platelet count is less than 20,000/mm^3. In the client with a solid (versus a hematologic) tumor, a platelet count greater than 10,000/mm^3 puts the incidence of bleeding at less than 12%; however, fatal CNS hemorrhage or massive GI hemorrhage can occur.[31] The platelet count usually recovers within 2 to 6 weeks after the recovery of the WBC count following chemotherapy. Chemotherapy is usually withheld until the platelet count rises to 100,000/mm.[3, 31]

Nursing measures to manage outcomes are utilized to prevent bleeding or detect early clinical manifestations of bleeding. Instruct the client to:

- Avoid injury, by being cautious with sharp objects and using an electric razor rather than a blade razor.
- Use lotions to prevent dryness and cracking of the skin
- Use lubrication (women) during sexual intercourse (if sexual activity is advisable during treatment).
- Maintain good oral hygiene and use either a soft toothbrush or, if the platelet count is very low, sponge oral swabs, and report excessive bleeding of gums.
- Avoid constipation; use stool softeners if needed.
- Avoid enemas or rectal suppositories, and report any rectal bleeding.
- Refrain from taking aspirin or nonsteroidal anti-inflammatory drugs (NSAIDs) without the doctor's permission.
- If nosebleeds or other external bleeding occurs, put pressure on the source of bleeding for 10 to 15 minutes.
- Avoid taking temperatures rectally at all times and orally if there is oral soreness or bleeding; take tympanic temperatures.
- Avoid intramuscular or subcutaneous injections; central lines can be used for parenteral medications.
- Notify the nurse or physician of manifestations of bleeding: petechiae (small red spots) or increased bruising, tarry stools, hypermenorrhea (heavy uterine bleeding), blood in urine or vomit, visual changes, and changes in level of consciousness (an early indication of intracranial hemorrhage).

Most oncologists use transfusions to keep a client's platelet count above 20,000/mm^3 unless the client is known to have a platelet antibody. As previously mentioned, the thrombopoietic growth factor oprelvekin (Neumega) is now available to prevent severe thrombocytopenia following myelosuppressive chemotherapy in patients with nonmyeloid malignancies.[82]

ANEMIA

Anemia in the client with cancer can have multiple causes. There may be blood loss secondary to the disease. Abnormal destruction of RBCs is commonly a secondary disorder, arising from such causes as liver or spleen disease, BMT, or drug toxicity. The most common cause of anemia in the client with cancer is inadequate production of RBCs. This can result from infiltration of the bone marrow by tumor or suppression of bone marrow production of RBCs by cancer therapy.[17] Anemia leads to an impairment of oxygen delivery that is a common and predictable sequela of many cancer therapies.[86] It may cause fatigue, headache, dizziness, fainting, pallor, dyspnea, palpitations, and tachycardia.

Anemia is an important component of cancer-related fatigue, which is one of the most common and distressing manifestations experienced by the oncology client. Fatigue is poorly understood; no one definition describes all experiences. Research on cancer-related fatigue is still in its infancy. It is difficult to predict with certainty which interventions will have therapeutic benefit for which clients.[97] As advances are made in the scientific understanding of cancer-related fatigue, recommendations for interventions will very likely be altered.

Careful evaluation of exacerbating and relieving factors, the effect of fatigue on daily life, and personal and cultural influences as well as review of laboratory data add depth to the assessment of a client's fatigue and help guide interventions.[17] Transfusions of packed RBCs may be utilized to relieve anemia that is producing manifestations. Erythropoietin may be prescribed to elevate or maintain the erythrocyte level and decrease the need for transfusions (see earlier). Other interventions can be grouped into three categories: (1) education, (2) exercise, and (3) attention-restoring activities. Clients who are taught that fatigue is expected report less fatigue than those who are not. Clients who balance exercise (such as walking) with rest report less fatigue. Engaging in activities that are interesting to the client may restore attention and the ability to think clearly.[17]

GASTROINTESTINAL EFFECTS

NAUSEA AND VOMITING

GI effects of chemotherapy include nausea and vomiting, anorexia, alteration in taste, weight loss, oral mucositis, diarrhea, and constipation. The vomiting center in the medulla can be stimulated by any of five different afferent pathways or by arousal of the chemotherapy trigger zone located in the fourth ventricle of the brain. The emetic potential of a particular chemotherapeutic regimen depends on the drugs given, the dose and route of administration, and the client's susceptibility to emesis. RT to the chest, abdomen, or back can stimulate afferent pathways. Radiation-related emesis is related to the area and size of the treatment field and the dose delivered.

Adequate control of nausea and vomiting is an essential factor in a client's compliance with treatment. Uncontrolled nausea and vomiting, among the most feared treatment-related side effects, is experienced by as many as 60% of people receiving chemotherapy. It can result in anorexia, malnutrition, dehydration, metabolic imbalances, psychological depression, and decreased immunity.

Three types of nausea and vomiting have been described. After the client has experienced nausea and vomiting, *anticipatory* nausea and vomiting may occur before the administration of further therapy. *Acute post-therapy* nausea and vomiting occur within minutes of the first 24 hours following therapy. *Delayed* nausea and vomiting consist of manifestations that persist or develop 24 hours after chemotherapy.[75]

Management of nausea and vomiting has greatly improved during the 1990s because of heightened interest and research. The drug armamentarium now includes premedication for chemotherapy regimens known to be highly emetogenic (causing nausea and vomiting). Newer serotonin receptor antagonists (5-HT_3) (e.g., ondansetron [Zofran], granisetron [Kytril], dolasetron [Anzemet]) are particularly useful for acute nausea and vomiting in the first 24 hours to control afferent pathway stimulation from the effects of the chemotherapy on the GI tract. Ongoing evaluation is essential to find the most effective dose, schedule, and combination of drugs for each client.

Nonpharmacologic interventions for nausea and vomiting related to chemotherapy include adjustment of oral and fluid intake, relaxation, exercise, hypnosis, biofeedback, guided imagery, and systemic desensitization. The client and caregivers should avoid offensive odors, such as those from flowers or foods. Food servings should be kept small and offered four to six times per day.

ANOREXIA

Anorexia and weight loss occur as a result of the disease process as well as the treatment. The client with cancer is at risk for protein-calorie malnutrition. Many variables, in addition to the effects of chemotherapy, may alter the client's ability to ingest food via the oral route. Common problems that may interfere with oral intake are anorexia, nausea and vomiting, early satiety, alterations in taste, dry mouth, stomatitis, esophagitis, viscous saliva, lactose intolerance, pain, diarrhea, and constipation.

Nursing management to prevent a compromised nutritional state is based on assessment. Weight loss of 5% or more in a 1-month period is considered significant. In assessing the client, you can begin by identifying potential interventions appropriate to the client's situation. If indicated, a referral can be made to a dietitian for a more comprehensive assessment. When medically appropriate, oral nutrition can be enhanced by relaxing dietary restrictions and emphasizing the need for a high-protein, high-calorie diet with fortification from natural food sources or commercial supplements. An excellent source of helpful tips and recipes for nutritious foods can be found in the booklet *Eating Hints*, which can be obtained free of charge from the NCI.[61] Enteral and parenteral feedings for the client with protein-calorie malnutrition are discussed in Chapter 29.

STOMATITIS

Stomatitis, or *oral mucositis*, is the term used to describe inflammation and ulceration of the mucosal lining of the mouth. The inflammation seen in the mouth is also present throughout the GI tract of a client with cancer or receiving cancer treatment. The severity of the stomatitis can affect the client's quality of life. Consequences of stomatitis include pain, decreased nutritional and fluid intake, infections, malabsorption, diarrhea, and delay of chemotherapy and radiation therapy treatments.

Nursing interventions should include teaching the client to clean and assess the mouth at least once daily and to report changes, including redness, extreme dryness, ulcers, blisters, white patches or bleeding in the mouth, difficulty swallowing, and temperature higher than 37.8° C (100° F).[7] An oral hygiene program should start before therapy and should continue throughout treatment. Such a program consists of:

- A dental examination and treatment prior to therapy
- Thorough and gentle cleaning to avoid further trauma
- Moisturization if saliva is scanty or absent
- Avoidance of alcohol and smoking
- Culture analysis and antimicrobial therapy for infections
- Topical anesthetics and analgesics for pain or discomfort

Dietary modifications include (1) avoiding extremely hot or cold foods, spices, and citrus fruits and juices, (2) eating soft foods, and (3) taking nutritional supplements.

DIARRHEA AND CONSTIPATION

Most clinicians define *diarrhea* as an increase in stool liquid or frequency.[56] It can result from GI mucosal damage secondary to RT or chemotherapy. A low-residue or liquid diet is usually advised. Electrolytes and intake and output should be carefully monitored. Scrupulous perineal hygiene is encouraged, especially in the client with neutropenia. Antidiarrheal agents may be prescribed.

Constipation is frequently described as hard, dry stool with straining, a decrease in the number of defecations, or both. Causes include (1) a decrease in either fluid and fiber intake or mobility of clients, (2) changes in usual bowel routines, (3) mechanical changes, such as tumor pressure on the bowel, and (4) metabolic changes, such as hypokalemia or hypercalcemia.[19] The vinca alkaloid chemotherapeutic agents (vinblastine, vincristine) can slow bowel peristalsis. Other causes of constipation are narcotic use, tumor invasion of the GI tract, and depression. Preventive measures may be taken for constipation, such as increasing fluid and bulk intake, using stool softeners prophylactically, increasing physical activity, and using laxatives when necessary.

■ INTEGUMENTARY EFFECTS

ALOPECIA

Alopecia is a common side effect of many antineoplastic agents. The extent of hair loss depends on the specific drug, dosage, and method of administration. Alopecia tends to begin 2 to 3 weeks after the first treatment. It is temporary. New hair growth tends to begin 4 to 6 weeks after the completion of chemotherapy, and 8 to 9 weeks following RT. Hair color and texture may change, but the hair usually returns to its former condition within a year.[93] There can also be loss of body hair, including eyelashes, eyebrows, and pubic hair.[39]

To help the client manage this side effect, which can be a traumatic change in body image and a constant reminder of the cancer, prepare the client for its occurrence. Begin by first allowing the client to grieve for the hair loss. Having information available about where to obtain attractive wigs or turbans is helpful. Many ACS units offer a wonderful program called "Look Good, Feel Better," which involves the assistance of a volunteer beautician. Remember, hair loss bothers many men more than they may be able to acknowledge. Wigs are available for men. Many men choose to wear baseball caps to conceal the hair loss and for warmth. Hearing the experience of others with hair loss can often be helpful to both men and women.

SKIN REACTIONS

The type of skin reactions that may occur in the client receiving chemotherapy depends on the drug administered. Red patches (*erythema*) or hives (*urticaria*) may appear at the drug injection site or on other body parts. (The extravasation of vesicant drugs was discussed earlier.) These reactions generally disappear within several hours.

Darkening of the skin (*hyperpigmentation*) in the nail beds and mouth, on gums or teeth, and along the veins used for IV chemotherapy usually occurs within 2 to 3 weeks after administration of chemotherapy and continues for 10 to 12 weeks after the end of therapy. Sensitivity to sunlight (*photosensitivity*) may result in an acute sunburn after just a short exposure to the sun. The sensitivity disappears once treatment stops. Teach the client to use sunscreen or protective clothing before sun exposure.

A skin reaction called *radiation recall* may occur in clients who received RT prior to the administration of chemotherapy. When chemotherapy is given several weeks or months later, a recall reaction occurs in the previously irradiated skin area. Skin effects range from redness, shedding, or peeling to blisters and oozing. After the skin heals, it is permanently darkened. It is important to maintain meticulous hygiene to avoid a superimposed infection in the area of radiation recall. Antibiotic therapy should be initiated at the first manifestation of infection.

■ EFFECTS ON THE REPRODUCTIVE SYSTEM

Surgery, RT, and chemotherapy each can have effects on sexual health and sexual self-image. Up to 25% of women undergoing modified radical mastectomy for breast cancer report problems with sexual functioning. Surgery can affect sexual functioning through impairment of the vascular supply, removal of organs, or reduction of circulating hormone levels. Fifty-five per cent to 78% of women treated with RT for cervical cancer report sexual impairments. Body image, sexual functioning, and fertility can be affected by chemotherapy.[4, 20] Not all clients experience these effects to the same degree, however. Preliminary studies suggest that the effects of chemotherapy on gonadal function vary with respect to the client's age at the time of therapy, the drugs administered, and the total drug dosage.[42]

Administration of antineoplastic agents during the first trimester of pregnancy increases the risk of spontaneous abortion and fetal malformations. Second- and third-trimester chemotherapy exposures may result in low birth weight or prematurity.[44] A pregnancy begun after cytotoxic chemotherapy has about the same chance of a successful outcome as a normal pregnancy.[4] However, the genetic effects of chemotherapy may not be evident for several generations of offspring. Therefore, you should discuss the unpredictability of occurrence, degree, and duration of genetic damage with the client and spouse or significant other.

Although you may initially not be comfortable with sexuality issues, you can still be an important source of support by giving the client permission to express concerns about this aspect of cancer therapy. Begin simply by asking open-ended questions about how the cancer experience has changed the client's relationships. Beyond providing information yourself, offer to seek out further information or to consult with a colleague who may have additional information or suggestions to alleviate or at least ease the concern.

The PLISSIT (*p*ermission, *l*imited *i*nformation, *s*pecific *s*uggestions, *i*ntensive *t*herapy) model for evaluation of sexual function can be used for assessment purposes.[12] Pretreatment sperm banking offers the possibility of retaining reproductive capacity for some clients. Use of vaginal lubricants, methods of dilating the vagina after RT for cervical cancer (see Chapter 39), and penile prostheses (see Chapter 38) are topics you can discuss with the client. Counseling with a sexual therapist may be indicated.

■ ONCOLOGIC EMERGENCIES

Infection, pain, spinal cord compression, hypercalcemia, SIADH, cardiac tamponade, superior vena cava syndrome, tumor lysis syndrome, and disseminated intravascular coagulation (DIC) are oncologic emergencies. If not identified early and treated, oncologic emergencies can result in severe morbidity and death. Each oncologic emergency is discussed only briefly here. The focus is on your role in appreciating and urgently reporting sometimes subtle manifestations to ensure the best possible outcome for the client. Consult other cancer nursing texts for further information on oncologic emergencies.

Oncologic emergencies can be grouped as follows:

- Metabolic (infection and pain, hypercalcemia, tumor lysis syndrome, SIADH, DIC)
- Structural (spinal cord compression, superior vena cava syndrome, cardiac tamponade)

INFECTION AND PAIN

Infection, which can quickly progress as a life-threatening emergency in the client with neutropenia, was discussed in the preceding section. Although pain does not usually arise suddenly or unexpectedly, it is often regarded as an oncologic emergency because it is such a pervasive problem. As many as a third of clients in active treatment and 60% to 90% of people with advanced cancer have pain.[84] Pain can interfere with a person's ability to enjoy activities and relationships that are meaningful. When pain is uncontrolled, the goal of enabling the client to live fully cannot be met. For nursing management of pain, see Chapter 23.

HYPERCALCEMIA

After infection, hypercalcemia is the most commonly occurring oncologic emergency and can be a potentially fatal condition. Hypercalcemia is due to bone resorption (demineralization) and is defined as a serum calcium level greater than 11 mg/dl. If the client also has decreased serum albumin, a common finding with cancer, a corrected serum calcium value should be used. Eighty per cent of cases of cancer-related hypercalcemia occur with solid tumors, including breast, lung, head, neck, and renal cancers. The other 20% of cases occur in hematologic cancers, such as multiple myeloma, leukemia, and lymphoma.

If the serum calcium level rises slowly, the client may be relatively asymptomatic for a time. When it rises swiftly, renal failure, coma, cardiac arrest, and death can result. Early manifestations may be difficult to distinguish from other cancer- or treatment-related manifestations: anorexia, fatigue, nausea and vomiting, constipation, excessive thirst, polyuria, poor skin turgor, and dry mucous membranes.[25, 43] Later manifestations include severe muscle weakness, diminished deep tendon reflexes, paralytic ileus, and electrocardiogram (ECG) changes.

Nursing management begins with the recognition of clients at risk for hypercalcemia, including people with (1) cancer of the breast, lung, head, neck, or kidney, (2) multiple myeloma, (3) leukemia, (4) lymphoma, and (5) potential or actual bone metastases. Maintaining adequate hydration and mobility are important preventive measures in the client at risk. Limiting dietary intake of calcium has little or no effect. Clients and family caregivers should be instructed on manifestations to report.

Medical management of hypercalcemia is aimed at controlling the growth of the tumor causing the hypercalcemia and, possibly, administration of drugs to lower serum calcium levels, such as calcitonin (Miacalcin) and oral glucocorticoids. For the client with advanced disease, for whom other interventions are no longer effective, treatment is aimed at comfort care.

Tumor Lysis Syndrome

Tumor lysis syndrome is a potentially fatal metabolic emergency that can develop as a tumor responds to treatment. When a large, bulky tumor is very responsive to treatment, especially chemotherapy, the destruction of a large number of malignant cells may rapidly release intracellular potassium, phosphorus, and nucleic acid into the circulation. Electrolyte imbalances and acute renal failure usually begin 1 to 2 days after treatment starts and end within a week following the completion of therapy. Clients with malignancies that are very responsive to treatment are at highest risk, especially if they have a very large tumor burden. Such malignancies include lymphomas, leukemias, and small cell carcinoma.

Medical management focuses on prevention in high-risk clients. Aggressive IV hydration is started before treatment begins and is continued until after treatment ends. Allopurinol (Zyloprim) is administered to decrease uric acid concentration. Sodium bicarbonate may be given in conjunction with the IV hydration to promote fecal excretion of excess phosphate.

Despite preventive measures, tumor lysis syndrome may occur. If so, the goal is to remove potassium from the extracellular fluid with medications, retention enemas, or IV 50% dextrose, which acts to increase plasma insulin and thereby forces potassium back into the intracellular fluid. When preventive and maintenance measures are not effective, the client requires renal dialysis.[43]

The most important nursing management responsibility is to recognize and report manifestations of tumor lysis syndrome immediately. Nursing management then focuses on maintenance of fluid and electrolyte balance by carrying out medical orders, including IV hydration, monitoring weight daily, and maintaining a record of intake and output. Clinical manifestations to observe for and report are (1) weakness, (2) nausea, (3) diarrhea, (4) flaccid paralysis, (5) ECG changes, (6) muscle cramps or twitching, (7) oliguria (diminished urine output), (8) hypotension, (9) edema, and (10) altered mental status. Especially when treatment is provided in the outpatient ambulatory setting, the client and family must be taught about which manifestations to report immediately.[43]

Syndrome of Inappropriate Antidiuretic Hormone

SIADH results from the abnormal production of antidiuretic hormone (ADH). The incidence of SIADH is relatively low, occurring in only about 1% to 2% of clients with cancer. Of clients with cancer-related SIADH, 80% have an underlying diagnosis of small cell lung cancer. Other causes of SIADH are infection, pulmonary disorders, emotional stress, CNS disorders, and some drugs, including such antineoplastic agents as cyclophosphamide (Cytoxan), vincristine (Oncovin), vinblastine (Velban), and cisplatin (Platinol-AQ). Manifestations, which are related to the rates of onset of the decrease in sodium and the increase in water retention, include (1) confusion, (2) irritability, (3) headache, (4) muscle weakness, (5) lethargy, (6) decreased urine output, (7) edema, (8) nausea and vomiting, and (9) anorexia.[26, 43]

SIADH is not a preventable complication. It is a medical emergency only when the hyponatremia is severe (<120 mEq/L) and the client experiences manifestations. Mild SIADH is treated conservatively with fluid restriction (<500 to 1000 ml/day). In about 7 to 10 days, the body should be able to normalize the serum sodium concentration and osmolality. An IV infusion of hypertonic saline (3% to 5%) is given in more severe cases to prevent pulmonary edema. Monitor intake and output. Pharmacologic agents given for SIADH include demeclocycline (Declomycin), lithium (Lithane), and urea. Beyond symptomatic treatment, the goal of medical management is to treat the underlying disease causing the SIADH.[26, 43]

Disseminated Intravascular Coagulation

DIC involves the development of extensive, abnormal clots throughout small blood vessels. The widespread clotting consumes all circulating clotting factors and platelets, leading to excessive bleeding from several sites. The bleeding can be minimal or life-threatening. Also, clots that are blocking blood vessels decrease blood flow to major organs, which can cause pain, stroke-like manifestations, dyspnea, tachycardia, oliguria, and bowel necrosis. The mortality rate is near 70% despite appropriate treatment.

In clients with cancer, DIC is often caused by gram-negative infection or sepsis, release of thrombin or thromboplastin (clotting factors) from cancer cells, or blood transfusions. DIC is most commonly associated with leukemia and adenocarcinomas of the lung, pancreas, stomach, and prostate. Management involves treating the cancer and other measures as discussed in Chapter 75.

Spinal Cord Compression

Even for the terminally ill client in a hospice setting, early detection of and intervention for spinal cord compression are vital. Failure to intervene in this emergency can leave the client with permanent neurologic disabilities. Spinal cord compression is caused by direct pressure on or compromise of vascular supply to the spinal cord. Back pain is often the only early presenting clinical manifestation, occurring in 95% of clients. Other early manifestations are motor weakness and decreased sensation.

Depending on the rate of tumor growth, it may take only hours or days for the spinal cord compression to progress to irreversible neurologic damage with paralysis and loss of bowel and bladder control. Late manifestations are motor loss, additional sensory loss, constipation, and urinary hesitancy.[85, 96]

In a client with known cancer, new-onset back pain should be a "red flag" signaling immediate evaluation. Pain localized over the involved area of the spine or radicular (belt-like) pain is present in more than 90% of clients with spinal cord compression. Carefully assess new-onset back pain; have the client point to the location of the pain and show you the areas of spread. Also carefully assess for any other clinical manifestations of neurologic deficit, such as numbness, tingling, constipation, and voiding hesitancy.

Data from the medical record can be helpful in determining whether the client has known bone metastasis. Give the physician a complete assessment of the pain, with a description of the location and characteristics. These data will provide the physician with the information needed to consider spinal cord compression in the differential diagnosis.

Treatment is usually with RT unless the tumor is resistant to RT or the client has already received the maximum RT dose in the involved area. A laminectomy for spinal cord decompression is an alternative. For the client in a hospice setting whose life expectancy is limited to days or weeks, administration of steroids to lessen the inflammation and swelling around the spinal cord can be a less aggressive but effective short-term alternative.

SUPERIOR VENA CAVA SYNDROME

Distressing but rarely life-threatening, superior vena cava (SVC) syndrome is a disorder resulting from internal or external obstruction of the superior vena cava. The obstruction reduces venous blood return to the heart and compromises cardiac output. SVC syndrome should be evaluated as an emergency because of concern for respiratory compromise. The onset of manifestations is usually gradual; however, if SVC syndrome was the presenting manifestation of cancer, time should be taken to accurately diagnose the underlying disease before treatment is initiated.

Typically, SVC syndrome is secondary to lung cancer, usually small cell carcinoma (65%), or lymphoma (8%). The classic presenting manifestations are dyspnea (63%) and facial swelling (50%) with jugular vein distention. The client is often sitting up and leaning forward to breathe. Other manifestations are swelling of the arms, pain in the chest, and dysphagia.

The goals of medical management are to provide rapid palliation of the distressing manifestations and to treat the underlying cancer. External-beam RT continues to be the standard of care for palliation. However, clients with small cell carcinoma of the lung or lymphoma may be palliated with the appropriate curative chemotherapy regimen with or without the addition of RT.[73]

CARDIAC TAMPONADE

With cardiac tamponade (acute compression of the heart), early detection and proper management are critical to preventing cardiovascular collapse and death. When fluid collects in the pericardial sac (pericardial effusion), it affects the heart's ability to function properly and leads to cardiac tamponade. Normally, the pericardium contains 15 to 50 ml of fluid; the pericardial sac may contain as much as 200 to 1800 ml of fluid before the heart begins to decompensate. The fluid prevents the heart from filling and contracting normally. The onset may be insidious.

The most common manifestations are tachycardia, severe dyspnea, cough, chest pain, edema, and hypotension. You may notice a narrowing of the pulse pressure (the difference between systolic and diastolic readings) or pulsus paradoxus (decreased or absent amplitude of the pulse with inspiration). Heart sounds may be muffled by the fluid. Jugular venous distention may be prominent. A chest x-ray is a cost-effective screening tool, although it cannot always visualize cardiac tamponade. An ECG shows a number of changes that could indicate tamponade.

Medical management of cardiac tamponade is individualized for the client. A pericardiocentesis (insertion of an 18-gauge needle into the chest to draw off the fluid) may be performed. Because the fluid can reaccumulate, a pericardiotomy may be performed; this surgical procedure creates a window or opening in the pericardial sac for subsequent drainage of fluid. Even then, the pericardial fluid can reaccumulate. Nursing management consists of carefully assessing clinical manifestations and teaching the client and family caregiver to watch for manifestations that may herald impending cardiac tamponade.[6]

PSYCHOSOCIAL ASPECTS OF CANCER CARE

When cancer becomes a part of life's journey, it is hard work. (See Bridge to Home Health Care: Dealing with Grief Related to a New Cancer Diagnosis.) The diagnosis of cancer affects not only the individual client but also the family. Because cancer is not just a physical disease it compels the clients—and health care professionals—to face the meaning of their lives and their relationships. Just as life experiences affect the perceptions a client brings to the cancer experience, so do your life experiences affect the perceptions you bring to the client's care. It is, therefore, valuable for you to reflect on your beliefs and values about life, death, and their meaning.

■ PROVIDING SUPPORT FOR CLIENTS

The most valuable intervention you can offer a client with cancer is your presence as a caring person. The dimensions of your presence consist of verbal expressions of empathy, positive regard, and availability of practical support.[99]

Hearing the stories of colleagues, clients, their families, and survivors can be a vehicle for a novice nurse to learn the art of cancer nursing.[89] Storytelling is becoming recognized for its value.[36, 49, 50] A story can be a means of providing comfort by offering social comparisons (helping clients know how others have fared and felt in a similar situation) or lessons from others' experiences. Using sailing as a metaphor for the teamwork that makes for a smoother journey, Janice Post-White[74] shares stories of her clients' journeys and her own family's journey with cancer. Through the stories, Post-White teaches nurses

BRIDGE TO HOME HEALTH CARE

Dealing with Grief Related to a New Cancer Diagnosis

Peoples' lives are changed forever by a new diagnosis of cancer. Grieving often begins with the news that an illness is cancer-related. When home health nurses or other nurses in the community start working with clients, they have many responsibilities in addition to meeting clients' physical needs; they also must (1) assess how the client, the family, and significant others are coping with the new diagnosis, (2) acknowledge the grief process as part of the illness, and (3) help them to express their feelings, needs, and concerns as they struggle with the process.

Consider what losses are contributing to the grief process. Losses are likely to include the sense of wellness, usual or anticipated family role, positive self-image, career, independence, and financial stability as well as the fear of loss of life. Feeling alone is not uncommon. Determine whether friends and family members are providing support for the person with cancer, or whether they need encouragement and suggestions about how to do so. Many people have difficulty knowing how to react or what to say, especially when the client is younger. Evaluate whether the client and the family feel overwhelmed as they face choices about treatment options, symptom management, and emotions that compound the reaction to the new diagnosis.

The feelings associated with a new cancer diagnosis can be very intense. Remember that feelings are not good or bad; they just are. By letting clients know that you are truly available to listen, you provide the opportunity for them to discuss various feelings that may be just under the surface. Sometimes it is easier to write about feelings rather than verbalize them. Encourage the client and others to write down questions, concerns, hopes, and fears in the form of a letter or a journal.

Teaching is an important responsibility of home health providers. Help the client, the family, and significant others learn about the disease to gain a sense of control during this time of chaos. If they know what to expect and what is "normal," they are less anxious. Provide information about the disease, treatments, management of side effects, and the dynamics of grief. The American Cancer Society is an invaluable resource for the client with a new cancer diagnosis; suggest additional resources, such as authenticated Internet sites, and support groups, such as I Can Cope and Reach to Recovery. Prepare the client and family for an information overload and for the numerous, questionable products and services that are for sale in the area.

When you help the client maintain a sense of normality, you also add to the sense of control. Work with the client to schedule daily activities and provide structure to help him or her cope with the changes that result from the illness or treatment. Encourage the client to participate in normal activities and relationships. For some clients, employment or volunteer activities are options. Planning for the future can give the client something positive to anticipate.

Remember that the grief process is very individualized. Wherever the client, family members, or significant others are in this process is the right place for them to be. Be careful to avoid a list of "shoulds" and "should nots." Validate them by acknowledging their feelings, and accept that they are real, being careful not to include bias in your acceptance. Your encouragement will help the grief process evolve in its own time and at its own pace. Teaching, listening, and offering support are critical interventions for managing the grief process.

Pamela K. Schaid, RN, MA, *Administrator, Seasons Hospice, Rochester, Minnesota*

that they can be the "wind behind the sails," empowering clients and their families by creating balance, uniting a team, and guiding them forward.

There is great variability in the distress, changes, and other effects of cancer in the lives of clients and their families. Responses to cancer depend on:

- The disease and the disabilities and disfigurements it may cause
- Pre-existing medical conditions that may limit treatment options
- The client's psychological make-up and spiritual well-being
- The client's family and social community
- Availability of medical and financial resources

■ PROVIDING SUPPORT FOR FAMILY

The diagnosis of cancer has an effect on the entire family as well. The daily life of the family is changed. Other family members may need to assume the role or responsibilities of the client or to serve as the family caregiver. Nursing often views the family as the context of caring for the client with cancer; the family needs to be the unit of care. A family's resources, perceptions of the cancer, functioning patterns, coping strategies, and stressors are factors affecting their ability to respond to the crisis of cancer.[79] Much of the distress for the client and the family can be lessened with minimal assistance from the health care team. Without these services, even highly functioning families struggle.[52]

■ PROMOTING POSITIVE SELF-CONCEPT

Cancer affects all levels of functioning. Physical and psychological distress, medication, or the disease itself can cloud the client's intellectual function. The client's self-concept is affected by physical changes as well as changes in role or function. A breadwinner in the family may become dependent on others and become a consumer of family savings and resources. The young adult, striving for independence, may need to revert to an earlier level of dependency.

Body image also changes for most clients. Weight loss, hair loss, and skin changes can result from treatment. Radical surgical procedures can make devastating and permanent changes in appearance and function. Procedures such as laryngectomy, glossectomy, mastectomy, and prostatectomy may result in physical changes that humiliate and overwhelm the client.

■ PROMOTING COPING THROUGHOUT THE CANCER CONTINUUM

Although each cancer experience is unique, people with cancer have some common problems. Strategies for outcome management to help clients cope with the disease and its treatment are addressed for each phase of the *cancer continuum:* diagnosis and treatment, survivorship, recurrent disease and progression, and terminal illness.

DIAGNOSIS AND TREATMENT

Clients reach the point of cancer diagnosis in many ways. A client may have had vague manifestations, such as weight loss and fatigue, that may have been ignored or a cause of some anxiety for weeks or months. Another client may have manifestations, such as pain or abdominal bloating, that evaded diagnosis. Many times, cancer is found incidentally during a routine examination. Often the client suspects cancer, but many people are shocked when the diagnosis is made. The diagnostic period may be long and extremely stressful. This period is filled with anxiety about each test result, especially when staging procedures are performed. More than 70% of clients consider the time of diagnosis and treatment as the most stressful in the cancer experience.[95]

Most clients fear death during the first few months of the cancer experience. Weisman[95] called this stage "the existential plight." Whether clients can express their fears or not, it is an underlying cause of distress. During diagnosis, the magnitude of the client's problems becomes apparent. The client wonders: Is my disease curable? Will my disabilities be temporary or permanent? What types of physical impairment will occur? What will be the side effects of treatment? Will my manifestations be relieved? Will I be able to return to work? What adjustments have to be made in family life or work? Will finances be adequate? What plans need to be abandoned? Which changes in lifestyle will be temporary and which permanent?

Clients must deal not only with specific problems but also with the emotional distress they experience throughout this time. They may feel angry and frustrated because their lives have been changed; they may feel isolated or may worry about being abandoned by family and friends. They may be shocked and unbelieving that they are the ones with cancer. They may also feel guilty if they believe that they have contributed to their disease through behavior, such as by smoking, drinking, or putting themselves at risk for sexually transmitted diseases (see Chapter 18, Tables 18–3 and 18–4).

Clients' reactions vary greatly. Initial response to the diagnosis of cancer may be profoundly influenced by previous life experiences with the disease. When the disease is advanced at the time of diagnosis, the client and family are likely to experience more psychological distress because they are confronted with the dual stressors of a cancer diagnosis and a terminal illness.[69] Some have minimal distress, whereas others may be overwhelmed and devastated. You may sometimes feel, on the basis of your own personality and experience, that a client is responding inappropriately (i.e., too little or too much) to a cancer diagnosis. It is very important, however, to acknowledge every client's mode of response as acceptable and unique for that client.

Weisman[95] identified coping styles used by many clients with cancer (Box 19–3). *Denial,* which is a part of coping, allows a client to "repudiate what cannot be avoided, by substituting a more favorable or agreeable idea."[59] Denial can be useful as a healthy coping mechanism in the diagnostic phase, when the number of problems may be overwhelming. Denial is harmful when it prevents the client from seeking appropriate treatment. Awareness and denial can exist at the same time.

Clients who are good problem-solvers or who cope effectively tend to confront reality, avoid excessive denial, remain flexible, accept support, and remain hopeful and optimistic. Clients who cope poorly use avoidance and excessive denial; they are pessimistic and feel hopeless.[59] Box 19–4 lists factors that enable or hinder a client's ability to cope. Every client uses a variety of strategies to cope with cancer.

Families also should be assessed for their coping abilities. Use of a specific family assessment tool may not be possible, but often you will be readily able to identify "high-risk" families from your interactions with them. Unresolved past problems may affect a family's ability to cope with cancer in the present. Families who use excessive denial, exhibit strong anger and guilt, or are unreasonably demanding may be at increased risk for dysfunction. When the client is the pivotal person in the family or when the family has had a previous experience of cancer with a negative outcome, their need for ongoing psychosocial support systems may be increased.

Actively listen for remarks that describe the meaning and effect of cancer as experienced by the client. Often, time limitations may not permit you to provide support separate from physical caregiving. Consequently, while giving care, take the opportunity to initiate social interactions, such as chatting about family, sharing stories, or greeting visitors. Consider these actions a professional

BOX 19–3 General Coping Strategies

- Seek more information (rational inquiry).
- Share concern and talk with others (mutuality).
- Laugh it off; make light of the situation (affect reversal).
- Try to forget; put it out of your mind (suppression).
- Do other things for distraction (displacement, redirection).
- Take firm action on basis of present understanding (confrontation).
- Accept but find something favorable (redefinition, revision).
- Submit to the inevitable (fatalism, passive acceptance).
- Do something, anything, however reckless or impractical (impulsivity).
- Consider or negotiate a feasible alternative (if *x*, then *y*).
- Reduce tension with excessive drink, drugs, danger (life threats).
- Withdraw into isolation; get away (disengagement).
- Blame someone or something (externalization, projection).
- Seek direction; do what you are told (cooperative compliance).
- Blame yourself; sacrifice or atone (moral masochism).

Modified from Weisman, A. (1979). *Coping with cancer* (p. 23). New York: McGraw-Hill.

BOX 19–4 Enabling and Hindering Factors in Coping with Cancer

Enabling Factors	Hindering Factors
Social support systems	Denial
Perception of control	Avoidance
Hardiness	Helplessness
Humor	Powerlessness
Positive appraisal	Hopelessness or despair
Hopefulness	Depression
Positive comparisons	Guilt
Religiosity	Erosion of autonomy
Self-esteem	Isolation or withdrawal
Information-seeking	Wishful thinking
Open communication	Anger or hostility
Social skills	Blaming others
Problem-solving ability	Noncompliance

From Jalowiec, A., & Dudas, S. (1991). Alterations in patient coping. In S. Baird, R. McCorkle, & M. Grant (Eds.), *Cancer nursing: A comprehensive text* (pp. 806–820). Philadelphia: W. B. Saunders.

intervention. What did you learn about the client's perceptions of cancer? What coping mechanisms did the client or significant others use with past lifestyle changes? How will the client's and the family's life be affected? What needs for teaching or community resources did you note? Would referrals to other members of the health care team, such as the chaplain and social worker, be helpful?

Providing social support and improving the client's sense of control help reduce anxiety. Stress reduction or relaxation techniques can be taught. Speaking with cancer survivors encourages many clients. Support groups and one-to-one visitation programs such as Reach to Recovery or CanSurmount (ACS) provide this opportunity. Internet support groups offer the same opportunity for clients who are uncomfortable with the face-to-face interactions of a traditional support group.

Informational needs of the client and family are very great during the diagnostic and treatment periods. Tests, procedures, and treatments, which are often very technical and complicated, must be explained. Present consistent, accurate information in as much detail as the client wants. Be sure all health care providers are telling the client the same thing. When clients from a cancer clinic were surveyed, information and support from family, friends, and caregivers was identified as a high-priority need (Box 19–5).[32]

Address specific problems by (1) helping the client identify them, (2) providing information when necessary, and (3) referring the client to appropriate resources. Both the NCI and the ACS provide useful written materials to reinforce teaching. Site-specific information can be obtained from the NCI via the Internet *(www.nci.nih.gov* or *www.cancernet.nci.nih.gov),* Fax (301-402-5874), or telephone (1-800-4-CANCER). Other key Internet Web sites may be bookmarked on a computer in the clinical area or in a patient library.

SURVIVORSHIP

Clients who have completed successful treatment enter an indeterminate period of long-term survivorship. Survivorship has been divided into a time of acute survival followed by a period of extended survival. Transition between these periods is not precise but evolves as time passes and the cancer does not recur.

Depending on the extent of treatment, the period of extended survival may still be one of physical fatigue and limitation. Physical rehabilitation to improve functioning may dominate the client's energy in this early period. Efforts focus on restoring the client's previous level of functioning.

The long-term physical effects of cancer treatment are now becoming apparent as data accumulate, especially from clients with pediatric cancer. The physical effects may range from minimal restriction to life-threatening complications. The effects can be organ-specific, such as cardiomyopathy or pulmonary fibrosis, or general, such as fatigue.

The potential for development of a second malignancy as a result of primary treatment is always a possibility. Although this possibility is usually rare, some studies have reported up to a 20% occurrence of another cancer after treatment of Hodgkin's disease and other cancers with alkylating agents.

Psychologically, the period of extended survival is one in which clients must take up previous roles or adjust and reorganize their lives. The possibility of recurrence may dominate their lives. Plans may be suspended. Decisions about changing jobs, buying a house, starting a family, or beginning retirement may be difficult in the face of the uncertainty of recurrence or concerns about insurance coverage.

Making sure the client carries through with routine follow-up and long-term health care with attention to prevention and early detection (health promotion) is vital to early detection of recurrent cancer and second primary sites as well as early intervention for late effects of treatment. Follow-up appointments and events such as National Cancer Survivors Day celebrations (which are held in many communities each June) are opportunities for obtaining emotional support, alleviating fears of recurrence, and enabling clients to know that they are not alone in their feelings and concerns.

BOX 19–5 Needs of Clinic Patients with Cancer

The following needs were identified and rank-ordered by a sample of clinic patients. The last three items were ranked of equal importance.

- Information about operating special equipment
- Information about radiation
- Information provided in a way that is understandable
- Ways to be active in decision-making
- Adequate preparation before discharge from hospital
- Support from family
- Support from friends
- Information about chemotherapy
- Time off from work to recuperate
- Information about what to expect in the future
- A patient caregiver
- Time off work for treatment

Modified from Gates, M. F., Lackey, N. R., & White, M. R. (1995). Needs of hospice and clinic patients with cancer. *Cancer Practice, 3*(4), 226–232.

Employment discrimination has been a problem for cancer survivors. Clients with a cancer history have proved themselves to be dependable and productive. Yet studies show that as many as 84% of blue-collar workers and 38% of white-collar workers with cancer experience some type of discrimination in employment.[34] Over the years, these issues have been partially rectified by state laws protecting the rights of the disabled.

Obtaining insurance coverage for a client with a history of cancer has also been difficult, ruinously expensive, and sometimes impossible. Legislative efforts have corrected some of these problems. Insurance discrimination can be legally appealed. Federal programs such as COBRA (Consolidated Omnibus Budget Reconciliation Act) protect the insurance coverage of an employee for 18 months following employment termination, but at an increased monthly premium. A client, spouse, or parent may be trapped in an unrewarding job to maintain the employer-funded group insurance. Direct clients who have difficulty with insurance coverage to contact the National Coalition for Cancer Survivorship (Box 19–6), the ACS, their state department of human rights, or their state insurance department. The NCI booklet *Facing Forward* provides detailed information about resources.[92]

With time, these problems usually recede and clients move into a period of extended survival. The experience of cancer is nonetheless indelibly imprinted on their lives. Amazingly, most clients cope very well and face the difficulties in their lives with courage. For many, the experience brings about a reappraisal of goals and values, making life richer and more meaningful.

BOX 19–6 Cancer-Related Resources

The following are a few key resources for the nurse to obtain information and share with the client with cancer.

Oncology Nursing Society (ONS)
501 Holiday Dr.
Pittsburgh, PA 15220-2749
(412) 921-7373
http://www.ons.org

Office of Cancer Communications
National Cancer Institute
Building 31, Room 11A52
Bethesda, MD 20892-4200
1-800-4-CANCER
http://www.nci.nih.gov
http://cancernet.nci.nih.gov

American Cancer Society (ACS)
1599 Clifton Rd. NE
Atlanta, GA 30333-3329
1-800-ACS-2345
http://www.cancer.org/frames/html

National Coalition for Cancer Survivorship
1010 Wayne Ave., 5th Floor
Silver Spring, MD 20910
(301) 650-8868
http://www.cansearch.org

Oncolink University of Pennsylvania
http://www.oncolink.upenn.edu

National Library of Medicine
http://www.nlm.nih.gov

RECURRENT DISEASE AND PROGRESSION

Most clients with cancer live with the threat or reality of recurrent disease. Weisman[95] describes the effect that this phase has on the client as "the hope for a cure" becoming the "struggle for existence." With recurrent cancer, therapy may once again be used to eradicate or stabilize the disease process.

Although subsequent recurrent disease may occur, it is usually the first recurrence that causes surprise, shock, and disbelief in the client. Physical impairment may be greater, and quality of life may be limited because of disease or treatment. The client who previously projected an optimistic outlook may now express a more guarded attitude. Maintain open communication and be sensitive to the informational and support needs of the client and family.

Palliative treatment and palliative care are two distinct options for the client whose cancer persists. *Palliative care* is the provision of manifestation management and psychosocial support, best offered by a multidisciplinary health care team. In the past, palliative care was linked solely to terminal care. Increasingly today, professionals are recognizing the role of palliative care for incorporating quality-of-life outcomes for clients throughout the course of their illness.[70] Surgery, RT, or chemotherapy may be used to palliate complications caused by persistent tumor growth. For example, surgery may be used to manage a malignant obstruction, or RT to prevent paralysis from spinal cord compression. Palliative treatment is not curative but, rather, is aimed at improving the quality of the remainder of the client's life, however long or short.

Communicate to the client that disease manifestations can be managed successfully and that resources are available to assist in providing supplies and support. Palliative care is effective in decreasing the stress and discomfort related to advanced cancer and offers the client and family options to help them as the disease enters the terminal phase.

TERMINAL ILLNESS

About 50% of clients with cancer still eventually die of their disease. The time from diagnosis to death ranges from weeks to years. Not all clients with cancer become terminally ill. Some clients die during the initial treatment; others die of complications of treatment. Many, however, reach an end-point at which their cancer no longer responds to treatment and progression of the disease cannot be controlled. Then, the goal of treatment is directed toward providing supportive care and minimizing distress until death occurs.

In the United States since the mid-1970s, hospice care has become the standard of care for terminally ill clients with cancer. The philosophy of hospice care emphasizes symptom control and pain management, providing comfort and dignity to enable the client to live fully until death.

In medieval times, hospices were way stations for travelers and pilgrims. Most were run by Christian religious orders. The Irish Sisters of Charity opened the first hospice specifically for the dying in the mid-19th century in London. However, it was not until 1967, when Dame Cicely Saunders opened the St. Christopher's Hospice in

London and pioneered techniques for adequate pain control, that the modern concept of hospice care emerged.[71]

The first hospice in the United States was established in 1974 in New Haven, Connecticut. Since that time, more than 1600 hospice programs have been established in the United States. A hospice can be affiliated with a hospital, community, home care agency, or skilled nursing facility. Care can be provided in the home, an inpatient hospital, or a separate facility such as a nursing home. The basic characteristics of a hospice program are:

- Control of manifestations, including pain relief
- Treatment of the client and family as a unit
- Provision of care by an interdisciplinary team
- 24-hour, 7-day-a-week services
- Coordinated home care with back-up inpatient services
- Use of trained volunteers to augment staff services
- Spiritual support
- Bereavement follow-up
- Services given on the basis of need and not ability to pay
- Structured systems of staff support

Community-based hospices also incorporate services such as nursing care, educating the family in basic nursing skills, family respite care, running errands, shopping, light housework, transportation, provision of medical equipment, and assistance to enable the client to choose to die at home. To qualify for hospice services, clients must have a life expectancy of less than 6 months and must be receiving supportive treatment only.

Clients approach death in as many ways as they approach life. Some try to remain active despite tremendous physical limitations. Others may withdraw into depression. This period is a time of suffering for both client and family as the physical loss of function and the psychological pain of anticipated and real losses in relationships and roles are intensified. See Chapter 22 for an in-depth discussion of end-of-life nursing care for the terminally ill client.

Masterful use of basic nursing skills, combined with creative management of manifestations and compassion for the client and family, is the essence of hospice nursing care. Nursing care remains the mainstay for the client and significant others. Beyond what machines and medicines and procedures can do for the client, the act of caring remains a powerful weapon in the fight against disease. It is the one thing that technology can never replace. When everything is done that can be done, compassion is the only thing that brings beauty and meaning to our lives. It is the irreplaceable gift.

CONCLUSIONS

Cancer therapy has progressed rapidly in the last half of the 20th century. Many cancers once considered incurable are now controlled with a variety of combination therapies. Even when cancer is not cured, length of life may be extended. Importantly, the quality of the extended length of life has also greatly improved. Professionals have greater knowledge of and skills in controlling pain and managing nausea and vomiting due to chemotherapy, and there are more options for helping clients cope with hair loss.

The hospice movement has demonstrated that there is still much that can be done for a client with cancer, even when cure is no longer possible. The survivorship movement has made visible the hopeful side of cancer as well as being a resource to clients in dealing with insurance, workplace, and other issues.

New treatment modalities are showing promise in clinical trials, with some already becoming standard care. The nurse in the 21st century needs to stay abreast of new developments in this rapidly expanding field.

THINKING CRITICALLY

1. **You are a nurse working in a health clinic that focuses on prevention of disease. This month, the featured goal is cancer prevention. How will you assess each client for cancer risk factors?**

Factors to Consider. How would you develop an assessment tool for the clinic nurses to use? How would you adapt teaching strategies to the cultural group being served? What teaching can help clients avoid factors that increase their risk for cancer?

2. **The client is a 22-year-old man who comes to the neighborhood health clinic with concern that his companion, who has pain and a lump in the right testicle, may have testicular cancer. The companion is at home. What teaching should be completed during this visit? What psychosocial concerns would the client and the companion have?**

Factors to Consider. What diagnostic studies should you anticipate? What care should be given to the client awaiting diagnosis after cancer testing?

3. **C. H. is a 54-year-old engineer responsible for grading, paving, and asphalting of county road surfaces. He is admitted for evaluation of chest pain and increasing shortness of breath. Because of a history of quadruple bypass surgery when he was 44, he assumes that he has additional coronary artery blockage. He has continued to smoke despite his cardiac history. Several members of his mother's family and his father died of cancer. He has lung cancer that has metastasized to the brain. He will be treated with chemotherapy and RT. What risk factors did C. H. have for lung cancer? What teaching should the nurse plan for him? What long-term plans should the nurse consider for him?**

Factors to Consider. How will this client's cardiac history affect his chemotherapy regimen? What oncologic emergencies does C. H. face? Why is he not a surgical candidate?

BIBLIOGRAPHY

1. Abel, L. J., et al. (1999). Nursing management of patients receiving brachytherapy for early stage prostate cancer. *Clinical Journal of Oncology Nursing, 3*(1), 7–15.
2. Almadrones, L., Campana, P., & Dantis, E. C. (1995). Arterial, peritoneal, and intraventricular access devices. *Seminars in Oncology Nursing, 11*(3), 194–202.

3. American Cancer Society. (2000). *Cancer facts and figures—2000.* Atlanta: Author.
4. Averette, H. D., et al. (1990). Effects of cancer chemotherapy on gonadal and reproductive capacity. *CA: A Cancer Journal for Clinicians, 40*, 199–209.
5. Bailey, S. S. (1997). The arts in spiritual care. *Seminars in Oncology Nursing, 13*(4), 242–247.
6. Beauchamp, K. A. (1998). Pericardial tamponade: An oncologic emergency. *Clinical Journal of Oncology Nursing, 2*(3), 85–95.
7. Beck, S. L. (1996). Mucositis. In S. L. Groenwald, et al. (Eds.), *Cancer symptom management* (pp. 308–324). Boston: Jones & Bartlett.
8. Berger, A., Portenoy, R. K., & Weissman, D. E. (1998). *Principles and practice of supportive oncology.* Philadelphia: Lippincott-Raven.
9. Boyle, D. M., & Engelking, C. (1995). Vesicant extravasation: Myths and realities. *Oncology Nursing Forum, 22*(1), 57–66.
10. Brown-Saltzman, K. (1997). Replenishing the spirit by meditative prayer and guided imagery. *Seminars in Oncology Nursing, 13*(4), 255–259.
11. Bruner, D. W. (1998). Cost-effectiveness and palliative care. *Seminars in Oncology Nursing, 14*(2), 164–167.
12. Bruner, D. W., & Iwamoto, R. R. (1996). Altered sexual health. In S. L. Groenwald et al. (Eds.), *Cancer symptom management* (pp. 523–551). Boston: Jones & Bartlett.
13. Bruner, D. W., et al. (1992). *Manual for radiation oncology nursing practice.* Pittsburgh, PA: Oncology Nursing Press.
14. Burke, M. B., et al. (Eds.). (1996). *Cancer chemotherapy: A nursing process approach* (2nd ed). Boston: Jones & Bartlett.
15. Camp-Sorrell, D. (1996). *Access device guidelines: Recommendations for nursing practice and education.* Pittsburgh, PA: Oncology Nursing Press.
16. Cartmel, B., & Reid, M. (1997). Cancer control and epidemiology. In S. Groenwald, et al. (Eds.), *Cancer nursing: Principles and practice* (4th ed., pp. 50–74). Boston: Jones & Bartlett.
17. Clark, P. M., & Lacasse, C. (1998). Cancer-related fatigue: Clinical practice issues. *Clinical Journal of Oncology Nursing, 2*(2), 45–53.
18. Cohen, R., & Frank-Stromberg, M. (1997). Cancer risk and assessment. In S. Groenwald, et al. (Eds.), *Cancer nursing: Principles and practice* (4th ed., pp. 108–132). Boston: Jones & Bartlett.
19. Curtiss, C. P. (1996). Constipation. In S. Groenwald, et al. (Eds.), *Cancer symptom management* (pp. 484–497). Boston: Jones & Bartlett.
20. Dockery, V. G., & Ellis, C. (1999). Sexual dysfunction. *American Journal of Nursing,* April Supplement, 28–30.
21. Dow, K. H. (1992). Principles of brachytherapy. In K. H. Dow & L. J. Hilderley (Eds.), *Nursing care in radiation oncology* (pp. 16–29). Philadelphia: W. B. Saunders.
22. Dow, K. H., & Hilderley, L. J. (Eds.) (1992). *Nursing care in radiation oncology*. Philadelphia: W. B. Saunders.
23. Eisenberg, D. M., et al. (1998). Trends in alternative medicine use in the United States, 1990–1997. *JAMA, 280*(18), 1569–1575.
24. Ezzone, S., et al. (1998). Music as an adjunct to antiemetic therapy. *Oncology Nursing Forum, 25*(9), 1551–1556.
25. Finley, J. P. (1998). Hypercalcemia. In C. R. Ziegfeld, B. G. Lubejko, & B. K. Shelton (Eds.), *Manual of cancer care* (pp. 425–430). Philadelphia: Lippincott–Williams & Wilkins.
26. Finley, J. P. (1998). Syndrome of inappropriate ADH (SIADH). In C. R. Ziegfeld, B. G. Lubejko, & B. K. Shelton (Eds.), *Manual of cancer care* (pp. 431–435). Philadelphia: Lippincott–Williams & Wilkins.
27. Fischer, B., et al. (1998). Tamoxifen for prevention of breast cancer: Report of the National Surgical Adjuvant Breast and Bowel Project P-1 study. *Journal of the National Cancer Institute, 90*, 1371–1388.
28. Fisher, G. (1997). Bone metastases: Part I—pathophysiology. *Clinical Journal of Oncology Nursing, 1*(2), 29–35.
29. Fleming, I. D., et al. (Eds.). (1997). *AJCC cancer staging manual.* (5th ed.). Philadelphia: Lippincott-Raven.
30. Frank-Stromberg, M. (1997). Cancer screening and early detection. In C. Varricchio, et al. (Eds.), *A cancer source book for nurses* (7th ed., pp. 56–66). Boston: Jones & Bartlett.
31. Fukuyama, S. N., & Itano, J. (1999). Thrombocytopenia secondary to myelosuppression. *American Journal of Nursing*, April Supplement, 5–12.
32. Gates, M. F., Lackey, N. R., & White, M. R. (1995). Needs of hospice and clinic patients with cancer. *Cancer Practice, 3*(4), 226–232.
33. Greco, F. A. (Ed.). (1996). *Handbook of commonly used chemotherapy regimens.* Chicago: Precept Press.
34. Groenwald, S., et al. (Eds.). (1997). *Cancer nursing: Principles and practice* (4th ed). Boston: Jones & Bartlett.
35. Groenwald, S. L., et al. (Eds.). (1996). *Cancer symptom management.* Boston: Jones & Bartlett.
36. Groopman, J. (1997). *The measure of our days: New beginnings at life's end.* New York: Viking.
37. Heusinkveld, K. B. (1997). Cancer prevention and risk assessment. In C. Varricchio, et al. (Eds.), *A cancer source book for nurses* (7th ed., pp. 35–42). Boston: Jones & Bartlett.
38. Hood, L. A., & Abernathy, E. (1996). Biological response modifiers. In R. McCorkle, et al. (Eds.), *Cancer nursing: A comprehensive text* (2nd ed., pp. 434–457). Philadelphia: W. B. Saunders.
39. Howser, D. M. (1996). Alopecia. In S. Groenwald, et al. (Eds.), *Cancer symptom management* (pp. 261–268). Boston: Jones & Bartlett.
40. Ignatavicius, D., Workman, M. L., & Mishler, M. (1999). *Medical-surgical nursing across the health care continuum* (3rd ed). Philadelphia: W. B. Saunders.
41. Ingle, R. (1995). Rare complications of vascular access devices. *Seminars in Oncology Nursing, 11*(3), 184–193.
42. Jassak, P. F. (1997). Biotherapy. In S. Groenwald, et al. (Eds.), *Cancer nursing: Principles and practice* (4th ed., pp. 366–392). Boston: Jones & Bartlett.
43. Jones, L. A. (1996). Electrolyte imbalances. In S. Groenwald, et al. (Eds.), *Cancer symptom management* (pp. 415–432). Boston: Jones & Bartlett.
44. Kaempfer, S. H., et al. (1985). Fertility considerations and procreative alternatives in cancer care. *Seminars in Oncology Nursing, 1*(1), 25–34.
45. Klemm, P., & Nolan, M. T. (1998). Internet cancer support groups: Legal and ethical issues for nurse researchers. *Oncology Nursing Forum, 25*(4), 673–676.
46. Kosier, M. B., & Minkler, P. (1999). Nursing management of patients with an implanted Ommaya reservoir. *Clinical Journal of Oncology Nursing, 3*(2), 63–67.
47. Kolcaba, K., & Fox, C. (1999). The effects of guided imagery on comfort of women with early stage breast cancer undergoing radiation therapy. *Oncology Nursing Forum, 26*(1), 67–72.
48. Larouere, E. (1999). The art of accessing an implanted port. *Nursing 99, 29*(5), 56–58.
49. Lehna, C. (1999). Storytelling in practice: Part one—mother's stories. *Journal of Hospice and Palliative Nursing, 1*(1), 21–25.
50. Lehna, C. (1999). Storytelling in practice: Part two—professional storytelling. *Journal of Hospice and Palliative Nursing, 1*(1), 27–30.
51. Lerner, M. (1996). *Choices in healing: Integrating the best of conventional and complementary approaches to cancer.* Cambridge: The MIT Press.
52. Lewis, F. M. (1998). Family-level service in oncology nursing: Facts, fallacies, and realities revisited. *Oncology Nursing Forum, 25*(8), 1377–1388.
53. Loescher, L. (1997). Dynamics of cancer prevention. In S. Groenwald, et al. (Eds.), *Cancer nursing: Principles and practice* (4th ed., pp. 94–107). Boston: Jones & Bartlett.
54. Lucas, A. B. (1992). A critical review of venous access devices: The nursing perspective. *Current Issues in Cancer Nursing Practice, 1*(7), 1–10.
55. McNally, J. C., et al. (Eds.). (1991). *Guidelines for oncology nursing practice*. Philadelphia: W. B. Saunders.
56. Martz, C. H. (1996). Diarrhea. In S. Groenwald, et al. (Eds.), *Cancer symptom management* (pp. 498–520). Boston: Jones & Bartlett.
57. Mayer, D. K. (1997). Bone metastases: Part II. Nursing management. *Clinical Journal of Oncology Nursing, 1*(2), 37–44.
58. Moore, K. (1998). Out-of-pocket expenditures of outpatients receiving chemotherapy. *Oncology Nursing Forum, 25*(9), 1615–1622.
59. Mullan, F. (1985). Seasons of survival: Reflections of a physician with cancer. *New England Journal of Medicine, 313*, 270–273.
60. National Cancer Institute. (1997). *Chemotherapy and you: A guide to self help during treatment.* (NIH Pub. No. 97–1136). Washington, D.C.: U.S. Government Printing Office.
61. National Cancer Institute. (1997). *Eating hints for cancer patients.* (NIH Pub. No. 97–2079). Washington, D.C.: U.S. Government Printing Office.

62. National Cancer Institute. (1997). *Radiation therapy and you: A guide to self-help during treatment.* (NIH Pub. No. 97–2227). Washington, D.C.: U.S. Government Printing Office.
63. National Cancer Institute. (1997). *Taking time: Support for people with cancer and the people who care about them.* (NIH Pub. No. 97–2059). Washington, D.C.: U.S. Government Printing Office.
64. National Cancer Institute. (1998). *Taking part in clinical trials: What cancer patients need to know.* (NIH Pub. No. 98–4250). Washington, D.C.: U.S. Government Printing Office.
65. Nelson, N. J. (1997). Studies show prophylactic surgeries seem to reduce cancer risk. *Journal of the National Cancer Institute, 89*(11), 762–763.
66. Nunez, A. M., & Liebman, M. C. (1999). Febrile neutropenia. *American Journal of Nursing,* April Supplement, 9–12.
67. Oncology Nursing Society. (1992). *Cancer chemotherapy guidelines: Recommendations for the management of vesicant extravasation, hypersensitivity, and anaphylaxis.* Pittsburgh, PA: Author.
68. Occupational Safety and Health Administration. (1995). *Workplace guidelines for personnel dealing with cytotoxic (antineoplastic) drugs.* (OSHA Instruction CPL 2–2.20B CH-4, 21-1–21-34). Washington, D.C.: U.S. Government Printing Office.
69. Pasacreta, J. V., & Pickett, M. (1998). Psychosocial aspects of palliative care. *Seminars in Oncology Nursing, 14*(2), 110–120.
70. Phillips, J., Belcher, A., & O'Neil, J. A. (1997). Special populations. In C. Varricchio, et al. (Eds.), *A cancer source book for nurses* (7th ed., pp. 56–66). Boston: Jones & Bartlett.
71. Pickett, M., Cooley, M. E., & Gordon, D. B. (1998). Palliative care: Past, present, and future perspectives. *Seminars in Oncology Nursing, 14*(2), 86–94.
72. Pickett, M., et al. (2000). Prostate cancer elder alert: Living with treatment choices and outcomes. *Journal of Gerontological Nursing, 26*(2), 22–34.
73. Pinover, W. H., & Cioa, L. R. (1998). Palliative radiation therapy. In A. M. Berger, R. K. Portenoy, & D. E. Weisman (Eds.), *Principles and practices of supportive oncology* (pp. 618–623). Philadelphia: Lippincott-Raven.
74. Post-White, J. (1998). Wind behind the sails: Empowering our patients and ourselves. *Oncology Nursing Forum, 25*(6), 1011–1017.
75. Potter, K. L., & Schafer, S. L. (1999). Nausea and vomiting: One of the most distressing chemotherapy-related symptoms. *American Journal of Nursing,* April Supplement, 2–4.
76. Powel, L. L. (1996). *Cancer chemotherapy guidelines and recommendations for practice.* Pittsburgh, PA: Oncology Nursing Press.
77. Pruett, J. (1996). Bleeding. In S. L. Groenwald, et al. (Eds.), *Cancer symptom management,* (pp. 269–288). Boston: Jones & Bartlett.
78. Rieger, P. T. (1996). Biotherapy: The fourth modality. In M. B. Burke, et al. (Eds.), *Cancer chemotherapy: A nursing process approach* (2nd ed., pp. 43–73.) Boston: Jones & Bartlett.
79. Robinson, D. (1997). Family stress theory: Implications for family health. *Journal of the American Academy of Nurse Practitioners, 9*(1), 17–23.
80. Rumsey, K. A., & Rieger, P. T. (Eds.). (1992). *Biological response modifiers: A self-instruction manual for health professionals.* Chicago: Precept Press.
81. Rumsey, K. A., & Richardson, D. K. (1995). Management of infection and occlusion associated with vascular access devices. *Seminars in Oncology Nursing, 11*(3), 174–183.
82. Rust, D. M., Wood, L. S., & Battiato, L. A. (1999). Oprelvekin: An alternative treatment for thrombocytopenia. *Clinical Journal of Oncology Nursing, 3*(2), 57–62.
83. Schulmeister, L. (1997). Preventing chemotherapy dose and schedule errors. *Clinical Journal of Oncology Nursing, 1*(3), 79–85.
84. Sheidler, V. R. (1998). Pain. In C. R. Ziegfeld, B. G. Lubejko, & B. K. Shelton (Eds.), *Manual of cancer care* (pp. 369–385). Philadelphia: Lippincott–Williams & Wilkins.
85. Shelton, B. K. (1998). Spinal cord compression. In C. R. Ziegfeld, B. G. Lubejko, & B. K. Shelton (Eds.), *Manual of cancer care* (pp. 410–419). Philadelphia: Lippincott–Williams & Wilkins.
86. Shelton, B. K. (1998). Anemia. In C. R. Ziegfeld, B. G. Lubejko, & B. K. Shelton (Eds.), *Manual of cancer care* (pp. 231–243). Philadelphia: Lippincott–Williams & Wilkins.
87. Sigley, T. (1998). Nutritional problems. In C. R. Ziegfeld, B. G. Lubejko, & B. K. Shelton (Eds.), *Manual of cancer care* (pp. 349–368). Philadelphia: Lippincott–Williams & Wilkins.
88. Somerville, E. T. (1991). Knowledge deficit related to chemotherapy. In J. C. McNally, J. Campbell Stair, & E. T. Somerville (Eds.), *Guidelines for cancer nursing practice* (2nd ed., pp. 36–39). Philadelphia: W. B. Saunders.
89. Taylor, E. J. (1997). The story behind the story: The use of storytelling in spiritual caregiving. *Seminars in Oncology Nursing, 13*(4), 252–254.
90. Tenenbaum, L., Leshin, D., & Hydzik, C. (1994). Other systems affected by chemotherapy and biotherapy. In L. Tenenbaum (Ed.), *Cancer chemotherapy and biotherapy: A reference guide* (2nd ed., pp. 371–408). Philadelphia: W. B. Saunders.
91. Tortorice, P. T. (1997). Chemotherapy: Principles of therapy. In S. Groenwald, et al. (Eds.), *Cancer nursing: Principles and practice* (4th ed., pp. 283–316). Boston: Jones & Bartlett.
92. U.S. Department of Health and Human Services. (1996). *Facing forward: A guide for cancer survivors.* (NIH Pub. No. 96–2424). Washington, D.C.: National Cancer Institute.
93. Vanderhoof, D. D., & Brant, J. M. (1999). Alopecia: The forgotten side effect? *American Journal of Nursing,* April Supplement, 17–19.
94. Varricchio, C., et al. (1997). *A cancer source book for nurses* (7th ed). Boston: Jones & Bartlett.
95. Weisman, A. (1979). *Coping with cancer.* New York: McGraw-Hill.
96. Wilkes, G. M. (1996). Neurological disturbances. In: S. Groenwald, et al. (Eds.), *Cancer symptom management* (pp. 324–363). Boston: Jones & Bartlett.
97. Winningham, M. L. (1996). Fatigue. In S. Groenwald, et al. (Eds.), *Cancer symptom management* (pp. 42–54). Boston: Jones & Bartlett.
98. Wujcik, D. (1996). Infection. In S. Groenwald, et al. (Eds.), *Cancer symptom management* (pp. 289–302). Boston: Jones & Bartlett.
99. Zewekh, J. V. (1997). The practice of presencing. *Seminars in Oncology Nursing, 13*(4), 260–262.
100. Ziegfeld, C. R., Lubejko, B. G., & Shelton, B. K. (1998). *Oncology fact finder: Manual of cancer care.* Philadelphia: Lippincott–Williams & Wilkins.

CHAPTER 20

Clients with Psychosocial and Mental Health Concerns: Promoting Positive Outcomes

Nancy Shoemaker

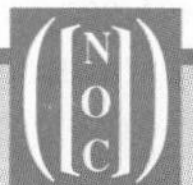

NURSING OUTCOMES CLASSIFICATION (NOC)
for Nursing Diagnoses—Clients with Psychosocial and Mental Health Concerns

Altered Thought Processes
Cognitive Ability
Cognitive Orientation
Communication Ability
Concentration
Decision Making
Distorted Thought Control
Identity
Information Processing
Memory
Risk Control: Alcohol Use
Risk Control: Drug Use
Safety Behavior: Personal

Anxiety
Acceptance: Health Status
Aggression Control
Anxiety Control
Coping
Impulse Control
Psychosocial Adjustment: Life Change
Self-Mutilation Restraint
Social Interaction Skills
Symptom Control

Body Image Disturbance
Acceptance: Health Status
Distorted Thought Control
Self-Esteem
Self-Mutilation Restraint
Social Involvement

Hopelessness
Comfort Level
Coping
Decision Making
Depression Control
Depression Level
Hope
Mood Equilibrium
Quality of Life
Sleep
Spiritual Well-Being

Ineffective Individual Coping
Aggression Control
Caregiver Emotional Health
Caregiver-Patient Relationship
Caregiver Well-Being
Depression Control
Depression Level
Family Coping
Family Environment: Internal
Family Normalization
Family Health Status

Knowledge Deficit
Cognitive Ability
Communication Reception: Receptive Ability
Concentration
Information Processing
Knowledge: Disease Process
Knowledge: Health Resources
Knowledge: Medication
Knowledge: Treatment Regimen
Memory

Risk for Self-Directed Violence
Cognitive Ability
Depression Control
Depression Level
Distorted Thought Control
Impulse Control
Loneliness
Mood Equilibrium
Quality of Life
Risk Control
Risk Control: Alcohol Use
Risk Control: Drug Use
Risk Detection
Self-Mutilation Restraint
Suicide Self-Restraint
Will to Live

Risk for Violence Directed at Others
Abuse Protection
Abusive Behavior Self-Control
Aggression Control
Cognitive Ability
Depression Control
Distorted Thought Control
Impulse Control
Quality of Life
Risk Control
Risk Control: Alcohol Use
Risk Control: Drug Use
Risk Detection

Self-Care Deficit
Self Care: Activities of Daily Living (ADL)
Self Direction of Care

Self-Esteem Disturbance
Body Image
Hope
Mood Equilibrium
Role Performance
Self-Esteem
Social Interaction Skills

Spiritual Distress
Anxiety Control
Hope
Quality of Life
Spiritual Well-Being
Suicide Self-Restraint
Well-Being
Will to Live

A sound knowledge base for responding to psychosocial and mental health concerns of clients and their families is vital in all settings where medical-surgical nursing is practiced. Psychosocial components are defined as the psychological and social aspects of the client's health status. Psychological factors include thinking, feelings, motivation, and personal strengths and weaknesses. Social issues are related to patterns of interaction with others (see also Chapter 9). For all clients seeking health care for a physical problem, there is a potential for alteration in their mental or emotional status because of the stress of illness and navigating the health care system. The North American Nursing Diagnosis Association (NANDA) currently lists 149 approved nursing diagnoses; approximately 41% are related to psychosocial functioning (see Box 20–1). To promote successful health outcomes, the nurse must address the psychosocial and mental health concerns of each client.

Some clients have a pre-existing mental disorder that may complicate or adversely affect the outcome of their medical treatment. At least 50 million Americans live with a mental illness at any given time.[23] In any one year, 23 million people suffer from anxiety disorders; 8 million more are affected by major depression; and 2.5 million are afflicted with schizophrenia.[8, 10, 25] For these clients, nursing attention to psychosocial needs makes the difference between compliance with treatment and noncompliance with resulting complications.

This chapter focuses on the psychosocial concerns of clients and families that require nursing care across various treatment settings. Basic principles regarding communication are outlined, and nursing interventions to reduce anxiety are presented. Concepts of anxiety, stress, coping mechanisms, and self-esteem are reviewed. Five clients with concurrent medical disorders and serious mental illness are discussed in order to illustrate the challenge that these individuals present for holistic nursing care. In each case, the role of the medical-surgical nurse is presented along with a suggested nursing care plan. Finally, the dimensions of culture, spirituality, and sexuality are addressed in relation to specific clients. Chapter 9 describes how to obtain a psychosocial history as part of the comprehensive nursing assessment.

Client Scenarios

Picture yourself as the nurse responsible for the clients in the following scenarios. These scenarios will help illustrate the later discussion of psychosocial and mental health issues and their application in nursing care across a variety of clinical settings.

1. You work the 3 to 11 PM shift in the emergency department (ED). You are assigned to Mrs. Barbara James, a 51-year-old black woman admitted several hours ago with acute chest pain and respiratory distress. Initial diagnostic tests to rule out myocardial infarction are negative, but final laboratory re-

BOX 20–1 NANDA 1998–2000 Nursing Diagnoses Related to Adult Psychosocial Concerns

Adjustment, Impaired
Anxiety
Body Image Disturbance
Caregiver Role Strain
Caregiver Role Strain, Risk for
Communication, Impaired Verbal
Coping, Community: Potential for Enhanced
Coping, Defensive
Coping, Family: Potential for Growth
Coping, Ineffective Community
Coping, Ineffective Family: Compromised
Coping, Ineffective Family: Disabling
Coping, Ineffective Individual
Death Anxiety
Decisional Conflict (Specify)
Denial, Ineffective
Energy Field Disturbance
Family Processes: Altered
Family Processes, Altered: Alcoholism
Fatigue
Fear
Grieving, Anticipatory
Grieving, Dysfunctional
Health Maintenance, Altered
Health Seeking Behaviors (Specify)
Home Maintenance Management, Impaired
Hopelessness
Loneliness, Risk for
Noncompliance
Parental Role Conflict
Parenting, Altered
Parenting, Risk for Altered
Personal Identity Disturbance
Post-Trauma Syndrome
Post-Trauma Syndrome, Risk for
Powerlessness
Rape-Trauma Syndrome
Rape-Trauma Syndrome: Compound Reaction
Rape-Trauma Syndrome: Silent Reaction
Relocation Stress Syndrome
Role Performance, Altered
Self Esteem Disturbance
Self Esteem, Chronic Low
Self Esteem, Situational Low
Self-Mutilation, Risk for
Sensory Perceptual Alterations (Specify: visual, auditory, kinesthetic, gustatory, tactile, olfactory)
Sexual Dysfunction
Sexuality Patterns, Altered
Social Interaction, Impaired
Social Isolation
Sorrow, Chronic
Spiritual Distress
Spiritual Distress, Risk for
Spiritual Well-Being, Potential for Enhanced
Therapeutic Regimen: Community, Ineffective Management
Therapeutic Regimen: Families, Ineffective Management
Therapeutic Regimen: Individuals, Ineffective Management
Thought Processes, Altered
Tissue Perfusion, Altered (cerebral)
Violence, Risk for: Self-Directed or Directed at Others

NANDA, North American Nursing Diagnosis Association.

sults are pending. When you introduce yourself to Mrs. James, she is crying and states, "I can't believe my heart is okay. This must be a heart attack. It can't be my nerves."

2. While on duty in a busy university medical clinic, you see a client with a recently diagnosed first-time hiatal hernia. Gregory Barnes is a 32-year-old, slightly obese black man who smiles pleasantly as you introduce yourself and shakes your hand. When you ask Mr. Barnes to describe his problem, he responds, "I don't get enough food. My stomach is connected to the elves in my basement, and they take all of my food as soon as I eat it." You notice Mr. Barnes' elderly mother sitting in the waiting room.
3. You are a staff nurse on a medical acute care unit. Returning from 2 days off, you are assigned to Mrs. Mary Conners, a 59-year-old West Indian woman admitted the previous day with diabetic ketoacidosis. Entering her room, you notice that the lights are off. She does not look up when you speak to her. When Mrs. Conners answers your second greeting, her voice is in a monotone and she quickly looks away. You observe several jars of food on her table. The admitting nurse states that Mrs. Conners had been verbal on admission and that her daughter seems very concerned about her.
4. As a home care nurse, you have recently started caring for Mr. John Moore, a 66-year-old white man who has had a second stroke. You completed his medication teaching quickly because he was familiar with most of his medicines. For the past few weeks, you have been supervising the home health aide while the physical therapist works on gait training. Today, you receive a call from the physical therapist who reports, "I don't know what to do with Mr. Moore. He has the strength to do his exercises, but he just won't try. I may have to discharge him for noncompliance."
5. You are the charge nurse in a long-term skilled nursing facility. As you are making morning rounds, one nursing assistant stops you to complain about Miss Celia Howard. She is a 75-year-old white woman who has been in your facility for 2 years because of multiple cardiac problems and the inability to care for herself. Recently hospitalized for acute dehydration, she returned 3 days ago. There has been a change in her behavior. Miss Howard is cursing and spitting at staff, and today she pushed her roommate out of the room. You remember that she was seeing the consultant psychiatrist in the past, but when you examine the chart, you note that her psychotropic medications have been discontinued.

UNIVERSAL ISSUES

Universal psychosocial concepts include anxiety, stress, coping mechanisms, and self-esteem. Additional factors that influence reactions to stress are cultural and family background, exposure to similar stressors, and repeated exposure to stressors.

■ ANXIETY

Before addressing the psychosocial concerns of clients with concurrent mental disorders, the nurse must first develop skills to manage the anxiety that is common to all clients. *Anxiety* is a universal human phenomenon, defined as a strong feeling of fear or dread with an unknown cause. All clients (and their loved ones) are vulnerable to feeling anxiety as they seek care for medical problems. Not only clients but everyone may feel anxiety at times, especially when facing an unknown situation (changing schools, starting a new job). Under normal conditions, this discomfort is short-lived and may be helpful for problem solving. Box 20–2 describes possible emotional, physical, and spiritual manifestations of anxiety.

■ STRESS

Anxiety is part of the human reaction to stress. *Stress* is defined as "a particular relationship between the person and the environment that is appraised by the person as taxing and/or exceeding his or her resources and endangering his or her well-being."[20] Resources can include one's coping skills. In the case of potential physical danger, one is mobilized for self-protection with the fight-or-flight response. Most people would experience strong reactions in the face of crisis situations such as an imminent car accident or a tornado. In addition to external stressful events, people may define stress in different ways because it is the perception of the event, not the event itself, that stimulates the response. For example, one student may feel extreme stage fright when giving a speech, whereas another may feel only mild tension. Table 20–1 describes the levels of anxiety with implications for client teaching.

BOX 20–2 Emotional, Physical, and Spiritual Manifestations of Anxiety

Emotional

Fearful
Helpless
Sense of impending doom
Insecure
Irritable
Fatigued
Lack of self-confidence

Physical

Increased blood pressure
Increased pulse
Increased respirations
Chest pain or tightness
Muscle tension
Excessive sweating
Dry mouth or nausea
Diarrhea or increased urination

Spiritual

Hopeless
Feeling abandoned by God
Blaming God for the suffering

TABLE 20–1 MANIFESTATIONS OF FOUR LEVELS OF ANXIETY

Anxiety Level	Physical Manifestations	Emotional Manifestations	Cognitive Manifestations
Mild	Increased pulse and blood pressure	Positive affect	Alert, can solve a problem, prepared to learn new information
Moderate	Elevated vital signs, tense muscles, diaphoresis	Tense, fearful	Attention focused on one concern, may be able to concentrate with direction
Severe	Fight-or-flight response, dry mouth, numb extremities	Distressed	Decreased sensory perception, can focus only on details, unable to learn new information
Panic	Continued as in severe level	Totally overwhelmed	Ignores external cues, focused only on internal stimuli, unable to learn

Regardless of the source of the stressor, a person's reaction to acute stress follows a predictable course.[15] When the brain perceives a threat, the sympathetic nervous system releases epinephrine and norepinephrine within 2 or 3 seconds. The hypothalamus responds by secreting corticotropin-releasing hormone (CRH), which activates the pituitary gland to secrete adrenocorticotropic hormone (ACTH). ACTH stimulates the adrenal glands to produce the steroid hormone cortisol (the "stress hormone"). Throughout this process, various organs are affected throughout the body, creating physical effects such as elevated vital signs and dry mouth. Within 10 minutes, usually the high level of cortisol triggers the hypothalamus and pituitary to cease production of CRH and ACTH to end the acute stress response.

■ COPING MECHANISMS

Most people respond to anxiety by using *coping skills* that are learned external behaviors or internal thought processes consciously used to decrease discomfort. Coping behavior can be classified as follows[30]:

- *Emotion-focused* behaviors include thinking, saying, or doing something to make oneself feel better (crying, sharing feelings with someone)
- *Problem-focused* behaviors include seeking facts about a problem, making a plan, or studying how others have overcome similar obstacles.

Chapter 1 discusses these behaviors in more detail.

Another common response to anxiety is the use of *ego defense mechanisms,* originally defined by Freud.[31] These thought processes are not deliberate or voluntary, like coping mechanisms. Instead, they exist at an unconscious level to disguise the real threat, protecting the person from feeling anxious about the real issue. One defense mechanism frequently seen in clients with serious illness is *denial.*[29] Use of denial allows one to ignore the problematic issue and its negative consequences. For example, after hearing the diagnosis of a heart condition, a client tells the nurse that he plans to exercise as soon as he is discharged and shows no interest in learning about diet and activity limitations. Momentarily, he is protected against the distress of facing the reality of permanent changes in lifestyle. Failure to cope effectively can increase anxiety levels. See Box 20–3 for definitions and examples of selected defense mechanisms.[31]

BOX 20–3 Selected Defense Mechanisms: Definitions and Examples

Definition	Example
Denial—avoidance of a problem by ignoring or refusing to recognize it	A client with a cardiac condition tells his family that he has a "little problem" after the physician explains his diagnosis of heart attack.
Displacement—transferring feelings for a threatening topic or person to another more neutral topic or person	After a client is told that he cannot be discharged today as planned, he spends the whole shift complaining that his breakfast was cold.
Intellectualization—showing excessive thinking and logic in order to avoid uncomfortable feelings	After a leg amputation, a client shows great interest in the details of the surgery and even requests a textbook to identify the muscles and bones, but he does not watch while the nurse changes the dressing.
Projection—assigning one's own uncomfortable feelings or motivation to another person	A client tells the nurse, "Please explain about the operation again to my wife, she is so afraid that I won't wake up."
Rationalization—giving an apparently logical and acceptable explanation to cover up a feeling or motive that may not be socially acceptable	The nurse finds a client eating breakfast when he is on NPO status (nothing by mouth) for a diagnostic test. The nurse specifically told him about the procedure yesterday: when asked what happened, the client states, "Well, the aide brought me this tray so I thought it was okay."
Regression—demonstrating behavior characteristics of an earlier stage of development	An adult client insists on keeping multiple stuffed animals on her bed and bursts into tears when the nurse moves one to check her arm for intravenous access.

Assess the level of anxiety in all clients, and intervene as early as possible to try to reduce the anxiety to a manageable level. To achieve desired outcomes such as cooperation with care and compliance with discharge instructions, the client or family must be calm enough to understand the teaching. A person's anxiety level beyond the moderate range poses an emotional barrier to learning new information.[18] You can use several simple communication techniques to decrease anxiety in clients, thereby increasing the likelihood that they will benefit from health instructions. Box 20–4 lists nursing interventions that may help reduce anxiety in non-psychiatric clients.

You must also be able to recognize and support positive coping efforts by clients and their families. As noted previously, these behaviors may be emotion-focused or problem-focused, but they function to decrease anxiety. Failure to understand these behaviors may lead to nontherapeutic staff reactions. For example, a client with a new diagnosis of cancer has a wife who never leaves his bedside. She studies every action by the nurses and constantly asks questions. In addition, the client has been observed tearfully talking about his father who died of colon cancer. Several staff members have suggested that the wife have limited visiting hours because she is upsetting the client. By considering her behavior as problem-focused coping, you might involve her in teaching and allow her to participate in care as much as possible. You might also realize the client is using emotion-focused coping skills by crying and expressing his feelings of loss.

BOX 20–4 Nursing Interventions to Decrease Client Anxiety

Nonverbal Interventions	Verbal Interventions
Listen with full attention, looking at the client with unbroken eye contact.	Answer questions honestly.
Maintain a calm, unhurried approach.	Explain all procedures in simple terms.
Speak slowly in a clear, firm voice (not loud).	Give reassurance based on the data.
Offer or use touch, e.g., holding a hand or giving a back rub.	Give information about tests, medicines, and treatments as requested.
If possible, decrease the noise and bright light.	Explain the reasons for limitations on activity or other restrictions.
	Acknowledge clients' anxiety, and encourage them to explore the reasons.
	Include family members in discussions unless the client requests otherwise.
	If necessary, repeat directions patiently.

■ SELF-ESTEEM

Another universal concern that affects the client's reaction to the stress of illness is self-esteem. *Self-esteem* is defined as "the degree of worth and competence one attributes to oneself."[4] The client's pre-existing level of self-esteem strongly contributes to successful or maladaptive adjustment to illness. A person with high self-esteem shows self-confidence and positive expectations in new situations. A new medical problem may be seen as just another challenge, and the client will actively participate in learning new health behaviors. In contrast, a person with low self-esteem consistently demonstrates negative feelings about oneself and is pessimistic in new situations. The same medical diagnosis may be met with a helpless, indecisive attitude that poses a barrier to teaching and developing alternative health behaviors. Table 20–2 presents characteristics of self-esteem with implications for nursing care.

ADDITIONAL NEEDS OF CLIENTS WITH CONCURRENT MENTAL ILLNESS

After recognizing the psychosocial concerns of clients in general, you should become aware of additional needs for successful care of clients with concurrent mental illness. These needs consist of (1) comprehensive nursing assessment, (2) your self-awareness regarding communication, (3) basic mental health teaching for the client and family, and (4) referral for specialized services.

■ COMPREHENSIVE NURSING ASSESSMENT

As soon as you realize that the client is presenting with an altered mood or thought process, review the nursing database to ensure that it is complete. In many admission situations, limited data are obtained before treatment is initiated because of the severity of the manifestation or time constraints. When developing a care plan for the client with coexisting mental illness, make sure that you gather a complete psychosocial history (see Chapter 9). Significant facts concerning motor activity, mood, affect, and speech must be documented and communicated objectively. Table 20–3 lists definitions of commonly used terms to describe abnormal findings.

Psychosocial risk factors, such as a history of self-destructive, aggressive, or socially inappropriate behavior, must also be identified and documented. Secondary sources, such as family and medical records, are often helpful. Information about the client's social support system and history of mental health treatment is necessary to ensure appropriate immediate intervention and discharge planning.

In addition to the psychosocial assessment, a complete medication history provides valuable data. Some clients under treatment for anxiety or depression may not demonstrate active manifestations on admission. They usually do not volunteer that information until they are asked about the reason for taking psychotropic medications.

On the other hand, remain alert to the possibility that medication can sometimes produce psychiatric manifestations in clients without a formal diagnosis. If a client adamantly denies an emotional problem and the manifestations are of an acute onset, carefully examine prescrip-

TABLE 20–2 CHARACTERISTICS OF PEOPLE WITH HIGH AND LOW SELF-ESTEEM

Characteristic	High Self-Esteem	Low Self-Esteem
Overall self-evaluation	Positive, "I am a good person"	Negative, "I am worthless"
Verbalization about self	Feelings of strength, pride	Feelings of weakness, shame
Perception of problem-solving ability	Self-confident, recalls past success	Insecure, dwells on past failures
Response to feedback from others	Accepts praise or criticism	Rejects praise and exaggerates criticism
Implications for nursing care	Requests active participation in care, information-seeking, makes prompt decisions	Passive involvement in care, may not ask questions, indecisive and dependent with decisions

tion and over-the-counter medication usage. Table 20–4 lists selected medicines that may cause psychiatric manifestations.[1]

■ AWARENESS OF COMMUNICATION

The second requirement in caring for psychiatric clients is to pay extra attention to all communication with them. Under ordinary circumstances, the nurse assumes that communication with clients is fairly routine and predictable, including necessary physical procedures and verbal questions, instructions, or explanations. In response, the nurse expects reactions from clients to fall within a range showing agreement, questioning, or refusing care. In essence, this is the model for daily communication that many nurses take for granted.

Human communication is complex and built upon many assumptions and unspoken rules inherent in a given culture. Communication between two participants involves all of the verbal and nonverbal behavior that they perceive in each other.[38] In addition to sending words, which are carefully selected, we are simultaneously sending nonverbal signals, which are largely involuntary. Nonverbal communication includes tone and volume of voice, eye contact, facial expression, body posture, and other body language. We expect to find congruence between the words and nonverbal cues; the words match the feeling

TABLE 20–3 COMMONLY USED TERMS TO DESCRIBE ABNORMAL MENTAL STATUS FINDINGS

Term	Mental Status Findings
MOOD	
Depressed	Feeling sad, decreased energy and interest in usual activities
Elated	Feeling euphoric, overly optimistic, and energetic
Labile	Rapidly changing from one state to another, e.g., happy to sad or irritable
AFFECT	
Blunted	Overall decrease in emotional tone compared with a normal reaction to a situation
Flat	No expression of feelings, regardless of variation in topics
Inappropriate	Nonverbal signs of feelings do not match the verbal report of the person, e.g., person smiles when reporting sad event
MOTOR ACTIVITY	
Agitation	Physically restless, unable to sit still
Psychomotor retardation	Physically slowed down, including all movements and speech
PERCEPTION	
Hallucination	Sensory perception originating from within the brain but attributed to external sources, e.g., hearing voices
Illusion	Incorrect interpretation of external sensory input, e.g., seeing a shadow in the closet and thinking it is a person
SPEECH	
Loose association	Speech pattern where the listener cannot follow the connections between the speaker's ideas, seems illogical to listener
Pressured speech	Rapid flow of speech with intense undercurrent of feeling, may refuse to be interrupted
THOUGHT PROCESS	
Delusion	A fixed, false belief that is strongly defended by the individual, e.g., may be paranoid (suspicious) or grandiose (unrealistically wonderful)
Psychosis	Severe impairment in reality testing, with distortion in perception and analysis of external and internal stimuli

TABLE 20–4 MEDICATIONS AND SUBSTANCES THAT MAY CAUSE PSYCHIATRIC MANIFESTATIONS

Medication	Psychiatric Manifestations
Anticholinergics	Disorientation, visual hallucinations, paranoia
Baclofen	Hallucinations, confusion, anxiety
Beta-adrenergic blockers	Depression, psychosis
Caffeine	Anxiety, psychosis
Calcium-channel blockers	Depression
Cephalosporins	Delusions, euphoria
Corticosteroids	Depression, mania, psychosis
DEET (diethyltoluamide [OFF])	Mania, hallucinations
Digitalis glycosides	Depression, mania, hallucinations
Fluoroquinolone antibiotics	Psychosis, agitation, depression
Histamine H_2-receptor antagonists	Confusion, aggression, psychosis
Narcotics	Dysphoria, anxiety, hallucinations
Salicylates	Agitation, confusion, paranoia
Thiazide diuretics	Depression

and tone of the body. For example, a client tells the nurse that he is in pain, and he is frowning. Another client says that she is happy about the discharge, and she is smiling. The nurse would respond to these two clients without hesitation because the verbal and nonverbal behaviors match. See Diversity in Health Care: The Significance of Cultural Assessment.

When the words and the nonverbal signs from a sender do not match, the receiving person must pause to analyze the situation. Often, this incongruent communication is the first clue that a client has a psychiatric disorder. Normal people may sometimes send a mixed message, but psychiatric clients consistently have difficulty with communicating their needs. It is generally agreed that when the verbal and the nonverbal communication are incongruent, the nonverbal communication reflects the person's true feelings.

First interactions with all clients are important. Recall Mrs. Conners' first interaction with the nurse. Looking at the words alone, the nurse greeted her and Mrs. Conners answered. The nonverbal cues—sitting in a dark room, delaying her response, and speaking in a monotone—conveyed to the nurse that this client was in an altered mental state. Conversely, Mr. Barnes' initial nonverbal communication—smiling and offering a handshake—is in stark contrast to his comment about elves in his basement.

When communicating with clients who have concurrent psychiatric problems, pay attention to the communication process for two reasons. First, thorough data must be collected to determine the nursing diagnoses and to communicate with the treatment team. Second, monitor your own nonverbal behavior to prevent sending negative nonverbal messages to the client. All clients are sensitive to the nonverbal communication of health care staff, and psychiatric clients often expect rejection. Mental illness in our society still carries a stigma shared by clients and staff alike. Clients feel ashamed because they have an emotional problem; staff may have biases based on personal experience.[5] Recall that Mrs. James would rather believe that she has a life-threatening cardiac problem instead of an emotional problem. To communicate acceptance to these clients and to help them to overcome their self-criticism, your verbal and nonverbal communication must be congruent.

■ CLIENT AND FAMILY TEACHING

The third important requirement for all clients with concurrent psychiatric disorders is basic client and family teaching. Certainly, for the client who is receiving a new diagnosis (Mrs. James), there are many questions. Even for those who are already in treatment, their understanding about the illness and its treatment must be assessed. Basic teaching for all clients includes a definition of the illness, medications and treatment options, and relapse prevention.[26] This information is readily available in written teaching materials, which can be kept on file along with medical-surgical teaching guides. Whenever possible, include a family member in the instruction. Families often play a significant caregiver role for these clients. Repeated studies have shown that they are desperately in need of education.[40] Box 20–5 lists resources to educate and support clients and their families.

■ SPECIALIZED REFERRALS

The fourth important requirement to consider when caring for clients with concurrent mental disorders is the need for specialized referrals. Once the nursing assessment is complete, the current problems and risk factors can be analyzed. If manifestations are severe or risk factors are significant, additional evaluation is necessary. At times, this evaluation is urgent and immediate, such as when a client shows self-destructive or aggressive behavior. You are in a key position on the health care team to advocate for appropriate services. In the hospital or institutional environment, consulting psychiatric staff (nurse, social worker, psychologist, or psychiatrist) can usually be called for an in-depth assessment and disposition. Likewise, in the community setting, referrals can be made to outpatient or home care services to provide specialized care.

■ SUMMARY

The medical-surgical nurse has a clear role to play with clients who have concurrent psychiatric disorders. The four steps just outlined do not require training beyond a generalist level. They do require a professional commitment to provide holistic care to all clients and to fully utilize the multidisciplinary team available in the health care setting. There is an inherent reward in providing excellent care for clients, but the nurse is also preventing potentially serious adverse outcomes. In the managed care environment, the front-line nurse must function as the clinical manager for the client by identifying the risk for complications and coordinating efficient use of resources.[14] For example, a client with a panic disorder (such as Mrs. James) must have the diagnosis clarified on the first trip to the ED with a clear plan for follow-up. If

DIVERSITY IN HEALTH CARE

The Significance of Cultural Assessment

It is important for a nurse not only to gain adequate cultural knowledge about particular ethnic groups but also to gather information about each client's cultural background in order to provide competent care. The major focus of a cultural, or "culturalogical," assessment is to identify "culture care patterns, expressions, and meanings that reflect the client's care needs and well-being or that influence the client's patterns of illness, disabilities, or death."[5]

Nurses as well as other health caregivers must use every effort to avoid projecting onto clients their own world views and should remember that every client is a unique person who may or may not be following the beliefs and practices of his or her ethnic group. There is as much diversity within a cultural group as across cultural or ethnic groups.[3]

In performing a cultural assessment, nurses become aware of the client's beliefs and practices in health and illness and how they may enhance or interfere with an intervention or a treatment regimen. Data from a cultural assessment provide meaning to behaviors that otherwise might be judged by the caregiver as negative or confusing. Both content and process are part of a cultural assessment; the *content* covers the actual categories in which data about clients are gathered, whereas the *process* includes the techniques by which data are gathered (e.g., nonverbal and verbal communication, approach to the client, and order of elicitation of information).[1]

Various nursing authors have identified models or guides for cultural assessments.[1–3, 5–7] A helpful addition to these models is the elicitation of the client's explanatory model of his or her illness, developed by Kleinman and co-authors,[4] in which the following questions are used:

- What do you think caused your problem?
- Why do you think it started when it did?
- What do you think your sickness does to you? How does it work?
- How severe is your sickness? Will it have a short or long duration?
- What kind of treatment do you think you should receive?
- What are the most important results you hope to receive from this treatment?
- What are the chief problems your sickness has caused for you?
- What do you fear most about your sickness?

The data gathered from these questions help the nurse or other health caregiver negotiate with the client and the family about acceptable treatment and expected outcomes.

Leininger[5] noted some guidelines for an effective assessment. For instance, the nurse must maintain a role of an active listener and refrain from expressing professional opinions about the client's beliefs and practices during the assessment process. The nurse should obtain a holistic picture of the client and convey respect for beliefs. Unless the nurse can be trusted to not demean the client's beliefs, the client will not be willing to share information.

A cultural assessment, optimally, is a means to help nurses and clients communicate more effectively, to show clients that the nurse is interested and respectful of their beliefs, and to provide information that enables nursing and health care interventions to be more relevant for clients and their lifestyles. Any health teaching or treatment instructions directed toward a client must be as compatible as possible with the client's beliefs and practices if the client is expected to adhere to the treatment regimen. The client's increased adherence and satisfaction as well as the nurse's success in this endeavor are the intermediate steps desired toward the overall goal of improved client health and well-being.

References

1. Andrews, M. M., & Boyle, J. S. (1999). *Transcultural concepts in nursing care.* (3rd ed.). Philadelphia: Lippincott–Williams & Wilkins.
2. Bloch, B. (1983). Bloch's assessment guide for ethnic/cultural variations. In M. S. Orque, B. Bloch, & L. S. A. Monrroy (Eds.), *Ethnic nursing care: A multi-cultural approach* (pp. 49–75). St. Louis: C. V. Mosby.
3. Giger, J. N., & Davidhizar, R. E. (1999). *Transcultural nursing: Assessment & intervention.* (3rd ed.). St. Louis: Mosby.
4. Kleinman, A., Eisenberg, L., & Good, B. (1978). Clinical lessons from anthropological and cross-cultural research. *Annals of Internal Medicine, 88,* 251–258.
5. Leininger, M. (1995). *Transcultural nursing: Concepts, theories, research and practices* (p. 118). New York: McGraw-Hill.
6. Purnell, L. D., & Paulanka, B. (1998). *Transcultural health care: A culturally competent approach.* Philadelphia: F. A. Davis.
7. Sharma, S. (1993). Promoting cultural sensitivity in nursing practice. *Practicing Anthropology, 15*(1), 31–32.

Sandra Sharma, PhD, ARNP, CS, *James A. Haley Veterans Hospital, Tampa, Florida*

not, she is likely to return for multiple visits and even go through expensive, dangerous diagnostic tests. In the cases of Mrs. Conners and Mr. Moore, who are suffering from depression, depending on their past history of manifestations and current support systems, they may be at risk for suicide as a desperate solution to their problems.

In the sections that follow, these five psychiatric clients will be revisited in more detail. An overview of their psychiatric disorders is presented along with specific nursing care plans for management in the medical-surgical setting. For a discussion on the importance of spirituality and health, see the Alternative Therapy feature.

ANXIETY

Mrs. James presents with a classic case of panic attack. The acute manifestations can strike unexpectedly and create severe physical distress: palpitations, chest pain, elevated vital signs, dizziness, nausea, and distinct fear that one is dying. The cardiac work-up does not reveal abnormal cardiac enzymes or electrocardiogram (ECG), and the manifestations subside spontaneously. After careful diagnostic testing to rule out other medical disorders such as thyroid disease, hypoglycemia, and pheochromocytoma, panic disorder can be identified.[8]

ALTERNATIVE THERAPY

Spirituality and Health

There is a growing awareness of the importance of spirituality in health and of the need for health care providers to acknowledge this. Many clients in the health care system consider spiritual issues important and feel that such issues are too often neglected in our modern technological medical environment. A growing body of research is showing that spiritual or spiritually related activities may in fact be protective of health.[6]

For many people, spirituality may mean their particular religious practice; for others, it may be their own personal views and beliefs or the way they feel connection to something beyond themselves. In fact, connectedness may be an important component of spirituality and its positive health benefits. The social and communal aspects of many religions and spiritual practices may be a common denominator in the health benefits seen. Conversely, social isolation is considered a factor in poor health.[4]

Some authors and researchers feel that love (and the perception of being loved) is very important in health and that love may be the essence of the benefits of spirituality and connection. Author and researcher Jeff Levin states that "love indeed has everything to do with our health and well-being." Levin has researched the epidemiology of religion and found that people who were more religious or spiritual also had better health, greater well-being, and less depression.[3]

Research into the effects of intercessory prayer (prayers said on someone else's behalf), sometimes without their being aware of it consciously, is both intriguing and controversial. Preliminary data from a pilot study of a number of interventions, including intercessory prayer, in a group of clients with unstable angina and infarction showed the least adverse outcomes when they were mentioned in the prayers of others.[2] Such studies are difficult to conduct and to evaluate. Yet other research has shown that when a certain percentage of a population is engaged in Transcendental Meditation, the incidence of violence decreases in surrounding populations.[5] Such research leads some to speculate that there is a field of consciousness that we are all a part of.

Some studies have shown that clients with cancer who participate in support groups show improvement in quality of life and in survival time.[4] Perhaps this is because "all relationships are spiritual." The more intimate and loving one's relationships, the better this is for one's health.[4]

What are we, as nurses, to make of the information regarding spirituality and health? One thing we must not do is draw the wrong conclusions. As Larry Dossey points out,[1] we must not assume that being religious or spiritual is a guarantee of good health or that poor health or illness implies spiritual shortcomings in someone. "Sickly saints and healthy sinners show us that there is no invariable, linear, one-to-one relationship between one's level of spiritual attainment and the degree of one's physical health. It is obvious that one can attain immense spiritual heights and still get *very* sick." We must also not equate our own particular religion or spiritual practice as being one that others *should* follow. Each person's spirituality should be authentically his or her own, emerging "from the center of one's being."[1]

What we can do is assess each client's degree of isolation or connectedness and encourage moves toward the latter. This may mean providing information about support groups for people with various illness or putting a client in touch with a chaplain or pastoral counselor. Our interest, concern, and sharing with clients in these areas serves to deepen our relationship with them, which may in itself be healing.

References

1. Dossey L. (1993). *Healing words: The power of prayer and the practice of medicine.* San Francisco: Harper San Francisco.
2. Horrigan, B. (1999). Mitchell W. Krucoff, MD, The Mantra Project. *Alternative therapies in health and medicine. 5*(3):75–82.
3. Horrigan B. (1999). Jeff Levin, MPH, PhD, The Power of Love. *Alternative Therapies in Health and Medicine, 5*(4): 78–86.
4. Ornish D. (1998). *Love and survival.* New York: HarperCollins.
5. Sharma, H. & Clark, C. (1998). *Contemporary ayurveda.* Philadelphia: Churchill Livingstone.
6. Ziegler, J. (1998). Spirituality returns to the fold in medical practice. *Journal of the National Cancer Institute, 90,*1255–1257.

James Higgy Lerner, RN, LAc, *Private practice of acupuncture, traditional Oriental medicine, and biofeedback*

Panic disorder is one of the eight subtypes of anxiety disorders identified by the *Diagnostic and Statistical Manual of Mental Disorders,* fourth edition (*DSM-IV*).[2] Anxiety disorders as a group are the most common psychiatric disorders in the United States and affect one out of four people in a given year.[8] The eight major categories are:

- Panic Disorder
- Generalized Anxiety Disorder (GAD)
- Phobias
- Obsessive-Compulsive Disorder (OCD)
- Post-traumatic Stress Disorder (PTSD)
- Acute Stress Disorder
- Anxiety Disorder due to Medical Condition
- Anxiety Disorder Not Otherwise Specified

Manifestations may range from mild to severe. Many of these clients never request treatment because of their feelings of shame. Box 20–6 describes each diagnosis. Whereas health care professionals often joke about obsessive-compulsive traits in themselves, clients with OCD (e.g., hand-washing 50 times each day) rarely admit that they have a problem. OCD, phobias, or Generalized Anxiety Disorder may come to the attention of the nurse only accidentally while the client is being treated for another condition. However, clients with panic disorder, PTSD, or acute stress disorder frequently seek urgent care because of severe distress. One survey estimated that as many as 8% of Americans 15 to 54 years of age suffer from PTSD as a result of witnessing a tragedy, domestic violence, or sexual abuse.[11]

BOX 20–5 Resources for Mental Illness Education

Alzheimer's Disease Education and Referral
www.alzheimers.org
Web site sponsored by National Institute on Aging with educational and research information related to Alzheimer's disease.

Anxiety Disorders Association of America
301-231-9350
www.adaa.org
Information and support groups for clients with anxiety disorders.

Depression and Related Affective Disorders Association (DRADA)
Johns Hopkins Hospital
600 N. Wolfe Street
Baltimore, MD 21287-7381
410-955-4647
www.med.JHU.edu/drada
Information, support groups, and research for clients with mood disorders and their families.

National Alliance for Research on Schizophrenia and Depression (NARSAD)
60 Cutter Mill Road, Suite 404
Great Neck, NY 11021
516-829-0091
www.mhsource.com
Supports research into mental illness and offers free information and a newsletter regarding schizophrenia and mood disorders.

National Alliance for the Mentally Ill (NAMI)
200 N. Glebe Road, Suite 1015
Arlington, VA 22203-3754
800-950-NAMI (800-950-6264)
www.nami.org
Provides information, support groups, and advocacy for clients and their families.

National Depressive and Manic-Depressive Association
730 N. Franklin Street, Suite 501
Chicago, IL 60610
800-82NDMDA (800-826-3632)
Information and support for clients with bipolar illness and their families.

National Institute of Mental Health
888-8ANXIETY (888-826-94389)
www.nimh.nih.gov/anxiety
Free information and educational material on anxiety disorders.

National Mental Health Association
1021 Prince Street
Alexandria, VA 22314-2971
703-684-7722
Information and support for clients with mental illness and their families.

The WEBster
www.cyberspy.com/~webster/index.html
Web site established by a pediatric nurse to provide support to clients and their families coping with death and dying, including suicide.

■ POSSIBLE CAUSES

There is no single known cause for anxiety disorders, and research is ongoing. Three major approaches have been proposed to explain the illness: (1) biologic, (2) psychodynamic, and (3) behavioral.

BIOLOGIC VIEW

From the biologic viewpoint, there is some evidence supporting a genetic influence for Generalized Anxiety Disorder, Panic Disorder, and phobias. First-degree relatives (parents, siblings, children) of clients with these disorders have an increased risk of the same manifestations compared with normal controls.[7] Anxiety disorders often coexist with other psychiatric problems that seem to run in families, such as depression or substance abuse.[8]

Evidence from drug studies and diagnostic imaging techniques, such as computed tomography (CT) or positron emission tomography (PET), and magnetic resonance imaging (MRI) has shown definite brain structures and neurotransmitters that are involved in the experience of anxiety. The limbic system of the brain is activated during the stress response (see the feature on anatomy and physiology of the neurologic system introducing Unit 15). The neurotransmitters epinephrine, norepinephrine, dopamine, serotonin, and gamma-aminobutyric acid (GABA) all are involved in regulating anxiety. Thus, disturbances in nerve structures or in levels of brain chemicals appear to be underlying causes of anxiety disorders.[8]

BOX 20–6 Key Features of the Anxiety Disorders

Panic Disorder—recurrent panic attacks followed by change in behavior to try and avoid another attack persisting over more than 1 month

Generalized Anxiety Disorder (GAD)—excessive anxiety for 6 or more months that is uncontrollable, often focused on health or money concern

Phobia—severe, persistent fear of an object or situation that the person recognizes as irrational but cannot overcome

Obsessive-Compulsive Disorder (OCD)—preoccupation with disturbing thoughts (obsessions) or repetitive actions (compulsions) that interferes with normal activities of daily living

Post-traumatic Stress Disorder (PTSD)—reexperiencing a real, horrifying event in nightmares or flashbacks, with a duration of manifestations more than 1 month that may be immediate or a delayed reaction

Acute Stress Disorder—similar to PTSD except that the manifestations occur within 1 month of the event and last only for approximately 1 month

Anxiety Disorder due to General Medical Condition—severe anxiety in the presence of clear physical findings of a somatic disorder, e.g., hypoglycemia

Anxiety Disorder Not Otherwise Specified—showing some anxiety or phobic manifestations but not severe enough to warrant a specific diagnosis

PSYCHODYNAMIC VIEW

Psychodynamic explanations point toward faulty psychological defenses or thinking processes. *Psychoanalytic* theory proposes that anxiety results from inability to repress (unconsciously inhibit) painful impulses, thoughts, or memories. Manifestations of anxiety are considered to be disguised forms of these repressed thoughts. *Intellectual theory* suggests that the problem is intellectual distortion; a person consistently distorts reality to see the world in a negative way. In the case of panic, the person incorrectly interprets the manifestations as impending death rather than as a reversible stress response.[31]

BEHAVIORAL VIEW

Behavioral theory views anxiety as a learned or conditioned response. A person who has experienced fear and all of its physical manifestations in a certain situation may learn to feel the same effects in a similar situation just because of past association. For example, one painful visit to the dentist as a child may condition a person to always feel anxious with a dentist even for routine, painless procedures.

■ OUTCOME MANAGEMENT

All of the anxiety disorders can be effectively treated through a combination of medication and psychotherapy. Several different classes of drugs that alter levels of neurotransmitters can be helpful. Benzodiazepines seem to increase the action of GABA. Buspirone is thought to affect serotonin receptors. Antidepressants alter the levels of serotonin or norepinephrine. Box 20–7 lists commonly prescribed anti-anxiety medications. These medicines may be prescribed for short-term or long-term use but usually are not needed permanently.

Medication may offer some immediate benefit to reduce the discomfort of anxiety, but some form of psychotherapy (individual, group, or family) is necessary to achieve lasting positive outcomes. Clients, and sometimes their loved ones, have usually tried to cope with their manifestations for a long time before seeking help. Often, they have adopted negative patterns of thinking or avoidance behaviors that are not easily given up despite serious impairment. For example, consider the limitations of a phobic person who cannot cross bridges. This person cannot work or socialize in any location that requires going over a bridge and probably invents excuses to hide the real reason from friends or family. In the context of a therapy relationship, the client works to identify and revise dysfunctional behavior.

BOX 20–7 Medications for Anxiety Disorders

- Benzodiazepines
  - Alprazolam
  - Clonazepam
  - Diazepam
  - Lorazepam
  - Oxazepam
- Buspirone
- Selective serotonin reuptake inhibitors (approved for treatment of anxiety)
  - Fluoxetine
  - Paroxetine
  - Sertraline
- Tricyclic antidepressants
  - Amitriptyline
  - Clomipramine
  - Desipramine
  - Imipramine
  - Nortriptyline

■ INTERVENTION

Returning to Mrs. James, the ED nurse needs to devise a care plan with a discharge plan quickly (see Care Plan). When the nurse sits down to talk with Mrs. James, she is not surprised to find that the psychosocial history is incomplete. This client had presented with potentially life-threatening manifestations, and the admitting nurse focused on selected, pertinent data such as medications and allergies. The database shows that Mrs. James has a history of hypertension and degenerative joint disease affecting her right knee, forcing her to use a cane.

COMPREHENSIVE ASSESSMENT

As the nurse explores the client's current psychological and social functioning, Mrs. James reports that this is not the first time that she has had respiratory distress. Over the past 6 months, she has had one or two episodes each month. Before this episode, they were milder and she did not have chest pain. She cannot relate the attack to any particular stressor but has learned to limit her outside activities to avoid all places where she feels anxious. Mrs. James depends on her daughter who lives with her to do all the shopping. She also describes difficulty sleeping and increased appetite. She feels she is worthless and has crying spells several times per week. She even confides that she has lost all sexual interest and that her boyfriend is starting to think that she does not love him anymore.

When asked about her past level of functioning, Mrs. James states that until 1 year ago she was working as a nurse's aide and was independent. She drove, helped to care for her mother, and enjoyed going out with friends to church and social events. After a fall resulting in a knee injury, she never recovered full ambulation and eventually applied for disability. Her daughter moved in with her to help with financial obligations. In relation to her family history for emotional problems, Mrs. James explains that her mother is alcoholic and her daughter takes antidepressants, but she has always been "too strong for that kind of problem."

COMMUNICATION AWARENESS

Throughout the interview, the nurse provides a private, supportive atmosphere. Initially, the nurse closes the curtain and moves the chair so that there is continuous eye contact. It is explained that they may have only 15 minutes before an interruption, but the nurse wants to learn as much as possible about Mrs. James. As the client talks, the nurse encourages her with nonverbal cues such as nodding her head. When the client becomes tearful at times, the nurse calmly pauses and offers her a tissue. The nurse shows no surprise or disapproval when Mrs. James mentions mental illness in her family. At the end of the assessment, the nurse tells the client that sharing this information will assist the treatment team to plan an

■ THE CLIENT WITH DEGENERATIVE JOINT DISEASE AND CONCURRENT PANIC DISORDER: MRS. JAMES

Nursing Diagnosis. Anxiety as evidenced by panic attacks related to physical loss of independence with associated changes in social and economic functioning.

Outcomes. Mrs. James will verbalize understanding that her manifestations may be caused by an emotional disorder, will consent to evaluation by a psychiatric consultant, will accept referral to psychiatric aftercare, and will receive appropriate psychiatric treatment to resolve panic attacks and to improve her level of functioning (long-term).

Interventions	Rationales
1. Assess for other emotional problems such as depression and substance abuse and include family history.	1. Panic Disorder frequently runs in families and may coexist with other mental disorders.
2. Assess for stressors and previous level of functioning.	2. Data provide a functional baseline so that the nurse can encourage the client to set realistic goals for change.
3. Assess for family support system and acceptance of problem.	3. Family involvement increases the likelihood of follow-up with recommended treatment.
4. Demonstrate acceptance of the client's feelings and distress.	4. Manifestations of emotional illness are just as important as physical distress.
5. Educate the client and family about anxiety as a treatable illness, and explain the role of the psychiatric consultant.	5. Preparation helps the client accept mental health services.
6. Communicate the history to the social worker, including the incomplete sexual assessment.	6. Ensures continuity of care and enables the social worker to focus on the client's key issues.

Evaluation. Accomplishment of short-term outcomes should be evident before discharge from the emergency department. Accomplishment of long-term outcome may require considerable time.

effective treatment regimen; the next step is to consult with the physician for recommendations. The nurse asks Mrs. James to call a family member to come and stay with her pending her discharge.

Client and Family Teaching

The nurse reports the findings on Mrs. James' anxiety and mood to the attending physician and recommends that the psychiatric social worker or psychiatric nurse practitioner for the ED be called. The physician agrees, noting that all laboratory findings are normal. The probable diagnosis is Panic Disorder. As the physician goes to speak with the client, the nurse accesses the client education file or on-line library and obtains material on panic attack, depression, and coping skills for families. The nurse gives these pamphlets to Mrs. James and her daughter, telling them that anxiety is a common, treatable problem. The nurse also explains the role of the psychiatric consultant and asks them to wait to talk with her. The client is uncertain, but the daughter encourages her to agree.

Specialized Referrals

In choosing the appropriate referrals for discharge planning for Mrs. James, the nurse is aware that the medical center offers several levels of psychiatric care (see Table 20–5). Because the client is not at immediate risk to harm herself or others, referral to the inpatient unit is not indicated. Yet, the risk exists that if she is given an appointment to go to the outpatient clinic next week, she may not follow through. Mrs. James has already suffered for 6 months and is still resisting the idea that her manifestations may be due to emotional issues. Thus, the nurse selects the resource who can make an immediate, specialized assessment and disposition—namely, the ED consultant.

The psychiatric consultant (social worker, advanced practice nurse, or psychologist) will perform a full, diagnostic interview, including appropriate standardized tests for anxiety and depression. Box 20–8 lists commonly used rating scales for mental health assessment. The ED nurse shares the nursing database with the psychiatric health care worker, noting the client's report of sexual difficulties, which needs further evaluation. Box 20–9 presents the psychosocial dimension of sexuality related to the nursing assessment and intervention.

After meeting with the client and her daughter, the psychiatric consultant recommends referral to the Partial Hospital Program on the following day because of the severity of manifestations. The nurse communicates this recommendation to the physician in order to coordinate the final discharge plan for Mrs. James. In reviewing the discharge instructions, the nurse strongly recommends that the daughter accompany the client to the intake appointment, and she agrees. Upon discharge, Mrs. James is no longer crying and states, "If all of you think that I should go, then I will."

Schizophrenia

Mr. Barnes demonstrates clear manifestations of *schizophrenia* with fixed delusions and hallucinations. He represents a generation of young, chronically mentally ill people who have been cared for primarily in the community instead of being institutionalized. Schizophrenia is an incurable, severe mental illness that usually strikes between the ages of 15 and 25.[24] *DSM-IV* lists five subtypes (Box 20–10).

In all cases, a person's thinking and communication skills are profoundly affected. Manifestations are generally classified as positive or negative.[22] *Positive* manifestations include the most obvious signs of psychosis (auditory or visual hallucinations, delusions, disorganized

TABLE 20–5 LEVELS OF PSYCHIATRIC TREATMENT SERVICES

Level of Care	Intensity of Psychiatric Treatment
Inpatient unit	Most intensive level of care for clients considered dangerous to self or others; admission may be voluntary or involuntary; brief length of stay, 1 week or less
Partial hospitalization	One step below inpatient, to prevent hospitalization or stabilize after a brief hospital stay; voluntary admission; short length of stay, from 1 to 4 weeks, with attendance 5 to 7 days per week
Psychosocial day program/rehabilitation	Structured daily activity for clients who need moderate, long-term supervision; voluntary admission; promotes socialization and vocational skills; indefinite length of stay
Mobile treatment	Outreach program to follow clients who require medication and case management but refuse to attend outpatient centers; voluntary admission; intermittent visits; indefinite length of stay
Psychiatric home care	Home visits by psychiatric nurse or social worker to treat homebound clients with an exacerbation of a *DSM-IV* diagnosis; voluntary participation; requires physician orders; length of stay 4 to 8 weeks
Outpatient clinic or private clinician	Least intensive level of care for clients following a more intensive level of treatment or for crisis, short-term treatment; voluntary participation; length of stay indefinite

DSM-IV, Diagnostic and Statistical Manual of Mental Disorders, 4th ed.

thinking and speech). *Negative* manifestations refer to the lack of usual emotional or social responses (blunted affect, avoidance of social contact, lack of attention to hygiene).

Schizophrenia affects at least 2.5 million people in the United States and about 1% of the world population.[24] As with other chronic illnesses such as cancer or heart disease, there are periods of exacerbation and remission. The devastating toll on clients and their families is not easily measured, but the financial cost each year in the United States for treatment, disability payment, and lost wages is approximately $48 billion.[24]

■ POSSIBLE CAUSES

In the 1960s, communication theorists and family therapists focused on disturbed patterns of communication in families with a schizophrenic member. They proposed that faulty communication and anxiety caused the illness and invented the term "schizophrenogenic mother."[32] This theory was never supported with controlled studies, but it had an unfortunate effect on therapeutic relationships with families. Many parents and family members felt blamed for their relative's illness and learned to distrust the mental health system.

Today, it is well recognized that schizophrenia is a biologic brain disorder. Repeated studies show a genetic influence, suggesting that the first-degree relatives of schizophrenics have 18.5 times the risk for the illness compared with relatives of controls.[7] CT and MRI scans have identified certain structural abnormalities in the brain, including enlargement of the ventricles and reduced size of the hippocampus.[24] The prefrontal cortex, which governs thinking and abstract mental functions, shows a decrease in the number of neurons and connections among regions.[15] It is not known whether these changes are caused by genetic, in utero, or environmental influences such as viruses, but research is ongoing.

Drug studies indicate that the neurotransmitter dopamine is implicated in schizophrenic manifestations. All of the medicines currently used for treatment are dopamine receptor blockers.[39] Dopamine is involved in mood and motivation and helps to regulate movement. Sophisticated PET scans can track the increased level of dopamine released in the brain at the same time that psychotic manifestations are observed.[34]

■ OUTCOME MANAGEMENT

The positive manifestations of schizophrenia can be controlled by antipsychotic medication, but the negative manifestations and severe social impairment require supportive psychotherapy. Antipsychotic medicines have been

BOX 20–8 Selected Standardized Tools for Assessment of Psychiatric Disorders

Psychiatric Disorder	Assessment Tool
Anxiety	Modified Spielberger State Anxiety Scale Sheehan Patient-Rated Anxiety Scale
Cognitive status	Mini-Mental State Examination (MMSE)
Depression	Beck Inventory Geriatric Depression Scale Hamilton's Depression Scale Zung Self-Report Inventory
Mania	Mania Rating Scale
Schizophrenia	Scale for Assessment of Negative Symptoms (SANS)
General functioning	Brief Psychiatric Rating Scale (BPRS) Global Assessment of Functioning Scale (GAF)

BOX 20–9 Psychosocial Dimension: Sexuality and Mental Illness

Issues related to sexuality may affect every client suffering with physical or mental illness, yet nurses often minimize or avoid this aspect of health. Human sexuality is broader than just physical sexual activity and includes gender identity, gender role, and sexual orientation. To provide holistic care, you must learn to be comfortable in promoting sexual health, "the physical and emotional state of well-being that enables us to enjoy and act on sexual feelings."*

Clients often worry about their sexual role following the effects of physical illness. There may be obvious disfigurement because of surgery or new activity restrictions resulting from compromised cardiac or respiratory status. Clients with mental illness may also suffer from altered sexual expression. In an effort to hide their feelings of anxiety or depression, some clients withdraw from intimate relationships. Loss of sexual desire is a frequent manifestation of depression, along with altered appetite and sleep. Even when clients acknowledge an emotional problem and seek treatment, they often complain of side effects from medication that alter their desire or performance.

Many clients do not volunteer their concerns but are eager to discuss questions when asked. One study showed that 76% of patients preferred the nurse to initiate discussion of sexual issues, but only 15% of the nurses included this in their assessment.[37] Common barriers that prevent nurses from exploring sexual issues include (1) not seeing the relevance to the admitting problem, (2) inadequate training, (3) embarrassment, and (4) fear of offending the client.

Sexual assessment refers to more than the client's sexual practices (see the Sexual Health Assessment tool in Chapter 37). The concepts of gender identity and gender role are important aspects. *Gender identity* refers to one's internal sense of being feminine or masculine, and *gender role* is the public expression of these beliefs. Attitudes about gender are learned in a specific sociocultural context. Learning takes place starting in early childhood in the home and in institutions such as school. By 3 years of age, children have an understanding of being male or female. Each family or community may have specific sexual values, with effects from religious and legal forces to control sexual expression.

Sexual orientation is another aspect of sexual health. About 90% of the population define themselves as *heterosexual* (preferring the opposite sex). Approximately 10% define themselves as *homosexual* (preferring the same-sex partner). A small number of people report themselves to be *bisexual* (interested in both sexes) or *transsexual* (feeling dissatisfied in their physical body because it does not match the internal view of their sexual identity).

To help the client communicate sexual concerns, the nurse must be competent in four areas: (1) knowledge about sexual function; (2) skills in assessment and intervention, including sex education and anticipatory guidance; (3) personal awareness of one's own values; and (4) awareness of the effect of one's attitude in delivering care. Becoming aware of your own values enables you to accept and respect the client's sexuality without imposing judgment. Sexual health issues should be considered part of the comprehensive nursing assessment, thus allowing clients to disclose their fears or questions in order to get resolution.

*See Edmisson (1997).[13]

used since the 1950s, and several classes of drugs have evolved over time in an effort to reduce unpleasant side effects (Box 20–11). These medications must be taken for a lifetime in order to control the manifestations. With medication, some clients report a total absence of hallucinations. For other clients, internal voices (auditory hallucinations) become a permanent experience. Not all voices or delusions are frightening; clients may learn to accept them as unusual but pleasant.

A major concern for most clients is the presence of side effects related to sedation and abnormal movements. Because typical antipsychotics target all dopamine receptors, including those affecting movement, muscle side effects known as *extrapyramidal symptoms* (EPS) are extremely common.[24] Manifestations of EPS may include stiffness or tremor in arms and legs, extreme restlessness with subjective discomfort, drooling, and acute muscle spasms of the tongue, neck, or face. These side effects are usually short-term and treatable with an anticholinergic agent such as benztropine or trihexyphenidyl. However, a long-term side effect of typical antipsychotics, called *tardive dyskinesia* (TD), occurs in approximately one third of clients and is usually irreversible. Common manifestations of TD are obvious, involuntary movements of the tongue, face, hands, or legs. The main benefit of the newer, atypical antipsychotics is the lower incidence of EPS and TD because the drugs are more selective in affecting neurotransmitters.

BOX 20–10 Types of Schizophrenia and Manifestations

Type	Manifestations
Paranoid	Presence of hallucinations and delusional thinking; fairly organized in speech and behavior, and may show some range in affect
Disorganized	Dominant manifestations of disorganized speech and behavior, with flat or inappropriate affect; may also have hallucinations and delusions
Catatonic	Presence of bizarre motor activity, either excessive and purposeless or immobilized as if in a stupor; may be mute or show incoherent speech
Undifferentiated	Presence of two or more of the following manifestations, but without a dominant feature as in the above three types: hallucinations, delusions, disorganized speech or behavior, and flat affect
Residual	Behavior does not show obvious hallucinations, delusions, or disorganization, but alterations persist in range of affect and thinking patterns

BOX 20–11 Medications for Schizophrenia

- Atypical antipsychotics
  - Clozapine
  - Olanzapine
  - Quetiapine
  - Risperidone
  - Ziprasidone
- Typical antipsychotics—phenothiazines
  - Chlorpromazine
  - Fluphenazine
  - Mesoridazine
  - Perphenazine
  - Thioridazine
  - Trifluoperazine
- Haloperidol
- Loxapine

One final side effect of typical antipsychotics should be noted. *Neuroleptic malignant syndrome* (NMS) is a rare but serious condition that may appear suddenly with extreme muscle rigidity, high fever, sweating, and fluctuations in consciousness. The client requires emergency hospitalization with supportive treatment to prevent seizures, coma, or even death.

Treatment of impaired social functioning involves long-term supportive therapy and psychosocial rehabilitation. Social withdrawal and lack of interest in school or work often signal the onset of the illness and may persist throughout treatment. To develop and maintain maximal level of functioning, schizophrenic clients need individual counseling and support, psychoeducation, organized rehabilitation services, and family psychoeducation.[32] Clients and families need education about the illness and coping skills to manage manifestations and prevent relapse. Rehabilitation efforts help the client complete basic schooling and learn job skills.

As with any chronic illness, the client experiences episodes of remission and exacerbation. Medication noncompliance, denial of illness, and stressful events may lead to multiple, short-term hospitalizations over a lifetime. With the consistent support of family and community resources, however, many clients can progress toward higher levels of independence and avoid long-term hospitalization.

■ INTERVENTION

Returning to the case of Mr. Barnes, the nurse immediately recognizes that the client has abnormal thinking (see Care Plan). The nurse notes that he is well groomed and shows appropriate social skills for the clinic environment; he demonstrates polite manners during the introduction. Uncertain about his reliability as a historian, the nurse asks Mr. Barnes whether his mother can be invited to join them as they complete his assessment and examination. He readily agrees.

Comprehensive Assessment

While completing the nursing assessment, the nurse evaluates the client's knowledge of his medical illness, his psychosocial functioning, and his current level of compliance with psychiatric care. Despite his bizarre speech, Mr. Barnes offers accurate dates and descriptions of his medical manifestations and doctor appointments. He shows some awareness of his diet and casually remarks, "I have this illness called schizophrenia. It makes me talk stupid sometimes." He firmly repeats his belief in the elves in the basement that talk to him at night and cause him to feel hungry all the time.

His mother adds that Mr. Barnes' mental illness was first diagnosed in his last year of high school. Before that, she had not noticed any problems. He had been a typical child who enjoyed school and was close to his older brother. He has been hospitalized 10 times for severe paranoia and hostile threats toward his family. The most recent stay was 6 months ago. He is compliant with his medication and has been going to the same psychiatrist for 5 years. Mr. Barnes expresses satisfaction with his doctor: "He is good. He tries to give me the right medicine, but sometimes it doesn't work."

Exploration of daily activities reveals that Mr. Barnes stays home with his mother, watching television, reading, and doing chores. He does not have any contact with peers and does not work. He states, "My brother and his friends don't like me anymore." His mother comments that his brother visits him regularly and tries to take him out, but sometimes the client refuses to go. She adds that he tried to work once at a "fast food" restaurant, but people made fun of him. Now she does not allow him to go outdoors alone.

Communication Awareness

Throughout the interview, the nurse takes care to include Mr. Barnes in the conversation even though his mother tends to dominate. The nurse maintains a calm facial expression when the client discusses his delusions and respectfully records his answers. No attempt is made to challenge the reality of his remarks, but the nurse does not communicate agreement with his distortions. The nurse is also careful not to invade the client's personal space, explaining all physical procedures and asking for permission before touching him.

Client and Family Teaching

Although the client and his mother seem to be familiar with the term *schizophrenia,* it is not clear how much teaching they have received about managing the illness. Neither mother nor son is involved in a community support group, and the client is socially isolated without any prospect of increased independence because of his mother's overprotective stance. Before giving them material about hiatal hernia, the nurse asks whether they would like to read more about schizophrenia. They both are interested. The nurse explains that schizophrenia is a chronic illness that can be controlled and praises the client for his knowledge of his medication and medical care. As Mr. Barnes proudly gathers up all of the teaching materials to take home, his mother smiles and says, "He always was a good reader."

Specialized Referrals

Before setting up the next clinic appointment, the nurse considers whether any other mental health resource is indicated. Mr. Barnes is in remission at this time, showing compliance with medications and monthly psychiatrist

C A R E   P L A N

THE CLIENT WITH HIATAL HERNIA AND CONCURRENT SCHIZOPHRENIA: MR. BARNES

Nursing Diagnosis. Altered thought processes and altered perception, as evidenced by auditory hallucinations and delusions related to paranoid schizophrenia.

Outcomes. Mr. Barnes will establish trust with the nurse and agree to return to the medical clinic, he and his mother will accept referral to the psychiatric clinical specialist to promote access to community resources, and he will remain in the community with outpatient services, which will help him develop to his maximal functioning (long term).

Interventions	**Rationales**
1. Assess for current compliance with psychiatric care and history of aggressive or self-destructive behavior.	1. Successful outcomes with medical condition depend on psychiatric stability; when decompensating, a schizophrenic client distorts reality and may become threatening to others or self.
2. Assess for current level of psychosocial functioning.	2. Chronic mental illness impairs social and vocational functioning even when target manifestations are under control.
3. Assess Mr. Barnes' mother's knowledge of the illness and impact on the family.	3. Families may alter their entire structure around an ill member, cutting off outside support.
4. Ask the client's permission before touching him for physical procedures.	4. A client with schizophrenia may misinterpret actions by strangers and become defensive.
5. Respond to the reality aspects of the client's speech.	5. The client is still cognitively intact and shows readiness to learn new information despite delusions.
6. Describe the role of the psychiatric nurse as just another member of the health care team.	6. The familiar environment of the medical clinic will help to reduce the client's anxiety about a new mental health provider.

Evaluation. Accomplishment of the expected outcomes will require time and a trusting relationship with the clinic nurse. Reassessment must be ongoing, with revision in the plan as necessary.

appointments; however, he feels stigmatized and has not accomplished the developmental tasks of young adulthood. He is totally dependent on his mother and experiences repeated relapses with his current living situation. To promote the best overall health outcomes for Mr. Barnes, the nurse must consider *tertiary prevention* with regard to his mental illness. (See Chapter 1 for a review of primary, secondary, and tertiary prevention.) The nurse sees that he needs additional professional support, such as participation in a structured day program, or even a part-time job to attain his maximal level of community functioning.

The nurse recommends a referral to the psychiatric clinical specialist in the outpatient clinic at the medical center. The purpose of referral is to explore community resources to support Mr. Barnes and his family. To increase the probability of their follow-up with an appointment, the nurse offers to introduce them to the psychiatric nurse at their next clinic visit. They hesitantly agree. The nurse calls the clinical specialist, who explains that one of several referrals can be made for Mr. Barnes: to a young adult supportive therapy group, a psychosocial rehabilitation program, or a mental health support group for clients and families. The clinical specialist will also call the attending psychiatrist to coordinate the treatment plan.

MOOD DISORDERS

Mrs. Conners, Mr. Moore, and Miss Howard represent clients with various mood disorders. Mood disorders are classified into three major categories: (1) Depressive Disorders, (2) bipolar disorder (formerly called manic depressive illness), and (3) Mood Disorder due to General Medical Condition or Substance Use.[3] Manifestations of all depressions include a sad mood, which may be accompanied by crying spells; persistent negative thinking with hopelessness; possible suicidal thinking; decreased energy and motivation; and changes in sleep, appetite, and sexual interest.

In clients with bipolar disorder, mood can fluctuate from depression to the other extreme, mania. *Manic symptoms* include excessive cheerfulness or irritability; an unrealistic, optimistic attitude toward one's accomplishments; overabundance of energy; and decreased sleep with increased physical appetite. Box 20–12 describes mood states.[12]

The key element in mood disorders is that the person cannot control the severity of the feeling. There may or may not be a clear precipitant for the reaction. Unlike a healthy person with transient mood changes, a depressed person cannot "just get over it" and the client with mania does not wish to give up the euphoria that characterizes this mood.

Up to 15% of adults may suffer from a mood disorder at any given time, and more than 4 million Americans may have a major depressive disorder. The age of onset is usually in the 20s and 30s, and the recurrent nature of the illness impacts productivity and quality of life. Up to 70% of the people with depression experience a relapse. Women are two times more likely to have depression, but bipolar illness affects men and women equally.[28]

Mood disorders frequently co-occur with other psychiatric or medical illnesses. Clients may show depression

BOX 20–12 Manifestations of Mood Disorders

Depression (major or bipolar)

Sad mood, but may be irritable
Crying spells
Negative thinking, continuously pessimistic
Feelings of guilt and hopelessness
Preoccupation with usually minor somatic complaints
Loss of pleasure in usual activities and decreased socialization
Decreased ability to concentrate and remember current events
Decreased energy level
Change in sleep, increased or decreased
Change in appetite, increased or decreased
Decreased libido and sexual activity
May feel suicidal
May develop psychosis with delusions about a negative future, e.g., fatal illness

Mania

Elated mood, not attributable to a reality event
Denial of having an emotional problem
Impulsive acts that may be dangerous or socially inappropriate, e.g., promiscuity
Increased energy level
Increased socialization to the point of becoming intrusive
Excessive, rapid speech
Change in appetite, increased or decreased
Decreased need for sleep
Increased libido

with substance abuse, an anxiety disorder, or an eating disorder. Medical problems often associated with depression include stroke, diabetes, coronary artery disease, cancer, chronic fatigue syndrome, and fibromyalgia.[35] Some prescription drugs cause depressed mood as a side effect (see Table 20–4.) Whenever depressive manifestations are mixed with somatic (physical) complaints, close collaboration between a psychiatrist and primary care provider is necessary to clarify the correct diagnosis and treatment plan.

The most serious adverse outcome for mood disorders is suicide. Take all verbal expressions of suicide intent or threat seriously and act accordingly (see later in this chapter). Up to 15% of clients who are hospitalized for major depression eventually commit suicide. For clients with bipolar disorder, 10% to 15% of untreated clients commit suicide, 20 times the rate in the general population.[35] The period of greatest risk is during psychiatric hospitalization or just after release. There are known risk factors associated with suicide in the United States (see Box 20–13).[36] Older adults are at special risk; each year, more than 6300 older adults commit suicide. White men over age 80 years have the highest suicide rate. It is notable that 75% of these older suicide victims have visited their primary care physician within the month preceding their death.[9] Chapter 3 discusses depression in older people.

■ POSSIBLE CAUSES

As with anxiety and schizophrenia, there is no clear cause of mood disorders. Biologic and psychodynamic theories are offered to explain the illness, and the answer is probably a combination of both. From the biologic point of view, there are several significant findings from research. First, the genetic influence is undeniable: 25% of clients with major depression and 50% of clients with bipolar disorder have a relative with a mood disorder. Evidence from studies of families with multiple affected members indicates sections of chromosomes 6 and 11 are linked to bipolar illness.[28]

Twin and adoption studies support a genetic link.[12] Children of parents with affective (mood) illness who are adopted into families without a history of affective disorder show three times as many depressive disorders as biologic children in the same family. Twin studies reveal that genes are not the sole cause of affective illness. With identical twins, if one twin has an affective illness, the chance of a disorder developing in the other twin ranges from 50% to 90%. Thus, other biologic or environmental factors must interact with the genetic predisposition.

Data from antidepressant drug studies point to abnormalities in the level of neurotransmitters and other brain chemicals. Antidepressant drugs bring about increased levels of serotonin or norepinephrine.[17] Research with lithium for bipolar disorder indicates that it corrects an imbalance in the compound glutamate.[16] In 1998, a brain chemical called substance P was identified with mood regulation, and drug manufacturers are developing new antidepressants to block its receptors.[19]

Abnormalities in brain structure or in the endocrine system can also lead to depression. People with brain damage from Parkinson's disease, Huntington's disease, or stroke often experience depression. Similarly, people with hypothyroidism or Cushing's disease are at risk for depression.[28]

There are multiple psychodynamic explanations for depression.[31] Historically, the *psychoanalytic view* considers depression as internalized anger about the loss of a loved person or an object with symbolic meaning. It is triggered by the loss of something or someone for whom the person felt ambivalence, a mixture of positive and negative feelings. *Object loss theory* postulates that a person is predisposed to depression because of early, traumatic separation from a loved one during childhood. Thereafter, every separation in adult life recalls the initial reaction. More recently, *cognitive theory* suggests that the person has distorted thinking that defines the world in a negative way. Any disappointment or painful experience is blamed on one's own shortcomings, and life experiences reinforce a self-image of inadequacy.

BOX 20–13 Risk Factors for Suicide

Depressed mood
Psychosis
Hopelessness
Serious medical disorder
Substance abuse
Male gender
Caucasian race
Family history of substance abuse
Living alone
Previous attempted suicide

The behaviorists use *social learning theory* to explain depression.[31] People constantly receive feedback or reinforcement as they interact with their environment (people or events). Positive reinforcement makes a person repeat behaviors and generally feels like a reward. Lack of positive reinforcement leads a person to feel sad and starts a cycle of increasing withdrawal from social interaction. For example, lack of rewards from friendships or work decreases a person's attempts to try new social situations, further decreasing the opportunity for positive experiences. Even though medications may be needed to address altered neurotransmitters, therapists still use a theoretical model to guide their therapy to help clients examine and revise behavior that has been affected by the biochemicals.

OUTCOME MANAGEMENT

Mood disorders can almost always be managed effectively through a combination of medication and psychotherapy. In some cases, electroconvulsive therapy may be indicated. Antidepressant medication may be needed for up to 1 year or for a lifetime, depending on the client's potential for relapse.[36] Particularly for bipolar disorder, mood stabilizers may be needed for long-term treatment.[6] Several classes of antidepressant drugs affect neurotransmitters in different ways (see Box 20–14). If a client does not respond to the medication after a fair trial, the physician may switch to another class or try a combination. Antidepressants and mood stabilizers do not produce effects immediately, as the anti-anxiety drugs do. Thus, the depressed client often suffers for 3 to 6 more weeks when starting treatment. Hopelessness about treatment, especially if the first medication is ineffective, compounds the risk for suicide.

Several types of psychotherapy may be helpful for mood disorders. In all cases, client education is important to explain the course of the illness and the benefits of treatment despite the delay in improvement. Often, short-term therapy is beneficial with a focus on learning to manage current stressors and relationships. Marital therapy may be indicated because a mood disorder frequently causes marital discord, and conflict with loved ones often precipitates a depressive episode.[36]

Electroconvulsive therapy (ECT) is a viable treatment alternative for some clients with depression and may be provided in an inpatient or outpatient setting. An electrical shock is administered to a specific region of the brain to induce a seizure. General anesthesia is required, and the client does not remember the experience. The mechanism of action is not entirely understood but its effect on the neurotransmitter receptors may be similar to that of the tricyclic antidepressants. The client experiences short-term memory loss, but improvement is faster than with medication treatment.[28]

Although it is not usually a first-line treatment, ECT may be superior to medication under the following circumstances: psychotic manifestations with active suicidal risk; severe psychomotor retardation and vegetative symptoms; lack of response to multiple medication trials; and concurrent medical condition that poses a serious risk with psychotropic medicines.[36]

The discussion that follows illustrates the variety of manifestations found with mood disorders.

BOX 20–14 Medications for Mood Disorders

Antidepressants

Monoamine Oxidase Inhibitors (MAOIs)

Isocarboxazid
Phenelzine
Tranylcypromine

Selective Serotonin Reuptake Inhibitors (SSRIs)

Citalopram
Fluoxetine
Fluvoxamine
Paroxetine
Sertraline
Trazodone

Tricyclics

Amitriptyline
Clomipramine
Desipramine
Doxepin
Imipramine
Nortriptyline

Other

Bupropion
Methylphenidate
Mirtazapine
Nefazodone
Reboxetine
Venlafaxine

Anti-manic agents

Carbamazepine
Gabapentin
Lamotrigine
Lithium
Valproic acid

INTERVENTION: MAJOR DEPRESSION

After meeting Mrs. Conners (in diabetic ketoacidosis), the nurse is concerned about two major problems. First, the client's mental status appears altered and she is in distress. Second, the average length of stay for this medical diagnosis is only 1 more day, and much teaching must be done before discharge. Returning to the nursing database, the nurse notes that the psychosocial section is incomplete. It is documented that the client is a native West Indian, lives with her daughter, and has a history of major depression. She has been hospitalized three times in the past year, twice on the psychiatric unit and once for ketoacidosis (see Care Plan).

COMPREHENSIVE ASSESSMENT

The nurse decides to attempt completion of the psychosocial history, even though Mrs. Conners may not be spontaneously verbal. The assessment is explained to the client, and she is asked whether her daughter may also be contacted. Mrs. Conners agrees and states that her daughter will be visiting at lunch time. She speaks in a soft voice, with just a few words at a time, and the nurse

CARE PLAN

THE CLIENT WITH DIABETIC KETOACIDOSIS AND CONCURRENT DEPRESSION: MRS. CONNERS

Nursing Diagnosis. Altered thought processes with self-care deficit, as evidenced by sad mood, tearfulness, and decreased grooming and eating related to depression.

Outcomes. Mrs. Conners will cooperate with the evaluation by her psychiatrist, will agree to a safe discharge from the medical unit to an appropriate level of psychiatric care, and will be able to return to her previous level of function and remain at home with her daughter (long term).

Interventions	Rationales
1. Assess psychological and physical effects of low mood, including suicidal thoughts, and effect on diabetes management.	1. Depression causes sleep and eating disturbance, and risk of suicide must always be evaluated; irregular sleep and eating patterns affect ability to safely manage glucose levels and insulin regimen.
2. Assess the previous level of functioning and pattern of medication compliance.	2. Prior treatment history can be used to reassure the client about this episode; medication noncompliance is the major cause of relapse.
3. Accept family input regarding the client's dress and food preferences.	3. Acceptance shows respect for the client's cultural needs and promotes collaboration with the family.
4. Teach about depression and the medications, offering as a review in view of long history.	4. Teaching emphasizes that no stigma is attached to the client because of mental illness and offers hope for the current episode.
5. Explain the role of the utilization review coordinator to coordinate a safe discharge plan.	5. Contact with team members is necessary for a timely, appropriate discharge plan for complex clients.

Evaluation. Accomplishment of these expected outcomes will ensure that the client receives adequate services upon discharge from acute medical care.

notices a slight accent. The client says that she has had diabetes for 15 years and depression for 35 years, since the birth of her daughter. She has been going to the same psychiatrist for 20 years and asks the nurse to notify him. When asked about her medication, Mrs. Conners knows the name and dosage of all four (two antidepressant and two antipsychotic agents) and admits that she occasionally misses a dose. She does not have suicidal thoughts and has never attempted suicide.

The client describes her mood as sad, and she becomes tearful. She states that she gets along fine with her daughter and then abruptly says that she is too tired to talk to the nurse anymore. The nurse defers the rest of the interview until the daughter arrives. When the nurse returns at lunch time, she finds Mrs. Conners dressed in a long gown and wearing a colorful turban wrapped around her hair. Her daughter is coaxing her to eat some homemade soup, and she is refusing the hospital food. The daughter mentions that she suspected that her mother was depressed again but that she did not expect her to become this sick. The client has a pattern of medication noncompliance, followed by diet noncompliance with overeating, which results in rehospitalization. The daughter explains that she is aware of the client's 1800-calorie diet, but she works and the client is alone during the day. When she is well, the client enjoys cooking and dressing according to her native custom.

COMMUNICATION AWARENESS

During the interview, the nurse is careful to respect Mrs. Conners' low energy level. The nurse uses questions that require only short answers and speaks clearly and softly. When the client talks about feeling sad, the nurse does not try to cheer her up but reminds her that her depression has been successfully treated in the past.

After the input from the daughter, the nurse realizes how important the client's cultural background is for the care plan (see Box 20–15). In the West Indian culture, an older person may be uncomfortable around authority figures and may avoid eye contact. Respect and good manners are important; people expect to be greeted with "Good morning" or "Good afternoon" and are always addressed by the last name. Privacy is important, and personal issues are discussed only with family members. Mental illness is seen as a weakness and carries a strong stigma. Elderly parents are usually cared for at home by an adult daughter. Food tastes are very specific, and home-brewed teas are considered medicinal.[21] At the end of the conversation, the nurse compliments Mrs. Conners on her appearance and does not try to interrupt the daughter feeding her the homemade soup.

CLIENT AND FAMILY TEACHING

Although the client and her daughter openly discuss the diagnosis of depression, the nurse emphasizes that this is a medical illness that can be treated just like the diabetes. The fact that the client takes multiple medications suggests that this depression is probably difficult to control. Reassurance may be needed about another possible change in medication or dosage. The nurse collects information on depression, the medications, and community support groups. This information is given to the client and her daughter to review and see whether they have any questions.

SPECIALIZED REFERRALS

As soon as the nurse observes that the depression is complicating the client's medical condition, the discharge

BOX 20–15 Psychosocial Dimension: Culture and Mental Illness

Cultural background plays an important role in a person's perception of illness and participation in treatment. *Culture* is defined as the beliefs, values, patterns of behavior, customs, and language of a group of people. To provide holistic care, nurses must be sensitive to the cultural needs of clients, and must be aware of their own cultural perspective.

Nurses need to understand several concepts regarding culture. *Cultural diversity* refers to the difference between different groups of people (e.g., from different countries or even different regions of one country). *Cultural imposition* is the process of the dominant culture imposing its beliefs on a less dominant group. *Cultural sensitivity* is an awareness and acceptance of different cultures.

As you encounter clients from various cultures, it is important to be aware of both Western and non-Western health care beliefs. In American society, the following ideas are taken for granted:

- Illness is considered to have a specific cause that is discoverable and treatable.
- It is important to prevent or reduce signs of illness, and there is a focus on wellness promotion.
- Clients are seen as partly responsible for their health behavior and partly as victims of disease.
- People value cleanliness and are time-conscious, expecting immediate or rapid relief from discomfort.
- The physician is the primary practitioner who treats illness.

In non-Western cultures, illness is defined by personalistic or naturalistic viewpoints. In the *personalistic* view, illness is caused by an agent, such as a deity, ghost, or witch, and is seen as a punishment or attack. In the *naturalistic* framework, illness is due to a failure in equilibrium among opposing elements. For example, Latin Americans believe in four humors, or fluids, in the body: blood (hot and moist), phlegm (cold and moist), black bile (cold and dry), and yellow bile or choler (hot and dry). Major body organs must possess certain quantities of dry, moist, hot, and cold fluids in order to be healthy. Illness is caused by disequilibrium of these forces and is treated through foods and other means to restore balance. People seek out indigenous (local or native) healers as the primary practitioner.

In providing holistic care to clients of different cultures, be sensitive to their needs and avoid cultural imposition (see cultural assessment as part of health assessment in Chapter 9). Ask clients and their families to explain their specific needs. Whenever possible, incorporate client and family customs into the treatment plan, such as dietary preferences. If there are significant points of conflict, carefully explain the clinical rationale and convey respect for the client's choices about treatment. In addition to these nursing interventions, help link the client to community resources with similar cultural background in order to reduce feelings of isolation in our predominantly Western culture.

planner/utilization review coordinator is contacted along with the attending physician. Discharge planning for Mrs. Conners requires a coordinated effort between medical and psychiatric clinicians. The client has already asked that her psychiatrist be called, and the attending physician asks the discharge planner to arrange for a consultation.

When the discharge planner calls the psychiatrist, he states that he can visit the client this evening. He adds that he may need to transfer her to the psychiatric unit because she has a history of becoming psychotic when she relapses, refusing to eat or care for herself. The nurse introduces the discharge planner to the client and her daughter and explains the role: to ensure a timely, appropriate discharge plan that considers all of the client's needs before returning home. When Mrs. Conners hears that her psychiatrist is coming to see her, she smiles and her daughter looks relieved. The daughter states, "Maybe he will admit her to the psych unit. She always gets better there."

INTERVENTION: DEPRESSION

After being notified by the physical therapist about Mr. Moore's condition (second stroke), the home care nurse makes an appointment and reviews the nursing and physical therapy database. The nurse recalls that Mr. Moore quickly recovered from his first stroke with minimal residual symptoms. He had returned to his previous level of function, such as driving and doing chores (see Care Plan).

When the nurse arrives at the home, Mr. Moore is sitting in the living room with the shades drawn. As the nurse starts to say that the therapist is concerned about his status, he gruffly states, "I won't use that stupid walker. What good is it to walk like a cripple?" The nurse notes that he looks thinner, and the chart shows that he refused to allow the aide to shave him this morning. Mrs. Moore calls the nurse into the kitchen and bursts into tears, saying, "I don't know what's wrong with him. He is so negative about everything. He was never like this before."

COMPREHENSIVE ASSESSMENT

The nurse decides to repeat the entire nursing assessment. Physically, there is no improvement in Mr. Moore's walking or balance compared with 6 weeks ago. He has lost 5 pounds and blames the loss on his wife's "lousy cooking." He reports that he cannot sleep at night because the sofa is uncomfortable and he cannot go upstairs to his bedroom. He refuses to allow the therapist to order a hospital bed for downstairs.

When the nurse asks about his mood, Mr. Moore pauses and says, "What does it matter?" When the nurse persists, he finally says that he feels useless. He cannot perform any of his previous activities or household responsibilities. Knowing that he and his wife used to attend church regularly, the nurse asks whether he has tried to go out or have the minister visit. Mr. Moore snorts and says, "I'm never going back there. At first I prayed, but what good did it do?" Noting these signs of spiritual distress, the nurse further assesses his beliefs and feelings about spirituality. See Box 20–16 for a guide to spirituality and Alternative Therapy: Spirituality and Health earlier.[33]

CARE PLAN

THE CLIENT WITH STROKE AND CONCURRENT DEPRESSION: MR. MOORE

Nursing Diagnosis. Hopelessness with risk of self-directed violence, as evidenced by depressed mood and passive death wish related to loss of independence due to stroke.

Outcomes. Mr. Moore will agree to a no-harm contract, will accept referral for more intensive evaluation and treatment of his depression, will experience improved mood, and will cooperate with his physical therapist to attain maximal rehabilitation goals (long term).

Interventions	Rationales
1. Assess for psychological and physical signs of depression, including suicidal thoughts.	1. Depression is a common complication with stroke and can interfere with physical rehabilitation.
2. Assess risk for suicide and ability to contract for safety; inform the wife.	2. Older, white men with concurrent medical problems are at high risk for suicide, and emergency department referral may be required.
3. Listen nonjudgmentally as the client expresses anger about loss and abandonment by God.	3. Listening shows acceptance of the client's feelings of distress and may reduce the client's feelings of guilt.
4. Expect the client to make decisions and take responsibility for treatment.	4. The nurse's confidence in the client shows respect for his abilities and counteracts feelings of helplessness and powerlessness.
5. Teach that depression is a treatable illness and about the need for regular eating, sleeping, and exercise.	5. Teaching offers information and hope that the current condition can be improved with the client's active participation.
6. Explain roles of the psychiatric nurse, social worker, and physical therapist to assist in his fullest recovery.	6. Multidisciplinary services are required for this client to prevent self-harm and promote recovery.

Evaluation. Accomplishment of the expected outcomes will establish a plan for safety and offer the best opportunity for physical and emotional healing.

BOX 20–16 Psychosocial Dimension: Spirituality and Mental Illness

Spirituality is a significant aspect of humanness made up of values and beliefs about the meaning and purpose of life and may or may not include a specific religion. Suffering experienced with physical or mental illness often leads a person to question beliefs about God or a higher power; such distress can have a serious effect on recovery. As part of holistic care, assess spiritual needs in order to support the client's internal forces for healing.

Spirituality is more than religion. A religion is an organized set of practices based on specific beliefs. The human spiritual dimension is closely linked to the mind and body. When one part of the system is jeopardized, by illness for example, the other parts are also affected. When clients suffer intense, persistent pain or experience hopelessness and despair, they may begin to doubt their former spiritual support system. This state of uncertainty weakens one's resolve to improve or to survive the stressful situation.

To assist the client through this crisis, you must be able to recognize and intervene in spiritual distress. As a nursing diagnosis, Spiritual Distress is defined by expressions of anger toward a deity or questions related to the meaning of suffering. Collect the following data in a spirituality assessment.*

Subjective

- Does the client verbalize feelings about God or spiritual concerns?
- Does the client feel the illness has changed feelings about God?
- Does the client feel abandoned or separated from spiritual support?
- Does the client question the validity of faith and the religious system?
- Does the client say that the illness is a punishment from God?

Objective

- Does the client pray or read religious material?
- Does the client keep religious material nearby (e.g., rosary, medal)?
- Does the client refuse to participate in spiritual or religious rituals?

The interventions for Spiritual Distress sound simple. Provide support through active listening (i.e., giving full attention and time to accept the client's verbal and nonverbal communication). By showing patience and concern, you can encourage clients to explore their feelings and questions. At the same time, be aware of your own spiritual beliefs and be careful not to impose these on the client. Finally, encourage the client and family to seek support from the appropriate clergy person or spiritual leader of their choice.

*See Edmisson (1997).[13]

In view of his depressed mood, hopelessness, and spiritual isolation, the nurse asks whether Mr. Moore has had any thoughts about hurting himself or ending his life. Initially, he looks away and refuses to answer. But then he admits he has dreams about his death, and he thinks his wife would be better off without him.

Communication Awareness

When talking with Mr. Moore, the nurse is careful not to react to his negative comments or irritable mood. The nurse asks about physical or emotional issues in a matter-of-fact tone of voice. In response to his pattern of avoiding a direct answer, the nurse rephrases the question and waits for a response. Noting that Mr. Moore may feel uncomfortable talking in front of his wife, the nurse asks her to wait in the kitchen during the interview.

When Mr. Moore states that he has thoughts of death, the nurse calmly asks specific questions to assess the risk for suicide (Box 20–17). Because the client verbally promises that he will not take action to harm himself (a verbal contract for safety), the nurse does not take emergency action.

Client and Family Teaching

Because Mr. Moore and his wife report no history of mental illness in the family, it is clear that they have no experience with mood disorders. The nurse defines the manifestations of depression and how depression can affect a person physically, emotionally, and spiritually. The nurse describes the effect on the family when one member is depressed. It is noted that depression often affects people who have suffered a stroke and that it is highly treatable. Briefly, the nurse explains medication and counseling treatment options and offers the home care resources of the psychiatric nurse and the social worker. Mr. Moore continues to say that nothing will help, but his wife requests assistance.

Specialized Referrals

Before leaving the house, the nurse telephones the attending physician to report the findings and to request orders. The psychiatric nurse will further evaluate the client, offer psychoeducation, and monitor the effectiveness of medication treatment. The social worker will evaluate the need for community resources and make the necessary referrals. The physician is surprised because he had not seen the signs of depression, but he is cooperative and asks that the team members report their findings to him.

The nurse contacts the office to arrange for the referrals. Both the psychiatric nurse and the social worker are informed of Mr. Moore's passive death wish and contract for safety. The nurse also informs them of his spiritual distress at this time, since spirituality can play a significant role in physical and psychological healing. After all the arrangements are made, the nurse calls Mr. Moore to tell him of the dates for their visits. He is pessimistic but agrees to talk with them. Later, the nurse also calls the physical therapist to explain the change in treatment plan and the need to continue physical therapy despite the client's depression.

■ INTERVENTION: BIPOLAR DISORDER

Upon hearing the staff complaints about Miss Howard (dehydration with change in behavior), the nurse again reviews the medical record. It is noted that the client was admitted to the facility 2 years ago because she was unable to manage her multiple medications for heart failure. Miss Howard also has digestive problems, with a

BOX 20–17 Screening Assessment of Suicidal Risk

Interview Questions

1. Have you been thinking about death or hurting yourself?
2. If yes, do you have a plan?
3. Have you ever tried to hurt yourself before?
4. If yes, what did you do?
5. What would stop you from hurting yourself now?
6. Can you sign a written contract with me that you will not harm yourself for the next ________ (time period until next evaluation)?

Additional Indications of Higher Risk for Suicide

1. Has a specific plan that is available and dangerous (e.g., hanging, shooting, or jumping from a high location)
2. History of previous attempts
3. Cannot identify person or religious belief that would prevent action
4. Refusal to sign a safety contract
5. Living alone or estranged from loved ones
6. Use of alcohol or drugs
7. Presence of psychosis with command hallucinations to harm self (cannot safely contract)

Results of Screening

1. If the client shows no positive risk factors, no action is necessary except continued monitoring of behavior.
2. If the client shows positive risk factors but agrees to a written contract not to harm self, the nurse:
   a. Co-signs the contract, defining the time period from now until the next visit
   b. Notifies the attending physician (e.g., by telephone) in front of the client to report the assessment and request a psychiatric nurse evaluation; if the physician orders other actions, these are shared with the client
   c. Strongly seeks the client's permission to share the contract with a family member, if available
   d. Contacts the psychiatric nurse to give a report and schedule a visit for the following day
3. If the client shows positive risk factors but refuses to sign a "no harm contract," the nurse must take emergency action. The nurse:
   a. Instructs the client, and family if available, that this condition is a mental health emergency and requires immediate evaluation by a physician in an emergency department
   b. Calls 911 for assistance, explaining that there is a psychiatric emergency
   c. Provides brief information to the police and emergency medical team upon arrival, with a follow-up telephone report to the appropriate emergency department
   d. Notifies the attending physician of the emergency actions

CARE PLAN

THE CLIENT WITH DEHYDRATION AND CONCURRENT BIPOLAR DISORDER: MISS HOWARD

Nursing Diagnosis. Altered Thought Processes with risk for violence directed at others, as evidenced by agitation, verbal threats toward others related to bipolar disorder, and mania.

Outcomes. Miss Howard will not harm self or others, will eat three small meals and drink adequate fluids daily, will sleep at least 6 hours each night, will experience a stabilized mood, and will return to her previous level of functioning (long term).

Interventions	Rationales
1. Assess for mood, nutrition, sleep, and activity level.	1. Clients in a manic phase disregard sleep and food, and their hyperactivity places them at risk for physical complications.
2. Assess for safety and assign staff to observe the client; move her roommate to another room temporarily.	2. The client has decreased impulse control and the potential to hurt others or self.
3. Reduce stimuli, and assign one staff member to offer food and fluids frequently.	3. One consistent staff member reduces the opportunity for staff conflict and supports adequate nutrition.
4. Accept verbalization of anger, but set limits on cursing and aggression.	4. Letting the client "ventilate" and setting limits show acceptance of the client's feelings and maintain safety for the client and others.
5. Maintain privacy and prevent socially inappropriate behavior.	5. The client needs assistance to preserve her dignity while she has decreased control of impulses.
6. Involve the client in her plan of care, offering realistic choices in the daily schedule.	6. This step promotes the client's responsibility for self and counteracts her feelings of fear and helplessness.
7. Coordinate communication among staff and family members regarding the plan of care.	7. The client has impaired communication skills and may distort information from caregivers.

Evaluation. Accomplishment of the expected outcomes will preserve the safety of the client, peers, and staff. Reassessment must be made daily, and plan will need revision in first week if not effective.

family history of pancreatic cancer. Her recent hospitalization was related to uncontrolled diarrhea with dehydration. Apparently, her psychotropic medications were discontinued at the acute care hospital and she has not received them in 8 days. Her diagnosis list shows a history of bipolar disorder (see Care Plan).

The psychosocial history is sparse except to note that she lived alone before admission and has never been married. A niece is listed as the next of kin, and staff members report that she visits monthly. She received outpatient psychiatric treatment and has current orders for valproic acid and lithium. The nursing home psychiatric consultant visits monthly.

When the nurse interviews Miss Howard, the client is pacing around her room wearing only her nightgown. She has a large bruise over her right eye from falling out of bed. The chart shows that she has slept 2 to 4 hours for the past three nights. Before the nurse can greet her, Miss Howard says loudly, "I'm glad you are here. These dumb staff of yours can't even get my breakfast right. I want another roommate; that old bag snores. Call the hairdresser. I need my hair done." Her speech is rapid, and her tone of voice is insulting. This behavior is unlike that of her baseline assessment; she tends to be outgoing, with a sarcastic sense of humor, and neatly groomed.

Comprehensive Assessment

In view of the significant change in behavior, the nurse updates the nursing assessment. When the nurse tells Miss Howard that she would like to talk about her recent hospitalization, the client eagerly offers her a chair. As the nurse asks about her current mood and activities, the client talks incessantly and frequently interrupts. She does not always answer the question, but from her speech and nonverbal behavior, the nurse gathers the following information. Miss Howard says she feels scared, lonely, and misunderstood. She fears that she has pancreatic cancer and does not trust that the doctors have ordered the right tests. She starts to cry as she describes her niece, who does not visit as often as she once did. She gives numerous complaints about the staff and her roommate and threatens to hit her roommate the next time she snores.

When asked about her psychiatric history, Miss Howard is vague about her problem and complains that even the psychiatrist does not come to see her anymore. She knows that she takes two psychotropic medications but does not know their names. Seeing that the client is an unreliable historian, the nurse asks permission to call her niece for information. Miss Howard agrees and tells the nurse to order her niece to buy her five more robes.

The niece is surprised to hear about Miss Howard's behavior. She reports that her aunt has been stable for years while taking her medication for bipolar disorder. She states that the client has a history of mood swings and becomes very irritable and demanding in the manic phase. Miss Howard has received outpatient psychiatric treatment for 40 years, and the nursing home psychiatrist observes her monthly. The nurse notes that the client was hospitalized when her monthly appointment was due this month. The niece promises to visit the next day and asks the nurse to notify the psychiatrist.

Before calling the psychiatrist, the nurse informs the attending physician about the client's status. The physician agrees that her behavior is altered but refuses to order any psychotropic medication, referring her to the psychiatrist. The nurse consults with the psychiatrist, who immediately orders resumption of lithium and valproic acid, with blood levels to be assessed in 1 week. A sleeping medication is also ordered for 1 week. The psychiatrist speculates that Miss Howard suffered a manic relapse because of the stress of hospitalization and lack of medication. He asks the nurse to reduce stimuli for the client to maintain her safety and the safety of others.

Communication Awareness

When communicating with Miss Howard, the nurse pays close attention to verbal and nonverbal behavior in order to avoid escalation of tension in the client. As the client talks rapidly and sometimes raises her voice, the nurse maintains a calm tone of voice and normal speed. When Miss Howard approaches the nurse too closely, the nurse moves beyond arm's reach and sets a limit on personal space. Even though the client does not seem to pose a high risk for physical harm, the nurse firmly tells her that physical aggression toward peers or staff will not be tolerated. (Miss Howard had verbally threatened her roommate.)

At the same time, the nurse acknowledges Miss Howard's fear and responds to the legitimate complaints. The nurse explains each diagnostic test and the negative results. The nurse listens seriously to the client's concerns about cold food and her roommate interfering with her sleep. The nurse suggests that part of the client's distress is due to a relapse in her mood disorder and expresses hope that she will feel better once her medications are resumed.

At the end of the interview, the nurse helps Miss Howard to put on her robe, slippers, and underwear. Together, they write a plan for the client's schedule for the rest of the day, including meals, medication, and exercise. The nurse explicitly directs Miss Howard not to threaten or hit anyone and gives her a notebook in which to write down any new complaints. The nurse promises to return at the end of the shift to reevaluate the plan.

Client and Family Teaching

The nurse believes that Miss Howard is not amenable to comprehending her illness while she is in a manic condition. Responding to the client's sleep complaint, the nurse shows her teaching materials on her medications. The nurse uses brief, simple terms to describe the desired therapeutic effects of the medication and leaves the material with the client to review.

In a 24-hour care facility, caregivers need the same information that would be given to family members in the community. Especially if physical violence is threatened, the nursing staff must have clear guidelines about communication techniques to reduce agitation. Staff members must know that the client is showing manifestations of her mental illness and that she temporarily does not have adequate impulse control. They must be cautioned not to argue with her or laugh at her behavior. It is likely that the client will recall some of her behavior and will feel guilty and embarrassed later. Efforts to preserve her dignity are just as important as attention to her safety.

Specialized Referrals

Knowing that time is limited for direct nursing intervention, the nurse considers the available resources of the facility. The physician, consultant psychiatrist, and family have already been called to contribute to the treatment plan. Other appropriate referrals include the facility in-service educator and social worker. The in-service instructor can present written and videotape material to the staff on how to communicate with agitated clients. In particular, the floor manager needs to know how to interact with the client so that a strong role model can be presented for the staff. The social worker can meet with the client to give her needed attention and to reassure her about her safety. If the plan does not succeed in calming the client, the nurse can recommend a referral to a partial hospital program to the psychiatrist to readjust the medication in a controlled environment.

The nurse returns to Miss Howard 3 hours later and tells her about the contacts with her niece and the staff. Miss Howard has already taken her medication and has eaten lunch. She has a new list of minor complaints but speaks with less pressure and hostility. She thanks the nurse and promises not to hit anyone.

CONCLUSIONS

The medical-surgical nurse has a vital role in caring for the psychosocial needs of all clients. Sensitivity to client and family anxiety improves the nurse's communication skills and increases the probability that clients will achieve the desired outcomes. For clients who have concurrent mental illness, the nurse must consider several additional needs in order to provide comprehensive nursing care:

- Increased attention to completing the comprehensive nursing assessment
- Heightened awareness of verbal and nonverbal communication
- Basic teaching about illness and treatment options
- Referral to appropriate specialized resources available in the health care system

To provide holistic care to clients with concurrent mental illness does not require specialized training beyond the generalist level, but nurses must learn about the range of multidisciplinary services available at the health care facility in a particular community. The nurse is in a prime position in the health care team to advocate for appropriate mental health services for clients. Recognition of mental health needs supports the accomplishment of general health outcomes while reducing the pain and suffering of preventable adverse events.

BIBLIOGRAPHY

1. Abramovitz, M. (1998). Some drugs that cause psychiatric symptoms. *Medical Letter on Drugs and Therapeutics, 40*(1020), 21–24.
2. American Psychiatric Association. (1994). *Diagnostic and statistical manual of mental disorders* (4th ed., rev.). Washington, DC: Author.
3. American Psychiatric Association. (1994). *Diagnostic criteria from DSM-IV.* Washington, DC: Author.
4. Anderson, K. N., & Anderson, L. E. (1994). *Mosby's pocket dictionary of medicine, nursing and allied health* (2nd ed.). St. Louis: Mosby–Year Book.
5. Andruzzi, E. A., & Carson, V. B. (1996). Highways for the journey: The mental health system. In V. B. Carson & E. N. Arnold

(Eds.), *Mental health nursing: The nurse-patient journey* (pp. 33–50). Philadelphia: W. B. Saunders.
6. Brightman, H. (1998). Manic and depressive recurrences: The search for mechanisms and treatments. *NARSAD Research Newsletter, 10*(2), 1–4.
7. Brown, A. (1995). Advances in genetics of psychiatric disorders. *NARSAD Research Newsletter, Fall,* 9–13.
8. Brown, A., & Lempa, M. (1996). Update on potential causes and new treatments for anxiety disorders. *NARSAD Research Newsletter, Fall/Winter,* 13–18.
9. Brown, A., & Lempa, M. (1997). Late-life depression. *NARSAD Research Newsletter, Winter Supplement,* 10–15.
10. Brown, A., & Weaver, R. (1998). Schizoaffective disorder: Just a set of symptoms or a separate disease? *NARSAD Research Newsletter, 10*(4), 25–29.
11. Clark, C. C. (1997). Posttraumatic stress disorder: How to support healing. *American Journal of Nursing, 97*(8), 27–32.
12. DePaulo, J. R., & Ablow, K. R. (1989). *How to cope with depression.* New York: Fawcett Crest.
13. Edmisson, K. W. (1997). Psychosocial dimensions of medical-surgical nursing. In J. M. Black & E. Matassarin-Jacobs (Eds.), *Medical-surgical nursing: Clinical management for continuity of care* (5th ed.). Philadelphia: W. B. Saunders.
14. Elder, K. N., et al. (1998). Managed care: The value you bring. *American Journal of Nursing, 98*(6), 34–39.
15. Fitzgerald, L. W. (1997). Explorations along the stress axis. *NARSAD Research Newsletter, 9*(2), 1–3.
16. Hall, A. (1998). A disorder yields its secrets: Breakthrough in study of manic-depression. *NARSAD Research Newsletter, 10*(3), 7–8.
17. Isaacs, A. (1998). Depression and your patient. *American Journal of Nursing, 98*(7), 26–31.
18. Katz, J. R. (1997). Providing effective patient teaching. *American Journal of Nursing, 97*(5), 33–36.
19. Langreth, R. (1998). Drug makers attack depression on a new front. *NARSAD Research Newsletter, 10*(3), 9–10.
20. Lazarus, R., & Folkman, S. (1984). *Stress, appraisal and coping.* New York: Springer.
21. Lipson, J. G., Dibble, S. L., & Minarik, P. A. (1997). *Culture and nursing care: A pocket guide.* San Francisco: University of California, San Francisco, Nursing Press.
22. Littrell, S. H., & Littrell, K. H. (1997). Recent advances in understanding negative symptoms in schizophrenia. *Journal of the American Psychiatric Nurses Association, 3*(4), 111–117.
23. ———. (1995). Mental health: Does therapy help? *Consumer Reports, 60*(11), 734–739.
24. NARSAD Research. (1997). *Understanding schizophrenia.* Great Neck, NY: Author.
25. Nemeroff, C. B. (1994). Contemporary issues in the management of depression—Introduction. *American Journal of Medicine, 97*(suppl. 6A), 15–25.
26. Rankin, E. A. D. (1996). Patient and family education. In V. B. Carson & E. N. Arnold (Eds.), *Mental health nursing: The nurse-patient journey* (pp. 503–522). Philadelphia: W. B. Saunders.
27. Reinhard, S. C. (1994). Perspectives on the family's caregiving experience in mental illness. *IMAGE: Journal of Nursing Scholarship, 26*(1), 70–73.
28. Resnick, W. M., & Carson, V. B. (1996). The journey colored by mood disorders. In V. B. Carson & E. N. Arnold (Eds.), *Mental health nursing: The nurse-patient journey* (pp. 759–792). Philadelphia: W. B. Saunders.
29. Robinson, A. W. (1999). Getting to the heart of denial. *American Journal of Nursing, 99*(5), 38–42.
30. Scherck, K. A. (1999). Recognizing coping behaviors. *American Journal of Nursing, 99*(4), 24AAA–24DDD.
31. Stuart, G. W., & Sundeen, S. J. (1991). *Principles and practice of psychiatric nursing* (4th ed.). St. Louis: Mosby–Year Book.
32. Sullivan, P. D., & Carson, V. B. (1996). Highways for the journey: The mental health system. In V. B. Carson & E. N. Arnold (Eds.), *Mental health nursing: The nurse-patient journey* (pp. 33–50). Philadelphia: W. B. Saunders.
33. Sumner, C. H. (1998). Recognizing and responding to spiritual distress. *American Journal of Nursing, 98*(1), 26–30.
34. Talan, J. (1997). Schizophrenia triggers described. *NARSAD Research Newsletter, 9*(2), 20–21.
35. U.S. Department of Health and Human Services. (1993). *Depression in primary care: Volume 1.* Rockville, MD: Agency for Health Care Policy and Research.
36. U.S. Department of Health and Human Services. (1993). *Depression in primary care: Volume 2.* Rockville, MD: Agency for Health Care Policy and Research.
37. Warner, P. H., Rowe, T., & Whipple, B. (1999). Shedding light on the sexual history. *American Journal of Nursing, 99*(6), 34–40.
38. Watzlawick, P., Beavin, J. H., & Jackson, D. D. (1967). *Pragmatics of human communication.* New York: W. W. Norton.
39. Worthington, J. F. (1995). From cause to treatment: Attacking schizophrenia from all sides. *NARSAD Research Newsletter, Summer,* 1–4.
40. Yamashita, M., & Forsyth, D. M. (1998). Family coping with mental illness: An aggregate from two studies, Canada and United States. *Journal of the American Psychiatric Nurses Association, 4*(1), 1–7.

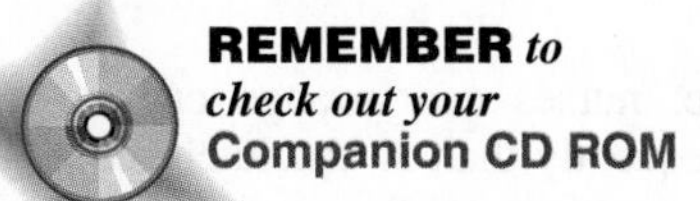

CHAPTER

21

Clients with Sleep and Rest Disorders and Fatigue: Promoting Positive Outcomes

Marlene Reimer

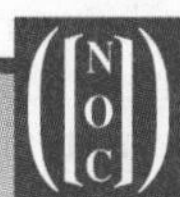

Nursing Outcomes Classification (NOC) for Nursing Diagnoses—Clients with Sleep and Rest Disorders and Fatigue

Sleep Pattern Disturbance
Anxiety Control
Rest
Sleep
Well-Being
Fatigue
Activity Tolerance
Endurance
Energy Conservation
Nutritional Status: Energy
Psychomotor Energy

Most of us experience occasional problems of disturbed sleep, unwanted drowsiness, fatigue, overstimulation, or understimulation. As a nurse, you will frequently be involved with clients in whom these disturbances interfere with health, healing, and daily activities. Contributing factors may include personal lifestyle habits, environmental features, internal rhythms, and changes associated with episodic illness or chronic illness.

SLEEP AND SLEEP PATTERN DISTURBANCES

Sleep can be defined as a normal state of altered consciousness during which the body rests; it is characterized by decreased responsiveness to the environment, and a person can be aroused from it by external stimuli. Almost a third of the general population has some problems with sleep during any given year.[51] More than half of the 9000 participants in a study of sleep in elderly persons (65 years or older) reported the following as sleep pattern disturbances that they experience most of the time[29]:

- Trouble falling asleep
- Frequent awakening
- Waking too early
- Needing to nap
- Not feeling rested

These disturbances may be secondary to situational, environmental, or developmental stressors, or they may be associated with illness or with pre-existing disorders. The relationship is often reciprocal, in that the disorder decreases sleep and the decreased sleep affects the disorder. Sleep pattern disturbance also contributes to sensory disorders, such as intensive care unit psychosis.

Sleep pattern disturbance is a nursing diagnosis that is defined as a disruption of sleep time that causes discomfort or interferes with a desired lifestyle.[17, 52] A sleep pattern disturbance may be related to one of more than

80 sleep disorders identified in the International Classification of Sleep Disorders, a partial list of which is presented in Box 21–1. Intermittent sleep-related problems are also of concern for nursing diagnosis and intervention.

CHRONOBIOLOGY

Chronobiology refers to the study of biologic changes as they occur in relation to time. Knowledge of chronobiology as it relates to sleep is important to nurses in planning client care and teaching.

The *sleep-wake cycle* is one of the circadian rhythms of the body. Circadian rhythms follow an approximate 24-hour cycle through a complex process linked to light and dark. The effects of illness and hospitalization may disrupt these rhythms, particularly in older persons, who are especially vulnerable to such changes.[6] Nurses can minimize this effect by encouraging a regular schedule with appropriate environmental cues.

Ultradian cycles are circadian rhythms of less than 24 hours. The recurrent pattern of sleep stages, repeating approximately every 90 minutes in adults, is an example. Recognizing this cycle, nurses can arrange care to avoid waking clients more frequently than is absolutely necessary.

Chronopharmacology refers to the study of how biorhythms affect the absorption, metabolism, and excretion of drugs. As an example, the blood level achieved by a continuous infusion of heparin varies throughout the day. The risk of clotting is greater in the morning, and the risk of bleeding is greater in the evening. Effectiveness of anticancer drugs varies according to the time of administration. Further, steroid medications should be administered in the morning to approximate most closely the natural elevation in cortisol levels.

BOX 21–1 International Classification of Sleep Disorders*

I. Dyssomnias
   A. Intrinsic sleep disorders
      1. Psychophysiologic insomnia
      2. Narcolepsy
      3. Obstructive sleep apnea syndrome
      4. Central sleep apnea syndrome
      5. Periodic limb movement disorder
      6. Restless legs syndrome
   B. Extrinsic sleep disorders
      1. Inadequate sleep hygiene
      2. Environmental sleep disorder
   C. Circadian rhythm sleep disorders
II. Parasomnias
   A. Arousal disorders
      1. Sleepwalking
      2. Sleep terrors
   B. Sleep-wake transition disorders
   C. Parasomnias usually associated with REM sleep
      1. Nightmares
      2. Sleep paralysis
   D. Other parasomnias
      1. Sleep bruxism
      2. Sleep enuresis
      3. Primary snoring
III. Sleep disorders associated with medical or psychiatric disorders
   A. Associated with mental disorders
   B. Associated with neurologic disorders
   C. Associated with other medical disorders
IV. Proposed sleep disorders

* This is a partial listing of common sleep disorders.
REM, rapid eye movement.
From the Diagnostic Classification Steering Committee, Thorpy, M. J., Chairman. (1997). *International classification of sleep disorders: Diagnostic and coding manual* (Rev. ed.). Rochester, MN: American Sleep Disorders Association.

PHYSIOLOGY OF SLEEP AND AROUSAL

The timing of the sleep-wake cycle and other circadian rhythms, such as body temperature, is controlled, at least in part, by the suprachiasmatic nucleus in the anterior hypothalamus. Located above the optic chiasm, this area receives input from the retina, which provides information about darkness and light. The suprachiasmatic nucleus controls the production of melatonin, which is believed to be a potent sleep inducer.[10]

Arousal from sleep, wakefulness, and the ability to respond to stimuli rely on an intact *reticular activating system* (RAS).[18] The RAS is located in the brain stem and contains projections to the thalamus and cortex. The diffuse network of neurons in the RAS is in a strategic position to monitor ascending and descending stimuli through feedback loops.[18]

Although the RAS provides the anatomic framework for arousal, it is the neurotransmitters that serve as the chemical messengers.[18] The onset of sleep and of each subsequent sleep stage is an active process involving delicate shifts in the balance of several of these neurotransmitters.

The transition from the awake state to *non–rapid eye movement* (NREM) sleep is marked by decreases in the concentrations of serotonin (5-hydroxytryptamine [5-HT]), norepinephrine, and acetylcholine. The later transition to *rapid eye movement* (REM) sleep is marked by a dramatic increase in acetylcholine and further decreases in serotonin and norepinephrine.[18, 35, 68] As REM sleep continues, the concentrations of serotonin and norepinephrine increase, eventually stopping REM sleep. Cholinergic activation with the release of acetylcholine seems to reestablish REM sleep.[35] The continuous interaction of these two systems is thought to produce the normal alterations between NREM and REM sleep.[35] Other neurotransmitters, such as gamma-aminobutyric acid (GABA) and dopamine, are also believed to have a part in the reciprocal processes involved in shifts in sleep state.

All of these neurotransmitters are actively involved in waking processes as well. For example, neurons that produce serotonin and norepinephrine play a role in the modulation of sensory input, mood, energy, and information processing, including attention, learning, and memory.[35] Thus, imbalances in these neurotransmitters induced through sleep pattern disturbances, medications, or diseases may reciprocally affect not only sleep but also aspects of sensory processing, mood, and cognition.

The Need for Sleep

Much is known about the architecture of the sleep cycle, but much less is known about the need for sleep. It is commonly held that sleep has a restorative and protective function.[36] In sleep, sympathetic activity decreases whereas parasympathetic activity may increase. Hormonal shifts facilitate anabolic processes. Selective deprivation of "slow-wave sleep" (see later) is associated with vague physical complaints.

REM sleep may be especially important for maintaining mental activities, such as learning, reasoning, and emotional adjustment. Sleep also appears to serve as an energy-conserving measure for most of the body except the brain.[37]

Sleep Stages

Sleep can be defined behaviorally, functionally, and electrophysiologically. Electrophysiologic monitoring of sleep, called *polysomnography,* includes at least three parameters: (1) brain wave activity, (2) eye movements, and (3) muscle tone. Polysomnography shows that sleep can be divided into REM and NREM. NREM sleep can be further divided into stages 1 through 4. The stages vary in depth but are characterized by slow rolling eye movements, low-level and fragmented cognitive activity, maintenance of moderate muscle tone, and slower but generally rhythmic respirations and pulse rate. As a person progresses from stage 1 to stage 4 sleep, the waveforms recorded by electroencephalography (EEG) become more synchronized, slower, and higher in amplitude (Fig. 21–1).

NREM sleep is characterized as follows:

Stage 1 is very light. Respirations begin to slow, and muscles relax. At sleep onset, some erratic breathing may occur as well as sudden myoclonic jerks (sleep starts) as the body shifts from an awake to a sleep state. Stage 1 is such a light stage of sleep that persons wakened from it often claim that they were not asleep at all.

Stage 2 is still light sleep. The brain waves are frequently mixed and low voltage in pattern, with bursts of activity called *sleep spindles* and large-amplitude waves called *K complexes.* More than 50% of sleep occurs as stages 1 and 2.

Stages 3 and 4 are known as *slow-wave sleep,* named for the characteristic high-voltage, low-frequency delta waves. Respirations become slow and even. The pulse and blood pressure fall. Oxygen consumption by muscle tissues and urine formation decrease. Dreams that occur during the NREM stages of sleep are generally thought-like ruminations about recent events and current concerns with little story line.[35]

REM sleep is characterized by low-voltage, random fast waves, as in stage 1 NREM. People in REM sleep

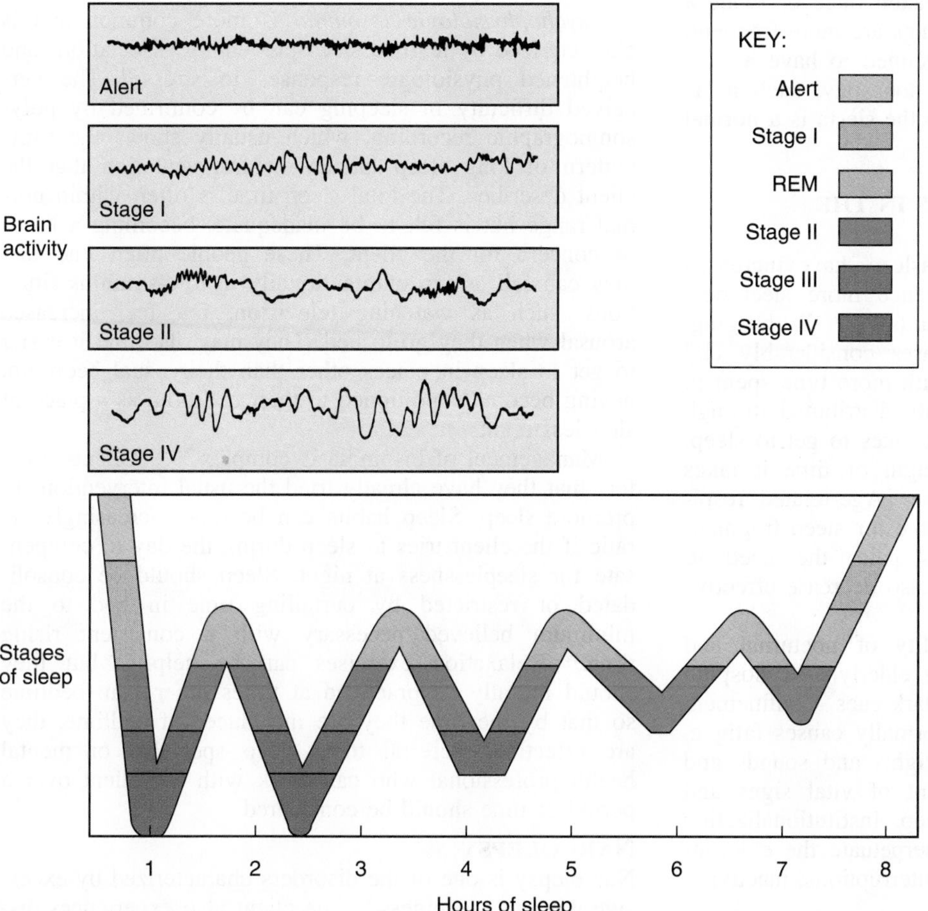

FIGURE 21–1 The electrical activity of the brain during various stages of sleep can be shown on electroencephalograms. During the night, people go through three to five sleep cycles. Each cycle includes a sequence of sleep stages. REM, rapid eye movement. (From Solomon, E. P., Schmidt, R. R., & Adranga, P. J. [1990]. *Human anatomy and physiology* [2nd ed.]. Philadelphia: Saunders College.)

have characteristic rapid eye movements, erratic respirations, changes in heart rate, and very low muscle tone (see Fig. 21–1). During REM sleep, ventilation depends primarily on the movement of the diaphragm because intercostal and accessory muscle tone is markedly diminished and all postural and nonrespiratory muscles are essentially paralyzed.[61] The ventilatory response to hypoxia and hypercapnia is decreased, and thermoregulation is significantly reduced. Dreams in REM sleep are vivid, story-like, emotional, and bizarre.

Most people move through an orderly progression of NREM sleep from stages 1 to 4 and back through stages 3 to 2 before initiating a period of REM sleep (see Fig. 21–1). Although this is the typical progression, it is not essential or always seen. Atypical progressions are characteristic of some sleep disorders, such as narcolepsy, in which REM sleep is entered almost immediately after sleep onset.

In adults, each sleep cycle through the various stages lasts about 90 minutes. During the first few cycles, more time is spent in slow-wave sleep, and the percentage of REM sleep increases later in the sleep period.

Wide variations in sleep patterns exist among individuals. By explaining the range of these variations, the nurse can help clients seek a pattern that leaves them feeling reasonably refreshed and alert. Eight hours of undisturbed sleep at night with no daytime naps has become the assumed ideal pattern in North American society. However, some adults do well with 6 hours or less and other healthy adults require 10 hours or more of nighttime sleep. Even young adults often awaken once or twice a night, and, with aging, such wakenings are more frequent. Humans may be physiologically inclined to have a long and a short sleep period each 24-hour day, such as is common in warmer climates, where the siesta is a normal part of the day's schedule.[22]

Changes in Sleep Patterns in the Elderly

Older people take longer to fall asleep, have increased nocturnal wakefulness, and experience more sleepiness during the day than do younger adults.[6, 9, 25] With aging, the percentage of stage 4 decreases considerably and REM sleep decreases somewhat, with more time spent in stage 1. REM sleep is more evenly distributed through the night. *Sleep latency,* the time it takes to get to sleep, increases, as does the average length of time it takes to get back to sleep after arousal.[5] Age-related respiratory dysfunction may be responsible for sleep fragmentation.[4] Other problems, such as pain, the need to void, and nocturnal dyspnea, may also decrease effective sleep.

Hospitalization affects the quality of nocturnal and other sleep time, especially for the elderly. The hospital environment often lacks light and dark cues. Confinement curtails activity or exercise that normally causes fatigue. In addition, there are unfamiliar sights and sounds and frequent awakenings for assessment of vital signs and other interventions that disturb sleep. Institutionalization in a long-term care facility may perpetuate the environmental impact of noise, caregiver interruptions, inactivity, and lack of day-night cues.[63]

SLEEP DISORDERS

Dyssomnias

The dyssomnias include sleep disorders characterized by difficulty initiating or maintaining sleep (insomnia) or by excessive sleepiness. These disorders may arise predominantly from within the body (*intrinsic*), from external sources (*extrinsic*), or from disruptions of circadian rhythm.[2, 21]

■ INTRINSIC SLEEP DISORDERS

Insomnia

Many people experience transitory periods during which they have difficulty initiating or maintaining sleep. The onset or exacerbation of illness, with or without hospitalization, may precipitate such difficulty. These sleep pattern disturbances are most often associated with disrupted or inconsistent sleep habits (*inadequate sleep hygiene*) or environmental disruptions. These disorders do not constitute insomnia, but they do predispose individuals to insomnia.

A much smaller proportion of the population has developed persistent difficulty in initiating or maintaining sleep. For them, the difficulty does not respond readily to improved sleep habits or removal of precipitating factors.[21]

Idiopathic insomnia is a rare disorder characterized by a lifelong history of inability to obtain adequate sleep. Its cause is thought to be an abnormality in the neurologic control of sleep.

Psychophysiologic insomnia is more common and is characterized by learned sleep-preventing associations and heightened physiologic responses to stress.[21] The perceived difficulty in sleeping can be confirmed by polysomnographic recording, which usually shows the same pattern of long sleep latency or fragmentation that the client describes. The total sleep time is often within normal range but is felt to be inadequate, becoming a focus of concern for the client. These people often find that they can fall asleep unintentionally in low-stimulus situations, such as watching television, but feel increased arousal when they go to bed. They may also find it easier to get to sleep in places other than their usual bedroom, having become conditioned to their bedroom as a place of sleepless nights.

Management of insomnia is complex.[27, 33] Clients often feel that they have already tried the usual interventions to promote sleep. Sleep habits can become increasingly erratic if the client tries to sleep during the day to compensate for sleeplessness at night. Sleep should be consolidated or restricted by curtailing time in bed to the minimum believed necessary with a consistent rising time.[34] Relaxation exercises can be helpful, but they should initially be practiced at times other than bedtime so that by the time they are introduced at bedtime, they are effective. Referral to a sleep specialist or mental health professional who can work with the client over a period of time should be considered.

Narcolepsy

Narcolepsy is one of the disorders characterized by excessive daytime sleepiness.[13] The client also experiences disturbed nocturnal sleep and repeated episodes of almost irresistible daytime drowsiness followed by brief periods of sleep, especially when engaged in monotonous activities. Many narcoleptic clients also experience *cataplexy,* a sudden loss of muscle tone at times of unexpected emotion (e.g., fright). Several other sleep-related abnormalities are commonly experienced by clients with narcolepsy. On initial wakening, they may experience *sleep paralysis* for one to several minutes, during which time they cannot move. This condition, like the other manifestations of narcolepsy, is thought to be linked to malfunctioning of the mechanism controlling REM sleep. The REM sleep that is experienced is normal, but it occurs at different times.

Another REM-like manifestation is *hypnagogic hallucinations,* hallucinatory experiences that occur at sleep onset or awakening.[13] Some people experience sleep paralysis or one of the other associated manifestations without narcolepsy. However, when these manifestations are seen together with excessive sleepiness, they constitute the narcolepsy tetrad.[21] Automatic behaviors during which there is a lapse of awareness are also frequent.

On polysomnography, the most characteristic finding is sleep-onset REM periods. A multiple sleep latency test, to measure how long it takes to fall asleep during normal waking hours, shows a sleep latency of less than 5 minutes over four or five testing periods. Occurrence of REM periods at sleep onset at least twice during the test periods is another criterion for the diagnosis.[3, 21, 32]

Narcolepsy is a genetically related condition with autosomal dominance in some cases. The prevalence is about 1 in 1000 people in the United States.[51] Genetic transmission of narcolepsy may be multifactorial and may involve a human leukocyte antigen (HLA) and another gene that is not HLA-related.[32] Environmental factors may also have a role.

The effects of the disease on lifestyle are significant, with 60% to 80% of clients reporting episodes of having fallen asleep at work, while driving, or both. The associated disruption of social and occupational roles and self-esteem may be a major factor contributing to the depression and personality disorders frequently seen in clients who have narcolepsy.[31]

Impaired release of neurotransmitters such as dopamine may also be a factor in both the narcolepsy and the associated depression.[3] Medical management of narcolepsy usually consists of low doses of stimulants to improve alertness and tricyclic antidepressants to control cataplexy.[3]

Emphasize good sleep hygiene in counseling clients who experience narcolepsy, It is important that they maintain a regular schedule with adequate nocturnal sleep. Recommend regular naps at times when clients are prone to increased sleepiness.[13] Safety is a major issue for these clients. Assistance may be needed in coping with the disruptive effects of narcolepsy on family, work, and social roles.

SLEEP APNEA SYNDROME

Sleep apnea is characterized by cessation of breathing for 10 seconds or longer occurring at least five times per hour.[21] Sleep apnea can be classified as obstructive and central nervous system (CNS) apnea. A combination of the two may be seen.

OBSTRUCTIVE SLEEP APNEA SYNDROME. In obstructive sleep apnea syndrome, respiratory efforts of the diaphragm and intercostal muscles are apparent but ineffective against a collapsed or obstructed upper airway.[28] Snoring indicates partial obstruction. Escalating snoring followed by a silent pause that ends with a gasp or snort probably indicates complete airway obstruction. As hypoxia ensues, the person eventually awakens to breathe. The frequent awakenings impair the normal sleep cycle. With sleep, the muscles of the upper airway relax and may occlude an airway that is already narrowed by enlarged soft tissue structures, jaw structure, or obesity. Partial obstruction may result in upper airway resistance syndrome with or without snoring. Repeated microarousals lead to excessive daytime sleepiness in most clients. A few, particularly older people, may present with insomnia.

Obstructive sleep apnea syndrome affects more than 1% of the adult population.[56] Prevalence may be as high as 5% in middle-aged men and much higher in people in certain occupational groups, such as truck drivers. Women are less likely than men to develop obstructive sleep apnea syndrome, particularly before menopause.[21] A much smaller percentage progress to the classic pickwickian syndrome, characterized by obesity, severe sleep apnea, daytime hypercapnia, and cor pulmonale.

Consider referral to a sleep disorders center for clients observed to have repeated periods of apnea (one a minute or more than 15 to 20 periods an hour) lasting longer than 10 seconds, whether or not these periods are associated with snoring. Because obstructive sleep apnea syndrome is particularly common among males who are obese with short, thick necks and who are heavy snorers, these clients should be observed during sleep for apneic periods. During assessment, question clients regarding the degree of daytime sleepiness experienced, and sudden nighttime awakening, with particular concern about safety in relation to driving and occupational activities.

Milder cases of obstructive sleep apnea syndrome, in which excessive daytime sleepiness is not yet a concern, may respond to weight reduction, measures to promote sleeping in positions other than supine, and avoidance of alcohol. However, once the apneic episodes are observed to occur on most nights and in all body positions, more definitive treatment is usually required.

The application of continuous positive airway pressure (CPAP) by means of a face mask covering the nose is the treatment of choice for clients with moderate to severe obstructive sleep apnea syndrome.[15] The CPAP device provides room air under increased pressure, essentially providing a pressure splint to keep the upper airway open. Bilevel positive airway pressure (BiPAP) operates by the same principle but uses lower pressure during expiration.

The CPAP mask should be applied securely over the nose and held in place by the head gear. It should be turned on whenever the client is ready to go to sleep and should be maintained throughout the sleep period. Additional humidification may be necessary, especially in dry environments. Clients may experience nasal congestion, air leaks, pressure marks on the face, or pressure intolerance. Such problems are not uncommon and may lead to discontinuation of the therapy if they are not effectively managed. It is therefore important that nurses have a working knowledge of the therapy, the importance of regularity in its use, and sources available for technical assistance (e.g., sleep disorders center, respiratory equipment supplier). CPAP units are portable and have features such as battery operation and voltage conversion to accommodate travel requirements.

People who regularly use CPAP should bring their units into the hospital with them. These clients need to be closely monitored when recovering from anesthesia and when receiving narcotics because they are at risk for ineffective breathing patterns.

A note should be made on the health record at the time of admission that the client has obstructive sleep apnea syndrome. If the client is scheduled for surgery, the anesthetist and recovery room staff must be alerted. The CPAP unit may be requested to accompany the client to the recovery room.

Question any order for benzodiazepines or other hypnotic drugs for clients with obstructive sleep apnea syndrome, chronic obstructive pulmonary disease (COPD), or loud snoring because of possible respiratory depression.[42] Teach clients with such conditions that alcohol may also worsen their manifestations because of its selective effect in relaxing the muscles of the upper airway and depression of arousal (see the Client Education Guide).

Uvulopalatopharyngoplasty (UPPP) is a common surgical procedure for reducing snoring. Resecting the uvula, the posterior portion of the soft palate, tonsils, and any excessive pharyngeal tissue, can reduce the propensity to obstruction in some clients.[24] Concern has arisen, however, that reducing or eliminating snoring may place clients at unknown risk for obstructive sleep apnea syndrome. Therefore, preoperative assessment, including respiratory pattern during sleep, is recommended before UPPP or the newer laser-assisted UPPP procedure, which is done in stages in a physician's office.[67] Somnoplasty is another surgical procedure for removal of excessive tissue through the use of high radiofrequencies that spare the mucosa. Tracheostomy may be required in severe obstructive sleep apnea syndrome.

Oral or dental appliances are being used increasingly as another treatment for sleep apnea.[62] Essentially, they act by keeping the jaw forward and the upper airway open.

CLIENT EDUCATION GUIDE

Living with Obstructive Sleep Apnea Syndrome

1. Avoid sleeping on your back because that is the position in which the syndrome tends to be worse. Try sleeping with pillows at your back, wearing a small backpack, or sewing a tennis ball into the back of pajamas or nightgown.
2. Aim to reduce or stabilize your weight so that body mass index (weight in kilograms divided by height in square meters) is 27 or less. Even a small weight loss may decrease the number of episodes of apnea or upper airway resistance. Increasing the amount of aerobic exercise is the most effective strategy.
3. Avoid alcohol, hypnotics, and other central nervous system depressants because of their relaxing effect on the upper airway.
4. Get adequate sleep. Chronic sleep deprivation can potentiate the effects of the syndrome.
5. Have your blood pressure checked regularly. Hypertension is often associated with this syndrome.
6. Try to limit driving to times when you feel well rested. If feeling drowsy, get someone else to drive or stop to have a nap. Snacks and caffeine drinks may provide temporary stimulation, but they cannot overcome physiologic sleepiness.
7. Carry an identification card or bracelet to alert emergency personnel to your problem.
8. If continuous positive airway pressure or an oral appliance is prescribed, use it regularly.

CENTRAL SLEEP APNEA SYNDROME. Central sleep apnea is characterized by apneic periods during which no apparent respiratory effort occurs.[21] It may be seen with CNS lesions, such as in stroke or brain stem involvement, but it is most commonly mixed with obstructive sleep apnea. Cheyne-Stokes respirations are common with this syndrome, and CPAP is the usual treatment. As with obstructive sleep apnea, sedative-hypnotic drugs should be avoided. In severe cases with CNS involvement, use of diaphragmatic pacemakers or mechanical ventilation may be required.

PERIODIC LIMB MOVEMENT DISORDER

Periodic limb movement disorder may also contribute to daytime sleepiness and frequent nocturnal wakenings. Originally described as nocturnal myoclonus, it is characterized by periodic episodes of repetitive, stereotypic leg (or arm) movements that occur during sleep, causing partial arousals.[8, 21] The diagnosis can be confirmed during polysomnography with surface electromyography (EMG) of the anterior tibial muscles.

Periodic limb movement disorder is common in the elderly population. Clonazepam, a benzodiazepine, or baclofen, a skeletal muscle relaxant, may be ordered to diminish the magnitude of the movement and the frequency of arousals. The antiparkinsonian drug carbidopa-levodopa (Sinemet) and the tricyclic antidepressant imipramine seem to act more directly and almost eliminate the movements. Most of the other tricyclic antidepressants aggravate the condition. For some clients, the use of transcutaneous electrical nerve stimulation (TENS) before sleep has been helpful.[8]

RESTLESS LEGS SYNDROME

Restless legs syndrome involves annoying "crawling," itching, or tingling sensations of the legs while at rest and causes an almost irresistible urge to move.[8, 21] The syndrome is often most severe before sleep onset. Clients almost always have periodic limb movements during sleep. Treatment is similar to that for periodic limb movements.

■ EXTRINSIC SLEEP DISORDERS

The extrinsic sleep disorders encompass a range of factors, from environmentally to chemically induced. Some environmental factors temporarily present during hospitalization are discussed under Hospital-Acquired Sleep Disturbances.

■ CIRCADIAN RHYTHM SLEEP DISORDERS

In the general population, the circadian rhythm sleep disorders, such as *time zone change syndrome* and *shift work sleep disorder,*[2] are not uncommon. In taking a nursing history, be alert to a history of long-time shift work.

Elderly and chronically ill clients who live alone may be vulnerable to *irregular sleep-wake patterns.* In this disorder, prolonged ignoring or absence of external cues to time, such as regular mealtimes, work periods, and daylight, leads to erratic periods of sleeping and wakefulness. Internal circadian cues may also be damped as a result of aging or diffuse brain disease.[21, 25]

Management strategies for circadian rhythm disorders include maintenance of a regular schedule (e.g., people who regularly work night shift are encouraged to maintain the same sleep schedule on nights off) and exposure to natural sunlight. Light therapy is being used to facilitate adjustments in circadian rhythms as well as in the treatment of *seasonal affective disorder* (SAD).[6, 44, 46]

SAD refers to the onset of a major depressive episode corresponding to a particular period of the year, usually late fall and early winter. Some seasonal variation in mood, activity level, and appetite is common in latitudes where climate and length of daylight change markedly.

Administration of bright light in the early morning is most effective in treating SAD or resetting habitual wakening to an earlier hour.[19, 70] Exposure to bright sunlight at those times can also be effective, but conventional indoor lighting is inadequate. Dosage of light is measured in units of illuminance (lux).[46] The usual dosage is about 5000 lux-hours, which may be taken as 2500 lux for 2 hours, 5000 lux for 1 hour, or 10,000 lux for 30 minutes. This level of illumination requires special light boxes, a variety of which are now available.

Help clients to realize that light therapy should begin only under the guidance of a clinician experienced in its use. Teaching should include appropriate positioning of the head in relation to the light source. The most common side effects are eyestrain and headache. Too much light may contribute to irritability and insomnia.[46, 70] The long-term risk of exposure of the eyes to bright light therapy is under investigation. Until more is known, the presence of retinopathy, glaucoma, or cataract is generally considered a contraindication.[46, 70]

PARASOMNIAS

The parasomnias are disorders that occur during sleep but that usually do not produce insomnia or excessive sleepiness.[21] The underlying pathologic mechanism may involve partial arousal or abnormalities in sleep-wake transition.

■ AROUSAL DISORDERS

Partial arousals typically occur during slow-wave sleep.[24] *Sleepwalking,* also known as *somnambulism,* may include semi-purposeful behavior, such as dressing. However, the behavior may be lacking in coordination and appropriateness, such as voiding in the closet. The occurrence of sleepwalking in adults is often associated with anxiety. *Sleep terrors* are sudden arousals from slow-wave sleep accompanied by screaming, tachycardia, tachypnea, diaphoresis, and other manifestations of intense fear.[21] If awakened, the person is often disoriented and has little recall of the nature of the dream image. Sleep terrors typically occur in young children but may develop in adults.

■ SLEEP-WAKE TRANSITION DISORDERS

Sleep-wake transition disorders are common in the general population, rarely causing enough disruption to be legitimately called disorders. As mentioned earlier, *sleep starts* refer to the sudden jerking movement of the legs that often occurs just as a person is falling asleep. Nocturnal leg cramps are also common. The frequency and intensity may be greater with high caffeine intake, stress, or intense physical activity before going to bed. *Sleeptalking* may also occur more frequently during times of stress.

■ PARASOMNIAS ASSOCIATED WITH RAPID EYE MOVEMENT SLEEP

Like the other parasomnias, those associated with REM sleep may be distressing but are seldom serious. *Nightmares* are frightening dreams that arise in REM sleep and are often vividly recalled on awakening. In contrast to night terrors, these dreams occur in slow-wave sleep and there is little recall. *Sleep paralysis* is one of the classic signs of narcolepsy but can occur in isolation. At sleep onset or on awakening, people experience episodes of one to several minutes during which they are unable to move.[24] This effect may be an extension of the normal state of low muscle tone during REM sleep.

■ OTHER PARASOMNIAS

Other parasomnias are not specifically associated with a particular sleep stage. *Sleep bruxism* refers to grinding of the teeth during sleep and may lead to dental damage. *Sleep enuresis,* or bed-wetting, may occur in adults in association with other disorders, such as obstructive sleep apnea syndrome.[21] *Primary snoring* is distinguished from obstructive sleep apnea syndrome by its rhythmic nature without episodes of apnea or hypoventilation.

SLEEP DISORDERS ASSOCIATED WITH MEDICAL AND PSYCHOLOGICAL DISORDERS

Secondary sleep disorders are of particular relevance in considering problems common to medical-surgical clients. Whereas some clients have a pre-existing sleep disorder of the dyssomnia or parasomnia type, others develop a sleep disorder secondary to disease or its manifestations. By remaining aware of the physiology of normal sleep, you can anticipate the risk of sleep pattern disturbances in medical-surgical clients.

■ NEUROTRANSMITTER IMBALANCES

Neurotransmitter imbalances predispose to sleep pattern disturbances.[60] These imbalances may be disease-related or drug-induced.

More than 70% of people being treated for Parkinson's disease, which results from a deficiency of the neurotransmitter dopamine, report sleep pattern disturbances.[21, 48] Insomnia is the most frequent initial concern, followed by sleep fragmentation, disturbances in the sleep-wake schedule, and visual hallucinations.

Depression is accompanied by sleep disturbance in at least 90% of people who suffer from it.[21] Milder forms of depression and those that occur in young people are often associated with sleep-onset insomnia; more severe depressions are characterized by broken sleep and early-morning wakening. Some relationship appears to exist between the pathogenesis of depression and REM sleep mechanisms in that depressed people who are deprived of REM sleep often show improved mood.[31, 40] The action of tricyclic antidepressants in suppressing REM sleep has been proposed as the primary mechanism underlying their effectiveness in treating depression.[57]

Neurotransmitter imbalances may also contribute to the sleep disturbances frequently seen with Alzheimer's disease and other dementias. The most typical pattern with dementias is frequent awakenings, with agitation progressing to loss of sleep-wake consolidation.[58] Assessing sleep patterns, minimizing caregiver-initiated awakenings (e.g., for toileting), and ensuring a regular bedtime may help to reduce nocturnal and daytime agitation.[14] The sleep-wake cycle may be completely reversed in a client with Alzheimer's disease. The client may nap during the day and be awake all night, restless, agitated, and wandering. The incidence of sleep apnea is higher in people with Alzheimer's disease, possibly as a result of associated neuronal degeneration in the brain stem. Therefore, the nocturnal respiratory patterns of these clients should be carefully assessed, with referral to a sleep disorders center if apnea is suspected.

■ HEAD INJURY

Head injury of all degrees of severity affects sleep patterns. The appearance of differentiated sleep stages on electroencephalography (EEG) in comatose clients with severe head injuries is a favorable prognostic indicator. Sleep stages indicate that connections between the brain stem, diencephalon, and telencephalon are intact and allow shifts to occur between NREM and REM sleep. Even after mild head injury, however, some degree of sleep disturbance may persist for several months.[20] Teaching clients and their families that this unsettled sleep is a typical part of *postconcussion syndrome* can allay anxiety and hasten functional recovery.

For clients in the confused, agitated stage of recovery that results from more severe head injury, use of environmental cues (e.g., light and darkness), regularity of daily schedule, and appropriate daytime exercise and activity can help to restore the sleep-wake cycle. Haloperidol (Haldol), which is often given to confused, agitated clients, blocks the activity of dopamine. This disruption of the delicate neurotransmitter balance may lead to insomnia. Thus, the health care team must balance the option of controlling agitated behavior—and its associated high consumption of energy—with the undesirable side effect of increasing sleep fragmentation through medication.[59]

■ HORMONAL IMBALANCES

Hormonal imbalances also contribute to sleep pattern disturbance. *Hyperthyroid* clients tend to have fragmented, short sleep periods with an excess of slow-wave sleep. *Hypothyroidism* is characterized by excessive sleepiness, and polysomnographic recordings show a reduction in the proportion of slow-wave sleep.

Clients with *diabetes mellitus,* particularly type 1, may experience hypoglycemic attacks during the night. Besides the usual clinical manifestations of sweating, palpitations, hunger, and anxiety, which the client may recognize as a hypoglycemic reaction, be alert to complaints of nightmares and early morning headaches. If these manifestations are present, check blood glucose levels at regular intervals during the night. Insulin dosage or timing may need to be changed. Diabetic clients who have autonomic neuropathy have a higher prevalence of breathing abnormalities during sleep because of the associated dysfunction of autonomic respiratory control; thus, their nocturnal breathing patterns should be assessed.

Sleep patterns normally vary across the menstrual cycle in response to estrogen and progesterone levels.[23] During the latter part of the cycle, when progesterone levels are higher, the first REM sleep period occurs earlier, and some studies have shown sleep disturbances to be more frequent.[45] Women with *premenstrual syndrome* tend to have less slow-wave sleep throughout the menstrual cycle than their asymptomatic peers. With *menopause,* many women experience poorer sleep quality that may result in mood changes.[7] Estrogen replacement therapy may help to reduce these symptoms. *Postmenopausal* women are also at higher risk for experiencing snoring and obstructive sleep apnea.[43]

■ RESPIRATORY DISORDERS

Nocturnal asthma attacks are common in cases of poorly managed asthma, contributing to frequent awakenings in up to 70% of people with asthma.[21] Bronchial resistance increases during the early morning hours, even in healthy people, as does sensitivity to histamine.

Chronic airway limitations, such as asthma and emphysema, contribute to difficulty initiating sleep, frequent arousals with shortness of breath or cough, and chronic fatigue. Oxygen saturation may fall, particularly during REM sleep, when ventilation depends on the diaphragm, which is often flattened and inefficient in clients with advanced chronic airflow limitation.[39, 55] In addition, ventilation and perfusion are altered. Dysrhythmias are common during sleep in clients with advanced respiratory disease, especially when oxygen saturation falls below 60%.[21] Pulmonary artery pressure increases as a result of the pulmonary vascular constriction induced by the low oxygen desaturation and the destructive processes of the underlying disease.

Ventilatory responses to hypoxia and hypercapnia are decreased during sleep, even in people with normal respiratory functioning.[4] Clients with advanced respiratory disease are even more vulnerable; therefore, hypnotics and other CNS depressants that damp arousal should be given with greater caution.

Some of the medications used in the treatment of chronic airway limitations, such as theophylline preparations, may contribute to insomnia. Anxiety and depression associated with effects of the disease may exacerbate the tendency toward fragmented sleep. Try to provide a calm, secure, and relaxed environment for clients. Stimulants such as caffeine may need to be avoided.

The recumbent posture for sleeping is problematic for many people with respiratory disorders. Encourage clients to use several pillows or to have the head of the bed elevated; during acute episodes, they may find it more comfortable to sleep in a reclining chair.

■ CARDIOVASCULAR DISORDERS

Up to 25% of people with hypertension have been found to have obstructive sleep apnea.[66] An association between snoring and hypertension has also been documented.[56] Thus, it is important that you assess clients who have hypertension or who snore while having repeated apneic periods during sleep.

In clients with severe heart failure, periodic breathing of the Cheyne-Stokes type occurs. This pattern may result in significant hypoxemia, frequent arousals, increased stage 1 sleep, and reduced total sleep time.

The variability of heart and respiratory rates during REM sleep may be a factor in nocturnal angina.[66] Clients recovering from myocardial infarction are often deprived of sleep during their stay in a critical care unit and may experience REM rebound on transfer to a step-down or standard unit. The greater cardiac demands during REM sleep may put some additional strain on the recovering heart, making continued nursing surveillance during this period particularly important.[47]

■ GASTROINTESTINAL DISORDERS

Gastric acid secretion normally decreases during sleep, but people with duodenal ulcers have higher than average levels of secretion.[66] Recurrent awakenings with epigastric pain are common, especially in the first 4 hours after sleep onset,[21] and antacids or histamine antagonists may need to be administered.

Gastroesophageal reflux (heartburn) can be more serious when it occurs during sleep, because the longer exposure of the esophagus to gastric acid can lead to esophagitis. Hypnotics should be used cautiously with such clients because the suppression of arousal makes them more vulnerable to esophagitis and pulmonary aspiration. You may suggest that these clients avoid eating within 3 hours of bedtime, consider use of antacids or histamine antagonists, and raise the head of the bed on blocks (reverse Trendelenburg position) to decrease the likelihood of reflux and subsequent aspiration.[54]

■ OTHER DISORDERS

Numerous other disorders seem to have an effect on or an association with sleep. Any condition that results in pain, discomfort, or impaired mobility has the potential to disrupt sleep.[53] Various skin conditions, such as atopic eczema, are associated with decreased REM sleep. Unrefreshing sleep, chronic fatigue, and diffuse musculoskeletal pain are among the diagnostic criteria for fibromyalgia. The EEG tracing of clients with this condition often shows a unique pattern of intrusion of alpha waves into slow-wave sleep, producing *alpha-delta activity*.[21] The clinical manifestations tend to be vague, and clients are often discouraged about the inability of health care professionals to diagnose and treat this condition. The nurse may be in a position to encourage referral to a sleep disorders center.

The effect of sleep or sleep deprivation on some disorders can be useful for diagnostic purposes. For example, the typical occurrence of erections in healthy males during REM sleep is being used as a diagnostic measure in differentiating sources of impotence.[71] REM-associated erections are also the reason that the nurse must be careful when securing an indwelling urinary catheter in a male client and allow a sufficient amount of loop to accommodate an erection.

Sleep deprivation and erratic sleep patterns reduce the seizure threshold, which you should consider in assessment and teaching of clients with seizure disorders. Seizure activity may also be a cause of sleep disturbance.[49] Partial and focal seizures can arise in all phases of sleep, including REM; generalized tonic-clonic seizures are more likely to occur during slow-wave sleep than during REM.[64] The tendency of sleep deprivation to trigger seizure activity is used diagnostically, in that clients may be required to stay awake all night before they undergo sleep-deprivation EEG. Some treatment regimens for clients susceptible to nocturnal seizures involve selective medication-induced suppression of sleep stages in which the client's seizures most frequently occur.

HOSPITAL-ACQUIRED SLEEP DISTURBANCES

Clients in the hospital may report difficulty getting to sleep, awakening frequently with difficulty getting back to sleep, or early morning awakening. The etiologic mechanism and interventions differ from each other.

■ SLEEP ONSET DIFFICULTY

Sleep onset difficulty is a common problem in hospitals because of the strange environment and the anxieties associated with illness and hospitalization. A sleep latency time of 20 to 30 minutes is within the normal range for most adults. Environmental control, such as reduction of noise and interruptions, and conservative relaxation measures, such as a back rub, should be tried before resorting to a hypnotic agent. The rapid-acting hypnotics, such as zolpidem (Ambien), are most effective with this type of insomnia.

If a hypnotic is given, monitor the client's safety in getting up at night. Most hypnotics cause some degree of antegrade amnesia, meaning that otherwise cognitively intact clients may become disoriented and forget where they are. The longer-acting hypnotics also result in some hangover effect. An increased risk of hip fractures from falls has been documented in people who are taking long-acting benzodiazepines.[59]

■ SLEEP MAINTENANCE DISTURBANCE

Sleep maintenance disturbance may be associated with sustained use of or withdrawal from a variety of medications and related substances. Alcohol hastens sleep onset but leads to awakening later in the night. In acute intoxication, REM sleep is suppressed. Abrupt withdrawal, as occurs with hospitalization, may trigger massive REM rebound. In chronic alcoholics, sleep architecture remains disturbed even several years after abstinence. Sustained use of or withdrawal from antidepressants, monoamine oxidase inhibitors, propranolol, and phenytoin can also contribute to insomnia.

Other factors that contribute to sleep fragmentation include stimuli that tend to awaken people in the middle of the night. Internal stimuli, such as pain, discomfort, and the urge to void, are frequent disturbers of sleep. Sleep disorders, such as sleep apnea and periodic limb movement, are more frequently associated with excessive somnolence, but they do trigger awakenings, after which some people have difficulty getting back to sleep. Hospitalization provides an opportunity for nursing surveillance, which may be instrumental in detecting these disorders as distinct from disturbances triggered by natural or transitory stimuli.

External stimuli include environmental factors, such as light, noise, and temperature, as well as disruptions by other people. You can reduce nocturnal stimuli by darkening the client's room; turn lights off, except for a small night light for safety purposes, and close curtains. To reduce nocturnal stimuli, reduce as much noise as possible by avoiding unnecessary conversation, minimizing equipment noise, and closing the client's door, if possible. You can adjust the temperature by providing bed coverings according to the client's preference and by modifying room temperature (directly, by adjusting the thermostat or air conditioner, or indirectly, by closing curtains and adjusting ventilation). Remove disturbing objects to create a pleasant, tidy environment, for example, removing equipment associated with painful procedures.

You can also reduce nocturnal stimuli by spacing necessary caregiving activities (e.g., turning, taking vital signs) to allow periods of 90 minutes or more of undisturbed sleep and, when possible, synchronizing these activities with periods during which the client is already awake. Finally, coordinate the nature and timing of interruptions by other caregivers (e.g., for laboratory testing or chest physiotherapy) to preserve periods of undisturbed sleep.

■ EARLY-MORNING AWAKENING

Early-morning awakening occurs frequently among the elderly. Sensitivity to environmental disturbances increases toward morning in people of all ages but even more so in older adults. Clients who are disturbed by early-morning awakening should be screened for indications of depression.

Sleeplessness and agitation may be associated with an acute confusional state (i.e., delirium). Especially among elderly people, this transient cognitive disorder may be associated with acute illness and admission to the hospital. Unlike that of dementia, the onset is rapid and is associated with a fluctuating level of consciousness. Thinking is disorganized and fragmented, memory is impaired, and delusions and hallucinations are common. Sleep is grossly disturbed with frightening dreams, disorientation, and restlessness. Delirium is usually precipitated by a treatable systemic illness such as dehydration, infection, drug toxicity, or renal failure. It is important that you identify delirium and pursue treatment possibilities. When the cause is removed, recovery is rapid.

■ SLEEP DEPRIVATION

Sleep deprivation is of particular concern for clients in critical care units. The noise level, 24-hour lighting, and frequency of caregiver interruptions create sensory overload and sleep deprivation, which is thought to be a major factor contributing to postoperative psychosis.[5]

Clients who have had surgery are also at risk for sleep pattern disturbance because of disruptions in circadian rhythms. The cause is unclear, but the disruptions may be related to the length and type of anesthesia, postoperative analgesia, or mechanisms associated with the procedure itself. REM sleep and slow-wave sleep are suppressed. It may take 4 to 6 weeks for the client's sleep patterns to return to normal after open heart surgery with cardiopulmonary bypass. Specific assessment of sleep quality and quantity should be incorporated into the care of all surgical patients.

DIAGNOSTIC ASSESSMENT

The primary diagnostic test for sleep disorders is polysomnography (Fig. 21–2). Clients may be referred to a sleep disorders center for overnight EEG, electro-oculography (EOG), and submental EMG with surface electrodes. Clients may also have continuous recording of arterial oxygen saturation by ear or finger oximeter, air flow as detected by monitoring expired carbon dioxide, respiratory movements by means of transducers placed around the chest and abdomen, and an electrocardiogram (ECG) and heart rate determination with standard limb leads. Ambulatory monitoring systems are also available to facilitate studies in the natural home environment.

A multiple sleep latency test (MSLT) may also be performed to assess impairment of daytime alertness. The MSLT is performed the day after a standard overnight polysomnogram. The time required for clients to fall asleep when in a relaxed state is evaluated at 2-hour intervals, with each nap limited to 20 minutes. The type of sleep is also assessed, making the test particularly useful in diagnosing narcolepsy, a condition in which clients typically have sleep-onset REM periods.[13]

Nursing Management

ASSESSMENT

Include a brief assessment of the client's usual sleep habits and recent sleep quality as part of the initial nursing history. On the care plan, note usual bedtime and rising times as well as preferences or rituals that may enhance sleep quality. For example, clients with ineffective breathing patterns associated with conditions such as COPD and hiatal hernia may be accustomed to sleeping with several pillows or with the head of the bed elevated.

If sleep quality is reported to be poor, explore the nature of the disturbance by noting the following:

- Usual activities in the hour before retiring
- Sleep latency
- Number and perceived cause of awakenings
- Regularity of sleep pattern (e.g., shift work)
- Consistency of rising time
- Frequency and duration of naps
- Events associated with initial onset of sleep disturbance
- Ease of falling asleep in places other than the usual bedroom
- Situations in which client fights sleepiness
- Daily caffeine intake
- Use of alcohol, sleeping pills, and other medications
- Incidence of morning headache
- Frequency of snoring, apparent pauses in breathing (apneas), and kicking movements; the latter information is

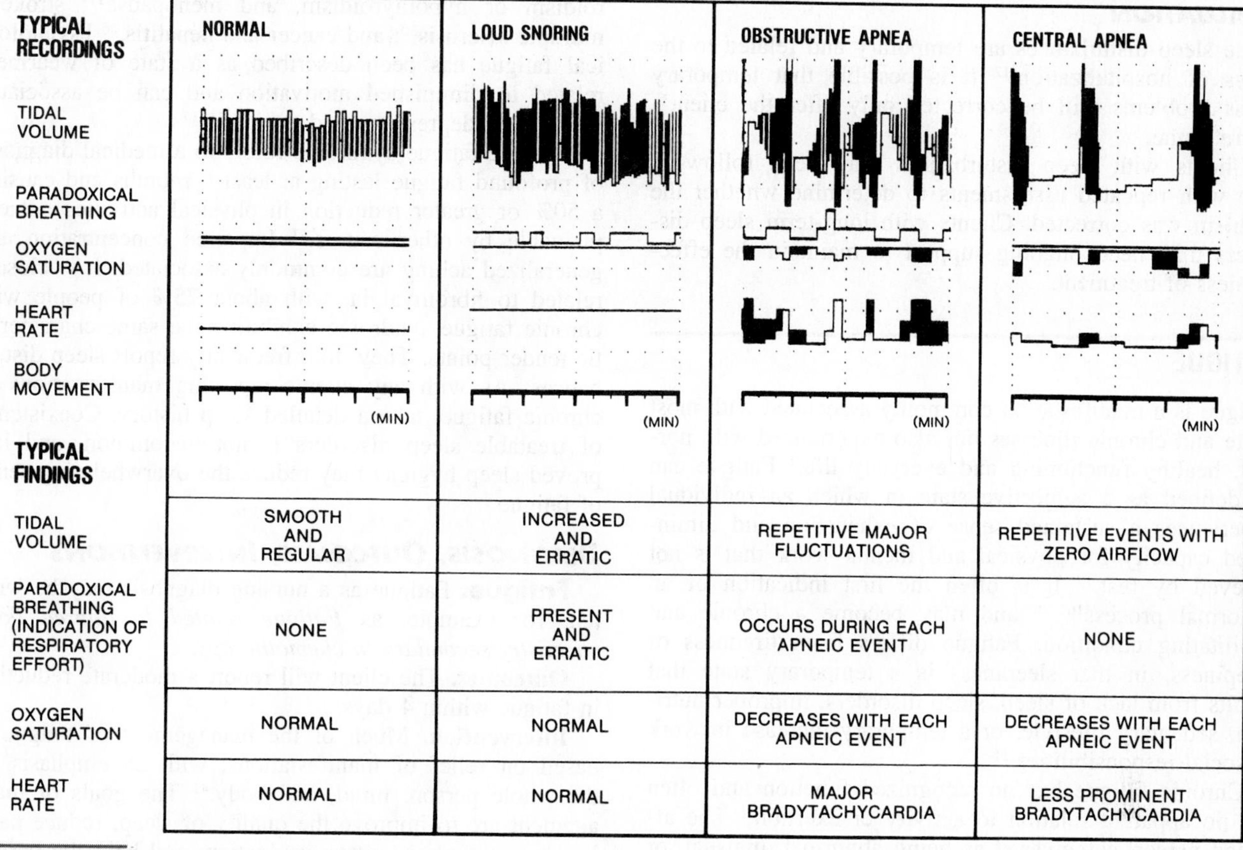

	NORMAL	LOUD SNORING	OBSTRUCTIVE APNEA	CENTRAL APNEA
TIDAL VOLUME	SMOOTH AND REGULAR	INCREASED AND ERRATIC	REPETITIVE MAJOR FLUCTUATIONS	REPETITIVE EVENTS WITH ZERO AIRFLOW
PARADOXICAL BREATHING (INDICATION OF RESPIRATORY EFFORT)	NONE	PRESENT AND ERRATIC	OCCURS DURING EACH APNEIC EVENT	NONE
OXYGEN SATURATION	NORMAL	NORMAL	DECREASES WITH EACH APNEIC EVENT	DECREASES WITH EACH APNEIC EVENT
HEART RATE	NORMAL	NORMAL	MAJOR BRADYTACHYCARDIA	LESS PROMINENT BRADYTACHYCARDIA

FIGURE 21–2 Polysomnography is used to determine the presence of sleep disorders. These examples are taken from a screening system that may be used in a person's home (in contrast to a laboratory), where sleep patterns are more typical. Screening studies can differentiate between obstructive sleep apnea and central sleep apnea as well as between loud snoring and normal sleep patterns. When a sleep disorder is identified, further assessment is needed, including electroencephalographic and electrocardiographic readings to elucidate the cause of the problem. (Courtesy of Vitalog, Mountain View, CA.)

best obtained from the sleeping partner or from your observation while the client is in the hospital

Objective data may include visible signs of fatigue and lack of sleep, such as circles under the eyes, lack of coordination, drowsiness, and irritability.

DIAGNOSIS, OUTCOMES, INTERVENTIONS

Sleep Pattern Disturbance. Sleep pattern disturbance is a common nursing diagnosis (e.g., *Sleep Pattern Disturbance related to changes in routine due to hospitalization and pain*). It may be related to change in sleeping environment, shift work schedule, recurrent pain, or many other possibilities. Other nursing diagnoses may also be applicable (e.g., *Risk for Injury related to excessive daytime sleepiness*).

Outcomes. The client will have improved sleep patterns within three nights as evidenced by sleeping for 6 to 8 hours at one time, stated feeling of lessened fatigue, and decreased irritability.

Intervention. The client's usual bedtime routine should be followed as closely as possible. For example, if the client usually watches television before sleeping, attempt to make this possible. Schedule nursing assessments and interventions in blocks of time to allow 90 to 120 minutes of uninterrupted sleep. The environment should mimic nighttime, with lights dimmed and quiet maintained. Offer extra blankets for external warmth. Provide a light complex carbohydrate snack, such as whole wheat crackers, if the client's condition allows.

Other techniques used to promote sleep include back massage, relaxing music, and progressive relaxation techniques. Medications to promote sleep should be used judiciously because they can alter the architecture of sleep, often reducing the REM sleep and eventually leading to REM rebound. If the client is in pain, analgesics rather than sleeping medications should be given. Clients in pain do not sleep restfully.

Sleep medications may be useful during short periods of sleep disturbance (e.g., hospitalization, bereavement, relocation). These medications are usually given at bedtime, and administration may be repeated once if they are not effective. Consider the drug's half-life and the time of night before repeating administration. To avoid prolonged drowsiness, do not repeat sleeping medications after 3 AM. In this case, you might try other measures to promote sleep, such as offering milk, analgesia, music, and back massage.

The client should be awakened with the least obtrusive stimulus possible, such as a soft touch or a soft voice. Startling the client may make it difficult for the client to go back to sleep. Many assessments and interventions can be performed without the client's being completely awake.

EVALUATION

Some sleep disturbances are temporary and related to the stress of hospitalization.[12] It is possible that temporary stress problems will be corrected only after the client's return home.

Clients with sleep disturbances may need follow-up care with repeated assessments to determine whether the problem was corrected. Clients with long-term sleep disorders may need ongoing support to maintain the effectiveness of treatment.

FATIGUE

Fatigue is a manifestation commonly associated with most acute and chronic illnesses but also experienced with normal, healthy functioning and everyday life.[1] Fatigue can be defined as a subjective state in which an individual experiences a sustained sense of exhaustion and diminished capacity for physical and mental work that is not relieved by rest.[17] It is often the first indication of an abnormal process[16, 26] and may become a chronic and debilitating condition. Fatigue differs from tiredness or sleepiness, in that sleepiness is a temporary state that results from lack of sleep, sleep disorders, improper nutrition, sedentary lifestyle, or a temporary increase in work or social responsibilities.[11]

Chronic fatigue has no recognized function and often has no apparent relation to activity or exertion.[1] The affected person perceives it as being abnormal, unusual, or excessive. It typically has an insidious onset, persists over time, and is not generally relieved by usual restorative techniques. Fatigue has a major effect on one's activities of daily living and quality of life.

Nurses have an important role in helping fatigued clients manage and cope effectively, whether they are in the hospital or in their own home. Understanding the debilitating effects of fatigue on individuals is an important component of effective nursing care.[16]

ASSESSMENT

The major defining characteristics of fatigue are as follows[17]:

- Verbalization of an unremitting and overwhelming lack of energy
- Inability to maintain usual routines
- Perceived need for additional energy to accomplish routine tasks
- Increase in physical complaints
- Emotional lability or irritability
- Impaired ability to concentrate and decreased performance
- Lethargy or listlessness
- Disinterest in surroundings
- Decreased libido
- Accident proneness

Fatigue, like pain, must be understood as multidimensional aspects that include physiologic, psychological, social, and spiritual components.[24]

Physiologic fatigue has been associated with sleep disturbances, infection, fever, pregnancy, and anemia[1]; acquired immunodeficiency syndrome (AIDS), hyperthyroidism or hypothyroidism, and menopause[17]; stroke[38]; multiple sclerosis[30]; and cancer and hepatitis.[26] Psychological fatigue has been described as a state of weariness related to diminished motivation and can be associated with stress, depression, and anxiety.[1, 17]

Chronic fatigue syndrome refers to a medical diagnosis of profound fatigue lasting at least 6 months and causing a 50% or greater reduction in physical activities not explainable by other causes.[41] Impaired concentration and generalized aching are commonly associated. It is closely related to fibromyalgia, with about 75% of people with chronic fatigue syndrome exhibiting the same characteristic tender points. They, too, frequently report sleep disturbances. As with any clients reporting manifestations of chronic fatigue, take a detailed sleep history. Coexistence of treatable sleep disorders is not uncommon, and improved sleep hygiene may reduce the overwhelming sense of fatigue.

DIAGNOSIS, OUTCOMES, INTERVENTIONS

Fatigue. Fatigue as a nursing diagnosis may be written, for example, as *Fatigue related to altered body chemistry secondary to chemotherapy.*

Outcomes. The client will report a moderate reduction in fatigue within 4 days.

Intervention. Much of the management of fatigue is based on relief of manifestations, with an emphasis on the whole person, mind, and body.[41] The goals of management are to improve the quality of sleep, reduce pain, increase neurotransmitter production, and help the person regain control of his or her life.[41]

You can support clients in understanding the causes of their fatigue and offer support in identifying energy patterns and the need for scheduling activities.[11] An understanding of the effects of conflict and stress on energy levels can help the individual learning new fatigue coping skills. Allowing the expression of feelings regarding the effects of fatigue on one's life is important. Monitor for factors contributing to fatigue on a daily basis, and intervene in a timely manner. Intervention may include carefully planning activities of daily living and daily exercise schedules with appropriate rest periods.[11] Assistance with self-care activities should be offered when needed, and attempts should be made to minimize sensory overload or sensory deprivation.

EVALUATION

Fatigue may not resolve completely, depending on the underlying factors. Thus, evaluation of outcomes and revisions to interventions should be based on mutual planning with the client and family to reduce manifestations and to improve management and quality of life. Balance is needed, so that strategies to reduce fatigue, such as avoidance of stress, do not preclude activities that are important to the client.

SENSORY DISTURBANCES

Each person has an optimal level of sensory input that facilitates a sense of well-being and optimal cognitive and motor performance. Sensory input comes from environmental and internal sources. Sensory input is received through peripheral receptors, transmitted via afferent neurons up the spinal cord, and channeled through the hypothalamus to the cerebral cortex, where it is interpreted in relation to previous patterns of experience.

People at risk for sensory overload or deprivation include those who are experiencing a new or unfamiliar environment, altered sensory input, altered cognitive processing, or impaired mobility.

It has been suggested that people with dementia have a progressively lowered stress threshold because of declining cognitive and functional abilities.[69] Other situations, such as acute illness or losses, may also reduce the ability to cope with a new or challenging environment.

CLASSIFICATION

SENSORY OVERLOAD

Sensory overload is a state in which the degree and nature of sensory input exceed the tolerance level of the individual, resulting in feelings of distress and hyperarousal with impaired thinking and problem-solving ability.

SENSORY DEPRIVATION

Sensory deprivation is a state in which the overall quantity or diversity of sensory input is decreased. People often compensate for an overall reduction in stimuli by increasing internal stimuli, such as by daydreaming or reminiscing.

DIAGNOSIS AND PREVENTION

DIAGNOSIS

Sensory/perceptual alterations is the nursing diagnosis relevant to sensory disturbances.[17] It is defined as a state in which the individual experiences a change in the amount or pattern of incoming stimuli accompanied by a diminished, exaggerated, distorted, or impaired response to such stimuli.

PREVENTION

You can minimize the risk of sensory disturbances by modifying the environment to prevent overstimulation and by enhancing orientation, meaning, and pattern. Practical interventions include reducing noise and glare and explaining not only procedures but also sights and sounds in the environment (e.g., the intercom).

Clients who have had limited prior experience with hospitalization or with health technology are at particular risk for sensory overload because they lack memories and knowledge to make sense out of much of their changed environment. In addition, clients whose sensory input is restricted or distorted are at risk for sensory deprivation in the sense that the stimuli are inappropriate to their needs. For example, a client with a spinal cord injury may be kept in a supine position initially, limiting the field of vision to the ceiling and the portions of the room that can be seen from each side.

Another major high-risk group of clients are those experiencing alterations in thought processes such as those that occur with stroke, head injury, schizophrenia, or dementia (e.g., Alzheimer's disease). Keep explanations to these clients simple and concrete. The environment should be structured and simplified, incorporating normalizing cues (e.g., drapes open to sunlight, familiar pictures and objects). Agitation can be decreased through choice of colors, reducing television or visitor noise, and creating stability and predictability in the immediate environment.[50, 65, 69]

Associated factors that can increase the risk of sensory overload include confinement, lack of ability to control the environment, and pressures related to time, decision-making, and complex task performance.

The inability to integrate incoming stimuli may be exhibited as confusion.[58] Sensory overload caused by an excess of poorly understood environmental stimuli may be superimposed on disturbed cerebral metabolism resulting from electrolyte disturbance, drugs, organic brain disease, and cardiopulmonary problems. The nurse should monitor the client for abnormal laboratory values and possible toxic responses to drugs or drug interactions, with particular attention to implications of slower metabolic processes in elderly people.[69] (For more information on assessing the confused client, see Chapter 68.)

Modification of the environment also has the potential to enhance the client's psychological well-being. The intervention called *environmental structuring* is defined as "an assortment of nurses' actions that directly or indirectly affect environmental features or conditions."[50] As more has been learned about psychoneuroimmunology, increasing evidence suggests that environmental conditions can be modified in ways that facilitate healing. Music therapy is an example of one such intervention that you can use to reduce psychophysiologic stress and to improve breathing patterns and the ability to communicate.[72]

CONCLUSIONS

The adequacy of sleep and rest and the appropriateness of sensory stimulation are important factors to consider in caring for clients with acute or chronic illness. Disorders of sleep, fatigue, and sensory stimulation have been discussed with consideration of the reciprocity among these processes, illness, and hospitalization. The nurse can play a pivotal role in environmental modification and client teaching to minimize the impact of sleep, fatigue, and sensory disturbances.

THINKING CRITICALLY

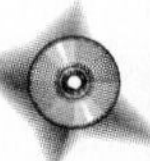

1. **The client has just been given a prescription for zolpidem (Ambien) to treat insomnia. She confides in you that she has been using a product from a health food store, recommended by a friend. Now she asks you whether it is safe to continue taking the herbal remedy as well as her new prescription.**

Factors to Consider. What is zolpidem? Can it interact with other medications? How could you find more information about the herbal medication the client is taking?

2. **A late-middle-aged client who has had a cerebrovascular accident and is unable to move or speak is placed in a room at the end of the hall, away from the nurses' station. This client was**

assigned a window bed. He has few visitors. His roommate is a young man recovering from a mild head injury. The roommate has many visitors and uses the radio and television loudly and frequently. Which client is more likely to develop sensory deprivation? Sensory overload? What nursing assessments and interventions would help prevent sensory disturbances?

Factors to Consider. What factors (age, environmental, physical, psychological) affect sensory functioning? How do clients receive and interpret incoming stimuli? Does the room assignment contribute to the development of sensory disturbance in either client?

3. **A young adult comes to the neighborhood health clinic. She is unkempt, has circles under her eyes, and yawns frequently. She gives a history of being unable to sleep for any length of time since she gave birth recently to twin sons. She took a variety of prescription "sleeping pills" before she became pregnant and wants a new prescription to help her sleep. What might be causing her sleeplessness? What sleep assessments should be completed? What impact may lack of sleep have?**

Factors to Consider. What measures might help this young mother sleep naturally? How would her lack of sleep affect the health of her children? How normal is it for a young adult to experience difficulty with sleep and to take medications to assist with sleep?

BIBLIOGRAPHY

1. Aaronson, L. S., et al. (1999). Defining and measuring fatigue. *Image: Journal of Nursing Scholarship, 31*(1), 45–50.
2. Akerstedt, T. (1998). Shift work and disturbed sleep/wakefulness. *Sleep Medicine Reviews, 2*(2), 117–128.
3. Aldrich, M. S. (1990). Narcolepsy. *New England Journal of Medicine, 323*(6), 389–394.
4. Ancoli-Israel, S., et al. (1991). Sleep disordered breathing in community dwelling elderly. *Sleep,* 14, 486–495.
5. Ancoli-Israel, S. (1997). Sleep problems in older adults: Putting myths to bed. *Geriatrics, 52*(1), 20–30.
6. Ancoli-Israel, S., et al. (1997). Identification and treatment of sleep problems in the elderly. *Sleep Medicine Reviews, 1*(1), 3–17.
7. Baker, A., Simpson, S., & Dawson, D. (1997). Sleep disruption and mood changes associated with menopause. *Journal of Psychosomatic Research, 43*(4), 359–369.
8. Beck-Little, R., & Weinrich, S. P. (1998). Assessment and management of sleep disorders in the elderly. *Journal of Gerontological Nursing, 24*(4), 21–29.
9. Bliwise, D. L. (1994). Normal aging. In M. H. Kryger, T. Roth, & W. C. Dement (Eds.), *Principles and practice of sleep medicine* (2nd ed., pp. 26–39). Philadelphia: W. B. Saunders.
10. Cardinali, D. P., & Pevet, P. (1998). Basic aspects of melatonin action. *Sleep Medicine Reviews,* 2(4), 175–190.
11. Carpenito, L. J. (1999). *Handbook of nursing diagnosis* (8th ed). Philadelphia: J. B. Lippincott.
12. Cohen, F. L., & Merritt, S. L. (1992). Sleep promotion. In G. M. Bulechek & J. C. McCloskey (Eds.), *Nursing interventions: Essential nursing treatments* (2nd ed., pp. 109–119). Philadelphia: W. B. Saunders.
13. Cohen, F. L., Nehring, W. M., & Cloninger, L. (1996). Symptom description and management in narcolepsy. *Holistic Nursing Practice, 10*(4), 44–53.
14. Cohen-Mansfield, J., & Marx, M. S. (1990). The relationship between sleep disturbances and agitation in a nursing home. *Journal of Aging Health,* 2(1), 42–57.
15. Collard, P., et al. (1997). Compliance with nasal CPAP in obstructive sleep apnea patients. *Sleep Medicine Reviews, 1*(1), 33–44.
16. Cook, N. F., & Boore, J. R. P. (1997). Managing patients suffering from acute and chronic fatigue. *British Journal of Nursing, 6*(14), 811–815.
17. Cox, H. C., et al. (1997). *Clinical applications of nursing diagnosis* (3rd ed.). Philadelphia: F. A. Davis.
18. Curtis, S. M. & Porth, C. M. (1998). Disorders of brain function. In C. Porth (Ed.), *Pathophysiology of altered health states* (5th ed., pp. 879–920). Philadelphia: J. B. Lippincott.
19. Czeisler, C. A., & Shapiro, C. M. (1995). Circadian rhythm disorders. In C. M. Shapiro (Ed.), *Sleep solutions manual* (pp. 190–207). Pointe Claire, Quebec: Kommunicom Publications.
20. Deb, S., Lyons, I., & Koutzoukis, C. (1998). Neuropsychiatric sequelae one year after a minor head injury. *Journal of Neurology, Neurosurgery and Psychiatry, 65*(6), 889–902.
21. Diagnostic Classification Steering Committee, Thorpy, M. J., Chairman. (1997). *International classification of sleep disorders: Diagnostic and coding manual* (Rev. ed.). Rochester, MN: American Sleep Disorders Association.
22. Dinges, D. F., & Broughton, R. J. (1989). *Sleep and alertness: Chronobiological, behavioral and medical aspects of napping.* New York: Raven Press.
23. Driver, H. S., & Baker, F. C. (1998). Menstrual factors in sleep. *Sleep Medicine Reviews, 2*(4), 213–229.
24. El-Ad, B., & Korczyn, A. D. (1998). Disorders of excessive daytime sleepiness: An update. *Journal of Neurological Sciences, 153*(2), 192–202.
25. Evans, B. D., & Rogers, A. E. (1994). 24-hour sleep-wake patterns in healthy elderly persons. *Applied Nursing Research, 7*(2), 75–83.
26. Ferrell, B. R., et al. (1996). "Bone tired": The experience of fatigue and its impact on quality of life. *Oncology Nursing Forum, 23*(10) 1539–1547.
27. Fleming, J. A., & Shapiro, C. M. (1995). Insomnia management. In C. M. Shapiro (Ed.), *Sleep solutions manual* (pp. 34–49). Pointe Claire, Quebec: Kommunicom Publications.
28. Flemons, W. W., & McNicholas, W. T. (1997). Clinical prediction of the sleep apnea syndrome. *Sleep Medicine Reviews, 1*(1), 19–32.
29. Foley, D. J., et al. (1995). Sleep complaints among elderly persons: An epidemiologic study of three communities. *Sleep, 18*(6), 425–432.
30. Ford, H., Trigwell, P., & Johnson, M. (1998). The nature of fatigue in multiple sclerosis. *Journal of Psychosomatic Research, 45*(1), 33–38.
31. Fredrickson, P. A., et al. (1990). Sleep disorders in psychiatric practice. *Mayo Clinic Proceedings, 65,* 861–868.
32. Guilleminault, C. (1994). Narcolepsy syndrome. In M. H. Kryger, T. Roth, & W. C. Dement (Eds.), *Principles and practice of sleep medicine* (2nd ed., pp. 549–561). Philadelphia: W. B. Saunders.
33. Hauri, P. J. (1994). Primary insomnia. In M. H. Kryger, T. Roth, & W. C. Dement (Eds.), *Principles and practice of sleep medicine* (2nd ed., pp. 494–499). Philadelphia: W. B. Saunders.
34. Hauri, P. J., & Linde, S. (1991). *No more sleepless nights.* New York: John Wiley & Sons.
35. Hobson, J. A. (1988). *The dreaming brain.* New York: Basic Books.
36. Hodgson, L. A. (1991). Why do we need sleep? Relating theory to nursing practice. *Journal of Advances in Nursing, 16,* 1503–1510.
37. Horne, J. A. (1988). *Why we sleep.* New York: Oxford University Press.
38. Ingles, J. L., Eskes, G. A., & Phillips, S. J. (1999). Fatigue after stroke. *Archives of Physical Medicine and Rehabilitation, 80,* 173–178.
39. Johnson, M. W., & Remmers, J. E. (1984). Accessory muscle activity during sleep in chronic obstructive pulmonary disease. *Journal of Applied Physiology, 57*(4), 1011–1017.
40. Kaplan, H. I., Sadock, B. J., & Grebb, J. A. (1994). *Kaplan and Sadock's synopsis of psychiatry* (7th ed.). Baltimore: Williams & Wilkins.
41. Kenner, C. (1998). Fibromyalgia and chronic fatigue: The holistic perspective. *Holistic Nursing Practice, 12*(3), 55–63.
42. Kryger, M. H. (1994). Management of obstructive sleep apnea: An overview. In M. H. Kryger, T. Roth, & W. C. Dement (Eds.), *Principles and practice of sleep medicine* (2nd ed., pp. 736–747). Philadelphia: W. B. Saunders.
43. Krystal, A. D., et al. (1998). Sleep in peri-menopausal and post-menopausal women. *Sleep Medicine Reviews, 2*(4), 243–253.
44. Lahaie, U. (1991). Shift-workers and seasonal affective disorder. *Canadian Nurse, 87*(5), 33–34.

45. Lee, K. A., et al. (1990). Sleep patterns related to menstrual cycle phase and premenstrual affective symptoms. *Sleep, 13*(5), 403–409.
46. Levitt, A., & Shapiro, C. M. (1995). Seasonal affective disorder. In C. M. Shapiro (Ed.), *Sleep solutions manual* (pp. 126–146). Pointe Claire, Quebec: Kommunicom Publications.
47. Littrell, K. D., & Schumann, L. L. (1989). Promoting sleep for the patient with a myocardial infarction. *Critical Care Nurse, 9*(3), 44, 46–49.
48. Lowe, A. D. (1998). Sleep in Parkinson's disease. *Journal of Psychosomatic Research, 44*(6), 613–617.
49. Lugaresi, E., et al. (1988). Sleep in clinical neurology. In R. L. Williams, I. Karacan, & C. A. Moore (Eds.), *Sleep disorders: Diagnosis and treatment* (2nd ed., pp. 245–263). New York: John Wiley & Sons.
50. Mion, L. C. (1992). Environmental structuring. In G. M. Bulechek & J. C. McCloskey (Eds.), *Nursing interventions* (2nd ed., pp. 254–264). Philadelphia: W. B. Saunders.
51. National Commission on Sleep Disorders Research. (1993). *Wake up America: A national sleep alert* (Executive summary and executive report, Report of the National Commission on Sleep Disorders Research. National Institutes of Health, January, Vol. 1, pp. 1–76. DHHS Publication, Washington, DC: Supervisor of Documents, U.S. Government Printing Office).
52. North American Nursing Diagnosis Association (NANDA). (1999). *Nursing diagnoses: Definitions and classification 1999–2000.* Philadelphia: Author.
53. Ohayon, M. M., et al. (1997). How sleep and mental disorders are related to complaints of daytime sleepiness. *Archives of Internal Medicine, 157*(22), 2645–2652.
54. Orr, W. C. (1994). Gastrointestinal disorders. In M. H. Kryger, T. Roth, & W. C. Dement (Eds.), *Principles and practice of sleep medicine* (2nd ed., pp. 861–869). Philadelphia: W. B. Saunders.
55. Parkosewich, J. A. (1986). Sleep-disordered breathing: A common problem in chronic obstructive pulmonary disease. *Critical Care Nurse, 6*(6), 60–64.
56. Partinen, M. (1994). Epidemiology of sleep disorders. In M. H. Kryger, T. Roth, & W. C. Dement (Eds.), *Principles and practice of sleep medicine* (2nd ed., pp. 437–452). Philadelphia: W. B. Saunders.
57. Partonen, T. (1998). A developmental approach to severe depression. *Medical Hypotheses, 51*(2), 165–166.
58. Rasin, J. H. (1990). Confusion. *Nursing Clinics of North America, 25*(4), 909–918.
59. Ray, W., Griffen, M., & Downey, W. (1989). Benzodiazepines of long and short elimination half-life and the risk of hip fracture. *JAMA, 262*(23), 3303–3307.
60. Reimer, M. (1989). Sleep pattern disturbances related to neurological dysfunction. *Axon, 10*(3), 65–68.
61. Remmers, J. E. (1990). Sleeping and breathing. *Chest 97,* 77S–80S.
62. Schmidt-Nowara, W., et al. (1995). Oral appliances for the treatment of snoring and obstructive sleep apnea: A review. *Sleep, 18*(6), 501–510.
63. Schnelle, J. F., et al. (1998). Sleep hygiene in physically dependent nursing home residents: Behavioral and environmental intervention implications. *Sleep, 21*(5), 515–523.
64. Shouse, M. N. (1994). Epileptic seizure manifestations during sleep. In M. H. Kryger, T. Roth, & W. C. Dement (Eds.), *Principles and practice of sleep medicine* (2nd ed., pp. 801–814). Philadelphia: W. B. Saunders.
65. Sloane, P. D., & Mathew, L. J. (1990). The therapeutic environment screening scale. *American Journal of Alzheimer's Care and Related Disorders and Research, 5*(6), 22–26.
66. Smith, R. P., et al. (1998). Obstructive sleep apnea and the autonomic nervous system. *Sleep Medicine Reviews, 2*(2), 69–92.
67. Standards of Practice Committee of the American Sleep Disorders Association. (1994). Practice parameters for the use of laser-assisted uvulopalatoplasty. *Sleep, 17*(8), 744–748.
68. Steriade, M. (1994). Brain electrical activity and sensory processing during waking and sleeping states. In M. H. Kryger, T. Roth, & W. C. Dement (Eds.), *Principles and practice of sleep medicine* (2nd ed., pp. 105–124). Philadelphia: W. B. Saunders.
69. Stolley, J. M., & Buckwalter, K. C. (1992). Confusion management. In G. M. Bulechek & J. C. McCloskey (Eds.), *Nursing interventions* (2nd ed., pp. 120–134). Philadelphia: W. B. Saunders.
70. Terman, M. (1994). Light treatment. In M. H. Kryger, T. Roth, & W. C. Dement (Eds.), *Principles and practice of sleep medicine* (2nd ed., pp. 1012–1029). Philadelphia: W. B. Saunders.
71. Ware, J. C., & Hirshkowitz, M. (1994). Monitoring penile erections during sleep. In M. H. Kryger, T. Roth, & W. C. Dement (Eds.), *Principles and practice of sleep medicine* (2nd ed., pp. 967–977). Philadelphia: W. B. Saunders.
72. Wiens, M., Reimer, M., & Guyn, H. L. (1998). Music therapy as a treatment method for improving respiratory muscle strength in advanced multiple sclerosis: A pilot study. *Rehabilitation Nursing, 24*(2), 74–80.

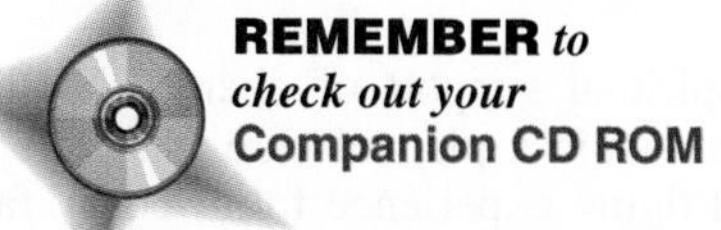

CHAPTER 22

Perspectives on End-of-Life Care

Kim K. Kuebler
Debra E. Heidrich

Nurses caring for clients with advanced diseases will ultimately witness the final stage of life—dying. The dying process is often accompanied by many different psychological, spiritual, and physical needs, and nurses are in the ideal position to identify and address them. Nurses must be knowledgeable about the normal dying process, the control of pain and other symptoms, and the role of the interdisciplinary team in order to provide optimal support and symptom management for dying clients and their families.

Note: In this chapter, *symptom* is used instead of *clinical manifestations,* the term used elsewhere in the text. The symptoms associated with dying differ from manifestations described with specific medical problems discussed in other chapters. *Symptom management* is the preferred term often used in the care of those clients with advanced illness and is the primary focus within the specialty of palliative care.

END-OF-LIFE CARE

The terms *hospice care*, *palliative care*, and *end-of-life care* sometimes are used interchangeably and at other times are used to differentiate various models of care. The following discussion briefly identifies the evolution of the hospice movement and the development of palliative care programs.

■ HOSPICE

The hospice movement began in the late 1960s in the United Kingdom. Dame Cicely Saunders established that the complex needs of dying clients were not being addressed in the traditional health care system. Her vision and understanding of the unmet needs of the dying prompted the first modern hospice, St. Christopher's Hospice in London, England.[14] Saunders believed that the dying required the multiple skills of an interdisciplinary team to provide "patient-centered care." The precepts of the hospice movement in the United States are a direct result of the work at St. Christopher's Hospice.[6, 17]

Another pioneer whose work greatly influenced the hospice movement was Elizabeth Kübler-Ross. Her theoretical framework for the death and dying process brought forth recognition of the psychological and existential needs of the dying.[24] Her life work was to help clients and society to view terminal illness not as a destructive, negative force but as one of the "windstorms" in life that can enhance inner growth.[24, 25] Kübler-Ross is most noted for identifying and defining the phases of the normal death and dying experience: (1) denial, (2) anger, (3) bargaining, (4) depression, and (5) acceptance.[24, 25] After spending many years at the bedsides of the dying, Kübler-Ross recognized the importance of the interdisciplinary team in providing support to the client and family as they experience the various phases of the dying process.[24, 25]

While Kübler-Ross was advocating for the dying and St. Christopher's Hospice was successfully caring for terminally ill clients, Florence Wald, then the dean of graduate nursing studies at Yale University, expressed interest in bringing the hospice movement to the United States. Wald recognized the tremendous need in America to improve the care of the dying. She helped integrate the British hospice movement into the first home care hospice in New Haven, Conn., in 1974.[6, 17]

At the same time, people in Canada were recognizing a need to provide better care at the end of life. Balfour Mount, the first to define *palliative care*, opened the first hospital-based palliative care service at the Royal Victoria Hospital of McGill University in Montreal in 1975.[14] The McGill model followed the interdisciplinary team approach of client-centered and family-centered care and was the first program to include research and education in the area of pain management.[6, 17]

All of these pioneers advocated for improved care of the terminally ill and their families. They believed that professionals trained to provide physical comfort through pain and symptom management as well as psychosocial and spiritual support could promote a healthy, normal dying experience.

During the 1970s, the hospice concept of care continued to grow as a grassroots movement throughout the United States. Citing the cost-effectiveness of and client and family satisfaction with this level of care, Congress approved a Medicare Hospice Benefit in 1982.[31] With a solid source of reimbursement available, the number of hospice programs grew markedly over the next several years.[6, 22, 31]

■ CONTINUED UNMET NEEDS OF THE DYING

The growth of hospices did not, however, address the needs of people dying in other health care settings. In 1995, findings of SUPPORT (Study to Understand Prognoses and Preferences for Outcomes and Risks of Treatments),[50] revealed that Americans were continuing to die in pain and without dignity. This $28 million dollar study, funded by the Robert Wood Johnson Foundation and conducted at five medical centers nationwide over 10 years, found that 80% of Americans die in institutional settings, often with unmanaged pain, in isolation, connected to mechanical ventilators, and in intensive care units. The utilization of living wills, health care proxies, and communication efforts between clients and their physicians often proved futile.[29, 35, 50]

The findings of SUPPORT stirred a massive interest in improving the care of the dying in America. Although hospice care was acknowledged as successful in addressing the concerns identified in the study, hospice care was not being accessed by the majority of dying people. Only about 17% of the American population receive hospice services.[50] There are several reasons for the underutilization of hospice services:

- Our society's being a "death-denying" one, in which many clients and health care professionals desire life-prolonging care
- Lack of knowledge regarding the availability of services
- Difficulty in determining prognoses in terms of 6 months or less

These issues, along with increasingly strict admission criteria enforced by the Health Care Financing Administration (HCFA) for Medicare clients, changed the view of hospice care from a "concept" of care to a system that pays for the care of the dying.

Thus, the benefits of hospice care for the client and family are available to only a small percentage of the population who have a limited prognosis, who elect hospice care, and who meet the highly regulated, stringent admission criteria.[53] The concept of palliative care developed from the desire to broaden the whole-person, comfort-care approach of the hospice concept and to make it available to more people in all health care settings.[14]

■ PALLIATIVE CARE

Palliative care is defined by the World Health Organization (WHO)[2] as follows:

> the active total care of patients whose disease is not responsive to curative treatment. Control of pain, of other symptoms, and of psychological, social and spiritual problems, is paramount. The goal of palliative care is achievement of the best quality of life for patients and their families. Many aspects of palliative care are also applicable earlier in the course of the illness in conjunction with therapies such as anticancer treatment.

Like hospice care, palliative care recognizes that dying is a normal process that should be neither hastened nor postponed. The provision of symptom management and both emotional and spiritual support of clients and their families are considered while a plan of care is developed to promote an optimal dying experience followed by family bereavement.[14, 29, 35] Unlike clients qualifying for hospice care, clients who receive palliative care are not required to have a 6-month or shorter prognosis, making palliative care available to more people. See Bridge to Home Health Care.

DISEASE TRAJECTORY

The time from the onset of a terminal diagnosis until death is considered the *disease trajectory*. Some terminal diagnoses have a long disease trajectory with a gradual decline in functional status over time; others have a very short trajectory with a sharp decline; still others have variable trajectories with periods of remission and exacerbation.

Determining specific interventions to improve each client's quality of life is largely determined by his or her position on the disease trajectory. An example is a client who suddenly experiences spinal cord compression. If the client is not imminently dying and is considered to be active and somewhat mobile (i.e., early in the disease trajectory), it is appropriate for the client to undergo magnetic resonance imaging (MRI) with the possibility of radiation therapy. If the client is actively dying (i.e., late in the disease trajectory), he or she would not be able to tolerate a hospital admission, MRI, and radiation therapy; this client may benefit from aggressive use of corticosteroids in the home.

A comprehensive assessment is essential in determining the client's disease trajectory in order to guide identification of appropriate palliative interventions. This assessment comprises the following actions[9, 29]:

1. Define the nature of the clinical finding and symptom.
2. Perform a thorough history and physical examination, review current and tried medications, and evaluate a minimal set of diagnostic procedures to differentiate underlying pathophysiologic disorder from a reversible symptom.
3. Evaluate the problem within the context of the client's situation and allowing for prioritization. For example, the priority assigned a urinary tract infection (UTI) in a cognitively impaired, dehydrated, and bedridden client will be different from that given to a UTI in a cognitively intact client with good symptom control.
4. Define the "cost" of diagnostic and therapeutic interventions and the varying differences between clients. For example, what may be considered appropriate therapy for one client may be inappropriate for another—when evaluating the risk versus benefit of treatment and the financial burden of unnecessary interventions.
5. Discuss the various care options with the client and the family, and encourage informed decision-making.

QUALITY OF LIFE

Palliative care is offered toward the end of client's life, when a progressive illness is symptomatic and interferes with the quality of life. Many variables go into defining quality of life, including (1) socioeconomic status, (2)

BRIDGE TO HOME HEALTH CARE

Providing Hospice Care

The focus of care shifts from cure to comfort when the decision is made to use hospice and remain at home. The hospice team allows clients to maintain independence and to make informed choices about caregiving, pain control, nutrition, elimination, and skin care during frequent home visits and phone calls. The team explores and clarifies spiritual beliefs, helps clients and family members resolve estrangement and conflict, and offers information about funeral planning.

The goal of the hospice program is to achieve around-the-clock pain control by following the National Hospice Organization guidelines for scheduling, titration, and use of breakthrough pain medications. When the oral route is no longer available because of weakness or coma, rectal, transdermal, sublingual, and intravenous medications can be used effectively. Consider adjuvant medications to enhance analgesia and address different types of pain. Benzodiazepams enhance the work of analgesics. Nonsteroidal anti-inflammatory drugs help to relieve bone pain. Tricyclic antidepressants and anticonvulsants are effective for pain of neuropathic origin.

It is normal for clients to lose their appetite during the terminal stages of illness. Encourage clients to eat what they can tolerate to reduce stress and provide comfort. Prevent nausea and vomiting by giving antiemetics regularly or as needed. Schedule meals at the time of day when the client's energy is the greatest. Clients and family members need to know that dehydration will occur, but usually with few manifestations. Offer small amounts of water frequently with a spoon, syringe, eye dropper, or sponge-tipped swabs.

It is important to anticipate when equipment will be needed and to have it delivered to the home. Such preparation decreases stress, prevents injuries, and helps maintain independence. Needed equipment includes beds, wheelchairs, commodes, and walkers. Reduce oxygen hunger by using a floor fan or providing supplemental oxygen. Prevent skin breakdown with foam mats for chairs or beds. Use a draw-sheet for turning and repositioning to decrease skin tears and shearing. Save energy and prevent accidents by having the client use a commode at the bedside.

Minimize distress and discomfort by anticipating bowel and bladder changes. Schedule the administration of stool softeners and laxatives, enemas, and suppositories to increase bowel regularity and comfort. Prevent unnecessary delays by having standing orders to insert straight or Foley catheters for bladder evacuation. Keep a supply of briefs and protective pads to use when the client's condition changes quickly.

As death approaches, increase physical and emotional care to ensure dignity. Give atropine ophthalmic drops to reduce lung congestion. Use repositioning, light massage, and gentle range-of-motion exercises. Promote calmness and serenity with quiet presence, hand-holding, soft music, or prayers. Give clients permission to "go," assure them that their loved ones will be all right, and offer words of love to help clients achieve a peaceful passage. Encourage family members to do the same. It is the responsibility of nurses on the hospice team to provide details about disease progression, manifestations of approaching death, and protocols at the time of death. A nurse visits at the time of death, makes the death pronouncement, and telephones the physician, coroner, and funeral home.

The decision to use hospice is not one of giving up hope. It is one of hoping for comfort and quality of life in the moments, hours, and days that remain for a client at the end of life.

Jane Allen Austgen, RN, BSN, CRNH, *Hospice Nurse Case Manager, Alegent Health Home Care and Hospice, Omaha, Nebraska*

physical health, (3) relationships with friends and family, and (4) satisfaction with self.[12, 45] See Alternative Therapy: Spirituality and Health in Chapter 20. Quality of life is defined as "a personal statement of the positivity or negativity of attributes that characterize life."[12]

A person's quality of life is often linked to the experience of symptom distress and the meanings that the person assigns to these physical sensations.[12, 45] Nurses caring for clients who are experiencing distressing symptoms, such as pain, fatigue, constipation, and nausea, should understand that each client responds differently. The effect of a symptom on life routines varies from client to client, depending on overall functional status, coping abilities, and social supports. In palliative care, the plan of care must be based not only on the symptom itself but also on the effect of the symptom on the client's overall quality of living.

SYMPTOMS AT THE END OF LIFE

Clients with advanced diseases experience multiple symptoms, some of which are more severe than others.[18, 43, 50] In one study, pain was found to be the most prevalent symptom among clients with advanced cancer (89% of respondents). In 87% of the clients with pain, the severity of the pain was rated to be moderate to severe. In addition to pain, the symptoms weakness, anorexia, dyspnea, constipation, early satiety, fatigue, and dry mouth were experienced by more than 40% of clients.[18, 43, 50]

Symptoms vary not only in frequency and intensity but also in the distress experienced by clients.[18, 50] Although pain may be very prevalent, it is not always identified as the most distressing symptom. Some studies have found that dyspnea, asthenia (lethargy, generalized weakness, and fatigue), dry mouth, anorexia, depression, and insomnia may actually be more distressing than pain for clients with terminal illnesses.[2, 9, 43, 50] The symptoms commonly experienced by the dying are discussed here.

■ PAIN

Pain is a multidimensional phenomenon. Not only is a person's pain experience a physical response to an underlying disorder or disease state; there are also emotional, intellectual, behavioral, sensory, and cultural dimensions.[42] When a client is nonresponsive and unable to report pain, the nurse should observe for the behavioral indicators of pain (Table 22–1). Communication within the entire health care team is essential for optimal pain management. Chapter 23 describes types of pain, subjective and objective assessment of pain, and pain management strategies.

Opioid Analgesics

Opioids are the mainstay of treatment for moderate to severe pain.[1] These medications bind with opiate receptors in the central nervous system (CNS) and block the transmission of the pain impulse to the higher brain centers.[42, 43] Most opioid medications bind to the mu receptor and are called *mu agonists*. Morphine (MS Contin), hydromorphone (Dilaudid), fentanyl (Duragesic), and oxycodone (Oxycontin) are examples of mu-agonist opioids frequently used in the treatment of pain.[42] There is no ceiling to the analgesic effect of mu-agonist opioids.[18, 42] See Chapter 23 for further discussion of opioids.

In addition to modulating the transmission and perception of the pain impulse, opioids may bind with receptors in other tissues, leading to the potential for side effects. There are, for example, opioid receptors in the gastrointestinal tract. When opioids bind with these receptors, intestinal motility is decreased and gastric emptying is delayed, leading to constipation. Prophylactic treatment of constipation with both a stool softener and a stimulant is essential and should be initiated along with the first opioid dose. The clinician should not wait for the client to complain of constipation before beginning treatment. Constipation is the only side effect of opioids to which a person does not develop tolerance. A bowel protocol must be continued for the duration of treatment with opioids.

Other potential side effects of opioids are respiratory depression, nausea and vomiting, and sedation. Clinically significant respiratory depression is rare during treatment of pain if the opioid dose is increased slowly and decreased if sedation is noted. In addition, people develop tolerance to the respiratory-depressive side effects of opioids after the first several days of treatment. The client who has taken the same dose of an opioid for several weeks is not at risk for a clinically significant opioid-induced respiratory depression.[42]

Although nausea and vomiting may not be a problem for all clients, many clients do experience this as a side effect of opioids. Nausea and vomiting occur when the chemoreceptor trigger zone (CTZ) of the brain is stimulated by these medications. A client is less likely to experience nausea when opioids are administered orally than parenterally. As with respiratory depression, tolerance to this side effect of opioids develops over time. Clients who experience nausea and vomiting should be treated with antiemetics for the first 2 to 3 days after the opioid is initiated until tolerance develops. A small number of clients may experience persistent nausea from the opioids. These clients may benefit from either changing to a different opioid or continuing to use antiemetics.[42]

A client who has been in pain and receives an initial dose of an opioid may experience some degree of sedation. This is due, in part, to the direct effect of opioids on the brain. In addition to the sedative side effect of the opioid, however, the client is probably exhausted from not sleeping well when in pain. Teach the client that some sleepiness is expected and that it is probably not all due to the new medication. As with the other side effects of opioids, tolerance to the sedation develops after the first 2 to 3 days. If, however, the client is difficult to arouse or the sedation lasts more than 2 to 3 days, the opioid dose may be too high for the intensity of the pain.

Clients who are sedated from an opioid and still experiencing pain probably have pain syndromes not completely responsive to opioids. These clients require the addition of adjuvant medications in order to achieve comfort. Recognize that *there is no ceiling to the amount of opioid analgesic* required for each client to achieve a satisfactory level of analgesia. Hence, clients may require very high doses of opioids to achieve pain relief.

TABLE 22–1 OBSERVATIONAL ASSESSMENT IN THE NONRESPONSIVE CLIENT

Restlessness	Agitation, frequent moving, an inability to get comfortable, fidgety, picking at things
Vocalizations	Moaning, groaning, crying out
Muscle tension	Tense muscles, not relaxed, clenched teeth, tightened fists, guarded movements
Facial expression	Frowning, grimacing, distressed
Physiologic indicators	Fast heart rate, frequent and labored breathing, sweating

Adjuvant Analgesics

Adjuvant medications have a primary action other than pain relief but can also serve as analgesics for some painful conditions. They are often used in combination with other analgesic medications. At each step of the WHO analgesic ladder (see Chapter 23), adjuvant medications may be added, depending on the type of pain experienced. Several classes of medications are essential to optimal management of pain (Table 22–2).

Nonsteroidal anti-inflammatory drugs (NSAIDs) can be very helpful when the inflammatory process is involved and is initiating the pain impulse, such as in bone or soft tissue damage. Clients with metastatic bone disease often require the combination of an opioid and an NSAID for comfort.

Tricyclic antidepressants (TCAs) and anticonvulsants can be effective analgesics in the management of pain syndromes that have a neurologic component.[18, 42] TCAs appear to be most helpful for pain described as burning or aching; anticonvulsants are useful in the treatment of shooting and shock-like neurologic pains. The effective analgesic dose of a TCA is much lower than the dose required for an antidepressant effect.[1, 42] Some clients are aware that these medications are used to treat depression and may be suspicious that the clinician "thinks the pain is in my head." Explain to clients that these medications are used to manage pain at low doses. Because it takes 5 to 7 days for TCAs to reach the desired plasma level, inform the client that it may take several days for this new medication to be effective.

TABLE 22–2 ADJUVANT ANALGESICS

Pain Source	Pain Character	Medication Class	Examples
Bone or soft tissue	Tenderness over bone or joint Pain on movement	Nonsteroidal anti-inflammatory drugs	Ibuprofen Naproxen Indomethacin
Nerve damage/neuropathic	Burning, shooting, shock-like, or aching pain	Tricyclic antidepressants	Amitriptyline Doxepin
		Anticonvulsants	Carbamazepine Phenytoin Valproic acid Gabapentin
Smooth muscle spasms	Cramping or grabbing pains (intermittent)	Anticholinergics	Scopolamine Hyoscyamine Oxybutynin Dicyclomine
Anxiety	Generalized restlessness and discomfort	Benzodiazepines	Lorazepam Diazepam
		Butyrophenones	Haloperidol

People who report "colicky" pain may be experiencing the discomfort of smooth muscle spasm. This type of pain is best treated with an anticholinergic medication.

Anxiety is a complex symptom caused by physical, emotional, and spiritual concerns. People who are in pain often experience some anxiety, and it may be helpful to treat the anxiety in order to achieve comfort.[1, 11, 38] Benzodiazepine medications are frequently used for anxiety in the palliative care setting. Haloperidol, a butyrophenone, may also be used. Management of anxiety is covered in Chapter 20.

Analgesic Dosing

Most analgesic medication doses must be titrated up or down to achieve effectiveness, both at the beginning of therapy and during the course of treatment. For example, a client receiving morphine for bone pain may find that a lower dose of morphine is possible when an NSAID is added to the regimen. The goal is to use the smallest dose that relieves the pain so that it causes the fewest side effects.

Dose increases are usually made at the time the medication reaches its peak effect in the body. For orally administered morphine, the peak effect is generally at 60 to 90 minutes. Therefore, if a client is not comfortable 1 to 1½ hours after the last dose of the morphine, the dose can be safely increased. The peak effect of amitriptyline (Elavil) is 4 to 5 days, and dose increases should occur only every 4 or 5 days if needed.[42]

Therapeutic levels of analgesics must be maintained at all times for clients with persistent or chronic pain in order to manage the pain. Therefore, an around-the-clock (ATC) schedule (see next section) is most appropriate.[1, 18, 41] The frequency of doses to maintain therapeutic levels is determined by the route of administration and the duration of action of the medication. *Immediate-release* (short-acting) oral morphine requires dosing every 4 hours; oral hydromorphone (Dilaudid) may need to be given every 3 hours. *Sustained-release* medications offer the benefit of more convenient dosing schedules (every 8, 12, or 24 hours).

Rescue Dosing

The goal of ATC dosing is to keep the level of the analgesic in a range high enough to manage the pain but below the point at which a client experiences avoidable or unmanageable side effects. Unfortunately, pain does not stay at the same intensity 24 hours a day. Many clients experience pain above the normal baseline pain; this pain is often labeled "breakthrough pain." The pain may spike above (break through) the therapeutic blood level of analgesia, and additional medications are required to manage such episodes. A short-acting (or immediate-release) dose of an opioid should be administered to "cover" the spike in the client's pain.[1, 42]

For clients taking oral opioids, the recommended rescue dose is in the range of 10% to 20% of the total daily ATC dose of opioid.[1] The rescue dose should be made available every 1 to 2 hours because most immediate-release opioids reach peak effectiveness in 60 to 90 minutes. After that point, the level of the opioid in the system begins to decrease. A client experiencing pain 2 hours after a rescue dose should not be made to wait for additional medication because the level of analgesia will continue to decrease and the client will become more and more uncomfortable. As a rule, a client who requires more than two rescue doses during a 12-hour period or is awakened from sleep experiencing pain should have the pain experience reevaluated. An increase in the ATC dose is often appropriate under these circumstances.

■ DYSPNEA

Dyspnea is a subjective experience described as difficult breathing or an "uncomfortable awareness" of breathing that accounts for a high proportion of the client's inability to carry out activities of daily living (ADL) and gravely affects the perceived quality of life.[3, 15, 16] Dyspnea occurs in as many as 50% to 70% of people at the end of life.[3, 15, 16] Clients also mention labored breathing, shortness of breath, and feelings of suffocation.[1] The continuous exhaustion that accompanies breathlessness can be one of the most devastating symptoms for both the client and the observing family members.[15]

Etiology

Dyspnea generally results from a greater awareness of normal breathing, an increased workload of breathing, or abnormalities in the ventilatory system.[3, 19, 40] In a 1999 consensus statement, the American Thoracic Society[5] emphasized that many factors may contribute to the symptom of breathlessness, including pathophysiologic changes as well as clients' emotional and spiritual evaluation of the changes in their functional status and quality of living.

Disease processes commonly associated with dyspnea include (1) acute and chronic pulmonary disorders, (2) heart failure, and (3) neuromuscular disorders. In the terminally ill population, anemia and generalized weakness may also contribute to dyspnea. In addition, emotions play a major role. The fear associated with the inability to "catch one's breath" can lead to panic and worsen the sensation of dyspnea.[3, 5, 19, 40]

Assessment

Assessment of clients with dyspnea includes subjective and observational data. Clients should be asked to rate dyspnea on a scale. The scale must make sense to the client, and all people caring for that client must use the same scale. This information can help determine the severity of the symptom and provides a baseline to evaluate the effectiveness of interventions. Clients' evaluations of their own functional status and the effect of dyspnea on ADL provide helpful information about both the physical and emotional responses to dyspnea.[5, 52]

An objective assessment of the client, particularly the nonresponsive client, provides additional information about dyspnea.[26] Observe for an increased respiratory rate, use of accessory muscles, gasping or labored breathing, restlessness, and diaphoresis.

Management

The underlying cause of dyspnea should be treated as appropriate for the client's position in the disease trajectory. For example, pneumonia in a client who is alert and oriented and has a good quality of life (as determined by the client) should be treated. However, it may be appropriate to *not* treat pneumonia in a client who is clearly near the end of the disease trajectory if treatment of the pneumonia will not improve the quality of life. All treatment options should be reviewed with the client and family, including the option of *no* treatment.[2, 3]

Although it may not be possible to treat the underlying cause of dyspnea at the end of life, many effective interventions can be used to manage the distress and uncomfortable sensations associated with dyspnea.[3, 40] Interdisciplinary team support is essential in the management of dyspnea. The psychosocial and existential issues contributing to the symptom of dyspnea require the support of professionals trained in these areas.

Opioids. Morphine is widely used for the relief of dyspnea.[3, 5, 40] Data from several clinical studies reveal that 80% to 95% of clients with terminal cancer find significant relief from the utilization of morphine. Exactly why opioids alleviate dyspnea is not known, but they are believed to blunt the perceptual response to dyspnea or to reduce the respiratory drive.[15, 16] There is no standard optimal dose of morphine for the treatment of dyspnea. Twycross[52] proposed the following recommendations based on clinical experience:

- For the client who is already taking morphine for pain and who is dyspneic, the morphine dose should be increased by 50%.
- The dyspneic client who has not been receiving morphine should be started on 2.5 to 5 mg of morphine every 4 hours as needed.

It may be appropriate to consider ATC dosing of morphine if the client is requiring frequent "as needed" doses. Sustained-release preparations may prove to be convenient and effective in this situation.[3, 15, 16]

Anti-Anxiety Agents. Both benzodiazepines and phenothiazines have been effective in the management of dyspnea. Each class of drugs has the potential to depress hypoxic or ventilator responses and to alter the emotional responses to dyspnea.[45, 50] Both classes of medications have the potential for side effects, but given the prevalence of anxiety associated with the experience of breathlessness, it is considered good palliative care to try anxiolytic therapy on an individual basis.[19]

Bronchodilators. Bronchodilators help to decrease the effort of breathing, and several studies cite its effects on breathlessness. The significant decrease in dyspnea after theophylline use is believed to result from an improvement in the length-tension relationship in the diaphragm.[19, 52]

Corticosteroids. Corticosteroids are commonly used in the palliative care setting to treat dyspnea. These medications are believed to influence the symptom of dyspnea by decreasing inflammation in the pulmonary tissue and increasing bronchodilation.[3, 19] Corticosteroid therapy is indicated when bronchodilators have been ineffective. Ahmedzai[3] states that a trial of corticosteroids is justified in almost all clients with problematic chronic airway disease, pointing out that the dose of steroid should be high enough to work efficiently but low enough not to cause potential gastric irritation or fluid retention.

Oxygen Therapy. Palliative care literature does not support the use of oxygen therapy for relief of dyspnea. Oxygen (O_2) therapy should only be used for clients who are hypoxic or tend to have pulmonary hypertension. If O_2 saturation is less than 90% with room air, the clinician may want to (1) consider O_2 by nasal cannula at 1 to 3 L/min, (2) recheck the client's O_2 saturation in 20 to 30 minutes, and (3) titrate the O_2 therapy up to 6 L/min by nasal cannula if necessary.[3, 26, 52]

Nonpharmacologic Interventions. Nurses are frequently the care providers who introduce nonpharmacologic interventions to clients and families and ensure, through education and support, that the interventions are being used to maximal effectiveness. Some interventions that nurses can initiate that contribute to comfort in clients experiencing dyspnea are (1) pursed-lip breathing, (2) breathing exercises, (3) positioning, (4) having a fan blowing in the room, (5) coping techniques, (6) a calming presence, (7) relaxation therapy, (8) massage, (9) acupuncture, (10) hypnosis, and (11) visualization.[26]

■ DELIRIUM

Delirium has been found in up to 77% to 85% of terminally ill clients with cancer and in 57% of terminally ill clients with acquired immunodeficiency syndrome (AIDS).[7, 8] Some clinicians consider delirium the "hallmark" of dying. Studies have indicated, however, that 25% to 35% of episodes of delirium are reversible.[7, 11] In the palliative care setting, early detection and assessment are likely to improve outcomes.[8]

A variety of terms have been used to describe delirium, such as acute brain failure, acute confusional state, acute secondary psychosis, exogenous psychosis, sundown syndrome, and organic brain syndrome.[7, 37] According to the American Psychiatric Association's *Diagnostic and Statistical Manual of Mental Disorders (DSM-IV)* criteria,[4] *delirium* is defined as "an etiologically non-specific, global, cerebral dysfunction characterized by concurrent disturbances of level of consciousness, attention, thinking, perception, memory, psychomotor behavior, emotion, and the sleep-wake cycle." It is often identified as a sudden and significant decline in a previous level of functioning and is conceptualized as a reversible process. Delirium can also affect sleep, psychomotor activity, and emotions.[8, 21, 22, 37]

DSM-IV criteria for delirium are as follows[4]:

1. Disturbance of consciousness with reduced ability to focus, sustain, or shift attention.
2. A change in cognition (such as memory deficit, disorientation, language disturbance) or the development of a perceptual disturbance that is not better accounted for by pre-existing, established, or evolving dementia.
3. Development of the disturbance over a short time (usually hours to days) and a tendency to fluctuate over the course of the day.

ASSESSMENT

The diagnosis of delirium is based on careful observation and awareness of its key features. Because the clinical manifestations are nonspecific, the clinician must (1) look for manifestations of a disturbance in consciousness and a change in cognition, (2) identify the rapidity of onset, and (3) assess for associated medical and environmental risks that lead to a definitive diagnosis. Delirium is commonly unrecognized by clinicians and hence is misdiagnosed.[21, 22]

The most commonly used assessment instrument for identifying cognitive changes is the Mini-Mental State Examination (MMSE). The MMSE is a systematically scored method of evaluating cognitive function. The examination can indicate early changes in cognition as it relates to the cortical function of the brain.[11] The MMSE evaluates orientation, attention, recall, and language. Scores below 24, out of a maximum of 30, are indicative of cognitive changes.[11] The MMSE relies heavily on client cooperation, however, and does not account for the abrupt changes that may often occur in a client's cognitive status.[11]

MANAGEMENT

The prognosis for the client experiencing delirium is often poor. This fact, however, should not deter the clinician from looking for the underlying cause because a significant number of cases are reversible.[37, 38] Bruera and colleagues[10] were able to determine cognitive failure in 80% to 90% of clients prior to death and identified a reversible cause of delirium in 44% (29 of 66) of clients studied. Frequently cited reversible causes of delirium are (1) medications (e.g., opioids, sedatives, anticholinergics, and steroids), (2) hypoxia, (3) dehydration, (4) metabolic causes (e.g., hypercalcemia), and (5) sepsis.[21, 22] Potentially helpful interventions for these reversible causes are listed in Table 22–3.

■ DEPRESSION

The prevalence of depression in clients with cancer ranges anywhere from 10% to 25%; the prevalence appears to increase in the presence of functional losses, advancing illness, and unmanaged symptoms.[8, 49] It is believed that many cases of depression in the terminally ill go unrecognized by clinicians because many of the clinical manifestations of depression (e.g., fatigue, anorexia or weight loss, insomnia) can be attributed to the disease process itself. Key indicators of clinical depression in the terminally ill are (1) alterations in mood, (2) feelings of hopelessness, worthlessness, or excessive guilt, and (3) recurrent death wishes, including thoughts of suicide.[41]

ETIOLOGY

A terminal diagnosis potentiates both anxiety and depression. People with a family or personal history of previous depressive episodes are at even higher risk for depression than the general population. Interestingly, some cancer diagnoses, such as pancreatic cancer, have been more strongly associated with depression. It is not clear whether psychological or physiologic factors are involved in this higher risk.[4, 7]

TABLE 22–3 REVERSIBLE CAUSES OF DELIRIUM

Cause	Intervention
1. Medications	
a. Opioid metabolites may accumulate, especially in the presence of renal insufficiency.	a. Consider switching to an equianalgesic dose of a different opioid.
b. Benzodiazepine metabolites may accumulate in the presence of hepatic disease.	b. Hydration may be helpful to assist in eliminating these metabolites. If antianxiety medications are needed, consider switching the client to a butyrophenone.
2. Hypoxia	2. Intervene to improve oxygenation with bronchodilators, mucolytics, and breathing techniques. Consider oxygen therapy if O_2 saturation is <90%
3. Dehydration	3. Consider oral or parenteral hydration.
4. Hypercalemia	4. Evaluate the benefits of hydration and use of bisphosphonates.
5. Sepsis	5. Consider anti-infective therapy.

It is thought that depression is a direct result of abnormal serotonin (5-hydroxytryptamine [5-HT]) neurotransmission in the CNS. This abnormal secretion may be genetic or may be induced by some unknown mechanism. Other neurotransmitters, such as gamma-aminobutyric acid (GABA) and norepinephrine, have also been closely linked in anxiety and may be associated with depression.[48]

ASSESSMENT

Nurses play a pivotal role in identifying people with depression. An important question you can ask is "Are you depressed?" or "How has your mood been lately?" Although feeling sad and anxious at times is a normal response to a terminal diagnosis, do not ignore these symptoms. People with clinical depression should be referred to skilled health care professionals for evaluation and treatment.

MANAGEMENT

Optimal therapy is achieved with the combination of supportive psychotherapy, cognitive-behavioral techniques, and pharmaceutical management. This approach requires coordination of the interdisciplinary team.

Antidepressant medications can be very effective in treating depression. There are several classes of antidepressants. The newer selective serotonin re-uptake inhibitors (SSRIs) cause fewer side effects and are at least as effective as the TCAs.[48] A trial of antidepressant therapy is warranted in the terminally ill client because it may greatly enhance the quality of life. See Chapter 20 for further discussion of anxiety, depression, medications, and treatments.

■ FATIGUE AND WEAKNESS

Fatigue is among the most prevalent symptoms of people with advanced illnesses and is universally associated with advanced malignancy. It is a distressing, subjective experience that impedes functioning and impairs quality of life. Clients describe fatigue as tiredness, exhaustion, generalized weakness, diminished energy, increased need to rest or sleep, diminished motivation, diminished capacity to pay attention, or a disturbed mood.[39, 44]

Although the etiology of fatigue is not clearly understood, many physiologic, psycho-emotional, and spiritual factors are recognized as contributing factors to the phenomenon of fatigue.[39, 44] Fatigue may result from any one or combination of the following problems:

Disease/treatment-related: Disease process, disease treatments (surgery, radiation therapy, chemotherapy, biologic therapy), infection, anemia, malnutrition or cachexia, chronic hypoxia, metabolic or electrolyte disorders, endocrine disorders, neuromuscular disorders, medication side effects (e.g., excessive sedation from opioids).

Physiologic: Over-exertion, immobility or lack of exercise, poor sleep, pain, or other discomfort.

Psycho-emotional: Stress, anxiety, grief, depression.

Spiritual: Fear, distress.

Because of the multidimensional nature of fatigue and the potential for several contributing factors to be present at any one time, a comprehensive assessment is required. It is important to identify and treat reversible causes of fatigue. All medications should be reviewed, and any unnecessary centrally acting drugs eliminated. If the clinician suspects that opioids are contributing to fatigue, reduction of the opioid dose by 25% should be considered, followed by evaluation of the client's cognition if pain is still controlled and fatigue is lessened.[44] If pain returns with the reduction in dose, the opioid dose should be returned to the previous level.

Note: The client who is still in pain and is sedated from opioids has an opioid-resistant pain syndrome; an adjuvant medication will be required (see Adjuvant Medications). Stress, fear, and spiritual distress may be best addressed through counseling.

Nurses can initiate many interventions to help clients cope with fatigue. Strategies to manage stress include counseling, education, relaxation, and massage. Instituting a regular exercise program can be effective in lessening fatigue in clients undergoing chemotherapy. Although no studies on the effect of an exercise program on fatigue in the palliative care setting have been published, this strategy should be considered for clients who are able to participate in some form of exercise. In addition, for clients who can eat and take in fluids, you can encourage adequate nutrition and hydration.[39, 44]

One helpful strategy is to help clients modify their activity and rest patterns. Encourage clients to (1) incorporate rest times into their daily schedules, (2) plan their most strenuous activities for the time of day when energy levels are highest, and (3) capitalize on saving energy by accepting the assistance of others, delegating tasks, and using equipment such as a bedside commode or a portable telephone.

Medications may be helpful to treat fatigue in some clients. Corticosteroids are sometimes used to treat fatigue in people with advanced cancer. The exact mechanism of action is not clear, but some researchers believe that corticosteroids may lessen fatigue by inhibiting tumor and tumor-induced substances that contribute to the symptom. Others suggest that fatigue is relieved by the central euphoric effect of these medications. If anorexia or cachexia is a contributing factor in fatigue, the appetite-stimulating effect of corticosteroids may be helpful.

Psychostimulants have also been used to treat people with fatigue (see Chapter 21). There have not been any controlled comparisons of these medications, but the largest experience in people with cancer has been with methylphenidate (Ritalin). Dextroamphetamine (Dexedrine) and pemoline (Cylert) have also been used.[39, 44]

■ SLEEP DISTURBANCES

Impaired sleep is a common, and often overlooked, problem in people with advanced illnesses. Many times, a disturbance in sleep is accepted as "part of being sick." However, it is important to recognize the importance of sleep. Sleep is associated with tissue restoration; sleep deprivation alters immune function. Although people with a terminal illness are not going to "recuperate" from their underlying disease, they can benefit from the healing and protective functions of sleep when dealing with tissue injury and infection. Excessive sleepiness is also emotionally disabling, resulting in an inability to participate in treatment, comprehend information, and share in social interactions. Furthermore, impairment of sleep may lead to depression, irritability, and withdrawal.[46]

An evaluation of the amount and quality of sleep is an important component of the overall assessment of a client in the palliative care setting.[46] This evaluation covers:

- Usual bedtime
- How long it takes to fall asleep
- Any wakefulness during the night
- Usual waking time
- Subjective feeling of being "refreshed" in the morning
- Frequency and length of daytime naps
- Use of sleep medications
- The cause of any sleep problems as identified by the client

There are many potential causes of sleep disturbances. Physiologic factors contributing to impaired sleep include pain, nausea and vomiting, respiratory problems, medications (e.g., corticosteroids, bronchodilators, antihypertensives), metabolic disturbances, and delirium. Psycho-emotional factors, such as depression and anxiety, also interfere with sleep. The client's environment definitely influences the amount and quality of sleep; unfamiliar surroundings, frequent interruptions, noise, bright lighting, and unpleasant odors can all lead to a disturbance in sleep. In addition, lack of exercise, inactivity, and boredom may lead to excessive napping during the day, resulting in poor sleep at night.

Treatable causes of sleep disturbance must be addressed with appropriate interventions and discontinuation of medications that interfere with sleep when possible. General sleep hygiene strategies include[46]:

- Establishing a regular sleep schedule
- Staying out of bed during the day
- Napping only when necessary
- Keeping active (mentally and/or physically) during the day
- Minimizing nighttime disruptions
- Avoiding stimulants at night (caffeine, nicotine)

One advantage of long-acting medications is a decreased need to awaken during the night for dose administration.

People who have difficulty falling asleep may benefit from establishing a relaxing bedtime routine. Depending on individual preferences, this relaxation routine may consist of massage, progressive muscle relaxation, imagery, music, and warm milk or herbal tea.

When other interventions are not effective in promoting or maintaining sleep, medications may be appropriate. Benzodiazepines are the main group of medications used to promote sleep. There is some controversy regarding the long-term effectiveness of the benzodiazepines, and most are recommended for short-term use. Thus, the need for sleep medications must be reevaluated on a regular basis. Benzodiazepines used for sleep disturbances include the following:

Short half-life (2 to 4 hours): Triazolam (Halcion), zolpidem (Ambien). Because of their quick onset of action, these medications are helpful for people who have difficulty falling asleep. However, they do not benefit people with sleep maintenance problems. Rebound insomnia is common if the medication is abruptly stopped. Triazolam, which is associated with adverse drug reactions, has been removed from the market in some countries.

Intermediate half-life (6 to 15 hours): Lorazepam (Ativan), oxazepam (Serax), temazepam (Restoril). These medications are helpful for promoting sleep onset and maintenance.

Long half-life (29 to 100 hours): Flurazepam (Dalmane), quazepam (Doral). Although these agents help promote sleep onset and maintenance, daytime sedation is common because of their long half-lives. Also, drug accumulation may occur in the elderly. (See Chapter 21 on sleep management.)

■ CACHEXIA-ANOREXIA SYNDROME

Cachexia is derived from the Greek words *kakos and hexis,* meaning "poor condition." The term "cachexia-anorexia syndrome" is often used loosely to define weight loss, wasting, or loss of appetite.[33] However, cachexia-anorexia syndrome is one of the most common problems afflicting clients with advanced cancer and AIDS. The incidence in clients with cancer varies with the type of primary tumor. The client who has adenocarcinoma of the breast is less likely to exhibit cachexia-anorexia syndrome than the client who has adenocarcinoma of the lung or pancreas. Wasting is not commonly observed in clients with a hematologic malignancy yet is very prevalent in clients with myelodysplastic syndromes.[33]

Several studies have identified chemical factors (due to tumor burden) that contribute to cachexia-anorexia syndrome. A number of cytokines have been identified to produce this syndrome, including tumor necrosis factor, interleukin-1 and interleukin-6, and interferon. Other causes are metabolic abnormalities, a decrease in nutritional intake, and eventual loss of appetite.[33] Correctable causes are found in clients who have obstruction of the upper or lower bowel as a result of tumor invasion. Simple starvation, which can often be corrected with parenteral or enteral nutrition (see Chapter 29), must also be considered in this client population.

Other contributing factors in cachexia-anorexia syndrome are presented in Table 22–4. Clinical manifestations commonly observed in this syndrome are (1) muscle loss, (2) impaired immunity, (3) loss of body fat, (4) glucose intolerance, (5) fluid retention, and (6) vitamin deficiencies.

Interventions are as varied as the contributing factors. Some clients may not respond favorably to the replacement of dietary supplements and require more aggressive intervention, such as a progestational (hormonal) agent. Scientific research has concluded that pharmacologic therapy alleviates cachexia-anorexia syndrome. The use of progestational agents in combination with other medications or with special diets achieves improved outcomes.

The following pharmacologic strategies are suggested for the client with cachexia-anorexia syndrome:

1. Progestational agents
2. Anabolic steroids
3. Dietary interventions involving omega-3 fatty acids and branched-chain amino acids
4. Combination approaches:
   a. Cannabinoids
   b. Dietary supplements
   c. Prokinetic agents
   d. CNS stimulants (methylphenidate)

Remember, the loss of appetite often assessed in the dying client is a normal process that should not be confused with cachexia-anorexia syndrome.

TABLE 22–4 FACTORS CONTRIBUTING TO CACHEXIA-ANOREXIA SYNDROME

Tumor involvement of gastrointestinal tract
Antitumor therapy
Infections
Taste change
Medications
Food aversions
Pain
Psychological factors
Changes in metabolism
Hormonal changes
Fatigue, weakness
Increased metabolic rate; altered fat, protein, or carbohydrate metabolism; fluid-electrolyte abnormalities; hormonal changes
Malabsorption
Tumor metabolism

INDICATORS OF IMMINENT DEATH

Certain physical, cognitive, and behavioral changes occur as a person enters the active dying process. The human body, like any other living organism, seeks survival; in doing so, it often alters normal physiology. As the body begins to die, blood is commonly shunted to the brain and the heart, the two most important organs. Thus, peripheral circulation is limited, leading to mottling and cyanosis. Because the kidneys are no longer perfused adequately, there is a decrease in urine output. Slowly, all body systems become involved in the dying process.

Tachycardia and diminished blood pressure are observed in the acute phase of decompensation (organ shutdown) of the cardiovascular system. The respiratory system works to compensate for metabolic deficiencies, causing tachypnea, dyspnea, or both. Table 22–5 highlights indicators of impending death.

COMMUNICATION

The dying process can be a time of emotional crisis for many families. You can help lead clients and families down a less threatening path to what is often termed "the unknown." In order to do so, however, you must develop a level of comfort in communicating with dying clients and their families. You will need to examine their personal feelings about death and dying before you can provide emotional support and guidance to the dying. If you are uncomfortable in this care setting, you may impede the ability of clients and families to finish their important business.

Clients and families facing the last days of life should be given the opportunity to express any or all of their concerns about issues that matter the most to them. The nurse acts as a listener, a friend, and an advocate for the client. Being available in a nonjudgmental and nonthreatening manner allows the client and family to trust the nurse. Once trust is established and the client believes that the nurse will effectively manage his or her symptoms, the client may begin to open up emotionally and discuss many concerns about the illness and death. Each client is unique, and so are the conversations that occur between nurse, client, and family. As professionals who have the most contact with clients, you are sometimes the only person with whom clients share thoughts and feelings. Emphasize to the client that the nurse is a member of a health care team and that sharing of some information with other members of the team, who can provide additional support, may be beneficial.

Communicating with dying clients and their families takes into account the multidimensional nature of people. See Diversity in Health Care: Cultural Aspects of Death and Dying. Your sensitivity to culture, spirituality, lifestyle, and emotional connections is essential for clients to feel supported.

One of the most important tasks of the bedside nurse is to empower clients and families to participate in the final act of living. Through ongoing assessment, communication, and skilled physical care, you can communicate reassurance, confidence, and support for the vulnerable client and family. The seasoned hand of a skilled professional supporting and guiding the client can change the journey through dying and death from a frightening process to one of peace and comfort.

CARE FOR THE CAREGIVERS

The families of terminally ill clients commonly serve as primary caregivers in the home care environment and are often highly involved in providing care in other palliative care settings. This "intensive caring" is physically and emotionally exhausting. In order to provide and maintain this level of care, these caregivers need education and support from all members of the interdisciplinary health care team. Coping tasks for families caring for a loved one who is dying and suggested interventions are described in Table 22–6.

Even though this intensive caring is very difficult,

TABLE 22–5 COMMON OBJECTIVE BODY SYSTEM INDICATORS OF IMMINENT DEATH

Cognition/orientation	Not always nonresponsive, may be agitated or restless, cannot subjectively respond to verbal stimuli
Cardiovascular	Tachycardia, irregular heart rate, lowered blood pressure or significant widening between systolic and diastolic, pressures, dehydration
Pulmonary	Tachypnea, dyspnea, use of accessory muscles, acetone breath, Cheyne-Stokes breathing, pooling of secretions or noisy respirations
Gastrointestinal	Diminished appetite, smaller amounts of feces (despite not eating), incontinence
Renal	Diminished urinary output, incontinence, concentrated urine
Mobility	Limited, bedbound, and requires frequent position changes

DIVERSITY IN HEALTH CARE

Cultural Aspects of Death and Dying

Death is a universal experience. Beliefs and behaviors regarding death, however, are highly personal and vary according to culture. The influx of many different cultural groups into the United States means that nurses are challenged to become knowledgeable about unique cultural beliefs and traditions related to death, dying, and bereavement.

The Problem

Nurses all too often avoid the death process because they have been educated to focus on restoring health or fostering environments in which the client returns to a previous state of health or adapts to physical, psychological, or emotional changes. Nursing education takes place within the Western view of health and illness. The U.S. health care system fosters the idea that with advanced technology, death can be controlled and postponed. Death is viewed as a medical and technological failure. This view of death as a failure of technology varies greatly from the view of cultures that perceive death as a natural part of the life cycle.[4]

"White" society is by and large viewed as a death-defying, death-denying society, whereas clients from immigrant communities may view the dying process very differently. For example, a comparison between most white and immigrant communities reveals that white society is often "I" centered; many immigrant communities are "we" centered, particularly in regard to decision-making.[6] For the client from another culture, there may be cultural conflict concerning who makes decisions about the client's impending death. Who is the decision maker—the client, the family, or the physician?

Cultural Perceptions of Death and Grieving

The way in which a family views life and death is a belief system with its core in the cultural heritage of the family. The family's basic disposition toward the meaning of life and death is expressed behaviorally.[2] For example, traditional Muslims believe that whatever happens in life is a result of destiny, or God's will. Consequently, a traditionally oriented Muslim client may believe that the time of death is predetermined and nothing can change it.[3] Such a client would not be interested in a technological intervention to prolong life. Navajos believe that speaking of the dead or expressing their emotions about the loss of a loved one can be detrimental to the living because of the power of the deceased. The Chinese view a sudden, unexpected, untimely, or violent death as a "bad" death. Such a death places shame on the family because it is thought to be caused by the transgressions of ancestors. Consequently, mourning is discouraged and grieving does not occur.[2]

Interventions

Nurses should become aware of cultural variations about grieving and perceptions of death because clients and their families are greatly in need of culturally sensitive care at this vulnerable time. Because there are many cultural variations of the perceptions about and behaviors that accompany death, dying, and bereavement, you are not expected to be knowledgeable about all of them.[4] It is important to talk with clients and families about cultural aspects of death and dying. The following guidelines to be used by the nurse for assessing death beliefs and rituals provides the structure for identifying a client's important cultural beliefs[5]:

1. Death rituals and expectations:
   a. Identify culturally specific death rituals and expectations.
   b. Explain the purpose of death rituals and mourning practices.
   c. What are specific burial practices, such as cremation?
2. Responses to death and grief:
   a. Identify cultural expectations of responses to death and grief.
   b. Explore the meaning of death, dying, and the afterlife.

Even though dying is a universal experience, its meaning varies greatly from one culture to another. Nurses are challenged to familiarize themselves with the death rituals and responses of terminally ill clients and their families. The preceding guidelines help in gathering this information. Having this knowledge enhances your ability to provide culturally competent care to clients and families when they are very vulnerable and in need of compassionate care—when they are experiencing death, dying, and bereavement.

References

1. Andrews, M. & Boyle, J. (1999). *Transcultural concepts in nursing care.* Philadelphia: Lippincott–Williams & Wilkins.
2. Esposito, L., Buckalew, P., & Chukunta, T. (1996). Cultural diversity in grief. *Home Health Care Management and Practice, 8*(4), 23–29.
3. Leininger, M. (1995). *Transcultural nursing: Concepts, theories, research and practices.* New York: McGraw-Hill.
4. O'Connell, L. (1996). Changing the culture of dying. *Health Progress, 77*(6), 16–20.
5. Purnell, L., & Paulanka, B. (1998). *Transcultural health care: A culturally competent approach.* Philadelphia: F. A. Davis.
6. Smith, J. (1996). Cultural and spiritual issues in palliative care. *Journal of Cancer Care, 5*(4), 173–178.

Joyce Larson-Presswalla, PhD, RN, *President, "Culture Counts," Marketing Coordinator, James A. Haley Veterans Hospital, Tampa, Florida*

most family caregivers are able to provide appropriate levels of care for their loved ones. Nurses play a pivotal role in assessing their educational and support needs, providing information and support, and referring caregivers to other team members and community agencies to address their needs.

Support of the Grieving Family

Bereavement care is an important component of any palliative care program.[54] Providing bereavement care requires an understanding of the normal grieving process and the tasks of grief work. Grief is a normal and expected reac-

TABLE 22–6 FAMILY COPING TASKS IN TERMINAL ILLNESS

Coping Task	Support or Interventions
1. Acceptance versus denial	1. Provide realistic information about the illness and treatment options. Encourage open and honest communication among family members.
2. Establish a relationship with the health care team	2. Explain the roles of all interdisciplinary team members. Establish trust, maintaining open lines of communication.
3. Meet the needs of the dying person	
a. Physical needs	a. Provide information about pain and symptom management, use of equipment, skin care/position, rest and nutrition, infection control, safety. Reassure caregivers that they are doing a good job. Assess need for assistance, such as home health aide. Assess need for transfer to a different care setting.
b. Emotional needs	b. Encourage caregivers to take time to sit and listen to loved one and to share each other's feelings and concerns. Assess need for additional support/counseling from the interdisciplinary team.
4. Maintain functional equilibrium (i.e., the family must maintain some sense of normalcy to continue to function as a family unit)	4. Assist family to identify and prioritize activities that must be continued (e.g., going to work or school, doing laundry, buying groceries). Assist family to identify support persons to help with these tasks. Encourage caregivers to use respite care services to care for selves and to attend family events outside of direct caregiving.
5. Regulate family affect	5. Allow the caregivers the opportunity to express their feelings. Give them permission to have whatever feelings they have (i.e., "feelings just are—there's no right or wrong") Acknowledge that normally joyful times, like holidays, may not feel as joyful. Encourage formal counseling, if needed. Encourage the caregivers to address their own needs and to care for themselves, too.
6. Negotiate relationships outside the family	6. Give permission to take time to maintain friendships. Discuss options for maintaining jobs while caring for a dying loved one.
7. Cope with the post-death phase (healthy grieving)	7. Support family while they accept the finality of their loss. Discuss the functioning of the family unit without the loved one. Encourage using available bereavement supports/counseling.

Adapted from Cohen, M. S., & Cohen, E. K. (1981). Behavioral family systems interventions in terminal care. In H. J. Sokel (Ed.), *Behavioral therapy in terminal care* (pp. 177–204). Cambridge, MA: Ballinger Publishing Co.; and Ferrell, B. R. (1998). Home care. In A. Berger, R. Portenoy, & D. Weissman (Eds.), *Principles and practice of supportive oncology.* Philadelphia: Williams & Wilkins.

tion to a loss. Family members will grieve the loss of their loved ones. One role of the health care team is to reinforce the understanding that grieving is healthy, a necessary process that the family must to through to be able to move on in their lives. Nurses need to validate as normal the manifestations that the bereaved may be experiencing (Table 22–7).

In addition to knowing the normal responses to grief, it is helpful for those working with the bereaved to understand the tasks of the grieving process. Four tasks of mourning that must be accomplished in order for the bereavement to reach a satisfactory conclusion include[54]:

- Accepting the reality of the loss
- Experiencing the pain of the loss
- Adjusting to the environment in which the deceased is missing
- Finding a way to remember the deceased while moving forward with life

Most people adjust to bereavement adequately, but for some, bereavement can be complicated. It is important for health care providers to identify people with abnormal or

TABLE 22–7 MANIFESTATIONS OF GRIEF

Psychological	Social	Physiological
1. *Avoidance phase:* Shock, denial, disbelief 2. *Confrontation phase:* Extremes emotions as person deals with the loss and its implications 3. *Reestablishment phase* Gradual decline in grief	Restlessness, inability to sit still Inability to initiate and maintain organized patterns of activity Social withdrawal	Anorexia/gastrointestinal disturbances Weight loss Sleep disturbances Crying Tendency to sigh Fatigue, lack of strength, lack of energy Heart palpitations, nervousness, tension Loss of sexual desire or hypersexuality Shortness of breath

From Rando, T. (1984). Grief, dying and death. In *Clinical interventions for caregivers.* Champaign, IL: Research Press Co.

complicated grieving and refer them for skilled counseling and support. Examples of complicated grieving are[54]:

- *Chronic grief:* prolonged grieving; the sense that person is "stuck" in the grieving process.
- *Delayed grief:* a previously insufficiently mourned loss that becomes evident at a later time.
- *Exaggerated grief:* intensification of the normal grief response to the point of dysfunction.
- *Masked grief:* grief that is hidden at the time of loss and manifests itself later as a physical or psychiatric problem.

Health care providers can assist families in their grieving process before the client dies by encouraging and supporting anticipatory grieving and by encouraging communication between client and family. As death becomes imminent, it is often helpful to encourage the family to be present with their loved one, if possible. Encouraging the family to reminisce and helping people deal with their feelings are important interventions after the death of the client.

CONCLUSIONS

The nurse caring for the dying client and family requires many skills. The nurse must possess the ability to offer compassion, assess the multitude of symptoms that occur at the end of life, and participate in symptom management. The nurse is also a member of the health care team whose focus is to help promote a healthy and positive dying experience for all involved.

THINKING CRITICALLY

1. **T. S., a 57-year-old man, has stage IV squamous cell carcinoma of the right lung with metastatic bony involvement. You find that he is in excruciating pain and is so sedated that he is unable to subjectively rate his pain. He is nauseated, has not had a bowel movement in 6 days, and is anorexic and dehydrated. His current medications include sustained-release morphine 60 mg every 6 hours, a transdermal opioid of 75 μg, and immediate-release morphine 20 mg every 2 hours, which have not provided relief. What can you do to make this client more comfortable?**

Factors to Consider. Besides poor pain control, what other problems need attention? Consider the addition of an adjuvant analgesic, the dosing of the opioids, and the client's hydration status.

2. **F. T., a 43-year-old man, entered the emergency department with complaints of severe dyspnea. The chest x-ray revealed pleural effusion of the right lung. The results of the thoracentesis, which drained 1500 ml of fluid, were positive for adenocarcinoma. After several diagnostic studies were performed, no primary site for the tumor was identified. He was referred to an oncologist for palliative chemotherapy. You are asked to make a home visit to change the dressing on his chest tube. Your first assessment reveals a very cachectic, dehydrated, constipated, dyspneic client whose pain was well managed. The chest tube drainage totals 450 ml daily. The client and his wife are questioning the relevance of the chemotherapy, given the poor prognosis as well as his continued weight loss, loss of appetite, and weakness. He informs you that he does not want to be hospitalized and would like to remain at home and comfortable. After learning about this client's status and wishes, what actions should you take?**

Factors to Consider. What actions should be taken to facilitate the client's request? Is 24-hour care needed now or in the future? What additional needs might the client or his wife have?

3. **J. K. is a 38-year-old, single teacher who has diabetes mellitus and polycystic kidney disease (PKD). Her most recent kidney-pancreas transplant has been rejected, and she is undergoing hemodialysis again. She has not been compliant with her diet and fluid restrictions, and multiple dialysis access sites have become infected. She states that she does not want to continue dialysis. What should you do next? Should her parents be told of her request?**

Factors to Consider. How can you be certain that the client understands the ramifications of ending the hemodialysis? What can you do to keep her comfortable once dialysis is discontinued?

BIBLIOGRAPHY

1. Agency for Health Care Policy and Research (1994). *Managing cancer pain.* Washington, DC: Department of Health and Human Services.
2. Ahmedzai, S. (1996). Making a success out of life's failure. *Progress in Palliative Care, 4,* 1–3.
3. Ahmedzai, S. (1998). Palliation of respiratory symptoms. In D. Doyle, G. Hanks, & N. MacDonald (Eds.), *Oxford textbook of palliative medicine* (2nd ed., pp. 583–616). Oxford: Oxford University Press.
4. American Psychiatric Association. (1994). *Diagnostic and statistical manual of mental disorders (DSM-IV)* (4th ed). Washington, DC: Author.
5. American Thoracic Society Standards. (1999). The diagnosis and care of patients with chronic obstructive pulmonary disease. *American Journal of Respiratory Critical Care Medicine, 159,* 321–340.
6. Bennahum, D. (1996). The historical development of hospice and palliative care. In D. Sheehan & W. Forman (Eds.), *Hospice and palliative care* (pp. 1–10). Sudbury, MA: Jones & Bartlett.
7. Brietbart, W., Chochinov, M., & Passik, S. (1998). Psychiatric aspects of palliative care. In D. Doyle, G. Hanks, & N. MacDonald (Eds.), *Oxford textbook of palliative medicine* (2nd ed., pp, 923–954). Oxford: Oxford University Press.
8. Brietbart, W., & Jacobson, P. (1996). Psychiatric symptom management in terminal care. *Clinics in Geriatric Medicine, 12,* 329–347.
9. Bruera, E., & Lawlor, P. (1998). Defining palliative care interventions. *Journal of Palliative Care, 14,* 23–24.
10. Bruera, E., et al. (1995). Frequency of alcoholism among patients with pain due to terminal cancer. *Journal of Pain and Symptom Management, 10,* 599–603.
11. Caraceni, A. (1995). Delirium in palliative medicine. *European Journal of Palliative Care, 2,* 62–67.
12. Clinch, J., Dudgeon, D., & Schipper, H. (1998). Quality of life assessment in palliative care. In D. Doyle, G. Hanks, & N. MacDonald (Eds.), *Oxford textbook of palliative medicine* (2nd ed., pp. 83–96). Oxford: Oxford University Press.
13. De Stoutz, N., & Stiefel, F. (1997). Assessment and management of reversible delirium. In R. Portenoy & E. Bruera (Eds.), *Topics in palliative care* (pp. 21–43). Oxford: Oxford University Press.
14. Doyle, D., Hanks, G., & MacDonald, N. (1998). Introduction. In D. Doyle, G. Hanks, & N. MacDonald (Eds.), *Oxford textbook of palliative medicine* (2nd ed., pp. 3–8). Oxford: Oxford University Press.
15. Dudgeon, D. (1997). Dyspnea clinical perspectives. In Symptoms in terminal illness: A research workshop treating symptoms at the end-of-life. Rockville, MD: National Institutes of Health.
16. Dudgeon, D., & Rosenthal, S. (1996). Management of dyspnea and cough in patients with cancer. *Hematology/Oncology Clinics of North America, 10,* 151–171.
17. Finn-Paradis, L. (1985). *The development of hospice in America: The hospice handbook.* Rockville, MD: Aspen.
18. Foley, K. (Ed.). (1996). Palliative medicine, pain control, and symptom assessment. In *Caring for the Dying,* pp. 11–18. Philadelphia: American Board of Internal Medicine.
19. Gift, A. (1997). Dyspnea methods perspective. In Symptoms in terminal illness: A research workshop treating symptoms at the end-of-life. Rockville, MD: National Institutes of Health.
20. Harwood, K. (1999). Dyspnea. In C. Yarbro, M. Frogge, & M. Goodman (Eds.), *Cancer symptom management* (2nd ed., pp. 45–55). Sudbury, MA: Jones & Bartlett.
21. Haskell, R., Frankel, H., & Rotondo, M. (1997). Agitation. *AACN Clinical Issues, 8,* 335–350.
22. Ingham, J., & Caraceni, A. (1998). Delirium. In A. Berger, R. Portenoy, & D. Weissman (Eds.), *Principles and practice of supportive oncology* (pp. 477–495). Philadelphia: Lippincott–Williams & Wilkins.
23. Kinzbrunner, B. (1998). Hospice: 15 years and beyond in the care of the dying. *Journal of Palliative Medicine, 1,* 127–137.
24. Kübler-Ross, E. (1969). *On death and dying.* New York: Macmillan.
25. Kübler-Ross, E. (1995). *Death is of vital importance: On life, death and life after death.* New York: Station Press.
26. Kuebler, K., et al. (1996). *Hospice and palliative care practice protocol: Dyspnea.* Pittsburgh, PA: Hospice Nurses Association.
27. Kuebler, K., & Ogle, K. (1998). Psychometric evaluation of an objective assessment instrument to measure pain, dyspnea and restlessness (Abstract). *Journal of Palliative Care, 14,* 125.
28. Leung, R., Hill, P., & Burdon, J. (1996). Effect of inhaled morphine in the development of breathlessness during exercise in patients with chronic lung disease. *Thorax, 51,* 596–600.
29. Lo, B. (1995). End-of-life care after termination of SUPPORT. *Hastings Center Report Special Supplement 25,* S6–S8.
30. Lynn, J. (1997). An 88-year-old woman facing the end-of-life. *Journal of the American Medical Association, 277,* 1633–1640.
31. Lynn, J. (1998). Complaints about hospice: Growing up or going wrong? *ABCD Exchange, 1,* 2–7.
32. Lucas, B. (1999). Coping with psychiatric emergencies in the office: Patient care for the nurse practitioner. *Clinician Reviews, 2,* 31–42.
33. MacDonald, N., Alexander, R., & Bruera, E. (1995). Cachexia-anorexia-asthenia. *Journal of Pain and Symptom Management, 10,* 151–155.
34. Mahoney, J. (1998). The Medicare hospice benefit—15 years of success. *Journal of Palliative Medicine, 1,* 139–146.
35. Marshall, P. (1995). The SUPPORT Study: Who's talking? *Hastings Center Report Special Supplement 25,* S9–S11.
36. McGuire, D. (1998). The multiple dimensions of cancer pain: A framework for assessment and management In D. McGuire, C. Yarbo, & B. Ferrell (Eds.), *Cancer pain management.* Boston, MA: Jones & Bartlett.
37. Milisen, K., et al. (1998). Delirium in the hospitalized elderly: Nursing assessment and management. *Nursing Clinics of North America, 33,* 417–439.
38. Minagawa, H., et al. (1996). Psychiatric morbidity in terminally ill cancer patients: A prospective study. *Cancer, 78*(5), 1131–1137.
39. Neuenschwander, H., & Bruera, E. (1998). Asthenia. In D. Doyle, G. Hanks, & N. MacDonald (Eds.), *Oxford textbook of palliative medicine* (2nd ed., pp. 573–581). Oxford: Oxford University Press.
40. Pereira, J., & Bruera E. (Eds.)(1997). Dyspnea. In *The Edmonton aid to palliative care.* Edmonton, Alberta, Canada: Division of Palliative Care, University of Alberta.
41. Pollack, M. (1999). New treatments for panic disorders, psychiatric illness in primary care. *Clinician Reviews, 9*(3), 4–9.
42. Portenoy, R. (1997). *Contemporary diagnosis and management of pain in oncologic and AIDS patients.* Newton, PA: Handbooks in Health Care Company.
43. Portenoy, R. (1997). Symptoms commonly experienced in terminal illness. In Symptoms in terminal illness: A research workshop treating symptoms at the end-of-life. Rockville, MD: National Institutes of Health.
44. Portenoy, R. K., & Miaskowski, C. (1998). Assessment and management of cancer-related fatigue. In A. Berger, R. Portenoy, & D. Weissman (Eds.), *Principles and practice of supportive oncology* (pp. 109–118). Philadelphia: Lippincott–Williams & Wilkins.
45. Rhodes, V., & McDaniel, R. (1999). The symptom experience and its impact on quality of life. In C. Yarbo, M. Frogge, & M. Goodman (Eds.), *Cancer symptom management* (pp. 3–8). Sudbury, MA: Jones & Bartlett.
46. Sateia, M. J., & Silberfarb, P. M.(1998). Sleep. In D. Doyle, G. Hanks, & N. MacDonald (Eds.), *Oxford textbook of palliative medicine* (2nd ed., pp. 751–767). Oxford: Oxford University Press.
47. Shepherd, S., & Geraci, S. (1999). The differential diagnosis of dyspnea: A pathophysiological approach. *Clinician Reviews, 9*(3), 52–71.
48. Sterling, L. (1999). Pharmacological review of SSRIs in panic disorder: Psychiatric illness in primary care. *Clinician Reviews, 9*(3), S10–S13.
49. Story, P. (1998). Symptom control in the dying. In A. Berger, R. Portnoy, & D. Weissman (Eds.), *Principles and practice of supportive oncology* (pp. 741–748). Philadelphia: Lippincott–Williams & Wilkins.
50. The SUPPORT Principal Investigators. (1995). A controlled trial to improve care for seriously ill hospitalized patients: The Study to Understand Prognoses and Preferences for Outcomes and Risks of Treatments (SUPPORT). *Journal of the American Medical Association, 274,* 1591–1598.
51. Trzepacz, P., et al. (1999). American Psychiatric Association Guidelines: Practice guidelines for the treatment of patients with delirium. *American Journal of Psychiatry, 156,* S1–S20.
52. Twycross, R. (Ed.) (1997). Respiratory symptoms. In *Symptom management in advanced cancer* (pp. 143–148). Abdingdon, UK: Radcliff Medical Press.
53. Walsh, D. (1998). The Medicare hospice benefit: A critique from palliative medicine. *Journal of Palliative Medicine, 1,* 147–149.
54. Weaver, S., & Eutsey, D. E. (Eds.) (1998). *Palliative care: Patient and family counseling manual.* Gaithersburg, MD: Aspen.

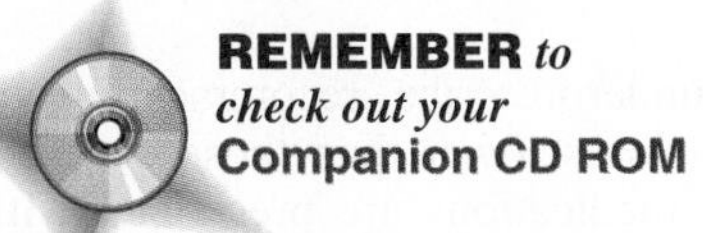

CHAPTER 23

Clients with Pain: Promoting Positive Outcomes

Juanita Fogel Keck
Susan Baker

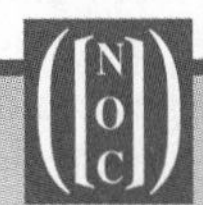

NURSING OUTCOMES CLASSIFICATION (NOC) for Nursing Diagnoses—Clients with Pain

Activity Intolerance
Endurance
Energy Conservation
Self-Care; Activities of Daily Living
Anxiety
Anxiety Control
Coping
Symptom Control Behavior
Fear
Fear Control
Comfort Level
Ineffective Individual Coping
Coping
Decision-Making
Quality of Life
Knowledge Deficit
Knowledge: Health Behaviors
Knowledge: Treatment Regimen
Pain
Comfort Level
Pain Control
Pain: Disruptive Effects
Pain Level
Symptom Control
Symptom Severity
Well-Being
Powerlessness
Health Beliefs: Perceived Control
Sleep Pattern Disturbance
Comfort Level
Pain Level
Rest
Sleep
Well-Being

Pain is a complex, multifaceted phenomenon. It is an individual, unique experience that may be difficult for clients to describe or explain and often difficult for others to recognize, understand and assess. Pain often leads to debilitation, diminished quality of life, and depression. Pain management challenges every health care team member, for there is no single, universal treatment.

Nurses are probably the most important component of the team, for they are the client's primary advocate for pain relief. Listening to concerns, assessing pain intensity and distress levels, planning for care, educating the client about pain, promoting use of nonpharmacologic pain techniques, and evaluating the process for promoting positive outcomes are nursing responsibilities. An attentive nurse can identify discomfort in clients often without verbal confirmation from the client (Fig. 23–1). Nurses have the capability to relieve pain merely by acknowledging the discomfort and confirming that measures will be taken to relieve the pain. This commitment and statement of caring establish trust and rapport with the client.

This chapter summarizes what is currently known about the physiology of pain, how to assess and diagnose aspects of pain, how to implement a variety of both pharmacologic and nonpharmacologic techniques to manage the discomfort, and how to evaluate outcomes appropriately.

The Problem of Pain

In the natural environment, pain serves as a mechanism to warn us about the potential for physical harm. Thus, pain is the body's protective mechanism to prevent further tissue damage by providing the impetus to withdraw from the pain-producing situation. The discomfort and distress associated with pain often last far beyond the tissue-damaging experience. Pain is the primary reason people seek health care and is associated with increased length of hospital stay, longer recovery time, and poorer client outcomes.[1, 59] Pain is typically undertreated.[58, 75] In the early 1970s, researchers reported that pain was seriously undertreated after surgery.[73] Thirty years later, this situation has changed little, even though there have been immense advances in knowledge of the causes of pain and the mechanisms that contribute to pain relief. New medications and the recognition of complementary pain

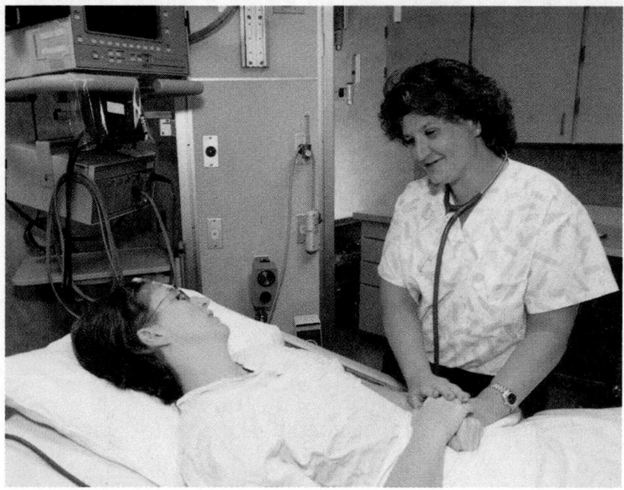

FIGURE 23–1 The nurse asks the client about pain. The client is the expert regarding her pain.

management strategies have contributed to the improved ability to manage pain and to provide satisfactory pain relief. If the existing knowledge and resources were utilized to manage pain, 90% of people with pain would receive satisfactory pain relief.[75, 116] Barriers to adequate pain management may involve health care professionals, including nurses; clients, physicians, and the health care system.[35, 52, 75] These barriers are presented in Box 23–1.

BOX 23–1 Barriers to Pain Management

Problems Related to Health Care Professionals

Inadequate knowledge of pain management
Poor assessment of pain
Concern about regulation of controlled substances
Fear of client addiction
Concern about side effects of analgesics
Concern about clients becoming tolerant to analgesics

Problems Related to Clients

Reluctance to report pain
Concern about distracting physicians from treatment of underlying disease
Fear that pain means disease is worse
Concern about not being a "good" client
Reluctance to take pain medications
Fear of addiction or of being thought of as an addict
Worries about unmanageable side effects
Concern about becoming tolerant to pain medications

Problems Related to the Health Care System

Low priority given to cancer pain treatment
Inadequate reimbursement (the most appropriate treatment may not be reimbursed or may be too costly for clients and families)
Restrictive regulation of controlled substances
Problems of availability of treatment or access to it

Modified from Jacox, A., et al. (1994). *Management of cancer pain. Clinical practice guidelines No. 9.* AHCPR Pub. No. 94-1592. Rockville, MD: Agency for Health Care Policy and Research, U.S. Department of Health and Human Services, Public Health Service.

Physicians tend to underprescribe, recommending over longer periods of time doses lower than those considered therapeutic. Typically, medications are prescribed with a range of allowable doses and time periods. For example, acetaminophen with codeine may be prescribed as one or two tablets taken every 3 to 4 hours. Many nurses tend to routinely administer the smallest prescribed dose of medication over the widest time frame (e.g., one tablet every 4 hours). Health care providers need to learn more about the mechanisms of pain. A nurse's inaccurate beliefs or expectations lead to misunderstandings about the client's pain experience. Often a client's complaint of pain is ignored or not believed if that client's experience does not match the nurse's expectation.

Clients may contribute to the problem of inadequate pain management. They may be reluctant to take pain medications due to fear of addiction, they may fear being labeled a "drug user," or they may worry that taking strong medications will render them unable to be adequately medicated in the future should their pain become worse. They may believe that some degree of pain is normal and cannot be relieved. Health care providers and people in pain may believe that some degree of pain is expected and is not treatable, especially after surgery and in the presence of cancer. Pain can be totally relieved, or nearly so, with appropriate strategies.

Nurses and clients do not know enough about combination drugs for pain relief. These situations generated by nurses can lead to frustrated, angry, uncooperative clients as a result of unrelieved pain. Education is a primary action to begin to remedy the problems.

DEFINITION OF PAIN

How is *pain* defined? Does the definition include feelings of agony, distress or suffering? Is pain defined in a structural, physiologic manner only? Does the definition include individual perception of the painful stimulus? Do cultural and ethnic backgrounds, gender, or age affect pain perception?

Pain is a multidimensional phenomenon and is thus difficult to define. It is a personal and subjective experience, and no two people experience pain in exactly the same manner. You may find pain control a difficult task when caring for individual clients; however, it is one of the most important areas of care because people cannot function adequately when they are in pain. Pain is best viewed as an experience, not merely as a manifestation of a medical condition.

Health care practitioners have defined pain in many ways. It is generally related to some type of tissue damage, which serves as a warning signal, but it is much more. The International Association for the Study of Pain (IASP) offers the accepted medical definition of pain as "an unpleasant sensory and emotional experience associated with actual or potential tissue damage, or described in terms of such damage."[58]

Sternbach[115] defined pain as "an abstract concept which refers to (1) a personal, private sensation of hurt; (2) a harmful stimulus that signals current or impending tissue damage; and (3) a pattern of responses to protect the organism from harm." This definition helps the nurse's understanding of the client's pain. It focuses on pain as something that belongs to the person, because pain is both personal and private. Sternbach's definition also reminds the nurse that pain may have a protective function.

McCaffery defined pain as "whatever the experiencing person says it is and existing whenever the person says it does."[75] This definition makes each person the expert about his or her own pain. Because clinical pain is subjective, the only people who can accurately define their own pain are those who are experiencing that pain. Despite its subjective nature, the nurse is charged with accurately assessing and helping to relieve pain and McCaffery's definition helps nurses achieve this goal. Remember, all pain is real even if the cause cannot be ascertained.

PERCEPTION OF PAIN

Pain *perception,* or *interpretation,* is an important component of the pain experience. Because we perceive and interpret pain based on our own individual experience, pain is different for each person. Pain perception does not depend solely on the degree of physical damage. Both physical stimuli and psychosocial factors can influence our experience of pain. Although few agree about the specific effects of these factors, *anxiety, experience, attention, expectation,* and the *meaning of the situation* in which injury occurs affect pain perception. Cognitive functions, such as distraction, may also affect the severity and quality of the pain experience.

In the past, pain was viewed primarily as a sensation, with motivational and cognitive processes believed to influence only the reaction to pain. However, it is now apparent that mechanisms within the pain pathway can modify pain-related neural impulses before they are transmitted to the brain. Thus, pain perception is likely to be determined by a relative balance between sensory peripheral input and mechanisms of central control in the brain.

Pain perception is influenced by one's tolerance for pain. To understand tolerance, we must differentiate between *pain threshold* and *pain tolerance.* The pain threshold is defined as the lowest intensity of a painful stimulus that is perceived by a person as pain. The pain threshold may vary according to physiologic factors (such as inflammation or injury near pain receptors), but essentially it is similar for all people if the central nervous system (CNS) and peripheral nervous systems are intact.

Tolerance is defined as the amount of pain a person is willing to endure. It is different for each person who experiences pain, based on subjective factors such as the meaning of the pain and the setting. Some people have a high tolerance; that is, they can tolerate a lot of pain without distress, whereas others have a very low tolerance. Tolerance also varies for a given person, depending on a variety of factors associated with each specific pain incidence, such as nausea, fatigue, meaning of the pain, coping ability, and sensory input. Only the person, not the health care team, can determine the person's tolerance level.

Another aspect that can alter our perception of pain is our past experience with pain. Expectations regarding the new pain experience may be based on previous pain episodes. For example, when a person has had a bad experience with pain, the anticipation that future pain may be as bad can make subsequent pain episodes worse. If the person has had a good experience with pain management, future pain episodes may be more positively experienced. Therefore, it is important for nurses to facilitate adequate pain control that will result in positive client outcomes.

MISCONCEPTIONS AND MYTHS

Many misunderstandings exist about pain (Table 23–1). If nurses continue to believe these myths, adequate pain assessment and relief are hampered. For example, many health care providers believe that it is possible to predict the amount of pain people should have, based on their medical condition. However, the diagnosis or type of surgery is *not* an effective fundamental basis for determining the amount of pain the person should be experiencing or the analgesic required to relieve that pain.

Both children and older adults experience unrelieved pain because health professionals incorrectly assume that age predicts pain.[116] The fact that clients do not visibly exhibit physiologic or behavioral signs of pain often leads to the belief by the health care provider that they do not have pain. A more likely explanation is that the client has adapted to the pain. The adaptive psychological responses include:

- A shifting away from the pain
- Reporting pain only if asked directly
- Exhibiting sleepiness (which may also be due to insomnia secondary to the pain)
- Exhibiting decreased physical activity
- Showing a blank facial expression

These signs do not mean that the person is not experiencing pain but that the person is exhibiting adaptive responses to pain that continues to be present.

A major barrier to adequate pain management is concern about addiction to pain medications, particularly to opioids, which results in undermedication for clients.[116] *Addiction* is a behavioral pattern of drug use characterized by (1) overwhelming involvement with the use of a drug (compulsive use) and securing a supply of it and (2) a tendency to relapse after withdrawal from the drug (to begin taking it again whether or not pain is present). This behavior is sometimes described as the "three Cs": *c*ompulsive, *c*raving for the drug, and seeking and using the drug despite the *c*onsequences. Most people who take opioid analgesic medication for pain do not become addicted; in actuality, psychological addiction rarely occurs. (The incidence of addiction is less than 0.1%.[67]) Never use the term *addict* unless a medical diagnosis has been established, since many individuals exhibiting "drug-seeking behavior" are simply seeking better pain relief, not the medication itself (see also Chapter 24).

Education is the primary means of removing the effect of these myths on pain management. By knowing the facts about pain, pain assessment, pharmacology and pain treatment, you can provide more complete care.

■ MISINFORMATION ABOUT PAIN

One of the major blocks to accurate assessment of a person's pain is the person. If the health care team members still believe myths and have misconceptions about pain, it is likely that the client as well has been misin-

TABLE 23–1 **COMMON MISCONCEPTIONS ABOUT PAIN**

Myth or Misconception	Fact
▪ Addiction occurs with prolonged use of morphine or morphine derivatives	▪ The incidence of addiction is less than 0.1%
▪ The nurse or physician is the best judge of a client's pain	▪ Only the client can judge the level and distress of the pain; pain management should be a team approach that includes the client
▪ Pain is a result, not a cause	▪ Unrelieved pain can create other problems, like anger, anxiety, immobility, respiratory problems, and delay in healing
▪ It is better to wait until a client has pain before giving medication	▪ Playing "catch-up" is not an effective way to manage pain; it is better to routinely administer analgesia, thus maintaining a low pain level
▪ Real pain has an identifiable cause	▪ There is always a cause of pain, but it may be very obscure and must be assessed carefully. Pain of a psychological origin is just as real as pain of physiologic origin
▪ The same physical stimulus produces the same pain intensity, duration, and distress in different people	▪ Intensity, duration, and distress vary with each individual
▪ Some clients lie about the existence or severity of their pain	▪ Very few people lie about pain
▪ Very young or very old people do not have as much pain	▪ All clients with an intact neurological system experience pain; age is not a determinant of pain, but it may influence expression of pain
▪ Pain is a part of aging	▪ Pain does not accompany aging unless a disease process or ailment is present
▪ If a person is asleep, they are not in pain	▪ People in pain become exhausted and may truly be asleep or merely trying to sleep. Some people sleep as an escape mechanism
▪ If the pain is relieved by nonpharmaceutical pain relief techniques, the pain was not real anyway	▪ Nonpharmaceutical pain relief methods can be effective. A client's method of relief should be acknowledged as long as it does not harm
▪ Nurses should rely on their own definitions of pain and cultural beliefs about pain	▪ It is a mistake to impose one's own definitions, cultural beliefs, and values to another person's pain. Let the client tell you what the pain means

formed about pain and pain control. People sense the expectations of the health care team about their own pain. They have learned that they are expected to tolerate certain levels of pain and not to complain excessively. People have also learned to be afraid of pain medications, especially opioids. A major nursing responsibility, therefore, is to educate clients about pain and pain control. The nurse needs to help people understand that they, not the health care team, are the true experts about their pain. The nurse is also responsible for helping clients provide an accurate pain history and assessment data.

When documenting pain, avoid saying that the client "complains" of pain. This term tends to invalidate or minimize the client's experience, as if the client is fussing unnecessarily. It is more accurate and helpful simply to use the word "states" or "reports." When discussing pain (e.g., with clients) or when documenting pain, avoid using the phrase *pain attack.* Feeling that one is "under attack" may increase the feeling of powerlessness, creating the perception that the client is a victim. Use the term "episode" to promote self-control and a sense of an ability to do something to manage the episode.

TYPES OF PAIN

■ ACUTE PAIN

Acute pain is usually of short duration (<6 months) and has an identifiable, immediate onset, such as incisional pain after surgery. It is also regarded as having a limited and often predictable duration, such as postoperative pain, which usually disappears as the wound heals. Acute pain is often described in sensory terms, such as "sharp," "stabbing," and "shooting." It is considered a useful and limiting pain, in that it indicates injury and motivates the person to obtain relief by treatment of the cause. Acute pain is usually reversible or controllable with adequate treatment. People suffering from acute pain often come to terms with it because of the meaning or the limited nature of the pain, as in the pain of childbirth. When the pain is relieved, the person returns to the pre-pain state.

Acute pain may be accompanied by observable physical responses, including (1) increased or decreased blood pressure, (2) tachycardia, (3) diaphoresis, (4) tachypnea, (5) focusing on the pain, and (6) guarding the painful part. The cardiovascular and respiratory responses are due to stimulation of the sympathetic nervous system as part of the *fight or flight response.* These responses are often interpreted as positive evidence of a person's pain. Such interpretation is not reliable, however, because these sympathetic responses are temporary and may not be present in clients with continuing acute pain.

In 1992, the Agency for Health Care Policy and Research (AHCPR)[1] released its first set of Clinical Practice Guidelines for acute pain resulting from surgery or trauma. The guidelines were intended to serve as a resource to help health care providers and clients facilitate positive pain management outcomes. The four major pain management goals are to:

- Reduce the incidence and severity of acute postoperative or post-traumatic pain
- Encourage clients to communicate unrelieved pain so that they can receive prompt evaluation and effective treatment
- Enhance comfort and satisfaction
- Contribute to fewer postoperative complications and shorter stays after surgical procedures

These guidelines were designed to help the individual, family, and health care professionals work *together* to promote better relief of acute pain. You can obtain valuable information from these guidelines, including using them to guide pain assessment and management to improve control of acute pain for all clients. The guidelines emphasize the following[1]:

- A collaborative, interdisciplinary approach to pain control, including all members of the health care team and input from the client and client's family, when appropriate
- An individualized proactive pain control plan developed preoperatively by clients and practitioners (since pain is easier to prevent than to bring under control, once it has begun)
- Assessment and frequent reassessment of the client's pain
- Use of both drug and non-drug therapies to control or prevent pain
- A formal, institutional approach to management of acute pain, with clear lines of responsibility

■ CHRONIC PAIN

Chronic pain is a major health concern. The pain may have originally been acute in nature or may have been so obscure that the person does not know when it first developed. Chronic pain syndromes are often defined in vague terms, and many of their causes remain unknown.[120] Therefore, a diversity of treatment modalities has been used to treat the symptoms.

Chronic pain may be divided into three types:

- Chronic nonmalignant pain, such as from low back pain or rheumatoid arthritis
- Chronic, intermittent pain, such as from migraine headache
- Chronic malignant pain, from cancer

Chronic pain lasts for long periods of time and is not readily treatable.[79] A person's mental response to pain depends on its duration and, possibly, its intensity. Pain that is constant, continuous, and moderate is often described as far more difficult to bear than pain that is intense but relatively short in duration. The course of chronic pain includes months and years of pain, not minutes or hours.

Chronic pain is associated with withdrawal and despair. Anxiety may give way to depression. Some clients learn to adapt and cope with the pain, adjusting their lives. Remember, however, that absence of the expected expression of severe pain does not mean that the pain is gone; therefore the client's description of pain, not the manifestations one expects to see, is very important. Intractable, prolonged, and intense pain is very difficult to bear. Most people undergo major affective and behavioral changes when experiencing pain for prolonged periods. Such changes may be compounded, and chronic pain syndrome can develop. Characteristics of clients experiencing chronic pain syndrome include:

- Depressed mood
- Increased or decreased appetite and weight
- Drastically restricted activity level, leading to reduced work capacity, poor physical tone, and increased depression
- Social withdrawal
- Preoccupation with physical manifestations
- Poor sleep and chronic fatigue, which may result from inactivity, analgesics, and depression as well as from pain

Some clients may not exhibit any of these manifestations or may exhibit only a few. Once these changes take place, however, the pain may become more difficult to treat than the pain's original physical source.

CHRONIC NONMALIGNANT PAIN

Chronic pain is usually considered pain that lasts more than 6 months (or 1 month beyond the normal end of the condition causing the pain) and has no foreseeable end unless it is associated with very slow healing, as with burns. It is continuous or persistent and recurrent. Some disagree about whether acute recurrent pain (as in migraine and sickle cell crisis) should be classified as chronic pain, but it is usually referred to as chronic.

Chronic pain may have an identifiable cause, although the cause may be difficult to determine. It is often described in affective terms, such as "hateful," or "sickening" and it is typically much more difficult than acute pain to treat. Chronic pain is frequently associated with concomitant disability as a result of the pain experience. For example, a client immobilized by the pain of severe rheumatoid arthritis may be further compromised by the effects of the immobility.

Chronic pain is a frustrating condition, making it difficult for the person to live a normal life. Clients experiencing continuous or continually recurring chronic pain tend to become increasingly engrossed in their illness. They may seem fearful, tense, fatigued, tending to become withdrawn and isolated. Their pain is exhausting both physically and emotionally for themselves and their families. Health care providers may also feel frustrated and incompetent when their attempts to relieve chronic pain are ineffective. However, if nurses understand the anatomy, physiology, and psychosocial aspects of chronic pain, they can be very helpful to the the client and family. Professionals may be able to intervene before extreme suffering occurs.

Chronic Intermittent Pain

Chronic intermittent pain refers to exacerbation or recurrence of the chronic condition. The pain occurs only at specific periods; at other times, the client is free from pain. Typical, conditions include migraine and cluster headache, sickle cell crisis, and the intermittent abdominal pain associated with chronic gastrointestinal disorders, such as irritable bowel syndrome and Crohn's disease. Pain management is directed toward control of pain in much the same manner as that for individual acute pain episodes. However, chronic recurrences render the condition more difficult to control. The client anticipates continual exacerbation of the situation and is intensely influenced by psychosocial factors that are difficult to manage.

Chronic Malignant (Cancer-Related) Pain

Malignant pain is considered to have qualities of both acute and chronic pain. The category encompasses neuropathic, deep visceral, and bone pain, among others (Table 23–2). Each type of pain is best managed by strategies specific to it. Therefore, the nurse needs to carefully assess each type of pain and treat it appropriately. A diagnosis of cancer adds an additional psychological component associated with potential physical deformity and the potential for impending death, preceded by agonizing suffering. The mental anguish may intensify the perception of pain.

TABLE 23–2 SOURCES OF NOXIOUS STIMULI FOR CLIENTS WITH CANCER

Source of Stimuli	Cause
▪ Cell destruction	Cell necrosis Ulceration Tumor invasion Tissue injury
▪ Inflammation	Products of cell destruction
▪ Infection	Bacterial invasion
▪ Nerve injury	Direct injury through incising nerve structures Tumor invasion of peripheral nerves, plexes, spinal cord, brain Chemotherapy/radiation injury
▪ Ischemia/hypoxia	Edema Hematoma Occlusion of vessels by tumor
▪ Noxious stretch or pressure	Distention of thoracic and abdominal viscera, fascia, periosteum Occlusion of gastrointestinal and genitourinary structures Obstruction of ducts and viscus

PHYSIOLOGY

■ PHYSIOLOGIC BASIS OF PAIN PERCEPTION

To understand the mechanisms by which pain relief might be facilitated, we must understand the neurologic contributions to pain perception. Pain is a perceptual interpretation of nerve activity that reaches consciousness. The sensation of pain depends on activation of neurons that transmit the noxious information to the CNS. Pain perception is initiated by activation of neurons along a pathway, which eventually terminates in a sensory cortex in the brain. The pathway involves both peripheral nervous system and CNS components and can be activated at any point along its path.

The typical initiation of pain producing nerve transmission begins with activation of receptors by chemical or mechanical stimuli. Receptor activation is followed by transduction of the stimulus to an electrical impulse that is transmitted from nerve cell to nerve cell along the pathway. The neuron responsible for transmitting the electrical signal is composed of three primary components: the cell body, dendrites, and an axon. Dendrites receive the signal and transmit it toward the cell body, where it is directed along the axon to activate the dendrites of the next neuron. Dendrites of the next neuron come in contact with the axon of the transmitting neuron at a synapse, a microscopic cleft at the contact area. The ends of the axons are configured with specialized structures (terminal boutons). The electrical signal is transmitted to the next neuron when specialized chemicals (*neurotransmitters*) are released by the terminal bouton. The neurotransmitter must diffuse across the synaptic cleft and attach to receptors on the dendrites of the next neuron.

Neurons involved in pain perception are A-delta (Aδ) and C fibers.[40, 44, 130] A-delta fibers transmit a signal more rapidly than C fibers do. They deliver information that allows us to recognize a pain-producing stimulus and to determine its relevant characteristics, such as location, severity, and type. A-delta fiber-mediated pain is perceived as sharp, cutting, or stabbing sensations, reflective of tissue damage. A-delta fiber activity typically results in activation of the sympathetic nervous system to prepare us to engage in fight or flight behaviors that allow us to react to the pain-producing event.[40] As a result, heart rate, respiratory rate, and blood pressure may be increased. These sympathetic reactions may or may not be observed in people with pain, since they are relatively rapidly adapting, often short-lived, responses.

C-fiber-mediated pain is conducted more slowly along the pain pathway and is characterized by dull, burning, sensations associated with suffering. C-fiber activity engages various brain stem and cerebral regions that contribute to the emotional, cognitive, and situational components of pain.

The first synapse in the pain pathway for both A-delta and C fibers occurs in the dorsal horn of the spinal cord, the area of the cord that receives all incoming sensory information[9, 40, 52] Here the nociceptive signal is transferred to the next neuron in the pain pathway and transmitted to the thalamus and brain stem structures by means of *spinal tracts.* The thalamic signal is involved in the ability to determine the location and intensity of the pain producing event. The signal is transmitted from the thalamus to the sensory cortex, where the pain as a sensation is perceived.

Secondary responses to the signal are initiated throughout the brain, including the limbic system, where the emotional response to pain is generated. Signals transmitted to brain stem structures contribute to the response we have to the pain experience and to endogenous (naturally occurring) pain modulation systems (Fig. 23–2).

Receptor Activation

Pain perception depends on the generation of an electrical signal within the pain pathway. The electrical signal most often begins with activation of a receptor by high-intensity chemical, thermal, or mechanical stimuli.[40, 69, 100] Receptors associated with pain perception are found on specialized dendrites called *free nerve endings.* These receptors are categorized as *nociceptors* and are found throughout the body in the periphery in skin, fascia, bone periosteum, skeletal muscle, ligaments, and mucous membranes. In the viscera, nociceptors are found in the capsules of most organs.[40, 116]

Chemically mediated activation of nociceptors can be initiated by (1) cell wall destruction as a result of events such as tissue injury, ulceration, tumor invasion and cell necrosis, (2) inflammation, (3) infection, (4) nerve injury, and (5) extravasation of plasma from the circulatory system associated with edema, ischemia, or occlusion of vessels. Mechanically mediated activation of nociceptors is accomplished by noxious stretch or pressure due to (1) distention of viscera, fascia or periosteum, (2) occlusion of gastrointestinal or genitourinary structures, or (3) obstruction of ducts/viscus.[40, 52]

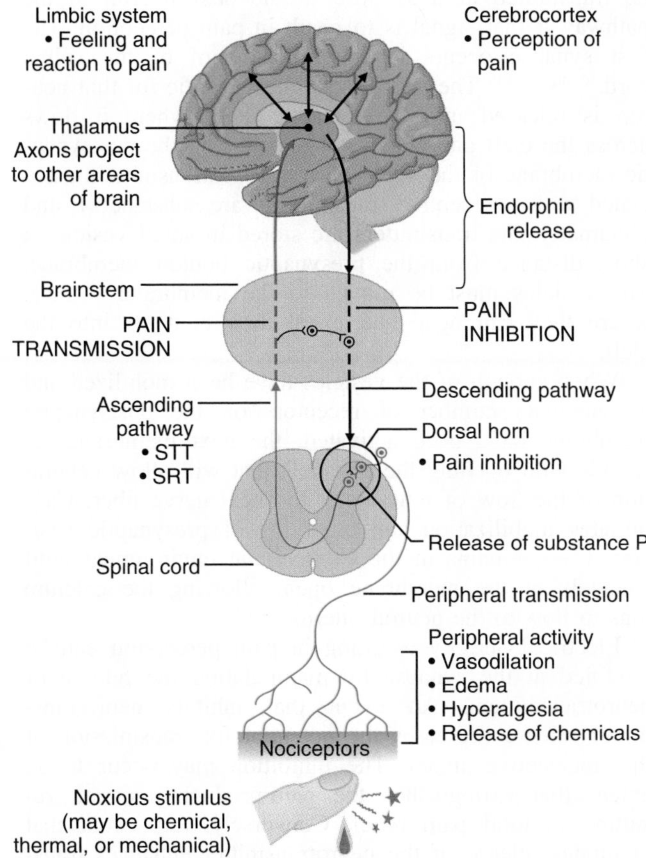

FIGURE 23–2 Ascending and descending nociceptive pain. (From Banasik J. *Perspectives on Pathophysiology Instructor's Manual,* 1995.)

The nociceptors are at rest until they are stimulated by an event in the receptor's environment. The stimulus causes a change in the receptor membrane, which generates the electrical signal. The electrical signal is transmitted along the nerve dendrites and axon by modification of the electrical charge of the nerve cell membrane. Movement of the signal along the membrane requires that positively and negatively charged ions flow from one side of the membrane to the other.[4, 54, 75]

When at rest, the extracellular surface of the neuron membrane maintains a positive charge (the intracellular surface a negative charge). The positive charge is a result of a higher concentration of positively charged ions, primarily sodium (Na^+), in the extracellular environment, in contrast to the intracellular surface. The intracellular charge is maintained by a higher concentration of negatively charged ions, such as chloride (Cl^-), and large anions along the interior cell membrane. Potassium ions (K^+) aid in maintenance of the resting membrane charge. A change in the charge of the membrane surfaces is necessary to initiate the electrical signal. The interior must become more positive, the exterior more negative. The change is achieved by allowing Na^+ to flow into the cell and Cl^- to flow out of the cell. The addition of positively charged Na^+ inside the cell makes the inside more positive. The outward flow of Cl^- causes the extracellular surface to be less positive.

Channels in the cell membrane maintain the charge difference. The channels provide the only route for ions to move across the membrane. The nociceptive signal cannot be generated or maintained unless the channels are induced to open. When a stimulus is strong enough to initiate receptor activation, events are put into play that cause channels to open and the charged ions to move across the nerve cell membrane. This causes a change in the electrical charge of the membrane known as *depolarization* of the membrane.[4, 54, 65, 75]

Pain-producing events may initiate the nociceptive electrical signal directly, or they may sensitize the receptor, rendering it more susceptible to nociceptive activation—depending on the degree to which the ions move across the membrane. If the flow of ions is of sufficient intensity, the nerve membrane reaches threshold and "fires" initiating the electrical signal. The flow may be sufficient to change the charge of the membrane, rendering it close to threshold (partially depolarized) but not strong enough to cause the membrane to fire.[4, 44, 103] The depolarized membrane now fires in response to stimuli less intense than those originally needed.

Sensitizing chemicals are released into tissues as a result of cell wall destruction, release of plasma from the circulatory system as seen with edema, inflammation, ischemia, and infection.[114] Cells may be damaged by trauma and by the events that accompany inflammation and infection, including mast cell destruction during the release of histamine in inflammation and the effect of neutrophil activity in the presence of infection.

Chemicals sensitize receptors and nerve fiber membranes that do not typically produce pain sensations making them capable of initiating pain-producing signals. Sunburned areas produce a burning sensation when one showers with water, which normally produces a pleasant, warm sensation. Injured areas are painful in response to touch and mild pressure that normally would not be painful. Normal peristalsis of the gut, which is typically undetectable, produces painful abdominal cramping in the presence of inflammation within the abdominal cavity.

The need for the flow of ions across the membrane provides a mechanism for pain to be intensified or decreased, depending on the activity of the membrane channels. Events or chemicals that cause channels to open and allow ions to flow across the membrane contribute to an increase in pain. Events that prevent channels from opening decrease the ability of pain-producing neurons to fire, resulting in decreased pain.

Chemicals that mediate nociception in the periphery include bradykinin, prostaglandins, substance P (sP), histamine, serotonin, leukotrienes, hydrogen ions, and nerve growth factor (NGF).[11, 55, 72, 100, 117]

Bradykinin, the most potent pain-producing chemical,[100, 135] is released into tissues when cell walls are destroyed and when plasma leaks from the vasculature.[15, 31, 69, 82] Bradykinin initiates a pain-producing signal by increasing the ability of Na^+ to flow across the membrane.

Prostaglandins result from cell wall destruction. They appear to contribute to the pain experience by sensitizing receptors, making them more responsive to other chemical, thermal, and mechanical stimuli.[24, 57, 129] They are also potent vasodilators, resulting in an increased release of bradykinin into the tissues.[24] The resulting edema may also contribute by stimulating pressure receptors. Pressure from edema typically is not painful, because the pressure is usually not strong enough to stimulate nociceptors. Prostaglandins depolarize these receptors, making them responsive to the relatively weak stimulus provided by the swelling of edema.

Substance P is released into peripheral tissues when nociceptive neurons are activated.[23, 46, 69, 129] The chemical facilitates the release of plasma by increasing vascular permeability, resulting in availability of bradykinin.[9, 69] Substance P further enhances pain responses by contributing to prostaglandin release.[23, 42, 122]

Histamine is released from mast cells when inflammation is a component of the pain-producing event. In the periphery, histamine increases vascular permeability, contributing to bradykinin activity and edema.[100] Substance P facilitates the release of histamine from mast cells.[23, 69, 129]

Serotonin is released in the periphery by platelets and mast cells.[104, 129] Therefore, any event that influences the presence of blood products in tissues or inflammation contributes to serotonin release. Serotonin causes pain directly by altering Na^+ flow in the receptive neuron membrane, causing the neuron to fire.[9, 104] Receptors are indirectly facilitated by serotonin as the chemical also sensitizes receptors to the effect of bradykinin.[15, 82]

Leukotrienes are produced by cell wall destruction during the same process that produces prostaglandins. They contribute to pain perception by attracting neutrophils to an area of injury.[65, 69] Cell wall destruction is a component of neutrophil activity to combat infection, resulting in bradykinin release. Thermal and mechanical receptors are also sensitized by leukotrienes.

Hydrogen (H^+) ions are released as a result of ischemia and hypoxia. They cause sodium channels to open, resulting in activation of neurons in the pain pathway. H^+ also facilitates calcium (Ca^{2+}) channel opening, enhancing neurotransmitter release.

Nerve growth factor is released when neurons are injured. NGF is similar to bradykinin in activating nociceptive neurons.[32, 65] NGF causes injured nerves to sprout new axons and dendrites in greater numbers than existed before the injury. As a result, the area responsive to nociceptive activation is increased in the periphery.[33] Substance P production is also increased by NGF increasing the nociceptive effect of the neurotransmitter. In addition, the number of Na^+ and K^+ channels are increased, making it easier to generate an ion flow, which will cause the neuron to "fire."

We respond to a pain-producing event with unique combinations of chemicals that modify the pain experience. For some, the combination of chemical mediators evoked may increase pain perception; for others, pain perception is limited. The multifaceted character of events that generate pain-producing signals accounts, in part, for variability in response to situations among people with similar tissue injury. Remember, we cannot predict the amount of pain a person might have in response to tissue injury or insult.

Transmission of Pain-Producing Activity to the Brain

An electrical signal generated in the periphery must be transmitted at a synapse to the next neuron in the pathway if that signal is to result in pain perception. The first synapse occurs in the dorsal horn of the spinal cord.[30, 40, 52, 135] The neurotransmitter specific for that neuron is released into the synaptic cleft, where it flows across the cleft and engages a receptor on the postsynaptic membrane of the next neuron. Neurotransmitters associated with nociceptive transmission are substance P and glutamate. The transmitters are stored in small vesicles a short distance from the presynaptic bouton membrane. The vesicles must be moved to the membrane surface, where they can open and expel their contents into the cleft.

When enough of the vesicles have been mobilized and an adequate number of receptors on the postsynaptic membrane have been activated, the next membrane responds with opening the channels that will allow generation of the flow of ions along the next nerve fiber. Ca^{2+} initiates mobilization and emptying of presynaptic vesicles. Ca^{2+} remains in the extracellular environment until channels in the membrane open, allowing the calcium ions to flow to the neuron interior.[44, 64]

Electrical activity resulting in pain perception can be modified at the synapse by manipulating the release of neurotransmitters. An event that inhibits neurotransmitter release decreases the potential for transmission of the nociceptive signal. The inhibition may occur to an extent that extinguishes the pain-producing signal, resulting in total pain relief. Conversely, any event that facilitates release of the neurotransmitter enhances transmission of the signal. For example, an event that prohibits the opening of the Ca^{2+} channels inhibits the pain response.

INHIBITION OF PAIN-PRODUCING NEURAL ACTIVITY

Pain relief can be accomplished by (1) preventing activation of nociceptive receptors in the periphery, (2) preventing transmission of the electrical signal along the neurons in the pain pathway, and (3) preventing transfer of the signal from one neuron to the next at the synapse. Events that inhibit factors that contribute to pain (including inflammation, edema, and infection) lessen the pain experience by decreasing the availability of pain-producing chemicals.

Medications provide a primary means of modifying receptor activation. Nonsteroidal anti-inflammatory drugs (NSAIDs), for example, aspirin and ibuprofen, contribute to pain relief by preventing the production of prostaglandins and decreasing the effect of inflammation on the facilitation of pain-producing activity. Preventing unnecessary stimulation of receptors by mechanical events helps to control the pain event. Examples include controlling excess pressure on painful areas by proper positioning, avoiding pressure-producing events, and splinting an incision.

Transmission of the pain-producing signal can be inhibited by conditions that prevent opening of Na^+, Cl^-, or K^+ channels along the fiber. Some medications act directly on these channels, leading to the inability of the neuron membrane to maintain electrical activity.

A primary avenue for pain inhibition is found at the synapse in the spinal cord.[40, 42, 122] Peripheral sensory nerve cells extend from the receptor to the dorsal horn of the cord. The first synapse in the pain pathway occurs here. The dorsal horn is subdivided into layers, or *laminae.* A-delta fibers terminate in lamina I, the marginal layer, and laminae II and V. They synapse with *nociceptive-specific* (NS) neurons that transmit the signal to the thalamus. C fibers terminate primarily in laminae I, II, IV, and V.[9, 40, 130] They may activate NS neurons or *wide dynamic range* (WDR) neurons that respond to both nociceptive and non-nociceptive stimuli. These neurons extend to the brain through spinal tracts that terminate in the thalamus, the reticular formation, or the mesencephalon.

Interneurons are located in laminae II, III and IV.[40, 130] These neurons have extensively branched axons and dendrites, which may project through several laminae. They do not project beyond the dorsal horn however, suggesting that they serve a modifying function in the pain pathway. The location of the neurons, combined with their dense and extensive branching, render them capable of interacting with numerous sensory neurons. Some interactions occur with the peripheral neuron prior to the synapse. Others occur with the second neuron at postsynaptic sites. The presynaptic interactions facilitate pain relief by preventing an adequate release of nociceptive neurotransmitters. The postsynaptic interactions render the membrane less responsive to the incoming signal by modifying the electrical charge of the membrane, preventing the opening of ion channels, or by modifying the ability of receptors to receive the nociceptive neurotransmitters.[12, 55, 71]

Enkephalin and gamma-aminobutyric acid (GABA) are the primary inhibitory neurotransmitters released by dorsal horn interneurons.[3, 86, 107, 135] GABA acts to prevent "firing" of the postsynaptic membrane.[86] GABA inhibits neurotransmitter release from the presynaptic membrane by interfering with the membrane's ability to mobilize Ca^{2+}.[86] Enkephalin is one of the body's endogenous opiates. A number of opiate receptor types exist within the CNS, including mu, delta, and kappa.[3, 135] Opiates that activate mu and delta receptors initiate activity that hyperpolarizes the neuron membrane by modifying the ability of K^+ to flow across the membrane. As a result, nociceptive neurons require stronger stimuli in order to "fire." The effect occurs at both presynaptic and postsynaptic levels. When kappa receptors are engaged, Ca^{2+} channels cannot open, preventing neurotransmitter release. Enkephalin inhibits release of substance P from presynaptic terminals.

Inhibitory neurons in the dorsal horn can be activated by peripheral, mechanical and thermal stimuli, which are perceived as nonpainful. Nonpainful stimuli are transmitted to the CNS by A-beta fibers. Activation of A-beta fibers results in sensations perceived as touch, pressure, warmth, coolness, and vibration. The fibers also transmit proprioceptive information from muscle spindles and tendon insertions. These neuron fibers enter the dorsal horn and send their primary projections to the brain by means of the spinothalamic tract. Collaterals of these nerve fibers project to the dorsal horn laminae, where they terminate on enkephalin-producing interneurons. Activation of the A-beta fibers contributes to pain relief by stimulating the release of enkephalin.[3, 12, 42] One can observe the result of A-beta activity mediated by activation of peripheral skin receptors when one places a finger, mildly burned while cooking, in cold tap water. The burning sensation is extinguished while the finger is in the water. The ability of muscle contraction and joint movement to decrease pain perception is evidenced by shaking the hand when a part of the extremity has been injured.

Additional neurotransmitters are found in the dorsal horn. The cell bodies of the neurons that release these transmitters are located in areas of the brain stem. Their axons project to the spinal cord, where they synapse with the interneurons that release the inhibitory neurotransmitters. Serotonin is produced in the nucleus raphe magnus. Norepinephrine is produced by neurons in the locus ceruleus. The mechanisms by which these supraspinal nuclei contribute to pain relief are still being determined. They appear to stimulate neurons that release enkephalin, resulting in release of the inhibitory neurotransmitter.

Neurons in the raphe and ceruleus nuclei are activated by both peripheral nervous system and CNS activity. Neurons ascending to the brain in spinal tracts make connections with areas of the brain known to be involved in pain inhibition. The primary sites are the periaqueductal (PAG) and periventricular gray (PVG) areas that line the ventricles and the aqueduct of the cerebrospinal fluid (CSF) system. Enkephalin and the neurohormone endorphin are produced by PAG/PVG cell bodies. Collateral projections of the spinal tracts terminate in PAG/PVG. Nociceptive information being transmitted to the brain also activates the endogenous pain inhibition pathway by stimulating PAG/PVG neurons. Axons of these neurons project to both nucleus raphe and locus ceruleus initiating the release of serotonin and norepinephrine in the dorsal horn.[38, 42, 104, 130]

Brain areas responding to cognitive, emotional, and situational stimuli can also activate PAG/PVG, nucleus raphe magnus and locus ceruleus neurons. These nuclei receive projections from the limbic system, various cortical association areas, the hypothalamus, the basal ganglia, the auditory system, and the reticular activating system, among others.[25, 28, 38] These interconnections allow for numerous factors to contribute to pain perception through their influence on endogenous inhibitory activity. They may also serve to increase pain perception through activity that enhances the nociceptive signal or prevents the inhibitory system from operating. Figures 23–3 and 23–4 illustrate these inhibitory mechanisms.

■ GATE CONTROL THEORY OF PAIN

Historically, the gate control theory of pain has been included throughout the nursing literature as the theoretical explanation of the ability of pain management interventions to provide pain relief. Melzack and Wall posited the theory in 1965 on the basis of what was then known about the dorsal horn.[78] They proposed that pain could be inhibited by non-noxious peripheral stimuli and by brain activity associated with meaning of the experience, past pain experience, emotional arousal, cognitive activity (such as distraction), and motivational aspects of the situation. They described a gate in the dorsal horn that allowed transmission of nociceptive information when the gate was open and that prevented transmission if the gate was closed (Fig. 23–5). They suggested that interneurons in the substantia gelatinosa (SG) of the spinal cord were involved in closing the gate. When these neurons were stimulated, events occurred that rendered the transmission neuron incapable of receiving the signal. They also proposed that supraspinal activity originating in the brain and brain stem could contribute to opening or closing the gate.

The theory provided the first conceptualization of pain as a multidimensional experience. Prior to publication of the theory, the primary explanation was based on the

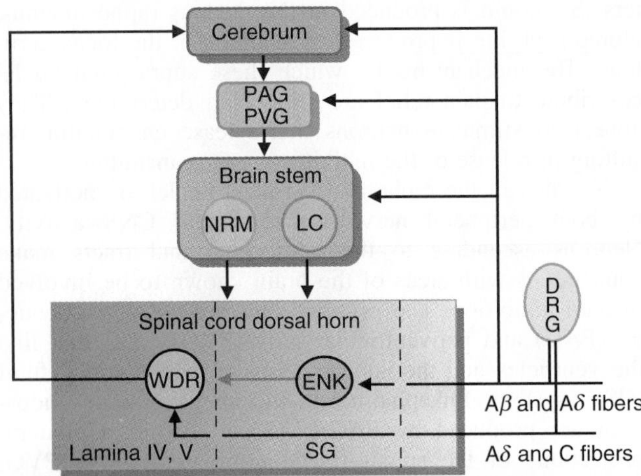

FIGURE 23–3 Schematic representation of pathways involved with pain transmission and its modulation in the dorsal horn of the spinal cord. (PAG = periaqueductal gray; PVG = periventricular gray; NRM = nucleus raphe magnus; LC = locus ceruleus; WDR = wide dynamic range neuron; ENK = enkephalin releasing neuron; SG = substantia gelatinosa.

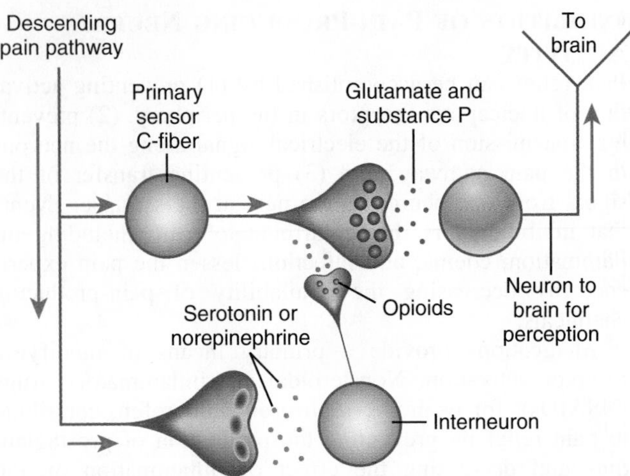

FIGURE 23–4 Endogenous inhibition in a synapse in the spinal cord. As the pain impulse enters the dorsal horn, it has the potential of being modified by interneurons in the synapse containing endogenous opioids.

belief that pain was a "straight through" stimulus-response phenomenon. When tissue damage occurred, specific nerve fibers were activated and the information was transmitted directly to the thalamus and then to the sensory cortex. The resulting pain perception could be accurately predicted based on the degree of tissue damage. The theory did not allow for pain inhibition by mechanisms other than interrupting the pain pathway or removing the pain-producing stimulus. The gate control theory replaced this conceptualization.

Although the theory has been helpful in bringing about a more realistic explanation of the human pain experience

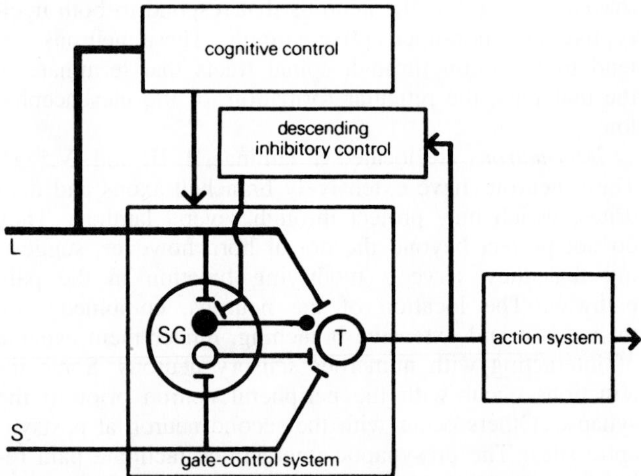

FIGURE 23–5 The gate-control theory: Mark II. The new model includes excitatory (*white circle*) and inhibitory (*black circle*) links from the substantia gelatinosa (SG) to the transmission (T) cells as well as descending inhibitory control from brain stem systems. The round knob at the end of the inhibitory link implies that its action may be presynaptic, postsynaptic, or both. All connections are excitatory, except the inhibitory link from SG to T cell. L, large-diameter fibers; S, small-diameter fibers. (From Melzack, R., & Wall, P. D. [1988]. *The challenge of pain* [2nd ed.]. New York: Penguin Books.)

at the time, it is less helpful today. Research over the past 30 years has delineated the actual mechanisms occurring in the spinal cord and has shown that the "gate" conceptualization is no longer tenable. In addition, inhibition activity is not limited to the SG. The SG is composed of dorsal horn laminae II and III. Inhibitory interneurons and their projections have been found beyond these two laminae. The theory was correct in predicting that nociceptive information was modifiable in the dorsal horn. Melzack and Wall proposed that nonpainful peripheral stimuli could initiate activation of events in the dorsal horn that would inhibit transmission of pain-producing signals beyond the spinal cord. The theory is now out of date, as subsequent research has more fully delineated the physiologic mechanisms underlying pain inhibition.

SOURCES OF PAIN

■ CLASSIFICATION

The human body is typically classified by systems. Systems involved in pain production include:

- *Superficial cutaneous* regions encompassing skin and subcutaneous tissues
- *Somatic* tissues of the body wall, including muscle, bone, periosteum, cartilage, tendons, deep fascia, ligaments, joints, blood vessels, and nerves
- *Visceral* structures, including organs and their capsules

The characteristics of a person's pain experience depends, in part, on the source of the noxious stimulation. Therefore, it is helpful to understand the typical characteristics of each pain type.

CUTANEOUS (SUPERFICIAL) PAIN

Cutaneous pain may be characterized by an abrupt onset and a sharp or stinging quality or by a slower onset and a burning quality, depending upon the type of nerve fiber involved. Cutaneous pain tends to be easily localized. The skin surface is readily divided into areas called *dermatomes.* Each dermatome is served by one spinal nerve and dorsal root. When the skin is stimulated by a noxious stimulus, the nerve serving that dermatome is activated. The signal is transmitted to the one specific area of the sensory cortex serving the dermatome. As a result, the stimulus is perceived to occur within that dermatome. The boundaries of dermatomes may appear to be distinct in anatomic drawings, but nerve distribution actually overlaps. Excitation of one nerve may produce pain that is perceived to originate from adjacent dermatomes.

DEEP SOMATIC PAIN

Somatic structures are those of the body wall, such as muscles and bone. Table 23–3 displays a comparison of deep somatic pain with cutaneous pain. Deep somatic pain is poorly localized, may produce nausea, and may be associated with sweating and blood pressure changes. Deep somatic pain is generally diffuse and less localizable than cutaneous pain. Pain from deep structures frequently radiates from the primary site (e.g., pain from a lumbar disc is felt along the sciatic nerve).

Somatic structures vary in their sensitivity to pain. Highly sensitive structures include tendons, deep fascia, ligaments, joints, bone periosteum, blood vessels, and

TABLE 23–3 CUTANEOUS AND DEEP PAIN

Characteristic	Cutaneous Pain	Deep Pain
Quality	Sharp, bright sensation or burning; felt superficially	Primarily dull and aching; may be described as boring, crushing, throbbing, or cramping; if less intense, described as soreness
Duration	Typically short	Often fairly long
Localization	Tends to be precise Pain is often experienced as a point, surface, or line	Often diffuse and inaccurate; seems to originate in a fairly broad area Pain frequently felt as if it were three-dimensional and occupying space
Hyperalgesia (excessive sensibility to pain)	May occur as a primary problem	May exist as secondary problem; occurring at a distance from the original noxious stimulus In referred pain, a superficial hyperalgesia may be associated with deep pain
Nausea	Rarely occurs	Sickening pain found only when deep structures are involved, as in renal and intestinal colic, gallstones, and angina
Associated symptoms	May be hyperalgesia, paresthesia, tickling, burning, or itching Also associated with brisk movements, a quick pulse, and a sense of invigoration	Resulting from autonomic responses, including pallor, sweating, nausea, vomiting, bradycardia (at times), lowering of blood pressure, syncope, faintness, and perhaps even death in shock Muscle contraction and tenderness often present Segmental spread of pain frequently noted; pain may not remain confined to original spinal segment but may spread into one or more adjacent segments

nerves. Skeletal muscle is sensitive only to stretching and ischemia. Bone and cartilage respond to extreme pressure and chemical stimulation (e.g., rheumatoid arthritis, osteomyelitis).

Visceral Pain

Visceral pain refers to pain coming from body organs. It tends to be a diffuse, poorly localized, vague, dull pain. Nerve fibers innervating body organs follow the sympathetic nerves to the spinal cord. This may be the reason why autonomic manifestations (e.g., diarrhea, cramps, sweating, hypertension) frequently accompany visceral pain. Visceral pain typically includes acute appendicitis, cholecystitis, and inflammation of the biliary and pancreatic tracts, gastroduodenal disease, cardiovascular disease, pleurisy, and renal and ureteral colic. Often visceral pain is manifested as sweating, restlessness, nausea, emesis, pallor, and agitation.

Most viscera are not sensitive to stimuli that cause pain in somatic structures (such as cutting, burning, or pressure). This is understandable, because viscera are not normally exposed to such traumas, and the body thus does not "need" a response system. Although these types of stimuli do not produce pain in most viscera, other stimuli may cause severe pain, for example, violent or abnormal contractions of hollow viscera, such as the ureters and alimentary tract.

In the chest, the parietal pleura is richly supplied with pain endings through the intercostal nerves and through the phrenic nerve, on the surface of the diaphragm. The visceral pleurae in the chest, however, are insensitive to pain. The bronchi, on the other hand, are sensitive to pain. Elsewhere and throughout its serous surfaces, the visceral pericardium is insensitive to pain, except for the lower portion of the fibrous pericardium, which appears to have pain fibers from the phrenic nerve.

Pain in the gastrointestinal tract is common. It appears to arise mainly from the tract's muscular and serous lining. Gastrointestinal pain seems to occur when intestinal mucosa is inflamed, ulcerated, or otherwise abnormal or when the visceral muscles contract strongly or develop spasm. While the wall of the intestine is not sensitive to cutting, burning, or crushing, it does produce pain under other conditions, such as widespread ischemia and distention. Abdominal pain may also occur when body organs are perforated and their contents drain into the peritoneal cavity.

Visceral pain differs from cutaneous pain, in that highly localized damage to the viscera rarely causes severe pain but such damage to the body surface would cause pain. For example, a surgical cut in the gut does not cause pain but a cut in the skin would cause severe pain. If the stimulus to the viscera causes diffuse stimulation of nerve endings, the resulting pain is severe, as in ischemia (lack of oxygen) of the gut. Visceral pain is known to produce referred pain.

■ REFERRED PAIN

Referred pain is felt in an area distant from the site of the stimulus. It occurs when nerve fibers serving an area of the body distant from the site of the stimulus pass in close proximity to the stimulus. The referred pain sensation may be intense, and there may be little or no pain at the point of noxious stimuli. For example, myocardial ischemia typically is not felt as pain in the heart but most often as left arm, shoulder, or jaw pain. The fibers innervating these areas are close to those innervating the myocardium, resulting in the referred pain.

Identification of the segment of the spinal cord that is involved in transmitting referred pain is helpful diagnostically. Pain arising from a deep structure, whether a viscus or a deep somatic structure, has a referred segmental distribution, or a pattern of pain, determined according to the spinal cord segment supplying the structure. Referred pain is often baffling, warranting careful assessment. Examples of common patterns include pleural pain from the diaphragm referred to the shoulder, and the pain of cholecystitis referred to the back and in the angle of the scapula. Figure 23–6 illustrates common sites of referred pain.

■ INFLAMMATION

Inflammation is one of the most common pathologic conditions influencing pain sensitivity. Numerous harmful

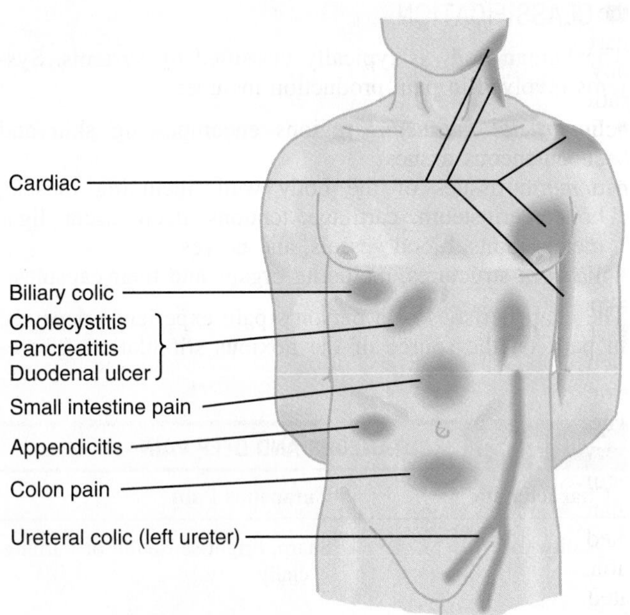

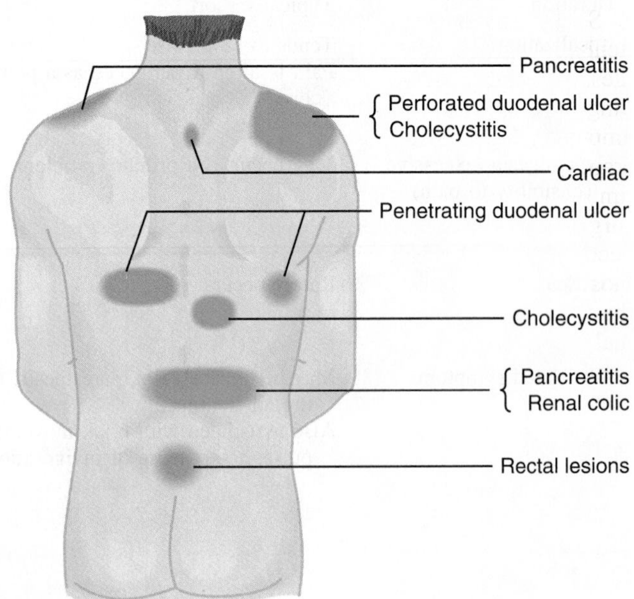

FIGURE 23–6 Areas of referred pain.

substances, such as bacterial and chemical agents, can cause inflammation. Inflammatory responses may result from stressors, such as heat, cold, or trauma. Gross assessment findings associated with the inflammatory process are redness, swelling, heat, and pain. Inflammatory pain is secondary to the distention of stretch-sensitive tissue (i.e., periosteum, pleura) and the direct effect of released neuroregulators on afferent nerve endings. Principal chemical mediators of the inflammatory response are histamine, substance P, bradykinin, prostaglandins, and leukokinins.

■ NEUROPATHY

Neuropathic pain is caused by damage or injury to nerve fibers in the periphery or by damage to the CNS. Noxious electrical impulses are generated at the site of the injury. The pain is perceived to occur in the area served by the nerve. For example, an injury to a nerve that serves the hand would be perceived as pain in the hand even though the injury may be at the spinal cord level. Such pain is particularly problematic for the individual, as there is no obvious pathologic process corresponding to the pain sensation (e.g., the hand). Therefore, the person may not be believed. Neuropathic pain is also difficult to manage because it responds poorly to typical pain medications, particularly to NSAIDs[133] and opioids.[94, 133]

■ PHANTOM LIMB SENSATION

Following amputation of a body part (e.g., limb, breast), a person may continue to experience sensations in the part amputated as if that part were still present or attached. The nerve fibers that served the part continue to extend to the periphery, ending now at the incision site. The nerves have been injured by the surgery. As the cut nerve endings attempt to regenerate, they may form small neuromas at the incision cite. When nerve fibers are stimulated as a result of injury or neuroma, they continue to mediate the sensations associated with their original location. As a result, neuropathic sensations may be generated. These abnormal sensations may be perceived as presence of the limb, paresthesia, or pain.

Sensations associated with paresthesia may consist of itching, pressure, tingling, numbness, or "pins and needles." Painful sensations include throbbing, burning, stabbing, boring, and vise-like sensations experienced in the amputated area. Phantom pain also may be experienced as cramped, twisted, and abnormal posturing of a phantom limb. As a result of the nerve injury associated with the surgery, a formerly painless phantom area may gradually become painful. Phantom limb sensation is limited for most clients, resolving as the brain adapts to the loss of the amputated part. For some clients, however, the abnormal sensations persist over the long term. Fatigue, excitement, sickness, weather changes, emotional stress, or other stimuli may exacerbate the condition.

■ HEADACHE

Headache results in the most common type of pain. Many causes exist, involving both intracranial and extracranial structures. The brain itself is almost insensitive to pain, although the venous sinuses, tentorium, dura, some of the cranial nerves, and associated vasculature are pain-sensitive. Headache is discussed in Chapter 69.

■ MALIGNANCY

Pain occurs in 40% to 70% of people with solid tumors.[5, 41, 106] The Oncology Nursing Society issued a three-part position paper on cancer pain addressing the scope of nursing practice regarding cancer pain, ethical issues, practice issues, education of staff and clients, research recommendations, and sections on nursing administration, social policy, and pediatric cancer pain.[110, 111, 112] The paper also lists cancer and pain management resources and is an excellent reference for the nurse caring for clients with cancer.

Treatment of cancer pain is difficult because of its many causes. Bone pain usually responds to a combination of radiation therapy and NSAIDs, whereas other pain may require opioid analgesics, such as morphine. The client and the nurse must believe that cancer pain is controllable if correct medications are used in adequate amounts and in adequate combinations. In 1994, the AHCPR developed clinical practice guidelines with 10 goals for the management of cancer pain (Box 23–2).[59]

■ HUMAN IMMUNODEFICIENCY VIRUS INFECTION

Pain is common in clients with active human immunodeficiency virus (HIV) infection. Reports on the prevalence

BOX 23–2 Clinical Practice Guidelines for the Management of Cancer Pain

1. Inform clinicians and clients and their families that most cancer pain can be relieved by available methods.
2. Dispel unfounded fears that addiction results from the appropriate use of medications to control cancer pain.
3. Inform clinicians that cancer pain: (a) accompanies both disease and treatment, (b) changes over time, (c) may have multiple simultaneous causes, (d) if unrelieved, can affect the physical, psychological, social, and spiritual well-being of the client.
4. Promote prompt and effective assessment, diagnosis, and treatment of pain in clients with cancer.
5. Strengthen the ability of clients with cancer and their families to communicate new or unrelieved pain in order to secure prompt evaluation and effective treatment.
6. Provide clinicians with a synthesis of the literature and expert opinion for application to the management of cancer pain.
7. Familiarize clients and their families with options available for pain relief and to promote their active participation in selecting among these.
8. Provide a model for cancer pain management to guide therapy in selected painful, life-threatening conditions such as AIDS.
9. Provide information and guidelines on the use of controlled substances for the treatment of cancer pain that distinguishes the use of these drugs for legitimate medical purposes from their abuse as illegitimate drugs.
10. Identify health policy and research issues that affect cancer pain management.

AIDS, acquired immunodeficiency syndrome.

Modified from Jacox, A., et al. (1994). *Management of cancer pain. Clinical practice guidelines No. 9.* AHCPR Pub. No. 94-1592. Rockville, MD: Agency for Health Care Policy and Research, U.S. Department of Health and Human Services, Public Health Service.

of pain in this population range from 25% to 40% in early and ambulatory stages to 60% to almost 100% in end-stage disease.[59] The sources of pain in this population include (1) gastrointestinal or abdominal pain from colitis, esophagitis, gastritis, herpes, and cytomegalovirus (CMV); (2) peripheral neuropathy; (3) headache; (4) pleuritic pain from pneumonia; (5) oropharyngeal pain from oral candidiasis or herpes; and (6) pain from Kaposi's sarcoma lesions, which causes lymphatic obstruction. Approximately 40% of clients with HIV experience neuropathic pain, which is particularly difficult to manage pharmacologically.

Pain management is made more difficult in this population by the psychosocial correlation of the pain experience. Clients often lack the social support and resources of persons with chronic, malignant pain in other populations.[114] The multidimensional character of the pain in HIV infection and the client's personal situation requires a multidisciplinary team that can establish an open, trusting relationship in order to provide the best pain relief.[68]

Pain associated with HIV infection is usually undertreated, even in late stages.[1, 68, 114] A health care provider's opinion about the client with HIV and acquired immunodeficiency syndrome (AIDS) may be negative, resulting in lack of desire to help manage pain. The health care professional may believe that pain is an appropriate punishment for the behavior that led the person to contract HIV. Clients may be reluctant to report pain, fearing that increasing pain indicates a worsening of disease. Pain management may be complicated by a previous history of drug abuse or addiction. Prior addiction should not alter the way in which pain is treated. Clients may require higher doses of analgesics because they may have a high tolerance to opioids. Third-party payers present an additional barrier because they have considered pain management a low priority.[68]

Pain management for clients with HIV/AIDS is often difficult. It has been recommended that pharmacologic treatment be accomplished using cancer pain as a model incorporating the World Health Organization (WHO) cancer management "ladder."[59, 68] However, caution must be taken with the use of NSAIDs because of reports of cross-reaction between acetaminophen and drugs used to treat HIV infection. In addition, clients with cancer are at risk for gastrointestinal and renal diseases, which contraindicate the use of NSAIDs.[68] Recommended oral analgesics for mild to moderate pain in AIDS include aspirin and ibuprofen, choline magnesium trisalicylate (Trilisate), and weaker opioids (codeine, oxycodone, propoxyphene [Darvon]).[68] Adjuvant medications are also suggested for this population at any step in the WHO ladder.[68] It is imperative that pain of HIV/AIDS be treated vigorously, using the model of cancer pain treatment as the foundation and giving attention to the unique aspects of pain associated with this disease.

FACTORS AFFECTING PAIN

A client's reaction to pain is intensely personal and accounts for the great variability in pain experiences from person to person. Numerous factors contribute to this variability (Fig. 23–7). Some of these are discussed as examples to indicate the means by which one person's pain experience can be expected to differ from that of another person's.

■ SITUATIONAL FACTORS

The situation associated with the pain influences the person's response to it. A response to pain experienced in a formal or crowded situation may differ greatly from the response of a client who is alone or in a hospital. A woman who has had a hysterectomy for cancer may perceive her pain as more severe than that of a woman who has undergone removal of a benign cyst even though the surgical trauma is similar. Pain perception is influenced by the diagnosis in addition to the tissue trauma. A woman with a cancer diagnosis may require more aggressive pain management and additional emotional support than a woman with a benign diagnosis.

■ SOCIOCULTURAL FACTORS

Race, culture, and ethnicity are critical factors in one's response to pain.[10, 26, 36, 45, 61, 63, 89] These factors influence all sensory responses, including responses to pain. We learn how to respond to pain and other experiences from our family and ethnic group. Pain responses tend to reflect the mores of our culture. Within this framework, we

FIGURE 23–7 Considerations of the pain experience.

PHYSIOLOGIC FACTORS

Organic origin
Integrity of nervous system, including endogenous opioids
Concomitant physical influences (stress, fatigue)
Age
Type of pain
Location
Intensity
Duration
Frequency
Quality
Threshold
Tolerance

AFFECTIVE FACTORS

Distress of pain
Depression
Mood
Anxiety, fear, worry

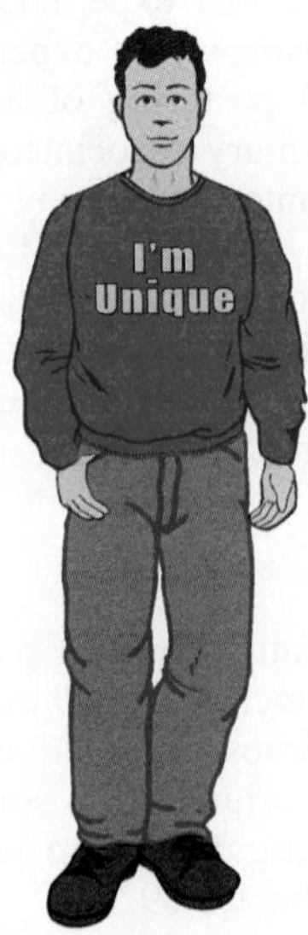

PSYCHOSOCIAL INFLUENCES

Family and occupational roles
Personal beliefs
Spiritual belief system
Cultural/societal influences
Sexual identity and stereotypes
Demographic factors

COGNITIVE

Past experience
Meaning of pain experience
Attention paid to sensation/distraction
Expectations
Coping mechanisms
Knowledge
Values/attitudes
Communication skills

learn what is appropriate and acceptable for our peer group. For example, verbally voicing pain may be considered appropriate within the Italian community and unacceptable within the German community, which values stoicism. In the Mexican culture, moaning or crying is used to help alleviate the pain rather than communicating a need for intervention.[22, 62] Cultural mores of some Hispanic groups view health as the absence of illness. If a person is not convinced that the pain is related to an illness, he or she might refuse treatment for it. The Diversity in Health Care feature discusses cultural aspects of pain response.

DIVERSITY IN HEALTH CARE

Cultural Perspectives on Pain

Anyone who has experienced severe pain understands that people are very vulnerable when they are in pain. Disease ravages the body, but pain ravages the soul. Pain is believed to be the main reason that a person initiates contact with the health care system. Nurses are responsible for evaluating clients' pain and making appropriate interventions. Consequently, nurses must realize that the meanings and expressions of pain are inextricably connected to cultural health beliefs and behaviors.[5]

Culture and Pain: Research Findings

The recognition that meanings and expressions of pain are colored by culture was first identified in the 1950s. It was reported that some patients experiencing pain were stoic and that others were expressive. For example, Americans of Northern European descent were likely to react to pain with stoicism but Italians and Jews tended to display high emotional responses to pain.[10] This research was the first to suggest that pain might be influenced by culture; however, the characterizations resemble stereotypes rather than generalizations.

Further research into how the context of culture shapes pain continues to suggest that an individual's experience of pain cannot be explained in simple physiologic terms—it is a product of culture. For example, the Navajo believe that pain is to be expected—a part of life.[2] Many Filipinos regard pain as part of life and view it as an opportunity to atone for transgressions.[6] Most Hispanics and Latinos are Catholic and consequently turn to religious practices to cope with pain. It is common for Hispanics-Latinos to believe that pain may be due to punishment and that suffering must be endured to enter heaven.[3, 4]

Another example of how culture influences the experience of pain involves African Americans, who may perceive that pain is a sign of illness or disease. This group may not take routinely prescribed medication unless pain is present (e.g., may take antihypertensive medication when they experience head or neck pain). This cultural practice interferes with effective management of hypertension.[8]

The Chinese generally believe the pain is caused from an illness that is due to a bodily imbalance. Consequently, the appropriate intervention becomes one that restores balance to the body.[8]

Mexican Americans have been shown to (1) accept pain as part of life, (2) feel obligated to "put up with" pain in the performance of their duties, (3) feel obligated to suffer stoically, and (4) feel that the type and amount of pain experienced are divinely predetermined. Their methods to alleviate pain are directed toward restoring and maintaining balance with the individual and the environment.[9]

Recognizing That Pain Is Influenced by Culture

Unfortunately, some nurses still question the importance of understanding the client's culture. Americans have been socialized to believe that the United States has the best health care system in the world. This ethnocentric attitude interferes with nurses' recognition and appreciation of culture. This is particularly troublesome because nursing supports the concept that holistic care is central to the practice of nursing. To not recognize the importance of culture is to truly miss the point of holistic care. Pain must be assessed within the context of culture.

Equally troublesome is the fact that within the subculture of nursing, it is expected that clients will be objective about the intensely subjective experience of pain. When clients are experiencing pain, they are expected to describe it in detail, but *not* to display emotional responses (i.e., to suffer in silence).[1] It has been suggested that silent suffering is probably the most valued response to pain in the United States.[7] If so, nurses are faced with the major challenge of *not* allowing their own ideas about pain to interfere with the care they give to clients in pain.

Finally, pain management is a major problem within health care. Although our communities are rich in cultural diversity, little emphasis has been devoted to pain management among culturally diverse populations. Nurses caring for clients with pain need to understand how culture influences pain. Health care providers need to be aware that their own values and perceptions may affect how they evaluate their clients' responses to pain and how they treat pain. It is important to validate the level of pain, pain intensity, and pain relief by involving the client and family. Understanding the health beliefs of different cultures regarding pain is crucial to providing culturally sensitive care.[3]

References

1. Andrews, M., & Boyle, J. (1999). *Transcultural concepts in nursing care.* Philadelphia: Lippincott.
2. Bell, R. (1994). Prominence of women in Navajo healing beliefs and values. *Nursing and Health Care, 15*(5), 232–240.
3. Juarez, G. (1997). Culture and pain. *Quality of life: A nursing challenge. 4*(4), 86–90.
4. Kumasaka, L., & Miles, A. (1996). 'My pain is God's will.' *American Journal of Nursing 96*(6), 45–47.
5. Leininger, M. (1997). Understanding cultural pain for improved health care. *Journal of Transcultural Nursing, 9*(1), 32–35.
6. Matson, S., & Lew, L. (1991). Culturally sensitive prenatal care for Southeastern Asians. *Journal of Obstetric, Gynecological, and Neonatal Nurses, 12*(1), 48–54.
7. McCaffery, P. (1979). *Nursing management of the patient with pain* (2nd ed.). Philadelphia: J. B. Lippincott.
8. Purnell, L., & Paulanka, B. (1998). *Transcultural health care: A culturally competent approach.* Philadelphia: F. A. Davis.
9. Villarruel, A., & Montellano, B. (1992). Culture and pain: A Mesoamerican experience. *Advances in Nursing Science, 15*(1), 32–38.
10. Zborowski, M. (1952). Cultural components in response to pain. *Journal of Social Issues, 8,* 16–30.

Joyce Larson-Presswalla, PhD, RN, *President, "Culture Counts," Marketing Coordinator, James A. Haley Veterans Hospital, Tampa, Florida*

Problems may also arise because of a person's view of health care team members. Members of various cultural groups may have difficulty communicating feelings to physicians and nurses who are from different backgrounds or ethnic groups.[10, 26] Health care providers may have difficulty appreciating the pain experiences of clients from unfamiliar cultural groups, because they tend to adopt white, middle-class cultural mores surrounding pain expectations and avenues for treatment.

Remember, people from different cultures may handle pain in various ways. A problem arises when the nurse does not recognize the person's way of dealing with pain or when the nurse does not accept it. Researchers found that nurses' judgments about pain their clients experienced was affected by the nurses' own beliefs and those of their culture.[22, 26] Nurses may also misinterpret expressions of pain from clients who do not speak English as a first language.[70] Health care providers must be sensitive to the contribution of cultural factors and language barriers in order to facilitate adequate pain management.

■ AGE

Age may play a significant role in perception and expression of pain. There are some variations in threshold associated with chronologic age, but no clear trends have been established.[43, 105] For example, infants perceive pain and respond to it with increasing sensitivity. Toddlers may respond to pain with crying and anger because they perceive it as a threat to security or sense that pain is a punishment. School-aged children may try to be "brave" and not cry or express much pain so that parents or nurses will not be angry with them. Adolescents may not want to report pain in front of peers, because they may perceive complaints of pain as weakness. Adults may not report pain for fear that it indicates a poor diagnosis. Pain may also mean weakness or failure for the adult.

There is controversy about pain in the elderly population. There is no reason to assume that pain perception is altered in older adults unless some damage has occurred in the CNS. The transmission and perception may be slowed with aging, but intensity of the pain is not diminished. Health care providers may underestimate the pain of older people as a result of impaired ability to express pain. Physical factors, such as paralysis and aphasia, may interfere with the ability to communicate.[115] Confused elderly clients may be unable to articulate their pain experience. Remember, altered expression does not mean absence of pain.

Age is considered an important factor in dosing of medications. Metabolic changes in the elderly affect their response to opioid analgesics. Drugs are metabolized and excreted more slowly in older people. In addition, elders frequently take combinations of medications for a variety of ailments, making them more susceptible to drug interactions.

Older people may assign different meanings to their pain. Pain may be considered a natural manifestation of aging. This may be interpreted in two ways. First, older people may think pain is simply something to be endured as a normal part of the aging process. Second, it may be seen as a sign of aging and, therefore, something to be denied because it means they are getting old. Many older people are hesitant to express pain for fear of being labeled as a "complaining" elder. These misconceptions serve to cause these people to experience pain unnecessarily. Careful assessment of the older person's pain is essential to prevent unnecessary suffering.

Few assessment instruments have been tested in the geriatric population, and visual, auditory, and motor impairments, common among elders, make typical assessment tools difficult to use.[1] Therefore, pay particular attention to verbal and nonverbal clues of pain in this population. Pain may be indicated by lack of appetite, sleeping disorders, tearing of the eyes, moaning, or splinting of a body part.

■ GENDER

Gender is an important factor in response to pain.[12, 14, 37, 123] In one study gender was a significant factor in the pain response, with men reporting less pain than women regardless of ethnicity. In some cultures in the United States, boys and men are expected to express pain less than women do. This does not mean that men feel pain less, only that they are assumed to show it less. Yet, health care providers who value bearing pain without complaint may view women as "complainers" and may ignore or devalue their pain expressions. Both men and women may experience pain unnecessarily if the nurse is not aware of gender biases in pain expression.

■ MEANING OF PAIN

The meaning of a person's pain influences his or her response to the pain.[19, 70, 128, 130] Pain caused by childbirth may be responded to differently than pain caused by surgery. If the cause of pain is known, the person may be better able to interpret meaning and to deal with the experience. If the cause is unknown, more negative psychological factors (e.g., fear, and anxiety) may be evoked, intensifying the degree of pain perceived. Pain may be perceived more intensely if the meaning of the experience is negative than pain perceived in situations with positive outcomes. For example, pain that is associated with a threat to body image may be much worse than pain that is not associated in this way. If the meaning of pain is not considered, you may make inappropriate assessments of the client's pain experience, resulting in inadequate pain control.

■ ANXIETY

The degree of anxiety experienced by the client may also influence the response to pain. Anxiety intensifies pain perception.[60] Anxiety is often related to the meaning of the pain. If the cause is unknown, anxiety is likely to be higher and the pain worse.

■ PAST EXPERIENCE WITH PAIN

Our past experience with pain affects the way we perceive our current pain. People who have had negative experiences with pain as children have reported greater difficulties with managing pain.[6, 96] The impact of past experiences, however, is not predictable. The person with a miserable experience in the past may perceive the next episode more intensely even though the medical conditions may be similar. Conversely, a person may view the next experience more positively because it is not as bad as the previous one. However, it is *not* true that the more pain we experience, the more accustomed we become to it. One might expect that the more pain we have experienced, the less anxious and more tolerant we may be. In actuality, we may be more anxious and desire rapid pain relief to avert a familiar and unpleasant painful experience.

Earlier pain experience allows us to adopt coping mechanisms that we may or may not use with subsequent episodes with pain. Discuss your clients' past experiences with pain, including how they managed the pain. In addition to methods that provided pain relief in the past, assess which measures did not have a positive outcome. Allow the client to use familiar positive intervention when possible.

EXPECTATION AND THE PLACEBO EFFECT

Client expectations play a major role in a person's pain experience, including perception of pain and the effectiveness of pain relief interventions.[2, 27, 119, 127] The severity of pain experienced, in addition to the emotional and cognitive overtones generated by the experience, is influenced by the client's expectations. Positive expectations engender positive outcomes; negative expectations lead to negative outcomes. Similarly, one's belief in the ability of an intervention to be effective affects the degree of pain relief attained. For example, it is not uncommon for a client to proclaim that the pain reliever Motrin is effective while Advil is not, even though the two medications are pharmaceutically identical.

You must realize that you can affect your clients' expectations by the messages you deliver regarding pain and pain management strategies. The confidence that you display regarding potential effectiveness of intervention strategies will have a significant effect on the client's ability to obtain positive pain relief outcomes.

Placebos have been administered when health care providers doubted that clients were truly in pain. Placebos are pills that look like medications but that have no medicinal properties. Historically, they have been made of sugars and inert materials. When clients are given placebos, they are told that the pills contain pain medication. It was not uncommon for these clients to obtain pain relief. It has been reported that 30% to 70% of people receiving placebos report short-lived pain relief which, in some research studies, has been reversed by naloxone (Narcan).[2, 127] The most likely explanation for the effect of placebos is the initiation of the body's endogenous opiate systems activated by the expectation of relief.[2] The response tends to be temporary, since the endogenous response is brief. A placebo response does not indicate absence of real pain; it indicates a person's ability to produce a positive pain relief outcome internally via a real physiologic mechanism.

Health care providers have incorrectly concluded that positive responses to placebos indicate that clients did not have real pain. However, a placebo response indicates that the client believes that the pill will "work" and has responded to the positive attitude portrayed by the nurse administering the pill. *Placebos should not be given.*[5, 59, 75, 134] The client's response to placebos provides no data about the nature or severity of pain. Placebo use is deceitful and unethical. It compromises the nurse-client relationship and the confidence the client has in the nurse's ability and desire to help with pain relief. Use of placebos is costly because the client is charged for an ineffective medication, which often needs to be followed with a true pain relief preparation. Clients receiving placebos may be reluctant to report continued pain or to ask for additional pain medication, leaving them at risk for the negative physical effects of unrelieved pain.

Nursing Management of the Client in Pain

ASSESSMENT

The primary goals of pain assessment are to identify the cause of the pain, to understand the client's perception of the pain, and to measure the characteristics of the pain to implement pain management techniques. To assess a client's pain, obtain a pain history, a daily account of the current pain history, and a collection of subjective and objective data through use of measurement tools. Perform the assessment in an unbiased, caring manner. Assessment is a constant and ongoing task, which may occur every 15 minutes for the acute, postoperative client to every four hours for the acute, stable client with adequate pain relief. The AHCPR Clinical Guidelines for acute pain management recommend that pain be assessed every 2 hours for the first 48 hours after surgery or trauma and every 4 hours thereafter as a standard routine and more often if indicated. In addition, assessment should occur within 20 to 30 minutes after administration of any medication given for pain relief.[1]

HISTORY AND PHYSICAL EXAMINATION. A complete medical history and physical examination (H&P) focuses on basic questions about physical, behavioral, and psychological factors (Box 23-3). This H&P helps the nurse to understand the unique pain experience of the client and to formulate a plan to resolve the pain. The H&P also provides baseline data to allow assessment of the client's progression through a pain experience.

Data Collection. Data collection by use of well-tested measurement tools is essential in assessing pain for appropriate management interventions.[77, 108] Multidimensional assessment tools (e.g., McGill-Melzack Pain Questionnaire, Initial Pain Assessment Tool by McCaffery and Beebe[1]) are useful to obtain the initial H&P data and to provide information regarding the multifaceted nature of the pain experience (Figs. 23–8 and 23–9).

Single-item assessment tools include the Visual Analog Scale (VAS), numerical scales, and visual descriptor scales. These scales can be used to measure both physical pain intensity and psychological distress (Figs. 23–10 and 23–11). The tools are easy to use and provide the client and nurse with a simple means to quantify pain. They are also cost-effective when used in clinical settings because they are easily copied and can be reproduced cheaply. They do require a relatively high level of cognitive ability.

Pictorial scales measure pain in small children, such as the widely used FACES scale developed by Wong and Baker[132] (Fig. 23–12). Clients with impaired cognitive ability may be better able to report their pain with the use of pictorial scales.

Clients may experience several types of pain during one medical episode. After surgery, one may experience pain due to poor body position, incisional pain, and deep

BOX 23–3 Subjective and Objective Assessment Data

History

Age
State of consciousness
Medications currently taken/ medication for allergies
Physical state (fatigue, debility, lack of sleep, and prolonged suffering all reduce a client's ability to tolerate pain)
Emotional state (worry, fear, and anxiety reduce a person's ability to tolerate pain)
Pain expectancy (the anticipation of pain)
Pain acceptance (willingness to experience pain)
Pain apprehension (generalized desire to avoid pain)
Pain anxiety (the anxiety pain provokes because of its associated mystery, loneliness, helplessness, threat)
Effects on activities and quality of life
Methods of Pain Relief

What do you do to relieve the pain?
What has *not* worked to relieve your pain?

Physical Examination

Sympathetic Responses

Pallor
Increased blood pressure
Increased pulse
Increased respiration
Skeletal muscle tension
Dilated pupils
Diaphoresis

Parasympathetic Responses

Decreased blood pressure
Decreased pulse
Nausea, vomiting
Weakness
Pallor
Loss of consciousness

Behavioral Characteristics

Assumes a posture that minimizes pain (lying rigidly, guarding, drawing up the legs, or assuming the fetal position)
Moans, sighs, grimaces, clenches the jaws or fist, becomes quiet, or withdraws from others
Blinks rapidly
Crying, appears frightened, exhibits restlessness
Has a drawn facial expression
Has twitching muscles
Withdraws when touched
Holds or protects affected area or remains motionless

visceral pain. The client may also have a condition that produces chronic pain such as arthritis, that continues to be painful, or a secondary complication may be developing, such as pain due to myocardial infarction or pulmonary emboli. When planning interventions, learn to distinguish among the causes of pain. Each pain assessment includes location, intensity, quality, and pattern to aid in making intervention decisions.

Intensity. The single most important indicator of pain intensity is the client's self-report of the pain. Many health care facilities have incorporated *pain rating scales* for use with standard practice. These scales are used to assess current levels of pain but can be used to determine the amount of pain the client finds acceptable. This information is essential for both the client and nurse in planning and evaluating pain interventions. The AHCPR recommends the Brief Pain Inventory (Short Form) (Fig. 23–13) as a means of conducting ongoing assessments of pain intensity.[59]

You can obtain the client's self-report of pain intensity by asking clients to rate pain on a scale that they must mentally visualize or by showing the scale to the client. People in pain may have trouble concentrating on mental tasks and may find it particularly difficult to respond to a scale they must visualize. In some hospitals, it has been beneficial to provide a copy of the intensity scale in plain view of each client, typically taped to the bedside wall.

Location. Location of pain may be ascertained by verbal description or by marking the location on a drawing of the body. Use of body drawings provides an opportunity for the client to report multiple sites of pain using a self-report document that can be included in the medical record. The document is then available for use by any member of the health care team caring for that client.

Quality. Quality of the pain is typically indicated by descriptive adjectives such as "stabbing like a knife" or "throbbing" (Box 23–4). Some clients may have difficulty describing the quality of painful sensations, or they may have problems using the term "pain" to indicate their discomfort. Showing clients a list of words to describe pain may facilitate their ability to report pain quality.

Pattern. Pattern refers to the time of onset, duration, and intervals of the pain. Terms used to classify the pattern include "constant, steady, intermittent, periodic, brief, or momentary."

Distress. The psychological reactions to pain contribute to the overall pain experience. The emotional component may serve to intensify or diminish pain perception. Pain management strategies may need to be directed toward modifying the distress aspect of a pain episode.

DIAGNOSIS, OUTCOMES, INTERVENTIONS

The primary nursing diagnosis is *Pain related to tissue injury from an incision, ischemia, tumor encroachment in organs or bone.* Nurses have an impact on pain, discomfort, or suffering, no matter what the cause. In some situations, the client may be experiencing unrelieved pain. Unrelieved pain may be related to:

- Underadministration of ordered medication doses
- Administering medications in inappropriate time frames
- Not providing stronger medications when indicated
- Not providing combinations of medications when indicated
- Inadequate use of nonpharmaceutical management strategies

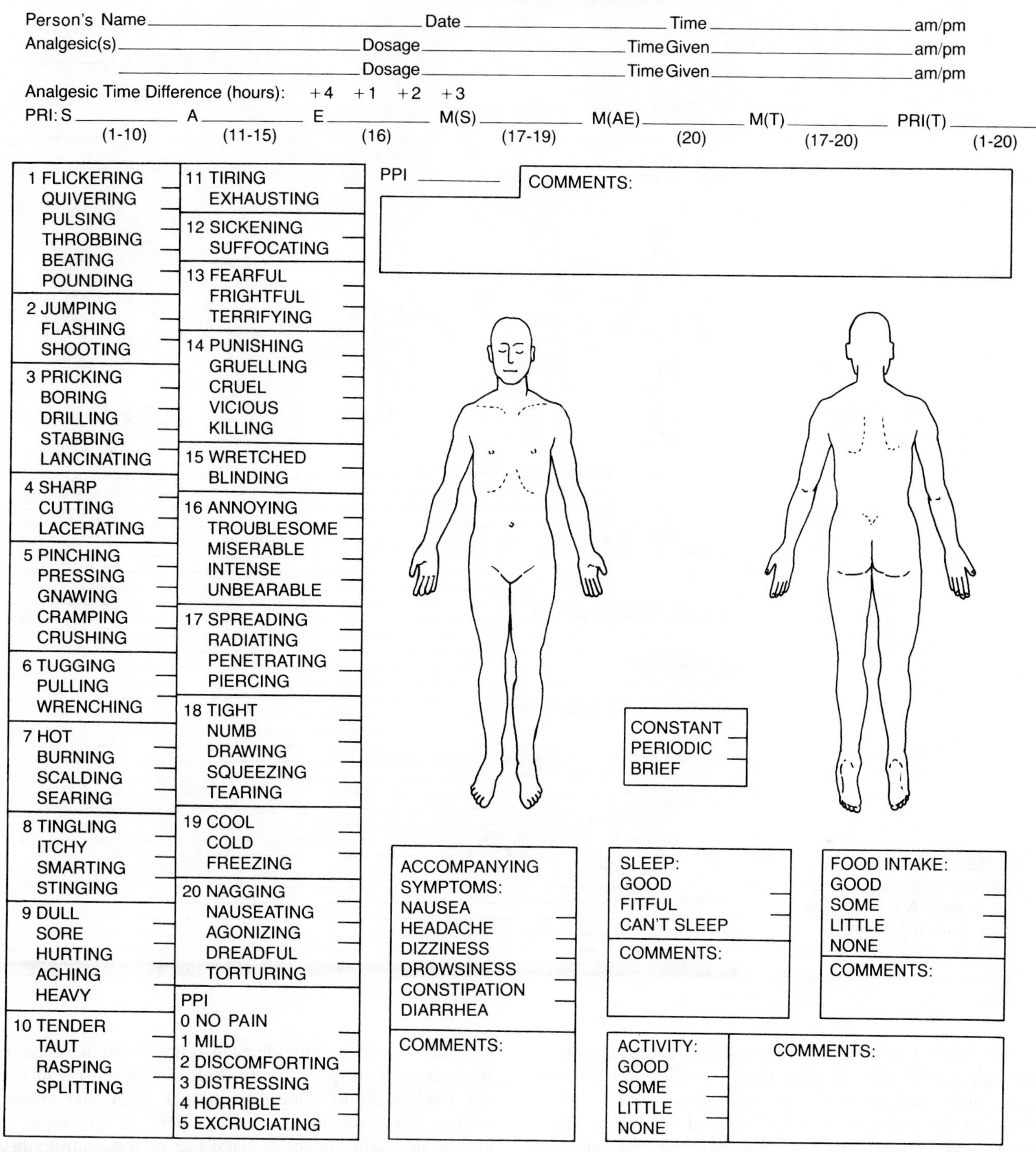

McGill - Melzack Pain Questionnaire

Person's Name ________ Date ________ Time ________ am/pm
Analgesic(s) ________ Dosage ________ Time Given ________ am/pm
________ Dosage ________ Time Given ________ am/pm
Analgesic Time Difference (hours): +4 +1 +2 +3
PRI: S ________ (1-10) A ________ (11-15) E ________ (16) M(S) ________ (17-19) M(AE) ________ (20) M(T) ________ (17-20) PRI(T) ________ (1-20)

1 FLICKERING, QUIVERING, PULSING, THROBBING, BEATING, POUNDING
2 JUMPING, FLASHING, SHOOTING
3 PRICKING, BORING, DRILLING, STABBING, LANCINATING
4 SHARP, CUTTING, LACERATING
5 PINCHING, PRESSING, GNAWING, CRAMPING, CRUSHING
6 TUGGING, PULLING, WRENCHING
7 HOT, BURNING, SCALDING, SEARING
8 TINGLING, ITCHY, SMARTING, STINGING
9 DULL, SORE, HURTING, ACHING, HEAVY
10 TENDER, TAUT, RASPING, SPLITTING
11 TIRING, EXHAUSTING
12 SICKENING, SUFFOCATING
13 FEARFUL, FRIGHTFUL, TERRIFYING
14 PUNISHING, GRUELLING, CRUEL, VICIOUS, KILLING
15 WRETCHED, BLINDING
16 ANNOYING, TROUBLESOME, MISERABLE, INTENSE, UNBEARABLE
17 SPREADING, RADIATING, PENETRATING, PIERCING
18 TIGHT, NUMB, DRAWING, SQUEEZING, TEARING
19 COOL, COLD, FREEZING
20 NAGGING, NAUSEATING, AGONIZING, DREADFUL, TORTURING

PPI
0 NO PAIN
1 MILD
2 DISCOMFORTING
3 DISTRESSING
4 HORRIBLE
5 EXCRUCIATING

PPI ________ COMMENTS:

CONSTANT, PERIODIC, BRIEF

ACCOMPANYING SYMPTOMS: NAUSEA, HEADACHE, DIZZINESS, DROWSINESS, CONSTIPATION, DIARRHEA
COMMENTS:

SLEEP: GOOD, FITFUL, CAN'T SLEEP
COMMENTS:

FOOD INTAKE: GOOD, SOME, LITTLE, NONE
COMMENTS:

ACTIVITY: GOOD, SOME, LITTLE, NONE
COMMENTS:

FIGURE 23–8 The McGill-Melzack Pain Questionnaire, adapted for the study of narcotic drugs. The descriptors listed at left comprise four groups: 1 to 10, sensory; 11 to 15, affective; 16, evaluative; 17 to 20, miscellaneous. The rank value for each descriptor is based on its position in the words set. Total rank values comprise the pain-rating index (PRI). The present pain intensity (PPI) is based on a scale from 0 to 5. The drawings are used to designate the site of pain (From Bonica, J. J. [1980]. *Pain* [p. 145]. New York: Raven Press.)

Pain may contribute to additional diagnoses as clients respond to the pain episode. Examples of such diagnoses are presented in Table 23–4.

Outcomes. Outcomes should be determined as a team with the client, physicians, nurses, and often the extended family. A realistic outcome should be established to control or maintain the client at desired levels of pain and functioning. Desirable outcomes are that the client will (1) report freedom from pain, (2) request analgesia, and (3) perform daily activities without limitation related to pain. The goals should be those of the client, not those of the health care team.

Initial Pain Assessment Tool

Date ______

Patient's Name ______ Age ______ Room ______

Diagnosis ______ Physician ______

Nurse ______

I. Location: Patient or nurse mark drawing.

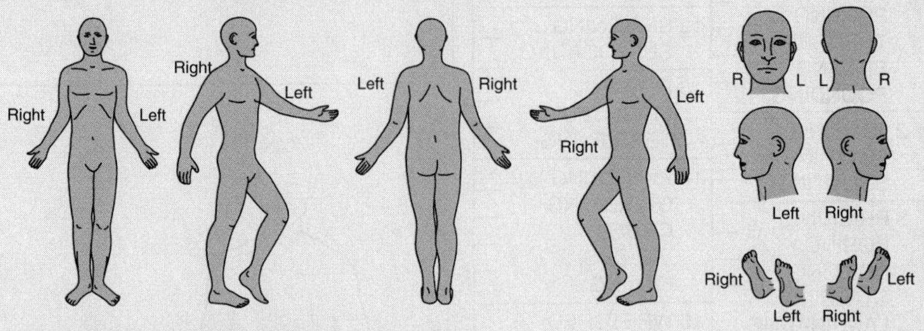

II. Intensity: Patient rates the pain. Scale used ______

Present: ______

Worst pain gets: ______

Best pain gets: ______

Acceptable level of pain: ______

III. Quality: (Use patient's own words, e.g., prick, ache, burn, throb, pull, sharp) ______

IV. Onset, duration variations, rhythms: ______

V. Manner of expressing pain: ______

VI. What relieves the pain? ______

VII. What causes or increases the pain? ______

VIII. Effects of pain: (Note decreased function, decreased quality of life.) ______

Accompanying symptoms (e.g., nausea) ______

Sleep ______

Appetite ______

Physical activity ______

Relationship with others (e.g., irritability) ______

Emotions (e.g., anger, suicidal, crying) ______

Concentration ______

Other ______

IX. Other comments: ______

X. Plan: ______

FIGURE 23–9 Initial pain assessment tool. (From McCaffery M., & Beebe., A [1989]. *Pain: Clinical manual for nursing practice.* St. Louis: Mosby–Year Book.)

A widely used method of providing effective care is through use of clinical care plans or clinical pathways. Care plans and pathways provide nurses with aids to diagnose the problem, plan for expected outcomes, implement interventions, state the rationale for the interventions, and evaluate the outcome. Many health care facilities provide standard care plans or clinical pathways that are part of the department protocol. Standard plans provide the beginning basis for client care. They are then modified as indicated based on the needs of each client.

Interventions. Effective pain control is best achieved through the combination of both pharmaceutical and nonpharmaceutical therapies. Historically, pharmaceutical management has been the primary means of providing relief from pain, particularly acute pain. Although medications continue to serve as a major contributor to pain management, nonpharmaceutical techniques are being increasingly used to provide pain relief. Nonpharmacologic interventions are particularly useful (1) when medications are inadequate to control pain, (2) while the client is waiting for medications to take effect, or (3) when side effects or client concerns make use of medications problematic.

ADMINISTRATION OF PAIN-RELIEVING MEDICATION. Numerous medications are used for pain relief. They are administered in a variety of ways; by mouth, rectally, topically, sublingually, by inhalation, or by injection. Medications may be injected by subcutaneous, intramuscular, or intravenous routes. Some medications may be injected spinally or paravertebrally or into selected nerves to produce nerve blocks. Physicians perform the latter types of injections, with nurses assisting with the procedures and providing aftercare. Too often nurses view the administration of pain-relieving medications as all

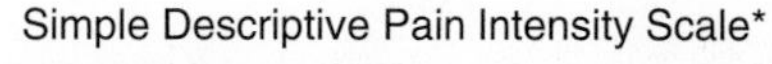

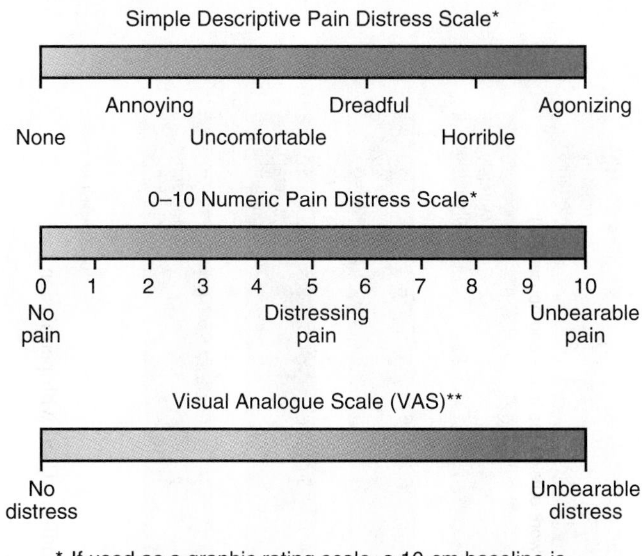

* If used as a graphic rating scale, a 10-cm baseline is recommended.

** A 10-cm baseline is recommended for VAS scales.

FIGURE 23–10 Pain distress scales.

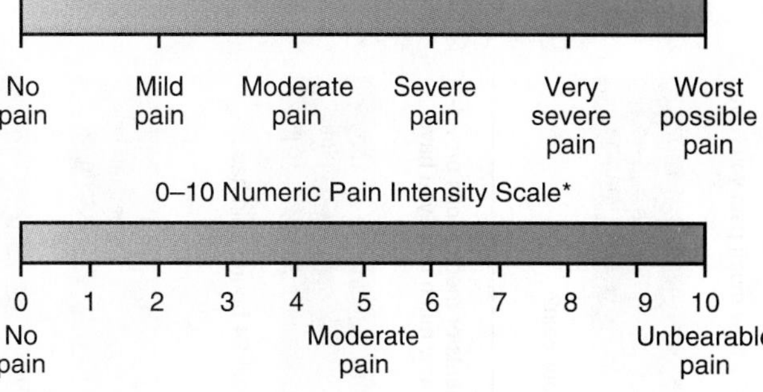

Visual Analogue Scale (VAS)**

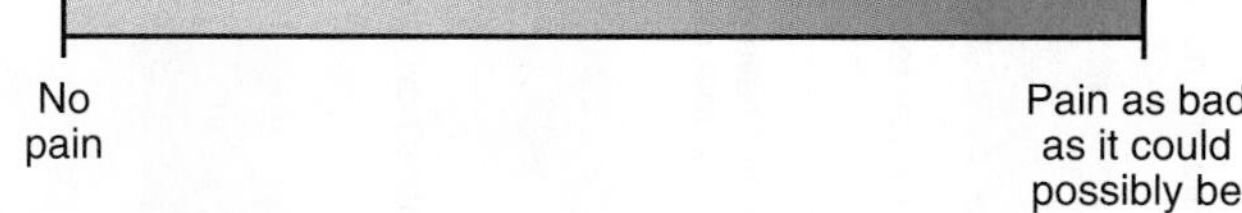

* If used as a graphic rating scale, a 10-cm baseline is recommended.

** A 10-cm baseline is recommended for VAS scales.

FIGURE 23–11 Pain intensity scales.

they need to do for pain management. However, medication may be more effective when combined with other pain relief techniques. When you administer medication and reposition the client, give a back rub, or simply interact with a client, the effectiveness of the drug may be increased. Simply giving an injection or a pill does not replace thoughtful, comprehensive pain management.

Therapeutic interaction with someone experiencing pain may include:

- Facilitating the client's expression of feelings, which imparts a sense of being cared for
- Providing support, reassurance, and understanding, which allows the client to develop confidence in the nurse
- Teaching the client self-management strategies to relieve pain

Pain management strategies, including medications, have been found to be more effective when clients believe that

PAIN INTENSITY MEASURES

Faces:

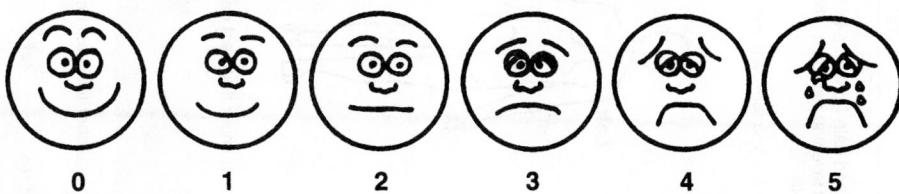

When using the Faces, explain to the person that each face is for a person who feels happy because he has no pain (hurt for young children) or sad because he has some or a lot of pain. Face 0 is very happy because he doesn't hurt at all. Face 1 hurts just a little bit. Face 2 hurts a little more. Face 3 hurts even more. Face 4 hurts a whole lot. Face 5 hurts as much as you can imagine, although you don't have to be crying to feel this bad.

Word:

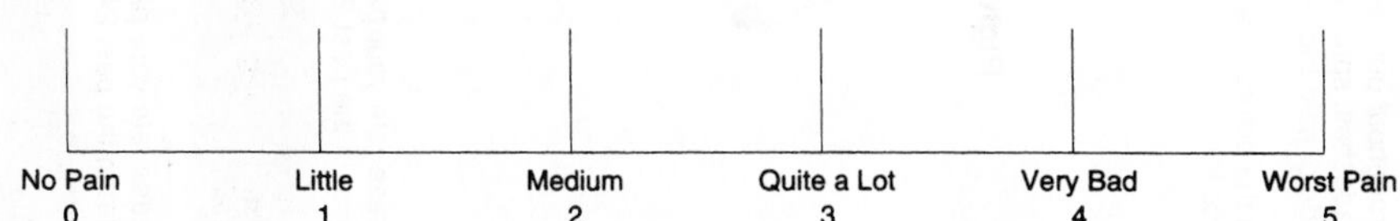

FIGURE 23–12 Faces Pain Rating Scale. Explain to the person that each face is for a person who feels happy because he has no pain (hurt) or sad because he has some or a lot of pain. Face 0 is very happy because he doesn't hurt at all. Face 1 hurts just a little bit. Face 2 hurts a little more. Face 3 hurts even more. Face 4 hurts a whole lot. Face 5 hurts as much as you can imagine, although you don't have to be crying to feel this bad. Ask the person to choose the face that best describes how he is feeling. This rating scale is recommended for persons age 3 years and older. (From Wong, D., & Baker, C. [1988]. Pain in children: Comparison of assessment scales. *Pediatric Nursing, 14*[1]: 9–17, 1988.)

Pain Inventory

Date: ____/____/____ Time: ________

Name: __________ Last __________ First ______ Middle Initial

1) Throughout our lives, most of us have had pain from time to time (such as minor headaches, sprains, and toothaches). Have you had pain other than these everyday kinds of pain today? 1. Yes 2. No

2) On the diagram, shade in the areas where you feel pain. Put an X on the area that hurts the most.

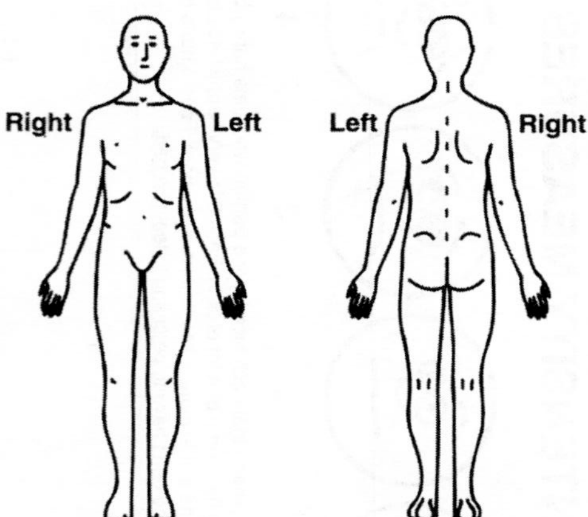

3) Please rate your pain by circling the one number that best describes your pain at its **worst** in the past 24 hours.

0 No pain	1	2	3	4	5	6	7	8	9	10 Pain as bad as you can imagine

4) Please rate your pain by circling the one number that best describes your pain at its **least** in the past 24 hours.

0 No pain	1	2	3	4	5	6	7	8	9	10 Pain as bad as you can imagine

5) Please rate your pain by circling the one number that best describes your pain on the **average**.

0 No pain	1	2	3	4	5	6	7	8	9	10 Pain as bad as you can imagine

6) Please rate your pain by circling the one number that tells how much pain you have **right now**.

0 No pain	1	2	3	4	5	6	7	8	9	10 Pain as bad as you can imagine

7) What treatments or medications are you receiving for your pain?

____

8) In the past 24 hours, how much **relief** have pain treatments or medications provided? Please circle the one percentage that most shows how much relief you have received.

0% No relief	10%	20%	30%	40%	50%	60%	70%	80%	90%	100% Complete relief

9) Circle the one number that describes how, during the past 24 hours, pain has **interfered** with your:

A. General activity

0 Does not interfere	1	2	3	4	5	6	7	8	9	10 Completely interferes

B. Mood

0 Does not interfere	1	2	3	4	5	6	7	8	9	10 Completely interferes

C. Walking ability

0 Does not interfere	1	2	3	4	5	6	7	8	9	10 Completely interferes

D. Normal work (includes both work outside the home and housework)

0 Does not interfere	1	2	3	4	5	6	7	8	9	10 Completely interferes

E. Relations with other people

0 Does not interfere	1	2	3	4	5	6	7	8	9	10 Completely interferes

F. Sleep

0 Does not interfere	1	2	3	4	5	6	7	8	9	10 Completely interferes

G. Enjoyment of life

0 Does not interfere	1	2	3	4	5	6	7	8	9	10 Completely interferes

UC9503409EN NP-2395EN

FIGURE 23–13 Pain Inventory, Short Form. (From Pain Research Group, Department of Neurology, University of Wisconsin-Madison. Used with permission.)

BOX 23–4 Descriptive Terms for Pain

Descriptive Word	How Pain Makes Person Feel
▪ Sharp	▪ Horrible
▪ Piercing	▪ Annoying
▪ Shooting	▪ Agonizing
▪ Crushing	▪ Killing
▪ Tender	▪ Miserable
▪ Hurting	▪ Unbearable
▪ Aching	▪ Frightening
▪ Dull	▪ Suffocating
▪ Sore	▪ Tortured
▪ Cramping	
▪ Prickly	

they are in control of the situation. A nurse who actively involves the client in the planning, intervention, and assessment of pain management strategies provides the client with enhanced potential to obtain satisfactory pain relief.

MANAGING CHRONIC INTRACTABLE PAIN. Chronic intractable pain (pain that cannot be satisfactorily relieved by typical pharmaceutical means) causes additional difficulties for those experiencing it. Clients may require a combination of nursing interventions (cognitive, behavioral, physical, pharmaceutical). Nursing and medical therapeutic regimens must be coordinated and consistent to ensure a unified approach. The client must not be promised complete pain relief, however, because this may be unrealistic.

MANAGING PROGRESSIVE PAIN. People with progressive pain, such as that seen in malignancies, may require pain-relieving medications routinely as a preventive measure, in the same way that vasodilators are regularly taken by people with ischemic heart disease. As the disease progresses, clients may require increasingly stronger drug doses. Some people hesitate to take pain-relieving medications routinely for fear of addiction. They may believe that they must avoid increasing dosages because they are afraid that they will "use up" the medication's pain relief potential and will not be able to obtained adequate medication in the future. They may also be concerned that they will be labeled as drug users if they take opioids over the long term.

In reality, people experiencing pain due to widespread cancer require routine pain-relieving medications in order to function. Help is needed for clients and their significant others to understand the need for regular, often strong medications. Reassurance that adequate pain relief will be possible in the future and that routine use of the medications means only that the condition warrants it, much like a client who requires the routine use of medication for hypertension.

Many conditions associated with pain are managed at home. The treatment of acute postoperative, chronic and malignant pain is often performed by clients and family members. The Bridge to Home Health Care discusses the nurse's role in home care for pain control.

TABLE 23–4 PAIN-RELATED NURSING DIAGNOSES

Diagnosis	Etiology
Activity Intolerance	related to Unrelieved pain
Ineffective Coping Strategies	related to Lack of knowledge of possible methods of coping
Powerlessness	related to Lack of participation in decision-making process
Anxiety	related to Past experiences of poor pain control
Sleep Pattern Disturbance	related to Unrelieved pain at night
Knowledge Deficit	related to Lack of exposure to informational resources
Fear	related to Anticipation of a pain experience

MEDICATIONS TO CONTROL PAIN

■ ANESTHETIC AGENTS

An *anesthetic* is a pharmacologic substance that, in addition to abolishing pain, generally causes loss of feeling and sensation. Many *analgesics* (pharmacologic substances that diminish or eliminate pain without producing unconsciousness), depending on their mode of action and route of administration, act as anesthetics when given in larger doses. There are many different types of anesthesia. *General anesthesia* is usually accompanied by loss of consciousness and reflexes along with amnesia regarding the experience. *Local anesthetics* produce anesthesia in a restricted area of the body without loss of consciousness.

A technique frequently used in minor surgery and other procedures is infiltration of a local anesthetic into the skin and subcutaneous tissue to produce loss of sensation, or local anesthesia. The same agent injected near a sensory nerve causes anesthesia in the distribution of the nerve (*regional anesthesia*). Nerves are often mixed in function; that is, they carry both sensory and motor fibers. Hence, a *nerve block* may cause motor weakness or paralysis, in addition to loss of sensation, in the innervated area. A nerve block is the application of a pharmacologic substance that inhibits nerve conduction (e.g., numbing the mouth for dental procedures).

Local anesthetic agents may be applied topically (on the skin or mucous membranes), infiltrated locally, used for specific nerve blocks (e.g., spinal anesthetic for surgery), or administered intravenously, depending on the reason for their use. Local anesthetic agents act by temporarily blocking nerve impulses between the peripheral structures and higher centers. Such blocks are reversible because the nerves regain their function over a period of minutes to hours.

Neurolytic agents (e.g., phenol, alcohol) produce prolonged nerve blocks, which destroy the nerves. Neurolytic blocks may not be truly permanent because nerve fibers regrow after several months. However, the growth is often disorganized. Hence, the sensation from these nerve fibers is often abnormal or painful. Consequently, neurolytic blocks are generally used only in terminally ill per-

BRIDGE TO HOME HEALTH CARE

Controlling Pain

To control the client's pain at home, you should be aware of many contributing factors. It is necessary to evaluate physical, social, emotional, and spiritual pain because each of these adds to the total pain experience. An effective plan of care should include a multidisciplinary approach to pain.

Pain control should be very individualized, and attention to age-specific needs must be considered in both assessment and treatment. A pain scale that includes pictures is effective for use with children. In addition, analgesic choices should be tailored to the age of the client, recognizing the special needs of the very young and the elderly.

Many times in the treatment of malignant pain (as with cancer), medication is given on a regular schedule to prevent exacerbations. This is in contrast to medications being taken at the time of pain or the prn (as needed) schedule used in acute care settings. This prophylactic scheduling is very effective but requires client education to ensure compliance. Scheduling may well be the single most important instruction in the use of analgesics for malignant pain. The use of adjuvant therapy, such as for pain control, should also be considered because this often increases the effectiveness of the analgesic. It is also important to consider various methods of analgesia, such as continuous, client-controlled analgesia pumps, time-released skin patches, sustained-released oral medications, and suppositories.

Fear of addiction is a major barrier for effective pain control. It is essential for the multidisciplinary team to explain that medication taken as directed will not cause addiction. For the pain of clients who are terminally ill, aggressive titration of medication is used until pain is relieved. The goal is pain control with minimal adverse reactions. When adverse reactions do occur, symptoms should be treated and the analgesic continued. Pain control is essential to quality of life and should be actively pursued. Clients should be assured that pain can and will be relieved. When the multidisciplinary team has an accurate assessment of the client's condition and home situation, the safest, most effective approach to pain management can then be determined.

Joanie J. Kush, RN, BSN, MS, *Director of Hospice, Visiting Nurse Association of Omaha, Omaha, Nebraska*

sons with a short life expectancy, such as those with cancer-related pain.

LOCAL ANESTHESIA

Chemically, local anesthetics are divided into two classes:

1. The *esters* (e.g., procaine [Novocain]) are metabolized in the plasma, are less heat-stable than the amides, and account for most of the rarely occurring allergic reactions to local anesthetics.
2. The *amides* (e.g., lidocaine [Xylocaine] and bupivacaine [Marcaine, Sensorcaine]) are metabolized in the liver.

Procaine produces analgesia in 3 to 10 minutes and lasts less than 1 hour. It is one of the least toxic of the local anesthetics, although allergies occur rarely. Procaine is not effective for topical use.

Lidocaine is one of the most commonly used local anesthetics. It acts within 5 to 10 minutes and lasts about 2 hours. It has a wide range of applications, including topical and intravascular block. Allergy to lidocaine is rare. A Bier block is an example of an intravascular block.

Bupivacaine is long-acting (4 to 8 hours) but has a slow onset. It is four times more potent than lidocaine and four to six times more toxic. Therefore, a lower concentration is used. Bupivacaine appears to block sensory nerves in preference to motor nerves when used in low concentration. Thus, effective analgesia may result without accompanying motor weakness.

Local anesthetics are usually vasodilators, increasing blood flow into the area in which they are injected. Thus, they shorten the duration of their own action by enhancing their own vascular absorption. Adding epinephrine, a vasoconstrictor, to local anesthetic solutions prolongs the anesthetic effect by decreasing the vascular uptake of the anesthetic, allowing it to stay in contact with the nerve tissue for a longer period. The recipient may sense an increased heart rate from the epinephrine.

Note: Epinephrine-containing solutions are *not* typically used for nerve blocks of the penis, fingers, or toes, where vasoconstriction could cause inadequate blood flow and necrosis of the distal extremity.

In addition to prolonging anesthesia, epinephrine-containing local anesthetic solutions offer other advantages. The supplementary use of a vasoconstrictor reduces the possibility of the anesthetic's reaching a toxic blood level. The toxicity of local analgesic medications depends on their concentration in the blood. This, in turn, depends on the speed of absorption. Vasoconstricting medications delay absorption of a local analgesic solution and thus prevent a suddenly high blood concentration, which gives the body more time to metabolize and detoxify them. Vasoconstrictors also inhibit bleeding in the area of the injection. Larger doses of epinephrine containing local anesthetic should be used cautiously in people with coronary artery disease. Care of clients who have anesthesia is discussed in Chapter 15.

TOPICAL LOCAL ANESTHESIA

Dilute solutions of local anesthetics may be applied topically in the form of pastes, sprays, or other preparations. They may reduce the severe pain of burns, abrasions, and necrosis of the mucous membranes and skin. Remember, once an area is anesthetized, it does not transmit painful sensation and the area is thus at greater risk for injury. If topical anesthetic agents are applied to burned or abraded skin or mucous membranes, absorption of the medication is almost as rapid as that following intravenous administration.

A relatively new agent, EMLA cream, is a mixture of lidocaine and prilocaine. It is useful in preventing pain from venipuncture, injections, heel sticks, and minor plastic surgery. It must be applied in advance to the area (45 minutes to 1 hour) and covered with an occlusive dressing. EMLA cream is an excellent strategy for eliminating the pain associated with penetration of the skin and should be encouraged.

■ ANALGESICS

Various factors are considered in selecting the most effective analgesic for a specific client. These factors include the cause, quality, intensity, duration, and distribution of the pain. The World Health Organization (WHO)[134] has suggested that decisions regarding pain medications may be aided by use of a "pain ladder" (Fig. 23–14). The ladder was originally designed to guide the care of persons with cancer pain, but its use has been extended to also apply to acute pain. Non-opioids, such as acetaminophen and NSAIDs, are suggested by the first ladder step. If the pain persists or increases, step 2 suggests mild opioids (such as codeine) plus non-opioid analgesics. If the pain continues to persist or increases, step 3 suggests strong opioids (such as morphine) with or without non-opioids. Adjuvant medications may be added at any step in the ladder.

Systemic analgesic medications are the most frequently used means of pain control. Analgesics are the most commonly prescribed, and thus widely used, medications. They are also purchased extensively over the counter. This is not unexpected, because pain is usually the first manifestation of injury, and most diseases begin with or include pain at some time during their course.

PHARMACEUTICAL CONSIDERATIONS

Some analgesics have a *ceiling effect,* which occurs when medications have a maximum effective dose; increasing the dose cannot increase pain relief but may increase side effects. Medications with a ceiling effect may be combined with other analgesics when additional pain relief is needed.

Tolerance

Tolerance occurs when larger doses of medications are needed to provide the same amount of pain relief as the previous smaller dose. It is common among people who require long-term pain management with opioids. The person becomes tolerant to these medications because the opiate receptors become less sensitive to them. Tolerance may be managed by continuing the dose of the opioid and adding a non-opioid analgesic or adjuvant medication or by switching to an alternate drug.

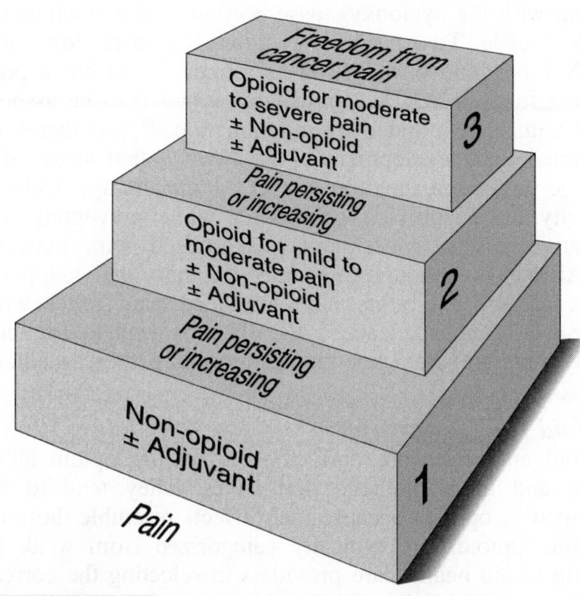

FIGURE 23–14 World Health Organization (WHO) analgesic ladder describes the steps in treating cancer pain. (From World Health Organization. [1996]. *Cancer pain relief* [2nd ed.] Geneva: Author.)

Tolerance should not be confused with *addiction,* which is extremely rare. Concern about addiction in cases of tolerance has led health care providers to modify opioid prescriptions by ordering smaller doses over longer periods of time. Client response to the modification may lead one to conclude that addiction was the underlying problem, as these people may be forced to display behaviors often associated with psychological addiction.[5] They no longer receive adequate pain relief and may attempt to manipulate the provider into providing adequate medication. Such behavior is understandable but is often viewed as "medication-seeking," a classic definition of one psychologically addicted. Clients may "act out" their pain in the belief that if they look as if they have severe pain, their need for medication will be recognized by the health care provider. The client does not receive adequate pain relief in response to these behaviors and rationalizes that health care providers are no longer dependable. The health care provider concludes that the client's behavior is inappropriate and no longer values or believes the client. This atmosphere of mistrust creates a situation in which adequate pain relief for the client becomes increasingly unlikely. Addiction is fully discussed in Chapter 24.

Dependence

Physical dependence commonly occurs when medications are taken over a long term. Physical manifestations associated with withdrawal of the medication include anxiety, irritability, chills alternating with hot flashes, salivation, lacrimation, rhinorrhea, diaphoresis, piloerection, nausea and vomiting, abdominal cramps, and insomnia.[5] The most common example of physical dependence is seen among coffee drinkers. Their bodies become dependent on the caffeine ingested. The most common manifestation is headache when caffeine is withheld.

Physical dependence is not a problem unless opioids are to be discontinued. The effects of withdrawal can be avoided by weaning the client from the medication slowly. It is essential that health care providers, clients, and their significant others realize that physical dependence is not synonymous with psychological addiction. Client and family education regarding this matter is an expected nursing function.

TYPES OF ANALGESICS

Analgesics are medications developed to provide pain relief. The discussion is organized according to the WHO analgesic ladder,[134] which is based on the notion that pain medication decisions are based in part on the intensity and controllability of the pain. The three steps reflect mild, moderate, and severe degrees of pain intensity.

Non-opioid Analgesics

Non-opioid analgesics fall into four primary categories[5]:

- Aspirin
- Salicylate salts
- Acetaminophen
- NSAIDs

As a group, these drugs have a ceiling effect but do not cause physical dependence or tolerance. Their site of action is primarily in the periphery at the receptor site, where they serve an anti-inflammatory function and prevent the production of prostaglandins. They may have a central role in pain relief, as prostaglandins inhibit the production or the release of serotonin, removing the pain relief effect of the neurotransmitter. Preventing prostaglandin production would maintain the inhibitory effect of serotonin in the dorsal horn. An exception is acetaminophen, which produces pain relief but is not an anti-inflammatory agent and does not appear to affect prostaglandins. The physical means by which acetaminophen produces pain relief is not known.[5]

The American Pain Society recommends that a non-opioid medication be included with any analgesic regimen, even when opioids are prescribed.[5] Opioids act centrally, within the brain and spinal cord. Non-opioids add peripherally mediated pain relief to the central effects of opioids when they are given in combination. Parenteral and rectal forms of non-opioids have been developed for individuals who cannot take oral medications. Refer to Table 23–5 for dosing information for non-opioid medications.

ASPIRIN. Historically, aspirin (acetylsalicylic acid, ASA) has been the primary non-opioid medication for pain. It is one of the most effective non-opioid medications available. Aspirin is available in many forms, including tablets (plain, chewable, enteric coated, sustained-release), capsules, rectal suppositories, and topical creams. As with most nonsteroidal analgesics, aspirin has an antiplatelet effect and is a gastric irritant. Side effects include bleeding associated with prolonged clotting time and gastric disturbances. Enteric-coated tablets reduce the gastric reactions because the coating remains intact until the product reaches the small intestine, where the tablet dissolves and is absorbed. Because of the association of aspirin with Reye's syndrome, a potentially fatal condition seen primarily in young children, it is not used for children under age 12 with viral illnesses. Recent cases of adults with Reye's syndrome-like symptoms and negative outcomes suggest that aspirin may pose a risk for people of any age when administered to those with viral infections.

SALICYLATE SALTS. These salts are similar to aspirin but produce fewer gastric side effects. Choline magnesium trisalicylate (Trilisate) and diflunisal (Dolobid) are typical examples. Platelet aggregation does not result when salicylate salts are used in people with normal clotting abilities.

ACETAMINOPHEN. Acetaminophen is similar to aspirin in its ability to provide pain relief, but it does not affect the gastric mucosa. It has no effect on platelet aggregation and does not affect bleeding time. Its anti-inflammatory effect is much less than that of other non-opioids. It is tolerated well by most people of any age, and it is the drug of choice when given for pain to people with viral infections.

NSAIDS. NSAIDs are nonsteroidal anti-inflammatory agents other than aspirin and acetaminophen. NSAIDs are present in numerous preparations, providing alternative medication choices. If one form is ineffective, another can be tried. NSAIDs were originally developed to treat arthritis, but they are also effective for mild to moderate pain of nonarthritic origin. NSAIDs act to decrease inflammation, but it is their ability to block prostaglandin synthesis that is credited for most of their pain-relieving properties.[21, 24, 57, 91, 102] NSAIDs are particularly helpful for clients with cancer or postoperative pain, since a major contributing factor to pain in these clients is cell destruction.

NSAIDs potentiate the effects of opiates and are often given in combination preparations that incorporate codeine or codeine derivatives. Tylenol with codeine is used widely for moderate pain. NSAIDs are particularly effective for pain resulting from bone insult, including bone metastases of malignancy and fractures. Degradation of bone tissue in these conditions produces prostaglandins. The ability of NSAIDs to prevent prostaglandin production significantly decreases pain produced by these lesions.[92] Ketoprofen and ketorolac (Toradol) also block production of leukotrienes.[57, 91]

The most common side effects associated with NSAIDs are gastrointestinal upset and possible bleeding. These agents also inhibit platelet aggregation, increasing the risk of hemorrhage. Clients taking NSAIDs must be monitored closely for the development of peptic ulcers. In clients who are taking high doses for long periods of time (as for arthritis) a histamine H_2-receptor antagonist such as ranitidine (Zantac) or misoprostol (Cytotec) may be used.

NSAIDs may also have negative effects on the renal system, particularly in clients with heart failure, chronic renal disease, lupus, blood volume depletion, diuretic use, atherosclerosis, and multiple myeloma.[5] Clients may experience sudden decreased urine output associated with water and sodium retention. These renal side effects quickly abate on discontinuance of the NSAID.

New forms of NSAIDs appear to prevent the negative side effects and to broaden the routes available for administration. For example, ketorolac was developed to provide an injectable form. The recently available cyclooxygenase (COX-2) inhibitors were developed in response to the negative gastrointestinal side effects of aspirin and NSAIDs.[51] Celecoxib (Celebrex) and meloxicam (Vioxx) disrupt the synthesis of prostaglandins by interfering with the cyclooxygenase portion of the arachidonic acid cascade. Two types of cyclooxygenase predominate. COX-1 is found primarily in the stomach and has a protective function. COX-2 is usually assumed to be associated with pain initiated by inflammation. It was therefore assumed that development of an NSAID that spares the gastric protection function of COX-1 but disrupts COX-2 activity would provide pain relief while preventing the negative gastric consequences associated with existing NSAIDs.[51, 93] Although this concept is not totally supportable, COX-2 inhibitors have provided pain relief with little gastric consequence.[46, 47, 51] Nurses need to continuously upgrade their knowledge regarding these medications.

Opioid Analgesics

Opioid analgesics are derived from natural opium alkaloids and their synthetic derivatives. They tend to be grouped as opioids because their effects resemble those of opium. Opioids are typically categorized from weak to strong to aid health care providers in selecting the correct medication (Table 23–6). Opioids are added to the medication regimen when pain is moderate to severe and non-opioids are insufficient to manage pain effectively. Tolerance and physical dependence seen in long-term

TABLE 23–5 DOSING INFORMATION FOR ACETAMINOPHEN AND NONSTEROIDAL ANTI-INFLAMMATORY DRUGS (NSAIDS)*

Chemical Class	Generic Name	Half-Life (hr)	Dosing Schedule	Recommended Oral Starting Dose (mg)	Maximum Oral Dose Recommended (mg/day)	Comments
P-Aminophenol derivatives	Acetaminophen	2	q4–6hr	650	6000	Overdosage produces hepatic toxicity. No GI or platelet toxicity. Available as liquid and for rectal administration.
Salicylates	Aspirin	3–12	q4–6hr	650	6000	Standard for comparison. May not be as well tolerated as some of the newer NSAIDs. Available for rectal administration.
	Diflunisal	8–12	q12hr	500	1500	Less GI toxicity than aspirin.
	Choline magnesium trisalicylate	9–17	q12hr	500–1000	4000	Minimal GI toxicity. No effect on platelet aggregation. Available as liquid.
	Choline salicylate	2–3	q3–6hr	870	5352	Liquid. Minimal effect on platelet function.
	Magnesium salicylate		q4–6hr	1000	4000	
	Salsalate	16	q12hr	500–1000	4000	
Proprionic acids	Ibuprofen	2	q6hr	400	3200	Available as a suspension.
	Naproxen	13	q12hr	250	1025–1375	
	Fenoprofen	2–3	q6–8hr	200	3200	
	Ketoprofen	2–3	q6–8hr	25	300	Available for rectal administration and as a topical gel.
	Flurbiprofen	5–6	q12hr	100	300	
	Oxaprozin	400	q24hr	600	1800	
Acetic acids	Indomethacin	4–5	q8hr	25	150	Higher incidence of GI and CNS side effects than proprionic acids. Available in slow-release preparations, and for rectal administration.
	Tolmetin	2–5	q8hr	200	2000	
	Sulindac	14	q12hr	150	400	Not recommended for prolonged use because of increased risk for GI toxicity.
	Diclofenac	2	q8hr	25	150	
	Ketorolac	4–7	q6hr	10	40	Use limited to 5 days. Recommended parenteral dose ≤30 mg; total daily dose ≤120 mg.
Oxicams	Piroxicam	50	q24hr	20	40	
Fenamates	Mefenamic acid	2	q6hr	250	1000	Use limited to 7 days.
	Meclofenamate	2	—	—	400	Not recommended for analgesia.
Pyranocarboxylic acids	Etodolac	7	q8hr	200	1200	
Other	Nabumetone	24	q24hr	1000	2000	Minimal effect on platelet aggregation.

*May be duplicated for use in clinical practice.
GI, gastrointestinal; CNS, central nervous system.
From McCaffery, M., & Pasero, C. (1999). *Clinical manual* (pp. 139–140). St. Louis: Mosby.

TABLE 23–6 ANALGESIC STEP PAIN LADDER

Step One	Step Two	Step Three
NSAIDs and Others	**Opioid-Agonist Drug**	**Agonist Drugs**
Acetaminophen	Codeine	Morphine sulfate
Acetylsalicylic acid (aspirin)	Oxycodone (w/aspirin and w/acetaminophen)	Methodone
Ibuprofen	Hydrocodone	Hydromorphone
Choline magnesium trisalicylate	Meperidine	Oxymorphone
Diflunisal	Propoxyphene HCl	Levorphanol
Ketoprofen	Propoxyphene napsylate (w/aspirin and w/acetaminophen)	Fentanyl
Naproxen	**Agonist-Antagonist Drugs**	**Agonist-Antagonist Drugs**
Ketorolac tromethamine	Pentazocine HCl	Butorphanol
Piroxicam		Nalbuphine
Sulindac		Dezocine
Indomethacin		**Partial Agonist Drugs**
Carbamazepine		Buprenorphine
Celecoxib		
Meloxicam		
Phenytoin		
Amitriptyline		
Doxepin		
Imipramine		
Trazodone		
Hydroxyzine		
Lidocaine		
Mexiletine		
Tocainide		
Dexamethasone		
Dextroamphetamine		
Methylphenidate		

From the World Health Organization (1996). *Cancer pain relief* (2nd ed.). Geneva: Author.

administration are not associated with short-term opioid treatment.

Opioids bind with receptors that can be engaged by endogenous opioids, including mu (μ), kappa (κ), and delta (δ) receptor types.[94, 107] Binding with receptors in the spinal cord renders the presynaptic membrane of nociceptor fibers incapable of opening Ca^{2+} channels, inhibiting nociceptive neurotransmitter release. Opiate binding with the postsynaptic membrane hyperpolarizes the membrane by altering the ability of K^+ ions to flow across the membrane.[3, 107] Opiate receptors are found in PAG/PVG. Activation of these receptors by opioids initiates the descending effect of serotonin and norepinephrine.[28, 38, 135]

All opioids produce side effects to some degree. The side effects are determined, in part, by the receptor type engaged by the medication and by the location of the receptor. The three receptor types have very different distributions and locations with the CNS. Side effects may be managed by discontinuing one form of opiate medication with untoward side effects, and replacing it with another that binds to a different receptor type.

OPIOID AGONISTS. Opioid agonists are opiate derivatives that bring about pain relief by producing the maximum degree of receptor binding. Agonists bind fully to their corresponding receptor type and do not affect the ability of other opioid preparations to engage their specific receptor. They are typically associated with mu receptors and have no ceiling effect.

Examples of opioid agonists are displayed in Table 23–7. They include morphine-like medications, which differ from morphine in rate of onset, duration of action, route of administration, adverse side effects, and chemical configuration. The mechanisms by which they produce pain relief are similar.

OPIOID ANTAGONISTS. These agents reverse the side effects and analgesia of opioids. They have no agonist effects and thus produce no analgesia. They are used to counteract a negative effect of an opioid, typically respiratory depression. Naloxone is the most common example.

OPIOID AGONIST-ANTAGONISTS. These medications engage one receptor type while inhibiting receptor binding of another. When they are given following use of the opioid they inhibit, they precipitously reverse the medication's effects and can precipitate acute withdrawal. When the combination agents are given alone, they produce analgesia and the positive effects of opioids with fewer side effects. Respiratory depression is a less likely effect, although psychomimetic effects are more probable. Examples are displayed in Table 23–7.

METHADONE. A potent, long-acting opioid analgesic, methadone gained popularity in the management of cancer pain before the development of the long-acting forms of morphine. Unlike most morphine preparations, methadone has a long plasma half-life. This long plasma half-life, when repeated doses are given, may account for methadone's longer duration of analgesic action, but it also poses certain problems. This medication is not recommended for older people and people with compromised hepatic and renal function. The long plasma half-

TABLE 23–7 EQUIANALGESIC DOSE CHART FOR SELECTED OPIOID DRUGS

A Guide to Using Equianalgesic Dose Charts

- Equianalgesic means approximately the same pain relief.
- The equianalgesic chart is a guideline. Doses and intervals between doses are titrated according to individual's response.
- The equianalgesic chart is helpful when switching from one drug to another or switching from one route of administration to another.
- Dosages in this equianalgesic chart are not necessarily starting doses. They suggest a ratio for comparing the analgesia of one drug to another.
- The longer the client has been receiving opioids, the more conservative the starting doses of a new opioid.

Opioid	Parenteral (IM/SC/IV) (Over ~ 4 hr)	Oral (PO) (Over ~ 4 hr)	Onset (min)	Peak (min)	Duration[1] (hr)	Half-life (hr)
MU AGONISTS						
Morphine	10 mg	30 mg	30–60 (PO) 30–60 (CR)[2] 30–60 (R) 5–10 (IV) 10–20 (SC) 10–20 (IM)	60–90 (PO) 90–180 (CR)[2] 60–90 (R) 15–30 (IV) 30–60 (SC) 30–60 (IM)	3–6 (PO) 8–12 (CR)[1,3] 4–5 (R) 3–4 (IV) 3–4 (SC) 3–4 (IM)	2–4
Codeine	130 mg	200 mg NR	30–60 (PO) 10–20 (SC) 10–20 (IM)	60–90 (PO) UK (SC) 30–60 (IM)	3–4 (PO) 3–4 (SC) 3–4 (IM)	2–4
Fentanyl	100 μg/hr parenterally and transdermally ≅ 4 mg/hr morphine parenterally; 1 μg/hr transdermally ≅ morphine 2 mg/24 hr orally	—	5 (OT) 1–5 (IV) 7–15 (IM) 12–16 h (TD)	15 (OT) 3–5 (IV) 10–20 (IM) 24 h (TD)	2–5 (OT) 0.5–4 (IV) 0.5–4 (IM) 48–72 (TD)	3–4 13–24 (TD)
Hydrocodone (as in Vicodin, Lortab)	—	30 mg[5] NR	30–60 (PO)	60–90 (PO)	4–6 (PO)	4
Hydromorphone (Dilaudid)	1.5 mg[6]	7.5 mg	15–30 (PO) 15–30 (R) 5 (IV) 10–20 (SC) 10–20 (IM)	30–90 (PO) 30–90 (R) 10–20 (IV) 30–90 (SC) 30–90 (IM)	3–4 (PO) 3–4 (R) 3–4 (IV)[1,3] 3–4 (SC) 3–4 (IM)	2–3
Levorphanol (Levo-Dromoran)	2 mg	4 mg	30–60 (PO) 10 (IV) 10–20 (SC) 10–20 (IM)	60–90 (PO) 15–30 (IV) 60–90 (SC) 60–90 (IM)	4–6 (PO) 4–6 (IV)[1,3] 4–6 (SC) 4–6 (IM)	12–15
Meperidine (Demerol)	75 mg	300 mg NR	30–60 (PO) 5–10 (IV) 10–20 (SC) 10–20 (IM)	60–90 (PO) 10–15 (IV) 15–30 (SC) 15–30 (IM)	2–4 (PO) 2–4 (IV)[1,3] 2–4 (SC) 2–4 (IM)	2–3
Methadone (Dolophine)	10 mg[7]	20 mg[8]	30–60 (PO) UK (SL) 10 (IV) 10–20 (SC) 10–20 (IM)	60–120 (PO) 10 (SL) UK (IV) 60–120 (SC) 60–120 (IM)	4–8 (PO) UK (SL) 4–8 (IV)[1,3] 4–8 (SC) 4–8 (IM)	12–190
Oxycodone (as in Percocet, Tylox)	—	20 mg	30–60 (PO) 30–60 (CR)[9] 30–60 (R)	60–90 (PO) 90–180 (CR)[9] 30–60 (R)	3–4 (PO) 8–12 (CR)[9] 3–6 (R)	2–3 4.5 (CR)
Oxymorphone (Numorphan)	1 mg	(10 mg R)	15–30 (R) 5–10 (IV) 10–20 (SC) 10–20 (IM)	120 (R) 15–30 (IV) UK (SC) 30–90 (IM)	3–6 (R) 3–4 (IV)[1,3] 3–6 (SC) 3–6 (IM)	2–3
Propoxyphene[10] (Darvon)	—	—	30–60 (PO)	60–90 (PO)	4–6 (PO)	6–12

Table continued on following page

TABLE 23–7 EQUIANALGESIC DOSE CHART FOR SELECTED OPIOID DRUGS *Continued*

Opioid	Parenteral (IM/SC/IV) (Over ~ 4 hr)	Oral (PO) (Over ~ 4 hr)	Onset (min)	Peak (min)	Duration[1] (hr)	Half-life (hr)
AGONIST-ANTAGONISTS						
Buprenorphine[11] (Buprenex)	0.4 mg	—	5 (SL) 5 (IV) 10–20 (IM)	30–60 (SL) 10–20 (IV) 30–60 (IM)	UK (SL) 3–4 (IV)[1, 3] 3–6 (IM)	2–3
Butorphanol[11] (Stadol)	2 mg	—	5–15 (NS)[12] 5 (IV) 10–20 (IM)	60–90 (NS) 10–20 (IV) 30–60 (IM)	3–4 (NS) 3–4 (IV)[1, 3] 3–4 (IM)	3–4
Dezocine (Dalgan)	10 mg	—	5 (IV) 10–20 (IM)	UK (IV) 30–60 (IM)	3–4 (IV)[1, 3] 3–4 (IM)	2–3
Nalbuphine[11] (Nubain)	10 mg	—	5 (IV) <15 (SC) <15 (IM)	10–20 (IV) UK (SC) 30–60 (IM)	3–4 (IV)[1, 3] 3–4 (SC) 3–4 (IM)	5
Pentazocine[11] (Talwin)	60 mg	180 mg	15–30 (PO) 5 (IV) 15–20 (SC) 15–20 (IM)	60–180 (PO) 15 (IV) 60 (SC) 60 (IM)	3–4 (PO) 3–4 (IV)[1, 3] 3–4 (SC) 3–4 (IM)	2–3

[1]Duration of analgesia is dose-dependent; the higher the dose, usually the longer the duration.
[2]As in, e.g., MS Contin.
[3]IV boluses may be used to produce analgesia that lasts approximately as long as IM or SC doses. However, of all routes of administration, IV produces the highest peak concentration of the drug, and the peak concentration is associated with the highest level of toxicity (e.g., sedation). To decrease the peak effect and lower the level of toxicity, IV boluses may be administered more slowly (e.g., 10 mg of morphine over a 15-minute period) or smaller doses may be administered more often (e.g., 5 mg of morphine every 1–1.5 hours).
[4]At steady state, slow release of fentanyl from storage in tissues can result in a prolonged half-life of up to 12 h.
[5]Equianalgesic data not available.
[6]The recommendation that 1.5 mg of parenteral hydromorphone is approximately equal to 10 mg of parenteral morphine is based on single-dose studies. With repeated dosing of hydromorphone (e.g., PCA), it is more likely that 2 to 3 mg of parenteral hydromorphone is equal to 10 mg of parenteral morphine.
[7]In opioid-tolerant clients converted from continuous IV hydromorphone to continuous IV methadone, start with 10% to 25% of the equianalgesic dose.
[8]In opioid-tolerant clients converted to methadone, start PO dosing PRN with 10% to 25% of the equianalgesic dose.
[9]As in OxyContin (oxycodone), for example.
[10]65–130 mg = approximately one-sixth of all doses listed in this chart.
[11]Used in combination with mu agonists, may reverse analgesia and precipitate withdrawal in opioid-dependent clients.
[12]In opioid-naive clients who are taking occasional mu agonists, such as codeine or oxycodone, the addition of butorphanol nasal spray may provide additive analgesia. However, in opioid-tolerant clients, such as those receiving ATC morphine, the addition of butorphanol nasal spray should be avoided because it may reverse analgesia and precipitate withdrawal.
ATC, around-the-clock; CR, oral controlled-release; h, hour; IM, intramuscular; IV, intravenous; μg, microgram; mg, milligram; min, minute; NR, not recommended; NS, nasal spray; OT, oral transmucosal; PO, oral; R, rectal; SC, subcutaneous; SL, sublingual; TD, transdermal; UK, unknown.
Modified from McCaffery M., Pasero C. (1999). *Pain: Clinical manual* (pp. 241–243). St. Louis, Mosby.

life necessitates close monitoring of any client receiving repeated doses because cumulative effects develop over 1 to 2 weeks. If the client becomes oversedated, the dosage should be reduced or the intervals between administration lengthened.

MEPERIDINE. Meperidine (Demerol) is a popular analgesic medication but has many limitations. It should not be used on a prolonged basis (more than a few doses) because of the potentially toxic breakdown product normeperidine, produced during its biotransformation. Meperidine does not provide effective pain relief with repeated doses and causes untenable CNS side effects. The metabolic by-product is toxic to the CNS and can lead to anxiety, tremors, myoclonus, and seizure activity. Nerve injury from diffusion of medication can also occur. Meperidine should not be used in clients with altered renal function.

Adverse Effects of Opioid Analgesics

Some side effects of opioid analgesics—constipation in particular—last as long as the medication is administered. Others, such as nausea and vomiting and drowsiness, decrease as the administration is continued. Other side effects (e.g., respiratory depression) are rare, and the incidence decreases precipitously with longer administration.

CONSTIPATION. Constipation is the most common side effect seen with opioid use[76, 127, 135] and results from increased smooth muscle tone and decreased motility of the gastrointestinal tract. Opioids diminish the propulsive peristaltic contractions in the small and large intestine and delay the passage of gastric contents through the duodenum. Tolerance does not develop to constipation as it does to the other side effects of opioids. Clients taking opioid analgesics need to follow a bowel regimen to prevent constipation. A diet high in fiber with plenty of fluids and stool-softening medications, such as docusate sodium (Colace) or docusate sodium casanthranol (Peri-Colace), is a common prophylactic treatment. A senna-based bulk laxative, such as Senokot-S, is also often needed.[75, 127] Constipation is treatable and is not a side effect mandating that opioid medications be discontinued.

NAUSEA AND VOMITING. Opioids may precipitate nausea and vomiting because of their action on the brain stem centers. Morphine-like medications also affect the vestibular system, which can produce these manifestations. Changing the type of opioid used may eliminate the side effect. Antiemetic agents may also be administered. Remember, this side effect decreases with analgesic use. Clients should not be denied pain relief because of this effect. Instead, they should receive treatment for the nausea and vomiting until it subsides.

RESPIRATORY DEPRESSION. Respiratory depression is caused by diminished sensitivity of the respiratory center to carbon dioxide. All opioids have the potential to produce respiratory depression, which can be rapidly reversed with an opioid antagonist, typically naloxone. The reaction is relatively rare, occurring primarily following the initial doses of opioid among those who never received the medication or whose last dose was a long time ago. It rarely occurs in awake individuals.[5]

This potential for respiratory depression should not discourage the proper use of opioids to relieve pain in people of all ages. The development of respiratory depression is not necessarily dose-related. Most clients do not respond with depressed respiratory rates regardless of dose. Another person may react with decreased respiration to relatively small doses. Rather than limit the use of opioid analgesics, carefully assess each client after giving the medication for the occurrence of respiratory depression.

Deaths that occur secondary to opioid overdose are usually due to respiratory depression and usually occur in people who have not received opioids in the past. With morphine, maximal respiratory depression usually occurs within 15 minutes of intravenous (IV) administration, within 30 minutes of intramuscular (IM) administration, within 90 minutes of subcutaneous (SC) administration, and within 4 to 12 hours of epidural administration. Remember these time ranges when assessing the respiratory status following administration of opioids. For an overdose to occur, however, doses well above the therapeutic level would have to be given. Accumulated doses, especially in clients with liver or renal failure and elderly clients, can cause an overdose.

It is also important to clearly diagnose respiratory depression. The presence of pain may result in increased respiratory rates among clients taking frequent, shallow breaths. Providing a opioid may relieve the pain allowing one's respiratory pattern to return to a more normal breathing pattern. A respiratory rate of 30 breaths per minute may be reduced to 15. This drop has been interpreted as medication-caused respiratory depression, and the pain relief achieved has been reversed by naloxone administration. Remember to assess respiratory depression in conjunction with normal functioning rather than the decrease in breaths per minute. Is the resulting respiratory rate life-threatening?

Treatment of respiratory depression includes arousing the client, establishing a patent airway, administering an opioid antagonist such as naloxone, and providing artificial ventilation as necessary.

CIRCULATORY DEPRESSION. In some clients, circulatory depression may produce hypotension.[71] In a supine client, therapeutic dosages of morphine or synthetic opioids have little effect on blood pressure and cardiac rate or rhythm. However, some people experience orthostatic hypotension when moving from a supine position to a head-up or standing position. This hypotension is secondary to a direct dilating action on the peripheral blood vessels, caused by the opioids, which reduces the capacity of the cardiovascular system to respond to gravitational shifts. Advise the client to avoid abrupt body position changes. For this reason, opioids are used very cautiously in people with reduced blood volume, since the effect is more pronounced. Increasing fluid volume decreases the orthostatic changes.

PARESTHESIAS. Paresthesias may complicate the use of intramuscular opioid analgesics. The intramuscular injection is generally not irritating to the local tissues; however, two exceptions are meperidine and methadone. SC methadone may cause local tissue irritation. Both SC and IM meperidine cause local painful tissue irritation and induration, and frequent administration can lead to severe fibrosis of muscle tissue and should be avoided when possible. If an analgesic is deposited in the region of a nerve after intramuscular injection, paresthesia and paresis may result along the course of the nerve. Proper injection techniques prevent direct nerve injury.

CUTANEOUS EFFECTS. Opioid medications may facilitate histamine release resulting in pruritus, flushing, and sweating. The client becomes tolerant to this effect with repeated administration of the opioid.[88] In the meantime, the clinical manifestations may be alleviated by ingestion of antihistamines.

URINARY RETENTION. Urinary retention may occur due to the increase in smooth muscle tone of the detrussor muscle of the bladder and the bladder sphincter.[75] The hypertoned muscle fibers resist opening preventing adequate bladder emptying. Urinary retention and urgency result. In severe cases, catheterization may be necessary.

Adjuvant Medications

Adjuvants are medications developed for other conditions but have been found to have pain reducing properties as well. Adjuvant medications may be used in combination with analgesics or may be used alone. A wide variety of medications can be classified as adjuvant analgesics.[32, 75, 87, 91, 93, 102] Tricyclic antidepressants (TCAs), such as amitriptyline (Elavil), are very effective for neuropathic pain. They can be given daily at bedtime, so that the drowsiness associated with them promotes sleep. Other effective medications for neuropathic pain are phenytoin (Dilantin), carbamazepine (Tegretol), and gabapentin (Neurontin). Nerve compression and bone pain may respond to dexamethasone (Decadron). Muscle relaxants, such as baclofen (Lioresal) and diazepam (Valium), are used to treat muscle spasm associated with pain.

Phenothiazines are not appropriate for pain relief. They are good antiemetics, but, when given for pain, phenothiazines simply increase sedation, hypotension, and respiratory depression. A phenothiazine such as promethazine (Phenergan) should never be used for pain relief. Promethazine actually increases the perception of pain.[128]

ANTIDEPRESSANTS. TCAs contribute to pain relief via the descending pain inhibitory system by blocking cellular re-uptake of serotonin and epinephrine. They may also potentiate the effect of opiates at synapses and increase their plasma bioavailability. The analgesic effect occurs with doses lower than needed to produce an antidepressant effect. TCAs are used to enhance pain relief regardless of a depression diagnosis. However, relief of depression in clinically depressed clients with pain is a positive outcome. TCAs can be given as a single daily dose at bedtime or in divided doses. Analgesic effects usually begin within a week of initiation of the TCA.

ANTI-ANXIETY AGENTS. Drugs such as diazepam and chlordiazepoxide (Librium) are believed to mediate pain by contributing to Cl^- channel opening. Movement of Cl^- ions hyperpolarizes the postsynaptic membrane, making it less receptive to incoming nociceptive stimuli. Diazepam is particularly effective for relief of painful muscle spasm.

ANTICONVULSANTS. Anticonvulsant agents are used in situations associated with nerve injury. Nerve fibers may generate electrical activity at the site of injury causing the nerve membrane to fire with a pain-producing signal. Agents such as phenytoin (Dilantin) and gabapentin (Neurontin), which stabilize the membrane, help to prevent the ectopic generation of pain-producing activity resulting in lancinating, shooting, shock-like pain.

CORTICOSTEROIDS. These drugs are used to facilitate relief for various types of pain. In the periphery, they reduce edema and inflammation, reducing the compression caused by swelling and the availability of chemical mediators of nociception. They may also inhibit the production of prostaglandins and leukotrienes. In the CNS, they function similarly to anti-anxiety agents by modifying the flow of Cl^- ions.

LOCAL ANESTHETIC AGENTS. Local anesthetics, when administered orally, are membrane stabilizers that produce analgesia by suppressing aberrant electrical activity in central neurons or peripheral axons. Membrane-stabilizing agents include mexiletine (Mexitil), lidocaine, bupivacaine, and tocainide (Tonocard). These agents appear to be effective against lancinating and continuous neuropathic pain. They operate to inactivate Na^+ or K^+ channels, preventing generation of the electrical pain-producing signal. Membrane-stabilizing agents are used primarily for their antiarrhythmic effect, and clients with heart disease must be carefully assessed before these medications are started.

MISCELLANEOUS AGENTS. *Baclofen,* a GABA antagonist, is used as an analgesic for lancinating or paroxysmal neuropathic pain. *Capsaicin* is a topical medication that depletes peptides (such as substance P) in small primary afferent neurons that mediate nociceptive transmission. It appears useful for postherpetic neuralgia and for postmastectomy pain in some clients.

FACTORS INFLUENCING THE EFFECTIVENESS OF ANALGESICS

Relative Analgesic Potency

Relative analgesic potency refers to the ratio of the doses of two analgesics required to produce the same effect. Analgesics are compared with therapeutic doses of morphine. Estimates of relative analgesic potency provide a basis for prescribing the dose when the client is being switched from one analgesic to another or from one route of administration to another. The route used to provide pain relief affects the potency of the medication.

The availability of the analgesic is determined in part by the events encountered before the drug enters the circulatory system. Orally administered medications must be dissolved in stomach contents and absorbed by the gut before the agent can contribute to pain relief. Using the IM or SC routes necessitates that the medication be absorbed from muscle or subcutaneous tissues before it becomes available. IV medications enter the circulatory system directly. Oral, IM, and SC doses must be higher than IV doses.

Duration of Action

The duration of action of an analgesic agent is the result of factors such as pain intensity, dose size, and the client's ability to absorb, biotransform, and eliminate the medication. The duration of action for the analgesics (see Table 23–7) is based on a dose that produces a peak effect equivalent to that of morphine. The time of peak effect and the duration of action of a particular opioid vary with the route of administration. For instance, the peak analgesic effect of IM morphine occurs between 30 minutes and 1 hour after administration. The peak analgesic effect of orally administered morphine occurs from 2 to 12 hours after administration. The duration of action of orally administered opioids is usually somewhat longer than that of IM analgesics. *Duration* of analgesia may not be the same as the *effect* of analgesia. Learn about peak and duration of analgesic effect so that activities that might produce pain can be planned to coincide with peak periods of action. For example, if you know that a client will be going for physical therapy at 10:00 AM, you will want to provide pain medication that will reach its peak effect around 10:00 AM.

Several new forms of morphine have been developed. An oral liquid can be given for more rapid but short-acting effects. A controlled-release form is also available. With long-acting morphine, the onset is somewhat slower but the duration ranges from 8 to 12 hours. Fentanyl is available as a patch for transdermal delivery of medication, effective for 48 to 72 hours. Fentanyl is also available for transmucosal delivery. Oral transmusocal fentanyl citrate is available in lollipop form. The medication is delivered systemically directly through the transmusocal route and partially by the amount of the medication that is swallowed.

Oral Potency

As opioids are absorbed from the intestine and pass through the liver and into the systemic circulation, they differ in the degree to which they are active. This difference in absorption accounts, in part, for the oral doses listed in Table 23–7 for various forms of oral morphine. Preparations with lower bioavailability require higher doses per pill. More recently developed forms of morphine have greater bioavailability, and therefore the dosages of these are lower than those of the older oral form. Because opioids are available in various forms, with varying onset, peak effect, duration, and half-lives, become aware of these variations. The different equianalgesic doses are based on a single dose of IV morphine (see

Table 23–7). An equianalgesic dose is expected to provide the same degree of pain relief as the single IV morphine dose. Dose requirements may decrease after the client has received a loading dose. Failure of health care providers to recognize differences in the oral and intramuscular potencies of opioids and the concept of equianalgesic doses can lead to undertreatment of a person's pain.

ADMINISTRATION OF ANALGESICS

Principles of administration of analgesics are shown in Box 23–5. The goal of analgesic administration is to provide pain relief while maintaining the ability of the client to be in control of the environment, participate in care, and reduce side effects. Assessment of the client before and after analgesic administration is necessary to ensure safe and adequate pain relief. Assess the following factors before analgesic administration:

- Medication allergies or sensitivities
- Previous response to analgesics
- Other medications being taken
- Body weight
- Individual pain experience
- Age, general state of health, mental status
- Cardiac, respiratory, renal, hepatic, and CNS

Allergies or Sensitivities to Medications

Before administering an analgesic such as morphine, ensure that the client does not have a history of untoward reactions to the medication. When possible, ask the client or significant others, and review the chart or other documentation for such information.

Concomitant Medications

Clients taking monoamine oxidase (MAO) inhibitor antidepressants should not receive meperidine. Medications that cause sedation, constipation, or orthostatic hypotension must also be considered when the client is receiving opioids.

Body Weight

The standard morphine dose is 10 mg parenterally. This dose produces satisfactory analgesia in approximately 70% of people with moderate to severe postoperative pain. The analgesic effect is dose-related. Analgesics tend to be prescribed according to a standard protocol applied to all clients with similar disease, however, rather than being based on physical characteristics, including body weight. Therefore, the standard dose may be too high for small adults and too low for obese adults. Remember, one cannot assume that the standard dose will produce adequate pain relief in all adults. You must routinely assess degree of pain relief to ensure that adequate doses are being delivered.

Individual Differences

Given the multitude of factors that contribute to any one person's pain experience, the characteristics of one client's pain may differ from those of another client. It is not possible to design a pain management regimen that will be equally effective for all people with similar pathologic processes. For example, a person's age determines, to some extent, the length of time during which an analgesic will be effective. Age may influence the amount of relief obtained from medications. While there is most likely little difference in the ability of the CNS of an older adult to respond to stimuli, decreases in muscle mass, increases in gastric pathology, and changes in circulatory characteristics may result in a decreased ability to absorb and utilize analgesics. An older person tends to receive pain relief from an opioid for a longer time compared with a younger person. This difference in duration of action may relate to the speed with which an opioid is cleared from the body. Opioid clearance is faster in younger people than in older people.

People with debilitating diseases, regardless of age, also have a heightened sensitivity to the effects of opioids. Because of individual differences in responses to

BOX 23–5 Principles of Pharmaceutical Pain Management

- Provide medications in adequate doses.
- Utilize a preventive approach to pain relief. Predictable and chronic pain is managed more effectively if the client maintains a therapeutic blood level of analgesics.
- Closely assess clients with particular diligence with first doses or when the medication dose or the type is changed.
- Medication doses are specific as to type and route. For example, the dose for an oral preparation is higher than that for an intravenous dose of the same medication.
- Combinations of analgesics may be more effective than those given singularly.
- Additions of adjuvant medications enhance pain relief produced by analgesics and are not intended to replace analgesics.
- Understand and be prepared to treat side effects of medications.
- Do not consider avoidance of non–life-threatening side effects (such as constipation, nausea, pruritus) more important than providing pain relief. These concomitant conditions are easily treated.
- Recognize that respiratory depression is a rare occurrence, occurring most commonly among clients who are sedated. Respiratory depression rarely occurs after the first few doses of an opioid.
- Asking for pain medication reflects need for pain relief in 99.9% of people with pain and does not reflect an addictive personality.
- Do not use placebos for pain. The placebo response usually indicates that the responder has a effective endogenous opiate system and had obtained opiate-mediated pain relief.
- Believe the client's report of pain.
- Maintain a therapeutic relationship that facilitates mutual trust. Your attitudes and beliefs do affect the client's ability to respond to pain management strategies.
- Incorporate the goal of total pain relief into the pain management regimen for most clients.
- Operate as a team to provide the most effective pain relief outcomes. Include the client and significant others in pain interventions, allowing the client to maintain an adequate degree of personal control in the experience.
- *Only the client, and no one else, can determine the amount of pain experienced. There is no objective indicator of pain that can be observed by another.*

pain medications, you must become diligent in assessing the client's responses to the medications.

Body System Assessment

Because all analgesics have the potential to produce mild to severe side effects, it is important to assess a client's cardiac, respiratory, renal, and CNS status before administering analgesics. Hepatic function is also assessed because of the important role of the liver in detoxifying analgesics. The presence of increased intracranial pressure is cause for concern. The physician typically conducts a body system assessment prior to ordering a specific medication regimen. You will need to report changes in physical status, which may place the client at risk if given the analgesic. The physician may then determine that an alternative regimen is needed.

METHODS OF ADMINISTRATION

Nurse-Administered (Demand) Analgesia

The traditional method of treating pain is by nurse-administered pain medication on a schedule, or on a *PRN* (as needed) basis. This system has several advantages:

- It allows you to assess the pain and evaluate effectiveness of the medication
- It facilitates your ability to detect or avoid untoward reactions or side effects
- It permits dose adjustment as necessary

Unfortunately, pain is often significantly undertreated with the PRN system.

Undertreatment may occur because (1) nurses assume authority for pain management, including determination of the amount of pain experienced by the client, and (2) overconcern about possible opioid side effects and fear of inducing opioid addiction by the nurse, the client, or their significant others. The concern about negative effects of pain results in medications ordered in inadequate doses in overly long intervals. When given a range of doses over a range of times, nurses tend to give the smallest dose over the longest time.

The primary inhibitory factor is couched in the belief by the nurse that he or she is in the best position to determine pain medication needs. However, studies have shown that nurses routinely underestimate the amount of pain being experienced. Since there is no objective indicator of pain, the only one who can determine pain medication needs is the client. We as nurses have been uncomfortable with this situation because we have been taught to treat medication-seeking behavior as a sign of addiction. The problem is particularly severe when medications are ordered on a PRN basis. We have typically interpreted the order as "when the client asks for medication." When the client does ask, our fears about addictive personalities surface and the client is seen as medication-seeking and may be labeled as a potential addict. The situation is especially severe when the client is young or belongs to a social or ethnic group devalued by the nurse.

Remember, *asking for nonscheduled medications is often the only means provided clients to obtain pain medications.* In most cases, the request is based on need for pain relief and nothing else. Clients must be valued and believed in order to receive adequate pain relief. The PRN system also deprives the client of the ability to control the situation. Lack of control over pain experiences increases the pain endured during the episode. The pain may be worsened by anxiety about whether you will give the next dose in time to prevent the return of severe pain.

Intermittent dosing, such as occurs with PRN medication orders, causes wide swings in the client's blood levels of the analgesic, which may result in sedation following one dose and unacceptable pain levels preceding the next dose. PRN dosing leads to a "hill and valley" pattern of pain relief. Clients receive a dose of medication sufficient to produce adequate pain relief. They are then expected to wait until the pain is again intense before asking for the subsequent dose.

We have been encouraged by values germane to our work environment to encourage clients to hold out as long as they can so as not to risk addition and undesirable side effects. The hill and valley approach requires that each succeeding dose be maximum strength to bring the client's blood level back to a therapeutic level. Pain relief is more efficiently and effectively achieved if the valleys are avoided. If the PRN schedule is to be maintained, clients need to be encouraged to request pain medication when their pain begins to return. This problem is lessened if we can offer PRN medications on a regular, scheduled basis for clients with acute pain. If the medication is administered regularly, by the clock, pain relief is enhanced.

Patient-Controlled Analgesia

Patient-controlled analgesia (PCA) entails use of an IV or SC infusion pump that contains the analgesic and that is controlled by the client. A bolus dose may be given at the onset of PCA use to provide immediate pain relief. The client can then self-administer subsequent doses by pressing a button that releases a preset dose delivered intravenously. The pumps are programmed to deliver preset demand doses of analgesic until a maximum dose is reached. Then there is a minimal interval during which no further analgesic can be administered (i.e., a lock-out period). With this system, clients control the administration of their own pain medication within the limits prescribed by the physician.

There are many advantages to PCA:

1. The client usually reports good pain control.
2. PCA helps to relieve the client's anxiety about waiting for the nurse to administer the medication, thereby lowering the dose needed to relieve pain.
3. PCA promotes the client's independence and control over the situation.
4. Clients administer lower doses of opioids compared with traditional PRN formats.
5. Clients can adjust their analgesic doses to a near-constant blood concentration.
6. Clients report superior analgesia with a lower incidence of side effects compared with the traditional nurse-administered method.
7. As the pain lessens, clients adjust themselves to lower doses and eventually stop taking the analgesic.

Some problems are associated with PCA. Some clients complain of inadequate analgesia at night, requiring frequent wakening to redose themselves. At some institutions, a basal rate is added at night by continuous delivery at a low but constant dose through the PCA pump to avoid this situation. The success of this method depends on your understanding of the system and on how well the client is taught to use it. Failure can often be traced to a poor understanding on the part of the client, the nurse, or both.

ORAL ROUTE. Oral (PO) dosing is usually preferred. It is noninvasive, convenient, and cost-effective and allows for the greatest flexibility in medication choices. Oral preparations may be in tablet, capsule, liquid, or sublingual forms. Some tablet preparations can be crushed and added to suspensions (e.g., to applesauce) that are more easily swallowed. Oral opioids are available in immediate and sustained-release forms. Sustained-release medications are constructed to be degraded slowly in the gastrointestinal system and must not be crushed or modified. The entire dose will be released at one time if the integrity of the tablet is compromised. The peak effect of oral medications is 1½ to 2 hours for immediate-release preparations. Availability of the medication is delayed until the tablet is degraded and the medication is absorbed, passed through the liver, and made available to the circulatory system.

INTRAMUSCULAR ROUTE. IM dosing is common but is the least desirable route and should be avoided. IM injections are painful, and some people find the injections so objectionable that they are reluctant to seek relief for their pain if the medications are to be administered this way. Additional disadvantages include wide variability and unreliable absorption from muscle and subcutaneous tissues. Peak effects occur within 30 to 60 minutes and are accompanied by a rapid "fall-off" of medication effectiveness. Additional side effects of IM injections include trauma-induced fibrosis of muscle and soft tissues, nerve damage from chemical injury, and development of sterile abscesses.[4]

INTRAVENOUS ROUTE. IV dosing provides the most rapid pain relief. Medications may be provided in bolus doses or by continuous infusions. Bolus doses are given in one administration and provide the most rapid onset of pain relief. Bolus fentanyl reaches peak effect in 1 to 5 minutes, morphine in 15 to 20 minutes.[4] Continuous infusion provides a steady delivery of IV pain medication. It is usually preferred because plasma levels of the medication are maintained and the occurrence of side effects is lessened. Bolus doses may be needed is pain relief falls below acceptable levels with continuous infusion. The infusion dose may then need to be increased to maintain adequate relief.

RECTAL ROUTE. Rectal suppositories provide an alternative route to parenteral administration for people unable to take oral medications. They are provided in doses similar to those of oral preparations. Medications appropriate for the rectal route include morphine, hydromorphone (Dilaudid), oxycodone (Percocet), methadone, and oxymorphone (Numorphan).

TRANSDERMAL ROUTE. Transdermal analgesia is provided by means of a skin patch. The most common opioid administered transdermally is fentanyl, which is very potent. It is available in a variable-dosing transdermal application system that the client or family member can apply independently. The patch is designed to deliver specified amounts of medication over 48 to 72 hours. This system provides an easy means of maintaining independence and avoids the inconveniences of frequent dosing.

Analgesia from the first application may take up to 24 hours to reach an adequate blood level. During this period, supplemental analgesia is maintained. The patch is typically applied to clean, dry skin on the chest or upper back. These areas are less vulnerable to dislodgment of the patch compared with other areas. The patch may be applied to any convenient location with intact skin as long as the client can protect it. Excessive hair should be carefully clipped before application. The patch should not be applied over irritated or broken skin. The patch is left in place for up to 72 hours, when it is removed. A new patch is applied at a different site to prevent skin irritation.

TRANSMUCOSAL ANALGESIA. Transmucosal analgesia is achieved either sublingually (methadone and buprenorphine (Buprenex) or by means of a lozenge (Oralet) or a lollipop (Actiq). The transmucosal route is particularly effective for breakthrough pain in clients with scheduled opioid medications around the clock. Up to two thirds of clients with chronic or malignant pain who are treated around the clock with opioids have episodes of breakthrough pain.[95]

CONTINUOUS SUBCUTANEOUS ANALGESIA. Pain relief is achieved through an infusion setup using a pump device. A 25- or 27-gauge needle is used, or a special SC needle device can be implanted subcutaneously. The client wears a medication reservoir that can be refilled as needed. The needle site is rotated every 3 to 7 days according to the type and volume of medication administered. The volume delivered ranges from 2 to 4 ml/h.

Observe the site for redness, excessive swelling, leakage of fluid around the infusion site, or edema. If an extremity is used, carefully assess it for the presence of edema, which interferes with absorption of the medication. Closely monitor the client for adequacy of analgesic effect. If the medication is ineffective and sufficient medication is available in the reservoir, a higher concentration may be required.

INTRASPINAL ANALGESIA. Opioids are injected intrathecally or epidurally. The epidural space is outside the dura mater of the spinal cord and brain; the intrathecal space is inside the dura mater and contains the spinal fluid. The dorsal horns of the spinal cord contain receptors for endogenous opioid substances. By means of the intraspinal analgesia route, medication is delivered directly into the areas with the intended receptor sites. These receptors bind opioids and provide excellent pain relief of long duration (8 to 24 hours) without causing sympathetic and motor nerve blockade. Relatively small doses provide high opioid concentrations in the spinal fluid that bathes the dorsal columns. These concentrations are far higher than those in the spinal fluid after similar doses given by standard parenteral routes.

Repeated bolus doses, PCA, or a constant infusion via an implanted refillable infusion pump of the opioid may be given through a small catheter placed in the epidural or intrathecal space. Catheters have been left in place for days to months without adverse effects.

Possible side effects include pruritus, urinary retention, and delayed respiratory depression occurring 6 to 12 hours after a dose. Low doses of naloxone may reverse these side effects without reducing analgesia.

Nerve Blocks. Neuroblockade is achieved through injection of various substances (e.g., local anesthetics) close to the nerves, thereby blocking their conductivity. Blockade may be used to produce a complete, reversible interruption of nerve pathways for the following purposes:

- To eliminate a local focus of pain-producing stimulation or nervous irritation
- To interrupt the perception of pain, either at the source of the pain or anywhere along the peripheral afferent neurons
- To interrupt reflex mechanisms that are maintaining abnormal activity in blood vessels, glands, or skeletal or smooth muscle
- To eliminate reflex responses to pain (e.g., tachycardia, hypertension) by directly infiltrating skeletal muscle and other involved structures

Irreversible nerve-blocking procedures, which permanently block the pain pathway, are often used in managing pain associated with cancer. The effect of the block may be short-lived, however. The nerves may regenerate to some extent, with an associated return of sensory and motor functions.

Nerve blocks given for pain relief are called *analgesic blocks*. The analgesia is generally produced by injection of a local anesthetic agent. The anesthetic agent relieves pain and thus allows treatment that might otherwise be extremely uncomfortable, such as manipulation of a painful joint or wound debridement. Sometimes, by interrupting reflexes that are causing sustained pain, analgesic blocks can produce a beneficial effect that is prolonged beyond the effective duration of the agent injected.

Analgesic blocks are useful in various acute and chronic disorders. They often reduce the amounts of analgesic medication that might otherwise be needed. Injecting local anesthetics into tender points of muscle or skin (*trigger point injection*) causes a type of analgesic block that may modify pain and break the pain cycle, allowing manipulation and stretching of a joint. However, the pain may not be permanently eliminated unless the primary afferent impulses are either chemically or surgically terminated or until the underlying pathologic condition causing the pain is corrected.

■ NEGATIVE EFFECTS OF PAIN

A barrier to adequate pain management has been the belief that pain, while uncomfortable, has few negative physiologic effects. Unrelieved pain can affect the major organ systems—pulmonary, cardiovascular, gastrointestinal, endocrine, and immune. Unrelieved pain has resulted in untoward effects that have resulted in increased costs that affect all of society. Costs are increased because of longer hospital stays, the need to treat the negative effects of pain, and the client's loss of productivity. Pain prevents coughing, deep breathing, and sighing, leading to pulmonary complications with significant morbidity and mortality. Pain may also prevent ambulation, contributing to the development of deep vein thrombosis and potential pulmonary emboli. Pain of any type induces release of catecholamines and stress hormones. Cardiovascular complications (tachycardia, hypertension) and decreased immune activity may result.

Reflex muscle contraction may be enhanced, resulting in increased muscle tension and spasm. Abdominal wall muscle tension and spasm reduce the ability of the chest wall to expand. As a result, clients take short, shallow, frequent breaths. Oxygen and carbon dioxide exchange is less effective with this breathing pattern. Vital capacity has been reported to fall to 40% of presurgery capacity when pain was not relieved and to only 70% of presurgery values when pain was totally relieved. Although respiratory depression in response to opioids is rare, hypoventilation resulting from untreated pain is not.

Intestinal and bladder smooth muscle tone is affected such that peristalsis and bladder motility are decreased. Bowel and bladder distention may result. The decreased motility of the bowel contributes to constipation. If distention is severe enough, the abdominal contents may interfere with the ability of the diaphragm to expand. It appears as though constipation may be a complication of either opioid administration or unrelieved pain. Given the negative effects of pain, it is better to give the opioid and treat the constipation.

Catecholamine secretion in response to pain leads to increased myocardial oxygen demand and consumption. Clients with atherosclerosis may be impaired to the point of myocardial ischemia, dysrhythmias, infarction, cardiac failure, and death. Unfortunately, the elderly population—at greatest risk for atherosclerotic vascular changes—are at greatest risk for receiving inadequate pain relief. On the basis of the negative effects of pain, a reasonable goal of pain management programs is the total relief of pain.

NONPHARMACEUTICAL INTERVENTIONS

Activities such as cutaneous stimulation, acupuncture, acupressure, massage, listening to music, progressive relaxation, guided imagery, rhythmic breathing, meditation, hypnosis, humor, biofeedback, Therapeutic Touch, distraction, and magnets have been used clinically with positive results. The therapies are thought to cause physiologic changes. For example, peripheral blood vessels may be dilated, muscle tension is decreased, the immune systems is strengthened, and brain chemicals are activated or modified. Techniques such as these can be used to manage pain and to promote healthy living. It may be possible to teach clients a combination of these techniques to maximize their opportunities for self-control over manifestations of pain. Figure 23–15 presents modalities for pain relief.

■ CUTANEOUS STIMULATION

Cutaneous stimulation activates the large-diameter (A-beta) fibers, which stimulate inhibitory neurons in the spinal cord and engage the descending analgesic system. Pain relief is achieved by endogenous opiate activity.

Cutaneous stimulation can decrease the intensity of pain the client perceives and, in some instances, may eliminate it.[76, 83] It also can help in changing the sensation in a painful or noxious area to a more pleasant sensation, such as warmth. This process may also be seen as a form

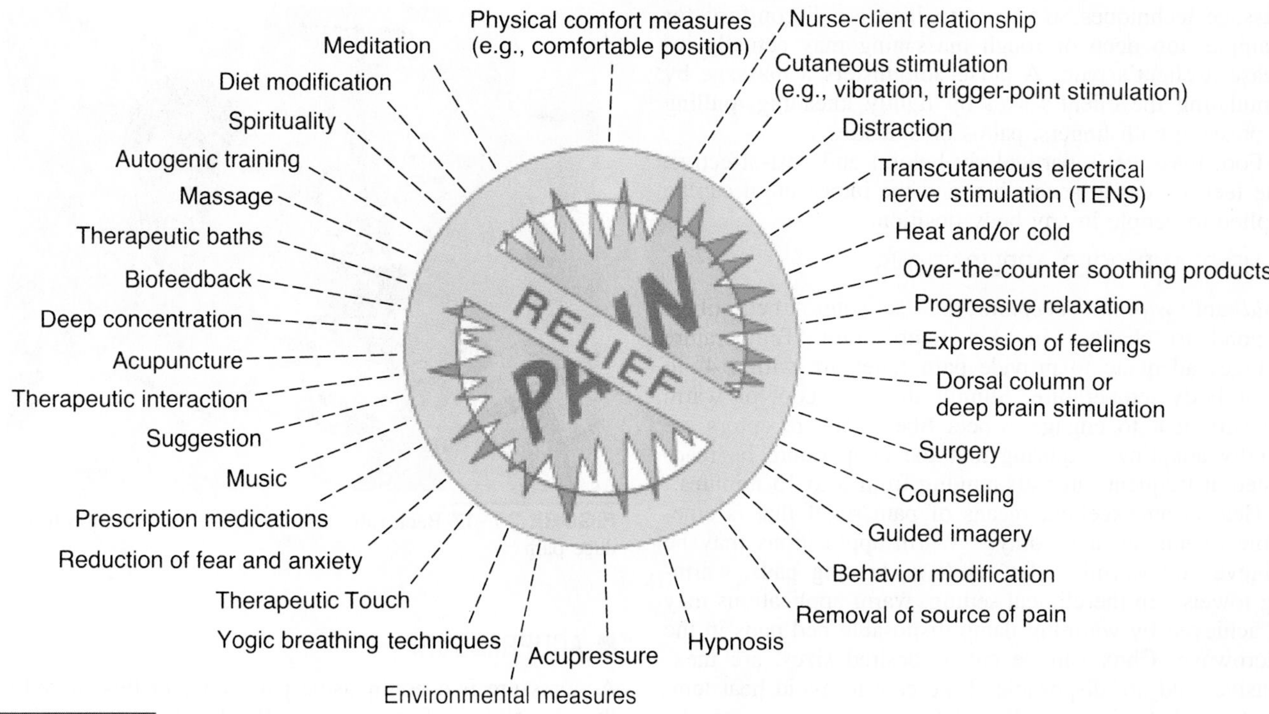

FIGURE 23–15 Pain relief measures.

of distraction because the client may focus on the sensation being created rather than the pain. Cutaneous stimulation can be applied to the unaffected side and still elicit positive benefits because the stimulated fibers cross within the spinal cord. This method is particularly useful when an area is too painful to be directly stimulated, as with burns.

■ TRANSCUTANEOUS ELECTRICAL NERVE STIMULATION (TENS)

TENS delivers electrical bursts through the skin to superficial and deep nerves. TENS is used most often for clients with chronic pain, such as muscle pain from arthritis.

TENS has been shown to relieve pain effectively in many people.[133] Success with TENS depends on the client's understanding of, interest in, and motivation to use the apparatus as well as the clinician's skillfulness in applying the device. The client needs to learn to adjust placement of the surface electrodes and the intensity and timing of the stimuli to maximize pain relief (Fig. 23–16). Involve significant others as appropriate in learning and teaching sessions. The client may need their help in applying the electrodes to areas that are difficult to reach. Electrode placement depends on the site of the pain. Positive and negative poles are usually placed within several inches of each other. Voltage and pulsation are controlled by the person wearing the device. Battery packs make the device portable.

■ MASSAGE

Massage may be effective when applied to various sites. A back rub is a good method of providing cutaneous stimulation (Fig. 23–17). It is particularly relaxing at bedtime and may block pain so as to promote more comfortable sleep. However, you should be knowledgeable in

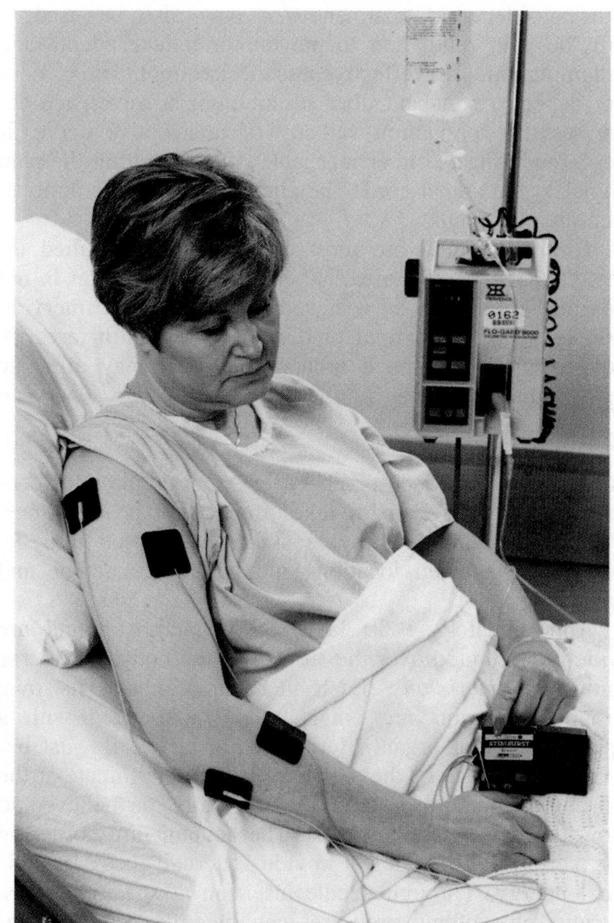

FIGURE 23–16 Surface patches are used for transcutaneous electrical nerve stimulation (TENS) treatment.

massage techniques so as not to increase discomfort; for example, too deep or rough massaging may actually increase a client's pain. A nurse administers a massage by stimulating the client's skin by lightly kneading, pulling or pressing with fingers, palms or knuckles.

Foot massage is particularly helpful and cost-effective. The feet are easily accessible, and the intervention can be applied to people in any body position.

HEAT AND COLD APPLICATIONS

Cold and *warmth receptors* that activate A-beta fibers respond to changes in skin temperature. Temperature changes adequate to provide pain relief are within 4° to 5° of body temperature. Stimuli that feel cool or warm are sufficient to engage A-beta fibers. The receptors are rapidly adapting, requiring that the temperature be readjusted at frequent intervals ranging from 5 to 15 minutes.

Heat is an excellent means of pain relief that is amenable to nursing autonomy.[80] Warm applications may be achieved by warming devices (e.g., heating pads, warming towels). In the clinical setting, warm applications may be achieved by warming damp disposable bed pads in the microwave. Chux can be cut to desired sizes, are inexpensive, and are disposable. Take care to avoid heat temperatures that will burn. Remember, painful areas may be hypersensitive to skin stimuli. Heat temperatures that are typically perceived as nonpainful may become painful when applied to the sensitive area.

Cold application also brings pain relief,[81] and nurses can consider this treatment. *Ice* may also be used to provide pain relief and to prevent or reduce edema and inflammation. The effectiveness of ice applications does not depend on A-beta fiber stimulation; however, ice decreases the conduction velocity of nociceptive nerve fibers, rendering the fiber incapable of transmitting the pain signal to the spinal cord. The client perceives the application area as numb.

Thermal stimuli are most effective when applied directly to the painful area. When direct application is not possible, relief may be achieved by applying the intervention to a point proximal or distal to the painful area. A cold compress wrapped around the wrist may alleviate pain in the hand.

ACUPUNCTURE

Acupuncture has been practiced in Asian cultures for centuries and produces pain relief in modern health care.[39] Very thin metal needles are skillfully inserted into the body at designated locations and at various depths and angles.

Approximately 1000 known acupuncture points are widely distributed over the surface of the body in patterns known as *meridians*. Each meridian contains its own group of acupuncture points and is associated with a specific visceral organ. Meridians run bilaterally just beneath the surface of the skin and begin or terminate at the tips of the fingers or toes. "Vital energy" is believed to flow through these meridians. The acupuncture points on the surface of the body provide external access to this vital energy. Through needle insertion at specific points, various physiologic processes can be influenced or controlled and are determined by the specific pathologic condition and the desired physiologic effect.

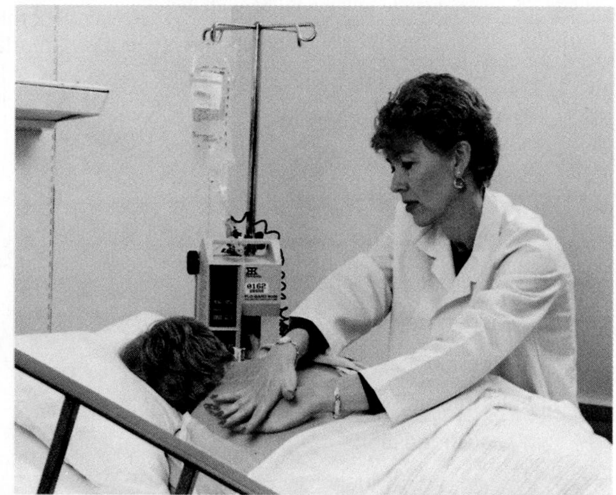

FIGURE 23–17 Back rub provides cutaneous sensation to reduce pain.

ACUPRESSURE

Acupressure is a noninvasive pain relief method based on the principles of acupuncture.[66] Pressure, massage, or other cutaneous stimulation, such as heat or cold, is applied over acupuncture points.

MUSIC

Music has been used to relieve pain in a number of settings.[11, 48, 49, 50, 53, 118, 125] The exact physiologic mechanisms have not been determined; however, several possible theories include distraction, release of endogenous opioids, or disassociation. All three mechanisms are probably involved. Music clearly provides distraction and disassociation by focusing on the characteristics of the musical selection. The auditory pathway interacts with endogenous opiate systems at several foci within the brain, including the hypothalamus and the limbic system. These areas are known to project to PAG/PVG, providing a mechanism to contribute to pain relief through both cerebral activity and spinal cord responses mediated by descending fibers from nucleus raphe and locus ceruleus.

People in pain may find music to be relaxing. Pain relief may also be achieved through physiologic responses to relaxation. The relaxation response is mediated through the hypothalamus.

When using music for pain relief, allow clients to choose the type of music most suited to them. Some people find the use of a radio, cassette, or compact disc players with headphones a quiet way to listen to music without bothering others. This allows the client to increase the music volume or to play it softly. Encourage the family members to bring in the client's favorite selections. This also gives the family a sense of doing something to help.

PROGRESSIVE RELAXATION TRAINING

Progressive relaxation training is used to treat various physical and psychosocial problems, including pain.[8, 85] The client is taught to gradually tighten, then deeply relax, various muscle groups, proceeding systematically from one area of the body to the next. The deep relaxation produced by this method can decrease anxiety and excessive muscle contraction and promote the onset of sleep. Audiotape cassettes are available.

■ DEEP BREATHING FOR RELAXATION

Deep breathing for relaxation is easy to learn and contributes to pain relief by reducing muscle tension and anxiety.[75] First, the client clenches the fists while taking a deep breath. The client then holds his or her breath for a moment, and exhales while letting oneself "go limp." The cycle is followed by a slow, deep breath mimicking a yawn.

■ GUIDED IMAGERY

Guided imagery helps a client to visualize a pleasant experience. The client is coached to visualize a scene (e.g., relaxing on a beach). The coach instructs the client to imagine the sensory aspects of the scene, the sounds, sights, and emotions expressed. The more vivid the image, the more effective the intervention. Visualization may be combined with soft, lyrical, relaxing music. Audiotapes for guided imagery are available.

Imagery relieves pain through several mechanisms.[121] It is a way to help people distract themselves from their pain, which may increase their pain tolerance. Imagery may also produce a relaxation response, thus relieving pain. Last, the image can be a healing one, designed not only to relieve the pain but possibly to diminish the source of the pain,[116] (e.g., a tension headache may be alleviated).

Imagery is often combined with relaxation and biofeedback to produce a multifocal pain relief technique. The image used in this technique can be a complex scene that requires the person to think of each detail. This image would increase distraction. The image might be a relaxing scene, such as a beach or meadow, which would help with the relaxation response, or the image might consist of visualizing the pain being worn away until it is so small that it can be "blown away." When introducing an image setting, ask the client what setting is relaxing for him or her. Avoid using an image that may provoke anxiety, such as using a beach for someone who is afraid of water or a meadow for someone with severe allergies to pollen.

■ RHYTHMIC BREATHING

Rhythmic breathing is typically considered a method of both relaxation and distraction. It may also provide effective pain relief by stimulating baroreceptors in the atria and carotid sinuses. Stimulation of these receptors initiates activity in a neuropathway that sends projections to the periaqueductal and periventricular gray matter, resulting in opioid-mediated pain inhibition. This method can be combined with rhythms such as music, a ticking clock, or a metronome. Little concentration is necessary because once the individual begins the process, it takes on an automatic quality. This method focuses attention away from the pain and on the breathing and the rhythm. The Lamaze method of childbirth is a good example of a pain control method that incorporates this technique.

■ MEDITATION

Meditation focuses one's attention away from pain. It also provides energy and peace to the meditator. The client simply sits comfortably and quietly with focused attention. The focus may vary. Examples include flow of the breath, a mantra, and a picture or mental image of a great spiritual being or peaceful place. Sometimes the meditator communicates with a spiritual being. There are many meditation techniques, some with a spiritual base, such as Siddha meditation. Meditation is easily practiced anywhere, and no special equipment is required. The positive experiences available through meditation are available to anyone, including people in pain.

■ HYPNOSIS

A person's reaction to pain can be significantly altered by hypnosis. Hypnosis is based on suggestion, dissociation, and the process of focusing attention.[97, 98]

Various procedures may be used to relieve pain following induction of a hypnotic state including:

- Suggestion to alter the character of the pain or one's attitude toward it
- Body disorientation and dissociation
- Anesthesia and analgesia for superficial and deep sensation

In situations of chronic pain, a posthypnotic suggestion may be used in combination with *autohypnosis* (self-hypnosis) to provide prolonged relief. Many hypnotic subjects successfully learn to use deliberate spontaneous trance induction or autohypnosis.

Although hypnosis cannot change organic lesions that are producing pain, it can often reduce discomfort.[97, 98] The procedure itself is fairly simple and innocuous compared with the administration of many anesthetic and analgesic medications; however, take care not to probe any fears or unpleasant memories. A hypnotherapist must be skilled and informed and the client carefully selected to avoid negative effects. Increasingly nurses are being certified to provide clinical hypnotic therapies in the United States.

Hypnosis may be used as an adjunct to other pain-relieving therapies. Alteration of pain by hypnosis should be performed by those who are aware of the possible diagnostic implications of pain in the medical management of disease.

■ HUMOR

Research in the use of humor in the clinical setting has revealed that the intervention actually increases the number of NK (natural killer) cells of the immune system.[7, 17, 74] This is particularly important for implementation in clients with cancer. It has been postulated that humor elevates endogenous opioids or endorphins. Regardless of the physiologic advantages, use of humor simply makes people feel better, more relaxed, and in less pain. Clients may find some degree of pain relief by watching comedic videotapes, listening to audiotapes and compact discs they find funny or reading humorous books. You may want to suggest that hospitalized clients might bring humorous materials with them to utilize during their inpatient experience.

■ BIOFEEDBACK

Biofeedback refers to a wide variety of techniques that provide a client with information about changes in bodily functions of which the client is usually unaware, such as blood pressure. Biofeedback equipment provides immediate, continuous information. Some people learn to use this information to control previously involuntary functions. The purpose of biofeedback in pain management is to teach self-control over physiologic variables that relate to the pain, such as muscle contraction and blood flow.

Information used to reduce muscle contraction is obtained by an electromyogram (EMG) recorded from body surface electrodes. (Needle EMG electrodes are not used.) Changes in blood flow are produced by monitoring skin temperature, which increases with increased blood flow. Depending on the equipment used, clients can self-monitor their changes through *auditory displays* (decreases in muscle contractions are heard as decreases in the pitch of a tone) or *visual displays* (increases in skin temperature are seen as increases on a dial). The client tries to change the display of information in the desired direction, such as to reduce muscle contraction (relax muscle tension) and reduce blood flow. The continuous, precise information received shows the effectiveness of the effort and often helps the client learn physiologic control of these functions.[109]

Biofeedback can be performed at home with purchased or rented equipment under the guidance of a suitably prepared health care worker. Alternatively, it may be performed in an office or clinic setting with a biofeedback therapist or other specialist, such as a nurse trained in biofeedback. The equipment is expensive.

■ THERAPEUTIC TOUCH

Therapeutic Touch is a type of pain management that has been used for disorders such as tension headaches.[34, 56, 101] It is a derivative of the "laying on" of hands. The human body is believed to have energy fields that express aberrant patterns when body systems are insulted. Therapeutic Touch is thought to realign aberrant fields. Education and practice are required on the part of the nurse.

Therapeutic Touch involves three steps.

1. Become centered or focused in a meditative state. This helps you become aware of the vibrations in the surrounding energy fields.
2. Assess the client's energy field. Pass your hands over the client's body at a distance of 2 to 6 inches to sense changes in the field.
3. During the treatment step, use your hands to rearrange the client's energy field and return it to normal.

■ DISTRACTION

Cognitive strategies to modify pain perception have been effective in numerous research studies. The most effective cognitive strategy involves distraction. Attention is directed away from the painful sensation or the negative emotional arousal associated with the pain episode. The primary theoretical explanation is that a person is able to focus attention on a limited number of foci. Actively focusing attention on a cognitive task is thought to limit one's ability to attend to the noxious sensation.

To be effective, the distraction task requires considerable cognitive effort. Distraction exercises that are too easy rapidly become automatic or engage monotonous repetitive responses and are likely to be ineffective.

Interventions may be administered by a multitude of modalities that require the client to engage in highly focused interesting mental exercises. Typical techniques utilized in hospital settings include videotapes of favorite movies, audiotapes of favorite music, craft activities, and interacting with others. The distraction technique may be more effective if it involves action on the client's part. For example, listening to music and tapping one's fingers to the rhythm may be more effective than passive listening alone. Cognitive strategies need to be tailored to the client's personal preferences. Techniques used should be self-selected. People may want to bring their own tapes, videos, books, or craft items. If the items are supplied by an agency, a library of materials will be needed to allow clients to select what will be pleasing to them.

■ MAGNETS

Magnets have been used to relieve a variety of painful disorders.[90, 124] It is speculated that the pull of the magnet increases blood flow to the region, opening the Na^+ and Cl^- channels in the cells. Magnet therapy has been a mainstay in pain management in Eastern Asian countries and is gaining popularity in Western medicine.

EVALUATION AND DOCUMENTATION

■ EVALUATION

Evaluation is most effective when a formal evaluation protocol is used throughout a health care agency "across all stages of the disease and across all practice settings."[59] A formalized process within the institution provides a unified methodology that can be learned and used by every member of the health care team. According to the Clinical Practice Guidelines,[59] key items to consider include:

- Client satisfaction with pain management and its impact on their quality of life
- Satisfaction with pain management and its impact on their quality of life (particularly in chronic illness or when clients require home health care)
- The designation of who is responsible for pain management
- The systematic assessment of pain in all settings where people receive care
- The accuracy of diagnostic approaches for common pain syndromes
- The range and appropriateness of pain management options available within a particular practice setting
- The effectiveness of pain management options utilized to prevent and treat pain
- The prevalence and severity of side effects and complications associated with pain management
- The quality of pain management across points of transition in the provision of services

The effectiveness of pain management protocols needs to be evaluated frequently and throughout the course of treatment. Figure 23–18 illustrates a sample plan used to determine pain management needs for clients having sur-

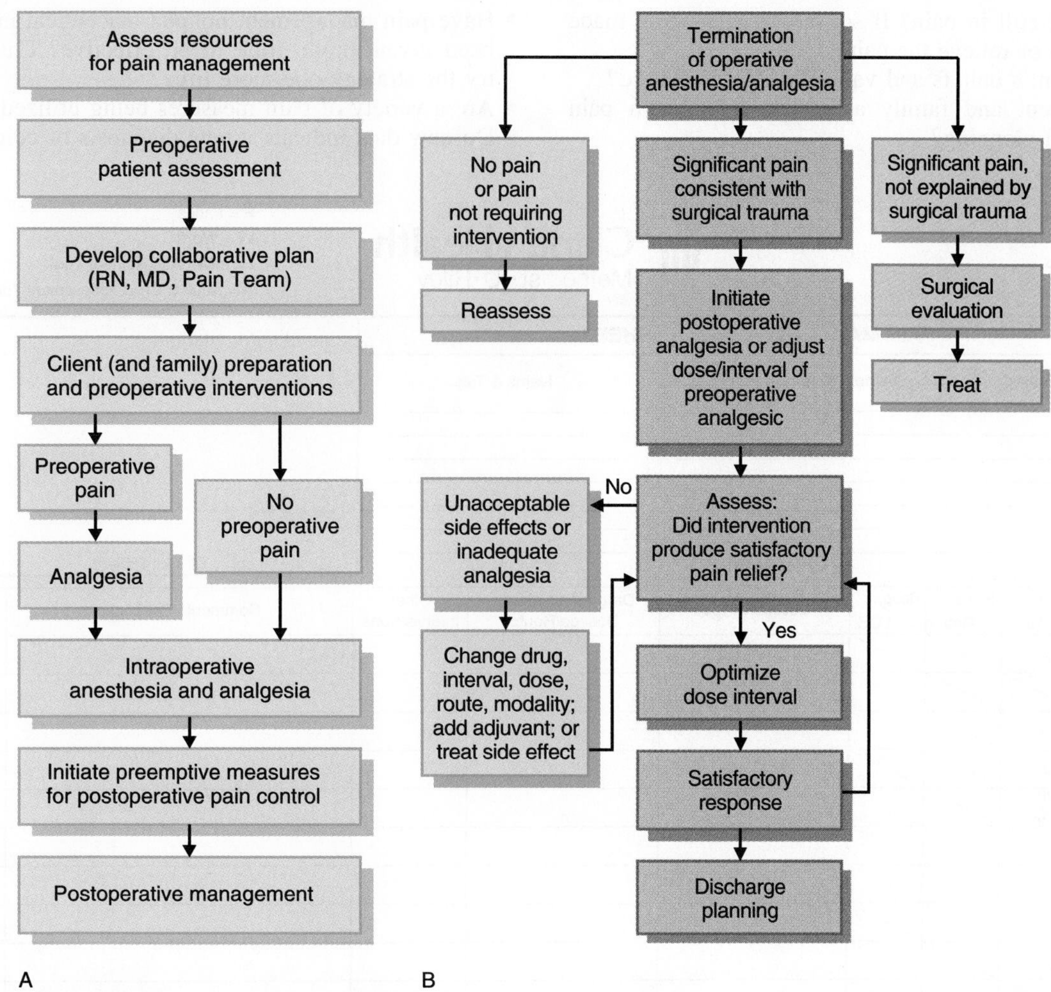

FIGURE 23–18 *A* and *B,* Pain treatment flow chart.

gery.[1] The example includes the three phases of a surgical experience (preoperative, intraoperative, and postoperative).

During an evaluation, both the process used to manage pain and the outcomes achieved are assessed. Assessment and evaluation are ongoing components of the plan. Remember, there are no objective indicators of a person's pain. The only means to determine pain intensity and associated emotional discomfort accurately is to ask the person. Sometimes direct measurement of a client's report of pain is not possible, and someone else must estimate pain by observation. These assessments may or may not be accurate. Ongoing evaluation of the effectiveness of pain management interventions is essential when the client is not verbal. The pain management strategy employed for the client is based on an interpretation of need. These clients cannot provide data regarding effectiveness of the strategy. The health care provider must ascertain whether the pain was indeed relieved by the intervention they selected.

Evaluation requires the identification of a standard against which practice process and outcomes can be compared.[59] For example, the health care provider consults with the client to determine the degree of pain relief desired by the client. An evaluation criterion will consider whether the desired outcome has been achieved. If the criterion is not met, the evaluation will try to determine the reason. Modifications in the pain management program may be needed to achieve the desired outcome. These modifications should be documented to allow for evaluation of outcomes achieved by the new interventions. Some institutions have employed a standard for all clients based on the knowledge that unrelieved pain has negative physical effects. For example, a standard may mandate that medication for pain be administered if a client reports a pain intensity of 3 or greater on an 11-point numerical scale.

While the primary focus of evaluation is directed toward effectiveness of management strategies for clients, it will also be necessary to periodically evaluate the treatment protocols incorporated into hospital procedure manuals and pain management standards accepted by the clinicians. As the knowledge base underlying practice interventions increases, the standard procedures for pain management may also need to change. Conducting periodic evaluation of practice, based on research, enhances the potential for providing the best care possible. A few questions to consider are as follows:

- Is the client still in pain? If so, is progress being made to minimize or relieve the pain?
- Are the client's beliefs and values being considered?
- Are the client and family active participants in pain management planning?
- Have pain management nonpharmaceutical interventions been given ample time to be effective? Can the client try the strategy one more time?
- Are a variety of pain measures being utilized?
- Do new data indicate a new diagnosis or complication?

MM#17986

3/97

Clarian Health
Methodist·IU·Riley

F = Faces
W = Word
I = Infant Assessment Tool
A = Adult & Child Assessment Tool

PAIN MANAGEMENT FLOW SHEET

Initials	Name & Title	Initials	Name & Title

☐ In-Patient ☐ Out-Patient

Date / Time	Scale / Rating	Resp. / LOS	Location/Type	Drug Administered Dosage/Route	Other Interventions	Comments/Response	Initials

LEVEL OF SEDATION	DEGREE OF SOMNOLENCE (Patient Awakens/Responds to:)
0	Caregiver entering room
1	Soft verbal stimulation
2	Loud Verbal Stimulation
3	Mild Physical Contact
4	Vigorous Physical Contact

Adapted from: Gwirtz, K.H. (1992). Single dose intrathecal opiods in the management of acute postoperative pain. In Sinatra, R., Hord, A., Ginsberg, R., & Preble, L. (Eds.). Acute Pain: Mechanisms and Management (pp.253-268). St. Louis: Mosby Publishing

INTERVENTIONS		COMMENTS EXAMPLES
R = repositioning	M = massage	diarrhea
F = feeding	CS = cutaneous stimulation	constipation
VS = verbal support	GI = guided imagery	depressed
HR = holding/rocking	MT = music therapy	crying
T = toileting/diapering	HA = hot application	vomiting
D = distraction	CA = cold application	nausea
A = adjust environment	SO = significant other present	anxious
E = emotional support	=	agitated
P = play	=	itching
S = sucking/pacifier	=	

19058

MEDICAL RECORDS COPY

PAIN MANAGEMENT FLOWSHEET W-37

B-CLIN. NOTES	E-LAB	G-X-RAY	K-DIAGNOSTIC	M-SURGERY	Q-THERAPY	T-ORDERS	W-NURSING	Y-MISC.

FIGURE 23–19 Pain management flow sheet. (Courtesy of Clarian Health Partners, Indianapolis.)

■ DOCUMENTATION

Data gathered through evaluation must be documented. Documentation data are to be recorded in a manner that makes the information available to all members of the health care team. This may be best done by means of a pain document record or flow sheet (Fig. 23–19) that allows visualization of the client's pain experience throughout a hospitalization experience and that can follow the client from one health care setting to another. The flow sheet should be entered into the client's permanent hospital record.

CONCLUSIONS

The most effective pain management program may depend on use of a combination of medications and nonpharmaceutical interventions. Clients may benefit from the incorporation of several nonpharmaceutical interventions utilized simultaneously. Research has supported the efficacy of numerous nonpharmaceutical techniques. These findings plus the wide variability in the strength and types of medications makes it possible (1) to design a pain program that can be individualized and (2) to modify a pain management protocol if one finds that a component of the program is ineffective. One ineffective strategy can be replaced by another until a successful combination of treatments is determined.

The variety of potential treatments also benefits clients for whom progression of the pain experience is a component. The protocol can be modified to meet changing needs when the pain increases or abates. Box 23–2 summarizes possible interventions posited by the Clinical Practice Guidelines for Management of Cancer Pain and Pain due to Trauma, Surgery, and Painful Procedures.[59]

THINKING CRITICALLY

1. A 33-year-old woman, Miss Brown, arrives in the emergency department with a severe headache. She has vomited twice. She states, "This is the worst headache I have ever had." The headache has lasted for about 6 hours, and two doses of acetaminophen have given no relief. Miss Brown cannot lift her head off of the pillow and cannot position herself for comfort. Her pupils are equal, and there is no diaphoresis. What further nursing history and assessments should be done? How soon can medication to alleviate the headache be administered?

Factors to Consider. How crucial is a thorough pain assessment? How can a migraine headache mimic manifestations of a cerebral disorder? Would it be advisable to delay giving analgesia? Why? Why not?

2. A 80-year-old client, Mrs. Parker, is terminally ill with cancer. An opiate analgesic has been prescribed for her pain. She is being cared for at home by family members who are concerned about pain control for their loved one. What should the client and family be taught about complications associated with use of opiate analgesia? Who would be the ideal client to assess and coordinate the client's response to dosing of a particular opiate or combination of opiate and non-opiate medications?

Factors to Consider. What complications are associated with use of opiate analgesia? What factors contribute to the dosing schedule of a client with cancer-related pain? How much control over analgesia is given to the client? How should the caregiver and family monitor the response of the individual to the prescribed medication regimen?

BIBLIOGRAPHY

1. Acute Pain Management Guideline Panel. (1992). *Acute pain management in adults: Operative procedures. Quick reference guide for clinicians.* AHCPR Publ. No. 92-0019. Rockville, MD: Agency for Health Care Policy and Research, Public Health Service, U.S. Department of Health and Human Services.
2. Ader, R. W. (1997). The role of conditioning in pharmacotherapies: The placebo effect? *Proceedings of the American Pain Society, 16th* Annual Scientific Meeting, New Orleans, p. 53.
3. Akil, H., et al. (1998). Endogenous opioids: Overview and current issues. *Drug and Alcohol Dependence, 51*(1–2), 127–140.
4. Albers, R. W., & Siegal, G. J. (1999). Membrane transport. In G. J. Siegal, et al. (Eds.), *Basic neurochemistry: Molecular, cellular, and medical aspects* (6th ed., pp. 95–118). Philadelphia: Lippincott–Williams & Wilkins.
5. American Pain Society. (1999). *Principles of analgesic use in the treatment of acute pain and cancer pain* (4th ed.). Skokie, IL: Author.
6. Anand, K. J. S. (1998). Clinical importance of pain and stress in preterm neonates. *Biology of the Neonate, 73,* 1–9.
7. Anderson, D. L. (1997). Nurses: act now. *Journal of Practical Nursing 47*(1), 16–18.
8. Atsberger, D. B. (1995). Relaxation therapy: Its potential as an intervention for acute postoperative pain. *Journal of Post Anesthesia Nursing, 10*(1), 2–8.
9. Basbaum, A. I., & Jessell, T. (2000). The perception of pain. In E. R. Kandel, J. H. Schwartz, & T. M. Jessell (Eds.), *Principles of neural science* (4th ed., pp. 441–429). Norwalk, CT: Appleton & Lange.
10. Bates, M. S., Rankin-Hill, L., & Sanchez-Ayendez, M. (1997). The effects of the cultural context of health care on treatment of and response to chronic pain and illness. *Social Science and Medicine, 45*(9), 1433–1447.
11. Beck, S. L. (1991). The therapeutic use of music for cancer related pain. *Oncology Nursing Forum, 18,* 1327–1337.
12. Bennett, G. J. (2000). Update on the neurophysiology of pain transmission and modulation: Focus on the NMDA receptor. *Journal of Pain and Symptom Management, 19*(1 suppl), 52–56.
13. Berkley, K. J. (1997). Sex differences and pain. *Behavioral and Brain Sciences 30*(3), 371–380, 435–513.
14. Berkley, K. J., & Holdcroft, A. (1999). Sex and gender differences in pain. In P. D. Wall & R. Melzack (Eds.), *Textbook of pain* (4th ed., pp. 951–965). Edinburgh: Churchill Livingstone.
15. Bevan, S. (1999). Nociceptive peripheral neurons: Cellular properties. In P. D. Wall & R. Melzack (Eds.), *Textbook of pain* (4th ed., pp. 85–104). Edinburgh: Churchill Livingstone.
16. Bonica, J. J. (1990), *The management of pain* (Vols. 1 and 2, 2nd ed.). Philadelphia: Lea & Febiger.
17. Botterff, J., Gogag, M., & Engelberg-Lotzkar, M. (1995). Comforting: Exploring the work of cancer nursing. *Journal of Advanced Nursing, 22,* 1077–1084.
18. Brander, B., et al. (1997). Evaluation of the contribution to postoperative analgesia by local cooling of the wound. *Anesthesia, 51*(11), 1021–1025.
19. Breitbart, W., Passik, S. D., & Rosenfield, B. D. (1999). Cancer, mind and spirit. In P. D. Wall & R. Melzack (Eds.), *Textbook of pain* (4th ed., pp. 1065–1112). Edinburgh: Churchill Livingstone.
20. Breitbart, W., et al. (1996). The undertreatment of pain in ambulatory AIDS clients. *Pain, 65,* 243–249.

21. Brune, K., & Zeilhoffer, H. U. (1999). Antipyretic (non-narcotic) analgesics. In P. D. Wall & R. Melzack (Eds.), *Textbook of pain* (4th ed., pp. 1139–1153). Edinburgh: Churchill Livingstone.
22. Calvillo, E. R., & Flaskerud, J. H. (1991). Review of literature on culture and pain of adults with focus of Mexican-Americans. *Journal of Transcultural Nursing, 2,* 16–23.
23. Cao, Y. Q., et al. (1998). Primary afferent tachykinins are required to experience moderate to severe pain. *Nature, 392,* 390–394.
24. Cashman, J., & McAnulty, G. (1995). Nonsteroidal anti-inflammatory drugs in perisurgical pain management: Mechanisms of action and rationale for optimum use. *Drugs, 49,* 51–70.
25. Chapman, C. R. (1998). Psychological interventions for pain: Potential mechanisms. In R. Payne, et al. (Eds.), *Assessment and treatment of cancer pain: Progress in pain research and management* (Vol. 12, pp. 109–131). Seattle: IASP Press.
26. Cleeland, C. S., et al. (1997). Pain and treatment of pain in minority patients with cancer: The Eastern Cooperative Oncology Group minority outpatient pain study. *Annals of Internal Medicine, 127,* 813–816.
27. Cousins, M., & Power, I. (1999). Acute and postoperative pain. In P. D. Wall & R. Melzack (Eds.), *Textbook of pain* (4th ed., p. 447). Edinburgh: Churchill Livingstone.
28. Craig, A. D., & Dostrovsky, J. O. (1999). Medulla to thalamus. In P. D. Wall & R. Melzack (Eds.), *Textbook of pain* (4th ed., pp. 183–214). Edinburgh: Churchill Livingstone.
29. Craig, K. D. (1999). Emotions and psychobiology. In P. D. Wall & R. Melzack (Eds.), *Textbook of pain* (4th ed., pp. 331–343). Edinburgh: Churchill Livingstone.
30. Doubell, T. P., Mannion, R. J., & Woolf, C. J. (1999). The dorsal horn: State-dependent sensory processing, plasticity and the generation of pain. In P. D. Wall & R. Melzack (Eds.), *Textbook of pain* (4th ed., pp. 165–182). Edinburgh: Churchill Livingstone.
31. Dray, A. (1997). Kinins and their receptors in hyperalgesia. *Canadian Journal of Pharmacology, 75,* 704–712.
32. Dray, A., & Urban, L. (1996). New pharmacological strategies for pain relief. *Annual Review of Pharmacological Toxicology, 36,* 3–80.
33. Dyck, P. J., et al. (1997). Intradermal recombinant human nerve growth factor induces pressure allodynia and lowered heat-pain threshold in humans. *Neurology 48*(2), 501–505.
34. Eckes Peck, S. D. (1997). The effect of therapeutic touch for decreasing pain in elders with degenerative arthritis. *Journal of Holistic Nursing, 15,* 176–198.
35. Edwards, M. (1998, March/April). Barriers to effective pain/symptom control. *American Journal of Hospice and Palliative Care, 15*(2), 107–111.
36. Edwards, R. R., Fillingim, R. B., & Roger, B. (1999). Ethnic differences in thermal pain responses. *Psychosomatic Medicine, 61*(3), 346–354.
37. Ellermeier, W., & Westphal, W. (1995). Gender differences in pain ratings and pupil reactions to painful pressure stimuli. *Pain, 61,* 435–439.
38. Fields, H. L., & Basbaum, A. I. (1994). Central nervous system mechanisms of pain modulation. In P. Wall & R. Melzack (Eds.), *Textbook of pain* (3rd ed., pp. 243–257). New York: Churchill Livingstone.
39. Filshie, J., et al. (1996). Acupuncture for the relief of cancer-related breathlessness. *Palliative Medicine, 10*(2), 145–150.
40. Fine, P. G., & Ashburn, M. A. (1998). Functional neuroanatomy and nociception. In M. A. Ashburn and L. J. Rice (Eds.), *The Management of Pain* (pp. 1–16). New York: Churchill Livingstone.
41. Foley, K. M. (1995). Pain relief into practice: Rhetoric without reform. *Journal of Clinical Oncology, 13,* 2149–2151.
42. Furst, S. (1999). Transmitters involved in antinociception in the spinal cord. *Brain Research Bulletin, 48*(2), 129–141.
43. Gagliese, L., Katz, J., & Melzack, R. (1999). Pain in the elderly. In P. D. Wall & R. Melzack (Eds.), *Textbook of pain* (4th ed., pp. 991–1006). Edinburgh: Churchill Livingstone.
44. Gardner, E. P., & Martin, J. H. (2000). Coding of sensory information. In E. R. Kandel, J. H. Schwartz, & T. M. Jessell (Eds.), *Principles of neural science* (4th ed.). Norwalk, CT: Appleton & Lange.
45. Garro, L. C. (1990). Culture, pain and cancer. *Journal of Palliative Care, 6*(3), 34–44.
46. Geiss, G. S., et al. (1998). Safety and efficacy of celecoxib, a specific COX-2 inhibitor. *Rheumatology Europe 27(suppl 1),* 118.
47. Geis, G. S. (1999) Update on clinical developments with celecoxib, a new specific COX-2 inhibitor: What can we expect? *Journal of Rheumatology, 26*(Suppl 56), 31–36.
48. Gerdner, L. A., & Buckwalter, K. C. (1999). Music therapy. In G. M. Bulecheck & J. C. McCloskey (Eds.), *Nursing interventions: Effective nursing treatments* (3rd ed., pp. 451–468). Philadelphia: W. B. Saunders.
49. Good, M. (1995). A comparison of the effects of jaw relaxation and music on postoperative pain. *Nursing Symptom Management, 11*(4), 52–57.
50. Good, M. (1996). Effects of relaxation and music on postoperative pain: A review. *Journal of Advanced Nursing, 24,* 905–914.
51. Hawkey, C. J. (1999). COX-2 inhibitors. *The Lancet, 353,* 307–314.
52. Hawthorn, J., & Redmond, K. (1998). *Pain, causes and management.* Oxford, England, Blackwell Science.
53. Heitz, L., Symreng, T., & Scamman, F. L. (1992). Effect of music therapy in the postanesthetic care unit: A nursing intervention. *Journal of Post Anesthesia Nursing, 7,* 22–31.
54. Hille, B., & Catterall, W. A. (1999). Electrical excitability and ion channels. In G. J. Siegal, et al. (Eds.), *Basic neurochemistry: Molecular, cellular, and medical aspects,* (6th ed., pp. 119–138). Philadelphia: Lippincott–Williams & Wilkins.
55. Holz, R. W., & Fisher, S. K. (1999). Synaptic transmission and cellular signaling: An overview. In G. J. Siegal, et al. (Eds.), *Basic neurochemistry: Molecular, cellular and medical aspects* (pp. 191–212). Philadelphia: Lippincott–Williams & Wilkins.
56. Hutchison, C. P., et al. (1999). Body-mind-spirit: Healing touch: An energetic approach. *American Journal of Nursing, 99*(4), 43–48.
57. Insel, P. A. (1996). Analgesics-antipyretics and anti-inflammatory agents; Drugs employed in the treatment of gout. In J. G. Hardman & L. E. Limbird (Eds.), *The pharmacological basis of therapeutics* (9th ed., pp. 617–658), New York: Pergamon Press.
58. International Association for the Study of Pain (1986). Pain terms: A current list with definitions and notes on usage. *Pain, 3,* S216–S221.
59. Jacox, A., et al. (1994). *Management of cancer pain. Clinical practice guidelines No. 9.* AHCPR Publication No. 94-1592. Rockville, MD: Agency for Health Care Policy and Research, U.S. Department of Health and Human Services, Public Health Service.
60. Janssen, S. A., & Arntz, A. (1996). Anxiety and pain: Attentional and endorphinergic influences. *Pain, 66,* 145–150.
61. Jordan, M. S., Lumley, M. S., & Leisen, J. C. (1998). The relationships of cognitive coping and pain control beliefs to pain and adjustment among African-American and Caucasian women with rheumatoid arthritis. *Arthritis Care and Research, 11*(2), 80–88.
62. Juarez, G., Ferrell, B., & Borneman, T. (1998). Influence of culture on cancer pain management in Hispanic patients. *Cancer Practice, 6*(5), 262–269.
63. Juarez, G., Ferrell, B., & Borneman, T. (1999). Cultural considerations in education for cancer pain. *Journal of Cancer Education, 14*(3), 68–73.
64. Kandel, E. R., & Siegelbaum, S. A. (2000). Transmitter release. In E. R. Kandel, J. H. Schwartz, & T. M. Jessel (Eds.), *Principles of neural science* (4th ed., pp. 253–277). Norwalk, CT: Appleton & Lange.
65. Koester, J., & Siegelbaum, S. A. (2000). Membrane potential. In E. R. Kandel, J. H. Schwartz, & T. M. Jessel (Eds.), *Principles of neural science* (4th ed., pp. 125–139). Norwalk, CT: Appleton & Lange.
66. Kovacs, F. M., et al. (1997). Local and remote sustained trigger point therapy for exacerbations of chronic low back pain: A randomized, double-blind, controlled, multicenter trial. *Spine, 22*(7), 786–797.
67. Lander, J. (1990). Fallacies and phobias about addiction and pain. *British Journal of Addiction, 85,* 803–809.
68. Lefkowitz, M. (1998). Pain management in the HIV-positive patient. In M. A. Ashburn and L. J. Rice (Eds.), *The Management of Pain,* New York: Churchill Livingstone.
69. Levine, J. D., & Reichling, D. B. (1999). Peripheral mechanisms of inflammatory pain. In P. D. Wall and R. Melzack (Eds.), *Textbook of pain* (4th ed., pp. 59–84). Edinburgh, Churchill Livingstone.
70. Linton, S. J. (1999). Psychological factors. In I. K. Crombie, et al. (Eds.), *The epidemiology of pain.* Seattle: IASP Press (pp. 25–42).
71. Lundeberg, T. (1995). Pain physiology and principles of therapy. *Scandinavian Journal of Rehabilitation Medicine Supplement, 32,* 13–42.

72. Mains, R. E., & Epper, B. A. (1999). Peptides. In G. J. Siegal, et al. (Eds.), *Basic neurochemistry: Molecular, cellular and medical aspects.* Philadelphia: Lippincott–Williams & Wilkins.
73. Marks, R. M., & Sacher, E. J. (1973). Undertreatment of medical inpatients with narcotic analgesics. *Annals of Internal Medicine, 78,* 173–181.
74. Matz, A., & Brown, S. T. (1998). Humor and pain management. *Journal of Holistic Nursing, 16*(1), 68–75.
75. McCaffery, M., & Pasero, C. (1999). *Pain. Clinical Manual* (2nd ed). St. Louis, Mosby.
76. McCaffery, M., & Wolf, M. (1992). Pain relief using cutaneous modalities, positioning and movement. *Hospice Journal, 8,* 121–153.
77. Melzack, R., & Katz, J. (1999). Pain measurement in persons in pain. In P. D. Wall & R. Melzack (Eds.), *Textbook of pain* (4th ed., pp. 409–426). Edinburgh: Churchill Livingstone.
78. Melzack, R., & Wall, P. D. (1965). Pain mechanisms: A new theory. *Science, 150*(3699), 971–979.
79. Merskey, H., & Bogduk, N. (1994). *Classification of chronic pain: Descriptions of chronic pain syndromes and definitions of pain terms.* Seattle: IASP Press.
80. Michlovitz, S. (1996). The use of heat and cold in the management of rheumatic diseases. In S. L. Michlovitz (Ed.), *Thermal agents in rehabilitation* (2nd ed., pp. 258–274): Philadelphia: F. A. Davis.
81. Michlovitz, S. (1996). Cryotherapy: The use of cold as a therapeutic agent. In S. L. Michlovitz (Ed.), *Thermal agents in rehabilitation* (2nd ed., pp. 88–108). Philadelphia: F. A. Davis.
82. Millan, M. J. (1999). The induction of pain: An integrative review. *Progress in Neurobiology, 57*(1), 1–164.
83. Mobily, P. R., Herr, K. A., & Nicholson, A. C. (1994). Validation of cutaneous stimulation interventions for pain management. *International Journal of Nursing Studies, 31,* 533–544.
84. Moore, R., & Brodsgaard, I. (1999). Cross-cultural investigations of pain. In I. K. Crombie, et al. (Eds.), *Epidemiology of pain* (pp. 53–80). Seattle: IASP Press.
85. *NIH [National Institute of Health] Technological Assessment Statement* (1995, October 16–18). Integration of behavioral and relaxation approaches into the treatment of chronic pain and insomnia. 1–34.
86. Olsen, R. W., & DeLorey, T. M. (1999). GABA and glycine. In G. J. Siegal, et al. (Eds.), *Basic neurochemistry: Molecular, cellular and medical aspects* (pp. 335–346). Philadelphia: Lippincott–Williams & Wilkins.
87. Page, G. G., & Ben-Eliyakie, S. (1998). Pain kills: Animal models and neuroimmunological links. In R. Payne, et al. (Eds.), *Assessment and treatment of cancer pain: Progress in pain research and management* (Vol. 12, pp. 135–143). Seattle: IASP Press.
88. Paice, J. A. (1999). Pain. In C. H. Yarbo, et al. (Eds.), *Cancer symptom management* (2nd ed., pp. 118–144). Boston: Jones & Bartlett.
89. Palos, G. (1998). Culture and pain assessment in Hispanic patients. In R. Payne, et al. (Eds.), *Assessment and treatment of cancer pain: Progress in pain research and management* (Vol. 12, pp. 35–51). Seattle: IASP Press.
90. Papi, F., et al. (1995). Exposure to oscillating magnetic field influences sensitivity to electrical stimuli: II. Experiments on humans. *Bioelectromagnets, 16,* 295–300.
91. Payne R. (1998). Nonopioid analgesics for cancer pain: Update on clinical pharmacology. In R. Payne, et al. (Eds.), *Assessment and treatment of cancer pain: Progress in pain research and management* (Vol. 12, pp. 289–307). Seattle: IASP Press.
92. Payne, R., & Janjan, N. (1998). Management of metastatic bone pain. In R. Payne, et al. (Eds.), *Assessment and treatment of cancer pain: Progress in pain research and management* (Vol. 12, pp. 269–273). Seattle: IASP Press.
93. Perkins, M., & Dray, A. (1996). Novel pharmacological strategies for analgesia. *Annals of the Rheumatic Diseases, 55,* 715–722.
94. Portenoy, R. K. (1996). Opioid therapy for chronic nonmalignant pain: A review of the critical issues. *Journal of Pain and Symptom Management, 11,* 203–217.
95. Portenoy, R. K., & Lesage, P. (1999). Management of cancer pain. *The Lancet, 353,* 1695–1700.
96. Porter F. L., Grunau R. E., & Anand K. J. (1999). Long-term effects of pain in infants. *Journal of Developmental and Behavioral Pediatrics, 20*(4):253–261.
97. Price, D. D. (1996). Hypnotic analgesia: Psychological and neural mechanisms. In J. E. Berber (Ed.), *Hypnosis and suggestion in the treatment of pain: A clinical guide* (pp. 67–84). New York: W. W. Norton.
98. Price, D. D. (1999). Mechanisms of hypnotic analgesia. In *Psychological mechanisms of pain: Progress in pain research and management* (Vol. 15, pp. 183–204). Seattle: IASP Press.
99. Puntillo, K., & Weiss, S. J. (1994). Pain: Its mediators and associated morbidity in critically ill cardiovascular surgical clients. *Nursing Research, 43*(1), 31–36.
100. Raja, S. N., et al. (1999). Peripheral neural mechanisms of nociception. In P. D. Wall & R. Melzack (Eds.), *Textbook of pain* (4th ed., pp. 11–58). Edinburgh: Churchill Livingstone.
101. Ramnarine-Singh, S. (1999). The surgical significance of therapeutic touch. *AORN Journal, 69*(2), 358, 360–365, 367–369.
102. Rummans, T. A. (1994). Nonopioid agents for treatment of acute and subacute pain. *Mayo Clinic Proceedings, 69,* 481–490.
103. Shapiro, S. (1997). Neurotransmission by neurons that use serotonin, noradrenaline, glutamate, glycine and gamma-aminobutyric acid in normal and injured spinal cord. *Neurosurgery 40*(1), 168–177.
104. Siegelbaum, S. A., & Koester, J. (2000). Ion channels. In E. R. Kandel, J. H. Schwartz, & T. M. Jessell (Eds.), *Principles of neural science* (4th ed., pp. 104–124). Norwalk, CT: Appleton & Lange.
105. Simmonds, M. A. (1997). Pharmacotherapeutic management of cancer pain: Current practice. *Seminars in Oncology, 24*(5) *Suppl 16,* 516-1–516-6.
106. Simons, W., & Malabar, R. (1995). Assessing pain in elderly clients who cannot respond verbally. *Journal of Advanced Nursing, 22,* 663–669.
107. Singh, V. K., et al. (1997). Molecular biology of opioid receptors: Recent advances. *Neuroimmunomodulation, 4*(5–6), 285–297.
108. Sloan, P. A., et al. (1996). Cancer pain assessment and management by housestaff. *Pain, 67,* 475–481.
109. Spence, S. H., et al. (1995). Effects of EMG biofeedback compared to applied relaxation training with chronic, upper extremity cumulative trauma disorders. *Pain, 63*(2), 199–206.
110. Spross, J. A., McGuire, D. B., & Schmitt, R. M. (1990). Oncology Nursing Society position paper on pain: Part 1. *Oncology Nursing Forum, 17*(4), 595–614.
111. Spross, J. A., McGuire, D. B., & Schmitt, R. M. (1990). Oncology Nursing Society position paper on pain: Part 2. *Oncology Nursing Forum, 17*(5), 751–760.
112. Spross, J. A., McGuire, D. B., & Schmitt, R. M. (1990). Oncology Nursing Society position paper on pain: Part 3. *Oncology Nursing Forum, 17*(6), 943–947.
113. Staats, P. S. (1998). The pain mortality link: Unraveling the mysteries. In R. Payne, et al. (Eds.), *Assessment and treatment of cancer pain: Progress in pain research and management* (Vol. 12, pp. 145–156). Seattle: IASP Press.
114. Stephenson, J. (1996). Experts say AIDS pain 'dramatically undertreated.' *Journal of the American Medical Association, 276,* 1369–1370.
115. Sternbach, R. (1968). *Pain: A psychophysiological analysis.* New York: Academic Press.
116. Stimmel, B. (1997). *Pain and its relief without addiction: Clinical issues in the use of opioids and other analgesics.* New York, Haworth Medical Press.
117. Strand, F. L. (1999). *Neuropeptides: Regulators of physiological procedures.* Cambridge, MA: MIT Press.
118. Taylor, L. K., et al. (1998). The effect of music in the postanesthesia care unit on pain levels in women who have had abdominal hysterectomies. *Journal of Perianesthesia Nursing, 13*(2), 88–94.
119. Turk, D. C. (1999). A cognitive behavioral approach to pain management. In P. D. Wall & R. Melzack (Eds.), *Textbook of pain* (4th ed.), Edinburgh: Churchill Livingstone.
120. Turk, D. C., & Okifuji, A. (1998). Directions in prescriptive chronic pain management based on diagnostic characteristics of the client. In P. J. Vincent (Ed)., *American Pain Society Bulletin, 8*(5), 5–11.
121. Tusek, D., Church, J. M., & Fazio, V. W. (1997). Guided imagery as a coping strategy for perioperative clients. *AORN Journal, 66*(4), 644–649.
122. Urban, M. O., & Gebhart, G. F. (1999). Central mechanisms in pain. *Medical Clinics of North America, 83*(3), 585–596.
123. Vallerand, A. H. (1995). Gender differences in pain. *Image: Journal of Nursing Scholarship, 7*(3), 235–237.

124. Varcaccio-Garofalo, G., et al. (1995). Analgesic properties of electromagnetic field therapy in clients with chronic pelvic pain. *Clinical and Experimental Obstetrics and Gynecology, 22*(4), 350–354.
125. Watkins, G. R. (1997). Music therapy: Proposed physiological mechanisms and clinical implications. *Clinical Nurse Specialist, 11*(2), 43–50.
126. Watling, C. J. (1998). Management strategies for pain in the cancer patient. In M. A. Ashburn & L. J. Rice (Eds.), *The Management of Pain.* New York: Churchill Livingstone, 473–488.
127. Wall, P. (1999). Placebos. In P. D. Wall & R. Melzack (Eds.), *Textbook of pain* (4th ed., pp. 1419–1430). Edinburgh: Churchill Livingstone.
128. Weisenberg, M. (1999). Cognitive aspects of pain. In P. D. Wall & R. Melzack (Eds.), *Textbook of pain* (4th ed., pp. 345–358). Edinburgh: Churchill Livingstone.
129. Wilkie, D. J. (1995). Neural mechanisms of pain: A foundation for cancer pain assessment and management. In D. B. McGuire, C. H. Yarbro, & B. R. Ferrell (Eds.), *Cancer pain management* (2nd ed., pp. 61–87). Boston: Jones & Bartlett.
130. Williams, A. C., (1999). Measures of function and psychology. In P. D. Wall & R. Melzack (Eds.), *Textbook of pain* (4th ed., pp. 427–446). Edinburgh: Churchill Livingstone.
131. Willis, W. D., & Westlund, K. N. (1997). Neuroanatomy of the pain system and of the pathways that modulate pain. *Journal of Clinical Neurophysiology, 14*(1), 2–31.
132. Wong, D., & Baker, C. (1988). Pain in children: Comparison of assessment scales. *Pediatric Nursing, 14*(1), 9–17.
133. Woolf, C. J., & Mannion, R. J. (1999). Neuropathic pain: Aetiology, symptoms, mechanisms, and management. *The Lancet, 353,* 1959–1964.
134. World Health Organization (WHO). (1990). Cancer pain relief and palliative care. *Report of a WHO expert committee. Technical report series 804.* Geneva, Author.
135. Yaksh, T. L. (1999). Central pharmacology of nociception. In P. D. Wall & R. Melzack (Eds.), *Textbook of pain* (4th ed., pp. 253–308). Edinburgh: Churchill Livingstone.

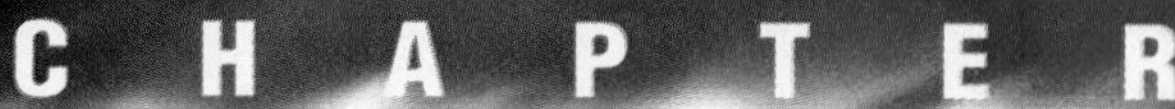

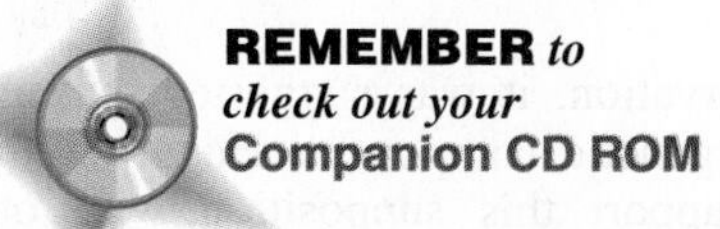

CHAPTER

24

Clients with Substance Abuse Disorders: Promoting Positive Outcomes

Linda Carman Copel

NURSING OUTCOMES CLASSIFICATION (NOC)
for Nursing Diagnoses—Clients with Substance Abuse Disorders

Acute Confusion
Cognitive Ability
Distorted Thought Control
Information Processing
Memory
Neurologic Status: Consciousness
Altered Family Processes
Family Coping
Family Environment: Internal
Family Functioning
Family Normalization
Altered Nutrition: Less Than Body Requirements
Nutritional Status: Nutrient Intake
Altered Role Performance
Abuse Protection
Altered Sexuality Patterns
Abuse Recovery: Sexual
Body Image
Self-Esteem
Sexual Identity: Acceptance
Altered Thought Processes
Cognitive Orientation
Concentration
Decision-Making
Identity
Information Processing
Memory
Anxiety
Aggression Control
Anxiety Control
Coping
Impulse Control
Self-Mutilation Restraint
Chronic Low Self-Esteem
Self-Esteem
Body Image
Dysfunctional Grieving
Concentration
Coping
Family Coping
Grief Resolution
Psychosocial Adjustment: Life Change
Fatigue
Activity Tolerance
Endurance
Fear
Fear Control
Hopelessness
Decision-Making
Hope
Mood Equilibrium
Quality of Life
Impaired Social Interaction
Role Performance
Social Interaction Skills
Social Involvement
Impaired Verbal Communication
Communication Ability
Communication: Expressive Ability
Communication: Receptive Ability
Ineffective Denial
Fear Control
Health Beliefs: Perceived Threat
Coping
Ineffective Individual Coping
Aggression Control
Depression Control
Depression Level
Knowledge Deficit
Knowledge: Substance Abuse Control
Communication: Receptive Ability
Concentration
Noncompliance
Adherence Behavior
Compliance Behavior
Treatment Behavior: Illness or Injury
Pain
Personal Identity Disturbance
Identity
Self-Mutilation Restraint
Powerlessness
Depression Control
Depression Level
Family Participation in Professional Care
Risk for Impaired Skin Integrity
Self-Mutilation Restraint
Risk for Injury
Risk Control
Safety Behavior: Personal
Safety Status: Physical Injury
Risk for Poisoning
Risk Control: Drug Use
Risk for Trauma
Risk Control
Safety Status: Physical Injury
Risk for Violence
Abuse Protection
Abusive Behavior Self-Control
Aggression Control
Distorted Thought Control
Impulse Control
Risk Control: Alcohol Use
Risk Control: Drug Use
Risk Detection
Sensory and Perceptual Alterations
Anxiety Control
Body Image
Distorted Thought Process
Sleep Pattern Disturbance
Sleep
Social Isolation
Loneliness
Mood Equilibrium
Social Interaction Skills
Social Involvement
Social Support
Spiritual Distress
Hope

As the client passed through the hospital door, it was the beginning—the first step of many on the journey back from the world of drugs and alcohol. No longer need this person be entangled in the cycle of pain, ineffective coping with addictive substances, more pain, and more drugs. The client, struggling to think clearly, had the following thoughts: "I must be dying. My body hurts. Where am I? What is going on here? How did this happen? I can't stand it. What are they doing to me? They can't help me. I can't help me. No one can help me. My life has always been a mess. There is nothing I can do."

Clients with psychoactive substance abuse disorders struggle with an inability to solve problems. They are unable to use adaptive behaviors to handle life stresses, traumas, and demands. *Ineffective Coping, Defensive Coping, Denial, Altered Nutrition, Risk of Injury,* and *Risk for Infection* are a few of the nursing diagnoses specific to the assessment data obtained from these clients. Nurses are challenged by the myriad of physical and emotional health problems faced by clients with addiction. Their health histories and at-risk behaviors culminate in problems ranging from liver and cardiovascular disease to depression and human immunodeficiency virus (HIV). The client's physical condition is further compromised by nutritional deficits and fluid and electrolyte imbalances. In addition, many clients suffer from injuries, either self-inflicted trauma or violence at the hands of others. Often, multiple injuries in various stages of healing are evident upon examination.

Underlying the physical problems are the emotional wounds from both past and present life situations. Without effective coping skills, clients tend to repeat their self-destructive pattern of behavior over and over. The inability to perceive reality accurately and to develop and maintain supportive relationships hinders successful lifestyle changes. Accelerating bouts of depression and feelings of powerlessness continue, perpetuating a sense of incompetence. A pervasive sense of failure may be overwhelming.

Studies consistently show that substance-abusing clients need both medical and psychiatric nursing care to achieve their highest level of functioning and to maintain sobriety. Nurses have the challenge of dealing not only with the addicted client's many physiologic problems but also with the effects and withdrawal symptoms of the drugs involved. Even as you seek to assess and diagnose the physiologic effects of abused substances, clients typically offer defensiveness and may remain in denial. These clients' lack responsibility for their personal behavior. Constantly blaming and manipulating of others are typical behaviors that require your attention and intervention along with the physiologic issues. As much as any client population, this one challenges the entire health care team to provide holistic treatment for physical, emotional, and spiritual needs.

FRAMEWORKS FOR EXPLAINING ADDICTIVE BEHAVIORS

Over the past 100 years, clinicians and researchers have attempted to develop and refine the knowledge base on substance-abusing people. Early studies of alcoholism noted generational patterns of alcoholism in families. On the basis of this observation, it was suggested that alcoholism might have a genetic component. However, there is no evidence to support this supposition with other commonly abused drugs.[11, 19, 22, 31]

Various explanations of the causes of substance abuse have focused on three conceptual frameworks:

- Biologic
- Psychological
- Sociocultural

However, there is no one identifiable cause of substance use. Rather, a combination of factors typically coalesces to produce drug use patterns. A person may be at risk for substance abuse because of a complex combination of biologic, psychological, and sociocultural variables. All aspects of the client's background must be considered when treatment is initiated. In addition to what the client brings to the treatment setting, the theoretical approach used by the team to view the underlying dynamics of substance abuse influences the process of recovery.

■ BIOLOGIC FRAMEWORK

The biologic theory, or disease concept, of substance abuse views addiction as a physiologic condition that can be identified and treated. The emphasis is on a physiologic cause, such as genetic predisposition, defects in metabolism, neurobiologic abnormalities, or abnormal levels of chemicals in the body.[38] Historically, studies attempting to link genetic transmission of alcoholism have been unable to find a target gene.

Present research focuses on examining the inherited biochemical abnormalities that may predispose an individual to alcoholism.[5] It is now believed that alcohol dependence is a combination of interwoven social and psychological variables in people who are physiologically vulnerable.[30] For example, people of East Asian ancestry tend to experience a physical reaction to alcohol characterized by tachycardia, a sensation of warmth and flushing, and generalized discomfort. The response is believed to be related to the lack of activation of the enzyme aldehyde dehydrogenase, resulting in the accumulation of acetaldehyde, a toxic product of alcohol metabolism.[5, 37] This physiologic process may be the reason that Asian Americans tend to have the lowest rate of alcohol consumption and associated substance use problems compared with other racial groups.[34] Hence, an examination of biologic differences associated with the use of alcohol warrants continued investigation.

■ PSYCHOLOGICAL FRAMEWORK

Psychological theories attempt to explain the variables that may predispose someone to substance use. According to the psychoanalytic model, the person is viewed as being fixated at the oral stage of development, seeking gratification of needs through behaviors such as drinking. With the psychodynamic approach, a person experiences both interpersonal and intrapersonal difficulties that provide the foundation for the addiction.

Behavioral theories regard addiction as a learned behavior that can be unlearned in a manner similar to that of changing negative habits or dysfunctional behaviors. A *family systems approach* emphasizes that relationships, roles, and unhealthy communication patterns among family members contribute to addictive behaviors; this dysfunctional lifestyle is transmitted to future generations.[14]

For years, researchers and clinicians have sought, without success, to discover an addictive personality type. Some common characteristics noted in clients who abuse substances are low self-esteem, low frustration tolerance, inability to cope with physical and emotional pain, depression, lack of healthy relationships, and involvement in high-risk behaviors. Proponents of the psychological theories believe that people engage in substance use in an attempt to feel better about themselves and to meet their emotional needs. Thus, the use of a psychoactive substance becomes reinforced and eventually evolves into an addiction.

■ SOCIOCULTURAL FRAMEWORK

With the sociocultural theories, substance use is viewed from the perspective of cultural and social norms within various groups in society. The issues of whether to use drugs, what type of drugs to use, and how and when to use them are determined by factors in a person's background. Such factors may include values, belief systems, spiritual orientation, ethnicity, sex, family standards, or the contemporary social environment. The relationships between these variables can contribute to a person's susceptibility to drug use and potential for addiction treatment and ongoing recovery.

DEFINITIONS AND TERMINOLOGY

According to the *Diagnostic and Statistical Manual of Mental Disorders,* fourth edition (*DSM-IV*),[2] the substance-related disorders comprise the range of substance use from taking a drug of abuse, to the adverse effects of any medication, to exposure to toxic substances. *DSM-IV* lists 11 types of substances commonly abused: alcohol, amphetamines, caffeine, cannabis, cocaine, hallucinogens, inhalants, nicotine, opioids, phencyclidine (PCP), and the group "sedatives, hypnotics, or anxiolytics."[2] Polysubstance dependence and other substance-related disorders, particularly toxins or prescribed and over-the-counter medications, are also included.[2]

To understand and assess substance abuse, you must learn the associated terminology (Table 24–1). In working with clients who are actively using substances, you must also know the types of drugs commonly used, the major routes of administration, and side effects (Table 24–2). The order and severity of manifestations are influ-

TABLE 24–1 SUBSTANCE ABUSE TERMS AND DEFINITIONS

Term	Definition
Psychoactive substance	A substance that affects a person's mood or behavior
Substance abuse	Continued use of a psychoactive substance despite the occurrence of physical, psychological, social, or occupational problems
Substance dependence	A range of physiologic, behavioral, and cognitive symptoms indicating that a person persists in using the substance, ignoring serious substance-related problems
Physiologic dependence	The body's physical adaptation to a drug, whereby withdrawal symptoms occur if the drug is not used
Psychological dependence	The emotional need or craving for a drug either for its effect or to prevent the occurrence of withdrawal symptoms
Addiction	A compulsion, loss of control, and progressive pattern of drug use, characterized by behavioral changes, impaired thinking, unkept promises to stop usage, obsession with the drug, neglect of personal needs, decreased tolerance, and physiologic deterioration
Polysubstance abuse	Concurrent use of multiple drugs
Intoxication	An altered physiologic state resulting from the use of a psychoactive drug
Overdose	Accidental or deliberate consumption of a drug in a dose larger than is ordinarily used, resulting in a serious toxic reaction or death
Tolerance	State resulting from metabolic changes in cell functions, whereby the tissue reaction to a drug declines and the person needs to take increasing amounts to achieve the same effect
Cross-tolerance	State whereby the effect of a drug is decreased and greater amounts are required to achieve the desired effect because the person has become tolerant to a similar drug
Predisposition	Any factor that increases the likelihood of an event occurring
Potentiation	The ability of one drug to increase the activity of another drug when taken at the same time
Drug misuse	Any use of a drug that deviates from medical or socially acceptable use
Dual diagnosis	The coexistence of a major psychiatric illness and a psychoactive substance abuse disorder
Blackout	An acute situation in which a person experiences a period of memory loss for actions as a direct result of using drugs or alcohol
Withdrawal	Discontinuation of a substance by a person who is dependent on it
Detoxification	The process of withdrawing a person from an addictive substance in a safe manner
Toxic dose	The amount of a drug that produces a poisonous effect
Recidivism	The tendency to relapse into a former pattern of substance use and associated behaviors
Recovery	Return to a normal state of health, whereby the person does not engage in problematic behavior and continues to meet life's challenges and personal goals
Sobriety	Complete abstinence from drugs while developing a satisfactory lifestyle
Abstinence	Voluntarily refraining from activities or use of substances that cause problems in the physiologic, psychological, social, intellectual, and spiritual arenas of a person's life

TABLE 24–2	CHARACTERISTIC EFFECTS OF ABUSE OF MAJOR SUBSTANCES
Drug Classification and Street Names (Route of Administration)	**Effects***
Alcohol (Oral)	Relaxation and sedation Decreased inhibition Lack of coordination Unsteady gait Slurred speech Nausea and vomiting Transient visual, tactile, or auditory hallucinations Anxiety Psychomotor agitation High risk of permanent liver or brain damage
Amphetamines (Oral, injected, smoked) Dexedrine Methamphetamine "Ice" "Uppers" "Crank" "Speed"	Grandiosity Hypervigilance Hypertension or hypotension Tachycardia or bradycardia Mydriasis (dilated pupils) Euphoria Appetite suppression Personality changes Antisocial behavior Psychosis similar to paranoid schizophrenia
Caffeine (Oral)	Stimulation of senses Alertness and enhanced performance Anxiety and restlessness Flushed face Talkativeness Tremors or muscle twitching Tachycardia or cardiac arrhythmias Insomnia Irritation of the stomach
Cannabis (Smoked, oral) Marijuana "Grass" "Pot" "Hash" "Weed"	Mild intoxication Increased appetite Dry mouth Lack of coordination Impaired judgment and memory Sexual arousal Tachycardia Visual hallucinations
Cocaine (Oral, injected, inhaled) "Coke" "Crack" "Snow" "Blow" "Lady" "Powder"	Talkativeness Grandiosity Hypervigilance Anxiety Impaired judgment Tachycardia or bradycardia Hypertension or hypotension Mydriasis Muscle twitching Respiratory depression Hallucinations, paranoid delusions, or paranoia Formication (sensation of insects crawling on the skin) Personality changes Antisocial behavior Euphoria followed by depression and feeling let down
Hallucinogens (Oral, inhaled) Lysergic acid diethylamide (LSD) "Acid" Peyote Psilocybin Mescaline	Intensified perceptions and feelings Synesthesia (seeing sounds or hearing colors) Visual, auditory, or tactile hallucinations Fear of losing one's mind Mydriasis Tachycardia Palpitations Blurred vision Dizziness, weakness, and tremors Altered perceptions (flashbacks) Impaired judgment and bizarre behavior Mood swings and psychosis-like symptoms

TABLE 24–2 CHARACTERISTIC EFFECTS OF ABUSE OF MAJOR SUBSTANCES *Continued*

Drug Classification and Street Names (Route of Administration)	Effects*
Inhalants (Inhaled)	Euphoria and giddiness
Spray can propellants	Headache
Paint	Dizziness, fatigue, or drowsiness
Paint thinner	Nystagmus (involuntary rapid eye movements)
Glue	Unsteady gait or tremors
Gasoline	Slurred speech
Cleaning fluid	Blurred vision or diplopia (double vision)
	Damage to major organs: lungs, liver, and kidneys
	Cardiac arrest
Nicotine (Inhaled, oral)	Tachycardia
	Vasoconstriction
	Irritation of oral mucosa
	Persistent cough
	Damaged alveoli and bronchioli
	Emphysema
	High risk of oral, laryngeal, or lung cancer
Opioids (Oral, injected, inhaled)	Immediate euphoria followed by dysphoria
Morphine	Psychomotor retardation or agitation
Codeine	Slurred speech
Methadone	Impaired judgment and memory
Hydromorphone (Dilaudid)	Sedation and respiratory depression
Heroin	Constricted pupils
"Smack"	Decreased sexual and aggressive drives
"Horse"	
Phencyclidine (PCP) (Oral, injected, inhaled)	Grandiosity and illusions of strength
"Angel dust"	Impulsiveness
"Hog"	Psychomotor agitation
	Assaultive behavior
	Decreased sensory awareness
	Hypertension and tachycardia
	Unsteady gait and lack of coordination
	Nystagmus
	Mood swings and paranoia
Sedatives, Hypnotics, and Anxiolytics (Oral, injected)	Incoordination and unsteady gait
Benzodiazepine (e.g., diazepam (Valium), alprazolam (Xanax), chlordiazepoxide (Librium))	Slurred speech
	Nystagmus
Secobarbital (Seconal)	Sedation
Pentobarbital (Nembutal)	Inappropriate sexual behavior and aggressive drives
Methaqualone (Quaalude)	Impaired judgment
	Mood swings

*Drug effects are arranged in order of severity of effect, with prolonged use or a high dose of the drug associated with appearance of the later effects.

From Copel, L. C. (2000). *Nurses' clinical guide to psychiatric and mental health care.* (2nd ed.). Springhouse, PA: Springhouse.

enced by the size of the dose and the length of time the drug has been used.

GENERAL ASSESSMENT

The purposes of a drug and alcohol assessment are to:

- Determine whether substance abuse exists
- Evaluate the relationship between substance abuse and other health care problems
- Implement effective health promotion and health restoration interventions

All clients must be assessed for the use and misuse of chemical substances. Clients who struggle with addiction are found at all stages of life and therefore in all clinical specialties. It is common for a client who abuses drugs to be hospitalized for an injury, illness, or surgical procedure. The nurse-generalist must identify clients with actual or potential substance problems (see Bridge to Home Health Care: Addressing Substance Use) and institute a collaborative team approach to provide health care.

The ability of nurses to provide care is influenced by the personal thoughts and feelings about substance abuse and the people who become addicts. Self-awareness about substance use and abuse is essential if the nurse is to establish a therapeutic relationship and provide treatment. The Seaman-Mannello Scale, a Likert-type scale that assesses nurses' attitudes toward alcohol and alcoholism, and the National Council on Alcoholism and Drug Dependence Scale can provide insight about personal values

BRIDGE TO HOME HEALTH CARE

Addressing Substance Use

Substance use is a prevalent problem, regardless of a person's age, gender, and social, economic, professional, or educational status. Nurses in community settings must collaborate with clients to prevent, screen, detect, and deal with abuse. Examples of strategies include the use of direct conversation, monitoring behavior changes, observing the environment, and providing education and referrals.

Use active listening skills consistently when you meet with clients in their homes or other informal community settings. By asking clients about their past use of substances and about substances used by their family and friends, you can gain accurate information about the client's history and current status. Often, you will be able to note changes in the client's behavior, social interactions, and lifestyle. Alcohol containers and the odor of marijuana are additional signs. When substance use is confirmed by the client and when it is suspected but denied, reassess frequently and ask questions that address the behaviors or signs observed.

It is even more critical to identify people who have substance use problems when the quality of life for others is endangered. Directly asking a pregnant woman, "How much alcohol have you consumed during the past month of your pregnancy?" allows a straightforward, honest answer. If alcohol use is detected, first give a clear message that there is no safe level of alcohol use during pregnancy, then offer assistance. When pregnant women consume alcohol, they expose their unborn children to potential birth defects, permanent brain damage, and a lifetime of physical, mental, and emotional impairments. Provide detailed information about the effects of substances on their unborn child, such as abnormal facial features, slow growth, mental retardation, attention deficit and hyperactive disorders, learning disabilities, and problems with daily living skills. The effects of substance use are clearly seen in children growing up with *fetal alcohol syndrome* (FAS) and *fetal alcohol effects* (FAE).

School-aged children give signals that substance use is present in the home. Identify children who are often late to school or absent, whose parents miss appointments with teachers or physicians, and who may be withdrawn or show a sudden behavior change. Collaborate with the school social worker or school nurse, arrange a meeting with the parents, and assess the home situation further.

Often, adolescents use substances habitually because of peer pressure. Assist schools in writing and promoting curricula that incorporate clear and consistent messages about the dangers of drinking and driving.

The community health nurse is a source of ongoing support who can provide reassurance, education, information, and home visits for clients. When substance use is detected, offer clients appropriate resources and counseling services. Examples of resources include local inpatient or outpatient treatment programs and Alcoholics Anonymous. Suggest specific programs, such as classes for pregnant women using alcohol and support groups for families who have children with FAS. In addition, become informed about and follow mandatory reporting statutes that apply to pregnant women using substances. Such laws exist in many states.

Jill E. Timm, RN, PHN, BAN, *Public Health Nurse II, Washington County Department of Public Health and Environment, Sillwater, Minnesota*

and beliefs regarding substances.[29] Nurses can also examine their attitudes and their own use of drugs and alcohol by considering the questions of how, when, where, and under what conditions they use them.

Individual beliefs about drug and alcohol use come from the nurse's family background and previous knowledge about and experience with addicted people. This information allows nurses to anticipate their response patterns toward this group of clients. If nurses know their feelings and beliefs, they will be able to recognize a judgmental attitude, rejecting behaviors, or enabling behaviors. This knowledge can prevent the nurse from being drawn into power struggles regarding the client's manipulative behavior.

In addition to self-assessment measures for nurses some instruments allow the nurse to gain information about the client's drug and alcohol use (Box 24–1). To use a tool as part of the assessment process, the nurse must know how to score the instrument and how to correctly interpret the findings.

Interviewing the substance abuse client presents a challenge because of the client's tendency to deny or minimize the problem. A comprehensive assessment includes the client's history and physical examination. The previously mentioned screening tools can be helpful. Laboratory studies address cardiac, liver, kidney, and respiratory functioning as well as urine toxicology. A thorough mental status assessment is a requisite part of the examination. The major components of this assessment are listed in Table 24–3.

BOX 24–1 Examples of Substance Use Screening Tools

For Use with Adults

- Michigan Alcoholism Screening Test (MAST)[33]
- Short Michigan Alcoholism Screening Test (SMAST)[34]
- Addiction Severity Index[24]
- CAGE Questions[12]
- T-ACE (a modified version of the CAGE used with pregnant women)[36]
- Alcohol Use Disorders Identification Test (AUDIT)[28]
- Alcohol Dependence Scale[35]
- Self-Administered Alcoholism Screening Test (SAAST)[39]
- Alcohol Use Inventory[18]

For Use with Adolescents

- Guided Rational Adolescent Substance Abuse Profile (GRASP)[1]
- Problem Severity Scales for Assessment of Alcohol and Drug Abuse[17]

TABLE 24–3 COMPONENTS OF THE MENTAL STATUS ASSESSMENT

General appearance	Appearance versus stated age Grooming and hygiene Posture, gait, and station Interaction during the interview Facial expressions Orientation or level of consciousness
Motor behavior	Restlessness Agitation Lethargy Tremors
Speech	Clarity and coherence of speech Rate of speech Volume and intonation Barriers to communication, such as confusion or delusions Vocabulary appropriate to socioeconomic background
Affect	Flat or labile
Mood	Euphoric, anxious, fearful
Thought processes	Thoughts presented as normal, concrete, scattered, or illogical Delusions—a false belief that is firmly maintained despite evidence to the contrary
Perception	Awareness of self and environment Illusions—misinterpretation of external stimuli Hallucinations—sensory experiences with no external stimuli present
Memory	Memory for remote, recent, and immediate past General knowledge level Ability to calculate Ability to think abstractly Insight Judgment or problem-solving ability

Attention is paid to the psychosocial evaluation, especially the components that address difficulties in family, occupational, social, or leisure functioning. Some clinicians recommend that after the history and physical examination are completed, the health care provider should take a specific drug and alcohol history that asks about drug usage for the 11 major psychoactive substances in addition to other prescription and over-the-counter substances.[10] Components of a drug and alcohol history are listed in Box 24–2.

Although all clients need to be assessed for substance abuse, of special concern are those who by virtue of lifestyle or social conditions may be at increased risk. Adolescents, women (particularly pregnant women), racial and ethnic minorities, homosexual women and men, clients with HIV infection or acquired immunodeficiency syndrome (AIDS), homeless people, older adults, and health care professionals are identified as populations requiring special prevention, treatment, and education about substance abuse.[4, 7] Extra attention must be given to clients with chronic physical or mental illnesses.

Self-medication can occur in vulnerable populations as a coping strategy to relieve physical and emotional pain associated with a chronic illness. After obtaining a comprehensive assessment, you may discover that a client struggles with polysubstance abuse. Such clients require specialized care during the withdrawal process according to the combination of drugs used.

Assessment and Management of Substance-Abusing Clients

The immediate result of overconsumption of any psychoactive substance is acute intoxication. Nurses in an emergency department or a medical-surgical setting may care for clients suffering from trauma as a direct result of acute intoxication. In addition to treating the client's injuries, the nursing care of intoxication consists of monitoring vital signs, especially respiratory status, because respiratory depression or arrest can occur. Be vigilant for manifestations of shock, cardiac dysrhythmias, electrolyte imbalances, or subdural hematomas. Typically, intravenous (IV) fluids are given to prevent dehydration. Some people become intoxicated but do not seek medical intervention because no injuries or emergencies bring them to health care facilities.

When a person sharply reduces or stops use of a psychoactive substance, the process of *withdrawal* occurs. Depending on the drug, withdrawal may begin within 8 to 12 hours or be delayed for 1 to 3 days. Prompt recognition of withdrawal symptoms can promote client safety and prevent complications. Factors that influence the withdrawal process include (1) the specific drug used, (2) the dose taken, (3) the method of intake, (4) the time of last use, and (5) the length of time during which the drug has been used. You must also consider the client's overall health, particularly the functioning of the kidneys, lungs, and liver—the principal organs that metabolize and excrete drugs. An overview of common withdrawal symptoms for alcohol and other substances appears in Table 24–4.

■ ALCOHOL

Ethyl alcohol (ethanol), a central nervous system (CNS) depressant, is found in alcoholic beverages. The ingested alcohol is absorbed directly into the bloodstream from the

BOX 24–2 Components of a Drug and Alcohol History

- How often the drug was used (past and recent use)
- Age at first use
- Duration of use
- Age at last use
- Method of use
- Quantity used
- Initial and current reactions to the drug
- How the drug was obtained or how use of the drug was supported
- What has been done to reduce drug use
- Client's perception of use of the drug as a problem
- Use of drug related to any health problems

TABLE 24–4 **COMMON WITHDRAWAL SYMPTOMS ASSOCIATED WITH PSYCHOACTIVE DRUGS**

Drug Classification	Major Withdrawal Symptoms
Alcohol	Nausea and vomiting Tremors and weakness Sweating Tachycardia Hypertension Delusions Agitated behavior Hallucinations and nocturnal illusions
Amphetamines	Dysphoria Disorientation Fatigue and depression with suicidal potential Disturbed sleep and unpleasant dreams Hallucinations or delusions
Caffeine	Irritability and nervousness Inability to concentrate Headache Tremors Lethargy
Cannabis	No acute withdrawal symptoms; other symptoms appear over varying time periods following withdrawal Amotivational syndrome (inability to concentrate or complete tasks) Chronic respiratory problems Memory and learning difficulty Suppressed prolactin and testosterone levels
Cocaine	Severe craving for drug Severe depression ("postcoke blues") Fatigue Psychomotor agitation or retardation Anxiety Insomnia or hypersomnia Increased appetite
Hallucinogens	Symptoms appear over varying time periods following withdrawal Apprehension, fear, or panic Hyperactivity Sweating Tachycardia Altered perceptions (flashbacks) Perceptual distortions, especially hallucinations
Inhalants	Symptoms appear over varying time periods following withdrawal Central nervous system damage (cerebral atrophy or peripheral neuropathies) Acute or chronic renal failure Bone marrow depression Cardiac dysrhythmias Respiratory damage (lung or sinus damage, pneumonitis, emphysema, respiratory depression) Liver disease (hepatitis, cirrhosis)
Nicotine	Irritability and nervousness Headache Inability to concentrate Craving for cigarettes Fatigue and dizziness Tremors and palpitations
Opioids	Dysphoria Anxiety Insomnia Increased respirations and yawning Sweating Lacrimation and rhinorrhea (nasal discharge) Tremors and muscle twitching Mydriasis (dilated pupils) Piloerection (erection of the hair) Nausea, abdominal cramps, and vomiting

TABLE 24–4 **COMMON WITHDRAWAL SYMPTOMS ASSOCIATED WITH PSYCHOACTIVE DRUGS** *Continued*

Drug Classification	Major Withdrawal Symptoms
Phencyclidine (PCP)	Symptoms may appear over varying time periods following withdrawal Anxiety Withdrawn, catatonic state Hypertension Seizures Bizarre behavior and speech associated with temporary psychosis
Sedatives, hypnotics, and anxiolytics	Anxiety Sweating Tachycardia Tremors Nausea and vomiting Insomnia and disturbing dreams Transient visual, auditory, or tactile hallucinations Seizures

*See Box 24–6, Resources.
From Copel, L. C. (2000). *Nurses' clinical guide to psychiatric and mental health care.* (2nd ed.). Springhouse, PA: Springhouse.

stomach and proximal part of the small intestine. Because alcohol is water-soluble, it circulates easily throughout the body and readily passes through the blood-brain barrier. Approximately 95% of alcohol is metabolized in the liver, with the remaining 5% being excreted through the lungs, kidneys, and skin.[26] The body's mechanism for oxidizing alcohol is accomplished through the liver enzyme alcohol dehydrogenase. This process breaks down the alcohol to acetaldehyde, which is further broken down to acetic acid. Acetic acid then goes through the citric acid cycle to become carbon dioxide and water. From this chemical process, it is evident that alcohol can affect every aspect of the body. A growing number of young people may be using alcohol to enhance a drug's effect.

A blood alcohol level (BAL) test is used to measure the concentration of alcohol in the blood. The purpose of the test is to detect and estimate the level of alcohol in the brain. The legal intoxication level in most states is 100 mg/dl (0.10%); in a few states, it is 0.08%.

Although some studies suggest that small amounts of alcohol can be harmless or even healthful, large amounts produce a predictable series of deleterious effects. After drinking one or two alcoholic beverages, a person experiences a depression of the inhibitory regions of the brain that manage judgment, self-control, speech, and motor coordination. Alcohol is classified as a CNS depressant that affects all levels of the brain, starting with the reticular activating system and the cerebral cortex. Alcohol suppresses the inhibitory neurotransmitter gamma-aminobutyric acid (GABA). When the release of GABA is decreased, the initial results are an excitement or euphoric response.

With acute alcohol intoxication, alcohol continues to accumulate in the brain, resulting in depression of the cerebral cortex, cerebellum, and midbrain. In severe brain depression, disruption of the spinal reflexes, respiratory system, cardiac functioning, or temperature regulation occurs. At this point, the intoxicated person may become unconscious, and without treatment death may occur.

Early clinical manifestations of alcohol withdrawal (e.g., tremors, anorexia, anxiety, restlessness, insomnia) tend to occur within 6 to 8 hours after the last drink is ingested. During the next 2 to 3 days, the client may further experience disorientation, nightmares, abdominal pain, nausea, diaphoresis, and elevations in temperature, pulse, and blood pressure along with visual and auditory hallucinations. *Delirium tremens* (DTs) is a manifestation of severe alcohol withdrawal or its life-threatening complications. The client with DTs is at risk for cardiac dysrhythmias, hypertension, increased respirations, profuse sweating, delusions, and hallucinations.

Many clients are given medications to decrease the incidence of withdrawal manifestations and to prevent DTs. The benzodiazepines are commonly used because they cause less respiratory depression and hypertension compared with other drugs. Typically, the physician orders either a long-acting benzodiazepine (diazepam [Valium] or chlordiazepoxide [Librium]) or a short-acting benzodiazepine (lorazepam [Ativan] or oxazepam [Serax]). The long-acting benzodiazepines are often used to facilitate the withdrawal process; the short-acting benzodiazepines are used for clients with severe liver dysfunction or a high degree of cognitive impairment.

Since 1995, the drug naltrexone hydrochloride (ReVia) has been approved for the treatment of alcoholism. It has been successful in decreasing the craving for alcohol and, together with the client's participation in a recovery program, facilitates client compliance with treatment. The drug was originally intended to treat clients undergoing opioid detoxification. According to the manufacturer, the mechanisms of action for naltrexone in alcoholism are not completely known. However, because the drug is an opioid receptor antagonist, it blocks the effects of opioid drugs by its competitive site binding. The relatively few side effects of the drug are nausea, fatigue, dizziness, headache, anxiety, and insomnia. Contraindications include hepatitis, liver disease, and liver failure.[14]

Treatment with naltrexone is controversial because taking the drug conflicts with the Alcoholics Anonymous (AA) model of total abstinence from alcohol and being "drug-free." The use of any drug is seen as a "crutch" or a substitution for the alcohol. For philosophical and political reasons, some clients taking naltrexone are excluded from receiving support and the other benefits of participating in AA.

There are also nonpharmacologic approaches to treating withdrawal. The *social model,* or the nonmedicinal treatment model, incorporates the use of an extensive physical examination, followed by close medical supervision during therapy. Several studies have shown that approximately 75% of the clients enrolled in these programs improve.[27, 41]

The major nursing interventions for a client experiencing withdrawal focus on the continuous monitoring of manifestations and promoting a safe, calm, and comfortable environment. During the withdrawal period, clients need reassurance and support because they may feel that they will not survive the ordeal of detoxification. In the immediate period after the withdrawal syndrome has ceased, you can refer the client for further assessment and treatment of addiction or its complications. At this time, especially after what the client has been through, address with the client the relationship between drug use and the concomitant acute or chronic physical health problems. Common medical consequences of alcohol abuse are identified in Table 24–5.

TABLE 24–5 MEDICAL CONSEQUENCES OF ALCOHOL ABUSE

Body System	Consequences
Cardiac	Dysrhythmias Hypertension Cardiomyopathy Heart failure Beriberi heart disease
Gastrointestinal	Gastritis Gastric or duodenal ulcers Perforated gastrointestinal ulcers Esophageal varices Pancreatitis Interference with absorption of vitamin B_{12}, thiamine, and folic acid Malabsorption syndrome Alteration in nutrition, with potential for malnutrition Wernicke-Korsakoff syndrome Enlarged or fatty liver Liver enzyme changes Cirrhosis Alcoholic hepatitis Portal hypertension Ascites Hepatic encephalopathy
Hematopoietic	Anemia Thrombocytopenia Leukopenia Capillary fragility Spider nevi Palmar erythema
Neurologic	Peripheral neuropathy Brain atrophy
Musculoskeletal	Myopathy Decreased bone density with risk of fracture Fractured bones related to trauma
Immune	Depressed immune system Increased susceptibility to infections
Respiratory	Altered respirations Chronic obstructive pulmonary disease Pneumonia Tuberculosis
Endocrine	Testicular atrophy Gynecomastia Irregular menses Decreased libido Hypoglycemia Alcoholic ketoacidosis

■ AMPHETAMINES

Amphetamines have been used to treat *narcolepsy* (sudden sleep) and *attention deficit hyperactivity disorder* (ADHD). People often use amphetamines illegally to remain awake and alert, to increase their ability to perform physical tasks, or to produce a state of euphoria (a "high"). The abuse of amphetamines, according to the National Institute on Drug Abuse, is most common in the 18- to 34-year-old age group.[19] The pattern of abuse tends to be one of daily chronic use or periodic binges that end with the user overwhelmed by exhaustion ("crashing").

Amphetamines stimulate the CNS and accelerate heart and brain activity. Amphetamines block the reuptake of dopamine and norepinephrine by interfering with the transport protein, ultimately causing accumulation of dopamine and norepinephrine at the synapses.[20] Amphetamines are metabolized by the liver enzymes and excreted in the urine. In some cases, after continual drug use, half of the drug may be excreted from the body unchanged.[7]

With amphetamine intoxication, the clinical findings may include cardiac dysrhythmias, hypertension, fever, labile emotions, paranoia, delusions, panic reactions, and psychosis. For client management, perform frequent assessment of vital signs and basic body functioning and provide safe, supportive care. Closely monitor the client for changes in cardiac or neurologic status, because myocardial infarction and cerebral hemorrhage have occurred after amphetamine use. Antipsychotic agents may be used to decrease CNS stimulation, or sedatives may be given. IV amino acids may be given to speed up the detoxification process of stimulant drugs.[3]

Amphetamines commonly cause psychological dependence, often with craving behavior. Abrupt cessation of the drug can precipitate anxiety, agitation, severe depression, hyperphagia, and hypersomnolence. An amphetamine psychosis may occur after continuous high doses. Nursing care focuses on (1) providing rest, (2) orienting the client as necessary, (3) monitoring for both physical and emotional changes, and (4) intervening to prevent complications of adverse effects or withdrawal symptoms.

■ CAFFEINE

In the United States, caffeine—a CNS stimulant—is the most commonly used psychoactive substance. Products containing caffeine include coffee, tea, chocolate, cola beverages, and prescription and nonprescription medications. People rely on caffeine to promote wakefulness, elevate their sense of well-being, decrease fatigue, and facilitate motor activity.

The mode of action within the body is stimulation of the CNS, thereby exciting the respiratory system and increasing body metabolism.[5] Caffeine is absorbed from the gastrointestinal tract, broken down in the liver, and excreted in the urine. The intake of a large quantity of caffeine can cause intoxication, manifested by cardiac dysrhythmias, sleep disturbances, mood changes, increased production of urine, gastrointestinal discomfort, and anxiety, especially panic attacks. Caffeinism and caffeine withdrawal syndrome are seen only with long-term use of caffeine, usually a documented intake of more than 500 mg/day.[19] Lack of caffeine can lead to severe headache. This problem can be seen in clients placed on NPO status (e.g., for surgery).

Nursing care begins with recognition of the clinical manifestations of excessive caffeine use and withdrawal. Monitoring the manifestations and observing for additional problems (such as whether the caffeine is exacerbating known health problems) are appropriate.

■ CANNABIS

Marijuana, a cannabis derivative, is the most widely used illegal drug in the United States, with more than 55% of young adults reporting personal use.[19] The mode of action of marijuana is not clearly understood, and researchers continue to try to identify the mechanism that accounts for its effects on the CNS and cardiovascular system.[7, 23]

Tetrahydrocannabinol (THC) is the active ingredient in marijuana and the agent responsible for the psychological effects. The amount of marijuana that crosses the blood-brain barrier depends on the method of intake used. THC is absorbed in fatty tissues, primarily the brain and testes, and is slowly released back into the bloodstream, where it is eventually excreted in urine and feces.[19]

Clients who use marijuana experience manifestations of intoxication, such as euphoria, mood changes, memory impairment, tremors, decreased body temperature, dry mouth, lack of coordination, elevated blood pressure and heart rate, and injected conjunctivae (bloodshot eyes). The CNS and cardiac, immune, and reproductive systems are affected. Long-term use also influences respiratory functioning. Marijuana residues in the lungs are considered more carcinogenic than tobacco residues.

Withdrawal from marijuana is typically an uncomfortable but not a life-threatening process. Nursing care includes monitoring the client's physical and emotional responses to the drug. It is often helpful for a nurse, family member, or friend to stay with the client, provide reassurance, and talk the client through the anxiety. Usually the client is not hospitalized unless pre-existing medical conditions or the coexistence of another psychoactive substance complicates the withdrawal process. For most clients, the initial effects of the drug dissipate within 4 to 6 hours; however, the effects of drug intoxication may last as long as 5 days.[30]

■ COCAINE

Cocaine is a narcotic obtained from the leaves of the coca plant; it was originally used by the Indians of the Andes to alleviate feelings of hunger and fatigue and to promote endurance. Today cocaine is readily available on the illicit market in the form of cocaine hydrochloride, which is soluble in water and used intravenously, inhaled (snorted), or smoked as "crack," a form of concentrated (freebase) cocaine.

Cocaine stimulates the CNS and blocks the conduction of peripheral nerve impulses. Continued use of cocaine increases the amount of dopamine in the synapses of nerve cells by preventing dopamine reuptake. Cocaine also decreases the breakdown of dopamine and other catecholamines, thereby increasing the level of catecholamine activity at the nerve cell synapses. Cocaine is metabolized in the liver and excreted in the urine. Evidence of cocaine use can be extracted from a urine sample for up to 72 hours after use.

In assessing for the effects of cocaine, remember that cocaine stimulates the CNS and the cardiovascular system. Cocaine abuse has led to myocardial infarctions in young, presumably healthy individuals. An overdose causes tremors, seizures, and delirium. Death can also result from cardiac or respiratory failure. Intervention is based on treating these identified problems and acting to prevent cardiac and respiratory complications. Cocaine intoxication may not be common in medical-surgical settings, because the half-life of cocaine is approximately 60 minutes.[3] Nursing management of a cocaine overdose focuses on preventing or handling cardiovascular collapse, respiratory distress, delirium, and hyperthermia.

Withdrawal from chronic use of cocaine ("binging") results in an exhausted state known as crashing. Clients experience a profound sense of depression, have memories of the cocaine-induced feelings of euphoria, and have cravings for the drug. Often, clients are hospitalized if there is severe depression with suicidal risk, if coexisting medical problems necessitate intense monitoring or treatment, or if there are medical problems directly related to complications of IV use. Besides providing the physical care required for the cocaine-dependent client, the nurse helps the client become aware of the need to develop effective coping skills.

■ HALLUCINOGENS

Hallucinogens, also known as *psychedelic drugs,* are both natural and synthetic substances that produce illusions, delusions, hallucinations, and alterations in thoughts, perceptions, and feelings. The effects of hallucinogens differ among individuals and are therefore unpredictable. An individual's personality may influence the reaction that occurs after hallucinogen use. Characteristic of lysergic acid diethylamide (LSD) and other psychedelic drugs are a subjective sensation of heightened awareness, an ability to look inward, and a feeling of oneness with the universe.

The mechanism of action is unknown. Hallucinogens are usually ingested and then absorbed from the gastrointestinal tract, metabolized in the liver, and excreted in the bile and feces.[7] The length of action is usually between 6 and 12 hours.[19]

The effects of hallucinogens are similar to those of other stimulants. The user experiences euphoria, dilated pupils, anxiety, and increased respirations, blood pressure, and heart rate. Panic attacks occur while the user is in a state of intoxication, accompanied by feelings of paranoia, confusion, hallucinations, possible dissociation, and loss of contact with reality. The resulting inability to perceive the environment accurately, impaired judgment, and feeling of having special powers make the person prone to dangerous activities. Suicide, homicide, and other acts of violence have been reported in people under the influence of hallucinogenic drugs. Some users also experience flashbacks. During a period of intoxication, or because of a flashback experience or the reliving of a "bad trip," a person may be brought to a health care setting.

Carefully assess the client for both physiologic and psychological problems. Nursing care focuses on attending to the panic that the client is experiencing as well as providing for client safety and creating a nonstimulating environment. Someone should stay with the client until the side effects have worn off. In the case of a severe overdose, be prepared to intervene for possible seizures, extremely high temperatures, and cardiac distress.[33] Because withdrawal symptoms may occur over a period of time, be vigilant for possible neurologic abnormalities and psychiatric manifestations.

■ INHALANTS

Inhalants are chemicals that give off fumes or vapors that readily pass through the blood-brain barrier to produce an alteration in consciousness. Commonly used inhalants are (1) solvents (glue, gasoline, nail polish remover, lighter fluid, paint thinner), (2) aerosols (hair spray, insecticides), and (3) anesthetic agents used for recreational purposes (nitrous oxide, chloroform, ether).

The probable mechanism of action is that these volatile substances alter the biologic membranes of the cells of the CNS and affect the metabolism of neurotransmitters in the brain.[19] Inhalants are metabolized in the liver and kidneys. Low doses of inhalants cause initial CNS excitement within minutes of use. Immediately after inhaling a volatile substance through the nose or mouth ("huffing"), the user experiences a "high," accompanied by feelings of giddiness and euphoria. There is a decrease in inhibitions and a slowing of the heart rate, respiratory rate, and overall mental activity. With inhalant intoxication, physical manifestations include delirium, cardiac dysrhythmias, irritation of the mucous membranes of the nose and mouth, cough, and depression of brain waves. Depending on the substance inhaled, the effects may last from a few minutes to several hours.[19]

Continuous use of volatile substances results in brain, lung, liver, kidney, and bone marrow damage. Withdrawal symptoms associated with inhalants vary with the specific substance used. Sudden death related to the use of inhalants can occur from life-threatening dysrhythmias and hypoxia.

Nursing care concentrates on prompt intervention in emergency situations (seizures, loss of consciousness, respiratory arrest). Effective management of the client's acute and chronic physiologic problems remains your primary goal.

■ NICOTINE

Nicotine is an alkaloid substance present in tobacco leaves. Using nicotine in the form of cigarettes, cigars, or chewing or pipe tobacco is an addictive habit practiced throughout the world. It is the leading cause of preventable death in the United States. Nicotine is absorbed through the lungs and within seconds crosses the blood-brain barrier and acts to stimulate the CNS. It is metabolized in the liver and excreted in the urine. Nicotine adversely affects the cardiovascular, respiratory, and gastrointestinal systems.

An overdose of nicotine is not a common occurrence. If intoxication develops, administration of oxygen and the treatment of symptoms are the nurse's priorities. Nicotine withdrawal occurs within 24 hours of smoking cessation. The withdrawal symptoms are uncomfortable, and the nurse can support the client through this process and assist with developing effective strategies for dealing with the manifestations.

■ OPIOIDS

Opioids comprise drugs produced from opium along with manufactured or semisynthetic narcotics. The human body also produces natural opiates, which facilitate feelings of well-being. Chemicals known as *endorphins* are neurotransmitters that connect with opiate receptors in the brain. When a person uses opiates or other narcotics, an interference is created in the natural opioid system and the functions of the neurotransmitters in the brain are disrupted.[16] Opioids are metabolized in the liver and excreted in the bile and urine.

An opioid overdose constitutes a life-threatening situation due to seizures, shock, respiratory depression, or cardiac dysrhythmias. The client is usually in an unconscious or lethargic state and may die without appropriate medical treatment. The nurse assesses and intervenes with the health care team to provide the required emergency care. Establishing an airway, monitoring cardiac functioning and treating dysrhythmias, maintaining hydration, and administering a narcotic antagonist such as naloxone (Narcan) are the nursing care priorities. The client should be hospitalized, with close monitoring of all body systems, for at least 24 hours.

For the client experiencing opioid withdrawal, focus on assessing and intervening for a variety of physiologic, psychological, and behavioral symptoms; these tend to occur within 72 hours of last drug use. Nursing care consists of constantly monitoring withdrawal symptoms along with providing rest, nutrition, and a comfortable environment. The initiation of a methadone program as a useful approach for treating opioid addiction is now recommended by the National Institutes of Health (NIH). Methadone therapy is useful for both detoxification and maintenance therapy. Clients often are referred to residential treatment programs to learn how to develop new, drug-free lifestyles.

■ PHENCYCLIDINE

Phencyclidine (PCP) is a synthetic drug with stimulant, depressant, and hallucinogenic properties.[7] PCP not only increases the production of dopamine but also blocks its reuptake, thus causing an increased blood pressure, heartbeat, and respiratory rates. PCP also increases acetylcholine in the CNS, thereby generating cholinergic effects manifested as diaphoresis, drooling, and pupillary constriction. Serotonin is also believed to be altered by the presence of PCP, resulting in a lack of coordination, slurred speech, and nystagmus.[19] PCP is metabolized in the liver and excreted in the urine.

Intoxication from PCP lasts up to 6 hours, and the effects of the drug are unpredictable. A person may experience euphoria, disorientation, or the racing or slowing of thoughts. In emergency departments, the client may be confused, hostile, violent, paranoid, or panicked. Nursing assessment of PCP intoxication often reveals severe cardiac or respiratory distress, which can lead to cardiac arrest. Clients under the influence of PCP can be in a psychosis-like state and can have nystagmus, abnormal muscle movements, and severe hypertension.

Nursing care concentrates on the assessment of subtle changes in vital signs and level of consciousness, gastric lavage if PCP has been ingested, and acidification of the urine.[19] In PCP withdrawal, you may see variable presentations of manifestations, particularly abnormal muscle movements. Carefully monitor the client's physical and mental condition to minimize health problems.

SEDATIVES, HYPNOTICS, AND ANXIOLYTICS

Sedative, hypnotic, and anxiolytic agents are considered to be CNS depressants. These medications are directly absorbed from the gastrointestinal tract into the bloodstream, where they enter the brain, are metabolized in the liver, and are eliminated via the kidneys. In cases of overdose, clients experience decreased CNS functioning along with the slowing of the cardiac and respiratory systems. Monitor vital signs and initiate emergency procedures based on the clinical manifestations presented. An overdose of any of these depressant drugs constitutes a medical emergency, with some clients requiring hospitalization in an intensive care unit (ICU).

Nursing care focuses on maintenance of adequate respiratory and cardiovascular status, hydration, and possible gastric lavage if the drugs were taken within the previous 4 to 6 hours.[33] For clients undergoing withdrawal, promote safety and rest while treating both physical and emotional manifestations. Nursing care priorities are awareness of the possibility of delirium, seizures, fever, and changes in cardiac and respiratory status as well as the interaction between adverse effects of the drug and pre-existing medical problems. Table 24–6 summarizes common health problems observed in clients who abuse drugs other than alcohol.

Nursing Management of Substance-Abusing Clients

The nurse plays a vital role in the care of clients experiencing intoxication and withdrawal. Nurses also meet basic needs, develop a therapeutic relationship, and teach both the client and family about addiction and its effect on the entire family. Nursing strategies for meeting actual or potential health problems are implemented for nursing diagnoses generated from assessment data. Nursing diagnoses commonly applied to the substance abuse population are listed in Box 24–3.

Education is an essential component of care to help the client understand the need for lifestyle changes. The main components of a drug education plan for clients and families are outlined in Box 24–4. Sometimes clients who abuse alcohol are referred for various treatment options and given disulfiram (Antabuse) to deter drinking. Clients receiving disulfiram must be carefully instructed about the drug. Information to include in a teaching plan is provided in Box 24–5.

Substance abuse has a major impact on family members. The family often tries to deal with a substance-abusing member by altering his or her behavior and compensating for the addict's unfilled responsibilities. Often the family inadvertently isolates itself from others as it focuses most of its energy on the addict. Personal needs of the caregiver, other adults, and children go unmet. Family members are strongly affected by the addiction and must be involved in the recovery process. A caring, supportive, and educative response from the nurse conveys that the family's concerns are understood and will be included in the treatment program. A major role of the nurse is education of client and family. The educative responsive is detailed in Box 24–4.

DRUG AND ALCOHOL INTERVENTION

CONFRONTATION ABOUT DRUG ABUSE

In medical-surgical settings, nurses and other members of the health care team may receive a request for assistance from family members who believe that the client needs to obtain drug and alcohol treatment. To confront the client about drug abuse, a carefully orchestrated format (a *therapeutic intervention*) can be implemented to force the client to participate in treatment.[10] The intervention must be planned in advance and executed under the guidance of a health care provider with a drug and alcohol counseling background. To prepare for the intervention, all participants compose a list of situations in which they have personal knowledge about the client's drug and alcohol behaviors.

During the therapeutic intervention, a group of family and friends gather together and bring the client face to face with the addiction problem. In an objective and nonjudgmental manner, the group states its concerns about the client, its observations about the client's substance abuse behavior, and its overall caring about the client's well-being. A plan for obtaining help from these significant people is presented to the client. This plan includes treatment recommendations and may contain a reservation for a particular treatment facility. It is believed that this loving and open confrontation can break through the abuser's denial and defensiveness. The client's family and friends must also state the consequences that will immediately ensue if help is refused.

TREATMENT OPTIONS

After completing a comprehensive health history and providing care for the client, you are in an optimal position to recommend a treatment modality that corresponds to

TABLE 24–6 HEALTH CONSEQUENCES OF COMMONLY ABUSED DRUGS

	Amphetamines	Caffeine	Cannabis	Cocaine	Hallucinogens	Inhalants	Nicotine	Opioids	Phencyclidine (PCP)	Sedatives, hypnotics, and anxiolytics
Abrupt withdrawal symptoms (similar to alcohol withdrawal)										X
Agitation										
Angina		X					X			
Acquired immunodeficiency syndrome (AIDS)				X				X		
Anemia								X		
Atelectasis								X		
Arthritis								X		
Aspiration				X						
Bone marrow depression						X				
Brain damage						X				
Bronchitis				X			X			
Cancer (laryngeal)							X			
Cancer (lung)							X			
Cancer (oral cavity)							X			
Cerebrovascular accident (stroke)				X			X			
Confusion									X	
Dysrhythmias	X	X			X	X		X		
Emphysema							X			
Endocarditis (bacterial)				X				X		
Excoriations (from scratching nonexistent bugs)	X									
Flashbacks					X					
Gastrointestinal distress/ulcers						X	X			
Hallucinations									X	
Hepatitis (bacterial, viral)				X		X		X		
Hypergammaglobulinemia								X		
Hypertension	X	X		X	X				X	
Immune dysfunctions									X	
Insomnia		X								
Judgment, impaired									X	
Lung abscess								X		
Lung irritation			X			X				
Lymphadenopathy								X		

TABLE 24–6 HEALTH CONSEQUENCES OF COMMONLY ABUSED DRUGS *Continued*

	Amphetamines	Caffeine	Cannabis	Cocaine	Hallucinogens	Inhalants	Nicotine	Opioids	Phencyclidine (PCP)	Sedatives, hypnotics, and anxiolytics
Mental slowness										X
Motor function, impaired										X
Muscle weakness						X				
Myocardial infarction				X			X			
Myositis ossificans (drug user's elbow)								X		
Nasal septal damage				X						
Nephritis								X		
Neuropathy (peripheral)						X				
Osteomyelitis								X		
Paranoid psychosis	X									
Peptic ulcers		X								
Pharyngitis (chronic)			X							
Phlebitis								X		
Pneumonia								X		
Pulmonary emboli				X						
Pulmonary fibrosis								X		
Renal failure				X		X		X		
Respiratory arrest/failure						X				
Seizures	X			X					X	X
Skin ulcers or abscesses				X						
Sinusitis (chronic)			X							
Splenomegaly								X		
Testosterone (lowered levels)			X							
Tremors		X								
Tuberculosis								X		
Visual loss (from adulterants in street drugs)								X		

BOX 24–3 Common Nursing Diagnoses for Clients Who Abuse Substances

- *Acute Confusion*
- *Anxiety*
- *Impaired Verbal Communication*
- *Ineffective Denial*
- *Altered Family Processes*
- *Fatigue*
- *Fear*
- *Dysfunctional Grieving*
- *Hopelessness*
- *Ineffective Individual Coping*
- *Risk for Infection*
- *Risk for Injury*
- *Knowledge Deficit* (specify)
- *Noncompliance* (specify)
- *Altered Nutrition: Less than Body Requirements*
- *Pain*
- *Altered Parenting*
- *Personal Identity Disturbance*
- *Risk for Poisoning*
- *Powerlessness*
- *Altered Role Performance*
- *Chronic Low Self esteem*
- *Sensory/Perceptual Alterations* (*Specify:* visual, auditory kinesthetic, gustatory, tactile, olfactory)
- *Altered Sexuality Patterns*
- *Risk for Impaired Skin Integrity*
- *Sleep Pattern Disturbance*
- *Impaired Social Interaction*
- *Social Isolation*
- *Spiritual Distress*
- *Altered Thought Processes*
- *Risk for Trauma*
- *Risk for Violence (Self-directed or directed at others)*

the needs of the client and family members. Activities that you are involved in range from primary prevention (education), to secondary prevention (outpatient services), to tertiary prevention (inpatient or outpatient detoxification and rehabilitation). The common interventions for all three levels of care are listed in Table 24–7. A list of community resources that can provide education and support to substance-abusing clients and their families appears in Box 24–6.

BOX 24–4 Components of a Client and Family Education Plan

- Concept of addiction
- Physical health problems associated with addiction
- Nutritional status
- Feelings and behaviors of all family members associated with addiction
- Areas of life affected by substance use: family, social, spiritual, sexual, occupational, financial, legal, and leisure
- Roles family members play in addiction
- Treatment options and treatment process
- Aftercare and self-help support groups or 12-step programs
- Community resources
- Skill building in the areas of communication, expression of feelings, socialization, and coping strategies
- Impact of both addiction and the recovery process on the roles and responsibilities of all family members
- Client confidentiality and right to privacy protected under the 1975 Federal Drug and Alcohol Abuse Act

BOX 24–5 Information to Include in a Teaching Plan About Disulfiram (Antabuse)

- Inform the client that disulfiram is not a cure for alcoholism; it only discourages drinking.
- Before initiating disulfiram therapy, ask whether the client has had any allergic reactions to substances such as sulfites, preservatives, or dyes.
- Ask whether the client has a history of seizures; severe mental illness, particularly psychosis; serious cardiac disease; kidney disease; diabetes mellitus; hypothyroidism; or skin allergies.
- Ask whether the client is taking anticoagulants (↑ effects), isoniazid (INH) (↑ CNS effects), metronidazole (Flagyl) (↑ toxicity), or phenytoin (Dilantin) (↑ toxicity).
- Instruct the client not to ingest any alcohol or use any products containing alcohol within 12 hours before taking disulfiram, while taking disulfiram, and for at least 14 days after discontinuing disulfiram.
- Explain to the client that it is necessary to read the labels on all products because alcohol is found in many foods, medicines, and personal hygiene products (e.g., sauces, vinegars, cough syrups, tonics, elixirs, mouthwash, colognes, after-shave lotions).
- Tell the client not to inhale chemicals that may contain alcohol (e.g., paints, varnish, shellac).
- Encourage the client not to use alcohol-containing products that are applied topically. Alcohol absorbed through the skin can cause redness, itching, headache, and nausea.
- Identify common side effects (e.g., headache, fatigue, a metallic or garlic-like aftertaste, skin rash) that may be experienced during the first 2 weeks of taking disulfiram. Inform the client that these manifestations resolve as the body adjusts to the medication.
- If the client ingests alcohol while taking disulfiram, blurred vision, chest pain, confusion, dizziness or fainting, palpitations, flushing, diaphoresis, nausea, vomiting, headache, and dyspnea may occur. These symptoms last as long as alcohol is in the body. If the client drinks a large amount of alcohol, seizures, myocardial infarction, unconsciousness, or death may result.
- Instruct the client to carry a card specifying that he or she is taking disulfiram, listing side effects of alcohol, and stating whom to contact in an emergency.

PREVENTION OF RELAPSE

Clients in the recovery process may be at risk for relapse or a return to substance abuse. Anticipate the possibility of *relapse* (slipping back into substance use after a period of abstinence), and prepare clients with strategies that may prevent it. This regression can occur any time and may be defined as one-time use, brief intermittent use, or daily long-term use. Relapse should be viewed as a potential part of the illness process, much like the potential course of any other chronic illness. Seeing relapse as client failure sets the client up for defeat instead of recovery.

Physiologic, emotional, and social variables all contribute to relapse. Clients must be taught ways to assess their strengths and to identify situations that can distract them

TABLE 24–7 LEVELS OF TREATMENT STRATEGIES

Level of Prevention	Activities	Resources
Primary prevention	Education to prevent substance abuse Risk factor identification Lifestyle guidance	School programs Community programs Health promotion activities
Secondary prevention (outpatient)	Assessment and intervention of early physical and emotional issues and problems Educational interventions Pharmacologic interventions Self-management strategies Support and self-help groups Psychotherapy	Medical facilities as appropriate Individual, family, or group therapy Psychoeducational groups Self-help groups (e.g., AA, NA, CA, Al-Anon, Alateen, Naranon, ACOA)*
Tertiary prevention (inpatient or outpatient)	Interventions to monitor withdrawal and prevent or treat complications Focusing on relapse prevention Determining plan for aftercare and methods of obtaining support Individual, family, or group therapy	Medical services, such as detoxification Aftercare, such as partial programs, supervised living, or halfway house Individual, family, or group therapy Psychoeducational groups Self-help groups (e.g., AA, NA, CA, Al-Anon, Alateen, Naranon, ACOA)*

*See Box 24–6, Resources.
AA, Alcoholics Anonymous; ACOA, Adult Children of Alcoholics; CA, Cocaine Anonymous; NA, Narcotics Anonymous.

from their recovery. Peer pressure, stress, and negative feelings may trigger a relapse. Some relapse prevention strategies to include in educational programs are listed in Box 24–7.

■ SURGERY AND SUBSTANCE ABUSE

Clients who abuse substances often experience accidents, injuries, or illnesses that require surgical intervention. In fact, many injuries seen by nurses in emergency departments are directly related to drug and alcohol use. Become skillful in observing for subtle changes, and perform frequent assessments in order to intervene immediately and prevent the escalation of manifestations. Traumatized clients usually require immediate surgery; hence, a thorough drug and alcohol assessment may not be done. It is a challenge for the nurse to distinguish medical problems, psychiatric disorders, and substance abuse disorders in a timely manner.

BOX 24–6 Resources

Alcoholics Anonymous (look in the local telephone directory, or call New York, NY: 212-686-1100 for information throughout the United States); *www.alcoholics-anonymous.org*

Al-Anon (look in the local telephone directory, or call New York, NY: 212-254-7230 for information throughout the United States); Al-Anon and Alateen Family Group Headquarters, Inc.: 888-4AL-ANON (888-425-2666); *www.al-anon.org*

Adult Children of Alcoholics (look in the local telephone directory, or call Torrance, CA: 213-534-1815 for information); *www.info@adultchildren.org*

BACCHUS (Boost Alcohol Consciousness Concerning the Health of University Students) (call Denver, CO: 303-871-3068 for information)

Children of Alcoholics Foundation, Inc. (call New York, NY: 212-351-2680 for information); 800-359-2623; *www.coaf.org*

MADD (Mothers Against Drunken Driving) (call Austin, TX: 817-268-6233 for information)

Narcotics Anonymous (look in the local telephone directory, or call Van Nuys, CA: 818-780-3951 for information); *www.na.org*

Cocaine Anonymous (call Los Angeles, CA: 800-347-8998 or 213-559-5833 for information); *www.ca.org*

Marijuana Anonymous (look in the local telephone directory, or call 800-766-6779); *www.marijuana-anonymous.org*

Dual Recovery Anonymous (look in the local telephone directory, or call 888-869-9230); *www.dualrecovery.base.org*

National Clearinghouse for Alcohol and Drug Information (call Rockville, MD: 301-468-2600 for information)

National Asian Pacific American Families Against Drug Abuse (call Bethesda, MD: 301-530-0945 for information)

Hotline Numbers

Center for Substance Abuse Treatment
National Treatment Hotline: 800-662-HELP (800-662-4357)

Center for Substance Abuse Prevention Workplace
Hotline 800-WORKPLACE 800-967-5752

National Alcohol Hotline
HelpLine: 800-ALCOHOL (800-252-6465)

National Cocaine Hotline
800-COCAINE (800-2622-2463)

BOX 24–7 Strategies to Prevent Relapse

- Assess and build on the client's coping skills.
- Take opportunities, such as role-playing, that help the client practice coping methods.
- Assist the client in identifying personal risks of relapse.
- Identify people, places, and things that can interfere with maintaining sobriety and encourage the client to minimize contact with these obstacles and develop ways to handle them.
- Change environmental variables when possible.
- Discuss the concept of craving, how to identify it, what may trigger it, and how to handle it.
- Focus on the client's physiologic feelings and sensations, and develop methods to handle them.
- Teach strategies that promote a healthy lifestyle, such as exercise, nutrition, stress management, and relaxation techniques.
- Encourage participation in support groups or self-help groups.
- Recommend group or individual therapy if the client has problems with the family of origin, struggles with daily functioning, or mental illness.

Alcoholic clients who are admitted for a surgical procedure require special attention. They are told not to drink for several days before surgery, but in reality they may have been drinking up to the night before. Postoperatively, the client begins to develop withdrawal and must be actively restrained. The challenges facing the nursing staff caring for a postoperative client with DTs are great. Client safety is a serious matter, as are wound healing and adequate nutrition. The client may be treated to reduce symptoms. In other cases, the client may be simply left to detoxify "cold turkey," a method that stops the substance abruptly. Your role as a client advocate is imperative for these clients.

If a client is addicted to CNS depressant drugs, a larger amount of an anesthetic may be needed to produce the desired effects. This situation occurs because the client has a higher tolerance to the anesthetic drug. For clients with liver impairment and overall poor health, anesthetics cannot be properly metabolized and the effect of sedation is prolonged. While undergoing surgery, the addicted client is at risk for cardiac dysrhythmias, respiratory depression, hemorrhage, and depletion of catecholamines.

In the postoperative period, these clients are susceptible to cardiac, respiratory, urinary, hemorrhagic, and wound complications. The experience of pain may be intensified because the clients often have tolerance to the pain medication. Carefully assess whether the client requires increased doses of medication for pain relief and needs to be slowly weaned from the medication during recovery. Some addicted clients may experience drug withdrawal postoperatively because withdrawal has been delayed by the use of anesthetics.

The Impaired Health Care Professional

Just like other people, health care professionals can become addicted to drugs and alcohol. Research on the prevalence of substance abuse among nurses has revealed no difference between nurses and other health professionals. Further, the prevalence of substance abuse among health professionals overall does not differ from that in the general population.[40] Many addicted health care professionals first started using drugs and alcohol in response to physical illness and pain, emotional difficulties, or work pressures.

The requirements of the professional nurse's role make nursing a stressful occupation. On a daily basis, the nurse is responsible for coordinating and directly providing care for clients who are in pain and crisis. The pressure of handling resources; making decisions; interfacing with medical and other personnel; working long hours, often with inadequate staff; and being responsible for the daily operation of the medical-surgical unit can be overwhelming. In addition, nurses have access to narcotics and operate on the premise that medications are a useful vehicle for relieving pain and altering states of feelings. Specialized knowledge about drugs and experience with administering them and watching their efficacy may lead health care providers to view drugs as a "pharmacologic coping method."[9, 25] It is a method that can ultimately backfire.

The signs of a chemically impaired colleague are subtle and easily overlooked by peers and supervisors. Even other health care professionals may deny and avoid the problem rather than confront the person suspected of being chemically dependent. It is essential that nurses be aware of the signs of chemical dependence in peers (Box 24–8). Document questionable or problematic incidents, and be willing to participate in an intervention if deemed appropriate. Remember, a peer who suffers from addiction cannot meet the requirements of your state nurse practice act. Some states have a law that mandates reporting of an impaired colleague.

As with clients, steps must be taken to assist an impaired nurse to obtain treatment. The use of an employee assistance program (EAP) and peer support or assistance groups from the state nurses' association can facilitate referrals to treatment and can assist with recovery. Although peer assistance programs vary from state to state,

BOX 24–8 Signs of a Chemically Impaired Colleague

- Alcohol on breath
- Mood changes or confusion
- Difficulty making judgments and impaired memory
- Red eyes with flushed face
- Unsteady gait
- Tremors or impaired eye-hand coordination
- Irritability or hyperactivity
- Lethargy or dozing on breaks
- Disheveled appearance
- Wearing long sleeves or a sweater constantly, even in hot weather
- Incorrect drug counts
- Accidents, spillages, or drugs frequently being wasted
- Frequently found in the bathroom, nurses' lounge, or off the unit
- Recurrent unfinished assignments or client care mistakes

most programs offer support, referral services, monitoring during recovery, and educational programs targeted to the health care professional.

CONCLUSIONS

Substance abuse remains a major health issue, affecting clients, families, and communities. Despite this reality many clients with substance abuse disorders are not identified and, therefore, do not obtain treatment. A lack of knowledge about addiction can perpetuate stigmatization of the client. Your challenge is to become informed about both the effects of drugs and appropriate strategies for treatment. Keen assessment skills, decision-making skills, and compassion are the prerequisites for comprehensive nursing care of the myriad physiologic and psychological needs presented by these clients.

Nurses play a vital role in developing and implementing drug and alcohol prevention strategies. Teaching how to use effective coping strategies, how to handle crises, and how to develop support systems are the primary steps that must be incorporated into the care. For you, as a nurse, it is important to spend time cultivating relationships and to allow yourself to engage in leisure activities that decrease feelings of frustration, hopelessness, and burnout.

THINKING CRITICALLY

1. A group of young college students celebrated the end of the semester with a week-long party. Alcoholic beverages were plentiful; food was not a priority. A young couple brought their friend to the emergency department. They reported their suspicions that she might have a drinking problem (e.g., erratic behavior, presence of alcoholic beverages in the dormitory room, smell of alcohol on her breath). They were unable to awaken her for any length of time and are worried that she drank too much. She has not had a drink for about 6 hours. What assessment is required? What nursing actions are appropriate?

Factors to Consider. How likely is it for the client to experience delirium tremens (DTs)? How will the client be treated?

2. You are a Registered Nurse in the local "Driving Under the Influence of Alcohol" (DUI) teaching program. Your topic is "Alcohol and the Human Body." The audience is made up of clients mandated by the court to attend. After the presentation, which focuses on the complications associated with long-term drinking, the clients ask, "If alcoholism is a disease, why are we treated as criminals?" "I didn't drink so much, why did they pull me over?" What might these questions indicate?

Factors to Consider. Is alcoholism a disease of addiction? What psychological factor is evident in such questions?

BIBLIOGRAPHY

1. Addiction Research Corporation. (1986). *GRASP: Guide's rational adolescent substance abuse profile.* Piscataway, NJ: Rutgers University Center of Alcohol Studies.
2. American Psychiatric Association. (1994). *Diagnostic and statistical manual of mental disorders* (4th ed.). Washington, DC: Author.
3. American Psychiatric Association. (1995). Practice guidelines for the treatment of patients with substance use disorders: Alcohol, cocaine, opioids. *American Journal of Psychiatry, 152*(11), Supplement 4–19.
4. Bellenir, K. (Ed.). (1996). *Substance abuse sourcebook.* Detroit, MI: Omnigraphics.
5. Blum, K., et al. (1990). Allelic association of human dopamine D2 receptor gene in alcoholism. *Journal of the American Medical Association, 15*(263), 2055–2060.
6. Bond, A., et al. (1994). Systemic absorption and abuse liability of snorted flunitrazepam. *Addiction, 89*(7), 821–830.
7. Burns, E. M., Thompson, A., & Ciccone, J. K. (1993). *An addictions curriculum for nurses and other helping professionals* (Vol. 2). New York: Springer-Verlag.
8. Clayton, L. (1997). *Tranquilizers.* Springfield, NY: Enslow.
9. Coombs, R. H. (1997). *Drug impaired professionals.* Cambridge, MA: Harvard University Press.
10. Copel, L. C. (2000). *Nurses' clinical guide to psychiatric* and *mental health nursing* (2nd ed.). Springhouse, PA: Springhouse.
11. Doweiko, H. (1999). *Concepts of chemical dependency.* Pacific Grove, CA: Brooks/Cole Publishing.
12. Ewing, J. A. (1984). CAGE. *Journal of the American Medical Association 252*(14):1906.
13. Freed, P. E., & York, L. N. (1997). Naltrexone: A controversial therapy for alcohol dependence. *Journal of Psychosocial Nursing and Mental Health Services, 35*(7), 24–28.
14. Freeman, E. M. (Ed.). (1993). *Substance abuse treatment: A family systems perspective.* Newbury, CA: Sage.
15. Galanter, M., & Kleber, H. D. (1994). *Textbook of substance abuse treatment.* Washington, DC: American Psychiatric Press.
16. Goldstein, A. (1994). *Addiction: From biology to drug policy.* New York: W. H. Freeman.
17. Henly, G. A., & Winters, K. C. (1988). Development of problem severity scales for the assessment of adolescent alcohol and drug abuse. *International Journal of the Addictions, 23,* 65–85.
18. Horn, J. L., Skinner, H. A., Wanberg, K. W., & Foster, F. M. (1984). *Alcohol use questionnaire (AUQ).* Toronto, Canada: Addiction Research Foundation.
19. Jaffe, J. (Ed.). (1995). *Encyclopedia of drugs and alcohol.* New York, Macmillan.
20. Jefferson, L. V. (1995). Chemically mediated responses and substance-related disorders. In G. W. Stuart & S. J. Sundeen (Eds.), *Principles and practices of psychiatric nursing* (pp. 569–605). St. Louis: Mosby–Year Book.
21. Keller, C. M. (1994). Flumazenil: A new benzodiazepine-specific antagonist. *Journal of the American Academy of Physician Assistants, 7*(8), 595–598.
22. Lowinson, J., Ruiz, P., Millman, R., & Langrod, J. (Eds.). (1997). *Substance abuse: A comprehensive textbook* (3rd ed.). Baltimore, MD: Williams & Wilkins.
23. Marx, J. (1990). Marijuana receptor gene cloned. *Science, 249,* 624–626.
24. McLellan, A. T., et al. (1992). The fifth edition of the addiction severity index. *Journal of Substance Abuse Treatment, 9*(3), 199–213.
25. Mynatt, S. (1996). A model of contributing risk factors to chemical dependency in nurses. *Journal of Psychosocial Nursing and Mental Health Services, 34*(7), 13–22.
26. Nace, E. P., & Isbell, P. I. (1991). Alcohol. In R. J. Frances & S. I. Miller (Eds.), *Clinical textbook of addictive disorders* (pp. 43–68). New York: Guilford Press.
27. Naranjo, C. A., Sellers, E. M., & Chater, M. (1983). Nonpharmacologic intervention in acute alcohol withdrawal. *Clinical Pharmacology and Therapeutics 34,* 814–819.

27a. National Consensus Development Panel. (1998). Effective medical treatment of opiate addiction. *Journal of the American Medical Association, 280*(22), 1936–1943.

28. National Institute on Alcohol Abuse and Alcoholism. (1984). *Alcohol abuse curriculum guide for nurse practitioner faculty* (DHHS

Pub. No. ADM 84-1313, Vol. 3). Rockville, MD: Health Professions Education Curriculum Resources Series.

29. National Institute on Alcohol Abuse and Alcoholism. (1990). *Seventh special report to the U.S. Congress on alcohol and health: From the secretary of health and human services* (DHHS Pub. No. ADM 90-1656). Rockville, MD: Author.
30. Ott, P. J., Tarter, R. E., & Ammerman, R. T. (1999). *Sourcebook on substance abuse: Etiology, epidemiology, assessment, and treatment.* Boston, MA: Allyn & Bacon.
31. Peele, S. (1986). The implications and limitations of genetic models of alcoholism and other addictions. *Journal of Studies on Alcohol, 47,* 63–73.
32. Pokorney, A. D., Miller, B. A., & Kaplan, H. B. (1992). The brief MAST: A shortened version of the Michigan Alcoholism Screening Test. *American Journal of Psychiatry, 129,* 342–348.
33. Selzer, M. L. (1971). The Michigan Alcoholism Screening test: The quest for a new diagnostic instrument. *American Journal of Psychiatry, 127,* 1653–1658.
34. Selzer, M., Vinokur, A., & van Roojan, L. (1975). A self-administered short alcohol screening test (SMAST). *Journal of Studies on Alcoholism, 36*(1), 86.
35. Skinner, H. A., & Horn, J. L. (1984). *Alcohol Dependence Scale (ADS): User's guide.* Toronto, Canada: Addiction Research Foundation.

35a. Smith, D. E., Wesson, D. R., & Calhoun, S. R. (1995). *Rohypnol (flunitrazepam) fact sheet.* (Available from the Haight-Ashbury Free Clinics, Inc., 409 Clayton Street, San Francisco, CA 94117.)

36. Sokol, R. J., Martier, S. S., & Ager, J. W. (1989). The T-ACE questions: Practical prenatal detection of risk-drinking. *American Journal of Obstetrics and Gynecology, 160,* 863–870.
37. Sue, D. (1987). Use and abuse of alcohol by Asian Americans. *Journal of Psychoactive Drugs, 19,* 57.
38. Sullivan, E. (1995). Nursing care of clients with substance abuse. St. Louis: Mosby–Year Book.
39. Swenson, W., & Morse, R. (1973). The use of self-administered alcoholism screening test (SAAST) in a medical center. *Mayo Clinic Proceedings, 50,* 204–208.
40. Trinkoff, A. M., Eaton, W. W., & Anthony, J. C. (1991). The prevalence of substance abuse among registered nurses. *Nursing Research, 40*(3), 172–175.
41. Whitfield, C. L., Thompson, G., & Lamb, A. (1978). Detoxication of 1,024 alcoholic patients without psychoactive drugs. *Journal of the American Medical Association, 17*(239), 1409–1411.

Decision-Making: Withholding or Withdrawing Life Support

QUESTION

What client and family factors influence decisions for or against withholding and/or withdrawing of fluids and nutrition from terminally ill adults?

CITATION

Riley, J. M., et al. (1999). Factors related to adult patient decision making about withholding or withdrawing nutrition and/or hydration. *Online Journal of Knowledge Synthesis for Nursing, 6*(3).

STUDIES

A broad search of *CINAHL, MEDLINE,* and *BIOETHICLINE* databases revealed 16 published reports that addressed the question and that were truly research studies (1977 to 1997). Some findings were embedded in more general studies about end-of-life decisions. The studies were analyzed by four collaborators, including an Advanced Practice Nurse and a nurse-ethicist.

A wide range of people and settings were studied, including 418 hospitalized clients, 1047 clinic clients, 112 residents of long-term care facilities, 2536 community-dwelling elders, and 433 family members or surrogates. Data were collected via interviews (six studies), questionnaires (seven studies), and client record audits (three studies). Four studies used hypothetical vignettes to help understand clients' and families' preferences for or against life-sustaining treatment.

Summary of Findings

Identification of Treatment Preferences

The issue of how various groups of people view life support (e.g., intravenous [IV] fluids, tube feedings, mechanical ventilation) was examined in five studies. The results showed little consensus that would be helpful in predicting how a person might feel about a particular form of life support. However, several studies suggested that in general people did not want life-sustaining measures that would prolong a diminished quality of life,[2, 5, 12] especially if they anticipated a diminished cognitive state.

Stability of Treatment Preferences

Of the four studies that examined the stability of client treatment preferences, three found that these preferences remained fairly stable in most people for 1 to 2 years.[4, 5, 12] However, in a cohort of community-based elders, the preference to forgo certain treatments was more stable than the preference to receive them.[3] For example, 75% of the people who answered "no" to tube feeding at the initial interview gave the same response 2 years later, whereas only 43% of those who answered "yes" to tube feeding did so. Some findings show that hypothetical decision-making may not predict actual choice in the event of serious illness.[5, 12]

Factors Associated with Client Decisions

An array of factors that influence end-of-life decisions has been studied, including (1) the time sequence for decision-making, (2) the presence of underlying malignancy, (3) mental status, (4) age, and (5) ethnicity. Across studies, however, none stands out as more important than the others. In one study, 74% of hospitalized clients had some interventions withdrawn or withheld before death; typically, these decisions were made near the time of death.[6] During the final episode of illness, 89% of clients decided to have limitations in their care; feeding tube limitations accounting for 11% of the interventions.[7]

Emotional state was also studied.[8, 14] When given "good" prognosis scenarios, depressed older adults wanted fewer life-saving treatments compared with older non-adults who were not depressed. With "poor" prognosis scenarios, however, preferences were similar for depressed and non-depressed elders.[8] "Increasing severity of depression explained less than 5% of the variance in decision-making in any treatment situation" (p 41).[8] Surprisingly, disease-specific factors (e.g., limitations of activity by disease, duration of illness, and clients' perceptions of the prognosis) were not significantly associated with desire for life support, nor were demographic variables (e.g., age, marital status, religion, and education).[14] However, in two studies, race did influence decisions in that African Americans and Hispanic Americans desired life support more often than whites did.[1, 14]

Client values such as not wanting to be a burden on anyone, wanting to do the most for oneself, retaining the right to choose one's own medical treatment, and viewing quality of life as more important that preservation of life influenced the preferences of many clients.[2] Previous experiences with life support were common among clinic elders (82% had at least one such experience); in one study, people with a positive experience were more likely to desire more life support than those with a negative experience.[14] In contrast, another study indicated that prior experience with life support was not a factor in a client's preference.[1]

Surrogate Decision-Making

When clients are unable to take part in the decision-making process regarding life-sustaining measures and when they have not made their wishes known, a difficult situation ensues. The research suggests that it is not clear how accurately a surrogate (i.e., the designated health care proxy) chooses what a client would choose. In one study surrogates chose life support treatments in accord with the clients' wishes about 60% of the time—a rate no better than chance guessing.[14] In contrast, another study demonstrated high agreement in the decision to accept or decline tube feedings.[9] Two studies found that many clients, including those who had written advance directives, had not conveyed their wishes to their surrogates.[2, 13] This is unfortunate, given the finding in one study that specific discussion between client and surrogate about life support was the only predictor of accurate surrogate decision-making.[14]

Many adult children–surrogates chose to continue fluid and hydration even when a parent's wishes to the contrary were known.[13] Surrogates tended to overestimate the client's preference for life-sustaining interventions, including the use of tube feedings, and often decided based on their own preferences.

Bridge continued on following page

Decision-Making: Withholding or Withdrawing Life Support *Continued*

Deciding whether to withhold or withdraw tube feedings clearly makes surrogates uncomfortable, particularly if they think their decision is inconsistent with the client's decision.[10] Spouses of patients with Alzheimer's disease were more uncomfortable with decisions to forgo tube feeding than with decisions to accept it, although more of them decided to forgo it as severity of illness increased.[11]

Limitations/Reservations. The large number of studies employing hypothetical scenarios casts some doubt on how well these studies as a whole have captured clients' and families' thinking about these complex issues. The authors of the review believe that qualitative studies sensitive to the meaning of these decisions as they are anticipated, made, and lived with over time are needed (p 61). Also, little is known about the experience and sensations that accompany not receiving nutrition and hydration at the end of life; yet this is a chief source of concern for surrogates (p 63).

Research-Based Practice

There is strong societal support for a client's self-determination regarding the use of life-sustaining treatments. These studies show that such choices are highly individualized and depend on assumptions about the length and quality of life. Since these assumptions are often based on the estimations offered by physicians, surrogates often have to decide in the context of much uncertainty, which is why many people wait until a situation seems hopeless.

A person's preferences for life-sustaining interventions are relatively stable as long as his or her health state is stable but are likely to change when health status changes substantially. The likelihood that clients' preference will change as their condition worsens makes repeated discussions between clients, their surrogates, and their health care providers very important. Clients may feel one way about nutrition and another way about hydration or about cardiopulmonary resuscitation (CPR). The documented preference of many African Americans and Hispanic Americans for life support and the declining of these measures by whites should be kept in mind and respected.

The studies in this review reveal the difficulties associated with discussing end-of-life treatment decisions before illness occurs. Specific illness scenarios are a widely used tool and probably are better than discussions about options without presenting an illness context. However, the scenarios presented should be carefully chosen and carefully worded. When clients face high-risk surgery or are in a physically or mentally deteriorating state, they should discuss their treatment wishes with their surrogate or health care proxy to ensure that their wishes are known. Discussions at these times can often be more relevant in nature than when a client was well because the problems that are likely to occur and the decisions that need to be made are more predictable.

Just as clients who have a proxy should be encouraged to talk with their surrogate, surrogates should be encouraged to hold frank discussions with the client they may need to represent. Whoever begins the discussion may need guidance from a nurse. You might suggest the idea of using "what if" scenarios rather than just talking about CPR or tube feedings or IV fluids. You might also join or facilitate the discussion or request the physician to join the discussion.

You can assist patients at many points in the process of making decisions about withholding or withdrawing life-sustaining measures. As the authors of the review stated, "Nurses share in the responsibility to ensure that individual patient's personal treatment preferences are thoughtfully formulated, clearly identified, consistently communicated, and respectfully honored" (p 49).

Cited References

1. Caralis, P. V., et al. (1993). The influence of ethnicity and race on attitudes toward advance directives, life-prolonging treatments, and euthanasia. *Journal of Clinical Ethics, 4,* 155–165.
2. Cohen-Mansfield, J., et al. (1991). The decision to execute a durable power of attorney for health care and preferences regarding the utilization of life-sustaining treatments in nursing home residents. *Archives of Internal Medicine, 151,* 289–294.
3. Danis, M., et al. (1994). Stability of choices about life-sustaining treatments. *Annals of Internal Medicine, 120,* 567–573.
4. Emanuel, L. L., et al. (1994). Advance directives: Stability of patients' treatment choices. *Archives of Internal Medicine, 154,* 209–217.
5. Everhart, M. A., & Pearlman, R. A. (1990). Stability of patient preferences regarding life-sustaining treatments. *Chest, 97,* 154–164.
6. Faber-Langendoen, K., & Bartels, D. M. (1992). Process of forgoing life-sustaining treatment in a university hospital: An empirical study. *Critical Care Medicine, 20,* 570–577.
7. Fried, T. R., & Gillick, M. R. (1994). Medical decision-making in the last six months of life: Choices about limitation of care. *Journal of the American Geriatrics Society, 42,* 303–307.
8. Lee, M. A., & Ganzini, L. (1992). Depression in the elderly: Effect on patient attitudes toward life-sustaining therapy. *Journal of the American Geriatrics Society, 40,* 983–988.
9. Libbus, M. K., & Russell, C. (1995). Congruence of decisions between patients and their potential surrogates about life-sustaining therapies. *Image: Journal of Nursing Scholarship, 27,* 135–140.
10. McNabney, M. K., Beers, M. H., & Siebens, H. (1994). Surrogate decision-makers' satisfaction with the placement of feeding tubes in elderly patients. *Journal of the American Geriatrics Society, 42,* 161–168.
11. Mezey, M., et al. (1996). Life-sustaining treatment decisions by spouses of patients with Alzheimer's disease. *Journal of the American Geriatrics Society, 44,* 144–150.
12. Schneiderman, L. J., et al (1992). Relationship of general advance directive instructions to specific life-sustaining treatment preferences in patients with serious illness. *Archives of Internal Medicine, 152,* 2114–2122.
13. Sonnenblick, M., Friedlander, Y., & Steinberg, A. (1993). Dissociation between the wishes of terminally ill parents and decisions by their offspring. *Journal of the American Geriatrics Society, 41,* 599–604.
14. Suhl, J., et al. (1994). Myths of substituted judgment: Surrogate decision making regarding life support is unreliable. *Archives of Internal Medicine, 154,* 90–96.

UNIT 5

Mobility Disorders

Anatomy and Physiology Review
The Musculoskeletal System

David Porta
Joyce M. Black

Physiologically, the musculoskeletal system enables changes in movement and position. The bony skeleton provides support, protection, and movable parts. Muscles facilitate movement. Movement serves two general purposes: (1) movement is necessary to perform normal activities of daily living, and (2) movement itself is a source of pleasure. Physical activities that contribute to physical fitness and promote physical health are also enjoyable. People who participate in exercise programs describe feelings of well-being from regular physical activity.

STRUCTURE OF THE MUSCULOSKELETAL SYSTEM

MUSCLE

Muscles make up 40% to 50% of body weight. Muscles produce movement and heat by contraction. The body contains three types of muscles: (1) skeletal, (2) cardiac, and (3) smooth.

■ SKELETAL MUSCLE

Skeletal muscle attaches to bones of the skeleton. Skeletal muscles are named according to the following properties: (1) action (e.g., flexor, extensor), (2) shape (e.g., quadrilateral, pennate), (3) origin (i.e., stationary attachment of muscle to skeleton), (4) insertion (i.e., movable attachment of the muscle), (5) number of divisions, (6) location, or (7) direction of fibers (i.e., transverse). The principal muscle groups are shown in Figure U5–1.

The contraction of skeletal muscle exerts force on bones or skin and moves them (Fig. U5–2). Most skeletal muscles are under voluntary control of the nervous system, but some are controlled by the somatic division of the peripheral nervous system, such as those used to maintain balance. See detailed discussion of muscle movement on page 534.

Under microscopic examination, many nuclei of muscle cells are visible and are grouped into thread-like *myofibrils.* A close look at the myofibrils reveals alternating bands of light and dark *(striations).* Muscle cells can be further divided into smaller segments called *sarcomeres,* delineated by Z bands. The sarcomere is the structure in the muscle where the actual contraction occurs. Two primary myofilaments are present in the sarcomere: thick myosin filaments and thin actin filaments. The filaments are proteins that briefly attach and ratchet or slide across one another to cause the muscle to contract.

Skeletal muscle is composed of many individual muscle cells called *muscle fibers.* These fibers are held together by thin sheets of fibrous connective tissue *(fascia).* Fascia also penetrates the muscle, separating it into bundles *(fasciculi).* Skeletal muscle is attached to the bones of the skeleton by very thin extensions of fascia or by tendons. *Tendons* (fibrous cords) make strong connections to bone.

■ CARDIAC MUSCLE

Cardiac muscle *(myocardium)* is involuntary and exists only in the heart. It is composed of branched, striated muscle cells having only one nucleus. Cardiac muscle is controlled by intrinsic factors (e.g., the amount of venous return to the right atrium), hormones, and signals from the autonomic nervous system. Cardiac muscle is discussed in Unit 12.

■ SMOOTH MUSCLE

"Smooth" muscle has no striations. It is involuntary and is present in the walls of hollow organs (e.g., digestive tract, blood vessels, urinary bladder) and in other areas (e.g., the eye). It is controlled by the autonomic nervous system, hormones, and intrinsic factors in the organ (e.g., stretch due to food in the intestine).

SKELETAL SYSTEM

Humans have an *endoskeleton* (i.e., it lies *within* the soft tissues of the body). It is composed of living tissue that is capable of growth, adaptation, and repair. The adult body contains 206 bones, which are divided into two major categories by position: axial and appendicular. The *axial skeleton* (80 bones) consists of the skull, vertebral column, and thorax. The *appendicular skeleton* (126 bones) includes the bones of the extremities, shoulders, and pelvis (Fig. U5–3). Bones can also be classified by their shape:

1. *Long bones* are all longer than they are wide and are found in the upper and lower extremities. The humerus, radius, ulna, femur, tibia, fibula, metatarsals, metacarpals, and phalanges are the long bones.
2. *Short bones* (e.g., carpals, tarsals) do not have a long axis; they are cubical.
3. *Flat bones* (e.g., ribs, cranium, scapula, and portions of the pelvic girdle) protect soft body parts and provide large surfaces for muscle attachments.
4. *Irregular bones* have various shapes, such as vertebrae, ear ossicles, facial bones, and pelvis. Irregular bones are similar to other bones in structure and composition.

■ GROSS ANATOMY OF BONE

A typical long bone (Fig. U5–4) has a shaft *(diaphysis)* and two ends (*proximal* and *distal epiphyses*). The diaphysis is a hollow cylinder of compact bone that surrounds a medullary cavity *(marrow).* It is lined with a thin con-

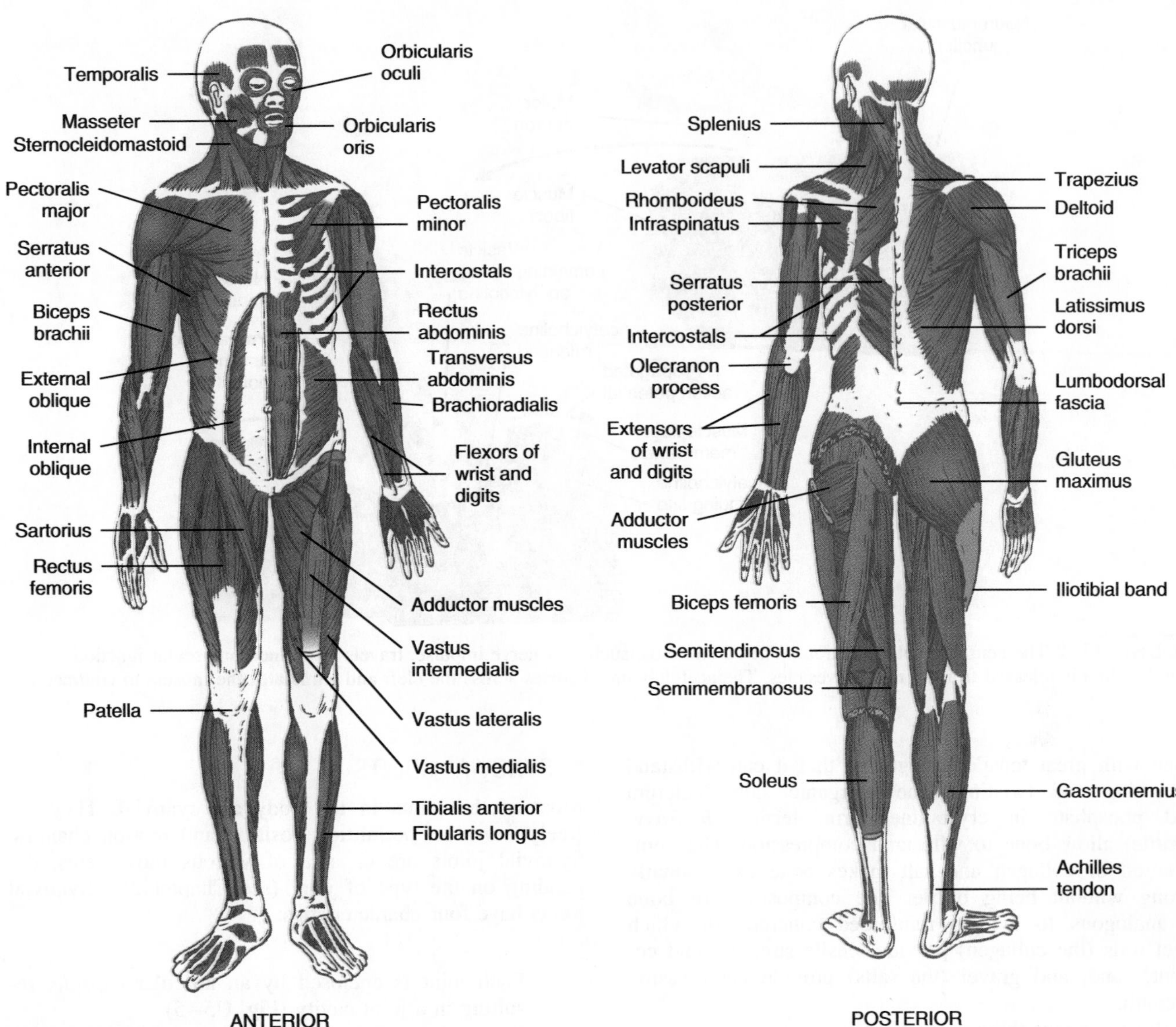

FIGURE U5–1 Principal muscles.

nective tissue layer called *endosteum.* In children and young adults, the epiphyses are separated from the diaphysis by *epiphyseal cartilage* or plates, where bone grows in length. When bone growth is complete, the epiphyseal cartilage is replaced with bone, which joins it to the diaphysis. Fractures of the epiphyseal plates in children can lead to slow bone growth or limb shortening.

Bones are covered with a layer of connective tissue called *periosteum.* The outer (fibrous) layer of periosteum is well supplied with blood vessels and nerves, some of which enter the bone through Volkmann's canals. This layer is very tough and can even hold fracture fragments in place with nondisplaced fractures. The inner (osteogenic) layer is anchored to the bone by bundles of collagen *(Sharpey's fibers).* There is no periosteum on articular surfaces of long bones; these areas are covered with articular cartilage.

■ MICROSCOPIC ANATOMY OF BONE

When viewed through a microscope, *compact bone* is highly organized and solid. It is organized into structural units, called *osteons* or *haversian systems.* An osteon is essentially a cylinder of bone. Each osteon contains (1) vessels in a central canal *(haversian canal);* (2) concentric layers of bone matrix *(lamellae);* (3) tiny spaces between the lamellae *(lacunae),* which contain osteocytes; and (4) small channels *(canaliculi).* The blood vessels transport nutrients to the bone and carry wastes away from the bone.

Spongy bone does not have such an organized structure. The lamellae are not arranged in concentric circles but, rather, in directions that correspond to the lines of maximum pressure or tension placed on the bone. Spongy bone has osteocytes embedded in lacunae, and lacunae intercommunicate via canaliculi. Blood reaches the osteocytes by passing through spaces in the bone marrow.

■ COMPOSITION OF BONE

Bone's organic framework is formed from protein complexes and fibers, especially collagen (similar to the collagen found in other connective tissues). *Collagen* provides

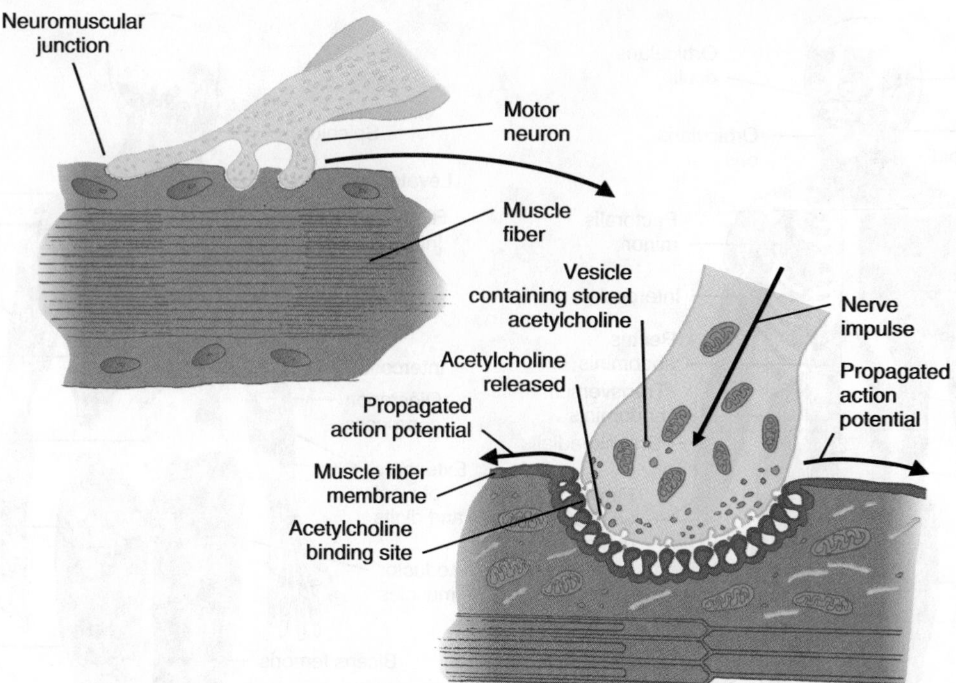

FIGURE U5–2 The neuromuscular junction. When a stimulus, such as a nerve impulse, travels to the neuromuscular junction, acetylcholine is released from storage in vesicles. The acetylcholine diffuses across the cleft and stimulates the muscle to contract.

bone with great tensile strength so that it can withstand stretching and twisting. The inorganic salts (calcium and phosphate in crystalline form, termed *hydroxyapatite*) allow bone to withstand compression. The combination of collagen and salt makes bone exceptionally strong without being brittle. The composition of bone is analogous to that of reinforced concrete, in which steel rods (the collagen) provide tensile strength, and cement, sand, and gravel (the salts) provide compression strength.

Bone contains three types of cells:

1. *Osteoblasts* are bone-forming cells; they lay down new bone by catalyzing reactions that take calcium and phosphate from the blood and form it into bone matrix in a collagen meshwork.
2. *Osteocytes* are osteoblasts that are found in the bone matrix.
3. *Osteoclasts* are cells that resorb (remove) damaged or old bone cells during periods of growth or repair. They are also critical in returning inorganic salts from bone to the bloodstream.

Bone cells allow bone to grow, repair itself, and change shape. Even mature bone constantly changes, with new cells being formed and old cells being destroyed.

ARTICULATIONS

Articulations (joints) are places of union between two or more bones. Not all joints permit movement. Joints may be synovial, fibrous, or cartilaginous.

■ SYNOVIAL JOINTS

Most of the joints in the body are synovial. They are freely movable, permitting position and motion changes. Synovial joints are capable of various movements, depending on the type of joint (see Chapter 25). Synovial joints have four characteristics:

1. Each joint is enclosed by an articular *capsule,* resulting in a joint cavity (Fig. U5–5).
2. Synovial membrane produces *synovial fluid,* which fills the cavity for lubrication and cartilage nourishment.
3. Bone surfaces in the joint are covered by *hyaline cartilage* (articular cartilage).
4. Synovial joints have additional *support* features. *Ligaments* and *tendons* reinforce the capsule and help to limit motion. *Articular discs* are located between the bones in some synovial joints to buffer forceful impact.

■ FIBROUS JOINTS

Fibrous joints are articulations in which bones are held together by fibrous connective tissue. Very little material separates the ends of the bone, and minimal movement is possible.

Suture Joints. Suture joints include the bones of the skull and sometimes the sutures between the ilium, ischium, and pubic bones. At birth, the bones of the skull are separated to facilitate birth. The bones usually fuse by 2 years. The edges of these bones have grooves *(interdigitations)* that fit firmly together and look somewhat like a suture.

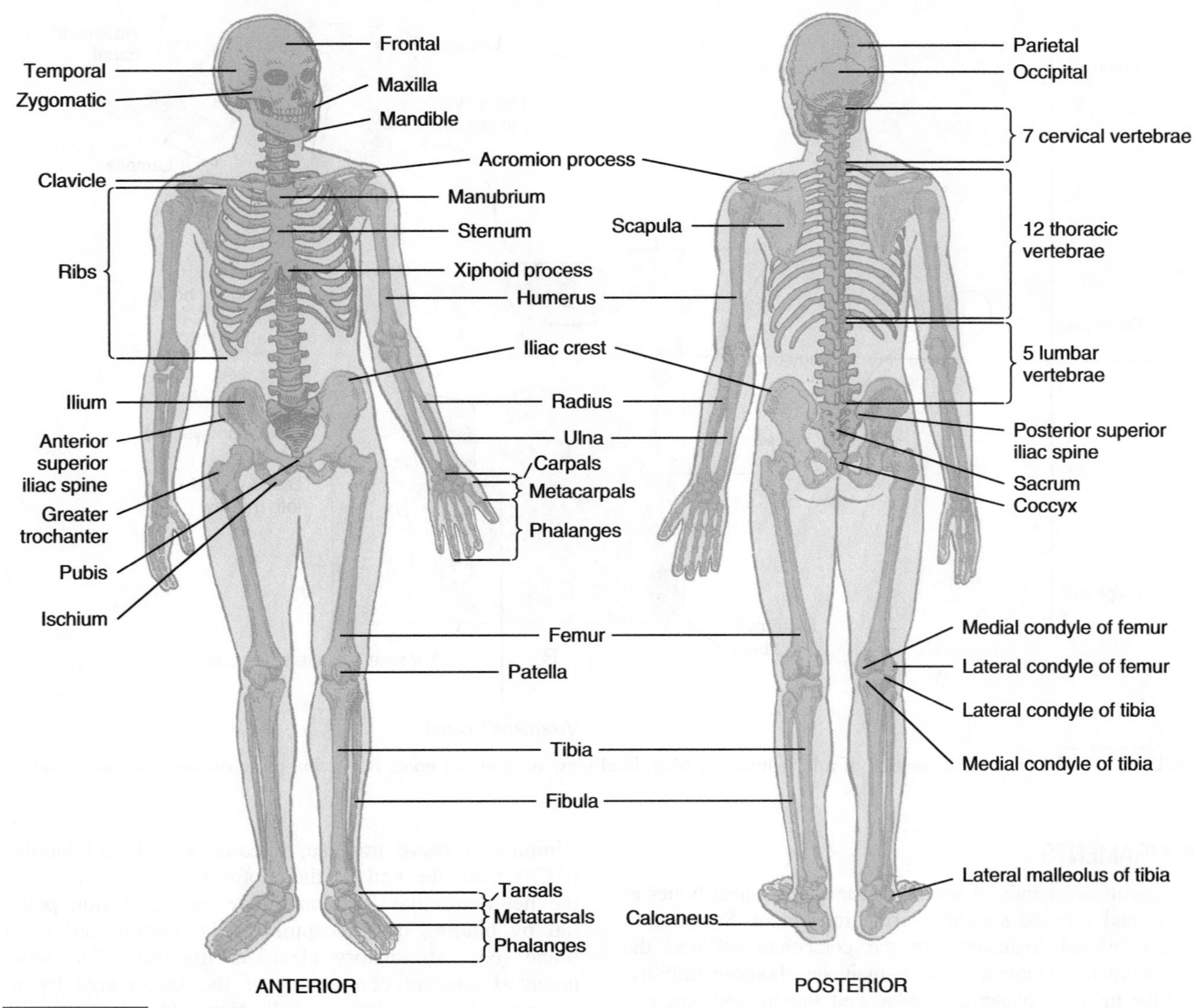

FIGURE U5–3 The adult human skeleton is composed of 206 bones. The axial skeleton is shown in blue, and the appendicular skeleton is shown in brown.

Syndesmosis Joints. Syndesmosis (ligamentous) joints are held together by ligaments (bands of fibrous tissue) or membranes. Syndesmosis joints allow some "give." The joints at the distal end of the tibia and fibula are examples of syndesmosis joints.

■ CARTILAGINOUS JOINTS

Bones are held together by cartilage (dense connective tissue; see later). Slight movement is possible in these joints. They are of two types.

Synchondroses. Synchondroses are held together by hyaline cartilage. Joints between the epiphyses and diaphyses of long bones are replaced by bone *(ossification)* at maturity. In the ribs, this form of cartilage also is temporary and is eventually replaced by bone. In the costal cartilages, synchondroses between ribs and sternum are not usually replaced by bone.

Symphyses. Symphyses are articular surfaces that have a fibrocartilaginous pad or disc connecting the articulating bones. Slight movement is allowed. Within the joint, the surfaces act as shock absorbers. The vertebrae are separated by symphyses.

Cushioning and Supportive Structures

■ BURSAE AND TENDON SHEATHS

Bursae are small sacs lined with synovial membrane and filled with synovial fluid (see Fig. U5–5). They act as cushions between structures. There are hundreds of bursae in the body. Some are subcutaneous, lying between bone and skin (e.g., the bursa between the olecranon process of the elbow and the skin).

Tendon sheaths are cylindrical synovial structures similar to bursae. They are found where tendons cross joints and may be subject to constant friction. The sheath wraps around the tendon, forming a fluid-filled cushion through which the tendon can slide.

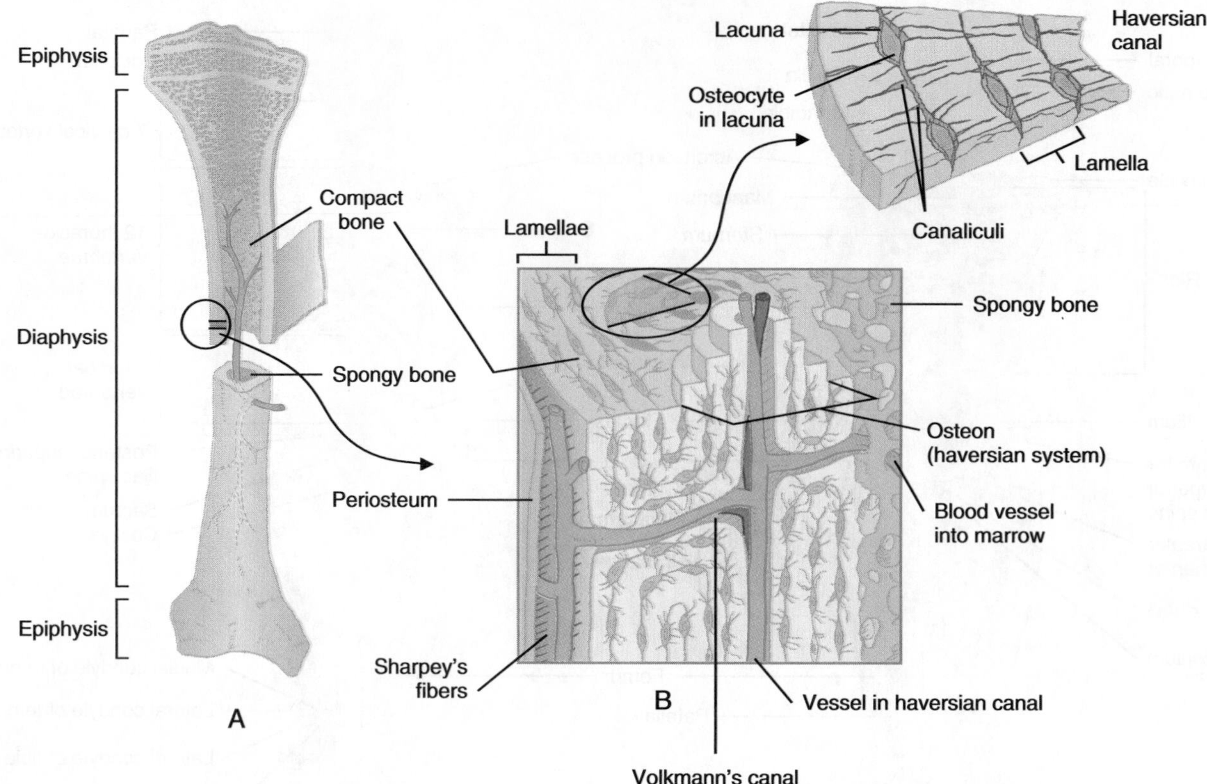

FIGURE U5–4 Longitudinal section of a long bone. *A,* Magnified view of compact bone. *B,* section of an osteon (haversian canal).

■ LIGAMENTS

Ligaments are bands of fibrous tissue that connect bones at joints and provide stability during movement. Some commonly injured ligaments are the coracohumeral and the glenohumeral ligaments, which maintain shoulder stability; and the medial, collateral, patellar, and anterior and posterior cruciate ligaments, which support the knee (Fig. U5–6).

■ CARTILAGE

Cartilage is a type of dense connective tissue that is prevalent throughout the musculoskeletal system. It can resist forces of tension and compression with considerable resilience. It is semi-opaque (bluish white or gray) and has limited nerve and blood supply. Most of the skeleton of an embryo is cartilage that gradually changes into bone *(ossification).*

Three types of cartilage are found in the body:

- *Hyaline cartilage,* in respiratory tract, developing bones, and ends of articulating bones
- *Fibrocartilage,* in ligaments and intervertebral discs
- *Elastin cartilage,* in the external ear

FUNCTION OF THE MUSCULOSKELETAL SYSTEM

Muscle

■ MOVEMENT

Skeletal muscle contraction occurs when a stimulus excites an individual muscle fiber (see Fig. U5–2). The stimulus, a nerve impulse, releases stored acetylcholine (ACh) from the end of the motor neuron. ACh crosses the neuromuscular junction and elicits an action potential by binding to a receptor on the muscle cell membrane (e.g., stimulatory electrical impulse). The action potential triggers contraction of the sarcomeres by releasing calcium inside the cell. Nerve fibers may supply more than 100 individual skeletal muscle cells. A continuous flow of stimuli maintains muscle tone (i.e., keeps muscles partially contracted, in a state of readiness for movement).

Muscle fibers relax between contractions because calcium ions that are released during the action potential are free only for a short time. Calcium quickly returns to storage in the sarcoplasmic reticulum in the muscle. If nerve impulses arrive in rapid succession so that calcium remains free, the muscle will continue to contract (called *spasm* or *tetany*).

To generate power, muscle cells require large amounts of oxygen and glucose. Muscles thus have a rich vascular supply. An oxygen debt develops during exercise if oxygen cannot be delivered to muscles in concentrations great enough to meet the immediate metabolic needs of the cell. After exercise, increased oxygen consumption is necessary to relieve oxygen debt.

■ PROPULSION

Smooth muscle is found in the walls of hollow conduits in the body and its contraction applies pressure that may mix, break up, or move substances forward. For example, smooth muscle of the gastrointestinal (GI) tract propels food through the tract during digestion. Smooth muscle in

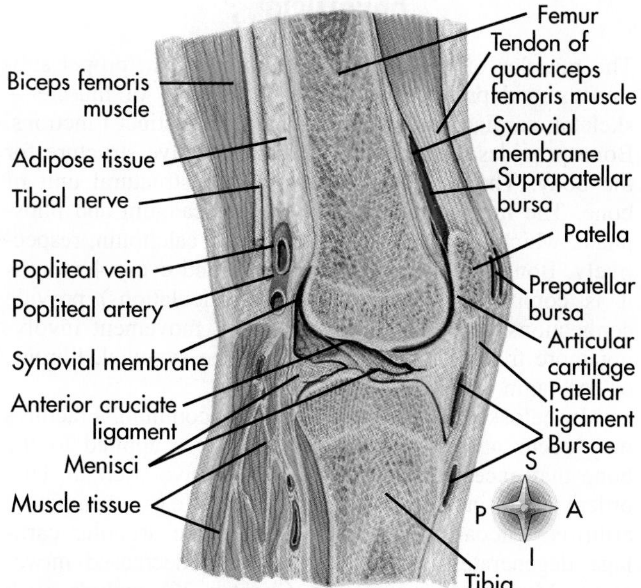

FIGURE U5–5 Anatomy of a synovial joint (knee). (From Thibodeau, G., & Patton, K. [1999]. *Anatomy and physiology* [4th ed.]. St. Louis: Mosby.)

arterioles regulates arterial blood flow by causing vasodilation and vasoconstriction. Smooth muscle in the uterus contracts during labor and smooth muscle in the airways can constrict *(bronchospasm)* or dilate to promote air movement.

■ HEAT PRODUCTION

The activity of skeletal muscle produces heat. Some of this heat can be used to maintain body temperature. During exercise, excess heat is released through sweating and vasodilation. When the body is cold, heat is generated by shivering.

SKELETAL SYSTEM

Bones give form to the body: they support various tissues and organs and permit movement by providing attachments for tendons and ligaments. The skeleton is also protective. The skull and rib cage, for example, protect the brain and special senses and the lungs, respectively.

■ HEMATOPOIETIC FUNCTION

Bone houses the hematopoietic tissues, which manufacture blood cells. In adults, blood cells form in marrow cavities in the skull, vertebrae, ribs, sternum, shoulder, and pelvis. There are two types of bone marrow: *yellow* and *red*. Some authors have noted a third type of bone marrow, brown. *Brown* marrow is generally found in older adults; it is similar to yellow marrow, in that it is inactive but lacks adipose tissue. *Yellow* marrow (connective tissue composed of fat cells) is found in the shafts of long bones and extends into the haversian systems. Yellow marrow does not produce blood cells except during times of increased blood cell need. *Red marrow* has a hematopoietic function; it manufactures red and white blood cells. It is located in the cancellous bone spaces, found in flat bones (see Unit 16).

■ ROLE OF BONE IN HOMEOSTASIS

Bones also provide a crucial portion of mineral balance; they store calcium, phosphorus, sodium, potassium, and other minerals and release them for cellular metabolism and use by other body systems. When blood levels of calcium fall, the parathyroid gland senses the decrease and releases *parathyroid hormone* (PTH). PTH increases the movement of calcium from bone into the extracellular fluids by stimulating the osteoclasts to break down bone and free calcium. PTH also decreases renal excretion of calcium, increases the excretion of phosphate, and increases the metabolic transformation of vitamin D_3 to its active form to increase calcium absorption from the intestine.

When serum calcium levels are high, *calcitonin* (a hormone from the thyroid gland) lowers plasma calcium by inhibiting calcium removal from bone (the opposite of the action of PTH).

■ BONE REMODELING

Throughout life, the bone mass continuously undergoes well-regulated processes of bone formation and bone resorption. The process of bone turnover is called *remodeling,* and it is one of the major mechanisms for maintaining calcium balance in the body. As much as 15% of the total bone mass normally turns over each year in a *three-phase process.*

Phase 1. The cycle begins when a stimulus (such as a hormone, drug, or stressor) activates the bone cell precursors to become osteoclasts.

Phase 2. Osteoclasts gradually resorb the bone. They leave behind an elongated cavity *(resorption cavity),* which matches the general structure of the haversian system or trabeculae.

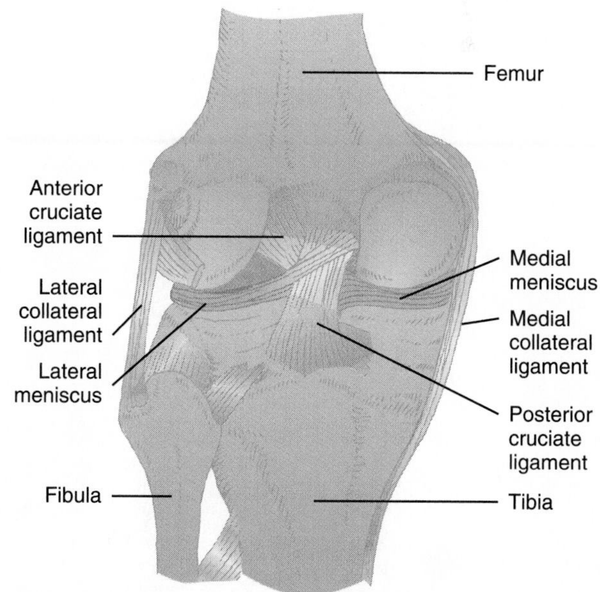

FIGURE U5–6 Posterior view of the knee. When the knee is extended, the taut anterior cruciate ligament prevents overextension. When the knee is flexed, the posterior cruciate ligament prevents the tibia from slipping posteriorly.

Phase 3. New bone is laid down by the osteoblasts. The osteoblasts follow the path of the osteoclasts to create new haversian systems and trabeculae.

The entire process takes about 4 months. Rebuilding of bone requires normal plasma concentrations of calcium and phosphate and is dependent on vitamin D.

■ BONE REPAIR

The remodeling process enables repair of small bony injuries, but breaks *(fractures)* and other wounds of bone heal in a different manner. Initially, the bone heals by forming a hematoma. The hematoma's fibrin provides a meshwork, which is the initial framework for healing. Granulation tissue *(pro-callus)* is produced, and a fibrocartilaginous callus develops prior to bony *(osseous)* depositions. Osteoblasts deposit disorganized clumps of bone matrix *(callus)*. The trabeculae and haversian systems follow. Finally, the bony edges are remodeled to the size and shape of the bone before injury.

EFFECTS OF AGING

Aging affects bone, muscle, and tendons. Bone tissue is lost because the rate of loss exceeds the rate of growth. The haversian systems in compact bone erode. The lacunae enlarge, and cortical bone becomes thin and porous. *Osteoporosis,* a condition of decreased calcium in bone, leads to weak and brittle bones and increased risk of fracture.

Eventually, cartilage becomes more rigid and fragile and muscle bulk decreases. As muscle mass decreases, so does maximal strength, which can decline by 50% between the ages of 20 and 50 years. Several theories have been offered to explain these changes, including changes in activity, reduced circulation, cardiovascular disorders, and nutritional problems.

CONCLUSIONS

The muscles of the body provide movement, propel substances, and produce heat. The three types of muscle—skeletal, cardiac, and smooth—perform distinct functions. Bone provides a framework and a protective structure for the body. The haversian system is the structural unit of bone. The major minerals in bone are calcium and phosphate, which are regulated by PTH and calcitonin, respectively. Bone is constantly remodeled, and every 4 months it is completely replaced. Joints (articulations) provide connections between bones and allow movement involving more than one bone. Joints may be synovial, fibrous, or cartilaginous.

Musculoskeletal disorders are very common. Fractures may occur at any age because of forces applied to the bone that exceed its tensile or compressive strength. Disorders seen in the articular surfaces (e.g., rheumatoid arthritis, osteoarthritis) develop when the articular cartilage degenerates, leading to pain and decreased movement. Muscle disorders (see Chapter 26) include such conditions as muscular dystrophy (progressive muscle degeneration) and myasthenia gravis (loss of receptors on the muscle for acetylcholine, leading to profound muscle weakness).

BIBLIOGRAPHY

1. Berne, R., & Levy, M. (1993). *Physiology* (3rd ed.). St. Louis: Mosby–Year Book.
2. Guyton, A. (1995). *Textbook of medical physiology* (9th ed.). Philadelphia: W. B. Saunders.
3. Heveron, B., & Kaempffe, F. (1995). Tears of the rotator cuff. *Orthopaedic Nursing, 14*(6), 38–41.
4. Thibodeau, G. & Patton, K. (1999). *Anatomy and physiology* (4th ed.). St. Louis: Mosby.

CHAPTER 25

Assessment of the Musculoskeletal System

Peggy Doheny
Carol Sedlak

Assessment of the musculoskeletal system begins with a health history, which provides direction for further assessment. The musculoskeletal physical examination can be either general (as in a screening examination) or local (for a specific problem or injury). Similarly, diagnostic tests can be either general or specific. The resulting data allow you to make judgments about the client's musculoskeletal status. Musculoskeletal assessment usually also includes the client's functional status and ability to perform activities of daily living (ADL) and to meet self-care needs. This aspect of the assessment involves evaluation of the client's exercise habits and leisure activities that promote health.

HISTORY

The musculoskeletal history consists of:

- Biographical and demographic data
- Chief complaint (including symptom analysis)
- Past health history
- Family history
- Psychosocial history
- Lifestyle data
- Review of systems

Collect information to help determine the nature and extent of the client's current disorder. If the chief complaint is related to trauma, keep the history interview brief and focus on the cause of injury. You may need to defer the interview, depending on the extent of the client's injury. Once the client's condition is stable, you can obtain a more complete history.

■ BIOGRAPHICAL AND DEMOGRAPHIC DATA

Personal information enables individualized care planning. For example, knowing where the client lives and the kind of transportation the client uses helps you understand the energy required for the client to keep an appointment. Getting to know the client's significant others is essential in planning care as well.

The client's age and sex may suggest possible causes of musculoskeletal problems. For example, 85% of people older than 70 years have some osteoarthritis. Osteoporosis (porous bone) occurs most often in postmenopausal women. Reiter's syndrome is most common in men between 20 and 40 years of age. Osteogenic sarcoma is rare after age 40. Carpal tunnel syndrome occurs more often in women than in men.

■ CURRENT HEALTH

Chief Complaint

Ask the client to describe the reason for seeking health care. Common clinical manifestations related to the musculoskeletal system are pain, tenderness, muscle tightness or weakness, joint stiffness, cramps, muscle spasms, swelling, redness, deformity, reduced movement or joint range of motion (ROM), sensory changes, and other abnormal sensations. ADL may be affected. Ask the client and significant others to recount their perceptions of the problem and its cause. Their answers often provide not only information about areas for further assessment but also clues about personal fears and concerns.

Symptom Analysis

Conduct a symptom analysis for each manifestation the client reports (see Chapter 9). Examples of assessment questions for typical musculoskeletal manifestations follow.

PAIN

Ask the client to point to the exact location of the pain. Poorly localized pain usually stems from problems in blood vessels, joints, fascia, or periosteum.

Ask the client to describe the pain: Is it an ache, a sharp pain, a throbbing? Throbbing pain is usually bone-related, and aches are commonly muscular. Sharp pain may be caused by a fracture or bone infection. Ask the client to rate the pain on a scale of 0 to 10, on which 0 is no pain and 10 is the worst pain possible.

What makes the pain worse: Temperature changes? Movement? Lifting or carrying something heavy? Pain from osteoarthritis is worse in cold, damp weather. Pain that occurs with movement is typical of joint problems.

Degenerative hip conditions produce pain during weight-bearing and during and after walking. Degenerative knee problems produce pain during and after walking. Vertebral disc herniation produces pain on bending or lifting and may radiate down one leg.

Is the pain worse at a particular time of day? Does it wake the client or prevent sleeping at night? Inflammation of bursae or tendons is worse at night. Degenerative joint pain is often worse at the end of a day.

Does rest relieve the pain? Most musculoskeletal pain is helped by rest.

Which medications help to relieve the pain? Pain from inflammation is usually helped by aspirin or nonsteroidal anti-inflammatory drugs (NSAIDs). Narcotic analgesics are usually required for traumatic injury.

Have there been any recent injuries? Sometimes a client does not associate a fall or other injury with current manifestations.

Is the pain associated with chills, fever, rash, or a sore throat? Joint pain occurring 10 to 14 days after a sore throat may be from rheumatic fever.

JOINT STIFFNESS

Ask the client to point to joints that are stiff. Are they always stiff? How long does the stiffness last? Some conditions, such as ankylosing spondylitis, have remissions and exacerbations.

At what time of day is the stiffness worst? With degenerative joint disease, stiffness is often most severe in the morning after a night in bed.

What relieves the stiffness? Temperature changes? Exercise? Coldness and lack of use typically increase joint stiffness. Heat may reduce muscle spasm. Heat applied to a recently injured joint may worsen stiffness by increasing bleeding into and swelling of the joint.

Does the joint lock so it cannot move? Does the client hear or feel bones rubbing together? Bone malalignment within a joint causes locking. *Crepitus* (the sound of bone ends rubbing together) indicates fractures or joint destruction.

Does the client have pain or weakness in muscles with certain movements? Weakness in muscles may result from various neuromuscular disorders. If weakness is present, does it interfere with the client's usual activities?

SWELLING

Ask how long the client has had the swelling. Is there pain? Swelling and pain commonly accompany bone and muscle injury. With degenerative joint disease, swelling may not develop for some time, maybe weeks, after pain is present—or it may not develop at all.

Does swelling limit the client's movement? Limited movement may stem from soft tissue damage and swelling in a joint.

Does rest or elevating the part give relief? Elevation reduces swelling in acute injuries.

Ask the client whether the body part was casted recently. Removing a cast can result in temporary swelling. A casted limb also may have muscle atrophy.

Has the area been hot or red? Redness and heat indicate inflammation, infection, or recent injury and are not usually present with degenerative conditions.

DEFORMITY AND IMMOBILITY

Has the deformity developed suddenly or gradually? A gradually developing mass may be a tumor.

Is movement limited? Is this limitation always present? Is it worse after activity? Does any body position make it worse or better? Immobility from degenerative joint disease varies with the severity of the condition.

Ask how the deformity affects the client's daily activities. Does the client use any supportive equipment, such as crutches, a walker, or bandages? Use of such aids offers clues to the severity of the disability.

SENSORY CHANGES

Does the client have a history of back pain or injury? If so, where is the pain located? Does the pain travel, for example, down the back of the leg? Does the client have trouble walking? Is there a loss of feeling anywhere? If so, is the loss of feeling associated with any pain? Does the client have any tingling or burning sensation? Pressure on nerves or blood vessels can occur from swelling, tumors, or fractures, causing loss of sensation. Sensory changes may be associated with pain in an arm or hand.

■ PAST HEALTH HISTORY

Carefully assess previous trauma, accidents, or surgery involving bones or joints. The client may have sustained fractures, dislocations, strains, or sprains. Previous accidents leading to bony fracture may predispose to degenerative changes.

Question the client about a range of past health problems because many diseases can affect the musculoskeletal system. Explore both childhood and adult-onset disorders because of their possible long-term effects.

Childhood and Infectious Diseases

Health conditions may affect the musculoskeletal system directly or indirectly. For example, diabetes mellitus may predispose a client to degenerative joint disease. Blood dyscrasias, such as hemophilia, may cause bleeding in joints that produces pain, swelling, tenderness, and deformity. Psoriasis may precede psoriatic arthritis. Cartilage damage from trauma may precipitate degenerative changes in a relatively young person. Ask about a history of tuberculosis, sickle cell disease, poliomyelitis, inflammatory or degenerative arthritis, scurvy, rickets, osteomyelitis, soft tissue infection, fungus infection of bones or joints, and streptococcal and neuromuscular disorders.

Major Illnesses and Hospitalizations

Besides inquiring about diseases, such as diabetes mellitus, tuberculosis, poliomyelitis, and arthritis, ask about hospitalizations related to musculoskeletal disorders or trauma. If the client or significant others cannot remember details, ask for permission to obtain the medical records. Ask about past or present minor and major injuries, including (1) circumstances of the injury, (2) diagnosis of the injury, (3) treatment received, (4) duration of treatment, and (5) current problems resulting from the injury.

Musculoskeletal injury involves fractures, sprains, strains, and joint dislocations. Minor injuries may be treated on an ambulatory basis, whereas major injuries may require prolonged hospitalization, surgery, or rest and immobilization. Ask whether the client has residual impairment from the injury, such as a need to use an assistive device (cane, crutches, or walker). Ask whether the client has had to change or adjust ADL because of lingering limitations.

Medications

Question the client about past and present prescription and over-the-counter medications as well as herbal remedies. For each medication, find out (1) the reason for taking it, (2) the dose and frequency, (3) how long the client has taken it, and (4) any observed side effects. Ask the client about specific medications used for musculoskeletal problems, such as muscle relaxants, salicylates, NSAIDs, and steroids, because some medications affect the musculoskeletal system.

For example, corticosteroid therapy can lead to necrosis of the femur head, septic arthritis, and muscle weakness. High doses of anticoagulants can produce hemarthrosis (blood in joints). Anticonvulsants may cause osteomalacia. Phenothiazines may produce gait disturbances. Potassium-depleting diuretics may produce cramps and muscle weakness. Amphetamines and caffeine cause a generalized increase in motor activity. Hormone replacement therapy with estrogen has been shown to modify the effects of osteoporosis in postmenopausal women.

Use of NSAIDs for more than 4 weeks can lead to bleeding problems—especially in the gastrointestinal (GI) tract—because of decreased platelet aggregation. Renal and hepatic changes can also develop. Long-term use of NSAIDs requires follow-up laboratory assessments to monitor for side effects. Complete blood count and serum assays of liver enzymes, potassium, and creatinine, and urinalysis are usually assessed.

The herb cayenne (*capsicum*) or capsaicin applied externally relieves the ache and pain of arthritis. If taken internally, however, capsaicin can cause GI distress and, at high doses, may damage unmyelinated and small-diameter myelinated nerve fibers. White willow (*Salix purpurea, S. fragilis, S. daphnoides, S. alba*) has analgesic properties. It contains salicin, which may have adverse effects similar to those of salicylate.

■ FAMILY HEALTH HISTORY

Some musculoskeletal problems with a familial predisposition are arthritis, osteoporosis, ankylosing spondylitis, gout, Heberden's nodes in osteoarthritis, muscular dystrophy, and scoliosis. Thirty per cent of people with psoriatic arthritis have a family history of psoriasis.

■ PSYCHOSOCIAL HISTORY

The integrity of the musculoskeletal system enables a person to function effortlessly. However, many problems can disrupt that integrity—and the coping ability of both client and significant others. Ask about the client's daily activities and habits. When assessing a client with a chronic illness or degenerative process, ask whether the disorder has affected the client's interactions with others or view of self and others. Crippling illnesses often curtail social activity and result in lower self-esteem.

Occupation

Ask whether heavy lifting or strenuous activity is common in the client's life. Such activity can cause muscle strain, degenerative vertebral disc problems, and other trauma. Low back pain can arise from jobs involving extensive driving. Habitually carrying heavy objects, such as a mailbag, shoulder bag, attaché case, or other equipment, places uneven pressure on the spinal column. Prolonged use of computers and keyboards can cause orthopedic injuries from repetitive strain (see Chapter 27).

Activities of Daily Living

Are there everyday activities that the client finds difficult or impossible, such as (1) opening containers, pouring liquids, and cutting up food, (2) dressing, using zippers, and fastening or unfastening buttons, snaps, or hooks, (3) grooming, combing hair, and applying makeup, (4) running a bath and testing water temperature, washing hair, and shaving, (5) writing, and (6) getting out of the house, climbing stairs, or getting in and out of chairs or cars?

Ask whether physical limitations prevent the client from performing any daily activities. Also assess the client's attention to safety. Ask about safety practices used at work and at home. Does the client use recommended equipment, such as safety shoes or safety guards on power tools? There is a high incidence of accidental injury among people who pay little attention to safety practices.

Exercise

Document the details of the client's typical recreational activities and exercise pattern. Lack of exercise produces poor muscle tone, which leads to muscle strain. Sporadic exercise of poorly toned muscles is more likely to cause muscle injury and spasm. Lack of warm-up exercises increases the likelihood of injury as well.

Fractures and other trauma can arise from contact sports. Achilles tendon damage can occur from improperly landing on heels while jogging. Pain in arm joints can be caused by racket sports, such as tennis and squash, which require a strong grasp, wrist extension, and forearm rotation.

Ask about typical footwear. High-heeled shoes can shorten the Achilles tendon and pitch the center of gravity forward, leading to lordosis.

Nutrition

A dietary history can provide clues to musculoskeletal problems as well (see Chapter 28). For example, obesity stresses weight-bearing joints and predisposes to ligament instability, particularly of the lower back. Poor calcium intake can lead to bone decalcification and fractures. Ask about foods eaten on a typical day. Adequate dietary intake of vitamins A and D, calcium, and protein is important for musculoskeletal health.

Inquire about recent weight changes. Excessive weight gain can place stress on the musculoskeletal system.

Habits and Safety

Health promotion habits and a positive lifestyle can reduce the risk for development of musculoskeletal disorders. Increasing dietary calcium and weight-bearing activities, such as walking, can help prevent osteoporosis and improve strength and flexibility. Maintaining musculoskeletal health enhances a person's ability to perform ADL. Moreover, early detection of conditions such as scoliosis through screening programs can help with early intervention.

■ REVIEW OF SYSTEMS

Ask about such musculoskeletal problems as (1) muscle pain, spasm, or tenderness, (2) joint pain, stiffness, pain, swelling, or redness, (3) weakness, (4) limited movement, (5) clumsiness, (6) crepitus, (7) backache, and (8) changes in joints or bones. Investigate each reported problem. Inquire about the effect of the problem on the client's ability to perform ADL.

Assessment findings from other body systems may indicate musculoskeletal problems. Examples are:

- Pain or burning when urinating, which is associated with Reiter's syndrome
- Tachycardia and hypertension, which may accompany gout
- Chronic diarrhea, which may occur when arthritis is associated with colitis or other GI problems
- Conjunctivitis, which may indicate Reiter's syndrome, and nongranulomatous uveitis, which may occur with ankylosing spondylitis
- Skin changes, which may indicate musculoskeletal problems (dry skin over the thumb and the first two fingers suggests carpal tunnel syndrome, for example)
- Cramping leg pain with activity, which may signal intermittent claudication
- Generalized muscle cramping, which may result from electrolyte imbalances
- Joint pain with recent chills, fever, or sore throat, which may result from rheumatic fever

Detailed questions for the review of systems are found in Chapter 9.

PHYSICAL EXAMINATION

Assessment of the musculoskeletal system should proceed systematically to avoid missing hidden problems. Use an examining room big enough for the client to move around. Natural lighting is best for assessing skin color changes and swelling. Artificial light distorts some assessment findings. During the examination, have the client sit, stand, and walk unless a position is contraindicated by the client's condition.

Musculoskeletal assessment consists of inspecting and palpating (1) *muscle masses* for symmetry, involuntary movements, tenderness, tone, and strength, (2) *joints* for symmetry, crepitus, tenderness or pain, and ROM, and (3) *bones* for deformity and leg length discrepancy. Assessment of muscle-stretch and deep tendon reflexes is discussed in Chapter 67.

PHYSICAL ASSESSMENT FINDINGS IN THE HEALTHY ADULT

Musculoskeletal System

Inspection

Joints in alignment; posture straight; gait smooth.
Extremities symmetrical and of equal length.
Muscle groups symmetrical, without atrophy or fasciculations.
Joints without erythema, swelling, or deformities.
Full range of motion (active and passive) in all major joints.

Palpation

Muscle groups firm, symmetrical, nontender; without masses or spasms.
Joints stable and nontender; without heat, crepitus (palpable or audible), bogginess, or nodules.
Muscle strength in all major muscle groups rated 5/5.

■ GENERAL MUSCULOSKELETAL EXAMINATION

Use inspection and palpation to examine each body part. First, examine the body at rest, then assess ROM and muscle strength. Look for normal findings such as those outlined in the accompanying Physical Assessment Findings in the Healthy Adult chart.

When the client enters the examination room, assess the gait, body mobility, posture, general joint motion, and balance. While observing movement and gait, watch for (1) gait patterns associated with specific disorders (see Chapter 67), (2) objective evidence of discomfort, and (3) indications of joint stiffness or muscle weakness, lack of coordination, and deformities. Then have the client sit on the edge of the examination table. Observe the client's general appearance and body build. Examine the head, neck, shoulders, and upper extremities.

Have the client stand, and examine the chest, back, and ilium. Observe posture, body build, body contours, body alignment, and the cervical, thoracic, and lumbar spine. Observe the relationships of various body parts to one another, such as the relationship of feet to legs, legs to hips, and hips to pelvis (Fig. 25–1).

Observe the client's stance, and note any spinal deformities or other abnormalities (Fig. 25–2), such as:

- *Kyphosis*, an abnormally increased roundness of the thoracic curve or hump-back
- *Scoliosis*, a lateral deformity of the spine
- *Lordosis*, an abnormal increase in the lumbar curve, or swayback
- *Genu varum*, or bowleg
- *Genu valgum*, or knock-knee

The terms *varus (varum)* and *valgus (valgum)* refer to the direction in which the deformity lies in relationship to the midline. With a varus deformity, the de-

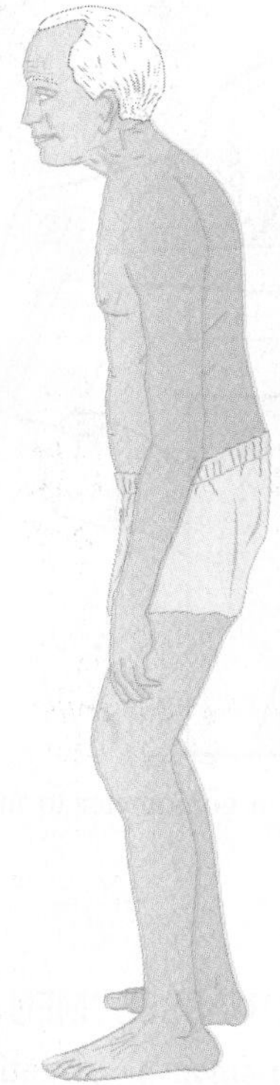

FIGURE 25–1 When performing a musculoskeletal assessment, have the client stand and walk if possible. Observe the client's stance, joint mobility, and posture. If you were to assess this man only while he was reclining, you might not notice his posture, the curvature of his spine, and his limited range of motion.

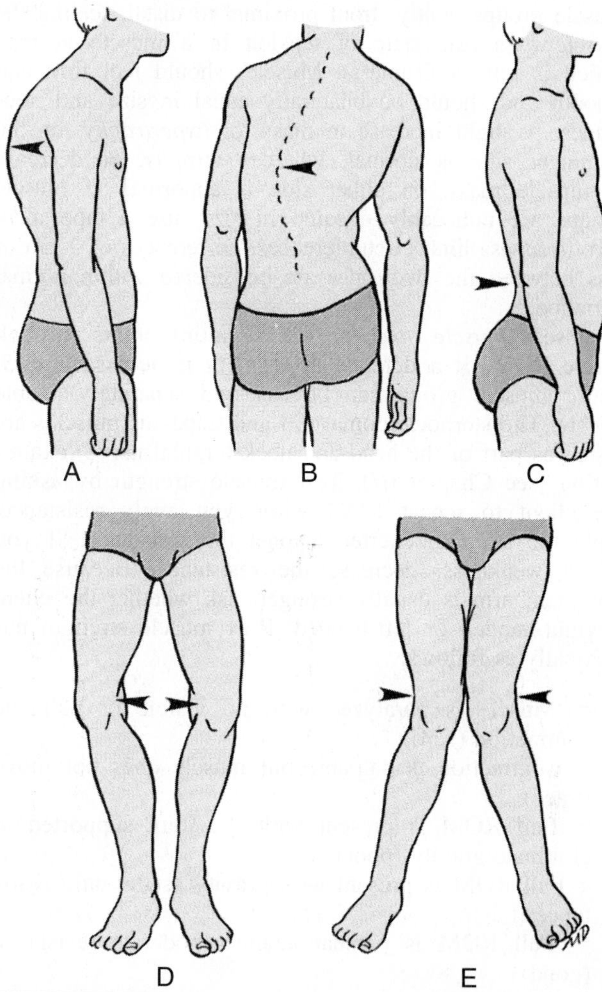

FIGURE 25–2 Musculoskeletal deformities observable during assessment. *A*, Kyphosis. *B*, Scoliosis. *C*, Lordosis. *D*, Genu varum. *E*, Genu valgum.

formity points toward the midline. With a valgus deformity, the deformity is bent or twisted away from the midline.

Last, with the client supine, examine the hips, knees, ankles, and feet for alignment, symmetry, and deformities. Determine any discrepancy between leg lengths by measuring from the anterior iliac spine to the medial malleolus. Measurements should be within 1 cm of each other. If a discrepancy is noted, determine whether it exists above or below the knee.

Muscles

Compare each muscle group with its contralateral side. Muscles should be free of *fasciculations* (fine muscle twitches) and smooth, without bulges or lumps. Palpate

TABLE 25–1 ASSESSING MUSCLE STRENGTH

Muscle Group	Technique
Deltoid	Push down client's arm while it is held up and client resists.
Biceps	Hold client's arm in extension while it is fully extended and client flexes arm.
Triceps	Keep client's arm in flexion while it is flexed and client extends arm.
Wrist and finger muscles	Push client's fingers together while client spreads them and resists.
Grip strength	Pull your own crossed index and middle fingers out from the client's grasp.
Hip muscles	Hold down client's leg while it is fully extended and while client lifts it off the table (client is supine).
Hip muscles (abduction)	Prevent client from spreading legs apart against resistance applied to the lateral surfaces of the knees (client is supine with legs extended).
Hip muscles (adduction)	Prevent client from bringing legs together against resistance applied to the medial surfaces of the knees (client is supine with legs extended).
Hamstrings	Straighten client's knees while client is supine with knees flexed and resists.
Quadriceps	Flex client's knee while client is supine with knee partially in extension and resists.
Ankle and foot muscles	Dorsiflex client's foot while client resists. Plantiflex client's foot while client resists.

muscle groups gently, from proximal to distal, feeling the *muscle tone* (the state of tension in a muscle at rest, which is felt as firmness). Muscles should feel firm and smooth and should be bilaterally equal in size and nontender. A slight increase in mass, or *hypertrophy*, on the dominant side is normal, whereas *atrophy*, or decrease in muscle mass, on either side is abnormal. If muscle groups are noticeably unequal in size, use a tape measure to assess limb circumferences. Differences of 1 cm or less between the two sides are considered within normal variation.

Assess *muscle strength* while putting joints through active ROM. If a detailed assessment is necessary, each major muscle group can be assessed separately (Table 25–1). The sternocleidomastoid and trapezius muscles are tested as part of the head and neck (cranial nerve) examination (see Chapter 67). Test muscle strength by asking the client to repeat ROM while you apply resistance. Note the strength exerted against the resistance. If you detect weakness, decrease the resistance. Because the dominant arm is usually stronger, ask whether the client is right-handed or left-handed. Rate muscle strength numerically as follows:

0 = Muscle is paralyzed with no visible or palpable contraction (zero)
1 = Contraction is palpable but muscle does not move (trace)
2 = Full ROM is present with the joint supported to eliminate gravity (poor)
3 = Full ROM is present with gravity as the only resistance (fair)
4 = Full ROM is present against moderate resistance (good)
5 = Full ROM is present against normal resistance and gravity (normal)

Include the muscle strength rating scale as part of the client's record to ensure understanding and consistency with other health care providers.

Joints and Bones

Inspect the client's joints and bones, and compare findings bilaterally. You should find symmetry without redness, swelling, enlargement, or deformity. Palpate each joint and bone for edema and tenderness, which should be absent. Palpate joints during movement for crepitus, which is abnormal. Joints should feel smooth as they move, and nodules should be absent.

ROM is the maximum range of movement attainable by a healthy joint. You can measure ROM with a goniometer, a flexible protractor-type instrument placed on a joint to measure the angles created by joint movement (Fig. 25–3). As needed, assess ROM in all the client's joints (Fig. 25–4).

Special Tests of Joint Function

Advanced practitioners may use special assessments to determine whether an injury has occurred in a joint. Some common tests are listed in Table 25–2. Two tests are shown in Figure 25–5.

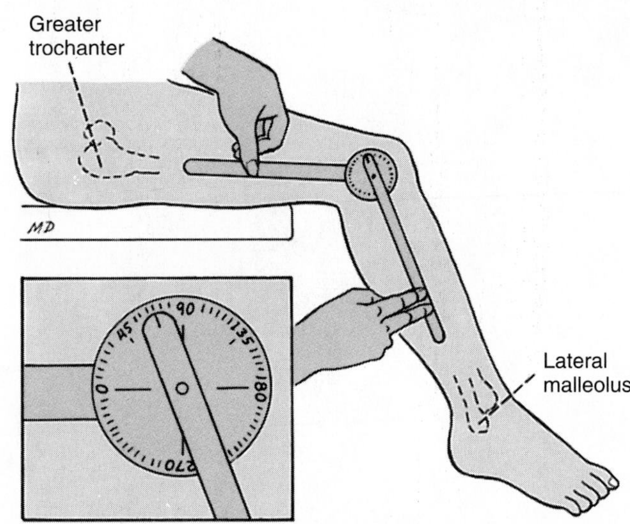

FIGURE 25–3 Use of a goniometer to measure joint range of motion.

■ NEUROVASCULAR ASSESSMENT

A neurovascular assessment is essential for clients with a past musculoskeletal injury because of the high risk of ischemia, deformity, or loss of function in the affected limb.

Components of Neurovascular Assessment

A neurovascular assessment involves checking for (1) pain, (2) pallor, (3) temperature, (4) pulses, (5) capillary refill, (6) paresthesia, and (7) mobility of affected joints.

If the client has pain, using an intensity rating scale of 0 to 10, as previously described, can help determine whether the pain is getting worse—a possible result of edema and nerve compression.

Pallor, coolness, or cyanosis can indicate circulatory compromise in the limb. Check pulses and capillary refill bilaterally to determine the adequacy of blood supply to small peripheral vessels. Capillaries should refill within 2 or 3 seconds.

Loss of sensation and motor function in a limb can signal nerve injury.

Peripheral Nerve Assessment

Test sensation and motor function in major peripheral nerves (Fig. 25–6). Check sensation with the client's eyes closed. Light touch should be perceptible if sensation is normal. If a "pins and needles" sensation is reported, assess further (see Chapter 67). The client should be able to demonstrate active motion of a specific joint upon request. Inability to move a joint and the presence of pain with passive ROM may indicate compartment syndrome.

Perform further assessments, such as of capillary refill, pulses, color, and warmth (see Chapter 27). When casts prevent full neurovascular assessment, observe for edema, capillary refill, and joint movement.

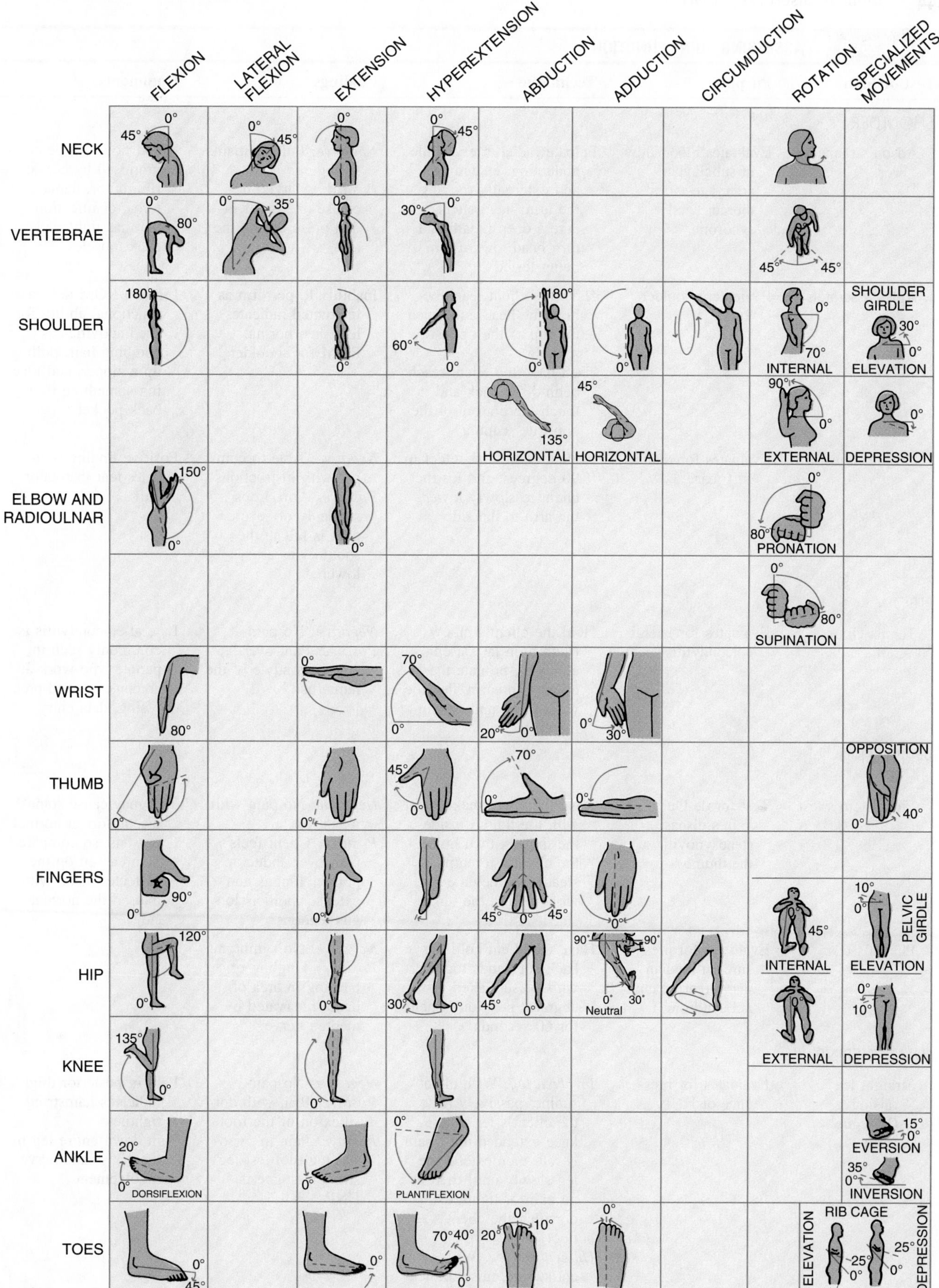

FIGURE 25–4 Joint range of motion (ROM). All joints are at 0 degrees when in anatomic position. ROM begins at 0 degrees, as shown by the *solid lines*. Attainment of average normal ROM is shown by *dotted lines* and the number of degrees in the angle formed by the two lines.

TABLE 25–2 ASSESSING JOINT FUNCTION

Test or Sign	Purpose	Technique	Findings	Comments
SHOULDER				
Adson's maneuver	Evaluates blood flow in subclavian artery; tests for thoracic outlet syndrome	Palpate radial artery while abducting, extending, and externally rotating the arm; have client take a deep breath and turn head toward arm being tested	*Negative:* Pulse remains strong *Positive:* Marked decrease or loss of radial pulse during the test	Blood flow can be compromised by cervical rib, tumor, hematoma, or infection that has tightened neck muscles
Apley's scratch test	Evaluates shoulder ROM	Have the client reach behind the head and touch the top of the opposite scapula Then have the client reach behind the back and touch the bottom of the opposite scapula	Inability to perform as instructed indicates less than normal ROM for shoulder	Limited ROM decreases functional ability for such activities as combing hair, pulling up a zipper, and placing something in a back pocket
Drop arm test	Evaluates for rotator cuff tear	Abduct client's shoulder to 90 degrees, and instruct client to slowly lower the arm to the side	*Negative:* Able to comply with instructions *Positive:* Arm drops suddenly or severe pain is felt in the shoulder as arm is lowered	Positive finding indicates tear in rotator cuff
ELBOW				
Tennis elbow test	Evaluates for lateral epicondylitis	Hold the client's elbow (thumb on lateral epicondyle), pronate the client's forearm, flex the wrist fully, and extend the elbow	*Negative:* No pain *Positive:* Pain over lateral epicondyle of the humerus	Lateral epicondylitis is commonly seen in people who work at computers (word processing, data entry)
WRIST AND HAND				
Finkelstein's test	Test for de Quervain's disease (tenosynovitis of the thumb)	Have the client make a fist with the thumb inside the fingers, then hold the client's forearm steady and deviate the wrist toward the ulnar side	*Negative:* No pain with maneuver *Positive:* Client feels pain over abductor pollicis longus and extensor pollicis longus tendons	Test may cause some discomfort in normal persons, so compare pain caused on the "affected" side with that on the normal side
Phalen's test	Evaluates for pressure on median nerve (carpal tunnel syndrome)	Have the client hold the backs of hands together with wrists flexed 90 degrees; position is held for 60 seconds	*Negative:* No symptoms *Positive:* Tingling or burning in area of hand innervated by median nerve	
LUMBAR SPINE				
Straight leg raising (Lasègue's sign)	Evaluates for presence of HNP	*Involved leg:* With client supine, passively raise the client's leg with knee extended until pain is felt, then extend the leg slowly until there is no pain or tightness; dorsiflex the client's floot *Uninvolved leg:* With client supine, raise the leg as described for the involved leg	*Negative:* No pain *Positive:* Pain with dorsiflexion of the foot *Positive:* Pain in opposite leg (not test leg) strongly suggests HNP	Pain in posterior thigh indicates hamstring tightness Pain down entire leg indicates sciatic nerve involvement

TABLE 25–2 ASSESSING JOINT FUNCTION *Continued*

Test or Sign	Purpose	Technique	Findings	Comments
KNEE				
Drawer test (anterior)	Evaluates stability of ACL	Have client lie on back with knee flexed to 90 degrees and hip to 45 degrees; hold the foot of the test leg in place, and then draw the tibia forward on the femur (Place your hands around the tibia with the thumbs on the medial and lateral joint lines of the knee, as shown in Fig. 25–5)	*Negative:* Movement 6 mm or less *Positive:* Movement more than 6 mm indicates tear in ACL	If PCL is injured, result may be false-positive If PCL injury is suspected, check for posterior "sag" sign (gravity and drawer test)
Drawer test (posterior)	Evaluates stability of PCL	Position client as described for anterior test and push tibia back on femur	*Negative:* Tibia does not move back *Positive:* Backward movement of tibia (felt or observed) indicates injury to PCL	
Gravity test (posterior sag sign)	Evaluates integrity of PCL	Have client lie supine with hips flexed to 45 degrees and knees to 90 degrees	*Positive:* Tibia "sagging" back on the femur indicates that PCL is torn	With minimal swelling, sag is very evident, as is obvious concavity distal to the patella
Lachman's test	Evaluates injury to the ACL	Have client lie supine with the knees between full extension and 30 degrees; then use one hand to stabilize the femur and the other hand to move the tibia forward (see Fig. 25–5*B*)	*Positive:* When tibia moves forward, the infrapatellar tendon slope disappears	This test is the best indicator of ACL injury
McMurray's test	Evaluates for medial and lateral meniscus injury	Have client lie supine with the injured leg fully flexed; then cup the heel with one hand and place your other hand on the knee (fingers on the medial joint line, thumb on the lateral joint line); first, rotate the tibia medially, changing degrees of flexion; then, rotate the tibia laterally, repeatedly changing degrees of flexion	*Positive:* If a snap or click is heard, there is probably a meniscal tear	Evaluation of meniscal injuries is difficult and requires considerable experience; because menisci have no blood or nerve supply, there may be no pain or swelling with injury

ACL, anterior cruciate ligament; HNP, herniated nucleus pulposus; PCL, posterior cruciate ligament; ROM, range of motion.
Adapted from Maher, A. B., Salmond, S. W., & Pellino, T. A. (1998). *Orthopaedic nursing* (2nd ed.). Philadelphia: W. B. Saunders.

DIAGNOSTIC TESTS

Diagnostic tests of musculoskeletal structures are grouped by whether they are invasive or noninvasive. See Chapter 11 for a more detailed discussion of many of these tests and the client preparation they require.

■ NONINVASIVE TESTS OF STRUCTURE

Radiography

Radiography (x-ray study) is the most widely used noninvasive musculoskeletal diagnostic procedure. X-ray examinations are used to:

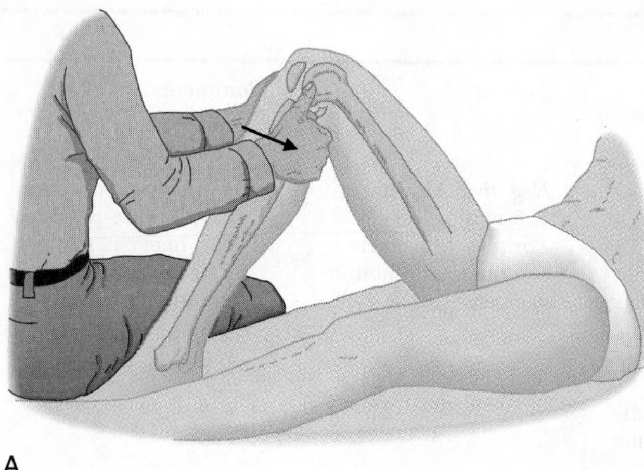

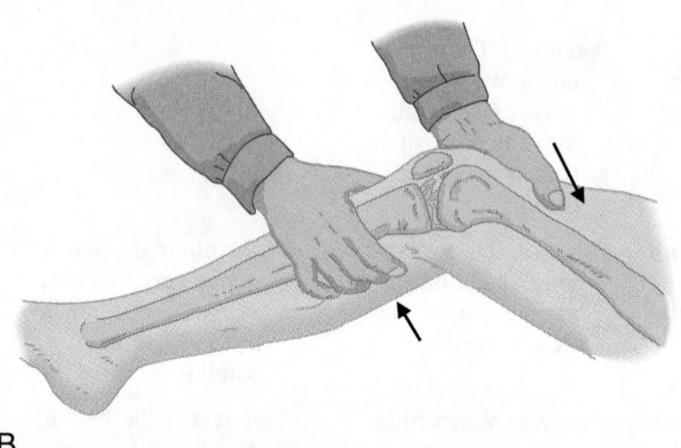

FIGURE 25–5 Special advanced tests of joint function. *A*, The drawer test for instability of the knee ligaments. *B*, Lachman's test for anterior cruciate instability.

- Establish the presence of a musculoskeletal problem
- Follow its progress
- Evaluate the effectiveness of treatment

A plain film is obtained, usually an anteroposterior (AP) or lateral view, possibly both. Other common views include a notch (posterior or less commonly anterior) view of the knee in flexion, an oblique (45-degree angle) view, and a sunrise or patella view of the underside of the patella.

TOMOGRAPHY. *Tomograms* (body-section radiographs) show tissue at various planes through the body as though slices had been made. Tomography can be used to locate bone destruction, small cavities, foreign bodies, and lesions overshadowed by other structures and to evaluate whether a bone graft has united.

FLUOROSCOPY. Fluoroscopy may be used in conjunction with myelography to verify the location of the lumbar puncture. Fluoroscopy also can be used to monitor the progress of contrast dye injected into the subarachnoid space during myelography. See Chapter 67.

DUAL-ENERGY X-RAY ABSORPTIOMETRY. Methods to measure bone density are performed to diagnose osteoporosis because the condition is not evident in x-ray studies until 30% to 50% of bone mass is lost. One method of measuring bone mass is with dual-energy x-ray absorptiometry (commonly called a DEXA scan). An x-ray tube is used to generate dual-energy photons. DEXA causes less radiation than an x-ray exposure and takes about 10 minutes. It can detect osteoporosis in sites such as the wrist, spine, and hips. No preparation is required, although the client may require teaching about osteoporosis once the findings are known.

COMPUTED TOMOGRAPHY. Computed tomography is useful for assessing some bone and soft tissue tumors and spinal fractures.

MAGNETIC RESONANCE IMAGING. Magnetic resonance imaging, or MRI, facilitates the early diagnosis of many conditions that affect tendons, ligaments, cartilage, and bone marrow (Fig. 25–7).

■ INVASIVE TESTS OF STRUCTURE

Specialized radiographic procedures that are invasive and allow more precise visualization include arthrograms, sinography, and myelography. Other invasive tests of structure are radionuclide scanning, arthrocentesis, arthroscopy, electromyography, and biopsy. All are discussed here.

Radiography

ARTHROGRAPHY

Arthrography is a radiographic examination of soft tissue joint structures. It is used to diagnose trauma to joint capsules or supporting ligaments, especially those of the shoulder, wrist, hip, ankle, and knee. After local anesthesia has been achieved, a contrast agent or air is injected into the joint cavity with the use of aseptic precautions. A series of x-ray films is taken as the joint is moved through ROM.

Before arthrography, explain the procedure, answer any questions, and obtain the client's informed consent to the procedure. Explain that the procedure may take up to an hour (follow-up x-rays are sometimes taken 30 minutes after the injection) and that the client must remain as still as possible except when asked to reposition. Ask whether the client has any allergies, especially to local anesthetics, iodine, or contrast dyes. Suggest that the client void before the procedure. Advise that the joint may be uncomfortable for 1 to 2 days afterward and the client should thus avoid strenuous exercise for that time.

SINOGRAPHY AND MYELOGRAPHY

Sinography and myelography are similar to arthrography, in that both modalities involve injection of contrast agents and the taking of x-ray films. Sinography is used to examine sinus tracts (deep draining wounds). Myelography is discussed in Chapter 67.

Radionuclide Imaging

BONE SCANS

In bone scanning, images of the skeleton are taken after a radioisotope (usually technetium 99m) is injected intravenously and allowed to migrate to bone. The whole

Peroneal Nerve

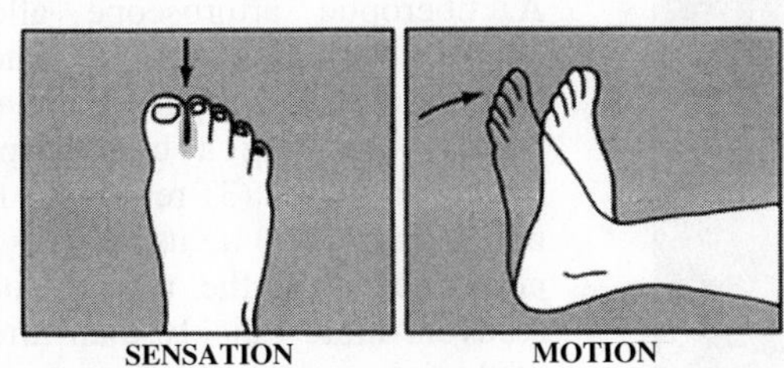

☐ **SENSATION**
Prick the web space between the great toe and second toe

☐ **MOTION**
Have client dorsiflex ankle and extend toes at the metatarsal phalangeal joints

Tibial Nerve

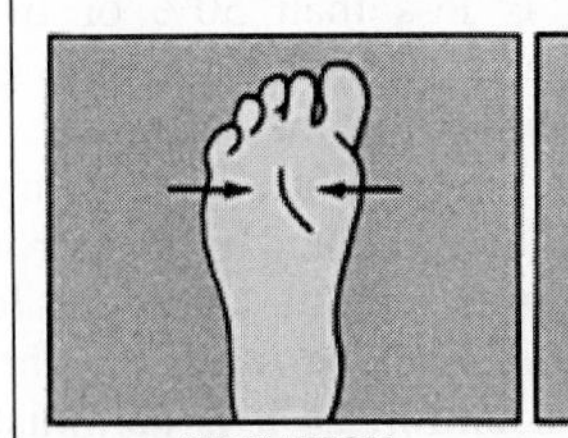

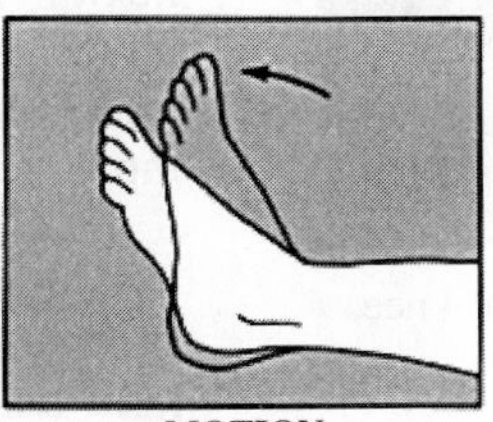

☐ **SENSATION**
Prick the medial and lateral surfaces of the sole of the foot

☐ **MOTION**
Have client plantar flex ankle and toes

Radial Nerve

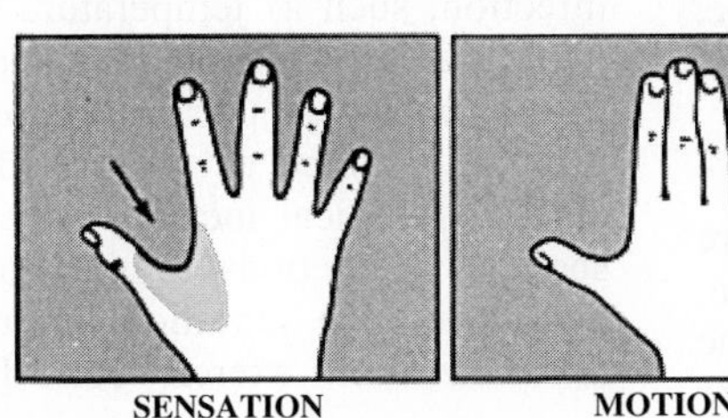

☐ **SENSATION**
Prick the web space between the thumb and index finger

☐ **MOTION**
Have client hyperextend thumb then wrist and hyperextend the four fingers at the MCP joints

Ulnar Nerve

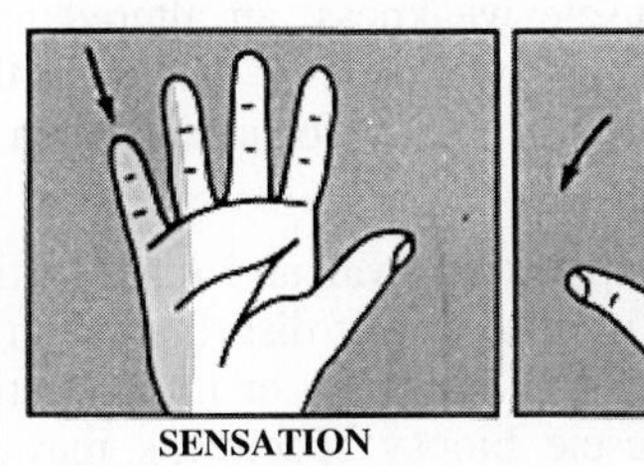

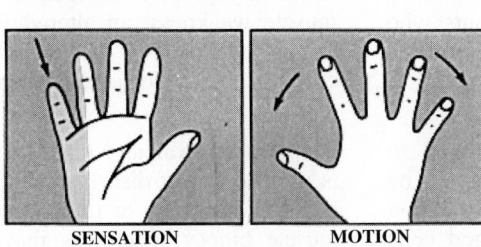

☐ **SENSATION**
Prick the distal fat pad of the small finger

☐ **MOTION**
Have client abduct all fingers

Median Nerve

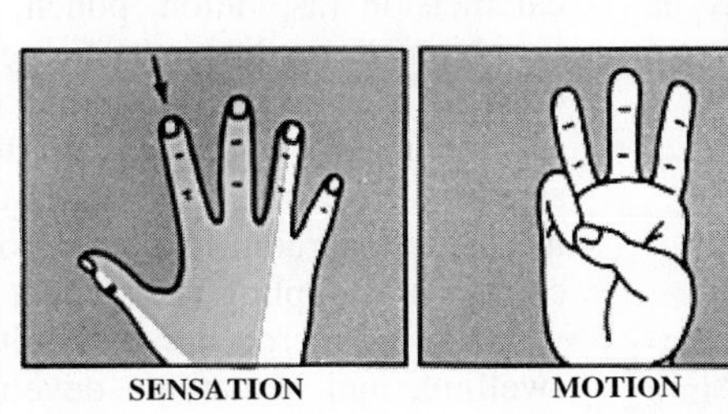

☐ **SENSATION**
Prick the distal surface of the index finger

☐ **MOTION**
Have client oppose thumb and small finger; note whether client can flex wrist

FIGURE 25–6 Neurovascular assessment of the peroneal, tibial, radial, ulnar, and median nerves. MCP, metacarpophalangeal. (Modified from Stearns, G. M., & Brunner, N. A. [1987]. *Operative care* [Vol. 1, p. 89]. Rutherford, NJ: Howmedica.)

body is usually scanned, although just a limb may be scanned (pinhole scan) if a stress fracture is suspected. Bone scanning is used to detect malignancies, osteomyelitis, osteoporosis, and some fractures, especially pathologic ones. The radioisotope concentrates in these areas, indicating abnormal bone metabolism. The radioisotope does not accumulate in poorly perfused bone.

Explain the procedure to the client and family, answer their questions, and obtain consent. The procedure takes about an hour, during which time the client lies supine. Reassure the client that the procedure is not painful and that there are no harmful effects from the isotopes. Suggest that the client void before the procedure.

After the scan, no special precautions are required ex-

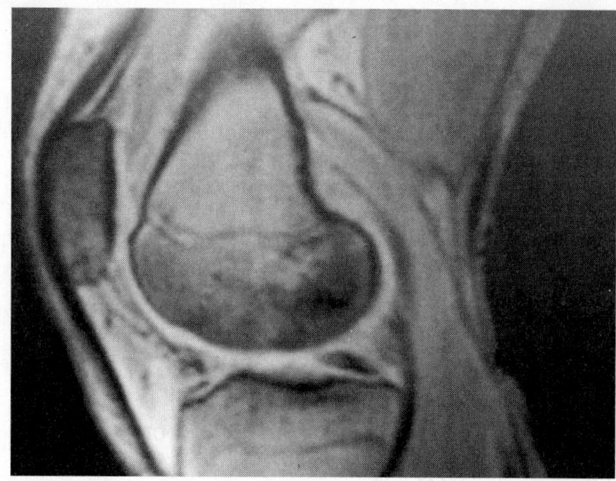

FIGURE 25–7 Magnetic resonance image of the right knee.

cept that the client should drink large amounts of water for 24 to 48 hours to help eliminate the radioisotope. Because the radioisotope carries minimal radioactivity, there is no hazard to others.

GALLIUM SCANS

Gallium scans are similar to bone scans but are more specific to bone disorders. Gallium also migrates to brain, liver, and breast tissue. Because it is taken up by bone more slowly than technetium 99, gallium is given to the client by a nuclear medicine technician 2 to 3 hours before the scan. The scan takes 30 to 60 minutes to complete. Mild sedation may be needed for clients who are in pain, are restless, or are elderly. No special follow-up care is required.

INDIUM IMAGING

Indium imaging is the use of indium 111, tagged to (connected to) leukocytes to detect bone infection. The client's leukocytes are separated from a sample of blood and labeled (tagged) with indium. Then the tagged cells are reinjected. Because leukocytes naturally accumulate in areas of bone infection, the tagged leukocytes can be detected by imaging. No special preparation or follow-up care is necessary.

Other Tests

ARTHROCENTESIS

Joint aspiration, or *arthrocentesis*, is a method of aspirating synovial fluid, blood, or pus via a needle inserted into the joint cavity. It is used to diagnose rheumatoid arthritis and other inflammatory conditions or to remove fluid to relieve pain. Normal synovial fluid is clear to straw-colored and is present in minute amounts. Inflamed joints produce increased amounts. In normal joints, synovial fluid is usually thick and has a string-like appearance when expressed from a syringe.

Arthrocentesis is performed with the use of aseptic precautions after local anesthesia has been achieved and with or without fluoroscopy. Medication may be instilled into the joint, if necessary, to alleviate inflammation in septic arthritis. Apply a compression bandage after arthrocentesis, and advise the client to rest the joint for 8 to 24 hours.

ARTHROSCOPY

A fiberoptic arthroscope allows endoscopic examination of various joints (hip, knee, shoulder, elbow, wrist) without making a large incision. Arthroscopy can be used for (1) obtaining a biopsy specimen, (2) assessing articular cartilage, (3) removing loose bodies, and (4) trimming cartilage. It usually is an outpatient procedure performed with the use of local anesthesia. The client recovers more quickly than after an *arthrotomy* (opening of the joint).

Arthroscopy is contraindicated in the client whose joint flexion is less than 50% or in whom a skin or wound infection is present at the site. Complications are rare but include infection, hemarthrosis (blood in the joint), swelling, synovial rupture, joint injury, and thrombophlebitis.

Instruct the client to fast from midnight the night before. Make sure that consent forms are signed. If local anesthesia is to be used, tell the client that there may be mild discomfort as it is administered and when the endoscope is inserted.

Teach the client to watch for signs of postprocedure infection, such as temperature elevation and local inflammation at the incision site, and to report them promptly. Ensure necessary postprocedure pain relief. A normal diet may be resumed as soon as desired. Tell the client that unless a surgical incision is made and the surgeon gives specific instructions to the contrary, walking is usually permitted once sensation has returned. The client should avoid strenuous exercise for a few days.

ELECTROMYOGRAPHY

Electromyography is used to assess such problems as muscle weakness, an altered gait, or lower motor neuron lesions. Chapter 67 discusses this test in more detail because it is used for clients with neurologic disorders.

BIOPSY

Biopsy (removal and examination of a sample of tissue) is used to detect disorders such as infection, cancer of the bone, and atrophy or inflammation of the muscle. Bone or muscle biopsy specimens may be collected either during surgery or through a needle or bore not requiring a surgical incision (aspiration, punch, or needle biopsy). Aspiration biopsy sampling may be performed under radiographic control, such as for sampling of the spine. Bone biopsy specimens are collected with the use of local anesthesia and aseptic technique in either the radiology department or the operating room to prevent osteomyelitis. Bone or muscle biopsy sampling takes about 30 minutes.

After the procedure, monitor the site for bleeding, swelling, and hematoma development. Because dressings usually cover the biopsy site, analyze the client's pain level to monitor for complications. Mild to moderate discomfort is expected; more severe levels of pain may signal complications. Elevate the biopsy site for 24 hours to reduce edema. Monitor the client's vital signs every 4 hours for 24 hours. Mild analgesia is often required. Instruct the client to assess the site on a regular basis (at least daily) for signs of infection when discharged.

■ LABORATORY STUDIES

Table 25–3 lists the most common laboratory tests for clients with musculoskeletal disorders. Chapter 77 describes laboratory tests specific for rheumatic problems.

TABLE 25–3 COMMON LABORATORY STUDIES USED IN DIAGNOSIS OF MUSCULOSKELETAL CONDITIONS

Test	Normal Value	Significance of Results
Antinuclear antibody (ANA)	Negative or at a titer ≤1:32	Positive results are associated with systemic lupus erythematosus, rheumatoid arthritis, rheumatic fever, and Raynaud's disease
C-reactive protein (CRP)	Trace amounts	Positive in acute inflammation, such as rhematoid arthritis
Erythrocyte sedimentation rate (ESR)	*Westergren method:* males, 0–15 mm/hr; females, 0–20 mm/hr *Wintrobe method:* males, 0–9 mm/hr; females, 0–15 mm/hr	Elevations common in arthritic conditions, infection, inflammation, cancer, and cell or tissue destruction
MINERAL METABOLISM		
Calcium	8.0–10.5 mg/dl or 4.5–5.5 mEq/L	Decreased levels found in osteomalacia, osteoporosis Increased levels found in bone tumors, Paget's disease, and healing fractures
Alkaline phosphatase	30–90 units/L	Elevations found in bone cancer, osteoporosis, osteomalacia, and Paget's disease
Phosphorus	2.5–4.0 mg/dl	Increased levels found in healing fractures and osteolytic metastatic tumor diseases
MUSCLE ENZYMES		
Aldolase A	1.3–8.2 units/dl	Elevations in muscular dystrophy and dermatomyositis
Aspartate aminotransferase	10–50 units/L	Found in skeletal muscle but primarily in heart and renal cells
Creatine kinase	15–150 units/L	Increased levels found in traumatic injuries, progressive muscular dystrophy, and polymyositis
Lactate dehydrogenase (LDH_4, LDH_5)	60–150 units/L	Elevations in skeletal muscle necrosis, extensive cancer, and progressive muscular dystrophy

CONCLUSIONS

Assessment of the musculoskeletal system begins with a complete history, including symptom analysis. Diagnostic studies commonly include x-rays and, in recent years, arthroscopy has evolved to allow the diagnosis and treatment of joint disorders during one procedure.

BIBLIOGRAPHY

1. Doheny, M., Linden, P., & Sedlak, C. (1995). Reducing orthopaedic hazards of the computer work environment. *Orthopaedic Nursing, 14*(1), 7–16.
2. Hunt, A. (1996). The relationship between height change and bone mineral density. *Orthopaedic Nursing, 15*(3), 57–66.
3. Jarvis, C. (2000). *Physical examination and health assessment* (3rd ed.). Philadelphia: W. B. Saunders.
4. Krowchuk, D. P. (1997). Preparticipation athletic examination (PAE): A closer look. *Pediatric Annals, 26*(1), 37–42.
5. Long, J. S. (1996). Shoulder arthroscopy. *Orthopaedic Nursing, 15*(2), 21–32.
6. Maher, A. B., Salmond, S. W., & Pellino, T. A. (1998). *Orthopaedic nursing* (2nd ed.). Philadelphia: W. B. Saunders.
7. Murray, W. J., & Gabel, T. L. (1998). *What about herbal medicine?* Unpublished Manuscript, University of Nebraska Medical Center, Omaha.
8. O'Hanlon-Nichols, T. (1998). Basic assessment series: A review of the adult musculoskeletal system. *American Journal of Nursing, 98*(6), 48–52.

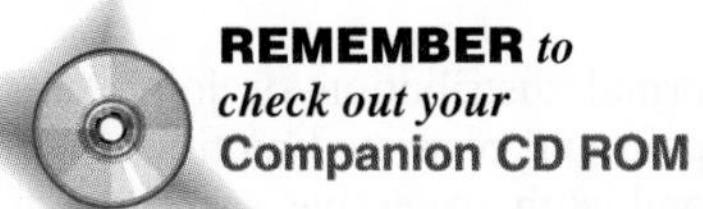

CHAPTER 26

Management of Clients with Musculoskeletal Disorders

Dottie Roberts
Joan Lappe

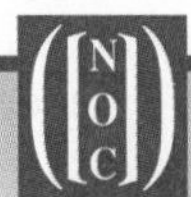

NURSING OUTCOMES CLASSIFICATION
for Nursing Diagnoses—Clients with Musculoskeletal Disorders

Impaired Physical Mobility
Ambulation: Walking
Joint Movement: Active
Mobility Level
Transfer Performance
Knowledge Deficit
Knowledge: Treatment Procedures
Pain
Comfort Level
Pain Control
Pain: Disruptive Effects
Pain Level

Risk for Altered Tissue Perfusion
Tissue Perfusion: Peripheral
Risk for Impaired Skin Integrity
Immobility Consequences: Physiological
Tissue Perfusion: Peripheral
Risk for Infection
Immobility Consequences: Physiological
Knowledge: Infection Control
Tissue Integrity: Skin and Mucous Membranes
Wound Healing: Primary Intention

Risk for Injury
Risk Control
Risk Detection
Risk for Peripheral Neurovascular Dysfunction
Circulation Status
Joint Movement: Active
Mobility Level
Muscle Function
Neurologic Status
Tissue Perfusion: Peripheral

The musculoskeletal system gives the body free movement and independent function. Bone is a vital, dynamic connective tissue that serves three major functions: (1) it provides mechanical integrity for movement and protection of internal organs, (2) it performs a major role in metabolism and mineral homeostasis, and (3) it serves as the primary site of hemopoiesis. Disorders of the musculoskeletal system cause considerable morbidity, lead to decreased quality of life, and often result in reduced life expectancy.

OSTEOARTHRITIS

Osteoarthritis (OA) is a chronic joint disease characterized by progressive degenerative changes in the articular cartilage that covers the joint surfaces. Although inflammation is not typical of OA, changes in the joint space may cause a localized inflammatory response.

Etiology and Risk Factors

OA has been classified by its cause as either primary or secondary. *Primary* OA is an idiopathic process found in people with no history of joint injury, joint disease, or systemic illness that might be associated with the development of arthritis. The most prevalent articular disease in adults age 65 years and older, primary OA occurs more commonly in women than in men. It accounts for substantial disability in the lower extremities as a result of its effects on the large weight-bearing joints. In the past, OA was accepted as an inevitable part of the aging process. Today we know that it is not a normal part of aging.

Although OA is not considered to be a genetic disease, a strong familial disposition exists for its development. A genetic link has been found in the occurrence of Heberden's nodes associated with OA of the distal interphalangeal (DIP) joints of the hands. In addition, sex hormones and other hormonal factors are believed to play an active part in the development and progression of OA.

Secondary OA occurs more frequently in men than in women and results from trauma, other inflammatory joint disease, avascular necrosis, or neuropathic disorders—such as Legg-Calvé-Perthes disease. Traumatic arthritis can develop after fracture or open joint injury. It can also stem from repetitive injury related to the person's occupation or sport (e.g., wrist arthritis in a keyboard operator, shoulder manifestations in a baseball pitcher).

Because OA has been traditionally considered an incurable disease process, much effort has been spent on identifying modifiable risk factors. For example, studies have consistently shown that overweight people have higher rates of OA of the knee than non-overweight peers. Although overweight people also appear to be at higher risk for OA of the hip, the association is not as strong or as consistent as for OA of the knee. This risk variation is due to the different amount of force exerted across these joints when a person stands or walks. Up to six times the body's weight is exerted across the knee, whereas only three times the body's weight is exerted at the hip.

Regular exercise decreases the risk for development of OA in several ways:

- Weight-bearing exercise leads to increased joint mobility and strengthens the joint's supporting muscles, tendons, and ligaments.
- Exercise stimulates cartilage growth by driving synovial fluid through the cartilage matrix. Because articular cartilage lacks blood vessels, the mechanical process of joint movement is essential to cartilage regeneration and continued joint mobility.
- Exercise protects joints indirectly by aiding in weight control.

Pathophysiology

Healthy articular cartilage appears smooth, glistening, and white. It is characterized by unique viscoelastic and compressive properties. *Chondrocytes,* the cellular components of cartilage, constantly remodel and maintain the integrity of this slippery, shock-absorbing pad in order to protect the bone ends in a joint. Chondrocytes actually create the cartilage matrix by producing type II collagen and proteoglycans. The hydrophilic (water-attracting) properties of the proteoglycans in particular add to the ability of cartilage to resist wear with heavy joint use.

In simplest terms, OA can be described as a process of cartilage matrix degradation accompanied by the body's ineffectual attempts at repair. Early pathologic changes include a decrease in proteoglycan content in the matrix, which leads to a softening and loss of elasticity by the cartilage. As the body attempts to compensate, chondrocytes initially proliferate and increase their synthesis of proteoglycans and collagen. Progressive destruction by lysosomal enzymes eventually outweighs production, however, and the cartilage becomes increasingly susceptible to joint friction. Changes in collagen synthesis also occur, minimizing the compressibility of the cartilage. Factors that cause these changes are not clearly understood, but the effect on cartilage is the loss of its ability to resist wear with heavy use.

Fibrillation, erosion, and cracking appear in the superficial layer of cartilage as collagen fibers rupture. While cartilage becomes yellowed and worn over articular surfaces, bone growth increases at the joint margins and bony outgrowths, or osteophytes, develop (Fig. 26–1). Central loss of cartilage, accompanied by buildup of cartilage and bone peripherally, produces inequality in the joint surfaces. The normal distribution of joint stress is changed, resulting in pain and restricted motion. The synovium may also respond with excessive secretion of synovial fluid, creating an inflamed distended joint capsule.

Clinical Manifestations

The diagnosis of OA may be confirmed by radiographic changes that include the presence of osteophytes and of a narrowed joint space caused by erosion of articular cartilage. However, the American College of Rheumatology (ACR) has established classification criteria for OA that do not rely solely on radiographic findings.

Typical clinical manifestations that help in the diagnosis of OA include worsening pain and stiffness that are increased with activity and relieved by rest. Affected joints may exhibit crepitus, mild tenderness in the area of joint wear, deficits in range of motion (ROM), and possibly some joint enlargement. One or more joints may be affected, but joint discomfort is not usually symmetrical. The client may describe weight-bearing joints that "lock" or "give way" as a result of advancing disease. New bone growth in the hands may be evident in the appearance of Heberden's nodes (DIP joints) or Bouchard's nodes (proximal interphalangeal [PIP joints]) (Fig. 26–2).

Although no laboratory test has the capacity to confirm the presence of OA, specific tests may be performed to rule out other conditions such as rheumatoid arthritis (RA), infection, gout, and tendinitis or bursitis. Differentiation between OA and RA is especially important (Table 26–1). Depending on the client's clinical presentation, orders may include a test for rheumatoid factor or a serum uric acid determination. Aspiration and analysis of synovial fluid allows the practitioner to role out infection or crystal deposition. An erythrocyte sedimentation rate

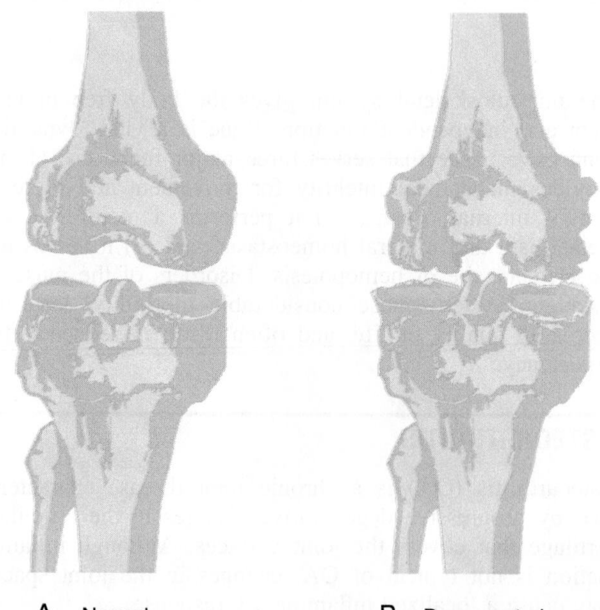

FIGURE 26–1 Pathologic changes seen with osteoarthritis. *A,* Normal bony surfaces for articulation. *B,* Surfaces are altered with loss of joint space and osteophyte formation.

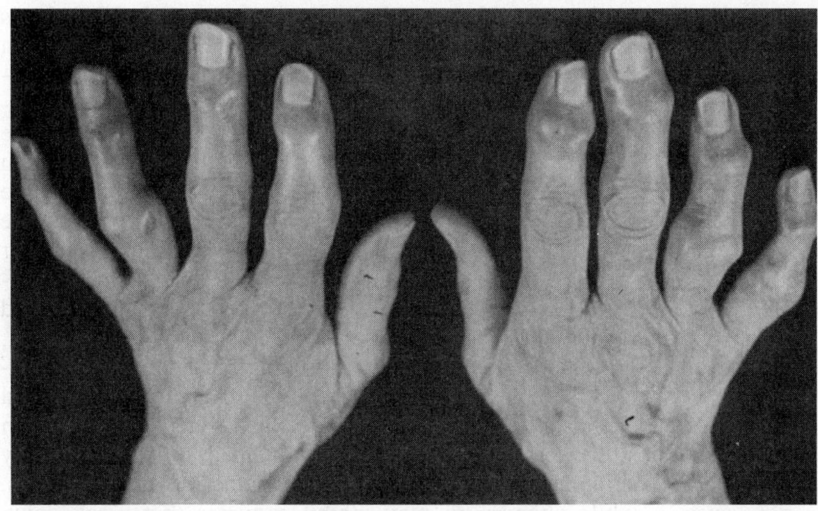

FIGURE 26–2 Osteoarthritis of the distal and proximal interphalageal joints. (From Moskowitz, R. W. & Bluestone, R. [1992]. General aspects of differential diagnosis. In R. W. Moskowitz et al. [Eds.], *Osteoarthritis: Diagnosis and medical/surgical treatment* [2nd ed., p. 475]. Philadelphia: W. B. Saunders.)

TABLE 26–1 DIFFERENTIATION OF OSTEOARTHRITIS AND RHEUMATOID ARTHRITIS

	Osteoarthritis	Rheumatoid Arthritis
Pathology	Progressive process of cartilage degeneration and bone degeneration (spurs)	Progressive process marked by exacerbations and remissions Inflammation of synovial membrane with cartilage damage and bone destruction Ligament, tendon, and joint capsule damage
Affected joints	Weight-bearing joints (hips, knees, ankles), spine, DIP and PIP joints Asymmetric	Small joints (PIP, MCP), wrists, knees Symmetric
Joint effusions	Uncommon	Common
Clinical manifestations	Localized pain and stiffness, usually without swelling Pain with activity, improves with rest Heberden's and Bouchard's nodules	Pain, swelling, tenderness, redness, and warmth Nodules Anemia, fatigue, and muscle aches Pain at rest, especially at night Elevated ESR, frequently positive rheumatoid factor
Other affected systems	None	Lung, heart, skin
Body size	Often overweight	Usually average to below average weight for size
Age at onset	Fourth to fifth decade of life	Young to middle age
Gender	2:1 female-to-male ratio	3:1 female-to-male ratio
Heredity	One form familial	Familial tendency
Diagnostic tests	X-rays	Rheumatoid factor (80% positive); x-rays; joint fluid analysis; negative Lyme disease titer
X-ray evidence	Osteophytes, subchondral cysts	Erosions, osteoporosis
Treatment	Exercise and weight control, maintenance of activity level with joint protection Heat or cold applications Relaxation strategies Medication and/or surgery	Inflammation reduction Balanced diet and exercise program with joint protection Relaxation strategies; heat or cold applications Medication and/or surgery

DIP, distal interphalangeal; ESR, erythrocyte sedimentation rate; PIP, proximal interphalangeal; MCP, metacarpophalangeal.
Adapted from Altizer, L. L. (1998). Degenerative disorders. In A. B. Maher, S. W. Salmond, & T. A. Pellino (Eds.), *Orthopaedic nursing* (2nd ed.). Philadelphia: W. B. Saunders.

(ESR) is of use only if systemic manifestations are present. In practice, the possible diagnoses are usually narrowed greatly after completion of the history and examination.

Outcome Management

Medical Management

Goals for medical management of OA include (1) pain relief with maintenance of mobility, (2) functional independence, and (3) maintenance of quality of life. Most people with OA can be successfully treated with a conservative approach that involves the simultaneous use of several modalities.

All clients benefit from a careful balance between rest and exercise. A sedentary lifestyle can lead to weight gain, which exacerbates arthritic symptoms. Low-impact aerobic exercise, such as brisk walking, does not cause further harm to damaged joints. In fact, walking can relieve pain and improve joint mobility. It also increases muscle tone and enhances joint stability. Exercise can help in weight loss, which should be encouraged in the obese client, who faces more rapid destruction of joints in the lower extremities.

The client with OA needs to understand the importance of rest if an affected joint becomes painful. A neoprene or elastic brace may reduce pain and help stabilize the joint during activity. Joints can also be rested when the client uses a cane in the contralateral hand during episodes of severe hip or knee pain. A collar, sling, or corset may be useful for manifestations in the neck, shoulder, or back.

Some clients also obtain relief by applying heat to affected joints or by alternating applications of heat and cold (contrast baths). Diathermy (deep heat therapy), ultrasound, or microwave treatments have not proved effective in clinical trials. Cold applications have proved beneficial for some people, especially immediately after exercise or in those with muscle spasms.

Many people with OA report good results from topical application of capsaicin cream to affected joints several times a day. The cream can be used alone or with oral medication. Capsaicin is especially effective for OA of the knees and hands. About 50% of capsaicin users describe a cutaneous burning, but this reaction usually declines with continued use.

Until recently, nonsteroidal anti-inflammatory drugs (NSAIDs) were the mainstay of pharmacologic management of OA. Because OA has only a minor inflammatory component, NSAIDs may not be the best first-line choice. Furthermore, research suggests that NSAIDs actually disrupt articular cartilage metabolism. Many deaths among older adults are also attributed to NSAID use each year, usually because of gastrointestinal bleeding. ACR guidelines recommend acetaminophen as the drug of first choice for those with hip or knee OA because of its effectiveness, safety, and low cost. It is less likely than NSAIDs to cause gastrointestinal, hepatic, or renal damage. The recommended maximum dose of acetaminophen is 1 g every 6 hours, or 4 g in a 24-hour period.

According to ACR guidelines, a person with OA should be switched to an NSAID when severe pain persists despite the maximum acetaminophen dose. Acetaminophen use often continues on an as-needed (PRN) basis as an adjunct to the NSAID, which should be started in an over-the-counter (OTC) strength. Progression to prescriptive strengths only occurs when clinical manifestations worsen. To minimize gastrointestinal effects, the NSAID can be prescribed with a synthetic prostaglandin such as misoprostol (Cytotec). Newer NSAIDs—the COX-2 selective agents—are now in use in prescriptive strength. While their analgesic properties initially appear greater than traditional NSAIDs, their long-term side effects have not been fully investigated. Medications used for OA are listed in Table 26–2.

Other compounds are also being considered as alternative therapies in the treatment of OA. Glucosamine and chondroitin appear to provide pain relief, perhaps even slowing the disease process. Glucosamine apparently stimulates cartilage cells to manufacture proteoglycans, while chondroitin may inhibit enzymes that break down cartilage. Recent research has examined only the short-term effects of these compounds. It is difficult to determine whether clients with OA will benefit over the long term or if they will experience adverse effects.

Nursing Management of the Medical Patient

The goal of nursing management is promotion of a healthy, positive adaptation in the client with OA. Education is the key to successful treatment of the disease, and the nurse plays a major role as a client educator. Clients and their families need accurate information about the disease and about steps to take to minimize its impact. Effective education can alter behavior, empowering clients to make a positive change in their health status. Important areas in client education include (1) pain management, (2) rest-activity balance, (3) nutrition and weight loss, and (4) self-care strategies.

Teaching clients about their medications is an important part of your role in successful long-term pain management. For example, a client who is taking an NSAID must be informed of the manifestations of gastrointestinal bleeding, such as abdominal pain, tarry stools, and hematemesis. Reinforce the client's need to notify the physician immediately if these manifestations occur. Also encourage the client to keep a pain journal to help focus on manifestations and identify cues that signal the need for rest or activity. Suggest nonpharmacologic pain management strategies (e.g., relaxation techniques, guided imagery) to decrease the feelings of anxiety or powerlessness that accompany disease progression. Other modalities, such as transcutaneous electrical nerve stimulation (TENS), can also be considered to reduce pain.

To assist with self-care deficiencies related to OA, collaborate with an occupational therapist in providing assistive devices that help the client maintain independence with dressing and hygiene. Self-fastening tape (Velcro) closures, zipper pulls, or elastic shoelaces can make dressing easier. Long-handled combs or thick-barreled toothbrushes can also help clients with basic self-care tasks. The client with OA can learn to maintain affected joints in a neutral position at rest in order to avoid flexion contractures that will affect functional ability.

Also recognize the possible influence of OA on the client's sexual role functioning. Pain and stiffness, along with limited ROM, can create problems with sexual ex-

TABLE 26–2 **MEDICATIONS FOR TREATMENT OF OSTEOARTHRITIS**

Category (Example)	Indications and Contraindications	Adverse Effects	Nursing Considerations
Analgesics (acetaminophen)	*Indications* Analgesia *Contraindications* Hepatic disease	Hepatic toxicity in excess doses	Maximum dose is 4 g in 24 hr. Avoid use in alcohol-abusing clients.
NSAIDs (ibuprofen)	*Indications* Analgesia Inflammation *Contraindications* Aspirin allergy	GI bleeding Injury to articular cartilage Sodium retention and hypertension Renal and hepatic damage, especially with long-term use	Administer with food. Observe for weight change. Observe for CNS changes, such as confusion, in older adults.
Prostaglandin synthesis inhibitor, or COX-2 inhibitor (rofecoxib [Vioxx])	*Indications* Osteoarthritis Acute postoperative pain Dysmenorrhea *Contraindications* Aspirin allergy Rofecoxib allergy	GI bleeding, ulceration Lower extremity edema Hypertension Epigastric pain Nausea Back pain	Absorption is not slowed by food. Calcium products reduce bioavailability. Monitor for GI bleeding, skin rash, unexplained weight gain or edema. Avoid administration with ACE inhibitors, aspirin, furosemide, lithium, rifampin, and warfarin.

ACE, angiotensin-converting enzyme; CNS, central nervous system; COX, cyclooxygenase; GI, gastrointestinal; NSAIDs, nonsteroidal anti-inflammatory drugs

pression. Joint deformities can also negatively affect self-image, leading to reduced libido and depression. Inform the client about alternative sexual positions (e.g., side-by-side) that promote comfort during intercourse, and encourage the client to use analgesics or to take warm baths to alleviate pain and stiffness before sexual activity.

Surgical Management

OSTEOTOMY

Osteotomy is a surgical fracture, a cut across a bone with resection of a bone fragment to either correct a deformity or to alter stresses on a joint. In early hip OA, when joint congruency still exists and motion is relatively normal, proximal femoral osteotomy may be performed. A wedge of bone is removed from the region of the lesser trochanter to realign the angle of the femoral neck and shaft. Partial weight-bearing is required for at least 3 months after surgery to allow healing of the osteotomy site. Because manifestations of OA generally progress despite this procedure, as many as 75% of clients treated with osteotomy require further surgery within 10 years.[2] Osteotomy is more frequently performed on clients in their 40s, with the full expectation that total joint replacement will be needed in the future.

ARTHRODESIS

In an arthrodesis (joint fusion) procedure, the surgeon removes articular joint surfaces and holds the bone ends together so that they unite like a fracture. Initial fixation may be provided with pins, braces, or casts. Arthrodesis is indicated for irreparable joint damage or instability. The procedure produces a sound, painless limb, but the resulting loss of movement may be a serious disadvantage in large joints such as the hip or knee.

Arthrodesis remains the operation of choice for the young client with advanced unilateral OA, severe post-traumatic arthritis, or septic arthritis. Hip fusion can result in shortening of the affected extremity by 1 to 1.5 inches, and the client commonly needs a shoe lift postoperatively to help maintain a normal gait. Knee fusion results in shortening of the affected leg by about 0.5 inch, which usually does not create significant postoperative dysfunction. Many clients resume a vigorous, active life following arthrodesis. After hip fusion in particular, they experience few of the initial limitations posed by hip replacement surgery.

TOTAL HIP REPLACEMENT (ARTHROPLASTY)

Total hip replacement (THR), or arthroplasty, is performed to restore joint motion by replacing arthritic bone with metal components. (See Chapter 77 for a discussion of shoulder, elbow, and hand arthroplasty.)

Indications

Indications for THR include (1) failure of conservative treatments, (2) severe compromise of the client's functional ability, and (3) significant pain. The client's subjective complaints frequently have a greater impact on the decision for surgery than radiologic changes do. Total hip replacement may also be performed for complications of femoral neck fractures, congenital disease or deformity, and failure of previous fixations or arthroplasties.

Both *cemented* and *noncemented* hip arthroplasties can be performed. Use of polymethyl-methacrylate (PMMA) bone cement allows immediate intraoperative fixation of femoral and acetabular components. Cemented prostheses are used for elderly clients or for those with compromised bone strength due to conditions such as osteoporosis. In younger, active, or heavier clients, cemented total hip replacements loosen at a rate of about 1% per year, usually from failure of the PMMA bone cement.[2] For these clients, use of prostheses with porous surfaces allows fixation without cement. Instead, bone grows into the porous surface as the client remains on limited weight-bearing status for a number of weeks following surgery. Although short-term outcomes of the two procedures are equivalent, long-term results must be determined in order to justify the cost of noncemented surgical technology. Many hospitals and orthopedic surgeons currently use a "demand matching" system to appropriately choose cemented or noncemented components based on client needs.

Contraindications

Contraindications to THR include (1) recent or active joint sepsis (except in joint revision due to infection), (2) neutrotrophic joints, or (3) an inability to cooperate with immediate postoperative requirements or long-term joint rehabilitation. In addition, the client's general health must allow tolerance of anesthesia, blood loss, and surgical stress. Heart, lung, liver, and metabolic disorders should be stable before surgery.

Surgical Techniques

Although a number of vendors have developed total hip prostheses, a common design currently in use is a three-component set: (1) the femoral neck and stem, (2) a slide-on femoral head, and (3) a metal acetabulum with or without fixation screw holes. Hip prostheses may be made of several different metal alloys that contribute to the relative lightness and durability of the components (Fig. 26–3).

Depending on physician preference and on the type of exposure needed for the procedure, the surgical approach may be (1) anterolateral, (2) direct lateral, (3) transtrochanteric, or (4) posterolateral. You must know the surgical approach in order to understand the leg position used to dislocate the operative hip. If that position is replicated after surgery, the client's risk for dislocating the hip prosthesis increases.

With an *anterolateral* position, the client lies supine on the table. The operative hip is externally rotated and extended, with the knee flexed. With the *posterolateral* position, the client lies on his or her side, with the operative hip internally rotated, flexed, and adducted. Many orthopedic surgeons use the posterolateral position for the anterior and posterior approaches.

Once the hip has been exposed, the surgeon performs an osteotomy of the femoral neck to expose the acetabulum. Osteophytes and cysts are removed from the acetabulum to prepare it for reaming and for the prosthesis. Trial prostheses are placed, and their fit is evaluated before final choice of appropriately sized components. If the prosthesis is to be *press-fit (noncemented),* the bone is prepared for pegs or spikes. The surgeon presses the cup firmly into place and evaluates its apposition to the bone. If a *cemented* prosthesis is used, anchor holes are drilled

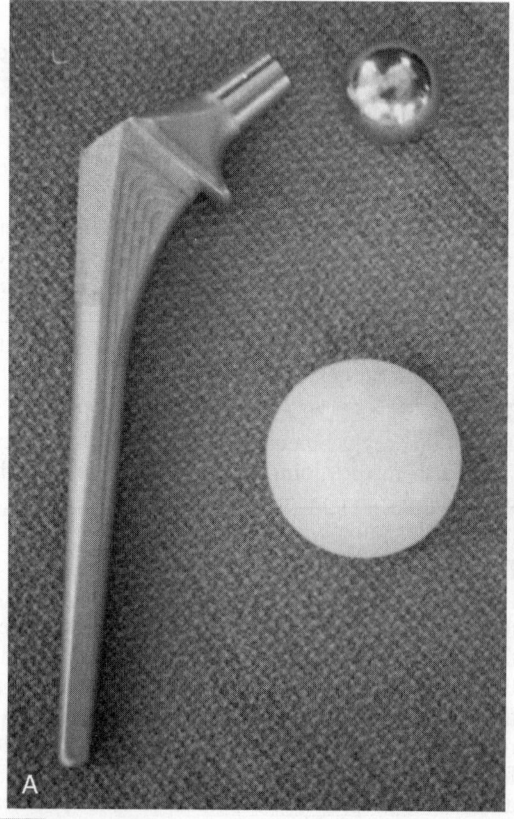

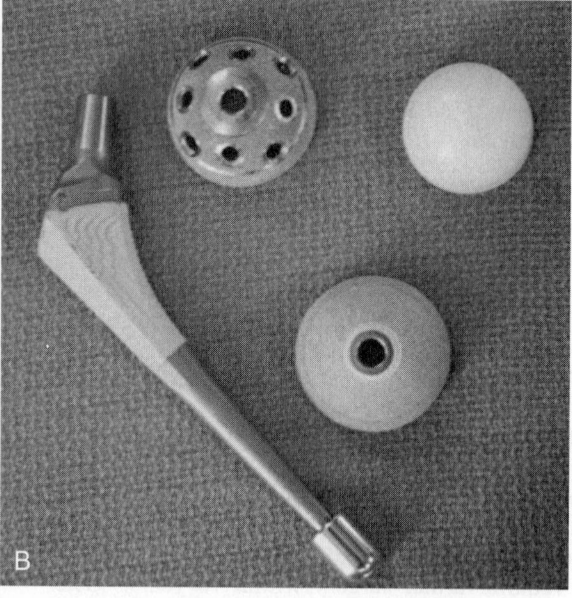

FIGURE 26–3 Hip prostheses. *A,* Coated femoral head and all-polyethylene acetabular cup for cemented total hip arthroplasty. *B,* Porous femoral and two types of acetabular components with femoral head for cementless total hip arthroplasty. (From Maher, A. B., Salmond, S. W., & Pellino, T. A. [Eds.] [1998]. *Orthopedic nursing* [2nd ed., p. 508]. Philadelphia: W. B. Saunders.)

into the iliac subchondral bone. After cleaning the bone thoroughly with pressure-pulsed lavage, the surgeon cements the cup into position.

To prepare the femur, the surgeon forms a tunnel by reaming the bone's intramedullary canal. After placement of a trial prosthesis, the hip is reduced to assess for motion, stability, and length. If results are acceptable, the surgeon removes the trial components. For a press-fit prosthesis, the femoral stem is pressed into the reamed intramedullary canal. For a cemented prosthesis, the femur is cleaned and the canal is plugged to prevent the cement from traveling too far distally. The surgeon fills the canal with cement, inserting the femoral stem and then placing the femoral head. After the hip is reduced, the surgeon evaluates the extremity for motion, stability, and length.

Before closing the incision (~10 inches long), the surgeon may place a closed wound drainage system, such as a Hemovac, to help prevent hematoma—which can increase the risk of infection. However, use of wound drainage systems has decreased in recent years as they have been found to be ineffective in preventing hematomas while possibly increasing the risk of blood loss and contamination of the surgical wound.

COMPLICATIONS

In-hospital mortality is only about 0.5%, but other postoperative complications can occur in as many as 25% of clients over 65 years of age after a THR.[2] While many complications are short-lived and reversible, others can have a great impact on the client's physical and psychological recovery from surgery. The most common and most serious complication is venous thromboembolism. Prevention of deep vein thrombosis (DVT) or pulmonary embolism (PE) requires early mobilization, often with a combination of pharmacologic and nonpharmacologic methods.

Infection following a THR is a serious concern because of the possible development of osteomyelitis. Prophylactic antibiotics are considered essential, and careful wound assessment must begin immediately after surgery. Bladder or urinary tract infection is also possible because of urinary stasis or the presence of an indwelling urinary catheter. Because any localized infection can also spread to the wound, prompt recognition and treatment of clinical manifestations is imperative.

Postoperative joint instability increases the risk for dislocation or subluxation. The risk is even greater following revision arthroplasty because of the extended surgical exposure and soft tissue deficiencies. Hip dislocation occurs in approximately 2% of clients who have undergone arthroplasty, with the greatest risk in the first 8 weeks after surgery.[2] All clients require a great deal of monitoring and education regarding the positions that should be avoided while soft tissues heal around the new joint. Positioning precautions are continued for about 6 weeks, until the surgical incision has healed and the client's periarticular muscle tone has improved.

After surgery with the commonly used posterolateral approach, the client must avoid positions of extreme hip flexion (>90 degrees), adduction, or internal rotation. Appropriate postoperative positioning requires an extended hip that is maintained in external rotation and abduction, often with a foam wedge. An anterolateral approach is used less often. The client must maintain the hip in hyperflexion, adduction, and internal rotation. After this surgical approach, the client can sit up at 90 degrees of hip flexion without increasing the risk of dislocation.

OUTCOMES

A THR commonly results in immediate reduction in the client's pain. Surgical or incisional pain is often described as substantially less than the bone-on-bone pain of OA, and it is frequently more manageable with postoperative analgesia. The client's functional status improves over the course of rehabilitation, with most clients achieving about 90% functional return by 1 year after surgery.[40] With the current emphasis on wellness, an increased number of clients now desire to resume sports activities after hip surgery. High activity levels are associated with decreased longevity for replacement components. However, low-impact activities, such as walking or hiking, swimming, bicycling, intermediate snow skiing, doubles tennis, golf, and bowling, are considered fairly safe for client participation and contribute greatly to improved quality of life after surgery.

Revision surgery may be needed for about 10% of clients because of prosthetic loosening or other complications.[2] However, improvements in component design and surgical technique help ensure that most older clients should never need revision.

Nursing Management of the Surgical Client

TOTAL HIP REPLACEMENT

In the current managed care environment, clients who have undergone THR do not typically remain in the acute care hospital setting for more than 4 or 5 days after a THR. They may be discharged to a rehabilitation unit, extended care facility, or even home. Although there is no universally accepted rehabilitation program after THR, coordination of care in the perioperative period speeds the client's recovery and return to independent living.

PREOPERATIVE CARE

ASSESSMENT

Because most clients are admitted to the hospital on the day of surgery, the preadmission assessment of their physical and psychological readiness is currently accomplished in a variety of ways. Telephone interviews may be used, but many hospitals invite clients into a preoperative clinic for nursing assessment and for laboratory tests or x-rays. Some programs also arrange home visits to allow a physical therapist or nurse to assess the client's ambulation and to introduce assistive devices. Discharge needs can often be identified based on the home environment and the extent of support available to the client.

DIAGNOSIS, OUTCOMES, INTERVENTIONS

Knowledge Deficit. The client's previous inexperience with hospitalization and surgery in general, or with THR and its postoperative restrictions, may be described with the nursing diagnosis of knowledge deficit. The diagnosis can be written *Knowledge Deficit related to prior inexperience with surgery (total hip replacement).*

Outcomes. The client will demonstrate understanding of the proposed surgery, postoperative restrictions, and rehabilitation, as evidenced by statements and adherence to the postoperative regimen.

Interventions. A common strategy for providing information about the details of hospitalization for THR is the use of a group class or "total joint camp." Clients receive information about various topics, from preoperative strengthening exercises and nothing by mouth (NPO) requirements to postoperative pain management and dietary advances. Topics include autologous blood donation and other transfusion options. Clients also often have the opportunity to use a walker or crutches for the first time as they are coached by a nurse or physical therapist. Instructors emphasize appropriate positioning precautions to prevent postoperative hip dislocation. Because poor dentition is also a potential infection source, the client should be encouraged preoperatively to achieve and maintain good oral hygiene.

EVALUATION

Clients will provide a simple explanation of the surgery and verbalize their role in recovery. Mild anxiety may heighten the client's receptiveness to information, but severe anxiety can be a powerful barrier to learning. Provide frequent reinforcement of teaching, and encourage the client to ask questions about unclear information.

POSTOPERATIVE CARE

General care of clients following THR does not differ greatly from the usual care provided for any postoperative client. (For a review of general postoperative care, see Chapter 15.) After a THR, however, the client cannot assist with turning and repositioning. Prop the client up with pillows to maintain a side-lying position, and then return the client to a supine position on a 2-hour schedule. Do not turn the client to the operative side unless ordered by the physician. Because of the client's impaired mobility, pay careful attention to maintenance of skin integrity. A pressure reduction mattress overlay may be indicated, especially if the client is frail or malnourished.

Indwelling urinary catheters are not routinely used because of the risk of infection, but women are still likely to have a catheter because of the difficulty of positioning on a bedpan or transferring to a bedside commode in the immediate postoperative period. Perform perineal and catheter care carefully, recognizing the client's surgical pain and positioning precautions. Men are less likely to have an indwelling urinary catheter, but they need assistance to sit or stand at the bedside in order to void.

ASSESSMENT

Frequent assessment of neurovascular status is imperative after a THR. Assess both legs according to hospital protocol for color, warmth, capillary refill, pedal pulses, movement, and sensation. Report any deficits promptly to the surgeon. Ensure that the client's postoperative position is maintained in accordance with specified hip precautions.

The surgical dressing applied at the end of the procedure, used to create pressure and promote hemostasis, is often bulky. It is left in place until removed by the surgeon, usually 2 to 3 days after surgery. However, it should be regularly assessed for excessive drainage and may be reinforced according to the surgeon's order. After removal of the original dressing, the wound is covered with a light dressing or left open to air according to surgeon order. If the surgeon also orders that the wound be kept dry, it should be covered with a transparent occlusive dressing when the client showers. Afterward, carefully examine the wound to be certain that no water has seeped through the dressing, since excessive wetness can interfere with wound healing.

In addition, a closed wound drainage system, such as a Hemovac, may be in place. Drainage is usually less than 200 ml per 8 hours (or 600 ml per 24 hours), but this amount can be increased if the client has been heavily hydrated. Measure drain output, and promptly report excessive drainage to the surgeon.

DIAGNOSIS, OUTCOMES, INTERVENTION

Pain. Acute pain is expected after any surgery, including THR. The diagnosis can be written as *Pain related to local tissue trauma from surgical incision.*

Outcomes. The client will demonstrate pain control after surgery, as evidenced by movement without grimacing, by requesting analgesics no more frequently than ordered, and by stating that the pain is tolerable and not interfering with rest or physical therapy.

Interventions. In the immediate postoperative period, the client may experience intense pain and require injected opioid analgesics to attain acceptable control. Common interventions include patient-controlled analgesia (PCA) or epidural analgesia. Within 24 to 48 hours, the client should be tolerating fluids and be able to take oral analgesics. Because pain is intensified with movement, the client may attempt to limit activity because of the expected increase in discomfort. Medicate the client before physical therapy or activities such as showering, and reinforce the importance of ambulation in decreasing the risk for postoperative complications. Although a THR can reduce pain in the operative joint, the client with arthritis in other joints continues to experience chronic pain. Use of opioid analgesics can help in reducing general discomfort.

Regularly assess for side effects of opioid analgesics. Respiratory depression is more likely with PCA or epidural analgesia than with oral opioids. Use pulse oximetry and regular assessment of vital signs to assess the client's respiratory status. Constipation, a very common problem following THR, is related to the client's impaired mobility, opioid use, and progression to a regular diet. Encourage the client's intake of fluids and dietary fiber. In addition, stool softeners or laxatives may be indicated. If the client regularly uses a bulk-forming laxative or other strategy to maintain bowel regularity at home, assist the client in continuing that program in the hospital. Regular assessment and implementation of a proactive bowel program are important to minimize client concerns about bowel elimination.

Impaired Physical Mobility. The client's degree of immobility following a THR will be affected by pain and fear of movement as well as by arthritic limitations in other joints. The diagnosis can be written as *Impaired Physical Mobility related to pain or fear of movement.*

Outcomes. The client will demonstrate improved physical mobility, as evidenced by the need for less assistance in transfers (bed to chair, bed to standing), by safe use of a walker or crutches, and by the ability to ambulate a functional distance (150 feet).

Interventions. Moving the client after a THR can create much anxiety for both the client and the nursing staff. First, be aware of any weight-bearing limitations ordered for the client before transfer. Following a THR with a cemented prosthesis, the client is often allowed to put as much weight as desired on the operative extremity. This order is written as WBAT (weight-bearing as tolerated) or FWB (full weight-bearing). Although incisional pain may keep the client from putting full body weight on the operative extremity, he can safely put weight through the leg without harming the prosthesis. If the surgery was accomplished with a noncemented prosthesis, the physician may order NWB (non–weight-bearing), TTWB (toe-touch weight-bearing), or PWB (partial weight-bearing with a percentage specified, as 25%). If the client is not allowed to bear full weight, pay careful attention to the operative extremity during transfers to be sure the client avoids passing any weight through the leg.

In addition to postoperative limitations, the client may suffer from arthritis in other joints that increases pain and affects the ability to transfer from the bed to the chair. While in-bed exercises may begin the day of surgery, the client is not usually ready to attempt transfer to a bedside chair until the morning after surgery. When the client stands and transfers for the first time, the assistance of at least two staff members will be required. Use of appropriate technique will ensure a safe transfer for the client and will minimize the risk of injury to the staff member's lower back.

Transfer the Client. All intravenous (IV) lines, urinary catheters, wound drains, and oxygen tubing should be freed for ready movement. Although you will typically determine the side of the bed for transfer, the client usually moves away from the operative side. If the bedside chair has brakes, they should be locked before client transfer is made. The client should also be wearing shoes or slippers with non-skid soles. Staff should assist the client to the edge of the bed, maintaining the operative leg position in accordance with appropriate hip precautions. Encourage the client to push off the bed with his or her arms to reach a sitting position. However, because of weakness in the hip abductors and upper arms, the client may need help to pivot in bed and to sit up.

Once the client is seated at the edge of the bed, apply a gait belt to the client's waist to help with transfer. Use of the gait belt allows you to help with standing and transfer without risking injury to yourself. If the client becomes dizzy or starts to fall, the gait belt also helps you control the client's movement to the floor or back onto the bed. Place the walker directly in front of the client, ready for use once he is standing. However, do not use it to help the client to a standing position because it will tip.

To help the client to stand, first position your foot in front of the client's foot to keep it from slipping on the floor. Standing close to the client, grasp the gait belt and encourage the client to push off the bed with his hands. Once the client is standing, he can grasp the walker and pause for a moment to take slow, deep breaths as needed.

Remain aware of the risk for falling, and ask the client about dizziness—a manifestation of orthostatic hypotension—before attempting the final transfer to the chair. To help increase awareness of surroundings, encourage the client to stand erect when using the walker rather than stooping over and looking at the floor. With coaching about weight-bearing status, the client should need no more than a few pivoting movements with the walker to reach the chair. Remind the client not to attempt to sit until he feels the chair seat against the back of his legs. Then the client should reach back to grasp the arms of the chair and lower himself slowly to a sitting position. You can assist the client by grasping the gait belt and guiding his descent into the chair. The client's legs can be elevated for comfort on a footstool or another chair, but pay close attention to maintaining flexion restrictions. For example, keeping the client's operative leg in a relaxed position, with the knee slightly lower than the hip, allows maintenance of precautions regarding hip flexion related to a posterolateral surgical approach. The gait belt can be loosened after the client is safely settled in the chair.

When the client is ready to return to the bed, coach him to slide forward to the edge of the chair and tighten the gait belt around the client's waist. Again, remind the client to keep the knee slightly lower than the hip as a positioning precaution. With the walker in position in front of the chair, the client uses the arms of the chair to push to a standing position before grasping the walker. Using the same ambulation process, return the client to bed and help him to a supine position. Maintain leg position according to individual hip precautions.

Introduce Additional Client Exercises. If the client is alert postoperatively, in-bed exercises are often begun the afternoon of surgery. Coach the client in ankle pumps and quadriceps and gluteal isometrics ("quad sets" or "glute sets"). Transfers and ambulation with a physical therapist generally begin the morning after surgery. In addition, the therapist may perform gentle active and assisted ROM exercises. The client will continue exercises that improve ROM and strengthen hip muscles, occasionally receiving physical therapy at home or on an outpatient basis after discharge from the acute hospital setting.

Because of its stability, a walker is often used by older clients to assist with ambulation. If the client has arthritis in the shoulders or hands, a special walker with arm platforms may be indicated. Walkers also necessitate less energy expenditure for the client who has respiratory disease. Crutches may be used if the client has no balance problems.

Risk for Peripheral Neurovascular Dysfunction. Surgery on any joint carries a risk for neurologic or vascular impairment. Be aware of the potential for compartment syndrome and nerve injury related to edema or extremity positioning that places pressure on the peroneal nerve. The diagnosis can be written as *Risk for Peripheral Neurovascular Dysfunction related to lower extremity edema or positioning.*

Outcomes. The client will demonstrate normal neurovascular status, as evidenced by adequate peripheral pulses with capillary refill time of less than 3 seconds and by absence of sensory impairments and motor weakness in the operative extremity.

Interventions. Assess the neurovascular status of the operative extremity at least every 4 hours or as directed by the surgeon. More frequent monitoring may be indicated by the client's condition. Assess the presence and quality of bilateral pedal pulses, skin color and temperature of the extremity, capillary refill in the toes, sensation and movement of the toes, and the client's ability to perform dorsiplantar flexion of the foot. Report any pallor or coolness, numbness or tingling, or inability to move the extremity promptly to the surgeon.

Risk for Injury. Because the hip is unstable as the surgical incision heals, the risk for dislocation of the prosthesis is a significant concern after a THR. Client education and attention to hip positioning precautions are essential. The diagnosis can be written as *Risk for Injury related to prosthesis dislocation.*

Outcomes. The client will demonstrate understanding of the risk for hip dislocation, as evidenced by an ability to verbalize positioning precautions and the use of precautions during ambulation or transfers.

Interventions. Following a THR, assess the client's position frequently to ensure that precautions related to the specific surgical approach are maintained. Remind the client of appropriate precautions through the use of instructional handouts or fliers that can be posted at the head of the bed. Performance of prescribed exercises such as gluteal isometrics also strengthens muscles surrounding the joint capsule and decreases the risk for dislocation.

If the surgeon has used a posterolateral approach, the client should not flex the hip beyond a 90-degree angle, should not bend over to tie or slip on shoes, and should not reach for sheets that are fan-folded at the bottom of the bed. Special attention should be paid to precautions when the client is getting in and out of bed or a chair. To avoid extremes of flexion, the client will need an elevated toilet seat (at least 21 inches high). The client should not cross his legs and should not inwardly rotate the operative leg.

To help maintain precautions after the posterolateral approach, the client may use a triangular foam abduction pillow placed between the legs and secured with straps (Fig. 26–4). Use of the pillow prevents adduction and flexion of the operative hip. However, you must carefully position the straps to avoid placing pressure on the client's peroneal nerve. Less commonly, balanced suspension or traction may be used to maintain the leg in abduction. If the client's leg is weak, a trochanter roll can be placed to maintain straight alignment. When using a walker, the client should be coached to point toes outward slightly. This position avoids internal rotation, particularly when the client is turning toward the operative side. Hip precautions must also be followed as the client is turned from back to side. The abductor pillow is left in place, and the client's side-lying position is maintained through the use of pillows at his back.

If the surgeon has used an anterolateral approach, precautions are almost the opposite of those for the posterolateral approach. Because the client should avoid active abduction, the legs should be maintained side by side without a pillow or wedge between them. When the client walks, he should avoid turning the toes and knee outward. The operative leg should not be extended backward. To help maintain anterolateral precautions, place the tray table and phone on the client's operative side.

To help the client maintain appropriate hip precautions, an occupational therapist may suggest several assistive devices. Long-handled shoe horns, sock donners, and

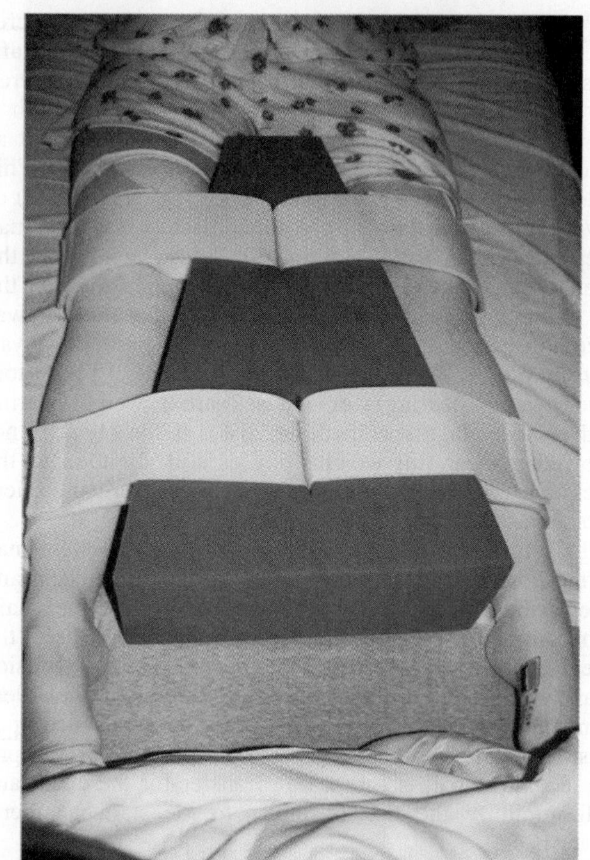

FIGURE 26–4 Abduction wedge is used to assist in maintaining the correct position of the hips after hip replacement. The main function is to prevent adduction and flexion of the hip.

reachers help the client avoid extreme hip flexion and provide more independence in dressing. The therapist or case manager can also assist the client in acquiring bathroom equipment, such as an elevated toilet seat and shower chair, for use after discharge. Reinforce the importance of using these devices to decrease the risk of hip dislocation.

Risk for Infection. Following a THR, the client is at increased risk for joint infection that may lead to the development of osteomyelitis. Although the incidence of infection is low (only 0.5% to 1%),[2] it is a great concern as a factor in possible surgical failure, leading to the removal of the prosthetic components. Joint replacements that are close to the skin surface or have poor soft tissue coverage, as in a thin patient, are more at risk for infection. *Revision* THR carries an increased infection rate compared to *primary* THR because of the longer operative time and the larger surgical exposure. The diagnosis can be written as *Risk for Infection related to surgical procedure (total hip replacement).*

Outcomes. The client will remain free from wound infection, as evidenced by normal temperature and white blood cell (WBC) count, absence of purulent drainage from the wound, and absence of redness or inflammation at the surgical site.

Interventions. Prophylactic IV antibiotics are routinely ordered immediately before surgery because of the risk of infection following a THR. The first dose is typically given 2 to 4 hours before surgery, and antibiotics are continued for 2 to 3 days postoperatively. If surgical drains are used to remove wound exudate, they should be emptied at least once a shift via aseptic technique. Because the drainage can harbor pathogens, note its color and odor and promptly report any abnormalities to the surgeon. Also routinely assess the surgical site for redness or purulent drainage. Use of staples is associated with a lower infection rate, but delays in wound healing can suggest superficial infection. Perform dressing changes using strict aseptic technique. Take the client's temperature at regular intervals, and perform careful assessments to determine the cause of any fever.

Increasing joint pain after superficial wound healing is also a possible sign of delayed, deep infection. Instruct the client to report this manifestation promptly to the physician and to inform other health care providers of the surgery.

Risk for Impaired Skin Integrity. Following a THR, the client is at high risk for pressure ulcers as a result of decreased physical mobility. Clients are often unable to change positions in bed without a great deal of assistance. Clients are also at risk for tape injury with dressing changes. This risk is due to (1) skin changes that occur in older adults, (2) intraoperative positioning and joint manipulation that lead to soft tissue edema, (3) the type of tape used to secure postoperative dressings, and (4) the method and direction of tape application. The diagnosis can be written as *Risk for Impaired Skin Integrity related to decreased physical mobility or to the application of tape with dressing changes.*

Outcomes. The client will demonstrate intact skin, as evidenced by absence of ulcers over bony prominences and absence of epidermal stripping beneath tape used to secure postoperative dressings.

Interventions. To decrease the risk of pressure ulcer development, assist the THR client with position changes on a regular schedule in the immediate postoperative period. As the client regains mobility, he will also regain independence in position changes. Carefully assess the skin over bony prominences such as the sacrum and coccyx, scapulae, elbows, and heels. In addition to using a regular turning schedule, place a pressure reducing mattress on the client's bed. Pressure on heels can be relieved using a towel roll for brief periods under the Achilles tendon. Examination gloves filled with water can also provide pressure relief under heels.

Avoid epidermal stripping by placing postoperative dressings over a skin sealant that is applied wherever the tape touches the skin. Elastic tape should be placed vertically (superior to inferior) without tension to allow for stretching related to postoperative edema. Evaluate any redness, blistering, or epidermal stripping, and consult an enterostomal nurse specialist about the client's care as appropriate.

Risk for Altered Tissue Perfusion. Venous thromboembolism, the most common complication after a THR, can be manifested as DVT. Risk factors include a surgical procedure of more than 30 minutes, advanced client age, previous history of thromboembolism, venous stasis, cardiac conditions such as heart failure or dysrhythmias, lower extremity trauma, obesity, use of oral contraceptives, sepsis, malignancy, long-term immobilization, stroke, and pregnancy. The client is most subject to development of blood clots in the thigh. The diagnosis can be written as *Risk for Altered Tissue Perfusion related to surgical procedure and immobility* (or other identified factors).

Outcomes. The client will remain free from thromboembolism, as evidenced by absence of calf or thigh pain, redness, or edema.

Interventions. Routinely assess the client for evidence of thrombophlebitis: excessive pain, unilateral edema, or a red vein track. Homans' sign is a more nonspecific indicator. The client may have thrombophlebitis but have a negative Homans' sign. Conversely, a positive Homans' sign can result from other conditions, such as shin splints. In reality, many clients have asymptomatic blood clots.

To decrease the risk of DVT, the surgeon may order various pharmacologic and nonpharmacologic interventions. Early mobilization is a key factor in decreasing DVT risk. Encourage the client to perform ankle pumps regularly because they contract the calf muscles, simulating the movements of ambulation and encouraging venous blood return. Physical agents such as pneumatic compression devices and elastic compression stockings are commonly used; they should be applied to both legs to promote adequate venous return. Compression devices or stockings should be worn until the client is fully ambulatory and should be removed only for brief periods to allow for showering or skin assessment. The pneumatic devices should be applied even when the client is sitting in a chair at the bedside because the dependent position of the lower extremities can contribute to increased venous stasis.

Pharmacologic agents used to decrease the risk of DVT include aspirin, low-dose heparin, low-molecular-weight heparin (LMWH), and warfarin sodium. These medications may be used singly or in combination, depending on surgeon preference and client risk. For example, a client may be started on both warfarin and LMWH on the evening after surgery. LMWH, which does not require laboratory monitoring, works quickly to bring about anticoagulation. Warfarin is slower to reach therapeutic blood levels but is less expensive and easier for the client to take after discharge. A prothrombin time or International Normalized Ratio (INR) is ordered to monitor the effects of warfarin, and the nurse promptly reports laboratory results to the surgeon to allow for timely ordering of the current day's dose.

Extensive education about anticoagulants is essential in order to maximize their effectiveness and to minimize the likelihood of complications. Inform the client of manifestations of internal bleeding, such as tarry stools, rust-colored or tea-colored urine, hematemesis, and abdominal or flank pain. Explain that even a minor cut will bleed for a longer period of time. Instruct the client to apply direct pressure, for example, following a shaving cut or a cut with a kitchen knife. Urge clients to seek immediate evaluation for any head injury because significant intracranial bleeding can occur in response to even minor trauma if an anticoagulant is being taken. If the client is to take warfarin, reinforce the importance of consistent intake of foods that contain vitamin K (e.g., green leafy vegetables). Many of these foods are nutritionally important and should not be totally avoided, particularly by clients with a history of heart disease who follow a low-fat diet. If the client will be discharged with a prescription for LMWH, start instruction on injection technique early enough in the hospital to allow ample time for practice and reinforcement.

If you suspect a blood clot, immediately notify the surgeon. Venography or Doppler ultrasound of the leg is commonly used in the diagnosis of DVT. If the test reveals the presence of a clot, the client will be placed on bed rest, with the leg elevated to promote venous return. A continuous heparin infusion and warfarin are often initiated at the same time, with the infusion continuing until a short time before discharge, and a warfarin prescription is written for home use. The surgeon may order calf measurements to aid in the detection of increased swelling related to DVT.

Because of the risk of pulmonary embolism, you must frequently assess the client's respiratory status. A clot in the leg can dislodge and move to the lung, typically causing dyspnea, anxiety, and a pleuritic chest pain. Because pulmonary embolism is often fatal, address suspicious manifestations promptly.

EVALUATION

Goals should be mutually established by the client and an interdisciplinary care team that includes surgeon, nurse, physical and occupational therapists, and case manager. A list of goals can be posted in the client's hospital room as a reminder of the focus for each postoperative day. Clinical pathways are commonly used to map the care of clients after a THR because of the consistent postoperative needs of this population (see Guide to Clinical Pathway: Total Hip Replacement). Pathways help providers limit the number of tasks, such as laboratory orders, that may be forgotten or overlooked. Outcomes are often also indicated on the clinical pathway to consistently track client progress. Pathways often extend from admission through acute care to client rehabilitation in another setting. They also allow for later review of discrepancies or "outliers," those clients whose experiences do not conform to the usual postoperative course.

Self-Care

The typical acute hospital stay after THR is 4 to 5 days. Because many clients require additional rehabilitation, they are sent from the hospital to rehabilitation centers or extended care facilities until they regain functional independence. Clients can be discharged home if they can transfer independently to and from the bed, walk alone a functional distance of 150 feet on a flat surface, and safely negotiate stairs.

Provide discharge instructions to the client and any family members or friends who will serve as support persons during the recovery period. The client must understand the hip precautions indicated by the surgical approach (anterolateral or posterolateral) in order to avoid dislocation. Precautions may continue for 6 months to a year after surgery, depending on the surgeon's assessment of soft tissue healing around the joint capsule.

Assistive devices, such as walker or crutches and bathroom equipment, should be available for immediate use at home. The client will progress from walker to crutches or cane as muscle strength increases, perhaps within 4 to 6 weeks after surgery if a cemented prosthesis was used. Clients with a noncemented prosthesis may have limited weight-bearing (e.g., TTWB) for 6 weeks, followed by WBAT with the use of a crutch for another 6 weeks.

Clients frequently have questions about driving or returning to work. Clients with sedentary occupations may be cleared by the surgeon to drive and to return to work within 6 to 8 weeks. However, they may be counseled to take regular breaks in order to avoid extended periods of sitting. It may be 3 months before a client can return to an occupation that requires lifting and bending, and activity will remain limited even after going back to work. Low-level physical activity, such as walking or swimming, is usually approved by the surgeon.

Depending on surgeon preference, the client may be allowed to shower after discharge. Safety measures, such as a nonslip mat and handrails in the shower area, are important. The client should not soak in a tub because water can enter the incision, increasing the risk of infection. Getting in or out of a tub may also violate hip precautions. The client can consume a regular diet but

GUIDE TO CLINICAL PATHWAY

Total Hip Replacement

The client undergoing a total hip replacement expects to be hospitalized about 4 days and then discharged home to complete rehabilitation on an outpatient basis. During the first 24 hours, pain management is important. Without adequate pain control, the goals of ambulation will not be met. Medicate the client before any movement.

The nursing goal on the first day after surgery is to have the client sitting up in the chair in the morning and again in the afternoon. Assess the degree of assistance the client needs to move from bed to chair. The rapid mobilization of the client is an interdisciplinary process. Note that on day 1, the goals of physical and occupational therapists are to have the client stand and sit at the bedside, ambulate 5 to 10 feet with the assistance of one to two people, and move in bed with the assistance of two people. Goals for ambulation continue to progress throughout the acute care stay. By the time the client is discharged, he or she should be able to ambulate 20 feet with the assistance of one person, move in bed with minimal assistance, and dress the lower extremities with adaptive equipment (the client cannot bend forward).

Thrombus remains a serious complication of orthopedic surgery and immobility. Baseline prothrombin time is assessed on admission, and anticoagulation begins on day 2. Warfarin (Coumadin) is ordered daily on the basis of International Normalized Ratio range.

The CareMap is reprinted with permission from Bergan Mercy Medical Center.

The CareMap shown is an excerpt of one that covers PO Day 1–4.

Helen Andrews, BSN, RN, *Care Manager, Alegent Health Bergan Mercy Medical Center, Omaha, Nebraska, and* **Linda R. Haddick, MSN, RN,** *Clinical Nurse Specialist, Alegent Health Home Care & Hospice, Omaha, Nebraska*

Bergan Mercy Medical Center CareMap®
Total Hip Replacement

—Addressograph—

Date or Time		
Time Frame	**PO Day 1** N D E	**PO Day 2** N D E
Assessments & Evaluations	Routine vital signs & neuro √ to affected leg **Pt reports pain 4 or < with PCA/PCEA/IM meds:** **Reported Level:** ___ ___ ___ Check BM - laxatives pm ______ Consider d/c drain Dry dressing to wound daily and as needed once initial dressing removed ______ **Pt demonstrates:** **- no excessive edema > 2+(>1")** ___ ___ ___ **- no numbness** ___ ___ ___ **- able to dorsi/plantar flex without pain** ___ ___ ___ **Wound/dressing clean and intact** ___ ___ ___	Routine vital signs & neuro √ to affected leg **Pt reports pain 4 or < with IM or oral meds with movement at rest** **Reported Level:** ___ ___ ___ Check BM Monitor hemovac exit site ___ ___ ___ Dry dsg to would daily & as needed once initial dsg removed ___ ___ ___ **Pt demonstrates:** **- no excessive edema >2+(>1")** ___ ___ ___ **- no numbness** ___ ___ ___ **- able to dorsi/plantar flex without pain** ___ ___ ___ **Wound/dressing clean and intact** ___ ___ ___
Consults	Anesthesia if epidural Pastoral Care as appropriate for spiritual needs R.D. nutritional evaluation	
Diagnostics	CBC Protime if on Coumadin	Protime if on Coumadin
Medications	DVT prophylaxis	DVT prophylaxis **Coumadin effective - INR range 1.8 - 2.5** ______
Diet/Fluid Balance	Intake and output IV & IV antibiotics Post-surgical diet - self feed B___ L___ D___ Ensure a.m. and HS snacks	IV intake and output if foley D/C IV if no foley/drains Post-surgical diet - self feed B___ L___ D___ Ensure a.m. and HS snacks ___ ___ ___
Activity/ Safety	Nsg: Encourage pt to use trapeze for repositioning **Nsg: Pt tolerates transfer activities with assist of one or two** ___ ___ ___ **Nsg: Up in chair a.m./p.m.** ___ ___ Nsg: Reinforce P.T. exercises ___ ___ ___ P.T.: BID, transfer train/exercise at bedside/ department ___ ___ **P.T.: Sit to stand with mod assist one or two** ______ **P.T.: Ambulated 5-10 ft with mod assist of two** ______ **P.T.: Bed mobility with mod assist of two** ______ Weight bearing to affected leg with walker or crutches ❑ as tolerated ❑ 50% ❑ 25% ❑ Touch ❑ NWB	Nsg: Encourage pt to use trapeze for repositioning **Nsg: Pt demonstrates transfer activities with assist of one or two** ___ ___ ___ **Nsg: Up in chair a.m./p.m.** ___ ___ Nsg: Reinforce P.T. exercises ___ ___ ___ **P.T.: BID, transfer train/exercise at bedside/department** ___ ___ **P.T.: Sit to stand with min assist of one** ______ **P.T.: Ambulated 15 ft with min assist of one** ______ **P.T.: Bed mobility with mod assist of one** ______ O.T.: Demonstrates understanding of precautions with minimal verbal cues ______ Weight bearing to affected leg with walker or crutches ❑ as tolerated ❑ 50% ❑ 25% ❑ Touch ❑ NWB
Education	CareMap® review ___ ___ ___ Hip film - O.T. remind pt to view ______ **O.T. & Nsg: Hip precautions teaching** ___ ___ ___ Verbal home assessment if not done pre-op ______ Have pt. view Coumadin film ______ O.T.: Lower extremity dressing, bathing options, adaptive equipment ______	**O.T. & Nsg: Hip precautions teaching** ___ ___ ___ O.T.: Lower extremity dressing, bathing options, adaptive equipment ______
Treatment Modalities	PCA/PCEA ___ ___ ___ Foley if hip revision Cath PRN Time:____ Time:____ Time:____ ↑ heels ___ ___ ___ Place two pillows between legs ___ ___ ___ Foot pump ___ ___ ___	D/C PCA/PCEA ______ D/C Foley catheter ______ ↑ heels ___ ___ ___ Place two pillows between legs ___ ___ ___ Foot pump ___ ___ ___
Discharge Planning	CM/MSS to see and make arrangements for home ❑ or subacute rehab ❑ ______ Team: Assess assistance at home vs. home care needs ______	Subacute evaluation completed ______ Obtain appropriate communication for discharge from MD

should also continue to be aware of any bowel elimination needs. Sexual activity can typically be resumed without discomfort as long as the client observes hip precautions.

The client should understand any medications, such as anticoagulants, that will be taken after discharge, and should note follow-up laboratory and surgeon appointments. If the surgeon has ordered home care services or outpatient therapy, provide agency telephone numbers or locations for appointments. After a THR, prophylactic antibiotics are recommended whenever a transient bacteremia is expected, such as with dental work or a minor surgical procedure. The health care provider prescribes oral antibiotic coverage before the procedure.

In addition to bathroom safety features, the client may need other home modifications to aid independent recovery. Ramps, for example, may allow easier access to entrances. If the client lives in a multilevel home, encourage him to remain on a ground level until recovery is complete.

Total Knee Replacement

After the hip and the spine, the knee is the third most common site of arthritic involvement. An extremely complex joint, the knee actually demonstrates movement in three separate planes (Fig. 26–5). Biomechanical stress during normal walking allows three times a person's body weight to be transmitted through the knee. Going up and down stairs increases the force to four or five times the body weight. The force is unevenly distributed, with the medial side of the knee often receiving the larger amount of stress. OA of the knee is better tolerated than OA of the hip, however, because the knee is not usually painful at rest.

Conservative treatment of OA of the knee is similar to that for the hip. Weight loss, activity modification, use of assistive devices, and use of analgesics or anti-inflammatory medications all help to decrease disease manifestations. Physical modalities such as ice or heat may also offer some pain relief.

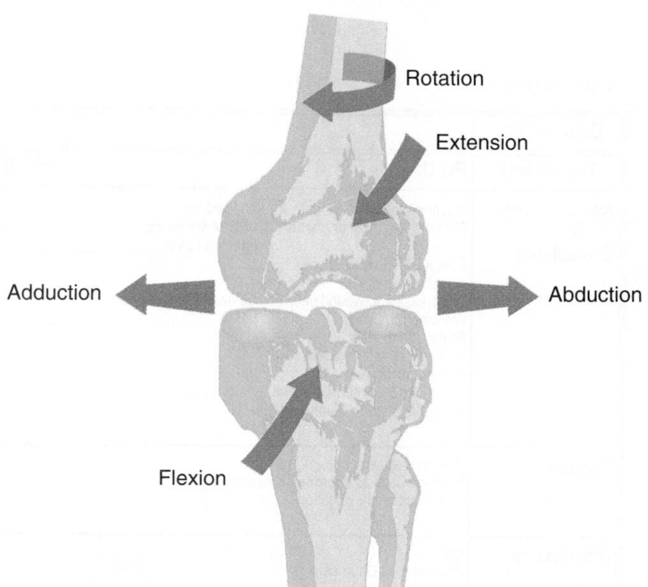

FIGURE 26–5 Movement of the knee occurs in three separate planes; the knee is not just a simple hinge joint. During normal gait, the knee moves through 70 degrees of flexion and extension, 10 degrees of abduction and adduction, and 10 to 15 degrees of internal and external rotation. (After Tooms, R. E. [1992]. Arthroplasty of the ankle and knee. In A. H. Chenshaw [Ed.], *Campbell's operative orthopaedics* [8th ed., p. 391]. St. Louis: Mosby–Year Book.)

Indications

If conservative interventions no longer control the client's symptoms, surgery may be appropriate. Options for OA management include (1) osteotomy, (2) fusion, and (3) arthroplasty. A tibial *osteotomy* may relieve the pain of knee OA by correcting the varus deformity (bow-leg) that follows wear of the medial compartment. Knee *fusion* is indicated for young, active clients who are poor candidates for joint replacement surgery; fusion results in an immobile joint fixed in extension.

Total knee replacement (TKR), or *arthroplasty,* allows resurfacing of the arthritic joint with the use of metal and polyethylene prosthetic components. The surgeon attempts to recreate the motions of flexion, extension, rotation, abduction, and adduction that may have been lost with progressive arthritis. TKR also relieves pain and corrects deformity.

Contraindications

Clients under 65 years of age who weigh more than 200 pounds or are extremely active may be better served by alternatives to TKR if possible. Improved prostheses and surgical techniques, however, are slowly extending the indications for this procedure with younger clients. Conditions such as diabetes mellitus and peripheral vascular disease increase the client's risk for infection and delayed wound healing. Other contraindications are similar to those for prospective THR candidates.

Surgical Technique

Knee prostheses most commonly include three components: the femoral component, the tibial plate, and the

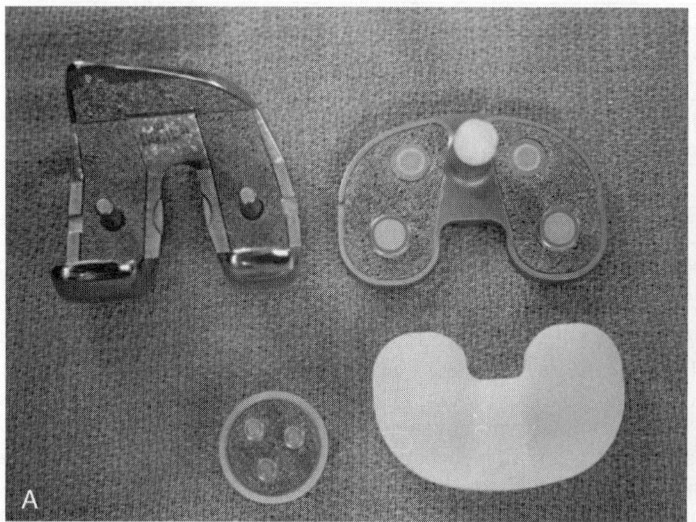

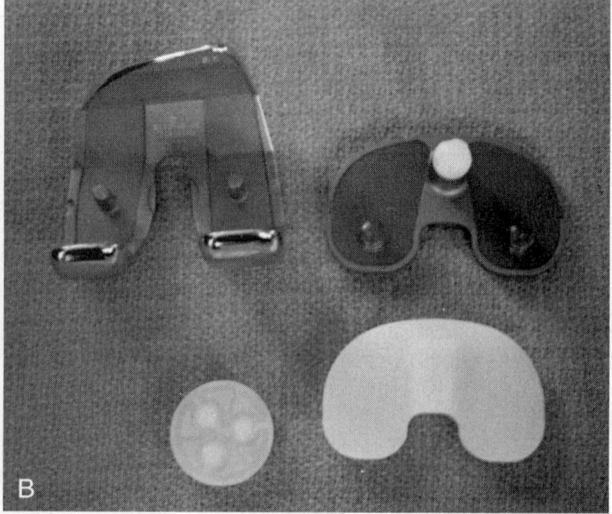

FIGURE 26–6 Total knee prostheses. This prosthesis consists of a femoral, a tibial, and a patellar component. *A,* A set of components for cementless arthroplasty of the knee. *B,* Components for a cemented total knee arthroplasty. (From Maher, A. B., Salmond S. W., & Pellino, T. A. [Eds.] [1998]. *Orthopedic nursing* [2nd ed., p. 521]. Philadelphia: W. B. Saunders.)

patellar button (Fig. 26–6). These tricompartmental prostheses vary in size to ensure the most accurate fit for each client. Some parts may also be specific for the right or left knee. A unicompartmental prosthesis, which is rarely used, replaces the femoral and tibial surfaces on only one side of the knee.

The surgical incision for TKR extends from 4 or 5 inches above the patella to 2 or 3 inches below it. Approach is either medial parapatellar or lateral parapatellar. Soft tissue is balanced across the joint, and the proximal tibia and distal femur are trimmed to fit the chosen prosthesis. Any flexion contractures or deformities (varus or valgus) may also be corrected. After osteotomy, the surgeon prepares the bone surfaces to accept the prosthesis based on use of cemented or press-fit (noncemented) components. The patella is resurfaced with a polyethylene button after the surgeon ensures that the patellar prosthesis will track normally during flexion and extension of the knee.

Wound drains may be placed prior to closure of the incision, and a bulky pressure dressing applied. If the client is to start *continuous passive motion* (CPM) immediately, a lighter dressing is used.

Complications

Infection, a potentially severe complication, occurs in about 2% of TKR clients.[2] Venous thromboembolism is also a serious possibility. Other complications may include patellar subluxation or dislocation, impaired wound healing, knee stiffness (inability to regain ROM), and loosening of the prosthesis.

Nursing Management of the Surgical Client

Preoperative assessment and care are the same as for the client undergoing THR. Postoperative care concerns are also similar, but there is more emphasis on knee exercise because dislocation is not a significant risk. The goal of knee rehabilitation—to obtain maximal ROM with good muscle control—can be accomplished with consistent physical therapy or use of a CPM machine (Fig. 26–7). This apparatus moves the knee slowly through its arc of motion, with settings determined by physician order. The machine, which is placed in a slightly abducted position on the bed, is frequently initiated at 0 degrees of extension and 10 to 40 degrees of flexion. Settings should be gradually and regularly increased, with the client and nurse working collaboratively to achieve the goal of 90 degrees of flexion.

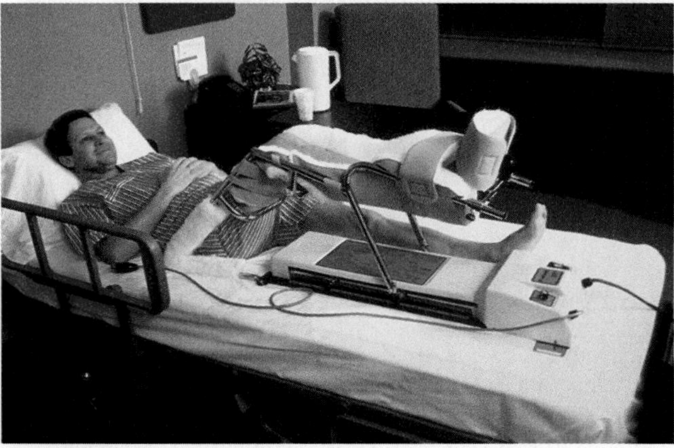

FIGURE 26–7 A continuous passive motion exerciser in use. (Courtesy of the Chattanooga Group, Inc., Hixson, TN.)

According to surgeon preference, the client may be placed in the machine immediately after surgery. Some physicians delay initiation of CPM until the evening of surgery or the morning after surgery. The CPM machine should be used a minimum of 6 to 8 hours a day. The client must be supine during use of the CPM machine, with the head of the bed elevated no more than 15 degrees, and should thus be removed from the machine for meals. The client may also find it uncomfortable to use the CPM machine during sleep; this concern should be discussed with the surgeon.

When the client is out of the CPM, a knee immobilizer may be ordered to promote knee extension. Make sure that the immobilizer is of the correct length for the client and it does not rub on the heel. No pillows should be placed under the client's knee when he is in bed because this promotes flexion contracture.

ROM and strengthening exercises are an important part of functional recovery following TKR. Ankle pumps decrease the risk for blood clots in the lower extremities. The physical therapist may lead the client in active ROM exercises or may perform gentle passive ROM and stretching to increase knee flexion or extension. Isometric exercises to strengthen the quadriceps, hamstrings, and gluteal muscles are an important part of the regimen. Straight-leg raises also help with muscle strengthening. A home exercise program after hospital discharge includes ROM exercises and isometrics, with weekly increases in resistance, as tolerated, without producing joint irritation. To obtain optimal knee function, the client should continue exercises for at least 6 weeks after surgery.

The client is usually allowed to transfer from bed to chair within 24 hours after TKR. Carefully supporting the operative extremity, nursing staff members help the client move to a sitting position on the side of the bed. Coach the client to push off from the bed to stand in front of the walker before gripping it. Weight-bearing status is determined by surgeon order based on the use of cemented or noncemented components. The client with a cemented prosthesis is often allowed to bear weight as tolerated, while NWB or TTWB is ordered for the client with a noncemented prosthesis. Once the client is in the chair, the operative leg can be elevated for comfort or gently flexed to the floor. When the client has regained enough muscle strength to move the operative leg without assistance, crutch-walking can begin if desired. Use of the assistive device continues until the client has sufficient quadriceps function to ambulate independently.

METABOLIC BONE DISORDERS

Inappropriate functioning of the metabolic processes results in disorders manifested by changes in both physical and chemical structure of the bone. Disorders that alter bony equilibrium and affect bone turnover can be due to estrogen deficiency, parathyroid gland abnormalities, vitamin deficiency, malabsorption, or physical inactivity.

OSTEOPOROSIS

Osteoporosis is defined as a systemic skeletal disease characterized by low bone mass and microarchitectural deterioration of bone tissue that leads to increased bone fragility and susceptibility to fracture. *Fragility fractures* result from low trauma, such as bending over to pick up a newspaper, which would not cause fractures in healthy bone. Fragility fractures due to osteoporosis most commonly involve the hip, vertebrae, and radius (Colles' fracture).

The term *osteopenia* refers to a low *bone mineral density* (BMD) compared with that expected for the person's sex and age. Persons with osteopenia have a greater risk for osteoporotic fracture than persons with normal or above-average density. Osteopenia is a risk factor for fracture just as hypertension is a risk factor for stroke.

In an attempt to assess the risk of osteoporotic fracture, the World Health Organization (WHO) has developed several general categories to clarify the definition of osteoporosis. These cut-offs are commonly used with table dual-energy absorptiometry (DXA) but cannot be universally applied to BMD measurements at all sites with all devices. The categories include:

1. *Normal*—a value for BMD or *bone mineral content* (BMC) that is not more than 1 standard deviation (SD) below the young adult mean value (Fig. 26–8*A*).
2. *Low bone mass (osteopenia)*—a value for BMD or BMC that lies between 1.0 and 2.5 SDs below the young adult mean value.
3. *Osteoporosis*—a value for BMD or BMC that is more than 2.5 SD below the young adult mean value (Fig. 26–8*B*).
4. *Severe (established) osteoporosis*—a value for BMD or BMC more than 2.5 SD below the young adult mean value *and* the presence of one or more fragility fractures.

Osteoporosis is a major public health problem in many parts of the world, and its scope will increase as the population ages. It affects between 13% and 18% of postmenopausal white women in the United States, and an additional 30% to 50% have osteopenia at the hip. One of every two women will experience a fracture at some point during her life. Nonwhite women and men are also at risk for osteoporotic fractures, although their risk is lower than that for white women.

Osteoporotic fractures also create a heavy economic burden; direct medical costs in 1995 were estimated at $13.8 billion. Hip fractures incur the greatest osteoporosis-related costs, and the number of these fractures may increase three-fold by the year 2040. Thus, any reduction in hip fractures would have a large impact on health care expenditures.

Etiology and Risk Factors

Many factors, both genetic and environmental, are involved in the development of osteoporosis. Bone mass, which is measured by bone densitometry and reported as BMC or BMD, is an important risk factor in osteoporosis. To understand the relationship of bone density and risk of fracture, it is helpful to review some facts about bone mass.

Peak bone mass is the highest bone mass attained. Although longitudinal growth usually is complete by about age 20 years, consolidation of bone continues so that peak bone mass is not attained until about age 30 years in both men and women. This is noteworthy because it indicates that interventions to increase peak mass can be effective up until about age 30.

What happens to bone mass in women between age 30 and menopause is uncertain. Most likely, bone mass plateaus until menopause or else decreases slightly during this period. Bone loss in the hip probably starts as early as age 20 years. Although it is debated as to when bone loss naturally begins, during perimenopause women experience a marked acceleration in bone loss due to the loss of natural estrogen. Women start to lose bone about 1.5 to 2 years before their last menstrual period and continue rapid loss until about 1.5 years after their last menses. They may lose as much as 15% of their total mass during the perimenopausal period, after which the rate of bone

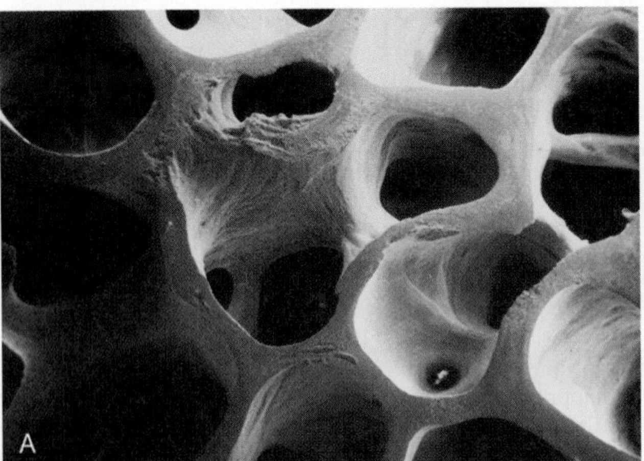

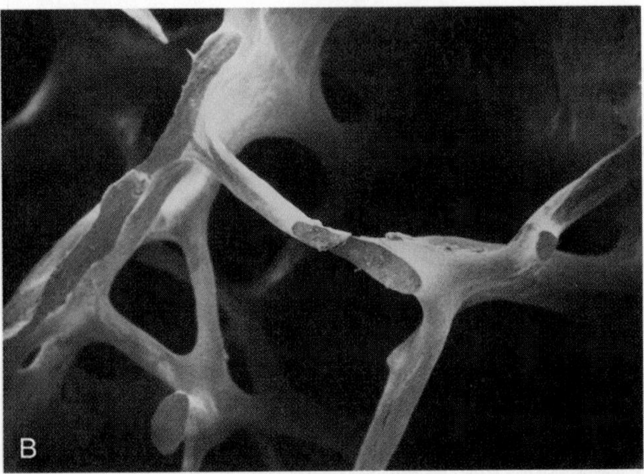

FIGURE 26–8 Electron micrographs of normal (*A*) and osteoporotic (*B*) bone. (From Dempster, D. W., et al. [1986]. A simple method for correlative light and scanning electron microscopy of human iliac crest bone biopsies: Qualitative observations in normal and osteoporotic subjects. *Journal of Bone and Mineral Research, 1,* 15–21.)

loss slows to a rate of about 1% per year. Rapid bone loss also occurs in women whose ovaries have stopped functioning, such as women being treated for prevention and treatment of ovarian and breast cancer.

Although men have larger and stronger skeletons than women, they can experience a marked loss of bone as they age, possibly resulting in fragility fractures. Bone loss in men starts later in life and progresses more slowly. Men do not experience the rapid bone loss associated with the perimenopausal decline in estrogen production seen in women. There are several reasons for loss of bone in men, including declining testosterone levels. In addition, estrogen may play a crucial role in men's bone health and changes in estrogen levels with age may be as important, if not more so, as changes in testosterone levels.

Those who have not gained their maximum peak bone mass have less bone "in the bank" to draw upon once the inevitable bone loss begins. Thus, peak bone mass as well as later bone loss is a major determinant of osteoporotic fracture. For this reason, osteoporosis has been described as a pediatric disorder. Strong adult skeletons are built during childhood.

From 60% to 80% of the risk for this disorder is inherited. A history of fracture in a first-degree relative is a risk for fragility fracture. Factors other than heredity known to influence development of osteoporosis include:

- Low body weight (< 127 pounds)
- Prolonged premenopausal amenorrhea or early menopause
- Inadequate physical activity
- Low intake of dietary calcium
- Suboptimal levels of serum vitamin D
- Cigarette smoking
- Excessive consumption of alcohol

Osteoporosis can also result from underlying medical conditions, such as thyrotoxicosis, hyperparathyroidism, anorexia nervosa, and Cushing's syndrome and from long-term use of medications such as thyroid hormone, anticonvulsants, furosemide, and corticosteroids. A person who has had one osteoporotic fracture is five times more likely to suffer another fracture than a person without a fracture. Thus, history of a low-trauma fracture is an important risk factor.

Pathophysiology

Bone is a dynamic tissue that undergoes continuous *remodeling,* the process by which old bone is replaced by new (Fig. 26–9). Bone remodeling serves two principal functions:

1. Replaces old bone with new so that the biomechanical properties of the skeleton are not compromised by continuous use
2. Plays a role in mineral homeostasis by transferring calcium and other ions into and out of the skeletal reservoir.

The remodeling sequence starts with activation of *osteoclasts,* which resorb a small portion of bone over a relatively short period of time (as short as 7 to 10 days). Bone formation then takes place as *osteoblasts* form an organic matrix that is subsequently mineralized.

Peak bone mass and the subsequent rate and duration of bone loss are important determinants of whether skeletal integrity will be compromised to the degree that a fragility fracture will result. In addition, as bone tissue is lost, other alterations in the skeleton (e.g., changes in architecture, aging of the bone tissue, accumulation of microdamage) contribute to fracture risk. The supporting structures become so weak that even minimal stress can cause fractures. Spinal fractures occurring with osteoporosis are usually compression fractures that occur when one or more vertebrae collapse from carrying the weight of the upright body (see Fig. 26–8*A* and *B*).

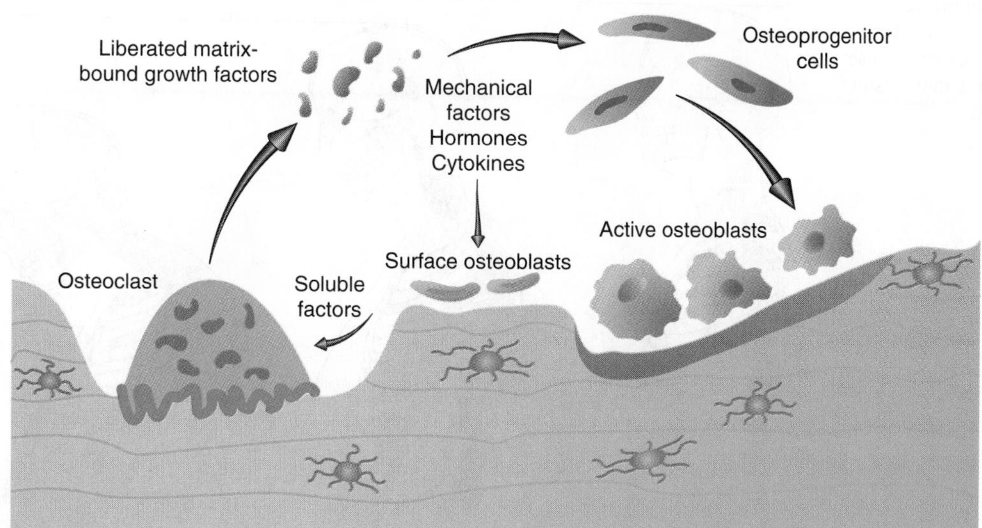

FIGURE 26–9 Bone remodeling is a process of bone resorption and bone formation. These two processes are controlled by systemic factors (the need for calcium) and local cytokines, some of which are found in the bone matrix. Cytokines are of key importance in communication between the osteoblasts and the osteoclasts. (Modified from Cotran, R. S., Kumar, V., & Robbins, S. L. [1994]. *Robbins pathologic basis of disease* [5th ed., p. 1217]. Philadelphia: W. B. Saunders.)

Clinical Manifestations

In many people, the diagnosis of osteoporosis is made after a fracture, often a vertebral compression fracture. Clinical manifestations of vertebral compression fracture include sudden onset of severe back pain that worsens on movement and is relieved by rest. This acute pain usually subsides within 2 to 6 weeks. Most compression fractures, however, are discovered accidentally on routine x-ray. Progressive vertebral deformities lead to shortened stature and progressive dorsal kyphosis (Fig. 26–10). The lower ribs eventually rest on the iliac crests, and downward pressure on viscera causes abdominal distention and bloating. Respiration may also be impaired by restricted lung expansion.

Bone loss can also occur in the mandible, which may lead to loss of teeth or poorly fitting dentures as well as changes in the appearance of the face. Unfortunately, fractures of the wrist in postmenopausal women are often not recognized as osteoporotic fractures.

The many changes in appearance and the difficulty in finding clothing that fits can have a profound negative effect on self-esteem. Quality of life may be affected by chronic pain and functional disability. Fear of subsequent fracture may cause people to reduce their activity.

The "gold standard" for measuring BMD is full-table DXA (Fig. 26–11). This technique carries low risk and takes only a few minutes. The most commonly measured sites with DXA are the spine and the hip. BMD is commonly reported as a "T-score," which is the difference between the patient's BMD and the BMD of "young normal adults" of the same gender. The difference between the patient's score and the young adult norm is expressed as SD below or above the average. (This is the basis for the WHO definition of osteoporosis discussed earlier.) Thus, a person with a T-score of −2.0 would have a BMD that is 2 SDs below the average for a young adult of the same gender. Under the WHO criteria, this person would be considered *osteopenic.*

In recent years, the number of peripheral densitometers has increased dramatically. These devices measure BMD at peripheral sites such as the heel or finger. They include *quantitative ultrasound* (QUS) devices and peripheral DXAs. These devices are smaller and less expensive than full-table DXAs, and the QUS devices involve no radiation exposure. However, criteria for interpreting results with peripheral devices are not well developed.

The National Osteoporosis Foundation (NOF) Guidelines for Treatment and Prevention of Osteoporosis recommend that the decision to test BMD should be based on a person's risk and that testing is not indicated unless the results of the testing would influence choices about treatment. According to NOF Guidelines, BMD testing should be performed for the following:

- All postmenopausal women under age 65 years who have one or more additional risk factors for osteoporosis (besides menopause)
- All women age 65 years and older regardless of additional risk factors
- Postmenopausal women who present with fractures (to confirm diagnosis and determine disease severity)
- Women who are considering therapy for osteoporosis if BMD testing would facilitate the decision
- Women who have been taking *hormone replacement therapy* (HRT) for prolonged periods of time

Laboratory tests may be performed to rule out secondary osteoporosis or other metabolic bone diseases. These

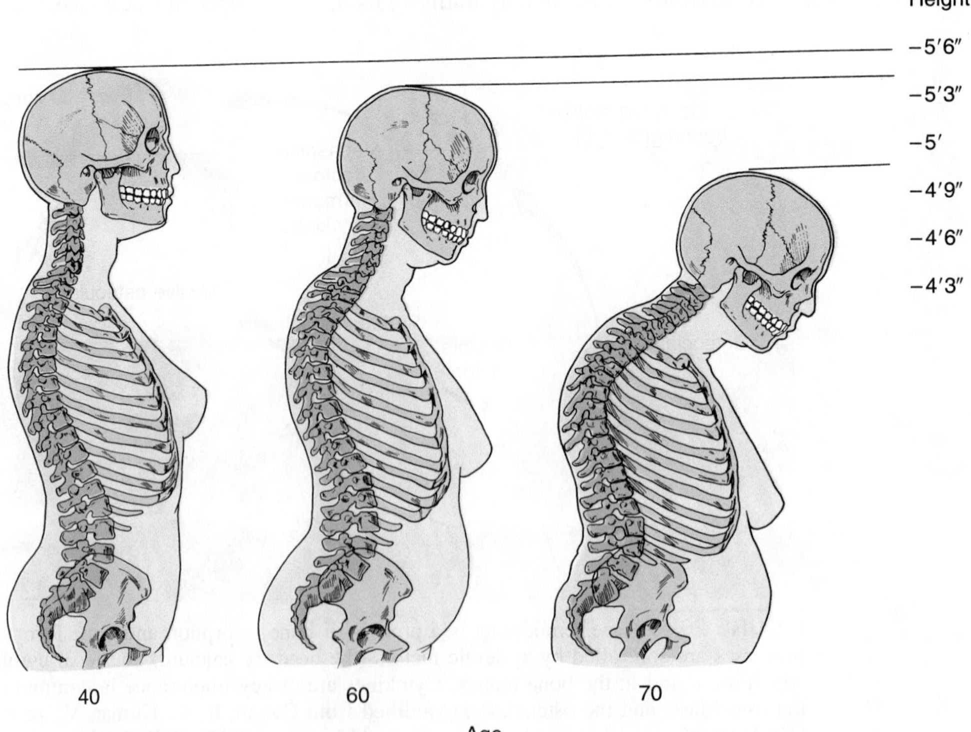

FIGURE 26–10 Osteoporotic changes: A normal spine at age 40 years and osteoporotic changes at ages 60 and 70 years. These changes can cause a loss of height and may result in dorsal kyphosis.

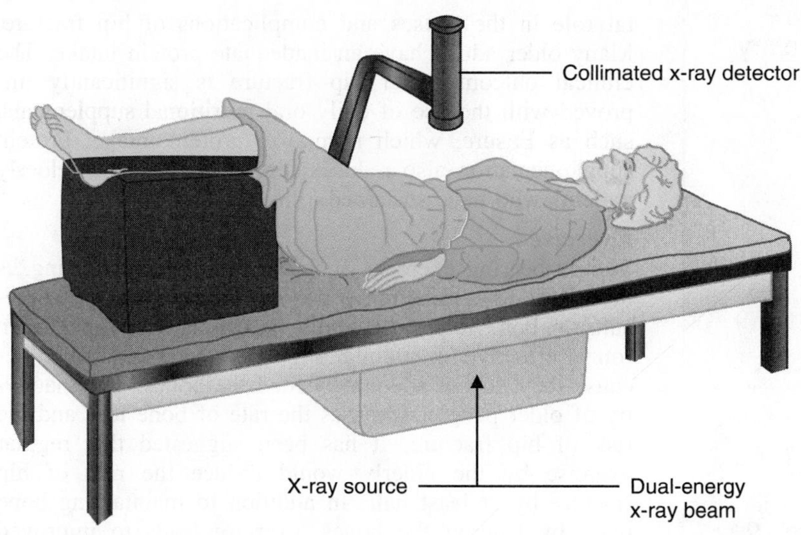

FIGURE 26–11 Dual-photon absorptiometry. (Adapted from an original illustration in *Clinical Symposia,* illustrated by Frank Netter, M.D., copyright by Ciba-Geigy Corporation.)

tests include blood count, urine calcium, multichannel screen, serum alkaline phosphatase, serum 25-hydroxyvitamin D, parathyroid hormone, ionized calcium, protein electrophoresis in urine and serum, and thyroid function. Biochemical markers of bone remodeling, such as urinary collagen cross-links, are sometimes used in conjunction with DXA or QUS to monitor effectiveness of therapy. However, biochemical markers alone are not appropriate for diagnosis of osteoporosis or for predicting the risk of fracture in the future.

Outcome Management

Medical Management

The goal of medical management is to prevent bone loss and fragility fractures. Lifestyle changes focused on dietary intake of adequate calcium and vitamin D and weight-bearing exercise are prescribed to prevent bone loss. *Estrogen replacement therapy* (ERT) is considered for women who are postmenopausal (see later discussion). Cigarette and alcohol cessation is advised.

Preventing Loss of Bone Mass

Osteoporosis is preventable. Strategies for prevention are most effective when they are started in childhood in order to maximize peak bone mass and to establish lifelong bone-healthy behaviors. Several interventions that maximize and preserve bone mass have general health benefits, including:

- Adequate intake of calcium and vitamin D
- Regular weight-bearing exercise
- Avoidance of tobacco and alcohol abuse

Calcium and Vitamin D Intake

A well-balanced diet containing the recommended level of calcium is an important component of bone health (Table 26–3). The major sources of dietary calcium are dairy products. Calcium can also be obtained from the wide range of calcium-fortified foods that are available (Box 26–1). National surveys of dietary intake indicate that many Americans are not consuming enough calcium. Most women consume less than half of the recommended daily levels. As early as age 10, the calcium intake of girls is considerably below that needed for optimal bone health.

People who have difficulty digesting milk due to a lack of the enzyme lactase, which breaks down the milk sugar lactose, may be able to tolerate acidophilus milk, yogurt, and hard cheeses; in addition, milk products may be tolerated if taken in small amounts. Skim milk and low-fat yogurt can be recommended for persons who are trying to maintain low-cholesterol diets. Diets high in dairy foods do not cause obesity; in fact, people who consume high amounts of dairy foods appear to have higher lean body mass.

TABLE 26–3 RECOMMENDED CALCIUM INTAKE LEVELS

Group	Calcium Intake (mg/day)
INFANTS	
Birth–6 mo	400
6 mo–1 yr	600
CHILDREN	
1–5 yr	800
6–10 yr	800–1200
11–24 yr	1200–1500
ADULTS	
Women 25–50 yr	1000
Postmenopausal women < 65 yr	
Taking estrogen	1000
Not taking estrogen	1500
Women > 65 yr	1500
Men < 65 yr	1000
Men > 65 yr	1500
PREGNANT WOMEN	
400 mg+ recommendation for age group	1400–1900

Data from National Institutes of Health Consensus Development Panel on Optimal Calcium Intake. (1994). Optimal calcium intake. *Journal of the American Medical Association, 272,* 1942–1948.

BOX 26–1 Calcium Equivalents of Dietary Sources (300 mg)

1 cup of milk
1 carton of low fat yogurt with fruit
1 ¼ cup frozen yogurt
1 cup vanilla pudding
1 cup baked egg custard
1 oz Swiss cheese
1 slice cheese pizza
½ cup ricotta cheese, part skim
1 ½ oz cheddar cheese
2 ¼ cup cottage cheese
11 dried figs
4 cups broccoli
7 oz baked wall-eyed pike fillet
¾ cup whole dried almonds

Prepared by Patricia T. Packard, R.D., C.N., Creighton University Osteoporosis Research Center, Omaha, NE.

Dietary calcium from a well-balanced nutritional plan is the preferred approach, but calcium supplements should be used when an adequate dietary intake cannot be achieved. All calcium supplements should be taken with food to enhance absorbability. Chewable supplements are preferred over those that are swallowed. Although a high dietary calcium intake is thought to increase the risk of renal calculi (stones), research findings suggest that high-calcium diets do not commonly result in renal calculi and may, in fact, protect against stone formation.

Vitamin D plays a major role in both calcium absorption and bone metabolism. Vitamin D is made in the skin in the presence of sunlight, or it may be obtained from food sources, primarily vitamin D–fortified milk. Although exposure to sunlight is necessary for cutaneous synthesis of vitamin D, prolonged exposure to sunlight does not necessarily increase the amount synthesized. An average of 15 minutes a day of sunlight exposure to hands, face, arms, and legs probably meets the requirements for most people. Although the use of sunscreen remains important to reduce photoaging and the risk of skin cancer, overuse of sunscreen is not advised. When sunscreen is applied so heavily that the skin receives no sunlight, vitamin D is not synthesized in the skin. Vitamin D supplementation (400 to 800 IU/day) is recommended for the institutionalized elderly, for persons living in high northern or southern latitudes, and for people who have limited sun exposure.

High dietary intake of sodium increases loss of calcium in the urine, and people who take in large amounts of sodium should increase their calcium intake accordingly. Although caffeine modestly increases calcium excretion in the urine, the loss is negligible compared with the effects of protein and sodium. The effect of caffeine can be offset by adding 40 mg of calcium to the diet for each cup of coffee. Phosphorus intake, as that in carbonated beverages, does not significantly affect calcium balance; however, people who drink a large number of carbonated beverages may not be consuming adequate calcium in the form of milk.

Low protein intake appears to play a distinct detrimental role in the causes and complications of hip fracture. Many older adults have an inadequate protein intake. The clinical outcome after hip fracture is significantly improved with the use of daily oral nutritional supplements, such as Ensure, which normalize protein intake. Protein supplementation also reduces further bone loss in elderly patients who have sustained a hip fracture.

Exercise

Weight-bearing exercise, such as walking and running, is necessary for maintaining bone mass because disuse results in bone loss. Swimming and biking have not been found effective in maintaining bone mass, probably because they do not adequately load the bones. The inactivity of older people increases the rate of bone loss and the risk of hip fracture. It has been suggested that regular exercise by the elderly would reduce the risk of hip fracture by at least half. In addition to maintaining bone mass by loading the bones, exercise leads to improved physical fitness, which is associated with improved muscle strength, stability, reaction time, balance, and coordination.

All of these factors help to decrease the risk of falling and subsequent fractures. Exercise regimens and weight training have been found to increase muscle strength even in persons older than 90 years of age. In light of the positive effects of exercise on bone and on health in general, nurses should recommend regular exercise for all clients. Previously sedentary clients who wish to start a more rigorous exercise program should undergo a physical evaluation before starting.

The American College of Sports Medicine recommends that at least 30 minutes of any physical activity be incorporated into daily schedules. Even activities such as walking, hiking, gardening, biking, and housework or yardwork increase daily energy expenditure and help promote muscular strength, flexibility, coordination, and endurance, which may ultimately decrease the number and severity of falls.

Alcohol and Tobacco

Alcohol abuse and smoking cigarettes increase the risk of osteoporosis. Current smokers have 2.1 times the risk of hip fractures as nonsmokers. If a woman quits smoking, she reduces her risk of hip fracture by 40%. Excessive alcohol intake reduces bone density and increases the risk of falls. Moderate alcohol intake has no known negative effect on BMD.

ESTROGEN REPLACEMENT AND PREVENTION OF BONE RESORPTION

Medications approved by the Food and Drug Administration (FDA) to prevent and treat osteoporosis include ERT, alendronate, raloxifene, risedronate, and calcitonin (Table 26–4). Clients receiving drug therapy for osteoporosis should be taught about the importance of calcium, vitamin D, physical activity, and avoidance of smoking and alcohol abuse as part of any treatment regimen. Treatment should not be limited to persons who have had a fragility fracture. Clients at high risk for osteoporotic fracture should be treated prophylactically. Clients receiving corticosteroid therapy are at very high risk of fracture and should always be treated prophylactically.

ERT has been effective in preventing and treating osteoporosis. In addition, it offers other health benefits, such

TABLE 26–4 MEDICATIONS FOR PREVENTION OF OSTEOPOROSIS

Category (Example)	Indications and Contraindications	Adverse Effects	Nursing Considerations
ESTROGEN (prevents bone loss, reduces risk of fracture, provides cardioprotective effects)			
Conjugated estrogens (Premarin)	*Indications* Early menopause Osteoporosis *Contraindications* Active thrombophlebitis Known or suspected estrogen-dependent cancers Known or suspected pregnancy Undiagnosed genital bleeding	Gallbladder disease Hypertension Hypercalcemia Vaginal candidiases Melasma (dark areas on the face) Hirsutism Headache, migraine	Teach the client to monitor for breast tenderness, mood changes, fluid retention and vaginal bleeding. Teach the client to report unilateral leg pain or swelling or any shortness of breath (signs of DVT). Teach the client to have regular mammograms and PAP smears. Monitor serum calcium level.
Selective estrogen receptor modulators (raloxifene [Evista])	*Indications* Prevention of osteoporosis in early menopause *Contraindications* Active thrombophlebitis Known or suspected pregnancy	Leg cramps Hot flashes Weight gain Peripheral edema Sinusitis Sweating	Avoid administration with ampicillin, indomethacin, naproxen, diazepam and clofibrate if possible. Do not administer with cholestyramine.
BISPHOSPHONATES (inhibit osteoclasts, reduce bone resorption)			
Alendronate (Fosamax)	*Indications* Osteoporosis Paget's disease *Contraindications* Delayed esophageal emptying Hypocalcemia	Gastric irritation, heartburn, dysphagia, flatulence, diarrhea, headache	Poorly absorbed: Administer on an empty stomach and do not eat or drink for 30 min. Take medication with water (not juice) and remain upright after swallowing. Do not chew or suck on the tablet. Monitor serum calcium levels. Monitor for gastric irritation for clients taking aspirin or NSAIDs.
Calcitonin (Miacalcin)	*Indications* Osteoporotic fractures Paget's disease Hypercalcemia *Contraindications* None known	Nausea, flushing, nasal irritation, serious allergic reactions	Administered by nasal spray Has analgesic effects also

as prevention of cardiovascular disease. ERT is most effective in maintaining bone health if it is started during the perimenopausal period, before rapid bone loss begins; however, it is also beneficial when started after menopause, even in women with established osteoporosis. The skeletal effects of estrogen are obtained with both oral and transdermal preparations. Rapid bone loss occurs if and when ERT is discontinued. Estrogen in lower doses (0.3 mg/day) is effective in maintaining bone mass and has fewer side effects than conventional doses.

Estrogen is usually given in combination with progesterone in women with an intact uterus to prevent uterine cancer. Administration of estrogen and progesterone continuously eliminates monthly bleeding in many women. Side effects of combined HRT include breast tenderness, mood changes, fluid retention, and vaginal bleeding. ERT also increases the risk of deep vein thrombosis and gallbladder disease. There is a perception that ERT causes weight gain; however, although postmenopausal weight gain may be common, women receiving ERT gain less weight than those not receiving ERT.

The major concern with prolonged ERT is the increased risk of breast cancer. After using ERT for 5 years or more, a woman's breast cancer risk has been found to increase by about 35%. However, more women in the United States die of heart disease than of all types of cancer combined. Thus, the benefits of ERT for heart and bone health may outweigh the risk of breast cancer. The decision to use ERT should be made by a woman in consultation with her primary care provider.

Marketed as Evista, raloxifene is a member of a class of drugs called *selective estrogen receptor modulators* (SERMs). SERMs provide the benefits of estrogen but avoid the risks. They prevent bone loss, reduce the incidence of osteoporotic fracture, and provide cardioprotective effects. They do not increase the risk of breast or uterine cancer. Evista increases the risk of DVT in a manner similar to that of ERT. Evista also increases hot flashes and is thus not effective in relieving menopausal symptoms.

Drugs that inhibit bone resorption are also prescribed. Alendronate and risedronate are bisphosphonates and are available as Fosamax and Actonil, respectively. Calcitonin, a hormone that slows bone resorption, is available as Miacalcin and is delivered as a single daily dose of nasal spray. Calcitonin is less effective than Evista or Fosamax in maintenance of bone mass. Interestingly, calcitonin has analgesic effects, which may help to relieve pain associated with fractures.

Promotion of Healing after Fracture

The goals of treatment after fracture are to manage pain, regain mobility and strength, promote healing, reduce bone loss, and prevent further fracture. Furthermore, treatment is directed toward limiting the disability associated with existing fractures.

Managing Pain. One of the most important interventions in the care of the client with an osteoporotic fracture is pain management. Often clients present with back pain resulting from vertebral crush fracture syndrome. Strict bed rest lasting between 5 and 7 days has been found to be most effective in relieving pain and shortening the course of pain. The client should lie supine or in a side-lying position. After 5 to 7 days of bed rest, the client is instructed to gradually increase activity.

Non-narcotic analgesics may be needed for 1 to 2 weeks to aid in relief of pain. If NSAIDs are used, protect the client from gastric ulceration by administering medications with food or antacids.

Flexible corsets with adjustable self-fastening tape (Velcro) may help to relieve back pain and fatigue. However, these corsets cannot correct the underlying problem of bone loss and spinal deformity. Corsets may be worn in bed but are most helpful if worn when the person is in the upright position.

Physical therapy is of utmost importance in the long-term treatment of back pain. Often chronic back pain is associated with decreased ROM, weakness, muscle spasm, postural change, muscle tenderness, and decreased endurance. Physical therapy should be started during the period of bed rest with ROM exercises and mild resistive exercises of the extremities in bed. Heat or ice, ultrasound, and TENS may be used for pain relief.

Regaining Mobility and Strength. After acute pain subsides, clients should carry out exercises specifically prescribed for them, such as stretching and strengthening. Water aerobics may be initiated early in the treatment before the client can tolerate weight-bearing exercise. A long-term physical activity program should include weight-bearing and aerobic exercise in addition to strengthening and flexibility exercise. Since osteoporotic clients are at risk for subsequent fractures, they should be taught how to move safely while maintaining or increasing physical activity. See the Management and Delegation feature for techniques on assisting with mobility.

Promoting Healing. Good general nutrition should be encouraged after fractures to promote healing. Optimal calcium and vitamin D intake continue to be important, and special attention should be given to adequate protein in the diet, especially in the elderly.

Preventing Further Fractures. Medications and treatments used to prevent osteoporosis are continued after a fracture to maintain and improve bone mass in existing bone.

Nursing Management of the Medical Client

Nursing management for the client with osteoporosis is detailed in the Care Plan.

Self-Care

Assess clients at high risk for fracture for activity level and dietary adequacy, and perform appropriate teaching to prevent fractures. In addition, assess the risk of falling in these clients. Assessment includes visual acuity, medications that may cause dizziness or postural hypotension, and difficulties with balance or coordination as well as the home environment for potential safety hazards. Evaluation of the home setting is performed via the admission assessment, discussions with the client, consultation with a specialist in social services, and home safety evaluation by a visiting nurse.

Discussion about fall prevention strategies is imperative. Instruct clients who are prone to dizziness to get up slowly from a lying position, sitting on the side of the bed first. Their eyeglass prescription may need to be updated to improve vision. An aid to ambulation, such as a cane or walker, may also be indicated to prevent falling. Alterations to the home may be recommended. Handrails in the bathroom, removal of scatter rugs, and increased lighting are some of the modifications that may be necessary.

Specific resources in the community that may be helpful to clients with osteoporosis include support groups and exercise programs. The National Osteoporosis Foundation (*www.nof.org*) is an excellent source of educational resources.

Paget's Disease

Paget's disease (osteitis deformans) is defined as an idiopathic bone disorder characterized by abnormal and accelerated bone resorption and formation in one or more bones. The normal bone is replaced by abnormal, structurally weaker bone that is prone to fractures. Paget's disease most frequently produces painful deformities of the femur, tibia, lower spine, pelvis, and cranium.

While the cause of Paget's disease is unknown, it is thought to be of viral origin. Laboratory data suggest involvement of the measles virus, respiratory syncytial virus (RSV), or canine distemper viruses, but these findings have not been confirmed. Although no definite hereditary pattern has been established, a familial clustering has been reported. However, only 4% to 5% of patients

MANAGEMENT AND DELEGATION

Assisting with Mobility and Use of Splints

Muscle overuse, traumatic injuries, and muscle disuse associated with prolonged bed rest can each contribute to complications of immobility. An important aspect of care is the prevention of these unnecessary complications. Interventions to minimize the complications of immobility include passive and active range-of-motion (ROM) exercises as well as the use of splints to maintain normal joint alignment and position. The performance of ROM exercises and the application and removal of splints may be delegated to unlicensed assistive personnel.

Although you may delegate these tasks, as the nurse, you remain responsible for assessment of the client's baseline level of function and development of a plan to prevent the complications associated with immobility. Interdisciplinary collaboration with physical and occupational therapists is often necessary to develop a comprehensive plan of care. Additionally, you will be monitoring the client's progress and response to these interventions and adjusting the plan of care in collaboration with the other involved disciplines.

When delegating these tasks to assistive personnel, emphasize the following:

- Specify any physical limitations that clients may have that would prohibit their ability to move an extremity through its normal range of motion.
- Identify the time at which this activity is best performed with a client. Establish a schedule of which the client and assistive personnel are aware. Often ROM activities are incorporated into the morning bath routine, which limits this activity to one time per day. Most clients, confined to bed, would be better served if passive or active ROM activities were performed two to three times per day, from the onset of illness. Plan these activity periods to allow for adequate rest intervals.
- Encourage or assist the client to be as independent as possible in performing activities of daily living. Haircombing, teeth-brushing, bathing, and eating are all good opportunities for clients to use their extremities through the normal ROM. Care providers are often tempted to do these things for a client to get the job done, but this does not enhance the client's independence, strength, or endurance.
- Remind assistive personnel to observe and report any signs of redness or deformity overlying a joint or extremity.
- Instruct assistive personnel that a new complaint of pain on movement is cause to cease the activity and report to you for further assessment. Delegated personnel should put no joint through its full range of motion if the client complains of pain.
- During removal and application of splints, observe the skin and involved bony prominence. Any signs of redness and irritation are cause for your examination. Revision of the splint, by the appropriate practitioner, may be necessary. Splints are often fitted by occupational therapists, although this may vary.
- Allow clients to stand to transfer from a bed to a chair rather than be slid from a bed to a stretcher chair. This action preserves and promotes the function of the quadriceps and lower leg muscles; these muscles are essential to the client's ability to resume walking activities. Standing, in contrast to sliding, the client also reduces the incidence of skin shearing that can occur via the slide method. Reserve sliding from bed to chair for clients who lack the mental capacity to follow instructions for standing or clients who are deemed too weak or unsafe to stand.
- Make sure that ambulation progresses from short to long distances. Assess the client's gait and balance. Instruct assistive personnel to monitor the client's balance and the ability to walk safely.

Verify the competency of assistive personnel in performing ROM exercises, transfer techniques, and splint application and use during orientation and annually thereafter.

Donna W. Markey, MSN, RN, ACNP-CS, *Clinician IV, Surgical Services, University of Virginia Health System, Charlottesville, Virginia*

with Paget's disease have a strong family history. Most cases are probably due to environmental causes.

Paget's disease increases in frequency with age in Western countries and is more prevalent in men than in women. It is seen infrequently in Africa and Asia. Epidemiologic studies suggest that Paget's disease is decreasing in both severity at the time of diagnosis and in prevalence.

In many instances, Paget's disease is diagnosed because the client has experienced trauma and x-rays demonstrate the characteristic changes of the disease. Ten per cent to 20% of persons with the disease are asymptomatic. Before clinical manifestations occur, x-ray films show increased bone expansion and density. After clinical manifestations have developed, the bone shows a characteristic mosaic appearance (Fig. 26–12). Bone scans are the most reliable means of identifying pagetic bone. Laboratory tests include urinary hydroxyproline and serum alkaline phosphatase (AP) that may be increased in active Paget's disease.

In symptomatic Paget's disease, the most common presenting complaints include one or more of the following: deep, aching bone pain; skeletal deformity, such as a barrel-shaped chest, bowing of the tibia or femur, or kyphosis; changes in skin temperature; pathologic fractures through diseased bone; and symptoms related to nerve compression. Diseased bone pressing on the cranial nerves may result in vertigo, hearing loss with tinnitus, and blindness. Rheumatoid arthritis, ankylosing spondylitis, and gout are commonly associated with Paget's disease.

NSAIDs, such as ibuprofen, and newer COX-2 inhibitors can often control bone pain. Pain may also be relieved with heat therapy, massage, and bracing. Further

THE CLIENT WITH OSTEOPOROSIS

Nursing Diagnosis. Altered Nutrition: Less Than Body Requirements, related to calcium imbalance

Outcomes. The client will meet U.S. Recommended Daily Allowances (RDA) requirements for calcium and vitamin D, will describe foods high in calcium and types of calcium supplements, will use less caffeine and alcohol, and will discuss ways to avoid the effects of lactose intolerance (as needed).

Interventions	Rationales
1. Teach the importance of diet to reduce the risk of further bone loss.	1. Dietary calcium is needed to maintain serum calcium levels, to maintain bone mass.
2. Refer to the dietitian for consultation.	2. Dietitians can offer assistance with food choices.
3. Encourage the client to eat foods high in calcium, such as plain yogurt, dairy products, seafood, sardines, green vegetables, calcium-fortified orange juice, and cereals.	3. These foods are excellent sources of calcium.
4. Provide current information about calcium supplements.	4. A calcium intake of 1000 to 1500 mg each day is easier to achieve with supplements.
5. Teach the need to reduce alcohol intake.	5. Excessive alcohol use increases bone resorption.
6. Teach ways to reduce risk of lactose intolerance, such as the use of acidophilus milk and commercially prepared lactase.	6. Lactose intolerance is caused by the inability to break down milk sugar lactose.

Evaluation. Changing nutritional habits takes time. Expect that this will be an ongoing problem for many weeks. Encourage small improvements.

Nursing Diagnosis. Impaired Physical Activity related to osteoporosis

Outcomes. The client will comply with the physical mobility plan to level of independent activities of daily living (ADLs), use assistive devices to perform independent ADL, and will identify and avoid potential hazards, thereby avoiding falls and fractures resulting from minimal injury.

Interventions	Rationales
1. Consult with physical therapist to develop an exercise program of weight-bearing exercises and strengthening exercises such as walking, tennis, hiking, and ballroom dancing. Discuss the benefits of walking at least ½ mile every day. Teach the importance of exercise in prevention of osteoporosis.	1. Weight-bearing exercises decrease bone loss. Strengthening exercises increase muscle tone and circulation. The National Institutes of Health (NIH) Consensus on Osteoporosis (1984) recommends walking, tennis, hiking, and ballroom dancing.
2. Assist with ADL allowing the client to remain independent.	2. Pain may limit the client's ability to perform ADL.
3. Evaluate the need for assistive devices for ADL and home use.	3. Devices may be needed for independent ADL.
4. Establish a hazard-free hospital environment: a. Provide adequate lighting b. Adjust bed to lowest position with side rails up when client is in bed c. Place necessary articles within client's reach d. Keep client area free of spills and clutter	4. A hazard-free environment reduces the risk of falls.

Evaluation. Increasing safe and weight-bearing activities will take several weeks. The client will be pain-free and develop muscle strength and flexibility before independence can be gained.

Nursing Diagnosis. Pain related to fracture (vertebral, Colles' wrist, hip)

Outcomes. The client will experience pain reduction or relief to perform independent ADL.

Interventions	Rationales
1. Assess the client's needs for pain medication. Plan a medication schedule with the client.	1. The client may not be receiving adequate medication because of inadequate dosing, need for around-the-clock administration, or iatrogenic causes of pain.
2. Administer non-narcotic analgesics.	2. Non-narcotic analgesics block production of chemical mediators of pain.
3. Monitor the effectiveness of analgesia.	3. Monitoring allows for revisions in the Care Plan.
4. Teach alternative modalities of pain relief, such as positioning, warm compresses, application of assistive devices, distraction, imagery, biofeedback, and hypnosis.	4. Alternative modalities can be effective in reducing pain.

Evaluation. Pain relief should be accomplished within a few days when the client is immobile. Expect to revise plans to control pain once the client is mobile or exercising.

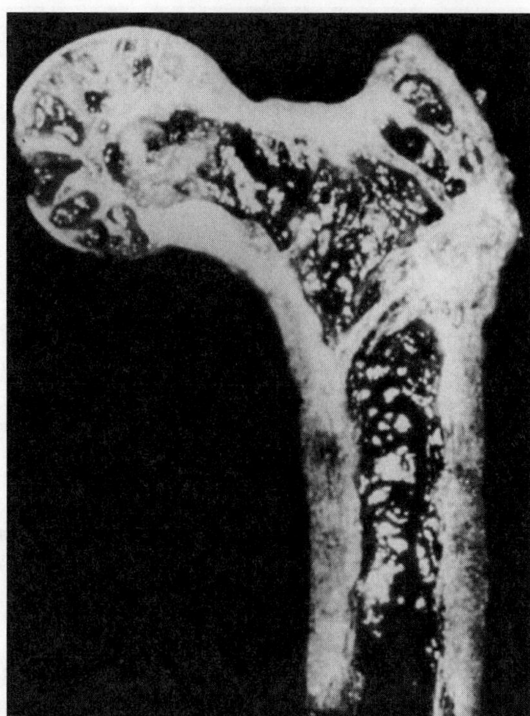

FIGURE 26–12 A pagetoid bone, demonstrating the characteristic mosaic pattern seen on x-ray. (From Merkow, R. L., & Lane, J. M. [1990]. Paget's disease of bone. *Orthopaedic Clinics of North America, 21*[1], 173.)

orthopedic treatment may be indicated for severe disabling arthritis, severe bowing deformities of the femur or tibia, and pathologic fractures.

The recent development of potent bisphosphonates, such as pamidronate (Aredia), alendronate (Fosamax), and residronate (Actonil), have greatly improved the treatment of Paget's disease. After a course of treatment, bone turnover indices such as AP return to normal in 60% to 70% of patients, reflecting suppression of abnormal bone turnover. Existing data suggest that effective disease suppression will likely reduce future disabling problems. Unfortunately, deformity and hearing loss are not corrected with these medications. Re-treatment is indicated if bone turnover markers exceed the upper limit of normal (once they had decreased to within normal limits).

OSTEOMALACIA

Etiology and Pathophysiology

Osteomalacia is a disease in which the bone becomes abnormally soft because of a disturbed calcium and phosphorus balance secondary to vitamin D deficiency. Osteomalacia is characterized by widespread decalcification and softening of bones, especially in the spine, pelvis, and lower extremities. Bones become bent and flattened as they soften. This leads to marked deformities of the weight-bearing bones and to pathologic fractures.

Osteomalacia mainly affects women, and it is endemic in Asia. It is also seen in Moslem women living in Western countries. Their style of dress prevents them from obtaining adequate vitamin D from sunlight exposure. Some causes are:

- Chronic use of anticonvulsants
- Strict vegetarianism
- Very-low-fat diets
- Renal osteodystrophy
- Hyperthyroid-induced osteopenia
- Fibrous dysplasia

Women who have had multiple pregnancies and who have breast-fed their children have a higher rates of the disease. Osteomalacia is similar to rickets, which occurs in children, and the condition is called *adult rickets.*

Clinical Manifestations

Clients generally report easy fatigability, malaise, and bone pain, which is diffuse, poorly localized, and accompanied by a general bony tenderness. Muscular weakness is often seen in severe cases. Serum calcium and phosphorus levels are reduced, and the AP level is moderately elevated. Radiographs indicate generalized demineralization with trabecular bone loss. Pseudofractures (Milkman's syndrome) and cyst formation are common. Bone biopsy is frequently necessary for diagnosis.

Outcome Management

Intervention for clients with osteomalacia includes daily vitamin D until signs of healing take place, when a daily low maintenance dose is continued. Adequate intake of calcium and phosphorus as well as protein should be ensured.

GOUT AND GOUTY ARTHRITIS

Gout is a metabolic bone disorder in which purine (protein) metabolism is altered and the by-product, uric acid, accumulates. Gout is classified as primary or secondary. *Primary* gout is caused by an inherited defect of purine metabolism, leading to increased or decreased renal excretion. Primary gout accounts for 85% of all cases, of which 95% affect males. The initial attack of gout occurs in the 30s or 40s.

Secondary gout is an acquired condition, following hematopoietic (multiple myeloma, polycythemia vera, and leukemia) or renal disorders. In hematopoietic disorders, there is an increase in cell turnover and increased uric acid production. In addition, gout may develop from the rapid induction of chemotherapy or radiation therapy when there is massive destruction of cells. Renal disorders that decrease the excretion of uric acid may lead to gout. Hyperuricemia may also result from use of aspirin, thiazide, and mercurial diuretics, and some antituberculosis medications. Alcohol intoxication and starvation increase serum urate levels by inhibiting renal excretion due to lactic acidosis and ketosis, respectively. In addition, alcohol ingestion increases urate production by stimulating purine breakdown. Prolonged use of diuretics and other medications (levodopa, nicotinic acid, low-dose salicylates) also reduce excretion of uric acid and precipitate gout.

In the body, uric acid is made by the enzymatic breakdown of tissue and dietary purines. Hyperuricemia develops because of underexcretion or overproduction of uric acid. In addition to accumulation in the blood, uric acid is concentrated in the synovial fluid, myocardium, kidneys, and ears. When uric acid levels reach a certain level, they crystallize, and the crystals (tophi) are deposited in connective tissue. Because the crystals are deposited in connective tissue, gout is classified as a form of arthritis (Fig. 26–13).

Clinical manifestations of gout develop in stages (Table 26–5). The diagnosis of gout is confirmed by the presence of persistent hyperuricemia (>7.0 mg/dl) in addition to the clinical manifestations. The presence of uric acid in an aspirated sample of synovial fluid confirms the diagnosis.

Outcome Management

The management of the client with gout has two components: (1) management of the *acute* attack and (2) *long-term* management of hyperuricemia.

Management of the acute attack includes the use of colchicine and NSAIDs to reduce pain and inflammation. Colchicine reduces the migration of leukocytes to the synovial fluids. The initial dose of colchicine is 0.6 to 1.0 mg followed by 0.5 mg/hr until pain is relieved or signs of toxicity develop. Use caution when giving colchicine because the therapeutic dose is close to the toxic dose. Signs of toxicity include nausea, vomiting, and diarrhea. Other NSAIDs can be used, such as indomethacin or naproxen. In resistant cases of gout, adrenocorticotropic hormone (ACTH) or steroids may be required. Ice over the inflamed joints may also relieve pain.

Medications to lower uric acid include allopurinol, which blocks formation of uric acid, and probenecid, which promotes resorption of uric acid deposits and excretion of uric acid. Long-term medication use is advised in clients who have more than two attacks of gout a year, secondary forms of gout, or persistent hyperuricemia. Salicylates (aspirin) antagonize the action of uricosuric agents and must not be used concurrently.

Opinions differ regarding dietary treatment for gout. In the past, a low-purine intake was used to eliminate many proteins from the diet. Some physicians have prescribed a decrease in red and organ meats; others prescribe no dietary changes at all. Encourage ample fluid intake (2000 to 3000 ml/day) to promote excretion of uric acid. A moderate intake of distilled forms of alcohol does not seem to precipitate gouty attacks. Beer, ale, and wine may precipitate them. Excessive alcohol in any form should be avoided.

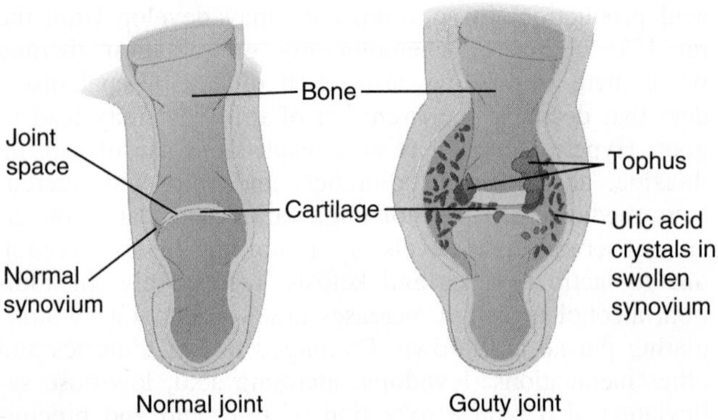

FIGURE 26–13 Comparison of a gouty joint and a normal joint.

TABLE 26–5 MANIFESTATIONS OF GOUT BY STAGE

Stage	Manifestations
Stage I	Asymptomatic hyperuricemia
Stage II	Asymptomatic hyperuricemia again; laboratory and x-ray findings are unchanged from stage II.
Stage III	Acute attack is accompanied by redness, swelling, and exquisite tenderness in one joint (toes, fingers, wrists, ankles, knees, or other joints). The great toe is the most common site. This first attack develops quickly, often overnight. Fever, tachycardia, malaise, and anorexia may be noted. The acute episode usually subsides within a week. As the edema subsides, pruritus and local desquamation (tissue loss) may be noted. After the initial attack the affected joint returns to normal and the client may be asymptomatic for years. Eventually, other attacks occur.
Stage IV	Permanent changes in multiple joints with restrictions in movement. Tophi may be detected on the ears, hands, elbows, feet, and knees. Renal and cardiac disorders may also develop. The client may have uric acid renal stones, renal colic, and hypertension. Atherosclerosis occurs in about 50% of all clients.

Gradual weight loss is encouraged after the initial attack. Weight loss alone may reduce the incidence of attacks and uric acid levels. However, a sudden loss of weight may precipitate an attack because of the destruction of cells, which release uric acid.

Clients who can recognize early manifestations of gout may be able to avert the attack by prompt use of colchicine or indomethacin. Long-term side effects (alopecia, bone marrow suppression, hepatic damage) from these agents, although rare, should be explained to the client.

Nursing management of the client with gout includes pain control. The client is usually placed at bed rest until pain subsides. Once ambulating, the client's need for crutches or a walker should be considered until gait is stable. Explain dietary restrictions, fluid requirements, and long-term self-management.

SPINAL COLUMN DEFORMITIES

The characteristic S curve of the lateral spine develops during fetal life and early childhood. Because other abnormal curves can occur due to defects in the bone, muscles, or nerves, every spinal problem must be considered from both an orthopedic and a neurologic viewpoint.

SCOLIOSIS

In the coronal plane, the spine should appear completely straight. Scoliosis is lateral curvature of the spine in any area—cervical, thoracic, thoracolumbar, or lumbar. It is important to distinguish curvature of *structural* origin from that of *nonstructural* origin. A structural curvature does not correct itself on forced bending against the curvature, and vertebral rotation is demonstrated. A nonstructural curvature is easily corrected on forced bending or in the supine position, and rotation of the vertebral bodies is not demonstrated.

Idiopathic scoliosis is the most common form, appearing in growing children with no other apparent health problems. The incidence is less than 1%,[43] occurring most often in preadolescents and adolescents. Scoliosis was once believed to be primarily a problem in girls, but school screening studies have shown small degrees of abnormal spinal curvature in equal numbers of boys and girls. Both boys and girls should be observed until it is proved that a curve is not progressive. Continued curve progression is possible even after skeletal maturity if the curvature is greater than 40 or 45 degrees, and excessive curvature can lead to cardiopulmonary problems and pain that prompt the client to seek medical care. The client may also seek help because of cosmetic deformity and loss in height. Skeletally mature clients with a curve less than 20 degrees do not require treatment. Skeletally immature clients with a curve between 20 and 40 degrees require brace management, while clients with curves greater than 45 degrees need surgical intervention.

Etiology

The cause of scoliosis can be congenital or neuromuscular. Congenital scoliosis results from a malformation of the bony vertebral segment of the spine, either because of failure of (1) formation (absence of a portion of a vertebra) or (2) segmentation (absence of normal separations between vertebrae). Neuromuscular conditions associated with spinal deformities include cerebral palsy, syringomyelia, polio, myelomeningocele, spinal muscle atrophy, spinal cord tumors, trauma, and myopathic conditions such as muscular dystrophy.

Clinical Manifestations

Clinical manifestations and a family history of spinal deformity are significant, but diagnosis is confirmed by upright posteroanterior and lateral radiographs that reveal a curvature of 10 degrees or more (Fig. 26–14*A*). X-rays are the only exact tool for monitoring changes in spinal deformity, but excessive radiation exposure is inappropriate in children. Two other noninvasive stereophotogrametic techniques—Moire topography and the integrated shape-imaging system (ISIS)—produce images on the back surface shape that can be correlated to underlying spinal deformities.

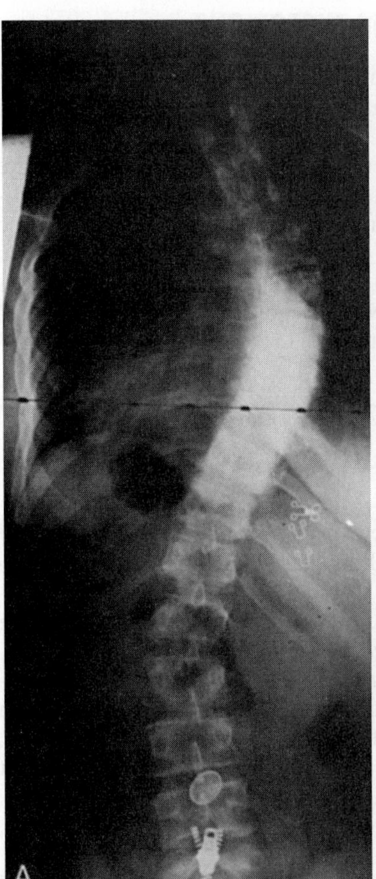

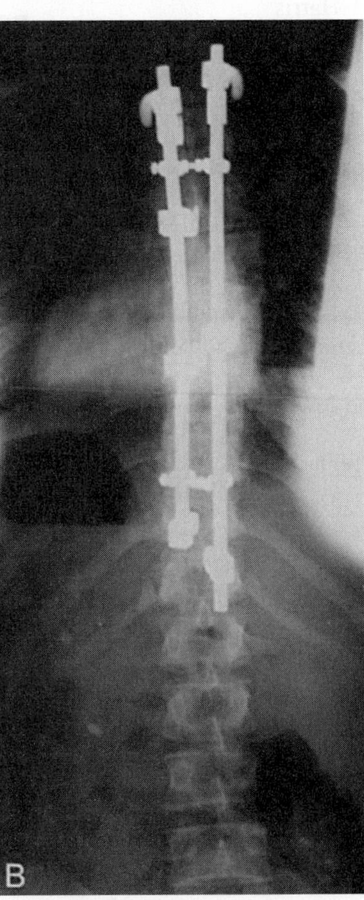

FIGURE 26–14 *A,* Scoliosis. *B,* Postoperative x-ray after correction with Cotrel-Dubousset instrumentation. (From Maher, A. B., Salmond, S. W., & Pellino, T. A. [Eds.]. [1998]. *Orthopedic nursing* [2nd ed., p. 557]. Philadelphia: W. B. Saunders.)

Outcome Management

Nonsurgical treatments for clients with spinal deformity consist of observation, bracing, and exercise. Each client needs to be individually evaluated, not only for the medical problem but also for willingness to participate in any suggested therapies. One client may refuse to wear a brace under any circumstances; another may insist on treatment for even a slight curvature.

The decision to proceed with surgical treatment is based not only on failure of conservative treatments but also on additional factors, such as the client's emotional stability and readiness to undergo a major procedure. Spinal fusion is the ultimate goal in many cases, attaching adjacent vertebrae to each other with a bone graft to prohibit motion between them. The surgical approach can be posterior or anterior, depending on the location of the deformity. A combined anterior-posterior approach has become increasingly popular for adults with severe thoracolumbar scoliosis.

Various types of instruments can be used to stabilize the spine and correct deformity. The choice of instrumentation is based on the diagnosis, the magnitude of the curvature and the flexibility of the curve, the client's age and inherent bone strength, and the client's ability to wear a postoperative immobilization device. The Cotrel-Dubousset (CD), Texas Scottish Rite Hospital (TSRH), Moss-Miami, and Luque systems are commonly used for a posterior approach (see Fig. 26–14). The Harrington rod system, developed in the 1960s, is still in use because of its availability and because many surgeons are very familiar with it. The most common types of instrumentation for an anterior approach are the Zielke and Harris systems.

COMPLICATIONS

Possible complications following scoliosis surgery include neurologic compromise, infection, respiratory problems, spinal fluid leakage, phlebitis, excessive blood loss, implant problems, and pseudarthrosis. The most devastating complications are paralysis and death.

POSTOPERATIVE CARE

Postoperative nursing management focuses on:

- Assessment of blood loss and maintenance of hemodynamic stability
- Assessment of motor and sensory function in the lower extremities
- Administration of adequate analgesia and fluid replacement
- Client education for effective pulmonary hygiene
- Wound and skin care
- Progressive ambulation

(Chapter 71 also discusses nursing management after lumbar fusion.)

KYPHOSIS

Also called "humpback" or "dowager's hump," the term kyphosis describes a posterior rounding of the thoracic spine. While a certain degree of kyphosis is considered normal, curvatures greater than 45 degrees are believed to be excessive and require additional evaluation as to the cause. Kyphosis is identified as *postural* if the client can voluntarily hyperextend the spine to correct the curvature and if there is no x-ray evidence of structural change. Kyphosis is common in metabolic disorders such as osteoporosis and osteomalacia, but it can also accompany neuromuscular diseases such as cerebral palsy and muscular dystrophy. Severe curvature can affect cardiopulmonary and gastrointestinal function, making intervention essential.

Kyphosis is most often treated with bracing or corsets to straighten the spine. Exercises to strengthen muscles and ligaments may also be encouraged. Spinal fusion with or without instrumentation may be required if response to other interventions is inadequate.

LORDOSIS

Lordosis is an excessive inward curvature of the lumbar spine sometimes seen in pregnant or obese clients or in those with large abdominal tumors. Extreme lordosis may lead to *swayback,* in which the lumbosacral spine curves sharply and the thoracolumbar spine exhibits kyphosis. Lordosis is often associated with sagging shoulders, an exaggerated pelvic angle, and medial rotation of the legs. If necessary, treatment may consist of bracing, spinal fusion, or osteotomy. Hyperlordosis in young children and prepubertal girls is a self-correcting problem thought to be related to rapid skeletal growth without corresponding soft tissue growth.

BONE INFECTIONS

Musculoskeletal system contamination can result either as infection spreads from other sites in the body or from external insults (e.g., puncture, surgery). Infections are often severe and difficult to treat because the bones are relatively inaccessible to protective macrophages and antibodies. Even a small number of microorganisms can be enough to establish a serious infection that can lead to loss of function or even death. For this reason, nurses should be diligent in wound care and alert to any symptoms that suggest infection.

OSTEOMYELITIS

Pathophysiology

Osteomyelitis is a severe pyogenic infection of bone and surrounding tissues. Although generally bacterial in origin, osteomyelitis can also be caused by a virus or fungus. *Staphylococcus aureus* is the most common infecting organism, but *Escherichia coli, Pseudomonas, Klebsiella, Salmonella,* and *Proteus* may also be found. Because osteomyelitis can be extraordinarily difficult to cure even with long-term antibiotics, prompt recognition is crucial. Delayed identification or inadequate treatment can result in a chronic infection accompanied by continuing pain, chronically draining sinuses, loss of function, amputation, or death.

Osteomyelitis occurs most frequently in the femur and

tibia. Males are affected more often than females, often as a result of trauma. Susceptibility to infection increases with intravenous drug use, diabetes, immunocompromising diseases, or a history of bloodstream infections. Limiting the spread of osteomyelitis may also be more difficult in clients with a disorder such as malnutrition, alcoholism, or liver failure.

Clinical Manifestations

Clinical manifestations may vary slightly according to the site of involvement. Infection in the long bones is accompanied by acute localized pain and redness or drainage, often with a history of recent trauma or newly acquired prostheses. Fever and malaise may be present, but adults do not always appear acutely ill with other systemic signs. Infection in the vertebrae usually brings pain and mobility difficulties. The client with vertebral osteomyelitis often reports a history of genitourinary infection or drug abuse. Osteomyelitis in the foot is most commonly associated with vascular insufficiency.

Laboratory studies and x-rays or bone scans are important in the definitive diagnosis of osteomyelitis. Elevated WBC and ESR, along with clinical manifestations, usually allow initial diagnosis and early treatment while the physician waits for further evidence from blood cultures or needle aspirate analysis. Radiographic changes related to osteomyelitis are generally evident within 7 to 10 days, but in some cases the diagnosis is not confirmed on x-rays until 3 to 4 weeks after infection develops. Early acute osteomyelitis is more efficiently identified by radionuclide bone scans, which can detect lesions within 24 to 72 hours after the onset of infection. Because of its ability to distinguish between soft tissue and bone marrow, magnetic resonance imaging (MRI) is also being used increasingly for definitive diagnosis of osteomyelitis.

Outcome Management

Elimination of the infecting organism, both locally from the bone and systemically from the body, is the major treatment goal for acute osteomyelitis. Prompt treatment also prevents further bone deformity and injury, increases client comfort, and avoids complications of impaired mobility. Surgery is initially performed on the adult client with osteomyelitis to ensure effective debridement and drainage, elimination of dead space, and adequate soft tissue coverage. Antibiotics alone rarely resolve infection in adults, but they do work more effectively after surgical preparation of the treatment area. High doses of parenteral antibiotics are frequently administered for 4 to 8 weeks to achieve a bactericidal level in the bone tissue. Oral antibiotics are continued for another 4 to 8 weeks, with serial bone scans and ESR measurements performed to evaluate the effectiveness of drug therapy. Open, draining wounds are packed with gauze to promote drainage. If initial treatment is delayed or inadequate, the necrotic bone separates from the living bone to form *sequestra,* which serve as a medium for additional microorganism growth. Chronic osteomyelitis can result.

SEPTIC ARTHRITIS

Etiology and Pathophysiology

Septic arthritis (also known as pyogenic arthritis, infectious arthritis, septic joint disease, bacterial arthritis, and suppurative arthritis) is a closed-space infection caused by invasion of the synovial membrane by pus-forming bacteria or other pathogens. Joints most commonly affected in adult clients are the knee, hip, shoulder, wrist, and ankle.

A variety of microorganisms may infect the joint, but *Neisseria gonorrhoae* is the most common causative pathogen in adults under age 30 years. A significant percentage of staphylococci, the second most common causative organism in adults, is methicillin-resistant. *Staphylococcus aureus* invades the joint through hematogenous spread, as an extension of adjacent soft tissue infection, or from direct inoculation following trauma or an invasive procedure.

Hematogenous spread, in which organisms reach the joint from a remote site, is the most common etiologic mechanism. Because the synovial membrane is very vascular, any microorganism that is circulating in the blood may be easily trapped in the synovial space. Upper respiratory infection, otitis media, furuncle, or impetigo may seed a susceptible site such as a previously traumatized or diseased knee joint.

The presence of septic arthritis typically reflects the failure of multiple defense mechanisms. In the early stages of infection, the synovial membrane swells and becomes infiltrated with neutrophils. A purulent effusion distends the joint as the neutrophils release lysosomal proteolytic enzymes that destroy the articular cartilage, subchondral bone, and joint capsule. Enzymatic cartilage destruction can actually occur in 3 to 24 hours, creating a medical emergency that requires prompt treatment to avoid permanent joint damage.

Clinical Manifestations

The client often presents with complaints of pain, swelling, warmth, and tenderness in a single joint and also generally experiences an acute systemic reaction. The adult client is more likely than the child to experience only a low-grade fever and malaise. However, high temperatures and shaking chills are generally present in the client who has positive blood cultures.

Assessment focuses on the presence of factors that may predispose the client to joint infection, such as recent surgery or injury, diagnostic procedures, intravenous drug abuse, or systemic disease. Because effective treatment requires accurate identification of the causative agent, initial laboratory studies attempt to differentiate septic arthritis from autoimmune diseases with joint involvement (such as rheumatoid arthritis). CBC, ESR, the antinuclear antibody (ANA) test, and rheumatoid factor (RF) measurements are often among studies that are ordered. In addition, joint fluid is aspirated for analysis, and a synovial biopsy is performed. Radioisotope scanning techniques may also be helpful in early detection of infection.

Outcome Management

Antibiotic therapy is a critical part of effective treatment of septic arthritis and must be promptly initiated to prevent permanent joint damage. Penicillin G, a bactericidal agent, is often administered initially because many common causative organisms are susceptible to the drug. After the specific organism and its sensitivities have been identified from synovial fluid cultures, the antibiotic therapy may be altered. Treatment time varies according to duration of clinical manifestations, the causative organism, and the status of the client's immune system. For most clients, parenteral antibiotics are administered for 2 to 3 weeks and oral antibiotics continue for another 1 or 2 weeks. However, elderly clients or those with more complex presentations may require parenteral therapy lasting 4 to 6 weeks. Decompression of the infected joint is also necessary, although controversy exists about the best methods. Open synovectomy and debridement or repeated joint aspirations and irrigations may be performed. Arthroscopic drainage and debridement have also been successful.

Effective nursing management requires scrupulous attention to the client's joint position, exercise, and rehabilitation. In the acute phase of septic arthritis, the client is likely to hold the joint in slight to moderate flexion as a position of comfort. Because this can lead to flexion deformities, slings, immobilizers, or splints may be used temporarily to hold the joint in an optimal position. As inflammation begins to resolve, passive ROM exercises are initiated to preserve joint function. CPM has also been used with some success. Active motion and weight-bearing may not be initiated until clinical manifestations and inflammation have almost totally disappeared. Pain management is also important for the client with septic arthritis to provide comfort and to allow greater ease in exercise participation.

BONE TUMORS

A bone tumor (neoplasm) may be benign or malignant (Table 26–6 and Fig. 26–15). Benign bone tumors may remain undiagnosed because they often cause no pain.

TABLE 26–6 PRIMARY BONE AND CARTILAGE TUMORS

Type	Description
BENIGN CARTILAGE-FORMING TUMOR	
Enchondroma	Lesion in mature cartilage but lacking histologic characteristic of chondrosarcoma; found in hands and feet; age range, 20–40 yr
Osteochondroma	Most frequent bone tumor; cartilage-capped bony projection on external bone surface; metaphyses of long bone, especially proximal tibia and distal femur; age range, 0–30 yr
BENIGN BONE-FORMING TUMOR	
Osteoid osteoma	Small osteoblastic lesion (less than 1 cm) with demarcated outline and reactive bone formation; femur and tibia; age range 10–20 yr
Osteoblastoma	Similar to osteoid osteoma but larger (>2 cm); spine
Giant cell tumor (osteoclastoma)	Aggressive benign bone tumor with richly vascularized tissue consisting of plump spindle-shaped cells and numerous giant cells; distal femur, proximal tibia, distal radius, proximal humerus; age range, 20–40 yr
MALIGNANT BONE-FORMING TUMOR	
Osteosarcoma	Most common primary malignant bone tumor; formation of bone or osteoid by tumor cell; metaphyses, especially of distal femur, proximal tibia, and proximal humerus; intramedullary region involved; age range, 10–30 yr
Ewing's sarcoma	Composed of densely packed small cells with round nuclei; often confused with osteomyelitis because it presents with fever, anemia, leukocytosis, increased ESR; diaphyseal regions of long and flat bones; age range, 5–15 yr
Fibrosarcoma	Formation of interlacing bundles of collagen fibers by spindle-shaped tumor cells; absence of other types of histologic differentiation; femur, tibia; age range, 5–80 yr
MALIGNANT CARTILAGE-FORMING TUMOR	
Chondrosarcoma	Formation of cartilage by tumor cells; higher cellularity and greater pleomorphism than in chondromas; femur, pelvis, ribs, scapula; age range, 30–60 yr

Adapted from Piasecki, P. (1996). Tumors. In S. W. Salmond, N. E. Mooney, & L. A. Verdisco (Eds.), *Core curriculum for orthopaedic nursing* (3rd ed.). Pitman, NJ: National Association of Orthopaedic Nurses.

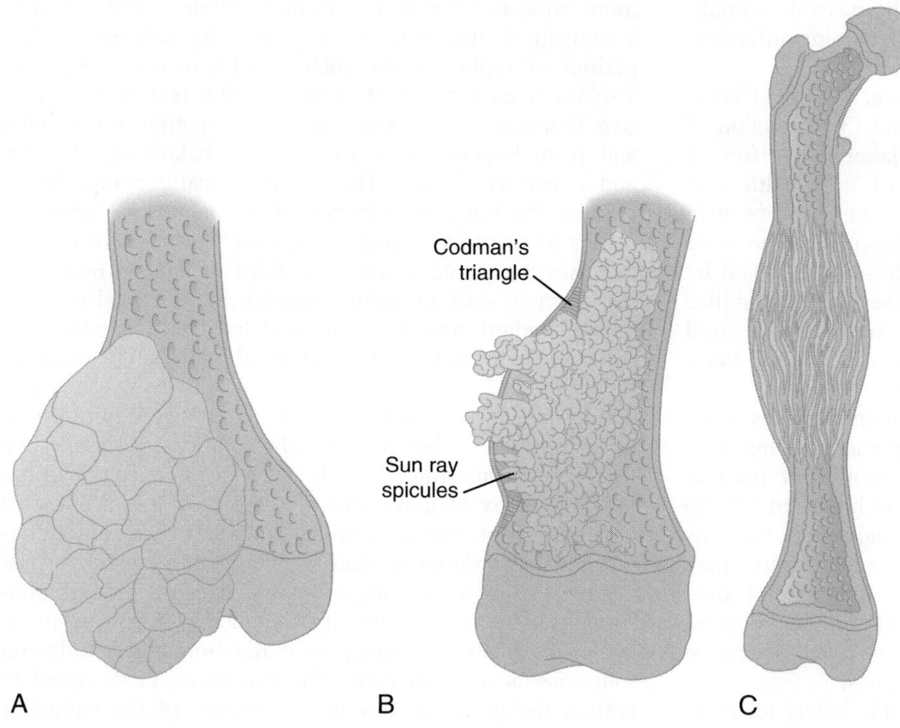

FIGURE 26–15 Bone tumors. *A,* A giant cell tumor. *B,* An osteogenic sarcoma. *C,* A malignant endothelioma (Ewing's sarcoma). (After Hughes, S. [1983]. *A short textbook of orthopedics and traumatology* [3rd ed.]. New York: ARCO.)

They may be noted as an incidental x-ray finding when the client is being evaluated for another complaint, such as fracture through a bone cyst. However, benign tumors that grow aggressively can cause bone pain, weakness, and destruction. In such a case, surgery is then indicated.

MALIGNANT BONE TUMORS

Primary malignant tumors originate in bone cells or form within the bone. Each year, about 2500 new cases of primary bone tumors are diagnosed, including osteosarcoma, chondrosarcoma, and Ewing's sarcoma.[24] Clients typically present with a mass or lesion, or a pathologic fracture. They may also report weight loss, fever, chills, or pulmonary manifestations.

The exact cause of primary bone tumors remains largely unknown, but several factors are believed to play a role in their development. Past trauma has been associated with tumor development, as has exposure to carcinogens such as asbestos, dioxin, and radium. Bone tumors may also develop from benign medical conditions (enchondromatosis, neurofibromatosis) or from metabolic conditions (Paget's disease). Fewer than 5% of clients with malignancies have a hereditary predilection to cancer.[24]

Metastatic bone tumors, winch are more prevalent than sarcomas, spread to the bone from primary carcinomas in sites such as the breast, prostate, lung, and kidney. Thyroid, bladder, uterine, colorectal, and vaginal cancers can also metastasize to bone. Cancer cells may spread directly within a body cavity, or they may metastasize by hematogenous or lymphatic spread.

Laboratory studies such as CBC, blood and urine calcium levels, and ESR assist in client evaluation, but they are not diagnostic themselves. Other laboratory tests, however, are used as tumor markers. An elevated serum AP level may be noted with osteoblastic tumors, for example, and lactate dehydrogenase (LDH) may mark tumor progression for Ewing's sarcoma. A plain radiograph in anterior and posterior views may provide an initial diagnosis, but other studies—such as a CT scan, MRI, or bone scan—are also commonly performed. A bone biopsy is needed for definitive diagnosis of metastatic bone disease.

Outcome Management

The treatment goal for the client with a primary tumor is to eradicate the tumor completely and promote long-term survival. *Chemotherapy* has dramatically increased the survival of clients diagnosed with primary bone tumors. *Radiation therapy* has become safer because of increased understanding of cancer and radiobiology; it is also now better tolerated through the use of radiation machines that reduce skin sensitivity. *Surgery* may be performed to eradicate the disease, either through excision of the tumor and a wide zone of surrounding normal tissue or through amputation. If the tumor is excised, the resulting defect is repaired by using a joint prosthesis or bone graft with internal fixation. The bone graft can be taken from the client at another anatomic site, or allograft (cadaver) bone may be used.

Pain management following surgery is a major focus. Opioids are often delivered by patient-controlled analgesia (PCA) pumps or via epidural catheter. Pain should be addressed aggressively and medication effectiveness assessed regularly. Frequent position changes and stimulation of non-tumor areas through heat, cold, or massage may be beneficial. Nonpharmacologic strategies, such as music therapy, imagery, and relaxation techniques, may provide powerful adjuncts to opioid administration. Postoperative nursing care also addresses the possible complications related to orthopedic surgery, including infection, DVT, and non-union of grafted bone.

For the client with metastatic disease, treatment goals include (1) palliation, (2) remission, and (3) extension of life. Pain management requires a collaborative effort of the client, family, and all members of the health care team. Because metastatic tumors can cause severe pain and have the potential to fracture, lesions in the long bones are commonly managed with excision, followed by intramedullary rodding and cement insertion to stabilize the weakened bone. Radiation therapy may also be used to decrease tumor size, improving bone strength and helping in pain management.

Pharmacologic treatment of pain often includes morphine. Oral administration facilitates home care management for the client with metastatic tumors, but intravenous or transdermal medications may be indicated for the client with gastric problems. Other analgesics, such as acetaminophen and anti-inflammatory medications, may also be used because they act on the peripheral pain mechanism. Adjuvant medications, including antidepressants and anticonvulsants, are frequently used to increase the effectiveness of conventional analgesics.

The key to pain management is to administer all analgesics on an around-the-clock (ATC) rather than on an as-needed (PRN) basis. Nonpharmacologic measures should also be employed to maximize pain relief.

As with postoperative treatment of the client with a primary tumor, pain should be addressed aggressively and medication effectiveness assessed regularly. Attempts at pain management for the client with a metastatic bone tumor may ultimately lead to a palliative neurosurgical procedure, such as a chordotomy, in which the anterolateral spinal cord tracts are severed to provide relief in the affected areas.

DISORDERS OF THE FOOT

HALLUX VALGUS (BUNIONS)

Bunions, a common foot deformity that involves the first metatarsal and the great toe (hallux), occur nine times more often in women than in men. Bunions may occur as a congenital disorder, or they may be acquired during periods of rapid growth, such as adolescence. They may also occur as a result of local irritation related to restrictive footwear. They result from a pronation abnormality and from hypermobility of the first metatarsal, phalanx, and cuneiform joints. The client typically complains of pain as the bony prominence of the metatarsal head becomes irritated from pushing against the inside of a shoe. *Calluses* under the second and third metatarsal heads occur from a shift in weight-bearing and may also cause pain. Standard anteroposterior and lateral x-rays show exostosis of the first metatarsal head with subluxation or dislocation.

To decrease pressure over the bunion and minimize the likelihood of bursitis, the client may try conservative treatment, consisting entirely of wearing shoes with a larger toe box to allow more space for the forefoot. If a change in footwear does not provide enough relief, orthoses may be ordered or steroid injections administered for acute inflammation. Surgery may be considered if conservative treatment fails, if the client desires cosmetic correction of the deformity, or if functioning of the lateral four toes is also affected. The procedure is designed to realign the great toe through osteotomy of the hallux or through fusion of the metatarsophalangeal joint (Fig. 26–16). Kirschner wires are inserted vertically through the involved toes, remaining in place for about 3 weeks after surgery. Bits of cork are placed on the wire tips for protection. In addition to routine care, the client who has undergone bunionectomy may use wooden postoperative shoes for ambulation.

MORTON'S NEUROMA (PLANTAR NEUROMA)

Athletes commonly experience Morton's neuroma because of excessive pressure placed on the branch of the medial plantar nerve between the third and fourth toes. The pressure causes a neuroma, or swelling of the nerve, that leads the client to complain of pain in the ball of the foot. Depending on the extent of the compression, pain may radiate into the toes and be accompanied by numbness. Pain may be increased if the client wears tight-

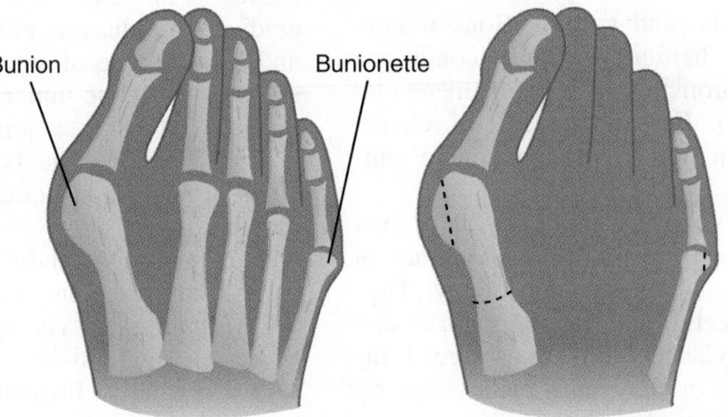

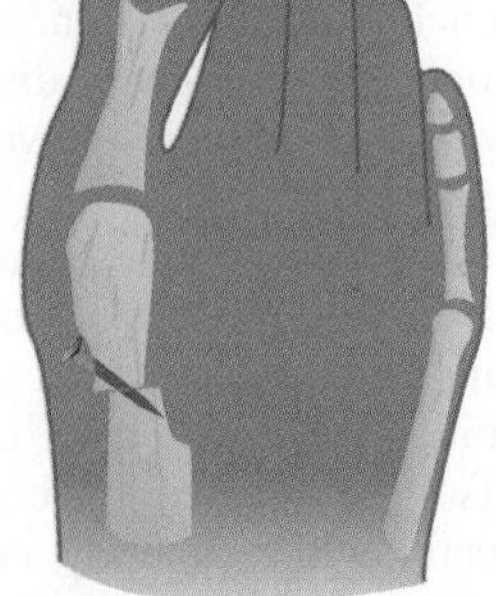

FIGURE 26–16 Bunions and their surgical correction.

fitting or high-heeled shoes. Hyperextension of the metatarsophalangeal joints or repetitive impact on the forefoot may also increase pain.

The usual treatment involves changing the type of shoe to one with a larger toe box that provides more room for the forefoot. Anti-inflammatory medications are often prescribed. If they are ineffective, steroid injections may be administered. Surgery to remove the neuroma may be considered if other treatments do not produce long-term relief.

HAMMER TOE

Hammer toe is a deformity caused by a flexion contracture of the proximal interphalangeal joint (PIP) with extension or slight hyperextension of the distal interphalangeal joint (DIP) (Fig. 26–17). This deformity often accompanies hallux valgus and may occur in clients with a family history of hammer toe, RA, and clawfeet. Hammer toe leads to improper fit of footwear, creating pain with walking and a change in gait patterns. Corns and calluses on pressure areas of the foot may need to be removed.

Treatment centers on choosing footwear with a wide toe box. Pads and inserts can help relieve pressure, but they can also cause previously unaffected areas of the foot to rub against the shoe. Osteotomy of the toe and resection of the proximal phalanx may be required for symptom relief.

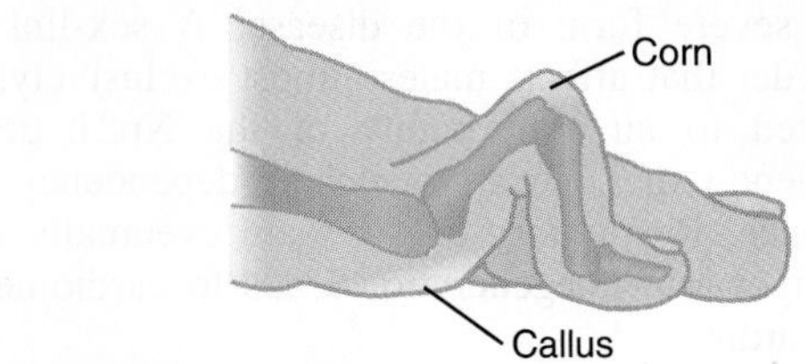

FIGURE 26–17 Hammer toe.

MUSCULAR DISORDERS

MUSCULAR DYSTROPHY

Muscular dystrophy (MD) is a term that generally designates a group of genetic disorders involving gradual degeneration of muscle fibers. The client experiences progressive weakness and skeletal muscle wasting, accompanied by disability and deformity. The various forms of MD are differentiated by the affected muscle groups, the client's age at onset of the disease, the rate of progression, and the inheritance mode (Table 26–7). *Pseudohypertrophic MD (Duchenne's MD)* is the most

TABLE 26–7 CLINICAL FEATURES IN MUSCULAR DYSTROPHY (MD)

	Duchenne's MD	Becker's MD	Limb Girdle MD
Incidence	Most common type of MD	Less common than Duchenne's MD	Less common than Duchenne's or Becker's MD
Age at onset	Usually <3 yr	Usually 5–15 yr	Usually by second decade
Inheritance	Sex-linked recessive gene, autosomal <10%	Sex-linked recessive gene	Usually autosomal recessive
Pattern of muscle involvement	Onset: Selected symmetrical weakness of proximal pelvic muscles, 3–5 yr Later: shoulder girdle muscle involvement	Similar to Duchenne's MD	Proximal shoulder and pelvic girdle
Late muscle involvement	Affects all muscles, including facial, oculopharyngeal, and respiratory	Face spared	Peripheral brachioradialis, hand, and calf
Pseudohypertrophy	Calf muscles	Calf muscles	Occurs in fewer than one third of cases
Contractural deformities	Common	Less common	Occurs in late disease; milder than Duchenne's MD
Scoliosis/kyphoscoliosis	Common in late disease	Not severe	Mild in late disease
Heart involvement	Yes	Uncommon in late disease	Rare
IQ	Decreased	Normal	Normal
Course	Steady progression	Slow progression	Slow progression, with greater variation among clients

IQ, intelligence quotient.

Adapted from Doleysh, N. (1996). Neuromuscular disorders. In S. W. Salmond, N. E. Mooney, & L. A. Verdisco (Eds.), *Core curriculum for orthopaedic nursing* (3rd ed.). Pitman, NJ: National Association of Orthopaedic Nurses.

common and severe form of the disease. A sex-linked recessive disorder that affects males almost exclusively, it has been linked to an abnormality of the Xp21 gene locus. The client experiences wheelchair dependency in early adolescence. Respiratory muscles are eventually involved, and myocardial degeneration leads to cardiomegaly and tachycardia.

Diagnosis of MD is accomplished through use of multiple modalities in an attempt to differentiate the disease from other disorders, such as myasthenia gravis and polymyositis. The most valuable laboratory test is serum creatine kinase analysis; levels are elevated in clients with MD because of an abnormality of striated muscle function. Enzyme levels do decrease, however, as muscle mass decreases. Muscle biopsy is essential to diagnosis of a neuromuscular disease such as Duchenne's MD. Muscle shows degeneration, with fibers replaced by connective tissue and fat in later stages of the disease.

Treatment is largely symptomatic and supportive because there is currently no cure for MD. Care is aimed at increasing the comfort and functional ability through corrective surgery for related deformities or use of braces for the spine or lower extremities. Breathing exercises may also be initiated for respiratory decompensation. More than 60% of clients with MD live to age 21 years, but survival beyond age 30 is unusual.[6] Death generally results from respiratory or cardiac failure.

CONCLUSIONS

The focus of this chapter has been musculoskeletal disorders, including metabolic bone diseases such as osteoporosis. Osteoarthritis is a common degenerative disorder that is often treated with joint replacement surgery. Special nursing care is required after such surgery to maximize the client's outcome. Benign and metastatic bone tumors, common foot disorders, and MD, a hereditary neuromuscular disorder, have also been discussed.

An understanding of these disorders is essential for the nurse who provides care for affected clients.

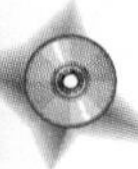

THINKING CRITICALLY

1. **You meet an older woman in the total joint class who is considering joint replacement surgery but has not yet scheduled the procedure with her orthopedist. She has osteoarthritis and, because of increasing pain in her hips, she now uses a wheelchair when she goes out in public. She tells you she also has diabetes mellitus. What would you discuss with her to help her prepare appropriately for surgery?**

Factors to Consider. What would be the benefit of increased upper arm strength for this client? Is she maintaining tight control of the diabetes? Is weight loss an issue before surgery?

2. **A middle-aged client is concerned about bone loss resulting from osteoporosis. She tells you that her mother has severe osteoporosis, and she realizes her lifestyle and family history are predisposing factors. She asks you to suggest a lifestyle program for her and her daughters. How should you proceed?**

Factors to Consider. What focused assessment should you complete? How should you complete teaching for the client and her daughters?

3. **An elderly woman tells you her physician wants her to eat a diet high in calcium. He wants her to consume 1500 mg of calcium without taking enriched antacids or calcium supplements. This woman is lactose-intolerant and has a hiatal hernia. She lives alone on a limited income. What problems might impair her compliance with the prescribed treatment regimen?**

Factors to Consider. What dietary sources of calcium are appropriate for the lactose-intolerant client? How does the presence of a hiatal hernia affect dietary intake?

BIBLIOGRAPHY

1. Altizer, L. (1995). Total hip arthroplasty. *Orthopaedic Nursing, 14*(4), 7–18, 63.
2. Altizer, L. L. (1998). Degenerative disorders. In A. B. Maher, S. W. Salmond, & T. A. Pellino (Eds.), *Orthopaedic nursing* (2nd ed.). Philadelphia: W. B. Saunders, pp. 480–544.
3. American College of Rheumatology Ad Hoc Committee on Clinical Guidelines. (1996). Guidelines for the initial evluation of the adult patient with acute musculoskeletal symptoms. *Arthritis and Rheumatology, 39,* 1–8.
4. Anderson, L. P., & Dale, K. G. (1998). Infections in total joint replacements. *Orthopaedic Nursing, 17*(1), 7–10.
5. Aubin, M., & Marks, R. (1995). The efficacy of short-term treatment with transcutaneous electrical nerve stimulation for osteo-arthritic knee pain. *Physiotherapy, 81*(11), 669–675.
6. Bender, L. H. (1998). Congenital and developmental disorders. In A. B. Maher, S. W. Salmond, & T. A. Pellino (Eds.), *Orthopaedic nursing* (2nd ed.). Philadelphia: W. B. Saunders, pp. 586–662.
7. Blaylock, B., et al. (1995). Tape injury in the patient with total hip replacement. *Orthopaedic Nursing, 14*(3), 25–28.
8. Bonatz, E. (1996). Overuse syndromes of the hand and wrist. In V. R. Masear (Ed.), *Primary care orthopaedics.* Philadelphia: W. B. Saunders, pp. 346–349.
9. Burrage, R. L., & Sutter, C. A. (1999). Arthritis. In J. T. Stone, J. F. Wyman, & S. A. Salisbury (Eds.), *Clinical gerontological nursing: A guide to advanced practice.* Philadelphia: W. B. Saunders, pp. 469–487.
10. Cerrato, P. L. (1998). Alternatives. Complementary therapies: Can these compounds curb arthritis? *RN, 6*(4), 57–58, 67.
11. Clough, J. D., Lambert, T., & Miller, D. R. (1996). The new thinking on osteoarthritis. *Patient Care, 30*(14), 110–113, 117–118, 121–124.
12. Crescimbeni, J. A. (1997). From bed to chair: Transferring the non–weight-bearing patient. *Orthopaedic Nursing, 16*(2), 47–50.
13. DiNubile, N. A. (1997). Osteoarthritis. How to make exercise part of your treatment plan. *The Physician and Sportsmedicine, 25*(7), 47–50, 52, 55–56.
14. Doleysh, N. (1996). Neuromuscular disorders. In S. W. Salmond, N. E. Mooney, & L. A. Verdisco (Eds.), *Core curriculum for orthopaedic nursing* (3rd ed.). Pitman, NJ: National Association of Orthopaedic Nurses, pp. 315–352.
15. Evans, J. A., & Madrid, C. L. (1995). High tibial osteotomy: Treatment for unicompartmental arthritis. *Operative Techniques in Sports Medicine, 3*(2), 112–116.
16. Facts and Comparisons (1998). The review of natural products: Chondroitin. St. Louis: Author.
17. Facts and Comparisons (1998). The review of natural products: Glucosamine. St. Louis: Author.
18. Felson, D.T. (1996). Weight and osteoarthritis. *American Journal of Clinical Nutrition, 63*(3S), 430S–432S.

19. Flynn, R. (1996). Arthritic disorders. In S. W. Salmond, N. E. Mooney, & L. A. Verdisco (Eds.), *Core curriculum for orthopaedic nursing* (3rd ed.). Pitman, NJ: National Association of Orthopaedic Nurses, pp. 217–263.
20. Fracaro, M. L. (1996). Infection. In S. W. Salmond, N. E. Mooney, & L. A. Verdisco (Eds.), *Core curriculum for orthopaedic nursing* (3rd ed.). Pitman, NJ: National Association of Orthopaedic Nurses, pp. 281–296.
21. Haynes, K. (1998). Neoplasms of the musculoskeletal system. In A. B. Maher, S. W. Salmond, & T. A. Pellino (Eds.), *Orthopaedic nursing* (2nd ed.). Philadelphia: W. B. Saunders, pp. 769–803.
22. Jaffe, K. (1996). Tumors of the musculoskeletal system. In V. R. Masear (Ed.), *Primary care orthopaedics.* Philadelphia: W. B. Saunders, pp. 263–288.
23. Jaffe, K., Greco, J., & Wade, J. (1996). Orthopaedic emergencies and infections. In V. R. Masear (Ed.), *Primary care orthopaedics.* Philadelphia: W. B. Saunders, pp. 35–49.
24. Kessenich, C. R. (1997). Myths & facts . . . about osteoarthritis. *Nursing97, 27*(8), 67.
25. Kettelman, K. (1998). Controlling bone pain: How to keep nausea and oversedation out of the picture. *Nursing98, 28*(11), 22.
26. Killian, J. T., & Coen, J. (1996). Developmental conditions in children. In V. R. Masear (Ed.), *Primary care orthopaedics.* Philadelphia: W. B. Saunders, pp. 289–303.
27. Kopp, M. (1997). Caring for the adult patient undergoing anterior/posterior spinal fusion. *Orthopaedic Nursing, 16*(2), 55–59.
28. Krug, B. (1997). Rheumatoid arthritis and osteoarthritis: A basic comparison. *Orthopaedic Nursing, 16*(5), 73–75.
29. Ling, S. M., & Bathon, J. M. (1998). Osteoarthritis in older adults. *Journal of the American Geriatrics Society, 46*(2), 216–225.
30. Lotkey, P. A. (1998). Knee arthroplasty: Alternatives, techniques, and management issues. DVT prophylaxis options: Facts and fictions. *Orthopaedics, 21*(9), 1025–1026.
31. Maher, A. B. (1998). Assessment of the musculoskeletal system. In A. B. Maher, S. W. Salmond, & T. A. Pellino (Eds.), *Orthopaedic - nursing* (2nd ed.). Philadelphia: W. B. Saunders, pp. 168–189.
32. Morris, N. S. (1999). Complications associated with orthopaedic surgery. In *An introduction to orthopaedic nursing* (2nd ed.). Pitman, NJ: National Association of Orthopaedic Nurses, p. 123–145.
33. Mosher, C. M. (1999). Total hip and knee replacement. In *An introduction to orthopaedic nursing* (2nd ed.). Pitman, NJ: National Association of Orthopaedic Nurses, pp. 67–81.
34. Osteoarthritis: Old scourge, new hope (1996). *Consumer Reports on Health, 8*(1), 3–5.
35. Pemberton, C. (1995). Diagnosing and treating bone metastases. *Nursing Times, 91*(3), 33–34.
36. Piasecki, P. (1996). Nursing care of the patient with metastatic bone disease. *Orthopaedic Nursing, 15*(4), 25–33.
37. Piasecki, P. (1996). Tumors. In S. W. Salmond, N. E. Mooney, & L. A. Verdisco (Eds.), *Core curriculum for orthopaedic nursing* (3rd ed.). Pitman, NJ: National Association of Orthopaedic Nurses, pp. 451–471.
38. Rodts, M. F. (1996). Spine. In S. W. Salmond, N. E. Mooney, & L. A. Verdisco (Eds.), *Core curriculum for orthopaedic nursing* (3rd ed.). Pitman, NJ: National Association of Orthopaedic Nurses, pp. 397–414.
39. Rodts, M. F. (1998). Disorders of the spine. In A. B. Maher, S. W. Salmond, & T. A. Pellino (Eds.), *Orthopaedic nursing* (2nd ed.). Philadelphia: W. B. Saunders, pp. 545–585.
40. Salmond, W. S. (1998). Infections of the musculoskeletal system. In A. B. Maher, S. W. Salmond, & T. A. Pellino (Eds.), *Orthopaedic nursing* (2nd ed.). Philadelphia: W. B. Saunders, pp. 804–858.
41. Schultz, D. L. (1995). The role of the neuroscience nurse in lumbar fusion. *Journal of Neuroscience Nursing, 27*(2), 90–95.
42. Stein, R. R. (1999). An overview of the lumbar spine. In *An introduction to orthopaedic nursing* (2nd ed.). Pitman, NJ: National Association of Orthopaedic Nurses, pp. 83–95.
43. Stephenson, S. (1996). Arthritis and degenerative conditions. In V. R. Masear (Ed.), *Primary care orthopaedics.* Philadelphia: W. B. Saunders, pp. 329–336.
44. U.S. Department of Health and Human Services, Public Health Service. (1991). *Healthy People 2000: National health promotion and disease prevention objectives.* Washington, DC: U.S. Government Printing Office.
45. What's new in drugs: Experts recommend acetaminophen for osteoarthritis (1996). *RN, 59*(3), 70.
46. Whittington, C. F. (1998). Exercise- and sport-related disorders. In A. B. Maher, S. W. Salmond, & T. A. Pellino (Eds.), *Orthopaedic nursing* (2nd ed.). Philadelphia: W. B. Saunders, pp. 746–768.

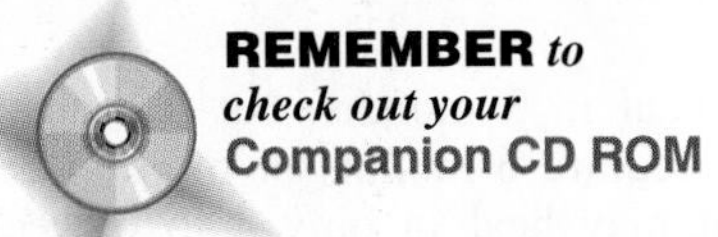

CHAPTER 27

Management of Clients with Musculoskeletal Trauma or Overuse

Dottie Roberts

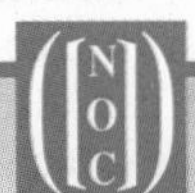

NURSING OUTCOMES CLASSIFICATION
for Nursing Diagnoses—Clients with Musculoskeletal Trauma or Overuse

Impaired Physical Mobility
Ambulation: Walking
Joint Movement: Active
Mobility Level
Pain
Comfort Level
Pain Control
Pain: Disruptive Effects
Risk of Constipation
Bowel Elimination
Hydration
Knowledge: Medication
Medication Response
Mobility Level
Self-Care: Nonparenteral Medication
Risk for Impaired Skin Integrity
Immobility Consequences: Physiological
Tissue Integrity: Skin and Mucous Membranes
Risk for Infection
Tissue Integrity: Skin and Mucous Membranes
Treatment Behavior: Illness or Injury
Risk for Peripheral Neurovascular Dysfunction
Joint Movement: Active
Mobility Level
Tissue Perfusion: Peripheral
Self-Care Deficit
Self-Care: Activities of Daily Living (ADL)
Self-Care: Bathing
Self-Care: Dressing
Self-Care: Grooming
Self-Care: Hygiene

Anyone who has experienced a broken bone or a ligament strain can appreciate the challenges facing a client who is recovering from musculoskeletal trauma or overuse. Activity restrictions and assistive devices both complicate and facilitate the healing process. Types of fractures and their medical and nursing management as well as common soft tissue injuries are discussed in this chapter.

FRACTURES

More than 58 million Americans experience injury from accidents each year. Trauma is the leading cause of death among people aged 1 to 37 years; motor vehicle accidents and falls are the most common causes of accidental death.[31] Because 4 million injured people are treated in hospitals each year, trauma also adds over $200 billion to the cost of health care in the United States.[36] Fractures account for a high percentage of traumatic injuries. Fractures occur in all age groups, but their incidence peaks in both males and females between the ages of 6 and 16 and in elderly people. Fractures can create significant changes in a person's quality of life by causing activity restrictions, disability, and economic loss.

A fracture is any disruption in the normal continuity of a bone. When fracture occurs, surrounding soft tissue is often damaged as well. A radiograph (x-ray) may confirm the bone injury, but it does not show evidence of the torn muscles or ligaments, severed nerves, or ruptured blood vessels that can complicate the client's recovery. To care appropriately for the client with a fracture, the nurse needs a concise and accurate description of the injury.

Etiology and Risk Factors

Fracture results from mechanical overload of the bone, when more stress is placed on the bone than it can absorb. The actual amount of force necessary to cause a fracture may vary greatly, depending in part on the characteristics of the bone itself. A client with a metabolic bone disease such as osteoporosis, for example, may experience fracture with even minor trauma because the bone is weakened by the pre-existing disorder. Fracture may result from direct force, as when a moving object strikes the body area over the bone. Force may also be applied indirectly, as when a powerful muscle contraction pulls against the bone. In addition, stress or fatigue can lead to fracture because of the bone's decreased ability to withstand mechanical force.

The two types of bone also respond differently to mechanical load. *Cortical* bone, the compact outer layer, is porous and can tolerate more stress along its axis (longitudinally) than across the bone. *Cancellous,* or *spongy,* bone is the dense inner bone material. It contains web-like formations and spaces filled with red marrow that make it better able to absorb force than is cortical bone. Bony projections, called trabeculae, separate the spaces and are arranged along lines of stress, making cancellous bone even stronger.

Predisposition to fracture results from biologic conditions such as osteopenia (caused by steroid use or Cushing's syndrome) or osteogenesis imperfecta, which alters the strength and composition of the bone. Neoplasms can also increase the risk for fracture. Postmenopausal estrogen loss and protein malnutrition lead to decreased bone mass. For persons with healthy bones, fractures can result from high-risk recreation or employment-related activities (e.g., skateboarding, rock climbing). Victims of domestic violence are also among people treated for traumatic injuries.

Pathophysiology

When fracture occurs, muscles that were attached to the ends of the bone are disrupted. The muscles can undergo spasm and pull the fracture fragments out of position. Large muscle groups can create massive spasms that displace even large bones, such as the femur. Although the proximal portion of the fractured bone remains in place, the distal portion can become displaced in response to both the causative force and the spasm in the associated muscles. Fracture fragments may be displaced sideways, at an angle (angulated), or as overriding bone segments. They may also be rotated or offset.

In addition, the periosteum and blood vessels in the cortex and marrow of the fractured bone are disrupted. Soft tissue damage frequently occurs. Bleeding occurs from both the soft tissue and from the damaged ends of the bone. In the medullary canal, a hematoma forms between the fracture fragments and beneath the periosteum. Bone tissue surrounding the fracture site dies, creating an intense inflammatory response. Vasodilation, edema, pain, loss of function, exudation of plasma and leukocytes, and infiltration of other white blood cells result. These processes serve as the initial step in bone healing.

Bone Healing

Unlike other specialized body tissues, bone healing occurs uniquely through tissue regeneration rather than scar tissue formation. Fracture repair occurs by the same mechanism as bone formation during normal growth and maintenance, with organized mineralization of newly synthesized bone matrix followed by remodeling to form mature bone. Adequate circulation to the fracture site and adequate fragment immobilization are crucial for effective bone healing. Factors such as the presence of systemic or bone diseases, the age and general health of the client, the type of fracture, and the treatment can also affect the speed and success of healing. For example, an impacted fracture may heal within several weeks but a displaced fracture may take months or even years to heal. A radial or ulnar fracture may heal in 3 months, but fractures in the tibia or femur may require 6 months or more to heal. A fracture in an infant may heal in only 4 to 6 weeks, but the same fracture in an adolescent may require 6 to 10 weeks to heal. The rate of fracture healing is not significantly decreased in older adults unless the client also has a metabolic disorder such as osteoporosis.

Fracture healing occurs in five stages (Table 27–1). These stages do not occur independently but tend to overlap as bone healing progresses. They are sometimes combined into a three-stage process.

Factors Affecting Bone Healing

If fracture healing is altered in any of the five stages, problems with bone union can result. Factors affecting bone healing are summarized in Box 27–1.

Most fractures heal adequately without any problems, but biologic interventions may be employed to stimulate fracture healing. For example, autogenous or allogeneic bone grafts can be used to stimulate bone growth. Injection or implantation of autogenous bone marrow is another intervention that is the subject of current research in fracture healing. A three-dimensional implant or graft can also be used as an aid to bone healing by supporting the attachment, spreading, division, and differentiation of bone cells. Osteoinduction involves the use of substances such as platelet-derived growth factor to stimulate bone healing.

Clinical Manifestations

Fracture diagnosis is based on the client's clinical manifestations and history, physical examination, and radiographic findings. Some fractures are immediately obvious; others are detected only on x-ray. Use of the correct radiologic view is essential for adequate evaluation of the suspected fracture. Two views (e.g., anteroposterior and lateral) taken at right angles are generally considered to be the minimal number needed for evaluation, and they should include the joints above and below the suspected fracture to identify additional dislocations or subluxations. Abnormal x-ray findings include soft tissue edema or displacement of air in relation to a shift of the bone after injury. Radiographs of the fractured bone show an alteration in its normal contour and a disruption of the normal joint relationship. The fracture line itself demonstrates increased radiolucency (Fig. 27–1). Radiographs are commonly taken before fracture reduction, after reduction, and then periodically during bone healing.

Physical assessment may reveal any of the following clinical manifestations:

Deformity. Swelling from local hemorrhage may cause deformity at the fracture site. Muscle spasms can cause limb shortening, a rotational deformity, or angulation. In comparison to the uninjured side, the fracture site may also have altered curves.

Swelling. Edema may appear quickly as a result of localization of serous fluid at the fracture site and extravasation of blood into surrounding tissues.

Bruising (ecchymosis). Bruising results from subcutaneous bleeding at the fracture site.

Muscle spasm. Frequently accompanying fractures, involuntary muscle spasm actually serves as a natural splint to decrease further motion of fracture fragments.

TABLE 27–1 STAGES OF BONE HEALING

Stage	Diagram	Description	Time
Stage I: Hematoma stage or inflammatory stage	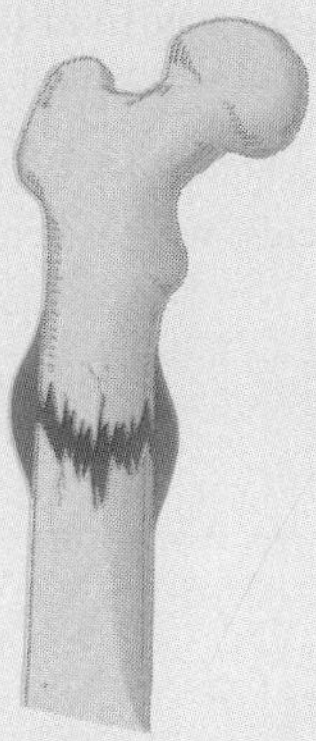	Immediate formation of a hematoma at the site of the fracture. The amount of damage to the bone, as well as to surrounding soft tissue and blood vessels, determines the size of the hematoma. The blood forms a clot among the fracture fragments, providing a small amount of stabilization. Necrosis of adjacent bone occurs in direct relation to the loss of blood supply to the affected region and will extend to the area where collateral circulation begins. Vascular dilatation occurs in response to the accumulation of dead cells and debris at the fracture site, and exudation of fibrin-rich plasma initiates the migration of phagocytic cells to the area of injury. If the vascular supply to the fracture site is inadequate, stage I healing will be greatly impaired.	1–3 days
Stage II: Fibrocartilage formation	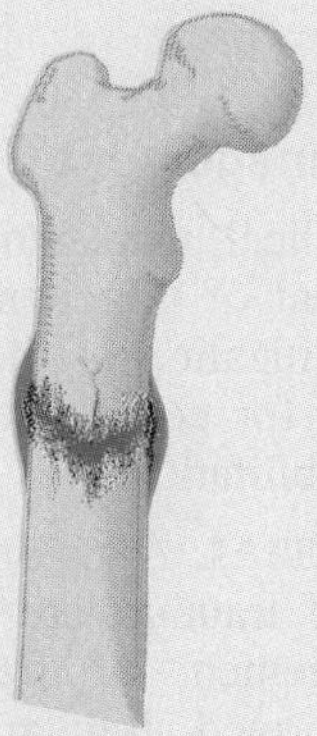	Fibroblasts, osteoblasts, and chondroblasts migrate to the fracture site as a result of the acute inflammation and form fibrocartilage. Organization of the hematoma then offers the foundation for stage II bone and tissue healing. Osteoblastic activity is stimulated by periosteal trauma, and bone formation occurs quickly. The periosteum is elevated away from the bone, and within a few days, the combination of periosteal elevation and granulation tissue formation creates a collar around the end of each fracture fragment. As the collars advance, they form a bridge across the fracture site. This early formation of fibrous tissue is sometimes called the *primary callus,* and it results in gradually increasing stability for the fracture.	3 days to 2 weeks
Stage III: Callus formation	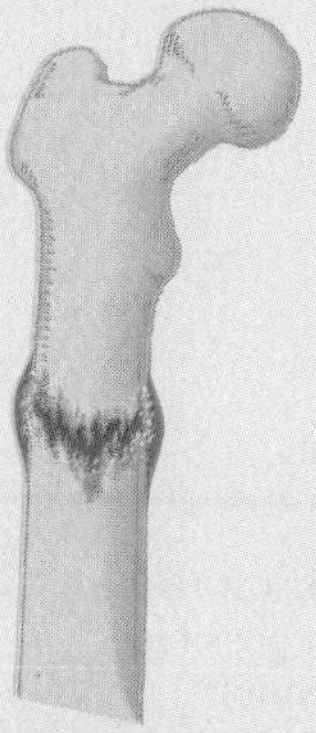	Granulation tissue matures into a provisional callus (procallus) as newly formed cartilage and bone matrix disperse through the primary callus. The procallus is large and loosely woven. It is generally wider than the normal diameter of the injured bone. The procallus secures the bone fragments, extending some distance beyond the fracture site to serve as a temporary splint, but it does not provide strength. If cells are distant from the blood supply and oxygen tensions are relatively low, cartilage is formed. When calcium is deposited in the collagen network of the granulation tissue, fibrous bone forms. Proper bone alignment is essential during stage III. This stage may be the most important in determining successful healing, and if it is slowed or interrupted, the final two stages cannot occur. Delayed union or non-union can then result.	2–6 weeks
Stage IV: Ossification	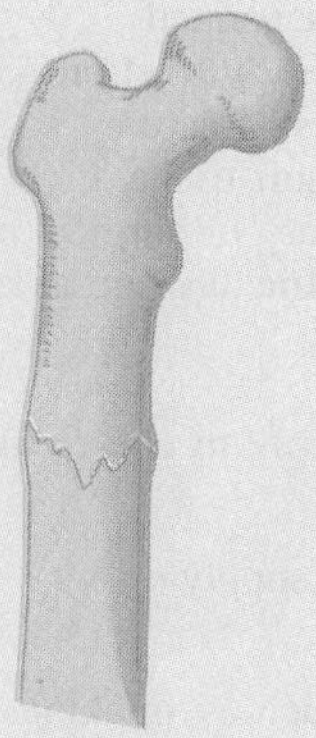	A permanent callus of rigid bone crosses the fracture gap between the periosteum and the cortex to join the fragments. In addition, medullary callus formation occurs internally to establish continuity between the marrow cavities. Trabecular bone gradually replaces the callus along stress lines. Bone union, which can be confirmed by x-ray, is said to have occurred when there is no motion with gentle stress and no tenderness with direct pressure at the fracture site. Weight-bearing in lower extremity fractures is also pain free after bone union.	3 weeks to 6 months

Table continued on following page

TABLE 27–1 STAGES OF BONE HEALING *Continued*

Stage	Diagram	Description	Time
Stage V: Consolidation and remodeling		Unnecessary callus is resorbed or chiseled away from the healing bone. The process of bone resorption and deposition along stress lines allows bone to withstand the loads applied to it. The actual amount and timing of remodeling depends on the stresses imposed on the bone by muscles, weight-bearing, and age.	6 weeks to 1 year

Pain. If the client is neurologically intact, pain always accompanies fracture; the intensity and severity of the pain differ from client to client. Pain is usually continuous, increasing in severity until the fracture is immobilized. It results from muscle spasm, overriding of fracture fragments, or damage to adjacent structures.

Tenderness. Tenderness over the fracture site is caused by underlying injuries.

Loss of function. Any loss of function results either from pain caused by the fracture or from loss of the lever-arm function in the affected extremity. Paralysis may be caused by nerve damage.

Abnormal mobility and crepitus. These manifestations are caused by motion in the middle of a bone or by fracture fragments rubbing together to create grating sensations or sounds.

Neurovascular changes. Neurovascular injury results from damage to peripheral nerves or to the associated vascular structures. The client may complain of numbness.

Shock. The client who experiences blood loss or other injuries may need treatment for shock.

FRACTURE CLASSIFICATION

More than 150 types of fractures have been identified according to various classification methods. See Table 27–2 for common descriptors.

The simplest classification method is based on whether the fracture is *closed* or *open* to the environment. A closed fracture has intact skin over the site of injury, whereas the open fracture is characterized by a break in the skin over the bone injury. Tissue damage can be extensive with open fractures, which are graded according to their severity:

Grade I. The wound is smaller than 1 cm; contamination is minimal.

Grade II. The wound is larger than 1 cm; contamination is moderate.

Grade III. The wound exceeds 6 to 8 cm; there is extensive damage to soft tissue, nerve, and tendon; and there is a high degree of contamination.

Because the wound communicates with the external environment, the risk of infection must be promptly recognized and addressed.

Outcome Management

Medical Management

The goals of medical management include prompt and thorough assessment of the client to discover all injuries, reduction and stabilization of the fracture with immobilization, monitoring for complications, and eventual remobilization and rehabilitation.

THOROUGH INITIAL ASSESSMENT

Basic principles of trauma care must be followed during emergency management of fractures. Assessment and treatment are performed simultaneously as the rescuer addresses the general condition of the injured client. During primary assessment, the rescuer focuses on airway man-

BOX 27–1 Factors Affecting Bone Healing

Favorable

Location

- Good blood supply at bone ends
- Flat bones

Minimal damage to soft tissue
Anatomic reduction possible
Effective immobilization
Weight-bearing on long bones

Unfavorable

Fragments widely separated
Fragments distracted by traction
Severely comminuted fracture
Severe damage to soft tissue
Bone loss from injury or surgical excision
Motion/rotation at fracture site as a result of inadequate fixation
Infection
Impaired blood supply to one or more bone fragments
Location

- Decreased blood supply
- Midshaft

Health behaviors such as smoking, alcohol use

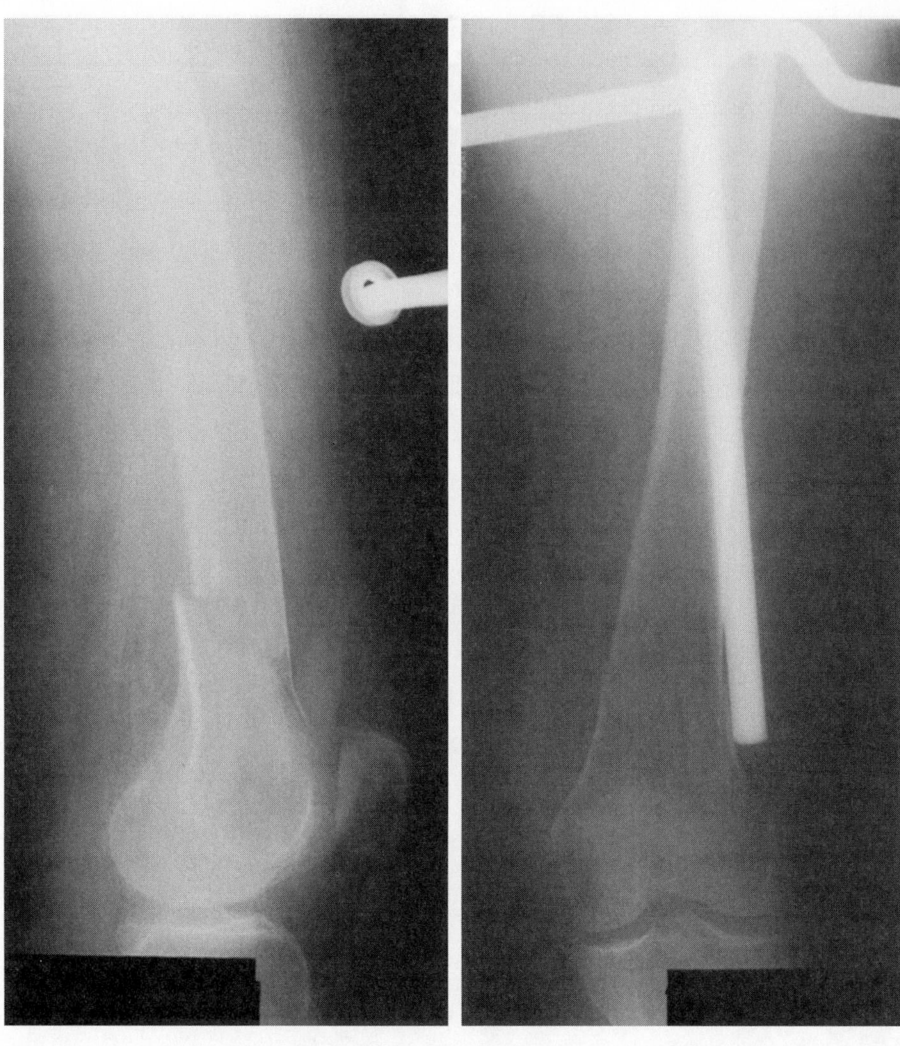

FIGURE 27–1 Fracture of the supracondylar femur. (Note radiolucency of fracture line.) Reduction of the fracture with traction. The fracture was eventually pinned.

agement, bleeding, and manifestations of shock. Any potentially life-threatening injuries must be stabilized immediately and emergency assistance summoned to transport the client to a medical facility for additional intervention. An injured client should not be moved unless the current location is not safe.

Because most fractures do not pose a serious threat to life, their management becomes a secondary priority in trauma care. Suspected injuries to extremities should be carefully splinted and moved as little as possible because multiple fractures frequently occur in the same limb. If the client complains of muscle spasm after a cervical spine or head injury, a fracture or dislocation is presumed to be present until radiographs can be performed and interpreted. The rescuer must stabilize the affected area and help the client remain still. An unconscious client should receive emergency management while the rescuer carefully notes any spontaneous movement as well as the client's position, head, and extremities. The rescuer performs a neurologic assessment that is based on the type of known or suspected injury. Any soft tissue damage must also be assessed because the injury may indicate a fracture site. Open fractures should be covered with sterile dressings and remain covered to prevent additional contamination until a thorough examination can occur in the nearest hospital.

When the client reaches the emergency department, the neurologic condition and vital signs are closely monitored, and the client is kept on *nil per os* (nothing by mouth; NPO) status in case surgery is indicated. Health care providers carefully examine the injured area and obtain the client's history. Details of the injury are very helpful in determining the probable type of fracture as well as associated injuries. If the client was in a motor vehicle accident, for example, was he or she sitting in the back or front seat? Was the client wearing a seat belt? What was the angle of impact? Was the client pulled from the car after a major collision? Or did the injury occur as a result of a fall on a hip or an outstretched arm?

Arterial damage is a possible early complication after fracture. The arteries may have been contused or lacerated, or they may have been constricted by tightly applied bandages or casts. With a displaced fracture, a hematoma may develop in the soft tissue as a result of damage to large blood vessels. Other indications of arterial damage include a variable pulse or absence of a pulse, poor capillary return, swelling, pallor or patchy cyanosis distal to the injury, pain, paresthesias, or coolness of an extremity as a result of poorly filled veins. Blood loss may be considerable, particularly with femur or pelvic fractures, and hypovolemic shock may become another complica-

Text continued on page 596

TABLE 27–2 COMMON TYPES OF FRACTURES

Name by Fracture	Description	Illustration
APPEARANCE		
Burst	Characterized by multiple pieces of bone; often occurs at bone ends or in vertebrae	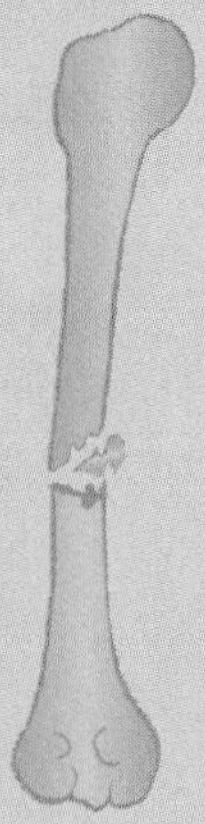
Comminuted	More than one fracture line; more than two bone fragments; fragments may be splintered or crushed	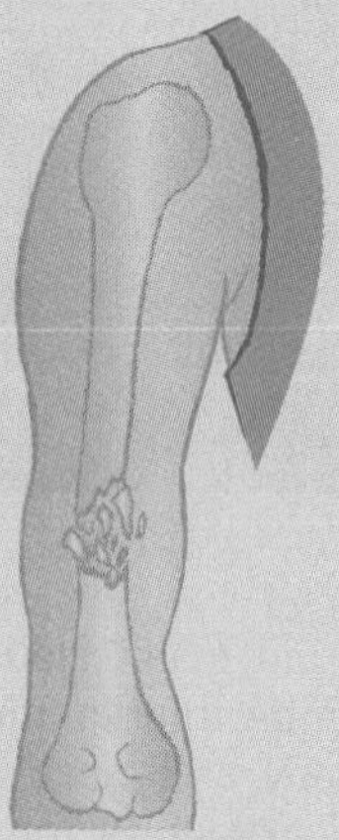
Complete	Break across the entire section of bone, dividing it into distinct fragments; frequently displaced	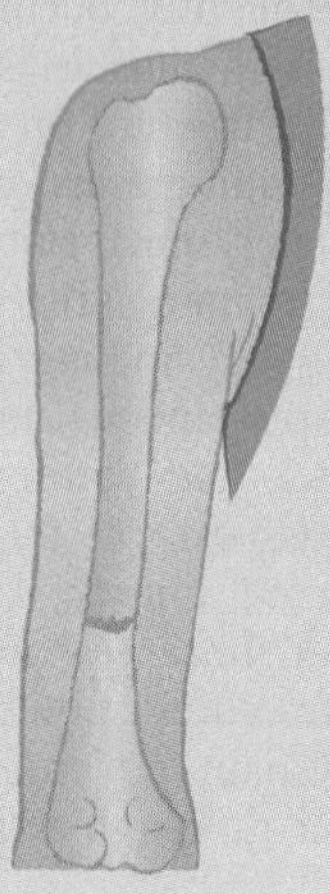

TABLE 27–2 **COMMON TYPES OF FRACTURES** *Continued*

Name by Fracture	Description	Illustration
Displaced	Fragments out of normal position at fracture site	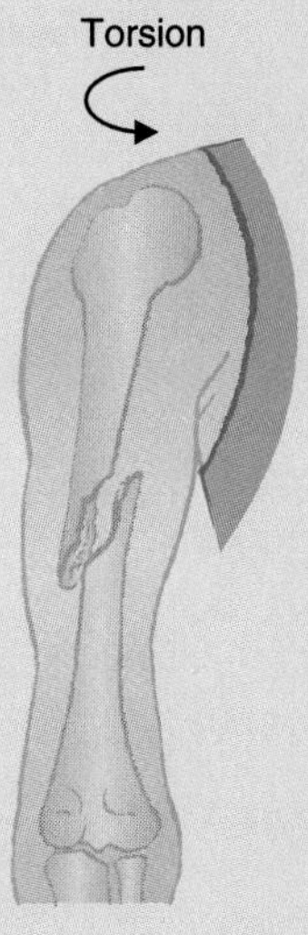 Torsion
Incomplete	Fracture occurs through only one cortex of the bone; usually nondisplaced	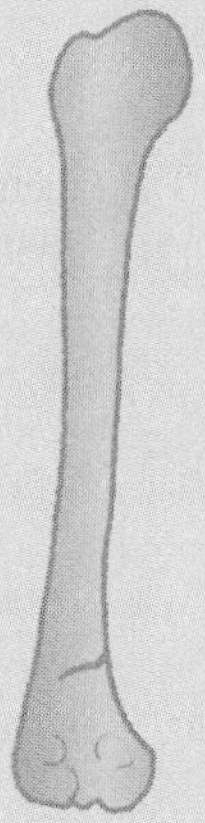
Linear	Fracture line is intact; fracture is caused by minor to moderate force applied directly to the bone	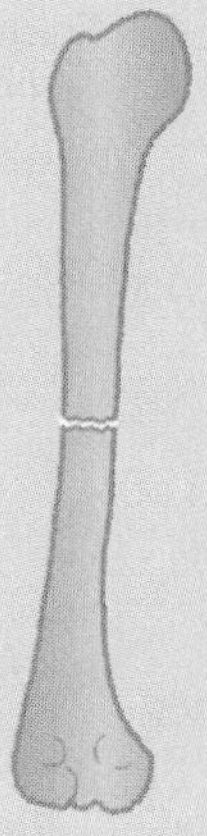

TABLE 27–2 COMMON TYPES OF FRACTURES *Continued*

Name by Fracture	Description	Illustration
Longitudinal	Fracture line extends in the direction of the bone's longitudinal axis	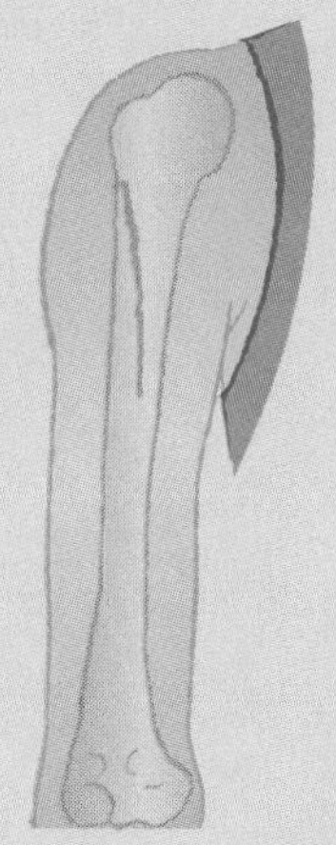
Nondisplaced	Fragments aligned at fracture site	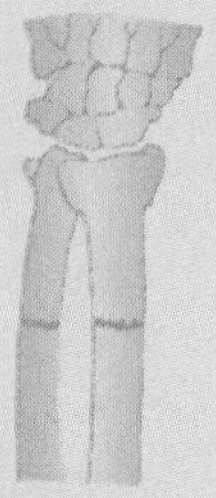
Oblique	Fracture line occurs at approximately 45-degree angle across the longitudinal axis of bone	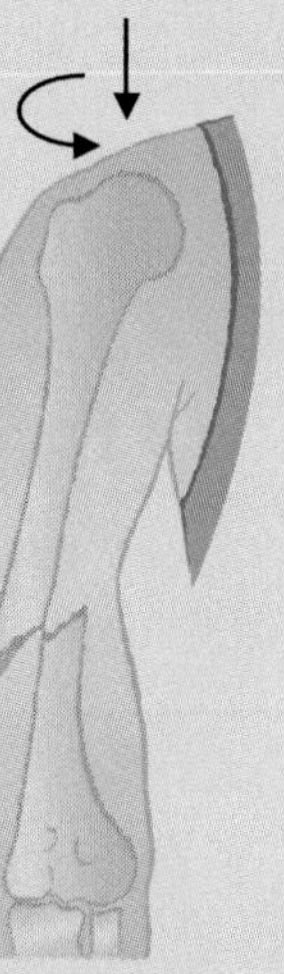
Spiral	Fracture line results from twisting force; forms a spiral encircling the bone	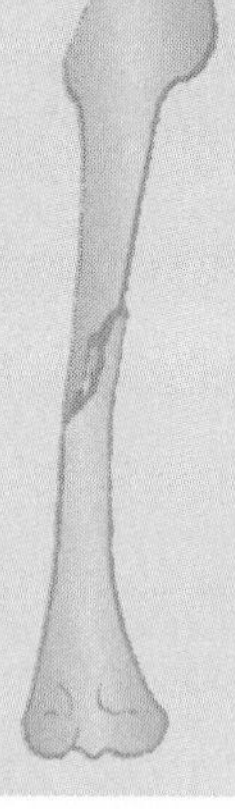

TABLE 27–2 COMMON TYPES OF FRACTURES *Continued*

Name by Fracture	Description	Illustration
Stellate	Fracture lines radiate from one central point	
Transverse	Fracture line occurs at 90-degree angle to longitudinal axis of bone	
GENERAL DESCRIPTION		
Avulsion	Bone fragments are torn away from body of the bone at site of attachment of a ligament or tendon	
Compression	Bone buckles and eventually cracks as the result of unusual loading force applied to its longitudinal axis	

TABLE 27–2 COMMON TYPES OF FRACTURES *Continued*

Name by Fracture	Description	Illustration
Greenstick	Incomplete fracture in which one side of the cortex is broken and the other side is flexed but intact	
Impacted	Telescoped fracture, with one fragment driven into another	
ANATOMIC LOCATION		
Colles'	Fracture within the last inch of the distal radius; distal fragment is displaced in a position of dorsal and medial deviation	
Pott's	Fracture of the distal fibula, seriously disrupting the tibiofibular articulation; a piece of the medial malleolus may be chipped off as a result of rupture of the internal lateral ligament	

tion. Extensive bleeding can occur even with closed fractures, and emergency surgery may become necessary; loss of blood supply to the fracture can result in areas of bone necrosis. Soft tissue infection can easily follow open fracture, and for optimal effectiveness, antibiotic therapy should begin as soon as possible after the injury.

Reducing Fractures

The first step in management of a displaced fracture is reduction: the manipulation of the fracture to restore alignment, position, and length by bringing the fragments into close approximation. Reduction, which is also called *bone setting,* alleviates compression or stretching of nerves and blood vessels. Because reduction is generally painful, sedation or local or general anesthesia may be needed.

Not all fractures require reduction. Fragments of a nondisplaced fracture, for example, are already in proper alignment. Splinting or casting allows the alignment to be maintained as the fracture heals. A few other fractures cannot be adequately splinted and instead are treated simply by resting the affected area until healing occurs (e.g., distal phalangeal fractures).

When a fracture of an extremity divides a bone into two fragments, the fragments are referred to as *proximal* (nearer the trunk) and *distal* (farther from the trunk).

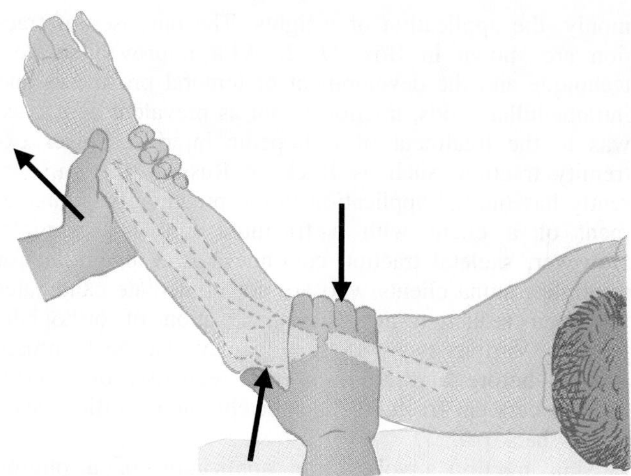

FIGURE 27–2 Closed reduction to realign a supracondylar fracture.

Because of its muscle attachment and location, the proximal fragment cannot be manipulated or moved when the fractured bone is being set. Instead, the distal fragment is moved to realign it with the proximal bone segment. Reduction methods can be used alone or in combination.

Closed Reduction

To perform closed reduction, a health care provider applies manual traction to move the fracture fragments and restore bone alignment (Fig. 27–2). Closed reduction should be performed as soon as possible after injury to decrease the client's risk for loss of function, to prevent or delay joint degeneration (traumatic arthritis), and to minimize the possible deforming effects of the injury.

Manual reduction is accomplished through four maneuvers, beginning with a longitudinal pull on the distal end of the fracture or extremity. Because it reverses the mechanism of injury, this pull overcomes any initial muscle spasm, any effects on limb length, and the overriding of bone fragments. Second, the bone ends of the fracture must be disengaged from each other. This is sometimes accomplished by rotating the distal portion of the fracture. In the third maneuver, the fracture fragments are realigned. This is a complex step because forces from various muscle groups have held the fragments in their new positions. Finally, the distraction force is released while alignment is maintained.

Because gravity, weight-bearing, and muscle contraction can again move the fragments, an immobilization device must be applied after x-ray studies have confirmed bone alignment. The immobilizer most commonly used after closed reduction is a cast, a temporary device made of plaster of Paris (anhydrous calcium sulfate) or synthetic materials such as fiberglass or thermoplastic polymer. Casts are used for several purposes in addition to immobilization: prevention or correction of deformity; maintenance, support, and protection of realigned bone; and promotion of healing in order to allow early weight-bearing for ambulation. Casts may be applied in a hospital emergency department, in the operating room, or at the client's bedside in the hospital. They are also commonly applied in a physician's office or clinic.

Synthetic materials are used to construct a strong, light-weight cast that sets in about 5 minutes. They also come in a variety of colors and patterns that can enhance self-esteem in both young and older clients after injury. Synthetic casts maintain their shape and firmness even if they become wet, but they must be dried thoroughly to prevent skin maceration. If there is no incision under the cast, synthetic materials can be dried with a hair blow dryer on a low setting; however, several hours are needed for the cast to dry thoroughly.

Plaster of Paris bandages are individual rolls of precut crinoline impregnated with plaster. They come in various sizes, and the body part to be casted determines the amount of plaster to be used. Plaster casts take at least 24 hours longer than synthetic casts to dry, and they lose their shape if they are allowed to get wet again.

Open Reduction and Internal Fixation

To perform open reduction, the surgeon makes an incision and realigns the fracture fragments under direct visualization. Open reduction is the treatment of choice for compound fractures that are comminuted or accompanied by severe neurovascular injury; it is also required if fracture fragments are widely separated or if soft tissue is interposed between pieces of bone.

Open reduction is usually performed in combination with internal fixation for femoral and joint fractures. Screws, plates, pins, wires, or nails may be used to maintain alignment of the fracture fragments (Fig. 27–3). Rods may also be placed through the fragments or fixed to the side of the bone, or they may be inserted directly

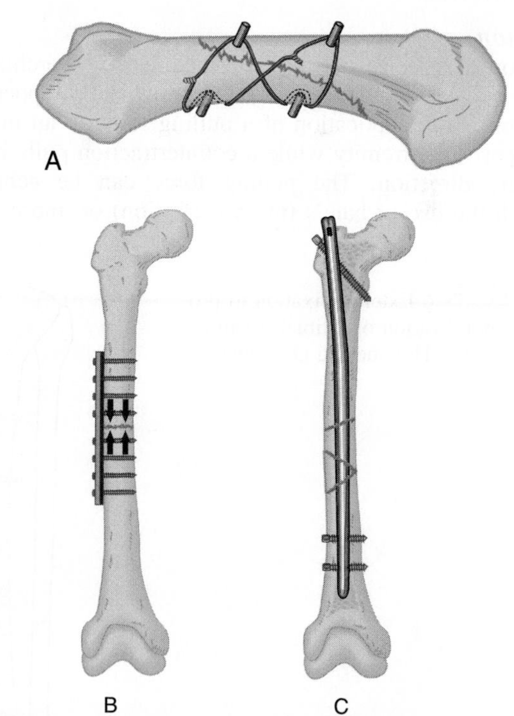

FIGURE 27–3 Examples of different types of internal fixation devices. *A,* Tension band wiring with Kirschner wires for a fracture of the phalanx. *B,* Compression plate and screws in the lateral aspect of the femur. *C,* Sliding hip screw. *D,* Intramedullary nail fixed to both the proximal and distal ends of the femur.

into the bone's medullary cavity. Internal fixation provides essential immobilization and helps prevent deformity, but it is not a substitute for bone healing. If proper healing fails to occur, the internal fixation device may actually loosen or break as a result of stress.

External Fixation

Depending on the client's condition and the physician's judgment, external fixation devices may be used for fracture fragment immobilization (Fig. 27–4). If, for example, soft tissue damage precludes the use of a cast, external fixation would be indicated for fracture immobilization. External fixation devices maintain position for unstable fractures and for weakened muscles, and they support areas with tissue or bone infection. They allow the client to use contiguous joints while the affected area remains immobilized. External fixation may also be indicated for bony non-union if fracture healing has not been successful after a certain time. Common sites for external fixation include the face and jaw, extremities, pelvis, ribs, fingers, and toes. Pins used in external fixation vary in number, length, and thickness on the basis of the treatment area.

Client selection is critical to the successful use of external fixation. Any potential problems with compliance should be thoroughly discussed with the client and family, including the effects of external fixation on the client's lifestyle. Noncompliance with the medical regimen can lead to pin loosening, loss of fracture stabilization, and infection. Specific activity orders are written after application of an external fixator, with special attention to weight-bearing status when the pelvis or a lower extremity is involved.

Traction

Traction has been used to treat fractures since prehistoric times, and its principles were well known to Hippocrates. Traction is the application of a pulling force to an injured body part or extremity while a countertraction pulls in the opposite direction. The pulling force can be achieved through the use of hands (manual traction) or, more commonly, the application of weights. The purposes of traction are shown in Box 27–2. With improved surgical technique and the development of femoral prostheses and intramedullary rods, traction is not as prevalent as it once was in the treatment of orthopedic injuries. Lower extremity traction, such as Buck or Russell traction, currently has limited application in the preoperative management of a client with a fractured hip, for example. However, skeletal traction continues to be an option for multiple trauma clients who are not immediate candidates for open reduction and internal fixation of orthopedic injuries. Various types of traction may also be treatment options before and after surgical reduction of injuries such as cervical fractures, and for chronic conditions such as low back pain.

Skin traction involves the application of a pulling force directly to the skin through the use of skin strips, boots, or foam splints. Cervical halters and pelvic belts allow traction to be applied to the neck or pelvis. Skin traction bears a low longitudinal force load (5 to 7 pounds), which gives it minimal effectiveness. Because of the risk of skin breakdown, this type of traction should be used only temporarily.

Skeletal traction uses pins to apply force to the bone. With skeletal traction, a direct force can be applied after the physician aseptically inserts stainless steel pins through the bone itself. The most common sites for pin insertion are the distal femur, the proximal tibia, and the proximal ulna. Skeletal traction can be tolerated for longer periods than can skin traction. Weights may reach 15 pounds, although 7 to 10 pounds are more commonly used.

In addition to the mode of application, traction can be categorized as *static* (continuous) or *dynamic* (intermittent). Suspension may also be running or straight (exerting a direct pull on the affected part) or balanced (exerting a pull on the affected part and also supporting the extremity in a splint). Table 27–3 describes major types of traction.

Major disadvantages include the potential need for pro-

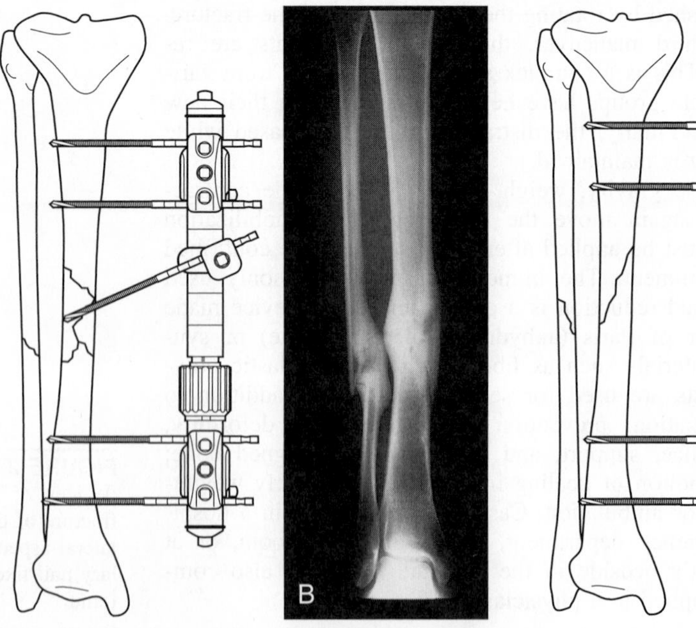

FIGURE 27–4 External fixation to provide immobilization of a tibial fracture. (From Stryker Howmedica Osteonics.)

BOX 27–2 Purposes of Traction

- Reduce, realign, and promote healing of fractured bones
- Decrease muscle spasms that may accompany fractures or follow surgical reduction
- Prevent soft tissue damage through immobilization
- Treat deformities
- Rest an inflamed, diseased, or painful joint
- Reduce an treat dislocations and subluxations
- Prevent the development of contractures
- Reduce muscle spasms associated with low back pain or cervical whiplash
- Expand a joint space during arthroscopy or prior to major joint reconstruction

From Ceccio, C. M. (1999). Key concepts in the care of patients in traction. In *An introduction to orthopaedic nursing* (2nd ed.). Pitman, NJ: National Association of Orthopaedic Nurses.

longed bed rest and the resulting effects of extended immobility. Long-term hospitalization is not always indicated if the client in traction can qualify for home care nursing services or, depending on the type of traction, receive additional treatment as an outpatient.

Complications After Fracture

Continuously assess the client with orthopedic trauma for potential complications and then intervene quickly to minimize effects. Certain client characteristics increase the likelihood of complications, particularly after surgical repair of fractures. These include age, the presence of other health problems (co-morbidities), and the client's use of medications that affect bleeding, such as warfarin, corticosteroids, and nonsteroidal anti-inflammatory drugs (NSAIDs).

Nerve Injury

Bone fragments and tissue edema associated with the injury can cause nerve damage. Be alert for pallor and coolness of the client's affected extremity, paralysis or paresthesia, complaints of increasing pain, or changes in the client's ability to move the extremity.

Compartment Syndrome

Muscle compartments in the upper and lower extremities are enclosed by tough, inelastic fascial tissue that does not expand if the muscle swells (Fig. 27–5). Edema that occurs in response to a fracture can lead to an increase in compartment pressure that reduces capillary blood perfusion. When the local blood supply is unable to meet the tissue's metabolic demands, ischemia begins. Compartment syndrome is a condition of compromised circulation related to progressively increased pressure in a confined space. It is caused by anything that decreases the compartment size, including external compression forces such as a tight cast or internal factors such as bleeding or edema. Continued ischemia results in histamine release by the affected muscles, leading to even greater edema and a further decrease in perfusion. An increase in lactic acid production causes more anaerobic metabolism and a sub-

TABLE 27–3 MAJOR TYPES OF TRACTION

Traction	Type	Common Conditions Treated	Duration
CERVICAL			
Chin halter	Skin	Severe strains or sprains; cervical trauma nerve root compression; torticollis	Intermittent
Skeletal tongs: Gardner-Wells, Crutchfield, Vinke	Skeletal	Fractures or dislocations of cervical or high thoracic vertebrae	Continuous
Halo traction	Skeletal	Fractures or dislocations of cervical or high thoracic vertebrae	Continuous
UPPER EXTREMITY			
Side-arm	Skin or skeletal	Vertical suspension to forearm	Continuous
Overhead/90-90	Skin or skeletal	Vertical traction to humerus; horizontal suspension to forearm	Continuous
Pelvic			
Pelvic belt or sling	Skin	Low back pain	Intermittent or continuous
LOWER EXTREMITY			
Buck	Skin	Hip and knee contracture; preoperative immobilization and muscle spasm relief for hip fractures	Continuous
Balanced suspension: Thomas ring and Pearson and Brady attachment	Skeletal	Used mainly with skeletal pins for supracondylar femur fracture; hip and knee contracture; postoperative positioning and immobilization	Continuous

Adapted from Bryant, G. G. (1998). Modalities for immobilization. In A. B. Maher, S. W. Salmond, & T. A. Pellino (Eds.), *Orthopaedic nursing* (2nd ed.). Philadelphia: W. B. Saunders; and from Ceccio, C. M. (1999). Key concepts in the care of patients in traction. In *An introduction to orthopaedic nursing* (2nd ed.). Pitman, NJ: National Association of Orthopaedic Nurses.

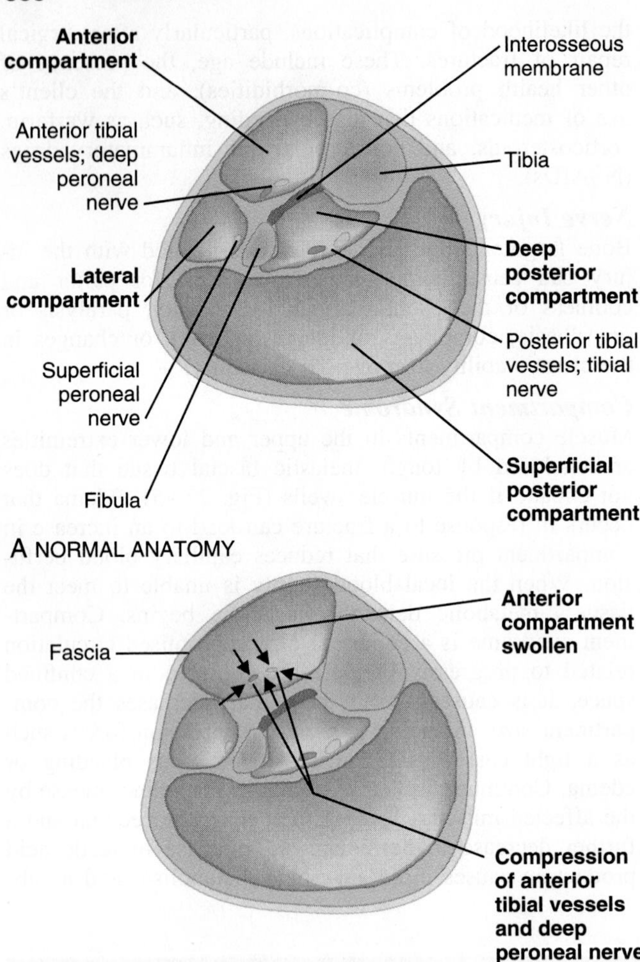

FIGURE 27–5 Compartments of the proximal third of the lower leg. The four compartments are (1) anterior, (2) lateral, (3) deep posterior, and (4) superficial posterior. As the compartment swells, it reaches its maximal size as a result of the inelastic fascia, which covers each compartment. As edema continues, pressure is exerted inward onto the nerves and vessels within the compartment.

sequent increase in blood flow that, in turn, increases the tissue pressure. This leads to a cycle of increasing compartment pressure. Compartment syndrome can occur anywhere in the body but occurs most often in the lower leg and forearm. If it goes unrecognized or untreated, the client can lose nerve and muscle function. Infection, myoglobinuria, and renal failure may follow, and amputation may be necessary.

Intracompartmental pressures can be measured by various monitors currently on the market. Normal compartment pressure is considered to be 0 to 8 mm Hg.[8] Although co-morbid conditions such as shock or compensatory hypertension can affect the client's response, compartment pressures ranging from 30 to 45 mm Hg have historically been considered high enough to cause tissue necrosis if treatment is not initiated. According to more recent medical consensus, imminent surgical intervention is not required for pressures greater than 40 mm Hg if the client's diastolic blood pressure remains high enough to perfuse the muscle compartment.[8]

The primary treatment of compartment syndrome is relief of the source of pressure. To accomplish this, the physician may order a constrictive bandage to be removed or a cast to be bivalved (to be described). The affected extremity should be kept at heart level because elevation above the heart actually decreases local arterial perfusion, further compromising blood flow. Adequate hydration is important for maintaining the client's mean arterial blood pressure. Pain should be managed to decrease the vasoconstrictive effects of the sympathetic nervous system.

If relief of external pressure is not enough to keep compartment pressures from rising, a fasciotomy may be necessary. An incision through the skin into the fascia of the muscle compartment allows for tissue expansion and restores blood flow by relieving pressure on the microcirculation. The incision is typically left open until the swelling decreases; the area is then loosely wrapped and the wrapping is left on for several days. The wound is closed by tertiary intention when edema has subsided.

Volkmann's Contracture

Volkmann's contracture is a limb deformity that results from unrelieved compartment syndrome. As prolonged pressure causes ischemia, muscle is gradually replaced by fibrous tissue that traps tendons and nerves. Tibial fractures have been linked to the development of this condition, which can lead to deformities such as cavus of the foot, equinus, and adduction of the forefoot with varus of the hindfoot. In the upper extremities, Volkmann's contracture most commonly occurs after fractures of the elbow and forearm or after crushing injuries of the forearm, or it is caused by tight bandages or casts. It can lead to a permanently stiff, claw-like deformity of the hand and arm. Contractures may be avoided through prompt recognition of manifestations of compartment syndrome, followed by limb splinting and compartment decompression as indicated.

Fat Embolism Syndrome

Fat embolism syndrome (FES) is a major cause of delayed recovery and mortality after fracture. The mechanical theory of FES origin describes the release of fat globules from the bone marrow into the venous circulation after fracture, particularly fractures of the long bones, pelvis, ribs, sternum, vertebrae, and clavicle. A biochemical or metabolic theory suggests that trauma leads to the release of fatty acids and neutral fats. Platelet aggregation and fat globule formation then occur. In reality, the pathophysiologic process of FES is unknown; it may include parts of both theories or reflect an entirely different, unknown etiology.

The deposit of embolic fat in the pulmonary circulation can lead to the rapid onset of a disorder similar to acute respiratory distress syndrome (ARDS). Perfusion pressure increases, and pulmonary vessels become engorged. As the lung becomes more rigid, the workload of the right side of the heart increases. The fat globules occluding the pulmonary circulation are hydrolyzed into free fatty acids that increase capillary permeability and activate lung surfactant. Hemorrhagic pulmonary edema and patchy alveolar collapse occur, leading to severe hypoxia. Diagnosis of FES is not made on the basis of a single manifestation, laboratory test, or radiologic study.

Instead, the client's presentation must be reviewed system by system.

While subclinical FES occurs in at least 50% of clients with pelvic or long bone fractures, the incidence of overt FES that necessitates intervention is only 1% to 5%.[32] FES varies with the number and type of fractures (open versus closed) and the treatment method. The syndrome occurs more often after closed fracture than after injury treated with external decompression. Clients who undergo open reduction with internal fixation (ORIF) within 24 to 48 hours of injury are at lower risk for FES than clients who are treated nonsurgically.

Prevention of FES begins with prudent treatment of long bone fractures, including careful handling, appropriate splinting, and avoidance of unnecessary manipulation of the injured area. In addition to prompt ORIF after injury, early aggressive resuscitation to prevent hypovolemic shock, adequate pain management, blood transfusion through a 20-μm filter, and prevention of sepsis are also considered standard preventive care.

Should FES occur, supportive treatment is directed at preserving the client's respiratory function. Oxygen is administered; intubation and continuous positive airway pressure (CPAP) are sometimes necessary. Steroids are commonly administered to decrease the inflammatory effects of the fatty acids on the alveolocapillary membrane. Hypotension is treated aggressively.

Deep Vein Thrombosis and Pulmonary Embolism

The client with orthopedic injuries is at high risk for thromboembolic conditions such as deep venous thrombosis (DVT) and pulmonary embolism (PE). DVT results from the formation of a blood clot (thrombus) in a deep vein in the lower extremity. If the thrombus travels into the pulmonary circulation, it is termed a PE.

Prevention of DVT is a primary goal. Clot prophylaxis is recommended through the use of pharmacologic agents such as subcutaneous fixed-dose low-molecular-weight (LMW) heparin or low-intensity oral anticoagulation. For appropriately selected clients, physical-mechanical measures such as intermittent pneumatic compression devices or elastic stockings may also have a role in DVT prevention. DVT is fully discussed in Chapter 53.

Infection

Infection continues to be a cause of morbidity among clients who have open or surgically repaired fractures. Pathogens can contaminate an open fracture or may be introduced at the time of surgery. Contamination during the postoperative period usually results from *Staphylococcus aureus* or *Staphylococcus epidermidis.* Osteomyelitis, a severe infection of the bone itself, can also result (see Chapter 26).

Cast Syndrome

Cast syndrome occurs when the duodenum is compressed between the superior mesenteric artery anteriorly and the aorta and vertebral bodies posteriorly (Fig. 27–6). Cast syndrome can develop weeks or even months after cast application; therefore, constant assessment of the limb is a priority. Because complete gastrointestinal obstruction can develop, immediate nursing intervention is needed. Untreated cast syndrome can be fatal because the obstruction of the superior mesenteric vein can lead to gastrointestinal hemorrhage and necrosis.

LONG-TERM COMPLICATIONS OF FRACTURES

JOINT STIFFNESS OR POST-TRAUMATIC ARTHRITIS. After injury or prolonged immobilization, joint stiffness may occur and can lead to joint contracture or muscle atrophy. Active range-of-motion exercises should be performed to the extent of client tolerance. Also perform passive range-of-motion exercises to decrease the risk for stiffness. The occurrence of post-traumatic arthritis, which can also lead to joint stiffness, is influenced by the severity of the initial injury and the success of bone reduction. Use of acetaminophen or NSAIDs may decrease joint discomfort. Exercise to tolerance may also ameliorate the symptoms of developing arthritis. However, surgical joint replacement may eventually be needed.

AVASCULAR NECROSIS. Avascular necrosis (AVN) of the femoral head occurs primarily in fractures proximal to the femoral neck. It results from local circulatory compromise. An x-ray film demonstrates collapse of the femoral head, and the client complains of pain that occurs months to years after fracture repair. Replacement of the femoral head with a prosthesis is required. The best chance for avoiding the development of AVN is prompt surgical repair after fracture diagnosis.

NONFUNCTIONAL UNION AFTER A FRACTURE. Several types of problems can result in regard to proper bony union.

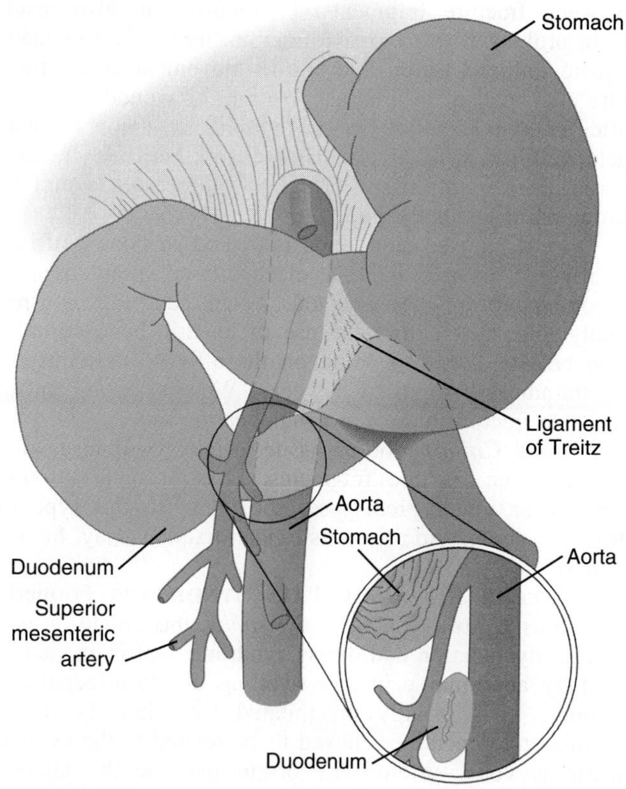

FIGURE 27–6 Cast syndrome results from the compression of the duodenum between the aorta and the superior mesenteric artery. The external compression is usually caused by a tight body cast. (After Cohen, L. B., Field, S. P., & Sachar, D. B. [1985]. The superior mesenteric artery syndrome: The disease that isn't, or is it? *Journal of Clinical Gastroenterology, 7,* 113.)

Malunion. Malunion results when fracture fragments heal in improper alignment as a result of unequal muscle pull and gravity. It can occur if the client bears weight on the affected extremity against medical advice or when an ambulatory device is applied before adequate healing has begun at the fracture site. The primary manifestation is external deformity of the involved extremity. Malunion is diagnosed by radiography. If it is identified early in the course of fracture healing, malunion can be corrected with adjustment of traction or remobilization. Malunion that is diagnosed after healing is complete must be surgically corrected. Prevention is accomplished by adequate fracture reduction and immobilization and by ensuring that the client understands the importance of any activity or position restrictions.

Delayed Union. Suspect delayed union if the client complains of continuation or increase in bone pain and tenderness beyond the healing period expected on the basis of the degree of trauma (3 months to 1 year). Healing is slowed but not completely stopped, possibly as a result of distraction of the fracture fragments or a systemic cause such as infection. If the cause can be identified and corrected early, the fracture usually heals.

Non-union. Non-union is identified when fracture healing has not occurred 4 to 6 months after the initial injury and when spontaneous healing is unlikely to occur. It is generally caused by insufficient blood supply and uncontrolled repetitive stress on the fracture site, possibly as a result of the presence of muscle, tendon, or soft tissue between fracture fragments. Non-union can also result from prolonged or excessive traction; insufficient or inadequate immobilization that allows movement at the fracture site; inadequate internal fixation; or wound infection after internal fixation. On radiograph, non-union is characterized by a relatively narrow gap between fracture fragments. A soft tissue bridge of fibrocartilage and fibrous tissue spans the gap.

Once diagnosed, non-union is treated by bone grafting, internal or external fixation, electric bone stimulation, or a combination of these methods. Client education is especially important before the use of electric bone stimulation because weight-bearing on the affected extremity is contraindicated for 6 to 8 weeks. Weight-bearing on an unstable fracture further prolongs healing time.

Fibrous Union. Fibrous tissue is interposed in a wide gap between fracture fragments. Loss of bone through surgery or injury predisposes the client to this type of fracture union. Additional surgical fixation may be required.

COMPLEX REGIONAL PAIN SYNDROME. Formerly known as *reflex sympathetic dystrophy,* this condition is a painful dysfunction and disuse syndrome that is characterized by abnormal pain and swelling of the affected extremity. It is usually precipitated by relatively minor trauma and generally believed to be related to the sympathetic nervous system. The origin may be the client's pain, fear, or anxiety. Symptoms may include disproportionate pain at the site of injury, edema, muscle spasm or vasospasm, stiffness and decreased joint mobility, increased sweating, atrophy, contractions, and loss of bone mass. Some treatment success has been experienced with sympathetic nerve blocks, especially in early stages of the syndrome. Drug therapies typically involve use of analgesics, muscle relaxants, and antidepressants. Physical therapy and transcutaneous electric nerve stimulation (TENS) may also be ordered. Psychological counseling is often suggested for the client living with this chronic condition.

Nursing Management of the Medical Client

CARE OF THE CLIENT IN A CAST

Closed reduction of fractures is followed by immobilization to relieve pain and to prevent rotation and shearing at the fracture site. Immobilization is most often accomplished through the use of a cast or splint (Fig. 27–7). Before application of a cast, the nurse's role may entail preparation of the client for casting, including a detailed explanation of the procedure. Skin preparation involves thorough cleansing and assessment of any lesions. Presence of unremovable dirt or foreign particles should be reported to the physician. After the skin preparation, padding or web-roll is applied to the extremity surrounding the fracture site. Additional padding made be indicated over bony prominences, but too much padding can actually increase pressure. Stockinette is applied over the padding and is cut several inches longer than the expected finished cast length so that excess portions can be pulled over exposed cast ends to protect the client's skin. Make sure that these coverings fit smoothly and without wrinkles, which could produce pressure areas on underlying tissues.

Rolls of casting materials, whether plaster or synthetic, are individually submerged in clean water in a bucket. Excess water is squeezed from the roll, and then the bandage is applied to encircle the injured body part. Assist during cast application by supporting the extremity from underneath, using only the palms of your hands to avoid applying pressure to any one area. Fingertips should not be pressed into the cast, and the cast should not be allowed to rest on a hard or sharp surface; these actions might cause flattening or indentations in the cast, which could create pressure. As soon as the casting procedure is complete, the client's skin must be cleansed of excess casting material. Plaster-laden water should never be emptied into an ordinary sink because the plaster sediment solidifies and plugs the plumbing. If a sink with a plaster trap is not available, wait for sediment to settle to the bottom of the bucket, and then drain off the water from the top. The remaining plaster sediment can be scraped from the bottom of the bucket and placed into the garbage container.

Drying a Cast

As the water from a newly applied cast eventually evaporates, a mature cast of full strength develops. Synthetic casts dry to the touch in a few minutes, but they take about 30 minutes to set completely and allow weight-bearing. Plaster casts set quickly but take hours to days to dry completely; a lower extremity plaster cast may not be totally dry for up to 48 hours, and larger casts can take even longer. Because both plaster and synthetic casts generate heat while drying; the client should be instructed to expect the sensation of heat. The cast should not be covered with a blanket or towel while it is drying because the retained heat can burn the client. Several towels may be placed under the cast on the pillow to absorb dampness. While the cast is still damp, the client may feel cold

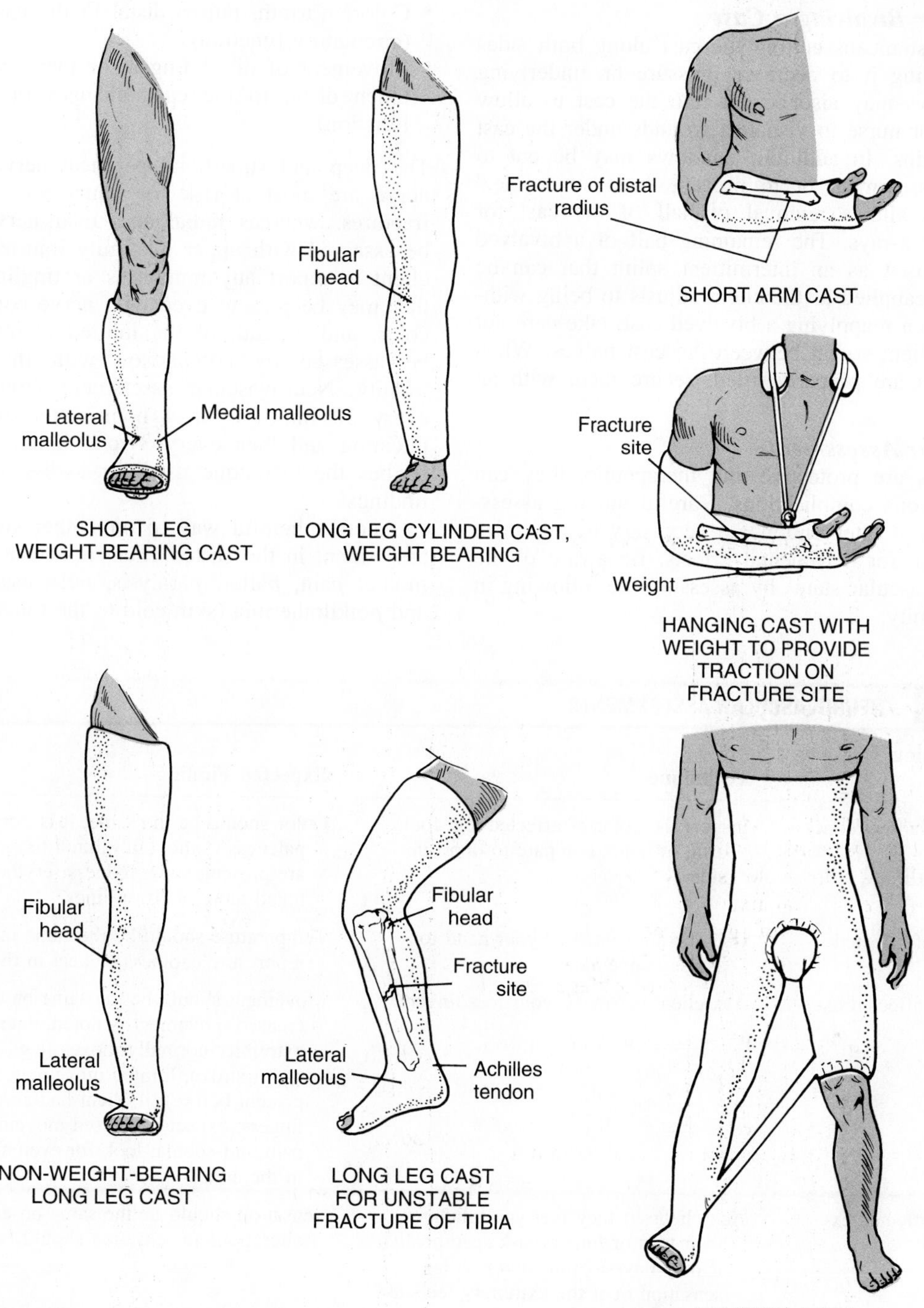

FIGURE 27–7 Common types of casts.

and may experience a decrease in body temperature. Adequate covering is provided for the client while dry, warm air is allowed to circulate around the damp cast. To avoid excessive chilling for the client who is in a large cast, sections of the cast should be exposed for brief periods of time alternately. Unless it is contraindicated, the client should also be turned regularly to expose more of the new cast to air. Rapid drying through use of a blow dryer is not advised because it can burn the client's skin under the cast and crack the cast.

A wet plaster cast smells musty and is dull on percussion, gray, and cold to the touch. When dry, the plaster cast is odorless, resonant, and white, and it feels close to room temperature when touched. Wet fiberglass casts feel hot and sticky to the touch. A wet fiberglass cast should not be placed over drainage-containing pads, such as incontinence pads, because paper and plaster adhere and the paper will become a permanent part of the cast. Once the cast is completely dry, it can safely be placed on a hard surface (e.g., a casted arm can rest on a table), but the client is usually more comfortable in continuing to rest the casted area on pillows.

Windowing or Bivalving a Cast

Bivalving a cast means cutting the cast along both sides and then splitting it to decrease pressure on underlying tissue. Windows may also be cut into the cast to allow the physician or nurse to visualize wounds under the cast or remove drains. In addition, windows may be cut to allow pulse assessment or to prevent "cast syndrome." Bivalving also allows removal of half of the cast for wound care or x-rays. The remaining half of a bivalved cast is often used as an intermittent splint that can be removed and reapplied as the client adjusts to being without a cast. When reapplying a bivalved cast, take care not to pinch the client's skin between the cast halves. When the cast halves are properly fitted, secure them with an elastic wrap.

Neurovascular Assessment

Although casts are protective and therapeutic, they can also cause serious complications. Careful nursing assessment and prompt intervention are necessary to minimize the client's risk for detrimental effects. Be aware of the client's neurovascular status by assessing the following in a casted extremity:

- Color, warmth, pulses distal to the cast, capillary refill (circulatory function)
- Movement of distal fingers or toes, awareness of light touch distal to the cast, changes in sensation (nerve function)

The deep and superficial peroneal nerves and the tibial nerve are most at risk for injury with lower extremity fractures, whereas radial and ulnar nerve function must be assessed with upper extremity injuries. Encourage the client to report any numbness or tingling, although neither may be present even with nerve compression. Pulse, color, and warmth of the injured extremity should also be assessed by comparison with the unaffected extremity. Neurovascular assessment should be performed every 30 minutes for 4 hours after cast or splint application and then every 3 to 4 hours. Table 27–4 describes the technique used for assessment and expected findings.

Another helpful way to remember significant areas of assessment in the casted client is to use the "6 Ps" mnemonic: *p*ain, *p*allor, *p*aralysis, *p*ulselessness, *p*aresthesia, and *p*oikilothermia (skin cold to the touch).

TABLE 27–4 NEUROVASCULAR ASSESSMENTS

Parameter Being Assessed	Technique	Expected Finding
Color of affected extremity	Inspect the color of affected leg, foot, arm, or hand; compare to opposite side	Color should be the same; it is normal to have some paleness (pallor) in injured tissues; if incisions are present, some redness (erythema) may be noted along incision lines
Temperature of affected extremity	Use dorsum (back) of your hand to assess temperature	Temperature should be the same in each extremity; report any coolness or heat in the extremity
Movement of affected extremity	Ask client to "move your toes/fingers"	Movement should be the same on each side; if decreased movement is noted, determine whether extremity normally moves (e.g., if the client has had a stroke, limited movement may have been present before); if client had surgery on toes or fingers, expect decreased movement as a result of pain and edema; look for even slight movement in the area
Sensation of affected extremity	Ask clients if they feel you touching their toes or fingers; ask specifically if they have a "pins and needles" sensation or if the extremity feels as if it is "asleep"	Sensation should be the same on each side; any alterations in sensation should be reported
Capillary refill in nail beds	Compress nail bed and measure time needed for refill (return of color)	Should be 2–4 sec; slowing to 4–6 sec should be reported
Edema	Inspect for edema in both extremities	No edema should be present; if edema is noted in affected extremity, consider whether it is caused by the trauma or surgery or thrombophlebitis; if present in both extremities, consider causes such as heart disease
Pain	Ask clients to rate pain on scale of 0–10, 0 being no pain and 10 being the worst pain they have ever felt	Pain is common in injured extremities; if no pain is reported, client may have recently had pain medication; uncontrollable pain usually signals compartment syndrome and should be reported
Pedal pulses	Palpate for pedal pulses on dorsum of foot	Pedal pulses should be present bilaterally; if absent, may be normal variation; absent pulses could also signal compression of vessels from edema

Assessment of Pain

Careful assessment of pain must be completed regularly, and the client must be encouraged to verbalize the degree of pain. Inadequate analgesic effects should be reported promptly to the surgeon because an increased dosage or change in medication may be indicated. Unrelieved pain is also a classic symptom of compartment syndrome; therefore, any complaint of pain should be given your full attention. Be especially alert to complaints of progressive pain or pain out of proportion to the injury or treatment.

Assessment of the Cast

The skin around the cast edges should be observed for damage or swelling. Also assess the cast itself. "Hot spots"—areas of the cast that feel warmer than other sections—may indicate tissue necrosis or infection under the cast. "Wet spots" may indicate drainage under the cast or a need for additional drying. Stains can indicate wound drainage or bleeding, and any stained areas should be carefully measured and documented. Also be aware of possible pressure points on underlying structures, such as the lateral malleolus under a short leg cast or the epicondyle under a short arm cast. Closely inspect areas of the cast that are known to cover wounds with the understanding that drainage on the surface of synthetic casts may not wick outward but may go to a dependent area determined by cast position (e.g., beneath the cast if it is flat, posterior and superior if the limb is elevated).

An older cast may develop a sour smell because of perspiration or normal sloughing of outer skin layers. Musty, offensive odors under the cast, however, may indicate tissue necrosis or infection. If the odor of mildew is present, the synthetic cast may have not been thoroughly dried after it became wet; notify the physician because the cast needs to be changed.

Assessment for Complications

COMPARTMENT SYNDROME Any client with an extremity fracture should be regularly assessed for compartment syndrome for the first week after injury. Traumatic injury and treatment such as closed reduction usually produces swelling, which progresses for the first 12 to 24 hours after injury. The greatest swelling is likely to be evident in the first 24 to 48 hours. Mild swelling is expected; however, moderate or severe swelling associated with pain or discoloration is abnormal. Excessive swelling constricts the enclosed soft tissues and introduces the risk for compartment syndrome.

The affected extremity should be regularly compared with the uninjured extremity, and current findings should also be compared with baseline assessment data. Manifestations of compartment syndrome can begin as early as 30 minutes after ischemic injury. The primary manifestation is increasing pain or pain that is out of proportion to the injury. Specifically, pain with passive stretching of the muscles in an affected compartment is one of the earliest indicators. Assess for the presence of tingling or paresthesia in the affected extremity; muscle strength and motion; and circulation, including the presence and quality of pulses distal to the injury, capillary refill, skin color, and temperature. Increased tenseness and erythema of the skin also suggest increasing compartment pressures. If the intracompartmental pressure increases to a level above the client's systolic blood pressure, pulses are absent, capillary refill is delayed, and pallor results. Paralysis is a very late sign of compartment syndrome. If compartment syndrome goes unrecognized and tissue pressures are not relieved, muscle damage becomes irreversible after 4 to 6 hours of ischemia; nerve damage becomes irreversible after 12 to 24 hours.[8] The physician must be notified immediately of assessment findings that suggest the development of compartment syndrome (see Critical Monitoring: The Client in a Cast).

FAT EMBOLI. Be alert to manifestations of hypoxemia, such as apprehension, anxiety, agitation, or acute confusion. The client with FES also exhibits fever (>103° F), dyspnea, tachypnea, and tachycardia. Diffuse rales and rhonchi may occur as late signs of FES. In 50% to 60% of clients, petechiae are noted on the chest, axillae, flanks, abdomen, clavicular fossae, and soft palate.[34]

INFECTION. The client may describe new pain or an increased level of pain and feelings of increased warmth under a bandage or cast. Your assessment may reveal fever or chills, an odor from the area of injury, erythema and warmth around the wound, purulent drainage, and poor wound healing.

DEEP VENOUS THROMBOSIS. The typical manifestations of DVT are unilateral edema, at or below the site of thrombosis, that results from venous inflammation or obstruction. Affected clients often complain of pain and tenderness at the site, which may also be red and warm. Homans' sign (in which dorsiflexion of the foot causes discomfort in the upper calf) is present in less than one third of symptomatic clients with DVT. Because Homans' sign is present in more than 50% of symptomatic clients who do not have DVT, it is not considered specific or sensitive to the condition. Venous ultrasonography is a

CRITICAL MONITORING

The Client in a Cast

Compartment Syndrome

- Pulselessness: slow nail bed capillary refill (longer than 3 sec)
- Skin pallor, blanching, cyanosis, or coolness
- Increasing pain, swelling, painful edema peripheral to cast, pain on passive motion
- Paresthesias (tingling, prickling), heightened sensitivity, numbness; hypesthesia (diminished sensitivity to touch); anesthesia (numbness)
- Motor paralysis of previously functioning muscles
- Hypesthesia (diminished sensitivity); anesthesia (numbness); paresthesias (tingling, prickling, heightened sensitivity, numbness)

Infection

- Musty, unpleasant odor over cast and/or at ends of cast
- Drainage through cast or cast opening
- Sudden unexplained body temperature elevation
- "Hot spot" felt on cast over lesion

Cast Syndrome

- Bloated feeling
- Prolonged nausea; repeated vomiting
- Abdominal distention; vague abdominal pain
- Shortness of breath

sensitive, accurate, noninvasive examination that has become the standard for diagnosis of DVT.

PE results if a thromboembolism lodges in the pulmonary circulation, leading to decreased or absent blood flow distal to the clot. Because manifestations of PE can be nonspecific and vary greatly, PE is often undetected or misdiagnosed. The most common clinical manifestations are sudden unexplained dyspnea and pleuritic chest pain. In the event of a massive PE, diagnosis and successful treatment may be extremely difficult because of the extensive loss of gas exchange area and the severe strain placed on the right chambers of the heart by pulmonary hypertension. Although pulmonary angiography is still considered the standard for diagnosis with a 98% sensitivity, the ventilation/perfusion ($\dot{V}/\dot{Q}$) scan is commonly ordered because it has a high sensitivity in ruling out PE. A chest radiograph can also be helpful in ruling out other pulmonary perfusion problems. (DVT is fully discussed in chapter 53, and PE is discussed in chapter 62.)

Cast Syndrome. If the client is in a body cast, closely attend to any complaints of nausea, abdominal pressure, vague abdominal pain, feelings of bloating or tightness, or inability to take a deep breath. These may be clinical manifestation of cast syndrome, a serious complication that can follow prolonged supine positioning, spinal surgery, or use of a body cast.

Management of suspected cast syndrome includes cutting a window or bivalving the cast to relieve pressure. Nasogastric intubation may be indicated to decompress the intestine, intravenous fluids may be ordered, and the client may be placed on NPO status. Antiemetics should be given sparingly to any client in a body cast because they can mask the manifestations of cast syndrome. The client who is discharged in a body cast should receive careful instruction about the clinical manifestations of cast syndrome and be encouraged to report any complaints promptly to the surgeon.

Interventions for Clients in Casts

To prevent or relieve swelling, the nurse typically elevates the entire casted extremity higher than the client's heart for the first 24 to 48 hours. The affected extremity may be placed on pillows. A casted arm may also be elevated in a sling attached to an intravenous (IV) pole. The entire arm, including the elbow, wrist, and hand, must be supported, and the fingers must be kept higher than the elbow to minimize swelling. Also apply ice bags around the cast, and exercise the client's fingers or toes to encourage circulation. Relieve pressure at the cast edges by petalling the cast or loosely padding an uncomfortable area. To prevent footdrop in a casted leg, splint or support the client's foot with the ankle in 90 degrees of flexion.

For the client in a hip spica or body cast, the buttocks should be exposed to prevent soiling or dampening of clothing during elimination and to provide adequate skin care. To further prevent soiling, incontinence pads can be tucked into the edge of the cast before the client uses a fracture bedpan. Slightly raising the head of the bed facilitates elimination and also prevents excrement from running under the cast; such raising is usually allowed unless the client is in shock, is hemorrhaging, or has a spinal injury. Dampness causes skin irritation and may increase the risk of infection if an open wound is present; therefore, thorough perineal care must be completed after elimination.

Position changes at least every 2 hours are needed to help prevent complications of immobility, and a turning schedule is useful for ensuring that the client does not remain in one position too long. Give instructions on turning to encourage client activity, but also provide assistance with bed mobility as needed. When mobility assistance is needed, always have adequate staff help to reposition a casted client. Three or four people may be needed to turn a client in a body or hip spica cast, for example. Roller boards or mechanical lifts may also be useful.

Clients in casts can often bear weight as soon as the cast is dry, depending on the nature of the injury and the physician's orders. Be aware of the client's weight-bearing status when attempting a transfer. For client safety, also use a transfer belt when getting the client out of bed. Weak, elderly, or debilitated clients may find the weight of the cast difficult to deal with and may tire rapidly with initial activity. The client should be instructed about the likelihood of increased pain when a casted leg is lowered to a dependent position with initial attempts at ambulation. Help the client lower the leg, encouraging him or her with regard to the decrease in pain as the leg becomes accustomed to the increased blood flow.

To ensure client cooperation, provide instruction on every aspect of care. Ensure that the client understands the availability of analgesics for treatment of pain and is allowed to voice any concerns about their use, such as fears of addiction. Initiate an honest discussion about any barriers to analgesic use if the client seems hesitant about taking or asking for medication. Administer analgesics as prescribed, and promptly inform the surgeon of inadequate effects. Client instruction should also include alternative methods of pain management, such as distraction, visualization, or massage, that may help the client relax.

Care of the Client in External Fixation

Assessment. The potential for neurovascular deficit or compartment syndrome is high when external fixation is used. The risk is increased because many clients with external fixation have extensive soft tissue injury. Even though the external fixator may be used for treatment of an open fracture, compartment syndrome can nonetheless develop in another compartment of the same extremity. Ongoing assessment of neurovascular status is critical. Current findings should be compared with baseline data, and the affected extremity should be compared with the unaffected extremity. Instruct the client to report any changes, and address any complaints promptly.

As with the client in a cast, careful assessment of pain must be completed regularly. Analgesia should be assessed, and inadequate effects should be reported promptly to the surgeon because an increased dosage or change in medication may be indicated. Unrelieved pain should raise suspicion of compartment syndrome, and any complaint of pain should be given full attention. Be especially alert to complaints of progressive pain or pain out of proportion to the injury or treatment.

Pin sites and wounds must be constantly assessed for signs of infection, and pins should be checked for loosening. A small amount of bleeding immediately after pin insertion is expected and can be controlled with small pressures dressings. However, bleeding that continues for more than 24 hours should be brought to the surgeon's attention. The progress of wound healing must be assessed, and changes must be carefully documented. The movement of adipose tissue at the pin sites may produce fatty drainage that looks a great deal like pus. Be alert to more specific signs of infection such as pin instability, drainage with odor or color, and skin tension or puckering at the insertion site (tenting). If tenting occurs, the surgeon should be notified so that the wound can be extended.

The client's nutritional status greatly affects bone and wound healing; pay attention to the adequacy of food intake as well as the client's ability to eat and swallow. Be aware of complaints of nausea or vomiting. Any abnormal laboratory values should also be assessed as possible evidence of poor nutrition.

INTERVENTIONS. Antibiotics may need to be administered prophylactically for 48 to 72 hours after application of an external fixator. Later, wound care may involve the application of wet-to-dry dressings. Because pin care methods still remain somewhat controversial, follow the surgeon's orders or institutional standards. Loose pins must be reported promptly to the surgeon; they will be removed to prevent osteomyelitis.

The client's sense of balance can be altered by the weight of a fixator frame on the lower extremity. Because the client often also has a prescribed weight-bearing status after application of a lower extremity external fixator, be scrupulous in assessing adherence to any weight-bearing restrictions and correct use of ambulatory aids. If the surgeon determines that the frame itself can be used to moved the affected extremity, the client should be instructed to move the extremity and the external fixator as a unit to avoid stress on the fracture site. The amount of support needed from the nurse is determined by the client's ability to control the extremity during movement.

Nausea or vomiting should be addressed aggressively with an antiemetic agent, as ordered, to decrease the risk for nutritional deficits or aspiration. Dietary supplements may be used, as needed. Client and family education is critical for achieving a successful outcome with use of external fixation. By the time of discharge, the client should have begun to accept the change in body image that accompanies use of external fixation. The client should also understand his or her responsibility for pin and wound care. He or she should be knowledgeable about manifestations of infection and should be aware of the significance of neurovascular or integumentary changes. The client must also receive instruction on use of analgesics and antibiotics as ordered by the surgeon. Instruction should include alternative methods of pain management, such as distraction, visualization, or massage, that may help the client relax.

Before discharge, teach the client how to meet hygiene needs and discuss any resumption of sexual activity. Clothing may need to be modified with snaps or self-fastening (Velcro) closures before discharge to fit over fixators. Advise the client with a pelvic fixator to reduce intake of gas-producing foods, which can lead to abdominal distention. Once the affected bone is healed, the fixator is removed.

CARE OF THE CLIENT IN TRACTION

ASSESSMENT. As with the other modalities for immobilization, the client in traction must be assessed for neurovascular compromise, pain, skin breakdown, nutrition deficit, and signs of infection. Pin tract infection and development of osteomyelitis are risks for the client in skeletal traction. Other complications of immobility such as constipation or respiratory compromise can also occur, especially in older clients and in clients with long-term traction use.

The client's position in bed, along with the traction positioning and alignment, requires constant vigilance. Bedside rounds between shifts may be useful to ensure proper positioning and alignment, especially if the client is active, confused, or noncompliant. Traction ropes and knots must be intact and secure. Ropes should move easily over pulleys and weights, which hang freely at the end or side of the bed. Traction mechanics should be checked at the beginning of each shift and after each application or position change; all clamps on the traction frame must be tight, and ropes should be unfrayed. A photograph or sketch of the correct traction setup may be useful for nursing staff.

INTERVENTIONS. If the client's nutritional status becomes a concern, dietary supplements may be ordered. Small, frequent meals may be indicated for the client in a halo vest to avoid a feeling of excessive fullness. Bent straws and adapted utensils may be indicated for clients who have limitations on head elevation.

To provide client comfort with elimination, provide a fracture bedpan and ensure privacy when the client needs to use it. The client's diet should include ample fluids and fiber if there are no contraindications. Stool softeners are often prescribed and should be administered regularly. Also determine whether the client has regular, effective strategies for previous treatment of constipation; those methods should be used to assist with elimination.

Encourage independence in client activities within the limitations of the traction. The client should be instructed on repositioning techniques, possibly using extended horizontal bars with roller traction to allow movement to a chair at the bedside. Unaffected joints should be exercised regularly through the use of free weights, foam balls, or elastic pull bands. A record book may be used to encourage the client to cross off the exercise session when it is completed.

Immediately after traction removal, the client is often weak and unsteady as a result of muscle atrophy or orthostatic hypotension. The client should be gradually assisted to a sitting position and then to a standing position later as tolerated. Movement of a previously bedridden client to a sitting or standing position may take several days, depending on the effects of previous immobility. Ensure adequate assistance and provide careful physical support when assisting the client with these position changes. An assistive device such as a walker or crutches may be needed for temporary support of weak muscles and stiff joints.

SPECIFIC FRACTURES

HIP FRACTURES

Hip fractures have become one of the leading causes of morbidity and mortality among the older population. The estimated occurrence is as high as 300,00 fractures each year, and more than 90% of those involve adults aged 70 years or older.[21, 44] Epidemiologists predicted a six-fold increase in the number of hip fractures worldwide between 1990 and 2050.[12] Hip fractures also have a significant impact on health care costs; the annual expense of medical and nursing services is estimated to be $7 billion to $10 billion. This amount is predicted to reach $16 billion by the year 2040 and, with 5% inflation, will approximate $240 billion.[27]

The first-year postfracture mortality rate ranges from 12%[44] to 24%.[21] Among the clients who survive the first year, most do not return to their prefracture functional status. Half of the affected persons become partially dependent, often requiring the care of a spouse or adult child as they continue to live in the community. They may remain unable to walk without an assistive device. One third of those with hip fractures require placement in a long-term care facility. In fact, up to 25% of previously independent clients remain in institutions for more than a year after a hip fracture.[6]

Etiology and Risk Factors

Numerous studies have associated low bone mass and increasing age with an increased risk of hip fracture. Women begin to lose bone about 1.5 years before the last menstrual period; the bone loss continues rapidly until about 1.5 years after the last menses. The rate of bone loss then slows, matching the rate of loss in men by age 65 or 70.[32] The development of low bone mass is known to be influenced by genetic factors. For example, women tend to have lower bone mass if their mothers or fathers have experienced vertebral fractures. Additional factors that can lead to the development of low bone mass include (1) low body weight, (2) physical inactivity, (3) low dietary calcium intake, (4) inadequate levels of serum vitamin D, (5) cigarette smoking, and (6) consumption of alcohol.

More than 90% of hip fractures are caused by falling. However, attempts to decrease the risk of falling through controlled trials have generally been ineffective. Some researchers have concluded that it is the dynamic interaction between the client's physical environment and intrinsic risk factors that actually increases the person's vulnerability to fall and injury.

Other factors have been associated with occurrence of falls that lead to hip fractures. These include the client's use of barbiturates or long-acting benzodiazepines, orthostatic hypotension, impaired vision, lower limb dysfunction, and neurologic conditions. Environmental hazards may also contribute to the elderly client's tendency to fall. These include loose carpeting or rugs, slippery floors, poor lighting, a slippery tub or shower, irregular pavement, and loose clothing or footwear.

Pathophysiology

Fractures of the hip are either *intracapsular* (located within the joint capsule) or *extracapsular* (located outside the joint capsule). Fractures are also described on the basis of their location in one of the four anatomic areas of the proximal hip (Fig. 27–8). Femoral neck fractures are more common in frail older persons, especially women, and are often associated with osteoporosis. They generally result from relatively mild trauma. Intertrochanteric fractures (between the femoral neck and the greater trochanter) and subtrochanteric fractures are more often seen in males and in vigorous older persons; they are likely to be associated with greater traumatic force.

Because blood flow to the hip is an important influence on fracture healing, delayed healing or non-union may occur in areas of the hip where circulation is impaired after injury. Healing of femoral head fractures, for example, is unlikely if AVN develops after local circulatory compromise.

Clinical Manifestations

Hip fracture is often caused by a fall at home that involves only a moderate amount of trauma, such as slipping out of a chair onto the floor. Immediately after the fall, the client is unable to bear weight on the affected leg. Objective findings include a shortened leg and an externally rotated hip. Deformity may also be evident in the lateral hip if the fracture is displaced. Ecchymosis at the hip is most likely to occur with subtrochanteric fractures. Location of pain depends on the specific fracture site (see Fig. 27–7*A, C, E, G*). A femoral neck fracture, for example, is characterized by groin and hip pain that increases with hip movement. Intertrochanteric fractures are accompanied by severe pain over the greater trochanter of the femur, whereas subtrochanteric fractures typically produce pain over the proximal thigh. Additional tissue trauma such as head or hand lacerations may also be evident.

Diagnosis of hip fracture is based on the client's clinical manifestations, history of trauma, and radiologic findings. The presence of a fracture is often confirmed by anteroposterior radiograph, although in some instances additional studies may be ordered. Computed tomographic (CT) scans, bone scans, fluoroscopy, myelograms, or magnetic resonance imaging (MRI) may be necessary to identify the fracture site.

Outcome Management

Medical Management

For a relatively few clients, nonoperative treatment is the best option following hip fracture. A client who cannot tolerate anesthesia or who was nonambulatory before the fracture may be treated with skeletal traction or spica casting. While the client remains in traction (approximately 8 to 12 weeks), develop a plan of care that will decrease the effects of immobility. For example, excellent skin care must be provided to reduce the risk of pressure ulcer development. Because older clients are at increased risk for skin impairment even before immobilization, a pressure-reducing mattress is essential. Perform careful daily assessment of bony prominences such as the heels, sacrum, scapulae, and vertebrae. In addition, instruct the client about leg exercises that will decrease the probability of thromboembolism; pneumatic compression devices or anticoagulant medications may also be used to lessen the likelihood of clot development. The Care Plan: The Client in Traction presents additional interventions.

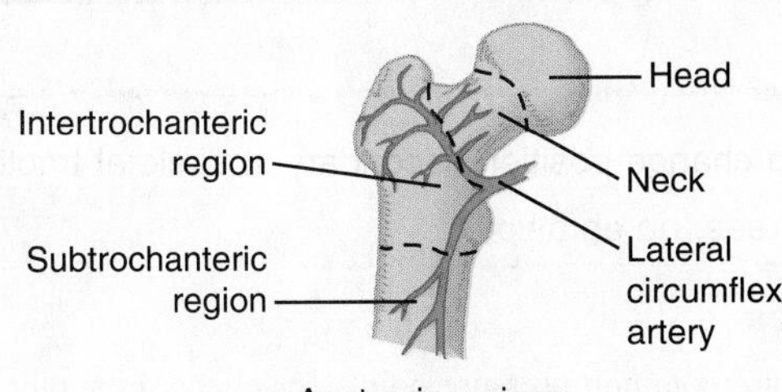

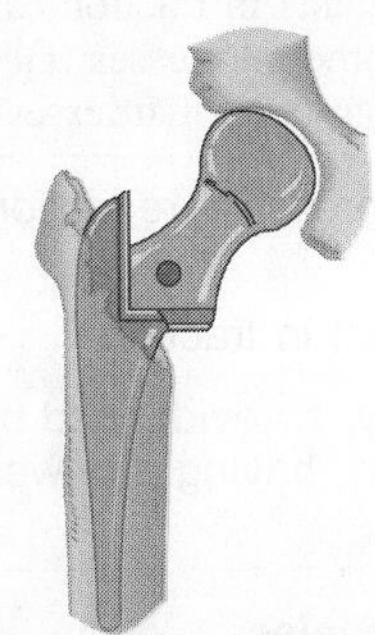
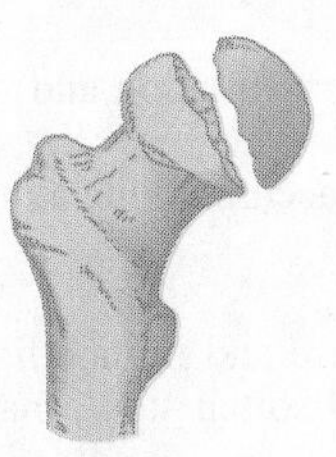

A Intertrochanteric fracture

B Repair of an intertrochanteric fracture with an endoprosthesis

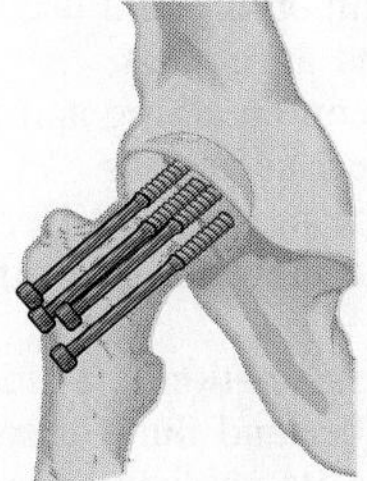
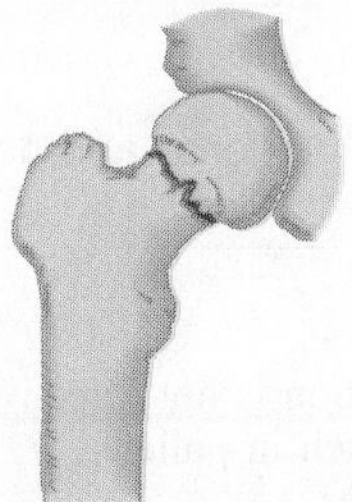

C Intracapsular fracture

D Repair of an intracapsular fracture with compression screws

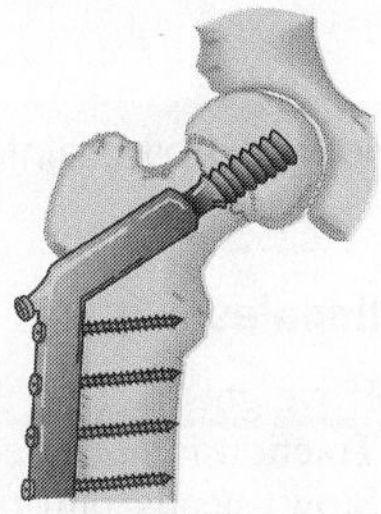
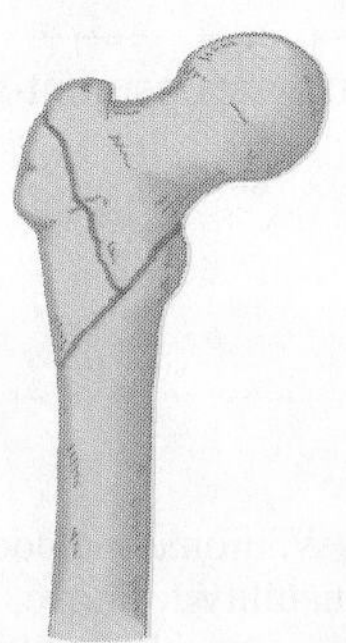

E Femoral neck fracture

F Repair of a femoral neck fracture with compression screws

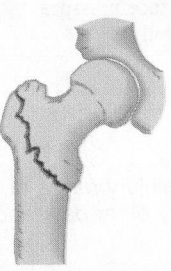

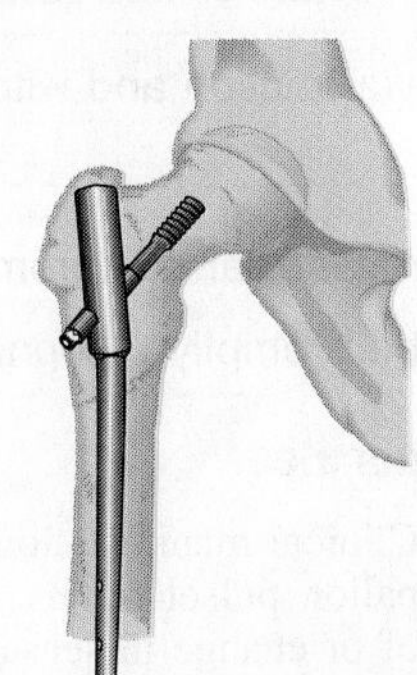

G Subtrochanteric fracture

H Repair of a subtrochanteric fracture with compression screws

FIGURE 27–8 Anatomic regions of the proximal femur and blood supply, and fracture patterns of the hip and surgical repairs.

THE CLIENT IN TRACTION

Nursing Diagnosis. Risk for Impaired Skin Integrity related to inability to change position secondary to skeletal traction

Outcomes. Client will retain intact skin, as evidenced by no reddened areas, no abrasions.

Interventions	Rationales
1. Assess pressure points (sacrum, heels, skin under ropes, and bones) every shift	1. These are common pressure points for clients in supine position
2. Provide skin care every shift by lifting client	2. Clients in traction cannot turn
3. Place therapeutic mattress on bed	3. Some mattresses (Geo-Matt) reduce surface pressure (egg-crate mattresses improve comfort only)

Evaluation. Expect the client's skin to remain intact with adequate pressure reduction interventions.

Nursing Diagnosis. Impaired Physical Mobility related to confinement in traction

Outcomes. The client will not experience complications of immobility, as evidenced by maintaining preinjury range of motion (ROM) in noninvolved joints, not developing thrombophlebitis, having a bowel movement every other day, and maintaining clear lung sounds.

Interventions	Rationales
1. Place all joints (except those immediately proximal and distal to fracture) through ROM every shift	1. ROM assists in maintaining muscle tone
2. Assess lung sounds every shift	2. Immobility and use of analgesia may cause hypoventilation and atelectasis
3. Teach client to deep breathe and cough every shift	3. Deep breathing and coughing cause hyperventilation and clear secretions
4. Assess for clinical manifestations of thrombophlebitis: unilateral leg edema or pain; do not rely on Homans' sign as an indicator	4. The presence of Homans' sign is not an accurate indicator of thrombophlebitis; other signs are assessed
5. Monitor bowel movements	5. Constipation is a side effect of narcotic use and immobility
6. Encourage the patient to consume fluids and food containing fiber	6. Fiber and fluids assist in adding bulk and soften stool, making its passage easier
7. Administer laxatives as needed	7. Laxatives irritate or stimulate the colon

Evaluation. After 3 to 5 days of immobility, clients may develop some of these complications. An aggressive prevention program should be effective.

Nursing Diagnosis. Risk for Injury related to traction

Outcomes. The client will sustain no injury while in traction, as evidenced by maintaining effective pulling force and desired vector of force.

Interventions	Rationales
1. Ensure that weights hang freely from pulleys	1. If weights rest on the bed or floor, traction is not effective
2. Ensure that knots in the rope do not catch in the pulleys	2. Traction is not effective when knots catch in pulleys
3. Add and remove weights slowly with physician's order	3. Slow, steady pull reduces muscle spasms
4. Assess skin at pin site daily or bid for signs of infection	4. Infection can develop in pin sites
5. Pin site care per agency policy	5. Reduces risk of infection
6. Adjust the position of the bed per physician's orders	6. Provides countertraction

Evaluation. Expect the client to maintain adequate pulling forces via traction and with adequate nursing assessment and care.

Collaborative Problem. Risk for compartment syndrome and neurovascular compromise

Outcomes. Clinical manifestations of compartment syndrome will be promptly recognized and reported.

Interventions	Rationales
1. Monitor color, warmth, movement, and sensation of extremity distal to traction every shift	1. Clinical manifestations of compartment syndrome include pallor, pulselessness, cool extremities, inability to move, loss of or change in sensation, and pain that is not relieved with usual analgesics.
2. Assess pedal radial pulse every shift	2. Distal pulses indicate peripheral blood flow.
3. Monitor reports of degree of pain and relief by analgesia	3. Pain that is increasing or beyond what is common with the injury may indicate ischemia.

continued

4. Immediately inform physician of changes in skin color, pulses, skin temperature, motion, sensation or an increase in pain | 4. Compartment syndrome mandates immediate medical intervention.

Evaluation. Risk of compartment syndrome exists until edema subsides (about 72 hours).

Nursing Diagnosis. Self Care Deficit related to inability to move in environment

Outcomes. The client will participate in self-care activities if possible, given sites of fractures.

Interventions	Rationales
1. Place necessary equipment and supplies within easy reach	1. Facilitates maximal self-care and independence
2. Allow client to schedule procedures, such as bath or linen changes	2. Provides client some control
3. Medicate for pain before movement	3. Movement increases pain and spasm in fracture site

Evaluation. The client should be able to assist with his or her own feeding, bathing, and dressing.

Nursing Diagnosis. Diversional Activity Deficit related to prolonged immobility, inadequate environmental stimulation, or lack of variation

Outcomes. The client will remain mentally and emotionally stable and will demonstrate interest in surroundings.

Interventions	Rationales
1. Plan varied activities of interest to the person to fill each day, such as reading, writing, listening to the radio, and watching television	1. Variety is a normal aspect of life
2. Be sure a telephone is convenient	2. Telephone can be used to maintain contact with significant others
3. Sit with, talk with, and touch the client as appropriate	3. Provides contact with nurses outside of usual activities (medications, cares)
4. Place the client's bed beside a window; keep the door open as possible	4. Allows passive interaction with outside
5. Provide accurate clock, current calendar and publications, clean eyeglasses and hearing aids, if worn by the client; obtain prism glasses if client is supine	5. Normal aids to orientation; prism glasses may help a person read more easily while lying flat
6. Have the radio and television clearly tuned, but do not leave them on continuously if the client cannot control them independently	6. Continuous noise can increase confusion

Evaluation. Problems with diversional activities develop after about 2 weeks, when pain is minimal and client must wait for bones to realign.

Surgical Management

Extensive blood loss can occur after hip fracture, particularly in older clients with other medical conditions. Additional deterioration can occur rapidly if the client is left on bed rest; therefore, prompt surgical intervention and early mobilization are keys to successful rehabilitation. The goal of surgical treatment is to achieve a stable reduction and fixation of the fracture segments internally to support early ambulation.

Open Reduction and Internal Fixation

Postoperative treatment goals include:

- Complete union of the fracture (4 to 8 months)
- Prevention of deformity and contractures to the hip, knee, or foot
- Restoration of weight-bearing ambulation with the use of assistive devices if needed
- Relief of pain and fear; prevention of complications
- Maintenance of optimal physiologic function

Fixation may be accomplished through the use of screws, plates, intramedullary pins or implants (see Fig. 27–8*B, D, F, H*). The term *open reduction* indicates that a surgical incision was made to expose the bone, in contrast to a closed reduction of a fracture (see earlier). *Internal fixation* indicates that instruments were used to hold the bones in alignment during healing. It may be difficult to achieve perfect anatomic reduction and fixation if the client has decreased bone density as a result of osteoporosis. If the fracture is highly comminuted or the head of the femur has been destroyed, use of an endoprosthesis to replace the entire head of the femur may be necessary. For the client who has an accompanying acetabular fracture, total hip arthroplasty may be indicated (see Chapter 26).

Nursing Management of the Surgical Client

Preoperative Care

Clients who require surgical reduction and fixation of hip fractures most often go directly from the emergency department to the operating room. Delay in repair not only places an elderly client at risk for additional effects of immobility but also increases the likelihood that AVN will develop as a result of inadequate blood supply to the fracture fragments. Assess routine blood work, and the client's baseline weight preoperatively. A bed scale should be used to minimize client discomfort with this procedure. Do not accept a stated weight from the client or family member, because accurate comparison with postoperative changes will be impossible.

Occasionally, a client may require stabilization of medical conditions before being cleared for surgery. Underlying disorders such as heart failure or malnutrition, for example, must be evaluated and controlled. In such cases, skin traction through use of a Buck's boot is commonly applied to decrease painful muscle spasms surrounding the hip joint.

Routine preoperative assessment is performed (see Chapter 15). For the client who has experienced a hip fracture, preoperative assessment also includes determination of preinjury level of functioning. Data should clearly address usual activities, ability to walk independently, and previous falls. Under the best of circumstances, the preoperative level of functioning is the level that the client can optimistically expect to achieve after surgery. Unfortunately, some loss of function is likely after fracture repair.

One significant factor in successful rehabilitation is the client's previous social functioning. The client who was previously independent and active and who enjoyed multiple social contacts is more likely to experience a full recovery than is the client who had restricted activity before injury.

POSTOPERATIVE ASSESSMENTS

After ORIF, the same basic nursing assessments are required as for any other surgical client (see Chapter 15). Additional assessment includes a comparison of the quality of peripheral pulses in the affected extremity with that in the unaffected extremity. Prompt recognition of abnormal data allows for early intervention for any neurovascular compromise. As the client progresses into rehabilitation, collaborate with physical and occupational therapists in assessing the client's mobility and self-care needs.

Complications seen after hip fracture repair include fat emboli and infection (see section on fractures). Complications specific to or of high incidence in clients with hip fractures are discussed here.

Deep Venous Thrombosis. Prevention of DVT is a primary goal for the client after ORIF of a hip fracture. Clot prophylaxis is recommended through the use of pharmacologic agents such as subcutaneous fixed-dose LMW heparin or low-intensity oral anticoagulation. For appropriately selected clients, physical-mechanical measures such as intermittent pneumatic compression devices or elastic stockings may also have a role in DVT prevention. DVT is discussed more fully in Chapter 53.

Pressure Ulcers. A pressure ulcer is tissue damage that results from unrelieved pressure, usually over a bony prominence. Its development may have begun as the injured client lay on a hard floor at home, on hard surfaces in an ambulance or in the emergency department, on a table for radiographs or surgery, or in the bed after surgery. Pressure ulcer development is compounded because the client is unable to turn independently after injury or surgery; without assistance, the client remains supine or in a semi-Fowler position for most of the hospitalization.

A turning schedule is essential for eliminating sustained pressure over bony prominences on the head, scapulae, vertebrae, coccyx, and heels. Other areas such as the elbows, ankles, and medial surfaces of the knee may also be affected by pressure that lasts as little as 15 minutes. Bony areas should be cushioned and supported with each position change. Heels should be elevated with calf pillows or foam boots. Prevention of ischemia can also be accomplished through the use of pressure-reduction bed overlays. An "egg-crate" mattress may contribute to client comfort in the bed, but it does not relieve pressure. Specialty mattresses or air beds are the only appropriate alternatives to assist in pressure reduction. The client who is using a specialty bed must still be turned on a regular schedule. Identification of the client's risk for skin impairment can be accomplished through use of an assessment tool such as the Braden Scale, presented in Chapter 49.

Acute Confusion. Confusion is characterized by an abrupt onset of numerous global, transient changes in a client's attention, cognition, psychomotor activity, or sleep-wake cycle or in several of these. The client may appear forgetful, inattentive, disoriented, or fearful. Daytime sleepiness and nighttime insomnia may be noticed. In the hospitalized client, confusion creates concerns about safety and dependence on others for self-care needs. It can greatly affect the emotional status of the client and family. It can also lead to prolonged hospitalization, possibly contributing to placement in a long-term care facility and definitely increasing costs. Some degree of confusion has been identified in up to 60% of hospitalized older clients.[29] The incidence of confusion after hip surgery may be as high as 42%.[29] Most affected clients have no history of confusion or mental impairment.

Consistent predictors of or risk factors for acute confusion have been difficult to identify clearly. The risk for development of confusion may in fact be a cumulative function of the client's biopsychosocial integrity, the level of illness and functional impairment, and the timing and magnitude of added stressors. Known contributors to confusion may be an unfamiliar environment; sensory overstimulation or deprivation; the client's loss of control and uncertain future; a disrupted routine, immobility and pain; and a disrupted elimination pattern. Because use of medications with anticholinergic effects has also been linked to client confusion, carefully monitor all medications.

Careful assessment of the client's attention, memory, orientation, psychomotor behavior, and sleep-wake cycle is needed. The risk for confusion may also be decreased by maintaining appropriate hydration, perfusion, and oxygenation in the client. Attention must be paid to managing pain, meeting nutritional requirements, and correcting metabolic imbalances. The client must have easy access to glasses, hearing aids, and other functional devices. Also address environmental factors by reorienting the confused client in a consistent way and minimizing disruption to the usual diurnal rhythms. Companionship of family members or volunteers is helpful, as is the use of calendars, clocks, and newspapers to provide a time reference for the client. Follow institutional guidelines for the use of restraints.

DIAGNOSIS, OUTCOMES, INTERVENTIONS

Risk for Impaired Skin Integrity. If the client has fallen while alone and experienced an extended time lying down before help arrived, even early assessment may show the development of pressure ulcers over bony prominences. After surgery, the client's mobility limitations and pain increase the risk for skin impairment. Malnutrition and dehydration, which may have existed before injury and may be exacerbated postoperatively, may also contribute. Older clients and clients receiving long-term corticosteroid therapy may have especially tissue paper–thin skin that is even more prone to breakdown and tears. Finally, the type of tape used to secure postoperative dressings and the method and direction of tape application can contribute to the development of skin blisters. An appropriate diagnostic statement may be *Risk for Impaired Skin Integrity related to mobility limitations or to the application of tape with dressing changes.*

Outcomes. The client will demonstrate intact skin, as evidenced by absence of ulcers over bony prominences and heels and absence of epidermal stripping beneath tape used to secure postoperative dressings.

Interventions. After ORIF of the hip, the client should be assisted with position changes at least every 2 hours. These clients can be turned to either side; however, they are usually most comfortable on the nonoperative side with a pillow to support the operative leg. Carefully assess the skin over bony prominences such as the sacrum, coccyx, scapulae, elbows, and heels. If areas of skin breakdown are noted, measure and describe them thoroughly. Treat the ulcer using institutional protocols or see Chapter 49.

In addition to using a regular turning schedule, place a pressure-reducing mattress on the client's bed. Pressure on heels can be relieved by placement of a towel roll for brief periods under the Achilles tendon. Examination gloves filled with water can also provide pressure relief under heels. Specific skin care products are available to be massaged gently into affected areas at the first sign of redness. Direct massage of stage I pressure ulcers is contraindicated.

Avoid epidermal stripping by placing postoperative dressings over a skin sealant that is applied wherever the tape would touch the skin. Elastic tape should be placed vertically (superior to inferior) without tension to allow for stretching that is related to postoperative edema. Any redness, blistering, or epidermal stripping should be evaluated, and an enterostomal nurse specialist should be consulted on the client's care as appropriate. Clients with thin skin should not have tape on their skin; use gauze wraps instead. Treatment of skin tears is discussed in Chapter 49.

Pain. Acute pain is expected after any surgery, including ORIF of the hip. The client may also have contusions or abrasions caused by the fall that led to hip fracture. The diagnosis can be written as *Pain related to local tissue trauma from surgical incision or other injuries.*

Outcomes. The client will demonstrate comfort after surgery, as evidenced by movement without grimacing, by requesting analgesics no more frequently than ordered, and by statements that the pain is tolerable and not interfering with rest or physical therapy.

Interventions. In the immediate postoperative period, the client may experience intense pain and require injectable analgesics to attain acceptable control. Common interventions include patient-controlled analgesia (PCA) or epidural analgesia. Ice application over the dressed surgical wound may also increase the client's comfort. See the Management and Delegation feature on safe use of ice. Within 24 to 48 hours, the client should be tolerating fluids and able to take oral analgesics. Because pain is intensified with movement, the client may attempt to limit activity because of the expected increase in discomfort. Medicate the client before physical therapy or activities such as transferring to the chair, and reinforce the importance of ambulation in decreasing the risk for postoperative complications. Use of non-narcotic analgesics can also help with acute pain management, muscle spasms, and other chronic medical problems such as arthritis.

Concerns about becoming addicted to narcotics should be addressed openly. Many older persons fear that they will become addicted quickly, and they may therefore tolerate unnecessary pain, delaying their recovery. Narcotic addiction is rare, but the fear is quite intense.

Regularly assess for side effects of narcotic analgesics. Respiratory depression is more likely to occur with PCA or epidural analgesia than with oral narcotics. Pulse oximetry and regular measurement of vital signs help you assess for hypoxemia that results from shallow or slow breathing. Most clients raise their oximetry readings with stimulation. Seldom is naloxone needed.

Constipation, a very common problem after hip fracture and repair, is related to the client's impaired mobility, narcotic use, and progression to a regular diet. Encourage the client's intake of fluids and dietary fiber. In addition, stool softeners or laxatives may be indicated. If the client uses a bulk-forming laxative or other strategy to maintain bowel regularity at home, assist in continuing that program in the hospital. Regular assessment and implementation of a proactive bowel program are important for minimizing clients' concerns about bowel elimination.

Impaired Physical Mobility. The client's degree of immobility after ORIF of the hip is affected by pain and fear of movement, as well as any limitations in other joints. If previous mobility limitations contributed to the fall, the client may have even greater problems with mobilization after surgery. The diagnosis can be written as *Impaired Physical Mobility related to pain or fear of movement.*

Outcomes. The client will demonstrate improved physical mobility, as evidenced by the need for less assistance in transfers (bed to chair, bed to standing), by safe use of a walker or crutches, and by the ability to ambulate a functional distance (150 feet). For the client with previous mobility limitations, outcomes may focus on bed mobility only.

Interventions. Moving the client after ORIF of the hip can create a great deal of anxiety for both the client and the nursing staff. First be aware of any weight-bearing limitations ordered for the client before transferring him or her (see Table 27–5 for a description of weight-bearing limitations). Non–weight-bearing orders are often received after hip fracture repair, and these must be strictly followed to avoid disruption to bone healing. If the client is not allowed to bear full weight, careful attention to the

MANAGEMENT AND DELEGATION

Application of Heat and Cold

Any equipment used to apply heat or cold may injure the client. Injury may result if the client is unable to perceive discomfort because of decreased peripheral circulation, decreased feeling, decreased sensorium, sedation, or agitation. The client may also be at risk if he or she cannot be left alone safely or if the client alters the controls of the heating pad or cooling device.

The application of heat or cold to an inflamed or painful area that is closed may be delegated to unlicensed assistive personnel. Before delegating the application of heat or cold, consider the following:

- What is the indication for the application of heat or cold? Check the physician's order. The order and indication may be sufficient to tell you whether you can delegate this task or not.
- What is the condition of the affected site? Assess for any areas of redness, swelling, breakdown, or scar tissue. It is important to know the baseline condition of the site before the application of heat or cold. There may be an indication to withhold this treatment or to confer with the physician about the order. You will also need to assess the condition of the site on completion of the treatment.
- What is the client's diagnosis? Is there any history of diabetes mellitus or impairment in sensorium or mentation? This may be an indication for you to perform this treatment yourself. If there is impairment of the client's mental or sensory status, it may be necessary for the unlicensed assistive personnel to remain with the client throughout the treatment.
- What is the competency level of the unlicensed assistive personnel who might perform this task?

Instruct the unlicensed assistive personnel providing the heat or cold application to do the following:

- Wash their hands
- Assemble the necessary equipment. Advise them as to which method of applying heat or cold is ordered.
- Check the temperature of the heat or cold device before applying it to the client's skin. A safe range for heat applications is 115° to 125° F for adults.
- Wrap any heat or cold application with a protective cover, such as a towel or a flannel sleeve.
- If using a heating pad, start with the device on the lowest setting to initiate treatment.
- Instruct the client not to adjust the heat setting.
- Check the client's response immediately. If the device is too hot or cold, an adjustment is necessary. Double the protective layer between the device and the skin or allow the temperature of the device to moderate slightly.
- Check the client's skin after 5 minutes. If it is tolerated, leave the heat or cold in place for 20 minutes. If it is not tolerated, the heat or cold should be removed immediately, and you should be made aware of this. Assess the situation and notify the physician as appropriate.
- Remove the heat or cold application at 20 minutes and to inform you that the treatment is complete.

You are responsible for examining the affected area and reassessing the client's skin at the completion of this treatment. You should document your findings and the client's response to treatment in the medical record. The unlicensed assistive personnel should immediately report any difficulty encountered during the course of treatment.

Donna W. Markey, MSN, RN, *Clinician IV, Surgical Services, University of Virginia Health System, Charlottesville, Virginia*

operative extremity is required while a transfer is made, to ensure that the client avoids passing any weight through the leg. Record the amount of assistance that the client requires for safe transfer. This information provides the benchmark that will determine whether the goal for increased mobility is being met. For example, the client may have needed the assistance of two staff members on the morning after surgery; by the next afternoon, increased mobility was demonstrated when only one nurse was needed to assist with transfer.

TABLE 27–5 WEIGHT-BEARING STATUS

Non-weightbearing	The client does not bear weight on the affected extremity; the affected extremity should not touch the floor
Touch-down weight-bearing	The client's foot of the affected extremity may rest on the floor, but no weight is distributed through that extremity
Partial weight-bearing	The client bears 30%–50% of weight on the affected extremity
Weight-bearing as tolerated	The client bears as much weight as he or she can tolerate on the affected extremity without undue strain or pain
Full weight-bearing	The client bears weight fully on the affected extremity

Adapted from Maher, A. B., Salmond, S. W., & Pellino, T. A. (1998). *Orthopaedic nursing*. Philadelphia: W. B. Saunders.

In addition to postoperative limitations, the client may suffer from arthritis in other joints or may have residual effects from a previous stroke. These conditions can increase pain and affect the ability to transfer from the bed to the chair. When the client stands and transfers for the first time, he or she will require the assistance of at least two staff members. Use of appropriate technique ensures a safe transfer for the client and also minimizes the risk of injury to the staff member's lower back (see Chapter 26 for additional information on requirements for appropriate mobility assistance). Make sure that the devices are on the client whenever he or she is in the bed or chair, which is when the legs are dependent and venous return may be affected.

Self-Care Deficit. After hip fracture and surgical repair, the client is likely to experience some degree of self-care deficit in hygiene and dressing. Limited mobility may decrease independence in self-care, and assistive devices may be required. The diagnostic statement may read

Self-Care Deficit: Bathing/Hygiene, Dressing/Grooming related to mobility impairment following hip fracture.

Outcomes. The client will resume pre-injury level of independence in meeting self-care needs.

Interventions. After ORIF of the hip, the client will be aided in recovery by physical and occupational therapists. Physical therapists assist with ambulation and strengthening. They offer instruction on climbing stairs and on getting in and out of a car. They also provide assistive devices that help in functional independence, including an elevated toilet seat and a walker. Occupational therapists instruct the client on bathing and dressing techniques. They may suggest use of a tub bench or a long-handled sponge. They may also provide long-handled reachers or sock aids to help the client dress with minimal assistance from others. Nursing staff will reinforce the use of techniques and assistive devices to encourage the client's optimal recovery.

Risk for Infection. Bone infection is a serious threat and can lead to loss of joint function. Pre-existent poor health status also contributes to risk. State this diagnosis as *Risk for Infection related to loss of primary defenses (skin) and malnutrition.*

Outcomes. The client will remain free of manifestations of infection, as evidenced by (1) white blood cell (WBC) count within normal limits, (2) an afebrile state, (3) absence of purulent wound drainage, (4) absence of increasing pain in wound, and (5) no inflammation in wound after 72 hours.

Interventions. Clients often receive prophylactic antibiotics during surgery and in the immediate postoperative period. After ORIF, the physician may prefer to perform the initial dressing change. Use strict aseptic technique in performing subsequent dressing changes, carefully assessing the wound each time for signs of healing or infection.

Risk for Peripheral Neurovascular Dysfunction. Be aware of the risk for neurologic or vascular impairment after surgery on any joint. Edema or extremity positioning can place pressure on adjacent nerves. The diagnosis can be written as *Risk for Peripheral Neurovascular Dysfunction related to lower extremity edema or positioning.*

Outcomes. The client will demonstrate normal neurovascular status, as evidenced by adequate peripheral pulses with capillary refill time of less than 3 seconds and by absence of sensory impairments and motor weakness in the operative extremity.

Interventions. Assess the neurovascular status of the operative extremity at least every 4 hours or as directed by the surgeon, and then compare findings to the unaffected extremity. More frequent monitoring may be needed if indicated by the client's condition. Assessment includes the presence and quality of bilateral pedal pulses, skin color and temperature of the extremity, capillary refill in the toes, sensation and movement of the toes, and the client's ability to perform dorsiplantar flexion of the foot. Any pallor or coolness, numbness or tingling, or inability to move the extremity should be reported promptly to the surgeon.

Risk for Constipation. Impaired mobility and the use of narcotic analgesics can lead to constipation. The risk is increased in older clients who have a pre-existing dependence on laxatives. The diagnosis could be written as *Risk for Constipation related to impaired physical mobility and side effects of narcotics.*

Outcomes. The client will maintain a pattern of regular bowel elimination by consuming adequate fluids and high-fiber foods and by having a bowel movement at least every 2 to 3 days.

Interventions. The client's diet should include ample fluids and fiber if not contraindicated. Stool softeners are often prescribed and should be administered regularly. Also, determine whether the client has regular, effective strategies for treating constipation and, if so, use those methods to assist with elimination. The client should be assisted to transfer to a bedside commode or ambulate to the bathroom whenever possible to meet elimination needs. To assist the bedridden client with bowel elimination, offer a fracture bedpan and ensure privacy when the client needs to use it.

Risk for Nutritional Deficit. After surgery, the client may experience nausea that delays the progression to a regular diet. Decreased activity may also lead to poor appetite. If the client has experienced blood loss, a nutritional deficit may also occur. Remember that the presence of obesity does not ensure that the client is well-nourished. This diagnosis may be stated as *Risk for Nutritional Deficit related to nausea or poor appetite following hip fracture.*

Outcomes. The client will maintain adequate dietary intake, as evidenced by energy for participation in physical therapy and by appropriate wound and bone healing.

Interventions. Stress the importance of a high-carbohydrate and high-protein diet for adequate healing, and then assist the client in making food choices as necessary. If the client's appetite remains poor, offer small, frequent meals. Encourage the client to eat at least some of every food at every meal to achieve balanced intake. After blood loss, increased dietary iron or iron supplements may be required. Encourage the client to eat foods high in iron, and administer a supplement as ordered. Inform the client that stool may appear black or tarry while he or she is taking an iron supplement.

EVALUATION

Clinical pathways or care maps are now often used to determine which outcomes have been met for the client with a hip fracture; they often suggest a time frame for each goal. Pain should decrease fairly soon after surgery. Injectable narcotic analgesics are not typically required after 24 to 36 hours. The client should advance to oral analgesics as soon as nausea is controlled and liquids are being taken freely. A regular diet should be offered by the first or second day after surgery, again on the assumption that nausea is controlled. Early feeding primes the gastrointestinal tract, helping the client avoid postoperative ileus. Adequate diet also contributes greatly to the client's physical stamina and to wound healing. If an indwelling urinary catheter has been used, it should be removed as soon as the client can transfer to a bedside commode, in order to decrease any risk for urinary tract infection (see Case Management: Hip Fracture).

A clinical pathway also often describes the involvement of a case manager or social worker in planning the client's discharge. In collaboration with the bedside nurse and the physician, the case manager assesses the client's

CASE MANAGEMENT

Hip Fracture

A hip fracture is an unexpected event, usually involving an older woman who falls at home. Sometimes the client is unable to summon help and is found after having fallen hours earlier.

The best case management is prevention of the fracture. Prevention of osteoporosis through good nutrition, exercise, and monitoring of bone density are important measures. Weight reduction and maintenance of optimum range of motion can also help to prevent bone problems. Correction of visual deficits and home safety (e.g., good lighting, elimination of throw rugs, safe footwear, grab bars) can also prevent accidents.

Assess

- What events led to the hip fracture?
- How long was it before help arrived?
- Are there underlying conditions that contributed to the hip fracture (osteoporosis, cancer, arthritis, incontinence, urinary tract infection)?
- Are there other chronic conditions that might inhibit recovery or make rehabilitation more difficult, such as anemia, heart disease, or a cognitive impairment?
- Are cognitive or sensory changes apparent? What is the client's pain status?
- If surgery is anticipated, what preparations are needed? Does the client have a health care proxy or advance directives?

Advocate

Take time to explain what is happening, taking into account cognitive and sensory deficits. If the client had to wait for assistance for some time after falling, consider dehydration, weakness, or even pneumonia as a consequence. Give the client and family information to help them make decisions about surgery or other treatments. Make sure that pain is managed. Frequently, older people do not ask for pain medication and suffer needlessly as a result. Inquire about the client's home situation and care needs; some assistance or change of residence may be required.

Prevent Readmission

Explain the surgical intervention and how to prevent dislocation. Many hospitals offer educational materials showing proper positioning and exercises. Physical and occupational therapists can aid the client in learning exercises, correct weight-bearing, and transfer and ambulation techniques as well as how to make changes in activities of daily living. Often short-term rehabilitation can assist the client, especially if no caregiver is available at home.

Monitor for manifestations of infection and teach the client to continue monitoring after discharge. Make sure that pain control is adequate and that the client understands necessary medication regimens, especially anticoagulants. Prevent complications, such as thrombophlebitis and bowel problems, through early mobilization. Refer appropriately for home nursing care, social services, physical therapy, and phlebotomy. Make sure that the client knows when follow-up appointments are scheduled and what to do if an emergency, especially dislocation, occurs.

Cheryl Noetscher, RN, MS, *Director of Case Management, Crouse Hospital and Community–General Hospital, Syracuse, New York*

discharge needs on the basis of information about the home environment and social support. An extended-care facility or rehabilitation unit may be one possible destination after acute care hospitalization. If the client can move from bed to chair with minimal or no assistance, he or she may instead go directly home with possible visits from a home health aide or nurse to meet other skilled needs, such as hygiene and mobility assistance. When the client is discharged directly to the home, the nurse must ensure that the family can safely assist the client with mobility needs and activities of daily living. The case manager assists the client in obtaining any durable medical equipment that may be needed, such as a walker or crutches, and finalizes discharge transportation if necessary (see Bridge to Home Health Care).

CONDYLAR FRACTURES

The condyles are bony prominences at the distal end of the femur. Condylar fractures occur most often with high-energy injuries in young clients. They may be among several injuries sustained in a motor vehicle accident, for example, when the client's flexed knee strikes the dashboard. Less severe condylar fractures are treated with knee immobilizers or casting. For more severe injury, ORIF is indicated. Bone grafting is used for comminuted fractures. Loss of knee mobility is a common outcome, and surgical revision may be needed to improve bony alignment. If the client develops severe pain and disability, arthrodesis (fusion) or arthroplasty (joint replacement) may be required.

PELVIC FRACTURES

The pelvis is a ring-like structure composed mostly of cancellous bone, with a thin cortex. This structure provides great strength, allowing the pelvis to offer structural support and also to serve as a shock absorber that protects the abdominal organs. Pelvic fractures have been on the rise since 1990 as a result of an increase in high-energy trauma, such as motor vehicle accidents and gunshot wounds. About two thirds of all pelvic fractures occur as a result of traffic accidents; pedestrians are injured more often than are the occupants of involved vehicles.[1]

Because fractures of the pelvic ring can vary in stability, their management depends on the severity of the injury. Most cases can be diagnosed correctly with an anteroposterior radiograph. If there is any indication of an unstable fracture, a urethrogram or intravenous pyelogram is used to assess for possible damage to the kidneys and lower urinary tract. Pelvic fractures also often result in hemorrhage, and the pelvis can hold as much as 4 L of blood. Unstable fractures have been treated aggressively since the mid-1990s with internal fixation in which plates and screws are used to achieve an intact pelvic ring. External fixation is also still used. Less severe pelvic fractures may be treated with bed rest alone. The client needs adequate pain management as well as assessment for neurovascular compromise or the development of complications such as thrombophlebitis or fat embolism.

PATELLAR FRACTURES

Fracture of the patella (kneecap) often results from a direct blow to the area. Some separation or splitting of the patella invariably occurs, and the client is unable to fully extend the knee because of pain and related damage to extensor mechanisms. Patellar fractures are usually more evident on a lateral radiograph than on other views. A stellate fracture (cracked patella without fragment displacement) can be managed conservatively by placing the client in a long leg cast for several weeks and then beginning mobilization. Indirect trauma, such as a forced flexion injury sustained in a fall, can result in a transverse fracture. ORIF is often necessary to minimize the potential for later problems with knee motion or chondromalacia. After a comminuted fracture, fragments may be difficult to reduce accurately, and removal of the patella may be best. Surgical repair of extensors such as the quadriceps tendon and the patellar tendon may also be needed.

TIBIAL AND FIBULAR FRACTURES

The fibula can be fractured alone in several ways: from direct trauma to the outer surface of the leg, producing a transverse or comminuted fracture; through twisting injuries, which produce a spiral fracture; or from repeated stress as in long-distance running, which can cause a fatigue fracture usually just above the inferior tibiofibular ligament. Fatigue fractures necessitate immobilization; for other nondisplaced fibular fractures, a cast may be needed to immobilize the ankle.

The tibia can also be broken, leaving the fibula intact. Fracture can result from direct trauma. Repeated stress can lead to a fatigue fracture at the junction of the middle and upper thirds of the tibia. This injury is commonly seen in long-distance runners, hurdlers, and ballet dancers who jump excessively. Twisting injuries rarely result in a lone tibial fracture. Tibial fractures are reduced and treated through cast immobilization, internal fixation, or external fixation. Although it may seem helpful to have the fibula intact, the undamaged bone actually holds the ends of the tibia apart and it may be necessary to cut the fibula in order to attain satisfactory alignment of the tibia.

Fractures of both the tibia and fibula are common results of motor vehicle accidents and sports injuries. Treatment concerns include possible problems with fracture union, vascular and soft tissue damage, skin loss, and the development of compartment syndrome. As with lone tibial fractures, fragments may be held in the reduced position through casting from groin to toe. Alternatively, internal fixation would be the treatment of choice for clients with unstable or multiple fractures. External fixation would be necessary if the wound is dirty or if there is skin loss.

If the knee is struck violently on the lateral surface, a tibial plateau fracture may result. Four fracture patterns can occur: the lateral tibial plateau may be split vertically; part of the tibial plateau may be thrust downward into the tibia to produce a depressed fracture; both of these can occur together; or the whole plateau may be depressed. Because the full extent of injury may not be apparent on radiographs, CT scanning or MRI may be needed to determine the fracture anatomy. Any large fragment split off the tibia must be secured back in place with screws to restore the contour of the bone. Large depressed fragments can be elevated to reconstitute the bone's surface, but the cavity that results below the fracture must be filled with a cancellous bone graft. If only a slight depression occurred in the tibial plateau, more conservative treatment with early mobilization may be appropriate.

FOOT FRACTURES

Because it provides a contact point with the ground and protrudes forward from the body, the foot is especially susceptible to injury. Fracture is most often caused by falls or jumps from great heights, running or twisting, motor vehicle accidents, or objects dropped on the foot. As with any other injury, the client with open fractures should be taken to the operating room for surgical debridement and repair. Closed fractures of the foot, however, can generally be treated conservatively through cast or brace immobilization or through the use of walking shoes. Weight-bearing is progressively resumed as tolerated.

UPPER EXTREMITY FRACTURES

Fractures of the proximal humerus are a common traumatic injury in older persons, often caused by a fall on an outstretched arm. A fall need not be serious to produce a humeral fracture in an osteoporotic client. Injury to the dominant arm of an older client can lead to dependence and immobility. The risk of falling also increases because the sense of balance is impaired as a result of loss of use of the arm. If the fracture is nondisplaced or minimally displaced, the extremity is usually immobilized with a sling. Gentle range-of-motion exercises can be started when shoulder discomfort subsides, usually within 2 or 3 weeks after injury. A displaced fracture is treated by ORIF. Prosthetic replacement is occasionally indicated for an intra-articular fracture or one that is severely comminuted. Prompt, appropriate treatment reduces the risk that AVN of the humeral head will develop.

Fractures of the humeral shaft usually result from a direct blow to the arm, a motor vehicle accident, a gunshot injury, or a crush injury. Humeral fractures can also result from indirect injuries such as a fall on an outstretched hand or on the elbow. Most humeral shaft fractures can be treated by initial immobilization with a U-shaped splint. Once the swelling has subsided, a commercially available humeral fracture brace may be used in conjunction with an arm sling. Heavy hanging arm casts should be avoided because they may contribute to a non-union. Surgery would be indicated for debridement of an open fracture. Surgical stabilization would also be required for any fracture associated with a vascular injury.

Intra-articular injuries of the elbow include condylar, olecranon, and radial head or neck fracture. These injuries frequently result from falls on or direct blows to the elbow. Because associated injuries to the three major peripheral nerves (radial, median, and ulnar) are possible, careful neurovascular assessment is critical. A high potential for compartment syndrome also exists after intra-articular fractures of the elbow. Most nondisplaced fractures can be treated with immobilization, followed by early range-of-motion exercises once acute discomfort has diminished (usually after 1 week). A posterior long arm splint may be used with a shoulder sling. Displaced fractures, especially supracondylar fractures, often necessitate ORIF. Repair of the brachial artery may also be necessary after traumatic injury. After surgery, immobilization can be accomplished with a posterior elbow splint, a cast, or traction.

Fractures of the shafts of the radius and ulna usually result from a direct blow to the forearm, a motor vehicle accident, or a fall on an outstretched arm. Associated injuries to the nerves (median, ulnar, and radial) and arteries (radial and ulnar) are possible. A sugar-tong splint can be used to provide initial immobilization of forearm fractures. Circumferential cast immobilization is generally not recommended in early treatment because fracture swelling in association with the constriction provided by the cast may lead to a compartment syndrome. Immobilization must include the wrist and the elbow to control rotation of the forearm. In adult clients, surgical treatment may be indicated for displaced or open fractures.

As with proximal humeral fractures, fractures of the distal radius are common injuries in older persons. Many older clients have a good outcome even with a residual deformity because their routine activities may not demand full use of the limb. However, deformity and possible resulting arthritic changes in younger clients may lead to inability to perform their current jobs. Colles' fracture is a common injury in which the distal radius fragment is displaced dorsally and proximally. Fracture reduction is

BRIDGE TO HOME HEALTH CARE

Managing the Immobile Client

To prevent skin breakdown and manage other physical and emotional effects of immobility, the multidisciplinary team must collaborate with clients who are paralyzed or have other desensitized areas, with their family members, and with their informal caregivers. The core team members are a nurse, a physical therapist, a social worker, and an occupational therapist.

If the person is chair- or wheelchair-bound, good seat cushions can be purchased from most pharmacies and vendors. Choose a cushion to match the client's seating problems. Some cushions are designed for active paraplegics that distribute pressure onto the posterior thigh. Heavy foam (4 inches thick) provides pressure reduction for clients with wheelchairs that have sling seats. Cushions of air can be inflated to reduce pressure and prevent posture problems. Pillows or gel should not be used: A pillow allows too much hip adduction and internal rotation and becomes uncomfortable; gel is expensive and heavy, breaks down, and makes it harder to move a wheelchair.

Evaluate how clients sit and use cushions. Inspect every cushion frequently for signs of wear. Avoid folds, wrinkles, or pockets on surfaces. The proper sitting position includes 90 degrees of flexion at the hips and knees. Clients should sit erect in chairs on their buttocks, not on the sacrum. Place pillows behind a client's back to promote more erect posture.

Teach clients to protect tissue, toughen skin, and avoid massaging lotion over bony prominences; massage makes skin soft and susceptible to breakdown or shearing. Minimize friction; avoid having tissue squeezed between two hard surfaces such as bedding and bony prominences. Teach clients, especially those with paraplegia, to use a mirror to check for friction or pressure. Clients who are confined to bed need to be repositioned at least every 2 hours, and use a footboard, a thoroughly padded plastic crate, or a box to prevent feet from being forced into extreme plantar flexion. Their heels, ankles, trochanters, sacrum, scapulae, elbows, and ears need to be checked at least daily. Pillows, blanket or towel rolls, balloons, foam, or rolled-up clothing are useful for padding and positioning. Sheepskin, elbow and heel protectors, and egg-crate cushions provide little protection; thick foam is better. Even though good-quality alternating pressure pads are best, there are other options, including waterbeds, silicon bead beds, and air mattresses. When alternating pads are used watch the skin for several days to ensure that the client is getting enough lift (see Chapter 49).

Daily exercise is essential. Passive exercise only increases flexibility, whereas active exercise increases circulation and air exchange, maintains joint lubrication and mobility, and helps prevent contractures. Provide all exercise gently to avoid joint or tissue damage. Movement of any kind can trigger spasms. Keep a firm hold on the extremity, moving it through the range of motion. Wait for any spasm to subside; then continue. If the spasticity is too strong or you feel uncertain about whether to continue the exercise, request assistance from a physical therapist.

After clients progress through the acute stage, they need to consider long-term issues and dramatic lifestyle changes. Provide information about alternative housing options, transportation, yard and housekeeping services, financial assistance, recreation, and stores that deliver prescriptions. Mental health and sexuality issues are important, too. Clients also need to consider and make decisions about nutrition, clothing, informal caregivers, and health care services. Some clients may be eligible for specially trained dogs or the Helping Hands Program that supplies capuchin monkeys for aid and companion assistance.

Mary E. McQuin, BSPT, *Physical Therapist, Visiting Nurse Association of Omaha, Omaha, Nebraska*

greatly enhanced by the use of a nerve block such as the Bier block. This fracture may be treated with 2 weeks of splinting followed by 3 weeks in a short arm cast. Comminuted fractures may necessitate external fixation or ORIF with bone grafting.

Fractures of the metacarpals and phalanges account for 10% of all hand fractures.[5] More than half of those fractures are work-related. A delay in seeking evaluation and diagnosis can make fracture reduction difficult because fractures in the hand form early callus within 7 to 10 days and become difficult to manipulate. Treatment involves accurate fracture reduction, movement of the uninvolved fingers to prevent stiffness, and elevation of the extremity to decrease edema. Simple measures such as "buddy taping" or splinting are usually sufficient treatment for stable fractures. Comminuted fractures and those necessitating open reduction take longer to consolidate and are not ready as quickly for mobilization. Client motivation plays a critical role in rehabilitation after hand injury and can often be enhanced by a brief course of physical therapy. Motion can typically be started about 21 days after injury for clients with closed, nondisplaced fractures.

Neurovascular assessment is critical for all clients with upper extremity fractures. Carefully compare the color, warmth, movement, sensation, and capillary refill of the affected extremity with those of the unaffected extremity. Elevation of the injured extremity is typically indicated. At night, the client should be observed frequently to be certain the arm does not move into a dependent position. If a cast or splint has been applied, the client and family should receive careful instruction about cast care and about the clinical manifestations of compartment syndrome.

DISLOCATIONS AND SUBLUXATIONS

Dislocation and subluxation both describe changes in joint relationships. In a dislocation, the opposing joint surfaces are no longer in contact. In subluxation, the joint surfaces are in partial contact, but their relationship is abnormal. Both injuries are caused by acute deforming forces applied to ligaments or tendons from a fall, a blow, or a strong muscle contraction. For example, the client who tries to break a fall down the stairs by holding on to the handrail may dislocate a shoulder.

After dislocation, the client often complains of severe pain that increases with attempted movement. Swelling around or below the joint is likely, along with complete or nearly complete loss of function and a visible deformity that may alter the length of the extremity. Fracture of the joint surface often accompanies dislocation. Neurovascular status of the affected extremity must be carefully assessed because the displaced bone may tear blood vessels and impede circulation, damage nerves, and rupture ligaments or muscle attachments. Immediate reduction is preferred before inflammation and spasm can become significant. If immediate reduction is not possible, analgesics and muscle relaxants must be given before any later attempt to reduce the dislocation. A splint, a harness, or padding should be used for 4 to 8 weeks after acute dislocation or until pain is significantly reduced and muscle function provides adequate support in cases of recurrent dislocation. Like fractures, dislocations are described in terms of the relationship of the distal bone to the proximal bone. In a posterior dislocation of the knee, for example, the tibia lies posterior to the femur.

After subluxation, the client experiences variable pain and the feeling that the joint was out of position briefly. The joint typically feels weak, and pain increases with attempted movement. Because radiographs are often normal with subluxations, the physician must rule out other possible injuries such as sprain, strain, muscle tear, and fracture. Muscle-strengthening exercises can help the client avoid future subluxations. Joint restrictive supports such as a shoulder harness may also be useful.

SPORTS INJURIES

OVERUSE SYNDROMES

Overuse syndromes are common sports-related problems. They begin insidiously as the result of microtraumas that often do not completely stop the affected person's activity. The client must understand that the manifestations of pain, tenderness, and swelling result from repeated stress on musculoskeletal structures. Eventual failure is likely because of fatigue or erosion if the client continues to exercise. Nonoperative treatment of stress injuries always includes relative rest. For example, the runner may be restricted from impact-loading activities but still allowed to cycle or run in the buoyancy of a swimming pool. Ice, compression (when swelling occurs), and NSAIDs are used routinely to reduce inflammation related to the injury. A supervised, stepped rehabilitation program is also helpful if the client plans to return to the athletic activity.

People who are at greatest risk for overuse include competitive athletes, first-time athletes, "born again" athletes (those who were once very active and now seek a return to athletics after a decade or more of sedentary living), and those recovering from injury. Other factors can contribute to an increased risk for injury (Box 27–3) and should be shared with clients who exercise regularly or are considering involvement in an exercise program. The risk for developing an overuse syndrome decreases if the client avoids the following:

- Training errors, such as progressing too fast or allowing inadequate time for conditioning

BOX 27–3 Factors that May Increase Risk for Injury

- Age over 40 yr
- Current inactive lifestyle
- Overweight by 20 lb or more
- Family history of cardiac disease
- Any past experience of pain or pressure in chest, arm, or throat
- Taking medications on a regular basis
- Documented high cholesterol level
- Smokes or has history of pulmonary disease
- History of diabetes or other chronic disorders
- History of joint disease

- Improper technique based on the individual activity (e.g., elbow problems from poor tennis technique)
- Improper equipment, such as incorrect shoes for the sport
- Unsafe environment, such as exercising on a slippery surface or experiencing repeated impact on a hard surface

Prevention, the key to overuse injuries, is enhanced by pre-participation assessment and client teaching. Rather than trying to ensure that the client is in optimal health, a pre-participation assessment allows recognition of potential problems that can occur as the client progresses in a sport. Client teaching should emphasize the importance of stretching to maintain joint flexibility and range of motion. Stretching exercises should be static (i.e., holding muscles in a stretched position for a few moments rather than repeatedly stretching and relaxing them). Static stretching reduces the danger of overstretching and tissue damage, causes less muscle soreness than a bouncing stretch, and relieves muscle soreness when it occurs. Box 27–4 presents additional information about injury prevention in fitness programs.

Overuse syndromes are classified according to severity of injury. Intervention generally depends on the sever-ity more than on the specific type of injury (Table 27–6).

BOX 27–4 Preventing Injuries in Fitness Programs

Lack of fitness is one of the main causes of sport injury.

Warm-up and Stretching Exercises

Always warm up and stretch before strenuous exercises. To warm up means to begin and finish exercises gradually. Stretching exercises increase muscle flexibility.

Pacing

Build up an exercise program gradually. It takes at least 6 to 8 weeks to get into strong condition. Add small, gradual increments of exercise. Proceed gradually and do not overdo. Tired muscles are prone to injury.

Intensity

When preparing for a specific event, plan training programs accordingly (e.g., a marathon demands a more intensive training program than does a 10-km race).

Capacity Level

Exercise to the capacity of physiologic limits.

Strength

Build strength gradually to gain greater endurance, speed, and power.

Motivation

Success in an exercise program depends on individual motivation.

Relaxation

Relaxation exercises relieve fatigue and tension.

Routine

Regular exercise is more valuable and less likely to lead to injury than bursts of activity followed by long periods of inactivity.

LOWER EXTREMITIES

Common overuse injuries of the lower extremities include the following.

Stress Fracture

The most common stress fracture occurs in the foot, in which fatigue or erosion commonly manifests as pain and swelling. Forces acting on the leg at heel contact during running are three to eight times an individual's body weight, repeated up to 2000 times.[18] Stress fractures commonly occur in the tarsal bones. Tarsal navicular stress fractures are fairly common in jumping athletes, but their recognition is frequently delayed. Once diagnosed, bone grafting and screw fixation may be necessary to obtain healing.

Plantar Fasciitis

One of the most common overuse syndromes of the foot results from repetitive strain to the plantar fascia, the long ligament that attaches to the plantar surface (sole) of the calcaneus (heel bone); its fibers fan out to attach to the forefoot. At times a bone spur is seen on radiographs at the plantar origin of the fascia as new bone forms, as a result of repeated tearing of the fascia. Plantar fasciitis can be very difficult to correct. Heel cups are used routinely, and arch supports may also be useful. Other standard modalities such as ice and ultrasonography with hydrocortisone cream can at times relieve pain. Direct injections of corticosteroid preparations may be indicated in resistant cases.

Shin Splints

A medial tibial stress syndrome results from excessive strain of the posterior tibial muscle origin. Shin splints are characterized by pain with activity and residual tenderness at the muscle origins for days after running or other repetitive activity. Shin splints are best treated by strengthening the involved muscles and by using orthotics to correct misalignment of the feet and reduce strain on injured muscles.

Patellar Tendinitis

Also known as "jumper's knee," patellar tendinitis results from repetitive loads placed on the knee's extensor mechanism through sports that require jumping, such as basketball and volleyball. The client complains of pain, tenderness, and sometimes swelling at either pole of the patella. The pain is aggravated by additional jumping. Patellar tendinitis is usually unilateral and rarely progresses to complete rupture. Treatment includes NSAIDs, reduction in the irritating activity, and improvement in the flexibility of the hamstrings and rectus femoris to improve efficiency of knee flexion and extension.

UPPER EXTREMITIES

Overuse injuries that occur in the upper extremities include:

Impingement Syndrome

Impingement syndrome is one of the most common problems encountered by the athlete involved in repetitive activity with arms upward over the client's head (e.g.,

TABLE 27–6 GRADES OF OVERUSE INJURIES

	Grade I	Grade II	Grade III	Grade IV
ASSESSMENT				
History	Hurts after, not during, activity	Hurts after and sometimes during activity	Hurts during and after activity	Hurts all the time
Physical examination	Generalized tenderness	Generalized tenderness over area	More localized tenderness	Localized tenderness
X-rays	Negative	Negative	Usually negative	May be positive
Bone scan	Negative	Negative	May be positive	Usually positive
TYPE OF TISSUE INJURED	Soft tissue	Soft tissue	Soft, hard, or bony tissue	Hard or bony tissue
MANAGEMENT	Ice Treat underlying problem	Ice Correct underlying problem Anti-inflammatory medication, e.g., aspirin Decrease exercise 25%–33%	Ice Correct underlying problem Anti-inflammatory medication, e.g., aspirin, NSAIDs; possibly prednisone Decrease exercise 50%–75%	Ice Correct underlying problem Anti-inflammatory medication, e.g., aspirin, NSAIDs; possibly prednisone Stop exercising altogether

NSAIDs, nonsteroidal anti-inflammatory drugs.
Adapted from The athlete's leg (1985). *Emergency Medicine, 17,* 83.

painters). Manifestations include pain and weakness associated with forward flexion or lateral abduction of the shoulder above 70 degrees. The subacromial bursa, long head of the biceps muscle, and the rotator cuff are the most frequently affected structures in the "painful arc." Initial treatment involves relative rest and NSAIDs. A subacromial injection of anesthetic and cortisone is also an accepted treatment. Physical therapy represents a major portion of recovery. Return to activity should be slow and progressive.

TENNIS ELBOW

Despite the common term "tennis elbow," lateral humeral epicondylitis is seen not only in tennis players but also in anyone involved in activities that require repetitive use of the wrist extensors or flexors. Most affected clients are 30 to 45 years of age. Nonoperative treatment to reduce inflammation is followed by a careful rehabilitation program that includes gradual stretching and isometric exercises. As the client returns to full activity, a counter-force brace can be worn to inhibit full muscle expansion and decrease tension on the injured tissue.

GOLFER'S ELBOW

The etiology and treatment of medial humeral epicondylitis are similar to those of tennis elbow.

TENDINITIS

Tendinitis involving the hand and wrist is quite common but usually transitory. When it persists, tendinitis may impair the client's ability to work. People at risk include those who engage in activities that require gripping, pinching, pulling, or lifting with repetitive wrist motion. Radiographs are obtained to rule out foreign bodies, arthritis, calcification, fractures, and other abnormalities.

STRAINS

Strains result from trauma to a muscle body or to the attachment of a tendon from overstretching, overextension, or misuse. They often arise from twisting or wrenching movements and may occur in any body part that contains muscles and tendons. Strains can occur *acutely* during unaccustomed vigorous exercise. They may also be *chronic,* developing after repetitive muscle overuse.

Strains are characterized by muscle spasm and discomfort; severity of clinical manifestations is related to the degree of injury. With more severe strains, ecchymosis and edema may be evident, and range of motion may be quite limited. Radiographs are necessary to rule out the possibility of fracture.

Acute strains necessitate rest and, if possible, splinting. The injured part should be elevated and ice should be applied for the first 24 to 48 hours to decrease swelling. Heat may be prescribed for comfort after 72 hours; it also hastens reabsorption of blood and fluid and promotes healing. Surgical repair may be needed if a rupture is present at the tendon-bone interface. During healing after strain (4 to 6 weeks), movement of the injured part should be minimized. Activity should never progress to the point that symptoms such as pain or swelling result. After mature scar tissue has formed, the injured part can be gradually and progressively exercised. Overactivity must absolutely be avoided during rehabilitation.

SPRAINS

A sprain is a ligamentous injury resulting from overstress that damages ligament fibers or their attachment to a bone. The ankle is the joint most frequently injured during sports participation. An ankle sprain most often occurs when the foot is forced inward to cause stretching or tearing of the ligaments that hold the joint in place. The greater the stress and the longer it is applied to the ankle, the more severe the sprain is. The severity of the swelling depends on the extent of tissue injury. However, ecchymosis does not always reliably indicate either the severity or the site of the injury. In order to plan treatment, it is important to determine the number of ligaments affected and the severity of injury to them.

Sprains may be *mild* (first degree), *moderate* (second degree), or *severe* (third degree) (Fig. 27–9). In a first-degree sprain, only a few ligament fibers are torn, with no loss of function and no weakening of the ligament. Appropriate treatment for this level of injury includes *r*est, *i*ce, *c*ompression, and *e*levation (RICE) for 3 to 5 days. Gentle range-of-motion and strengthening exercises can then be started. In a second-degree sprain, a portion of the ligament is torn, producing some loss of function. Protection is crucial to prevent further tearing. Immobilization with a splint or brace is indicated until initial swelling has diminished, usually 1 to 2 weeks. Pain and swelling typically mandate restricted weight-bearing as well, and the client may need instruction on walking with crutches. A brace such as an airsplint can be used to prevent ankle inversion and eversion. In a third-degree sprain, a ligament is completely torn, either from its attachment or within the ligament body itself. With complete ligament rupture, surgical repair is often required. Cast or brace immobilization is needed for 4 to 6 weeks after the injury.

Once the conventional immobilizer is removed, the injured ankle can be placed in an aircast to allow dorsiflexion and plantar flexion of the foot while restricting lateral movements of the ankle. At this point, gentle range-of-motion and strengthening exercises can be initiated. When the client returns to full exercise, adequate taping and protection are needed for the next 6 months. Sprains can also lead to avulsion fractures (Fig. 27–9*D*).

Client education following an ankle sprain is extremely important. Explain all phases of recovery, and offer strategies to prevent future injury to the ankle.

ROTATOR CUFF TEARS

Pathophysiology

Most shoulder injuries involve the soft tissues, and many result directly from repetitive activities such as throwing or overhead motion within the shoulder girdle. The shoulder girdle includes the sternoclavicular joint, the acromioclavicular joint, the glenohumeral joint, the subacromial space, and the scapulothoracic space. Movement at all of these articulations allows for the complexity of a pitcher's throwing motion. Four muscles also contribute to the shoulder's varied movements and form the rotator cuff: (1) the subscapularis (anterior), (2) the supraspinatus, (3) the infraspinatus, and (4) the teres minor (posterior).

Normal shoulder movement is a smooth, pain-free activity of the rotator cuff muscles. However, excessive joint activity can lead to repetitive trauma, or muscles can be injured by an external force. Careful history and appropriate examination by the physician often lead to a diagnosis of the extent of injury. If the rotator cuff is torn, the client is not able to perform abduction and external rotation. Activity at the glenohumeral joint is also painfully impaired. Confirmation can be gained through use of radiography, arthrography, CT scans, MRI, or arthroscopy.

Treatment of rotator-cuff injury often begins conservatively with rest and sling support for the shoulder. NSAIDs may relieve discomfort. Some physicians also advocate intra-articular injection of analgesics or steroids. When acute manifestations subside, the client should begin active exercises that address range of motion and strengthen the rotator cuff muscles. Any elastic graded equipment (e.g., TheraBand) can be used in a daily program of progressive gentle exercises. Exercise may be preceded by application of heat and followed by ice if discomfort occurs.

Surgery may be necessary to repair a tear in the rotator cuff. Repair may be performed on an outpatient basis, or the client may have a short hospital stay. Postoperative management includes instruction on the use of a shoulder immobilizer and introduction of a program of gentle exercises such as the pendulum shoulder movement. The neurovascular status of the affected arm should be assessed at regular intervals, and findings should be compared to

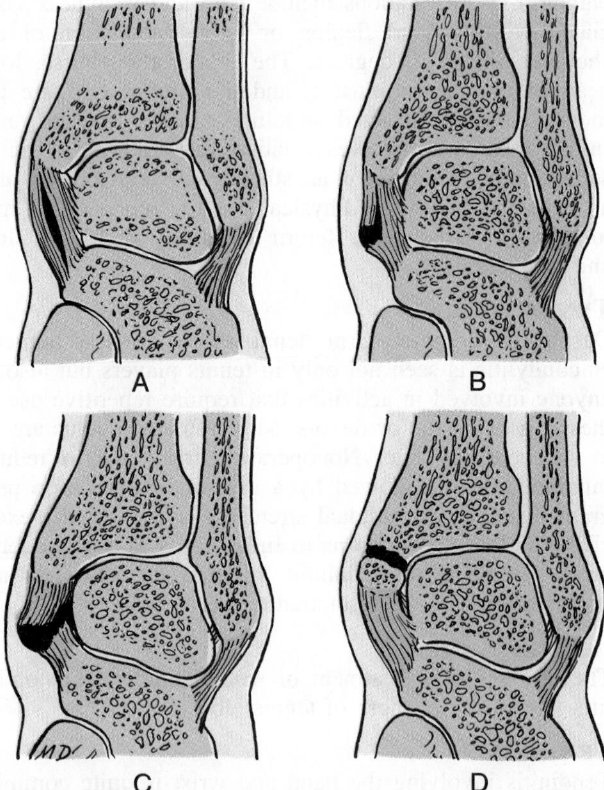

FIGURE 27–9 Various types of sprains (with the ankle as an example). *A,* Mild (first-degree) sprain is a small hematoma in a localized area. *B,* Moderate (second-degree) sprain is more severe, with more than half of the fibers torn. *C,* Severe (third-degree) sprains tear completely through the ligament.

the nonoperative arm. Pain management should also be a focus of postoperative care.

ANTERIOR CRUCIATE LIGAMENT INJURIES

One of the most common knee injuries in sports is a tear of the anterior cruciate ligament (ACL) (Fig. 27–10). For example, an estimated 80% of ski injuries involve the ACL. About 80% of the injured athletes are able to return to sports, but 50% to 65% are reinjured in 1 to 2 years; after 5 years, only 35% still participate. ACL injury also occurs in sports such as basketball, gymnastics, football, and soccer.

The ACL is usually injured as part of a complex mechanism of hyperextension, internal rotation, extremes of external rotation, and deceleration. The ligament may actually be torn from the femur or tibia. More commonly, however, the tear occurs in the midportion of the ACL. The injured client often describes hearing a loud pop. Severe swelling can occur in the first few hours after injury. The knee feels unstable ("gives way"), particularly in rotation, and full extension is difficult.

The physician may attempt to determine knee stability during examination by using the Lachman test, the most sensitive test for ACL insufficiency. The client rests in a relaxed supine position with the injured knee flexed at 15 to 30 degrees. Placing one hand around the client's distal thigh and the other around the client's proximal tibia, the physician attempts anterior-posterior translation. The test result is positive when anterior-posterior sliding occurs. Routine radiographs may also be used for diagnosis of ACL injury, but the MRI is especially sensitive and specific for difficult cases. Arthroscopy, the most important advance in the diagnosis of knee disorders, can enable the physician to confirm the degree of ACL damage and determine the extent of associated intra-articular injuries. Arthroscopy is also the surgical treatment of choice for ACL reconstruction.

Initial treatment focuses on decreasing pain and swelling and on protecting the joint from further injury by immobilization. ACL reconstruction can be accomplished within several weeks of injury and still allow a return of joint function and stability. Repair is often accomplished with the use of a portion of the client's patellar tendon. After ACL reconstruction, the surgeon often orders the use of a continuous passive motion (CPM) machine to help the client achieve rapid, satisfactory knee mobility. The CPM machine is generally applied in the recovery area and should be used at least 8 hours a day or until full range of motion is achieved. Some surgeons advocate the use of a long leg brace with fixed knee flexion, either alone or in combination with the CPM machine. After ACL reconstruction, the client receives instructions on performance of isometric exercises such as quadriceps setting, bent-knee leg exercises, and foot exercises. The exercise program is progressed over the next 4 to 6 weeks.

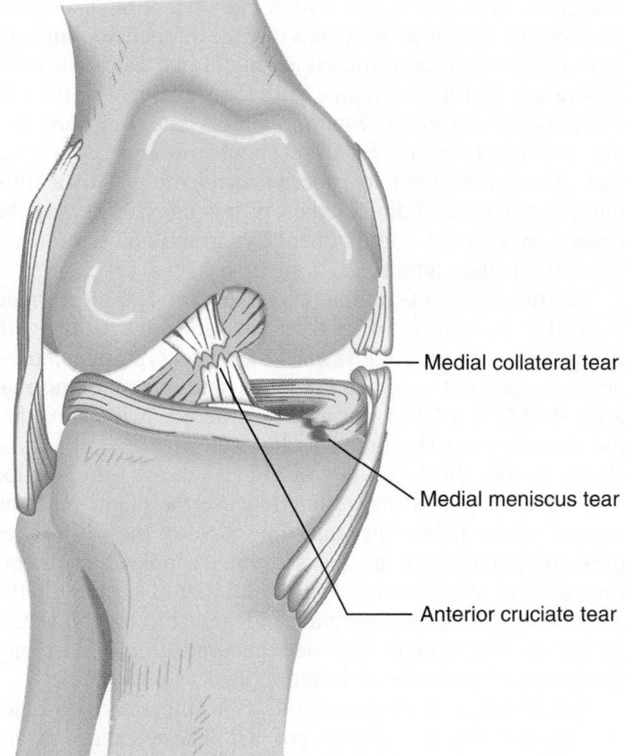

FIGURE 27–10 Common knee injuries: medial collateral tear, commonly caused by inversion and twisting. Anterior cruciate ligament injury, commonly caused by twisting a hyperextended knee. Medial meniscal injury, commonly caused by twisting an everted knee.

MENISCAL INJURIES

The meniscus is the fibrous cartilage that lies on top of the tibia, between the tibia and the femur, and acts as the shock absorber of the knee. It is torn less frequently than the ACL, but most longitudinal tears of the meniscus occur in conjunction with ACL or medial collateral ligament injuries (Fig. 27–10). Because the meniscus has very little blood supply, it heals very slowly, if at all, after injury.

Meniscal injuries often result from fixed-foot rotation in weight-bearing with the knee flexed. A combination of compression and rotational forces are thus exerted on the meniscus. Mild swelling may be evident, and the client may complain of joint-line pain. Popping, slipping, catching, or buckling of the knee can also occur, particularly if a piece of the cartilage is torn and floating within the knee capsule. Routine radiographs are usually normal, although some spurring may be evident if the tear has been present for a long time. Arthrography enables the physician to diagnose posterior tears, but MRI is a more sensitive and specific procedure for reliable diagnosis. Arthroscopy has an additional advantage as both a diagnostic and treatment option. After surgery, the leg is elevated and ice is applied. Effective pain management is an initial priority. An exercise program includes quadriceps strengthening and range of motion for the knee.

REMOBILIZATION AFTER TRAUMATIC INJURY

Strategies for remobilization include therapeutic exercise, use of CPM machines, passive and active range-of-motion exercises, and active resistive range-of-motion exercises. Therapeutic exercise programs are developed to improve joint range of motion, muscle strength, and cardiovascular endurance. Before beginning an exercise program, the client must be aware of limiting factors such as pain and the inability to relax. Exercise should progress at a pace that allows the client to experience no more than a little muscle soreness. Pain in the exercising client may be caused by chronic compartment syndrome and should receive immediate attention.

Passive range-of-motion exercises can be performed with the assistance of a therapist or a nurse or with equipment such as a CPM machine. This type of exercise helps to prevent joint contractures and maintain normal joint ROM. If a CPM machine is ordered, make sure that the device properly fits the client. If, for example, the client is too short for the machine settings, the device may be too tight in the groin. Because the client must be supine when using the machine, assess the skin over pressure points such as the sacrum, scapulae, and heels for signs of impairment. The client should be taught the purpose of the CPM machine and how to stop and start it. He or she should also be encouraged to report any symptoms of pressure or irritation.

Active range of motion results from the active contraction of the muscle against gravity. These exercises are part of a program that increases muscle strength and endurance. Examples include straight-leg raises and knee flexion and extension when the client is in a sitting position. In active assistive range of motion, the therapist, a mechanical device, or the opposite extremity provides an external force to the affected extremity during joint motion. This type of exercise is often a second step in rehabilitation. It includes isotonic exercise, such as weight lifting, or isokinetic exercise through use of equipment such as Cybex machines.

Difficulties with ambulation can occur as a result of disorders of the musculoskeletal, nervous, and cardiovascular systems. Cognitive awareness, balance, and coordination are also important for safe walking. After an orthopedic injury, the client should ambulate as soon as possible. The client who has been bedridden even for brief periods may exhibit muscle atrophy and weakness, decreased endurance and cardiovascular fitness, and decreased joint flexibility. Orthostatic hypotension is also common after bed rest. A gradual progression of exercise is needed to remobilize the client. Bed exercises may be the first intervention. If the client has been on extended bed rest, a tilt table can be used to assist him or her to an upright position.

Be aware of the client's weight-bearing status before attempting to assist with ambulation. The degree of protected weight-bearing is determined by the physician on the basis of the client's injury and any surgical procedure. Ambulatory assistive devices such as canes, a walker, or crutches can be used as needed.

CONCLUSIONS

Musculoskeletal trauma ranges from simple strains or sprains to complex, life-threatening injuries. Your role is to promote early mobility, prevent possible complications, and teach the client how to prevent further injury.

THINKING CRITICALLY

1. A young college student arrives in the emergency department holding his arm close to his body. His wrist is obviously misshapen, but swelling is minimal. He tells you he was playing basketball with friends and hit the gym wall after running toward the goal to attempt a lay-up shot. He complains of pain with attempted flexion or rotation of the wrist. A radiograph confirms a wrist fracture, and cast application is planned. What intervention should receive priority? What teaching about cast care should be completed?

Factors to Consider. How should you relieve the client's pain? What is involved in the healing process for a fracture? What complications might the client face because of the cast?

2. Friends of a 22-year-old woman assist her into the doctor's office. She twisted her knee on the pitcher's mound during a competitive softball game and says she heard a popping sound. Swelling over her knee is significant. The client states that her knee buckled when she attempted to walk off the field. What is your priority for care? What will be the long-range care goals?

Factors to Consider. What is the initial treatment for this type of injury? What postoperative treatments will be ordered?

3. An 80-year-old woman is brought to the nursing unit to await surgical repair of a femoral neck fracture. She is mildly confused. A neighbor says he found her on her kitchen floor after an apparent fall. What assessments should be performed on an ongoing basis? What will be the treatment goals after ORIF of the fracture?

Factors to Consider. What possible complications could result after hip fracture? How can they be prevented?

BIBLIOGRAPHY

1. Alonso, J. E. (1996). Pelvic and acetabulum fractures. In V. R. Masear (Ed.), *Primary care orthopaedics* (pp. 63–71). Philadelphia: W. B. Saunders.
2. Anders, R. L., & Ornellas, E. M. (1997). Acute management of patients with hip fracture: A research literature review. *Orthopaedic Nursing, 16*(2), 21–46.
3. Bonatz, E. (1996). Bone and soft tissue injuries of the hand. In V. R. Masear (Ed.), *Primary care orthopaedics* (pp. 185–198). Philadelphia: W. B. Saunders.
4. Bonatz, E. (1996). Overuse syndromes: Overuse syndromes of the hand and wrist. In V. R. Masear (Ed.), *Primary care orthopaedics* (pp. 246–249). Philadelphia: W. B. Saunders.
5. Bryant, G. G. (1998). Modalities for immobilization. In A. B. Maher, S. W. Salmond, & T. A. Pellino (Eds.), *Orthopaedic nursing* (2nd ed., pp. 296–350). Philadelphia: W. B. Saunders.
6. Buddenberg, L. A., & Schkade, J. K. (1998). Special feature: A comparison of occupational therapy intervention approaches for older patients after hip fracture. *Topics in Geriatric Rehabilitation, 13*(4), 52–68.
7. Cailliet, R. (1996). *Soft tissue pain and disability* (3rd ed.). Philadelphia: F. A. Davis.
8. Ceccio, C. M. (1999). Key concepts in the care of patients in traction. In *An introduction to orthopaedic nursing* (2nd ed., pp. 45–60). Pitman, NJ: National Association of Orthopaedic Nurses.

9. Childs, S. G. (1998). Anatomy and physiology of the musculoskeletal system. In A. B. Maher, S. W. Salmond, & T. A. Pellino (Eds.), *Orthopaedic nursing* (2nd ed., pp. 145–267). Philadelphia: W. B. Saunders.
10. Conklin, M. J. (1996). Orthopaedic evaluation. In V. R. Masear (Ed.), *Primary care orthopaedics* (pp. 1–34). Philadelphia: W. B. Saunders.
11. Cooper, C., & Campion, G. (1992). Hip fractures in the elderly: A world-wide projection. *Osteoporosis International, 2,* 285–289.
12. Eckhouse-Ekeberg, D. R. (1999). Care of the patient with an external ambulatory device. In *An introduction to orthopaedic nursing* (2nd ed., pp. 31–43). Pitman, NJ: National Association of Orthopaedic Nurses.
13. Fisher, M., & Mowatt, M. Fractured neck of femur: The role of the nurse. (1997). *Nursing Times, 93*(24), 5–8.
14. Fisher, M., & Mowatt, M. Fractured neck of femur: Professional issues. (1997). *Nursing Times, 93*(25), 9–12.
15. Garth, W. P., Jr. (1996). Overuse syndromes: Overuse syndromes of the upper and lower extremities. In V. R. Masear (Ed.), *Primary care orthopaedics* (pp. 236–246). Philadelphia: W. B. Saunders.
16. Hager, C.A., & Brncick, N. (1998). Fat embolism syndrome: A complication of orthopaedic trauma. *Orthopaedic Nursing, 17*(2), 41–46, 58.
17. Herzberg, M. A. (1997). *Osteoporosis independent study.* Pitman, NJ: National Association of Orthopaedic Nurses.
18. Johnson, J., et al. (1995). Roller traction: Mobilizing patients with acetabular fractures. *Orthopaedic Nursing, 14*(1), 21–24.
19. Jonas, G., & Masear, V. R. (1996). Fractures and ligament injuries of the wrist. In V. R. Masear (Ed.), *Primary care orthopaedics* (pp. 169–184). Philadelphia: W. B. Saunders Company.
20. Koval, K. J., et al. (1998). Predictors of functional recovery after hip fracture in the elderly. *Clinical Orthopaedics and Related Research, 348,* 22–28.
21. Lappe, J. M. (1998). Prevention of hip fractures: A nursing imperative. *Orthopaedic Nursing, 17*(3), 15–23.
22. Lee, D. H. (1996). Fractures and dislocations of the shoulder. In V. R. Masear (Ed.), *Primary care orthopaedics* (pp. 42–155). Philadelphia: W. B. Saunders.
23. Lee, D. H. (1996). Fractures of the forearm. In V. R. Masear (Ed.), *Primary care orthopaedics* (pp. 165–168). Philadelphia: W. B. Saunders.
24. Lee, D. H. (1996). Injuries to the humerus and elbow. In V. R. Masear (Ed.), *Primary care orthopaedics* (pp. 156–164). Philadelphia: W. B. Saunders.
25. Maher, A. B. (1996). Trauma. In S. W. Salmond, N. E. Mooney, & L. A. Verdisco (Eds.), *Core curriculum for orthopaedic nursing* (3rd ed., pp. 415–449). Pitman, NJ: National Association of Orthopaedic Nurses.
26. Masear, V. R. (1996). Fractures and dislocations of the foot. In V. R. Masear (Ed.), *Primary care orthopaedics* (pp. 128–141). Philadelphia: W. B. Saunders.
27. McAndrew, M. (1996). The treatment of geriatric hip fractures. *Topics in Geriatric Rehabilitation, 12*(1), 32–37.
28. Miller, J., et al. (1996). A study of discomfort and confusion among elderly surgical patients. *Orthopaedic Nursing, 15*(6), 27–34.
29. Morris, N. S. (1999). Complications associated with orthopaedic surgery. In *An introduction to orthopaedic nursing* (2nd ed., pp. 123–145). Pitman, NJ: National Association of Orthopaedic Nurses.
30. National Association of Orthopaedic Nurses. (1993). *The impact of orthopaedic conditions on the health and economy of the United States.* Pitman, NJ: Author.
31. Nye, P. J. (1996). Complications. In S. W. Salmond, N. E. Mooney, & L. A. Verdisco (Eds.), *Core curriculum for orthopaedic nursing* (3rd ed., pp. 147–163). Pitman, NJ: National Association of Orthopaedic Nurses.
32. Orwoll, E., & Klein, R. (1995). Osteoporosis in men. *Endocrine Review, 16,* 87–166.
33. Pellino, T. A., et al. (1998). Complications of orthopaedic disorders and orthopaedic surgery. In A. B. Maher, S. W. Salmond, & T. A. Pellino (Eds.), *Orthopaedic nursing* (2nd ed., pp. 212–295). Philadelphia: W. B. Saunders.
34. Rauscher, N. A. (1996). Musculoskeletal assessment. In S. W. Salmond, N. E. Mooney, & L. A. Verdisco (Eds.), *Core curriculum for orthopaedic nursing* (3rd ed., pp. 25–57). Pitman, NJ: National Association of Orthopaedic Nurses.
35. Roberts, D. (1999). Introduction to bone: Structure and function, fractures, and osteoporosis. In *An introduction to orthopaedic nursing* (2nd ed., pp. 3–16). Pitman, NJ: National Association of Orthopedic Nurses.
36. Rockwood, C., et al. (1996). *Fractures in adults* (4th ed.). Philadelphia: Lippincott-Raven.
37. Slauenwhite, C. A., & Simpson, P. (1998). Patient and family perspectives on early discharge and care of the older adult undergoing fractured hip rehabilitation. *Orthopaedic Nursing, 17*(1), 30–36.
38. Snyder, P. E. (1998). Fractures. In A. B. Maher, S. W. Salmond, & T. A. Pellino (Eds.), *Orthopaedic nursing* (2nd ed., pp. 663–717). Philadelphia: W. B. Saunders.
39. Stephenson, S. (1996). Fractures and ligamentous injuries of the knee: Fractures about the adult knee. In V. R. Masear (Ed.), *Primary care orthopaedics* (pp. 106–109). Philadelphia: W. B. Saunders.
40. Taggart, H. M. (1999). Caring for the elderly hip fracture patient. In *An introduction to orthopaedic nursing* (2nd ed., pp. 113–122). Pitman, NJ: National Association of Orthopedic Nurses.
41. Thompson, D. (1996). Therapeutic modalities. In S.W. Salmond, N.E. Mooney, & L.A. Verdisco (Eds.), *Core curriculum for orthopaedic nursing* (3rd ed., pp. 187–209). Pitman, NJ: National Association of Orthopaedic Nurses.
42. Whittington, C. F. (1998). Exercise- and sport-related disorders. In A.B. Maher, S.W. Salmond, & T. A. Pellino (Eds.), *Orthopaedic nursing* (2nd ed., pp. 746–768). Philadelphia: W. B. Saunders.
43. Williams, M. A., et al. (1996). Family caregiving in cases of hip fracture. *Rehabilitation Nursing, 21*(3), 124–138.
44. Wolinsky, F. D., Fitzgerald, J.F., & Stump, T.E. (1997). The effect of hip fracture on mortality, hospitalization, and functional status: A prospective study. *American Journal of Public Health, 87*(3), 398–403.
45. Zuckerman, J. D., et al. (1995). Postoperative complications and mortality associated with operative delay in older patients who have a fracture of the hip. *Journal of Bone and Joint Surgery, American Volume, 77*(10), 1551–1556.

BRIDGE TO EVIDENCE-BASED PRACTICE

Falls Among the Elderly

QUESTIONS

What factors predict falls among older adults?
What preventive interventions do these factors support?

CITATION

Rawsky, E. (1998). Review of the literature on falls among the elderly. *Image: Journal of Nursing Scholarship, 30,* 47–52.

STUDIES

More than 100 studies published between 1979 and 1996 were included in the analysis of this review. They were identified using a *MEDLINE* search; however, how the studies came to be included or excluded from the review analysis was not explained in the report. Many of the studies consisted of retrospective chart reviews, although some prospectively compared adults who had previously fallen with those who had not (i.e., a control group). The review includes studies of falls in hospitals, homes, extended-care facilities, and nursing homes.

Summary of Findings

Intrinsic Factors

Risk factors for falls can be classified as *intrinsic* (characteristics of individuals) or *extrinsic* (contextual and environmental in nature). Cognitive impairment and sensory deficit have been implicated in a few studies. In 16 studies, cognitive impairment was found to be associated with falls; in seven studies, sensory deficit was associated. A study of specific cognitive impairments and falling implicated poor problem-solving, general anxiety, and attention deficits.[15]

Another grouping of associated factors is mobility, gait, and balance problems; in 14 studies, at least one of them was found to be associated with falling. Other associated factors include a fall history (six studies), elimination patterns (six studies), and postural hypotension (four studies). It is not clear whether increased age itself should be considered a risk factor, although "older elderly" people experience more adverse sequelae from falls compared with "younger elderly" persons.[17, 19] Men have a higher incidence of falling than women,[3, 9] although the one study with a control group revealed that gender did not make a difference.[12]

An interesting issue is the extent to which falls result in injury.[7, 17, 20] A prospective, case-controlled study of community-dwelling elders found that falls occurring while a person was turning were more likely to result in a hip fracture.[4] One study found that women are more at risk than men for hip fracture as a result of falling.[21] In turn, hip fracture often leads to death, particularly in people over age 75.

Extrinsic Factors

Changes in physiologic adaptive abilities (such as balance, proprioception, and vestibular stability) make compensation for environmental irregularities more difficult.[1, 21] Hazards include poor lighting, slippery or uneven flooring, objects in path, stairs, and steps.[20] High-gloss floors have been associated with falling, and vinyl flooring is more likely to result in injury compared with carpeted surfaces.[7] A somewhat unexpected finding is that environmental hazards may be more likely to contribute to falls in elders who are in better health than in their more frail counterparts.[2, 13]

Ironically, assistive devices can actually contribute to falls.[12, 21]; mechanical restraints do not appear to reduce the incidence of falls and may actually worsen outcomes.[5, 6, 8, 22]

The extent to which staffing patterns and assignments affect the incidence of falls is uncertain, although in one hospital study a discrepancy between recommended and actual hours of staffing contributed to an increased number of falls.[24] Moreover, several studies have found that patients who had fallen had not asked for help.[26]

Interventions

"Anticipatory nursing" (e.g., routine assistance with toileting, and offering assistance for future activities rather than waiting for patients to ask for help) appears effective in reducing the frequency of falling.[3, 18] Providing appropriate footware[14] and treaded slipper socks can reduce the incidence of falls.[11] Various types of exercise programs, particularly those aimed at muscle strengthening and improving balance, have been effective in reducing the incidence of falls in older people in the community and in nursing homes.[10, 16, 23] Two studies have documented the benefits of *Tai Chi,* an ancient Chinese exercise form, in reducing falls.[16, 25]

Limitations Reservations: This review did not examine the effectiveness of assessment tools for fall risk and did not comprehensively address interventions to reduce the risk of falling or programs to prevent falls. There is considerable research on preventing falls among community-dwelling elders but much less among older people in hospitals and nursing homes. The most recent studies included in the review are from 1996.

Research-Based Practice

At the individual practice level, nurses should know how to assess clients for the presence of risk factors related to falling; these assessments should be done at the time of admission and whenever the client's condition changes. The cognitive part of this assessment should go beyond orientation to time, place, and person to include the abilities to problem-solve and to pay attention to tasks at hand; general anxiety should also serve as a "red flag" for fall risk. Assessing the person's balance, gait, vision, and hearing and identifying people with frequent or urgent urination or bowel needs are also important in identifying those at risk.

Once a person is identified as being at risk because of the presence of several of the factors just discussed, you will be able to decide on the appropriate level of intervention. Simple anticipatory actions, such as readily available call lights, assurances that you want to be called to help them get up, and uncluttered pathways to the bathroom (the most frequent destination), all help prevent falls. Wiping up liquids or urine on the

Falls Among the Elderly *Continued*

floor is another simple but effective action. Low bed positions and treaded slipper socks also help.

For higher-risk clients, bed alarms or door alarms can alert the staff that the client is getting up without assistance or is moving around. Another intervention for high-risk patients would be referral to physical therapy for gait and balance training.

At the institutional level, the physical characteristics of the environment can help lower the risk of falls and fall injuries. Good lighting, grab bars in bathrooms, handrails in halls (not blocked by equipment), and unslippery floor surfaces may help reduce adverse outcomes from falls. The maintenance of and use of wheel locks on over-bed tables and bedside cabinets also play a role because patients may lean on them, not realizing that the furniture is on wheels and will move. The choice of side rails is critical because their design can protect patients from falls or can increase the likelihood of their occurrence.

In all settings, prevention of falls is very effective when an organized fall prevention program is in place.[3, 18] Such a program can identify clients at risk and can set forth measures to be put in place. Intervention algorithms are helpful, providing quick guides to the measures that should be activated.

Some clients who have not exhibited any risk factors may fall, just as some who have several risk factors may not fall. Still, risk factors are useful in identifying those at risk for a fall. These risk factors cannot be converted to a simple formula, but you can keep in mind the many factors that are associated with falls and enact an individualized package of several interventions.

Cited References

1. Adler-Traines, J. (1994). Falls in the senior population. *Physical Therapy Forum, 9,* 14–17.
2. Baldwin, R., Craven, R., & Diamond, M. (1996). Falls: Are rural elders at greater risk? *Journal of Gerontological Nursing, 22*(8), 14–21.
3. Brady, R., et al. (1993). Geriatric Falls: Prevention strategies for the staff. *Journal of Gerontological Nursing, 19*(9), 26–32.
4. Cumming, R., & Klineberg, R. (1994). Fall frequency and characteristics and the risk of hip fractures. *Journal of American Geriatrics Society, 42,* 774–778.
5. Evans, L., & Strumpf, N. (1990). Myths about elder restraint. *Image: Journal of Nursing Scholarship, 22,* 124–128.
6. Gaebler, S. (1993). Predicting which patients will fall again . . . and again. *Journal of Advanced Nursing, 18,* 1895–1902.
7. Healey, F. (1994). Does flooring type affect risk of injury in older inpatients? *Nursing Times, 90,* 40–41.
8. Janken, J., Reynolds, B., & Swiech, K. (1986). Patient falls in the acute care setting: Identifying risk factors. *Nursing Research, 35,* 215–219.
9. Kilpack, V., Boehm, J., & Smith, N. (1991). Using research-based interventions to decrease patient falls. *Applied Nursing Research, 4,* 50–56.
10. McNeely, E., Clements, S., & Wolf, S. (1992). A program to reduce frailty in the elderly. In S. Funk, et al. (Eds.), *Key aspects of elder care* (pp. 89–96). New York: Springer.
11. Meddaugh, D., Friedenberg, D., & Knisley, R. (1996). Special socks for special people: Falls in special care units. *Geriatric Nursing, 17,* 24–26.
12. Morse, J., Tylko, S., & Dixon, H. (1987). Characteristics of the fall prone patient. *The Gerontologist, 27,* 516–522.
13. Northridge, M., et al. (1995). Home hazards and falls in the elderly: The role of health and functional status. *American Journal of Public Health, 85,* 509–515.
14. Orhon-Jech, A. (1992). Preventing falls in the elderly. *Geriatric Nursing, 34,* 43–44.
15. Persad, C., et al. (1995). Neuropsychological predictors of complex obstacle avoidance in healthy older adults. *Journal of Gerontology, Series B, Psychological Sciences & Social Sciences, 50*(5), P272–P277.
16. Province, M., et al. (1995). The effects of exercise on falls in elderly patients: A preplanned meta-analysis of the FICSIT trials. *Journal of the American Medical Association, 273,* 1341–1347.
17. Rhymes, J., & Jaeger, R. (1988). Falls: Prevention and management in the institutional setting. *Clinics in Geriatric Medicine, 4,* 613–622.
18. Ruckstuhl, M., et al. (1991). Patient falls: An outcome indicator. *Journal of Nursing Care Quality, 6,* 25–29.
19. Sattin, R. (1992). Falls among older persons: A public health perspective. *Annual Review of Public Health, 13,* 489–508.
20. Shroyer, J. (1994). Recommendations for environmental design research correlating falls and the physical environment. *Experimental Aging Research 20,* 303–309.
21. Tideiksaar, R. (1993). Falls in older persons. *Mount Sinai Journal of Medicine, 60,* 515–521.
22. Tinetti, M., Liu, W., & Ginter, S. (1992). Mechanical restraint usage and fall-related injuries among residents of skilled nursing facilities. *Annals of Internal Medicine, 116,* 369–374.
23. Tinetti, M., et al. (1994). A multifactorial intervention to reduce the risk of falling among elderly people living in the community. *New England Journal of Medicine, 331,* 821–827.
24. Whedon, M., & Shedd, P. (1989). Prediction and prevention of patient falls. *Image: Journal of Nursing Scholarship, 21,* 108–114.
25. Wolf, S. et al. (1993). The Atlanta FICSIT study: Two exercise interventions to reduce frailty in elders. *Journal of the American Geriatrics Society, 41,* 329–332.
26. Wright, B., et al. (1990). Frequent fallers: Leading groups to identify psychological factors. *Journal of Gerontological Nursing, 16*(4), 15–19.

Sarah Jo Brown, PhD, RN, *Principal and Consultant, Practice-Research Integrations, Norwich, Vermont*

UNIT 6

Nutritional Disorders

Anatomy and Physiology Review

The Nutritional (Gastrointestinal) System

Robert G. Carroll

The nutritional or gastrointestinal (GI) system is a long, hollow tube that passes through the body, providing an isolated environment for digestion and absorption of nutrients. Ingested contents pass sequentially through the following structures: mouth, esophagus, stomach, small intestine (duodenum, jejunum, and ileum), and large intestine (colon), before exiting the body at the anus.

GI tract function is regulated by a complex series of neural, hormonal, and local control systems. The *enteric nervous system* integrates motor and secretory activities along the GI tract. Ganglia have sensory neurons that respond to temperature, chemical agents, and mechanical deformation. Ganglia also have effector neurons to smooth muscle, secretory cells, endocrine cells, and autocrine cells. GI secretion and motility are enhanced by parasympathetic activity and inhibited by sympathetic activity.

GI hormones, which control and integrate both motility and secretion, are distributed in the stomach and small intestine. GI hormones are also important trophic factors, stimulating proliferation of the GI tract to enhance absorptive capacity.

Finally, the GI tract has an extensive *immune system.* Gut-associated lymphoid tissue (GALT) may account for up to 80% of the immunoglobulin-producing cells in the body. These cells are important because of the intimate association of the GI system and the "outside environment," the chyme in the lumen of the GI tract.

STRUCTURE OF THE GASTROINTESTINAL SYSTEM

In cross-section, the GI tract generally has four distinct layers (Fig. U6–1). The innermost layer is the *mucosa,* where epithelial cells contact ingested food. The mucosa often has microvilli to increase the surface area available for absorption. Beneath the mucosa is the *submucosa (lamina propria),* containing glands, blood vessels, and lymph nodules. Next is a *muscular layer,* with smooth muscle oriented either circularly or longitudinally. The outermost layer is the *connective tissue serosa layer.*

The entrance (mouth, upper esophagus) and exit (external anal sphincter) of the GI tract contain GI-associated skeletal muscle, which is partially under voluntary control. The remainder of the GI tract (Fig. U6–2) has smooth muscle, under involuntary control. GI smooth muscle is electrically connected by gap junctions, allowing a wave of depolarization and contraction to spread along the tract (see Motility).

Food is chewed *(masticated),* mixed with saliva in the mouth, and swallowed. It passes through the pharynx and into the *esophagus.* The upper third of esophagus has striated (voluntary) muscle, the middle third has both types of muscle, and the lower third has only smooth muscle. The vagus nerve innervates both the smooth and skeletal muscle of the esophagus. Sphincters isolate the esophagus from the remainder of the GI tract. The upper esophageal sphincter prevents entry of tracheal air, and the lower esophageal sphincter prevents reflux of gastric contents *(aspiration).* Acute failure of the lower esophageal sphincter causes *esophagitis* (heartburn), and chronic gastric reflux causes digestion of the esophagus. The opposite problem, *achalasia,* occurs if the lower esophageal sphincter does not relax sufficiently to allow food to pass into the stomach.

The *stomach* is divided into the *fundus, body,* and *antrum.* The fundus and body are highly distensible, and act as a reservoir for the ingested meal. Food can be stored unmixed in fundus and body for up to 1 hour. During this time, there may be a separation due to density, because fats float to the top and liquids accumulate on the bottom. Thus, liquids are the first to leave the stomach and to be absorbed through the intestine. Gastric contents empty from the antrum through the pylorus into the duodenum. The gastroduodenal junction is important in sequestering acid in the stomach and bile in the duodenum.

The *small intestine* is divided into *duodenum* (25 cm), *jejunum* (2.5 m), and *ileum* (3.6 m). The duodenum and jejunum are the major sites of digestion and absorption. Pancreatic and biliary ducts carry digestive enzymes, bicarbonate, and bile to the lumen of the duodenum. The continuous epithelial cell lining of the small intestine separates luminal contents from the body and provides a barrier across which nutrients must be absorbed. Epithelial cells reproduce rapidly and are lost (exfoliated) at the tip of the microvilli.

Chyme, the nonabsorbed component of the diet, passes through the *ileocecal valve* (a sphincter) to enter the *large intestine.* The large intestine (~1.5 m in length) includes the *cecum* (a pouch where small and large intestines join and from which the appendix projects); the *ascending, transverse, descending,* and *sigmoid colon;* and the *rectum* (anal canal). The large intestine contains mucus-secreting goblet cells and cells specialized for absorption; it lacks villi and does not produce digestive enzymes. An internal sphincter (smooth muscle) and an external sphincter (voluntary muscle) govern the expulsion of feces (defecation).

Gastrointestinal Blood Supply and Lymphatic Drainage

Arterial blood enters the GI tract by various branches of major arteries. Venous drainage, however, is unique in

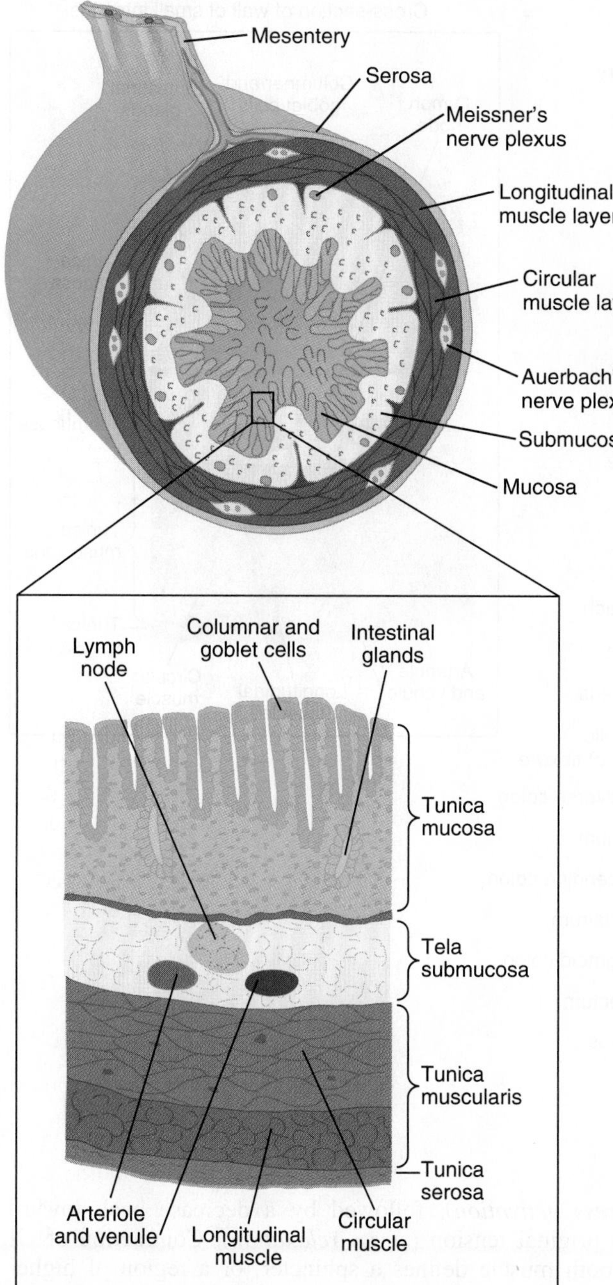

FIGURE U6–1 Typical cross-section of the gastrointestinal tract. *Inset* shows enlargement of a cross-section of the small intestine.

that the veins from the GI tract empty into the hepatic portal vein. Portal venous blood passes through the liver before entering the vena cava. This arrangement allows the liver to begin processing and detoxifying compounds absorbed across the stomach and intestines before those compounds enter the general circulation.

The esophageal arteries, the inferior thyroid artery, and the left gastric artery provide the esophagus with its arterial blood supply. The left gastric and inferior phrenic arteries supply the gastroesophageal area. Venous blood is returned via the azygos, thyroid, and left gastric veins. Lymphatic drainage from the cervical esophagus and from the tracheal and postmediastinal nodes flows to the internal jugular vein while intercostal nodes drain the thoracic esophagus. The lymphatic drainage of the lower esophagus occurs through the diaphragmatic, intracardiac, and left gastric lymph nodes.

The arterial blood supply to the stomach is derived from the celiac artery, which branches off the lesser and greater curvatures. Gastric arteries, from the splenic artery, supply the fundus. The portal vein provides the venous drainage of the stomach. The right and left gastroepiploic veins drain the greater curvature; the right gastric and coronary veins drain the lesser curvature. Lymph nodes of the stomach arise in the submucosa and drain into the thoracic duct.

Except in the duodenum, arterial blood supply to the small intestine is derived from the superior mesenteric artery. Arterial blood from the hepatic artery supplies the duodenum. Venous drainage is via the superior mesenteric vein, which unites with the inferior mesenteric, splenic, and gastric veins and then empties into the portal system.

NEURAL REGULATION

Enteric Nervous System

The enteric system regulates motility and secretion along the entire length of the GI tract. The enteric nervous system can function independently of the central nervous system (CNS). Enteric reflexes, originating from GI sensory nerves, synapse in either the submucosal plexus or the myenteric plexus. Efferent nerves then supply the smooth muscle or secretory glands. Enteric activity can be modulated by external inputs, particularly by the sympathetic and parasympathetic nerves.

Auerbach's plexus (motor function) and *Meissner's plexus* (sensory function) provide intrinsic innervation for the stomach. Both begin in the esophageal wall and extend the length of the gut. Stimulation of Auerbach's plexus (between the longitudinal and circular muscle layers) generates gastric motility, increasing the intensity and rate of contractions and the release of gastrin from the antrum. *Meissner's plexus* (in the submucosa) functions with Auerbach's plexus to coordinate the motor and secretory activity of the gastric mucosa.

Sympathetic and Parasympathetic Nervous Systems

Sympathetic nerves supplying the GI tract originate in the celiac, superior mesenteric, inferior mesenteric, and hypogastric ganglia. In general, *sympathetics* inhibit activity in enteric plexuses, constrict GI system blood vessels, and decrease glandular secretions. GI motility is also decreased through contraction of circular muscle and certain sphincters, and indirect inhibition of peristalsis.

The vagus is the primary parasympathetic nerve supplying the GI tract, innervating all structures from the salivary glands to the transverse colon. Nerves from the hypogastric plexus innervate the remainder of colon. Parasympathetic postganglionic neurons are located in intramural plexus. In general, *parasympathetics* stimulate motor activity, secretory activity, and endocrine secretions.

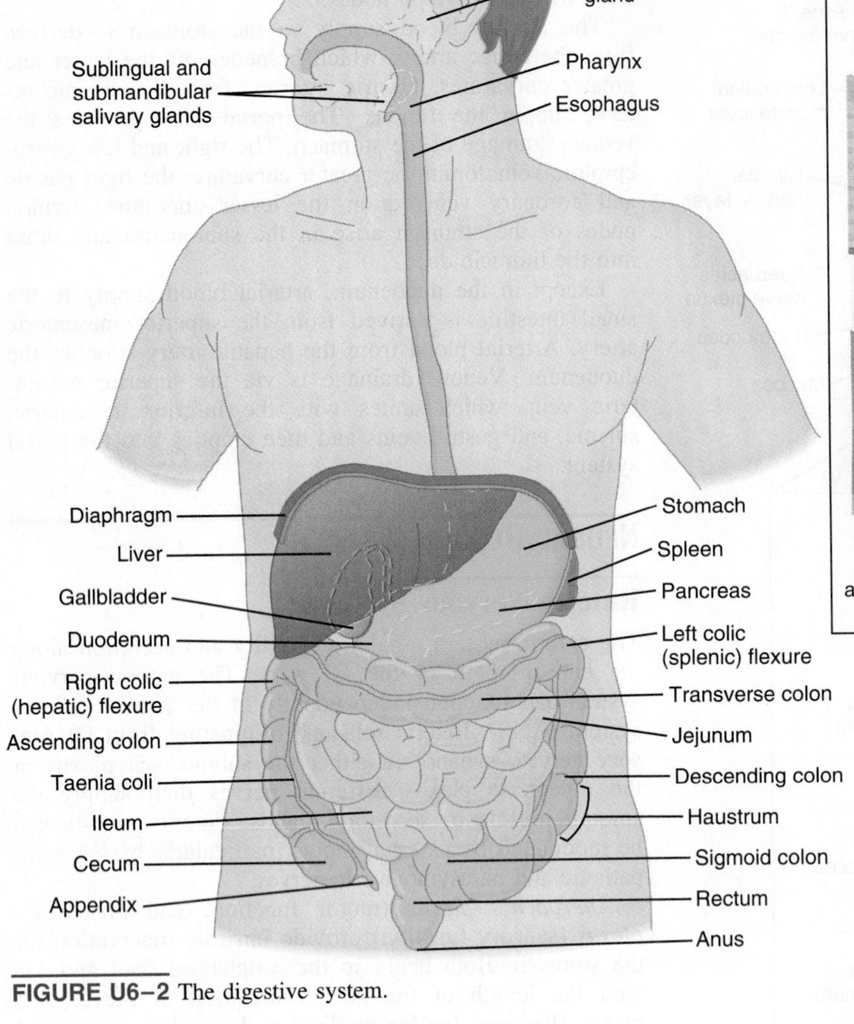

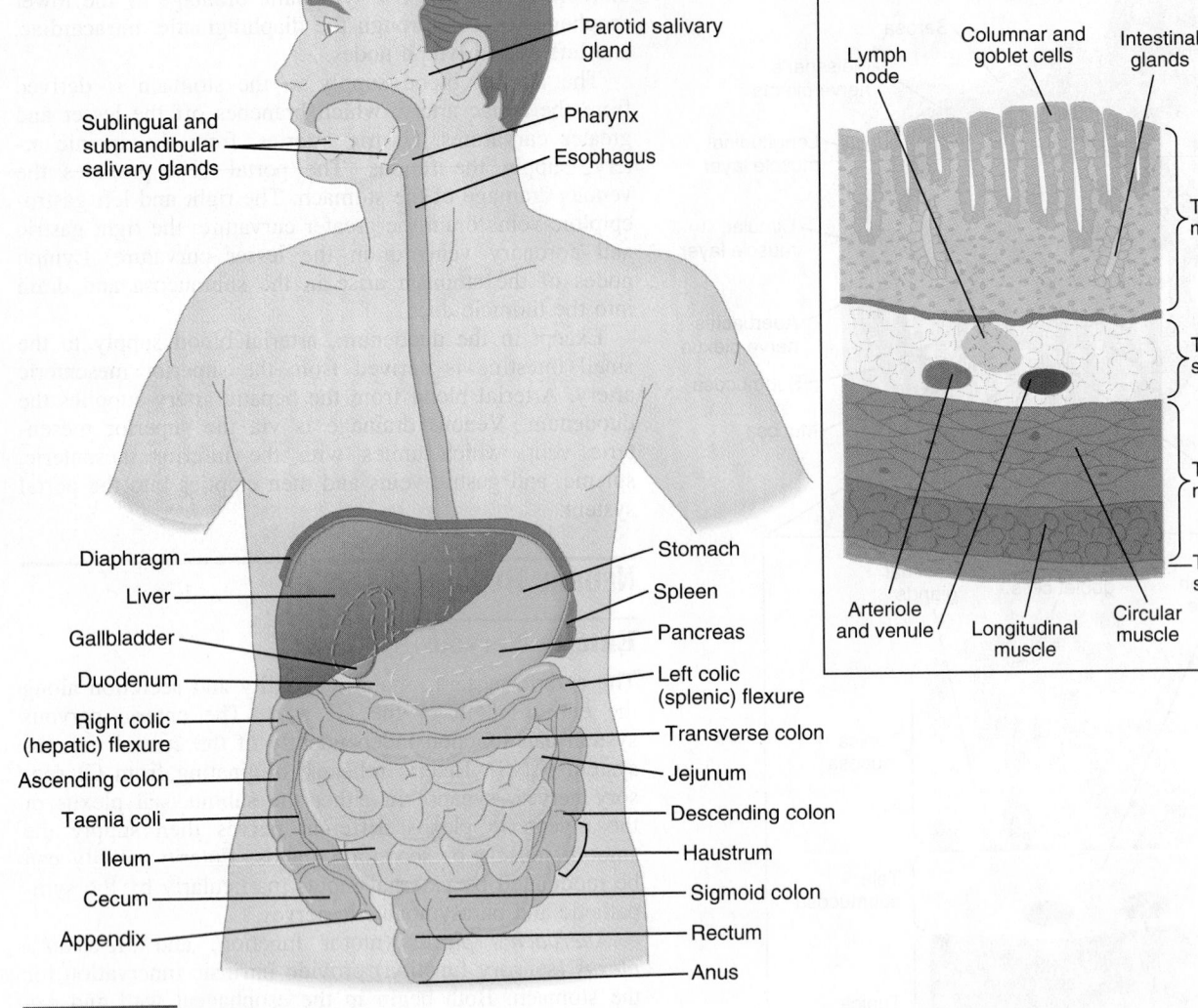

FIGURE U6–2 The digestive system.

FUNCTION OF THE GASTROINTESTINAL SYSTEM

The GI system isolates ingested food and provides an environment for digestion and absorption of nutrients. The major functions of the GI tract are (1) motility, (2) secretion, (3) digestion, and (4) absorption.

MOTILITY

Smooth Muscle

Smooth muscle of the GI tract is electrically connected by gap junctions, allowing a wave of depolarization and contraction to spread along the tract. Pacemakers along the length of the GI tract set the slow-wave contraction frequency. Nerves and hormones alter this rate and, therefore, GI motility.

GI smooth muscle produces long, strong contractions. Muscle basal tone provides some tension even at rest and is influenced by neurotransmitters, hormones, and drugs. Stretch of GI system increases action potential frequency *(stress activation),* followed by a decrease back toward the original tension *(stress relaxation).* Contraction of GI smooth muscle defines a sphincter, or a region of higher tone, which may not have any anatomic features.

Peristalsis is an organized wave of contraction of the longitudinal muscle layer that propels contents aborally (away from the mouth). Distention of a segment of intestine elicits a reflex contraction. The smooth muscle aboral to the contraction relaxes, and the contents move. This sequence is repeated, and contents are moved for a short distance before the wave diminishes and disappears. A descending wave of peristalsis initiates sphincter relaxation, mediated by vasoactive intestinal peptide (VIP) neurotransmitter in vagal nerves. Decreased vagal cholinergic activity also contributes to relaxation.

Intrinsic motility regulation uses interneurons to coordinate activity. The enteric nervous system has neuromodulators, similar to those in the brain. Intrinsic plexuses inhibit basal activity, and action potentials are thus elicited by fewer than half of the slow waves.

Contractions of the various layers of smooth muscle propel and mix luminal contents. Peristaltic contraction of the longitudinal muscle layer accomplishes aboral movement. Contraction of circular muscle mixes luminal contents (chyme) and increases contact with microvilli.

Mouth to Esophagus. The process of moving food from the mouth into the esophagus is illustrated in Figure U6–3. The esophageal phase of swallowing is involuntary. Contraction of the upper esophageal sphincter isolates the pharynx from the esophagus. A primary peristaltic wave, controlled by the swallowing center, moves food through esophagus in 10 seconds. Secondary peristalsis is initiated by esophageal distention (enteric nervous system); it propels any food still remaining in the esophagus into the stomach.

Stomach. Gastric contractions after feeding occur at a rate of three per minute. They begin in the middle of the body, increasing in force and velocity as they approach the antrum. The antrum produces strong contractions that fragment food into smaller particles and mix it

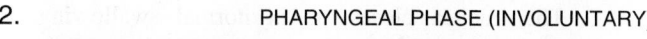

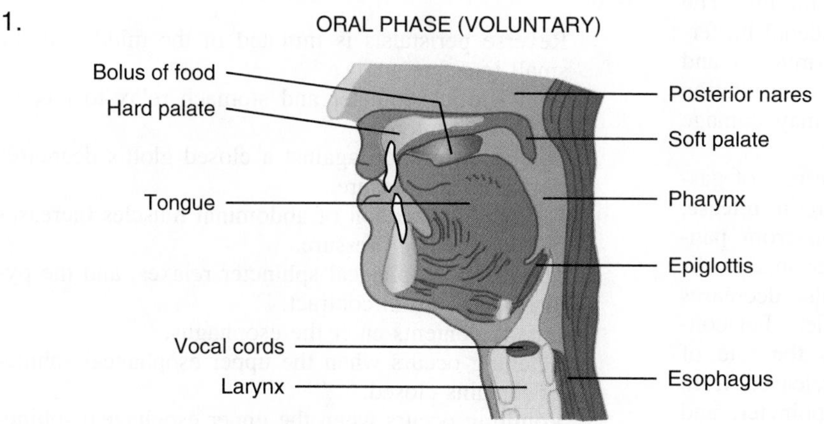

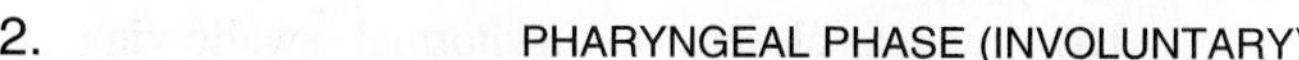

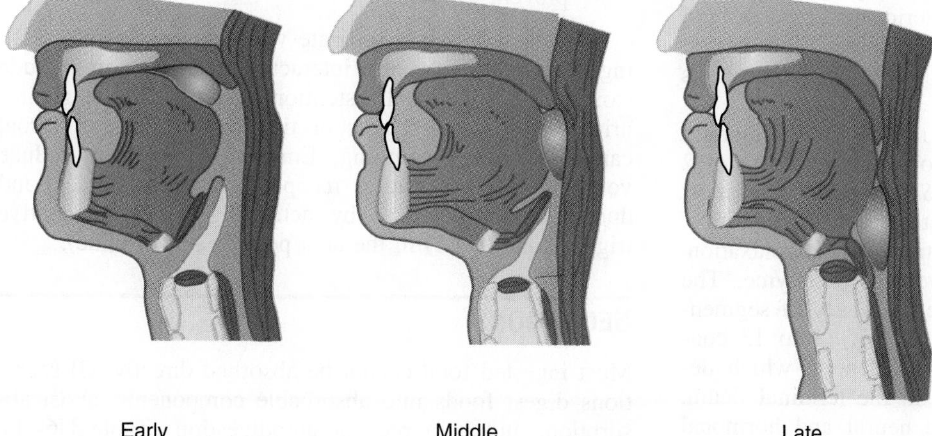

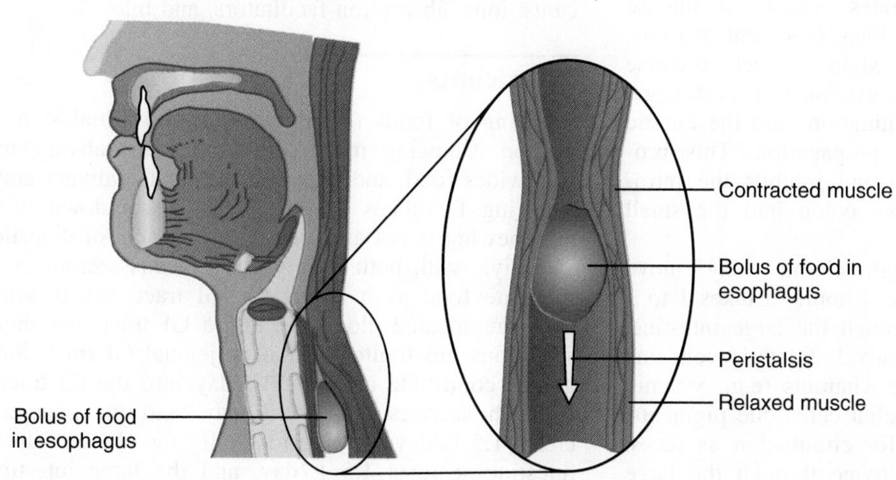

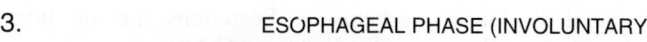

FIGURE U6–3 Swallowing occurs in three phases: (1) *Voluntary* or *oral* phase. The tongue presses food against the hard palate, forcing it toward the pharynx. (2) *Involuntary, pharyngeal* phase. *Early:* wave of peristalsis forces bolus between tonsillar pillars. *Middle:* Soft palate draws upward to close posterior nares, and respirations cease momentarily. *Late:* vocal cords approximate and larynx pulls upward, covering the airway and stretching the esophagus open. (3) *Involuntary, esophageal* phase. Relaxation of the upper esophageal (hypopharyngeal) sphincter allows a peristaltic wave to move the bolus down the esophagus.

with gastric secretions to initiate digestion. The rate of contractions is increased by gastrin and decreased by secretin. Sensory afferents from the stomach play a role in satiety. Increased intragastic pressure, gastric distention, gastric acidity, and pain all lessen the desire to ingest food.

Gastroduodenal Junction. Gastric contents empty into the duodenal bulb at a controlled rate. The pylorus and terminal end of antrum contract almost simultaneously *(systolic contraction),* allowing only a small amount of antral content to enter duodenum. The remainder of antral contraction moves antral contents backward *(retropulsion)* and causes further mixing. The rate of gastric emptying must match the duodenal buffering ability, or acid may damage duodenal mucosa and cause duodenal ulcers. The pylorus prevents regurgitation of duodenal contents into stomach, or bile may damage stomach mucosa, causing gastric ulcers.

Duodenal acidity (pH < 3.5) decreases the rate of gastric emptying. A neural reflex causes secretin release, which increases bicarbonate buffer secretion from pancreas and liver. Chyme becomes more hypertonic as digestion progresses. Duodenal hypertonicity also decreases the rate of gastric emptying by a neural reflex. Fat content in the duodenal chyme also decreases the rate of gastric emptying. Cholecystokinin (CCK) released from duodenum and jejunum contracts pyloric sphincter, and glucose-dependent insulinotropic peptide (GIP) may also have a role. Fatty acids (especially long-chain and unsaturated) decrease the rate of gastric emptying. Monoglycerides increase contractility of pyloric sphincter. Amino acids (tryptophan) and peptides in duodenum slow gastric emptying by promoting gastrin release, which constricts the pylorus.

Small Intestine. Peristalsis moves chyme aborally an average of 10 cm per contraction, and chyme takes 2 to 4 hours to move the 6 meters. *Segmentation,* the most frequent type of intestinal contraction, can be rhythmic, with adjacent sites alternating contraction and relaxation. Eating actually slows aboral movement of chyme. The enteric nervous system controls the frequency of segmentation and peristalsis. An intrinsic rate of 11 to 13 contractions per minute exists in the duodenum, which declines to eight to nine per minute in the terminal ileum. This rate is modified by extrinsic neural and hormonal inputs.

Migrating Myoelectric Complex. The migrating myoelectric complex generates periods of intense electrical activity, followed by long quiescent periods. The resulting contractions, initiated in stomach, traverse the entire small intestine. There is evidence for both vagal and hormonal (motilin) role in initiation, and the enteric nervous system is required for propagation. This process sweeps the intestines clean and inhibits the retrograde movement of bacteria from colon into the small intestine.

Large Intestine. Although chyme may move through the small intestine in 2 to 4 hours, it takes 1 to 3 days to complete its passage through the large intestine. Here sodium and water are absorbed. Bacteria consume more nutrients and release some vitamins (e.g., vitamin K). Solid wastes (sloughed epithelial cells, bile pigments, unabsorbed food) are prepared for elimination as feces. Abnormally fast movement of chyme through the large intestine results in diarrhea; abnormally slow movement results in constipation. Inflammation of the appendix *(appendicitis)* can lead to peritonitis and other complications.

Vomiting

Vomiting expels gastric (and sometimes duodenal) contents by mouth. Retching, an action in which gastric contents are forced into the esophagus, but not the pharynx, precedes vomiting. The vomiting reflex follows a set pattern:

1. Reverse peristalsis is initiated in the middle of the small intestine.
2. The pyloric sphincter and stomach relax to receive duodenal contents.
3. Forced inspiration against a closed glottis decreases intrathoracic pressure.
4. Forceful contraction of abdominal muscles increases intra-abdominal pressure.
5. The lower esophageal sphincter relaxes, and the pylorus and antrum contract.
6. Gastric contents enter the esophagus.
7. Retching occurs when the upper esophageal sphincter remains closed.
8. Vomiting occurs when the upper esophageal sphincter opens.
9. The trachea closes, as in normal swallowing, to prevent aspiration.

The medulla has a separate vomiting center and retching center that normally interact. Afferent inputs include stomach and duodenal distention, and pain in the genitourinary system. Dizziness or tickling the back of throat can also induce vomiting. Emetics are used to induce vomiting by stimulating receptors in the stomach and duodenum (ipecac), or by activating a chemoreceptive trigger zone (CTZ) in the area postrema (morphine).

SECRETIONS

Most ingested food cannot be absorbed directly. GI secretions digest foods into absorbable components, assist absorption, and help prevent autodigestion (Table U6–1). GI secretions are regulated by a series of hormonal and neural feedback mechanisms. Secretions include lubricants, ions, absorption facilitators, and bile.

Lubricants

Chewing of foods *(mastication)* is the initial step in digestion. Chewing mixes the food with salivary mucus, subdivides food, and exposes starches to salivary amylase. Chewing facilitates the mechanical breakdown of food, but chewing is not an essential component of digestion.

Saliva, with both watery and mucous secretions, helps lubricate food as it enters the GI tract. Mucus-secreting cells are located along the entire GI tract, but digestive secretions are limited to the prejejunal GI tract. Salivary glands contribute about 1.5 L/day into the GI tract. The stomach secretes about 2 L/day, and the pancreas secretes 1.5 L/day, helping to liquify the chyme. The small intestine secretes 1.5 L/day, and the large intestine secretes 400 ml/day. In addition, 0.25 to 1.5 L/day of hepatic secretions enter the duodenum.

Gastric secretions begin protein digestion and protect the gastric epithelium. After a meal, there are three distinct phases of gastric acid secretion.

1. The *cephalic phase* is caused by a neural reflex initiated by the sight, smell, or taste of food. The drop in antral pH acts directly on the parietal calls to attenuate the cephalic phase.
2. The *gastric phase* is due to gastric distention caused by food in the stomach.
3. The *intestinal phase* is initiated by chyme entry into duodenum.

Gastric parietal cell hydrochloric acid (HCl) secretion involves the interplay of acetylcholine, gastrin, histamine, and a second cell type, the enterochromaffin cell. A powerful synergistic interaction between these stimuli causes difficulty in diminishing acid secretion by blocking only one pathway. HCl secretion can be blocked by atropine (acetylcholine) or cimetidine (H_2 histamine), but a blocker for gastrin is not yet available. Ranitidine is more effective, producing fewer side effects, and is used to treat duodenal ulcers. Gastric ulcers, although associated with increased HCl secretion, involve a gram-negative bacterium, *Helicobacter pylori,* which damages the gastric mucosa. Other agents, such as aspirin and nonsteroidal anti-inflammatory drugs (NSAIDs) can damage the gastric mucosa and cause gastric ulcers.

Absorption Facilitators and Ions

Pancreatic enzymes are essential for the normal absorption of lipids, proteins, and carbohydrates. Table U6–1 lists the important enzymes and ionic pancreatic secretions.

Bile and the Enterohepatic Circulation

Bile acids are secreted by liver as bile, stored in the gallbladder, and released into the duodenum after a meal. Bile acids are reabsorbed by both diffusion and active transport in the terminal ileum and returned to the liver by the he-

TABLE U6–1 GASTROINTESTINAL (GI) SYSTEM–ASSOCIATED SECRETIONS

Class	Location	Secretion	Role
Lubricants	Entire GI tract	Mucus	Lubricant
	Salivary gland	Water	Lubricant, solvent
	Pancreas	Water	Lubricant
	Small intestine	Water	Lubricant
Digestive enzymes	Salivary glands	Amylase	Digestion of starch
		Lingual lipase	Digestion of triglycerides
	Stomach	Pepsin (pepsinogen)	Digest proteins
		Gastric lipase	Digest triglycerides
	Pancreas	Amylase	Digest starch
		Lipase	Digest triglycerides
		Colipase	Digest triglycerides
		Phospholipase	Digest phospholipods
		Trypsin	Digest peptides
		Chymotrypsin	Digest peptides
		Nucleases	DNA, RNA
	Intestinal epithelium	Disaccharidases	Disaccharides
		Peptidases	Peptides
Hormones and neurotransmitters	Stomach	Gastrin	Hydrochloric acid secretion
	Pancreas	Somatostatin	Inhibition of insulin, glucagon release
	Small intestine	Cholecystokinin	Pancreatic enzyme secretion
		Secretin	Pancreatic bicarbonate secretion
		Glucose-dependent insulinotropic peptide (GIP)	Pancreatic insulin release
		Motilin	GI smooth muscle contraction
		Enteroglucagons	Pancreatic insulin release
Enteric neurons		Vasoactive intestinal peptide (VIP)	GI smooth muscle relaxation
			Pancreatic secretion
		Bombesin	Gastrin release
Ionic secretions	Salivary glands	Sodium bicarbonate	Alkalinize ingested food
		Potassium chloride	Maintain secretion osmolality
	Stomach parietal cells	Hydrochloric acid	Activation of pepsin
	Mucus cells	Potassium bicarbonate	Protection of stomach from acid
	Pancreas	Sodium bicarbonate	Neutralization of gastric secretion
Absorption facilitators	Stomach	Intrinsic factor	Ileal absorption of vitamin B_{12}
	Liver	Bile acids	Small-intestine lipid absorption

DNA, deoxyribonucleic acid; RNA, ribonucleic acid.

patic portal vein. The liver then actively extracts bile acids from the portal venous blood and secretes the reabsorbed bile acids into bile, beginning the process anew. Only about 15% to 35% of the bile acid pool is lost in feces each day and is replaced by new synthesis of bile acids.

Bile acids are normally secreted conjugated to glycine or taurine and at neutral pH of small intestine are salts (bile salts).

With the sphincter of Oddi at the junction of the bile duct and duodenum normally contracted, bile is diverted to and stored in gallbladder between meals. The gallbladder extracts sodium ions (Na^+) actively, anions via electroneutrality, and water osmotically, concentrating bile. CCK is the primary stimulus for the gallbladder to contract (expel contents) into the duodenum. Vagal nerves also contract the gallbladder and relax the sphincter of Oddi, and sympathetics and VIP inhibit gallbladder emptying.

Disorders of bile secretions lead to crystal (stone) formation. Gallstones are primarily cholesterol crystals around a bilirubin crystal core. Bile pigment stones, a calcium salt of unconjugated bilirubin, can also form. If cholesterol content exceeds the dissolving capability of the micelles, cholesterol crystals form and act as a nucleus for gallstones.

DIGESTION AND ABSORPTION

Complex carbohydrates are broken down to absorbable monoglycerides. Poorly absorbed large proteins are broken down into monopeptides, dipeptides, and tripeptides. Pancreatic lipases digest lipids to components, which are absorbed primarily as bile acid micelles.

Carbohydrates

Digestion and absorption of carbohydrates occurs primarily in the duodenum and the jejunum. The ability to absorb carbohydrates greatly exceeds normal dietary intake. Occasionally, an inability to absorb dietary carbohydrates from the diet occurs because of deficiency of digestive enzymes or transport proteins. Microflora metabolize any carbohydrates that pass through to the colon, producing gas, increased motility, and diarrhea. The diagnosis of malabsorption is confirmed by exposure to a specific carbohydrate, such as an oral glucose tolerance test (GTT) or a biopsy of jejunal epithelial cells. Treatment involves dietary restriction or supplemental enzyme ingestion.

One common disorder, lactose malabsorption syndrome *(lactose intolerance),* is a genetic lactase deficiency that affects 50% of adults. This syndrome is almost universal in those of Asian ancestry, common in native Africans and those from Mediterranean areas but infrequent in those of Northern European backgrounds.

Proteins

A protein intake of 0.5 g/kg/day is necessary for normal balance, and a higher intake is required for growth. Dietary intake varies among cultures. Separately from ingestion, the body provides some protein for the intestines, mostly from digestive secretions (20 g/day) and desquamated epithelial cells (20 g/day). Fecal elimination is low and is due mostly to colonic bacteria, desquamated cells, and proteins in colonic mucous secretions.

Digestion occurs in the stomach and small intestine, and absorption occurs primarily in the duodenum and jejunum. Large proteins are poorly absorbed. L-isomers and single amino acids as well as dipeptides and tripeptides are absorbed by an Na^+-coupled process. Genetic malabsorption and intolerance affects intestinal and renal transport proteins. Hartnup's disease is a rare genetic defect in neutral amino acid transporter, and prolinuria is a rare defect in proline transporter.

Lipids

Triglycerides are the major component of dietary lipids; other components include sterols, sterol esters, and phospholipids. Lipids are hydrophobic and separate from the remainder of chyme as an oily phase in the stomach. In the duodenum, lipids are emulsified by bile acids and are digested to form micelles with bile acids. The micelles are absorbed at the intestinal brush border.

Some digestion occurs in the intestine and stomach, but the duodenum, as a result of pancreatic lipases, is the major site of lipid digestion.

Micelles are essential to increase contact area for absorption in the duodenum and jejunum. Lipophilic cholesterol, fatty acids, and lysophosphatides diffuse across the cell membrane. The lipids accumulate in smooth endoplasmic reticulum and are resynthesized to triglycerides, phospholipids, and cholesterol esters. They are then packaged in chylomicrons and extruded by exocytosis. After entering the lacteals, chylomicrons pass through the lymphatics to enter venous circulation at thoracic duct.

Fat lost in feces comes primarily from colonic microflora and desquamated cells. Malabsorption of lipids is tied to impaired digestion or absorption. Complete bile deficiency reduces absorption of fatty acids by 50% and impairs absorption of other lipids. Complete absence of pancreatic lipases impairs absorption of all classes of lipids. Impaired absorption can also result from epithelial cell damage, such as intestinal mucosal atrophy, tropical sprue, and gluten enteropathy. Note that the addition of nonabsorbable lipids (e.g., Olestra) and lipid absorption inhibitors impair absorption of fat-soluble vitamins (A, D, E, and K).

Water and Electrolytes

The GI tract absorbs 99% of ingested water. Absorption is greatest in the jejunum and least in the colon as a result of the tightness of the "tight junctions" on the epithelial cells. The GI tract receives 2 L/day from ingestion and 7 L/day from GI secretions and loses only 50 to 100 ml/day in feces. The colon absorbs 400 ml/day against an apparent osmotic gradient.

The jejunum is also the primary site of Na^+ absorption, secondary to amino acid and carbohydrate transport. The colon has an active Na^+ absorption. Potassium (K) is reabsorbed in jejunum and ileum, but net K balance is determined in the colon. The colon reabsorbs K^+ if the luminal K^+ concentration is high, and secretes K^+ if the luminal K^+ concentration is low. A significant K^+ loss accompanies water loss from diarrhea.

Intestinal chloride load is from ingestion and pancreatic secretions. Chloride is reabsorbed in jejunum, ileum, and colon. Bicarbonate intestinal load is from pancreatic secretions. It is absorbed in jejunum and may be secreted in the ileum and colon by a HCO_3^-/Cl^- exchange. There is a net secretion if HCO_3^- levels are high *(alkalosis)* and a net reabsorption if HCO_3^- levels are low *(acidosis)*.

Intestinal Ion and Water Balance

Sympathetic activity enhances water and sodium chloride (NaCl) absorption, and parasympathetic activity decreases water and NaCl absorption. Aldosterone provides the major hormonal control of absorption, causing Na^+ and water reabsorption and colonic K^+ loss. Enkephalin (opioid peptides) enhance NaCl and water absorption, and somatostatin enhances colonic NaCl and water absorption.

Excessive GI secretions are a clinically important problem. Na^+, Cl^-, and water secretion in crypts in the small intestine can exceed the absorptive capacity of the remainder of the GI tract. Cholera toxin stimulates crypt cell secretion, as do other cyclic adenosine monophosphate (cAMP) stimulators, such as VIP and prostaglandins. Pancreatic cholera results from a pancreatic tumor that secretes VIP.

Impaired nutrient absorption causes an excessive osmotic load and causes water and potassium loss in diarrhea. Carbohydrate malabsorption syndromes and fat malabsorption cause water loss in feces if colon absorptive capacity is exceeded.

Calcium absorption in the duodenum and jejunum is stimulated by vitamin D. Dietary iron is also reabsorbed primarily in the duodenum and jejunum, with about 20% of ingested heme iron absorbed. Approximately 50% of ingested magnesium is absorbed along the length of the intestine. Phosphate is also absorbed along the length of the intestine, possibly by active transport.

Flora

The flora of the small intestine are predominantly gram-positive lactobacilli, streptococci, and staphylococci. *Aerobacter aerogenes, Bacteroides, Candida albicans, Escherichia coli, Proteus, Pseudomonas,* and *Streptococcus faecalis* are also found. Bile acids and gastric acid may inhibit bacterial proliferation in the intestine.

Vitamins

Vitamins are essential amino acids that must be absorbed from a dietary source. Water-soluble vitamins can be absorbed by membrane transport proteins. Folic acid and nicotinic acid are absorbed by diffusion or facilitated diffusion. Diffusion causes absorption of pyridoxine and riboflavin. Secondary active transport causes absorption of vitamin C in the ileum, biotin in the duodenum and ileum, and folic acid and thiamine in the jejunum. Vitamin B_{12} absorption across the ileum requires intrinsic factor, a gastric secretion. Lipid-soluble vitamins (A, D, E, K) are absorbed in micelles. Compounds that diminish or impair fat absorption also impair absorption of fat-soluble vitamins.

EFFECTS OF AGING

Physiologic changes in the GI tract occur with aging. In the mouth, teeth may become loose from loss of supporting gums and bone. Circulation in the gums is reduced, and aging teeth may darken, become uneven, and fracture. Decreased output of the salivary glands leads to dryness of mucous membranes and increased susceptibility to breakdown. This decrease can cause difficulty in swallowing and decreased stimulation of taste buds.

Secretion of digestive enzymes and bile also decreases. In the stomach, atrophy of gastric mucosa leads to a decreased secretion of HCl. A decrease in HCl causes reduction in iron and vitamin B_{12} absorption and a proliferation of bacteria. This reduction leads to the development of anemia. Increased bacteria in the gut may result in diarrhea and infection. With a decrease in bile secretion, absorption of fats and fat-soluble vitamins becomes impaired. This decreased absorption of fat can lead to weight loss, and the decrease in fat-soluble vitamins can lead to various problems, such as altered calcium metabolism and bleeding from the decrease of vitamin K, which is needed to synthesize prothrombin.

CONCLUSIONS

A thorough knowledge of the structure and function of the GI system helps the nurse to provide knowledgeable care to clients. Medical disorders are related to the four major functions of the GI system: motility, secretion, digestion, and absorption. To provide effective interventions, the nurse must understand the normal physiology and the digestive organs.

BIBLIOGRAPHY

1. Guyton, A. C., & Hall, J. (1996). *Textbook of medical physiology* (9th ed.). Philadelphia: W. B. Saunders.
2. Fauci, A. S., et al. (1998). *Harrison's principles of internal medicine* (14th ed.). New York: McGraw-Hill.
3. Johnson, L. R. (1997). *Gastrointestinal physiology* (5th ed.) St. Louis: Mosby–Year Book.
4. Silverthorn, D. (1998). *Human physiology*. Upper Saddle River, NJ: Prentice Hall.

CHAPTER

28 Assessment of Nutrition and the Digestive System

Vicki M. Ross

Adequate and appropriate nutrition underlies the success of all medical therapies. Nutritional health requires a gastrointestinal (GI) tract that can receive, transport, absorb, and metabolize nutrients. Similarly, adequate and appropriate nutrition is necessary for the GI tract to function properly. Because of this interdependence, assessment of the GI tract and nutritional status occurs simultaneously or in close succession. Systematic and thorough assessment of nutritional status and the upper GI tract can detect a wide range of actual or potential health problems.

This chapter focuses on assessment of nutritional status and the upper GI tract, which we will consider to include the mouth, esophagus, stomach, and small intestine. Assessment of the large intestine (colon), rectum, and accessory organs (liver, pancreas, and gallbladder) are discussed in Chapters 32 and 42.

Screening and Assessment of Nutritional Status

■ NUTRITIONAL HEALTH

Nutritional health is the result of consistently meeting the body's nutrient requirements.[4] Because of the many variables that differ from person to person—such as gender, age, size, metabolism, activity level, and more—it is difficult, if not impossible, to determine the exact nutrients required. However, we can determine average nutrient requirements by comparing individual characteristics with published standards or reference groups, such as the *Recommended Dietary Allowances* (RDAs) or the *Food Guide Pyramid.*

RDAs were developed by the Food and Nutrition Board of the National Council/National Academy of Sciences and are commonly used to determine nutritional requirements for specific groups of people.[12] The RDA system lists specific types and amounts of nutrients (e.g., protein, vitamins, minerals, and trace elements) for average, healthy people of various ages and sizes. RDAs are set at levels that may exceed actual individual nutrient requirements. Assess the adequacy of a client's diet by having the client complete a food diary (Fig. 28–1) and by comparing nutrient intake to that listed in the RDAs for people with characteristics similar to those of the client. For example, the RDA for iron is 15 mg for a 30-year-old, nonpregnant woman. If a client with these characteristics consumes on average 7 mg of iron per day, she is at risk for anemia.

RDAs should not be confused with *Reference Daily Intakes* (RDIs) for specific nutrients. RDIs are based on the amount of essential nutrients required to meet the physiologic needs of people in specific age or gender groups. Although RDIs include some micronutrients that are also included in the RDAs, the recommended amounts may be larger. An RDI may list a tolerable upper intake level and an adequate intake level, or it may list an estimated average requirement. An RDA is calculated from the estimated average requirement; otherwise, the adequate intake level is used. The adequate intake level is a goal for nutrient intake, based on the consensus of experts. Clients who consume less than the RDI amount may or may not be receiving adequate amounts of micronutrients. Consistent consumption of a nutrient above the tolerable upper intake level increases risk of adverse effects.

Another standard for assessing dietary intake is the Food Guide Pyramid published by the U.S. Department of Agriculture. It is a graphic representation of the types and proportions of foods recommended for average, healthy persons (see Chapter 2, Fig. 2–1). The Pyramid may be used to compare the client's daily food intake with recommended servings and food groups. Clients who consistently omit foods from one or more of the food groups are at nutritional risk.[10]

Because the RDA system and the Food Guide Pyramid are based on average, healthy populations, it may not be appropriate to apply these standards to clients who are ill or outside the average height or weight range. Nutritional requirements differ if clients are ill or have underlying disease. Fever, for example, increases caloric requirements 7% for each degree Fahrenheit of temperature increase. Some specialty groups publish nutritional standards or recommendations for clients with specific

Record *all* foods and drinks that you had during the day and during the night.

Day of the Week (Mon Tues Wed Thurs Fri Sat Sun)

Breakfast

Foods and Drinks — Amounts (cups, tbsps)

Lunch

Foods and Drinks — Amounts (cups, tbsps)

Dinner

Foods and Drinks — Amounts (cups, tbsps)

Snacks

Foods and Drinks — Amounts (cups, tbsps)

Do you take vitamin or mineral supplements? Yes______ No_______

Please list kind and how many per day.

FIGURE 28–1 A food diary form. (From U.S. Senate Select Committee on Nutrition and Human Needs. [1977]. *Dietary goals for the United States.* Washington, DC: U.S. Government Printing Office.)

diseases or conditions.[1, 13] In general, protein requirements decrease and nonprotein calorie requirements increase if kidney or liver function is impaired. Dietary fats are restricted if a client has pancreatic exocrine dysfunction; carbohydrates are restricted if a client has pancreatic endocrine dysfunction.

The National Health and Nutrition Examination Surveys, National Food Consumption Survey, and the Continuing Survey of Food Intakes by Individuals are examples of population-based surveys that describe dietary intake, nutritional status, or health outcomes related to nutrition. Information from these studies may be used in assessments of similar populations. For example, data from such surveys indicate that the body weight of Americans continues to increase. In addition to changes in caloric intake, sedentary lifestyles appear to contribute to this weight gain. When conducting an assessment and using information from these surveys, include questions about the client's physical activity in addition to dietary intake (see Chapters 1 and 2).

■ MALNUTRITION

When nutrient availability is inadequate or excessive over an extended period, malnutrition occurs. Malnutrition incorporates both starvation and obesity.

Starvation, or the inadequate delivery of nutrients to the body, can be primary or secondary.

- *Primary* malnutrition occurs when adequate nutrition is not delivered to the upper GI tract over an extended period (e.g., famine, anorexia, mechanical obstructions of the GI tract, fad diets)
- *Secondary* malnutrition occurs when the upper GI tract fails to absorb, metabolize, or use nutrients (e.g., ischemic bowel or Crohn's disease).

Marasmus, kwashiorkor, or mixed-type malnutrition result when inadequate amounts of protein or calories are delivered or absorbed over an extended period (Table 28–1). The development of a specific type of malnutrition depends on a number of factors that are defined by clinical presentation and laboratory values.[11, 18]

TABLE 28–1 TYPES OF MALNUTRITION ASSOCIATED WITH PROTEIN AND CALORIE DEFICITS

Type of Malnutrition	Clinical History	Clinical Manifestations	Laboratory Results
Kwashiorkor	Inadequate protein intake with adequate calorie intake	Body weight at or above ideal range Edema sometimes present	Visceral proteins (albumin, prealbumin, transferrin) below normal
Marasmus	Inadequate calorie and protein intake	Cachectic appearance Body weight and anthropometric measurements below normal	Visceral proteins within normal range
Mixed	Inadequate calorie and protein intake with increased nutritional requirements	Cachectic appearance Body weight and anthropometric measurements below normal	Visceral proteins below normal

Inadequate food consumption rarely causes deficits of single nutrients. Instead, clients typically present with deficits of multiple nutrients. Micronutrient malnutrition occurs when vitamins, minerals, or trace elements are not delivered, absorbed, or used by the gut. Because vitamin, mineral, or trace element deficits occur in combination, it is difficult to identify deficits of single micronutrients. Laboratory tests designed to measure vitamin or trace element levels are rarely specific or sensitive enough to accurately determine if adequate amounts are available in the body.[14] The best method to identify actual or potential micronutrient deficits is with a thorough history and meticulous physical examination. Table 28–2 lists clinical manifestations of micronutrient deficits and foods that contain specific micronutrients.

In addition to protein or calorie malnutrition, suspect micronutrient malnutrition in clients who have had previous gastric surgery, chronic pancreatitis, short-bowel syndrome, pressure ulcers, various types of cancer, and acquired immunodeficiency syndrome (AIDS). Gastric surgery can impair absorption and use of vitamin B_{12}. Chronic pancreatitis can lead to fat malabsorption and decreased absorption of fat-soluble vitamins. Short-bowel syndrome results in decreased transit time and micronutrient absorption. Pressure ulcers can cause zinc and vitamin C deficits. Some drug therapies, especially those for cancer and AIDS, decrease the absorption or use of vitamins and minerals such as folate, potassium, and magnesium. If the client's dietary intake is inadequate or if the client presents with a clinical history such as these, suspect and assess for micronutrient malnutrition.

Although not commonly regarded as a type of malnutrition, *obesity* results from nutrient delivery that exceeds the client's nutrient requirements. In the United States, the incidence and prevalence of obesity are rising. Clients who consume recommended amounts of nutrients but have sedentary lifestyles are at risk for obesity, as are clients who consume excess calories[16] (see Chapter 2).

■ NUTRITION SCREEN OR ASSESSMENT?

Nutrition screening and nutrition assessment are not the same. Nutrition screening is a method of categorizing clients at high or low risk for malnutrition. Tools for nutrition screening usually contain a brief list of questions about changes in weight or dietary intake, any underlying disease or upper GI problems, and a comparison of the client's current weight to a standard. On the basis of the client's responses to nutrition-related questions, an assigned score determines whether the client is at low or high risk of malnutrition.[6, 9]

The Nutrition Support Screening Alert is one example of a nutrition screening tool. Developed by a multidisciplinary panel of experts, this tool is a tiered approach designed to identify older clients at risk for malnutrition (Box 28–1). Each tier, or level, of the instrument requires a more sophisticated assessment. The client or caregiver can perform the initial assessment for nutritional risk. *Level I* calls for additional information, including calculation of the client's body mass index, and *Level II* calls for information from the previous levels plus laboratory measurement of serum proteins. This instrument and all nutritional screening tools are used to identify clients at risk for malnutrition.

In general, nutritional screening takes place within the first few days of the client's encounter with the health care system and includes general questions about nutritional status and upper GI function. A client entering an inpatient setting should be assessed upon admission. When the nutritional screen indicates that a client is at risk for malnutrition, an in-depth nutrition and upper GI assessment are performed. Nutritional and upper GI assessments are client-centered and include an in-depth history, physical examination, and diagnostic testing to determine actual or potential problems involving the upper GI tract, nutritional status, or both. As needed, ask a dietitian to consult during this process.

HISTORY

Assessment of nutritional status and the upper GI tract begins with collection of history data. The historical account determines the direction and focus of the physical examination and the required diagnostic testing. Historical data include (1) biographical information, (2) chief complaint, (3) previous illness or hospitalization, (4) medications, (5) dietary supplements, (6) allergies, (7) family health, (8) psychosocial factors, and (9) a review of systems.

■ BIOGRAPHICAL AND DEMOGRAPHIC DATA

Analyze the client's demographic data (e.g., gender, age, religious affiliation, and marital status) within the context of nutritional status and upper GI function. For example, because women are more likely to experience problems related to calcium deficiency, include specific questions

TABLE 28–2 SOURCES OF MICRONUTRIENTS AND EVIDENCE OF DEFICIENCY

Micronutrient	Selected Foods with High Micronutrient Content	Evidence of Deficit
Vitamin A	Dark green, leafy or yellow-orange vegetables Milk fat Egg yolks	Loss of appetite and taste Night blindness Bumpy or scaly skin
Vitamin B_1 (thiamine)	Lean meats Egg yolks Legumes Enriched or whole grain cereals and breads	Paresthesias and peripheral neuropathies Mental confusion Heart failure Edema
Vitamin B_6 (pyridoxine)	Yeast Wheat germ Pork Liver Whole grain cereals Legumes	Sore, reddened tongue Seborrhea-like dermatitis Paresthesias
Vitamin B_{12} (cobalamin)	Beef Fish Milk Eggs Cheese	Sore, reddened mouth Atrophy of the tongue Megaloblastic anemia Paresthesias
Vitamin C (ascorbic acid)	Oranges Lemons Strawberries Tomatoes Cabbage Green peppers	Gingivitis Dry mouth Alopecia Pruritus (itching) Ecchymotic lesions on the skin
Calcium	Dairy products Sardines Salmon Dark green, leafy vegetables	Osteoporosis Osteomalacia
Copper	Organ meats Legumes Chocolate Nuts	Decreased absorption of iron Anemia Neutropenia Leukopenia
Vitamin D (calciferol)	Fish and fish oil Fortified dairy products	Softening of the bones Joint pain Fatigue Muscle tetany
Vitamin E (tocopherol)	Sunflower, corn, or soybean oil Wheat germ oils	Lipid absorption or transport abnormalities
Folate (folic acid)	Legumes Liver Dark green or leafy vegetables Lean beef Potatoes	Sore, reddened tongue and mouth Glossitis Megaloblastic anemia
Iodine	Seafood Iodized salt	Enlargement of the thyroid gland
Iron	Organ meats Shellfish Poultry Legumes Blackstrap molasses Fortified cereals	Hypochromic, microcytic anemia
Vitamin K	Broccoli Cabbage Turnip greens Green tea	Ecchymotic lesions Bruising

Table continued on following page

TABLE 28–2 SOURCES OF MICRONUTRIENTS AND EVIDENCE OF DEFICIENCY *Continued*

Micronutrient	Selected Foods with High Micronutrient Content	Evidence of Deficit
Manganese	Whole grains Legumes Nuts Tea	Magenta tongue Dermatitis
Niacin	Organ meats Brewer's yeast Peanuts Fish Poultry Whole grains Beans	Sore, reddened mouth Atrophy of the tongue Angular stomatitis Dermatitis
Riboflavin	Liver Milk Cheddar cheese Cottage cheese Yogurt Brewer's yeast	Sore, reddened tongue and mouth Angular stomatitis Seborrhea-like dermatitis
Zinc	Oysters Wheat germ Beef Cheese	Angular stomatitis Seborrhea-like dermatitis Alopecia (hair loss)

Adapted from Mahan, L. K., & Escott-Stump, S. (Eds). (2000). *Krause's food, nutrition, and diet therapy* (10th ed.). Philadelphia: W. B. Saunders.

about calcium intake in the history. Because older people who live alone face an increased risk of inadequate food intake, question them about how and what they eat. People in their teens or 20s may be at increased risk of duodenal ulcers or gastric cancers, whereas older clients are more are at risk for gastric ulcers and colon cancers. Women in their 20s and 30s are at risk for inadequate nutritional intake.

For clients in these age ranges, include specific questions about changes in GI function. Culture and ethnic origin also affect the type, amount, and frequency of dietary consumption (see Chapter 9).

BOX 28–1 Nutrition Support Screening Alerts

If an older person indicates that the following questions listed on the Nutrition Health Checklist, Level I and II screens are descriptive of their condition or life situation, nutrition counseling and support interventions may help them solve their nutritional problems and improve their nutrition status.

Determine Your Nutritional Health Checklist Alerts

I have an illness or condition that made me change the kind and/or amount of food I eat.
Without wanting to, I have lost or gained 10 pounds in the last 6 months.
I am not always physically able to shop for, cook for, or feed myself.

Level I Screen Alerts

Has lost or gained 10 pounds or more in the past 6 months
Body mass index < 22
Body mass index > 27
Is on a special diet
Has difficulty chewing or swallowing
Has pain in mouth, teeth, or gums
Usually or always needs assistance with preparing food or shopping for food

Level II Screen Alerts

In addition to Level I Screen Alerts:

Has pain in mouth, teeth, or gums
Midarm muscle circumference < 10th percentile
Triceps skinfold < 10th percentile
Triceps skinfold > 95th percentile
Serum albumin < 3.5 g/dl
Serum cholesterol < 160 mg/dl
Clinical evidence of mental/cognitive impairment
Clinical evidence of depressive illness
Clinical evidence of insulin-dependent diabetes, adult-onset diabetes, heart disease, high blood pressure, stroke, gastrointestinal disease, kidney disease, chronic lung disease, liver disease, osteoporosis, or osteomalacia.

Adapted from the Nutrition Screening Initiative, a project of the Amercian Academy of Family Physicians, the American Dietetic Association, and the National Council on Aging, Inc., and funded in part by a grant from Ross Products Divisions, Abbott Laboratories, Inc.

DIVERSITY IN HEALTH CARE

Cultural Influences on Nutrition

Probably no subject has intrigued human beings more universally and persistently than food. Food is more than a source of nutrition. Food has always served many functions and uses with culturally unique symbols and meanings. It is important that nurses understand their clients' food beliefs, functions, symbols and practices.[3] The nurse can obtain this knowledge by conducting a nutritional assessment. This information assists the nurse in providing nursing care that is safe and congruent with the client's culture.

The following case study provides a poignant example of the importance of understanding the client's cultural food beliefs and behaviors.

Case Study

Maria is a 17-year-old pregnant, English-speaking, Mexican American who comes for her prenatal appointment. Her blood pressure was significantly elevated, and she had a marked increase in weight. The examining physician admitted her to the hospital for tests. Maria had several consultations during her 3-day stay. It was a mystery why her hematocrit level ranged from 15 to 17 and her platelet and blood counts were dangerously low. Even a hematologist could not explain the abnormal blood levels.

The client received a pint of blood. An intern familiar with traditional health beliefs asked Maria one question: Was she eating anything other than her normal food? It was discovered that she was daily eating eight bars of Magnesia de Carbonate (chalk). She was experiencing heartburn and vomiting as well as craving dirt and ice (pica). She acknowledged that a family member had given her the chalk to cleanse her stomach. The family member also prevented her from eating ice because of the belief that eating ice would give her and the baby pneumonia and bronchitis.[2]

An assessment of the client's cultural influences on nutrition would have prevented this scenario and the resulting hospitalization.

The table identifies guidelines the nurse may use for assessing cultural influences regarding nutrition.

Guidelines for Determining Cultural Influences Regarding Nutrition

Meaning of Food

1. Explore the meaning of food to this group.

Common Foods and Food Rituals

1. Identify foods, preparation practices, and major ingredients commonly used by this cultural group.
2. Identify specific food rituals.

Dietary Practices of Health Promotion

1. Identify dietary practices used to promote health or to treat illness in this group.

Nutritional Deficiencies and Food Limitations

1. Identify enzyme deficiencies or food intolerances commonly experienced by this group.
2. Identify large-scale or significant nutritional deficiencies experienced by this group.
3. Identify native food limitations in America that may cause special health difficulties.[4]

Cultural Food Practices and Religion

Cultural food practices are often interconnected with religious practices. Most Americans have little knowledge about the cultural food practices of other religions. The following table summarizes the food-related practices of selected religious groups.

Food Restrictions for Selected Religions

Group Restrictions	Cultural Implications
Church of Jesus Christ of Latter-Day Saints (Mormonism)	
No alcoholic beverages	Avoid medicines containing alcohol (e.g., cough suppressants).
No stimulants (caffeinated beverages, such as coffee, tea, sodas)	For clients on liquid diets, substitute decaffeinated beverages for brewed and instant regular coffee, teas, cocoa, and carbonated beverages containing caffeine (e.g., colas). Avoid medicines containing caffeine, such as the following over-the-counter drugs: *Analgesics:* Anacin, Bromo-Seltzer, Cope, Empirin, Excedrin *Stimulants:* NōDōz, Vivarin, Caffedrine *Diet Pills:* Dexatrim, similar generic brands Many cold preparations
Observant Mormons fast on the first Sunday of each month. Fasting means refraining from food and liquids.	Fasting is not required during illness or in persons with diabetes, hypoglycemia, ulcers, or other medical condition for which fasting is contraindicated.

Chart continued on following page

DIVERSITY IN HEALTH CARE *Continued*

Group Restrictions	Cultural Implications
Judaism	
Three major groups: 1. Orthodox (strict observance) 2. Conservative (basic observance) 3. Reform (less ceremonial emphasis and observance of dietary laws)	
The dietary laws (Kashrut) dictate which foods are permissible under religious law: 1. Only meat from cloven-hoofed animals that chew cud (cattle, sheep, goat, ox, or deer) is allowed. These animals must be slaughtered ritually in a manner that results in minimal pain to the animal and maximal blood drainage. Two methods are used to prepare Kosher meats: a. The meat is soaked in cold water for 30 minutes, salted, and drained to deplete blood content. It is then washed under cold water and drained again before cooking, *or* b. The meat is first prepared by quickly searing or cooking over an open flame, which permits liver to be eaten. 2. Meat and dairy products cannot be served at the same meal, and they cannot be cooked or served in the same set of dishes. Milk or milk products may be consumed just before a meal but not until 6 hours after eating a meal in which meat has been consumed. Milk may not be used in coffee if served with a meat meal. Nondairy creamers can be substituted if they do not contain sodium caseinate, which is derived from milk. Fish, eggs, vegetables, and fruits are considered neutral *(parve)* and may be eaten with dairy products or meats. 3. Fish with fins and scales are allowed. No shellfish (crab, lobster, shrimp, clam, oyster) or scavenger fish (catfish, shark, porpoise) may be eaten. Crocodile, frog, snail, snake, and tortoise also are prohibited. *Note:* Kosher foods in stores are marked with one of two symbols: a. The letter "K" with a circle (Kosher) b. The encircled letter "U" (the seal of the Union of Orthodox Jewish Congregations of America) Additional dietary laws are followed during the week of Passover. No bread or product with yeast may be eaten; instead, matzah or unleavened bread is eaten. Products that are fermented or that can cause fermenting or souring may not be eaten.	*Kosher* (fit or proper to use) meals are available in hospitals and other health care settings. They usually are served on paper plates with plastic utensils that are sealed. Do not unwrap the utensils or transfer food onto another dish. Do not bring nonkosher foods into the home of a Jewish client who follows the laws of Kashrut. When teaching clients about special diets, be sure that sample menus are congruent with dietary laws. Be aware that keeping a kosher kitchen requires two sets of dishes, pots, and utensils.
There are a number of fast days in the Jewish calendar, with the holiest being Yom Kippur (Day of Atonement), during which Jews abstain from food and drink from sunset the evening before the holy day until after sunset the following day.	Encourage Jewish clients to consult with a rabbi if their insistence on fasting may be detrimental to health (e.g., those with insulin-dependent diabetes, hypoglycemia, or ulcers). Maintaining one's health supersedes the laws of fasting.
Islam	
Pork, pork products, animal shortening, and alcohol are strictly prohibited.	Clients in hospitals and other health care settings may need assistance in identifying foods that have been prepared using animal shortenings or pork seasonings. Clients should avoid regular gelatin made with pork, marshmallow, and other confections made with pork. Avoid medicines containing alcohol, such as some cough suppressants. Avoid extracts such as vanilla or lemon that contain alcohol.
The slaughter of poultry, beef, and lamb must be done ritually by a Muslim to ensure that it is *halal* (slaughtered in a prescribed way).	Although many health care settings do not routinely provide foods that are *halal,* these products are often available at specialty grocery stores, particularly in large urban areas.

DIVERSITY IN HEALTH CARE *Continued*

Group Restrictions	Cultural Implications
Fasting is common. During the month of Ramadan, no foods or beverages are consumed until after sunset. *Note:* Recent immigrants from the Middle East may eat and pass food with the right hand. Because the left hand is used for toileting, it is considered extremely impolite to eat with the left hand.	Fasting is not required for persons who are ill.
Roman Catholicism	
Abstinence from meat and meat products (gravy, soups) and fasting on Ash Wednesday and the Fridays during a 40-day period of religious observance called Lent.	Fish, cheese, or other meat substitutes are offered on these days.
Rules of fasting apply to those between the ages of 12 and 65 years. Fasting refers to eating one regular meal and two smaller meals per day.	Fasting is not required for children or the elderly or anyone who is ill.
Seventh Day Adventism	
Fermented or alcoholic beverages are prohibited.	Avoid medicines containing alcohol (e.g., cough medicines). Avoid vanilla and lemon extract.
Optional vegetarianism may take three forms: 1. Strict vegetarians (e.g., vegans): Include no animal-derived products in their diet 2. Ovolactovegetarians: Use milk, milk products, and eggs but no meats. 3. Semivegetarians: Refrain from pork or pork products, shellfish, and blood	Strict vegetarians may need assistance in selecting a balanced diet from the hospital menu.
Snacking between meals is discouraged.	Some clients with diabetes, hypoglycemia, or ulcers may require between-meal snacks.

Summary

Food has many uses and meanings.

Assess the role that food plays in keeping people well and in aiding in recovery from illness. Use the knowledge to provide safe and culturally competent care.

References

1. Andrews, M. (1999). Culture and nutrition. In M. Andrews & J. Boyle (Eds.) *Transcultural concepts in nursing care* (pp. 350–352). Philadelphia: J. B. Lippincott.
2. Cooper, T. (1996). Culturally appropriate care: Optional or imperative. *Advanced Practice Nursing Quarterly, 2*(2), 1–6.
3. Leininger, M. (1995). *Transcultural nursing: Concepts, theories, research and practices.* New York: McGraw-Hill.
4. Purnell, L., & Paulanka, B. (1998). *Transcultural health care: A culturally competent approach.* Philadelphia: F. A. Davis.

Joyce Larson-Presswalla, PhD, RN, *President, "Culture Counts," Marketing Coordinator, James A. Haley Veterans Hospital, Tampa, Florida*

■ CURRENT HEALTH

Chief Complaint

Chief complaints related to nutritional status and upper GI function include nausea and vomiting, indigestion, abdominal pain, diarrhea, and changes in weight or appetite from psychological, mechanical, or metabolic causes. When a client presents with these manifestations, conduct a symptom analysis.

Symptom Analysis

Include the following questions (see Chapter 9 for additional questions).

NAUSEA AND VOMITING. When does the nausea or vomiting occur? How long does it last? Is it related to food intake? Does food relieve or worsen the symptoms? Does the vomitus contain undigested food or bile? What does it look like? How much is vomited per episode? Is pain associated with the onset of nausea and vomiting?

INDIGESTION. Are the symptoms of indigestion related to food intake? Which foods worsen or relieve them? Does the client take any medications or antacids for the indigestion? How does the client describe the indigestion? Is it a "burping" or burning sensation?

ABDOMINAL PAIN. Did the pain begin rapidly or gradually? What is the intensity of the pain? Does the pain radiate? Does it worsen or improve with movement?

Does the client have a fever with the pain? Does food worsen or ease the pain? What specific foods alter the pain?

Abdominal pain is associated with a number of disorders, some of which are life-threatening (Table 28–3). Naturally, it is crucial to differentiate abdominal pain caused by a life-threatening condition from pain caused by a more minor condition.

WEIGHT AND APPETITE CHANGE. Ask specific questions about the client's usual appetite and weight and the amount of weight lost or gained and over what period of time. Was the weight gain or loss intentional? If so, ask about the diet. Does a specific weight loss organization or health club sanction the client's diet? Does the client take diet pills, such as appetite stimulants or suppressants?

Unintentional changes in weight may stem from psychological, physiological, or metabolic causes. Ask the following:

- Are weight changes associated with changes in mood?
- Does the client feel sad or depressed?
- Has there been a change in activity level?
- Has the client experienced early satiety, anorexia, or any changes in the taste of food?
- Does the client have trouble chewing or swallowing or problems with the teeth or gums? If the client wears dentures, ask how they fit. Ill-fitting dentures can decrease appetite and lead to weight loss.

DIARRHEA. How many stools does the client expel per day? Can the client describe the amount of stool (do feces fill the toilet or is the amount small)? Are stools liquid or solid? What color are they? Are they black or bloody? Do they sink or float? Does the client experience pain with defecation? Does abdominal bloating or cramping accompany the diarrhea? Does the diarrhea occur during the day, the night, or both day and night? Does the client experience fecal incontinence? How many days or weeks has the diarrhea persisted? Does the diarrhea decrease at certain times during the month (indicating a hormonal influence)? Does physical activity change the diarrhea symptoms?

Ask specifically about the relationship of stool output and dietary intake. Bloating and diarrhea that occur when the client consumes dairy products may signal lactose intolerance (see Allergies). High-fat diets that result in floating, greasy stools may indicate fat malabsorption. If there is copious or persistent diarrhea or vomiting, assess for fluid and electrolyte deficits (see Chapters 12 and 13).

Nonspecific GI problems, such as nausea, vomiting, and diarrhea, can result from food-borne poisoning (Table 28–4). When clients present with these manifestations, ask about the type of food consumed over the past 2 or 3 days, how the food was prepared, and whether anyone else who ate the same food also became ill.

TABLE 28–3 SOURCES AND CHARACTERISTICS OF ABDOMINAL PAIN

Source	Characteristics
Intestinal obstruction	Distended abdomen No bowel movements or flatus Intermittent or colicky pain Right upper quadrant pain radiating to shoulder associated with gallbladder Pain near umbilicus associated with small bowel Lumbar pain associated with colon
Peritoneal inflammation (perforated ulcer, ruptured spleen, ruptured appendix)	Steady, aching pain directly over area of inflammation Pain increasing with motion Intensity of pain varying with source of inflammation Gastric acid may produce more pain than alkaline content of small bowel Sometimes associated with manifestations of shock
Vascular obstruction	May be preceded by 2 to 3 days of mild to moderate pain and hyperperistalsis, followed by severe abdominal pain and manifestations of shock

PAST HEALTH HISTORY

Major Illnesses and Hospitalizations

The client's history of illnesses and hospitalizations can provide clues about nutritional status and the function of the upper GI tract. For example, a client with a history of bleeding is at increased risk for iron deficiency. A client with liver disease may have an increased risk for protein malnutrition. Has the client had or been hospitalized for peptic ulcer disease, vomiting blood (hematemesis), anemia, jaundice, gallbladder disease, pancreatitis, cancer, a change in bowel habits, tarry stools, or unexplained weight loss or gain?

Has the client had diagnostic tests of the upper GI system, such as a barium swallow, upper GI studies, endoscopic retrograde cholangiopancreatography (ERCP), or computed tomography (CT)? If the client has undergone previous diagnostic testing, the results may offer clues about current health problems in addition to providing baseline data. For example, for a client who reports having had a previous endoscopic procedure, ask about the purpose and results of the procedure.

Past surgical procedures also provide information about nutritional status and the structure and function of the upper GI tract. Ask specifically about any previous surgery of the mouth, throat, stomach, liver, pancreas, gallbladder, or abdomen. Include dates and outcomes for all tests, procedures, and operations.

Medications

Obtain detailed information about current or previous prescribed and over-the-counter medications (Table 28–5).

- Does the client use aspirin, aspirin compounds, or nonsteroidal anti-inflammatory drugs (NSAIDs) that may contribute to gastritis or bleeding?

TABLE 28–4 FOOD-BORNE POISONING: SOURCES AND MANIFESTATIONS

Organism	Associated Food	Clinical Manifestations
Bacillus cereus	Fried rice	Watery diarrhea
Campylobacter jejuni	Raw or undercooked poultry, unpasteurized milk, untreated water	Fever, headache, and myalgias, followed 2 to 4 days later by abdominal pain, cramping, and watery diarrhea
Clostridium botulinum	Improper canning of fruits and vegetables. Honey used as a sweetener in infant formulas	Mild to severe manifestations occur in 18 to 36 hours; nausea and vomiting with no fever; cranial nerve involvement results in ptosis, diplopia, dysarthria, and dysphagia
Enterotoxigenic *Escherichia coli*	Fecal-oral route (contaminated water, contaminated meat, uncooked vegetables, unpasteurized apple cider)	1- to 2-day incubation period, followed by watery explosive diarrhea and abdominal cramps
Salmonella (non-typhoidal salmonellosis)	Contaminated raw eggs, unpasteurized dairy products	24- to 48-hour incubation period, followed by nausea, vomiting, and abdominal cramps
Staphylococcus aureus	Ham, poultry, potatoes, egg salad, mayonnaise, cream pastries	Nausea, vomiting, watery diarrhea within hours of consuming contaminated food
Trichinella	Undercooked pork or meat from carnivores	Mild to severe abdominal pain, nausea, vomiting, diarrhea during first week and progressing over next 3 to 4 weeks to include edema, rash, and muscle weakness
Vibrio parahaemolyticus	Shellfish	Cramping and inflammatory diarrhea more than 6 hours after ingestion of contaminated food

- Does the client take antacids? If so, note the type and the frequency. Does the client use laxatives or stool softeners?
- Does the client take any vitamin or mineral supplements? Ask specifically about supplements containing iron, because iron can cause gastric irritation and can change stool color and consistency.

Nutritional Supplements

Nutritional supplements include vitamins, minerals, herbs used for medicinal purposes, amino acids, and meal supplements or replacements. Because nutritional supplements are sold over the counter, they are often viewed as harmless. Taken in excess or in combination with certain drugs or supplements, however, nutritional supplements can be harmful.

If the client takes a vitamin supplement, determine the amount of each vitamin, mineral, and trace element contained in each dose. Multivitamins contain differing amounts of individual micronutrients. Indeed, some vitamins contain more than 100% of the RDA for specific micronutrients; others contain less than 100% of the RDA. In excessive doses, some vitamins can produce toxic side effects. Excess amounts of vitamin A, for example, may cause yellowing of the skin and abnormal liver function test results.

Does the client consume any herbs or similar products? Because herbal products contain varying amounts of active ingredients, note the amount and brand of the herbal preparation (Table 28–6).

Various forms of amino acids and hormones are also gaining notoriety as nonprescription remedies. Does the client consume such preparations as glucosamine, melatonin, or dehydroepiandrosterone (DHEA)?

Meal supplements or replacements are usually purchased in a liquid form and provide a convenient means of increasing nutritional intake. Because of the wide variation in nutritional content and the potential for consuming inadequate or excessive amounts of specific micronu-

TABLE 28–5 DRUG-NUTRIENT INTERACTIONS

Drug Class	Possible Nutrient Interactions
Antacids	Decreased absorption of calcium, iron, magnesium, and zinc
Anticoagulants	Vitamin K antagonist
Anticonvulsants	Decreased folate and biotin
Antituberculosis drugs	Disrupted metabolism of vitamins B_6 and B_{12}
Cathartics	Non-renal losses of calcium, potassium, water
Cholesterol-reducing drugs	Inhibited fat digestion and absorption
Diuretics	Increased renal loss of potassium, calcium, magnesium, and zinc
Histamine H_2 blockers	Decreased vitamin B_{12} absorption
Monamine oxidase inhibitors	Interactions with tyramine-containing foods (cheese, smoked fish, wine, yeast)

TABLE 28–6 COMMON HERBAL SUPPLEMENTS

Herb	Common Name	Purported Indications	Form	Side Effect
Allium sativum	Garlic	Atherosclerosis Hypertension Anticlotting agent Increased peristalsis	Capsules, powder, liquid, bulb	Heartburn, flatulence, rare allergic reaction; caution needed if client is taking aspirin or anticoagulants
Echinacea angustifolia, E. purpurea, E. pallidus	Echinacea, purple coneflower, narrow-leaved echinacea	Immune stimulant Anti-infective Topical wound therapy	Capsules, tea, liquid	Potential for allergic reactions
Ephedra sinica Stapf, *E. equisetina* Bunge	Ephedra, *ma huang,* ephedrine (illegal in some areas)	Nasal decongestant Central nervous system stimulant Bronchodilator	Capsules, tea	Increased blood pressure, heart rate, irritability; avoid with hypertension, diabetes, and thyroid disease
Eleutherococcus senticosus Maxim, *Acanthopanax senticosus* Harms	Siberian ginseng, eleuthero	Increased mental alertness and physical endurance	Tea	Not related to Ginseng class but commonly confused with it
Ginkgo biloba Linneaus	Ginkgo	Vasodilatation Increased cerebral and/or peripheral blood flow	Leaf extracts in solid or liquid form	Headache, gastrointestinal upset, dizziness, nausea and vomiting, diarrhea, decreased clotting times
Hypericum performatum Linneaus	St. John's wort, klamath weed, amber touch-and-heel, goatweed, rosin rose	Treatment of depression, anxiety, bedwetting, diuretic, hemorrhoids, topical treatment for burns	Tea, capsules, tinctures, oil macerates	Fatigue, allergic reactions, photosensitivity
Panax ginseng C. A. Mey (Orient), *P. quinquefolium* Linneaus (American)	Ginseng	Strengthen body functions Increase vitality Aphrodisiac	Fresh dried roots, capsules, tablets, teas, gum	Nervousness, excitation, diarrhea, skin eruptions; avoid with hypertension

trients, ascertain the brand and amount of meal supplement consumed per day.

Allergies

Inquire about allergies to foods. Distinguish between actual allergic responses and food intolerances or preferences. Food allergies typically result in systemic types of responses, such as hives or dyspnea. If allergies are suspected, question the client about associated manifestations. How does the client describe an allergic reaction? What GI problems does the client have: cramping, flatulence, diarrhea?

Lactose intolerance is a common condition for many adults, because inadequate amounts of *lactase* (an enzyme in the small bowel) cannot break down large lactose molecules. As a result, fluid is drawn into the small bowel, resulting in abdominal cramping and diarrhea. If the client's manifestations result from lactose intolerance, eliminating lactose from the diet eases them. Some people benefit from taking lactase in tablet form before eating dairy products. Products such as Lact-Aid and dairy substitutes (e.g., lactose-free milk and ice cream) are also available.

■ FAMILY HEALTH HISTORY

A family history of certain GI problems may influence a client's current and past health problems. Inquire about the health status of family members. Is there a family history of cancer, ulcers, or colitis? Many diseases, such as ulcerative colitis and Crohn's disease, seem to have a familial component. Some diseases may result from genetic or environmental predisposition. Is there a family history of jaundice, alcoholism, hepatitis, pancreatitis, obesity, peptic ulcers, or irritable bowel syndrome?

■ PSYCHOSOCIAL HISTORY

Occupation

Ask about the client's occupation. Are toxic substances (e.g., arsenic, lead, mercury, carbon tetrachloride) present in the workplace? Does the client travel for work? The onset of GI problems, such as diarrhea or nausea, may be related to recent travel to foreign countries. For some travelers, invasion of the GI tract by bacteria, protozoa, helminths, or other parasites may cause nausea, vomiting, or diarrhea.

Nutrition

The type, amount, and time of food intake are heavily influenced by psychosocial factors, such as culture and ethnic origin (see the Diversity in Health Care feature). Social deprivation and institutionalization have been associated with decreased nutritional intake and malnutrition. Ask the client to describe a typical meal. Who purchases and prepares the meal? Who usually dines with the client?

Does the client consume alcohol? If so, ask how much, what type, and how frequently it is consumed?

Diet

How does the client describe her appetite (little, normal, ravenous)? Has there been any change in appetite? Ask the client to describe the usual foods and fluids (including coffee, colas, and alcohol) typically consumed in a 24-hour period. Has the client modified her usual diet and, if so, why?

Consider having the client complete a food intake record to determine dietary intake (see Fig. 28–1). Typically, a food intake record includes two weekdays and a weekend day. Because memory lapses decrease the reliability of information, instruct the client to record everything she ate immediately after she eats it. After the client completes the food intake record, consult a registered dietitian to collaborate in determining the adequacy of the diet. In general, the average, healthy person requires about 30 to 35 calories per kilogram and 0.8 to 1.2 g of protein per kilogram of body weight. For example, a woman weighing 55 kg (120 pounds) would require 1650 to 1925 calories and 44 to 46 g of protein.

■ REVIEW OF SYSTEMS

Inquire about the condition of the client's mouth, including the presence of dental caries, number and condition of teeth, condition of the gingivae, and use of dentures.

- Are there any oral lesions, halitosis, excessive salivation, or mouth dryness?
- How often does the client floss and brush?
- When was the last visit to the dentist for teeth cleaning?
- Does the client have trouble chewing or swallowing?
- If pain is reported with eating, is it related to specific foods or associated events?

Has the client had a change in bowel habits or stool characteristics? Are changes in appetite, upper GI symptoms, or bowel movements associated with menstrual cycles? Ask specifically about problems of the hepatic and biliary systems, such as jaundice, pruritus, ascites, dark-colored urine, pale stools, or bleeding problems. Detailed questions for the review of systems are found in Chapter 9.

PHYSICAL EXAMINATION

■ ANTHROPOMETRIC MEASURES

Anthropometric measures provide an assessment of body mass or body compartments. Height, weight, frame size, body mass index, midarm muscle circumference (MAMC), and waist-to-hip proportions are examples of anthropometric measures.

Height and Weight

Use a telescoping ruler and balance scale to measure height and weight. If the client cannot bear weight, consider using a calibrated sling or wheelchair scale. Describe clothing and other accessories (light clothing, shoes with or without heels, orthopedic casts, braces, and so on) worn by the client.

If the client cannot stand, use an arm span measurement to approximate height. To do so, extend the client's arms laterally and measure from the tip of the middle finger on one hand to the tip of the middle finger on the other hand.

Compare the client's current weight to her reported usual weight. Unintentional weight changes of less than 90% or more than 110% of the client's usual weight are considered significant. For example, for a client who usually weighs 100 pounds, a weight change of ±10 pounds (current weight $<$ 90 pounds or $>$ 110 pounds) would place the client at nutritional risk. To calculate the difference as a percentage of usual weight, divide the client's current weight by the usual weight and multiply times 100:

$$\%\text{ usual weight} = \frac{\text{current weight}}{\text{usual weight}} \times 100$$

Ideal Body Weight and Frame Size

Most methods for determining ideal or desirable body weight require an estimation of body frame size (Box 28–2). Calculate body frame size by measuring the client's wrist circumference and dividing it into the height. Compare the resulting r value with a chart to determine the client's body frame size. An alternative method for calculating body frame size is to measure the elbow breadth.

Ideal body weight may be calculated by several methods. A traditional method is to use a formula based on height, weight, and body frame size (Box 28–3). Factor the body frame size into the calculation for ideal body weight.

Another method is to compare the client's weight with the Metropolitan Life Insurance Company recommendations (Table 28–7). When using this table, adjust height and weight to account for the height of shoes and the weight of clothing. The client's weight should fall within the range for gender, height, and body frame size. A weight more than 20% above or 10% below the calculated ideal body weight indicates nutritional risk. This table is only a guideline and does not account for variations based on genetic or cultural factors.

Body Mass Index

An acceptable method of standardizing height-for-weight measurement is the body mass index (BMI). To calculate the BMI, divide the client's weight in kilograms by the height in meters squared as follows:

BOX 28–2 Calculating Body Frame Size

Wrist Circumference Method

1. Measure the client's right wrist (in centimeters) at the point of the smallest circumference, just distal to the styloid process of the radius and ulna.

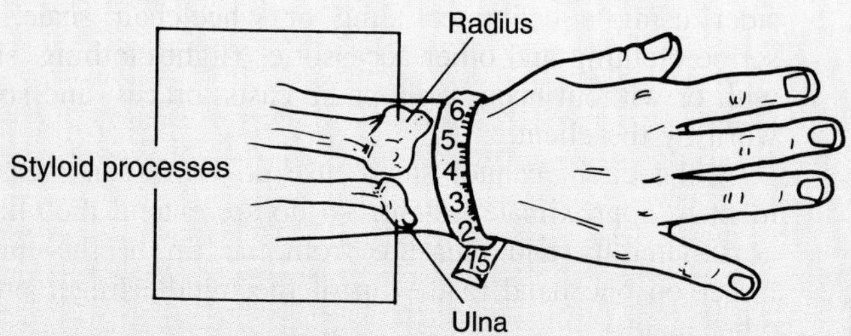

2. Obtain the client's height (in centimeters) without shoes.
3. Divide the client's wrist circumference into the client's height to obtain the *r* value:

$$r = \frac{\text{height (in cm)}}{\text{wrist circumference (in cm)}}$$

4. Use the chart below to determine the client's body frame size based on the calculated *r* = value and sex:

	Men	*Women*
Small frame	$r > 10.4$	$r > 10.9$
Medium frame	$r = 9.6–10.4$	$r = 9.9–10.9$
Large frame	$r < 9.6$	$r < 9.9$

Elbow Breadth Method*

1. Instruct the client to extend his or her right arm, then bend the forearm to a 90-degree angle with the fingers pointing straight up.
2. Measure the width of the client's right elbow (in inches) across the greatest breadth of the joint between the bony prominences of the lateral and medial epicondyles of the humerus. To measure, either use calipers or place your thumb and index finger on the epicondyles and measure the distance between the thumb and finger.
3. Use the chart below to determine the client's body frame size based on the client's elbow breadth, sex, and height in 1-inch heels. The values shown are for a medium body frame. Measurements less than the values shown indicate a small frame; greater values indicate a large frame.

Height	Elbow Breadth
Men	
5′2″–5′3″	2½″–2⅞″
5′4″–5′7″	2⅝″–2⅞″
5′8″–5′11″	2¾″–3″
6′0″–6′3″	2¾″–3⅛″
6′4″	2⅞″–3¼″
Women	
4′10″–4′11″	2¼″–2½″
5′0″–5′3″	2¼″–2½″
5′4″–5′7″	2⅜″–2⅝″
5′8″–5′11″	2⅜″–2⅝″
6′0″	2½″–2¾″

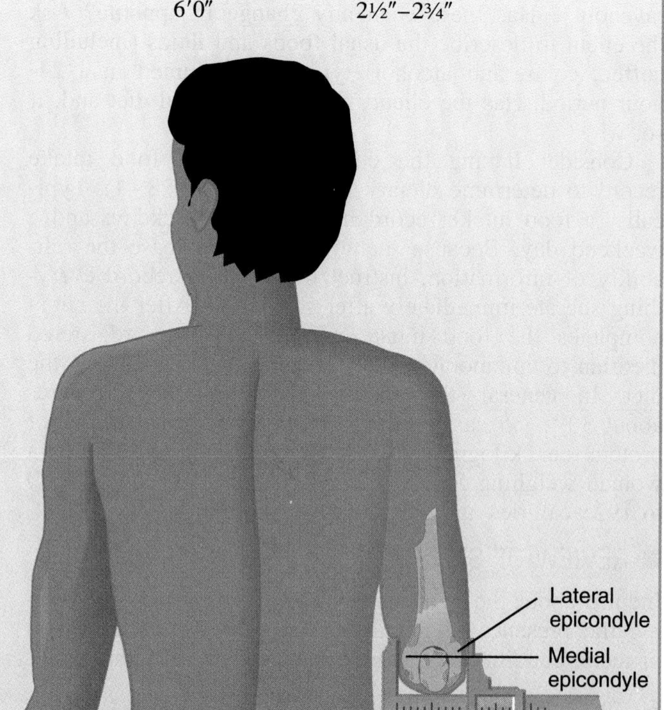

*Courtesy of Metropolitan Life Insurance Company.

$$\text{BMI} = \frac{\text{wt (kg)}}{\text{ht (m}^2)} \quad or \quad \frac{\text{wt (lb)}}{\text{ht (in.}^2)} \times 703$$

For example, a 60-kg (132 pounds) client with a height of 145 cm (57 inches) has a BMI of 28.5, putting the client in the overweight range. Figure 28–2 contains normal and abnormal ranges for different BMI values.

Circumferential Measurements

Circumference measurements assess muscle mass and body fat proportions and distribution. Midarm muscle circumference and waist-to-hip ratio are examples of circumferential measurements.

To obtain a client's midarm muscle circumference, measure the triceps skinfold (TSF) thickness and midarm circumference (MAC) and calculate the MAMC. Compare these measurements and calculated results with published standards for the client's gender and age (Fig. 28–3).

Determine waist-to-hip proportions by dividing the waist measurement at its smallest circumference by the hip measurement at its largest circumference. Waist-to-hip proportions greater than 0.8 for women and 1.0 for men indicate fat distribution that is associated with negative health outcomes.

■ MOUTH

Assessment of the oral cavity includes inspection and palpation. Good illumination is essential. A headlamp

BOX 28–3 Calculating Ideal Body Weight (IBW)

Adult Male*	Adult Female*
Take 106 lb for the first 5 ft of height; add 6 lb/inch for each additional inch over 5 ft	Take 100 lb for the first 5 ft of height; add 5 lb/inch for each additional inch over 5 ft

Small Frame Calculate 10% of the amount for medium frame and subtract it from the first amount (i.e., IBW is 10% *less* for persons with small frames)

Large Frame Calculate 10% of the amount for medium frame and add it to the first amount (i.e., IBW is 10% *more* for persons with large frames)

Example An adult male is 6′1″ tall with a large body frame. His IBW is calculated as follows:
6′1″ = 5 ft plus 13 inches
First 5 ft of height = 106 lb
Additional height over 5 ft = (13) × (6) = 78 lb
Medium frame IBW = 106 + 78 = 184 lb
Allowance for large frame = (10%) × 184 = 18.4 lb
Large frame IBW = 184 + 18.4 = 202.4 lb

*These formulas are for adults with a medium body frame. Adjust formulas for clients with small or large frames (adjustment is the same formula for both sexes).

Data from The American Dietetic Association. (1981). *Handbook of clinical dietetics.* New Haven: Yale University Press.

provides direct illumination, and a head mirror provides indirect lighting; both items keep your hands free for the physical examination. A penlight and tongue blade may also be used.

Inspection

Begin your assessment of the client's mouth by inspecting the lips for symmetry, color, hydration, lesions, or nodules. Put on clean gloves, and ask the client to remove any dentures. Note the symmetry of facial movements and the fit of the dentures as the appliance is removed. Instruct the client to open her lips while clenching her teeth. Inspect the position of the upper and lower teeth for malocclusion or missing teeth.

Next, ask the client to open her mouth wide, and inspect the structures inside (Fig. 28–4). Start at the left side of the mouth, and continue in a clockwise fashion. Note any evidence of dental caries, missing or broken teeth, or receding gums. Note the color of the mucosa and gums. Inspect for red lesions (erythroplakia), white lesions (leukoplakia), swelling, bleeding, or ulcers. Survey the pharynx for abnormalities of the tonsils, such as redness, swelling, lesions, ulcers, uvular deviations, drainage, or unusual mouth odor.

Inspect the tongue for symmetry, color, and moisture. Note any areas of atrophy, abnormal coatings, swelling, or lesions. Next, ask the client to stick out her tongue and move it from side to side, upward, and downward. Observe for symmetry of movement and voluntary or involuntary movement of the tongue. Abnormal tongue movement may be a result of infiltration of muscle by tumor or nerve entrapment.

Palpation

Palpate the client's lips, gingivae, and buccal mucosa. Check for loose teeth, masses, swellings, or areas of tenderness. If you find lesions, note the location, size, color, consistency, and presence or absence of tenderness.

Gently grasp the client's tongue with cotton gauze. Extend and lift it while inspecting and palpating the un-

TABLE 28–7 METROPOLITAN LIFE TABLE OF ADULT WEIGHT STANDARDS

Weights* for men (according to frame, ages 25–29) for greatest longevity†

Height‡ Feet	Inches	Small Frame	Medium Frame	Large Frame
5	2	128–134	131–141	138–150
5	3	130–136	133–143	140–153
5	4	132–138	135–145	152–156
5	5	134–140	137–148	144–160
5	6	136–142	139–151	146–164
5	7	138–145	142–154	149–168
5	8	140–148	145–157	152–172
5	9	142–151	148–160	155–176
5	10	144–154	151–163	158–180
5	11	146–157	154–166	161–184
6	0	149–160	157–170	164–188
6	1	152–164	160–174	168–192
6	2	155–168	164–178	172–197
6	3	158–172	167–182	176–202
6	4	162–176	171–187	181–207

Weights* for women (according to frame, ages 25–59) for greatest longevity†

Height‡ Feet	Inches	Small Frame	Medium Frame	Large Frame
4	10	102–111	109–121	118–131
4	11	103–113	111–123	120–134
5	0	104–115	113–126	122–137
5	1	106–118	115–129	125–140
5	2	108–121	118–132	128–143
5	3	111–124	121–135	131–147
5	4	114–127	124–138	134–151
5	5	117–130	127–141	137–155
5	6	120–133	130–144	140–159
5	7	123–136	133–147	143–163
5	8	126–139	136–150	146–167
5	9	129–142	139–153	149–170
5	10	132–145	142–156	152–173
5	11	135–148	145–159	155–176
6	0	138–151	148–162	158–179

* Weight in pounds (in indoor clothing weighing 5 lb for men, 3 lb for women).
† Metropolitan no longer labels these weights "ideal" or "desirable," because these adjectives mean different things to different people.
‡ In shoes with 1-inch heels.
Courtesy of Metropolitan Life Insurance Company, copyright 1983.

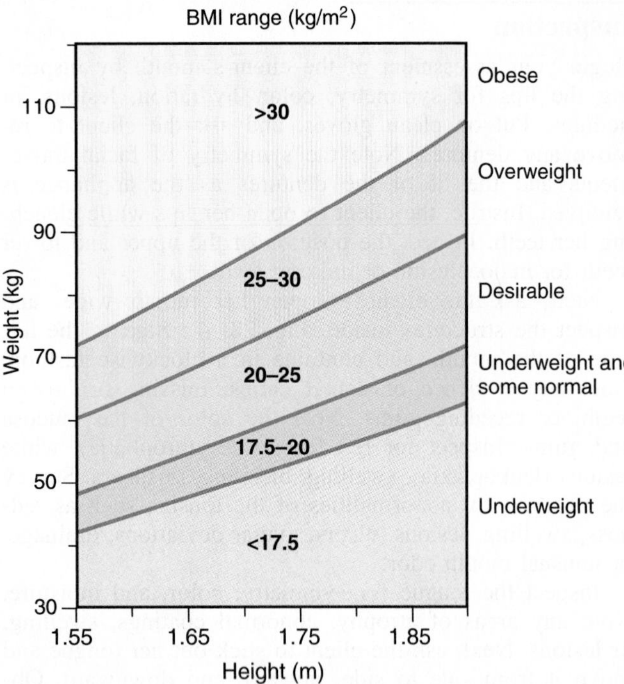

FIGURE 28–2 Weight and height for different ranges of body mass index (BMI). (From Elia, M. [1997]. Assessment of nutritional status and body composition. In G. L. Rombeau & R. H. Rolandelli [Eds.], *Clinical nutrition and enteral and tube feeding* [3rd ed.]. Philadelphia: W. B. Saunders.)

derside of the tongue and the floor of the mouth. Palpate all areas of the tongue and floor of the mouth for masses, swellings, or areas of tenderness. Note any lesions or areas of color changes. Many precancerous oral lesions are pain-free and asymptomatic. Clients with suspected lesions that do not clear within 2 to 3 weeks should be referred for further evaluation.[15]

Release the tongue, and depress it with a tongue blade. Ask the client to say "aah." Note the symmetry and movement of the uvula and soft palate. If there are no contraindications, give the client a sip of water. As the client swallows, observe for symptoms of difficulty in swallowing (*dysphagia*). Clients who exhibit difficulty with swallowing or asymmetrical movement of oral cavity structures should be evaluated for dysphagia and risk for aspiration. Oral-pharyngeal dysphagia typically presents as difficulty moving solid foods to the back of the mouth and indicates further assessment and evaluation to rule out cranial nerve involvement (see Chapter 67). Esophageal dysphagia presents as difficulty swallowing solids or liquids and indicates motor disease or obstruction of the esophagus. A speech therapist can evaluate further.

ABDOMEN

Because a full bladder can interfere with abdominal assessment, ask the client to void before the examination. Place the client in a supine position with her arms at her sides. Place a small pillow under the client's knees to relax the abdominal muscles. Because percussion and palpation can alter intestinal activity, assess the abdomen in the following sequence: inspection, auscultation, percussion, and palpation. Visualize the underlying organs as you assess, and describe the abdomen by anatomic regions, or quadrants (Fig. 28–5).

Inspection

Stand at the client's right side, and begin inspecting the abdomen by noting the condition of the skin and the abdominal contour. The skin should be smooth and intact, with varying amounts of hair. The contour should be flat, concave, or rounded, depending on the client's body type. Note any areas of distention or irregular contour, which may suggest obstruction, hernia, tumor, or previous surgery. Bulging flanks and glistening, taut skin are abnormal findings and suggest ascites (see Chapters 32 and 42).

Inspect the abdomen for rashes, discoloration, scars, petechiae, striae (stretch marks), and dilated veins. Scars on the abdomen should correlate with the client's history of past surgical procedures, and striae should correlate with reported changes in weight. The umbilicus should be concave, located at the midline, and the same color as the abdominal skin, with no evidence of drainage. Note the shape, position, color, and presence of any discharge at the umbilicus.

Next, sit at eye level to the client's abdomen and observe for peristaltic movement or abdominal pulsation. Normally, peristaltic movements are not visible but abdominal pulsations may be observed in a very thin client.

Diastasis recti is a separation of the rectus muscle that results from obesity, pregnancy, or other conditions in which the abdominal muscles are subjected to sustained increased intra-abdominal pressure. This condition is not a true hernia and, for most clients, of no clinical significance. If there are no contraindications, instruct the client to bear down and perform a Valsalva maneuver or attempt a sit-up. The increased intra-abdominal pressure enhances the separation of weakened rectus muscles at the midline, where a bulge appears.

Inspect the rectal area after the abdominal examination is completed. Chapters 32 and 37 explain the rectal examination.

Auscultation

Using the diaphragm of your stethoscope, begin auscultating the client's abdomen. Press the diaphragm lightly to the abdominal wall, beginning in the right lower quadrant at the area of the ileocecal valve. Continue in a clockwise fashion, auscultating each quadrant or region. As air and fluid move through the GI tract, soft clicks and gurgles can be heard every 5 to 15 seconds. Note the frequency and character of bowel sounds. Normal bowel sounds occur irregularly at a rate of 5 to 35 per minute.[8] Loud, high-pitched bowel sounds *(borborygmi)* represent hyperactivity of the GI tract. Borborygmi may be present in clients who are hungry or who have gastroenteritis, or they may be present in early intestinal obstruction.

Hypoactive bowel sounds occur at a rate of one or fewer every minute. To determine the absence of bowel

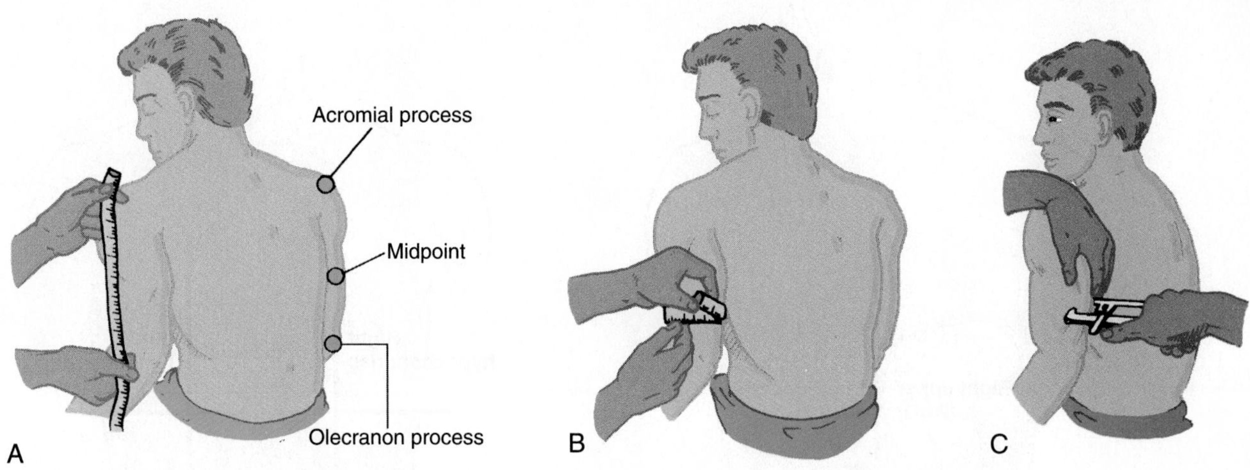

D Calculate the midarm muscle circumference (MAMC) using the following formula:
MAMC (in cm) = [MAC in cm] – [(0.314) × (TSF in mm)]

MEASUREMENT		STANDARD	90%	60%
Midarm circumference (MAC)	Men	29.3 cm	26.4 cm	17.6 cm
	Women	28.5 cm	25.7 cm	17.1 cm
Triceps skinfold (TSF)	Men	12.5 mm	11.3 mm	7.5 mm
	Women	16.5 mm	14.9 mm	9.9 mm
Midarm muscle circumference (MAMC)	Men	25.3 cm	22.8 cm	15.2 cm
	Women	23.2 cm	20.9 cm	13.9 cm

FIGURE 28–3 Measuring adipose and skeletal muscle tissue to estimate the client's reserves of protein and calories. *A,* Locate the *midpoint* of the client's relaxed, nondominant upper arm by palpating the acromial and olecranon processes and measuring the distance between the two points with a tape measure. Mark the posterior aspect of the arm at the midpoint with a pen. *B,* Measure *midarm circumference* (MAC) at the midpoint, keeping the tape measure level. *C,* Just above the midpoint at the posterior aspect of the arm, grasp the client's skin and subcutaneous tissue between thumb and index finger, freeing it from the underlying muscle mass. Place the calipers at the midpoint just below the fold of grasped tissue. Squeeze the calipers until they are equilibrated at the "measure" markings. Read the measurement to the nearest millimeter. Repeat the readings two more times, allowing a rest period of 3 seconds between readings. Calculate the average of the three readings for the *triceps skinfold thickness* (TSF). *D,* Compare the client's values for MAC, TSF, and *midarm muscle circumference* (MAMC) to the following standards to determine nutritional risk status. *Undernutrition* is indicated by a measurement below 90% of the standard. *Protein-calorie malnutrition* is indicated by a measurement of less than 60% of the standard, especially for MAMC. *Obesity* is indicated by a triceps skinfold measurement of 120% or more above the standard.

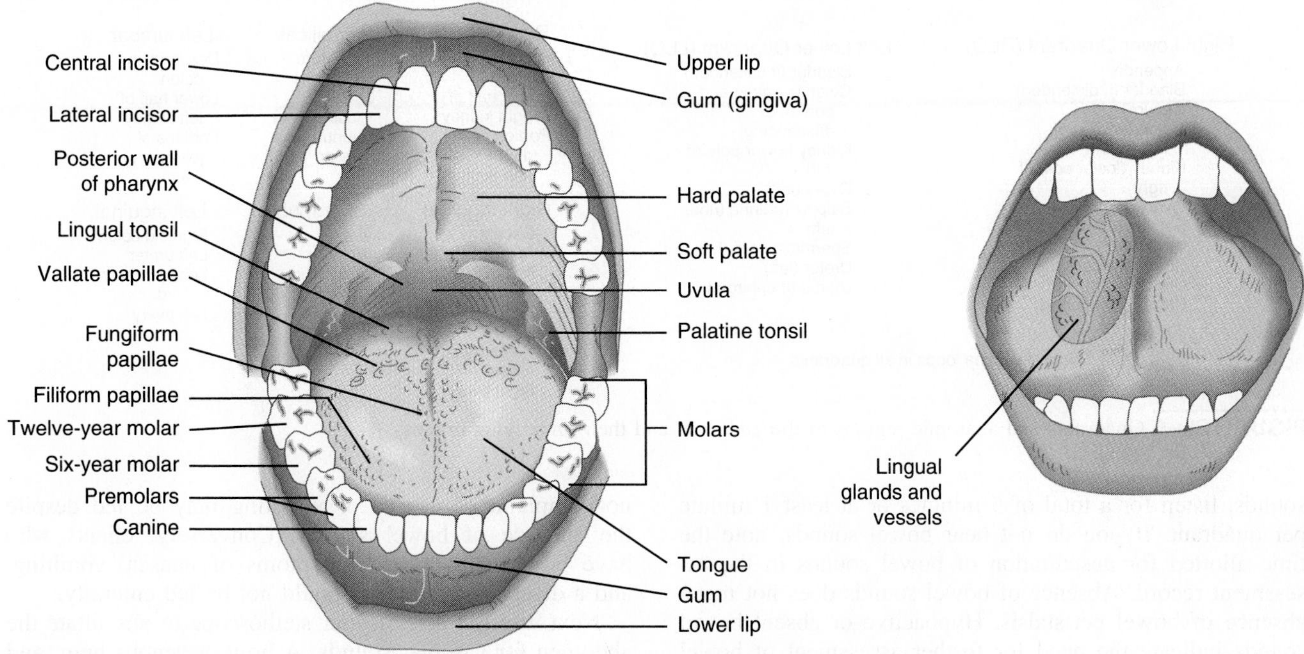

FIGURE 28–4 Assessment of the oral cavity: terminology and normal findings.

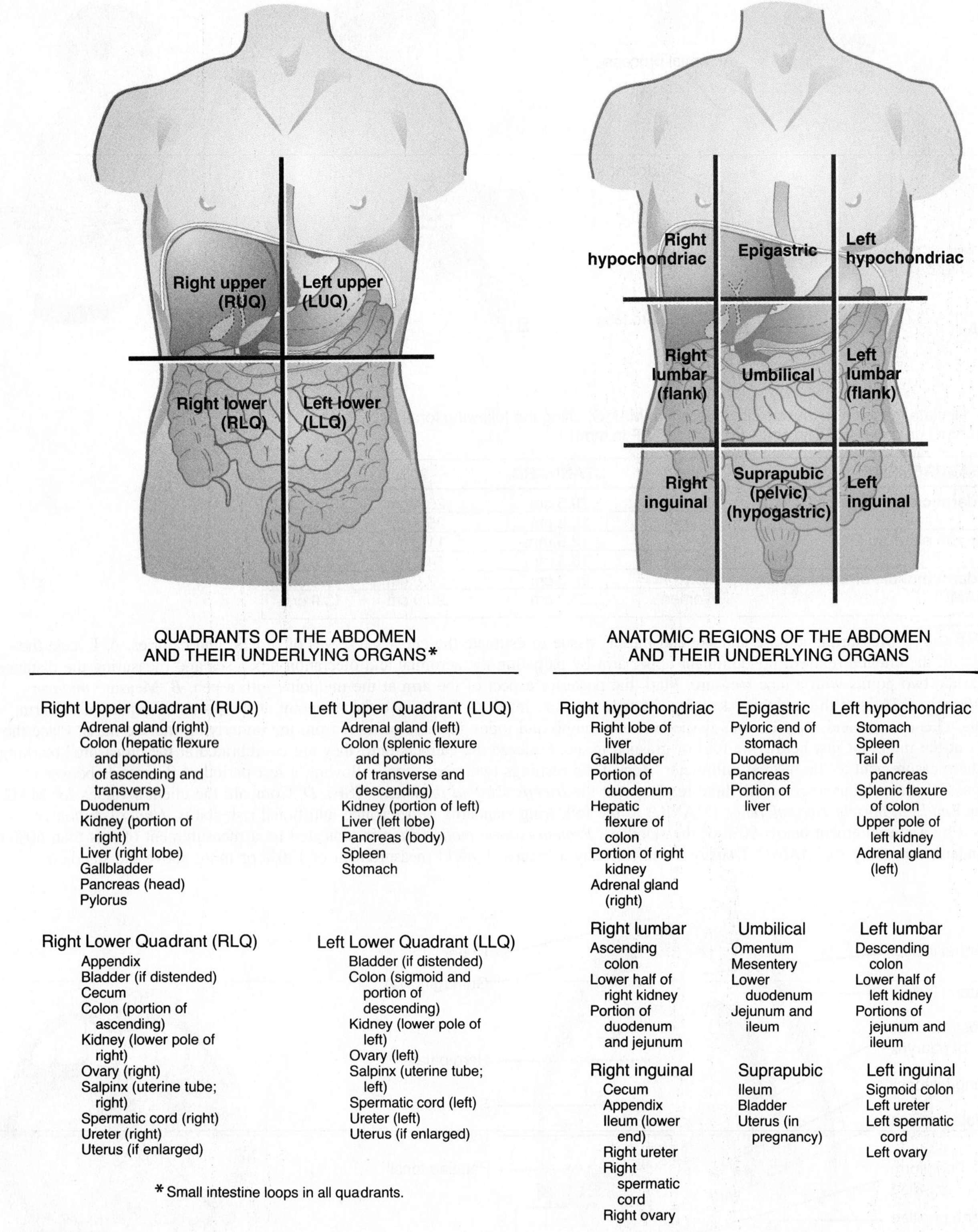

FIGURE 28–5 Quadrants and anatomic regions of the abdomen and their underlying organs.

sounds, listen for a total of 5 minutes or at least 1 minute per quadrant. If you do not hear bowel sounds, note the time allotted for auscultation of bowel sounds in the assessment record. Absence of bowel sounds does not mean absence of bowel peristalsis. Hypoactive or absent bowel sounds indicate the need for further assessment of bowel function. Clients who have a nondistended abdomen and no complaint of nausea or vomiting may be fed despite the absence of bowel sounds. Conversely, clients who have bowel sounds and symptoms of nausea, vomiting, and a distended abdomen should not be fed enterally.

Next, use the bell of your stethoscope to auscultate the abdomen for vascular sounds. A bruit, a venous hum, and a friction rub are examples of abnormal sounds that may be auscultated during the abdominal examination. Bruits auscultated over major blood vessels indicate turbulent blood flow, such as an aneurysm or partial obstruction of a vessel. A continuous venous hum heard in the periumbilical area indicates engorged liver circulation. Friction rubs sound like two pieces of leather rubbing together and suggest a hepatic tumor or splenic infarction.

Percussion

Percuss the abdomen to determine the size and location of abdominal organs and to detect fluid, air, or masses. Percuss all quadrants or regions, and compare the sounds to expected findings. Normally, percussion sounds over the abdomen are high-pitched, loud, or "musical" (tympanic) over gas and dull (thud-like) over fluid or solid organs. Percussion can be used to determine the size and position of the liver and spleen (see Chapter 42) and to assess the level of a distended bladder (see Chapter 32). If you suspect an abdominal aneurysm or if the client has undergone abdominal organ transplantation, percussion is contraindicated.

Palpation

Palpate the abdomen in a systematic, quadrant-to-quadrant or region-to-region manner, beginning with nontender areas and progressing to painful ones. Start with light palpation, depressing the abdomen 1 to 2 cm. Palpate for masses or areas of tenderness. Note any areas of involuntary abdominal rigidity or guarding. McBurney's point is located in the right lower quadrant midway between the umbilicus and the anterior iliac crest. Localization of pain in this area suggests appendicitis.

After lightly palpating all areas, use deep palpation to determine the size and shape of abdominal organs and masses. Use caution when examining any tender areas. Rebound tenderness suggests peritoneal inflammation. To elicit rebound tenderness, depress the abdomen deeply over the area of tenderness and then quickly release it. If rebound tenderness is present, the client will report an increase in pain and tenderness upon release.

Palpation of organs such as the kidney, liver, and spleen is discussed in Chapters 32 and 42, and techniques are described in Chapter 10. The Physical Assessment Findings in the Healthy Adult feature is an example of a recording of a normal abdominal physical examination.

PHYSICAL ASSESSMENT FINDINGS IN THE HEALTHY ADULT

Gastrointestinal System

Inspection

Mouth. Lips symmetrical, pink, moist, without lesions. Buccal mucosa and gingivae pink, moist, intact, without lesions. Hard and soft palates pink, intact. Tonsils behind pillars, without inflammation. Posterior pharynx pink, without exudate. Uvula rises midline with phonation. Tongue midline, mobile, without deviation or fasciculations.

Abdomen. Flat, symmetrical, with umbilicus inverted, centered, and midline. No scars, lesions, dilated veins, visible peristalsis or pulsations, or separation of rectus muscles at rest or with straining.

Anus and Rectum. Perianal area free of lesions, inflammation, fissures, bulges, or external hemorrhoids.

Auscultation

Abdomen. Bowel sounds present in all four quadrants.

Percussion*

Abdomen. General tympany throughout, with liver and splenic dullness. Liver span 10 cm at right midclavicular line.

Palpation*

Abdomen. Liver and spleen nonpalpable. Abdomen soft, nontender, no masses or rebound tenderness; muscle tone firm, relaxed.

Anus and Rectum. Anus and rectum without tenderness, masses, hemorrhoids, or prolapse. Rectal mucosa smooth. Stool negative for blood.

*In assessment of the abdomen, palpation is performed after auscultation so that the bowel is not stimulated.

DIAGNOSTIC TESTS

Diagnostic tests provide information about the nature and severity of upper GI tract or nutritional problems. Laboratory tests, radiography, ultrasonography, endoscopy, cytology, gastric analysis, and other tests are commonly used to identify and treat nutrition and upper GI tract problems.

■ LABORATORY TESTS

Nutritional Anemias

Normal hematologic function requires adequate intake, absorption, use, and storage of nutrients, such as protein, iron, vitamin B_{12}, and copper. Assessment of red blood cell function and iron stores is crucial to nutritional assessment. Chapter 74 describes assessment for hematologic disorders and anemias.

Serum Proteins

Serum proteins are important in maintaining fluid pressures and as carrier molecules. Tests for serum proteins include albumin, prealbumin, retinol-binding protein, and transferrin. Measurement of serum proteins calls for a venous blood sample to be drawn with the client in a fasting or nonfasting state. Obtaining blood samples for laboratory tests is discussed in Chapter 11.

Table 28–8 lists serum proteins, normal values, half-lives, and conditions associated with abnormal values. In general, serum proteins with long half-lives (e.g., albumin) tend to be global indicators of nutritional status. Serum proteins with shorter half-lives (e.g., prealbumin and transferrin) suggest acute changes in nutritional status.

Total Lymphocyte Count

Immune function and nutritional status are closely related. Consequently, total lymphocyte count (TLC), an indicator

TABLE 28–8 SERUM PROTEINS

Protein	Normal Range	Half-Life	Associated Conditions
Albumin	3.5–5.0 g/dl	14–20 days	Values increased in dehydration Values decreased in malnutrition, overhydration, trauma, protein loss, and liver disease
Prealbumin	20–40 mg/dl	3–5 days	Values increased in nutrition intake and renal failure Values decreased in poor dietary intake
Retinol-binding protein	3–6 mg/L	8–12 hr	Values decreased in overhydration, liver disease, zinc and vitamin A deficiency
Transferrin	200–400 mg/dl	8–10 hr	Values increased in pregnancy and iron deficiency Values decreased in chronic infection, cirrhosis

of immune function, provides a gross measure of nutritional status as well. To determine TLC, obtain a white blood cell (WBC) count with differential from the client's venous blood sample. Next, multiply the percentage of lymphocytes by the total WBC count. For example, a client with a WBC count of 7000/mm^3 and 30% lymphocytes would have a TLC of 2100.

TLCs below 1800/mm^3 suggest malnutrition. Keep in mind, however, that this count is a gross indicator of immune function and nutritional status. Clients who are not malnourished may have a low TLC after chemotherapy. Alternatively, an elevated TLC may be found in malnourished clients with sepsis.

D-Xylose Absorption Test

D-Xylose, a monosaccharide, is absorbed in the small intestine and is used to assess malabsorption. The client receives nothing by mouth (NPO) for 10 to 12 hours before the test. A blood sample and first-voided morning urine specimen are collected. After oral administration of a known quantity of D-xylose in water, blood and urine levels of D-xylose are measured. Blood is drawn 2 hours after D-xylose is given, and all urine is collected for a specified time. Instruct the client to remain in bed during the test because activity alters the results. Decreased values of absorbed D-xylose in blood and urine indicate possible malabsorption in the small intestine.

Nitrogen Balance

Nitrogen balance is a measure of one's anabolic or catabolic state. To determine the nitrogen balance, simultaneously record the amount and type of food consumed in a 24-hour period and obtain a 24-hour urine collection. The start and stop times for the food intake record and the 24-hour urine collection must be the same. Instruct the client about the procedure and about the importance of recording all food intake and saving all urine for 24 hours.

The 24-hour urine collection begins with discarding the first voided specimen, then collecting all urine for the next 24 hours in an iced, preservative-free container. After completing the 24-hour urine collection, send the urine to the laboratory for measurement of the urine urea nitrogen (UUN). Urine creatinine, sodium, and potassium may also be measured to determine the adequacy of the urine collection. Consult a registered dietitian to calculate the client's 24-hour protein intake from the food intake record. If the client received tube feedings or parenteral nutrition during the 24-hour test period, the amount of protein from these sources must be included in the calculation.

Protein is approximately 16% nitrogen. To determine the amount of nitrogen consumed over the 24 hours, multiply the amount of protein consumed (in grams) by 0.16. UUN is the major source of nitrogen excretion. Subtract the UUN (in grams) from the amount of nitrogen consumed. Because nitrogen is also lost through the skin, stool, and the GI tract, subtract a correction factor of 3 from the nitrogen consumed, as follows:

$$\text{nitrogen balance} = \text{nitrogen consumed (in grams)} - \text{UUN (in grams)} - 3$$

Normal nitrogen balance is positive and ranges from 4 to 6 g. Negative values indicate catabolic states or increased nutritional requirements.

Fecal Analysis

Fecal content is an indicator of the absorptive capacity of the gut. Chapter 32 presents laboratory tests for fecal lipids and stool cultures.

■ RADIOGRAPHY

General principles for the following radiographic tests are explained in Chapter 11.

Flat Plate of the Abdomen

A flat plate of the abdomen is an x-ray (radiograph) of the abdominal organs. This test can help identify abnormalities, such as tumors, obstructions, abnormal gas, fluid collections, and strictures.

Upper Gastrointestinal Series

An upper GI series, also known as a *barium swallow*, permits radiologic visualization of the esophagus, stomach, duodenum, and jejunum. It can aid in the detection of strictures, ulcers, tumors, polyps, hiatal hernias, or motility problems. The client drinks a radiopaque contrast medium (barium) while standing in front of a fluoroscopy tube. The client may also be asked to assume other positions, such as lying on the x-ray table. This test is usually done after a barium enema or gallbladder radiographic series to prevent the swallowed barium from interfering with other diagnostic images.

PREPROCEDURE CARE

The client cannot have food or fluids for 6 to 8 hours before the test. Instruct the client about the procedure and about the barium preparation. Barium has a thick consistency and a chalky taste. It may be necessary to drink up to 16 ounces for the procedure. The test lasts about 45 minutes.

POSTPROCEDURE CARE

A laxative is usually given to help expel the barium and to prevent a fecal impaction. Assess the abdomen for distention, and observe the stool to determine whether the barium has been eliminated. Initially, the stool is white, but it should return to its normal brown color within 72 hours. A distended abdomen and constipation may indicate a barium impaction. Clients with ostomies should be closely monitored for retained barium.

Because the barium swallow is commonly performed on an outpatient basis, inform the client that the stool may be white for up to 72 hours after the procedure. Instruct the client to contact the physician immediately if constipation and abdominal distention occur.

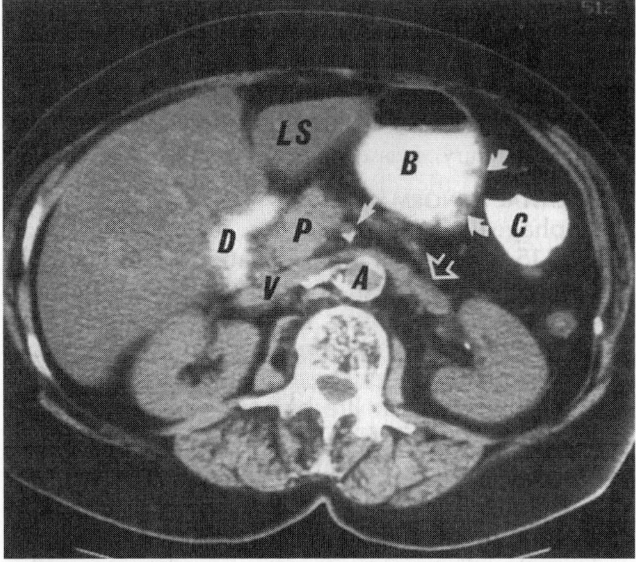

FIGURE 28–6 Normal computed tomography (CT) scan of the stomach. The CT scan is through the body of the stomach (B) at a level just below the spleen. The lateral segment of the left lobe of the liver (LS), head of the pancreas (P), and splenic flexure of the colon (C) are adjacent structures. A, aorta; D, duodenum; V, inferior vena cava. *Solid arrow* represents the superior mesenteric artery, and *open arrow* represents the vein. The rugae *(curved arrows)* are well visualized. (From Moss, A., Gamsu, G., & Genant, H. K. [1992]. *Computed tomography of the body: With magnetic resonance imaging* [Vol. 3, 2nd ed.]. Philadelphia: W. B. Saunders.)

Modified Barium Swallow

A modified barium swallow, also known as *videofluoroscopy* or an oropharyngeal motility study, is performed to assess swallowing and the risk of aspiration. While sitting in a chair equipped with videofluoroscopy, the client is given a small amount of barium to swallow in liquids and foods of various textures. During the procedure, a speech therapist or radiologist observes the client for difficulty with swallowing.

Clients are maintained on NPO status before the procedure. Maintain hydration with intravenous (IV) fluids if the client is expected to remain NPO for an extended period. After the procedure, nothing should be ingested by mouth until the speech therapist, radiologist, or physician has evaluated the test results. If diet alterations are required, consult a registered dietitian, speech therapist, or both to collaboratively develop an appropriate and adequate nutrition plan.

■ COMPUTED TOMOGRAPHY

CT scanning is used to identify masses, such as neoplasms, cysts, focal inflammatory lesions, and abscesses of the liver, pancreas, and pelvic areas (Fig. 28–6). CT also aids in evaluating local tumor spread, especially if barium studies suggest tumor growth beyond the bowel wall.[7] To distinguish normal bowel from abnormal intraperitoneal masses, dilute oral barium or other contrast media may be administered. The client is placed supine on the examination table and asked to lie still and hold her breath when instructed.

The client receives nothing by mouth for 6 to 12 hours before the procedure. Report any client allergies to iodine to the radiologist. Non-iodine contrast medium may be used when the client is allergic to iodine. No follow-up care is needed. Chapter 11 covers the general preparation and care of the client undergoing CT scanning.

■ ULTRASONOGRAPHY

Ultrasonography of the GI system helps to identify pathophysiologic processes in the pancreas, liver, gallbladder, spleen, or retroperitoneal tissues. Ultrasound studies can be used to identify fluid, masses (such as tumors), adipose tissue, abscesses, or hematomas. Physical examination is enhanced by ultrasound techniques because palpable masses and areas of tenderness can be correlated with anatomic structures while the client is on the examining table (see Chapter 11).

Because gas may interfere with the procedure, the client may take nothing by mouth for 8 to 12 hours beforehand. Reassure the client that the test is painless and safe. There are no specific postprocedure precautions or observations related to ultrasound.

■ ENDOSCOPY

Endoscopy is the direct visualization of the GI system by means of a lighted, flexible tube. It is more accurate than radiologic examination because the physician can directly observe sources of bleeding, surface lesions, or healing tissues.

PROCEDURE

Upper GI tract endoscopy includes esophagoscopy, gastroscopy, and esophagogastroduodenoscopy (Fig. 28–7). These procedures are useful for examining clients who have acute or chronic GI bleeding, pernicious anemia, esophageal injury, masses, strictures, dysphagia, substernal pain, epigastric discomfort, or inflammatory bowel disease. Conscious sedation with a sedative, narcotic, or tranquilizer (e.g., diazepam, midazolam, or meperidine) may be given before or during the procedure. Anticholinergic medications may be given to decrease oropharyngeal secretions and to prevent reflex bradycardia.

When the client is sedated, a local anesthetic is sprayed on the posterior pharynx to ease discomfort and prevent gagging during insertion of the endoscope. The anesthetic often tastes unpleasant and makes the tongue feel swollen. To reduce the risk of aspiration, the client is placed in the left lateral decubitus (Sims) position to allow saliva to drain from the side of the mouth.

After the client is positioned, sedated, and anesthetized, a flexible fiberoptic tube is passed orally into the esophagus, stomach, pylorus, and duodenum. Some endoscopes are equipped with a camera that allows the physician to obtain color photographs. If cancer is suspected, cells or tissue can be collected for cytologic examination. Small, single polyps may be removed.

During the procedure, monitor for cardiac or respiratory complications. Assess the client's heart rate, blood pressure, respiratory rate, and pulse oximetry frequently. Specific antagonists to benzodiazepines and narcotics should be available for emergency reversal of drug effects. Upper GI endoscopy should not be performed in clients with severe cardiovascular disease.

PREPROCEDURE CARE

Clients undergoing endoscopic procedures require a signed consent. If the client will be going home within 24 hours after the procedure, someone should be available to drive her home. For clients with a history of cardiac valve disease or replacement, administer antibiotic prophylaxis. To prevent aspiration of stomach contents into the lungs, keep the client NPO for 8 to 12 hours before the procedure. Assess the oral cavity, and report any loose teeth or lesions to the gastroenterologist. Remove the client's dentures and any removable bridges.

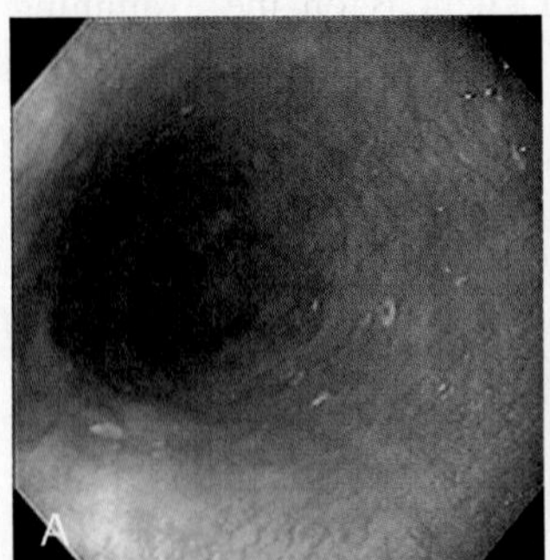

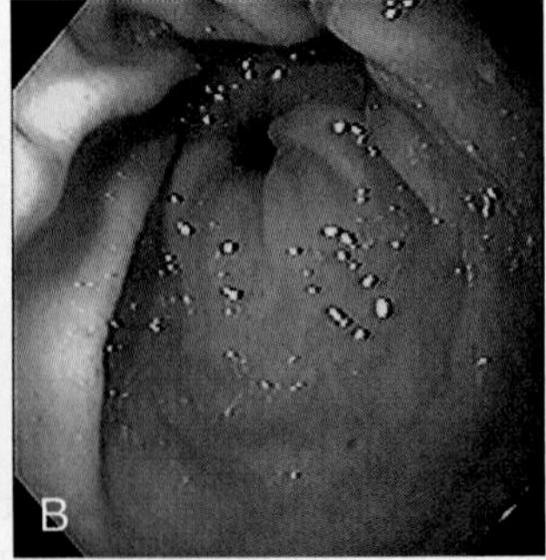

FIGURE 28–7 Endoscopy showing normal gastric mucosa *(A)* and normal duodenal mucosa *(B)*.

Even with anesthesia, the client may experience some discomfort, nausea, or pressure. Tell her to breathe through her nose during the procedure. Explain that the room will be cool and dark and that she will not be able to talk while the endoscope is in place.

POSTPROCEDURE CARE

To prevent aspiration, place the client in the Sims position until the sedation and local anesthesia wear off. Withhold fluids and solids for 2 to 4 hours after the procedure or until the gag reflex returns. Test for return of the gag reflex by stroking the back of the client's throat with a tongue blade to see if gagging occurs. Once the gag reflex returns, the physician may order anesthetic throat lozenges or normal saline gargles to ease throat irritation or hoarseness.

Monitor for bradycardia or other dysrhythmias that may occur as a result of sedatives or anesthetics. Assess for signs of esophageal or gastric perforation. Esophageal perforation may cause crepitus (crackling) in the neck (from air leakage), fever, bleeding, or pain. Neck and throat pain, aggravated by swallowing or moving, may also occur. Mid-esophageal perforation results in referred substernal or epigastric pain. Distal esophageal perforation results in shoulder pain, dyspnea, or manifestations similar to those of perforated ulcers. If you suspect perforation, an x-ray study should be obtained to confirm the presence of free air.[2]

Endoscopic examination of the lower GI tract is discussed in Chapter 32.

■ EXFOLIATIVE CYTOLOGIC ANALYSIS

Exfoliative cytologic analysis, developed by George Papanicolaou, is a study of cells that have sloughed off from a tissue. The examination is performed in an effort to distinguish benign from malignant lesions. Malignant cells exfoliate more readily than normal cells. Specific areas of the GI tract are lavaged, and cells are collected and sent to the laboratory for analysis. Cells of the esophagus, stomach, small intestine, and colon can be examined. Stomach contents are examined for the presence of *Helicobacter pylori*, a bacterium that can cause gastritis and peptic ulcer disease. In this procedure, a nasogastric tube is placed and cells are obtained by saline lavage through the tube.

Explain the procedure to the client and, if required, obtain a written consent. Keep the client NPO before the procedure. Afterward, the client rests and may resume eating.

■ GASTRIC ANALYSIS

Gastric analysis is performed to measure secretions of hydrochloric acid (HCl) and pepsin in the stomach. Analysis of gastric contents can aid in the diagnosis of duodenal ulcer, Zollinger-Ellison syndrome, gastric carcinoma, and pernicious anemia. Gastric analysis consists of (1) the basal cell secretion test and (2) the gastric acid stimulation test.

PROCEDURE

For the *basal cell secretion test*, a nasogastric tube is inserted and attached to suction. Stomach contents are collected every 15 minutes for 1 hour. Label specimens carefully with time, volume, and client identification. The specimens are analyzed. If abnormal gastric secretion is suggested, a gastric acid stimulation test is performed.

The *gastric acid stimulation test* measures the amount of gastric acid for 1 hour after subcutaneous injection of a drug that stimulates its secretion (pentagastrin and betazole). If results are abnormal, radiographic studies or endoscopy may be done to determine the cause. A markedly increased level of gastric secretion may indicate Zollinger-Ellison syndrome, whereas a moderately increased level suggests a duodenal ulcer. Decreased levels of gastric secretion may indicate gastric ulcer or carcinoma.

Preprocedure Care

The client ingests nothing orally for 12 hours before the test. Insert a nasogastric tube, and remove any contents left in the stomach. Do not administer drugs that interfere with gastric acid levels, such as cholinergics, histamine blockers, or antacids. If a client requires coronary vasodilator therapy, change the oral form to an ointment or sublingual preparation during the procedure.

Postprocedure Care

If the nasogastric tube is left in place, attach it to low intermittent suction. Record the amount and color of the drainage.

ACID PERFUSION TEST

The acid perfusion test, also known as the *Bernstein test*, determines whether a client's chest pain is related to acid perfusion across the esophageal mucosa. A nasogastric tube is inserted, and gastric contents are aspirated. Normal saline solution (0.9%) and 0.1% HCl are alternately instilled into the lower esophagus. If the client does not experience pain, the test is considered normal. If pain occurs, normal saline is administered until pain ceases. To ensure that the pain is caused by acid perfusion, 0.1% HCl is readministered. After the test, the nasogastric tube is withdrawn.

Keep the client NPO the night before the test. Instruction about the procedure includes preparing the client for insertion of the nasogastric tube. After the procedure, the client may receive an antacid.

ESOPHAGEAL MANOMETRY

Manometry is used to assess esophageal motor function and can be used to assess and diagnose dysphagia, esophageal reflux, spasm, motility disorders, and hiatal hernia. A special enteric tube with fused small-caliber catheters is inserted into the esophagus. The tube is designed to measure simultaneous pressures of the esophagus and lower esophageal sphincter by infusion of water into the catheters. The client is asked to swallow small amounts of water, and esophageal pressures are recorded during muscular relaxation and contraction.

Instruct the client about the procedure, and maintain NPO status for 6 to 8 hours before the procedure. The test takes about 15 to 20 minutes. After the test, remove the enteric tube. The physician may recommend medications or diet alterations based on the results.

AMBULATORY ESOPHAGEAL pH MONITORING

The relationship between pH changes in the esophagus and symptoms of chest pain and indigestion may be assessed by ambulatory esophageal pH monitoring. This test is used to distinguish chest pain caused by gastric acid reflux into the esophagus from chest pain caused by angina or myocardial infarction. Location of the lower esophageal sphincter (LES) is determined by esophageal manometry, and a nasoenteric tube with a pH sensor is inserted 5 cm above the LES. The enteric tube is secured to the client's face and attached to a battery-operated recorder. The client is then instructed to push a button on the recorder when she starts and ends specific activities, such as eating, sleeping, and smoking. She is told to note when chest pain or indigestion starts and ends.

Because the location of the LES must be determined, inform the client that esophageal manometry may be performed first after which a second enteric tube may be placed for the pH monitoring. You may need to stop giving the client drugs that affect the GI tract (e.g., H_2 histamine blockers and motility drugs) before the procedure. Instruct the client about the importance of recording activities and symptoms. The tube must remain securely taped. Tell the client to avoid bumping or pulling the tube when dressing or washing her face. After the procedure, remove the tube and advise the client that she may resume normal activities.

CONCLUSIONS

Nutritional health and a functional upper GI tract are basic to health. Systematic assessment of nutritional status and the upper GI tract can lead to prompt diagnosis and treatment of disorders. The diagnostic process is facilitated by performing a careful and thorough assessment and by properly preparing the client for procedures to maximize the potential for optimal health.

BIBLIOGRAPHY

1. A.S.P.E.N Board of Directors. (1993). Guidelines for the use of parenteral and enteral nutrition in adult and pediatric patients. *JPEN: J Parenteral and Enteral Nutrition, 17*, 1SA–25SA.
2. Barkin, J., & O'Phelan, C. A. (Eds.). (1994). *Advanced therapeutic endoscopy* (2nd ed.). New York: Raven Press.
3. Bartels, C. L., & Miller, S. J. (1998). Herbal and related remedies. *Nutrition and Clinical Practice, 13*(1), 5–19.
4. DeHoog, S. (1996). The assessment of nutritional status. In L. Mahan & S. Escott-Stump (Eds.). *Krause's food, nutrition, and diet therapy* (9th ed., pp. 361–386). Philadelphia: W. B. Saunders.
5. Fauci, A. S., et al. (Eds.). (1998). *Harrison's principles of internal medicine* (14th ed.). New York: McGraw-Hill.
6. Grindel, C. G., & Costello, M. C. (1996). Nutrition screening: An essential assessment parameter. *MEDSURG Nursing, 5*(3), 145–156.
7. Haubrich, W. S., Schaffner, F., & Berk, J. E. (Eds.). (1995). *Bockus gastroenterology* (5th ed.). Philadelphia: W. B. Saunders.
8. Jarvis, C. (2000). *Physical examination and health assessment* (3rd ed.). Philadelphia: W. B. Saunders.
9. Kovacevich, D. S., et al. (1997). Nutrition risk classification: A reproducible and valid tool for nurses. *Nutrition in Clinical Practice, 12*(1), 20–25.
10. Krebs-Smith, S. M., et al. (1997). Characterizing food intake patterns of American adults. *American Journal of Clinical Nutrition, 65*(suppl), 1264S–1268S.

10a. Mahan, L., & Escott-Stump, S. (Eds.). (2000). *Krause's food, nutrition, and diet therapy* (10th ed.). Philadelphia: W. B. Saunders.

11. Mitchell, M. K. (1997). *Nutrition across the life span*. Philadelphia: W. B. Saunders.

12. National Academy of Science. (1989). *Recommended dietary allowances* (10th ed.) Washington, DC: National Academy Press.

13. Schears, G., & Deutschman, C. (1997). Common nutritional issues in pediatric and adult critical care medicine. *Critical Care Clinics, 13*(3), 669–690.

14. Shenkin, A. (1997). Micronutrients and outcome. *Nutrition, 13*(9), 825–828.

14a. Shils, E., Olson, J. A., & Shike, M. (Eds.). (1999). *Modern nutrition in health and disease* (9th ed.). Baltimore: Williams & Wilkins.

15. Shugars, D. C., & Patton, L. L. (1997). Detecting, diagnosing, and preventing oral cancer. *The Nurse Practitioner, 22*(6), 105–132.

16. Solomon, C. G., & Manson, J. E. (1997). Obesity and mortality: A review of the epidemiologic data. *American Journal of Clinical Nutrition, 66*(suppl), 1044S–1050S.

17. Stone, R. (1996). Primary care diagnosis of acute abdominal pain. *The Nurse Practitioner, 21*(12), 19–41.

18. Torun, B., & Chew, F. (1994). Protein-energy malnutrition. In M. E. Shils, J. A. Olson, & M. Shike (Eds.), *Modern nutrition in health and disease* (8th ed.). (pp. 950–976). Philadelphia: Lea & Febiger.

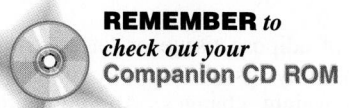

CHAPTER 29

Management of Clients with Malnutrition

Nancy Evans Stoner
Candace Cantwell

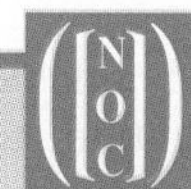

NURSING OUTCOMES CLASSIFICATION (NOC) for Nursing Diagnoses—Clients with Malnutrition

Altered Nutrition: Less Than Body Requirements
Nutritional Status
Nutritional Status: Food and Fluid Intake
Nutritional Status: Nutrient Intake
Weight Control

Altered Nutrition: More Than Body Requirements
Nutritional Status: Food and Fluid Intake
Nutritional Status: Nutrient Intake
Weight Control

Feeding Self-Care Deficit
Nutritional Status
Nutritional Status: Food and Fluid Intake
Self-Care: Eating
Swallowing Status

Impaired Swallowing
Swallowing Status

Risk for Injury: Dysrhythmias
Cardiac Pump Effectiveness
Circulation Status
Electrolyte and Acid-Base Balance
Tissue Perfusion
Vital Signs Status

Malnutrition can develop as a result of acute or chronic diseases and treatments that affect the ability to ingest or digest foods. In turn, it can cause such problems as delayed wound healing, impaired immune function, and a decreased functional status. Obesity, anorexia nervosa, and bulimia nervosa are eating disorders that alter nutritional health. Nursing diagnoses pertinent to malnutrition include *Altered Nutrition: Less than Body Requirements, Altered Nutrition: More than Body Requirements,* and *Feeding Self-Care Deficit.*

PROTEIN-ENERGY MALNUTRITION

Malnutrition broadly describes *undernutrition* or *overnutrition* related to excess or deficient dietary intake. Protein-energy malnutrition (PEM) results when the body's need for protein and/or energy (glucose and fat) is not supplied by dietary intake. Prolonged deficiencies in energy and protein can result in any of these clinical syndromes of malnutrition:

- Kwashiorkor, which reflects primarily a deficiency in protein
- Marasmus, which reflects primarily an energy deficit
- Marasmic kwashiorkor, which reflects both an energy and a protein deficit

PEM can be classified as *primary* when the deficits result simply from poor food intake. *Secondary* PEM refers to malnutrition associated with acute or chronic disease that causes one or more of the following: (1) decreased food intake, (2) decreased nutrient absorption, (3) increased nutrient losses, or (4) increased nutrient requirements.[6, 17, 20]

PEM is a significant problem in adult medical-surgical clients in both hospital and home settings. Initial studies of malnutrition found PEM in up to 40% of hospitalized medical and surgical clients.[3, 4] More recent studies have found similar rates of documented malnutrition on admission to the hospital in general medical clients (46%), clients with respiratory disease (45%), and geriatric clients (43%).[9, 13, 19]

Malnutrition was documented in 10% of 441 clients who lived at home with cancer and chronic disease.[6, 9] The elderly population is at particular risk for malnutrition; in one study of nursing home residents, 85% of those assessed had significant nutritional deficits.[6, 9] Among community-dwelling elderly, the prevalence of PEM may be 5% to 10%.[6, 9] Decreases in functional capacity, mobility, and independence, which are common in older adults, can result from malnutrition or may contribute to its development. The most important changes in body composition associated with aging are a loss of lean body mass and a gain in body fat. The loss of lean body mass is an important factor in the impairment of pulmonary function, immune function, and strength.[6, 9, 18]

The cost of treating malnutrition varies greatly, depending on the level of nutritional care, for example, simply providing supplemental formulas ($4 to $5 per six-pack). More sophisticated nutritional support therapies used to treat and prevent malnutrition are more expensive; *total enteral nutrition* (TEN) costs $30 to $40 per day, and *total parenteral nutrition* (TPN) costs $250 to $350 per day. Even so, these costs are small when compared to the costs of not using therapies to prevent or treat malnutrition. The consequences can include an increased length of stay, delayed wound healing, and prolonged infection. In the Veterans Affairs TPN Cooperative Study, the use of TPN in severely malnourished clients greatly reduced the number of complications related to surgery.[21]

Etiology and Risk Factors

The etiologic mechanism of PEM is multifactorial and is usually associated with the presence of acute or chronic disease. Causes of PEM can be related to social factors, economic factors, or physiologic changes in nutrient absorption or nutrient requirements. Socioeconomic factors that have a negative effect on nutritional status include:

- Social isolation
- Limited access to food
- Emotional depression
- Substance abuse
- Poverty

Physiologic factors leading to malnutrition usually result from other diseases that can cause compromised food intake, decreased absorption of nutrients, or increased demand for nutrients. Changes in nutrient intake can result from the disease or from its treatment.

Inadequate food intake is common in hospitals and can lead to malnutrition if diminished intake is prolonged or severe. Many disease processes affect the client's swallowing function and are common reasons for decreased food intake (see Chapter 30). Inadequate absorption of nutrients is the result of various disorders of the gastrointestinal (GI) tract, such as inflammatory bowel disease (see Chapters 31 and 33). In addition, the demand for nutrients increases in response to critical, chronic, and infectious illnesses

In your role of preventing and restoring nutritional status, you should take a multidisciplinary approach. Health *promotion* interventions include activities that support the client's knowledge of normal nutrition and provide nutritional information to maintain optimal health and prevent disease. Such strategies might include diet information related to decreasing cancer risk or identifying support for an elder who cannot prepare meals independently. Health *maintenance* interventions include targeting specialized diet therapy for a client with an illness (such as diet instruction for a client with Crohn's disease). Health *restoration* activities can include retraining a client to swallow after a stroke or administering TPN to a malnourished client with severe inflammatory bowel disease.

Pathophysiology

PEM can develop gradually over weeks to months, or quickly over days to weeks, when coupled with severe stress and illness. When the total supply of nutrients is less than the body's requirement, malnutrition can occur. When the primary deficit is in energy balance, the result is, first, the depletion of adipose tissue or fat stores, with eventual loss of lean body tissue (muscle mass). This deficit is reflected in weight changes. An unintentional weight loss of 5% in 1 month or 10% in 6 months suggests that the client is at significant risk for malnutrition.[13]

When the nutrient deficit is primarily in protein intake, the result is a depletion of nonessential tissue, such as skeletal muscle. When the client is hypermetabolic from severe illness, however, there is a marked depletion of the skeletal muscle and the visceral proteins, such as albumin, transferrin, and prealbumin. This depletion results from a decrease in the synthesis of visceral proteins, such as albumin, as well as from an increase in protein breakdown.[17] Starvation related to severe stress affects organ function at the cellular level by impairing specific biochemical functions, which increases the risk of mortality and morbidity.[6, 19]

Clinical Manifestations

Table 29–1 presents the pathophysiology and related clinical manifestations of malnutrition. In addition to these, you may also notice hair loss or hair that is dull and dry. The client's skin may be dry and bruised. Nails are brittle. Saliva production decreases. Periodontal disease and bleeding gums as well as cheilosis may be present. Most malnourished clients are also anemic. The client may have decreased neurologic reflexes, weakness, edema, increased sensitivity to cold, amenorrhea, impotence, and atrophied breasts. Most clients experience delayed wound healing.

Abnormal laboratory values that may indicate malnutrition include decreased hemoglobin, blood urea nitrogen (BUN), creatinine, albumin, total protein, transferrin, prealbumin, and lymphocyte proliferation. All of these findings are related primarily to a protein deficit.

Outcome Management

Medical Management

Management of PEM starts with identifying clients who are malnourished as well as clients at risk for malnutrition. Assess or screen all clients for nutritional problems. First-level screening can be done through admission forms or simple questionnaires. Nutritional screening generally focuses on a few key data points (such as a weight change, a change in dietary habits, and GI manifestations) to identify clients that require a more comprehensive nutritional assessment.

A comprehensive nutritional assessment includes a review of the medical history, weight and diet history, anthropometric measures, biochemical profiles, and physical examination (see Chapter 28 for an in-depth review of nutritional assessment).

Define Nutrient Outcomes

The outcomes for weight and fat stores and protein stores define the nutrient goals for each client. Weight maintenance is appropriate for clients within 90% to 120% of a reference weight, whereas depletion of fat stores and weight loss is appropriate for obese clients (>120% of reference weight). Clients with severely depleted fat stores and more than 10% weight loss need calories sufficient to replete these stores and to gain weight.

TABLE 29–1 CONSEQUENCES OF MALNUTRITION

Organ System	Pathophysiology	Clinical Manifestations
Cardiac	Decreased cardiac muscle mass	Postural hypotension Diminished venous return
Pulmonary	Decreased diaphragm strength Decreased respiratory strength Decreased endurance	Inability to clear secretions Decreased exercise tolerance Inability to wean from ventilator
Immune function	Decreased cell-mediated immunity Delayed cutaneous hypersensitivity	Increased incidence and severity of infection
Wound healing	Decreased collagen synthesis	Delayed wound healing
Skeletal muscle strength	Altered muscle contractions Relaxation response Decreased muscle endurance	Fatigue Inability to perform activities of daily living Risk of falling
Gastrointestinal function	Impaired intestinal absorption of lipids Decreased rate of glucose absorption Decreased gastric, pancreatic, and bile production	Diarrhea

Data from Kinney J. M., et al. (1988). *Nutrition and metabolism in patient care.* Philadelphia: W. B. Saunders.

The energy needs of most clients can be determined with formulas that estimate the basal energy expenditure (BEE). The Harris-Benedict equation is the most commonly used formula:

$$\text{BEE (men)} = 66 + (13.7 \times \text{weight in kg}) + (5 \times \text{height in cm}) - (6.8 \times \text{age})$$

$$\text{BEE (women)} = 655 + (9.6 \times \text{weight in kg}) + (1.7 \times \text{height in cm}) - (4.7 \times \text{age})$$

The BEE represents the basal metabolic rate and is multiplied by a factor that accounts for stress and activity. Table 29–2 outlines targets for daily energy requirements using predictive equations. These equations are most useful in mildly stressed clients and may overestimate or underestimate energy needs during critical illness. Indirect calorimetry can be used for severely stressed clients for a precise measurement of energy expenditure.

The protein needs of a hospitalized client are nearly twice those of normal needs. Protein repletion is necessary to maintain equilibrium when the client experiences increased protein breakdown and decreased protein synthesis. Protein requirements for the metabolically stressed client range from 1.5 g of protein per kilogram (kg) to as much as 2.5 g protein per kg of *ideal body weight* (see later discussion of obesity).

TABLE 29–2 DETERMINING DAILY ENERGY REQUIREMENTS

Goal for Fat Stores	kcal (in Hospital)	Requirement (kcal/kg/day)
Replete	BEE × 1.5	30–35
Maintain	BEE × 1.3	25–30
Reduce	<BEE	20–25

BEE, basal energy expenditure.
From Evans Stoner, N. (1997). Nutritional assessment. *Nursing Clinics of North America, 32*(4), 648.

DETERMINE ROUTE OF FEEDING

The goals to meet nutrient needs must be translated into a practical, safe, and medically appropriate nutritional plan of care. To prevent or correct existing malnutrition through oral dietary manipulation, a registered dietitian can assist in meal planning or can recommend diet modification to increase oral intake. Supplements to boost the oral intake of calories and protein are available in a variety of forms, such as liquid milk-like drinks, clear juice-like drinks, nutrient bars, and puddings (Table 29–3).

When the client is unable to eat or when oral intake is contraindicated, an alternate means of nutritional support is necessary, such as TPN or TEN. If the GI tract is functional, TEN should be used. If the GI tract is not functional, the client is a candidate for TPN. Figure 29–1 presents an algorithm for determining the appropriate route of feeding.

Nursing Management of the Medical Client

ASSESSMENT

Nurses play a vital role in identifying clients with nutritional problems. Of all the various health care providers that clients see, you are typically the first to assess clients as they enter a health system. You also have the most constant contact during a hospitalization. You are also the last to see clients before they leave. Naturally, you are in a key position to evaluate a client's nutritional intake.

Nursing admission forms should include questions regarding weight history, weight change, diet history, and food tolerances. Daily flow sheets or nursing records must include a section on nutrition, including weight measures and tolerance to nutritional therapy. Box 29–1 is an example of an admission nutrition screening tool that can be used to determine a client's nutritional risk.

DIAGNOSIS, OUTCOMES, INTERVENTIONS

Feeding Self-Care Deficit. The nursing diagnosis most appropriate for the intervention of feeding is *Feeding Self-Care Deficit related to impaired motor function, impaired cognitive function, sensory-perceptual altera-*

TABLE 29–3 ORAL NUTRITIONAL SUPPLEMENTS

Type of Product	Calories Per Serving	Protein (g Per Serving)	Features
MILK-BASED			
Nutra Shake (4 oz)	200	8	High-calorie/protein, lower-volume supplement
Carnation Instant Breakfast (8 oz) made with 2% milk	250	12	Widely available, economical, high-calorie/protein supplement
Ensure Pudding (5 oz)	250	6.8	Thicker consistency (dysphagia), low-volume supplement with added vitamins and minerals
LACTOSE-FREE			
Boost Plus (8 oz)	360	14.6	High-calorie/protein supplement with added vitamins and minerals
Probalance (8 oz)	300	13.5	High calorie/protein, fiber-containing supplement with added vitamins and minerals
DISEASE-SPECIFIC			
Nepro (8 oz)	475	16.6	Specialized for clients with renal failure who are receiving dialysis; low in electrolytes and volume
Resource Diabetic (8 oz)	250	15	High-calorie/protein, low-carbohydrate supplement, lactose-free
NUTRITIONAL BARS			
Boost Bar (44 g)	190	4	Candy bar appeal, convenient, with added vitamins and minerals; various flavors
Powerbar Essentials (65 g)	180	10	High-protein, low-fat supplement with added vitamins and minerals; various flavors

tions, or decreased appetite. Neuromuscular impairments, such as Parkinson's disease, muscular dystrophy, myasthenia gravis, muscular weakness, and central nervous system tumors, are contributing factors. Visual disorders can occur with glaucoma, cataracts, or a cerebrovascular accident. A situational factor may include immobility, trauma, or the placement of external fixating devices that restrict arm movement. Older clients may have decreased visual and motor abilities, increased muscle weakness, and altered taste and appetite.

Outcomes. The client will maintain an ideal body weight or will gain 1 to 2 pounds per week to return to an ideal body weight by overcoming decreased appetite or motor, sensory-perceptual, or cognitive impairments.

Interventions

Improve Nutritional Intake. General strategies to improve nutritional intake relate to choices of menu items and the accessibility of dietitians and food service personnel who can evaluate client food preferences and assist in meal planning. Clients should be able to choose from a menu in order to avoid food monotony. Dietitians should be accessible during mealtimes to help assess individual preferences. Kitchen facilities and supplies should be available at the unit level to increase client choices. Dedicated refrigeration and microwave equipment for client and family use may encourage the families to bring foods that are appealing to the client and may allow more flexible mealtimes that coincide with the client's appetite.

Increase Appetite. Appetite is often impaired in a hospital setting for a variety of reasons. Several strategies can be used to maximize or enhance a client's desire for food. First, you can create a pleasant environment during mealtime. Clear the area of unsightly bedpans, urinals, suctioning equipment, and dressing supplies. Ensure adequate pain relief before meals, and avoid invasive procedures just before a meal. Increased activity through regular exercise may also increase the client's appetite.

Appetite can be enhanced by taste, smell, and vision. Taste alterations can occur from injury after radiation to the oral cavity, surgical resection to the tongue, medications, and oral infections. Oral hygiene is important to support the optimal function of taste buds. Routine mouth care should include:

- Cleansing the mouth after each meal and at bedtime
- Using a soft-bristle toothbrush
- Rinsing with warm saltwater
- Avoiding alcohol-containing mouthwash
- Avoiding glycerin and lemon juice

The ability to smell prepared foods may also stimulate the appetite. Although clients cannot participate in food preparation, offering them a chance to smell food before a meal may be helpful. Reduce all noxious odors that might negatively affect appetite. Let the client see the food to help stimulate appetite, position the food to make it visible, and describe the different foods. Your description is especially important for clients with visual impairment.

Increase Social Interaction. Eating is ordinarily a time for social interaction, yet clients are usually given meals in their own rooms. Creating social contact by feeding clients in a central area or encouraging family and friends to visit during mealtimes may be an option. Client care assignments should be designed so that clients requiring feeding can be assigned to the same caregiver as much as possible. As the client and caregiver develop a therapeutic

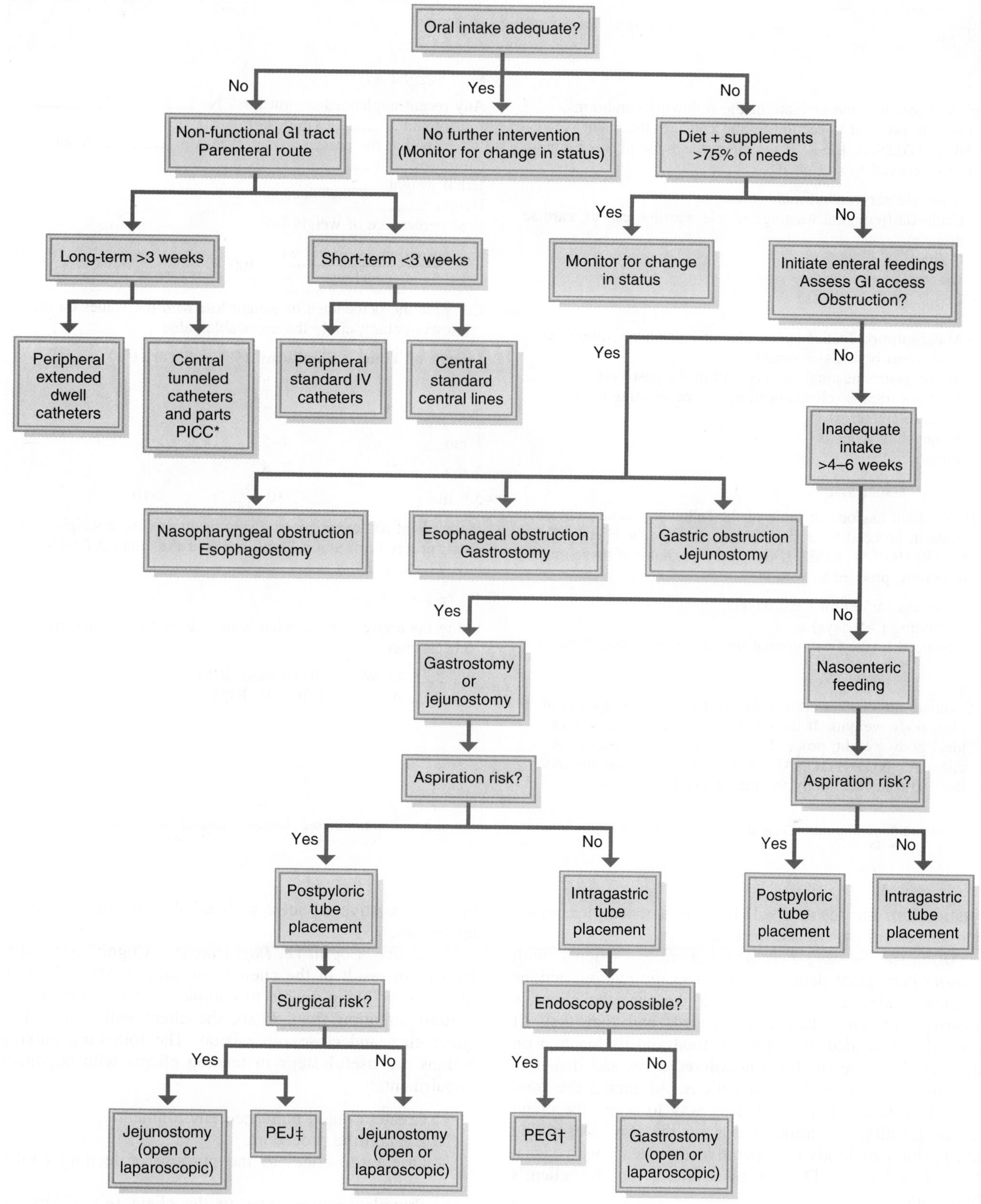

FIGURE 29–1 Algorithm to determine appropriate route of feeding. (Data from Mahan, L. K., & Escott-Stump, S. E. [2000]. *Krause's food, nutrition, & diet therapy* [10th ed., p. 467]. Philadelphia: W. B. Saunders; modified and adapted from Gorman R. C., Morris, J. B. [1997]. Minimally invasive access to the gastrointestinal tract. In J. L. Rombeau & R. H. Rolandelli [Eds.], *Clinical nutrition: Enteral and tube feeding* [p. 174]. Philadelphia: W. B. Saunders.)

BOX 29–1 Features of the Admission Nutrition Screening Tool

A. Diagnosis

If the client has one or more of the following conditions, circle it, proceed to section E, and consider the client AT NUTRITIONAL RISK. If the client has none of these conditions, proceed to section B.

- Anorexia nervosa/bulimia nervosa
- Cachexia (temporal wasting, muscle wasting, cancer, cardiac disease)
- Coma
- Diabetes
- End-stage liver disease
- End-stage renal disease
- Malabsorption (celiac sprue, ulcerative colitis, Crohn's disease, short-bowel syndrome)
- Major gastrointestinal surgery within the past year
- Multiple trauma (closed-head injury, penetrating trauma, multiple fractures)
- Nonhealing wounds
- Pressure ulcers

B. Nutrition Intake History

If the client has one or more of the following manifestations, circle it, proceed to section E, and consider the client AT NUTRITIONAL RISK. If the client has none of these manifestations, proceed to section C.

- Diarrhea (>500 ml for 2 days)
- Vomiting (>5 days)
- Reduced intake (<½ normal intake for more than 5 days)

C. Ideal Body Weight Standards

Compare the client's current weight for height to a chart of ideal body weights. If the client weighs less than 80% of ideal body weight, proceed to section E and consider the client AT NUTRITIONAL RISK. If the client weighs more than 80% of ideal body weight, proceed to section D.

D. Weight History

Any recent unplanned weight loss? No ________ Yes ________
Amount ________ (lb or kg)
If yes, within the past ________ weeks or ________ months
Current weight ________
Usual weight ________
Height ________
Find percentage of weight loss:

$$\frac{\text{usual wt} - \text{current wt}}{\text{usual wt}} \times 100 = \text{\_\_\_\_\_\_\_\_ \% wt loss}$$

Compare the percentage of weight lost with the values on the following chart; circle the applicable value.

Length of Time	Significant (%)	Severe (%)
1 wk	1–2	>2
2–3 wk	2–3	>3
1 mo	4–5	>5
3 mo	7–8	>8
5+ mo	10	>10

If the client has experienced a significant or severe weight loss, proceed to section E and consider the client AT NUTRITIONAL RISK.

E. Nurse Assessment

Using the above criteria, what is this client's nutritional risk? (check one)

________ LOW NUTRITIONAL RISK
________ AT NUTRITIONAL RISK

Adapted from Kovacevich, D., et al. (1997). Nutrition risk classification: A reproducible and valid tool for nurses. *Nutrition in Clinical Practice, 12,* 22.

relationship, the feeding will become a more pleasurable and successful experience for both.

Minimize Sensory-Perceptual Deficits. Clients with sensory-perceptual deficits require specific nursing actions to ensure adequate food intake. Make sure the client is wearing corrective lenses, if needed, and that they fit properly. If needed, describe the food and its location on the tray. The use of different-colored trays and dishes is helpful to clients with these deficits. Arranging the food in a clock-face pattern is an easy way to orient the client to the position of various foods on the tray. Describing the position of foods is imperative for clients with visual field disturbances. Do not place foods on the client's blind side.

Minimize Neuromuscular Impairments. Various neuromuscular impairments can make the seemingly simple task of eating difficult or impossible. The occupational therapy staff can help in planning the feeding intervention and teaching the correct use of assistive devices. For a client with physical impairment, ensure privacy, allow adequate time for eating, position the client at a 90-degree angle with the meal tray at elbow height, and provide assistive devices, such as plate guards and built-up spoons.

Minimize Cognitive Impairments. Cognitive impairments can result in the client's misunderstanding the task of eating or being unable to complete the task because of a short attention span. If so, the client will require frequent cues and close supervision. The following nursing actions are useful steps in feeding clients with cognitive impairments:

1. Create a quiet, unhurried environment.
2. Explain the procedure.
3. Orient the client to the purpose of feeding equipment.
4. Provide frequent cues to the client (e.g., "Mrs. S, pick up the toast" or "Mr. S, chew the food in your mouth").
5. Provide several small meals for clients with short attention spans.

Minimize Fatigue. Another physical factor that can affect a person's ability to feed oneself is endurance. The client may be able to start the task but becomes quickly fatigued and cannot complete it. The client's ability to maintain a level of performance is related to cardiovascular, respiratory, neurologic, and musculoskeletal function.

For a client with reduced endurance, plan rest periods before mealtimes, especially when the meal follows an activity, such as physical therapy or ambulation. Help the client conserve energy for eating by helping with meal setup, opening packages, and cutting food.

Impaired Swallowing. Chewing and swallowing dysfunction are frequent additional reasons for difficulties in eating. The client may experience malnutrition because of problems with swallowing. In this case, an appropriate nursing diagnosis is *Impaired Swallowing related to neuromuscular impairment (decreased or absent gag reflex), mechanical obstruction (edema, tracheostomy tube, tumor), fatigue, or limited awareness.*

Outcomes. The client will be able to freely swallow solids or liquids and will not experience any aspiration problems.

Interventions

Use a Team Approach. A team approach has been described in the literature in the successful management of clients with swallowing impairments.[6, 17] In addition to nurses, physicians, physical and occupational therapists, and speech pathologists can be helpful in localizing the impairment and suggesting useful strategies. You must also understand the complexity of normal swallowing mechanisms in order to plan appropriate interventions.

Assess Swallowing. Take these four steps before feeding to assess client readiness:

1. Assess level of consciousness; the client must be alert.
2. Assess the client's gag reflex by tickling the back of the throat.
3. Have the client produce an audible cough.
4. Have the client produce a voluntary swallow.

Implement Swallowing Techniques. Feeding should take place in a calm, adequately supervised environment. Place the client in a normal eating position with the feeder clearly visible. Some clients may have trouble moving the food bolus from the front to the back of the mouth. Food should be placed in the unaffected side of the mouth. If the tongue is damaged or impaired, assistive devices, such as adapted feeding syringes, can move food toward the pharynx, where the swallowing reflex (if intact) takes over.

Once the food bolus arrives at the pharynx, the client should tilt the chin down to decrease the risk of aspiration. Massaging the throat on the affected side helps stimulate the tactile areas that initiate the swallowing reflex. If the client has difficulty coordinating chewing, breathing, and swallowing, instruct the client to hold the head forward and to hold the breath before swallowing.

Watch the thyroid cartilage to see whether the client has swallowed, and inspect his or her mouth before placing more food in the oral cavity. Allowing sufficient time between each mouthful helps to ensure that the client adequately chews and swallows the food. Stay alert for signs that the client is becoming fatigued, restless, or agitated. Keep suction equipment available in case of an emergency. Also, know how to perform the Heimlich maneuver to prevent choking.

See Bridge to Home Health Care: Managing Swallowing Difficulties.

BRIDGE TO HOME HEALTH CARE

Managing Swallowing Difficulties

Swallowing difficulty (dysphagia) can vary in severity and duration. It can be mild to severe, short term (acute), or long term (chronic).

When you feed clients who have dysphagia, use good observational skills and plenty of communication and patience. Observe their responses to what you are doing. They may frown, spit, clamp their jaws together, or cough when food choices are not appealing. Try to adapt meals to their tastes. For example, if a client enjoys bananas, dice, mash, or blend them into a shake, or even freeze them to offer variety; select the consistency that your client tolerates best.

Promote use of the sense organs during mealtime. Encourage your clients to think or talk about their favorite foods before meals to stimulate saliva flow and to aid in chewing. Ask clients to close their eyes and to visualize tasting and chewing these foods. Provide mouth care before and after the client eats meals and swallows medications to keep the mouth and breath fresh and facilitate saliva production. If your clients find it pleasurable, have them watch the food being prepared, smell the food cooking, and participate in the meal preparation as much as possible. Use an activity such as folding napkins to begin involvement. Play the client's favorite music tapes during mealtime.

The home health nurse should schedule shared visits periodically with the speech or occupational therapist to promote continuity of care. Discuss strategies related to mealtime and food preparation. Work with the therapists to help clients strengthen their mouth muscles by practicing pushing their lips or "puckering," humming, or whistling. Demonstrate the techniques you are trying to teach; hold a mirror so that clients can see their own mouth.

A high Fowler's position with 90-degree flexion of the hips is usually the best position for mealtime. Position your client with shoulders back and torso erect. Slightly flexing the client's head forward may aid in swallowing. Placing a pillow at the lower back and a towel roll behind the neck can facilitate a smooth flow of food from the mouth into the stomach. Observe your clients closely to see which position makes them most comfortable. Cushions, pillows, or bedrolls are used to support any dependent limbs or "weak" sides. Increasing physical comfort decreases distraction and allows more focus on eating.

Maintaining the high Fowler's position, with at least 75- to 80-degree flexion at the hips for at least 30 minutes after a meal, helps reduce reflux and aspiration. Check your client's mouth carefully for lingering food pockets that may become dislodged and cause aspiration long after the meal. For your safety, never place your unprotected fingers in the client's mouth when teeth or dentures are in place.

Close observation, good communication, and a sense of humor will keep mealtime pleasurable for your client and you.

Bernice Christopher, RN, BSN, *Keystone Mercy Health Plan, Philadelphia, Pennsylvania*

Medical Management of the Client Receiving Parenteral Nutrition

PARENTERAL NUTRITION

TPN is indicated to maintain nutritional status and prevent malnutrition when the client cannot be fed orally or by tube feeding. TPN should not be used when the GI tract is functional. Box 29–2 outlines some common indications for the use of parenteral nutrition.

The TPN prescription is guided by the nutritional assessment and the definition of nutrient goals for calories and protein. The TPN solution contains carbohydrate and fat to meet the calorie goal and amino acids to meet the protein goal.

Carbohydrates

Glucose is the most commonly used carbohydrate to supply energy and calorie needs; it usually accounts for 50% to 70% of the nutrient prescription. At least 100 or 150 g of glucose (350 to 500 kcal) should be given daily to support the nitrogen-sparing effect of carbohydrate.

Fat Emulsions

Intravenous (IV) fat emulsions (lipids) generally provide about 10% to 30% of the daily nutrient prescription. Fat emulsions (1) provide a calorie-dense isotonic energy source and (2) supply fatty acids to prevent essential fatty acid deficiency.

Amino Acids

Crystalline amino acids of differing composition and a concentration varying from 3% to 15% are the source of protein in parenteral solutions. The standard commercially available solution is a mix of essential and nonessential amino acids. Some amino acid solutions have been developed to target specific clinical problems, such as renal failure and liver failure. However, the increase in efficacy over the general amino acid solution is not conclusive.

Fluids, Electrolytes, Vitamins, and Trace Elements

Fluids, electrolytes, vitamins, and trace elements are all equally important in the parenteral nutrient solution. The daily electrolyte regimen should be individualized and should reflect the client's clinical condition (including any ongoing losses) and the function of major organ systems. Table 29–4 outlines recommendations for daily electrolyte requirements and situations that can result in an increased or decreased need.

Vitamins and trace elements are needed to promote optimal nutritional repletion, and they support a variety of important metabolic pathways. One injectable multivitamin preparation contains both water-soluble and fat-soluble vitamins for daily use (Table 29–5). Vitamin K, a fat-soluble vitamin, is not contained in these commercial preparations and must be added to the TPN formula weekly (10 mg) or daily (1 mg). Other vitamins are sometimes added to the standard vitamin preparation, such as vitamin C, to promote wound healing, and vitamin B_{12}, thiamine, and folic acid to correct deficiencies commonly associated with alcohol abuse.

Guidelines for the administration of trace elements have been outlined by the American Medical Association's Nutritional Advisory Group (Table 29–6). Supplemental zinc may be indicated for clients with high-output fistulae, large wounds, or extreme catabolism.

BOX 29–2 Clinical Indications for Total Parenteral Nutrition

- Malabsorptive syndromes
  - Severe short-bowel syndrome
  - Severe, prolonged radiation enteritis
  - High-output fistulae that cannot be bypassed with small bowel enteral feeding
- Motility disorders
  - Persistent postoperative or disease-related ileus
  - Intestinal pseudo-obstruction
  - Severe persistent vomiting (as in hyperemesis gravidarum)
- Intestinal obstruction
- Perioperative nutrition for severe malnutrition
- Critically ill client when enteral therapy is contraindicated
- Low-flow state

Data adapted from Shils, M., & Brown, R. (1999). Parenteral nutrition. In M. Shils, et al. (Eds.), *Modern nutrition in health and disease* (p. 1658). Baltimore: Williams & Wilkins.

Combination Systems

A *total* nutrient admixture (TNA) is a single-bag TPN delivery system that contains glucose, lipids, amino acids, electrolytes, vitamins, and trace elements. The main advantages of the TNA are a shortened preparation and

TABLE 29–4 DAILY ELECTROLYTE RECOMMENDATIONS

Electrolyte	Daily Replacement	Factors Affecting Daily Requirement	Effect
Sodium	80–150 mEq	Diuretic therapy	↑
		Renal failure	↓
		Fluid overload	↓
Chloride	80–150 mEq	Gastric losses	↑
Potassium	80–100 mEq	Aggressive refeeding	↑
		Diuretic therapy	↑
		Gastrointestinal losses	↑
		Renal failure	↓
Calcium	10–20 mEq	Blood transfusions	↑
Magnesium	8–30 mEq	Aggressive refeeding	↑
		Gastrointestinal losses	↑
		Renal failure	↓
Phosphorus	15–45 mMol	Aggressive refeeding	↑
		Excessive antacid administration	↑
		Renal failure	↓
Acetate	0–60 mEq	Metabolic acidosis	↑
		Metabolic alkalosis	↓
		Sepsis	↑

↑, increased requirement; ↓, decreased requirement.

From Evans, N. (1994). The role of total parenteral nutrition in critical illness: Guidelines and recommendations. In M. Ackerman, K. Puntillo, & J. Clochesy (Eds.), *Clinical issues in critical care nursing*. Philadelphia: J. B. Lippincott.

TABLE 29–5 PARENTERAL MULTIVITAMIN SUPPLEMENTATION*

Vitamin	Amount Supplied
A	1 mg/3300 IU
D	5 μg/200 IU
E	10 mg/10 IU (as dl-α-tocopherol acetate)
B_1	3 mg
B_2	3.6 mg
B_3	40 mg
B_5	15 mg
B_6	4 mg
B_{12}	5 μg
C	100 mg
Biotin	60 μg
Folic acid	0.4 mg

*Roche and Astra products. Amounts of vitamins reflect the 1979 Nutritional Advisory Group recommendations of the American Medical Association.

From Galica, L. (1997). Parenteral nutrition. *Nursing Clinics of North America, 32*(4), 711.

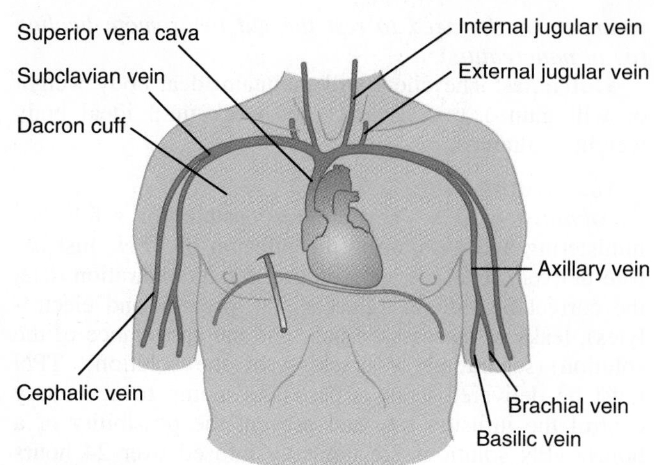

FIGURE 29–2 Insertion of catheter into superior vena cava via right subclavian vein. Once in place, this catheter may be used to administer total parenteral nutrition. (From Mahan, L. K., & Escott-Stump, S. E. [2000]. *Krause's food, nutrition, & diet therapy* [10th ed., p. 474]. Philadelphia: W. B. Saunders.)

administration time and possibly decreased contamination from fewer manipulations of the IV delivery system. The main disadvantage is that TNA supports the growth of some microorganisms better than a simple glucose–amino acid solution does.

VASCULAR ACCESS

TPN is infused into the central venous circulation. In contrast, nutrient solutions infused into a peripheral vein are known as *peripheral parenteral nutrition* (PPN). PPN generally results in underfeeding because, in order to keep the osmolarity of the solution under 1000 mOsm/L, glucose administration must be reduced. Its use should be limited to the client with adequate peripheral vascular access who needs parenteral therapy for 5 to 10 days. In the client with poor peripheral access or with severe hypermetabolism and hypercatabolism, TPN is recommended.

In central vascular access, the tip of the catheter must be positioned in a high-flow vein, such as the superior or inferior vena cava. Access to this central system can be achieved through several veins, such as a peripheral vein, the jugular vein, the subclavian vein, or the femoral vein (Figure 29–2). Temporary central venous catheters are percutaneous nontunneled catheters that are best used in an acute care setting for a short time.

More recently, the peripherally inserted central venous catheter (PICC) has offered an option for long-term use. For extended therapy (>3 months), external tunneled central venous catheters or totally implanted ports are the best option.

Nursing Management of the Client Receiving Parenteral Nutrition

ASSESSMENT

In addition to the nutritional assessment measures outlined earlier, you must check the infusion bag for correct ingredients and appearance of the solution, assess the condition of the venous access site, monitor blood glucose levels and the rate of infusion, and observe the client for untoward reactions to the solution.

DIAGNOSIS, OUTCOMES, INTERVENTIONS

Altered Nutrition: Less Than Body Requirements. The nursing diagnosis most appropriate for the client receiving TPN is *Altered Nutrition: Less Than Body Requirements related to the need for IV delivery of nutrients, fluids, and electrolytes to maintain nutritional status secondary to malabsorption problems of the GI tract, gastric cancer, cancer cachexia, anorexia nervosa, excessive metabolic needs (as in extensive burns or draining*

TABLE 29–6 DAILY PARENTERAL TRACE ELEMENT SUPPLEMENTATION

Trace Element	AMA Guidelines	M.T.E.-4	M.T.E.-5	M.T.E.-5 Concentrate
Zinc	2.5–4.0 mg	1 mg	1 mg	5 mg
Copper	0.5–1.5 mg	0.4 mg	0.4 mg	1 mg
Manganese	0.15–0.8 mg	0.1 mg	0.1 mg	0.5 mg
Chromium	10–15 μg	4 μg	4 μg	10 μg
Selenium	20 μg	—	20 μg	60 μg

AMA, American Medical Association; M.T.E., multiple trace elements.

From Galica, L. (1997). Parenteral nutrition. *Nursing Clinics of North America., 32,* 4, p. 711.

wounds), or the need to rest the gut to promote healing (as in pancreatitis).

Outcomes. The client will maintain ideal body weight or will gain 1 to 2 pounds per week until ideal body weight is attained.

Interventions

Administer TPN. You are responsible for safely administering and monitoring the infusion of TPN. Just before delivery, check every solution for its expiration date, the correct ingredients (glucose, fat, protein, and electrolytes), leaks or tears in the bag, and the appearance of the solution (separating or cracking of the solution). TPN must be delivered using a peristaltic pump to accurately control the infusion rate and prevent the possibility of a bolus. TPN solutions are typically infused over 24 hours in the acute care setting. In the home, clients often receive TPN while sleeping.

Monitor Serum Glucose Levels. The first time TPN is administered, serum glucose levels should be monitored every 6 hours to assess the client's response to glucose. If blood glucose is within the normal range for 24 hours, monitoring can be changed to daily. Persistent elevations of blood glucose are managed by delivering regular insulin in the TPN solution after the daily requirement for insulin is determined. If the client's clinical status is unstable, the insulin dose cannot be stabilized over a 24-hour period, or both, the insulin should be delivered outside of the TPN as an insulin drip or intermittent subcutaneous injections. Most clients can tolerate an acute discontinuation of TPN and therefore do not need to be weaned from TPN gradually.

Observe for Allergy to Lipids. TPN solution that contains lipids (fats) should be introduced slowly the first time to assess for reaction to the lipid. Although rare, allergic reactions to IV lipid preparations have been reported and usually present within 30 minutes. A clinical manifestation of reactions can be any of the following: fever, shaking chills, shortness of breath, chest pain, or back pain. If the client complains of any of these manifestations, stop the TPN infusion immediately and inform the health care team of the manifestations.

Maintain Vascular Access. You play a pivotal role in ensuring the proper functioning of the vascular access system and preventing catheter-related infection. Maintain catheter patency by following a routine heparin flush protocol. Table 29–7 outlines the suggested protocols for central catheters that deliver TPN.

Prevent Infection. Prevention of catheter-related infection is key to the successful use of parenteral nutrition. Most infections that do occur result from contamination of the exit site or catheter hub.[6, 7] You must follow strict guidelines/protocols for the care of the vascular access device before, during, and after its insertion. Although

TABLE 29–7 CENTRAL VENOUS CATHETER MAINTENANCE

Catheter Type	Site Care	Flushing
Nontunneled central venous catheter	▪ *Dressing:* Transparent or gauze ▪ Transparent dressing enhances catheter stability ▪ Performed as a sterile dressing ▪ Skin antisepsis protocols include one or a combination of the following: 70% alcohol (3 swabs), 10% povidone-iodine (3 swabs), chlorhexidine	*Internal volume:* 0.1–0.53 ml *Flush volume:* 1–2 ml *Frequency:* Usually daily
Tunneled, cuffed central venous catheter	▪ *Dressing:* Transparent or gauze until incision healed ▪ Dressing commonly discontinued when incision healed and suture removed ▪ Performed as an aseptic dressing (skin antisepsis as above) ▪ Hydrogen peroxide may be used to remove crusting at the site	*Internal volume:* 0.15–1.8 ml *Flush volume:* 3–4 ml *Frequency:* Usually daily *Groshong catheters:* 5 ml 0.9% normal saline solution weekly
Peripherally inserted central catheter	▪ *Dressing:* Transparent preferred to enhance catheter stability ▪ Performed as a sterile dressing (skin antisepsis as above) ▪ Dressings required as long as catheter is in place	*Internal volume:* 0.04–1.2 ml *Flush volume:* 2–3 ml *Frequency:* Daily
Ports	▪ *Dressing:* Transparent when port is accessed to stabilize needle ▪ Sterile gauze may be placed between needle and skin ▪ Huber needle changed at least every 7 days ▪ Sterile approach needle insertion and dressing recommended (skin antisepsis as above before needle placement) ▪ Dressing remains until healed (several days postoperatively)	*Internal volume:* 0.5–1.5 ml *Flush volume:* At least 3 ml *Frequency:* Every 4 weeks

From Krzywada, E., & Edmiston, C. (1998). Parenteral access/equipment. *The ASPEN nutrition support practice manual.* Silver Spring, MD: ASPEN Board of Directors, with permission.

catheter site care is somewhat varied and is controversial, strict adherence to hand-washing and aseptic technique is clearly the most important way to prevent infection. Dedicate (and mark) one lumen of a multilumen catheter to the infusion of TPN to minimize manipulations of the IV system. The most recent recommendations from the Centers for Disease Control and Prevention (CDC) are to change the tubing for lipid-containing TPN solutions every 24 hours.[7]

Provide Dressing Changes. The dressing change protocol for central venous access devices continues to be controversial. Various protocols exist for skin cleaning and the type and frequency of dressing change. The catheter exit site should be cleaned with an antiseptic agent, such as 70% alcohol and 10% povidone-iodine. Another product that has shown positive results in preventing catheter-related infections is chlorhexidine. Antibiotic ointments should not be applied to the catheter exit site.

The type of dressing applied over the catheter exit site should be either a sterile gauze or a transparent dressing. Frequency of dressing changes depends on client needs (e.g., more frequent changes are needed for a diaphoretic client) and the type of dressing. Gauze dressings typically are changed every 48 hours, transparent dressings every 3 to 7 days. The most important concept is that the dressing must remain adherent to be effective. Therefore, any dressing must be changed immediately if it becomes damp, soiled, or loose. Follow your agency's policy regarding dressing change protocols.

Medical Management of the Client Receiving Enteral Nutrition

ENTERAL NUTRITION

"Total enteral nutrition" (TEN) refers to a method of infusing nutrient solutions or formulas directly into the GI tract through tubes that enter through the nose, mouth, or abdominal wall. Enteral nutrition is indicated when the client has impaired ingestion but normal intestinal absorption.

Some common indications for enteral nutrition are listed in Box 29–3. Enteral feeding is contraindicated in clients with complete intestinal obstruction, ileus, severe pseudo-obstruction, severe diarrhea, intestinal ischemia, severe acute pancreatitis or malabsorption syndrome. In clients with impairments of the proximal GI tract, from fistulae or tumor, enteral feeding may be used if the tip of the tube is positioned distal to the impairment.

In clients with adequate GI tract function, *enteral* rather than *parenteral* nutrition should be used. One of the most important benefits of enteral nutrition relates to the importance of utilizing the GI tract to maintain and support gut integrity and function and prevent atrophy of the gut mucosa. The protection offered by using the GI tract can result in a reduction of infectious complications.[1, 2, 6] Other factors that make enteral therapy desirable include reduced cost and safer administration.

The TEN prescription is guided by the nutritional assessment and the definition of nutrient goals for calories and protein. The selection of an enteral formula is based on the client's nutrient needs, the absorptive function of the GI tract, the fluid status, and the level of stress. More than 100 enteral formulas are available on the market today. Most can be placed into one of the following three classifications:

- *Standard formula:* contains intact (nonhydrolyzed) protein; may be concentrated, high-protein, or fiber-enriched
- *Predigested elemental formula:* not in the "intact state"; instead, contains hydrolyzed protein in the form of dipeptides and tripeptides
- *Disease-specific formula:* contained in a standard or elemental form reported to enhance specific organ function, such as the kidneys, liver, pulmonary system, or immune system

Table 29–8 outlines the classification of enteral products and includes brief descriptions of formula characteristics. Standard formulas, which contain 1 kcal/ml, are used most often. Concentrated calorie-dense formulas, which contain 1.5 to 2.0 kcal/ml, are helpful for clients who are fluid-restricted or unable to tolerate high volumes of formula. High-protein formulas contain more than 50 g/L of protein and are useful for critically ill clients who are hypercatabolic and have a proportionally lower calorie and fluid need with high protein requirements. The addition of fiber to standard formulas can help regulate bowel function and prevent diarrhea and constipation.

Enteral formulas are designed to provide the recommended dietary allowance (RDA) of vitamins and trace

BOX 29–3 Indications for Enteral Feeding

Neurologic and Psychiatric

Anorexia nervosa
Cerebrovascular accident
Demyelinating disease
Failure to thrive
Inflammation
Cancer
Severe depression
Trauma

Oropharyngeal and Esophageal

Inflammation
Cancer
Trauma

Gastrointestinal

Fistula (not mid-gut)
Mild inflammatory bowel disease
Mild malabsorption
Mild pancreatitis
Preoperative bowel preparation
Short-bowel syndrome (later stages)

Miscellaneous

Acquired immunodeficiency syndrome (AIDS)
Burns
Chemotherapy
Organ transplantation
Radiation therapy

Adapted from Guenter, P., et al. (1997). Delivery systems and administration of enteral nutrition. In J. Rombeau & R. Rolandelli (Eds.), *Clinical nutrition: Enteral and tube feeding* (3rd ed., p. 240). Philadelphia: W. B. Saunders.

TABLE 29–8 CLASSIFICATION OF ENTERAL NUTRITION PRODUCTS

Classification	Formula Characteristics	Sample Products
Intact protein blenderized	Isotonic; nutritionally complete; containing fiber; lactose and lactose-free	Compleat Modified Formula Compleat Regular Formula, Vitaneed,
Low-residue standard protein	Isotonic; nutritionally complete; lactose-free	Entrition 1.0, Isocal, Isolan, Isosource, Osmolite, Resource
Intermediate, high-protein	Isotonic; nutritionally complete; lactose-free	Entrition 1.0, Isocal HN, Isosource HN, Osmolite HN
Concentrated	Calorically dense (1.5–2.0 cal/ml); lactose-free; nutritionally complete; hyperosmolar	Isocal HCN, Magnacal, TwoCal HN, Nutren 2.0
Fiber-supplemented	Isotonic; nutritionally complete; lactose-free; fiber range, 5–14 g/L; standard to intermediate protein	Fibersource, Jevity, Fiberlan, Ultracal
Disease-specific renal (pre-dialysis)	Low- and standard protein; low-mineral, vitamin A, and vitamin D content; lactose-free; calorically dense; hyperosmolar	Suplena
Glucose-intolerant	Low-carbohydrate, high-fat; lactose-free; isotonic; containing fiber; nutritionally complete	Glucerna
Pulmonary	Low-carbohydrate, high-fat; lactose-free; nutritionally complete; hyperosmolar; calorically dense	Nutrivent, Pulmocare, Respalor
Trauma/stress	High-protein; isotonic to hyperosmolar; lactose-free; nutritionally complete; some containing fiber, hydrolyzed protein, supplemental amino acids (BCAA, arginine, glutamine), and β-carotene; low-fat	AlitraQ, Impact, Impact w/Fiber, Immun-Aid, Isotein HN, Promote, Replete, Replete w/Fiber, TraumaCal
Hydrolyzed protein, very-low-fat	Nutritionally complete; lactose-free, fewer than 10% of calories from fat; hyperosmolar, varying in peptide length; containing amino acids	Accupep HPF, Criticare HN, Vital High Nitrogen
Low-fat	Nutritionally complete; lactose-free, 11%–30% of calories from fat; hyperosmolar; varying in peptide length; containing amino acids	Travasorb HN, Travasorb STD
Moderate-fat	Nutritionally complete; lactose-free, 30%–35% of calories from fat (high MCT); hyperosmolar, varying in peptide length; containing amino acids	Peptamen, Reabilan
Disease-specific; trauma	Nutritionally complete; lactose-free, intermediate to high in protein content; 25%–35% of calories from fat (high MCT); varying in peptide length; containing amino acids; sometimes containing supplemental arginine and β-carotene	Perative, Reabilan HN
Crystalline amino acids	Nutritionally complete; lactose-free, low-fat (1%–3% of total calories); low to standard protein content; hyperosmolar	Tolerex, Vivonex T.E.N.
Disease-specific; hepatic failure	High BCAA; nutritionally incomplete; lactose-free; low-fat	NutriHep
Renal failure (with dialysis)	Essential and nonessential amino acids: nutritionally incomplete but containing water-soluble vitamins; hyperosmolar; lactose-free; low-fat	Nepro

MCT, medium-chain triglyceride; BCAA, branched-chain amino acid; LCT, long-chain triglyceride.
Adapted from Hopkins, B. (1994). Enteral nutrition products. In G. Zaloga (Ed.), *Nutrition in critical care.* St. Louis: Mosby–Year Book, p. 447.

elements based on an intake of 1500 to 2000 calories/day. Clients receiving lower-calorie regimens may require supplemental vitamins during extended enteral nutrition.

The daily fluid needs of the client receiving enteral nutrition must be calculated to avoid overhydration or underhydration. The most vulnerable client is the one receiving a calorie-dense or concentrated formula, which contains less free water than that in a standard formula. Such a client may require additional water delivered as an intermittent flush or bolus throughout the day to meet fluid needs. A client with excessive GI losses may also require supplemental water to maintain hydration.

ENTERAL ACCESS

Enteral feeding requires the administration of a liquid solution through a tube into the GI tract. Enteral nutrients can be delivered into the stomach (intragastrically) or into the small intestine (postpylorically). Selection of the type of enteral access device depends on the functional status of the GI tract, the risk for aspiration, and the estimated length of therapy. Figure 29–3 depicts the various types of enteral access placements.

The functional status of the client's GI tract often defines the site of feeding. Resections, obstructions, motility disorders, or fistulae of the upper GI tract necessitate that the client be fed into the small bowel, distal to the impairment. A client who has aspirated or is at risk for aspiration may benefit from postpyloric feeding. The duration of enteral therapy defines the type of tube placed: temporary tubes for short-term therapy (<4 to 6 weeks) and permanent tubes for long-term therapy (>4 to 6 weeks).

For short-term feeding, nasogastric or nasoenteric tubes are the tubes of choice. Tubes varying in length and ranging in size from 5 to 16 French (Fr.) are placed into the stomach or small intestine at the bedside, and the tip position is then verified with an abdominal radiograph. If postpyloric feeding is indicated, the tip of the tube can be advanced under fluoroscopy, or via endoscopy, client positioning, or the administration of prokinetic agents (e.g., cisapride, metoclopramide, or erythromycin). Small-bore enteral feeding tubes are made of polyurethane or silicone plastic and are thus softer and more flexible than a standard nasogastric tube used for decompression.

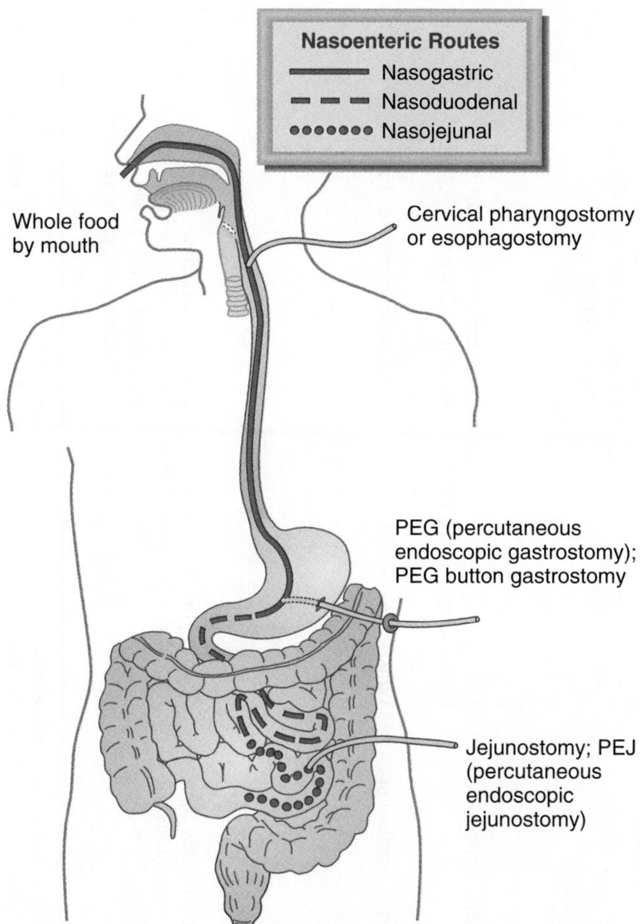

FIGURE 29–3 Placements for enteral access. (From Mahan, L. K., & Escott-Stump, S. E. [2000]. *Krause's food, nutrition, & diet therapy* [10th ed., p. 468]. Philadelphia: W. B. Saunders.)

For long-term enteral feeding, gastrostomy and jejunostomy tubes are indicated. These tubes can be placed surgically, endoscopically, or radiologically. Surgically placed devices (gastrostomy or jejunostomy tubes), are used most commonly in clients undergoing a laparotomy, and general anesthesia is required. More recently, the percutaneous endoscopic gastrostomy (PEG) or jejunostomy (PEJ) approach has become the most common method of placing a permanent long-term feeding device. This nonsurgical approach avoids the need for general anesthesia and can be performed on an outpatient basis.

Table 29–9 describes various enteral feeding devices and their indications. Various GI tubes and their placement and management are discussed in Chapters 30 and 31.

METHODS OF ADMINISTRATION

Enteral feeding can be administered by either an *intermittent* or *continuous* drip. The method of delivery is determined by (1) the location of the tube tip and (2) the client's tolerance. When the tube tip is located in the small intestine, continuous feeding is the desired choice. For gastric feedings, the type of administration can be (1) bolus, (2) intermittent, or (3) continuous.

In *intermittent* or *bolus* feedings, 300 to 500 ml of enteral formula are delivered several times per day. Bolus feedings are usually delivered via a syringe over 10 to 15 minutes.

In *intermittent* feeding, formula is placed into a gravity bag and dripped in over 30 to 60 minutes. An infusion pump may also be used. Intermittent feeding is a more common method than bolus feeding to deliver periodic feedings into the stomach in the acute care setting because of improved tolerance.

Continuous feedings are administered via an infusion pump to more closely control the rate of infusion. The feedings are generally infused over 24 hours at rates ranging from 50 ml to 150 ml. As clients are switched to cycled nocturnal feedings in preparation for discharge, they often require and can tolerate continuous rates slightly above 150 ml/hr. However, clients usually cannot tolerate continuous feeding into the small intestine at rates above 200 ml/hr.

Continuous feeding into the stomach has been associated with less gastric distention and aspiration compared with bolus or intermittent feeding into the stomach.[6, 10] In addition, continuous gastric feedings may reduce metabolic complications and protect against stress ulcers more effectively compared with intermittent gastric feedings.[6, 10]

Nursing Management of the Client Receiving Enteral Nutrition

ASSESSMENT

In addition to the nutritional assessment measures described earlier, you should review the type of formula being used; the time, frequency, and amount of feeding; the client's specific indications; and the placement and

TABLE 29–9 ENTERAL ACCESS DEVICES

Enteral Access	Tube Size and Length	Indications	Advantages	Disadvantages
Nasogastric (small-bore feeding tube)	8–12 Fr., 17–36 inches	Functional stomach Upper gastrointestinal tract obstruction Dysphagia to solids Not at risk for aspiration	Placed at bedside Low morbidity Easily inserted Continued use of GI tract	Client discomfort Risk of aspiration
Nasoduodenal	14–18 Fr., 35–45 inches	Gastric atony Risk of aspiration	Decreased risk of aspiration Continued use of GI tract	Client discomfort Difficult placement Easily malpositioned
Nasojejunal	14–18 Fr., 36–45 inches	High risk for pulmonary aspiration of gastric contents Functional small bowel	Decreased risk of aspiration Continued use of GI tract	Increased cost of tube and skilled professional to place tube Easily malpositioned
Gastrostomy, surgical	14–30 Fr.	Inability to use percutaneous placement GI surgery Long-term feeding	Continued use of GI tract Can be placed in clients with esophageal or pharyngeal cancers Used in obese clients when unable to transilluminate abdominal wall for PEG placement	General anesthesia Tube migration Easily obstructed Local stoma site complications
Gastrostomy, percutaneous	14–22 Fr.	Long-term feeding tube No history of aspiration	No surgical procedure needed Placement without general anesthesia Continued use of GI tract	Potential for aspiration Cannot be used in obese clients
Low-profile gastrostomy device (G-Button)	18–28 Fr.	Long-term feeding Ambulatory patients Disoriented patients who pull at the gastrostomy tube	Increased mobility Decreased cost over time because of device longevity Decreased nursing time compared with time needed for replacement tube change Continued use of GI tract	Skilled professional needed for placement Increased trauma to client compared with replacement tube Increased cost compared with cost of gastrostomy tube change Second procedure required after gastrostomy tube placement
Jejunostomy, temporary	5 Fr. Jejunostomy kit, 14 Fr.	Short-term enteral nutrition Usually ≤2 weeks	Continued use of GI tract	Surgical placement Tube easily obstructed Costly
Jejunostomy, permanent	Whistle tip, 14–18 Fr.	Long-term jejunal feeding	Silicone plastic Continued use of GI tract Easily replaced when fistulous tract is formed Larger-bore Location proximal jejunum, thus elemental products not required	Continuous or slow intermittent tube feeding required via a pump
Combination tubes for gastric decompression	Gastric port, 16–30 Fr. Jejunal feeding port, 9 Fr.	Long-term feeding Dysfunctional stomach Functional small bowel Short-term postoperative care	Can decompress a dysfunctional stomach and prevent regurgitation of gastric contents during small intestine feeding Continued use of GI tract	Skilled professional needed for placement Expensive process Jejunal feeding needed Can be dislodged from original position Placed during surgery

PEG, percutaneous endoscopic gastrostomy; Fr., French; GI, gastrointestinal.
Adapted from Shuster, M., & Mancino, J. (1994). Ensuring successful home tube feeding in the geriatric population. *Geriatric Nursing, 15,* 67–82.

patency of the tube. Monitor the client for aspiration of tube feeding or GI contents.

See Bridge to Home Health Care: Managing Tube Feedings.

DIAGNOSIS, OUTCOMES, INTERVENTIONS

Altered Nutrition: Less Than Body Requirements. The nursing diagnosis most appropriate for the client receiving enteral feeding is *Altered Nutrition: Less Than Body Requirements related to difficulty swallowing, esophageal or gastric resection or obstruction, or inability to ingest adequate calories and nutrients.*

BRIDGE TO HOME HEALTH CARE

Managing Tube Feedings

Home health agency nutrition support teams usually consist of a nurse, a registered dietitian, and a pharmacist. When these professionals regularly visit a client who has a new feeding tube, the chances for successfully managing the client and the tube feedings at home are greatly increased. In addition to providing direct care, the team provides instructions to the client and family, communicates with the client's physician, prevents problems if possible, and monitors any problems that develop.

Consistently flushing the tube with water before and after each feeding enhances the longevity of the tube. Although flushing the tube with carbonated beverages has been suggested, studies indicate few or no benefits over flushing with water. Flush all types of feeding tubes with a 50-cc syringe; smaller syringes can create pressure high enough to rupture a tube.

Teach the client and family to secure a nasogastric tube firmly to the nose and to either side of the face or to another position of comfort. To secure the tube, use tape, a transparent occlusive dressing, or a commercial tube holder with a hydrocolloid backing with a self-fastening tape (Velcro) closure.

When the client has a percutaneous endoscopic gastrostomy (PEG) or a percutaneous endoscopic jejunostomy (PEJ), observe daily for tube dislodgment, leaking, skin irritation, and clinical manifestations of infection. Clean the site daily with hydrogen peroxide followed by normal saline rinse. Slide the external bridge away for cleaning, then reposition. No dressing is required. Good hand-washing technique is essential for all personnel.

Management of tube feedings varies with the type of infusion: continuous infusion with a pump, bolus infusion, or infusion by gravity. Numerous commercial products are available to meet the client's nutritional needs. The physician and the registered dietitian are responsible for assessing the type of feeding and method of infusion. However, the client may tolerate one formula better than another. Positioning clients at a 45-degree angle or greater helps them tolerate the feeding. Changing the rate and frequency of infusion may decrease or eliminate nausea, diarrhea, or tube displacement. Successful tube feeding begins in the hospital and continues at home as the client, family, home care nurse, registered dietitian, pharmacist, and physician work together as a team.

Colette H. McVaney, RN, BSN, *Lead Nurse, Geriatric Clinic, Nebraska Health System, Omaha, Nebraska*

Outcomes. The client will maintain ideal body weight or will gain 1 to 2 pounds per week until ideal body weight is attained.

Interventions

Prevent Contamination of Formula and Delivery System. You are primarily responsible for administering and monitoring enteral feeding. The care and handling of the feeding formula and equipment is a key factor in the success of enteral feeding. To prevent contamination of the enteral formula, you must adhere to strict hand-washing before handling the feeding formula and equipment. *Open delivery systems,* which use cans and syringes and bags, are the most vulnerable because of the great degree of manipulation. Formulas administered via an open system should hang for only 4 hours before being changed and the tubing flushed or rinsed. The equipment should be changed every 24 hours. *Closed delivery systems,* which use a prefilled container, minimize the amount of preparation; thus, the chance of formula contamination is reduced and the hang time is extended (24 to 48 hours).

Assess Tube Location. Before administering an enteral feeding, ensure that the tube is positioned properly. If a nasoenteric tube is being used to feed a client for the first time, make sure that an abdominal radiograph has verified that the tip is located in the GI tract.

Routinely evaluate the position of the enteral feeding device, and be alert for the possibility of tube migration or dislodgment. Nasoenteric tubes can be marked to indicate the position so that it will be evident if the tube has moved. Nasoenteric tubes can easily migrate when the client coughs or vomits, but more often the tubes are dislodged when a confused or agitated client inadvertently removes the tube.

In addition to determining whether the tube has migrated, you may need to evaluate the location of the tube tip. Is the tube tip in the stomach, small intestine, or respiratory tract? Three methods can be used to evaluate tip location:

- *Auscultation:* injecting air into the feeding tube and listening with a stethoscope for the sound
- *Aspiration:* observing the fluid that is removed through the feeding tube
- *pH paper testing:* checking the pH of the fluid removed from the feeding tube

Auscultation is the least reliable method and should not be used to evaluate the tube tip position. Observing the aspirated fluid and checking its pH are more useful. However, aspiration should not replace a radiographic evaluation after the initial placement or when tube migration is suspected.

An enterostomy (e.g., gastrostomy, jejunostomy) tube can migrate in or out if it is not properly secured at the exit site with sutures or a tube attachment device. Enteral feeding tubes that are not well secured at the exit site can pivot, causing an accumulation of granulation tissue and a widening of the tract. If the tract becomes widened, formula and digestive enzymes can come up through it and excoriate the skin on the abdomen.

Administer Feedings. Starter regimens for enteral feedings differ according to tube tip location and the client's clinical status. Continuous feedings into the small intestine are usually started at 30 to 40 ml/hr and advanced as tolerated every 12 to 24 hours until the daily goal is reached. Intermittent feedings into the stomach are initiated at 100 to 120 ml every 4 hours and advanced every 12 to 24 hours as tolerated.

Prevent Aspiration. Preventing aspiration during enteral feeding is crucial. The use of postpyloric or small bowel feeding is recommended for a client with a high risk of aspiration. Proper administration and delivery techniques are especially important during gastric feedings. The head of the bed must be elevated 45 degrees for 1 hour before and 1 hour after gastric feeding. Continuous gastric feedings require that the head of the client's bed remain elevated. Gastric residuals can be monitored every 4 hours initially and then as needed to assess gastric emptying and to prevent aspiration. A significant gastric residual is approximately 100 to 150 ml. Feeding into the jejunum theoretically reduces the risk of aspirating enteral formula. However, the head of the bed should still be elevated about 30 degrees during continuous jejunal feeding.

Maintain Enteral Access. Maintenance of enteral access consists of caring for the external site, maintaining tube patency, and maintaining the correct tube position. Nasoenteric tubes most often exit the nose and are secured to the nose or cheek with tape or an adhesive attachment device. The nasoenteric tube should exit the nose, hang straight down, and then be gently looped up and secured to the cheek. Tubes that are sharply angled as they exit the nostril can cause necrosis or obstruct the flow of enteral formula through the tube. With any method of securing, the tube should be repositioned and resecured at least every other day to prevent skin irritation.

For tubes that exit the abdominal wall (e.g., PEG, gastrostomy, and jejunostomy tubes), a dressing is required for the first 24 hours after placement. The site care consists of a daily cleaning with mild soap and rinsing with warm water. Dressings are optional for healed enterostomy sites, but a light nonocclusive dressing may help secure the tube as well as contain mucus that commonly drains from the tube tract.

Maintaining the patency of the enteral feeding tube is a critical nursing intervention for the client receiving enteral feeding. Enteral feeding tubes clog for a variety of reasons, the most common of which is the improper administration of medications through the tube. Medication administration via enteral feeding tubes is probably the most poorly understood part of working with enteral feeding devices and thus highly prone to error. Medications should be given through an enteral access device only when there is an absolute contraindication to taking them by mouth. Problems that can result from incorrect medication administration via an enteral feeding tube include tube clogging, altered drug availability, and diarrhea. Box 29–4 lists some steps to follow for safe administration of medications via an enteral feeding tube.

Tubes of any diameter will clog without strict adherence to a flushing protocol. The most effective irrigant for flushing an enteral feeding tube is water. Flush the tube with at least 30 ml of warm water every 4 hours during continuous feedings and before and after each intermittent feeding or medication. Acidic flushing solutions, such as cranberry juice, may precipitate with protein and obstruct the tube; thus, they are not recommended.[6]

See the Management and Delegation feature.

BOX 29–4 Guidelines for the Administration of Medications via an Enteral Feeding Tube

- If possible, administer the medication by mouth.
- Use a liquid form of the medication if available.
- If the medication can be crushed, crush it to a fine powder and dissolve it in 30 ml of water.
- Do not crush enteric-coated or time-released tablets or capsules.
- Flush the tube with 30 ml of water before and after giving each medication.
- Do not mix multiple medications or give them together.
- Do not deliver a medication that must be absorbed in the stomach into the small intestine, such as sucralfate (Carafate) or antacids.
- Hold feedings 1 to 2 hours before and after giving a medication that might have drug-nutrient interactions, such as phenytoin (Dilantin).

EVALUATION OF NUTRITIONAL INTERVENTIONS

When caring for a client receiving TEN or TPN, you must regularly evaluate the client's response to therapy. Assessing the client's tolerance to the nutrient regimen includes evaluation of the fluid status (intake/output data and weights) and a thorough assessment of the GI system. Evaluation also includes monitoring vital signs, reviewing laboratory tests, and assessing the function of the nutritional access device. Together with a nutritional support team, you will be collecting pertinent data, such as weight and visceral protein measures, to assess the success of the nutrient prescription.

Table 29–10 outlines common parameters used to monitor clients receiving enteral or parenteral nutrition. Comprehensive and routine monitoring can prevent complications related to nutritional support therapies.

Self-Care

Nutritional support therapies, such as TEN and TPN, are routinely administered in the home setting. Nurses play a pivotal role in determining appropriate candidates for home nutrition support by helping to determine the plan of care and providing client and family education.

The nursing assessment includes a comprehensive review of the client and family or caregivers. The physical and cognitive abilities of the client or caregiver must be evaluated so that you can be sure of their ability to carry out complex procedures. Manual dexterity and eyesight are particularly important when care involves programming pumps for infusion and drawing up medication in syringes. The client's home environment must be evaluated to ensure that it is safe for home therapy. The client or caregiver education process should ideally start in the hospital and be reinforced after discharge. Clients receiving either TPN or tube feedings need to learn a wide range of related skills (Box 29–5).

MANAGEMENT AND DELEGATION

Care of Nasogastric Tubes, Small-Bore Feeding Tubes, and Gastrostomy and Jejunostomy Tubes

Nasogastric Tubes

Decompression relieves stomach pressure by removing gas and fluids from the stomach. It can be used to prevent nausea, vomiting and gastric distention when gastrointestinal (GI) motility is delayed or absent or when the client has a distal obstruction or has had recent GI tract surgery. Nasogastric tubes may also be used to initiate enteral feedings upon resumption of bowel motility.

The detailed assessment and potential risks associated with nasogastric tube insertion, maintenance, and removal prevent delegation of these procedures to unlicensed personnel. You may delegate the gathering of equipment and the measurement, recording, and testing of nasogastric drainage to assistive personnel. Delegation of short-term disconnection of nasogastric tubes (for the purposes such as toileting or ambulation) may be appropriate under the supervision of a Registered Nurse (RN). Reconnection of the nasogastric tube to suction requires the RN to verify pressure settings. You may delegate skin care of the client's nose and comfort care for the client's mouth to unlicensed personnel.

Nasogastric Tubes: Mouth and Nose Care

Instruct assistive personnel to:

1. Wash hands and don gloves.
2. For nasal care:
   a. Gently clean and lubricate the client's external nares to prevent buildup of crusted secretions and skin breakdown.
   b. Use a clean cotton-tipped swab and a water-soluble lubricant to clean the client's nostril.
   c. Make sure that the skin on the client's nose is clean and dry.
   d. Apply tincture of benzoin or other skin adhesive on the tip of the patient's nose and allow to dry
   e. Secure tube with hypoallergenic tape, taking care to avoid pressure on nares
3. For mouth care:
   a. Offer or administer frequent oral hygiene with non-alcohol containing solutions to remove debris, increase comfort and maintain a healthy oral cavity.
   b. Brush teeth or assist patient to do so.

Small-Bore Feeding Tubes and Gastrostomy and Jejunostomy Tubes

The most desirable and appropriate method of providing nutrition is via the oral route. For clients who are unable or unwilling to meet their nutritional needs orally, enteral tube feedings may be an option. Tube-feedings may be delivered through large-bore or small-bore gastric tubes that may be inserted by the RN with a physician's order, through gastrostomy tubes, or through jejunostomy tubes. A gastrostomy tube is large and is surgically or endoscopically placed directly into the stomach, exiting through an incision in the left upper quadrant of the abdomen. A jejunostomy tube is also placed surgically (directly into the jejunum for small bowel feedings), or endoscopically (into the gastrostomy tube and passed through to the jejunum).

A physician's order is required for placement of a small-bore nasogastric or nasointestinal feeding tube. Accuracy of feeding tube placement is confirmed by abdominal radiograph. Insertion of nasogastric tubes and verification of placement of nasogastric, gastrostomy and jejunostomy tubes require problem-solving and knowledge application unique to the professional nurse. For this reason, delegation of these skills is inappropriate. You may delegate skin care to the exit site of the tube to unlicensed personnel.

Gastrostomy and Jejunostomy Exit Site Care:

Exit site care is performed 24 hours after feeding tube insertion. Instruct assistive personnel to:

1. Wash hands and don gloves.
2. Remove the old dressing.
3. Clean around the tube insertion site with normal saline to remove exudate or dried blood.
4. Do not use hydrogen peroxide or any antiseptic cream unless specifically ordered by the physician.
5. Rinse the tube insertion site with clean water and dry thoroughly.
6. Apply a new split drain sponge dressing if needed.

Describe findings that are immediately reportable to you for assistive personnel, including redness, swelling, abnormal drainage (thick, foul-smelling, yellow or green color), or pain at the tube's insertion site. Have assistive personnel report any complaints of abdominal pain, bloating, cramping, or diarrhea. Verify the competence of assistive personnel in performing these tasks during orientation and annually thereafter.

Hilary S. Blackwood, MSN, RN, *Clinician IV, Surgical Nutrition Support Services, University of Virginia Health System, Charlottesville, Virginia*

EATING DISORDERS

OBESITY

Obesity is characterized by an excess accumulation of fat and reflects an overall imbalance between energy intake and expenditure.

Etiology and Risk Factors

The etiology of obesity is multifactorial, making effective treatment a challenge. When a positive energy balance occurs (more calories are consumed than expended), obesity or an accumulation of stored energy (fat) occurs. Causes of obesity can be related to either side of this energy equation. The most important factors[5] seem to be:

1. *Genetic tendency*. Genetic makeup determines the *basal metabolic rate* (BMR), defined as the energy required for basic maintenance of the body's cells and functions. The BMR can vary widely (as much as 30%) and is often higher in the obese client.[7] More recent studies of causes of obesity are focusing on other genetic factors, such as neurotransmitters and peptide levels, that may control and regu-

TABLE 29–10 SUGGESTED NUTRITION MONITORING PROTOCOL

Parameter	Frequency of Assessment
BIOCHEMICAL MEASURES	
Electrolytes	Daily
Magnesium, calcium, phosphorus	Daily
Glucose	Every 6 hours for 48 hours, then daily
Albumin, prealbumin, transferrin	Weekly
Triglyceride	Pre-infusion, post-infusion, then daily
Liver function tests	Pre-infusion, then weekly
Complete blood count, prothrombin time, partial thromboplastin time	Weekly
NURSING ASSESSMENT	
Weight	Daily
Intake/output	Hourly/every 8 hours
Infusion rate	Every 4 hours
Temperature	Every 8 hours
NUTRITIONAL MONITORING	
24-hour urine collection for urinary urea nitrogen	Weekly
Measured resting energy expenditure	Weekly

late food intake and affect the development of obesity.

2. *Environment.* The relationship between environmental factors and obesity is unclear. However, societal factors that may play a role include a more sedentary lifestyle, which is typical of our industrialized society. Much of our daily lifestyle no longer requires physical work. In addition, when food is plentiful, particularly high-fat alternatives, obesity can develop.

BOX 29–5 Teaching Topics for Clients Who Need Enteral or Parenteral Feedings at Home

Care of the Nutritional Access Device

- Flushing the venous access or feeding tube
- Changing the dressing
- Observing for evidence of infection

Formula Preparation

- Adding medication to the TPN formula
- Placing enteral formula in feeding bag
- Setting up enteral or parenteral feeding pump or bag
- Obtaining formula for TPN and related supplies

Monitoring for Complications

- Assessing temperature
- Monitoring weight

TPN, total parenteral nutrition.

3. *Diet.* The composition of diet is increasingly important and continues to receive public attention. The intake of a high-fat, calorie-dense diet can increase the likelihood of obesity.[16]

Pathophysiology

Obesity is a serious health risk and has been associated with increased mortality and morbidity. With obesity, the risk for cardiovascular disease is increased; with increasing weight, elevated blood pressure, blood lipids, and glucose levels have been documented.[8, 12, 15, 16]

A strong relationship between obesity and the development of type 2 diabetes mellitus has been known for some time. The cause is thought to be the increased amount of fat stores, which are associated with glucose intolerance and abnormal metabolism of insulin. Other serious health problems that occur more often in obesity include respiratory problems, gallbladder disease, and arthritis.

More recently, a relationship between obesity and cancer has been suggested. Some cancers, such as colorectal, breast, and prostate cancer, have been linked to obesity. However, whether this link between cancer and obesity is simply due to the excess weight or to specific dietary factors is unclear.

Clinical Manifestations

Obesity is a significant problem in the United States. Estimates from 1988 to 1991 indicated that approximately 33% of Americans are obese, an increase from 23% in 1971.[8] Obesity is defined as more than 45% above *ideal body weight* (IBW) for women and more than 35% above ideal body weight for men. *Body mass index* (BMI) is another way to quantify obesity. A BMI above 27 kg/m² is characteristic of obesity. To determine BMI, use the following formula:

$$\text{BMI} = \frac{\text{wt (kg)}}{\text{ht (m}^2\text{)}} \quad or \quad \frac{\text{wt (lb)}}{\text{ht (in.}^2\text{)}} \times 703$$

Outcome Management

Medical Management

The medical management of obesity should include a combination of diet and behavior modification, exercise, and occasionally medication. Diet instruction with a trained registered dietitian is the optimal intervention to encourage weight loss. A balanced hypocaloric diet in the range of 1100 to 1200 kcal is regarded as the most successful approach to long-term diet modifications. More severe calorie restrictions are difficult to maintain for longer periods and can result in severe vitamin and mineral deficiencies. Clients on low-calorie diets should consume about 60 g/day of protein (~25% of total calories).

An exercise program should be part of the overall care of the obese client. Exercise is an important way to increase the energy expenditure and to facilitate weight loss. Diet restriction in combination with an exercise program, compared with diet restriction alone, is a more successful way to lose weight and maintain the weight loss.

The role of medication in promoting weight loss is controversial, in part because of the known dangers of some regimens. Drugs used to treat obesity are categorized by the following three mechanisms: (1) reduction of food intake, (2) decrease in the absorption of nutrients, and (3) increase in energy expenditure.[15] Although various drugs have been effective in promoting weight loss, any prescribed drug therapy regimen should be under the strict supervision of a qualified health care team to prevent potentially life-threatening complications.

Surgical Management

Surgical treatment of obesity may be considered when the client has been unsuccessful after diet modification, behavioral therapy, exercise, and drug therapy. Two surgical approaches have been used.

JEJUNOILEAL BYPASS. A "shortened small bowel" is created, resulting in malabsorption of nutrients. However, severe metabolic complications—including hypokalemia, hypocalcemia, vitamin B deficiency, and hepatic toxicity—have made this procedure less than optimal.

GASTRIC STAPLING. The more favorable option is revision of the stomach to create a smaller pouch, which limits oral intake. Gastric stapling is the most common surgical approach for the morbidly obese client. This procedure involves creation of a small pouch (~50 to 60 ml) and an outlet to the small intestine. This surgical approach is associated with fewer complications than jejunoileal bypass. Diet instruction must be part of the postoperative care of these clients, focusing on the increased frequency and decreased size of meals. In addition, clients are instructed to take a multivitamin every day.

ANOREXIA NERVOSA AND BULIMIA NERVOSA

Anorexia nervosa and bulimia nervosa have become of increasing concern to nurses and other health care professionals. These abnormalities in eating behavior can result in life-threatening complications. Together, these disorders afflict about 1.2 million young women in the United States. Clients with these disorders are frequently seen by medical-surgical nurses for treatment of the nutritional problems. Mental health consultations are particularly important for these clients.

A client with anorexia nervosa intentionally imposes severe dietary restrictions, resulting in weight loss, endocrine dysfunction, and fluid and electrolyte imbalance. The client's body image is grossly distorted, and her attitude toward eating is impaired. Clients with bulimia nervosa have similar distortions in attitudes toward weight and eating; however, this disorder is characterized by frequent binge eating and purging (vomiting).

Etiology and Risk Factors

The etiology of eating disorders involves biologic, psychological, and social factors. Endocrine changes related to the onset of puberty may be the influencing biologic factor, since dramatic changes in physical appearance and weight gain are occurring. Psychological factors may play a contributing role, especially early sexual and/or physical abuse. The social aspects relate to our society's obsession with thinness. The group most at risk for development of eating disorders is young females 15 to 24 years of age. The incidence of bulimia nervosa is twice that of anorexia nervosa.

Early recognition can lead to treatment before the client's life is in jeopardy. Although the disorders are psychological in origin and not responsive to education, health promotion activities include instruction about avoidance of fad diets, proper nutrition, and ways to build self-confidence safely.

Pathophysiology

The pathophysiologic changes associated with severe eating disorders are similar to those seen in starvation. When nutrient intake is severely limited, the body adapts by utilizing the body's fat stores and sparing protein and glucose stores. With prolonged starvation, significant shifts in fluid and electrolyte balance can occur and can be life-threatening. Alterations in the metabolism of insulin, thyroid hormone, and catecholamines explain common clinical manifestations, including decreases in pulse, respiratory rate, blood pressure, cardiac output, and gut motility.[11] The hypothalamus responds to the lack of nutrient intake with changes in pituitary function, resulting in amenorrhea and infertility.

Clinical Manifestations

Clients with anorexia nervosa are usually first introduced to the health care system when the disordered eating behavior results in obvious weight loss. Clients may limit themselves to 200 to 500 kcal/day—only 60% to 70% of the amount needed for ideal body weight. Physical manifestations (Fig. 29–4) include dry skin, pallor, bradycardia, hypotension, intolerance to cold, constipation, and amenorrhea.

Clinical manifestations of bulimia nervosa include episodes of binge eating followed by self-induced vomiting. The eating and vomiting episodes occur most often in the late afternoon and evening and are done in secret. Some clients may abuse laxatives and diuretics as well. Personality characteristics typical of clients with bulimia are related to depression. Physical manifestations may not be as obvious, since the client with bulimia may be of normal weight without any depletion of fat stores. Less obvious clinical manifestations are erosion of tooth enamel, from frequent vomiting, and esophageal and throat irritation.

Outcome Management

Medical Management

The medical management of eating disorders must include physical and psychological components. Psychotherapy should focus on the underlying problems causing the disordered eating behavior. The physical rehabilitation of nutritional status targets ways to normalize the client's eating pattern and to help the client begin regaining weight, if needed. Excessive caloric intakes are not necessary in clients with anorexia and can actually be harmful in the severely malnourished client. A registered dietitian

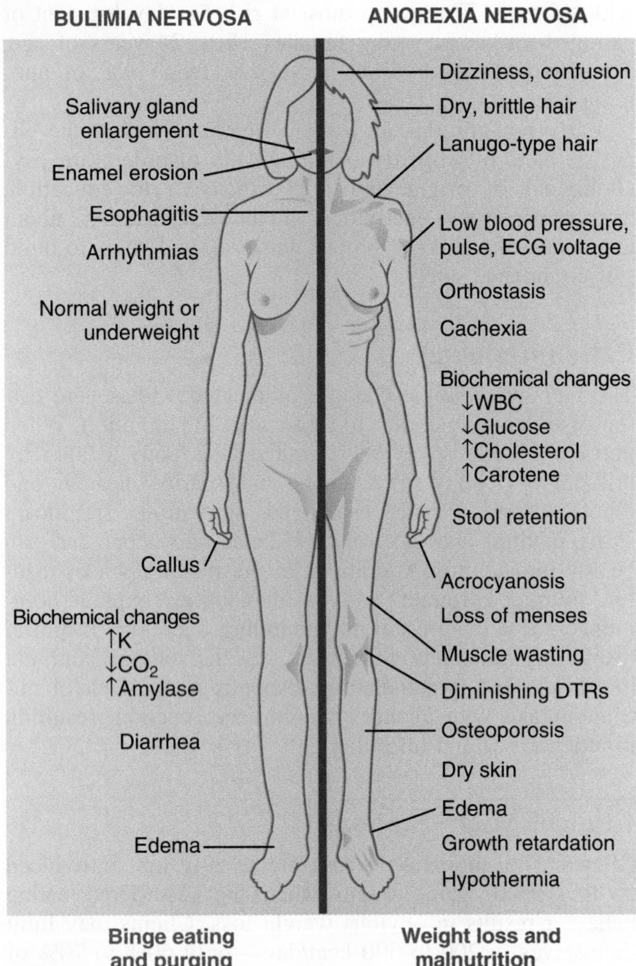

FIGURE 29–4 Physical manifestations of anorexia nervosa and bulimia nervosa. CO_2, carbon dioxide; DTRs, deep tendon reflexes, ECG, electrocardiographic; K, potassium; WBC, white blood cell. (From Mahan, L. K., & Escott-Stump, S. E. [2000]. *Krause's food, nutrition, & diet therapy* [10th ed., p. 521]. Philadelphia: W. B. Saunders.)

should be part of the treatment team and assist in the determination of caloric goals.

Hospitalization is necessary when malnutrition is severe enough to result in serious fluid and electrolyte disturbances. Enteral or parenteral therapy may be needed in extreme cases when the client has not responded to strategies to encourage and improve oral intake. Nutritional support therapies should be introduced slowly in severely malnourished clients to avoid complications of refeeding syndrome. Refeeding syndrome is characterized by precipitous drops in serum potassium, magnesium, and phosphorus when nutrients are administered to depleted clients.

Nursing Management of the Client with Eating Disorders

ASSESSMENT

A comprehensive history will help identify the type of eating disorder (see Chapter 28). Collect details of weight history and eating patterns to successfully identify the problem and help develop an appropriate plan of care. Have the client describe her typical pattern of eating, and ask about the use of appetite-suppressing medication, laxatives, and self-induced vomiting. Other pertinent data to gather include exercise patterns and menstrual history.

DIAGNOSIS, OUTCOMES, INTERVENTIONS

Altered Nutrition: Less Than Body Requirements. The client with anorexia nervosa often experiences *Altered Nutrition: Less Than Body Requirements related to inadequate food intake (anorexia nervosa).*

Outcomes. The client will be able to resume normal eating behaviors. In clients with severe nutritional depletion, the client will be able to regain weight at a safe rate (1 to 2 pounds/week).

Interventions. When caring for a client with anorexia nervosa, help the client select foods from the Food Guide Pyramid for a nutritionally balanced diet. The client is usually allowed to refuse a specific number of foods (such as two or three) so that some sense of control is felt. Observe the client during mealtimes. Be supportive during mealtimes and, if needed, stay with the client after she eats to prevent her from purging. Education related to nutrition must include the client's family, caregivers, or co-residents. An accurate calorie count and regular monitoring of weight are other important interventions. TPN or TEN may be required if the client is severely malnourished.

Altered Nutrition: More Than Body Requirements. Clients with bulimia nervosa and obesity often experience *Altered Nutrition: More Than Body Requirements related to increased food intake.*

Outcomes. The client will lose 1 to 2 pounds per week until ideal body weight is achieved and maintain ideal body weight thereafter.

Interventions. Teach the client how to use the Food Guide Pyramid to select a healthy diet with portions of appropriate size. Encourage the client to eat slowly and to develop a regular exercise pattern. Encourage the client to approach food, eating, and self-image in a new way. Provide emotional support and supervision for the client to overcome stressful periods and break the binge-and-purge cycle.

Body Image Disturbance. The client with an eating disorder often has a *Body Image Disturbance related to misconception of body size or negative feelings (all disorders).*

Outcomes. The client will develop a more normal image of self, as evidenced by statements concerning self and by the client's ability to overcome the eating disorder.

Interventions. Recognize that clients suffering from eating disorders typically have low self-esteem. These clients see the regulation of food and exercise of self-control in eating patterns and amounts as ways to prove themselves successful. It is important that the client's significant others help the client find other areas of self-regard.

Risk for Injury: Dysrhythmias. Both anorexia and bulimia lead to altered fluid and electrolyte balance. This puts them at *Risk for Injury: Dysrhythmias related to hypokalemia.*

Outcomes. The client will maintain normal cardiac output, as evidenced by the absence of cardiac dysrhythmias and adequate tissue perfusion.

Interventions. Monitor the client's serum potassium level at regular intervals. If the potassium level is low, administer potassium supplements as prescribed. If the level is dangerously low, IV replacement may be required.

EVALUATION

It is expected that the client will overcome the eating disorder with consistent and continued treatment and that weight will return to normal.

CONCLUSIONS

The nutritional care of the adult medical-surgical client is an important part of a comprehensive treatment plan. Preventing and treating malnutrition is just one way to facilitate recovery from acute and chronic illness. As a nurse, you have a vital role in nutritional assessment as well as in the prevention and treatment of malnutrition. Clients with eating disorders, such as obesity, anorexia nervosa, and bulimia nervosa, require both medical-surgical and psychological interventions.

THINKING CRITICALLY

1. **You are caring for a 62-year-old client in a nursing home. She has had a cerebrovascular accident and is paralyzed, sometimes confused, and incontinent. She refuses to eat and drink after many episodes of coughing and choking at mealtimes. A small-bore feeding tube has been inserted. When you check the tube for aspirate to confirm patency, you are unable to obtain any return aspirate. What nursing measures should be instituted to determine the problem? What is the priority nursing intervention?**

Factors to Consider. What conditions contribute to the lack of aspirate return? What is your decision if the tube remains occluded?

2. **You are assigned to care for two clients. One is an older man with a 6-month history of difficulty swallowing and a weight loss of 25 pounds. The other client, a woman in her mid-30s, has Crohn's disease and has been admitted with an exacerbation of the disease. How should nutritional needs be addressed for each client?**

Factors to Consider. How should nutritional needs be met for the client with an upper gastrointestinal tract disorder? With a lower gastrointestinal tract disorder?

3. **D. A. is a 20-year-old white woman who is a sophomore in college and living away from home. She is 5 feet 1 inch tall. She has been steadily losing weight, although she participates in the campus meal plan and takes her meals in the dormitory cafeteria. She plays on the college volleyball and basketball teams. Most of the students are excited about Thanksgiving holiday plans, but the dormitory counselor noticed that D. A. has not voiced any plans. She is found unconscious on the floor in the dormitory communal bathroom. She is taken by ambulance to the community hospital. Her college physical health record states that she weighed 98 pounds in June and had no known medical problems. On admission to the hospital, she weighs 79 pounds. What is her percentage of weight loss? What additional data need to be collected?**

Factors to Consider. What interventions can be used to increase D. A.'s food intake? Is it feasible for a nurse on a busy medical-surgical unit to stay with D. A. during and after her meals? What alternatives might be used?

BIBLIOGRAPHY

1. ASPEN Publications. (1998). *The ASPEN nutrition support practice manual*. Silver Spring, MD: Author.
2. ASPEN Publications. (1998). *Clinical pathways and algorithms for delivery of parenteral and enteral nutrition support in adults*. Silver Spring, MD: Author.
3. Bistrian, B., et al. (1974). Protein status of general surgical patients. *Journal of the American Medical Association, 230*, 858–860.
4. Bistrian, B., et al. (1976). Prevalence of malnutrition in general medical patients. *Journal of the American Medical Association, 235*, 1567–1570.
5. Blackburn, G., Miller, D., & Chan, S. (1997). Pharmaceutical treatment of obesity. *Nursing Clinics of North America 32*(4), 831–848.
6. Bowers, S. (1999). Nutrition support for malnourished acutely ill adults. *MEDSURG Nursing, 8*(3), 145–161.
7. Centers for Disease Control and Prevention. (1996). The Hospital Infection Control Practices Advisory Committee: *Guidelines for the prevention of intravascular device–related infections*. Atlanta: Author.
8. Centers for Disease Control and Prevention. (1997). Prevalence of overweight among children, adolescents, and adults—United States, 1988–1994. *Morbidity and Mortality Weekly Report, 46*(9), 198–202.
9. Edington, J., Kon, P., & Martyn, C. (1996). Prevalence of malnutrition in patients in general practice. *Clinical Nutrition, 15*, 60–63.
10. Guenter, P., et al. (1997). Delivery systems and administration of enteral nutrition. In J. Rombeau & R. H. Rolandelli (Eds.), *Clinical nutrition: Enteral and tube feeding* (3rd ed., pp. 240–267). Philadelphia: W. B. Saunders.
11. Huse, D., & Lucas, A. (1999). Behavioral disorders affecting food intake: Anorexia nervosa, bulimia nervosa and other psychiatric conditions. In M. Shils, et al. (Eds.), *Modern nutrition in health and disease* (9th ed., pp. 1513–1522). Baltimore: Williams & Wilkins.
12. Kannel, W., & Gordon T. (1979). Physiologic and medical concomitants of obesity: The Framingham Study. In G. Bray (Ed.), *Obesity in America*. National Institutes of Health, Pub. No.79. Washington, DC: Department Health, Education, and Welfare.
13. Metheny, N. (1997). *Minimum Data Set, version 2*. Des Moines, IA: Briggs Corporation.
14. Metheny N., et al. (1999). pH and concentration of bilirubin in feeding tube aspirates as predictors of tube placement. *Nursing Research, 48*(4), 189–197.
15. National task force on the prevention and treatment of obesity. (1996). Long term pharmacotherapy in the management of obesity. *Journal of the American Medical Association, 276*, 190–196.
16. Poppit, S., & Prentice, A. (1996). Energy density and its role in the control of food intake: Evidence from metabolic community studies. *Appetite, 26*, 153–156.
17. Rombeau, J. L., & Rolandelli, R. H. (1997). *Clinical nutrition: Enteral and tube feeding* (3rd ed.). Philadelphia: W. B. Saunders.
18. Saltzman, E., & Mason, J. (1997). Enteral nutrition in the elderly. In J. L. Rombeau & R. H. Rolandelli (Eds.), *Clinical nutrition: Enteral and tube feeding* (3rd ed., pp. 385–401). Philadelphia: W. B. Saunders.
19. Stoner, N. E. (1997). Nutrition assessment: A practical approach. *Nursing Clinics of North America, 32*(4), 637–650.
20. Torun, B., & Chew, F. (1999). Protein-energy malnutrition. In M. Shils, et al. (Eds.), *Modern nutrition in health and disease* (9th ed., pp. 963–988). Baltimore: Williams & Wilkins.
21. Veterans Affairs Total Parenteral Nutrition Cooperative Study Group. (1991). Perioperative total parenteral nutrition in surgical patients. *New England Journal of Medicine, 325*, 525–532.

REMEMBER *to check out your* **Companion CD ROM**

CHAPTER 30

Management of Clients with Ingestive Disorders

Elizabeth A. Murphy-Blake

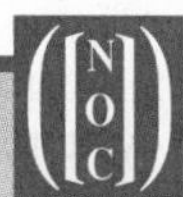

NURSING OUTCOMES CLASSIFICATION (NOC) for Nursing Diagnoses—Clients with Ingestive Disorders

Altered Nutrition: Less Than Body Requirements
Nutritional Status
Nutritional Status: Food and Fluid Intake
Nutritional Status: Nutrient Intake
Altered Oral Mucous Membrane
Oral Health
Tissue Integrity: Skin and Mucous Membrane
Impaired Swallowing
Swallowing Status
Swallowing Status: Esophageal Phase
Swallowing Status: Oral Phase
Swallowing Status: Pharyngeal Phase
Impaired Verbal Communication
Communication Ability
Communication: Expressive Ability
Knowledge Deficit
Knowledge: Illness Care
Knowledge: Treatment Procedure
Knowledge: Treatment Regimen
Pain
Comfort Level
Pain: Disruptive Effects
Risk for Impaired Skin Integrity
Nutritional Status
Nutritional Status: Biochemical Measures
Tissue Integrity: Skin and Mucous Membranes
Wound Healing: Secondary Intention
Risk for Ineffective Individual Coping
Coping
Decision Making
Information Processing
Role Performance
Social Support
Risk for Injury
Risk Control
Risk Detection

The client with an ingestive disorder, regardless of the cause, may have a problem in the oral cavity or esophagus that indicates a common nursing diagnosis, such as *Altered Oral Mucous Membrane; Pain; Altered Nutrition: Less than Body Requirements; Impaired Verbal Communication;* or *Impaired Swallowing.* Usually, the client first experiences pain in the mouth or esophagus or difficulty with swallowing. Shortly thereafter, oral communication and nutritional intake may be compromised. These complications may also result in the development of personal and family coping problems as well as a lack of knowledge related to the treatment required for the disorder.

DENTAL DISORDERS

A person must have healthy teeth and gums for good general health. Health care providers strive to preserve healthy gums and natural teeth for as long as possible for these reasons:

- Natural teeth are almost always more functional in masticating food than is a dental prosthesis.
- Effective mastication of food helps promote efficient digestion.
- Efficient digestion of food results in healthy gastrointestinal (GI) function and good general health.

The most frequent causes of tooth loss are dental decay and periodontal disease. Plaque is the major cause of both caries (decay) and periodontal disease. The best treatment for dental caries is prevention. Encourage clients to brush and floss regularly, eat a diet low in simple carbohydrates, use fluoride, and schedule regular visits to the dentist for examination, cleaning, and treatment of dental caries.

Increasing the resistance of the enamel also helps prevent caries. The resistance of enamel increases with the ingestion of fluoridated water during tooth formation and the continued use of fluoride throughout life. The daily use of fluoride rinses produces a more acid-resistant structure, enhances tooth mineralization, and interferes with bacterial growth. In addition, the dentist may apply topical fluoride to the teeth.

Treatment of dental caries may include drilling out cavities and filling them with material to restore the tooth, extraction (removal) of the entire tooth, and preservation of the tooth by *root canal therapy* (pulpectomy) followed by proper restoration. Any number of teeth can be removed because of disease. They are usually replaced with some type of dental prosthesis (crowns, dentures, dental implants). If only one tooth or a few teeth are removed,

This chapter incorporates material written for the fifth edition by Jane Hokanson Hawks.

local anesthesia is usually used. Removing several teeth or having a full-mouth extraction may require sedation or general anesthesia. Potential complications include hemorrhage and abscess formation.

During root canal therapy, the entire pulp of the tooth is removed. The canal space within the roots is filled aseptically and sealed to prevent infection. The tooth remains rooted in the gingiva and can still be used. Subsequent restoration of the tooth is essential to retain the tooth in a normal functional relationship with the rest of the teeth.

Periodontal disease, caused by plaque formation and bacterial colonization, results in gingival inflammation if the plaque is not removed by proper brushing and flossing. Eventually, inflammation destroys the underlying tissues and separates the gingiva from the tooth. In periodontitis, the inflammation extends from the gums into the alveolar bone and periodontal ligament, destroying the supporting structures of the teeth. As a result, the teeth loosen and extraction may be required.

Postoperative care of a tooth extraction includes assessing the oral cavity for bleeding and monitoring vital signs (if the client stays in an inpatient facility or recovery area). A gauze pad is usually placed over the extraction site, and the client is instructed to bite down gently on the pad to maintain pressure. Ice may be applied to the jaw over the site to decrease the blood flow and edema. Small amounts of bleeding may be normal, but you should notify the dentist or physician (or instruct the client to do so) if bleeding lasts longer than 1 hour.

The client usually requires analgesics to control pain. Instruct the client to eat soft foods and to avoid hot or cold foods for several days. The client should gently rinse the mouth with normal saline but should avoid brushing any remaining teeth for about 24 hours.

ORAL DISORDERS

STOMATITIS

Stomatitis, an inflammation of the oral cavity, may be of infectious origin or a manifestation of a systemic condition. It may be caused by *mechanical* trauma, such as injury, or *chemical* trauma, such as drugs given for cancer treatment. Jagged teeth, cheek-biting, and mouth-breathing also may result in mechanical trauma. Certain foods and drinks and sensitivity to mouthwashes or toothpaste may produce chemical trauma. The imflammatory sloughing of tissue allows organisms to multiply; thus, stomatitis may lead to infection by viruses, bacteria, yeasts, or fungus.

Stomatitis is classified as primary or secondary, depending on the cause. Primary stomatitis includes aphthous stomatitis (canker sore), herpes simplex, and Vincent's angina. Secondary stomatitis results when a client's lowered resistance allows an opportunistic infection to develop. Secondary stomatitis can be caused by a local or systemic disorder. Systemic disorders that can affect the oral mucous membranes include (1) allergies, (2) bone marrow disorders, (3) nutritional disorders, (4) immunodeficiency disorders, and (5) chemotherapy, radiation therapy, or immunosuppressive therapy.

■ APHTHOUS STOMATITIS

Commonly known as *canker sores,* the lesions caused by aphthous stomatitis are recurrent, small, and ulcerated. They develop in the soft tissues of the mouth, including the lips, tongue, and insides of the cheeks. Canker sores affect people of all age groups, although young adult women are more frequently affected. The cause of canker sores is unknown, but they may be related to emotional stress, trauma, vitamin deficiency, food and drug allergies, endocrine imbalances, and viral infections. Prevention is almost impossible because the exact cause is unknown.

These lesions start as small, reddened areas that undergo central necrosis and ulceration. The lesions are not infectious but are simply inflammatory. They heal within 1 to 3 weeks without treatment. Assessment usually reveals a well-circumscribed erythematous macule that undergoes necrosis, creating a well-defined pseudomembranous ulcer with an erythematous border.

Medical treatment involves topical application of amlexanox (Aphthasol) to the ulcer. Topical or systemic steroids may shorten the healing time. In addition, to suppress recurrence, teach clients prone to allergic reactions to avoid tomatoes, chocolate, eggs, shellfish, milk products, nuts, and citrus fruits.

■ HERPES SIMPLEX

Herpes simplex stomatitis is a form of inflammation and ulceration caused by the herpes simplex virus (HSV). By age 5 years, 90% of the population has been infected with *primary* herpes simplex. When the client is first infected with the primary herpes virus, lesions appear in the oral cavity. These vesicles, which can appear throughout the oral cavity, rupture to form ulcerated areas that resemble canker sores and heal within several weeks. The client's tongue has a characteristic heavy white coating. The client may have manifestations of generalized infection as well.

Secondary herpes is a recurrent infection that appears to lie dormant after the primary herpes infection. Secondary herpes takes the form of herpes labialis (fever blister, cold sore) and is often seen in clients receiving immunosuppressants and in those with human immunodeficiency virus (HIV) infection or acquired immunodeficiency syndrome (AIDS). Any infection, especially upper respiratory infections, fever, stress, or even sunlight, can reactivate the virus.

Assessment reveals clear, vesicular lesions, most often appearing at the mucocutaneous junction of the lips (Fig. 30–1) and face. The lesions are contagious, last about 1 week, and heal without scarring. Later in the course of the infection, the tongue may appear coated and the client may complain of a foul breath odor.

General pain may be treated with analgesics. Local ointments and anesthetics may soothe lesions. Clients who are immunocompromised are started on intravenous (IV) acyclovir (Zovirax). Clients with competent immune systems may be given acyclovir in oral or topical forms or penciclovir (Denavir) topical cream. Unless the ulcer is secondarily infected, antimicrobial treatment does not affect the progress of the ulcer.

■ VINCENT'S ANGINA

Vincent's angina (necrotizing ulcerative gingivitis, trench mouth) is an acute bacterial infection of the gingivae

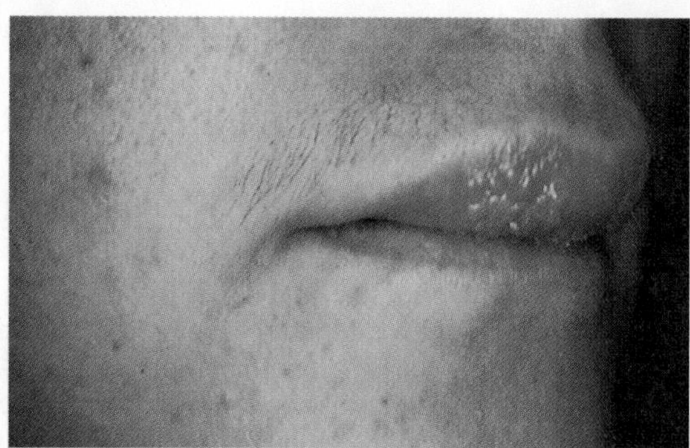

FIGURE 30–1 Herpes simplex of the lip. (From Hurwitz, S. [1993]. *Clinical pediatric dermatology* [2nd ed., p. 321]. Philadelphia: W. B. Saunders.)

caused by resident flora in the mouth, fusiform bacteria, and spirochetes. Precipitating factors include poor oral hygiene, increased age, nutritional deficiencies, lack of rest and sleep, local tissue damage, and debilitating diseases, such as infectious mononucleosis, nonspecific viral infections, bacterial infections, blood dyscrasias, and diabetes mellitus. Most of these factors are unavoidable and therefore unpreventable. This condition is not contagious.

The disease is of sudden onset, causes erythema and ulceration of the gingivae, and affects the entire oropharynx. Once the tonsils are removed, this disorder rarely recurs. Assessment reveals ulcers covered with a pseudomembrane. A smear from an ulcer exudate identifies the causative organisms. Clients often have an elevated white blood cell (WBC) count. The client may complain of a foul taste, pain, a choking sensation, fever, thick secretions, anorexia, and occasionally, lymphadenopathy.

Management consists of removing the devitalized tissue and correcting the underlying cause with rest, improved oral hygiene, a bland diet, and vitamins. Pain medications and saline, peroxide, or half-saline half-peroxide mouthwashes promote comfort.

CANDIDIASIS

Candidiasis (moniliasis, thrush) is caused by the organism *Candida albicans,* a yeast-like fungus that is part of the normal flora of the oral cavity. Candidiasis of the oral cavity is commonly seen in immunosuppressed clients, such as those receiving chemotherapy or those with HIV infection or AIDS. The incidence is also increased in clients with diabetes mellitus and those who are pregnant, under stress, receiving high-dose or long-term antibiotic therapy, or receiving long-term tube feeding.

Etiology and Risk Factors

When the client is in a state of immunosuppression or has decreased levels of some normal oral flora, an overgrowth of the normal flora *Candida* can occur. Candidiasis commonly occurs in critically ill clients with prolonged intubation. The major risk factors are immunosuppression and prolonged use of antibiotics that disrupts the normal flora. Clients with either risk factor should be monitored closely. Prophylactic treatment is often started for these high-risk clients.

Pathophysiology

Candidiasis is a secondary infection resulting from either an immunodeficiency or prolonged use of antibiotics. When the normal flora is disrupted, an overgrowth of the *Candida* organism may occur.

Clinical Manifestations

Assessment reveals white patches on the tongue, palate, and buccal mucosa (Fig. 30–2). These lesions adhere firmly to the tissues and are difficult to remove. The lesions are often referred to as "milk curds" because of their appearance. Clients describe the lesions as dry and hot. Clients who have recurrent candidiasis infections should be examined for a possible systemic cause.

Outcome Management

Medical Management

Medical management includes topical antifungal agents as well as other topical agents to alleviate the infection and provide pain relief. Analgesics, such as acetaminophen or aspirin, may also be administered to promote pain relief. Mouthwashes of warm saline (or water) or half warm saline (or water) and half hydrogen peroxide are often ordered as part of an oral hygiene regimen. A bland liquid or puréed diet may be necessary. Prophylactic use of antifungal agents is indicated for high-risk clients. Oral pharyngeal cultures should be taken if infection is suspected.

Nursing Management of the Medical Client

ASSESSMENT

Clients with the risk factors of immunosuppression or prolonged antibiotic use should be monitored closely. Assess whether the client has pain, tenderness, or bleeding in any part of the oral cavity or has had any febrile episodes. Ask about a history of previous infection elsewhere in the body and the use of any medications, especially antibiotics. Ask the client about a history of treatment with radiation or chemotherapy because both can

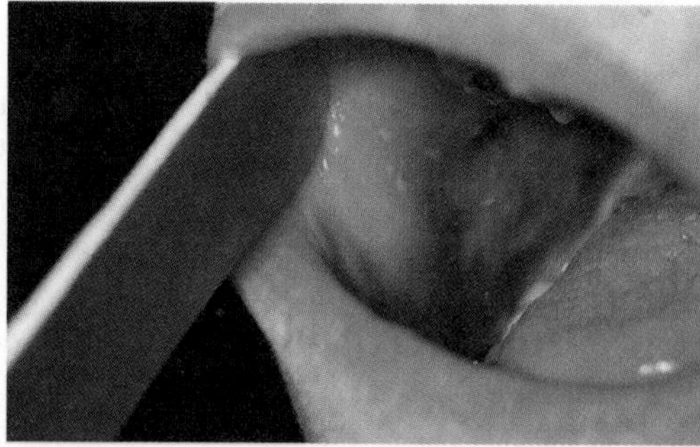

FIGURE 30–2 Oral candidiasis. Note the small white patches on the buccal mucosa. (From Moschella, S. L., & Hurley, H. J. [1992]. *Dermatology* [3rd ed., p. 231]. Philadelphia: W. B. Saunders.)

affect the oral mucosa. Prophylactic treatment for these high-risk clients may have been instituted.

To perform the oral assessment, have a tongue blade and good lighting and wear gloves. Inspect the oral cavity, noting any areas of inflammation, vesicular eruptions, ulcers, white patches, or erythema of the gingivae.

DIAGNOSIS, OUTCOMES, INTERVENTIONS

Pain. A common nursing diagnosis for the client with candidiasis is *Pain related to altered oral mucous membrane and ulcerations.*

Outcomes. The client's pain will be relieved or controlled, as evidenced by expressions of pain relief and demonstrating the ability to maintain normal nutrition.

Interventions

Minimize Pain. Assess for oral pain using a pain scale, and administer analgesics, such as aspirin or acetaminophen, as ordered. Topical agents and topical mouth rinses often provide pain relief. Antifungal agents to rinse with and swallow are used to alleviate the infection. A change in diet to liquid or puréed foods often eases the discomfort of eating. The client should avoid spicy foods, citrus juices, and hot liquids.

Provide Oral Care. Clients with painful lesions cannot tolerate commercial mouthwashes because of the high alcohol level in these products. A solution of warm saline (or water), half-strength hydrogen peroxide, or mouthwash formulas specific to many institutions are better tolerated and may promote healing. If painful oral lesions are present, suggest modifications in the client's oral hygiene regimen. Gauze pads may replace toothbrushes, and oral rinses may be needed to clean the area of debris and promote healing.

Promote Self-Care

Give the client oral and written instructions regarding a dental hygiene regimen, diet, medications, and manifestations of complications. The client should demonstrate proper techniques of dental hygiene. Minimal home health care preparation is required unless the client requires alternative feeding routes. If the client is receiving tube feedings, referral to a home health agency may be appropriate. If home care is not affordable, teach the client or significant other how to perform the tube feedings (see Chapter 29). The client should be scheduled for follow-up to assess for recurrence.

EVALUATION

The infection should clear up within a few days to a week in most clients. Assess the client for other risk factors if reinfection occurs. Educate the client about the signs of infection and what to report to the health care practitioner.

TUMORS OF THE ORAL CAVITY

BENIGN TUMORS OF THE ORAL CAVITY

The most common benign tumors of the mouth are fibromas, lipomas, neurofibromas, and hemangiomas. As with benign tumors in other parts of the body, oral tumors cause problems primarily by occupying space and causing pressure. Benign tumors are usually excised if they cause functional or cosmetic problems.

PREMALIGNANT TUMORS OF THE ORAL CAVITY

LEUKOPLAKIA. Leukoplakia, a potentially precancerous, yellow-white or gray-white lesion, may occur in any region of the mouth. The size and shape of lesions vary, but they are usually elevated and have a roughened or leathery surface and clearly defined borders (Fig. 30–3). Leukoplakia is a common disorder of the oral mucous membranes, usually seen in people in their 30s and 40s. Men are affected twice as often as women; however, the incidence in women is increasing because of the increasing number of women who smoke.

Leukoplakia results from chronic irritation of the mucosa by physical, chemical, or thermal factors. Physical factors include poorly fitting dentures, broken teeth, cheek nibbling, and occlusion problems. Chemical and thermal factors arise from the use of tobacco products, both inhaled and chewing products. Ingestion of excessively hot food and beverages also places the person at risk. This condition may also develop from systemic factors such as poor nutrition or syphilis.

ERYTHROPLAKIA. Erythroplakia is a red, velvety-appearing patch that commonly indicates early squamous cell carcinoma. It occurs most frequently in people ages 50 to 60, with men and women equally affected. Risk factors are the same as those for squamous cell carcinoma.

MALIGNANT TUMORS OF THE ORAL CAVITY

Cancers of the oral cavity account for fewer than 3% of total cases of body malignancies. Cancers in this area most frequently are seen in people in their 40s and 50s and in men more frequently than women. Cancers of the oral cavity are most often associated with alcohol consumption and tobacco use. With the increase of tobacco use by younger people, especially the use of smokeless (chewing) tobacco, and by women, the age and sex ratios are changing.

Health promotion actions are to teach clients to avoid excessive use of tobacco, alcohol, and very hot beverages and foods. Encourage clients to maintain meticulous oral hygiene, to eat a well-balanced diet, and to use sunscreen

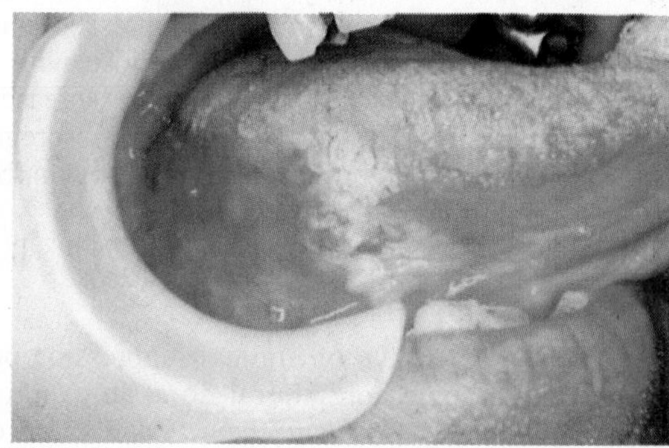

FIGURE 30–3 Leukoplakia of the lateral edge of the tongue. (From Sleisenger, M. H., & Fordtran, J. S. [1989]. *Gastrointestinal disease: Pathophysiology, diagnosis, and management* [4th ed.]. Philadelphia: W. B. Saunders.)

during exposure to sunlight. Health maintenance activities involve oral screening of smokers and drinkers of alcohol and teaching these high-risk people to observe for early manifestations of oral cancer. Health restoration interventions include the management of chemotherapy and radiation for clients after tumor excision and providing nutritional support as needed.

BASAL CELL CARCINOMA. Basal cell carcinoma of the oral cavity, the second most common oral cancer, occurs primarily on the lips. It starts as a small scab that develops into an ulcer with a characteristic pearly border. Basal cell carcinoma primarily occurs as a result of excessive exposure to sunlight, tending to occur more commonly in fair-skinned people who are exposed to sunlight.

SQUAMOUS CELL CARCINOMA. Squamous cell carcinoma is a malignant growth arising from tiny flat squamous cells that line mucous membranes. Squamous cell carcinoma is the leading type of oral cancer. Most tumors occur in clients older than age 45. Common sites include the lower lip and tongue. About 95% of cancers found on the tongue are squamous cell carcinomas. Malignancies of the tongue represent 1% to 1.5% of all malignancies in the United States.

The primary cause of squamous cell carcinoma is chronic irritation of the mucous lining of the mouth and oral cavity. Overuse of alcohol and tobacco is the primary cause of oral irritation. In combination, tobacco and alcohol are extremely destructive to the oral mucosa.

Squamous cell carcinoma develops from tiny cells that line the oral cavity. It can occur on the lips, buccal mucosa, tongue (Fig. 30–4), floor of the mouth, and tonsils. It is usually well differentiated, and the rate of metastasis is less than 10%. Cells metastasize by direct infiltration of local lymph nodes and can extend into the buccal fat and even to the mandible.

Manifestations may include a sore or lesion in the oral cavity. Red-appearing (erythroplakia) squamous cell carcinomas may not be well delineated and often bleed easily. Because squamous cell carcinomas usually grow slowly, they may be large before manifestations are detected. Other manifestations can include a mild irritation of the tongue, sore throat, trouble with wearing dentures, or pain in the tongue or ear.

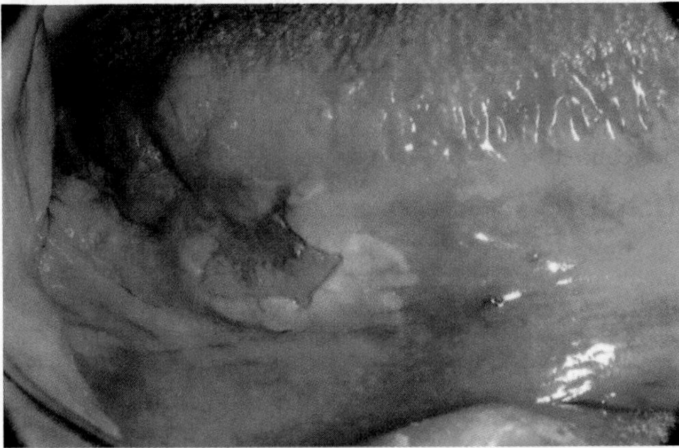

FIGURE 30–4 Oral squamous cell carcinoma. This is an ulcerated lesion with surrounding leukoplakia on the posterior lateral and ventral portions of the tongue. (From Neville, B. W., et al. [1995]. *Oral and maxillofacial pathology.* Philadelphia: W. B. Saunders.)

Only a biopsy of lesions positively confirms a diagnosis of oral cancer. Cytologic examination of mucosa thought to be malignant, while valuable in screening, unfortunately is not used widely enough to reduce the mortality rate. To be a valuable diagnostic aid, cytologic examination must be followed by biopsy when questionable cells are found. Biopsies may be performed with local or general anesthesia. To diagnose carcinoma at the base of the tongue, a laryngoscopic examination must be performed.

Outcome Management

Medical Management

INHIBIT TUMOR GROWTH

The survival rate of clients with oral cancer depends on the site and staging of the tumor. The tumor-node-metastasis (TNM) staging system (see Chapter 19) is used to stage oral cancers. Of the oral cancers, cancer of the lip carries one of the highest cure rates. Squamous cell carcinoma of the tongue carries the poorest prognosis because of the tongue's extensive vascular and lymphatic supply. Management of oral cancers includes radiation therapy, chemotherapy, and surgery and, again, depends on the site and staging of the tumor.

RADIATION THERAPY. Oral cancers can be treated with *external beam therapy* or *interstitial radiation therapy (brachytherapy).* The external beam passes through the skin or mucous membrane to the tumor. Interstitial radiation involves implanting radioactive seeds into the tissue for a prescribed period of time. Because interstitial radiation affects local tissue, it is used for small lesions that have not infiltrated the surrounding tissue. The client undergoing interstitial radiation is hospitalized and placed on radiation precautions (see Chapter 19) while the materials are active.

CHEMOTHERAPY. The effectiveness of chemotherapy for the treatment of oral cancers is unknown. Several drugs are used to treat head and neck cancers. They include bleomycin (Blenoxane), cisplatin (Platinol), cyclophosphamide (Cytoxan), doxorubicin (Adriamycin), 5-fluorouracil (5-FU), hydroxyurea (Hydrea), methotrexate (Folex), and vincristine (Oncovin).

Nursing Management of the Medical Client

ASSESSMENT

Carefully question the client about manifestations. A common finding is that of a painful ulcer. Assess the client for difficulty in swallowing, white or red patches on the oral mucosa, bleeding in the mouth, lumps in the neck, pain referred to the ear, foul odor, and hoarseness. Ask about the use of alcohol and tobacco, oral hygiene habits, and sun exposure. Assess the client's rehabilitative needs. Surgery can cause disfigurement and may alter speech; the client may experience depression from a change in body image and the diagnosis of cancer.

DIAGNOSIS, OUTCOMES, INTERVENTIONS

Altered Oral Mucous Membrane. A common nursing diagnosis for the client who has oral cancer or who is at risk for oral cancer is *Altered Oral Mucous Membrane related to irritants such as alcohol or tobacco, chemotherapy, radiation therapy, ill-fitting dentures, poor nutrition, and knowledge deficit of prevention and treatment of oral lesions.*

Outcomes. The client will understand and comply with measures to maintain the oral mucosa, as evidenced by statements of understanding of the substances and activities to avoid. The client will also be able to discuss the treatment regimen.

Interventions

Avoid Oral Irritants. Teach the client about the disease and treatment protocols. Advise the client to avoid chemical, physical, and thermal oral trauma; to perform careful, frequent oral hygiene, preferably three times daily; to see a dentist about ill-fitting dentures; and to see a physician about any mouth lesion that does not heal in 2 to 3 weeks.

Promote Comfort. If the client is receiving radiation therapy or chemotherapy, discuss possible side effects of these forms of treatment. Provide the client with comfort measures to minimize side effects, such as frequent oral hygiene and antiemetics to prevent nausea and vomiting.

Altered Nutrition: Less Than Body Requirements. Clients with oral cancers often have nutritional difficulties, and a usual nursing diagnosis is *Altered Nutrition: Less than Body Requirements related to oral pain and difficulty eating and swallowing.*

Outcomes. The client will maintain weight or show weight gain before surgery, as evidenced by an increase in intake, maintenance of weight, or a weight gain of 1 pound per week preoperatively.

Interventions

Promote Nutrition. The location and size of a tumor, and the pain it causes, commonly interfere with a client's ability to eat. Small, frequent feedings can promote intake. Giving an analgesic 30 to 45 minutes before a meal can decrease the pain associated with eating. Provide oral care before and after meals to remove debris and minimize oral odors. Give the client with poor nutrition guidelines for improving the diet. Supply pamphlets outlining the basic nutrients for good health, and refer the client to a dietitian as needed.

Relieve Mouth Dryness. Unfortunately, treatments such as radiation alter salivation and taste perception. Xerostomia (dryness of the mouth) usually lessens with the use of pilocarpine and artificial saliva. Suggest that the client chew sugarless gum or suck on sugar-free hard candy to increase moisture. The client should perform frequent oral rinses with cool water to reduce dryness.

EVALUATION

The best outcome is for the client to stop high-risk behaviors for oral cancer, undergo successful treatment, and maintain nutritional status.

Surgical Management

Surgical management of oral cancers can range from local excision of small tumors to extensive surgery for invasive tumors. Small tumors can be treated in outpatient facilities by local excision, radiation, or laser therapy. Small tumors of the floor of the mouth can be locally excised with or without removing a portion of the mandible. Small tumors in the anterior floor of the mouth can be excised, and the area can be reconstructed with the use of a split-thickness skin graft.

A thin layer of skin, usually from the anterior thigh, can line the surgical site, allowing the client to maintain good mobility and function of the tongue. Xeroform gauze is usually placed over the skin graft and sutured into place. This can restrict the tongue, causing aspiration of secretions. Because of this packing and as a result of postoperative edema, a tracheostomy tube (see Chapter 60) is usually placed until edema subsides and the oral airway is patent. The client receives nothing by mouth (NPO) for 7 to 10 days after surgery to allow for healing. A nasogastric (NG) feeding tube, gastrostomy, or percutaneous endoscopic gastrostomy (PEG) is used to provide nutrition until the client can resume oral feedings (see Chapter 29).

Clients with invasive tumors require extensive surgical excision, usually involving removal of associated lymph nodes. Depending on the location, glossectomy (removal of the tongue), mandibulectomy (removal of the mandible), hemiglossectomy (removal of part of the tongue), or radical neck dissection may be performed. A radical neck dissection is an extensive procedure that involves removal of all tissue under the skin, from the jaw down to the clavicle, and from the anterior border of the trapezius muscle to the midline. To remove the cervical lymph nodes in this procedure, the surgeon must remove the sternocleidomastoid muscle, the spinal accessory nerve, and the jugular vein. A modified radical neck dissection involves removal of the lymph nodes only and is preferred when the disease is confined to mobile lymph nodes (see Chapter 60 for surgical management of cancer of the larynx). The Commando procedure is an extensive oral operation in which part of the mandible is excised along with the oral lesion. This procedure is often combined with a radical neck dissection.

Nursing Management of the Surgical Client

ASSESSMENT

Assessment of the surgical client is similar to assessment of the medical client. Complete routine preoperative and postoperative assessments, and ensure that the client understands the implications of the selected surgical approach and the associated postoperative assessments and treatments. Assessment of rehabilitative needs, such as speech therapy and coping with disfigurement, may also be required.

DIAGNOSIS, OUTCOMES, INTERVENTIONS

Risk for Injury. Surgery for oral cancer involves many potential risks. *Risk for Injury related to surgical procedure, including hemorrhage, ineffective airway clearance and possible wound infection* is an appropriate nursing diagnosis.

Outcomes. The client will remain free from injury, as evidenced by absence of excessive bleeding, maintenance of a patent airway, and wound healing without manifestations of infection.

Interventions

Maintain Airway. The most critical postoperative intervention is to maintain a patent airway. If the surgical procedure has been extensive, a tracheostomy is usually in place to help prevent respiratory difficulty from edema of the oral and pharyngeal structures. Clients at risk for ineffective airway clearance should be in a semi-Fowler to a high Fowler position after surgery to promote venous lymphatic drainage. The client may have a dusky appearance about the face from venous congestion. Pulse oximeter readings also should be used to determine whether the client is sufficiently oxygenated.

For the client with a tracheostomy, some blood-tinged mucus is normal in tracheal secretions for the first 48 hours after surgery. Bright red bleeding from the tracheostomy tube or site is a manifestation of hemorrhage. Notify the physician immediately if this occurs.

Provide Wound Care. The amount of nursing care required by the client after surgery depends on the extent of the procedure. After local excisions, teach the client how to perform hygiene gently. If a dressing and packing are in place, monitor the amount of drainage. After the dressing and packing are removed, the client should rinse the oral cavity with a mild half-strength form of hydrogen peroxide and water or saline solution every 4 hours to remove debris and promote healing. If half-strength hydrogen peroxide and water is used, it should be followed with normal saline or water to prevent drying.

With more extensive surgery, the suture lines must be protected from trauma. Oral hygiene and oral suctioning are usually not implemented until healing has begun and the physician decides that this type of cleaning can be performed.

Monitor for Bleeding. Hemorrhage may occur at any time after surgery, especially with extensive resection of the tongue. Hemorrhage can be massive because of the large vessels that supply the mouth and oral area. If bleeding occurs, apply pressure on the site until the bleeding stops spontaneously or stops with medical or surgical intervention. Surgical repair may be required. If an extensive resection is performed requiring skin grafts, monitor the site every 4 to 8 hours for drainage and manifestations of infection.

Altered Nutrition: Less Than Body Requirements. After surgical intervention for oral cancers, the client often continues to have difficulties with nutrition. *Altered Nutrition: Less Than Body Requirements related to altered oral mucosa and surgical procedure* is an appropriate nursing diagnosis.

Outcomes. The client will maintain or gain weight after surgery, as evidenced by stabilization of weight and, possibly, a weight gain of 1 pound per week.

Interventions

Administer Supplemental Nutrition. Immediately after surgery, monitor IV hydration. Assess bowel sounds every shift. The return of bowel sounds is often an indication to begin tube feedings. When adding each feeding to the feeding bag, assess the client for proper tube placement and retention of stomach contents. Administer nutritional supplements by pump or bolus feedings. In addition, the physician may order total parenteral nutrition (TPN) as the first line of nutritional management (see Chapter 29 and the achalasia discussion in this chapter).

Discuss Eating Modifications. Once the edema has subsided, healing has occurred, and the tracheostomy tube has been removed, the client may resume oral feedings. Caution the client about a decrease in sensation in the oral cavity after surgery. Assess swallowing carefully before eating begins. Instruct the client to avoid putting food directly on the surgical resection site. After meals, the client should always perform oral hygiene to remove any particles that remain and that may cause problems with the incision.

Impaired Verbal Communication. When the client has a tracheostomy after surgery, a common diagnosis is *Impaired Verbal Communication related to the presence of tracheostomy.*

Outcomes. The client will use alternative forms of communication to communicate with staff and significant others.

Interventions

Promote Alternate Forms of Communication. Assess the client's literacy, and provide paper and pencil, magic slate, chalkboard or a marker board for the client to write on as a substitute for talking. An alternative is to provide the client with a picture board to use for communicating any needs. Ideally, the assessment and instruction are completed preoperatively. The client should be allowed to communicate by gestures or written notes if this approach puts the client at ease. Most important, your manner should communicate acceptance, compassion, and caring. It is common to treat clients who cannot talk as though they cannot hear or understand. Be alert to any tendency to treat these clients as though they were mentally incompetent or deaf. Help the client avoid social isolation by taking the client for walks and meeting others. Friendly social encounters and physical activity can help alleviate depression.

Relieve Anxiety. Help clients who cannot speak to express their needs, concerns, and feelings. Check on the client frequently to reduce anxiety and loneliness. Place the call light within easy reach, and respond to the light promptly. If an intercom is used, it should be appropriately labeled regarding the client's limited ability to speak.

EVALUATION

The most favorable outcome is that the client heals within 6 weeks to 3 months, according to the extent of the radical surgery, and without complications. If complications develop, provide the name of the person to call. Also evaluate the client's ability to maintain intake of nutrients. If the client can self-feed via a tube until healing occurs and then increase oral intake, nutritional status should remain adequate. All clients also need tremendous emotional support with this type of surgical intervention and need to be evaluated for possible complications related to lack of support from family or significant others.

Self-Care

On discharge, supply the client and family with complete instructions regarding diet, medications, manifestations of complications, and any treatments, such as care of the wound or tracheostomy. Explain how and when to contact health care practitioners. The client needs to be seen by the physician after discharge to ensure complete healing of any extensive surgical wounds. If the client has a tracheostomy, it may be permanent or may be closed at a later date. Clients who have undergone extensive surgery may need a referral to a home health agency for possible assistance with respiratory support (home oxygen), suctioning, nutritional support, and wound and tracheostomy care.

DISORDERS OF THE SALIVARY GLANDS

INFLAMMATION

Parotitis ("surgical mumps") is an inflammation of the parotid glands. It is the most common inflammatory condition affecting the salivary glands and probably results from inactivity of the glands caused by certain medications (such as diuretics), prolonged NG intubation, and lack of oral intake, such as that seen in postoperative clients. As secretions of the salivary gland diminish, oral bacteria have an opportunity to invade the gland and multiply. Interventions involve:

- Administering frequent oral hygiene to keep the bacterial count of the mouth low
- Keeping the client well hydrated
- Suggesting that the client use sugarless hard candies or chew sugarless gum to stimulate secretion of saliva

CALCULI

Stones, or calculi, form in the salivary glands when the glands are inactive and a metabolic condition favors the precipitation of salts. A nidus, or focus of origin, is necessary for stimulating salt precipitation. Assessment reveals that irritation from the stones causes local inflammation, swelling, and pain when the gland is stimulated to secrete, as during chewing. Intervention requires local excision by a physician. Stones occur most commonly in the submaxillary glands, probably because of the longer length of the duct and production of viscous alkaline secretions.

TUMORS

Most tumors in the salivary glands are benign. The most frequently seen malignant tumor is adenocarcinoma. Both benign and malignant tumors are characterized by enlargement of the gland. Pain occurs when expansion within the capsule of the gland creates pressure on sensory nerves. The treatment of choice for both benign and malignant tumors is usually surgical excision. If the tumor has recurred or is highly malignant, radiation therapy may also be used.

DISORDERS OF THE ESOPHAGUS

The most common manifestation of esophageal disease is dysphagia (difficulty with swallowing). Other manifestations include regurgitation, pain (which is probably linked with spasm), and heartburn.

DYSPHAGIA

Dysphagia can be caused by any esophageal disorder. Specific causes include neuromotor malfunction, mechanical obstruction, cardiovascular abnormalities, and neurologic diseases.

■ DYSPHAGIA CAUSED BY MECHANICAL OBSTRUCTIONS

Mechanical obstructions causing dysphagia include congenital defects, cancer, and acquired conditions such as hiatal hernia. When an obstruction narrows the esophageal lumen, clients first experience dysphagia only with solid foods. Later, dysphagia becomes associated with semisolid foods and liquids. Finally, clients are unable to swallow their own saliva. Obstructive disorders, particularly esophageal cancer, may be accompanied by weight loss and cachexia.

■ DYSPHAGIA CAUSED BY CARDIOVASCULAR ABNORMALITIES

Dysphagia also may result from cardiovascular abnormalities, particularly in older people. Specific conditions causing vascular dysphagia include an enlarged heart, an aortic aneurysm, and calcification of the descending aorta. Figure 30–5 shows the relationship of the heart and great arteries to the esophagus.

■ DYSPHAGIA CAUSED BY NEUROLOGIC DISEASES

Dysphagia also may be caused by certain neurologic diseases, such as cerebrovascular accident (CVA), multiple

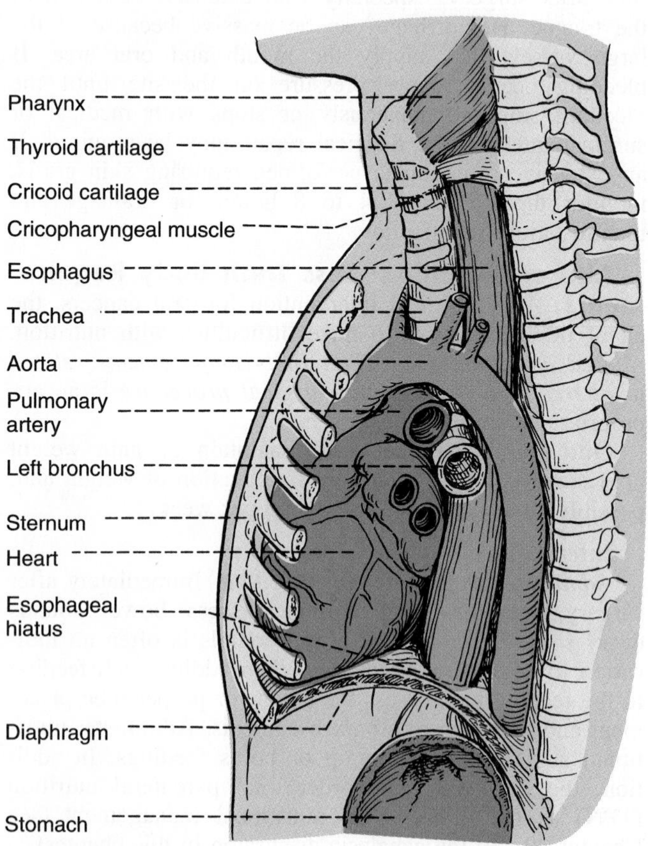

FIGURE 30–5 Relationship of the heart and great arteries to the esophagus.

sclerosis, poliomyelitis, and amyotrophic lateral sclerosis (ALS). CVA is the most frequent cause of dysphagia.

■ DYSPHAGIA FROM OTHER CAUSES

Dysphagia can be experienced after swallowing if food gets caught in the esophagus. Clients may obtain relief by drinking liquids to force the impacted bolus through the narrow segment or by retching to dislodge the food. If vomiting does not succeed, endoscopy may be used to remove food lodged in the esophagus.

REGURGITATION

Regurgitation is the ejection of small amounts of chyme or gastric juice from the mouth without antecedent nausea. It is usually caused by an incompetent lower esophageal sphincter (LES). Regurgitation occurring immediately after swallowing results from structural or motor abnormality in the LES. Contributing factors include abnormal motor activity, increased abdominal pressure, and sphincter abnormality. Regurgitation occurs with achalasia, pylorospasm, lesions proximal to the cardia, hiatal hernia, reflux esophagitis, and esophageal ulcer or cancer. Stooping or lying down facilitates the flow of gastric contents into the esophagus, thus exacerbating regurgitation.

PAIN

Pain, which may be constant or may occur only with swallowing, suggests diffuse esophageal spasm. Pain may result from alterations of the mucosa from reflux disease, radiation, or viral infection. Pain that affects the esophageal mucosa and occurs with swallowing is called *odynophagia.* The client usually describes the pain as sharp, constricting, sticking, crushing, stabbing, or knife-like. Odynophagia is usually severe, quite distressing, and often associated with a deep and long-lasting pain. The pain, located substernally, may radiate to the neck, back, and shoulder. Pain may occur throughout the day and can be confused with angina. Odynophagia can be triggered by a cold or carbonated beverage or by solid food passing through the esophagus. The most common cause is the reflux of gastric contents into the esophagus.

HEARTBURN

Heartburn (pyrosis, indigestion, or dyspepsia) is another common manifestation of esophageal disease. Generally, it is a painful sensation of warmth and burning in the lower retrosternal midline. Because clients may use the word "heartburn" to describe very different sensations, it is essential to find out exactly what this term means to the client using it. Heartburn usually means substernal, midline burning that tends to radiate, generally in waves, upward to the neck, resulting from abnormalities of the LES. Clients often describe this discomfort as cramping or knotting.

Heartburn is commonly experienced with postural changes (such as bending, stooping, and lifting) gulping of food or liquids, or ingestion of alcohol. Manifestations often are relieved by standing or eructing. Heartburn also arises in the presence of refluxed gastric or duodenal contents. Disorders most commonly associated with heartburn are reflux esophagitis, hiatal hernia, achalasia, and gastric stasis. Heartburn is common in people with pyloric or duodenal ulcers and LES disorders.

ACHALASIA

Achalasia is a disorder characterized by progressively increasing dysphagia, with the client eventually having great difficulty swallowing and expressing the feeling that "something is stuck in the throat." Achalasia commonly occurs in people in their 20s and 30s and appears equally often in men and women.

Etiology and Risk Factors

Achalasia is a chronic, progressive disease of unknown cause. Occasionally, the client can relate the onset to an episode of acute dysphagia, but usually the onset is obscure. The disease is noticed only when dysphagia becomes severe. Because achalasia is idiopathic, there are no identified risk factors. There may be a familial component.

Pathophysiology

Achalasia is characterized by impaired motility of the lower two thirds of the esophagus. The LES fails to relax normally with swallowing. Inadequate functioning occurs because nerve impulses cannot pass through the esophagus or sympathetic receptors are absent from the LES. There also may be degeneration of the ganglion cells or impairment of impulses from Auerbach's plexus. Impaired propulsion and a constricted LES result in accumulation of food and fluid within the lower esophagus. When hydrostatic pressure exceeds the force of resistance of the LES, the contents pass into the stomach. Reflux esophagitis with resultant ulceration (Fig. 30–6) is a possible complication (see Gastroesophageal Reflux Disease). Aspiration of regurgitated esophageal contents may result in atelectasis and other pulmonary problems.

Clinical Manifestations

The initial manifestation of achalasia is dysphagia. It is difficult for food and fluid to pass through the LES. In the early stages of achalasia, the client may have subster-

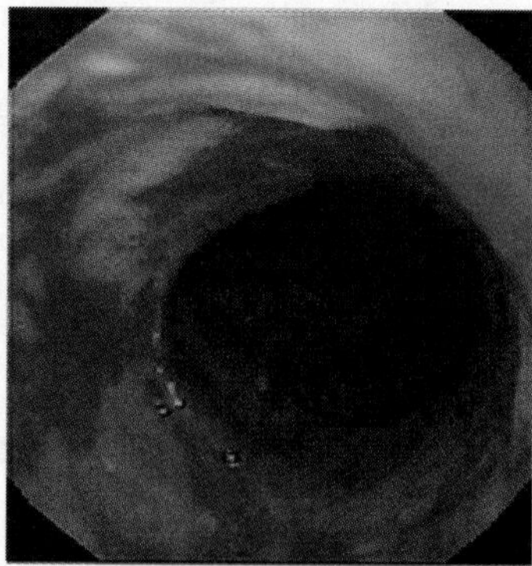

FIGURE 30–6 Endoscopic view of severe esophagitis.

nal pain because of spasms of the esophagus or may be unable to eructate (belch). The client may regurgitate undigested food eaten many hours earlier as well as large amounts of mucus that have been stimulated by esophageal irritation. As achalasia progresses, manifestations increase in frequency and severity. Upper respiratory infections, emotional disturbances, overeating, and pregnancy may exacerbate the problem.

Diagnostic tests used to determine the presence of achalasia include barium swallow, endoscopy, and manometry. The barium swallow is considered positive for achalasia if it reveals nonpropulsive waves and esophageal dilation. Barium may also be retained in the esophagus. Endoscopy helps determine the status of the LES, the amount of dilation, and the presence of food. Manometry (measurement of pressure in the esophagus) confirms the diagnosis with elevated resting pressures in the LES or slow, low-amplitude, or absent peristalsis.

Outcome Management

Medical Management

RELIEVE MANIFESTATIONS

Treatment of achalasia is aimed at relieving clinical manifestations. Management usually begins with medical treatment on an outpatient basis. Often, as the problem progresses, hospitalization is required for surgical procedures or for placement of a gastrostomy, PEG, or percutaneous endoscopic jejunostomy (PEJ) tube for nutritional support.

ADMINISTER MEDICATIONS

Medications that relax the LES or lower esophageal pressures (such as anticholinergic drugs, nitrates, gastrointestinal hormones, and calcium-channel blockers) have been studied, but none of them have proved to be of consistent value or effectiveness. Pain is managed with antacids, H_2 receptor antagonists, and proton pump inhibitors.

MODIFY DIET

Changes in diet may ease the pressure and reflux in the client with achalasia. Small, frequent feedings ease the passage of food, and semisoft, warm foods are better tolerated than cold, hard foods. The client should avoid hot, spicy, and iced foods as well as alcohol and tobacco. Foods should be chewed thoroughly to add saliva to the mixture for lubrication and allowing the bolus to pass more easily from the esophagus to the stomach.

ALTERNATE POSITIONS

The client should experiment with different positions to reduce pressure while eating. Some clients benefit from arching the back while swallowing. After eating, the client should remain upright by standing or sitting. Restrictive clothing, which may increase esophageal pressure and regurgitation, should be avoided.

To prevent nocturnal reflux of food, the client should sleep with the head of the bed elevated. You may place the client in a semi-Fowler position, using a wedge pillow to keep the head higher than the LES, or may elevate the head of the bed on 4- to 6-inch blocks.

Nursing Management of the Medical Client

ASSESSMENT

Obtain a history, noting the manifestations the client is experiencing, onset and duration of aggravating factors, and any methods the client uses for relief. Assess respiratory manifestations because reflux or regurgitation can affect the respiratory tract. Assess the client's nutritional status, noting any weight changes and the effects of esophageal manifestations on dietary habits.

DIAGNOSIS, OUTCOMES, INTERVENTIONS

Altered Nutrition: Less Than Body Requirements. The client with achalasia experiences a great deal of difficulty swallowing, leading to the diagnosis of *Altered Nutrition: Less Than Body Requirements related to dysphasia.*

Outcomes. The client will maintain an adequate nutritional intake, as evidenced by maintenance of ideal body weight or gaining back any weight lost at a rate of 1 pound per week.

Interventions. Consult with the client concerning dietary habits and daily intake of nutrients. Obtain a baseline weight and daily weights. Teach the client about changes in dietary habits that may relieve manifestations, as discussed under Medical Management. A gastrostomy tube, PEG tube, or PEJ tube may be used to provide adequate nutritional support if dysphagia continues to be a problem. Nursing management of feedings is discussed in Chapter 29 and later in this chapter under Nursing Management of the Surgical Client.

Pain. When the client experiences gastric reflux, the acid in the esophagus causes *Pain related to episodes of gastric reflux,* making this an appropriate nursing diagnosis.

Outcomes. The client will experience a decrease in pain or an absence of pain, as evidenced by verbalizing a reduction in or an absence of pain and an ability to maintain oral intake.

Interventions. Pain can be decreased or relieved through the use of medications (such as antacids, histamine H_2 receptor antagonists, and proton pump inhibitors), dietary changes, and repositioning. Assess the client every shift to determine whether medications, changes in diet, and repositioning are effective in controlling or relieving pain.

EVALUATION

The most appropriate outcome would be that the achalasia is controlled with medical treatment and the client's nutritional status is maintained. If the client's manifestations cannot be controlled with medical treatment, surgical intervention may be necessary.

Surgical Management

Surgical management of achalasia may involve dilating the LES (esophageal dilation) or enlarging the sphincter (esophagomyotomy). Esophageal dilation (bougienage) forcefully dilates the LES (Fig. 30–7). This procedure, which is usually done on an outpatient basis, is used to help correct not only achalasia but also esophageal spasms and strictures. Vigorous dilation is associated with a 75% success rate. Local anesthesia is used under radiologic guidance.

In the more complex procedure, esophagomyotomy (Heller's procedure), the surgeon enlarges the vestibule by incising the circular muscle fibers down to the mucosa

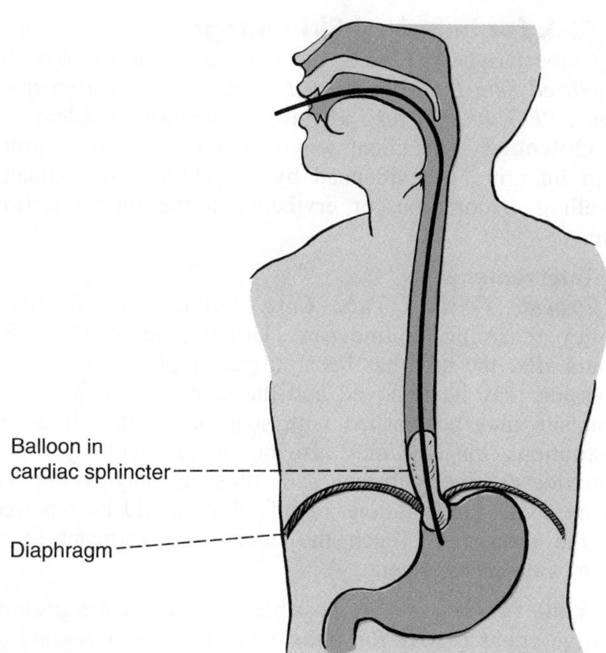

FIGURE 30–7 Bougienage (passage of a bougie) relieves dysphagia by dilating the lower esophageal sphincter.

(Fig. 30–8). Complications may include reflux esophagitis and restenosis.

If a client cannot swallow for long periods, a gastrostomy tube, PEG, or PEJ may be inserted. The tubes may be inserted surgically, laparoscopically or via percutaneous endoscopy.

For the laparoscopic or surgical method, the physician makes an incision in the wall of the abdomen and sutures the tube to the gastric wall.

For a percutaneous endoscopic approach, the physician uses local anesthesia and inserts a cannula into the stomach through a small abdominal incision. A suture is threaded through the cannula. A second physician uses an endoscope to pull the suture through the client's mouth. The PEG tube is attached and advanced down the esophagus, through the abdominal incision, where crossbars (Fig. 30–9) secure it internally and externally. Some tubes contain an internal balloon instead of an internal crossbar, while other tubes contain internal and external crossbars and an internal balloon. Skin care around the percutaneous site is necessary postoperatively. In the PEJ procedure, the tube is inserted into the jejunum instead of the stomach. See Chapter 29 for a comparison of enteral feeding routes.

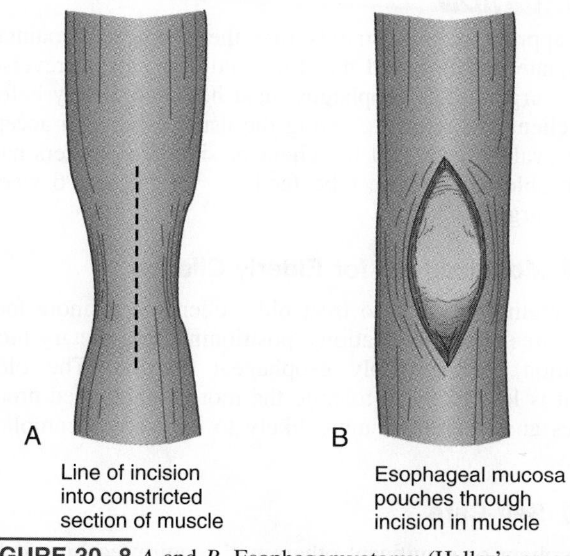

FIGURE 30–8 *A* and *B*, Esophagomyotomy (Heller's procedure) is the surgical procedure of choice when a segment of esophagus narrows and causes functional obstruction.

Nursing Management of the Surgical Client

PREOPERATIVE CARE

ASSESSMENT

Obtain a history, noting the onset and duration of manifestations the client is experiencing, aggravating factors, and any methods the client uses for relief. Assess the client's respiratory status and nutritional status in addition to the routine preoperative assessments.

DIAGNOSIS, OUTCOMES, INTERVENTIONS

Knowledge Deficit. To prepare the client for surgery, consider the nursing diagnosis *Knowledge deficit related to preoperative preparation and postoperative care.*

Outcomes. The client will understand and be prepared for surgery, as evidenced by asking questions and expressing statements of understanding.

Interventions

Teach about Esophageal Dilation. If your client is to undergo esophageal dilation, explain that the client will be awake during the procedure. A local anesthetic solution is sprayed on the throat, and an analgesic or tranquilizer may be given. The client should take long, slow breaths during passage of the bougies. As the bag is inflated, the client may feel brief discomfort. Weighted

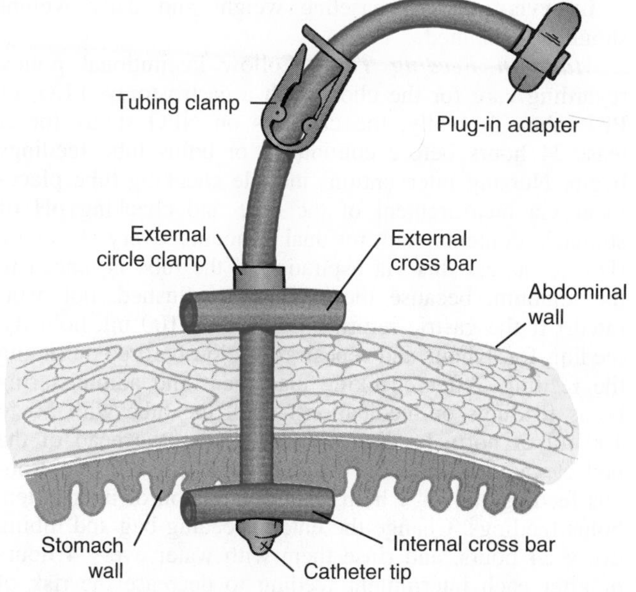

FIGURE 30–9 Percutaneous endoscopic gastrostomy tube in place for a client with achalasia.

bougies with increasing weight can also be used for dilation. Esophageal dilation is often performed on an outpatient basis.

Explain Esophagomyotomy. Esophagomyotomy is a more complex procedure. The client will require a general anesthetic and remain hospitalized for more than 24 hours. Instruct the client undergoing an esophageal procedure about the usual preoperative procedures, such as an NPO status after midnight, IV fluids, and preoperative medications. Discuss pain control, drains, surgical dressings, and the presence of an NG tube, a gastrostomy tube, a PEG tube, or a PEJ tube. The possibility of a thoracotomy approach being used to reach the esophagus requires instruction concerning chest tubes. Discuss manifestations of respiratory complications related to esophageal reflux and aspiration.

Instruct clients who have undergone an esophagomyotomy to sleep with the head of the bed elevated and to recognize manifestations of respiratory complications. Explain the manifestations of infection and esophageal perforation; urge the client to notify the physician if any of these problems occur.

POSTOPERATIVE CARE

ASSESSMENT

Routine postoperative assessments, such as monitoring vital signs, pain, and drainage tubes placed during surgery, are required. In addition, monitor the client's respiratory and nutritional status and the site of the feeding tube (if placed).

DIAGNOSIS, OUTCOMES, INTERVENTIONS

Altered Nutrition: Less Than Body Requirements. For the client experiencing dysphagia, the nursing diagnosis *Altered Nutrition: Less Than Body Requirements related to dysphagia and placement of a gastrostomy, PEG, or PEJ tube* is appropriate.

Outcomes. The client will maintain an adequate nutritional intake, as evidenced by maintaining ideal body weight or gaining weight at a rate of 1 pound per week to replace previous weight loss.

Interventions. A baseline weight and daily weight should be obtained.

Maintain Feeding Tube. Follow institutional policy regarding care for the client with a gastrostomy, PEG, or PEJ tube. Typically, the client is on NPO status for at least 24 hours before continuous or bolus tube feedings begin. Nursing interventions include checking tube placement via measurement of the tube and checking pH of stomach contents and residual amounts every 4 hours. (Do not assess this via aspiration if the tube is placed in the jejunum, because these tubes are flushed, not aspirated.) If the gastric return is more than 100 ml, hold the feeding for 1 hour and repeat aspiration before continuing the feeding. After checking placement and administering bolus feedings or medications, flush the tube with 50 to 100 ml of normal saline or water. Keep the head of the bed elevated at least 30 degrees at all times for continuous feedings or for 1 hour after completion of intermittent bolus feedings. Change the enteral feeding bag and tubing every 24 hours, and rinse them with water every 4 hours or after each intermittent feeding to decrease the risk of bacterial contamination. (See Chapter 29 for additional information about enteral feedings.)

Risk for Impaired Skin Integrity. When a feeding tube has been placed, the nursing diagnosis *Risk for Impaired Skin Integrity related to placement of a gastrostomy, PEG, or PEJ tube* identifies a potential problem.

Outcomes. The client will maintain or regain normal skin integrity, as evidenced by the absence of exudate, swelling, excoriation, or erythema at the tube insertion site.

Interventions

Provide Feeding Tube Care. Follow your facility's policy regarding routine care. Usually, about 12 to 24 hours after the tube has been surgically placed, the initial dressing may be removed and the skin around the insertion site may be washed with soap and water. In some institutions, the area may also be cleaned with hydrogen peroxide or other substances. A dressing may be applied as needed. Manifestations of infection should be reported to the physician. Teach the client or significant other home care management.

Risk for Injury. A possible problem in the postoperative client is *Risk for Injury: Pneumothorax related to surgical procedure and presence of chest tubes.*

Outcomes. Injury will be prevented, as evidenced by absence of hemorrhage, absence of manifestations of perforation, normal temperature, and absence of problems associated with chest tubes, such as respiratory distress.

Interventions

Monitor for Complications. After esophageal dilation, monitor the client for manifestations of perforation, such as elevated temperature, chest or shoulder pain, and subcutaneous emphysema. If any of these manifestations are noted, notify the physician immediately. The client will require an x-ray study to determine whether air is in the mediastinum, indicating perforation.

Maintain Chest Tubes. After an esophagomyotomy, a thoracotomy incision and chest tubes are in place. Maintain chest tube drainage and the NG or gastric drainage system, and manage the client's pain see Chapter 62 for care of the client with chest tubes.

EVALUATION

An appropriate outcome is that the client will maintain adequate nutrition and that the condition will be reversed with surgery. The esophagus must heal completely before the client can return to eating the usual foods. An acceptable evaluation is that the client or significant others have been able to continue tube feedings for at least 6 weeks after surgery.

Modifications for Elderly Clients

An attempt is made to treat older clients with more local measures (pain medications, positioning, and dietary modification) and possibly esophageal dilation. The older adult is less likely to tolerate the more complicated procedures and, therefore, more likely to experience complications.

Self-Care

The client or significant others will require teaching if the feedings are required after discharge. Initially, home visits by a nurse may be necessary to assist the client with any home care needs related to tube feedings, diet, medications, and wound care and to provide an ongoing evaluation of the client's condition. A referral to a social worker may be needed to assist the client with financial assistance, community resources, counseling, and specialized equipment (see Chapter 29).

GASTROESOPHAGEAL REFLUX DISEASE

Esophageal reflux is a backward flow of gastric contents into the esophagus. Gastroesophageal reflux disease (GERD) refers to a syndrome resulting from esophageal reflux. Reflux exposes the esophageal mucosa to the gastric contents, which gradually breaks down the esophageal mucosa. This condition, sometimes called *reflux esophagitis,* is often associated with a sliding hiatal hernia. However, complications causing reflux can occur without a hiatal hernia, and people with a hiatal hernia may not have manifestations of reflux.

GERD can occur in any age group. About 10% of the population have daily manifestations of GERD, and as much as one third of the population have monthly manifestations. Manifestations are often overlooked and attributed to stress.

Etiology and Risk Factors

The cause of GERD seems to be an inappropriate relaxation of the LES (Fig. 30–10). The exact cause of the relaxation is unknown, but reflux occurs with:

- An alteration in the innervation of the pressure zone in the region of the gastroesophageal sphincter
- Displacement of the angle of the gastroesophageal junction
- An incompetent LES

Risk factors and health promotion and maintenance behaviors are important teaching topics. These factors include obesity and weight gain, pregnancy, chewing tobacco, smoking, high-fat foods, theophylline, caffeine, chocolate, and high levels of estrogen and progesterone. Teaching clients to limit smoking, caffeine, chocolate, and high-fat foods helps to prevent GERD. Eating small meals and increasing dietary protein also helps. Losing weight, elevating the head of the bed for sleeping, and avoiding lifting, straining, bending, and tight or constrictive clothing can further help prevent the problem. Once GERD has developed, a health restoration action is to instruct the client on how to take prescribed medications.

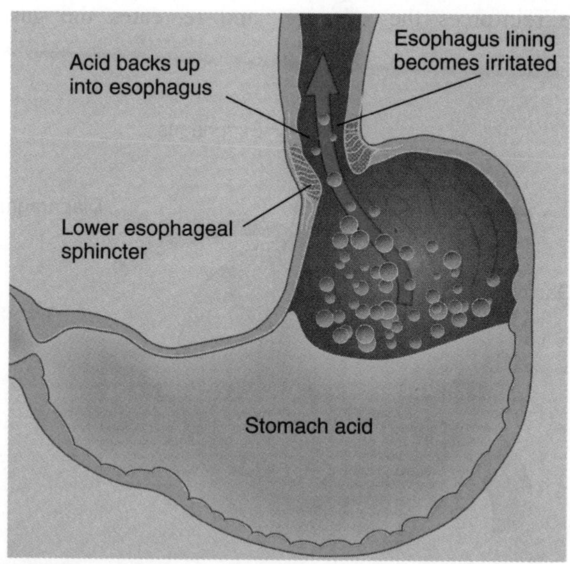

FIGURE 30–10 Anatomy of gastroesophageal reflux disease (GERD): Relaxed lower esophageal sphincter, displaced angle of the gastroesophageal junction, and altered nerve innervation in the region of the gastroesophageal sphincter.

Pathophysiology

Normally, a high-pressure zone exists in the region of the gastroesophageal sphincter. High pressure prevents reflux but permits the passage of food and liquids. When there is an alteration in this region, reflux occurs.

Reflux esophagitis may also occur with gastric or duodenal ulcer, after esophageal or gastric surgery, after prolonged vomiting, or after prolonged gastrointestinal intubation. The reflux most often consists of hydrochloric acid or gastric and duodenal contents containing bile acid and pancreatic juice. Frequent or prolonged reflux results in inflammation of the esophageal mucosa (esophagitis). The degree of reflux esophagitis present depends on (1) frequency of the reflux, (2) contents of the reflux, (3) buffering ability of the saliva and mucous secretion, and (4) rate of gastric emptying.

Clinical Manifestations

GERD may begin suddenly or gradually. The client may complain of heartburn, odynophagia, dysphagia, acid regurgitation, water brash (the release of salty secretions in the mouth), or eructation. Pain in GERD is typically described as a burning sensation that moves up and down. If the condition is severe, the pain may radiate to the back, neck, or jaw. Pain usually occurs after meals and is relieved with antacids or fluids. Discomfort sometimes accompanies activities that increase intra-abdominal pressure, such as lifting or straining. The client may state that discomfort occurs when lying supine or when the stomach is distended. Standing and walking may relieve it. Dysphagia resulting from edema, spasm, or a narrowed lumen is intermittent and worse at the beginning of meals. Responses to pain-relieving measures (such as nitroglycerin) help to differentiate between esophagitis and problems of cardiac origin (such as angina pectoris).

Diagnosis rests on the demonstration of reflux. Barium swallow, esophageal manometry, esophagoscopy, esophageal biopsy, cytologic examination, analysis of gastric secretions, and acid perfusion tests confirm the diagnosis of GERD (see Chapter 28).

Outcome Management

Medical Management

DECREASE REFLUX WITH MEDICATIONS

Of the many medications used to treat GERD, only one drug of its class is discussed. A more detailed description of these classifications of drugs is provided in Chapter 31. For people receiving long-term therapy with nonsteroidal anti-inflammatory drugs (NSAIDs), misoprostol (Cytotec) is useful for preventing gastric ulcer formation and, in some instances, GERD manifestations. Anticholinergic drugs, calcium-channel blockers, and theophylline should be avoided because they appear to decrease LES pressure or delay gastric emptying.

ANTACIDS. Drug therapy for GERD usually starts with an antacid, which commonly provides prompt relief. Typically, the client takes 30 ml of antacid 1 hour before and 2 to 3 hours after each meal to neutralize gastric acid secretions. Clients typically tolerate combination products such as calcium carbonate–magnesium carbonate (Mylanta) or magnesium hydroxide–aluminum hydroxide (Maalox). Aluminum hydroxide–magnesium carbonate (Gaviscon) is another excellent antacid because of its foaming action. A major disadvantage of antacids is that their effects last only about a half-hour.

HISTAMINE RECEPTOR ANTAGONISTS. If manifestations are severe or persist, the client may be prescribed histamine receptor antagonists such as ranitidine (Zantac) or famotidine (Pepcid) to decrease gastric acid secretions.

CHOLINERGICS. Bethanechol (Urecholine) may be added for clients with severe manifestations because it has been found to increase LES pressure and prevent reflux. Because bethanechol is a cholinergic drug, it is usually given with antacids and a histamine receptor antagonist because it can increase the secretion of gastric acid. It should be taken before meals.

GASTROINTESTINAL STIMULANTS. Metoclopramide (Reglan) may be prescribed because it increases LES pressure by stimulating the smooth muscle of the GI tract and increases the rate of gastric emptying. This medication is taken before meals.

Cisapride (Propulsid) was pulled in July 2000 by the FDA because of problems with dysrhythmias, and is used only when no other drug is effective and the client has no contraindications and is closely supervised.

PROTON PUMP INHIBITORS. Lansoprazole (Prevacid), a proton pump inhibitor, suppresses secretion of gastric acid. It has been effective for short-term treatment of GERD.

DECREASE REFLUX WITH LIFESTYLE AND DIET CHANGES

In mild GERD, diet and lifestyle changes may be sufficient to relieve manifestations. Instruct the client to follow this regimen:

- Restrict the diet to small, frequent feedings (four to six per day).
- Drink adequate fluids at meals to assist food passage.
- Eat slowly and chew thoroughly to add saliva to the food.
- Avoid extremely hot or cold foods, spices, fats, alcohol, coffee, chocolate, and citrus juices.
- Avoid eating and drinking for 3 hours before retiring to prevent the common problem of nocturnal reflux.
- Elevate the head of the bed 6 to 8 inches to prevent nocturnal reflux.
- Lose weight, if overweight, to decrease the gastroesophageal pressure gradient.
- Avoid tobacco, salicylates, and phenylbutazone, which may exacerbate esophagitis.

Nursing Management of the Medical Client

ASSESS MANIFESTATIONS

Identify specific manifestations the client has been experiencing. Document when manifestations started, their frequency and severity, and the relationship of manifestations to food and various food products. Assist in maintaining the client's general appearance and nutritional status. Help the client identify risk factors for GERD, and instruct the client about lifestyle changes to reduce those risk factors.

PROVIDE TEACHING

Instruct the client in the prescribed diet regimen, and evaluate both the client's understanding of treatment and its effectiveness. Administer medications ordered for the pain, and document their effectiveness. Instruct the client in the prescribed medication regimen, and evaluate the client's understanding of the treatment.

Surgical Management

Clients who do not respond to medical management undergo one of three surgical procedures: the Nissen fundoplication, the Hill operation, or the Belsey operation. The surgeon may use an open surgical approach or a laparoscopic approach to complete these procedures. Recovery is usually faster with the laparoscopic approach.

The *Nissen fundoplication* is most common and involves suturing the fundus around the esophagus (Fig. 30–11). An abdominal approach is usually used. An increase in pressure or volume in the stomach closes the cardia and blocks reflux into the esophagus. The surgeon creates a valve-like substitute sphincter with inherent contractility.

The *Hill operation* narrows the esophageal opening and anchors the stomach and distal esophagus to the median arcuate ligament (posterior gastropexy). This procedure reinforces the sphincter and recreates the gastro-

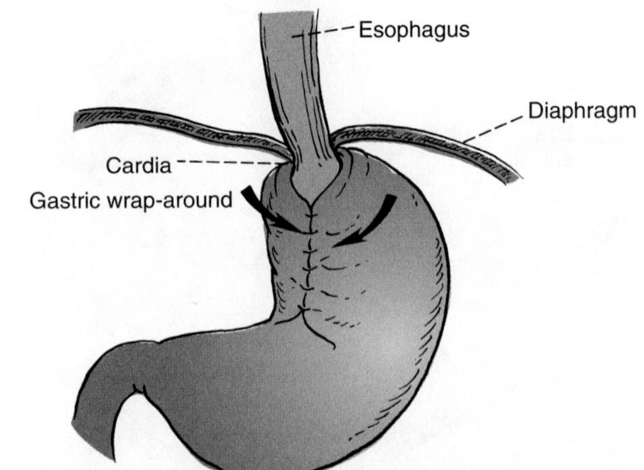

FIGURE 30–11 Nissen fundoplication for hiatal hernia. The gastric fundus is wrapped around the distal esophagus and sutured to itself.

esophageal valve. A partial wraparound (180 degrees) of the stomach around the esophagus is created via an abdominal approach.

The *Belsey (Mark IV) repair* consists of plication of the anterior and lateral aspects of the stomach onto the distal esophagus. The surgeon creates the esophagogastric angle without opening the esophagus or the diaphragm. A 280-degree esophageal wraparound is created via a thoracic approach.

In clients with severe reflux, an Angelchick prosthesis may be inserted. A laparotomy is performed, and a synthetic C-shaped silicone prosthesis is tied around the distal esophagus (Fig. 30–12). The prosthesis anchors the LES in the abdomen and reinforces sphincter pressure. The success of this procedure is variable, depending on the severity of the problem. In clients with severe reflux, this procedure may be unsuccessful.

Clients undergoing a surgical procedure are encouraged to follow the GERD antireflux medical regimen (medications, diet changes, lifestyle changes) because the recurrence rate is significant.

Nursing Management of the Surgical Client

COMPLETE POSTOPERATIVE ASSESSMENTS

The surgical client requires the same assessments as those for the medical client as well as routine preoperative and postoperative assessments. If chest tubes are placed postoperatively, monitor the client for respiratory distress. An abdominal incision results in a greater chance of a wound infection. Assess the wound drainage for signs of infection. The client will have an NG tube, and tube patency must be maintained to avoid stomach distention.

PREVENT RESPIRATORY COMPLICATIONS

Teach the client the importance of coughing and deep breathing after surgery to prevent respiratory complications. Because postoperative breathing can be painful, the client must cough and deep-breathe to avoid respiratory complications. The use of an incentive spirometer may be ordered by the surgeon. If a thoracic approach is used, explain the purpose of the chest tubes and the care needed (see Chapter 62).

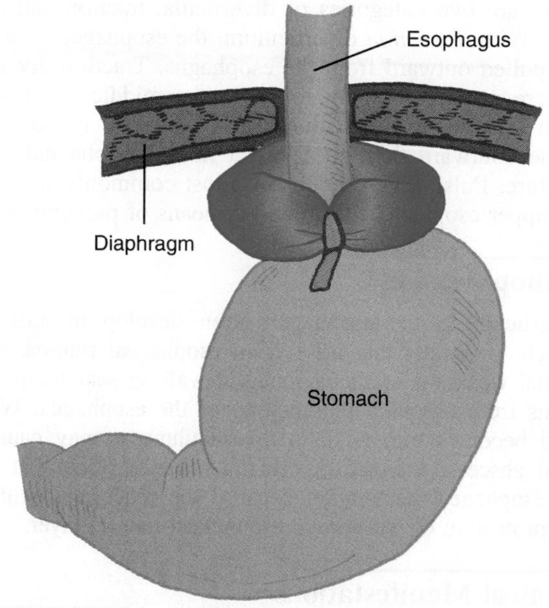

FIGURE 30–12 Angelchick antireflux prosthesis in place.

PREVENT GAS-BLOAT SYNDROME

Fluids are usually resumed after 24 hours, and the diet is progressively advanced as tolerated when peristalsis returns. Small, frequent meals are provided to avoid overloading the stomach. After fundoplication, the client may experience gas-bloat syndrome if the wrap of the fundus is too tight, causing bloating and an inability to eructate. Clients should avoid carbonated beverages and gas-producing foods and should drink with a straw. Ambulating can assist peristalsis in removing air from the GI tract. The condition is usually temporary. Instruct clients to report dysphagia, epigastric fullness, bloating, or excessive borborygmi to their physician or health care practitioner.

HIATAL HERNIA

A hiatal hernia (diaphragmatic hernia) is a condition in which the cardiac sphincter becomes enlarged, allowing a part of the stomach to pass into the thoracic cavity. There are two major types of hernias: *sliding* hernias (type I) and *rolling* or *paraesophageal* hernias (type II). In a sliding hernia, the upper stomach and the gastroesophageal junction are displaced upward into the thorax (Fig. 30–13). Sliding hernias account for about 90% of the total cases of esophageal hiatal hernias. With a rolling hernia, the gastroesophageal junction stays below the diaphragm but all or part of the stomach pushes through into the thorax (see Fig. 30–13).

The incidence of hiatal hernia is estimated as 5 per 1000 in the general population and may be as high as 60% in clients over age 60 years. Women tend to be affected more often than men, and the incidence increases significantly with age.

Etiology and Risk Factors

Hiatal hernias are related to muscle weakness in the esophageal hiatus, which loosens the esophageal supports and allows the lower portion of the stomach to rise into the thorax. As with other hernias, the muscle weakness is caused by a variety of conditions, such as aging, trauma, congenital muscle weakness, surgery, or anything that increases intra-abdominal pressure such as lifting or coughing.

Risk factors are those that weaken the diaphragm and increase intra-abdominal pressure. Pressure may be increased by conditions such as obesity, pregnancy, or ascites.

Health promotion behaviors to prevent or at least delay a hiatal hernia include avoiding any activities that increase intra-abdominal pressure. These activities include heavy lifting and wearing tight constrictive clothing, especially around the waist. Other than these measures, hiatal hernias are not preventable.

Pathophysiology

A hiatal hernia involves protrusion of part of the stomach through a weakness in the diaphragm. The resulting re-

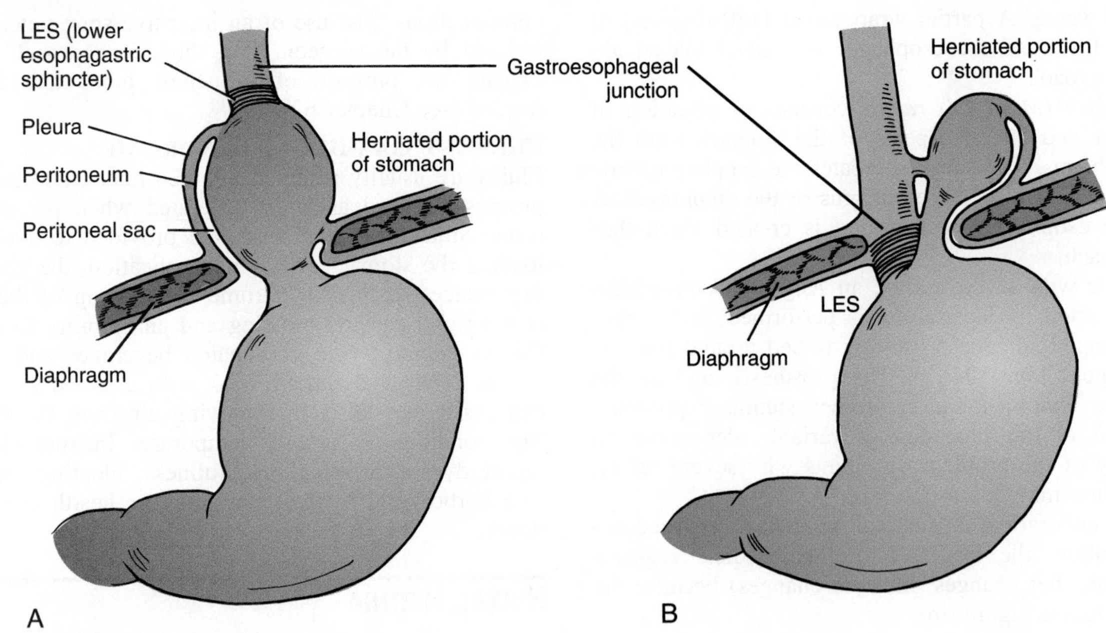

FIGURE 30–13 *A*, A sliding hiatal hernia. *B*, A rolling hiatal hernia.

gurgitation and motor dysfunction cause the manifestations associated with hiatal hernia. The major problem with a sliding hernia is reflux (GERD), which appears to be caused by the exposure of the LES to the low pressure in the thorax.

With a rolling hernia, the LES remains below the diaphragm and reflux is not a problem. Complications of a rolling hiatal hernia include obstruction, strangulation, and the development of a volvulus.

Clinical Manifestations

Manifestations of hiatal hernia vary in kind and severity. In sliding hiatal hernias, the client may experience heartburn 30 to 60 minutes after meals. Reflux may also result in substernal pain.

The client with a rolling hiatal hernia does not have manifestations of reflux. The client may complain of a feeling of fullness after eating or may have difficulty breathing. Some clients experience chest pain similar to that of angina. Pain is usually worse when the client lies down.

A barium swallow with fluoroscopy can reveal a hiatal hernia by showing the position of the stomach in relation to the diaphragm.

Outcome Management

Medical and Surgical Management

The medical and surgical management for the client with a hiatal hernia is the same as that for the client with GERD.

Nursing Management of the Medical or Surgical Client

The nursing care of the client with a hiatal hernia is the same as that for a client with GERD.

DIVERTICULA

An esophageal diverticulum is a sac-like outpouching in one or more layers of the esophagus. As food is ingested, it becomes trapped in a diverticulum and can later be regurgitated. The most common type of esophageal diverticulum is esophageal pulsion (Zenker's) diverticulum. Esophageal diverticula are considered rare. Zenker's diverticula occur three times more often in men as in women.

Etiology and Risk Factors

The cause of esophageal weakness may be a congenital defect, esophageal trauma, scar tissue, or inflammation. There are two categories of diverticula: traction and pulsion. With a *traction* diverticulum, the esophageal mucosa has pulled outward from the esophagus. Traction diverticula are most commonly found in the middle esophagus. With a *pulsion* diverticulum, the esophageal mucosa has pushed outward through a defect in the esophageal musculature. Pulsion diverticula are most commonly found in the upper esophagus. There is no means of prevention.

Pathophysiology

Diverticula in the esophagus often develop in areas of muscle weakness that arise from esophageal trauma, congenital weakness of the esophageal wall, or scar tissue that forms from chronic inflammation of the esophagus. When food becomes trapped in a diverticulum, it may cause a local abscess. Infected diverticula place the client at risk for esophageal perforation because the mucosa is without the protection of the normal esophageal muscle layer.

Clinical Manifestations

Initially, the client usually complains of difficulty swallowing. Other manifestations may include eructation, regurgitation of undigested food, halitosis, and a sour taste in the mouth. Coughing also may occur because of irritation of the trachea from regurgitated food.

A barium swallow is performed to locate the diverticulum. Endoscopy is usually contraindicated because the diverticulum may be perforated by the endoscope.

Outcome Management

Medical Management

Medical management of esophageal diverticula includes dietary management and positioning. Small, frequent meals of semi-soft foods often facilitate passage of food. The client should note which foods ease or worsen the manifestations.

To prevent reflux of food, the caregiver should raise the head of the bed for 2 hours after meals. Sleeping with the head of the bed elevated can often prevent nocturnal reflux. The client also should avoid constrictive clothes and vigorous exercise after eating.

Nursing Management of the Medical Client

Obtain a history from the client, noting the onset and duration of manifestations and whether they occur at mealtimes or at night. Assess the client's respiratory status because regurgitation can cause respiratory complications.

Teach the client how changes in diet and positioning can control manifestations. Encourage the client to try various foods and various positions to evaluate which are most effective.

Surgical Management

When manifestations become severe, surgery may be indicated. A cervical approach is used for Zenker's diverticulum, whereas a thoracic approach is used for diverticula located lower in the esophagus. In both procedures, the diverticulum is excised and the esophageal mucosa is reanastomosed.

Nursing Management of the Surgical Client

ASSESSMENT

Obtain a history, noting the onset and duration of manifestations, aggravating factors, and any methods the client uses for relief. In addition, routine preoperative and postoperative assessments are required.

DIAGNOSIS, OUTCOMES, INTERVENTIONS

Risk for Injury. When an esophageal diverticulum is treated surgically, the nursing diagnosis *Risk for Injury related to surgical procedure and presence of chest tubes* is appropriate.

Outcomes. Injury will be prevented, as evidenced by a normal temperature and an absence of hemorrhage, infection, and problems associated with the chest tubes, such as respiratory distress.

Interventions

Provide Teaching. Discuss the normal preoperative routines. Explain that the client will be taking nothing by mouth after surgery and that an NG tube will be present until healing occurs. If a thoracic approach is used, preoperative and postoperative nursing care is similar to that for clients having thoracic surgery and chest tubes (see Chapter 62).

Maintain the NG Tube. After surgery, the client's NG tube is attached to low intermittent suction to avoid trauma to the stomach lining. Assess the amount and color of drainage during each shift. Check for continued bloody NG drainage as well as for external bleeding. Do not irrigate or reposition the NG tube unless told to do so by the physician. Moving the NG tube can perforate the esophagus or stomach (see Chapter 31 on irrigation of tubes if ordered by the surgeon). Assess the client for manifestations of esophageal perforation, such as chest pain, fever, and subcutaneous emphysema. The client will receive IV fluids until tube feedings begin. Once fluids and supplemental feedings begin, record the client's response.

After surgery, the client may be discharged with an NG or a gastrostomy tube in place to allow for esophageal healing. Give the client written and verbal instructions about tube feedings, diet, and positioning. A visiting nurse should see the client at home to ensure that tube feedings are being tolerated well and should continue visits until the feeding tube is removed.

Promote Comfort. Assess the client's pain, and administer and evaluate prescribed analgesics. After surgery, the head of the bed should be elevated 30 degrees to reduce edema around the neck and upper chest. Frequent oral hygiene increases the client's comfort.

EVALUATION

An appropriate outcome for the client with a diverticulum is that the altered diet will control the problem. If surgery is required, the client's nutritional intake should return to normal after healing occurs.

Modifications for Elderly Clients

Older adults are treated more conservatively, with an emphasis on diet and positioning rather than surgery. Surgery may entail too much risk for older clients.

ESOPHAGEAL CANCER

Cancer of the esophagus takes the form of either squamous cell carcinoma or adenocarcinoma of the esophageal mucosa. An estimated 12,300 new cases of esophageal cancer are diagnosed each year in the United States.[1] The incidence is three times as high in men as in women, and it is higher in African American and Asian men than in white men. Adenocarcinoma of the esophagus occurs less often than squamous cell carcinoma and develops primarily in the distal esophagus.

Etiology and Risk Factors

The cause of esophageal cancer is unknown, but researchers are studying environmental differences between locations with a low and a high incidence. In the Western world, evidence points to heavy smoking, nutritional deficiencies, and habitual ingestion of alcohol, hot foods, and hot drinks as underlying etiologic factors.

In other parts of the world, contaminants in the soil and food, high levels of nitrosamines, smoking opium, and nutritional deficiencies (especially of fruits and vegetables) have been linked to the condition. Chronic irritation from other esophageal problems, such as achalasia, hiatal hernia, and stricture, plays a minor role in the development of esophageal cancer.

These are very preventable causes. Prevention should be targeted particularly toward the African American population because their risk is higher. Risk factors include smoking tobacco or opium, nutritional deficiencies, ingestion of hot foods and beverages, habitual ingestion of alcohol, ingestion of smoked meats or meats cooked over very high heat, irritation from GERD, hiatal hernia, or achalasia. Health promotion and maintenance behaviors involve limiting or stopping smoking and avoiding chronic ingestion of alcohol, hot foods, and hot beverages. Restorative behaviors include advising the client to follow the appropriate medical or surgical regimen for treatment of the specific condition.

Pathophysiology

Cancer of the esophagus begins as slow-growing benign tissue changes. Most of these cancers are squamous epidermoid tumors that are commonly found in the middle or upper third of the esophagus. Because the esophagus has no serosal layer to limit its extension, esophageal tumors expand locally and very rapidly. Early spread to the lymph nodes is common. The rich lymphatic supply to the mucosa provides an excellent means for the cancer to metastasize widely. The cancers are typically intraluminal, ulcerating lesions that encircle the esophageal wall and extend upward and downward.

The disease is progressive and almost always fatal. As it progresses, most clients experience some pulmonary complications because of the formation of tracheoesophageal fistulae that result in aspiration. If the condition is not treated, total esophageal obstruction is the inevitable outcome of the disease. Infiltration into blood vessels may predispose the client to hemorrhage. Metastasis is common because of the large supply of lymph channels in the area.

Clinical Manifestations

Typically, the first manifestations are dysphagia or odynophagia. Unfortunately, they are usually not apparent until the cancer involves the circumference of the esophagus. By the time the client becomes aware of a swallowing problem and seeks medical care, the cancer frequently has invaded the deeper layers of the esophagus and, sometimes, adjacent structures such as the bronchus.

At first, dysphagia is usually mild and intermittent, occurring only after ingestion of solid food (especially meat). Soon, dysphagia becomes constant and manifestations of esophageal obstruction appear. These manifestations include an increase in salivation and mucus in the throat, nocturnal aspiration, regurgitation, and an inability to swallow even liquids.

Barium swallow, endoscopy, cytologic examination, and direct biopsy confirm the diagnosis. Computed tomography (CT) scans provide an excellent definition of the size of the primary lesion and reveal the extent of nodal involvement.

Outcome Management

Medical Management

INHIBIT TUMOR GROWTH

Treatment of esophageal cancer depends on the tumor's location and size, metastases, and the condition of the client. If the cancer is found in an early stage, treatment is directed toward cure; however, it is usually detected in the late stages, when treatment becomes palliative, aimed specifically at allowing the client to continue eating.

RADIATION THERAPY. Radiation therapy can be used alone or before or after surgery. It provides palliation by reducing tumor size and slowing tumor growth. Because high-dose radiation therapy may cause stenosis of the esophagus, treatments are usually administered over 6 to 8 weeks to minimize this effect.

CHEMOTHERAPY. Chemotherapy, combining several drugs, provides symptomatic relief. Neoadjuvant chemotherapy with cisplatin (Platinol) and 5-fluorouracil (5-FU) before surgery can facilitate surgical resection by decreasing tumor size and invasiveness of the disease in about 50% of clients treated. Chemotherapy, combined with radiation and followed by surgery, shows promising early results.[3, 19]

PHOTODYNAMIC THERAPY. Photodynamic therapy is a relatively new therapy for palliative treatment of esophageal cancer in clients who are not surgical candidates. The client receives an injection of a light-sensitive drug (Photofrin), which is followed 2 days later with a special fiberoptic probe with a light-bearing tip placed in the esophagus. The light activates the Photofrin and kills only cancer cells. This outpatient procedure utilizes conscious sedation, takes about 13 minutes to perform, and enables about 1 inch of tumor to be removed. Clients return home the same day and resume their usual activities the next day.[19]

MAINTAIN NUTRITION

Maintaining nutrition is a major goal for the client with esophageal cancer. Early in the disease, the client may be able to tolerate small, frequent feedings of soft or semisoft foods. As the disease progresses, feeding tubes may be needed. If necessary, a feeding gastrostomy or jejunostomy may be created. Short-term TPN may be used to improve the client's nutritional status before surgery. Proper positioning after meals is necessary if the client is experiencing frequent regurgitation or wearing a prosthesis. The head of the bed should always be elevated 30 degrees.

Nursing Management of the Medical Client

ASSESSMENT

Obtain data concerning the client's nutritional status. Most clients complain of dysphagia that is both persistent and progressive. The client initially may have difficulty swallowing solid foods and then may have difficulty swallowing soft foods and liquids.

A careful assessment of dysphagia is important. Other manifestations, such as odynophagia, regurgitation, chronic cough, increased secretions, and hoarseness (from involvement of the larynx), also are important to assess.

DIAGNOSIS, OUTCOMES, INTERVENTIONS

Altered Nutrition: Less Than Body Requirements. Because of the progressively worsening dysphagia, the client with esophageal cancer exhibits the nursing diagnosis *Altered Nutrition: Less Than Body Requirements related to the client's inability to swallow.*

Outcomes. The client will maintain an adequate nutritional status, as evidenced by maintenance of stable body weight or slowed weight loss.

Interventions. Monitor the client's nutritional status throughout treatment, including daily weights, intake and output, and calories consumed. In the beginning, teach the client about diet changes that can make eating easier.

As the disease progresses, you may have to provide tube feedings. Assess the skin around the feeding tube for impairment of skin integrity caused by leakage of gastric juices. Wash the skin around the opening with a gentle soap and dry thoroughly twice daily or as needed. Apply a protective ointment, such as zinc oxide or karaya gum, to the skin for further protection.

Risk for Impaired Swallowing. The client with esophageal cancer experiences increasing dysphagia that may lead to the diagnosis *Risk for Impaired Swallowing related to esophageal obstruction from tumor.*

Outcomes. The client will not suffer from impaired swallowing, as evidenced by an absence of choking and maintenance of a patent airway.

Interventions. Many problems arise when the client is unable to swallow. The client can easily choke on saliva and mucous secretions and must spit frequently or drool. Constant wiping of saliva from the lips can cause irritation, cracking of the skin, and open lesions. Because it is impractical to collect this quantity of secretions in tissues, the client should carry a receptacle to receive the saliva. While hospitalized, clients are often taught to do self-suctioning. To prevent oral lesions and infections and to provide comfort, you should administer or assist with frequent oral care.

Risk for Ineffective Individual Coping. The client with cancer of the esophagus has many problems associated with both the disease and its treatment. This can lead to a nursing diagnosis of *Risk for Ineffective Individual Coping related to changes in body image and potentially terminal prognosis.*

Outcomes. The client will effectively cope with the alterations in body image and potentially terminal prognosis, as evidenced by maintenance of activities and continued social interaction.

Interventions. In addition to meeting the client's physical needs, you must provide emotional support. The gastrostomy tube may cause an alteration in body image and increased dependency. The drooling or need to spit constantly also may cause the client a great deal of emotional distress. The poor prognosis of esophageal cancer necessitates psychological support and interventions aimed at helping the client and significant others prepare for the client's death (see Chapters 19 and 22).

EVALUATION

Successful control of manifestations and prevention of extensive weight loss, as the client is supported to a peaceful death, may be the desired outcomes. Few clients survive for 5 years.

Surgical Management

Esophageal dilation may be necessary throughout the course of the disease to treat strictures and obstruction caused by the tumor. The physician should perform the treatment as often as needed to relieve dysphagia.

In advanced disease, a prosthesis may be inserted to bypass the tumor or to prevent aspiration in clients with fistulae. The prosthesis can maintain esophageal patency but can perforate the esophagus if it becomes dislodged or the tumor increases in size.

Surgery may be performed for prophylaxis, cure, or palliation, depending on the extent of the disease. For high-risk clients with Barrett's esophagus, a premalignant healing process that occurs in association with GERD, the lower third of the esophagus is removed prophylactically.[19] Three surgical procedures can be performed:

1. An *esophagectomy* consists of the removal of all or part of the esophagus. The resected esophagus is replaced with a polyester (Dacron) graft. This procedure is usually performed via a thoracotomy, but it may be performed transhiatally, which eliminates the need for a thoractomy.
2. An *esophagogastrostomy* involves resection of the lower portion of the esophagus and anastomosis of the remainder to the stomach, brought up into the thorax.
3. In an *esophagoenterostomy* (colon interposition), the esophagus is resected and replaced with a segment of the descending colon.

Nursing Management of the Surgical Client

ASSESSMENT

Obtain data about the client's nutritional status, ability to swallow, respiratory status, and ability to cope with the diagnosis. In addition, routine preoperative and postoperative assessments are required.

DIAGNOSIS, OUTCOMES, INTERVENTIONS

Risk for Injury. Surgery to treat esophageal cancer is often extensive, necessitating a thoracic approach and leading to the nursing diagnosis *Risk for Injury related to surgical procedure.*

Outcomes. Injury will be prevented, as evidenced by an absence of atelectasis, fever, wound infection, or problems associated with the chest tubes.

Interventions

Improve Nutritional Status before Surgery. Before surgery, clients usually require 2 to 3 weeks of nutritional support. Often, this support includes tube feedings or TPN. The client's weight and fluid and electrolyte status are monitored.

Provide Preoperative Teaching. Provide extensive instruction on postoperative respiratory care, including turning, coughing, deep breathing, and chest physiotherapy. Teach the client about all incisions, wound drainage tubes, feeding tubes, and chest tubes that may be present after surgery. Oral care should be performed four times a day to help prevent infection postoperatively. If an esophagoenterostomy is performed, a complete bowel preparation is performed before surgery.

Maintain Airway. After surgery, respiratory care is a high priority. The client may be placed on a ventilator in a critical care unit (see Chapter 62 for care of a client receiving mechanical ventilation). Otherwise, the client must turn, cough, and deep-breathe every hour. Carefully assess the client's respiratory status, report any manifestations of atelectasis or pneumonia, and administer supplemental oxygen. Administer pain medication frequently, and assist the client in splinting the incision while coughing. Place the client in a semi-Fowler position to prevent reflux. Continually monitor the chest tube drainage for amount, color, and patency.

Maintain Fluid and Electrolyte Balance. Assess the client's fluid and electrolyte status. Monitor drainage from the NG, gastric, and all drainage tubes at least every shift. The client will be NPO for 4 to 5 days until peristalsis returns. During the first 24 hours after surgery, NG or gastric drainage is bloody but should then change to a greenish yellow color. If bloody drainage continues, it may indicate bleeding at the suture line and should be reported.

Leakage at the site of anastomosis may appear about 5 to 7 days after surgery. Assess the client for early manifestations of shock as well as for fever, fluid accumulation at the wound site, and inflammation. Check all dressings for bleeding, drainage, or separation of the suture lines.

Advance Diet as Tolerated. The client should be started on small sips of water. If this intake is tolerated, the quantity is slowly increased. Supervise the client, making sure the client stays in an upright position, and monitor for manifestations of leakage at the anastomosis site. If this is tolerated, the client gradually progresses to puréed and semi-solid foods. Explain the importance of small, frequent feedings, and advise the client to sit upright at meals and for 1 hour after meals to prevent overdistention of the stomach and reflux.

EVALUATION

The poor prognosis associated with the illness means that successful control of manifestations and prevention of extensive weight loss may be the only reasonable outcomes for these clients. Few clients survive for 5 years. They should receive support during the process of dying.

Self-Care

Upon discharge, give the client and family written and oral instructions concerning wound healing, nutritional support, respiratory care, and medications. Teach the client about possible wound and respiratory complications, manifestations that should be reported immediately, and how to contact appropriate members of the health care team.

Make appropriate referrals to community agencies. Most clients need a great amount of assistance at home. Provide information about services offered by the American Cancer Society and local hospice (see Chapter 19), if it becomes apparent that hospice care is necessary. End-of-life care is discussed in Chapter 22.

VASCULAR DISORDERS

The principal vascular disorder of the esophagus is varices. Because esophageal varices result from portal hypertension, this condition is discussed with liver disorders in Chapter 47.

TRAUMA

Major traumatic conditions of the esophagus include chemical burns, the presence of foreign bodies, and injuries from external forces, such as endoscopic equipment. Chemical burns result from the ingestion of acids or alkalis and sometimes from highly spiced foods. Thermal burns can occur after drinking extremely hot liquids, accidental ingestion of foreign bodies that lodge in the natural narrow spots of the esophagus, and self-mutilation related to suicide attempts. Trauma can cause esophageal perforation, with resultant contamination of the mediastinum and stricture formation as a complication of the healing process. Treatment of esophageal strictures involves dilation of the esophagus or surgical excision of the diseased portion and reanastomosis or interposition of a piece of gut from the stomach or colon (see Esophageal Cancer).

CONCLUSIONS

Disorders of the mouth and esophagus range from fairly simple problems, such as dental caries, to complex and potentially lethal problems, such as cancer of the esophagus. No matter how minor, disorders throughout the oral-esophageal area can interfere with the client's nutritional intake. Always keep this fact in mind when assessing and caring for clients with these disorders.

THINKING CRITICALLY

1. **The client is a 72-year-old retired schoolteacher who lives with her 70-year-old sister. She is being evaluated for complaints of chest pain, which have become increasingly more frequent. Yesterday, while she was lifting flats of bedding plants to prepare for planting, she became dyspneic and collapsed. Her sister called the ambulance, and the client was admitted to a medical-surgical unit. This morning, she underwent an abdominal ultrasound prior to an upper GI series. An electrocardiogram (ECG) followed the tests. When the nurse last checked, the client was sleeping soundly. Now the client's call light is on. When entering the room, the client is gasping, clutching at her chest, and attempting to get out of bed, saying, "Please help me! I can't catch my breath!" What is your first priority?**

Factors to Consider. Is the client experiencing manifestations of a cardiovascular problem or a gastrointestinal one? How can the nurse tell the difference?

2. **A 61-year-old woman is being treated as an outpatient for gastroesophageal reflux disease. She tells the nurse that the doctor told her to take Maalox but did not tell her how else to treat her condition. What would you teach her?**

Factors to Consider. What lifestyle changes might help the client manage her condition?

3. An 18-year-old man is seen at a dental clinic following the blow of a soccer ball to the head. Several teeth were loosened by the impact. During the oral examination, the nurse notes that the gums are reddened and tender and bleed easily when probed with a tongue blade. The area under the left premolar is swollen, tender, and abscessed. The client pulls away and tells the nurse to stop because it hurts too much to touch that tooth and states, "It's been hurting for the past several weeks." When questioned, the client states that he brushes his teeth once a day or every other day, has never flossed, and usually eats several candy bars a day. What nursing interventions are appropriate?

Factors to Consider. What might be the problem with the client's tooth? What could be the cause of his gingival problems?

BIBLIOGRAPHY

1. American Cancer Society. (2000). *Cancer facts and figures.* Atlanta: Author.
2. Ault, D. L., & Schmidt, D. (1998). Diagnosis and management of gastroesophageal reflux. *Nurse Practitioner, 23*(6), 81–82, 88–89.
3. Cooper, J., et al. (1999). Chemoradiotherapy of locally advanced esophageal cancer. *JAMA, 281*(17), 1623–1627.
4. Copstead, L. (1999). *Perspectives on pathophysiology* (2nd ed.). Philadelphia: W. B. Saunders.
5. Feldman, M., Scharschmidt, B., & Sleisenger, M. (Eds.). (1997). *Gastrointestinal and liver disease: Pathophysiology/diagnosis/management* (6th ed.). Philadelphia: W. B. Saunders.
6. Gavaghan, M. (1999). Anatomy and physiology of the esophagus. *AORN Journal, 69*(2), 372–386.
7. Goldsmith, C. (1998). Gastroesophageal reflux disease. *American Journal of Nursing, 98*(9), 44–45.
8. Graling, P. R. (1998). Managing the patient with perforated intrathoracic esophagus. *AORN Journal, 68*(1), 56–58, 61–61, 67.
9. Hansen, M. (1998). *Pathophysiology: Foundations of disease and clinical intervention.* Philadelphia: W. B. Saunders.
10. Heuman, D., Mills, S., & McGuire, H. (1997). *Gastroenterology.* Philadephia: W. B. Saunders.
11. Lehne, R. (1998). *Pharmacology for nursing care* (3rd ed.). Philadelphia: W. B. Saunders.
12. McCorkle, R., et al. (1996). *Cancer nursing: A comprehensive textbook* (2nd ed.). Philadelphia: W. B. Saunders.
13. McHale, J. M., et al. (1998). Expert nursing knowledge in the care of patients at risk of impaired swallowing. *Image, 30*(2), 137–141.
14. Metheny, N., et al. (1997). pH and concentrations of pepsin and trypsin in feeding tube aspirates as predictors of tube placement. *Journal of Parenteral and Enteral Nutrition, 21,* 279–285.
15. Metheny, N., et al. (1999). pH and concentration of bilirubin feeding tube aspirates as predictors of tube placement. *Nursing Research, 48*(4), 189–197.
16. Mittal, R., & Balaban, D. (1997). The esophagogastric junction. *New England Journal of Medicine, 336*(13), 924–932.
17. Moody, F. (1999). *Atlas of ambulatory surgery.* Philadelphia: W. B. Saunders.
18. Pehl, C., et al. (1999). Effect of low and high fat meals on lower esophageal sphincter motility and gastroesophageal reflux in healthy subjects. *American Journal of Gastroenterology, 94*(5), 1190–1196.
19. Quinn, K. L., & Reedy, A. (1999). Esophageal cancer: Therapeutic approaches and nursing care. *Seminars in Oncology Nursing, 15*(1), 17–25.
20. Rombeau, J., & Rolandelli, R. (1997). *Clinical nutrition: Enteral and tube feeding* (3rd ed.). Philadelphia: W. B. Saunders.
21. Sabiston, D., & Lyerly, H. (Eds.). (1997). *Textbook of surgery: The biological basis of modern surgical practice* (15th ed.). Philadelphia: W. B. Saunders.
22. Schlomer, P. (1998). Using a prosthesis to treat gastroesophageal reflux. *AORN Journal, 68*(1), 93–96.
23. Spiess, A., & Kahrilas, P. (1998). Treating achalasia. *JAMA, 280*(7), 638–643.
24. Steele, G., & Katz, J. (1996). *Primary Care: Gastroenterology, 23*(3), 417–648.
25. Whitney, L. (1995). Vincent's angina, periodontitis, and stomatitis. *Nursing, 25,* 32.

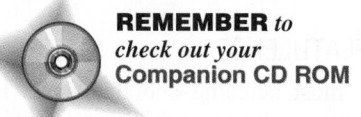

CHAPTER 31

Management of Clients with Digestive Disorders

Elizabeth A. Murphy-Blake

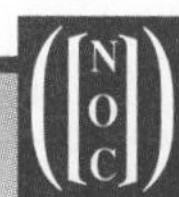

NURSING OUTCOMES CLASSIFICATION (NOC)
for Nursing Diagnoses—Clients with Digestive Disorders

Altered Nutrition: Less Than Body Requirements
Knowledge: Diet
Nutritional Status
Nutritional Status: Food and Fluid Intake
Nutritional Status: Nutrient Intake
Fear
Fear Control
Anxiety Control
Coping
Ineffective Management of Therapeutic Regimen (Individual)
Compliance Behavior
Knowledge: Treatment Regimen
Participation: Health Care Decisions
Treatment Behavior: Illness or Injury
Risk for Injury: Postoperative Complications
Circulation Status
Risk Control
Risk Detection
Safety Status: Physical Injury
Symptom Control
Tissue Perfusion: Abdominal Organs
Tissue Perfusion: Peripheral
Vital Signs Status
Pain
Comfort Level
Pain Control
Pain: Disruptive Effects
Pain Level

The client with a gastric disorder usually has a problem with nutritional intake. As a result, the most common nursing diagnoses are *Altered Nutrition: Less Than Body Requirements* and *Pain.* Additional nursing diagnoses (e.g., *Ineffective Management of Therapeutic Regimen [Individuals] related to dietary changes and pharmacologic management, Fear,* and *Risk for Injury related to complications)* are also possible.

GENERAL CLINICAL MANIFESTATIONS OF GASTROINTESTINAL DISORDERS

Manifestations of gastrointestinal (GI) tract dysfunction are caused by excessive gastric secretions that erode stomach mucosa, excessive motility, and retention of gastric contents. The most prominent clinical manifestations are pain, acid reflux, anorexia, belching and flatulence, nausea, vomiting, bleeding, indigestion, and diarrhea.

■ PAIN

Pain is the most characteristic clinical manifestation; it usually results from chemical irritation of nerve endings. Nerve irritation occurs when acid comes into contact with the eroded stomach mucosa. It also results from stretching and contracting of the stomach, caused in turn by increased motility and increased smooth muscle tension, as found in an obstruction.

■ ANOREXIA

Anorexia, or loss of appetite, is often experienced by clients with malignancy or various other disorders. Hunger is normally caused by several stimuli, including contraction of the empty stomach. When the stomach empties slowly or when gastric stasis occurs because of a gastric disorder, anorexia can result.

■ NAUSEA AND VOMITING

Nausea is a result of conditions that increase tension on the walls of the stomach, duodenum, or lower end of the esophagus. Unpleasant stimuli, distention, gastritis, and carcinoma of the stomach can produce nausea. Vomiting

---

This chapter incorporates material written for the fifth edition by Jane Hokanson Hawks.

may follow nausea or occur without it. Vomiting is caused by stimulation of the emetic center:

1. The chemoreceptor trigger zone (CTZ) in the fourth ventricle. The CTZ is stimulated by various drugs and body toxins. Conversely, medications of the phenothiazine derivative groups, such as chlorpromazine (Thorazine) and prochlorperazine (Compazine), depress vomiting caused by chemoreceptor stimulation. Serotonin antagonists, such as ondansetron (Zofran), block serotonin receptors in the vagus nerve and CTZ.
2. Nerve impulses, which can be excited by
   a. Direct mechanical stimuli, as in increased intracranial pressure
   b. Chemical stimuli from blood-borne metabolites or toxic substances
   c. Sympathetic and parasympathetic afferent nerve impulses through the vagus, glossopharyngeal, vestibular, and splanchnic nerves (the most sensitive receptors are located in the proximal duodenum)
3. Unpleasant odors, subjects, and sights that stimulate higher center impulses
4. Distention of stomach or duodenum
5. Decreased gastric motility
6. Pain, because the pain centers are close to the vomiting centers in the medulla
7. Increased intracranial pressure

BLEEDING

Bleeding results from local trauma or irritations that cause erosion or ulceration of the GI tract mucosa. The disorders involved include stomach neoplasms, gastric ulcer, gastritis, anastomotic (marginal) ulcers, and duodenal ulcers. Duodenitis can also cause bleeding. Although bleeding may have numerous causes, up to 75% of all cases of upper GI tract bleeding result from esophagogastric varices (venous), hemorrhagic gastritis (capillary), or peptic ulcer. Ulcers account for 80% of all upper GI tract hemorrhage.

DIARRHEA

Diarrhea can be caused by increased peristalsis resulting from an increased gastrocolic reflex or from the effort of the stomach and intestines to eliminate a local irritant.

BELCHING AND FLATULENCE

Swallowed air causes most belching and flatulence. It is easy to swallow air during eating and drinking, especially when food is ingested rapidly. Frequently, clients attempt to belch to relieve a vague feeling of distress in the stomach caused by swallowed air. Attempting to belch with the mouth closed sometimes adds more air to the stomach than it removes.

INDIGESTION

Indigestion or dyspepsia can be caused by such factors as strong emotions, GI tract disease, eating too rapidly, chewing inadequately, gas-forming foods (e.g., beans and cabbage), and food allergy.

GASTROINTESTINAL INTUBATION

Gastric and intestinal tubes are inserted for several purposes: (1) decompression, (2) lavage, (3) gastric analysis, and (4) tube feedings.

Decompression relieves the pressure caused by contents and gases that remain in the stomach or bowel because of some obstruction. Long intestinal tubes are sometimes used to dilate the lumen or to release an obstruction. Postoperative decompression removes secretions that cannot pass through the GI tract because of edema and decreased gastric motility. The placement of a tube (intubation) helps prevent vomiting, distention, and obstruction.

Lavage is the irrigation or washing out of an organ. Gastric lavage washes out the stomach. It is used most frequently as an emergency treatment in poisoning. Lavage is also used for exfoliative cytology to determine the presence of abnormal cells.

Tube feeding or *gavage feeding,* referred to as *enteral nutrition,* is a method of giving clients fluids and nutrients via a tube when oral intake is inadequate or impossible.

TYPES OF TUBES

Three types of tubes are used for decompression: (1) *short* nasogastric (NG) tubes are used for the stomach, (2) *medium* tubes extend into the duodenum or jejunum, and (3) *long* tubes are used for the rest of the GI tract (see Table 31–1).

TABLE 31–1 GASTRIC AND INTESTINAL TUBES

	Length	Size (French)	Lumen	Other Characteristics
SHORT TUBES				
Levin type (plastic or rubber)	125 cm (50 inches)	12, 16, 18	Single	
Salem sump	120 cm (48 inches)	12, 14, 16, 18	Double	Sump-type suction
MEDIUM TUBES				
Dobhoff (nasoduodenal or nasojejunal)	160–175 cm (60–66 inches)	8, 10, 12	Single	Radiopaque, tungsten-weighted
LONG TUBES				
Cantor	300 cm (10 feet)	16	Single	Mercury weighted
Harris	180 cm (6 feet)	14, 16	Single	Mercury weighted
Miller-Abbott	300 cm (10 feet)	12, 14, 16, 18	Double	Mercury weighted

Short Tubes

Short tubes include the Levin and Salem sump tubes. Short tubes are long enough to extend into the stomach but not into the bowel. These tubes are usually attached to suction. Occasionally, they may be used for short-term enteral feedings over a brief period. However, nasoduodenal tubes are preferred for feedings because of the high rate of aspiration pneumonia associated with NG tube feedings.

LEVIN TUBE. The Levin tube is a single-lumen tube used to remove fluid or gas or to obtain a specimen of gastric contents. Because the tube has only one lumen, low intermittent suction is required to minimize the irritation of the gastric mucosa. Levin tubes may be made out of plastic, rubber-like silicone (Silastic), or rubber.

SALEM SUMP TUBE. The Salem sump tube is a double-lumen tube used to empty and decompress the stomach. Low, continuous suction is used because the "pigtail" lumen on the Salem sump tube vents the tube and protects gastric mucosa from being sucked against the tube. The pigtail lumen should not be clamped or irrigated and should be kept higher than the client's stomach to prevent drainage.

Medium Tubes

Medium tubes include a variety of nasoduodenal (e.g., Dobhoff) tubes that extend into the duodenum and are designed for short-term feeding. They are less likely to cause aspiration pneumonia because of their small size and weighted tip. Placement is verified by abdominal x-ray study (radiography).

Long Tubes

The long tubes extend into the small bowel, sometimes for its entire length. They are between 1.8 and 3.0 m (6 and 10 feet) long and are used to prevent gas and fluid accumulation in the intestine, which is usually caused by intestinal obstruction. The more common long tubes are the Miller-Abbott, Cantor, and Harris tubes.

MILLER-ABBOTT TUBE. The Miller-Abbott tube is a double-lumen tube, 3 m (10 feet) long. One lumen is used to introduce mercury or to inflate the balloon at the end of the tube, and the other is used for aspiration. Markings on the tube indicate the distance the tube has been passed. Initial placement of the tube is completed by a physician. The nurse is responsible for advancing the tube as ordered.

CANTOR TUBE. The Cantor tube is used for aspirating intestinal contents and has only one lumen. It is 3 m (10 feet) long and is larger than the other tubes. It has 4 to 5 ml of mercury in a bag at the end, which is wrapped about the tube before insertion. For intestinal intubation, the tube is threaded through the nose into the stomach and then through the pylorus, where peristaltic activity of the bowel carries it to the desired intestinal area.

HARRIS TUBE. The Harris tube is a single-lumen, mercury-weighted tube, 1.8 m (6 feet) long. A metal tip is introduced into the nostril after it is lubricated. The weight of the mercury carries the tube by gravity. This tube is used for suction and irrigation.

Sometimes it is difficult to get intestinal tubes to pass through the pylorus. The client is instructed to lie on the right side in order to facilitate passage. When the tube has passed into the duodenum, it is advanced, as ordered, an additional 4.8 to 9.6 cm (2 to 4 inches) every hour or half-hour. When the tube has reached the desired location, tape it securely to the client's face to prevent further advancement.

Other Tubes

For long-term enteral feedings, gastrostomy tubes (GTs or G tubes) or jejunostomy tubes (JTs or J tubes) are often placed surgically. The GT and JT (see Chapter 29) can be inserted surgically or laparoscopically. The percutaneous gastrostomy (PEG), which is the most common, and the percutaneous jejunostomy (PEJ) have been discussed in Chapter 29.

■ INSERTING GASTROINTESTINAL TUBES

GI tubes are generally inserted through the nose into the stomach or small intestine; they are rarely inserted through the mouth. Explain each step of the intubation procedure at the client's level of understanding. Assist the client to assume a high Fowler's position, which makes intubation easier. Measure the distance on the tube from the tip of the nose to the ear lobe plus the distance from the ear lobe to the tip of the xiphoid process (the NEX measurement). This approximates the distance that the tube must be passed to reach the stomach. Mark this distance on the tubing with adhesive.

After measuring the tube, lubricate and gently insert the tube through the nares and posterior nasal pharynx and into the oropharynx. When the tube is in the oropharynx, instruct the client to swallow; sometimes the client is allowed to drink water at this point to help with tube passage. Having the client swallow is important, because the sphincter at the proximal end of the esophagus remains closed except during swallowing. The larynx rises during swallowing, stretching the cricopharyngeal muscle and causing it to relax, thus reducing resistance to the tube. Swallowing also enables the tube to enter the esophagus rather than the trachea. After the tube passes the sphincter, advance it into the stomach.

To verify placement, perform at least two of these activities:

1. Aspirate gastric contents.
2. Measure the pH of the aspirant; the pH of the stomach is less than that of the lungs.
3. Instill air into the tube with a syringe and listen with a stethoscope for air passing into the stomach.
4. Check with an x-ray study for the radiopaque lines on the tube.

After confirming placement, secure the tube to the nose with hypoallergenic tape. (This procedure is used for short tubes only; medium tubes are checked with an x-ray and long tubes need to be able to advance.)

■ SUCTIONING GASTROINTESTINAL TUBES

When suction is applied to a GI tube to remove accumulated gas and fluid, ensure that the GI mucosa is not traumatized. Excessive negative pressure causes the mucosa to be sucked into the openings on the tube, impairing suction and injuring the mucosa. Intermittent suction is used to avoid this problem unless a double-lumen tube, such as the Salem sump, is used. Mucus tends to plug the openings of these tubes, making it necessary to irrigate with saline as ordered to maintain or to check tube patency (usually every 4 hours).

■ NURSING MANAGEMENT OF CLIENTS WITH GASTROINTESTINAL TUBES

Maintain the client's comfort while the tube is in place. Some helpful nursing interventions include these steps:

1. Clean and lubricate external nares. The nares may become sore because of crusted secretions around the tube. Always use a water-soluble lubricant to avoid the possibility of lipid pneumonia when using an oil-based lubricant.
2. Tape the tube in a manner that prevents irritation of the nares.
3. Administer frequent oral hygiene to remove debris, increase comfort, maintain a healthy oral cavity, and stimulate saliva secretion. The client's mouth is usually dry because the absence of chewing prevents the normal stimulus to salivary secretions and the presence of the tube causes mouth breathing.
4. Permit the client, if possible, to chew gum or suck on sour candies or ice chips to help stimulate salivation. Excessive use stimulates gastric secretions and causes electrolyte loss through the suction.
5. Brush the client's teeth or assist the client in brushing teeth.
6. Request an order for anesthetic mouth rinses or lozenges because the presence of the tube frequently causes sore throat.

Placement of the tube in the throat may result in cricoid chondritis (irritation of the cricoid cartilage of the larynx) and laryngeal injuries. Presenting clinical manifestations include:

- Localized odynophagia
- Pain radiating to the ears
- Sore throat
- Stridor
- Bloody sputum
- Mild hoarseness

Assess for these potential complications and report the findings immediately. An order for anesthetic lozenges or gargles to relieve manifestations may be needed. Frequent assessment of secretions for color, odor, and quantity is essential. Report any changes to the physician. It may be necessary to send samples of these secretions to the laboratory for analysis. Measure the contents of the suction containers to maintain an accurate record of GI losses. Metabolic alkalosis may result from a major loss of water and electrolytes. Monitor potassium levels, since potassium is one of the major electrolytes lost through suctioning.

The irrigating solution instilled into a GI tube is counted as intake if it is not removed when contents are aspirated. Keep accurate records of the amount instilled and the amount aspirated from the tube during irrigations. Normal saline is the preferred irrigating solution because water, a hypotonic solution, increases electrolyte loss through osmotic action if the tube is irrigated frequently.

GASTRITIS

ACUTE GASTRITIS

Gastritis, an inflammation of the gastric mucosa, is classified as either acute or chronic. The incidence of gastritis is highest in the fifth and sixth decades of life; men are more frequently affected than women. The incidence is greater in clients who are heavy drinkers and smokers.

Etiology and Risk Factors

The acute form of gastritis may be seen with nausea and vomiting, epigastric discomfort, bleeding, malaise, and anorexia. It usually stems from ingestion of a corrosive, erosive, or infectious substance. Aspirin and other nonsteroidal anti-inflammatory drugs (NSAIDs), digitalis, chemotherapeutic drugs, steroids, acute alcoholism, and food poisoning (typically caused by *Staphylococcus* organisms) are common causes. In addition, food substances, including excessive amounts of tea, coffee, mustard, paprika, cloves, and pepper, can precipitate acute gastritis. Foods with a rough texture or those eaten at an extremely high temperature can also damage the stomach mucosa. Ingestion of corrosive agents, such as lye or drain cleaner, also causes acute gastritis.

Disorders linked with acute gastritis include uremia, shock, central nervous system lesions, hepatic cirrhosis, portal hypertension, and prolonged emotional tension. Acute gastritis is usually of short duration unless the gastric mucosa has suffered extensive damage.

Health promotion behaviors include limited use of NSAIDs, alcohol, and caffeine and avoidance of nicotine products. Health maintenance behaviors include use of enteric-coated aspirin, misoprostol (Cytotec) to protect against NSAIDs, histamine-receptor antagonists to decrease gastric acidity, or proton pump inhibitors to block gastric acid production. Clients with medical disorders that may lead to gastritis should follow orders for prescribed medications to minimize stomach irritation.

Pathophysiology

The mucosal lining of the stomach normally protects it from the action of gastric acid. This mucosal barrier is composed of prostaglandins. If this barrier is penetrated, gastritis occurs, with resultant injury to the mucosa. When hydrochloric acid comes into contact with the mucosa, injury to small vessels occurs with edema, hemorrhage, and possible ulcer formation. The damage associated with acute gastritis is usually limited.

Clinical Manifestations

Assessment typically reveals epigastric discomfort, abdominal tenderness, cramping, belching, reflux, severe nausea and vomiting, and sometimes hematemesis. Sometimes GI bleeding is the only manifestation. When contaminated food is the cause of gastritis, the client usually develops diarrhea within 5 hours of ingestion of the offending substance.

Diagnosis is based on a detailed history of food intake, medications taken, and any disorders related to gastritis. The physician may also perform a gastroscopic examination with a biopsy.

Outcome Management

Medical Management

Intervention involves removing the cause and treating the manifestations. Vomiting frequently responds to medications of the phenothiazine group; pain responds to antacids or histamine (H_2) receptor antagonists (see Table 31–2). If ingestion of NSAIDs is a problem, a prostaglandin E_1 (PGE_1) analog may be prescribed to protect the stomach mucosa and inhibit gastric acid secretion.

Initially, foods and fluids are withheld until nausea and vomiting subside. Once the client tolerates food, the diet includes decaffeinated tea, gelatin, toast, and simple, bland foods. The client should avoid spicy foods, caffeine, and large, heavy meals. In the continued absence of nausea, vomiting, and bloating, the client can slowly return to a normal diet.

Nursing Management of the Medical Client

Nursing management of the medical client with acute gastritis is described in the section on chronic gastritis.

CHRONIC GASTRITIS

This condition appears in three different forms:

- *Superficial gastritis,* which causes a reddened, edematous mucosa with small erosions and hemorrhages
- *Atrophic gastritis,* which occurs in all layers of the stomach, develops frequently in association with gastric ulcer and gastric cancer, and is invariably present in pernicious anemia; it is characterized by a decreased number of parietal and chief cells
- *Hypertrophic gastritis,* which produces a dull and nodular mucosa with irregular, thickened, or nodular rugae; hemorrhages occur frequently

Etiology and Risk Factors

Peptic ulcer disease (PUD), infection with *Helicobacter pylori* bacteria, or gastric surgery may lead to chronic gastritis. Other risk factors are similar to those for acute gastritis. Chronic gastritis is associated with atrophy of the gastrin glands. After gastric resection with a gastrojejunostomy, bile and bile acids may reflux into the remaining stomach, causing gastritis. *H. pylori* infection can lead to chronic atrophic gastritis, which predisposes to the development of gastric cancer. Age is also a risk factor; chronic gastritis is more common in older adults.

Pathophysiology

The initial pathophysiologic changes associated with chronic gastritis are the same as with acute gastritis. The stomach lining first becomes thickened and erythematous and then becomes thin and atrophic. Continued deterioration and atrophy lead to loss of function of the parietal cells. When the acid secretion decreases, the source of intrinsic factor is lost, which results in inability to absorb vitamin B_{12}; this leads to the development of pernicious anemia.

In chronic gastritis the mucosa usually heals without scarring, but ulcer formation and bleeding can occur. The atrophic changes eventually result in a minimal amount of acid being secreted into the stomach (achlorhydria), which is a major risk factor for the development of gastric cancer.

Clinical Manifestations

Manifestations are vague and may be absent (because the problem does not cause an increase in hydrochloric acid). Assessment may reveal anorexia, a feeling of fullness, dyspepsia, belching, vague epigastric pain, nausea, vomiting, and intolerance of spicy or fatty foods.

Complications of Gastritis

The clinical course of clients with chronic gastritis may include such complications as bleeding, pernicious anemia, and gastric cancer. Bleeding can be a complication of gastritis, especially when the stomach mucosa becomes denuded or erosive. Bleeding is common with use of alcohol, aspirin, or NSAIDs. The client should undergo an endoscopic examination to determine the source of the bleeding. Another possible complication of atrophic gastritis is diminished ability of the stomach to secrete intrinsic factor, resulting in malabsorption of vitamin B_{12}, which is confirmed by Schilling's test. Gastric cancer may be suspected in a client whose gastritis does not heal with therapy. (See Gastric Cancer later in this chapter.)

Outcome Management

Medical Management

Intervention begins when the health care provider rules out cancer as a causative factor. Discomfort may lessen with a bland diet, small frequent meals, antacids, anticholinergics, and sedatives and with avoidance of foods that cause manifestations.

If *H. pylori* bacteria are present, a combination of clarithromycin (Biaxin), metronidazole (Flagyl), and omeprazole (Prilosec) is administered to eliminate the bacteria. If 1 week of this regimen does not succeed eliminating the bacteria, it may be repeated for an additional week.

Medications used to treat chronic gastritis are the same as those given in Table 31–2 for treatment of PUD. Corticosteroids are sometimes prescribed in the hope of inducing some parietal cell regeneration. Intramuscular injections of vitamin B_{12} may be administered monthly if the client has pernicious anemia.

Nursing Management of the Medical Client

When assessing the client with acute or chronic gastritis, carefully focus on risk factors. Consider the client's diet, patterns of eating, use of prescription and over-the-

TABLE 31–2 MEDICATIONS COMMONLY USED TO TREAT PEPTIC ULCERS

Class	Action	Therapeutic Outcomes	Adverse Outcomes	Dosing
ANTIBACTERIAL REGIMEN TO ERADICATE *H. PYLORI*				
Clarithromycin (Biaxin); metronidazole (Flagyl); and omeprazole (Prilosec) or ranitidine (Zantac)	Eradicate *H. pylori* bacteria that cause peptic ulcer disease and gastritis	Reduced gastric pain and bleeding. Elimination of *H. pylori*	Diarrhea, suprainfection with *Clostridium difficile*	Instruct client to take as ordered (usually twice daily for 7 days); monitor for diarrhea and signs of suprainfection; encourage client to take entire prescribed regimen.
HYPOSECRETORY AGENTS				
Histamine (H_2) Receptor Antagonists				
Ranitidine hydrochloride (Zantac)	Inhibits gastric acid secretion by blocking H_2-receptors on parietal cells	Reduced gastric pain and bleeding. Short-term and maintenance treatment of duodenal and gastric ulcers. Prevention of PUD with NSAIDs and stress ulcers	All side effects rare including nausea, constipation, bradycardia, increased liver enzymes, and headache	Give IM, IV, or PO 1 hr before meals or as maintenance dose at bedtime. Give antacids at least 1 hr before or 2 hr after ranitidine; use cautiously in clients with liver or renal disorders; absorption not affected by food; interacts minimally with diazepam (Valium), glipizide (Glucotrol), theophylline, and warfarin (Coumadin).
Prostaglandin Analogs				
Misoprostol (Cytotec)	Suppresses secretion of gastric acid and stimulates production of cytoprotective mucus	Prevention of aspirin and NSAID-induced gastric ulcers. Relief of pain and bleeding for PUD	Diarrhea, nausea, abdominal discomfort, headache, and dizziness Cannot be used in pregnancy because it stimulates uterine contractions	Give with meals qid (last dose at bedtime). Avoid with Mg^+ antacids and pregnancy.
Anticholinergics				
Dicyclomine hydrochloride (Bentyl)	Muscarinic antagonist; inhibits secretion of gastric acid in large doses	Decreases motility and spasms of GI tract	Headache, palpitations, dizziness, constipation, paralytic ileus, urinary hesitancy and retention, and dry mouth	Give 1 hr before meals and at bedtime. Do not give if active bleeding. Do not use in clients with obstructive uropathy, gastrointestinal obstruction, ulcerative colitis, unstable cardiovascular status, or toxic megacolon; use carefully in clients with narrow-angle glaucoma, hyperthyroidism, hiatal hernia, congestive heart failure, hepatic or renal disease.

Proton Pump Inhibitors				
Omeprazole (Prilosec)	Suppression of acid secretion by inhibiting H^+, K^+-ATPase (the enzyme that makes gastric acid)	Short-term (4–8 weeks) treatment of active duodenal ulcer, active benign gastric ulcer, and heartburn associated with gastroesophageal reflux disease	Headache, diarrhea, nausea, vomiting. Gastric cancer is a risk factor with long term use	Give once a day for 4–8 weeks before breakfast or at bedtime.
Antacids				
Aluminum-magnesium combinations (Riopan, Maalox, Mylanta, Gelusil)	Increases gastric pH to reduce pepsin activity; strengthens gastric mucosal barrier and esophageal sphincter tone; direct H^+ ion buffering	Short-term treatment of duodenal ulcer. Hasten healing of gastric ulcers. Treatment of reflux disease	Mild constipation or diarrhea	Give 1 hr before meals and at bedtime. Do not use in clients with renal disease; monitor bowel movements and signs of hypermagnesemia; Riopan low in sodium; do not give within 1 to 2 hr of H_2-receptor antagonists, tetracycline; causes decreased absorption of many drugs.
MUCOSAL BARRIER FORTIFIERS				
Sucralfate (Carafate)	In presence of mild acid condition, forms viscid and sticky gel and adheres to ulcer surface, forming a protective barrier	Short-term treatment of active gastric ulcers Maintenance treatment of PUD	Dizziness, constipation, sleepiness, nausea, and gastric discomfort	Give on empty stomach 1 hr before meals and at bedtime. Do not give within 30 min of antacids. Urge client to take entire prescribed regimen.

ATP, adenosine triphosphate; GI, gastrointestinal; IM, intramuscularly; IV, intravenously; NSAIDs, nonsteroidal anti-inflammatory drugs; PO, orally; qid, four times a day; PUD, peptic ulcer disease.

counter drugs, and lifestyle, including alcohol consumption and cigarette smoking.

Reduce Pain

Focus on teaching the client about the causes of gastritis and foods that may worsen the disease. Help the client assess factors that increase manifestations, such as stress or fatigue, taking certain medications on an empty stomach, ingestion of foods and beverages, alcohol consumption, and smoking. Encourage the client to avoid these agents.

Aluminum hydroxide with magnesium trisilicate (Gaviscon), which produces a soothing foam, is the best antacid for gastritis. H_2-receptor antagonists, proton pump inhibitors, antisecretory agents, and drugs that enhance mucosal defenses also provide pain relief (Table 31–2).

If the nausea and vomiting are severe, the client may be given nothing by mouth until these problems decrease in severity. When the pain and nausea associated with gastritis have subsided, the client is instructed to have a well-balanced diet and avoid irritating foods and beverages.

Promote Self-Care

Clients with acute and chronic gastritis are managed at home unless complications develop. Instruct the client with chronic gastritis to see the health care provider at regular intervals. This is particularly important if the diagnosis is *H. pylori* infection and atrophic gastritis, because these problems are closely related to gastric cancer. Teach the client to use medications correctly, to maintain adequate nutrition, and to control risk factors that contribute to gastritis.

Surgical Management

If conservative measures have not controlled bleeding, surgery may be necessary. Subtotal gastrectomy, pyloroplasty, vagotomy, or total gastrectomy may be indicated with severe erosive gastritis. These procedures are discussed in the section on peptic ulcer disease.

PEPTIC ULCER DISEASE

Peptic ulcer disease (PUD) involves a break in continuity of the esophageal, gastric, or duodenal mucosa. It may occur in any part of the GI tract that comes into contact with gastric juices (hydrochloric acid and pepsin). The ulcer may be found in the esophagus, stomach, duodenum, or the jejunum after gastroenterostomy.

PUD occurs in approximately 10% of the population. Gastric ulcers are more likely to occur during the fifth and sixth decades of life; duodenal ulcers more commonly occur during the fourth and fifth decades for men. For women, the occurrence is about 10 years later in life. Men are more likely to have both gastric and duodenal ulcers.

■ DUODENAL ULCERS

Duodenal ulcers, which have a higher incidence than gastric ulcers, usually occur within 1.5 cm (0.6 inch) of the pylorus. These ulcers are usually characterized by high gastric acid secretion. Some are associated with normal gastric secretion associated with rapid emptying of the stomach. Hypersecretion of acid is attributed to a greater mass of parietal cells. Stimuli for acid secretion include protein-rich meals, alcohol consumption, calcium, and vagal stimulation.

Clients with a duodenal ulcer experience low pH levels in the duodenum for longer periods. The stomach lining is more sensitive to gastrin and secretes excess gastrin.

Finally, clients with duodenal ulcers have more rapid gastric emptying. The combined effect of hypersecretion of acid and rapid emptying of food from the stomach reduces the buffering effect of food and results in a large acid load in the duodenum. Within the duodenum, inhibitory mechanisms and pancreatic secretion may be insufficient to control the acid load.

■ GASTRIC ULCERS

Gastric ulcers, which tend to heal within a few weeks, form within 1 inch (2.5 cm) of the pylorus of the stomach in an area where gastritis is common. Gastric ulcers are probably caused by a break in the mucosal barrier. The barrier, which differs from the layer of glycoprotein mucus that overlies the gastric epithelium, normally allows hydrochloric acid to be secreted into the stomach without injury to the epithelial cells. An incompetent pylorus may decrease production of mucus, the usual gastric defense. The reflux of bile acids through an incompetent pylorus into the stomach may break the mucosal barrier. Decreased blood flow to the gastric mucosa may also alter the defensive barrier and may make the duodenum more susceptible to gastric acid and pepsin trauma. The recurrence rate of gastric ulcer is lower than that of duodenal ulcer.

Table 31–3 distinguishes gastric from duodenal peptic ulcers.

■ STRESS-INDUCED AND DRUG-INDUCED ULCERS

Besides peptic ulcers, acute gastric erosion, frequently called *stress ulcers* or *stress erosive gastritis,* can occur after an acute medical crisis. Major assaults that give rise to gastroduodenal ulcerations include:

- Severe trauma or major illness
- Severe burns (may cause what is known as Curling's ulcers)
- Head injury or intracranial disease (frequently called Cushing's ulcers)
- Ingestion of a drug (e.g., aspirin, NSAIDs, steroids, and alcohol) that acts on the gastric mucosa (Fig. 31–1)
- Shock
- Sepsis

Etiology and Risk Factors

The causal factor in more than 90% of all peptic ulcers has been attributed to *H. pylori.* Eradication of the organism usually results in resolution of gastritis and subsequent ulcer healing. Multiple studies support this finding, which calls into question earlier theories about the causes of PUD.

The occurrence of PUD depends on the defensive resistance of the mucosa in relation to the aggressive force of secretory activity. The defensive resistance of the mu-

TABLE 31–3 CLASSIFICATION OF PEPTIC ULCERS

Assessment Data	Duodenal Ulcers	Gastric Ulcers
Location of ulcer	¼ to 1 inch from pylorus	Junction of fundus and pylorus, some in antrum
Acid secretion	Increased	Normal to decreased
Serum pepsinogen I	Increased	Normal
Serum gastrin		
Fasting	Normal	Elevated
Postprandial	Elevated	
Blood group	Most frequently type O	No difference
Age at onset	25–50 years	Peaks at 45–54 years
Gender predominance	Men to women, 4:1	Men to women, 2:1
Associated gastritis	None	Common and increased
Pain	Occurs on empty stomach, 2–3 hr after meals or in middle of night; relieved by food and antacids	Variable pain pattern; may be made worse by food; antacids ineffective
Nutritional status	Usually well nourished	Probably malnourished
Malignancy potential	Rare, no increase in incidence	Occurs in approximately 10% of clients
Bleeding pattern	Melena more common than hematemesis	Hematemesis more common than melena
Recurrence	May occur as marginal ulcers after surgery	Recurrence unlikely after surgery

cosa depends on mucosal integrity and regeneration, presence of a protective mucous barrier, adequate blood flow to the mucosa, ability of the duodenal inhibitory mechanism to regulate secretion, and the presence of adequate gastromucosal prostaglandins. The aggressive factors of PUD are related to the presence of *H. pylori* and the volume of hydrochloric and biliary acids. Ulceration occurs when aggressive factors exceed the defensive barrier. The aggressive nature of the gastric juice may be the result of hypersecretion of gastric juices, increased stimulation of the vagus nerve, decreased inhibition of gastric secretions, increased capacity or number of the parietal cells secreting hydrochloric acid, or increased response of the parietal cells to stimulation.

Risk factors that contribute to PUD include smoking (nicotine), steroids, aspirin, NSAIDs, caffeine, alcohol, and stress. Certain medical conditions, including Crohn's disease, Zollinger-Ellison syndrome, and hepatic and biliary disease, may also play a role.

Health promotion and health maintenance actions for clients with PUD are the same as those discussed for acute gastritis. Health restoration for clients involves treating medical disorders that cause secondary PUD. Ensure that the client complies with the prescribed medication regimen to minimize stomach irritation. Treat aggressively any disorders that result in the development of PUD, for example, long-term use of steroids, severe burns, and chronic renal failure.

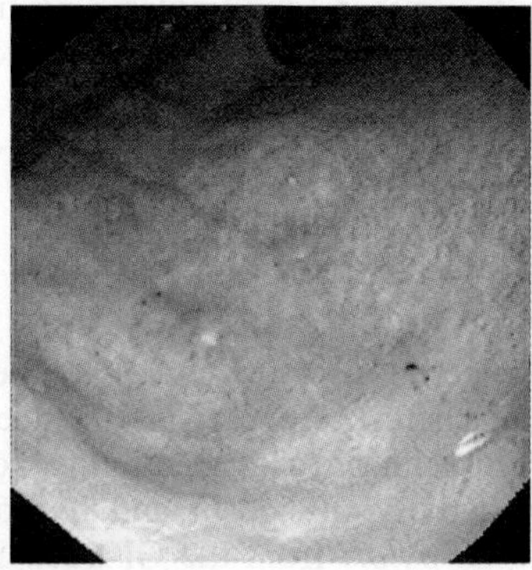

FIGURE 31–1 Gastric peptic ulceration caused by nonsteroidal anti-inflammatory drugs.

Pathophysiology

In addition to *H. pylori* inflammation as the primary pathophysiologic change, two different mechanisms for the development of PUD have been proposed. In the stomach, it is thought that a breakdown of the normally protective epithelial lining causes gastric ulcers. Under normal circumstances, flow of hydrochloric acid from the lumen of the stomach is prevented by the presence of tight, nonpermeable junctions between the epithelial cells and by the slightly alkaline layer of mucus that coats the surface of the gastric epithelium.

In the formation of a gastric peptic ulcer, this diffusion barrier may be interrupted by the chronic presence of such injurious substances as aspirin, NSAIDs, cortisone, adrenocorticotropic hormone (ACTH), caffeine, phenylbutazone (Butazolidin), alcohol, and chemotherapeutic agents. These substances may stimulate acid production, cause local mucosal damage, and suppress mucus secretion. The substances strip away surface mucus and cause degeneration of epithelial cell membranes with massive diffusion of acid back into the gastric epithelial wall.

The pathogenesis of duodenal peptic ulcers has a different proposed mechanism, as excess acid secretion is responsible for ulcer development. Activity of the vagus nerve is increased in people with duodenal ulcers, particularly during a fasting state and at night. The vagus nerve stimulates the pyloric antrum cells to release gastrin, which travels via the bloodstream and acts on the gastric parietal cells to stimulate the release of hydrochloric acid.

Another factor in PUD is emotional stress, which can cause an increase in gastric secretion, blood supply, and gastric motility by thalamic stimulation of the vagal nerves. Hormonal influence takes place via the hypothalamus through the pituitary adrenal route. In clients with stress reactions, the sympathetic nervous system causes the blood vessels in the duodenum to constrict, which makes the mucosa more vulnerable to trauma from gastric acid and pepsin secretion. On activation of the adrenal cortex, mucus production decreases and gastric secretion increases. Together, these factors result in increased vulnerability to ulceration. Stress reactions thus upset the aggressive-defensive balance. Prolonged stress associated with burns, severe trauma, and other conditions can produce stress ulcers, or stress erosive gastritis, in the GI tract.

Zollinger-Ellison syndrome is characterized by abnormal secretion of gastrin by a rare islet cell tumor in the pancreas. Pathophysiologic changes associated with this syndrome include hypergastrinemia and diarrhea secondary to fat malabsorption resulting from decreased duodenum-inactivating pancreatic lipase or acid-induced injury of the villi. In addition to increased gastric secretion, hyperplasia of the gastric mucosa is induced by the trophic effects of gastrin. Treatment of the Zollinger-Ellison syndrome is aimed at suppression of acid secretion.

Treated ulcers usually heal without difficulty. Untreated ulcers or those that do not respond to treatment can result in perforation, hemorrhage, or obstruction, which may require surgical treatment. Some ulcers recur after healing, particularly if the risk factors associated with their development are not modified.

Critically ill clients are susceptible to *stress ulcers*. For example, gastric mucosal changes caused by stress develop within 72 hours in 78% of clients with greater than 35% burns on their body. Stress ulcers manifest with superficial gastric erosions, often accompanied by painless massive gastric hemorrhage. The client characteristically has multiple lesions, usually small and superficial, that do not extend through the muscularis mucosae. These lesions may appear to ooze blood. The mechanism causing stress ulcerations is unknown, but it probably involves ischemia. In the presence of acid, ischemia can produce erosive gastritis and ulcerations. Increased hydrogen ion back-diffusion and decreased mucosal perfusion may also contribute to stress ulcer formation. Low gastric pH (high acidity) is necessary for development of stress ulcers.

Researchers continue to seek the precise mechanism by which stress ulcers occur. Few manifestations accompany stress ulcer. These ulcerations are typically painless unless perforation occurs, which is rare. Upper GI tract hemorrhage is the major manifestation of stress ulcers. About 10% of clients experience dyspepsia before hemorrhage, but typically there are no warning manifestations. When stress ulcers cause profound hemorrhage, the mortality rate rises to about 50%.

Clinical Manifestations

PAIN. The principal manifestation of ulcers is an aching, burning, cramp-like, gnawing pain. The pain has a definite relationship to eating. With gastric ulcers, food may cause the pain and vomiting may relieve it. Clients with duodenal ulcers have pain with an empty stomach, and discomfort may be relieved by ingestion of food or antacids. Clients usually describe the pain as circumscribed in an area 2 to 10 cm (0.8 to 4 inches) in diameter, between the xiphoid cartilage and the umbilicus. Gastric ulcer pain often occurs in the upper epigastrium, with localization to the left of the midline, whereas duodenal pain is in the right epigastrium. Ulcer pain also varies with the site, size, or penetration of the ulcer or the amount of surrounding fibrotic tissue.

In duodenal ulcers, steady pain near the midline of the back between the sixth and 10th thoracic vertebrae with radiation to the right upper quadrant may indicate perforation of the posterior duodenal wall. Fullness or hunger may also be present. Distention of the duodenal bulb produces epigastric pain, which may radiate to the back and thorax. Hydrochloric acid secretion may produce edema and inflammation, with resultant pain, or may activate motor changes with increased spasm, intragastric pressure, and increased motility, also with resultant pain. In addition, ulcer pain tends to occur in distinct periods (periodicity).

NAUSEA AND VOMITING. Clients with a duodenal ulcer usually have a normal appetite unless pyloric obstruction is present. Carcinoma, gastric ulcers, or gastritis may be associated with anorexia, weight loss, and dysphagia. Vomiting occurs more often with gastric ulcer than with uncomplicated duodenal ulcer. It also occurs more frequently when the ulcer is in the pylorus or antrum of the stomach. Vomiting results from gastric stasis or pyloric obstruction, and the client typically vomits undigested food. Severe retching and vomiting may suggest an esophageal tear.

BLEEDING. Clients with ulcers often bleed when the ulcer erodes through a blood vessel. Bleeding may occur as massive hemorrhage or may be occult, with slow oozing. Approximately 25% of clients with gastric ulcers may experience bleeding.

The diagnosis of ulcers is confirmed on the basis of manifestations, x-ray evidence, and endoscopy. The history and physical examination do not yield much significant information in a client with uncomplicated peptic ulcer. A complete blood count with decreased hematocrit and hemoglobin values may indicate bleeding. Stool testing for occult blood might also be positive if bleeding is present. Testing for the presence of *H. pylori* can be done via urea breath tests or identification of *H. pylori* serum antibodies in addition to esophagogastroduodenoscopy (EGD) with biopsy.

The major diagnostic tests include EGD and an upper GI tract x-ray series. The EGD has several advantages. It allows the physician to take tissue specimens and to treat the ulcer with either multipolar electrocoagulation (MPEC) or heater-probe therapy (see complications under Medical Management).

Outcome Management

Medical Management

The primary objective of intervention for peptic ulcer is to provide stomach rest. Approaches include neutralizing or buffering hydrochloric acid, inhibiting acid secretion, decreasing the activity of pepsin and hydrochloric acid, and eradicating *H. pylori* from the GI tract. Specific measures include medications, physical and emotional rest, dietary management, and stress reduction.

Response to the therapeutic program varies with clients' perception of their health status and the degree to which lifestyle influences the ulcer disease. The following list outlines the hallmarks of successful interventions:

- The client experiences a decrease in pain with eventual elimination of all ulcer pain and related manifestations.
- The client eats a nutritionally sound diet and reports increased tolerance of food.
- The client complies with the medication schedule (see Table 31–2).
- The client identifies stressors and develops ways to modify stress and make necessary lifestyle changes.

ELIMINATE *H. PYLORI* BACTERIA

The antibacterial regimen used for treatment of *H. pylori* consists of clarithromycin (Biaxin), 250 mg twice a day, plus metronidazole (Flagyl), 250 mg four times daily, plus omeprazole (Prilosec), 20 mg twice a day or ranitidine (Zantac) twice a day (see Table 31–2). More than 90% of clients are cured by using this protocol for 1 week. Fewer than 10% of clients require a second week of treatment or a variation of pharmacologic agents.

REDUCE GASTRIC SECRETIONS

Hyposecretory agents cause a reduction in acid secretions. These agents include H_2-receptor antagonists, prostaglandin analogs, anticholinergics, proton pump inhibitors, and antacids (the drugs are shown in Table 31–2).

STRENGTHEN MUCOSAL BARRIER

Mucosal barrier fortifiers prevent hydrogen ion back-diffusion into the mucosa and stimulate mucus production, which results in accelerated gastric ulcer healing (see Table 31–2). Prostaglandin analogs, in addition to decreasing acid secretion, stimulate production of cytoprotective mucus.

MODIFY DIET

For uncomplicated ulcer disease, few physicians or advanced practitioners favor strict dietary changes. There is scant evidence that diet treatment promotes or accelerates healing. Foods known to increase gastric acidity or cause discomfort should be avoided, such as coffee, alcohol, protein foods, and milk.

PREVENT AND TREAT COMPLICATIONS

Hemorrhage, perforation, and obstruction are the main complications that develop after PUD.

Hemorrhage

ASSESS BLEEDING. Hemorrhage varies in degree from minimal, manifested by the presence of occult blood in the stool (melena), to massive, manifested by vomitus containing bright red blood (hematemesis). The usual manifestation of GI tract bleeding is either vomiting of coffee ground–like material or passing of tarry stools. Acid digestion of blood in the stomach results in a granular dark emesis, whereas digestion in the duodenum or below may result in a black stool. Hemorrhage tends to occur more often with gastric ulcers (Fig. 31–2), especially in the elderly population. Although the onset of hemorrhage may be associated with fatigue, nervous tension, upper respiratory tract infection, dietary indiscretion, alcoholism, or irritating drugs, there may be no known precipitating factor.

Manifestations depend on the severity of the hemorrhage. With mild bleeding (<500 ml), the client may experience only slight weakness and diaphoresis. Severe loss of more than 1 L of blood per 24 hours may cause manifestations of shock (see Chapter 81).

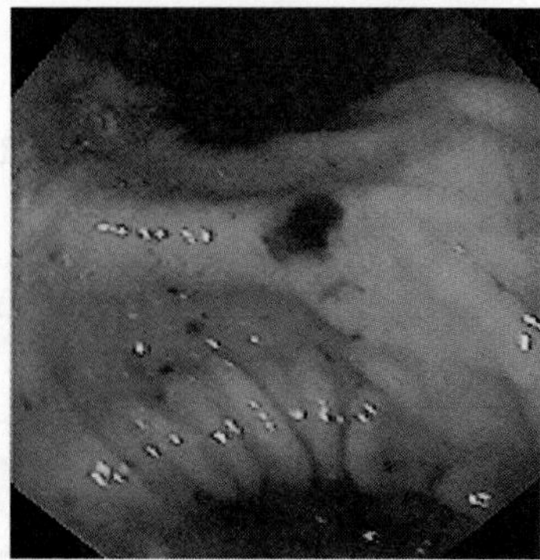

FIGURE 31–2 Bleeding ulcer on gastric mucosa.

PREVENT SHOCK. Intervention for massive bleeding aims to treat hypovolemic shock, prevent dehydration and electrolyte imbalance, and stop the bleeding. The client, who should be fasting, receives intravenous fluids until the bleeding subsides. The nurse or the physician may insert an NG tube in the presence or absence of blood in

GUIDE TO CLINICAL PATHWAY

GI Hemorrhage

GI hemorrhage is an acute condition that requires a complete assessment of the client. This care map indicates a 3 day hospital stay in order to diagnose and treat the bleeding. Some of the assessments are completed in the laboratory, where the client may undergo endoscopy to determine the cause and location of the bleeding. Ensure that the client will be ready for the endoscopy by maintaining NPO status.

A second major nursing focus is assessment of the influence of blood loss on activity and oxygenation. Note the client's hemoglobin levels, reports of fatigue at rest and during activity, and oxygenation levels at rest and during activity with and without oxygen (using pulse oximetry). If oxygen saturation cannot be kept above 92%, transfusion may be required. Blood loss may be occult, and the client should be assessed for changes in vital signs, and presence of blood in vomitus or stool.

Discharge to self-care is the goal, but only if the cause and location of the bleeding are determined and only if the client can provide self-care. If the bleeding is a result of suspected or confirmed alcohol abuse, consult the discharge coordinator or social worker early in the hospital stay to determine discharge needs.

The CareMap is reprinted with permission from Baptist Health Center–Montclair. The CareMap shown is an excerpt of one covering emergency department admission through discharge.

Helen Andrews, BSN, RN, *Care Manager, Alegent Health Bergan Mercy Medical Center, Omaha, Nebraska,* and
Linda R. Haddick, MSN, RN, *Clinical Nurse Specialist, Alegent Health Home Care & Hospice, Omaha, Nebraska*

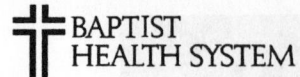

BAPTIST HEALTH SYSTEM

GI HEMORRHAGE CAREMAP

(Addressograph)

	Phase I - ER Adm 0-24 Hrs.: Date: ______	INITIAL Met	INITIAL Not Met	Phase II - 24-48 Hrs.: Date: ______	INITIAL Met	INITIAL Not Met
General Safety:	Bed rails up Fall precautions Bleeding precautions Airway precautions Call light within reach			Bed rails up Fall precautions Bleeding precautions Call light within reach		
Activity	Advance as tolerated.			Advance as tolerated.		
	Goal: Tolerates activity without SOB.	____	____	**Goal:** Tolerates activity progression.	____	____
Dietary: Consult Date/Time Completed ______	NPO except meds. Advance per orders			Advance as ordered.		
	Goal: Tolerates 50% of diet as ordered.	____	____	**Goal:** Tolerates po intake.	____	____
Respiratory: Consult Date/Time Completed ______	Check SaO2 on RA: if < 92%, start O2 at 2 L/M. Wean O2 per protocol.			Wean O2 per protocol as indicated.		
	Goal: SaO2 ≥ 92%; No SOB.	____	____	**Goal:** SaO2 ≥ 92% on RA.	____	____
Rehab: Consult Date/Time Completed ______	**Goal:**	____	____	**Goal:**	____	____
Discharge Planning: Consult Date/Time Completed ______	1. Identify DCP needs & initiate plan. Notify Social Worker if: • patient has HHC • patient is from a Nursing Home or Assisted Living facility • patient has other discharge/social needs 2. Initiate Teaching For: • Diet • NSAID use • ETOH use • Smoking cessation • Treatment for PUD 3. Discharge Instruction sheet (if discharged) 4. Distribute Patient/Family CareMap.			Continue DCP plan. Reinforce Teaching For: • Diet • NSAID use • ETOH use • Smoking cessation • Treatment for PUD Discharge Instruction sheet (if discharged)		
	Goal: DCP needs identified; plan initiated. **Goal:** Teaching plan initiated.	____ ____	____ ____	**Goal:** Discharge/Teaching Plan continued. **Goal:** Prepare for D/C in AM.	____ ____	____ ____
Nursing: Consult Date/Time Completed ______	Vital signs: frequency per MD orders. Assess GI function, bowel sounds, N/V/D. Document color/character of emesis/stool. Document use of NSAIDS, antiplatelets, anticoagulants. Have transfusion consent signed. I & O Q shift. Verify MD consults.			Assess GI function, bowel sounds, N/V/D. VS q shift. Document color/character/amount of aspirate, emesis, stool. I & O Q shift.		
	Goal: No signs/symptoms of GI bleeding. **Goal:** No vomiting or diarrhea **Goal:** VS stable.	____ ____ ____	____ ____ ____	**Goal:** No signs/symptoms of GI bleeding. **Goal:** No vomiting or diarrhea **Goal:** VS stable.	____ ____ ____	____ ____ ____
Tests:	CBC; Basic Metabolic Profile; PT with INR; Colonoscopy; Hemoccult Stool; Type & Screen; Hct now then Q 8 h x 24 hr then QD. Permit for EGD, Colonoscopy, Routine pre-post procedure orders. Transfuse per orders			HCT QD		
	Goal: Initial diagnostic test completed w/i 24 hours. **Goal:** Site identification via diagnostic procedure. **Goal:** No adverse reaction to blood components.	____ ____ ____	____ ____ ____	**Goal:** Hct stable and increasing.	____	____
Other:						
	Goal:	____	____	**Goal:**	____	____

GI HEMORRHAGE CAREMAP G-99-5149-2 PG REV. 9/22/99 P

the stomach to assess the rate of bleeding, prevent gastric dilation, and administer room temperature saline to remove blood from the stomach. The room temperature saline is cooler than the body temperature, which creates mild vasoconstriction. Gastric cooling may also be promoted by cool saline lavage, which, although controversial, further curtails hemorrhage through its vasoconstrictive effect. Iced saline is rarely used because it may lead to more mucosal damage by decreasing perfusion to the gastric mucosa and may cause a vagal response, decreasing systemic perfusion.

REPLACE FLUIDS. Blood volume depletion is a major problem for the client with severe hemorrhage. For those who have suffered a massive upper GI tract hemorrhage, a primary objective of intervention is to replace blood volume. Restlessness and tachycardia are the earliest manifestations of hypovolemia. The client also has a greatly decreased urine output, which should be monitored with a Foley catheter and hourly urine measurement. This is important because fluids must be replaced to prevent damage to the kidneys.

ADMINISTER VASOPRESSIN. Arterial administration of vasopressin (via an infusion pump) can also control acute hemorrhage. Vasopressin produces few complications if given intravenously for less than 36 hours to control bleeding.

INJECT ARTERY WITH EMBOLI. Another approach to control of bleeding is selective arterial embolization with angiography. The emboli may consist of autologous blood clots with or without an absorbable gelatin sponge. A modified clot may be made with a mixture of the client's own blood, aminocaproic acid, and platelets. Fibrin glue has also been used.

MAINTAIN REST. The client must have absolute bed rest for several days after bleeding has subsided. Rest decreases blood pressure and GI tract activity. When bleeding stops, the client is allowed bathroom privileges. If the client requires narcotics, administer with caution. Morphine sulfate can cause nausea and vomiting; however, the drug may calm the client who is extremely restless and apprehensive. A better alternative is to manage anxiety with non-narcotic alternatives.

MAINTAIN HIGH GASTRIC pH. During the first few days of hemorrhaging, gastric pH should be maintained between 5.5 and 7.0. To maintain the pH at this level, administer H_2-receptor antagonists intravenously for 4 days or as prescribed and advance to oral administration. Monitor gastric pH at least each shift. Anticholinergics are not recommended. Administer antacids for 1 week to complement the H_2-receptor antagonists. Give antacids 1 hour before or 2 hours after the H_2-receptor antagonists so that the antacids do not interfere with absorption of drugs. The client may require antacids every 30 minutes after starting intake of food or fluids.

STOP BLEEDING SURGICALLY. If bleeding continues beyond 48 hours, recurs, or is associated with perforation or obstruction, surgery may be indicated. Increased surgical risk is associated with prolonged bleeding, multiple transfusions, debilitation, electrolyte imbalances, and increased age. Surgical procedures include partial gastric resection, excision of the ulcer, and vagotomy and pyloroplasty.

PERFORM MULTIPOLAR ELECTROCOAGULATION OR HEATER-PROBE THERAPY. Two endoscopic procedures have been effective in treating bleeding ulcers: MPEC and heater-probe therapy. In MPEC, a bipolar electric current cauterizes the bleeding lesion; in heater-probe therapy, direct heat cauterizes the lesion.

Perforation

Perforation is usually a surgical emergency. When the ulcer perforates, gastroduodenal contents empty through the anterior wall of the stomach into the peritoneal cavity, resulting in chemical peritonitis, bacterial septicemia, and hypovolemic shock. Peristalsis diminishes, and paralytic ileus develops. Posterior perforation is not as clear and often results in pancreatitis, because the pancreas plugs the perforation.

ASSESS PAIN. Perforation occurs most frequently with duodenal ulcers (Fig. 31–3). It occurs when the ulcer erodes through the tunica muscularis. The client experiences sudden, sharp, severe pain beginning in the midepigastrium. As peritonitis develops, the pain spreads over the entire abdomen, which becomes tender, hard, and rigid. (See discussion of peritonitis in Chapter 33.)

The degree of pain depends on the amount and type of contents that are spilled. The pain often causes the client to bend over or draw the knees up to the abdomen in an effort to decrease the tension on the abdominal muscles. If the perforation occurs on the posterior gastric wall, it may erode through to adjacent organs and become sealed, causing few manifestations. When a perforation erodes into the pancreas, manifestations of pancreatitis (see Chapter 46) develop.

REPLACE FLUIDS. If perforation occurs, the client needs immediate replacement of fluids, electrolytes, and blood as well as administration of antibiotics. Nasogastric suction should be instituted to drain gastric secretions and thus prevent further peritoneal spillage. A small perforation that closes immediately by adhering to adjacent tissues causes only a small loss of gastric contents.

CORRECT PERFORATION SURGICALLY. When surgery is necessary, the surgeon evacuates the escaped gastric contents, cleans the peritoneal cavity by flushing it out with normal saline or an antibiotic or both, and closes the perforation by patching it with omentum. Vagotomy and hemigastrectomy or vagotomy and pyloroplasty provide definitive control of both the ulcer and the complications. The Case Study describes the treatment of a client whose perforated ulcer was surgically managed. After surgery, antibiotics are given to combat peritonitis. The NG tube remains in the stomach until peristalsis returns. Postoperative complications include subphrenic abscess, hemorrhage, duodenal or gastric fistula, atelectasis, and pneumonia.

Obstruction

Long-standing ulcer disease causes scarring because of repeated ulcerations and healing. Scarring at the pylorus frequently causes pyloric obstruction, manifested most often by pain at night, when the stomach cannot be emptied by peristalsis. Pyloric obstruction can also lead to vomiting. Surgery (pyloroplasty) is usually required to correct the problem.

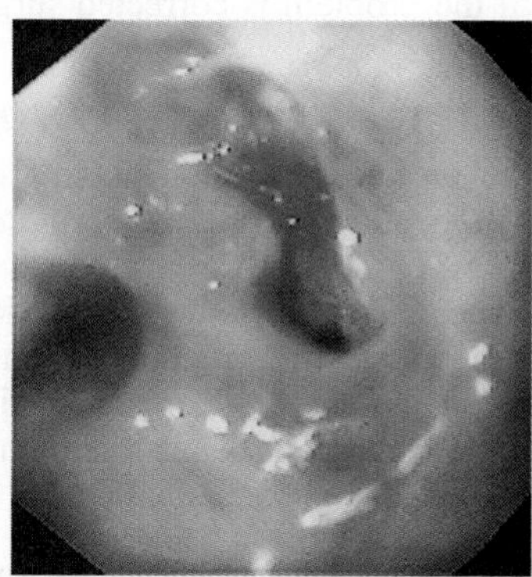

FIGURE 31–3 Perforation of a duodenal ulcer.

Nursing Management of the Medical Client

ASSESSMENT

Nursing assessment involves gathering both psychosocial and pathophysiologic data concerning the client. To assess psychosocial aspects of ulcer disease, ask the client about a familial incidence of ulcer, ingestion of medications that cause gastric irritation, cigarette smoking, alcohol intake, stressors, and coping patterns. Questions about lifestyle, occupation, work, and leisure activities can yield valuable information.

Physical assessment includes accurately observing and immediately reporting manifestations that help pinpoint the diagnosis or that might indicate the presence of a complication. Manifestations include pain, vomiting, and, occasionally, bleeding and changes in appetite. Always obtain a complete history of previous ulcer attacks, including frequency, duration, manifestations, and response to intervention.

Monitor for the development of complications of ulcers, such as hemorrhage, perforation, or obstruction. Assessment also involves describing the bleeding, including hematemesis and melena. Note such factors as color, amount, consistency, and frequency. Bright red blood usually signifies new bleeding; dark red blood indicates old bleeding. If bleeding is severe, always maintain a current and accurate record of the client's hemoglobin, hematocrit, red blood cell count, and fluid intake and output. Monitor the client closely for the development of manifestations of shock that might occur if bleeding is present.

Because of shock, the client may experience decreased renal blood flow, which causes a decrease in the glomerular filtration rate and in renal excretion. As the body absorbs the by-products of erythrocyte destruction and renal blood flow decreases, watch for an increase in blood urea nitrogen (BUN), creatinine, and ammonia levels. An elevated BUN may follow dehydration from vomiting. In addition, carefully assess the client for metabolic acidosis caused by vomiting.

Monitor the client for the development of perforation. Assess the abdomen for pain, tenderness, or rigidity. Report suspected perforation to the physician immediately, and prepare the client for possible surgery.

Monitor the client for the development of gastric obstruction. If the client vomits, record the frequency and the consistency (digested or undigested food or hematemesis) of the vomitus. If pyloric obstruction is present, nasogastric tube and intravenous fluids and electrolytes are needed until the problem is corrected surgically.

DIAGNOSIS, OUTCOMES, INTERVENTIONS

Pain. One of the most common nursing diagnoses for the client with a peptic ulcer is *Pain related to gastric mucosal injury.*

Outcomes. The client's pain will be relieved, as evidenced by healing of gastric or duodenal mucosal injury and the client's statement of decreased pain on a pain scale of 1 to 10 with the pain being less than 2 or 3.

Interventions

Administer Prescribed Medications. Administer medications as ordered to relieve the client's pain. The following medications may be used:

- Eliminate *H. pylori* (triple therapy)
- Neutralize gastric acids (antacids)
- Reduce secretions (H_2-receptor antagonists, prostaglandin analogs, proton pump inhibitors)
- Protect the gastric mucosa (mucosal barrier fortifiers, prostaglandin analogs)

Assess the effectiveness of the medications that the client is taking, and notify the physician if the pain is not relieved by the medications used in the treatment regimen.

Promote Rest and Relaxation. Avoidance of strenuous physical activity decreases gastric secretions and peristalsis. Help the client achieve rest, both physically and mentally. Be alert for factors that interfere with the client's rest. Arrange the environment to encourage relaxation. If certain visitors or telephone calls agitate the client, discourage these visits or calls until the client improves.

Encourage clients who attempt to carry on their normal work routine (despite prescribed rest) to schedule physical and mental relaxation. Explore with the client and significant others or co-workers ways to reduce work responsibilities temporarily.

Modify Diet. The diet must meet basic nutritional needs. Because an empty stomach stimulates gastric acid secretion, advise the client to eat small amounts at frequent, regular intervals. Discourage ingestion of alcohol, cola, tobacco, caffeine, milk, and foods that cause discomfort. The client may drink decaffeinated beverages.

During the acute phase, the client often requires a bland, nonirritating, low-fiber diet. Clients and their significant others need to learn the modifications in the diet. Also, have the dietitian review the home diet with the client or whoever will be cooking for the client.

Ineffective Management of Therapeutic Regimen (Individuals). For the client with an uncomplicated ulcer, most of the care must be done by the client at home. Write the nursing diagnosis as *Risk for ineffective management of therapeutic regimen (individual) related to lack of knowledge of cause of ulcer and measures to treat and prevent recurrence.*

Outcomes. The client will understand and be able to discuss the cause of the ulcer and the treatment and ways to prevent recurrence.

Interventions

Provide Teaching. Treatment of PUD places the responsibility for self-care on the client. To maintain good self-care, the client must understand the process underlying ulcer development and the rationale underlying interventions.

Help the client to:

- Understand the pathogenesis of the ulcer and the significance of the pain
- Realize that healing takes place rapidly when the irritating effect is removed
- Understand what caused the condition to develop and what must be done to lessen the stimulation
- Discover which substances cause pain by stimulating secretion of gastric juices and to eliminate the substances from the diet until the ulcer heals
- Understand the importance of continuing the medical regimen, although the pain is gone, until healing is completed

- Recognize that once maintenance therapy stops, the ulcer may recur

Instruct the client to use acetaminophen instead of aspirin preparations when these medications are needed. Teach the client to examine the labels of all nonprescription medications, particularly cold remedies, for aspirin (acetylsalicylic acid), other salicylates, NSAIDs (ibuprofen, phenylbutazone), adrenocorticosteroids, and ACTH. These medications are ulcerogenic (ulcer causing), particularly when combined. If any of these medications must be taken, advise the client to check with the physician first, to eat between meals, and to use H_2-receptor antagonists or antacids to protect the stomach lining.

Provide Support. Helping clients with PUD cope with psychosocial problems is a vital part of intervention. Encourage the client to learn about the stressors that may be causing the development of ulcers. Discussing coping and relaxation techniques may enable clients to better deal with problems.

EVALUATION

Medical management usually controls PUD, often within a few weeks. Many clients must continue treatment to remain ulcer-free. The client must follow the therapeutic regimen and practice good health maintenance and restoration behaviors in order to avoid complications and prevent future recurrence of PUD.

Surgical Management

GASTRIC SURGICAL PROCEDURES

INDICATIONS. Various types of gastric surgery are performed to reduce the stomach's acid-secreting ability, to remove a malignant or potentially malignant lesion, to treat a surgical emergency that develops as a complication of PUD, or to treat clients who do not respond to medical intervention. Most chronic, recurring ulcers are eventually managed surgically.

Surgery for prevention of ulcer recurrence is performed to:

- Facilitate enterogastric regurgitation of mucous secretions, bile, and pancreatic juice
- Decrease the secretory capacity of the stomach by removing parietal cells
- Remove stimuli for hydrochloric acid secretion by cutting the vagus nerve;
- Eliminate the gastrin hormone mechanisms by antrectomy

CONTRAINDICATIONS. Most contraindications to gastric surgery involve the client's age and physical condition. Any life-threatening disease process, such as chronic obstructive pulmonary disease (COPD) or heart failure, may be a contraindication to surgery.

COMPLICATIONS. Complications are discussed after the types of surgeries.

OUTCOMES. The outcomes desired from the various surgeries are that the client will survive and recover from the surgery without further injury related to surgery. After most procedures, the client will return home in 7 days or less and resume the previous lifestyle within 6 to 12 weeks. It may take 3 months to a year before the client can eat normally.

TYPES OF OPERATIONS

VAGOTOMY. Vagotomy is performed to eliminate the acid-secreting stimulus to gastric cells. There are three types of vagotomy (Fig. 31–4A):

1. *Truncal vagotomy.* Each vagus nerve is completely cut.
2. *Selective vagotomy.* The surgeon partially severs the nerves to preserve the hepatic and celiac branches.
3. *Proximal* vagotomy. Partial cutting is performed, but only the parietal cell mass is denervated; innervation of both the antrum and the pyloric sphincter is preserved. Cutting the vagal nerve fibers selectively avoids the problems of impaired emptying and diarrhea that follow the truncal vagotomy. It

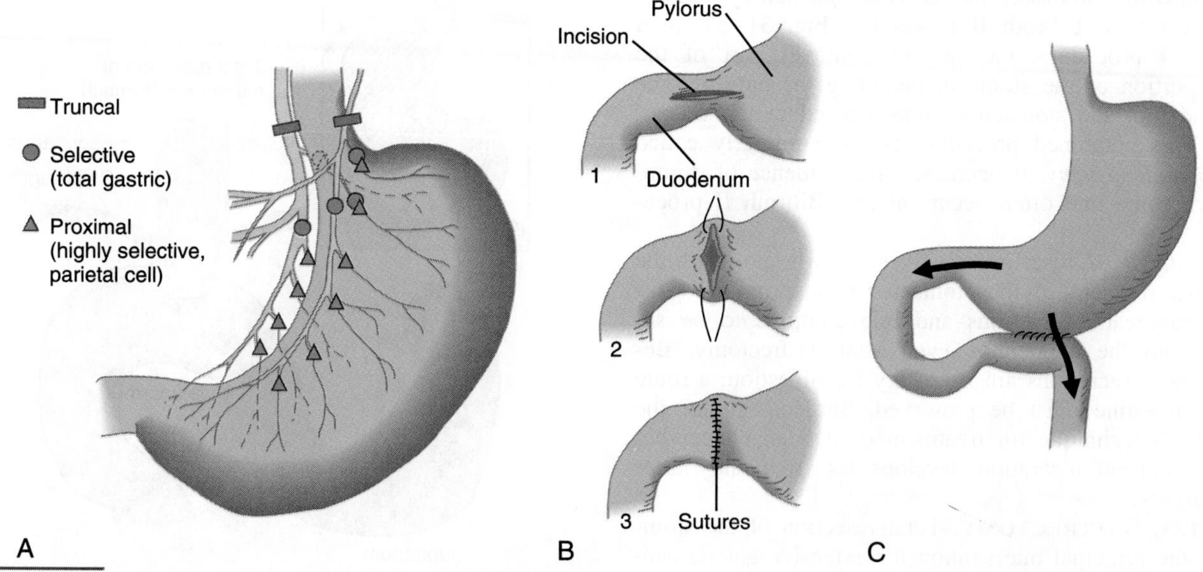

FIGURE 31–4 Vagotomy and drainage. *A,* Sites at which the three types of vagotomy are performed. *B,* Pyloroplasty provides a larger opening from stomach to duodenum to enhance emptying after vagotomy. *C,* Gastroenterostomy, another associated surgical procedure, creates a passage between the body of the stomach and the jejunum.

also eliminates the necessity for a drainage anastomosis to offset gastric stasis. Proximal vagotomy also reduces acid secretion and preserves the function of the antrum.

VAGOTOMY WITH PYLOROPLASTY. Vagotomy with pyloroplasty involves cutting the right and left vagus nerves and widening the existing exit of the stomach at the pylorus. This procedure prevents stasis and enhances emptying, thereby preventing belching, weight loss, and feelings of fullness (see Fig. 31–4*B*).

GASTROENTEROSTOMY. A simple gastroenterostomy (Fig. 31–4*C*) permits regurgitation of alkaline duodenal contents, thereby neutralizing gastric acid. A drain is made in the bottom of the stomach and sewn to an opening made in the jejunum. Because this neutralization interferes with the inhibition of gastrin release, a net increase in acid secretion may result. If the gastroenterostomy drains the stomach, it reduces motor activity in the pyloroduodenal area. Drainage also diverts acid away from the ulcerative area, which facilitates healing. A gastroenterostomy does not reduce the secretory capacity of the parietal cell mass, and the gastrin mechanism continues to function. Gastroenterostomy should be combined with vagotomy to reduce vagal influences.

ANTRECTOMY. Antrectomy is performed to reduce the acid-secreting portions of the stomach. The procedure removes the entire antrum of the stomach; thus, the cells that secrete gastrin are excised. This delays or eliminates the gastric phase of digestion by withdrawing the source of stimulation for acid release and slows the direct response to protein. The surgeon then anastomoses the remaining portion of the stomach to the duodenum.

Antrectomy is often accompanied by vagotomy; thus, the cephalic and gastric phases of gastric secretion are eliminated and GI tract motor activity is decreased. This surgical procedure usually prevents recurrence and is probably superior to more extensive operations.

SUBTOTAL GASTRECTOMY. Subtotal gastrectomy, a generic term referring to any surgery that involves partial removal of the stomach, may be accomplished by either a Billroth I or a Billroth II procedure (Fig. 31–5). In a *Billroth I* procedure, the surgeon removes part of the distal portion of the stomach, including the antrum. The remainder of the stomach is anastomosed to the duodenum. This combined procedure is more properly called *gastroduodenostomy.* It decreases the incidence of dumping syndrome that often occurs after a Billroth II procedure.

A *Billroth II* resection involves reanastomosis of the proximal remnant of the stomach to the proximal jejunum. Pancreatic secretions and bile continue to be secreted into the duodenum, even after gastrectomy. Because these secretions are necessary for digestion, a route to the intestine must be preserved. Surgeons prefer the Billroth II technique for treatment of duodenal ulcer because recurrent ulceration develops less frequently after this surgery.

TOTAL GASTRECTOMY. Total resection of the stomach is the principal intervention for extensive gastric cancer. This surgery involves removal of the stomach, with anastomosis of the esophagus to the jejunum, an esophagojejunostomy (Fig. 31–6). To perform total gastrectomy,

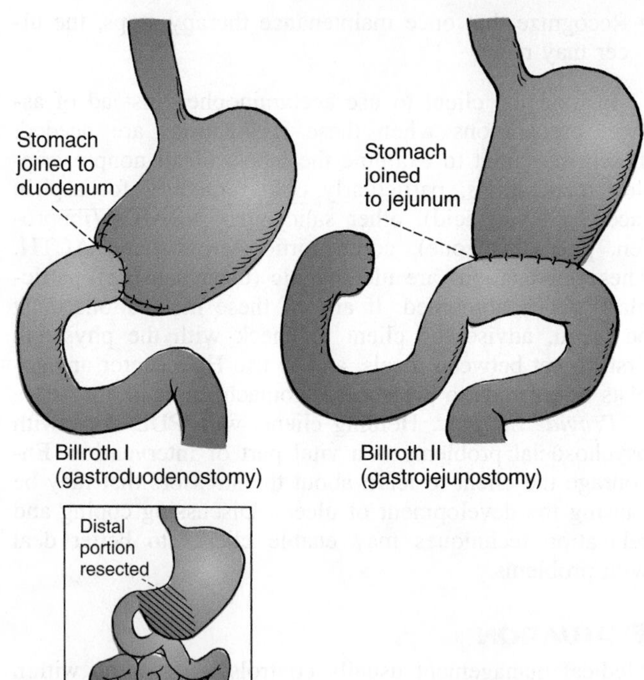

FIGURE 31–5 Subtotal gastrectomy removes acid-secreting portions of the stomach. After removing the distal stomach (*inset*), a surgeon sutures the remaining portion of the stomach to the duodenum (Billroth I procedure) or to the proximal jejunum (Billroth II procedure).

the surgeon enters the chest; thus, the client returns to the recovery room with chest tubes.

COMPLICATIONS OF GASTRIC SURGERIES

MARGINAL ULCERS. A marginal ulcer can develop where gastric acids come in contact with the operative site, either at the site of the anastomosis or in the jeju-

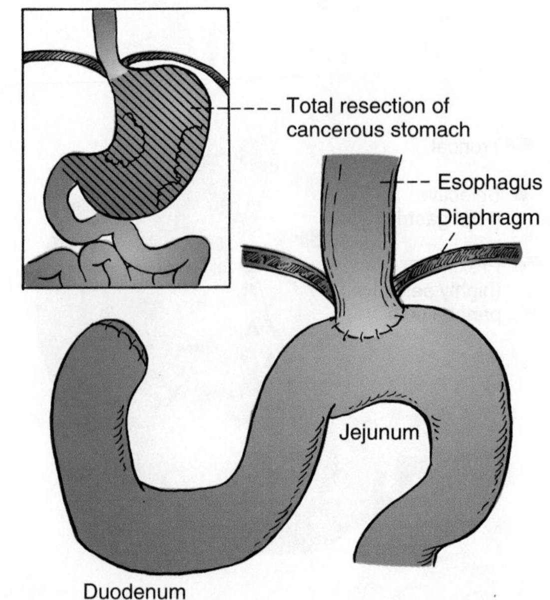

FIGURE 31–6 Total gastrectomy (*inset*) with anastomosis of esophagus to jejunum (esophagojejunostomy), which is the principal intervention for extensive gastric cancer.

num. Ulceration may cause scarring and obstruction. Hemorrhage and perforation can also occur at the surgical site.

Hemorrhage. The reported incidence of hemorrhage after gastric surgery is 1% to 3%. Bleeding is usually caused by a splenic injury or slippage of a ligature. Assess the client postoperatively for manifestations of bleeding and intraperitoneal hemorrhage.

Alkaline Reflux Gastritis. Alkaline reflux gastritis caused by duodenal contents occurs after gastric surgery in which the pylorus has been bypassed or removed. It also occurs after pyloroplasty and gastrojejunostomy. Usually, an associated vagotomy has been performed, which decreases gastric motility, allowing reflux of duodenal contents into the stomach.

Acute Gastric Dilation. In the immediate postoperative period, distention of the stomach produces epigastric pain, tachycardia, and hypotension. The client complains of a feeling of fullness, hiccups, or gagging. Gastric dilation rapidly improves after insertion of a nasogastric tube or clearing of a plugged nasogastric tube.

Nutritional Problems. Nutritional problems common after stomach removal include vitamin B_{12} and folic acid deficiency, calcium metabolism disorders, and reduced absorption of calcium and vitamin D. Such problems result from a shortage of intrinsic factor and inadequate absorption because of rapid entry of food into the bowel. With the Billroth II gastric resection, pancreatic juice and bile secretion are reduced because the usual stimulus of food passing through the duodenum is missing.

Dumping Syndrome. This postprandial problem occurs after gastrojejunostomy because ingested food rapidly enters the jejunum without proper mixing and without the normal duodenal digestive processing. It usually subsides in 6 to 12 months. Early manifestations, which occur 5 to 30 minutes after eating, involve the vasomotor disturbances of vertigo, tachycardia, syncope, sweating, pallor, palpitation, diarrhea, and nausea with a desire to lie down. The client's blood pressure and pulse may either rise or fall.

Dumping syndrome is most common after the Billroth II procedure. Intestinal manifestations include epigastric fullness, distention, abdominal discomfort, abdominal cramping, nausea (with only occasional vomiting), and borborygmi (rumbling sounds in the bowel). The client may experience tenesmus (ineffectual and painful straining to defecate). Pain is not present.

Early manifestations are probably caused by rapid movement of extracellular fluids into the bowel to convert the rapidly entering hypertonic bolus into an isotonic mixture. This rapid fluid shift decreases the circulating blood volume. A jejunum distended with food and fluid increases intestinal peristalsis and motility. Late manifestations, which occur 2 to 3 hours after eating, are a result of rapid entry of high-carbohydrate food into the jejunum, a rise in blood glucose level, and excessive insulin levels.

Management involves decreasing the amount of food taken at one time and maintaining a high-protein, high-fat, low-carbohydrate, dry diet. Gastric emptying can be delayed by eating in a recumbent or semi-recumbent position, lying down after meals, increasing the fat content in the diet, and avoiding fluids 1 hour before, with, or 2 hours after meals. The Client Education Guide provides a diet for clients with dumping syndrome.

The client may also be given sedatives and antispasmodic agents to delay gastric emptying. When manifestations persist, surgical intervention may include reducing the size of the gastroenterostomy or converting a Billroth II resection to a Billroth I by inserting a short segment of jejunum between the duodenal stump and the stomach.

Gastrojejunocolic Fistula. This postoperative complication follows recurrent PUD. The fistulae arise from perforation of a recurrent ulceration at the gastrojejunal anastomosis site. The perforation forms a fistula between the ulcer and adjacent bowel. Manifestations are variable but include fecal vomiting, diarrhea, weight loss, and anorexia. Belching of gas that has a fecal odor may also occur. The manifestations are caused by bacterial overgrowth in the small intestine.

Pyloric Obstruction. Pyloric obstruction, manifested by vomiting, occurs at the pylorus and is caused by scarring, edema, inflammation, or a combination of these conditions. When vomiting persists, alkalosis tends to develop because large quantities of acid gastric juice are vomited. A client who vomits persistently is usually hospitalized to receive intravenous fluids with electrolytes added.

Pyloroduodenal obstruction can cause gastric dilation, gastritis, and gastric stasis. These mechanisms create

CLIENT EDUCATION GUIDE

Diet for Dumping Syndrome

Client Instructions

Eat five to six small meals every day.

Eat high-fat, high-protein, low-carbohydrate foods.

Do not eat much roughage.

Avoid milk, sweets, and sugars.

Drink liquids between meals only (avoid liquids 1 hour before and 2 hours after meals).

Eat meat (beef, fish, pork, and poultry) and meat substitutes (cheese, peanut butter, and eggs); potatoes, rice, pasta, and starchy vegetables; white bread, rolls, muffins, cracker, and cereals; cooked vegetables; unsweetened cooked or canned fruits; dietetic drinks, jellies, and syrups; margarine, oils, butter, and salad dressings.

Eat the following foods with caution: Drink fluids 1 hour before and/or 2 hours after meals. Whole-grain breads, rolls, cereals, and pasta; foods made with milk; gas-producing vegetables (cabbage, onions, and broccoli); raw vegetables; fresh fruit; caffeinated beverages; mayonnaise; and salt.

Avoid spicy meats, soups, and potatoes; breads with frosting or jelly; sweetened fruit or fruit juice, cakes, pies, cookies; malts, milk shakes and milk products; carbonated beverages; alcoholic beverages; and spices, sugar, jelly, syrup, molasses, and honey.

manifestations that gradually make it more difficult for the stomach to empty. Assess the client for feelings of fullness, distention, or nausea after eating, with loss of appetite and weight loss.

Management of obstruction focuses on restoring fluid and electrolytes and decompressing the dilated stomach; if necessary, surgical intervention is instituted.

Nursing Management of the Surgical Client

PROVIDE SUPPORT

Surgical intervention for gastric and duodenal conditions may be either a planned procedure or an emergency. When emergency surgery is required (e.g., for acute obstruction, perforation, or hemorrhage), the client is very ill and is usually frightened. Provide calm, efficient, knowledgeable care, and explain what is being done. Note and respond to the client's nonverbal behavior. Help significant others provide the client with empathy and emotional support.

When cancer is suspected, the client may want to talk about fears and concerns. Listen to the client carefully, respond to cues, and offer support and understanding. The client may wish to attend to personal matters before surgery (e.g., review a will, see a clergyperson).

When elective surgery is done, the client will have an extensive series of preoperative tests, such as a GI tract x-ray series, endoscopy, and perhaps acid secretion studies (see Chapter 28).

PROVIDE TEACHING

Preoperative teaching should include an explanation of the surgery. Explain that the client will have either an NG tube or a gastrostomy tube with suction. An intravenous infusion line is placed in the client's hand or arm for fluids until the surgical site heals. Thoroughly demonstrate and discuss the importance of deep-breathing exercises or use of an incentive spirometer or both. Warn clients that the high abdominal incision makes deep breathing uncomfortable and that the high incision increases the risk of respiratory complications.

ASSESSMENT

Assess the client with surgical management of PUD in the same way as for the client being managed medically. In addition, perform routine preoperative and postoperative assessments (see Chapter 15).

DIAGNOSIS, OUTCOMES, INTERVENTIONS

Risk for Injury. After surgery, the client is susceptible to postoperative complications. The diagnosis is *Risk for Injury: Postoperative complications (immediate and delayed) related to bleeding, distention and atelectasis.*

Outcomes. The client will not suffer injury related to postoperative complications (immediate and delayed) as evidenced by decreasing bloody drainage from the NG tube, absence of abdominal distention, and normal breath sounds.

Interventions. Nursing care after gastric surgery is the same as postoperative care for any client recovering from major abdominal surgery.

Maintain Nasogastric Tube. In addition to general postoperative care, perform the following functions:

- Check drainage from the NG tube
- Maintain NG tube patency with saline irrigations, as ordered
- Ensure that the NG tube is attached to suction, as ordered
- Assess the operative site for excessive drainage; too much fluid in the remaining gastric stump may cause increased pressure and injury
- Note the color and consistency of drainage from the operative site, and report bleeding or hemorrhaging

The client will return from surgery with an NG or gastrostomy tube to prevent retention of gastric secretions. Carefully assess for abdominal distention. Do not reposition the NG or gastrostomy tube after gastric surgery because it is placed directly over the suture line. Gently irrigate with saline *only* if specifically ordered to do so by the physician.

The color of the drainage in the NG tube may be bright red during the early hours after surgery but should become dark red by the end of 24 hours. The drainage has the appearance of coffee grounds for several days after surgery.

Monitor for Complications. Immediate complications after gastric surgery include hemorrhage, gastric distention, obstruction, and disruption of the suture line. Also, observe for general surgical complications, such as shock, hemorrhage, pulmonary problems, thrombosis, infection (peritonitis), evisceration, and paralytic ileus. Nausea and vomiting should not occur if the nasogastric tube is patent. Carefully measure and document intake (oral and intravenous) and output (urine, suction and wound drainage).

Promote Comfort. Keep the client comfortable with liberal administration of pain medications; this helps the client to cooperate more fully during deep-breathing and coughing exercises. Give fluids by intravenous infusion, as ordered, until edema and swelling have diminished enough to allow fluids to pass the operative area (seen as a decrease in the gastric tube output and return of bowel sounds).

Altered Nutrition: Less Than Body Requirements. After surgery the client is at risk for *Altered Nutrition: Less Than Body Requirements related to decreased nutrient absorption secondary to dumping syndrome.*

Outcomes. The client will maintain adequate nutrition, as exhibited by maintaining weight and with no evidence of dumping syndrome.

Interventions. When healing has occurred, clamp the NG or gastrostomy tube and begin oral intake by giving the client clear water, usually 30 ml at a time. Aspirate the tube an hour or so later to see whether the fluid has been retained. When GI function has returned (e.g., active bowel sounds, passage of flatus) and the client tolerates clear water, the NG tube is usually removed and the diet progresses to soft foods; eventually, a regular diet of five or six small meals a day is given. The diet should not begin too early or progress too rapidly. At first, the client may experience discomfort if too much food is taken at one time.

EVALUATION

Postoperatively, some clients need help to reduce the number of stressors in their lives. Strategies for altering

Perforated Ulcer Managed Surgically

Mr. Fong is a 50-year-old, divorced, second-generation Asian American who is the chief executive officer of a local telecommunications firm. He has a history of peptic ulcer disease. Mr. Fong has been taking clarithromycin (Biaxin), 250 mg bid; metronidazole (Flagyl), 250 mg bid; and omeprazole (Prilosec), 20 mg bid, for 1 week. He reports that he has not been able to eat breakfast or lunch on a regular basis and has subsequently not taken sucralfate (Carafate) as ordered. He was taken to the emergency department today via rescue squad with complaints of sudden onset of severe abdominal pain accompanied by emesis of bright red blood at his office. He is admitted to the hospital unit for preoperative diagnostic evaluation and preoperative preparation.

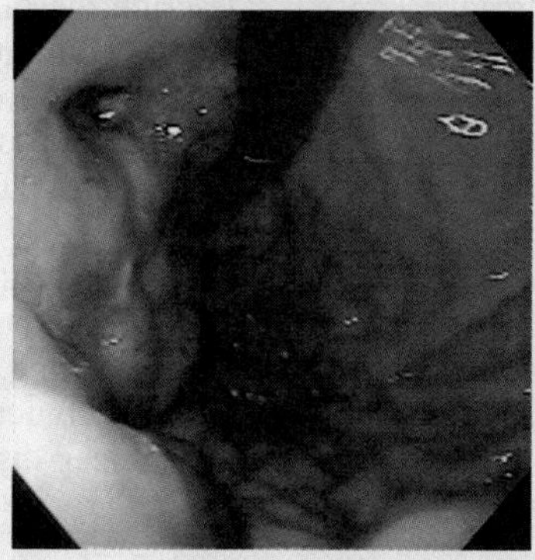

● Endoscopic view of a perforated peptic ulcer.

Nursing Admission

Assessment

Mr. Fong arrives at the unit accompanied by his girlfriend. He vomits bright red blood on admission and is unable to answer questions. He assumes the fetal position and clutches his abdomen.

Mr. Fong's girlfriend tells the nurse that she is not aware of any allergies. She states that he did take his medicine and ate breakfast this morning, but she is uncertain whether he ate lunch. Other pertinent preoperative assessment data include that Mr. Fong smokes two packs of cigarettes a day and drinks one or two alcoholic beverages every evening before dinner. He practices Buddhism.

In addition to his anti-ulcer medications, he has been taking ibuprofen-pseudoephedrine (Advil Cold & Sinus) three or four times a day for 5 days. Mr. Fong removed his partial bridge when he vomited the first time at the office. His contact lenses are still in place. Mr. Fong's girlfriend is concerned that his two teenage children will not arrive before their father goes to surgery.

Emergency Department Diagnostic Test Results

- Red blood cells (RBCs): 4.8 million/mm³ L
- Hemoglobin (Hg): 13.5 g/dl
- Hematocrit (Hct): 40%
- White blood cells (WBCs): 8000/mm³
- Sodium: 140 mEq/L
- Potassium: 4 mEq/L
- Chloride: 101 mEq/L
- Glucose: 90 mg/dl
- Prothrombin time (PT): 15 seconds
- Partial thromboplastin time (PTT): 40 seconds
- Electrocardiogram (ECG): Normal sinus rhythm (NSR)
- Chest x-ray: Within normal limits

Nursing Physical Examination

Assessment

- Height: 5 feet, 9 inches
- Weight: 150 lb (68.2 kg)
- Vital signs: Blood pressure, 90/50; temperature, pulse, and respirations, 99, 120, 22
- Level of consciousness (LOC): Awake, restless, complaining of severe abdominal pain
- Eyes, ears, nose, throat (EENT): Within normal limits
- Cardiac: Tachycardia, regular rate and rhythm without gallop or murmur
- Pulmonary: Lung sounds coarse and diminished bilaterally
- Abdominal: Rigid, board-like abdomen without bowel tones
- Genitourinary: No urine output since admission; client denies urge to void
- Peripheral pulses: 2/2 without edema

Initial Treatment Plan

- Medications: Preoperative medications per anesthesia
- Intravenous: D_5LR (lactated Ringer's) at 100 ml/hr
- Diet: nothing by mouth (NPO)
- Activity: bed rest
- Other: surgical permit for upper gastrointestinal endoscopy with possible gastric or duodenal resection

Mr. Fong's endoscopy revealed a perforated peptic ulcer and he was taken to the operating room for resection of the ulcer. He returns to the surgical unit after 2 hours in the postanesthesia care unit. Consider the postoperative orders and related assessments and interventions expected in the care of Mr. Fong.

Case Study continued on following page

Nursing Assessments and Interventions Expected in the Postoperative Care of Mr. Fong

Mr. Fong is reluctant to take his pain medication because he is afraid of addiction. Two days postoperatively, he has a temperature spike of 101.6° F. On occasion, his cough is productive of thick, white sputum. His lungs remain coarse and diminished with scattered rhonchi and occasional wheezes bilaterally. A chest x-ray film reveals bilateral atelectasis. Discuss how the nurse might have intervened to prevent this situation.

Mr. Fong's incision is clean, dry, and intact. His abdomen is tender but soft. Bowel sounds remain absent and Mr. Fong denies flatus. Nasogastric intubation returns moderate amounts of green drainage. Consider the pathophysiology related to the continued absence of bowel tones.

Three days after the surgery, Mr. Fong continues to receive an IV infusion and IV antibiotics. His hemoglobin is 7.6 g/dl, and hematocrit is 24%. He complains of being very thirsty and asks when he will be able to eat and drink. Discuss appropriate medical and nursing interventions.

Eight days after the surgery, Mr. Fong is taking a soft diet and ambulating in the halls with good tolerance. He is scheduled for discharge in the morning.

Discharge Criteria

- Average length of stay: 6.7 days without complications; 12.1 days with complications
- Complete discharge teaching (includes diet, medications, activity, stress management, and follow-up appointments)
- Community referral: smoking cessation program

Questions to Be Considered

1. Categorize Mr. Fong's surgeries according to the Categories of Surgical Procedures (Table 15–4). Define Mr. Fong's surgical procedures. Review the roles of the nurses on the perioperative team.
2. Compare and contrast local versus general anesthesia. Identify which type would be used for each of Mr. Fong's surgeries. Why?
3. Discuss the principles of surgical positioning. How would Mr. Fong be positioned for each of his surgical procedures? Include the rationale for your answer.
4. How is the routine preoperative abdominal surgery client prepared for surgery? Discuss how Mr. Fong's preparation was different and the implications this would have for his recovery.
5. Explain informed consent. Describe the nurse's role in obtaining and completing informed consent forms.
6. Discuss the nurse's role in the promotion of wound healing. Include dietary management, wound care, positioning, rest, pain management, and pulmonary hygiene.
7. Discuss the psychosocial, spiritual, and cultural factors that may influence clients' attitudes about surgery and recovery. Apply these factors to Mr. Fong.
8. Compare and contrast the etiology, clinical manifestations, and management of peptic ulcer disease (gastric versus duodenal).

lifestyle may be an important part of the rehabilitation and recovery plan. Clients need to know that convalescence after gastric surgery tends to be slow. It may be 3 months before they regain strength and even partial ability to eat in a more normal manner. It may take a year or so before clients can eat three normal meals a day, and they may need to eat five times per day to accommodate changes in the anatomic structures. When complications such as dumping syndrome occur, clients may feel disappointed. Many clients expect a rapid recovery and may be unprepared when complications develop. Most clients can learn to control manifestations and lead a fairly normal life.

GASTRIC CANCER

Gastric cancer refers to the malignant neoplasms found in the stomach, usually adenocarcinoma, although there may be malignant lymphomas. For unknown reasons, the incidence of stomach cancer in the United States has diminished steadily since 1960.

The American Cancer Society estimated that 21,500 new cases of gastric cancer would be diagnosed in 2000, with 13,000 deaths attributed to gastric cancer. Stomach cancer is twice as common in men as in women, more common in whites in the United States, and more frequent in clients who have pernicious anemia.

Etiology and Risk Factors

Although no specific cause of gastric cancer has been identified, several factors are associated with the development of the disease. The latest research indicates that the presence of *H. pylori* in the stomach increases the incidence of gastric cancer. Gastric cancer often develops in conjunction with chronic atrophic gastritis and affects individuals who live in urban areas, have a low socioeconomic status, eat smoked fish or meats, and have a history of exposure to background radiation or trace metals in soil. The changes in the mucosa may lead to an increase in absorption of carcinogens from the diet, such as pickled foods, salted fish, and nitrates. Other etiologic factors include achlorhydria, pernicious anemia, and smoking. There may also be a genetic factor because the disease seems to run in families. Metalcrafts workers, coal miners, bakers, and those working in dusty, smoky, and sulfur dioxide–containing environments are at increased risk. Wood or tobacco smoke, nitrite food preservatives, and overheated fat products may predispose clients to gastric cancer.

Avoidance of the carcinogenic agents is important, especially in clients with other risk factors, such as chronic gastritis, *H. pylori* infection, and pernicious anemia. Cessation of smoking is an excellent health promotion behavior. The American Cancer Society recommends screening for cag A strain of *H. pylori* bacteria in people with a family history of gastric cancer.

Pathophysiology

Gastric cancer most often arises from the mucous lining of the stomach. Most of these cancers occur in the lesser curvature of the stomach in the pyloric and antral regions. Prognosis is best for stomach cancer involving polypoid lesions; it is poor for ulcerating cancers and poorest for infiltrating forms. Stomach cancer spreads by direct extension into the pancreas via the lymphatics and by hematogenous infiltration of the liver, lungs, and bones. The particular route depends on the location and the type of tumor. Some tumors penetrate, some ulcerate, and some spread along the tissue planes.

Gastric cancer is staged using the tumor, nodes, and metastasis (TNM) classification with stages I to IV (see Chapter 19). The cancer is resectable in early stages before it has invaded the wall of the stomach. The 5-year survival rate is about 90% for local disease and drops below 10% for stage III disease. In advanced gastric cancer, the survival rate is almost zero.

Clinical Manifestations

Because clinical manifestations occur late in the course of the disease, stomach cancer is seldom detected in an early stage. Unless hemorrhage or perforation occurs, manifestations are vague and indefinite. The presence of a palpable mass, ascites, or bone pain caused by metastasis may be the first manifestation. Manifestations vary, depending on the location of the tumor in the stomach. If the cancer grows near the cardia, the client may experience dysphagia because of early involvement of the esophagus. If the cancer is near the pylorus, manifestations may result from obstruction.

Assessment reveals weight loss, vague indigestion, anorexia, or a feeling of fullness or mild discomfort so insidious that the client does not recognize it as abnormal or seek medical assistance. Discomfort may be brought on or relieved by eating. Anemia from blood loss commonly occurs, and occult blood may be present in the stool. The presence of lactic acid and a high lactate dehydrogenase (LDH) level in the gastric juice suggests carcinoma.

The diagnosis of gastric cancer is confirmed by upper GI tract x-ray examination and gastroscopy. Gastroscopy allows direct visualization and permits cytologic brushing or biopsies to facilitate retrieval of cells for cytologic examination.

Outcome Management

Medical Management

Little effective medical treatment is available for gastric cancer. Clients may receive chemotherapy and radiation therapy, but the primary treatment is surgical resection. At present, best results are achieved with multiple drug combinations. Drugs giving the best results are 5-fluorouracil, mitomycin C, cisplatin, etoposide, leucovorin, and doxorubicin (Adriamycin). A combination of radiation and chemotherapy after surgery may be used. Total parenteral nutrition (TPN) (see Chapter 29) is a method for providing nutrition to the client intravenously, bypassing the GI tract.

Surgical Management

Surgery is the only intervention that effectively treats stomach cancer. Unfortunately, because the diagnosis is usually late, surgery is more often palliative than curative. Gastrectomy, either partial (with Billroth I or II reconstruction) or complete depending on tumor location, is the usual procedure. Ideally, the surgeon removes all local growth and associated lymph nodes. When an extensive tumor makes resection impractical or impossible and the pylorus is obstructed, the surgeon may perform a palliative gastroenterostomy (surgical creation of a passage between the stomach and small intestine).

Nursing Management of the Surgical Client

ASSESSMENT

Clients may present with manifestations similar to those of PUD, but frequently manifestations are not present until the tumor is advanced. While assessing the client, note any history of risk or factors predisposing to the development of gastric cancer. These include a history of chronic gastritis, pernicious anemia, previous gastric surgery, presence of *H. pylori* infection, or smoking. Ask the client if there is a history of ingestion of large amounts of nitrates, smoked fish, salty foods, or pickled foods.

DIAGNOSIS, OUTCOMES, INTERVENTIONS

Pain. Both before and after surgery, a primary nursing diagnosis for the client is *Pain related to gastric erosion and postoperative pain related to high surgical incision.*

Outcomes. The client will have pain controlled or experience a reduction in pain, as evidenced by the client's use of a pain scale of 1 to 10 and stating a pain score of less than a 2 or 3.

Interventions. It is important that the client receive pain relief. Pain that is not controlled can interfere with sleep and eating and contributes to overall physical and mental deterioration. (Chapter 23 describes pain control in detail.) The client should have verbal and written instructions regarding medications, treatments, and follow-up care.

Altered Nutrition: Less Than Body Requirements. An important nursing diagnosis for the client with gastric cancer is *Altered Nutrition: Less Than Body Requirements related to decreased appetite, pain, possible gastric obstruction and nausea and vomiting.*

Outcomes. The client will maintain nutritional intake to meet metabolic requirements, as evidenced by maintenance of normal body weight.

Interventions. Nutritional therapy is an important aspect of management of the client with gastric cancer. TPN or jejunostomy tube feedings may be used postoperatively (or for clients with inoperable disease) to maintain the nutritional status (see Chapter 29).

Fear. Because of the uncertainty of the disease, an appropriate nursing diagnosis for the client with gastric cancer is *Fear related to knowledge deficit, body image changes, treatment and life-threatening illness.*

Outcomes. The client will have reduced or controlled fear, as evidenced by the client's ability to understand and discuss disease and treatment options.

Interventions. The client needs an explanation of the disease and all treatment options. Reinforce information to the client as needed. The client also needs information concerning operative procedures and postoperative interventions (nothing by mouth [NPO] status, NG tubes, other drains, intravenous infusions). This information will help decrease the client's fear.

Postoperative complications include hemorrhage, obstruction, anemia, nutritional deficiency, dumping syndrome, duodenal stump leakage, gastric dilation, and delayed gastric emptying. A home health care referral can assist the client with emotional support and treatments and provide an ongoing assessment of the client's condition. Referring the client to a dietitian, member of the clergy, and hospice team may also be necessary. Various community support groups are also available (e.g., I Can Cope). For terminal cancer care, see Chapters 19 and 22.

EVALUATION

The prognosis for clients with gastric surgery is poor. Generally, surgery is performed to provide a palliative means of assisting the client to be more comfortable rather than a cure of the stomach cancer. Therefore, the only appropriate outcome may be as good a quality of life as possible and adequate control of manifestations.

CONCLUSIONS

Gastric disorders are common; unless treated promptly and completely, they can continue to cause problems throughout the client's life. Assist clients to learn a new way of eating to achieve and maintain health and to make necessary lifestyle changes. This is a difficult task; however, unless the client modifies behavior, especially eating behaviors, many of the gastric disorders recur. The foci of nursing interventions are education and modifications of the client's behavior to promote a healthier lifestyle pattern.

THINKING CRITICALLY

1. A young female executive comes to the health clinic with complaints of epigastric pain and malaise. She works under stress and smokes heavily. She is in a hurry and wants quick action. The physician or advanced health practitioner recommends ranitidine (Zantac) for pain relief and an upper gastrointestinal x-ray film to rule out a duodenal ulcer. What further nursing assessment is required? What nursing interventions should be planned?

Factors to Consider. What places the client at risk for a duodenal ulcer? What teaching is required for medication and dietary management? How should changes in lifestyle be addressed?

2. A 43-year-old male client is being evaluated for intractable peptic ulcer disease. He has a history of recurrent duodenal ulcers. Last night he awakened at 2:00 AM and requested an antacid. This morning after breakfast, he passed a large, dark, liquid stool that tested positive for occult blood. Just before his 11:00 AM H_2-receptor antagonist, he turns on his call light. When the nurse enters the room, he is lying on his side with his knees drawn up, moaning and holding his pillow against his abdomen. He is diaphoretic, pale, and breathing rapidly and shallowly. The client states, "It's never hurt like this before. I feel as though I've been stabbed." What should the nurse's first actions be? What has probably happened to this client? Will he need surgery?

Factors to Consider. What type of surgery will be performed? What are the expected nursing assessments postoperatively? What complications is he at risk for? What discharge teaching will be needed to enhance his health maintenance and prevent recurrence of PUD?

3. A 52-year-old man who had a subtotal gastrectomy for stage III gastric cancer 10 weeks ago is having difficulty maintaining his body weight. His usual body weight is 190 pounds; he currently weighs 165 pounds. His wife reports that her husband is depressed, will not eat, and sleeps all day in his chair. She states, "I don't know what to do anymore! I think he just wants to die." She then starts crying. What should the nurse say to the client's wife? Whom should the nurse contact to assist the family?

Factors to Consider. Why is the client at nutritional risk? What is his percentage of weight loss? What measures might be initiated to facilitate nutrition?

BIBLIOGRAPHY

1. American Cancer Society. (2000). *Cancer facts and figures.* Atlanta: Author.
2. Aronson, B. (1998). Update on peptic ulcer drugs. *American Journal of Nursing, 98*(1), 41–47.
3. Bode, C., & Bode, J. C. (1997). Alcohol's role in gastrointestinal tract disorders. *Alcohol Health and Research World, 21*(1), 93–96.
4. Branicki, F., et al. (1998). Quality of life in patients with cancer of the esophagus and gastric cardia: A case for palliative resection. *Archives of Surgery, 133,* 316–322.
5. Brooks, M., Maxson, C., & Rubin, W. (1996). The infectious etiology of peptic ulcer disease: Diagnosis and implications for therapy. *Primary Care, 23*(3), 443–454.
6. Copstead, L. (1999). *Perspectives on pathophysiology* (2nd ed). Philadelphia: W. B. Saunders.
7. Djonret, L. L. (1998). Perspectives: An unexpected outcome after gastroesophagogastroduodenoscopy. *Gastroenterology Nursing, 21*(3), 29–30.
8. Erstad, B., et al. (1997). Impacting cost and appropriateness of stress ulcer prophylaxis at a university medical center. *American Journal of Industrial Medicine, 25,* 1678–1684.
9. Feldman, M., et al. (1998). Role of seroconversion in confirming cure of *Helicobacter pylori* infection. *Journal of the American Medical Association, 280*(4), 363–365.
10. Gillen, D., et al. (1999). Rebound hypersecretion after omeprazole and its relation to on-treatment acid suppression and *Helicobacter pylori* status. *Gastroenterology, 116*(2), 239–247.

11. Hansen, M. (1998). *Pathophysiology: Foundations of disease and clinical intervention.* Philadelphia: W. B. Saunders.
12. Hay, J., et al. (1997). Prospective evaluation of a clinical guideline recommending hospital length of stay in upper gastrointestinal tract hemorrhage. *Journal of the American Medical Association, 278*(24), 2151–2156.
13. Heslin, J. (1997). Peptic ulcer disease. *Nursing, 27*(1), 34–37.
14. Laine, L., et al. (1998). Has the impact of *Helicobacter pylori* therapy on ulcer recurrence in the United States been overstated? A meta-analysis of rigorously designed trials. *American Journal of Gastroenterology, 93,* 1409–1415.
15. Lehne, R. (1999). *Pharmacology for nursing care* (3rd ed.). Philadelphia: W. B. Saunders.
16. Levenstein, S., et al. (1999). Stress and peptic ulcer disease. *Journal of the American Medical Association, 281,* 10–11.
17. Lind, T., et al. (1999). The MACH2 study: Role of omeprazole in eradication of *Helicobacter pylori* with 1-week triple therapies. *Gastroenterology, 116*(2), 249–253.
18. McConnell, E. (1997). How to determine gastric pH. *Nursing, 27*(8), 26.
19. McCorkle, R., et al. (1996). *Cancer nursing: A comprehensive textbook* (2nd ed.) Philadelphia: W. B. Saunders.
20. Metheny, N., et al. (1994). Visual characteristics of aspirates from feeding tubes as a method for predicting tube location. *Nursing Research, 43*(5), 282–287.
21. Metheny, N., et al. (1993). Effectiveness of pH measurements in predicting feeding tube placement: An update. *Nursing Research, 42*(6), 314–331.
22. Metheny, N., et al. (1993). How to aspirate fluid from small-bore feeding tubes. *American Journal of Nursing, 93*(5), 86–88.
23. Miller, D., & Miller, H. (1995). Giving meds through the tube. *RN, 58*(1), 44–48.
24. Nardone, G., et al. (1999). Effect of *Helicobacter pylori* infection and its eradication on cell proliferation, DNA status, oncogene expression in patients with chronic gastritis. *Gut, 44*(6), 789–799.
25. O'Connor, K. (1999). Gastric cancer. *Seminars in Oncology Nursing, 15*(1), 26–35.
26. Ohkusa, T., et al. (1998). Disappearance of hyperplastic polyps in the stomach after eradication of *Helicobacter pylori:* A randomized, controlled trial. *Annals of Internal Medicine, 129,* 712–715.
27. Onishi, K., & Miaskowski, C. (1998). Mechanisms and management of gastric cancer. A comparison between the Japanese and U.S. experiences. *Cancer Nursing, 19*(3), 187–196.
28. Pehl, C., et al. (1999). Effect of low and high fat meals on lower esophageal sphincter motility and gastroesophageal reflux in healthy subjects. *American Journal of Gastroenterology, 94*(5), 1192–1196.
29. Peterson, W., & Cook, D. (1998). Antisecretory therapy for bleeding peptic ulcer. *Journal of the American Medical Association, 280*(10), 877–878.
30. Rutgeerts, P., et al. (1997). Randomized trial of single and repeated fibrin glue compared with injection of polidocanol in treatment of bleeding peptic ulcer. *Lancet, 350,* 692–696.
31. Sabiston, D. (1997). *Textbook of surgery: The biological basis of modern surgical practice* (15th ed.). Philadelphia: W. B. Saunders.
32. Smith, A. D., et al. (1999). Dyspepsia on withdrawal of ranitidine in previously asymptomatic volunteers. *American Journal of Gastroenterology, 94*(5), 1202–1213.
33. Soll, A., et al. (1996). Gastrointestinal Diseases. In J. Bennett & F. Plum (Eds.), *Cecil textbook of medicine* (20th ed.). Philadelphia: W. B. Saunders.
34. Vakil, N., & Cutler, A. (1999). Ten-day triple therapy with ranitidine, bismuth, amoxicillin, and clarithromycin in eradicating *Helicobacter pylori. Gastroenterology, 116*(3), 1197–1199.
35. Veldhuyzen van Zanten, S., et al. (1998). Adding once-daily omeprazole 20 mg to metronidazole/amoxicillin treatment for *Helicobacter pylori* gastritis: A randomized, double-blind trial showing the importance of metronidazole resistance. *American Journal of Gastroenterology, 93,* 5–10.
36. Wagner, S., et al. (1997). Regulation of gastric epithelial cell growth by *Helicobacter pylori:* Evidence for a major role of apoptosis. *Gastroenterology, 113,* 1836–1947.

BRIDGE TO EVIDENCE-BASED PRACTICE

Feeding Tube Placement Errors

QUESTIONS

What is the prevalence of feeding tube placement errors?

What are the risk factors associated with misplacement at the time of insertion and subsequent displacement from the intended site?

How accurate and reliable is gastric pH measurement as a method for verifying placement?

CITATIONS

Ellet, M. L. C. (1997). What is the prevalence of feeding tube placement errors and what are the associated risk factors? *Online Journal of Knowledge Synthesis for Nursing, 4*(5).

Chen, C. A., Paxton, P., & Williams-Burgess, C. (1996). Feeding tube placement verification using gastric pH measurement. *Online Journal of Knowledge Synthesis for Nursing, 3*(10).

STUDIES*

For the Ellet review, study reports were located by searching *MEDLINE* (1966–1996) and *CINAHL* (1982–1996) using the terms feeding tube, tube placement determination, risk factors, and enteral nutrition. Five studies addressed placement insertion errors, and two addressed tube displacement in adults. Six studies addressed risk factors associated with feeding tube placement errors.

For the Chen review, study reports were located by searching *MEDLINE* and *CINAHL* (1988–1995) using the terms feeding tube, feeding tube placement, gastric pH, nasogastric tube, pH measurement, pH sensor, and pH paper. Nursing, medical, and interdisciplinary studies were included.

Summary of Findings from the Ellett Review

Prevalence of Misplacement and Displacement

In two studies of small-bore feeding tubes in critically ill adults, the rates of misplacement at time of insertion were 4.4%[6] and 1.3%.[12] By radiologic detection, tubes were found to be inadvertently placed into the esophagus, lungs, pleural space, and brain.[7, 16] The latter errors occurred in clients with severe traumatic craniofacial injuries.[5, 10] The rate of displacement of gastric feeding tubes, after confirmation of correct original placement, was 15% in one study[14] and 18% in another[3]; most displacements involved upward migrations of the tube. The small-bore feeding tubes in use today are more prone to misplacement and displacement than the larger tubes formerly used.[8]

Feeding tubes intended to terminate in the small intestine are even more subject to placement errors.[9, 11, 14] The most common problems are that (1) the tubes never pass through the distal part of the stomach (i.e., the pylorus) into the small intestines, or (2) once in place they migrate upward (i.e., backward) into the stomach or esophagus.

In a comparison of weighted and unweighted duodenal tubes,[11] only 57% of the weighted tubes and 67% of the unweighted tubes were in the desired location. In another study of intestinal tubes,[14] 27% of the weighted tubes and 50% of the unweighted tubes were not in the correct position.

Risk Factors Associated with Placement Errors

Several factors are related to incorrect tube position and subsequent aspiration. One risk factor associated with misplacement into the tracheobronchial tree is the presence of a high-compliance, low-pressure cuffed endotracheal tube.[7, 15] During insertion, the feeding tube follows the endotracheal tube past the cuff and into the trachea.

Other risk factors include decreased levels of consciousness, impaired gag and cough reflexes, coughing, tracheal suctioning, retching, vomiting, failure to maintain elevation of the head of the bed, restlessness, and recent extubation.[1, 2, 4, 7, 14] In one study, 41% of clients with feeding tubes pulled out at least one tube[4]; restlessness and disorientation were significant associated factors.

Summary of Findings from the Chen, Paxton, & Williams-Burgess Review

Accuracy and Reliability of Placement Verification Methods

Various nonradiologic methods have been used to test feeding tube placement, including aspiration of recognizable gastric contents, auscultation of air introduced via syringe into the tube, and measurement of pH of fluid aspirated via syringe.

Inadvertent respiratory placement can also be ruled out by observing for coughing, choking, or cyanosis; asking the client to speak; and observing for bubbles caused by exhaled air when the end of the tube is held under water.

The research findings indicate a low level of accuracy in predicting feeding tube location[21–23]; however, several of these studies used simulations rather than actual clinical situations. In 1988, Metheny and coworkers[14] pointed out that many of the verification methods were developed for use with large-bore feeding tubes and thus might be inaccurate for use with the small-bore feeding tubes in use today.

*The findings of the two reviews are presented separately; the research-based care actions are combined.

Feeding Tube Placement Errors *Continued*

Use of Gastric pH Measurement

A study of gastric and intestinal readings demonstrated that the two placements could be differentiated based on pH values.[24] pH values below 4.0 indicated gastric placement, whereas pH values above 4.0 indicated intestinal placement; these parameters were adjusted if the patient was receiving medications to prevent gastric stress ulcers. In a follow-up study of 405 aspirates from nasogastric tubes and 389 aspirates from nasointestinal tubes, gastric placement was successfully distinguished from intestinal placement using pH meter readings in both the presence and absence of acid inhibitors.[25] Although it was hypothesized that gastric and respiratory aspirates could be differentiated based on pH levels, this hypothesis was not tested because of a very low number of readings from tubes in the respiratory tract; however, the average pH of tracheobronchial fluid aspirates was 7.81 (alkaline)—much higher than that of gastric contents.

The pH of aspirated gastric contents can be measured using pH paper or a tube having a built-in probe and pH meter. The accuracy of pH paper is not clear. In one study, paper determinations were accurate in obtaining both true low pH results and true high pH results.[20] In another study, however, in which the goal was to maintain a gastric pH of greater than 3.5 to prevent upper GI bleeding in critically ill clients,[19] the pH paper accurately determined the pH of gastric contents with values of less than 4 only 67% of the time; with pH values of 4 or more, the paper was accurate 95% of the time. It was concluded that using pH paper lacks accuracy and reliability in the clinical setting and may result in significant undertreatment.

Three studies have compared the values of pH determination by color-coded pH paper with the values produced by the pH probe and meter.[17, 18, 20] One study revealed that the pH probe and meter were more accurate, especially in clients with decreased amounts of gastric acid.[18] The other study[20] found a high correlation between the two measurements. One research group noted that differences between the two ways of measuring gastric pH may be related to the fact that the probe samples gastric contents right next to the mucosa, whereas the paper measures pooled gastric contents.[26] Use of the gastric pH probe and pH meter required less staff contact with gastric aspirates and required less time to perform than pH paper measurements.[26]

Limitations/Reservations: It was not clear whether all the studies examined small-bore tubes; it is possible that some of the older studies involved large-bore enteral tubes. Several studies demonstrated that what worked under controlled laboratory conditions did not necessarily work well in clinical situations; thus, research regarding accuracy of determinations at the bedside is needed. Studies differentiating respiratory from intestinal placement are also lacking; this is important because the pH levels of their aspirates overlap.

Research-Based Practice (From Both Reviews Combined)

It is evident that some feeding tubes either never reach their intended destination or become displaced after insertion. The tube can be placed or can migrate into the respiratory tract, the esophagus, or traumatized craniofacial spaces. After being placed, a tube can move back from the intestines into the stomach, or it can migrate from the stomach into the distal esophagus. Tubes passed with the aid of a guide wire tend to perforate the wall of the bronchus or the lung, causing a pneumothorax. The actual rate of insertion and displacement errors is not known.

Clients who are at risk for incorrect tube position include those who (1) have low-pressure cuffed endotracheal tubes, (2) cough a lot or have a depressed cough reflex, and (3) have a decreased level of consciousness. Elevating the head of the bed may help prevent tube displacement. Even though feeding tubes are often taped where they exit from the nose, this is not a guarantee that the end point of the tube is in the correct location. Check the location frequently to prevent aspiration or other problems associated with incorrect location.

Clearly, radiographic studies can accurately demonstrate the location of feeding tubes; however, clients should not be required to undergo repeated x-ray examinations for this purpose. An easy-to-use, accurate, and dependable bedside method is needed to monitor tube placement on an ongoing basis. Many of the commonly used monitoring signs and methods (e.g., coughing, auscultation of inserted air, and visual identification of gastric contents) are probably not dependable with small-bore tubes. At this point, small-bore tubes with a probe and pH meter provide the easiest and most accurate method of pinpointing the location of a tube. Advantages include the ability to continuously monitor tube location and to measure gastric pH right next to the mucosa rather than pooled gastric secretions, as with the aspirate method. The latter feature is a benefit when the client is receiving anti-ulcer therapy. Although using pH paper to determine gastric acidity may not be as accurate as using a pH probe and sensor, pH paper has been found to be more accurate than most of the other methods.

More recently, determining the pH of the aspirate combined with a laboratory measurement of pepsin and trypsin levels has been found to be very accurate in confirming the location of a tube. The pattern of presence or absence of the two enzymes and the pH level of the aspirate enable 100% accuracy in determining respiratory locations and a high level of accuracy in distinguishing between gastric and intestinal locations.[27] The ability to determine pepsin and trypsin levels as well as pH levels at the bedside would provide even better ongoing monitoring of feeding tube locations.

Cited References from the Ellet Review

1. Arms, R. A., Dines, D. E., & Tinstman, T. C. (1974). Aspiration pneumonia. *Chest, 65,* 136–139.
2. Bartlett, J. G., & Gorbach, S. L. (1975). The triple threat of aspiration pneumonia. *Chest, 68,* 560–566.
3. Crocker, K. S., Krey, S. H., & Steefee, W. P. (1981). Performance evaluation of a new nasogastric feeding tube. *Journal of Parenteral and Enteral Nutrition, 5,* 80–82.
4. Eisenberg, P., Spies, M., and Metheny, N. A. (1987). Characteristics of patients who remove their nasal feeding tube. *Clinical Nurse Specialist, 1,* 94–98.
5. Fletcher, S. A., et al. (1989). The successful surgical removal of intracranial nasogastric tubes. *Journal of Trauma, 27,* 948–952.
6. Ghahremani, G. G., & Gould, R. J. (1986). Nasoenteric feeding tubes: Radiographic detection of complications. *Digestive Diseases and Sciences, 31,* 574–585.
7. Harris, M. R., & Huseby, J. S. (1989). Pulmonary complications from nasoenteral feeding tube insertion in an intensive care unit: Incidence and prevention. *Critical Care Medicine, 17,* 917–919.

Bridge continued on following page

Feeding Tube Placement Errors *Continued*

8. Keohane, P. P., et al. (1983). Limitations and drawbacks of "fine bore" nasogastric feeding tubes. *Clinical Nutrition, 2,* 85–86.
9. Kiver, K. F., et al. (1984). Pre- and postpyloric enteral feeding: Analysis of safety and complications (Abstract). *Journal of Parenteral and Enteral Nutrition, 8,* 95.
10. Koch, K. J., et al. (1989). Intracranial placement of a nasogastric tube. *American Journal of Neuroradiology, 10,* 443–444.
11. Levenson, R., et al. (1988). Do weighted nasoenteric feeding tubes facilitate duodenal intubations? *Journal of Parenteral and Enteral Nutrition, 12,* 135–137.
12. McWey, R. E., et al. (1988). Complications of nasoenteric feeding tubes. *American Journal of Surgery, 155,* 253–257.
13. Metheny, N. A. (1993). Minimizing respiratory complications of nasoenteric tube feedings: State of the science. *Heart and Lung, 22,* 213–223.
14. Metheny, N. A., Spies, M., & Eisenberg, P. (1986). Frequency of nasoenteral tube displacement and associated risk factors. *Research in Nursing and Health, 9,* 241–247.
15. Scholten, D. J., Wood, T. L., & Thompson, D. R. (1986). Pneumothorax from nasoenteric feeding tube insertion: A report of five cases. *American Surgeon, 52,* 381–385.
16. Woodall, B. H., Winfield, D. F., & Bissett, G. S. III. (1987). Inadvertent tracheobronchial placement of feeding tubes. *Radiology, 165,* 727–729.

Cited References from the Chen, Paxton, & Williams-Burgess Review

17. Botoman, V. A., Kirtland, S. H., & Moss, R. L. (1994). A randomized study of a pH sensor feeding tube vs. a standard feeding tube in patients requiring enteral nutrition. *Journal of Parenteral and Enteral Nutrition, 18,* 154–158.
18. Caballero, G. A., et al. (1990). Gastric secretion pH measurement: What you see is not what you get. *Critical Care Medicine, 18,* 396–399.
19. Dobkin, E. D., et al. (1990). Does pH paper accurately eflect gastric pH? *Critical Care Medicine, 18,* 985–988.
20. Levine, R. L., et al. (1994). Equivalence of litmus paper and intragastric pH probes for intragastric pH monitoring in the intensive care unit. *Critical Care Medicine, 22,* 945–948.
21. Metheny, N., et al. (1990). Detection of inadvertent respiratory placement of small-bore feeding tubes: A report of 10 cases. *Nursing Research, 37,* 324–329.
22. Metheny, N., et al. (1990). Effectiveness of the auscultatory method in predicting feeding tube location. *Nursing Research, 39,* 262–267.
23. Metheny, N., et al. (1994). Visual characteristics of aspirates from feeding tubes as a method for predicting tube location. *Nursing Research, 43,* 282–287.
24. Metheny, N., et al. (1989). Effectiveness of pH measurement in predicting feeding tube placement. *Nursing Research, 38,* 280–285.
25. Metheny, N., et al. (1993). Effectiveness of pH measurements in predicting feeding tube placement: An update. *Nursing Research, 42,* 324–331.
26. Neill, K. M., Rice, K. T., & Ahern, H. L. (1993). Comparison of two methods of measuring gastric pH. *Heart and Lung, 22,* 349–355.

Added Reference

27. Metheny, N. A., et al. (1997). pH and concentrations of pepsin and trypsin in feeding tube aspirates as predictors of tube placement. *Journal of Parenteral and Enteral Nutrition, 21,* 279–285.

Sarah Jo Brown, PhD, RN, *Principal and Consultant, Practice-Research Integrations, Norwich, Vermont*

UNIT 7

Elimination Disorders

Anatomy and Physiology Review: *The Elimination Systems*

Robert G. Carroll

The urinary tract is composed of four structures:

- Kidneys
- Ureters
- Bladder
- Urethra

The *kidneys* balance the urinary excretion of substances against the accumulation within the body through ingestion or production. Consequently, they are a major controller of fluid and electrolyte homeostasis. The kidneys also have several nonexcretory metabolic and endocrine functions, including blood pressure regulation, erythropoietin production, insulin degradation, prostaglandin synthesis, calcium and phosphorus regulation, and vitamin D metabolism.

Filtration at the renal glomerulus is the first step in urine formation. Normally, a volume equal to plasma volume is filtered every 24 minutes and a volume equal to total body water is filtered every 6 hours. This glomerular filtrate is similar to plasma, but it lacks cells and large-molecular-weight proteins. The glomerular filtrate is modified by active transport, diffusion, and osmosis as it passes through the renal tubules. *Reabsorption* of filtrate components enhances conservation of glucose, amino acids, and electrolytes. *Secretion* of plasma components enhances elimination of organic acids and bases (and some drugs). The remnants of the glomerular filtrate exit the kidney through the ureters.

The *ureters* conduct urine from the kidneys to the bladder by peristaltic contraction. The *bladder* is a distensible chamber that stores urine until it is *excreted.* The *urethra* is the exit passageway from the bladder that carries urine for elimination from the body.

STRUCTURE OF THE ELIMINATION SYSTEM

KIDNEYS

The kidneys are located retroperitoneally, in the posterior aspect of the abdomen, on either side of the vertebral column (Fig. U7–1). They lie between the 12th thoracic and the third lumbar vertebrae. The left kidney is usually positioned slightly higher than the right. Adult kidneys average approximately 11 cm in length, 5 to 7.5 cm in width, and 2.5 cm in thickness. Affixing the kidneys in position behind the parietal peritoneum is a mass of perirenal fat (adipose capsule) and connective tissue called *Gerota's (subserosa) fascia.* A fi-

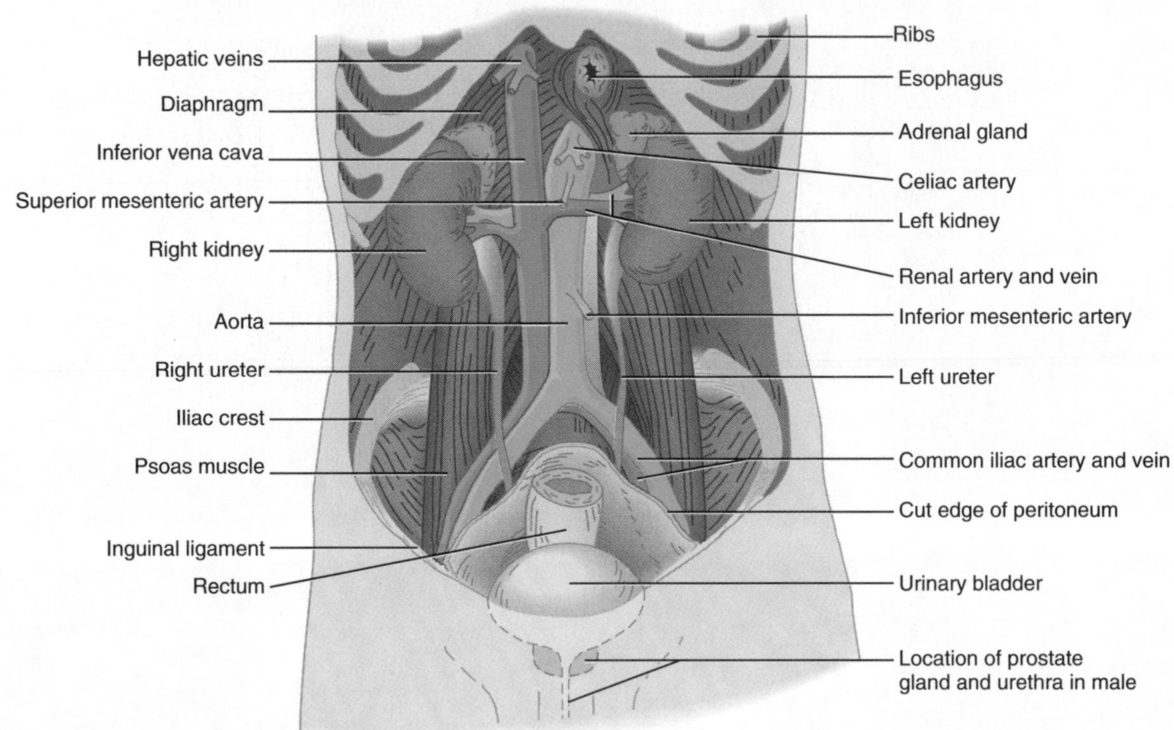

FIGURE U7–1 Anatomic relationship of the kidneys and related structures.

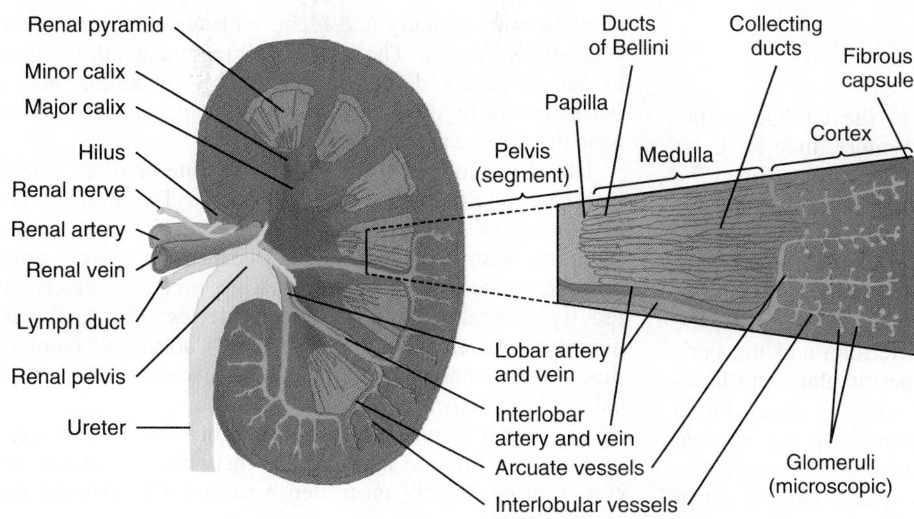

FIGURE U7–2 Anatomy of the kidney. *Inset,* Enlargement of a segment of the kidney.

brous capsule (renal capsule) forms the external covering of the kidney, except for the hilum. The kidney is further protected by layers of muscle of the back, flank, and abdomen as well as by layers of fat, subcutaneous tissue, and skin.

The kidney has a characteristic curved shape, with a convex distal edge and a concave medial boundary. In the innermost part of the concave section is the *hilus,* through which pass the renal artery, renal vein, lymphatics, nerves, and the renal pelvis (the natural upper extension of the ureter). A fibrous capsule surrounds each kidney and adheres to the renal parenchyma. Each kidney is divided into three major areas: (1) cortex, (2) medulla, and (3) pelvis (Fig. U7–2).

The *cortex* of the kidney lies just under the fibrous capsule, and portions of it extend down into the medullary layer to form the renal columns (columns of Bertin) or cortical tissue that separates the pyramids. The *medulla* is divided into eight to 18 cone-shaped masses of collecting ducts called the *renal pyramids.* The bases of the pyramids are positioned on the corticomedullary boundary. Their apices extend toward the renal pelvis, forming papillae. The papillae have 10 to 25 openings each on the surface, through which the urine empties into the renal pelvis (see *inset,* Fig. U7–2). Eight or more groups of papillae are present in each pyramid; each empties into a *minor calix,* and several minor calices join to form a *major calix.* The two to three major calices are outpouchings of the *renal pelvis* (the inner area of the kidney). They channel the urine from the pyramids to the renal pelvis. The *renal pelvis* is a cavity lined with transitional epithelium. The combined volume of the pelvis and calices is approximately 8 ml. Volumes in excess of this amount damage the renal parenchymal tissue. The renal pelvis narrows as it reaches the *hilus* and becomes the proximal end of the ureter.

Within the cortex lies the *nephron,* the functional unit of the kidney, consisting of both vascular and tubular elements (Fig. U7–3). Filtration begins at the renal *glomerulus.* The glomerular tuft (glomerulus) contains capillaries and the beginning of the tubule system, Bowman's capsule. Filtrate from the glomerulus enters Bowman's capsule and then passes through a series of tubule segments that modify the filtrate as it passes through the renal cortex and medulla and, finally, flows into the renal calices. A second capillary bed, the peritubular capillaries, carries the reabsorbed water and solutes back toward the vena cava.

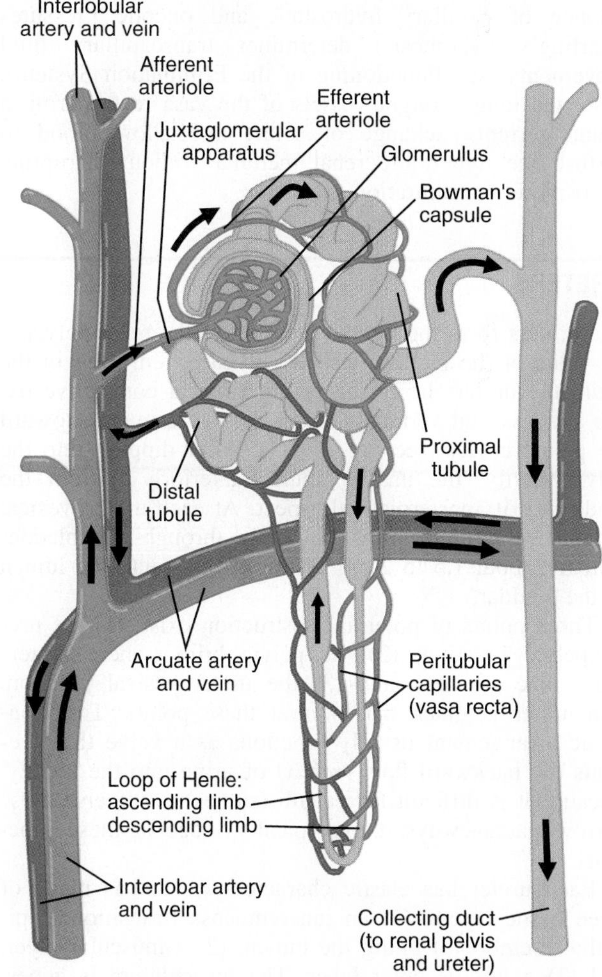

FIGURE U7–3 Diagram of a nephron and associated vascular structures.

Renal Blood Flow and Glomerular Filtration

The kidneys receive 20% to 25% of the cardiac output under resting conditions, averaging more than 1 L of arterial blood per minute. The renal arteries (see Fig. U7–2) branch from the abdominal aorta at the level of the second lumbar vertebra, enter the kidney, and progressively branch into lobar arteries, interlobar arteries, arcuate arteries, and interlobular arteries. Blood flows from the interlobular arteries through the afferent arteriole, the glomerular capillaries, the efferent arteriole, and the peritubular capillaries. Some of the peritubular capillaries carry a small amount of blood (~5% of renal blood flow) to the renal medulla in the vasa recta (long, straight blood vessels) before entering the venous drainage. The blood leaves the kidney in a venous system closely corresponding to the arterial system: interlobular veins, arcuate veins, interlobar veins, and the renal vein. The renal circulation then empties into the inferior vena cava.

The arrangement of the two capillary beds in series in the nephron allows most of the large volume of filtrate at the glomerular capillaries to be reabsorbed by the peritubular capillaries. The normal glomerular filtration rate (GFR) is 125 ml/min, but because of filtrate reabsorption at the peritubular capillaries only about 1 ml/min of urine flows from the kidneys. As with other capillaries, the balance of capillary hydrostatic and oncotic pressures (Starling's hypothesis) determines transcapillary fluid movements (see Functioning of the Elimination System). Also, the long, straight vessels of the vasa recta permit a countercurrent exchange of solute and allow blood to perfuse the hypertonic renal medulla without disrupting the osmotic concentration gradient.

URETERS

The ureters form the medial tapering of the renal pelvis at the hilus of the kidney. Usually 25 to 35 cm long in the adult, the ureters lie in the extraperitoneal connective tissue and descend vertically along the psoas muscle toward the pelvic cavity (see Fig. U7–1). After dipping into the pelvic cavity, the ureters course anteriorly to join the bladder in its posterolateral aspect. At each ureterovesical junction, the ureter runs obliquely through the bladder wall for about 1.5 to 2 cm before opening into the lumen of the bladder.

Three points of potential obstruction exist: (1) the ureteropelvic junction, (2) the pelvic brim (where ureters cross iliac arteries), and (3) the ureterovesical junction. The ureter is much narrower at these points. This anatomic arrangement usually functions as a valve that prevents the backward flow *(reflux)* of urine into the kidney. Because it is difficult for calculi (stones) to traverse these narrow passageways, they typically lodge at these junctions.

Each ureter has elastic characteristics and is made of three tissue layers: (1) an inner mucosa (transitional epithelial membrane) lining the lumen, (2) a muscular layer, and (3) a fibrous outer layer. The musculature is generally designated as *inner longitudinal* and *outer circular.* Along most of the ureter, however, the muscle fibers actually run obliquely and blend with one another to form a mesh-like tissue. The muscle arrangement allows urine to be propelled down the ureter by peristaltic action. Peristalsis is regulated by a myogenic pacemaker located near the renal calices.

Blood is supplied to the ureters by one or more vessels that run longitudinally along the tube. The number and assortment of arteries anastomosing with the ureteric vessels vary with each individual. Because the ureters travel through several anatomic areas, the ureteral vessels are fed by several of the following arteries: (1) renal (frequently), (2) testicular or ovarian, (3) aorta and common iliac, (4) internal iliac (frequently), (5) vesical, (6) umbilical, and (7) uterine.

The ureter's innervation comes from the 11th thoracic to the first lumbar nerves. The network of nerves becomes progressively more dense toward the terminal end of the ureters.

BLADDER

The *urinary bladder* is a hollow organ located in the anterior half of the pelvis behind the symphysis pubis (see Unit 8 review, Figs. U8–1*B* and U8–4, for a discussion of anatomic structures). The space between the bladder and the symphysis pubis is filled with a loose connective tissue that allows the bladder to stretch cranially as it fills. The peritoneum covers the top border of the bladder, and the base is held loosely in place by the true ligaments. The bladder is also enveloped by a loose fascia.

The bladder wall has several tissue layers. The internal lining of the vesical wall is transitional epithelium with some mucus-secreting glands. There are three ill-defined muscle layers: the inner and outer layers (longitudinal) and middle layer (circular). The fibers from these layers interweave to form a mesh-like muscle layer called the *detrusor muscle.* This arrangement allows the bladder wall to be elastic while maintaining strength. Bundles of these smooth muscle layers come together at the base of the bladder to form the internal sphincter, or opening into the urethra. The *trigone* is the triangular area formed by the ureterovesical junctions and the internal sphincter.

The superior and lateral aspects of the bladder are served by the superior vesical artery, which branches from the umbilical artery and internal iliac artery. The inferior vesical artery, which supplies the underside of the bladder, may arise independently or in common with the middle rectal artery. The veins draining the bladder pass to the internal iliac trunk.

Innervation for the bladder comes from the hypogastric sympathetic, pelvic parasympathetic, and pudendal somatic nerves. Ganglia are most commonly found in the bladder base and around the urethral orifice. These areas tend to act in continuity with each other, and their functions seem to be coordinated by both the sympathetic and parasympathetic nervous systems.

URETHRA

The urethra is a tube that extends from the base of the bladder to the surface of the body. The urethra differs greatly in females and males.

Female Urethra

The female urethra is approximately 4 cm long and curves slightly forward as it reaches the external opening, or *meatus,* located between the clitoris and the vaginal orifice. The urethra is lined with epithelium, which contains some mucus-secreting glands. The longitudinal muscle layer is a continuation of longitudinal layer of bladder muscle. The circular muscle fibers encompass the urethra and meet with the circular bladder muscle. This muscle thins out near the meatus. As the urethra passes through the urogenital diaphragm, the circular muscle fibers form the external sphincter.

Male Urethra

In males, the urethra is a common outlet for the reproductive system and urinary elimination. The *prostate gland,* although not a direct part of the urinary system, is a major cause of urinary dysfunction in men. Located below the bladder neck, the prostate completely surrounds the urethra. Normally, this relationship causes no problem, but if the prostate enlarges, it constricts the urethra and obstructs the outflow of urine (see Chapter 38).

The male urethra is about 20 cm long and is divided into three main sections. The *prostatic urethra* extends about 3 cm below the bladder neck, through the prostate gland, to the pelvic floor. The ejaculatory ducts of the reproductive system empty into its posterior wall. The *membranous urethra* is about 1 to 2 cm in length and ends where the muscle layer forms the external sphincter. The distal portion is the *cavernous (penile) urethra.* Approximately 15 cm long, it travels through the penis to the urethral orifice at the tip of the penis; it is also lined with epithelial cells.

FUNCTION OF THE ELIMINATION SYSTEM

Transcapillary Fluid Exchange

Fluid movement at each capillary bed depends on the balance of fluid pressures and osmotic pressures. Glomerular capillary blood pressure reflects resistance to flow at afferent and efferent arterioles. *Preglomerular contraction* (primarily afferent arteriole), such as caused by renal sympathetic nerves, decreases flow of blood into the glomerular capillaries and decreases glomerular capillary blood pressure and GFR. *Postglomerular contraction* (primarily efferent arteriole), such as caused by angiotensin II, traps blood in the glomerulus and increases glomerular capillary pressure and GFR. Peritubular capillary blood pressure, because the peritubular capillaries are located downstream of the glomerulus, decreases following either afferent or efferent arteriolar contraction. A decrease in peritubular capillary pressure facilitates reabsorption of glomerular filtrate.

Plasma oncotic pressure, due primarily to albumin, attenuates filtration at the glomerular capillaries. If the glomerular barrier is damaged, the permeability of the glomerular capillary to protein decreases the normal oncotic reabsorptive forces and GFR is increased. The primary barrier to protein filtration is the negatively charged endothelium and basement membrane of the glomerular capillaries. A loss of this negative charge, such as occurs in diabetes, allows some proteins to pass into the urine (proteinuria).

Tubular Mechanisms for Secretion and Reabsorption

The renal tubules are lined with epithelial cells that selectively secrete or reabsorb compounds (Table U7–1). This blind-ended tubular segment originates at the glomerulus. Transport proteins and tightness of tight junctions help define segments of the tubules. Because the renal tubules and urinary tract are lined with epithelial cells, tubular fluid is functionally outside of the body (as with the gastrointestinal tract).

Modification of ultrafiltrate occurs by *diffusion* and *selective transport* in tubules. Diffusion is quantitatively the most important process. Some compounds are absorbed by carrier-mediated transport, such as sodium (Na^+)-coupled glucose transport.

Glomerular filtrate travels progressively through Bowman's capsule, the proximal tubules, the loop of Henle, the distal tubules, the connecting segment, and the collecting duct; it then enters renal medullary space, passes into ureter, and is stored in the bladder before exiting body as urine. The tubule segments are anatomically adjacent to the vascular supply for that nephron. The juxtaglomerular apparatus consists of the glomerulus and the distal tubule that originated from that glomerulus. This arrangement allows negative feedback control of glomerular filtrate formation at the individual nephron level.

Water reabsorption is driven by osmotic gradients. The osmolality of the renal cortex is 300 mOsm, similar to that in most areas of the body. Osmolality of the renal medulla, however, can reach 1500 mOsm, as a result of the high concentrations of urea, Na^+ and chloride (Cl^-) in the intersitial spaces. Two tubular segments, the loop of Henle and the collecting ducts, pass through the renal medulla and, consequently, play a major role in determining urine volume and osmolality.

Renal Tubular Segments

The proximal tubules reabsorb 65% of filtered water, Na^+, Cl^-, and potassium (K^+). This segment also reabsorbs 100% of filtered hexoses (glucose), amino acids, and small peptides by Na^+-coupled co-transport. Because this mechanism exhibits saturation kinetics, glucose can pass into the urine if the filtered load (plasma concentration $\times$ GFR) exceeds the renal reabsorptive capacity (T_{max}). This situation occurs in diabetes mellitus, generally when the plasma glucose concentration exceeds 300 mg/dl.

The thin limb of the loop of Henle is water-permeable, allowing water to exit the tubule as the filtrate passes into the osmotically concentrated renal medulla. Sodium chloride (NaCl) and urea, the osmotic particles of the medulla, can also enter the tubule in this segment. The thick ascending limb of the loop of Henle is water-impermeable, as—in the absence of antidiuretic hormone (ADH)—are the remaining segments of the urinary system. The $Na^+/K^+/2Cl^-$ transporter reabsorbs electrolytes. This solute transport without water movement results in hypotonic filtrate (100 mOsm); thus, this tubule segment is sometimes called the *diluting segment.*

Transport in the distal tubule and collecting duct represents the final chance to modify the tubular fluid before it is lost from the body as urine. Aldosterone promotes K^+

TABLE U7–1 KIDNEY REABSORPTION AND SECRETION

Compound	Mechanism	Blocker
PROXIMAL TUBULE REABSORPTION		
Na^+	Facilitated diffusion	Amiloride
HCO_3^-	Na/H antiport	Carbonic anhydrase inhibitors
Cl^-	Diffusion	
K^+	Diffusion	
Water	Osmosis	
Glucose	Na-coupled transport	Phloritine
Amino acids	Na-coupled transport	
Urea	Diffusion	
Urate	Diffusion	
PROXIMAL TUBULE SECRETION		
Penicillin	Active transport	Probenecid
Para-amino hippuric acid (PAH)	Active transport	
Quinine, choline, thiamine, others	Active transport	
Creatinine	Active transport	
H^+	Na^+/H^+ antiport	Carbonic anhydrase inhibitors
THICK ASCENDING LIMB OF THE LOOP OF HENLE REABSORPTION		
Na^+	Na/K/2Cl transporter	Furosemide and bumetanide
K^+	Na/K/2Cl transporter	Furosemide and bumetanide
Cl^-	Na/K/2Cl transporter	Furosemide and bumetanide
Mg^{2+}	Electrochemical gradient	
NH_4	Na/K/2Cl transporter	Furosemide and bumetanide
THICK ASCENDING LIMB OF THE LOOP OF HENLE SECRETION		
H^+	H^+ ATPase	
DISTAL TUBULE REABSORPTION		
Na^+/Cl^-	NaCl symport	Thiazides
Na^+	Diffusion (aldosterone)	Amiloride, spironolactone
H^+ or HCO_3^-	Intercalated cells	Carbonic anhydrase inhibitors
DISTAL TUBULE SECRETION		
K^+	Aldosterone Na^+ reabsorption	Amiloride, spironolactone
H^+	H^+ ATPase	
COLLECTING DUCT REABSORPTION		
Urea	Transporters (ADH control)	
Water	Aquaporins, osmosis (ADH control)	
NaCl	NaCl symport	Thiazides

secretion in the distal tubule, and ADH increases water reabsorption. The filtrate that flows from the collecting duct into the ureter is the final excretory product or *urine*. The bladder stores urine for elimination but does not further modify urine composition.

Renal Mechanisms in Acid-Base Balance

Renal acid-base excretion complements pulmonary carbon dioxide (CO_2) elimination to regulate body acid-base status. Renal acids are hydrogen (H^+), ammonium, phosphate, and sulfate buffers. The renal base is predominantly bicarbonate (HCO_3^-). Because of the high HCO_3^- filtered load, reabsorption of HCO_3^- is the primary task of the tubule segments. This is accomplished in the proximal and distal tubules by H^+ secretion, and carbonic anhydrase–mediated CO_2 formation. Ultimately, urinary acid secretion is determined by plasma CO_2 levels.

Ammonium (NH_4^+) formation in the proximal tubule augments acid secretion, particularly in chronic acidosis. The proximal tubule cells metabolize glutamine to form ammonia (NH_3). NH_3 is uncharged and diffuses into tubular lumen, where it combines with secreted H^+ to form NH_4^+. Ionic NH_4^+ does not freely diffuse, and it remains in the lumen in a process termed *ammonia trapping*.

Distal nephron pH is regulated by intercalated cells. There are two populations of intercalated cells: one is oriented for HCO_3^- secretion, the other for H^+ secretion. Increased plasma CO_2 causes net sodium bicarbonate ($NaHCO_3$) reabsorption, correcting the acidosis. Decreased plasma CO_2 promotes net hydrochloric acid (HCl) reabsorption, correcting the alkalosis.

Clearance

The clearance principle assumes that the substance being cleared has been completely removed from a hypothetical amount of plasma. Clearance is the minimum flow of plasma required to deliver that substance to the kidney and is calculated as

$$C_x = \frac{U_x \dot{V}}{P_x}$$

$$\text{clearance} = \frac{\text{urine concentration} \times \text{urine flow rate}}{\text{plasma concentration}}$$

where U_x is urine concentration and $\dot{V}$ is urine minute volume.

Clearance of inulin or creatinine provides a noninvasive measurement of GFR, and clearance of para-aminohippurate (PAH) or Diodrast provides an estimate of renal plasma flow.

Free water clearance is the rate of solute-free plasma (water) added to or subtracted from urine flow necessary to make the urine isosmotic to plasma. It provides a measure of water balance. A client may be in *positive* free water clearance if urine osmolarity is less than plasma osmolarity or in *negative* free water clearance if urine osmolarity is greater than plasma osmolarity.

Urinary Concentration and Dilution

Urine osmolarity reflects the balance of water and solute reabsorption rates. It is determined by the medullary osmolarity and the amount of ADH acting on the collecting ducts. Glomerular filtrate is isosmotic with plasma (300 mOsm), and the filtrate osmolarity remains unchanged in the proximal tubule. Osmolarity increases in the descending loop of Henle. The ascending loop of Henle, where the Na/K/2Cl transporter removes ions but not water, causes the filtrate osmolarity to drop to 100 mOsm. This value is close to the lower limit of urine osmolarity, but some additional NaCl can be reabsorbed in the distal tubule and collecting duct. ADH acts on the distal tubule and collecting duct to increase water and urea permeability, allowing the filtrate to become isosmotic with the cortex (300 mOsm); if a large amount of ADH is present, filtrate becomes isosmotic with the inner medulla (1500 mOsm). The inner medulla osmolarity represents the upper limit on urine osmolarity.

Regulation of Urine Formation

Renal perfusion pressure is the dominant long-term regulator of glomerular filtrate formation and urine production (pressure diuresis and pressure natriuresis). However, other mechanisms also alter the rate of filtrate formation and the efficiency of filtrate reabsorption.

Tubuloglomerular feedback at the juxtaglomerular apparatus provides negative feedback control of filtrate formation. The juxtaglomerular apparatus is formed by the junction of the glomerular afferent arteriole and the macula densa of the distal convoluted tubule. A decrease in distal tubule NaCl delivery causes a reflex increase in GFR, both by afferent arteriolar dilation and an angiotensin II–mediated efferent arteriolar constriction. Blockade of angiotensin II formation reduces the effectiveness of this system and may cause a drop in GFR.

Neural regulation by the sympathetic nervous system also regulates urine formation. Sympathetic contraction of afferent arterioles reduces filtrate formation and enhances salt and water conservation. Renal sympathetics are activated in response to hypotension sensed by arterial baroreceptors and in response to hypovolemia sensed by cardiopulmonary volume receptors.

Renal Endocrine and Metabolic Actions

Most endocrine actions of the kidney are tied to the cardiovascular system. The kidneys synthesize and secrete *erythropoietin,* the hormone that increases blood cell synthesis in the bone marrow. *Renin* release from the afferent arteriole ultimately leads to formation of vasoconstrictor angiotensin II and release of aldosterone. *Intrarenal prostaglandin* production assists the regional distribution of renal blood flow. One exception to the renal-cardiovascular connection is vitamin D. Vitamin D_3 is activated to 1,25-dihydroxycholecalciferol by renal proximal tubules to enhance calcium (Ca^{2+}) absorption.

Second only to the liver, the kidney has a powerful capacity for *gluconeogenesis.* Urine represents a possible loss pathway for nutrients, especially in disease. Proteinuria may cause a greater loss of protein than may be offset by ingestion. The glucosuria of diabetes may also represent a significant loss of potential calories.

Micturition

Urine production by the kidneys is relatively constant (~1 ml/min) but can vary from 0.5 to 20 ml/min. Flow through ureters is intermittent and is controlled by the rate of peristaltic wave generation. The peristalsis that forces the urine into the bladder for storage occurs every 10 to 150 seconds. Parasympathetic activation increases frequency of peristalsis, and sympathetic stimulation decreases frequency. Afferent (pain) nerves initiate the *ureterorenal reflex.* This reflex, activated by obstruction, causes ureter constriction and also causes afferent arteriolar constriction to decrease urine production. Lodging of kidney stones in the ureter is a major cause of this response.

Both sensory and motor components of the pelvic nerves supply the bladder. Activation of the parasympathetic nerves causes a contraction of the detrusor muscle (bladder). The internal sphincter at neck of bladder is normally contracted, but it is relaxed when the bladder muscle contracts. The external sphincter is skeletal muscle under voluntary control, innervated by pudendal nerves. These nerves are tonically active, but activity can be decreased when controlled from higher central nervous system (CNS) centers.

The *micturition reflex* is initiated when bladder filling increases wall tension above a threshold point. Sensory nerves transmit tension information to the spinal cord, where an increase in parasympathetic activity causes contraction of the detrusor muscle. This contraction further increases wall tension, increasing reflex parasympathetic activity and enhancing the contraction. The process repeats until tension plateaus (for a minute or so), the reflex fatigues, or the external sphincter is relaxed and the bladder empties. If emptying does not occur, the process begins again after a few minutes.

Urination is facilitated by abdominal contraction, which compresses the bladder and increases wall tension, initiating the reflex. The micturition reflex is modulated by descending inputs from higher CNS structures. The pons has both strong facilitatory and inhibitory centers. The cerebral cortex also can modulate the reflex, allowing voluntary control of the timing of urination.

Effects of Aging and Nutrition

Aging causes atrophy of the kidneys and a progressive loss of renal function. This change is usually not critical, because the kidneys have an excess function capacity. Damage or loss of one kidney, however, may allow the age-related changes to impair renal function in the remaining kidney. The increased capillary hydrostatic pressure caused by hypertension or protein ingestion causes progressive damage to glomeruli and accelerates the age-related decrease in renal function. Low-protein diets attenuate the age-related decrease in renal function and are recommended for clients with damaged kidneys.

The aging process also affects micturition. The bladder becomes funnel-shaped as a result of alterations in the connective tissue and weakening of the pelvic floor muscles. Irritability of the bladder wall often increases, adding more urgency to the normal desire to void. Finally, impairment of the detrusor muscle's ability to elongate results in decreased bladder capacity. Because of these changes, older people may have problems with incontinence, frequency, urine retention, or dysuria.

Dietary components can alter renal function at the glomerular and tubular levels. Ingestion of a protein-rich meal dilates the afferent arteriole and increases renal blood flow. The increase in glomerular capillary pressure increases the GFR. These responses are termed *postprandial renal hyperemia.*

CONCLUSIONS

The four organs of the urinary elimination system—kidneys, ureters, bladder, and urethra—work together to filter liquids and to remove waste from the body in the form of urine. The kidneys control fluid and electrolyte homeostasis and play a role in blood pressure regulation, red blood cell production, insulin degradation, prostaglandin synthesis, calcium and phosphorus regulation, and vitamin D metabolism. The body can survive minimal kidney dysfunction because of its excess-function capacity. However, serious renal dysfunction is life-threatening, requiring dialysis or transplantation.

BIBLIOGRAPHY

1. Fauci, A. S. (1998). *Harrison's principles of internal medicine.* New York: McGraw-Hill.
2. Guyton, A. C., & Hall, J. (1996). *Textbook of medical physiology* (9th ed.). Philadelphia: W.B. Saunders.
3. Silverthorn, D. (1998). *Human physiology.* Upper Saddle River, NJ: Prentice Hall.
4. Valtin, H., & Schaffer, J. A. (1995). *Renal function* (3rd ed.). Boston: Little, Brown.

CHAPTER 32

Assessment of Elimination

Roberta Jorgensen
Karen A. Hanson

In spite of advanced technology for diagnosing problems of elimination, every diagnostic evaluation is guided by an accurate, thorough, and documented assessment. Assessment of elimination is fundamental to the evaluation of the client.

Taking a health history requires exceptional skills in speaking, listening, observing, and interpreting the client's communication because anxiety and embarrassment often accompany discussion of bowel, urinary, or genital problems. Language and semantic barriers can interfere with communication, especially with the variety of terms used to describe bowel and urinary elimination. Differences in educational background can result in fear and poor communication when the client has difficulty understanding medical terminology. A calm, caring, and accepting atmosphere during the interview promotes communication. The client may wish to have a family member present to assist with describing the details of the problem or health history.

BOWEL ELIMINATION

HISTORY

Assessment of the lower gastrointestinal (GI) system begins with the health history, followed by physical examination of the abdomen, anus, and rectum and diagnostic studies. Review previous hospitalizations, surgery, recent exposure to infection, recent travel, current medications, habits, and family history. Explore family risk factors for lower GI disorders, such as a history of colon cancer. Determine whether the client has regular screening for colon cancer.

■ BIOGRAPHICAL AND DEMOGRAPHIC DATA

A thorough review of biographical and demographic characteristics helps to elicit data related to disorders that are more likely to occur. Many lower GI disorders are associated with age and sex. For example, colorectal cancer is predominantly a disease of older adults, peaking in the seventh decade.[19] Ulcerative colitis occurs more frequently in whites and in those of Jewish descent. Diverticular disease is most common in individuals living in developed countries whose diets consist primarily of refined foods. Diverticular disease is also more common in older people. In the United States, diverticulitis develops in approximately one third of the population by age 50 and in almost two thirds by age 80.[13]

■ CURRENT HEALTH

A simple, open-ended question, such as "How are you feeling?" may elicit concerns about conditions that contribute to the current health problem. Explore potentially relevant areas such as the client's social situations, life events, and difficulties surrounding the health problem. Many lower GI manifestations are vague and have various causes.

Chief Complaint

Allow clients to describe the chief complaint in their own words. Elicit information about and learn to recognize a wide variety of manifestations that are potentially associated with a specific GI disorder. Manifestations include abdominal cramping, gaseousness, or rectal pain and may be influenced by socioeconomic status and culture. Objective findings, such as ascites and rebound tenderness, may be observed upon physical examination. For any lower GI disorder, some manifestations may occur together. With experience, you will learn to recognize these as they relate to a specific GI disorder.

Symptom Analysis

Obtain more specific information about the problem by means of a symptom analysis (see Chapter 9). Include the following.

TIMING. When was the problem first noticed? How long did it last? Was the onset abrupt or insidious? Where was the client when it occurred? Has the problem been present since that time? Abrupt onset of abdominal pain could indicate emergent conditions such as appendicitis, volvulus, or bowel obstruction. Pain of gradual onset may be related to acute inflammation of the colon or diverticula, severe gastroenteritis, or constipation and gas.

Is the problem related to food intake? If diarrhea is present, ask about awakening during the night because of diarrhea. If this is the case, it may indicate *inflammatory bowel disease* rather than *irritable bowel syndrome* (IBS).[22]

Quality and Quantity. Ask the client to describe the problem in detail. If the complaint is lower abdominal pain, determine whether it is sharp, dull, aching, burning, intermittent, or spasmodic. If the pain is deep, dull, and diffuse, it is probably visceral in origin, that is, the result of localized inflammation or ischemia. Pain that is sharp and more localized may be parietal or peritoneal pain that might be the result of generalized inflammation. If the client has noticed bloody stools, ask whether bleeding occurs with every bowel movement or only on occasion. Ask whether the blood is mixed in with the stool or present only on the surface.

Location. Assist the client in defining and locating abdominal pain. Does the pain radiate? The location of pain provides clues to common causes. Right upper quadrant pain may be hepatic in origin, resulting from disorders such as hepatitis, liver abscess, or perihepatitis. Right lower quadrant pain may indicate appendicitis. Left upper quadrant pain may result from splenic rupture, infarct, or abscess. Left lower quadrant pain suggests a left colon origin and may indicate diverticulitis or ischemic colitis.[22] Generalized abdominal pain suggests a number of possible causes such as appendicitis, intestinal obstruction, inflammatory bowel disease, or generalized peritonitis.

Precipitating Factors. Are there events that occur in relation to or before the problem onset, such as stress, specific foods, medications, or activity? Does the problem occur at a certain time of the day? In cases of suspected gastroenteritis, has the client's source of drinking water changed recently, or has the client eaten unusual foods such as wild mushrooms or improperly handled food?

Aggravating and Relieving Factors. Are there situations that worsen the problem? Are there particular medications or actions that have provided relief? What has the client done to make the situation better?

Associated Manifestations. Has the client noticed other manifestations that have become apparent recently? Disturbances in lower GI elimination may affect appetite, energy level, and weight. In addition to or in association with the problem, are there other GI manifestations such as nausea, vomiting, early satiety, anorexia, eructation (belching), flatulence, diarrhea, constipation, abdominal distention, heartburn, or indigestion? Does the client have food intolerances, abdominal cramping, weight gain or loss, hematemesis (vomiting of blood), melena (black, tarry stools), rectal pain, or anal pruritus? Other lower GI manifestations related to hepatic, biliary, or pancreatic disorders include jaundice, ascites, fatty stools, and colicky, abdominal pain. (Metabolic system assessment is discussed in Chapter 42.)

Abdominal pain that accompanies diarrhea is frequently associated with infectious gastroenteritis, inflammatory bowel disease, diverticulitis, and early intestinal obstruction. Constipation preceding abdominal pain by several days may be associated with diseases of the colon or rectum.

Explore all manifestations because a health problem related to the GI system rarely occurs in the absence of other manifestations or etiologic events. Clients may be aware of other relevant symptoms. Review the client's health status, discussing general health, diet, lifestyle, and health risk factors. It is an opportune time to assess the client's health awareness and implement health promotion teaching. (See Chapters 9 and 28 for discussions of diet history and nutritional assessment and this chapter for assessment of elimination patterns.)

PAST HEALTH HISTORY

The past health history includes information about the client's general state of health, past illnesses, immunizations, injuries, hospitalizations, surgeries, current medications, and allergies.

Childhood and Infectious Diseases

Inquire about both childhood and adult problems. In addition to asking about common childhood infectious diseases, specifically question the client about hepatitis, intestinal infections, encephalitis, sexually transmitted diseases, and human immunodeficiency virus (HIV) infection.

Immunizations

Record the immunization history. Inquire whether the client has received routine childhood immunizations including *Haemophilus influenzae* type b (Hib) conjugate. Everyone should be immunized against hepatitis B, particularly people whose lifestyles put them at risk. In addition, inquire about hepatitis A vaccination, which is indicated for international travelers or those employed in day care settings. Ask whether immunizations are current, and note dates of the last tetanus booster and influenza vaccination.

Major Illnesses and Hospitalizations

Note all hospitalizations and major illnesses. Has the client been hospitalized or treated for abdominal pain, anemia, GI bleeding, change in bowel habits, colitis, unexplained weight loss, or colon cancer? What was the plan of care, and what was found? Ask for a summary of the hospitalization experience, including laboratory tests, diagnostic procedures, and the results obtained. Ask about previous operations, particularly those involving the GI tract or accessory organs.

Try to determine what was found as a result of hospitalization. A discharge summary may be beneficial in treating the current health problem. How has the client been since having an operation performed? If the colon was resected, as for cases of severe chronic ulcerative colitis, the client may be functioning and feeling much improvement.

Medications

Note all current medications and how they are taken. Ask about over-the-counter medications, such as vitamins, antacids, laxatives, enemas, pain relievers, herbal remedies, and nutraceuticals (health food supplements). Often, clients consider these medications and natural remedies not worth mentioning. Be aware of potential relationships between what is taken and the client's current GI manifestations. For example, nonsteroidal anti-inflammatory drugs (NSAIDs) can contribute to epigastric pain, gastric ulcers, and bleeding. Calcium preparations can cause constipation, as can iron preparations. Magnesium preparations can contribute to diarrhea. Soluble fiber products such as oat bran, dried beans, and psyllium reduce fat absorption and have a laxative effect. Herbs that can cause GI upset include milk thistle (*Silybum marianum*), goldenseal (*Hydrastis canadensis*), ginger (*Zingiber officinale*), kelp (*Fucus vesiculosus*), comfrey (*Symphytum officinale*), chaparral (*Larrea divaricata*), cayenne (*Capsicum*), and alfalfa (*Medicago sativa*).

Allergies

Ask about allergies that are related to the environment, food, or drugs. Seek specific details to determine the client's allergic response. Be careful to distinguish between foods that are merely difficult to tolerate and those that induce an actual allergic reaction. Ask what types of lower GI problems occur when the client ingests a particular food. Note allergic manifestations such as abdominal cramping, belching, or diarrhea.

■ FAMILY HEALTH HISTORY

A number of GI disorders have a familial association. Inquire whether any family members have been diagnosed with Crohn's disease, chronic ulcerative colitis (CUC), intestinal polyps, or colon cancer. Information about the family incidence of other GI-related disorders such as jaundice, hepatitis or other liver disease, bleeding ulcers, or irritable bowel syndrome is also relevant.

■ PSYCHOSOCIAL HISTORY

The psychosocial history includes information on occupation, current environment, life experiences, personal relationships, and lifestyle habits. Determine the client's knowledge about the manifestations and illness. Has the illness caused the client to lose time from work? Does the client have insight into the symptoms? Are there environmental or psychosocial factors that have changed recently in the client's situation?

Occupation and Environment

Explore the client's occupational and environmental history to determine whether exposure to disease-provoking substances or environments has occurred. Ask about occupational exposure to substances that may be toxic if ingested or absorbed. If travel is a regular part of the client's job, has there potentially been exposure to unusual or improperly handled foods or contaminated water? Does the client have any hobbies that involve possibly hazardous materials? Has there been increased stress in the workplace?

Geographical Location

Has the client recently traveled abroad and been exposed to contaminated food or drink? The enteropathogens most commonly responsible for traveler's diarrhea are transmitted via contaminated food or drink. The most frequent causes are bacterial pathogens, of which *Escherichia coli* is the most common. The most common protozoal infectious agent in travelers is *Giardia intestinalis (Giardia lamblia)*. Protozoa and helminths account for a greater proportion of cases of prolonged diarrhea after travel abroad.[19]

Exercise

Ask whether the client has a regular exercise program or whether physical activity is part of the daily routine. A sedentary lifestyle can be a causative factor in certain types of lower GI disorders, particularly constipation.[23]

Nutrition

Thorough assessment of dietary habits is essential when evaluating GI elimination disorders. The diet may be a causative factor, or it may have been altered in an attempt to ameliorate the manifestations. GI disorders may cause significant impairment of normal digestive function. In addition, nutritive factors may be responsible for GI disease, as exemplified by the relationship between a high-fat diet and the development of colorectal cancer and that between lack of dietary fiber and the development of diverticulosis.[15]

When assessing the diet, ask the client to describe what was eaten the previous day, as this is usually easiest to recall. Ask about consumption of high-fiber foods such as fruits and vegetables, whole grains, breads and cereals, red meats, and saturated fats. Are most of the meals eaten at home or at a restaurant, where there is a greater likelihood of high fat and sodium content? Assess the client's knowledge of what constitutes a healthy diet. Are there dietary modifications that might be made to improve the client's nutritional intake?

What fluids are consumed in a day and in what amounts? Ask about water, coffee, cola, and alcohol intake in a 24-hour period. Many GI symptoms attributed to irritable bowel syndrome may be related to excess alcohol and caffeine intake.[19]

Assess the relationships between dietary intake and resultant GI manifestations. Excessive ingestion of synthetic, nonabsorbable sugars such as sorbitol may cause diarrhea. Lactose intolerance occurs when the intestine does not produce enough lactase to digest lactose (milk sugar), resulting in abdominal bloating and cramping. It is the most common cause of osmotic diarrhea.[13] Chapter 28 discusses nutritional assessment.

Habits

Certain lifestyle habits may contribute to GI manifestations. Lack of a regular bowel elimination routine in the daily schedule can lead to chronic constipation. Excessive alcohol consumption, if not curtailed, may lead to gastritis and eventual hepatic damage.

Inquire whether the client is experiencing increased stress either at home or at work. Altered stress levels can bring about GI-related manifestations such as epigastric pain, ulcers, and diarrhea.

■ REVIEW OF SYSTEMS

Review possible GI manifestations, and check each system to uncover additional symptoms of "unrelated" illness. Are there problems in chewing or swallowing food? Ask about the condition of the teeth or whether dentures (if worn) fit properly. Are there sores in the mouth or on the tongue, or has there been difficulty with mouth dryness and odor?

Determine whether there has been a change in appetite, either excessive hunger or anorexia, or problems with indigestion such as excessive belching or heartburn. Has the client experienced abdominal pain, nausea, or vomiting? If there was vomiting, what was the character of the vomitus? Has there been a change in bowel movements such as change in color, consistency, or caliber? Has there been rectal bleeding or black, tarry stools? Does the client experience rectal pain or pruritus? In addition, determine whether there have been any manifestations related to the accessory organs of digestion, such as the development of jaundice, ascites, peripheral edema, generalized intractable pruritus, clay-colored stools, or dark urine.

PHYSICAL EXAMINATION

Physical examination of the lower GI tract includes the abdomen, anus, and rectum. Discussions of upper GI tract, liver, and spleen assessment appear in Chapters 28 and 42. An example of an abdominal assessment recording is given in Chapter 28.

■ ABDOMEN

Lower GI tract assessment begins with the abdomen. The abdomen is divided into either four quadrants or nine regions for descriptive purposes. Be familiar with the abdominal structures located in each of these areas. Figure 28–5 shows the quadrants and anatomic regions of the abdomen and their underlying organs.

The equipment for the examination of the abdomen and rectum includes a stethoscope, gloves, lubricant, tissues, materials for occult blood testing, and reagent. The client should be supine, with the abdomen fully exposed from the sternum to the knees (see Fig. 10–6). A sheet or towel may be placed over the genitalia. The arms should be at the sides and the legs extended. A pillow under the knees aids in relaxing the abdominal muscles. Stand at the client's right side. If the current problem is one of abdominal pain, examine the area of pain last to avoid stimulating tightening of the abdominal muscles (guarding). Proceed as follows: inspection, auscultation, percussion, palpation, and rectal examination.

Inspection

Inspect the abdominal contour for evidence of distention, masses, asymmetry, or visible peristaltic waves, which are abnormal and should be reported. In addition, note scars, striae, petechiae, and the presence of dilated veins. Note the shape, position, and color of the umbilicus. A protruding umbilicus may indicate ascites, mass, or an umbilical hernia.

Assess for inguinal, umbilical, and femoral hernias by asking the client to cough. A sudden bulge may indicate a hernia. In addition, coughing may elicit localized pain. Lastly, ask the client to perform the Valsalva maneuver (if not contraindicated) or attempt a stomach curl. Look for a separation of the rectus muscles at the midline (*diastasis recti*), which may be accompanied by a bulge. This condition results from obesity, pregnancy, or problems in which sustained elevated intra-abdominal pressure weakens the muscles.

Auscultation

Auscultation of bowel sounds provides information about the motion of liquid and air through the intestinal tract. Perform auscultation before percussion and palpation. Palpation and percussion may affect intestinal motility and therefore alter bowel sounds.

While the client is supine, place the diaphragm of the stethoscope over the midabdomen. Normal bowel sounds are high pitched and heard every 5 to 10 seconds. If no sounds are heard after listening for at least 2 minutes, bowel sounds are considered absent. The absence of bowel sounds suggests a paralytic ileus that may be related to diffuse peritoneal irritation.[20] Rushes of rapid high-pitched bowel sounds or *borborygmi* are associated with hyperperistalsis and may be present in gastroenteritis or early intestinal obstruction.

Auscultation helps to determine whether an abdominal *bruit* is present. Place the diaphragm of the stethoscope in the midline of the abdomen 2 inches above the umbilicus, and listen carefully for an aortic bruit. Next, listen at a point 2 inches above the umbilicus and 1 to 2 inches laterally on both sides of midline for a renal bruit. A renal bruit may indicate renal artery stenosis. Bruit is discussed further in Chapter 51.

A *peritoneal friction rub*, like a pleural or pericardial rub, indicates inflammation. During respiration, a friction rub may be heard in the right or left upper quadrant, suggesting hepatic or splenic pathology.[20] A rub is described further in Chapter 10.

Percussion

Percussion is used to detect the presence of fluid, gaseous distention, or solid masses and to determine the location and size of abdominal organs, primarily the liver and spleen. At times, it may be preferable to palpate before percussion, especially if the client is complaining of abdominal pain.

The client should be supine. Evaluate all four quadrants. The most common percussion note heard in the abdomen is *tympany* (high pitched, loud, or musical), which is due to the presence of gas in the stomach, small bowel, and colon. If the bladder is full, the suprapubic area may sound *dull* (thud-like sounds over fluid or solid organs) when percussed (see the discussion of bladder percussion later). Percussion of the liver and spleen is discussed in Chapter 42.

If ascites is suspected, a special percussion test for *shifting dullness* may be performed by nurses who have advanced assessment skills. Ascitic fluid sinks to the lower abdomen as a result of gravity (when standing), shifts to the side of the abdomen (when lying on one's side), and bulges in the flanks (when supine). While the client is supine, the borders between the areas of tympany and dullness are percussed. The area of tympany is due to gas in the bowel present above the ascites and is located above the area of dullness. The client is then asked to turn on the side, and the nurse again percusses the abdomen. If ascites is present, the area around the umbilicus that was initially tympanic becomes dull because the ascites has shifted to the more dependent position.[20] Ascites may also be detected by determining the presence of a *fluid wave*. This advanced assessment technique is discussed in Chapter 42.

Palpation

Abdominal palpation usually proceeds from light to deep and then to the liver, spleen, and kidneys. The client is supine, and the examination begins with the area of the abdomen that is farthest from the area of pain, if present.

Light palpation is used to detect masses, areas of muscular spasm or rigidity, and areas of direct tenderness. Deep palpation is used to determine the size and shape of abdominal organs and masses. Deep palpation is used primarily by nurses in advanced practice areas. Palpation techniques are discussed in detail in Chapter 10.

If the abdominal rectus muscles do not relax and soften during expiration, abdominal *rigidity* is present. Rigidity may indicate peritoneal irritation if diffuse or an inflamed gallbladder if localized. In clients who complain of abdominal pain, palpation is performed gently.

Perform a test for *rebound tenderness* if the client has abdominal pain. Palpate slowly and deeply away from the area of suspected inflammation; then quickly withdraw the palpating hand. The feeling of pain on the side of the inflammation that occurs when the palpating hand is withdrawn is called rebound tenderness. Because this maneuver may induce generalized pain, perform this test at the end of the abdominal examination.

Palpation of the liver and spleen is discussed in Chapter 42, and palpation of the kidneys is discussed later in this chapter.

■ ANUS AND RECTUM

The abdominal examination concludes with examination of the anus and rectum. Maintain a calm, matter-of-fact approach because it is often embarrassing for the client.

Most nurses perform only a visual inspection of the perianal area, but advanced practice nurses can perform a complete digital examination of the rectum. Be familiar with rectal anatomy and expected physical findings. This information is necessary when digitally assessing for rectal impaction or administering rectal medications (Fig. 32–1).

Inspection

Perform the rectal examination with female clients in the lithotomy position immediately after the pelvic examination, in Sims' position, or in a dorsal recumbent position. Male clients may be examined either in Sims' position or standing and leaning across the examination table, which makes examination of the prostate gland easier. Spread the buttocks apart with the gloved nondominant hand, and examine the anus and surrounding tissue.

Inspect perianal skin for signs of inflammation, rashes, nodules, ulceration, fissures (cracks), fistulous openings, and hemorrhoids (dilated veins seen as reddened skin protrusions). Normally, the anus looks moist and hairless with coarse folded skin that is more darkly pigmented than the perianal skin. The anal opening should be tightly closed. No lesions should be present. Inspect the sacrococcygeal area, which is normally smooth and even. Ask the client to strain while you look for evidence of rectal prolapse (protrusion of rectal mucosa through the anal opening), internal hemorrhoids, polyps, or fissures. There should be no break in the skin integrity or protrusion through the anal opening.

Palpation

Inform the client that a rectal examination will be performed. Tell the client that there will be the sensation of a cool lubricant and a feeling as if having a bowel movement.

Use the gloved nondominant hand to spread the buttocks apart, and place the lubricated index finger of the other hand on the anus. Apply gentle pressure over the anus, thereby relaxing the sphincter. Instruct the client to take a deep breath as the index finger is inserted into the anal canal. The anal sphincter should close completely around the examining finger, at which time sphincter tone may be assessed. Advance the examining finger approximately 6 to 10 cm (2 to 4 inches) into the rectum in the direction of the umbilicus. The rectal mucosa should feel smooth and be nontender. Note irregularities such as polyps, masses, or undue tenderness, and describe their location and characteristics. Once the index finger is fully inserted, instruct the client to bear down again and feel for a mass descending from above against the palpating finger. A mass should be absent.

In a female client, the cervix of the uterus may be felt through the rectovaginal wall along the anterior rectum (see Chapter 37). The rectovaginal wall is firm, smooth, and resilient. In a male client, the prostate gland may be palpated through the anterior rectal wall. This part of the examination is discussed in Chapter 37.

Note the color of the fecal material present on the glove when you withdraw your finger. Mucus; blood; or tan, gray, or black tarry stool is abnormal. Test the fecal material for occult blood (described later in this chapter). If a sexually transmitted disease is suspected, obtain a rectal culture (see the discussion later in this chapter). Wipe the perianal area clean, and inform the client that the examination is completed.

DIAGNOSTIC TESTS

Diagnostic tests are performed to determine the nature of the lower GI disorder. The general methods of diagnosis include laboratory tests (Table 32–1), radiographic stud-

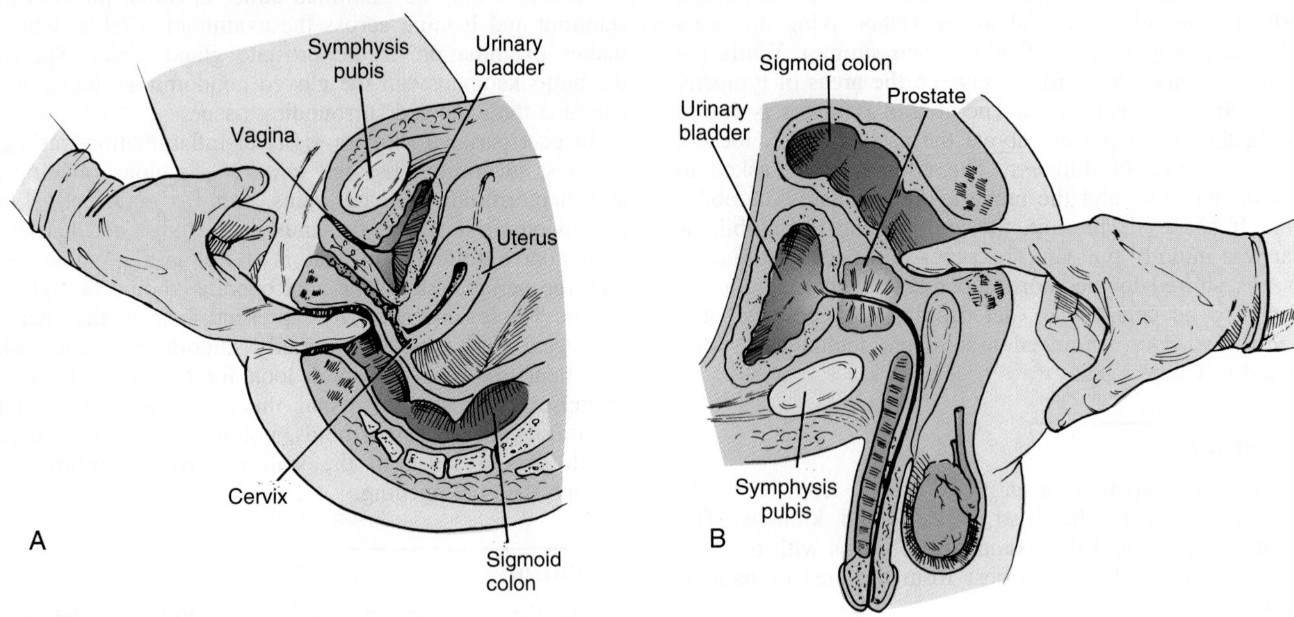

FIGURE 32–1 Palpation of the rectum in female *(A)* and in male *(B)* clients.

TABLE 32–1 LABORATORY TESTS USED TO ASSESS LOWER GASTROINTESTINAL (GI) FUNCTION

Test	Normal Findings	Abnormal Findings
COMPLETE BLOOD COUNT		
Red blood cells	4.2–5.4 million/mm³ (women) 4.5–6.2 million/mm³ (men)	Decreased values may indicate anemia or hemorrhage
Hemoglobin	12–16 g/dl (women) 14–18 g/dl (men)	Increased values indicate possible hemoconcentration, caused by dehydration
Hematocrit	38%–46% (women) 42%–54% (men)	
ELECTROLYTES		
Potassium	3.5–5.0 mEq/L	Decreased values indicate possible GI suction, diarrhea, vomiting, intestinal fistulas
Calcium	8.0–10.5 mg/dl	Decreased values indicate possible malabsorption
Sodium	135–145 mEq/L	Decreased values indicate possible malabsorption and diarrhea
CEA	<5 ng/ml (nonsmokers)	Increased values indicate possible colorectal cancer and inflammatory bowel disease
FECAL ANALYSIS		
Stool for occult blood	Negative	Presence indicates possible peptic ulcer, cancer of the colon, ulcerative colitis
Stool for ova and parasites	Negative	Presence of *Entamoeba histolytica* (amebiases) or *Giardia lamblia*
Stool cultures	No unusual growth	Presence of *Salmonella typhi* (typhoid fever), *Shigella* (dysentery) *Escherichia coli* (gastroenteritis), *Staphylococcus aureus* (food poisoning), *Clostridium botulinum* (food poisoning), or *Aeromonas*
Stool for lipids	2–6 g/24 hr (normal diet)	Steatorrhea (increased values) can result from intestinal malabsorption or pancreatic insufficiency

ies, ultrasonography, and endoscopy. Hematologic studies and electrolyte determinations offer additional information; however, these reflect primarily general health status.

LABORATORY TESTS

Carcinoembryonic Antigen

Carcinoembryonic antigen (CEA) is a glycoprotein secreted on the glycocalyx surface of cells lining the GI tract and is normally produced during the first or second trimester of fetal life. High CEA levels are characteristic of various malignant conditions such as cancer of the colon, lung, or breast and of certain nonmalignant conditions such as liver disease, cirrhosis, alcoholic pancreatitis, heavy smoking, and inflammatory bowel disease.

CEA levels cannot be used as a general indicator of cancer, but they are useful for preoperative staging of colorectal cancer and assessing the adequacy of surgical resection. Often called a tumor marker, CEA is used to monitor the effectiveness of colorectal cancer therapy. Serum levels usually return to normal within 6 weeks if cancer treatment is successful.

Perform venipuncture and collect the sample in a 7-ml red-top tube. Handle the sample gently to prevent hemolysis, which may alter test results. There is no postprocedure care.

FECAL ANALYSIS

Fecal analysis aids evaluation of digestive efficiency and the integrity of the stomach and intestines. Analysis begins with gross examination of stool color, consistency, odor, and other characteristics and concludes with microscopic, chemical, or bacterial analysis.[22]

If the colon is partially obstructed or loses its elasticity, stool in transit may cause bleeding. Blood in the stool also may result from hemorrhoids. A black, tarry stool can result from upper GI bleeding. A large, bulky, foul-smelling stool that floats in the toilet may indicate fat malabsorption. Diarrhea is a result of too rapid transit of food in the GI tract, often caused by a viral infection. Mucus or pus in the stool may be a result of rectal abscesses or ulcerative colitis. A stool specimen is often required for diagnosis of infectious diseases, GI bleeding, and other GI tract disorders. Because stool specimens cannot be obtained on demand, close cooperation is necessary to secure a suitable specimen.

Fecal Occult Blood Tests

Fecal occult blood tests are most useful in screening asymptomatic clients at risk for developing colorectal cancer or in detecting GI bleeding. The Hemoccult test is widely used to detect occult blood in the feces. It is based on the change in color of a guaiac-based colorless dye to blue caused by the peroxidase activity of hemoglobin.

The Hemoccult test has been used in screening programs for colon cancer. Annual fecal occult blood testing, in conjunction with flexible sigmoidoscopy every 3 to 5 years, has been recommended by the American Cancer Society for screening people between 40 and 50 years of age.[12]

The fecal occult blood test can be performed immediately after the rectal examination or on stool specimens collected over 3 days. Two samples from each of the consecutive stools are tested to avoid false-positives. A wooden applicator is used to apply stool to one side of guaiac-treated paper. Developing solution is applied, and the result is immediately noted. Blue indicates a positive reaction and should be reported.

The client should abstain from rare meat and peroxidase-rich foods such as raw fruits and vegetables for 3 days before the test. Aspirin and NSAIDs, which may increase GI bleeding, should be withheld, although clients with painful arthritis may find this difficult. There is no postprocedure care.

Stool Examination for Ova and Parasites

Examination of a stool specimen can detect intestinal infection caused by several types of parasites and their ova (eggs). Wear gloves, and collect the stool specimen directly in the container. Note the date and time of the collection, the consistency of the specimen, pertinent dietary history, and recent or current antimicrobial therapy. The specimen should be sent to the laboratory within 30 minutes of passage or refrigerated if it is not examined immediately.

Instruct the client to avoid treatments with castor oil or mineral oil, bismuth, magnesium or antidiarrheal compounds, barium enemas, and antibiotics for 7 to 10 days before the test. Three specimens should be tested by collection of a stool every other day or every third day. There is no postprocedure care.

Stool Cultures

Bacteriologic examination of the stool identifies pathogens that may be causing overt GI disease. Identifying these organisms is necessary to treat the client and thereby prevent potentially serious complications. A sensitivity test may follow isolation of the pathogen. Some viruses may also cause GI symptoms, but these viruses can be detected only by immunoassay or electron microscopy.

A stool specimen is collected on 3 consecutive days. Wear gloves to obtain the specimen, which is collected directly in the container. Stool may also be collected by means of a rectal swab inserted past the anal sphincter, rotated gently, and withdrawn. Place the swab in the appropriate container, and send immediately to the laboratory. Note the dietary history, recent antimicrobial therapy, and any recent travel that might indicate endemic infection or infestation. There is no postprocedure care.

Fecal Lipids

Dietary lipids, emulsified by bile, are almost completely absorbed in the small intestine provided that there are adequate biliary and pancreatic secretions. However, both digestive and absorptive disorders may cause *steatorrhea* (excessive secretions of fecal lipids). A quantitative test performed on stool collected over a 72-hour period confirms the presence of steatorrhea. Collect the stool in a non-wax container and keep refrigerated.

Instruct the client to abstain from alcohol and to consume a high-fat diet (100 g/day) for 3 days before the test and during the collection period. Drugs that may affect test results, such as mineral oil, potassium chloride, and neomycin, should be withheld. There is no postprocedure care.

■ RADIOGRAPHY

Flat Plate of the Abdomen

A flat plate of the abdomen is an x-ray film of the abdominal organs. It is used to help identify tumors, obstructions, abnormal gas collections, and strictures.

Lower Gastrointestinal Series (Barium Enema)

PROCEDURE

A barium enema is administered for the radiographic examination (with or without fluoroscopy) of the large intestine. Barium sulfate (single-contrast technique) or barium sulfate and air (double-contrast technique) are instilled rectally. The test is indicated for clients with a history of altered bowel habits, lower abdominal pain, or passage of blood, mucus, or pus in the stools. The test helps detect tumors, diverticula, stenoses, obstructions, inflammation, ulcerative colitis, and polyps.

PREPROCEDURE CARE

Adequate preparation is essential and varies among agencies. Typical preparation includes a low-residue or clear liquid diet for 2 days before the test to reduce feces volume. The client usually receives a potent laxative and an oral liquid preparation for cleaning the bowel the day before the test and has nothing by mouth (*nil per os*, NPO) after midnight. The morning of the examination, a suppository or cleansing enema may be administered. If the client has active bleeding or an ileostomy, different bowel preparations may be needed. *If ultrasonography, an abdominal scan, or colonoscopy is also indicated, it should be performed first because barium interferes with these tests.* The procedure is uncomfortable and takes 60 to 90 minutes.

POSTPROCEDURE CARE

Barium impaction is a serious complication after a lower GI series if the barium is not evacuated. A laxative or cleansing enema is often given after the test to empty the large bowel. Stools are white for 24 to 72 hours after the examination. Encourage the client to increase liquid intake to prevent fecal impaction. Instruct the client to report any pain, bloating, absence of stool, or bleeding.

Computed Tomography

Computed tomography (CT) is a complementary test in assessing acute diverticulitis and abscess formation, diagnosing colorectal cancer, and staging rectal tumors. CT is a useful alternative to barium enema for clients who are unable to retain barium. CT is used primarily to identify masses such as neoplasms, cysts, focal inflammatory lesions, and abscesses of the liver, pancreas, and pelvic areas (see Chapter 11).

Ultrasonography

Ultrasonography is used to identify pathophysiologic processes in the pancreas, liver, gallbladder, spleen, and retroperitoneal tissues. Gas in the abdomen may interfere with the ultrasound waves (see Chapter 11).

■ ENDOSCOPY

Endoscopy is the direct visualization of the GI system by means of a lighted, flexible tube. The physician can directly observe sources of bleeding and surface lesions and determine the status of healing tissues.

Proctosigmoidoscopy

PROCEDURE

Proctosigmoidoscopy is the endoscopic examination of the lining of the distal sigmoid colon, the rectum, and the anal canal using two instruments: a proctoscope and a sigmoidoscope. Indications include a recent change in bowel habits, lower abdominal and perineal pain, prolapse on defecation, anal pruritus, and passage of mucus, blood, or pus in the stool. This procedure involves three steps: a digital examination, sigmoidoscopy, and proctoscopy.

During digital examination, the anal sphincters are dilated to detect any obstruction that might hinder the passage of the endoscope. During sigmoidoscopy, a 25- to 30-cm (10- to 12-inch) rigid sigmoidoscope is inserted into the anus to allow visualization of the distal sigmoid colon and rectum. The flexible sigmoidoscope also permits visualization of the descending colon. During proctoscopy, a 7-cm (2-inch) rigid proctoscope is inserted into the anus to aid examination of the lower rectum and anal canal. Specimens may be obtained by biopsy, lavage, cytology brush, or culture swab at any point during the procedure from the mucosal areas under suspicion.

PREPROCEDURE CARE

Explain to the client that proctosigmoidoscopy allows visual examination of the lining of the distal sigmoid colon, the rectum, and the anal canal. Describe the preparation for the procedure and the position assumed (knee-chest or left lateral). In addition, explain that some colicky, abdominal pain may result from passage of the instrument and introduction of air into the intestines. Reassure the client that there will be adequate draping to avoid embarrassment during the procedure. Obtain consent.

Agencies may specify various dietary and bowel preparations for this procedure. Clients are usually required to maintain a clear liquid diet for 24 to 48 hours before the test and to fast on the morning of the procedure. If a special bowel preparation is ordered, explain that this clears the intestine to provide a better view. A warm tap water or Fleet enema may be administered as ordered on the morning before the procedure.

POSTPROCEDURE CARE

Observe closely for signs of bowel perforation (malaise, rectal bleeding, abdominal distention and pain, mucopurulent drainage, and fever) and for vasovagal attack related to emotional stress (depressed blood pressure, pallor, diaphoresis, and bradycardia). If the knee-chest position was used, instruct the client to rest supine for several minutes before standing to avoid postural hypotension. As ordered, the client is given nothing by mouth and vital signs are monitored every 30 minutes until the client is alert.

Colonoscopy

PROCEDURE

Colonoscopy is the visual examination of the lining of the large intestine with a flexible fiberoptic endoscope. This procedure is indicated for clients with a history of constipation and diarrhea, persistent rectal bleeding, or lower abdominal pain when results of proctosigmoidoscopy and a barium enema are negative or inconclusive. Colonoscopy is also used to screen clients at high risk for colon cancer.

PREPROCEDURE CARE

The client is sedated and placed on the left side. After the colonoscope is inserted through the anus, a small amount of air is insufflated to locate the bowel lumen. The scope is advanced through the rectum into the sigmoid colon under direct visualization. When the instrument reaches the descending sigmoid junction, the client may be assisted to the supine position to aid the scope's advance past the splenic flexure. After the scope has passed the splenic flexure, it is advanced through the transverse colon and past the hepatic flexure into the ascending colon and cecum. Abdominal palpation or fluoroscopy may help guide the colonoscope through the large intestine.

POSTPROCEDURE CARE

Observe the client closely for signs of bowel perforation (malaise, rectal bleeding, abdominal pain and distention, fever, and mucopurulent drainage). Monitor vital signs as ordered until they are stable.

URINARY ELIMINATION

HISTORY

Urologic assessment includes assessment of elimination as well as sexual and reproductive function. This chapter describes urologic assessment, and Chapter 37 describes reproductive assessment.

■ BIOGRAPHICAL AND DEMOGRAPHIC DATA

Biographical and demographic data, such as age, gender, marital status, race, occupation, and geographical location, provide the framework for the health history. Gather specific information regarding sexual preference or practices to assess the client's risk of venereal disease or HIV infection. Certain diseases and health states are more common in specific groups of people. For example, urinary incontinence affects approximately 13 million Americans, with the highest prevalence in the elderly population. It is more common in women than in men (10% to 30% versus 1.5% to 5%) and often affects older multiparous women (who have had multiple pregnancies) in the form of stress incontinence.[3]

Benign prostatic hyperplasia (BPH), a benign growth of the prostate, occurs in men older than 50 years and often coincides with prostate cancer, possibly because of a common hormonal cause.[18] BPH is usually the cause of irritative and obstructive voiding manifestations in older adult men. Prostatitis can mimic some of the manifestations of BPH but is more likely to be the diagnosis if the client is younger than 40 years of age.

Black males and men older than age 40 are at risk for adenocarcinoma of the prostate. The incidence of prostate cancer doubles with each decade of life after age 40.[18] Testicular cancers most often occur in young men between ages 25 and 35. Bladder cancer occurs more often in men than in women and in white than in black males. Bladder cancer has been linked to a variety of environmental factors, such as aromatic amines in certain dyes and organic chemicals such as pesticides.[18]

■ CURRENT HEALTH

Clients with urologic complaints may find it embarrassing to discuss their problems. Establish a private, confidential, unhurried atmosphere when obtaining the history. Continually assess verbal and nonverbal feedback, evaluate nonjudgmentally and objectively, and provide information using language and diagrams that the client understands.

Chief Complaint

Upon identifying the chief complaint, ask specific questions about common urologic manifestations. Clients who have a urologic chief complaint describe manifestations in the categories of disturbances of voiding, alterations in urine characteristics, pain or referred pain, and systemic or GI manifestations.[24] More than one manifestation may be present. Explore each one.

Symptom Analysis

DISTURBANCES IN URINATION

Disturbances in urination include changes in urinary volume, irritative or obstructive manifestations, and urinary incontinence. Normal adult bladder capacity is about 300 to 500 ml. Adults normally void five or six times per 24 hours, more during the day than at night. Total daily urine output ranges between 800 and 1800 ml.[2] This amount varies with changes in the amount and type of fluid intake, amount of perspiration, environmental or ambient temperature, and the presence of vomiting or diarrhea. It may also be affected by pathologic changes in the urinary system.

CHANGES IN URINARY VOLUME. *Anuria* refers to a total urine output of less than 100 ml per 24 hours, and *oliguria* refers to a total urine output of 100 to 600 ml per 24 hours. Anuria and oliguria are associated with acute or chronic renal failure secondary to systemic events (shock, dehydration, reduced cardiac output), renal injury (glomerulonephritis, acute interstitial nephritis, renal artery aneurysms or emboli), or postrenal obstruction (ureteral, bladder outlet, or urethral).[10] *Polyuria* (voiding in unusually large daily amounts) may be associated with systemic disease (diabetes mellitus or diabetes insipidus, adrenal insufficiency), diuretic medication, or chronic renal disease resulting in electrolyte imbalance.

Review the client's health history to determine any known precipitating medical causes of urine volume changes. Inquire about the onset and duration of the urinary volume change to establish whether it is acute or chronic in nature or reflects an acute exacerbation of a chronic disease. Assess fluid intake, noting the amount and timing of consumption, especially of caffeinated and alcoholic beverages.

IRRITATIVE AND OBSTRUCTIVE MANIFESTATIONS. Irritative voiding symptoms of urgency, frequency, nocturia, and dysuria can occur with infection, inflammation, calculus, cancer, obstruction, or neurogenic dysfunction of the lower urinary tract (bladder, prostate, and urethra). Urgency and frequency are often present regardless of etiology and often appear in combination.

Urinary frequency, voiding more often than every 2 hours, is a common manifestation. It can occur because of changes in urine volume, decreased bladder capacity (such as with prostatic enlargement or detrusor instability), increased postvoid residual urine, inflammatory irritability of the bladder mucosa, and psychological disorders.

Urgency is a sudden strong desire to void that can usually be controlled. Urgency is caused by irritation of the lower urinary tract secondary to inflammation, calculus, bladder cancer, or neurogenic dysfunction.

Nocturia is excessive urination during the night (awakening with the need to urinate more than twice nightly). Nocturia may be related to the same urinary conditions listed for urinary frequency. It may also occur in clients who have circulatory problems that result in dependent edema during the day. The recumbent position helps to mobilize the sequestered fluids, resulting in increased venous return to the circulatory system and subsequent increased renal perfusion.

Dysuria, described as a burning sensation on initiation of, during, or at the end of urination, is usually associated with infection, inflammation, or, rarely, cancer of the bladder or urethra. It is usually accompanied by urgency and frequency.

Irritative manifestations may be accompanied by obstructive manifestations, such as hesitancy, straining to begin urination, intermittency, decreased force and caliber of the urinary stream, high postvoid residual, and urine retention. The cause is usually bladder outlet obstruction secondary to prostatic enlargement (in men), congenital urethral valves, urethral meatal stenosis, or urethral stricture. Symptom severity can be established for BPH by reference to the American Urologic Association (AUA) symptom index (Fig. 32–2). Neurologic diseases may mimic obstructive symptoms by affecting the innervation of the striated or smooth muscle components of the bladder and external sphincter, thereby impairing bladder contractility.

Hesitancy refers to delay in initiation of urination of at least 10 seconds. It is not associated with "bashful bladder," which can occur when urinating in a public restroom. It often leads to straining or pushing, which voluntarily increases intra-abdominal pressure to start the *urinary stream*. With prostatic obstruction or urethral stricture, straining is rarely helpful in initiating the stream.

When the client presents with obstructive manifestations, ask for a description of the urinary stream. Note whether (1) there is decreased force and caliber, (2) the stream is intermittent or interrupted (bladder stones or impaired bladder contractility), and (3) the stream is bifurcated or spraying (commonly seen with urethral stricture or meatal stenosis).

AUA Symptom Index

Name: ____________ Date: ________

Clinic #: ____________

A description of what each number represents is located at the top of each column. Circle the number in the column which best describes your situation.	Not at all	Less than 1 time in 5	Less than half the time	About half the time	More than half the time	Almost always
1. Over the past month or so, how often have you had a sensation of not emptying your bladder completely after you finished urinating?	0	1	2	3	4	5
2. Over the past month or so, how often have you had to urinate again less than two hours after you finished urinating?	0	1	2	3	4	5
3. Over the past month or so, how often have you found you stopped and started again several times when you urinated?	0	1	2	3	4	5
4. Over the past month or so, how often have you found it difficult to postpone urination?	0	1	2	3	4	5
5. Over the past month or so, how often have you had a weak urinary stream?	0	1	2	3	4	5
6. Over the past month or so, how often have you had to push or strain to begin urination?	0	1	2	3	4	5
	None	1 Time	2 Times	3 Times	4 Times	5 Times
7. Over the past month, how many times did you most typically get up to urinate from the time you went to bed at night until the time you got up in the morning?	0	1	2	3	4	5

AUA Symptom Score: ________

(Sum of all numbers circled in questions 1–7)

FIGURE 32–2 American Urologic Association (AUA) Symptom Index. (Modified from Barry, M. J., et al. [1992]. The American Urologic Association symptom index for benign prostate hyperplasia. *Journal of Urology, 148,* 1549–1557.)

Clients who have significant amounts of *postvoid residual* urine or *urinary retention*, usually greater than 100 ml, may describe a sense of incomplete bladder emptying. This is noted either as bladder fullness after urinating or more commonly as "double voiding," a second urination necessary within 5 to 15 minutes after the initial void. When clients experience long-standing high residual urine volumes, sometimes more than 1000 ml, they are considered to have *chronic urinary retention*. These clients experience little or no pain but may demonstrate other obstructive manifestations. Continual overflow incontinence is common because the bladder remains full to capacity at all times.

Acute retention is a sudden inability to void, accompanied by severe suprapubic pain (which distinguishes it from anuria) and urgency. It may occur postoperatively or post partum (after delivery), with use of certain medications, or with worsening of bladder outlet obstruction. It is a medical emergency requiring immediate intervention (e.g., urethral or suprapubic catheterization).

URINARY INCONTINENCE. *Urinary incontinence* refers to involuntary loss of urine. According to the Agency of Health Care Evaluation Clinical Practice Guidelines, urinary incontinence plagues 10% to 35% of adults and is widely underreported and underdiagnosed.[3] The social stigma and embarrassment of urinary incontinence result in loss of self-esteem and decreased ability to maintain an independent lifestyle. Decreased social interactions and decreased sexual activity are commonly reported. Considering the impact on one's quality of life, thoroughly investigate any mention of urinary incontinence by the client.

Urinary incontinence can be divided into several types: urge, reflex, stress, mixed, overflow, and functional.

Urge incontinence is the involuntary loss of urine associated with a strong desire to void. It is present with *detrusor instability* (DI) and normal bladder sensation.

Urge incontinence resulting from DI that is present without normal bladder sensation is considered *reflex incontinence*. Diseases of the spinal cord above the sacral micturition center (S2-4) produce reflex incontinence. DI with a neurologic cause is commonly referred to as *detrusor hyperreflexia*. It may also be accompanied by poor detrusor contractility and thus may contribute to difficulty emptying the bladder completely. Ask, "Are you able to feel when your bladder is full?" "Are you aware of urinary leakage when it happens?" "Do you still feel fullness in the bladder after you urinate?"

Stress incontinence is the leakage of urine with physical exertion or with an increase in intra-abdominal pressure but without actual detrusor contraction. Stress incontinence in women is most often due to urethral hypermobility associated with the pelvic descent that occurs after childbearing. In both sexes, it may be due to intrinsic urethral sphincter deficiency (ISD), congenital or acquired, in which the sphincter cannot create enough resistance to retain urine. Ask when the urine loss occurs. Is it with coughing, sneezing, laughing, or other physical activity?

A combination of stress and urge incontinence, or *mixed incontinence*, typically occurs in older women. Urge incontinence is more distressing for the client, probably because there is less control in social situations.

Overflow incontinence is associated with chronic overdistention of the bladder secondary to impaired bladder contractility or bladder outlet obstruction. Clients present with frequent or constant dribbling or may have stress or urge incontinence.

Functional incontinence is associated with cognitive or physical impairments outside the lower urinary tract and is often seen in nursing home clients. It can often be remedied, even when it coexists with other types of incontinence, by changes in medications, improvements in hydration status, and removal of environmental barriers to toileting.

A careful interview and health history are instrumental in differentiating between the types of incontinence so that the appropriate diagnostic evaluation can be performed.

ALTERATIONS IN URINE CHARACTERISTICS

When evaluating urine characteristics, ask the client to describe (1) the color, (2) the clarity, and (3) the odor of the urine.

Urine *color* is affected by blood, changes in hydration status, certain diseases, and ingestion of certain foods or medications (Table 32–2). Color can be clinically significant, especially if the client reports even a single episode

TABLE 32–2 CAUSES OF URINE DISCOLORATION

Color	Disease Etiology	Medication, Dyes, Dietary
Colorless	Chronic glomerulonephritis Diabetes mellitus Diabetes insipidus	Excessive fluid intake, alcohol, diuretics
Cloudy white	Phosphate in alkaline urine Epithelial cells Bacteria, pus, chyle	
Yellow	Concentrated urine	Tetracycline, rifampin
Dark yellow	Urobilinogen	Santonin, phenindione, rhubarb (in acid urine), nitrofurantoin, sulfasalazine, docusate calcium, thiamine (multivitamins)
Pink or red	Red blood cells Hemoglobin Urate excretion Myoglobin *Serratia marcescens* Menstrual contamination	Beet ingestion, vegetable dyes, phenolphthalein laxatives (in alkaline urine), cascara (in alkaline urine), senna (X-Prep, Senokot), rhubarb (in alkaline urine)
Brown	Highly concentrated urine Red blood cells	Metronidazole (left standing), porphyrin
Dark brown or black	Highly concentrated urine Bilirubin Melanin Red blood cells (old)	Porphyrin (after standing), tyrosine, phenacetin, quinine, senna, methyldopa
Blue-green	Bilirubin *Pseudomonas*	Methylene blue, indigo carmine, thymol, phenol, amitriptyline

of "bloody urine" (*hematuria*), which can be pink, red, tea colored, dark brown, or maroon and may or may not be accompanied by blood clots. Gross hematuria is often the only presenting manifestation of bladder cancer. If clots are present, question the client regarding their appearance. Clots from the ureter or kidney are often long and stringy, whereas those from the bladder or prostate are large and amorphous. Further define the hematuria by asking at which point during voiding it occurs. *Initial* hematuria indicates a urethral, prostatic, or seminal vesicle origin. *Terminal* hematuria indicates bleeding from the bladder neck, trigone, or posterior urethra. Hematuria throughout the stream may indicate glomerulonephritis. *Total* hematuria indicates profuse bladder, ureteral, or kidney hemorrhage. Rule out menstrual contamination in female clients. Urinary tract infection is a common cause of hematuria in women.

Urine *clarity* is affected by infection or inflammation of the urinary tract that results in bacteriuria and *pyuria* (white blood cells in the urine). Most typically, cloudy urine is due to amorphous phosphates in alkaline urine. Other causes of hazy or cloudy urine are epithelial cells from the lower urinary tract (contamination only), yeast, crystals, mucus, or fecal material. Milky urine results from prostatic fluid or semen, lipids, lymphatic fluid (chyle), or blood. Microscopic urinalysis determines the cause of the cloudiness. Figure 32–3 depicts examples of urine casts and crystals.

Urine *odor* is rarely of clinical significance, but strong-smelling or foul-smelling urine may indicate infection, and a sweet or fruit-like odor can be due to ketonuria. A strong ammonia odor may occur if the urine is left standing too long. Medications and dehydration can also affect urine odor.

Pneumaturia is the presence of gas in the urine during voiding. Pneumaturia suggests fistula formation between the bladder and bowel.

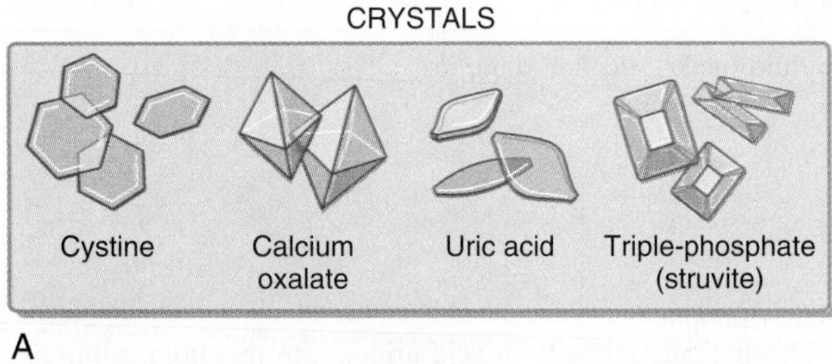

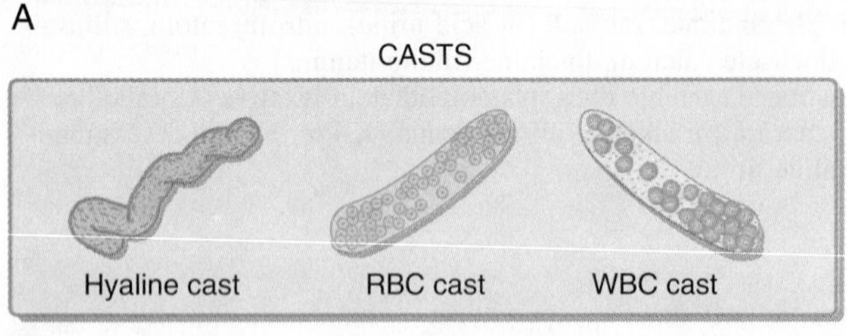

FIGURE 32–3 Urine clarity can be affected by crystals *(A)* and casts *(B)*. RBC, red blood cell; WBC, white blood cell. (400× magnification.) (Modified from Walsh, P. C., et al. [Eds.]. [1998]. *Campbell's urology* [7th ed.]. Philadelphia: W. B. Saunders.)

Pain or Referred Pain

Urinary tract disease does not always cause pain. When pain is present, ask the client to describe the location, intensity, onset, and duration to define the etiologic mechanism further. What seems to alleviate or worsen the pain? Is the pain affected by bladder fullness or urination? Is it better or worse with position change, ejaculation, or bowel movement?

Pain in the upper urinary tract (kidney and ureter) is frequently felt locally as a dull, constant ache in the costovertebral angle just lateral to the sacrospinal muscle and beneath the 12th rib posteriorly. Sudden distention of the renal capsule secondary to acute pyelonephritis or ureteral obstruction is typically the cause of renal pain. Renal distention may refer pain to the epigastric area as well as to the subcostal area toward the umbilicus and lower abdominal quadrant. Ask when the pain occurs. Costovertebral pain caused by mechanical back pain and radiculitis differs from renal pain in that it becomes worse with heavy physical work and position changes of the spine.

If the pain is colicky in nature, the ureter is probably involved. Ureteral colic may radiate to the bladder, scrotum, and testicle in a male and to the vulva in a female. Colicky pain can be continuous, spasmodic, severe, and unbearable. If ureteral stones are suspected, ask the client to identify the site of referred pain to help identify the location of the stone. Upper ureteral stones result in pain referred to the testicles, midureteral stones cause pain referred to the intestine, and stones near the ureteral orifices in the bladder cause irritative bladder symptoms. Manifestations tend to be localized in adults but are more generalized in children, who often present with only GI symptoms of abdominal pain, nausea, and vomiting.

Bladder pain is usually associated with acute overdistention, infection, or irritation of the bladder wall. Acute urinary retention causes agonizing suprapubic pain and sometimes bladder spasms, which are experienced as intermittent, cramping, severe pain in the bladder. Bladder spasms also result from irritation of the bladder wall by a foreign body, such as an indwelling urinary catheter, infection, or bladder tumors. With bladder infections there may be only pain referred to the distal urethra, causing dysuria while voiding.

In the absence of a bacterial infection, symptoms of urgency and frequency can be caused by *interstitial cystitis*, a type of local autoimmune disorder that occurs most often in middle-aged women. Interstitial cystitis is often debilitating and poorly understood.[10] Pain in the spine or bony structure of the pelvis or pain that radiates down one or both legs may be due to metastasis of prostate, kidney, or bladder cancer.

Prostate pain is not common. Men with acute prostatitis may feel fullness in the rectum or perineum, have irritative voiding manifestations, and have postejaculatory pain. Testicular pain secondary to orchitis, trauma, or torsion of the spermatic cord is usually localized and severe and may radiate along the spermatic cord to the lower abdomen. Pain may be referred to the testicle from an inguinal hernia or upper ureteral stone.

Epididymal pain results from acute infection and initially occurs as local pain and swelling in the scrotum.

The pain can progress to an exquisitely painful mass involving the entire hemiscrotum, possibly radiating to the groin and lower abdomen. Epididymal pain is relieved by elevating the scrotum (Prehn's sign).

Pain in the urethra is localized and results from inflammation and irritation of the urethral mucosa. It occurs with urethral stricture, urethritis, or urethral cancer. Urethral pain may be more apparent before and after voiding.

SYSTEMIC MANIFESTATIONS

Fever and chills are usually associated with acute, not chronic, infectious processes in the urinary tract such as cystitis, pyelonephritis, prostatitis, and epididymitis. GI manifestations such as nausea, vomiting and diarrhea, abdominal distention, and pain commonly occur with many urinary tract disorders. With "silent" urologic disease, GI manifestations may be the only presenting complaint.

Renal pathology causes GI symptoms for several reasons. The renointestinal reflexes, which arise from common autonomic and sensory innervations of the urinary and GI tract, can trigger pylorospasm or changes in the smooth muscle of the GI tract when there is distention of the renal capsule. The kidneys are anatomically related to the colon, duodenum, liver, spleen, pancreas, diaphragm, and psoas muscle; inflammation of the kidney may create manifestations in any of these intraperitoneal or retroperitoneal organs. Anteriorly, the kidneys are covered by the peritoneum; thus, renal inflammation may provoke muscle rigidity and rebound tenderness.

Evaluate the client carefully for signs of infection if renal failure is suspected or confirmed. Sepsis is the most common cause of death in clients with renal failure.[11] Observe for manifestations of end-stage renal disease, such as edema, confusion, lethargy, weakness, and muscle twitching or cramps. Weight loss and lethargy can occur with advanced stages of urinary cancer.

■ PAST HEALTH HISTORY

In obtaining the past health history, inquire about coexisting systemic disease. Many disorders affect urinary function. Because urinary tract infection, retention, urinary calculi, or incontinence can be chronic or recurrent, explore any history of these disorders, including treatments implemented and their outcomes.

Childhood and Infectious Diseases

Congenital anomalies of the urinary tract are common but range in severity from being incidental radiologic findings to being incompatible with life. The kidney may be absent *(renal agenesis)*, dysplastic or atrophic, ectopic (located outside the flank position), or fused (joined, as in "horseshoe" kidney). Note when a client has a solitary kidney because treatment must be tailored to preserve optimal renal function. Children with ectopic or fused kidneys are likely to have other genitourinary, skeletal, GI, or cardiovascular anomalies. When ectopia or fusion occurs alone, it is often asymptomatic. Ureters can be ectopic, incomplete, or absent (agenesis); duplicated; or markedly dilated *(megaureter)*. Bladder extrophy, persistent urachus, and epispadias are congenital anomalies that require reconstructive surgery and potentially lead to long-term problems with urinary incontinence.

Malformations of the spinal cord, such as meningomyelocele and spina bifida, can cause neuropathic voiding disorders. Childhood streptococcal infections, mononucleosis, mumps, measles, and cytomegalovirus infections can result in acute glomerulonephritis.

Trauma

Is there a history of a motor vehicle accident, falls, straddle injury, penetrating abdominal injury, or contact sports injury? Assess the injury, how long ago it occurred, and the medical or surgical management that followed. The most frequent renal injury is blunt trauma, which is often managed conservatively, whereas penetrating trauma is usually explored surgically. Assessment of blunt or penetrating renal injury involves observing for a flank mass, tenderness, or bruising, especially when there is visible evidence of abdominal trauma. Long-term complications are rare with early intervention and careful follow-up.

Injury to the ureters is rare and most often occurs after penetrating wounds or complicated pelvic surgery. If ureteral injury is promptly corrected surgically, long-term complications are rare. When treatment is delayed, the client may experience flank or abdominal pain, peritonitis, paralytic ileus, fever, and possibly fistulae. Delayed diagnosis increases the risk of renal damage secondary to infection, hydronephrosis, abscess formation, and ureteral stricture.

Bladder trauma is related to the amount of urine in the bladder at the time of the injury; the bony pelvis protects the empty bladder. Suspect trauma anytime a pelvic fracture has occurred. If the bladder wall is ruptured by a penetrating or blunt injury to the lower abdomen, urine may extravasate into the peritoneal cavity and cause an acute abdomen or peritonitis if the urine is contaminated. Typically, the client has suprapubic pain or is unable to void. Gross hematuria is usually present. Complications of bladder injury are rare if it is treated promptly but can include temporary incontinence.

Urethral injuries are more common in males than females and can occur with instrumentation such as endoscopy or catheterization, straddle injury of the anterior urethra (distal to the urogenital diaphragm), or pelvic fracture in the posterior urethra (proximal to the urogenital diaphragm). In females, urethral injury is sometimes seen after traumatic intercourse, childbirth, or vaginal surgery. Assess for blood at the meatus, urinary retention, and bladder distention. Partial or complete disruption of the urethra may lead to urethral stricture, which can restrict urinary flow and predispose to urinary tract infections.

Major Illnesses and Hospitalizations

Ask about recent illnesses, including diarrhea, vomiting, trauma (abdominal, pelvic, or vascular), and any associated manifestations such as visual disturbances or excessive thirst. Include chronic diseases that may affect urinary function. Hypertension, diabetes, electrolyte imbalance, coronary artery disease, heart failure, and anemia worsen renal disease. Diabetes mellitus and multiple sclerosis can impair urinary and erectile function by interfering with autonomic function of the bladder.

A history of tuberculosis is significant when a client reports manifestations of renal insufficiency or failure, ureteral obstruction, or chronic urinary tract infections. *Mycobacterium tuberculosis* may travel from the lungs to the genitourinary organs and cause a chronic granulomatous infection. A history of tuberculosis helps to differentiate between tuberculosis of the bladder and interstitial cystitis.

Clients with a history of sickle cell anemia are at risk for papillary necrosis of the kidney and erectile dysfunction secondary to recurrent priapism. If renal neoplasm is suspected, inquire whether the client has von Hippel–Lindau syndrome, an autosomal dominant disorder that causes angiomatous cerebellar cysts, angiomatosis of the retina, and tumors of the pancreas; it is associated with cysts or adenocarcinoma of the kidneys. Disorders of the central nervous system can also affect innervation of the bladder. Disorders leading to hypercalcemia, such as hyperparathyroidism, limited mobility, and excessive vitamin D intake, can predispose to renal stones, obstruction, and subsequent renal failure. External beam radiation therapy for bladder or prostate cancer can cause radiation cystitis.

Scleroderma, an autoimmune disorder characterized by massive deposits of collagen, may involve the kidneys. Erythema multiforme, an inflammatory disorder of the skin associated with allergic or toxic reactions to drugs or microorganisms such as *Mycoplasma pneumoniae* and herpes simplex virus, can involve the kidneys of young adults and children in its most severe form (Stevens-Johnson syndrome). Systemic lupus erythematosus may lead to glomerulonephritis with hypertension and nephrotic syndrome.

Operations

Previous abdominopelvic or genitourinary procedures can affect urinary function through accidental trauma to the ureters and bladder. Document all invasive procedures, especially if the client may need surgery again. Ask about previous surgery for urinary calculus, obstruction, or incontinence. Surgical management of urologic cancers includes radical nephrectomy, transurethral resection and fulguration of bladder tumors, radical cystectomy with urinary diversion, and radical prostatectomy with pelvic lymphadenectomy. Has the client had a hysterectomy? Other operations that may interfere with the innervation of the urinary tract include neurosurgical and orthopedic procedures of the spine. Colon and rectal surgery can lead to a neurogenic bladder or erectile dysfunction.

Medications

Many medications can affect urinary function. Obtain a complete history of prescription and nonprescription medications, including herbs and nutraceuticals. Medications that can worsen some urinary conditions may be helpful in others. For example, anticholinergics and alpha-sympathomimetics can relieve urinary incontinence in some clients but may lead to urinary retention in others. If the client presents with urinary calculi, inquire about antihypertensives, diuretics, or silica antacids. Prolonged consumption of analgesics containing acetaminophen, aspirin, caffeine, and phenacetin may be associated with an increased risk of upper tract urothelial cancers. Determine the medication, dose, dosage changes, length of time taken, type, and frequency to ascertain a possible relationship to the onset of the chief complaint. Medications that are known to alter urinary function are listed in Table 32–3.

Allergies

Document allergies to antibiotics. Penicillin, cephalosporins, sulfonamides, and quinolones are often used in treatment of urinary tract infections. Aminoglycosides are used when less toxic antibiotics are ineffective or contraindicated; however, they pose a greater risk of allergic reaction. Inquire about allergies to radiographic contrast dyes as well as to iodine, as iodine dyes are used in some of the radiologic diagnostic tests routinely performed in a urologic evaluation.

■ FAMILY HEALTH HISTORY

Ask about a family history of urinary calculi and renal or sickle cell disease when clients present with pain or hematuria or both. The client who has stones is twice as

TABLE 32–3 MEDICATIONS THAT AFFECT URINARY ELIMINATION

Medication Type	Effect on Urination
Anticholinergics	Decreased detrusor contractility (oxybutynin, methantheline), urinary retention, hesitancy
Antispasmodics	Decreased detrusor contractility (dicyclomine, belladonna), urinary retention, urinary hesitancy
Tricyclic antidepressants	Decreased detrusor contractility (imipramine), urinary retention, less incontinence
Cholinergics	Increased detrusor contractility (bethanechol chloride), incontinence, urgency
Alpha-sympathomimetics	Increased sphincter resistance (pseudoephedrine), urinary retention, dysuria
Alpha-blockers	Reduced sphincter resistance (prazosin, terazosin), frequency, incontinence
Estrogens (women)	Increased urethral muscle tone (progestin, estriol), reduced incontinence
Antiandrogens (men)	Improved urinary flow (flutamide, bicalutamide)
Sedatives-hypnotics	Urinary incontinence
Nonsteroidal anti-inflammatories	Renal papillary necrosis (long term)
Diuretics	Polyuria, urinary incontinence (hydrochlorothiazide)
Aminoglycoside antibiotics	Nephrotoxicity (gentamicin, amikacin)
Calcium channel blockers	Urinary retention (diltiazem, verapamil)
Alcohol	Polyuria, frequency, urgency

likely as one who does not to have a first-degree relative with renal stones.[24] Certain other diseases, such as prostate or testicular cancer and BPH, tend to be familial.[18] Hypertension and diabetes are often inherited and can have a significant effect on renal function. Well-known genetic urinary disorders include adult polycystic kidney disease, tuberous sclerosis, von Hippel–Lindau disease, renal tubular acidosis, and cystinuria.

■ PSYCHOSOCIAL HISTORY

Psychosocial assessment is ongoing throughout the interview. Observe and assess for impairments in vision, hearing, or speech. Assess the level of mobility and social factors of living and work environment, caregivers, social contacts, and family. For clients who report (or you suspect have) involuntary incontinence, evidenced as wetness of clothing or odor, assess access to toilets and overall hygiene. Ask about positive or negative childhood experiences with toilet training that may have had a long-term effect on urination patterns.

Assess the client's knowledge of variables in daily life at home and at work that may contribute to the urinary problem. Is the client anxious about urinating in a public place? Anxiety and stress can stimulate or inhibit urination and provoke urgency and frequency. Establish how the client recognizes and manages stress, particularly when the presenting manifestation is worsened by anxiety and stress. Clients may be unaware of lifestyle changes that they might make to improve their urinary problem.

Ascertain the client's knowledge and anxiety about a potential cancer diagnosis. Provide information and feedback according to the client's educational and emotional needs. Some clients have misconceptions or fears regarding their problem and treatments available. Address fear of surgery and changes in body functions, which can seriously alter body image, so that support can be provided throughout the treatment process.

Occupation

Occupation can play a role in urinary function. Exposure at work to toxic chemicals (e.g., aniline dyes in the automobile industry, polycyclic aromatic hydrocarbons in motor exhaust, and benzidine in paint) can lead to bladder cancer. The prevalence of bladder cancer is significant enough in some occupational groups to warrant closer surveillance and possible screening of such populations.[18] Assess the accessibility of toilets in the workplace, especially for clients who have urgency and urge incontinence. Prolonged exposure to heat or cold can affect urination. An increased risk of renal adenocarcinoma has been reported among shoe workers, leather tanners, and those exposed to cadmium, petroleum products, and asbestos.[18]

Geographical Location

Hot climates can lead to chronic dehydration if fluid intake is inadequate. This, along with increased exposure to sunlight, can increase the risk of urinary calculi. People who live in warm climates are at increased risk for infection in larva-infested water used for swimming, bathing, and farming. Larvae may cause the disease schistosomiasis, which predisposes to urinary obstruction and bladder cancer.

Exercise

The positive effects of regular exercise on physical and psychological well-being cannot be overstated. What type of exercise does the client participate in regularly? How strenuous is the exercise? Does exercise affect the urinary problem in any way, or does the urinary problem prohibit participation? Does the client become rehydrated as needed after heavy physical exertion? Long-distance runners sometimes have hematuria, which may originate from the kidney or bladder or may be a sign of underlying glomerular disease.

Nutrition

Nutritional status can have a significant impact on urinary elimination. Diets rich in saturated and unsaturated fats, animal protein, and sugar and deficient in vegetable protein and unrefined carbohydrates (as seen in more affluent countries) can increase the risk of renal stone formation. Ask about dietary habits that may increase the risk for urinary stones, such as dairy products; purine in meats, fish, and poultry; and oxalate in tea, chocolate, and nuts. Excessive dietary intake in obesity may predispose the client to urinary tract carcinogenesis by promoting hormonal changes and arteriosclerosis of the renal arteries.[18]

Ingestion of spicy foods and caffeine can lead to bladder irritation and may exacerbate conditions such as interstitial cystitis (Table 32–4). For the client who complains of nocturia, assess when and what type of fluids are consumed during the evening. Coffee, tea, and caffeinated sodas can have a diuretic effect on the urinary tract. Some studies have linked coffee consumption, diuretic use, and obesity to renal cell adenocarcinoma. High-fat diets have been implicated in increased risk of prostate cancer in the United States.[18]

Habits

Obtain a history of tobacco, alcohol, and recreational drug use. Cigarette smoking has been consistently shown

TABLE 32–4 DIETARY IRRITANTS OF THE URINARY TRACT

Irritant*	Possible Substitutes
Alcohol	Late harvest dessert wines
Apples, apple juice	Apricot or pear nectar, papaya juice
Coffee, tea	Kava, cold brewed coffee, herbal tea
Chocolate	Carob
Carbonated beverages	
Chilies, spicy foods	
Aspartame (NutraSweet)	Fructose
Strawberries, cranberries	
Grapes, guava, cantaloupe	
Peaches, pineapples, plums	
Tomatoes, onions	
Vinegar	

*Not all irritants have a corresponding substitute.

to be a risk factor for urothelial cancers, increasing the risk two or three times over a nonsmoker's risk.[18] Smoking can also lead to peripheral vascular disease and to subsequent erectile dysfunction. The risk associated with cigarette smoking declines significantly with years of smoking cessation.

Alcohol can irritate the bladder and increase urinary output. Chronic alcoholism may lead to autonomic and peripheral neuropathy that impairs urinary and sexual function and to decreased serum testosterone, testicular atrophy, and decreased libido. If the client is scheduled for surgery, heavy tobacco and alcohol use can increase the risk of perioperative complications significantly. (See Chapter 15 for a discussion of the effects of tobacco and alcohol on perioperative outcomes.)

■ REVIEW OF SYSTEMS

Ask about symptoms such as GI complaints, blood pressure changes, weight loss or gain, edema, fatigue, lethargy, headaches, blurred vision, changes in mentation, numbness or tingling of the extremities, pruritus, bleeding tendencies, exposure to infectious disease, and allergies that may be associated with urologic disorders. See Table 9–2 for additional questions to include in the review of systems.

PHYSICAL EXAMINATION

The urologic physical examination typically includes:

- Temperature, pulse, blood pressure, height, and weight
- General inspection of the skin for integrity, color, and peripheral edema
- Examination of the abdomen, pelvis, genitalia, and rectum

The examination may be tailored to the client's specific complaint or condition. Instruct the client to empty the bladder before the examination. When the physical examination is completed, document findings using the Physical Assessment Findings in the Healthy Adult feature as a guide.

PHYSICAL ASSESSMENT FINDINGS IN THE HEALTHY ADULT

Urinary System

Inspection

Lower abdomen flat, nondistended. External urethral orifice pink without discharge.

Auscultation

No renal bruit noted anteriorly or posteriorly over the right or left costovertebral angle.

Percussion

Flat note over symphysis pubis and tympany over lower abdomen. No tenderness posteriorly over the right or left costovertebral angle.

Palpation

Lower pole of right kidney palpable, smooth, nontender. Left kidney nonpalpable.

■ ABDOMEN

Inspection

Have the client lie in a supine position with arms at the sides and knees slightly flexed to relax the abdominal muscles. If the client has complained of abdominal, back, or flank pain, note whether there is guarding or restlessness in this position. Inspect the abdomen for symmetry and contour. Asymmetry or a mass in the upper quadrants may indicate a renal tumor or hydronephrosis, although only a very large renal or adrenal mass in a very thin client would potentially be visible. Fullness in the suprapubic area may indicate a distended bladder.

Note any surgical or traumatic scarring that may have affected the urinary or GI tract or caused adhesions, especially if the client presents with abdominal complaints. Also note any herniation, either at the site of surgical scarring, around a stoma, or in the ventral area (epigastric or umbilical region), particularly with straining (see discussion under lower GI elimination physical examination).

For clients who have had previous urologic surgery, note the presence of a stoma, the type, whether it is a continent urinary diversion, and the appearance of the stoma and surrounding skin. Observe the size and contour of the stoma, and note the color of the mucosa. Observe for abnormal findings such as retracted or prolapsed stomal mucosa, lesions, inflammation, or macerated skin. Document the type of ostomy appliance or stomal covering, if used. Also note the presence of an indwelling urethral or suprapubic catheter, its patency, and the color and odor of the urine. Document the presence of sediment in the drainage collection system. Evaluate the drainage system for cleanliness and closed system integrity.

Auscultation

Auscultation is performed before palpation to avoid disruption of vascular murmurs and bowel sounds. Renal artery bruits are most commonly heard just above and slightly left of the umbilicus and can indicate renal artery stenosis or aneurysm or arteriovenous malformation. If a bruit is heard, avoid deep palpation. Evaluate bowel sounds in all four quadrants for frequency, intensity, and pitch, especially in the presence of GI manifestations (see lower GI tract physical examination earlier).

Percussion

Percussion is valuable in identifying a bladder containing at least 150 ml of urine. The percussion sound changes from tympanic to dull over a full bladder. Blunt percussion can also be valuable if performed anteriorly and posteriorly to identify renal masses or tenderness when renal trauma and hemorrhage prevent deep palpation. With the client sitting, place one hand over the costovertebral angle on the left side and strike the hand lightly with the opposite fisted hand. The effect is perceived as a dull thud in a normal kidney but as sharp pain or tenderness in a distended kidney. Repeat for the right kidney. Figure 32–4 illustrates this maneuver, and Chapter 10 describes the blunt percussion technique.

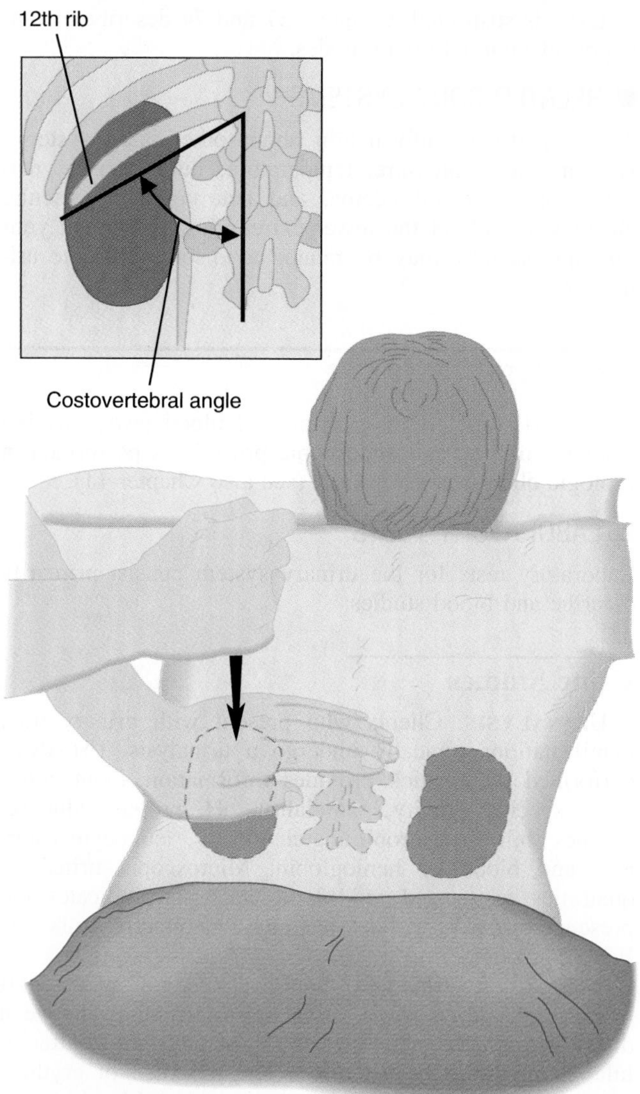

FIGURE 32–4 Percussion over the costovertebral angle.

Palpation

Begin palpation with a *light* touch, depressing the skin no deeper than 1 to 2 cm, to assess tenderness and muscle resistance or guarding, which might be a sign of peritoneal irritation. Light palpation allows examination of tender abdominal areas with minimal production of pain. Such pain may cause voluntary muscle rigidity and reduce the effectiveness of deep palpation.

Examine each of the four quadrants noting areas of muscle resistance, which may indicate a superficial or large pelvic mass, either infectious or neoplastic, or bladder distention if it is in the suprapubic area. Involuntary muscle rigidity is usually unilateral, whereas voluntary rigidity is symmetrical. To differentiate between a rigid muscle and a mass, note whether the area of resistance follows an abdominal muscle or is lobular in shape.

Last, palpate any region under suspicion on the basis of the health history and previous inspection.

Deep palpation follows light palpation and is used primarily to detect renal enlargement or masses. The technique is similar to that of light palpation, but the depth is 4 to 5 cm. Reinforced (bimanual) palpation is used in cases of more resistant muscle tone. (See Chapter 10 and Figure 10–3 for a discussion of bimanual palpation.)

Describe identified masses in terms of location, size, consistency, surface characteristics, tenderness, mobility, and pulsation. Assess rebound tenderness to determine the presence of peritoneal inflammation. Deep palpation should never be used in cases of known renal trauma, polycystic kidneys, abdominal aortic aneurysm, kidney transplantation, or appendicitis.

The kidneys are normally well protected by the diaphragm and lower ribs and cannot be palpated easily. The right kidney is slightly lower than the left because of the presence of the liver. In a thin client, the lower pole of the right kidney can sometimes be detected with deep palpation. Palpate the kidney bimanually, with one hand on the costovertebral angle posteriorly and the other hand pushing firmly and deeply under the costal margin anteriorly, while instructing the client to inhale deeply. As the client inhales, the right kidney descends and may be felt by the anterior hand as it slides between the hands. A normal kidney feels smooth, firm, and rounded (Fig. 32–5). The left kidney is usually not palpable because it lies higher up under the rib cage. In older adults, the kidneys may be palpated more readily because of loss of abdominal muscle firmness.

An empty bladder cannot be palpated. In acute or chronic urinary retention, the bladder rises up out of the pelvis at the midline toward the umbilicus. It may be seen and usually felt. When there is chronic urinary retention, the bladder is atonic and difficult to palpate.

■ GENITALIA

Use inspection and palpation to examine the genitalia. Clients tend to be more anxious about examination of the genitalia. Therefore, remain straightforward and professional and perform this part of the examination after establishing rapport.

MALE CLIENTS

While the male client lies supine, inspect the perineum and groin area for signs of skin irritation or excoriation, especially if he has reported urinary incontinence. Examine the glans meatus. Circumcised males have a dry glans, whereas uncircumcised males have a relatively moist and pink glans. Examine the urethral meatus after carefully retracting the foreskin (in uncircumcised males).

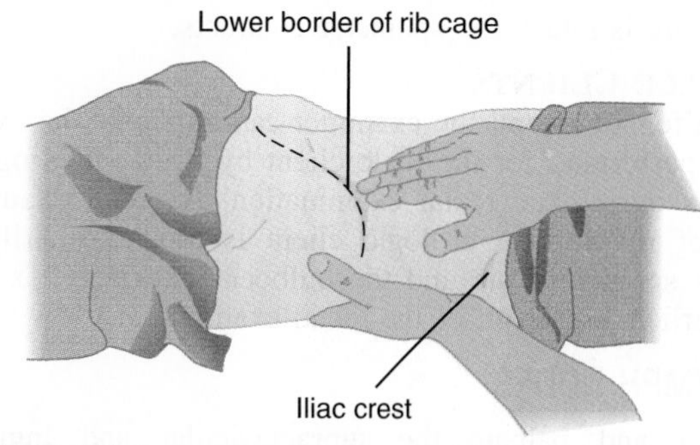

FIGURE 32–5 Palpating the kidneys.

The foreskin should retract easily. Normally, the meatus is located centrally on the glans and the mucosa is pink and moist, readily separating when the glans is pressed between the thumb and forefinger.

A meatus opening dorsally on the glans, penile shaft, or penoscrotal junction indicates *epispadias*. *Hypospadias* is an anomaly in which the urethra opens on the ventral aspect of the glans, penile shaft, or penoscrotal junction. Malposition of the urethral meatus can interfere with normal voiding and can be associated with curvature of the penis that is called *chordee*. Note the presence of any urethral discharge or reddened edematous meatal edges that indicate urethritis. Difficulty exposing the distal meatal mucosa (fossa navicularis) may indicate stenosis. Next, palpate the penile shaft ventrally along the urethra for tenderness, swelling, or mass. (Chapter 37 covers the examination of the genitalia.)

Female Clients

Urologic examination of the female genitalia includes examination of the external genitalia and in some cases a complete pelvic examination (see also Chapter 37). For an examination of the external genitalia, position the client in a supine recumbent position with knees and feet apart and knees flexed. Examine the urethral meatus for eversion or redness, which may indicate urethritis.

Palpate the urethra by inserting a gloved index finger into the vagina and palpating the anterior vaginal wall for induration or mass from the bladder to the meatus. Inspect for the presence of urethral discharge indicative of infection.

Ask the client to cough or strain, and note any bulging of the vaginal walls. Bulging of the anterior vaginal wall can indicate a *cystocele* and that of the posterior wall a *rectocele*. Cystocele is seen with relaxation of the pelvic floor musculature and may be the source of irritative voiding symptoms and stress incontinence.

■ RECTUM

Male Clients

The urologic digital rectal examination of the male client is done to evaluate the prostate gland. Although the prostate is primarily a reproductive organ, disorders of the gland can affect urination. Disorders include BPH, prostatitis, prostatodynia, and prostate adenocarcinoma. Examination of the prostate is discussed in Chapter 37.

Depending on the skill of the examiner, the bulbocavernosal reflex can be assessed for neurologic abnormalities. Evaluate the reflex by gently compressing the glans penis with the thumb and forefinger of the opposite hand while the index finger remains in the rectum. When the reflex arc is intact, the sphincter contracts.

Female Clients

In the female client, the examiner can duplicate the evaluation performed for the male client by gently flicking the clitoris during the rectal examination. A rectal examination of the female urologic client is done primarily to assess sphincter tone and the bulbocavernosal reflex (see the earlier discussion of the rectal examination).

■ LYMPH NODES

Inspect and palpate the supraclavicular and inguinal groups of lymph nodes if metastatic cancer of the prostate or testis is suspected. Chapters 37 and 74 describe examination of inguinal lymph nodes.

■ RELATED BODY SYSTEMS

Assess pertinent information about other body systems, such as blood pressure, temperature, fluid balance, evidence of peripheral edema, and neurologic or vascular changes that affect the lower extremities. Document your findings, as they may be related to disorders of the urinary tract.

Diagnostic Tests

An overview of common urine and blood tests, imaging studies, voiding, and endoscopic procedures performed in urologic clients, is given next (see also Chapter 11).

■ LABORATORY TESTS

Laboratory tests for the urinary system consist primarily of urine and blood studies.

Urine Studies

Urinalysis. Clients who present with urinary tract manifestations typically undergo a urinalysis. Urinalysis performed by dipstick provides information about color, odor, specific gravity, osmolality, pH, protein, glucose, ketones, bilirubin, urobilinogen, nitrites, leukocyte esterase, and blood or hemoglobin. Microscopic urinalysis quantifies white and red blood cells and indicates the presence of casts, crystals, bacteria, or epithelial cells (see Fig. 32–3).

Microscopic urinalysis should always follow a report of red urine. Microscopic urinalysis differentiates between discoloration related to ingested substances and extracellular hemoglobin in the urine. The presence of erythrocyte casts indicates a renal origin of the blood. Gross hematuria and microscopic hematuria, defined as more than three red blood cells per high-power field (HPF), can indicate trauma, infectious processes, toxicity, calculus, and benign and malignant neoplasms (Table 32–5).

Specific gravity indicates the concentration of urine and reflects the client's hydration status as well as renal function. For example, clients who have diabetes insipidus consistently have specific gravity values less than 1.010. Clients with extensive tubular damage or endocrine disease involving antidiuretic hormone (ADH) insufficiency have specific gravity fixed at 1.010, the level of the plasma.

Osmolality is a measure of the concentrating ability of the kidney. Osmolality increases in hypernatremia, acidosis, and shock. It decreases in diabetes insipidus, hypercalcemia, excessive hydration, and renal tubular acidosis.

Urine pH can fluctuate with fluid intake but is important in a few specific clinical situations. Clients with uric acid stones usually have more acidic urine with a pH less than 6.5. In clients who have renal tubular acidosis, the pH of the urine cannot be less than 6.0. Urinary tract infections caused by urea-splitting organisms (e.g., *Proteus*) cause the urinary pH to rise above 7.0. Urine left standing more than 2 hours or collected after a large meal may be more alkaline.

TABLE 32–5 **UNDERSTANDING URINALYSIS**

Variable	Normal Values	Causes of Abnormal Values
Specific gravity	1.001–1.035	Decreased: increased fluid intake, diuretics, decreased renal concentration, diabetes insipidus Increased: dehydration, diabetes mellitus, increased ADH secretion, iodine contrast
Osmolality	50–1200 mOsm/L	Varies with hydration
pH	5.5–6.5	<5.5: metabolic or respiratory acidosis, renal tubular acidosis type II >7.5: presence of urea-splitting organism *(Proteus),* renal tubular acidosis type I
Blood	None	Carcinoma, renal lithiasis
Protein	<20 mg/dl	Glomerular disease, nephropathy, interstitial disease, strenuous exercise, multiple myeloma
Glucose	Negative	Diabetes mellitus
Ketones	Negative	Diabetic ketoacidosis
Bilirubin	Negative	Intrinsic hepatic disease, bile duct obstruction
Urobilinogen	Trace	Hemolysis, hepatocellular disease
Nitrites	Negative	Bacteriuria
Leukocyte esterase	Negative	Bacteriuria
Red blood cells	<3 RBCs/HPF	Urinary tract cancer, IgA nephropathy, lithiasis, prostate enlargement, menstrual contamination, infection, papillary necrosis, renal artery embolism or thrombosis
White blood cells	0–5 WBCs/HPF	Infection
Bacteria	None	Urinary tract infection
Casts	0–4 hyaline/HPF	Red blood cell casts: glomerular bleeding White blood cell casts: glomerulonephritis Fatty casts: nephrotic syndrome
Crystals	Varies	Significant in renal lithiasis

ADH, antidiuretic hormone; HPF, high-power field; IgA, immunoglobulin A; LPF, low-power field; RBC, red blood cell; WBC, white blood cell.

Proteinuria or persistent elevation of protein in the urine may be glomerular, tubular, or overflow in origin. Glomerular proteinuria occurs with immunoglobulin A (IgA) nephropathy or diabetes mellitus. Tubular proteinuria results from failure to resorb immunoglobulins because of defective tubular function. Overflow proteinuria is due to an increase in abnormal immunoglobulins and is often seen with multiple myeloma. Prolonged fever and excessive physical exertion can cause a transient elevation of urinary protein levels. Orthostatic proteinuria occurs occasionally when the client has been standing for several hours. A false-positive result for urine protein may be obtained when the urine is concentrated or contains white blood cells or vaginal secretions.

Glucosuria (glucose in the urine) most often occurs in clients with diabetes mellitus, which may result in renal papillary necrosis and recurrent urinary tract infections. Glucosuria occurs when the serum glucose level exceeds the resorptive capacity of the kidneys, a level of 180 mg/dl. *Ketonuria* (ketones in the urine) occurs when body fat is metabolized for energy, as in cases of diabetic ketoacidosis, fasting, pregnancy, vomiting, and diarrhea.

Direct bilirubin is made in the hepatocyte and appears in the urine only when extrahepatic biliary tract obstruction or intrinsic hepatic disease is present. *Urobilinogen* is the end product of conjugated bilirubin metabolism, and a small amount, 1 to 4 mg/day, is excreted in the urine.

Leukocyte esterase indicates white blood cells in the urine. *Nitrites* in the urine strongly suggest bacteriuria. Epithelial cells are often present in urinary sediment. Renal tubular cells are least often seen but are indicative of renal disease.

Casts are formed in the distal tubules and collecting ducts of the kidneys and signify renal disease when found in the urine. Red blood cell casts indicate glomerulitis or vasculitis. White blood cell casts indicate bacterial infection but are often difficult to distinguish from epithelial casts. Granular casts often represent disintegrated epithelial cells, leukocytes, or protein associated with renal tubular disease. Hyaline casts represent a mixture of mucus and globulin from the tubules and are not significant in small numbers.

Depending on the test ordered, urinalysis may be performed on a clean catch specimen, midstream specimen, fresh urine specimen, first morning specimen, 12- or 24-hour collection, multiple bottle voidings (serial urine collections), or a specimen obtained with a catheter. First voided morning specimens are helpful in evaluation of renal function. Ideally, the urine should be obtained several hours after eating because postprandial specimens may contain lysed blood cells and disintegrated casts. Clean catch continues to be the standard method for obtaining urine specimens. Several studies have shown that there is little difference in contamination levels between a clean catch and a midstream urine specimen collected without previous cleansing with an antiseptic towelette.[17]

Instruct female clients to separate the labia and uncircumcised males to retract the foreskin. For a catheterized client, collect urine from the port on the tubing, not the urinary drainage bag, because this urine may be contaminated. Use a drip method to collect urine from a urostoma. Approximately 10 ml is required. In some situations, catheterization for a urine sample may be required. In these cases, follow universal precautions and maintain sterile technique (see Chapter 11 for additional discussion of urinalysis). Refer to a nursing fundamentals textbook for specific information about the techniques for collecting urine specimens (random, clean catch, catheterized, timed, and from a urostomy). Always follow protocol for specimen collection and handling.

URINE CULTURE. When urinary tract infection is suspected from the client's history or the presence of bacteria or significant white blood cells on urinalysis, a urine culture is necessary. This test identifies the offending organism and quantifies the amount of colonization. Generally, the presence of organisms in a concentration greater than 100,000/ml indicates infection, although the value may vary, depending on the method of collection and symptoms of infection.

Collection technique is as for midstream clean catch or catheter specimens for urinalysis. Determining the sensitivity of the organism to specific antibiotics is not usually necessary because *E. coli,* known to cause 85% of routine infections, is sensitive to most oral antibiotics. Identifying the drugs to which the bacteria are sensitive is done in cases with recurrent or persistent symptoms of urinary tract infection.

URINE CYTOLOGY. When urinary tract carcinoma is known or suspected, urine cytologic evaluation is performed. The specimen may be voided or a bladder washing obtained either by catheterization or cystoscopically. Transitional cell carcinoma of the bladder typically sheds cells into the urine more than upper tract carcinomas, but the amount of cells retrieved for study depends on the adequacy of the specimen and the grade and volume of the tumor.

CLEARANCE STUDIES. Urine clearance studies determine the glomerular filtration rate and tubular excretion ability of the kidney. Creatinine clearance is the most accurate measure of glomerular filtration rate, although urea, insulin, para-aminohippuric acid, and phenolsulfonphthalein can also be measured. Radioisotopes may also be used to determine clearance rates. Renal excretory function is measured as the difference between the filtration rate of a substance and the rate of excretion in the urine.

For a creatinine clearance test, collect the urine specimen for 12 or 24 hours as ordered (see Chapter 11). A blood sample is drawn at any point during the collection period in a 7-ml red-top tube. There is no postprocedure care.

CONCENTRATION AND DILUTION STUDIES. Loss of ability to concentrate and dilute urine indicates significant renal tubular damage. Several tests can be performed to evaluate the ability of the kidneys to concentrate and dilute the urine. Many of these tests can be risky for clients who have compromised renal or cardiac function because of the severe fluid loading or fluid deprivation that is part of the procedure. Carefully assess and monitor the client's fluid balance and cardiovascular status (pulse, blood pressure, lung sounds) during urine concentration and dilution testing.

Blood Studies

BLOOD UREA NITROGEN. Blood urea nitrogen (BUN) is a measure of renal function because urea is the primary end product of protein metabolism and is excreted by the kidneys. An elevated BUN level may indicate impaired renal function, although it is not specific for the kidneys. BUN may be elevated because of systemic factors such as sepsis, excess protein consumption, starvation, dehydration, and cardiac failure.

SERUM CREATININE. Serum creatinine is more specific for renal function because it is not affected by dietary intake or hydration status. It can be elevated in cases of glomerulonephritis, pyelonephritis, acute tubular necrosis, nephrotoxicity, renal insufficiency, and renal failure. Elevations are also seen in clients who have renal failure secondary to outlet obstruction. Some studies suggest that the elevated serum creatinine levels seen with urinary obstruction are related to coexisting hypertension or diabetes rather than the obstruction.[17] The normal ratio of BUN to creatinine is 10 : 1.

■ RADIOGRAPHY

Kidney-Ureter-Bladder X-ray Study

The kidney-ureter-bladder (KUB) x-ray study provides an anteroposterior film of the kidneys, ureters, and pelvis taken without contrast medium. It is used to evaluate suspected radiopaque urinary calculi or masses and as a preliminary study for other radiologic tests of the abdomen.

Client preparation includes bowel preparation if the KUB study is done as a preliminary evaluation test. Advise the client that the x-ray procedure is painless.

Intravenous Pyelography or Excretory Urography

Intravenous pyelography (IVP) or excretory urography (EXU) is a study in which a series of radiologic films are obtained after intravenous injection of contrast medium. IVP or EXU provides information about the entire urinary tract because films are taken at regular intervals as the contrast medium moves through the tract. The final film is taken after the client voids to evaluate the ability of the bladder to empty. Pressure applied across the client's lower abdomen to compress the ureters allows enhancement of the renal pelvis and proximal ureters. This test is used to evaluate renal stones, masses, hematuria, obstructive uropathy, congenital anomalies, infection, and renal function.

PREPROCEDURE CARE

Client preparation includes careful screening for potential allergies or sensitivity to contrast medium and iodine. A steroid may be given before injection of contrast medium in cases of sensitivities. Instruct clients about the necessary bowel preparation. This includes a liquid meal before 6 PM the preceding evening, followed by a laxative such as senna extract (X-Prep). Fluids are withheld after 10 PM the evening before the procedure to promote greater concentration of the contrast medium in the kidneys.

Explain that there may be a sensation of flushing and warmth, an unpleasant or salty taste in the mouth, or nausea when the contrast dye is administered. Allergic reactions (e.g., urticaria, itching, and respiratory distress or failure) occur in about 5% of clients. Because reactions happen immediately after injection of the contrast medium, antihistamines, steroids, and an emergency cart must be readily available. IVP or EXU is not recommended for clients who have renal insufficiency or failure.

Postprocedure Care

Monitor the hydration status of the client after IVP or EXU to reduce the risk of renal failure in susceptible clients. Unless there is a contraindication, force fluids to promote renal clearance of the contrast medium. Monitor output.

Retrograde Urography

For clients who are allergic to iodine-based contrast media, a *retrograde pyelogram* can be obtained. Contrast medium is administered directly into the urinary tract (rather than intravenously) during endoscopic visualization via cystoscopy. (Cystoscopy is discussed later in this chapter.) A retrograde pyelogram details the ureter, ureteropelvic junction, renal pelvis, and calices.

A *cystogram* is obtained after instillation of contrast medium directly into the bladder via a catheter. Cystographic studies are used to evaluate recurrent urinary tract infections, vesicoureteral reflux, hematuria, trauma, postsurgical healing, and stress urinary incontinence.

A *voiding cystourethrogram* is similar to a cystogram, except that films are taken while the client is voiding. A *retrograde urethrogram* is indicated when there is suspicion of urethral stricture, fistula, trauma, diverticulum, or tumor. Oblique x-ray films are taken after instillation of 15 to 30 ml of contrast medium into the urethra via a catheter in the fossa navicularis or a catheter-tip syringe.

Urinary tract infection should be ruled out before any of these procedures. Instruct clients to watch for and report symptoms of infection, which may occur for up to 24 to 48 hours after the procedure (flank pain, dysuria, chills, fever). Encourage consumption of fluids. Transient flank pain, bladder, or urethral discomfort may occur but should resolve in 24 to 48 hours.

Computed Tomography

CT is used in urology to evaluate the kidneys, major renal vessels, ureters, and bladder as well as the abdominal and pelvic contents for malignant masses, metastases, or lymphadenopathy. It is used primarily for tumor staging and identifying abscesses. Other uses for CT are to evaluate a nonfunctioning kidney, urinary tract trauma, a transplanted kidney, renal calculi, and infections. Clients should fast for 4 hours before the procedure. (See Chapter 11 for general care of the client having a CT scan.)

Magnetic Resonance Imaging

Magnetic resonance imaging (MRI) is used to visualize the kidneys, retroperitoneum, bladder, prostate, testes, and penis. It is used in urology to stage cancers of the kidney, bladder, and prostate. MRI has become increasingly useful when gadolinium, an extracellular contrast agent, is used.[24] (See Chapter 11 for general care of the client undergoing MRI.)

Renal Angiography

Angiography is the visualization of blood vessels by the use of radiopaque contrast media. This modality is used to visualize renal and penile structures but has little use in evaluation of the ureter, bladder, and prostate. Renal arteriography is used to evaluate renal tumors, to obtain vascular maps preoperatively, or to evaluate potential kidney donors. Angiography is rarely used in urology for strictly diagnostic purposes because it is expensive and invasive compared with other imaging procedures. A safer technique, *digital angiography*, uses computerized radiographic subtraction to obtain images of renal arteries with an intravenous injection of contrast medium instead of femoral artery puncture and catheterization. (Chapter 11 describes general care of the client undergoing angiography.)

■ ULTRASONOGRAPHY

Ultrasonography is used in urology to evaluate the kidneys, ureters, bladder, prostate, testes, and penis. In a renal scan, the client's abdomen and back are scanned in the longitudinal and transverse planes. The kidneys can be evaluated for size, hydronephrosis, calculi, solid tumors, and cysts. Renal ultrasonography is used to differentiate simple cysts from other types of mass lesions in the kidney. Other uses include localizing and mapping the kidneys before biopsy and evaluating transplanted kidneys.

The bladder may be scanned for residual urine volume, bladder wall thickness, bladder calculi, tumors, and diverticula with an ultrasound probe over the suprapubic area. A portable ultrasound instrument exists that computes bladder volume from 12 cross-sectional readings. It is used to determine postvoid residual accurately and has been shown to reduce the risk of nosocomial (hospital-acquired) urinary tract infection associated with catheterization for postvoid residual.[16]

Prostate ultrasonography is performed transrectally with a transducer probe inserted 4 to 5 inches into the rectum. Images are obtained in the anterior-posterior (AP), coronal, and sagittal planes to approximate size with an ellipsoid volume equation:

$$\text{volume} = \text{AP} \times \text{coronal} \times \text{sagittal} \times 0.5236$$

Prostate ultrasonography is also used to evaluate the peripheral zone for hypoechoic areas that may be associated with prostate cancer. (Chapter 37 describes ultrasonography of the testes and penis.)

Reassure clients that ultrasonography is painless and not invasive. An exception is transrectal ultrasonography, which can cause discomfort and pressure when the anus is dilated. For prostate ultrasonography, instruct the client to evacuate the rectum by administering a Fleet enema about 45 minutes before the procedure. No colon or proctologic examinations should be performed on the same day.

■ RADIONUCLIDE STUDIES

Nuclear medicine studies are performed in urology to evaluate renal failure, masses, hydronephrosis, and renal blood flow and to rule out metastatic bone disease in genitourinary cancers. Clients receive an injection of a technetium-based isotope. This is followed by a nuclear scan 3 hours later when the radioactive tracer has concentrated in the target organ. Encourage clients to force fluids before the scan. (See Chapter 11 for a general discussion of radionuclide studies.)

■ ENDOSCOPY

Cystourethroscopy and Urethroscopy

Endoscopy (see Chapter 11) is utilized in urology most commonly in *cystourethroscopy*. This endoscopic study is used to evaluate the anterior and prostatic urethra, bladder urothelium and trigone, and the ureteral orifices in the bladder. The procedure is performed transurethrally, by either a rigid or flexible cystoscope (Fig. 32–6). Cystoscopy allows diagnostic inspection of the urinary tract for evidence of urinary calculi, infection, vesicoureteral reflux, prostatic obstruction, bladder tumor, and urethral stricture. A variation of cystourethroscopy is *urethroscopy*, in which only the urethra is visualized.

Preprocedure Care

Before the procedure, a urine culture or Gram stain must be negative because an active urinary tract infection is a contraindication to the test. The procedure is usually performed with the client in the lithotomy position, and the urethra is prepared with a water-soluble lubricant containing 2% lidocaine. A spinal or general anesthetic is administered if the cystoscopy is done before a surgical procedure such as transurethral resection of the prostate (TURP) or bladder tumor. Instruct the client in the preoperative protocol for spinal or general anesthesia and obtain consent (see Chapter 15). Clients who have artificial joints, cardiac valvular disease, or valve replacement require prophylactic antibiotic therapy before the procedure to prevent the development of subacute bacterial endocarditis.

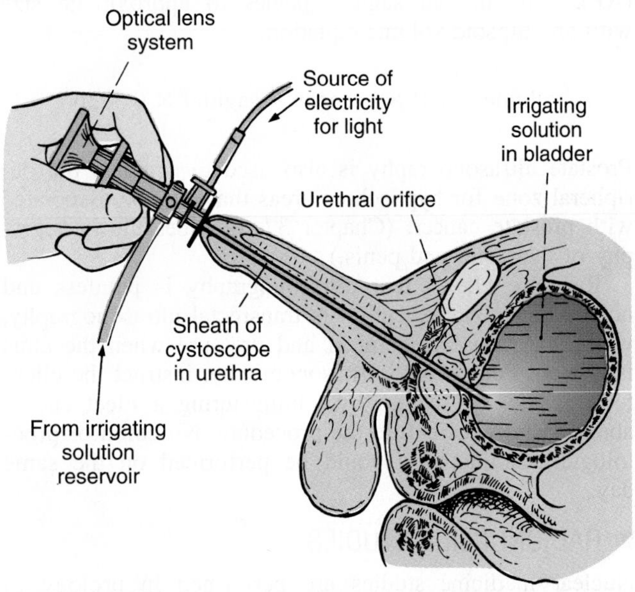

FIGURE 32–6 Cystoscope in the male bladder.

Postprocedure Care

Hematuria (pink-tinged urine) is expected after cystoscopy. Instruct the client to force fluids and to report any frank bleeding or clots in the urine or symptoms of urinary tract or systemic infection (e.g., dysuria, fever, or chills). Warm baths and NSAIDs may relieve dysuria. If acute urinary retention occurs after cytoscopy, intermittent bladder catheterization is required. Belladonna and opium suppositories or antispasmodics, such as propantheline bromide, may relieve bladder spasms.

Ureteroscopy, Nephroscopy, and Ureterorenoscopy

Endoscopic procedures for the upper urinary tracts (see Chapter 34) include the following:

- *Ureteroscopy,* performed for diagnostic as well as therapeutic purposes, is used to evaluate radiologic filling defects, gross hematuria, and malignant cytology. Additional information regarding the grade and extent of malignant tumors can be obtained with ureteroscopic biopsy.
- *Nephroscopy* is used to evaluate the renal pelvis for abnormalities.
- *Flexible deflectable ureterorenoscopy* is used for biopsy of interstitial lesions in the outflow tract as well as to retrieve stones up to the level of the calices.

These procedures are performed transurethrally with a flexible or rigid ureteroscope and allow direct visualization of the ureter and renal pelvis. The client is placed in a Trendelenburg position, and general or regional anesthesia or intravenous sedation is administered. Manipulation of the lower urinary tract, especially dilation of the ureteral orifice, can cause discomfort.

Preprocedure Care

Client preparation includes ensuring sterile urine, administering a perioperative broad-spectrum antibiotic, giving the client nothing by mouth, and obtaining consent. A history of previous radical surgery or ureteral manipulation should be known before ureteroscopic examination because it may make the procedure more difficult or impossible to complete successfully.

Postprocedure Care

Because of the ureter's smaller anatomic size, observe for possible complications including perforation and urinary extravasation into the abdomen, which occur in about 4% of clients, as well as infection, renal colic, and bleeding. Typically, a ureteral stent or temporary diversion catheter is left in place for at least 48 hours. The time may be extended if minor perforations have occurred with urinary extravasation. Encourage the client to force fluids, and continue prophylactic antibiotics as ordered after the procedure.

■ BIOPSY

Biopsies for malignancy in the urinary tract can be done transurethrally (kidney, ureter, bladder, and urethra) and percutaneously (prostate). Biopsy of the kidney can be performed by either a percutaneous or an open surgical approach.

Transurethral Biopsy

Biopsy of a suspicious lesion in the bladder that is discovered during cystourethroscopy is done with the client under regional or general anesthesia. Biopsy specimens of surrounding bladder tissue are also taken randomly to evaluate the rest of the bladder. Care of the client is the same as for the client undergoing endoscopy but also involves preparation for anesthesia (see Chapter 15).

Intervention includes assisting the client in anesthesia recovery as well as using comfort measures for urethral pain, bladder spasms, flank pain, and dysuria, which are commonly experienced after biopsy. Instruct the client to watch for signs of urinary tract infection or infection of the puncture site and to report these promptly after the procedure.

Transrectal Prostate Biopsy

Biopsy of the prostate gland is performed via a rectal approach. The biopsy specimen is usually obtained with a multiple-core biopsy needle guided by ultrasonography. The procedure is done in an outpatient setting when preliminary tests indicate the presence of prostate cancer. Before the procedure, instruct the client to avoid aspirin for 10 days and NSAIDs for 24 hours. A urine specimen is obtained for culture to ensure sterile urine. Prophylactic antibiotics are given.

Instruct clients that they may experience dysuria, hematuria, hematospermia, rectal bleeding, or urinary retention for 24 to 48 hours after the procedure. (See Chapter 37 for additional discussion of prostate biopsy.)

Percutaneous Renal Biopsy

Percutaneous biopsy of the renal pelvis is used to diagnose benign and malignant masses, establish a prognosis, and follow progression and response to treatment. Renal biopsy is contraindicated for clients who have a solitary kidney, malignant tumors, hydronephrosis, infection or abscess, serious hypertension, or coagulation disorders. Small-gauge (21- to 25-gauge) needles are used for cytologic examination, and larger-gauge (14- to 20-gauge) needles are used to obtain tissue cores for histopathologic examination (Fig. 32–7). Guided imaging such as fluoroscopy, ultrasonography, CT scanning, or MRI is used to help avoid large blood vessels. The physician inserts the biopsy needle as the client inspires deeply, and the client must be able to cooperate. Complications after biopsy include pneumothorax, hemorrhage, infection, and laceration or perforation of the kidney.

Brush biopsies of lesions of the upper tract urothelium are performed with a steel or nylon brush inserted via a ureteral catheter with endoscopic guidance. Biopsies of the renal pelvis, calices, and ureter can be obtained with this approach (see earlier discussion of ureteroscopy).

Preprocedure Care

Prepare the client for local anesthesia (see Chapter 15), obtain consent, and give nothing by mouth. Determine that results of coagulation studies are in the client's record. Obtain and record baseline vital signs. Clients are often managed in an outpatient setting with conscious sedation.

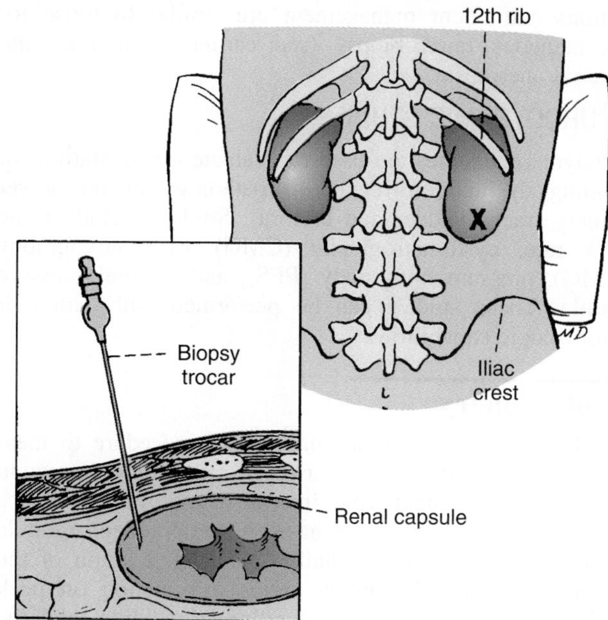

FIGURE 32–7 Percutaneous renal biopsy showing location of the trocar.

Postprocedure Care

Immediately after the biopsy, apply pressure to the puncture site for 20 minutes. Apply a sterile dressing. Pressure may be maintained by having the client lie on a sandbag placed against the biopsy site. Check the puncture site for bleeding and monitor vital signs according to agency protocol. Force fluids to promote urination and to prevent clot formation, which can lead to urine obstruction.

Observe each voiding for hematuria; protocol may require checking each specimen with a dipstick for microscopic blood. Postbiopsy hematocrit levels are usually monitored.

The time for bed rest varies; clients may be discharged between 4 and 24 hours after biopsy. Encourage limited activity for the first 24 hours to prevent bleeding.

Complications after renal biopsy include gross hematuria, pain, infection, decreased hematocrit, and hypotension indicative of hemorrhage. Instruct the client to report immediately fever, increasing pain levels (back, flank, or shoulder), bleeding from the puncture site, weakness, dizziness, grossly bloody urine, or dysuria. Activity should be restricted if blood is seen in the urine. Advise the client to avoid strenuous lifting, physical exertion, or trauma to the biopsy site for up to 2 weeks after discharge.

Open Renal Biopsy

An open biopsy approach is indicated for diagnosis of renal diseases when tissue sampling by other methods is inadequate. The client requires preparation for general anesthesia (see Chapter 15) as well as renal function and coagulation studies. The procedure requires a nephrotomy via a flank incision to permit direct visualization of the kidney.

After surgery, monitor vital signs, fluid balance, wound hemostasis, urine color, and pain levels. Complications and client management are similar to those for percutaneous renal biopsy (see earlier discussion) and general anesthesia.

■ URODYNAMIC STUDIES

Urodynamic studies are used to evaluate manifestations of voiding dysfunction related to pathology of the lower urinary tract (bladder and urethra). Studies include urine flow rate, cystometrography (CMG), electromyography (EMG), pressure flow study (PFS), and urethral pressure profile. These studies can be performed with video or fluoroscopic capabilities.

Uroflowmetry

Uroflowmetry is a simple noninvasive procedure to measure the peak flow rate of urine in milliliters per second by having the client void into a special funnel device with a spinning disc at the base. A computerized module attached to the device digitally calculates a graph of the voiding episode. The graph yields information on peak and mean urine flow rates, duration of voiding, and the volume voided (Fig. 32–8). Peak flow may be diminished in clients with bladder outlet obstruction or poor detrusor contractility.

Instruct the client to prepare for the test by having a full bladder. Accuracy of the measurement depends on a voided volume of at least 125 ml, although clients should avoid overfilling the bladder. Complications or risks associated with this test are minimal. The bladder may be further evaluated for postvoid residual volume with ultrasonography (see earlier discussion of ultrasonography of the bladder).

Cystometrography

CMG involves the use of at least one urethral catheter to measure bladder pressure and a second catheter in the rectum or vagina to measure intra-abdominal pressure. The abdominal pressure measurement is then subtracted from the bladder pressure measurement to obtain an accurate representation of the detrusor pressure and the reaction of the smooth muscle of the bladder wall during filling and voiding. CMG is performed in both the filling and voiding phases to evaluate bladder compliance, capacity, stability, and sensation. CMG is indicated for evaluating bladder outlet obstruction and urinary incontinence.

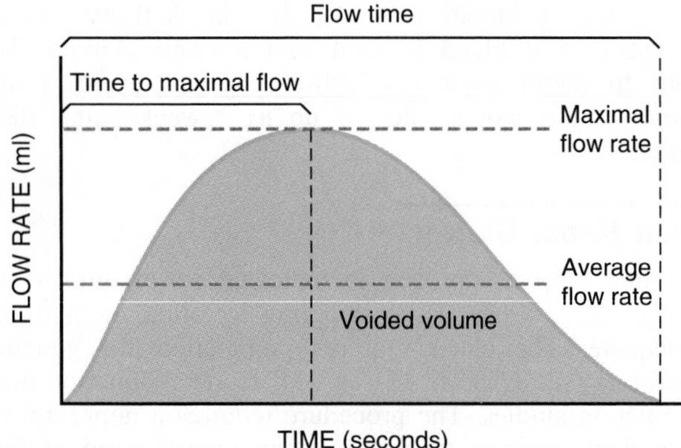

FIGURE 32–8 Diagram of terminology used in urodynamic studies. *Shaded area* shows voided volume. *Dotted lines* show how voided volume is divided into time and flow rate.

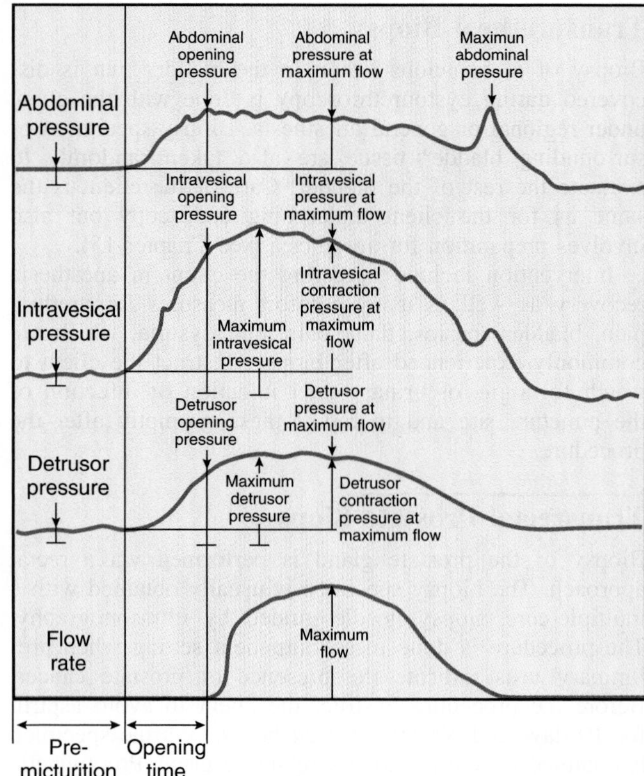

FIGURE 32–9 Diagram of a pressure flow study graph. (Modified from Walsh, P. C., et al. [Eds.]. [1998]. *Campbell's urology* [7th ed.]. Philadelphia: W. B. Saunders.)

Sphincter Electromyography

EMG is performed at the same time as CMG. EMG evaluates for detrusor or sphincter dyssynergia, which occurs when the sphincter cannot relax or becomes overactive during detrusor contraction with voiding. This disorder can cause elevated postvoid residual volumes, urinary tract infection, or urinary retention and occurs in neurologic disorders.

Patch, wire, or needle electrodes are positioned on the perineum to monitor the response of the pelvic floor muscles to bladder filling and voiding. The patch and wire electrodes are painless but are prone to recording artifact. The needle electrodes provide detailed information but can cause discomfort and limit mobility. The integrity of the sacral reflex arc may be tested by eliciting the bulbocavernosal reflex during EMG (see earlier discussion of assessment of this reflex).

Pressure Flow Study

The pressure flow study is performed with the voiding cystometrogram and simultaneously illustrates graphically a comparison of the detrusor pressure, abdominal pressure, urine flow rate, and electromyogram. It can help to distinguish between poor detrusor contractility and bladder outlet obstruction (Fig. 32–9).

Video-Fluoroscopic Urodynamics

The lower urinary tract can be directly visualized during CMG and EMG by filling the bladder with a radiologic contrast medium instead of sterile water, saline, or carbon dioxide. This technique provides more information about voiding disorders. Results can be recorded on videotape for later evaluation.

Urethral Pressure Profile

The urethral pressure profile measures sphincter closure pressure and evaluates urethral incompetence. The urethral length and continuous urethral response to filling, voiding, and provocative measures, such as coughing, may be assessed. A specialized catheter, either a membrane catheter or a catheter mounted with microtransducers, is withdrawn slowly through the urethra while recording pressure readings at every level. This test can be done in cases of sphincter dysfunction, urinary incontinence, or detrusor or sphincter dyssynergia.

Preprocedure Care

All urodynamic testing except uroflowmetry requires a negative Gram stain or urine culture. Advise clients to force fluids and to abstain from voiding approximately 1 to 2 hours before the procedure if possible. Clients may be advised to discontinue any medications that may affect urinary function before the study. The study should not be performed after recent cystoscopy or prostate biopsy. Clients who have artificial joints or cardiac valvular disease or replacements should have appropriate prophylactic antibiotics.

Explain how the procedure is performed, the catheters and equipment used, the client's role in the study, and what the client can expect to feel during and after the study. If videourodynamics are measured, explain the need to have two or three people in the room (the nurse or technician performing the study, a radiologic technician, and possibly a urologist). Reassure the client that every effort will be made to preserve privacy.

Postprocedure Care

Teach the client to watch for and report manifestations and symptoms of urinary tract infection, urgency, and frequency persisting after 24 hours. Encourage the client to drink at least two 8-ounce glasses of water each hour for 4 hours after the procedure. A warm bath or washcloth applied to the perineum may help alleviate the urethral irritation that is common after the procedure.

CONCLUSIONS

A thorough knowledge of the potential causes of elimination disorders is essential in order to obtain a pertinent health history and to perform an accurate physical assessment. Careful assessment facilitates formulation of accurate nursing and medical diagnoses and planning for the optimal treatment of the client. Knowledge of diagnostic testing is necessary to prepare the client for the tests and to facilitate the diagnostic process.

BIBLIOGRAPHY

1. Chiverton, P. A., et al. (1996). Psychological factors associated with urinary incontinence. *Clinical Nurse Specialist, 10*(5), 229–233.
2. DeGowin, E. L., & DeGowin, R. L. (1971). *Bedside diagnostic examination*. New York: Macmillan.
3. Fantl, J. A., et al. (1996). *Urinary incontinence in adults: Acute and chronic management* (Clinical Practice Guideline No. 2, AHCPR Publication No. 96-0682). Rockville, MD: Agency for Health Care Policy and Research, Public Health Service, U.S. Department of Health and Human Services.
4. Gallo, M. L., Fallon, P. J., & Staskin, D. R. (1997). Urinary incontinence: Steps to evaluation, diagnosis, and treatment. *The Nurse Practitioner, 22*(2), 21–42.
5. Goroll, A. H., May, L. A., & Mulley, A. G. (Eds.). (1995). *Primary care medicine: Office evaluation and management of the adult client* (3rd ed.). Philadelphia: J. B. Lippincott.
6. Gray, M. (1992). *Genitourinary disorders*. St. Louis: Mosby–Year Book.
7. Hanson, K. A., & Blute, M. L. (1994). Endourologic diagnosis and conservative management of upper tract urothelial cancer. *Urologic Nursing, 14*(4), 159–163.
8. Heitkemper, M., et al. (1995). Interventions for irritable bowel syndrome: A nursing model. *Gastroenterology Nursing, 18*(6), 224–230.
9. Holmes, H., et al. (1998). *Illustrated guide to diagnostic tests* (2nd ed.). Springhouse, PA: Springhouse Publishing.
10. Karlowitz, K. A. (1995). *Urologic nursing: Prevention and practice*. Philadelphia: W. B. Saunders.
11. Kelly, M. (1996). Chronic renal failure. *American Journal of Nursing, 96*(1), 36–37.
12. Khullar, S., & DiSario, J. (1997). Colon cancer screening: Sigmoidoscopy or colonoscopy. *Gastrointestinal Endoscopy Clinics of North America, 7*(3), 365–386.
13. McCance, K., & Huether, S. (1994). *Pathophysiology: The biologic basis for diseases in adults & children* (2nd ed.). St. Louis: Mosby–Year Book.
14. McConnell, J. D., et al. (1994). *Benign prostatic hyperplasia: Diagnosis and treatment* (Clinical Practice Guideline No. 8, AHCPR Publication No. 94-0582). Rockville, MD: Agency for Health Care Policy and Research, Public Health Service, U.S. Department of Health and Human Services.
15. McQuaid, K., & Friedman, S. (1996). *Current diagnosis and treatment in gastroenterology*. Norwalk, CT: Appleton & Lange.
16. Moore, D. A., & Edwards, K. (1997). Using a portable bladder scan to reduce the incidence of nosocomial urinary tract infections. *MEDSURG Nursing, 6*(1), 39–43.
17. Prandoni, D., et al. (1996). Assessment of urine collection technique for microbial culture. *American Journal of Infection Control, 24*(3), 219–221.
18. Schottefeld, D., & Fraumeni, J. F. (1996). *Cancer epidemiology and prevention*. New York: Oxford University Press.
19. Shearman, D., et al. (1997). *Diseases of the gastrointestinal tract and liver* (3rd ed.). New York: Churchill Livingstone.
20. Swartz, M. (1994). *Textbook of physical diagnosis, history and examination* (2nd ed.). Philadelphia: W. B. Saunders.
21. Tanagho, E. A., & McAninch, J. W. (1995). *Smith's general urology*. Norwalk, CT: Appleton & Lange.
22. Uphold, C., & Graham, M. (1994). *Clinical guidelines in family practice* (2nd ed.). Gainesville, FL: Barmarrac Books.
23. Vickery, G. (1997). Basics of constipation. *Gastroenterology Nursing, 20*(4), 126–128.
24. Walsh, P. C., et al. (1998). *Campbell's urology* (7th ed.). Philadelphia: W. B. Saunders.
25. Wozniak-Petrofsky, J. (1997). Urodynamic tests: Client preparation, assessment, and follow-up. *The Nurse Practitioner, 22*(3), 70–91.

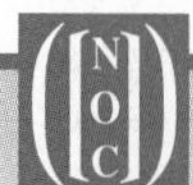

REMEMBER *to check out your* **Companion CD ROM**

CHAPTER 33

Management of Clients with Intestinal Disorders

Helen Murdock Rogers

NURSING OUTCOMES CLASSIFICATION (NOC) for Nursing Diagnoses—Clients with Intestinal Disorders

Altered Nutrition: Less Than Body Requirements
Nutritional Status
Bowel Incontinence
Bowel Elimination
Bowel Continence
Tissue Integrity
Constipation
Bowel Elimination
Hydration
Diarrhea
Fluid Balance
Hydration
Symptom Severity
Fluid Volume Deficit
Bowel Elimination
Fluid Balance
Hydration
Knowledge Deficit
Knowledge: Treatment Procedures
Pain
Comfort Level
Pain: Disruptive Effects
Risk for Body Image Disturbance
Grief Resolution
Psychosocial Adjustment: Life Change
Self-Esteem
Risk for Ineffective Individual Coping
Coping
Decision-Making
Role Performance
Social Support
Risk for Ineffective Management of Therapeutic Regimen (Individuals)
Health Beliefs: Perceived Ability to Perform
Knowledge: Treatment Regimen
Participation: Health Care Decisions
Risk for Infection
Risk Detection
Risk for Injury
Risk Control
Safety Status: Physical Injury
Risk for Sexual Dysfunction
Sexual Functioning
Body Image
Self-Esteem

The client with an intestinal disorder usually has a problem with bowel elimination. Hence, the most common nursing diagnoses are *Constipation, Bowel Incontinence,* and *Diarrhea.* Additional nursing diagnoses are *Pain, Altered Nutrition: Less Than Body Requirements, Fluid Volume Deficit,* and *Body Image Disturbance.*

General Clinical Manifestations

Disorders of the intestine disrupt one or more of its functions. They can slow, obstruct, or accelerate the movement of intestinal contents (*chyme*) through the intestine, or they can disrupt secretion, motility, and absorption of intestinal contents. Disorders occur in response to inflammation, tumors, infections, obstructions, and changes in the structure of the intestine. Manifestations of intestinal disorders vary according to which function (motility, digestion, or absorption) is disturbed. The major manifestations of dysfunction are hemorrhage, pain, nausea and vomiting, distention, constipation, diarrhea, and abnormal fecal contents.

Hemorrhage. Bleeding may be caused by trauma, ulceration, inflammation, or a growth that erodes through a blood vessel. The usual manifestation is blood in the stool (*hematochezia*) rather than in vomitus (*hematemesis*). The amount of bleeding varies from a minute quantity that is invisible except by testing (*occult blood*) to large quantities that cause stools to be bright red to tarry-black (*melena*). The stool color is affected by (1) the digestive processes acting on the blood and (2) the rapidity with which chyme passes through the bowel. For instance, slow bleeding from the duodenum may not increase peristalsis and may produce a tarry stool. If the rate of bleeding or of peristalsis increases, subsequent stools may become brighter red.

Pain. Mechanical, inflammatory, or ischemic changes cause pain by stimulating the nerve endings in the muscular or submucosal layers of bowel wall. Mechanical factors cause pain by stretching and distending the bowel; these actions then activate nerve endings. For example, edema and vascular congestion cause painful stretching. Biochemical mediators that are released during the inflammatory process cause pain by stimulating nerve endings.

Obstruction of blood supply to the intestine (*ischemia*) also can cause pain. Acute or partial occlusion of the mesenteric artery causes intermittent pain during digestion because of the greater need for blood at that time. Occlusion can occur in the major artery or one of the smaller branches.

Discomfort occurs in various places and is characterized as three types:

- *Visceral pain* arises from a stimulus acting on the involved portion of the bowel. It results in a diffuse, poorly localized pain that clients describe as gnawing, burning or cramping.
- *Somatic pain* arises from the parietal peritoneum and is more localized and intense than visceral pain.
- *Referred pain* is visceral pain felt at a distance from an affected organ.

Nausea and Vomiting. In intestinal disorders, nausea results from distention of the duodenum. Vomiting may occur from changes in the integrity of the intestinal wall (as in gastroenteritis) or from changes in the motility of the bowel (such as caused by an obstruction). Vomitus that contains fecal matter usually indicates a distal obstruction in the small intestine.

Distention. Distention is caused by excessive gas in the intestines. It may be due to the inability to adequately digest a specific nutrient, such as lactose, or may result from a defect in intestinal motility. *Flatus* (passing of bowel gas) may be another clinical manifestation.

Diarrhea. *Diarrhea* is defined as an increase in the frequency, volume, and fluid content of stool. Rapid propulsion of intestinal contents through the small bowel results in diarrhea and may lead to a serious fluid volume deficit. Common causes are infections, malabsorption syndromes, medications, allergies, and systemic diseases.

Constipation. *Constipation* is the infrequent or difficult passage of stools. It is a very common manifestation that can be caused by inadequate fluid or bulk, mechanical blockage of the passage of intestinal contents (by a tumor), or slow peristalsis.

Abnormalities in Fecal Content. The presence of fats or other abnormal constituents, normally absorbed from the stool, indicates malabsorption. Other fecal abnormalities that may aid in diagnosis are bacteria, parasites, pus, blood, and abnormal quantities of mucus from the colon.

DISORDERS OF THE LARGE AND SMALL BOWEL

INFLAMMATORY DISORDERS

Inflammation can occur in any portion of the bowel and can be caused by organisms, toxins produced by organisms, infiltration of the bowel wall by granulomatous processes, injury from radiation, trauma, and medications.

Infections and Infestations

■ VIRAL AND BACTERIAL INFECTIONS: GASTROENTERITIS

Gastroenteritis is an inflammation of the stomach and intestinal tract that primarily affects the small bowel. The major clinical manifestations are diarrhea of varying degrees and abdominal pain and cramping. Associated clinical manifestations are nausea, vomiting, fever, anorexia, distention, *tenesmus* (straining on defecation), and *borborygmi* (hyperactive bowel sounds).

Gastroenteritis occurs throughout the world, often in epidemic outbreaks. Contaminated food and water are major sources of these diseases and cause thousands of deaths yearly. The incidence of infections caused by food-borne diseases is rising; only respiratory infections are more common. Eighty million cases of food-borne disease occur annually in the United States, costing society billions of dollars each year. *Campylobacter* causes an estimated 2 million illnesses each year. Another bacteria, *Escherichia coli 0157:H7*, causes an estimated 30,000 infections and 250 deaths annually.

Infection with *Clostridium difficile,* also known as pseudomembranous colitis, is a bacterial dysentery commonly seen in clients who have been receiving large doses of antibiotics or who have taken antibiotics for a long time. The condition is becoming more common in hospitalized clients.

Etiology and Risk Factors

Pathogens that cause gastrointestinal (GI) disease are transmitted by the fecal-oral route, from person to person, and through ingestion of fecally contaminated food and water. GI infections are often referred to as "food poisoning" because food is frequently the vehicle for transmission of actively growing microbes or their toxins. Common bacterial sources of contaminated foods are eggs (*Salmonella*), raw or undercooked meat (*E. coli*), and chicken (*Campylobacter*). Outbreaks of food-borne viral infections are almost entirely caused by fecally contaminated shellfish. Unpasteurized milk, apple juice, and ice cream are also sources of food-borne infection. Other causative organisms are *Vibrio cholerae* (cholera), *Shigella* bacilli (dysentery) and *Staphylococcus aureus* (staphylococcal food poisoning). The incubation period for all viral and bacterial infections ranges from 6 hours to 3 or 4 days.

Health promotion actions for avoiding such GI infections involve instructing clients about (1) good handwashing technique after defecation and before handling food and (2) obtaining available vaccinations against bacterial and viral gastroenteritis. Encourage cleanliness and sanitation as well as proper food handling, preparation. and storage techniques, such as cooking meats to 150° F, cooking chicken to 170° F, and not allowing food to sit at room temperature for long periods. Advise clients to avoid the use of antibiotics over a long time. Teach travelers going to developing countries about safe food practices, such as avoiding tap water, milk products, raw seafood, and foods that cannot be cooked or peeled.

Health maintenance activities include the assessment of clients who are receiving high or continued doses of antibiotics for manifestations of *C. difficile* infection and other manifestations of GI infection secondary to antibiotic use. Health restoration interventions involve client self-management of manifestations. Instruct clients to follow their medication regimen and to call their health care provider if (1) manifestations continue for several days, (2) they might be dehydrated, or (3) body temperature is higher than 100° F. Promote bowel rest and replacement of fluids and electrolytes as needed.

Pathophysiology

Normally, human intestinal flora protect the bowel from colonization of pathogens. However, the intestinal flora can be (1) disrupted by harmful bacteria and viruses that cause tissue damage and inflammation or (2) depressed by antibiotic therapy. Antibiotics most often implicated in the depression of normal flora are clindamycin, penicillins, cephalosporins, and aminoglycosides.

Pathogens cause tissue damage and inflammation by releasing endotoxins that stimulate the mucosal lining of the intestine, resulting in greater secretion of water and electrolytes into the intestinal lumen. The active secretion of chloride and bicarbonate ions in the small bowel leads to inhibition of sodium reabsorption. In order to balance the excess sodium, large amounts of protein-rich fluids are secreted in the bowel, overwhelming the large bowel's ability to reabsorb the fluid and leading to diarrhea. Pathogens also cause damage and inflammation by invading and destroying the mucosal lining of the bowel, resulting in bleeding and ulceration. When the integrity of the GI tract is impaired, its ability to carry out digestive and absorptive functions may be affected.

Clinical Manifestations

The universal manifestation of gastroenteritis is diarrhea, which occurs in varying intensity depending on the organism involved and the health status of the individual. The diarrhea may be mild (two to three stools per day) or intense (>10 watery stools per day). Nausea, vomiting, and anorexia may occur from abdominal distention caused by increased fluid content and undigested food. Abdominal pain, cramping, and borborygmi may occur from gas released from undigested food, irritation of bowel mucosa, and distention of the intestines. The client may have a fever, depending on the causative organism. The stool may test positive for leukocytes and may contain the causative organism as well as mucus and varying amounts of blood.

Prognosis

Most cases of gastroenteritis are temporarily disabling and self-limiting, with resolution in 1 to 5 days. However, gastroenteritis can be fatal in debilitated, older, or very young people. Early detection and treatment with fluids and electrolytes are critical to prevent death or disability in such cases. Up to 10% of clients infected with *E. coli 0157:H7* develop hemolytic uremic syndrome (HUS), which causes death in 3% to 5% of the people it affects and chronic renal failure in 10% to 30% of those who survive it.

■ PARASITIC INFECTIONS

PROTOZOA

Protozoa are parasites that replicate in the intestines of infected hosts and are excreted in the feces. They are transmitted in the same way as bacterial and viral pathogens; however, fewer numbers or organisms are needed to produce clinical manifestations. Enteric protozoa are the leading cause of water-borne disease and are becoming more frequently implicated as causes of food-borne infections. Several new protozoa have been identified; for example, *Cyclospora,* which has been linked to contaminated raspberries. Some protozoa are becoming resistant to methods used to eliminate them, such as chlorination.

Giardiasis, the most common protozoal diarrheal illness in the United States, is caused by the protozoan *Giardia lamblia.* It generally spreads through the water system or spoiled food. Most infected people are asymptomatic. However, those with manifestations may present several weeks after exposure with nausea, vomiting, excessive foul flatulence, and malabsorption, which results in weight loss and copious, foul-smelling, greasy stools. Organisms infect the small intestine mucosa and submucosa and are found in the stool. The medications used for treatment include metronidazole (Flagyl), quinacrine (Atabrine) and furazolidone (Furoxone). A new vaccine may be available in the near future; however, at present, no agent is effective in preventing giardiasis.

Cryptosporidium is associated with water-borne and food-borne outbreaks in nursing homes and day care centers. It is spread by drinking contaminated water or swimming in infected lakes or swimming pools. The organism attaches itself to the intestinal epithelium, causing surface damage, inflammation, and watery diarrhea.

Amebiasis produces diarrhea when a protozoan *(Entamoeba histolytica)* invades the lining of the colon. Manifestations include rectal inflammation as well as blood, pus, and amebae in the stool. Metronidazole (Flagyl) is the drug of choice for treatment.

HELMINTHS

The intestinal tract may be infested with any of several species of helminths or parasitic worms, including *Ascaris* (roundworms), *Enterobius* (pinworms), *Trichinella spiralis* (which causes trichinosis), and various species of *Cestoda* (tapeworms). These parasites are found worldwide. Worm infestations, contracted through the skin or from ingesting contaminated food or water, can cause serious and even fatal disease if the parasites are not eradicated from the intestinal tract. Worms also may cause urinary tract infections or pruritus ani. Fortunately, most of these parasites are susceptible to medications such as mebendazole and pyrantel pamoate. Piperazine and quinacrine hydrochloride also may be used, but they have more side effects. Treatment of all household members may reduce reinfection.

Schistosomiasis is caused by a blood fluke (a parasitic flatworm). The infection is prevalent worldwide, occurring in about 1 in 30 people. The cercariae (larvae) of the parasite penetrate the skin, migrate to the liver via the lungs, and remain in intrahepatic portal venules until the worm matures. The mature worm, which does not multiply within humans, then moves into its final habitat. Depending on the species involved, the worm may settle in the veins of the large bowel, small bowel, or bladder, where it lays eggs. These eggs, which form pseudotubercles (small, nobby prominences), have been found in every system of the body. Schistosomiasis may have mild or severe manifestations, depending on the species of worms involved and the number present. Laboratory studies to identify the species are completed before pharmacologic treatment with oxamniquine, metrifonate, praziquantel, or niridazole is started.

Outcome Management for Viral, Bacterial, and Parasitic Infections

Medical Management

REST THE BOWEL

Rest, with nothing by mouth (NPO [from the Latin *nil per os*]) until the vomiting has stopped, is the best intervention.

DECREASE DIARRHEA

When diarrhea is severe and does not resolve within 2 to 3 days, the infecting organism needs to be identified from stool specimens and blood samples. Medications to decrease intestinal motility are usually not administered because the infecting agents need to be eliminated; this is particularly true with *C. difficile* infection because the bacteria multiply if GI motility is slowed and the bacteria are retained. Anti-infective agents are chosen on the basis of the organism identified.

RESTORE FLUIDS AND ELECTROLYTES

The client is started on small amounts of clear liquids as tolerated. An electrolyte replacement beverage may be given. The diet is advanced after 24 hours as tolerated. If the client has a severe fluid depletion, an intravenous (IV) agent such as 0.45% sodium chloride may be required. A potassium supplement may be ordered if the client's serum potassium level is low.

Nursing Management of the Medical Client

Most clients present with an acute onset of diarrhea. Carefully note a description of the diarrhea, including (1) onset, (2) number, color, and consistency of stools, and (3) accompanying manifestations, such as nausea and vomiting. Ask the client about recent foreign travel, eating habits, and antibiotic use.

Assess the client's abdomen. Examination may reveal hyperactive bowel sounds, distention, and tenderness. Dehydration and electrolyte imbalance may be present, depending on the amount of fluids and electrolytes lost. Assess muscle weakness and fatigue due to hypokalemia. Metabolic alkalosis from bicarbonate loss is also a potential problem. Carefully examine all stool for blood and mucus, and record intake and output. Examine the client's anal area for irritation. After cleaning the area, apply a protective moisture barrier product for clients with irritation.

Administer anti-infective medications, such as antibiotic and antiparasitic agents, to treat the specific cause of the diarrhea. Antidiarrheals may be ordered if the diarrhea is uncontrollable. If there are manifestations of fluid and electrolyte imbalance, start IV fluids until oral fluids are tolerated. Begin clear liquids with electrolytes in small amounts until the client can tolerate toast and crackers. Advance the diet as tolerated.

Provide written and oral instructions regarding medications, diet, and rest as well as about when and how to report any continued problems. If other family members are sharing the bathroom, the client must be reminded to wash the hands well and to maintain absolute cleanliness.

APPENDICITIS

Appendicitis is an inflammation of the vermiform appendix that develops most commonly in adolescents and young adults. It can occur at any age but is rare in clients younger than 2 years and reaches a peak incidence in clients between 20 and 30 years. It is not common in older adults; however, when it does occur in such clients, rupture of the appendix is more common. Appendicitis affects 7% to 12% of the population.

Etiology and Risk Factors

Appendicitis can be caused by:

- A fecalith (a fecal calculus, or stone) that occludes the lumen of the appendix
- Kinking of the appendix
- Swelling of the bowel wall
- Fibrous conditions in the bowel wall
- External occlusion of the bowel by adhesions

There are no particular risk factors for appendicitis. Because it is not preventable, early detection of the condition is important.

Pathophysiology

When the appendix becomes obstructed, the intraluminal pressure increases, leading to decreased venous drainage, thrombosis, edema, and bacterial invasion of the bowel wall. After the initial obstruction, the appendix becomes increasingly hyperemic, warm, and covered with exudate, progressing to gangrene and perforation.

Clinical Manifestations

The classic manifestations of appendicitis begin with acute abdominal pain that comes in waves. At first, the pain may be perceived merely as discomfort that makes the client feel that passing flatus or having a bowel movement will bring relief. Unfortunately, many clients take a laxative during this period, which may lead to rupture of the appendix and peritonitis.

The pain typically starts in the epigastrium or periumbilical region. It then shifts to the right lower quadrant as the inflammatory process spreads to involve the serosal layers of the bowel, thereby bringing the inflammatory process into contact with the peritoneum. The pain becomes steady rather than intermittent, and the client often *guards* or protects the area by lying still and drawing the legs up to relieve tension on the abdominal muscles.

Assessment also may reveal vomiting that begins after the pain starts, loss of appetite, low-grade fever, coated tongue, and bad breath. Mild leukocytosis is usually present, with the white blood cell (WBC) count between 10,000 and 15,000/mm^3. Pain at McBurney's point, which lies midway between the right anterior superior iliac crest and the umbilicus, confirms the diagnosis.

Outcome Management

Surgical Management

APPENDECTOMY

There is no medical treatment for appendicitis. Preoperatively, IV fluids and antibiotics are administered. Pain medication is withheld until the diagnosis is confirmed.

INDICATIONS. Surgical intervention involves removal of the appendix (*appendectomy*) within 24 to 48 hours of onset of the manifestations. The surgery can be performed through a small open incision or a laparoscope (a lighted scope used to visualize and remove the appendix). When the operation is performed in time, the mortality rate is less than 0.5%. Delay usually causes rupture of the organ and resultant peritonitis (see "Peritonitis").

COMPLICATIONS. Perforation of the bowel is the most common complication. Antibiotics and surgical drainage are required if perforation occurs. Peritonitis may develop after perforation.

OUTCOMES. Following a laparoscopic procedure, the client is usually discharged in 24 to 48 hours. Another day of hospitalization may be indicated after an open surgical procedure. Lifting is restricted for 2 to 4 weeks. The client can resume all activities 4 to 6 weeks after surgery.

Nursing Management of the Surgical Client

ASSESSMENT

The client is usually admitted with severe abdominal pain. Carefully assess the pain, especially to determine its location. Also assess the client for rebound tenderness (sharp pain when pressure is released on abdomen after deep palpation) and the presence of peritonitis (see "Peritonitis"). Carefully assess the client's vital signs, fluid and electrolyte status, and laboratory data. The client with appendicitis should fast preoperatively.

DIAGNOSIS, OUTCOMES, INTERVENTIONS

Pain. One of the most appropriate nursing diagnoses for the client with acute appendicitis is *Pain related to inflammation.*

Outcomes. The client describes decreased postoperative pain.

Interventions. An abrupt change in the character of the pain preoperatively may indicate perforation. Postoperatively, pain control, as described in Chapters 15 and 23, should be practiced. Sometimes, pain medication is not given until the client is actually ready for surgery. Never give an enema or a laxative or apply heat to the abdomen of the client with appendicitis, because any one of these actions may lead to bowel perforation.

Risk for Fluid Volume Deficit. Another appropriate nursing diagnosis for the client with acute appendicitis is *Risk for Fluid Volume Deficit related to vomiting.*

Outcomes. The client maintains fluid and electrolyte balance, as evidenced by balanced intake and output and electrolyte levels within normal limits.

Interventions. As soon as the client is admitted, IV fluids are started to maintain fluid balance, with electrolytes added as needed. If the client is vomiting, a nasogastric (NG) tube may be inserted. Carefully measure intake and output.

Risk for Infection. The diagnosis *Risk for Infection related to rupture of appendix* is common.

Outcomes. An infection will not develop, or rupture will be diagnosed early, as evidenced by (1) removal of the appendix before rupture or (2) prompt treatment of the rupture.

Interventions. Check the client's vital signs regularly, monitoring closely for an increase in temperature and a change in pulse and blood pressure, which may signify a ruptured appendix. Preoperative antibiotics are usually administered to reduce the infection. Monitor pain closely. If the pain becomes generalized throughout the abdomen and the abdomen becomes rigid and board-like, the appendix may have ruptured.

After surgery, monitor vital signs, urine output, level of consciousness, and IV therapy and assess the client's respiratory status and the surgical wound. The client may have a drain, and if the appendix ruptured, packing may be present. Assess the dressings, provide wound care, reposition the client approximately every 2 hours, and adequately manage the client's pain.

The client who has had a ruptured appendix with an infected wound needs to be taught the proper way to care for the wound. Wound care usually involves irrigation of the wound with sterile saline and application of a sterile dressing at least several times a day. Assess the client's ability to function at home and to care for the wound. A home health care referral may be needed to assist the client with physical needs and to ensure that the wound is healing properly.

EVALUATION

The usual outcome after an uncomplicated appendectomy is healing within a few weeks. If the appendix has ruptured, however, healing takes longer. With a ruptured appendix, healing cannot occur until the infection has cleared and the wound is clean. A secondary closure may be required after the wound is clean. Some incisions are left open to heal through granulation (regeneration) of tissue.

PERITONITIS

Peritonitis is inflammation of the peritoneal membrane. The *peritoneum* is a semipermeable two-layered sac filled with approximately 1500 ml of fluid. This sac covers all the organs in the abdominal cavity. Because it is well supplied with somatic nerves, stimulation of the parietal peritoneum that lines the abdominal and pelvic cavities causes sharp, well-localized pain. The visceral peritoneum is relatively insensitive.

Etiology and Risk Factors

Peritonitis can be primary or secondary. Major sources of inflammation are from the gastrointestinal tract, from the external environment, and through the bloodstream. Normal flora of the intestine become a source of infection when they enter the sterile peritoneal cavity. The most common organism is *E. coli,* although streptococci, staphylococci, and pneumococci also may be involved. The peritoneum may produce an inflammatory reaction and wall off (prevent the spread of) a localized process to combat an infection if the stimulus is not too massive and if the source of infection does not continue.

There are no risk factors for peritonitis because the condition is a result of another problem. Causes include ruptured or gangrenous gallbladder, perforated peptic ulcer, perforated stomach or intestine secondary to cancer or inflammatory bowel disorders, bowel obstruction, penetrating wounds, and other conditions (such as acute pancreatitis and mesenteric thrombosis). The major preventive measures are early diagnosis of clients at risk for peritonitis and initiation of early treatment help to prevent spread of the infection.

Pathophysiology

Peritonitis produces severe systemic effects. Circulatory alterations, fluid shifts, and respiratory problems can cause critical fluid and electrolyte imbalances. The inflammatory response shunts (diverts) extra blood to the inflamed area of the bowel to combat the infection. Peristaltic activity of the bowel ceases. Fluids and air are retained within its lumen, raising pressure and increasing fluid secretion into the bowel. Thus, circulating blood volume diminishes. The inflammatory process increases oxygen requirements at a time when the client has difficulty ventilating (breathing) because of abdominal pain and increased abdominal pressure, which elevates the diaphragm.

Clinical Manifestations

Manifestations of peritonitis vary according to the cause. Pain may be localized or generalized. Well-localized pain that causes rigidity of abdominal muscles and pain that increases with any pressure or motion of the abdomen are characteristic of peritonitis. Also, the client usually experiences nausea, vomiting, and, possibly, a low-grade fever. Assessment reveals absence of bowel sounds and shallow respirations because the client is trying to avoid the pain caused by body movement.

The client with peritonitis commonly has an elevated WBC count (20,000/mm^3) with a high neutrophil count. Abdominal x-ray studies are performed, which may show dilation and edema of the intestines or free air or fluid in the abdominal cavity. If the client is vomiting, manifestations of altered fluid and electrolyte balance also may be present.

Outcome Management

Medical Management

Maintain Fluid and Electrolyte Balance

If peritonitis is advanced and if surgery is contraindicated by shock and circulatory failure, oral fluids are prohibited. IV fluids are necessary for replacement of electrolyte and protein losses. An NG tube or a long intestinal tube may be inserted to reduce pressure within the bowel. See Chapter 31 for nursing care of a client with an NG or intestinal tube.

Control Infection

Once the infection has been walled off and the client's condition improves, surgical drainage and repair can be attempted. The other major treatment of peritonitis is IV antibiotic therapy with potent broad-spectrum agents.

Surgical Management

Surgery may be performed to prevent peritonitis, such as an appendectomy for an inflamed appendix or a colon resection (surgical removal) for inflamed diverticulum. If the perforation is not prevented, the major surgical intervention is incision and drainage of the abscess once it is walled off.

Nursing Management of the Surgical Client

Preoperatively, obtain a thorough history, including specific information about the client's pain. Assess the abdomen, noting the presence or absence of bowel sounds. Palpate the abdomen, noting whether the abdomen is firm, distended, or rigid. Note areas of rebound tenderness.

Clients with peritonitis are acutely ill and are given broad-spectrum antibiotics immediately. The perforated organs are usually repaired as soon as the client is stable enough to withstand the stress of surgery. During surgery, any leakage can be sampled for culture so that specific antibiotic therapy can be implemented. The peritoneal cavity is irrigated with an antibiotic solution to reduce the bacterial count. Often, the wound is packed open or drains are placed so that infection can be treated.

Postoperatively, carefully monitor clients for the development of postoperative complications, such as adult respiratory stress syndrome (ARDS), sepsis, and shock. Closely monitor the client's fluid balance by assessing vital signs, bowel sounds, urine output, skin turgor, mucous membranes, and weight. Immediately report any manifestations of sepsis, such as a drop or rise in temperature or a drop in blood pressure. IV fluids are administered along with antibiotic therapy. Upon discharge, provide the client with oral or written instructions regarding wound care, medications, activity restrictions, and follow-up visits.

Inflammatory Bowel Disease

Inflammatory bowel disease (IBD) affects approximately 2 million Americans, or 1 of every 125 people. Each year, 30,000 people learn that they have this chronic disease. It is estimated that IBD costs between $1.8 and 2.6 billion annually in lost wages and disability and health care payments. Relatives of clients with IBD are 10 times more likely to experience IBD than the general population.

IBD consists of two chronic inflammatory disorders: Crohn's disease (regional enteritis) and ulcerative colitis. These chronic, recurrent diseases predominantly affect younger people. Treatment is symptomatic, and responses are often unpredictable. Frequently, clients with IBD require surgery, which may be followed by recurrence. Because of the similarities between Crohn's disease and ulcerative colitis, the two conditions are compared throughout the following discussion and in Table 33–1.

Crohn's Disease

Crohn's disease is a chronic relapsing disease that may develop discontinuously (without sequence and skipping

TABLE 33–1 **DIFFERENTIATION BETWEEN CROHN'S DISEASE AND ULCERATIVE COLITIS**

Characteristic	Regional Enteritis (Crohn's Disease)	Ulcerative Colitis
GENERAL DESCRIPTION		
Age at onset	Young	Young to middle age
PATHOLOGY AND ANATOMY		
Depth of involvement	Transmural (all layers of submucosa)	Mucosa and submucosa
Rectal involvement	50%	95%
Right colon involvement	Frequent	Occasional
Small bowel involvement	Involved, ileum narrow	Usually normal
Distribution of disease	Segmental	Continuous
Inflammatory mass	Chronic and extensive	Rare (crypt abscess)
Cobblestone-like mucosa and granuloma	Common	Absent
Mesentery lymph involvement	Edema and hyperplasia	Not involved
Toxic megacolon	Occasional	Occasional
Steatorrhea	Frequent	Absent
Malignancy results	Rare	After 10 years
Fibrous stricture	Common	Absent
CLINICAL CHARACTERISTICS		
Course of disease	Slowly progressive	Remissions and relapses
Rectal bleeding	Occasional	Common (90%–100%)
Abdominal pain	Colicky (45%)	Predefecation (60%–70%)
Hematochezia	Unusual or absent	Almost always present
Diarrhea	Present (65%–85%)	Early and frequent (80%–95%)
Vomiting	Present (35%)	Present (15%)
Nutritional deficit	Common	Common
Weight loss	Present (60%–70%)	Present (10%)
Fever	Present (35%)	Present (10%)
Anal abscess	Common (75%)	Occasional (10%)
Fistula and anorectal fissure fistula	Common (80%)	Rare (10%–20%)
SYSTEMIC MANIFESTATIONS		
Arthritis	20%	Uncommon (10%)
Peripheral sacroiliitis	18%	18%–20%
Hepatobiliary involvement	Uncommon	15% cholestatic dysfunction 19%–38% fatty liver 30%–50% pericholangitis
Skin: erythema nodosum, pyoderma gangrenosum	Common	Present (5%–10%)
Nephrolithiasis	Occasional	Rare

sections) in any segment of the alimentary tract. The most common location is the terminal ileum. Crohn's disease more characteristically involves the entire thickness of the bowel wall (*transmural*), particularly the submucosa. The mortality rate is not high, but recurrences and complications can result in disability. Crohn's disease is more common in whites and among Ashkenazi Jews. There is a higher incidence within families. The disorder occurs at all ages but more often in people between 20 and 30 years old. The two sexes are affected equally.

Ulcerative Colitis

Ulcerative colitis is a disease that spans the entire length of the colon and involves only the mucosa and submucosa. The disease usually starts in the rectum and distal colon, spreading upward beyond the rectosigmoid valve to involve most of the sigmoid and descending colon. Ulcerative colitis causes inflammation, thickening, congestion, edema, and minute lacerations that ooze blood and eventually develop into abscesses. The edema may lead to extreme friability of the mucosa, and bleeding can thus occur from any minor trauma. Ulcerative colitis is more common than Crohn's disease. It occurs at all ages, but the incidence is higher among young adults, women, and Jews. The disorder has demonstrated a familial tendency.

Etiology and Risk Factors

Crohn's Disease

The cause of Crohn's disease is unclear, although there may be a genetic or hereditary basis. It is also considered an autoimmune disease. The only risk factors identified for Crohn's disease are genetic. There are no preventive measures.

Ulcerative Colitis

Several theories have been advanced to explain the cause of ulcerative colitis. One theory is that the disease is of bacterial origin, because many clients have a history of bacterial infection before the onset of the condition. Researchers have also suspected an allergic reaction as a basis of the disease. Others believe that ulcerative colitis may be due to an altered immune status because antibodies have been found in the colon. Still others suggest that destructive enzymes and a lack of protective substances in the bowel wall cause the inflammatory process. An emotional disturbance can precipitate an exacerbation or prolong an attack of the disorder, but it is not the primary cause.

No preventable risk factors are associated with ulcerative colitis. Once the client has the disease, controlling stress can help keep the disease in remission.

Pathophysiology

Crohn's Disease

Lesions typically develop in several separated segments of bowel. They are visible on gross examination (without aid of a microscope), and their color is dramatically different from that of normal tissue. Examination of the bowel tissue by endoscopy reveals edematous, heavy, reddish purple areas. Granular spots also may be present. Enlarged lymph nodes appear in the submucosa, and Peyer's patches are seen in the intestinal mucous membrane. These areas undergo small superficial ulcerations with granulomas and fissures. Fissures may completely penetrate the bowel wall, leading to fistulas and abscesses. Collections of lymphocytes throughout the mucosa, submucosa, and serosa are the only microscopic features of Crohn's disease. The small bowel wall becomes congested and thickened, narrowing the lumen.

Small bowel–related complications include malabsorption, kidney stones, gallstones, and hydronephrosis. Anorectal problems include internal fistulae and abscesses. Anal fissure (see later) is common and is directly related to the severity of the diarrhea, which produces ulceration of the perianal skin. Pain is aggravated by walking, sitting, and defecation.

Ulcerative Colitis

The appearance of the colon depends on the stage, activity, and severity of the disease. The most characteristic lesion of ulcerative colitis is an inflammatory infiltrate called a *crypt abscess*. This abscess consists of polymorphonuclear leukocytes, lymphocytes, red blood cells, and cellular debris appearing at the base of the crypts of Lieberkühn. Secretions from crypt abscesses result in purulent discharge from the bowel mucosa. Abscesses may become necrotic and may ulcerate.

Infections secondary to ulcerative colitis produce further inflammatory reactions in the mucosa and submucosa. When the inflammatory lesions heal, scarring and fibrosis, with narrowing, thickening, and shortening of the colon and loss of haustral folds, may follow.

Cancer of the colon is more common among clients with ulcerative colitis than in the general population. The incidence is greatly increased when ulcerative colitis develops before the client is 16 years of age and in clients who have had the condition for more than 20 years.

Toxic megacolon is an extreme dilation of a segment of the diseased colon (often the transverse segment) that results in complete obstruction. Toxic megacolon usually occurs during an acute exacerbation of ulcerative colitis, and it may follow hypokalemia, a barium enema, or the use of anticholinergics, narcotics, corticosteroids, or antibiotics. Bacterial overgrowth contributes to this complication. Perforation and peritonitis may complicate the condition.

Clinical Manifestations

Crohn's disease and ulcerative colitis produce similar manifestations. Clients suffer from abdominal pain, diarrhea, fluid imbalances, and weight loss. Severe diarrhea or vomiting may cause metabolic acidosis. Remissions are followed by exacerbations of acute disease. When the disease is acute, the client has a fever. The general appearance of clients with IBD varies from reasonably healthy to wasted, drawn, and malnourished, with varying degrees of pallor. They usually report a steady and progressive weight loss. Inspection reveals a flat or concave shape to the abdomen, with visible peristaltic activity. Palpation of the abdomen reveals tenderness over the area of inflamed bowel. Increased bowel sounds are heard on auscultation. Hemorrhoids and, in Crohn's disease, perianal abscess, fistula, and ulcers may be apparent.

Hematocrit and hemoglobin values are usually decreased. A barium enema study with air contrast is often performed to differentiate ulcerative colitis from Crohn's disease. The client with suspected IBD routinely undergoes colonoscopy. Biopsy and cytologic studies also help distinguish among carcinoma, ulcerative colitis, and Crohn's disease. The clinical manifestations of Crohn's disease and ulcerative colitis are compared in Table 33–1.

Crohn's Disease

Diarrhea in Crohn's disease is usually less severe than that in ulcerative colitis. Stool consistency is typically soft or semiliquid. Urgency to expel stools may awaken the person at night. The client rarely passes gross blood unless ulceration is present. Malabsorption, associated with steatorrhea, may develop. If so, stools may be foul-smelling and fatty.

The client with severe steatorrhea, diarrhea, or long-standing enteritis may have associated nutritional deficits, weight loss, anorexia, pain, anemia, debility, fatigue, and metabolic disturbances. Nutritional deficits arise from (1) a reduction in the intestinal absorptive surface, (2) malabsorption of protein and carbohydrates, and (3) impaired absorption of fat, folic acid, iron, calcium, and vitamins A, B_{12}, C, D, E, and K. Alterations in bile salt and vitamin metabolism may result from surgery or mucosal defects. Metabolic requirements increase because of the inflammatory process and infection, the decrease in food intake, and the loss of nutrients in the feces due to rapid gastrointestinal transit time. Electrolytes lost from diarrhea include sodium, potassium, chloride, the trace elements (magnesium, zinc, copper), and minerals. Nitrogen excretion remains normal if there is no loss of protein from the inflammatory exudate. The consequences of malnutrition include:

- Loss of immunocompetence
- Decreased resistance to infection
- Diminished wound healing
- Reduced pancreatic enzyme output
- Impaired healing (fistula and surgical wounds)
- Decreased iron-binding capacity resulting from chronic infection or blood loss

Ulcerative Colitis

The predominant manifestation of ulcerative colitis is rectal bleeding. Clients often experience diarrhea, possibly

20 or more stools per day. The severity and frequency of diarrhea depend on the extent of involved colon. Severe diarrhea can cause a loss of 500 to 17,000 ml of water in 24 hours. Liquid stools occur with tenesmus and may contain blood, mucus, and pus. A sense of urgency and cramping abdominal pain may occur with the diarrhea. The client typically experiences colicky pain in the lower left quadrant.

Nausea, vomiting, anorexia, weight loss, and decreased serum potassium concentration may occur with severe disease. In addition, the client loses plasma proteins, prothrombin, and fluids. Anemia may develop with severe blood loss and decreased dietary iron intake.

Physical findings include tenderness in the lower left quadrant, guarding, and (in severe ulcerative colitis) abdominal distention. Following remissions, ulcerative colitis may recur after bouts of emotional stress, dietary indiscretion, or the ingestion of irritants such as laxatives and antibiotics. Physical exertion, respiratory infections, and overfatigue also may cause an attack.

Prognosis

Remissions and exacerbations characterize both types of IBD. The only known cure for ulcerative colitis is surgical removal of the colon. Surgical procedures and medication therapy can control the manifestations in Crohn's disease, but currently there is no known cure.

Outcome Management

Medical Management

Decrease Diarrhea

Medical treatments, which primarily aim to control the manifestations, are similar for ulcerative colitis and Crohn's disease. Because the inflammatory process in Crohn's disease involves deeper layers of the bowel wall and is more chronic, healing may occur more slowly than in ulcerative colitis. Thus, anti-inflammatory therapy, including steroids, is required for longer periods in Crohn's disease than in ulcerative colitis.

Fluids, electrolytes, and blood are replaced as needed to maintain the client's homeostasis. Physical activity should be kept to a minimum during an acute attack to decrease intestinal motility. The client with a mild attack may work but needs extra rest. The client with fever, toxemia, frequent bowel movements, bleeding, or pain requires bed rest. Failure of the inflamed colonic mucosa to reabsorb water and electrolytes, bile salts, and lactose interferes with control of diarrhea. The extent of large bowel involved by the disease influences the severity of diarrhea. The client should keep a record of the number of stools, their consistency and color, and the presence or absence of blood.

Bowel rest and parenteral hyperalimentation may result in restored immunocompetence, greater resistance to infection, correction of nutritional deficiencies, and relief of edema and bowel inflammation.

Pharmacologic Agents

Antidiarrheal Medications. Antidiarrheal preparations may provide symptomatic benefit. Loperamide (Imodium) is superior to atropine-diphenoxylate (Lomotil) in controlling the diarrhea of Crohn's disease, with fewer side effects. Use of opiates for diarrhea control may cause distention and megacolon. Hydrophilic mucilloids, such as psyllium (Metamucil), may improve consistency of stools and control incontinence. Antispasmodic medications, such as propantheline bromide, glycopyrrolate, and dicyclomine hydrochloride, may reduce postprandial (after-meal) pain and diarrhea.

Aminosalicylates. Diarrhea associated with IBD may be treated successfully with agents that inhibit prostaglandin synthesis and reduce inflammation. Examples are sulfasalazine (Azulfidine), mesalamine (5-ASA), and olsalazine (Dipentum). Mesalamine is available orally as Asacol and Pentasa and rectally as Rowasa. The oral tablets should not be crushed because they are coated for release of the drug in the colon. Rowasa suppositories and rectal suspension are used when disease is contained in the rectum or distal colon. The suppository should be retained in the rectum for 1 to 3 hours, and the suspension should be retained for 8 hours.

Corticosteroids. Clients whose IBD fails to respond to the previously discussed measures may require corticosteroid medications. Adrenal steroids and corticotropin may be used with other therapy to reduce the body's response to inflammation. Steroids may be given orally, intravenously, intramuscularly, or rectally. Oral forms include hydrocortisone, prednisolone, and prednisone. Hydrocortisone also can be administered rectally as an enema or suppository. Steroids do not cure IBD, but they modify its course. Long-term complications associated with steroid use must be weighed against the relief of manifestations of IBD. Antacids or histamine receptor antagonists should be given during steroid therapy to prevent gastric ulceration. Steroids reduce adrenal function and may impair resistance, causing defective healing of abscesses and fistulas.

Immunosuppressive Agents. 6-Mercaptopurine (Purinethol) is used when other treatment modalities fail and can be effective against chronic, unrelenting Crohn's disease. Methotrexate (Folex) and azathioprine (Imuran) are now widely accepted as therapies for IBD. Cyclosporine (Sandimmune) is an effective agent but is associated with much toxicity. Infliximab (Remicade) is a new drug for Crohn's disease that blocks the action of tumor necrosis factor—a natural protein that causes intestinal inflammation. This agent is given by a single IV infusion that may be repeated every 2 to 3 months. Several new drugs, currently in clinical trials, are the selective cytokine-inhibiting drug CDC 801 (SelCID) and two successor compounds to SelCID called inflammation modulator imidazoles (IMIDs).

Anticholinergic Medications. During acute exacerbations, the client is given anticholinergic medications to relieve abdominal cramps and help control diarrhea. Anticholinergic, antidiarrheal, and antispasmodic agents allow the colon to rest. Withhold these medications if there are manifestations of obstruction.

Anti-Infective Medications. Medications commonly used to prevent or control infections include sulfonamides and antibiotics such as metronidazole (Flagyl) and ciprofloxacin (Cipro). Antibiotics may be given to control secondary bowel inflammation and infection.

INCREASE NUTRITIONAL INTAKE

Nutritional deficiencies are the most common complications of IBD. These deficits derive from decreased intake, increased losses, greater nutritional requirements, and side effects of certain medications. Diarrhea leads to fluid and electrolyte losses with resultant muscle wasting and edema. Malabsorption due to bacterial overgrowth or mucosal involvement of the bowel may cause further problems. Deficiencies of fat-soluble vitamins (A, D, E, and K) and folate may develop. Vitamin K deficiency causes bleeding tendencies.

DIET AND SUPPLEMENTS. A diet high in protein and calories is given in an attempt to restore normal nutritional levels but is not always well tolerated. Liquid supplements are residue free, low in fat, and digested mainly in the upper jejunum.

Anemia and vitamin deficiencies should be corrected nutritionally or with supplements. Folate deficiency, which may be due to the therapeutic use of sulfasalazine, may be prevented by (1) increasing dietary intake of folate, (2) having the client take sulfasalazine between meals, or (3) supplementing the intervention regimen with folic acid.

TOTAL PARENTERAL NUTRITION. Total parenteral nutrition (TPN) is indicated when a client has not responded to medical intervention, is being prepared for surgery, or has undergone intestinal resection. TPN provides bowel rest by removing all stimulation of secretion and by decreasing fecal bulk. Weight gain, positive nitrogen balance, and a temporary remission of manifestations can occur. TPN appears to be more useful in Crohn's disease than in ulcerative colitis.

When oral food and fluids are resumed, they should be chemically and mechanically nonirritating and high in calories, protein, and minerals. The client should avoid cocoa, chocolate, citrus juices, cold or carbonated drinks, nuts, seeds, popcorn, and alcohol.

Nursing Management of the Medical Client

ASSESSMENT

Assess the client's bowel elimination pattern, noting the number of stools, their color and consistency, and the presence or absence of blood or steatorrhea. Also assess the client's abdomen. Note bowel sounds and the location of pain. Complete a nutritional assessment, as directed in Chapter 29.

DIAGNOSIS, OUTCOMES, INTERVENTIONS

Diarrhea. Diarrhea is the most common manifestation of IBD, so the primary nursing diagnosis is *Diarrhea related to inflamed intestinal mucosa.*

Outcomes. The client will experience a decrease in diarrhea, as evidenced by a decrease in number and a more solid consistency of stools.

Interventions. Antidiarrheal medications may be administered to control the client's diarrhea. Perianal excoriation often occurs with diarrhea. After every bowel movement, gently clean the skin with warm water and apply a protective moisture barrier product.

See the Management and Delegation feature (p. 799).

Altered Nutrition: Less Than Body Requirements. The client with inflammatory bowel disease has many difficulties with nutrition, making *Altered Nutrition: Less Than Body Requirements related to diarrhea and malabsorption* a common nursing diagnosis.

Outcomes. The client will increase nutritional intake to meet metabolic requirements, as evidenced by weight stabilization and, possibly, weight gain.

Interventions. Monitor the client's nutritional intake. The type of diet ordered depends on the client's condition. If the client can tolerate a diet, encourage intake of fluids and food. Because eating stimulates the gastrocolic reflex and the urge to defecate, many people are afraid to eat; small servings may enable the client to avoid this problem. Foods should be easily digested to promote absorption during the short time the food remains in the bowel.

Clients with Crohn's disease are often receiving home TPN because they cannot tolerate foods for long periods as a result of disease exacerbation (see Chapter 29). These clients also may have undergone multiple bowel resections, resulting in short-bowel syndrome and problems of malabsorption.

Pain. Another common nursing diagnosis for the client with inflammatory bowel disease is *Pain related to inflamed mucosa.*

Outcomes. The client will experience a relief in abdominal pain, as evidenced by the client's statement of pain relief.

Interventions. Assess the client's pain, and give pain medications as ordered. Note any changes in the client's complaints of pain because they may indicate the development of complications. Narcotics are generally used sparingly so that they do not mask manifestations.

Risk for Ineffective Individual Coping. Stress is associated with inflammatory bowel disease. Write the nursing diagnosis as *Risk for Ineffective Individual Coping related to stress of disease and exacerbations related to stress.*

Outcomes. The client will cope effectively with the disease, as evidenced by fewer exacerbations and an improved coping style.

Interventions. Although emotional factors may not contribute to the cause of the disease, they do influence its course. Prolonged stress often precedes the onset of IBD and exacerbations. Recommend that the client schedule a follow-up physical examination and colonoscopy every 1 to 2 years. Refer clients with IBD to the Crohn's and Colitis Foundation of America (386 Park Ave. S., New York, NY 10016-8804) to learn about the condition and about meetings of local support groups. Instruct the client to call the physician at the first manifestation of IBD recurrence.

EVALUATION

It is hoped that the client's disease will respond to medical management and that the client will achieve remission, improved coping, and adequate nutritional intake. If the client's IBD does not respond to medical management, surgical intervention may be required.

Surgical Management

Surgery, the only cure for ulcerative colitis, is usually indicated when medical management fails and the condition is intractable. Twenty-five per cent to 40% of clients with ulcerative colitis must undergo surgical removal of the colon with a permanent ileostomy or a restorative procedure, such as an ileal pouch–anal anastomosis (suturing two loops of bowel together) or a Kock pouch, or continent ileostomy. Surgery is not indicated in Crohn's disease except to treat complications. An operation may be indicated in either or both conditions, however, for complications, such as perforation, hemorrhage, obstruction, toxic megacolon, abscess, fistula, and disease intractability.

Total Proctocolectomy

In a total proctocolectomy, the colon and rectum are removed and the anus is closed. The terminal ileum is brought out through the abdominal wall, and a permanent ileostomy is formed.

Ileorectal Anatomosis

Ileorectal anastomosis is another form of surgical management. The colon is resected, leaving a rectal stump. The terminal ileum is then anastomosed to this stump. The client has diarrhea postoperatively; in time, however, the stool usually becomes more solid.

Ileorectal anastomosis, an early alternative to total proctocolectomy, is associated with several problems, however. The remaining rectum is often still affected by the disease, and further treatment, even eventual resection, is often required. There is also a significant incidence of rectal cancer among clients who have undergone this procedure. The need for ileorectal anastomosis has essentially been eliminated because safer, more effective procedures are now available.

Continent Ileostomy

Indications. A continent ileostomy, or Kock pouch, is a procedure in which a reservoir or pouch is constructed from a loop of ileum. This allows stool to be stored intra-abdominally until it is drained through a nipple valve made from an intussuscepted portion of ileum (prolapse of one part of intestine into an adjacent section) (Fig. 33–1). The client has a flat stoma on the right side of the abdomen. Advantages of the continent ileostomy are (1) no need to wear an external pouch, (2) minimal skin problems, and (3) usually, no flatus or leakage of stool. The client drains the pouch several times a day using a catheter, usually in response to a feeling of fullness.

Contraindications. A continent ileostomy should not be performed for Crohn's disease. If the client has malnutrition, TPN may be required to improve the outcome of surgery and promote wound healing.

Complications. After the formation of the Kock pouch, suture line leakage with local or generalized peritonitis may occur in the early postoperative period. Other complications, including fistula formation, sliding of the valve, and obstruction by food residue, may occur late in the recovery period.

Outcomes. The client resumes usual activities within 4 to 6 weeks. Nutritional status also improves. The client experiences improved quality of life without the necessity of frequent trips to the bathroom.

Ileal Pouch–Anal Anastomosis

Indications. Ileal pouch–anal anastomosis is the preferred surgical procedure for clients with ulcerative colitis. The procedure (the J pouch) avoids an ostomy and preserves the rectal sphincter muscle.

The rectal mucosa is excised, and the colon removed. An ileoanal reservoir is then created in the anal canal, and a temporary loop ileostomy is formed. After healing has taken place, usually in 2 to 3 months, the ileostomy is reversed, so that stool drains into the reservoir, which is created by suturing two loops of bowel together (Fig. 33–2). Some surgeons are completing this procedure in one operation so that a temporary ileostomy is not required.

Contraindications. This anastomosis should not be performed for Crohn's disease. If malnutrition is a problem, TPN may be needed to improve the outcome of surgery and promote wound healing.

Complications. Complications include anastomotic leakage, pouchitis (inflammation of the pouch), and bowel obstruction.

Outcomes. The client resumes regular activities in 4 to 6 weeks after the second procedure or after the first procedure if a temporary ileostomy has not been performed. Nutritional status improves, and the client experi-

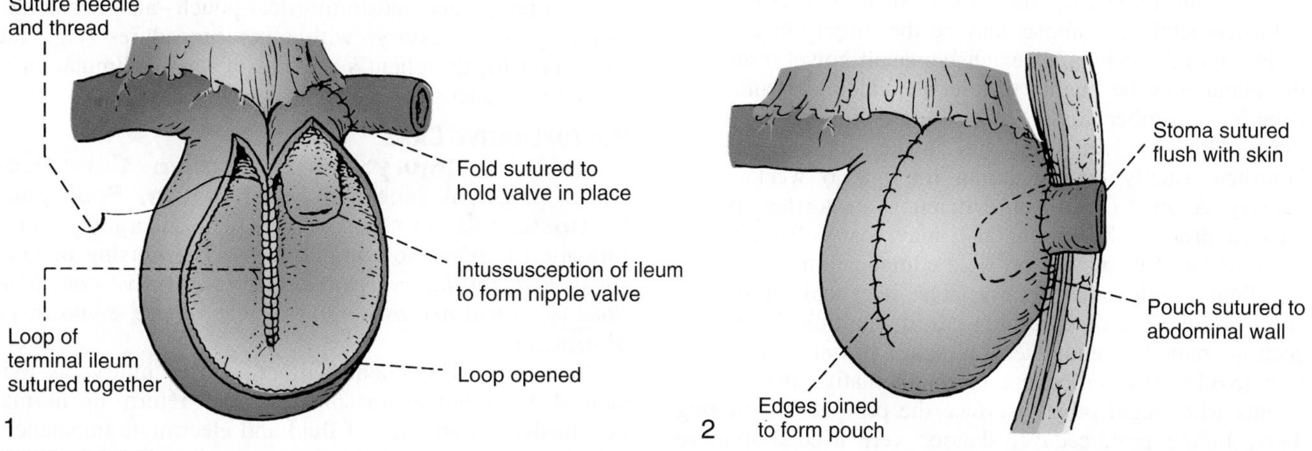

FIGURE 33–1 Continent ileostomy (Kock pouch). *1,* Loop of terminal ileum is sutured together and cut open. Using forceps, the surgeon intussuscepts the distal ileum to form a nipple valve. *2,* Free edges are sutured together to form the reservoir, the stoma is sutured flush with the skin, and the pouch is sutured to the abdominal wall.

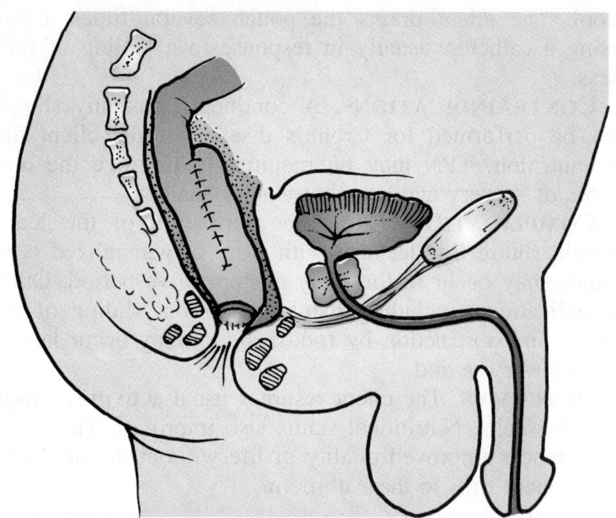

FIGURE 33–2 Ileal J pouch–anal anastomosis. The two-loop ileal pouch is simple to construct, provides adequate storage capacity, and is evacuated spontaneously and fully.

ences improved quality of life with nearly normal bowel movements and fewer trips to the bathroom.

SURGICAL RESECTION OF SMALL BOWEL

INDICATIONS. In Crohn's disease, surgery is used only to treat the complications, because even when the diseased portion is removed, the incidence of recurrence is 50%. The physician may prescribe antibiotics to control infection. During surgical resection for Crohn's disease, attempts are made to preserve as much of the small intestine as possible. Two thirds of the small intestine may be removed with no ill effects if the remaining portion is normal.

CONTRAINDICATIONS. Clients may be too malnourished to undergo surgery. TPN is needed to prepare the client for surgery and to improve wound healing.

COMPLICATIONS. With resection of the distal ileum, the client cannot absorb vitamin B_{12} and removal of more than 6 to 8 feet results in impaired absorption of glucose, fat, and protein. If the colon is diseased, an ileotransverse colectomy (right colon and ileum), segmental colectomy, or total colectomy may be performed. A total colectomy with ileorectal anastomosis may be the surgery of choice.

For 1 to 3 weeks after extensive small bowel resection, the client may be unable to tolerate oral intake and may experience further losses in body protein or lean body mass. TPN is given until oral intake can be resumed. Diarrhea usually occurs during the first 6 weeks after surgery. Anemia (from iron deficiency, steatorrhea, or decreased protein absorption) also may ensue. Paralytic ileus (see later) is another possible complication.

Clients with either irreversible intestinal failure or short-bowel syndrome resulting from multiple bowel resection, may be candidates for small bowel transplantation (SBT). This procedure is an alternative therapy for clients who might otherwise face the prospect of lifelong TPN. In the past, cadaver donors were used, but more recently a living-related intestinal transplantation has been accomplished. Clients undergoing SBT have a difficult postoperative course and long-term complications of immunosuppression, and they are at risk for graft rejection (see Chapter 80).

OUTCOMES. It is hoped that the client can return to regular activities with complete wound healing and adequate nutrition 4 to 6 weeks after surgery.

Nursing Management of the Surgical Client

ASSESSMENT

Assessment of the surgical client is similar to assessment of the medical client. However, routine preoperative and postoperative assessments as discussed in Chapter 15 are also necessary. If the client is malnourished, TPN may be required preoperatively to improve nutritional status.

DIAGNOSIS, OUTCOMES, INTERVENTIONS

PREOPERATIVE CARE

Knowledge Deficit. The client who is to undergo surgical resection for inflammatory bowel disease has many learning needs. The nursing diagnosis is *Knowledge Deficit related to surgical procedure and possible ileostomy or other bowel resection.*

Outcomes. The client will understand the surgical procedure and implications of bowel resection, as evidenced by the ability to describe the procedure and perform a demonstration of ileostomy care.

Interventions. Describe the anticipated postoperative course, including types of tubes that will be in place. Ostomy care must be fully explained to the client scheduled for ileostomy surgery. A preoperative visit from a member of any ostomy association may be helpful. An enterostomal therapy nurse should assist with the preoperative preparation. Before surgery, the site of the ileostomy is selected, with consideration being given to the location of the disease, body contours, convenience, and type of clothing the client wears. The client may wear the pouch for 1 to 2 days before surgery to ensure comfort with the site selected. In order to provide assistance and support, assess the client's body image as well as feelings about loss of a major body part and wearing a pouch for a lifetime.

If the client is having a continence-sparing surgery, extensive teaching is still required. The client needs to understand the type of bowel resection to be performed and the implications of the surgery. With some procedures, a temporary ileostomy (ileal pouch–anal anastomosis) may be necessary; with other procedures (e.g., the Kock pouch), the client's method of waste elimination is altered permanently.

POSTOPERATIVE CARE

Risk for Injury: Postoperative Complications (Stomal Necrosis, Retraction, Prolapse, Stenosis, Obstruction). The client undergoing stoma formation is prone to complications. The nursing diagnosis is *Risk for Injury related to postoperative complications of stomal necrosis, retraction, prolapse, stenosis, or obstruction.*

Outcomes. The client will not suffer injury, as evidenced by minimal distention, rapid return of normal peristalsis, and absence of fluid and electrolyte imbalance.

Interventions

Monitor Stoma. Monitor the stoma after surgery. Ensure that there is no pressure on the stoma that could interfere with circulation. Assess the color of the stoma frequently (see Fig, 33–7 for appearance of a normal stoma). If the stoma becomes pale, dusky, or cyanotic, notify the physician immediately. When blood supply to the stoma is compromised, surgical revision is required.

Advance Diet. An NG tube is in place for several days after surgery to remove gases and fluids that would increase intestinal distention and put pressure on the suture line. The drainage must be accurately noted. The passage of flatus indicates return of peristalsis. As bowel sounds return, clamp the tube as prescribed, and give the client ice chips and water. When the client has tolerated ice chips and water for a minimum of 24 hours, the tube is usually removed, and clear liquids are given.

Monitor for Complications. Although the postoperative course for most clients with ileostomies is uneventful, several complications can occur. The most common is an intestinal obstruction, which may be caused by obstruction of the lumen, adhesions, food, or stomal edema. Early manifestations of obstruction are (1) anorexia, (2) abdominal cramps, (3) absence of ileostomy drainage or a foul, brown, watery discharge in the pouch, and (4) visible peristalsis. Other early postoperative complications are hemorrhage, hypoxia, and fluid and electrolyte imbalance. If there are severe or prolonged problems with absorption, parenteral nutrition may be necessary.

Risk for Body Image Disturbance. The client with an ostomy has to face alterations in self-concept and body image. Write the nursing diagnosis as *Risk for Body Image Disturbance related to alteration of lifestyle secondary to ostomy.*

Outcomes. The client experiences a positive body image and self-concept, as evidenced by the client's statements and the ability to care for the ostomy without embarrassment.

Interventions. A few days after surgery, the client needs to begin to (1) confront the stoma and (2) integrate its function and appearance into his or her body image. Help the client look at and touch the stoma as soon as possible. Always use proper terms for the stoma and equipment.

Because clothing can be a concern for the client with an ostomy, clothing options should be discussed. Discourage the client from wearing a tight waistband, which might rub on the stoma. Encourage the client to try on various outfits to ensure that the stoma and pouch are not visible. A visit from another person with an ostomy, usually available through the local chapter of the American Cancer Society, often helps the client realize that the ostomy is easily hidden beneath clothing.

Encourage the client to verbalize feelings about the stoma and its appearance. The client may be very accepting of the stoma because the illness (ulcerative colitis) is now gone and his or her life may be more normal and productive than it had been with the disease. Young men and unmarried women may express the greatest concern about body image. Find out how family or significant others now view the client. Their response might be positive because the client may have been chronically ill prior to surgery and now appears much healthier.

Risk for Ineffective Management of Therapeutic Regimen (Individuals). The client with a new stoma has much to learn about self-care. The nursing diagnosis is *Risk for Ineffective Management of Therapeutic Regimen (Individuals) related to ileostomy care, care following ileorectal anastomosis, care of an ileal pouch–anal anastomosis, or care of a continent ileostomy.*

Outcomes. The client will understand proper care of the chosen surgical procedure, as evidenced by (1) the ability to apply the appliance correctly, without leakage, and to empty the pouch appropriately, and (2) absence of perianal breakdown.

Interventions

Ileostomy

Teach ostomy care. The client must master the skills needed to provide self-care. Stoma care is the area of greatest concern to the client with an ileostomy. Consultation with an enterostomal therapy nurse, if available, may enhance teaching and care (see Management and Delegation: Stoma Care). Initially, the client can simply observe care of the stoma. Begin by telling the client what the stoma looks like; that it extends ½ to ¾ inch beyond the abdominal wall, is 1 to 1½ inches in diameter, and is very red and swollen at first. Assure the client that permanent changes in stoma size occur within the first 3 months after surgery as the swelling subsides.

The frequency with which the ileal pouch needs to be emptied varies with each client. It should be emptied whenever it is approximately one-third to one-half full. Instruct the client to empty the pouch during times of low output, usually before meals, at bedtime, and upon arising in the morning. It is best to change the pouch when the ileostomy is the least active, usually first thing in the morning.

When changing the pouch, have all equipment ready before removing the old pouch. Remove the old pouch carefully using a moist cloth. A piece of gauze may be held over the stoma until the new pouch is attached. Encourage the client to inspect and touch the stoma at this time. Remind the client with a new ileostomy to take ostomy supplies along when traveling. The client may want to keep supplies handy in a shaving or cosmetic case instead of a suitcase. Many different types of pouches are available (Fig. 33–3). Clients should try to find the best pouch for their needs.

Teach stoma assessment. When changing the pouch, the client should learn to check the size and color of the stoma, assess the odor of the drainage, and observe for manifestations of irritation. When the ileostomy begins to function, the output is minimal. As the client takes in more food, the drainage becomes thicker and has a weak odor. Because an ileostomy may drain continuously (drainage is related to eating patterns), a pouch must be worn continuously, and the stoma must be covered with gauze when the pouch is being changed.

Prevent skin irritation. The pouch should be cut to fit the stoma, allowing only 1/16 inch of room around the stoma. If the pouch does not fit well, severe skin irritation can occur because of the alkalinity of the effluent. Skin irritation can vary from redness to weeping dermatitis or ulceration. Irritation also can result from adhesives or frequent removal of the appliance. The skin should be washed and rinsed thoroughly between removing one pouch and applying another. With a two-piece setup, a pouch is snapped onto the faceplate, which is applied to

MANAGEMENT AND DELEGATION

Stoma Care and Application of Ostomy Appliances

The care of a mature stoma and the application of an ostomy appliance may be delegated to unlicensed assistive personnel. The assessment and care of a newly created ostomy, however, should be performed only by a Registered Nurse. Before delegating stoma care and applying an ostomy appliance, consider the following:

- The age of the ostomy. Is this a postsurgical client with a new ostomy, or a client with an ostomy that is several weeks, months, or years old? For the client with a new ostomy, you or a trained ostomy nurse should provide care. For the client with a long-standing ostomy, assess the ostomy to ensure that the client is caring for it properly and that the stoma and surrounding skin are intact before you delegate ostomy care to assistive personnel.
- The client's need to learn self-care of the stoma and ostomy. You or a trained ostomy nurse should provide this instruction for a client needing to learn self-care.
- The client's acceptance of the ostomy, altered appearance, and bowel function. Clients having difficulty accepting their altered body image would benefit from having you or an ostomy nurse help them increase the acceptance and their ability to cope with the new ostomy.
- The competency level of the unlicensed assistive personnel who will potentially perform this task.

The assistive personnel providing stoma care and applying ostomy appliances should be instructed to:

1. Provide privacy for the client.
2. Place a waterproof pad around the ostomy or under the client, to protect the skin and bed linens.
3. Empty the contents of the ostomy bag prior to removing the bag, noting the consistency, color, volume, and odor of the feces.
4. Loosen the skin barrier with alcohol or another adhesive.
5. Gently remove the barrier and bag while supporting the client's skin.
6. Place a gauze pad or tissues over the exposed stoma to avoid soiling from leakage.
7. Wash the skin around the stoma with warm water and a mild soap, and wash the stoma with clear water.
8. Rinse the area with water and pat it dry.
9. Note the color, moisture, and protrusion of the stoma and the condition of the surrounding skin.
10. Create a circle 14 to 18 inches larger than the size of the stoma on the back of the appliance. A stoma-measuring guide may be helpful for this procedure.
11. Prepare the barrier and appliance as a unit.
12. Smooth the barrier to remove all air bubbles.
13. Fill in irregular stoma borders with skin paste.
14. Apply the unit, skin barrier, appliance, and bag around the stoma. Position the bag to hang in a dependent position. If the client is ambulatory, remember to position the bag for optimal drainage while the client is upright.
15. Dispose of the soiled bag and appliance properly. Do this outside the client's room to prevent embarrassment about any odors.

Assistive personnel should also be taught to report immediately to you if they find black, tarry stools or overt signs of blood in the bag or bleeding from the stoma. Reddened, inflamed skin surrounding the stoma should also be brought to your attention. Information pertaining to the care and condition of the stoma should be recorded.

Donna W. Markey, MSN, RN, ACNP-CS, *Clinician IV, Surgical Services, University of Virginia Health System, Charlottesville, Virginia*

the skin. This arrangement allows for easy emptying of the pouch. The faceplate usually remains adherent to the skin for 5 to 7 days. It may need to be changed sooner if it becomes loose or if leakage occurs.

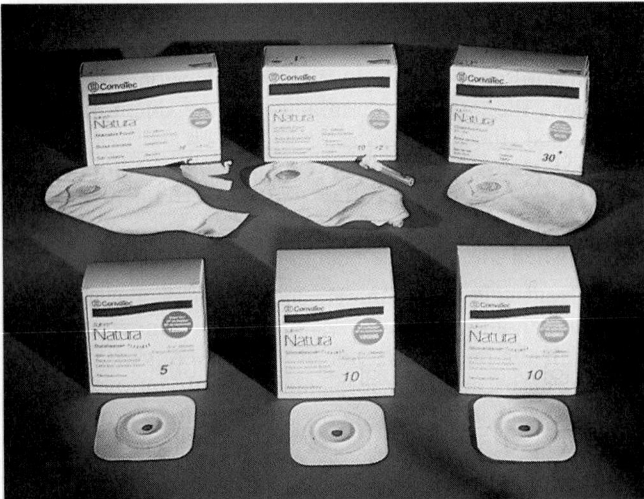

FIGURE 33–3 Natura brand ostomy products. (Courtesy of ConvaTec, Bristol-Myers Squibb, Skillman, NJ.)

Treat skin problems. If skin irritation does occur, first check the fit of the pouch. The best initial treatment for this problem would be to reapply the ostomy appliance, ensuring a proper fit and seal. The skin barrier of the appliance is usually sufficient to protect and heal the skin. If this method does not work, other barriers must be used. A wide variety of skin care products are available. If the problems continue, consult an enterostomal therapy nurse for further assistance.

Skin infection also can occur. *Candida* is the most common cause. The peristomal skin takes on a rash-like appearance. An antifungal powder should be rubbed onto the affected skin area. The barrier can then be applied over the powder.

Reduce odor. Foods such as eggs, fish, onions, cabbage, and some greens cause stool odor; therefore, deodorizing solutions and tablets may be placed in the pouch. Spinach, parsley, yogurt, and buttermilk reduce drainage odor.

Discuss medications. The client also needs special instructions regarding prescription and over-the-counter medications. Enteric-coated tablets, such as iron preparations, vitamins, and hormones, multilayer tablets, timed-release capsules, and gelatin capsules may not be absorbed in the small intestine. The client should note whether any medications are obvious in pouch drainage;

if so, the physician must prescribe different medications or different forms of medication.

Emphasize fluid intake. The client who has had an ileostomy needs to pay close attention to fluid intake. It is very easy for such a client to become dehydrated. The approximate output from an ileostomy is 1200 to 1500 ml/day. The client must monitor this output for any increase that could lead to severe fluid and electrolyte imbalance.

Explain dietary recommendations. A low-residue diet that is high in protein, carbohydrates, and calories is recommended after ileostomy surgery. Supplemental vitamins A, D, E, K, and B_{12} may be needed. Berries, whole-grain cereals, and raw fruits and vegetables can cause problems for the client with an ileostomy. Any foods that cause discomfort or diarrhea should be omitted. Ingested foods pass through the ileostomy within 4 to 6 hours. It is not advisable to eat a large meal close to bedtime.

The client with an ileostomy must learn to chew food well because the shortened bowel transit time would caused poorly chewed food to be passed undigested. High-fiber and high-cellulose foods may absorb excessive moisture, leading to swelling and possibly constipation or even obstruction. Foods that should be avoided or limited, at least initially, include popcorn, peanuts, tough fibrous meats, vegetables with skins, rice, bran, and coconuts.

Clients may find that the postoperative diet is less restrictive than the diet they followed before the operation. The diet required by the presence of the disease was often very restricted because so many foods increased the diarrhea and other manifestations. Clients with ileostomies often gain weight after surgery, sometimes to the point of having to restrict caloric intake.

Prevent urolithiasis. Some clients with ileostomies tend to have calcium oxalate, uric acid, or urinary calculi because greater amounts of fluid are lost through the ileostomy, leading to decreased urine output. Uric acid stones tend to form when urine volume is low and the urine is persistently acidic. Ingestion of sodium bicarbonate or potassium citrate alkalinizes the urine. Allopurinol may be used if uric acid levels remain elevated. Fluid intake should be at least 2000 ml/day.

Ileorectal Anastomosis. The client with an ileorectal anastomosis does not have to learn about stoma or pouch care unless a temporary ileostomy is present. The major goal of teaching centers on the importance of defecating before the rectum becomes overly distended. Most clients find that they have four to five stools per day once their bodies have adjusted to the surgical alteration. The feces of these clients are often described as pasty in consistency, and they appear to contain fewer electrolytes than the drainage from a traditional ileostomy. It may take up to 1 year for the client's altered bowel to adapt.

Encourage follow-up. Clients with ileorectal anastomoses must understand the importance of follow-up meetings with the physician. They must understand that the remaining mucosa can become diseased with ulcerative colitis or Crohn's disease, requiring further resection and, possibly, formation of an ileostomy. They also need to know that they are at increased risk for development of rectal cancer. Such clients must undergo regular proctoscopic examinations following surgery.

Avoid irritating foods. The client should learn to avoid foods that may cause diarrhea. It is best to try new foods one at a time so the effect can be determined. The diet is usually not limited; however, it should include adequate fluids to avoid dehydration.

Ileal Pouch–Anal Anastomosis. The client with an ileal pouch–anal anastomosis also has no need to learn about stoma or pouch care unless a temporary ileostomy was created. The client will learn to respond to the sensation to defecate so that spillage does not occur. After the bowel adapts to the surgical alteration, the stool becomes more formed, and many clients have only five or six stools per day. The client should maintain an adequate fluid intake.

Continent Ileostomy (Kock Pouch)

Maintain ileal drainage. During surgical formation of the Kock pouch, an evacuation catheter is inserted. A skin barrier and special gauze dressing are then applied. These hold the catheter in an upright position to avoid stress on a healing nipple valve. It is imperative to avoid distention of the ileostomy reservoir in the early postoperative period because of the pressure it would put on the suture line. Thus, the reservoir is attached to straight drainage for several days after surgery. Then it is emptied every 2 hours for about 2 weeks.

Carefully observe for the start of ileal drainage, which usually begins 3 or 4 days postoperatively. About 2 weeks after surgery, the catheter is removed from the pouch. The catheter may then be used to drain the pouch. The intervals between drainings are gradually increased each week until the ileostomy is emptied four to six times per day and once or not at all at night.

Teach Reservoir Catheterization. Explain the following procedure for emptying the reservoir, which should be performed with the client sitting on the toilet:

1. Lubricate the catheter with a water-soluble lubricant, and insert it into the stoma through the valve.
2. Allow the contents to drain by gravity through the catheter into the bathroom toilet; drainage should be complete in 3 to 5 minutes.
3. Apply a small gauze dressing over the stoma.
4. Clean the equipment with mild soap, and rinse it; the equipment can be carried in a plastic case.

The reservoir volume continues to increase to a maximum of around 600 ml in 6 months.

Explain dietary recommendations. The client needs an oral intake of at least eight 8-oz glasses of fluid per day. Foods that could cause a blockage of the valve and the stoma, including mushrooms and nuts, may need to be avoided. All foods need to be chewed thoroughly because partly digested food may occlude the stoma.

Risk for Sexual Dysfunction. In the client with an ileostomy, there are no physiologic reasons for sexual dysfunction; however, psychological changes may lead to sexual dysfunction. In this case, the nursing diagnosis is *Risk for Sexual Dysfunction related to concern about ileostomy and altered body image and self-concept.*

Outcomes. The client will not have a sexual dysfunction, as evidenced by the ability to resume pre-ileostomy sexual functioning and role.

Interventions. The client with an ileostomy may be concerned about sexual activity and pregnancy. Encourage the client to express any such concerns and to discuss them with the sexual partner. Clients can be taught activities to lessen the intrusiveness of the pouch during intercourse, such as emptying the pouch before intercourse, wearing a soft flannel pouch cover, and being open to using different positions for intercourse. If there are problems, a sexual therapist should be consulted for further information and assistance. Impotence is uncommon; psychological reasons should be explored if it does occur.

Pregnancy and normal vaginal delivery are possible for a client with an ileostomy. The United Ostomy Association has a wide variety of booklets available for clients with an ostomy. Titles include *Sex, Pregnancy and the Female Ostomate; Sex, Courtship and the Single Ostomate; Sex and the Male Ostomate;* and *Insight into the Emotional Aspects of Ileostomies and Colostomies*. Similar resources are available from the American Cancer Society.

EVALUATION

If teaching was adequate, the client should be able to care for the ostomy and to handle the altered elimination. Preoperative activities may be resumed within 6 weeks.

Self-Care

Postoperative care and care of the stoma or diversion should be reinforced before the client is discharged. The client with an ileostomy should be encouraged to join the United Ostomy Association. This organization often helps clients regain self-esteem and improve self-concept and body image. The successful rehabilitation of others helps clients believe that they, too, can return to a normal lifestyle.

The Client Education Guide: Ostomy Supplies mentions the equipment needed to care for an ileostomy. The client should be aware of the nearest ostomy supply center so that equipment will be easy to obtain. If the client experiences difficulty with self-care, a visiting nursing or enterostomal therapy nurse should visit the client at home to follow up on learning needs.

No long-term restrictions are placed on physical activities. Tell the client to wear a medical alert identification bracelet and to carry a brief description of the pouch and drainage procedure in case of emergency.

NEOPLASTIC DISORDERS

BENIGN TUMORS OF THE BOWEL

Various kinds of benign tumors are found in the bowel. Polyps are the most commonly found benign tumor of the large bowel. A *polyp* is a lesion that projects into the lumen of the bowel. Some polyps have stems (*pedunculated*), whereas others do not (*sessile*). Polyps are usually benign lesions, but some types are precursors of cancer (i.e., premalignant tumors). Polyps are dangerous because (1) they can mask the presence of a malignant tumor and (2) they may serve as the focus for bowel obstruction or intussusception. Benign bowel tumors have clinical manifestations similar to those of malignant tumors. Some benign tumors bleed profusely and cause abdominal discomfort. Bleeding benign tumors are usually removed surgically.

CANCER OF THE BOWEL

■ CANCER OF THE SMALL BOWEL

Fewer than 5% of all gastrointestinal cancers involve tumors of the small bowel. It was estimated that, in 2000, 4700 people would have cancer of the small bowel and 1200 will have died of it.[1] The average age of onset is 53 to 58 years. Most tumors are in the ileum, with the remainder almost equally divided between the duodenum and jejunum. Manifestations are vague and nonspecific; they include weight loss, pain, anemia, nausea, vomiting, obstruction, a palpable mass, and hemorrhage.

Surgery is the only intervention that offers hope of cure. Unfortunately, even with early diagnosis and bowel resection, only about 20% of clients small bowel cancer survive 5 years. With late diagnosis, the 5-year survival rate decreases to about 5%.

■ COLORECTAL CANCER

More than 95% of cancers of the colon are adenocarcinomas. In both sexes, colon and rectal (colorectal) cancer is the third most common cause of death from cancer in the United States.[1] Men are more likely to have colorectal cancer than women. In 2000, it was estimated that about 130,200 new cases of colorectal cancer, including 93,800 of colon cancer and 36,400 of rectal cancer, will have been diagnosed. About 56,300 people will have died from colorectal cancer, accounting for about 11% of all cancer deaths. The incidence rates have been declining in the last 20 years, a trend most likely attributable to increases in screening and polyp removal. Likewise, mortality rates have also been declining, most likely a reflection of falling incidence rates and rising survival rates from early diagnosis and treatment.

Most tumors are found in the distal portion of the large bowel, from the sigmoid colon to the anus. In the 1990s, the incidence of carcinoma of the right colon increased, whereas that of the rectosigmoid area decreased.

Survival following diagnosis correlates with the stage of tumor invasion (Fig. 33–4). The 5-year survival rate for colorectal cancer is 90% when disease is diagnosed and treated in the early stage. Once the cancer has spread to other organs, the 5-year survival rate decreases to 65%. For clients with metastasis to distant organs, the 5-year survival rate is 8%.

Etiology and Risk Factors

The cause of colorectal cancer is not definitely known. It may be related to low-residue, high-fat diets and highly refined foods with an inadequate intake of fruits and vegetables. There is a higher incidence in cities and industrialized countries. Genetic mutations are involved in hereditary forms of colorectal cancer; there also is a familial tendency. Gene mutations found in people with hereditary nonpolyposis colorectal cancer (HNPCC) suggest a lifetime risk of colon cancer of 80% to 85%. The risk of cancer increases with age and in those who have ulcerative colitis or familial polyposis.

Epidemiologic studies indicate that diet may be a major factor in the development of cancer of the large bowel. Studies on bulk in stool and the rate of transit of fecal matter have so far given mixed results. Some re-

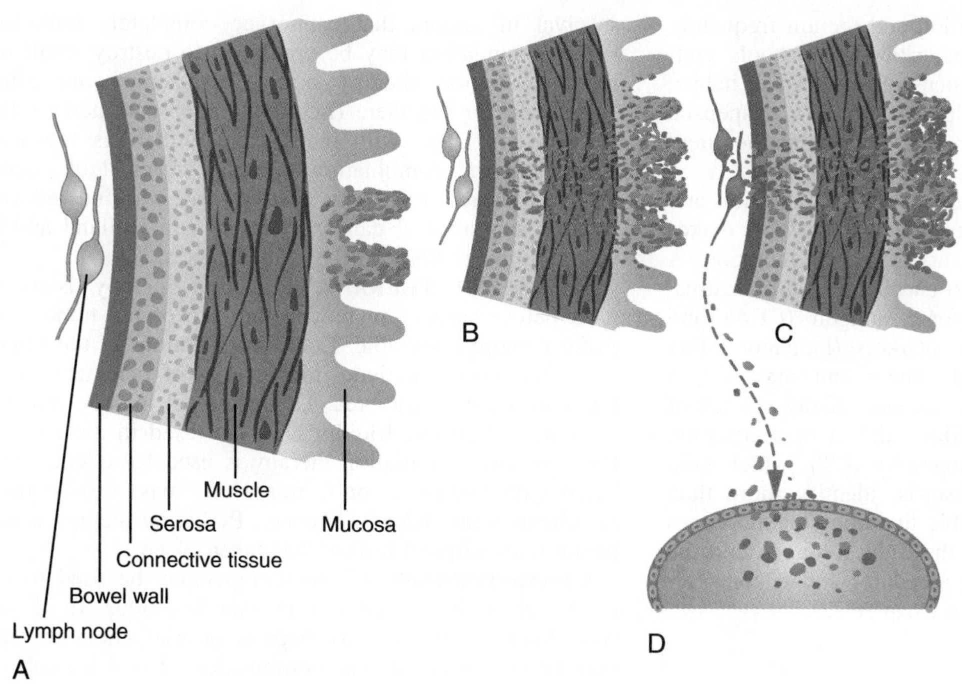

FIGURE 33–4 Stages of colon cancer, tumor (T), node (N), metastasis (M) system. *A,* Dukes' A or TNM I. Cancer is confined to bowel mucosa. *B,* Dukes' B or TNM II. Cancer extends into muscle, serosa, and connective tissue or adheres to or invades adjacent organs. *C,* Dukes' C or TNM III. Cancer penetrates the bowel wall and adheres to or invades adjacent organs; lymph nodes are positive. *D,* Cancer metastasizes to distant organs.

searchers propose that metabolic and bacterial end products are carcinogenic and that constipation allows a longer contact with the bowel wall, thus raising the probability that cancer will develop. Increasing fiber in the diet may reduce exposure to carcinogens by speeding stool transit through the intestines. Folate and selenium have been found to possibly prevent colon cancer.

Some studies have indicated that hormone replacement therapy and regular use of nonsteroidal anti-inflammatory drugs (NSAIDs) may reduce the risk of colon cancer. Uses of these agents are health promotion actions, as are regular physical activity and the identified diet changes.

Health maintenance activities include yearly screening with fecal occult blood test (FOBT) and digital rectal examination (DRE) for people at average risk for colorectal cancer who are older than 50 years of age. A flexible sigmoidoscopy, colonoscopy, or double-contrast barium enema study should be performed every 5 to 10 years in clients with normal screening results and more frequently in clients from whom polyps have been removed. Clients should begin colorectal cancer screening at a younger age, should undergo screening more frequently, or both if they have a family or personal history of colorectal cancer, polyps, or IBD, or genetic indicators for colorectal cancer. It is vital to explain to all clients the necessity for early detection and the importance of reporting manifestations such as rectal bleeding and a change in bowel habits to a health care provider.

Pathophysiology

Most malignant tumors (at least 50%) occur in the rectal area; another 20% to 30% are found in the sigmoid colon and descending colon. The remainder are found in the transverse colon and ascending colon, with twice as many found in the ascending colon as in the transverse colon.

Cancers of the colon almost always develop from adenomatous polyps. As a polyp becomes malignant, it increases in size within the lumen and begins to invade the bowel wall. Tumors in the right intestine tend to be bulky and to cause necrosis and ulceration. Tumors in the left intestine start as small, button-like masses that cause ulceration of the blood supply.

Colon cancer is staged using the TNM (tumor-node-metastasis) or Dukes' classification system. The TNM system is described in Chapter 19. Figure 33–4 compares the TNM system with the Dukes system, the system most commonly used for colon cancer. Dukes' classifications (A, B, C, D) correlate with the TNM stage groupings (I, II, III, IV).

Malignant bowel tumors spread by (1) direct extension to a nearby organ, such as to the stomach from the transverse colon, (2) lymphatic and hematogenous channels, usually to the liver, and (3) seeding of, or implanting of cells into, the peritoneal cavity. The urinary bladder, ureters, and reproductive organs are frequently involved by direct extension. Blood-borne metastasis extends most commonly to the liver but also may involve the lungs, kidneys, and bones.

Clinical Manifestations

Manifestations of colon cancer include rectal bleeding, changed bowel habits, abdominal pain, weight loss, anemia, and anorexia. In general, tumors in the small bowel and right colon are more likely to cause abdominal pain and cramping, nausea, and vomiting. Because the large intestine distends, cancer located there has fewer early manifestations. At this location, lesions often ulcerate, resulting in anemia and dark, reddish brown stools. Anorexia, weight loss, weakness, debility, and a palpable mass in the right lower quadrant may be present at the time of diagnosis. Lesions of the ascending colon and transverse colon often manifest as progressive obstruction.

Tumors in the descending colon and rectum frequently cause obstructive manifestations, ribbon-like stools containing bright red blood and mucus, altered bowel habits, and tenesmus, but not weight loss, anemia, or dyspepsia. Bleeding is the manifestation that often prompts the client to seek health care.

One third of malignant tumors of the distal colon and rectum can be felt with an examining finger. This makes DRE one of the more important diagnostic methods. A stool guaiac test is performed to check for gastrointestinal bleeding. Serum carcinoembryonic antigen (CEA) and cancer antigen (CA) 19–9 are markers (indicators) that may be elevated in colorectal cancer and may aid in determining the progress of the disease. X-ray studies of the colon may show either a filling defect or a stricture. Ultrasound and computed tomography (CT), which help establish tumor size and metastasis, identify more than half of colorectal tumors. Flexible fiberoptic colonoscopes permit better visualization into the right colon, extend the diagnostic capabilities of the procedure, and enable collection of biopsy specimens (see Chapter 32).

Prognosis

The prognosis in colorectal cancer depends on (1) the health of the client, (2) how early the disease is diagnosed, and (3) how effective the treatment is. The 5-year survival rates, listed according to Dukes' classification, are as follows: Dukes' A, 80% to 90%; Dukes' B, about 60%; Dukes' C, 25% to 40%; Dukes' D, less than 5%. Overall, 51% of clients with a diagnosis of colorectal cancer survive for 10 years. Early diagnosis and treatment are essential for a good outcome. However, only 37% of colorectal cancers are identified in the early stages.

Outcome Management

Medical Management

DECREASE TUMOR GROWTH

The primary treatment for colon cancer is surgery; however, medical treatment is used as an adjunct to improve survival in tumors that cannot be completely removed. Electrocoagulation may be employed to destroy small tumors. Radiation therapy and chemotherapy are often given alone or together. The combination can increase the survival of clients with rectal cancer; there is less evidence that the combination increases survival of clients with colon cancer. A new custom-made vaccine reduced stage B postsurgical cancer recurrence in Holland and is currently under study in the United States.

RADIATION THERAPY. Radiation therapy is often used before surgery to reduce the size of the tumor and make it more resectable. Local interventions at the tumor site after surgery include implantation of radioactive isotopes into the tumor area. Isotopes used include radium, cesium, and cobalt. Iridium has been used in the rectum. Postoperatively, radiation therapy is used for clients classified with Dukes' B or C tumors. It may also be used for clients with Dukes' D cancer. Radiation therapy is not begun until surgical healing has taken place.

CHEMOTHERAPY. Chemotherapy may be used to reduce metastasis and control its manifestations. In clients with liver metastasis, intrahepatic arterial chemotherapy may be administered. The combination of oral levamisole (Ergamisol) and IV 5-fluorouracil (5-FU) has improved survival in Dukes' C tumors. Leucovorin (folinic acid) also may be given with 5-FU, with or without levamisole, to increase its effects. Irinotecan (Camptosar) has been effective when colorectal cancer recurs after treatment with 5-FU.

Nursing Management of the Medical Client

Care of the client undergoing medical treatment for colon cancer revolves around care of a client undergoing chemotherapy and, occasionally, radiation therapy. See Chapter 19 for further information on the care of these clients.

Surgical Management

Intervention depends on the type of tumor, its location and stage, and the client's general condition. A variety of surgical procedures are performed to treat colorectal cancer (Figs. 33–5 and 33–6). Early colorectal cancers can

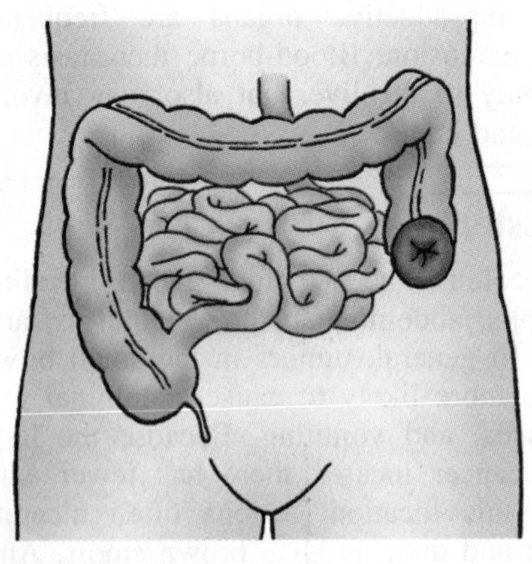
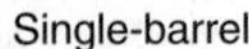
Single-barrel

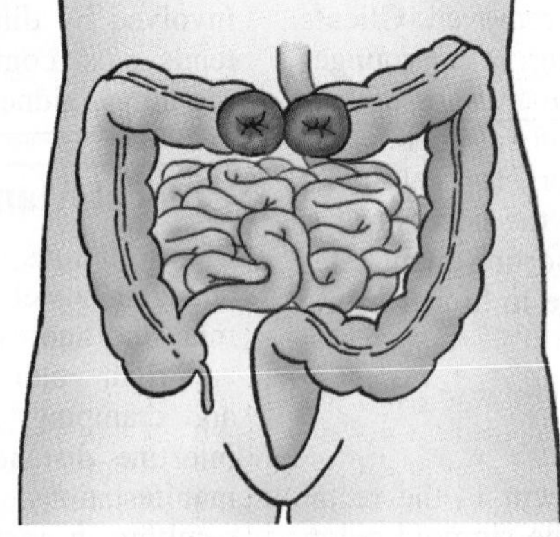
Double-barrel

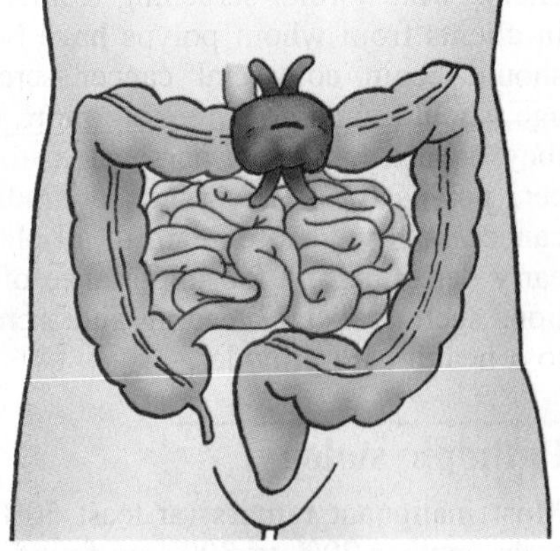
Loop

FIGURE 33–5 Types of colostomies. Single-barreled colostomies are usually permanent. Double-barrel colostomies are usually temporary, and stomas may be adjacent or several inches apart. Loop colostomies are temporary and are formed by bringing a loop of colon through the abdominal wall and supporting it with a plastic brace.

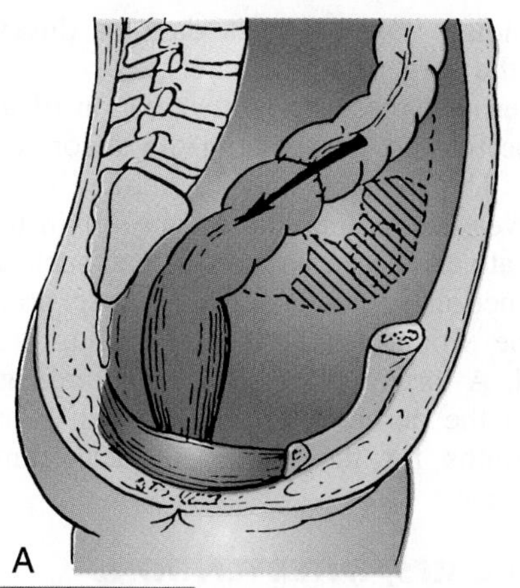

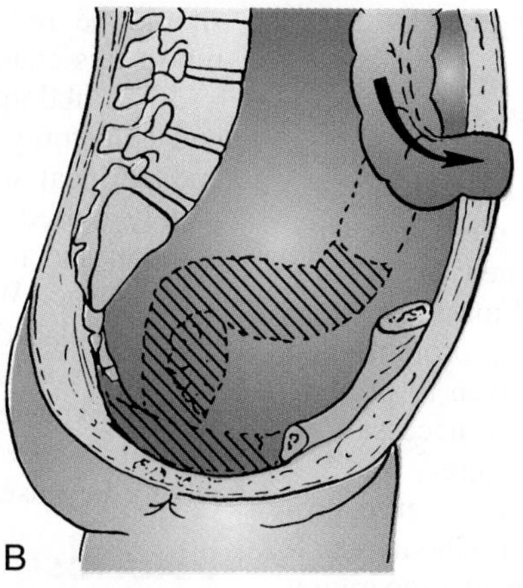

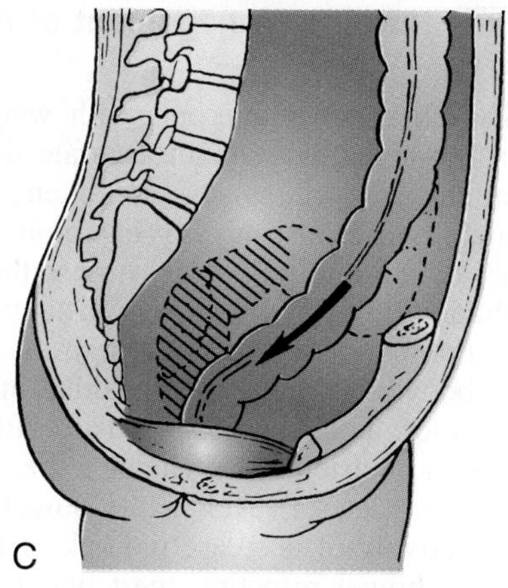

FIGURE 33–6 Resecting malignant tumors in the rectosigmoid segment of the bowel. *A,* Anterior resection with primary anastomosis is used for cancer at any point in the bowel except the terminal rectum. Associated lymph nodes are resected, *B,* Abdominoperineal (anteroposterior) resection with formation of permanent colostomy (Miles' operation) for cancer involving the anus and terminal portion of the rectum. *C,* Proctosigmoidectomy with pull-through and preservation of external sphincter muscles is appropriate when the tumor is in the proximal rectum and unlikely to metastasize further.

be excised and removed through a colonoscope; however, most procedures entail colon resection. The tumor is removed with several inches of colon on either side of the tumor. An end-to-end anastomosis is performed, if possible. A sleeve resection may be performed for clients with advanced disease; it is a less involved procedure in which segments of the intestine are resected to relieve obstruction and bleeding.

Several different procedures are used for rectal cancer, depending on tumor location. It may be possible to preserve sphincter function by resecting tumors located in the proximal area. However, sphincter function may not be preserved if tumors are less than 2 to 2.5 cm from the anal opening.

Colostomy

Indications. A colostomy may have to be performed for colorectal cancers. This procedure involves creating an opening between the colon and abdominal wall, from which fecal contents will pass. Because the main function of the large bowel is to absorb water, the colostomy is easier to manage nearer the sigmoid colon, because the stool is more formed here than in the transverse or right colon. A colostomy can be located in the ascending, transverse, descending, or sigmoid colon and can be permanent or temporary.

A temporary colostomy allows the bowel to rest and may later be reanastomosed. The temporary colostomy also can be used to treat inoperable bowel cancer, with the ostomy placed proximal to the cancer. A temporary colostomy is made most commonly at the midpoint of the left colon or transverse colon, whereas a permanent colostomy is usually placed in the sigmoid colon. When creating a temporary loop colostomy, the surgeon brings a loop of bowel out through a wound that is separate from the surgical incision. To keep the loop from slipping back into the abdominal cavity, the surgeon places a rod or bridge beneath it. Although the bowel is usually opened with a cautery in surgery, the surgeon may wait 2 or 3 days postoperatively to open the bowel. Because there are no sensory nerve endings in the bowel wall, this procedure is essentially painless, except for some cramping. The surgeon usually indicates which is the proximal loop and which is the distal loop.

A colostomy may also be single-barreled or double-barreled. When only one loop end of bowel is opened onto the abdominal surface, the result is called an *end* or *single-barreled colostomy*; the client has only one stoma. An end colostomy is permanent if the bowel distal to it has been resected. A *double-barreled colostomy* is one in which both loops, distal and proximal, are open onto the abdominal wall. It may be closed later, depending on the disease present. A double-barreled colostomy can be two separate stomas, a loop with one stoma and two openings, or one stoma and a mucus fistula. The fistula expels mucus and is covered with a gauze dressing or pouch.

Contraindications. Any health condition that makes the client a poor surgical risk is a contraindication to a colostomy procedure.

Complications. Suture line leakage with local or generalized peritonitis may occur in the early postoperative period. Other complications are hemorrhage and stomal necrosis, retraction, prolapse, and stenosis. Stomal complications may require additional surgery to revise the stoma.

Outcomes. The client resumes usual activities within 4 to 6 weeks and is able to perform self-care of the stoma. If needed, radiation therapy and chemotherapy are initiated.

Abdominal-Perineal Resection

Rectal tumors may require an abdominal-perineal resection, with the formation of a permanent or end colostomy. The affected colon and entire rectum are excised, and the anus is closed. The colon is removed through an abdominal incision, and the rectum through a perineal incision. Newer surgical techniques allow removal of low sigmoid tumors while leaving the rectal sphincter intact; normal bowel elimination is maintained.

Nursing Management of the Surgical Client

PREOPERATIVE CARE

The client often presents with weight loss and a change in bowel habits. Obtain accurate descriptions of manifestations as well as an assessment of major risk factors, such as a family history of colon cancer, ulcerative colitis, or familial polyposis. Assess the abdomen, noting any abnormalities, such as pain, distention, and masses.

Preoperatively, a diet high in calories, protein, and carbohydrates but low in residue may be given to provide nutrition and reduce peristalsis. TPN may be necessary to provide nutrients and vitamins the client requires.

The bacteria level in the bowel must be lowered preoperatively to decrease the risk of infection. Clients needing a bowel resection must undergo a bowel preparation to minimize bacterial growth in the bowel and postoperative wound infection. This preparation usually involves:

- A low-residue or liquid diet to reduce the fecal contents of the bowel
- Oral administration of cathartics, such as polyethylene glycol–electrolyte solution (GoLYTELY) or a pre-procedure bowel evacuator (Fleet Prep Kit No. 2), which is started at least 12 to 24 hours preoperatively
- Administration of antibiotics, such as sulfonamides and possibly neomycin and cephalexin, usually by mouth, for 12 to 48 hours preoperatively
- Administration of enemas to clean the bowel (the inside of the bowel lumen should be as clean and as bacteria-free as possible)
- Blood transfusions to correct severe anemia

Identify the client's level of anxiety and provide supportive efforts. Explain all treatments and procedures fully. Clarify and reinforce the information provided by the physician. Encourage clients to ventilate their feelings and meet with health team members to discuss treatments and prognosis. The client also needs to know how treatment decisions will be made when the results of pathologic study are available and what to expect after the operation, such as placement of tubes and measures to prevent postoperative complications.

If a colostomy is necessary, an enterostomal therapy nurse should be asked to educate the client about the ostomy, answer questions, and advise on optimal placement of the stoma. If an enterostomal therapy nurse is not available, assume the responsibility for teaching the client about the stoma. The risk of sexual dysfunction should be explained to the client in a supportive atmosphere.

POSTOPERATIVE CARE

ASSESSMENT

Immediate postoperative assessments are as discussed in Chapter 15. Assess for the return of peristalsis; indications are passage of flatus and return of bowel sounds, heard during auscultation of the abdomen. Gastric suction may be continued until peristalsis returns. Make sure the NG tube is patent.

Additionally, if a colostomy was created, monitor the colostomy output, and use special care to keep fecal contents from the colostomy (which contain bacteria) away from the surgical incision. Assess the client's stoma closely for the presence of stomal ischemia. The stoma should be red and moist. If it becomes dark or dusky, report this change to the surgeon immediately.

If an abdominal-perineal resection with creation of an end colostomy was performed, assess both the abdominal and perineal wounds. The incision may be sutured completely closed. However, sometimes drains are left in the incision and may be attached to a suction device such as a Hemovac. When suction is not used, a Penrose drain may be placed in the wound; change the dressing frequently or as ordered. A large amount of serous drainage can be expected from the perineal wound. It often takes several weeks to months for the wound to heal completely because of its size.

DIAGNOSIS, OUTCOMES, INTERVENTIONS

Risk for Injury. The postoperative client is at risk for the development of postoperative complications. The nursing diagnosis is *Risk for Injury related to postoperative complications, including infection, hemorrhage, wound disruption, thrombophlebitis, and abnormal stomal function.*

Outcomes. The client does not experience an injury, as evidenced by absence of manifestations of infection, bleeding, and evidence of wound disruption, thrombophlebitis, stomal ischemia, and bowel spillage.

Interventions

Monitor Vital Signs. Immediate postoperative interventions are the same as those used for any major abdominal procedure; they involve monitoring vital signs for manifestations of infection and shock.

Advance Diet as Tolerated. An NG tube is usually in place until peristalsis returns. It is usually several days before the NG tube is discontinued and the client begins to consume fluids and food. As the client tolerates food, he or she is slowly advanced to a regular diet.

Decrease Cramping. Abdominal cramps commonly occur after surgery, as does distention of the bowel. Distention is uncomfortable and may put pressure on suture lines. The insertion of a rectal tube for 20 to 30 minutes per physician order will help if the rectum contains gas. Early ambulation helps relieve distention and promotes peristalsis.

Apply Rectal Dressing. Prepare the client to wear a rectal dressing throughout the healing period. The character, volume, and odor of the drainage should be assessed. If the drainage in any way suggests a developing infection, arrange for a culture of the wound to identify the organism.

Occasionally, in the immediate postoperative period, sump drainage is placed in the perineal wound. This is also indicated if the wound becomes infected. The sump tube is attached to suction, allowing the wound to heal from its deepest portion without forming an abscess.

Reduce Pain. The perineal wound can be very painful, and the client should receive sufficient medication to control the pain. Once the packing is removed, the wound is irrigated, and the client should take a sitz bath three or four times a day. The client will find a side-lying position in bed most comfortable.

Monitor Stoma Drainage. There may be a colostomy pouch over the stoma. Make sure that this pouch is not applying pressure to the stoma, which would interfere with its blood supply. When changing or emptying the pouch, prevent contamination of the surgical wound by fecal discharges. Monitor the return of bowel function by observing the type and quantity of discharges from the stoma.

Prevent Thrombophlebitis. The high lithotomy position associated with the abdominal-perineal resection is associated with an increased risk of development of postoperative phlebitis. To prevent this problem, subcutaneous injections of heparin, usually 5000 units every 12 hours after surgery, are often prescribed. Sequential pressure stockings or thigh-high antiembolic hose also must be worn. The client must perform leg exercises before and after surgery. Monitor the client for manifestations of thrombophlebitis.

Risk for Body Image Disturbance. The client with an ostomy must face alterations in self-concept and body image. Write the nursing diagnosis as *Risk for Body Image Disturbance related to colostomy and lifestyle changes.*

Outcomes. The client adjusts to changes in body image, as evidenced by the ability to identify and use effective coping methods in dealing with the disease and losses experienced.

Interventions. Give emotional support while the client begins the process of adjusting to the colostomy. It is also important to provide extensive teaching about how to care for the colostomy. The client's significant others also must adjust to the colostomy; help them by listening to their reactions and explaining the client's problems to them.

A client's reactions to a new colostomy may range from apparently easy acceptance to total withdrawal from social contacts. How well clients adjust depends partly on their attitudes toward excretory functions, previous knowledge about colostomies, and general ability to adjust to stressful situations.

Some clients refuse to look at the stoma and find it very difficult to accept its presence, whereas others begin to participate in stoma care almost immediately. Your reactions to and manner toward the client and the care required can affect the client's adjustment. For some clients, the colostomy represents a "cure"; for others, it is palliation when the cancer has spread.

Continuing sexual relationships is a major concern for the client with a colostomy and the significant other. There is no physical reason that a client cannot enjoy normal sexual relations, although a small number of men become impotent after a radical perineal dissection. If this complication occurs, the physician may recommend a urology consultation to discuss treatment options for impotence (see Chapter 38). Psychological barriers may cause problems. With love, patience, understanding, and good hygienic practices, there should be no problem. However, it may be several months after surgery before a couple manages to reestablish a satisfactory sexual relationship. Referral to a social worker, counselor, psychiatric liaison, sex therapist, or registered nurse with a counseling background may be beneficial.

Risk for Ineffective Management of Therapeutic Regimen (Individuals). The client with a colostomy needs to learn about self-care. The nursing diagnosis is *Risk for Ineffective Management of Therapeutic Regimen (Individuals) related to colostomy care, irrigation, and possible complications associated with colostomies.*

Outcomes. The client understands care of the colostomy, as evidenced by the ability to (1) apply the pouch, (2) care for peristomal skin, (3) irrigate the colostomy, if applicable, and (4) prevent or treat any associated problems.

Interventions. Carefully assess the client's physical condition and emotional and mental attitude toward the colostomy before attempting to teach ostomy self-care. Pace the teaching to the client's level of acceptance of the colostomy and ability to manage it.

Teach Ostomy Care. Teach the client how to correctly apply the pouch to the stoma. The client first should be taught how to examine the stoma. A healthy stoma is red and slightly raised. (Figure 33–7 shows a colostomy during application of an appliance.) The skin around the stoma (*peristomal skin*) should be clear, without evidence of irritation. The peristomal area should be cleaned well with a mild soap and water and dried well before the new pouch is applied. The skin should be treated with a skin barrier and the new pouch applied, cut about 1/16 to 1/8 inch larger than the stoma. The pouch should be changed every 4 to 5 days or when leakage occurs. If a two-piece system is used, the faceplate may stay in place for 7 days. Types of pouches are shown in Figure 33–3.

Teach the client to empty the pouch when it is about half full and how to clean out the pouch when emptying it. The client should demonstrate the ability to empty and change the pouch independently before being discharged. See the discussion of ileostomy care for further information.

Teach Stoma Irrigation. Clients with end sigmoid colostomies can be taught to regulate the colostomy through regular irrigation. Clients who are physically, mentally, and emotionally capable should be encouraged to attempt irrigation and regulation. Some clients, in spite of irrigation, may never achieve regularity of elimination. If they have not achieved regularity within 6 months, they probably never will.

The Client Education Guide: Colostomy Irrigation lists the steps involved in irrigation. The best time for irriga-

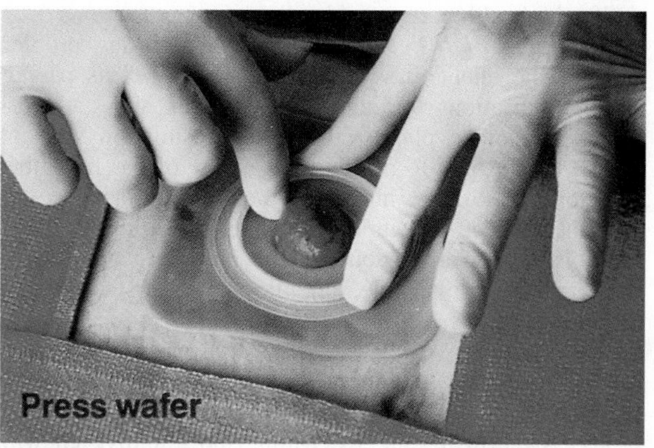

FIGURE 33–7 Healthy stoma during application of wafer. (Courtesy of ConvaTec, Bristol-Myers Squibb, Skillman, NJ.)

CLIENT EDUCATION GUIDE

Colostomy Irrigation

1. Assemble all the irrigation equipment and skin care products, and new colostomy pouch.
2. Remove and discard the old pouch.
3. Clean the peristomal skin.
4. Apply the irrigating sleeve, and close off the distal end or place it in the toilet.
5. Using 500 to 1000 ml of warm tap water, suspend the solution container about 18 inches above the stoma. Clear the air from the irrigation tubing. Insert the lubricated cone (water-soluble lubricant) 2 to 4 inches into the stoma (*never force the cone*), and allow the solution to flow gently into the colon.
6. Once all solution has been instilled for 6 to 8 minutes, either allow most of the stool to pass into the toilet and then close off the pouch for another 30 to 45 minutes, or simply close off the end of the pouch until the bowel has evacuated.
7. Once the bowel has emptied, simply remove the sleeve, clean the stoma, and cover it with a small pouch or gauze pad.

tion is when the client formerly had a daily bowel movement, because the bowel is already "trained" to evacuate at this time. If there is difficulty inserting the catheter, let a little solution flow in, and rotate the catheter. If the catheter will not go in, teach the client to apply gloves or a finger cot, lubricate the finger, and gently pass it into the stoma. This method often dislodges any feces that may be near the stoma. If the client cannot pass a catheter and no obstruction is felt digitally, the client should notify the health care provider.

If cramping occurs, the client should stop the solution temporarily, take a few deep breaths, and restart the solution slowly. The client should *never* (1) use more than 1000 ml, (2) irrigate the colostomy more than once a day, or (3) irrigate the colostomy if diarrhea is present.

If there is no return after irrigation, the client should ambulate, gently massage the abdomen, and try drinking some warm water. If there is still no return, the client should apply a pouch and try the irrigation again the next day. If there is no return the second day, the client should notify the health care provider.

Minimize Flatus. Flatus is an embarrassing problem because the client may have no control over its passage and no sensations to indicate when it is about to pass. Flatus can make clients avoid social situations. Clients can be taught how to muffle the passage of gas from their colostomies. Women may hold their purses or arms, and men their folded jackets or hats, over the stoma to muffle the noise. Odor-proof pouches and pouches with charcoal filter discs are available, but the most satisfactory way to control flatus is through diet. Because everyone is different, clients must learn by trial and error which foods cause gas. In general, nuts, corn, cabbage, sauerkraut, broccoli, cauliflower, and legumes are gas-forming foods. Swallowing air by eating too rapidly, chewing gum, and drinking carbonated beverages also cause intestinal gas.

EVALUATION

The client should recover from surgery without complications and should resume usual activities within 6 weeks. When a colostomy has been performed, the client should be able to manage it within 2 months. If the client is unable to accomplish self-care, the need for further teaching should be explored.

Self-Care

In preparation for discharge, clients need support and knowledgeable advice as they learn to live with their colostomies. The client needs to know the nearest location for purchase of ostomy supplies (see Client Education Guide: Ostomy Supplies). Immediately after dismissal, home delivery of supplies may be necessary. The enterostomal therapy nurse can help the client learn to manage and accept the ostomy and to achieve a smooth transition from the health care facility to the home. Some cities have established ostomy rehabilitation clinics to help clients, and most large communities have an ostomy association that maintains contact with the American Cancer Society. These support groups are helpful because clients can share their ostomy concerns with others who have similar problems. A home health care referral can add to the client's peace of mind, identify problems that might not otherwise be known, and ensure necessary follow-up care. See to Bridge to Home Health Care.

Before discharge, advise clients that it may take several weeks for them to regain their strength after major bowel surgery; further, when segments have been removed from the bowel, bowel habits may alter until the body adjusts to the situation. You may need to teach the client and significant others how to change dressings at home, because wounds may not be healed totally by the time the client is discharged. In general, teaching should cover (1) dressing changes, (2) dietary or activity restrictions, (3) colostomy care if applicable, and (4) manifestations of intestinal obstruction and perforation.

CLIENT EDUCATION GUIDE

Ostomy Supplies

Before you leave the hospital, find out where to purchase supplies for your ostomy. Obtain written instructions, including the brand name, order number, size of pouch, skin barrier, and pouch deodorants, as well as the name, address, and telephone number of a local medical supply facility. Ostomy supplies are very expensive; the following resources may help you obtain them more economically:

- *Ostomy Quarterly*, which lists mail order houses selling equipment at a discount (telephone: 1-800-826-0826)
- Talking with other ostomates at a local meeting of the United Ostomy Association (telephone: 1-800-826-0826)
- *The Ostomy Book*, by Barbara Dorr Mullen and Kerry Anne McGinn, an excellent publication written especially for clients and their families (Palo Alto, CA, Bull Publishing Co., 1992).

BRIDGE TO HOME HEALTH CARE

Adjusting to Life with a Colostomy

When you visit a client who has a new colostomy, assess the stoma and peristomal skin thoroughly before selecting a pouch. The stoma should be beefy red; a pale red or pale pink stoma indicates a limited blood supply. A healthy stoma is moist; dryness suggests dehydration. Note whether the outer edges are intact and attached to the peristomal skin. The stoma should be round and raised; it will shrink during the next 4 to 6 weeks. Assess the stoma when the pouch is off and the client is lying down; repeat when the client sits. Watch for (1) changes in stoma shape, (2) skin folds, (3) creases, and (4) dimpling of the peristomal skin.

Clients and caregivers are more likely to manage a colostomy independently if they understand and follow your instructions and participate in care. Demonstrate how to clean the stoma; request return demonstrations. Some bleeding is normal; applying pressure should stop the bleeding. Excessive bleeding is abnormal; if this happens, they should call the physician immediately. Tell client and caregiver to expect output (effluent) daily. The effluent will by runny initially but will thicken within 2 to 4 weeks. Expect excessive flatulus (bowel gas) for 4 to 8 weeks. Teach clients and caregivers to watch for manifestations of intestinal obstruction that require immediate medical care, such as nausea or vomiting, body temperature exceeding 101° F, severe abdominal pain, distention, limited or no output, and decreased bowel sounds.

Leakage is a common problem. To minimize leakage, provide detailed instructions about pouch fit and care; the pouch should be changed twice a week. *Do not* assume that the appliance the client took home from the hospital will fit when the stoma shrinks. If the peristomal skin retracts, the client needs a pouch with a convex wafer, not a flat wafer. If the stoma is round, you may use a precut pouch; if it is not round, use a cut-to-fit pouch. Make and date a pattern of the stoma by tracing the outline of the stoma on a clear piece of rigid plastic with an indelible marker. Cut out the pattern and check it for proper fit against the stoma; it may not fit when the stoma shrinks. Use an ostomy belt that is snug but not tight to improve the bond between the pouch and peristomal skin. If the client is using a two-piece pouch system, make sure that there is a good seal between the pouch and the wafer.

To reinforce instructions between your visits, leave simple, step-by-step directions for pouch changing for clients and caregivers. Also leave written details about purchasing ostomy supplies locally or by mail order. Provide verbal and written diet and hydration information. Suggest that the client avoid foods high in fiber initially, such as corn, popcorn, mushrooms, peanuts, and Chinese foods; these foods can cause the bowel to swell and become obstructed. When the swelling decreases in 4 to 8 weeks, clients should be able to gradually resume eating a regular diet and to increase fluid consumption to prevent constipation at resumption of regular diet.

Refer clients with a colostomy and their family members to organizations that can help them cope with the colostomy diagnosis and changed body image, such as the United Ostomy Association (1-800-826-0826), the American Cancer Society (1-800-227-2345), and the National Wound, Ostomy, and Continence Nurses Association (1-888-224-9626). Nurse members of the last group can provide valuable information about resuming a normal lifestyle and can help manage complicated ostomies.

James McLean, RN, BSN, WOCN, *Enterostomal Therapist, Fort Worth, Texas*

The client who is having a problem with the colostomy should see an enterostomal therapy nurse. The client with an abdominal-perineal resection needs follow-up from the surgeon to ensure that the perineal wound is healing properly.

OTHER DISORDERS OF THE LARGE AND SMALL BOWEL

HERNIATIONS

A *hernia* is the abnormal protrusion of an organ, tissue, or part of an organ through the structure that normally contains it. Hernias most commonly occur in the abdominal cavity when a section of the bowel protrudes through as a result of a congenital or acquired weakness of abdominal musculature. Hernias can occur at any age and in either sex. Approximately 700,000 inguinal herniorrhaphies are performed in the United States each year. Indirect inguinal hernias, the most common type, typically occur in men. Direct inguinal hernias are found more commonly in older people. Incisional or ventral hernias occur most often in clients who had poor wound healing after surgery. Obese or pregnant clients are more likely to develop umbilical hernias.

Etiology and Risk Factors

Hernias develop when there is a defect in the integrity of the muscular wall accompanied by increased intra-abdominal pressure. Congenital muscle weakness is one risk factor as are any factors that increase intra-abdominal pressure. The muscle weakness cannot be prevented, but exercises can be performed to strengthen weak muscles. Because obesity is one cause of increased intra-abdominal pressure, such an increase can be prevented by weight control. Avoiding heavy lifting and straining also reduces intra-abdominal pressure. Early diagnosis is important to prevent incarceration and strangulation of the herniated tissue.

Pathophysiology

Defects in the muscular wall may be congenital and due to weakened tissue or a wide space at the inguinal ligament or may be caused by trauma. Intra-abdominal pressure increases with pregnancy, obesity, heavy lifting, coughing, and traumatic injuries from blunt pressure. When two of these factors coexist with some tissue weakness, a hernia may occur. Increased pressure without a weakness is not likely to cause a hernia. Weakness, in addition to being present from birth, is acquired as part of the aging process. As clients age, muscular tissues become infiltrated and are replaced by adipose and connective tissues.

When the contents of the hernial sac can be replaced into the abdominal cavity by manipulation, the hernia is said to be *reducible. Irreducible* and *incarcerated* are terms that refer to a hernia in which the contents of the sac cannot be reduced or replaced by manipulation. When pressure from the hernial ring (the ring of muscular tissue through which the bowel protrudes) cuts off the blood supply to the herniated segment of bowel, the bowel becomes *strangulated.* Incarcerated hernias usually become strangulated. This situation is a surgical emergency because unless the bowel is released, it soon becomes gangrenous because of the lack of blood supply.

Hernias may penetrate through any defect in the abdominal wall, through the diaphragm, or through some internal structure within the abdominal cavity (Fig. 33–8). This discussion covers only the more common types of hernias: inguinal (both indirect and direct), femoral, umbilical, and incisional. (Hiatal hernia is discussed in Chapter 30.)

INDIRECT INGUINAL HERNIA. An indirect inguinal herniation occurs through the inguinal ring and follows the spermatic cord through the inguinal canal. It is more common in males than females because of the space allowed for the testicles to descend. There is a high incidence of indirect inguinal hernia in young people. The incidence is also high among clients 50 to 60 years of age and then gradually decreases in older age groups. These hernias can become extremely large and often descend into the scrotum.

DIRECT INGUINAL HERNIA. In a direct inguinal hernia, bowel passes through the abdominal wall in an area of muscular weakness, not through a canal as do indirect inguinal and femoral hernias. This type of hernia is more common in the elderly. Direct inguinal hernia gradually develops in an area that is weak owing to a congenital deficiency in the number of fibers it contains.

FEMORAL HERNIA. A femoral hernia occurs through the femoral ring and is more common in females than in males. It begins as a plug of fat in the femoral canal that enlarges and gradually pulls the peritoneum, and almost inevitably the urinary bladder, into the sac. There is a high incidence of incarceration and strangulation with this type of hernia.

UMBILICAL HERNIA. Umbilical herniation in the adult is more common in women and is due to increased abdominal pressure. It usually occurs in obese clients and in multiparous women.

INCISIONAL OR VENTRAL HERNIA. The incisional or ventral hernia occurs at the site of a previous surgical incision that has healed inadequately because of a postoperative problem, such as infection, inadequate nutrition, extreme distention, or obesity.

Outcome Management

Medical Management

Hernias that are not strangulated or incarcerated can be mechanically reduced. A truss, a firm pad held in place by a belt, also can be used to keep the hernia reduced. The pad is placed over the hernia after it has been reduced and is left in place to prevent the hernia from recurring. The client is taught to apply the truss daily before arising. The client should carefully inspect the skin under the truss for any manifestation of breakdown.

Surgical Management

A hernia repair is performed using a small incision directly over the weakened area. The intestine is then returned to the perineal cavity, the hernia sac is excised, and the muscle is closed tightly over the area. Hernias in the inguinal region are usually repaired with the use of

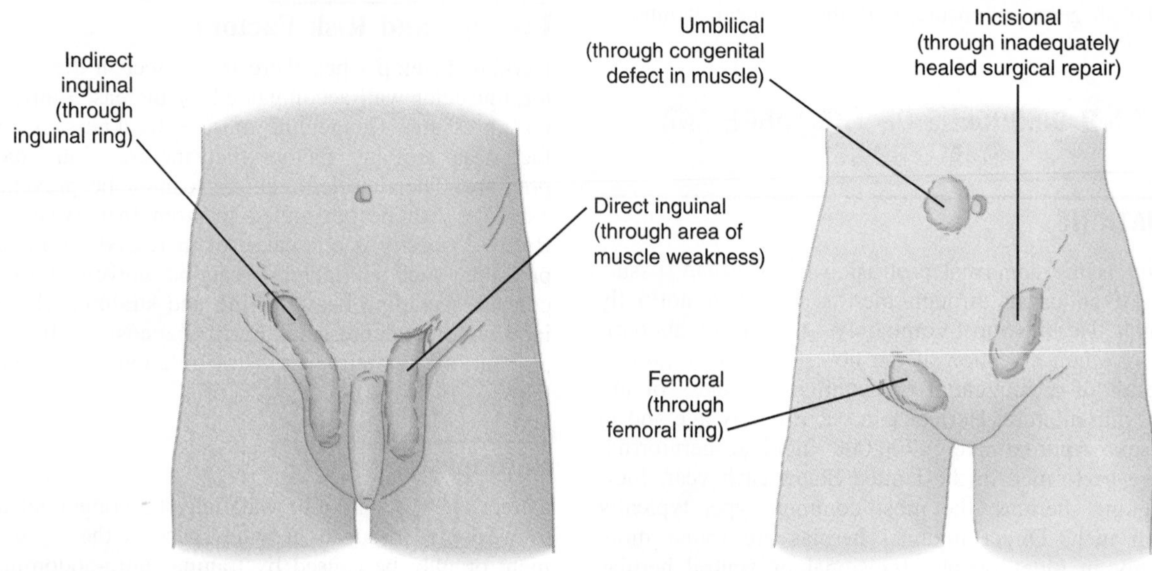

FIGURE 33–8 Common types of herniation.

spinal or local anesthesia. Most hernia repairs are now performed as outpatient procedures. Laparoscopic extraperitoneal (LEP) herniorrhaphy is a newer technique that results in higher success rates with less recurrence, less pain, and shorter postoperative recovery periods.

Some repairs are difficult because there is insufficient muscle mass to keep the intestines in place. In this case, mesh grafts are used to reinforce the area of herniation. Clients with difficult repairs are usually hospitalized for 1 to 2 days to receive prophylactic antibiotics.

Nursing Management of the Surgical Client

Make certain the client voids after hernia surgery, because urinary retention is a common problem, especially in males. Return the client to a general diet as soon as he or she tolerates food. When general anesthesia is used, postoperative progress is slower. Assure the client that during the immediate postoperative period, the hernia will not recur. Some clients hesitate to become active because of this fear. The client should be told not to engage in any lifting for 4 to 6 weeks after surgery. Obese clients progress more slowly, heal more slowly, and may need more encouragement to participate in postoperative activities.

Following an inguinal hernia repair, an ice pack is usually applied to the incisional area to control pain and reduce swelling. In males, the scrotal area should be carefully assessed for swelling. An ice pack also can be applied to the scrotal area. To reduce scrotal swelling, position the client so as to elevate the scrotum and have the client wear a scrotal support when out of bed.

DIVERTICULAR DISEASE

Diverticular disease refers to two disorders, diverticulosis and diverticulitis. A *diverticulum* is a blind outpouching or herniation of intestinal mucosa through the muscular coat of the large intestine, usually the sigmoid colon. *Diverticulosis* is the presence of non-inflamed diverticula. *Diverticulitis* is inflammation of a diverticulum. Diverticular disease is common in men and women older than 45 years and in the obese. It is present in approximately one third of the population older than 60 years.

Etiology and Risk Factors

Low-fiber diets have been implicated in the development of diverticula, because such diets decrease bulk in the stool and predispose to constipation. In the presence of muscle weakness in the bowel, this increase in intraluminal pressure can lead to the formation of diverticula.

Diverticulitis occurs when undigested food blocks the diverticulum, leading to a decrease in blood supply to the area and predisposing the bowel to invasion of bacteria into the diverticulum.

Pathophysiology

Diverticula have a narrow neck like that of a flask that communicates with the bowel lumen. Weak points in the bowel musculature exist where branches of the blood vessels penetrate the colonic wall. These weak points create areas for bowel protrusion when there is increased intraluminal pressure. Diverticula frequently develop in the sigmoid colon because of the high pressures required in this area to move the stool into the rectum.

Diverticulitis may be acute or chronic. If the diverticulum is not infected, it causes few problems. However, when fecaliths do not liquify and drain from the diverticulum, they may become trapped, causing irritation and inflammation (diverticulitis). The inflamed area becomes congested with blood and may bleed or perforate. Chronic diverticulitis results in increased scarring and eventual narrowing of the bowel lumen, potentially causing obstruction.

Clinical Manifestations

The manifestations of diverticulitis depend on the extent of the inflammation and the site of occurrence. Discomfort consists of dull, episodic or steady, left quadrant or midabdominal pain. Assessment also reveals alteration in bowel habits (constipation, diarrhea, or both), increased flatus, anorexia, and low-grade fever. The inflammatory process usually subsides within several weeks. If the infection penetrates the pelvic floor or retroperitoneal tissues, abscesses may result. Extension of the inflammation to adjacent organs can lead to fistulas of the bladder or vagina and peritonitis. Repeated inflammation can result in narrowing and obstruction of the bowel.

Rectal bleeding occurs in about 15% of clients. Stools also may contain mucus. Urinary frequency can occur if the inflammation is in the proximity of the bladder. Straining, coughing, or lifting causes an increase in intra-abdominal pressure and manifestations such as diarrhea, constipation, pain, mucus and flatus. The clinician may palpate a tender mass on digital rectal examinations.

Outcome Management

Medical Management

Asymptomatic diverticular disease requires no specific therapy other than diet modification. Mild disease can be treated by adherence to a high-fiber diet and prevention of constipation with bran and bulk laxatives (hydrophilic colloids). Advise clients to notify the physician of any change in bowel movement pattern (constipation or diarrhea) or character (presence of mucus or blood), or if fever, abdominal pain, or urinary manifestations develop.

Diverticulitis may be treated conservatively with medical intervention by allowing the colon to rest. Clients with acute diverticulitis are assigned to NPO status, may have an NG tube, and receive parenteral fluids and antibiotics until pain, inflammation, and temperature decrease. When the acute episode subsides, oral liquids and, later, a progressively more inclusive diet can be added. Nursing care involves the preceding interventions and client teaching about diet changes.

Surgical Management

Surgery is indicated for diverticular disease with complications, such as hemorrhage, obstruction, abscesses, and perforation. Surgical procedures usually involve ligation and removal of the sac or resection of involved bowel if there are complications. With abscess or obstruction, the surgeon performs a colon resection with a temporary colostomy, which is left in place until the client's condition improves. For some clients, the temporary colostomy alone allows the bowel to rest and heal. For nursing care, see the earlier discussion of bowel resection.

MECKEL'S DIVERTICULUM

Meckel's diverticulum, an outpouching of the bowel, is a vestige of embryonic development found on the ileum within 10 cm of the cecum. The pouch may be lined with gastric mucosa or may contain pancreatic tissue. The gastric mucosal lining sometimes ulcerates and bleeds or perforates. In addition, the diverticulum may become inflamed and may mimic appendicitis. Meckel's diverticulum is sometimes attached to the umbilicus by a fibrous band and may be the focus around which the bowel twists, causing obstruction. Treatment involves surgical excision of the diverticulum.

OBSTRUCTION

Partial or complete impairment of the forward flow of intestinal contents is known as an intestinal obstruction. Approximately 90% of bowel obstructions occur in the small bowel, especially in the ileum, which is the narrowest segment. Obstructions of the small intestine are a common surgical emergency. Obstruction produces nausea, vomiting, dehydration, and severe pain. Intestinal obstruction has a high mortality rate if it is not diagnosed and treated within 24 hours.

Etiology and Risk Factors

Obstruction of the small intestine may be caused by narrowing of the intestinal lumen due to inflammation, neoplasms, adhesions, hernia, volvulus, intussusception, food blockage, or compression from outside the intestine. Paralytic ileus (see later discussion), vascular problems such as mesenteric embolus and thrombus, and hypokalemia from diuretics or antihypertensive agents also may result in small bowel obstructions. Lobar pneumonia, peritonitis, and pancreatitis frequently produce an ileus (see later discussion) of infectious origin.

Cancer accounts for approximately 80% of obstructions of the large intestine, most occurring in the sigmoid colon. Other causes are diverticulitis, ulcerative colitis, and previous abdominal surgery. Factors causing intestinal obstructions may be mechanical, neurogenic, or vascular.

Mechanical Factors

ADHESIONS. Adhesions are probably the most common cause of obstruction in both the small and large intestines. Adhesions form after abdominal surgery, and for unknown reasons, some clients have massive adhesions. Irritants that remain in the abdomen following surgical procedures enhance the formation of adhesions. These fibrous bands of scar tissue can become looped over a portion of the bowel. The loops can then become either the focus around which the bowel can twist (*volvulus*) (Fig. 33–9) or the band that mechanically obstructs

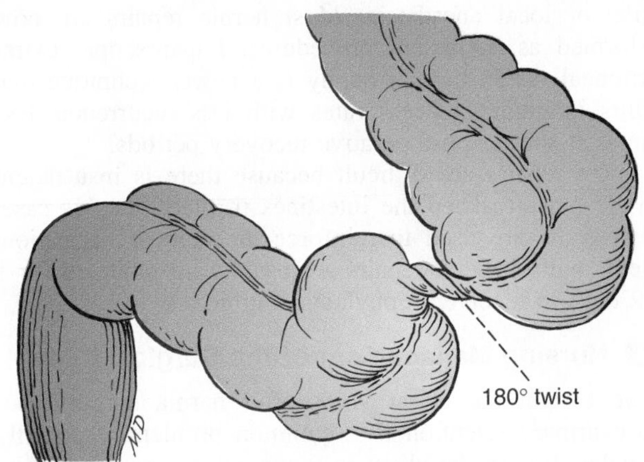

FIGURE 33–9 Volvulus. Intestine twists at least 180 degrees, causing obstruction and ischemia.

the bowel by external pressure. The presence of multiple adhesions increases the risk of obstruction.

HERNIA. An incarcerated hernia may or may not cause obstruction, depending on the size of the hernial ring. However, the potential for obstruction is always present in any hernia. A strangulated hernia is always obstructed, because the bowel cannot function when its blood supply is cut off.

VOLVULUS. Volvulus is a twisting of the bowel that commonly occurs about a stationary focus (e.g., tumor or Meckel's diverticulum) in the abdominal cavity (see Fig. 33–9). It can cause infarction of the bowel and can occur in either the large or small bowel. Volvulus can sometimes be corrected without surgical intervention. Successful decompression of the bowel with a long tube (Cantor or Miller-Abbott tube) releases pressure against the proximal end of the loop, thus allowing a small bowel volvulus to relax.

INTUSSUSCEPTION. *Intussusception*, which sometimes complicates IBD, is a telescoping of the bowel (slipping of a section of bowel into an adjacent section) (Fig. 33–10). The condition is often associated with tumor of the large bowel. Peristaltic action telescopes the proximal bowel into the bowel distal to it. Intramural lesions often cause intussusception.

CANCERS. In the large bowel, cancer is the chief cause of obstruction. Carcinogenesis is slow and, because of the large lumen of the bowel, may become advanced before a fecal mass lodges at the constricted site and

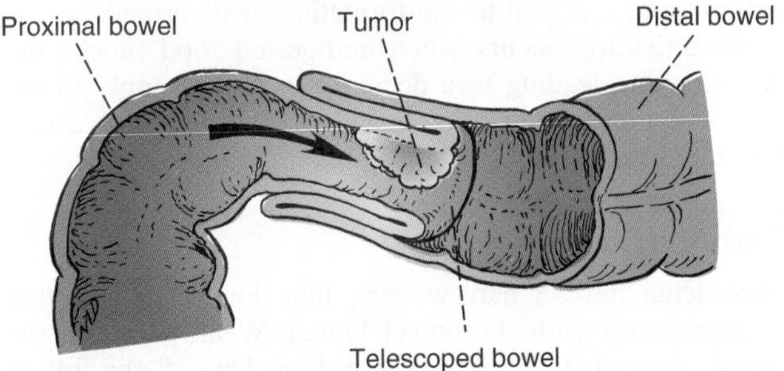

FIGURE 33–10 Intussusception. A portion of bowel telescopes into adjacent (usually distal) bowel.

precipitates an acute obstructive process. In the small bowel, obstructive manifestations are frequently the first indication of a tumor. Even though the lumen of the small bowel is smaller, manifestations do not appear early in the process because the intestinal contents are liquid.

Neurogenic Factors

An *adynamic* (or functional) obstruction, sometimes called a *paralytic ileus*, is caused by lack of peristaltic activity. Paralytic ileus commonly occurs after abdominal surgery. The bowel ceases to function for a few hours to several days. Extensive surgical procedures in the bowel and in the retroperitoneal area may cause a postoperative neurogenic problem. Treatment involves aspiration of secretions by NG suction until the bowel begins to function.

Vascular Factors

When the blood supply to any part of the body is interrupted, the part ceases to function, and pain occurs. Blood is supplied to the bowel by way of the celiac and superior and inferior mesenteric arteries. These vessels have anastomotic intercommunications at the head of the pancreas and along the transverse bowel. Obstruction of blood flow can arise as a result of complete occlusion (mesenteric infarction) or partial occlusion (abdominal angina).

COMPLETE OCCLUSION (MESENTERIC INFARCTION). Any occlusion of arterial blood supply to the bowel, as in mesenteric thrombosis, effectively stops bowel function. The usual cause is an embolus. An acute occlusion, at its onset, causes intense abdominal pain. Usually, there are no manifestations of advanced intestinal obstruction because the pain results from ischemic tissue rather than from obstruction. As the process advances, fever, leukocytosis, shock, and other manifestations of bowel gangrene appear. Acute mesenteric obstruction constitutes a surgical emergency and carries a high mortality rate (approximately 75%). Surgical intervention must be initiated early. Sometimes, an embolectomy can restore circulation. The surgeon also must resect necrotic (dead) segments of the bowel.

PARTIAL OCCLUSION (ABDOMINAL ANGINA). Abdominal angina usually results from atherosclerosis of the mesenteric arteries. It is a common, although often asymptomatic, problem, being found in 33% of routine autopsies. Because there is a greater need for oxygenation during the digestive process, pain may develop 15 to 30 minutes after eating in a client with abdominal angina. Initially, pain may occur only after ingestion of a large meal. However, as the arterial process extends, it may occur even after a small meal, and eventually, the pain becomes almost continuous.

Manifestations arise only when interruption of blood supply is sufficient to compromise bowel function. At this time, in addition to pain after eating, assessment reveals a change in bowel habits, nausea and vomiting, and weight loss due to the client's restriction of intake to avoid the discomfort of eating. Vascular or bypass grafts can sometimes improve the blood supply to the affected portion of the bowel.

Pathophysiology

Normally, 7 to 8 L of electrolyte-rich fluid is secreted by the bowel, and most of the fluid is reabsorbed. When the bowel is obstructed, this fluid is partially retained within the bowel and partially eliminated by vomiting, causing severe reduction in circulating blood volume, which results in hypotension, hypovolemic shock, and diminished renal and cerebral blood flow. Because fluid is lost but blood cells are not, hematocrit and hemoglobin values rise, thus increasing the potential for vascular occlusive disorders, such as coronary, cerebral, and mesenteric thromboses.

For instance, with the onset of an obstruction, fluids and air collect proximal to the site of the problem, causing distention. Manifestations occur sooner and are more intense in a small bowel blockage because the small bowel is narrower and normally more active. The large volume of secretions from the small bowel adds to the distention. The only significant secretion from the large bowel is mucus.

Distention causes a temporary increase in peristalsis as the bowel attempts to force the material through the obstructed area. Within a few hours, the increased peristalsis ends and the bowel becomes flaccid, thus reducing pressure within the lumen and slowing the process caused by the obstruction. Greater pressure within the bowel reduces its absorptive ability, which increases the fluid retention still further. Soon the intraluminal pressure reduces venous return, increasing venous pressure, congestion, and vessel fragility. This process, in turn, raises capillary permeability and allows plasma to extravasate (escape) into the bowel lumen and the peritoneal cavity. The bowel wall becomes permeable to bacteria, and bowel organisms enter the peritoneal cavity. Rising pressure in the bowel wall soon slows arterial blood flow, causing necrosis and, in some cases, toxemia and peritonitis.

Strangulation of the bowel results in decreased arterial blood supply. Necrosis and perforation may force the intestinal contents into the peritoneal cavity, causing peritonitis. Bacteria proliferate in the strangulated bowel and may form endotoxins. When the endotoxins are released into the peritoneal cavity or systemic circulation, there is rapid circulatory collapse with endotoxic shock, accounting for the high mortality rate associated with this condition. These complications are especially likely to occur in older adults, who tend to have atherosclerotic narrowing of these vessels, making thrombosis more likely.

Clinical Manifestations

Manifestations of intestinal obstruction depend on the level and length of bowel involved, the extent to which the obstruction interferes with blood supply, the completeness of the obstruction, and the type of lesion producing the obstruction. Local changes in the bowel wall include congestion, fragility, reduced circulation, and increased pressure. Increased pressure leads to reverse peristalsis, producing vomiting that helps prevent overdistention of the bowel. These local effects result from (1) loss of fluids, electrolytes, and plasma, (2) bacterial proliferation, and (3) perforation. Systemic effects include a reduction in extracellular fluid and circulating blood volume, toxemia, and peritonitis.

The client with small bowel obstruction typically experiences abdominal pain in rhythmically recurring waves. The pain results from distention and the small intestine's peristaltic efforts to push its contents past the obstruction. Small intestinal pain is felt in the upper and midabdomen, whereas colonic pain is experienced in the lower abdomen. Soon after the small intestine becomes distended, the peristaltic waves are visible, accompanied by high-pitched tinkling sounds. The client usually becomes nauseated and vomits, bringing some relief from the pain if the obstruction is high or proximal to the ileum.

If the obstruction is distal to the ileum, vomiting fails to empty the bowel completely, allowing the accumulation of fluids, residue, and gases. As the muscles become atonic, loops of small bowel dilate, compounding the problem of distention. Eventually, severe distention may raise the diaphragm, thereby inhibiting respirations. Hypoxia (due to inadequate respirations, decreased circulating blood volume, and hypotension) often develops. Vomiting is more severe if the obstruction is located high in the small bowel. At first, vomitus is composed of semidigested food and chyme; later, it becomes watery and contains bile. Finally, the client vomits dark fecal material, the result of bacterial growth in the fluid that has stagnated in the obstructed bowel.

When the colon is obstructed, the competent ileocecal valve prevents regurgitation (and vomiting), and pressure within the lumen increases, resulting in distention. The cecum may perforate. Obstruction of the colon results in altered bowel habits, lower abdominal pain, a desire to defecate, distention, and borborygmi. In the presence of an incompetent ileocecal valve, distention progresses to the small intestine. Vomiting that accompanies large intestine obstruction is a very late manifestation, and occurs only from a distended small intestine.

Clients with vomiting may experience severe fluid and electrolyte imbalances. They lose not only water but also sodium, chloride, potassium, and bicarbonate. The result is an acute extracellular volume deficit (dehydration), which in turn lowers the circulating blood volume. Hydrogen ion imbalances frequently occur in intestinal obstructions, with metabolic acidosis being the most common problem.

Specific diagnostic tests for possible bowel obstruction consist of a plain x-ray film, which shows gas shadows, barium or radiopaque x-ray studies, and complete blood studies. Increased hemoglobin and hematocrit values may indicate dehydration. Leukocytosis may point to a strangulated bowel. A decrease in sodium, potassium, and chloride levels and a rise in nonprotein nitrogen and blood urea nitrogen (BUN) levels may indicate small bowel obstruction.

Outcome Management

Medical Management

Decompress the Bowel

The major treatment for an intestinal obstruction is the insertion of an intestinal tube (see Chapter 31). Often, an intestinal tube both decompresses the bowel and breaks up the obstruction.

In adynamic ileus, the best intervention is bowel rest and prevention of distention by gastric suction. Medications are not effective in stimulating bowel activity. The bowel will respond when it recovers completely from the effects of obstruction.

Nursing Management of the Medical Client

Assessment

Obtain a complete history of the onset of manifestations, eating patterns, food tolerance, vomiting episodes, stools (number per day and appearance), distention, and factors that increase or decrease pain.

During physical assessment, note abdominal distention, quality of bowel sounds, presence and extent of dehydration, and manifestations of abdominal pain, such as muscle guarding. A lack of bowel sounds indicates peritoneal irritation or adynamic ileus. Usually, in the case of bowel obstruction, auscultation reveals high-pitched peristaltic rushes with high, metallic tinkling sounds.

Diagnosis, Outcomes, Interventions

Fluid Volume Deficit. A priority nursing diagnosis for the client with an intestinal obstruction is *Fluid Volume Deficit related to vomiting, decreased intestinal reabsorption of fluid, and decreased intestinal secretions.*

Outcomes. The client maintains fluid balance, as evidenced by balanced intake and output, no manifestations of dehydration, and blood pressure within the client's normal range.

Interventions

Maintain Fluid Balance. Maintain good fluid balance in the client with an obstruction by carefully replacing fluids and electrolytes. Administer parenteral fluids with sodium chloride, bicarbonate, and potassium added as ordered.

Decompress the Bowel. An intestinal tube is inserted and attached to suction to relieve the vomiting and distention. If the obstruction is not mechanical, an intestinal tube can achieve decompression. If the obstruction is due to adhesions, hernia, or tumors, the tube stops at the point of obstruction and keeps the bowel decompressed above the obstruction.

Note the progress of an intestinal tube, the amount and type of drainage, and whether or not relief of distention and nausea occurs. Assess and measure drainage from the intestinal tube; document color, odor, consistency, and volume. Inform the physician of blood levels of sodium, potassium, and bicarbonate, and the pH of the blood, all of which reflect fluid and electrolyte balance.

Provide Discharge Teaching. For dismissal following medical resolution of the obstruction, the client needs to learn ways to prevent recurrence and to maintain bowel elimination. The client must be seen by a primary health care provider at intervals after the obstruction is relieved to confirm that it has not recurred. The client's nutritional status also should be monitored to ensure that adequate nutrition is maintained.

Evaluation

Once the obstruction is relieved medically, bowel function should return to normal within a matter of days. If the obstruction cannot be relieved medically, surgery is required.

Surgical Management

If intestinal intubation does not relieve the obstruction, surgery is the only remaining option. The major objective in treating bowel obstruction is to relieve the cause and thus eliminate the problem. However, the cause is not always immediately obvious. Diagnosis of the cause of the acute abdominal condition may be difficult and commonly can be made only during surgery. Document specific observations to aid in the diagnosis.

In most vascular and mechanical obstructions, surgical excision of the cause is the only intervention. Surgery relieves the obstruction and removes any ischemic bowel. Relieving the obstruction should reestablish bowel patency. The type of surgery depends on the location and type of obstruction. The surgeon may perform bowel resection, colostomy, or a bypass procedure.

Nursing Management of the Surgical Client

Assessment of the surgical client is the same as assessment of the medical client. In addition, routine preoperative and postoperative assessments are required. Additional nursing interventions are the same as those discussed for other GI procedures.

IRRITABLE BOWEL SYNDROME

Irritable bowel syndrome (IBS) is a functional disorder of motility in the intestines. There is no organic disease or anatomic abnormality. Other descriptive names for this condition are: spastic colon, irritable colon, nervous indigestion, spastic colitis, intestinal neurosis, and laxative or cathartic "colitis." IBS is the most common gastrointestinal disorder in Western society, accounting for 50% of subspecialty referrals. It is more common in women than men and occurs during middle age. It is estimated to affect 17% to 20% of the American population.

Etiology and Risk Factors

Clients at risk for IBS are those who consume diets high in fat, fresh fruits, gas-producing foods, carbonated beverages, and alcohol. Also at risk are clients who smoke, are lactose intolerant, have high stress in their lives, or complain of alterations in sleep and rest.

Health promotion strategies are to instruct clients to consume a high fiber, low-fat, well-balanced diet that avoids problematic foods and carbonated beverages. Also encourage clients to reduce stress, limit smoking and alcohol consumption, engage in regular exercise, and get 8 hours of sleep each night. To promote health maintenance, advise clients to stop smoking and to follow diet and fluid recommendations previously described. Encourage clients to practice stress relaxation techniques. Health restoration actions are to administer sedative and antispasmodic medications. Encourage clients to follow diet, exercise, and relaxation regimens and to increase fiber in their diets.

Pathophysiology

IBS appears to be a disorder of gastrointestinal motility. Motility may be altered by any number of factors, including diet and emotions. The alteration in motility can cause diarrhea, constipation, or alternating diarrhea and constipation. The structure of the bowel mucosa is not changed, although the disease continues whenever the client is exposed to the causative agents. Causative agents vary among clients; however, most clients can clearly identify them.

Clinical Manifestations

The client with IBS is usually found to have some combination of the following manifestations: abdominal pain, altered bowel function, constipation or diarrhea, hypersecretion of colonic mucus, dyspeptic manifestations (flatulence, nausea, anorexia), and some level of anxiety or depression. Manifestations vary in intensity. Fiber, fruits, alcohol, and fatigue may aggravate or precipitate manifestations.

Emotional disturbances affect the autonomic nervous system (ANS) and its innervation of the bowel. Disturbances of ANS function probably alter motor activity and bowel transit time. Manifestations may mimic various organic and systemic diseases. Pain may be steady or intermittent, and there may be a dull deep discomfort with sharp cramps in the morning or after eating. The typical pattern consists of lower left quadrant abdominal pain and constipation or diarrhea. There may be tenderness over the sigmoid area.

Diarrhea tends to be the major problem but does not usually occur at night; nocturnal diarrhea tends to be associated with organic disease of the bowel. Examination of the stool reveals mucus but not blood. Eating may aggravate pain and defecation, and passing flatus or stool may provide temporary relief. Spastic contractions sometimes occur with stools that are small, dry, hard, and pellet-like. Other manifestations are abdominal disturbances such as nausea, distention, dyspepsia, eructation (belching), and borborygmi due to aerophagia (swallowing of air) and decreased gas motility. Anorexia, foul breath, sour stomach, flatulence, and cramps also may be present. Associated behavioral disturbances are anxiety, tension, nervousness, depression, sleep disturbances, weakness, and difficulty concentrating.

Because there are no confirmatory diagnostic tests for or histologic features of IBS, diagnosis generally is made by excluding other diseases. Diagnostic techniques, therefore, must eliminate the possibility that the client has organic GI disease.

Clients older than 50 years in whom IBS is suspected must be carefully evaluated to rule out malignancy and diverticular disease. When functional bowel disease develops, the client usually gives a history of nervousness and emotional disturbance. The client also may be bowel-conscious and a frequent user of cathartics and enemas. Palpation may demonstrate abdominal tenderness, particularly along the course of the colon.

Sigmoidoscopy or colonoscopy may reveal spasm and mucus in the colonic lumen. A barium enema study is usually performed. A complete blood count and stool examination are needed to rule out occult blood, ova, parasites, and pathogenic bacteria.

Outcome Management

Medical Management

ENCOURAGE LIFESTYLE CHANGES

Treatment is supportive. Advise the client to limit responsibilities, seek rest, and adopt measures to reduce stress, such as progressive relaxation, biofeedback, and a regular exercise routine. The client can control manifestations through diet, medication, and regular physical activity. The client must continue with routine follow-up assessment and care.

Administer Medications

Sedative and antispasmodic medications may help the client feel more relaxed. Vegetable mucilages, such as psyllium hydrophilic mucilloid (Metamucil), can increase stool bulk.

Modify Diet

A high-fiber diet helps control IBS through the production of bulkier stools and reduction of tension in the walls of the sigmoid colon. Fiber helps manage both constipation and diarrhea. In constipation, the softer, bulkier, and heavier stools produced by dietary fiber tend to decrease transit time. In diarrhea, the fiber diet helps absorb water, giving form to the stool and increasing transit time.

Sources of fiber include unprocessed miller's bran, bran cereals, whole wheat, other whole grains such as brown rice, and fresh vegetables. Clients should drink six to eight 8-oz glasses of water daily, because water helps regulate stool consistency and frequency. If diarrhea is a problem, the client needs to avoid foods that may cause it, such as carbonated beverages, and to drink liquids between meals rather than at mealtime.

Nursing Management of the Medical Client

Reinforce the physician's explanation of the nature of the disorder, the intervention plan, and the prognosis. Make it clear to the client that the bowel responds to stress, foods, and medications. Emphasize the importance of regular hours, nourishing meals, and adequate sleep, exercise, and recreation. Help the client establish a regular bowel routine. Advise the client with diarrhea to limit foods that are gas-producing or irritating and to avoid (1) caffeinated and carbonated beverages, (2) alcohol, (3) foods containing nondigestible carbohydrates, such as beans, and (4) milk and milk products. Provide empathy and support.

For alternative therapeutic interventions, see the Alter-

ALTERNATIVE THERAPY

Alternative Treatments for Irritable Bowel Syndrome

The pathophysiology, incidence, and medical and nursing treatments of irritable bowel syndrome (IBS) have been discussed in this chapter. A number of alternative treatments may be helpful for this condition. *Traditional Chinese medicine* has long been used to treat a variety of gastrointestinal complaints.[2] Herbal formulas are generally administered, being chosen according to the specifics of the diagnostic patterns of traditional Chinese medicine. Most of the literature about such usage appears either in Chinese or Japanese journals or in textbooks of Chinese medicine, some of which are now available in English translations. As the number of English language journals of traditional Chinese medicine increases, articles on disorders such as IBS are appearing.[1]

Results of a randomized, double-blind, placebo-controlled trial appeared in *JAMA* in late 1998. This trial, conducted in Australia, showed that Chinese herbal formulations were able to offer improvement in manifestation management for clients with IBS.[3] Participants, other than those receiving placebos, received herbs for 16 weeks. Interestingly, some experienced relief of symptoms for up to 14 weeks after completing the herb therapy. Also of note is that two groups in the study received herbs: one received a standardized formula for that group, and the second received herbs chosen on the basis of individual traditional Chinese medicine diagnoses. The researchers noted that although there was no significant difference in outcome between the two groups at the end of the treatment period, the group receiving individually prescribed herbs maintained the greatest improvement at the 14-week follow-up.

Peppermint oil, an herbal extract, has also been studied for its use in IBS. A meta-analysis of prior trials showed that there was a significant improvement in IBS manifestations with peppermint oil preparations,[7] but the researchers cautioned that study design flaws make a fully positive conclusion difficult. They judged that further well-designed trials were necessary to determine the true effectiveness of peppermint oil for IBS. A later randomized, double-blind, placebo-controlled trial not included in their analysis concluded that peppermint oil capsules were both effective in treating IBS manifestations and well tolerated.[6]

Another area of research that has shown good results in the treatment of IBS is biofeedback. Also called "psychophysiologic self-regulation," biofeedback is a relaxation training method that gives individuals a greater degree of awareness and control of physiologic function. Usually, computer-based biofeedback equipment is used, which gives immediate feedback to the client as to progress in influencing certain parameters, such as muscle electrical activity and skin temperature. Numerous studies have shown that biofeedback training leads to reduction in IBS manifestation scores, even in cases refractory to medical therapy.[5, 8]

Other similar interventions have utilized variously psychotherapy, stress management, and relaxation exercises, often in combination. As many as two thirds of participants in some studies achieved some relief of their IBS manifestations.[4, 9]

References

1. Bean, J. (1999). Irritable bowel syndrome. *California Journal of Oriental Medicine, 10*(2), 30–34.
2. Bensky, D., & Barolet, R. (1990). *Chinese herbal medicine—formulas and strategies.* Seattle: Eastland Press.
3. Bensoussan, A., et al. (1998). Treatment of irritable bowel syndrome with Chinese herbal medicine—a randomized controlled trial. *Journal of the American Medical Association, 280,* 1585–1589.
4. Guthrie, E., et al. (1991). A controlled trial of psychological treatment for the irritable bowel syndrome. *Gastroenterology, 100,* 739–740.
5. Leahy, A., et al. (1998). Computerised biofeedback games: A new method for teaching stress management and its use in irritable bowel syndrome. *Journal of the Royal College of Physicians of London, 32,* 552–556.
6. Lilu, J. H., et al. (1997). Enteric-coated peppermint-oil capsules in the treatment of irritable bowel syndrome: A prospective, randomized trial. *Journal of Gastroenterology, 32,* 765–768.
7. Pittler, M. H., & Ernst, E. (1998). Peppermint oil for irritable bowel syndrome: A critical review and meta-analysis. *The American Journal of Gastroenterology, 93,* 1131–1135.
8. Schwarz, S. P., et al. (1990). Behaviorally treated irritable bowel syndrome. A four-year follow-up. *Behavioral Research and Therapy, 28,* 331–335.
9. Shaw, G., et al. (1991). Stress management for irritable bowel syndrome: A controlled trial. *Digestion, 50,* 36–42.

James Higgy Lerner, RN, LAc, *Private practice of acupuncture, traditional Oriental medicine, and biofeedback*

native Therapy feature, Alternative Treatments for Irritable Bowel syndrome.

DISORDERS OF THE ANORECTAL AREA

The major function of the rectum is to store feces until evacuation. When feces enter the rectum, peristalsis occurs. Many disorders in the rectal area result from constipation or failure to empty the rectum when peristalsis occurs.

At the mucocutaneous border of the anal canal, the mucous membrane changes to skin that has cutaneous somatic nerve endings. Because of this anatomic structure, lesions of the external anal canal are very painful. The two most common manifestations are bleeding and pain. Drainage of mucus and fecal matter and irritation of the skin by organisms can cause intense itching.

Hemorrhoids and skin tags may protrude from the anal opening, and there may be drainage of pus from abscesses. Bright-red blood per rectum usually indicates a lesion of the left colon or anorectal region. Blood on the toilet paper alone usually indicates perianal disease, whereas blood on the surface of a formed stool may suggest a polyp or carcinoma of the left colon or rectum. Blood mixed with the stool suggests inflammatory bowel disease or carcinoma of the proximal colon. Blood in the toilet bowl after the passage of formed stool suggests hemorrhoidal bleeding, the most common source of bright-red blood in the stool. All rectal bleeding must be evaluated by a physician.

HEMORRHOIDS

Hemorrhoids are perianal varicose veins. Hemorrhoids may be internal or external (Fig. 33–11). Internal hemorrhoids are varicosities of the superior hemorrhoidal plexus occurring above the mucocutaneous border (pectinate line); they are covered by mucous membrane and are innervated by the autonomic nervous system. Hemorrhoids are a common disorder, affecting both men and women of any age, but the incidence is higher in people between 20 and 50 years old.

Etiology and Risk Factors

Enlargement of hemorrhoids is caused by increased intra-abdominal pressure. Pregnancy, constipation with prolonged straining, obesity, congestive heart failure, prolonged sitting or standing, and cirrhosis with portal hypertension also raise the incidence of hemorrhoids. Any condition that increases constipation, intra-abdominal pressure, or hemorrhoidal venous pressure raises the risk of development of hemorrhoids. Prevention of constipation through more fiber in the diet is an excellent measure to reduce the risk of hemorrhoids.

Pathophysiology

Tenesmus increases intra-abdominal and hemorrhoidal venous pressures, leading to distention of the hemorrhoidal veins. When the rectal ampulla (pouch) is filled with formed stool, venous obstruction is believed to occur. As a result of the repeated and prolonged increase in this pressure and the obstruction, hemorrhoidal veins become permanently dilated. As a result of the distention, thrombosis and bleeding also may occur.

Clinical Manifestations

The major manifestation of external hemorrhoids is an enlarged mass at the anus. Internal hemorrhoids are characterized by bleeding and prolapse (protrusion outside the

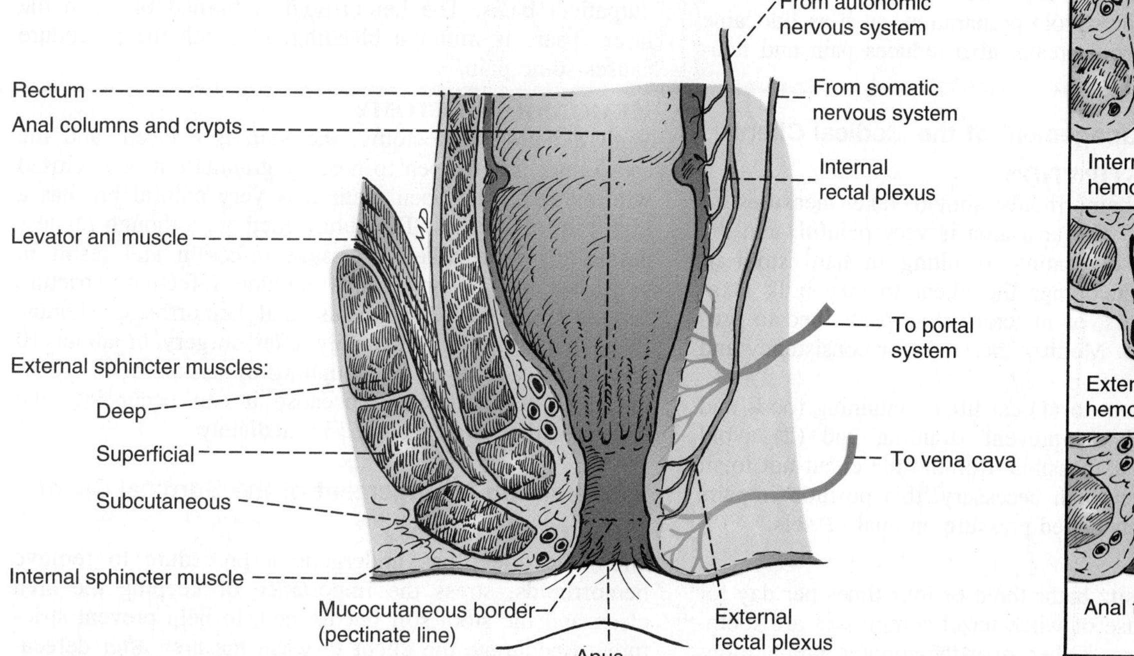

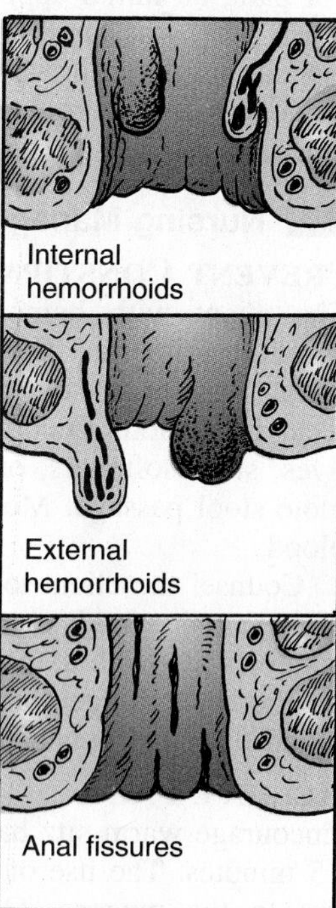

FIGURE 33–11 Structure of the anus and common disorders: internal hemorrhoids, external hemorrhoids, and anal fissures.

anus). Other manifestations are rectal itching and constipation. Pain may be present if there is associated thrombosis. The blood is bright red and may be seen in the stool or on toilet tissue. A prolapse may occur in severe cases after exercise or after prolonged standing. Hemorrhoids may prolapse during defecation and spontaneously return, or the client may need to replace them manually. In some clients, hemorrhoids are prolapsed at all times.

External hemorrhoids are diagnosed by visual examination; internal hemorrhoids are diagnosed through history, digital palpation, and proctoscopy. Asking the client to strain during assessment causes the veins to enlarge, thus aiding diagnosis.

Complications of hemorrhoids are bleeding, thrombosis, and hemorrhoidal strangulation. Severe bleeding from prolonged trauma to the vein during defecation can cause iron deficiency anemia. Blood oozes or may even spurt out following a bowel movement. Thrombosis within the hemorrhoids can occur at any time and manifests as intense pain. Strangulated hemorrhoids, prolapsed hemorrhoids in which the blood supply is cut off by the anal sphincter, can result in thrombosis when blood within the hemorrhoid clots. Assessment reveals severe pain, extreme edema, and inflammation.

Outcome Management

Medical Management

Medical therapy is used for small, uncomplicated hemorrhoids with mild manifestations.

Prevent Constipation

Dietary changes used to treat constipation include increasing fluids and fiber in the diet. Constipation unrelieved by diet may require use of a stool softener (docusate sodium) or a hydrophilic psyllium preparation (e.g., Metamucil).

Relieve Pain

For pain, an initial application of cold packs, followed by warm sitz baths three or four times a day, should help. A topical anesthetic or steroid preparation, such as lidocaine (Xylocaine) or steroid cream, also reduces pain and itching.

Nursing Management of the Medical Client

Prevent Constipation

The client with hemorrhoids should take measures to avoid constipation. The anal area is very painful, and the client may avoid defecating, resulting in hard stool or fecal impaction. Encourage the client to take bulk laxatives, stool softeners, or mineral oil as prescribed to promote stool passage. Monitor the stool for consistency and blood.

Counsel the client to (1) eat fiber-containing foods and drink ample fluids to prevent straining and (2) avoid laxatives as much as possible. Remind the client not to sit on the toilet longer than necessary; this position impairs blood flow and puts added pressure on anal vessels.

Relieve Pain

Encourage warm sitz baths three or four times per day for 15 minutes. The use of witch hazel compresses are soothing to the mucosa. Other over-the-counter preparations may temporarily relieve pain.

Surgical Management

Several surgical procedures are used to treat hemorrhoids. Most are performed as outpatient or clinic procedures.

Sclerotherapy

Sclerotherapy is performed by the injection of a sclerosing agent (substance that causes formation of scar tissue) between and around the veins. This produces an inflammatory reaction that leads to thrombosis and fibrosis. This procedure can be performed on an outpatient basis but requires one to four injections 5 to 7 days apart. The sclerosing agent can scar the anal canal.

Ligation

Ligation, a common procedure for internal hemorrhoids, is performed in the office setting. The client can usually resume normal activities immediately after the treatment. Unfortunately, the procedure cannot be used for external hemorrhoids and may be only temporarily effective. The surgeon inserts a ligator, a small, double-lumen cylinder with a small rubber band on the inner layer, through an anoscope. The hemorrhoid is then grasped with forceps and pulled through the ligator. The rubber band is placed around the neck of the hemorrhoid. Although bleeding can occur, the most common problem is some pain during ligation. The client takes a bulk laxative after the procedure to avoid local trauma from a hard fecal mass. In 8 to 10 days, the rubber band cuts through the neck of tissue, and the tissue sloughs.

Cryosurgery

Cryosurgery (freezing) of hemorrhoids is performed less commonly today. It is also an outpatient procedure. The freezing of the tissue leads to necrosis and sloughing of the hemorrhoids. The problems associated with this procedure are the prolonged periods of drainage, the amount of foul drainage, the presence of large residual skin tags, and possibly, incomplete destruction of the hemorrhoids.

Laser

Laser removal of hemorrhoids is also is performed on an outpatient basis. The hemorrhoid is burned off with the laser. There is minimal bleeding, although the procedure causes some pain.

Hemorrhoidectomy

With a hemorrhoidectomy, the vein is excised, and the area either is left open to heal by granulation or is closed with sutures. The open method is very painful but has a high rate of success. The suture method, although far less painful, is more likely to cause infection and result in poor healing. Complications include infection, stricture formation as the lesion heals, and hemorrhage. Hemorrhage may occur immediately after surgery or about 10 days later as a result of sloughing of tissue. Also, bleeding may not be evident because it can occur into the rectum without being passed immediately.

Nursing Management of the Surgical Client

Promote Healing

After the client has undergone a procedure to remove hemorrhoids, stress the importance of keeping the area clean and the stool soft but formed, to help prevent strictures. Encourage the client to wash the area after defecation and to pat it dry. Local moist heat, applied with a washcloth or piece of cotton to the anal opening for a few minutes, cleans, soothes, and promotes healing. Never apply heat in the immediate postoperative period because of the increased risk of hemorrhage. Beginning 12 hours after surgery, sitz baths three or four times a day, as the client desires, and after each bowel movement are encouraged. A sanitary napkin is the most convenient perianal dressing if one is required.

Prevent Complications

Postoperative complications requiring nursing assessment include hemorrhage and urinary retention. The proximity of the bladder and tenderness in the area sometimes make urination difficult. Reestablishment of bowel habits is another potential postoperative problem. The client may need instruction on the relationship of proper diet and adequate fluid intake to bowel regularity, the physiology of defecation, and the importance of establishing a regular bowel routine.

Relieve Pain

Postoperative pain can be controlled with parenteral and then oral analgesics. Warn the client to avoid vigorous perianal wiping during the immediate postoperative period. The client is usually given a stool softener and mineral oil to soften and lubricate the first stool. Warn clients that fainting can occur, from pain and vagal stimulation, during the first postprocedure bowel movement.

Pilonidal Cyst

A *pilonidal cyst* occurs at the base of the sacrum, usually contains hair, and becomes infected, forming an abscess and then a sinus tract. It is most common in young adults, especially men. It may result from hairs that penetrate the skin and cause sinus tracts to form. Constant irritation (e.g., from clothing and perspiration from activity) can cause hairs to become embedded and then infected. Acute pain and swelling result, followed by a discharge. Treatment involves surgical excision of the abscess. Healing is slow, and if the infectious process is not completely removed, the condition may recur. The client also may receive antibiotics.

Anal Fissure

An *anal fissure* is an ulceration or tear of the lining of the anal canal, usually the posterior wall, that occurs as a result of excessive tissue stretching and possibly from passage of a hard or large stool. The skin tear is tender and tends to reopen at subsequent defecation.

Chronic fissures are usually secondary to infectious material retained in the anal crypts. Sharp pain accompanies defecation, followed by burning. Severe muscle spasm of the sphincter usually accompanies chronic conditions. The client may try to avoid defecation, aggravating the conditions.

If the acute lesion does not heal with local dilations, cleaning, and control of constipation, the tract can be excised surgically. A chronic fissure usually does not heal spontaneously and requires surgery.

Advise the client to (1) keep the stool soft with psyllium hydrophilic mucilloid (Metamucil), mineral oil, or docusate sodium, as prescribed, (2) have a bowel movement daily, and (3) clean the area after defecation, preferably with warm water. Sitz baths aid healing and may relieve pain. Suppositories with a local anesthetic may relieve constipation.

Anal Fistula

A *fistula* is a sinus tract that develops between two body cavities or between a body cavity and the surface of the body. A rectal fistula is a tract that leads from the anal canal to the skin outside the anus, or from an abscess to either the anal canal or the perianal area. It usually is preceded by an abscess. A fistula may heal over temporarily and then open and drain periodically.

Anal fistula is a chronic condition for which surgery is the only cure. The surgeon excises the tract and cleans the area, leaving it open to heal by granulation. It may heal very slowly and be very painful. Advise the client to keep the area clean, especially after a bowel movement.

Anorectal Abscess

Anorectal abscesses form in several locations. Most abscesses begin as cryptitis, with the formation of cysts that extend through the tubular ducts into the submucosal spaces. They also may originate from abrasions of the local tissues, with entry of a virulent organism. Anal intercourse may also cause a rectal abscess. Treatment involves drainage of the abscess and surgical excision of any associated fistulas. Two stages of surgery may be required to accomplish the needed resection.

Cancer

Carcinoma and melanoma can occur at the anus but are rare, constituting less than 5% of anorectal cancers. They spread by local extension into the perirectal spaces and then to the inguinal nodes. Cancer of the anal canal or lower rectum can coexist with other rectal conditions, and the client may falsely attribute bleeding to a hemorrhoid instead of carcinoma. Anal cancers are more common in blacks and usually occur in clients with preexisting anal and perianal problems, such as fistula.

Bleeding, pain, and tenesmus are characteristic manifestations. The client is usually aware of a lump near the anus that has bled and gradually becomes more and more painful, particularly during or just after a bowel movement. Many cancers are not diagnosed until they are large, and by then the prognosis is poor. Some tumors are treated with radiation and chemotherapy, whereas others may require surgical excision. Surgical intervention involves excision of the anus with an abdominoperineal resection.

Bowel Incontinence

Bowel incontinence may develop in clients as a result of aging, trauma, diabetes, rectal prolapse, or childbirth injuries or a neurogenic cause, such as spina bifida. Clients with cancer in the lower pelvic and rectal areas or with a history of radiation therapy to the rectal region are also at risk for bowel incontinence.

As an aid to promote continence, a new device called an artificial rectal sphincter (ARS) has been used successfully to promote bowel continence in almost all clients except those who have a history of cancer or radiation and who would be unable to activate the pump. The device mimics the natural process of bowel control and elimination.

The ARS consists of three parts: (1) a cuff, placed under the skin to fit around the anal canal for an artificial rectal sphincter, (2) a pressure-regulating balloon, placed in the abdominal wall and filled with liquid such as a contrast agent that can be seen on x-ray, and (3) a control pump, placed in the scrotum or labia to inflate the cuff. The cuff inflates like a balloon to prevent passage of stool and to promote continence. To evacuate the rectum, the client deflates the plastic ring and stool is able to pass through. After a bowel movement, the cuff automatically inflates in 10 minutes.

General or spinal anesthesia is used for surgical implantation of the ARS, and the procedure takes about 1 hour. The bowel is cleaned with antibiotics, laxatives, and enemas (see preparation for bowel surgery).

Postoperatively, the client is given IV antibiotics for several days to prevent infection. The nurse teaches the client how to deflate the cuff for bowel evacuation and monitors the client's bowel patterns as well as for complications such as mechanical failure, infection, and ulceration. If mechanical failure is suspected, manometry is used to measure the closing pressure of the ARS. Client satisfaction has been reported.

(See also the Management and Delegation feature on rectal pouches for clients with diarrhea.)

BLUNT OR PENETRATING TRAUMA

Blunt or penetrating trauma to the abdomen refers to accidental or intentional trauma causing internal injuries. Most blunt abdominal trauma is caused by automobile steering wheel or pedestrian accidents, whereas most penetrating trauma is caused by gunshot wounds or stabbings.

Etiology and Risk Factors

Almost any kind of injury can cause blunt trauma to the abdomen. In automobile accidents, rapid, uncontrolled deceleration is the force that produces the trauma, when the client's body hits the steering wheel or some other object. Penetrating trauma commonly results from gunshot wounds, which cause a great deal of internal damage. Stabbings are the next most common cause of penetrating abdominal wounds, although the wounds are less traumatic.

Trauma is the leading cause of death in adults younger than 40 years and the fifth leading cause of death in all adults. Although not all cases of trauma involve abdominal trauma, abdominal injuries are common with motor vehicle accidents. One method of prevention is wearing seat belts, which could decrease abdominal trauma during accidents.

Pathophysiology

Blunt trauma to the abdomen can cause shearing, crushing, or compressing forces that rupture the bowel and other abdominal structures. Gunshot wounds can damage every structure in the abdomen. The bullets may perforate the stomach or bowel, causing peritonitis and sepsis.

Stab wounds produce less trauma to internal abdominal structures because the abdominal organs have more time to shift out of the way of the penetrating instrument.

Clinical Manifestations

Assessment of the client first involves obtaining a thorough history of the accident so that the extent of blunt trauma can be estimated. For penetrating trauma, careful assessment of the position of entry and possibly exit wounds is vital.

The client may show manifestations of an acute abdomen with either type of trauma. With both injuries, either internal or external hemorrhage may occur. If the bowel is ruptured, manifestations of peritonitis are present. All abdominal drainage is closely assessed for the presence of bowel contents.

Abdominal lavage is commonly used to assess the presence of bleeding in all abdominal wounds. This procedure involves instillation of a crystalloid solution into the peritoneal cavity followed by paracentesis (drainage of contents). Note and record the color and amount of the drainage.

A CT scan of the abdomen is now considered the base assessment of intra-abdominal injury. Angiography, intravenous pyelography (IVP), and other studies may be performed to assess different organs and the degree of trauma suffered.

Outcome Management

Medical Management

If minimal blunt trauma was sustained without severe injury to any abdominal organs, the client may simply be observed for problems once the diagnostic tests have been performed. Penetrating trauma always requires surgical intervention. The major complications of trauma are hemorrhage, shock, peritonitis, and sepsis.

The client's pain is treated conservatively until the severity of trauma has been determined. If the bowel has been ruptured, large doses of IV antibiotics are given to control infection. If hemorrhage and shock are present, IV fluids, colloids, and vasopressors may be used. The client is assigned to NPO status until the abdomen has been assessed and found to be intact.

Surgical Management

The treatment of choice for abdominal trauma with injury is an exploratory laparotomy. Depending on the injury, the surgery may be as simple as a closure of tears or as complex as a bowel resection and even a temporary colostomy.

Nursing Management of the Medical-Surgical Client

Careful assessment of the client's injury is vital. The client often must be prepared for immediate emergency surgery. Prepare the client as quickly as possible, knowing that postoperatively, much more teaching and support will be required.

MANAGEMENT AND DELEGATION

Application and Care of Rectal Pouches and Rectal Tubes

Diarrhea is the rapid movement of fecal matter through the gastrointestinal (GI) tract, resulting in poor absorption of nutrients, water and electrolytes. Because of this rapid transit, the client experiences frequent evacuation of watery, liquid, or unformed stools. The stool in diarrhea is usually alkaline because it contains digestive enzymes. Skin breakdown results if there is prolonged or frequent cutaneous contact. A rectal pouch may be applied to collect feces, to protect the skin from prolonged contact with fecal material, and to prevent subsequent skin breakdown.

You may delegate the application and care of rectal pouches to unlicensed assistive personnel.

Application of Rectal Pouches

Instruct assistive personnel to:

- Wash hands and don gloves.
- Provide privacy for the client.
- Wash and dry the rectal area thoroughly with soap and water.
- Assist the client to a side-lying position, with upper knee drawn to the chest to expose the perineal area.
- Remove the rectal pouch from packaging, and enlarge the opening in the skin barrier with scissors if necessary.
- Remove paper backing from the skin barrier.
- Spread the patient's buttocks, then apply the adhesive backing to the perineal area; apply firm, gentle pressure to ensure adherence.
- Release the buttocks, allowing them to assume a relaxed position.
- Assist the client to a comfortable position, returning the bed to its lowest position.
- Remove gloves and wash hands.

Emptying the Collection Bag

- Wash hands and don gloves.
- Empty the collection bag by opening the cap on the drain and by directing stool into a collection container or bedpan.
- Remove gloves and wash hands.
- Record stool volume per physician's order.

Removing the Rectal Pouch

- Wash hands and don gloves.
- Empty and reseal the collector bag.
- Gently ease the skin barrier away from the client's skin.
- Discard the pouch into an appropriate receptacle.
- Wash and dry the perineal area thoroughly with soap and water.
- Assist the client to a comfortable position, returning the bed to its lowest position.
- Remove gloves and wash hands.

Rectal Tubes

Flatulence (presence of abnormal amounts of gas in the GI tract) may occur any time peristalsis is decreased or absent. Excess gas may lead to a bloated feeling, abdominal distention, and cramping pain. A rectal tube may be inserted and left in place for 20 to 30 minutes to facilitate the client's passage of excessive flatus. You may delegate the skin care and positioning of a client with a rectal tube to unlicensed assistive personnel.

Skin Care and Positioning of a Client with a Rectal Tube

- Wash hands and don gloves.
- Provide privacy for the client.
- Wash the patient's rectal area with soap and water.
- Place a water proof pad under the client's hips and buttocks.
- Assist the patient to a left Sims position.
- Assist the Registered Nurse with insertion of the rectal tube as needed.
- Instruct the client to remain in a side-lying position to prevent dislodgment of the tube.
- Wash hands and don gloves before assisting with removal of the rectal tube after 20 to 30 minutes.
- Wash and dry the perineal area thoroughly with soap and water if needed.
- Assist the client to a comfortable position, returning the bed to its lowest position.
- Remove gloves and wash hands.

Describe findings that are immediately reportable to you for assistive personnel, including any difficulty with application of the rectal pouch, continued complaints of abdominal pain or discomfort by the client, and any areas of skin breakdown.

Verify competence of assistive personnel in performing these tasks during orientation and annually thereafter.

Hilary S. Blackwood, MSN, RN, *Clinician IV, Surgical Nutrition Support, Services, University of Virginia Health System, Charlottesville, Virginia*

Usually, once the injuries and repair have had sufficient time to heal and the infection has been adequately treated, the client returns to the hospital so that the temporary ostomy may be closed and the bowel returned to normal.

Discharge Teaching

Prior to discharge, the client may need education regarding home health care, which may include ostomy care and extensive wound care. The client or significant others may have to learn to change dressings and to care for an open, draining wound. Follow-up care from a visiting nurse may also be required for the administration of antibiotics at home, further ostomy teaching, or wound care for an open draining wound.

CONCLUSIONS

Intestinal disorders are common and may cause problems for the client throughout life if they are not treated promptly and completely. Even with early treatment, many clients require ostomies for treatment of large and small bowel disorders. The resultant body image changes are the focus of nursing interventions to educate the client and facilitate modifications in behavior to promote health and adaptation to the changes.

THINKING CRITICALLY

1. A young man is admitted with an exacerbation of inflammatory bowel disease. He reports frequent watery stools, general weakness, lack of appetite with a loss of 5 lb in a week, and cramping abdominal pain. What nursing history and physical assessment are required? How will his exacerbation be treated?

Factors to Consider. What are the clinical manifestations of inflammatory bowel disease? What are priority nursing interventions?

2. An elderly client has undergone a bowel resection with placement of a temporary transverse colostomy for treatment of colon cancer. He lives with his wife of 25 years. She is very interested in learning how to help her spouse manage care for the stoma and how to change the colostomy bags. What is your priority assessment? What teaching methods should you use to teach the client and his wife?

Factors to Consider. What is the appearance of a healthy stoma and healthy skin around the stoma? What dietary management is important?

3. A young man arrives in the emergency department in a highly anxious state. He has a history of numerous abdominal operations and now eliminates fecal material through a colostomy. He is handsome, appears very thin, and cannot sit still. He has a paper bag which he says contains a gun. He wants to shoot the doctor who did this to him. He wants to be admitted for a revision and asks that his bowel be "reconnected." What is your priority intervention? What psychosocial assessment should you pursue?

Factors to Consider. How is the client coping with his changed body function? What are relationships with others his age, especially women?

BIBLIOGRAPHY

1. American Cancer Society. (2000). *Cancer facts and figures.* Atlanta: Author.
2. Botoman, V., Bonner, G., & Botoman, D. (1998). Management of inflammatory bowel disease. *American Family Physician, 57*(1), 57–68, 71–72.
3. Bradley, M., & Pupiales, M. (1997). Essential elements of ostomy care. *American Journal of Nursing, 97*(7), 38–46.
4. Carlson, E. (1998). Irritable bowel syndrome. *Nurse Practitioner, 23*(1), 82–91.
5. Cavalieri, J., & Franklin, B. (1998). Hereditary nonpolyposis colon cancer. *American Journal of Nursing, 98*(10), 42–43.
6. Climo, M., et al. (1998). Hospital-wide restriction of clindamycin: Effect on the incidence of *Clostridium difficile*-associated diarrhea and cost. *Annals of Internal Medicine, 128,* 989–995.
7. Crohn's & Colitis Foundation. (1998). *Crohn's disease and ulcerative colitis.* New York: Author.
8. Dunn, D. (1997). Common questions about ileoanal reservoirs. *American Journal of Nursing, 97*(11), 67–75.
9. Fathi, J., Isler, J., & Billingham, R. (Eds.). (1999). *Primary care: Office management of common anorectal problems, 26*(1), 1–187.
10. Ferzoco, L., Raptopoulos, V., & Silen, W. (1998). Acute diverticulitis. *New England Journal of Medicine, 338*(21), 1521–1526.
11. Gastrointestinal illness appears to be increasing. (1999). *Infectious Disease News* (On-line). Available: *http://www.slackinc.com.*
12. Gefland, D. (1997). Colorectal cancer: Screening strategies. *Radiology Clinics of North America, 35*(2), 431–438.
13. Giovannucci, E., et al. (1998). Folate: Is there a colon cancer connection? *Annals of Internal Medicine, 129,* 517–524.
14. Glaser, E., & Grogan, L. (1999). Molecular genetics of gastrointestinal malignancies. *Seminars in Oncology Nursing, 15*(1), 3–9.
15. Gruessner, R., & Sharp, H. (1997). Living-related intestinal transplantation: First report of a standardized surgical technique. *Transplantation, 64* 11), 1605–1607.
16. Guyton, A. C., & Hall, J. E. (1996). *Textbook of medical physiology* (9th ed.). Philadelphia: W. B. Saunders.
17. Hansen, M. (1998). *Pathophysiology: Foundations of disease and clinical intervention.* Philadelphia: W. B. Saunders.
18. Held, J. (1997). Caring for a patient with colon cancer. *Nursing, 27*(4), 34–39.
19. Howe, J., & Guillem, J. (1997). The genetics of colorectal cancer. *Surgical Clinics of North America, 77*(1), 175–195.
20. Klonowski, E., & Masoodi, J. (1999). The patient with Crohn's disease. *RN, 62*(3), 32–37.
21. Lehne, R. (1998). *Pharmacology for nursing care* (3rd ed.). Philadelphia: W. B. Saunders.
22. Lerman, C., et al. (1999). Genetic testing in families with hereditary nonpolyposis colon cancer. *Journal of the American Medical Association, 281*(17), 1618–1622.
23. Levin, T., et al. (1999). Predicting advanced proximal colonic neoplasia with screening sigmoidoscopy. *Journal of the American Medical Association, 281*(17), 1611–1617.
24. Mamounas, E., et al. (1997). Future directions in the adjuvant treatment of colon cancer. *Oncology, 11*(9 Suppl 10), 44–47.
25. McCorkle, R., et al. (1996). *Cancer nursing* (2nd ed.). Philadelphia: W. B. Saunders.
26. Moody, F. (1999). *Atlas of ambulatory surgery.* Philadelphia: W. B. Saunders.
27. Newland, J. (1997). Traveler's diarrhea. *American Journal of Nursing, 97*(4), 161–162.
28. Outbreak of *Campylobacter* reported in Oklahoma. (1998). *Infectious Disease News* (On-line). Available: *http://www.slackinc.com.*
29. Pastore, R., Wolff, B., & Hodge, D. (1997). Total abdominal colectomy and ileorectal anastomosis for inflammatory bowel disease. *Diseases of the Colon and Rectum, 40*(12), 1455–2464.
30. Sabiston, D. C., Jr. (1997). *Textbook of surgery* (15th ed.). Philadelphia: W. B. Saunders.
31. Saddler, D., & Ellis, C. (1999). Colorectal cancer. *Seminars in Oncology Nursing, 15*(1), 58–69.
32. Schoemaker, D., et al. (1998). Yearly colonoscopy, liver CT, and chest radiography do not influence 5-year survival of colorectal cancer patients. *Gastroenterology, 114,* 7–14.
33. Warmkessel, J. (1997). Caring for a patient with colon cancer. *Nursing, 27*(4), 34–39.
34. Wellwood, J., et al. (1998). Randomized controlled trial of laparoscopic versus open mesh repair for inguinal hernia: Outcome and cost. *British Medical Journal, 317,* 103–110.
35. Wyngaarden, J. B., et al. (Eds.). (1996). *Cecil textbook of medicine* (20th ed.). Philadelphia: W. B. Saunders.

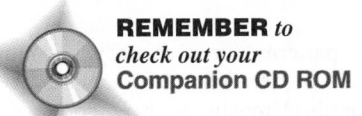

CHAPTER 34

Management of Clients with Urinary Disorders

Francie Bernier

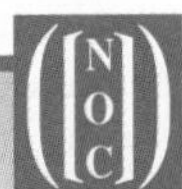

NURSING OUTCOMES CLASSIFICATION (NOC) for Nursing Diagnoses—Clients with Urinary Disorders

Altered Urinary Elimination
Urinary Continence
Urinary Elimination
Effective Management of Therapeutic Regimen
Adherence Behavior
Compliance Behavior
Family Participation in Professional Care
Knowledge: Treatment Regimen
Participation: Health Care Decisions
Risk Control
Symptom Control
Functional Urinary Incontinence
Urinary Continence
Urinary Elimination
Knowledge Deficit
Knowledge: Disease Process
Knowledge: Health Behaviors
Knowledge: Health Resources
Knowledge: Illness Care
Knowledge: Medication
Knowledge: Prescribed Activity
Knowledge: Treatment Procedure
Knowledge: Treatment Regimen
Pain
Comfort Level
Pain Control
Pain: Disruptive Effects
Pain Level
Powerlessness
Depression Control
Depression Level
Family Participation in Professional Care
Health Beliefs
Health Beliefs: Perceived Ability to Perform
Health Beliefs: Perceived Control
Health Beliefs: Perceived Resources
Participation: Health Care Decisions
Reflex Urinary Incontinence
Neurologic Status: Autonomic
Urinary Continence
Urinary Elimination
Risk for Body Image Disturbance
Body Image
Grief Resolution
Psychosocial Adjustment: Life Change
Self-Esteem
Risk for Injury
Risk Control
Risk Detection
Symptom Control
Risk for Impaired Skin Integrity
Nutritional Status
Risk Detection
Tissue Integrity: Skin and Mucous Membranes
Tissue Perfusion: Peripheral
Wound Healing: Primary Intention
Wound Healing: Secondary Intention
Risk for Sexual Dysfunction
Body Image
Role Performance
Self-Esteem
Stress Incontinence
Urinary Continence
Urinary Elimination
Total Incontinence
Tissue Integrity: Skin and Mucous Membranes
Urinary Continence
Urinary Elimination
Urge Incontinence
Tissue Integrity: Skin and Mucous Membranes
Urinary Continence
Urinary Elimination
Urinary Retention
Urinary Continence
Urinary Elimination

Nurses commonly provide the initial assessment, diagnosis, and outcome management of altered urinary elimination and related nursing diagnoses. *Altered urinary elimination* is a nursing diagnosis used for dysfunction involving the urethra, bladder, or ureters. More specific nursing diagnoses include *Stress Incontinence, Reflex Urinary Incontinence, Urge Incontinence, Functional Urinary Incontinence, Total Incontinence,* and *Urinary Retention*. Several additional nursing diagnoses are discussed throughout the chapter.

Because of the personal nature of the urinary system, its proximity to the reproductive system in females, and the shared urinary and reproductive system of males, urinary disorders commonly lead to feelings of shame, isolation, and embarrassment. It is vital that you be sensitive to the psychosocial needs of any client with a urinary disorder.

It is also important to recognize that urinary diagnoses may signal other medical conditions as well. Long-term sequelae or conditions occurring as a consequence of altered urinary elimination may include such problems as impaired kidney function, changes in fluid volume and electrolytes, skin breakdown, changes in quality of life, and other associated conditions.

INFECTIOUS AND INFLAMMATORY DISORDERS

CYSTITIS

The diagnosis of a *urinary tract infection* (UTI) is typically confirmed on the basis of a certain number of microorganisms in the urinary system (usually 10^5 organisms), although manifestations may begin with many fewer organisms than that. The infectious process usually affects the bladder, but the urethra, ureters, and kidneys may be involved. *Cystitis,* the most common type of UTI, is an inflammation of the bladder wall, usually caused by ascending bacteria or obstructive voiding patterns that lead to decreased flow or stasis of urine. *Urethritis*, inflammation of the urethra, may cause the same manifestations as cystitis.

UTI is one of the most common infections treated by primary care providers. Untreated, it has the potential for serious consequences, such as pyelonephritis (inflammation of the kidney) (see Chapter 35) and bacteremia (bacteria in the blood). On rare occasions, complications of a UTI can lead to death.

The prevalence of UTIs is about eight times higher in women than in men, probably because the female urethra is shorter and lies closer to the anal and vaginal openings. This position increases the risk of bacterial contamination of the lower urinary tract. About 6 to 7 million young women see physicians for UTIs each year, second in frequency only to upper respiratory infections.[22] In 5% to 10% of cases, the UTI recurs after initial treatment.

UTIs rarely develop in men before age 50 years because of the length of the male urethra and the antibacterial properties of prostatic fluid. The incidence of UTIs in men rises with age, as does the incidence of prostate disease. This medical problem leads to dysfunctional voiding patterns with incomplete emptying of the bladder. Stasis of urine in the bladder raises the risk of cystitis.

The incidence of UTIs increases during hospitalization, usually from catheterization procedures and possibly from inadequate catheter care. Nosocomial (hospital-acquired) UTIs occur in about 2% of inpatients. About 1% of nosocomial UTIs (5000 each year) become life-threatening.[29]

Etiology and Risk Factors

The most common UTI-causing bacteria are gram-negative organisms found in the intestine. *Escherichia coli* probably causes about 80% of UTIs, and *Klebsiella* causes about 5% of reported UTIs. *Enterobacter* and *Proteus* are found in about 2% of reported cases.[22]

Women with vaginal *candidiasis* commonly complain of UTI manifestations. Other causative organisms, such as *Chlamydia trachomatis, Trichomonas vaginalis, Neisseria gonorrhoeae,* and herpes simplex, may be responsible for UTI manifestations as well. Therefore, ask female clients about any gynecologic manifestations when clients present with potential UTIs.

Besides the shorter urethra and its proximity to the vagina and anus, other risk factors for women may be related to sexual intercourse, pregnancy, poor hygiene, dysfunctional voiding patterns, or a history of female genital mutilation (see Chapter 39). Colonization of the vaginal opening and urethral meatus with *E. coli* is characteristic of women who have recurrent UTIs. Hormonal changes in pregnant and postmenopausal women alter the vaginal pH, change the vaginal flora, and may allow abnormal levels of normal bacteria to grow.

In addition, shrinkage of the mucosal layer of the lower urogenital system of postmenopausal women increases the risk of urethral irritation during intercourse. In fact, sexual intercourse may increase the risk of UTI in all women. The thrusting motion during coitus can push organisms up the urethra and into the bladder, which can lead to cystitis if the woman does not void after intercourse. The term "honeymoon cystitis" is frequently used to describe this phenomenon.

A poorly fitting contraceptive diaphragm or pessary may lead to recurrent UTI as well. Pressure against the urethra may obstruct the flow of urine, leading to irritation and incomplete emptying of the bladder. Spermicides are also associated with increased UTIs. They seem to increase the vaginal pH, alter the normal vaginal flora, and increase colonization of *E. coli.*

In women, synthetic underwear and pantyhose, tight jeans, and wet bathing suits can also foster the development of cystitis. Allergens or irritants—such as feminine hygiene sprays, bubble baths, perfumed toilet paper, sanitary napkins, and soaps—contribute to the development of cystitis in some women.

Indwelling urethral catheters dramatically increase the occurrence of UTIs. Indeed, UTIs are the most common nosocomial infection. Among catheterized clients, the rates for UTIs in most hospitals are well above 50%, with some rates reported as high as 100%. Indwelling catheters can introduce bacteria into the urinary tract, possibly from poor insertion technique, irritation and consequent inflammation of the urethra, and ascension of bacteria along the length of the catheter. The rate of infection rises significantly if the drainage system does not remain closed.

Diabetic clients are at increased risk for UTIs because increasing neuropathy can keep the bladder from emptying completely. Anything that interrupts the integrity of the bladder lining opens the way to possible infection. Loss of integrity of the mucosal lining may be caused by an indwelling catheter, calculus, tumor, or diminished estrogen levels. In addition, anything that contributes to urinary stasis significantly increases the risk of UTI.

In older men, obstructive uropathy, loss of the bactericidal properties of prostatic secretions, poor bladder emptying, and other medical disorders contribute to the development of UTIs. The incidence of UTI in older men is about 15%.

Health promotion and health maintenance strategies are discussed under Nursing Management of the Medical Client.

Pathophysiology

The most common mechanism by which a UTI develops is via ascending and invading bacteria. The organism triggers an inflammatory response in the lining of the urinary tract. This irritation leads to pain, frequent voiding, and other clinical manifestations.

Clinical Manifestations

Any change in a client's voiding habits should alert you to a possible UTI. The most common clinical manifestations of cystitis are burning pain on urination (dysuria), frequency, urgency, voiding in small amounts, an inability to void, incomplete emptying of the bladder, cloudy urine, and hematuria (blood in the urine). Lower back or suprapubic pain may be present as well. Other manifestations may include malaise and abdominal and flank pain related to upper tract infection. Manifestations of ureteral involvement may include abdominal distention, nausea, and diarrhea.

Asymptomatic bacteriuria (bacteria in urine) is seen in about 10% of cases, most often in older adults. The only reported manifestation of asymptomatic bacteriuria in an older client may be a change in the mental status with or without fever.

A urine culture is the most accurate diagnostic tool. Initially, a dipstick test for leukocyte esterase and nitrite activity may detect bacteriuria, allowing for immediate broad-spectrum antibiotic therapy to begin. However, the dipstick test should not be used as the exclusive diagnostic tool for a UTI. Some bacteria, such as enterococci, do not convert from nitrates to positive nitrites. Therefore, a urine culture is essential for all clients with evidence of cystitis or a positive dipstick test. Sensitivity testing can determine which antibiotics the bacteria will respond to. A urine specimen drawn by catheter yields a more accurate test than a voided specimen does.

An area of controversy arises in asymptomatic clients with indwelling urinary catheters and a high bacterial count. Some believe that the UTI should not be treated until the catheter is removed or manifestations develop. Others say that the infection should be treated when a culture is found to grow bacteria. However, most clinicians believe that specimens must be obtained for culture before antibiotics are started.

Traditionally, a bacterial count above 100,000/ml for voided specimens has been considered appropriate for antibiotic intervention. However, symptomatic clients may need treatment even with bacterial counts as low as 1000 to 10,000/ml.

Diagnostic testing, such as an intravenous pyelogram (IVP), voiding cystourethrogram (VCUG), retrograde pyelogram, or cystoscopy, may be used to evaluate clients with recurrent UTIs or clients at risk for strictures from previous interventions that have been used to identify structural abnormalities, stones, tumors, or foreign bodies in the lower urologic tract. The VCUG detects obstructive voiding patterns, as from an enlarged prostate, that increase the client's risk for recurrent cystitis.

Outcome Management

Medical Management

INHIBIT BACTERIAL GROWTH

To promote comfort and decrease complications, broad-spectrum antibiotics typically begin before the culture and sensitivity results are known. Later, on the basis of the sensitivity report, a more specific antibiotic may be prescribed. Fosfomycin (Monurol), a single-dose medication, is commonly used for an initial uncomplicated infection of the lower urinary tract. Single-dose therapy does not suppress the client's normal flora, including altered vaginal flora leading to yeast infections, to the same degree as long-term therapy, and it reduces the development of resistant organisms.[22] Other commonly used pharmacologic agents include urinary antiseptics, sulfonamides, fluoroquinolones, and other antibiotics, such as aztreonam (Azactam), ampicillin (Omnipen), and cephalexin (Keflex). Medications containing azo dyes, such as phenazopyridine (Pyridium), have an anesthetic effect on the urinary tract mucosa and are used to treat the burning sensation often felt with cystitis (Table 34–1).

Simple, acute bacterial cystitis may also be treated with a 3-day course of antibiotic therapy. Treatment failures and recurrences are treated with a 7- to 10-day antibiotic regimen. Some clients may be treated for 14 days if they are medically compromised, such as a hospitalized client with an indwelling catheter or a client with a history of diabetes or immunosuppression.

A client who reports continued manifestations after completing an antibiotic course or who complains of recurrent UTIs should return for a follow-up culture after antibiotic therapy. If the urine is not yet sterile, antibiotic therapy may be continued with the same or another antibiotic, based on the sensitivity report of the repeated culture.

Chronic or recurrent infections are a frustrating problem. Each infection must be treated with antibiotics. Persistent infections may call for suppression to keep the urine sterile. This measure consists of a small dose of antibiotic taken once daily or several times a week. Clients should be educated to avoid self-diagnosis and self-treatment with over-the-counter products, such as phenazopyridine. Each infection necessitates culture and sensitivity testing with specific treatment. The primary caregiver either may prescribe continuous suppression therapy or may continue episodic administration of antibiotics when a UTI recurs.

There is a growing trend to provide self-care for medication administration in clients with chronic infections. For example, women who experience UTIs in relation to sexual activity may receive a prescription for an antibiotic and instructions to take the medication after coitus. Other clients with frequent recurrences are:

- Given a prescription for medication
- Taught to recognize early manifestations of a UTI
- Instructed to begin antibiotic therapy at the first hint of infection
- Reminded to complete the full course of antibiotics even if the manifestations disappear

Treating the client with asymptomatic bacteriuria is yet another problem. Some clinicians suggest that an asymptomatic infection be treated only if intervention is certain to prevent further morbidity or if the client is medically compromised. Others suggest immediate antibiotic treatment to reduce the risk of damage to the upper urinary tract.

MODIFY DIET

Certain foods are known to irritate the bladder, such as caffeine, alcohol, tomatoes, spicy food, chocolate, and

TABLE 34–1 **MEDICATIONS USED TO TREAT CYSTITIS**

Class	Action	Therapeutic Outcome	Adverse Outcome	Dosing
URINARY ANTISEPTICS				
Cinoxacin (Cinobac)	Antibacterial action in urine with little or no systemic action. Effective against *Escherichia coli, Klebsiella, Enterobacter, Pseudomonas mirabilis,* and other gram-negative organisms.	Reduce or eliminate bacteria for treatment of initial, uncomplicated acute UTI. Sometimes used to prevent reinfection with persistent bacteriuria.	Monitor for photosensitivity, GI upset, and rash.	Administer 2–4 times daily P.O. for 7–14 days with meals. Maintain urine output of at least 2500 ml/day. Avoid sunlight. Most antiseptics require acidic urine for best effectiveness. Some antiseptic drugs discolor urine, such as nitrofurantoin (Macrobid).
SULFONAMIDES				
Trimethoprim-sulfamethoxazole (Bactrim, Septra)	Antibacterial action. Effective against *E. coli, Morganella morganii, Pseudomonas mirabilis, Pseudomonas vulgaris, Enterobacter,* and other organisms.	Reduce or eliminate bacteria for treatment of initial, uncomplicated acute UTI. Sometimes the drug is used to treat reinfection or as prophylactic treatment of bacteriuria.	Monitor for photosensitivity, GI upset, and rash.	*Acute UTI:* Administer 2 double-strength (DS) tablets P.O. × 1 or 1 DS tablet P.O. every 12 hours for 3 days. *Persistent UTI or reinfection:* 1 DS tablet P.O. every 12 hours for 7 days. *Prophylaxis:* ½ single strength tablet at bedtime or after intercourse. Give with large amounts of water to maintain urine output >2500 ml. Monitor serum glucose. Avoid sunlight. Most sulfonamides require alkaline urine for best effectiveness. Some may discolor urine, such as sulfisoxazole (Gantrisin).

berries. Cranberry juice and ascorbic acid (vitamin C) have been used to acidify the urine. However, research findings disagree as to whether these remedies adequately reduce the urinary pH and suppress infection. Although cranberry juice can acidify the urine, some commercial products do not contain a high enough concentration of pure juice to reduce the pH. In addition, the effectiveness of some antibiotics, such as nitrofurantoin (Macrodantin), is diminished by acidic urine.

Increase Fluid Intake

To treat and prevent UTI, encourage increased fluid intake, especially water, if the client is not required to restrict fluids. The desired amount is 3 to 4 liters per day (L/day). Research suggests that calculating ½ ounce of fluid per pound of body weight (or dividing body weight in half to find the ounces of fluid needed) is an easy way to individualize fluid intake. Increased fluids flush the urinary system and are important in preventing *urolithiasis* (urinary calculi, or stones) in clients treated with sulfa drugs. Fluids containing alcohol and caffeine should be avoided because they increase mucosal irritation.

Prevent Complications

Broad-spectrum antibiotic therapy may destroy normal flora in the body and allow an overgrowth of opportunistic organisms. On occasion, diarrhea, associated bowel problems, and vaginal candidiasis may develop. Some antibiotics may reduce the effectiveness of oral contraceptives and estrogen, whereas sulfa drugs increase sensitivity to the effects of the sun.

Complications can also occur if the infection is not completely eradicated. An ascending infection can migrate from the bladder to the kidneys, resulting in pyelonephritis. Recurrent pyelonephritis can predispose the client to renal scarring and chronic renal failure if damage to the

TABLE 34–1 MEDICATIONS USED TO TREAT CYSTITIS *Continued*

Class	Action	Therapeutic Outcome	Adverse Outcome	Dosing
FLUOROQUINOLONES				
Ciprofloxacin (Cipro)	Antibacterial action. Effective against Enterobacteriaceae staphylococci, some enterococci, *Pseudomonas aeruginosa.*	Reduce or eliminate bacteria for treatment of complicated UTI or when parenteral treatment is needed. (To prevent organism resistance, use the drug rarely for uncomplicated UTI.)	Monitor for GI upset, dry mouth, and oral and vaginal fungal infections.	Give P.O. every 12 hours for 3 days for uncomplicated UTI and every 12 hours P.O. or IV for 7–10 days for complicated UTI. Avoid aluminum antacids, which may hinder fluoroquinolone absorption. Avoid in pregnancy. Give with large amounts of water to maintain urine output >2500 ml/day.
ANTIBIOTICS				
Aztreonam (Azactam)	Antibacterial action. Effective against *E. coli, Klebsiella, Serratia, Enterobacter, Shigella, Providencia.*	Reduce or eliminate bacteria for treatment of complicated, drug resistant UTI.	Monitor for GI upset and rash.	Give IM or IV every 8–12 hours for 7–14 days. Contraindicated in clients allergic to penicillins and cephalosporins or if creatinine clearance <30 ml/min. Probenecid and furosemide increase effects of aztreonam.
URINARY ANALGESICS				
Phenazopyridine (Pyridium)	Topical analgesic and anesthetic	Relieves pain, itching, burning, urgency, and frequency associated with UTI.	Monitor for GI upset, rash, and blue to purple skin discoloration.	Give P.O. 3 times daily for 2 days. Teach to not self-medicate when manifestations appear. Causes bright red-orange urine that stains clothing. Interferes with urine tests based on color reactions. Avoid in renal insufficiency.

UTI, urinary tract infection; GI, gastrointestinal.

kidneys is severe enough. In clients with a history of recurrent or chronic infections, diagnostic testing is necessary to prevent complications associated with recurrent UTIs.

Nursing Management of the Medical Client

ASSESSMENT

Direct the initial nursing assessment at the history and clinical manifestations, as described earlier, to determine whether the problem is acute or chronic in nature. Also take a gynecologic, sexually transmitted disease (STD), and contraceptive history from female clients. Question male clients about presenting manifestations, and take an STD history.

A key nursing responsibility is to instruct the client about clean-catch urine collection to minimize contamination from surface organisms. Appropriate collection of a clean catch urine specimen for a dipstick test and culture and sensitivity should be included in the assessment. The urine specimen should initially be checked for leukocytes, blood, and nitrites. Color, odor, and clarity should also be evaluated. The urine specimen should then be sent for culture and sensitivity testing. If a client presents with chronic manifestations, additional radiologic diagnostic testing may be ordered to locate the origin of the disease process.

DIAGNOSIS, OUTCOMES, INTERVENTIONS

Altered Urinary Elimination. The primary nursing diagnosis when a client is experiencing problems related to cystitis is *Altered Urinary Elimination related to irritation and inflammation of the bladder mucosa.*

Outcomes. The client will have return of normal voiding habits within 3 days of starting antibiotic treatment, as evidenced by an absence of fever, pain, burning, frequency, and urgency.

Interventions

Inhibit Bacterial Growth. Give adequate instructions to the client regarding antibiotic therapy and dietary and activity restrictions needed during antibiotic therapy. Make sure the client understands the drug, its side effects, and the importance of taking the full course of the drug even after manifestations disappear. Have the client restate the antibiotic instructions by asking questions to ensure that the instructions have been understood.

Modify Diet. Provide information about dietary changes needed to keep the urine acidic and to reduce bladder irritation, such as avoiding alcohol and caffeinated beverages. Caffeine is found in coffee, tea, chocolate, some carbonated beverages, and some over-the-counter medications. Spicy foods and tomatoes are also associated with increased irritation.

Increase Fluid Intake. In an effort to control the urgency and frequency caused by a UTI, clients may limit rather than increase fluid intake. Instruct your client to eliminate fluids that increase urgency and frequency, such as caffeinated beverages, and to increase the intake of other fluids to 3 to 4 L/day to flush the urinary system. To treat infection and prevent recurrence, teach the client how to calculate an appropriate fluid intake: ½ ounce of fluid per pound of body weight per day unless this amount is contraindicated.

Prevent Complications. Tell the client about the increased manifestations that might result from infection of the upper urinary tract and what to do if those manifestations occur. You should maintain a closed urinary drainage system and provide meticulous perineal care with mild soap and water for clients with an indwelling catheter. Keep the catheter bag below the level of the bladder at all times.

Teach Health Promotion Strategies. Encourage the client to engage in health promotion activities to prevent UTIs. For example, encourage a fluid intake of at least 3 L/day, especially of water and acid-ash items to acidify the urine (such as cranberry juice and vitamin C). Advise clients to avoid caffeinated and alcoholic beverages that may irritate the bladder lining.

An important health promotion activity centers on client teaching to prevent recurrence of UTI. Female clients should learn the risks associated with chemical irritants, intercourse, poorly fitted vaginal devices, and the additional risk of lowered estrogen levels associated with menopause. A review of correct hygienic practices should also be included. Alert both male and female clients that STDs can cause manifestations similar to those of a UTI. Inform male clients about obstructive voiding problems, caused by benign prostatic hypertrophy (BPH), that lead to urinary stasis.

Emphasize the importance of increased fluids and avoidance of foods and fluids that increase irritation. Also remind the client to void every 2 to 4 hours during the day (unless the bladder program is planned otherwise) to keep the urinary system flushed. Pregnant women should void every 2 hours.

Encourage women to void before and after coitus. Suggest that sexually active women use positions that minimize pressure on the anterior vaginal wall during intercourse. Also emphasize the need to maintain good perineal hygiene. For example, instruct women to wipe the urinary meatus from front to back. Encourage women who experience frequent UTIs to shower rather than take tub baths, and urge them to avoid bubble baths, salts, and scented feminine hygiene products. Wearing cotton underpants, which are more absorbent and breathable or porous than synthetic undergarments, and avoiding pantyhose with slacks, a practice that can trap moisture in the perineal region, are additional ways to lower the risk of UTI in women.

The application of vaginal estrogen increases circulation to the lower urogenital system and increases the mucosal layer of atrophic tissues commonly seen in postmenopausal women. Since the lower urogenital system is heavily enriched with estrogen receptors before menopause, women should be informed about the need for topical estrogen and systemic estrogen in the postmenopausal period. Using a vaginal lubricant during intercourse is helpful as well.

Health maintenance activities include (1) monitoring pregnant women and older male clients (especially those with BPH) for the presence of UTI, (2) teaching high-risk clients the clinical manifestations of infection, and (3) monitoring clients with an indwelling catheter for the presence of infection. Many postoperative clients receive prophylactic antibiotics while an indwelling catheter is in place.

Finally, clients with a UTI are managed with antibiotics and increased fluid intake. To restore health, clients should be taught ways to prevent recurrence and the importance of taking all antibiotics, followed with repeated cultures and sensitivity testing as ordered.

Pain. Another common nursing diagnosis for clients with cystitis is *Pain related to irritation and inflammation of bladder and urethral mucosa.*

Outcomes. The client will be able to urinate without discomfort within 24 hours after treatment begins and will return to normal voiding habits within 3 days, as evidenced by an absence of pain and burning on urination.

Interventions. Medications prescribed specifically to treat pain, such as phenazopyridine (Pyridium), should be administered. Other comfort measures include forcing fluids to dilute urine and taking a warm sitz bath to decrease urethral smooth muscle spasms. Some clients find a heating pad applied to the suprapubic area helpful in reducing bladder spasms and suprapubic pain.

EVALUATION

After the first 24 hours of treatment, the client should be able to report a reduction in pain, burning, urgency, and frequency. Antibiotic therapy usually brings about complete resolution of irritation and pain within 3 days. If indicated, urine culture specimens should be negative after 1 week of treatment or after the course of antibiotics is completed.

Surgical Management

The need for surgery is rare, and operations are performed only to address structural anomalies that cause repeated infections. Strictures of the bladder neck or urethra are the most common problems requiring surgical intervention. BPH may also be treated surgically (see Chapter 38). Correction of structural abnormalities or obstruction should resolve recurrent UTIs. Nursing care of clients after surgery is discussed under the specific disorder. Chapter 38 describes nursing care of men after surgery for BPH.

Self-Care

Promotion of self-care for a client with a UTI includes recognition of lifestyle changes needed to decrease risk factors, the ability to restate the medication protocol, and return for follow-up urine cultures, if indicated. Explain risk factors for UTIs and health promotion strategies to prevent recurrence. These strategies include increased fluid intake, fluid and diet modifications, voiding every 2 hours, and lifestyle modifications, as previously discussed. Advise the client to seek care if manifestations recur.

Modifications for Elderly Clients

In older people, cystitis may occur more often than in younger people but for different reasons. Such a cause might be immobility, constipation, fecal and urinary incontinence, urinary retention (incomplete voiding), altered mental status, or systemic disease.

In older women, atrophic changes resulting from decreased estrogen affect the vagina and urethra. This alteration causes bladder dysfunction, which may predispose this population to infection.

In older men, BPH is one of the main risk factors for UTIs. BPH becomes more common with increased age. Management of recurrent UTIs in men involves treatment of BPH. Once BPH is treated, the infections should diminish.

When administering medications to older or compromised clients, you must consider their renal and hepatic status. Many drugs used to treat UTIs necessitate that the client have adequate renal and hepatic function, particularly with long-term administration. Also, consider any changes in cardiovascular status that might prevent an increase in fluid intake.

INTERSTITIAL CYSTITIS

Cystitis may be noninfectious or abacterial. One type, interstitial cystitis (IC), is also called painful bladder disease (PBD), Hunner's ulcer, urethral syndrome, pseudomembranous trigonitis, and other names. This greatly underdiagnosed condition involves urgency, frequency, and a painful bladder despite a lack of bacteria in the urine culture. The most severe forms of this disease involve ulcerations and hemorrhages in the bladder wall. The cause of these ulcers is unknown, but the ulcers may stem from a defect in the epithelial molecular layer of the bladder wall.

Etiology and Risk Factors

IC occurs mainly in young women (90% to 95% of all cases), usually white but occasionally African American. The disease is increasing significantly among Jewish women, which may be somehow related to the increase in inflammatory bowel disease associated with autoimmune disorders in this population.[25]

Pathophysiology

IC is a poorly understood disorder with an unclear pathophysiology. It may be a local autoimmune phenomenon. Despite clinical manifestations, the urine is usually sterile. The most current theory seems to be associated with a breakdown in the permeability of the glycosaminoglycan layer of the bladder mucosa, which is usually impermeable to urea and bacteria. This theory has been questioned in some studies, which suggest that the permeability of the bladder in clients with IC is no greater than that in normal people.[25]

Characteristic pathologic changes are found in more severe forms of IC, including nonspecific chronic inflammatory infiltrate, edema, vasodilation, and eventually fibrosis of the submucosa and detrusor layers of the bladder wall. The fibrosis of the submucosa seems to decrease the elasticity of the detrusor muscle, which decreases bladder capacity.

Mast cell infiltrates have been identified in the bladders of clients with IC, particularly in the detrusor layer. Because mast cells are associated with allergic reactions, it is worth noting that about half of clients with IC are reported to have allergies and 30% have inflammatory bowel disease.[25] Finally, another hypothesis is that bacteria are found only in the wall of the bladder and not in the urine.[25]

Clinical Manifestations

The clinical manifestations of IC are tenderness in the area of the bladder trigone during anterior palpation during a vaginal examination, complaints of lower abdominal or pelvic pain, urinary urgency, and frequency (up to 60 times a day), *nocturia* (excessive urination at night), and, in some women, dyspareunia (painful intercourse). Presenting manifestations and their severity vary from client to client. Some women find the disorder debilitating. Manifestations may be present for years and treated as bacterial cystitis before an appropriate diagnosis is made.

The National Institute of Arthritis, Diabetes, Digestive, and Kidney Diseases recommends specific diagnostic criteria for identifying clients with clinical manifestations. These criteria include:

- A detailed client history
- A completed bladder diary
- Urine cytology
- Urodynamic evaluation to determine bladder capacity and evaluate bladder function
- Cystoscopy with the client under anesthesia and with hydrodistention of the bladder
- Bladder biopsy

During cystoscopy and hydrodilation of the bladder, the presence of outpouches in the bladder wall, Hunner's ulcers, and a severely decreased bladder capacity is considered by many physicians to be the clinical diagnostic feature of IC. Others believe that IC may be present even without these findings.

Outcome Management

Medical Management

Reduce Pain

The treatment of IC is controversial, with no single accepted treatment. Anti-inflammatory, antispasmodic, antidepressant, and antihistamine medications and, occasionally, tranquilizers or narcotics may be used.

Pentosan polysulfate sodium (Elmiron) is the newest oral medication of choice. This drug increases the bladder defense mechanism or detoxifies irritants in urine that might break down the bladder lining. The mechanism of action is like heparin, with anticoagulant and antifibrin effects. Relief of manifestations may take up to 3 months.

Other treatments include instillation of a variety of agents into the bladder to promote healing and pain relief, such as sodium oxychlorosene (Clorpactin), silver nitrate, and dimethyl sulfoxide (DMSO). Heparin itself has been instilled in the bladder, initially daily for 3 to 4 months. Therapy is continued three times a week for 3 to 6 months. Some clients may not notice any improvement in manifestations until after the first 2 to 4 months of treatment.[25] All of these treatments are designed to decrease the permeability of the bladder mucosa so that the causative agent has more difficulty penetrating the lining.

Although the mechanism of action is unclear, bacille Calmette-Guérin (BCG) has been effective as an intravesical agent administered weekly. BCG instillations for 6 weeks have led to a decreased need for pain medications, a doubling of cystometric capacity, and sometimes a decrease in client discomfort.[25]

Referrals to centers providing conservative management programs with behavioral intervention, electrical stimulation, and biofeedback to the pelvic floor musculature may also alleviate manifestations of IC. Because of the chronic nature of the disorder, physicians are reluctant to offer narcotics for pain relief. During severe exacerbations, however, narcotics may be appropriate.

Improve Coping

Many clients with IC complain of exhaustion and depression. The exhaustion usually stems from poor sleep patterns caused by nocturnal urgency, frequency, and pain. Depression can result from frustration, exhaustion, chronic pain, and difficulty in obtaining effective medical care.

During the acute phase, these clients may require medications to improve sleep as well as antidepressant therapy to increase coping ability. Referrals to social workers or other health care professionals to improve coping strategies and mental status may be needed. You also may need to refer the client to a center that specializes in treating IC.

Nursing Management of the Medical Client

Reduce Pain

Nurses provide a great deal of education about drug therapy. Many of the medications have a cumulative effect, making long-term therapy necessary for maximal results. You may need to continuously reinforce this point if the client grows frustrated with pharmacologic intervention. You also should counsel the client before narcotic intervention. Because IC is a chronic problem, inform the client about risk factors associated with narcotic drugs.

Improve Coping

Your major responsibility is to support the client through diagnosis and treatment. Because the cause of IC is unclear, few nursing interventions are aimed at prevention. IC is a chronic disorder requiring long-term client support. Clients may need additional psychological counseling to help with stress-related coping strategies. Become familiar with national and local resources for clients with IC or painful bladder disease (Interstitial Cystitis Association), and refer clients as appropriate.

Bladder retraining with conservative management programs can help to reduce clinical manifestations. Teaching clients to void by the clock rather than by urge will gently and slowly increase bladder capacity. Biofeedback-directed pelvic floor exercises teach the client the urge suppression technique. This process decreases episodes of urgency and frequency and promotes control of manifestations. The additional use of transvaginal or transanal electrical stimulation may help to override bladder spasms and can increase the quality of pelvic floor contractions.

Surgical Management

Surgery is rarely used to manage the client with IC. The traditional therapy is hydraulic distention of the bladder, with or without instillation of DMSO to increase the bladder's functional capacity. Clients with severely reduced bladder capacity and incapacitating manifestations may be candidates for a transurethral resection (TUR), laser surgical resection of the lesions, a partial or complete *cystectomy* (resection of the bladder), and *urinary diversion* (surgical rerouting of the normal urinary flow) (see bladder cancer later).[55]

UROSEPSIS

Urosepsis is a gram-negative bacteremia originating in the genitourinary tract. The most common predisposing factor is an indwelling catheter or an untreated UTI in a medically compromised client. Other primary risk factors include immunosuppression therapy and chemotherapy. The most common organism responsible for gram-negative bacteremia is *E. coli,* which has the ability to develop resistant strains.

The pathophysiologic mechanisms of urosepsis are complex and not fully understood. The disorder can lead to septic shock if it is not treated immediately and aggressively (see Chapter 81). The cell wall of the gram-negative bacillus is composed of a lipid-carbohydrate complex. Bacteria release endotoxins, which damage cells. The cells release lysosomes, which further damage tissues and set off the kinins and complement cascade. Cellular metabolism becomes anaerobic, and lactic acidosis develops. Fever is the most common early manifestation; in older adults, however, fever and altered mental status are the first clinical signs.

To prevent sepsis and shock, treatment of gram-negative urosepsis must be instituted right after specimen collection for culture and sensitivity testing. Initial treatment consists of intravenous (IV) aminoglycosides, beta-lactam antibiotics (such as aztreonam), or third-generation cephalosporins until culture results are available. As soon as culture and sensitivity results are available, the antibiotic may be changed if necessary. IV treatment is directed by the status of the client and continued for 3 to 5 days once the client becomes afebrile. Oral antibiotics are continued for the duration of therapy.

URETHRITIS

Urethritis, or inflammation of the urethra, is commonly associated with STDs or sexually transmitted infections (see Chapter 41) and is an associated manifestation of cystitis. The most common causes of urethritis are gonorrhea, chlamydial infection, and other bacterial infections. Among women, common causes also include feminine hygiene sprays, scented toilet paper, sanitary napkins, spermicidal jellies, UTIs, and changes in the vaginal mucosal lining. In short, any irritant that comes into contact with the urethra can cause urethritis.

Exposure to irritants causes the mucosal lining of the urethra to become inflamed. The mucosal lining becomes swollen, painful, red, and irritated. Pus may be produced. *Pyuria*, the presence of pus in the urine, is a common indication of urethritis. Manifestations are similar to those described for cystitis. Frequently, women reveal a history of chemical irritant exposure. Male clients frequently exhibit a urethral discharge.

The diagnosis is often confirmed on the basis of the client's history and clinical manifestations. Culture and sensitivity testing of the urine should be performed, and culture specimens should be obtained to exclude STDs if indicated.

Management of urethritis includes removing the etiologic mechanism. If a microorganism is the cause, administration of systemic and topical antibiotics is essential. Sitz baths and an increased fluid intake are also encouraged. Advise the client to avoid coitus until the manifestations subside or treatment of the STD is completed. The use of lubricants with intercourse decreases irritation in women who have had frequent episodes. Common medications are the same as those used to treat cystitis. The physician may also prescribe topical estrogens for a menopausal woman.

Prevention of urethritis by decreasing exposure to STDs is essential. Inform women about the increased risk of urethritis from spermicides and about the need to avoid feminine hygiene sprays, perfumed toilet paper, and scented sanitary napkins.

URETERITIS

Ureteritis, or inflammation of the ureter, is commonly associated with pyelonephritis (see Chapter 35). Once the kidney infection is treated, ureteral inflammation usually subsides. Chronic pyelonephritis can cause the ureter to become fibrotic and narrowed by strictures, which in turn can continue to foster this condition.

OBSTRUCTIVE DISORDERS

BLADDER CANCER

Most bladder cancers are transitional or papillary tumors in the bladder urothelium. These tumors may infiltrate the bladder wall. Bladder cancer is the most frequent neoplasm of the urinary tract, accounting for about 6% of all cancer cases in men and 2.5% in women. It is rarely seen in adults younger than 40 years of age and occurs most frequently in 50- to 60-year-old adults. Now the fourth most common cancer in men and the eighth most common cancer in women,[1] it affects whites twice as often as blacks. Bladder cancer is more common in people living in urban, industrialized northern states than those living in southern states.[32] In addition, the incidence is higher in people of Jewish descent than in non-Jewish persons. Heredity has not been linked to the development of bladder cancer.

Etiology and Risk Factors

The disease process has several possible causes. There is a strong correlation between cigarette smoking and bladder cancer. Hence, a health promotion and health maintenance strategy is to encourage smokers to stop smoking and to be screened regularly after age 50 years for hematuria and other manifestations of bladder cancer.

Industrial exposure to certain substances, such as aniline dyes, asbestos, and aromatic amines (e.g., benzidine and 2-naphthylamine) may also result in bladder cancer. The latency period of industrial exposure can be as long as 18 to 45 years. Workers in this high-risk group should also be screened regularly after age 50 for hematuria and other manifestations of bladder cancer.

Artificial sweeteners have been weakly linked to the development of bladder cancer. Attempts to connect coffee consumption and bladder cancer have produced contradictory findings because of the increased use of artificial sweeteners and cigarettes associated with coffee consumption. Use of the drug phenacetin has also been debated. Other risk factors may be chronic cystitis, pelvic radiation, and the chemotherapeutic drug cyclophosphamide (Cytoxan).

Clients who have undergone transurethral resection or removal of superficial bladder cancer should return for regular cystoscopic follow-up as a health maintenance and restoration activity. Teaching clients to care for a urinary diversion is a health restoration activity provided by nurses.

Pathophysiology

Bladder cancer appears to result from exposure of the bladder wall to a *carcinogen* (a cancer-causing agent). Cigarette smoking or second-hand smoke may result in carcinogenic metabolites produced by abnormal tryptophan metabolism, with the metabolite excreted in the urine. Cigarette smoke also contains nitrosamines as well as 2-naphthylamine (both carcinogens), which are also excreted in the urine.

Premalignant proliferative changes are often found in the transitional cell layer. These changes are called *dysplasia* and refer to abnormal cell configuration found in several degrees of severity. The extent of dysplasia may be described as mild, moderate, or severe, leading to carcinoma in situ (localized).[44] Most bladder cancers start as papillary or transitional cell tumors and account for 70% of bladder tumors. These tumors are most commonly found in the trigone of the bladder and lateral wall of the bladder.

Staging of a tumor indicates the depth of penetration into the bladder wall and degree of *metastasis*. Staging must be done to determine the treatment modality. Clinical staging includes the results and review of an excretory urogram, cystoscopy, biopsy, and bimanual examination with the client under anesthesia. For evaluation of specific areas of metastasis as well as for staging, chest radiography, lymphangiography, isotope bone scans, computed tomography (CT), and liver function analysis are needed. The most frequently used staging systems are the Jewett-Marshall-Strong System and the tumor-node-metastasis (TNM) classification.[17] The stages refer to the depth of invading tumor found during biopsy (Fig. 34–1).[17]

Metastasis to other organs begins once the invading cancer penetrates the submucosal and muscular layer of the bladder. The invasion progresses through pelvic lymph nodes and spreads to liver, bones, and lungs. As metastasis progresses, it can extend into the rectum, vagina, other pelvic soft tissues, and retroperitoneal structures. The prognostic "dividing line" lies between stages B1 and B2; stage C and D tumors portend a much poorer prognosis. Clients with superficial bladder tumors have a survival rate of 70% after 5 years. Other clients with muscle invasive disease experience tumor recurrence within 18 to 24 months of the diagnosis.[17, 44]

Superficial tumors have a good chance of being eradicated or stabilized; however, recurrence is frequent. Therefore, it is crucial to do follow-up cystoscopic examinations every 3 months for 2 years, with additional cystoscopic examinations every 6 months for 2 years, then yearly.[17, 44] In a study of 114 clients, the interval between the original intervention and recurrence ranged from 3 months to 27 years. Nineteen per cent involved a new tumor of a higher grade, and 22% of the tumors were of a more advanced stage. Most recurrences of superficial tumors represent lesions that can be controlled by transurethral resection.[17, 44]

Clinical Manifestations

Gross painless hematuria is most frequently the first manifestation of bladder cancer, occurring in 85% of all cases. Unfortunately, the bleeding is usually intermittent initially, which may often lead a client to delay seeking health care. As the disease becomes more invasive, the client may experience frequent bladder irritability with dysuria, frequency, and urgency. Frequently, gross hematuria or obstruction in voiding forces the client to seek help. The amount of hematuria does not correlate with stage of disease.

When gross or microscopic hematuria is identified without any known etiologic agent, an extensive evaluation is necessary. Cystoscopy is indicated to identify and visualize the tumor directly and to obtain a biopsy specimen of the lesion for cytologic study. Flow cytometry can be done to examine the deoxyribonucleic acid (DNA) content of the cells in the urine. Bladder washings during cystoscopy produce more accurate specimens compared with a voided specimen. The mechanical action resulting from saline washings enhances tumor shedding, with better-quality specimens sent for cytologic study.

Another examination, IVP, is a dye-enhanced x-ray examination that allows one to evaluate not only the bladder but also the ureters and kidneys. CT, magnetic resonance imaging (MRI), and ultrasonography also may be done to assess the bladder and surrounding structures, such as the rectum or uterus, possible sites of spread. A tumor marker, serum carcinoembryonic antigen (CEA), which is present with adenocarcinomas of the bladder, can also be evaluated.

Outcome Management

Medical Management

The outcome desired with medical management is to eradicate the bladder of transitional or papillary cell carcinoma in situ in the early stages. This is best achieved with alkylating intravesical chemotherapy or BCG instillations, which are the first-line and most common therapies. Advanced cancer that has invaded muscle is usually treated surgically with a radical cystectomy. Radiation therapy is rarely used except for advanced disease or as palliative treatment.

Chemotherapy Administration

Intravesical therapies can be administered for superficial tumors, such as transitional cell, papillary cell, or Stage

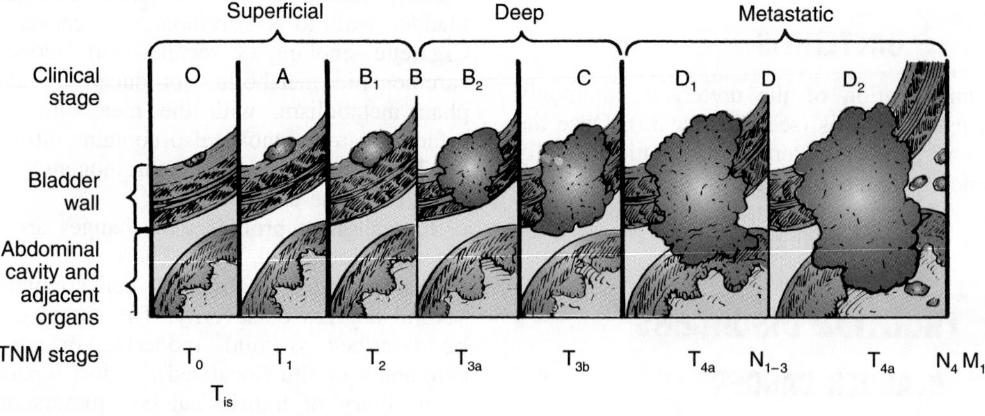

FIGURE 34–1 The Jewett-Marshall-Strong clinical staging of bladder cancer. The diagram shows the degree of tumor infiltration at each stage and compares it with the tumor, node, metastasis (TNM) system. (Adapted from K. Karlowicz (Ed). [1995]. *Urologic nursing: Principles and practice.* Philadelphia: W. B. Saunders.)

0-A tumors. Intravesical BCG therapy appears to be quite successful in treating carcinoma in situ. The best results have been obtained with BCG as an intravesical agent for transitional cell tumors, although it has also been used for papillary tumors, adenocarcinoma, and squamous cell carcinoma.

Usually, BCG is instilled into the bladder through a urethral catheter. The catheter is clamped or removed. The client is directed to retain the fluid for 2 hours, with side-to-side position changes or supine-to-prone changes required every 15 to 30 minutes. Once the 2 hours have passed, the client voids in a sitting position or the catheter is unclamped to allow drainage. Finally, the client is instructed to drink two glasses of water to help flush the bladder. Steroids and ciprofloxacin (Cipro) have sometimes been given after intravesical BCG treatment to prevent recurrence. If two treatments of intravesical BCG have been ineffective, most urologists recommend a cystectomy.

Intravesical instillation of an alkylating chemotherapeutic agent, another common practice, provides concentrated topical treatment with relatively little systemic absorption. Thiotepa, mitomycin, doxorubicin (Adriamycin), and cyclophosphamide (Cytoxan) are all used for low-grade, superficial, papillary tumors. Systemic chemotherapy drugs are used for more advanced disease, to treat the metastasis of the bladder tumor, and to prolong life. However, surgical removal of the bladder is the most common approach in advanced disease when tumor has invaded muscle.

The major side effects or complications of intravesical chemotherapy or BCG instillation include bladder irritation, frequency, urgency, and dysuria. These manifestations usually resolve within 1 or 2 days. Occasionally, hematuria, fever, malaise, nausea, chills, arthralgia (joint pain), and pruritus (itching) are reported. These manifestations are more representative of systemic reaction and should be reported to the physician.

RADIATION THERAPY

Radiation therapy alone is not as effective a treatment for bladder cancer as surgery and chemotherapy; the 5-year survival after radiation alone is less than 40%. Radiation therapy is rarely used except as palliation for advanced disease that cannot be eradicated by intravesical chemotherapy or radical surgery. Most bladder cancers are poorly radiosensitive, and high doses of radiation are necessary.

External supervoltage radiation, somewhat unsuccessful by itself, is effective when used in combination with surgery or chemotherapy. Hyperbaric radiation therapy increases the oxygen tension of the tumor cells and their radiosensitivity. Palliative radiation may be used to relieve pain, to prevent and relieve bowel obstruction, to control potential hemorrhage, and to alleviate leg edema secondary to venous or lymphatic obstruction.

The major side effects of radiation are hemorrhagic cystitis and bladder irritation. Local instillation of formalin may control bladder hemorrhaging resulting from the cancer or the treatments. Hemorrhagic cystitis may occur even as late as 10 years after pelvic radiation. Other complications include manifestations of cystitis and proctitis, such as dysuria, frequency, urgency, nocturia, and diarrhea. Delayed adverse effects, such as ileitis, colitis, persistent cystitis, bladder ulceration, and fistula formation, may occur as late as 6 to 12 months after radiation.

A *fistula* is an abnormal passage between two organs or between an organ and the skin. It allows for intercommunication of secretions and other substances. After radiation to the bladder, a vesicovaginal fistula may be found in women or a colovesical fistula may develop. A fistula is suspected when urine leaves the body from an unnatural site, such as the vagina, when fecal material or air appears in the urine, or when the client has recurrent UTIs. Diagnosis is confirmed by IVP, cystography, cystoscopy, or sigmoidoscopy. To further delineate the path of a fistula, a dye, such as Congo red or indigo carmine, is instilled into the bladder and all outlets are identified.

Before surgical repair of a fistula, the client must maintain a continuous flow of urine from the kidney through temporary urinary diversion, either externally or with a catheter. Surgical repair often requires a long and slow surgical procedure and may require several procedures. The primary goals are to excise the fistula and to reestablish tissue integrity.

Nursing Management of the Medical Client

ASSESSMENT

Begin your assessment of a client being evaluated for bladder cancer with a careful health, medical, and surgical history. Because this client will be undergoing extensive diagnostic evaluation, be sure to collect additional information about drug, chemical, and food allergies. Explain risk factors from exposure to known carcinogens. Ask the client about changes in urine or urination patterns, noting changes in color, frequency, and amount.

DIAGNOSIS, OUTCOMES, INTERVENTIONS

Powerlessness. The client with bladder cancer will experience *Powerlessness related to lack of knowledge of disease process, options, treatment, and side effects of therapy; fear of the disease process and treatment; and loss of control following the diagnosis and decisions regarding treatment offered.*

Outcomes. The client will learn about the medical management of the disease process, with a full understanding of client responsibilities during the treatment. The client and family will be involved with decisions about therapies and care. The client will also be encouraged to help direct care with involved health care professionals.

Interventions

Provide Education. To increase knowledge, educate the client and family about the use, rationale, risks, side effects, and expected outcomes of intravesical chemotherapy, BCG instillation, radiation, and surgery. You play an important role in client education of treatment modalities and complications that may accompany them.

Encourage Decision-Making. Encourage the client to discuss and make decisions about care. Provide opportunities for the client to express desires for care as well as time to discuss what the diagnosis and treatment mean personally.

Altered Urinary Elimination. *Altered Urinary Elimination related to urgency, frequency, dysuria, and* *hematuria resulting from chemotherapy, radiation, or BCG instillation for treatment of bladder cancer.*

Outcomes. Normal voiding will resume by day 3 after removal of the catheter, and the client will not experience sequelae to BCG instillation, chemotherapy, or radiation therapy.

Interventions. Nursing management of intravesical chemotherapy includes client education, administration of the chemotherapy agent, care of the client throughout the procedure, and monitoring for complications after administration.

Provide Education. Preparation before BCG or chemotherapy bladder instillation requires fluid restriction for 4 hours before the procedure to decrease the need to void for 2 hours afterward. Tell the client that a catheter will be inserted before the instillation and that it will be necessary to rotate and change positions every 15 to 30 minutes during treatment. After the 2-hour instillation, fluids are encouraged to flush the urinary system. Explain that treatments are typically repeated weekly for 4 to 8 weeks and then monthly for varying periods. Follow-up cystoscopy is required to monitor tumor growth.

Promote Safety. Because of the toxicity of the intravesical chemotherapy or BCG instillation, it is important to provide a safe environment for health care workers who may come in contact with the chemotherapeutic agent. For 6 hours after treatment, urine and the toilet bowl must be disinfected with bleach.

Promote Comfort. Dysuria or irritation while voiding may result from the side effects of chemotherapy, placement of an indwelling catheter, and the presence of the tumor, and it must be managed. Tumor pain is managed with analgesics. Irritative problems of dysuria, frequency, and urgency from the catheter will diminish when the catheter is removed. Irritation from the chemotherapy will decrease after about 2 days.

Reassure the client that dysuria, frequency, and urgency from catheter placement and intravesical treatment will diminish over 2 days. Discuss prescribed analgesics, antispasmodics, or anticholinergics, and explain how they should be taken.

Risk for Injury. The client who undergoes chemotherapy, BCG instillation, or radiation therapy is at *Risk for Injury from side effects of these treatments.*

Outcomes. Complications resulting from these treatments will be minimized. The client will verbalize an understanding of risk and side effects following the selected treatment option.

Interventions. Explain expected and unexpected outcomes of BCG instillation, chemotherapy, or radiation therapy. Inform the client and family how and when to alert medical staff to potential complications. Interventions for side effects include administration of antispasmodics, increasing fluid intake, and administering urinary tract antiseptics or analgesics.

If a high fever develops after BCG instillation, treatment with isoniazid or other medications used to treat tuberculosis may be indicated.

For radiation proctitis, the client will require a low-residue diet and drugs to decrease intestinal motility. For complete information on nursing care for clients receiving radiation therapy, see Chapter 19.

Urine from a client undergoing this intervention should be sent to the radioisotopes laboratory for monitoring. A client with radioactive implants is typically placed in a private room with limited visitation, but hospital policies may vary.

EVALUATION

Complications that arise from medical treatment may be difficult to manage, but they typically resolve after the treatment has ended. Evaluation of the nursing management of radiation therapy and intravesical BCG and chemotherapy will be based on the client's ability to restate personal responsibilities, to verbalize an understanding of the disease process, and to participate in care.

Because clients with bladder cancer require long-term follow-up care and continuous evaluation, they must understand the disease process and long-term follow-up responsibilities needed to maintain optimal health. If medical therapies are unsuccessful, surgical removal of the bladder may be required.

Surgical Management

Several surgical options may be used to treat bladder cancer that has not responded to medical therapies or that has invaded the bladder muscle. Surgical intervention ranges from local resection and fulguration of the tumor (destruction of tissue by electrical current through electrodes placed in direct contact with the growth) to total cystectomy, which requires diversion of normal urinary flow.

TRANSURETHRAL RESECTION

The simplest procedure is transurethral resection of the bladder tumor and fulguration done for low-grade, superficial, isolated papillary tumors or, sometimes, for inoperable tumors for palliation. The bladder is accessed through a cystoscope, which has been inserted through the urethra (see Chapter 38). This procedure is commonly followed by intravesical BCG or chemotherapy to prevent recurrence from reattachment of loose bladder cancer cells.

PARTIAL CYSTECTOMY

A segmental or partial cystectomy may be done if the client cannot tolerate a radical cystectomy and for isolated tumor which cannot be treated by transurethral resection. Up to half the bladder can be removed. This procedure is appropriate for 10% to 15% of clients. The recurrence rate can be high.

During the initial postoperative period, bladder capacity is markedly reduced. The postoperative bladder may be able to hold no more than 60 ml. Over several months, bladder tissue expands, increasing its capacity from 200 to 400 ml.

RADICAL CYSTECTOMY AND URINARY DIVERSION

A radical cystectomy with urinary diversion is the procedure of choice when potentially curable stage B disease is too advanced for transurethral resection or intravesical chemotherapy. The procedure may also be performed for treatment of:

- Neurogenic bladder (see Neurogenic Bladder Dysfunction later on)

- IC or radiation-induced cystitis with severely reduced bladder capacity
- Congenital anomalies of the lower urinary tract, such as bladder exstrophy

Radical cystectomy entails removal of the bladder, urethra, uterus, fallopian tubes, ovaries, and anterior segment of the vagina in women. In men, the bladder, urethra, and usually the prostate and seminal vesicles are removed. Cystectomy also involves removal of perivesical fat and dissection of the pelvic lymph nodes. This procedure is necessary when the tumor has invaded the bladder wall, involves the trigone, or cannot be treated adequately by less radical methods. When the bladder and urethra are removed, permanent urinary diversion is required. The entire surgical procedure is done in one step, with urinary diversion and cystectomy performed at the same time.

Ileal Conduit

An ileal conduit (also called ureteroileostomy, ileal bladder, or Bricker's procedure) is one type of urinary diversion. Using a segment of the intestine as a conduit, the surgeon constructs a system in which urine empties through an artificial opening in the skin called a *stoma* (Fig. 34–2). Usually, a portion of the terminal ileum, which has the least reabsorptive power, is used for the conduit. After the continuity of the remaining intestine is reestablished with end-to-end anastomosis, the proximal end of the segment is closed. The distal end is brought out through a hole created in the abdominal wall, folded back, and sutured to the skin to form a stoma. The ureters are then implanted into the ileal segment. Urine flows into the conduit and is continually propelled out through the stoma by peristalsis. Mucous shreds will always be present in the urine because of the mucus produced by the lining of the bowel.

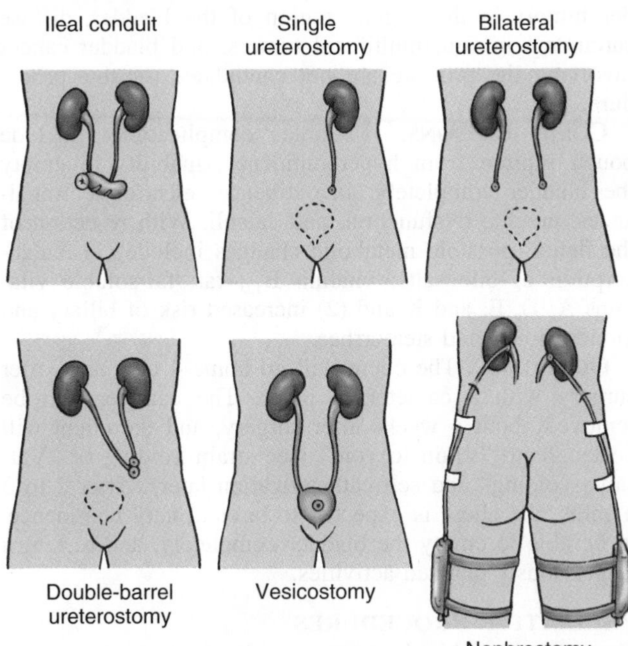

FIGURE 34–2 Some older surgical alternatives for urinary diversion.

INDICATIONS. The client who has undergone an ileal conduit must wear an appliance over the stoma to collect the urine. This treatment is rarely selected for clients with a life expectancy of more than 1 to 2 years. The procedure involves less time, and the conduit is easier to construct compared with other diversion procedures, which makes it an excellent choice for older clients who are unable to tolerate a lengthy surgery because of other medical conditions. Because the ileal segment is not a reservoir, absorption of electrolytes and the frequency of other complications are minimal.

CONTRAINDICATIONS. Clients who cannot maintain follow-up care or treatment because of physical limitations or mental impairment are not candidates for an ileal conduit; clients with chronic bowel disease or colon cancer may not be candidates either. Any medical condition that prevents a major surgical procedure would also be a contraindication.

COMPLICATIONS. Several complications related to stoma management (e.g., skin irritation, stomal defects, and stomal pouching problems) may arise. Leakage at the anastomosis site, stenosis, peristomal hernia, ulceration, and obstruction at the ureteroileal anastomosis may develop. Finally, clients who have undergone an ileal conduit procedure are at increased risk for pyelonephritis, hydronephrosis (distention of renal pelvis and calices with urine), and formation of calculi.

OUTCOMES. Eight weeks after surgery, it is expected that the client will adjust to the stoma and appliance, maintain stoma and appliance care, have a urine output of ½ ml/kg/hr, and return to most previously enjoyed activities.

Indiana Pouch

Other diversionary procedures are the Indiana pouch, Florida pouch, Kock pouch, and continent internal ileal reservoir. A reservoir is created from the ascending colon and terminal ileum. The Indiana pouch is an improved and larger version of the original Kock pouch (Fig. 34–3). Other continent reservoir operations vary slightly regarding surgical technique and the portion of the colon and ileum used.

Once the reservoir has been created, the ureters are implanted into the side of the diversion. A special nipple valve is then constructed and used to attach the reservoir to the skin. Several weeks after surgery, the client is taught to use a catheter to drain the reservoir at 3- to 4-hour intervals. Internal storage of up to 800 ml of urine is possible, with a daytime continence rate of up to 93% and a nighttime continence rate of up to 76%.

INDICATIONS. Because this procedure involves no appliance for collecting urine, it is preferred for clients with a life expectancy of more than 2 years. Creation of the reservoir and nipple valve requires 1 to 3 more hours more surgical time compared with the time needed to construct an ileal conduit. The client's serum creatinine level should be 2.5 mg/dl or less. The client will need gross and fine motor coordination to catheterize the nipple valve and must be willing and able to participate in self-care. Electrolyte reabsorption is minimal with this diversion technique as long as the urine is drained regularly.

CONTRAINDICATIONS. Clients with a history of significant bowel resection and malabsorption related to diar-

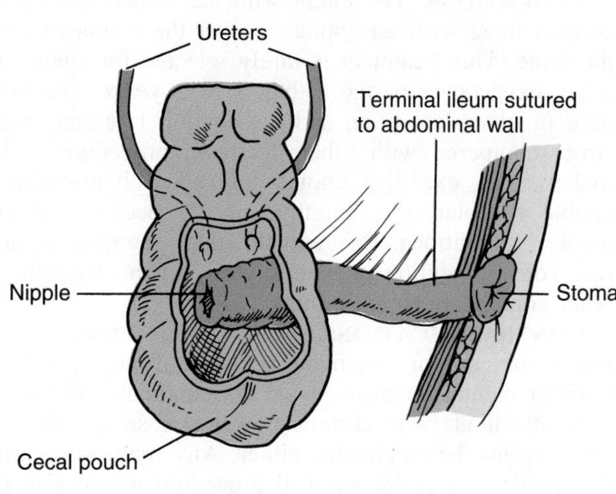

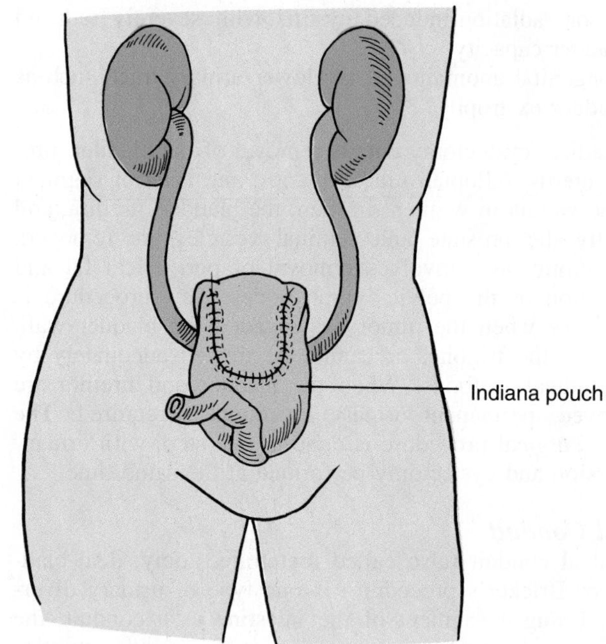

FIGURE 34–3 Indiana pouch procedure.

rhea, irritable bowel syndrome, ulcerative colitis, diverticular disease, bowel cancer, Crohn's disease, progressive neurologic disorders, morbid obesity, kidney disease (creatinine > 2.5 mg/dl) and pelvic radiation are not candidates for an Indiana pouch.

COMPLICATIONS. Possible complications include incontinence, difficult catheterization, urinary reflux, anastomotic leaks, pyelonephritis, obstruction, bacteriuria, calculi, erectile dysfunction, electrolyte imbalances, and rupture of the reservoir.

OUTCOMES. About 8 to 10 weeks after surgery, the client will have urinary continence, will remain free of urinary tract infection, and will return to activities pursued before surgery. Self-catheterization should begin 3 weeks postoperatively.

Neobladder

Sometimes the urethra can be spared, allowing the creation of a *neobladder,* also known as an ileal W-bladder. This operation is the treatment of choice for a client with bladder cancer that has invaded the bladder muscle. Although this procedure differs from one in which the reservoir empties through an abdominal stoma, a neobladder empties via a pelvic outlet to the urethra. Maintaining continence can be a problem unless the lower portion of the bladder can be spared.

Some surgeons believe that the urethra should be removed because of the risk of tumor recurrence. If the urethra is resected, a reconstructed neourethra together with an artificial sphincter is created. This procedure is more successful in males because of the longer urethra.

Several weeks after surgery, the catheter is removed and the client empties the neobladder by relaxing the external sphincter and creating abdominal pressure. The client will have to learn intermittent self-catheterization to cope with any voiding difficulties. Even with the potential postoperative problems that may be encountered, acceptance of this procedure is very high because it allows a more normal anatomy to be maintained for the client. Total continence is achieved in 84% to 96% of clients at 5 years.

INDICATIONS. Because an appliance is not required and normal anatomy is maintained, the neobladder technique is the preferred urinary diversion for clients with a life expectancy of more than 2 years and with no contraindications. Other indications are as described for an Indiana pouch.

CONTRAINDICATIONS. In addition to the contraindications listed for an Indiana pouch, the client with bladder tumors in the trigone region of the bladder, diffuse carcinoma in situ, multifocal tumors, and bladder cancer involving the prostate are not candidates for this procedure.

COMPLICATIONS. Possible complications include pouch rupture from hypercontinence, inability to empty the bladder completely, incontinence, electrolyte imbalances, erectile dysfunction, and calculi. With resection of the ileum, possible metabolic changes include (1) malabsorption of bile salts; vitamin B_{12}; fat; fat-soluble vitamins A, D, E, and K and (2) increased risk of biliary and kidney stones and steatorrhea.

OUTCOMES. The client will go home 4 to 8 days after surgery with a catheter in place. The catheter will be removed about 4 weeks after surgery, and the client will be taught to "strain to void" (see strain voiding or "Valsalva voiding" and self-catheterization later). After 2 to 3 months, the client is expected to have urinary continence, to be able to empty the bladder completely, and to return to previously pursued activities.

PALLIATIVE PROCEDURES

Percutaneous Nephrostomy or Pyelostomy

For the client with inoperable bladder cancer, a percutaneous nephrostomy (see Fig. 34–2) or pyelostomy may be performed to prevent obstruction. A catheter is inserted into the renal pelvis by surgical incision or, more likely, a percutaneous puncture procedure. In the surgical approach, a balloon-tipped or mushroom-tipped catheter is connected to an external drainage system.

In the percutaneous nephrostomy procedure, a trocar is inserted under fluoroscopy by direct puncture into the renal pelvis or calix. A flexible small-gauge needle is then used to instill contrast material to verify proper location. Using angiographic wire as a guide, the surgeon places the nephrostomy tube and connects it to a closed drainage system. The entire procedure is done with the client under local anesthesia. It is important to stabilize the tube to prevent dislodgment.

Ureterostomy

A ureterostomy may be performed as a palliative procedure if the ureters are obstructed by tumor. During a cutaneous ureterostomy, the surgeon attaches the ureter to the surface of the abdomen where urine flows directly into a drainage appliance without an intermediary conduit. For clients with ureterostomies, infection, obstruction to urine flow secondary to strictures at the opening, and skin irritation are potential problems. This procedure includes several variations (see Fig. 34–2).

Nursing Management of the Preoperative Client

ASSESSMENT

Preoperative nursing management of the client with bladder cancer is directed at educating the client and family. Assess the client and family's understanding of pending diagnostic testing, bladder cancer, and proposed surgical procedure. Evaluate the client's anxiety level by providing opportunities to talk about feelings and to ask questions about the upcoming surgery, potential for distorted body image, and support systems outside the hospital.

In addition to educating and counseling the client, obtain physical assessment findings. Check for (1) costovertebral tenderness and masses in the upper abdomen and flank, (2) distention before and after urination, (3) vaginal or rectal masses, and (4) signs of discharge in urethral meatus and perianal areas. Assessment of other body systems includes (1) monitoring vital signs; (2) measuring intake and output; (3) examining skin for color, bruises, petechiae, and hydration; and (4) auscultating heart and lung sounds.

Complete a self-care or functional assessment to determine whether the client can manage drains and indwelling catheters and is able to catheterize a continent stoma or urethra. Finally, determine whether a family member can provide care or whether home health care is available to the client.

DIAGNOSIS, OUTCOMES, INTERVENTIONS

Knowledge Deficit. The most common nursing diagnosis preoperatively is *Knowledge Deficit related to bladder cancer and diagnostic testing, possible bowel preparation prior to surgical intervention, and surgical intervention with associated expected course of treatment.*

Outcomes. Preoperative education will bring about an increased awareness of the procedure and lowered anxiety preoperatively and postoperatively. The client will understand diagnostic tests, bowel preparation, surgical intervention, and the anticipated postoperative course, as evidenced by statements and demonstrations of self-care.

Interventions

Provide Preoperative Teaching. Assess the client's educational deficits surrounding bladder cancer, proposed treatment, and expected outcomes by encouraging discussion. Include the family in the discussion to review diagnostic evaluation, preoperative treatment, and postoperative expectations. Explain the purpose of various tubes, such as IV lines, the nasogastric (NG) tube, stents, drains, and catheters that will be present after surgery and when they will be discontinued. As needed, discuss support services available after discharge.

Discuss Bowel Preparation. If a diversion or pouch procedure has been chosen as the appropriate surgical intervention, discuss the preoperative bowel preparation ("bowel prep"). Because a segment of bowel will be used to create the conduit or reservoir, this measure relates to the segment of intestine to be used in the procedure.

Bowel preparation calls for a clear liquid diet for 1 to 3 days, laxatives and enemas to clear the bowel, and antibiotics to lower the bacterial count in the bowel. Because this step takes several days and includes enemas, dietary restrictions, and medications, it is extremely important to teach the client and family to strictly adhere to the directions.

Provide Enterostomal Nurse Visitation. If the client will have a pouch or diversion procedure, a visit from an enterostomal nurse may be reassuring for the client and family. This visit allows the client and family to interact and learn the expected postoperative course with a nurse with expertise in this field.

Before surgery, the enterostomal nurse selects and marks the best site for ostomy placement if the surgeon plans to construct a stoma. The main criterion for stomal placement is finding a site that allows the faceplate of the drainage appliance to bind securely to the surface of the abdomen.

The stoma must be clearly visible to the client. This means that the surgeon should avoid the umbilicus, rib margins, pubis, iliac crests, and pre-existing scars, wrinkles, or crevices. Placing the stoma directly on the client's waistline can cause excessive pressure from clothing.

The client is observed in the supine, standing, and sitting positions during the selection process. Stoma placement is usually on the right lower quadrant of the abdomen, in the abdominal rectus muscle, about 2 inches below the waist and 2 inches from the midline. Explain the proper way to care for the urinary diversion.

Risk for Body Image Disturbance. The client is at *Risk for Body Image Disturbance related to surgery, possible stoma formation, possible sexual dysfunction, and potential change in urinary elimination.*

Outcomes. The client will not experience body image disturbance postoperatively, as evidenced by the ability to discuss concerns regarding altered body image, stoma placement, change in urination pattern, risk of sexual dysfunction, and verbalization of fears.

Interventions. Identify factors that reveal the client's difficulty in coping with anticipated changes in body image. Should a diversion procedure be necessary, in addition to a preoperative visit from an enterostomal nurse, you may want to suggest a visit from a client with a similar diagnosis and procedure. These visits provide the client with a comfortable opportunity to ask questions, to experience a sense of comfort and support, and to receive information.

Preoperative teaching should include explanations of the expected anatomic and physiologic alterations and possible effects for the client. Because of the lifestyle changes that are required by diversion or pouch surgery, be sure to offer support and refer the client for additional counseling if indicated. Community associations, such as the United Ostomy Association and the American Cancer Society, provide tremendous help for clients undergoing urinary diversion.

Radical bladder surgery may cause a disturbance in sexual function. Because of the private and personal nature of this surgery, you should use this opportunity to discuss potential sexual dysfunction following radical surgery for bladder cancer. Although nerve sparing procedures and vaginal reconstruction procedures can reduce sexual dysfunction, clients should be prepared to take advantage of available resources in case impotence or difficulty with intercourse develops after surgery.

EVALUATION

It is expected that the client will be prepared for and will undergo the selected surgery successfully. The client will restate information about bladder cancer, diagnostic testing, the bowel preparation, and surgical intervention. In addition, the client will be able to voice concerns about body image disturbance and sexual dysfunction after surgery. The client will be aware of outside resources available following discharge.

Nursing Management of the Postoperative Client

ASSESSMENT

Routine postoperative evaluation and care involve the usual assessments for a client after major abdominal surgery. The stoma, if present, should be inspected hourly for 24 hours after surgery, then every 4 hours for 24 hours, then every 8 hours. The stoma should be red and moist at all times and will be edematous just after surgery. The edema will diminish by 200% to 500% within a few weeks. Peristomal sutures may be seen adhering to the skin and mucosal bowel edge. Any sign that the stoma is becoming pale, dark, dusky, gray, or cyanotic may mean loss of vascular supply; this event must be corrected immediately to avoid necrosis.

Peristalsis in the intestinal tract will be absent for several days because of the manipulation and resection of the bowel. The client will continue to receive nothing by mouth (i.e., will remain on NPO status) with IV lines and a nasogastric tube in place until peristalsis returns. Assessment of bowel sounds and nasogastric contents is required.

Urine flow never stops after surgery. Ureteral stents originating in the renal pelvis extend through the ureters and through the reservoir, conduit, or neobladder. The stents that exit through a stoma are contained in the pouch. With continent reservoirs, a catheter is placed through the nipple valve to drain the internal reservoir for 2 to 3 weeks until healing occurs. For a neobladder, a suprapubic catheter may be placed through the abdominal wall into the reservoir to keep it drained while another catheter is placed through the urethra and used as a stent. This protects the anastomosis of the urethra and neobladder.

In some instances, ureteral stents or catheters may drain urine after neobladder or continent reservoir surgery. The stents and catheter are removed once adequate healing has occurred; this is usually in 3 to 4 weeks. The catheter is usually the last tube to be discontinued. Constantly monitor the tubes for patency and continuous drainage, usually in separate closed gravity systems. For the first 24 to 48 hours, hourly intake and output records may be required. Clients should be kept from manipulating tubes immediately after surgery.

HEMATURIA. Assess for hematuria, stenosis, and other complications after surgery. Hematuria, a common problem after transurethral resection, is controlled with a three-way indwelling catheter and, if necessary, bladder irrigation. The greatest potential problems after any diversion or pouch procedure are infection, wound dehiscence, skin irritation, ulceration, and stomal defects. Later complications are renal deterioration caused by reflux, stenosis of the stoma, strictures at the site of the anastomosis, hydronephrosis, calculi, and peristomal hernia.

STENOSIS. Stenosis of the stoma may occur from scarring during stomal maturation. If the opening on the faceplate is too large, epithelial hyperplasia or thickening of the peristomal skin may contract the stoma. Clients with urinary diversion are also susceptible to uric acid and calcium stone disease. The onset of urinary stone development usually occurs at least 2 years postoperatively and sometimes as long as 5 to 10 years later. UTI is a perpetual threat because of the exposure of the urinary tract. Obstruction anywhere in the urinary tract may interfere with normal urine flow.

OTHER COMPLICATIONS. The potential complications of continent reservoirs or pouch procedures include incontinence, difficult catheterization, urinary reflux, and possible pyelonephritis, obstruction, bacteriuria, electrolyte imbalances, urolithiasis, or absorptive problems. The reservoir may rupture if the client does not comply with the self-catheterization protocol.

Monitor the client for other complications as well following a radical cystectomy. Cystectomy is a very invasive surgery that puts the client at risk for most of the usual postoperative complications, including shock and hemorrhage. The extensive pelvic dissection associated with this surgery can increase the risk of thrombophlebitis. Additionally, pelvic lymph node dissection can predispose the client to lymphedema in the lower limbs. You may need to assess calf circumference during each shift.

DIAGNOSIS, OUTCOMES, INTERVENTIONS

Risk for Injury: Occlusion of Urinary Drainage. A potential problem for the postoperative client is *Risk for Injury: Occlusion of urinary drainage device related to hematuria, clot formation, and swelling following the surgical procedure.*

Outcomes. Catheters and other drainage tubes will not become obstructed, and urine will flow freely.

Interventions. After transurethral resection of the bladder, the client will usually have hematuria. A three-lumen, indwelling urethral catheter will be attached to a continuous or intermittent closed bladder irrigation system to facilitate urine flow, minimize blood clots, and monitor for postoperative bleeding. Nursing care is similar to that after transurethral resection of the prostate (see Chapter 38). Bright red or pink urine will fade to clear in about 3 days.

Nursing care after segmental bladder resection centers on maintaining constant urinary drainage to ensure that the remaining bladder does not become distended, putting strain on the suture line. The client usually has both urethral and suprapubic catheters. The client is discharged with the catheter in place, and it remains in place for about 2 weeks or until complete healing has occurred.

As with any major abdominal surgery, clients who undergo a radical cystectomy and urinary diversion are at an increased risk for hemorrhage. Monitor the client's vital signs, the incision, and the drainage tubes closely for early signs of excessive bleeding. If an ileal conduit is formed, the client will have a pouch in place to collect urine from the ileal conduit or ureteral catheters or stents.

After a continent diversion, make sure that the catheter is draining urine freely. If any obstruction occurs, the newly created reservoir can become damaged and internal leakage along the suture line can occur. Monitor the catheter output closely, and perform irrigations at regular intervals as directed. Perform catheter irrigation gently in the immediate postoperative period, using about 60 ml of normal saline solution. Irrigation is necessary to help prevent obstruction from clots or mucus.

After neobladder surgery, one or two catheters will be in place to prevent overdistention of the newly created bladder. These catheters are treated as closed drainage systems. Carefully monitor the neobladder for possible obstruction. Regular irrigation is needed to rid the neobladder of mucus.

When ureteral stents or catheters are placed, patency is very important to prevent hydronephrosis and pyelonephritis. Because there is no mucus in urine from the kidney, irrigation is usually not required and is kept to a minimum to prevent pyelonephritis and hydronephrosis. In fact, do not irrigate ureteral catheters unless you have a specific order to do so, and then only with 5 to 10 ml of sterile saline solution. Urine output from each ureteral catheter should be ¼ ml/kg/hour or roughly half of the ½ ml/kg/hr normally expected from a urethral catheter. Ureteral catheters may drain into a pouch when a stoma is present (see Critical Monitoring feature).

If the client has a stoma, a temporary, clear urostomy pouch over the stoma will be connected to a gravity drainage system. Sometimes ureteral catheters are used to splint the ureters while they heal. These catheters, usually removed before the client is discharged, may extend through the stoma.

Label all catheters, stents, and drainage tubes to prevent errors in irrigation and output calculations. Secure all tubes. Use a separate closed gravity drainage system for each tube unless, as with an ileal conduit, ureteral catheters exit into the pouching system until they are discontinued. A separate system for each tube minimizes the risk and extent of bacterial infection.

CRITICAL MONITORING

Postoperative Monitoring After Urinary Diversion Procedures

- Measure urine output every hour for the first 24 hours, and at least every 8 hours thereafter; report any amount less than ½ ml/kg/hour (~30 ml/hr) or no output for more than 15 minutes.
- Check the ostomy pouch for leaks and the skin under it for irritation every 4 hours initially, then every 8 hours.
- Inspect the stoma every hour for the first 24 hours after surgery. (This will give you a baseline from which you can quickly detect deviations. The stoma should be red and moist.) If you find no problems, extend intervals to every 4 hours, then to every 8 hours.
- Note the stoma's size, shape, and color. Expect it to be edematous in the immediate postoperative period. However, other changes may indicate complications, warranting action from the physician. A dusky or cyanotic stoma color may denote an insufficient blood supply and the onset of necrosis. This is an emergency. The reduced blood supply may result from surgical technique, from an appliance faceplate that is too small or improperly centered, or from peristomal protective materials that have been poorly applied. Other complications with the stoma include prolapse (protrusion from the skin) or retraction into the abdomen beneath the skin.
- Watch for manifestations of peritonitis, such as fever and abdominal pain and rigidity. Leakage at the site of the anastomosis or ureteral separation from the conduit may allow urine to seep into the peritoneal cavity, leading to peritonitis.
- Observe for bleeding. Although bleeding from the stoma may indicate a surgical defect, it is also common for the intestinal mucosa, which is very fragile, to bleed during a change of appliance or because of a poorly fitted collection pouch.

Effective Management of Therapeutic Regimen. Clients undergoing any type of urinary diversion need to learn new self-care strategies. The nursing diagnosis of *Effective Management of Therapeutic Regimen related to complexity of therapeutic regimen* is applicable for this client.

Outcomes. The client will effectively manage the urinary diversion or neobladder, as evidenced by the ability to describe the regimen and to perform the required care successfully.

Interventions

Ileal Conduit. For a client with an ileal conduit, teach stoma care and skin care, promote self-care of the collection device, prevent odor, promote independence, and encourage follow-up.

Teach stoma care. The client will need to learn to care for the stoma and skin with proper application of a urinary pouch (see Bridge to Home Health Care). An opening must be cut in the skin barrier just large enough to fit over the stoma. The barrier is then applied to the

BRIDGE TO HOME HEALTH CARE

Managing an Ileal Conduit

When clients first come home from the hospital, they need your help to get organized and feel in control. Use a small plastic basket, such as one purchased at a discount store, to store small supplies, such as adhesive tape, stoma adhesive, a pen, and a small scissors. A wash basin, a small box, or a small organizer on wheels works well for the larger items, such as faceplate or wafers, skin barriers, pouches, and paper towels.

Typically, clients are taught about stoma care before discharge, but they may have been so overwhelmed that they did not hear or remember instructions. Once home, they may have many questions. While you change the appliance, have your clients lie down with a mirror positioned so they can become accustomed to seeing the stoma and can learn to care for the stoma without experiencing side effects such as faintness or dizziness. Eventually, the client should face the toilet while sitting comfortably on a stool or chair.

Before removing the original wafer, cut the new faceplate or wafer to size, snap it on the pouch, and make certain that everything is ready. Some clients may need a circular insert in the wafer to form a convex angle that makes a tighter seal around the small stoma. Once you take off the old appliance, cover the stoma; peristalsis causes urine to squirt out spontaneously.

Do not make your client laugh; pressure will cause urine to leak out. It is frustrating to repeatedly reclean the area. Use thick, absorbent paper towels to cover the stoma; they are also inexpensive and readily available.

Before cleaning the skin surface, make sure that the stoma is open and not becoming filled with mucus from the bowel. Use a small amount of lubricating jelly (e.g., K-Y) on your little finger, and gently enter the stoma. Quickly cover the stoma with a paper towel to absorb urine. To keep the skin healthy, wash around the stoma with soap and water, and prepare the skin with a skin barrier. Cover the stoma, and allow the skin barrier to dry. Once you are ready to secure the appliance, remove the paper towel quickly and apply the wafer.

Place your warm hands on the faceplate or wafer for a few minutes to help it adhere to the skin. You may need to apply an extra piece of adhesive tape in the corner or side to prevent leaking. Assess skinfolds before applying the wafer; consider shifting the wafer to a diamond position to decrease the bend at the fold and the potential for leaking.

Leakage is one of the most distressing aspects of the ileal conduit. Instruct clients to attach an overnight Foley bag to the pouch at bedtime and to be sure that there are no kinks in the tubing. Back-pressure and overflow into the pouch will cause the faceplate or wafer to pop off or leak. Until they feel confident, clients may decide to awaken about 2:00 AM to check the pouch. During the day, they need to empty the pouch often because the tension of a full pouch will cause a leak. Clients should change the pouch every 3 to 4 days, the faceplate or wafer once a week to 10 days to avoid odor problems and to decrease the risk of a UTI. The pouch is made with a hard plastic ring that snaps onto the faceplate or wafer because frequent changes are necessary.

Clients may call on enterostomal nurses at local hospitals, the United Ostomy Association, and the American Cancer Society for help in adjusting to an ileal conduit.

Mary M. Stasiak, RN, BSN, PHN, MA, *Case Manager, Allied Health Alternatives, Inc., Rochester, Minnesota*

skin before attaching the pouch or faceplate. A skin cement or adhesive disc may help the faceplate stick more securely to the skin. A non–water-soluble adhesive spray allows the client to go swimming. Most pouches come as two pieces, a faceplate or wafer and a removable pouch. Not having to remove the faceplate or wafer as frequently makes care much easier for many clients.

Teach skin care. Skin irritation or breakdown is a constant threat to a client with a urinary diversion. Advise the client to prevent urine from contacting the skin. This can be achieved in part when a well-fitted and properly attached appliance is used (Fig. 34–4). The opening in the adhesive backing of the faceplate or wafer should be cut no more than 3 mm larger than the stoma. This opening needs to be remeasured after the edema in the stoma recedes.

Each time the faceplate or wafer is changed, the skin around the stoma should be cleaned with a mild, nonresidue soap and water, and thoroughly dried. A gauze pad, absorbent paper towel, or tampon should be held over the stoma during cleaning to prevent urine from flowing out over the skin. Remove this pad or tampon just as the appliance is reapplied. The appliance should be changed early in the morning because urine production is slowest at this time.

Promote self-care of the collection device. Urine pouches have a valve in the bottom for intermittent urine drainage. Alternatively, the pouch may be drained by gravity into a leg or bedside bag, especially at night. The self-contained pouch drainage system allows the client to resume most, if not all, former activities with little or no change in style of dress.

However, instruct clients to empty the pouch when it is one-third to one-half full. The weight of accumulating urine may pull the faceplate away from the skin and cause leakage. Advise clients to check the seal often if they are perspiring heavily.

Prevent odor. Urine odor is a common problem with urinary stomas. Noxious odors result mostly from poor hygiene, alkaline urine, normal breakdown of urine (ammonia), concentrated urine from insufficient fluid intake, and the ingestion of certain foods, such as asparagus.

Because diluted urine has less odor, adequate fluid intake is very helpful. Reusable appliances can be washed with soap and lukewarm water. The pouch can also be soaked in diluted white vinegar or in a commercial deodorant product for 20 to 30 minutes. Rinse the pouch, and allow it to dry. Deodorant tablets are available for placement in the pouch while it is being worn.

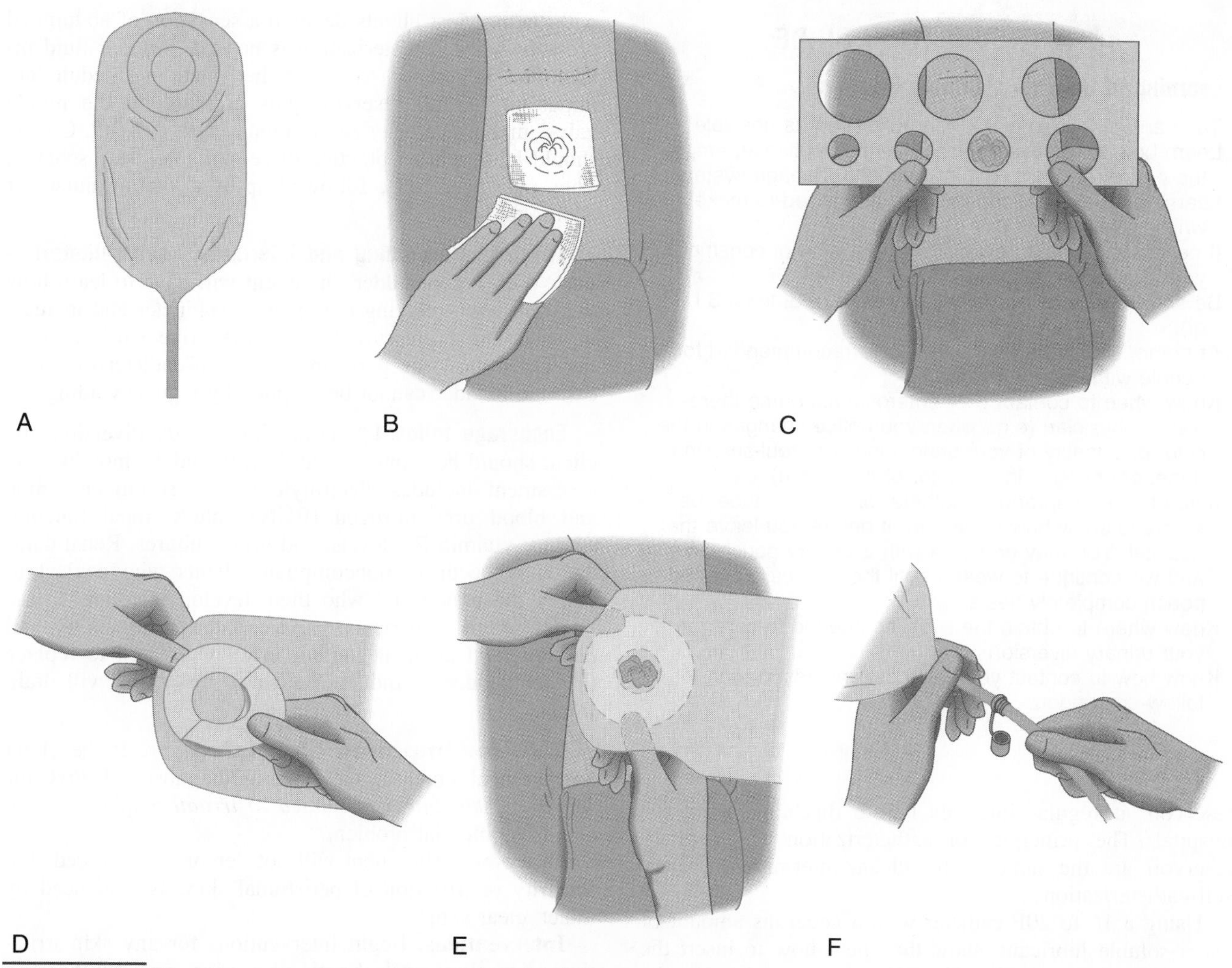

FIGURE 34–4 Applying a disposable ostomy pouch. *A,* Gather supplies: ostomy pouch, ostomy belt, skin barrier, stoma template, gauze pads, pouch clip or rubber band, safety pin, and clean gloves. Clamp or wrap rubber band around the end of the pouch to prevent leakage during the procedure. Make sure that lighting is adequate and that the client is comfortable and understands the procedure. Wash your hands, and don clean examining gloves. *B,* Gently remove the old pouch, using warm water or an adhesive solvent around the seal if necessary. Place the gauze pad over the stoma to prevent leakage as you gently clean peristomal area with moist gauze. *C,* Measure the stoma with the stoma template. Trace the shape onto the skin barrier and adhesive, using the template. Cut openings no more than 3 mm larger than the stoma. *D,* Remove backing from the adhesive surface of the disposable ostomy pouch. *E,* Center a pouch opening over the stoma with the pouch drain pointing to floor. (If the client ambulates frequently, the pouch drain should point to the client's feet.) Make sure that the seal is complete. *F,* Connect drainage tubing to the ostomy pouch if appropriate. Secure tubing; with a rubber band around the tubing, pin a rubber band to the sheets if the client is immobile.

Promote independence. Long-term nursing intervention aims to maintain a functional urinary system and prevent complications. It takes time for clients and significant others to adjust to a urinary diversion. Even though counseling may have been excellent during the preoperative period, the reality of the diversion commonly produces anxiety, depression, and anger. The client may need help at first to look at or even talk about the stoma. As soon as possible after surgery, the client must begin to help care for the stoma, peristomal skin, and drainage system, gradually assuming more responsibility until achieving independence (see Client Education Guide).

Encourage follow-up. A client with bladder cancer must receive follow-up at regular intervals to assess for a recurrence of the cancer. The client should also continue to be seen by an enterostomal therapy nurse to check for problems with the ostomy.

Continent Diversion. Postoperative care for the client with an Indiana pouch is similar to that for any client with a urinary diversion, except there is no external pouch. The client will have a 24 French (F) to 26F or Medina catheter in place to drain urine continuously until the pouch has healed. The reservoir is irrigated through the catheter with about 50 to 60 ml of normal saline every 4 hours to wash out clots or mucus, which may cause obstruction.

Teach reservoir catheterization. After a radiographic study, remove the catheter at 3 to 4 weeks after surgery to make sure that the continent reservoir is functioning properly. The client must learn to empty and irrigate the

CLIENT EDUCATION GUIDE

Learning to Care for a Urinary Diversion

Take an active role in your care as soon as possible.
Learn how to remove and reapply the appliance, empty the pouch, and attach it to the night drainage system.
Learn about adaptations that you may need to make while traveling.
If necessary, select new clothing that will not constrict your drainage pouch.
Be sure to maintain a daily fluid intake of at least 3 L (3 qt).
At home, select the foods and fluids recommended for people with urinary diversions.
Know when to contact your enterostomal nurse therapist or physician (e.g., when you notice changes in the color or quantity of your urine, cloudy or foul-smelling urine, or changes in the color of the stoma).
If you have a suprapubic catheter or Medena tube, be sure you know how to care for it before you leave the hospital. You may go home with a urinary pouch on and will continue to wear it until the surgically created pouch completely heals.
Know where to obtain the supplies needed to care for your urinary diversion.
Know how to contact your local ostomy association for follow-up support.

reservoir at regular intervals before discharge from the hospital. The principles of catheterization of a urinary reservoir are the same as for clean, intermittent urinary self-catheterization.

Using a 16 to 20F catheter with a generous amount of water-soluble lubricant, show the client how to insert the catheter into the nipple valve. Warn against forcing the catheter into the reservoir. If resistance occurs, tell the client to pause and apply only gentle pressure while slightly rotating the catheter. If this does not work, the client should call the physician. Advise the client to insert the catheter every 2 to 3 hours to drain the reservoir. Each week thereafter, the interval is increased by 1 hour, until finally catheterization is completed every 4 to 6 hours during the day.

Teach reservoir irrigation. Once the urine has stopped flowing, the client should take several deep breaths and move the catheter in and out 2 to 3 inches to be sure that the pouch is fully emptied. The catheter should be withdrawn slowly so additional urine can drain.

After urine has been drained from the reservoir, tell the client to leave the catheter in place and to use 50 to 60 ml of normal saline solution to irrigate the reservoir and to prevent excess mucus buildup, which may cause obstruction. The fluid can either be gently aspirated or allowed to drain from the catheter. Once the irrigant is drained, the catheter is removed and the end of the catheter is pinched before removal to prevent dripping. The irrigations may be repeated until the drainage returns free of mucus. If the mucus is very viscous (thick), increasing fluid intake and drinking cranberry juice can decrease the viscosity. Usually, mucus production lessens over time.

Because the catheterization procedure can be unpredictable, advise clients to carry catheterization supplies with them. Most clients develop a sensation of abdominal pressure when catheterization is needed. Regular fluid intake and adherence to the catheterization schedule are important. A full reservoir puts pressure on the nipple valve, making catheterization much more difficult. Clients should be taught to practice these skills before discharge. They may need to be followed up by a visiting nurse for additional help.

Teach strain voiding and intermittent self-catheterization. With a neobladder, the client will have to learn how to *strain void*, relaxing the external sphincter and increasing abdominal pressure to start the urine stream. Show the client how to perform clean self-catheterization in case the bladder cannot be emptied by regular voiding.

Encourage follow-up. Following urinary diversion, the client should be monitored at 3, 6, 9, and 12 months. The assessment includes electrolyte values, serum creatinine and blood urea nitrogen (BUN) values, renal function studies, vitamin B_{12} levels, and urine cultures. Renal damage may occur in noncompliant clients who neglect to empty the pouch and who then develop infection. These clients often experience severe kidney infections and damage, and an ileal conduit must be created to replace the neobladder or Indiana pouch so that urine will drain freely.

Risk for Impaired Skin Integrity. If the client has an ileal conduit, the nursing diagnosis of *Risk for Impaired Skin Integrity related to irritation of peristomal skin* is a potential problem.

Outcomes. The client will not demonstrate altered skin integrity or irritation of peristomal skin, as evidenced by intact, clear skin.

Interventions. Begin interventions for any skin irritation promptly. Check the pH of a urine specimen because strongly alkaline urine irritates the skin and facilitates crystal formation. Encourage the client to drink cranberry juice to help acidify the urine. Any positive urine culture result requires treatment. Check appliances carefully to identify leakage and to detect skin sensitivity.

Skin irritation may result from changing the pouch too frequently. A general recommendation is to leave the pouch in place as long as it is not leaking. During appliance changes, leave the skin open to the air as much as possible. Apply a pouch with a non-karaya (sterculia gum) skin barrier. Karaya cannot be used with urinary pouches because urine erodes karaya.

Skin irritation around the stoma commonly results from a yeast infection. Nystatin creams or powders are effective against topical yeast. Nystatin powder is applied directly over the irritated skin area and sealed to the skin with a liquid skin barrier.

Risk for Sexual Dysfunction. Extensive surgical dissection may alter the reproductive anatomy and may result in *Risk for Sexual Dysfunction related to potential postoperative impotence in men or painful intercourse in women following a radical cystectomy and changes in body image affecting sexuality.*

Outcomes. The client will accept and adopt alternative methods of sexual expression and will obtain additional information about sexuality through questions and statements.

Interventions. Male clients have a risk of impotence after a radical cystectomy related to the resection. Offer counseling both before and after the surgery to help the client adjust to any alterations (see Chapter 38 for information about alterations in male sexuality). Sildenafil (Viagra), 50 to 100 mg three times weekly, is being offered to most male clients immediately after the catheter is removed to maintain blood flow to the corpora cavernosa, so that when sexual intercourse can be resumed the client will have fewer problems with impotence.

For women who have had a total abdominal hysterectomy, bilateral salpingo-oophorectomy, and anterior vaginal resection, the result can be shortening and tightening of the vagina, leading to painful intercourse. Alternative positions, lubricants, topical estrogen, and vaginal dilators may decrease the discomfort. Booklets discussing both female and male sexual dysfunction are available from the American Cancer Society.

For partners of any client, encourage holding, touching, kissing, and other activities to promote intimacy. Partners are often afraid to touch the client for fear of inflicting hurt; embarrassment may also be an issue. Encourage open discussions.

EVALUATION

Carcinoma in situ is considered curable with a simple transurethral resection. Intravesical chemotherapy or BCG may be combined to decrease the risk of recurrence. If the postoperative care of the client has been successful, the client will be able to make the transition to self-care with minimal difficulty. Even with a radical cystectomy, however, the 5-year survival rate for clients with muscle invasive tumor (stage C or greater) is only 40% to 50%.

Self-Care

Motivation to promote preoperative self-care may influence the postoperative course. Direct the client toward self-care by improving knowledge, encouraging independence, and fostering participation in care and treatment. When the client increases self-care, there will be a decreasing need for nursing care and an increase in health promotion activities.

The client will need referrals to durable medical equipment companies for ostomy supplies or catheters for reservoir irrigation or intermittent self-catheterization if needed. These items can be delivered to the client's home. If the client lives alone, it may be necessary to arrange home delivery of groceries and medications.

Housekeeping and lifting are limited for the first 6 to 8 weeks after surgery. Evaluate the client's ability to engage in self-care, and identify the need for additional care from home health nurses. If the client cannot provide care and if a family member is involved with care, respite services may be required. Also consider directing the client and family to local support groups.

Modifications for Elderly Clients

The major modification for older clients with urinary diversion stems from difficulties with self-care. Changing an appliance is one area of difficulty because some dexterity is required. Older clients commonly have arthritis and other disabilities, including decreased visual acuity, that may limit their ability to manipulate catheters and pouches. These concerns must be closely assessed and appropriate assistance offered.

URETERAL TUMORS

Primary tumors of the ureter are rare. In men, ureteral cancer occurs mainly during one's 50s and 60s. This form of cancer rarely affects women. Ureteral neoplasms usually extend from renal or bladder neoplasms or from tumors originating in the bowel, uterus, or ovary. Those primary neoplasms usually occur first as a papillary, transitional cell, or squamous cell carcinoma. These tumors are most frequently found in the lower third of the ureter. In later stages of ureteral cancer, the tumor extends outside the ureter to adjacent structures and regional lymph nodes or to distant sites. Common sites for metastasis include the lungs and liver.

Usually, the first manifestation of ureteral malignancy is gross hematuria. The tumor normally develops painlessly until obstruction occurs. At this point, the client may experience flank pain. Diagnosis is made through urine cytology, IVP, cystoscopy, ultrasonography, and CT scanning.

Treatment of ureteral cancer almost exclusively involves surgical excision and resection. Radiation may also be used in advanced cases with local extension. When the lesion is located in the middle or proximal third of the ureter, the surgical procedure usually involves nephroureterectomy, removal of the kidney, ureter, and attached segment of the bladder on the affected side. If the tumor is in the distal third of the ureter and noninvasive, a more conservative procedure may be used; in this case, just the distal portion of the ureter is resected with ureteral reimplantation.

Silicone rubber (Silastic), polytetrafluoroethylene (Teflon), polytetrafluorourethane, and bovine carotid heterograft are used to replace the resected ureter, facilitating reimplantation in the bladder. A ureter-ureter anastomosis also may be performed. Preoperative and postoperative intervention is similar to that for clients undergoing nephrectomy, ureteral reimplantation, or segmental resection of the bladder.

If the decision is made not to perform any of these procedures, some palliative measure may be needed to prevent or alleviate ureteral obstruction. Urinary diversion may be performed, as described previously, or a ureteral stent catheter may be placed into the ureter during cystoscopy to maintain its patency. The older catheter, a flanged, winged stent (Gibbon's stent), or the newer double J stent is made to prevent migration up the ureter or dislodgment by ureteral peristaltic waves or gravity.

URINARY CALCULI

Urinary calculi *(urolithiasis)* are calcifications in the urinary system. Commonly called stones, calculi form primarily in the kidney *(nephrolithiasis)*, but they can form in or migrate to the lower urinary system. They are typically asymptomatic until they pass into the lower urinary tract. Stones are usually managed by a urologist. Primary bladder calculi are rare and usually develop from a history of urinary stasis from obstruction or chronic infection.

Up to 4% of the population in the United States have urolithiasis. About 12% of the male population have a renal stone by age 70. More than 200,000 Americans require hospitalization for treatment of stones each year. Many more people pass stones spontaneously with only minor manifestations that require no treatment, whereas others are treated in an ambulatory setting. The recurrence rate for calcium oxalate stones is about 50% within 5 years.[43]

Etiology and Risk Factors

The two primary causative factors are (1) urinary stasis and (2) supersaturation of urine with poorly soluble crystalloids. Increased solute concentration occurs because of fluid depletion or an increased solute load. This increased concentration leads to the precipitation of crystals, such as calcium, uric acid, and phosphate. Urinary pH influences the solubility of certain crystals, with some crystal types precipitating readily in acid urine and some in alkaline urine. Abnormal pH levels occur in renal tubular acidosis with the administration of carbonic anhydrase inhibitors, in the presence of urea-splitting bacteria, and in severe, chronic diarrhea. Stasis of urine from bladder neck obstruction, continent urinary diversion, and immobilization increases the risk for development of stones because the crystals in unmoving urine precipitate more readily.

Infection, foreign bodies, failure to empty the bladder completely, metabolic disorders, and obstruction in the urinary tract contribute to the formation of calculi as well. The presence of precipitators has been noted in the urine (such as protein matrix and bacteria or inflammatory elements).

Inhibitor substances, such as citrate and magnesium, appear to keep particles from aggregating and forming crystals; a lack of inhibitors increases risk of stone development. Not only does the deficiency of inhibitors predispose the client to calculi, but there may be "anti-inhibitors" in the urine, such as aluminum, iron, and silicone. Certain medications may induce calculus formation, such as acetazolamide, absorbable alkalis (e.g., calcium carbonate and sodium bicarbonate), and aluminum hydroxide. Massive doses of vitamin C increase urinary oxalate levels.

There is an increased risk of calculus formation in the southeast part of the United States—an area known as "the stone belt." Men between ages 30 and 50 years have three times the risk of calculi.[26] Stones are also more common among people of European or Asian descent. Once a client has had calculi, there is an increased risk of additional ones.

Urolithiasis results not from any single factor but from multiple phenomena. One unanswered question is why some clients form calculi whereas others do not. This problem is particularly important with recurrent "stone formers."

Risk factors for stone formation include anything that either causes stasis or supersaturation of the urine, including:

- Immobility and a sedentary lifestyle, which increase stasis
- Dehydration, which leads to supersaturation
- Metabolic disturbances that result in an increase in calcium or other ions in the urine
- Previous history of urinary calculi
- Living in stone-belt areas
- High mineral content in drinking water
- A diet high in purines, oxalates, calcium, animal proteins
- UTIs
- Prolonged indwelling catheterization
- Neurogenic bladder
- A history of female genital mutilation

Health promotion and health maintenance activities are discussed under Nursing Management of the Medical Client.

Pathophysiology

The exact mechanism of stone formation has not been clearly defined. In fact, some researchers believe that a low calcium intake contributes whereas others contend that a high calcium intake contributes. Both groups agree on the role of supersaturation, however. Crystallization appears to be the primary factor in calculus development from[19, 30]:

- Supersaturation of urine with increased solutes
- Matrix formation caused when mucoproteins bind to the mass of the stone
- Lack of inhibitors caused by increased or absent protectors against stone formation
- A combination of these conditions

Generally, crystal growth involves *nucleation*, in which crystals are formed from supersaturated urine. Growth continues by aggregation to form larger particles. One of these particles may travel down the urinary tract until it is trapped at some narrow point where it becomes the nidus for stone formation.

Inhibitor substances (e.g., citrate, pyrophosphate, and magnesium) have been identified as *chelating agents*. When present in adequate amounts, they act to keep crystals from aggregating and forming stones. When inhibitors are absent, stone formation following crystal aggregation is more likely. Also, a fibrous matrix of urinary organic material (mostly mucoproteins) may form in the kidney or bladder, producing a substance into which crystallites are deposited and trapped. This, then, becomes the nidus of the stone. The excessive production of this mucoprotein may, in part, account for a family history of urolithiasis in clients with calculi.

TYPES OF CALCULI

Stones may be of one crystal type or a combination of types.

Calcium

Calcium is the most common substance and is found in up to 90% of stones.[26] Calcium stones are usually composed of calcium phosphate or calcium oxalate. They may range from very small particles, often called "sand" or "gravel," to giant staghorn calculi, which may fill the entire renal pelvis and extend up into the calyces (Fig.

34–5). The peak onset is during a person's 20s, and these stones affect primarily males.

Hypercalciuria (an increased solute load of calcium in the urine), is caused by four main components:

- A high rate of bone reabsorption, which liberates calcium, as in Paget's disease, hyperparathyroidism, Cushing's disease, immobility, and osteolysis caused by malignant tumors of the breast, lung, and prostate
- Gut absorption of abnormally large amounts of calcium, as in milk-alkali syndrome, sarcoidosis, and excessive intake of vitamin D
- Impaired renal tubular absorption of filtered calcium, as in renal tubular acidosis
- Structural abnormalities, such as "sponge kidney"

About 35% of all clients with calcium stones do not have high serum levels of calcium and demonstrate no apparent cause of hypercalciuria.

There are two variants of hypercalciuria:

1. The primary abnormality is increased intestinal absorption of calcium or increased bone reabsorption. The resulting higher serum calcium level triggers increased renal filtration of calcium and parathyroid hormone (PTH) suppression. This in turn decreases tubular reabsorption, thereby increasing the concentration of calcium in the urine.
2. "Renal leak" of calcium, the other abnormality, is caused by a tubular defect. The resulting hypocalcemia stimulates PTH production, which increases intestinal absorption of calcium. This cycle fits into the previous one, causing an increased solute load of calcium. Clients with this problem are often called "calcium wasters."

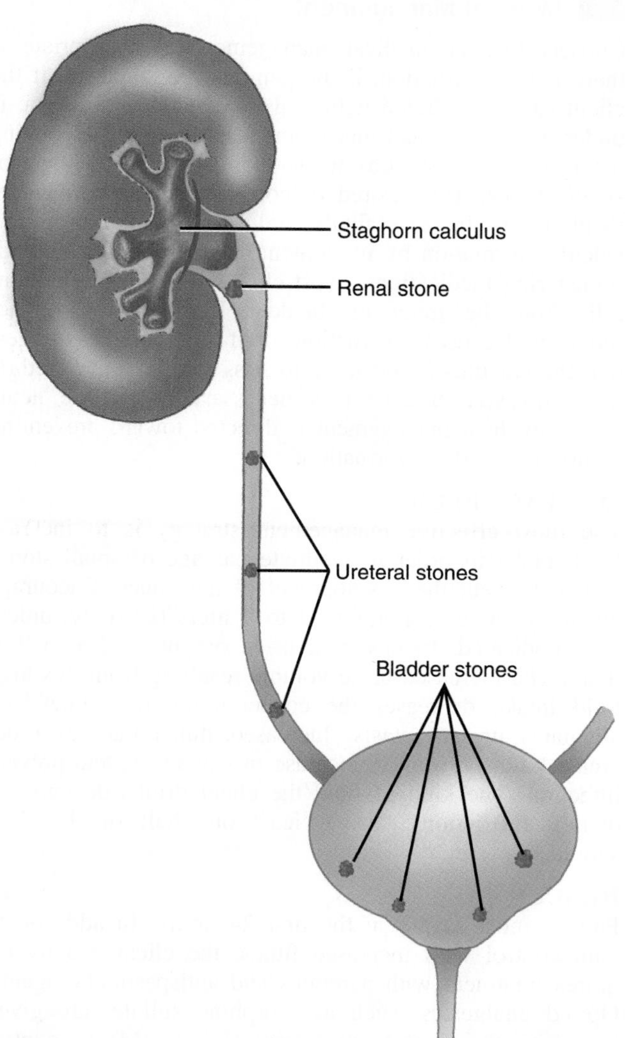

FIGURE 34–5 Staghorn calculus (stone) and other locations of calculi in the urinary tract.

Oxalate

The second most frequent stone is oxalate, which is relatively insoluble in urine. Its solubility is affected only slightly by changes in urinary pH. The mechanism of oxalate availability is unclear but may be closely related to diet. The disease is most common in areas where cereals are a major dietary component and least common in dairy-farming regions.

An increased incidence of oxalate stones may be related to:

- Hyperabsorption of oxalate, seen with inflammatory bowel disease
- Postileal resection or small-bowel bypass surgery
- Overdose of ascorbic acid (vitamin C), which metabolizes to oxalate
- Familial oxaluria (oxalate in the urine)
- Concurrent fat malabsorption, which may cause calcium binding, thus freeing oxalate for absorption

Struvite

Struvite stones, also called triple phosphate, are composed of carbonate apatite and magnesium ammonium phosphate. Their cause is certain bacteria, usually *Proteus*, which contain the enzyme urease. This enzyme splits urea into two ammonia molecules, which raises the urine pH. Phosphate precipitates in alkaline urine. This action is responsible for the label "urea-splitter" characterizing these organisms.

Stones formed in this manner are staghorn calculi (see Fig. 34–5). Abscess formation is common. Struvite stones are difficult to eliminate because the hard stone forms around a nucleus of bacteria, protecting them from antibiotic therapy. Any small fragment left after surgical removal of the stone begins the cycle again.

Uric Acid

Uric acid stones are caused by increased urate excretion, fluid depletion, and a low urinary pH. *Hyperuricuria* is the result of either increased uric acid production or the administration of uricosuric agents. Approximately 25% of people with primary gout and about 50% of persons with secondary gout develop uric acid stones. A high dietary intake of food rich in *purine* (a protein) may predispose clients to uric acid stone formation. Also, treating neoplastic disease with agents that cause rapid cell destruction may increase the urinary uric acid concentration. Moreover, a link between hyperuricuria and calcium stone formation may exist. It is hypothesized that uric acid crystals absorb some of the crystal inhibitors normally found in urine.

Cystine

Cystinuria is the result of a congenital metabolic error inherited as an autosomal recessive disorder. Cystine stones typically appear during childhood and adolescence; development in adults is very rare.

Xanthine

Xanthine stones occur as a result of a rare hereditary condition in which there is a xanthine oxidase deficiency. This crystal precipitates readily in acid urine.

SUMMARY

Despite the type of stone that forms, the potential damage is essentially the same: (1) pain, spasm, or colic from peristalsis movements of the ureter contracting on the stone; (2) obstruction with possible hydronephrosis or hydroureter; (3) tissue trauma with secondary hemorrhage; and (4) infection.

Clinical Manifestations

The most characteristic manifestation of renal or ureteral calculi is a sharp, severe pain of sudden onset caused by movement of the calculus and consequent irritation. Depending on the site of the stone, this pain may be either *renal colic* or *ureteral colic*. Renal colic originates deep in the lumbar region and radiates around the side and down toward the testicle in the male and the bladder in the female. Ureteral colic radiates toward the genitalia and thigh.

When the pain is severe, the client usually has nausea, vomiting, pallor, grunting respirations, elevated blood pressure and pulse, diaphoresis, and anxiety. Visceral pain such as renal colic is mediated by the autonomic nervous system via celiac ganglia, which causes nausea, vomiting, decreased intestinal motility, and possibly paralytic ileus. Some people, especially those with bladder stones, experience manifestations of urgency, frequency, hematuria, and chronic cystitis. Pressure against the bladder neck during micturition (voiding) may cause a heavy feeling in the suprapubic region, obstruction in voiding, a decreased bladder capacity, and an intermittent urinary stream. If the stone enters the urethra, urine flow will be obstructed. The pain lasts for minutes to days and can be somewhat resistant to narcotic intervention.

Pain may be intermittent, which usually means that the stone has moved. Physicians hypothesize that the ureter dilates just proximal to the calculus, which allows urine to pass, relieving the ureteral distention. Then, as the stone moves into a new obstruction site, the pain returns. The pain subsides when the stone reaches the bladder.

Pain caused by renal stones is not always severe and colicky. It may be dull or aching or may be experienced as a heavy feeling. This is particularly true during the early stages of hydronephrosis. Sometimes, there may be no sensation, and the first clue the client has is seeing blood in the urine or hearing a "clink" against the toilet when the stone passes.

Other manifestations of calculi include infection with an elevated temperature and white blood cell (WBC) count and urine obstruction that causes hydroureter, hydronephrosis, or both. A flat plate of the abdomen and an x-ray study of the kidney, ureter and bladder (commonly called a KUB) are the standard diagnostic tools. These studies should reveal radiopaque stones and aid in the evaluation of stone size.

Determining the size of the calculus is essential in selecting the treatment. Stones smaller than 4 or 5 mm can pass without intervention. Because some stones, such as uric acid stones, are not radiopaque and not visible on x-ray, it is crucial to note when a client presents with manifestations of calculi. Elevated serum uric acid levels may confirm a suspicion of urinary calculi. In addition, an IVP may show a filling defect at the site of the stone or ultrasonography may reveal the stone. Diagnosis of a bladder stone is confirmed by direct visualization through cystoscopy. Once the stone is retrieved, its components must be analyzed.

Additional studies of blood and urine may be required to determine whether metabolic problems predispose the client to stone formation. Other possible disease processes, such as metastatic bone cancer, must be ruled out as possible causes of calculi.

Outcome Management

Medical Management

Conservative or medical management is appropriate if there is no obstruction, if the pain can be managed, if the client can be hydrated with oral fluids, and if the stone is under 5 mm. Medical management is directed at relieving the acute manifestations while facilitating the passage of small stones. The desired outcomes of medical management are to increase fluids, reduce pain, and minimize calculus formation by implementing diet changes and administering medications. Most clients pass the stone naturally from the ureter and bladder. If the stone does not move, if it causes obstruction, or if x-ray studies suggest that the calculus is too large to pass safely to the urethra, more invasive treatment is necessary. After the acute phase, medical management is directed toward preventing recurrence of stone formation.

INCREASE FLUIDS

The most effective management strategy is to increase fluid intake in order to facilitate passage of small stones and to prevent the development of new ones. Encourage clients to increase fluids to 3 to 4 liters (L) daily, unless contraindicated, to ensure a urine output of 2.5 to 3 L daily. The increased urine volume resulting from this high fluid intake decreases the concentration of solutes and alleviates urinary stasis. Increased fluids may also decrease pain, prevent an increase in stone size, and prevent infection. The kind of fluid the client drinks depends on dietary restrictions, but at least one half of the fluid should be water.

REDUCE PAIN

Pain is most severe in the first 24 hours. In addition to pain control with increased fluids, the client usually requires treatment with narcotics and antispasmodic agents. Opioid analgesics, such as morphine sulfate, are given intravenously or intramuscularly (IV or IM) to control moderate to severe pain. Nonsteroidal anti-inflammatory drugs (NSAIDs) may also be effective.

Antispasmodic agents, such as oxybutynin chloride (Ditropan), are very effective for relieving and controlling colic pain associated with spasms of the ureter. Clients with repeated stone formation may have a family member drive them to a clinic, ambulatory care center, or emergency department for administration of opioid analgesics and antispasmodic agents so that they can relax, go home, and pass the stone naturally. Other clients may require admission to an acute care setting for administration of these medications. For nausea and vomiting associated with colic, antiemetics may also be necessary.

PREVENT STONE RECURRENCE

Diet modifications and medications may be required to prevent further calculus formation in clients who return with repeated stones. Increased fluid intake is still the primary prevention measure. Results of a stone analysis are essential before these recommendations are implemented.

IMPLEMENT DIETARY CHANGES. Some controversy exists over dietary restrictions because of their uncertain effectiveness and the problems clients experience in following the regimen. Calcium stones and hypercalciuria may be controlled by limiting excessive calcium intake, although it should be maintained at about 800 mg daily.

Clients with oxalate stones should avoid high-oxalate foods, such as tea, tomatoes, instant coffee, cola drinks, beer, rhubarb, green beans, asparagus, spinach, cabbage, celery, chocolate, citrus fruits, apples, grapes, cranberries, peanuts, and peanut butter. Megadoses of vitamin C increase oxalate excretion in the urine and should be avoided. If the stone is composed of uric acid, the client should follow a low-purine diet, which involves limiting such foods as aged cheeses, wine, bony fish, and organ meats.

ADMINISTER MEDICATIONS. Following recurrent stone formation, analysis of the stone, or abnormal metabolic findings, medications may be required. For hypercalciuric clients, a thiazide diuretic such as hydrochlorothiazide (HydroDIURIL) will promote calcium resorption from the renal tubules, thereby preventing excess calcium loads in the urine. Potassium citrate is commonly added to the thiazide diuretic to replace potassium as needed.

For low urine citrate levels, potassium or sodium citrate may be ordered. Since these medications can be expensive, many urologists encourage the client to drink a quart of lemonade for both the increased fluid and citrate benefits.

Calcium oxalate stones may be treated with vitamin B_6 (pyridoxine), magnesium oxide, or cholestyramine. For clients with hyperuricosuria and calcium oxalate stones, allopurinol (Zyloprim) is prescribed only if a reduced purine diet fails and stones persist.

Uric acid stones are treated with drugs to lower uric acid, such as allopurinol. In addition, sodium bicarbonate or citrate may be indicated to raise urinary pH because uric acid stones form in acidic urine. This treatment is also effective for xanthine stones, which are inhibited in alkaline urine. Cystine stones are treated with tiopronin (Thiola) and d-penicillamine, which make cystine more soluble for excretion. Long-term antibiotics are used to control the infection that leads to struvite stone formation.

Nursing Management of the Medical Client

ASSESSMENT

Ask the client about any family history of calculi, previous UTIs, immobility, and recent dietary habits. For instance, a large intake of purines may be significant, as would drinking a large amount of fruit juice or tea, which could cause oxalate precipitation. Also assess the amount, pattern, and types of fluids consumed.

Assess the client for the clinical manifestations described earlier. Use rating scales to measure the severity of pain. Many clients describe renal or ureteral colic as "the worst pain I've ever had." Vital signs should be monitored. A decreasing blood pressure may indicate severe pain and impending shock; increased pulse and temperature may result from infection. A sudden onset of little or no urine output suggests obstruction, which is an emergency that must be treated immediately to preserve kidney function. Frequency and dysuria commonly occur when a stone reaches the bladder.

All urine voided should be strained through several layers of gauze or through a commercial urine strainer. Carefully examine all debris caught by straining. Save any stone material so that the stone's composition can be analyzed as a basis for treatment and to show how much has passed through the urinary tract. A routine urinalysis, urine for culture and sensitivity testing, and a 24-hour urine specimen may be needed.

DIAGNOSIS, OUTCOMES, INTERVENTIONS

Pain. The priority nursing diagnosis is *Pain related to irritation and spasm from stone movement in the urinary tract.*

Outcomes. The client will report pain relief or control.

Interventions. During the acute phase of treatment, offer pain medications, antispasmodics, and antiemetics, if necessary. For severe pain, give the medications on a regular schedule. Use a rating scale to help evaluate the client's pain.

Once pain is controlled, the client will be able to force fluids and ambulate, which will facilitate passage of the stone. Relaxation techniques, such as guided imagery or therapeutic or healing touch, can help to relieve pain. Help the client find a comfortable position to alternate with ambulation.

Effective Management of Therapeutic Regimen. More than half of clients with a urinary calculus experience another within 5 years. As a result, an important nursing diagnosis is *Effective Management of Therapeutic Regimen related to prevention of recurrent calculi.*

Outcomes. The number of recurrences will be reduced, and the interval between stones will increase.

Interventions

Increase Fluids. Teach the client to drink 3 to 4 L of fluid daily to flush the urinary system. At least half the fluid consumed should be water. Intake should be as consistent as possible throughout the 24-hour period.

As a rule, encourage the client to drink a full glass of water every hour during the day and two large glasses just before going to bed. This schedule will probably create the need to void during the night, at which time the client should drink another glass of water.

Teach Stone Prevention Measures. Besides increased fluid intake, teach the client other measures to prevent stone recurrence, such as diet modifications, medications if required, and avoidance of urinary stasis (see Client Education Guide). Prompt treatment of urinary tract infections and early recognition of manifestations of stone recurrence are also important.

Health promotion activities include frequent turning and range of motion for immobilized clients, increased fluid intake, and decreased intake of stone-forming solutes in the diet, such as oxalates, purines, and animal proteins. Health maintenance interventions include monitoring high-risk clients with indwelling catheters or obstructions for calculi.

EVALUATION

If medical management is successful, the client's pain will be controlled, the stone will pass unaided, and the client will have no complications of obstruction or infection. The client will be able to describe factors that increase the risk of developing stones and will be able to identify self-care strategies to prevent stone recurrence.

Surgical Management

About 20% of stones require additional treatment with shock wave lithotripsy or endourologic or surgical procedures. Open surgery is used only for the small percentage of clients who cannot be successfully treated with lithotripsy or endourologic procedures.

ENDOUROLOGIC PROCEDURES

Depending on the position of the calculus, cystoscopy may be done. Small stones may be removed transurethrally with a cystoscope, ureteroscope, or ureterorenoscope. Additionally, one or two ureteral catheters or stents may be inserted past the stone. From this point, several different interventions are appropriate. The catheters may be left in place for 24 hours or longer to drain urine trapped proximal to the stone and to dilate the ureter, which may prompt spontaneous movement of the calculus. Otherwise, the catheter may mechanically guide the stone downward as it is removed.

At times, a continuous chemical irrigation may be used to dissolve uric acid, struvite, and cystine stones. Finally, an attempt may be made to manipulate or dislodge the stone with a variety of special catheters with loops and expanding baskets used to snare the stone. Care of these clients is the same as that following cystoscopy.

Larger stones may be crushed with an instrument called a *lithotrite* (stone crusher) to facilitate removal. *Cystolitholapaxy* is performed when a bladder stone is soft enough to be crushed. In cystoscopic lithotripsy, an ultrasonic lithotrite is placed to pulverize the stone, followed by extensive flushing of the bladder. Possible complications associated with this procedure include hemorrhage, urinary retention, infection, bladder perforation, and possibly retained stone fragments.

A flexible ureteroscope, passed through a cystoscope, is used to collect stones in the ureter. This procedure, called *ureteroscopy*, is used to retrieve 4- to 5-mm stones or, combined with ultrasonic lithotripsy, to remove fragments after treatment. Minimal sedation or anesthesia is necessary, and postoperative complications are usually few.

A flexible ureterorenoscope can be passed for access to the entire upper urinary tract, including the distal ureter and intrarenal collecting system so that stones or lesions in the lower pole or lateral calices can be reached.

A nephroscope may be inserted to retrieve free-lying renal stones. Figure 34–6*A* shows a nephroscope in place. The stone may be removed with alligator forceps or a stone basket followed by irrigation. Electrohydraulic, laser, or ultrasound lithotripsy may be completed through the nephroscope. After this procedure, a nephrostomy tube remains in place for 1 to 5 days. The client can go home with it in place. Increased fluids are essential to achieve a urine output greater than 3000 ml (3 L). The tube is removed after diagnostic studies determine that all stone fragments have been removed.

LITHOTRIPSY

LASER LITHOTRIPSY. A newer treatment for calculi is laser lithotripsy. Lasers are used together with a ureteroscope to remove or loosen impacted stones. Constant water irrigation of the ureter is required to dissipate the heat. Complications resulting from this procedure are the same as those of any endourologic procedure.

EXTRACORPOREAL SHOCK WAVE LITHOTRIPSY. *Extracorporeal shock wave lithotripsy* (ESWL) is the use of sound waves applied externally to break up stones in

CLIENT EDUCATION GUIDE

Preventing Recurrence of Urinary Stones

Increase your fluid intake to at least 3 L (3 qt) every day.
Be sure to urinate at least every 2 hours.
Remember the early manifestations of urinary stones. If the symptoms occur again, see your physician promptly.
Monitor the pH of your urine with pH paper. If you had calcium stones, keep your urine acidic. If you had uric acid stones, keep your urine basic. Keep urine acidic with high-protein diet. Keep urine basic with a low-protein diet, plenty of vegetables, and citrus fruits.
Be sure to follow your physician's instructions for follow-up urinalysis and blood tests to detect factors that can cause urinary stones.
If manifestations of urinary tract infection develop, see your physician promptly for diagnosis and treatment. Manifestations include pain and burning when you urinate, a sense of urgency to urinate, having to urinate frequently, and a fever.

Stones Other than Uric Acid Stones

Follow your physician's instructions for keeping your urine acidic.

Calcium Stones

Follow an 800-mg calcium diet.

Uric Acid Stones

Follow a low-purine diet.
Take the medications, such as allopurinol (Zyloprim), prescribed to improve your excretion of uric acid.

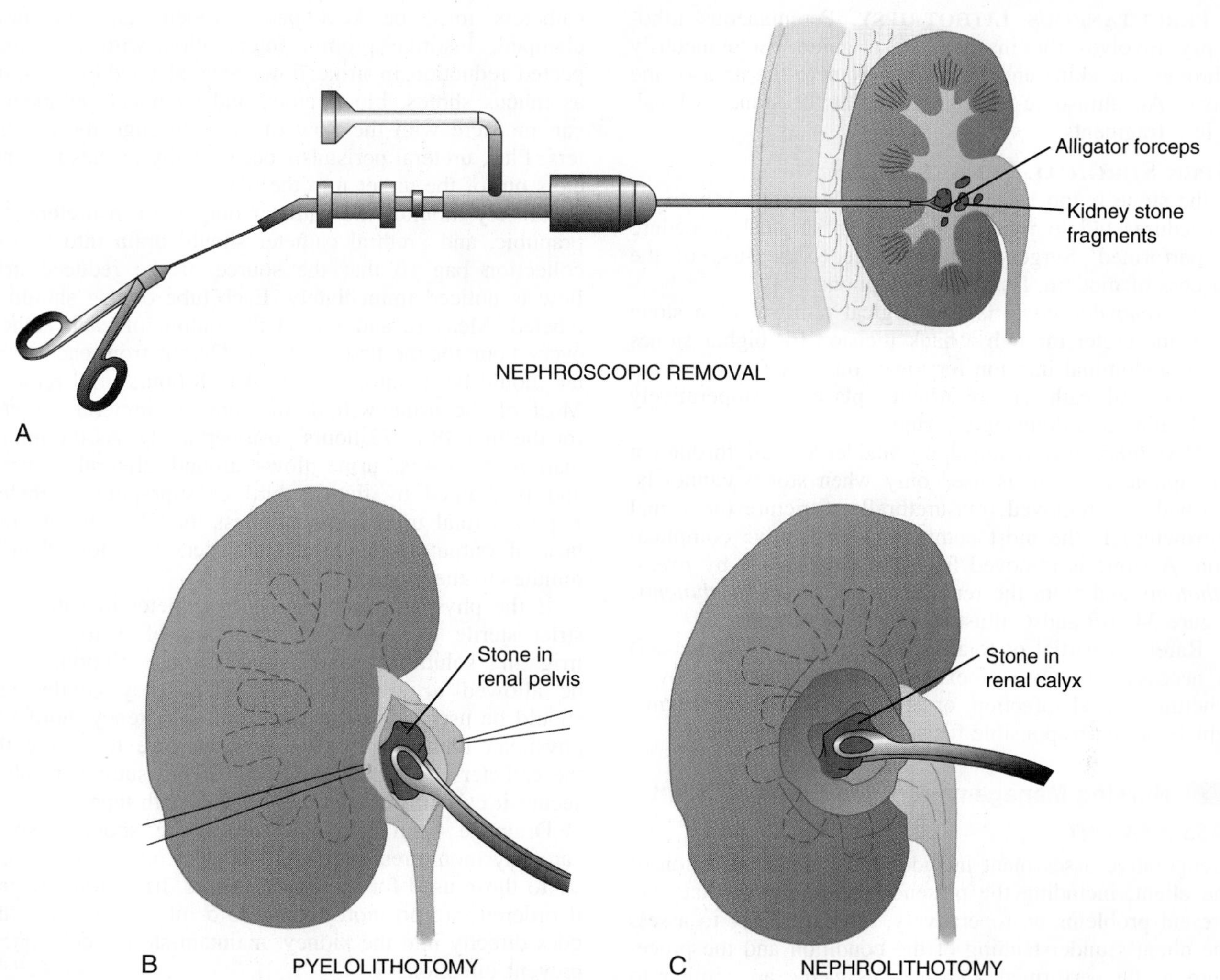

FIGURE 34–6 *A–C,* Surgical techniques for removal of kidney stones.

the kidney or ureter (Fig. 34–7). High-energy shock waves, aimed by fluoroscopy, are transmitted to the stone. The shock waves break the stones into small fragments, which are passed or retrieved endoscopically. The client may be strapped to a frame in a water bath or secured on a table, depending on the type of lithotripsy equipment selected or available. The client is usually sedated with regional or general anesthesia.

The procedure lasts 30 to 50 minutes with administration of 500 to 1500 shock waves. Cardiac monitoring is required to synchronize shock waves with the R wave to prevent cardiac dysrhythmias. Complications of ESWL include ecchymosis on the affected flank, retained fragments, urosepsis, perinephric hematoma, and hemorrhage.

Stone fragments may bunch up in the distal ureter, obstructing the kidney. To prevent this accumulation and obstruction, a double J stent is commonly placed via cystoscopy before ESWL for stones larger than 6 mm. The stent is removed during a follow-up visit.

After ESWL, the client may experience renal or ureteral colic that needs to be treated with antispasmodics. Early ambulation and increased fluid intake are important for flushing out stone fragments. The fragments may be passed for up to 3 months after the procedure.

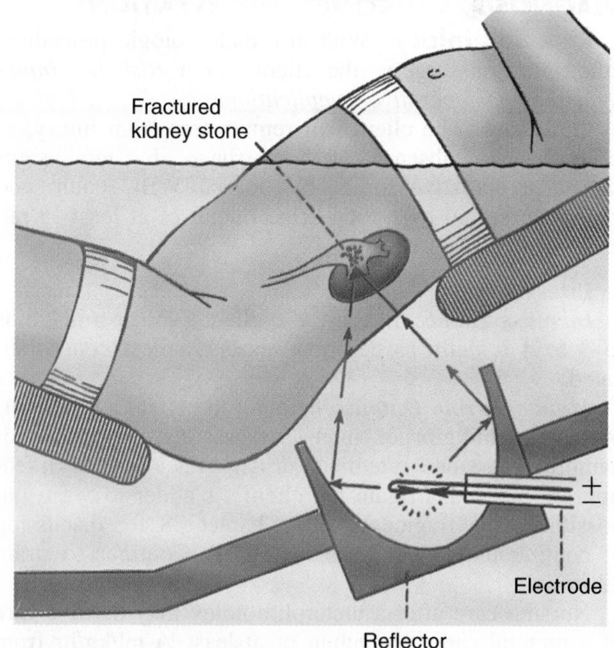

FIGURE 34–7 Water bath extracorporeal shock wave lithotripsy. Electrically generated shock waves fracture kidney stones.

Percutaneous Lithotripsy. Percutaneous lithotripsy involves the insertion of a guide percutaneously (through the skin) under fluoroscopy near the area of the stone. An ultrasonic wave is aimed at the stone to break it into fragments.

Open Surgical Procedures

If the stone is too large or if endourologic and lithotripsy procedures fail to remove it, an open surgical procedure is performed. Surgery is rarely needed because of the success of modern, less invasive options.

A *ureterolithotomy* is the surgical removal of a stone from the ureter through a flank incision for higher stones or an abdominal incision for lower ones. A Penrose drain and ureteral catheter are usually placed postoperatively for healing and drainage of urine.

Cystolithotomy, removal of bladder calculi through a suprapubic incision, is used only when stones cannot be crushed and removed transurethrally. Stricture (abnormal narrowing) is the most common postoperative complication. A stone is removed from the renal pelvis by *pyelolithotomy* and from the renal calyx by a *nephrolithotomy*. Figure 34–6*B* and *C* illustrates these procedures.

Rarely, a partial or total *nephrectomy* (see Chapter 35) is necessary because of extensive kidney damage, overwhelming renal infection, or abnormal renal parenchyma, which can be responsible for stone formation.

Nursing Management of the Surgical Client

Assessment

Preoperative assessment includes the general condition of the client, including the presence of conditions that may present problems postoperatively. It is a priority to assess the client's understanding of the condition and the procedure to be performed. Other assessments are similar to those described under Nursing Management of the Medical Client.

Diagnosis, Outcomes, Interventions

Risk for Injury. With any endourologic procedure, lithotripsy, or surgery, the client has a *Risk for Injury related to postoperative complications.*

Outcomes. The client will remain free from injury, as evidenced by absence of hemorrhage, by vital signs within preoperative limits, by normal WBC count and temperature, and by a total urine output of at least ½ ml/kg/hr from all sources.

Interventions

Increase Fluids. Increase the client's IV or oral fluids to 3 to 4 L daily as described earlier, unless contraindicated.

Monitor Urine Output. Maintain the client's urine output at ½ ml/kg/hr or more. Assess any indications of hemorrhage, stone retention, urinary retention, or infection. As needed, irrigate the client's bladder to wash out possible stone fragments. See Chapter 38 for discussion of continuous bladder irrigation (CBI). Continue to strain all urine.

Nursing care after a ureterolithotomy may involve care of a ureteral catheter. Output of at least ¼ ml/kg/hr from the ureteral catheter should be expected and closely monitored. Because the renal pelvis holds only 5 ml, ureteral catheters must be kept patent (open) and are never clamped. Institute prompt intervention with any unexpected reduction in urine flow. Several conditions—such as mucus shreds, blood clots, and chemical sediment—can interfere with the flow of urine through these catheters. Plus, ureteral peristalsis occasionally pushes the catheters out of the ureter into the bladder.

Closely monitor the catheter output. Each ureteral, suprapubic, and urethral catheter should drain into its own collection bag so that the source of the reduced urine flow is noticed immediately. Each tube or bag should be labeled. Measure and record the output of each catheter every hour for the first 24 hours. Output from each catheter should be monitored every 4 to 8 hours until removal. Most of the urine will drain from the ureteral catheters for the first 48 to 72 hours postoperatively. As the inflammation decreases, urine flows around ureteral catheters and is drained by the urethral or suprapubic catheters. Report a total urine output of less than ½ ml/kg/hr or a lack of output from ureteral catheters for more than 15 minutes to the physician immediately.

If the physician orders ureteral catheter irrigation, use strict sterile technique. A maximum of 3 to 5 ml of irrigating solution, usually sterile saline solution, should be allowed to flow in by gravity. Very gentle force should be used. If you cannot confirm patency, notify the physician immediately. Use extreme care to ensure that the catheter is not dislodged. If it is not sutured in place, secure it carefully to the client's skin with tape.

Drainage from a nephrostomy tube should also be carefully monitored and cared for with interventions similar to those used for ureteral catheters. Irrigation amounts, if ordered, are no more than 3 to 5 ml. Because the tube goes directly into the kidney, maintain sterile technique to prevent infection.

Clients with any type of catheter must be taught how to care for them before returning home. They should learn how to clean around them, empty them, prevent kinking, and irrigate them if necessary. A home health nurse may be required to assist with these activities.

Prevent Complications. If a the client has a flank incision, care is similar to that needed after nephrectomy (see Chapter 35). To prevent pneumonia, the client will need to cough and deep breathe 10 to 20 times each hour. To facilitate this, administer opioid narcotics regularly to control incisional pain. Other postoperative interventions are similar to those for a client with any major abdominal incision, such as monitoring bowel sounds, vital signs, and output from drains and nasogastric tube. Antibiotics may be given prophylactically or at the first sign of infection.

Evaluation

It is expected that surgical intervention for stone removal is completed with the least invasive procedure possible and before renal damage occurs. In most instances the client can go home the day of the procedure and does not need to be hospitalized. Clients may go home with catheters in place for about a week and will need to learn catheter care or have home health follow-up. For major surgical intervention, the client is dismissed 3 to 4 days after the procedure.

Self-Care

A client with urolithiasis is at risk for recurrence. You have a major role in helping the client develop and maintain an effective, individual regimen to prevent stone recurrence. The main components of prevention are (1) increased fluids, (2) dietary modifications, (3) medications as ordered, and (4) prompt treatment of UTIs. The client must understand that these are lifelong changes in lifestyle. If catheters are in place after surgical intervention, client management of the tubes is necessary before discharge from the hospital.

URINARY REFLUX

Urinary reflux is the backward flow of urine in the urinary tract. It usually begins at the vesicoureteral junction. Urine flows back into the ureter and upward into the renal pelvis. The severity of vesicoureteral reflux is stated as grade I, which is least severe, through grade V, which is most severe. There is an increase in the development of reflux in men over 50 years of age because of chronic bladder neck obstruction from BPH. Reflux typically occurs in younger children or in young adults from congenital abnormalities of the vesicoureteral junction.

Etiology and Risk Factors

Reflux can be caused by a congenital abnormality, such as ectopic ureter, chronic bladder infections secondary to dysfunctional bladder, or outlet obstruction in the bladder neck. Urinary reflux is more frequently seen as a result of another condition. Reflux contributes to the increase of intravesical pressure (within the bladder) until it finally overwhelms the resistance of the intramural ureteral sphincters, allowing reflux to occur. Clients with obstructions must be evaluated to have the cause identified and treated to prevent and relieve intravesical pressure.

Pathophysiology

In bladder outlet obstruction, the main result is the continuous presence of residual urine, which leads to chronic UTIs. Continual overdistention of the bladder can also decrease detrusor tone, increasing the bladder's capacity and raising the threshold needed to start the micturition reflex.

Renal damage and pyelonephritis are the two primary problems resulting from vesicoureteral reflux. Because the capacity of the renal pelvis is only 5 ml, larger amounts of urine can cause renal parenchymal changes, hydronephrosis, or hydronephroureterosis if they result from ureteral obstruction or reflux. The increased hydrostatic pressure leads to renal cortical atrophy from ischemia and hypoxia and then to calicectasis (dilation of the renal calices). The destruction of kidney tissue, often asymptomatic and undetected, can progress to end-stage renal disease. The kidneys are usually protected from ascending infections by the intramural portion of the distal ureter. With reflux, however, any pathogens in the bladder are carried through the ureters to the kidney. This problem leads to recurrent pyelonephritis. Chronic pyelonephritis leads to renal failure.

Clinical Manifestations

The major manifestation of reflux in the bladder neck is pyelonephritis. When the obstruction is in the vesicoureteral junction or higher, renal failure may be clinically evident. The major diagnostic studies are (1) the VCUG to visualize the lower urinary system during voiding, (2) cystoscopy to evaluate manifestations of obstruction, (3) ureteroscopy to assess the vesicoureteral junction, (4) ultrasound to assess for hydronephrosis, and (5) IVP to evaluate the entire collecting system. Blood studies of BUN and creatinine levels are also done to assess renal function.

Outcome Management

Surgical Management

Because there are no medical regimens to prevent or treat reflux caused by ectopic ureter, the primary therapy is surgical. Renal damage from the reflux usually calls for surgical intervention. Surgery is also indicated for obstruction at the ureteropelvic junction, for intractable infection, and for a problem not resolved by maturation. Because the most common causes of reflux are ureteral defects, surgical procedures focus on reimplantation or other treatments for the ureter.

Postoperatively, a urethral or suprapubic catheter keeps the bladder empty to reduce tension on the suture line. A ureteral catheter is also inserted into the ureter involved in the surgical procedure. The tip of this tiny, semi-rigid catheter usually rests in the renal pelvis. The distal end extends through the bladder and out through the urethra or through an abdominal incision.

A ureteral catheter provides three benefits: it splints the ureter to facilitate healing, it prevents obstruction from edema after surgery or other trauma in the area, and it drains urine.

Nursing Management of the Surgical Client

Carefully assess any client with a high risk of obstruction for any manifestation of urinary reflux. The client being evaluated for urinary reflux requires support during this diagnostic process. Preoperative preparation for ureteral surgery is similar to that required by any client who needs surgery (see Chapter 15).

Postoperative care is similar to that discussed earlier for urinary calculi. Assess the color of the client's urine frequently. Expect it to progress from bright red to clear yellow over a matter of days. Discharge teaching depends on a variety of factors, including the cause of the reflux, the treatment or procedure done, and the amount of renal damage present. For the client with kidney damage, renal function must be monitored at regular intervals to evaluate any changes in status.

VOIDING DISORDERS

URINARY RETENTION

Urinary retention is the inability of the bladder to empty partially or completely during voiding. Treatment is directed at relieving the cause of the problem.

Etiology and Risk Factors

Detrusor failure is the most common cause of urinary retention in women. Failure of the bladder to contract, demonstrated on urodynamic evaluation, is often associated with neurologic conditions. In men, obstructive voiding due to an enlarged prostate is the frequent cause of retention. Other disorders, urethral strictures, medications, detrusor-sphincter dyssynergia, calculi, blood clots, tumors, bladder neck contractures and history of female genital mutilation may also cause retention. Neuropathies affecting bladder function include diabetes, strokes, and spinal cord injuries. These long-term problems affect the neurologic status of the bladder and interfere with the micturition reflex. Remember, urinary retention is a manifestation of another pathologic condition.

Retention may be caused by decreased sensory input to and from the bladder, muscle tension, anxiety, or other neurologic conditions affecting the bladder. Surgery has traditionally been a factor; spinal anesthesia causes retention more often than general anesthesia does. After surgery, 10% to 15% of clients who received general anesthesia require catheterization because of an inability to void, and 20% to 25% of those who received spinal anesthesia require a catheter.

In women, prolapse of the back wall of the vagina (rectocele or enterocele) increases the risk of retention by exerting pressure against the urethra. Also, a large cystocele may cause kinking of the bladder neck, decreasing the bladder's ability to empty.

More than half of men older than age 50 experience BPH, a common cause of retention. This is not a preventable problem, although the client with an enlarged prostate should be monitored closely for obstruction secondary to the enlargement. Neurologic injury or disease, such as diabetes mellitus, spinal cord injuries, or multiple sclerosis, may lead to urinary retention as well. Other risk factors are a history of structural abnormalities and use of certain medications, such as tricyclic antidepressants. In some clients, a psychogenic origin may be found.

Pathophysiology

Retention of urine is hazardous because the resulting urinary stasis contributes to UTIs, stone formation, and eventual complications of long-term structural damage to the bladder, ureters, or kidneys. Additionally, continued bladder distention leads to loss of bladder tone.

The pathologic process of retention produces a snowball effect. Retained urine increases hydrostatic pressure against the bladder wall, which results in hypertrophy of the detrusor muscle, formation of trabeculae (connective tissue in the bladder wall), or development of diverticula. At the same time, peristalsis in the ureteral musculature increases against the pressure of the accumulating urine. The ureter may gradually become elongated, tortuous, and fibrotic. Increasing pressure is also transmitted through the renal pelvis and calices into the renal parenchyma. The resulting hydronephrosis exerts pressure on the blood vessels, causing ischemia and increasing the renal damage. If the process is not interrupted, it can proceed to renal failure and death. Figure 34–8 demonstrates the sequence. Even after the retention is relieved, when the alterations caused by increased pressure reach the renal parenchyma, the damage may be permanent and irreversible.

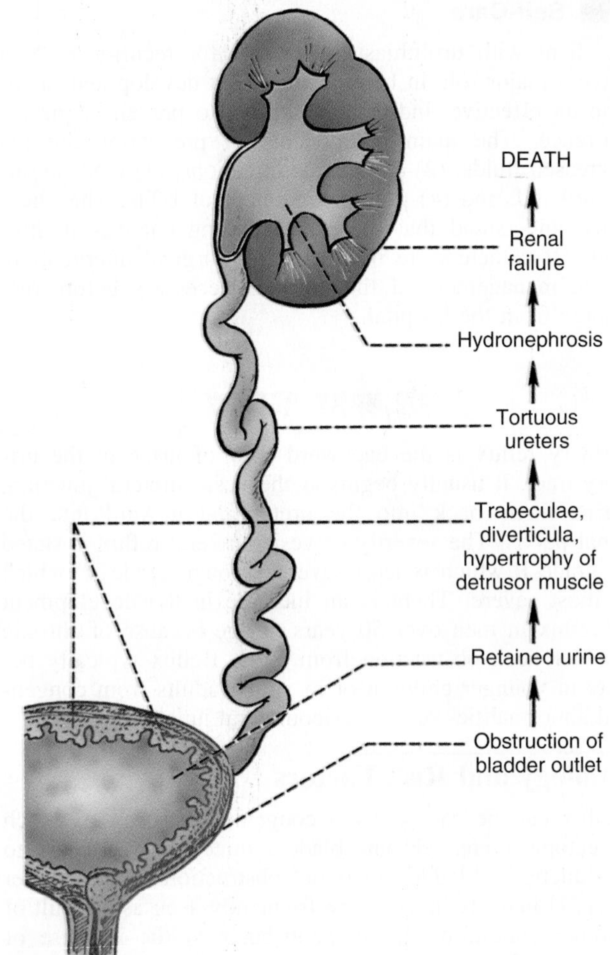

FIGURE 34–8 Potential effects of urinary tract obstruction.

Medications, such as opiates, tricyclic antidepressants, sedatives, antispasmodics, anti-Parkinson drugs, beta-adrenergic blockers, and psychotropic agents, can interfere with normal neurologic function and the micturition reflex. Diseases with neurologic effects, such as stroke, multiple sclerosis, diabetes mellitus, tabes dorsalis, and spinal cord lesions, also disrupt the micturition reflex.

Urinary retention may result in chronic UTI or a series of UTIs and dysfunctional voiding. Conversely, chronic UTIs and dysfunctional voiding may result in urinary retention. The detrusor muscle may become irritated and fail to function correctly, leading to incomplete bladder emptying. Irritation and scarring of the bladder neck or urethra may develop, thus placing these clients at greater risk for urinary retention.

A disorder of psychogenic origin, such as anxiety or fear of voiding in a public restroom, may lead to distention of the bladder and urinary retention. Inability to relax the urethra because of anxiety or neurologic deficit may lead to urinary retention as well.

Anorectal problems, such as hemorrhoids, abscess, fecal impaction, and vaginal prolapse, can be contributing factors, either from obstruction or from secondary spasms of the perineal musculature that interfere with the urethra during voiding.

Decreased oral or IV fluid intake reduces the glomerular filtration rate (GFR). This causes very slow urine production and overfilling of the bladder. The slow increase allows the detrusor muscle to accommodate the increased volume until the muscle's fibers are stretched beyond their ability to contract, hampering micturition.

Urinary retention with overflow incontinence results from the following events. As the bladder continues filling, the intravesical pressure rises. Eventually, this pressure overcomes the resistance of the sphincter. Urine flows out of the bladder until it reduces the intravesical pressure, but only to the level at which the external sphincter can again control the flow of urine. Most clients report that the bladder does not feel empty. It overfills again, and the cycle is repeated.

Prolonged obstruction leads to increased pressures in the urinary tract and may predispose the client to bladder diverticula. A *diverticulum* is a pouch or sac resulting from the herniation of the mucous membrane lining caused by weakness in the muscular wall of an organ. Bladder diverticula are most common in men. Many diverticula are asymptomatic and are usually discovered by chance during assessment of other conditions.

Bladder diverticula can cause two major problems: (1) UTIs, resulting from stasis of urine, and (2) malignancies, probably a result of chronic irritation by persistent infection. Intervention involves removing the obstruction and relieving the retention, followed by surgical excision of the pouch and reestablishment of normal patency of the urinary tract. Postoperatively, catheter drainage of urine is required to allow complete tissue healing. Clients who have had chronic or recurring infections usually require long-term antibiotic therapy after surgery.

Clinical Manifestations

The primary manifestation of urinary retention is a distended bladder or an inability to empty the bladder completely. Voided amounts of 25 to 50 ml one or more times an hour may indicate retention with overflow. The major diagnostic test is catheterization. A post-void residual amount greater than 100 ml after an attempt to void signals retention. Other diagnostic measures, such as cystoscopy and urodynamic testing to include pressure voiding studies, help to identify the cause of the retention.

Outcome Management

Medical Management

Identifying the cause of urinary retention is the first step in determining treatment. Finding the underlying neurologic problem or obstructive disorder is crucial in selecting a treatment plan.

Administer Medications

In some cases, cholinergic medications have been known to help stimulate bladder contractions. If a mechanical obstruction is present, however, cholinergic drug therapy should not be used. In this instance, intravesical pressure increases against an obstructed outlet, causing ureterovesical reflux or a ruptured bladder.

Although their effects are somewhat controversial, bethanechol (Urecholine) and neostigmine (Prostigmin) are commonly given. Bethanechol improves detrusor tone but also increases bladder outlet and urethral resistance. To counteract this, bethanechol is sometimes combined with phenoxybenzamine (Dibenzyline), prazosin (Minipress), and terazosin (Hytrin), which are potent alpha-adrenergic blockers.

Urethral Dilations

In some instances, urinary retention is relieved by dilation of the urethra by means of the placement of progressively larger urethral sounds. Local or sometimes general anesthesia is used.

Nursing Management of the Medical Client

Interventions described next are appropriate for the nursing diagnosis *Urinary Retention.*

Assess Urine Output Patterns

It is important to distinguish retention from *oliguria* (diminished urinary secretion) and *anuria* (complete suppression of urinary secretion). In urinary retention, the kidneys are producing a normal amount of urine but the bladder does not function properly. It fills with urine and rises above the level of the pubic symphysis, sometimes being displaced to either side of midline. Percussion over the bladder produces a dull sound. The client may experience increasing discomfort and the need to urinate. The client also may complain of restlessness, sweating, anxiety, bladder pain, and feelings of bladder fullness.

Implement Measures to Stimulate Independent Voiding

Nursing interventions may be used initially to treat retention. Provide privacy, and place the client in a normal sitting or standing position, using gravity and increased intra-abdominal pressure to help relieve an acute problem. Running the water or flushing the toilet within earshot of the client may encourage voiding. Tape-recorded aquatic sounds may be effective. A warm bath or pouring warm water over the perineum often promotes muscle relaxation. Immersing the client's hands in water sometimes works. Applying ice or gently stroking the inner thigh sometimes works as well. These measures may stimulate trigger points of the micturition reflex. If the client is tense and anxious, any measure that induces relaxation may aid in relieving the situation, even a back rub or soothing music.

Catheterize the Client

For clients with persistent urinary retention, a straight or retention catheter may be inserted through the external meatus, into the urethra beyond the internal sphincter, and into the bladder. A straight catheter is removed after the bladder drains. An indwelling (Foley) catheter is kept in place for continuous or intermittent drainage by inflating a balloon near the catheter's tip. Strict sterile techniques are used for insertion except for clients on an intermittent self-catheterization program; these clients may use clean technique.

The indwelling catheter is attached to either a bedside drainage bag or a leg bag. A leg bag is commonly used for long-term catheterization, especially for a client going home with the catheter in place. This device allows the client more mobility and eliminates the embarrassment of carrying a drainage bag in public view (Fig. 34–9).

Because of the bag's small capacity, it must be emptied frequently. A conventional drainage system is used at night to avoid the need to empty the bag at night. Instruct the client to avoid attaching the rubber straps too tightly, because doing so may cause skin irritation, thrombophlebitis, and ulcer formation. Loose straps tend to tighten as the bag fills. Recent improvements have lead to the use of nylon self-fastening tape (Velcro) leg straps for clients with circulatory problems, latex allergy, and at high risk for skin breakdown. Meticulous skin care and periodic removal of the bag help prevent these problems. Cleanliness and odor control are managed by washing the apparatus with soap and water and soaking the bag in a 1% acetic acid (white vinegar) solution overnight.

PREVENT INFECTION

Prolonged use of an indwelling catheter increases the risk of UTI and tissue trauma. More than 80% of people who develop nosocomial (hospital-acquired) UTIs have undergone urologic instrumentation. Bacteriuria increases in direct relationship to duration of catheter placement; estimates of infection rates range from 4% (within 24 hours) to 95% (within 4 weeks). Organisms enter the catheter through any contamination or break in the system or intrude via the thin layer of fluid and exudate that forms around the outside of the catheter.

Catheter insertion should be avoided unless necessary to monitor urine output. Wash your hands thoroughly before and after handling a catheter or drainage system. In addition:

1. Maintain a closed drainage system.
2. Avoid backflow of urine.
3. Avoid unnecessary manipulation of the catheter during perineal cleaning.
4. Prevent microbial invasion and colonization in the urine collection bag.
5. Maintain patency of the catheter.
6. Encourage a high fluid intake.

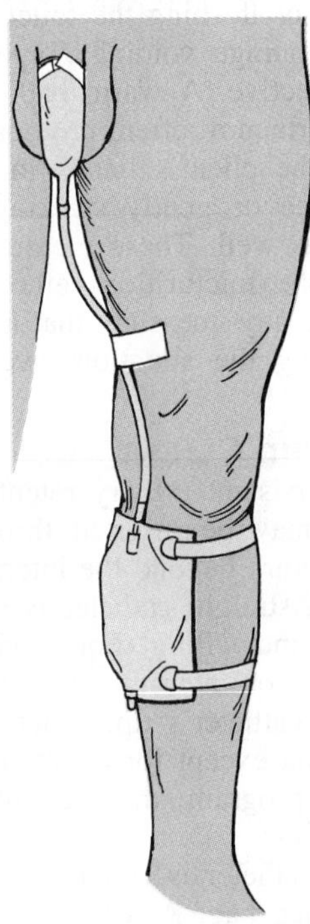

FIGURE 34–9 Condom drainage and leg bag. The bag may be attached to the calf of the leg, as shown, or to the thigh.

On occasion, prophylactic antibiotics are given to clients with catheters in place. The practice is not routine, however, because of the threat of resistant organisms and possible adverse reactions.

PREVENT TISSUE INJURY

Tissue trauma may occur during catheterization. Tissue irritation or necrosis may result from:

- Using an oversized catheter
- Continuous pressure and pulling of the catheter between the meatus and the site of taping on the leg or abdomen
- Friction caused by the continuous movement of the catheter, causing tissue breakdown and enhancing encrustation on the outside of the catheter
- Local or systemic allergic reactions to rubber in clients with a history of latex allergy; silicone catheters are available for these clients

The subject of bladder decompression drainage is still misunderstood. In the past, it was incorrectly assumed that rapid emptying of a distended bladder through a catheter could result in bladder hemorrhage and hypotension. Consequently, the catheter was clamped after 1000 ml of urine had been drained, reopened after an hour to drain another 1000 ml, and clamped and reopened again until the bladder was decompressed. Cystometric studies have shown that this problem does not occur with retention. It is now thought that any amount of urine can be drained.[49] Drainage does not occur rapidly, because the usual size of a catheter does not allow rapid drainage.

Surgical Management

Surgical intervention is usually employed if a structural defect is found. Intervention may include (1) removal of an enlarged prostate gland or urethral stricture or (2) correction of a structural abnormality.

BLADDER NECK REPAIR

Surgical intervention is sometimes needed for obstructions below the bladder. If the bladder neck becomes rigid as a result of inflammation, cystoplasty may be done by insertion of an elastic wedge into the area. A transurethral incision of the bladder neck might also be done. Excision of urethral strictures, sometimes with a *urethroplasty* (plastic repair of the urethra), helps return proper functioning. Alternatively, a meatotomy may be performed to open the urethral meatus.

SUPRAPUBIC CYSTOTOMY

INDICATIONS. Suprapubic catheterization is sometimes used to relieve urinary retention. Placement of the catheter allows postoperative clients to begin a bladder training program. The catheter is placed when urethral catheterization is difficult, as in clients with a severely enlarged prostate, urethral strictures, or quadriplegia. Local anesthesia is used, although general anesthesia may be used if another surgical procedure is also performed. To facilitate proper placement of the catheter, the bladder must be distended with urine or water before insertion. If the bladder is insufficiently distended with urine, additional fluid is instilled through a catheter or cystoscope.

The suprapubic skin is prepared. Under sterile technique, the suprapubic catheter is inserted through a small surgical incision or by passing a trocar through the skin into the bladder. Once the trocar is in place, the pointed core of the cannula is removed. The catheter is threaded through the cannula and attached to a closed drainage system. The catheter is commonly sutured in place or secured with a commercially made retention seal. When the catheter is removed, the muscle layers of the bladder immediately contract over the puncture site and shrink the surface wound.

CONTRAINDICATIONS. Short-term catheter placement may be a possible contraindication.

COMPLICATIONS. Potential complications of a suprapubic catheter include dislodgment of the catheter, hematuria (especially after the use of a large-bore catheter), bowel perforation during trocar insertion, and failure of the wound to close, which results in a urinary fistula.

OUTCOMES. When a suprapubic catheter is used instead of a urethral catheter, a lower rate of UTIs, increased comfort, and easier implementation of a bladder training protocol are expected.

Nursing Management of the Surgical Client

The client with a suprapubic catheter requires care similar to that needed for clients with a urethral catheter. The most frequent problem is catheter obstruction caused by (1) twisting or kinking or (2) sediment or clots. Disconnecting the catheter from the drainage tubing can disrupt the siphon drainage. When the catheter is removed, dressing changes may be needed to protect the skin from urinary leakage from the site. The suprapubic catheter site usually closes completely immediately or within 24 hours of removal.

Self-Care

The client who is discharged with an indwelling suprapubic or urethral catheter needs to know how to care for the catheter at home. The family and significant others should learn how to empty the drainage bag and how to prevent infection. They should also be taught the clinical manifestations of UTI and instructed to call the physician if they occur. When the client is discharged with a catheter in place, follow-up care is required. Removal of the catheter will depend on the cause of the retention.

Modifications for Elderly Clients

Older clients are more susceptible to urinary retention because of a chronic decrease in bladder tone. Retention leading to infection may also be worse in older clients. Treatment, however, remains the same.

URINARY INCONTINENCE

Urinary incontinence has been defined by the International Continence Society (ICS) as "a condition in which involuntary loss of urine is a social or hygienic problem and is objectively demonstrable."[64] The Agency for Health Care Policy and Research (AHCPR) published a collection of booklets on urinary incontinence in 1996.

Some 10% to 35% of noninstitutionalized adults over age 60 years and at least half of nursing home residents have problems related to incontinence.[60] The annual cost

ALTERNATIVE THERAPY

Urinary Disorders

Two common urinary problems that affect women, especially older women, may be helped by relatively simple interventions.

Urinary Tract Infection

Cranberry juice has been used as a folk remedy for prevention and treatment of urinary tract infection (UTI). Initially thought to be of benefit for its acidifying effect on the urine, cranberry seems to prevent microbial adherence to the epithelial cells lining the urinary tract.[3, 5] A randomized, double-blind, placebo-controlled trial using a commercially available cranberry beverage at a dosage of 300 ml/day in a group of older women showed a reduction in bacteria in the urine.[1] Tyler[5] recommends 90 ml/day as a preventive dose, with one third of that being pure cranberry juice, with an increase to 360 to 960 ml/day for UTI treatment. In light of the problem of microbial resistance, cranberry, which has no direct antimicrobial effect, may be a good choice for prevention and initial treatment of UTI.

Urge Incontinence

Urge urinary incontinence is characterized by urgency, frequency of urination, and dysuria. Acupuncture performed at a point approximately 3 inches above the internal malleolus can be effective in reducing manifestations. In a report of urodynamic studies, 22 of 26 women receiving acupuncture at the point known as Spleen 6, traditionally used for genitourinary complaints, showed improvement, with 17 women showing increased bladder capacity and marked reduction of manifestations after a single treatment.[2] While this report used standard acupuncture, a later one utilized electrical stimulation through needles at the same location, stating that this area is where "nerves that affect bladder control could be stimulated."[4] The authors claim good results in treating urge incontinence in many patients, from children to older adults.

References

1. Avorn, J., et al. (1994). Reduction of bacteriuria and pyuria after ingestion of cranberry juice. *Journal of the American Medical Association, 271*:751–754.
2. Chang, P. L. (1988). Urodynamic studies in acupuncture for women with frequency, urgency and dysuria. *Journal of Urology, 140*:563–566.
3. Kerr, K. G. (1999). Cranberry juice and prevention of recurrent urinary tract infection. *The Lancet, 399*:673.
4. Stoller, M. L., & Harris, M. G. (1998). Needle stimulation (through the skin) for the treatment of incontinence. *Quality Care, 16*(1):1–2.
5. Tyler, V. E. (1994). *Herbs of choice.* Binghamton, NY: Pharmaceutical Products Press.

James Higgy Lerner, RN, LAc, *Private practice of acupuncture, traditional Oriental medicine, and biofeedback*

of incontinence exceeds $15 million.[60] Yet most people avoid seeking treatment because they feel shame and embarrassment, which means that the problem is severely underreported and underdiagnosed. Many health care providers do not understand the effects of urinary incontinence on quality of life. Affected people may forfeit their active lifestyles and turn to a reclusive existence because they fear embarrassment.

There are three major types of incontinence: (1) *stress incontinence*, (2) *urge incontinence*, and (3) *overflow incontinence*. Under each of these types are many subtypes that may present in clients as an individual diagnosis or a combination of diagnoses.

Etiology and Risk Factors

Urinary incontinence commonly results from many factors, including anatomic defects and physical, physiologic, psychosocial, and pharmacologic factors. Anatomic and physiologic incontinence results from sphincter weakness or damage, urethral deformity, altered muscle tone at the urethrovesical junction, and detrusor instability.

Stress incontinence is an involuntary loss of urine that occurs without detrusor (bladder) contraction when intravesical pressure exceeds urethral pressure.[9] It commonly results from obstetric or surgical trauma, repeated straining, urogenital prolapse, and congenital weakness. After a suprapubic prostatectomy and transurethral prostatectomy, men may experience some exertional urine loss after the postoperative catheter is removed. Surgical interventions may cause bladder neck damage, with possibly permanent incontinence. A radical perineal or retropubic prostatectomy may cause permanent incontinence if the bladder neck is partially damaged during surgery.

Dysfunction of the urethrovesical junction (the area where the bladder meets the urethra) occurs mainly in women. Common causes include pregnancy, vaginal delivery, menopause, and surgical procedures that damage nerves leading to muscles of the pelvic floor. These injuries may lead to stress incontinence of varying degrees. A change in the angle of greater than 30 degrees from a horizontal plane during straining indicates hypermobility due to relaxation of the urethrovesical junction.

A simple diagnostic test for a hypermobile urethrovesical junction is a *Q-tip test*. A sterile, well-lubricated cotton applicator is placed in the urethra. The client is asked to strain as if to have a bowel movement. More than a 30-degree difference in a horizontal plane indicates a positive result or urethral hypermobility of the urethrovesical junction (Fig. 34–10).

Detrusor instability has many possible causes, although in many cases the cause remains unknown. On occasion, the cause can be identified as a bladder lesion, lower or upper spinal cord lesion, complication of pelvic surgery, or neurologic deficit. The International Continence Society offers two descriptions to characterize detrusor instability. In the first, the bladder contracts either spontaneously or with provocation while the client attempts to inhibit micturition. These contractions are seen during the filling phase of a cystometrogram in a neurologically intact client. In the second, detrusor overactivity results from disturbances of the nervous control mechanism. These clients have objective evidence of bladder dysfunction from a neurologic disorder. This type of detrusor instability, known as *detrusor hyperreflexia*, is commonly seen in the client with a history of a stroke or neurologic impairment.

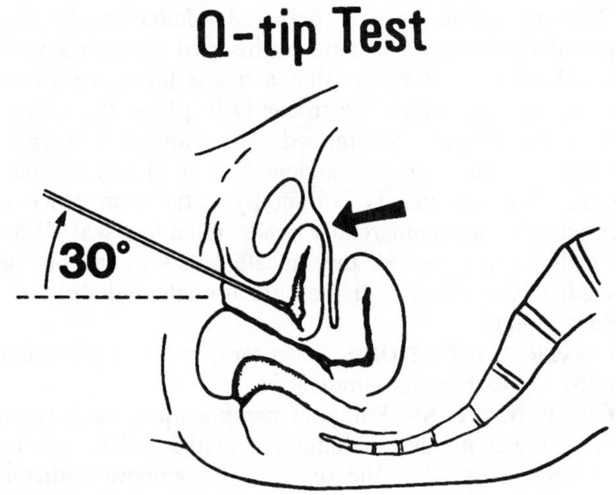

FIGURE 34–10 Diagnostic "Q-tip test" determines the descent of the normal urethrovesical junction contributing to stress incontinence in women. More than a 30-degree increase during exertional activities indicates a hypermobile urethrovesical junction.

Urge incontinence occurs randomly when involuntary urination is preceded by the warning of a few seconds to a few minutes. It is caused by uncontrolled contraction or overactivity of the detrusor muscle seen with central nervous system disorders (Alzheimer's disease, brain tumor, Parkinson's disease, multiple sclerosis), bladder disorders (interstitial cystitis, radiation effects, carcinoma in situ), and spinal cord interference with spinal inhibitory pathways (spondylosis, cancer growth in spinal cord).

Overflow incontinence, as defined by International Continence Society, is an involuntary urine loss associated with overdistention of the bladder.[9] The bladder is able to store urine but does not empty completely, causing urine loss as a result of diminishing resistant pressures.

Physical causes of incontinence independent of disorders of the urinary tract are often related to physical immobility, especially with older adults. These clients are often physically unable to get to the toilet independently because of stroke, fractures, or weakness. Failing vision and distances from the bathroom can also contribute to incontinence if the client cannot see the commode or bedpan.

Psychosocial causes of incontinence range from true psychological problems, such as dementia, to simple confusion. Clients may be unaware of the need to void or may be unable to respond appropriately when they feel the urge to empty the bladder. Other possible causes include regression, dependence, insecurity, sensory deprivation, and the disturbance of conditioned reflexes.

Drugs can also contribute to incontinence, especially overflow incontinence. Examples include:

- Narcotics, tranquilizers, sedatives, and hypnotic agents, all of which may affect sensory perception

- Alcohol
- Rapid-acting diuretics
- Antihistamines
- Atropine and atropine-like substances
- Hypotensive agents
- Alpha-adrenergic blockers
- Beta-adrenergic agents
- Ganglionic blockers

Other causative factors include fecal impaction, bladder scarring, urethral adhesions, diabetes mellitus, and obesity. Frequent voiding by clients who fear "accidents" leads to decreased bladder capacity, increased detrusor tone, and thickening of the bladder wall, which only fosters the dysfunction.

Incontinence health promotion activities involve prevention of impaired mobility and UTIs, exercise to minimize muscle weakness, and assisting clients to the bathroom by the clock to prevent accidents. Health maintenance measures are to thoroughly assess clients who report incontinence and monitor high-risk clients for development of incontinence. Teaching clients to perform pelvic muscle exercises (Kegel exercises) to improve muscle tone, follow bladder training protocols, and decrease incontinence by regulating fluid intake (e.g., not drinking large amounts of fluid at bedtime) are examples of health restoration interventions.

Pathophysiology

Pathophysiologic changes associated with incontinence vary with the specific cause of the disorder. In *stress incontinence*, increased vesical pressure commonly stems from such activities as sneezing, coughing, laughing, and exertion. There may be some dysfunction of the urethral sphincter or, in women, changes in the urethrovesical junction caused by weakness of periurethral muscles. Muscle weakness from childbirth, menopause, or other problems loosens the pelvic floor. In addition to the loss of muscle tone supporting the urethrovesical junction, there is increased descent, with a funneling effect of the bladder neck during exertion. In men, the pathophysiologic change usually results from BPH, which causes retention, overflow, and stress incontinence.

Urge incontinence is associated with several pathophysiologic changes. One problem is uninhibited detrusor contraction associated with motor disorders. Another cause is decreased mobility from an upper motor neuron spinal lesion combined with an inability to stop voiding once the impulse is felt.

Overflow incontinence stems from overdistention of the bladder and eventual overflow of the excessive amount of urine. Usually, this problem results from obstruction at the bladder outlet, as with BPH.

If incontinence is not controlled, it can lead to both psychological and physical problems. The psychological consequences of incontinence are serious. Clients may isolate themselves, and the fear of embarrassment may lead to depression. Incontinence is also a leading cause of nursing home admissions. The physical complications of incontinence include infection, skin breakdown, and permanent voiding dysfunctions.

Clinical Manifestations

The major manifestation of urinary incontinence is involuntary urine loss. Manifestations vary from client to client. An excellent diagnostic tool, the *bladder diary*, reveals voiding frequency, fluid intake, patterns of urinary urgency, and number and severity of incontinent episodes. A 7-day diary reveals patterns of incontinence and may be helpful before a diagnostic evaluation.

Urodynamic evaluation provides the best diagnostic information in determining the precise cause of the client's incontinence. The purpose of urodynamics is to reproduce the manifestations. The information collected is used to determine and guide treatment. Additionally, an evaluation of pelvic floor prolapse in women can reveal other contributing factors of urogenital dysfunction.

The variety of urodynamic examinations, including cystometrography and electromyographic (EMG) monitoring, are described in Chapter 32. Urine flow rate studies help identify hypotonic detrusor or an obstructional or dysfunctional voiding mechanism. A urethral pressure profile helps to determine pressure in the urethra, which may contribute to a severe type of stress incontinence *(intrinsic sphincter deficiency)* (see Bladder Neck Suspensions later on). Ultrasonography or catheterization of the bladder can detect elevated residual urine levels. Additionally, cystoscopy can be used to diagnose tumors, foreign bodies (such as stones or sutures), trabeculations, or structural abnormalities in the bladder and urethra.

Outcome Management

Successful management of urinary incontinence requires appropriate diagnostic testing. Treatments include pelvic floor behavioral interventions, drug therapy, and surgery. Naturally, the least invasive treatment should be tried first.[63] Many therapies aimed at improving incontinence can be implemented without risk to the client. Success is based on motivation, competency, and willingness to add these changes to one's lifestyle. Surgery should be performed only when a structural or anatomic defect is found.

The goals of treatment for a client with urinary incontinence include the following:

- Careful evaluation
- Treatment decisions based on the specific abnormalities identified for each client
- Treatment modalities that coordinate with the client's personality, expectations, environment, and clinical status
- A treatment plan that includes ways to circumvent environmental constraints
- Ability of the client to make an informed choice among treatment options

Medical Management

Many noninvasive, behavior-based therapies may be effective in controlling some types of incontinence. The AHCPR guidelines provide numerous algorithms that detail the diagnosis and treatment of various forms of incontinence.[63]

Pelvic Muscle Exercises

Originally designed for postpartum women, these exercises—commonly known as Kegel exercises—have long been the technique of choice for reducing urinary incontinence. Reports of success range from 30% to 90%. New devices have improved the success rate by fostering the correct use of these exercises.

The vaginal cone has been successful in enhancing awareness and in improving the effectiveness of pelvic muscle exercise. The client inserts the cone into the vagina and is instructed to hold the cone in place for 15 minutes twice a day. Correct muscle contraction is required to keep the cone in position. The client advances to a heavier cone once she can retain the lighter cone for the 15 minutes twice a day.

Pelvic Floor Reeducation

Biofeedback has been used for clients with incontinence to help them learn to reuse the pelvic floor musculature. Clients are educated to control incontinence by isolating and contracting the pelvic floor muscles. The use of biofeedback has been successful in eliminating incontinence in about 54% to 77% of clients who try it.

Biofeedback provides a "relay-like" system by which the client can visualize the isolation and contraction of the pelvic floor musculature. The muscle activity is recorded by either pressure manometry or EMG monitoring.

Clients are taught to use the pelvic floor muscles to override the sense of urgency in an effort to retrain the bladder. They can also be taught to contract the correct muscle group to inhibit urine loss caused by exertion. Biofeedback can also be used to teach clients to relax the pelvic floor if they have problems with urinary retention.

Electrical Stimulation

Electrical stimulation of the pelvic floor can be used to inhibit the micturition reflex and to contract the pelvic floor muscles. Delivery of a weak electrical current helps to close the urethra more tightly by direct and reflexogenic contraction of the striated periurethral muscles. Electrical stimulation also helps to increase bladder volume through bladder inhibition and stabilized detrusor activity.

The most common method of delivery is by insertion of a vaginal or anal probe. The procedure can be done in a physician's office or at home. The client inserts the internal device, and the stimulation level is directed at maintaining a synchronous pelvic floor contraction during an on-and-off cycle. Figure 34–11 shows the computerized systems used for biofeedback and electrical stimulation.

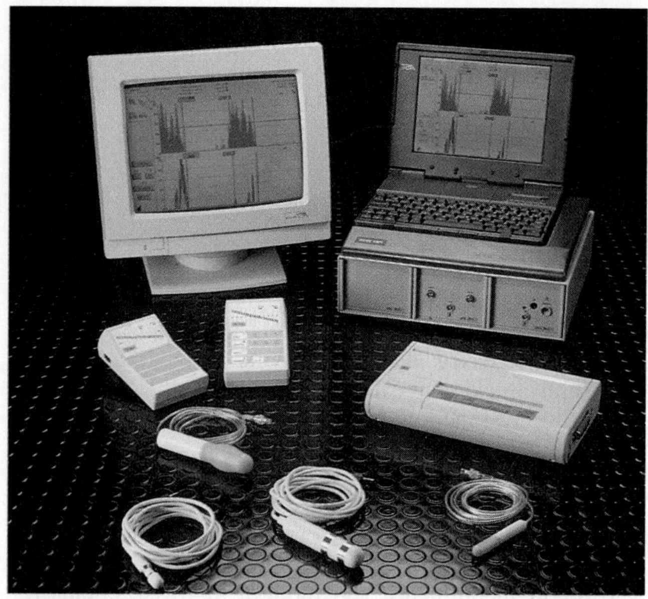

FIGURE 34–11 An electrical stimulation and biofeedback system can be used to treat men and women with incontinence. This system is called the InCare PRS 9500 (Hollister Incorporated, Libertyville, IL.)

Bladder Training and Behavioral Training

The client who uses bladder and behavioral training to address incontinence first voids at short intervals throughout the day—once an hour or less, if necessary. The client then tries to gradually lengthen the time between voiding up to 3 hours. This method seems to benefit 10% to 15% of clients with urge and stress incontinence, and most clients find at least some improvement.

Institutionalized clients can also use a form of bladder training. With these clients, health care workers encourage voiding at hourly intervals and give positive feedback. The time between voiding can then be gradually increased to 2 hours.

Administer Medications

Drug therapy for incontinence is guided primarily by the following events. During the bladder filling phase, the detrusor relaxes because of beta-adrenergic activity. At the same time, the bladder outlet contracts in response to alpha-adrenergic stimulation. If these actions are insufficient to keep urine in the bladder, drugs can be prescribed to supplement or replacement them (Table 34–2).

Medications are used mainly for urge (overactive bladder) to relax the bladder and, possibly, to increase bladder capacity. The most commonly used medications are anticholinergics and antispasmodics. These medications are contraindicated in clients with bladder outlet obstructions or a weak detrusor muscle. A new antispasmodic medication, tolterodine (Detrol), is reported to produce significantly fewer side effects and to be extremely effective for overactive bladder.

Alpha-adrenergic drugs may alleviate stress incontinence because they tend to increase the uptake of the alpha receptors in the urethra, thus increasing urethral resistance and urinary control.

By increasing circulation to the urogenital system, topical and systemic estrogens can improve function and help relieve manifestations of estrogen deficiency in postmenopausal women.

Fluid Intake and Dietary Changes

The major nutritional aspect of management involves controlling fluid intake. Decreasing fluid intake, especially after dinner, may help decrease nocturia. For obese clients, weight reduction may help decrease stress inconti-

TABLE 34–2 MEDICATIONS USED TO TREAT VOIDING DISORDERS

Class	Action	Therapeutic Outcome	Adverse Outcome	Dosing
ANTISPASMODICS				
Oxybutynin (Ditropan, Ditropan XL) tolterodine (Detrol)	Inhibits muscarinic action of acetylcholine on bladder smooth muscle.	Decreases bladder contractility and promotes urine storage by delaying urge to void and increasing bladder capacity for treatment of urge incontinence (overactive bladder).	Monitor for dry mouth, dry eyes, constipation, headache, drowsiness, tachycardia, blurred vision, and urinary retention.	Give 1 hour before meals. Avoid alcohol and other sedatives that potentiate antispasmodic actions. Avoid with obstructive uropathy. Give hard candy or gum for dry mouth.
ANTICHOLINERGICS				
Propantheline bromide (Pro-Banthine)	Blocks effects of acetylcholine at muscarinic receptors	Decreases bladder contractility and promotes urine storage by delaying urge to void and increasing bladder capacity for treatment of urge incontinence (overactive bladder)	Monitor for dry mouth, dry eyes, constipation, urinary retention, and glaucoma.	Give 1 hour before meals, avoid in clients with glaucoma, ulcerative colitis, heart disease, hypertension, and obstructive uropathy. Give hard candy or gum for dry mouth.
ALPHA-ADRENERGICS				
Pseudoephedrine hydrochloride (Sudafed)	Exaggerates alpha response in bladder neck and urethra to increase bladder outlet resistance.	Increases bladder outlet resistance for relief of stress incontinence and postprostatectomy incontinence.	Monitor for hypertension, tachycardia, urinary retention, insomnia, and restlessness.	Give PO every 4 hours or every 12 hours if extended release form used.
CHOLINERGICS				
Bethanechol (Urecholine)	Stimulates muscarinic cholinergic receptors in bladder to increase bladder tone and sensations to bladder filling.	Stimulates detrusor contractility and promotes bladder emptying for acute postoperative or other urinary retention and neurogenic atony of bladder with retention.	Monitor for increased GI motility, decreased pulse, hypotension, and vasodilation (atropine is antidote).	Give PO 1 hour before meals or SC if client is in NPO status. Contraindicated with bladder obstruction and IM or IV routes.
HORMONES				
Estrogen	Strengthens periurethral blood flow and tissues.	Increases bladder outlet resistance for treatment of incontinence in postmenopausal women.	Monitor for breast tenderness, hypertension, weight changes, and vaginal bleeding.	*Oral:* Once a day cyclically. *Intravaginal:* Daily at bedtime for 12 weeks, then 1–3 times per week. *Topical:* Replace patch weekly.

GI, gastrointestinal; IM, intramuscular; IV, intravenous; NPO, nothing by mouth; PO, by mouth; SC; subcutaneous.

nence by decreasing pressure against the bladder neck during exertion. The client should also avoid bladder irritants, such as alcohol, chocolate, and caffeinated drinks.

Bladder Neck Support Prosthesis

A bladder neck support prosthesis, a Silastic vaginal device, offers an easy and inexpensive alternative to surgery for certain women with stress incontinence (Fig. 34–12). This ring-shaped device is fitted into the vagina, and the ridges elevate the urethrovesical junction in a manner similar to that of a Burch colposuspension (see Bladder Neck Suspensions later on). The prosthesis reduces incontinence by elevating and supporting the urethrovesical junction during exercise. Every woman requires proper sizing, fitting, and instruction.

Nursing Management of the Medical Client

Multiple nursing diagnoses can be used, depending on the specific type of incontinence: *Stress Incontinence, Reflex Urinary Incontinence, Urge Incontinence,* and *Functional*

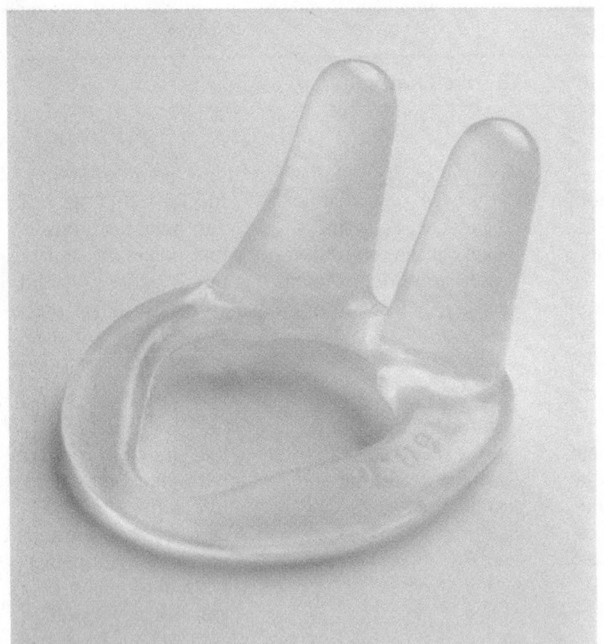

FIGURE 34–12 The bladder neck support prosthesis (Introl). A rubber-like silicone (Silastic) vaginal device supports the urethrovesical junction in women with stress incontinence. The two ridges support the urethrovesical junction during exertional activities.

Urinary Incontinence. All of the following interventions may be implemented as appropriate. Nurses often offer the first intervention for the client with urinary incontinence. The primary intervention is asking about bladder health with sensitivity. Remember, many clients feel shame and embarrassment about incontinence, and they may be reluctant to acknowledge the existence of a bladder control problem.

Implement a Bladder Training Program

A successful bladder training program requires much patience on everyone's part. The client must accept the program and be a willing and active participant. The first step is to discuss all procedures, expectations, and anticipated outcomes with the client. Do your best to inspire a sense of hope and a positive attitude when discussing the client's prognosis.

A bladder training program involves (1) adequate fluid intake, (2) accessibility to a toilet, (3) muscle-strengthening exercises, and (4) carefully scheduled voiding times. Implementing the program also requires well-organized teaching guidelines. The client also may need behavioral modification or intermittent catheterization.

Monitor Fluid Intake

Many clients with incontinence reduce their fluid intake in an effort to decrease urine production and increase control. Actually, adequate fluid intake and adequate urine production are necessary to stimulate the micturition reflex. Unless the client's physical status is a contraindication, encourage a daily fluid intake of ½ ounce of fluid for every pound of body weight. Carefully space these fluids throughout the day, limiting fluids in the evening to allow longer sleep periods at night. Fluids should be free of caffeine and alcohol, both of which may irritate the bladder.

Teach Kegel Exercises

Performed diligently, Kegel exercises strengthen the pubococcygeal muscle, help resolve stress incontinence, and decrease urgency and frequency. Instruct the client to contract the pelvic floor muscles as if to hold back intestinal gas. Do not ask the client to start and stop the urine stream as a way to isolate the correct muscle group. Stopping and starting the urine stream may cause dysfunction of the micturition reflex and may encourage urinary retention.

Once the client can isolate the correct muscle group, he or she should contract these muscles 10 times in sitting, standing, and lying positions, three times a day, working up to 10-second contractions. Then encourage the client to contract the pelvic floor muscles to learn the urge suppression technique or before any exertion that might cause incontinence. As with any exercise program, the program takes a conscious effort and may take months for the muscles to become adequately toned.

Develop a Voiding Schedule

At the same time that the client is strengthening pelvic floor muscles, the nurse should develop a voiding schedule with the client. Determine how often the client urinates during the day by asking her to maintain a voiding record. Depending on the voiding pattern, help the client to the toilet or commode every 30 minutes, increasing the time to 2 hours. As the program progresses, encourage the client to hold the urine longer. This increases voiding intervals, which increases bladder capacity.

Implement Biofeedback Techniques

Biofeedback and behavior modification may improve the outcome of the bladder training program. Use biofeedback techniques to help the client regain control over the external urethral sphincter and pelvic floor musculature. An internal probe is placed to measure the pelvic floor muscle activity. As the client contracts the pelvic floor, a Visual Analogue Scale or video graphs indicate the activity, strength, and duration of the muscle contraction. The system gives immediate feedback of progress. The therapy can be offered in the practitioner's office or with the use of a home unit.

Use Behavior Modification

Behavior modification is a variation of the voiding schedule. This program conditions the bladder to empty when the client attempts to void. The client is encouraged to void by the clock rather than by urge. The initial time between voiding is based on a completed bladder diary before therapy is begun. The time between voiding may be as little as every 30 minutes, with weekly increases of 15 to 30 minutes between. The gradual increase in time between voiding helps to decrease urge incontinence and to increase bladder capacity.

Explore Obstructive Devices

Obstructive devices are sometimes used to interfere with the outflow of urine. For example, certain types of vaginal pessaries can reduce incontinence by obstructing the urethra. Removing the device allows complete emptying of the bladder. Women using such devices must have the dexterity to remove the device for voiding.

A penile clamp can compress the urethra in a male client, but its use is controversial (Fig. 34–13). The clamp should be used only rarely and for short intervals. It must be removed and repositioned frequently to prevent pressure sores and ischemia of the penis.

RECOMMEND COUNSELING

A mental health consultation may help clients with depression that stems from incontinence. Talking to a counselor can help clients manage the fear of embarrassment, sense of increased dependence, and self-image problems accompanying incontinence. Avoid medications such as antidepressants because of the potential for more bladder dysfunction.

USE OTHER INCONTINENCE PRODUCTS

Disposable Pads

Sometimes none of the measures described are effective. Nursing interventions must then be aimed at protecting the client's skin, clothing, and bed linen. Adult-sized disposable pads or briefs help protect and increase the social mobility of clients with chronic incontinence. These commercially available undergarments have elastic legs and cellulose padding that draws fluid away from the skin by capillary action. Some brands include an odor-reducing agent.

Skin Care

If the skin becomes wet, it must be meticulously cleaned with a pH-balanced cleaner and dried to prevent serious rashes and skin breakdown from maceration and ammonia. The skin should then be carefully moisturized. Indwelling catheters to drain urine should be used only in an effort to avoid skin breakdown.

Condom Systems

External condom catheter drainage involves placing a thin rubber or plastic sheath over the penis and connecting it to either a leg bag or a bedside drainage bag (see Fig. 34–9). When the bladder releases urine, it runs down the tube into the collecting device. Problems include leakage (with or without detachment of the condom), twisting of the condom, and stasis of urine, which can macerate the penis.

Select the correct size of sheath, attaching it to stay in place without compromising circulation to the distal penis. Make sure that the sheath is not too tight, particularly at the ring. You may need to remove some of the client's pubic hair before preparing the skin. Wash the penis with soap and water and allow it to dry thoroughly to remove skin oils. If appropriate, apply an adhesive paste or commercial skin barrier.

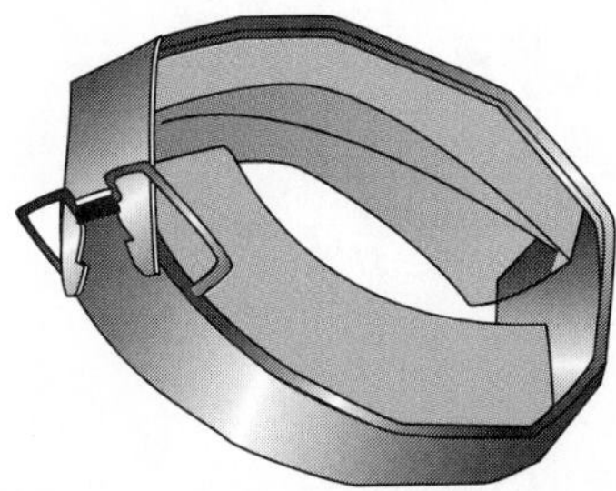

FIGURE 34–13 A penile clamp compresses the urethra to prevent incontinence.

Many commercially prepared condom systems contain a double-sided adhesive liner that is applied to the penis before the condom. Many newer devices are self-adhesive.

When rolling the condom sheath over the penis, allow at least 1.5 cm between the distal end of the penis and the internal end of the sheath. This reduces skin irritation. Make sure that the foreskin is over the glans.

Use only elastic tape to allow for expansion or erection. Apply this tape in a spiral only. To avoid impaired circulation, never encircle the penis completely with tape. Frequently monitor the patency of the system, and remove the condom daily to clean and dry the skin.

ENCOURAGE FOLLOW-UP

The client should be seen at regular intervals to make sure that interventions are adequate and continence is improved. Referral to a continence clinic may sometimes be appropriate to ensure close follow-up of continuing problems. The National Association for Continence and the Simon Foundation for Continence both publish newsletters containing important information for the incontinent client and family (see Management and Delegation).

Surgical Management

Surgical procedures are performed only to correct or compensate for anatomic defects leading to incontinence. After an injury to the bladder neck, the surgeon can resuspend the bladder neck and attempt to recreate normal anatomy. Implantation of an artificial sphincter can bring about opening and closing of the urethra to allow voiding. Other procedures, such as collagen or fat injections, are used to attempt to fill or occlude a urethra that cannot close completely.

BLADDER NECK SUSPENSIONS

Bladder neck suspensions are surgical procedures intended to restore the normal urethrovesical junction or to lengthen and support the urethra. Resuspending the bladder neck allows the urethrovesical junction to function correctly.

The *Burch colposuspension* is a popular surgical procedure for women with stress incontinence. This surgical intervention is a modification of an older procedure known as the MMK (Marshall, Marchetti, Krantz). In the Burch procedure, a surgeon fixes the periurethral tissue to Cooper's ligament, whereas in the MMK procedure, the surgeon sutures the periurethral tissue to the symphysis pubis. After surgery, a suprapubic catheter must usually be in place for up to 14 days. The drainage system must remain patent because the pressure of a filling bladder can inhibit the healing process.

A *sling procedure* is used for intrinsic sphincter deficiency, a severe type of stress incontinence. Material is placed beneath the urethra to elevate it and to increase urethral compression. The sling material may be synthetic or autologous (from one's self), such as fascia from another part of the client's abdomen. There are many variations of the procedure; some present a significant risk of voiding dysfunction.

Other surgical procedures aim to provide an intact, patent route for the transport of urine. Scar tissue that interferes with normal bladder neck function must be removed.

MANAGEMENT AND DELEGATION

Helping Clients with Urinary Incontinence

Various underlying conditions can result in urinary incontinence. Although women are at greater risk than men, incontinence also affects men. You and the physician assess and evaluate the client to determine the appropriate interventions to manage incontinence and may use a bladder record or voiding diary to document patterns and trends. Pelvic muscle rehabilitation, behavior therapy, pharmacologic interventions, and surgical procedures are the recommended treatments. For many, incontinence is an acute problem; for others, it is a chronic one.

Bladder training, assistance with toileting, and providing good skin care are duties that may be delegated to unlicensed assistive personnel. These measures are necessary for improving continence and for keeping clients dry and clean to prevent complications associated with skin irritation and ulceration.

Helping the incontinent client who cannot get out of bed is crucial in preventing skin breakdown and pressure ulcers. Utilizing a bedpan, a bedside commode, or a raised toilet seat may be helpful at times. If the client uses a walking aid to ambulate, ensure that the wheelchair, walker, or cane is near the bed and that the pathway to the bathroom is well lit and clear. Indicate which modality is appropriate for each patient.

Instruct unlicensed assistive personnel to:

- Respond promptly to all call lights in their assigned area.
- Closely measure and record urine output. Cloudy, foul-smelling, or dark urine should be reported immediately to you.
- Give each client plenty of time to void. Create privacy by closing the door or pulling the bedside curtain.
- Never scold a client who is wet. The client may be upset or feel ashamed about incontinence.

With bladder training instruction, direct unlicensed assistive personnel to:

- Assist or prompt the client to the bathroom on a scheduled interval, usually every 1 to 2 hours at the beginning of the training period.
- Increase the interval of time to assist or prompt the client to the bathroom as the client begins to achieve dryness.

Ask unlicensed assistive personnel to:

- Explain when the next bathroom time will be before they leave the room.
- Offer positive reinforcement to the client who can successfully void or asks for assistance to the bathroom to urinate, or has a dry absorbent pad.
- Assist clients with exercises to strengthen pelvic muscles to help minimize incontinence, reinforcing your previous instruction.

Direct unlicensed assistive personnel about which toileting methods to use:

- *Scheduled toileting:* Assist the client to the bathroom every 2 to 4 hours whether or not the client is wet or dry.
- *Prompted voiding:* Check whether the client is wet or dry; ask the client whether he or she needs to void, and help the client to the bathroom if the client answers "yes."
- *Habit training:* Once the client's voiding times each day are determined, help the client to the bathroom at the same times each day.

Maintaining clean, dry, and intact skin is necessary to prevent skin breakdown and unnecessary complications associated with wet skin. Instruct unlicensed assistive personnel to provide proper skin care and to identify any changes such as red, excoriated, or tender skin to you. The regimen may include:

- Cutting back on evening or night fluid intake to decrease voiding accidents during the night.
- Changing disposable wet pads or diapers every time the client is wet.
- Utilizing ointments or creams to protect the skin and to serve as a barrier after cleaning the client.
- Applying absorbent pads or diapers that are not chafing to the skin.

Have unlicensed assistive personnel communicate and report (1) any changes in skin or urine, (2) the client's inability to follow the toileting plan, and (3) any other questions that arise. Remember, you are responsible for assessing, implementing, evaluating, and making all changes to the client's plan of care.

References

1. Agency for Health Care Policy and Research (1996). *Clinical practice guideline: Urinary incontinence in adults: Acute and Chronic Management* (AHCPR Pub. No. 96-0682). Rockville, MD: U.S. Department of Health and Human Services.
2. Agency for Health Care Policy and Research (1996). *Clinical practice guideline: Caregiver guide: Helping people with incontinence* (AHCPR Pub. No. 96-0683). Rockville, MD: U.S. Department of Health and Human Services.

Elizabeth W. Good, MSN, RN, C, *Clinician IV, Urology Care Coordinator, Surgical Services, University of Virginia Health System, Charlottesville, Virginia*

IMPLANTATION OF AN ARTIFICIAL URINARY SPHINCTER

Implantation of an artificial urinary sphincter may help some clients achieve continence. This procedure usually is avoided until all other treatments have failed. Figure 34–14 shows a sphincter device, which consists of an inflatable cuff, a reservoir, and a control pump. The surgeon implants the cuff around the bladder neck or urethra, the deflation (or control) pump in the scrotum or labia, and the fluid reservoir in the abdomen.

The cuff keeps the urethra closed until the client manually squeezes the pump. This moves the fluid from the cuff to the reservoir. The bladder will then drain. The cuff automatically refills after 3 to 5 minutes, again occluding the urethra.

Candidates for this treatment must not have an obstructed lower urinary tract, detrusor hyperreflexia, or progressive neurologic disease affecting bladder function. Clients must have adequate manual dexterity and motivation to manage the system. Failure of the device poses a long-term risk that the client will need more surgery. Clients must be absolutely compliant, or the upper tracts of the urinary system can be damaged by obstruction.

Nursing Management of the Surgical Client

Nursing care of clients undergoing surgery focuses on maintaining adequate urinary drainage. With bladder suspension, preventing distention is a priority to help avoid excessive pressure on the healing surgical site. During the immediate postoperative period, a bladder training program is initiated to help the client regain detrusor muscle tone. Clamp the catheter for lengthening intervals while urine collects in the bladder, unclamping it periodically to empty the bladder. If the client reports severe pressure, the catheter should be unclamped immediately.

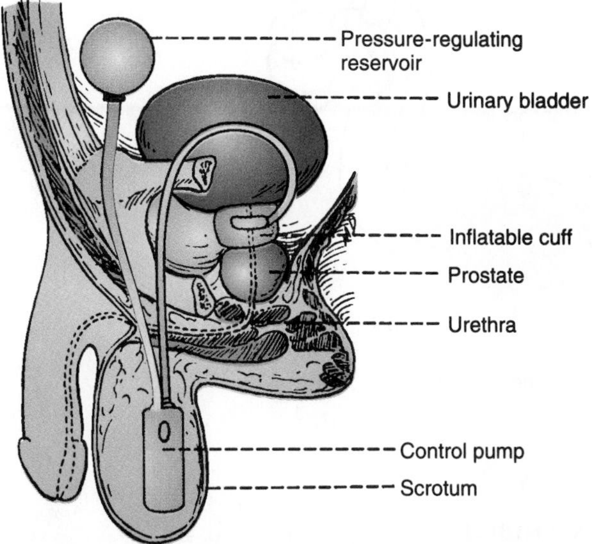

FIGURE 34–14 Artificial urinary sphincter. This surgically implanted urethral sphincter restores continence. To urinate, the client deflates the cuff around the bladder neck by squeezing the control pump within the scrotum. The cuff reinflates automatically.

If a suprapubic catheter is used, the client should try to void every 2 to 3 hours. After voiding is attempted, the catheter is drained to measure the residual urine and determine the effectiveness of bladder emptying.

Self-Care

The expected outcome is that the client will resume control over bladder function. Many strategies to achieve continence may be tried, and the client will select what is most comfortable and best able to support preferred activities. Management options can be expensive, such as multiple biofeedback sessions. If continence is achieved with any of the described therapies, however, treatment to achieve continence is cheaper than the purchase of adult briefs for daily use; in addition, the client would be free to engage in desired activities. Teach the client about continence options, and help the client make decisions about treatment options.

Modifications for Elderly Clients

Incontinence is not a normal part of the aging process, but it is a common problem among older adults. The elderly can be treated with any of the previously mentioned treatments. Because older people are more sensitive to many medications, care should be used when drugs are administered.

NEUROGENIC BLADDER

The term "neurogenic bladder" refers to several bladder dysfunctions caused by lesions of the central or peripheral nervous systems (Fig. 34–15). Their manifestations depend on the site of the lesion. A neurogenic bladder may involve a combination of one or more nervous system dysfunctions. There are five major types of neurogenic bladder dysfunction:

- Uninhibited
- Sensory paralytic (detrusor muscle hyperreflexia)
- Motor paralytic (detrusor muscle areflexia)
- Autonomous
- Reflex

Neurogenic bladder dysfunctions may also be classified according to the level of the lesion in the central nervous system.

Upper motor neuron lesions occur above the sacral segments of the spinal cord. They produce bladders that are spastic or characterized by exaggerated reflexes (hyperreflexia).

Lower motor neuron lesions occur at or below the sacral vertebrae. They produce bladders that are lacking reflexes (areflexic) or tone (atonic).

The incidence of neurogenic bladder dysfunction reflects the incidence and etiology of neurologic injuries or disorders. With certain disorders, a neurogenic bladder may develop in 100% of clients, as with transection of the spinal cord. Clients with conditions such as multiple sclerosis are affected with varying degrees of manifestations.

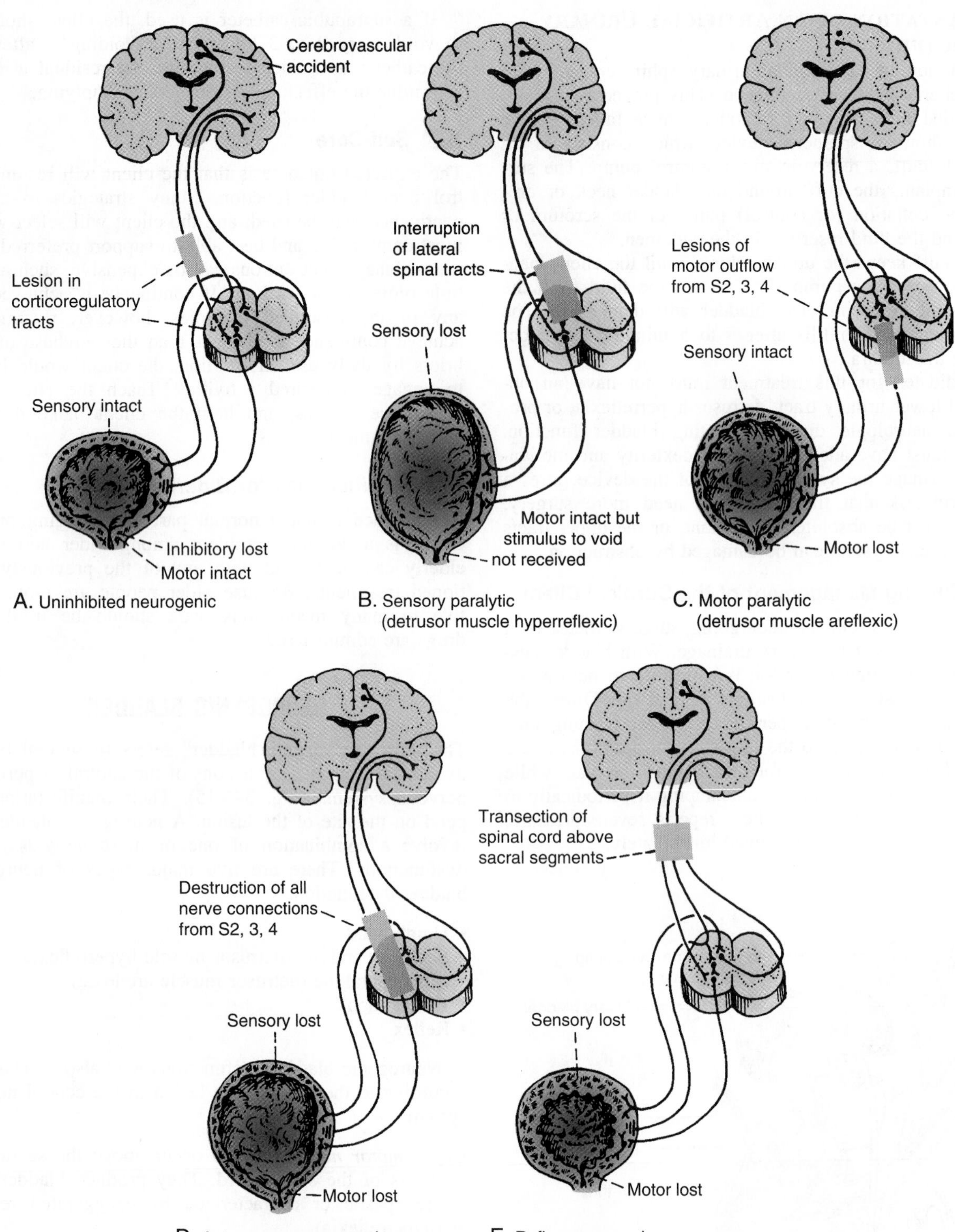

FIGURE 34–15 Types of neurogenic bladder dysfunction.

Etiology and Risk Factors

Risk factors for neurogenic bladder disorders include tumors, neurologic disorders, and trauma to the nervous system. Accidents are the only preventable cause of this problem.

UNINHIBITED

The uninhibited neurogenic bladder produces "infantile" or uninhibited voiding. The urge to void causes urine to flow. The primary cause is a lesion in the corticoregulatory tracts, as from a cerebrovascular accident or multiple sclerosis.

SENSORY

A sensory paralytic bladder results from an interruption in the lateral spinal tracts, as occurs in tabes dorsalis, diabetic neuropathy, and pernicious anemia. Because of the sensory loss, the client cannot sense the bladder filling. This lack of perception leads to atonic bladder, retention with possible overflow incontinence, and upper tract involvement.

MOTOR

A motor paralytic bladder is the most uncommon type and is caused by lesions in the motor outflow from vertebrae S2 to S4. Disease processes causing this dysfunction include poliomyelitis, tumor, trauma, spina bifida, and infection. This dysfunction may be temporary if a bacterial or viral infection is the cause. Although there is full sensation of bladder filling, even to the point of pain, the client cannot initiate micturition.

AUTONOMOUS

Clients with an autonomous neurogenic bladder cannot perceive bladder fullness, or they cannot start and maintain urination without some type of exertional pressure. Retention and incontinence are common problems. The autonomous type of dysfunction occurs after destruction of all nerve connections between the bladder and the central nervous system at vertebrae S2, S3, or S4 following trauma, inflammatory processes, spinal anesthesia, or malignancy.

REFLEX

Transection of the spinal cord above the sacral segments causes a reflex neurogenic bladder. There is no sensation, and the bladder contracts reflexively but does not empty completely.

Pathophysiology

Lesions at the lower motor neuron level of the spinal cord often directly interfere with the reflex arc leading to inappropriate interpretation of efferent and afferent impulses. When the bladder fills, the message is transmitted through afferent fibers to the brain cortex. The injury keeps these impulses from being correctly interpreted, leading to loss of the micturition reflex. A flaccid bladder with urinary retention is the result.

With upper motor neuron lesions, impulses are not transmitted to or from the lower spinal areas to the cortex. When the bladder distends, no sensation is transmitted. Because the lower cord is intact, activity of the reflex arc can occur. The client would have reflex incontinence as a result.

When the damage is to the cortical area itself, as with a stroke or trauma, the client cannot correctly interpret the impulses that are being transmitted. Unless the client is evaluated and treated appropriately, serious UTIs, skin breakdown associated with incontinence, and even renal failure due to chronic overdistention of the bladder are more likely to develop.

Clinical Manifestations

The major clinical manifestation of neurogenic bladder dysfunction is retention with or without incontinence. The client may or may not feel a need to void or feel a sense of bladder distention. The diagnosis is made from the location of neurologic dysfunction. Urodynamic studies, including EMG monitoring, should be done to determine the extent of neurologic involvement to guide an appropriate treatment plan.

Outcome Management

Medical Management

BLADDER TRAINING

If possible, some form of bladder training should be attempted for a client with neurogenic bladder dysfunction. This measure includes a bladder training program, medication, possible intermittent catheterization, and sometimes surgical intervention.

ADMINISTER MEDICATIONS

A number of medications are used to treat neurogenic bladder dysfunction (see Tables 34–1 and 34–2). Antispasmodics and anticholinergics (such as dicyclomine, propantheline, and flavoxate) are given to relieve uninhibited or reflex bladder contractions. Phenoxybenzamine and other alpha-adrenergic blockers may be used. Bethanechol may help stimulate an atonic bladder. Other medications described in the discussion of incontinence may be useful as well.

PREVENT COMPLICATIONS

Autonomic dysreflexia is a serious, potentially life-threatening complication affecting clients who have spinal cord injuries. It may occur during bladder training programs if the urinary system or bowel becomes obstructed. The most frequent cause is bladder distention or feces in the rectum, although autonomic dysreflexia can be triggered by visceral distention or stimulation of pain receptors in the skin. This condition results from an excessive autonomic response to normal stimuli and affects primarily clients with upper motor neuron lesions.

The most common manifestations are severe hypertension, bradycardia, a throbbing headache, flushing, diaphoresis above the level of the lesion, blurred vision, nasal congestion, nausea, and pilomotor spasm ("goose bumps") above the lesion. If left untreated, this problem can lead to retinal hemorrhage, seizures, or stroke. It is important for the client to recognize the earliest manifestations and summon help immediately. Preventing bladder distention is one way to prevent this emergency. If stool is accumulating in the rectum, careful evacuation should be done to avoid either overdistention or overstimulation.

Medications such as diazoxide (Hyperstat), phenoxybenzamine (Dibenzyline), guanethidine monosulfate (Ismelin), propantheline bromide (Pro-Banthine), phentolamine mesylate (Regitine), and mecamylamine (Inversine) relieve both acute manifestations and the chronic recurrence of episodes.

Nursing Management of the Medical Client

PREVENT AUTONOMIC DYSREFLEXIA

Always be prepared for the development of autonomic dysreflexia. If severe hypertension (sometimes 300/180 mm Hg), flushing, and a pounding headache suddenly develop, you must address the manifestations immediately.

Nursing interventions involve removal of the triggering stimuli by reestablishing urine flow or removing the fecal impaction. Remove any fecal impaction only after a topical anesthetic agent has been inserted into the rectum to avoid further stimulation. In addition, a catheter may be necessary; if one is already in place, restore its patency by irrigation or by removing kinks and obstructions. Monitor the client's vital signs every 5 minutes, and raise the head of the bed to the semi-Fowler's position. Administer medications as ordered.

Teach Methods to Stimulate Micturition

Neurogenic bladders are difficult to control, but you can teach many clients how to stimulate the micturition reflex and maintain urination. Assist the client by providing external pressure on the abdomen. The client can lean forward or press on the abdomen. Have the client breathe deeply to push the diaphragm downward. Wearing a corset or girdle can provide an extra source of external pressure. The Valsalva maneuver is another method of increasing intra-abdominal pressure on the urinary bladder.

Another method that helps the client learn to empty the bladder is the Credé maneuver. The client places the fingers over the bladder and presses downward slowly toward the symphysis pubis, as though "milking" the urine out of the urinary system. This should be done with great caution. If the client has sphincter dyssynergia (failure of muscle coordination) or if the sphincter does not readily relax, the Credé maneuver can lead to sphincter damage and may cause ureteral reflux if there is any obstruction of outflow. The Credé maneuver is often combined with intermittent self-catheterization.

The client can use several other methods to initiate and maintain micturition. Locate trigger points on the body (lower abdomen, inner thighs, and pubic area), and explain how to stimulate them by stroking, pinching, or applying ice. Stretching the anal sphincter also relaxes the reflexes of the external urethral sphincter because they are both innervated by the pudendal nerve. The client leans forward while sitting on the toilet and inserts two gloved fingers into the anus. The fingers are then either widened apart or pulled posteriorly. Men must be careful to avoid touching the glans penis, which stimulates the bulbocavernosus reflex, contracting the external sphincter.

Perform Intermittent Catheterization

For the treatment of long-term or short-term bladder atony (lack of tone), an intermittent catheterization program is an alternative to indwelling catheterization. A straight urethral catheter is inserted into the bladder at specified intervals, the urine is drained, and the catheter is removed. This may be done in a health care facility or in the client's home (see Bridge to Home Health Care).

Teach Intermittent Self-Catheterization

Clients with bladder atony should be encouraged to learn self-catheterization because it increases independence and mobility. The client or any other person who has been properly educated about the technique may insert the catheter.

Sterile technique is necessary in health care facilities because of the high risk of nosocomial infections. At home, *clean technique* can be used for catheterization without increasing the rate of UTIs. Clean technique is also easier and less expensive for the client. To reduce the risk of bacteriuria, urinary antiseptics and acidification or bladder irrigation with antibiotics and antiseptics are used with each catheterization.

There are several procedural differences between clean and sterile techniques. For clean technique:

1. Gloves are not worn. The client must perform thorough hand-washing before starting.
2. A clean (rather than a sterile) catheter is used.
3. The catheter can be washed and reused indefinitely.
4. Lubricant should be used because the urethra is susceptible to traumatic urethritis.

The catheter should be washed thoroughly after use with soap and water and stored in a clean sandwich-size plastic bag or other clean container.

During self-catheterization, the client may sit or stand. When a female client stands, she should separate her legs or place one leg on a toilet seat. After separating the labia, she can use a mirror to find the meatus.

Timing is important for successful catheterization programs. Catheterization should be carried out at specified intervals throughout the day until bedtime. The interval between catheterization is set according to the degree of continence. The average interval for adults is every 3 to 4 hours, but the client usually has to start at intervals of 2 to 3 hours. Clients should use the catheter to remove 350 to 400 ml each time. A client who cannot follow a schedule is not an appropriate candidate for the program.

The amount of fluid intake allowed is under debate. Some programs allow fluid as desired; others restrict fluid intake to varying degrees. This aspect of the program requires systematic investigation. Clinicians generally recommend that the client drink about 250 ml of fluid at about 2-hour intervals. Ingestion of large amounts of fluid within a short period can cause bladder distention and reflux. Most clients are urged to drink up to 2 L of fluid daily at regular intervals.

A catheter-free bladder and absence of bacteriuria indicate a successful intermittent catheterization program. Controversy exists about the treatment of asymptomatic bacteriuria. A successful catheterization program may be due to several factors, including intermittent bladder distention, which causes stimulation of the normal micturition reflex and reactivation of the bladder's normal antibacterial properties. Other advantages include continence, independence, good hygiene, prevention of complications arising from urinary stasis or a retention catheter, decreased cost, and comfortable sexual relations.

Intermittent catheterization is not a panacea. The program requires the client to assume a great deal of personal responsibility. Some clients are not sufficiently motivated to fulfill the responsibilities involved in self-catheterization. Also, some problems can occur when the client is away from home.

Clients with high resting pressures in the bladder that are incontinent between catheterizations are likely to have difficulty with intermittent self-catheterization. All clients should be evaluated before starting the program. If urodynamic evaluation reveals high resting pressures, anticholinergic medications are administered.

BRIDGE TO HOME HEALTH CARE

Inserting Urinary Catheters

Indwelling catheters may be inserted to treat urinary incontinence. Indications include pressure ulcers or surgical wounds that do not heal, overflow incontinence associated with obstructions that cannot be removed, and decisions of the client or family that dryness and comfort outweigh the risks, especially in cases of serious or terminal illness.

Catheters affect the client's quality of life and self-esteem and are frequently accompanied by recurrent urinary tract infections (UTIs) that can lead to more serious complications and hospitalization. Therefore, you must evaluate whether a catheter is in the clients' best interest and will adequately meet their needs. Catheters should be the last treatment option; consider a referral to a continence care nurse or continence clinic first. You are responsible for providing instructions about daily cleansing, adequate fluid intake, manifestations of UTI, and indications to call the nurse or physician.

Use the smallest French (F) size catheter to meet the client's needs. A 14F to 16F catheter may be the best size for a woman; a 16F to 18F catheter may be best for a man. The balloon should hold 5 to 10 ml of fluid. A catheter that is too large or is overinflated will cause bladder spasms and urine to leak around the catheter. Men who have an enlarged prostate may need a coudé tip catheter.

Adequate lighting is often a challenge in the home. Consider using a flashlight or small lamp. It may be necessary to ask a family member or informal caregiver to help position the client and to hold the light.

When inserting a urinary catheter, place a female client in the supine position with her knees flexed and separated. Arrange pillows laterally under her knees to provide comfort and increase relaxation. Consider using the posterior approach if the client is obese or has severe lower extremity contractures; turn her on her side facing the other way.

Using sterile technique, check the catheter balloon for appropriate filling, deflate, and set aside on the sterile field. Cleanse the labia and meatal opening one side at a time, using downward stokes; discard the swabs after each stroke. The last swab may be left slightly inside the vagina as a marker.

Ask the client to breathe deeply, and insert the well-lubricated catheter into the meatal opening. When urine returns, insert the catheter another inch and inflate the balloon with the preattached saline syringe; gently pull back to seal the catheter. If no urine returns, gently insert the gloved little finger into the vagina to assess for slippage of the catheter into the vagina.

If a catheter is accidentally inserted into the vagina, leave it in place as a marker. Never reuse a catheter. Obtain a new catheter, and insert with sterile technique as before.

Place male patients in a supine position. Using sterile technique, check the balloon for appropriate filling, then deflate and set aside on the sterile field. Retract the foreskin, and hold the penis at a 60- to 90-degree angle. Clean the glans penis in circular motion, starting at the meatus and working outward. Using a rotating motion, insert the well-lubricated catheter into the meatus. Do not force the catheter if resistance is met, but maneuver it gently as the client breathes deeply, coughs, or bears down.

When urine returns, inflate the catheter balloon with the saline-filled syringe. If placement cannot be verified, notify the physician. Always hang the drainage bag below the bladder level. Many clients prefer to hang the drainage bag on a clean wastepaper can to prevent urine from leaking on the floor.

Kimberly Stallo, RN, BSN, CETN, *Wound, Ostomy, and Continence Nurse, Fort Worth, Texas*

Surgical Management

Surgery is not the primary treatment option for the client with neurogenic bladder. However, if conservative measures are ineffective in treating the neurogenic bladder, surgical intervention may be necessary. External sphincterotomy or incision of the bladder neck may restore normal bladder emptying. Interrupting innervation to the bladder reflex can aid an uninhibited bladder. Injection of alcohol into the subarachnoid space or rhizotomy (cutting) of the sacral nerves increases bladder capacity by inhibiting reflex bladder contractions, without interfering with normal sphincter function. Sometimes a temporary sacral nerve block is performed before surgery to evaluate the potential candidate. Electrodes may be implanted at thoracic or cervical levels of the spinal epidural space and attached to a percutaneous stimulator. As soon as the client learns to regulate the electrical stimulation properly, the device can be used to inhibit or interrupt reflex bladder contractions.

Continuous intrathecal baclofen administered through an implanted infusion pump is another method of treating a neurogenic bladder. Baclofen helps decrease spasms and detrusor sphincter dyssynergia. Clients report improvement in bladder compliance and capacity. Finally, if all else fails, urinary diversion may be performed to provide the client with a more manageable urinary system.

Nursing Management of the Surgical Client

Nursing care of the client undergoing surgery for a neurogenic bladder with either an external sphincterotomy or a revision of the bladder outlet is the same as for any client undergoing bladder surgery. Urinary output maintenance is the priority of these clients. A suprapubic or urinary catheter may be needed until healing occurs.

As with the other surgical procedures, focus care on teaching the client self-care. The client needs to learn to regulate electrical stimulation appropriately to inhibit or interrupt the reflex bladder contractions.

Proper care of the implantable infusion pump is another important area of client education. Care of clients undergoing urinary diversion has been discussed under Bladder Cancer.

Self-Care

The focus of discharge teaching for the neurogenic bladder client is intermittent self-catheterization. Teach the client and significant others a bladder training program and, possibly, a catheterization program. Assess the client's ability to understand and perform self-care procedures, and ensure that the client understands the self-catheterization program. Written materials, teaching videos, and diagrams can be used to reinforce the teaching.

Clients need to be assessed in the home setting to make sure they can function as well as in the hospital. A visiting nurse may be included to help in the discharge planning of the self-catheterization or bladder training program. The client's urinary function should be monitored at regular intervals, including renal function tests and yearly renal ultrasound studies. Teach the client to call the health care provider if manifestations of a UTI develop.

Modifications for Elderly Clients

Older clients are more likely to have other medical problems, such as arthritis and visual changes, that can interfere with their ability to use the self-catheterization program. However, they may still be able to use this method if they have adequate help.

TRAUMATIC DISORDERS

BLADDER TRAUMA

Bladder trauma is defined as a blunt or penetrating injury to the bladder that may cause bladder rupture. Bladder trauma often results from automobile accidents, when the seat belt compresses the bladder. A bladder distended by urine can rupture with a direct blow to the lower abdomen. The bladder may also be punctured by a bullet, knife, bony splinter from a fractured pelvis, or internal medical instrumentation. When the bladder ruptures, urine spills into the peritoneal cavity. Complications of peritoneal urine accumulation from a ruptured bladder are peritonitis and pelvic cellulitis.

Clinical Manifestations

Bladder injuries usually produce hematuria and pain low in the abdomen or pain referred to a shoulder. The client also may have trouble voiding. Manifestations of peritonitis may develop as well. Fever is usually present as the peritonitis and pelvic cellulitis continue to develop. If the client has had an injury or blow to the abdomen, suspect bladder injury as the cause of the manifestations.

Diagnostic tests include an IVP with lateral views or a CT scan with the bladder full and empty, a cystogram, and a voiding cystourethrogram. If blood is flowing from the meatus, urethral disruption may be present. In this case, catheterization should be avoided until the urethra is evaluated. This allows assessment of both bladder integrity and the bladder's ability to empty.

Outcome Management

Medical Management

The first treatment for suspected bladder injury is insertion of an indwelling or suprapubic catheter to monitor for hematuria or urine production and to keep the bladder decompressed during healing. Any injury other than a simple contusion or very small perforation will require surgical repair.

Nursing Management of the Medical Client

Immediately assess for a suspected bladder injury if the client has had blunt trauma to the lower pelvis or abdomen. Closely monitor the client's urine output for both amount and the presence of hematuria. Report any decrease in urine output in relation to fluid intake to the physician immediately. Careful catheter insertion is necessary for the client with suspected bladder trauma.

Surgical Management

Clients with bladder injuries usually require surgical intervention. After a urethral or suprapubic catheter has been inserted, surgical repair of the damaged bladder wall is performed. The extravasated urine in the perivesical area is drained. It is important to maintain urinary drainage through a patent catheter to promote healing and to avoid the potential development of fistulas or leakage.

Nursing Management of the Surgical Client

Postoperatively, maintain urinary drainage to prevent tension on the sutures in the bladder. A Penrose drain is left in place to allow drainage of any urine remaining in the pelvis. This may necessitate dressing changes.

Because the client may be discharged with an indwelling or suprapubic catheter, teach catheter care to the client and significant others. Assess the client's self-care abilities to determine a possible need for assistance at home. If the client or significant others cannot care for the catheter, arrange for a home health visit.

Follow-up care is essential after discharge to assess healing. A cystogram may be done before the catheter is removed. If a suprapubic catheter has been placed, the client can begin bladder training before the catheter is removed. If the client has a urethral catheter, the catheter is removed before the client can attempt to void. If clients do not void within 4 to 6 hours after removal, the catheter will need to be reinserted.

URETHRAL TRAUMA

The urethra as well as the bladder may be injured in a pelvic fracture. Falling astride an object, such as the bar on a boy's bike, with sudden force to the groin may cause urethral contusion and laceration. Injury may also occur during medical or surgical interventions, may be self-inflicted, or may occur after female genital mutilation (see Chapter 39). Penetrating wounds also cause urethral damage.

Evaluation of urethral damage is indicated if the client cannot void, has an altered urine stream, or has visible blood at the meatus. Even if the client can pass some urine through the urethra, voiding will cause urinary extravasation, resulting in swelling of the scrotum or inguinal areas, which can lead to sepsis and necrosis. Blood may appear at the external meatus and may also extravasate into the surrounding tissues, giving the area an ecchymotic appearance.

The two most common complications of urethral trauma are (1) development of urethral strictures and (2) risk of impotence in men. Impotence occurs because the corpora cavernosa of the penis, blood vessels, or nerves supplying this area are damaged.

Proper management of urethral injuries is controversial. Clinicians generally agree that urinary drainage must first be established with either a urethral or suprapubic catheter. Some physicians suggest an immediate primary surgical repair of the urethra. Others prefer to wait 2 to 3 weeks to see whether the urethra will heal around the urethral catheter without surgery. During any waiting period, the client must be monitored for developing infection and continuing extravasation of urine.

URETERAL TRAUMA

The ureters are located deep within the abdomen and are protected by the spine and surrounding musculature. Thus, most ureteral trauma takes place accidentally during surgery. Perforation or tearing may occur during manipulation of intraureteral catheters or other instruments. The ureters may be occluded by ligating sutures or a misplaced clamp, or they may be transected during pelvic surgery. Many surgeons insert ureteral stents before pelvic procedures to easily identify the ureters and prevent trauma. Gunshot and stab wounds may also traumatize the ureters. On occasion, blunt trauma from a car accident can tear these structures.

Trauma is often not discovered until a clinical manifestation develops, such as hematuria, flank pain, or the presence of extravasated urine. As the urine seeps out into the tissues, pain may occur in the lower abdomen and flank. As extravasation continues, there may be sepsis, paralytic ileus, a palpable intraperitoneal mass, and the appearance of urine in an external wound. An IVP and ultrasonography are the most definitive means of diagnosis.

Surgical intervention is used to repair the defect, preferably with end-to-end anastomosis. More radical procedures may be needed, such as cutaneous ureterostomy, transureteroureterostomy, and reimplantation. The surgeon may use prosthetic ureteral implants. A nephrectomy is performed if obstruction or sepsis causes severe renal damage. It is essential to treat sepsis aggressively. Significant extravasation of urine may require the surgeon to open the abdomen and drain the urine.

CONGENITAL ANOMALIES

A congenital anomaly of the bladder is exstrophy of the bladder that develops when the symphysis pubis fails to close in utero. The lower anterior abdominal wall and anterior bladder wall are absent, allowing the bladder to protrude through the defective abdominal wall. These conditions are often treated with urinary diversion in childhood, but additional revisions may be needed as the child grows. Children who have had a diversion may be candidates for continent reservoir revisions.

Although congenital anomalies of the ureter are uncommon, several types are described.

1. *Ectopic ureter* occurs when a ureter follows an abnormal course or has an abnormal distal opening. It is the most common congenital ureteral anomaly. An ectopic ureter occurs as a result of the abnormal embryologic development of the ureter. During micturition, this anomaly often results in a back-flow of urine. Misplacement of the meatus (hypospadias and epispadias) is discussed in Chapter 38.
2. *Duplicate ureters,* arising from the same renal pelvis, may develop when the ureters on one side unite at some point, both may open in the normal portion of the trigone or when both may open into the urethra or vagina. This anomaly is not usually recognized unless a radiographic study is done for another reason. Pyelonephritis develops, and an evaluation reveals the anomaly. Surgical intervention is usually not necessary unless complications occur.
3. *Abnormal dilation of the ureter (megaureter)* is characterized by dilation and pouching of the ureteral wall just adjacent to the vesicoureteral junction. Resulting manifestations are seen as reflux or obstructive effects, which predispose the client to recurrent UTIs.
4. *Congenital ureteropelvic obstruction* occurs at the junction of the renal pelvis and the ureter. This anomaly is usually bilateral. A mild obstruction may never cause manifestations of a urinary tract disorder. As long as the kidney produces urine at a rate below 6 ml/minute, the ureter can generally handle the flow; however, urine production above this rate causes urinary stasis in the kidney, which results in hydronephrosis. If the condition is symptomatic, treatment consists of surgical repair of the narrowed section at the ureteropelvic junction.

CONCLUSIONS

Urinary system disorders can be extremely problematic for clients. Nurses play a major role in the diagnosis, prevention, and treatment of these disorders. Many of the disorders of the urinary system are chronic or become chronic problems, leading to renal disease or incontinence. Some of the manifestations of these disorders can drastically alter the client's self-concept and lifestyle. Problems of the lower urinary tract may become life-threatening, and the nurse must ensure that the client receives prompt and adequate treatment of disorders within the lower urinary system.

THINKING CRITICALLY

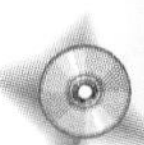

1. A 28-year-old newlywed woman has been experiencing pain and burning with urination for the past 24 hours. This is the third episode of urinary manifestations she has had in the past 3 months. What is the probable cause of the urinary manifestations? What further information do you need to assess her problem? What can you do to help her treat this problem and prevent further difficulties?

Factors to Consider. For what urinary tract problems does the client's status as a newlywed place her at risk?

Which tests would help differentiate an infectious problem from a noninfectious one?

2. **The client had a radical cystectomy with formation of an Indiana pouch 12 hours ago. He has a catheter in place, which has drained 10 ml in the last hour. The stoma is a very pale pink. His vital signs are elevated from their preoperative levels. His pulse rate is 100 beats per minute, and his temperature is slightly increased. What actions would be appropriate at this point in the client's care?**

Factors to Consider. Is the client's urinary output within expected limits? What color should a fresh stoma normally be?

3. **A 69-year-old man with diabetes is admitted with severe left flank pain, nausea, vomiting, and diarrhea. His abdomen is soft and only slightly tender. His urinalysis reveals increased red blood cells, and his KUB shows a large staghorn calculus in the left kidney with hydronephrosis of the left kidney. What would be a priority assessment for this client?**

Factors to Consider. What other diagnostic tests should be done? What are the treatment options for large renal stones?

BIBLIOGRAPHY

1. American Cancer Society. (1999). *Cancer facts and figures—1999.* Atlanta: Author.
2. Andriole, V. (1997). Urinary tract infections. *Infectious Disease Clinics of North America, 11*(3).
3. Appell, R. (1998). Periurethral injection therapy. In P. Walsh, et al. (Eds.), *Campbell's urology* (7th ed., pp. 1109–1120). Philadelphia: W. B. Saunders.
4. Atala, A., & Keating, M. (1998). Vesicoureteral reflux and megaureter. In P. Walsh, et al. (Eds.), *Campbell's urology* (7th ed., pp. 1859–1916). Philadelphia: W. B. Saunders.
5. Barrett, D., & Licht, M. (1998). Implantation of the artificial genitourinary sphincter in men and women. In P. Walsh, et al. (Eds.), *Campbell's urology* (7th ed., pp. 1121–1134). Philadelphia: W. B. Saunders.
6. Benson, M., & Olsson, C. (1998). Continent urinary diversion. In P. Walsh, et al. (Eds.), *Campbell's urology* (7th ed., pp. 3190–3246). Philadelphia: W. B. Saunders.
7. Bernier, F., & Harris, L. (1995). Treating stress incontinence with the bladder neck support prosthesis. *Urologic Nursing, 15*(1), 5–9.
8. Bernier, F., & Jenkins, P. (1997). The role of vaginal estrogen in the treatment of urogenital dysfunction in postmenopausal women. *Urologic Nursing, 17*(3), 92–95.
9. Blaivas, J., Ramanzi, L., & Heritz, D. (1998). Urinary incontinence: Pathophysiology, evaluation, treatment overview, and nonsurgical management. In P. Walsh, et al. (Eds.), *Campbell's urology* (7th ed., pp. 1007–1043). Philadelphia: W. B. Saunders.
10. Bowers, V., Hannigan, K. F., & Kushner, K. L. (1995). Bladder exstrophy and epispadias. In K. Karlowicz (Ed.), *Urologic nursing: Practice and principles* (pp. 565–592). Philadelphia: W. B. Saunders.
11. Burgio, K., et al. (1998). Behavioral vs drug treatment for urge urinary incontinence in older women. *Journal of the American Medical Association, 280*(23), 1995–2000.
12. Burton, D. S., et al. (1995). Urinary calculi. In K. Karlowicz (Ed.), *Urologic nursing: Practice and principles* (pp. 177–198). Philadelphia: W. B. Saunders.
13. Button, D., et al. (1998). Consensus guidelines for the promotion and management of continence by primary health care teams: Development, implementation and evaluation. *Journal of Advanced Nursing, 27*, 91–99.
14. Clayman, R., McDougall, E., & Nakada, S. (1998). Endourology of the upper urinary tract: Percutaneous renal and ureteral procedures. In P. Walsh, et al. (Eds.), *Campbell's urology* (7th ed., pp. 2789–2874). Philadelphia: W. B. Saunders.
15. Curhan, G., et al. (1998). Beverage use and risk for kidney stones in women. *Annals of Internal Medicine, 128*, 534–540.
16. Davila, G., & Bernier, F. (1995). Multimodality pelvic physiotherapy for urinary incontinence in women. *International Urogynecology Journal, 6*(4),185–194.
17. Droller, M. (1998). Bladder cancer: State-of-the-art care. *CA: A Cancer Journal for Clinicians, 48*(5), 269–284.
18. Engberg, S., et al. (1998). Treatment of urinary incontinence among caregiver-dependent adults. *Urologic Nursing, 18*(2), 131–136, 155.
19. Fabrizio, M., Behari, A., & Bagley, D. (1998). Ureteroscopic management of intrarenal calculi. *The Journal of Urology, 159*, 1139–1143.
20. Fantl, J. A., et al. (1996). *Urinary incontinence in adults: Acute and chronic management.* AHCPR Publication No. 96-0682. Clinical Practice Guideline, No. 2 (update). Rockville, MD: Agency for Health Care Policy and Research, Public Health Service, U.S. Department of Health and Human Services.
21. Getliffe, K., & Dolman, M. (1997). *Promoting continence: A clinical and research resource.* London: Bailliere Tindall.
22. Giroux, J. A. (1995). Urinary tract infections in adults. In K. Karlowicz (Ed.), *Urologic nursing: Principles and practice* (pp. 141–175). Philadelphia: W. B. Saunders.
23. Ghoniem, G., Elsergany, R., & Lewis, V. (1998). The evolving role of submucosal injectables for treating internal sphincteric deficiency. *Urologic Nursing, 18*(2), 125–130.
24. Gow, J. (1998). Genitoruinary tuberculosis. In P. Walsh, et al. (Eds.), *Campbell's urology.* (7th ed., pp. 807–836). Philadelphia: W. B. Saunders.
25. Hanno, P. (1998). Interstitial cystitis and related diseases. In P. Walsh, et al. (Eds.), *Campbell's urology* (7th ed., pp. 631–662). Philadelphia: W. B. Saunders.
26. Hanson, M. (1998). *Pathophysiology: Foundations of disease and clinical intervention.* Philadelphia: W. B. Saunders.
27. Hinman, F. (1998). *Atlas of urologic surgery* (2nd ed.). Philadelphia: W. B. Saunders.
28. Huffman, J. (1998). Ureteroscopy. In P. Walsh, et al. (Eds.), *Campbell's urology* (7th ed., pp. 2755–2785). Philadelphia: W. B. Saunders.
29. Karram, M. M. (1996). Lower urinary tract infection. In D. Ostergard & A. Bent (Eds.), *Urogynecology and urodynamics: Theory and practice* (4th ed., pp. 387–408). Baltimore: Williams & Wilkins.
30. Karlowicz, K., & Meredith, C. (1995). Adult voiding disorders. In K. Karlowicz (Ed.), *Urologic nursing: Principles and practice* (pp. 377–408). Philadelphia: W. B. Saunders.
31. Kuo, R., et al. (1998). Impact of holmium laser settings and fiber diameter on stone fragmentation and endoscope deflection. *Journal of Endourology, 12*, 523–527.
32. Leek, C., et al. (1996). In R. McCorkle, et al. (Eds.), *Cancer nursing: A comprehensive textbook* (2nd ed., pp. 677–697). Philadelphia: W. B. Saunders.
33. Leonetti, F., et al. (1998). Dietary and urinary risk factors for stones in idiopathic calcium stone formers compared with healthy subjects. *Nephrology, Dialysis, and Transplantation, 13*(3), 617–622.
34. Lingeman, J., et al. (1999). Divergence between stone composition and urine supersaturation: Clinical and laboratory implications. *Journal of Urology, 161*, 1077–1081.
35. Lingeman, J., et al. (1998). Medical reduction of stone risk in a network of treatment centers compared to a research clinic. *Journal of Urology, 160*, 1629–1634.
36. Loughrey, L. (1999). Taking a sensitive approach to urinary incontinence. *Nursing, 29*(5), 60–61.
37. Marchiondo, K. (1998). A new look at urinary tract infection. *American Journal of Nursing, 98*(3), 34–39.
38. Marshall, F. (1998). Surgery of the bladder. In P. Walsh, et al. (Eds.), *Campbell's urology* (7th ed., pp. 3274–3298). Philadelphia: W. B. Saunders.
39. Martin, T., & Sosa, R. (1998). Shock-wave lithotripsy. In P. Walsh, et al. (Eds.), *Campbell's urology* (7th ed., pp. 2735–2752). Philadelphia: W. B. Saunders.
40. Massey, L., & Kynast-Gales, S. (1998). Substituting milk for apple juice does not increase kidney stone risk in most normocalciuric

adults who form calcium oxalate stones. *Journal of the American Dietetic Association, 98*(3), 303–308.

41. McDougall, W. (1998). Use of intestinal segments and urinary diversion. In P. Walsh, et al. (Eds.), *Campbell's urology* (7th ed., pp. 3121–3161). Philadelphia: W. B. Saunders.
42. McGuire, E., & O'Connell, H. (1998). Pubovaginal slings. In P. Walsh, et al. (Eds.), *Campbell's urology* (7th ed., pp. 1103–1108). Philadelphia: W. B. Saunders.
43. Menon, M., Parulkar, B., & Drach, G. (1998). Urinary lithiasis: Etiology, diagnosis, and medical management. In P. Walsh, et al. (Eds.), *Campbell's urology* (7th ed., pp. 2661–2734). Philadelphia: W. B. Saunders.
44. Messing, E., & Catalona, W. (1998). Urothelial tumors of the urinary tract. In P. Walsh, et al. (Eds.), *Campbell's urology* (7th ed., pp. 2327–2382). Philadelphia: W. B. Saunders.
45. Montagnino, B., Welch, V., Hoyler-Grant, C. (1995). Congenital anomalies that affect the kidney, ureter, and bladder. In K. Karlowicz (Ed.), *Urologic nursing: Principles and practice* (pp. 526–564). Philadelphia: W. B. Saunders.
46. Moody, F. (Ed). (1999). *Atlas of ambulatory surgery*. Philadelphia: W. B. Saunders.
47. Morris, R. (1999). Female genital mutilation: Perspectives, risks, and complications. *Urologic Nursing, 19*(1), 13–19.
48. Nicolle, L. E. (1996). Uncomplicated urinary tract infection in women. In W. R. Cattel (Ed.), *Infections of the kidney and urinary tract*. New York: Oxford University Press.
49. Nyman, M., Schwenk, N., & Silverstein, M. (1997). Management of urinary retention: Rapid versus gradual decompression and risk of complications. *Mayo Clinic Proceedings, 72*, 951–956.
50. Parsons, C. L. (1996). Interstitial cystitis. In D. Ostergard & A. Bent (Eds.), *Urogynecology and urodynamics: Theory and practice* (4th ed., pp. 409–425). Baltimore: Williams & Wilkins.
51. Raz, S. (1996). *Female urology* (2nd ed.). Philadelphia: W. B. Saunders.
52. Raz, S., Stothers, L., & Chopra, A. (1998). Vaginal reconstructive surgery for incontinence and prolapse. In P. Walsh, et al. (Eds.), *Campbell's urology* (7th ed., pp. 1059–1094). Philadelphia: W. B. Saunders.
53. Reilly, N. J. (1995). Cancer of the bladder. In K. Karlowicz (Ed.), *Urologic nursing: Principles and practice* (pp. 243–270). Philadelphia: W. B. Saunders.
54. Reilly, N. J. (1995). Genitourinary trauma. In K. Karlowicz (Ed.), *Urologic nursing: Principles and practice* (pp. 411–435). Philadelphia: W. B. Saunders.
55. Rondorf-Klym, L., Colling, J., & Simonson, W. (1998). Medication use by community-dwelling elderly with urinary incontinence. *Urologic Nursing, 18*(3), 201–206.
56. Schaeffer, A. (1998). Infections and inflammations of the genitourinary tract. In P. Walsh, et al. (Eds.), *Campbell's urology* (7th ed., pp. 531–614). Philadelphia: W. B. Saunders.
57. Society of Urologic Nurses and Associates. (1997). *Scope and standards of urologic nursing practice*. Pitman, NJ: Author.
58. Steers, W. (1998). Physiology and pharmacology of the bladder and ureter. In P. Walsh, et al. (Eds.), *Campbell's urology* (7th ed., pp. 870–916.). Philadelphia: W. B. Saunders.
59. Stockert, P. (1999). Getting UTI clients back on track. *RN, 62*(3), 49–52.
60. Stone, J., Wyman, J., & Salisbury, S. (1999). *Clinical gerontological nursing: A guide to advanced practice* (2nd ed.). Philadelphia: W. B. Saunders.
61. Swibold, L. (1999). Maintenance therapy with bacillus Calmette-Guérin in clients with superficial bladder cancer. *Urologic Nursing, 19*(1), 38–41.
62. Urinary Incontinence Guideline Panel. (1992). *Urinary incontinence in adults: A client's guide*. AHCPR Publication No. 92-0040. Rockville, MD: Agency for Health Care Policy and Research, Public Health Service, U.S. Department of Health and Human Services.
63. Urinary Incontinence Guideline Panel. (1992). *Urinary incontinence in adults: Clinical practice guideline*. AHCPR Publication No. 92-0038. Rockville, MD: Agency for Health Care Policy and Research, Public Health Service, U.S. Department of Health and Human Services.
64. Urinary Incontinence Guideline Panel. (1992). *Urinary incontinence in adults: Quick reference guide for clinicians*. AHCPR Publication No. 92-0041. Rockville, MD: Agency for Health Care Policy and Research, Public Health Service, U.S. Department of Health and Human Services.
65. Walsh, P., et al. (Eds). (1998). *Campbell's urology* (7th ed.). Philadelphia: W. B. Saunders.
66. Webster, G., & Khoury, J. (1998). Retropubic suspension surgery for female sphincteric incontinence. In P. Walsh, et al. (Eds.), *Campbell's urology* (7th ed., pp. 1095–1102). Philadelphia: W. B. Saunders.
67. Wein, A. (1998). Neuromuscular dysfunction of the lower urinary tract and its treatment. In P. Walsh, et al. (Eds.), *Campbell's urology* (7th ed., pp. 953–1006). Philadelphia: W. B. Saunders.
68. Wein, A. (1998). Pathophysiology and categorization of voiding dysfunction. In P. Walsh, et al. (Eds.), *Campbell's urology* (7th ed., pp. 917–926). Philadelphia: W. B. Saunders.
69. Wein, A. (1998). Physiology and pharmacology of the renal pelvis and ureter. In P. Walsh, et al. (Eds.), *Campbell's urology* (7th ed., pp. 839–869). Philadelphia: W. B. Saunders.
70. Wolfish, N. (1997). Caring for the renal client. In D. Levine (Ed.), *Pediatric nephrology* (3rd ed., pp. 108–130). Philadelphia: W. B. Saunders.

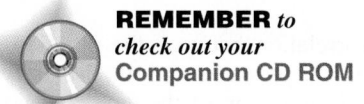

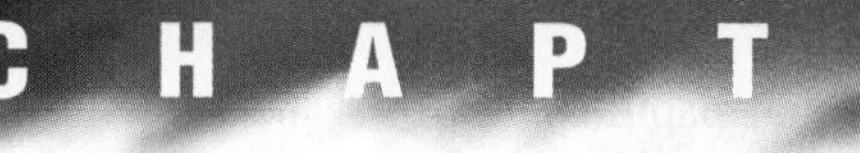

CHAPTER 35

Management of Clients with Renal Disorders

Anita E. Molzahn

NURSING OUTCOMES CLASSIFICATION (NOC)
for Nursing Diagnoses—Clients with Renal Disorders

Altered Health Maintenance
Health-Promoting Behavior
Health-Seeking Behavior
Knowledge: Health Behaviors
Knowledge: Health Promotion
Self-Direction of Care
Altered Nutrition: Less Than Body Requirements
Nutritional Status: Food and Fluid Intake
Anxiety
Anxiety Control
Coping
Fatigue
Activity Tolerance
Endurance
Energy Conservation
Nutritional Status: Energy
Fluid Volume Excess
Fluid Balance
Hydration
Pain
Comfort Level
Pain Control
Pain: Disruptive Effects
Pain Level
Risk for Fluid Volume Deficit
Bowel Elimination
Fluid Balance
Hydration
Knowledge: Medication
Knowledge: Treatment Regimen
Urinary Elimination
Risk for Impaired Skin Integrity
Nutritional Status
Tissue Integrity: Skin and Mucous Membranes
Tissue Perfusion: Peripheral
Risk for Infection
Immune Status
Risk Control
Risk Detection
Risk for Injury
Risk Control
Risk Detection
Symptom Control

The kidneys regulate the body's fluid, electrolyte, and acid-base balances while removing toxic substances from the blood and excreting them in urine. The kidneys also play a significant role in erythropoietin and prostaglandin synthesis, in insulin degradation, and in the renin-angiotensin-aldosterone system.

This chapter identifies the common disease processes and injuries that can interfere with normal renal function. Although the effects of extrarenal influences on the kidneys are briefly described, the primary purpose of this chapter is to discuss specific renal pathologic processes. Some of these disorders can result in renal failure (see Chapter 36). Because of the potential seriousness of any renal problem, the client and significant others have physical as well as psychological needs. You need to know about both aspects and should maintain a consistent awareness of the need for appropriate intervention.

EXTRARENAL CONDITIONS

Many conditions primarily located in other parts of the body affect the kidneys, such as diabetes mellitus, hypertension, and sepsis. This chapter provides a brief description of the renal implications of these extrarenal conditions. For further discussion, see Chapters 45, 52, and 81.

DIABETES MELLITUS

One of the most common extrarenal diseases affecting the kidney is diabetes mellitus. *Diabetic nephropathy*, a progressive process, commonly leads to renal failure. About 30% of clients with end-stage renal disease (ESRD) have diabetes mellitus. Researchers estimate that 25% to 50% of clients with insulin-dependent diabetes mellitus (IDDM, or type 1 diabetes) have end-stage renal disease within 10 to 20 years of beginning insulin therapy. Renal disease can also occur in the non–insulin-dependent diabetic client. The incidence of proteinuria is about 25% after 20 years of diabetes.

Several pathologic changes lead to renal failure in clients who have diabetes mellitus. The most common is a characteristic intercapillary *glomerulosclerosis*, or scarring of the capillary loops. Progressive microangiopathy, called *nephrosclerosis*, affects the afferent and efferent arterioles and eventually scars the glomerulus, tubules, and interstitium. *Pyelonephritis* (kidney infection) can scar the renal parenchyma and lead to ischemia. It may also lead to renal papillary necrosis and sloughing of the papillae. *Neurogenic bladder* dysfunction may contribute to renal failure. The high incidence of urinary tract infection or the increased pressure in the kidney caused by the back-up of urine may also contribute to renal dysfunction.

Initially, the sclerotic, or hardening, process of glomerulosclerosis increases renal vascular resistance, contributing to systemic hypertension. This does not cause renal insufficiency. Indeed, the glomerular filtration rate (GFR) may increase as much as 20% to 50% above the normal GFR during this early "silent" phase. It is now recognized that microalbuminemia (measurable by assay) occurs quite some time before clinical proteinuria. If it is diagnosed, it may be a much earlier indicator of eventual renal failure. As more nephrons are destroyed, available functioning renal tissue decreases and the client begins to show clinical proteinuria (a key manifestation), hypertension, edema, and evidence of renal failure.

The kidney metabolizes 30% to 40% of insulin, and as renal function declines, the degradation of insulin also decreases, resulting in a lower insulin requirement. Renal failure may be initially identified when the client is evaluated for recurrent insulin reactions. Researchers hope the sclerotic process can be slowed by:

- Carefully controlling hypertension
- Adjusting insulin therapy and carefully monitoring blood glucose to maintain euglycemia
- Restricting dietary protein

Regardless of diabetic control, however, renal failure inevitably develops within 5 to 10 years after the appearance of significant proteinuria.

HYPERTENSION

Because the kidneys receive quite a large share of cardiac output, renal function can affect or be affected by cardiovascular changes. Renal blood flow determines the GFR, which directly affects renal function. Hypertension is one condition that can either cause or be affected by renal disease. For example, renovascular hypertension results from renal artery stenosis or renal infarction. The reduction in renal blood flow activates the renin-angiotensin-aldosterone system and increases systemic blood pressure.

Renal hypertension associated with parenchymal renal disease (e.g., glomerulonephritis, polycystic disease, pyelonephritis) usually results from the kidney's decreasing ability to excrete salt and water. Other causes include increased renin release from increased glomerular perfusion and inadequacy of renal vasodilating substances, as occurs with analgesic nephropathy. Among clients with renal failure, 80% to 85% of hypertension results from excess salt and water retention; renovascular hypertension accounts for up to 15% of all systemic hypertension.

On the other hand, sustained systemic high blood pressure adversely affects the kidneys. Researchers report that nephrosclerosis can be seen microscopically in clients who have had uncontrolled hypertension for more than 5 years, although all other renal diagnostic tests may be normal. Kidney damage is the direct result of degenerative changes in the arterioles and interlobular arteries caused by increased blood pressure.

There is a direct correlation between the duration and degree of elevated blood pressure and the severity of renal vascular disease. Progression of the disease can usually be halted or slowed by controlling blood pressure. Client teaching is vital to managing the hypertension and preventing renal failure.

HYPOTENSION

Cardiovascular shock, or hypotension, also affects renal function. Renal vasoconstriction reduces renal blood flow. However, because of the autoregulation capabilities of the kidneys (see Chapters 12, 32, and 81), GFR remains at a functional level until the advanced stages of systemic shock, at which time acute renal failure develops. Restoring systemic blood pressure usually reverses the renal vasoconstriction, and kidney function returns, typically within 2 to 8 weeks as long as prolonged ischemia has not occurred. A period of polyuria (excessive urination) may follow the correction of hypovolemia, although the mechanisms for this are unclear.

Before renal function returns to normal, another oliguric period may occur, followed by a "mobilization phase" in which sequestered fluid is shifted into the intravascular space. The shift may cause some hypertension until the kidneys can remove the extra fluid. Careful assessment of the client's fluid status and meticulous fluid management are crucial during these recovery phases.

RHABDOMYOLYSIS

Rhabdomyolysis is a disorder usually associated with traumatic injury of skeletal muscle tissue, which releases myoglobin and intracellular substances into the blood. It can also occur after serious crush injuries, strenuous exercise, seizures, heat stroke, prolonged coma, and drug overdose. The resulting acute renal failure is usually reversible with treatment.

Clinical evidence of rhabdomyolysis includes fever, malaise, nausea, vomiting, muscular weakness, pain, and swelling. The release of substances from damaged muscles results in myoglobinemia, myoglobinuria (which can be seen as brown urine and confirmed through urinalysis), hyperkalemia, hyperphosphatemia, hyperuricemia, and elevated creatine kinase. Hypocalcemia occurs initially because of the precipitation of calcium with phosphate. Later, in the diuretic phase of acute renal failure, hypercalcemia can occur as calcium is mobilized.

Treatment is typically symptomatic, including bed rest to reduce muscle metabolism and steps to correct acidosis and maintain normal fluid volume.

CARDIOVASCULAR DISEASE

Cardiac disease influences kidney function primarily through its effect on cardiac output and circulating blood volume. The hemodynamic and hormonal changes of cardiac disease may decrease the kidneys' ability to excrete sodium and water. This, in turn, increases intravascular congestion and edema and establishes a pathologic cycle.

Hemodynamic changes also occur with normal aging. Blood flow to the kidneys decreases by up to half by age

70 years, and GFR can decrease by 40% to 50% as well. Renal function deteriorates as glomeruli become sclerotic and atrophy.

PERIPHERAL VASCULAR DISEASE

Thromboembolic disease can affect the renal circulation and cause infarction of the tissue supplied by the affected blood vessel. In clients with sickle cell disease, the interstitial hypertonicity and low oxygen pressure found in the renal medulla seem to favor sickling of red blood cells in the kidney's juxtamedullary region. These cell masses cause gross hematuria as venules rupture, papillary necrosis, renal infarction, concentrating disturbances resulting from interference with the countercurrent mechanism, nephrotic syndrome, pyelonephritis, and, finally, renal failure.

In disseminated intravascular coagulation, in which diffuse clotting consumes clotting factors and causes hemorrhage in affected areas throughout the body, the kidney is the organ most affected.

SEPSIS

Extrarenal sepsis may affect kidney function either through its effect on systemic circulation or by stimulating the immune system. Renal reactions to septic shock are similar to those in hypotension. Immunologic injury can lead to glomerulonephritis (see later). Occasionally, pathogens may break away from extrarenal foci of infection and travel to the kidney to establish additional sites.

PREGNANCY

Pregnancy has a definite influence on kidney function. During the first trimester, the collecting system dilates and the kidneys enlarge, a condition that may persist 9 to 12 weeks after delivery. Renal blood flow and GFR increase by 30% to 50% during pregnancy, contributing to increased creatinine clearance and decreased uric acid excretion. These normal changes (such as lower serum creatinine) must be taken into account in interpreting laboratory findings for pregnant women. Pregnancy also increases the likelihood of proteinuria (usually transient), polyuria, and nocturia (excessive urination at night). These disorders may be caused by external bladder compression and alterations in antidiuretic hormone metabolism.

OTHER CAUSES

Kidney function is influenced by many other extrarenal disease processes, such as cancer, connective tissue disorders, and metabolic disturbances. Many systemic diseases produce clinical manifestations like those of glomerulonephritis, although they typically have other systemic features characteristic of the disease (see glomerulonephritis later). These diseases include systemic lupus erythematosus, systemic scleroderma, polyarteritis nodosa, thrombocytopenic purpura, Wegener's granulomatosis, hemolytic-uremic syndrome, gout, amyloidosis, and Henoch-Schönlein syndrome. Diagnosis can be confirmed by renal biopsy.

Renal disease has become an increasingly common complication for people infected with the human immunodeficiency virus (HIV). Among the several renal disorders associated with HIV and acquired immunodeficiency syndrome (AIDS) are renal tuberculosis and cytomegalovirus, such malignancies as lymphoma and Kaposi's sar coma, and HIV-associated nephropathy, a focal glomerulosclerosis that is manifested by nephrotic syndrome (see later).

NEPHROTOXINS

Nephrotoxins have specific, destructive effects on renal cells. They can cause the following types of renal injury:

- Acute tubular necrosis
- Defects in the tubular transport system
- Interstitial nephritis
- Vasculitis
- Nephrotic syndrome

Nephrotoxic substances in the environment include heavy metals, such as mercurial compounds, lead, cadmium, bismuth, arsenic, copper, and phosphorus; carbon tetrachloride; ethylene glycol; trichloroethylene; carbon monoxide; and chlorinated hydrocarbons. Exposure to many of these substances occurs in industrial locations. Other environmental nephrotoxins include snake venom and certain mushrooms. Acute tubular necrosis is the most frequent injury resulting from exposure to nephrotoxins. Some nephrotoxins also cause tubular transport defects and nephrotic syndrome. Box 35–1 presents some common nephrotoxic substances.

All five types of kidney damage may result from nephrotoxic reactions to medications. Two types of medications well known to cause renal damage are antibiotics and certain analgesics. Because the kidneys are the major

BOX 35–1 Nephrotoxins

Antibiotics

Aminoglycosides
Tetracyclines
Amphotericin B
Cephalosporins
Sulfonamides
(co-trimoxazole)
Bacitracin
Polymyxin
Colistin

Heavy Metals

Lead
Mercury
Arsenic
Copper
Gold
Lithium

Poisons

Mushrooms
Insecticides
Herbicides
Snake bites

Anesthetics

Contrast Dyes

Organic Solvents

Glycols
Gasoline
Kerosene
Turpentine
Tetrachloroethylene

Other Drugs

Acetaminophen
Nonsteroidal anti-inflammatory
medications
Salicylates
Heroin
Dextran
Mannitol
Interleukin-2
Cisplatin
Amphetamines

route of excretion for many antibiotics, renal tissue is directly exposed to these compounds. The longer the exposure, the higher the risk of renal toxic effects. Pre-existing renal disease, decreased renal blood flow, electrolyte imbalances, and concurrent use of other nephrotoxic medications enhance a medication's nephrotoxic effect.

High-risk antibiotics include cephalosporins, sulfonamides, polymyxins, aminoglycosides, and amphotericin B. Carefully monitor renal function tests to identify early nephrotoxic reactions so that causative medications can be discontinued or the dose decreased. Closely monitor drug levels to make sure that dosages stay in the therapeutic range. Besides using these medications as briefly as possible and at as low a dose as possible, maintaining a high fluid intake may help prevent nephrotoxic effects. A high urine output keeps the medication diluted in the kidney and helps prevent crystallization.

The risk of renal damage caused by excessive use of certain analgesics has been receiving more attention. Salicylates, acetaminophen, phenacetin, and nonsteroidal anti-inflammatory drugs (NSAIDs) are the most common nephrotoxic agents. Short-term overdose or long-term consistent use of these medications may cause acute tubular necrosis or chronic renal failure. Researchers estimate that 5% to 10% of clients with end-stage renal disease have analgesic nephropathy.

Anesthesia reduces the kidney's vasoconstrictive ability, which helps protect it against systemic blood pressure drops; thus, the kidney is made more vulnerable to the effects of shock. In addition, certain anesthetics, particularly methoxyflurane, have a direct nephrotoxic effect. Administration of this general anesthetic agent can cause acute tubular necrosis and has been associated with fatal acute renal failure. Halothane may also adversely affect renal function.

Diuretics may have nephrotoxic effects as well and, when used aggressively, can cause hypovolemia. Other common medications that may have nephrotoxic effects include probenecid, phenytoin, low-molecular-weight dextran, rifampin, phenindione, lithium, and gold. You must know about the possible adverse effects of any medication a client takes so that you can assess and intervene appropriately.

Radioiodinated contrast agents used in radiographic and computed tomographic (CT) studies have been associated with acute tubular necrosis. Risk factors include:

- Age older than 60 years
- Pre-existing renal insufficiency, especially diabetic nephropathy
- Dehydration
- Low cardiac output with pre-existing renal disease
- Proteinuria
- Hypoalbuminemia
- Multiple myeloma
- Multiple contrast studies within a 24-hour period

Using non-dye studies whenever possible and keeping the client well hydrated throughout the test reduce the risk of acute renal failure. Baseline renal function tests before the contrast study should be available to compare with post-test findings. Monitor the client's urine output carefully for several hours after the study is completed.

ACQUIRED DISORDERS

NEPHROLITHIASIS

Although calculi (stones) can form anywhere in the urinary tract, the most frequent site is the kidney. These stones may travel down the urinary tract, lodge anywhere along the tract, and cause obstruction and tissue damage. Or they may stay in the kidney. Urolithiasis is described in detail in Chapter 34.

Treatment and nursing care of clients with renal calculi are similar to those of people with calculi lower in the urinary tract. However, damage to the kidney caused by calculi can be permanent and may require nephrectomy (described later).

PYELONEPHRITIS

Pyelonephritis is an inflammation of the renal pelvis and parenchyma caused by a bacterial infection. The cause may be an active infection in the kidney or the remnants of a previous infection. There are two main types of pyelonephritis: acute and chronic. They differ primarily in their clinical picture and long-term effects.

Etiology and Risk Factors

Sometimes an infection may be a primary disease, as happens with reduced host resistance (e.g., calculi, malignancy, hydronephrosis, or trauma). Most kidney infections, however, are extensions of infectious processes located elsewhere, especially the bladder. Chapter 34 discusses the etiologic mechanism and pathogenesis of infections in the lower urinary tract.

The bacteria spread to the kidney primarily by ascending the ureter to the kidney. Blood and lymphatic circulation also provide channels for the organisms. Ureteral reflux, which allows infected urine back into the ureter, and obstruction, which causes urine to back into the ureter and allows organisms to multiply, are the most common causes of ascending urinary tract infections. *Escherichia coli* is the most common bacterial organism causing pyelonephritis.

Health promotion is key to preventing recurrence of infection and further renal damage. The nurse provides information to clients about health and lifestyle measures to prevent urinary tract infections, including (1) perineal hygiene measures such as wiping from front to back, (2) acidification of the urine (by drinking cranberry juice or taking ascorbic acid), and (3) ensuring adequate fluid intake. Early detection and adequate treatment of lower urinary tract infections greatly reduce the incidence of pyelonephritis.

After infection, health maintenance includes education about the importance of completing the course of antibiotics. Follow-up cultures are important with recurrent pyelonephritis to ensure that the infection has been eradicated. Health restoration measures depend on the extent of renal damage and the cause of the disease. If obstruction precipitated the infection, the cause of the obstruction must be treated.

ACUTE PYELONEPHRITIS. Acute pyelonephritis often occurs after bacterial contamination of the urethra or after introduction of an instrument, such as a catheter or a cystoscope.

CHRONIC PYELONEPHRITIS. Chronic pyelonephritis is more likely to occur after chronic obstruction with reflux or chronic disorders. It is slowly progressive and usually associated with recurrent acute attacks, although there may be no history of acute pyelonephritis.

Pathophysiology

Pyelonephritis occurs when bacteria enter the renal pelvis, causing an inflammatory response and an increase in white blood cells (WBCs). The inflammation leads to edema and swelling of the involved tissue, beginning at the papillae and sometimes spreading to the cortex. The infection can be either ascending, as occurs after cystitis or prostatitis, or descending, as from a streptococcal infection in the bloodstream.

As the infection is treated and the inflammation recedes, fibrosis and scar tissue may develop. The calices become blunted with scarring in the interstitial tissues. If the infection recurs, more and more scar tissue develops; fibrosis and altered tubular reabsorption and secretion lead to decreased renal function.

ACUTE PYELONEPHRITIS. Acute pyelonephritis is associated with the development of renal abscesses, perinephric abscesses, emphysematous pyelonephritis, and chronic pyelonephritis that can lead to renal failure.

Acute pyelonephritis is usually brief. It often recurs, however, either as a relapse of a previous infection not eradicated or as a new infection; 20% of these recurrences take place within 2 weeks after completion of therapy. A client must be treated adequately to prevent the development of chronic pyelonephritis. The infection may also progress to bacteremia.

CHRONIC PYELONEPHRITIS. This disease is characterized by a combination of caliceal abnormalities and overlying cortical scarring. The kidney becomes contracted, and the number of functioning nephrons decreases as they are replaced by scar tissue. Renal failure may ensue, although uremia is less common than once thought.

Clinical Manifestations

ACUTE PYELONEPHRITIS. Acute pyelonephritis is characterized by enlarged kidneys, focal parenchymal abscesses, and accumulation of polymorphonuclear lymphocytes around and in the renal tubules. Typically, the client seems to be in acute distress, although the disorder may cause minimal or no manifestations.

Assessment usually reveals high fever, chills, nausea, flank pain on the affected side (costovertebral angle [CVA] tenderness), headache, muscle pain, and general prostration. The pain commonly radiates down the ureter or toward the epigastrium and may be colicky if the infection is complicated by calculi or sloughed renal papillae. Percussion or deep palpation over the CVA elicits marked tenderness. Commonly, the client has experienced dysuria, frequency, urgency, and other evidence of cystitis for several days. The urine may be cloudy or bloody, is foul smelling, and shows a marked increase in WBCs and casts. Chapter 32 describes assessment of the renal system.

Urine culture and sensitivity studies, along with a physical examination, are the primary diagnostic tests. Studies may be done to detect calculi, especially with recurrent infections, because calculi may seed and cause reinfection, particularly with *Proteus*. X-ray studies, as of the kidney, ureter, and bladder (a KUB study), and intravenous pyelography (IVP) are commonly done. A cystourethrogram may be obtained, especially after an initial episode of pyelonephritis, to look for underlying defects, particularly any cause of reflux. Magnetic resonance imaging (MRI) or a CT scan may also be used to evaluate the kidney size or the presence of other problems.

CHRONIC PYELONEPHRITIS. This disease has no specific manifestations of its own. Thus, it is usually discovered incidentally when the client is being evaluated for hypertension or its complications. Hypertension itself is the most frequent manifestation of the disease.

Abnormal laboratory studies may show azotemia, pyuria, anemia, acidosis, and proteinuria. They may also demonstrate poor urine-concentrating ability.

Outcome Management

Medical Management

ACUTE PYELONEPHRITIS

Ideal outcomes of medical management include:

- Elimination of the pathogenic organisms with appropriate antibiotics, as identified by urine culture and sensitivity studies
- Removal of any factor or disease contributing to decreased host resistance

If calculi or other obstructions are found to be the cause of recurrent infection, appropriate treatment is instituted.

INHIBIT BACTERIAL GROWTH. Antibiotic therapy is based on the results of urine culture and sensitivity tests. Typically, a broad-spectrum antibiotic is prescribed; it may be changed after the results of the culture are available. Sulfonamides or the combination of sulfamethoxazole and trimethoprim is commonly used as first-line therapy unless the client is allergic to one of these drugs. Typically, antibiotic therapy continues for 10 days to 2 weeks.

Antibiotics may be administered orally or by the single large-dose method described in Chapter 34. In severe cases of acute pyelonephritis, intravenous antibiotics may be administered. With oral therapy, the client must understand that completing the full course of antibiotic therapy is important to prevent recurrence of the infection. Recurrent infections are commonly treated with long-term prophylactic antibiotic therapy. Additional pharmacologic therapy may be needed to correct any predisposing factors.

RELIEVE PAIN. Analgesic or urinary antiseptic medications can be prescribed to reduce discomfort. Antibiotics quickly reduce discomfort as well.

CHRONIC PYELONEPHRITIS

The desired outcome of medical management is prevention of further renal damage. If bacteria are found, appropriate antibiotics are given, as in acute pyelonephritis. Chronic pyelonephritis tends to be less painful. Above all, hypertension must be controlled. Additional intervention depends on the degree of renal failure that has already occurred. Although high fluid intake may be advisable in acute pyelonephritis, it may be contraindicated in chronic pyelonephritis if the degree of renal dysfunction is significant.

INHIBIT BACTERIAL GROWTH. Antibiotics specific to the bacteria present are given to treat chronic pyelonephritis (see Chapter 34 and Acute Pyelonephritis).

CONTROL HYPERTENSION. Renal damage can cause hypertension, which can cause further renal damage. Thus, it is important to control the client's blood pressure. Reduction of dietary sodium and pharmacologic therapy may be indicated. Management of hypertension is discussed in Chapters 34 and 52.

Nursing Management of the Medical Client

ASSESSMENT

Assessment of the client with pyelonephritis begins with a thorough history and physical examination, with close attention to the presence of risk factors, previous urinary tract infections, hypertension, and CVA tenderness. Look for evidence of pyelonephritis.

DIAGNOSIS, OUTCOMES, INTERVENTIONS

Risk for Fluid Volume Deficit. A common diagnosis is *Risk for Fluid Volume Deficit related to fever, nausea, vomiting, and possible diarrhea.*

Outcomes. The client will remain free from fluid volume deficit, as evidenced by balanced intake and output, maintenance of adequate hydration, and an absence of signs or symptoms of dehydration.

Interventions. Prepare the client for the diagnostic tests and probable antibiotic therapy. Clients with severe nausea and vomiting may require intravenous fluids. Keep in mind that overhydration may dilute antimicrobials, diminishing their effectiveness. See Chapter 34 on the nursing care of the client with cystitis.

Pain. Another common diagnosis is *Pain related to an inflammatory process in the kidney and possible colic.*

Outcomes. The client will report no pain or will report that pain is controlled.

Interventions. Medications can be given to control pain caused by calculi. CVA tenderness should decrease as the antibiotics control the infection. Medication for nausea can be given as needed with antipyretics for high fevers. Adequate treatment of the infection quickly reverses the dysuria, pyuria, and frequency. Urinary analgesics (see Chapter 34) can also help the client with these problems. Fluid intake of 3 to 4 L/day is recommended. This fluid helps to dilute the urine and to reduce irritation and burning. The continual flow of urine serves to prevent stasis and discourage multiplication of bacteria in the urinary tract.

Altered Health Maintenance. Client teaching is important to promote self-care and prevent recurrent infections. Write the diagnosis *Altered Health Maintenance related to prevention of recurrent infections.*

Outcomes. The client will understand how to prevent recurrent infections, as evidenced by the client's statements and no recurrence of infection.

Interventions. The preventive measures for acute and chronic pyelonephritis are similar to those for cystitis (see Chapter 34). It is important to prevent permanent renal damage. Make sure that the client can recognize the manifestations of a urinary tract infection and knows to seek prompt medical attention when they occur.

When the acute infection subsides, instruct the client to continue follow-up care. This care includes completing the full course of antibiotic therapy and having repeated urine cultures. Also, teach ways to prevent further infections in the urinary tract, including ensuring a high fluid intake (see Chapter 34).

It is vital that the client return for follow-up urine cultures and possibly other diagnostic tests if the cause of the pyelonephritis is not clear. Emphasize that follow-up cultures are important because bacteriuria may be present but may produce no manifestations. Advise the client to report any manifestations of recurrence immediately so that retreatment can begin.

EVALUATION

The infection should subside with adequate antibiotic treatment. Successful management results in reduced pain and negative findings on follow-up urine cultures. The client must also be made aware of the cause of this infection and ways to prevent further infections (see Chapter 34).

Self-Care

The focus of client self-care is to maintain high levels of fluid intake and prevent recurrence of infection. If manifestations arise, the client must report them promptly and begin treatment to prevent further renal damage.

Modification for Elderly Clients

In older clients, the kidneys may be less able to recover from a severe infection. Antibiotic therapy should be monitored closely because older adults may vary in their sensitivity and response to the medication. Older adults may also have altered blood levels of antibiotics because renal perfusion decreases with age, reducing the kidney's ability to excrete drugs.

RENAL CANDIDIASIS

Bacteria cause most cases of pyelonephritis, but the incidence of renal candidiasis, a fungal infection, is increasing. Primary renal candidiasis is most common in women with diabetes mellitus. Clinical manifestations include ureteral obstruction secondary to a bezoar (tangled hyphae or clumps of yeast cells); progressive oliguria, sometimes alternating with episodic diuresis; ureteral colic; passing tissue or stone-like material; pyuria; and progressive renal failure. Diagnosis is based on the presence of fungi in several properly collected urine cultures; the presence of serum *Candida* precipitins; and selected radiologic findings, such as hydronephrosis, caliceal erosion, and filling defects called fungus balls.

Amphotericin B and flucytosine are the keys to medical management, although these medications require careful administration and monitoring of dosage to prevent nephrotoxicity. In clients with severe disease, surgery or nephrectomy may be needed to remove the obstruction.

RENAL TUBERCULOSIS

Tuberculosis of the kidney, which affects men more than women, occurs when the causative organism, *Mycobacterium tuberculosis*, reaches the kidney via the bloodstream from another source in the body, usually the lungs. In the kidney, the organism may become dormant for many years. By the time it again becomes active, the original infection is often well healed. Frequently, the primary tubercular site is asymptomatic, which makes it difficult to identify renal tuberculosis on the basis of history.

Clinical Manifestations

The clinical course of renal tuberculosis is generally indolent, and clinical manifestations often do not become evident until the later stages of the disease. Early disease involves the renal cortex or medulla. Tissue destruction extends in all directions, eventually eroding into a calix at the tip of the papilla and progressing to rupture into the renal pelvis. When the infection reaches the pelvis, it spreads along the mucosa. The causative organisms then have full access to the rest of the kidney and can move down the urinary tract and infect any of the urinary organs. If untreated, this destructive process continues to form large, caseating masses that coalesce and destroy kidney tissue. X-ray examination at this time shows a moth-eaten appearance of the kidneys.

Organisms that reach the lower urinary tract usually cause fibrosis, stricture formation, and destruction of the ureterovesical valve. If these processes result in stenosis (narrowing) of the ureter, reducing the exit for pus and urine from the infected kidney, renal destruction accelerates. Descending tubercle bacilli may also lodge in the male reproductive organs, causing reduced function.

When renal tuberculosis becomes evident, assessment findings are often nonspecific. Renal manifestations may be preceded by general malaise, weight loss, low-grade fever, and night sweats, but these are not as frequent as with pulmonary tuberculosis. Manifestations of cystitis, as described in Chapter 34, commonly form the client's chief complaint. Flank pain may be present, and hematuria and pyuria are common. Males frequently have evidence of epididymitis.

Growth of *M. tuberculosis* in a culture of the urine confirms the diagnosis. Culture specimens are collected on at least three successive mornings. Because tubercle bacilli are shed intermittently, three to 12 negative cultures are needed to rule out active renal tuberculosis.

Outcome Management

Medical Management

Chemotherapy with antitubercular agents has reduced the need for surgical intervention. Therapy that combines several medications (rifampin, ethambutol, isoniazid, and pyridoxine, for example, or streptomycin, cycloserine, and sodium para-aminosalicylate) is the most common intervention. Because tubercle bacilli divide slowly, the medications are usually given in a single daily dose. If side effects develop, the day's dose may be divided. See Chapter 62 for further information on antitubercular medications.

Nursing Management of the Medical Client

During the acute phase, nursing interventions involve assisting with diagnostic procedures, protecting against the spread of causative organisms, providing relief of manifestations, and assisting the client with the medication regimen. Because tuberculosis arouses a great deal of fear and a feeling of social isolation, expect your nursing diagnoses to include fear and anxiety for the client as well as for significant others. Help the client discuss and work through feelings. Listen to the client's concerns, and make a referral for additional counseling if necessary.

Surgical Management

Surgical intervention includes total or partial nephrectomy (discussed later) or cutaneous ureterostomy (see Chapter 34). Permanent urinary diversion may be necessary if strictures are severe or bladder damage is irreparable (see Chapter 34). Indications for surgery include persistent infection that fails to respond to chemotherapy, intractable pain, hemorrhage, uncontrollable hypertension, renal malignancy, and progressive strictures.

If surgery is needed, perioperative nursing intervention is similar to that for any client having major surgery (see Chapter 15).

Self-Care

Renal tuberculosis is a prolonged illness that requires long-term care and support. Because the client is usually seen on an outpatient basis, instruction in self-care is important in maintaining and restoring health. One of the biggest challenges with clients recovering from renal tuberculosis is ensuring that they continue with the prescribed medical and nursing regimens, particularly when they begin to feel better. Help the client understand the need for continuing medication therapy and continuing follow-up examinations.

Explain the importance of maintaining general good health, such as proper nutrition, adequate rest, and good hygiene. Work in partnership with the client during recovery, and give the client positive feedback for taking medications regularly, if appropriate. If the client is not taking medications, help develop strategies that facilitate willingness to take medications.

RENAL ABSCESS

A renal abscess (renal carbuncle) is a localized infection in the cortex of the kidney. It can form when smaller infectious foci or microabscesses combine in the renal parenchyma. It is usually secondary to urinary tract infection with a species of Enterobacter and is often complicated by renal calculi and obstruction. Organisms from extrarenal sites may also cause this infectious process. For example, many clients report a history of recent cutaneous furuncles (boils).

Clients with renal abscess typically have high fever and moderate to severe pain. The pain is usually constant and located in the upper abdomen or the costovertebral area; it sometimes resembles renal colic. Unlike the findings in pyelonephritis, the urine is usually sterile because the abscess does not reach into the urinary collecting system. Other manifestations of this infectious process include weakness, anorexia, weight loss, night sweats, and leukocytosis.

Medical and nursing interventions for renal abscess resemble those for acute pyelonephritis. Aggressive antibiotic therapy is usually successful. Needle aspiration of the abscess may be done for culture and sensitivity studies, which help identify appropriate antimicrobial therapy. Surgical incision and drainage of the abscess are sometimes necessary. If incision and drainage are performed, nursing intervention expands to include postoperative care of the incision. A drain is left in place for some time.

PERINEPHRIC ABSCESS

A perinephric abscess involves the fatty tissue surrounding the kidney. It may be an extension of a renal infectious process (most common), or the organism may have spread in the bloodstream from an extrarenal site. The abscess may spread in several directions, extending to the peritoneal cavity, chest, or skin.

Assessment findings are the same as for a renal abscess—fever, tenderness, flank or loin pain, and other manifestations of sepsis—with the possible addition of swelling over the site.

Medical and nursing interventions are almost identical to those for renal abscess. Appropriate antibiotics are administered and symptomatic interventions undertaken. Because of the nature of a perinephric abscess, incising and draining are more likely than with a renal abscess. After this surgical procedure, there may be profuse drainage from the wound; frequent dressing changes and nursing interventions are required to prevent or treat skin excoriation.

HYDRONEPHROSIS

Hydronephrosis is distention of the renal pelvis and calices caused by an obstruction of normal urine flow. Urine production continues, and the urine is trapped proximal to the obstruction. Causes of occlusion include calculus, tumor, scar tissue, congenital structural defects, and a kink in the ureter.

Whatever the cause, the accumulating urine exerts pressure on the renal pelvis wall. At low to moderate pressures, the kidney may dilate with no obvious loss of function. Over time, sustained or intermittent high pressure causes irreversible nephron destruction. In addition to pressure-related problems, pyelonephritis is always a risk because of urinary stasis.

Outcome Management

Medical Management

Treatment aims to relieve the obstruction and prevent infection. Depending on the location of the obstruction, it may involve placement of a ureteral catheter or stent above the point of obstruction. Typically, surgery is required (see Chapter 34) to relieve the obstruction and restore adequate drainage of the urinary system.

Removal of the obstruction results in sudden release of the pressure on the renal parenchyma caused by the trapped urine, which leads to diuresis. Thus, postobstructive diuresis occurs and can lead to fluid and electrolyte imbalances, including dehydration. The kidney gradually begins to concentrate urine appropriately.

Nursing Management of the Medical Client

ASSESSMENT

Assessment of a client with hydronephrosis includes monitoring for the presence, location, intensity, and character of pain. Monitor urine output, and report manifestations of renal failure (oliguria, anorexia, lethargy), hematuria, and dysuria. Reduced urine output could indicate obstruction. Palpate the client's bladder to assess for any manifestations of distention. The kidneys, if palpated, may be tender.

DIAGNOSIS, OUTCOMES, INTERVENTIONS

Risk for Fluid Volume Deficit. *Risk for Fluid Volume Deficit related to increased urine output* is the most important nursing problem. Because of the dangers involved in postobstruction diuresis, it is crucial to monitor the client closely after an obstruction is released.

Outcomes. The client will remain free of a fluid volume deficit, as evidenced by balanced intake and output, maintenance of adequate hydration, and no manifestations of dehydration.

Interventions. Make frequent assessments, including hourly outputs; daily weights; vital signs every 30 minutes for the first 4 hours and then every 2 hours; urine for specific gravity, albumin, and glucose; and edema. Make periodic serum electrolyte and glucose determinations as well. Consider the expected presence of severe fatigue caused by urinary losses and the need for frequent observation. Fluid management during this period is crucial; hourly fluid replacement is based on the previous hour's output.

EVALUATION

The client with hydronephrosis must understand the importance of fluid balance, the need to monitor urinary output, and the need to report any changes in condition. Specific evaluation criteria will vary depending on the cause of obstruction.

Surgical Management

Surgery is commonly required to relieve the obstruction causing hydronephrosis. Management of the surgical client is discussed under urolithiasis in Chapter 34.

Self-Care

Clients who have had hydronephrosis should watch for signs of infection and obstruction, such as pain and reduced urine output. Avoiding urinary tract infections is important in preventing pyelonephritis and preserving renal function (see Chapter 34).

RENAL CANCER

Benign kidney tumors are rare. Classifications include lymphangioma, lipoma, medullary fibroma, adenoma, leiomyoma, and oncocytoma. When large benign tumors occur, it is relatively impossible to distinguish them from a malignant tumor by x-ray examination.

At least 85% of all renal tumors are malignant, and approximately 12,000 people die of kidney cancer each year. The tumors are most common in people between ages 50 and 70. They affect men more than women. Approximately 31,200 new cases of renal cancer were expected to be diagnosed in the United States in the year 2000.[2]

Etiology and Risk Factors

The exact cause of renal tumors is unknown. Some links have been established between renal cancer and tobacco, lead, cadmium, and phosphates. A genetic link has also been postulated.

Because of the possible association between smoking and renal cancer, one means of avoiding renal cancer may be to quit or not start smoking; avoiding exposure to chemicals such as lead, phosphate, and cadmium may also prevent some renal cancers. However, the cause of many renal cancers is not established and prevention may not be possible.

After surgery, most people have difficulty in dealing with cancer and the risk of recurrence. If nephrectomy is required, clients are often concerned about living with only one kidney. Assure them that one kidney can meet the body's needs but that care should be taken to protect that kidney. The care includes preventing injuries and infections, controlling blood pressure if necessary, and maintaining overall health and well-being by getting adequate nutrition, rest, and so on.

Pathophysiology

Renal cell carcinoma, or adenocarcinoma, is the most common tumor type; it accounts for 90% of all kidney neoplasms. Tumor growth begins in the renal cortex and usually continues for some time before it produces manifestations. The tumor can grow very large and tends to compress the adjacent renal parenchyma rather than infiltrate it. The tumor, usually avascular, tends to surround blood vessels and constrict them. The lungs and mediastinum are the most frequent metastatic sites of occurrence. Liver, bone, skin, spleen, renal vein, and brain are other common sites.

Other types of renal cancer include (1) nephroblastoma, (2) sarcoma, and (3) epithelial tumors in the renal pelvis.

Nephroblastoma, or Wilms' tumor, is primarily a childhood disease, although it occasionally occurs in adults. The prognosis for adults is worse than for children, with some sources reporting only a 25% survival rate.

Sarcoma is infrequent and typically arises in the renal capsule.

Most tumors of the renal pelvis are primarily urothelial in origin and include three tissue types: transitional cell, squamous cell, and adenocarcinoma.

Spontaneous regression of renal adenocarcinoma reportedly occurs in fewer than 1% of all cases. Most of these regressions occur after nephrectomy and involve metastatic areas. Authorities consider these episodes as more evidence that the disease is associated with immunologic or hormonal factors.

Clinical Manifestations

Manifestations of renal malignancies vary, and tumor growth may advance significantly before the disease is discovered. It is not uncommon for the client to have clinical manifestations apparently unrelated to renal disease. Frequently, a palpable abdominal mass found during a routine physical examination arouses the first suspicion. The average time between the onset of hematuria and the onset of pain is 9 months, and that between initial pain and diagnosis is 14 months. Extrarenal manifestations are commonly found before a diagnosis of renal cancer is confirmed. As many as 35% of clients have metastasis when the final diagnosis of a renal neoplasm is made.

The common triad of manifestations consists of hematuria, flank pain, and a palpable abdominal or flank mass. The hematuria is usually gross and intermittent, which helps explain the client's delay in seeking medical advice. The clinical picture also contains a combination of the following usual findings: fever, weight loss and cachexia, fatigue, hypertension, amyloidosis, thrombophlebitis, anemia, erythrocytosis, hypercalcemia, abnormal serum liver profile, and an elevated erythrocyte sedimentation rate (ESR). Less frequent findings include peripheral neuropathy, inferior vena cava obstruction, priapism, and varicocele. Hydronephrosis may occur if the tumor obstructs the ureteropelvic junction. The incidence of pulmonary embolus as a presenting manifestation may be higher than previously thought because of the high rate of vena cava and renal vein involvement. Plasma erythropoietin, renin, and chorionic gonadotropin levels are elevated, and prostaglandin production increases in renal cell carcinoma.

Several diagnostic tests help confirm a diagnosis of renal cancer. IVP is probably the most helpful in identifying a space-occupying lesion. Ultrasonography helps differentiate a cyst from a solid mass. Other noninvasive procedures include CT scan, nephrotomography, and radioisotope studies. Arteriography is used to evaluate the renal vascular system. Renal biopsy, usually done percutaneously, provides definitive data about the lesion.

Outcome Management

Staging of the tumor helps delineate the appropriate treatment and can suggest the client's prognosis (Fig. 35–1). Five-year survival rates for stage I are about 65%; for stage II, about 40%; 10-year rates drop to 40% and 35%, respectively. Five-year survivals are rare in stages III and IV.

Medical Management

Radiation Therapy

Radiation may be used as an adjunct with chemotherapy and surgery. Irradiation is most useful in preoperative preparation of the tumor. It is sometimes also used postoperatively to destroy residual or recurrent tumor cells, treat lymphatic involvement, and treat metastatic sites, such as bones, palliatively.

Chemotherapy

Clinical investigators continue to search for an effective chemotherapeutic regimen. Medroxyprogesterone and testosterone have been used as hormonal therapy, but their

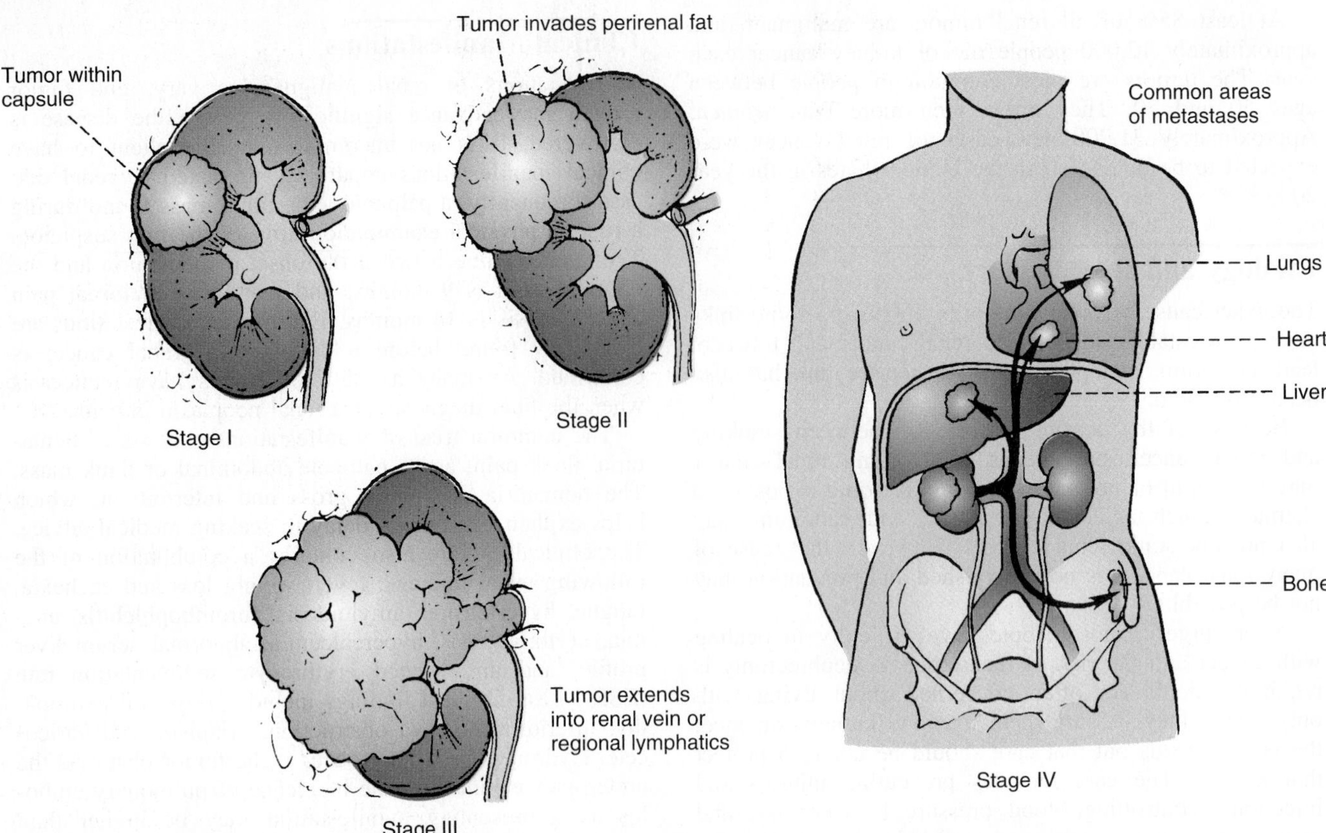

FIGURE 35–1 Staging system for renal carcinoma. Stage I tumor is confined within the renal capsule. Stage II tumor extends beyond the renal capsule to invade local perinephric fat but has no metastasis. Stage III tumor extends into the renal vein or involves local lymphatics. Stage IV tumor has metastasized to other parts of the body.

effectiveness has been limited. Vinblastine seems to be the most effective single agent, with response rates of 25%. Combination regimens seem to increase toxic effects without improving response rates. Many agents are being studied, but renal cancer cells seem insensitive to chemotherapeutic or hormonal agents, possibly because of their slow growth rate.

IMMUNOTHERAPY

Immunotherapy holds some promise in the treatment of renal cancer. Stimulants of the immune system have led to some positive results as long as the tumor is not too large and the immunosuppression not too severe. There has also been some response to natural and recombinant interferon-alfa. Interleukin-2 has been approved by the Food and Drug Administration for treating renal carcinoma.

Nursing Management of the Medical Client

Nursing management of the client with renal cancer must include general aspects of care for any cancer (see Chapters 18 and 19).

Surgical Management

NEPHRECTOMY

For renal cell carcinoma, the surgical procedure of choice is generally radical nephrectomy, which includes removal of the kidney, the adrenal gland, and perinephric fat with the retroperitoneal lymphatics. Several surgical approaches can be used to remove the diseased kidney. Transabdominal and thoracoabdominal approaches are preferred to secure the renal artery and vein and to prevent the spread of malignant cells.

A retroperitoneal approach is also possible. An incision of 6 to 10 inches is made, usually in the flank area; muscle layers are divided; and tissues are excised. The renal artery and vein are clamped and cut, and the ureter is dissected. When the tumor is in the renal pelvis, a nephroureterectomy is usually performed because of a tendency for transitional cell cancer to "seed" down the ureter into the bladder. With nephroureterectomy, a cuff of the adjacent bladder is removed.

Lymphadenectomy remains controversial. Even in advanced cases, when the prognosis is poor, nephrectomy may be done to relieve pain and hematuria.

If the neoplastic disease is bilateral or if there is a solitary functioning kidney, a partial nephrectomy may be done on at least one kidney, leaving enough renal tissue to support life without long-term dialysis. If partial nephrectomy is not possible in either instance, the entire kidney is removed and the client is given dialysis. These clients may be candidates for renal transplantation, but they are usually maintained with dialysis for about a year to watch for recurrence of the disease.

Although open nephrectomy tends to be the procedure of choice for many urologists, laparoscopic nephrectomy is being performed in a number of centers with considerable success. Four small incisions are made, through fewer muscle layers. A special laparoscope is inserted through one of the incisions, and laparoscopy instruments are placed in the others. Carbon dioxide is passed through a tube in one incision to inflate the abdominal cavity, which enables the surgeon to see the organs and provides room for manipulation of instruments. At the end of the procedure, the kidney is removed through a small 2- to 3-inch incision below the navel.

The surgical procedure tends to be longer (6.9 versus 2.2 hours), but clients undergoing the laparoscopic procedure require fewer analgesics, resume oral intake earlier, are discharged home earlier, and return to work sooner than those undergoing open surgery. Increasingly, even removal of a kidney for organ donation is being performed laparoscopically.

INDICATIONS. Nephrectomy or heminephrectomy is indicated with tumors of the kidney. Other treatments are not successful.

CONTRAINDICATIONS. As with any surgery, nephrectomy is contraindicated in clients with systemic or respiratory infections. General health must be satisfactory to withstand anesthesia, blood loss, and surgical stress. Any metabolic and systemic disorders should be stabilized before surgery.

COMPLICATIONS. Because the kidney is a very vascular organ, the risk of hemorrhage is high. Renal artery embolization of the affected kidney may be done to obstruct the tumor's blood supply and reduce its vascularity, thereby reducing the risk of hemorrhage. Embolization is usually accomplished by occluding the renal artery using an absorbable gelatin sponge (Gelfoam), metal coil, barium, subcutaneous fat, isobutyl-2-cyanoacrylate, absolute ethanol, or a balloon. This procedure may also be performed to control hemorrhage in an inoperable kidney. In addition, some researchers believe that embolization may stimulate an immune response against the dying cancer cells.

Other possible complications include those associated with any major surgery, such as atelectasis, pneumonia, thromboembolism, and infection of the surgical wound.

OUTCOMES. Nephrectomy reduces pain and hematuria caused by the tumor. The hospital stay is typically 4 to 6 days, with a return to work in 4 to 8 weeks. With laparoscopic nephrectomy, hospitalization is reduced and return to work after 2 to 4 weeks is not uncommon. Living with one kidney has few, if any, negative effects. Long-term outcomes, however, depend on the stage of the cancer.

Nursing Management of the Surgical Client

PREOPERATIVE CARE

Preoperative preparation of the client having renal surgery includes the general guidelines described in Chapter 15. Increase fluid intake, if indicated, to ensure adequate excretion of waste products before surgery. Give emotional support because the client may be anxious, not only about the surgery but also about postoperative renal function and possible recurrence of the disease. If the remaining kidney functions adequately, assure the client that this kidney can fully meet the body's needs.

POSTOPERATIVE CARE

ASSESSMENT

Postoperatively, monitor the client's vital signs frequently and watch for any manifestations of bleeding or hemorrhage. Bleeding may be through the incision or internal.

Surgically induced or spontaneous pneumothorax occurs occasionally after nephrectomy; monitor for this complication by assessing for sudden shortness of breath and loss of breath sounds on the affected side.

DIAGNOSIS, OUTCOMES, INTERVENTIONS

Risk for Injury: Postoperative Complications. The nursing diagnoses are likely to include *Risk for Injury: Postoperative complications related to surgical procedure.* Although postoperative care is similar to that for laparotomy, one of the biggest challenges is reestablishing effective breathing patterns. Deep breathing and coughing are difficult because the incision is very close to the diaphragm. Also, assuming the jackknife position on the surgical table increases pain and soreness in the thoracic region, limiting respiratory excursion. Paralytic ileus is a common problem. Urine output must be maintained.

Outcomes. The client will maintain normal respiratory excursion and have no additional breath sounds and no signs of atelectasis or infection. There will be normal bowel sounds within 2 to 3 days. Urine output will be at least ½ ml/kg/hr.

Interventions. Liberal use of narcotics (including patient-controlled analgesia) to relieve pain and external mechanical support of the chest and abdomen with pillows or hands help the client to perform deep-breathing and coughing exercises more effectively. An incentive spirometer provides immediate feedback about the effectiveness of deep breathing.

Other interventions include carefully assessing the client's urine output and gastrointestinal status postoperatively and beginning oral intake only after adequate bowel function has resumed. Total urine output from all urine collection tubes should total ½ ml/kg/hr. Notify the physician of lesser amounts. Other wound drainage tubes also need to be monitored. Early ambulation is indicated.

Pain. A diagnosis of *Acute Pain related to surgery* is common because the nephrectomy incision is extensive and causes significant discomfort. Muscle pain may develop from the prolonged position maintained during surgery.

Outcomes. Pain will be controlled, as indicated by the client's reports of reduced discomfort as well as by nonverbal indications of reduced discomfort, particularly during movement.

Interventions. The pain may be relieved by narcotic analgesics (including the use of patient-controlled analgesia) and proper positioning. Epidural fentanyl or morphine sulfate can provide effective analgesia.

Anxiety. People with cancer and people undergoing surgery experience anxiety because of uncertainty about the future. A diagnosis of *Anxiety related to disease and surgery* is probable.

Outcomes. Ideally, the client will report having the information needed to reduce uncertainty and will report that the information reduced anxiety.

Interventions. To help reduce feelings of anxiety, continue to keep the client and significant others informed about the progress made. Encourage them to express their concerns and to talk with one another. This need for support continues throughout the follow-up period.

EVALUATION

The client should be able to resume regular activities within 6 to 8 weeks after surgery. Long-term survival is dependent upon the stage of cancer diagnosed.

Self-Care

With shorter hospitalizations, clients who have undergone nephrectomy may require home care and support. Clients are weakened by surgery and possibly by other treatments. Activity should increase gradually; typically, 6 weeks must elapse before clients are ready to return to work or lift more than 10 pounds.

Concern about recurrence of the cancer is common. The American Cancer Society and other support groups may by helpful in the client's adjustment to cancer. People with one kidney can lead normal lives. There is, however, a need to protect the remaining kidney by prevention of infection and trauma.

TUBULOINTERSTITIAL DISEASE

Traditionally, the term "interstitial nephritis" has been applied to renal disease characterized by the presence of inflammatory cells in the spaces between the renal tubules. However, not all disease processes included in this classification are inflammatory. Therefore, the term *tubulointerstitial disease* is being advocated for this category of renal disorders.

Tubulointerstitial diseases are commonly classified as either acute or chronic. The acute form usually represents an allergic reaction and has a rapid onset. Assessment findings are typically related to tubular injury. Manifestations often include fever, skin rash, eosinophilia, oliguric renal failure, and occasionally gross hematuria. The disease may progress along any of three courses:

- Complete recovery
- Rapid progression to renal failure and death
- Movement to the chronic form

Although corticosteroids are commonly prescribed, their value is unclear. Treatment is similar to that for acute renal failure.

Chronic tubulointerstitial disease is characterized by progressive interstitial fibrosis and usually chronic inflammatory cell infiltration with tubular atrophy. In the terminal stages, the altered renal vasculature and renal structure make the disease virtually indistinguishable from chronic pyelonephritis.

Morphologic findings in tubulointerstitial disease include interstitial edema, cellular infiltration of the interstitium, tubular cellular atrophy and flattening, and interstitial fibrosis. As the disease progresses, renal involvement extends beyond the tubules to progressive fibrosis of Bowman's capsule with secondary involvement of the glomeruli.

Potential causes of this pathologic process are many:

- Acute pyelonephritis
- Septicemia
- Analgesic abuse, especially with phenacetin, aspirin, and acetaminophen
- Immunologic mechanisms, for example, renal allograft, systemic lupus erythematosus, and Sjögren's syndrome
- Heavy metal toxicity
- Drug toxicity
- Hypercalcemia
- Hypocalcemia

In addition, several medication hypersensitivities may contribute. The medications involved include rifampin, penicillin and its analogs, sulfonamides, cephalosporins, allopurinol, captopril, cimetidine, azathioprine, phenytoin, thiazide, lithium, NSAIDs, and possibly furosemide.

An early manifestation of tubulointerstitial disease is a sudden, unexplained decrease in renal function that may be mild to severe. Specifically, there may be inability to concentrate urine, salt wasting, and poor acidification of the urine leading to metabolic acidosis. Finding a variety of urine sediment abnormalities is also common. Because glucose, uric acid, phosphates, amino acids, and bicarbonate are not effectively reabsorbed in the tubules, they appear in the urine. Severe bicarbonaturia is an indicator of renal tubular acidosis. Proteinuria is less severe than with other renal disease. Systemic hypertension is a common finding.

GLOMERULONEPHRITIS

Glomerulonephritis encompasses a variety of diseases, most of which are caused by an immunologic reaction that results in proliferative and inflammatory changes in glomerular structure. Glomerulonephritis can be acute or chronic. It is usually manifested by either a nephrotic syndrome or a nephritic syndrome. Percutaneous renal biopsy is typically used to identify the type of glomerulonephritis, and the findings assist in planning interventions and determining the prognosis.

NEPHROTIC SYNDROME

Nephrotic syndrome is a set of clinical manifestations caused by protein wasting secondary to diffuse glomerular damage. Manifestations include proteinuria (>3.5 g/day), hypoalbuminemia, and edema. Abnormal permeability of the glomerular basement membrane (especially to albumin) results in loss of protein in the urine. The resulting hypoalbuminemia alters oncotic pressure in the vascular tree, and fluid moves into the interstitial spaces, causing edema. This movement stimulates plasma renin activity and augments aldosterone production; as a result, the kidney retains sodium and water, thus adding to the accumulation of extracellular fluid.

Hyperlipidemia usually occurs as well, probably because of increased hepatic lipoprotein synthesis in response to decreased serum albumin. Depending on the degree of renal failure, some level of normocytic anemia is common.

The causes of nephrotic syndrome are numerous. Besides glomerulonephritis, certain systemic disorders can cause it, such as diabetes mellitus, systemic lupus erythematosus (SLE), amyloidosis, hepatitis B, syphilis, carcinoma, leukemia, infectious disease, and preeclampsia. Other predisposing factors include:

- Allergic reactions
- Reactions to such drugs as penicillamine, anticonvulsants, probenecid, captopril, gold salts, heroin, and NSAIDs
- Renal vein thrombosis
- Sickle cell disease
- Heart failure

Potential complications of nephrotic syndrome include the effects of extracellular fluid accumulation and the progressive development of renal failure. The client may also experience severe hypovolemia, thromboembolism, secondary aldosteronism, abnormal thyroid function, osteomalacia, and increased susceptibility to infections.

Usually, edema is the client's chief problem. Although its onset may be insidious, it becomes massive. The client's skin typically takes on a characteristic waxy pallor, resulting from the edema rather than anemia. Other manifestations include anorexia, malaise, irritability, and abnormal or absent menses. Large amounts of protein appear in the client's urine along with granular and epithelial cell casts and fat bodies; proteinuria may account for losses of 4 to 30 g/day. Some hematuria may be present. Serum albumin concentrations may drop as low as 1.0 to 2.5 g/dl.

The primary aim of treatment for nephrotic syndrome is to heal the leaking glomerular basement membrane, stop the loss of protein in the client's urine, and break the cycle of edema. Interventions typically include maintaining the client's fluid and electrolyte balance, reducing inflammation, preventing thrombosis, and minimizing protein loss.

MAINTAIN FLUID AND ELECTROLYTE BALANCE. Unless the client is hyponatremic, fluids are not usually restricted. The client's fluid balance should, however, be carefully monitored via daily weights, girth measurements, and intake and output determinations. These data are important because weight loss may represent true tissue loss involving protein rather than fluid.

Loop diuretics (i.e., those that work on the loop of Henle), such as furosemide (Lasix), are typically prescribed. Plasma volume expanders, such as albumin, plasma, and dextran, may be administered to raise the oncotic pressure in the vascular tree. The increased pressure pulls fluid from the extracellular spaces, making it available for kidney filtration. Diuresis in older clients must be handled with particular caution because of their reduced ability to tolerate sudden shifts in intravascular volume.

Because the kidneys have a reduced capacity to excrete sodium, mild sodium restriction is usually instituted. The diet should be as palatable as possible, however, because the client must consume adequate protein and calories. Potassium may also be restricted as serum potassium levels rise.

Because edema disrupts cellular nutrition, the client is at increased risk for skin breakdown. Thus, skin care is vital. Interventions include good hygiene, massage, position changes, and possibly special mattresses. Use research-based tools to assess the client's risk of breakdown (see Chapter 16).

REDUCE INFLAMMATION. Steroid therapy helps some clients, depending on the cause of disease. Cytotoxic agents such as cyclophosphamide and chlorambucil, indomethacin, anticoagulants, and antiplatelet agents may be used as well.

PREVENT THROMBOSIS. Because clients with nephrotic syndrome are vulnerable to renal vein thrombosis, some are given long-term anticoagulation therapy. Teach such clients how to monitor for hemorrhage, and encourage them to carry identification that lists the drugs they take.

MINIMIZE PROTEIN LOSS. For clients with nephrotic syndrome, most physicians recommend a protein intake of 1.0 to 1.5 g/kg/day with more than 35 kcal/kg/day to prevent further protein breakdown. Twenty-four-hour urine collections are used to measure urinary protein losses and monitor the success of treatment. Treatment to reduce inflammation ultimately reduces protein loss.

An important nursing role is to help the client with nephrotic syndrome maintain health and cope with the illness. Teach the client to take prescribed medications regularly, follow the prescribed diet, and report changes in health status, such as increasing edema, reduced urine output, weight gain, respiratory distress, and signs of infection. Explain that the amount of exercise allowed is based, at least in part, on the severity of the edema. Bed rest is imposed only during severe edema. As the fluid level moves toward normal, the client is allowed more activity. Other important areas of teaching include nutrition, prevention of infection, and methods of careful self-assessment.

■ NEPHRITIC SYNDROME

Nephritic syndrome refers to a set of clinical manifestations that include hematuria and at least one of the following: oliguria (urine output <400 ml/24 hours), hypertension, elevated blood urea nitrogen (BUN), or decreased GFR. Nephritic syndrome is common with many types of glomerulonephritis, including immunoglobulin A (IgA) nephropathy and Henoch-Schönlein purpura. Treatment includes management of the underlying disease (usually through immunosuppressive drugs, as noted later) and symptomatic treatment of blood pressure and uremia.

TYPES OF GLOMERULONEPHRITIS

There are many types of glomerulonephritis, most of which involve either nephrotic syndrome or nephritic syndrome. The diagnosis of the specific type can be made by assessment of clinical manifestations and through renal biopsy. Box 35–2 presents a classification system based on

BOX 35–2 Classification of Glomerulonephritis Based on Etiology

Primary Glomerulonephritis—Immune Response to Pathogens

- Acute glomerulonephritis
- Postinfectious glomerulonephritis
- Group A beta-hemolytic streptococcus
- Other infectious conditions such as cytomegalovirus infection, measles, mumps, staphylococcus, or pneumococcal bacteremia
- Infectious glomerulonephritis
- Membranoproliferative glomerulonephritis
- Rapidly progressive glomerulonephritis
- Idiopathic membranous glomerulonephritis
- Immunoglobulin A (IgA) nephropathy
- Chronic glomerulonephritis
- Lipoid nephrosis
- Focal glomerular sclerosis

Secondary Glomerulonephritis—Related to Systemic Disease

- Goodpasture's syndrome
- Hemolytic-uremic syndrome
- Henoch-Schönlein purpura
- Polyarteritis
- Progressive systemic sclerosis
- Systemic lupus erythematosus
- Wegener's granulomatosis
- Thrombocytopenic purpura
- Postpartum renal failure

TABLE 35–1 TYPES OF GLOMERULONEPHRITIS: ONSET, FINDINGS, AND PROGNOSIS

Type	Onset	Diagnostic Findings	Prognosis
Poststreptococcal glomerulonephritis	1 to 3 weeks after beta-hemolytic streptococcal infection of throat or skin Nephritic syndrome	Underlying infection Elevated antistreptolysin O titer Microscopic urinalysis, urine with many casts	Variable Complete recovery to end-stage renal disease
Membranoproliferative glomerulonephritis	Nephrotic syndrome sometimes preceded by a streptococcal infection	Proteinuria Hematuria (microscopic or gross)	Gradual progressive chronic renal failure
Rapidly progressive glomerulonephritis	Nephritic syndrome Sudden May follow antigen or infection Peak ages 40–60 yr	Hematuria Edema Hypertension Proteinuria Oliguria Acidosis	Progresses to renal failure within weeks or months
Idiopathic membranous glomerulonephritis	Insidious Peak ages 40–70 yr Unknown antigen	Asymptomatic proteinuria or nephrotic syndrome	Mixed: 25% have spontaneous remission, 25% have renal failure, 25% have persistent proteinuria, 25% have deteriorating renal function
Immunoglobulin A (IgA) nephropathy (also called Berger's disease)	Most frequent in young adults Nephritic syndrome	Hematuria Red blood cell casts on microscopic urinalysis	Usually progresses slowly over 10–20 yrs. A small proportion progress to renal failure.
Lipoid nephrosis (also called minimal change glomerulonephritis)	Nephrotic syndrome	Found on biopsy	Generally good May be relapses and spontaneous remission
Focal glomerular sclerosis	Peaks between ages 30 and 50 yr Nephrotic syndrome	Found on biopsy May be few symptoms	Poor, although rate of deterioration varies widely Recurs after transplantation
Membranous glomerulonephritis	Commonly secondary to drug therapy toxins or systemic autoimmune disease Nephrotic syndrome Insidious onset	Heavy proteinuria	Variable 30% have spontaneous remission
Hemolytic-uremic syndrome	Follows infection with *Escherichia coli* (01571 H7 serotype) History of eating undercooked hamburger Children and older adults particularly vulnerable	Hemorrhagic manifestations, such as bleeding and bruising Purpura manifestations, such as acute renal failure, hemolytic anemia, and thrombocytopenia	Recovery rate 95% but may leave residual renal damage

etiology. Table 35–1 describes the onset, diagnostic findings, and prognosis for various types of glomerulonephritis.

Pathophysiology

Glomerulonephritis is an immunologic disorder that causes inflammation and increased cells in the glomerulus. Because the primary function of the glomerulus is to filter blood, most cases result when antigen-antibody complexes produced by an infection elsewhere in the body become trapped in the glomerulus. This entrapment causes inflammatory damage and impedes glomerular function, reducing the glomerular membrane's capacity for selective permeability. The source of the antigens may be either *exogenous* (e.g., after streptococcal infection) or *endogenous* (as in systemic lupus erythematosus). Evidence also indicates that some antigen-antibody complexes may form in the kidney itself.

Glomerulonephritis may also result from antibodies affixed to the glomerular basement membrane. For example, Goodpasture's syndrome involves pulmonary hemorrhage and glomerulonephritis.

The primary pathologic processes in glomerulonephritis, lipoid nephrosis, and focal glomerular sclerosis are proliferation and inflammation. However, lipoid nephrosis and focal glomerular sclerosis are characterized by degeneration. Figure 35–2 depicts the pathophysiologic mechanisms of glomerulonephritis.

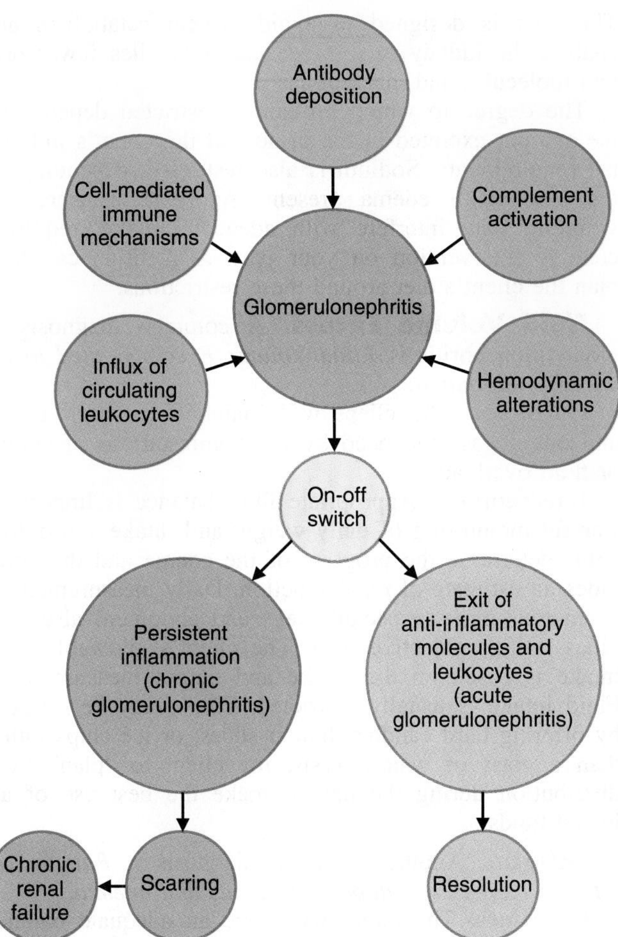

FIGURE 35–2 Pathophysiologic mechanism of glomerulonephritis.

Clinical Manifestations

Acute glomerulonephritis may develop insidiously or suddenly, varying considerably with the pathophysiology involved. Classic manifestations of sudden onset include hematuria with red blood cell casts and proteinuria. Fever, chills, weakness, pallor, anorexia, nausea, and vomiting may be present. Generalized edema, particularly facial and periorbital swelling, is a typical finding. The client may have ascites, pleural effusion, and heart failure.

The client is likely to have a headache and moderate to severe hypertension. Visual acuity may be reduced because of retinal edema. Abdominal or flank pain may develop, probably because of kidney edema and distention of the renal capsule. Oliguria, even anuria, may be present for several days; the longer it persists, the more irreversible the kidney damage. In contrast, the disease may be so mild that the client reports only vague weakness, anorexia, and lethargy.

Acute glomerulonephritis can become a fulminant process, proceeding quickly to uremia or chronic glomerulonephritis. Most clients, however, start to recover within 14 days. Most clinical manifestations disappear within several weeks, although hematuria and proteinuria may be present for longer periods. If complete recovery does not occur within 2 years, it probably will not occur at all.

Some clinicians use the term *subacute glomerulonephritis* to describe disease persisting more than 6 to 8 weeks. Although most of the manifestations of the acute disease have disappeared, the client is still at high risk for exacerbation of glomerulonephritis. The term *latent glomerulonephritis* refers to an asymptomatic condition characterized by significant albumin levels and casts in the urine for more than 1 year after acute onset. These findings indicate continued but slow parenchymal changes.

Most types of glomerulonephritis can progress to a chronic state. Sometimes, glomerulonephritis is first seen as a chronic process. Chronic glomerulonephritis progresses over an extended period, often as long as 30 years. When it progresses to end-stage renal failure, dialysis must begin or the client will die.

As the glomeruli and tubules are destroyed by the pathologic process, the kidneys shrink and become severely contracted. Fibrous and scar tissue replaces functioning renal tissue. Sclerosis of renal blood vessels also occurs. The destruction rates vary.

Common manifestations include malaise, weight loss, edema, increasing irritability and mental cloudiness, a metallic taste in the mouth, polyuria and nocturia resulting from the kidney's inability to concentrate urine, headache, dizziness, and digestive disturbances. As the disease progresses, these manifestations intensify, and the client may experience respiratory difficulty and angina.

The cardinal manifestation of this disease is hypertension. It is not uncommon for the client to experience such complications as nosebleed, manifestations of arteriosclerosis, cardiomegaly, and hemorrhage into the kidneys, lungs, retina, or cerebrum. Edema increases as heart failure becomes more severe and the serum albumin decreases. Examination of the eyegrounds shows vascular changes and edema of the discs. Urinalysis shows a fixed specific gravity, small amounts of proteinuria except during exacerbation, casts, WBCs, renal tubular cells, and consistent hematuria. Anemia tends to be severe.

Examining the urine usually provides the information necessary for a diagnosis of glomerulonephritis (see Chapter 32). Gross hematuria and proteinuria are the cardinal findings. The client's urine, which may be scant, usually has a dark, smoky, cola-colored, or red-brown hue. The proteinuria produces a persistent and excessive foam. The urine may have a low pH and a specific gravity in the midnormal to high-normal range if there is enough renal damage to affect the kidneys' ability to concentrate.

Other studies may assist in the diagnosis as well. Serum urea nitrogen and creatinine levels may be elevated, and creatinine clearance rates may be decreased. C-reactive proteins and antistreptolysin O titer are usually elevated in poststreptococcal glomerulonephritis, and the serum complement level is low in many forms of glomerulonephritis. Hematocrit and hemoglobin studies may indicate anemia, particularly if renal failure is imminent.

Outcome Management

Medical Management

Medical intervention aims to eliminate antigens, to alter the client's immune balance, and to inhibit or alleviate inflammation to prevent further renal damage and improve kidney function. Although some clients may require initial hospitalization, treatment is typically on an outpatient basis.

REDUCE INFLAMMATION

Plasmapheresis has been used in some research protocols to reduce the number of antigens in certain types of glomerulonephritis, including rapidly progressive glomerulonephritis. This intervention is usually administered in conjunction with corticosteroids and immunosuppressive agents (azathioprine, cyclophosphamide). The technique is designed to remove the specific circulating antibody or mediators of the inflammatory response. Large volumes of the client's plasma are cyclically removed and replaced with fresh frozen plasma through a continuous-flow blood cell separator.

Antibiotic therapy (such as penicillin for streptococcal organisms) is used to treat poststreptococcal glomerulonephritis. It is also used prophylactically after streptococcal infections to prevent further damage.

MAINTAIN FLUID AND ELECTROLYTE BALANCE

Volume overload and hypertension are treated with diuretics, antihypertensives, and restriction of dietary sodium and water. Common complications of fluid overload include heart failure with pulmonary edema and increased intracranial pressure. Renal failure may develop (see Chapter 36). Appropriate monitoring is essential and should include vital signs, intake and output, and weight. Recognizing complications early facilitates prompt medical intervention.

Nursing Management of the Medical Client

ASSESSMENT

For any client with suspected glomerulonephritis, take a comprehensive history that includes upper respiratory tract infection (such as strep throat), skin infections, scarlet fever, or a history of glomerulonephritis. Also question the client about systemic disorders that might be present, such as SLE, scleroderma, amyloidosis, and hypertension. Any recent invasive procedures should also be noted.

Physical examination may reveal ascites, pleural effusion, and manifestations of heart failure with pulmonary edema. Examine the urine closely for color, amount, and abnormal substances. In particular, microscopic analysis of the urine can be a valuable diagnostic tool with glomerulonephritis; urinary casts are commonly seen under high magnification (see Chapter 32). Check the client's vital signs closely, especially blood pressure.

DIAGNOSIS, OUTCOMES, INTERVENTIONS

Altered Nutrition: Less Than Body Requirements. If the client has a reduced appetite or an aversion to food, the diagnosis *Altered Nutrition: Less than body requirements related to anorexia and increased metabolic demands* is appropriate.

Outcomes. The client will maintain adequate nutritional intake, as evidenced by no weight loss, absence of a negative nitrogen balance, and normal electrolytes.

Interventions. It is important to protect the kidneys while they are recovering their function. The prescribed diet is likely to be high in calories and low in protein. This diet is designed to avoid protein catabolism and enables the kidney to rest because it handles fewer protein molecules and metabolites.

The degree to which protein is restricted depends on the amount excreted in the urine and the client's individual requirements. Sodium is also restricted, depending on the amount of edema present. Anorexia, nausea, and vomiting may interfere with adequate intake, requiring creative intervention on your part. A dietitian can help plan the client's diet around these restrictions.

Fluid Volume Excess. A common diagnosis in glomerulonephritis is *Fluid Volume Excess related to reduced urine output.*

Outcomes. The client will maintain balanced intake and output, as evidenced by no manifestations of edema or fluid overload.

Interventions. Appropriate fluid balance is important. Careful monitoring of daily weight and intake and output helps determine the progress of the edema and thus provides an estimate of renal function. Daily measurement of edematous parts (especially legs and abdomen) also provides useful, objective data. The client's allowable fluid intake is based on the intake and output measurements. Fluid intake is usually restricted. Thirst may be relieved by offering hard candies, lemon slices, or ice chips rather than a glass of water. Assist the client to "plan" fluid distribution during the day to make the best use of allowed fluids.

Fatigue. Another common diagnosis is *Fatigue related to increased metabolic demands and anemia.*

Outcomes. The client will have an adequate balance of rest and activity, as evidenced by absence of complaints of fatigue.

Interventions. Rest is essential—both physical and emotional. As mentioned, activity level correlates directly with the amount of hematuria and proteinuria. Exercise also increases catabolic activity. The allowable amount of activity depends on the results of serial urinalyses. Bed rest interspersed with periods of limited activity may continue for several weeks to months. Therefore, the client may need help in arranging personal matters, such as family, home, job, finances, and community responsibilities.

Encourage the client to talk about any fears or concerns, and, if necessary, help the client deal with the emotional reactions expected during a long-term illness with a questionable prognosis. Only after handling these problems can the client rest emotionally. Appropriate diversionary activities may help the client cope with prolonged physical immobility.

Risk for Impaired Skin Integrity. A typical diagnosis is *Risk for Impaired Skin Integrity related to edema.*

Outcomes. The client will remain free of skin breakdown, as evidenced by continued intact skin.

Interventions. Edema interferes with cellular nutrition, which makes the client more susceptible to skin breakdown. Take precautions to prevent this complication. Interventions include good hygiene, massage, and position changes as well as other prophylactic measures, such as mattress devices. Use research-based tools to assess the client's risk of breakdown (see Chapter 16).

Risk for Infection. Another diagnosis after immunosuppressive therapy is *Risk for Infection related to altered immune response secondary to treatment.*

Outcomes. The client will remain free of infection, as evidenced by normal temperature and an absence of local or systemic manifestations of infection.

Interventions. Glomerulonephritis markedly diminishes a client's natural defenses to infection, especially to streptococcal organisms. Immunosuppressives and corticosteroids further reduce host resistance. Although isolation is not necessary, take care to protect the client from people with obvious infectious processes. General supportive measures help boost the client's defense mechanisms. Client teaching should involve appropriate ways to avoid infections, especially respiratory and urinary tract infections.

EVALUATION

The client must be able to understand the condition and the reasons for limitations, including dietary and fluid restrictions. Stress the importance of follow-up treatments to minimize the risk of recurrence.

Self-Care

Clients with glomerulonephritis are followed as outpatients, often for many years. Self-care activities should include regular follow-up, recommended medications and dietary restrictions, and monitoring for changes in condition. It is vital that blood pressure be controlled to prevent further renal damage; many clients learn to monitor their own blood pressure at home. Because the disease may progress to renal failure, there are numerous quality-of-life issues, as discussed in Chapter 36.

Modification for Elderly Clients

The older client is at greater risk for renal damage because of the pre-existing effects of age on the kidneys. The older client is also more likely to have concurrent chronic diseases—such as hypertension and diabetes—that may have affected the kidneys, although treatment is the same.

Renal Trauma

Serious kidney injury is relatively rare because of the protection afforded by the rib cage, the heavy muscles of the back, and the tough capsule surrounding the kidney. Traffic accidents and falls in which the client lands on the abdomen, flank, or back are the most common cause of injury, usually from blunt trauma. Kidney lacerations can result from fractures of the spine and ribs as well as penetrating injuries from bullets and knives.

Pathophysiology

Five categories of traumatic injury can affect the kidney:

- Contusion with intrarenal hemorrhage
- Minor laceration (rupture with subcapsular hemorrhage)
- Major laceration (rupture into the renal pelvis)
- "Fractured" kidney (shattered rupture)
- Vascular (pedicle) injury, which damages renal blood supply (Fig. 35–3)

In a contusion, a hematoma develops and remains confined within the renal parenchyma. Rupture of the kidney may cause hemorrhage between the capsular walls; bleeding may or may not reach into the renal pelvis. A shattered or fractured kidney causes hemorrhage throughout the renal tissue. The pedicle holds the renal artery and other vital circulatory and nervous system connections to the kidney. Injury to the pedicle may jeopardize the life of the kidney and may occur with or without intrarenal hemorrhage.

Clinical Manifestations

The type of injury the client has suffered gives the first real key to identifying renal trauma. Commonly, the client has multiple serious injuries, and renal trauma may not be immediately apparent. Hematuria (gross or microscopic) is a cardinal manifestation and is found in about 80% of cases. However, serious renal injury can occur without hemorrhage and clear urine does not automatically rule out renal trauma. Other findings include shock, flank pain, and a palpable mass in the affected flank area or over the 11th or 12th rib. Paralytic ileus may also occur. You may see bruises over the client's flank and lower back secondary to retroperitoneal hemorrhage, a development known as Grey Turner's sign. A KUB film, IVP, retrograde pyelography, renal scan, ultrasonography, CT scan, and renal arteriography all help confirm the type and degree of kidney injury.

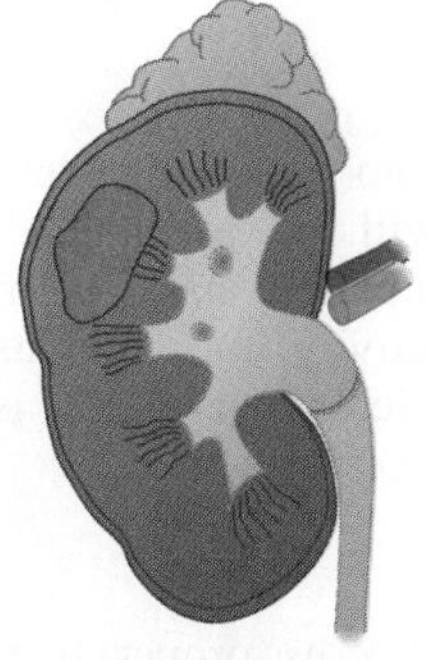

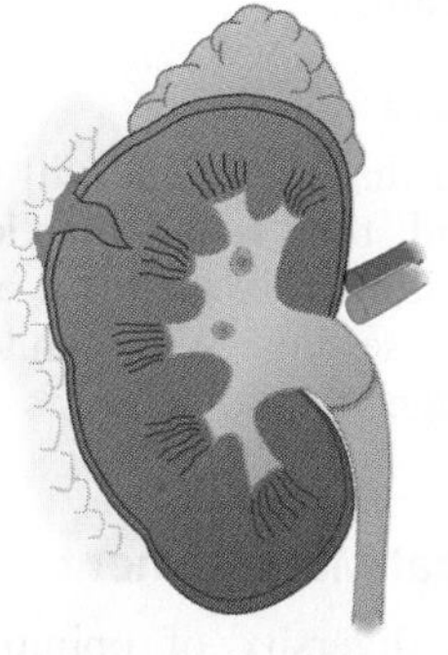

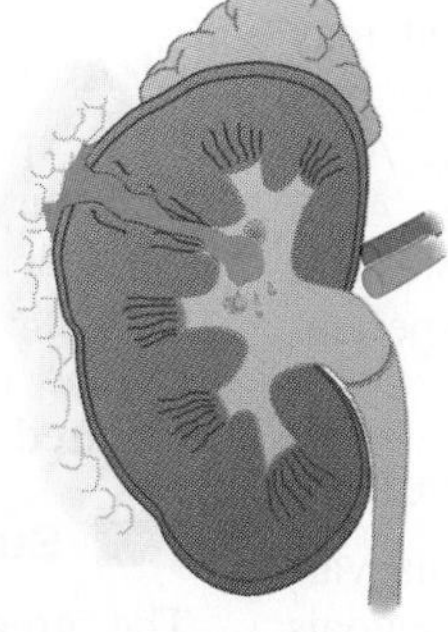

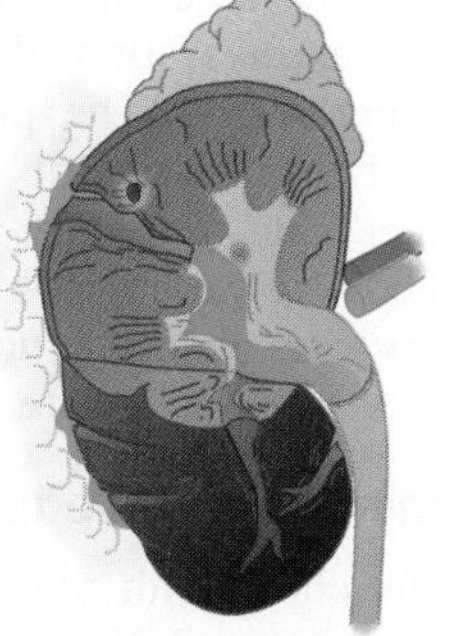

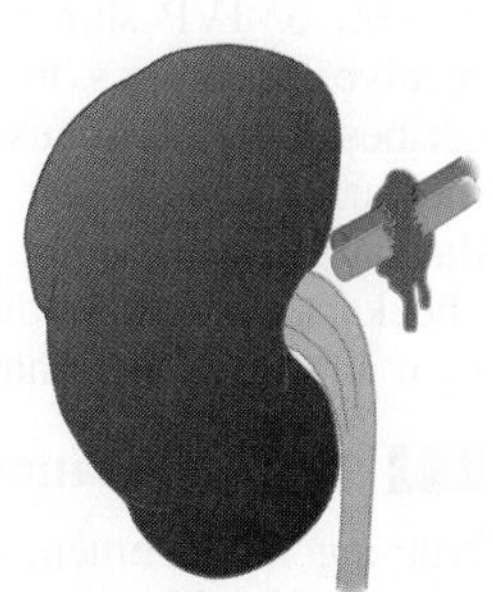

FIGURE 35–3 Categories of renal trauma.

Complications

In addition to the immediate problems of hemorrhage and loss of functioning renal tissue, kidney trauma makes the client highly susceptible to a number of other problems. Even in closed injuries, there is a high risk of sepsis leading to kidney and perinephric abscesses. Secondary hemorrhage is not uncommon. Other complications include hypertension resulting from fibrosis and ischemic kidney, renal artery thrombosis, arteriovenous aneurysms, fistula formation from extravasation of urine, urinomas, and pseudocysts.

Outcome Management

Whether conservative or surgical treatment should be used for renal trauma is controversial. Most physicians agree that kidney contusion calls for conservative treatment. Other minor injuries, such as small subcapsular hematomas and minor lacerations without extravasation, may also be better followed conservatively.

Clients with major injuries (e.g., renal fracture, parenchymal injury with major arterial occlusion, avulsion injuries, tears in the renal artery or vein, and parenchymal lacerations with extending perirenal hematomas or urinary extravasation) may require surgical exploration. Possible indications include continued moderate to severe hemorrhage and continued urinary extravasation. Urinary extravasation itself is not a definite reason for surgery because sterile urine usually resolves or is encapsulated spontaneously. However, it sometimes produces a severe tissue reaction and causes fistula formation. The pocket of extrarenal urine may also become obstructive.

Medical Management

Medical management, which primarily involves waiting and watching, is possible because the retroperitoneal space allows tamponade. In the absence of other injuries, a client with microscopic hematuria and normal findings on IVP may be observed on an ambulatory basis with careful instructions about activity restrictions and the need for adequate hydration. If there is gross hematuria, bed rest is required until the urine clears. Serial observations of the urine, hematocrit, and vital signs are made to watch the progress of the hemorrhage. Sequential urine specimens may be collected to compare current and previous urine color and turbidity.

Even if replacement fluids are not needed, a prophylactic intravenous line may be established, and a type and crossmatch for blood may be done. If a hematoma is present or IVP shows urine extravasation, the client may receive antibiotics to prevent sepsis. The physician prescribes blood transfusions if the hematocrit is low. After the urine clears, the client can be more active. After discharge, the client needs follow-up blood pressure checks and IVP studies to rule out secondary hypertension and anatomic changes in the renal system.

Nursing Management of the Medical Client

Nursing management of the client with renal trauma varies considerably, depending on extent of injury. The goals of nursing care are to prevent further bleeding and injury and to alleviate the client's anxiety.

ASSESSMENT

Assessment includes checking for tenderness at the CVA. Watch for bleeding, which may occur as hematuria or may be internal, depending on the nature of the injury. Assess the client's vital signs for evidence of shock. Make serial observations of urine, hematocrit, and vital signs to watch the progress of hemorrhage. Sequential urine specimens may be collected to compare current and previous urine color and turbidity.

DIAGNOSIS, OUTCOMES, INTERVENTIONS

Risk for Injury: Hemorrhage. The goals of nursing after renal trauma are related to monitoring for shock and minimizing the risk of further bleeding. For this reason, the nursing diagnosis is *Risk for Injury: Hemorrhage related to blood loss, further injury, and hypovolemia.*

Outcomes. The client will not experience shock, and bleeding will stop, as evidenced by a decrease in hematuria, pain, or other bleeding.

Interventions. Nursing interventions during conservative treatment center on monitoring urinary elimination patterns and helping the client to cope and comply with the medical regimen. If there is gross hematuria, bed rest is required until the urine clears. Monitoring includes assessment of vital signs as well as intake and output. Notify the physician if urine output drops below ½ ml/kg/hr. Because bed rest can cause problems with bowel elimination and adequate fluid intake, circulation, and respiratory function, take appropriate measures to minimize the risk of these complications (passive exercise, for example). A client with microscopic hematuria and normal IVP results who is observed on an ambulatory basis should be given careful instructions about activity restrictions and the need for adequate hydration.

Anxiety. Renal trauma can cause considerable anxiety over the possible loss of renal function and possible shock. Hence, a nursing diagnosis of *Anxiety related to injury* is highly likely.

Outcomes. The client will report less anxiety and will have the information needed to understand the situation and prognosis.

Interventions. Nursing care related to anxiety involves providing information about the plan of care, including activity restrictions. The client is concerned about the progress, and you may be in a position to facilitate communication between the patient and other members of the health care team.

EVALUATION

It is expected that the client will have no further bleeding or injury and that renal function will be maintained, whether monitoring is done on an outpatient basis or in an acute care setting. With limited activity, most clients can be managed at home unless surgical intervention is required.

Surgical Management

The greatest diversity of opinion concerns proper handling of the renal damage discovered during exploration. When the other kidney is functioning effectively, some physicians recommend free use of nephrectomy to avoid later sequelae, whereas others believe that the goal should be salvaging maximal renal function. The latter group advocates giving the conservative approach a fair trial and, if surgery is necessary, attempting to repair the kidney before deciding to remove it. With renal vascular injury, fewer than half of kidneys can be salvaged if the injury is 18 hours old; there is virtually no chance of renal recovery after 24 hours.

Renal hemorrhage may be controlled by injection of an autologous clot into the secondary arteries supplying the bleeding site. Blood is drawn from the client and allowed to clot. The clot is then injected angiographically. Because normal endothelium has a strong clot-lysing effect, the clot disappears from the normal adjacent vasculature after several hours and affects only the damaged portion.

If kidney repair is attempted rather than nephrectomy, the surgical procedure is designed to debride devitalized tissue, achieve hemostasis, establish a watertight seal of the collecting system, approximate the renal parenchymal edges, and drain the renal fossa.

Two surgical techniques improve the outcome of repair:

- *Extracorporeal,* or *bench, surgery* allows the kidney to be removed from the body for better visualization and manipulation of the organ during the repair process; the kidney is returned by autotransplantation. During its time outside the body, the kidney is maintained by hypothermia or by a perfusate mechanically pulsed through it.
- The *slush technique*, in which the kidney is immersed in iced saline slush, slows the metabolism and oxygen requirement of the renal tissue, allowing longer intraoperative ischemic times. This technique causes some systemic hypothermia, but it is not significant. Pedicle vascular injury may also be repaired.

If either technique fails, nephrectomy is necessary.

Nursing Management of the Surgical Client

Nursing management of the client undergoing surgery for renal trauma is similar to that for other surgical procedures on the kidney (see nephrectomy in this chapter).

Self-Care

The client being observed on an ambulatory basis requires an appropriate teaching plan covering health maintenance activities and the need for a follow-up program. The client should promptly report any change in condition or recurrence of bleeding or pain to the physician. Strenuous activity should be avoided for several weeks or more, depending on the extent of the injury. The client must also maintain adequate hydration.

RENAL VASCULAR ABNORMALITIES

The kidneys depend on adequate blood circulation to nourish tissues and provide blood for filtration so that they can perform their intended functions. Anything that interferes with the normal circulatory flow significantly reduces renal function.

Renal Artery Disease

Etiology and Risk Factors

Ninety per cent of all renal artery disease is caused by atherosclerosis or fibromuscular dysplasia. Atherosclerosis affects males more often than females and usually involves the proximal third of the artery. Health promotion activities are the same as those for atherosclerosis as discussed with circulatory and cardiac disorders. Fibromuscular dysplasia is an alternating stenosis and dilation; arteriographic studies demonstrate a "string-of-beads" appearance of the artery. This condition affects females four to five times as often as males. Because the cause is unknown, there are no health promotion actions.

There are several other, less common, causes of renal artery disease. Cancer may obstruct the vessels. Embolism or thrombosis can cause acute obstruction. Trauma, as described earlier, can interrupt blood flow. The renal artery may be purposely occluded to produce a "medical nephrectomy" or total renal infarction; the occlusion may be done preoperatively in the case of renal adenocarcinoma or to control proteinuria or hypertension. Shredded Gelfoam may be used, or a liquid substance that polymerizes instantly when it comes in contact with blood may be injected into the renal artery. A dissecting aneurysm in the renal artery may also interrupt renal circulation.

Pathophysiology

The end result of any of these conditions, if severe enough, is reduced renal blood flow. The reduced flow causes renal parenchymal ischemia and, finally, renal atrophy. The role of renal artery disease in renovascular hypertension is also well documented, and hypertension alone may indicate treatment of the condition.

Clinical Manifestations

Because of the kidney's compensatory mechanisms, the gradual development of renal artery stenosis from atherosclerosis and cancer may give rise to very few manifestations, at least until the resulting hypertension and decreasing renal function become evident. Acute obstruction makes itself known relatively quickly, however. Manifestations of this sudden episode include flank pain over the affected kidney or abdominal pain and fever. Atrial dysrhythmias are a frequent finding; however, because they commonly alternate with periods of normal sinus rhythm, this manifestation can be missed. Urinalysis may be normal, and blood chemistry profiles may show elevated aspartate aminotransferase and lactic dehydrogenase. IVP shows a nonfunctioning kidney, and a renal scan shows no arterial blood flow.

In response to reduced renal circulation, collateral circulation helps preserve the kidney if sufficient development takes place before total obstruction. Collateral circulation, in addition to a marked reduction in filtration, renal work, and oxygen requirements, allows the kidney to tolerate ischemic periods for up to several weeks. In acute total occlusion, a normal kidney can remain viable for about 2 hours before infarction and tissue necrosis begin.

Outcome Management

Surgical Management

Treatment of the ischemic kidney usually involves surgical revascularization. Arterial endarterectomy may be done with follow-up anticoagulant or antiplatelet therapy. In the technique known as *percutaneous transluminal renal angioplasty* (PTRA), the vessel is cleared with a balloon catheter. If it cannot be recanalized, a renal artery resection with end-to-end anastomosis or an aortorenal bypass graft procedure may be performed.

Percutaneous Transluminal Renal Angioplasty

In clients undergoing PTRA, a balloon-tipped catheter is inserted, usually through the femoral artery, and threaded under radiologic guidance to the obstructed renal artery. The physician inflates the balloon and pulls it through the obstructed area, stretching it and increasing the size of the arterial lumen. A stent may be placed at the site of occlusion to maintain the size of the lumen, prevent restenosis, and minimize the risk of abrupt vessel reclosure. If a stent is placed, antiplatelet agents or anticoagulants may be prescribed to minimize the risk of acute thrombosis.

Indications. Renal artery angioplasty is usually the first intervention for renovascular hypertension. If angioplasty is unsuccessful or if the condition recurs, more invasive surgical approaches are considered.

Contraindications. Angioplasty may be contraindicated if there is previous damage to the femoral artery or severely impaired circulation to the limb.

Complications. Renal artery angioplasty is considered a relatively safe procedure. The overall complication rate is about 10%. The most common complications include renal artery dissection, renal artery thrombosis or occlusion, segmental renal infarction, and hematoma formation or puncture trauma.

Outcomes. About one third of clients with renovascular hypertension do not respond to this therapy. A significant number are cured, and about half improve significantly. The treatment can be repeated if necessary. Clients usually return home in 24 to 48 hours.

Nursing Management of the Surgical Client

Preoperative Care

Because the length of stay is limited for most clients undergoing PTRA, it is a challenge to coordinate their care during the diagnostic and intervention phases of treatment. Typically, diagnostic tests such as angiograms and blood work are completed during the week before the procedure. Teaching about angioplasty and discharge instructions must be provided in a short time period.

Postoperative Care

Care after PTRA is similar to other care after any angioplasty. Just after the procedure, vital signs are monitored every 15 minutes for 1 hour, every 30 minutes for 2 hours, hourly for 3 hours, and then regularly according to the established protocol. Check the dressing at these times for manifestations of bleeding or hematoma formation, and check peripheral pulses to assess circulation in the affected limb. Bed rest for up to 24 hours may be ordered.

In the longer term, the client's blood pressure should be monitored because hypertension can indicate recurrence of the lesion. Control of hypertension is crucial to preserving renal function.

After renal artery bypass graft surgery, nursing care is similar to other care after any kidney surgery, such as nephrectomy (see earlier). However, in the postoperative period after an aortorenal bypass graft procedure, the client may experience an initial exacerbation of hypertension. Its cause is unclear, but it is thought to be related to systemic vasoconstriction secondary to general anesthesia and intraoperative hypothermia, severe pain, or transient renin secretion caused by clamping the aorta and manipulating the kidney. This episode usually lasts no more than 48 hours, but it can be significant and may require medical intervention. You must monitor blood pressure frequently.

Renal Vein Disease

The primary pathologic process involving the renal vein is thrombosis. Obstruction of venous drainage increases interstitial pressure, which reduces renal function. Findings include severe lumbar pain, renal enlargement, proteinuria, and hematuria. If the obstruction is bilateral, oliguria and azotemia occur. Contributing factors include diabetic nephropathy, chronic glomerulonephritis, and renal amyloidosis.

Kidney survival depends largely on the development of collateral circulation before the vessel is fully occluded. Embolectomy or ligation of the renal veins may be done, and anticoagulants may be prescribed. Intravenous streptokinase is used to lyse the occluding clot. If enough renal damage has occurred, nephrectomy is an option.

CONGENITAL DISORDERS

Renal congenital anomalies usually involve abnormalities in the number, position, form, size, or structure of the kidneys. Blood supply may be abnormal, although malformations that significantly affect renal function are rare. Anomalies of the ureteropelvic junction usually obstruct at that point and result in hydronephrosis. Typically, this situation is discovered and treated during childhood.

Anomalies Involving Kidney Number and Position

Renal agenesis is the absence of one or both kidneys. Having only one kidney presents no difficulty if this kidney functions adequately. A client can live normally with one properly functioning kidney, as kidney donors aptly demonstrate. Bilateral agenesis, however, is fatal. Even in unilateral agenesis, the functioning kidney is at high risk for development of additional anomalies.

Supernumerary kidneys (more than two kidneys) are usually asymptomatic and are discovered during IVP. The extra ureter enters either the ipsilateral ureter or the bladder.

Ectopic, or malpositioned, kidneys are usually found in the pelvis, although thoracic kidneys have been docu-

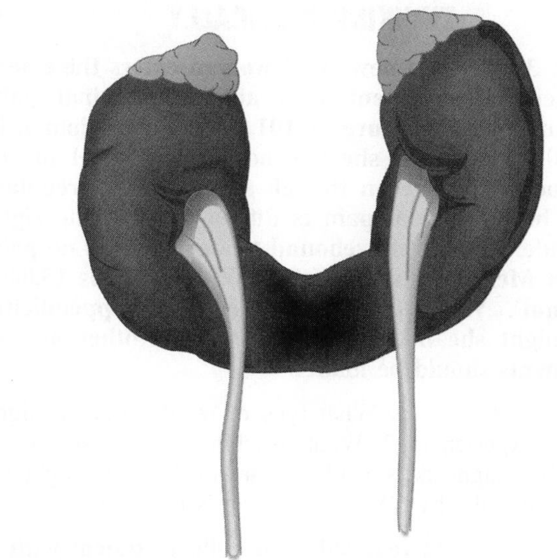

FIGURE 35–4 Horseshoe kidney.

mented. Problems associated with this anomaly include respiratory difficulties, pain caused by pressure on nerves or surrounding structures, and difficulty in childbirth.

Occasionally, one kidney may be across the midline, so that both kidneys are on the same side. This condition usually remains undiscovered until infection or obstruction indicates a need for x-ray examination.

ANOMALIES INVOLVING KIDNEY FORM AND SIZE

Anomalies of kidney form and size include aplasia, hypoplasia, dysplasia, and *horseshoe kidney*. Aplastic kidneys are small and contracted and contain no functioning renal tissue. Renal hypoplasia produces miniature kidneys with some functioning tissue. Although clinically this condition may be asymptomatic, it may cause hypertension and recurrent urinary tract infection.

Horseshoe kidney results when two kidneys are joined into a single organ whose shape somewhat resembles that of a horseshoe (Fig. 35–4). The kidneys are connected, usually at the lower poles, by an isthmus of tissue. Because the developmental error interferes with normal ascent and medial rotation, the kidney is usually located in the lower lumbar region with its pelvis facing anteriorly. Although clients with horseshoe kidney may be asymtomatic, they are susceptible to hydronephrosis, infection secondary to ureteropelvic junction obstruction, and calculus formation.

ANOMALIES INVOLVING CYSTIC DISEASE

Cystic disease in renal tissue can range from a simple, solitary fluid-filled mass to almost complete replacement of renal structures by cystic tissue. A simple renal cyst commonly originates superficially in the renal parenchyma. It grows slowly and usually produces no manifestations until adulthood, when it may cause heaviness and pain in the abdomen and become a palpable mass. Arriving at a diagnosis may be complicated because renal cysts closely resemble malignant tumors; naturally, differentiation between the two is vital. As long as a simple renal cyst remains asymptomatic, intervention usually is unnecessary. If intervention is necessary, the cyst may be aspirated with a needle or a partial nephrectomy may be performed to remove it.

■ POLYCYSTIC KIDNEYS

Polycystic disease of the kidney is a hereditary disorder in which grape-like cysts containing serous fluid, blood, or urine replace normal kidney tissue (Fig. 35–5). The condition may develop at any age.

Infantile polycystic kidney disease is inherited as an autosomal recessive trait, and both parents must have carried the gene. It is a rare disorder that affects both kidneys and often the liver. In an infant, the disease usually causes death within days. Milder forms of the disease do not appear until childhood.

Adult polycystic disease accounts for about 10% of the clients receiving dialysis or transplantation. It is inherited as an autosomal dominant trait. It usually appears after age 40 years, although it may begin as early as age 20 or as late as age 80. There are diverse manifestations; the most common are dull, aching lumbar or flank pain, which may be colicky, and hematuria. Other common findings are proteinuria, palpable kidney masses, pyuria, calculi, and uremia (see Chapter 32). Early in the disease, the ability to concentrate urine decreases. Hypertension develops along with cardiac enlargement and heart failure.

Polycystic liver disease occurs in about one third of cases, and cystic lesions are sometimes found in the thyroid, lung, pancreas, spleen, ovary, testis, epididymis, uterus, and bladder. Cerebral aneurysms occur in about 2% of clients with polycystic kidney disease.

The cystic kidney can become so enlarged that it causes severe pressure on other organs, with production of additional extrarenal manifestations. The ultimate result of this disease is chronic renal failure (see Chapter 36). As the disease slowly progresses, renal nephrons are de-

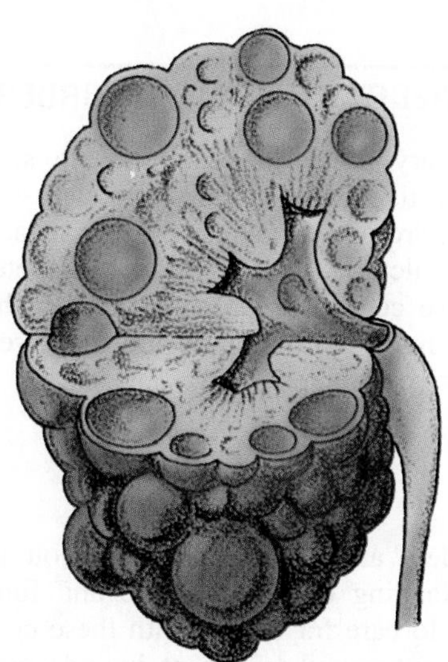

FIGURE 35–5 Polycystic kidney disease.

stroyed, renal function deteriorates, and uremia ultimately results. The mean duration of polycystic kidney disease from onset of manifestations to development of uremia varies a great deal and may be 15 to 30 years or more.

Because there is no known way to arrest the progress of the destructive cysts, conservative medical treatment is designed to preserve kidney function. Urinary tract infection is the most common complication because of the distorted renal architecture; chronic infection may occur if resistant bacteria develop. Aggressive control of hypertension is essential.

Unlike clients with decreasing creatinine clearance rates caused by other kidney diseases, those with polycystic kidney disease seem to waste rather than retain sodium. Thus, they need an increased sodium and water intake. When end-stage renal disease develops, dialysis or renal transplantation is required. Nursing interventions for clients with renal failure are discussed in Chapter 36.

Genetic counseling is advisable because of the hereditary nature of the disease—especially if the disease is diagnosed during childbearing years. However, because the disease typically appears after the childbearing period, the likelihood of transmitting the disease to another generation is high. Therefore, counseling the extended family is essential when the disease has been identified.

■ ADULT-ONSET MEDULLARY CYSTIC DISEASE

Adult-onset medullary cystic disease, sometimes called *uremic sponge kidney* or *medullary polycystic disease*, is also an autosomal dominant disorder. It is similar to polycystic disease in all aspects except that it progresses to uremia rapidly after its onset in the teenage years or in one's 20s. Hemodialysis and renal transplantation are likely to be required.

■ MEDULLARY SPONGE KIDNEY

Medullary sponge kidney is a cystic disorder in which spaces are produced at the apex of the renal pyramids. Onset peaks during adolescence or between ages 30 and 40 years. Infection, calculi, pain, and hematuria are potential complications. Renal function usually remains adequate unless the client has uncontrolled infection or calculi.

OTHER HEREDITARY RENAL DISORDERS

Other hereditary renal disorders include some types of chronic nephritis (such as Alport's disease), congenital nephrotic syndrome, distal renal tubular acidosis, idiopathic hypercalciuria, and nephrotic diabetes insipidus. Many of these conditions are fatal during childhood, but some persist into adulthood and are discussed in the appropriate parts of this text.

CONCLUSIONS

Renal disorders are highly complex. You must have a clear understanding of the structure and function of the renal system to care for clients with these conditions. The outcomes of successful treatment include preservation of renal function.

THINKING CRITICALLY

1. A 35-year-old newlywed woman enters the emergency department with acute abdominal pain and a temperature of 101.8° F. Her abdomen is distended, and she has not had a bowel movement today, even though she is usually regular. The abdominal pain is diffuse and on the right side. She has no rebound tenderness and no pain at McBurney's point. Her WBC count is 15,000/mm^3. What problems other than appendicitis might she be experiencing? What other assessments should be made?

Factors to Consider. What type of renal problem might she be experiencing? What teaching would she need when the diagnosis is made? What medication might be prescribed and why? What follow-up is needed?

2. L. S. is a 22-year-old male college student with a diagnosis of acute glomerulonephritis. Three weeks ago, he received oral antibiotic therapy for strep throat. He is scheduled for a renal biopsy to confirm a diagnosis of acute poststreptococcal glomerulonephritis. What other diagnostic assessments should be made? What is the expected course of treatment?

Factors to Consider. What teaching does this client need when the diagnosis is confirmed? What medication might be prescribed, and how will it be delivered? What follow-up is needed?

3. C. H. is a 68-year-old retired mail carrier who lives with his wife. They spend 6 months living in their midwestern home state and spend the winter months in Arizona. The client is admitted with a diagnosis of suspected renal cell carcinoma. Diagnostic tests confirm the diagnosis. What surgical procedure will be scheduled? What nursing interventions are associated with this procedure?

Factors to Consider. What diagnostic tests were used to confirm the diagnosis of renal carcinoma? What tests will be used to determine whether radiation, chemotherapy, and immunotherapy are needed? Describe the postoperative assessments you should make for pain management, vital signs, surgical dressings, drainage tubes, and urine output. If Mr. and Mrs. H. plan to drive to Arizona a month after surgery, what should you discuss with them about their travel plans?

BIBLIOGRAPHY

1. Ambrus, J., & Nagaraja, N. (1997). Immunologic aspects of renal disease. *Journal of the American Medical Association, 278*(22), 1938–1945.
2. American Cancer Society. (2000). *Cancer facts and figures—2000.* Atlanta: Author.
3. Bennett, J. C., & Plum, F. (Eds.). (1996). *Cecil textbook of medicine* (20th ed.). Philadelphia: W. B. Saunders.
4. Breisch, A. J., & Perez, J. A. (1995). The cardiovascular clinical nurse specialist as case manager during endovascular revascularization of renal artery stenosis. *Journal of Vascular Nursing, 13*(1), 14–20.
5. Brenner, B. M. (Ed.). (1996). *Brenner and Rector's the kidney* (5th ed.). Philadelphia: W. B. Saunders.

6. Burrows-Hudson, S. (Ed.). (1999). *Standards and guidelines of clinical practice for nephrology nursing*. Pitman, NJ: American Nephrology Nurses Association.
7. Chow, W., et al. (1999). Rising incidence of renal cell cancer in the United States. *Journal of the American Medical Association, 281*(17), 1628–1631.
8. Clark, P. (1999). 13-year experience with percutaneous management of upper tract transitional cell carcinoma. *Journal of Urology, 161,* 772–776.
9. Diamond, G. L., & Zalups, R. K. (1998). Understanding renal toxicity of heavy metals. *Toxicology and Pathology, 26*(1), 92–103.
10. Dickson, C. (1995). Treatment of renal carcinoma. *Nursing Times, 91*(34), 29–31.
11. Eggena, P. (1996). *Renal physiology*. Rensselaerville, NY: Novateur Medmedia.
12. Fong, K. Y., et al. (1998). Systemic lupus erythematosus: Initial manifestations and clinical features after 10 years of disease. *Annals of the Academy of Medicine, Singapore, 26*(3), 278–281.
13. Gill, I. (1995). Advances in urological laparoscopy. *Journal of Urology, 154*(10), 1275–1294.
14. Glassock, R. J. (1998). *Current therapy in nephrology and hypertension* (4th ed.). St. Louis: Mosby–Year Book.
15. Gunnarsson, I., et al. (1997). Occurrence of anti-C1q antibodies in IgA nephropathy. *Nephrology Dialysis and Transplantation, 12*(11), 2263–2268.
16. Guyton, A. C., & Hall, J. E. (1996). *Textbook of medical physiology* (9th ed.). Philadelphia: W. B. Saunders.
17. Guyton, A., & Hall, J. (1997). *Human physiology and mechanisms of disease* (6th ed.). Philadelphia: W. B. Saunders.
18. Hansen, M. (1998). *Pathophysiology: Foundations of disease and clinical intervention*. Philadelphia: W. B. Saunders.
19. Hiller, J., et al. (1997). Functional advantages of laparoscopic live donor nephrectomy versus open nephrectomy. *Journal of Transplant Coordination, 7*(3), 134–140.
20. Hinman, F. (1998). *Atlas of urologic surgery* (2nd ed.). Philadelphia: W. B. Saunders.
21. Hricik, D., Chung-Park, M., & Sedor, J. (1998). Glomerulonephritis. *New England Journal of Medicine, 339*(13), 888–899.
22. Karlowicz, K. A. (Ed.). (1995). *Urologic nursing: Principles and practice*. Philadelphia: W. B. Saunders.
23. Koeppen, B. M., & Stanton, B. A. (1997). *Renal physiology* (2nd ed.). St. Louis: Mosby–Year Book.
24. Krivak, L. (1995). Laparoscopic transperitoneal nephrectomy. *Canadian Operating Room Nursing Journal, 13*(2), 21–24.
25. Lancaster, L. E. (Ed.). (1995). *Core curriculum for nephrology nursing* (3rd ed.). Pitman, NJ: American Nephrology Nurses Association.
26. Levine, D. Z. (Ed.). (1997). *Caring for the renal patient* (3rd ed.). Philadelphia: W. B. Saunders.
27. Loeb, W. F. (1998). The measurement of renal injury. *Toxicology and Pathology, 26*(1), 26–28.
28. Lubkin, I. (1998). *Chronic illness: Impact and interventions* (4th ed.). Boston: Jones & Bartlett.
29. Mansi, M. K., & Alkhudair, W. K. (1997). Conservative management with percutaneous intervention of major blunt renal injuries. *American Journal of Emergency Medicine, 15*(7), 663–637.
30. Massry, S. G., & Glassock, R. J. (Eds.). (1995). *Massry and Glassock's textbook of nephrology* (3rd ed.). Baltimore: Williams & Wilkins.
31. Matthews, L. A., & Spirnak, J. P. (1995). The nonoperative approach to major blunt renal trauma. *Seminars in Urology, 13*(1), 77–82.
32. McCarthy, S., & McMullen, M. M. (1997). Autosomal dominant polycystic kidney disease: Pathophysiology and treatment. *ANNA Journal, 24*(1), 45–56.
33. McCorkle, R., et al. (1996). *Cancer nursing: A comprehensive textbook* (2nd ed.). Philadelphia: W. B. Saunders.
34. McDougall, E., & Clayman, R. (1994). Advances in laparoscopic urology. Part I: History and development of procedures. *Urology, 43*(4), 420–426.
35. McKinney, B. (1996). When this rare cancer strikes . . . renal cell carcinoma. *RN, 59*(12), 36–41, 51.
36. McKinney, B. (1998). Softening the edge of radical nephrectomy. *Nursing 98, 28*(7), 32hn1–32hn4.
37. Moody, F. (1999). *Atlas of ambulatory surgery*. Philadelphia: W. B. Saunders.
38. Morey, A. F., & McAninch, J. W. R. (1996). Renal trauma: Principles of evaluation and management. *Trauma Quarterly, 13*(1), 79–94.
39. Motzer, R., Bander, N., & Nanus, D. (1996). Renal cell carcinoma. *New England Journal of Medicine, 335*(12), 865–874.
40. Muehlbauer, P. (1998). Are you prepared for interleukin-2? *RN, 68*(2), 34–39.
41. Ritchie, W. (1999). Interferon and survival in metastatic renal carcinoma: Early results of a randomized controlled trial. *Lancet, 353,* 14–17.
42. Sansevero, A. C. (1997). Dehydration in the elderly: Strategies for prevention and management. *Nurse Practitioner, 22*(4), 41–42, 51–52, 54–57.
43. Schrier, R. W. (Ed.). (1995). *Manual of nephrology*. Boston: Little, Brown.
44. Schrier, R. W. (1997). *Renal and electrolyte disorders* (5th ed.). Boston, Little, Brown.
45. Schrier, R. W., & Gottschalk, C. W. (Eds.). (1997). *Diseases of the kidney* (6th ed.). Boston: Little, Brown.
46. Segal, S. (1996). Nursing rounds: Radical nephrectomy. *Nurse Practitioner, 96*(7), 37.
47. Staudenherz, A., et al. (1999). Is there a diagnostic role for bone scanning of patients with a high pretest probability for metastatic renal cell carcinoma? *Cancer, 85,* 153–155.
48. Stone, J., Wyman, J., & Salisbury, S. (1999). *Clinical gerontological nursing: A guide to advanced practice* (2nd ed.). Philadelphia: W. B. Saunders.
49. Tanagho, E. A., & McAninich, J. W. (1995). *Smith's general urology* (14th ed.). Norwalk, CT: Appleton & Lange.
50. Thumboo, J., et al. (1998). Clinical predictors of nephritis in systemic lupus erythematosus. *Annals of the Academy of Medicine, Singapore, 27*(1), 16–20.
51. Valtin, H., & Schafer, J. A. (1995). *Renal function: Mechanisms preserving fluid and solute balance in health* (3rd ed.). Boston: Little, Brown.
52. Vander, A. (1995). *Renal physiology* (5th ed.). New York: McGraw-Hill.
53. Walsh, P., et al. (1998). *Campbell's urology* (7th ed.). Philadelphia: W. B. Saunders.

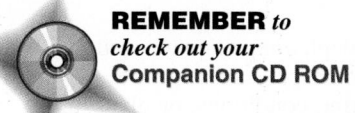

CHAPTER 36

Management of Clients with Renal Failure

Anita E. Molzahn

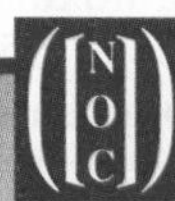

NURSING OUTCOMES CLASSIFICATION (NOC)
for Nursing Diagnoses—Clients with Renal Failure

Altered Nutrition: Less Than Body Requirements
Nutritional Status
Nutritional Status: Food and Fluid Intake
Anxiety
Anxiety Control
Coping
Constipation
Bowel Elimination
Hydration
Fatigue
Activity Tolerance
Endurance
Energy Conservation
Nutritional Status: Energy
Fluid Volume Deficit
Electrolyte and Acid-Base Balance
Fluid Balance
Hydration
Fluid Volume Excess
Electrolyte and Acid-Base Balance
Fluid Balance
Hydration
Risk for Impaired Skin Integrity
Dialysis Access Integrity
Nutritional Status: Biochemical Measures
Risk Control
Risk Detection
Self-Mutilation Restraint
Tissue Integrity: Skin & Mucous Membranes
Tissue Perfusion: Peripheral
Risk for Ineffective Breathing Pattern
Respiratory Status: Ventilation
Risk for Ineffective Family Coping: Compromised
Family Coping
Family Normalization
Risk for Ineffective Individual Coping
Coping
Decision-Making
Role Performance
Risk for Ineffective Management of Therapeutic Regimen: Families
Family Functioning
Family Health Status
Family Participation in Professional Care
Risk for Ineffective Management of Therapeutic Regimen: Individuals
Family Functioning
Family Health Status
Family Participation in Professional Care
Risk for Infection
Dialysis Access Integrity
Immune Status
Risk Control
Risk Detection
Tissue Integrity: Skin and Mucous Membranes
Risk for Injury
Risk Control
Risk Detection
Symptom Control

A disruption in renal function impairs the body's ability to maintain fluid, electrolyte, and acid-base balance. Reduced renal function interferes with erythropoietin and prostaglandin synthesis. Insulin degradation and the renin-angiotensin-aldosterone system are also affected by decreased renal function.

The diseases and problems that cause renal failure are described in Chapter 35. This chapter identifies common manifestations of acute and chronic renal failure and outlines treatments used to replace or restore renal function, such as dialysis and transplantation. For clients and families, psychosocial needs may arise from the physiologic problems caused by renal failure. You have a key role in helping to promote quality of life and rehabilitation for these clients.

UREMIC SYNDROME

The terms uremia, uremic syndrome, and renal failure are used synonymously. *Uremia* literally means "urine in the blood." This term and the term *uremic syndrome* describe a set of manifestations that result from loss of renal function. This loss may be of sudden onset or may develop over a long period. It may be self-limiting or irreversible. Sudden loss of kidney function, as occurs with damage from trauma, shock, toxins, or acute glomerulonephritis, brings on uremia rapidly and usually causes severe deterioration of the client's condition. Gradual loss of kidney function over an extended period may occur with glomerulonephritis, hypertension, chronic pyelonephritis, and other diseases.

Because the kidneys perform a wide variety of functions, the effects of uremia occur not only in the kidneys but also in other organ systems. Because of the time involved, chronic renal failure causes more degenerative changes throughout the body than acute uremia does. However, both types of renal failure have many of the same consequences. Unless the process can be halted or replacement therapy initiated, coma, seizures, and death result.

ACUTE RENAL FAILURE

Acute renal failure (ARF) refers to the abrupt loss of kidney function. Over a period of hours to a few days, the glomerular filtration rate (GFR) drops. Serum creatinine and urea nitrogen rise. A healthy adult who eats a normal diet needs a minimum urine output of about 400 ml over 24 hours to excrete the body's waste products through the kidneys. An amount lower than this indicates a decreased GFR. *Oliguria* refers to daily outputs of urine between 100 and 400 ml; *anuria* refers to urine output of less than 100 ml.

Etiology and Risk Factors

There are many possible causes of ARF, the most common of which are hypotension and prerenal hypovolemia. The etiologic mechanism of these disorders is discussed in Chapter 35.

CLASSIFICATION

The numerous causes of ARF can be categorized into three major areas: prerenal, renal, and postrenal (Fig. 36–1).

Prerenal Causes

Prerenal causes of ARF are those that interfere with renal perfusion. The kidneys depend on adequate delivery of blood to be filtered by the glomeruli. Therefore, reduced renal blood flow lowers the GFR and can lead to ARF. Conditions that contribute to decreased renal blood flow include the following:

- Circulatory volume depletion, as may occur with diarrhea, vomiting, hemorrhage, excessive use of diuretics, burns, renal salt-wasting conditions, or glycosuria
- Volume shifts, as from third-space sequestration of fluid, vasodilation, or gram-negative sepsis
- Decreased cardiac output, as during cardiac pump failure, pericardial tamponade, or acute pulmonary embolism
- Decreased peripheral vascular resistance, as from spinal anesthesia, septic shock, or anaphylaxis
- Vascular obstruction, such as bilateral renal artery occlusion or dissecting aneurysm

Intrarenal Causes

Intrarenal (or renal) causes of ARF involve parenchymal changes caused by disease or nephrotoxic substances. Acute tubular necrosis is the most common intrarenal cause of ARF and accounts for about 75% of cases. This destruction of the tubular epithelial cells results from impaired renal perfusion or direct damage by nephrotoxins. In addition to the nephrotoxins described in Chapter 35, acute tubular necrosis may be caused by heme pigments, such as myoglobin and hemoglobin, which are liberated from damaged muscle tissue. This release may result from trauma (rhabdomyolysis), such as surgery, crush injury, and electric shock, or from nontraumatic conditions, such as severe muscle exertion, genetic conditions (such as diabetes mellitus or malignant hyperthermia), infectious disease, metabolic conditions (such as hypokalemia, phosphatemia, or heat stroke), and rejection of a transplanted kidney.

Other intrarenal causes of ARF include glomerulonephritis; microvascular and large vascular lesions, as in hemolytic-uremic syndrome; thrombosis; vasculitis; scleroderma; trauma; atherosclerosis; tumor invasion; and cortical necrosis, which is caused by prolonged vasospasm of the cortical blood vessels.

Postrenal Causes

Postrenal causes of ARF arise from an obstruction in the urinary tract, anywhere from the tubules to the urethral meatus. Common sources of obstruction include prostatic

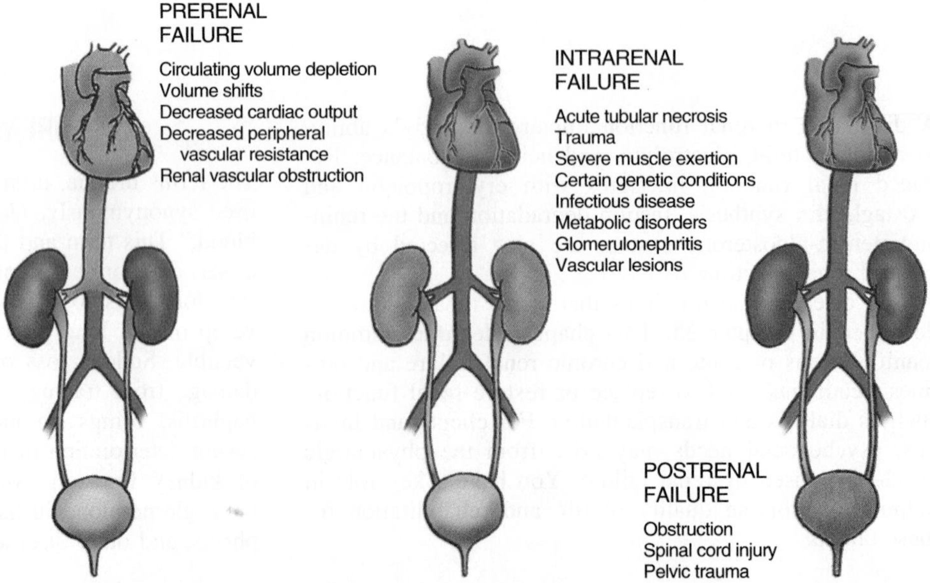

FIGURE 36–1 Causes of acute renal failure: prerenal, intrarenal, and postrenal.

hypertrophy, calculi, invading tumors, surgical accidents, ureteral or urethral strictures or stenosis, and retroperitoneal fibrosis. Spinal cord injury may lead to decreased bladder emptying and a functional obstruction.

General Considerations

In management of the client with ARF, it is important to determine whether the disorder originates from prerenal, intrarenal, or postrenal causes before intervention begins. Appropriate interventions require determining the cause of the disorder.

One health promotion strategy is to teach clients about the risks of nephrotoxic agents identified in Chapter 35. Other health promotion and health maintenance actions include monitoring of vital signs and urine output and early identification and reversal of hypotension and hypovolemia, the two causes of ARF associated with the highest mortality rates. Prevention of urinary obstruction is another health promotion and maintenance action.

Pathophysiology

The pathogenesis of ARF is not clear. One hypothesis is that the damaged tubules cannot conserve sodium normally, which activates the renin-angiotensin-aldosterone system. The effect is to redistribute the renal vascular supply by increasing the tone of both the afferent and efferent arterioles. The resulting ischemia may cause an increase in vasopressin, cellular swelling, inhibition of prostaglandin synthesis, and further stimulation of the renin-angiotensin system. The reduced blood flow decreases glomerular pressure, GFR, and tubular flow; thus, oliguria occurs.

Another theory is that cellular and protein debris in the tubule obstruct the lumen, which raises the intratubular pressure. The increasing oncotic pressure opposes filtration pressure until glomerular filtration stops. A biochemical theory claims that decreased renal blood flow leads to decreased oxygen delivery to the proximal tubules; this causes a reduction in cellular adenosine triphosphate, which increases cytosolic and mitochondrial calcium concentrations. The result of this process is cell death and tubular necrosis. Vasomotor nephropathy, which causes spasms of peritubular capillaries, may result in tubular damage. Other possible pathogenic mechanisms include leakage of filtered urine through damaged tubules back into the peritubular capillaries and chemical or morphologic changes in the basement membrane of the glomerular capillary, which decrease nephron filtration. The reversibility of this mechanism depends on the level of destruction of the basement membrane.

Clinical Manifestations

The clinical course of ARF is marked by several phases. The onset (or initiating) phase covers the period from the precipitating event to the development of renal manifestations. Manifestations may begin immediately or up to a week after the precipitating event. The oliguric-anuric (or nonoliguric) phase lasts 1 to 8 weeks. The longer this phase, the poorer the prognosis. Dialysis may be required during the oliguric-anuric phase.

A gradual or abrupt return to glomerular filtration and leveling of the blood urea nitrogen (BUN) signal the diuretic phase. Urine output may be 1000 to 2000 ml/day, which may lead to dehydration; 25% of the deaths from ARF occur during this phase.

The recovery phase lasts 3 to 12 months. During this time, the client commonly returns to an activity level similar to that before the onset of the illness. Mild tubular abnormalities, including glycosuria and decreased concentrating ability, may continue for years, and the client is continually at risk for fluid and electrolyte imbalance, especially during times of stress.

The effects of ARF are widespread. The major consequences include the following:

- Fluid and electrolyte imbalances (fluid overload or depletion, hyperkalemia, hyponatremia, hypocalcemia, and hypermagnesemia)
- Acidosis
- Increased susceptibility to secondary infections
- Anemia
- Platelet dysfunction
- Gastrointestinal complications (anorexia, nausea, vomiting, diarrhea or constipation, and stomatitis)
- Increased incidence of pericarditis
- Uremic encephalopathy characterized by apathy, defective recent memory, episodic obtundation, dysarthria, tremors, convulsions, and coma
- Impaired wound healing

Other manifestations are usually a result of these sequelae. The most common overall manifestation of ARF is alteration of the expected urine output. Usually, oliguria or anuria is found, but polyuric ARF accounts for 30% of the cases. There are two varieties of ARF: nonoliguric and oliguric.

Nonoliguric Renal Failure

Although nonoliguric, or polyuric, ARF is being recognized more often, its status remains controversial. It may be an independent entity, or it may be a phase of oliguric ARF.

Clients with nonoliguric renal failure may excrete as much as 2 L/day, and this must be recognized as a possible sign of ARF. The urine produced is dilute and nearly isosmolar, reflected in a low urine specific gravity indicating that not all nephrons have stopped filtering. Hypertension and tachypnea, with manifestations of fluid overload, are comonly found. The client may also demonstrate manifestations of extracellular fluid depletion, such as dry mucous membranes, poor skin turgor, and orthostatic hypotension. Nonoliguric renal failure is usually associated with less morbidity and mortality than the oliguric form, probably because of the lesser degree and shorter duration of azotemia.

Oliguric Renal Failure

In oliguric ARF, urine production usually falls below 400 ml/day. However, the aging kidney normally loses its concentrating ability, and renal function becomes more susceptible to insult. Therefore, an older client may have had oliguria even at urine volumes of 600 to 700 ml/day.

The clinical manifestations of oliguric ARF depend on the cause. In prerenal failure, assessment findings are quite diverse, depending on the underlying condition. The client commonly has a history of a precipitating event, such as hemorrhage or cardiac insult. The urine has a high specific gravity and osmolarity, and there is little or no proteinuria. Urine sediment is usually normal, although it may contain a few hyaline and granular casts. There is very little urinary sodium excretion. The BUN-creatinine ratio is significantly elevated, reaching levels between 10:1 and 40:1.

Systemic manifestations of intrinsic renal failure may include edema, weight gain, hemoptysis resulting from elevated left ventricular end-diastolic pressure, weakness from anemia, and hypertension. The urine has a fixed specific gravity, a high sodium concentration, and definite proteinuria. The client with glomerulonephritis has hematuria and red blood cell and hemoglobin casts. Acute tubular necrosis causes muddy brown granular casts. If there has been significant tissue damage, expect elevated levels of serum creatinine, phosphokinase, and potassium.

Urine produced in postrenal failure may have fixed specific gravity and elevated sodium concentration with little or no proteinuria. Urine sediment is generally normal. The most definitive manifestations are those indicating obstruction, as described with calculi and neoplasms. Wide fluctuations between anuria and polyuria may indicate intermittent urinary tract obstruction.

Urinalysis and determinations of urine specific gravity and sodium levels, serum creatinine, and urea nitrogen are common diagnostic tests for ARF. The amount of urine in relation to intake is also important in formulating the diagnosis. To measure the exact urine output or to obtain a specimen for culture and sensitivity, the client may need to be catheterized one time only (with a straight catheter).

Prognosis

The mortality rate in ARF may be as high as 50%; the highest mortality rates occur when failure is caused by trauma or surgery. The lowest mortality rate is in ARF caused by nephrotoxic substances (see Chapter 35). When obstruction or glomerulonephritis is the cause, the mortality rate is low.

Outcome Management

Medical Management

Prevent Acute Renal Failure

The medical management of ARF is largely based on preventing and treating its effects. As with any disease process, prevention is the primary intervention. Attaining and maintaining adequate hydration and diuresis in high-risk clients is crucial, as is the prevention of contributing factors.

Once ARF has developed, prompt recognition and action facilitate restoration of optimal renal function. Correction of the underlying condition, such as hydration for a client with hypovolemic shock, may be all that is necessary in ARF caused by prerenal disorders. Postrenal causes must be rectified. In the meantime, the sequelae of ARF require specific intervention.

Maintain Fluid and Electrolyte Balance

In ARF, maintenance of fluid and electrolyte balance is key to survival. Imbalances are common and pose significant challenges to the clinician.

Fluid replacement must be done carefully to avoid fluid overload. Fluid replacement volumes are usually calculated on the basis of some fraction of the previous day's urine output plus an amount (commonly 400 ml) to account for the usual insensible losses that occur during a 24-hour period. Amounts lost in other ways, such as vomiting and diarrhea, are added to the daily allotment. Unless the client is receiving total parenteral nutrition (TPN), some physicians use a daily weight loss of 0.2 to 0.5 kg/day as a measure of the success of the fluid replacement program. This amount represents the usual daily weight loss through catabolism and loss of lean body mass.

Diuretic therapy may be used cautiously. Furosemide and mannitol are the drugs used most often, but furosemide can be nephrotoxic, increasing the risk of further renal damage. It is also important to avoid dehydration, and fluids should be replaced as needed to maintain adequate blood flow to the kidneys.

Electrolyte replacement is based primarily on urine and serum electrolyte concentrations. Hyperkalemia is probably the most dangerous imbalance because of its contribution to cardiac arrhythmias and arrest. In addition to the kidney's inability to excrete potassium, this electrolyte is released in greater quantities from the body cells when acidosis is present and is further increased by rapid tissue catabolism.

Electrocardiographic monitors are commonly used to check for effects of hypokalemia or hyperkalemia. Cation exchange resins may be administered orally or rectally to facilitate excretion of potassium through the gastrointestinal tract. Sorbitol, an osmotic cathartic, is given with cation exchange resins to induce a diarrhea to eliminate the potassium ions that were exchanged for sodium ions in the resins. Sorbitol can be given orally, as an enema, or by nasogastric tube. Potassium-containing foods and medications should be avoided. In an emergency, administration of 50% glucose and regular insulin, with sodium bicarbonate if necessary, can temporarily prevent cardiac arrest by moving potassium into the cells and reducing serum potassium levels.

Hyponatremia usually results from dilution rather than true lack of sodium. Therefore, intervention is a matter of proper fluid replacement (i.e., fluid restriction and self-correction).

Because magnesium is normally excreted by the kidneys, it can accumulate in renal failure. Dark green vegetables, unrefined grains, seeds, nuts, legumes, and antacids and osmotic laxatives containing magnesium should be avoided because they increase serum magnesium levels.

Metabolic acidosis usually results from the accumulation of acid waste products. Sodium bicarbonate, sodium lactate, or sodium acetate may be used in the short term to correct this condition. Dialysis is usually used for severe acidosis.

Low doses (1 to 5 μg/kg/min) of dopamine hydrochloride (Intropin) may be given to activate dopamine receptors in the kidney. Dopamine, a sympathomimetic, can dilate renal blood vessels, which improves renal function, increases urine flow, and increases sodium excretion to improve renal function.

Replace Renal Function

Dialysis (detailed later in the chapter) is frequently required for treatment of ARF. Indications for dialysis include:

- Significant volume overload
- Uncontrolled hyperkalemia or acidosis
- Progressive uremia, as evidenced by rising BUN and creatinine concentrations
- Altered central nervous system function
- Pericarditis

There are some special considerations for dialysis of clients with ARF. First, heparin is generally decreased to reduce the risk of bleeding. Because hypotension is common, clients must be carefully monitored and replacement fluids provided as appropriate.

For clients with ARF, continuous renal replacement therapy (CRRT) has benefits. There are several types of CRRT, including (1) continuous arteriovenous hemofiltration (CAVH), (2) continuous venovenous hemofiltration (CVVH), (3) continuous venovenous hemodialysis (CVVHD), (4) continuous arteriovenous ultrafiltration (CAVU), and (5) slow continuous ultrafiltration (SCUF). In essence, these methods involve removal of plasma water and dissolved contents from the client's blood across a membrane. In contrast, in dialysis, particles are removed by diffusion. Slow continuous removal of waste products and water through CRRT is less stressful to the client than shorter, more efficient dialysis treatments.

Prevent Infections

Secondary infections are a significant cause of death in clients with ARF. The client must be monitored carefully for infectious processes; if these occur, they should be treated aggressively. Except to monitor urine output during ARF, indwelling urethral catheters are usually avoided because of their great potential for introducing infection. If a catheter is placed, meticulous catheter care is essential.

Monitor the Client

Treatment of ARF may take place in an intensive care unit or other critical care unit, depending on the cause. Much of the care consists of physiologic monitoring and assessment. In addition to monitoring fluid and electrolyte balance, you should monitor the progression of manifestations associated with renal failure. Pericarditis occurs in as many as 18% of clients with renal failure. Assessment findings include pleuritic pain (which may subside when the client assumes an upright position), pericardial friction rub, tachycardia, and fever. Treatment usually starts with steroids or nonsteroidal anti-inflammatory drugs (NSAIDs). Pericardiocentesis and pericardiectomy may be necessary if cardiac function is compromised.

Other problems call for relief of manifestations. The rising BUN decreases the seizure threshold, resulting in a rise in the number of seizures. These seizures may be relieved by intravenous phenytoin or phenobarbital. Anemia is treated by transfusions or the use of recombinant erythropoietin. Erythropoietin is a hormone produced by the kidney that stimulates red blood cell production. Erythropoietin is used in chronic renal failure, but its use in ARF has not been studied extensively. Bleeding tendencies may be minimized by correcting vitamin K deficiencies as well as by lowering the serum BUN level, because BUN interferes with platelet aggregation.

Maintain Nutritional Status

Proper nutrition is crucial. A high-calorie, low-protein diet is usually prescribed. The diet may also be low in sodium, magnesium, phosphate, and potassium. The protein must be of high biologic value (complete), containing the essential amino acids to reduce nitrogenous waste products. Adequate carbohydrate intake reverses the process of gluconeogenesis. During the acute phases, intake should be 135 to 150 nonprotein kilocalories (kcal) for each 6.25 g of protein ingested; this ratio is considered adequate for preventing protein catabolism. Liquid supplements, low in potassium, may also be used. If oral intake is not sufficient to meet requirements, tube feedings or total parenteral nutrition, including lipids, may be instituted.

Nursing Management of the Medical Client

Assessment

Carefully monitor any client with risk factors for ARF. In fact, it is important to assess fluid balance in any hospitalized or seriously injured client. Because hypovolemia is a common cause, assess the client closely for this problem. When the diagnosis is ARF, carefully assess for such complications as pleural effusion, pericarditis, acidosis, and uremia. See the Case Study on acute renal failure.

Diagnosis, Outcomes, Interventions

Fluid Volume Deficit or Fluid Volume Excess. A common diagnosis in ARF is *Fluid Volume Deficit related to fluid loss from a variety of causes.* Another common nursing diagnosis is *Fluid Volume Excess related to inability of the kidneys to produce urine secondary to ARF.*

Outcomes. The client will not have fluid volume deficit and ARF; if ARF does occur, fluid volume excess will not develop or it will be managed with dialysis or CRRT, as evidenced by a return to balanced intake and output (I & O).

Interventions. Careful monitoring of fluid balance indicators is crucial to the management of ARF. Accurate intake and output measurements guide the fluid replacement regimen. Compare these values, and look for 24- to 48-hour trends. Check the client's vital signs (including postural blood pressures and apical pulses), skin turgor, and mucous membranes about every 4 hours, depending on the severity of the illness. Carefully obtain daily weights using the same scale at the same time of day. Obtain blood pressure measurements via an arterial line, if one is in place.

Urine specific gravity, usually an indication of fluid balance, may not be useful with intrinsic renal disease. Abnormalities in heart sounds, breath sounds, and mental status may indicate the presence of fluid and electrolyte imbalances.

When the physician has determined the client's fluid allotment, make sure that intake amounts for each shift are followed. This means carefully monitoring fluid intake to ensure that the prescribed amount is taken. Often, this amount represents a significant fluid restriction for the client, which causes a problem with thirst. Help the client stay within the prescribed restriction with careful oral hygiene and judicious use of ice chips, lip ointments, and appropriate diversionary activities. Placing the allotted water in a spray bottle may help to spread out the amount

Acute Renal Failure and Abdominal Aortic Aneurysm Resection

Mr. Carlson is a 70-year-old retired farmer who is brought in by squad to a small rural hospital complaining of boring abdominal pain that radiates through to the back. A CT scan of the abdomen reveals a dissecting abdominal aneurysm. Mr. Carlson is subsequently flown to an urban hospital for emergency resection of the aneurysm. Complications encountered in surgery require that the aorta be cross-clamped for a number of hours. Multiple blood products are administered to replace those lost through hemorrhage. Mr. Carlson is admitted to the surgical intensive care unit for postoperative care and monitoring.

Initial Postoperative Orders

Routine postoperative vital sign monitoring
Monitor urine output every 1 hour and call if less than ½ ml/kg/hr
5% dextrose in 0.2% normal saline (D_5¼ NS) at 150 ml/hr
Cefazolin sodium (Ancef) 1 g IV every 6 hours
Morphine sulfate 1 to 4 mg IV every 1 hour as needed (prn) for pain
Check metabolic chemistry panel and CBC in AM
Turn, cough, and deep-breathe every 2 hours
Incentive spirometer every 1 hour while awake
NG tube to low intermittent suction, irrigate prn

Nursing Admission Assessment

Mr. Carlson is groggy but easily arousable. His wife of 45 years is at his bedside. She relates that Mr. Carlson expressly told her not to let them keep him alive if anything "bad" should happen. She reports that her husband previously had been in good health and was enjoying his retirement and their grandchildren. He was a coffee drinker but did not use tobacco.

Nursing Physical Assessment

Height: 6 ft
Weight: 175 lb (79.5 kg)
Vital signs: BP, 100/50; TPR, 96.8, 112, 14
LOC: groggy but arousable
EENT: PERLA
Cardiac: sinus tachycardia, S_1 and S_2 readily audible without rubs or murmurs
Pulmonary: breath sounds diminished throughout
Abdominal: NG tube in place and draining small amounts of brown drainage. Large abdominal dressing in place. Abdomen flat; bowel tones absent
Genitourinary: Foley catheter in place draining clear straw-colored urine
Peripheral pulses: 2/2, without edema noted

Throughout the night, Mr. Carlson's urine output dropped and the color changed to dark amber. By 6 AM Mr. Carlson was averaging 30 to 40 ml/hr. He was cooperating well with turning and had received morphine on an hourly basis which was controlling his pain. His dressings remain dry and intact and the NG drainage had changed to golden bile colored liquid. Mr. Carlson's abdomen remains flat and without bowel sounds. The AM laboratory specimens were drawn as ordered, revealing the following pertinent values:

AM Laboratory Values

RBCs: 3.0 million/mm^3
Hb: 10.0 g/dl
Hct: 30%
WBCs: 13,000/mm^3
Sodium: 145 mEq/L
Chloride: 105 mEq/L
Potassium: 4.8 mEq/L
Creatinine: 2.6 mg/dl
BUN: 47 mg/dl

Consider the pathophysiologic causes of the abnormalities noted in the AM laboratory values. In the next 48 hours. Mr. Carlson's urine output continued to dwindle and his potassium, creatinine, and BUN continued to rise. Mr. Carlson has become increasingly confused and the doctors have turned to Mrs. Carlson to give consent for various treatments. Mr. Carlson's surgeon ordered a nephrology consultation, and the decision has been made to start hemodialysis. A dopamine infusion has been started at the renal perfusion dosage, and intravenous steroid therapy has been initiated. Consider Mr. Carlson's wishes to have no heroic measures.

Dialysis is performed in Mr. Carlson's room every day for the first 3 days and then every other day for the next week. Mr. Carlson's urine output increases, and his blood and urine chemistry values reflect return of marginal renal function. Furosemide (Lasix) at 80 mg twice a day is instituted, and hemodialysis is discontinued. Mr. Carlson is transferred to a medical surgical nursing unit. Mr. Carlson's bowel tones have returned, but he reports a lack of appetite and that food tastes "funny." Mr. Carlson's medications have been converted to oral dosages. It is expected that he will be discharged to his home in his wife's care tomorrow.

Discharge and Post-treatment Considerations

Average length of stay for abdominal aortic aneurysm repair without complications, 5.7 days; with complications, 12.4 days
Complete discharge teaching (including diet, wound care, medications, activity, and follow-up appointments)
Community referral: nutrition and postoperative care support to home nursing service

Questions to Be Considered

1. Compare and contrast the ethical considerations related to treatment options for clients with acute renal failure

and for those with chronic renal failure. Discuss the nurse's role in assisting clients and families with resolution of ethical dilemmas regarding treatment options.

2. Discuss the nutritional and fluid replacement considerations necessary for a postoperative client who develops acute renal failure. Identify nutritional and fluid replacement considerations that are necessary for clients receiving diuretic therapy.
3. Compare and contrast the causes, clinical manifestations, and management of acute renal failure versus chronic renal failure. Identify nursing care and monitoring of the catheters or arteriovenous fistulas used for the various types of dialysis.
4. Identify the nursing measures used to monitor client's fluid and electrolyte status (i.e., fluid balance, sodium, potassium, calcium, chloride, magnesium, and phosphorus).
5. Discuss the nursing measures used to prevent secondary infections for clients with acute renal failure. Identify the factors that place these clients at greater risk for secondary infections.
6. Compare and contrast hemodialysis and peritoneal dialysis. Identify factors that made Mr. Carlson ineligible for peritoneal dialysis.
7. Identify classes of drugs that may be nephrotoxic. Discuss the rationale and implications for the use of these drugs for patients with renal failure.

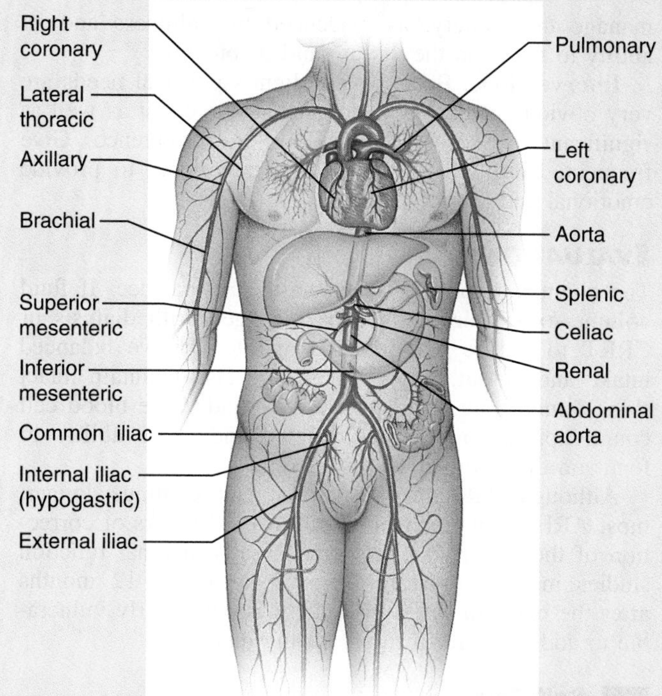

● Major arteries of the chest and abdomen. (Modified from Thibodeau, G. A., & Patton, K. T. [1999]. *Anatomy and physiology* [3rd ed.]. St. Louis, Mosby–Year Book. Illustrated by Barbara Cousins.)

BP, blood pressure; BUN, blood urea nitrogen; CBC, complete blood count; CT, computed tomography; EENT, eyes-ears-nose-throat; Hb, hemoglobin; Hct, hematocrit; IV, intravenous; LOC, level of consciousness; NG, nasogastric; prn, as needed; PERLA, pupils equal and reactive to light and accommodation; RBCs, red blood cells; TPR, temperature, pulse, respirations; WBCs, white blood cells.

taken. Fluid from foods must be taken into account as well. To conserve fluids for the client, administer medications with meals, if possible.

Altered Nutrition: Less Than Body Requirements. Another common diagnosis for clients with this disorder is *Altered Nutrition: Less Than Body Requirements related to anorexia and altered metabolic state secondary to renal failure.*

Outcomes. The client will maintain adequate nutrition, as evidenced by sufficient intake to prevent protein catabolism and laboratory values within safe levels.

Interventions. A client with renal failure commonly experiences anorexia, nausea, stomatitis, and taste changes. These, combined with a generally less palatable diet, make adequate nutrition a challenge for nurse and client. Work with the client to plan a diet that is most acceptable. The therapeutic dietitian is a good resource.

Provide a pleasant environment at mealtime. Preparing foods in an attractive manner and presenting them in small amounts may help. Medications to alleviate the discomfort of nausea and stomatitis may be useful. Enteral or parenteral nutrition may be instituted if the client's nutritional status cannot be maintained with oral intake.

Risk for Impaired Skin Integrity. You may need to use the diagnosis *Risk for Impaired Skin Integrity related to poor cellular nutrition and edema.*

Outcomes. The client will not develop impaired skin integrity, as evidenced by intact skin.

Interventions. The poor systemic nutrition and edema that accompany renal failure may cause skin breakdown. Meticulous skin care, frequent turning, and special mattresses are important. Range-of-motion exercises facilitate movement and increase circulation.

Risk for Infection. Acute or chronic renal failure makes clients more susceptible to infection, resulting in a diagnosis of *Risk for Infection related to lowered resistance.*

Outcomes. The client will not develop infection, as evidenced by normal vital signs, a normal white blood cell count, and no outward manifestations of infection.

Interventions. The client with ARF is immunocompromised and very susceptible to secondary infection, a stress that the kidneys cannot handle. Nursing intervention must be designed to prevent infection in the usual high-risk sites (e.g., respiratory tract, wounds, central catheters, and mouth). Urethral catheters are avoided if possible. If they must be used, provide meticulous catheter care. Also, be alert to early manifestations of infection so that aggressive medical treatment may be instituted.

Anxiety. Inevitably, the client will experience *Anxiety related to unknown outcome of disease process.*

Outcomes. The client will demonstrate an ability to

manage the anxiety, as evidenced by calmness and an ability to focus on the disease and its outcome.

Interventions. Because the client's physical needs are very obvious, it is easy to forget that the client as well as significant others will be anxious and frightened. Give frequent, careful explanations, and remember to provide emotional and psychological support.

EVALUATION

The client is expected to maintain fluid balance. If fluid volume excess develops, it is managed with dialysis or CRRT to reduce body weight and to achieve balanced intake and output. The client should also maintain intact skin, demonstrate normal vital signs and white blood cell count, appear to be less anxious, and show ability to focus on the information provided.

Although ARF manifestations may continue longer, most ARF clients recover within 4 to 10 weeks of correction of the underlying problem. Results of renal function studies may continue to improve for up to 12 months after the onset of ARF. The client is particularly vulnerable to additional renal injury during this time.

Self-Care

It is important for the client to understand the implications of ARF and the importance of following the therapeutic regimen. The client and significant others have to understand which manifestations might indicate further renal damage or chronic renal failure (CRF). The client must be closely observed by a nephrologist for at least a year after ARF is reversed so that deterioration of renal function can be monitored. The client and significant others require knowledge of renal failure and an understanding of the possible need for ongoing treatment.

Modifications for Elderly Clients

Older clients are at increased risk for ARF because of reduced cardiac contractile function, vascular compliance, renal plasma flow, and renal mass. The older adult has more difficulty maintaining a homeostatic fluid balance. The ability to retain sodium declines with age, as does the ability to concentrate urine. Older clients are also more likely to have pre-existing renal damage from such diseases as hypertension, diabetes, and benign prostatic hypertrophy in men. Therefore, dosages of medications that are nephrotoxic or excreted by the kidney may need to be adjusted.

CHRONIC RENAL FAILURE

Chronic, or irreversible, renal failure is a progressive reduction of functioning renal tissue such that the remaining kidney mass can no longer maintain the body's internal environment. CRF can develop insidiously over many years, or it may result from an episode of ARF from which the client has not recovered.

The incidence of CRF varies widely by state and country. In the United States, the incidence is 268 new cases per million population. According to the U.S. Renal Data System, at the end of 1997, more than 300,000 people were being treated for CRF or end-stage renal disease (ESRD). More than 191,000 people were receiving hemodialysis and 86,000 people had functioning renal transplants.[45]

Etiology and Risk Factors

The causes of CRF are numerous. Chapter 35 discussed various injuries and disease processes that may end in renal failure. Chronic glomerulonephritis, ARF, polycystic kidney disease, obstruction, repeated episodes of pyelonephritis, and nephrotoxins are examples of causes. Systemic diseases, such as diabetes mellitus, hypertension, lupus erythematosus, polyarteritis, sickle cell disease, and amyloidosis, may produce CRF. Diabetes is the leading cause and accounts for more than 30% of clients who receive dialysis. Hypertension is the second leading cause of CRF.

To reduce the risk of CRF, the client should be closely observed and should receive adequate treatment to control or slow the progress of these problems before they progress to ESRD. Some conditions, such as lupus and diabetes, can progress to renal failure despite close treatment.

Pathophysiology

The pathogenesis of CRF involves deterioration and destruction of nephrons with progressive loss of renal function. As the total GFR falls and clearance is reduced, the serum urea nitrogen and creatinine levels rise. Remaining functioning nephrons hypertrophy, as they are required to filter a larger load of solutes. A consequence is that the kidneys lose their ability to concentrate urine adequately. In an attempt to continue excreting the solutes, a large volume of dilute urine may be passed, which makes the client susceptible to fluid depletion. The tubules gradually lose their ability to reabsorb electrolytes. Occasionally, the result is salt wasting, in which the urine contains large amounts of sodium, which leads to more polyuria.

As renal damage advances and the number of functioning nephrons declines, the total GFR decreases further. Thus, the body becomes unable to rid itself of excess water, salt, and other waste products through the kidneys. When the GFR is less than 10 to 20 ml/min, the effect of uremic toxins on the body becomes evident. If the disease is not treated by dialysis or transplantation, the outcome of CRF is uremia and death.

Clinical Manifestations

The clinical manifestations of the early stages of renal failure depend on the disease process and contributing factors. As the destruction of nephrons progresses to ESRD, the manifestations become similar and are described as uremic syndrome. The clinical course of irreversible renal disease and uremic syndrome follows a pattern:

- *Reduced renal reserve* refers to the state in which BUN is high-normal but the client has no clinical manifestations. Normal functioning is evident as long as the client is not exposed to unusual physiologic or psychosocial stress.

- *Renal insufficiency* reflects a more advanced pathologic process with mild azotemia when the client is receiving a general diet. Impaired urine concentration, nocturia (excessive urination at night), and mild anemia are common findings. Renal function is easily impaired by stress.
- *Renal failure* is indicated by severe azotemia, acidosis, impaired urine dilution, severe anemia, and a number of electrolyte imbalances, such as hypernatremia, hyperkalemia, and hyperphosphatemia.
- *ESRD* is characterized by two groups of clinical manifestations: deranged excretory and regulatory mechanisms and a distinctive grouping of gastrointestinal, cardiovascular, neuromuscular, hematologic, integumentary, skeletal, and hormonal manifestations. The kidneys can no longer maintain homeostasis.

The clinical manifestations of CRF are present throughout the body. No organ system is spared. Renal alterations (described previously) include the kidney's inability to concentrate urine and regulate electrolyte excretion. Polyuria progresses to anuria, and the client loses normal diurnal patterns of voiding. In addition, all normal functions of the kidney, such as regulation of acid-base balance, regulation of blood pressure, synthesis of 1,25-dihydroxycholecalciferol, biogenesis of erythropoietin, degradation of insulin, and synthesis of prostaglandins, become curtailed and are eventually lost.

See the algorithm Understanding Chronic Renal Failure and Its Treatment.

Electrolyte Imbalances

Electrolyte balance may be upset by impaired excretion and utilization in the kidney. Although many clients maintain a normal serum sodium level, the salt-wasting properties of some failing kidneys, in addition to vomiting and diarrhea, may cause hyponatremia. Apparent hyponatremia may be a dilutional effect of water retention. Late in the disease, salt and water retention often contributes to hypertension and heart failure.

Because the kidneys are efficient at excreting potassium, potassium levels usually remain within normal limits until late in the disease. However, hyperkalemia then becomes a challenging problem. Catabolism, potassium-containing medications, trauma, blood transfusions, and acidosis contribute to potassium excess.

Several mechanisms contribute to hypocalcemia. Conversion of 25-hydroxycholecalciferol to 1,25-dihydroxycholecalciferol (necessary to absorb calcium) is decreased, which results in reduced intestinal absorption of calcium. At the same time, phosphate is not excreted, which causes hyperphosphatemia. Because calcium and phosphate are inversely related, a high phosphate level results in a reduced calcium level. This combination stimulates the parathyroid glands to secrete parathyroid hormone in an attempt to facilitate phosphate excretion and raise the serum calcium level by resorbing calcium from bone. Osteomalacia, osteitis fibrosa, and osteosclerosis are commonly seen in clients with CRF as a result of these metabolic alterations in calcium, phosphorus, parathyroid hormone, and vitamin D. In some clients, hypercalcemia may develop because of persistent secretion of parathyroid hormone.

Mildly elevated serum magnesium levels are found early in the disease. Magnesium does not usually reach a dangerous level unless the client is receiving magnesium-containing laxatives or antacids.

Metabolic Changes

In advancing renal failure, BUN and serum creatinine rise as waste products of protein metabolism accumulate in the blood. The serum creatinine level is the most accurate measure of renal function. The normal ratio of BUN to creatinine is 10:1, and it remains the same as both the creatinine and BUN rise.

The proteinuria accompanying renal disease and sometimes inadequate dietary intake of proteins cause hypoproteinemia, which lowers the intravascular oncotic pressure. Serum uric acid is often high but is not commonly associated with manifestations of gout.

Carbohydrate intolerance results from impaired insulin production and metabolism. Four mechanisms are responsible:

- Peripheral insulin antagonism
- Impaired insulin secretion
- A prolonged insulin half-life, which is directly related to kidney malfunction
- Abnormalities in circulating insulin

Therefore, special care is needed in adjustment of insulin doses for clients with diabetes mellitus complicated by renal failure. Even short-acting regular insulin functions as a longer-acting insulin, resulting in a need for lower dosages or fewer injections per day. Serum glucose levels must be monitored closely.

Elevated triglycerides are found almost universally. This type IV hyperlipidemia is thought to be caused by increased production of lipids by the liver in response to elevated blood glucose and insulin levels. At the same time, assimilation of lipids in the peripheral tissues appears to be reduced, possibly because of the blockage of lipoprotein lipase activity. This contributes to a secondary complication of cardiovascular disease.

Metabolic acidosis occurs because of the kidney's inability to excrete hydrogen ions. Decreased reabsorption of sodium bicarbonate and decreased formation of dihydrogen phosphate and ammonia contribute to this problem. Acidosis accentuates hyperkalemia and the reabsorption of calcium from the bones.

Pericarditis is usually related to the accumulation of uremic toxins, rarely to infection. Manifestations include pericardial pain (often relieved by an upright position), tachycardia, pleural friction rub, and fever. The condition may progress to pericardial effusion and cardiac tamponade, a life-threatening complication.

Hematologic Changes

The primary hematologic effect of renal failure is anemia, usually normochromic and normocytic. It occurs because the kidneys are unable to produce erythropoietin, a hormone necessary for red blood cell production. If it is left untreated, hematocrit levels can drop below 20%. Frequently, the fatigue, weakness, and cold intolerance accompanying the anemia lead to a diagnosis of renal failure.

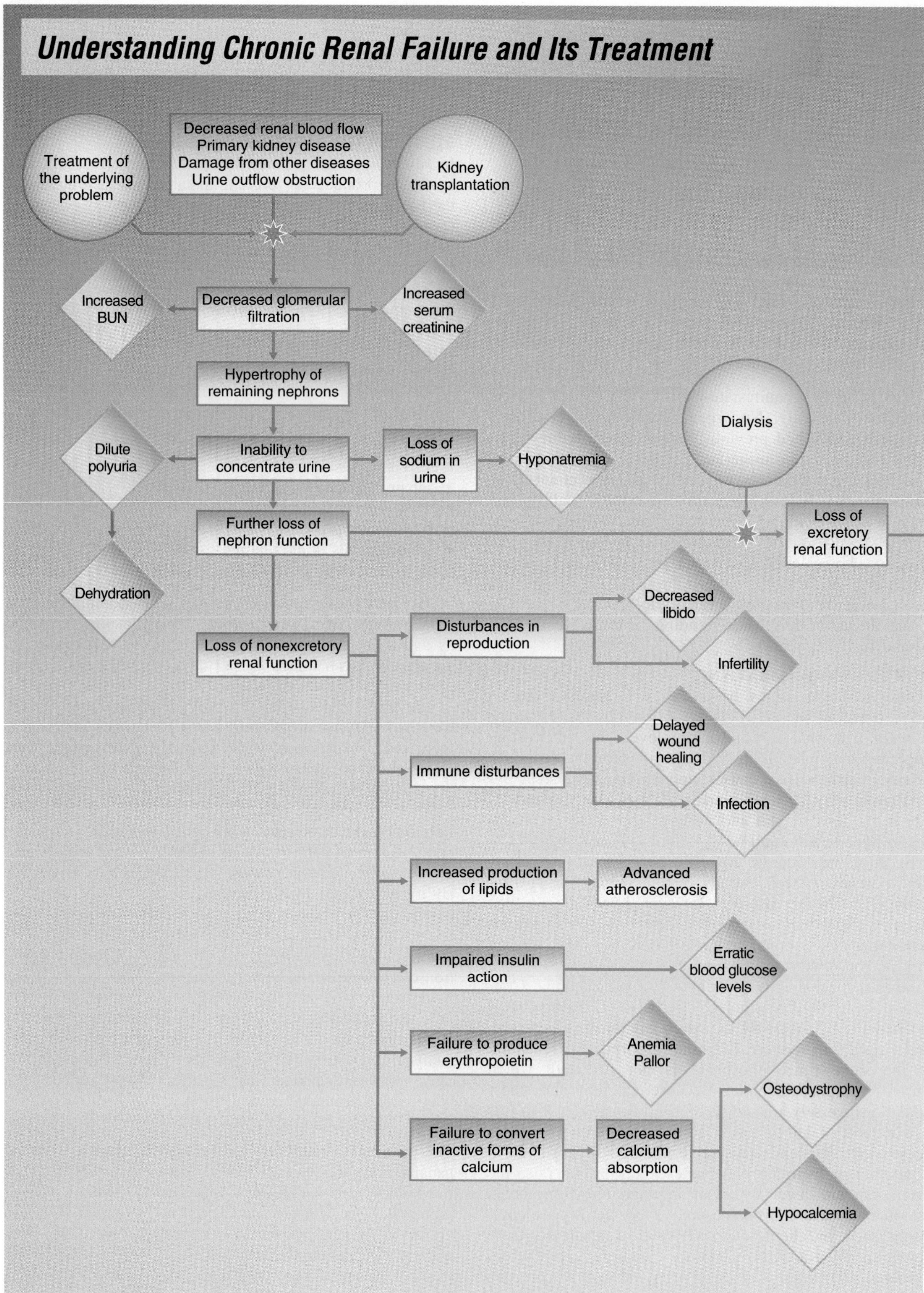
Understanding Chronic Renal Failure and Its Treatment
Treatment of the underlying problem
Decreased renal blood flow
Primary kidney disease
Damage from other diseases
Urine outflow obstruction
Kidney transplantation
Increased BUN
Decreased glomerular filtration
Increased serum creatinine
Hypertrophy of remaining nephrons
Dialysis
Dilute polyuria
Inability to concentrate urine
Loss of sodium in urine
Hyponatremia
Further loss of nephron function
Loss of excretory renal function
Dehydration
Decreased libido
Loss of nonexcretory renal function
Disturbances in reproduction
Infertility
Delayed wound healing
Immune disturbances
Infection
Increased production of lipids
Advanced atherosclerosis
Impaired insulin action
Erratic blood glucose levels
Failure to produce erythropoietin
Anemia
Pallor
Osteodystrophy
Failure to convert inactive forms of calcium
Decreased calcium absorption
Hypocalcemia

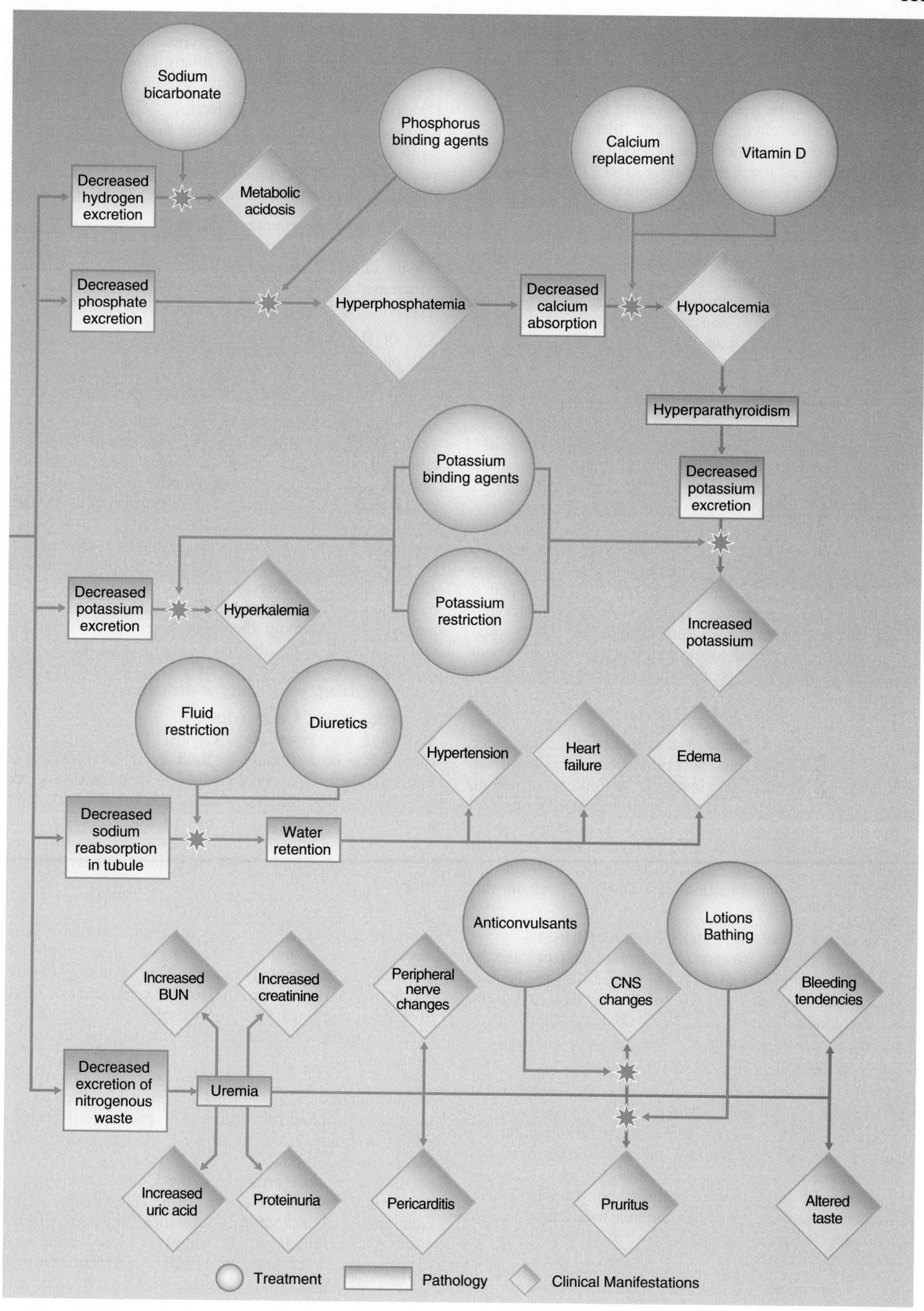

■ BUN, blood urea nitrogen; CNS, central nervous system.

The mild anemia found in the early stages is usually due to reduced production of the hormone, erythropoietin, which results in decreased production of red blood cells. Later, hemolysis, gastrointestinal losses, and clotting abnormalities contribute to the severity of the condition. Occasionally, the client has iron or folate depletion because of nutritional deficiencies. Bleeding tendencies become apparent as the disease progresses. Platelet abnormalities are the primary defect responsible for bleeding in the uremic client. The accumulation of uremic toxins interferes with platelet adhesiveness.

Gastrointestinal Changes

The entire gastrointestinal system is affected. Transient anorexia, nausea, and vomiting are almost universal. Clients often experience a constant bitter, metallic, or salty taste, and their breath commonly smells fetid, fishy, or ammonia-like. Stomatitis, parotitis, and gingivitis are common problems because of poor oral hygiene and the formation of ammonia from salivary urea. Accumulations of gastrin (from increased secretion of gastric acid) may be a major cause of ulcer disease. Esophagitis, gastritis, colitis, gastrointestinal bleeding, and diarrhea may be present. Serum amylase levels may be increased, although they do not necessarily indicate pancreatitis.

Constipation is a common problem. It often results from phosphate-binding agents; restriction of fluids and high-fiber foods, many of which are rich in potassium and phosphorus; and decreased activity. Constipation is a particular challenge because many of the usual interventions to prevent it (i.e., adding fruits, vegetables, and grains to the diet) and to treat it (e.g., magnesium-containing laxatives) are contraindicated for a client with renal failure.

Immunologic Changes

Impairment of the immune system makes the client more susceptible to infection. Several factors are involved, including depression of humoral antibody formation, suppression of delayed hypersensitivity, and decreased chemotactic function of the leukocytes. Immunosuppression is an important part of the medical management of renal diseases such as glomerulonephritis. Immunosuppression after transplantation is discussed later in this chapter.

Changes in Medication Metabolism

CRF has a serious effect on the metabolism of medications. The uremic client is at high risk for medication toxicity because of the effect of renal changes on the pharmacokinetics (absorption, distribution, metabolism, and excretion) of otherwise therapeutic medications. There are three main causes of this toxicity:

- A high plasma level of the medication caused by low serum albumin, decreased binding sites, impaired renal excretion, or impaired hepatic metabolism of the drug
- Increased sensitivity to the medication because of uremia-induced changes in the target organ
- A metabolic load due to administration of the medication; for example, hypoalbuminemia means less protein available for binding

Various tables and formulas are available to help guide dosage decisions. Remember, medication dosages must be altered and the usual dosage ranges are not safe for a client with CRF. Assess the client carefully for toxic reactions. Keep in mind that many medications, particularly water-soluble ones, are removed by dialysis.

Cardiovascular Changes

Between 50% and 65% of deaths that occur during CRF result from cardiovascular complications. The most common clinical manifestation is hypertension (which may also be the cause of renal failure), produced through:

- Mechanisms of volume overload
- Stimulation of the renin-angiotensin system
- Sympathetically mediated vasoconstriction; for example, increased levels of dopamine β-hydroxylase
- Absence of prostaglandins

Any of the many systemic complications of prolonged high blood pressure may be found.

The effects of volume overload on the heart are seen, including left ventricular hypertrophy and congestive heart failure. Heart failure may also result from anemia, vascular access, complications of coronary artery disease, electrolyte imbalance, acidosis, myocardial calcification, and thiamine depletion. Dysrhythmias may be caused by hyperkalemia, acidosis, hypermagnesemia, and decreased coronary perfusion.

Atherosclerosis is accelerated because of abnormal carbohydrate and lipid metabolism; impaired fibrinolysis, which leads to the development of microemboli; and hyperparathyroidism. Arterial calcifications have been identified, the ankles being the most common early location. Other sites include the abdominal aorta, feet, pelvis, hands, and wrists. These vascular calcifications also occur within the heart, particularly at the mitral valve.

Respiratory Changes

Some of the respiratory effects, such as pulmonary edema, can be attributed to fluid overload. Pleuritis is a frequent finding, especially when pericarditis develops. A characteristic condition called *uremic lung* is a type of pneumonitis that responds well to fluid removal. Metabolic acidosis causes a compensatory increase in respiratory rate as the lungs try to eliminate excess hydrogen ions.

Musculoskeletal Changes

The musculoskeletal system is affected fairly early in the disease process, and up to 90% of clients with CRF experience renal osteodystrophy. This condition develops insidiously and takes several forms: osteomalacia, osteitis fibrosa, osteoporosis, and osteosclerosis. The etiologic mechanism involves the kidney-bone-parathyroid and calcium-phosphate-vitamin D connections. As the GFR decreases, phosphate excretion decreases and calcium elimination increases. Abnormal levels of calcium and phosphate stimulate the release of parathyroid hormone, which mobilizes calcium from the bones and facilitates phosphate excretion.

As renal failure progresses, the kidney no longer converts vitamin D to its active form, 1,25-dihydroxycholecalciferol. The lack of this substance interferes with calcium absorption from the intestine and paradoxically facilitates phosphate retention. Thus, mineralization of the bone with calcium and phosphate is impaired. Demineralization of the bone frees more calcium and phosphorus into the blood. As the disease progresses, the parathyroid gland may become unresponsive to the normal feedback system and continue to produce parathyroid hormone, accelerating renal osteodystrophy. Partial parathyroidectomy is the treatment of choice when hypercalcemia and high plasma levels of parathyroid hormone cannot be controlled with medication.

In addition to bone demineralization, this process leads to deposition of calcium in subcutaneous, vascular, and visceral tissues throughout the body. In advanced stages, joint pain is severe. The client may also report diffuse and generalized bone and muscle pain. Bone deformities and frequent fractures are common. In children, bones fail to calcify, causing growth retardation. Tissue calcifications may be lethal if they develop in vital tissues, such as cerebral, coronary, or pulmonary vessels.

Some clients complain of muscle cramps. These may result from osmolar changes in the body fluids or sometimes hypocalcemia.

Integumentary Changes

Integumentary problems are particularly uncomfortable for some clients with CRF. The skin is also often very dry because of atrophy of the sweat glands. Severe and intractable pruritus may result from secondary hyperparathyroidism and calcium deposits in the skin. Pruritus can lead to excoriated skin because of continued scratching.

Several color changes affecting the skin are found in clients with renal failure. A bleeding tendency often results in increased braising, petechiae, and purpura. These do not usually cause problems themselves, but their presence may be alarming to the client. The pallor of anemia is evident. The cause of retained urochrome pigments, making the skin orange-green or gray in color, is not clear.

Hair is brittle and tends to fall out; nails are thin and brittle as well. Characteristic red bands that develop on the nails are called Muercke's lines. Another nail pattern that has been observed is a "half-and-half" nail, with the proximal half normally white and the distal portion brown.

Neurologic Changes

Although dialysis has reduced the incidence of neurologic changes, some clients experience these problems early in the disease process. Peripheral neuropathy causes many manifestations, such as burning feet, inability to find a comfortable position for the legs and feet (restless legs syndrome), gait changes, footdrop, and paraplegia. These manifestations move up the legs and may extend to include the arms. Initially, it is primarily a problem of the sensory system; however, if left untreated, it may progress to the motor system. Nerve conduction becomes slower, and deep tendon reflexes and vibratory sense are diminished.

Central nervous system involvement is demonstrated through forgetfulness, inability to concentrate, short attention span, impaired reasoning ability and judgment, impaired cognitive functioning, increased nervous irritability, nystagmus, twitching, dysarthria, seizures, central nervous system depression, and coma. Involvement of the cranial nerves may alter any of the senses. Hearing threshold levels show a high-frequency deficit early in the disease, and hearing progressively deteriorates. Uremic amaurosis is the sudden onset of bilateral blindness, which seems to be reversed in hours to days. The eyes often contain calcium salts, which give them an irritated appearance.

Reproductive Changes

Reproductive system changes can be alarming. Women commonly experience menstrual irregularities, particularly amenorrhea (absence of menstrual periods), and infertility. However, some women with CRF have conceived and had successful term pregnancies. Men commonly report impotence of both physiologic and psychological causes. They may also experience testicular atrophy, oligospermia (decreased sperm count), and reduced sperm motility. Both sexes report decreased libido, possibly from both physiologic and psychological factors.

Endocrine Changes

CRF also affects the endocrine system, such as the insulin utilization and parathyroid function discussed already. Pituitary hormones, such as growth hormone and prolactin, may be increased in some people. The levels of luteinizing hormone and follicle-stimulating hormone vary greatly from client to client. Thyroid-stimulating hormone is usually normal, but it may show a blunted response to thyrotropin-releasing hormone; this commonly results in hypothyroidism.

Psychosocial Changes

Psychosocial changes probably result from both the physiologic alterations and the extreme stress experienced by a client who has a chronic, life-threatening disease. Common stressors include feelings of powerlessness and lack of control over the illness and treatment, intrusive therapy, restrictions imposed by the medical regimen, changes in body image, and changes in sexuality.

Clients commonly suffer from role reversal, loss or reduction of work, financial strain, and many lifestyle changes. Scheduling dialysis can create many difficulties. The client's self-concept and body image may be altered, leading to further problems with work and relationships.

People cope with these stressors in various ways, and not all coping strategies are positive. They can range from obtaining support from family and friends and seeking more information about the condition to depression and thoughts of suicide. Indeed, helping a client cope with psychosocial changes will be one of the hardest nursing challenges you face.

Prognosis

The survival rate of people with CRF has improved with the advent and improvement of dialysis and transplantation. At 1 year after dialysis begins, the survival rate is about 79%. After 5 years, it drops to 33%.[16, 45]

Outcome Management

Medical Management

Conservative intervention does not cure CRF, but it may slow the progress of the disease. Eventually, most clients need renal replacement therapy. However, even successful dialysis and transplantation do not preclude the potential for death from complications of renal failure or its treatment.

After correcting contributing factors, control of blood pressure and fluid and dietary adjustments are the mainstays of conservative intervention for a client with CRF. The five goals of medical management are:

- To preserve renal function
- To delay the need for dialysis or transplantation as long as feasible
- To alleviate extrarenal manifestations as much as possible
- To improve body chemistry values
- To provide an optimal quality of life for the client and significant others

Preserve Renal Function and Delay Dialysis

Preservation of renal function can delay the need for dialysis therapy. It can be accomplished by controlling the disease process (see Chapter 35), by controlling blood pressure, and by reducing dietary protein intake and catabolism.

CRF commonly causes hypertension, which accelerates kidney damage. Good blood pressure control helps to preserve renal function. Blood pressure can be controlled through diet, weight control, and medications (see Chapters 35 and 52).

Specific adjustments of dietary elements often depend on the results of the client's blood chemistry studies. Although there is some debate over whether and how to restrict proteins, keeping the daily intake of protein of high biologic value below 50 g may slow the progression of renal failure. Generally, recommendations range from no restriction other than avoiding high-protein fad diets to a restriction to 1 g/kg/day. This protein must be of high biologic value so that the essential amino acids can be used more efficiently with less nitrogenous waste. This restriction of proteins also limits accumulation of acid, potassium, and phosphate.

It is also important to provide adequate nonprotein calories to prevent or reduce catabolism. One recommendation is a carbohydrate and fat intake of 40 to 50 kcal/kg/day. As the renal disease progresses, the client's ability and willingness to take in adequate nutrition diminish and the challenge becomes not only to maintain appropriate intake of nonprotein calories but also to satisfy protein needs. In these instances, elemental diets, enteral feedings, or TPN may be used instead of or in addition to regular food intake.

Alleviate Extrarenal Manifestations

Pruritus can be very annoying. Many interventions have been tried, including topical emollients and lotions, antihistamines, intravenous lidocaine, and ultraviolet B light, but relief has been inconsistent and usually temporary. Subtotal parathyroidectomy has sometimes helped, but there have been reports of recurrence. Effective dialysis seems to relieve the manifestations for many clients.

Neurologic manifestations require safety measures to protect the client from injury. Anticonvulsants and sedatives may be used. Phenothiazines are potentiated by uremia and should be avoided. The rise of uremic toxins causes a reduction in cognitive functioning, and patience is required in explaining things to the client.

The hematologic changes can also be treated medically. Therapy with epoetin alfa three times a week helps to stimulate the production of red blood cells. Supplemental iron, vitamin B_{12}, and folic acid are usually administered as well.

Improve Body Chemistry

The client's body chemistry can be improved through dialysis, medications, and diet. Dialysis removes excess water and nitrogenous wastes, reducing the manifestations of renal failure. Dialysis can be used temporarily if the client has ARF or as a permanent, life-sustaining treatment if the client has CRF. In the latter case, dialysis must continue for the rest of the client's life unless a successful kidney transplantation is performed.

Dialysis is also used to control uremia and to physically prepare the client to receive a transplanted kidney. Dialysis is usually necessary to keep the client alive until a suitable donor kidney is found. If the transplanted kidney does not immediately function adequately, dialysis may help prevent uremia until the kidney begins functioning sufficiently.

The four basic goals of dialysis therapy are:

- To remove the end products of protein metabolism, such as urea and creatinine, from the blood
- To maintain a safe concentration of serum electrolytes
- To correct acidosis and replenish the blood's bicarbonate levels
- To remove excess fluid from the blood

Principles of ultrafiltration and diffusion are used to accomplish the goals of dialysis. *Ultrafiltration* refers to removal of fluid from the blood using either osmotic or hydrostatic pressure to produce the necessary gradient. *Diffusion* is the passage of particles (ions) from an area of high concentration to an area of low concentration. Both processes occur across a semipermeable membrane with pores large enough to allow certain particles (such as urea, creatinine, and electrolytes) to pass through but too small to allow the passage of larger particles (such as protein and red blood cells). When the two solutions are separated by a semipermeable membrane, solute particles move toward the solution of lower concentration. Simultaneously, water moves toward the solution of higher solute concentration.

Solute particles and water can move freely across the membrane in either direction between the blood and the dialysate. Thus, if the blood has a higher concentration of urea, creatinine, and certain electrolytes than does the prepared dialysate solution, these particles move into the dialysate solution, lowering the level in the blood. If the blood is deficient in a substance, such as bicarbonate, the higher concentration of this substance in the dialysate causes it to move into the blood, raising the blood level.

There are two types of dialysis: *peritoneal dialysis* and *hemodialysis.* The semipermeable membrane in the dialyzer or "artificial kidney" used is either the peritoneal membrane (for peritoneal dialysis) or an artificial membrane (for hemodialysis). The blood and a specially prepared electrolyte solution, called the *dialysate,* are placed in compartments on opposite sides of the membrane. The tendency is always toward equalization of the concentrations of the two solutions.

Peritoneal Dialysis

Peritoneal dialysis involves repeated cycles of instilling dialysate into the peritoneal cavity, allowing time for substance exchange, and then removing the dialysate. The procedure is useful for both ARF and CRF and for fluid and electrolyte imbalances. It has been used to treat overdoses of drugs and toxins, but because its clearance is much slower than that with hemodialysis, it may not be satisfactory for this purpose.

One of the primary advantages of peritoneal dialysis is its relative ease, which allows it to be used in community health care facilities without all the sophisticated equipment needed for hemodialysis. It can be easily managed at home and commonly allows the client more independence and mobility than hemodialysis does.

Peritoneal dialysis is typically used for clients with severe cardiovascular disease, especially those whose problems would be worsened by the rapid changes in urea, glucose, electrolytes, and fluid volume that occur during hemodialysis. Some physicians prescribe peritoneal dialysis for diabetic clients to reduce the risk of retinal hemorrhage associated with the heparin used during hemodialysis and because good blood glucose control can be achieved by adding insulin to the dialysate. Peritoneal dialysis is the dialysis treatment of choice for children because it seems to have less effect on growth.

Contraindications to peritoneal dialysis include hypercatabolism, in which peritoneal dialysis cannot adequately clear uremic toxins, and poor condition of the peritoneal membrane because of adhesions or scarring. Relative contraindications to peritoneal dialysis include obesity, a history of ruptured diverticula, abdominal disease, respiratory disease, recurrent episodes of peritonitis, abdominal malignancies, severe vascular disease, back problems (because the increased weight of fluid may increase back strain), and extensive abdominal surgery with drains or tubes that may increase the risk of infection.

TYPES OF PERITONEAL DIALYSIS. Several types of peritoneal dialysis are in use today. The most common are continuous ambulatory and automated peritoneal dialysis.

Continuous Ambulatory Peritoneal Dialysis (CAPD). In the continuous type of peritoneal dialysis, 1.5 to 3.0 L of dialysate is instilled into the abdomen and left in place for a prescribed period of time. The empty dialysate bag is folded up and carried in a pouch or pocket until it is time to drain the dialysate. The bag is then unfolded and placed lower than the insertion site so that the fluid drains by gravity flow. When full, the bag is changed and new dialysate is instilled into the abdomen as the process continues.

Another version of this procedure is the disconnect system. With this system, the client removes the empty dialysate bag after inflow and attaches a protective cap to the dialysis catheter. A new sterile bag is used for each drainage and infusion, which eliminates the need to wear the tubing and bag between exchanges.

CAPD usually uses four dialysis cycles every 24 hours, including an 8-hour dwell overnight. There are two major advantages. First, because there is no need for machinery, electricity, or a water source, the client can go about almost any desired activity during dialysis. Second, because the continuous exchange process closely resembles normal renal function, the body more easily maintains homeostasis, allowing fewer dietary and fluid restrictions. For management of diabetic clients, insulin can be added to the dialysate.

See Bridge to Home Health Care.

Automated Peritoneal Dialysis. Automated peritoneal dialysis necessitates use of a peritoneal cycling machine. This method can be performed as continuous cyclic, intermittent, or nightly intermittent peritoneal dialysis.

Continuous cyclic peritoneal dialysis. In this variation, there are usually three cycles at night and one cycle with an 8-hour dwell in the morning. The advantage of this procedure is that the peritoneal catheter is opened only for the on-and-off procedures, which reduces the risk of infection. Another advantage is that the client does not require exchanges at work or school.

Intermittent peritoneal dialysis. This is not a continuous dialysis procedure. Instead, dialysis is performed for 10 to 14 hours, three to four times a week, by the same peritoneal cycling machine as in continuous cyclic peritoneal dialysis. Hospitalized clients may be dialyzed for 24 to 48 hours at a time if they are catabolic and require additional dialysis time.

Nightly intermittent peritoneal dialysis. Dialysis is performed for 8 to 12 hours each night with no daytime dwells.

PERITONEAL DIALYSIS PROCEDURES. Several steps are involved.

Peritoneal Catheter Insertion. For a client who needs peritoneal dialysis, one of several types of soft catheters is inserted through the abdominal wall and into the peritoneal cavity. Usually, the catheter is inserted in the operating room, with the client under local anesthesia, although it may be inserted at the client's bedside. The client is medicated before the procedure to provide relaxation and to reduce discomfort.

The preferred insertion site is 3 to 5 cm below the umbilicus, an area that is relatively avascular and has relatively low fascial resistance. Figure 36–2 illustrates three types of peritoneal catheters. The Tenckhoff catheter has two polyester (Dacron) felt cuffs bonded to the catheter. Over a period of 1 to 2 weeks, there is an ingrowth of fibroblasts and blood vessels into the cuffs, which fix the catheter in place and provide an effective barrier against dialysate leakage and bacterial invasion. Note in Figure 36–2 that a subcutaneous tunnel is created for the catheter to reduce direct bacterial invasion into the peritoneum. The other catheters illustrated have cuffs to provide stability.

Dialysate. The dialysate is usually allowed to run into the peritoneal cavity by gravity flow. It is warmed slightly to avoid chilling the client and to dilate the peritoneal blood vessels, thus facilitating substance exchange. In an adult 2 L is usually instilled, although smaller amounts may be needed at first until the client adjusts. Throughout the procedure, care must be taken to prevent air from entering the peritoneal cavity.

The *dwell time* is the period during which the dialysate is left in the peritoneal cavity. In intermittent peritoneal dialysis, equilibrium between the dialysate and the body fluids usually occurs within 15 to 30 minutes, with the maximum exchange during the first 5 minutes. Therefore, the solution is typically left in place 30 to 45 minutes for manual dialysis or 10 to 20 minutes when an automatic

BRIDGE TO HOME HEALTH CARE

Living with Peritoneal Dialysis

When you admit clients to home health services who have end-stage renal disease, are starting peritoneal dialysis, and have Medicare benefits, you will be collaborating with physicians and the staff of the peritoneal dialysis unit. The unit staff is the designated provider of total services, including nursing services. Clinic nurses can and do make limited visits; a peritoneal dialysis nurse is on 24-hour call.

You are involved when clients need Medicare-reimbursed services in addition to dialysis treatments. While you provide care, it is important to discuss what the life of your client and the client's family was like before the recent hospitalization, what they know about dialysis, and how long they expect the client to receive dialysis. Share both physical and psychosocial information with the other health care team members to help clients and their families consider their options and adapt their lifestyles and home to the requirements of peritoneal dialysis.

Hospitals have sophisticated equipment readily available and are treatment oriented. When clients return home, home health nurses can suggest ways to improve the quality of daily life and decrease the focus on technology. For example, the nurse may suggest an alternative way to hang the bags for the dialysis solution, such as hooking the bag on a hanger and a door frame or using a floor-style plant hanger rather than a pole for intravenous solutions. When clients have continuous ambulatory peritoneal dialysis (CAPD), the solution runs for 4 to 10 hours four times per day. Because no machinery, electricity, or water source is required, clients can go about most of their daily activities. Clients have fewer dietary and fluid restrictions, and they maintain better homeostasis. When clients have ambulatory peritoneal dialysis (APD), the solution dwells for 4 to 10 hours before being changed four times per day. Often a dwell time of 8 hours is used during the daytime with three shorter cycles being completed during the night. Clients have less freedom to move about and go about daily activities. Although APD requires a peritoneal cycling machine, it can be scheduled as a continuous, intermittent, or nightly procedure.

Instruct clients and their families to watch for untoward manifestations. A drop in blood pressure can cause dizziness or faintness, and elevated blood pressure can cause headaches. Fluid overload can cause shortness of breath. If clients experience any of these manifestations, they should notify the nurse or physician immediately.

When assessing psychosocial issues, the home health nurse should identify barriers to care and determine how much responsibility clients can assume for self-care and how much assistance they need. If clients feel depressed or lack confidence, they may not follow instructions involving the dialysis procedure, their diet and fluid intake, or their medications. The nurse needs to offer support and allow the client and family members to ask questions and verbalize concerns. The entire dialysis process might involve much more than clients and family had expected. Suggest involving friends or neighbors who can be taught about peritoneal dialysis and become part of the client's and family's support system. Discuss other appropriate community resources such as spiritual and financial counselors. Provide information about resources and support groups available through the National Kidney Foundation (1-800-622-9010) or the American Kidney Fund (1-800-638-8299).

Shawnda M. Braun, RN, *Case Manager, Allied Health Alternatives, Inc., Faribault, Minnesota*

cycler is used. The fluid is then allowed to run out through the catheter by gravity. In continuous ambulatory and automated peritoneal dialysis procedures, the dwell time is prolonged to 4 to 8 hours with a solution that allows continuous exchange and better clearance of certain elements.

Cycles. The number of dialysis cycles depends on the normalization of body fluids and blood chemistries, as indicated by laboratory studies. Peritoneal clearance is influenced by several factors, including the size of the membrane area, blood flow to the peritoneum, and alterations in the permeability of the peritoneal membrane.

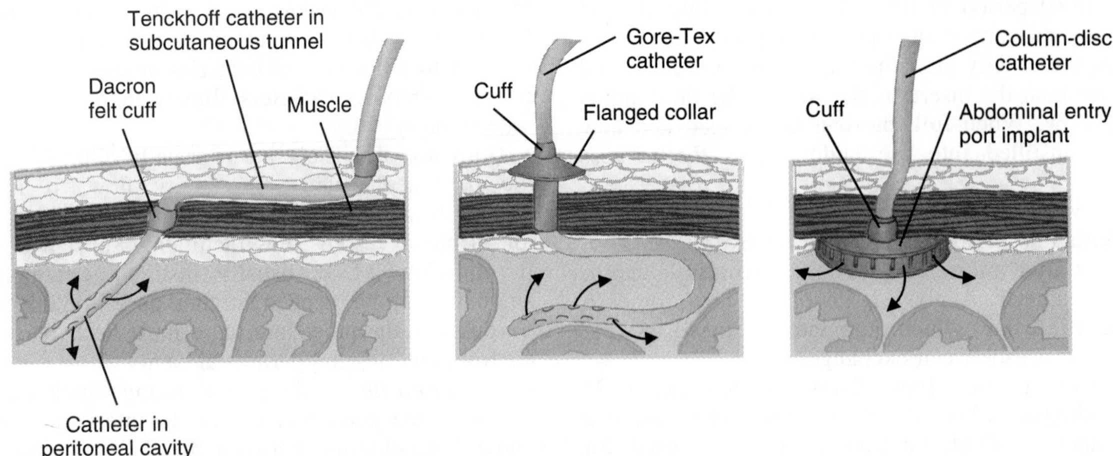

FIGURE 36–2 Three types of peritoneal dialysis catheters. The Tenckhoff catheter has two polyester (Dacron) felt cuffs that hold the catheter in place and prevent dialysate leakage and bacterial invasion; a subcutaneous tunnel also helps to prevent infection. The Gore-Tex catheter has a Dacron cuff above a flanged collar. The column-disc catheter has a cuff and a large abdominal entry port implant.

Complications of Peritoneal Dialysis. Although peritoneal dialysis is considered a safe procedure, a number of complications can be attributed to it.

Peritonitis. Peritonitis is the major concern; therefore, meticulous aseptic technique must be maintained during handling of the catheter, tubing, and dialysate solution. Bacteria may enter the peritoneal cavity through contaminated dialysis fluid, a contaminated catheter lumen, or the catheter insertion site.

Clinical evidence of peritonitis includes fever, rebound abdominal tenderness, nausea, malaise, and a cloudy dialysate output. Laboratory tests routinely used to diagnose peritonitis include white blood cell counts with differential, culture, and sensitivity and Gram's stain of the peritoneal fluid. Peritonitis is the diagnosis when the dialysate white blood cell count is above 100/mm^3 and neutrophils are above 50%. The causative organism does not always grow in routine cultures, but Gram's stain is positive in up to 40% of the samples.

If peritonitis develops, appropriate antibiotics are added to the dialysate; in addition, systemic antibiotics may be used.

Catheter-Related Complications. Catheter problems include displacement and obstruction. Obstruction may be due to malposition, adherence of the catheter tip to the omentum, or infection. Constipation can reduce catheter flow, possibly because peristalsis facilitates outflow. A bisacodyl suppository may be used prophylactically even if the client is not constipated. Fluid leakage may indicate improper catheter function, incomplete healing of the insertion site, or excessive instillation.

Especially in the early stages, it is sometimes necessary to use small-volume instillations. Bloody effluent is usually insignificant and disappears spontaneously. Heparin may be added to the dialysate to prevent fibrin clot formation in a new catheter or after treatment for peritonitis. Also be aware of the possibility of bowel perforation, which is most likely to occur in cachectic (profoundly ill and malnourished) clients or those who have abdominal adhesions. Fecal material returned in the dialysate or massive diarrhea after instillation may also signal perforation. Bladder perforation can also occur if the bladder has not been emptied before catheter insertion.

Dialysis-Related Complications. Pain during dialysis may result from rapid instillation, incorrect dialysate pH or temperature, dialysate accumulation under the diaphragm, or excessive suction during outflow. Some pain is expected in the early stages but should disappear after 1 to 2 weeks. Low back pain may develop with continuous dialysis procedures because the abdominal weight affects posture; appropriate exercises help relieve this problem. Hernia may occur. Systemic cardiovascular and neurologic effects are usually the result of fluid and electrolyte imbalances. Especially during small-volume exchanges, a significant amount of dialysate fluid may be absorbed by the body.

Hypotension may result from too rapid removal of fluid. Overhydration, from insufficient fluid removal, may be manifested as heart failure and pulmonary edema. Hypoalbuminemia leading to hypovolemia often occurs because the peritoneal membrane allows the passage of albumin, as much as 100 g/day if the client is infected. It is especially a problem if dietary intake of protein is poor, the client is infected, or dialysis treatment is used for several consecutive days. Hyperglycemia may occur in diabetic clients as a result of absorption of glucose from the dialysate and electrolyte changes. These clients require extra insulin. Respiratory difficulties may occur during dwell time because of pressure on the diaphragm. Weight gain may occur because of the high concentration of glucose in the dialysate.

Outcomes. Long-term outcomes associated with peritoneal dialysis are considered good. The treatment is usually effective for years. However, scarring of the peritoneum and repeated infections may require a change to hemodialysis.

Hemodialysis

Hemodialysis is used for clients with acute or irreversible renal failure and fluid and electrolyte imbalances. It is usually the treatment of choice when toxic agents, such as barbiturates after an overdose, need to be removed from the body quickly.

Historical Overview. The first artificial kidney was developed in 1943 in The Netherlands. In 1960, the first successful treatment of clients with CRF was reported. In the early years, although the technology was available, the exorbitant cost and lack of equipment required a stringent selection process in choosing clients for hemodialysis. Clients were screened on the basis of their motivation, intelligence, emotional stability, and rehabilitative potential. In essence, it had to be decided who among the many potential candidates would best be able to cope with the program and who would make the biggest contribution to society.

In 1972, an amendment to the Social Security Act required that anyone with CRF be able to have any lifesaving treatment needed. In 1973, Medicare took over the financial responsibility for many clients receiving hemodialysis. Thus, availability of this treatment for clients with end-stage renal failure has become more prevalent. Generally, self-selection is the only criterion used now. As a result, the population receiving hemodialysis now represents a wide cross-section of age, rehabilitative potential, and socioeconomic status. There continue to be problems with selection of appropriate candidates, when to start, and when and how to stop. With the reduction in available health care dollars, the problems associated with selection criteria will only increase.

Hemodialysis Procedure. In hemodialysis, the client's toxin-laden blood is diverted into a dialyzer, cleaned, and then returned to the client (Fig. 36–3). While the blood is in the dialyzer, a mechanical proportioning pump causes dialysis fluid to flow on the other side of the membrane (Fig. 36–4). Toxins diffuse across the membrane from the blood to the dialysate. Strict asepsis must be maintained throughout the procedure.

One of the vital aspects of hemodialysis is the establishment and maintenance of adequate blood access. Without it, hemodialysis cannot be done. The major routes of access are external arteriovenous shunts and subclavian catheters for acute dialysis and internal arteriovenous fistulas and grafts for chronic dialysis.

The external arteriovenous shunt requires surgical placement of two rubber-like silicone (Silastic) cannulas into the forearm or leg. The two cannulas are connected

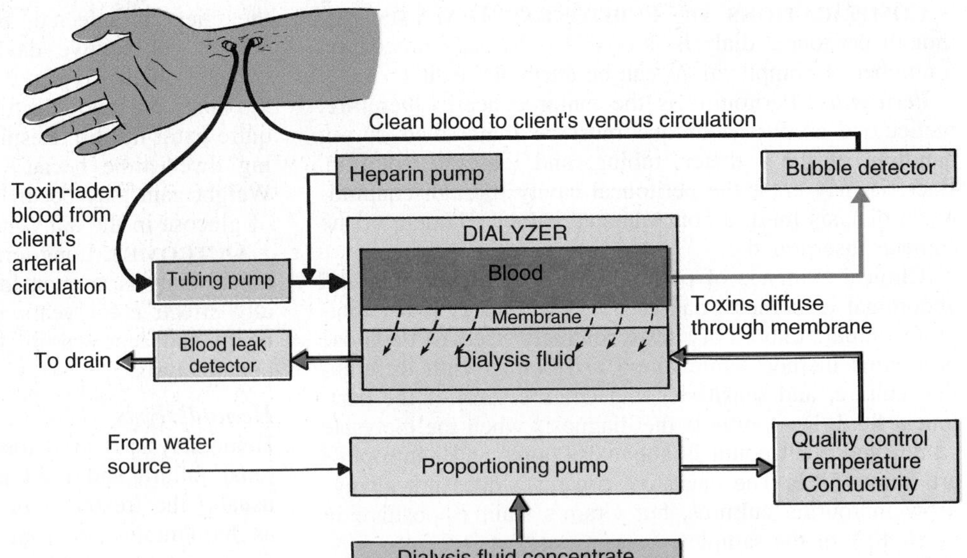

FIGURE 36–3 Typical hemodialysis system. Toxin-laden blood from the client diffuses across the membrane within the dialyzer into the dialysis fluid. Clean blood is returned to the client.

to form a U shape. Blood flows from the client's artery through the shunt into the vein.

When the client is to be connected to the hemodialyzer, a tube leading to the membrane compartment is connected to the arterial cannula. Blood then fills the membrane compartment and flows back to the client by way of a tube connected to the venous cannula. When dialysis is completed, the arterial cannula is clamped. Once the blood in the membrane compartment has been returned to the body, the venous cannula is clamped and the ends of the two cannulas are reattached to form their U. This access can be created quickly and thus is particularly suitable when dialysis must be started immediately.

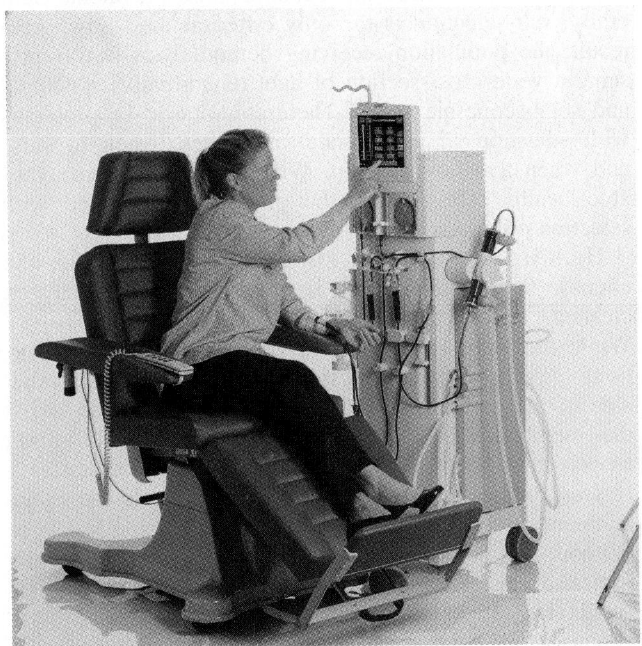

FIGURE 36–4 A client undergoing outpatient hemodialysis. (Reprinted with permission from Althin Medical, Inc., Miami Lakes, FL.)

Infection at the insertion site and clotting are complications that often necessitate moving the cannula sites. Other problems that occur with shunts are accidental dislodgment, hemorrhage, and skin erosion.

The internal arteriovenous fistula is the access of choice for clients receiving chronic dialysis. The fistula is created through a surgical procedure in which an artery in the arm is anastomosed to a vein in an end-to-side, side-to-side, side-to-end, or end-to-end fashion (Fig. 36–5*A*). The result is an opening or fistula between a large artery and a large vein. The flow of arterial blood into the venous system causes the veins to become engorged (Fig. 36–5*B*). These fistulae require up to 6 weeks to mature before they can be used, which makes this approach inappropriate for immediate hemodialysis. Peritoneal dialysis or large venous access catheters may be used while the fistula is maturing. External arteriovenous shunts are rarely used.

The internal arteriovenous graft is used primarily for chronic dialysis. In this approach, an artificial graft made of water-repellent fabric (Gore-Tex) or a bovine carotid artery is used to create an artificial vein for blood flow. The graft is used in clients who do not have adequate blood vessels for surgical creation of a fistula. One end of the artificial graft is anastomosed to an artery, tunneled under the skin, and anastomosed to a vein. The graft can be used 2 weeks after insertion. Complications include clotting, aneurysms, and infection.

Once the fistula graft is placed and ready for use, two 15- or 16-gauge needles are placed in the access at each dialysis treatment (Fig. 36–5*C*). A pump pulls arterial blood out by way of the fistula and into the hemodialyzer. Blood returns to the client by a tube connected to the other needle. Alternatively, single-needle dialysis may be used. With this device, only one puncture is required each time, but there may be significant recirculation of dialyzed blood, meaning that clearance rates are decreased. Internal arteriovenous grafts may cause hand swelling or ischemia (steal syndrome), carpal tunnel syndrome, hemorrhage, thrombosis, and aneurysms. Besides the arm, the subclavian, thigh, and ankle areas may be used as sites for hemodialysis access.

Subclavian, jugular, and femoral catheters can be inserted at the bedside for vascular access or surgically placed in the operating room. Double-lumen catheters are usually used to provide access for both removal and return of blood. These catheters are usually a temporary source of vascular access and must be replaced frequently to prevent infection. Strict aseptic technique must be used during insertion, and dressing changes are usually performed by a limited number of trained nurses. Thrombosis and infection are the most common complications.

DIALYZERS. Several types of dialyzers are available, including flat plate and hollow fiber mold devices. Choice of a particular system is mostly a matter of preference. There are differences in urea and creatinine clearance rates as well as ultrafiltration rates. Many centers that perform chronic dialysis now reprocess and disinfect the unit and reuse it for the same client to reduce costs. The dialysate solution is altered to fit the client's need.

HEMODIALYSIS SCHEDULES. Hemodialysis as a treatment for CRF must be continued intermittently for the client's lifetime unless successful kidney transplantation is performed. A typical schedule is 3 to 4 hours of treatment 3 days per week. This schedule varies with the size of the client, the type of dialyzer used, the rate of blood flow, the personal preference of the client, and other factors.

THERAPEUTIC EFFECTS OF HEMODIALYSIS. The overall therapeutic effects of hemodialysis are to (1) clear waste products from the body; (2) restore fluid, electrolyte, and acid-base balances; and (3) reverse some of the untoward manifestations of irreversible renal failure. Success is varied. Excess fluid, potassium, urea nitrogen, and acid ions are removed but only temporarily; between dialyses, these elements build up again. Nutritionally, carbohydrate intolerance is usually reduced. Amino acids, protein, glucose, and water-soluble vitamins are lost. Anemia generally worsens because of blood loss associated with the therapy. The predialysis causative factors are still present, and additional losses occur during dialysis because of blood sampling, residual blood left in the dialyzer, and bleeding secondary to anticoagulation during dialysis. Serum iron stores are also further depleted.

Hyperlipidemia (elevated serum lipid levels) seems to increase and is associated with accelerated atherosclerosis. Renal osteodystrophy usually improves, and this can be further enhanced by adding calcium to the dialysate. Pruritus may occur for reasons not yet understood. Men who have maintenance dialysis often have low testosterone levels and develop gynecomastia, which is usually transient. Many other sexual manifestations of uremia are reversed after a period of adaptation.

The usual effect of hemodialysis on serum concentration of medications is increased clearance, which is therapeutic in the case of overdose. Dosage schedules are

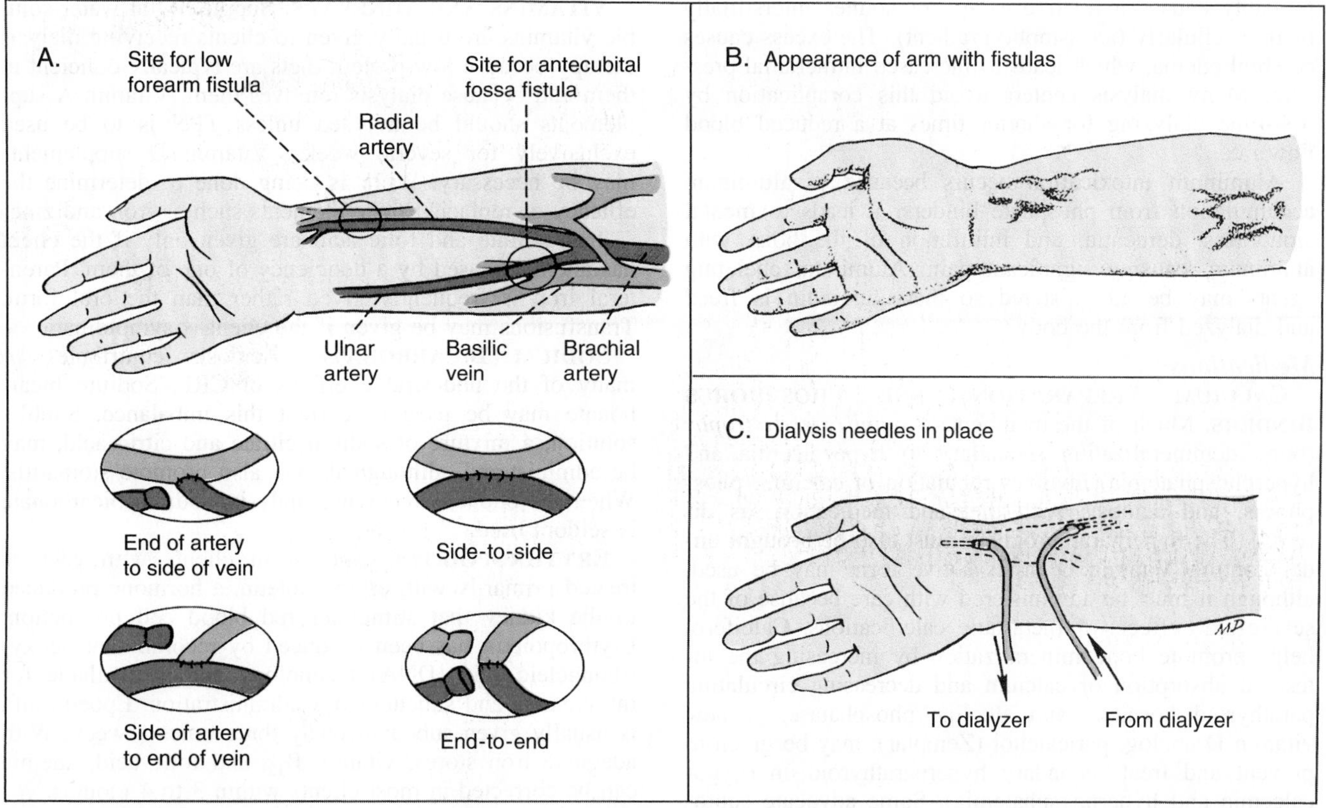

FIGURE 36–5 Internal arteriovenous fistula. Surgical creation of an arteriovenous anastomosis provides easy access to blood for hemodialysis. This method reduces the risk of infection and makes external shunts unnecessary except during hemodialysis. The internal fistula must be created 2 to 6 weeks before it can be used. In this illustration, arteries, not veins, are toned. *A,* Types of fistulas. *B,* Appearance of arm with fistulas. *C,* Dialysis needles in place.

altered to prevent, as much as possible, loss of medications through dialysis. Supplemental doses may be necessary to maintain therapeutic levels of certain medications.

COMPLICATIONS OF LONG-TERM HEMODIALYSIS. In addition to its therapeutic effects, chronic hemodialysis can cause a number of complications:

- Technical problems, such as blood leaks, overheating of the dialysate solution, insufficient loss of fluid, improper concentration of salts in the dialysate, and clotting
- Hypotension or hypertension
- Cardiac dysrhythmias from potassium imbalance
- Air embolus
- Hemorrhage resulting from heparinization with particular concern for subdural, retroperitoneal, pericardial, and intraocular bleeding
- Restless legs syndrome
- Pyrogenic reactions

Gastrointestinal ulcer disease is often complicated by hemorrhage. Muscle cramps may occur as a result of hyponatremia or hyposmolality and too rapid removal of fluid. Infection is a significant complication, with hepatitis B being a significant risk. Frequent infectious processes include local access infection, bacteremia, and infectious endocarditis.

Dialysis disequilibrium syndrome can occur, particularly during the client's first few dialysis episodes. It is characterized by mental confusion, deterioration of the level of consciousness, headache, and seizures. It may last for several days. Rapid solute removal from the blood probably causes a relative excess of solutes interstitially or intracellularly (an osmotic gradient). The excess causes cerebral edema, which leads to increased intracranial pressure. Many dialysis centers avoid this complication by first-time dialyzing for shorter times at a reduced blood flow rate.

Aluminum intoxication occurs because of aluminum accumulation from phosphate binders. It leads to mental cloudiness, dementia, and infiltration of the bone with aluminum, causing significant pain. Aluminum chelating agents may be administered so that aluminum is freed and dialyzed from the body.

Medications

CALCIUM PREPARATIONS AND PHOSPHORUS BINDERS. Much of the treatment of *renal osteodystrophy* (bone demineralization secondary to hypocalcemia and hyperphosphatemia) involves regulation of calcium, phosphorus, and acidosis with diet and medication, as directed. The hyperparathyroidism must also be brought under control. Vitamin D in its active form may be used, although it must be administered with care because of the severe side effects of metastatic calcifications. Calciferol helps promote bone mineralization by increasing the intestinal absorption of calcium and decreasing circulating parathyroid hormone and alkaline phosphatase. A new vitamin D analog, paricalcitol (Zemplar), may be given to prevent and treat secondary hyperparathyroidism (hypocalcemia and hyperphosphatemia). Some advocate subtotal parathyroidectomy if all other methods fail.

Phosphorus intake is usually limited to less than 1000 mg/day. To improve excretion of phosphorus, the client is given calcium-based phosphate binders such as calcium acetate or calcium carbonate. Aluminum-based antacids such as Alu-Cap, Amphojel, and Basaljel were formerly used to bind phosphorus so that it could be excreted in the feces. These medications are seldom used now because they increase the risk of dementia related to excessive absorption of aluminum.

ANTIHYPERTENSIVE AGENTS. Fluid regulation and sodium regulation are the major interventions in heart failure. Other cardiovascular manifestations are managed in much the same way as for clients without CRF, but diuretics are not used except in the early stages of conservative management. Hypertension must be aggressively controlled with stronger medications such as angiotensin-converting enzyme inhibitors and calcium-channel blockers. Antihypertensive drugs are administered as necessary in relation to renal function and nephrotic response.

DIURETICS. Diuretics may be used early to stimulate excretion of water by the kidneys. The appearance of edema indicates fluid overload, but some physicians prefer to have a little end-of-the-day edema so that it is more evident that fluid depletion is not a danger. Thirst is not a reliable indicator; if thirst were used as a guide, fluid overload would be inevitable. As renal failure progresses, diuretics are not effective and it usually becomes necessary to restrict fluid intake. Although authorities differ in the exact amounts, daily fluid allowances may be 400 to 1000 ml plus measured output. Diuretics are not given before dialysis because of potential problems with hypotension. Antihypertensive medications are also often withheld until after dialysis.

VITAMINS AND MINERALS. Supplemental water-soluble vitamins are usually given to clients receiving dialysis therapy because low-protein diets are typically deficient in them and because dialysis removes them. Vitamin A supplements should be avoided unless TPN is to be used exclusively for several weeks. Vitamin D supplements may be necessary. Work is being done to determine the efficacy of replacing trace elements such as iron and zinc.

Iron sulfate and folic acid are given only if the client has anemia caused by a deficiency of one of them. Parenteral iron is frequently given rather than the oral form. Transfusions may be given if the client is symptomatic.

SODIUM BICARBONATE. Acidosis contributes to many of the undesirable effects of CRF. Sodium bicarbonate may be used to correct this imbalance. Shohl's solution, a mixture of sodium citrate and citric acid, may be administered, although it may also promote stomatitis. When the client is receiving dialysis, sodium bicarbonate is seldom used.

ERYTHROPOIETIN. Anemia in clients with CRF is treated primarily with erythropoietin, a hormone produced in the kidney that stimulates red blood cell production. Erythropoietin has been produced by recombinant deoxyribonucleic acid (DNA) technology and is available for intravenous and subcutaneous administration. Epoetin alfa is usually given subcutaneously three times a week. With adequate iron stores, vitamin B_{12}, and folic acid, anemia can be corrected in most clients within 3 to 4 months.

Diet

Dietary adjustment is dictated by many components of CRF, including accumulation of nitrogenous waste products, impaired excretion of electrolytes, vitamin deficiencies, and continued catabolism. The wasting syndrome is a major problem. The client with renal failure constantly loses body weight, muscle mass, and adipose tissue.

Dietary intake of electrolytes may be encouraged or restricted. The regulation of sodium is a delicate matter. At times the kidneys waste salt, and sodium intake must be encouraged to replace it. More frequently, however, the kidneys retain sodium. Some believe that there should be moderate restriction with careful monitoring of urinary sodium excretion as a guideline. Serial monitoring of fluid status also gives important information about sodium needs. Many regimens are used.

Potassium is frequently restricted. Clients must be reminded not to use salt substitutes because they contain potassium chloride. When hyperkalemia becomes evident, restriction of potassium in food and fluids is instituted. In an emergency situation, when the serum potassium is above 7.0 mEq/L, the client may receive intravenous glucose (50% dextrose in water, $D_{50}W$) and insulin; oral or rectal sodium polystyrene sulfonate (Kayexalate), which is a cation exchange resin; or both. Dissolving the resin in ginger ale helps to prevent it from sticking to the client's teeth and helps to mask its gritty texture. Sorbitol is usually given with the resin to avoid constipation and counteract the sodium retention that can occur. Dialysis is also effective in removing potassium from the blood.

If serum calcium levels are low, adequate calcium intake is important. Dietary sources may be supplemented with calcium carbonate, calcium lactate, or calcium gluconate. Supplements are definitely needed for clients receiving dialysis therapy. If serum calcium levels are high, however, dietary restriction may be recommended. Phosphorus is restricted. In addition, calcium carbonate may be used to reduce phosphorus levels further. Finally, mild magnesium restriction may be imposed.

PROMOTE QUALITY OF LIFE

Renal failure and its therapies significantly affect the quality of life of the client and family members. As noted earlier, there are numerous stressors and life changes. Much of the care required by clients receiving chronic peritoneal dialysis and hemodialysis and their significant others concerns the psychosocial aspects of dialysis.

Clients receiving maintenance dialysis often have ambivalent feelings. They realize that dialysis therapy is their tie to life, but the many restrictions and lifestyle changes it imposes make continuation of the program extremely difficult. Clients often report that they feel in limbo between the worlds of life and death.

The process of adaptation to loss is part of adjustment. It is not uncommon for clients to feel grateful and optimistic at the start of dialysis treatments. Usually, they have felt ill for some time, and they view the intervention as a route to survival and feeling well again. It takes a few days or weeks for them to realize fully the permanent place of dialysis in their lives. Depression during this period is expected. The suicide rate among clients receiving dialysis has been estimated as 100 times that of the general population.

Common psychosocial problems include changes in body image, dependence on technology, and uncertainty regarding the future. The client's own feelings of weakness and illness and the presence of the arteriovenous fistula and dialysis equipment are constant reminders that the client is no longer a "whole person." These clients often play one of three roles:

- Professional client, in which all of life revolves around the dialysis
- Rebel, in which the client acts noncompliant or mischievous
- Adult, in which the client uses appropriate coping skills and is able to focus outward

Relationships with relatives and friends, job, and community roles and responsibilities are probably altered. The client's normal need for independence is continually threatened by dependence on the dialysis equipment and care providers. This is especially true of adolescents and young adults. Other emotional problems include the need for identity, safety, control of the environment, love, esteem, and communication. The stress on marital relationships and significant others is extreme.

Research suggests that the quality of life of people with ESRD is influenced positively by transplantation, erythropoietin therapy, social support, a positive outlook on life, and the ability to function (including work and activities of daily living). Providing an optimal quality of life involves a concerted effort by all members of the health care team with the client and family members as active partners. Many dialysis facilities have established active rehabilitation programs. Elements of these programs include education, exercise, encouragement, employment, and evaluation.[12, 26, 27]

Nursing Management of the Medical Client

ASSESSMENT

When a client is thought to have CRF, take a complete history and look closely for risk factors. Question the client about past and present medications, diet and weight changes, energy levels and unexplained fatigue, and the pattern of urinary elimination.

Assess the client for the multiple effects of CRF on all body systems, such as the presence of cardiovascular or respiratory abnormalities, neurologic changes, gastrointestinal problems, or skin changes.

Assess the client's understanding of CRF, the diagnostic tests that will be done, and the possible treatment regimens. Evaluate the client's level of anxiety and ability to cope. Involve the family in the assessment to determine their ability to cope with the disease and treatments.

When a client has CRF, the client, significant others, the nephrologist, and the nephrology nurse discuss the use of dialysis and decide which type best meets the client's needs. If the client is to receive dialysis, assess the client's and significant others' understanding of the treatment regimen and the client's ability to cope with the treatment regimen. The family's ability to cope and their ability to support the client are also vital.

When the client begins peritoneal dialysis, the first assessment is for infection. Inspect the insertion site carefully for redness or other problems. Carefully assess the drained dialysate or effluent for cloudiness, fibrin streaks, or blood. Monitor the client's vital signs and weight closely.

If the client is undergoing hemodialysis, the first assessment is for the patency of the venous access site. In a patent arteriovenous fistula or graft, a "thrill" or vibrating sensation should be palpable and a bruit should be audible with a stethoscope. It is vital that this site be assessed for possible occlusion or, if it is an external site, for infection. Also ascertain the client's understanding of the access site and its care.

DIAGNOSIS, OUTCOMES, INTERVENTIONS

Fluid Volume Deficit or Fluid Volume Excess. As with all renal disorders, a common diagnosis is *Fluid Volume Deficit or Fluid Volume Excess related to impaired renal function, fluid shifts between dialysate and blood, and blood loss during hemodialysis.*

Outcomes. Neither a fluid volume deficit nor an excess will occur, as evidenced by the absence of edema or dehydration.

Interventions

Monitor Fluid Volume Status. A fluid volume deficit or overload is a serious problem. The current fluid status must be known and fluid intake carefully regulated in keeping with it. Monitor the client's fluid status by observing daily weights, orthostatic blood pressure, skin turgor, and mucous membrane moistness and by meticulous intake and output comparisons.

Give written instructions to outpatients that explain how to weigh themselves properly and how to interpret the relationship of daily weight loss or gain to their need for sodium and water. Help the client understand that vomiting, diarrhea, and working or playing in a hot environment may cause excessive fluid loss and must be prevented or controlled. Teach the client how to take his or her blood pressure and record it daily.

Follow Fluid Restrictions. When the fluid allowance for the day has been determined, help the client follow the recommendation. Fluid restrictions are difficult for most clients. Offer suggestions about reducing thirst and moistening lips with lip balms, frequent oral hygiene, and taking ice chips or spray bottles rather than drinking. Spread out fluid intake over a longer period of time. If intravenous fluids are used, carefully attend to them to ensure proper administration rates. Water may be restricted so that the client can drink more nutritious liquids, such as apple juice, cranberry juice, or milk.

Monitor Fluid Status During Dialysis. During dialysis, carefully monitor the client's vital signs, including postural blood pressure, pulse, weight, and intake and output. Watch for hypovolemia and retention of dialysate. The amount of desired fluid loss may be ordered by the dialysis physician. Alternatively, a "dry" or "ideal" weight is established and you select appropriate solutions to remove additional fluid.

If fluid does not drain properly during peritoneal dialysis, check the system for kinks or other obstructions. Inform the physician about fluid accumulations that exceed the limit set in the dialysis orders. If the client is undergoing hemodialysis, hypotension and excess fluid removal are risks; monitor carefully.

Altered Nutrition: Less Than Body Requirements. Yet another common diagnosis in CRF is *Altered Nutrition: Less Than Body Requirements, related to anorexia and nausea.*

Outcomes. The client will maintain adequate nutrition, as evidenced by maintenance of weight without loss of muscle mass.

Interventions. Dietary management is vital to the conservative management of CRF. Anorexia results from many of the manifestations of irreversible renal failure, emotional depression, and a frequently unpalatable diet. Thus, a major nursing challenge is to help the client take in adequate nutrition while minimizing uremic toxicity. This problem grows as the disease progresses, and the client may develop an aversion to meat and other sources of protein.

To help stimulate the client's appetite, take measures to relieve nausea and vomiting, stomatitis, and other gastrointestinal manifestations. Diet counseling is essential. Teaching aids (such as those in Fig. 36–6) may be helpful. Arrange for dietary consultation if possible. The client needs to know how to translate the dietary regimen into a palatable, understandable food program. Help the client select and prepare foods and learn where to obtain special foods if necessary. Exercise may also improve appetite.

Constipation. The treatment of CRF leads to the predictable diagnosis of *Constipation related to medications, fluid and dietary restrictions, and decreased activity level.*

Outcomes. The client will remain free of constipation, as evidenced by a bowel movement at least every other day.

Interventions. Constipation is a major problem for clients with CRF. Because of fluid restrictions, inability to eat most high-fiber foods, and limited activity, it is difficult to use customary measures for preventing constipation. Phosphate-binding agents contribute to the problem as well.

Bran, which is not rich in potassium or phosphorus, can be used. Stool softeners are often administered regularly, although care should be taken to avoid those that contain calcium and sodium. If necessary, bulk laxatives (such as psyllium hydrophilic mucilloid) may be given. The recommended amount of fluid should be taken with the powder and subtracted from the day's fluid allotment.

Stimulant and lubricant laxatives should be used only if necessary, especially compounds containing magnesium or phosphorus, such as sodium biphosphate–sodium phosphate (Fleet) enemas. If none of these measures is effective, small-volume, gentle stimulant enemas may be used sparingly, but large-volume enemas should be avoided because of possible fluid and saline absorption. Clients with renal failure are at risk for diverticular disease because of the constipation and straining.

Fatigue. Physiologic alterations can ensure a diagnosis of *Fatigue related to anemia and altered metabolic state.*

Outcomes. The client will have a balance of rest and activity, as evidenced by the client's statement of decreased fatigue.

Interventions. Rest is important to any client whose body is under a great deal of stress. Encourage frequent naps. Insomnia is frequently a problem, and you may

TIPS ON PROTEIN INTAKE
THERE ARE TWO DIFFERENT TYPES OF PROTEIN

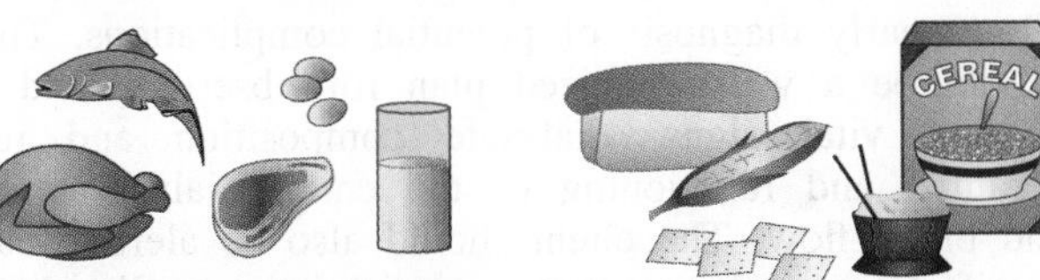
CEREAL
One is called animal or high biological protein, which contains ALL essential amino acids.
The other kind is vegetable or low biological protein, which contains SOME amino acids.
THE HEMODIALYSIS AND THE PERITONEAL MEMBRANE ARE NOT SELECTIVE, WHICH MEANS THAT VITAL AMINO ACIDS AND VITAMINS AS WELL AS UNWANTED WASTES ARE REMOVED

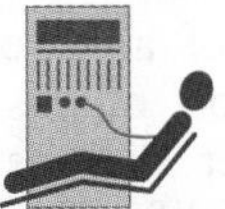
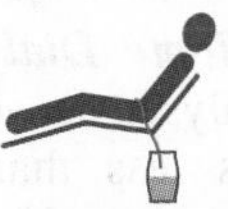
If you are on HEMODIALYSIS, you should aim for **1.2 grams of protein per kg of body weight.** E.g., if you weigh 65 kg (143 lb), your protein intake should be about 78 grams per day.
If you are on PERITONEAL DIALYSIS, you should aim for **1.3 grams of protein per kg of body weight.** E.g., if you weigh 70 kg (154 lb), your protein intake should be about 91 grams per day.
EXAMPLES OF PROTEIN SOURCES

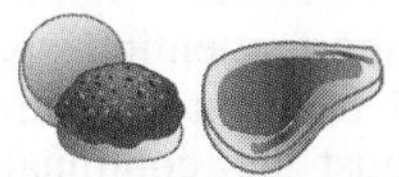
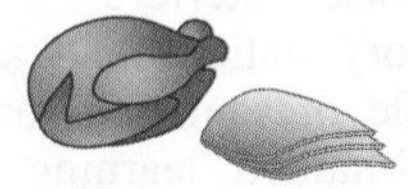
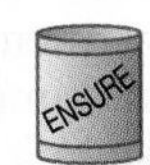
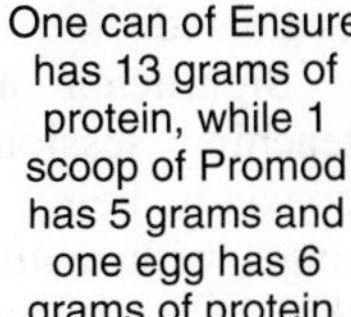
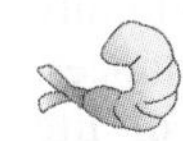
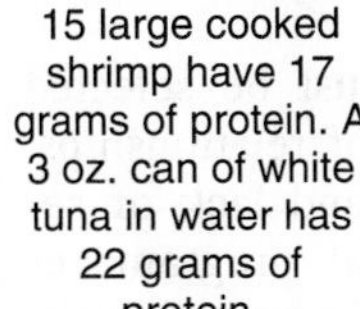
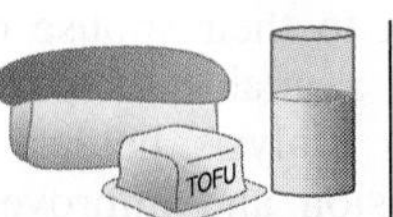
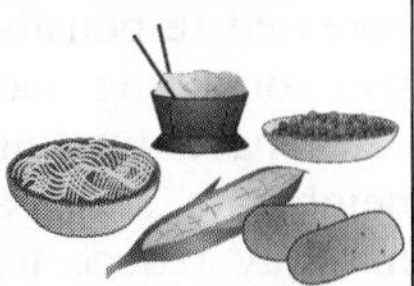
ENSURE
PROMOD
TUNA
TOFU
3.5 oz. of extra lean ground beef has 24 grams of protein, while rib eye has 28 grams of protein.
Half of a chicken breast (3.5 oz.) has 29 grams of protein. Turkey light meat (3.5 oz) has 30 grams of protein.
One can of Ensure has 13 grams of protein, while 1 scoop of Promod has 5 grams and one egg has 6 grams of protein.
15 large cooked shrimp have 17 grams of protein. A 3 oz. can of white tuna in water has 22 grams of protein.
One cup of milk has 8 grams of protein, while ½ cup of regular tofu has 10 grams and one slice of white bread has 2 grams of protein.
One cup of cooked corn, peas, potato, pasta or rice has about 4 grams of protein.

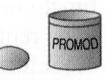

FIGURE 36–6 Renal teaching aids: Tips on Protein Intake. (Modified from Darlene Michl, Sidney, British Columbia.)

need to make suggestions about how to solve this problem (as by observing a presleep quiet time and establishing a presleep routine). Assessment in a sleep center may be helpful.

Hypnotics and sedatives must be used cautiously because they may alter mentation and may be metabolized differently by a client with renal failure. The client also needs to establish and maintain an appropriate exercise program. Anemia should be treated with iron and erythropoietin therapy to increase energy levels.

Risk for Impaired Skin Integrity. Edema and skin changes create a *Risk for Impaired Skin Integrity related to edema, dry skin, and pruritus.*

Outcomes. The client will not develop impaired skin integrity, as evidenced by intact skin.

Interventions. Dry skin is a common problem. Use of soap may need to be eliminated. Because of the increased risk of secondary infection, however, the client's skin still needs to be kept clean. Moisturizing oils in the bath water or applied directly to the skin help to correct dryness. Avoid any products that contain alcohol or perfumes; they increase dryness and pruritus. If edema is present, avoid sustained pressure on the area. The potential for skin breakdown is particularly acute in clients with diabetes. Observe for poor circulation and areas of breakdown or infection.

Risk for Ineffective Individual and Family Coping. An important diagnosis is *Risk for Ineffective Individual and Family Coping related to chronic illness, uncertain future for the client, role reversal, and effects of long-term dialysis.*

Outcomes. The client and family will cope with the client's chronic illness and future deterioration, as evidenced by acceptance of the client's problems and ability to support the client. The client and family will cope effectively with the effects of long-term dialysis, as evidenced by the client's level of activity, feelings of self-worth, and participation in dialysis treatment.

Interventions

Involve in Decision-Making. Assistance for the client and significant others must begin before dialysis is started. A client with CRF faces a future of continued deterioration but with an unknown course and timetable. In addition, the disease itself produces behavioral manifestations that contribute to the client's susceptibility to stress.

Many such clients must make important decisions about the choice of treatment modes at a time when they do not feel well. It is often difficult for the client to voice concerns about discontinuing dialysis, and it may be difficult for care providers and families to accept the client's decision to stop treatment and choose death instead. For these reasons, you need to assess how the client handled change and stress before the illness began. The client and significant others need to be actively involved in the care planning process because they will be living with the disease for many years.

Provide Support. The client and significant others will have many questions about such issues as family functioning, job or school demands, dependence, and sex. The client may experience reduced self-esteem. Significant others commonly report a decline in their quality of life that correlates directly with changes in the client's quality of life. Encourage the client and significant others to discuss their feelings and concerns, together and individually, using therapeutic communication techniques. Support groups and peer counseling programs are often helpful.

Offer Home Dialysis. About 15% of all clients who receive dialysis do so at home. The cost of this type of program is less than that of in-center dialysis, and it usually improves the client's quality of life. Home dialysis offers the client more access to significant others and greater feelings of independence and control. However, this type of treatment also produces stress on personal relationships, especially on the person who becomes the "dialysis helper" during home hemodialysis. Some spouses have voiced concern about lack of free time and increased responsibility; others see it as an opportunity to give something back to their spouse or loved one. Some states have funding available to pay for a non–family member to serve as dialysis helper. In some instances, this may reduce tension and improve the quality of life for the family.

Clients for home dialysis programs must be selected carefully. Criteria might include stability of relationships, psychological stability, financial support, and lack of severe physical complications. A successful program requires care providers who are advocates of home dialysis, a good training program, and good support services, possibly including nursing, medical, and social services; provision of supplies; equipment maintenance; dietary counseling; home visits; and retraining as necessary.

Risk for Ineffective Management of Therapeutic Regimen: Individuals and Families. There is *Risk for Ineffective Management of Therapeutic Regimen: Individuals and Families related to lack of knowledge of the disease process and treatment.*

Outcomes. The client will understand the disease process and treatment regimen as evidenced by ability to describe the disease and treatment and participate in the treatment regimen.

Interventions

Provide Information. Teaching is a crucial part of the nursing management plan. Most of the time, the client is observed on an outpatient basis and is responsible for following the recommended treatment regimen. The client and significant others must know about normal renal function and how the disease has altered it, the details of the management protocol and how to follow it, a number of self-assessment skills as described earlier, and when to seek professional consultation for possible complications. Teaching aids are available from many sources, such as the National Kidney Foundation, the National Association of Patients on Hemodialysis and Transplantation, various corporations, and the Internet. The American Nephrology Nurses Association regularly publishes a directory of educational resources.[2]

Explain Dialysis. The client and significant others need to know about dialysis and how to work with its ramifications. With peritoneal dialysis, most clients continue the treatment mode in their homes; hence, their knowledge needs to be complete and detailed. They participate in a complete training program so that they can handle the entire dialysis process independently.

Continuous monitoring during hemodialysis provides vital information about the progress of the treatment and allows early diagnosis of potential complications. There should be a well-organized plan for observing and recording vital signs, dialysate composition and temperature, and functioning of the entire dialysis system and blood flow. The client should also be alert to early manifestations of potential complications, as listed earlier. The nurse often serves as case manager and coordinates the services provided by the nephrology team, which includes the physician, nurses, social worker, and dietitian.

Reduce Anxiety. Although clients with renal disease must learn about their disorder, they may not always be ready to learn. Anxiety itself interferes with learning. In addition, the disease interferes with normal cognitive functioning; memory deficits and a short attention span may require simple presentations and frequent repetition of information. Retained learning must be continually evaluated.

Significant others may be especially frustrated during teaching sessions by the client's inability to grasp the concepts being presented. The client may seem out of touch with reality. Significant others need reassurance that this is an effect of the disease and that the client will become more capable of learning, especially after institution of dialysis.

Risk for Infection. Indwelling catheters carry a high *Risk for Infection related to the presence of an indwelling peritoneal catheter and instillation of dialysate or related to venipuncture and connection of tubing during hemodialysis.*

Outcomes. The client will remain free of infection, as evidenced by a normal white blood cell count, absence of fever, and clear dialysate.

Interventions. Because peritonitis is the main complication of peritoneal dialysis, strict aseptic technique must be used throughout the procedure. Masks are worn by the nurse and client when the peritoneal dialysis circuit is opened. Gloves are worn by anyone touching the catheter during all connection and disconnection procedures. The catheter is soaked before and after these procedures in a povidone-iodine solution. Dressing changes around the catheter site are performed according to the specific unit protocol. Be sure dressings are kept dry at all times.

With hemodialysis, use strict aseptic technique during venipuncture and when attaching the tubing and solution.

Risk for Ineffective Breathing Pattern. Peritoneal dialysis also creates a *Risk for Ineffective Breathing Pattern related to pressure from dialysate.*

Outcomes. The client will have an effective breathing pattern, as evidenced by an absence of shortness of breath.

Interventions. Because dialysate presses on the diaphragm, its full excursion may be reduced and an immobilized client may be at risk for respiratory problems. Encourage the client to cough and deep-breathe regularly. Keep the client in the semi-Fowler position to ease breathing. Also, remind the client to stay alert for early manifestations of compromised respiratory function.

Risk for Injury. Trauma and complications associated with the vascular access for hemodialysis may occur, leading to the diagnosis *Risk for Injury related to trauma to hemodialysis venous access site.*

Outcomes. The client will not experience injury to the venous access site, as evidenced by continued patency of the site.

Interventions. Careful attention to the access site—to prevent infection and clotting—is important to its life expectancy. A dressing is used to protect cannulas and subclavian catheters from infection. The access site must also be protected from trauma that could cause clotting, bleeding, or physical disruption of the site. For example, warn the client against wearing tight sleeves or carrying a purse over the access site. The limb that contains the access site should not be used to take blood pressure or to draw blood.

Between dialysis periods, the skin over the fistula or graft requires only routine care with soap and water. The site of a fistula should be carefully assessed. To assess patency, palpate over the fistula for a thrill and auscultate for a bruit at regular intervals. The client must also learn to assess the access site for patency.

EVALUATION

The client is expected to improve physically and mentally when dialysis begins. The client's weight and blood pressure should begin to stabilize if dietary and fluid restrictions are followed and as fluid balance stabilizes.

Normal electrolyte and albumin levels reflect adequate nutrition and compliance with diet. The client should report regular, normal bowel movements. The client should report less fatigue and increased energy and activity as hematocrit values approach normal levels. Skin should remain intact.

The client should understand and adapt to the treatment regimen and be successfully maintained with peritoneal dialysis or hemodialysis. Clients receiving peritoneal dialysis (and some receiving hemodialysis) should be able to demonstrate successful performance of the dialysis procedure and care of the vascular access site or peritoneal catheter. They should remain free from complications associated with dialysis. As long as venous or peritoneal access can be maintained, the client can be managed with dialysis until transplantation (if the client is a candidate) is completed, the client elects to stop dialysis, or other complications result in death.

Significant others should cope with the client's chronic illness and dialysis, show acceptance of problems, support the client, and report improved satisfaction with their own quality of life. The family and significant others should assist the client with treatment as needed.

Self-Care

Clients must comply with dietary and fluid intake modifications and take prescribed medications as ordered. They must monitor and record weight and blood pressure daily and care for the venous access or peritoneal catheter as ordered. Noncompliance with the regimen leads to complications. The client or family must perform dialysis at home or keep scheduled dialysis appointments.

Modifications for Elderly Clients

The types of dialysis for older clients are evaluated on the basis of the presence of other chronic disorders that would limit the ability to comply with any treatment.

Older clients may have had multiple abdominal surgical procedures with the development of adhesions that limit the usefulness of peritoneal dialysis. They are more likely to have pre-existing cardiovascular problems that may limit the usefulness of many venous access sites.

Surgical Management

RENAL TRANSPLANTATION

INDICATIONS. Renal transplantation is the surgical implantation of a human kidney from a compatible donor in a recipient. This procedure is performed as an intervention in irreversible kidney failure. The kidney is surgically placed extraperitoneally in the iliac fossa. The renal artery is anastomosed to the recipient's hypogastric internal or external iliac artery (occasionally the aorta) and the renal vein to the recipient's iliac vein (Fig. 36–7). Usually, the kidney begins to function immediately.

Selection of a transplant recipient is based on careful evaluation of the client's medical, immunologic, and psychosocial status (see Chapter 80). Usually, a recipient is younger than age 70, has an estimated life expectancy of 2 years or more, and is expected to have an improved quality of life after transplantation. Conservative management and dialysis should have made the client's state as nontoxic as possible. Bilateral nephrectomy may be performed before the transplantation procedure for persistent or active bacterial pyelonephritis, uncontrolled renin-mediated hypertension, polycystic kidneys, or rapidly progressive glomerulonephritis.

Successful transplantation prolongs life and markedly improves its quality. The client is freed from the restrictions of dialysis and from the reversible manifestations of uremia.

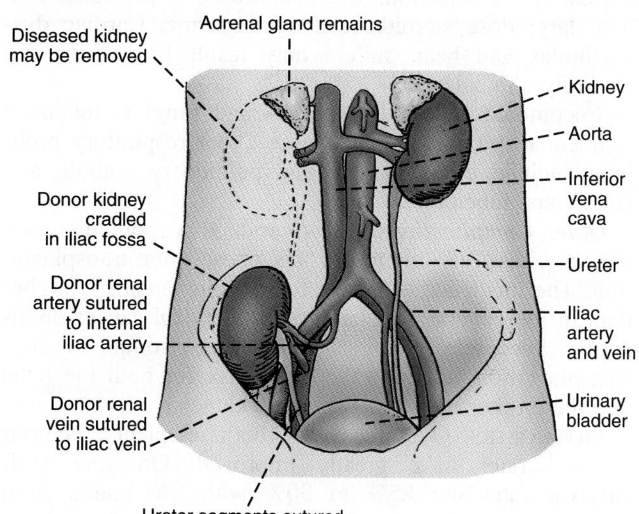

FIGURE 36–7 Transplanted kidney placement in the right iliac fossa.

Because graft survival rates are higher, the most desirable source of kidneys for transplantation is a living related donor who matches the client closely. Willing family members are evaluated for physical and mental health and screened for ABO blood group, tissue-specific antigen, and human leukocyte antigen histocompatibility (see Chapter 80). Consideration has been given to transplanting kidneys from emotionally related donors, such as friends or spouses. Nevertheless, most transplanted kidneys are cadaver organs.

CONTRAINDICATIONS. Infection and active malignancy are the only absolute contraindications to transplantation. Some physical conditions markedly increase the risk for the client, however, primarily because long-term immunosuppressive medications are necessary to avoid graft rejection. Clients with liver disease, psychological disorders, advanced atherosclerosis, hypertension, respiratory disease, and gastrointestinal bleeding need particular consideration. The primary factor limiting the number of transplantations done is the availability of kidneys.

COMPLICATIONS. Major complications of transplantation, such as graft rejection (and antirejection therapy), infection, skin and gastrointestinal problems, and other complications, are discussed in Chapter 80.

Graft Rejection. The manifestations of renal transplant rejection include fever, graft tenderness at the site of the transplanted kidney, anemia, and malaise.

Urinary Tract Complications. Several complications may occur in the urinary tract. Although it is rare, spontaneous rupture of the kidney may occur because of rejection or ischemic damage. Leaking of urine from the ureter-bladder anastomosis causes the development of a urinoma, which eventually puts pressure on the kidney and ureter, reducing renal function. Long-term uremia and steroid therapy may predispose the client to ureteral, bladder, or caliceal-cutaneous fistulas. Other urinary tract complications include ureteral, bladder, or pelvic leaks; obstruction; reflux; and lymphoceles.

Cardiopulmonary Complications. Hypertension occurs in 50% to 60% of adult recipients and may be caused by renal artery stenosis, acute tubular necrosis, acute and chronic graft rejection, hydronephrosis, hyperaldosteronism, large-dose steroids, and cyclosporine. Cardiac dysrhythmias and heart failure may result from fluid and electrolyte imbalances.

Pneumonia caused by bacteria and fungi is the most frequent respiratory complication. Other respiratory problems include pulmonary edema, pulmonary emboli, and reactivated tuberculosis.

Other Complications. The reproductive problems associated with CRF commonly disappear after transplantation. The incidence of gynecologic malignancies is higher than in the general population, with cervical cancer dominating. Successful pregnancies have been completed after transplantation, although there is a risk for both the fetus and the mother with a transplanted kidney.

OUTCOMES. Over the years, both recipient and graft survival rates have greatly improved. One-year graft survival rates are 85% to 90% with transplants from living related donors and 75% to 80% with cadaver kidneys. The overall mortality rate 2 years after transplantation is about 10%.[21] This represents a dramatic decrease; two decades ago, the 2-year survival was 40% to 50%.

In particular, the decrease in the death rate related to infection in the first 2 years after transplantation has been dramatic. Advances in immunosuppressive therapy and the treatment of infectious diseases have contributed to the overall improvement. Cardiovascular problems remain the leading cause of death in the late transplantation period. Myocardial infarction, stroke, and heart failure are the primary causes of death.

Nursing Management of the Surgical Client

PREOPERATIVE CARE

Before kidney transplantation, assess the client's understanding of the procedure and follow-up regimen. Also, assess the client's ability to cope with a complex medication regimen after transplantation. The client needs to understand the transplantation and therapeutic regimen. Preoperative preparation of both the living donor and the recipient includes all aspects of general preoperative care as outlined in Chapter 15.

POSTOPERATIVE CARE

Assessment for renal transplant recipients is similar to that for most other postoperative clients (see Chapter 15), with the exception of the focus on renal function. Give particular attention to fluid balance, and carefully monitor intake and output (every 30 to 60 minutes) and weight (daily). To monitor renal function and maintain electrolyte balance, obtain serial laboratory determinations of hemoglobin, hematocrit, BUN, creatinine, electrolytes, white blood cell count, and platelets. Auscultate the kidney regularly to check for bruits, which might indicate stenosis. Monitoring of vital signs is key, because even a slight temperature increase may indicate an infection.

The function of the transplanted kidney is a primary concern after surgery. A kidney from a cadaver may not function immediately, and the client may be maintained with hemodialysis until it functions adequately. Postoperatively, manage intravenous fluids carefully; the amount of fluid infused is typically based on the previous hour's output. A high urine output is usually desired. The additional care required by the recipient is related to potential complications. Care of the client with a transplant is discussed in more detail in Chapter 80.

Psychologically, the client must be helped to incorporate the new kidney as a part of the whole being. Provide education and counseling to enhance changes in lifestyle that promote health-seeking behaviors and compliance with transplantation medications. If the graft fails, expect the client to feel anger, hostility, guilt, and a helplessness-hopelessness syndrome. Relatives and friends may mirror these feelings. Role changes that were well established during the chronic illness may lead to problems, as with the family member who no longer feels needed as the caregiver. Likewise, the client may have difficulty giving up the sick role.

Self-Care

Failure to follow the prescribed regimen is a major problem after transplantation, and your knowledge and creativity are needed to help the client follow the recommended regimen. Many clients—particularly adolescents—miss doses of their immunosuppressive medications (see Chapter 80). This practice contributes to early loss of renal function and possible graft loss.

Clients may be reluctant to take medications for many reasons. For some, the side effects disrupt their lives. Others may believe that they no longer need the medications because they are stable. Economic concerns also need to be addressed. Immunosuppressive medications, particularly cyclosporine, are expensive. Currently, Medicare covers payment of these drugs for up to 48 months after transplantation. After that time, other sources of funding need to be explored to ensure compliance with medications. Work with the client to provide needed information and to develop strategies that fit the client's lifestyle.

Overall, transplantation offers clients with CRF a much better quality of life than does dialysis therapy. Renal function returns, and many of the clinical manifestations of CRF disappear. Complications do occur, and care must be taken to prevent graft loss. Renal transplant recipients are monitored regularly at transplantation clinics. The visits become less frequent as renal function stabilizes and time passes. Blood tests are taken regularly to monitor serum creatinine levels and cyclosporine levels. Every transplantation center has protocols for routine follow-up tests.

Modifications for Elderly Clients

One of the major modifications for older clients may be fewer options available for treatment. Renal transplantation is not routinely done for elderly clients. Clients older than 60 years are evaluated on an individual basis; clients as old as 75 years of age have had successful transplantations. One problem for elderly clients is that a less effective immune system in conjunction with immunosuppressants can lead to further complications.

CONCLUSIONS

Caring for the client with renal failure involves many challenges. There are numerous physical and psychosocial manifestations associated with renal disease and its treatment. The nurse can significantly impact the client's quality of life through the provision of education, encouragement, promotion of exercise, and ongoing assessment of the client and family as well as evaluation of programs offering treatment for end-stage renal disease. The nurse, in collaboration with the multidisciplinary team, can facilitate positive outcomes.

THINKING CRITICALLY

1. **You are caring for a 74-year-old man 1 day after coronary artery bypass surgery. His urine output is about 15 ml/hr. He has a long history of hypertension (controlled), and his blood pressure usually ranges from 180 to 190 over 90 to 100 mm Hg. His blood pressure since surgery has ranged from 120 to 130 over 70 to 76 mm Hg. His serum sodium concentration is 145 mEq/L and potassium is 4.9 mEq/L. His skin turgor is poor, and mucous membranes are dry. What is your first assessment and action?**

Factors to Consider. What has his intake been since surgery? What are the possible causes of his low blood pressure, increased electrolytes, and decreased urine output? If he has renal failure, what is the probable cause? What other assessments should you make?

2. **You are caring for a 60-year-old woman with diabetes, hypertension, and chronic renal failure. She has had hemodialysis for over a year and has decided that she no longer wants to continue living this way. She has informed her physician and family that she no longer wishes to continue dialysis. Her family is trying to persuade her that she should go for her next treatment. She asks you your opinion, "Would you want to live this way?" How would you respond? How would you ensure that she is making the right decision?**

Factors to Consider. What is the client's cognitive and emotional status? How have the client and her family members coped with the illness and its treatment? Given the information you have, what is her prognosis? Do people have the right to refuse life-sustaining therapy? Knowing that health care resources are finite, what is the best use of resources for all members of society?

BIBLIOGRAPHY

1. Abuelo, J. G. (Ed.). (1995). *Renal failure: Diagnosis and treatment.* Norwell, MA: Kluwer.
2. American Nephrology Nurses Association. (1997). 1997 educational resource directory. *ANNA Journal, 24*(4), 427–440.
3. Arnold, R. M. (Ed.). (1995). *Procuring organs for transplant: The debate over non–heart-beating cadaver protocols.* Baltimore: Johns Hopkins University Press.
4. Bach, F. H., & Auchincloss, H., Jr. (1995). *Transplantation immunology.* New York: Wiley-Liss.
5. Badzek, L., Hines, S. C., & Moss, A. H. (1998). Inadequate self-care knowledge among elderly hemodialysis patients: Assessing its prevalence and potential causes. *ANNA Journal, 25*(3), 293–300.
6. Bennett, J. C., & Plum, F. (Eds.). (1996). *Cecil textbook of medicine* (20th ed.). Philadelphia: W. B. Saunders.
7. Binik, Y. M., & Mah, K. (1994). Sexuality and end-stage renal disease: Research and clinical recommendations. *Advances in Renal Replacement Therapy, 1*(3), 198–209.
8. Brenner, B. M. (Ed.). (1996). *Brenner and Rector's the kidney* (5th ed.). Philadelphia: W. B. Saunders.
9. Burrows-Hudson, S. (Ed.). (1999). *Standards and guidelines of clinical practice for nephrology nursing.* Pitman, NJ: American Nephrology Nurses Association.
10. Busson, M., et al. (1995). Analysis of cadaver donor criteria on the kidney transplant survival rate in 5,129 transplantations. *Journal of Urology, 154*(2, Pt. 1), 356–360.
11. Corbett, J., & Ross, K. (1998). Neoral: The new cyclosporine. *ANNA Journal, 25*(1), 71–72.
12. Crampton, K., et al. (1998). Renal rehabilitation programs: Keys to success. *ANNA Journal, 25*(2), 248–251.
13. Flye, M. W. (Ed.). (1995). *Atlas of organ transplantation.* Philadelphia: W. B. Saunders.
14. Glassock, R. J. (1998). *Current therapy in nephrology and hypertension* (4th ed.). St. Louis: Mosby–Year Book.
15. Guyton, A. C., & Hall, J. E. (1996). *Textbook of medical physiology* (6th ed.). Philadelphia: W. B. Saunders.

16. Health Care Financing Administration. (1998, October). HCFA research report provides ESRD facility data. *Contemporary Dialysis and Nephrology, 19*(10), 18.
17. Headley, C. M. (1998). Hungry bone syndrome following parathyroidectomy. *ANNA Journal, 25*(3), 283–292.
18. Headley, C. M. (1998). Osteitis fibrosa: Treatment trends. *ANNA Journal, 25*(1), 21–30.
19. Horsburgh, M. E., Rice, V. H., & Matuk, L. (1998). Sense of coherence and life satisfaction: Patient and spousal adaptation to home dialysis. *ANNA Journal, 25*(2), 219–230.
20. Jacobs, C., et al. (1996). *Replacement of renal function by dialysis.* Norwell, MA: Kluwer.
21. Karlowicz, K. A. (Ed.). (1995). *Urologic nursing: Principles and practice.* Philadelphia: W. B. Saunders.
22. Kinzer, C. L. (1998). Warfarin sodium (Coumadin) anticoagulant therapy for vascular access patency. *ANNA Journal, 25*(2), 195–209.
23. Koeppen, B. M., & Stanton, B. A. (1997). *Renal physiology* (2nd ed.). St. Louis: Mosby–Year Book.
24. Lancaster, L. E. (Ed.). (1995). *Core curriculum for nephrology nursing* (2nd ed.). Pitman, NJ: American Nephrology Nurses Association.
25. Lev, E. L., & Owen, S. V. (1998). A prospective study of adjustment to hemodialysis. *ANNA Journal, 25*(1), 495–506.
26. Levine, D. Z. (Ed.). (1997). *Caring for the renal patient* (3rd ed.). Philadelphia: W. B. Saunders.
27. Life Options Rehabilitation Advisory Council. (1997). *Building quality of life: A practical guide to renal rehabilitation.* San Francisco: Amgen.
28. Long, J. M., et al. (1998). Medication compliance and the older hemodialysis patient. *ANNA Journal, 25*(1), 43–56.
29. Massry, S. G., & Glassock, R. J. (Eds.). (1995). *Massry and Glassock's textbook of nephrology* (3rd ed.). Baltimore: Williams & Wilkins.
30. Molzahn, A. E., & Kikuchi, J. F. (1998). Reported quality of life of children and adolescents with parents on dialysis. *ANNA Journal, 25*(6), 411–418.
31. Molzahn, A. E., Northcott, H. C., & Dossetor, J. B. (1997). Quality of life of individuals with end stage renal disease: Perceptions of patients, nurses, and physicians. *ANNA Journal, 24*(3), 325–336.
32. Neyhart, C. D. (1998). Contraception in ESRD and immunosuppression for the pregnant transplant patient. *ANNA Journal, 25*(3), 345–348.
33. Nolan, M. T., & Augustine, S. M. (Eds.). (1995). *Transplantation nursing: Acute and long-term management.* Norwalk, CT: Appleton & Lange.
34. Parker, J. (Ed.). (1998). *Contemporary nephrology nursing.* Pitman, NJ: American Nephrology Nurses Association.
35. Parker, K. P. (1997). Sleep and dialysis: A research-based review of the literature. *ANNA Journal, 24*(6), 626–639.
36. Redman, B. K., Hill, M. N., & Fry, S. T. (1997). Ethical conflicts reported by certified nephrology nurses practicing in dialysis settings. *ANNA Journal, 24*(1), 23–34.
37. Richbourg, M. J. (1997). Vision screening in older adults on dialysis: Do nephrology nurses have a role? *ANNA Journal, 24*(3), 541–544, 549.
38. Rodriguez, D., & Lewis, S. L. (1997). Nutritional management of patients with acute renal failure. *ANNA Journal, 24*(2), 232–241.
39. Rogers, A. E. (1997). Nursing management of sleep disorders. Part 1: Assessment. *ANNA Journal, 24*(6), 666–671.
40. Rogers, A. E. (1997). Nursing management of sleep disorders. Part 2: Behavioral interventions. *ANNA Journal, 24*(6), 672–675.
41. Schlatter, S., & Ferrans, C. E. (1998). Teaching program effects on high phosphorus levels in patients receiving hemodialysis. *ANNA Journal, 25*(1), 31–42.
42. Schrier, R. W. (Ed.). (1995). *Manual of nephrology.* Boston: Little, Brown.
43. Schrier, R. W., & Gottschalk, C. W. (Eds.). (1997). *Diseases of the kidney* (6th ed.). Boston: Little, Brown.
44. Wicks, M., et al. (1997). Subjective burden and quality of life in family caregivers of patients with end stage renal disease. *ANNA Journal, 24*(5), 527–540.
45. United States Renal Data System. (1999). *Annual data report.* Washington, DC: United States Department of Health and Human Services, Health Care Financing Administration, Bureau of Data Management and Strategy.

UNIT

8

Sexuality and Reproductive Disorders

Anatomy and Physiology Review

The Reproductive Systems

Robert G. Carroll

The human reproductive system is specialized for the production and joining of *germ cells*—the ovum, or egg (female) and the sperm (male). The female reproductive system is also specialized to nurture and protect the fertilized ovum during the 9-month gestation period. Gonadal development begins in utero, but maturation of the reproductive system *(puberty)* is delayed until adolescence. At 45 to 60 years of age, fertility gradually decreases, ending at *menopause* (permanent cessation of menstruation) in women.

GONADAL DEVELOPMENT

The *gonads* are the sex glands of the female *(ovaries)* and male *(testes)*. Their primary function is to form germ cells, which have half the normal number of chromosomes. The ovaries produce ova; the testes produce spermatozoa (sperm).

Gonadal development begins during the 5th week of fetal life, and gonadal differentiation occurs in the 7th and 8th weeks of gestation. Human chorionic gonadotropin (HCG) is released from the placenta, stimulating the ovaries to release estradiol and progesterone and the testes to release testosterone. In males, the Wolffian ducts develop into the epididymis, vas deferens, and seminal vesicles, and the Müllerian ducts regress. In females, the Wolffian ducts regress and the Müllerian ducts develop into fallopian tubes, uterus, and upper vagina. The external genitalia—the glans penis and scrotum—are complete in boys by 14 weeks of gestation. The clitoris, labia majora, and labia minora are complete in girls by 11 weeks of gestation.

FEMALE REPRODUCTIVE SYSTEM

GENITAL STRUCTURES

■ EXTERNAL STRUCTURES

The female reproductive organs consist of both external and internal structures. The external structures, collectively termed the *vulva* or *pudendum,* play a role in sexual stimulation and provide a barrier to protect the body from foreign materials (Fig. U8–1*A*). External female genital structures consist of the mons pubis, labia majora and minora, clitoris, vestibular bulbs, and vestibule (Table U8–1). The *perineum* is the area posterior to the vestibule, between it and the anus.

The *hymen,* a fold of mucous membrane that is sometimes present, partially covers the opening to the vagina. In the past, the presence or absence of a hymen was used as proof of a woman's virginity or sexual activity. However, the hymen may be ruptured in various ways (e.g., during exercise, sexual activity, surgery, vaginal examination, tampon insertion). Pregnancy has even been known to occur with an intact hymen.

■ INTERNAL STRUCTURES

The internal female genital structures produce and release the reproductive cell or ovum, transport ova to the potential site of fertilization, and provide an appropriate environment for the implantation, growth, and delivery of the fetus (see Table U8–1).

Ovaries are the female gonads, producing both the female germ cell (ovum) and hormones (estrogen and progesterone). Normally two ovaries are located in the pelvis, one on either side of the uterus and below the fallopian (uterine) tubes (Fig. U8–1*B*). The ovaries are contained in the posterior surfaces of the broad ligaments. They are also supported by the suspensory ligament (to the side of the pelvis) and by the utero-ovarian ligament (to the uterus). In young females, ovaries are smooth; with age, they become pitted.

Ova, in various stages of development in addition to their surrounding tissue, make up the *ovarian follicles.* Each follicle contains a developing ovum; it grows and matures in the stroma, close to an abundant blood and lymphatic supply. A mature follicle (a mature ovum and its surrounding tissues) is an endocrine gland secreting estrogen hormones (see Estrogens). At birth, several hundred thousand follicles, each containing an oocyte or end-stage ovum, are present. They decrease in number as puberty (the onset of functional reproductive capability) approaches, and they gradually disappear around menopause.

The *corpus luteum* is a glandular body that produces the hormones progesterone and estrogen. It develops from a graafian follicle after ovulation (see Secretory Phase).

Two *fallopian tubes* connect the uterus to the ovaries and are the usual site of fertilization (Fig. U8–1*C*). They convey the ovum to the uterus. Each fallopian tube is about 10 cm long.

The *uterus* is located in the pelvic cavity slightly below and between the fallopian tubes, almost at a right angle to the vagina. The normal uterus is movable in all directions, but maintains its normal position in the body cavity through the action of various ligaments and the pelvic floor. The cardinal (lateral cervical) ligaments run between the pelvic wall and the cervix and vagina and provide the most support. If these ligaments are weak, the uterus is likely to prolapse (drop) into the vagina.

The uterus has three functional layers: (1) the *parametrium,* the thin peritoneal and fascial covering of the uterus; (2) the *myometrium* (bulk of the uterus), a muscular layer composed of three layers, mainly of involuntary

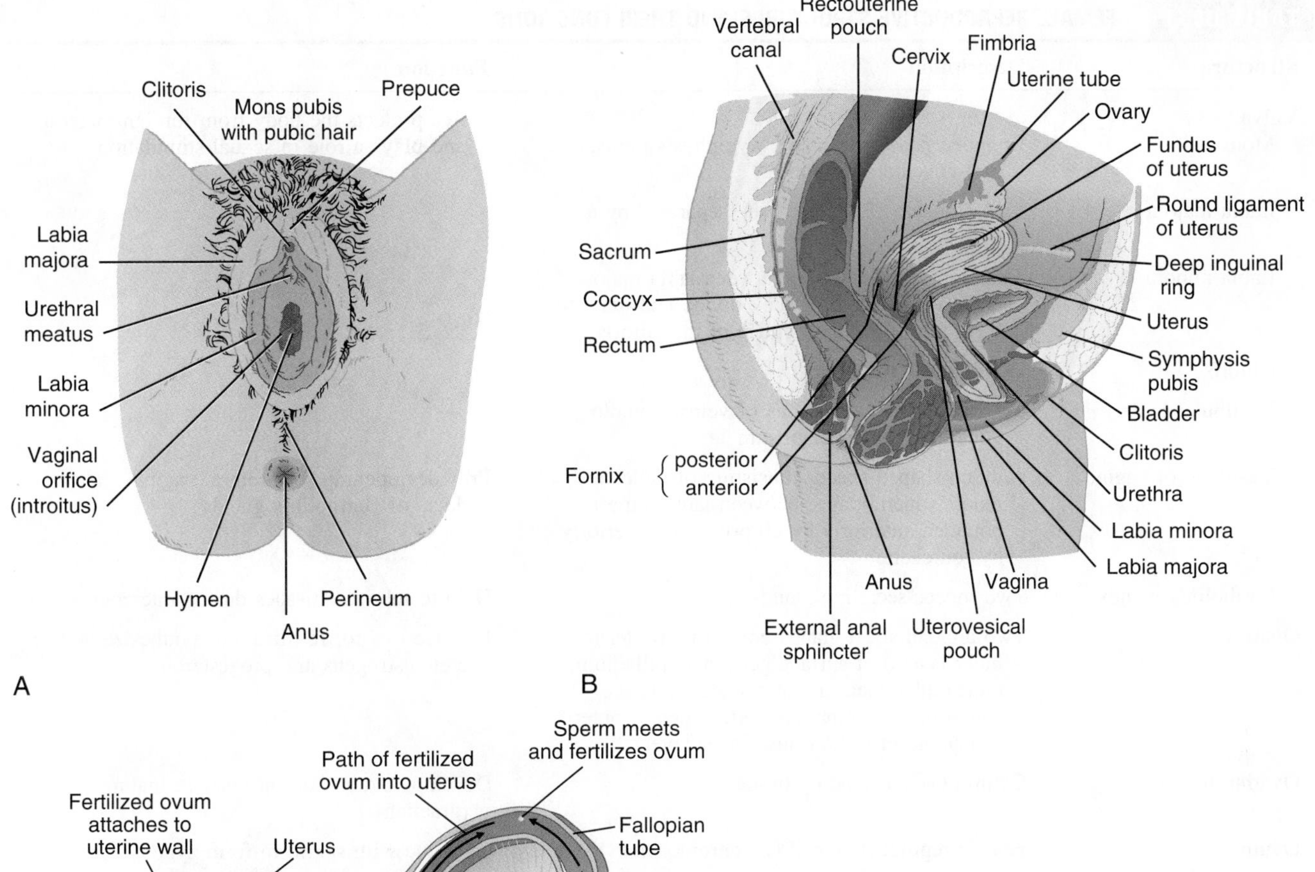

FIGURE U8–1 *A,* Anatomic landmarks of external female genitalia. *B,* Midsagittal section of the female pelvis. *C,* Pathways of sperm and ovum in the female reproductive organs. (Modified from Miller, B. F., & Keane, C. B. [1992]. *Encyclopedia and dictionary of medicine, nursing and allied health* [5th ed., p. 1085]. Philadelphia: W. B. Saunders.)

muscles; and (3) the *endometrium,* the mucous membrane lining the inner surface of the uterus. The superior two thirds of the endometrium responds cyclically to hormones. A fertilized ovum implants in the endometrium. When the ovum is not fertilized, the endometrial lining is shed (see Menstruation).

The *vagina* is a musculomembranous canal connecting the uterus with the external genitalia. The mucosa of the inner surface of the vaginal wall folds over in small ridges (rugae) extending laterally upward. This rugal pattern adds to the vagina's elasticity, making it very distensible. The rectum is posterior to its lower two thirds. The vagina's smooth rugal pattern and elasticity diminish during the menopausal and postmenopausal years. The vagina can easily become infected from urethral or rectal secretions.

■ PELVIC BLOOD SUPPLY, INNERVATION, AND LYMPHATIC DRAINAGE

Blood Supply

The most important *blood supply* to the external genitalia comes from the internal iliac (hypogastric) artery. This artery branches to supply the pelvic floor, pelvic walls, and pelvic viscera. The principal vessels supplying the internal genitalia are the *uterine arteries,* from the internal iliac artery, and the *ovarian arteries,* which stem directly from the aorta. The uterine artery provides a rich vascular bed to the uterus, and anastomoses the arterial supply to the vagina (vaginal arteries). The ovarian artery supplies blood to the ovaries, fallopian tubes, and body of the uterus. Venous drainage roughly parallels the arterial supply.

TABLE U8–1 FEMALE REPRODUCTIVE STRUCTURES AND THEIR FUNCTIONS

Structure	Description	Function
Vulva		Vulva protects the body from foreign materials and plays a role in sexual stimulation
Mons pubis	Rounded pad of flesh over symphysis pubis; hair-covered after puberty	
Labia majora	Two elongated folds of tissue separated by a cleft	
Labia minora	Two thin folds of tissue between labia majora and vaginal opening; they divide and unite to form the hood-like prepuce of the clitoris	
Clitoris	Homologous to penis	
Vestibular bulbs	Two sacculated collections of veins; homologous to corpus spongiosum	
Vestibule of vagina	Almond-shaped space, consisting of delicate mucous membranes, between labia minora; bounded anteriorly by clitoris and posteriorly by fourchette	Provides opening for urethra, vagina, and two ducts of Bartholin's glands
Bartholin's glands	Two mucus-secreting glands	Help to lubricate tissues during intercourse
Ovaries	Two almond-sized glands consisting (outer to inner layers) of surface germinal epithelium, tunica albuginea (dense connective tissue), and stroma. Stroma has cortex (dense, outer layer) and medulla (loose inner layer).	Produce ova for fertilization, synthesize and secrete estrogens and progesterone
Ovarian follicle	Ovum plus surrounding tissue	Develops ovum from primary to mature (graafian)
Ovum	Female reproductive cell (23 chromosomes)	Combine with sperm to form zygote
Fallopian tubes	Thin-walled tubes with serosal covering, muscular layer, and ciliated mucous lining	Transport ova to uterus for implantation
Uterus	Pear-shaped, hollow muscular organ in pelvic cavity (2–5 cm thick, 5 cm long, 5 cm at widest to 2 cm at narrowest point with opening to vagina (cervix)	Environment for implantation, development, and delivery of fetus; cervix allows entry of sperm for fertilization
Vagina	Canal between uterus and vestibule having three layers: epithelium, fibrous connective tissue, and muscular layer	Route of entry for sexual intercourse. Exit for menstrual blood and birth canal
Breasts	Modified sebaceous glands and skin appendages lying within superficial fascia of anterior chest wall (vertically from second to sixth rib, horizontally from sternum to midaxillary line). Parenchyma consists of ductular, lobular, and acinar epithelial structures; stroma is made of fibrous and fatty tissue.	Produce milk to feed infants

INNERVATION

Both the sympathetic and parasympathetic autonomic nervous systems provide innervation to the pelvic structures. Sexual arousal is controlled by the parasympathetic dilatation of blood vessels in the vestibular bulbs and clitoris. The uterine myometrium is innervated only by the sympathetic nerve fibers. The perineum is supplied principally by the pudendal nerve.

LYMPHATIC DRAINAGE

The pelvic *lymphatics* are a rich network of superficial and deep systems that roughly parallel the blood supply. The intermingling of the pelvic lymphatics and blood vessels is significant for the potential spread of cancer.

THE BREASTS

■ FEMALE BREASTS

Structures of the Breast

Breasts play an important role in our culture. Because breasts are visible, their size and shape are often mistakenly viewed as a measure of sexuality, femininity, and attractiveness. However, breasts are a secondary sexual characteristic; that is, reproduction can occur without them. The physiologic function of female breasts is secretion of milk to feed infants. An average nonlactating breast weighs between 150 and 250 g, and a lactating breast weighs 400 to 500 g.

The *parenchyma* of a breast consists of ductular, lobular, and acinar epithelial structures. The stroma of a breast is made of fibrous and fatty tissue. The upper lateral quadrant of the breast, which is mostly glandular, is the most common site of tumor occurrence. A breast consists of 12 to 20 *lobes,* subdivided into *lobules,* made up of acini. Breast lobes are arranged like the spokes of a wheel around the nipple. Each lobe is drained by a duct, 12 to 20 of which open independently on the surface of the nipple.

The *nipple,* located at the fourth intercostal space, is surrounded by a circular pigmented area called the *areola.* Estrogen increases pigmentation of the areola at any age. The areolar epithelium contains some small hairs and sebaceous glands, sweat glands, and accessory mammary glands. The sebaceous glands (Montgomery's glands) enlarge to lubricate the nipple during pregnancy and lactation.

BLOOD SUPPLY

The two main sources of the breast's blood supply are the lateral mammary artery and the lateral thoracic artery. These arteries form an extensive network of anastomoses. The main veins follow the arterial pattern.

LYMPHATIC DRAINAGE

Lymphatic pathways generally follow the pathways of the veins. There are three types of lymphatic drainage of the breast (Fig. U8–2):

- Cutaneous or superficial lymphatic drainage from the skin
- Areolar lymphatic drainage from the areola and nipple
- Glandular lymphatic drainage from deep glandular tissue

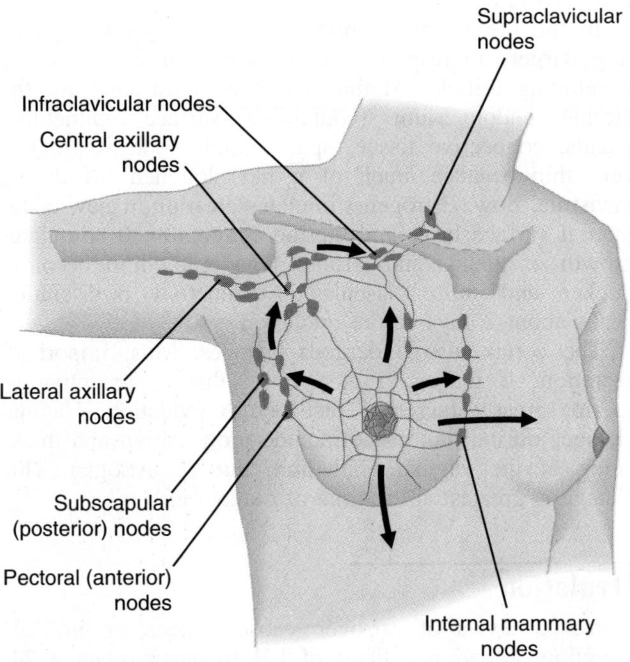

FIGURE U8–2 Routes of lymphatic drainage from the breast. These routes are very important in the spread of breast cancer.

Lymphatic drainage pathways and lymph nodes are important in the prognosis and treatment of breast cancer (see Chapter 40). The nerve supply is derived from the anterior and lateral branches of the fourth to sixth intercostal nerves.

Functions of the Breast

The physiologic changes that affect the breast are:

- Growth and development
- The menstrual cycle
- Pregnancy and lactation

Estrogen and progesterone act synergistically with the pituitary growth hormones prolactin and corticotropin to produce breast development and function. Breast development usually occurs between 9 and 16 years of age and takes 4 to 5 years. Estrogen is responsible for the growth of the breast and periductal stroma. Progesterone promotes the development of lobular and acinar structures.

After menopause, the ovaries stop producing estrogen and progesterone. Estrogen is then produced by the adrenals through stimulation from the anterior pituitary. During this life stage, there is a continuous involution of the breast with loss of glandular elements and tissue atrophy.

During pregnancy, estrogen, progesterone, and pituitary hormones increase, increasing breast vascularity and the permeability and dilation of breast lymphatics. When pregnancy ends, prolactin initiates lactation. Prolactin and corticoptropin help maintain lactation. The "letting down" (flow) of milk is a complex response involving a mother's subjective response and the mechanical stimulation of suckling. Suckling releases the pituitary hormone oxytocin into the bloodstream. This causes the mammary acini to contract and release milk into the duct system.

■ MALE BREASTS

The male breast is similar to that of a preadolescent girl. It contains a few ducts surrounded by connective tissue. Estrogen can cause a man's breast to enlarge *(gynecomastia)* (see Chapter 83). Accumulation of fat in obese men can also make the breasts appear large.

FEMALE REPRODUCTION

■ ROLE OF HORMONES

Under control of the hypothalamic releasing factors and anterior pituitary FSH and LH, the ovaries manufacture estrogens and progestins. These hormones accomplish the following functions:

- Stimulate sexual desire
- Interact with the hypothalamic-pituitary unit and the uterus for (1) ovarian changes (follicular development, ovulation, corpus luteum formation), (2) pregnancy (implantation of a fertilized ovum), or (3) menstruation
- Exert additional effects elsewhere in the body

Estrogens

Estrogens (female sex hormones) produce cyclic changes in the uterine endothelium and vaginal epithelium. Estrogens are steroids that are secreted in both males and females by the adrenal cortex and in females by the ovary (main source) and placenta. Natural estrogens include estradiol, estrone, and estriol. Estrogens in low doses may be used therapeutically as a replacement hormone during menopause.

The main effects of estrogenic stimulation on the body occur at puberty and include breast growth (fatty tissue deposition, pigmentation), fat deposition in the vulva, pubic and axillary hair growth, bony pelvis growth and broadening, closure of the epiphyseal plates of long bones, vaginal epithelial changes, and general growth. The effects of hormones on menstruation are discussed later.

It is not known precisely how the trophic actions of estrogen interact with other endocrine systems. Thus, whether estrogen replacement should be given during menopause is under investigation. Osteoporosis (increased bone porosity) is associated with estrogen deficiency in adult women.

Progesterone

Progesterone is a steroid hormone that helps prepare the endometrium to receive and implant the fertilized ovum; it also promotes development of the placenta (a spongy structure in the uterus that provides nourishment for a developing fetus) and the mammary glands.

Progesterone is used therapeutically to treat threatened abortion and such menstrual problems as dysmenorrhea or amenorrhea. It is secreted from the placenta and the corpus luteum under control of the anterior pituitary hormone luteinizing hormone (LH). Progesterone plays a minor role in sodium and water balance. It also influences nitrogen balance, breast function, and body temperature during the menstrual cycle, raising body temperature by 1° F in the postovulatory phase of the cycle.

■ MENARCHE

The beginning of menstrual life (menarche) is a biologic, psychological, and social milestone. Psychosocial support, education about the physical changes that are happening, and knowledge about self-care are essential to a young woman at this stage of life.

The average age for menarche in the United States is now 12.8 years. Menarche is preceded by characteristic body changes (such as breast development) that occur between ages 9 and 16 years.

The age at which menarche occurs is affected by genetic factors. Menarche may be delayed by poor nutrition, high levels of exercise (athletes or dancers), and several medical conditions, such as diabetes mellitus, congenital heart disease, and ulcerative colitis. Early menarche may occur with other conditions, such as hypothyroidism, central nervous system (CNS) tumors, and head trauma. Girls usually show an increase in height of only 2 to 3 inches after the onset of menstruation.

Early menstrual cycles are often irregular and anovulatory (not preceded by ovulation and discharge of an ovum). Although menstrual cycles may not be regular for several years, the woman is still potentially fertile.

■ MENSTRUAL CYCLE

The menstrual cycle is a complex set of recurrent changes in the uterus, ovaries, cervix, and vagina. The cycle consists of:

- Proliferation
- Secretion
- Premenstrual phases

■ MENSTRUATION

Each phase is characterized by specific histologic changes in the endometrium. The length of the menstrual cycle is calculated from the first day of menstrual flow. The cycle generally runs about 25 to 32 days but can vary from month to month, even in the same woman.

The menstrual cycle depends on interactions between the CNS, anterior pituitary, ovaries, and uterus. Variations in the length of the proliferative phase (which ends with ovulation) typically cause a change in the length of the entire cycle. Environmental influences, climatic changes, emotionally traumatic experiences, stress, or acute or chronic illness also may affect the menstrual cycle.

Proliferative Phase

The proliferative phase of the menstrual cycle depends on the ratio of follicle-stimulating hormone (FSH) to LH. In the ovary, after menstrual flow has begun, primary follicles (containing oocytes, or primitive ova) and follicular cells begin to develop under the influence of FSH from the anterior pituitary gland (Fig. U8–3). The thecal (stromal) cells surrounding ova produce estrogens. The increased level of estrogen signals the pituitary to inhibit FSH production and to stimulate secretion of LH. Acting together, the two pituitary hormones then stimulate further estrogen production. Estrogens further inhibit FSH release from the anterior pituitary. LH becomes dominant, stimulating maturation of the follicle.

About 2 days before ovulation, a graafian follicle reaches full maturity and the remaining primary follicles degenerate. Ovulation occurs when the graafian follicle migrates to the ovary's cortex and ruptures through the ovary's wall.

In the uterus, meanwhile, related changes are occurring, largely in response to increased estrogen from the developing follicle. At the end of a menstrual flow, the uterine endometrium (containing surface epithelium, glands, connective tissue, spaces, and blood vessels) is very thin because much of it has sloughed off during menstrual flow. Estrogen stimulates creation of new endometrial surface layer and uterine epithelium. It stimulates growth of glands and stroma. The epithelium becomes thicker and more vascular. Endometrial proliferation peaks about 2 days before ovulation.

The cervix also undergoes changes. Most important, secretion of mucus, a clear fluid that is receptive to sperm, greatly increases just before ovulation. Vaginal changes during this phase include proliferation and thickening of the vaginal epithelium due to estrogen. This change is greatest at the time of ovulation.

Ovulation

Increased levels of estrogen cause a decrease in FSH secretion, allowing a flood of LH to occur. Over a 24-hour period, this process causes the thecal and granulosa cells lining the follicle to hypertrophy and proliferate.

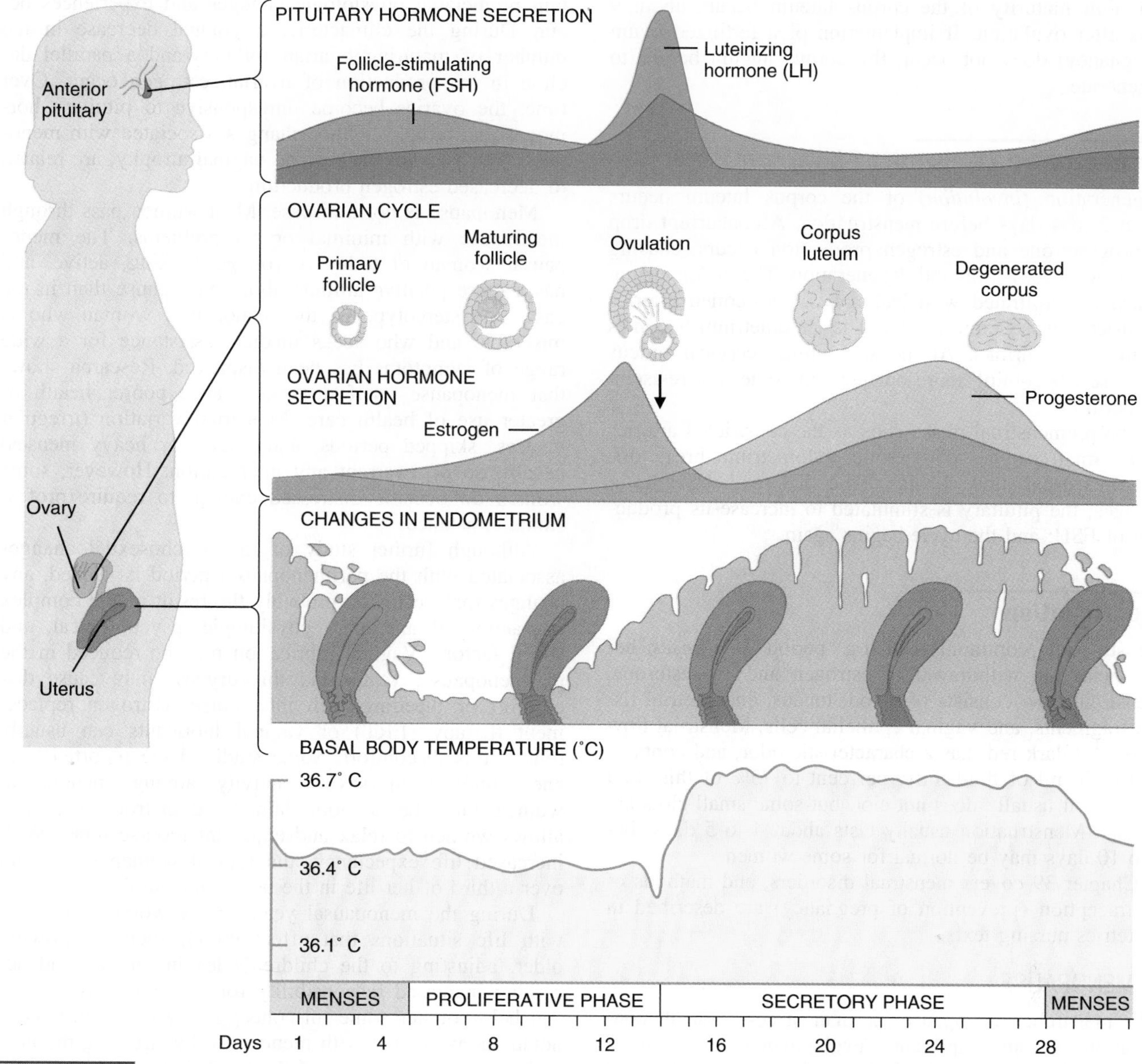

FIGURE U8–3 Menstrual (uterine) cycle. Note hormonal control of the menstrual cycle and the effects on ovaries *(center)* and endometrium *(bottom).*

When ovulation occurs, the ovarian follicle collapses and estrogen production temporarily drops.

At ovulation, the graafian follicle breaks through the ovary's wall and passes into the abdominal cavity. Some hemorrhage occurs into the center of the ruptured follicle, where a clot quickly forms. This may produce a transient abdominal pain *(mittelschmerz).*

Once in the abdominal cavity, the graafian follicle is usually picked up by the fimbriated ends of the fallopian tube and is slowly transported to the uterus. Unless it is fertilized, it eventually passes out of the body with the menstrual flow.

Ovulation occurs 12 to 15 days before the onset of the next menstrual period. It is almost impossible to determine exactly when ovulation will occur, even if one counted from the first day of the preceding menstrual period.

Secretory (Luteal) Phase

During the secretory phase (lasting 10 to 14 days), progesterone and estrogen promote marked changes in the endometrium. Connective tissue hypertrophies. The arteries coil and become tortuous. The glands become larger and more tortuous and abundantly secrete a substance containing glycogen. The endometrium becomes edematous, compact, and thickened. Development peaks 7 to 8 days after ovulation. This is the most favorable time for implantation of a fertilized ovum.

In the ovary after ovulation, the corpus luteum (yellow body) develops within the ruptured ovarian follicle. First, the clot that developed in response to follicular hemorrhage is replaced with yellowish luteal cells containing lipids. These cells eventually form the *corpus luteum,* an endocrine body that secretes progesterone and some estrogen. Full maturity of the corpus luteum occurs about 9 days after ovulation. If implantation of a fertilized ovum (pregnancy) does not occur, the corpus luteum begins to degenerate.

Premenstrual (Ischemic) Phase

Degeneration *(involution)* of the corpus luteum occurs about 2 to 4 days before menstruation. A concurrent drop in progesterone and estrogen production occurs, causing endometrial retraction and degeneration. The endometrium is heavily infiltrated with leukocytes. The coiled arteries constrict and ischemia results. The endometrium becomes anemic and shrinks. At the same time, cervical mucus decreases, becoming more opaque and somewhat resistant to sperm.

The premenstrual phase ends as the constricted arteries open. Small patches of necrotic endometrium break off, and menstrual flow begins. The LH and FSH ratio changes; the pituitary is stimulated to increase its production of FSH; and the cycle begins again.

Menstruation

Menstruation, commonly called a "period" or *menses,* begins with the withdrawal of estrogen and progesterone. Menstrual flow consists of blood, mucus, endometrial tissue fragments, and vaginal epithelial cells. Menstrual flow is usually dark red, has a characteristic odor, and contains 60 to 150 ml of fluid. Fifty per cent to 75% of this fluid is blood; it usually does not clot, but some small clots are normal. Menstruation usually lasts about 4 to 5 days, but 1 to 10 days may be normal for some women.

Chapter 39 covers menstrual disorders, and methods of contraception (prevention of pregnancy) are described in obstetrics nursing texts.

■ MENOPAUSE

Like menarche, menopause (permanent cessation of menstruation) is an important developmental event in a woman's life, having physical, psychological, and social implications for the woman. Menopause is one event of a complex biologic aging sequence of the *climacteric,* or *perimenopausal,* period. This period lasts about 15 to 20 years (ages 40 to 60); during this time, the body makes the transition from fertility to infertility. Menopause usually occurs between the ages of 48 and 54, but it may occur as early as age 35. The average age at menopause appears to be increasing in industrialized countries.

Menstrual cessation may be abrupt, but usually it occurs over 1 to 2 years. Periodic menstrual flow gradually lessens, occurs less frequently, and becomes irregular. Anovulatory cycles are common, and occasional episodes of profuse bleeding may be interspersed with episodes of scant bleeding. Menopause is said to have occurred when there have been no menstrual periods for 12 consecutive months. Because unplanned pregnancy may occur during the premenopausal period, sexually active women should use contraception for at least 6 months after menses have ceased. Any spontaneous uterine bleeding after menopause is abnormal and should be investigated.

Although the cause of menopause is not known, certain predictable physiologic changes and experiences occur. During the climacteric, a gradual decrease in the number of maturing ovarian follicles and a parallel decline in the production of ovarian estrogen occur. Over time, the ovaries become unresponsive to pituitary hormones and atrophy. Other changes associated with menopause, such as hot flashes and vaginal atrophy, are related to decreased estrogen production.

Menopause is not a disease. Most women pass through menopause with minimal or no problems. The menopausal woman of today is younger-looking, active, and has a more positive attitude about menopause than in the past. The stereotype of the menopausal woman who is miserable and who seeks medical assistance for a wide range of symptoms has been disproved. Research shows that menopause itself does not cause poorer health or greater use of health care. Menstrual variation (irregular menses, skipped periods, and scanty or heavy menses) usually do not warrant any intervention. However, some women do become distressed enough to require professional assistance.

Although further study of the psychosexual changes associated with the perimenopausal period is needed, any changes that occur are probably the result of the complex interaction of anatomic, physiologic, psychological, and social factors. Vaginal lubrication may be reduced in the perimenopausal years, and this dryness may cause discomfort or bleeding with intercourse. Estrogen replacement therapy (ERT) or vaginal lubricants can usually relieve this discomfort. Some studies have reported lessened interest in sexual activity among menopausal women, but other authors claim freedom from pregnancy allows women to relax and enjoy intercourse more. With increased life expectancy, the typical woman can spend over a third of her life in the postmenopausal years.

During the menopausal years, many women are faced with life situations that affect mood, such as growing older, adjusting to the children's leaving home, and accepting increased responsibility for aging parents. Nurses can help counter some misconceptions and negative connotations associated with menopause by stressing the normal and positive aspects of the experience, clarifying misconceptions about menopause, and differentiating the physiologic manifestations of menopause from midlife developmental changes.

MALE REPRODUCTIVE SYSTEM

STRUCTURES

The male reproductive organs consist of paired *testicles,* lying within the scrotum; epididymides; seminal ducts; spermatic cords; seminal vesicles; ejaculatory ducts; bulbourethral (Cowper's) glands; the prostate gland; and the penis (Table U8–2 and Fig. U8–4). The penis and scrotum are external, visible genitalia, whereas the other structures are internal. The male perineum is the external area between the scrotum and the anus.

■ PENIS AND RELATED STRUCTURES

The *penis* is both a sexual organ (organ of copulation) and an organ for urination. This cylindrical, pendulous

TABLE U8–2 MALE REPRODUCTIVE STRUCTURES AND THEIR FUNCTIONS

Structure	Description	Function
Penis	Erectile tissue arranged in three columns, each enclosed in a fascial sheath (tunica albuginea): two lateral columns (corpora cavernosa) and a median column (corpus spongiosum) that contains the urethra. All are surrounded by a thick, fibrous envelope (Buck's fascia)	Ejects semen for fertilization; excretes urine
Bulbourethral (Cowper's) glands	Two small glands above the corpus spongiosum; homologous to Bartholin's glands	Enhances lubrication during intercourse
Scrotum	Double pouch of muscular contractile tissue between the root of the penis and the perineum. It is bisected by a ridge. Each half contains a testicle and epididymis, and part of a spermatic cord made up of nerves, testicular vessels (spermatic artery, vein, lymph vessels), and vas deferens	Provides protective environment for production of sperm
Testicles	Two smooth, solid, ovoid structures (4 cm × 2 to 2.5 cm) with outer coat of inelastic fibrous tunica albuginea. Lobules in testicles contain tubules composed of germ cells (develop into sperm) and Sertoli cells (support spermatogenesis). Between the tubules are Leydig cells (source of testosterone)	Produce testosterone and sperm
Sperm	Germ cell with flattened, broad, oval head with a nucleus, protoplasmic middle piece or neck, and a hair-like tail (flagellum); has 23 chromosomes	Fertilizes ovum
Epididymis	Small oblong structure consisting of a convoluted tube 3.96 to 6.1 m long; attaches to upper end of testicle	Transports sperm
Vas deferens	Smooth muscle tube about 46 cm long	Stores and transmits sperm from testicles
Prostate gland	Partly muscular, partly glandular structure posterior to the symphysis pubis; urethra and ejaculatory ducts pass through it	Contributes to liquefaction of semen
Seminal vesicles	Two sac-like structures 5 cm long; they connect to the vas deferens	Secretions contribute to sperm nutrition and activation

structure suspends from its attachment to the pubic arch. The skin of the penis is dark, hairless, thin, and loose (permitting considerable distention).

The portion of the penis between its end or head and its attachment to the pubic bone is the *shaft.* In males, the urethra's external opening *(meatus* or orifice) is in the glans *(glans penis),* the cone-shaped end or head of the penis. The glans is the conical expansion of the corpus spongiosum. The expanded posterior border of the glans is the *corona.* At its junction with the shaft is the *coronal sulcus.* A flap of movable skin *(foreskin* or *prepuce)* covers the glans. *Smegma* is a cheesy, thick, odoriferous secretion of sloughed-off epithelial cells that collects under the prepuce. (In females, smegma is the secretion of the apocrine glands of the clitoris together with epithelial cells.)

The penis is homologous to the female clitoris. Usually, the penis is flaccid, but, when stimulated (physically or during sexual excitement), it becomes rigid. An *erection* occurs when the corpora cavernosa fill with blood. The tissue becomes congested (hyperemic) with blood. Following *orgasm* (climax of sexual excitement) and *ejaculation* (emission of semen), the blood leaves. An erect penis may differ in size from a flaccid penis. Penis size, however, does not physically influence sexual pleasure. The secretion of the *bulbourethral (Cowper's) glands* forms part of the semen.

■ SCROTUM AND TESTES

The *scrotum* is a double pouch hanging from the root of the penis. It is separated into halves internally by muscular contractile tissue *(tunica dartos)* and externally by a *raphe* (ridge) that runs over the scrotum from the root of the penis to the anus. Each half of the scrotum contains (1) a testicle with its epididymis and (2) part of a spermatic cord held together by spermatic fascia.

The *vas deferens (ductus deferens, seminal duct)* is the testicle's excretory duct. It is the continuation of the epididymis and it conveys sperm from the testicle to the prostatic urethra (from the epididymis to the ejaculatory

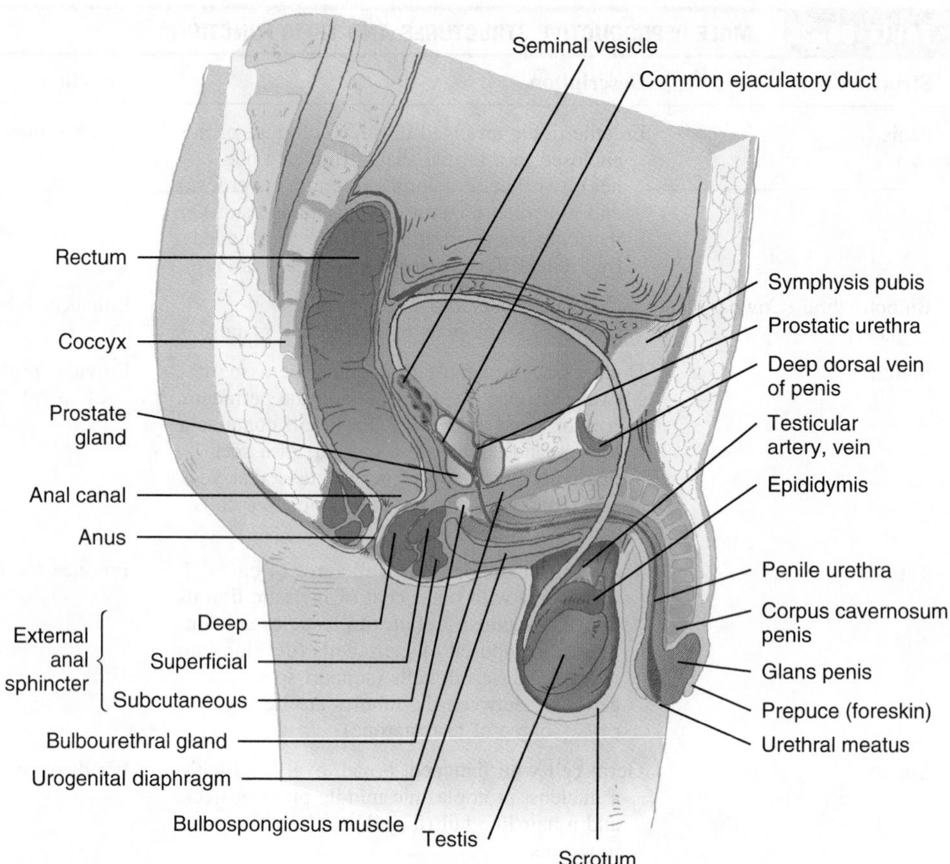

FIGURE U8–4 Midsagittal section of the male pelvis and external genitalia.

duct). The *ejaculatory duct* then conveys semen to the urethra.

The *spermatic cord* goes through the inguinal canal, and the vas deferens continues into the abdominal cavity. It passes behind the bladder, anterior to the rectum, to join the duct of the seminal vesicle, becoming the ejaculatory duct. The spermatic cord is movable for protection from trauma and facilitates optimal production of mature, functional sperm.

Testicles produce the male hormone *(testosterone)* and the male reproductive cells *(sperm).* Many lobules, separated by septa, divide a testicle. Each lobule contains one to three seminiferous tubules where sperm are produced. There are 600 to 1200 seminiferous tubules (90% of the mature testis) in each testicle. Between the seminiferous tubules are interstitial cells called *Leydig cells,* the source of testosterone, the male hormone. The lobules of the testicles lead to straight ducts that join a plexus, from which efferent ducts lead to the epididymis.

The *epididymis* rests on and beside the posterior surface of the testicle. Its head caps the upper end of the testicle and its tail becomes continuous with the vas deferens, which joins other vessels to form the spermatic cord. The head of the epididymis contains 12 to 20 testicular efferent ducts.

■ SPERM

Sperm are mature male sex or germ cells that develop after puberty. Resembling tadpoles, sperm propel themselves by hair-like tails like *flagella.* A normal sperm has a flattened, broad, oval head with a nucleus. A middle piece or protoplasmic neck connects to the tail. During fertilization, the sperm's head pierces an ovum. The sperm's tail is lost when fusion of two cells occurs. Sperm are produced in the seminiferous tubules of the testicles. Sperm develop in great quantities from spermatids (spermoblasts) and are stored in the vas deferens.

■ PROSTATE GLAND AND RELATED STRUCTURES

The prostate gland surrounds the neck of the male urinary bladder and urethra. In childhood the prostate is small, but during puberty it grows to the size of a chestnut. The adult prostate gland lies like a flattened cone in the pelvis, about 2 cm posterior to the symphysis pubis. In a normal adult man, the prostate weighs 15 to 20 g and is 4 to 6 cm long. The prostate is inverted, so that its apex is inferior, and it is suspended by the urogenital diaphragm. The base of the prostate is superior and at the bladder neck, anterior to the rectum. A firm fibrous capsule, containing smooth muscle fibers in its inner layer, encloses the prostate. The bladder overlies the prostate's basal surface.

The posterior surface of the prostate is in close contact with the rectal wall. This is the surface of the prostate that is available for digital examination.

The portion of the urethra that passes through the prostate is called the *prostatic urethra.* Prostatic muscle fibers encircle the urethra and separate the prostate's glandular tissue.

The *seminal vesicles* are sac-like structures whose secretion, a component of *semen* (seminal fluid, or ejaculate), may contribute to sperm nutrition and activation. They lie behind the bladder and connect to the vas deferens on each side.

Male Sexual Development and Function

Development of the male genitalia requires two hormones: (1) müllerian duct inhibitory factor, secreted by *Sertoli cells,* and (2) testosterone, secreted by Leydig cells (see gonadal development earlier). Germ cells develop into spermatozoa, and Sertoli cells support spermatogenesis.

The hypothalamus and pituitary gland regulate testicular function. The hypothalamus secretes gonadotropin-releasing hormone (GnRH) in a pulsatile fashion. GnRH stimulates the anterior pituitary gland to produce LH and FSH. LH stimulates Leydig cells to produce testosterone, which modulates the secretion of GnRH and therefore LH through negative feedback to the hypothalamus and pituitary gland. FSH and testosterone stimulate Sertoli cells and germ cells to start and complete spermatogenesis. *Inhibin,* released from Sertoli cells, provides a negative feedback on FSH release by the anterior pituitary.

Testosterone is the primary androgen secreted by the testis. The testis also secretes androstenedione and estradiol. Estradiol may be important for skeletal maturation in the male.

■ SPERMATOGENESIS

Spermatogenesis is the process of sperm production and development that occurs within the seminiferous tubules during active sex life. It begins at puberty as a result of stimulation by the gonadotropic hormones from the anterior pituitary.

Spermatogonia are the germinal epithelial cells found in the outer border of the tubular epithelium. These cells are continually formed to replenish themselves while a portion continue to develop into sperm. During the first stage of spermatogenesis, the spermatogonia divide and migrate toward the Sertoli cells. The spermatogonia penetrate the membranes of Sertoli cells and become enveloped within the cytoplasm of these cells. The spermatogonia continue this close relationship with Sertoli cells throughout their development.

During the 24 days when it is in contact with Sertoli cells, the spermatogonium changes and enlarges to form a primary *spermatocyte.* After this development, the spermatocyte splits into two secondary spermatocytes, each with only 23 chromosomes. After 2 to 3 days, the spermatocytes undergo a second division to form four *spermatids,* again with 23 chromosomes. The sperm that eventually fertilizes the female ovum contains half the genetic material; the ovum contains the other half.

The period of spermatogenesis from germinal cell to sperm takes about 74 days. During this time, the spermatocytes lose some cytoplasm, the chromatin material of the head reorganizes to form a compact head, and the remaining cytoplasm and cell membranes collect at one end of the cell to form the tail of the sperm.

■ ROLE OF HORMONES

Testosterone is essential to the growth and division of the germinal cells that form the sperm. LH stimulates Leydig cells to secrete testosterone. FSH stimulates Sertoli cells to promote spermatogenesis. Estrogens, formed from testosterone when Sertoli cells are stimulated by FSH, appear to be essential in spermatogenesis. Growth hormone (GH) promotes early division of spermatogonia.

■ MATURATION IN THE EPIDIDYMIS

After the sperm are formed in the seminiferous tubules, they spend several days passing through the epididymis. After about 24 hours in the epididymis, they become motile and capable of fertilization (i.e., they are mature).

Sperm are stored in small amounts in the epididymis but are mainly stored in the vas deferens and the ampulla of the vas deferens. With low levels of sexual activity, the sperm can be stored there up to a month, maintaining their motility and fertility. When sexual activity is frequent, sperm may be stored only a few days.

■ PROSTATIC FLUID

The prostate gland secretes a milky fluid that forms part of the semen. This fluid aids the passage of sperm and helps keep them alive, supplying them with food, if needed. Prostatic secretion is manufactured in a network of branching glands embedded in muscle within the prostate. This muscle contracts during ejaculation, and prostatic secretions are ejected through the ejaculatory ducts into the urethra.

■ SEMEN

Semen is a viscid, thick, opalescent secretion discharged by males through the urethra at the climax of sexual excitement or orgasm. It contains sperm and other secretions. About 10% of the semen is composed of sperm and fluid from the vas deferens, with about 60% made up of fluid from the seminal vesicles. The remaining 30% is composed of prostatic fluid and small amounts of mucoid secretion from the bulbourethral glands.

Semen is slightly alkaline, with a pH of about 7.5. The prostatic fluid contains a clotting enzyme, causing the fibrinogen of the seminal vesicle fluid to form a weak coagulum. This coagulum holds the semen near the uterine cervix. The coagulum dissolves in about 15 to 30 minutes, at which time the sperm become highly motile. The sperm can live within the vagina for 24 to 48 hours after ejaculation.

CONCLUSIONS

The human reproductive system is tremendously complex, and reproductive and sexual characteristics can have a great physical and emotional impact on our lives from conception. Changes initiated at the fetal stage cause differentiation between male and female. Sexual maturation, starting between the ages of 9 and 13 years, alters both external and internal structures. A thorough knowledge of the structure and function of the female and male reproductive systems is important so that the nurse will be able to provide safe, effective care for clients with associated problems. The nurse must be sensitive to the delicate nature of reproductive problems because many disorders affect sexuality.

BIBLIOGRAPHY

1. Fauci, A. S., et al. (1998). *Harrison's principles of internal medicine* (14th ed.). New York: McGraw-Hill.
2. Guyton, A. C., & Hall, J. E. (1996). *Textbook of medical physiology* (9th ed.). Philadelphia: W. B. Saunders.
3. Silverthorn, D. (1998). *Human physiology*. Upper Saddle River, NJ: Prentice Hall.

CHAPTER 37

Assessment of the Reproductive System

Rhonda Holloway

Your ability to assess the reproductive system competently and compassionately is important to your clients on both physical and psychosocial levels. To perform this task well, you will need a combination of sound assessment skills and a nonjudgmental attitude that is both professional and empathic.

Because of the close association between the reproductive, urinary, and bowel elimination systems, you must be prepared for some overlap in their assessment (see also Chapter 32.) You also must be prepared for some difficulty in discussing reproductive and elimination topics. Many clients are uncomfortable talking about them. Language and semantic barriers may interfere with communication as well, in part because of the many words and slang terms used to describe reproductive anatomy, function, and problems. Educational or cultural barriers also can inhibit a client from discussing a problem. Remain sensitive and nonjudgmental, and do your best to put the client at ease.

Clients have the right to be informed and to actively participate in decisions about their health. A supportive, respectful attitude on your part promotes comfort, cooperation, and participation in health care. Be alert to sexist attitudes in yourself and the health care system, either of which may lead to ignored health complaints, unnecessary or inappropriate prescriptions, and unneeded procedures. Be an advocate, and positively influence the client's perception of health care and the importance of health maintenance.

Especially when assessing the reproductive system, provide privacy and create an environment conducive to the expression of feelings. Encourage the client to voice concerns and ask questions. Assess the client's understanding of health care information, and explore what the client perceives as needs and problems. You may need to repeat information, especially if the client is anxious or feeling stressed, for example, during a pelvic or prostate examination. Provide a sensitive, humane orientation to reproductive health care. Teaching and counseling promote health maintenance.

Besides providing a history and physical examination, an adequate reproductive assessment should include an in-depth review of the client's lifestyle, health habits, self-perception, body image, and developmental stage along with cultural, religious, socioeconomic, and educational factors. These factors influence the client's health and health-seeking behaviors. Throughout your assessment, you will find that a respect for others' values facilitates effective care. Cultural or ethnic background, socioeconomic status, and sexual preference should never limit a client's access to, or quality of, health care.

THE FEMALE REPRODUCTIVE SYSTEM

Many women receive most, if not all, of their primary health care from obstetric and gynecologic health care providers—not only for gynecologic conditions but also for general health. An annual gynecologic examination provides opportunity to discuss health maintenance activities. For example, during a client's health visit for a Papanicolaou (Pap) smear, take the opportunity to teach breast self-examination and discuss risk factors associated with gynecologic cancer and heart disease. Explain developmental changes (e.g., adolescence, menarche, or menopause) and menstrual hygiene and symptom management. Discuss lifestyle factors that affect health maintenance, such as diet, exercise, adequate sleep and rest, stress management, cessation of smoking, and general risk factor identification. If appropriate, provide information about protection against sexually transmitted diseases (STDs).

After establishing rapport, perform a comprehensive gynecologic nursing assessment appropriate to the situation. (For a review of a comprehensive history and psychosocial assessment, see Chapter 9). Follow the health history with a systematic physical examination. Diagnostic tests may be ordered, some of which you will perform. The resulting data are the basis for nursing intervention.

HISTORY

The health history for the female reproductive system includes data related to the genitals, the reproductive system, the breasts, and the woman's overall health status. Conduct the interview in private while the woman is clothed to maintain her level of comfort.

BIOGRAPHICAL AND DEMOGRAPHIC DATA

Biographical and demographic data can help to establish the client's health risk status. The incidence of some gynecologic cancers is higher in certain age groups. For example, the risk of breast cancer rises with age. Ethnicity may also be a risk factor for certain gynecologic cancers, such as cancer of the cervix. Because controversy exists about the influence of environmental factors in the development of reproductive disorders, the client's living and working environments may prove to be important.

CURRENT HEALTH: THE CHIEF COMPLAINT

Ask the client to describe her reason for seeking gynecologic care. Be alert to the possible nature of the problem as well as to the level of the woman's understanding of the problem. This information will direct the health history interview and your health teaching. If the client's visit is for a specific problem rather than for a routine examination, ask her to relate the history of the problem and conduct a symptom analysis (see Chapter 9).

PAST HEALTH HISTORY

To investigate the client's past health history, review her childhood and infectious illnesses, major illnesses and hospitalizations, medications, and allergies.

Childhood and Infectious Diseases

The most serious childhood infectious illness that may affect a woman of childbearing age is *rubella.* Maternal rubella during the first trimester increases fetal risk for congenital disorders. Ask the client if she has had rubella or has immunity to it. If she is contemplating pregnancy, suggest that a rubella titer be drawn to determine her immunity status. If the titer is negative, indicating that immunity is lacking, encourage the woman to be vaccinated. Advise the newly immunized woman to avoid pregnancy for at least 3 months. A pregnant woman should not be vaccinated.

Ask the client about her history of STDs and STD exposure. Many of these diseases, left unrecognized or untreated, can damage the reproductive system, particularly the fallopian tubes. The result may be problems with fertility and achieving pregnancy.

Major Illnesses and Hospitalizations

Ask about major illnesses. For instance, diabetes is associated with increased maternal and fetal morbidity and mortality. Pregnancy and oral contraceptive use are also linked with higher morbidity and mortality rates in women who have a history of cardiovascular disease, such as angina, hypertension, and thrombophlebitis. Anemia can result from menstrual disorders, such as dysfunctional uterine bleeding. Hypothyroidism and hyperthyroidism can affect the menstrual cycle, as can other endocrine disorders.

Urinary tract disorders can interfere with sexual function. Women who have migraine headaches or seizure disorders may need to avoid oral contraceptives because of the increased risk of migraines and seizures associated with their use. Oral contraceptives, pregnancy, dietary changes, or a high-fat diet may worsen cholecystitis. Hepatitis and other liver disorders contraindicate estrogen use because of its route of metabolism. Estrogens are usually contraindicated in women who have had breast cancer or cancers of the reproductive tract.

Ask about surgery involving the reproductive system. Specific surgical procedures include dilation and curettage (D&C), tubal ligation, cryosurgery or cryotherapy, cystocele and rectocele repair, hysterectomy, oophorectomy, salpingectomy and salpingotomy. Inquire about interrupted pregnancies, including both elective and spontaneous abortions.

Medications

Collect a complete medication history, including prescription and over-the-counter medications, vitamin and mineral supplements, and recreational or illegal substances. Contraceptive medications can include oral contraceptive pills, medroxyprogesterone injections, and vaginal preparations. Ask about episodic medications, such as those used for premenstrual syndrome (PMS) and menstrual discomforts (e.g., diuretics), and the use of herbal or other "natural" substances. These may include:

- Black cohosh (*Cimicifuga racemosa*) for menstrual irregularity, PMS, and menopausal problems
- Chamomile (*Martricaria recutita, Chamaemelum nobile*) for menstrual cramps
- Chaste tree (*Vitex agnuscastus*) for PMS and menopausal problems and possibly for mastalgia
- Evening primrose (*Oenothera biennis*) for PMS
- Feverfew (*Tanacetum parthenium*) for menstrual problems
- Sage (*Salvia officinalis*) for menstrual irregularity
- Soybeans and other legumes for their phytoestrogens that may help prevent breast cancer

Ask specifically about hormone replacement therapy (including estrogen, progesterone, thyroid hormones, and corticosteroids). Recreational or illegal substances, such as alcohol, amphetamines, barbiturates, marijuana, and hallucinogens, may affect sexual behavior and risk status for exposure to an STD, among other problems.

Allergies

Ask the client about all allergies, including allergic reactions. Antibiotics are used to treat genitourinary infections. Latex and rubber are used in contraceptive devices such as condoms, cervical caps, and diaphragms, some of which are used in conjunction with spermicides. Some intrauterine contraceptive devices contain copper. Allergies to these substances eliminate their use for contraception. Use vinyl gloves instead of latex while examining the client, if necessary.

GYNECOLOGIC HISTORY

A gynecologic history includes questions about breasts, menstruation, contraceptives, sexual practices, obstetric problems, genitourinary problems, and reproductive health practices. For a menopausal or older woman or a woman who has had a hysterectomy, ask only the appropriate questions.

Breast History

Ask the client about breast pain or tenderness and its occurrence in relation to the menstrual cycle. Many women experience breast tenderness before menstruation in relation to hormonal changes. Ask whether the woman has had or currently has breast lumps or masses. If a lump is present, ask the woman to describe its location, onset, and size and whether it is painful. Determine whether the lump has changed shape, size, consistency, or degree of tenderness since it was first noticed. Does the lump change during the menstrual cycle? Because the breasts become more firm and cystic during the luteal phase, the best time to perform breast palpation is 7 to 10 days after onset of menses.

Ask about any nipple discharge, which would be abnormal in women who are not pregnant or lactating. If discharge is present, determine the color, consistency, amount, and odor.

Ask whether the woman performs a monthly breast self-examination (BSE). Ask about frequency of examination and the technique used so that you can decide whether the client needs a review of the procedure and supervised practice. Note whether the woman includes the axillary nodes in the BSE (see Chapter 2.)

Finally, ask whether there is a history of breast cancer in the client's blood-related female relatives, including mother, sisters, maternal grandmother, or maternal aunts. Breast cancer in these relatives indicates an increased risk of breast cancer for the client.

Menstrual History

Ask the woman at what age she started menstruating. Determine the first day of her last menstrual period. Ask the number of days per cycle and the regularity of cycles. Assessing the amount of menstrual flow is difficult. Knowing whether more than one pad or tampon per hour becomes saturated helps to determine whether the flow is unusually profuse. Are there clots in the flow? How long does the menstrual period last?

Does the woman experience pain during menstruation? If so, have her describe the pain, its duration, whether it occurs with every cycle, and what she uses for relief. Does she experience midcycle bleeding, spotting, or pain. Are there any moliminal (premenstrual discomfort) manifestations? Are there any menopausal manifestations, including menstrual cycle changes?

Contraceptive History

Document the current contraceptive method (if any), satisfaction with the method, duration of use, any contraceptive problems, and any desire to change methods. Ask about previous contraceptive methods, problems encountered, and reason for discontinuation. Provide contraceptive information if appropriate. For a woman of reproductive age who is not sterilized and who is heterosexually active, determine whether she wants to become pregnant.

Sexual History

Obtain a sexual history using a direct approach and terms the woman understands. The purpose of a sexual history is to identify sexual problems and to give the woman an opportunity to ask questions or express concerns (Table 37–1). To help put the client at ease, explain why you are asking for this information and assure her that it will be kept confidential.

Begin with general questions about whether the woman is satisfied and comfortable with her current sexual activity. A nonjudgmental approach is essential; make no assumptions about anything, including the sex or number of partners. Follow up on any concerns or issues she raises. Of particular importance are difficulties or concerns she may have. Be alert for any risk-taking behaviors, including those that put her at risk of STDs. See Chapter 9 for further information on sexuality assessment.

Obstetric History

If the woman is in her childbearing years, ask if she thinks she may be pregnant. (Pregnancy may contraindicate mammography or other radiologic studies as well as certain medications.) If the woman has been pregnant, obtain information about each pregnancy, including the delivery and postpartum period. Document details of any difficulties or complications (physical or psychosocial). Record any spontaneous or planned abortions. If the woman has never been pregnant, ask whether children were or are desired. If the woman has relinquished a child for adoption, explore the circumstance and her feelings about it. See Chapter 9 for detailed questions to assess the obstetric history.

Genitourinary History

Ask about previous problems with genitourinary infections and vaginitis. Determine whether the woman has had a previous pelvic infection or STD, treatment, or complications. Determine whether the woman experiences urinary or fecal incontinence and the circumstances surrounding the incontinence. (Chapter 34 discusses urinary incontinence, and Chapter 33 discusses fecal incontinence.)

Reproductive Health Practices

Seek information about menstrual, sexual, and gynecologic hygiene, including douching. Ask about the frequency of gynecologic examinations. If appropriate, ask the client whether she uses protection against STDs and unwanted pregnancy.

■ FAMILY HEALTH HISTORY

A family history of diabetes, cardiovascular disease, or cancer of a reproductive organ may indicate a higher risk for development of those diseases. If the woman's mother received diethylstilbestrol (DES) while pregnant with the client, the woman may be at risk for reproductive tract cancer or structural and functional abnormalities.

■ PSYCHOSOCIAL HISTORY

Occupation and Environment

Ask the woman about any exposures to hazards encountered at work, including toxins or radiation. Many sub-

TABLE 37–1 SEXUAL HEALTH ASSESSMENT

Sexual health assessment may include consideration of the client's current

- Knowledge about sexuality
- Attitudes about sexuality and toward sexual partner(s)
- Level of comfort and feelings of adequacy regarding own sexuality
- Concerns about sexuality of significant others
- Perception of own sex role and that of sexual partner(s)
- Sexual self-concept as a female or male
- Fears and anxiety about intimacy and other aspects of sexuality
- Self-perception of own body (body image)
- Ability to function sexually (e.g., to obtain an erection and control ejaculation, to please sexual partner, to achieve pain-free orgasm, to reproduce, to obtain adequate contraception, to obtain sufficient vaginal lubrication, to give and receive effective sexual stimulation and pleasure)
- Typical sexual patterns and activities (e.g., partner choice [female, male, spouse, extramarital, multiple, single, same partner, different partners], frequency of sexual activity, type of sexual activity [vaginal, anal, oral, masturbation], partner satisfaction, self-satisfaction)
- Level of interest in sexual activity (sex drive)
- Level of satisfaction regarding current sexual opportunity and activity
- Physical health problems affecting sexuality (e.g., menstrual problems, pregnancy, medication, surgery [colostomy, surgical amputation, recent heart surgery or brain surgery], paralysis, illness [hypertension, diabetes, recent myocardial infarction, cerebral vascular accident, injury [recent spinal cord injury, recent head injury, burns, traumatic amputations], sexually transmitted disease, genitourinary problems)

Sexual History

There is no single approach to taking a sexual health history. Information obtained may relate to historical (past) information about the following:

BOTH FEMALES AND MALES

- Pregnancies (information about unplanned pregnancies)
- Fertility management
- Genitourinary problems
- Sexually transmitted disease
- Sexual abuse (e.g., incest, rape, pedophilia, battering)
- Relationship-partner history (e.g., number of sexual partners, sexual orientation [bisexual, homosexual, heterosexual])
- First experience of sexual activity
- Early sexual development and influences
- Adolescent sexual experiences
- Sexual techniques used (e.g., masturbation, intercourse ([oral, vaginal, anal])
- Role models for sexuality (e.g., peers, parents, guardians, famous people, advertising models)
- Spiritual-philosophical models influencing the client's sexuality

FEMALES

- History specific to menstruation, abortion, pregnancy

MALES

- History specific to impotence, nocturnal emissions

stances can affect overall health status generally and reproductive function specifically.

Habits

Ask whether the client smokes cigarettes. Smoking is associated with an increase in morbidity, especially when used in conjunction with oral contraceptives, and also may be related to an earlier than normal onset of menopause. Note the use of alcohol and recreational drugs, habits that increase risk of acquiring STDs.

Domestic Violence

In private, ascertain whether the woman is a victim of domestic violence. Ask every client about violence in her life. Explain that the same question is asked of all women and that she is not being singled out. (She might assume that you ask the question because of her race, nationality, or socioeconomic status.) Clients frequently deny domestic violence many times before acknowledging it; consequently, repeated questioning in a variety of ways may help determine whether the client is a victim. Be alert to physical and behavioral manifestations that are inconsistent with the explanation of their cause. Also be aware of an overprotective significant other. This is also a good time to educate women about options available should violence be or become a problem.

Psychosocial Factors

Because the genital organs and their reproductive capacity have symbolic significance for many women, problems in this area can affect a woman's sexuality and sense of femininity. Gynecologic problems may be associated with changes in self-concept, body image, personal identity, and role performance. Reproductive capabilities, the expression of sexuality, and sexual activities may be affected. In short, gynecologic disorders may result in psychological consequences. For this reason, psychological assessment is especially important. A woman's outward reaction to gynecologic problems does not necessarily correspond with either her inner experience or the seriousness of the condition.

Be sensitive when interviewing and examining a woman. Do not insist on information that she is hesitant to reveal. The woman herself may not understand her responses. Empathic listening is supportive and may lessen the stress the woman feels.

The woman may express fear because of a suspected unhealthy change in the genitals or of unwanted pregnancy. She may feel anxious and embarrassed before undergoing a pelvic examination. Many women consider the pelvic examination unpleasant despite its minimal risk of injury or physical pain. Other feelings that may be expressed include humiliation, guilt, or anger. Deep, powerful feelings may prevent women from seeking gynecologic care. Intrusive gynecologic procedures may evoke memories or strong reactions in women who have experienced sexual abuse or assault. The opportunity to express and discuss feelings with a nurse skilled in therapeutic communication may help these women cope more effectively and follow through with appropriate care. A therapeutic conversation can provide opportunities for clarifying a woman's misconceptions about her diagnosis, proposed treatment, and preventive care. Many women have never received accurate information about reproductive problems.

■ REVIEW OF SYSTEMS

Review the client's physical health history, proceeding from head to toe. Note especially (1) cardiovascular disorders (hypertension, angina [pain], myocardial infarction [MI], thrombophlebitis), (2) endocrine disorders (hypothyroidism, hyperthyroidism), (3) disorders of the pituitary gland, (4) liver disorders, and (5) cholecystitis. Ask about problems involving the urinary tract and reproductive system, such as urinary tract infection, urinary incontinence, vaginitis, and any bleeding disorders associated with menstruation (e.g., amenorrhea, dysmenorrhea, breakthrough bleeding, menorrhagia, or postcoital bleeding). Detailed questions for the review of systems are found in Chapter 9.

PHYSICAL EXAMINATION

Elements of a standard gynecologic examination can vary slightly but usually include the following physical assessment and laboratory data:

- Vital signs (temperature, pulse, respiration, blood pressure)
- Height
- Weight
- Hematocrit (or complete blood count)
- Urinalysis
- Pelvic examination and Pap smear
- Physical assessment of skin, heart, lungs, breasts and axillae, thyroid, and abdomen
- Periodically, lipid profile and thyroid-stimulating hormone (TSH) level
- As appropriate for age and history, colorectal sigmoidoscopy, fecal occult blood testing, and mammography

If unusual or abnormal findings are obtained during the gynecologic history or physical examination, additional data must be sought.

■ BREASTS AND AXILLAE

Examination of the breasts and axillae is an important part of the gynecologic examination. Good lighting is essential. Some examiners complete this portion of the examination before assessing the anterior lungs and heart. Because the breasts are sensitive and closely associated with sexuality, some examiners delay this portion until there has been more hands-on interaction with the client during assessment of the lungs and heart. Others integrate assessments so that the client is sitting for those portions of the heart, lungs, breasts, and axillae examination before being helped to a supine position for the remaining portions. Any sequence is acceptable as long as you are thorough, you maintain the client's privacy, and the client can tolerate the position changes. Instruct the client in BSE while examining the breasts. (See Chapter 2.)

Ask the client when her last menstrual period began. Breasts are usually tender the week before onset of menses and least tender the week after menses has ceased. If the client reports that one breast is tender, begin palpation with the opposite breast. Thorough examination requires exposure of both breasts for comparison.

Inspection

Begin breast inspection while the client is seated with her arms at her sides. Ask her to raise her hands over her head. Finally, ask her to press her hands firmly on her hips or together to tighten the pectoral muscles. Examine women who have large or pendulous breasts while they bend at the waist and face forward with the breast hanging down (Fig. 37–1). In all positions, inspect the breasts for symmetry, size, shape, contour, and skin characteristics, including the vascular pattern.

Breasts are symmetrical, although it is not unusual for one breast to be slightly larger than the other. The breasts should hang evenly between the third and fourth ribs with the nipples about level with the fourth intercostal space when the client sits with her arms at her sides. With aging and loss of tissue elasticity, the breasts hang lower, especially after pregnancy and breast-feeding. The contour is even. Dimpling (retraction), masses, or surface flattening are abnormal. Skin color is the same as that of the abdomen. *Striae* (stretch marks from rapid skin stretching) may be present; recent striae are reddened and become paler with time. Venous patterns, if noticeable, should be symmetrical. Local areas of hyperpigmentation or edema should be absent.

Ask the client to raise her arms over her head while you examine the lateral and undersurfaces of each breast. Contraction of the pectoral muscles exaggerates signs of retraction or skin flattening. Note areas of redness or excoriation from poorly fitting brassieres. The breasts

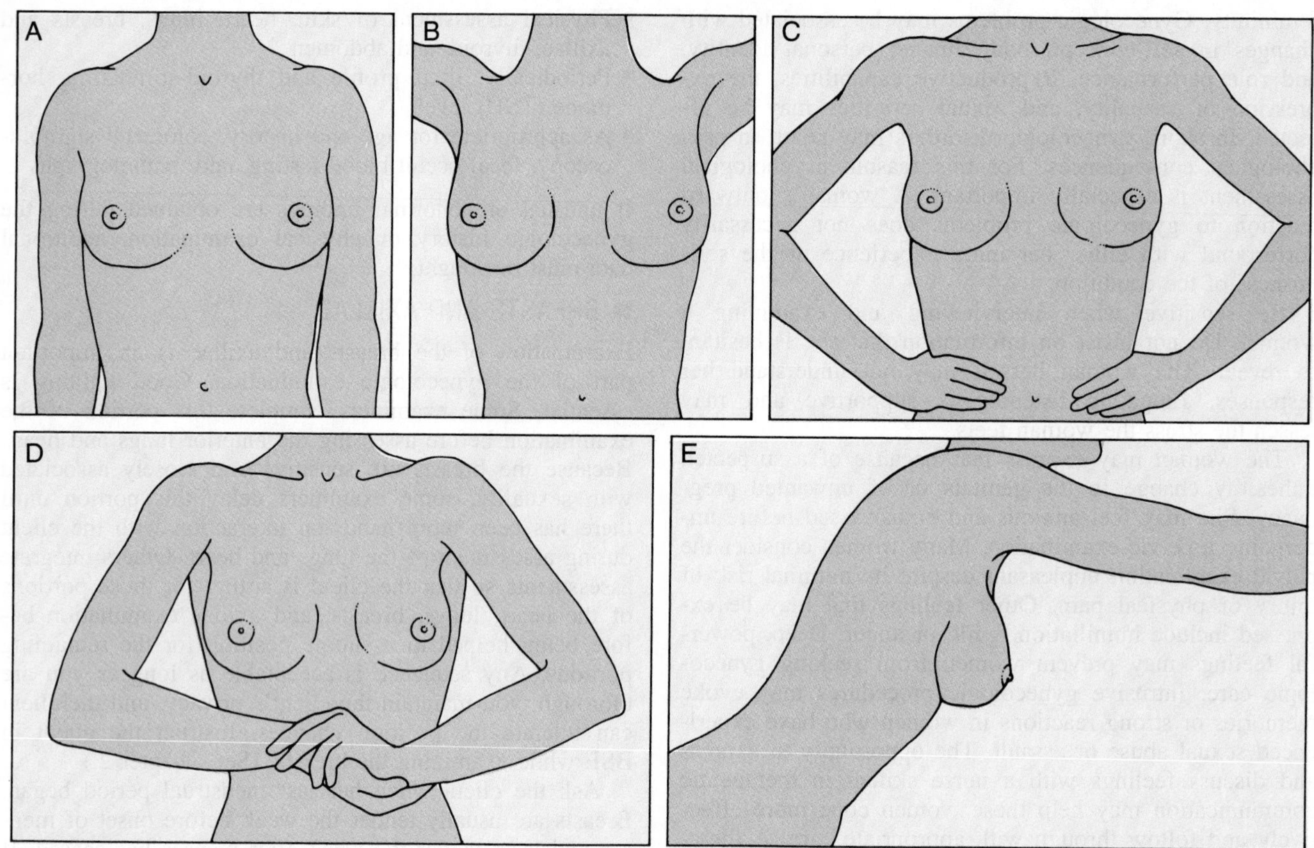

FIGURE 37–1 Positions for breast examination. *A,* Arms at side. *B,* Hands raised over head. For tightening pectoral muscles, the examiner asks the client to press hands firmly on hips (*C*) or to press hands together (*D*). *E,* Breasts may also be examined with the woman leaning forward at the waist, allowing the breasts to hang down.

should elevate evenly so that the areolae remain at the same level. Then ask the client to put her hands on her hips and press inward firmly while you repeat the inspection for masses, retraction, or skin flattening.

Inspect the areolae and nipples for size, shape, contour, symmetry, surface characteristics, and masses or lesions. Areolae are pink in fair-skinned women and darker in dark-skinned women. Slight asymmetry is common, but the nipples should point in symmetrical directions. Masses or lesions are abnormal. Montgomery's tubercles may be prominent around the nipple, which is normal. The nipples are round or oval, equal in size, of the same color, soft, and smooth. If one or both nipples are inverted, ask whether this is a recent occurrence or has been present for a while and how long. Recent nipple inversion is abnormal, and the client should be referred to an appropriate health care provider for follow-up. Rashes, crusts, or discharge should be absent unless the client is in the late stages of pregnancy, when colostrum (a yellowish fluid) may leak from the nipples.

Inspect the axillae for rashes, masses, and areas of unusual pigmentation, which should be absent. Axillary hair should be present unless the client removes it.

Palpation

Palpation of axillae is usually done while the client is seated; breast palpation is facilitated with the client supine. For clients who have large and pendulous breasts or a history of breast masses or cancer or who are at increased risk for breast cancer, the breasts should be palpated in both positions.

Palpation of the axillae includes examination of five sets of lymph nodes (Fig. 37–2). Encourage the client to relax her arm; this relaxes the chest muscles and eases palpation. Begin by palpating the edge of the pectoralis major muscle along the anterior axillary line, using a bimanual technique if necessary, to examine the pectoral (anterior) nodes. Then reach high up into the axilla at the midaxillary line to palpate the midaxillary (central) nodes against the ribs and serratus anterior. Palpate the subscapular (posterior) nodes along the posterior axillary fold along the anterior edge of the latissimus dorsi. Palpate the brachial (lateral) nodes along the humerus in the upper inner arm.

Last, palpate the infraclavicular area. The supraclavicular nodes, which also receive lymphatic drainage from the breasts, are usually examined with the neck nodes. All the nodes should be nonpalpable, although detection of one or two small, nontender, mobile central nodes is often a normal finding. Abnormal findings include firm, fixed nodes that may or may not be tender. If nodes are palpated, note the number of nodes felt, their location, size, shape, mobility, tenderness, and consistency.

Conduct breast palpation systematically to examine all breast tissue, including the tail of Spence in the upper outer quadrant. Any one of several approaches may be used as long as each portion of the breasts, areolae, and

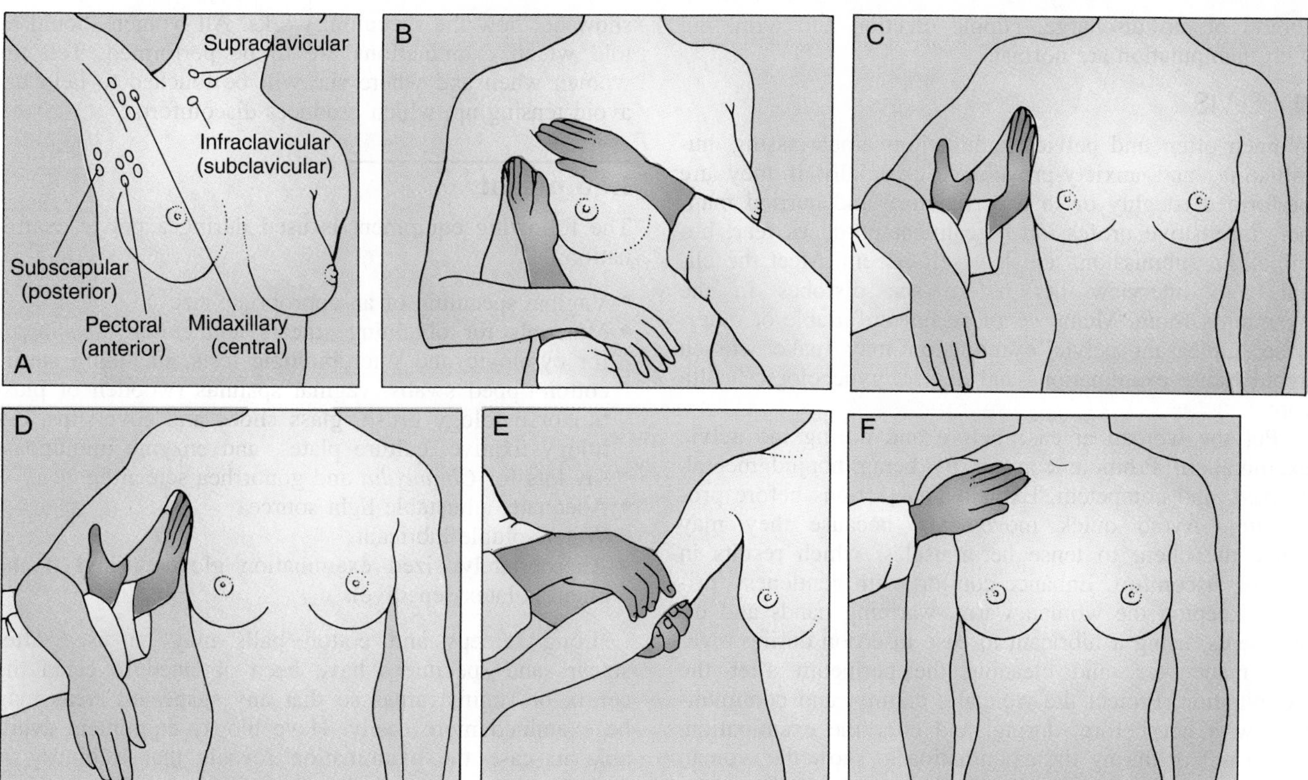

FIGURE 37–2 Assessment of axillary lymph nodes. *A,* Location of the groups of nodes examined. *B,* Pectoral (anterior) nodes. *C,* Midaxillary (central) nodes. *D,* Subscapular (posterior nodes). *E,* Brachial (lateral) nodes. *F,* Infraclavicular (subclavicular) nodes. Axillary nodes are also palpated for male clients.

nipples is palpated. The breast and areola may be palpated in concentric circles, in a wheel-and-spokes pattern, or back and forth from superior to inferior. When the client is sitting, you may prefer to use a bimanual technique, especially if the breasts are large. When the client is supine, place a small folded towel under her shoulder to enhance breast flattening against the chest wall. Have her place her arm behind her head. Slide your fingers along the tissue using a rotary motion to press the breast against the chest wall. Your fingers remain in contact with the skin surface. The firm, curved ridge along the inferior breast is the inframammary ridge.

Breast consistency varies from firm and elastic in young women to stringy and nodular in older women. If the client reports a mass, begin palpation with the unaffected breast so that you have a basis for comparison. Pay particular attention to the upper outer quadrant and tail of Spence, where most of the glandular tissue is located and 50% of breast lesions are found. There should be no masses or local areas of warmth. If you feel a lump or mass, note its characteristics. Include the exact location (and the position the client is in for the palpation), using the areola for a reference point. Note size, shape, contour, consistency, mobility, tenderness, and discreteness. Visualize the breast as having four quadrants plus the tail; the location of lesions can be diagramed in the written record. See the feature Physical Assessment Findings in the Healthy Adult for a recording example.

Palpate the areola and nipple gently. Compress the nipple between your thumb and index finger. There

PHYSICAL ASSESSMENT FINDINGS IN THE HEALTHY ADULT

Female Reproductive System

Inspection

Breasts and Axillae: Breasts symmetrical, full, rounded, smooth in all positions, without dimpling, retractions, or masses. Faint, even vascular pattern and striae noted. Nipples everted, areolae even. Axillae even color, without masses or rash.

Genitalia: Pubic hair distribution varies with stage of sexual development; clean, coarse. Labia majora covered with pubic hair in adult women; may gape open slightly. Labia minora pink, smooth. Clitoris midline, smooth. Urethral meatus pink, discharge absent. Vaginal orifice clean, without bulges. Vaginal walls intact, pink, glistening, rugae present; discharge, bulges, and masses absent. Cervix round with os round or oval in nulliparous women and slit-like in parous women; discharge absent.

Palpation

Breasts and Axillae: Breasts firm without masses, lumps, local areas of warmth, or tenderness. Nipples without discharge. Axillae smooth, nodes nonpalpable.

Genitalia: Pelvic floor musculature firm. Skene's glands without discharge or tenderness. Bartholin's glands without masses or tenderness. No bulges in vaginal wall with straining. Uterus anteverted, firm, smooth, mobile, nontender, without masses. Ovaries oval, firm, movable, nontender.

should be no discharge. Nipple erection and wrinkling with manipulation are normal.

■ PELVIS

Women often find pelvic examinations embarrassing, humiliating, and anxiety-provoking, especially if they are performed roughly or in a perfunctory and hurried manner. Insensitive professional treatment produces fear, humiliation, submission, and low self-esteem. Meet the client, and interview her before she disrobes in the examining room. Memories of an uncomfortable or otherwise unpleasant pelvic examination may make women avoid future examinations and neglect gynecologic health care.

Put the woman at ease before and during the pelvic examination. Promote comfort by being nonjudgmental, relaxed, and competent. Explain your actions before proceeding. Avoid quick movements, because they may cause the client to tense her muscles, which results in greater discomfort. Enhance comfort with gentleness, privacy, keeping the woman warm, warming hands and instruments, using a lubricant to ease insertion during invasive maneuvers, and cleaning the perineum after the examination. Protect the woman's dignity, and communicate with her before, during, and after the examination. Use a mirror during the examination to show the woman her anatomic structures, if she desires, to facilitate the learning process.

A pelvic examination is less dreaded when a woman can participate and learn while retaining a sense of power and self-control. Encourage questions and expression of concerns, feelings, and wishes. Some women are afraid that the examiner will detect their sexual "secrets" from a pelvic examination. Provide these clients with a sense of control over self-disclosure so that they do not feel you are prying or able to "read their past."

Remain professional, and avoid actions or remarks that may be misconstrued by the client as demeaning or sexually provocative. For example, use a firm touch instead of gentle stroking. Be aware that the client may become sexually stimulated; alter the sequence of the examination, if necessary, but continue in a professional manner. Some facilities mandate that a female assistant be present when an examiner performs a pelvic examination to both comfort the client and discourage accusations of sexual impropriety.

Preparation

Instruct the woman not to douche, have intercourse, or use any vaginal products for 2 to 3 days before a pelvic examination. If a Pap smear is to be obtained, the woman should not be menstruating. Just before the examination, ask the woman to empty her bladder and bowels to to enhance comfort and accuracy. If necessary, collect a urine specimen at this time.

Ask the woman to remove enough clothing to allow examination of the abdomen and perineum. If a breast examination is planned, request that the woman disrobe completely and have her put on a gown. Ask about previous experiences with pelvic examinations, and acknowledge any feelings the woman may have. If this is the client's first examination, explain the procedure fully and show her how the speculum works. All women should be told which examinations are to be performed. Tell the woman when and where she will be touched to help her avoid tensing up, which produces discomfort.

Equipment

The following equipment is used during a pelvic examination:

- Vaginal speculum of an appropriate size
- Materials for obtaining smears and culture specimens for cytologic and microbiologic tests, including sterile cotton-tipped swabs, vaginal spatulas (wooden or plastic) or cytology brush, glass slides and coverslips, cytology fixative, culture plates, and enzyme immunoassay kits for *Chlamydia* and gonorrhea screening
- Adequate, adjustable light source
- Water-soluble lubricant
- Appropriately sized examination gloves (vinyl if the client is latex-sensitive).

Long forceps and cotton balls may be used after smears and specimens have been obtained to clean the cervix or vaginal areas so that any suspected areas may be examined more easily. Have biopsy equipment available in case the examination reveals that a biopsy is necessary.

Position

Help the client to assume a dorsal recumbent or lithotomy position, and keep her draped until it is time for the examination. In the lithotomy position, the buttocks should be aligned with the end of the table. The client may not have to put her feet into stirrups if only the external genitalia are examined. Help the client to flex and abduct her hips and knees with her arms at her sides or crossed over the chest. Adjust the stirrups to accommodate the woman's height.

The lithotomy position, with the perineum exposed, may be uncomfortable and embarrassing. Do not keep a woman exposed any longer than necessary. Elevate the client's head on a small pillow to aid abdominal muscle relaxation and facilitate the examination. Low back pain or a hip deformity may contraindicate this position; an alternative position, such as Sims, might be necessary (see Fig. 10–6), or an assistant can help the client abduct one or both legs. There must be an adjustable light source. Wear nonsterile, disposable examining gloves (latex or vinyl).

External Genitalia

Inspect the external genitalia and perineum (Fig. 37–3*A*). Assess secondary sexual characteristics, such as pubic hair distribution and developmental stage of external genitalia, during examination of the external genitalia and rectum while these areas are uncovered. Before touching the client's perineum, place one hand on the client's thigh to avoid startling her.

The mons pubis is a mound of tissue superior to the labia. In adults, it is usually covered by pubic hair distributed as an inverse triangle over the mons, anterior

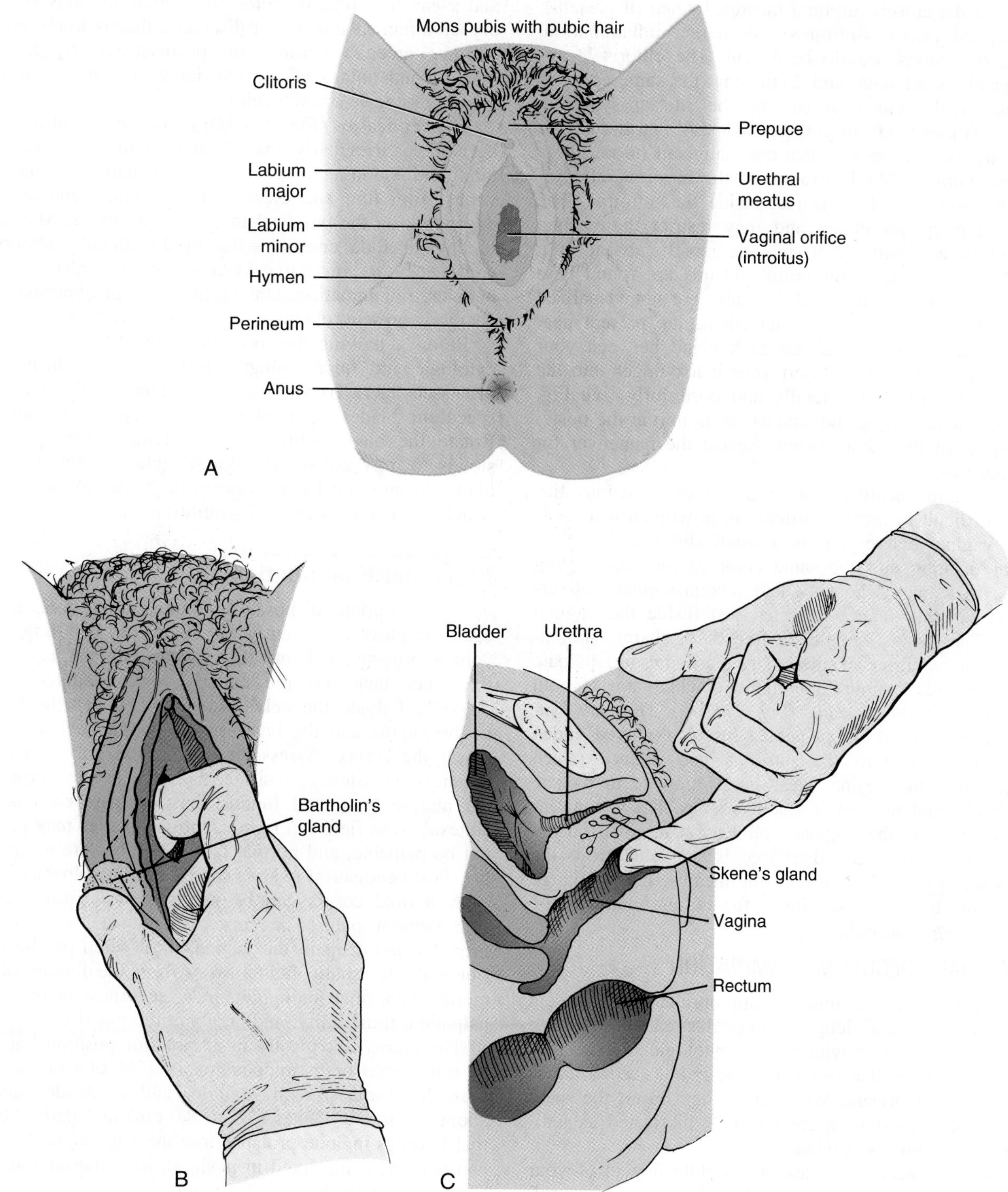

FIGURE 37–3 *A,* Anatomy of the female perineum and external genitalia. *B,* Palpation of Bartholin's glands. *C,* Palpation of Skene's glands.

perineum, and medial aspects of the upper thighs. Inspect the hair for nits and the skin for parasites, irritation, inflammation, edema, and lesions. An offensive odor should not be present. Any discharge should be scanty and clear to white in color.

Perineal skin is slightly darker than the rest of the body. The labia majora are symmetrical, rounded, and full. If the client has had a previous vaginal delivery, the labia majora gape slightly and the labia minora are evident. After menopause, the labia majora slowly atrophy. They should be free of edema, inflammation, and lesions. The labia minora are thinner than the labia majora, and one side may be larger than the other side. Gently separate the labia to inspect the vulva and remaining external structures. Place the thumb and index finger of your nondominant hand inside the labia minora, and retract the tissues laterally. Maintain a firm hold to avoid unnecessary manipulation of sensitive tissues.

Inspect the clitoris, urethral meatus, hymen (if present), and vaginal orifice (introitus); discharge, inflammation, edema, or lesions, should be absent. The clitoris is approximately 1 cm wide and 2 cm long, the same color as the rest of the vulva. It can be the site of syphilitic chancres (more likely in younger women), and the site of dry, scaly, nodular lesions that are malignant (more likely in older women). While examining the introitus, also inspect the hymen, which is just inside the introitus. The hymen may be prominent and may restrict the vaginal opening in a virgin, or it may be mostly absent in a sexually active client. Bartholin's glands are found near the base of the introitus and normally are not visualized or palpable. If inflammation and edema are present near the posterior introitus, palpate each gland between your thumb and index finger. Insert your index finger into the introitus, and rotate it laterally and posteriorly (see Fig. 37–3*B*). Palpate the gland against the thumb at the posterior aspect of the labia majora. Repeat the maneuver for the other side.

The urethral meatus, between the clitoris and introitus, can be difficult to locate, particularly in women who have had a vaginal delivery. It is a small slit just above the vaginal opening and the same color as the surrounding tissues. In women who have had several vaginal deliveries, the opening may be located just inside the vaginal orifice. The meatus should be free of discharge, inflammation, or swelling. If these signs are present, palpate Skene's glands (paraurethral glands), which are at both sides of the urethral meatus (Fig. 37–3*C*). They are usually not visualized or palpable. Insert a gloved index finger palm up into the introitus and about 1 inch (2.5 cm) into the vagina. Press gently upward to palpate the glands, and note their characteristics. Draw your index finger along the vaginal wall as you remove it from the vagina so that any discharge is "milked" from the glands into the urethra and out the meatus. If a discharge is present, collect a specimen for culture and change gloves before proceeding.

■ VAGINAL SPECULUM EXAMINATION

Select a vaginal speculum of appropriate size; specula differ in width and length. Lubricants cannot be used because they interfere with various cytologic studies, such as the Pap smear. If a cervical smear is not needed, use a water-soluble lubricant. Wear gloves, and insert the speculum, either rinsed in warm water or lubricated as indicated, gently into the vagina.

To do so, place the index and middle fingers of your nondominant hand in the vaginal orifice and gently pull posteriorly. Insert the closed speculum at a 45-degree angle, with the tip pointing downward into the vaginal orifice over your fingers (Fig. 37–4*A*). Withdraw your fingers while slowly rotating the speculum downward into the vagina until the handle is in a vertical position and the blades are fully inserted (Fig. 37–4*B*). Open the blades to observe the vaginal walls and cervix (Fig. 37–4*C* and *D*). You may need to make several gentle attempts to correctly position the cervix between the blades of the speculum. Offer the woman a mirror if she wants to see her cervix.

Vaginal mucous membranes are moist and pink, without discharge. If a discharge is present, it should be thin and clear to white in color. Abnormal findings include dry or inflamed mucosa; a discharge that is thick, curdy, yellow, green, odorous, or profuse; ulcers; lesions; masses; and bulges of the vaginal wall (which could be from a cystocele or rectocele).

The cervical os (Fig. 37–4*D*) is usually round but may be a slit or irregularly shaped after vaginal delivery. It is pink and smooth. A discharge is usually present that varies from thin and clear to thick, white, and stringy, depending on the phase of the menstrual cycle. Abnormal findings include unusual color of the mucosa, abnormal consistency of discharge, ulcerations, growths, masses, nodules, inflammation, and bleeding. If an abnormal discharge is present, obtain a specimen for culture.

Before removing the speculum from the vagina, obtain cytologic and microbiologic specimens, if indicated, as discussed later. To visualize the vaginal walls, leave the speculum blades open slightly as they are withdrawn. Rotate the blades obliquely, and remove the speculum slowly to fully assess the vaginal walls. Do not allow the blades to press on the urethra or the blades to close fully, which can cause extreme discomfort.

Bimanual Examination

Wear appropriate disposable examination gloves. Lubricate the glove and gently insert one or two fingers of your dominant hand into the vagina, palm up, and place the other hand on the client's lower abdomen (Fig. 37–4*E*). Palpate the pelvic contents between the fingers in the vagina and the hand on the abdomen. Locate and assess the cervix. Assess the size, shape, surface characteristics, consistency, position, mobility, and tenderness of the uterine body and fundus. Last, palpate each of the adnexal areas (left and right). Normal ovaries may or may not be palpable, and normal fallopian tubes are not palpable. Postmenopausal ovaries should not be palpable.

A normal cervix can be gently moved from side to side without pain. The cervix should feel smooth and firm, located deep in the vagina, most often on the anterior wall. It usually points away from the fundus of the uterus. Abnormal findings include tenderness or pain with palpation, immobility, and an abnormal position.

The uterus is typically in an anterior position but may be retroverted or in midposition in 15% of women. It is normally firm, smooth, mobile, and nontender and is about 2⅛ to 3⅛ inches (5.5 to 8.0 cm) in length. Abnormal findings include prolapse into the vagina, hard or soft consistency, being fixed in position, irregular contour, enlargement, or tenderness.

A normal ovary is 4 to 6 cm in diameter and feels smooth, firm, and oval. Slight tenderness on palpation is normal, but extreme tenderness, pain, or masses are not.

Withdraw your hand, palm up, halfway from the vaginal orifice, and assess the integrity of the pelvic floor musculature. Ask the client to contract her pelvic floor muscles as if trying to stop the flow of urine. The muscles will constrict around your fingers with more tone in a nulliparous client than in a client who has had a vaginal delivery. Next, ask the client to bear down as if straining to void. Feel for bulging of the vaginal walls pressing down against the introitus. If the anterior wall of the vagina bulges, the client probably has a *cystocele* (pro-

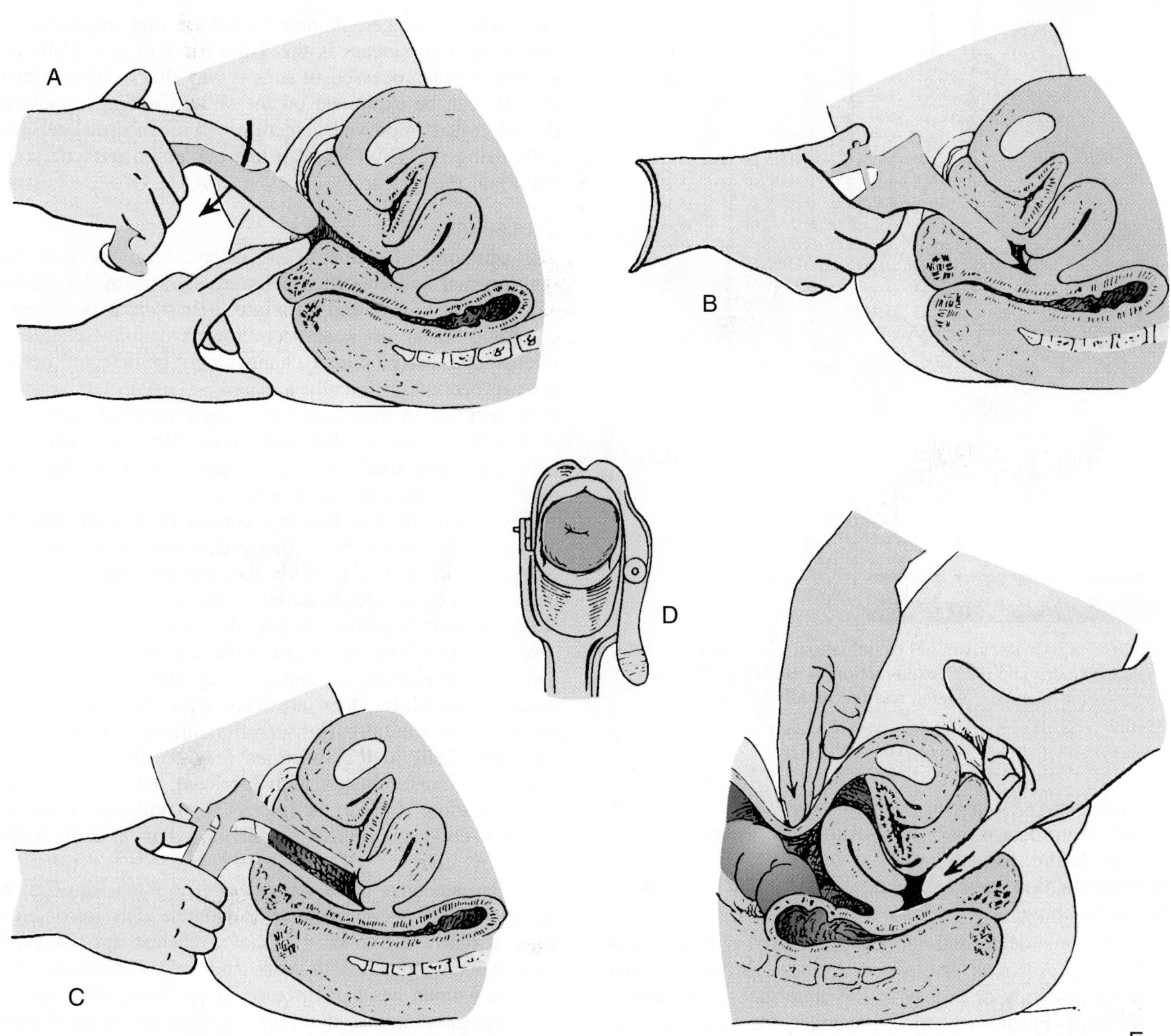

FIGURE 37–4 Pelvic examination and insertion of the vaginal speculum. *A,* The speculum blades are turned obliquely, and any pressure is directed downward onto the perineum. *B,* After full insertion, the blades are rotated to a horizontal position. *C,* Squeezing the speculum handles opens the blades. *D,* A full view of the cervix and cervical os. *E,* The bimanual examination. The abdominal hand presses the pelvic organs to be palpated toward the intravaginal hand.

lapse of the urinary bladder). A posterior vaginal wall bulge is often the result of a *rectocele* (rectal wall prolapse). Both of these are common in multiparous or obese clients.

Rectovaginal Examination

Insert your lubricated middle finger into the rectum and the index finger into the vagina (Fig. 37–5) to assess the rectal tissues for abnormalities, such as hemorrhoids (see Chapter 32). Ask the woman to bear down in order to ease insertion of your finger into the rectum. Rectal examination also confirms uterine position. If the uterus is retroverted, palpate the body and fundus. Reassess the adnexal areas, and palpate the rectovaginal septum and cul-de-sac. Normal pelvic organs can be palpated through the posterior cul-de-sac. Abnormal masses or normal ovaries are often felt in the cul-de-sac.

Assess anal sphincter tone and the rectal wall, which should be smooth. Assess the rectovaginal wall, which should be smooth, firm, and resilient (see Chapter 32). If the uterus is retroverted, it may be felt through the rectovaginal wall. The cervix feels smooth, round, firm, and movable without tenderness. Do not mistake the cervix or a vaginal tampon (if one is left in place) for a rectal mass.

If a stool specimen is needed for occult blood testing, obtain it at this time. When the examination is completed, help the client sit up and offer her tissues or wipes to clean the perineum.

If it has been well performed, a vaginal examination in women who have no pathologic conditions usually causes no or minimal discomfort. Some discomfort may occur during palpation of the ovaries during the bimanual and rectal examinations. Acknowledge this, and help the

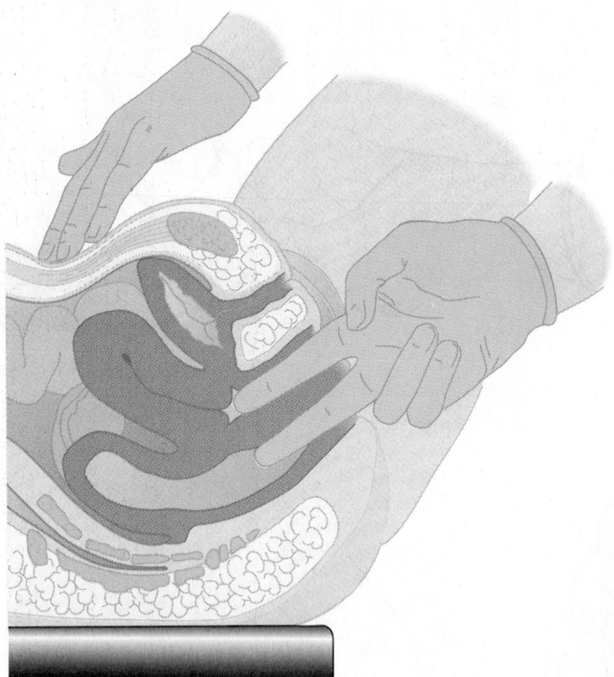

FIGURE 37–5 Rectovaginal examination. The examiner combines bimanual and rectal examination by inserting the index finger in the woman's vagina and the middle finger in the rectum.

woman relax by asking her to bear down during the rectal examination and to breathe deeply through her mouth during palpation of the ovary. After completing the examination, give instructions and conduct appropriate health teaching.

Sometimes abnormal cervical or vaginal tissue, a mass, or other problem is discovered during a pelvic examination. Colposcopy or biopsy of the abnormal tissue may be performed. Further examination under anesthesia may be necessary for exploration of a mass or unexplained tenderness. A pelvic examination is conducted before various other gynecologic tests (such as a Pap smear, colposcopy, hysterosalpingogram) and before surgery (such as laparoscopy or laparotomy).

DIAGNOSTIC TESTS

■ GYNECOLOGIC STUDIES

Laboratory Studies

The most common gynecologic laboratory studies are the Pap smear, wet smear, and cervical culture. The woman should not be menstruating at the time specimens are collected. Instruct her to avoid douching or using vaginal hygiene sprays or deodorants for at least 24 hours before a test.

PAPANICOLAOU SMEAR

Cytology is examination of the structure, function, pathology, and chemistry of the cell (Fig. 37–6). In gynecology, the most common cytologic test is the Pap smear, named after George Papanicolaou, the physician who devised it. The Pap smear identifies preinvasive and invasive cervical cancer. A new technique that improves the quality of Pap smears is the ThinPrep Pap test. Cells are collected and processed in such a way that a thinner layer of cells can be examined on the slide. Clinical trials have demonstrated improved detection of precancerous cervical cells using the ThinPrep Pap test compared with the conventional Pap smear.

PROCEDURE

The principle of the Pap test is based on the fact that both normal and abnormal cells are shed from the uterine and cervical linings and pass into their secretions. When a cytologic smear of these secretions is examined under a microscope, early cellular changes may be detected before disease becomes clinically apparent. The Pap test is up to 95% accurate in the diagnosis of early cervical carcinoma provided, of course, that correct sampling and handling techniques are used. It is only about 40% accurate in detecting endometrial carcinoma.

Specimens for the Pap test consist of a small amount of secretions taken from the endocervix and exocervix (Fig. 37–6*B* and *C*). With the conventional Pap test, these secretions are smeared separately on clean, dry slides or may be placed on one slide divided into sections (Fig. 37–6*E*). The slides are marked with "C" for cervix and "E" for endocervix. Immediately after the smears are made on the slides, they are fixed with either a commercial spray or solution. The secretions must be fixed before they dry. Cells in the specimen may be distorted if they dry or are contaminated with lubricant, which makes accurate reading difficult or impossible. With the ThinPrep test, the collected secretions are placed in a small bottle of preservative.

A Pap smear is usually painless. The American Cancer Society (ACS) recommends that women who are or have been sexually active or who have reached age 18 years should have annual Pap tests and pelvic examinations. After a woman has had three or more consecutive normal annual examinations, the Pap smear may be performed less often at the discretion of the health care provider. Many health care providers, however, continue to recommend annual examinations. The Pap test should be continued after menopause. Vaginal smears are obtained for Pap smear in women who have had a hysterectomy with removal of the cervix (see Chapter 39). Secretions are obtained from the vaginal pool, located in the posterior fornix (Fig. 37–6*D*).

In the past, reported findings were classified numerically. Descriptive reports are preferred because they are more useful in clinical decision-making. Reports either classify findings as normal or describe more fully the cellular changes seen. Specific infections may also be identified, and hormonal assessment may be done.

An abnormal Pap smear does not always mean malignancy. There is about a 5% false-positive or false-negative rate for the Pap test, and this rate is much higher if the specimen has been incorrectly collected or handled. However, having an abnormal Pap smear can be a frightening experience. Careful interpretation of cytologic findings is very important. The woman needs an opportunity to ask questions, to discuss concerns and feelings, and to participate in follow-up care planning.

If the cervix appears abnormal to the naked eye during

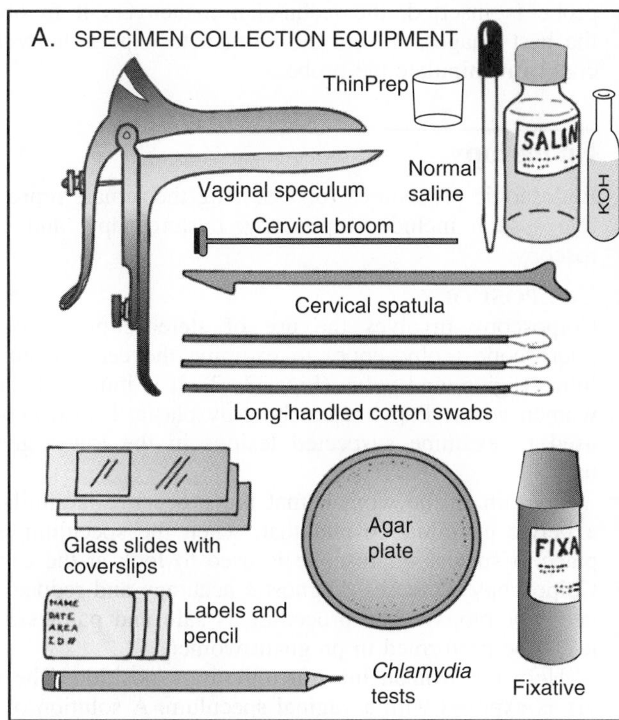

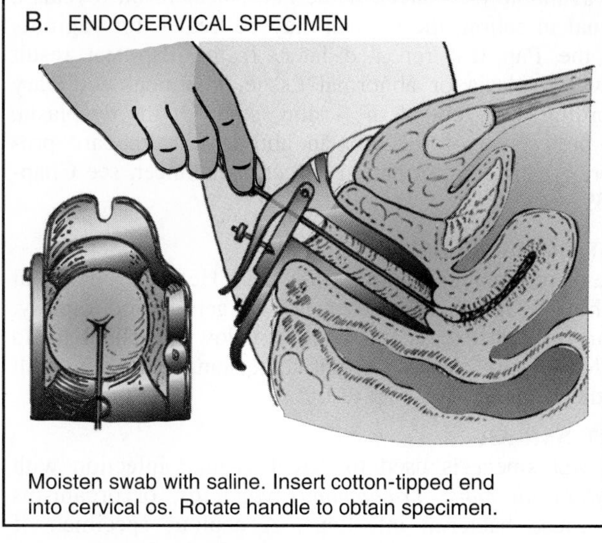

Moisten swab with saline. Insert cotton-tipped end into cervical os. Rotate handle to obtain specimen.

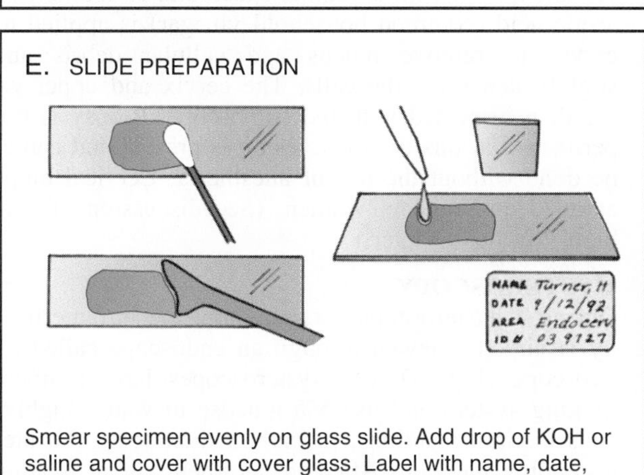

Smear specimen evenly on glass slide. Add drop of KOH or saline and cover with cover glass. Label with name, date, area of sample, identification number.

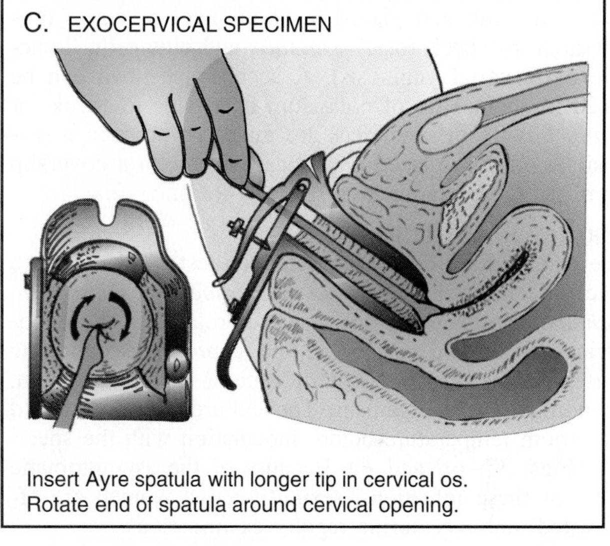

Insert Ayre spatula with longer tip in cervical os. Rotate end of spatula around cervical opening.

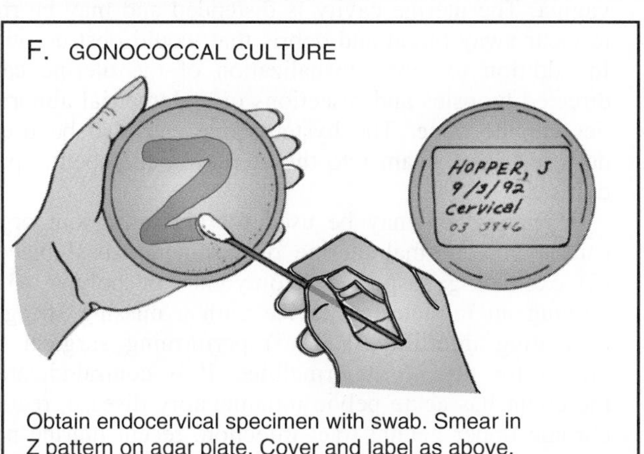

Obtain endocervical specimen with swab. Smear in Z pattern on agar plate. Cover and label as above.

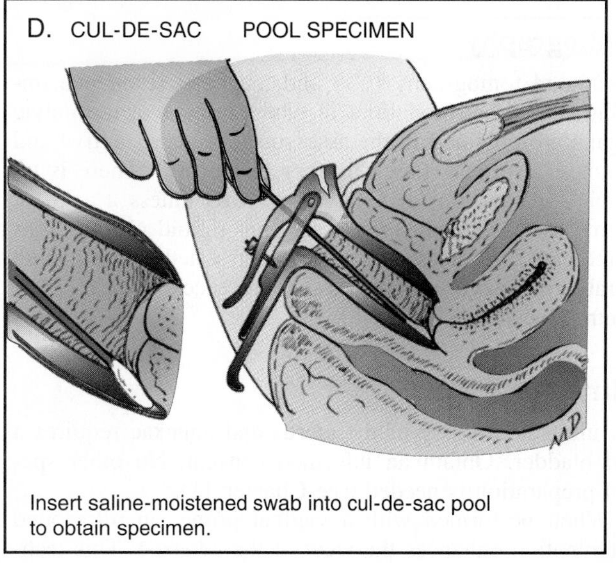

Insert saline-moistened swab into cul-de-sac pool to obtain specimen.

FIGURE 37–6 *A–F,* Collection of cervical cytocology specimens.

the examination, colposcopy may be done at that time if it is available (see later). If the Pap smear result reveals a vaginal infection, the woman may be treated for vaginitis and the Pap test repeated later. If the Pap test result shows dysplasia or abnormal tissue, treatment will vary according to extent of the lesion, grade of the dysplasia, and preference of the woman and her health care provider. For more information on cervical cancer, see Chapter 39.

Postprocedure Care

Care is minimal following a Pap test. Help the client out of the stirrups, and tell her not to get up too rapidly. Clean off any excess lubricant, or allow the client to do so. Make sure that the client understands how she will get the results of her Pap test.

Wet Smear

The wet smear is used to detect vaginal infection with *Candida albicans, Trichomonas vaginalis,* or organisms that cause bacterial infections. A copious specimen of discharge from the vaginal vault is obtained with a cotton-tipped swab and placed in about 1 ml of warm normal saline to check for *T. vaginalis* and clue cells (indicative of bacterial vaginosis). A second specimen can be placed in about 1 ml of potassium hydroxide to check for *C. albicans.* Both specimens are mixed to produce a suspension and then placed on a glass slide with a coverslip for microscopic examination (Fig. 37–6*E*).

Cervical Culture

A cervical culture or antigen detection test can be done to detect infection with *Neisseria gonorrhoeae* or *Chlamydia trachomatis.* A cotton-tipped swab is rotated in the endocervical canal and placed in the appropriate culturette tube or rolled in a Z pattern onto a culture medium, depending on the organism. The culture medium should be at room temperature before inoculation with the specimen (Figs. 37–6*B* and *F*). Because of the asymptomatic nature of these infections, sexually active women are often tested routinely during regular examinations.

Radiography

Computed tomography (CT) and magnetic resonance imaging (MRI) are modalities in which images of the pelvic organs are obtained in the assessment of reproductive and urologic disorders. (see Chapters 11 and 32). There is no special preparation for CT scan or MRI unless a contrast agent (dye) is given. Pregnancy and morbid obesity contraindicate both tests. Ask the woman whether she has an intrauterine device in place, the presence of which may contraindicate MRI.

Ultrasonography

An ultrasound study of the uterus and adnexae requires a full bladder. Obtain an informed consent. No other special preparation is needed (see Chapter 11).

When performed with a vaginal probe, an ultrasound examination enhances the view of the adnexae. This technique is used to evaluate ovarian cancer and cysts and ovaries that have been stimulated with fertility-enhancing drugs. For this approach, the bladder must be empty to promote comfort. The woman inserts the vaginal probe (sheathed in a protective, lubricated cover). Once the probe is inserted, the technician maneuvers it to obtain the best images. Inform the woman to expect the technician to manipulate the probe.

Endoscopy

Endoscopic procedures for assessing the female reproductive system include colposcopy, hysteroscopy, and laparoscopy.

Colposcopy

Colposcopy involves the use of stereoscopic binocular microscope (colposcope) to examine the cervical epithelium, vagina, and vulva (Fig. 37–7). It is indicated for all women whose Pap smears show dysplasia. It also may be used to examine suspected lesions in the lower genital tract.

Explain to the woman that the procedure is similar to a pelvic examination and that, when the speculum is in place, a special microscope is used to look at the cervix. Colposcopy increases diagnostic accuracy and reduces the need for biopsy. The procedure is safe and painless, and it can be performed in pregnant women.

Help the woman into the lithotomy position. The cervix is exposed with a vaginal speculum. A solution of 3% acetic acid (common household vinegar) is applied to the cervix to remove mucus and cellular debris and to slightly dehydrate the cells. The cervix and upper vagina are then inspected with the colposcope. Biopsy is usually performed at this time if a lesion is present and can easily be done without the use of anesthesia. Cervical biopsy is avoided on pregnant women. (See discussion of cervical biopsy in this chapter.)

Hysteroscopy

During a hysteroscopic examination, the intrauterine cavity is directly viewed through an endoscope called a hysteroscope (Fig. 37–8). Hysteroscopes have a fiberoptic lighting system and use 5% glucose in water, highly viscous dextran solutions, or carbon dioxide as the uterine-distending medium. After an anesthetic agent is administered, the hysteroscope is passed into the uterus via the vagina. The uterine cavity is distended and may be rinsed to clear away blood and debris that would obstruct vision. In addition to direct visualization of the uterine cavity, directed biopsies and resections of endometrial abnormalities can be done. The hysteroscope can also be used to deliver a laser beam into the uterus for therapeutic procedures.

Hysteroscopy may be used for (1) ruling out organic causes in abnormal uterine or postmenopausal bleeding, (2) examining suspected leiomyomas or polyps, (3) removing an intrauterine device with a missing string, (4) evaluating infertility, and (5) performing surgical techniques for uterine abnormalities. It is contraindicated if the client has acute pelvic inflammatory disease, recurrent chronic upper genital tract infection, recent uterine perforation, or suspected or known cervical malignancy. It also is contraindicated in pregnancy.

Explain the procedure to the client, and obtain an informed consent. Position the client in the lithotomy position, as for a pelvic examination. Complications of the procedure may include bleeding, uterine perforation,

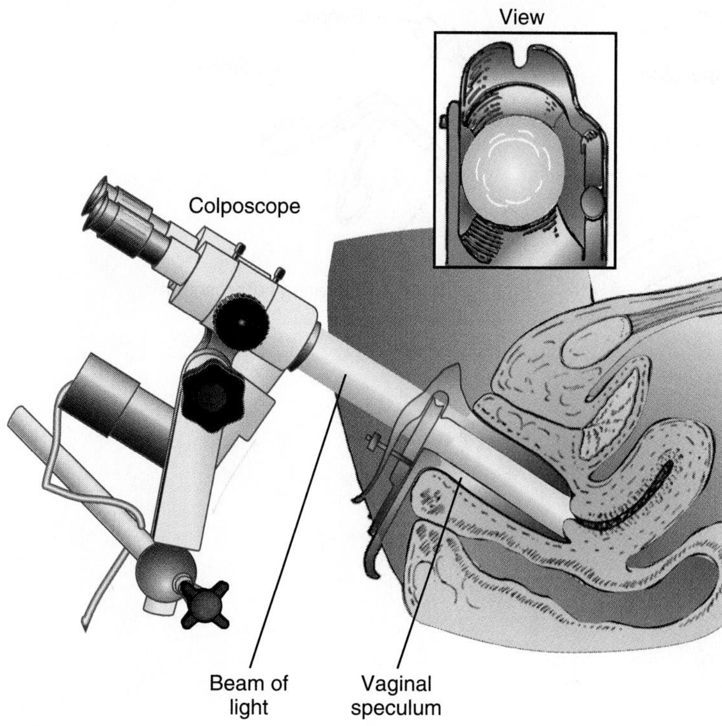

FIGURE 37–7 A colposcope is used to evaluate clients with an abnormal Papanicolaou smear and a grossly normal cervix. (From Hacker, N. F., & Moore, J. G. [1998]. *Essentials of obstetrics and gynecology* [3rd ed.]. Philadelphia: W. B. Saunders.)

infection, and rarely, bowel injuries. The woman may have referred shoulder pain if carbon dioxide was introduced into the pelvic cavity during the procedure; it usually resolves within 24 hours. Monitor the client's vital signs, and assess pain levels and location carefully.

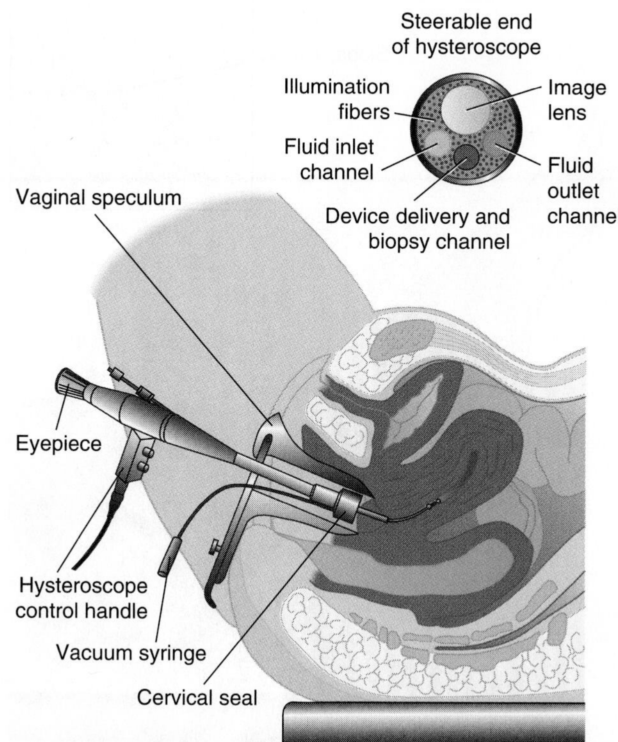

FIGURE 37–8 Hysteroscopy.

LAPAROSCOPY

A laparoscope, a common diagnostic and therapeutic tool (Fig. 37–9), is a telescope with an illuminated optical system. It is inserted into the abdomen through a small incision in or near the umbilicus to visualize abdominal and pelvic organs. Laparoscopy is a safe, convenient procedure that can be performed in hospitals, offices, or clinics equipped for outpatient surgery. The postprocedure recovery period is short, and the scar is small.

Laparoscopy may be performed diagnostically for conditions such as pelvic pain, pelvic masses, infertility, suspected ectopic pregnancy, and endometriosis. It also may be performed therapeutically for such procedures as tubal ligation, lysis of adhesions, treatment of endometriosis, drainage and removal of cysts, and for laparoscopic-assisted hysterectomy.

The main contraindication to laparoscopy is serious cardiac or pulmonary disease, although severe obesity may preclude its use. Previous lower abdominal surgery is not a contraindication, but it should be considered.

To prepare a client for laparoscopy, explain the procedure and inform the client how she can expect to feel afterward. Tell her to take nothing by mouth past midnight on the night before the procedure. Someone else should drive her to the health care facility because she should not drive after the procedure. Suggest that she wear loose-fitting clothes because it will be easier to dress after discharge. Typically, women who have laparoscopy in a same-day surgery setting can go home 2 to 4 hours after the procedure.

After laparoscopy, take the client's vital signs every 15 minutes for the first hour or until they are stable. If local anesthesia has been used, the woman can have fluids and a light snack as soon as she wants. After general anesthesia, the woman may have fluids and a light snack as soon as she is fully awake and has no nausea.

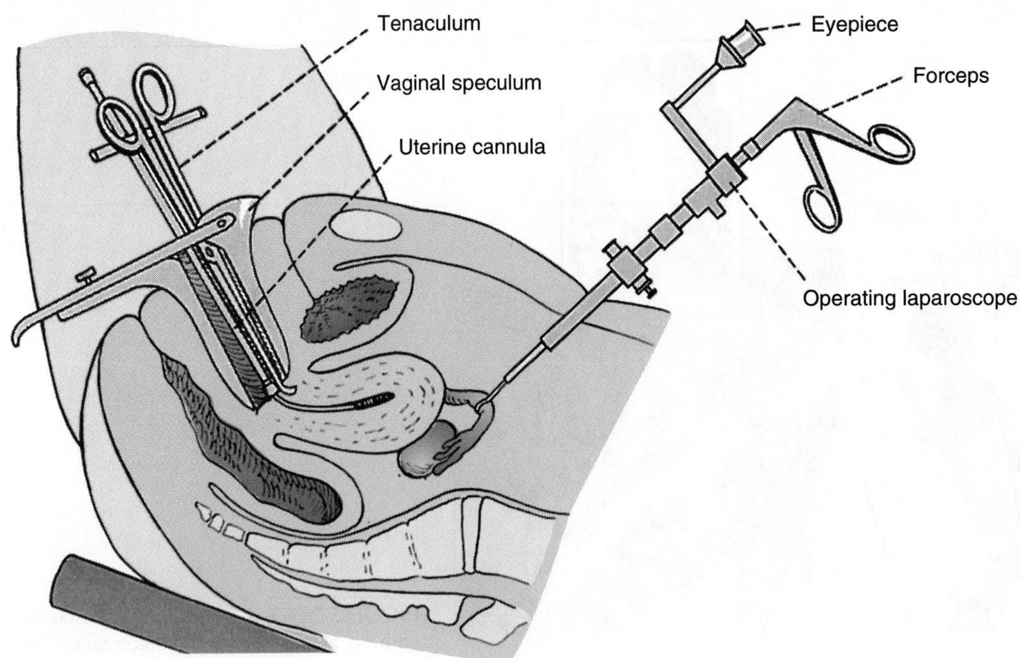

FIGURE 37–9 Laparoscopy.

Explain that she may experience mild-to-moderate transient shoulder pain or a feeling of bloating as a result of the carbon dioxide or nitrous oxide that was used to distend the abdomen, separate the organs, and allow better visualization during the procedure. The discomfort usually lasts only a few hours and may be relieved by positioning or mild analgesics. The woman may also experience mild incisional pain or abdominal cramping for the first few hours or days after the procedure, which is usually relieved by rest.

If general anesthesia was used, the client might have a sore throat from intubation. Soreness should disappear within 48 hours.

Teach her how to keep the incision clean and dry. After it heals, the scar will be barely noticeable. Sexual intercourse can be resumed within a week or less.

Biopsy

Cervical Biopsy

Cervical biopsy is performed to rule out malignancies. A specimen of the cervical lesion that has been identified with the naked eye or with colposcopic magnification is usually obtained in the outpatient setting with little or no anesthesia. A solution of 3% acetic acid can be applied to the cervix to identify areas suspected to be dysplasia, metaplasia, or malignancy. These areas undergo a color change and appear white after acetic acid is applied.

When colposcopy cannot identify an abnormal lesion on the cervix or vagina, Schiller's test may be performed. Lugol's iodine solution is applied to the vagina and cervix. Normal tissue takes up the stain and appears as a homogeneous mahogany-brown color. Usually, abnormal tissue does not take stain as well and may appear light yellow instead. This is a positive finding and can indicate areas necessitating biopsy. A biopsy may be done when a cervical lesion is first noted, or it may be delayed until about 1 week after the menstrual period, when the cervix is least vascular. Multiple biopsy specimens are usually obtained at specific sites with biopsy forceps (Fig. 37–10). Hemostasis is achieved with topical application of Monsel's solution or silver nitrate. For ruling out

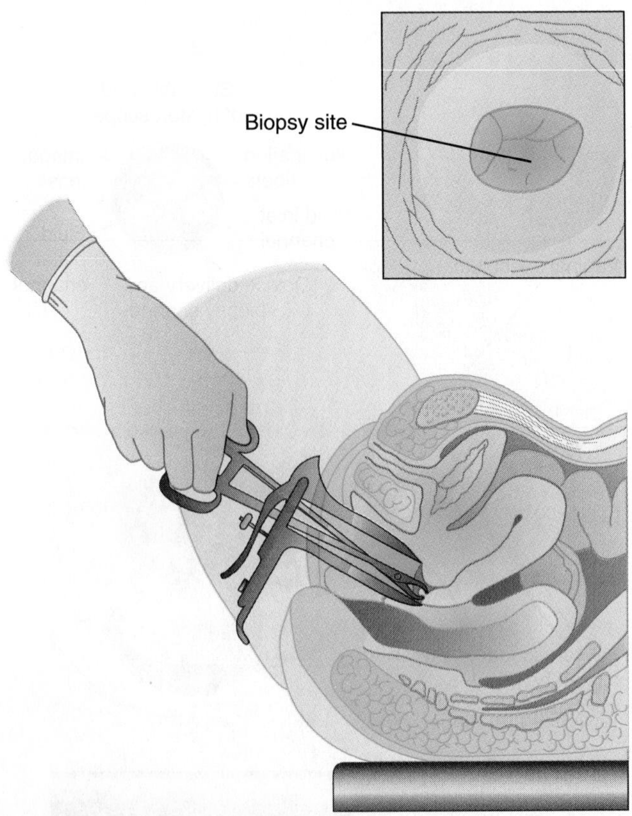

FIGURE 37–10 Cervical biopsy.

disease in the endocervical canal, endocervical curettage may be performed.

Before a cervical biopsy, explain the purpose of the test and obtain the client's informed consent. The test is usually not done while the client is menstruating. The lithotomy position is assumed.

After a cervical biopsy, allow the client to rest for a short time before she goes home. Although she may note a small amount of blood-tinged vaginal discharge or the mustard and blackish discharge from the Monsel's solution, tell her to report any excessive bleeding immediately. Advise her to abstain from vaginal sexual activity and to avoid tampons and douching until the bleeding has completely stopped, in order to achieve hemostasis, to lessen trauma, and to promote healing.

Endometrial Biopsy

An endometrial tissue sample is obtained for histologic study through the technique of endometrial biopsy. Tissue may be analyzed for endometrial cancer, dysfunctional uterine bleeding, and occasionally, for infertility. The biopsy is performed after bimanual examination of the uterus. Because the biopsy procedure may result in cramping, the woman may receive a nonsteroidal anti-inflammatory drug, a paracervical block, or both to relieve the discomfort.

The cervix is dilated under sterile conditions, and a uterine sound is inserted to measure the depth of the uterine cavity. An aspirating instrument is passed into the uterus, and a small amount of tissue is removed from the endometrium for examination (Fig. 37–11).

Explain the purpose of the test and the procedure, including the use of an anesthetic block. Obtain an informed consent. Position the client as for a pelvic examination.

If cramping persists after the procedure, administer analgesics as ordered or apply heat to the lower abdomen.

■ BREAST STUDIES

Laboratory Studies

No laboratory tests can screen for breast cancer. Some progress has been made in identifying biologic tumor

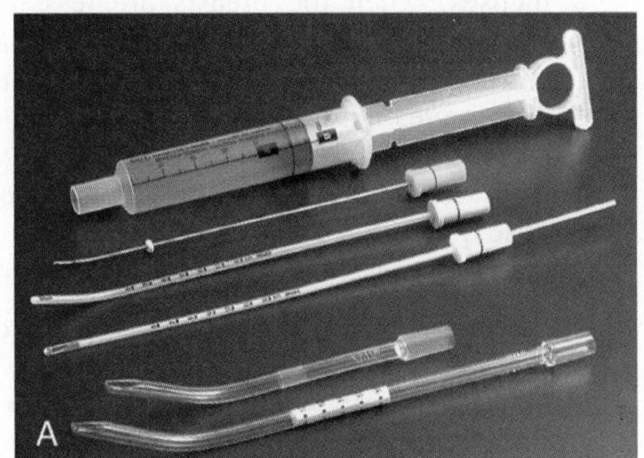

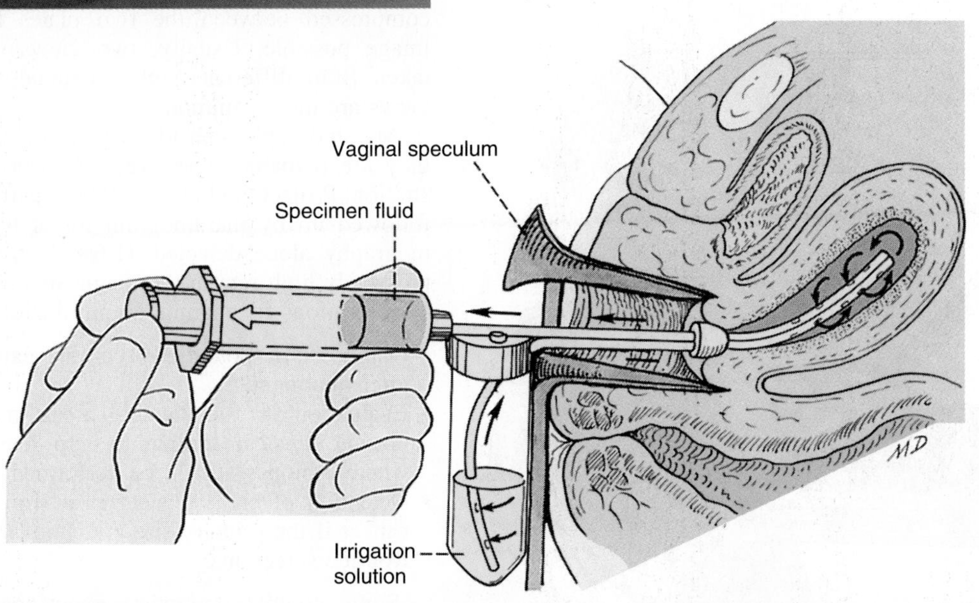

FIGURE 37–11 *A,* Endometrial sampling devices for uterine cancer screening. Endometrial curets range in size, composition (stainless steel, plastic), and flexibility (rigid, semirigid, flexible) and may be used with a vacuum collection syringe or with an irrigation system and suction syringe. The uterus is sounded for position and depth to determine the size of the curet to be used. Loosened cells collected in the syringe are transferred to a specimen jar with fixative for cytopathologic examination. (Courtesy of Milex Products, Inc.) *B,* Endometrial uterine lavage using sterile normal saline and negative pressure. *Arrows* indicate the flow of the irrigating solution and collection of the specimen. Fluid does not enter the fallopian tubes. A plug at the cervical os helps maintain negative pressure within the uterus. (From Boone, M. I., et al. [1984]. Uterine cancer screening by the family physician. *American Family Physician, 30,* 157.)

markers for breast cancer that detect metastatic disease. Elevations in carcinoembryonic antigen (CEA), alkaline phosphatase, ferritin, and gamma-glutamyltransferase seem to be associated with the recurrence of breast cancer. Other possible tumor markers that have been studied include C-reactive protein, acid glycoprotein, sialyltransferase, the urinary hydroxyproline-creatinine ratio, and gross cystic disease fluid protein.

Radiography

Various techniques have been tried to identify early-stage breast cancer in women accurately and safely when assessment indicates breast lesions. Such techniques are also important in finding an effective method to screen women without clinically apparent manifestations. At present, only mammography has been shown to be useful for widespread screening. While ultrasonography is not specific enough to identify lesions suggestive of cancer, it does differentiate cystic from solid lesions. Other methods of testing are being investigated.

Mammography

A mammogram is a soft tissue radiographic breast examination used to detect small invasive and noninvasive tumors and benign lesions. Two common methods of obtaining mammograms are *film-screen mammography* (Fig. 37–12) and *xeromammography* (Fig. 37–13). The film-screen method uses x-ray film. Xeromammography produces an electrostatic image on plastic-coated paper. Each technique has strengths and limitations and involves acceptably low radiation doses.

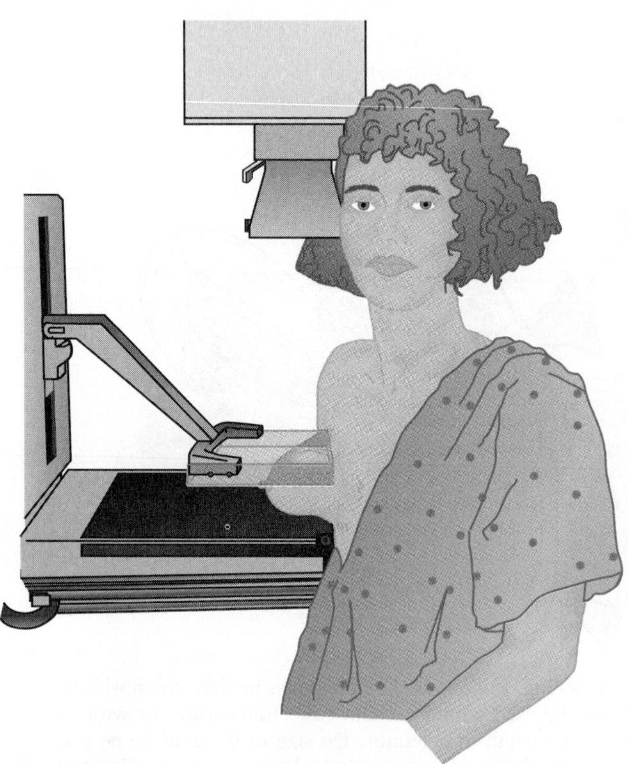

FIGURE 37–12 Mammography, a technique for obtaining an x-ray image of the breast, is the most reliable mechanical method of detecting a breast cancer before it can be felt. This technique is also used to help diagnose breast cancer.

Common questions and possible answers about mammography include the following:

1. *How often should I have a screening mammogram?* Use the ACS or National Cancer Institute (NCI) guidelines for the age and risk group.
2. *What is the cost?* Prices vary. Inquire at the facility where the mammogram will be performed. Tell the client that while it is worthwhile to compare prices, ensure that the facility meets the necessary quality standards.
3. *How much time is involved?* About 15 to 30 minutes. Results are usually available within 1 to 21 days, depending on the facility.
4. *What preparation is required?* The woman should not wear any body powder, creams, or deodorant on the torso the day of the procedure.
5. *Is there pain?* Discomfort may be experienced because of the compression needed to obtain the best image. Some women find it helpful to schedule a mammogram for the week after the end of their menses, when the breasts are less tender. Women who have tender breasts may take a nonsteroidal anti-inflammatory drug, if not contraindicated, about 30 minutes before the procedure.
6. *Is there a risk in the exposure to the radiation?* Both methods of mammography use the smallest dose possible. The long-term effects of an annual mammogram are considered to be harmless.

During a mammogram, the woman disrobes from the waist up and her gown is separated to expose one breast at a time. The breast is placed between an x-ray plate and a compression paddle that is adjusted so the breast is compressed between the two plates to obtain the best image possible. Usually, two views of each breast are taken from different angles. Cranial-caudal and oblique views are most common.

Mammography can identify some breast cancers before they are palpable. The Breast Cancer Detection Demonstration Project included 280,000 participants who were followed up by mammogram for at least 5 years. Mammography alone detected 41.6% of the cancers—an impressively high rate in the diagnosis of small cancers.[18]

Indications for mammography include:

- Diagnosis of potentially curable cancer and follow-up after treatment
- Evaluation of questionable breast masses or other abnormal physical findings to help determine whether and where a biopsy should be performed
- Detection of breast cancer in a woman with metastatic cancer if the primary site is unknown
- Routine screening

Some controversy exists about the age at which to begin routine screening mammograms. The ACS recommends a baseline mammogram for all women by age 40 and mammography screening of asymptomatic women ages 40 to 49 at intervals of 1 to 2 years and annually over age 50.[1] The NCI no longer recommends routine screening of women under age 50 years. Until there is further evidence, the decision when to begin may be

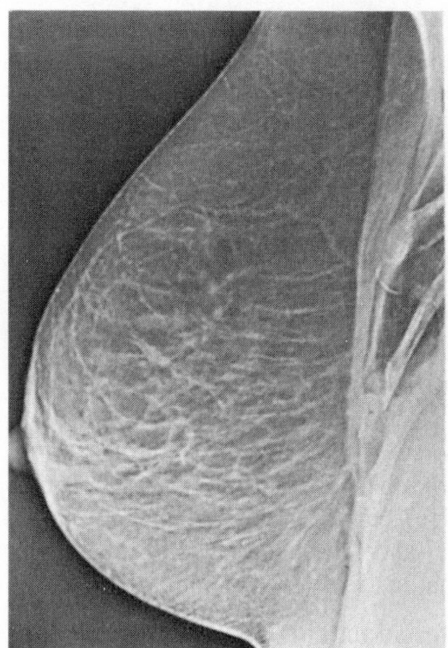
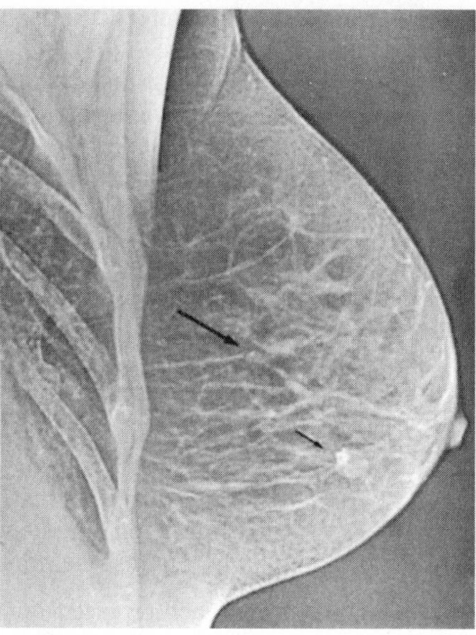

FIGURE 37–13 A xeromammogram, performed before a planned biopsy of a palpable mass that proved to be benign (*small arrow*), revealed the presence of a hidden cancerous lesion (*large arrow*). (From Lippman, M. E., et al. [1988]. *Diagnosis and management of breast cancer.* Philadelphia: W. B. Saunders.)

made on an individual basis, with the woman and her health care provider together evaluating her risk for breast cancer as well as the possible risks and benefits of the screening test. A woman who is at high risk for breast cancer should follow the recommendations of her health care provider.

Ultrasonography

An ultrasound study of the breast involves scanning with an automated whole breast scanner and a hand-held real-time sector scanner. Ultrasonography is useful in determining the consistency of breast masses and differentiating cystic (fluid-filled) from solid lesions; however, it cannot differentiate solid benign from solid cancerous lesions. Ultrasound is useful in confirming the fluid consistency of cystic-appearing lesions seen on a mammogram. It is also useful in guiding fine-needle aspiration of cysts and other breast masses. No special preparation is needed, and the procedure is painless; no radiation risk is involved.

Biopsy

Biopsy is essential to the diagnosis of breast cancer. No treatment should be undertaken without an unequivocal histologic diagnosis of cancer. A *core needle biopsy* and a *fine-needle aspiration* (FNA) biopsy may be performed with local anesthesia during an office visit.

Core needle biopsy, a simple procedure, takes just a few minutes. After the site is cleaned and prepared with povidone-iodine, a small core of tissue is obtained with a special needle (e.g., Vim-Silverman). The core of tissue removed is placed in formalin and sent to the pathologist for histologic diagnosis. Occasionally, a suture is needed to close the skin.

With a fine-needle aspiration biopsy, a needle and syringe are used to aspirate cells from a breast mass or fluid from a cyst. The cells are fixed on a slide (as in a Pap smear), and a cytologic diagnosis is made. Mammography is used to guide the needle for aspiration of nonpalpable lesions. The cytologic examination is useful for confirming the diagnosis of clinical and mammographic findings of fibroadenoma (a fibrocystic condition), intramammary lymph nodes, fat necrosis, subareolar papillomatosis, chronic subareolar abscess, and cancer. If the cytologic findings suggest that the specimen is acellular or that only blood and adipose cells are present, a biopsy or further evaluation is needed to rule out breast cancer.

Both fine-needle aspiration and core needle biopsy involve taking only a small amount of cells and tissue from a lesion. Because false-negative results are possible, an *open biopsy* may still need to be performed.

Incisional or *excisional* open biopsies are usually performed in an operating room or a minor surgical suite with the use of local anesthetic or intravenous (IV) sedation. About 35% of clients who require an open biopsy for a breast lesion have a malignancy. Excisional biopsy involves removal of the entire palpable mass, incisional biopsy only a portion of the mass. In both cases, the tissue removed is sent to the pathologist for histologic assessment. The incision is closed with sutures, and a dressing (sometimes a pressure dressing) is placed over the site. Typically, the dressing is in place for 24 to 48 hours before it is removed.

Percutaneous needle localization determines the area for an open biopsy if a mass is very small, for example, those detected by a mammogram alone. The lesion is localized in the radiology department. A thin needle is passed into the area in question that has been identified by mammography. A second mammogram confirms the position of the lesion. The needle is secured in place with tape, and the woman is taken to the operating room, where an open biopsy is immediately performed. Frozen section examination may be done for rapid diagnosis.

Before a breast biopsy, explain the purpose of the biopsy to the client and obtain her consent. Restrict food and fluids if IV sedation is to be used. Discuss the post-procedure self-care activities that the client should follow. Most women fear that the biopsy will result in a finding of cancer; some clients may ask about what will happen if cancer is found (see Chapter 40).

After the biopsy, instruct the woman to report any bleeding, swelling, or evidence of infection. After a needle biopsy, normal activity can be resumed as soon as it is comfortable to do so. Vigorous activity should be avoided for 1 to 2 weeks after an open biopsy. The woman may find it more comfortable to wear a supportive brassiere 24 hours a day until the site is healed, as long as the wires and elastic do not rub on the incision.

THE MALE REPRODUCTIVE SYSTEM

Disorders of the male reproductive and urinary tract (which is closely associated with the reproductive tract) occur in men of all ages. Assessing these disorders requires expertise in conducting the health history interview and physical examination. Be sensitive and tactful because many men are uncomfortable discussing issues associated with these disorders. Discuss lifestyle factors that affect health maintenance, such as diet, exercise, adequate sleep and rest, stress management, smoking cessation, and individual risk factor identification. If appropriate, provide information about protection against STDs. Explain what is involved in the physical examination, use easily understood terms, and discuss any diagnostic tests that may be indicated.

HISTORY

A complete health history, including sexual and reproductive systems, and physical examination are necessary for men experiencing reproductive disorders. History-taking provides an opportunity to:

- Allow men to express sensitive concerns
- Identify and dispel myths and misinformation
- Teach health information
- Offer referrals
- Facilitate further communication

The following discussion addresses the major risk factors pertinent to men's reproductive health history.

BIOGRAPHICAL AND DEMOGRAPHIC DATA

Review the client's biographical and demographic data to determine his health risk status. Age, race, and occupation all have health risk implications. Men over age 50 years may have benign prostatic hypertrophy (BPH), an enlargement of the prostate gland. Men younger than age 40, who have manifestations that resemble those of BPH, are more likely to have prostatitis. African American men and those over age 40 are at increased risk for adenocarcinoma of the prostate. Younger men, particularly those between ages 25 and 35, have a higher incidence of testicular cancer. Occupations and activities that involve prolonged, strenuous lifting or straining can provoke hernias. Exposure to some chemicals and pesticides may be linked to fertility and reproductive disorders.

CURRENT HEALTH: THE CHIEF COMPLAINT

The client may present with problems related to the genitourinary or reproductive system or to sexuality. A chief complaint may include the following areas:

- Systemic disturbances, such as weight loss, fever, and malaise
- Voiding disturbances, such as frequency, polyuria, oliguria, nocturia, pyuria, enuresis, dysuria, urgency, or incontinence
- Disturbances in urine characteristics, such as hematuria and pyuria
- Gastrointestinal disturbances, such as nausea, vomiting, anorexia, abdominal discomfort, constipation, or diarrhea
- Reproductive disturbances, infertility, history of STDs, genital lesions, or genital discharge in self and partner; genital trauma
- Sexual functioning (whether the client is sexually active or celibate), such as changes in libido; changes in erectile ability; decreased ejaculatory ability; gynecomastia (breast enlargement); and the effects of disability, chronic disease, trauma, surgery, or treatment

For each reported manifestation, conduct a symptom analysis (see Chapter 9).

PAST HEALTH HISTORY

Significant health history for the male reproductive system includes childhood and infectious diseases, immunizations, major illnesses and hospitalizations, medications, and allergies.

Childhood and Infectious Diseases

The most significant childhood infectious illness to affect male fertility is mumps. Its occurrence in young men is associated with sterility. Ask whether the client has ever had mumps or been immunized against it. Question the client also about the presence of cryptorchidism at birth and the age at which the testicles descended or were brought down surgically.

Major Illnesses and Hospitalizations

Ask about major illnesses, such as diabetes, hypertension, cerebrovascular accident (CVA), and MI. Men who have diabetes commonly have problems with potency related to the accompanying neurologic and vascular changes. Hypertension and CVA can cause impotence related to physiological or psychological factors. Impotence may also occur in men who have had an MI because they may fear having another episode as a result of sexual excitement and activity.

Urinary tract disorders can interfere with sexual functioning because of the close proximity of anatomic structures. Endocrine disorders can also affect sexual performance. Be alert to the man's concerns and fears, remain nonjudgmental, and offer the support of counseling and referral to peer groups established for this purpose.

Ask the client about any previous surgery involving the reproductive system, such as herniorrhaphy, vasectomy, prostatectomy, varicocelectomy, orchiopexy, and testicular torsion repair.

Medications

Obtain a complete medication history for prescription, over-the-counter, and recreational drugs; nutritional supplements; and herbal remedies. Some medications prescribed for hypertension (e.g., methyldopa, clonidine, guanethidine, and hydralazine) may cause impotence. Tranquilizers can interfere with sexual performance. Other medications can decrease sperm count and motility. Recreational drugs (e.g., marijuana and hallucinogens) that alter behavior can also affect physiologic reproductive function and may raise the risk of STDs. Herbs frequently used to treat reproductive disorders include saw palmetto (*Seronoa repens*) for BPH and yohimbe (*Pausinystalia yohimbe*) for erectile dysfunction and impotence.

Allergies

Ask the client about any allergies to antibiotics, rubber, or latex. Male genitourinary disorders are often treated with antibiotics, and latex and rubber are found in condoms as well as in examination gloves commonly worn during the physical examination. If the man is allergic to latex, wear vinyl gloves.

■ SEXUAL AND REPRODUCTIVE HISTORY

A sexual and reproductive history includes questions about breasts, contraceptives, sexual practices, genitourinary problems, and reproductive health practices (see Chapter 9).

Breast History

Collect data about the breasts and axillae. Ask about breast pain, masses, skin changes, and nipple discharge. Ask whether the man has noticed any changes in breast tissue, such as enlargement. *Gynecomastia* can occur in obese or older men and as a side effect of some medications. Ask whether the client performs BSE, similar to the technique taught to women.

Contraceptive History

Document the man's current contraceptive method (if any), his satisfaction with the method, the effect of contraception on sexual function, and any desire to change methods. Has the man used contraceptive methods previously? If so, did any problems lead to their discontinuation?

Sexual History

Inquire about the client's patterns of sexual relationships. Can the man relate the total number of sexual partners he has had and the frequency of sexual activity? Multiple partners and contacts increase the client's risk of STDs. Does the man use condoms during sexual intercourse? Does he have homosexual or bisexual relationships, both of which increase the risk of human immunodefciency virus (HIV) infection.

Does the client have any sexual concerns, such as an inability to attain or maintain an erection? If so, does this problem occur frequently or occasionally? Is the client able to discuss sexual concerns with his partner? Have he and his partner developed ways to cope with or adjust to disturbances in sexual function? If sexual dysfunction exists, does the client want a referral to, or consultation with, a sex counselor?

Throughout the interview, ask questions directly. Phrase questions in a neutral, nonjudgmental way. This interview technique helps preserve dignity and self-esteem instead of fostering guilt or shame. Chapter 9 provides further information on sexuality assessment.

Genitourinary History

Ask about past problems with genitourinary infections, such as prostatitis. Determine whether the client has had a previous pelvic examination. Does he have such problems as urinary incontinence, dribbling, hesitancy, a weak urinary stream, or other manifestations? Chapter 32 describes assessment of the urinary system.

Reproductive Health Practices

Inquire about sexual and reproductive hygiene. How often does the man examine his breasts and testes? (See Chapter 2.) Does he protect himself against STDs? Chapter 9 discusses health risk management.

■ FAMILY HEALTH HISTORY

Ask whether the client has a family history of infertility, diabetes, hypertension, CVAs, or endocrine disorders. As with women whose mothers took DES during pregnancy, men who have been exposed to DES in utero are at increased risk for congenital anomalies, including structural defects of the genitourinary system and reduced semen levels.

■ PSYCHOSOCIAL HISTORY

Assess the client's occupation, environment, habits, and psychosocial factors.

Occupation and Environment

Determine the client's type of work and recreational activities to identify any exposure to chemicals, pesticides, heat, heavy metals, hormones, and radiation. These materials can directly affect the number and integrity of sperm and the quality of germinal tissue.

Habits

Assess the client's use of caffeine, alcohol, tobacco, and recreational drugs, including marijuana. These substances may affect the sperm count, contribute to impotence, decrease libido, or encourage risk-taking behaviors. Physical and recreational sports can put the client at risk for genital trauma if protective gear is not used.

Psychosocial Factors

Review the following subjects when conducting a health history interview with a man who has a reproductive disturbance. You may not be able to obtain detailed information in each of these areas, but the outline should help you to view each man and his significant others as individuals and to avoid stereotypical and, possibly, judgmental nursing care. Note:

1. *Self-concept.* How has the client's health affected how he feels about himself? How do his partner and significant others feel about him? What is his

posture, dress, grooming? What is his emotional response? What is his mood? His tone?

2. *Role relationships.* Who are the important people in this client's life? Who accompanied him to the health care facility? Who is his most significant other? How is he able to carry out his various social roles (partner, husband, friend, father, worker)? How has his health affected his economic situation and his partner or significant others?
3. *Communication.* How does the client communicate, both verbally and nonverbally, with you and his significant others? Does he maintain eye contact? Does he use gestures or touch? How does he speak (volume, tone, vocabulary, repetition)?
4. *Value system.* What values, opinions, and beliefs does the client hold? What is his predominant lifestyle? What is his cultural or subcultural background?
5. *Coping and stress tolerance.* Who supports and nurtures the client? Does he experience intimacy with anyone? How connected is the client with significant others? What supports and resources does he have? How does he spend his leisure time? To what extent does he engage in physical activity or exercise?
6. *Cognitive-perceptual.* How does the client use words? Can he read? What is his level of comprehension? What is his major source of information about reproductive health?

■ REVIEW OF SYSTEMS

Ask about diabetes, hypertension, CVA, angina, MI, endocrine disorders, renal disorders, and urinary tract problems. Detailed questions for the review of systems may be found in Chapter 9.

PHYSICAL EXAMINATION

Skillful history-taking helps to establish a therapeutic relationship that facilitates physical examination. Many men find physical examination of the reproductive system stressful and embarassing. Some men may view the genitals as private or unclean.

Help the client become more comfortable by sharing normal findings while you proceed. Explain each step. Increase the client's comfort by maintaining eye contact, proceeding in an unhurried manner, and involving the client in self-examination. Occasionally, a man will have an erection during an examination. A kind, professional manner and a firm, yet gentle touch lessen this possibility. If the man does have an erection, explain that this is normal and does not have sexual connotation.

The physical examination focuses on findings that may be associated with reproductive or sexual disorders. These may include the following disorders:

- Inflammatory, such as enlarged, tender, movable, or fixed lymph nodes in the inguinal region
- Endocrine and genetic, including indications of such conditions as Cushing's syndrome or acromegaly, hair distribution, and gynecomastia
- Neurologic, including a gross neurologic examination of the legs
- Vascular, including the femoral and pedal pulses
- Traumatic, such as a hernia

Follow an orderly sequence for the physical examination, and teach the client how to perform similar self-examinations regularly. The male breasts and axillae are included here as part of the reproductive system examination.

■ BREASTS AND AXILLAE

Examine the client's breasts and axillary nodes. Although the incidence of breast cancer in men is low, it can occur because men have glandular tissue beneath each nipple.

Inspect and palpate the breasts and axillae while the man is sitting, following the same guidelines as for the female breast examination. The male breast is flat and symmetrical, without nodules, edema, or ulceration. One-sided (unilateral) breast enlargement that persists beyond puberty is abnormal. Palpation reveals a small, flat disc of glandular tissue under the areola. There should be no masses or discharge. Axillary nodes should be nonpalpable (see Fig. 37–2).

■ EXTERNAL GENITALIA

The client's urinary bladder should be empty. The client may be supine or lying on his side with his legs spread slightly for the first portion of the genital examination; ask him to stand during the assessment for inguinal herniation. Alternatively, the client might stand for the entire examination of the genitals while you remain seated. Because the male urethra is the common conduit for both urine and semen, examination of the male reproductive tract also includes assessment of the urinary system. Wear nonsterile, disposable examining gloves.

Inspect the external genitalia and perineum (Fig. 37–14), observing the pubic hair and skin. You must be familiar with normal growth and development of the male genitalia. Observe general appearance and body build. Note the hair distribution. Pubic hair distribution in men is triangular, with hair covering the symphysis pubis, base of the penis, and inner aspects of the thighs. Hair distribution may also spread toward the umbilicus in a diamond pattern. Inspect hair for nits and the skin for parasites, rashes, excoriation, and lesions. Masses, lesions, edema, and offensive odors should be absent. Scrotal skin is darker than other skin surfaces and is loose and wrinkled.

The penis includes the penile shaft, prepuce (foreskin), glans, and urethral meatus (Fig. 37–15). Inspect and palpate these structures for lesions, nodules, swelling, inflammation, atrophy, and discharge. Penile skin in a flaccid penis is wrinkled. The foreskin, if present, covers the glans. The foreskin is absent in a circumcised client. Instruct the client to retract the foreskin to expose the glans, which is easily accomplished. You may see a small amount of cheesy, thick, white, odoriferous *smegma* between the glans and the foreskin; it is normal. If other discharge is noted, obtain a specimen for culture. The area between the glans and foreskin is a common site of venereal lesions. The area is normally free of lesions; if any are present, palpate them for tenderness, size, shape, and consistency, then change gloves before proceeding.

Next, inspect the urethral meatus, located at the tip of the penis. It looks like a slit. Malposition of the meatus

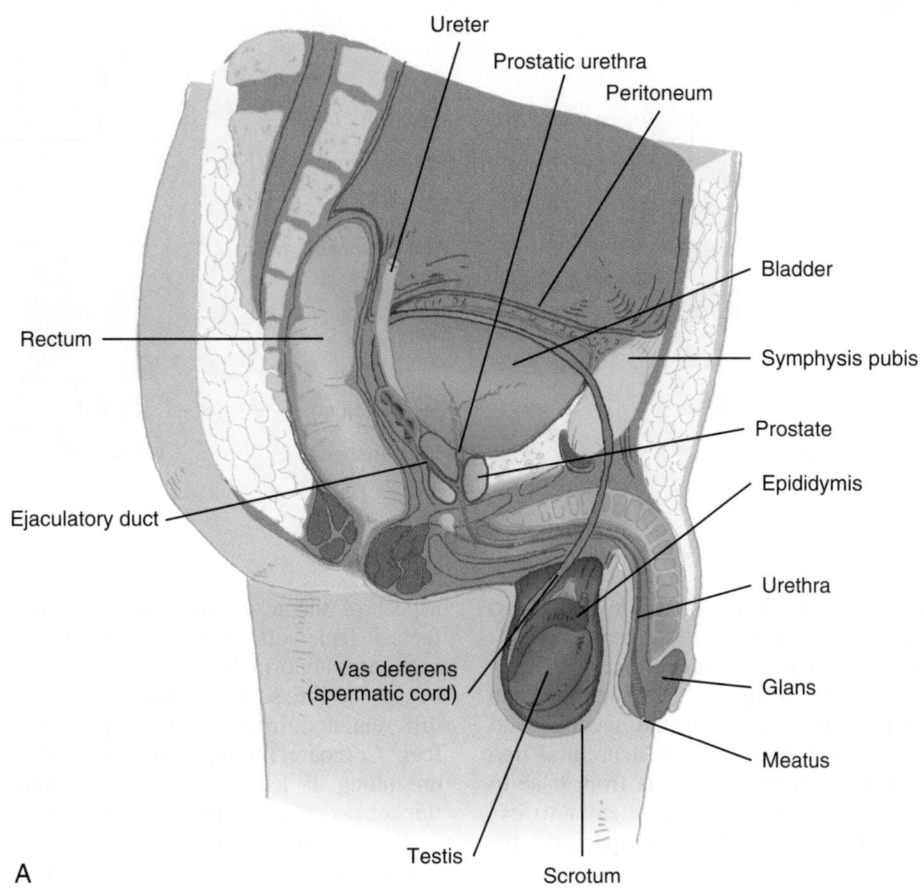

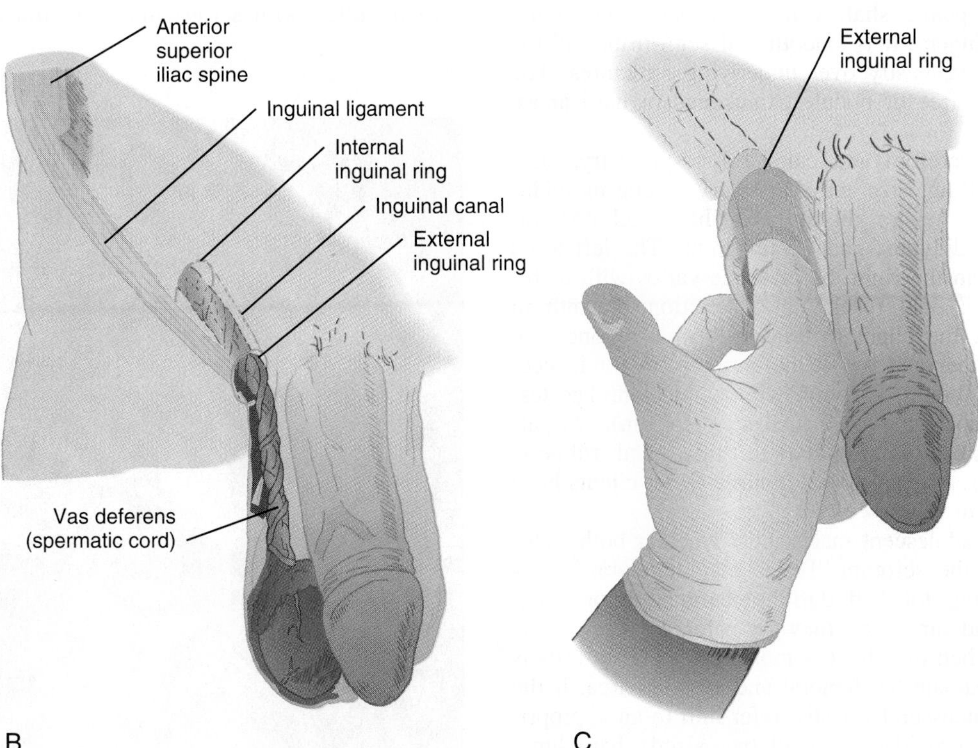

FIGURE 37–14 *A,* Male genitourinary anatomy. *B,* Anatomy of male inguinal structures. *C,* Palpation to detect an indirect hernia.

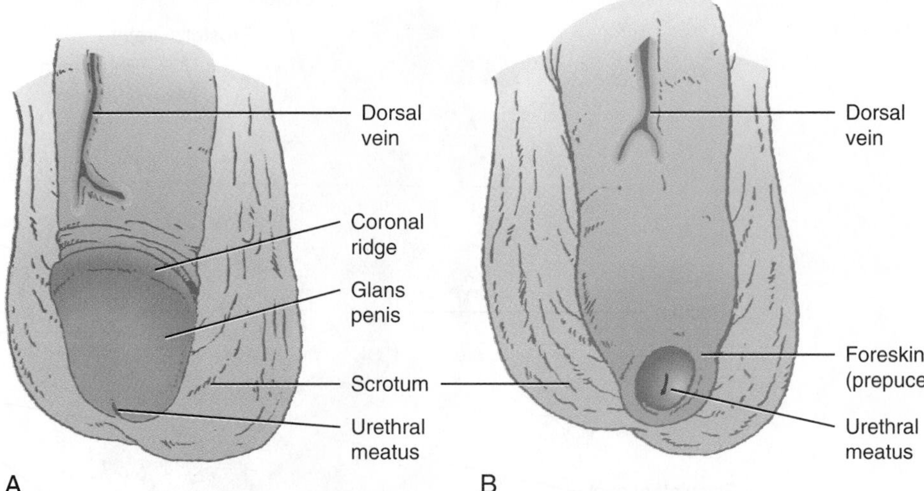

FIGURE 37–15 Appearance of a circumcised (*A*) and an uncircumcised (*B*) penis.

on either the underside of the penile shaft *(hypospadias)* or upper side *(epispadias)* is usually a congenital condition. The meatus is pink and without ulcers, scars, inflammation, or discharge. Gently compress the glans between your thumb and index finger to open the meatus, and inspect for discharge. If the client reports a urethral discharge, ask the client to compress the penis from base to tip between his thumb and fingers in an attempt to express a discharge. If one appears, obtain a specimen for culture or microscopic examination. You may need to change gloves again before continuing with the examination.

Palpate the penile shaft gently between your thumb and first two fingers. It is smooth and semi-firm, and the skin should move easily over underlying structures. The normal penis is free of nodules, thickened or hard areas, and tenderness.

Inspect the scrotum and palpate for symmetry, size, shape, and swelling. Size and shape vary among individuals. The scrotum has a right and a left half, each containing a testis, epididymis, and vas deferens. The left testis hangs lower than the right. Scrotal size varies with ambient temperature; cold results in contraction, warmth in relaxation. Ask the client to hold the penis to one side and then the other and to lift the scrotum up for inspection. The skin should be loose, without tension. The testes are ovoid, about ⅘ × 1⅗ inches (2 × 4 cm). On palpation, they are normally smooth, firm, and rubbery, without nodules, masses, or tenderness. Older clients have smaller, less firm testes.

In younger, adolescent males, note whether both testes are present in the scrotum. Testes may temporarily migrate from being touched during examination or being exposed to cold air. They may be palpable later in the examination, when the client is more relaxed. If a testis is not apparent, palpate the femoral and inguinal area. If the client has an undescended testis, refer him to an appropriate health care provider. A small (pea-sized), hard lump located on either the anterior or lateral aspect of a testis suggests a malignancy; again, refer the client for follow-up. Compare testes bilaterally for similarity.

Palpate each epididymis between your thumb and index finger. The epididymis is located on the superior aspect of the testis and extends down the posterior surface. It feels soft, resilient, and tender. Swelling and hardness are abnormal. The vas deferens (spermatic cord) begins at the superior, lateral aspect of the testis. It is differentiated from the epididymis by its firmer, tubular feel. Compare findings bilaterally. Palpate the vas deferens along its length toward the inguinal canal. Note any thickening or asymmetry, which is abnormal.

If you find swelling, nodules, or other abnormalities during the scrotal examination, perform transillumination of the scrotum (Fig. 37–16). Darken the room, and shine a flashlight through the scrotum from behind the mass. A scrotum filled with serous fluid will transilluminate as a

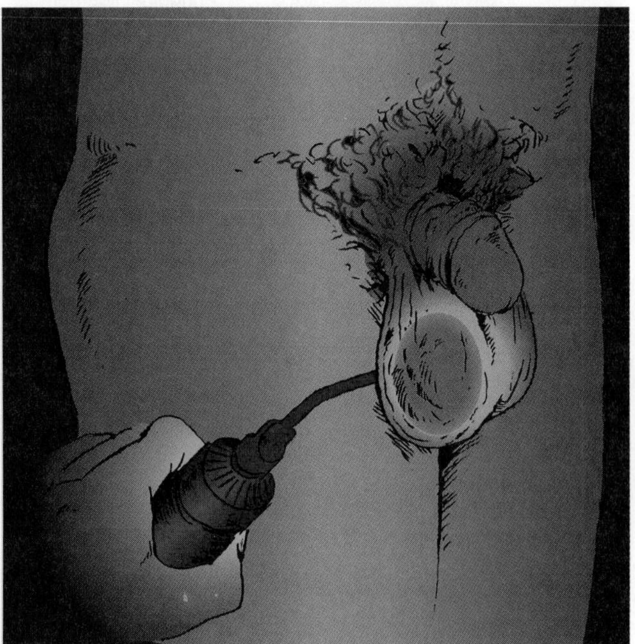

FIGURE 37–16 Transillumination of the scrotum. In a darkened room, place a strong, lighted flashlight or transilluminator next to the scrotum, as shown. Light normally passes through the scrotum (transillumination), but this does not occur with testicular tumor. A hydrocele shines red.

red glow. More solid lesions, such as a hematoma or mass, do not transilluminate and may be seen as a dark shadow. Record the characteristics of the abnormality, including whether it transilluminates.

While the client is standing, examine for an inguinal *hernia* (a prolapse or protrusion of a loop of intestine through the inguinal wall or canal). Inspect the inguinal areas for bulges while the client stands quietly and again after he bears down and strains, as though attempting a bowel movement. Bulges should be absent.

A *direct* inguinal hernia enters the inguinal canal behind the external ring because of a weakened abdominal wall; it does not pass through the inguinal canal. Assess for a direct hernia by gently inserting an index finger into the loose scrotal skin over the external inguinal ring; the finger does not enter to the external ring. Use the left index finger to palpate the client's right side and the right finger for the client's left side while the client faces you. Instruct the client to bear down while you feel for a bulge, which should be absent.

An *indirect* inguinal hernia enters the inguinal canal through the internal ring and can remain in the canal or pass down through the external ring and into the scrotum. To palpate for an indirect hernia, gently invaginate the scrotal skin with the index or little finger, following the vas deferens to where it passes into the external ring (Fig. 37–14*C*). Ask the client to flex the knee on that same side to help relax the muscles so that the finger can be inserted through the external ring and into the inguinal canal. Advance the palpating finger as far as possible, and instruct the client to bear down while you feel for a tissue mass touching the finger. The mass retreats up the canal when the client relaxes.

A *femoral* hernia, which is more common in women, occurs inferiorly and more laterally compared with an inguinal hernia; it often has the appearance of an enlarged inguinal lymph node. Palpate the inguinal area directly for a femoral hernia while the client is relaxed and again after instructing him to bear down. A palpable mass should be absent.

■ PROSTATE

After examining the anterior genitalia, assess the anus, rectum, and prostate gland. A rectal-prostatic examination should be performed annually in men over age 40 years to look for signs of an STD, changes in the size and consistency of the prostate gland, and evidence of a tumor or acute or chronic infection. Emphasize the importance of regular examinations as the best way to detect prostatic cancer for effective treatment.

Just before the examination, ask the client to empty his bladder, and collect a urine specimen at this time if one is needed. Explain that an empty bladder makes the examination more comfortable and more accurate. Also explain that it is normal to experience sensations of having to urinate or defecate during the examination.

Two possible positions for the client during the rectal examination are the knee-chest position, with the buttocks elevated, or bending over from the hip, with elbows placed either on the knees or on the examining table. (Positions are discussed in Chapter 10, and the anal and rectal examination is discussed in Chapter 32.)

Wear gloves, and apply water-soluble lubricant to the examining finger. Place your dominant hand on the client's hip to stabilize his position and to reassure him. Gently spread his buttocks with the nondominant hand. Observe the perineum and perianal areas for lesions, hemorrhoids, inflammation, or discoloration. Ask the client to bear down. Explain that this helps relax the anal sphincter and makes it easier to insert the examining finger.

Insert the ball of the finger toward the anterior wall of the rectum. The normal prostate is located 2 to 5 cm beyond the anal sphincter along the anterior wall of the rectum. It is normally about 4 cm long and 5 cm wide (Fig. 37–17*A* and *B*). The prostate is shaped like a doughnut wrapped around the neck of the urethra (Fig. 37–17*C*). Only the posterior and lateral lobes can be felt through the rectal wall (Fig. 37–17*D* and *E*). The lateral lobes should be symmetrical. A normal prostate feels smooth, rubbery, and firm, somewhat like the base of the thumb. In a man with BPH, the prostate feels larger than normal, with a firmer consistency, like that of the chin. Tenderness and bogginess (like the cheek of the face) may indicate acute or chronic prostatitis. Carcinoma feels like a stone or hard nodule, that is, a circumscribed area of induration. Any induration is abnormal. The seminal vesicles (superior and lateral to the prostate) are normally nonpalpable.

Prostatic massage may be indicated even when the client is asymptomatic to aid in the detection of prostatitis. Roll the pad of your index finger across the prostate gland, starting laterally and superiorly and moving toward the midline of the prostate (Fig. 37–17*F*). Then strip (or "milk") the area of the seminal vesicles, starting laterally and superiorly, toward the midline (Fig. 37–17*G*). Send the resulting meatal secretions for microscopic examination. A large number of pus cells suggests prostatitis. Staining may identify acid-fast organisms. Cultures may be needed to identify organisms such as gonococcal, chlamydial, or tubercous bacilli. If a culture is required, the glans of the penis must be cleaned and the bladder emptied to clear the urethra before prostatic massage. Collect meatal secretions in sterile culture media.

Withdraw your finger from the rectum, and observe for stool on the glove. Feces, if present, are normally brown. Mucus or blood and black, tarry, light-tan, or gray stools are abnormal. Test the stool sample for occult (hidden) blood, which should be absent (see Chapter 32). If you suspect an STD, obtain a rectal swab for culture. Wipe the perianal area, and inform the client that the examination is completed. See the Physical Assessment feature for an example of a recorded examination of the male reproductive tract.

DIAGNOSTIC TESTS

Various diagnostic tests may be done to assess for disorders of the male reproductive system. Men and their significant others are often anxious about diagnostic tests. You can help to reduce anxiety by giving careful explanations before and during the tests. It is much less frightening if a client knows what to expect and what is included in the process. Sedation or pain relief may be required before a test. An informed consent may be necessary. Physiologic preparations may be required, such as fasting or an enema. During the test, tell the client what

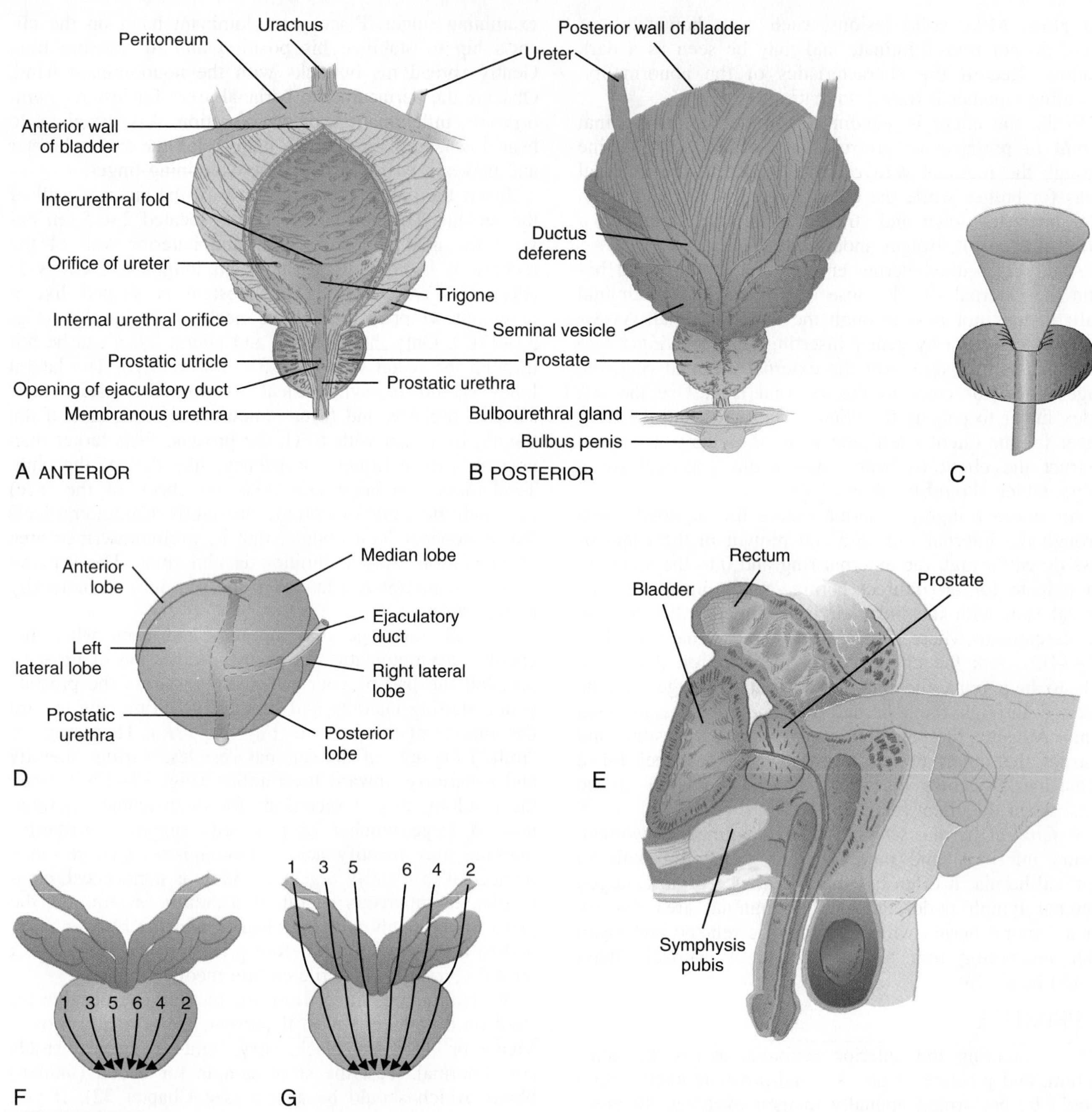

FIGURE 37–17 Rectal-prostatic assessment. *A* and *B,* Anterior and posterior views of the prostate gland. *C,* Diagrammatic representation of the anatomic position of the prostate gland. The gland surrounds the urethra rather like a doughnut wrapped around the outlet of a funnel. *D,* Posterior and lateral lobes of the prostate. *E,* Rectal examination. Insert a gloved index finger into the anus while the client is bearing down. Palpate all surfaces. *F,* Prostatic massage. Roll the pad of the index finger across the prostate, starting laterally and superiorly and moving toward the midline of the prostate. *G,* Seminal vesicles and prostatic massage. Use the same technique as for prostatic massage, but extend the finger over the area of the seminal vesicles.

is happening. Help him maintain the required positions. Observe him during and after the test for adverse reactions, such as pain, excessive anxiety, pallor, or nausea.

■ LABORATORY STUDIES

Blood Studies

PROSTATE-SPECIFIC ANTIGEN

Prostate cancer screening has been revolutionized by the prostate-specific antigen (PSA) assay. PSA, a substance found in prostatic fluid, aids the liquifaction of semen. PSA serum levels in men without prostate cancer are very low. The PSA level increases with age, and some controversy exists over the normal level. A level of 4.0 ng/ml or higher may be normal only for men over age 65, with a lower level being normal for younger men. Prostatic massage or rectal examination within 48 hours before the assay can cause elevated PSA levels. The PSA test has largely replaced the measurement of serum acid phosphatase as a screening tool for prostate cancer.

PHYSICAL ASSESSMENT FINDINGS IN THE HEALTHY ADULT

Male Reproductive System

Inspection

Breasts and Axillae: Breasts symmetrical, smooth in all positions, without retractions or masses. Vascular pattern and striae absent. Nipples everted and areolae even. Axillae even color, without masses or rash.

Penis: Penis size and shape vary among individuals. Foreskin may or may not be present. Head of penis slightly rounded without discharge (if client is circumcised). Smegma under the foreskin (normal if client is uncircumcised). Urinary meatus at the tip of the head of the penis, free of discharge or drainage. Shaft smooth.

Scrotum: Scrotal size and shape vary normally. Hangs below the penis with the left side lower than the right. Scrotal skin thin and rugose. Sparse hair on the scrotum. Transillumination shows no masses or areas of thickness.

Inguinal-Femoral Area: Coarse hair covers symphysis pubis, inner thighs, extending toward umbilicus. No bulges over the inguinal or femoral area, either at rest or with coughing or straining.

Palpation

Breasts and Axillae: Breasts firm without masses, lumps, local areas of warmth, or tenderness. Nipples even, without discharge. Axillae smooth, nodes nonpalpable.

Penis: Masses along the penile shaft and head of the penis absent. Firm, nontender.

Testis: Two testicles present, smooth, oval, and similar in consistency. Mobile and equal in size. Slight tenderness with palpation.

Epididymis: Present at the posterior of the scrotum (found in the anterolateral or anterior area of the testis in a small percentage of men). No tenderness.

Vas Deferens: Cord-like, mobile, smooth, and nontender. No masses.

Inguinal Canal: No bulge or mass in inguinal canal either at rest or with straining.

To further clarify the meaning of the PSA level, there are two additional tests: (1) PSA *density* (PSAD) and (2) PSA *velocity* (PSAV). PSA density relates PSA level to prostate size. PSA velocity involves the rate of change in PSA level over time. The PSA density test is combined with transrectal ultrasonography to determine the volume of the prostate. Clients who have PSA density levels less than 0.10 ng/ml are considered unlikely to have significant prostate cancer. As PSA levels rise, however, the presence of cancer cells is more likely. Clients who have a PSA velocity that rises more than 0.7 ng/ml per yr or that increases 20% or more a year are considered at high risk of having prostate cancer.

Alkaline Phosphatase

Alkaline phosphatase is present ubiquitously and is particularly associated with a variety of bone diseases. It is used as a diagnostic test in men with prostate cancer as a measure of possible bone metastasis. With higher levels in clients with known prostate cancer, the probability of bone metastasis is higher. However, many medications can artificially raise or lower the level.

Semen Examination

Semen testing is used to evaluate fertility. One to three samples of semen, collected at intervals of 2 to 4 weeks, are examined to accommodate for normal variations. To provide an adequate sample, the client should abstain from ejaculation for 2 to 5 days before the test. Prolonged abstinence may decrease sperm quality and motility, whereas more frequent ejaculations reduce sperm concentration and volume.

In the laboratory or office, the client masturbates into a clean, dry specimen container. Ordinary condoms or coitus interruptus is not an appropriate method because contamination or loss of the specimen is likely. If the client must collect the specimen outside the laboratory or office, the specimen should be kept at room temperature and brought to the laboratory within 30 minutes of collection.

Sperm analysis is used to assess infertility and to evaluate the effectiveness of a vasectomy. Tests for infertility include a sperm count, morphology, and motility along with semen pH, viscosity, appearance, and volume. If abnormalities are found, further analysis for the presence of antibodies can also be performed. If the test is being done to evaluate the effectiveness of a vasectomy, the presence or absence of sperm is sufficient.

Secretion Analysis

Secretions from the throat, penis, and anus or lesions from the oral, pharyngeal, and perineal areas may be examined for microorganisms. A sterile, cotton-tipped applicator is placed on or in the affected area, and the specimen is transferred to a sterile tube or slide. Be careful not to touch any other surface with the applicator.

■ RADIOGRAPHY

CT scanning and MRI are used to assess male reproductive and urologic disorders. Procedures include clinical staging of testicular and prostate cancers and imaging of pelvic organs for epididymitis, hydrocele, spermatocele, scrotal hernia, or testicular torsion and infarction. Chapter 11 covers these diagnostic procedures.

■ ULTRASONOGRAPHY

A transrectal approach is used in prostatic ultrasonography. The rectum must be free of feces. Help the client into a left lateral Sims' position. After a rectal examination, a well-lubricated transducer is inserted. The probe is covered with a water-filled condom to enhance sound wave transmission; a full bladder may also improve sound transmission. The examiner moves the probe along the prostate to complete the scan. Tell the client that some discomfort may be felt with probe insertion and manipulation. Once the probe has been removed, there should be no further discomfort.

■ RADIONUCLIDE IMAGING

Radioisotope scans may be used to assess testicular abnormalities, such as torsion, epididymitis, abscess, tumors, hydroceles, varicoceles, and spermatoceles. A radioactive substance is administered intravenously, and several scans are taken. Before a scan is taken, ask the client whether he has any history of allergies.

■ CYSTOSCOPY

Cystoscopy is indispensable for assessing and treating prostate and urologic problems. It is used to determine the cause of urinary manifestations, such as those related to prostatic hypertrophy, and to obtain specimens, such as in a transurethral prostatic biopsy. Cystoscopy may be done in a urologist's office or in an operating room before surgery. Inspection of the bladder interior includes looking for trabeculation, diverticula, and bladder neck contracture and checking the size and contours of the prostatic lobes. Chapter 32 describes the procedure and client care in detail.

■ URODYNAMIC ASSESSMENT

Urodynamic studies measure pressure from the bladder or urethra, urinary flow, and striated muscle activity. Common tests include uroflometry, cystometrography, electromyography, and a urethral pressure profile. They are useful in determining the cause of frequency and decreased urinary stream in men (as from prostatic obstruction). Chapter 32 describes urodynamic testing in detail.

■ PROSTATIC BIOPSY

Areas of the prostate that suggest a problem are assessed by biopsy after abnormal findings in PSA level, transrectal ultrasonography, or digital rectal examination. Biopsy of the prostate allows cytologic examination for the presence of cancer. The tissue may be obtained by a transurethral, transrectal, or perineal approach. The client must understand the approach to be used, the preparation, and the procedure for it. Obtain an informed consent. Physical preparation often includes an enema for the transrectal or perineal approach. The client must void before the procedure.

For the *transurethral* approach, place the client in the lithotomy position. Local anesthesia is used. The biopsy tissue is removed through transurethral endoscopy. Even though direct visual guidance is used in this approach, malignant tissue may be missed. This is partly because prostate cancer commonly begins in the posterior lobe, making it more difficult to obtain a specimen by this approach.

For the *perineal* approach, the lithotomy position is usually used; a jackknife position is an alternative. After the perineal area is cleaned and anesthetized, one or more biopsies are taken. This approach allows direct access to the posterior lobe of the prostate. Direct pressure is applied to the area. If there is no bleeding, a sterile dressing is applied.

For a *transrectal* approach, place the client in Sims' position. A rectal examination is performed to identify any hard nodules. The biopsy is performed with the examiner's finger as a guide. Some think that this approach is inappropriate because malignant cells from the nodule may be seeded into the rectal mucosa.

After the procedure, monitor the client's vital signs at regular intervals to detect signs of hemorrhage. If a transurethral approach was used, some hematuria is normal, although frank bleeding should be reported. The client must be able to void after the procedure. With the perineal approach, carefully assess the dressing for blood. After a transrectal approach, monitor for bleeding or infection.

PREVENTION OF MALE REPRODUCTIVE PROBLEMS

Primary prevention (preventing a problem before it occurs) includes genetic counseling, immunization against infectious diseases, good nutrition, careful genital hygiene, the use of condoms to prevent STDs, knowing one's partner, avoiding multiple sex partners, and avoiding sexual intercourse (oral, anal, or genital) with a person who has genital lesions.

Secondary prevention (detecting and treating a problem early) includes screening activities, such as serum PSA levels in men over age 50 and testicular self-examination (TSE). See Chapter 2 for discussion of BSE and TSE.

Tertiary prevention (avoiding complications and rehabilitation) is health care provided for clients experiencing acute and chronic disorders. For example, teaching perineal exercises after a prostatectomy helps men regain urinary control.

CONCLUSIONS

Assessment of the female and male reproductive systems requires knowledge of the physiologic and psychological implications associated with reproductive disorders. Exhibit a concerned, caring attitude when assessing any client with a reproductive disorder because these disorders are laden with psychosocial overtones. Assess the client in a thorough but matter-of-fact manner to put the client at ease and to expedite a complete assessment.

BIBLIOGRAPHY

1. American Cancer Society (1997). *Special touch: A personal plan of action for breast health.* Publication No. 97-500M-No. 2095-CC. Atlanta: Author.
2. American Cancer Society. (1997). *Guidelines for the early detection of cancer.* Publication No. 97-700M-No. 2070-CC. Atlanta: Author.
3. American Cancer Society. (1999). *Cancer facts and figures, 1999.* Publication No. 99-300M-No. 5008.99). Atlanta: Author.
4. Bickley, L. S. (1999). *Bates' guide to physical examination and history taking* (7th ed.). Philadelphia: J. B. Lippincott.
5. Benign Prostatic Hyperplasia Guideline Panel. (1994). *Benign prostatic hyperplasia: Clinical practice guideline.* AHCPR Publication No. 94-0583. Rockville, MD: Agency for Health Care Policy and Research, Public Health Service, U.S. Department of Health and Human Services.
6. Benign Prostatic Hyperplasia Guideline Panel. (1994). *Benign prostatic hyperplasia: Diagnosis and treatment.* AHCPR Publication No. 94-0582. Rockville, MD: Agency for Health Care Policy and Research, Public Health Service, U.S. Department of Health and Human Services.
7. Benign Prostatic Hyperplasia Guideline Panel. (1994). *Benign prostatic hyperplasia: Patient guide.* AHCPR Publication No. 94-0584. Rockville, MD: Agency for Health Care Policy and Research, Public Health Service, U.S. Department of Health and Human Services.

8. Bobak, I. M., & Jensen, M. D. (1997). *Maternity and women's health care* (6th ed.). St. Louis: Mosby–Year Book.
9. Grimes, J., & Burns, E. (1996). *Health assessment in nursing practice* (4th ed.). Boston: Little, Brown.
10. Hacker, N. F., & Moore, J. G. (1998). *Essentials of obstetrics and gynecology* (3rd ed.). Philadelphia: W. B. Saunders.
11. Jarvis, C. (2000). *Physical examination and health assessment* (3rd ed.). Philadelphia: W. B. Saunders.
12. Karlowicz, K. A. (Ed.). (1995). *Urologic nursing: Principles and practice.* Philadelphia: W. B. Saunders.
13. Kee, J. L. (1999). *Laboratory and diagnostic tests with nursing implications* (5th ed.). Stamford, CT: Appleton & Lange.
14. Kirby, R., & Christmas, T. (1997). *Benign prostatic hypertrophy* (2nd ed.). Chicago: Mosby International.
15. Mashburn, J., & Scharbo-DeHaan, M. (1997). A clinician's guide to Pap smear interpretation. *The Nurse Practitioner, 22*(4), 115–143.
16. McCorkle, R., et al. (1996). *Cancer nursing: A comprehensive textbook.* Philadelphia: W. B. Saunders.
17. Reeder, S., Mattin, L., & Koniak-Griffin, D. (1997). *Maternity nursing* (18th ed.). Philadelphia: J. B. Lippincott.
18. Seidman, H., et al. (1987). Survival experience in the breast cancer detection demonstration project. *CA: A Cancer Journal for Clinicians, 37*(5), 258–291.
19. Smith, D. R. (1996). *General urology* (14th ed.). Norwalk, CT: Appleton & Lange.
20. Star, W., Lommel, L., & Shannon, M. (Ed.). (1998). *Women's Primary Health Care Protocols for Practice.* Washington, DC: American Nurses Publishing.
21. Weber, E. S. (1997). Questions and answers about breast cancer diagnosis. *American Journal of Nursing, 97*(10), 34–38.
22. Youngkin, E. Q., & Davis, M. S. (1998). *Women's health* (2nd ed.). Stamford, CT: Appleton & Lange.

CHAPTER 38

Management of Men with Reproductive Disorders

Patricia McCallig Bates

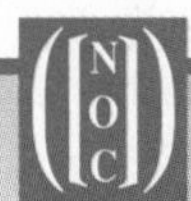

NURSING OUTCOMES CLASSIFICATION (NOC) for Nursing Diagnoses—Men with Reproductive Disorders

Altered Urinary Elimination
Urinary Continence
Urinary Elimination
Ineffective Management of Therapeutic Regimen (Individuals)
Compliance Behavior
Knowledge: Treatment Regimen
Participation: Health Care Decisions
Treatment Behavior: Illness or Injury

Pain
Comfort Level
Pain Control
Pain: Disruptive Effects
Pain Level
Risk for Injury: Postoperative Complications
Circulation Status
Electrolyte and Acid/Base Balance
Fluid Balance

Risk Control
Risk Detection
Safety Status: Physical Injury
Symptom Control
Tissue Perfusion: Abdominal Organs
Tissue Perfusion: Peripheral
Urinary Continence
Urinary Elimination
Vital Signs Status

Today, men are more actively involved in health maintenance. This is evidenced by their increased interest in fitness and exercise, increased attainment of lifestyle factors related to fitness (such as smoking cessation), and increased participation in childbirth and parenting. As men learn to express their interest in general health maintenance, you can extend these interests to reproductive and urinary health maintenance. Often, knowledge about risk factors, preventive measures, and improved disease management encourages men to make changes in lifestyles and attitudes and to see health care providers for counsel or early detection of reproductive disorders.

Reproductive and genital disorders are significant, and their incidence is being increasingly recognized. Because the male urinary and reproductive systems involve the same structures, men may have mixed problems. Men are often reluctant to ask for help because they see such problems as a potential threat to their sexuality and are embarrassed to talk about them. Some men may also fear negative reactions from their health care providers because of their age or sexual preference.

Because of this reluctance to seek help, skillful therapeutic interaction is essential to help men express their concerns. Sensitivity to fear and embarrassment, respect for privacy and confidentiality, careful history-taking, and addressing information needs help put these clients at ease. When the client allows, partners should be brought into management plan discussions because most reproductive and genital disorders affect relationships.

Statements such as "Many men are concerned about how this problem will affect their sex lives," "It is common to worry about how your partner might feel about this problem," and "What are some of your concerns?" may help the client begin to talk about his concerns.

Giving men permission to express their feelings and their health-related concerns draws them and their significant others into the process of health care. Having topic-related brochures visible may provide the impetus for a man to ask questions.

PROSTATE DISORDERS

BENIGN PROSTATIC HYPERPLASIA

The prostate is the genital organ most commonly affected by benign and malignant neoplasms. Enlargement of the prostate gland with aging is called *benign prostatic hypertrophy* or *hyperplasia* (BPH). Hyperplasia (an increase in the number of cells) is the more acceptable term. BPH becomes a disorder when enlargement obstructs the urinary channel and causes changes in the urinary tract with associated manifestations.

Prostatic enlargement eventually occurs in 80% of men. By age 50, about 50% of men have some degree of BPH. The incidence is increased in African American men and is lower in Asians.

Etiology and Risk Factors

The exact cause of BPH is not known. Because BPH is a universal disorder in older men, several theories concerning the cause have been examined. Diet, effects of chronic inflammation, socioeconomic factors, heredity, race, body build, and sexual activity have been investigated, but no significant relationships have been found. It is thought that hormonal alteration is responsible. Testicular androgen appears to be the hormone suspected as the cause. BPH rarely occurs in men who are castrated or who have permanent hypogonadism before puberty or in early adulthood.

Because aging is the major risk factor for the development of BPH, little can be done for health promotion and prevention. Dietary factors have been examined, and it has been concluded that lycopene in cooked tomatoes and in green and yellow vegetables and other elements of the traditional Japanese diet appear to provide some protection against BPH. Early detection can lead to early treatment, which can prevent complications related to urinary obstruction. Men should be encouraged to discuss changes in urinary patterns and to have a digital rectal examination (DRE) annually if they are older than 40 years of age.

Pathophysiology

Benign prostatic enlargement refers to an abnormal increase in the number of normal cells (hyperplasia) in the prostate along with increased contraction of the smooth muscle elements of the prostatic stroma. These processes are often referred to as *static* and *dynamic* processes in the development of BPH. Many theories have been postulated, but the pathophysiology may be complex and is not clearly understood.

The pituitary secretes luteinizing hormone (LH) in response to changes in serum levels of LH, testosterone, and luteinizing hormone–releasing hormone (LHRH) produced by the hypothalamus. LH causes the testes to produce testosterone, which combines with an enzyme in the prostate, 5α-reductase, to form dihydrotestosterone (DHT). DHT influences prostatic cellular production. Simultaneously, alpha-adrenergic receptors in the smooth muscle of the prostate, along with the smooth muscle of the bladder neck and rhabdosphincter, cause contraction. This muscle contraction may cause enough resistance to restrict urine flow.

In response to increasing *bladder outlet obstruction* (BOO), urinary tract changes occur (Fig. 38–1). Urine remains in the bladder after urination. The detrusor muscle compensates by thickening to increase pressure against the outlet's resistance to empty the bladder. When it can no longer compensate, trabeculation (banding of fibromuscular tissue that appears thick in some places and thinner in others) and bladder diverticula (outpouchings in the bladder wall) may occur. Diverticula may retain urine, causing infection and stones.

Compensation and decompensation can also cause reflux (backflow of urine past the ureterovesical junction [UVJ]) and upper urinary tract infection (UTI). "Fishhooking" of the ureters is common (i.e., ureters looping downward like a fishhook as they enter the bladder). Compensation and decompensation processes may also occur in the ureter and kidney, causing conditions of hydroureter and hydronephrosis. Eventually, the renal parenchyma atrophies, resulting in irreversible loss of kidney function.

Clinical Manifestations

BPH usually develops slowly and may persist in a silent state without creating a major problem. As a man becomes older, he may assume that increasing frequency of

ALTERNATIVE THERAPY

Benign Prostatic Hyperplasia

Benign prostatic hyperplasia (BPH) is a common problem in men after 50 years of age. Enlargement of prostatic tissue often leads to a variety of manifestations, including urinary frequency, hesitancy in voiding, decreased force of urine flow and postvoid dribbling. For many years, an herb known as saw palmetto (the fruit of the scrub palm *Serenoa repens* which grows on the southeastern Atlantic coast) has been used to treat this condition.

Saw palmetto seems to be effective in a number of ways. It appears to block the conversion of testosterone to 5α-dihydrotestosterone (DHT) by the enzyme 5α-reductase. It is DHT that stimulates growth of prostatic tissue. The herb apparently also has an anti-inflammatory effect that, when combined with the anti-androgenic effect, helps to reduce manifestations of BPH.[2] In one review,[3] saw palmetto produced similar positive benefits as the drug finasteride with fewer side effects.

The German Commission E monograph on saw palmetto recommends a daily dosage of 1 to 2 g of the berry, or 320 mg of a lipophilic extract.[1] The latter amount is necessary for proper extraction of the active constituents, which cannot be extracted in water. The herb does not shrink the prostate but only relieves the manifestations associated with BPH.[1]

Another herb, stinging nettle root (*Urtica dioica L.* or *U. urens L.*) has also been effective.[1, 2] Unlike saw palmetto, the root of stinging nettle may be prepared as a tea because the active ingredients appear to be water-soluble. To date, however, less research is available regarding this plant for the treatment of BPH.

References

1. Blumenthal, M. (1998). *The complete German Commission E monographs.* Austin, TX: American Botanical Council.
2. Tyler, V. (1994). *Herbs of choice.* Binghamtom, NY: Pharmaceutical Products Press.
3. Wilt, T. J., et al. (1998). Saw palmetto extracts for treatment of benign prostatic hyperplasia: A systematic review. *Journal of the American Medical Association, 280,* 1604–1609.

James Higgy Lerner, RN, LAc, *Private practice of acupuncture, traditional Oriental medicine, and biofeedback*

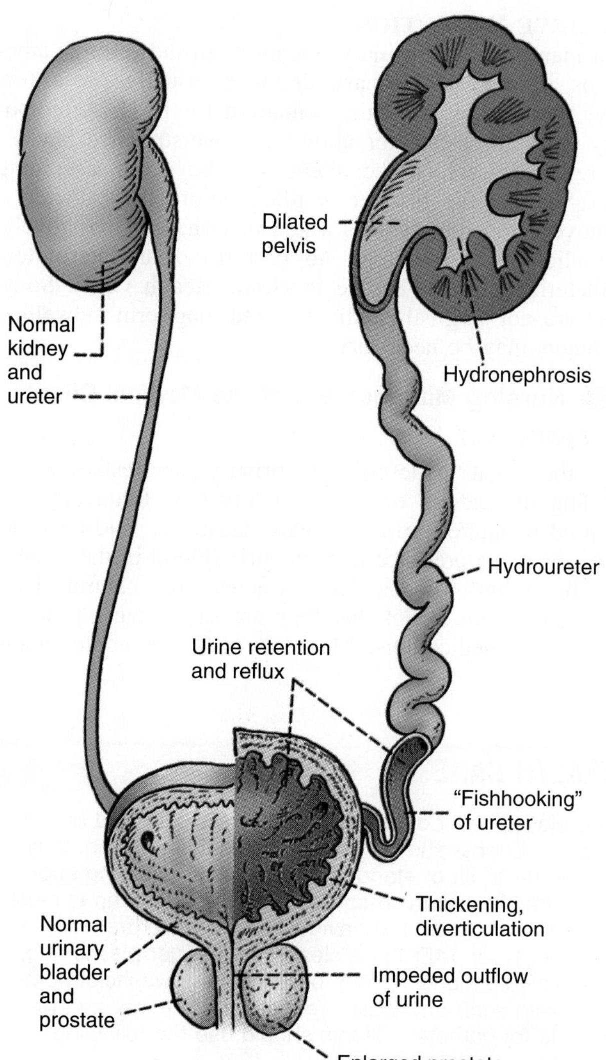

FIGURE 38–1 Complications of benign prostatic enlargement. *Left,* Normal kidney, ureter, bladder, and prostate. *Right,* Potential complications.

urination is part of aging. He may wait until he is bothered by retention before seeking medical care. Acute urinary retention in the client with BPH is often precipitated by cold weather, alcoholic beverages, infection, a delay in voiding, or bed rest. Some medications, such as decongestants, anticholinergics, and antidepressants, may also precipitate retention.

The severity of manifestations caused by BPH varies and is not related to the size of the enlargement. For example, a man with mild BPH may have strong stromal resistance and may experience severe bladder outlet obstruction. Another man may have enlargement of a median lobe of the prostate that grows up toward the bladder. This type of enlargement would not be detected by rectal examination. He, too, may experience moderate to severe bladder outlet obstruction. In contrast, another man may have a very large prostate with minimal manifestations.

History-taking includes specific questions about the size and force of the urine stream, hesitancy, need to strain, frequency, intermittency, urgency, nocturia (excessive urination at night), incomplete emptying, and urinary leakage. The American Urological Association's International Prostate Symptom Score Index (IPSS) is a short questionnaire commonly used by urologists to assess the client's opinion about the severity of these manifestations. The client scores manifestations from "not at all" to "almost always." The client also rates his quality of life from "delighted" to "terrible." The IPSS may also be used to evaluate treatment effectiveness.

A digital rectal examination is performed to evaluate size and tissue consistency and to rule out nodules or a tender, boggy prostate. Urinalysis, urine culture, blood tests for kidney function, and a *prostate-specific antigen* (PSA) test may be done to exclude accompanying urologic diseases. Chemistry panels, such as electrolyte, liver function, and blood coagulation studies, may be added if surgery is being considered.

Uroflowmetry is used to estimate the pattern and force of voiding. A man starts this test with a full bladder, voids into a specific toilet or container, and empties his bladder to the best of his ability. Residual urine is determined after the urine flow either by catheterization or by ultrasonography. A normal urine flow is considered to be 20 to 25 ml/second, but the figure may be lower for older men. BPH may cause decreased flow and a long, weak flow pattern with evidence of starts and stops or strained voiding. Depending on the severity of the client's manifestations and general medical condition, cystourethroscopy, intravenous pyelography (IVP), or urodynamic studies may be done.

Outcome Management

Medical Management

Medical management has become a common initial approach for BPH because it is noninvasive and can be effective. "Watchful waiting" is a relatively new approach to BPH, particularly for the client who has few or mild manifestations. Periodic reassessment is necessary to reassess the severity of manifestations and to detect developing complications. Treatment is instituted if significant changes occur.

Definitive treatment is aimed at prostatic muscle relaxation or at androgen deprivation, which slows growth of the prostate and reduces its size. Relief of lower urinary tract manifestations is the subjective tool used to evaluate the effectiveness of treatment.

Slow Prostate Growth

Finasteride (Proscar), a 5α-reductase inhibitor, blocks the conversion of testosterone to DHT and thus reduces BPH. Because finasteride is metabolized mostly in the liver, liver function tests are important before therapy is started. Side effects include a decrease in ejaculatory semen, decreased libido, and *erectile dysfunction* (inability to achieve or maintain an erection), although the latter two effects occur in only about 1% to 5% of men taking this drug. Finasteride may have to be taken for 6 to 12 months before any improvement in lower urinary tract manifestations occurs. Finasteride lowers the level of PSA (a glycoprotein) and can mask the occurrence of prostate cancer. Because finasteride can cause abnormal development of a male fetus, pregnant women should not come in contact with the semen of a man taking this drug.

Antiandrogens and LHRH antagonists (testosterone-ablating agents), agents used to treat prostate cancer, have been tried in the treatment of BPH, but side effects outweigh the benefits for most men. Side effects include loss of libido, hot flashes, gynecomastia (breast enlargement), and impotence. These agents are used on occasion.

Relax Prostate Muscle

Alpha-adrenergic blocking medications act on receptors in prostatic muscle tissue and seem to be effective in reducing manifestations. This group of drugs includes terazosin (Hytrin), phenoxybenzamine (Dibenzyline), prazosin (Minipress), doxazosin (Cardura), and tamsulosin (Flomax). The major side effects are orthostatic hypotension, dizziness, and tachycardia. Dry mouth, nasal congestion, palpitations, blurred vision, headache, and fatigue may also occur. Clients are started at a lower dose, which is increased if the medication is tolerated. Clients should not adjust the dosage without permission of the physician because serious cardiovascular consequences can occur. Several weeks of treatment may be necessary before improvement of lower urinary tract manifestations can be evaluated.

Relieve Retention

If a man has acute urinary retention, an indwelling catheter is inserted for urinary drainage, usually for a few days, before any urologic evaluation for BPH. A temporary indwelling catheter allows the overstretched bladder to rest, after which the client may be given a voiding trial; that is, the bladder is filled before the catheter is removed, and the client is asked to urinate. Alternatively, the client may be taught to perform clean intermittent catheterization (see Bridge to Home Health Care). Some men are not surgical candidates, and long-term indwelling catheters may be necessary.

Nursing Management of the Medical Client

Assessment

Ask the client to describe all urinary manifestations, including the pattern of urination, urgency, frequency, decreased or altered urinary stream, hesitancy, and nocturia. Ask about the presence of hematuria (blood in the urine).

Clients have used agents extracted from natural plants for years in the belief that they are safer than physician-prescribed medications. Men may tell you about taking

BRIDGE TO HOME HEALTH CARE

Intermittent Self-Catheterization for Men

Intermittent self-catheterization is indicated for transient or persistent urinary retention. Retention occurs when clients are unable to empty their bladders completely as a result of neurologic conditions such as spinal cord injury, multiple sclerosis, or brain injury. An obstructive condition such as an enlarged prostate is another common cause of retention. The amount of residual urine that clients retain can vary greatly.

When intermittent self-catheterization is used to manage urinary retention, an indwelling catheter is not needed and the risk of infection is decreased. The procedure can be used as a temporary measure, for example, for the development of temporary bladder atony after bladder surgery. Before self-catheterization is selected for long-term management, a thorough assessment should be completed and noninvasive methods should have been attempted without success.

To use intermittent self-catheterization successfully, clients should have sufficient manual dexterity and cognitive ability, and they should follow guidelines. Because they must not overfill their bladders, it is essential that clients be motivated to catheterize four or five times daily. The goal is to obtain a quantity of urine that does not exceed 500 ml per catheterization. Most physicians recommend a moderate daily fluid intake. They tell clients to establish a consistent plan that includes the time and amount of their intake so that they do not overfill their bladders. It is also important that clients understand that poor or inconsistent technique increases the risk of complications. Infection is the most frequently occurring complication; persistent overfilling of the bladder can cause ureterovesical reflux with subsequent renal damage.

Clean self-catheterization is acceptable in the home setting. Using clean technique implies that clients do not wear gloves and do not need to use a sterile field or supplies. Clients should use a comfortable position; they may prefer to sit or stand. They need the following supplies: straight or curved-tip Tiemann (the Tiemann is most common and desired to navigate in the male urethra) catheter (12 or 14Fr.) in a clean container or plastic bag, water-soluble lubricant (K-Y or Surgilube), washcloth prepared with soap and water, receptacle for urine, and receptacle for catheter. Clients should use the following procedure:

1. Wash hands and gather equipment. (Storing all equipment in one easy-to-carry container simplifies the procedure.)
2. Assume desired position. If sitting on bed, place plastic under a towel to protect bedding.
3. Retract foreskin if present, and wash tip of penis thoroughly with soap and water.
4. Remove catheter from container and lubricate first 4 to 6 inches with lubricant; place other end over receptacle or toilet to catch urine.
5. Hold penis at right angles to the body, keeping foreskin retracted.
6. Insert catheter 7 to 10 inches into penis or until urine flows; then insert one more inch.
7. Allow catheter to drain while pressing down with abdominal muscles to promote complete emptying.
8. After drainage is complete, gently withdraw catheter.
9. Wash and dry area.
10. Wash catheter in warm soapy water, rinse with clear water, shake dry (to eliminate excess water in lumen), and dry outside with paper towel. Place in a plastic bag for storage. (Use catheters for 2 to 4 weeks; then discard.)
11. Wash hands.

Eleanor M. Stockbridge, CRRN, MS, FNP, *Community Nurse Case Manager, Poudre Valley Health System, Fort Collins, Colorado*

saw palmetto, *Serenoa repens, Echinacea,* or pollen to lessen BPH manifestations.

DIAGNOSIS, OUTCOMES, INTERVENTIONS

Ineffective Management of Therapeutic Regimen (Individuals). The nurse has a major teaching role to help the client avoid *Ineffective Management of Therapeutic Regimen related to lack of understanding of disease, manifestations, and medical treatments.*

Outcomes. The client will understand disease, manifestations, and medical treatment, as evidenced by client statements, increased fluid intake, and ability to follow medication regimen.

Interventions

Provide Teaching About BPH. Men often have only a vague understanding of what an enlarged prostate is, much less where the gland lies. Many men fear they have prostate cancer or that BPH is a precursor of prostate cancer. Beliefs about treatment affecting their sexual functioning are also a concern. Show the client and significant other a picture of the reproductive organs and prostate, and explain the effects of enlargement on urine excretion.

Encourage Fluids. Many clients limit their fluid intake to combat the manifestations of BPH. Explain that concentrated urine acts as an irritant to the bladder. Caffeine, alcohol, acidic juices, and spicy foods may also irritate the bladder and should be avoided. Clients increase their risk of UTI with limited fluid intake. Unless it is otherwise contraindicated, the client should maintain an intake of at least 2000 ml/day to prevent UTI.

Explain Medications. If medications are being used to treat BPH, men need a thorough explanation of how the medications work, their side effects, and precautions. Warn the client to increase dosage only under the physician's orders because more medication may not help manifestations and may cause serious cardiovascular problems. Encourage clients to be patient, as effects of medication on the prostate may take time. Discourage clients from taking medications that contain alpha-adrenergic agonists, such as cold medicines and diet pills, because they can cause a man with BPH to experience acute urinary retention.

Altered Urinary Elimination. The client with BPH usually experiences manifestations such as frequency, urgency, hesitancy, change in stream, incontinence, retention, and nocturia. Write the nursing diagnosis as *Altered Urinary Elimination related to increasing urethral occlusion.*

Outcomes. The client will remain free of manifestations of BPH or those manifestations will decrease with treatment, as evidenced by absence of frequency, urgency, hesitancy, change in stream, incontinence, retention, or nocturia.

Interventions

Catheterize. When the client has urinary difficulties, such as obstruction, urinary retention, or diminished renal function, some form of catheterization may be necessary. Table 38–1 shows various types of urethral catheters, and the Bridge to Home Health Care feature explains intermittent self-catheterization for men. Never force a urinary catheter. If it cannot be inserted with gentle pressure, notify a urologist, who may need special instruments to get the catheter past the obstruction. Bladder spasms are common with indwelling catheters. If bladder discomfort and leakage are significant, medications can be ordered to reduce them (see Chapter 34). Clean the meatus several times a day with water and mild soap.

Monitor Urine Output. If an indwelling catheter is placed for acute retention, observe the client for hourly urinary output (should be at least ½ ml/kg/hr), hematuria, and shock caused by postobstructive diuresis. Hematuria can occur because of the sudden release of pressure on the blood vessels supplying the bladder. Postobstructive diuresis means increased urine output caused by inability of the renal tubules to absorb water and electrolytes after prolonged urinary obstruction. It is usually self-limiting but can cause sodium depletion in some clients, which leads to vascular collapse and death if not detected and treated.

EVALUATION

The client should be able to manage the manifestations of the disease and to take the medication appropriately. Clients should also continue follow-up so that the usefulness of the medical treatment can be assessed. Surgical intervention may be needed if medical management fails.

Surgical Management

Surgery is indicated for severe obstruction, recurrent UTIs, hematuria, bladder stones, changes in the upper urinary tract, or severe discomfort and inconvenience of the client. The part of the gland causing the obstruction is removed in a procedure called a *prostatectomy*. The term prostatectomy is a misnomer because the procedure is actually removal of new tissue growth. The true prostate and fibrous capsule are not removed. Figure 38–2 illustrates various surgical approaches. The method used depends on the size of the prostate and the general health of the client.

Regrowth of prostate tissue after prostatectomy for BPH may require a second operation, but this is rare. Prostate cancer may still develop because the total prostate is not removed. These clients need the same follow-up as other men who have not had prostate surgery.

OPERATIVE TECHNIQUE

Transurethral Resection

Transurethral resection of the prostate (TURP) is the most widely used of all prostatic surgical techniques. Newer surgical procedures are also used for treating BPH, but TURP is still the "gold standard" with which they are compared. TURP is especially suitable for men who have relatively small prostatic enlargements or are poor surgical risks. No incision is made.

A resectoscope is inserted through the urethra (Fig. 38–2*A*). The surgeon is able to visualize the inside of the bladder by inserting a telescope through the resectoscope. A movable loop is inserted through the resectoscope that cuts tissue and coagulates bleeding vessels with high-frequency electric current. (A cold-punch resectoscope that punches out tissue, piece by piece, with a circular knife blade is rarely used today.)

In a new procedure, transurethral electrovaporization of the prostate (the Vapor-Trode procedure), an electrova-

Text continued on page 954

TABLE 38–1 UROLOGIC INSTRUMENTS MOST COMMONLY ENCOUNTERED IN A CLINICAL SETTING

Name	Appearance	Purpose or Use	Remarks
URINARY CATHETERS			
1. Nélaton red rubber urethral catheter	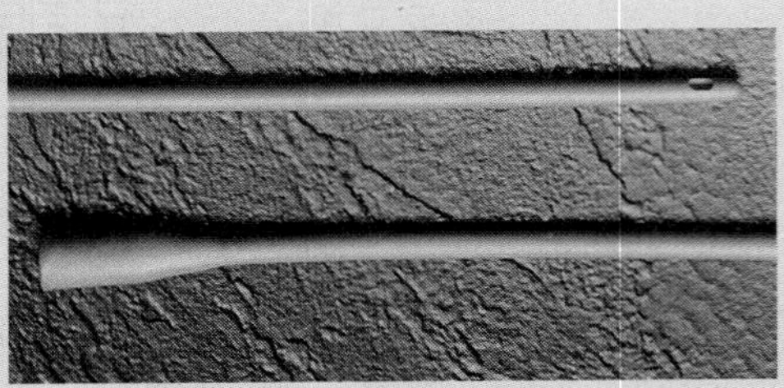	One-time, immediate drainage of the bladder; used when indwelling catheter is not needed	Blunt, round-tip straight catheter with one eye
2. Robinson red rubber urethral catheter	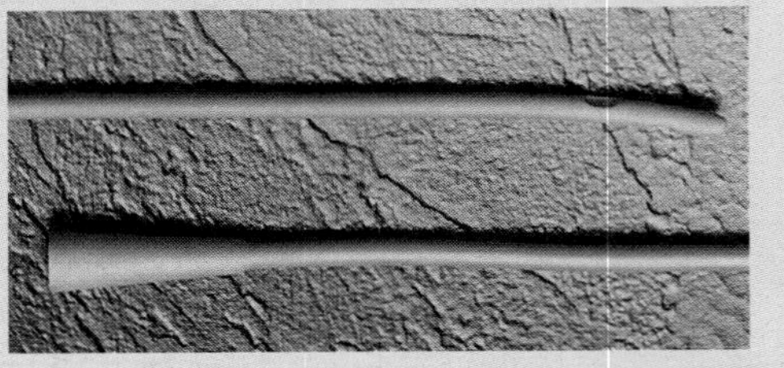	Same as No. 1	Round, hollow-tip straight catheter with two eyes
3. Councill red rubber urethral catheter (5-ml balloon)	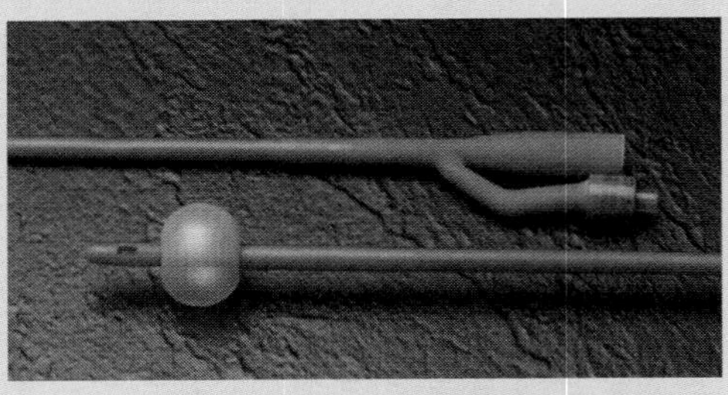	Used when passage of a filiform or guide wire is required	Hole at tip
4. Tiemann coudé red rubber urethral catheter	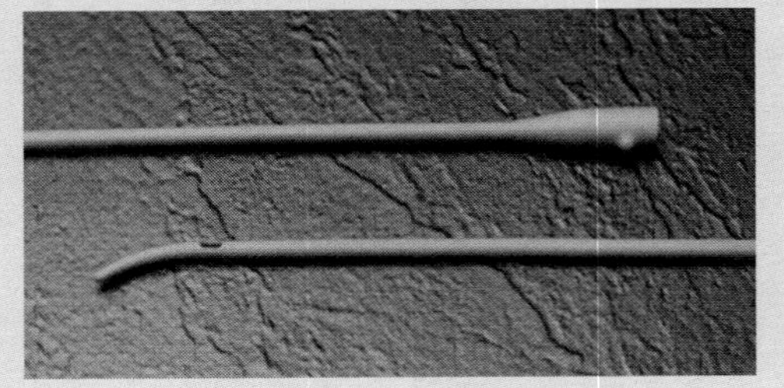	Used when a catheter must be negotiated through a urethral, prostatic, or bladder neck blockage	Curved, olive-tip catheter with two eyes

5. Indwelling Foley urethral catheter	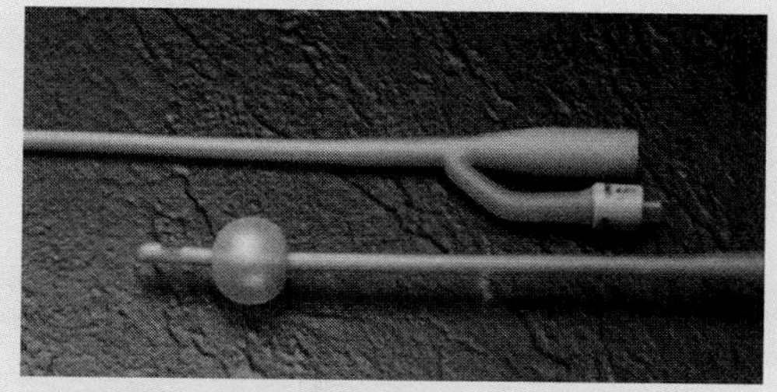	Used when a catheter must be retained in the bladder for continuous drainage	Various French sizes of catheters with 5- or 30-ml balloon
6. Three-way Foley urethral catheter	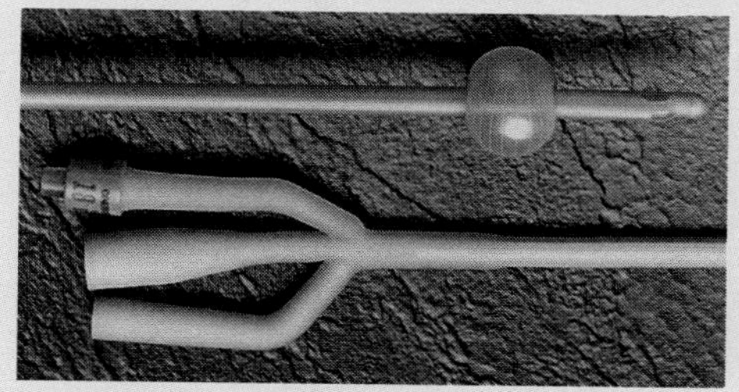	Used when irrigation of a retention catheter may be needed (e.g., after transurethral resection of the prostate)	Various French sizes of catheters with 5- or 30-ml balloon and a third port for irrigation
7. Coudé round-tip Foley urethral catheter	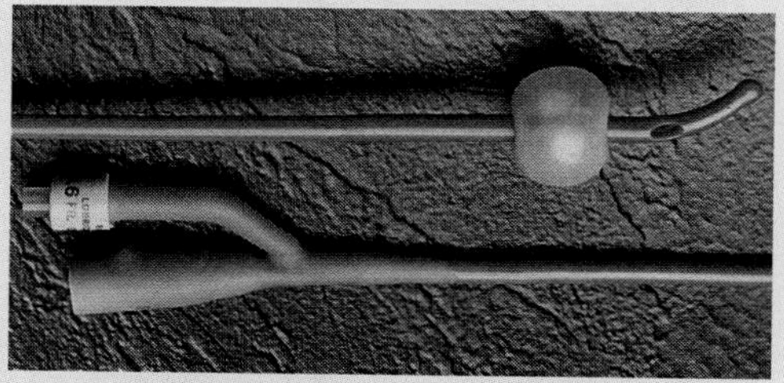	Used when retention catheter must be passed through urethral, prostatic, or bladder neck blockage	Curved tip; various French sizes of catheters with 5- or 30-ml balloon
8. Double-balloon Foley urethral catheter	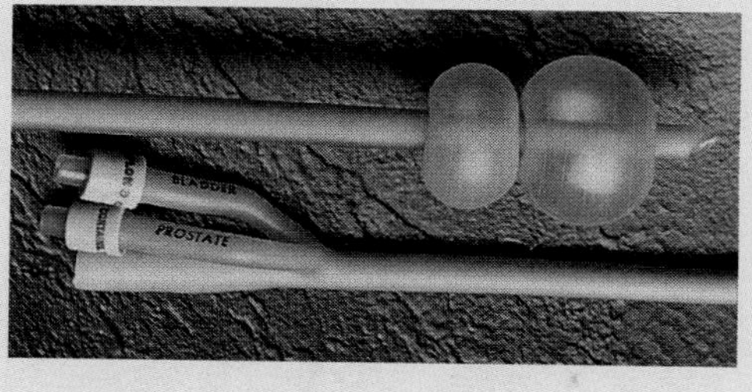	Used when bladder drainage and pressure on a resected area must be accomplished simultaneously	

Table continued on following page

TABLE 38–1 UROLOGIC INSTRUMENTS MOST COMMONLY ENCOUNTERED IN A CLINICAL SETTING *Continued*

Name	Appearance	Purpose or Use	Remarks
9. Malecot catheter		Sometimes used to drain and irrigate continent reservoirs; for temporary or continuous suprapubic drainage	Self-retaining winged catheter; design may have two or four wings; Stamey type used for suprapubic puncture
10. Otis bougie à boule		Catheter-like device used to dilate urethra; used to calibrate urethral passage	Olive tip; usually available in even sizes from 8 to 40 F
11. Walther sound. *A*, Dilator. *B*, Tapered dilator		Metal instrument used to dilate female urethra	Tapers toward handle
12. Béniqué sound		Used to dilate male urethra	Curve in tip is more pronounced than in other sounds
13. LeFort sound		Often used to dilate severe (usually trauma-induced) urethral strictures in males	Threaded tip for attachment of woven filiform

14. Catheter stylet or guide	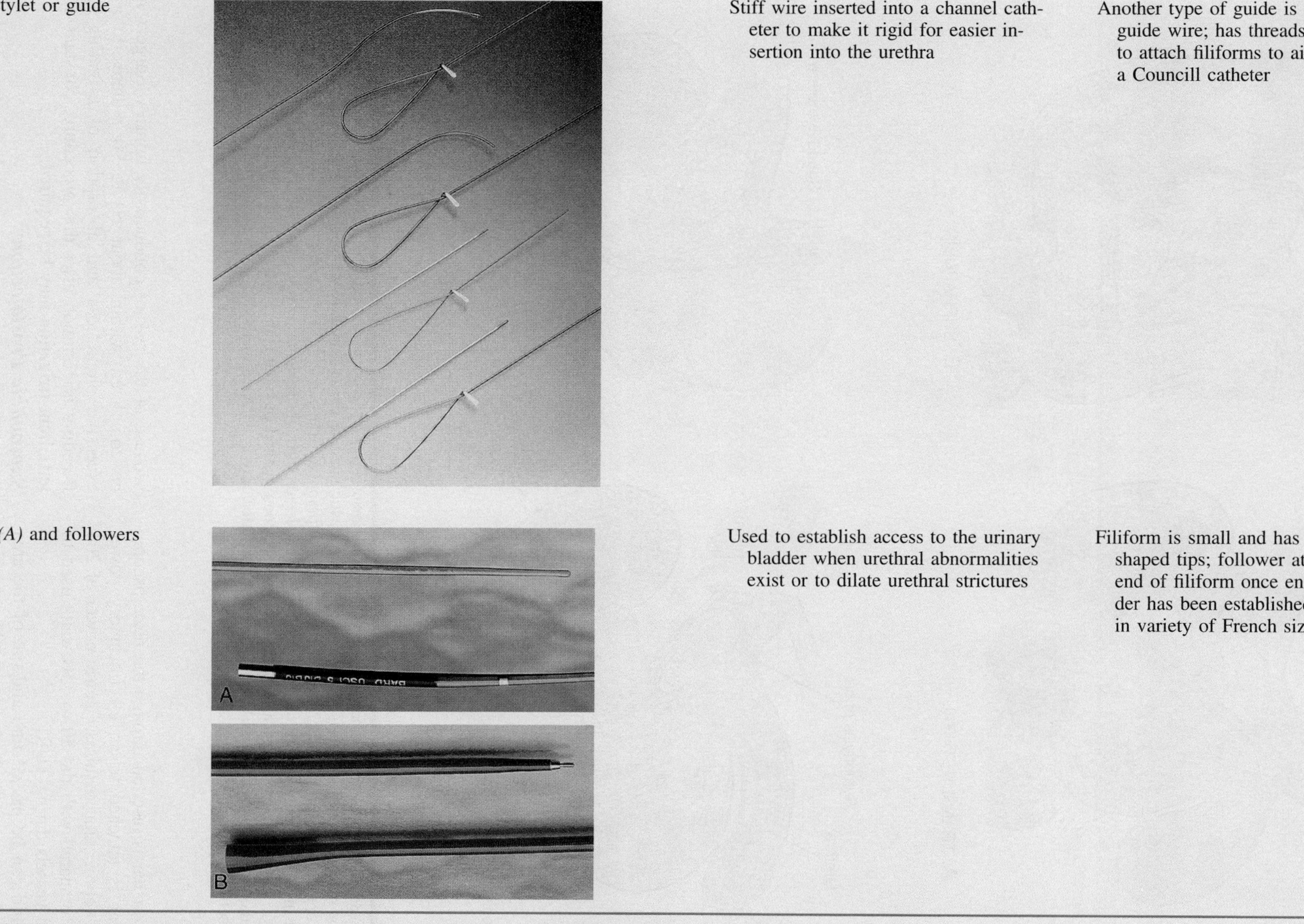	Stiff wire inserted into a channel catheter to make it rigid for easier insertion into the urethra	Another type of guide is the filiform guide wire; has threads at the end to attach filiforms to aid in inserting a Councill catheter
15. Filiforms *(A)* and followers *(B)*		Used to establish access to the urinary bladder when urethral abnormalities exist or to dilate urethral strictures	Filiform is small and has different shaped tips; follower attaches to end of filiform once entry to bladder has been established; available in variety of French sizes

From Karlowicz, K. A. (Ed.). (1995). *Urologic nursing: Principles and practice* (p. 660). Philadelphia: W. B. Saunders.

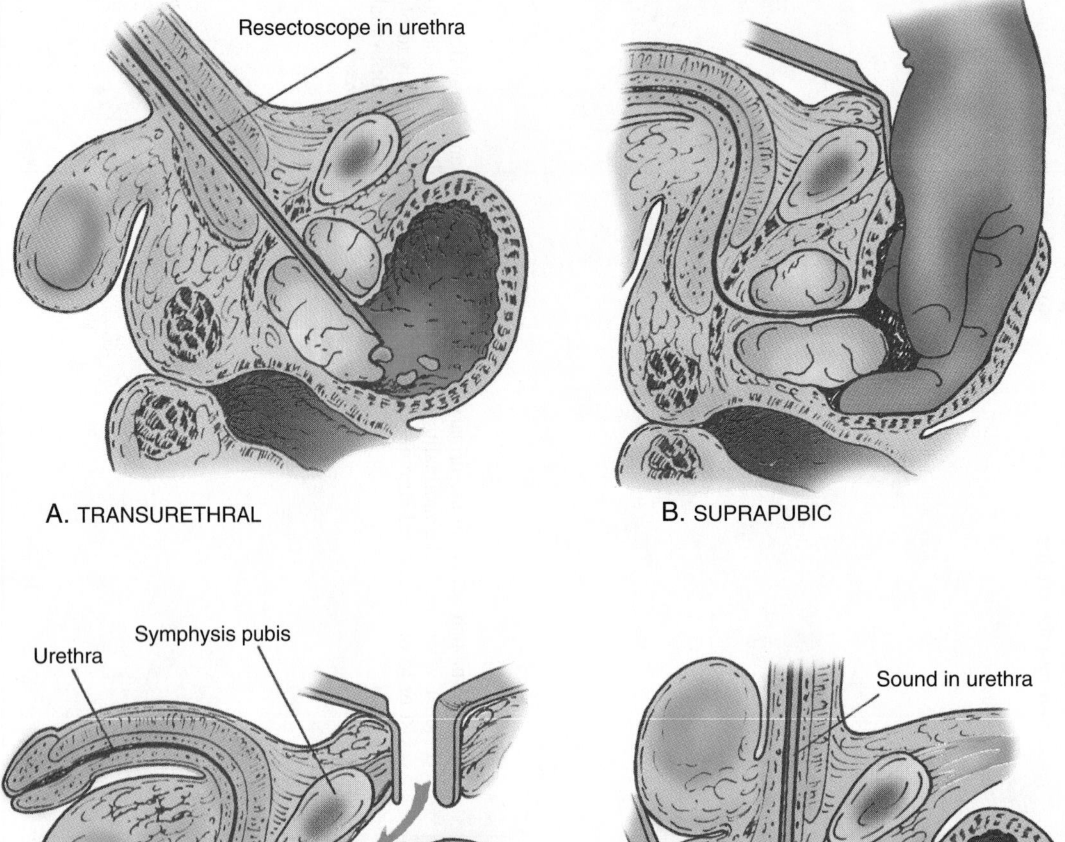

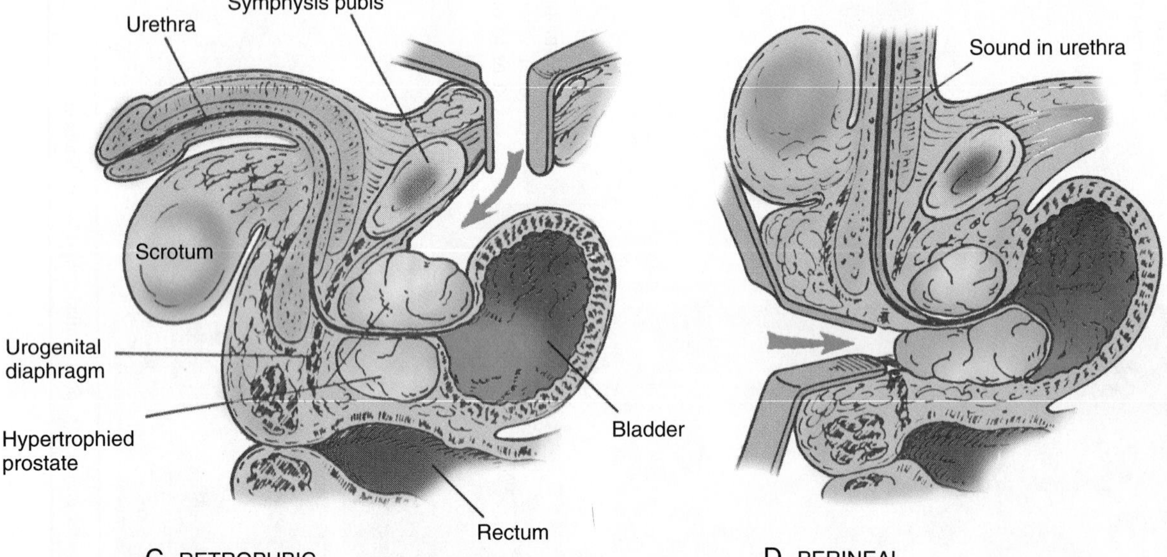

FIGURE 38–2 Surgical approaches to the prostate. *A,* Transurethral resection of the prostate (TURP) is a closed method of treatment; no incision is made, and the hyperplastic prostate tissue is removed through a resectoscope (like a cystoscope), which is inserted through the urethra. *B,* Suprapubic (transvesical) prostatectomy is an open method of treatment in which the hyperplastic prostatic tissue is enucleated through the anterior walls of the abdomen and bladder. *C,* Retropubic (extravesical) prostatectomy is an open method of treatment; a low abdominal incision is made between the pubic arch and the bladder. *D,* Perineal prostatectomy is an open method of treatment involving an incision between the anus and the scrotum.

porization ball or bar is inserted through the resectoscope. The ball or bar is attached to an electrocautery power source. Tissue vaporization requires electric power of 200 to 300 watts, compared with the 80 to 150 watts used to cauterize blood vessels during TURP.

Irrigating fluid can be passed into and out of the area through the scope; debris falls back into the bladder and is washed out. Closed-system, sterile gravity irrigation is used with an isotonic fluid solution. Water is never used because it is hypotonic, is absorbed into the bloodstream, and can precipitate hyponatremia, hypervolemia, hemolysis, and acute renal failure. Normal saline is also not used because of the risk of conductivity injuries. Surgery must be completed within about 60 to 90 minutes to avoid excessive blood loss and absorption of irrigating fluid. Bleeding is common after this procedure; constant or intermittent irrigation may be required.

Suprapubic Prostatectomy

Suprapubic prostatectomy is a surgical approach that involves a lower abdominal incision (Fig. 38–2*B*). It may be the operation of choice when (1) the prostate is too large to be resected transurethrally; (2) a large, pedunculated middle prostatic lobe or later lobes are present; (3) a bladder abnormality needs correction; or (4) an abdominal surgical exploration is necessary. An incision is made into the bladder, and the enlarged tissue is enucleated by blunt dissection. Both suprapubic and urethral catheters are inserted. Bladder abnormalities can be treated concurrently with this procedure, and complete tissue removal is facilitated; however, hemostasis can be difficult to achieve.

The client may experience more bladder spasms, urinary leakage into the abdominal wound around the suprapubic catheter, and a relatively prolonged and uncomfortable convalescence. Incontinence and *erectile dysfunction* (impotence) can occur after this procedure.

Retropubic Prostatectomy

In the retropubic prostatectomy (Fig. 38–2*C*), the surgeon approaches the prostate through a low abdominal incision without entry into the bladder. This is the operation of choice when the prostate is very large and a severe urethral stricture is present. Advantages include direct visualization of the prostate and direct hemostasis in the prostatic fossa. Disadvantages are that associated bladder problems cannot be treated and osteitis pubis (pubic bone inflammation) may occur.

Perineal Prostatectomy

An incision is made into the perineum between the anus and the scrotum (see Fig. 38–2*D*). This operation is rarely used for treating BPH because of the great potential for erectile dysfunction. The client must be in a lithotomy position, which is contraindicated for people with severe arthritis or cardiopulmonary disease. Other complications include rectourethral fistula, UTIs, epididymitis, and urinary retention.

Transurethral Incision of the Prostate

Transurethral incision of the prostate (TUIP) is an option for men with a small prostate that is causing outlet obstruction. Incisions are made into the prostatic tissue to enlarge the lumen of the prostatic urethra. This procedure is associated with relatively few postoperative complications and can be performed with local anesthesia for high-risk clients. High client satisfaction has also been reported with this procedure; many clients report no change in ejaculation, which makes this an excellent procedure for younger men with a small prostate gland.

Transurethral Balloon Dilation of the Prostate

Transurethral balloon dilation of the prostate has become a popular technique (Fig. 38–3). The concept of dilating the prostate is not new—sounds, bougies, and other dilators have been used in the past—but use of the balloon is fairly new. The procedure is actually not surgical, but it is invasive.

A small catheter is inserted into the urethra. The balloon is positioned within the prostatic urethra and is inflated for 15 minutes. This measure applies pressure to the enlarged gland, which causes the prostatic urethra to dilate. Care is taken to ensure that the balloon does not migrate downward, which can damage the sphincter, or upward into the bladder, which can negate the effect of the procedure.

The client has a urethral catheter at least overnight. There is no blood loss, and postprocedure complications are few. There are two major concerns: (1) the duration of effectiveness of the procedure and (2) the possibility that prostate cancer will be missed because no tissue is removed. Manifestations may return in as little as 3 months, but some clients have gone without manifestations for more than 3 years.

Transurethral Ultrasound-Guided Laser Incision of the Prostate

Transurethral ultrasound-guided laser incision of the prostate (TULIP) is a newer procedure in which a laser is used to make the incision into the prostate. The procedure causes minimal blood loss, no irrigation is necessary, and the client does not need a catheter after surgery. This procedure is usually done in an ambulatory or outpatient setting.

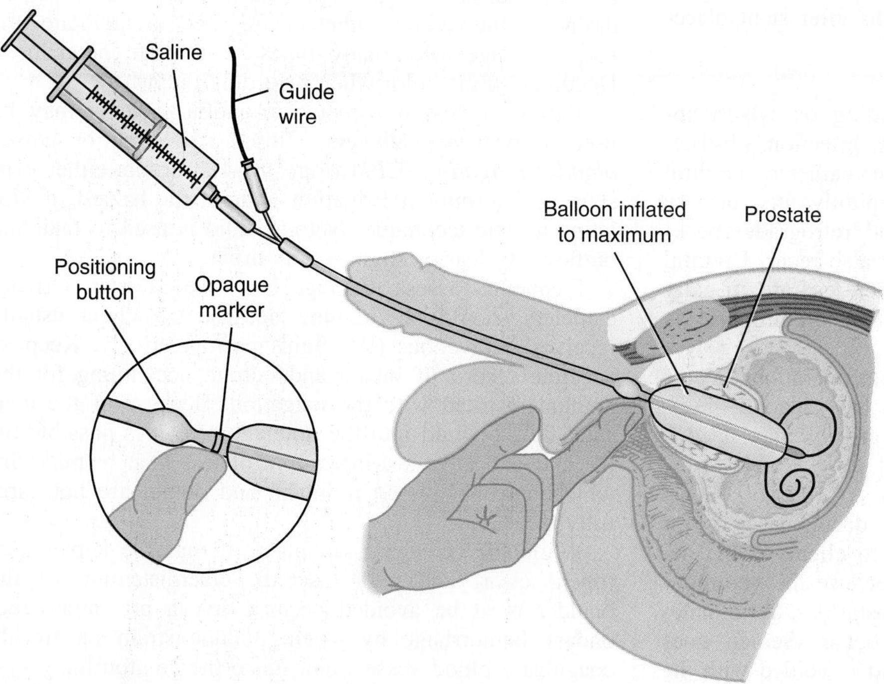

FIGURE 38–3 Balloon dilation of the prostate. (After Dowd, J. B., & Smith, J. J. [1990]. Balloon dilation of the prostate. *Urologic Clinics of North America, 17*[3], 673.)

Visual Laser Ablation of the Prostate

Visual laser ablation of the prostate (VLAP) has become more successful since the development of right-angle laser fibers. Neodymium–yttrium aluminum garnet (YAG) is the medium that produces the energy to destroy tissue through a special endoscope. Sloughing of tissue may be delayed, but blood loss is minimal. Dysuria (painful urination) and the need for longer catheterization have been noted.

Hyperthermia and Thermal Therapy

Hyperthermia and thermal therapies are new procedures. Hyperthermia refers to administration of temperatures below 45° C; thermal therapy refers to administration of higher temperatures. Microwave, radiofrequency, or high-intensity ultrasound waves are used to heat prostate tissue. Microwave hyperthermia is delivered via a rectal probe over four to 10 treatments. Each treatment lasts about 60 minutes. Transurethral thermal therapy is showing more promising short-term results, but postprocedure urinary retention and urinary discomfort are significant side effects.

The transurethral needle ablation (TUNA) system uses radiofrequency energy to destroy prostatic tissue. All of these procedures are performed without anesthesia on an outpatient basis. The ultimate efficacy of these approaches has not been determined.

Prostatic Stent

Prostatic stent insertion, another new treatment, at first was used for clients who were extremely poor operative risks. The mesh-like tube (a coil-shaped device has also been used) can be inserted through an endoscope into the prostatic urethra, where it holds the urethra open mechanically. Over time, usually about 3 to 6 months, epithelial cells grow over the stent, which is permanent in most cases. Irritative voiding problems seem to be common but subside within several months. The stents have had to be removed when they migrate, become encrusted or infected, or cause persistent perineal discomfort. To prevent complications, clients should be cautioned not to be catheterized through the stent for 3 months after stent placement.

COMPLICATIONS

Complications after treatment, depending on which approach is used, may include bleeding, infection, obstruction, accidental displacement of the catheter, urethral stricture, bladder neck contracture, epididymitis, urinary incontinence, erectile dysfunction, and retrograde (backward) ejaculation. Manifestations may also recur. Urethral strictures and bladder neck contractures are usually treated with dilation. If this is ineffective, urethroplasty is a surgical option.

Persistent incontinence after prostate operations occurs in 2% to 4% of clients. Clients who have bladder instability along with obstruction preoperatively may need a year to attain complete urinary control.

Erectile dysfunction occurs in 5% to 10% of clients and only when nerves are damaged during surgery for prostate resection. Of major concern to clients is the occurrence of retrograde ejaculation. Because the verumontanum is destroyed during most prostate surgery, antegrade (forward) ejaculation cannot occur. Semen goes into the bladder during ejaculation and is voided with the next urination. The urine is cloudy. This effect is harmless, and the ability to have an erection or experience orgasm is not affected.

OUTCOMES

It is expected that the client will achieve significant improvement in manifestations without complications. Although many of these procedures are completed in an outpatient setting, the full benefits of the procedure may not be known for several weeks or months.

Nursing Management of the Surgical Client

PREOPERATIVE CARE

Assess the client's ability to empty his bladder. The bladder should be palpated for distention. If the client cannot void, a urethral catheter may have to be placed. Clients receiving anticoagulants should have stopped taking them, as ordered, before the procedure. Careful preoperative assessment in both physical and psychosocial areas is important. Assess the client's knowledge about the surgery and its outcomes.

You may be able to lessen the client's fear and anxiety by taking a nursing history and giving appropriate explanations. Respond to the concerns of the client and significant others with empathic listening, accurate information, and ongoing support. Restating the explanations given by the surgeon and anesthetist when securing informed consent may be necessary because stressed clients frequently forget what they have been told.

Informed consent requires that the man understand the risks (e.g., possible sexual dysfunction, including erectile dysfunction; retrograde ejaculation; and infertility) and short-term and long-term benefits (e.g., relief of urinary manifestations and arrested reduction of renal function). It is important for the client to receive honest answers to questions concerning sexuality and reproduction.

POSTOPERATIVE CARE

ASSESSMENT

Immediately after surgery, your major task is postoperative observation of vital signs and maintenance of urinary drainage. Indwelling catheters are used to facilitate urinary drainage after many types of prostate procedures. Document urine color when recording output.

Various types of catheter irrigation systems may be used with these catheters. Closed irrigation, or *closed bladder irrigation* (CBI) (Fig. 38–4), permits either constant or intermittent irrigation without the hazard of violating aseptic technique. Isotonic fluid is used to maintain outflow of clear or slightly pink urine.

Frequently assess drainage from the catheter. Urinary catheters should be draining because the client usually receives intravenous (IV) fluids postoperatively. Keep an accurate record of intake and output, accounting for the amount instilled with the irrigation. Because of the constant flow of fluid into the drainage bag, it is possible for the client to have a urine output of less than ½ ml/kg/hr, which may be missed if intake and output are not carefully measured.

While the catheter is in place, it must be kept patent (open, clear, and unobstructed). Overdistention of the bladder must be avoided because it can precipitate secondary hemorrhage by placing undue strain on freshly coagulated blood vessels and make the genitourinary sys-

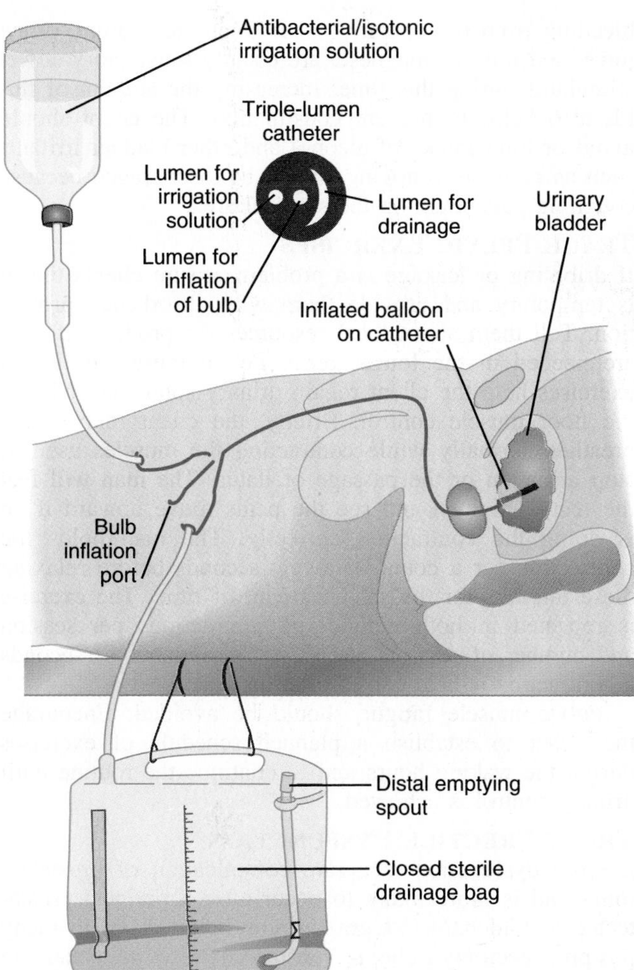

FIGURE 38–4 A closed bladder irrigation system.

tem more prone to infection. Proper positioning of the catheter and drainage system is important to maintain good drainage and prevent obstruction of the system. Blood clots, prostatic debris, mucus plugs, kinked tubing, or catheter displacement may obstruct urinary flow. Assess catheter patency frequently to make sure the catheter is draining.

DIAGNOSIS, OUTCOMES, INTERVENTIONS

Risk for Injury. A common problem after all procedures is *Risk for Injury related to presence of urinary catheters, hematuria, irrigation, or suprapubic drains.*

Outcomes. The client will not experience hemorrhage, as evidenced by absence of gross bleeding, infection, catheter obstruction, and water intoxication and maintenance of urine output of at least ½ ml/kg per hour.

Interventions

Maintain Irrigation. Closed bladder irrigation decreases the development of obstruction. If obstruction is suspected, manual (hand) irrigation may be necessary. After prostatectomy for BPH, at least 60 ml of irrigant must be used, with some force, to dislodge and evacuate blood clots and other debris. If there is resistance to the introduction of irrigating fluid into the catheter or if there is no return of irrigating fluid, *do not force the fluid.* Notify the surgeon immediately. If a catheter cannot be cleared, it may have to be removed and a new one inserted. In such cases, the surgeon usually performs this procedure.

Catheters and the procedures themselves cause increased urethral mucus production. Practice good meatal care. Keep the penis and meatal area clean by washing them with soap and water at least twice a day. Antibacterial ointments were formerly used, but they are no more effective than cleansing. Antibacterial soaps or antiseptics may dry out skin.

Monitor for Bleeding. Some hematuria is usual for several days after surgery. However, frank bleeding, arterial or venous, may occur during the first day after surgery. Arterial blood is bright red, has numerous clots, and is viscous. Blood pressure may fall, and emergency surgical intervention may become necessary. Venous bleeding in the prostatic area may be controlled by increasing the pressure (adding fluid) in the balloon end of the urethral catheter, pulling the catheter tightly to move the balloon into the prostatic fossa, and taping or using a Velcro device (self-fastening tape) to secure the catheter to the thigh (called *applying traction*). Traction is left in place for 24 hours or more and is released by the physician when the bleeding has stopped. The surgeon can also remove fluid slowly from the balloon as the bleeding decreases.

Prevent Catheter Dislodgment. The client may be confused immediately after surgery or may forget he has a catheter and accidentally pull out the catheter. Show him how to get in and out of the bed or chair without pulling on the catheter. Remind the client that he has a tube in his bladder through his penis or abdomen (whichever it is), and instruct him not to touch it. A displaced or removed urinary catheter after prostatic surgery is painful and disrupts recovery. Securing the catheter with a wide catheter holder, tape, or stockinette may be necessary. If the client does pull the catheter out, notify the surgeon immediately.

Prevent Infection. Observe the client carefully for local or systemic indications of infection. Handle catheters, drainage apparatus, and urine collection carefully to avoid introducing microorganisms into the urinary tract. Maintain a closed urinary drainage system unless manual irrigation is absolutely required. Encourage increased fluid intake, ambulation, and deep-breathing exercises.

Wound drains are usually removed earlier than suprapubic catheters. Keep skin around drain and catheter sites clean, dry, and protected. Observe for redness, edema, or infection.

The suprapubic catheter is left in place until voiding function has returned. When the client is voiding well, the suprapubic catheter can be removed. Expect urinary leakage from the suprapubic catheter site, mostly on the day the catheter is removed, until the wound is completely healed. Frequent dressing changes are necessary at first. If a suprapubic catheter is removed before the client has returned to normal voiding, the wound may not heal properly, leading to fistula formation.

Monitor for Retention. The length of time urethral catheters are left in place varies according to the surgeon's preference, the client's recovery, and the type of surgery. After a urethral catheter is removed (and after a transurethral resection), monitor the client closely for manifestations of urinary retention or difficulty.

Manage Temporary Incontinence. Advise the client that irritative manifestations such as frequency, urgency, leakage, and dysuria are natural until complete healing occurs. Keep reminding him that these problems are temporary and may take some time to resolve. Be understanding of the man's feelings, and keep him dry without embarrassing him. Absorbency products may be needed temporarily. They vary in size, shape, and absorbency capacities. Pelvic muscle exercises may help to reduce this problem. Additional surgery is sometimes required for persistent incontinence.

Pain. A common nursing diagnosis is *Pain related to surgery and bladder spasms.*

Outcomes. The client's pain will be under control, as evidenced by the client's report.

Interventions. Pain control after surgery is discussed in Chapters 15 and 23. Bladder spasms frequently occur after prostate procedures. Be sure that the drainage system is not obstructed, because obstruction as well as bladder irritation causes bladder spasms. Antispasmodic medications, such as belladonna and opium suppositories, propantheline bromide (Pro-Banthine) or oxybutynin (Ditropan), may be prescribed. They may cause complications, however. Clients with severe cardiac disease or glaucoma should not receive these agents. Since antispasmodic drugs can cause constipation and straining at stool can precipitate bleeding from the operative site, stool softeners such as docusate sodium (Colace) are often given.

EVALUATION

It is expected that the client will be discharged without complications and resume regular activities within 4 to 6 weeks. Depending on the procedure performed, some clients return home the same day. The client who has undergone TURP is usually discharged about 2 to 3 days after the operation. Clients who had open procedures are discharged after 4 to 6 days. Voiding of urine improves, and complications such as urgency, frequency, and dribbling end within 3 months.

Self-Care

PROVIDE TEACHING

In addition to teaching the client verbally, give him written materials to take home after discharge. If applicable, review catheter and wound management. Clients who go home with a catheter have leg bags for day use and a Foley bag for use at night.

Some activities are limited after prostatectomy. The surgeon's orders should be followed regarding heavy lifting, strenuous activity, prolonged sitting, sexual activity, and driving or riding in an automobile. Because prolonged sitting increases intra-abdominal pressure and may precipitate bleeding, the man should avoid sitting except during meals. Clients should avoid driving an automobile or taking prolonged automobile rides until at least 2 weeks after surgery, when the risk of bleeding lessens. Strenuous exercise is also contraindicated for 4 to 6 weeks.

PREVENT INJURY

Advise the client not to strain during defecation for at least 6 weeks after surgery, because this can lead to bleeding from the operative site. Docusate sodium, prune juice, and milk of magnesia are usually satisfactory bowel stimulants during this time. Increasing the amount of fluids also helps to prevent constipation. The client should avoid or limit intake of alcohol and other bladder irritants such as caffeine. Smoking should be discouraged because coughing puts strain on the surgical area.

TEACH PELVIC EXERCISES

If dribbling or leakage is a problem, assure clients that it is temporary and provide them with absorbency protection. Tell them about local resources for products if they are needed in the longer term. Pelvic muscle or Kegel exercises help the client regain urinary sphincter and pelvic floor muscle control. Briefly, the client relaxes and breathes normally while contracting the muscles used to stop urination or the passage of flatus. The man will feel the rectum tighten and see the penis move upward if he is doing the contraction correctly. The man holds the contraction for a count of a few seconds before relaxing these muscles for the same amount of time. The exercise is repeated in both number of contractions per session and number of sessions per day. The number of seconds a contraction is held can also be increased.

Pelvic muscle fatigue should be avoided. Encourage the client to establish a planned schedule of exercises during the waking hours and to continue the routine until urinary control is achieved.

TREAT ERECTILE DYSFUNCTION

Erectile dysfunction is a rare complication of prostatectomy and is more likely to occur after a perineal prostatectomy. Sildenafil (Viagra) is now being given to many postprostatectomy clients postoperatively to maintain blood flow to the corpora cavernosa during the recovery period. As a result, fewer men are experiencing erectile dysfunction.

Information and supportive care of the significant other are extremely important. Referral for sexual counseling may be helpful. The man needs to know that he can still please a partner and that lovemaking techniques other than intercourse may be necessary. The couple may need information about alternatives to intercourse, such as cuddling, stroking, or manual or oral stimulation to orgasm. Vacuum erection devices, intracorporeal injections, and intraurethral or oral medications are also topics that sexual counselors can discuss. A penile implant may be considered (see Erectile Dysfunction later).

ARRANGE FOLLOW-UP

Be sure the client knows when and where to reach the surgeon and how to get in touch with health care professionals if he has concerns. He should especially report any elevated temperature, unusual bleeding, signs of wound infection or UTI, and obstructed urinary flow. He should know the date and time of his follow-up appointment with the surgeon.

PROSTATE CANCER

Prostate cancer is the most common cancer among men and the second most common cause of cancer death among men in the United States. The American Cancer Society has estimated that 180,400 new cases of prostate cancer would be diagnosed in the United States in the year 2000.[1] The risk for development of prostate cancer increases with age, and the disease typically occurs in men at age 50 years and older. Younger men tend to have more aggressive disease. African American men have a higher rate of prostate cancer. The diagnosis of prostate cancer is more common today because of the development of better screening tools.

Etiology and Risk Factors

The cause of prostate cancer is unknown, but epidemiologic studies suggest several associated factors. BPH does not lead to the development of prostate cancer.

Men with a family history of prostate cancer are at greater risk. Research has identified a gene on the X chromosome that appears more often in men with prostate cancer who have strong family histories. The gene, called human prostate cancer on the X chromosome (*HPCX*), is in the early stages of investigation.

Because the risk of prostate cancer increases with age, it may be associated with the hormonal shifts that accompany aging. It is rarely found in men younger than 40 years of age. Occult prostate cancer has been demonstrated at autopsy in 95% of men older than 90 years who died of other causes.

Diet may also be a factor. Asians have a lower rate of prostate cancer, but the rate is increased in those who move to the United States. High fat consumption (typical of American diets) can alter cholesterol and steroid metabolism, which may increase the risk of cancer. Green and yellow vegetables (typical of Japanese diets) and lycopene in cooked tomatoes may have a protective effect against prostate cancer. Some studies have postulated that a vitamin D deficiency may play a role. People who received more sunlight exposure had a lower incidence of and lower death rate from prostate cancer.

Occupational and environmental exposure to carcinogens may be risk factors. A higher incidence of prostate cancer is found in men living in urban areas. Occupations linked to higher rates of prostate cancer include employment in fertilizer, textile, and rubber industries and work with batteries containing cadmium.

Sexually transmitted virus-like organisms have been found in prostate cancer tissue, suggesting that viruses may be associated with the disease. High levels of testosterone have also been linked to development of prostate cancer.

Questions have arisen regarding a relationship between vasectomy and the development of prostate cancer, although the National Institutes of Health (NIH) has concluded that a relationship could not be proved. The NIH recommended further study but suggested no change in practice for providing vasectomies. The NIH also recommended that prostate cancer screening be the same for men who have and have not had vasectomies.

It is hoped that late prostatic cancer will become rare as increasing emphasis is placed on early diagnosis through routine rectal examinations, rectal ultrasound studies, measurements of PSA, and prompt intervention.

Except for diet, not much has been discovered in relation to prevention of prostate cancer. Reducing saturated fats and increasing the intake of lycopene (found in tomatoes) seem to reduce the incidence of the disease. Other dietary ingredients being investigated are genistin and diadzien (found in soy products), selenium, and vitamin E.

Health maintenance activities include annual digital rectal examinations and determination of serum PSA levels for early detection. Health restoration includes teaching pelvic muscle exercises to improve return of urinary control in postoperative clients and sexual counseling after radical perineal prostatectomy.

Pathophysiology

Prostate tumors are usually adenocarcinomas that begin in the periphery of the posterior lobe of the gland, whereas BPH occurs centrally and the gland is large by the time it restricts urination. The tumor may appear as normal prostatic tissue, which delays diagnosis. Typically, such lesions grow slowly and remain confined to the prostatic capsule, and if they occur late in life, the client may die of other causes. Sometimes, however, the tumor grows rapidly and metastasis has occurred by the time a diagnosis is made.

When prostate cancer metastasizes (spreads), it does so mainly through direct extension to the bladder neck and seminal vesicles. Other spread occurs through lymphatic and hematogenous routes. Obturator and iliac nodes are commonly positive. With advanced disease, metastasis to the bone is common, as is spread to the lungs and liver.

Clinical Manifestations

Men with prostate cancer commonly have no manifestations. Manifestations are usually related to other prostate conditions such as BPH and prostatitis. Early diagnosis through PSA measurement and digital rectal examination is essential. These tests are recommended for men between 50 and 70 years of age and younger men if they are African American or have a family history of the disease. The benefit of PSA screening after a man is 70 years old with a life expectancy of less than 10 years is questionable.

PSA, a glycoprotein produced by the prostate gland, may be elevated in men with prostate conditions. The detection rate of PSA screening for prostate cancer is about 55%. Normal PSA levels are below 4.0 ng/ml, but some variation is allowed for age and other conditions. A PSA level below 4.0 ng/ml is of concern if there is a rapid rise (i.e., 2.0 to 3.5). A hard nodule, asymmetry, or induration felt on digital rectal examination raises the suspicion of malignancy.

Other specialized tests that may be performed when PSA levels and digital rectal examination findings are normal but prostate cancer is suspected measure *prostate-specific antigen density* (PSAD) and *free PSA*. These tests seem to be more useful as part of the screening process when the PSA value is moderately elevated (4 to 10 ng/ml).

- The PSAD is calculated by dividing the PSA by the prostatic volume, as determined on ultrasonography. Men with PSAD scores above 0.15 are more likely to have cancer than men with lower PSAD scores.
- Free PSA is PSA that is not bound to proteins in the blood. Prostate cancer cells secrete more bound PSA than normal or noncancerous cells. Therefore, a lower ratio of free PSA to total PSA suggests prostate cancer and the need for further tests.

If the PSA is elevated or an abnormal prostate is felt, or both, the client undergoes a transrectal prostate biopsy with ultrasound imaging. The client must not take aspirin-containing medications or anticoagulants for several days before prostate biopsy in order to prevent bleeding at the biopsy sites. Premedication with diazepam or similar medications should be offered.

A probe is inserted into the rectum so that the prostate can be visualized and measured. Small cores of tissue are taken from different areas of the prostate for pathologic examination. Ultrasound visualization cannot confirm the presence or absence of cancer; it helps guide the needle to selected areas. The client and physician wait for the pathology report. Complications include bleeding, infection, and a missed cancer. Biopsies are also performed by a transperineal approach in some institutions.

Prostate cancer is graded according to the differentiation of tumor cells. Differentiation is directly related to the cancer's aggressiveness. *Well-differentiated* cancer cells differ only slightly from normal cells and tend to grow slowly. *Poorly differentiated* cancer is characterized by very abnormal, disorganized cells that tend to grow more rapidly. A Gleason score on a scale of 1 to 5 is given to the tissues examined on the basis of primary and secondary tumor patterns. The Gleason score is the sum of two grades assigned to the different areas:

- Well differentiated, a score of 2 to 4
- Moderately well differentiated, a score of 5 to 7
- Poorly differentiated, a score of 8 to 10

A premalignant condition that may appear on a prostate pathology report is *prostatic intraepithelial neoplasia* (PIN). Close surveillance is necessary and may include repeated prostate biopsies throughout the gland.

If prostate cancer is found, additional tests are ordered to stage the cancer and to determine how far it has spread. Staging is done through bone scans, computed tomography (CT), or magnetic resonance imaging (MRI). Two main classification systems are used to stage prostate cancer: the Whitmore-Jewett A-B-C-D system and the tumor, nodes, and metastasis (TNM) system. These classifications are outlined in Box 38–1.

BOX 38–1 Staging and Grading of Prostate Tumors

Stage A: Tumor Microscopic (T1 N0 M0)

A1: Microscopic focus

A2: Diffuse

Stage B: Tumor Macroscopic (T1–2 N0 M0)

B1: One lobe involved, nodule ≤ 1.5 cm

B2: Both lobes involved, nodule ≥ 1.5 cm

Stage C: Tumor Extracapsular (T3 N0 M0)

C1: Localized, nodule ≤ 70 g

C2: Pelvic sidewall fixation, nodule ≥ 70 g

Stage D: Metastatic Disease (T4, N1–3, M)

D1: Confined to pelvis

D2: Extrapelvic

A specific imaging scan can be used to locate metastases of prostate cancer in soft tissue. Capromab pendetide (ProstaScint) targets prostate-specific membrane antigen (PSMA), which is found in prostate cancer cells. Two sessions 4 days apart are required. The ProstaScint scan is especially useful in finding "skipped" metastases (i.e., abdominal lymph node involvement without pelvic lymph node involvement), but it is expensive.

Outcome Management

Nursing Management of Clients Undergoing Diagnosis

Provide Support

Men with prostate cancer and their significant others need ongoing sensitive support and accurate information to make the difficult decisions required of them. Their concerns are considerable and may include the choices of available treatments, fear of death, anxiety about residual disability and illness, feelings of loss of control, and the possible effects of the illness on people in their social network and in their marriage. After diagnosis, prostate cancer can affect their masculinity and self-esteem. Depression and fatigue are common after many treatments for prostate cancer.

Suggest Resources

Increased awareness of prostate cancer has led to the development of many resources, including books, articles, and Internet Web sites in the public sector. Local and national prostate cancer support groups have organized. Information is also available from the American Cancer Society (Man to Man program), the American Foundation for Urologic Disease in Baltimore (800-242-2383), and US TOO International in Hinsdale, Ill. (800-808-7866).

Be sure to include the client's partner or spouse in planning care at the time of diagnosis and when the client is choosing treatment as well as when he is adapting to the treatment. The partner usually takes on essential support responsibilities when the client is gathering information and coping with the disease and treatments.

Surgical Management

Radical Prostatectomy

Radical prostatectomy is the treatment of choice for cancer confined within the prostate if the client is in good enough health to undergo surgery and has a life expectancy of 10 to 15 years. Radical surgery involves removing the entire prostate gland (rather than just enucleation), the outer capsule, the seminal vesicles, sections of the vas deferens, adjacent lymph nodes, and portions of the bladder neck. Bilateral prostatic lymph node dissection (BPLND) is not done as much today in health care institutions, especially when PSA values and Gleason scores are low. Laparoscopic lymph node dissection is performed when required.

Surgical approaches include retropubic (see Fig. 38–2*C*) and perineal (see Fig. 38–2*D*) approaches. Radical retropubic surgery is the procedure most commonly performed. Today techniques are used to preserve the neurovascular bundles, which reduces the consequences of permanent erectile dysfunction or incontinence. Bladder neck contracture occurs in about 5% of clients.

In some institutions, radical perineal prostatectomy is an alternative approach. The rates of seminal vesicle and rectal injury are higher, but the incidence of incontinence and erectile dysfunction is about the same when surgeons are experienced with the two techniques. After this procedure, less blood is lost during surgery and less postoperative pain occurs.

CRYOSURGICAL ABLATION

In cryosurgical ablation of the prostate, the surgeon uses guided transrectal ultrasonography to insert cryoprobes into desired areas of the prostate to freeze and thereby destroy the tissue. A warming tube in the urethra keeps the urethra from freezing. Cryosurgery may be an option for clients with localized cancer and other serious medical conditions that preclude them as candidates for radical surgery. Although the technique is less invasive and causes less pain and bleeding than radical surgery, it is considered investigational.

Nursing Management of the Surgical Client

PREVENT INJURY

The physical nursing care for the client with prostatic cancer is essentially the same as that for clients undergoing other major surgery (see Chapter 15) and similar to that for the client undergoing surgery for BPH. A few special exceptions are observed:

1. The catheter stays in at least 2 to 3 weeks after the surgery while the anastomosis of bladder and urethra heals.
2. Securing the catheter to prevent accidental removal is imperative.
3. Enemas and rectal thermometers are avoided in most hospitals and used with extreme caution in others.

A midline lower incision is closed with staples and drains are in place when a retropubic approach is used. Regularly observe drainage, and change or reinforce dressings as ordered. If a perineal approach is used, aseptic technique is especially important because of the high possibility of infection in a wound close to the anal area. Sitz baths or heat lamps may be ordered to facilitate perineal wound healing. A double-tailed T binder, mesh pants, or scrotal support may be used to secure perineal dressings.

PROVIDE SUPPORT

The psychosocial and emotional care of these clients differs from care of clients with BPH because issues such as cancer and sexual image must be addressed. Thoughts of postoperative self-care at home are overwhelming. Both the client and significant other need detailed instructions, much reassurance, and resources for supplies and advice should concerns surface at home. Sildenafil (Viagra) is given to many clients after prostatectomy to maintain blood flow to the corpora cavernosa during recovery. As a result, fewer men are experiencing erectile dysfunction.

Medical Management

Medical management of prostate cancer is approached in several ways: radiation, hormonal manipulation, watchful waiting, and, sometimes, chemotherapy. One of these approaches is always chosen for cancer that has spread outside the prostate. Controversy exists regarding the most effective management of prostate cancer.

Watchful waiting is a reasonable choice only when a client has a very low-grade, low-stage prostate cancer. Many physicians add the criterion that life expectancy should be less than 10 years. Mortality in older clients is often due to other causes. Routine follow-up and PSA determinations are very important. If there are changes in the digital rectal examination or PSA elevation, treatment should be initiated.

DECREASE TUMOR GROWTH

RADIATION THERAPY. Radiation therapy is an alternative choice for cancer confined to the prostate. Treatment can be in the form of external beam radiation, interstitial seed implantation, or a combination of both methods. Radiation therapy can be used to reduce bone pain when prostate cancer has metastasized. Strontium 89 (Metastron) and samarium 153 lexidronam (Quadramet) are radioactive agents that are injected to help control pain related to bone metastases. Men usually begin to notice a reduction in pain 10 to 20 days after the injection. Pain reduction lasts for 4 to 15 months but usually only about 6 months. If pain returns, the injection can be repeated every 3 months with no limit on the number of injections given.

External beam radiation is administered to the prostate and surrounding tissue daily for several weeks (see Chapter 19).

In the technique of interstitial seed implantation (*brachytherapy*), special needles are used to insert radioactive isotopes directly into the prostate. Because the radioactive focus of the seeds is more controlled than in external beam radiation, surrounding tissues are usually not as affected. Radioactive palladium, iodine, or gold seeds are used for this procedure. The long half-life of these seeds allows delivery of an effective radiation dose for 1 year. Temporary irritative and obstructive voiding manifestations are common after implantation.

HORMONAL THERAPY. Hormonal manipulation blocks androgen (testosterone) production and includes a selection or combination of bilateral orchiectomy, estrogens, gonadotropin-releasing hormone analogs, and antiandrogens. The greatest amount of androgen is produced in the testicles, and small amounts are produced in the adrenal glands.

Orchiectomy (removal of testicles) is a minor surgical procedure that removes the source of androgen. Local anesthesia is usually used. Because the procedure is irreversible, the psychological impact on a man is great. Most men want medications to control their prostate cancer.

Estrogen. Estrogen (diethylstilbestrol) suppresses the release of pituitary gonadotropin and reduces serum testosterone levels. Side effects can be serious and include edema, myocardial infarction, cerebrovascular accident, hypertension, thrombophlebitis, and pulmonary embolism. Gynecomastia and abdominal discomfort are other side effects.

Gonadotropin-Releasing Hormone (GnRH) Analogs. GnRH analogs, commonly called luteinizing hormone–releasing hormone (LHRH) agonists, stimulate and then suppress pituitary gonadotropins, which interferes with androgen production in the testicles. Leuprolide (Lupron) and goserelin acetate (Zoladex) are injected every 1 to 4 months, depending on the time-released dosage. Hot flashes, erectile dysfunction, loss of libido, and minor weight gain caused by water retention are common side effects. The client with metastasis and bone pain may experience an initial increase in pain or voiding manifestations.

Antiandrogens. Antiandrogens such as flutamide (Eulexin) and bicalutamide (Casodex) block androgens produced by the adrenal glands. These medications are often combined with LHRH therapy. Gynecomastia, diarrhea, and erectile dysfunction are common side effects. Finasteride is also used.

Intermittent Hormonal Therapy. Use of intermittent hormonal therapy is a newer concept for control of disease and prevention of hormonal side effects or resistance to hormonal treatment. It is being investigated as a safe alternative to continuous hormonal therapy for prostate cancer.

CHEMOTHERAPY. Chemotherapy is used for palliation (alleviation of manifestations) when prostate cancer is hormone-resistant. Chemotherapeutic agents may be given singly or in combination, depending on protocols. Examples of agents sometimes used are cyclophosphamide (Cytoxan), fluorouracil, estramustine phosphate (Emcyt), doxorubicin (Adriamycin), and mitomycin (Mutamycin), taxol, and VP-16 or etoposide (Etopophos). Mitoxantrone (Novantrone) is a chemotherapeutic drug used in combination with corticosteroids to relieve pain in hormone-resistant prostate cancer. This treatment is often successful after just one dose.

Nursing Management of the Medical Client

PROVIDE EDUCATION

Nursing care depends on the type of medical therapy. Explain how treatments help prostate cancer, their side effects, and expected outcomes. Repetitive explanations are often necessary because clients must absorb much information and make decisions during a period when they may be in a state of shock. Provide information in a variety of formats, and include telephone numbers to be called when the client or partner has questions.

EXPLAIN SIDE EFFECTS

Common side effects of external beam radiation to the pelvic area include irritable voiding problems, diarrhea, and dermatitis. If a client is undergoing brachytherapy, specific safety precautions should be followed. These entail how close family members can be to the client for the first week after therapy and how to retrieve and return expelled seeds.

Clients receiving hormonal manipulation therapy must comply with medication directions in order to maintain therapeutic blood levels. Clients need a great deal of support to help them cope with erectile dysfunction and hot flashes. With all approaches used for hormonal manipulation, the importance of follow-up cannot be overstressed.

PROVIDE SUPPORT

Encourage men with prostate cancer and their significant others to attend relevant support groups or to subscribe to publications by organizations mentioned earlier. The best ways for clients to control fear and to keep a positive attitude are to learn as much as they can about treatments and to meet other men with prostate cancer. A health care provider who specializes in erectile dysfunction can best counsel a couple about ways to achieve sexual satisfaction.

RELIEVE PAIN

When a client has metastases, assess pain levels (see Chapter 23) as well as activities of daily living. Keeping a pain diary is useful for the client's and provider's awareness. Men tend to be stoic about pain and may have misconceptions about taking narcotics. Carefully explain that addiction and decreasing drug effectiveness are not problems when cancer pain is being treated. Better pain control helps a man stay active and in control of his life.

PROSTATITIS

Prostatitis (inflammation of the prostate gland) is a common and often perplexing problem. As many as 50% of men experience manifestations of prostatitis in their lifetime. Traditionally, prostatitis is categorized as acute bacterial prostatitis, chronic bacterial prostatitis, nonbacterial prostatitis, or prostatodynia (painful prostate without a cause). Nonbacterial prostatitis is the most common form of the disease.

Etiology and Risk Factors

Gram-negative bacteria such as *Escherichia coli*, *Klebsiella,* and *Enterobacter* are the usual cause of acute and chronic prostate infections. *Enterococcus*, a gram-positive organism, can also cause chronic prostate infection. Other organisms, such as *Chlamydia, Ureaplasma,* gonococci, and cytomegalovirus, are less common causes. It has also been proposed that nonbacterial prostatitis is an autoimmune disease.

Factors predisposing to chronic prostatitis are those that cause prostatic congestion, such as perineal trauma, excess alcohol intake, and certain sexual practices. Inadequately treated acute prostatitis may also predispose to chronic prostatitis. Muscle spasms in the prostate and bladder neck are believed to be the cause of prostatodynia, which occurs more frequently in younger and middle-aged men.

Pathophysiology

Routes of infection (Fig. 38–5) include urethral ascent, descent from the urinary bladder or kidneys, direct extension or lymphatogenous spread from the rectum, and hematogenous spread.

Marked inflammation occurs in acute prostatitis. Small abscesses or spread to the periprostatic space can occur if the condition is untreated. Repeated bouts of acute prostatitis may cause fibrosis within the gland and can be confused with prostate cancer on digital rectal examination. Small calculi (stones) commonly form in the prostate after chronic infections and are rarely significant.

Clinical Manifestations

The client's manifestations depend on the type of prostatitis he has. The client with acute bacterial prostatitis presents with abrupt onset of urinary urgency, frequency,

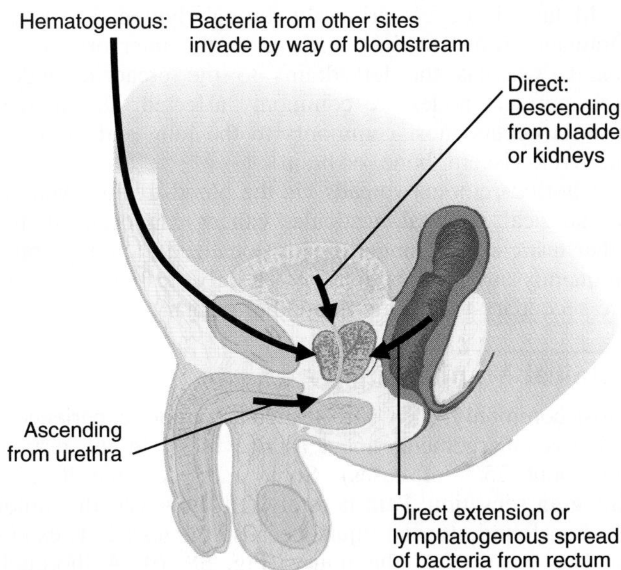

FIGURE 38–5 Postulated pathways of infection to the prostate gland.

nocturia, and dysuria, and he may have urinary retention. Fever, chills, and malaise are present, and the client complains of low back and perineal pain. He appears quite ill and may be experiencing nausea and vomiting. The prostate is extremely tender and boggy when examined. Prostate massage (expression of prostate secretions via digital rectal examination) is usually not performed because it is painful to the client and can precipitate bacteremia. Urine is usually infected.

Manifestations may or may not be present in chronic bacterial prostatitis. Episodes of urinary infection may occur intermittently. Asymptomatic bacteriuria may be an incidental finding in some clients. Usually, voiding problems and pain are mild to moderate and rectal examination is normal or shows slight tenderness. Microscopic examinations of expressed prostatic secretions (EPSs) along with segmented urine cultures help to differentiate this condition from nonbacterial prostatitis, urethritis, and prostatodynia.

It is best if the client has a full bladder when segmented urine specimens are collected. The technique is as follows:

1. The client washes the glans and retracts the foreskin (if uncircumcised). He keeps the foreskin retracted throughout the entire urine collection procedure.
2. He voids about the first 10 ml of urine into a sterile container. This is the urethral specimen and is labeled VB1.
3. He then voids about another 200 ml of urine, and a specimen is obtained. This is the bladder specimen and is labeled VB2.
4. The client stops voiding after the second specimen, and a prostatic massage is performed to obtain prostatic secretions. This specimen is labeled EPS.
5. The client voids about another 10 ml. This specimen has prostatic secretions mixed in it and is labeled VB3.

All specimens are checked for the presence of white blood cells (WBCs) and are sent for culture analysis. If the VB1 and VB2 specimens have greater bacterial colony counts, urethritis and bladder infection, respectively, are the diagnoses. If the EPS and VB3 specimens have significantly greater colony counts, the diagnosis is bacterial prostatitis.

The manifestations of nonbacterial prostatitis are similar to those of chronic prostatitis. WBCs are found in the EPS, but no organism is found on culture analysis. Digital rectal examination findings are normal.

Men with prostatodynia complain of similar manifestations, but they have no history of UTI and have normal segmented urine specimens and EPS. Fever is never present. Pelvic and perineal pain is the major complaint.

Outcome Management

Medical Management

REDUCE INFLAMMATION

Clients with *acute* bacterial prostatitis may be so ill that they need hospitalization and IV antibiotics. Practically all antibiotics diffuse into the prostate when it is inflamed. Quinolones are the drugs of choice. Levofloxacin (Levaquin) is a newer quinolone drug that has less bacterial resistance potential than other drugs in this class. An alternative antibiotic is sulfamethoxazole-trimethoprim (Bactrim). Transurethral instrumentation is avoided unless absolutely necessary for urinary retention. The client should have at least 4 weeks of antibiotic therapy to eradicate the infection completely and to prevent chronic prostatitis.

The same antibiotics are used for *chronic* bacterial prostatitis because they can penetrate the noninflamed gland. Doxycycline (Vibramycin) is also used for both chronic and nonbacterial prostatitis. Clients with chronic bacterial prostatitis are treated longer with antibiotics, usually 3 months, and often given lower suppressive doses.

Because no bacteria are found in nonbacterial prostatitis, doxycycline may be ordered for 2 weeks to see whether there is any improvement in manifestations. It is not continued if there is no improvement.

Clients with prostatodynia are treated with alpha-blockers. Nonsteroidal anti-inflammatory drugs (NSAIDs), hot sitz baths, and regular sexual activity (ejaculation) may be ordered as adjunctive treatment.

Surgery may be considered for the client with chronic bacterial prostatitis when medical therapy does not improve manifestations that affect the man's quality of life; however, surgery is rarely performed because of the potential for surgical complications.

Nursing Management of the Medical Client

In all cases of prostatitis, rest, increased fluids, and analgesics are important. Sometimes alcohol or spicy foods exacerbate (worsen) manifestations. Be aware of manifestations of bacteremia. Constipation can be a painful problem for clients with prostatitis. Often, stool softeners are ordered.

The client may be uncomfortable, frustrated, and fearful that the manifestations will never go away or may lead to something more serious than infection. He may have sexual or fertility concerns or may believe that the infection can be sexually transmitted. Clients need much reassurance and teaching. They should understand the importance of complying with the total treatment course and know the side effects of prescribed medications. Clients should also be taught that increasing sexual activity or masturbation may help decrease prostatic gland congestion.

TESTICULAR AND SCROTAL DISORDERS

TESTICULAR CANCER

Testicular cancer is the most common and serious solid tumor cancer in men between the ages of 15 and 35 years. It rarely occurs in men younger than age 15 or older than age 40. In broad perspective, it is rare, with approximately 3.7 cases per 100,000 cases diagnosed in the United States and European countries each year. In many cases it is curable, sometimes even in an advanced stage.

Testicular cancer is less common in African American and Asian men. The incidence is about the same in Hispanic men as in white men. In Israel, the rate is three times higher in Jewish men than non-Jewish men. Testicular cancer is about twice as frequent in high socioeconomic groups.

Etiology and Risk Factors

The cause of testicular cancer is unknown. Family history, exogenous estrogen, and cryptorchidism (undescended testicles) are known risk factors. Cryptorchidism is the major risk factor. Surgery (orchiopexy) is recommended soon after birth, but it does not completely eliminate the risk of cancer.

The male offspring of women who used estrogen in the form of diethylstilbestrol (DES) during the first trimester of pregnancy (called *DES sons*) or who were exposed to estrogen-progestin combinations frequently used in diagnostic tests to confirm pregnancy are at greater risk for testicular cancer. Between 1940 and 1970, DES was given to pregnant women who had a high risk of spontaneous abortion. DES sons also have an increased risk of genitourinary abnormalities such as micropenis, meatal stenosis, varicocele, hypoplastic testicles, infertility, and abnormal semen.

Children with an undescended testicle should be closely observed. Men 15 to 45 years of age should practice monthly testicular self-examination (TSE) (see Chapter 37). Men at high risk for testicular cancer should see a physician for yearly examinations. Early detection can lead to early diagnosis and cure.

Pathophysiology

Most testicular cancers (90% to 95%) are germinal cell tumors, such as seminoma (about 30% to 40% of all tumors), embryonal carcinoma (about 20%), teratocarcinoma, or choriocarcinoma. Seminomas generally carry a favorable prognosis (about a 90% 5-year survival rate) because they are usually localized, metastasize late, and are radiosensitive.

Nongerminal tumors make up the remainder of testicular tumors and are classified as either interstitial cell tumors or testicular adenomas. They arise from interstitial cells or cells that compose the fibrous and vascular networks. They are usually benign.

Metastasis occurs primarily through lymphatic spread. Drainage from the right testis is to the interaortal caval nodes, whereas the left drains to the preaortic nodes. Retroperineal nodes are commonly affected. Distant metastasis occurs most commonly to the lung and rarely to the liver, viscera, bone, or brain.

Choriocarcinoma spreads via the bloodstream. Even after surgical removal, testicular cancer can occur in the other testicle. Carcinoma in situ (localized), although rare, frequently involves both testes. Rarely, testicular tumors are secondary to cancers in another primary site.

Clinical Manifestations

Most commonly, men with testicular tumors experience a painless enlargement, noted as heaviness, in the testicle (in about 75% of cases). Some men describe it as a dragging sensation. Pain is rarely felt; however, the tumor is often found after an injury because the testicle is examined as a result of the injury (Fig. 38–6). A thorough description of family and birth histories and manifestations is the first step in assessment.

Assessment findings suggesting metastasis to the retroperitoneal lymph nodes include back pain, vague abdominal pain, nausea and vomiting, bowel and bladder changes, anorexia, and weight loss. If the lungs are involved, manifestations may include cough, dyspnea, and hemoptysis.

The next step is physical examination of the scrotum and testicles, in which the health care provider determines the location and size of any nodule. If there is a nodule, a light may be held against the scrotum to see whether it is transilluminated (to see whether light passes through). Whereas cysts and hydroceles are transilluminated, tumors and hernias are not.

Ultrasonography of the testes follows. If tumor is suspected, chest x-ray studies and CT scans are ordered to detect metastases. An IVP may be ordered to detect urinary tract involvement.

Tumor usually asymptomatic.
Found on testicular self-examination.
Scrotal discomfort may result from hemorrhage within tumor.
Pain is not usually elicited by squeezing. However, some men have testicular pain.
Testis does not transilluminate.
Testis may be irregular or ovoid.
Hydrocele or hematocele may develop.
Painless enlargement or heaviness of testicle.

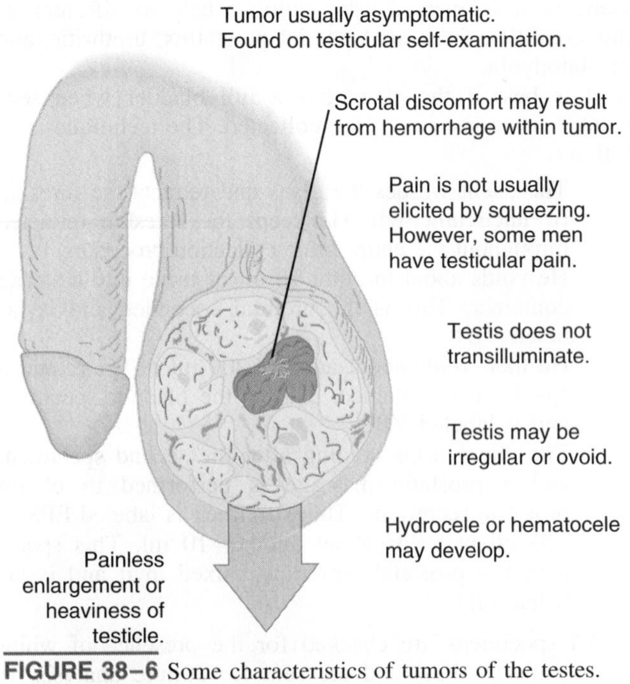

FIGURE 38–6 Some characteristics of tumors of the testes.

Blood tests are ordered. Alpha-fetoprotein (AFP), beta human chorionic gonadotropin (beta-HCG), and lactic acid dehydrogenase (LDH) are the tumor markers used to detect testicular cancer. Elevated AFP is not seen in clients with testicular seminomas. Beta-HCG can be elevated in either seminomas or nonseminomas and, when elevated, may cause gynecomastia in men with testicular cancer. LDH is often elevated in germinal testicular cancers because of the cancer's cell activity, and this elevation also suggests metastasis because LDH is produced in the liver, kidney, and brain.

Testicular cancer is verified by inguinal exploration. If a definite mass is not found, a frozen biopsy may be done. If there is still suspicion, a radical orchiectomy is performed. The testis, epididymis, and vas deferens are removed. The spermatic cord is ligated just inside the internal inguinal ring to prevent seeding of the cancer. Any testicular mass is considered malignant until proved otherwise.

Staging testicular tumors helps to guess at prognosis and to determine treatment options. Testicular tumors are staged as follows:

Stage I_a: Tumor confined to testicle (T1 N0 M0)

Stage I: Metastasis to para-aortic or iliac nodes (T1 N1 M0)

Stage II: Tumor spread to retroperitoneal nodes but disease limited to below the diaphragm (T23, N2, M0)

Stage III: Tumor above the diaphragm or spread to body organs (usually the lungs) T4, N3–4, M+)

Outcome Management

Surgical Management

Radical orchiectomy, performed to diagnose testicular cancer, is also the primary treatment. *Retroperitoneal lymph node dissection* (RPLND) may be done when there is lymph node involvement. The primary use of this procedure is controversial in advanced-stage cancer because treatment with chemotherapy for nonseminomas is very successful. Impotence rates are high after RPLND because many of the autonomic nerves necessary for ejaculation are located in this area. RPLND is performed when testicular cancer is embryonal because this type of cancer metastasizes rapidly.

In other types of testicular cancer, surgeons who perform RPLND believe that it limits the amount of chemotherapy needed. This approach may be used as an adjunct to chemotherapy when only a partial response is achieved. A thoracoabdominal or transabdominal incision is made, and modified dissection techniques are used. The newest approach is a *laparoscopic node dissection.* A smaller incision and fewer complications (especially retrograde ejaculation) result after laparoscopic surgery.

Nursing Management of the Surgical Client

Clients undergoing radical orchiectomy usually require a short hospital stay and experience few complications. The scrotal area is tender and slightly swollen after surgery. Ice bags are applied to the scrotum, and a scrotal support is worn when the client is ambulating. Teach the client self-care strategies and how to monitor for the development of complications. Provide written instructions, a resource he can call should questions or concerns arise, and a follow-up appointment with the surgeon. The client needs to be aware that testicular cancer can recur in the other testicle, and he should know how to do testicular self-examination.

If the client undergoes RPLND, hospitalization is longer, depending on the approach used. Counseling about potential infertility problems and sperm banking takes place before the procedure.

Postoperatively, the client must be monitored closely for possible problems associated with major abdominal surgery. The client requires adequate pain control to comply with ambulation and vigorous coughing and deep breathing to prevent respiratory complications. Anxiety and fear about cancer, sexuality, quality of life, and life expectancy are issues that must frequently be addressed. Be sure that follow-up appointments are made with the surgeon and oncologist for further treatment if appropriate.

Medical Management

Medical management follows radical orchiectomy during the treatment of testicular cancer. A period of close follow-up and observation is necessary to detect recurrence and plan future care.

Destroy Cancer Cells

Radiation Therapy. Low-grade seminomas are particularly radiosensitive. The perineum and pelvis are irradiated, as are the mediastinal and supraclavicular nodes if peritoneal nodes are positive for cancer. Side effects include common complications associated with pelvic radiation: irritable bowel and bladder problems, skin reactions, fatigue, nausea, and anorexia. Radiation may also cause temporary or permanent infertility. Side effects are usually minimal because the dose and number of treatments required are low. Almost 95% of clients with low-stage seminomas survive more than 5 years.

Chemotherapy. Nonseminomatous tumors are not radiosensitive, and they and high-grade seminomas are therefore treated with chemotherapy. The major agent used is cisplatin in combination with vinblastine and bleomycin. Cisplatin in combination with other agents dramatically increases the long-term survival rate for men with testicular cancer. These agents, in combination with a variety of others, have been used to treat metastatic disease or refractory tumors with some success. (Complications of these chemotherapeutic agents are covered in Chapter 19.) Cisplatin has nephrotoxic effects, bleomycin causes pneumonitis, and vinblastine causes peripheral neuropathy.

Nursing Management of the Medical Client

During assessment of a man born between 1940 and 1971, ask whether his mother took any medication during pregnancy to prevent pregnancy or miscarriage. If he appears at particular risk but does not know these details, it may be necessary to obtain the mother's medical history. Information and referral are available through DES Action, Long Island Jewish-Hillside Medical Center, New Hyde Park, NY 11040.

Supportive nursing care for these young men is important during both diagnosis and treatment. Be aware of the threat to sexuality that this condition and its treatment pose to young men. Chapter 19 reviews the care of clients undergoing chemotherapy and radiation therapy.

TESTICULAR TORSION

Testicular torsion (Fig. 38–7*A*) occurs when a testicle is mobile and the spermatic cord twists, cutting off the blood supply. It is the most common testicular disorder in children. It can occur at any age but is most usual at puberty, and about 30% of cases occur in men in their 20s. Manifestations usually arise suddenly, with acute scrotal swelling and severe pain as blood supply to the testicles is interrupted.

If testicular torsion is suspected, a testicular scan and Doppler ultrasonography are performed to assess the blood supply. Torsion causes a decrease (blood supply would be increased with epididymitis).

Testicular torsion is an emergency requiring immediate surgical intervention. The spermatic cord is untwisted and the testicle immobilized by suturing it to the scrotum (orchiopexy). Without prompt surgery, the testicle may atrophy or develop an abscess. If the testicle is necrotic, it is removed. Because there is a risk that the other testicle will be prone to torsion, it is also affixed to the scrotum at the time of surgery.

ORCHITIS

Orchitis is a rare, acute testicular inflammation. It may be associated with trauma or an infection elsewhere in the body, such as mumps, pneumonia, tuberculosis, and syphilis. Mumps orchitis, which occurs in about 30% of men who develop mumps after puberty, is usually bilateral.

Assessment reveals edematous and extremely tender testicles, reddened scrotal skin, fever, and prostration. Treatment includes bed rest, scrotal support, local heat to the scrotum, and medications for pain relief, fever, and infection. An acute phase may last about a week. Permanent sterility may occur if both testicles are affected, whereas decreased fertility may result if only one is affected.

EPIDIDYMITIS

Epididymitis is more common than orchitis. Infections in the urethra, prostate, or bladder can spread along the vas deferens; infections also spread through the lymphatic and vascular systems. Bladder outlet obstruction can cause reflux of infected urine. Epididymitis can occur as a complication related to urethral instrumentation, such as catheterization or instrumentation in transurethral surgeries, but its frequency has decreased since prophylactic antibiotics have been prescribed after such procedures. Sexually transmitted organisms frequently cause the condition in younger men, and urinary pathogens cause epididymitis in older men. Trauma is a noninfectious cause.

Epididymitis is almost always unilateral. Early in the disease, a client has local pain and swelling. As epididymitis progresses, the testicle becomes involved (epididymo-orchitis), the entire scrotum becomes reddened and painful, and an inflammatory hydrocele can occur. After the acute phase, fibrosis and occlusion may result, with subsequent sterility. Recurrences are common when other conditions are unresolved. Treatment is the same as for orchitis.

HYDROCELE, HEMATOCELE, AND SPERMATOCELE

Hydrocele (Fig. 38–7*B*) is a painless collection of clear, yellow fluid in the scrotum caused by an opening between the peritoneum and the tunica vaginalis or by an imbalance in production and reabsorption of fluid within the tunica vaginalis. The soft intrascrotal mass is translucent to light. Often, if the hydrocele is due to a communication with the peritoneum, it decreases in size when the man lies down. If constant discomfort, embarrassment, or impaired circulation occurs, aspiration or surgical drainage may be performed. Hydroceles can conceal a testicular tumor or inguinal hernia.

A hematocele is a collection of blood in the tunica vaginalis caused by trauma. Hematoceles are less likely than hydroceles to be transilluminated on light examination. They require only drainage.

A spermatocele is a cystic dilation of part of the epididymis that contains a milky fluid and dead spermatozoa. It is painless, and surgery is usually not required.

VARICOCELE

Varicocele (Fig. 38–7*C*) is a dilation and varicosity of the pampiniform plexus (the network of veins supplying

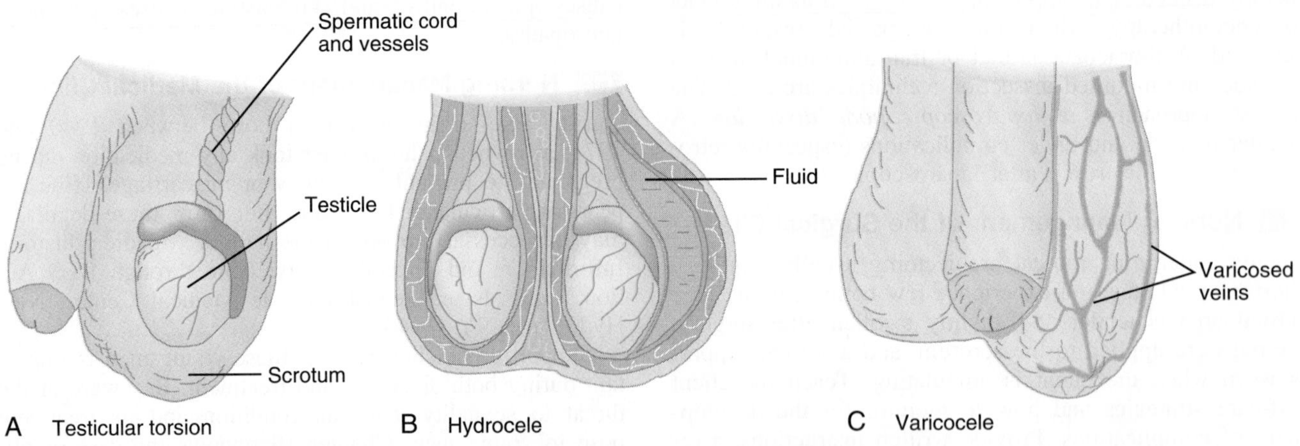

FIGURE 38–7 Disturbances of the testicles.

the testicles) within the scrotum. They usually arise slowly. Ninety per cent of varicoceles are left-sided because the left spermatic vein enters the renal vein at a 90-degree angle, causing back-pressure. Pain may be relieved by masturbation or sexual intercourse. Varicoceles are found in 19% to 41% of men who are evaluated for infertility. A right-sided varicocele suggests tumor or retroperitoneal fibrosis.

On palpation, with the man standing, a varicocele feels like a mass of tortuous veins above and posterior to the testicle. When the man lies down, the mass abates. Treatment includes the use of a scrotal support. Surgery is performed if there is severe pain or if the varicocele is thought to contribute to infertility.

VASECTOMY (ELECTIVE STERILIZATION)

A vasectomy is an elective surgical procedure to ensure a permanent method of contraception. It is sometimes performed after a prostatectomy to prevent retrograde epididymitis. The surgery is usually performed in the urologist's office or in an outpatient setting with the use of local anesthesia. The procedure, performed through a small incision in the scrotum, involves cutting out a segment of the vas deferens, ligating the ends, and tucking them into different tissue planes to prevent reanastomosis (Fig. 38–8).

Slight pain, swelling, and bruising occur postoperatively, but discomfort is controlled with ice, a mild analgesic such as acetaminophen (aspirin is avoided to prevent bleeding), and rest for a few days. A scrotal support also increases client comfort. The client can resume heavy lifting and sexual intercourse about a week after surgery. The client must continue to practice other means of birth control until the follow-up semen analysis shows azoospermia (absence of sperm), because live sperm are left in the ampulla of vas deferens. Bleeding, infection, and mild chronic pain (rare) are complications that can occur after vasectomy.

The client must consider vasectomy a permanent means of contraception. Vasovasostomy, which is a surgical reversal of a vasectomy, can be done; however, it is expensive and fertility is not guaranteed.

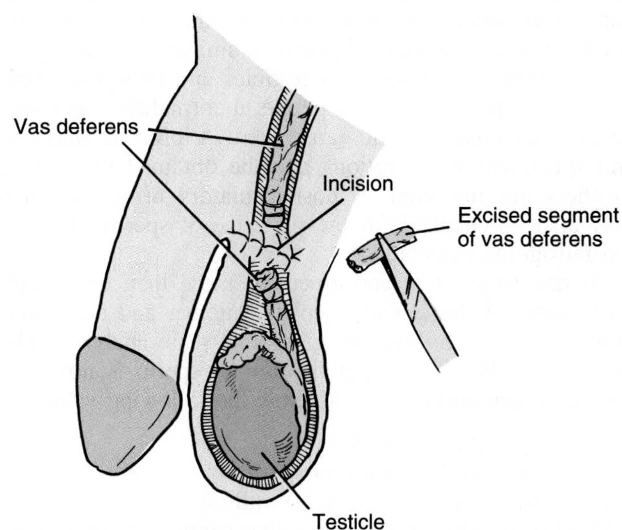

FIGURE 38–8 Vasectomy.

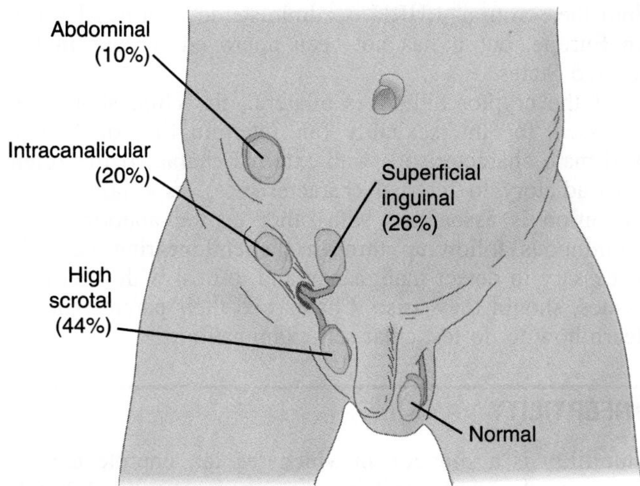

FIGURE 38–9 Undescended or mispositioned testis (cryptorchidism).

UNDESCENDED OR MISPOSITIONED TESTICLES

The most common congenital testicular condition is that of mispositioned undescended testes (cryptorchidism) (Fig. 38–9). Testes normally descend from the abdomen into the scrotum before birth, but sometimes they do not. One or both testicles may be arrested in the abdomen, inguinal canal (canalicular), low pelvis, or high scrotum. An ectopic testicle descends to the wrong area outside the normal path of decent (e.g., perineum). A retractile testicle descends into the scrotum but pulls back into the inguinal canal because of a hyperactive cremasteric reflex. Complete absence of a testicle may also occur.

Undescended testicles occur in about 4% of full-term male infants and are more common in premature infants. Many resolve by the first year of life. Inguinal hernias and torsion commonly occur with undescended testicles.

Cryptorchidism is associated with infertility. High body temperature, endocrine understimulation, and an abnormal epididymis that seems to accompany an undescended testicle cause changes that prevent normal fertility in the future. The incidence of testicular cancer is high in men with undescended testes if the condition is not corrected before puberty. A man with an undescended testicle has a 1 in 80 chance of testicular cancer development. Correction, however, does not guarantee prevention.

Treatment, which is surgical, is performed when the child is between 9 and 12 months old, and certainly by 18 months, not only to allow time for spontaneous descent but also to decrease the risk of total infertility and testicular cancer. An inguinal incision is used so that additional repair (i.e., hernia repair or excision of connective tissue bands) or orchiectomy (should the testicle look abnormal) can be done.

Retractile testes usually descend and stay in the scrotum by puberty, but surgery is not required. HCG has sometimes been used to promote passage of the testicle into the scrotum. LHRH is administered as a nasal spray in Europe, but it has not been approved for use in the United States.

If the cryptorchidism is bilateral, the child should be assessed for intersexuality (an intermingling of female and male characteristics with external characteristics often contradictory to internal characteristics), especially if the condition is associated with other genital abnormalities. Continuous follow-up through the childbearing years is necessary to detect malignancy and to deal with infertility issues, should they arise. Clients and their parents should learn how to do testicular self-examination.

INFERTILITY

Infertility is a situation in which regular, unprotected intercourse does not result in a pregnancy over a 12-month period. Infertility affects 20% to 35% of couples in the United States who are trying to have children, and requests for infertility services are increasing rapidly.

A male factor contributes partially or totally to the couple's inability to conceive in about 50% of the cases. However, it is best that the two partners be treated together. Minimal fertility *(subfertility)* in one partner can be offset by strong fertility in the other. If both partners are minimally fertile, infertility is more likely. Awareness of these statistics alerts health care professionals to clients who may have concerns about infertility but who have difficulty expressing them. Male factors for infertility are discussed in this chapter.

Etiology and Risk Factors

Pretesticular (hormonal) causes involve endocrine dysfunction and account for approximately 3% to 25% of cases. Examples are pituitary and adrenal tumors, thyroid disorders, diabetes, and cirrhosis.

Testicular causes are most common. Varicoceles are found in 19% to 41% of infertility cases. Other testicular causes include congenital abnormalities, torsion, genitourinary infection, trauma, and exposure to substances known to interfere with spermatogenesis (sperm formation). Cryptorchidism is directly related to infertility.

Post-testicular causes include congenital blockage of the vas deferens and other malformations of structures distal to the testes. Epididymitis, emotional factors, surgical procedures that cause retrograde ejaculation, and some medical conditions such as renal disease or paraplegia are additional causes.

Infection of the prostate, epididymis, or testicle can affect fertility. The mumps virus attacks the testicle in 5% to 37% of adults who acquire the infection. Of these men, 16% to 65% have bilateral involvement. Although rare in the Western world, tuberculosis is a genital infection seen in other countries and in immigrants to the United States.

Whether testicular trauma and infertility are related is a matter of controversy. The formation of anti-sperm antibodies is one theory. Some surgical procedures cause retrograde ejaculation.

Chemicals, drugs, and other substances that affect spermatogenesis are called *gonadotoxins* (e.g., heavy use of alcohol, marijuana, and anabolic steroids). Many medications, including allopurinol, cimetidine, nitrofurantoin, sulfasalazine, and chemotherapeutic drugs, have been related to infertility. Alpha-adrenergic blockers and ganglion blockers may cause retrograde ejaculation and may thus be a secondary cause of inability to conceive. Exposure to agricultural, industrial, and warfare agents is an increasing concern. Lead, Agent Orange (a herbicide used as a defoliant in Vietnam), and some pesticides affect fertility. Tobacco smoke has been investigated as a cause of infertility, but a clear link has not been established; data suggest that smoking may be involved in subfertility. Radiation and hyperthermia also affect fertility.

Problems with intercourse are responsible for infertility in about 5% of couples. These include erectile dysfunction, premature ejaculation, unfavorable timing or frequency of intercourse, excessive masturbation, and aberrant sexual behaviors. Many water-soluble lubricants used during intercourse can be toxic to sperm.

Pathophysiology

The pathophysiologic mechanisms involved in infertility vary, and the problem is often a complex one. Hormonal imbalance between the hypothalamus, pituitary gland, and testicles can interfere with the production and maturation of sperm. Hypoxia of the testicle and elevated scrotal temperature cause germ cell damage. Seminal WBCs present in genitourinary infections are believed to release bioactive cytokines that affect spermatogenesis.

Some viruses and bacteria directly destroy cells or cause enough inflammation to cause tissue necrosis. Sexually transmitted diseases, particularly gonorrhea and infection with *Chlamydia trachomatis*, may account for cases of infertility because they can cause testicular atrophy, but a clear relationship has not been proved. Immune responses may prevent the formation of normal sperm. Gonadotoxins can decrease the number of sperm, decrease motility (the forward movement of sperm), or cause abnormal morphology. Congenital factors and trauma can impair patency of the ductal system that extends from the testicles through the prostate.

Clinical Manifestations

Assessment of infertility includes obtaining a detailed occupational, sexual, medical, and reproductive history and conducting a thorough physical examination. During an examination, the presence of testicles and their size, varicocele or other scrotal and penile abnormalities, and secondary sex characteristics are noted. A prostate massage and specimens of secretions may be obtained for culture to check for infection. A postejaculatory urine specimen may also be checked for the presence of sperm, suggesting retrograde ejaculation.

Semen analysis is performed on more than one specimen. Semen volume and viscosity, number and concentration of sperm, motility, and morphology are analyzed. The presence of WBCs or agglutination of sperm is noted. A normal semen analysis would show the following values:

- Semen volume, 1.5 to 5.0 ml
- Concentration, >20 million sperm/ml
- Total sperm count, >50 to 60 million
- Motility, ≥60% grade 2 or higher (on a scale of 1 to 4)
- Morphology, ≥60% normal

Motility refers to the forward movement of sperm; *morphology* refers to sperm form and size. Normally, sperm have one head and one tail. Abnormal sperm may be immature, may have misshapen heads, or may have two tails. Some infertility specialists consider slightly lower percentages for sperm count, motility, and morphology to be adequate when evaluating semen quality. Other more specific tests may be done to evaluate semen, such as checking for viscosity, coagulation, and the presence of fructose.

Serum endocrine studies are conducted to assess testosterone, prolactin, LH, and follicle-stimulating hormone (FSH). For example, if testosterone levels are normal, nonhormonal causes are pursued. If testosterone levels and prolactin levels are low but LH levels are high, primary testicular disease may be suspected. If FSH levels are high, spermatogenesis is probably arrested. If FSH levels are normal, *azoospermia* (absence of sperm) or *oligospermia* (scarcity of sperm) is probably caused by obstruction in the post-testicular ducts, which may be corrected by microsurgery.

If anatomic abnormalities are suspected, imaging techniques such as Doppler ultrasonography, MRI, cavernosography, and color flow Doppler imaging are ordered. A testicular biopsy may be performed if sperm are absent or scarce along with normal hormone levels. Clients are carefully selected for such studies because the tests are costly and, when invasive, may cause testicular damage.

Outcome Management

Medical Management

Pretesticular Causes

Treatment of male infertility with pretesticular causes varies. No treatment is available for primary testicular failure or hypogonadism. Testosterone may be prescribed to correct low testosterone levels. A testosterone patch is applied directly to the scrotum (Testoderm) or to the torso or extremities (Androderm). Scrotal skin is five times more permeable, and there is concern about too much absorption and side effects. With both transdermal methods, skin irritation or contact dermatitis is experienced in about 9% of clients. Testosterone is contraindicated for men with prostate cancer or severe bladder outlet obstruction. Hyperprolactinemia may be treated by surgical removal of a pituitary tumor or by administration of bromocriptine (Parlodel).

Treatment of male sexual dysfunction is discussed under Erectile Dysfunction. For oligospermia caused by excessive frequency of ejaculation, recommend that the couple have intercourse only once every 36 hours during the woman's periovulatory period, because it takes 24 hours for a normal sperm count to be generated after ejaculation.

Testicular Causes

Treatment of male infertility with testicular causes also varies. Instruct the client to avoid factors that depress spermatogenesis such as heat, drugs, alcohol, and marijuana. He should keep the testicles cool by avoiding hot baths and tight clothing or by using a commercially prepared, water-dampened scrotal cooling device; keeping the testes cool appears to improve the sperm count. Advise the client to maintain good nutrition. Medications such as HCG or testosterone (Depo-Testosterone) are sometimes prescribed as hormonal treatments. Nonhormonal therapy may consists of kallikrein, steroids, indomethacin, arginine, zinc, or vitamins. Varicocele is treated surgically.

Post-Testicular Causes

Treatment of male infertility with post-testicular causes involves correcting ejaculatory abnormalities and obstruction. Ejaculatory abnormalities may be corrected by the split-ejaculate technique. The first half of the ejaculate contains more sperm than the second half. The first half may be used for artificial insemination or may be deposited in the vagina during intercourse, followed by withdrawal of the penis. Absence of ejaculation or retrograde (backward) ejaculation may be treated with drugs such as ephedrine, imipramine, or antihistamines. When the client experiences retrograde ejaculation, artificial insemination may be performed using sperm from urine obtained by centrifugation. Obstructive infertility is treated by surgery.

Appropriate antimicrobial drugs are used to treat genitourinary infections. Male infertility with immunologic causes may be treated with steroids and artificial insemination of sperm that have been washed to remove antibodies contained in the sperm.

Nursing Management of the Medical Client

Provide Support

The client and his partner are often highly emotional in the diagnostic phase, and your sensitivity can ease their concerns somewhat. Both may need help and support to express their feelings and concerns about infertility. Failure to conceive may make several demands on the couple, threatening their individual self-concepts, sex roles, relationship, and sexual interaction. Guilt and blame about previous sexual activity, sexually transmitted diseases (STDs), or abortion may come between them. Some men find masturbation (necessary to obtain a semen sample) difficult for personal, cultural, or religious reasons. Many men do not know what chemicals they have been exposed to at the workplace or elsewhere. Fear and anxiety may be lessened during your assessment and teaching sessions. This provides you with the opportunity to support, respond to questions, and explain diagnostic and treatment procedures. Emphasize the need for consistent follow-up to evaluate progress.

Referral for counseling or support groups, or both, for infertile couples may be appropriate. A nationally known support group in the United States is RESOLVE (Department P, Box 474, Belmont, MA 02178).

Provide Education

Because thorough and complete fertility assessment is expensive and can be ineffective, the client needs to understand the testing and the reasons for the various examinations. Explain fully how to collect a specimen for sperm analysis so that results are accurate. Written as well as verbal instructions are important because anxiety levels may be high. The man should refrain from sexual activity for 3 days before collecting a semen sample and should take the specimen immediately (within 1 hour) to the laboratory for analysis. Masturbation is the preferred method because some semen is lost during intercourse. Condoms and lubricants may make the sperm immotile. The specimen should be kept close to the body to maintain normal temperature. Two to three interval specimens are required for evaluation because results can vary. Ensure that the client understands the medical regimen suggested and the importance of following it closely.

Prevent Infertility

If possible, it is more effective to prevent infertility than to treat it. Clients who want to conceive at present or in the future can try to prevent infertility by:

1. Avoiding gonadotoxins, as discussed earlier.
2. Decreasing exposure to occupational and environmental hazards.
3. Keeping the scrotum cool by avoiding excessive heat, hot baths, and tight clothing.
4. Avoiding transmission of STDs by limiting the number of sexual partners and by using condoms.
5. Developing effective means of stress reduction.
6. Eating a well-balanced, nutritious diet.

PENILE DISORDERS

Phimosis

Phimosis occurs when the penile foreskin (prepuce) is constricted at the opening, making retraction difficult or impossible. The condition can be congenital or a result of inflammation, infection, or local trauma. It is not usually painful, but it can lead to obstructive uropathy if it is severe enough. Prolonged phimosis, caused by chronic inflammation and irritation, predisposes to penile cancer. Assessment reveals edema, erythema, tenderness, and purulent discharge. Intervention includes controlling infection with local treatment and broad-spectrum antimicrobial drugs.

Effective genital hygiene is essential to prevent acquired penile disorders. In uncircumcised males, the man cleans the penis by pulling the foreskin back gently and washing the area with a washcloth (Fig. 38–10). This technique should be done daily to eliminate the normally accumulated smegma, and the foreskin should be returned to its normal position.

Routine *circumcision* (surgical removal of the foreskin) of male infants has not been considered medically necessary by the American Academy of Pediatrics and other health professionals and health organizations. Some parents have religious or cultural reasons for continuing the practice of circumcision. The operation may be indicated for clients with penile infection, phimosis, or paraphimosis. The rate of penile cancer is almost nil in circumcised men. The procedure should be done with the client under general anesthesia. Potential risks include excessive bleeding, infection, and penile trauma.

Paraphimosis

Paraphimosis (Fig. 38–11) occurs when a tight foreskin, once retracted, cannot be returned to its normal position. This sometimes happens after rigorous cleaning, masturbation, sexual intercourse, catheter insertion, or cystoscopy if the foreskin is not returned to its normal position. Circulation is thus impeded, and the glans swells rapidly. It is painful and edema is common. The foreskin can be gently compressed either manually or with an elastic wrap. The client can then attempt manual reduction by gently pulling the foreskin. Surgical incision of the foreskin with local anesthesia may be necessary if the condition does not resolve.

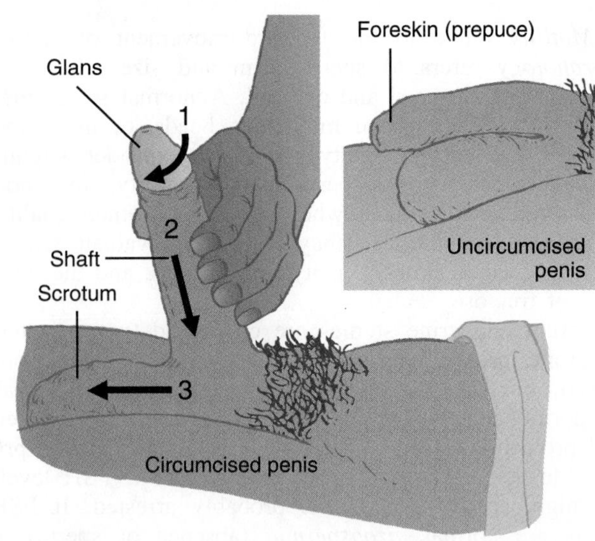

FIGURE 38–10 A circumcised penis and an uncircumcised penis. The foreskin of an uncircumcised penis should retract easily. During physical examination, ask the man to retract his foreskin himself. Effective genital hygiene is essential to prevent acquired penile problems. Many men have never been taught how to do this. *1,* Begin washing at the tip of the penis. For an uncircumcised penis, gently retract the foreskin and wash. *2,* Proceed down the penis shaft toward the body. *3,* Next wash the scrotum. Wash the anal area last.

Posthitis and Balanitis

Posthitis (foreskin inflammation) and balanitis (inflammation of the glans penis and the mucous membrane beneath it) (Fig. 38–12) are caused by irritation and invasion of microorganisms. Good hygiene and thorough drying of the penis are recommended. It is important to assess for diabetes, which predisposes the client to secondary infection. Antibiotics may help control local infection. Circumcision may be necessary.

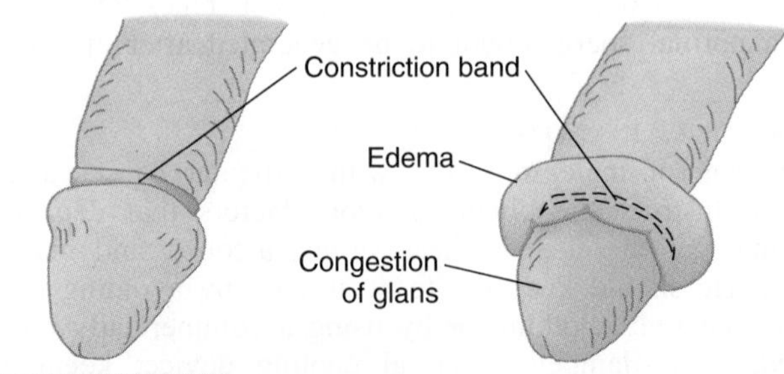

FIGURE 38–11 Paraphimosis.

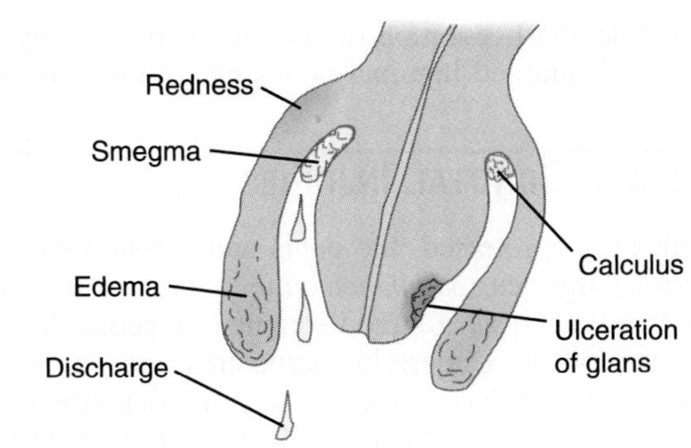

FIGURE 38–12 Posthitis and balanitis.

URETHRITIS

Urethritis, an acute urethral inflammation, is discussed under STDs and urinary disorders (see Chapters 34 and 41). It is mentioned throughout this chapter because it predisposes to other genitourinary disorders.

URETHRAL STRICTURE

Urethral stricture is caused by urethral scarring or narrowing. It may be congenital or caused by untreated or severe urethritis or urethral injury (including urologic instrumentation, e.g., cystoscopy). Manifestations are caused by obstruction: small-caliber urinary stream, hyperdistended bladder, infection, fever, and dysuria. Urethral strictures are released surgically by urethral dilation or urethroplasty. See Chapter 34 for further information.

EPISPADIAS

Epispadias (Fig. 38–13*A*) is a rare congenital condition in which the urethral meatus opens dorsally on top of the penis, proximal to the glans, most commonly at the abdominal-penile junction. Surgery is required to correct urinary incontinence and to return the urethra to a normal position in the penis.

HYPOSPADIAS

Hypospadias (Fig. 38–13*B*) is a congenital condition in which the urethral meatus opens on the ventral side of the penis. Common locations include the glans penis, penile shaft, penoscrotal junction, and perineum. *Chordee* (curvature of the penis) is often associated with hypospadias. Hypospadias occurs in about two to eight per thousand live male births.

Early assessment of internal reproductive organ development is necessary to confirm the child's sex. For psychological reasons, hypospadias should be repaired before the child starts school. It is important to ask about this condition when taking the history.

PEYRONIE'S DISEASE

Fibrous plaques develop in the connective tissue in Peyronie's disease, usually near the dorsal midline of the penile shaft in middle-aged and older men. Although the etiologic mechanism is unknown, one theory is that the disease is caused by an abnormal fibrotic reaction to trauma. The disease has two phases: acute and chronic. Pain is more likely during the initial phase, and plaques begin to develop. This phase can last about 1 to 1½ years. Pain usually subsides during the chronic phase, but fibrosis is increased.

Diagnosis may be made during history-taking, although men usually seek a physician because of concern about penile lumps (fear of cancer), painful erection, or erectile dysfunction. The man may have penile curvature on erection, painful erection, and unsatisfactory vaginal penetration. Peyronie's disease is often associated with Dupuytren's contracture of the hand tendons.

Some cases improve spontaneously. Reassure the client that this is not a malignant condition and does not lead to development of cancer. If a client is not having discomfort and has soft plaques and minimal curvature, the physician may advise waiting several months before instituting therapy. Medical treatment includes vitamin E,

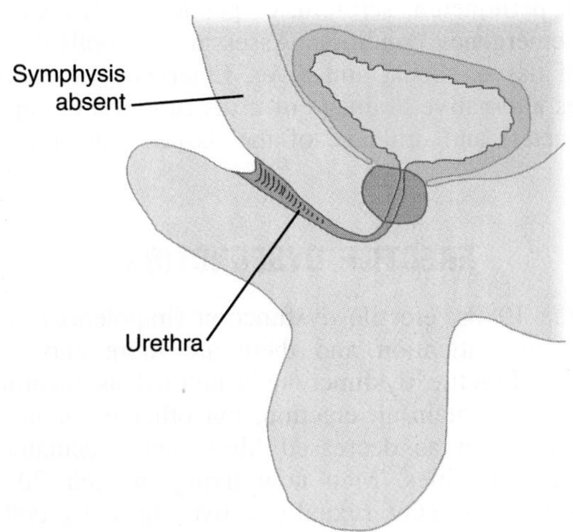

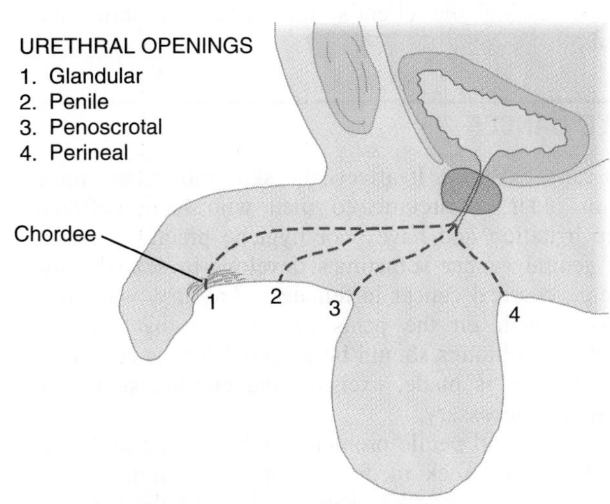

FIGURE 38–13 Epispadias *(A)* and hypospadias *(B)*.

para-aminobenzoic acid, tamoxifen, and colchicine. Intralesional injections, local radiation, and ultrasonography have also been used. Surgical correction is necessary when previous treatments have failed and the client is unable to perform sexually.

PRIAPISM

Priapism is a prolonged, persistent penile erection without sexual desire. It can last hours or even days and may be very painful. The condition is sometimes associated with leukemia or sickle cell anemia. Self-injection of medications (mainly papaverine) to treat impotence is the other common cause. It may also result from some medications, such as anticoagulants, alcohol, phenothiazines, alpha-adrenergic blockers, and marijuana.

Two major types of priapism have been defined according to a physiology-based system. *High-flow* arterial priapism, the less common type, usually occurs after trauma and is less painful. *Low-flow* veno-occlusive priapism, the more common form, is an emergency situation and is extremely painful.

In the client with low-flow priapism, circulation to the penis is compromised, predisposing to ischemia and permanent erectile dysfunction. The client may also be unable to void. Treatment in most cases consists of aspiration of blood from the penis followed by serial intracavernosal injections of phenylephrine.

Low-flow priapism must be resolved within 24 hours to prevent penile ischemia, gangrene, fibrosis, and erectile dysfunction. If the more conservative treatments are unsuccessful, more invasive therapy is required to prevent permanent damage. Surgical treatment is designed to drain the congested blood from the corpora cavernosa.

High-flow priapism can often be treated with ice and compression. If these measures are not successful, the client may require selective embolization or ligation of the traumatized artery.

Be sensitive to the embarrassing nature of this problem. Men are often reluctant to admit that this problem has occurred and yet may be in severe pain. Be understanding, and try to make the client comfortable while decreasing the client's embarrassment about the problem.

PENILE CANCER

Penile cancer is rare. It affects the skin and occurs most often in older, uncircumcised men who have suffered chronic irritation and have poor hygiene practices. Associated genital cancer sometimes develops in sexual partners (e.g., cervical cancer in females). Any dry, wart-like, painless growth on the penis or foreskin that fails to respond to antibiotics should be assessed for cancer. If an early diagnosis is made, excision and circumcision may be all that is necessary.

Many men find penile problems embarrassing and consequently do not seek medical attention for months. By this time, a lesion may be ulcerated, involve the foreskin and penile shaft, and have metastasized to the inguinal nodes. Penile shaft resection or sometimes penectomy and dissection of enlarged inguinal nodes may be necessary.

PENILE AND SCROTAL INJURIES

Although fairly protected, the penis and scrotum can sustain various injuries. *Nonpenetrating* injuries result from sudden force, such as a straddle injury or penile fracture during intercourse. Underlying structures can be bruised or ruptured. Items placed around the penis that strangulate may also cause significant tissue damage. *Penetrating* injuries usually involve knife or gunshot wounds but also include self-emasculation attempts and amputation. The male genitalia can also be injured by radiation, chemical or electrical burns, and avulsion (from accidents caused by working with machinery).

Hemorrhage is immediate, whether microscopic or obvious. Pain and edema accompany bleeding. Minor hemorrhage is controlled by ice packs, bed rest, analgesia, and scrotal elevation. Direct compression and pressure dressings may be needed if bleeding is worse. For penile injury, a retrograde urethrogram is obtained to rule out urethral injury. If the urethra is intact, an indwelling catheter is inserted. If bleeding from the penis is noted, urethral disruption is assumed and instrumentation is contraindicated. For scrotal injury, scrotal ultrasonography is performed.

Surgery is necessary to drain a hematoma, to debride necrotic tissue, or to repair damage, including reanastomosis if appropriate. Microsurgical techniques are used. Postoperative antibiotics are given, and catheterization continues until penile injuries are healed. Often, further operations are required for repair of strictures, skin grafting, or reconstruction. If scrotal skin is avulsed, the remaining scrotal skin is usually replaced over the scrotal organs; scrotal skin regenerates. When this is not possible, surgeons may perform skin grafts and temporarily reimplant the testes into subcutaneous thigh pouches. These clients need professional approaches and much explanation and reassurance to reduce anxiety. If the client has sustained self-inflicted injuries, psychological referral is part of the care.

When the urinary tract is disrupted, urine can escape into the peritoneum, scrotum, or penile tissue, thus creating an emergency condition. Assessment reveals discoloration of tissue, shock, and fever. Emergency intervention includes alternative drainage of urine (urethral or suprapubic catheter) and drainage of the tissues with a Penrose drain.

ERECTILE DYSFUNCTION

Since the 1980s, erectile dysfunction (impotence) has received more attention and there are more choices for treatment. Erectile dysfunction is defined as inability to achieve or maintain an erection, but other problems may contribute, such as decreased libido and ejaculatory or orgasmic difficulties. Men now living in their 70s and beyond want to stay sexually active. In most cultures, sexual performance is a measure of manhood. Erectile dysfunction was once thought to be psychogenic in origin, but physiologic causes are found in more than 50% of the cases.

Etiology and Risk Factors

Both psychological and physiologic factors may contribute to erectile dysfunction, such as performance anxiety, stress and fatigue, low self-esteem, depression, and changes in a relationship. After experiencing failure once, a man may be so anxious that he "fails" again and again, worsening the problem. Stress caused by psychological factors can increase catecholamine levels and can block sympathetic response, causing a physiologic dysfunction.

True psychogenic erectile dysfunction is distinguished by the following:

- Normal and sustained erection during foreplay but loss of erection at the moment of intromission (penetration)
- Normal erection with some sexual partners but not with others
- Normal erection with masturbation but not with partners
- Sudden onset of total impotence in a man younger than 40 years of age
- Alternating periods of normal function and total impotence

Physiologic causes include diseases, interruption related to surgery, anatomic abnormalities, and medications or substance abuse. Erectile dysfunction may be partial or total. Vascular conditions, such as arteriosclerotic changes, trauma to the penile blood supply, hypertension, stroke, diabetes mellitus, sickle cell anemia, leukemia, Hodgkin's disease, and aortic aneurysms, are common causes. Neurologic causes include interference with sympathetic or parasympathetic innervation, degenerative diseases, and spinal cord injury. Endocrine disorders that lower testosterone also cause erectile dysfunction. Peyronie's disease, prostatitis, and prolonged priapism are genitourinary causes.

Congenital anomalies of the penis, chordee, and a short penis are anatomic factors. Surgical disruption may occur during radical prostatectomy, pelvic lymph node dissection, radical cystectomy, and, of course, bilateral orchiectomy. Numerous medications can affect erection, libido, orgasm, and ejaculation, but erectile problems do not always arise in men who take the medications. Recreational drugs, alcohol, and smoking also cause erectile dysfunction.

Pathophysiology

A normal erection requires desire, sensual stimulation, release of LH, arterial engorgement of the corpora cavernosa (and venous constriction), and an intact nervous system from the brain to the penile nerves. Anything that interferes with this process can cause erectile dysfunction.

Clinical Manifestations

A detailed medical and sexual history is the first step in determining the cause of erectile dysfunction. A limited physical examination is performed to rule out obvious genitourinary causes. Laboratory tests may include determinations of serum testosterone, LH, FSH, and prolactin levels and thyroid function. Increased prolactin blocks testosterone effectiveness and decreases the desire for sexual activity. Both hyperthyroidism and hypothyroidism may cause erectile dysfunction, usually affecting libido.

When erectile function is normal, men have involuntary erections during times of deep sleep when rapid eye movement (REM) occurs. Nocturnal penile tumescence (NPT) studies help to determine the presence of these erections; some tests can evaluate the quality. The least expensive test employs a snap gauge device with pressure bands wrapped around the penis. The bands break at increasing pressures during nocturnal erections. NPT monitors can also be used to evaluate several nocturnal erections during a night's sleep. A special monitor, called a Rigiscan, records nocturnal erections and their quality (duration, rigidity, and changes in circumference of the penile shaft during each erection). Other tests include penile Doppler ultrasonography, penile angiography, and dynamic infusion cavernosometry (DICC). DICC provides information about arterial inflow, cavernous sinoid compliance, and venous leakage.

Outcome Management

Medical Management

Correct Psychological Problems

Sometimes just giving accurate information about normal sexual function, alternative sexual activity, and dispelling myths is all that is necessary for a client to deal with erectile dysfunction. Myths about sexual activity greatly influence outcome success. Behavioral modification techniques (the best known were developed by Masters and Johnson in the 1960s) may be used when psychogenic causes are determined. Psychologists and sexual therapists may use psychometric testing, including the Minnesota Multiphasic Personality Inventory (MMPI), the Derogatis Sexual Function Inventory, or the Walker Sex Form, to assess psychological functioning.

Correct Physiologic Problems

When physiologic causes are involved, several approaches may be used. Medications used for diseases may need to be changed or habits (use of recreational drugs or alcohol and smoking) eliminated. Medical conditions causing erectile dysfunction need to be treated if possible. Low testosterone levels, once treated by intramuscular injection of testosterone, is now more commonly treated with testosterone dermal patches that can be placed on several areas of the body. Testosterone can increase libido but does not necessarily help erectile dysfunction. Administration of testosterone is contraindicated for men with prostate cancer and those with normal testosterone production (suppresses natural production).

Stimulate Erection

Medications. Yohimbe, an adrenergic blocking medication, may cause vasodilation in the corpora cavernosa. It is usually ordered three times a day. It can cause side effects such as fluid retention, nausea, orthostatic hypotension, and diaphoresis or may not be effective at all.

Intracavernosal vasodilating drugs such as papaverine, phentolamine, and prostaglandin E_1 (PGE_1) can be injected. Combinations of these drugs may be given in a single injection. Because pain, bruising, or fibrosis at the injection site and priapism are possible side effects, it is recommended that injections be given not more than two or three times per week.

Intraurethral instillation of an alprostadil (PGE_1) pellet has been successful. This approach eliminates injection of the penis, but the technique must be accurately performed in order to achieve the erection. This can be a good approach for a client who is obese or has problems with dexterity or vision. The dosage varies from 125 to 1000 μg and can be given no more than twice in a 24-hour period. Side effects are the same as described before; intraurethral pain and minor bleeding may occur. PGE_1 administration is contraindicated if penile anatomy is abnormal or the client has urethritis.

Sildenafil (Viagra), an oral agent, is the newest medication for treatment of erectile dysfunction. It inhibits an enzyme in the corpora cavernosa that chemically ends the erection. This drug does not produce the erection; direct penile stimulation is required to release nitric oxide in the penile nerves, which activates another enzyme to relax the corporeal blood vessels. Side effects may include headache, a flush feeling, dyspepsia, nasal congestion, and a color tinge or other mild visual disturbances. Sildenafil is contraindicated for any client taking nitrates in any form. Caution must be observed when men are taking alpha-adrenergic blockers or have a peptic ulcer. The dosage is usually 25 to 100 mg taken no more than once a day.

Vacuum Erection Devices. Vacuum erection devices are legitimate medically prescribed pumps that mechanically achieve an erection. A cylinder is placed over the penis and a pump is used to create vacuum suction, thus drawing blood into the corpora cavernosa. When an erection is achieved, a compression ring is applied to the base of the penis and the cylinder is removed for intercourse. The ring must be removed within about 30 minutes to prevent tissue damage caused by interrupted circulation. Bruising and cold penile skin as well as lack of spontaneity are minor problems that may result. Priapism can also occur.

Nursing Management of the Medical Client

Provide Support

A sensitive, caring approach is vital for nurses who work with these clients because embarrassment may cause many men to avoid treatment. Just knowing that erectile dysfunction is common and treatment alternatives are available can be reassuring to the client. Involve the sexual partner when the client permits. Erectile dysfunction is a "couple" problem.

Provide Education

Teach the client about normal erectile physiology, factors that interfere, and how different approaches correct the problem. Inform the client about public or community resources. If medication is used, explain how to administer the medication and caution the client to follow directions as prescribed and not to use the medication more often then directed. Some men erroneously believe that if a little does work, more would be better.

The client who must use intracorporeal injections needs to know how to draw up medication into a syringe, cleanse the site, inject the medication, and safely dispose of equipment. He should know that bruising may occur. Injections should be given at the 2 o'clock or 10 o'clock position, and sites should be rotated to minimize fibrotic changes. Intraurethral pellets require using the applicator correctly, careful insertion, and waiting about 10 minutes for an erection to occur. Standing or walking during this time and stimulation are important.

Surgical Management

Surgical management of erectile dysfunction includes implantation of a penile prosthesis, revascularization procedures, and incision of Peyronie's plaques. Penile prostheses are the most common if medical therapy is not effective and if the client is a good surgical candidate.

Penile Prosthesis

There are two basic categories of penile prostheses (Fig. 38–14):

1. *Inflatable* prostheses come in one-piece, two-piece, and three-piece units that are hydraulic devices. In the one-piece prosthesis, the reservoir, pump, and cylinders fit within the penis. Two-piece units have a reservoir-pump system within the scrotum. The reservoir on the three-piece devices is implanted in the abdominal cavity and the pump is implanted in the scrotum.
2. *Semi-rigid* prostheses can be malleable, with spring-like mechanisms that help make the penis more erect for intercourse, or mechanical, with cable strands in the device that can be bent to make the penis more erect.

Ice and penile or scrotal elevations are used postoperatively to minimize swelling. Pain should be well controlled with medication. Sexual activity can usually be resumed 6 to 8 weeks after surgery when healing is complete and pain is controlled. Infection, extrusion of the prosthesis, and mechanical failure are some of the complications after surgery.

Revascularization

Revascularization surgical procedures attempt to restore circulation to the corpora cavernosa. Techniques involve reanastomosis, angioplasty, endarterectomy, and grafts. Venous ligation is used to treat penile vein incompetence. Over time, collateral veins form and "leakage" recurs.

Nursing Management of the Surgical Client

Care of the client having surgery for erectile dysfunction is the same as that of any surgical client. Penile circulation and dressing should be observed consistently as ordered. Encourage the client to use pain medication before the pain becomes severe. All clients are given antibiotics before and after surgery. The client is taught preoperatively how to use the prosthesis and cautioned not to use it before healing has occurred. These men need a great deal of emotional support because of secrecy with friends, emotional issues with partners, and sometimes doubt about the decision to have surgery related to pain.

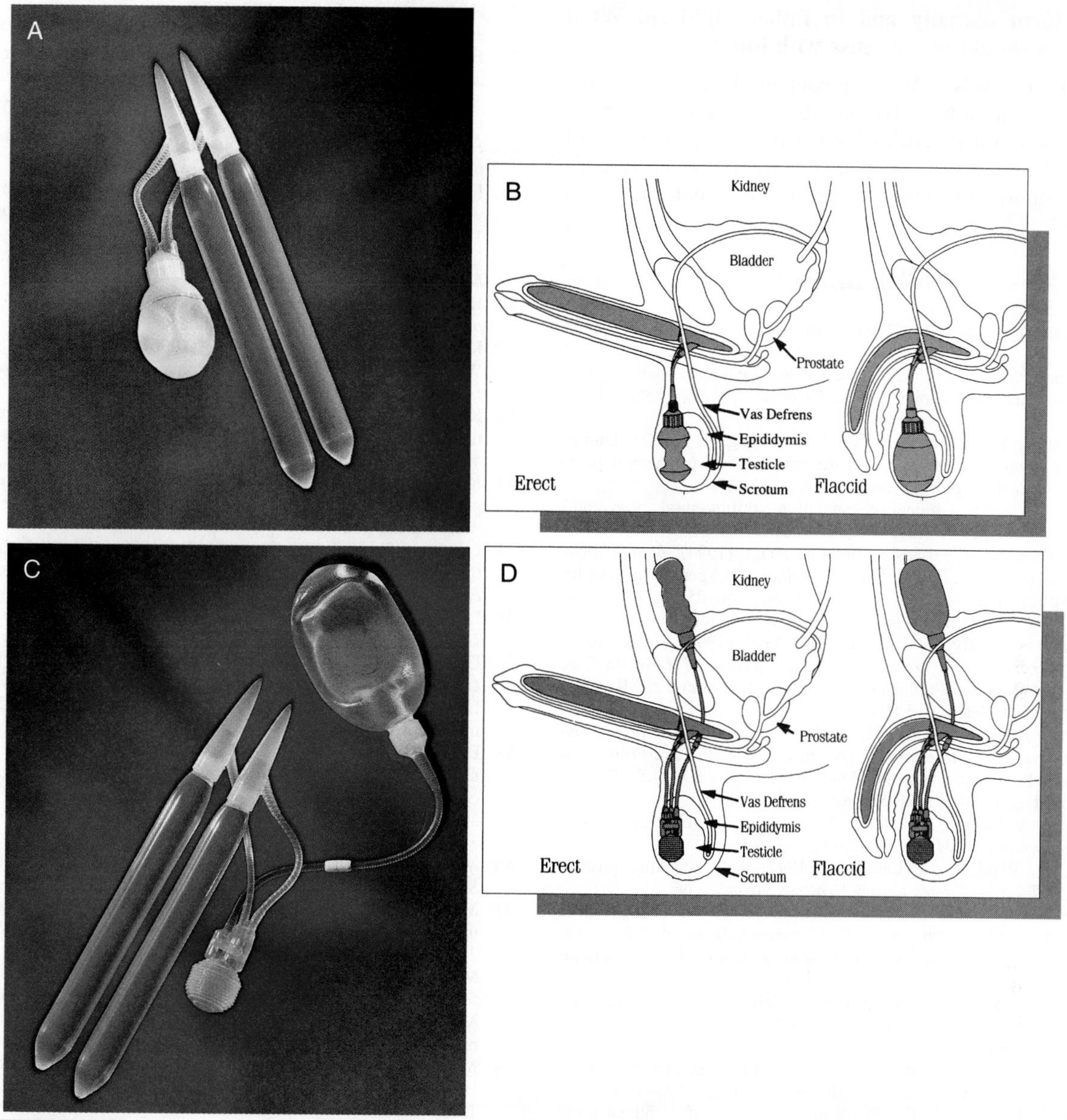

FIGURE 38–14 Penile prostheses. *A,* Mark II (two-piece inflatable penile prosthesis). *B,* Mark II prosthesis erect and flaccid. *C,* Alpha I (three-piece inflatable penile prosthesis). *D,* Alpha 1 prosthesis erect and flaccid. (Courtesy of Mentor, Santa Barbara, CA.)

CONCLUSIONS

Male genital and reproductive disorders can be complex problems for the client and the nurse. The client often finds that these disorders threaten sexuality and sexual function or normal urinary elimination. These effects may be physiologic, but complex psychosocial problems also arise.

Prostate disorders are among the most common problems experienced by clients throughout their lifetime. Cancers of the male reproductive tract can be life-threatening, but if they are detected early, they can be cured or at least controlled for long periods. Problems such as erectile dysfunction and infertility directly affect both partners, who experience the diagnostic and treatment phases together. The nurse acts as a caregiver, educator, support, and resource person.

THINKING CRITICALLY

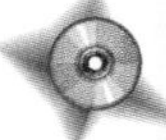

1. **Your client underwent a laser-assisted TURP yesterday. Closed bladder irrigation is being used, and his urine is dark to bright red with multiple clots. He is complaining of intense cramping pain in the lower abdomen. What further assessments should you make? What could be causing the cramping pain? What nursing action should you take?**

Factors to Consider. Is the dark to bright red urinary output normal at this stage? What does the nature of the client's pain tell you about its likely cause?

2. **A young man in his early 20s is given a diagnosis of testicular cancer, and he is very concerned about the treatment's effects on his ability to**

perform sexually and to father children. What issues should you discuss with him?

Factors to Consider. What impact might a bilateral orchiectomy or a radical lymph node dissection have on erectile function and fertility? What might be the effect of a unilateral orchiectomy? What options for fathering children are important to consider before the client undergoes treatment?

BIBLIOGRAPHY

1. American Cancer Society. (2000). *Cancer facts and figures.* Atlanta: Author.
2. Anderson, P., et al. (1998). Prostate disease patients: Planning services to meet their coping needs. *Urologic Nursing, 18*(3), 195–197.
3. Bartkiw, T., Kraetschmer, N., & Trachtenberg, J. (1997). Understanding microwave therapy as a treatment option for benign prostatic hyperplasia. *Urologic Nursing, 17*(2), 53–57.
4. Bates, P. (1997). Clinical conversation: Intraurethral alprostadil (MUSE). *Urologic Nursing, 17*(4), 159–161.
5. Benign Prostatic Hyperplasia Guideline Panel. (1994). *Benign prostatic hyperplasia: Clinical practice guideline* (Agency for Health Care Policy and Research Publication No. 94–0583). Rockville, MD: U.S. Department of Health and Human Services.
6. Benign Prostatic Hyperplasia Guideline Panel. (1994). *Benign prostatic hyperplasia: Diagnosis and treatment* (Agency for Health Care Policy and Research Publication No. 94-0582). Rockville, MD: U.S. Department of Health and Human Services.
7. Benign Prostatic Hyperplasia Guideline Panel. (1994). *Benign prostatic hyperplasia: Patient guide* (Agency for Health Care Policy and Research Publication No. 94-0584). Rockville, MD: U.S. Department of Health and Human Services.
8. Bosl, G., & Motzer, R. (1997). Testicular germ-cell cancer. *New England Journal of Medicine, 337*(4), 242–253.
9. Bruce, R., Waid, T., & Lucas, B. (1997). Understanding postobstructive diuresis. *Contemporary Urology*, *9*(6), 53–66.
10. Catalona, W., Smith, D., & Ornstein, D. (1997). Prostate cancer detection in men with serum PSA concentrations of 2.6 to 4.9 ng/ml and benign prostate examination. *Journal of the American Medical Association, 277*(18), 1452–1455.
11. Chin-A-Loy, S., & Fernsler, J. (1998). Self-transcendence in older men attending a prostate cancer support group. *Cancer Nursing, 21*(5), 358–363.
12. Colpo, L. (1998). Evaluation, treatment, and management of erectile dysfunction: An overview. *Urologic Nursing, 18*(2), 100–106.
13. D'Amico, A., et al. (1998). Biochemical outcome after radical prostatectomy, external beam radiation therapy, or interstitial radiation therapy for clinically localized prostate cancer. *Journal of the American Medical Association, 280*(11), 969–974.
14. Ebersole, M. (1996). Hormonal administration in prostate cancer: A caring approach. *Urologic Nursing, 16*(1), 23–26.
15. Elder, J., & Shapiro, E. (1998). Undescended testes. *Family Urology, 3*(1), 13–16.
16. Fox, S., et al. (1999). Male genitourinary cancer sexuality questionnaire. *Urologic Nursing, 19*(2), 101–107.
17. Gallo, M., & Fallon, P. (1996). Evaluation of a pelvic floor treatment plan for patients undergoing radical prostatectomy. *Urologic Nursing, 16*(1), 9–13.
18. Gordon, S., et al. (1997). When the dx is penile cancer. *RN, 60*(3), 41–45.
19. Gray, M. (1992). *Genitourinary disorders.* St. Louis: Mosby–Year Book.
20. Gray, M., & Allensworth, D. (1997). Medical management of benign prostatic hyperplasia. *Urologic Nursing, 17*(4), 137–141.
21. Gray, M., & Allensworth, D. (1999). Electrovaporization of the prostate: Initial experiences and nursing management. *Urologic Nursing, 19*(1), 25–31.
22. Gregoire, I. (1995). Pharmacologic erection program: An alternative solution for the man with erectile dysfunction. *Urologic Nursing, 15*(1), 10–13.
23. Gregoire, I., Kalogeropoulis, D., & Corcos, J. (1997). The effectiveness of a professionally led support group for men with prostate cancer. *Urology Nursing, 17*(2), 58–66.
24. Hanson, K., & Lieber, M. (1996). Role of a urology nurse in evaluating patients with prostatism. *Urologic Nursing, 16*(3), 108.
25. Harris, J. (1997). The prevalence of impotence after radical prostatectomy. *Urologic Nursing, 17*(4), 142–145.
26. Heyman, E., & Rosner, T. (1996). Prostate cancer: An intimate view from patients and wives. *Urologic Nursing, 16*(2), 37–44.
27. Hinman, F. (1998). *Atlas of urologic surgery* (2nd ed.). Philadelphia: W. B. Saunders.
28. Intili, H., & Nier, D. (1998). Self-esteem and depression in men who present with erectile dysfunction. *Urologic Nursing, 18*(3), 185–187.
29. Intili, H. (1998). Impotence and perceived partner support. *Urologic Nursing, 18*(4), 279–280, 287.
30. Karlowicz, K. A. (Ed.). (1995). *Urologic nursing: Principles and practice.* Philadelphia: W. B. Saunders.
31. Keetch, D. W., & Andriole, G. L. (1996). Prostate cancer screening: What are physicians to do? What have we learned? *Monographs in Urology, 17*(3), 31–48.
32. Kennedy, W., Huff, D., & Snyder, H. (1998). The value of testis biopsies in cryptorchidism. *Contemporary Urology, 10*(4), 46–57.
33. Kletscher, B., & Osterling, J. (1995). Prostatic stents: Current prospectives for the management of BPH. *Urologic Clinics of North America, 22*, 423–430.
34. Laumann, E., Paik, A., & Rosen, R. (1999). Sexual dysfunction in the United States: Prevalence and predictors. *Journal of the American Medical Association, 281*(6), 537–544.
35. Lipshultz, L. (1996). Is semen quality declining? *Contemporary Urology, 8*(9), 50–62.
36. Lipshultz, L. (1997). Medical therapies for erectile dysfunction. *Contemporary Urology, 9*(12), 34–45.
37. Lipshultz, L., & Meacham, R. (1998). Male infertility: Causes and management. *Family Urology, 3*(2), 19–22.
38. Lipski, B., Garcia, R., & Brawer, M. (1996). Prostatic intraepithelial neoplasia: Significance and management. *Seminars in Urologic Oncology, 14*(3), 149–155.
39. Maffeo, R. (1997). Managing testicular cancer. *Nursing, 27*(5), 32hn6–32hn8.
40. Moody, F. (1999). *Atlas of ambulatory surgery.* Philadelphia: W. B. Saunders.
41. Moore, K., & Estey, A. (1999). The early postoperative concerns of men after radical prostatectomy. *Journal of Advanced Nursing, 29*(5), 1121–1129.
42. Moore, R., Partin, A., & Marshall, F. (1997). LPLND or mini-lap for lymphadenectomy. *Contemporary Urology, 9*(4), 39–50.
43. Moul, J. (1998). Pelvic muscle rehabilitation in males following prostatectomy. *Urologic Nursing, 18*(4), 296–301.
44. Moul, J., & Lipo, D. (1999). Prostate cancer in the late 1990s: Hormone refractory disease options. *Urologic Nursing, 19*(2), 125–132.
45. Newton, M., & Kosier, J. (1998). Nonsteroidal anti-androgens: Role in treating advanced prostate cancer. *Urologic Nursing, 18*(1), 56–57, 83.
46. Ortega, A., & Cunha, B. (1997). The perplexing nature of prostatitis. *Contemporary Urology, 9*(5), 73–80.
47. Padma-Nathan, H. (1997). The future of pharmacological management of impotence. *Family Urology, 2*(1), 13–15.
48. Partin, A., et al. (1997). Combination of prostate-specific antigen, clinical stage, and Gleason score to predict pathological stage of localized prostate cancer. *Journal of the American Medical Association, 277*(18), 1445–1451.
49. Pound, C., et al. (1999). Natural history of progression after PSA elevation following radical prostatectomy. *Journal of the American Medical Association, 281*(17),1591–1597.
50. Prostate Health Council of the American Foundation for Urologic Disease. (1998). Survey on BPH awareness. Baltimore: Author.
51. Raper, J. (1995). Priapism: Causes and treatment. *Urologic Nursing, 15*(3), 75–79.
52. Ross, S. (1995). Getting beyond chronic nonbacterial prostatitis. *Urologic Nursing, 15*(2), 61–63.
53. Sabiston, D. (Ed.). (1997). *Textbook of surgery* (15th ed.). Philadelphia: W. B. Saunders.
54. Shipley, W., et al. (1999). Radiation therapy for clinically localized prostate cancer: A multi-institutional pooled analysis. *Journal of the American Medical Association, 281*(17), 1598–1604.
55. Sprouse, D. (1994). Fertility issues and anejaculation. *Urologic Nursing, 14*(2), 62–65.

56. Sprouse, D. O. (1995). Sexual rehabilitation of the prostate cancer patient. *Cancer Supplement, 75*(7), 1954–1956.
57. Stamey, T., et al. (1999). Biological determinants of cancer progression in men with prostate cancer. *Journal of the American Medical Association, 281*(15), 1395–1400.
58. Thompson, I., et al. (1995). Chemoprevention of prostate cancer. *Seminars in Urology, 23*(2), 122–129.
59. Tingen, M., et al. (1998). Perceived benefits: A predictor of participation in prostate cancer screening. *Cancer Nursing, 21*(5), 349–357.
60. Walsh, P., et al. (Eds.). (1998). *Campbell's urology* (7th ed.). Philadelphia: W. B. Saunders.
61. Watt, E., & Lillibridge, J. (1998). Time of day urinary catheters are removed. *Urologic Nursing, 18*(1), 23–25.
62. Witt, T., et al. (1998). Saw palmetto extracts for treatment of benign prostatic hyperplasia. *Journal of the American Medical Association, 280*(18), 1604–1608.
63. Witte, M., & Morton, R. (1997). Prostate cancer in high-risk groups: Searching for explanations. *Contemporary Urology, 6*(7), 52–63.
64. Zaccagnini, M. (1999). Prostate cancer. *American Journal of Nursing, 99*(4), 34–35.

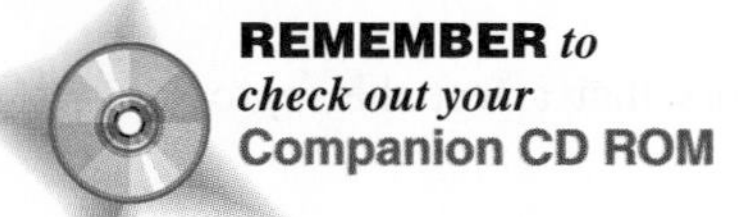

CHAPTER 39

Management of Women with Reproductive Disorders

Francie Bernier

NURSING OUTCOMES CLASSIFICATION (NOC)
for Nursing Diagnoses—Women with Reproductive Disorders

Constipation
Bowel Elimination
Hydration
Risk for Dysfunctional Grieving
Concentration
Coping
Family Coping
Grief Resolution
Psychosocial Adjustment: Life Change
Role Performance
Risk for Infection
Immune Status
Knowledge: Infection Control
Risk Control
Risk Control: Sexually Transmitted Diseases
Risk Detection
Tissue Integrity: Skin and Mucous Membranes
Treatment Behavior: Illness or Injury
Wound Healing: Primary Intention
Wound Healing: Secondary Intention

The major themes of all gynecologic disorders are sexuality and self-concept, including body image and self-esteem. Any disorder of the reproductive tract may lead to changes in sexual functioning or sexual identity. Change in sexual habits, such as abstinence from sexual activities or use of different positioning during vaginal intercourse, can be related to this diagnosis as well. The disorders and their treatments have the potential to change a woman's perceived or actual body structure, possibly leading to shame, embarrassment, and other negative emotions.

Alterations in sexuality and body image have a major effect on some women's feminine identity. Even in the 19th century, the common medical view was that the reproductive organs dominated a woman's body. Some aspects of this view, which reduces women's identity to the functioning of their body parts, persist in our culture today.

Contraception is a major health issue in various religious groups. Many religions, such as the Church of Jesus Christ of Latter-Day Saints (Mormons), the Roman Catholic Church, some Orthodox Jewish groups, and Baha'i, encourage followers to be fruitful and multiply. Sterilization and abortion are opposed by religious doctrine in many groups.

This chapter incorporates material written for the fifth edition by Elizabeth Carlson.

MENSTRUAL DISORDERS

CULTURAL INFLUENCES

Attitudes toward menstruation are often culturally based, and adolescent girls may be taught a variety of folk beliefs and practices at the time of puberty. Among Hispanic Americans, for example, menstruating females are not permitted to walk barefooted, wash their hair, or take showers or baths. Some Hispanic Americans believe that sour or iced foods cause menstrual blood to coagulate. Some Puerto Rican women have been taught that drinking lemon or pineapple juice will increase menstrual cramping. The nurse should be aware of these beliefs and respect cultural practices.

Some Arab women who practice Islam, such as Palestinians, Lebanese, Jordanians and Saudi Arabians, and some African women have ethnoreligious prohibitions and duties during and after menstruation. In Islam, blood is considered to be unclean (*najis*). The blood of menstruation, as well as blood lost during childbirth, renders the woman ritually impure. In Islamic legal language, the term used for menstruation is *hayz* and the menstruating woman is called *ha'iz*. Because one must be in a pure state in order to pray, the *ha'iz* are forbidden to perform certain acts of worship, such as touch the Koran, enter a mosque, pray, and participate in certain feasts. During the menstrual period, sexual intercourse is forbidden for both men and women. When the menstrual flow stops, the woman performs *ghusl*, a washing ritual to purify herself.

In the Navajo culture, a ceremony called the *kinaalda* announces the achievement of menarche (beginning of menstruation). Although fertility was the goal of the ceremony in the past, the most common reason for the *kinaalda* today is educational, to equip the girl to participate in society as an adult female. Menstruating Navajo women may not look at sand painting, enter a ceremonial *hogan*, attend or lead a sing, or join in the dancing that occurs at certain ceremonies.

In various cultures, menstruating women may be subject to restrictions on work and physical activities as well as rules related to the disposal of menstrual fluid and the proper disposal of sanitary napkins. Attitudes toward intercourse during menstruation are variable. Many religions also require or encourage women to engage in certain practices during and after menstruation. It is easy to understand why reproductive disorders can have such far-reaching effects on women.

REACTIONS TO MANIFESTATIONS

Women may experience some menstrual problems during their 30 or more years of menstruating. They tend to seek professional help for obvious abnormalities, such as excessive and irregular vaginal bleeding; however, they may not bring other menstrual problems to the attention of health care providers.

Women react to menstrual problems individually. Although some promptly seek health care, others do not, for various reasons. For example, one woman may hesitate and may be unable to discuss menstruation. She may view the subject as a personal and intimate problem that should be kept private. Another woman may have low self-esteem or may have been told that problems are to be expected. Therefore, she may dismiss her own complaints as unimportant or may not seek help, expecting the problems will disappear in time. Others may desire a relief of manifestations or may fear that the treatment will be worse than the problem. It is not uncommon for menstrual problems to remain undetected unless the nurse is skillful and sensitive in assessment. The nurse may identify a menstrual problem during a discussion of contraception or other needs. Some of the most common menstrual problems are dysmenorrhea (painful menstruation), premenstrual syndrome (PMS), and abnormal uterine bleeding.

DYSMENORRHEA

Dysmenorrhea is estimated to affect 30% to 75% of women. *Primary* dysmenorrhea is believed to be caused by either a prostaglandin excess or an increased sensitivity to prostaglandins with no underlying pathologic pelvic disorders. Prostaglandins are hormone-like secretions which cause smooth muscle contraction. *Secondary* dysmenorrhea begins with an underlying disease condition.

Etiology and Risk Factors

There are no preventive measures for dysmenorrhea, which has a variety of causes. The causes can be grouped according to five factors that affect the reproductive system in various ways:

- Elevated levels of uterine prostaglandins
- Endocrine factors
- Myometrial factors
- Biochemical factors
- Psychosocial factors

Secondary dysmenorrhea is suspected when pain is concentrated in a specific area, is unilateral, or begins after age 20 years. It may be caused by:

- Pelvic inflammatory disease (PID)
- Endometriosis
- Adenomyosis (invasion of uterine myometrium by endometrial tissue) (see Anatomy and Physiology Review at the beginning of this unit)
- Uterine prolapse
- Uterine myomas
- Polyps

Pathophysiology

Prostaglandin synthesis at the time of menstruation appears to produce strong myometrial contractions. The severe muscle spasms constrict blood vessels supplying the uterus, causing ischemia and pain. The excess prostaglandins in smooth muscle also help explain the presence of gastrointestinal (GI) manifestations, headache, and other manifestations.

Clinical Manifestations

Primary dysmenorrhea characteristically begins 1 to 2 months after menarche (onset of menses) in conjunction with ovulatory cycles. Generally, it increases in severity over several years with a decline when the woman reaches her mid-20s. Primary dysmenorrhea often decreases significantly after childbirth.

The discomfort of primary dysmenorrhea commonly begins 1 to 2 days before the onset of menstrual flow. The more severe discomfort is usually experienced during the first 24 hours of flow and typically subsides by the second day. More than half of the women experiencing dysmenorrhea also have systemic manifestations, such as nausea and vomiting, diarrhea, syncope, headache, and back pain.

Diagnosis is based on a thorough history, including medications used for symptomatic relief. A physical examination is performed to rule out underlying pathologic causes of dysmenorrhea.

Outcome Management

Medical Management

The current approach to primary dysmenorrhea emphasizes prevention and education. For women with mild manifestations who want to avoid medication, nonpharmacologic remedies might be effective. For example, biofeedback, Therapeutic Touch, or acupuncture might be helpful. Nutritional measures include decreasing the intake of sodium and increasing the intake of vitamin B_6, calcium, magnesium, and protein.

Administer Oral Contraceptives

If contraception as well as relief of dysmenorrhea is desired, combination oral contraceptives may relieve menstrual pain. The combination inhibits ovulation, resulting in decreased endometrial prostaglandin production and a concurrent reduction of uterine activity. For the woman with a contraceptive *intrauterine device* (IUD), removal of the IUD may lead to relief. Another form of contraception may be desired.

Promote Exercise

Exercise, such as aerobic exercise and swimming, has also been used as a remedy for dysmenorrhea. Exercise increases blood flow of beta-endorphins, the body's endogenous opiates, making them available for pain relief. The exact mechanism responsible for pain relief is not known.

Administer Prostaglandin Synthesis Inhibitors

Prostaglandin synthesis inhibitors (antiprostaglandin agents) may provide relief by decreasing prostaglandin activity, even in the presence of ovulatory cycles. Some commonly prescribed medications in this group are ibuprofen (Motrin), mefenamic acid (Ponstel), indomethacin (Indocin), and naproxen (Naprosyn). Ibuprofen (Advil) and naproxen (Aleve) are available as nonprescription drugs in lower doses, which makes them easy to obtain.

These medications may have GI side effects. Other possible side effects are sodium and water retention, rashes, and potential allergic reactions. For maximum effectiveness, the medications should be administered either before or at the onset of menses. Sometimes a client may have to try several prostaglandin synthesis inhibitors to find the one with maximum effectiveness for her.

Treatment of secondary dysmenorrhea is directed toward the underlying cause, such as endometriosis or PID (see later). Antiprostaglandin agents may provide some relief.

Nursing Management of the Medical Client

Education and supportive reassurance are important nursing interventions for clients with primary dysmenorrhea. Provide information about the mechanisms involved in dysmenorrhea and the actions and possible side effects of any prescribed medications. Assess the client's general health status. Encourage adequate nutrition, decreased caffeine intake, and appropriate rest, sleep, and exercise. Assess stress, which may increase manifestations, and explore methods of stress management.

Premenstrual Syndrome

Premenstrual syndrome is defined as a combination of emotional and physical manifestations that occur cyclically in the female before menstruation and regress or disappear during menstruation. PMS is somatic (a physical syndrome), not psychic, in origin. It is a complex mechanism involving not only the endocrine system but the autonomic and central nervous systems as well. A predominant alteration is the retention of body fluids.

The incidence of PMS is difficult to determine because of its variable manifestations and the lack of a clear understanding about the syndrome. PMS manifestations peak in women 30 to 40 years old. Variable reports in the literature indicate that 20% to 60% of all women experience some form of PMS.

Etiology and Risk Factors

The cause of PMS is unclear. However, neuroendocrine mechanisms appear to be involved. It is not clear whether PMS is a single syndrome or a group of separate disorders. Some suggested causes of PMS are as follows:

- Estrogen-progesterone imbalance, especially in estrogen excess and a progesterone deficiency, or estrogen deficiency at time of manifestations
- Interaction among estrogen, progesterone, and aldosterone
- Excess of prolactin, hypothyroidism, or hypoglycemia
- Dietary factors, such as deficiency of vitamin B_6, magnesium, or both
- Lifestyle factors, such as increased stress and poor diet

Health promotion and health maintenance activities include good nutrition, vitamin and mineral supplements, stress management, exercise, and rest.

Clinical Manifestations

Typically, manifestations of PMS appear during the last few premenstrual days and are relieved suddenly with full menstrual flow. However, manifestations may begin with ovulation and may not be relieved until during or toward the end of menses. Characteristically, manifestations gradually worsen until menses begin.

Various manifestations are attributable to PMS, including altered emotional states, behavioral changes, somatic problems, changes in appetite, and motor effects. Different sets of manifestations are experienced by individual women. Emotional manifestations may include tension, depression, irritability, hostility, insomnia, loneliness, a tendency to cry easily, and indecision. Forgetfulness and mental confusion may occur. Psychosis and suicidal tendencies are rare.

Somatic problems are headache, breast tenderness and abdominal bloating, peripheral edema, joint pain and backache, hives, constipation, and exacerbation of preexisting conditions, such as migraine and herpes. Because PMS manifestations usually do not occur during the menstrual flow, women may not associate them with the menstrual cycle.

To date, there is no objective method of diagnosing PMS. The diagnosis is usually made by documenting the cyclic nature of the manifestations on a menstrual calendar. A diary of manifestations and menstrual periods is an essential part of the assessment when PMS is suspected. Manifestations must occur for a minimum of three menstrual cycles. The diagnosis is confirmed according to the timing of manifestations rather than on the presence of particular manifestations.

Outcome Management

Medical Management

Relieve Manifestations

Vitamins and Minerals. Daily intake of vitamin B_6 and elimination of caffeine have improved some premenstrual manifestations. Nonprescription over-the-counter medications include calcium, vitamins A and C, magnesium, and trace elements. Essential fatty acid supplements are often recommended.

MEDICATIONS. Prescription medications commonly include oral spironolactone (Aldactone), progesterone, oral contraceptives, and anti-anxiety agents.

Spironolactone is a synthetic steroid aldosterone antagonist that inhibits the physiologic effect of aldosterone on the distal renal tubules. It is commonly used to treat the edema associated with excessive aldosterone secretion.

Progesterone may relieve physiologic and psychological manifestations. Bromocriptine (Parlodel) reduces serum prolactin concentrations by inhibiting prolactin release from the anterior pituitary gland. It has been used successfully to reduce breast pain in some cases of PMS.

Sedatives and analgesics, including antiprostaglandin agents, are often prescribed. Antidepressants may be prescribed for severe PMS.

See Alternative Therapy feature, p. 1009.

Nursing Management of the Medical Client

Nurses are in a key position to help women identify and cope with PMS when it is present. Clients who are in poor physical condition may be particularly susceptible to premenstrual difficulties. Thus, the nursing assessment includes general lifestyle, sleep and dietary habits, and overall health maintenance.

PROVIDE EDUCATION

Once the diagnosis of PMS is confirmed, the client needs accurate information about the syndrome and reassurance about the physiologic basis of the manifestations. Women often benefit from the opportunity to talk about their feelings and experiences with PMS, especially because of the confusion and misconceptions surrounding the syndrome. Instructions on how to take medications, if ordered, are important.

ENCOURAGE LIFESTYLE MODIFICATIONS

Suggested dietary modifications include reducing intake of salt and refined carbohydrates. Eating small, frequent meals to stabilize blood glucose levels can decrease fatigue, irritability, and craving. A calcium intake of at least 1000 mg/day may also decrease manifestations. Other vitamins and minerals have already been discussed along with medical management.

It may also be helpful to reduce alcohol and caffeine intake and to stop smoking. Give careful attention to stress management and reduction.

Weight reduction, if applicable, may decrease manifestations. Daily exercise (such as aerobics, jogging, or swimming) has been recommended to improve circulation, reduce stress, and promote a sense of well-being.

IMPROVE COPING

Another major nursing responsibility is helping the client and her significant others cope with the manifestations of PMS. Keep in mind the client's particular lifestyle and preferences. For example, a reallocation of responsibilities within the family might help to reduce her stress. If the client prefers to retain her current responsibilities, explain how she might manage them in ways that minimize stress.

Support groups or educational sessions may be helpful as well. These sessions can serve as a forum for sharing information, providing mutual support, and discussing feelings. You can help form such a group if none exist in the area.

ABNORMAL UTERINE BLEEDING

Abnormal uterine bleeding encompasses a wide variety of menstrual disorders, such as lack of menstrual flow and irregular or excessive uterine bleeding. Changes in menstrual patterns can create anxiety in any woman. Associated manifestations disrupt activities of daily living. Sometimes abnormal uterine bleeding indicates an underlying pathologic disease. The term *dysfunctional uterine bleeding* refers to abnormal uterine bleeding for which no organic cause can be found through the usual assessment techniques. The presence of abnormal uterine bleeding necessitates careful assessment by a qualified health care provider.

AMENORRHEA

Amenorrhea means the absence of menses. *Primary* amenorrhea occurs if a woman has not begun to menstruate by the age of 16. *Secondary* amenorrhea is the absence of menses for 6 months in a woman who previously had regular cyclic bleeding or 12 months in a woman with a history of irregular bleeding.

Etiology and Risk Factors

There are many causes of amenorrhea, and they may appear alone or in combination (Fig. 39–1).

Clinical Manifestations

Results of the physical examination are usually normal. Laboratory tests and on occasion, endometrial biopsy may be used to identify and treat amenorrhea.

Outcome Management

Medical Management

Treatment depends on the woman's needs and the cause of the amenorrhea. Particularly important are her wishes regarding childbearing. If pregnancy is not desired at this time, progesterone may be prescribed. If pregnancy is desired, ovulation induction with clomiphene citrate (Clomid) may be undertaken.

Nursing Management of the Medical Client

RULE OUT PREGNANCY

The absence of spontaneous menstrual flow in a female older than 16 years requires careful assessment, including history and physical examination. Pregnancy also must be ruled out for any woman of childbearing age experiencing secondary amenorrhea. Ask about the presence of manifestations of pregnancy, such as breast tenderness, nausea, urinary frequency, weight gain, fatigue, and changes in food tolerance. Even if the client has been consistently using birth control, pregnancy must be considered.

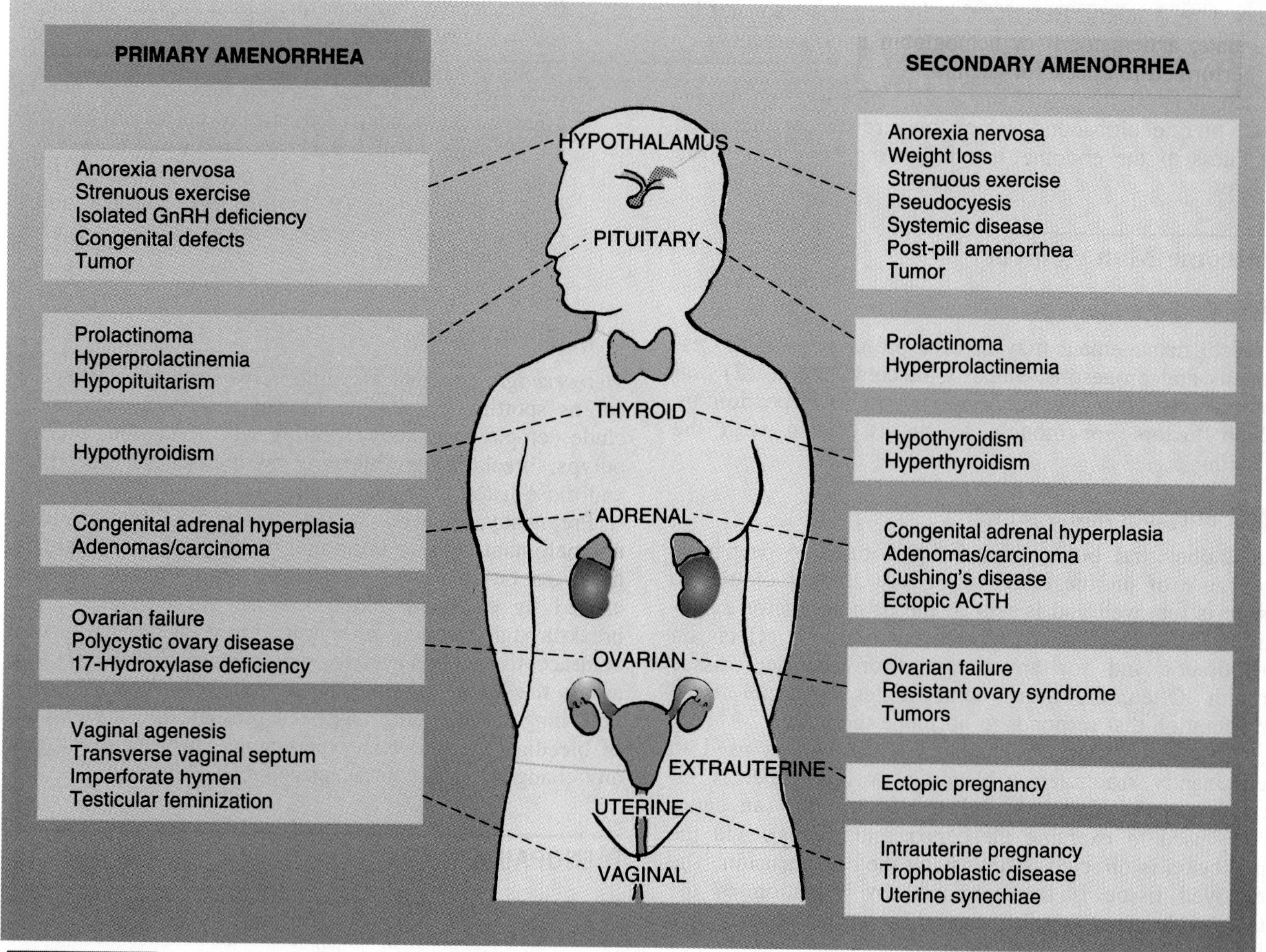

FIGURE 39–1 Causes of amenorrhea. GnRH, gonadotropin-releasing hormone; ACTH, adrenocorticotropin-releasing hormone.

Young girls may deny having had sexual intercourse (penile penetration), but may admit, on careful questioning, that they have engaged in sexual play involving ejaculation between the thighs or near the introitus (opening into the vagina). Pregnancy can result from the migration of sperm in these situations, and a pregnancy test is necessary. If the pregnancy test result is positive, an ultrasound study should be performed to determine fetal size and to confirm estimated date of confinement (EDC). Additionally, if the test result is positive, the client should be offered appropriate opportunity to discuss her wishes about continuing or terminating the pregnancy.

Provide Teaching

Teaching opportunities are an important part of nursing care. Depending on the cause of amenorrhea, the client may need help in reducing energy drain from excessive physical activity and in controlling stress. Assess her general health, and help her plan and make changes as indicated.

■ MENORRHAGIA

The term *menorrhagia* means excessive vaginal bleeding at normal intervals.

Etiology and Risk Factors

There are a number of causes of menorrhagia, including:

- Anovulatory menstrual cycles
- Uterine fibroids and adenomyosis
- Anatomic lesions
- Spontaneous abortion
- Inflammatory processes (e.g., endometritis and salpingitis)
- Blood dyscrasias (disordered cellular elements)
- Hypothyroidism
- Use of an IUD
- Endometrial carcinoma
- Medications (e.g., anticoagulants)

Clinical Manifestations

Assessing the amount of blood loss can be difficult. Many women are unable to give a reliable history of blood loss. Asking the client to compare the number of pads or tampons used during the abnormal period with the number used during a normal cycle is a way of determining abnormality. Significant blood loss may be considered if the client is changing her pad or tampon every 1 to 2 hours. Because this information may not be adequate, a hematocrit or hemoglobin measurement may be performed to check for anemia.

Another test for significant uterine bleeding is transvaginal uterine ultrasound, which may reveal an increased thickness of the endometrium indicating abnormal tissue growth.

Outcome Management

Medical Management

Medical management may involve prescription of (1) estrogens and progestins, alone or in combination, (2) oral contraceptives, or (3) antifibrinolytic agents, depending on which factors are thought to be associated with the bleeding.

Surgical Management

An endometrial biopsy may be performed to determine the cause of uterine bleeding. A tiny amount of uterine tissue is removed and is sent to the pathologist for evaluation. The specimen is analyzed for hormone effects on the tissues and for any irregular or abnormal tissue growth. Often, the tissue demonstrates abnormal tissue proliferation that responds to hormone therapy.

Outpatient endometrial ablation (removal) is used to permanently stop uterine bleeding. A laser fiber is inserted into the uterus through a hysteroscope (an endoscope used to examine the cervix and uterus), and the laser beam is directed at destroying the endometrium. The destroyed tissue is then removed by irrigation of the uterus with saline. Sterility caused by uterine scarring is a likely consequence of the procedure.

Nursing Management of the Surgical Client

Other than an explanation of biopsy and the obtaining of informed consent for the procedure, no preoperative care is required before an endometrial biopsy, although emotional support is indicated. For an ablation, preoperative care includes having the client restrict food and fluid intake for anesthesia. The client is placed in the lithotomy position for this procedure.

Postoperatively, a perineal pad is in place. The pad should be checked and changed frequently. There may also be vaginal packing, which is usually removed within 24 hours.

During the first few hours, monitor vital signs and assess for excessive vaginal bleeding. Assess the client's ability to urinate. Urination may be difficult, especially if vaginal packing is exerting pressure on the urethra. Report excess bleeding, inability to void, or excessive pain. The client usually experiences only minimal uterine cramping postoperatively. Mild analgesics, such as acetaminophen and codeine (Tylenol No. 3) usually relieve any discomfort. The client should avoid aspirin for the first 24 to 48 hours to prevent excessive bleeding.

Follow-up instructions are as follows:

1. Avoid strenuous activity for about 1 week.
2. Do not douche or engage in vaginal or rectal intercourse until your physician judges that healing is complete.
3. Expect a small amount of pinkish vaginal discharge, followed by a dark red or dark brown discharge, during the healing process.
4. Subsequent menstrual periods may or may not be affected. Your next menses may not occur, may be on schedule, or may vary from the usual time.
5. Call your physician if any complications such as excessive bleeding (more than one pad per hour), excessive pain, or temperature elevation of greater than 100° F occur.
6. Return for a follow-up appointment.

METRORRHAGIA

Metrorrhagia (vaginal bleeding between menses) may occur as spotting or outright bleeding. Possible causes include ectopic pregnancy, spotting with ovulation, cervical polyps, breakthrough bleeding with oral contraceptives, and those listed for menorrhagia.

Pregnancy, as well as the presence of malignant or nonmalignant cells or hormonal or physical abnormalities, needs to be ruled out or treated appropriately. Anemia caused by excessive blood loss should be treated. For breakthrough bleeding in conjunction with the use of oral contraceptives or *hormone replacement therapy* (HRT), assess the length of time the hormones have been given, how long the bleeding has been present, and the amount of bleeding the client is experiencing in order to suggest any change in oral contraceptive or HRT dosing.

MENOPAUSE

Physiologic menopause (cessation of menstruation) is discussed in the Anatomy and Physiology Review.

SURGICAL MENOPAUSE

Menopause may be induced at any age by surgical removal of the ovaries, ablation with chemicals, or pelvic irradiation. *Hysterectomy* is the removal of only the uterus, not the ovaries, and does not usually cause surgical menopause. On occasion, the surgical intervention may have menopausal manifestations. In these instances, it is possible that blood vessels supplying the ovaries have been injured. The resulting loss of blood supply causes the ovaries to atrophy. Another possible cause is the hormone imbalance produced by removal of the uterus and its loss as a hormone receptor.

PERIMENOPAUSAL CHANGES

A wide variety of physical and psychosocial manifestations have been attributed to the perimenopausal period, but the only manifestations due to menopause itself (not the associated changes that are due to aging or stressful life events) are vasomotor instability, menstrual irregularities, and vaginal changes. A positive clinical manifestation is a follicle-stimulating hormone (FSH) level greater than 40 mIu/ml, indicating the intense attempt of the pituitary gland to stimulate the ovaries to produce estrogen, with the subsequent low serum estradiol level.

VASOMOTOR INSTABILITY. Manifestations of vasomotor instability, such as "hot flashes," night sweats, and the occasional palpitations and dizziness associated with menopause, appear to be caused by hormonal changes.

Hot flashes are sudden involuntary waves of heat that begin in the upper chest or neck and proceed up the face and head. These sensations last from a few seconds to an hour and are exacerbated by anything that increases heat production in the body. A hot flash may or may not be accompanied by a *hot flush,* which consists of a measurable change in skin temperature, a visible pink to bright red change in the skin, and perspiration.

A *night sweat* is a hot flash with or without a hot flush that occurs in the night, is accompanied by perspiration, which can be profuse, and is often followed by chills. Voda[37] describes the following types of hot flashes:

1. *Mild hot flash.* A warm feeling, often so fleeting it is barely noticeable. May or may not be accompanied by dampness and slight flushing.
2. *Moderate hot flash.* A warm to extremely warm feeling, that lasts longer and is more noticeable than a mild hot flash. Often accompanied by sweat and sometimes by flushing.
3. *Severe hot flash.* An intense or extremely hot feeling, usually accompanied by profuse and very uncomfortable sweating or flushing. The thermal discomfort of a severe hot flash may lead a woman to stop her activity at the time of the hot flash and to seek relief by using a fan, showering, removing or changing clothes, or lying down. Other bodily sensations associated with a severe hot flash are feelings of waves of heat, dizziness, a feeling of suffocation, inability to concentrate, and chest pain.

Generally, the manifestations of the hot flash occur about 45 seconds before the hot flush. In perimenopausal women, the reported incidence of the hot flash varies from 68% to 92%. There is a great variance in both the quantitative and qualitative aspects of women's experiences of hot flashes. Women in other cultures do not all report experiencing hot flashes; thus, the hot flash may not be a universal manifestation, or it may not be culturally acceptable for women to discuss menopausal manifestations.

Atrophic Vaginitis and Other Changes. The vaginal mucous membrane is especially responsive to low estrogen levels. When these levels remain low both during and following menopause, the vaginal walls become thinner and drier, with greater sensitivity and susceptibility to infection. These changes lead to the manifestations of atrophic vaginitis in menopausal women. Other manifestations are vaginal irritation, burning, pruritus, increased leukorrhea (vaginal discharge), bleeding, and dyspareunia (difficult or painful intercourse).

Vaginal epithelium loses its elasticity and subcutaneous fat after menopause. Pubic hair may become thinner. As the epidermal layer thins, the labia minora flatten and become flush with the labia majora. Other urogenital changes may be related to the loss of the estrogen-rich mucosal layer of the urethra and urethral atrophy associated with a higher incidence of cystitis and urethritis. In addition, these manifestations may also be confused with a urinary tract infection (UTI) or vaginitis.[4]

The pubococcygeus muscles tend to lose their tone, and stress urinary incontinence (see Chapter 34) also may occur. In addition, manifestations of urge incontinence, such as urgency, frequency and urine loss, may increase and may be confused with persistent UTI.

Some women experience difficulty sleeping. Others have backache, joint pain, and other manifestations of osteoporosis (a skeletal disorder characterized by the loss of bone mass and bone calcium). The calcium loss leads to an increased predisposition to bone collapse or fracture. Estrogen has been clinically proven to inhibit bone breakdown and loss. A decrease or absence of estrogen in conjunction with other risk factors may lead to osteoporosis.

Many myths abound about the occurrence of depression at the time of menopause, but no relationship between depression and menopause has been demonstrated. Some women appear to complain of depression or emotional changes at menopause more than at any other time in their lives. A woman's experience of menopause is affected not only by hormonal changes but also by her life circumstances and relationships. Psychosocial stress at the time of menopause, however, may affect menopausal manifestations.

Outcome Management

Medical Management

Replace Hormones

Hormone replacement therapy (estrogen plus progesterone) may be part of the medical management of perimenopausal, menopausal, and postmenopausal manifestations. Women must be informed of the advantages and risks of HRT so that they can make informed decisions about treatment. Some studies of the benefits and risks of the long-term use of HRT have demonstrated a decrease in incidence of cardiovascular disease, osteoporosis, Alzheimer's disease, and urogenital dysfunction.

It is often difficult for women to decide to begin and continue HRT because of conflicting information and fears related to a rise in the incidence of breast and uterine cancer associated with the treatment. Some researchers have claimed that the risk of breast cancer actually decreases with HRT, although further study is necessary to support this claim. HRT alleviates vasomotor instability, vaginal and urinary tract atrophy, and dyspareunia. It is also a preventive measure against osteoporosis and, possibly, cardiovascular disease.

In the middle to late 1970s, evidence of an association between *estrogen replacement therapy* (ERT) and endometrial cancer was discovered. In subsequent years, this association has been studied extensively. Today, estrogen is given with a progestational agent to simulate normal endometrial tissue. The progestin provides a protective effect against endometrial cancer. *Unopposed ERT* (estrogen without progestin) is no longer recommended for a woman with an intact uterus. It is generally accepted that estrogens should not be given to women with the following features:

- Known or suspected breast or uterine cancer or any estrogen-dependent cancer (or a strong family history of the same)
- Undiagnosed abnormal uterine bleeding
- Previous or present thrombophlebitis
- Acute liver disease
- Risk factors such as obesity, varicosities, hypertension, and heavy smoking, which become even more significant when they occur in combination
- Additional risk factors related to uterine fibromyomas,

severe varicose veins, chronic hepatic dysfunction, and diabetes mellitus, which require thorough assessment before estrogen is prescribed

The use of ERT or HRT should be individualized according to the client's needs and wishes, individual manifestations, and risks. The risk for women with fibrocystic breast disease is unclear, but careful assessment must be made. Risks should be assessed for endometrial cancer, osteoporosis, cardiovascular disease, and breast cancer. Both ERT and HRT are effective against perimenopausal hot flashes, atrophic vaginitis, and urinary tract changes. Unless otherwise indicated, HRT or ERT should be considered lifelong replacement therapy. Dosage may decrease with the client's age. Some recent research suggests that hormone replacement therapy be taken for only 5 years.

Both ERT and HRT decrease the risk of osteoporosis. The optimal duration of therapy for osteoporosis prevention is not known but is considered lifelong. Raloxifene (Evista) is a medication that prevents osteoporosis and may provide cardioprotective effects without increasing cancer risk. The possible cardioprotective effects of ERT, HRT, and raloxifene are being investigated. Hormone therapy is considered replacement of female hormones and should be discussed as such with the client before it is started.

If a client opts for ERT or HRT, she should be monitored for the development of breast cancer or any complication with annual breast examinations and mammography. Women must receive adequate education regarding the risk factors and anticipated effects of HRT as well as signals of impending problems it may cause.

Treatment regimens vary for estrogen-progesterone combinations. In some cases, estrogens may be used for 25 days each month or continually, whereas progesterones may be prescribed for 10 to 14 days a month. A low-dose continuous progesterone therapy may be given along with continuous ERT. The advantage of continuous combined therapy is the elimination of withdrawal bleeding. Bleeding usually ceases in about 4 months.

Side effects of high-dose progesterone therapy include bloating, depression, acne, breast tenderness, and premenstrual tension; however, these effects can generally be lessened by adjusting the dose, as with continuous therapy, or lengthening the duration of therapy. Side effects of progesterone may unfavorably alter the ratio of high-density-lipoprotein (HDL) and low-density-lipoprotein (LDL) cholesterol. Therefore, unopposed estrogen has been recommended for the client whose uterus has been surgically removed.

Transdermal estrogen patches are an alternative when oral estrogens cannot be tolerated or when the hepatic effects of estrogen (increased secretion of renin substrate causing hypertension and increased clotting factors as a result of liver stimulation) are a problem.

Vaginal estrogen is indicated for any woman experiencing urogenital manifestations of menopause (e.g., atrophic vaginitis, incontinence, and vaginal dryness). Vaginal estrogen can be delivered in continuous dosing, such as in a vaginal ring that is changed every 3 months. A small amount of vaginal cream, 0.5 to 1 g, can be inserted into the vagina at bedtime, several times per week.

Nursing Management of the Medical Client

PROVIDE EDUCATION

Nurses have a unique role in providing education for women undergoing menopause and their partners or significant others. The role involves providing support, education, and assistance in moving through this normal life experience as comfortably as possible. Accurate information about menopause and what to expect can be helpful and reassuring. Provide educational information about the risks and benefits of estrogen therapy.

To help clients cope with the minor discomforts of menopause, you may recommend the following self-care advice:

1. *Relief of vaginal dryness.* Intercourse and masturbation aid circulation and keep tissues flexible; use water-soluble vaginal lubricants as often as needed. Topical estrogen cream or other vaginal estrogen preparations eliminate manifestations.
2. *Prevention of osteoporosis.* Take part in weight-bearing exercises; increase calcium intake; stop smoking; reduce alcohol and caffeine intake.
3. *Prevention of UTIs.* Increase fluid intake (six to eight glasses of water per day; attempt to void every 2 to 3 hours; maintain good perineal hygiene; wear cotton underwear.
4. *Pelvic relaxation.* Perform Kegel (pelvic floor) exercises to increase muscle tone (see later and Chapter 34); lose weight if appropriate.

Remind women experiencing menopause of the value of good health habits. Balanced nutrition and adequate sleep and rest are important. Phytoestrogens (plant estrogens), found in soy products, flaxseed oil, nuts, and brown rice, have a very mild estrogenic effect that may reduce vaginal dryness. Exercising at least three to four times per week for 45 minutes improves bone and cardiovascular health.

See Alternative Therapy feature, p. 1009.

POSTMENOPAUSAL BLEEDING

Postmenopausal bleeding (vaginal bleeding occurring after menopause) is a manifestation, not a diagnosis (Fig. 39–2). Careful assessment is necessary because it may be a manifestation of many conditions of the lower reproductive tract: atrophic vaginitis, cervical polyps, uterine fibroids, endometrial hyperplasia, cervical erosion, and uterine or cervical cancer.

PELVIC INFLAMMATORY DISEASE

The term *pelvic inflammatory disease* refers to ascending pelvic infection that involves the upper genital tract.

Etiology and Risk Factors

Chlamydia trachomatis, gonococci, staphylococci, streptococci, and other pus-producing (pyogenic) organisms commonly cause PID. A common risk factor is an untreated bacterial infection. Most of these infections are sexually transmitted. The lack of condom use increases the risk of passing the bacteria between partners.

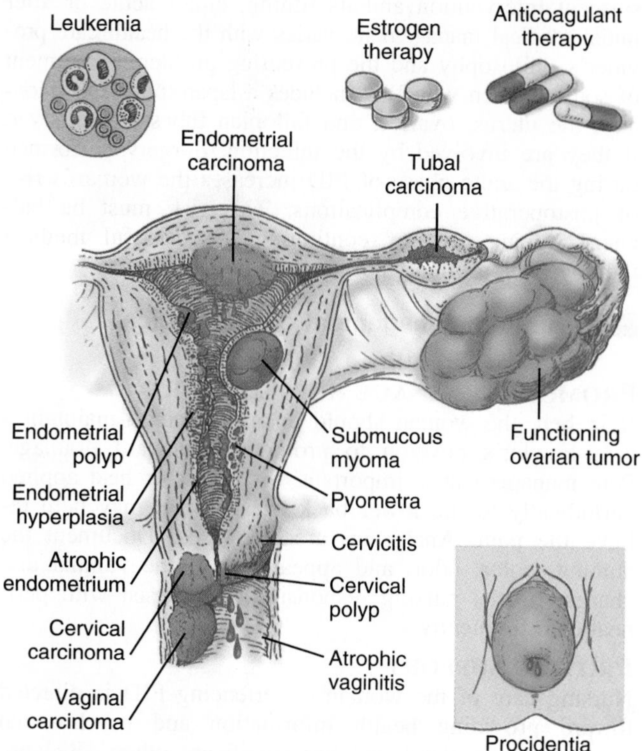

FIGURE 39–2 Causes of postmenopausal bleeding.

Health promotion actions are to advise clients to avoid (1) unprotected intercourse, (2) sex with multiple partners, especially with use of an IUD, (3) IUD for birth control, and (4) douches. To maintain health, clients should seek treatment immediately when manifestations of PID appear and if a sexual partner has a sexually transmitted disease (STD).

Health restoration activities include advising clients to complete the full course of medications used to treat a PID and to follow health promotion recommendations to prevent reinfection.

Pathophysiology

Once an infection is in the upper genital tract, the bacteria may travel along several routes (Fig. 39–3). Tuberculosis (TB), a rare cause of PID, travels through the blood and affects the fallopian tubes and sometimes the ovaries, uterus, and pelvic peritoneum. The woman's excreta are contaminated until the antituberculin medications have taken effect.

C. trachomatis and gonococcal and staphylococcal organisms spread along the uterine endometrium to the fallopian tubes, where an acute *salpingitis* (inflammation of the fallopian tubes) occurs. The tubes become partially occluded and may drain pus, leukocytes, and other debris into the pelvic cavity, causing pelvic peritonitis, or the material may form a pocket around the ovary, causing a tubo-ovarian abscess.

Streptococci spread similarly, but they tend to travel via the uterine or cervical lymphatics across the parametrium to the tubes or ovaries. Pelvic cellulitis and occasional thrombophlebitis of the major pelvic veins with additional risk of the development of emboli may occur. Another route of infection is from the pelvic cavity itself. Organisms such as *Escherichia coli* may be extruded from a ruptured bowel, causing peritonitis.

Although septic shock and other complications may appear, the most common is a pelvic abscess.

More than 50% of women with a history of PID have difficulty becoming pregnant or experience an ectopic pregnancy after the infection has cleared. These problems are due to scarring by the inflammatory process and subsequent closing and scarring of the fallopian tubes.

Clinical Manifestations

PID may be "silent" (asymptomatic), especially in the early stage. Clinical manifestations of PID include malaise, fever, chills, anorexia, nausea and vomiting, aching and tachycardia. In addition, the woman usually experiences acute, sharp, severe aching pain on both sides of the abdomen or pelvis. Pain is worsened by urination or defecation and may be accompanied by a heavy, purulent, and, possibly, odorous discharge. Occasionally, vaginal bleeding occurs. The rapidity of onset of PID depends on (1) the virulence (degree of severity) of the infecting organism, (2) the status of the client's pelvic organs, and (3) the client's general health.

Other helpful clues to PID are obtained from the history. A history of acute lower genital tract infection is significant. Other data, including a thorough sexual history, are important. A history of contraceptive use is established because the presence of an IUD correlates with a higher incidence of PID.

The long-term sequelae of untreated, silent PID may be detected when attempts to achieve a pregnancy have proved unsuccessful. During a clinical evaluation of the client, routine screening tests, such as cultures, may yield

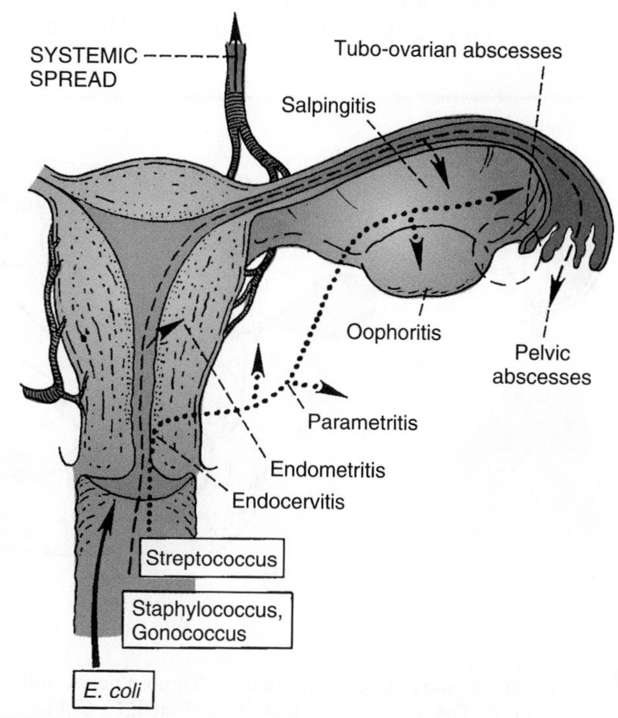

FIGURE 39–3 Routes of spread of pelvic inflammatory disease.

positive results. The usual laboratory tests for infection, including multiple cultures (Fig. 39–4), are performed. Some practitioners perform a culture of any evident drainage and obtain specimens from various sites, such as the cervix, vagina, and urethra. Additional specimens from the vagina and the adjacent structures may be obtained to evaluate for bacterial infection of the genital tract. If multiple organisms are found, several types of antibiotics may be necessary to treat the infection.

Histologic examination of endometrial biopsy specimens, colposcopy (examination with use of a large color-filtering, magnifying instrument), or ultrasonography to identify an abscess may also be used in the diagnosis of PID.

Outcome Management

Medical Management

ELIMINATE CAUSATIVE ORGANISM

Most clients with PID are treated as outpatients, receiving antibiotics appropriate to the specific organism causing the infection. They are cautioned to avoid sexual activity, douching, and other activities that might enhance the infectious process. With improvement, the client should return to the clinic in a week for reevaluation of status. Advise the client being treated at home for PID to return sooner if her condition deteriorates or if manifestations increase.

Hospitalization may be necessary for a client with PID who is acutely ill. During hospitalization, antibiotics are administered in maximal doses if the cause of PID is bacterial; PID resulting from TB is treated with antituberculosis medications. Treatment with medication is aimed at removing or destroying the causative organism.

Surgical Management

Some abscesses must be removed by surgical intervention. Others may rupture, causing peritonitis. The type of surgical intervention and its timing, either acute or after initial medical management, varies with the health care provider's philosophy and the presenting problem. Treatment of some women with PID includes a laparotomy. Occasionally, the uterus, ovaries, and fallopian tubes are removed if they are involved by the infection. Surgery performed during the acute phase of PID increases the woman's risk of postoperative complications. This risk must be balanced against that of continuing unsuccessful medical therapy, which often leads to chronic PID.

Nursing Management of the Medical-Surgical Client

PROMOTE DRAINAGE AND COMFORT

If in bed, the woman should be instructed to maintain a semi-Fowler's position to promote downward drainage. Pain management is important. Sitz baths or heat applied periodically to the lower back or abdomen may help relieve the pain. Analgesics are also used. Document the amount, color, odor, and appearance of the vaginal discharge. It is a nursing responsibility to assist with perineal care frequently.

PROVIDE SUPPORT

Nursing care of the woman experiencing PID is directed toward providing health information and psychosocial support to the client and her significant others. Because PID is often caused by STDs, there may be guilt feelings and emotional stress within the relationship. Usually, the woman's sexual partner requires treatment whether symptomatic or not.

Some women are infertile after PID. This loss of fertility may be difficult for the client and her significant other to accept. Plan and provide time for the expression of such feelings.

PROVIDE EDUCATION

Education is important for the client with PID. Women with PID can benefit from factual discussion about the

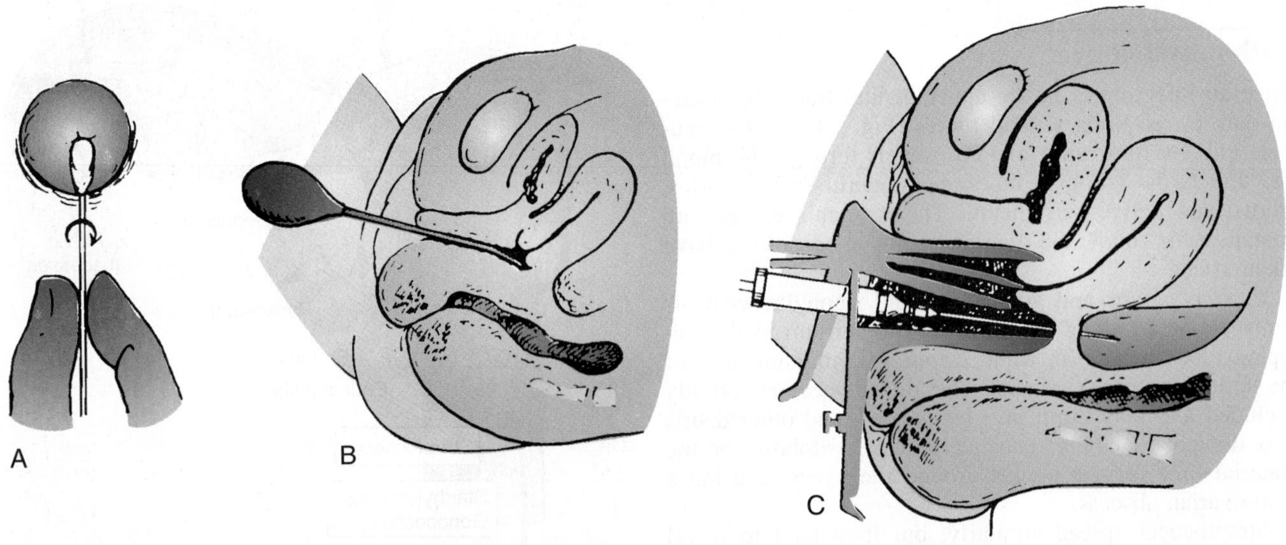

FIGURE 39–4 Some procedures used to diagnose pelvic inflammatory disease. *A*, Swabs may be obtained from the cervix, urethra, and rectum. *B*, The vaginal pool may be aspirated. *C*, Culdocentesis may be performed. Gram's stains of cervical secretions show gram-negative intracellular diplococci. Cultures are placed on Thayer-Martin medium. Negative stains and cultures do not rule out gonococcal disease.

infection, recognizing the manifestations of recurrences, and general hygienic and sexual measures to help prevent new infections. The client should be instructed to wash the perineal area regularly with soap and water, to wipe the perineum from front to back after elimination, to change tampons and pads several times a day during menses, and to wash hands before and after changing tampons or pads.

Balanced nutrition, adequate rest, sleep, and exercise can improve general health and reduce the risk of infection. Inform clients when sexual activity can be resumed, how to ensure the safety of sexual encounters, and when other restrictions can be lifted.

CHRONIC PELVIC INFLAMMATORY DISEASE

Chronic PID can occur if the acute phase of the illness does not respond to treatment or if treatment is inadequate. Clinical manifestations of chronic PID include chronic pelvic discomfort, menstrual disturbances or dysfunctional uterine bleeding, constipation, malaise, and periodic return of acute manifestations. Sterility, one of the more serious complications, results from destruction of part of the fallopian tubes and loss of their patency (their being wide open).

Treatment of chronic PID is aimed at removing the offending organism and improving the client's general health. If treatment is unsuccessful, surgical removal of the pelvic organs may be necessary.

UTERINE DISORDERS

ENDOMETRIOSIS

Endometriosis is an abnormal condition in which *endometrium*, the tissue that normally lines the uterus, is located in internal sites other than in the uterus. Endometriosis most commonly affects women in their mid-30s. It occasionally occurs in women younger than 20 years of age. There is a familial predisposition, and the highest incidence is in white women who are nulliparous (have not given birth).

Etiology and Risk Factors

The cause of endometriosis is unknown, although a few theories have been proposed, for instance:

1. *Retrograde menstruation theory.* Menstrual secretions flow backward through the fallopian tubes and deposit particles of viable endometrial tissue outside the uterine cavity. Spread then occurs as endometrial tissue reproduces itself, a process called *metaplasia.*
2. *Vascular and lymphatic dissemination theory.* Spread (metastasis) of endometrial tissue occurs through the lymphatic and vascular systems to locations outside the uterus. This may explain some of the distant sites of metastasis, such as the lungs and kidneys.

Pathophysiology

Although the abnormally located endometrial tissue is usually confined to the pelvic cavity, it may be found in other areas. The most common sites are the ovary and the dependent portion of the pelvic peritoneum. Rarely, tissue may lie outside the pelvis, such as in surgical scars, lungs, and extremities. Possible sites are shown in Figure 39–5.

Regardless of the site, this misplaced endometrial tissue responds to hormonal stimulation and bleeds, producing a variety of manifestations. Scarring and inflammation occur at these extrauterine sites. Repeated episodes of intraperitoneal bleeding, due to hormonal stimulation of the endometrial tissue, cause adhesions. Scarring and adhesions cause the organs and peritoneal surface to become fixed to each other.

Because endometrial tissue is hormone-dependent, the tissue usually atrophies with the normal ovarian regression associated with menopause; it also regresses during pregnancy.

Infertility is a major complication of endometriosis. Usually, the infertility is due to scarring, leading to obstruction of the fallopian tubes.

Clinical Manifestations

Manifestations of endometriosis relate more to the *site* than to the *extent* of disease present. Pain is the most characteristic manifestation; however, about 25% of women with this condition are asymptomatic. Pain typically begins before the menstrual period, lasting for the duration of menstruation and sometimes for several days afterward. The intensity of pain is not correlated with the extent of endometriosis. Pain usually reaches its peak just before the onset of menstrual flow and during the first 1 or 2 days of the menstrual period. The pain may be located in several areas, making the diagnosis more difficult to confirm. Unfortunately, some health care providers may view some women with endometriosis as having psychosomatic complaints and drug-seeking behaviors.

Other manifestations of endometriosis are dyspareunia, menstrual irregularities, and infertility in the absence of tubal obstruction. When the condition occurs inside the ovary, it can produce a "chocolate" cyst, or *endometrioma.* Severe pain is associated with the presence or rupture of this cyst. Implants of endometrium on the ureters may cause obstruction. Rectal implants may be associated with bleeding, diarrhea, or obstruction. Bowel involvement may cause painful defecation.

The diagnosis is generally made from the history, a pelvic examination, and observation of lesions either by laparoscopic examination or pelvic surgery. Direct observation of lesions is necessary for a definitive diagnosis.

Outcome Management

Medical Management

Appropriate treatment of endometriosis depends on the client's manifestations, age, number of children (parity), and extent of disease. When manifestations and extent of disease are mild, the client is given support, information, and coping strategies for pain management. Mild analgesics may be helpful. If manifestations become severe or the disease progresses, additional treatment is generally necessary.

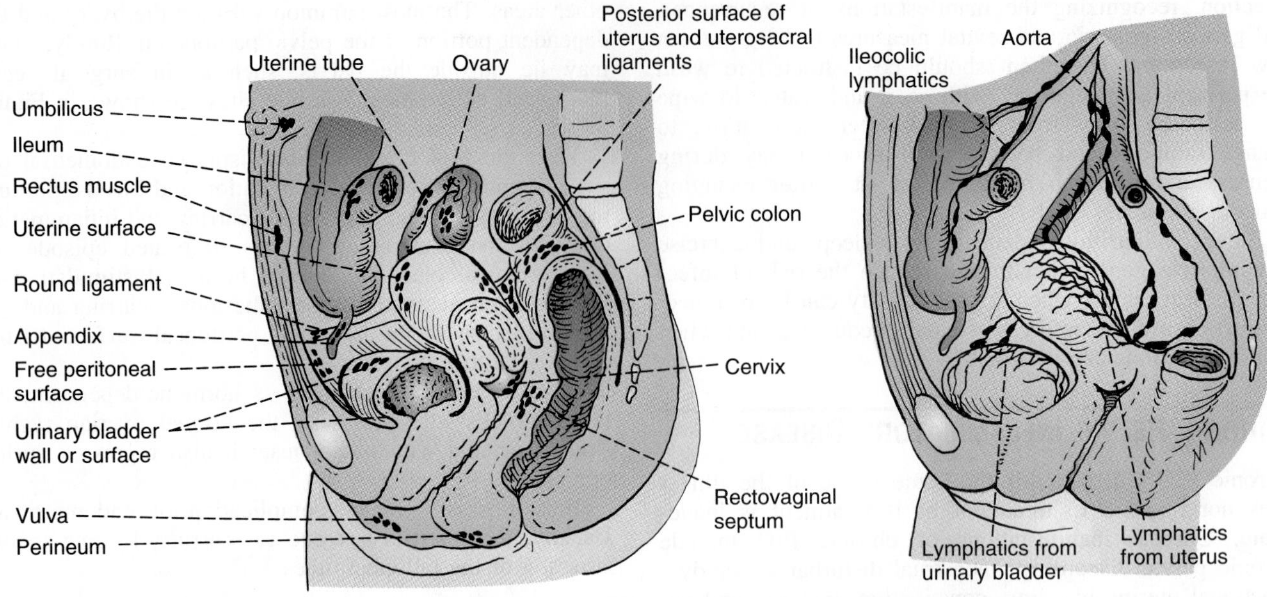

FIGURE 39–5 Endometriosis. *A*, Sites of endometriosis. The locations most frequently affected are the ovaries and the dependent pelvic peritoneum. However, many other sites may be involved. *B*, Pelvic and lymph nodes are important.

REDUCE MANIFESTATIONS

Medication may inhibit endometriosis enough to allow pregnancy or, at least, relieve manifestations. Hormonal intervention includes inducing a *pseudopregnancy* (false pregnancy) with oral contraceptives, progesterone, or both. During the course of this treatment, progestins cause the endometrial implants to slough off. Thus, theoretically, the endometrial tissue no longer functions in abnormal sites. This type of treatment is not successful in all women.

The other hormonal treatment is to induce *ovarian suppression* or *pseudomenopause* (false menopause). Danazol (Danocrine) is an antigonadotropin testosterone derivative that inhibits gonadotropin release, causing ovarian suppression and regression of endometriosis. The medication provides rapid and safe relief of manifestations. Side effects may include acne, hirsutism (excess hair), weight gain, decreased breast size, hot flashes, and vaginal dryness.

Leuprolide (Lupron), a synthetic analog of luteinizing hormone (LH), reduces endometrial pain and lesions. The client can administer it herself monthly in an intramuscular (IM) injection or daily in a subcutaneous (SC) injection. This medication also carries associated menopausal side effects.

Nafarelin (Synarel) acts as a synthetic analog of gonadotropin-releasing hormone (GnRH). Lesions are reduced because endometrial lesions are sensitive to ovarian hormones. It is administered intranasally twice a day and may create menopausal side effects.

Hormonal treatments are very expensive, costing from $100 to more than $300 per month.

Surgical Management

Exploratory or therapeutic surgery directed at endometriosis may make pregnancy possible. Conservative surgical intervention involves restoring normal anatomy and removing or destroying endometriotic foci. A carbon dioxide laser may be used to vaporize adhesions and endometrial implants. Even if the client claims that pregnancy is not desirable at this time, conservative surgery should be considered.

More radical surgery involves removing the uterus, as many implants as possible, and, possibly, the ovaries. This procedures has wide-reaching consequences for affecting sexuality, cardiovascular health, and the risk of osteoporosis unless HRT is also given. This surgical intervention is used only when other measures have failed and the client does not wish to preserve fertility. It causes surgically induced menopause and permanent sterility.

Controversy exists about the use of HRT after such an extensive surgical procedure. The client with a history of endometriosis who undergoes surgically induced menopause may be at risk for induction of additional growth of endometrial implants if she is given some form of HRT after the procedure, particularly in the first few months postoperatively. Conservative surgery is effective for most women. More radical surgery is almost completely effective.

Nursing Management of the Medical-Surgical Client

Nursing care of the woman with endometriosis is individualized and depends on (1) severity of manifestations, (2) extent of disease, (3) age, and (4) childbearing status. Nursing care consists of support during the diagnostic process as the client considers the various treatment options.

Nursing interventions should include discussion of information about the nature of endometriosis, its treatment, and ways to cope with the manifestations. Yoga and relaxation techniques may provide relief. If infertility is an issue, provide information and support in decision-making in this area as well.

Surgical management is similar to that discussed for abdominal hysterectomy, tubal ligation, or laparoscopy (see later).

BENIGN UTERINE TUMORS (LEIOMYOMAS)

Leiomyomas are the most common tumors of the female genital tract. They occur in more than 20% to 30% of all women during the menstrual years. The incidence is two to three times greater in African American women than in white women. Leiomyomas are more common in women approaching menopause.

Leiomyomas are known by various names related to the tissue involved such as fibroids, fibromas, fibromyomas, fibroleiomyomas, myomas, and fiber balls. Leiomyomas are composed mainly of muscle and fibrous connective tissue.

Etiology and Risk Factors

The cause of leiomyomas is unknown. Their growth seems to be related to estrogen stimulation because the fibroids often enlarge with pregnancy and shrink with menopause. A leiomyoma begins as a simple proliferation of smooth muscle cells. It has been suggested that this type of proliferation is stimulated by physical or mechanical means and may occur at points of maximal stress within the myometrium. Because there are many points of stress within the uterus resulting from contractions, fibroids are often multiple (Fig. 39–6).

Pathophysiology

Leiomyomas develop from the uterine myometrium. Growth is usually associated with proliferation of the smooth muscle cells. Estrogen and other hormones influence growth of the muscle cells. Manifestations usually decrease after menopause.

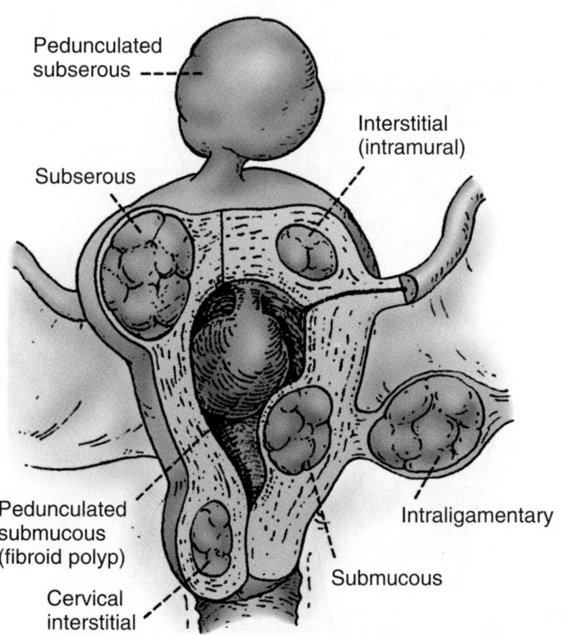

FIGURE 39–6 Some sites of leiomyomas (fibroids). Uterine leiomyomas, depending on their location and size, may interfere with passage of sperm and implantation of a fertilized ovum.

Classification

Leiomyomas may be classified according to their location (those occurring in the uterine body are most common; see Fig. 39–6):

1. *Intramural.* Found in the uterine wall, surrounded by myometrium. Clinical manifestations include increased uterine size, vaginal bleeding between menses, and dysmenorrhea.
2. *Submucosal.* Located directly under the endometrium, involving the endometrial cavity. May become pedunculated (grow on a stalk). Clinical manifestations include prolonged vaginal bleeding and cramps, and the tumor may be seen protruding through the cervix.
3. *Subserosal.* Found on the outer surface (under the serosa) of the uterus. Tends to become pedunculated, to wander (see later), and to be multiple and large. Clinical manifestations include backache, constipation, and bladder problems.
4. *Wandering or parasitic.* A pedunculated leiomyoma that twists on its pedicle, breaks off, then attaches to other tissues, particularly the omentum.
5. *Intraligamentary.* Implants on the pelvic ligaments. May displace the uterus or involve the ureters.
6. *Cervical.* Occur infrequently and may obstruct the cervical canal.

Clinical Manifestations

Frequently, leiomyomas are asymptomatic. Manifestations relate to tumor size, location, and number. Additionally, abnormal bleeding, often resulting in hypermenorrhea (excessive uterine bleeding), is frequently related to the fibroid's hormone dependence.

Manifestations vary widely and occur in about half of clients with leiomyomas. When present, manifestations often relate to the size, location, and number of leiomyomas. The onset of manifestations most commonly occurs in a client's late 40s and early 50s, just before menopause. Once menopause begins, manifestations often cease. It is rare for manifestations to begin after menopause, when leiomyomas tend to regress with decreasing estrogen stimulation. If new manifestations develop during these years, other diagnoses, such as cancer, need to be ruled out.

The most common clinical manifestation is abnormal uterine bleeding, which may be excessive in either amount or duration. Additionally, it may accompanied by anemia, with manifestations of tiredness, weakness, and lethargy. Dysmenorrhea and a sense of pelvic pressure are often present. Urinary frequency is common when the tumor presses on the bladder. Urinary retention also may occur when bladder function is compromised by tumor size. Constipation, hydroureter (abnormal distention of ureter with urine), hydronephrosis (distention of kidney due to abnormal accumulation of urine in the kidney pelvis), abdominal pain, and dyspareunia are less common manifestations.

Occasionally, the client may have vaginal discharge, which may be foul or water-tinged and blood-tinged. Abdominal pressure occurs if the leiomyoma is large enough to cause abdominal distention. The tumor may be palpable. Also, the client may experience sterility or have a history of one or more spontaneous abortions.

A characteristic history, confirmed by findings of abdominal and pelvic examinations, usually establishes the diagnosis. Ultrasonography may demonstrate an abnormal uterine shape. Various disorders, such as cancer and a problem pregnancy, must be ruled out before treatment is planned.

Outcome Management

Medical Management

A plan of treatment for leiomyomas depends on manifestations, age of the client, location and size of the tumors, onset of complications, and client's desire to preserve fertility. Leiomyomas can be assessed every 6 months by a practitioner if the client is not pregnant; if there is no excessive bleeding or pressure on the bladder, bowel, or ureters; and if the tumor is not rapidly growing.

GnRH analogs (see Endometriosis earlier) may be administered to reduce size and inhibit growth of tumors. Malignant degeneration is rare. A rapid increase in the size of the leiomyoma, as indicated by manifestations or detected on examination, should be thoroughly evaluated, and aggressive therapy should be considered.

Surgical Management

Surgical treatment may involve cutting off the blood supply to the fibroid or *myomectomy* (removal of a tumor without removal of the uterus). Both procedures preserve the reproductive organs and reproductive capability. However, because of the increased risk that additional leiomyomas may develop later, a hysterectomy may be the preferred procedure.

HYSTERECTOMY

INDICATIONS. Three types of hysterectomy may be performed:

Total hysterectomy—removal of the uterus and cervix. Can be performed either abdominally or vaginally.

Total hysterectomy with bilateral salpingo-oophorectomy (TAH-BSO)—removal of uterus, cervix, fallopian tubes, and ovaries. Can be performed vaginally or abdominally (Fig. 39–7).

Radical hysterectomy—same as a TAH-BSO plus removal of the lymph nodes, upper third of the vagina, and parametrium. Usually performed if a malignant tumor is found.

CONTRAINDICATIONS. The only contraindication to hysterectomy is any health condition that prevents surgery.

COMPLICATIONS. Hemorrhage and infection are the primary complications.

OUTCOMES. It is expected that the client will return home in 2 to 4 days and resume regular activities within 4 to 6 weeks, depending on the type of hysterectomy performed. Pain, abnormal bleeding, and anemia, if present, will cease. For all procedures except myomectomy, menstruation ends.

Nursing Management of the Surgical Client

PREOPERATIVE CARE

The client seeks medical help because of some form of abnormal uterine bleeding, dyspareunia, or pelvic pain. Obtain a thorough history from the client, especially if there are complaints of irregular bleeding. It is also important to assess the client's knowledge of her condition and the surgery. Listen carefully for any questions she has about sexuality after treatment.

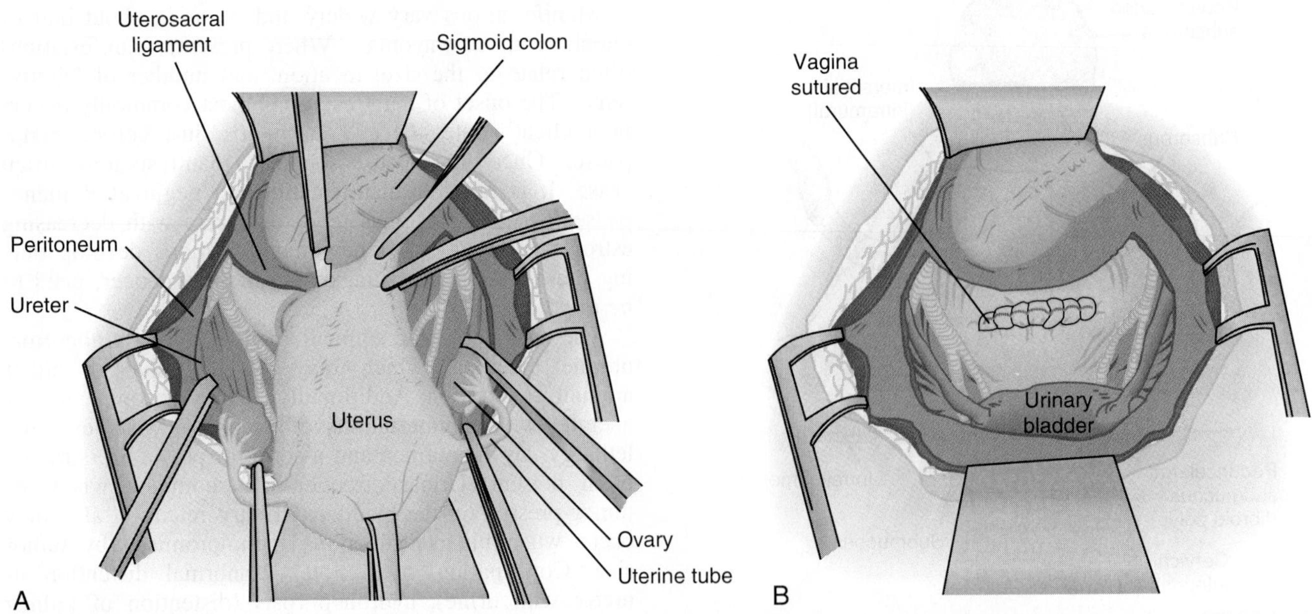

FIGURE 39–7 Total abdominal hysterectomy with salpingo-oophorectomy. *A*, The uterus with attached uterine tubes and ovaries is lifted out after it has been freed from the ligaments holding it. *B*, After the specimen has been removed en masse, the vagina is sutured closed.

Reduce Pain. Before surgery is performed, the client can be taught ways to reduce pain associated with intercourse, such as assuming positions in which leiomyomas are not pressed on during intercourse and using water-soluble lubricants. Pain medications can be used for severe pain. Sometimes, sitz baths or the application of heat to the lower abdomen may be helpful.

Provide Education. The client undergoing a hysterectomy has many learning needs. Frequently, a woman undergoing gynecologic surgery needs help understanding the problem and the proposed operation. She needs to understand her options and the differences among the procedures proposed.

If a hysterectomy is planned, inform the client about the loss of fertility. If the ovaries are to be removed in conjunction with the hysterectomy, discuss surgical menopause and HRT. Some women are relieved that the operation will remove the risk of unwanted pregnancy and monthly menstrual manifestations.

Discuss how sexual intercourse may change after a hysterectomy. Although the client's ability to achieve orgasm should not change, the vagina will be shortened and there may be scar tissue.

The client whose ovaries are removed may complain of a decrease in *libido* (sexual desire). This is due to the loss of testosterone that is normally produced by the ovaries. HRT may include a small daily dose of testosterone. Tell the client that once healing has occurred, intercourse should be pain-free. Answer any questions asked, and encourage the client and her significant other to express their feelings and concerns about sexuality.

Postoperative Care

Assessment

Perform the usual postoperative assessments. Evaluation of psychological manifestations is also important.

The proximity of the bladder to the female reproductive organs increases the risk of urinary problems, which must be monitored postoperatively. A Foley catheter is usually inserted at the time of surgery to prevent bladder distention and injury during surgery; the catheter is often left in place for 24 hours postoperatively. Potential postoperative problems related to the placement of a Foley catheter are UTI and temporary urinary retention due to voiding dysfunction.

Assess GI function by listening for bowel sounds, noting distention and seeing whether the abdomen is soft or firm. Passing of flatus (bowel gas) indicates the return of GI function. After an abdominal hysterectomy, assess the abdominal incision for bleeding and intactness.

Assess vaginal bleeding. One saturated pad should be necessary in 4 hours after abdominal or vaginal hysterectomy. Excessive bleeding should be considered if one sanitary napkin is saturated in one hour or less.

Diagnosis, Outcomes, Interventions

Risk for Dysfunctional Grieving. Some women experience grief about their loss of the female reproductive organs, making *Risk for Dysfunctional Grieving related to loss of reproductive capacity and perceived loss of femininity* an appropriate nursing diagnosis for a client undergoing hysterectomy.

Outcomes. The client can be expected to go through a grieving process over her loss after hysterectomy and may express her feelings about the loss.

Interventions. When reproductive ability is lost, the client may undergo a grief response. It is important for the nurse to understand the grieving process and to be able to help the woman understand that this response is normal. Some women experience relief rather than grief. Support normal grieving, including temporary denial, which is a part of the grieving process. If the client continues to experience grief beyond the normal degree or time expected, she may require counseling.

Risk for Infection. During surgery for a hysterectomy, a Foley catheter is inserted, leading to the nursing diagnosis *Risk for Infection related to surgical intervention and presence of a urinary catheter.*

Outcomes. The client will remain free of infection, or will report any infection immediately for proper diagnosis and treatment.

Interventions

Prevent Urinary Infection. When a Foley catheter is in place, instruct the client to keep the urinary drainage catheter below the level of the bladder, drink at least 2 to 4 L of liquid daily, and report any urinary pain or discomfort. Check the urinary drainage system closely for leaks and kinks in the system, provide complete perineal care every shift, and report any change in color or odor of the urine. When a Foley catheter is discontinued, monitor the client for the first void. Voiding frequently in small amounts, inability to void, and bladder distention or hematuria should be reported to the physician.

Prevent Retention. Often, a suprapubic catheter is placed instead of a Foley catheter. This allows the client to clamp the catheter and attempt to void as soon as she is ambulatory. If the suprapubic area becomes distended when the catheter is clamped and the client is unable to void, the suprapubic catheter can be opened and drained. Using a suprapubic catheter avoids the need for recatheterization of a client who cannot void.

Constipation. Because of bowel manipulation during surgery, the nursing diagnosis *Constipation related to bowel manipulation during surgery* is appropriate.

Outcomes. The client will not become constipated, and bowel distention will be treated, as evidenced by return to a normal bowel pattern and absence of abdominal distention.

Interventions

Promote Peristalsis. Pain and discomfort after abdominal hysterectomy usually center on the incision and postoperative gas pains. After abdominal hysterectomy, GI functioning returns slowly. Uncomfortable gas pains are often experienced during the early postoperative period. Early, frequent ambulation helps to improve GI function. If gas pains persist, a small enema may be prescribed to facilitate peristalsis and to prevent constipation. Continue to encourage frequent ambulation to facilitate the return of normal GI functioning. Drinking warm fluids may encourage the return of peristalsis.

Evaluation

It is expected that the client will recover from a hysterectomy without complications. She can return to normal activities within 4 to 6 weeks without permanent problems.

Self-Care

The client should understand the type of surgery she has had and the follow-up needed. If she has had a myomectomy, pregnancy is still an option. She must continue to have routine gynecologic examinations and to use birth control measures until her physician judges that she can attempt a pregnancy. If she has undergone TAH-BSO, discuss menopause and HRT with her. Discharge teaching should also include the following instructions:

1. Eat a well-balanced diet, drink six to eight glasses of water daily, and get plenty of rest.
2. Avoid heavy lifting for about 6 weeks, to prevent straining on the abdominal muscles and surgical sites.
3. Avoid activities that increase pelvic congestion, such as aerobic activity, horseback riding, and prolonged standing. Optimal circulation is necessary to promote healing of pelvic tissues.
4. Avoid vaginal and rectal intercourse and douching until healing is complete, usually in about 6 weeks. These activities can interfere with healing of the vaginal cuff or other healing tissues and can introduce infection.
5. Report any fresh bleeding and any abnormal vaginal discharge to the surgeon.
6. Return for follow-up care as requested by the surgeon.

ENDOMETRIAL (UTERINE) CANCER

Endometrial cancer is the most common malignancy of the female genital reproductive system. In 2000, it was estimated that 36,100 new cases of uterine cancer would be diagnosed in the United States. The 5-year survival rate is 95% if the cancer is discovered at an early stage and 64% if the cancer is identified at a regional stage.[1]

Etiology and Risk Factors

Endometrial cancer is thought to be related to overstimulation of the endometrium from excessive circulating estrogen. Common sources of excessive estrogen are successive anovulatory menstrual cycles and unopposed ERT (estrogen without progestin) in a woman who still has her uterus. Other factors are history of pelvic radiation, other reproductive cancer, family history, history of diabetes or hypertension, obesity, and hyperestrogenism (early menarche, late menopause, dysfunctional uterine bleeding, delayed onset of ovulation).

Health promotion actions include advising overweight women to lose weight and use of HRT (estrogen and progestin) or raloxifene (Evista) instead of estrogen therapy. Health maintenance actions are to advise women to have yearly pelvic examinations even after menopause, ensure that high-risk women undergo endometrial biopsy at regular intervals, and inform the client to have postmenopausal bleeding assessed.

Pathophysiology

In women with endometrial cancer, the cell type is usually adenocarcinoma, a tumor that involves the glands. This relatively slow-growing tumor metastasizes late in its course and tends to spread slowly to other organs. Most commonly, the carcinoma invades the uterus, causing uterine enlargement. The cancerous process may extend along the endometrial surface to the cervix or fallopian tubes and ovaries. It can spread to other peritoneal structures, including the lymphatics and blood vessels. It can then spread to the vagina, through the lymphatics to other areas, and, occasionally, to distant sites such as the brain and lungs.

Clinical Manifestations

Because there is no practical, accurate method of screening for endometrial cancer, the cancer is usually discovered after the first manifestations appear. The most significant manifestation is some type of abnormal uterine bleeding, especially in the postmenopausal woman. Other manifestations relate to invasion, metastasis to other organs, or both (Fig. 39–8).

A diagnosis of endometrial cancer is usually established by pelvic examination and pathologic analysis of an endometrial biopsy specimen. Women at high risk may undergo endometrial biopsy at each annual or biannual pelvic examination. An endovaginal ultrasound study of the endometrium may be used to detect a thickened endometrium, or a hysteroscope (a small intrauterine instrument that visualizes uterine contents) with biopsy may be used to assist in the diagnosis.

Outcome Management

Surgical Management

Endometrial cancer is generally treated with surgery, radiation, or a combination. Early endometrial cancer is sur-

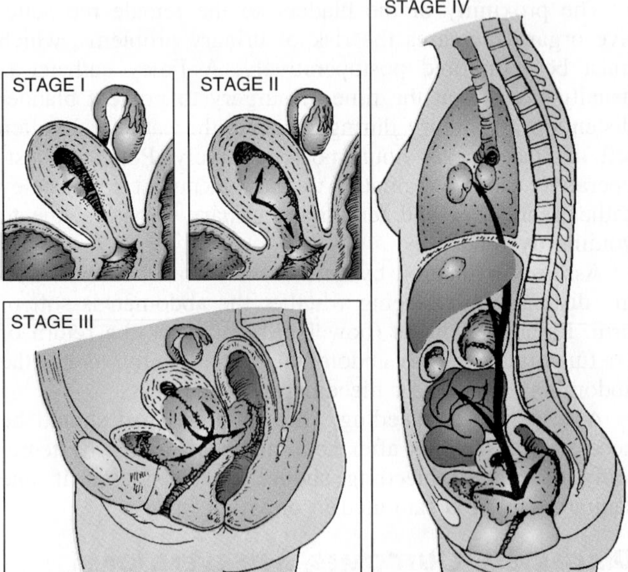

FIGURE 39–8 Staging uterine cancer. *Stage 1,* The tumor is confined to the uterine corpus. *Stage 2,* The cancer has also invaded the cervix. *Stage 3,* The cancer has spread beyond the uterus but remains confined to the pelvis, such as in the bladder or rectum. *Stage 4,* Highest level of invasiveness since the cancer has spread beyond the pelvis, causing metastatic disease and large masses, such as in the liver or lungs.

gically treated with a TAH-BSO. Surgery may be preceded or followed by irradiation, either external of internal. Surgical management is the same as for benign uterine tumors (leiomyomas).

Medical Management

External irradiation is discussed in Chapter 19. If intracavity (internal) radiation therapy (IRT) or brachytherapy is selected, an applicator is placed through the vagina into the uterus with the use of anesthesia. Correct placement is verified by x-ray study, and the client is taken to a hospital room. A radiologist places a radioactive isotope in the applicator, which remains for 1 to 3 days.

Precancerous endometrial changes may be treated with the hormone progesterone. Chemotherapy and hormonal therapy with tamoxifen (Nolvadex) are used to treat late stages of endometrial cancer.

Nursing Management of the Medical-Surgical Client

Nursing care of the surgical client is the same as described for the client with benign uterine tumors (leiomyomas).

While the radioactive implants are in place, the client is strictly isolated in a private room. She must remain at bed rest, with the head of the bed flat or elevated no more than 20 degrees. Movement is restricted except for deep breathing and leg exercises. A Foley catheter is inserted to prevent dislodgment of the implants, and the client is given a low-residue diet to prevent bowel movements, which may dislodge the implant. Increased fluid intake, to prevent urinary stasis, is encouraged. You may also administer antiemetics, broad-spectrum antibiotics, sedatives, analgesics, antidiarrheal medications, and heparin (to prevent thrombophlebitis).

Radiation precautions are enforced while a radioactive implant is in place. Pregnant nurses or female nurses attempting to become pregnant must not be assigned to care for such a client. Organize care so that you spend minimal time at the client's bedside. Give care from as far away as possible, behind lead shields when possible. Visitors should keep visits brief. Radiation therapy is detailed in Chapter 19.

The high dose of radiation may cause vaginal shrinkage, because exposure thins the vaginal epithelium and reduces vaginal lubrication. It may also cause vaginal adhesions and stenosis. Such changes can make vaginal sexual activities uncomfortable or painful. Vaginal penetration, with water-soluble lubrication as needed, during the course of irradiation and in subsequent months minimizes the possibility of vaginal stenosis and contracture. Depending on personal preference, vaginal penetration and dilation can be accomplished with the woman's own fingers, a vaginal dilator, or her sexual partner's fingers or penis. Vaginal dilators can be used for 10 minutes per day with water-soluble lubricants until sexual activity is resumed in 2 to 6 weeks. Support for the woman experiencing body image changes is extremely important.

CERVICAL CANCER

The incidence of invasive cervical cancer has steadily decreased over the years, whereas that of cervical carcinoma in situ (localized) has risen. The decrease is largely attributed to the prevalence of screening with the Papanicolaou test (Pap smear). About 12,800 new cases of invasive cervical cancer were expected to have been diagnosed in 2000, with approximately 4600 cervical cancer deaths expected.[1] The incidence in African American and Native American women is nearly twice as high as in white women. Spanish-speaking women younger than 39 years are the least likely to have Pap smears.

Etiology and Risk Factors

The exact cause of cervical cancer is unknown, although chronic irritation is often present prior to diagnosis of cervical cancer. There is a strong relationship between the presence of the human papillomavirus (HPV), types 16 and 18, and cervical intraepithelial neoplasia (CIN). CIN has increasingly progressed to carcinoma in situ and invasive cervical cancer. Other risk factors are:

- Having multiple sexual partners or a partner who has had multiple sexual partners
- Early age of first intercourse
- Smoking tobacco
- Low socioeconomic status
- Untreated chronic cervicitis
- STDs
- Having a sexual partner with a history of penile or prostate cancer

Health promotion actions involve instructing clients (1) to avoid and to seek early treatment of vaginal or cervical infection, (2) to limit the number of sexual partners, and (3) to use condoms to limit the transmission of STDs and HPV. Yearly Pap smears for high-risk women is a health maintenance activity. After three or more consecutive annual examinations with normal results of Pap smears, the client with average risk may undergo Papanicolaou testing less frequently, at the discretion of the health care provider. Pap smears are important because cervical carcinoma in situ is potentially 100% curable.

Pathophysiology

Cervical dysplasia (an abnormal alteration in cell structure), the earliest premalignant change noted in cervical epithelium, is now further divided into several levels:

- Mild dysplasia, or CIN 1
- Moderate dysplasia, or CIN 2
- Severe dysplasia, or CIN 3
- Carcinoma in situ

Potentially, all women with carcinoma in situ and 91% of women with nonmetastatic disease can be cured. Five to 10 years may elapse between the preinvasive and invasive stages of cervical cancer. Most cervical cancers are of the squamous cell type. Squamous cell carcinoma usually begins at the squamocolumnar junction, near the external end of the cervix. The spread of squamous cell cervical cancer occurs first by direct extension to the vaginal mucosa, the lower uterine segment, parametrium, pelvic wall, bladder, and bowel. Distant metastasis occurs mainly through lymphatic spread, with some spread occurring through the circulatory system to the liver, lungs, or bones.

On occasion, cervical adenocarcinomas occur, but they are more difficult to identify. Adenocarcinoma generally involves the endocervical glands.

Clinical Manifestations

There are no early indications of carcinoma in situ or early cervical cancer. An abnormal Pap smear result, however, indicates the need for further assessment. Abnormal Pap smear results may be followed by HPV deoxyribonucleic acid (DNA) testing to confirm malignancy or repeating of the Pap smear. Another effective diagnostic test involves swabbing the cervix with vinegar; a flashlight then illuminates abnormal cells.

Assessment findings in late stages of cancer include the presence of vaginal discharge and bleeding, especially after intercourse. Metrorrhagia, postmenopausal bleeding, and *polymenorrhea* (increased frequency of menstrual bleeding) may be present. Early bleeding also may occur as spotting or contact bleeding from cervical trauma secondary to sexual intercourse or douching. This early minimal bleeding increases in amount and duration as the cancer progresses.

Vaginal discharge, which is normally watery, becomes dark and foul-smelling as the disease advances. With infection of the neoplastic area, the discharge becomes more profuse and malodorous. Concurrent bleeding makes this condition more unpleasant.

Other assessment findings that develop as the disease progresses relate to the areas involved in the malignant process. They include (1) pressure on the bowel, bladder, or both, (2) bladder irritation, (3) rectal discharge, (4) manifestations of ureteral obstruction, and (5) heavy, aching abdominal pain. Fistulae may form as the malignancy erodes through the walls of adjacent organs.

Pain is another late manifestation. It usually becomes a difficult problem with the onset of *cachexia*, or general wasting syndrome. This syndrome often accompanies the terminal stage of cervical cancer.

Pap Smear

The Pap smear is the primary diagnostic tool for cervical cancer. Further assessment of an abnormal Pap smear result typically includes repetition of cytologic and pelvic examinations. Colposcopic examination can often locate lesions for biopsy. Biopsy specimens are collected with the aid of a colposcope. After the cervix is wiped clean of any mucus or discharge, acetic acid is placed on it. The practitioner views the cervix through the colposcope, looking for abnormalities of color and cell formation. Tiny biopsy specimens are collected from any areas under suspicion. Colposcopy is an office procedure that causes mild discomfort.

Cold Conization

Occasionally, biopsy specimens may be obtained by cold conization, a procedure that may be performed when colposcopic examination is not considered adequate and a larger specimen is necessary. A cone-shaped section of the cervix is obtained with a scalpel. This procedure enables more tissue to be provided for analysis, thus increasing the chances of identifying an area of invasive carcinoma or carcinoma in situ. The procedure is particularly helpful if areas such as the endocervical glands are involved and are not readily visualized.

Sometimes analysis of the tissue removed during a cold conization demonstrates that a wide area of normal tissue surrounds an excised malignancy. When this situation occurs, conization serves not only serves as the diagnostic procedure but may also be the only treatment needed. This procedure allows the woman to maintain reproductive capacity. Cautery (burning of abnormal cervical tissue) or *cryosurgery* (freezing of cervical tissue) may be performed instead of cold conization.

Loop Electrocautery Excision Procedure

A loop electrocautery excision procedure (LEEP) is the newest and most common procedure. A LEEP is performed to excise the cervical areas causing concern. Once the clinician has identified the lesions with colposcopy, a paracervical nerve block is administered for anesthesia, and the lesion or lesions are totally removed by a low-voltage diathermy loop (an electrical current causing burning). There is less risk with this procedure because it is performed in the ambulatory setting without general anesthesia.

Outcome Management

Medical Management

Irradiation is used as primary therapy for early cervical cancer. It is usually curative, but it induces menopause. Intracavity radiation has been described previously (see uterine cancer), and external irradiation is discussed in Chapter 19. In 1999, cancer experts recommended a change in the treatment of advanced surgical cancer, urging that chemotherapy be added to the standard treatment using irradiation.

Treatment of clients with cervical cancer during pregnancy varies, depending on the stage of the cancer, the duration of the pregnancy, and the client's wish to preserve fertility. A client can usually complete the pregnancy if CIN or carcinoma in situ is diagnosed. She may then be treated with cold conization or a LEEP 2 to 3 months post partum if she desires further childbearing. If a pregnant woman has invasive cervical carcinoma, however, abortion is recommended up to 24 weeks into the pregnancy. After 24 weeks, therapy is delayed until the fetus is viable (28 to 32 weeks), and a cesarean section is performed. The client may then be treated with either hysterectomy or irradiation in the postpartum period.

Nursing Management of the Medical Client

Prevent Complications

For the care of a client with radiation implants, see uterine cancer earlier; external radiation is covered in Chapter 19.

Prevent Recurrence

All clients who have been treated conservatively for cervical cancer need information about recurrence. Encourage clients who have been treated for cervical cancer to have frequent health examinations to identify manifestations of recurrence of the cancer. Pelvic examinations and Pap smears should be scheduled every 3 months for the first 2 years, as advised by the physician.

Surgical Management

Treatment may range from cryosurgery, conization, laser therapy, or LEEP for localized tumors to a radical hysterectomy for invasive cancer:

1. *Cryosurgery* is the local freezing of abnormal cells and tissues with volatile gases such a nitrous oxide or carbon dioxide. Cell death results from dehydration and cell membrane destruction; dead tissue then sloughs off with a heavy discharge for 2 to 3 weeks.
2. *Conization* is the removal of a small cone of tissue with a sharp instrument (see earlier).
3. *Laser therapy* or *LEEP* (see earlier) may also be performed to remove abnormal tissue. Laser therapy causes a burn of the tissues, leading to an increase in sloughing discharge for several weeks. There may also be minimal bleeding.

A total abdominal hysterectomy can be used to treat carcinoma in situ in women who have finished childbearing or to treat invasive cancer. *Pelvic exenteration* (Fig. 39–9), an extremely radical procedure, is performed if the cancer has spread. This procedure involves removal of all pelvic organs, including the uterus, fallopian tubes, ovaries, vagina, bladder, rectum, and colon. In addition, an ileal conduit and ileostomy may be performed if removal of the bladder or colon is indicated.

Nursing Management of the Surgical Client

For care of the client with a hysterectomy, see benign uterine tumors (leiomyomas). For care of the client with an ileal conduit, see Chapter 34. For care of the client with a colostomy or ileostomy, see Chapter 33.

CRYOSURGERY, LASER THERAPY, LEEP

EXPLAIN PROCEDURE. Nursing preparation of a client for cryosurgery, laser therapy, or a LEEP involves informing the client that a surgical incision will not be made. Explain that the procedure is performed with a vaginal speculum in place, as during a routine pelvic examination. During treatment, a few clients experience headaches, dizziness, flushing, and some cramping.

PROVIDE SUPPORT. During the procedure, provide psychological support by (1) staying with the client, (2) informing her of what is to be done, (3) talking with her, listening to her, and facilitating her expression of concerns, (4) continuing to acknowledge her presence during

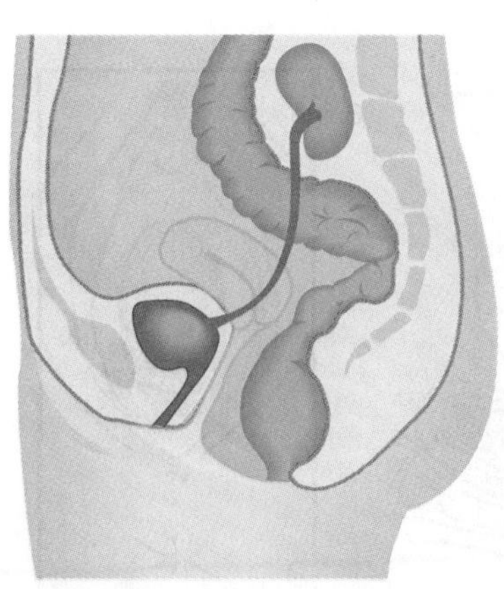

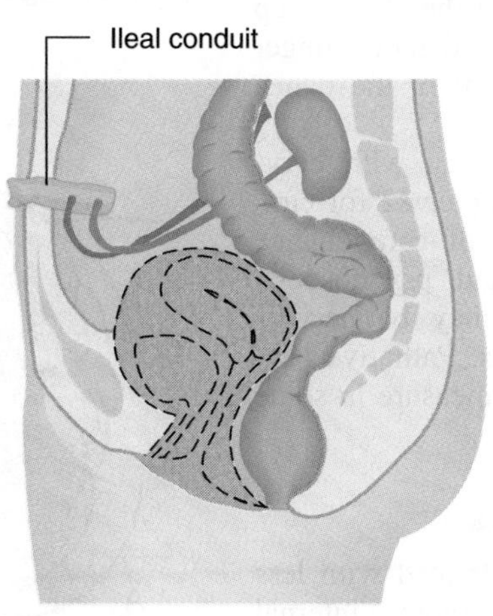

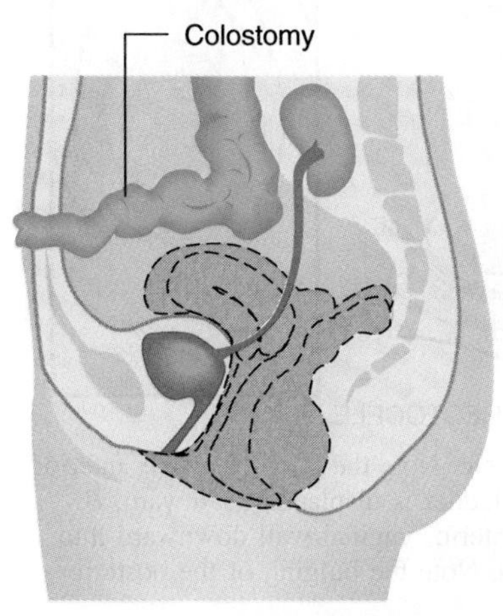

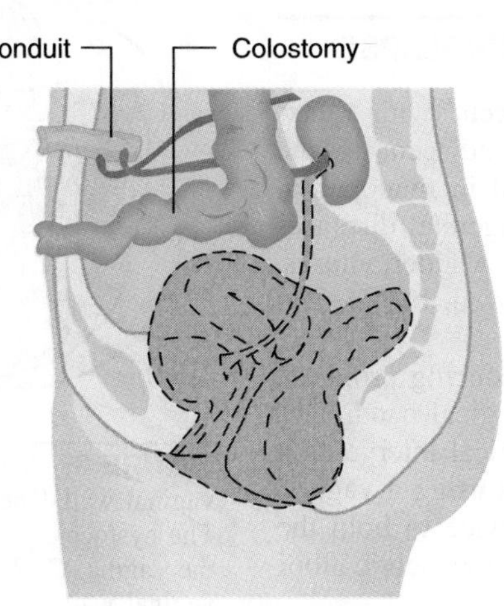

FIGURE 39–9 Pelvic exenteration. *A*, Natural pelvic structures. *B*, Anterior exenteration: formation of the ileal conduit. *C*, Posterior exenteration: formation of colostomy. *D*, Total exenteration: formation of both ileal conduit and colostomy.

the procedure rather than excluding her, and (5) allowing her to retain as much self-control as possible. For example, tell her what she can do during the procedure to help it move along quickly and smoothly.

PROMOTE COMFORT. Assess the client's discomfort during the procedure. A mild analgesic may be prescribed for pain following the procedure. Discuss how she can help manage postprocedure discomfort, such as performing slow, deep breathing. Tell the client what to expect afterward; mild cramping may continue for several days.

ENCOURAGE PERINEAL HYGIENE. A clear, watery discharge usually occurs for up to several weeks. This is followed by a malodorous discharge containing debris from the sloughing of dead cells. If the discharge continues longer than 8 weeks, an infection is suspected.

Meticulous perineal hygiene minimizes the risk of infection and makes the client more comfortable. Healing takes about 6 weeks. The client should take showers during this time, avoiding tub and sitz baths.

RADICAL HYSTERECTOMY

After a radical hysterectomy, the vagina is shortened and the trigone region of the bladder and the sigmoid colon may adhere to the vaginal apex. This may cause dyspareunia, the pain of which may be felt deep in the pelvis. Recommend that during penile penetration the client keep her thighs adducted and use her thumb and index finger at the vaginal opening to encircle the shaft of the penis, providing some extra length to the vagina.

Despite vigorous treatment, some women with cervical cancer become terminally ill (see Chapter 22 for end-of-life care) In this situation, the goals of care change and are directed toward physiologic and psychosocial comfort. Pain relief (see Chapter 23) may be accomplished through use of narcotic analgesics. Palliative irradiation may also be used as a pain relief measure in some cases.

Modifications for Elderly Clients

In older clients, cervical cancer may be treated with less invasive methods. The older client undergoing internal irradiation treatments should be monitored closely after treatment for development of fistulae.

UROGENITAL DISPLACEMENT AND PROLAPSE

Urogenital displacement and prolapse occur with relaxation and descent of the pelvic organs adjacent to the vagina. This is a common problem found in menopausal women. The organs that descend with urogenital displacement and then prolapse are the urethra, bladder, uterus, vaginal apex if the uterus has been removed, bowel, and rectum.

Surgery has been very successful in reducing prolapse. However, some women who are poor surgical candidates or who choose not to proceed with a surgical intervention may elect a nonsurgical approach, such as using a vaginal support device known as a *pessary* (a device to hold the organs in correct position) or increasing the pelvic floor support with Kegel exercises.

Etiology and Risk Factors

Menopause causes a decrease in circulating estrogens. With a decrease of estrogen, the supporting structures of the pelvic floor lose their elasticity and ability to support, causing relaxation and prolapse of the urogenital organs.

Additional factors that put a woman at risk for development of prolapse are multiparity, childbirth trauma, chronic straining, and inability to maintain the perineal musculature. The occurrence of prolapse has decreased with improved obstetric care. Better preparation of women for labor and the rare use of forceps during delivery have helped. Help prevent prolapse by encouraging pregnant clients to seek qualified obstetric care and instructing them to perform Kegel exercises before and after delivery.

CYSTOCELE AND URETHROCELE

A *cystocele* involves a descent of the urinary bladder because of weakened pelvic floor muscles; it is seen as a protrusion of the anterior part of the vaginal wall (Fig. 39–10*A* and *B*). A *urethrocele* (prolapse of the urethra) often accompanies a cystocele as the bladder descends into the vagina. Urinary difficulties caused by the cystocele and urethrocele include incontinence, urinary tract infections, and urinary retention. Additionally, the client may complain of vaginal pressure with or without pelvic discomfort.

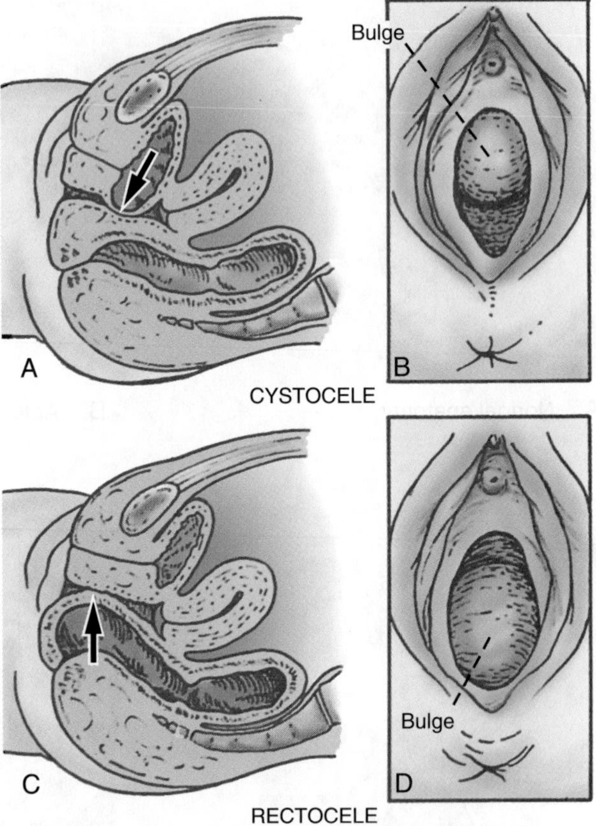

FIGURE 39–10 *A*, Cystocele. Note the bulging of the anterior vaginal wall. The urinary bladder is displaced downward. *B*, The cystocele pushes the anterior vaginal wall downward into the vagina. *C*, Rectocele. *D*, Note the bulging of the posterior vaginal wall.

■ RECTOCELE AND ENTEROCELE

A *rectocele* is the protrusion of the vaginal wall musculature that supports the rectum (Fig. 39–10*C* and *D*). A rectocele can produce constipation, incomplete emptying of the rectum, fecal incontinence, and rectal or vaginal pressure. To completely empty the rectum, some women find it necessary to support the posterior wall of the vagina with a finger while having a bowel movement.

An *enterocele* is the descent of the bowel and protrusion of the upper portion of the posterior wall of the vagina. It often accompanies a rectocele and is usually without manifestations when it is seen alone.

■ VAGINAL OR UTERINE PROLAPSE

Vaginal or uterine prolapse is the descent of the uterus into the vagina (Fig. 39–11). The associated manifestations are increasing vaginal pressure, dyspareunia, and backache. As the prolapse descends through the vagina, there may be bleeding from irritation and ulcerations on the prolapsing cervix.

Clinical Manifestations

Manifestations of displacement and prolapse often depend on the level of descent and clinical signs. Some clients present with significant descent but have no manifestations. Clinically, prolapse should be assessed by the level of the descent. The grading scale is as follows[29]:

Grade 0: No descent
Grade 1: Descent half way between the ischial spines and the hymenal ring
Grade 2: Descent to the hymenal ring
Grade 3: Descent halfway beyond the hymenal ring
Grade 4: Descent fully outside the hymenal ring

Outcome Management

Surgical Management

Treatment of prolapse depends on the extent of prolapse and the client's health status. The most effective treatment is reconstructive surgery. A vaginal pessary may be used if surgery is not desired or the health status of the client is less than optimal.

The cystocele is often corrected by a procedure called an *anterior colporrhaphy*; an additional procedure called a *Burch colposuspension* may be included if a urethrocele is present (see Chapter 34). The rectocele is usually corrected with a *posterior repair.* The accompanying enterocele is often corrected at the same time by one of various enterocele reconstructive procedures. Hence, an anterior and posterior (A & P repair) involves both procedures.

A hysterectomy may be performed at the same time as the reconstructive surgery if the client does not want to preserve fertility and if the uterus has descended into the vagina. The hysterectomy is performed by way of incisions through the vaginal wall into the pelvic cavity and supportive structures. The uterus is removed from its supporting broad, round, and uterosacral ligaments. The supporting ligaments are then attached to the vaginal cuff to maintain vaginal length.

Nursing Management of the Surgical Client

PREVENT BLADDER DISTENTION

During the operation and for at least the first 24 hours afterward, the bladder is kept decompressed. If a Foley catheter is placed, it is usually removed as soon as the client is ambulatory. When the catheter is removed, the client must be taught to keep her bladder empty by voiding every 2 hours to avoid placing pressure along the suture line. If a suprapubic catheter is placed, bladder retraining is begun once the client is ambulatory.

MONITOR BLEEDING

Postoperatively, monitor the client closely for excessive vaginal bleeding. There is normally a small to moderate amount of frank vaginal bleeding. If heavy vaginal bleeding is accompanied by a rapidly distending, rigid abdomen, referred shoulder pain, and indications of shock, immediate surgery may be indicated. Other times of potential bleeding are the 4th, 9th, 14th, and 21st days after surgery as sutures dissolve. If vaginal packing, a drain, or both are in place, the surgeon usually removes them after 24 to 48 hours.

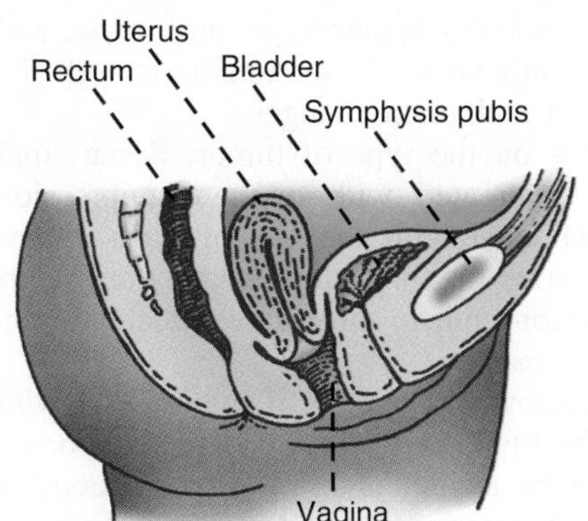

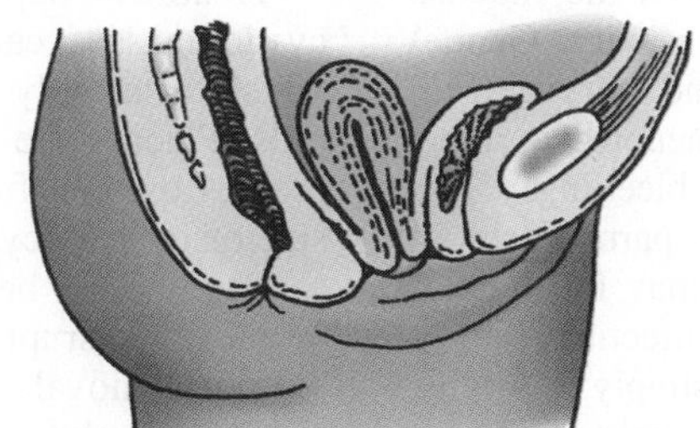

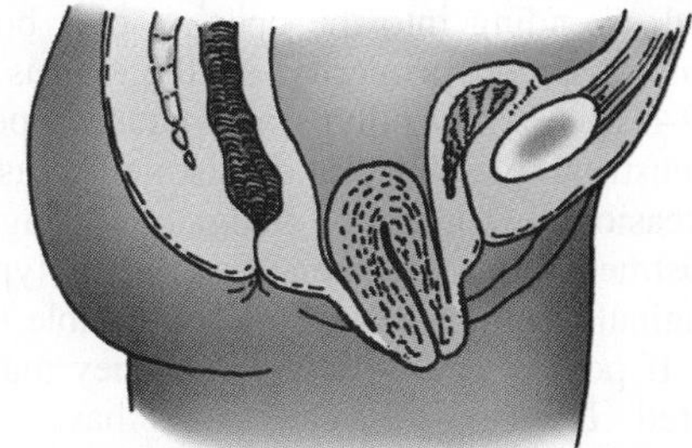

FIGURE 39–11 Uterine prolapse.

Medical Management

The vaginal pessary has been used more successfully over the last few years as an alternative to surgery or as a comfort measure during the wait for surgery. This device holds the prolapsing vaginal organs in the correct position. Pessaries come in different sizes and styles. A well-fit pessary should be comfortable. Therefore, for proper compliance, the client should not experience any discomfort from the pessary during activities. She should be able to void normally with the pessary in place and should be comfortable inserting and removing it.

Nursing Management of the Medical Client

TEACH PELVIC FLOOR (KEGEL) EXERCISES

Mild manifestations may be relieved by pelvis-strengthening Kegel exercises. These exercises may be prescribed to help a client achieve pubococcygeal muscle control. Instruct the client to practice alternately tightening and relaxing her rectal and vaginal muscles. She tightens these muscles as if she were trying to hold back a bowel movement or a stream of urine. She holds this tightened position for a few seconds and then relaxes the muscles. Over time, she should hold the contraction for a longer period. Kegel exercises can be performed frequently during the day, whenever the clients thinks of them, or for a specified number of times two or three times a day.

TEACH PESSARY CARE

Because a pessary has the potential to irritate the vaginal mucosa, instruct the client to remove the device daily and to reinsert it after cleaning it with a mild, unscented soap and water.

Follow-up care is important. Within 2 weeks after fitting and insertion of the pessary, the client needs professional reassessment. At that time, the clinician performs a pelvic examination to assess the vaginal mucosa for irritation. The pessary may be changed or removed as indicated. Estrogen cream is often inserted into the vagina at bedtime two times a week in an effort to maintain tissue integrity.

If a pessary is left in place too long, it may erode the tissues and adhere to the mucosa. It is important for the client to understand the need for follow-up care. Most clients can care for a pessary without assistance, but some clients with poor manual dexterity need help with its removal and cleaning.

POLYPS

Polyps are pedunculated tumors arising from the mucosa and extending into the opening of a body cavity. Genital polyps occur primarily in the uterus and cervix (Fig. 39–12). Uterine polyps may cause hypermenorrhea, intermenstrual bleeding, and postmenopausal bleeding. They occasionally undergo malignant changes, particularly in postmenopausal women. Cervical polyps may bleed after vaginal intercourse and are susceptible to infection.

If polyps are asymptomatic, they may simply be monitored. Because cervical polyps have a pedicle, they are easily removed by ligation. This procedure is usually performed in the physician's office. Uterine polyps are not easily removed because of their location within the uterus. Uterine polyps do not usually need to be removed

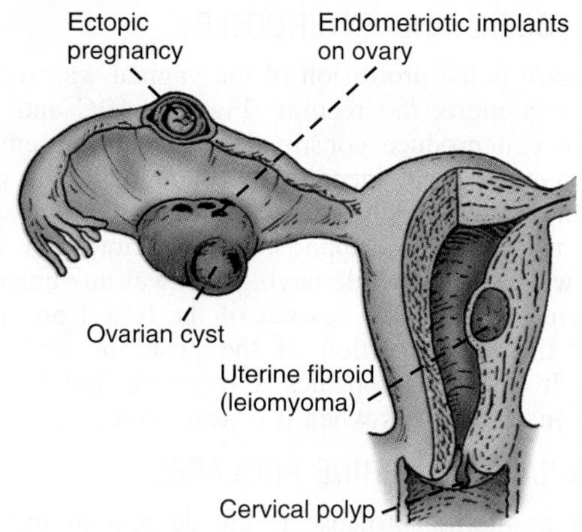

FIGURE 39–12 Common sites of some common benign gynecologic lesions.

unless they become symptomatic; if they must be removed, hysteroscopy is usually performed.

OVARIAN DISORDERS

BENIGN OVARIAN TUMORS

Benign ovarian tumors are either solid or cystic. Ovarian tumors are often asymptomatic until they are large enough to cause discomfort associated with pressure; this characteristic makes their early detection difficult. Typical manifestations associated with pressure are constipation, urinary frequency, a full feeling in the abdomen, vague pelvic aching and sensations of heaviness, painful defecation, and dyspareunia. Acute pain may be experienced during menses or with rupture. With an increasing growth, the client's abdominal girth increases, and her clothes may not fit as well. Generally, the client is unable to become pregnant.

Late and rare manifestations of a benign tumor include marked abdominal distention with dyspnea, peripheral edema, and anorexia. Pelvic pain may be present as a later manifestation if the ovarian tumor is growing rapidly. If the tumor produces hormones, menstrual irregularities and masculinizing or feminizing effects may be seen.

Complications include (1) hemorrhage into a cyst, with rupture and possible infection, (2) torsion (twisting) of a cystic pedicle, and (3) malignant changes.

Treatment depends on the type of tumor. Some small cystic masses can be treated with ovarian suppression, which is usually achieved with the use of birth control pills. Placing the ovaries in a pseudopregnancy state suppresses ovarian function and, in most cases, decreases the size of ovarian cystic masses.

Tumors can be removed surgically if they are growing rapidly or disrupt the function of the pelvic organs or the ovary. Removal can be achieved through laparoscopy or with open abdominal surgery. Surgery may include removal of (1) only the tumor, (2) the tumor and the ovary or ovaries, or (3) the tumor, both ovaries and tubes, and the uterus. The type of nursing care needed depends on the extent of surgery performed.

Ovarian cysts are physiologic tumors of ovaries. They are common and may or may not have manifestations. When manifestations do occur, the women may experience pelvic pain that is often worse on one side, pressure in the lower abdomen, backache, and menstrual irregularities.

A client with an ovarian cyst may be monitored for a month or two to determine whether the cyst might regress without intervention. If the cyst does not regress but is small, oral contraceptive therapy may provide a noninvasive therapy. Explain the treatment plan and condition to the client, and provide information about follow-up health care appointments and how to seek emergency care if needed.

A *follicular cyst* is caused by an unruptured follicle at the time of ovulation. It is often asymptomatic and frequently disappears without intervention. Sometimes, however, a cyst continues to enlarge as a result of hormone stimulation. Oral contraceptive therapy may be used if the cyst is small. Surgical intervention is required if the cyst increases in size and does not respond to medical management.

Corpus luteum cysts form when the corpus luteum fails to regress after discharging the ovum. Oral contraceptive therapy may be helpful for small cysts. However, surgical excision of the corpus luteum may be necessary. The remainder of the ovary can usually be saved.

OVARIAN CANCER

Ovarian cancer, although not the highest in incidence among reproductive tumors, is the leading cause of death from genital reproductive malignancies. The death rates have risen over time, probably because of a lack of early detection methods. An estimated 23,100 new cases of ovarian cancer were expected to have been detected in the United States in 2000, with 14,000 deaths.[1] White women show higher rates of ovarian cancer than African American women do.

Etiology and Risk Factors

The cause of ovarian cancer is unknown. Risk factors include:

- Age above 40 years
- Family history of ovarian or breast cancer (mutations in *BRCA1* or *BRCA2* genes have been observed in families)
- Family history of hereditary nonpolyposis colorectal cancer (HNPCC)
- Nulliparity
- History of infertility
- History of dysmenorrhea
- Use of ovulation-stimulating medications (a high number of ovulations increases the chances that a tumor suppressor gene called p53 can be mutated)

Pregnancy and the use of oral contraceptives appear to reduce the risk of ovarian cancer.

Health promotion factors include telling clients that ovarian cancer may be prevented by anything that interrupts constant ovulatory cycles, such as more than one full-term pregnancy, oral contraceptive use, breast-feeding, and bilateral oophorectomy. Health maintenance activities include routine pelvic examinations, determinations of CA-125 antigen levels in high-risk women, and performance of transvaginal ultrasound combined with bimanual pelvic examination and Doppler studies for lesions in question. Prophylactic mastectomy and oophorectomy may be performed in women with *BRCA1* or *BRCA2* mutations as a way of increasing life expectancy.

Pathophysiology

Most ovarian cancers are epithelial tumors, although some are adenocarcinomas. Ovarian cancer tends to grow and spread silently until manifestations of pelvic pressure on adjacent organs or abdominal distention cause the woman to seek medical care. When these pressure-related manifestations finally appear, the malignancy has usually spread to the fallopian tubes, uterus, and ligaments. Ovarian cancer often spreads to the other ovary and associated structures. The cancer may invade bowel surfaces, the omentum, liver, and other organs. When the pelvic blood vessels become involved, distant metastasis occurs. The usual routes of spread are lymphatic spread, hematogenous spread (through blood), local extension, and peritoneal seeding.

Clinical Manifestations

Clinical manifestations of ovarian cancer include (1) abdominal distention with increasing abdominal girth, (2) urinary frequency and urgency, (3) pleural effusion, (4) malnutrition with weight loss, (5) pain from pressure caused by the growing tumor and the effects of urinary or bowel obstruction, (6) constipation, (7) ascites with dyspnea, and (8)ultimately, general severe pain. Indications of ovarian cancer do not typically appear until the malignancy is well established, which is often not until it has spread. Unfortunately, unless the malignancy is diagnosed early, when it is most likely asymptomatic, most affected clients eventually have terminal cancer.

Identification of a pelvic mass by palpation is usually the first assessment finding. However, detecting such a mass may be difficult in a woman who is obese or who cannot relax during the examination. Palpation of the ovary in postmenopausal women should always be considered an abnormal finding and should be followed up with pelvic sonogram to rule out abnormalities.

When an ovarian mass is suspected, a complete evaluation is performed. This includes an intravenous pyelogram (IVP), computed tomography (CT) scan, and, possibly, a barium enema study. Ultrasonography can determine whether the mass is solid or cystic. Generally, after the evaluation, exploratory surgery is performed to directly visualize the ovaries, obtain biopsy specimens of the adjacent structures, and perform a resection if the mass is malignant.

A serum CA-125 determination may be performed to be used as a tumor marker to track tumor growth and regression. This test should not be the only one used to determine the presence of ovarian cancer because it can give false-positive and false-negative results.

A new diagnostic blood test may soon be available that measures levels of a chemical in the body called lysophosphatidic acid (LPA), which stimulates the growth of ovarian cancer cells. Elevated levels of LPA would indicate that a woman has ovarian cancer. This test is more precise than CA-125 measurement. Further research is needed before the LPA test becomes readily available.[41]

Outcome Management

Surgical Management

The extent of an ovarian malignancy is determined by exploratory surgery. Ovarian cancer is usually treated aggressively. A young woman with a borderline malignancy may be treated conservatively with a TAH-BSO. The surgery of choice is a TAH-BSO, partial or complete omentectomy, and removal of all visible tumor. The less residual tumor left, the better the prognosis.

Some women with ovarian cancer recover following treatment. Oncologists may recommend a second-look laparotomy in women who are clinically free of disease and who have received chemotherapy for 6 to 24 months to aid in the decision whether to continue treatment. During this procedure, multiple biopsy specimens are collected and analyzed to determine the presence or absence of residual tumor.

Medical Management

Adjuvant therapy varies with the stage of the disease. With stage I ovarian cancer, women typically receive irradiation or chemotherapy after surgery to destroy cancer cells that may have spread into the abdominal cavity. Systemic chemotherapy may be administered (see Chapter 19). Women with stage II or higher ovarian cancers typically receive the same treatment as those with stage I disease, with the inclusion of pelvic and, possibly, abdominal radiation.

Nursing Management of the Medical-Surgical Client

For the nursing care of the client who has undergone TAH-BSO, see earlier in this chapter; for care of the client with ovarian cancer, see Chapter 19.

VAGINAL DISORDERS

VAGINAL DISCHARGE AND PRURITUS

The female reproductive tract maintains its integrity through various natural defense mechanisms. Inflammation and infection occur when organisms disrupt or overcome these natural defenses. The resulting manifestations, although usually not life-threatening, can be uncomfortable and annoying. Vaginal discharge and itching are among the most common problems women mention to health care providers.

All women have normal, nonbloody, asymptomatic vaginal discharge called *leukorrhea.* This discharge, secreted by the endocervical glands, is a clear or white exudate that keeps vaginal mucous membranes moist and clear. As this exudate passes through the vagina, it may become cloudy and acquire a slight odor as desquamated epithelial cells, leukocytes, and normal vaginal flora are added.

The amount of vaginal discharge often varies in relation to the menstrual cycle. It is greatest at ovulation and just before menses. Pregnancy, sexual stimulation, and oral contraceptives tend to increase the discharge. Changes in the amount, color, character, or odor of vaginal discharge may indicate a problem.

Some women view normal vaginal discharge and odor as offensive and go to great lengths to eliminate it. However, use of douches or vaginal deodorants may disrupt the normal vaginal bacterial flora, causing vaginal irritation and infection. The consensus in the medical literature holds that periodic douching is unnecessary. There is evidence that douching may actually be detrimental. Douching washes away protective mucus and normal bacterial flora of the vagina and may cause overgrowth of undesirable bacteria and yeast.

The most common causes of vaginal discharge and irritation are (1) vaginal infections, (2) parasites, such as pinworms, (3) STDs (see Chapter 41), and (4) mechanical or allergic irritants. An example of a mechanical irritant is a tampon left in place too long. Some forms of contraceptive creams or foams may be allergenic irritants for some clients.

Most inflammatory and infectious vaginal problems are accompanied by pathologic vaginal discharge, which may be copious, malodorous, and abnormal in color. The discharge frequently causes itching, irritation, and redness of the vulva and surrounding areas. It may be accompanied by burning and frequency of urination, anal discomfort, and pain in the lower abdominal region.

VAGINITIS

Vaginitis is inflammation of the vagina, a common problem experienced by most women at some time in their life. Causes of vaginitis include change in normal vaginal flora, change in vaginal pH, and invasion of the vagina by virulent organisms. These conditions can be caused by congestion of the pelvic organs, mechanical irritation, vaginal infection, overmedication with antibiotics, long-term steroid therapy, uncontrolled diabetes, and acquired immunodeficiency syndrome (AIDS). Candidiasis (*Candida albicans* infection) is one of the most common causes of vaginitis. Health promotion actions related to vaginitis are described in the accompanying Client Education Guide: Preventing Vaginitis

The vagina is a cavity with a normal protective population of flora, including various bacteria. The adult vagina is normally acidic because of lactic acid formed from the glycogen in desquamating vaginal epithelium. Normal vaginal function depends on a delicate balance between hormones and bacteria. Disturbance of this balance can precipitate infection.

Vaginitis is characterized by a change in vaginal discharge. It may become profuse, odorous, and purulent. The diagnosis is confirmed by a speculum examination and microscopic examination of the discharge. Specimens may be obtained for culture if manifestations indicate an STD or bacterial infection. As a result of edema and tenderness in the vagina, the examination may be painful

CLIENT EDUCATION GUIDE

Preventing Vaginitis

Client Instructions

- Take care of yourself to prevent infection. Get enough rest, eat nutritious meals, and exercise at least three times a week.
- After using the toilet, always wipe yourself from front to back to avoid spreading germs.
- Change tampons or sanitary pads at least four times a day during your menstrual period, and wash your hands before and after each change.
- Avoid feminine hygiene sprays, which can be irritating. Soap and water are best for keeping yourself clean.
- Avoid tight-fitting jeans, pants, pantyhose, non-cotton (e.g., nylon) underwear, and any garment restricting ventilation.

and must be performed as gently as possible. Some bleeding may occur during and after the examination. Inform the client beforehand about the potential for pain and possible bleeding from the intrusion of the examination.

Vaginitis can be a stubborn, discouraging problem. Early, vigorous treatment may be necessary to prevent chronicity. Treatment is aimed at correcting the cause of the vaginitis. Attention must be given to the client's overall health.

TOXIC SHOCK SYNDROME

Toxic shock syndrome (TSS) is an acute condition caused by the toxin of a local infection with *Staphylococcus aureus*, which can develop into a systemic infection. It usually occurs in women who are menstruating and are using tampons or who have chronic vaginal infections.

TSS begins suddenly with a high fever, vomiting, and severe, watery diarrhea. Within 48 hours, a characteristic rash and hypotensive shock develop. Once the diagnosis is confirmed, antistaphylococcal antibiotics and fluid replacement therapy are begun.

Advise women to change tampons several times daily or to alternate tampons with sanitary napkins and to practice good hand-washing techniques to prevent development of TSS. If a vaginal sponge or diaphragm is used for contraception, it should be removed within 24 (diaphragm) to 30 (vaginal sponge) hours after intercourse. The diaphragm should not be used during menstruation.

ATROPHIC VAGINITIS

Atrophic vaginitis occurs in postmenopausal women. Atrophic, thin, vaginal mucosa and increased watery alkaline vaginal discharge provide an environment conducive to invasion by pyogenic bacteria. Assessment findings include a discharge with or without a bloody tinge, a vaginal burning sensation, itching of the vagina and vulva, and dyspareunia. If secondary infection is present, vulvar excoriation and burning with urination often occur. Long-term use of estrogen cream is the usual medical treatment. If a secondary infection is present, therapy with an appropriate antibiotic is added.

VAGINAL FISTULAE

Vaginal fistulae are abnormal tube-like passages from the vagina to the bladder *(vesicovaginal),* rectum *(rectovaginal),* or urethra *(urethrovaginal)* (Fig. 39–13). Fistula formation is an extremely distressing problem in the genitourinary tract.

Etiology and Risk Factors

Fistulae may be congenital or may result from injury or surgery. About 10% of all fistulae occur in the female reproductive area. Vaginal fistulae may occur because of the spread of a malignant lesion, after irradiation for cancer, as a result of inflammatory disease, and after a prolonged, difficult labor and traumatic delivery.

Clinical Manifestations

Urine or flatus and feces leak into the vagina. Vaginal and vulval tissues become excoriated and irritated. Chronic urinary tract infection may result. Rectovaginal fistulas may cause an offensive, particularly unpleasant odor. The client experiences wetness and a sensation of feeling unclean.

In addition to their unpleasant physical manifestations, vaginal fistulae produce severely distressing psychosocial problems. Clients often become social recluses. Fistulae greatly disrupt intimate relationships and social activities. Clients often do not seek professional health care until the problem becomes severe. Even then, they may be embarrassed and reluctant to discuss it.

A simple diagnostic test is the instillation of methylene blue dye into the bladder or rectum via Foley catheter and placement of a tampon in the vagina. The woman is asked to walk and perform exertional exercise for a short while. The tampon is then removed and evaluated for color and absorption. The test is considered positive if blue dye is found on the tampon. A *fistulogram* (injection of dye into the vagina) can be performed to assess the location and extent of the fistula.

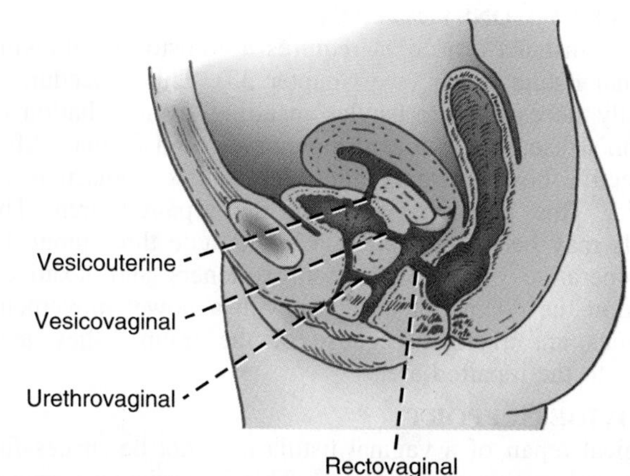

FIGURE 39–13 Locations of main types of vaginal fistulas.

Outcome Management

Medical-Surgical Management

The diagnosis and treatment of a vaginal fistula may be difficult. Treatment varies with the fistula's location, extent, and cause and the client's general health. Occasionally, a fistula heals spontaneously. Medical management is used first to treat infection because surgical management is rarely successful, especially when an infection is present. The client must be in optimal physical condition before surgery is attempted.

On occasion, a temporary colostomy may be necessary to treat a rectovaginal fistula (see Chapter 33), and a suprapubic catheter must be inserted to prevent bladder distention after a repair of a vesicovaginal fistula. Excision of either of these fistulae is difficult with a high rate of recurrence.

Nursing Management of the Medical-Surgical Client

An accepting attitude of health professionals to a client with a vaginal fistula is essential to help her comfortably accept and follow through with needed treatments. Help the client to minimize the manifestations and care for herself.

PREVENT INFECTION

Some clients unadvisedly restrict their fluid intake in an attempt to decrease the drainage. This action may actually increase the size of the fistula and raise the chance of infection. Make sure the woman understands the importance of increasing her fluid intake to reduce the risk of infection. Perineal hygiene measures may include cleansing the perineum every 4 hours, taking sitz baths, and changing perineal pads frequently.

If surgery is used to repair the fistula, care is directed at avoiding physical stress on the repaired area and preventing infection. A Foley or suprapubic catheter is used after a vesicovaginal or urethrovaginal fistulectomy to drain the urinary bladder. Careful attention is necessary to keep the catheter patent and draining. Provide and encourage enough fluid intake so that internal catheter irrigation is accomplished. It is a nursing responsibility to monitor the catheter for patency. If the catheter becomes obstructed, the increased bladder pressure could adversely affect the surgical sites and cause the fistula to reopen.

PREVENT CONSTIPATION

In rare instances, a client requires a colostomy following vaginal fistula repair (see Chapter 33). This procedure is usually necessary for fistulas resulting from radiation or Crohn's disease and for postoperative rectal fistulas. After corrective bowel surgery, the client's first stools may be liquid. This prevents stress on the repaired area. The stools may be maintained in a liquid state throughout the postoperative period with stool softeners and laxatives. Caution the client not to strain with a bowel movement. Enemas are avoided because of the trauma they may cause to the repaired area.

PROVIDE SUPPORT

Surgical repair of a vaginal fistula may not be successful, even under optimal conditions. This is particularly true if a client has extensive tissue damage from tumors or irradiation. Supportive nursing care is extremely important for women experiencing this distressing disorder and for their significant others as well.

VAGINAL CANCER

Primary invasive vaginal cancer is a rare lesion, typically occurring in women over 50 years old. However, it is seen in younger women whose mothers took diethylstilbestrol (DES) during pregnancy. DES was widely prescribed in the United States from 1940 to 1970 for threatened miscarriage and other high-risk pregnancy problems. Among women who have not been exposed to DES, vaginal cancer is rare in African Americans and almost nonexistent in Jews.

Etiology and Risk Factors

The risk factor for vaginal (clear cell) cancer is maternal ingestion of DES. Other potential causes of vaginal cancer are (1) exposure to the drug in utero in girls and women between menarche and age 30 (adenocarcinoma), (2) repeated pregnancies, (3) a history of STD, herpes virus, or HPV, (4) prior irradiation, (5) immunosuppressive therapy, and (6) significant irritation due to a poorly fitting pessary. Leukoplakia and leukorrhea are often associated with vaginal cancer.

Pathophysiology

The staging of vaginal cancer is similar to that used for other pelvic malignancies. The primary lesion and involvement of adjacent structures are considered. Primary invasive cancer tends to involve the anterior or posterior vaginal walls, or both. Complications may involve the urinary bladder or bowel, as in fistula formation.

Despite active treatment, the prognosis for vaginal cancer is generally poor. The overall cure rate reported by the American Cancer Society is about 35%. Half of women with vaginal cancer die within 18 months of diagnosis.[1] Low survival rates are due to the rarity of the cancer (2100 cases per year in the United States), which makes it difficult to identify, the typically advanced stage of the cancer when it is diagnosed, and the difficulty in treating this cancer with radiation or surgery because of the proximity of important structures.

Clinical Manifestations

Indications of vaginal cancer include foul vaginal discharge, painless vaginal bleeding, pruritus, pain (not associated with bleeding), and the presence of a vaginal mass or lesion. Urinary bladder manifestations, such as pain and frequency, may occur if a vaginal mass compresses the bladder.

Women exposed to DES in utero should receive careful examination of the cervix, along with cytologic examination of the cervix and any questionable area in the vagina. Colposcopy may be used to identify areas to be sampled for biopsy. During pelvic examination, Lugol's solution may be applied to any vaginal areas that appear abnormal. Lack of staining identifies suspect areas. Unfortunately, the lesions of vaginal cancer are often well advanced before manifestations appear. Earlier lesions might be missed during pelvic examination.

Outcome Management

Medical Management

The usual treatment for vaginal cancer is either external or intravaginal radiation therapy or, less often, surgery. External radiation therapy is used for all stages of vaginal cancer. Internal radiation is generally used only in the earlier stages. The difficulty of applying radiation to the vagina without causing harm to the bladder and rectum has led some physicians to prefer surgical intervention.

Surgical Management

For earlier stages, radical hysterectomy, lymphadenectomy, and vaginectomy are performed. *Partial vaginectomy* refers to removal of the upper third to half of the vagina as part of the procedure in a radical hysterectomy. Pelvic exenteration is used in more advanced cancer if the bladder or rectum is involved; it is also indicated in a client with recurrent metastases.

Nursing Management of the Medical-Surgical Client

During assessment, ask young women born between 1940 and 1970 about medications their mothers may have taken during pregnancy. All those whose mothers took DES when pregnant with them should have a gynecologic examination at least twice yearly beginning at menarche, or at age 14, whichever comes first.

PROVIDE SUPPORT

Vaginal surgery may be anxiety-promoting and frightening. Ostomies (see Chapters 33 and 34) also may need to be performed, adding to the client's fears and problems.

DISCUSS SEXUALITY

Sexuality is an important nursing consideration in the care of women with vaginal cancer. Postoperatively, vaginal sexual activity is not possible unless vaginal reconstruction has been performed. Vaginal sex may be difficult after surgery or radiation therapy because of changes in the size and shape of the vagina. Assess the client's previous sexual history and her self-esteem to identify possible problems. Create a therapeutic environment that allows her to feel comfortable discussing sexual concerns.

Discuss the potential impact of the disease process and treatment on sexuality, as appropriate. Potential problems include fatigue, pain, dyspareunia, decreased libido, and altered body image. If a partial vaginectomy is performed, the client can probably still enjoy normal vaginal sexual activity, using large amounts of lubricant and modified positioning, because the vaginal tissue will stretch.

PROMOTE REST

To help the client cope with fatigue and pain, suggest that she schedule sexual activity after resting. Also, schedule pain medication so that the peak of action coincides with sexual activity. A warm bath, a back rub, alternate positioning, or relaxation techniques might also help. Advise the client to use a water-soluble lubricant during intercourse and, perhaps, a vaginal dilator at other times to prevent vaginal fibrosis and tightening.

VULVAR DISORDERS

VULVITIS

Vulvitis (inflammation of the vulva) is caused by direct irritation of vulvar tissues or by direct extension of irritation from the vagina to the vulva that results in itching. Risk factors associated with vulvitis include skin disorders, inflammatory problems, infection, allergies, postmenopausal atrophy and dryness, uncontrolled diabetes, pediculosis, scabies, cancer, incontinence, and poor perineal hygiene.

Medical treatment is based on the specific cause of the condition. Itching, the most common manifestation associated with vulvitis, can be severe. A local or systemic antipruritic or antihistamine agent, such as hydrocortisone cream, diphenhydramine hydrochloride (Benadryl), or hydroxyzine hydrochloride (Atarax), may be given to relieve the itching.

Teach the client the following measures to relieve itching:

1. Apply cold compresses.
2. Wear light, nonrestrictive clothing, including well-washed and well-rinsed cotton underpants. Synthetic underpants tend to keep the vulvar area warm and moist.
3. Avoid feminine hygiene sprays.
4. Apply prescribed hydrocortisone ointment or anesthetic sprays.
5. Keep the vulva clean and dry. Clean after elimination by washing the vulva with very mild soap and water; wiping with toilet tissue or a washcloth from front to back; rinsing and drying the area well; and applying cornstarch to maintain dryness.

VULVAR CANCER

Vulvar cancer is found mainly in women older than 50 years of age. It accounts for about 3400 cases of female genital carcinoma each year in the United States.[1]

Etiology and Risk Factors

Vulvar disorders (e.g., lichen sclerosus, previously called kraurosis vulvae or atrophic leukoplakia, and diabetic vulvitis) increase the risk of vulvar cancer. Contracting certain STDs, such as HPV, also raises the risk.

Pathophysiology

Vulvar cancer arises from skin, urethra, glands, or subcutaneous tissues. Approximately 90% to 95% of vulvar cancers are squamous cell carcinoma. The remaining 5% to 10% are adenocarcinoma, Paget's disease, malignant melanoma, or sarcoma.

Vulvar cancer grows slowly and remains localized for a long time. Most lesions are located in the labia, primarily the labia majora. Some are on the clitoris. Local spread may occur to the urethra, vagina, anus, and rectum. Lymphatic spread is to the inguinal, femoral, pelvic, and finally, periaortic nodes. The usual causes of death from widespread vulvar cancer are distant metastasis, urethral obstruction, infection, uremia, and hemorrhage.

The prognosis is poor with vulvar invasive lesions. Five-year survival rates for clients who have undergone vulvectomy and lymphadenectomy are approximately 65%. Recurrence as well as distant metastasis may appear in the first 2 years. When lesions are diagnosed in an advanced stage with node involvement, the survival rate is only 8% to 10%.

Clinical Manifestations

Lichen sclerosus is characterized by thickened gray patches of epithelium scattered over the vulva and perineum. Cracked areas in these patches provide an ideal medium for infection, which causes the tissues to ulcerate and macerate. Eventually, these areas may become malignant.

Secondary infection is characterized by a bright red, smooth, almost transparent vulvar epithelium. Lichen sclerosus is most common in postmenopausal women. With its progression, the vulvar tissues shrink and constrict the vaginal opening.

Initially, lichen sclerosus causes itching and soreness or pain but may be asymptomatic. Clinical manifestations of early vulvar cancer include pruritus, minimal vulval soreness, dyspareunia, and tissue irritation with some bleeding. The potential seriousness of these relatively mild problems may not be appreciated by women or their health care providers because the manifestations are similar to those of nonmalignant vulvar lesions. As the vulvar cancer progresses, clinical manifestations of vulvar edema and pelvic lymphadenopathy develop. Secondary infection may cause a foul-smelling discharge. Biopsy of the affected area confirms the diagnosis.

Outcome Management

Medical Management

When lichen sclerosus is present, a biopsy to rule out cancer is indicated. Infection is treated with an appropriate systemic or topical antibiotic, steroid creams, and hormone cream. Other manifestations are treated symptomatically.

Irradiation and chemotherapy are used less often than surgical therapy. Irradiation is not generally used because the involved tissues do not tolerate it well. Chemotherapy is typically not given unless metastasis has occurred. The agent of choice is then selected according to the extent of metastasis.

Nursing Management of the Medical Client

Nursing management of the client with lichen sclerosus is mainly supportive care throughout the diagnostic period. Itching can be treated symptomatically with antipruritic creams such as hydrocortisone.

Surgical Management

A vulvectomy is performed to remove abnormal tissue through procedures such as a skinning technique, local wide excision, or a simple or radical vulvectomy. A laser may be used in conjunction with these procedures to destroy specific abnormal tissue.

A *simple vulvectomy* involves removal of the labia majora, labia minora, and sometimes the glans clitoris. Occasionally, the perineal area is also removed, requiring plastic surgery to cover the vulvar area. However, extensive surgery is avoided if the client's condition allows a simpler procedure.

A *radical vulvectomy* (Fig. 39–14) consists of excision of tissue from the anus to a few centimeters below the symphysis pubis (skin, labia majora, labia minora, and clitoris). Bilateral dissection of groin lymph nodes, such as the superficial groin and deep inguinal, femoral, iliac, hypogastric, and obturator nodes, also may be performed.

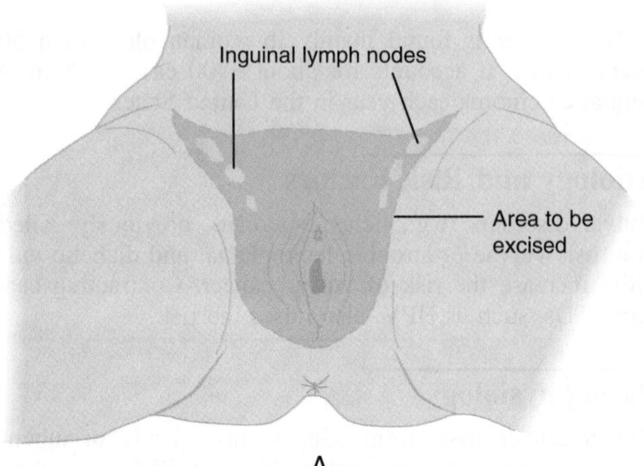

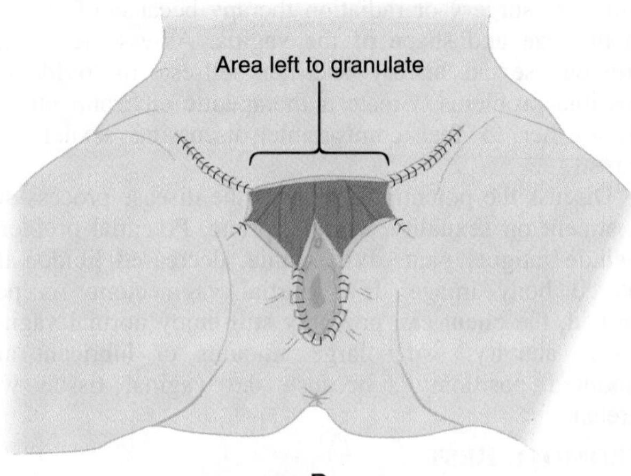

FIGURE 39–14 Radical vulvectomy. *A*, Area to be excised and line of incision *(dashed line).* The vulvar skin, underlying subcutaneous tissue and muscles, and regional lymph nodes are excised. If the anus is involved, the incision also continues around it. Inguinal and femoral lymph nodes are resected en bloc. *B*, Completed surgery. Perineal skin is approximated to the vagina, and a large area is left open to heal gradually by filling in with granulation tissue. A simple vulvectomy (not shown) does not remove the lymph nodes. Hence, the incision does not extend into the groin.

Full recovery is possible but may take 6 months or longer. Wound infections and delayed wound healing may lead to numerous problems. The long recovery and potential complications further impair the client's body image.

Nursing Management of the Surgical Client

PREOPERATIVE CARE

For a woman experiencing vulvar surgery, psychosocial support is especially important and should begin preoperatively. Some problems you might anticipate are fear of disfigurement, grief over the loss of a body part, fear of death, and sexual concerns.

Preoperative preparation is similar to that for other gynecologic procedures. The client scheduled for a vulvectomy must understand what the surgery entails, know what preoperative procedures will be performed, and have an idea of what to expect in the postoperative period. See the Client Education Guide: Recovering from Radical Vulvectomy.

POSTOPERATIVE CARE

The client undergoing a radical vulvectomy is susceptible to many postoperative complications because of the extensive nature of the operation. In addition to routine postoperative care, a suction device (e.g., Hemovac), tubes, or drain must be placed in the incision to remove drainage and to reduce the risk of infection. Carefully monitor the amount of bleeding. A bed cradle is helpful in keeping bed linens away from the incision.

CLIENT EDUCATION GUIDE

Recovering from Radical Vulvectomy

Client Instructions

- Avoid strenuous exercise involving the legs and pelvis.
- Gradually resume normal physical activities.
- Resume sexual activity, if desired, when the surgeon indicates. If intercourse is resumed, top or side positions are preferable to avoid direct pressure on the operative area. Water-soluble lubricants can be used for comfort.
- Take showers rather than tub baths. Showers reduce the likelihood of postoperative wound infection. Gentle, thorough washing of the genital area is important. Wipe gently from front to back after bowel movements and urinating. Do not douche without permission from the surgeon.
- Notify the surgeon if any of the following problems occurs:
  - Perineal pain unrelieved by prescribed medication
  - Foul-smelling perineal discharge
  - Heavy perineal bleeding or clots
  - Foul odor from the incision
  - Change in color of the incision (especially manifestations of decreased circulation)
  - Swelling of the groin or genital area
  - Frequent urination, urinating in small amounts, or discomfort or burning on urination
  - Temperature of 100° F (37.8° C) or higher
  - Pain, tenderness, or redness in the calves

PREVENT THROMBOPHLEBITIS. The client wears antiembolism or sequential compression stockings to prevent leg edema and thrombophlebitis, which constitutes a postoperative and a long-term problem. Keep the legs elevated as much as possible. Resuming ambulation postoperatively as early as possible helps to decrease leg edema and thrombophlebitis. The client should perform leg exercises to prevent circulatory problems. Teach the client to avoid sitting with the legs dependent, standing, and crossing the legs. A low-dose anticoagulant, such as heparin, warfarin (Coumadin), or aspirin, may be used prophylactically (as prevention) to reduce the risk of phlebitis and subsequent pulmonary embolism.

Lower extremity lymphedema can cause a change in clothing size and an upsetting change in appearance. In addition, some clients have difficulty sitting for long periods, making activities such as long automobile trips difficult.

PREVENT INFECTION. Prevent infection in the incisional area through frequent dressing changes, perineal care or sitz baths after voiding and bowel movements, and meticulous wound care. A Foley catheter is usually in place for 7 to 14 days or until healing is adequate. If the catheter is removed, carefully monitor urination with supportive care to prevent infection and voiding dysfunction. Additionally, it is important to monitor bowel movements. Once healing has occurred, the client may require reconstructive surgery.

PROVIDE SUPPORT. Psychosocially, a vulvectomy may be a devastating experience for a woman because of its direct effect on the external genitalia. The surgery, especially a radical vulvectomy, may compromise the client's physical integrity and her sense of wholeness. Some important issues for a woman are fear of recurrence and metastasis, disfigurement, concern about future sexual activity, and fear of her partner's rejection.

Nursing care involves helping the woman redefine her self-image to include the physical changes of vulvectomy. Try to create an environment in which she can express her feelings. Provide opportunities for her to mourn the loss and its effect on her sexuality. Encourage her to resume her normal activities as soon as possible to reinforce her feelings of self-worth.

Stress in social relationships is common after this radical surgery. The client and her significant other may benefit from counseling aimed at developing healthy coping skills.

The effect of a vulvectomy on female sexuality has not been well described. The disfigurement secondary to the surgery can lead to body image distortion, which affects sexual functioning. Physical changes, such as removal of the clitoris, result in loss of the ability to experience orgasm. The client may experience loss of sensation within the vagina. Also, stenosis of the introitus may follow surgery, making intercourse painful or difficult; this can have a major impact on sexuality. If stenosis occurs, it can be treated with vaginal dilators. If dilation is unsuccessful, plastic surgery should be considered.

Sexual counseling should be considered for all women undergoing vulvectomy and their partners. Assist the client and her sexual partner by communicating openly with them, answering their questions, explaining structural vulvar changes, and suggesting alternative forms of sexual arousal for the client.

PROMOTE VOIDING. Some women experience unpredictable voiding difficulties following a radical vulvectomy. A client may present with complaints of incontinence, retention, or a dysfunctional voiding pattern (see Chapter 34).

BARTHOLINITIS

Inflammation of Bartholin's glands can be caused by various organisms, including gonococci, streptococci, staphylococci, and *E. coli.* The infection involves the duct of the gland, producing edema and, eventually, obstruction. Because the inflamed gland cannot drain, it swells, and an abscess forms. Cellulitis develops in the surrounding tissues, producing more pain and systemic manifestations. The abscess may rupture spontaneously or may require incision and drainage.

After the acute episode, occlusion of the duct by fibrosis and scarring causes retention of secretions and dilation of the duct. It then becomes a palpable, mobile cyst, which usually is not painful. Manifestations, which relate to the size of the cyst, include dyspareunia and pain on walking.

Systemic antibiotics specific for the causative organism are prescribed. Local heat with hot packs or sitz baths may help promote drainage. Surgery may be necessary, such as an incision and drainage or removal of the gland if cancer is suspected or for repeated infections with abscess formation.

FEMALE GENITAL MUTILATION

Female genital mutilation (FGM), often called *female circumcision,* is a medically unnecessary surgical modification of the female genitalia practiced in several African, Asian and Middle Eastern countries. It may be seen in female immigrants from these areas. The procedure is performed on girls between ages 4 and 12 years old. Globally, FGM is estimated to affect 130 million girls and women, with approximately 2 million new FGM procedures performed yearly. About 120,000 immigrants to the United States between 1991 and 1995 originated from countries in which FGM is practiced.[24]

There are four major types, and types 1 and 2 are performed in 85% of cases[24]:

Type 1, Sunna: excision of the clitoral prepuce only, or *clitoridectomy* (partial or complete removal of the clitoris).

Type 2, Excision: removal of prepuce and clitoris along with adjoining parts of labia minora.

Type 3, Infibulation: removal of parts described in type 2 and parts of interior labia majora. The raw surfaces of the two sides of the vulva are then sutured together, obliterating the introitus. A small opening is left to allow for urine and menstrual flow.

Type 4, Other: burning of instead of cutting of the clitoris, stretching labia minora to enhance sexual pleasure, or making cuts into the vagina.

Etiology and Risk Factors

The FGM procedure originated from the belief that women are highly sexual and promiscuous. Type 3 FGM is performed to isolate women from sexual desires and temptation. Other factors are (1) religious influences, (2) promotion of social and political cohesion, (3) distinguishing chaste from adulterous women, (4) distinguishing indigenous from non-indigenous women, and (5) economic benefits for the father are additional reasons. Some practitioners of FGM believe that removal of the external genitalia makes the woman cleaner and more sexually attractive. Others believe that the clitoris generates additional excitement for the male, leading to early ejaculation, so that removal of the clitoris limits sexual excitement for both sexes. Still others believe that FGM after childbirth ensures fidelity in a marriage. Finally, some ethnic groups believe that the clitoris can kill a child if it touches the child's head during birth.

The decision to perform FGM is left to mothers, grandmothers, and elderly women. The rationale for disfavoring the practice includes marriage complications, labor complications, psychosexual beliefs, abandonment because of sterility, and the effects of the traumatic experience. Despite these problems, many ethnic groups, including men and women, continue to support the practice of FGM even while living in the United States.

Clinical Manifestations

Complications from FGM include:

- High infant mortality rate
- Hemorrhage, shock, and death during the procedure
- Keloid formation
- Chronic vaginal and pelvic infections
- Acute urinary retention
- Recurrent urinary tract infections
- Urolithiasis
- Urinary, rectal, and vaginal fistulas
- Damage to the urethra
- Prolonged labor and problems with delivery
- Psychological trauma

Clinical manifestations of these complications may lead the woman to seek health care.

Outcome Management

Management of the client with FGM is directed toward relief of clinical manifestations related to the complications. Some of these conditions have been discussed earlier in this chapter and in Chapter 34. To enable childbirth, a cesarean section or *deinfibulation* (opening of the incisional area anteriorly) may be required.

When caring for a woman with FGM, remain sensitive and nonjudgmental to gain her confidence and establish a trusting, therapeutic relationship. Teach her about the complications of the procedure; this issue is extremely important if she has daughters, who may be at risk for FGM. Unresolved grief and low self-esteem after the trauma of the experience or sterility caused by chronic PID may require supportive intervention or counseling.

Health care providers must act as advocates for women and girls affected by FGM by increasing professional and public awareness of the practice and its existence in the United States. Report FGM involving a girl younger than 18 years, because it is considered child abuse.

ALTERNATIVE THERAPY

Female Reproductive System: Premenstrual Syndrome and Menopause

Premenstrual Disorders

For the 20% to 50% of women who suffer from premenstrual tension or premenstrual syndrome (PMS) at some point in their lives, nutrient and herbal remedies may also be helpful. One review of vitamin B_6 in treating PMS found that although many studies were not of good quality, thus warranting further research, vitamin B_6 at doses up to 100 mg/day appeared to be helpful in treating PMS and premenstrual depression.[11]

Even more effective than vitamin B_6, in a comparison trial, was the herb chaste tree berry (*Vitex agnus-castus*). Several studies have found chaste tree berry beneficial in treating PMS.[7] Although more side effects were seen in the chaste tree berry group than in the vitamin B_6 group, no serious side effects were observed.

As with the treatment of menopausal manifestations, Chinese herbs are commonly used in treating PMS.[3] Aside from anecdotal reports, however, there is a lack of controlled studies using these therapies.

Menopause

Although a normal, natural and asymptomatic process for many women, menopause can be an uncomfortable transition time for others. There seem to be cultural and geographic differences in menopausal manifestations reported around the world, perhaps in part related to dietary variations. Some have suggested that there has been a "medicalization" of menopause, a focus on "the change" as a pathologic condition requiring treatment rather than as a normal healthy process.[9]

Chinese herbal therapies are widely used by practitioners of Asian (Oriental) medicine for treating the manifestations of perimenopause and menopause. Although such use is detailed in the Asian medical literature, Western research in this area remains inconclusive. Interestingly, in Japan the main manifestation reported by perimenopausal women is stiffness of the neck and shoulders, with hot flashes low on the report list of manifestations.

The herb black cohosh (*Cimicifuga racemosa*), originally used by native Americans, has been extensively studied in Europe in more than 1700 clients, over 3 to 6 months, showing benefits in treating hot flashes, sweating, and sleep disturbances related to menopause.[5] Such preparations of black cohosh have been used for more than 40 years in Europe. More recently, black cohosh has been combined with St. John's wort for concomitant treatment of depressive manifestations during menopause and to enhance its effect for clients with sleep disturbances.[8]

Phytoestrogens (plant hormones) have been studied for their potential effects in treatment of menopausal manifestations and for their longer-term effects in preventing both heart disease and osteoporosis. Phytoestrogens from soy products have been studied extensively, and it is speculated that intake of soy products in Asia may account for differences in menopausal manifestations reported there compared to the West. Phytoestrogens may help as many as two thirds of women with hot flashes, although there is little evidence that they help with vaginal dryness, another complaint of menopausal women.[4] Soy products have been shown to reduce total and low-density lipoprotein cholesterol levels, to lower diastolic blood pressure, and to decrease the severity of vasomotor manifestations.[10] In rat studies, soy isoflavones have conserved bone. Research in postmenopausal women has been limited but has shown small, positive effects only in lumbar vertebrae.[2]

The importance of lifestyle factors in the prevention of heart disease and osteoporosis is well known. With newer evidence for antioxidant vitamins in the prevention of heart disease and calcium for delaying osteoporosis, women have a number of choices of treatment of menopausal symptoms and of longer-term prevention of osteoporosis and heart disease.[1, 6]

References

1. Adams, A. K., Wermuth, E. O., & McBride, P. E. (1999). Antioxidant vitamins and the prevention of coronary heart disease. *American Family Physician, 60,* 895–904.
2. Anderson, J. J., & Garner, S. C. (1998). Phytoestrogens and bone. *Baillieres Clinical Endocrinology and Metabolism, 12,* 543–557.
3. Bensky, D., & Barolet, R. (1990). *Chinese herbal medicine-formulas and strategies.* Seattle: Eastland Press.
4. Eden, J. (1998). Phytoestrogens and the menopause. *Baillieres Clinical Endocrinology and Metabolism, 12,* 581–587.
5. Foster, S. (1999). Black cohosh: *Cimicifuga racemosa,* A literature review. *HerbalGram, 45,* 35–49.
6. Keller, C., Fullerton, J., & Mobley, C. (1999). Supplemental and complementary alternatives to hormone replacement therapy. *Journal of the American Academy of Nurse-Practitioners, 11(5),* 187–198.
7. Klepser, T., & Nisly, N. (1999). Chaste tree berry for premenstrual syndrome. *Alternative Medicine Alert, 2,* 64–67.
8. Liske, E., Gerhard, I., & Wustenberg, P. (1997). Phytocombination alleviates psychovegetative disorders. *TW Gynakologie, 10,* 172–175.
9. Locke, M. (1993). *Encounters with aging: Mythologies of menopause in Japan and North America.* Berkeley, CA: University of California Press.
10. Washburn, S., et al. (1999). Effect of soy protein supplementation on serum lipoproteins, blood pressure, and menopausal symptoms in perimenopausal women. *Menopause, 6,* 7–13.
11. Wyatt, K. M., et al. (1999). Efficacy of vitamin B_6 in the treatment of premenstrual syndrome: Systematic review. *British Medical Journal, 318,* 1375–1381.

James Higgy Lerner, RN, LAc, *Private practice of acupuncture, traditional Oriental medicine, and biofeedback*

CONCLUSIONS

Female reproductive disorders can occur throughout a woman's life. These problems range from menstrual disorders to life-threatening malignancies. Nurses can provide much of the needed education to help clients become more aware of preventive measures. The physical and psychosocial care of these clients is important. The skillful and empathic nurse can assist the woman through what is often an extremely distressing diagnosis and treatment.

Nurses who need more information on reproductive issues should consult a women's health (obstetrics and gynecology) textbook. Information on contraception, tubal ligation, abortion, and other issues can be found there.

THINKING CRITICALLY

1. **The client, a 52-year-old woman, comes into the clinic stating, "I can't put up with it any longer!" Her last menstrual period was 4 months ago, and she has had severe hot flashes and night sweats for almost 6 months with no abatement. Vaginal intercourse has become so painful that she and her husband have refrained from sexual activity for 3 months. She states that the night sweats are so bad that she has had very few nights of uninterrupted sleep.**

Factors to Consider. What are your priorities for her care? What interventions might be used?

2. **A 38-year-old woman enters the clinic with a complaint of acute, sharp, severe bilateral pelvic pain. She has a temperature of 102.2° F, a pulse rate of 100 beats/min, a respiratory rate of 20 breaths/min, and chills. Her cervical culture shows gonococcal infection. She uses oral contraceptives for birth control.**

Factors to Consider. Besides teaching her about antibiotic medication, what is your priority in caring for her, and what interventions are necessary?

3. **The client, a 61-year-old woman, had a TAH-BSO 2 days ago for early endometrial cancer. Her Foley catheter was removed yesterday. Her temperature is 101.1° F, her pulse rate is 96 beats/min, and her respiratory rate is 16 breaths/min. Her blood pressure is 128/74 mm Hg. She complains of flank pain and urinary hesitancy. Her urine output for the past 4 hours is 120 ml, which is the total from three separate voidings. Her urine is cloudy and has a slightly foul odor.**

Factors to Consider. What is your priority, and what interventions are needed?

BIBLIOGRAPHY

1. American Cancer Society. (2000). *Cancer facts and figures.* Atlanta: Author.
2. Avis, N. E., & McKinlay, S. M. (1995). The Massachusetts Women's Health Study: An epidemiologic investigation of the menopause. *Journal of the American Medical Women's Association, 50*(2), 45–49.
3. Baker, V., & Deppe, G. (1997). *Management of perioperative complications in gynecology.* Philadelphia: W. B. Saunders.
4. Bernier, F., & Jenkins, P. (1997). The role of vaginal estrogen in the treatment of urogenital dysfunction in postmenopausal women. *Urologic Nursing, 17*(3), 92–95.
5. Bobak, I. M., & Jensen, M. D. (1997). *Maternity and women's health care* (6th ed.). St. Louis: Mosby–Year Book.
6. Compston, J., & Marsh, M. (1999). *HRT and the menopause: Current therapy.* London: Martin Dunitz.
7. Cunningham, G., & Williams, J. (1997). *Williams' obstetrics* (20th ed.). Stamford, CT: Appleton & Lange.
8. DiSaia, P., & Creasman, W. (1997). *Clinical gynecologic oncology.* St. Louis: Mosby–Year Book.
9. Fogey, C. I., & Woods, N. F. (Eds.). (1995). *Women's health care: A comprehensive handbook.* Thousand Oaks, CA: Sage Publications.
10. Fontana, P. (1998). Endometrial cancer, cervical cancer, and the adnexal mass. In B. Agar (Ed.), *Primary Care: Oncology, 25*(2), 433–458.
11. Griffith, C. (1997). *Gynecologic oncology.* London: Mosby-Wolfe.
12. Hansen, M. (1998). *Pathophysiology: Foundations of disease and clinical intervention.* Philadelphia: W. B. Saunders.
13. Hopkins, W., Perez, C., & Young, R. (1997). *Principles and practice of gynecologic oncology* (2nd ed.). Philadelphia: Lippincott-Raven.
14. Howell, D. (1999). *The unofficial guide to coping with menopause.* New York: Macmillan.
15. Hulley, S., et al. (1998). Randomized trial of estrogen plus progestin for secondary prevention of coronary heart disease in postmenopausal women. *Journal of the American Medical Association, 280*(7), 605–613.
16. Kolander, C., Ballard, D., & Chandler, C. (1999). *Contemporary women's health: Issues for today and the future.* Boston: WCB McGraw-Hill.
17. Lichtman, R. (1996). Perimenopausal and postmenopausal hormone replacement therapy: I. An update of the literature on benefits and risks. *Journal of Nurse-Midwifery, 41*(1), 3–28.
18. Manos, M., et al. (1999). Identifying women with cervical neoplasia using human papillomavirus DNA testing for equivocal Papanicolaou results. *Journal of the American Medical Association, 281*(17), 1605–1610.
19. McCorkle, R., et al. (1996). *Cancer nursing: A comprehensive text* (2nd ed.). Philadelphia: W. B. Saunders.
20. Mills, D. (1999). *Endometriosis: A key to healing through nutrition.* Boston: Shaftesbury Dorset.
21. Mishell, D., et al. (1997). *Comprehensive gynecology.* (3rd ed.). St. Louis: Mosby–Year Book.
22. Mogus, M. (1997). Pelvic floor surgery? *RN, 67*(4), 36–41.
23. Moody, F. (1999). *Atlas of ambulatory surgery.* Philadelphia: W. B. Saunders.
24. Morris, R. (1999). Female genital mutilation: Perspectives, risks and complications. *Urologic Nursing, 19*(1), 13–19.
25. Ozols, R. (Ed.). (1998). *Gynecologic oncology.* Boston: Kluwer Academic Publishers.
26. Raz, S. (1996). *Female urology* (2nd ed.). Philadelphia: W. B. Saunders.
27. Sabiston, D. (1997). *Textbook of surgery: The biological basis of modern surgical practice* (15th ed.). Philadelphia: W. B. Saunders.
28. Schrag, D., et al. (1997). Decision analysis: Effects of prophylactic mastectomy and oophorectomy on life expectancy among women with *BRCA1* or *BRCA2* mutations. *New England Journal of Medicine, 336*(20), 1565–1471.
29. Schull, B. (1996). Initial evaluation and physical examination. In L. Brubaker & T. Sacharides (Eds.), *The female pelvic floor* (pp. 41–49). Philadelphia: F. A. Davis.
30. Selleck, C. (1997). Identifying and treating bacterial vaginosis. *American Journal of Nursing, 97*(9), 16AAA–16DDD.
31. Seltzer, V., & Pearse, W. H. (Eds.). (1995). *Women's primary health care.* New York: McGraw-Hill.
32. Shurpin, K. (1997). Ovarian cancer. *American Journal of Nursing, 97*(4), 34–35.
33. Smith, A., & Hughes, P. (1998). The estrogen dilemma. *American Journal of Nursing, 98*(4), 17–20.
34. Smith-Bindman, R., et al. (1998). Endovaginal ultrasound to exclude endometrial cancer and other endometrial abnormalities. *Journal of the American Medical Association, 280*(17), 1510–1517.
35. Star, W. L., Lommel, L. L., & Shannon, M. T. (Eds.). (1995). *Women's primary health care: Protocols for practice.* Washington, D.C.: American Nurses Publication.
36. Teaffy, N. (1999). *Perimenopause: Preparing for the change: A guide to the early stages of menopause and beyond* (2nd ed.). Rocklin, CA: Prima.
37. Voda, A. M. (1994). Risks and benefits associated with hormonal and surgical therapies for healthy midlife women. *Western Journal of Nursing Research, 16*(5), 507–523.
38. Walsh, B., et al. (1998). Effects of raloxifene on serum lipids and coagulation factors in healthy postmenopausal women. *Journal of the American Medical Association, 279*(18), 1445–1451.
39. World Congress on Endometriosis. (1998). *Understanding and managing endometriosis: Advances in research and practice*: Proceedings of the Sixth World Congress on Endometriosis, June 30–July 4, 1998. Quebec City, Canada: Author.
40. Wright, S., et al. (1995). Short-term Lupron or danazol therapy for pelvic endometriosis. *Fertility and Sterility, 63*(3), 504–507.
41. Xu, Y., et al. (1998). Lysophosphatidic acid as a potential biomarker for ovarian and other gynecologic cancers. *Journal of the American Medical Association, 280*(8), 719–723.

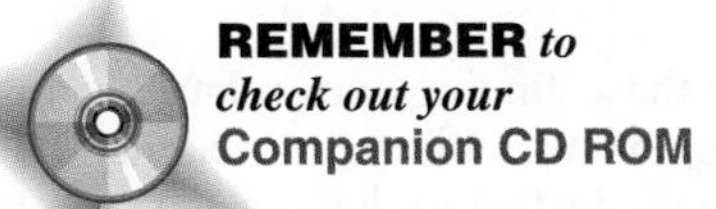

CHAPTER 40

Management of Clients with Breast Disorders

Michelle Goodman
Stephanie Mellon-Reppen

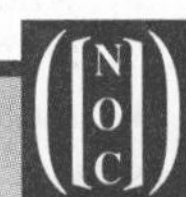

NURSING OUTCOMES CLASSIFICATION (NOC)
for Nursing Diagnoses—Clients with Breast Disorders

Altered Nutrition: Less Than Body Requirements
Nutritional Status: Food and Fluid Intake
Nutritional Status: Nutrient Intake
Body Image Disturbance
Grief Resolution
Psychosocial Adjustment: Life Change
Self-Care: Activities of Daily Living (ADL)
Self-Esteem
Effective Management of Therapeutic Regimen and Knowledge Deficit
Decision-Making
Family Participation in Professional Care
Knowledge: Diet
Knowledge: Disease Process
Knowledge: Medication
Knowledge: Treatment Regimen
Knowledge: Treatment Procedures
Participation: Health Care Decisions
Risk for Impaired Skin Integrity
Tissue Integrity: Skin and Mucous Membranes
Treatment Behavior: Illness or Injury
Wound Healing: Primary Intention or Secondary Intention
Risk for Ineffective Individual Coping and Risk for Ineffective Family Coping
Caregiver Emotional Support
Coping
Decision-Making
Family Coping
Family Normalization
Family Participation in Professional Care
Information Processing
Role Performance
Social Support
Risk for Injury
Symptom Control

A woman who finds a breast lump or other breast problem will probably first suspect cancer, even though eight of 10 lumps are benign. Despite many misconceptions regarding the etiology of breast cancer, public awareness about this health threat has grown dramatically. In the past, the subject was avoided, or if information was shared, it was often inaccurate. Now breast cancer is openly discussed, and information about this topic is frequently presented in mass media. With the recent media focus on breast cancer awareness and early detection, the public is becoming more aware of the role that breast self-examination, clinical examination, and especially routine mammograms have in the early detection of a breast mass.

Nurses have a responsibility to teach the public about breast lesions and cancer, to correct misconceptions, and to provide accurate information concerning normal breasts and breast disease, detection, and treatment. Facts about the disease, treatment, and prognosis need to be shared openly with all members of society, particularly the underserved. If women understand the importance of early detection and treatment, they are more likely to have regular mammograms and less likely to delay seeking medical care when an abnormality is found. Delay in seeking medical care is often due to (1) fear that the problem is cancer and (2) lack of knowledge that breast cancer can be curable if caught early.

BREAST CANCER IN WOMEN

Breast cancer is the most common malignancy in women in the United States and is second only to lung cancer as a cause of cancer death.[1] The incidence of breast cancer in the United States has been increasing gradually for the past 30 years. In 2000, the number of new cases of breast cancer diagnosed in the United States was estimated at 182,800, with 40,800 deaths caused by the disease.[1] At age 85, a woman's risk for breast cancer is one in eight, depending on where she lives. The highest incidence of breast cancer is found in the United States and Europe.

Before 1990, there had been little evidence of any decrease in the United States age-standardized death rate from breast cancer. Currently, breast cancer mortality appears to be declining among white women but increasing among African American women, especially those who are premenopausal. (Breast cancer in men is rare and is discussed later in this chapter.) The decrease in mortality may be ascribed to the combined benefits of early detection and better treatment (particularly with adjuvant chemotherapy and tamoxifen) during the 1980s.[28, 39] The increase in early diagnosis due to mammography and the generally increased awareness of breast cancer among women and their physicians have resulted in detection of smaller tumors, which are more likely to be localized and to be treated successfully.[10]

Probably the most important encouragement to breast cancer detection has been the discovery that screening mammography reduces breast cancer deaths by 30%.[2, 32] The Breast and Cervical Cancer Mortality Act of 1990 was enacted to ensure that underinsured or uninsured women receive mammograms and appropriate treatment services.[3] Women need to understand the importance of mammography in detecting breast cancers while the tumors are small. Likewise, they should understand that the treatment is less toxic and more effective for all modalities used when the disease is detected early, even before the tumor is palpable. With regard to surgery, less tissue is removed when the tumor is small; therefore, better cosmesis is possible. With irradiation of a smaller volume of diseased tissue, cure is more likely and a lower dose is needed for cure by radiation therapy. With adjuvant treatment, a small tumor burden means that systemic therapy may not be needed; if it is needed, drug treatment will be more successful. Smaller tumors also mean less regional node involvement and fewer complications associated with axillary node dissection.[25]

Nurses need to provide current and accurate information concerning the latest approaches to breast cancer treatment and related complications. Encouraging the client to participate in research, if appropriate, is especially important, so that critical questions regarding breast cancer therapy can be addressed. Clients and their families are required to make many difficult decisions. The nurse can be especially helpful by ensuring that the client understands treatment options and by providing clarification when appropriate.

Etiology and Risk Factors

The cause of breast cancer is not known. Many women are anxious about their risk for breast cancer, and many tend to overestimate their risk. Although genetic, hormonal, or biochemical factors are likely to be involved, 70% of women with breast cancer had no known risk factors.

Age and Ethnicity

All women are at risk for breast cancer, and the most important single risk factor is age. Risk increases with age, although the rate of increase slows after menopause. The annual incidence of breast cancer in American women 80 to 85 years of age is 15 times higher than that in women 30 to 35 years of age. African American women under age 50 years have a higher age-specific incidence of breast cancer than that in Caucasian women.

Edwards and colleagues, in their examination of the impact of race on survival in breast cancer, found that not only are African American women less likely to be cured than their non–African American counterparts, but they also survive for a shorter time until death from breast cancer.[20] Even when matched for tumor stage, they are more at risk for micrometastatic disease and early death. It is not clear whether these findings are related to tumor biology, host response, or variability in treatment. Psychosocial and socioeconomic factors have a major role in governing access to medical care. Uninsured clients and those insured by Medicaid present with more advanced disease, have a higher risk of death, and have lessened survival compared with privately insured clients.[20]

Breast cancer incidence among Hispanic women living in North America is only 40% to 50% as great as that among non-Hispanic white women. Asian women born in Asia have a very low lifetime risk of breast cancer, but their daughters born in North America have the same lifetime risk of breast cancer as for American white women.[3]

Ovarian and Hormonal Function

Early menarche (first menses) and late menopause (cessation of menses) lead to an increased total lifetime number of ovulatory menstrual cycles and a corresponding 30% to 50% increase in breast cancer risk. The woman who experiences natural menopause before age 45 years has a risk for breast cancer that is half that of the woman whose menopause occurs after age 55 years.[2] Likewise, oophorectomy before a woman reaches menopause lowers her risk of breast cancer by approximately two thirds. Both nulliparity (no births) and age over 30 years at first live birth are associated with a nearly doubled risk of subsequent breast cancer.[48] The use of hormone replacement therapy (HRT) has also demonstrated a small but significant increase in risk for breast cancer in women who used it for more than 10 years. The Women's Health Initiative study, which includes women who are randomized to receive hormones or placebo, should ultimately answer the question of the effect of other hormonal factors. Definitive findings are expected to be available in the year 2005.

At present there is no convincing evidence that oral contraceptive use affects the risk of breast cancer. The question is difficult to address because the oral contraceptives in use today are vastly different (in that dosages are much lower) from those used 15 and 20 years ago. Even if oral contraceptives influence the incidence of breast cancer, it would be only of historical interest because the drugs used years ago are not comparable to those used today.

Benign Breast Disease

Benign breast disease is not more common in women with other risk factors for breast cancer. Nonproliferative lesions (such as cysts, duct ectasia, mild hyperplasia, and fibroadenoma) do not increase the risk of breast cancer; however, cellular atypia or atypical hyperplasia (a proliferative disease) is an example of a histologic change associated with a higher risk. Sclerosing adenosis increases the risk of breast cancer by approximately 70%.[2] Nearly 40% of women with a family history of breast cancer and atypical hyperplasia subsequently have breast cancer.

Family History

Family history is one of the known risk factors for breast cancer. Breast cancer due to the inheritance of a specific germline mutation from either maternal or paternal relatives is rare. In fact, the breast cancer susceptibility gene *BRCA1* and *BRCA2* and the p53 tumor suppressor gene have been identified in fewer than 10% of all women with breast cancer. Certain populations have a higher incidence of *BRCA* mutations than the general population (e.g., native Icelanders and Ashkenazi Jews).[8]

Depending on the familial context, the lifetime risk of breast cancer, ovarian cancer, or both associated with carrying a mutation ranges from 50% to 85%.[2, 8] Families with several affected first-degree relatives and clients with early-onset disease have been found to harbor mutations at a higher frequency. Women who have the *BRCA2* mutation tend to have early-onset (before age 50) breast cancer but not ovarian cancer. Identification of the *BRCA1* gene makes it possible to identify women who have a 90% to 95% lifetime likelihood of developing breast cancer (with a 70% risk of breast cancer by age 60).[8] Tests for these mutations exist, and research efforts to develop comprehensive genetic screening and counseling programs are ongoing.

ENVIRONMENTAL AND DIETARY FACTORS

An increased incidence of breast cancer has been reported in women who received mantle radiation for the treatment of Hodgkin's disease, particularly if they were younger than 20 years of age.[14] The latency period is between 10 and 25 years. The disease in this group typically presents more aggressively, with a high rate of nodal involvement and bilaterality. It is for this reason that all persons who receive mantle radiation for Hodgkin's disease, especially those treated prior to age 20, receive a regular mammography follow-up examination in order to detect these lesions early.[14]

Alcohol intake is the best-established dietary risk factor for breast cancer in epidemiologic studies. The positive correlation of alcohol intake with breast cancer risk has been established, and it appears that moderate alcohol intake (two drinks per day) increases the risk of breast cancer by altering estrogen metabolism.[30]

As is commonly observed, Japanese women living in Japan have a very low incidence of breast cancer. When they move to the United States, their risk for breast cancer approximates that of native white women within one generation. In a large study involving nearly 338,000 women, there was no apparent correlation between breast cancer risk and dietary intake of fat.[30] If fat intake is relevant to breast cancer, it is probably early in life, perhaps at adolescence. Epidemiologic evidence does not support any substantial increase in breast cancer risk associated with caffeine consumption.

Nurses have a unique role in fostering health promotion and in teaching women about breast cancer as well as in identifying a woman's individual risk for breast cancer. Because most women—especially those with any family history of breast cancer—greatly overestimate their risk for breast cancer, it is helpful to instruct women about the known risk factors and, as indicated, provide support to lessen some of their fears (Table 40–1). Counseling, with appropriate referrals when required, should always accompany specific recommendations for clients with significant risks.

HEALTH PROMOTION ACTIVITIES

Although no known agent or practice guarantees that a woman will remain free of breast cancer, methods are

TABLE 40–1 BREAST CANCER RISK ASSESSMENT AND RECOMMENDATIONS

	Recommendations	
Risk Factors	*Low Risk (<15%*)*	*Moderate to High Risk (15%–>30%*)*
Gender: Women are affected far more often than men, in a ratio of 99:1	Mammogram: Baseline at age 35; every other year ages 40–50; every year after age 50	Mammogram: Baseline at age 30; frequency of subsequent mammograms depends on findings and on recommendations of radiologist
Age: Risk increases with age	Clinical breast examination every year	Clinical breast examination every 6 months
Place of birth: North America; northern Europe	Breast self-examination every month	Breast self-examination every month
Socioeconomic status: High		For known *BRCA1* or *BRCA2* mutation carriers, possible prophylactic mastectomy, prophylactic oophorectomy, or both after childbearing.
Age at first full-term pregnancy: Older than 30 years		
Menstrual history: Early menarche; late menopause		
Health history: History of breast cancer; diagnosis of atypical hyperplasia; exposure to radiation		
Family history: Mother or sister with history of breast cancer; any first-degree relative with breast cancer; *BRCA1* gene carrier		

*Lifetime cumulative risk.

under investigation that may alter the risk and therefore can be considered health promotion activities.

Chemoprevention

Chemoprevention is the use of a drug to prevent the development of a certain malignancy. Two agents have been found to decrease the risk of breast cancer: tamoxifen (Nolvadex) and raloxifene (Evista).

Tamoxifen is an agent commonly used in clients who have breast tumors with receptors for estrogen. Fisher and colleagues[22] looked at tamoxifen and its role in decreasing the incidence of breast cancer in high-risk clients. In this study, 13,388 high-risk women were randomized to receive either placebo or tamoxifen 20 mg/day. Tamoxifen reduced the risk of invasive breast cancer by 49% overall; however, endometrial cancer developed in twice as many women in the tamoxifen group as in the placebo group. In another study, 7705 women with osteoporosis were randomized to receive either placebo or raloxifene.[13] Through a period of 33 months, nearly twice as many invasive breast cancers were seen in the placebo group as in the raloxifene group.

In contrast to the tamoxifen trial, there was no increase in the incidence of endometrial cancer in women who received raloxifene. Because raloxifene has never been compared with tamoxifen as a chemopreventive agent and has not been studied in women at high risk for breast cancer, the National Surgical Adjuvant Breast Project (NSABP) is conducting a double-blind study that will compare these two drugs in 22,000 high-risk women. Tamoxifen is currently the more widely used of the two drugs; it costs approximately $75 in the United States for a month's supply and is covered by most insurance plans.

Prophylactic Mastectomy

The only other measure that may predictably prevent the occurrence of breast cancer and be considered a method of health promotion is prophylactic mastectomy. All of the breast tissue is removed in a woman who does not have evidence of breast cancer. Women who may benefit from this procedure are those who have a strong family history of breast cancer, a history of breast cancer in the other breast, a history of atypical hyperplasia on repeated surgical biopsies, or presence of a mutated *BRCA1* or *BRCA2* gene.

Lifestyle Changes

Women can also be encouraged to make changes in lifestyle to lower their potential risk for breast cancer. For instance, they can decrease their consumption of alcohol. Although a moderate decrease in dietary fat intake does not reduce appear to reduce the risk of breast cancer, decreasing fat intake to 20% of dietary calories is a worthwhile goal.[30]

Exercise may have an indirect role in the prevention of breast cancer. Exercise leads to a decrease in body fat, thereby reducing the amount of free estrogen stored in body fat. Hence, it is another health promotion activity.

HEALTH MAINTENANCE ACTIVITIES

Health maintenance involves optimal screening and early detection of breast cancer. Regardless of the method used, regular and careful physical examination is the key to identifying asymptomatic cancerous lesions. When combined with mammography, physical examination decreases mortality, especially in women over age 50. According to the National Cancer Advisory Board (NCAB), a committee that advises and consults with the director of the National Cancer Institute (NCI), data presented at the Consensus Development Conference showed that regular screening mammography of average-risk women in their 40s reduces deaths from breast cancer by about 17% to 24%.[10, 46] On the basis of this finding, the NCAB recommended to the NCI that women between the ages of 40 and 49 years have screening mammograms every 1 to 2 years if they are at average risk for breast cancer.

For women 50 years and older, a mammogram is recommended every 1 to 2 years regardless of risk. However, the American Cancer Society, the American College of Radiology, and the American College of Obstetrics and Gynecology recommend a mammogram every 1 to 2 years for women between ages 40 and 50 and then annually after the age of 50. In addition, the American Cancer Society advises that a baseline mammogram be obtained between ages 35 and 40.

The currently available data do not warrant a universal recommendation for mammography for all women in their 40s. The decision to have a screening mammogram in the absence of risk factors in this age group is based on the woman's personal wishes and the recommendation of her primary health care provider. Cost is an important issue in the use of mammography screening in younger women; the cost of screening younger women may approach $1 billion annually.

Once a mammogram reveals an area suggestive of cancer, an ultrasound study is a useful complement to diagnostic mammography as a means for distinguishing cystic from solid masses. For women with particularly dense breasts or with implants, magnetic resonance imaging (MRI) scanning and digital mammography provide improved sensitivity. It is hoped that better mammography technology, including digitized radiography, routine use of magnified views, and greater skill in interpretation, combined with MRI and positron emission tomography (PET) scanning will make it possible to identify breast cancers at an earlier stage.

Health care professionals and health care advocates have for many years promoted breast self-examination (BSE) as a key component of early cancer detection because most breast cancers are detected by the woman herself, usually after the mass has grown to the size of 2.5 cm or larger. The only reason the cancer is detected then is that the mass is large enough to be felt. A better goal would be to detect the cancer while it is still small, before it can be felt (Fig. 40–1). The only way to do this is by regular mammography and physical examination by a trained clinician (see Chapter 37). BSE has not been proven to save lives or to increase survival. There is insufficient evidence to recommend for or against the teaching of BSE.[24] Of course, teaching a woman to examine her breasts is an important strategy for increasing her awareness of the risk of breast cancer. See Chapter 37 for a discussion of BSE.

HEALTH RESTORATION ACTIVITIES

Arm exercises and positioning after surgery to prevent lymphedema, obtaining a prosthesis, and breast reconstruction are health restoration activities. If lymphedema

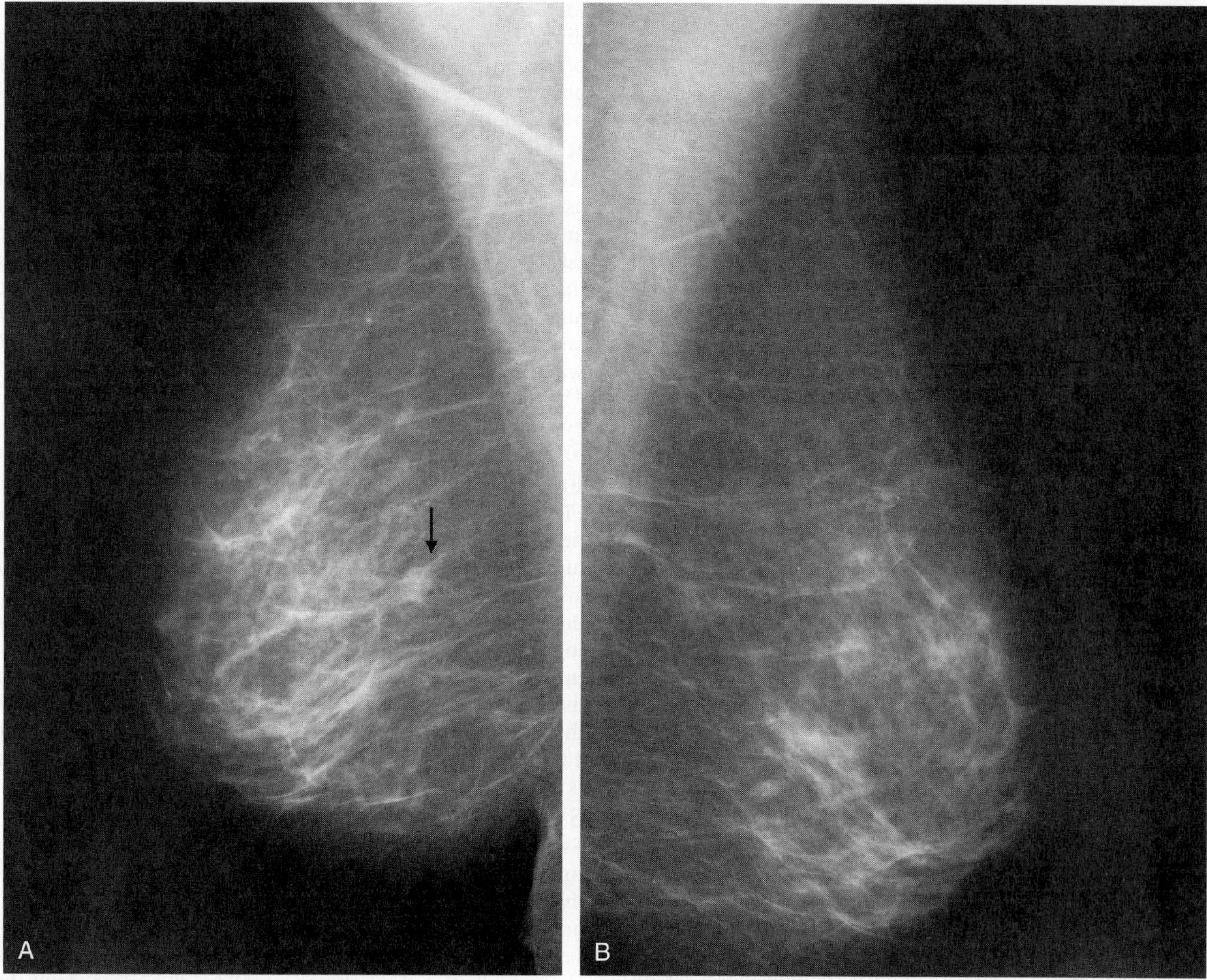

FIGURE 40–1 *A,* Screening mammogram of a 56-year-old woman with a strong family history of breast cancer, right mediolateral oblique view. The mammogram shows a small, irregular, nonpalpable mass *(arrow)*, which was highly suggestive of malignancy. *B,* The left mediolateral oblique view shows a normal breast.

develops despite exercises and positioning, referral to a physical therapist or specialized nurse for lymphedema management is recommended.

Pathophysiology

Breast cancers are malignant tumors that typically begin in the ductal-lobular epithelial cells of the breast and spread via the lymphatic system to the axillary lymph nodes. The tumor may then metastasize to distant regions of the body, including lungs, liver, bone, and brain. The finding of breast cancer in the axillary lymph nodes is an indicator of the tumor's ability for potential distant spread and is not merely contiguous growth into the adjacent region of the breast. Most primary breast cancers are adenocarcinomas located in the upper outer quadrant of the breast (Fig. 40–2).

Carcinoma in Situ

Malignant-appearing cells confined to the ductal or lobular units without permeation of the basement membrane are considered to represent carcinoma in situ. *Ductal carcinoma in situ* (DCIS) is considered a precursor of infiltrating carcinoma. Pathologists classify DCIS as high-intermediate-grade or low-grade according to the growth pattern of cells occupying the ducts, their nuclear features, mitotic activity, presence of necrosis, and type of microcalcifications. Low-grade DCIS tends to be the most common and is typically multifocal; high-grade DCIS is second in prevalence and tends to be architecturally contiguous and associated with prominent microcalcifications. High-grade DCIS tends to be estrogen receptor–negative, shows increased expression for human epidermal growth factor receptor (HER-2)/Neu protein (c-erbB2), and has a mutated p53 tumor suppressor gene.

Ipsilateral (affecting the same side) invasive carcinoma develops within 10 years in approximately 30% of cases of DCIS. Left untreated, intraductal carcinoma will be transformed into invasive ductal carcinoma.

Lobular carcinoma in situ (LCIS) is characterized by a solid proliferation of atypical cells expanding lobular units. In contrast to DCIS, LCIS is usually found incidentally and is not typically associated with microcalcifica-

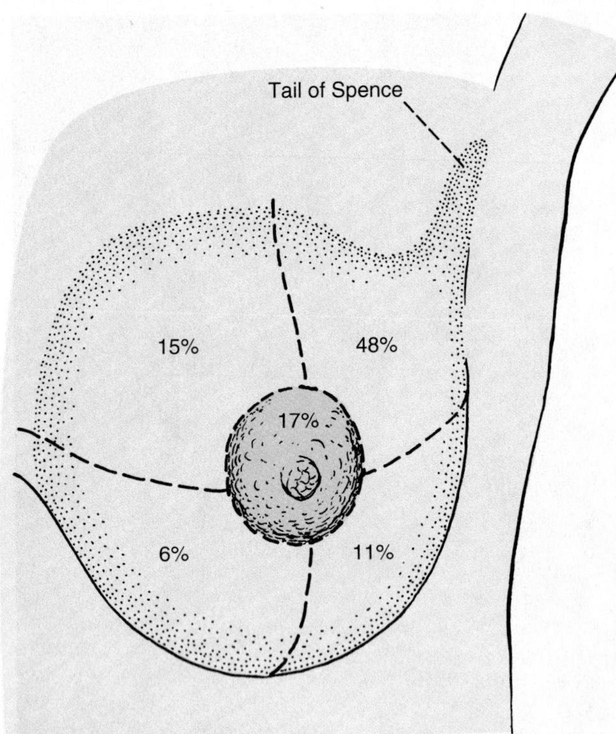

FIGURE 40–2 Frequency of occurrence of breast cancer according to location. The highest occurrence is in the upper outer quadrant and in the tail of Spence.

tions. LCIS has a lower tendency to develop into infiltrating carcinoma.

Invasive Breast Cancer

The majority of breast cancers (75%) are infiltrating ductal carcinomas. They typically metastasize to regional lymph nodes and beyond. Lobular carcinomas account for about 5% to 10% of cases and usually present as a generalized thickening. Tumor types that are associated with a favorable prognosis include tubular (accounting for 2% of cases), medullary (5% to 7%), and mucinous (colloid) carcinoma (3%). These histologic types tend to have low-grade histology, positive estrogen and progesterone receptors status, diploid deoxyribonucleic acid (DNA) content, low S phase fraction (discussed later under Prognosis and Defining Extent of Disease), and no oncogenic markers. Tumors with poor clinical prognosis are those associated with high-grade histology and dermal lymphatic invasion designated as "inflammatory carcinoma." Inflammatory breast cancer is characterized by skin redness and induration. Edema and warmth are other common associated findings. Frequently, palpable axillary and supraclavicular nodes and distant metastases are involved.

Clinical Manifestations

Most breast cancers present as painless, nontender, hard, irregularly shaped, nonmobile masses. About 60% of cancers are somewhat movable, 40% have regular borders by palpation, and 40% can feel soft or cystic. Even when no mass is present, other physical findings, such as nipple discharge, induration, and dimpling, can suggest malignancy. Heat and erythema of the breast skin may be related to inflammation but may also indicate inflammatory carcinoma. Skin edema is characteristic of malignant disease. The edema is due to the invasion and obstruction of dermal lymphatics by the tumor. If a tumor is suspected on the basis of the physical findings, a diagnostic mammogram is indicated.

Radiographic Findings

Additional diagnostic films of the affected breast, as well as localized compression and magnification views, increase the specificity of identifying the abnormality. Digital mammography and computer-assisted diagnosis (CAD) may be useful to evaluate the lesion, because these tests allow more variations in exposure and show the differences in tissue contrast more clearly. CAD utilizes a software program to target lesions suspected to be malignant. The specificity of the image is enhanced by on-screen evaluation that allows manipulation of contrast, which improves detection.

Fine-Needle Aspiration

Fine-needle aspiration (FNA) is performed on an outpatient basis. The purpose is to determine whether a solid lump is a cyst or to confirm a clinically apparent diagnosis. If the mass turns out to be a cyst, the lump should disappear after the aspiration. If a lump is solid, a cytologic specimen may be obtained by making several passes into the lesion to retrieve small cell samples; this technique can reduce the incidence of false-negative results. If the FNA results are negative and the physician suspects cancer from the clinical findings, excisional biopsy (open) is indicated.

Stereotactic Needle-Guided Biopsy

Stereotactic needle-guided biopsy (SNB) is used mainly to target and identify nonpalpable lesions in the breast that have been detected with mammography. The basic goal is to immobilize the breast from fixed horizontal and vertical coordinates to calculate the exact position of the lesion within a three-dimensional field. SNB permits biopsy diagnosis of benign disease without the trauma or scarring of an open biopsy.

Open Biopsy

Excisional or open biopsy is chosen when the lesion is determined to be solid and indeterminate in nature, when results of cytologic or histologic analysis are insufficient, or when the clinical or mammographic findings suggest malignancy. A wire-localized biopsy procedure similar to the stereotactic method can be used; the aim of this procedure is to assist the surgeon in locating the nonpalpable lesion for the purpose of excisional biopsy and to minimize the volume of tissue removed to avoid unnecessary deformity.

Prognosis and Defining Extent of Disease

Once a diagnosis of cancer is made, the cancer needs to be evaluated further to determine the most appropriate therapy. For example, if breast-conserving surgery (lumpectomy) is being considered, the presence of microcalcifications would need to be evaluated further to determine whether the disease in the breast is multifocal.

The tumor is staged according to the extent of local, regional, and distant spread. *Staging* permits an accurate definition of the extent of the disease and therefore a more accurate prognosis. The American Joint Committee on Cancer (AJCC) staging system for breast cancer is based on the tumor-node-metastasis (TNM) system, presented in Table 40–2. Prognosis for breast cancer is associated primarily with the extent of disease at detection. The tumor staging is based on (1) the size of the primary tumor; (2) whether it extends to the chest wall or skin; (3) the presence of axillary lymph nodes; (4) whether they are matted, fixed, or mobile; and (5) the presence of distant metastases (Fig. 40–3). The 5-year survival rate for breast cancer based on stage of disease is presented in Table 40–3.

Prognostic factors are used to determine prognosis or the natural history of breast cancer. At present, only pathologic lymph node status, tumor size, estrogen and progesterone receptor status, histologic grade, and histopathology are considered to be independent prognostic indicators and therefore appropriate to consider in determining therapy and prognosis. Another factor that is often taken into consideration is the DNA content of the tumor. *DNA ploidy* refers to the degree of multiplication of chromosome sets. *Diploid* and *euploid* signify an exact multiple of the haploid number of chromosomes. *Aneuploid* indicates a deviation from an exact multiple of the haploid number and a poorer prognosis. The S phase index identifies the percentage of tumor cells in S phase (start of DNA synthesis) of the cell growth cycle. The higher the percentage of cells in S phase, the more aggressive the cancer.

TABLE 40–2 TNM STAGING SYSTEM FOR BREAST CANCER

Primary Tumor (T)

TX	Primary tumor cannot be assessed
T0	No evidence of primary tumor
Tis	Carcinoma in situ: intraductal carcinoma, lobular carcinoma in situ, or Paget's disease of the nipple with no tumor
T1	Tumor 2 cm or less in greatest dimension
T1mic	Microinvasion 0.1 cm or less in greatest dimension
T1a	Tumor more than 0.1 cm but not more than 0.5 cm in greatest dimension
T1b	Tumor more than 0.5 cm but not more than 1 cm in greatest dimension
T1c	Tumor more than 1 cm but not more than 2 cm in greatest dimension
T2	Tumor more than 2 cm but not more than 5 cm in greatest dimension
T3	Tumor more than 5 cm is greatest dimension
T4	Tumor of any size with direct extension to (a) chest wall or (b) skin, only as described below
T4a	Extension to chest wall
T4b	Edema (including peau d'orange) or ulceration of the skin of the breast or satellite skin nodules confined to the same breast
T4c	Both T4a and T4b
T4d	Inflammatory carcinoma

Regional Lymph Nodes (N)

NX	Regional lymph nodes cannot be assessed (e.g., previously removed)
N0	No regional lymph node metastasis
N1	Metastasis to movable ipsilateral axillary lymph node(s)
N2	Metastasis to ipsilateral axillary lymph node(s) fixed to one another or to other structures
N3	Metastasis to ipsilateral internal mammary lymph node(s)

Distant Metastasis (M)

MX	Distant metastasis cannot be assessed
M0	No distant metastasis
M1	Distant metastasis (includes metastasis to ipsilateral supraclavicular lymph node[s])

Stage Grouping

0	Tis	N0	M0
I	T1*	N0	M0
IIA	T0	N1	M0
	T1*	N1†	M0
	T2	N0	M0
IIB	T2	N1	M0
	T3	N0	M0
IIIA	T0	N2	M0
	T1†	N2	M0
	T2	N2	M0
	T3	N1	M0
	T3	N2	M0
IIIB	T4	Any N	M0
	Any T	N3	M0
IV	Any T	Any N	M1

*T1 includes T1mic.
†The prognosis for patients with N1a cancers is similar to that for patients with N0 cancers.
Adapted, with permission, from Fleming I. D., Cooper J. S., Henson D. E., et al. (Eds). *AJCC Cancer staging manual* (5th ed.). Philadelphia, Lippincott-Raven, 1997.

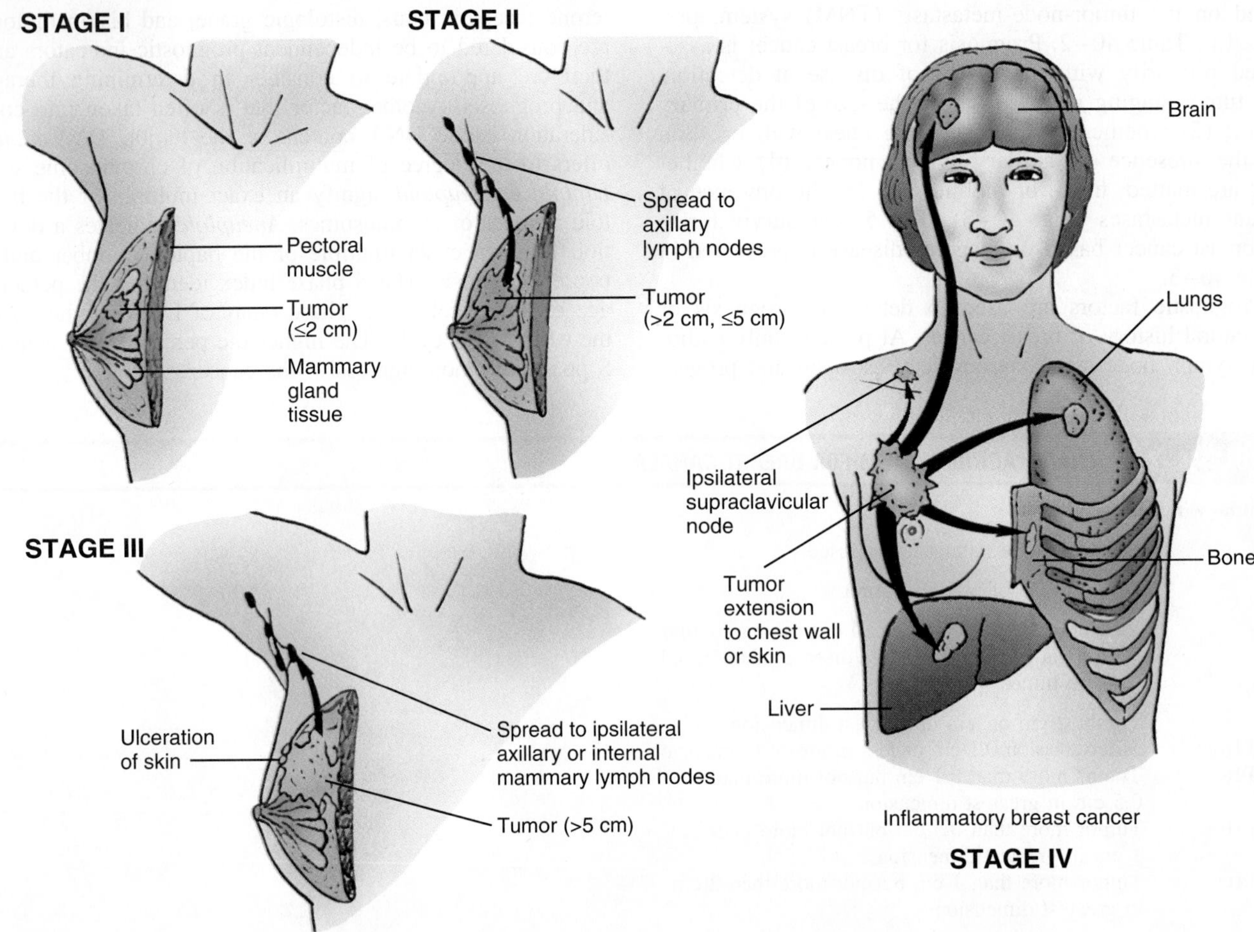

FIGURE 40–3 Clinincal staging of breast cancer. *Stage I,* Tumor 2 cm or less in diameter and confined to the breast. *Stage II,* Tumor up to 5 cm, or early metastasis to axillary lymph nodes. *Stage III,* Tumor larger than 5 cm with involvement of the ipsilateral axillary or internal mammary lymph nodes. *Stage IV,* Distant metastasis, such as to brain, bone, or liver; ipsilateral supraclavicular lymph node; skin and/or extension to chest wall; or inflammatory breast cancer.

The tumor is generally graded to determine the degree of differentiation and therefore prognosis. Tumors are classified as *well differentiated* (grade I), *moderately well differentiated* (grade II), or *poorly differentiated* (grade III) according to the degree of anaplasia observed. Other factors identified on the pathology report include nucleus size and shape, presence or absence of mitotic figures, and degree of tubule formation. Dermal lymphatic invasion and microvascular invasion may also be predictive of metastatic disease.

Although the prognostic significance of HER-2/Neu protein (c-erbB2) remains under investigation, it appears that overexpression of this protein in the primary tumor correlates with less favorable prognostic indicators and may be predictive of response to chemotherapy, especially paclitaxel (Taxol). Post-chemotherapy c-erbB2 levels are also a prognostic indicator of disease-free survival.[4] Steroid receptor status is an accepted predictive factor for response to endocrine therapies. If the tumor is determined to be estrogen receptor–positive and progesterone receptor–positive, antiestrogen therapy would be an appropriate therapeutic option with or without chemotherapy.

Tumor markers are not considered useful preoperatively when adjuvant therapy for cure is planned. Tumor markers are assessed as part of the work-up of advanced disease and generally have significance only in a woman with metastatic disease. Carcinoembryonic antigen (CEA), CA-125, and CA 15-3 are substances that are produced by the tumor and are present in the serum of the woman with breast cancer. A tumor marker would be expected to be present only in metastatic disease, in which case it is assessed on a monthly basis to monitor response to therapy.

TABLE 40–3 FIVE-YEAR SURVIVAL RATE FOR BREAST CANCER BY STAGE

Stage	5-Year Survival (% of Patients)
0	99
I	92
IIA	82
IIB	65
IIIA	47
IIIB	44
IV	14

Data from Surveillance Epidemiology End Results (SEER), National Cancer Institute, *http://www.seer.ims.nci.nih.gov.,* April 25, 2000.

Pretreatment assessment also includes a metastatic work-up to determine extent of disease. Tests are selected according to the clinical presentation and the likelihood of metastatic disease. A chest x-ray film and a bone scan are possible useful baseline studies. A bone scan is usually not indicated unless the client has invasive breast cancer that is at least stage II or III. Only 30% to 60% of clients with a true-positive bone scan have increased alkaline phosphatase levels, and only 20% of clients with elevated alkaline phosphatase levels are disease-free. If the bone scan is abnormal, then radiographs of the affected sites are necessary to confirm metastatic disease and to exclude a benign etiologic mechanism.

A complete metabolic panel and physical examination will detect any liver dysfunction and may identify the need for a liver scan. The liver scan is usually not done unless there is reason to suspect that the disease has spread or except in the presence of stage III disease. When metastatic disease is strongly suspected, an MRI study or a computed tomography (CT) scan may be ordered to further define and measure the extent of disease. A PET scan is not usually indicated unless results of the MRI or CT scan are indeterminate and metastatic disease is strongly suspected. PET may also be used to determine whether a sentinel node biopsy is appropriate.

Outcome Management

In the past, management of the client with breast cancer typically included a modified radical or a radical mastectomy. Postoperatively, the surgeon would assure the woman that all the cancer was removed, and that would be the end of her treatment. Today the management approach to localized breast cancer is much more complicated, because much more is known about the systemic nature of breast cancer and the need for local control as well as appropriate adjuvant therapy. Historically, it was believed that cancer spread locally to the lymph nodes in an orderly, defined manner. If this were true, radical mastectomy should eliminate the disease. It is now known that breast cancer does not spread in an orderly manner and that cancer cells metastasize through the bloodstream and lymphatic system to other tissues and organs such as skin, regional lymph nodes, or more distant sites, including bone, lung, liver, and brain. Because breast cancer is now considered a systemic disease, less radical, more breast-conserving surgical procedures are done in combination with radiation therapy, hormonal therapy, or chemotherapy.

Soon after a biopsy-proven diagnosis of breast cancer, the client should consult with a team of interdisciplinary consultants who are part of a comprehensive breast center, before deciding on the definitive approach to management of her breast cancer. Most insurance companies encourage this consultation because there are numerous approaches to the management of breast cancer and an interdisciplinary approach is not only most advantageous for the client but also most efficient and cost-effective. The interdisciplinary team generally includes a medical oncologist, a radiation oncologist, and a surgical oncologist. An oncology nurse practitioner, a nutritionist, and a psycho-oncologist are also vital members of the team, because many clients have questions concerning quality of life, how to maintain nutrition, and ways to promote communication among family members. Another advantage to evaluation at a comprehensive breast center is that such centers usually have the most advanced diagnostic tools, offer the most current research protocols, and can provide a comprehensive breast cancer risk assessment, genetic evaluation, and appropriate counseling.

■ PRIMARY BREAST CANCER

Carcinoma in situ (meaning that it has not invaded the tissue of origin) is becoming more of an issue in local control of breast cancer, owing to the success of mammography in detecting these small cancers. DCIS is generally managed by local excision with or without radiation. The risk of local recurrence following breast-sparing surgery is approximately 10% at 10 years. Whether radiation therapy is necessary for all clients is uncertain. The addition of tamoxifen as therapeutic as well as prophylactic treatment following local treatment is gaining acceptance. Obviously, women require scheduled diagnostic follow-up mammograms along with physician examination every 6 to 12 months.

LCIS is considered a risk factor for breast cancer rather than a precursor lesion. Because of the bilateral multifocal nature of LCIS, options for management range from careful observation and mammography at 6- to 12-month intervals to bilateral prophylactic mastectomy—options that for many women appear either too conservative or too extreme. The physician-nurse team needs to explain the options carefully and permit time for the client to understand her risks and choices for management.

The management of localized invasive breast cancer has changed dramatically since the mid-1980s. Approximately 30% of women with breast cancer are now managed with breast-conserving surgery. Many more women are candidates for this procedure, but unfortunately surgeons are reluctant to change, and research takes many years and thousands of clients to prove that one form of therapy is superior to another. However, several studies have indicated that breast-conserving treatments, consisting of the removal of the primary tumor by some form of lumpectomy with or without irradiation to the breast, may result in survival that is equal to that of more extensive procedures, including mastectomy and modified radical mastectomy.[34, 35] Similarly, the addition of radiation therapy to mastectomy does not improve 10-year survival rates and is not indicated if the surgical margins are clear and if no other factors place the client at high risk for local recurrence.

At the time of the initial consultation, a plan of care is devised and the goal of therapy is determined. It is crucial to identify clients at substantial risk for recurrence because they do benefit from systemic therapy. Likewise, in a woman with a tumor smaller than 1 cm with no evidence of axillary node involvement, there is little justification for adjuvant chemotherapy. When the tumor is larger than 1 cm and there is evidence of axillary lymph node involvement, other parameters are assessed, such as estrogen receptor status and measures of tumor growth rate. These help determine not only the need for adjuvant chemotherapy but also whether a doxorubicin-containing regimen is appropriate.

For example, tumors with a high proportion of cells in the S phase of cell division are associated with a greater risk of relapse, and chemotherapy offers a greater survival benefit. Cancers that lack either estrogen or progesterone receptors are more likely to recur than those that are estrogen receptor–positive and progesterone receptor–positive. Tumors with a poor nuclear grade have a higher degree of recurrence than tumors with a good nuclear grade.

Tumors that overexpress HER-2/Neu protein (c-erbB2) or that have a mutated p53 gene have a poor prognosis. Tumors that overexpress HER-2/Neu protein are more likely to respond to higher doses of doxorubicin. (The presence of c-erbB2 is determined at the time of surgery and usually appears on the pathology report.) HER-2/Neu status (positive or negative) is usually considered in therapeutic decisions about the use of a doxorubicin- or taxane-containing regimen.

Surgical Management

The extent of the surgical intervention is determined by the clinical presentation and by the possibility of resecting the tumor with clean margins. The goal today is to preserve the breast, because there is no evidence that a mastectomy is more beneficial than lumpectomy plus radiation therapy. However, because of size or the multifocal or multicentric extent of disease, a mastectomy may be necessary to provide adequate tumor removal.

Breast-Preserving Procedures

Indications. Breast-preserving procedures are selected for stage I and stage II breast cancers. Such conservative surgical approaches may be appropriate, depending on the size of the primary tumor. Clients with small invasive cancers generally require a wide local excision under local or general anesthesia for partial mastectomy involving removal of the tumor plus a 1- to 2-cm margin of normal tissue (lumpectomy). A variation of the procedure is the quadrantectomy (removal of the quadrant of the breast in which the cancer is located).

Radiation therapy is begun once healing is confirmed, provided that the client is not receiving a doxorubicin- or taxane-containing regimen. If the individual is to receive either of these two chemotherapeutic agents plus radiation, then the radiation therapy commences 3 weeks after the last course of chemotherapy. If the client is to receive methotrexate (Mexate) and 5-fluorouracil (5-FU) with or without cyclophosphamide (Cytoxan), the radiotherapy may begin with the chemotherapy, may be sandwiched in after the third course and continue for 5 to 6 weeks, or may begin a few weeks after the last course of chemotherapy.

Contraindications. Breast-conserving surgery is not performed when women cannot tolerate irradiation because of pregnancy or pre-existing rheumatic disorders, such as arthritis, lupus, and scleroderma. Other contraindications are extensive intraductal involvement requiring a wide incision, the presence of two cancers simultaneously in the same breast, diffuse malignant microcalcifications throughout the breast, and large, aggressive tumors. Client preference for a complete breast removal, client fear of radiation burns or other cancer development following irradiation, and inability to travel to and from a radiation therapy facility are additional contraindications.

Complications. Although rare, infection, cellulitis, hematoma, and, less commonly, lymphedema may occur after the surgery.

Outcomes. After breast-conserving surgery with radiation therapy or chemotherapy or both, the the client will remain free of cancer and its recurrence.

Mastectomy

Indications. Mastectomy is the treatment of choice when the following apply:

- The tumor involves the nipple-areola complex
- The tumor is larger than 7 cm
- The tumor exhibits extensive intraductal disease involving multiple quadrants of the breast
- The woman cannot comply with daily radiation therapy

A *modified radical mastectomy* is an en bloc removal of the breast, axillary lymph nodes, and overlying skin, with the muscles left intact. Owing to more sophisticated diagnostic techniques that detect breast cancers of a smaller size and at an earlier stage, this procedure is done much less frequently now than 10 years ago. In a *total* or *simple* prophylactic *mastectomy,* used most commonly to prevent cancer in high-risk women, breast tissue and some skin are removed.

Contraindications. Although not contraindicated for treatment of small tumors, mastectomy is usually not used for stage I and stage II tumors unless the client prefers this approach.

Complications. Possible complications of breast surgery include lymphedema, infection, seroma, hematoma, and cellulitis. Because clients are often discharged from the hospital within a few days of surgery, they should be taught to report any unusual manifestations early. Any evidence of infection, such as fever, chills, or an area of redness or inflammation along the incision line, should be reported to the physician. Any increase in drainage, foul odor, or separation at the incision site should be reported immediately.

Outcomes. After surgery and adjuvant chemotherapy or radiation therapy, the client will remain free of cancer and its recurrence. If a cancer-free state cannot be achieved, the focus is on promoting quality of life for the client. See Guide to Clinical Pathway.

Axillary Dissection

The role of axillary dissection is in transition. In women with clinically negative node disease and a primary tumor that is 1 to 2 cm in size, a node dissection is probably not necessary.[2] When more extensive surgery is required (e.g., if disease is multicentric or the primary tumor is larger than 5 cm), a mastectomy and axillary dissection are done using two incisions. Except when it is necessary to remove obvious tumor, the axillary dissection is not a therapeutic procedure but, rather, is a diagnostic procedure. The number of axillary nodes involved has in the past helped to determine the need for chemotherapy as well as whether more aggressive therapy is required. Information regarding nodal status is also valuable in determining prognosis and eligibility for research protocols and high-dose chemotherapy regimens.

Recognizing that most women with breast cancer benefit from adjuvant chemotherapy, hormonal therapy, or

GUIDE TO CLINICAL PATHWAY

Mastectomy

The woman having mastectomy expects to be hospitalized only 24 hours, and nursing care must therefore be very organized to meet all the goals. In addition to the usual postoperative care, the client is taught the care of her incisions and how to strip the drainage tubes, empty drains, and record the amount of drainage. The operative arm is elevated to reduce edema, and use of the arm is limited to allow for incisional healing. Because the client is going home in the morning, ambulation the night of surgery is important.

The CareMap focuses on education. Teach the client and family how to care for the incision, begin exercising the arm, and recognize the manifestations of infection. Some clients do not know their cancer diagnosis, yet the use of "Reach to Recovery" is discussed. Because of the fear of cancer, it is important to develop a therapeutic relationship with the client. Even after only a few hours of nursing care, the client may be comfortable enough to discuss fears and concerns with you. Needs may be modified upon discharge from the hospital, with additional referrals based on these fears or concerns.

Helen Andrews, BSN, RN, *Care Manager, Alegent Health Bergan Mercy Medical Center, Omaha, Nebraska,* and **Linda R. Haddick, MSN, RN,** *Clinical Nurse Specialist, Alegent Health Home Care & Hospice, Omaha, Nebraska*

both, some authorities claim that it is no longer necessary to determine the status of the axillary lymph nodes in clients with breast cancer. However, the lymph node status in clients with early breast cancer remains the most powerful predictor of recurrence and survival. The 5-year survival rate for clients with nodal metastasis is about 40% less than that for clients who are free of nodal disease. Further, nearly a third of clients with clinically negative nodes are found to have pathologically involved nodes. Information obtained from pathologic examination of axillary lymph nodes frequently changes the adjuvant therapy plan for women with nonpalpable axillary lymph nodes.[16]

In some cases, axillary node dissection is not necessary because its findings would not affect the choice of therapy. For example, a client presenting with a large primary cancer or evidence of metastatic disease that requires extensive surgery does not need an axillary dissection, nor does a client undergoing mastectomy for a tumor greater than 5 cm or a client in whom the surgical margins are positive for residual tumor. In both of these cases, the risk of local recurrence is sufficiently high to warrant the use of post-mastectomy radiotherapy to the chest wall and supraclavicular areas. Women who have four or more positive axillary lymph nodes also are at increased risk for local recurrence; chest wall and supraclavicular radiotherapy is usually considered even though it is not certain that prophylactic chest wall radiotherapy would improve overall survival.

Sentinel Node Biopsy

Nodal assessment may be conducted using the sentinel node biopsy, a diagnostic test to determine the status of regional lymph nodes. The sentinel node is the first lymph node to receive lymphatic drainage from a tumor. The node can be detected by injection of a blue dye or radioactive colloid around the primary tumor, which travels to and identifies the first draining (sentinel) node. The sentinel lymph node can reveal whether there are lymphatic metastases, making extensive axillary dissection obsolete.[36]

The procedure is technically challenging. Although it is still undergoing clinical investigation, the possibility that this procedure may replace axillary dissection and reduce the potential for lymphedema is encouraging.[33]

Nursing Management of the Surgical Client

Preoperative Care

Assessment

The preoperative time, before the biopsy for breast cancer and before a woman knows whether she has cancer in her breast or not, is extremely stressful, constituting a psychological emergency. To put off the biopsy for more than just a few days is often impossible for the woman once a cancer is suspected. Once the diagnosis is established, the woman can return to the routines of her life, or if the biopsy result is positive, she can begin to mobilize her resources to determine the next step. Initially, the woman may be in shock and perhaps even denial, because her decision to undergo the biopsy procedure may have been based largely on her recognition that 8 out of 10 breast masses are benign. A few days are often needed for her to recover from the diagnosis of cancer before beginning the consultation process.

Most women do not sign a consent for an immediate surgical resection or mastectomy upon evidence of a positive biopsy result. Generally, women are given ample time to evaluate the options for management once the diagnosis is confirmed. Most authorities recommend that definitive surgery be performed within 2 weeks of the biopsy, but some women need more time to sort through the copious literature before deciding on a course of treatment. Physicians are required to present the risks and benefits of each of the numerous treatment options for breast cancer and to allow the woman to choose her course of treatment. The options include (1) mastectomy alone, (2) mastectomy with immediate reconstruction, and (3) breast-preserving treatment. Because there is no absolute right answer for many women, each option must be fully considered. Every woman with breast cancer deserves time to deliberate and to participate actively in the decision-making process. Because the possibilities for treatment may be overwhelming, it is appropriate to refer the woman to a comprehensive breast center in which all disciplines are available to address her concerns regarding therapy.

The plan for treatment, which may include surgery, radiation therapy, chemotherapy, hormone therapy, and/or biologic immunomodulation therapy, is laid out before treatment is begun. In addition, clients should be offered a research protocol if there is one for which they are eligible. Be familiar with these multimodality protocols

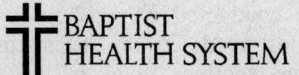

MASTECTOMY CAREMAP

(Addressograph)

	Pre-Admit/Pre-Op Date: ______	INITIAL Met	INITIAL Not Met	Day of Surgery Date: ______	INITIAL Met	INITIAL Not Met
General Safety:	Home activity			Bed rails up x 2 Fall precautions Call light within reach Post sign in room: **NO BP/IV IN R/L ARM**		
Activity	Ad Lib			1. OOB/BRP with assistance 2. Limited use of arm on affected side		
	Goal:			**Goal:** Tolerates ambulation		
Dietary: Consult Date/Time Completed ______	NPO at MN day prior to surgery			1. Clear liquid post-op 2. Reg/Home diet for dinner		
	Goal: Verbalizes understanding of NPO after MN			**Goal:** Tolerates > 50% of diet		
Respiratory: Consult Date/Time Completed ______	Incentive Spirometer Instruction **Goal:** Pt. verbalizes and is able to demonstrate use of Incentive Spirometer			Incentive Spirometer q2H WA **Goal:** Lungs clear to auscultation		
Rehab: Consult Date/Time Completed ______	**Goal:**			**Goal:**		
Discharge Planning: Consult Date/Time Completed ______	1. Assess for D/C needs and support system 2. SWS for HHC if indicated 3. Notify Case Management Dept. for anticipated D/C delays			1. SWS for HHC if indicated 2. Notify Case Mgmt Dept. for anticipated D/C delays		
	Goal: Potential D/C needs identified			**Goal:** Potential D/C needs identified		
Nursing: Consult Date/Time Completed ______	1. Pre-op & Post-op Instructions 2. Consult Anesthesia for pre-op assessment and instruction 3. Have pt. sign appropriate consents 4. Notify Reach to Recovery (American Cancer Society) 5. SCD Hose (Order for day of surgery) if ordered 6. Have pt. view Mastectomy Video 7. Provide written handouts for pre-op/post-op instruction 8. Instruct in technique of emptying, measuring and recording JP drainage 9. Review hospital plan of care with patient and family 10. Review Patient/Family CareMap and give copy to patient 11. Evaluate pre-op emotional status regarding surgery			1. Give pt. Mastectomy Information Bag & review contents with pt./family 2. Show Mastectomy Video if not viewed in PAT 3. No BP/IV in affected arm 4. Empty and record JP drainage 5. Keep drains stripped and compressed 6. Keep affected arm up on pillow 7. Notify MD for excessive JP drainage 8. Apply SCD Hose while in bed (if ordered pre-op). D/C when up ambulating 9. Encourage to Turn, Cough & Deep Breathe q 2 H while in bed 10. Review expectations of care progress with pt./family		
	Goal: Pt./Family verbalizes understanding of pre-op & post-op care			**Goal:** Pt./Family verbalizes understanding of drain and arm care **Goal:** No lymphadema		
Tests:	Labs as ordered					
	Goal: MD notified of any abnormal results			**Goal:**		
Other:				Consult Chaplain if needed		
	Goal:			**Goal:** Pt. able to verbalize fears and concerns regarding surgery		

MASTECTOMY CAREMAP G-99-5137-2 PG REV. 8/17/99

for treating breast cancer. It is an enormous challenge to help clients understand and feel confident in their decisions regarding therapy. To be knowledgeable about the client's options for therapy, make every effort to be present for the initial discussion between the physicians and the client and family. Then clarify any misconceptions the client and family members may have, and reinforce what they have been told regarding the therapy.

DIAGNOSIS, OUTCOMES, INTERVENTIONS

Knowledge Deficit. The nursing diagnosis may be expressed as *Knowledge Deficit related to inexperience*

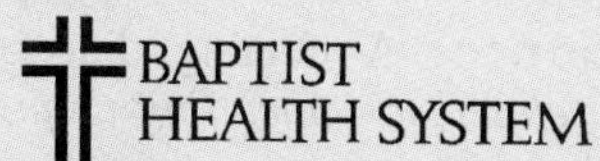

BAPTIST HEALTH SYSTEM

MASTECTOMY CAREMAP

(Addressograph)

	Post-Op Day 1 (D/C Day) Date: ______	INITIAL Met	INITIAL Not Met	Date: ______	INITIAL Met	INITIAL Not Met
General Safety:	Bed rails up x 2 Fall precautions Call light within reach Post sign in room: **NO BP/IV IN R/L ARM**			Bed rails up x 2 Fall precautions Call light within reach Post sign in room: **NO BP/IV IN R/L ARM**		
Activity	1. Up ad lib 2. Limited use of affected arm (Do not raise arm above shoulder level					
	Goal: Tolerates ambulation **Goal:** Verbalizes understanding of limited use of affected arm	____ ____	____ ____	**Goal:**	____	____
Dietary: Consult Date/Time Completed ______	Regular or Home diet					
	Goal: Tolerates > 50% of diet	____	____	**Goal:**	____	____
Respiratory: Consult Date/Time Completed ______	Incentive Spirometer q 2-4 WA **Goal:** Lungs clear to ausculatation	____	____	**Goal:**	____	____
Rehab: Consult Date/Time Completed ______	**Goal:**	____	____	**Goal:**	____	____
Discharge Planning: Consult Date/Time Completed ______	1. Assess for D/C needs and support system 2. SWS for HHC if indicated 3. Notify Case Management Dept. for anticipated D/C delays					
	Goal: Potential D/C needs identified	____	____	**Goal:**	____	____
Nursing: Consult Date/Time Completed ______	1. Notify Reach to Recovery if not done pre-op 2. Ensure pt. has Mastectomy Information Bag and Mastectomy Video 3. Instruct pt./caregiver in emptying, measuring & recording JP drainage 4. Review Mastectomy Discharge Instructions and give copy to pt. 5. No BP/IV in affected arm 6. Empty & record JP drainage & keep drains stripped and compressed 7. Notify MD for excessive drainage 8. Keep affected arm up on pillow					
	Goal: Pt. has viewed and has copy of Mastectomy Video **Goal:** Pt. has received Mastectomy Information Bag **Goal:** Pt./Caregiver demonstrates ability to empty, measure and record JP drainage **Goal:** Pt. verbalizes understanding & has copy of Mastectomy Discharge Instructions **Goal:** Pt. verbalizes understanding of bringing drainage record to MD on first post-op visit **Goal:** Pt. has prescription for pain meds prior to discharge **Goal:** Pt. verbalizes understanding of when to follow-up with MD **Goal:** Pt./Caregiver verbalizes understanding of rehab exercises & has copy of instructions **Goal:** Pt./Caregiver verbalizes understanding of signs & symptoms to report to MD **Goal:** Pt. has been contacted or visited by Reach to Recovery Volunteer prior to discharge	____	____	**Goal:**	____	____
Tests:	Labs as ordered					
	Goal: MD notified of any abnormal results	____	____	**Goal:**	____	____
Other:						
	Goal:	____	____	**Goal:**	____	____

MASTECTOMY CAREMAP

G-99-5137-3 PG REV. 8/17/99

and new information regarding available options for treatment.

Outcomes. The client will understand the available treatment options, as evidenced by her questions and statements concerning options and her ability to explain her choice.

Interventions

Explain Options. The woman should receive information about recommendations and treatment options before surgery or treatment is initiated. The nurse can help women understand treatment options.[2, 9, 35]

Initiate Teaching Plan. Because the typical hospital

stay for a modified radical mastectomy or lumpectomy and axillary node dissection surgery is 1 to 3 days, preoperative teaching is done on an outpatient basis, usually in the physician's office. Give clients written instructions regarding postoperative care, including wound care and hand and arm care.

Nursing assessment provides data about knowledge deficits for use in formulating a teaching plan. This plan includes preoperative activities, explanations of surgery, postoperative care, discharge planning, and a discussion of any limitations the woman may have as a result of surgery. Encourage the woman to question her physicians about lymph node dissection versus lymph node sampling. Alert her to the possibility of radiation therapy modification in order to preserve the lymphatics and minimize underlying tissue scarring.[29, 41] Because the woman's anxiety level may be so high that she cannot remember new information, it is important to provide written as well as oral instructions. Give instructions in the presence of a family member. Because clients are discharged early postoperatively, they also need emergency phone numbers and instructions regarding whom to call if they have a question or a problem after discharge. Evaluate the client's and family members' learning, and repeat information as often as is necessary.

Risk for Ineffective Individual Coping and Risk for Ineffective Family Coping. The nursing diagnosis may be expressed as *Ineffective Individual Coping and Ineffective Family Coping related to diagnosis of cancer and surgical changes in breast.*

Outcomes. The client will cope with the diagnosis of cancer and surgical changes in the breast, as evidenced by her statement of acceptance and decisions about treatment. Family members will also cope effectively, as evidenced by support given to the client.

Interventions. Preoperatively or before any treatment, assess the client's and significant others' coping ability and concerns. Do not rush the assessment. Identify the coping mechanisms usually used by the client and her significant others. Are there any potentially disabling coping patterns? Use this information as the basis of support. The woman may fear pain, mutilation, death, loss of control, and the hospital environment. Use these findings to establish a plan of care to help the client use positive, growth-producing coping and to avoid disabling coping.[9, 11]

EVALUATION

For a positive outcome, the client will be adequately prepared for surgery and its outcomes. Recovery from the surgical procedure is usually uncomplicated. Delayed grieving, even for months following mastectomy, is not uncommon, because intellectually the woman knows the surgery is necessary and because her grief is overshadowed at first by fear of dying.

POSTOPERATIVE CARE

ASSESSMENT

Assess the client's psychological reaction to the surgery. Also, inspect the wound and drains, assess for the presence of clinical manifestations of infection and pain, and perform routine postoperative assessments as discussed in Chapter 15.

DIAGNOSIS, OUTCOMES, INTERVENTIONS

Body Image Disturbance. A nursing diagnosis of *Body Image Disturbance related to impending changes in breast and sexuality* may be appropriate.

Outcomes. The client will begin to exhibit her presurgical or baseline positive body image, as evidenced by wearing usual make-up and using her own nightgown or other feminine attire after surgery.

Interventions

Initiate Referral. Because the hospital stay is usually only 1 to 3 days, there may be little opportunity for the woman to express her usual feelings regarding her femininity and the manner in which she might display a positive adaptation to her surgery. In this case, it is appropriate merely to ask the woman if she feels that she or family members might benefit from a consultation with the psycho-oncologist, social worker, or sex therapist. Ask if she would like to talk to someone who has had a similar surgical procedure, possibly someone from the American Cancer Society's Reach for Recovery program. (See the Case Study: Breast Cancer with Mastectomy.)

Assess Coping Strategies. Women who undergo surgery for breast cancer experience a sense of loss—changes in life routines, social interactions, self-concept, and body image—and fear of death. Recovery during the postoperative period after mastectomy requires a great deal of energy. Fatigue is a persistent complaint for 6 months or more after surgery. A client's usual coping strategies may not be effective. Not everyone perceives or handles stress in the same way. Displacement, projection, denial, hope, prayer, meditation, stoicism, fatalism, and any combination of these reactions may be used as coping mechanisms. Clients who have surgically lost a breast may adapt in the same way as they would to any loss.

Encourage Self-Care Activities. Effective postoperative care is essential for successful psychosocial and physical rehabilitation. During the 1- to 3-day hospital stay, the focus of nursing care is on recovery from surgery and anesthesia as well as on discharge planning for self-care postoperative management. The client's self-image improves with self-care activities.

Explain Possible Body Image Concerns After Discharge. The full impact of losing a breast or having breast cancer may not be felt until a while after the client goes home. Many women are surprised by events such as the amount of pain and discomfort, marked fatigue, slow incision healing, and arm swelling. Ordinary motions, such as shifting to a comfortable position in bed, may be difficult and painful. As time passes, however, the woman and her significant others reorganize and restructure their lives. During this time, the woman resumes her role in society. Important changes in this role may be necessary. Individual women cope differently; feelings of sexual inadequacy, poor body image, and loss of a sense of femininity are common. Because body image is further altered by weight gain and alopecia if the woman is undergoing chemotherapy, she should be encouraged to purchase a wig and other hair coverings prior to hair loss. Fatigue, decreased libido, and periods of depression are common in women receiving chemotherapy and radiation therapy.

Discuss Strategies to Improve Body Image. Gradually the woman will decide whether to conceal her incision from significant others or let it be seen. The incision may be camouflaged for a woman by an appropriately fitted brassiere or a special bathing suit or evening dress, but doubts and fears about her attractiveness may affect even the most secure woman. You can offer understanding and facilitate communication between the client and significant others. The woman may wish to talk with other breast cancer survivors who have faced similar problems due to breast cancer. Breast cancer support groups may also be beneficial, but, they should be composed of women in similar stages of illness. A woman who is undergoing adjuvant therapy for curative breast cancer, for example, may be overwhelmed and frightened by the discussions and concerns of women with advanced metastatic breast cancer.

Risk for Impaired Skin Integrity. The nursing diagnosis may be expressed as *Risk for Impaired Skin Integrity related to surgery or radiation therapy.*

Outcomes. The client will remain free of impairment in skin integrity after surgery or radiation therapy, as evidenced by healing skin without redness, infection, hematoma formation, or breakdown.

Interventions

Provide and Explain Dressing and Drain Care. Postoperatively, a pressure dressing is usually used initially. Explain that a drain, connected to gentle suction, prevents blood or serum collection in the operative space after a modified radical mastectomy or axillary node dissection. Instruct the woman about emptying the drain and recording the amount of drainage. Advise her to notify the physician if the drain becomes plugged or dislodged or shows any sign of infection or if frank bleeding develops.

When changing the dressing, gently encourage the woman to look at the incision. Seeing the incision for the first time is often difficult, but the nurse's matter-of-fact approach can help. In future dressing changes, teach methods of cleaning the incision at home and of watching for manifestations of infection.

Prevent Skin Complications Following Radiation Therapy. During radiation therapy, scaling, flaking, dryness, itching, erythema, hair loss, rash, or dry desquamation of the involved skin may occur. Careful treatment of the skin is important in minimizing the skin effects of radiation therapy. Instruct women not to wash the area with soap but to rinse it with water only. No lotion or powder is to be put on the skin that overlies the radiation port. If the area under the arm becomes reddened because of friction, moisture, or radiation damage, place a soft, clean gauze pad between skinfolds to prevent skin breakdown.

Risk for Injury. The nursing diagnosis may be expressed as *Risk for Injury related to increased risk of infection and lymphedema secondary to axillary node dissection.*

Outcomes. The client will not experience injury, as evidenced by absence of infection or lymphedema.

Interventions

Arm edema (e.g., lymphedema) occurs less commonly today owing to the performance of less extensive mastectomy procedures and less extensive axillary dissection. Lymphedema results from insufficient transport of water and protein from the skin and subcutaneous tissue because of an inadequate development or eradication of lymphatic vessels. Lymphedema following axillary dissection has been reported in as many as 70% of cases, although probably a more accurate estimate of the average occurrence of lymphedema as a significant consequence of local therapy for breast cancer is 20% in the United States and Europe.[2] Clearly, the major risk for lymphedema exists when complete axillary dissection with stripping of the axillary vein and nodal irradiation is combined with mastectomy.

Older age, obesity, and lifting of heavy objects such as grocery bags and suitcases are also thought to increase the risk of lymphedema. Arm edema, stiffness, pain, and numbness have been reported in 40% to 50% of clients approximately 1 month after beginning radiation therapy to the axilla.[32] Lymphedema occurring years after surgery or radiation therapy is generally the result of infection, inflammation, or recurrent tumor.

Prevent Lymphedema. In the early postoperative period, encourage arm exercises, described in the Client Education Guide: Postmastectomy Exercises; elevate the arm on a pillow so that the elbow is level with the heart and the hand rests just higher than the elbow. The goal is to promote lymphatic drainage and prevent infection.

Administer Antibiotics for Infection. If a woman complains of redness, swelling, and a generalized area of warmth on the affected arm with or without fever, she should be examined for possible infection in the hand or arm. If an infection is present, the woman may need to be admitted to the hospital for intravenous antibiotics to treat the infection. Such infections can occur from a slight cut on the hand, and though they may seem innocuous, they pose a serious threat to these clients.

Minimize Lymphedema. Wearing an elastic bandage or a custom-fitted pressure-gradient elastic sleeve may be helpful in the months following surgery if lymphedema is present. Some women feel that wearing a sleeve while they are on an airplane minimizes swelling due to pressure changes in the airplane, although no studies have confirmed the efficacy of this practice.

Emphasize that it is important to prevent lymphedema. Once lymphedema occurs, it is more likely to occur again and be progressive. This is because the tissue, like a balloon, is a potential space that, once expanded, will expand again to that size and beyond at the least provocation.

Available treatments include application of compression garments, intermittent pneumatic compression, and massage by a trained physiotherapist.[45] Clients can obtain more information from the National Breast Cancer Coalition, the International Society of Lymphology, and the Oncology Nursing Society.

EVALUATION

The client who has undergone breast surgery for cancer will be discharged from the hospital 24 to 72 hours postoperatively. The surgical wounds may be healed within 4 weeks. Regaining complete use of the affected arm and shoulder may take as long as 6 weeks to several months, depending on the extent of the surgical procedure, rate of healing, compliance with exercises, and the degree of postoperative complications.

Breast Cancer with Mastectomy

Samantha Guern is a 33-year-old African American who presents to a free health care clinic with complaints of a painless rash on her left breast. She indicates that she does not perform breast self-examination and has not noticed any pain or tenderness in either breast. A mammogram is ordered, and Samantha is informed that a follow-up ultrasound examination and biopsy of the lump may be necessary. Samantha is tearful and asks: "How will I pay for these tests? What if you find something awful?!" Consider appropriate responses that the nurse might make.

The mammogram reveals a 3.5-cm solid lesion in the left breast. A follow-up ultrasound examination confirms that this is a solid lesion. A fine-needle aspiration of the lesion is performed, and the pathology report confirms the diagnosis of poorly differentiated breast cancer. A chest radiograph and bone scan are subsequently ordered. Results indicate no gross indications of metastasis at this time.

Samantha is referred to an oncologist to receive consultation about her treatment options. Because Samantha's lesion is a stage III carcinoma, she is advised to consider a modified radical mastectomy with a possible stem cell transplant procedure after the mastectomy. Samantha also meets with a social worker to determine whether there are any financial or other entitlements for which she would be eligible. In addition, the social worker assists Samantha in drafting a medical power of attorney that would provide the father of her children with authority to make decisions for her if necessary. Samantha is relieved to find that she qualifies for Medicaid.

Samantha's mastectomy is scheduled for the following day. Consider the behaviors that Samantha would exhibit that indicate she has been properly educated and prepared for the procedure.

Nursing History

Samantha is alert and cooperative. Samantha reports that she works full-time for a small local business that does not offer health benefits and that she has three school-aged children. Samantha is not married and mentions that occasionally the father of her three children stays at their house. She denies any known health problems, stating, "When you're a single parent and don't have health insurance, you can't afford to be sick." She says she has no allergies. Samantha indicates that she drinks iced tea and caffeinated sodas but states that she does not use alcohol, tobacco, or any other controlled substances. Samantha states that one of her mother's sisters had breast cancer and that she is not aware of any other cancer history in her family. Samantha's current method of birth control is a Depo-Provera injection, which she receives at the clinic every 3 months. Consider factors that place Samantha at risk for breast cancer.

Nursing Preoperative Physical Assessment

Height: 5′8″ Weight 130 lb (59.1 kg)
Vital Signs: BP 140/90, TPR 98.6, 84, 22
LOC: Alert and cooperative
EENT: WNL
Cardiac: Heart tones are regular. S_1 and S_2 are readily audible with no murmurs or rubs noted; *nontender walnut-sized lump noted in upper outer quadrant of left breast during auscultation of heart tones.*
Pulmonary: Lung sounds are clear bilaterally.
Abdominal: Abdomen is flat and nontender with normal, active bowel tones.
Genitourinary: Deferred
Peripheral pulses: 2/2, without edema

Samantha returns to the nursing unit from the recovery room. Her initial postoperative treatment orders include the following:

Meds: Cefazolin 1 gm IVPB every 6 hours
Morphine by PCA pump with basal rate of 1 mg per hour and 1 mg available per patient demand with a 15-minute lockout; no 4-hour limit is specified
Compazine 25-mg suppository PR every 6 hours as needed for nausea
Percocet 1 or 2 tabs every 4 to 6 hours as needed for less severe pain
D_5/½NS with 20 mEq KCl at 150 ml/hr
Clear liquids this evening progressing to DAT
Routine postoperative vital signs
Dangle patient this PM and to chair as tolerated in AM
No blood pressures, IV lines, or venous laboratory draws in patient's left arm
Call physician for urine output of less than 1 ml/kg/hr
Empty and record drain outputs every 4 hours
Reinforce dressings as needed

Samantha progresses satisfactorily and is scheduled for hospital discharge tomorrow. The surgical drains will be left in place after discharge.

Discharge Criteria

Average LOS: 2.1 days without complications, 2.9 days with complications
Initiate "Reach to Recovery" referral. What other community referrals would you make? Why?
Initiate instructions for home care and follow-up appointments with surgeon and oncologist.

Questions to Be Considered

1. A home health nurse is scheduled to visit Samantha to empty the surgical drains and to assess her ability to perform this procedure herself. What information should be taught and what behaviors might Samantha display that would indicate her ability or inability to empty her own drains?
2. Discuss the usual postoperative treatment course for a client with a stage III carcinoma considering a stem cell transplant procedure. Compare these treatment options with those for a client with a stage I or II carcinoma. What are the risks and benefits of each treatment option? What side effects might be expected by the client?

3. Three weeks postoperatively, Samantha returns to the clinic and reports that she is concerned about the recurrent swelling in her left arm and hand. Explain the physiologic basis for the swelling. What instructions should the nurse give Samantha to aid in reducing this problem?
4. Compare and contrast bone marrow transplantation and stem cell transplantation in the treatment of malignant breast cancer. What are the risks and benefits of transplant procedures for breast cancer clients?
5. Impaired body image is a concern for mastectomy clients. Outline the nursing interventions that could be used to assist the client to improve her body image. What behaviors would indicate that a client is successfully coping with her altered body image? Discuss the options that Samantha would have, if she elected to have breast reconstruction completed.

BP, blood pressure; D_5, 5% dextrose; DAT, diet as tolerated; EENT, eye-ear-nose-throat; IV, intravenous; IVPB, intravenous-piggyback; KCl, potassium chloride; LOC, level of consciousness; LOS, length of stay; NS, normal saline; PCA, patient-controlled analgesia; PR, per rectum (rectally); TPR, temperature-pulse-respirations; WNL, within normal limits.

CLIENT EDUCATION GUIDE

POSTMASTECTOMY EXERCISES:

When to Begin	Purpose	Exercises: Perform Exercises 5–10 Times Each, Three Times a Day
Postoperative days 1–5	Prevent and/or reduce swelling	▪ Position arm against your side in a relaxed position. Elbow should be level with your heart, and the wrist just above the elbow when resting. ▪ Rotate wrist in a circular fashion. ▪ Touch fingers to shoulder and extend arm fully.
After drains are removed	Promote muscle movement without stretching	▪ While standing, brace yourself with your other arm and bend over slightly, allowing your affected arm to hang freely. Swing the arm in small circles and gradually increase in size. Make 10 circles—rest—repeat in the opposite direction. ▪ Swing arm forward and back as far as you can without pulling on the incision. ▪ While standing, bend over slightly and swing arms across the chest in each direction. ▪ While sitting in a chair, rest both arms at your side. Shrug both shoulders, then relax. ▪ While sitting or standing, pull shoulders back, bring the shoulder blades together.
After sutures are removed	To stretch and regain full range of motion. To gain mobility of your shoulder, you must move it in *all* directions, several times a day	▪ While lying in bed with arm extended, raise arm over your head and extend backwards. ▪ While lying in bed, grasp a cane or short pole with both hands across your lap. Extend arms straight up and over your head and return. ▪ Repeat, rotating the cane clockwise and then counterclockwise while over your head. ▪ While standing, extend arm straight over your head and down. ▪ Extend your elbow out from your side at a 90° angle—hold it for 10 seconds—relax. ▪ Extend your arm straight out from your side even with your shoulder—extend arm straight up toward the ceiling. ▪ Stand at arm's length facing a wall. Extend arms so your fingertips touch the wall. Creep fingers up the side of the wall, stepping forward as necessary. Repeat the procedure going down the wall—keep arms extended. ▪ Stand sideways to the wall. Extend arm out so fingers touch the wall. Creep up the wall a little more each day. ▪ Use hand and arm normally.
After 6 weeks	To strengthen arm and shoulder and to regain total use of arm and shoulder	▪ Begin water aerobics. ▪ Begin overall fitness program. ▪ Begin aerobics, Jazzercise, or other resistive exercises. ▪ Avoid using weights, as these may increase arm edema and subsequent swelling.

Reprinted with permission from Chapman, D., & Goodman, M. (1997). Breast cancer. In S. Groenwald, M. Frogge, & M. Goodman (Eds.), *Cancer nursing principles and practice* (4th ed.), pp. 916–979. Boston: Jones & Bartlett.

Self-Care

To promote self-care, the client will need to learn about postoperative arm exercises, postoperative care, and care of the breast prosthesis. A referral to Reach for Recovery may also be helpful.

Teach Arm Exercises

In the early postoperative period (days 1 and 2), encourage the client to focus on the elbow, wrist, and hand of the affected side. The client performs active elbow flexion and extension, gently squeezes a soft rubber ball, and does deep breathing to facilitate lymph flow. Shoulder shrugs and active range of motion, including flexion and abduction, can be added on the second postoperative day. Encourage self-care activities (e.g., feeding, combing hair, washing face) and other activities that use the arm, with care taken not to abduct the arm or to raise the arm or elbow above shoulder height until the drains are removed.

Approximately 10 days after surgery, the client can begin active assisted range of motion exercises (see Client Education Guide: Postmastectomy Exercises). Tell the client to do these exercises at least twice a day as tolerated. Provide pain medication 30 minutes before exercises to permit the client to perform exercises without pain. Women who do not carry out these exercises as instructed are at greater risk for lymphedema and loss of shoulder joint mobility. (Arrangements for a physical therapist to assist with range of motion and strengthening exercises may need to be made at the same time surgery is planned because of the shortened hospital stay.) Always provide written and oral instructions about arm precautions after axillary node dissection, as shown in the Client Education Guide for arm care.

Refer to Reach for Recovery

The Reach for Recovery program of the American Cancer Society is a rehabilitation program for breast cancer survivors, specifically those who have had breast surgery. This program is designed to help women meet common psychosocial, physical, and cosmetic needs. With authorization of the physician and the client's permission, volunteers from this program visit the hospital or the home and give the woman information and help, including:

1. A kit, ball, book, rope, and temporary soft cotton prosthesis for women who have had a mastectomy
2. Instruction sheet for and demonstration of postoperative axillary node dissection exercises
3. Discussion of brassiere comfort, various breast prostheses, clothing adjustments, and personal problems as appropriate

Provide Breast Prosthesis

Women who have had a mastectomy may wear a temporary lightweight prosthesis immediately after the sutures and drains are removed. This may facilitate adjustment to the loss of the breast. A soft cotton breast form may be supplied by the Reach for Recovery visitor; cotton padding inserted into a pocket sewn into a lightweight brassiere is also a good temporary substitute. A permanent prosthesis should not be purchased until the wound has healed completely because the contours of the incision site may change. Cocoa butter may be rubbed into the incision once healing has occurred to help soften the scar and prevent scar contracture.

Because breast prostheses are expensive and not very comfortable, many women choose breast reconstruction. If a woman chooses to have a prosthesis, even temporarily while considering breast reconstruction, she should choose one that is appropriate for her. A breast prosthesis may be purchased in foundation departments in most large stores or at medical-surgical supply stores that sell durable medical equipment. Most of these stores have experienced sales associates to help women obtain the

CLIENT EDUCATION GUIDE

Arm Care After Axillary Lymph Node Dissection

Because you have had an axillary node dissection, the affected arm may swell and is less able to fight infection. Use your arm normally, following these recommendations.

Avoid burns while cooking or smoking.
Wear a long-length oven mitt.
Do not reach into a hot oven with this arm.
Do not hold a cigarette in the affected hand.
Avoid sunburn and insect bites.
Wear long-sleeved shirts and gloves.
Use sunscreen.
Use insect repellent to avoid bites and stings.
Avoid cuts, pinpricks, and scratches.
Wear gloves when gardening.
Do not work near thorny plants or dig with your hands.
Use a thimble when sewing.
Use an electric razor with a narrow head for underarm shaving to reduce the risk of nicks or scratches.
Never cut or pick at cuticles; use hand cream or lotion.
Wash cuts promptly; treat them with antibacterial medication and cover them with sterile dressing, and check often for redness, soreness, pus, or other manifestations of infection.
Avoid strong detergents, harsh chemicals, and abrasive compounds.
Wear protective gloves while doing dishes and cleaning.
Avoid other trauma.
Have all injections, vaccinations, blood samples, and blood pressure tests done on the other arm whenever possible.
Wear a medical identification tag that cautions against test injections or blood pressure readings on the affected arm.
Carry your handbag and other heavy objects on the other arm.
Wear watch or jewelry loosely, if at all, on the operated arm.
Avoid elastic cuffs on blouses and nightgowns.
Use a lanolin hand cream a few times each day.
Wear an elastic sleeve if recommended by your physician.
Contact your physician if the arm or hand becomes red, is swollen, or feels hot; in the meantime, try to keep your arm over your head and periodically pump your fist.

Adapted from National Cancer Institute. (1987). *After breast cancer: A guide to follow-up care* (NIH Publication No. 87–2400). Washington, DC: Author.

proper fit. Most private and government insurance plans pay for at least the first breast prosthesis and brassiere, provided that a written prescription from the physician accompanies the receipt. Many plans also pay for yearly replacements.

BREAST RECONSTRUCTION

Many women have feelings of loss, depression, and alterations in body image after mastectomy. Breast reconstruction is an accepted component of the treatment plan. In the 1990s, improvements were made to surgical prostheses and surgical techniques, helping women become more confident in their choice to have reconstructive surgery and retain their self-confidence and body image, thereby enhancing their quality of life. The goal for clients having reconstructive surgery is to "feel whole again." This includes appearing "normal" in a bathing suit as well as in the nude.

The only contraindications to breast reconstruction are the client's need for chest wall irradiation and the physical inability to withstand additional surgery due to a co-morbid condition. Breast reconstruction is not contraindicated by a woman's age, her need for adjuvant chemotherapy, a poor prognosis, or even the presence of metastatic disease. The timing of the breast reconstruction may be immediate (at the time of the mastectomy) or delayed, even until years after mastectomy. When adjuvant chemotherapy is planned, the surgeon may prefer to wait until the chemotherapy is completed to begin reconstructing the breast.

Several surgical techniques can be used to reconstruct the breast mound and nipple-areola complex. The choice of technique is based upon the client's wishes, the amount of tissue available, and whether the woman has had radiation therapy in the past. The simplest method of reconstruction involves the insertion of an implant into a pocket of skin purposely left by the surgeon. This approach is best for women with small or moderate-size breasts, in whom the implant is of a size similar to the remaining breast. Other methods of reconstruction include the following.

Tissue Expanders

A tissue expander is a deflated silicone envelope that is inserted under the chest muscles and expanded slowly over 6 to 8 weeks by adding 60 to 200 ml of saline per week via a remote percutaneous injection port. When the skin overlying the breast mound is sufficiently overinflated to accommodate the implant comfortably, the expander is removed and the implant is inserted. Many times the expanded implant is expanded to become the permanent implant.

Transverse Rectus Abdominis Muscle Flap

The transverse rectus abdominis muscle (TRAM) flap procedure is commonly referred to as the "tummy tuck." A low transverse elliptical incision is made, and abdominal muscle and fat are tunneled under the abdominal skin to the mastectomy site. Tissue viability and perfusion are retained by the superior epigastric vessel. The tissue can also be transferred as a free flap. The donor site in the abdomen is closed as for a modified abdominoplasty (Fig. 40–4). Contraindications to the TRAM flap are the presence of abdominal scars and inadequate abdominal tissue.

Latissimus Dorsi Muscle Flap

The latissimus dorsi muscle, a large fan-shaped muscle beneath the scapula, is used when inadequate skin is available at the mastectomy site. It is considered an expendable muscle because alternative muscle groups are able to adduct the humerus and rotate the shoulder posteriorly. An ellipse of skin along with the latissimus dorsi muscle is tunneled through the axilla and rotated onto the mastectomy site. The viability of the tissue is maintained through the thoracodorsal vessels (Fig. 40–5).

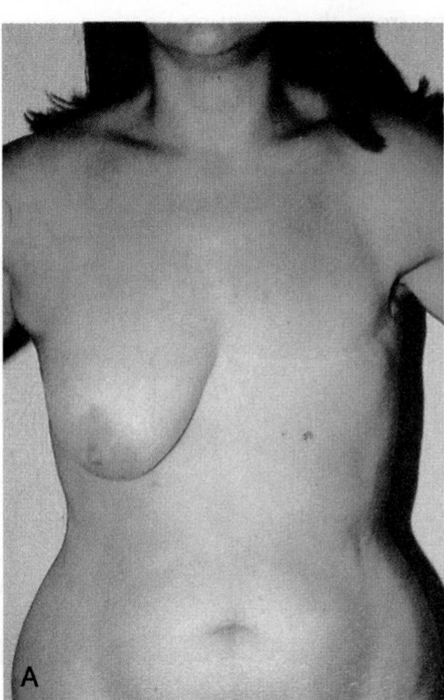

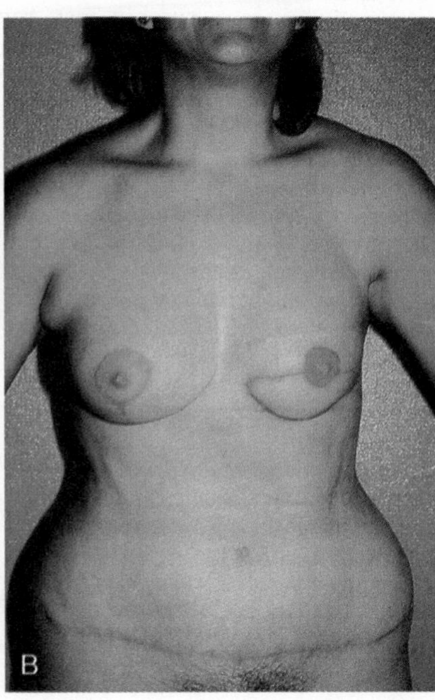

FIGURE 40–4 Breast reconstruction using transverse rectus abdominis myocutaneous flaps. *A,* Preoperative appearance. *B,* Postoperative appearance.

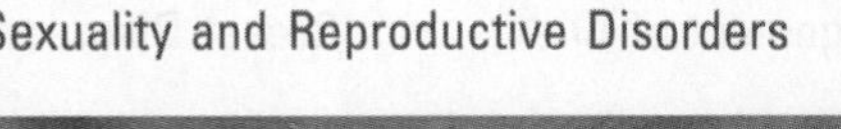

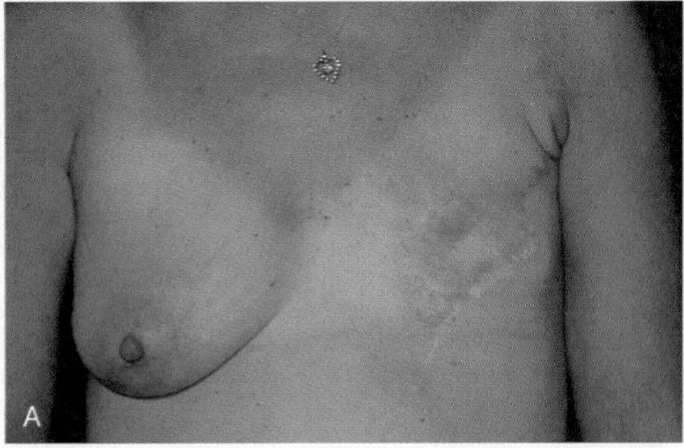

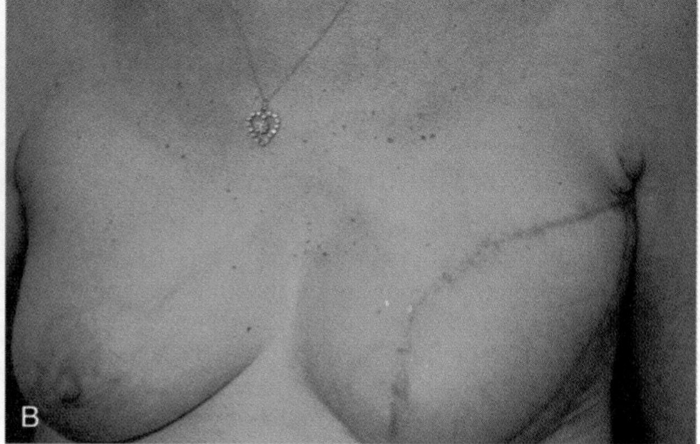

FIGURE 40–5 An ideal result of reconstructive surgery using a latissimus dorsi myocutaneous flap and an implant. *A,* Preoperative appearance. *B,* Postoperative appearance. A subpectoral implant is used in the right breast for symmetry.

GLUTEAL MUSCLE FREE FLAPS

A much less common form of breast construction involves the use of the gluteus muscle. The muscle and overlying skin are lifted from their bed and connected to the chest wall using an operating microscope.

NIPPLE-AREOLA RECONSTRUCTION

Some women elect also to have the nipple-areola reconstructed. To achieve symmetry, nipple reconstruction should be delayed for several months following breast reconstruction. During the healing process, the contour of the reconstructed breast may change as the incisions heal and edema subsides. Areola can be reconstructed with a tattoo or by nipple sharing. The dark tissue of the areola is most commonly reconstructed by tattooing. Nipple projection is constructed with a skate flap (Fig. 40–6). Many years ago, the nipple was removed from the breast before amputation and stored ("banked") on the inner thigh. This procedure is no longer performed because of the risk of cancer spread.

Nursing Management of the Client with Breast Reconstruction

PREOPERATIVE CARE

Preoperatively, the nurse reinforces the physician's instructions regarding the goals of reconstruction and any postoperative care needs. It is important that the client have realistic expectations of the outcome of the surgery. The client may be shown pictures of reconstructed breasts to familiarize her with what can be achieved. The client may express anger, disbelief, and fear related to the surgery, especially if the reconstruction is being combined with a mastectomy for a known carcinoma. Many women will at the same time express relief that the cancer surgery is being done and the cancer is being removed. Some will find comfort in discussing their feelings of disbelief at this time. Periods of depression are normal.

Encourage clients to express their feelings and fears with family members and to seek assistance from the psycho-oncology service or chaplain should this be appropriate. Assess risks for anesthesia-related problems and operative blood loss prior to surgery. Advise any client who smokes cigarettes to stop, because smoking compromises flap and skin circulation.

POSTOPERATIVE CARE

In addition to providing the postoperative nursing care required by any person having surgery, after reconstructive breast surgery you will assess the flap or breast area for color, temperature, and capillary refill. If any area appears dusky and congested with blood, the flap may be suffering from venous obstruction. A flap that is pale is not receiving blood and may be experiencing arterial constriction. Whenever circulation or perfusion is in question, notify the physician immediately. The success of this surgical procedure is directly dependent on astute nursing assessment and proper physician notification of complications. Laser Doppler flow may be used to monitor skin perfusion after free flap transfer.

Inform a woman with a recent subpectoral implant that initially the implant feels very firm and is higher on the chest than a normal breast. Over time, the muscle stretches, allowing the implant to drop and soften. Women with subpectoral implants do not wear bras, because the implant needs to move into the pocket created in the chest wall. Women who undergo other types of surgery may return from the operating room wearing a bra to support the breasts. A front-closing support bra without underwires is preferred. Wearing a bra also helps some women feel more normal, encouraging a return to

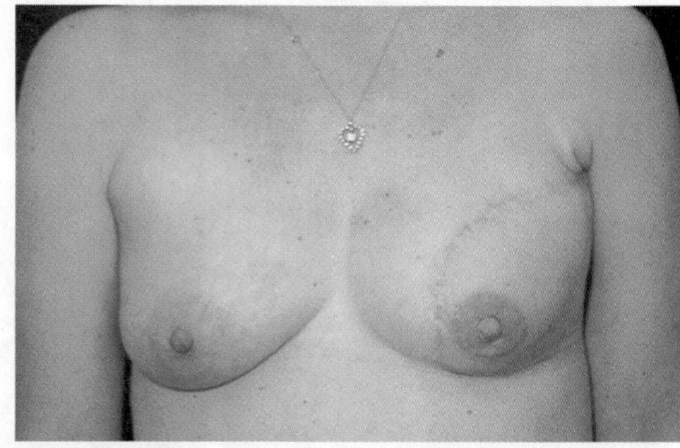

FIGURE 40–6 Nipple-areola reconstruction.

wellness. Psychosocial readjustment to breast reconstruction, including incorporation of the reconstructed breast into the woman's body image, usually occurs 3 to 4 months after surgery.

Medical Management

ELIMINATE OR PREVENT SPREAD OF CANCER

After surgery or instead of surgery, it may be possible to prevent further extension of cancer or to completely eliminate the cancer cells by using radiation therapy, chemotherapy, and/or hormonal therapy modalities.

Radiation Therapy

Radiation therapy is used in breast cancer treatment as follows:

- The breast and underlying chest wall are irradiated after lumpectomy or quadrantectomy as adjuvant therapy for stage I or II breast cancer.
- Women who are poor surgical candidates because of health problems such as heart disease typically receive radiation therapy to the affected breast.
- The chest wall is irradiated if it is involved or for local control after mastectomy with positive margins.
- The axilla is irradiated in women at high risk for axillary metastases who are poor surgical candidates for axillary dissection or who have gross disease that was not surgically excised.
- The supraclavicular region is irradiated if positive axillary nodes are found.
- Additional areas are irradiated for management of metastatic disease to the brain, bone, or skin.

Radiation in combination with lumpectomy or quadrantectomy is an accepted treatment for early-stage breast cancer. An axillary dissection or a sentinel node biopsy is usually done for staging purposes. Radiation therapy, when used to treat micrometastatic disease following mastectomy, successfully reduces the risk of local recurrence and therefore of distant metastases. The utility of radiation therapy following mastectomy or modified radical mastectomy comes into question when the client is also receiving adjuvant chemotherapy, tamoxifen, or both. Although it may decrease local recurrence, the addition of radiation therapy does not influence survival unless there is microscopic disease in the margins. Therefore, the use of postoperative radiation therapy is not indicated in clients with negative axillary nodes except when there is evidence of disease at the deep margins of the tumor.[2] Where axillary nodes are positive, radiation therapy is useful to reduce the likelihood of local recurrence and to improve survival.

When chemotherapy is given with radiation therapy, the radiotherapy may be given concomitantly or sandwiched with the chemotherapy, or given sequentially after completion of the chemotherapy. Concomitant therapy results in a greater incidence of skin reactions than has been reported with sequential treatment. The only situation in which radiation therapy might be given prior to chemotherapy is in a case in which there are negative axillary nodes (and therefore low risk for distant disease) and positive surgical margins, when the risk for local recurrence is great. The real risk to women with breast cancer is that it is a systemic disease. Therefore, chemotherapy is critically important to eradicate any micrometastatic disease wherever it may be, including the chest.

Radiation therapy can be administered through an external beam or via iridium implants. For external beam irradiation, the radiation is administered on an outpatient basis 5 days a week for 5 to 6 weeks to the entire breast (and possibly the lymphatics), usually with a boost to the tumor bed. The total dose of radiation is approximately 5000 rad. Regional lymph nodes may be treated if they have not been removed.

Interstitial implant therapy using iridium^{192} (^{192}Ir) is an in-hospital procedure. The insertion of the iridium implant may be done using local anesthesia. Stainless steel guide needles are threaded through the tumor area at l-cm intervals. Flexible plastic tubes are inserted in the guide needles. The guide needles are then removed, leaving the tube in place. Strands of radioactive iridium seeds are threaded through each tube (Fig. 40–7). The seeds, at 1-cm intervals, form a grid with those above and below to cover the tissues evenly with radiation.

At the end of the insertion procedure, a button is attached to the end of the tubes and the ends are crimped and cut to prevent the seeds from falling out. An x-ray film confirms the implant's location. The implant usually must remain in place for 2 or 3 days. The procedure is mildly uncomfortable. The woman is able to be up and about in her room. Radiation precautions related to time, distance, and shielding are maintained (see Chapter 19). Because of the excellent results from breast reconstruction, most women opt for complete tumor removal rather than the use of implants, which potentially leave residual disease behind.

Side effects of radiation therapy to the breast include:

- Temporary skin changes such as itching, dryness, tenderness, redness, swelling, and/or dry desquamation
- Moist desquamation, especially in skinfolds
- Fatigue
- Dry throat may occur owing to radiation scatter, especially if the supraclavicular area is irradiated
- Pneumonitis (rare); may present as a dry cough and dyspnea; a result of inflammatory changes in the irradiated underlying lung
- Arm edema (rare), occurring more commonly with axillary irradiation
- Increased susceptibility to rib fracture in the irradiated field
- Difficulty in obtaining optimal doses of chemotherapy in women receiving chemotherapy concurrently with radiation therapy because of the effect of radiation on bone marrow

Radiation therapy can be emotionally taxing and physically fatiguing. Nursing support is needed during the 5- to 7-week treatment period. Women receiving radiation therapy have many of the same fears as those having a mastectomy: fear of death, fear of mutilation, and feelings of sexual inadequacy. These are compounded by the stress of daily treatment and the fatigue that occurs with coping with a chronic illness, often while recovering from the side effects of chemotherapy.

Systemic Chemotherapy

LOCALIZED BREAST CANCER. Adjuvant systemic chemotherapy for early stage I and stage II breast cancer gener-

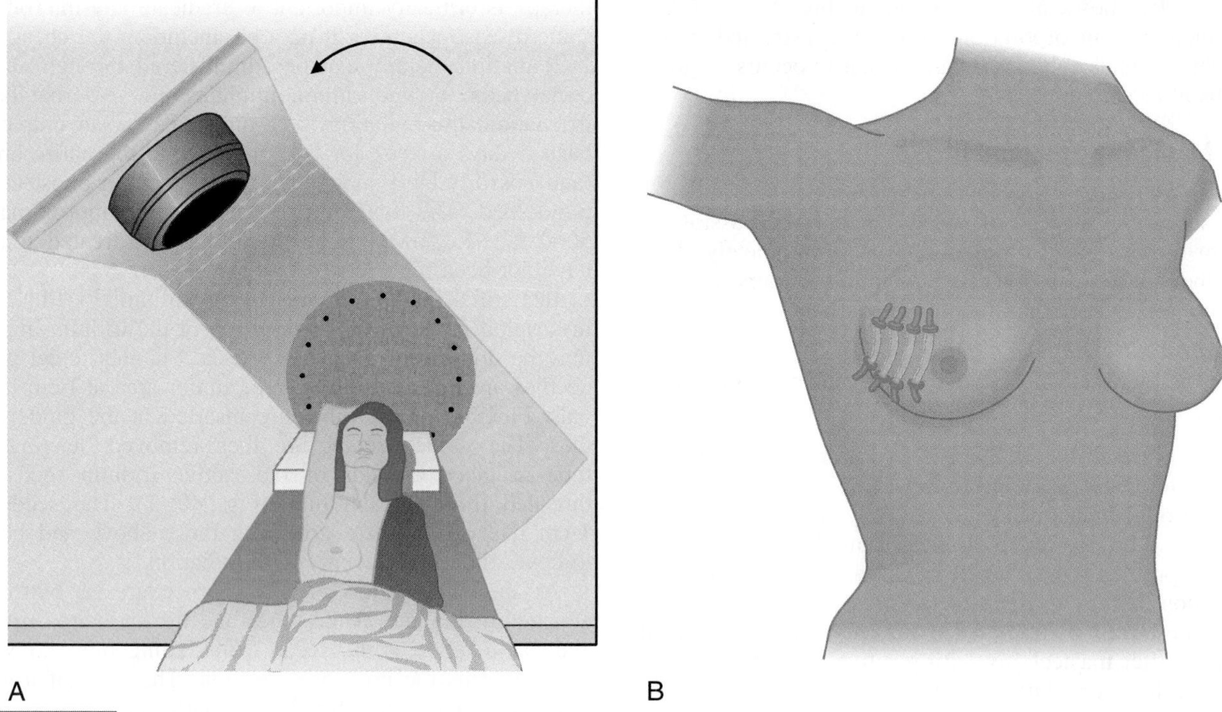

FIGURE 40–7 Radiation therapy is given via an external beam (*A*) or iridium implants (*B*).

ally follows local surgical intervention and includes combinations of cyclophosphamide (Cytoxan), doxorubicin (Adriamycin), methotrexate (Mexate), 5-fluorouracil (5-FU), paclitaxel (Taxol), and docetaxel (Taxotere), with or without tamoxifen (Nolvadex). Six cycles of cyclophosphamide, methotrexate, and 5-fluorouracil (CMF) and four cycles of doxorubicin and cyclophosphamide with methotrexate, 5-fluorouracil, or leucovorin (Wellcovorin) all are standard adjuvant (curative) therapy for breast cancer.

For the most part, clients are divided into three groups: those who have no involved axillary lymph nodes, those with one to three involved nodes, and those with four or more involved nodes. Adjuvant systemic therapy is usually not given to women whose tumors are 0.5 cm or less in greatest diameter and without lymph node involvement. Clients whose tumors are larger than 0.5 cm but less than 1.0 cm and without lymph node involvement may be divided into those with a low risk of recurrence and those who have unfavorable prognostic features that warrant consideration of adjuvant therapy. Unfavorable prognostic features include lymphatic invasion, high S phase fraction, high nuclear and histologic grades, and HER-2–positive status.

Clients with lymph node involvement or with tumors larger than 1.0 cm in diameter are appropriate candidates for adjuvant systemic therapy. Cytotoxic chemotherapy using CMF or a regimen of cyclophosphamide, doxorubicin, and 5-FU (CAF) is appropriate for women younger than 50 years of age (or premenopausal) and for those 50 years of age or older (or postmenopausal) with hormone receptor–negative tumors.

For women who are 50 years of age or older and have receptor-positive tumors, tamoxifen therapy for 5 years is recommended. The addition of tamoxifen therapy significantly improves the 10-year survival for this population.[18] The benefit of the addition of tamoxifen therapy to chemotherapy is less clear for women younger than 50 years of age and those with hormone receptor–positive tumors. The addition of chemotherapy to tamoxifen therapy for women 50 years of age or older with hormone receptor–positive, pathologic stage II cancers is somewhat controversial.

The decision to use tamoxifen with or without chemotherapy in women with estrogen receptor–positive disease should be based on the absolute magnitude of risk reduction expected with the systemic therapy and the individual client's willingness to experience toxicity in order to achieve that incremental risk reduction. Obviously, for women with estrogen receptor–negative disease, the choice is for adjuvant chemotherapy. A meta-analysis has shown that combination chemotherapy on the average produces an absolute improvement of 7% to 11% in 10-year survival for women younger than 50 years of age and of 2% to 3% for those aged 50 to 69.[18]

Because there is little agreement about optimal chemotherapy regimens, it is particularly difficult for clients to choose their treatment. For some, the decision is based on whether they will lose their hair and be finished after four injections over 9 weeks, or perhaps whether they will keep their hair but take treatment that lasts for 6 months and requires 12 visits to complete.

In some instances, the physician may recommend primary, induction, or "neoadjuvant" chemotherapy (i.e., given before surgery). Primary chemotherapy is beneficial because the physician can evaluate response to chemotherapy directly, which is impossible once the cancer is removed. Therefore, the physician can know whether the choice of chemotherapy is optimal. In addition, the tumor may actually shrink so much that the disease may be "downstaged," permitting a breast-preserving procedure.

Because induction therapy is given promptly after a diagnosis of breast cancer, the treatment of potential micrometastases, without delays related to surgery, theoretically could result in higher cure rates.[7]

However, although preoperative chemotherapy was as effective as postoperative chemotherapy NB, the results have not demonstrated higher cure rates or influenced survival for stage I and II breast cancers. It does, however, offer the opportunity to observe the biologic response of the tumor to the effects of chemotherapy.[5, 21] When given to clients with inflammatory breast cancer, primary chemotherapy permits shrinkage of the tumor and possible mastectomy, whereas without prior chemotherapy, it might not have been possible to obtain clear surgical margins.

ADVANCED LOCALIZED BREAST CANCER. When a client has more extensive (stage III) yet curable disease, her options and decisions for therapy are even more difficult and controversial. Women with unfavorable stage IIIA or IIIB breast cancers generally require a more aggressive management approach. Affected women typically have larger tumors (>5 cm), direct invasion of the skin of the breast or the chest wall, or fixed or matted axillary lymphadenopathy. Usually, these women undergo preoperative chemotherapy, with or without hormone therapy, followed by surgery and radiotherapy. An alternative approach involves the use of high-dose combination chemotherapy, followed by an additional combination of agents that are also active in breast cancer. The concept is to minimize the risk of drug resistance and to attempt to kill cells before they have an opportunity to mutate to resistance. The addition of paclitaxel every three weeks for four cycles following the standard doxorubicin (Adriamycin) and cyclophosphamide regimen every three weeks for four cycles for women with node-positive breast cancer is associated with increased relapse-free survival.[26]

Other adjuvant treatments under investigation include the combination of paclitaxel and the monoclonal antibody trastuzumab (Herceptin). When these two agents are combined, there appears to be significant synergy without increased toxicity.[44] HER-2 is overexpressed in 25% to 30% of human breast cancers and indicates a worse prognosis in clients who have positive axillary lymph nodes. Despite the association of HER-2 overexpression with poor prognosis, a clinical response to taxanes was three times more likely to occur in HER-2–positive clients than in HER-2–negative clients.[4, 43]

A multicenter research trial combining trastuzumab, doxorubicin, and cyclophosphamide with paclitaxel is being proposed by the NCI. All women with stage III breast cancer who enter the research study would receive all four drugs plus dexrazoxane (Zinecard)—a drug to prevent cardiac damage, included because all four drugs are associated with cardiac toxicity. Once the chemotherapy treatment is complete, the women would then be randomized either to continue trastuzumab for a year or to have no further chemotherapy.[27]

Dose intensification requiring the use of colony-stimulating factors or autologous hematopoietic support is not considered standard therapy in adjuvant breast cancer. Research conducted by the National Surgical Adjuvant Breast Project included two randomized trials (NSABP B22 and NSABP B25) of dose intensification, and neither one to date has demonstrated that higher doses of drug given in a compressed time period are superior to standard dosing of the same drugs (doxorubicin and cyclophosphamide).[23] Furthermore, the toxicity associated with dose intensification is significant.[15] Although pilot trials of autologous bone marrow transplant procedures for women with multiple positive nodes have shown some success, more research is needed to demonstrate the efficacy of bone marrow transplantation in breast cancer.

Nursing Management of the Medical Client

ASSESSMENT

Nursing management of the woman receiving chemotherapy for breast cancer centers on her need for information and instructions regarding self-care procedures. Because in most cases the woman undergoes her breast surgery in the hospital and goes home 1 to 3 days later, there is often little time to discuss her concerns regarding chemotherapy and radiation therapy. Even though the client does not start these treatments until complete healing has taken place (usually 3 to 4 weeks after surgery), the nurse has an important role in providing the client and family members with information regarding the side effects of chemotherapy and radiation therapy. In planning care, be sure to consider the emotional, social, cognitive, spiritual, and physical impact of the diagnosis and treatment on the woman and her family.

DIAGNOSIS, OUTCOMES, INTERVENTIONS

Effective Management of Therapeutic Regimen. The nursing diagnosis may be expressed as *Effective Management of Therapeutic Regimen related to chemotherapy and radiation therapy.*

Outcomes. The client will understand the purpose and goals of chemotherapy and radiation therapy as evidenced by her statements concerning the necessity for treatment and possible side effects associated with that treatment.

Interventions

Teach About Radiation Therapy. Teaching is a major role of the nurse who is caring for clients receiving radiation therapy.

Include in the teaching plan instructions regarding skin care, sun protection, and management of fatigue. If the client is receiving chemotherapy concurrently, there is heightened risk for infection due to neutropenia. Therefore, instruct clients to report any evidence of infection. Monitor blood counts on a weekly basis. Tell the client that written materials, including the booklet *Radiation Therapy and You,* are available from the NCI free of charge by calling 1-800-4-CANCER. See Chapter 19 for further information on radiation therapy.

Teach About Chemotherapy. Nurses are responsible for teaching clients about the side effects of chemotherapy. The booklet *Chemotherapy and You* (also available free of charge from the NCI) explains the purpose of chemotherapy and possible side effects. Once the regimen is selected, discuss side effects. Teach the client the names of the drugs, how the drugs are given, expected side effects and their management, preventive measures, and complications that need to be reported to the physician or nurse (e.g., infection, fever, bruising, bleeding, mouth sores).

You should vary the teaching plan, depending on the drug regimen selected, because the side effects are different for each of the drugs. For example, not all chemotherapy agents cause hair loss. Women receiving methotrexate and 5-FU will not experience hair loss, whereas women receiving doxorubicin and cyclophosphamide will have complete hair loss at 2½ weeks after their first injection. Cyclophosphamide taken orally for 14 days and methotrexate and 5-FU given by injection twice a month will cause a gradual thinning of the hair, but generally the woman can get by without a wig, especially if her hair is kept short. Methotrexate and 5-FU can cause diarrhea and stomatitis, which may interrupt therapy. Advise women taking cyclophosphamide by mouth for the 14-day regimen to drink eight glasses of water a day to prevent hemorrhagic cystitis.

Altered Nutrition: Less Than Body Requirements. The nursing diagnosis may be expressed as *Altered Nutrition: Less Than Body Requirements related to nausea, vomiting, and stomatitis secondary to chemotherapy.*

Outcomes. The client will maintain adequate nutrition, as evidenced by absence of nausea and vomiting, control of stomatitis, intake of adequate calories daily, and no or minimal weight loss.

Interventions. Nausea, vomiting, anorexia, stomatitis, and taste change are common side effects of chemotherapy agents. Some drugs, specifically doxorubicin and methotrexate, will cause stomatitis 4 to 5 days after the injection.

Provide Oral Hygiene. To minimize the severity of the stomatitis, the client is instructed to perform oral hygiene three to four times a day and to rinse with baking soda and water to maintain a basic environment in the oral cavity. Bacteria thrive in an acid environment. If a client experiences any mouth soreness, she should suck on ice during injection of the chemotherapy agent. This simple form of cryotherapy helps to minimize exposure of the oral cavity to the irritating effects of chemotherapy agents.

Prevent Nausea and Vomiting. Nausea and vomiting are usually preventable when antiemetic medications are taken on a schedule rather than just as needed. A combination of a dopamine antagonist, a serotonin antagonist, and a steroid is usually adequate to prevent nausea and vomiting from chemotherapy. Because chemotherapy slows colonic transit time, clients often experience epigastric distress and bloating after administration of these agents. In addition, the serotonin antagonists can be constipating. For these reasons, encourage clients to eat lightly, taking primarily liquids for the 3 days following chemotherapy. Drugs such as metoclopramide (Reglan) or cisapride (Propulsid) are useful to enhance gastric emptying and to reduce bloating. Most women who receive chemotherapy for breast cancer do not lose weight; in fact, they gain weight. Women receiving CMF therapy may gain between 15 and 25 pounds during their therapy. Counsel clients to control their weight and to watch what they are eating.

EVALUATION

Many factors affect the duration of the chemotherapy regimen. Some considerations are:

- Whether the chemotherapy is adjuvant
- Stage at which the breast cancer was diagnosed
- Co-morbidities
- Whether the disease remains stable during chemotherapy

Self-Care

TEACH ABOUT FOLLOW-UP SURVEILLANCE

The highest risk factor for breast cancer is a history of breast cancer. Therefore, instruct clients that they require follow-up cancer surveillance for the rest of their lives. Most women are emotional and apprehensive after completing their adjuvant therapy. For the most part, they are happy to be finished but nervous that they are no longer receiving any therapy to oppose the cancer. If they are receiving tamoxifen, remind them that it is treatment for their cancer as well as a medicine to help prevent breast cancer. Women express fear that the cancer will come back, and many wonder whether they could ever endure chemotherapy again if the disease did come back. It is important to acknowledge and discuss the fact that they will worry and feel afraid, so that they can realize that such feelings are normal.

Explain that the physical examination by the physician every 3 to 4 months is designed to detect any problem early and that they should make every effort to keep their appointments. The surveillance schedule involves a physical examination every 3 to 4 months for 3 years, every 6 months for 2 years, and then once a year. A mammogram and a chest film (optional) are obtained every 12 months. Routine chemistry screening is done every year. For women on tamoxifen who still have their uterus, a pelvic examination is done every year.

Routine liver, bone, and brain scans are not indicated as surveillance tests for recurrent disease.[42] Until research determines that early institution of therapy is critical to the outcome, the goal of surveillance is to detect the disease just as the disease begins to be symptomatic.[2]

PROMOTE ACCEPTANCE OF BODY IMAGE

For the woman who has had a mastectomy (a less common procedure today), acceptance of the change in body image takes time. Evaluate adaptation to this loss by asking the woman how she feels about the loss and whether she thinks it would be helpful to see a social worker or psycho-oncologist to discuss strategies for coping. Adaptation and acceptance of the loss may be evident by her ability to discuss plans for a permanent prosthesis or by her questions regarding breast reconstruction. Do not insist that a woman look at her incision; she needs to wait until she is ready. A woman's reluctance to look at the incision is in no way evidence of inability to accept her loss.

Inform women of outside resources that can help them adapt to the changes imposed by the disease. For example, breast cancer support groups and other resources are designed to help the woman and her significant other learn to cope. Information about where to buy a prosthesis and a wig is helpful. Even having the telephone number and name of a person who can help with a wig or prosthesis can make a difficult time more bearable.

LOCAL RECURRENCE

Nearly 80% of local recurrences appear within 5 years of mastectomy.[2] Local recurrence after mastectomy generally presents as an isolated nodule in or under the skin of the chest wall, usually near the mastectomy scar. Breast reconstruction does not interfere with early detection of a local recurrence. A complete staging work-up is conducted to define the extent of recurrence. Wide local excision and radiation therapy have been the standard form of local treatment for clients with local recurrence after mastectomy. Hormone therapy is appropriate if the tumor is estrogen receptor–positive, or chemotherapy is recommended in view of the very high risk for distant metastases. The goal of therapy is control of local and distant disease.

Local recurrence after breast-preserving surgery and radiation therapy carries a better prognosis than that associated with local recurrence after mastectomy. Mastectomy is the standard form of therapy for local recurrence, provided that there is no evidence of supraclavicular node involvement or distant metastases. After a mastectomy, many women have breast reconstruction with a myocutaneous flap, which is psychologically important but also improves healing.

■ METASTATIC BREAST CANCER

Medical Management

DETERMINE EXTENT OF DISEASE

Despite adjuvant therapy, after varying periods of disease-free survival, nearly half of clients who have received treatment for apparently localized breast cancer develop metastatic disease. The majority of cases occur within 2 years of definitive surgery, but several initial breast cancer recurrences occur more than 5 years after initial therapy.[34] In general, the clinical course and presentation of metastatic disease are variable in terms of growth rate and responsiveness to systemic therapy. As a result of the heterogeneous nature of breast cancer, the disease may present as aggressive visceral disease in multiple organs, as a small skin recurrence such as in a supraclavicular lymph node, or as metastatic bone disease.

Selection of therapy depends on the extent of disease and whether any visceral organs are involved. The goal of therapy is control of disease and optimal palliation with prolongation of life and minimal disruption of the woman's lifestyle and quality of life. Life expectancy after breast cancer recurrence is variable. If disease recurs in the liver, most women die within 3 years of the recurrence. Others with disease in bone or skin may survive for many years. Women with more aggressive disease tend to be *premenopausal,* with estrogen receptor–negative, HER2–positive disease that recurs in liver or lung. Women with less aggressive disease tend to be *postmenopausal,* with estrogen receptor–positive disease that is HER-2–negative and recurs in bone and skin.

All clients with suspected metastatic disease undergo a metastatic work-up to determine the extent of disease. Typically, a physical examination, serum chemistry profiles, a complete blood count, chest radiograph, and a bone scan are obtained initially. If the client has clinical manifestations associated with organ dysfunction, a CT scan of the area is appropriate. A CT scan or MRI study of the chest, abdomen, or pelvis may also be done if the client is being considered for a research protocol. Serum markers include CEA, CA-125, and CA 15-3. Serum markers that are elevated are monitored monthly to evaluate response to therapy.

PREVENT FURTHER EXTENSION OF CANCER

Once extent of disease is determined, an overall therapeutic approach is established based on the client's age, disease-free interval, hormone receptor status, and location and extent of disease. For older women with limited and non–life threatening disease, no significant manifestations of disease, and estrogen receptor–positive tumors, hormone therapy is the initial treatment of choice. If the disease involves liver or lung or if the tumor is estrogen receptor–negative, the choice of treatment is chemotherapy, with or without trastuzumab if the tumor is HER-2–positive. Radiation therapy is instituted only if the disease is symptomatic.

The basic philosophy of management of the woman with metastatic breast cancer is to use all therapies to their fullest worth, but not to the point of toxicity, when the treatment becomes worse than the disease. A treatment that creates a stable condition is still a worthwhile treatment. Treatments are not abandoned until their utility is fully spent. The emphasis is on the need for therapeutic options.

Endocrine Therapy

As stated earlier, when a woman is known to have breast cancer, her tissue sample is tested for the presence of estrogen and progesterone receptors. Estrogen and progesterone receptor assays are performed using radioimmunoassay and immunohistochemical techniques. The more strongly estrogen receptor–positive the tumor, the more likely it is that the disease will respond to hormone therapies. Yet although more than 60% of human breast cancers are estrogen receptor–positive, no more than two thirds of them will respond to endocrine therapy.

Hormone therapies are generally classified as *ablative* (removal of the hormone) or *additive* (addition of a hormone changes the hormonal environment sufficiently to affect tumor growth). The response rates for all hormonal manipulations are basically similar. Women who have a response to one hormonal intervention often have a response to a second after the first becomes ineffective.

In general, the least toxic intervention is chosen first. Once the disease is no longer controlled with a specific approach, the next least toxic agent is selected, and so forth. With the exception of tamoxifen, which is an antiestrogen, hormone therapies are reserved for women with metastatic disease. There is no therapeutic benefit to combining hormone therapies. It is generally accepted practice to continue each therapy for as long as it provides benefit before instituting other therapy. Even withdrawing a hormone manipulation may result in a therapeutic response.

Antiestrogens

If the woman has not previously received tamoxifen, it is typically the first hormonal agent given because of its limited toxicity. Tamoxifen works in premenopausal women, but it is more active in the absence of ovarian function and is therefore especially effective in postmenopausal women. Tamoxifen is a partial estrogen agonist that has mixed estrogenic and antiestrogenic properties; it has a favorable effect on cardiac status and opposes calcium loss as women age. Side effects include nausea, hot flashes, weight gain, menstrual irregularities, and thromboembolic events in 1% to 2% of cases. The risk of endometrial cancer is minimal (2 cases per 1000 women annually in postmenopausal women).[12] Other antiestrogens include toremifene (Fareston), raloxifene, and long-acting ICI 182,780 (Faslodex).

Ablative Endocrine Procedures

Ablative endocrine procedures have been replaced by specific, well-tolerated hormone treatments. In premenopausal women, it is possible to administer goserelin (Zoladex), a luteinizing hormone–releasing hormone (LHRH) agonist that causes a medical oophorectomy. Injections are given every 1 to 3 months depending on the preparation. The only difference between surgical oophorectomy and medical oophorectomy is that results with surgical intervention are immediate and permanent.

For women in whom initial hormone ablation therapy fails, administration of either megestrol acetate (Megace) or an aromatase inhibitor is an option. Aromatase inhibitors prevent the peripheral conversion or aromatization of other steroids (namely, androgens to estrogen), primarily in body fat. The efficacy of aromatase inhibitors is limited to postmenopausal women. In clinical trials it appears that anastrozole (Arimidex) and letrozole (Femura) as aromatase inhibitors are associated not only with less toxicity but also with greater efficacy and even survival than have been reported for megestrol acetate.[40]

Chemotherapy

Eventually, all hormone-responsive tumors become refractory to hormone manipulation, and chemotherapy becomes the treatment of choice. The selection of combination chemotherapy again is guided by the toxicity of the regimen and the extent of disease. A doxorubicin-containing regimen is usually selected if the client has lung or liver disease, because the response is usually prompt and durable. CMF is also a good option and is somewhat less toxic. The taxanes with or without trastuzumab are excellent options, as is vinorelbine (Navelbine). All of these drugs and drug combinations are options for the woman with metastatic disease, and each offers some degree of response and tumor control.

For the most part, metastatic breast cancer is considered an incurable disease. However, long-term responses have been seen with aggressive high-dose chemotherapy regimens, including autologous stem cell transplantation. This latter procedure involves having the woman donate her own bone marrow, either through bone marrow aspiration or through peripheral stem cell pheresis. The client then is given very-high-dose chemotherapy, followed by reinfusion of her own marrow or stem cells after the chemotherapy has destroyed her own marrow. Further information on bone marrow transplantation can be found in Chapter 78. These high-dose therapies are associated with increased expense and toxicity of therapy.[6]

Another important option for treatment in women with bone metastases is a bisphosphonate added to the chemotherapeutic or hormonal therapy regimen. Pamidronate (Aredia) and clodronate (Ostac) not only reduce pain and incidence of complications but also help the bone to heal and prolong survival of the client without complications associated with bone metastases. Pamidronate is given intravenously over 2 hours every month. Adjuvant clodronate therapy has been shown to decrease the risk of bone metastases.[17, 40]

BREAST CANCER IN MEN

Breast cancer in men is rare, with approximately 1400 new cases diagnosed and nearly 400 deaths due to breast cancer each year.[1] The average age at onset is about 60 years (10 years older than the average for women). Factors associated with an increased risk of breast cancer in men include:

- A first-degree male or female relative with breast cancer
- Presence of the *BRCA2* gene
- Klinefelter's syndrome
- Hepatic schistosomiasis
- Exposure to ionizing radiation

Breast cancer in men tends to be identified at a more advanced stage, possibly because of the unexpected nature of the disease and the fact that the mass is usually painless and located beneath the nipple-areola complex. Generally, the mass is detected when it becomes large, ulcerates, or becomes fixed to underlying muscle. Assessment findings indicating male breast cancer include a painless lump beneath the areola or, more often, nipple discharge, retraction, crusting, or ulceration.

Biopsy is necessary for diagnosis of male breast cancer. The most common histologic type is infiltrating ductal carcinoma. Most male breast cancers are estrogen receptor–positive and respond to endocrine therapy. Staging of disease is the same as for women. Axillary dissection is done to determine nodal status and prognosis.

A modified radical mastectomy is usually required to obtain clear margins. Radiation therapy may be indicated, depending on the size of the primary tumor. Chemotherapy, usually a doxorubicin-containing regimen, is administered as adjuvant therapy and followed by radiation. Tamoxifen therapy is appropriate for adjuvant therapy. In the presence of metastatic disease, an LHRH agonist (goserelin) is appropriate hormonal manipulation and takes the place of orchiectomy. The pattern of metastasis is similar to that of female breast cancer.

BENIGN BREAST DISEASE

Most women have a profound underlying fear of breast cancer. For some women the fear is so great that they are immobilized, and ignore the problem altogether. This is why some women who see a physician because of a lump, pain, or nipple discharge present with breast cancer at an advanced stage. Mastalgia, or breast pain, is frequently linked emotionally to the fear of breast cancer. Become sensitive to the emotional aspects associated with breast problems, take clients' fears seriously, provide reassurance through discussion, and perform appropriate evaluation.

The basic techniques of breast evaluation consist of:

- A breast-oriented medical history, including the woman's age, menstrual history, family and personal history of breast cancer, last mammogram, and current or past history of hormone therapy

- Clinical breast examination
- Mammography
- FNA of a persistent palpable mass

FIBROCYSTIC BREASTS

Fibrocystic breasts are the most frequently occurring pathologic problem in the female breast.[35] The exact cause is unknown, although some evidence indicates hormonal imbalance and even high caffeine consumption may be associated with it. The fibrocystic condition typically improves during pregnancy and lactation. It occurs during the reproductive years and disappears with menopause.

Typical fibrocystic lesions are fluid-filled cysts that are round, well circumscribed, and movable. Depending on the amount of fluid in the cyst, the cyst may feel soft or hard. Assessment findings may include nodularity and tenderness. Pain is common, and the cysts frequently increase in size premenstrually. Cysts are generally aspirated rather than undergo surgical biopsy. If there is any question, however, a biopsy is done. A biopsy is necessary if the cyst keeps recurring after being aspirated. Fibrocystic disease is considered a risk factor for breast cancer when it is accompanied by cellular proliferation and atypia.

HYPERPLASIA AND ATYPICAL HYPERPLASIA

Ductal hyperplasia is found in 20% of all breast biopsy specimens.[35] Atypical lobular hyperplasia is found in 1% of breast biopsy specimens. The diagnosis of hyperplasia and atypical hyperplasia can be confirmed only by pathologic examination of breast tissue from a biopsy. The presence of hyperplasia or atypical hyperplasia indicates an increased risk for breast cancer.

FIBROADENOMA

Fibroadenoma is a common breast tumor that usually occurs in young women, most frequently between ages 15 and 30 years.[35] This tumor is generally a nontender, round, firm, or rubbery mass 1 to 3 cm in diameter. Movability of the adenoma in the breast tissues is one of its most distinctive characteristics. Fibroadenomas are readily diagnosed by FNA cytology.

PAPILLOMA

Intraductal papillomas are lesions growing in the terminal portion of a duct (solitary) or throughout the duct system of a sector of breast (multiple or intraductal). Papillomas typically occur in women in their 40s. Solitary intraductal papillomas are usually not precancerous. Multiple papillomas may occasionally be cancerous. Intraductal papilloma is usually identified as a serous, serosanguineous, or bloody discharge from the nipple. Often, no mass is palpable, although a small soft tumor in a central or periareolar portion of the breast is usually present. Examination by FNA or excision is necessary to determine whether the lesion is benign or malignant.

DUCT ECTASIA

Duct ectasia, a disease of ducts in the subareolar zone, occurs in aging breasts, usually in perimenopausal or postmenopausal women. Manifestations may include a palpable dilated duct; a thick, sticky nipple discharge; and burning pain, itching, and inflammation. There appears to be no association with cancer. However, biopsy is performed because on physical examination it is difficult to differentiate duct ectasia from cancer.

MASTODYNIA AND MASTALGIA

Mastodynia and mastalgia refer to breast pain. Breast pain is the most common breast complaint. Pain is not usually associated with breast cancer. Many women have cyclic premenstrual mastodynia. Women with cyclic premenstrual mastodynia usually have lumpy breast (nodularity) and pain for the week before menses. After any other problems have been ruled out, treatment is symptomatic. Wearing a well-fitting brassiere for support, particularly during jogging and other bouncing exercise, may be helpful. Decreasing caffeine intake may also be helpful.

GYNECOMASTIA

Gynecomastia (hypertrophy of one or both male breasts) is common at puberty and in older men. The hormonal mechanism causing gynecomastia is not well understood, although several drugs, an increase in estrogen levels, tumors, and thyroid and hepatic problems may contribute. Usually the situation is temporary. If the gynecomastia causes severe psychosocial trauma, reduction mammoplasty can be performed, or antiestrogen (tamoxifen) or synthetic androgen (danazol [Danocrine]) medications may be administered.

MAMMAPLASTY

Mammaplasty is the surgical revision in the size or shape of the breast. It is often performed electively for cosmetic reasons to enlarge or reduce breast size.

BREAST AUGMENTATION

Clients seeking breast augmentation are often young women who have had chronic feelings of inadequacy and self-consciousness because of small or undeveloped breasts. Some clients are mature women who have postpartum breast atrophy. Current prostheses are durable, seamless, silicone rubber envelopes filled with saline. The prosthesis is inserted beneath existing breast tissue or the pectoralis muscle (called subpectoral placement) through an inframammary (under the breast), transaxillary (through the axilla), or periareolar (around the nipple) incision (Fig. 40–8).

Thorough preoperative breast assessment is essential to rule out breast cancer. Mammography is generally not recommended in women younger than 35 years of age unless they have a positive family history of cancer or a suspicious lump. Surgery is performed on an outpatient basis. Nurses provide teaching and support, mostly over the telephone.

Early complications of breast augmentation include changes in breast or nipple sensation, hematoma (collection of clotted blood), infection, or leakage from the prosthesis. The most frequent complication is capsule formation (development of fibrous sacs of scar tissue enclosing the implant), followed by contracture of the scar. These complications cause excessive breast firmness and distortion of the breast into a hard, round ball. Possible causes of capsular contracture include infection and formation of a seroma (a collection of serosanguineous fluid) or hema-

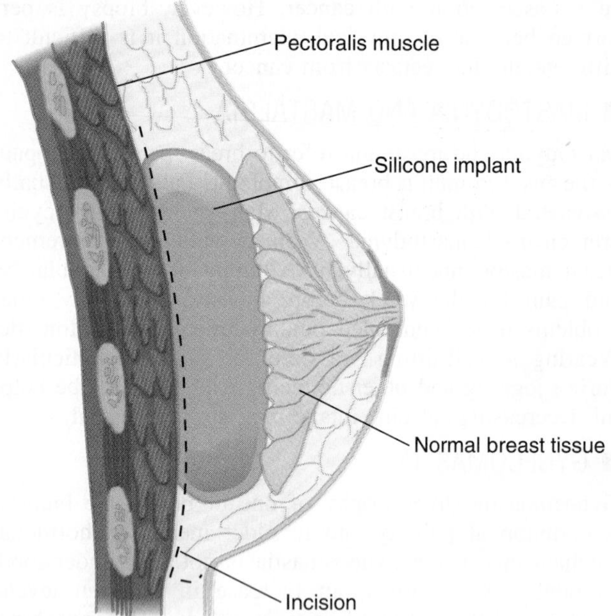

FIGURE 40–8 Augmentation mammaplasty is achieved by insertion of a saline-filled implant beneath normal breast tissue or beneath the pectoral muscle. An inframammary approach is illustrated. Before beginning the retromammary dissection, the surgeon creates a subcutaneous flap. The incision is represented by a *dashed line.*

toma. The basic problem in these processes is that the body's defense mechanisms respond to the prosthesis as a foreign body, and scar tissue forms around the prosthesis to wall it off. Capsule formation is usually treated with open (surgical) capsulotomy. Open capsulotomy, performed under general anesthesia, involves incising the capsule.

Breast massage may be prescribed postoperatively with smooth-walled implants or after capsulotomy to reduce capsule formation. Breast massage typically begins postoperatively according to the surgeon's instructions. Teach the woman to push each breast up, to the side, and toward the middle of the chest, supporting the breast in each position for a count of 10. Discharge instructions usually include the following:

- To reduce edema, maintain a head-elevated position for a week when in bed.
- To reduce hematoma formation, get plenty of rest for a week (no excessive activity, take it easy).
- To avoid moving the pectoralis muscle and irritating the surgical site, do not raise the arms above the head for 3 weeks (e.g., while washing or brushing hair), do not play golf or tennis or swim for 6 weeks, sleep on the back and not on the stomach or sides, and be careful when closing car doors.
- Because of their anticoagulant effect, do not use aspirin or aspirin-containing compounds.
- Notify the physician if bleeding occurs or if a fever with temperature higher than 37.6° C (99.6° F) develops.

REDUCTION MAMMAPLASTY

Reduction mammaplasty surgically reduces the size of large, pendulous breasts. Women usually seek such surgery to reduce the physical and psychosocial discomforts of large breasts, such as back pain, the presence of bra strap indentations in the shoulders, inability to wear normal clothing styles, intertriginous dermatitis (skin breakdown under large breasts), and distress from others' comments about breast size.

Excess breast tissue is removed through incisions under the breast (Fig. 40–9). The nipple is transposed on a pedicle of tissue or grafted onto the newly formed breast. A possible complication is loss of blood supply to the nipple-areola complex. Any duskiness or pallor around the nipple-areola complex should be reported to the physician. Altered sensation and the inability to perform breast-feeding are common findings after this procedure.

FIGURE 40–9 Reduction mammaplasty, in which breasts are surgically reduced. Excess breast tissue is removed, and the breast is recontoured. The nipple is relocated (e.g., moved higher) on a pedicle of tissue. The pedicle supplies the nipple with blood until new blood vessels form.

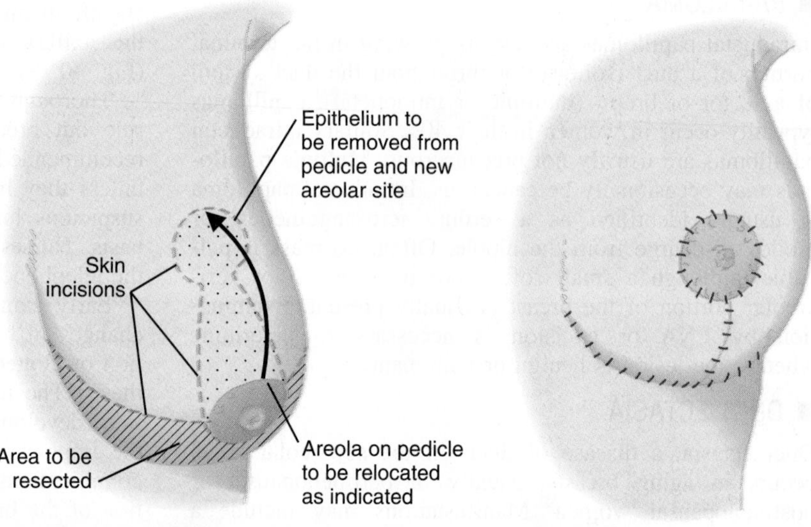

■ MASTOPEXY

Mastopexy is the correction of mammary ptosis (drooping), to achieve an improved breast contour and position. Mastopexy may be performed with subcutaneous mastectomy or on normal breasts to improve contour. Postoperative care is similar to that with other types of breast surgery.

CONCLUSIONS

Diseases of the breast are usually benign conditions that occur throughout the life cycle. Breast cancer, however, has greatly increased in incidence over the last 30 years. The nurse has a vital role in teaching clients early detection methods so that breast cancer can be detected at a curable stage.

All diseases of the breast potentially pose problems in body image and sexuality. Even benign fibrocystic disease can cause breast tenderness and possibly interfere with sexual functioning. Breast cancer and the possibility of mastectomy as treatment can be extremely threatening to a woman's body image. The nurse can help the client cope with these potential threats and successfully adapt to any changes that occur.

CRITICALLY THINKING

1. The pathology report of your client's breast biopsy reads: "8 mm invasive ductal carcinoma, invasive carcinoma to the margins, estrogen receptor– and progesterone receptor–positive." The client is considering further treatment and asks you what her options are. How would you respond?

Factors to Consider. What treatment options might the client have? What interventions might be required?

2. Your client has come to the surgery clinic 10 days after a modified radical mastectomy. The breast incision line is clean and intact. A Jackson-Pratt drain is sutured in place in the axilla. The skin around the drain is clean and intact. Drainage is serosanguineous, and the client has recorded 25 ml and 20 ml, respectively, of drainage per 24 hours for the last 2 days. The client looks at the incision and the drain and asks questions while you examine her incision and drainage site. She asks when the drain will come out, when she can drive her car, when she can shower and resume her normal activities, and when she can be fitted for a prosthesis. What would you tell her? What else should you assess? What medical and nursing care does this client need during her appointment? What other teaching needs does she have?

Factors to Consider. Think about what structures are removed as part of the modified radical mastectomy. What are the functions of these structures? What functional limitations can be expected to affect the client's self-care needs? Consider the client's needs in this immediate postoperative period, in a few months, and over the long term.

3. Two years ago, your client's stage II cancer of the right breast was treated with a quadrantectomy (margins negative), axillary lymph node dissection (8 of 19 nodes positive), radiation therapy of the chest and axilla, and six courses of CAF (Cytoxan [cyclophosphamide], Adriamycin [doxorubicin], 5-fluoruracil) chemotherapy. Today, she presents with pain, tingling, and swelling of her right hand and arm. She states that although she noticed intermittent problems with slight swelling over the past 6 months, it has become severe over the past 2 weeks and is affecting her ability to work as a court stenographer. What further information should you assess? What are your priority interventions?

Factors to Consider. What do pain, tingling, and swelling of the hand and arm suggest in a client who has undergone lymph node dissection? Should a referral to a physical therapist for lymphedema management be made?

REFERENCES

1. American Cancer Society. (2000). *Cancer facts and figures.* Atlanta: Author.
2. Abeloff, M., et al. (2000). Breast. In M. Abeloff, et al. (Eds.), *Clinical oncology* (2nd ed., pp. 2051–2159). New York: Churchill Livingstone.
3. Anonymous. (1998). Use of cervical and breast cancer screening among women with and without functional limitations—United States, 1994–1995. *Morbidity and Mortality Weekly Report, 47*(40), 853–856.
4. Baselga, J. B., et al. (1997). HER2 overexpression and paclitaxel sensitivity in breast cancer: Therapeutic implications. *Oncology, 11* (3), 43–48.
5. Bear, H. D. (1998). Indications for neoadjuvant chemotherapy for breast cancer. *Seminars in Oncology, 25*(2), 3–12.
6. Bezwoda, W. R., Seymour, L., & Dansey, R. D. (1995). High-dose chemotherapy with hematopoietic rescue as primary treatment for metastatic breast cancer: A randomized trial. *Journal of Clinical Oncology, 13,* 2483–2489.
7. Brenin, D. R., & Morrow, M. (1998). Breast-conserving surgery in the neoadjuvant setting. *Seminars in Oncology, 25*(2), 13–18.
8. Brody, L. C., & Biesecker, B. B. (1998). Breast cancer susceptibility genes. *BRCA1* and *BRCA2. Medicine, 77*(3), 208–226.
9. Chapman, D., & Goodman, M. (1997). Breast cancer. In S. Groenwald, et al. (Eds.), *Cancer nursing principles and practice* (4th ed., pp. 916–979). Boston: Jones & Bartlett.
10. Chu, K. C., et al. (1996). Recent trends in U.S. breast cancer incidence, survival, and mortality rates. *Journal of the National Cancer Institute, 88*(4), 1571–1579.
11. Cohen, M. Z., Kahn, D. L., & Steeves, R. H. (1998). Beyond body image: The experience of breast cancer. *Oncology Nursing Forum, 25*(5), 835–841.
12. Cuenca, R. E., Giachino, J., Arredondo, M. A., et al.(1996). Endometrial carcinoma associated with breast carcinoma: Low incidence with tamoxifen use. *Cancer, 77,* 2058–2063.
13. Cummings, S. R., et al. (1999). The effect of raloxifene on risk of breast cancer in post menopausal women: Results from the Multiple Outcomes of Raloxifene (MORE) trial. *Journal of the American Medical Association, 281,* 3, 2189–2197.
14. Cutuli, B., et al. (1996). Breast cancer after treatment for Hodgkin's disease. Analysis of clinical and pathological characteristics in 54 cases [Abstract]. *Proceedings of the Annual Meeting of the American Society of Clinical Oncology, 15,* A1299.
15. Decillis, A. (1997). Acute myeloid leukemia (AML) and myelodysplastic syndrome (MDS) in NSABP B-25: An update (Abstract). *Proceedings of the Annual Meeting of the American Society of Clinical Oncology, 16*;130a.
16. Dees, E. C., et al. (1997). Does information from axillary dissection change treatment in clinically node-negative patients with breast cancer? An algorithm for assessment of impact of axillary dissection. *Annals of Surgery, 226,* 279–286.

17. Diel, I. J. (1998). Reduction in new metastases in breast cancer with adjuvant clodronate treatment. *New England Journal of Medicine, 339,* 357.
18. Early Breast Cancer Trialists' Collaborative Group. (1998). Tamoxifen for early breast cancer: An overview of the randomized trials. *Lancet, 351,* 1451–1467.
19. Early Breast Cancer Trialists' Collaborative Group. (1998). Polychemotherapy for early breast cancer: An overview of randomized trials. *Lancet, 352,* 930–942.
20. Edwards, M. J., et al. (1998). Infiltrating ductal carcinoma of the breast: The survival impact of race. *Journal of Clinical Oncology, 16*(8), 2693–2699.
21. Fisher, B., Bryant, J., & Wolmark, N. (1998). Effective preoperative chemotherapy on the outcome of women with operable breast cancer. *Journal of Clinical Oncology, 16*(8), 2672–2685.
22. Fisher, B., et al. (1998). Tamoxifen for prevention of breast cancer. Report of the National Surgical Adjuvant Breast and Bowel Project: Project P-1 Study. *Journal of the National Cancer Institute, 90,* 1371–1388.
23. Fisher, B. (1997). Increased intensification and total dose of cyclophosphamide in a doxorubicin-cyclophosphamide regimen for the treatment of primary breast cancer: Finding from the National Surgical Adjuvant Breast and Bowel Project B-22. *Journal of Clinical Oncology, 15,* 1858–1863.
24. Frykberg, E. R. (1996). Screening mammography in women under fifty years of age. *Breast, 2,* 221–225.
25. Heimann, R., & Hellman, S. (1998). Aging, progression, and phenotype in breast cancer. *Journal of Clinical Oncology, 16*(8), 2686–2692.
26. Henderson, I. C. (1998). Improved disease-free survival (DFS) and overall survival (OS) from the addition of sequential paclitaxel (T) but not from the escalation of doxorubicin (A) dose level in the adjuvant chemotherapy of patients (pts) with node-positive primary breast cancer (BC) (Abstract). *Proceedings of the Annual Meeting of the American Society of Clinical Oncology, 17,* 101a.
27. Herceptin raises its sights beyond advanced breast cancer. (1998). *Journal of the National Cancer Institute, 90*(2), 882–883.
28. Hortobagyi, G. N. (1998). Treatment of breast cancer. *New England Journal of Medicine, 339* (14), 974–984.
29. Humble, C. A. (1995). Lymphedema: Incidence, pathophysiology, management, and nursing care. *Oncology Nursing Forum, 22*(10), 1503–1509.
30. Hunter, D., & Willett, W. C. (1996). Nutrition and breast cancer. *Cancer Causes and Control, 7,* 56–68.
31. Hunter, D., et al. (1996). Cohort studies of fat intake and the risk of breast cancer: A pooled analysis. *New England Journal of Medicine, 334,* 356.
32. Knobf, M. T. (1996). Breast cancer. In R. McCorkle, et al. (Eds.) *Cancer nursing: A comprehensive textbook* (2nd ed., pp. 547–610). Philadelphia: W. B. Saunders.
33. Krag, D., et al. (1998). The sentinel node in breast cancer. *New England Journal of Medicine, 339*(14), 941–946.
34. Lippman, M. E. (1998). Breast cancer. In A. S. Fauci, et al. (Eds.), *Principles of Internal Medicine* (14th ed., pp. 562–568). New York: McGraw-Hill.
35. Marchant, D. J. (1997). *Breast disease.* Philadelphia: W. B. Saunders.
36. McMasters, K. M., et al. (1998). Sentinel-lymph node biopsy for breast cancer—not yet the standard of care. *New England Journal of Medicine, 339*(14), 990–995.
37. Mehta, R. R., et al. (1998). Plasma c-erbB-2 levels in breast cancer patients: Prognostic significance in predicting response to chemotherapy. *Journal of Clinical Oncology, 16*(7), 2409–2416.
38. Parker, S. L., et al. (1997). Cancer statistics. *CA: A Cancer Journal for Clinicians, 47*(1), 5–27.
39. Peto, R. (1996). Five years of tamoxifen—or more? *Journal of the National Cancer Institute, 88*(24), 1791–1793.
40. Powles, T. J. (1998) Oral clodronate reduces the incidence of bone metastasis in patients with operable breast cancer (Abstract). *Proceedings of the American Society of Clinical Oncology, 17,* 123a.
41. Price, J., & Purtell, J. R. (1997). Prevention and treatment of lymphedema after breast cancer. *American Journal of Nursing, 97*(9), 34–37.
42. American Society of Clinical Oncology. Recommended breast cancer surveillance guidelines. (1997). *Journal of Clinical Oncology, 15,* 2149–2156.
43. Seidman, A. D., et al. (1997). Paclitaxel for breast cancer: The Memorial Sloan-Kettering Cancer Center experience. *Oncology, 11*(3), 20–28.
44. Slamon, D., et al. (1998). Addition of Herceptin to first-line chemotherapy for HER2 overexpressing metastatic breast cancer markedly increases anticancer activity: A randomized multinational controlled phase III trial [Abstract]. *Proceedings of the American Society of Clinical Oncology, 17,* 98a.
45. Smith, J. (1998). The practice of venipuncture in lymphedema. *European Journal of Cancer Care, 7*(2), 97–98.
46. Tabar, L. (1996). Breast-cancer screening with mammography in women aged 40–49 years. *International Journal of Cancer, 68,* 693–699.
47. Thomas, D. B., et al. (1997). Randomized trial of breast self-examination in Shanghai: Methodology and preliminary results. *Journal of the National Cancer Institute, 89,* 335–340.
48. Vogel, V. G. (1996). Assessing women's potential risk of developing breast cancer. *Preventive Medicine, 10*(10), 1451–1463.

REMEMBER *to check out your* Companion CD ROM

CHAPTER 41

Management of Clients with Sexually Transmitted Diseases

Meg Blair

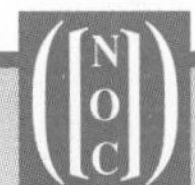

NURSING OUTCOMES CLASSIFICATION (NOC)
for Nursing Diagnoses—Clients with Sexually Transmitted Diseases

Altered Health Maintenance	Knowledge: Treatment Regimen	**Anxiety**
Health Belief: Perceived Resources	Participation: Health Care Decisions	Anxiety Control
Health Promoting Behavior	Psychosocial Adjustment: Life Changes	Coping
Health Seeking Behavior	Risk Detection	Impulse Control
Knowledge: Health Behaviors	Self-Direction of Care	Social Interaction Skills
Knowledge: Health Promotion	Social Support	
Knowledge: Health Resources	Treatment Behavior: Illness or Injury	

SEXUALLY TRANSMITTED DISEASES: AN OVERVIEW

The term *sexually transmitted disease* (STD) refers to any infection contracted primarily through sexual activities or contact. *STD* has replaced the older term *venereal disease* (VD), which referred to diseases transmitted only by sexual intercourse. STD is also known as sexually transmitted infection (STI). More than 50 organisms are known to spread through sexual activity. The five most widely known STDs are chlamydial infection, gonorrhea, syphilis, genital herpes, and genital warts (see later). Other infections are chancroid, lymphogranuloma venereum, granuloma inguinale, trichomoniasis, acquired immunodeficiency syndrome (AIDS), and some enteric and ectoparasitic infections. The number of STDs is increasing as new agents are implicated in the sexual transmission of disease.

STDs share the following characteristics:

1. STDs can be transmitted by any sexual activity between opposite-sex or same-sex partners (not only vaginal-penile sex but also oral and anal sex).
2. Having one STD confers no immunity against future reinfection with that STD or with any other STD (except, possibly, for hepatitis B).
3. Sexual partners of infected clients need to be assessed for treatment (see individual diseases for specific recommendations).
4. STDs affect people from all socioeconomic classes, cultures, ethnicities, and age groups.
5. Women bear a disproportionate number of the effects of STDs.
6. Frustration, anger, anxiety, fear, shame, and guilt are emotions commonly associated with an STD diagnosis.
7. STDs frequently coexist in the same client (for example, a client may have both chlamydial infection and gonorrhea).

The last fact may be responsible for some treatment failures. Current treatment guidelines for STDs are available in the United States from the Centers for Disease Control and Prevention (CDC) in Atlanta.

STDs are a very serious public health problem. Recognized since the beginning of recorded history, these diseases are associated with substantial morbidity and, in some cases, mortality. The incidence of STDs continues to increase worldwide, and infections are becoming more severe. STDs also facilitate the development of human immunodeficiency virus (HIV) infection and AIDS. Thus, the scope of the health problem they create is increasing

This chapter incorporates material written for the fifth edition by Patricia E. Downing.

rather than decreasing. It is a matter of public concern that treatments for STDs be safe, inexpensive, and effective.

Except for the common cold and influenza, STDs are the most prevalent communicable diseases in the United States, which has the highest STD rate in the industrialized world. Most sources describe STD rates as epidemic. Symptomatic STDs are diagnosed in more than 13 million people in this country annually, not including HIV infection and AIDS, and 86% of affected people are between 15 and 29 years of age. Another 40 million people are infected with human papillomavirus (HPV), which causes genital warts. It is estimated that 50% of all Americans will have had an STD by age 30 years. Although AIDS is probably the best publicized and most dangerous, the most common STDs are chlamydial infection, gonorrhea, genital herpes, genital warts, and syphilis.

Official national incidence statistics for STDs are published by the CDC and by local health authorities, but the actual incidence is unknown. Accurate statistics are difficult to compile for a number of reasons. Statistics reflect the accuracy of case reporting, and reporting is not mandatory for all STDs. Rates for some STDs, such as genital herpes and genital warts, are based on estimates derived from local studies and physician reports. These estimates are thought to be low. Even rates developed from mandatory case reporting are believed to be low.

The costs of STDs are staggering, both in medical expense and in emotional suffering. Up to $10 billion a year is spent to treat STDs and their sequelae (consequences), including at least $1 billion a year to treat subsequent infertility. These figures, like statistics, can be misleading. For instance, women, who are two times more likely to be infected with an STD than men, are less likely to receive treatment, often because the STD is asymptomatic. Also, STDs can lead to infertility. The cost of treating infertility due to STDs is an indirect cost of the STD. Many couples in lower socioeconomic classes cannot afford infertility treatments. Hence, infertility services are used most often by middle-class and upper-class couples. The true cost of STDs that result in infertility cannot be accurately estimated.

BOX 41–1 Etiology of Sexually Transmitted Diseases

STDs Caused by Bacteria

Gonorrhea
Chlamydial infection
Syphilis
Bacterial vaginosis
Nongonococcal urethritis
Chancroid
Lymphogranuloma venereum
Granuloma inguinale
Sexually transmitted enteric infections

STDs Caused by Viruses

Acquired immunodeficiency syndrome (AIDS)
Genital herpes
Genital warts
Hepatitis B
Hepatitis A
Hepatitis C (possible sexual transmission)

STD Caused by Protozoa

Trichomoniasis

STD Caused by Fungi

Vulvovaginal candidiasis

STDs Caused by Ectoparasites

Scabies
Pediculosis pubis

Etiology and Risk Factors

STDs can be caused by bacteria, viruses, protozoa, fungi, and ectoparasites (Box 41–1). Anyone who engages in intimate physical contact can contract and transmit an STD. Many health care providers do not always acknowledge that fact, especially in regard to middle-class, upper-class, or older clients. Although younger people have the highest rates for STDs (86%), all age groups are at risk. The fetus or neonate can be infected across the placenta or during vaginal birth. Infants and children can be infected through child abuse. Older adults can be infected or can experience residual sequelae from infections contracted earlier in their lives. When a client complains of manifestations that might be those of an STD, STDs should always be part of the differential diagnosis.

The worldwide increase in the incidence of STDs is a result of many factors. STDs due to antibiotic-resistant strains of bacteria have become more common. For example, the incidence of gonorrhea has risen since the evolution of penicillinase-producing *Neisseria gonorrhoeae*. The use of intrauterine devices (IUDs) and oral contraceptives may lower women's resistance to infection and facilitate transmission of STDs. Women may not think to use an infection barrier *in addition to* effective contraception. Sterilized women often do not use condoms.

Lack of knowledge also plays a role in the incidence of STDs. Clients may find it difficult to obtain accurate information, even from health professionals. Politics and religion continue to affect the controversy over sex education in schools. Accurate information about sex and STDs is not always presented in a manner designed to appeal to, and therefore influence the behavior of, young people.

Specific risk factors for acquiring STDs are:

- Intravenous (IV) drug use
- Other substance abuse
- High-risk sexual activity (use of prostitutes, multiple or casual sexual partners, sex with IV drug users and infected people, unprotected sex, exchanging sex for money or drugs)
- Younger age
- Younger age at *sexarche* (the beginning of sexual activity)

- Inner city residence
- Poverty
- Poor nutrition
- Poor hygiene

The young are particularly at risk; immaturity of the immune system, cervical differences, peer group pressure, and the belief that they are invincible all combine to make young people particularly susceptible to STDs. Many people have a cavalier attitude about infection and illness in general because of the advances that have been made in antimicrobial therapy. Many people think any infection can now be easily cured, and thus they do not consider STDs to be serious diseases with possible complications.

According to the CDC, STD prevention and health promotion should focus on five major concepts:

- Education
- Detection of active disease (including asymptomatic infections)
- Effective diagnosis and treatment
- Evaluation and treatment of sexual partners
- Pre-exposure vaccination if available

Sex education in schools, risk-reduction counseling, promotion of safer sex, and an open, accepting attitude from health professionals can increase knowledge levels. Health professionals must be comfortable asking clients about sexual activity and practices and must provide information in a way that does not "turn off" the client or cause embarrassment.

Health maintenance consists of:

- Screening high-risk people
- Maintaining a high index of suspicion for asymptomatic infections
- Providing accurate, timely diagnosis and treatment
- Performing follow-up after treatment when indicated
- Reporting cases of STDs
- Identifying and treating sexual partners of clients with STDs

Health restoration includes measures to reverse the effects of disease, such as infertility (see Chapters 38 and 39). Although some STDs can be passed nonsexually, most are transmitted sexually because the causative organisms thrive in a warm, dark, moist environment within the body and survive only very briefly outside that environment. Therefore, their transmission requires intimate contact. Prevention and control must concentrate on breaking the chain of sexual transmission of disease.

Pathophysiology

An STD occurs when an individual is infected by an organism through sexual contact. Some STDs remain localized; others spread and become systemic. Some STDs are seen in an acute episode; others are chronic illnesses. See discussions of specific STDs for more detailed information.

Clinical Manifestations

Clinical manifestations vary among the STDs and depend on the organism involved and the location of the infection (local or systemic). Diseases may be grouped according to their primary manifestation (e.g., those that cause vaginal discharge). Diagnostic testing is individualized for each condition. See specific STDs for more detailed information.

Outcome Management

Medical Management

Medical management focuses on eradicating the offending organism, if possible, or managing a chronic condition. Table 41–1 provides a concise overview.

Nursing Management of the Medical Client

Nursing outcomes are similar to medical outcomes. The following discussion of nursing care can be generalized to all STDs. Specific details are provided in the discussion of each STD.

ASSESSMENT

A thorough nursing assessment consists of (1) general health assessment and examination, (2) sexual history, preference, and practices, (3) previous history of STDs, (4) specific complaints (60% to 80% of STDs are asymptomatic), (5) genital hygienic practices (douching), (6) contraceptive history, and (7) infection barriers used. A holistic approach also includes lifestyle, nutrition, stress, and sexuality. High-risk clients should be screened for STDs regardless of whether manifestations are present at the time of a visit to a health care provider. Never assume that a client is not sexually active and at risk, and make sure that the client understands questions exactly.

Nurses need to know about the variety of sexual activities, their effect on transmission of STDs, and the common manifestations for which to assess. Examine your own attitudes about sexuality and sexual behavior. Separate your personal views of morality from appropriate nursing activities. Judgmental attitudes may deter clients from seeking care and may interfere with therapeutic professional relationships. Bias and prejudice can be communicated in obvious and subtle ways that make the client feel uncomfortable, judged, and discounted. A prejudiced health professional cannot provide comprehensive care. An accepting attitude may ensure treatment and prevent disease transmission.

STDs are associated with a social stigma. Ashamed, many clients try to keep the diagnosis secret. Many relate STDs with low social status and immorality, and many have misconceptions and fears about the dangers of STDs. Other problems may surface with discovery of an STD. For example, a newly infected client may be angry at the responsible sexual partner or may hesitate to identify or inform the sexual partner or partners about the STD. When a marital or committed relationship is involved, questions about infidelity or infertility may arise.

Clients can seek treatment from various sources: health department STD clinics, physician offices, Planned Parenthood clinics, and other community-based clinics. Such clinics frequently deal with STDs and have staff especially sensitive to the needs of clients with STDs. Strict confidentiality is essential. It is especially, but not exclusively, important to gay men and lesbians, who may be at

TABLE 41–1 TREATMENT OF COMMON SEXUALLY TRANSMITTED DISEASES (STDs)

Condition (Causative Organism)	Diagnostic Methods	Manifestations	Treatment	Management of Sexual Partner
Gonorrhea (*Neisseria gonorrhoeae*)	Smear Culture	Incubation period: 3–8 days *Female* Asymptomatic or thick, purulent vaginal discharge Genital irritation Urinary symptoms Pelvic pain (PID) May be asymptomatic *Male* Urethral discharge Urinary manifestations Scrotal pain (epididymitis) Perineal pain (prostatitis) *Either sex* Pharyngeal infection Conjunctivitis	Ceftriaxone, IM once *or* Cefixime, PO once *or* Ciprofloxacin, PO once *or* Ofloxacin, PO once *plus* Doxycycline, PO for 7 days *or* Azithromycin, once	Treat if sexual contact occurred in last 60 days *or* Treat *most recent* partner
		Disseminated infection Bacteremia Arthritis-dermatitis syndrome	Ceftriaxone, IM or IV q 24 hours; continue for 24–48 hours after improvement then switch to PO to complete 1 full week of treatment	
Chlamydial infection (*Chlamydia trachomatis*)	Culture Antigen-antibody DFA, ELISA	Incubation period: 7–21 days *Female* Asymptomatic or pelvic pain (PID) *Male* Asymptomatic or mild dysuria White or clear urethral discharge Scrotal pain	Azithromycin, PO once *or* Eythromycin ethylsuccinate, PO for 7 days or doxycycline bid for 7 days *or* Ofloxacin, PO for 7 days	Treat if sexual contact occurred in last 60 days
Syphilis (*Treponema pallidum*)	Dark-field microscopy Serology Nonspecific (e.g., VDRL test) Specific (e.g., FTA-ABS test)	Incubation period: 10–90 days *Primary stage* Painless chancre at site of exposure Regional lymphadenopathy *Secondary stage* Maculopapular rash Generalized lymphadenopathy Mucous patches Condylomata lata Fever, malaise Alopecia *Latent stage* Asymptomatic *Tertiary stage* Cardiovascular changes *Neurosyphilis* Central nervous system changes	*Primary, secondary, and early latent stages* Benzathine penicillin G, IM once *Late latent stage and tertiary stage* Benzathine penicillin G, IM weekly for 3 weeks *Neurosyphilis* Aqueous penicillin G, IV q 4 h for 10–14 days *or* Procaine penicillin, IM daily for 10–14 days *plus* Probenecid, PO for 10–14 days	See CDC guidelines

TABLE 41–1 TREATMENT OF COMMON SEXUALLY TRANSMITTED DISEASES (STDs) *Continued*

Condition (Causative Organism)	Diagnostic Methods	Manifestations	Treatment	Management of Sexual Partner
Genital herpes	Culture Pap smear Visual examination	Incubation period: 3–7 days *Acute phase* Paresthesia/burning Painful genital ulcers Fever/chills/muscle pain *Latent phase* Asymptomatic	*Initial episode* Acyclovir, PO for 7–10 days *or* Famciclovir *or* valacyclovir, PO for 7–10 days	All contacts should be evaluated and treated if symptomatic
Genital warts, human papillomavirus	Pap smear Colposcopy Biopsy	Incubation period: 1–2 months Single or multiple genital or anal warts	Topical podophyllin or podofilox *or* Topical trichloroacetic acid *or* Cryotherapy *or* Electrocautery *or* CO_2 laser *or* Surgical excision	All contacts should be evaluated and treated if symptomatic Female partners need Pap smear at diagnosis and at least annually

The CDC considers the following diseases reportable: gonorrhea; syphilis; chlamydial infection; chancroid; granuloma inguinale; lymphoma inguinale; and acquired immunodeficiency syndrome (AIDS). However, laws vary from state to state. Nurses working with clients who have STDs should know their state's reporting requirements.

bid, twice a day; CDC, Centers for Disease Control and Prevention; CO_2, carbon dioxide; DFA, direct fluorescent antibody; ELISA, enzyme-linked immunosorbent assay; FTA-ABS, fluorescent treponemal antibody absorption tests; IM, intramuscularly; IV, intravenously; Pap, Papanicolaou; PID, pelvic inflammatory disease; PO, orally; VDRL, Venereal Disease Research Laboratory.

risk for discrimination if their sexual orientation is disclosed.

DIAGNOSIS, OUTCOMES, INTERVENTIONS

Altered Health Maintenance. The client with an STD needs to improve health behaviors, which makes *Altered Health Maintenance related to lack of understanding of the causes, treatments, and prevention of STDs* the priority nursing diagnosis.

Outcomes. The client will understand the cause, treatment, and prevention of specific STDs, as evidenced by client's statements, the client's avoidance of STDs, successful treatment of an STD, and, if possible, the absence of recurrence of the STD.

Interventions

Teach About STDs. Provide accurate, factual information about the transmission, prevention, and treatment of STDs (see the Client Education Guide on STDs). Myths about STDs abound; for example, many people erroneously believe that oral contraceptives protect them against STDs. Promote the use of condoms in conjunction with nonbarrier contraceptives, even though clients regard using two methods as difficult. Teaching methods should consider religious and cultural concerns. Include the following topics in teaching sessions about STDs:

1. Name, nature, and seriousness of the condition
2. Mode of transmission
   a. Any sexual activity can spread STDs, not just intercourse.
   b. High-risk activities include new or multiple partners.
3. Actions the client should take to prevent the spread of infection to others

CLIENT EDUCATION GUIDE

Sexually Transmitted Diseases

Treatment will not protect you from getting this disease again. Having a sexually transmitted disease (STD) will not keep you from getting the same disease again or from getting another STD. You must take precautions and use a condom with every sexual encounter to avoid getting STDs.

It is best to wait until you and your sexual partner have finished all your medications before you resume sexual activity. If you wait, you will not be in danger of spreading the infection to your sexual partner or, possibly, of getting the disease again yourself. If you feel that you cannot wait, be sure to use barrier protection, such as a condom.

We would like to see you again if (1) the manifestations do not go away after you have finished your medication, (2) the manifestations return, or (3) you think you may have been exposed to another infection. Be sure to call us if you have any questions.

For women: You should have yearly gynecologic examinations. Along with the Pap smear, ask your doctor to check for STDs. You may have an STD even if you do not have any manifestations.

a. Always use a new latex condom for each sexual act (male and female condoms are available).
b. Finish all the medication given to you.
c. Ensure that your partner is evaluated and treated if needed.
d. Do not have sex until you and your partner have been treated.
e. Do not have sex if you or your partner have any manifestations of an STD.

4. Incubation periods
5. Manifestations of infection
6. Asymptomatic problems
7. When and how to seek treatment
   a. Be sure the client understands the difference between Papanicolaou (Pap) smears and STD examinations; both are not always done at the same time.
8. Treatment methods
   a. Teach client about medication or other treatments.
9. Follow-up care (when and how to obtain it)
10. Consequences of not completing treatment
    a. Infertility
    b. Chronic abdominal pain
    c. Higher risk of ectopic pregnancy or spontaneous abortion
11. Risks and consequences of recurrent infections
    a. STDs increase the risk of acquiring AIDS

Teach Condom Use. The latex condom (called a *rubber* in lay terms) is the most effective mechanical barrier to STDs and its use by sexually active people who are at risk should be promoted. Sexually active men and women should learn to use condoms properly, effectively, and consistently.

There are several barriers to the use of condoms by sexually active people. Women may not believe that they are empowered to make healthy choices. Condoms require male cooperation; unfortunately, many women are in relationships defined by an imbalance of power in which they believe they cannot insist on condom use. Some studies have shown that the fear of losing a sexual partner is greater for some women than the fear of contracting an STD, even AIDS. Condoms may not be acceptable to some clients for religious, social, cultural, or ethnic reasons.

Condom failure is primarily due to improper or inconsistent use rather than to product defect. The Client Education Guide on how to use a condom provides instructions for correct condom use.

Use Therapeutic Communication. When caring for clients with STDs, you obtain privileged or private information and provide instruction about these diseases. Both activities require sensitivity and skillful interaction. You need to be very adept in interpersonal communication to help clients seeking counsel or treatment for STD. Such clients need encouragement, support, and accurate information.

Identify Resources. Nurses play a pivotal role in identifying community and national resources available to clients. Most public health agencies have STD education, prevention, and treatment programs that are open to the public. Clients can also obtain information anonymously from the National STD Hotline (1-800-227-8922) or the National HIV/AIDS Hotline (1-800-342-AIDS).

Anxiety. The client with an STD often experiences a great deal of uncertainty, which makes *Anxiety related to threat to biologic integrity and threat to self-concept* an important nursing diagnosis.

CLIENT EDUCATION GUIDE

How to Use a Condom

Client Instructions

Before Intercourse

- Talk to your partner about using condoms *before* you begin to have sex.
- Decide that you will have sex *only* with a condom.
- Before you have sex, practice using a condom.
- Keep condoms in a handy place.

To Use a Male Condom

- Use a *new latex* condom *each time* you have sex. Do not use natural membrane condoms.
  - Put the condom on before your genitals touch your partner's genitals.
  - Place a spermicide with nonoxynol 9 inside the condom, unless you or your partner is allergic to it. You can buy spermicides in a drug store without a prescription.
  - Place the rolled-up condom on the head of the erect penis.
  - Pinch the end of condom to create a little space to catch what is ejaculated.
  - Unroll the condom until your fingers reach the base of the penis. The condom should unroll easily. If it doesn't, replace it with a new one.
  - Right after ejaculation, hold the condom firmly at the base of the penis and withdraw the penis from the vagina before the erection goes away.
  - Throw the condom away in a safe place. *Never* reuse a condom.
- If you use a lubricant, use only a water-soluble lubricant. Never use oil-based lubricants such as petroleum jelly, baby oil, cooking oil, or shortening, which would destroy the condom.

To Use a Female Condom

- Squeeze the inner ring of the pouch between your fingers, and insert it into the vagina.
- Advance the inner ring until the ring is just behind the pubic bone.
- Leave 1 inch (2.25 cm) of the pouch's open end (the outer ring) outside the vagina.
- Immediately after ejaculation, twist the outer ring and gently pull out the pouch.
- Throw the condom away. *Never* reuse a condom.

Adapted from The American College of Obstetricians and Gynecologists (1995). *ACOG patient education: Gonorrhea and chlamydia* (Pamphlet AP071). Washington, DC: Author.

Outcomes. The client will experience a decrease in anxiety, as evidenced by verbal statements, showing acceptance of the condition, and demonstrating appropriate coping methods.

Interventions

Provide Support. STDs can threaten a client's self-concept and pose potential physical problems, such as infertility and fetal damage. The client may express guilt, apprehension, and fear of rejection. Help the client reduce anxiety by being warm and supportive, facilitating the expression of feelings, and encouraging effective coping strategies.

Help with Problem-Solving. Assist the client with learning and problem-solving once anxiety is reduced. Role-playing and practicing negotiation skills may help a woman become more assertive in being able to ensure her sexual health.

EVALUATION

It is expected that the STD will be succesfully treated and, if possible, eradicated. The client will be able to state the cause, manifestations, treatment, and prevention of STDs and to remain free of STDs.

DISEASES CHARACTERIZED BY URETHRITIS OR CERVICITIS

CHLAMYDIAL INFECTIONS

Chlamydial infection is the nation's most common bacterial STD (see Table 41–1). The number of new cases per year is estimated to be at least 4 million.

Etiology and Risk Factors

The causative organism, *Chlamydia trachomatis,* is a nonmotile, gram-negative bacterium. This organism is the most common cause of what was previously diagnosed as nonspecific vaginitis in women and of nongonococcal urethritis (NGU) in men.

C. trachomatis is always transmitted by intimate sexual contact. Women usually acquire the infection during intercourse with an infected man. Homosexual males can also transmit the infection through oral-anal contact or anal penetration. The infection does not cross the placenta, but passage through the birth canal of an infected mother can cause conjunctivitis and pneumonia in a newborn.

Pathophysiology

Chlamydial infection is known as "the great sterilizer." Undetected and untreated cases can progress to have serious, irreversible consequences. *C. trachomatis* causes inflammation that leads to scarring and ulceration of involved tissue. In women, the infection can extend to the endometrium and salpinx (fallopian tube); the major consequence is salpingitis (inflammation of the fallopian tubes) with subsequent infertility or high risk of ectopic (tubal) pregnancy. Secondary extension to the peritoneum can cause *pelvic inflammatory disease* (PID) (see Chapter 39). In men, the infection can cause a urethral stricture that may extend to the *epididymis*. Sterility can result from the ensuing epididymitis. A serious systemic complication more common in men is Reiter's syndrome, which consists of urethritis, polyarthritis, and conjunctivitis.

Clinical Manifestations

Chlamydial infections primarily affect the cervix, urethra, and rectum. In most cases, the infection is asymptomatic for an extended period. When present, manifestations closely resemble those of gonorrhea but are less severe. In women, the primary site of infection is the endocervix. The cervix becomes edematous and produces a yellow, mucopurulent vaginal discharge. This discharge may be accompanied by spotting at menstrual midcycle or with sexual intercourse. *C. trachomatis* also causes urethritis with dysuria (painful or difficult urination) and urinary frequency in women. One study found that in 65% of women who had urinary manifestations and negative urine culture results, results of culture for *C. trachomatis* were positive. Involvement of Bartholin's duct produces a purulent discharge.

In males, the chief manifestation is urethritis with dysuria (painful and difficult urination) and clear to mucopurulent discharge. In both sexes, proctitis (rectal inflammation) and pharyngitis (inflammation of the pharynx) may develop with rectal and orogenital contact.

Because chlamydial infection may produce few or no manifestations, clients tend not to seek medical treatment and the diagnosis is difficult and often missed. Because chlamydial and gonorrheal infections often coexist, diagnostic tests are recommended for both when either condition is suspected. Presumptive treatment for chlamydial infection in clients being treated for gonorrhea is appropriate, particularly when testing for *C. trachomatis* is not performed.

The definitive test for the fast and accurate diagnosis of chlamydial infection has yet to be developed. The best and most sensitive diagnostic test is tissue culture of cellular material from the urethra, endocervix, or rectum. This test, however, is expensive and technically difficult.

Rapid nonculture detection tests performed on urogenital secretions are readily available, including direct fluorescent antibody (DFA), microscopy and enzyme-linked immunosorbent assay (ELISA), and monoclonal antigen-antibody tests to detect *C. trachomatis* antigens. Although less accurate than cultures, these tests are more convenient, less expensive, and quicker. For men who refuse insertion of a cotton applicator 2 to 4 cm into the urethra to obtain an adequate specimen of urogenital secretions, the ELISA test can be used to detect *C. trachomatis* antigen in the initial 10 to 20 ml of voided urine. These tests are recommended for screening of asymptomatic, high-risk clients in whom chlamydial infection might otherwise go undetected. Priority groups for testing are (1) high-risk pregnant women, (2) adolescents, and (3) women aged 20 to 24 years who have new or multiple sexual partners or who do not use condoms routinely. Many sources also recommend testing any woman with a history of infertility, ectopic pregnancies, or spontaneous abortions.

Outcome Management

Medical Management

ERADICATE DISEASE AND MANIFESTATIONS

The treatment of choice for chlamydial infection is doxycycline (Vibramycin) given orally for 7 days or one dose of azithromycin (Zithromax). To prevent salpingitis and other serious sequelae, it is imperative that treatment be aggressive and started early and that the entire course of antibiotics be completed. Antichlamydial therapy is almost always effective; therefore, test of cure is not necessary unless manifestations persist or reinfection is suspected.

All partners with whom the client has had sexual contact within 60 days before diagnosis should be examined and treated. When the client's last sexual contact occurred more than 60 days before diagnosis, the last partner should be treated. If testing for chlamydial infection is not available, treatment is often prescribed on the basis of clinical diagnosis only or as co-treatment for gonorrhea. The Bridge to Home Health Care provides information on teaching clients about STDs in a holistic, sensitive manner.

Nursing Management of the Medical Client

ERADICATE DISEASE AND MANIFESTATIONS

Instruct clients about the greater risk of infection with multiple sexual partners and inform them of the serious danger of sterility, particularly for women. Infected clients should scrupulously avoid all sexual activity until both partners are cured, and they should use condoms thereafter.

To increase the efficacy of doxycycline, advise clients to space the pills equally throughout each 24-hour period and to avoid iron, dairy products, and antacids during treatment. Clients should report manifestations of superinfection (such as yeast infection, thrush).

GONORRHEA

Gonorrhea (also known as *clap, white, drips, strain*, and *dose* in lay terms) can be divided into two categories: local and disseminated. *Local infection* can involve the mucosal surfaces of the cervix, urethra, and rectum; vestibular glands; pharynx; or conjunctiva. *Systemic infection (disseminated gonococcal infection)* involves bacteremia

BRIDGE TO HOME HEALTH CARE

Teaching About Sexually Transmitted Infections

When you are working with people who have sexually transmitted infections, it is important to consider the whole person in relation to their history and development. The infection may be symptomatic of an underlying pattern of risk behavior, such as chemical or alcohol use; such patterns impair your clients' judgment. Adolescents may believe that they are invincible to the risks of these behavior patterns.

Unless you, as the nurse, address the underlying cause of risk behaviors and your clients take action, the chance of recurrent infection remains unchanged. Talk about testing even when manifestations are not present, especially if your client changes partners. The most prevalent sexually transmitted organism, *Chlamydia trachomatis,* is easily transmitted and may not produce manifestations that make intercourse painful or prompt people to seek treatment. If chlamydial infection is detected early in asymptomatic clients, transmission and future problems with infertility can be prevented. Women can be tested easily when they have their Pap smear. When your client has one infection, be alert to the possibility of others. The risk of reinfection continues if the client's partner is not treated at the same time.

Become informed about community resources that offer testing for sexually transmitted infections and contraceptive care. As part of your health education, help clients identify needed resources. Many young adults are uninsured. Adolescents do not want the charges for tests to appear on their parents' bills. Often, community clinics provide testing and treatments at reduced rates and ensure confidentiality for adolescents and young adults. A list of community clinics can be obtained from your state's public health department.

The concept of safer sex is an important focus of preventive education. The only sure protection is a monogamous relationship with a low-risk partner, one who has not used intravenous drugs and has not had previous partners. Although it is advisable to use condoms, they can also give a false sense of security. Genital herpes and warts can be spread to the partner if the lesions are on the perineum and not covered by condoms. Condoms can also break or slip off. Provide information about the correct use of condoms. Instruct clients that irritation from condom latex and spermicides may produce vaginitis that appears to be an infection in sensitive individuals. The irritation increases tissue vulnerability to infection.

Teaching about sexually transmitted infections should include:

- Anticipatory guidance to reduce high-risk behaviors
- Manifestations of infection and consequences of transmission and untreated infection
- Facts about incidence and risk to help clients make informed decisions
- Community resources that offer low-cost, confidential testing and treatment of infections
- Responsibility to inform others who may be exposed to the infection
- Pamphlets about sexually transmitted infections
- Anatomic illustrations and models

As nurses, we can help prevent unnecessary human suffering, birth defects, preterm labor, loss of fertility, premature death, and costly treatments if we provide education and facilitate access to early diagnosis and treatment.

Susan Flannigan, RNC, ANP, MPH, *Adult Nurse Practitioner, Fairview Lakes Medical Center, Chisago City, Minnesota*

with polyarthritis, dermatitis, endocarditis, and meningitis. Systemic infection is more common in women.

Etiology and Risk Factors

Gonorrhea is one of the most prevalent STDs in the United States; more than 600,000 new cases are reported each year. It is widely believed that the incidence of gonorrhea is underreported and that the actual number of cases is much greater. Teenagers and young adults are at highest risk. Most cases of gonorrhea occur in people age 15 to 29 years, with the highest rate in those age 20 to 24 years.

Pathophysiology

Gonorrhea is caused by the gram-negative diplococcus *Neisseria gonorrhoeae*. The causative organism does not survive long outside the body. Gonorrhea, therefore, is almost always transmitted by direct sexual contact. The few rare exceptions are infection in infants, who can contract gonorrhea during vaginal birth, and infection of medical personnel through broken skin.

Clinical Manifestations

The endocervical canal is the primary site of gonorrheal infection in women. In most women, the urethra is also infected. Infection can also involve the vestibular glands and anus. The vagina is resistant to the infection in adulthood but not before puberty. The disease may be asymptomatic in women. There is a large *carrier population* (people who carry the organism and have no manifestations but can transmit the disease) for gonorrhea. Manifestations of gonorrhea include (1) heavy, yellow-green, purulent vaginal discharge, (2) cervical erythema, (3) a red, swollen, sore vulva, (4) abnormal menstrual bleeding, and (5) dysuria and urinary frequency.

The most common complication of gonorrhea in women is salpingitis, which can progress to PID. Both PID and salpingitis can produce infertility secondary to scarring and occlusion of the fallopian tubes. The first recognizable manifestations of gonorrhea in women may arise from PID.

Manifestations of gonorrhea are usually evident earlier in men than in women. The infection is principally one of the anterior urethra that produces a purulent discharge, dysuria, and urinary frequency. Complications include epididymitis and prostatitis, but these are not common with early and complete antibiotic therapy.

In addition to the gender-specific manifestations, both men and women may have conjunctivitis or pharyngitis due to orogenital contact or proctitis from anal contact.

Disseminated infection, the most serious form of gonorrhea, results from gonococcal bacteremia and is often manifested by septic arthritis, skin lesions, asymmetrical arthralgias, and tenosynovitis (inflammation of the tendon and synovial membrane). Rarely, hepatic adhesions (Fitz-Hugh–Curtis syndrome), endocarditis, or meningitis may occur.

Diagnosis of gonorrhea is made through history, physical examination, identification of the gonococcus on a smear, and culture of the exudate from infected areas. Culture with selective culture media remains the cornerstone of diagnosis.

Outcome Management

Medical Management

Eradicate Disease and Manifestations

All sexually active women in high-risk groups should be screened for gonorrhea on a regular basis. All clients in whom gonorrhea is detected should also be tested for chlamydial infection.

Gonorrhea is treated aggressively with antibiotics. Before the advent of resistant organisms, penicillin was the treatment of choice. The current recommended regimen for uncomplicated gonorrhea is a single intramuscular (IM) dose of ceftriaxone (Rocephin), or a single oral dose of cefixime (Suprax), ciprofloxacin (Cipro), or ofloxacin (Floxin). Any of these single doses is followed by oral doxycycline (Vibramycin) for 7 days for the presumptive treatment of co-infection with *C. trachomatis* (chlamydial infection commonly coexists with gonorrhea). A single IM injection of spectinomycin (Trobicin) plus oral doxycycline can be used for clients who cannot tolerate ceftriaxone.

For clients with disseminated gonococcal infection, the recommended regimen is administration of ceftriaxone, given IM or IV every 24 hours and continued 24 to 48 hours after improvement begins, followed by cefixime or ciprofloxacin, given orally for a full week.

After therapy for uncomplicated gonorrhea is completed, a follow-up examination and culture are not necessary. Treatment failure following combined ceftriaxone-doxycycline therapy is rare. Manifestations that persist after treatment should be evaluated with a follow-up culture. Any gonococcal organisms appearing on the second culture should be tested for antibiotic sensitivity to identify possible resistant organisms.

Nursing Management of the Medical Client

Eradicate Disease and Manifestations

Discuss the importance of identifying and treating all sexual partners, as there seems to be a reservoir population of asymptomatic men. Recurrence due to reinfection may indicate the need for improved client education and sexual partner referral.

Warn pregnant clients of the danger of infecting their newborns during delivery. Clients receiving treatment for gonorrhea must understand the importance of taking the *complete* course of prescribed medication. Common side effects of treatment are pain at the injection site and yeast infection. Clients should understand that because of its long half-life, azithromycin is given only once.

Investigation of the client's sexual contacts is essential for the prevention and control of gonorrhea. All sexual partners who were exposed to the client's gonorrhea within the 60 days before the diagnosis should undergo examination, culture, and presumptive treatment. Reporting sexual contacts can be difficult and frightening for an infected client. Ask for contact information in a positive, nonthreatening, sensitive way during the initial treatment visit.

DISEASES CHARACTERIZED BY ULCERATIONS

SYPHILIS

Syphilis (lay terms are *bad blood, lues, pox,* and *syph*) is a systemic, highly infectious STD (see Table 41-1). It became less prevalent after the advent of penicillin, but the disease has not been eradicated. The incidence of syphilis has been rising since about 1960, and it is one of the most commonly reported communicable diseases in the United States.

Etiology and Risk Factors

Syphilis is caused by the delicate motile (self-moving) spirochete *Treponema pallidum.* Although *T. pallidum* cannot survive long outside the body, syphilis is highly infectious. Sexual transmission of *T. pallidum* occurs only when the mucocutaneous lesions of primary and secondary syphilis are present. Adolescents, young adults, African American men, and homosexual men are at greatest risk.

Pathophysiology

T. pallidum enters the body through intact mucous membranes or abraded skin, almost exclusively by direct sexual contact. After entry, the organisms multiply locally and disseminate systemically through the bloodstream and lymphatics. The infection can also be passed transplacentally from an untreated pregnant woman to her fetus during any stage of the disease (*congenital syphilis*).

In rare instances, syphilis has been contracted through nonsexual personal contact, accidental inoculation, or blood transfusion from a syphilitic donor. Syphilis can progress to irreversible blindness, mental illness, paralysis, heart disease, and death.

Clinical Manifestations

STAGES

Syphilis is characterized by well-defined sequential stages that occur over years: primary, secondary, latent (early latent and late latent), and late or tertiary.

PRIMARY STAGE. The principal manifestation of primary syphilis is the appearance of a genital chancre. A *chancre* is an oval ulcer with a raised firm border that does not bleed readily and is painless unless infected (Fig. 41-1). The chancre develops at the site of inoculation, usually the genitalia, anus, or mouth. Most commonly, a single chancre occurs about 4 weeks after initial infection. Chancres in women often remain unnoticed. Lymphadenopathy may occur as lymph glands near the chancre become enlarged. Nodes are painless, firm, and discrete. If untreated, a chancre heals spontaneously in 4 to 6 weeks, leaving a thin, atrophic scar.

SECONDARY STAGE. If the primary disease is untreated, secondary syphilis develops 6 to 8 weeks after infection. Indications of the second stage are:

1. *Generalized rash.* Typically, a maculopapular and nonpruritic rash appears on the palms of the hands and soles of the feet (few other diseases cause a rash in these locations).

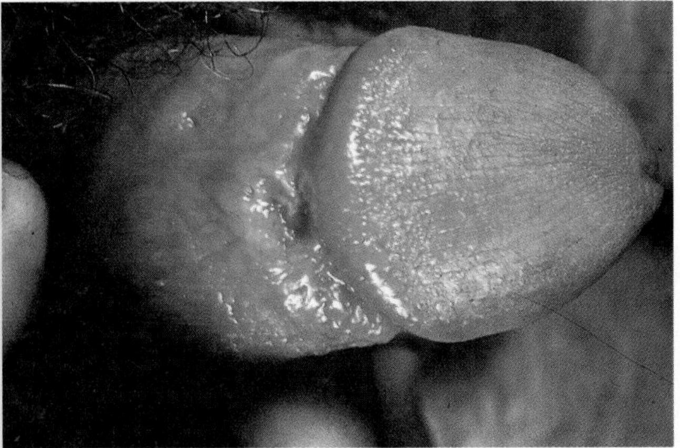

FIGURE 41-1 Ulcer of primary syphilis. (Courtesy of Dr. Rodney M. S. Basler.)

2. *Generalized, nontender, discrete lymphadenopathy.*
3. *Mucous patches.* Gray, superficial patches occur on the mucous membranes in the mouth and may be accompanied by a sore throat.
4. *Condylomata lata.* Broad-based, flat papules, these lesions usually can be easily distinguished from the typical narrow-based, pedunculated growth of condylomata acuminata (genital warts). Condylomata lata may develop in warm, moist body areas—most commonly on the labia or anus or at the corners of the mouth. They are highly contagious.
5. *General flu-like manifestations,* including nausea, anorexia, constipation, headache, muscle, joint, and bone pain, and a chronically elevated temperature.
6. *Patchy hair loss* from eyebrows and scalp (alopecia).

Secondary stage manifestations usually disappear after 2 to 6 weeks. A latency period then begins.

LATENT STAGE. The latent stage of syphilis typically produces no manifestations. *Latent syphilis* is defined as that period after infection with *T. pallidum* when a client is seroreactive (with a positive blood test) but shows no other evidence of disease. During this stage, syphilis is noninfectious except via transplacental spread or blood transfusion. Syphilis is not transmitted by sexual contact during the latent phase unless a secondary syphilitic mucocutaneous skin lesion reoccurs during early latent syphilis. Latent syphilis usually occurs 1 to 2 years after the primary lesion and can last as long as 50 years. About 66% of infected clients remain in this stage without further problems.

TERTIARY STAGE. In 1 to 35 years after the primary infection, about 33% of clients with untreated syphilis experience devastating, irreversible complications, such as chronic bone and joint inflammation, cardiovascular problems (for example, valvular involvement, aneurysms), granulomatous lesions (*gummas*) on any part of the body, and ophthalmic, auditory, and central nervous system problems. This stage, although not infectious, may be terminal if untreated (see Chapter 69 for manifestations of neurosyphilis [syphilis affecting the central nervous system]).

DIAGNOSIS

The diagnosis of syphilis is based on health assessment and various direct and indirect laboratory studies. A *direct test* identifies the causative organism; an *indirect test* identifies antibodies of the causative agent. *T. pallidum* cannot be grown in culture. Primary or secondary stage lesions can be scraped and the causative organism identified directly with dark-field microscopy or DFA testing. Dark-field examination must be done by an expert, because other spirochetes closely resembling *T. pallidum* are present in oral and genital mucosa. This test confirms a diagnosis of syphilis in the primary stage (when other tests are generally negative) and the secondary stage.

Serologic tests for syphilis are indirect tests that detect antibodies. These antibodies are not present in the serum until 4 weeks *after* the appearance of the chancre. Such tests include:

- The Venereal Disease Research Laboratory (VDRL)
- Rapid plasma reagin (RPR), which uses an antigen to detect the antibody relatively specific for *T. pallidum*
- Fluorescent treponemal antibody absorption (FTA-ABS) tests

The VDRL test for nonspecific antibodies is the most commonly used screening test. Results are negative in the early primary stage, before antibodies to *T. pallidum* are formed and are present in the circulation. Results may be falsely positive if the VDRL test is performed during the early stages of several common viral illnesses (mumps, measles, hepatitis, chickenpox, infectious mononucleosis). Results are given as "nonreactive," "borderline," "weakly reactive," or "reactive." Reactive and weakly reactive results are considered to be positive.

The FTA-ABS serologic test is more specific because it measures antibodies specific to *T. pallidum.* It is used when the VDRL result is positive but the diagnosis of syphilis is still uncertain. In clients who have mononucleosis or systemic lupus erythematosus, a false-positive test result is possible. The FTA-ABS test result usually becomes positive 3 to 4 weeks after infection. Once positive, FTA-ABS test results usually remain positive for the client's life, regardless of treatment or cure. Cerebrospinal fluid may be examined for characteristic findings in late neurosyphilis.

Syphilis often coexists with other infections. The CDC recommends that all clients with syphilis be counseled on the risks of HIV infection and AIDS and encouraged to undergo HIV testing.

Outcome Management

Medical Management

ERADICATE DISEASE AND MANFESTATIONS

Parenteral penicillin remains the treatment of choice for all stages of syphilis; however, the structural changes present in late syphilis are irreversible despite successful treatment. The dosage schedule and length of therapy are determined by the stage of the disease and current guidelines for treatment. For primary, secondary, and early latent syphilis, the treatment of choice is benzathine penicillin G, given IM in one dose. Late latent syphilis is treated with three weekly penicillin injections. Neurosyphilis is treated with IV aqueous crystalline penicillin G.

Use of penicillin to treat syphilis in clients with penicillin allergy is a complicated issue. Clients who are pregnant or noncompliant with therapy or who have neurosyphilis should undergo desensitization and treatment with penicillin. Desensitization guidelines are available from the CDC. For nonpregnant clients who are allergic to penicillin, oral doxycycline or tetracycline for 2 weeks may be given, but they are not as effective as penicillin.

Treatment failure can occur with any given regimen. Compliance is often a problem. Clients should be reexamined clinically and evaluated with serologic testing at 6, 12, and 24 months after treatment. No definitive criteria for cure exist. With successful treatment, ideally, no evidence of disease should be present and serial serologic test values should decline.

Treating sexual partners is also a complex issue; treatment is best guided by information available from the CDC. All people who have had sexual contact with the client who has primary syphilis must be identified and evaluated. Most practitioners treat sexual contacts as if they have primary syphilis whether or not they show evidence of infection.

Nursing Management of the Medical Client

ERADICATE DISEASE AND MANIFESTATIONS

A client with syphilis needs information and psychosocial support to deal with this complex illness. Individualize health teaching to meet the client's particular needs and psychosocial situation. A diagnosis of syphilis can be frightening and difficult to accept.

Clients with primary or secondary syphilis should abstain from sexual contact for at least 1 month after treatment. Adequate treatment should be curative, but reinfection is possible and can be detected with clinical examinations and monitoring of serologic test values. Proper follow-up, although essential, is time-consuming and difficult. Many clients do not understand the severe consequences of not obtaining adequate treatment.

GENITAL HERPES

Genital herpes is a recurrent, systemic viral infection (see Table 41–1). Although recognized for centuries, genital herpes has received renewed attention because of its epidemic incidence. Now one of the most common STDs (45 million cases in the United States), it is the most frequent cause of genital ulceration. Its peak incidence is among adolescents and young adults.

Etiology and Risk Factors

Caused by herpes simplex virus (HSV) type 2, the infection is closely related to other herpes infections, such as the classic cold sore caused by HSV type 1. HSV type 1 infection is mainly nongenital, occurring above the waist (often on the lips or nose). HSV type 2 infection occurs primarily below the waist as a sexually transmitted genital infection. It is possible for HSV type 1 to cause genital infections and for HSV type 2 to cause oral lesions (Fig. 41–2).

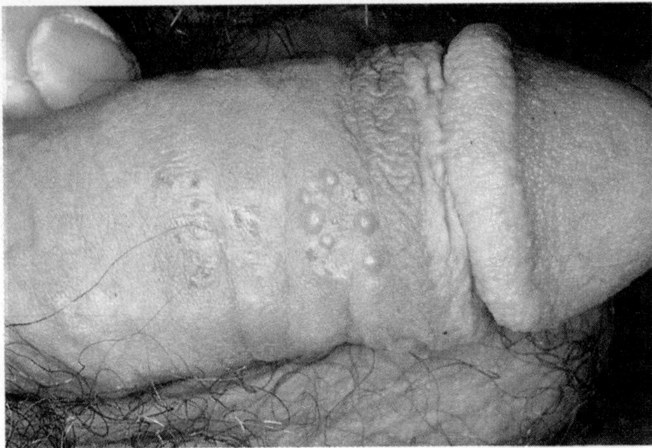

FIGURE 41–2 Typical herpes vesicles. (Courtesy of Dr. Rodney M. S. Basler.)

Pathophysiology

The HSV organism is present in the exudate of the lesion. Herpes can be transmitted while a lesion is present and for 10 days after a lesion has healed. Genital herpes is usually transmitted by direct contact with the exudate during sexual activity, but transmission is possible by *fomites* (objects that can harbor pathogenic microorganisms), such as towels used by an infected person. Many cases of genital herpes are acquired from people who do not know they have an infection or who are asymptomatic at the time of sexual contact. Newborns can be infected during vaginal delivery when active genital lesions are present. Birth by cesarean section prevents this transmission.

Clinical Manifestations

Many people with HSV type 2 infection have mild or unrecognized disease. Manifestations of genital herpes usually occur 3 to 7 days after contact. Initially, a burning sensation (paresthesia) is noted at the site of inoculation. Next, numerous small vesicles with an erythematous border form painful, shallow ulcers that then crust and heal with a scar in about 2 to 4 weeks.

The major problem with HSV is recurrence. Up to 75% of clients have a recurrent infection within 1 year of the first episode. The virus is believed to lie dormant in the body, probably in nerve ganglions, until it is activated, at which point another episode of genital herpes, with characteristic lesions, occurs. Stress, infection, trauma, menses, or sexual activity may trigger recurrent episodes.

Characteristically, recurrent genital herpes causes local, but not systemic, manifestations. Prodromal (pre-onset) manifestations of a burning sensation may occur before the vesicles erupt. The vesicles tend to reappear at the sites of previous infection, but they can involve new sites. Manifestations are similar to, but usually less severe than, those in the primary infection. Vesicles rupture in 24 to 48 hours, and the syndrome generally lasts 7 to 10 days.

Potential complications of HSV infections include disseminated infections, meningitis, and transverse myelitis. Women are at risk for spontaneous abortion, and it has been suggested that HSV type 2 predisposes to carcinoma of the cervix.

A diagnosis of genital herpes is often made visually. The diagnosis is confirmed by a viral culture, direct immunofluorescence staining, or antigen detection testing of the vesicular exudate. A Pap smear can also be performed; the presence of multinucleated giant cells in the Pap smear, with or without inclusion bodies, is characteristic of a herpes infection.

Outcome Management

Medical Management

Reduce Manifestations

Genital herpes is a chronic disease without a cure. Management is geared toward preventing or lessening occurrences and giving palliative care. The recommended treatment for an acute primary infection is acyclovir (Zovirax), an antiviral agent, taken orally for 7 to 10 days. Episodic recurrences are treated with acyclovir, valacyclovir (Valtrex), or famciclovir (Famvir) taken for 5 days.

Clients with frequent recurrences (six or more episodes in 1 year) take daily suppressive therapy. Daily acyclovir taken for 4 months to 3 years may prevent or reduce the frequency and severity of recurrence in most clients. After 1 year, the acyclovir should be discontinued to assess the need for continued suppressive therapy. If genital herpes recurs, daily therapy is resumed.

Severe disease is treated with IV acyclovir for 5 to 7 days.

Nursing Management of the Medical Client

Prevent Reinfection

When the vesicles of herpes rupture, they release a highly contagious exudate. Clients as well as health care personnel must observe strict medical asepsis in the presence of HSV infection. Clients should wash their hands thoroughly after any contact with the herpetic lesions to avoid *autoinoculation* (spread of the disease to another part of their own bodies). HSV infections of the eye are particularly serious. Advise infected clients to have separate towels and other personal items and to avoid touching their eyes. Clients should use condoms during latent periods because the possible risk of transmission exists even when lesions are not present. Women should have annual pelvic examinations and Pap smears because of the association of HSV with cervical cancer.

Provide Support

Coping with genital herpes may cause tremendous psychosocial stress. Although recurrence cannot always be predicted, nurses can help clients identify possible triggers. Reappearance of the disease can significantly affect sexual activity. Support groups may help clients deal with the anger, guilt, and shame that many commonly feel. Stress reduction techniques may be helpful. Sexual partners should be offered counseling, evaluation, and treatment if needed.

Relieve Pain

The pain of herpes lesions is problematic. Palliative measures include (1) keeping the involved area clean and dry,

(2) wearing loose-fitting, nonsynthetic undergarments, and (3) using sitz baths, cooling applications, and analgesic medications, such as aspirin, for pain relief.

Clients should understand that acyclovir does not cure HSV infection or prevent its spread. Clients should begin oral suppressive therapy when they first recognize the prodromal sensations or first become symptomatic. Topical acyclovir ointment should be applied with a glove and should never be put in or around the eyes.

CHANCROID

Chancroid is a highly contagious infection caused by the gram-negative bacillus *Haemophilus ducreyi*. The initial papules or pustules produce multiple painful, irregular, and deep genital ulcers, often accompanied by tender inguinal lymphadenopathy (Fig. 41–3). Although chancroid is more common in the tropics, the incidence is endemic in many areas of the United States. Chancroid is well established as a cofactor for HIV transmission. There is a high rate of HIV infection in clients with chancroid.

Definitive diagnosis requires the culture of *H. ducreyi.* It is difficult to isolate the organism, and culture of *H. ducreyi* is not widely available. A probable diagnosis may be made if the client has one or more painful genital ulcers and regional lymphadenopathy (especially tender inguinal adenopathy) without clinical or serologic evidence of syphilis or genital herpes. People with whom the client has had sexual contact within 10 days before the onset of manifestations should be examined and treated. Clients with chancroid should also be tested for HIV infection, HSV infection, and syphilis.

Recommended treatment is oral azithromycin or ceftriaxone given IM in a single dose; alternatively, ciprofloxacin or erythromycin may be given orally.

LYMPHOGRANULOMA VENEREUM

Lymphogranuloma venereum is a systemic infection that is rare in the United States. It is caused by certain strains of *C. trachomatis*. The primary lesion is a small, painless papule on the glans penis or the vaginal mucosa that heals spontaneously and may go unnoticed.

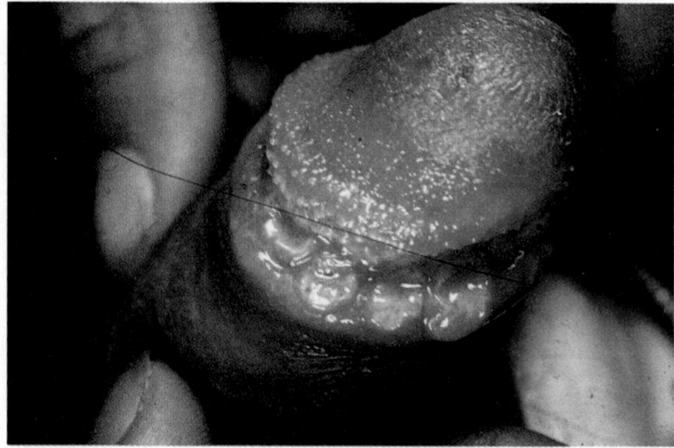

FIGURE 41–3 Chancroid lesions. (Courtesy of Dr. Rodney M. S. Basler.)

The most common clinical manifestations are markedly tender, enlarged, and inflamed inguinal lymph nodes (*buboes*), which are usually unilateral and appear 2 to 6 weeks after the primary lesion. Eventually, draining ulcerations, scarring, lymphatic obstruction, and marked external genital deformity may occur. Rectal fibrosis and strictures are late sequelae.

Definitive diagnosis is made with a positive culture for *C. trachomatis.* Recommended therapy is doxycycline, given orally for 21 days. Oral erythromycin is an alternative.

GRANULOMA INGUINALE

Granuloma inguinale (donovanosis) is a chronic infection endemic in some tropical and developing areas but rare in the United States. It is caused by the small gram-negative bacillus *Calymmatobacterium granulomatis.*

Granuloma inguinale is characterized by genital and perianal papular lesions without lymphadenopathy. These become painless, gradually enlarging, ulcerating granulomatous lesions that cause tissue destruction that is difficult to differentiate from cancer. The lesions are highly vascular, bleed easily, and have a beefy-red appearance. Diagnosis is made by microscopic identification of Donovan's bodies (inclusion bodies of the causative organism) in a smear taken from edge scrapings of the lesion.

Treatment consists of a long course of an antibiotic such as trimethoprim-sulfamethoxazole or doxycycline. Relapses can occur despite adequate treatment. IV aminoglycosides are given for infections that do not improve with first-line antibiotics. All partners who have had sexual contact with an infected client within 60 days before diagnosis need evaluation and treatment.

INFECTION WITH HUMAN PAPILLOMAVIRUS

GENITAL WARTS (CONDYLOMATA ACUMINATA)

Etiology and Risk Factors

Genital warts, the fourth most common STD, are caused by HPV; they are usually transmitted by sexual contact (see Table 41–1). Factors that may favor their development include HIV, pregnancy, smoking, drug or alcohol use, poor nutrition, and fatigue.

Pathophysiology

More than 20 types of HPV affect the genital tract. The natural history of HPV is complex and poorly understood. Infection with certain strains of HPV is strongly associated with carcinomas of the genitals, including the cervix.

Clinical Manifestations

Genital warts are benign growths that typically occur in multiple, painless clusters on the vulva, vagina, cervix, perineum, anorectal area, urethral meatus, or glans penis 1 to 2 months after exposure (Fig. 41–4). Oral, pharyngeal, and laryngeal lesions can also occur. HPV can cause

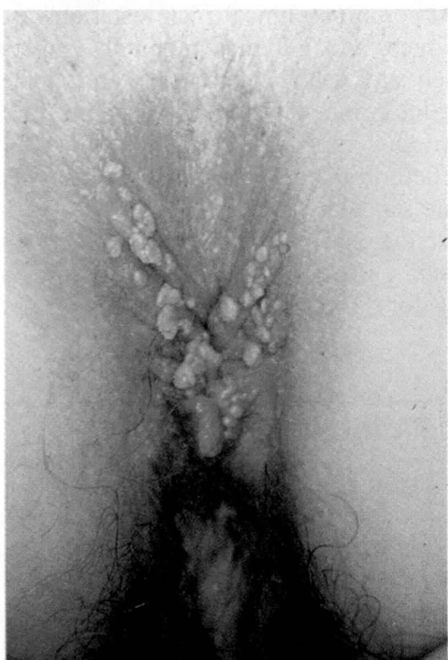

FIGURE 41–4 Genital warts (condylomata acuminata). (Courtesy of Dr. Rodney M. S. Basler.)

laryngeal papillomatosis in infants born to mothers with vaginal warts.

Diagnosis is typically made visually. Subclinical (asymptomatic or not visible) warts can be identified through Pap smear and colposcopy (examination of vagina and cervical tissues with a scope containing a magnifying lens) of the cervix. Biopsy of lesions may be performed to differentiate warts from carcinoma or condylomata lata of the secondary stage of syphilis.

Outcome Management

Medical Management

REMOVE VISIBLE WARTS

There is no cure for genital warts. A variety of chemical, mechanical, and ablative techniques are used for visible lesions, but no specific antiviral therapy for the HPV is available. Treatment varies according to the site and severity of the warts and is also guided by client preference. Treatment is more successful if the warts are small and have been present for less than a year.

TOPICAL THERAPY. The most common pharmacologic treatment is podophyllin in compound tincture of benzoin or trichloroacetic acid (TCA) applied topically to the warts *only*. Treatments are repeated weekly until all the lesions have disappeared and the skin is healed. Podophyllin is contraindicated during pregnancy because of its *abortifacient* (abortion-causing) properties.

Topical podofilox is the only agent approved for self-application by clients at home. For safe application, the client must be able to see and reach the warts easily. Podofilox is also contraindicated during pregnancy. If warts persist, other modes of therapy should be considered.

OTHER TREATMENT. Warts can be treated with cryotherapy using liquid nitrogen or a cryoprobe. Carbon dioxide lasers, electrocautery, and simple surgical excision can be used on extensive warts. The antiviral drug interferon has also been used, but it is expensive and is associated with a high rate of adverse side effects. Remember, genital warts are not cured, and recurrence is very common.

It is not necessary to evaluate and treat sexual partners of clients with genital warts, since treatment is not effective in eradicating the disease or its spread. Female partners should be referred for a Pap smear, and all sexual partners should be offered the opportunity to be examined and tested for other STDs.

Nursing Management of the Medical Client

Inform clients with genital warts that no cure exists. Clients must be warned that they are at increased risk for genital malignancy. HPV infections are strongly associated with cancer of the cervix and vulva in women and squamous cell carcinoma of the penis in men. All women with genital warts should receive a Pap smear *at least* every year and, when indicated, cervical colposcopy and biopsy. Encourage condom use. Improved detection and treatment of HPV infection in men may be important to prevent genital carcinoma in women.

DISEASES CHARACTERIZED BY VAGINAL DISCHARGE

Infections manifested by vaginal discharge include trichomoniasis and vaginitis (bacterial and yeast). Though occasionally transmitted sexually, candidiasis (vaginal yeast infection) is generally not considered an STD. Recurrent vaginal yeast infections are a common manifestation of HIV infection in women (see Chapter 39 for discussion of vaginitis).

TRICHOMONIASIS

Etiology and Risk Factors

Trichomoniasis is a protozoal infection causing vulvovaginitis. Although not life-threatening, the incidence is very high worldwide and the disease remains a major health problem. Often asymptomatic, trichomoniasis affects 3 million people annually, and its role in PID and infertility may be greatly underestimated.

Pathophysiology

Trichomoniasis is caused by the anaerobic, flagellated, parasitic protozoan *Trichomonas vaginalis.* The organism is almost always transmitted sexually. *T. vaginalis* prefers an alkaline environment (pH 6 to 7), and alterations in the vaginal *flora* (the usual bacteria and fungi) make a woman more susceptible to infection. Trichomoniasis can be very resistant to treatment, and recurrence is common.

Clinical Manifestations

Manifestations may be minor, especially in men. In women, manifestations include a copious, malodorous, yellow-green vaginal discharge. This is irritating to the vulva and causes severe itching, burning, and excoriation and maceration of the vulvar tissues. Occasionally, the cervix is covered with punctate (point-like) hemorrhages ("strawberry cervix"). The vaginal mucosa appears reddened and slightly edematous. Some women experience dyspareunia (pain during sexual intercourse).

If trichomoniasis extends to the urethra, urinary frequency and burning with urination may occur. This is the most common manifestation in a man. Anal involvement may also occur, either asymptomatically or with a slight discharge. Bladder and anal involvement are more common when the infection has become chronic.

The diagnosis can be made immediately in the health care facility after a fresh, warm specimen of vaginal exudate in a saline wet mount is examined under a microscope and the highly motile organisms are identified. Cultures are an option but are rarely necessary. A wet mount is obtained by placing a drop of vaginal exudate on a glass slide, mixing in a drop of saline, and covering it with a cover slide. The vaginal speculum used to obtain the exudate must be inserted without lubrication to avoid destroying the organism. If possible, instruct the client not to douche before the vaginal examination.

Outcome Management

Medical Management

ERADICATE DISEASE AND MANIFESTATIONS

The preferred treatment of trichomoniasis is a single oral dose of metronidazole (Flagyl) with simultaneous treatment of all sexual partners for a cure. Metronidazole should not be taken during the first trimester of pregnancy because it may adversely affect fetal development. *T. vaginalis* does not affect the fetus. Single-dose metronidazole therapy is usually curative, but recurrence is common.

Instruct clients to seek prompt treatment if manifestations return. Metronidazole may be given in a 7-day regimen for recurrent infection.

Nursing Management of the Medical Client

Advise clients taking metronidazole not to drink alcoholic beverages, because doing so might cause nausea, vomiting, and headaches. This prohibition includes all alcohol-containing products, such as cough syrup. Emphasize the importance of good perineal hygiene.

Treatment should continue through the client's menstrual period because the vagina is more alkaline during this time and a flare-up is more likely to occur. Metronidazole can be taken without regard to meals. Advise clients that urine may turn dark, reddish brown.

BACTERIAL VAGINOSIS

Bacterial vaginosis (BV), formerly known as nonspecific or *Gardnerella* vaginitis, is a common condition in adults.

Etiology and Risk Factors

Bacterial vaginosis is linked to sexual activity, although not all cases are caused by sexual activity.

Pathophysiology

Like the organisms responsible for vulvovaginal *Candida* (yeast) infections, the causative bacteria are found in the normal vagina. The infection is thought to be caused by the overgrowth of a number of different organisms, including *Gardnerella vaginalis* and vaginal anaerobes. Overgrowth may occur when the normal flora and pH of the vagina are altered.

Clinical Manifestations

The vulvovaginitis produced by bacterial vaginosis is mild or asymptomatic. The main manifestation is a mild to moderate, malodorous vaginal discharge. The discharge is usually thin, watery, and grayish white and tends to adhere to the vaginal wall. The odor is described as "fishy," and is often more noticeable after sexual intercourse. Manifestations are almost always confined to the vulvovaginal area. Mild vaginal burning and irritation may occur, but redness and pruritus are not common.

Evaluation is mainly by physical examination of the vagina, microscopic examination of the discharge, and determination of the pH of the discharge. The diagnosis is determined by the presence of at least three of the following manifestations:

- A homogeneous gray or white discharge that adheres to the vaginal wall
- Vaginal fluid pH higher than 4.5 (normal pH is 4.0 to 4.5)
- Positive result of the "whiff" test—a fishy odor elicited when potassium hydroxide (KOH) is added to the vaginal fluid
- Presence of *clue cells* (desquamated vaginal epithelial cells characteristically stippled by the adherence of coccobacilli to their surfaces) on either a saline wet mount or a Gram's stain of vaginal fluid

Outcome Management

Medical Management

The recommended treatment of bacterial vaginosis in nonpregnant women is metronidazole (Flagyl), given orally for 7 days. Single-dose regimens can be used to improve compliance, but they are less effective than the 7-day regimen. Pregnant women are treated with lower doses of metronidazole to minimize exposure to the fetus. Alternative treatment includes metronidazole in a high, single dose, clindamycin orally, or metronidazole vaginal gel (data are limited on metronidazole gel use during pregnancy).

Nursing Management of the Medical Client

BV is not necessarily transmitted sexually, though its occurrence is associated with sexual activity. Treatment of male partners is recommended only with recurrent or resistant infection. Recurrence is common.

ACQUIRED IMMUNODEFICIENCY SYNDROME

AIDS is a viral STD that has reached epidemic proportions worldwide. HIV infection has had an effect on the transmission of STDs, and vice versa. People with AIDS are more susceptible to other STDs. These coexistent STDs require more aggressive therapy and tend to recur. Conversely, people infected with an STD, especially those with genital ulcerations, are more susceptible to AIDS. On the positive side, national campaigns to prevent and control the transmission of HIV have had a beneficial effect on the incidence of some STDs (e.g., reduced incidence of hepatitis B in the homosexual population). AIDS is discussed in Chapter 79.

VACCINE-PREVENTABLE DISEASES

Vaccines for STDs are receiving attention as possible strategies for control of STDs. Currently, vaccines are available for hepatitis B and hepatitis A. Trials are under way for vaccines against other STDs.

Hepatitis A and Hepatitis B

Sexual contact is the most frequently reported mode of transmission for the hepatitis B virus (HBV) (30% to 60% of all cases), although blood-borne and perinatal transmission also occur. Clients at high risk for sexually transmitted hepatitis B are (1) heterosexuals with multiple sexual partners, (2) sexual partners of IV drug users, and (3) homosexual men. Sexually transmitted hepatitis B has decreased dramatically in the homosexual population, probably as a result of the modification of high-risk sexual behaviors to prevent AIDS.

Hepatitis A is caused by a virus shed in the stool. The virus is also found in serum and saliva. Risk factors for hepatitis A include (1) sexual contact with people who have the virus, (2) homosexual activity, and (3) IV drug abuse or sexual contact with an IV drug user. Vaccination is recommended for gay and bisexual men and for sexual partners of IV drug users if a local outbreak occurs within this population. See Chapter 47 for further discussion of hepatitis A and B.

DISEASES CAUSED BY INFESTATIONS

Pediculosis Pubis and Scabies

Cutaneous infestation with pubic lice (pediculosis pubis) or mites (scabies) results either from close physical contact with an infected person or from contact with contaminated objects of an infected person, such as linens and clothing. Because sexual transmission is possible, these conditions are included in any list of STDs. For further discussion, see Chapter 49.

SEXUALLY TRANSMITTED ENTERIC INFECTIONS

Gastroenteritis caused by enteric pathogens are typically acquired from food or water contaminated with fecal matter. Since the mid-1970s, it has been recognized that these pathogens can also be transmitted by oral and anal sexual contact. Sexually transmitted enteric infections include shigellosis, salmonellosis, amebiasis, and giardiasis. Homosexual men are at highest risk for these infections. See Chapter 33 for discussion of gastroenteritis.

MANAGEMENT OF CLIENTS REPORTING SEXUAL ASSAULT

Victims of sexual assault need immense support from health care professionals, a discussion of which is beyond the scope of this chapter. Regarding STDs, a sexual assault victim needs an immediate physical examination, including tests for pregnancy, gonorrhea, chlamydial infection, trichomoniasis, HIV, hepatitis A and B, and syphilis. Follow-up testing should be repeated in 2 weeks; syphilis and HIV testing should also be repeated at 6, 12, and 24 months. Prophylaxis for HIV infection is described in Chapter 79.

CONCLUSIONS

STDs are more prevalent now than ever before. This phenomenon is attributable to many factors. The improper and indiscriminate use of antibiotics has produced a number of resistant organisms. Sexual activity, especially among adolescents and young adults, has increased. Many STDs are asymptomatic and go undetected. As a nurse, you are in a unique position to help clients salvage or restore their sexual health and have an ever-increasing responsibility and role in the prevention, early detection, and treatment of STDs.

THINKING CRITICALLY

1. **A 20-year-old unmarried man comes to a walk-in STD clinic with a purulent urethral discharge. The diagnosis is uncomplicated gonorrhea. The client has no known allergies. He is sexually active with multiple partners. He gives a temporary address. What are the priorities of care? What are the priority interventions?**

Factors to Consider. What effect would the client's status as a walk-in client have on your planning? Consider the fact that gonorrhea often leads to PID in women. What effect would the client's temporary address have on your planning and need for identification of partners? What diseases are likely to coexist with gonorrhea?

2. **Your client is a 65-year-old widowed woman who comes for treatment of acute, symptomatic genital herpes. Her male sexual contact told her when their sexual relationship began that he had a history of genital herpes but that, because he had no active lesions, there was no risk of her becoming infected. She is humiliated by having contracted herpes and tells you that she feels dirty and contaminated. She also states that she "knows nothing" about condoms, and, furthermore, that she "wouldn't be caught dead buying them." What are the goals of her care? What interventions might be used?**

Factors to Consider. How accurate is the client's knowledge about the transmission of genital herpes? What are the client's psychosocial needs? What obstacles to buying condoms can you identify, and how will you help this client control her sexual health?

3. **A 25-year-old monogamous woman seeks outpatient treatment for the irritating, malodorous vaginal discharge of trichomoniasis. She has had trichomoniasis before, and metronidazole (Flagyl) was prescribed. What interventions should the care of this client include?**

Factors to Consider. Knowing that metronidazole is usually curative, consider what might have caused the client's recurrence.

BIBLIOGRAPHY

1. Able, E., Hilton, P., & Miller, I. (1996). Sexual risk behavior among urban women of childbearing age: Implications for clinical practice. *Journal of American Academy of Nurse Practitioners, 8*(3), 115–124.
2. Borchardt, K., & Noble, M. (Eds.). (1997). *Sexually transmitted diseases: Epidemiology, pathology, diagnosis, and treatment.* Boca Raton, FL: CRC Press.
3. Buzby, M. (1996). Viral hepatitis: A sexually transmitted disease? *Nurse Practitioner Forum, 7*(1), 10–15.
4. Carson, S. (1997). Human papillomatous virus infection update: Impact on women's health. *Nurse Practitioner: American Journal of Primary Health Care, 22*(4), 24–5, 28, 30, 35–37.
5. Centers for Disease Control and Prevention. (1998). 1998 guidelines for treatment of sexually transmitted diseases. *Morbidity and Mortality Weekly Report (Suppl.), 47*(RR-1), 1–116.
6. Dienstag, J. L. (1997). Sexual and perinatal transmission of hepatitis C. *Hepatology, 26*(3, suppl. 1), 66S–70S.
7. Ferreira, N. (1997). Sexually transmitted *Chlamydia trachomatis. Nurse Practitioner Forum, 8*(2), 70–76.
8. Fleming, D., et al. (1997). Herpes simplex virus type 2 in the United States, 1976–1994. *New England Journal of Medicine, 337*, 1105–1111.
9. Ford, K., & Norris, A. E. (1996). Sexually transmitted diseases: Experience and risk factors among urban low income, African American and Hispanic youth. *Ethnicity and Health, 1*(2), 175–184.
10. Fugate, K. A., & McClusky, M. M. (1996). The impact of sexually transmitted diseases on fertility. *Infertility and Reproductive Medicine Clinics of North America, 7*, 521–534.
11. Gorbach, S., Bartlett, J., & Blacklow, N. (1998). *Infectious diseases* (2nd ed.). Philadelphia: W. B. Saunders.
12. Gunn, R., et al. (1998). The changing paradigm of sexually transmitted disease control in the era of managed health care. *JAMA, 279*, 680–684.
13. Hiltabiddle, S. J. (1996). Adolescent condom use, the health belief model, and the prevention of sexually transmitted disease. *Journal of Obstetric, Gynecologic, and Neonatal Nursing, 25*, 61–66.
14. Jackson, S., & Soper, D. (1997). Sexually transmitted diseases in pregnancy. *Obstetrics and Gynecology Clinics of North America, 24*, 631–644.
15. Kenney, J., Reinholtz, C., & Angelini, P. (1998). Sexual abuse, sex before age 16, and high-risk behaviors of young females with sexually transmitted diseases. *Journal of Obstetric, Gynecologic, and Neonatal Nursing, 27*, 54–63.
16. Lappa, S., Coleman, M.T., & Moscicki, A. B. (1998). Managing sexually transmitted diseases in adolescents. *Primary Care, 25*(1), 71–110.
17. O'Connell, M. (1996). The effect of birth control methods on sexually transmitted disease/HIV risk. *Journal of Obstetric, Gynecologic, and Neonatal Nursing, 25*, 476–480.
18. Pagana, K., & Pagana, T. (1998). *Mosby's diagnostic and laboratory test reference.* St. Louis: Mosby–Year Book.
19. Roe, V., & Gudi, A. (1997). Pharmacological management of sexually transmitted diseases. *Journal of Nurse-Midwifery, 42*, 275–289.
20. Rooney, G., & Robinson, A. (1997). Look out for the hidden STD. *The Practitioner, 241*, 372–382.
21. Sharts-Hopko, N. (1997). STDs in women: What you need to know. *American Journal of Nursing, 97*(4), 46–55.
22. Skidmore-Roth, L. (1998). *Mosby's drug guide for nurses.* St. Louis: Mosby–Year Book.
23. Urban, M., Coury-Doniger, P., & Reichman, R. (1997). Results of a screening program for *Chlamydia trachomatis* infection in men attending a sexually transmitted diseases clinic. *Sexually Transmitted Diseases, 24*, 587–592.

UNIT

9

Metabolic Disorders

Anatomy and Physiology Review

The Metabolic Systems

Robert G. Carroll

Metabolism depends on the availability of fuel (glucose and fatty acids), oxygen, and the balance of *anabolic* (building) against *catabolic* (break-down) processes. The regulation of this balance is dynamic and is one function of the endocrine and neuroendocrine systems. Metabolic processes affect all cells of the body, and whole-body metabolic regulation involves numerous endocrine structures, the liver, muscle, and fat cells.

Endocrine secretions, together with the nervous system, coordinate the balance of metabolism, reproduction, water and electrolyte balance, and nutrient absorption. Metabolism is closely regulated by thyroid hormone, with some influence exerted by cortisol and epinephrine. Growth and development are regulated by growth hormone (also called somatotropin), with thyroid hormone, insulin-like growth factors, and the sex hormones providing significant effects. Plasma glucose is closely regulated by insulin, with glucagon and the metabolic hormones cortisol, growth hormone, and epinephrine having a role. Endocrine agents involved in water and electrolyte balance, nutrient absorption, and reproduction are described in Units 6 and 8.

The liver and pancreas have both endocrine and exocrine roles. The exocrine secretions assist the digestion and absorption of the diet (see Unit 6). The endocrine role is tied closely to metabolism, particularly the regulation of plasma glucose. Plasma glucose represents the balance of glucose absorption from the diet, movement into and out of storage pools, new glucose synthesis from amino acids *(gluconeogenesis),* and, finally, glucose consumption by the tissues. The liver plays a central role in these processes and is a good point to begin the discussion of metabolism.

STRUCTURE OF THE METABOLIC SYSTEMS

LIVER

The liver is the largest gland in the body, representing about 2.5% of body weight. It lies in the upper right quadrant of the abdomen, just below the diaphragm. The rib cage encloses the liver except for the lower margin. The lungs extend over the liver's upper portion. The lower portion of the liver provides a "roof" for the stomach and intestines. A peritoneal covering blankets most of the liver and also the adjacent gallbladder. The liver divides at the falciform ligament into two major lobes, right and left (Fig. U9–1). These two lobes, in turn, divide into superior and inferior portions of the posterior, anterior, medial, and lateral segments.

Liver blood flow represents about 20% of the cardiac output, about 1 L/min. The hepatic artery supplies the liver with about one third of its blood, and the portal vein supplies the other two thirds (see *inset,* Fig. U9–1). The hepatic artery carries oxygenated blood; the portal vein carries deoxygenated blood. The superior and inferior mesenteric veins and the splenic vein, which receive blood from the pancreas, spleen, stomach, intestines, and gallbladder, join to form the portal vein. The portal vein carries nutrients, metabolites, and toxins from the digestive organs to the liver for processing, detoxification, or assimilation. Blood pressure in the hepatic sinuses is low; hence, any process elevating central venous pressure causes liver engorgement. Similarly, any process impeding blood flow through the liver causes engorgement of vessels draining the digestive organs. The liver is an important reservoir for blood, with contraction of the hepatic venules and veins moving about 500 ml into the circulation.

The functional unit of the liver is the *lobule,* and the *hepatocyte* is the major cell. Hepatocytes are arranged in a hub-like fashion around a central vein. One side of the polyhedral hepatocyte faces the *hepatic sinusoids* (the capillary system of the liver); another faces the bile canaliculi. As incoming blood from the portal vein and the hepatic artery enters the sinusoids and passes through the liver lobules, many substances are exchanged between the blood and the hepatocytes. Lymphatic ducts drain excess interstitial fluid. Bile is formed in the hepatocytes, is secreted into the *bile canaliculi,* and travels through bile ductules to the gallbladder. Endothelial and *Kupffer's cells* form the walls of the sinusoids.

Kupffer's cells are an important part of the mononuclear phagocyte system (formerly, the reticuloendothelial system). This system is so effective that fewer than 1% of the bacteria entering the portal system from the intestine pass through the liver. After leaving the sinusoids, blood flows into the central vein, the hepatic veins, and the inferior vena cava.

ENDOCRINE SYSTEM

The endocrine glands are distributed throughout the body. *Endocrine* tissues (*endo,* within) secrete a compound (hormone) that is carried by the blood to act on a target tissue. This is in contrast to *exocrine* (*exo*, outside) tissues, which secrete across an epithelium, such as sweat and pancreatic peptidases (the lumen of the gastrointestinal [GI] tract is "outside" the body), and *paracrine* (*para*, around) cells, whose secretions do not need to be transported in the blood to reach their target tissue.

Hormones are generally classified on the basis of molecular structure as follows:

1. *Steroids.* Steroids are derived from cholesterol, and are consequently poorly soluble in water. After secretion, steroids are transported in the blood by

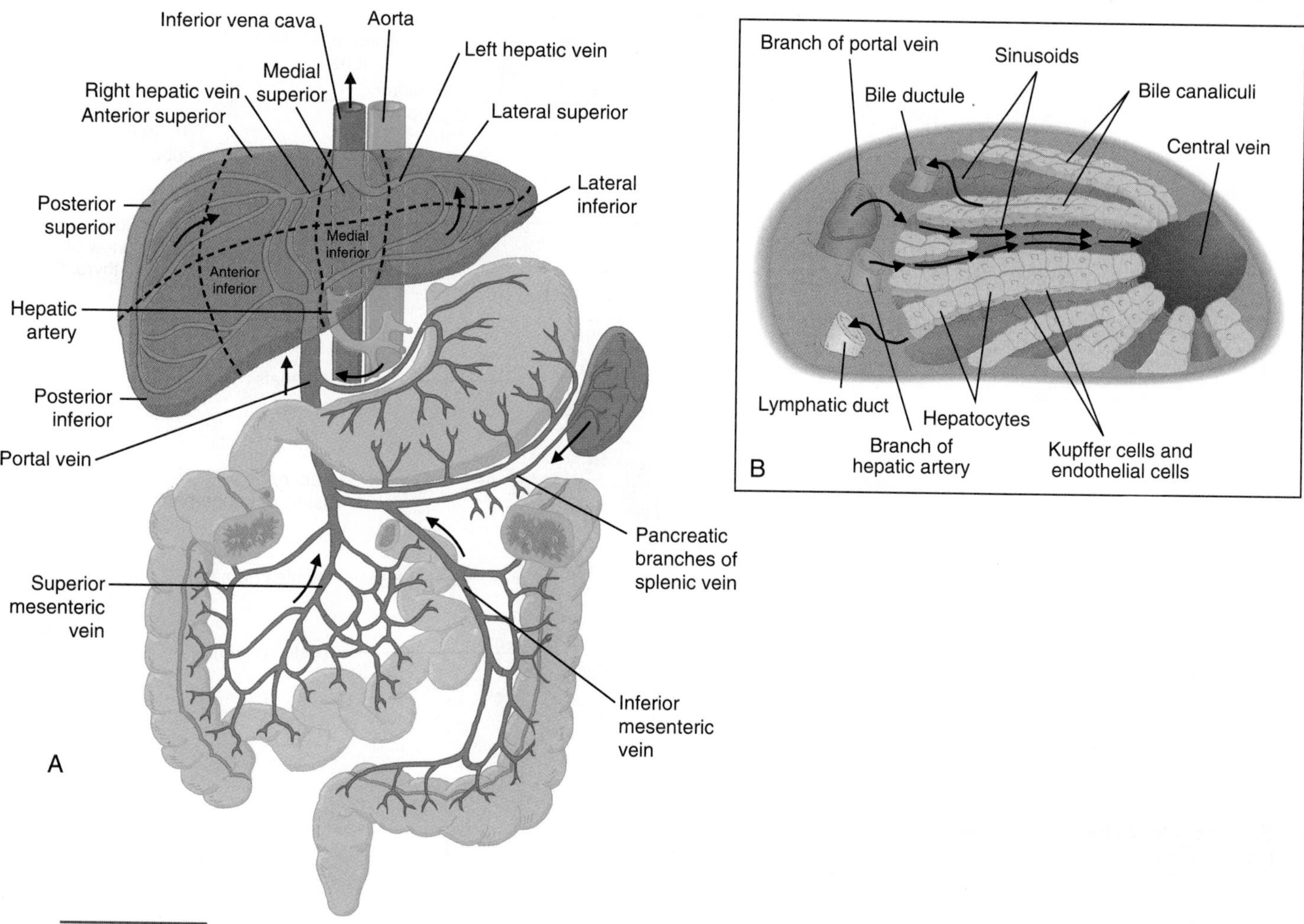

FIGURE U9–1 The liver and vascular drainages. Blood enters the liver from the hepatic artery, and the hepatic portal vein supplies the liver with blood from the digestive organs. *Inset,* Liver lobule. Blood from the hepatic artery and portal vein is processed by the hepatocytes as it flows through the sinusoids into the central vein. Lymphatics and bile ducts leave the liver through separate pathways.

carrier proteins. Steroids diffuse across the cell membrane of the target tissue, bind to a cytoplasmic-binding protein, and the steroid-binding protein complex enters the nucleus where it alters deoxyribonucleic acid (DNA) transcription. There is usually a time lag of minutes to hours before steroids exert their effects.

2. *Peptides. Proteins* and *polypeptides* are synthesized in the endoplasmic reticulum of the endocrine tissue and are secreted in vesicles. After transport in the blood, they bind to cell membrane receptors on the target tissues and activate either second messenger systems or ion channels. Peptide hormones generally have rapid response times.
3. *Amino acid derivatives.* The derivatives of tyrosine include thyroid hormone and the catecholamines epinephrine, norepinephrine, and dopamine. Thyroid hormone alters DNA synthesis through a pathway similar to that for steroids, but the catecholamines bind cell membrane receptors, similar to the mechanism of peptides.

The major endocrine organs described in this review include the pituitary, the thyroid, the parathyroid, the pancreas, the adrenal, and, to a lesser extent, the gonads (Fig. U9–2). Other organs have important endocrine secretions, including the kidney (renin and erythropoietin), the heart (atrial natriuretic peptide), and the placenta of a pregnant female (human chorionic gonadotropin [HCG], estrogen, progesterone, and the growth hormone somatomammotropin). See Units 7, 8, and 12.

Hypothalamus and Pituitary Gland

The pituitary gland *(hypophysis)* is a small (1 g) extension on the dorsal surface of the hypothalamus, connected to the hypothalamus by the hypophyseal stalk (Fig. U9–3). The pituitary has three histologically distinct sections, two of which secrete hormones in humans:

1. The *anterior pituitary (adenohypophysis)* is glandular tissue, containing a variety of secretory cell types.
2. The *posterior pituitary (neurohypophysis)* is neural tissue, containing glia cells and terminal axons from cells of the hypothalamus.
3. The *pars intermedia* is a vestigial remnant in humans, with little physiologic significance.

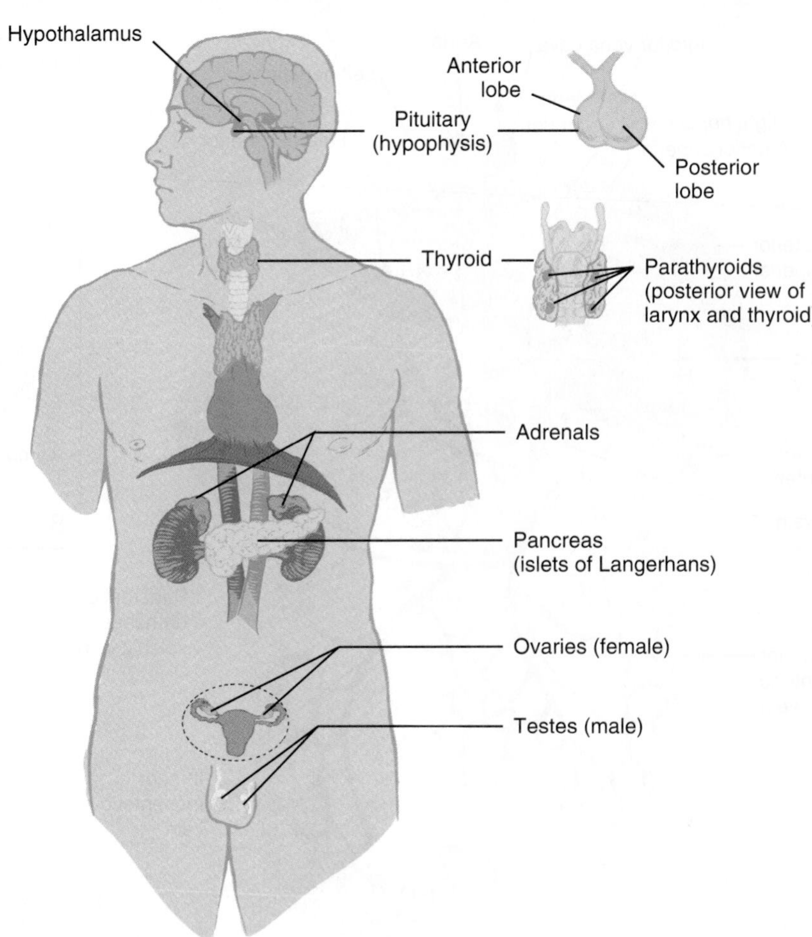

FIGURE U9–2 Organs of the endocrine system.

The hypothalamus lies dorsal to the pituitary gland and regulates secretion of both the anterior and the posterior pituitary hormones. The hypophyseal stalk has two distinct pathways leading from the hypothalamus to the pituitary.

The *neural stalk* contains axons originating in the hypothalamus that terminate in the posterior pituitary. Cell bodies are in the supraoptic and paraventricular nuclei, and axons terminate in the posterior pituitary, where the synaptic terminals secrete hormones, rather than make synaptic connections with another neuron.

The *hypothalamo-hypophyseal portal system* provides a vascular connection between the median eminence of the hypothalamus and the anterior pituitary. Arterial blood enters the capillaries of the hypothalamus. Blood flows through portal vessels in the hypophyseal stalk, before entering a second set of capillaries (sinuses) in the anterior pituitary. Blood then exits the anterior pituitary and joins with other venous drainages. This vascular supply ensures that releasing and inhibiting hormones secreted in the median eminence of the hypothalamus remain concentrated until delivered to the target cells of the anterior pituitary.

The *anterior pituitary* is the end organ for growth hormone and prolactin secretion. The other anterior pituitary hormones act on endocrine target organs to stimulate the release of additional hormones. In the *posterior pituitary* are glia-like cells, which support and nourish the nerve endings. Oxytocin and antidiuretic hormone (ADH) are synthesized in the hypothalamus and transported to the posterior pituitary gland for secretion.

Thyroid and Parathyroid

The thyroid gland is located in the neck, just below the cricoid cartilage, somewhat H-shaped (Fig. U9–4). The right and left lateral lobes lie on either side of the trachea. The lobes are connected by a thin mass of tissue (the *isthmus*), which stretches over the surface of the trachea. Each lobe is composed of irregularly shaped lobules, which consist of a multitude of tiny sacs (follicles) filled with a jelly-like, iodine-containing substance called *colloid* (see *inset,* Fig. U9–4). The main component of colloid is thyroglobulin—the storage form of the hormone thyroxine. The *parathyroid glands* are four small glands near, attached to, or embedded in the thyroid gland.

Endocrine Pancreas

The pancreas (see Fig. U9–2) contains islets of Langerhans, which secrete three hormones that regulate blood glucose: (1) *alpha* cells secrete *glucagons,* (2) *beta* cells secrete *insulin,* and (3) *delta* cells secrete *somatostatin,* identical to the growth hormone inhibitory hormone secreted by the hypothalamus. The close proximity of these

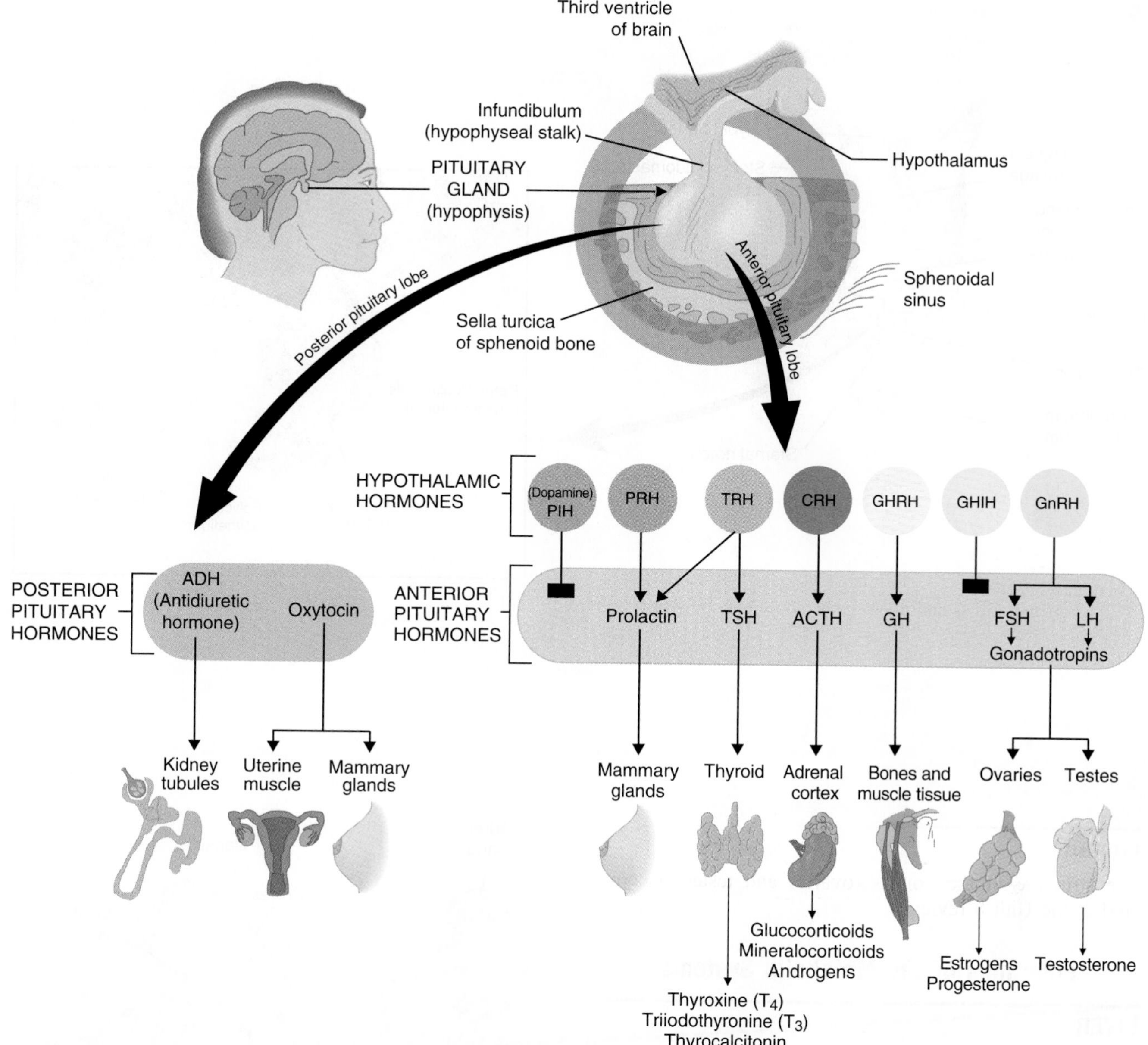

FIGURE U9–3 Hypothalamus, pituitary gland, and target tissues. The pituitary gland is suspended from the hypothalamus by the infundibular or hypophyseal stalk. Hormones released from the hypothalamus travel in a portal vascular system to the anterior pituitary gland, where they stimulate (or inhibit) the release of anterior pituitary hormones. Posterior pituitary hormones are synthesized in the hypothalamus and are released from axons in the posterior pituitary gland.

cells within the islets allows a coordinated paracrine regulation of pancreatic secretion, as insulin inhibits glucagon release, and somatostatin inhibits both insulin and glucagon release.

Adrenal Glands

The adrenal glands are paired endocrine organs situated at the superior poles of the kidneys. The adrenal gland is divided into an outer cortex and an inner medulla (Fig. U9–5). The *cortex* has three zones. The outer *zona glomerulosa* secretes the mineralocorticoids aldosterone and corticosterone. The inner *zona fasciculata* and *zona reticularis* secrete the glucocorticoids cortisol and corticosterone as well as androgen sex hormones. Corticosterone and deoxycorticosterone are secreted in small amounts and exert both glucocorticoid and mineralocorticoid effects. Adrenal cortical hormones are steroids formed from a cholesterol nucleus. Deficits in synthetic enzymes often lead to overproduction of other adrenal hormones. Stimuli that enhance adrenal cortical secretions also cause hypertrophy of the appropriate cortical zones.

The *adrenal medulla* functions as a postganglionic sympathetic nerve, secreting the catecholamines epinephrine and norepinephrine. About 80% of the basal (resting) catecholamine secretion is epinephrine, but this ratio varies with adrenal stimulation.

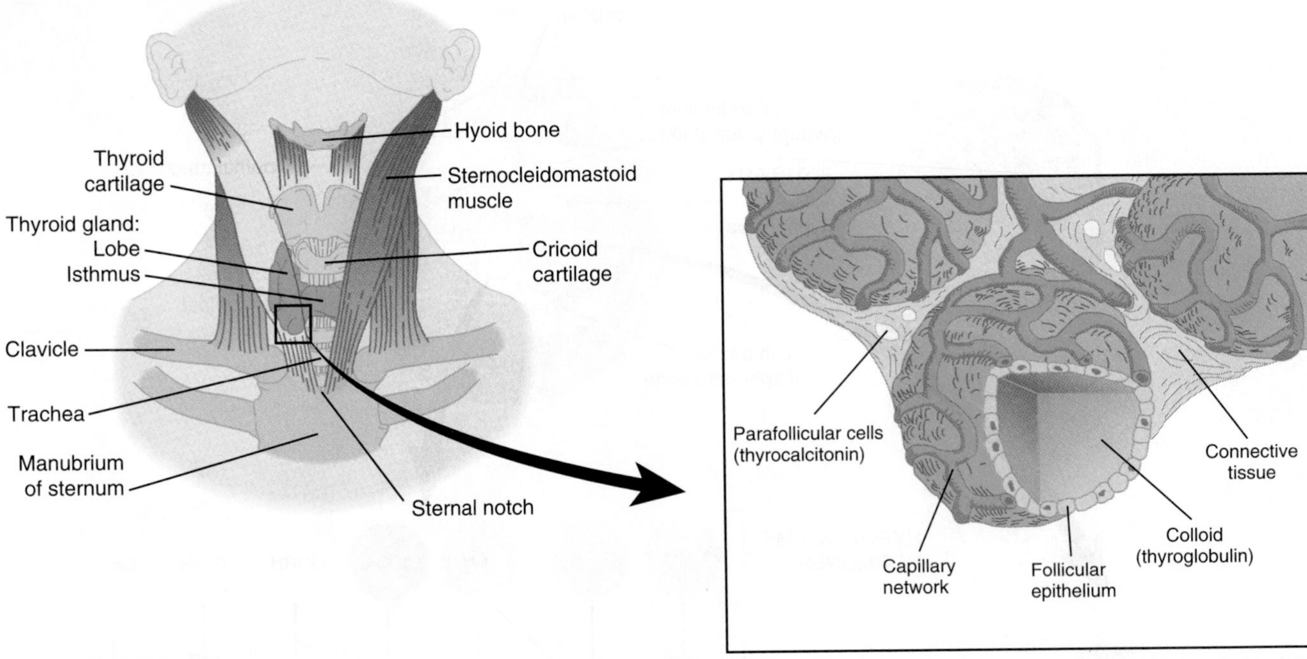

FIGURE U9–4 Gross and microscopic *(inset)* anatomy of the thyroid gland.

Gonads

The structure of the gonads (ovaries and testes) is covered in the Unit 8 review.

Functions of the Metabolic Systems

LIVER

The liver plays a central role in the regulation of metabolic substrates, glucose, and fatty acids. Additionally, hepatic synthesis provides most of the proteins circulating in the plasma.

The liver is the major storage organ for *glycogen,* a polymer of glucose. In addition to storage, the liver converts glucose to glycogen *(glycogenesis),* breaks down glycogen into glucose *(glycogenolysis),* and forms glucose from other sugars (galactose and fructose) or amino acids *(gluconeogenesis).* The regulation of these processes is discussed later.

The major functions of the liver in relation to fat metabolism are as follows:

- Oxidation of fatty acids for energy
- Formation of most lipoproteins
- Synthesis of cholesterol and phospholipids
- Synthesis of fat from proteins and carbohydrates

The liver provides energy from fats by splitting them into glycerol and fatty acids; when the fatty acids are oxidized, tremendous amounts of energy are released.

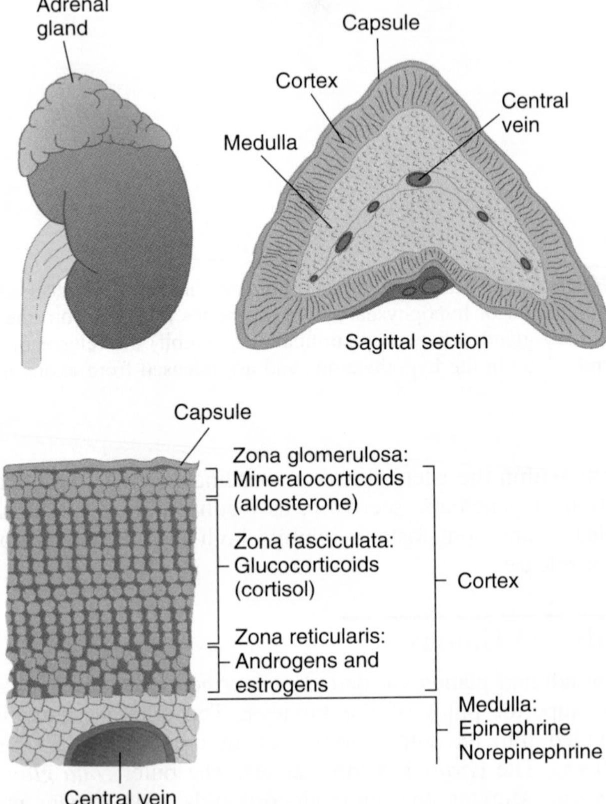

FIGURE U9–5 Gross and microscopic anatomy of the adrenal gland.

Most of the cholesterol synthesized in the liver is converted into bile salts; the remainder is transported in the lipoproteins throughout the body. Phospholipids are also synthesized in the liver and transported in lipoproteins. The cholesterol and phospholipids help form cell membranes and intracellular structures and are involved in cellular function.

The primary functions of the liver in relation to protein metabolism are as follows:

- Deamination of amino acids
- Formation of urea for removal of ammonia from the body
- Formation of plasma proteins
- Biotransformation of hormones, drugs, and other substances

Degradation is the process of excess amino acid catabolism. This process begins in the liver with deamination, the removal of amino groups ($—NH_2$). Ammonia (NH_3), which results from deamination, is converted into urea by the liver and is excreted by the kidneys and intestines. Ammonia can also be formed in the intestines by bacterial action. In severe liver disease or damage, ammonia that is normally converted to urea by the liver accumulates to dangerously high levels in the blood. As a result, a severe toxic state *(hepatic encephalopathy)* develops.

The liver also synthesizes plasma proteins, such as albumin, prothrombin, fibrinogen, and clotting proteins (factors V, VI, VII, IX, and X). Albumin is essential for maintaining plasma oncotic pressure, while the other proteins contribute to blood clotting. Plasma oncotic pressure prevents intravascular fluid from moving out into the extravascular spaces, where it manifests as *ascites* and varying degrees of peripheral edema. Vitamin K, a fat-soluble vitamin, must be present for synthesis of several clotting proteins. Assimilation of vitamin K depends on the presence of bile in the intestine. Gamma globulins are the only plasma proteins not synthesized by the liver.

The liver primarily detoxifies and biotransforms hormones, drugs, and other chemicals. Some substances are deactivated by deamination, hydroxylation, oxidation, or reduction. Through conjugation, other substances become soluble in water, resulting in their excretion through the bile and, therefore, in feces or urine.

Clients with compromised liver function are at high risk for untoward reactions to many medications, all opiates, and many chemicals. The two major problems that result are prolonged action and increased potency of the substance.

ENDOCRINE SYSTEM

Regulation of endocrine secretions is generally by a negative feedback loop, linking the hormone to a response, to another hormone, or to glucose of some other plasma compound. Endocrine agents also have significant trophic effects on the target tissues, with high hormone levels often causing hypertrophy, and inadequate hormone levels causing atrophy, of the target tissues. Regulation of endocrine systems is often integrated with the nervous system. When the distinction between endocrine and nervous systems is blurred, the system is described as the *neuroendocrine system.*

Hypothalamus and Pituitary Gland

The hypothalamus regulates secretion of anterior and posterior pituitary hormones. Five hypothalamic-releasing hormones and two hypothalamic inhibitory hormones regulate secretion of the six anterior pituitary hormones (see Fig. U9–3).

GROWTH HORMONE (SOMATOTROPIN)

The anterior pituitary is the end organ for secretion of growth hormone, which exerts several effects:

- Stimulates growth in almost all body tissues, causing both an increase in cell size *(hypertrophy)* and an increase in cell number *(hyperplasia)*
- Diverts amino acids into protein synthesis *(anabolism)* and decreases protein breakdown *(catabolism)*
- Enhances use of free fatty acids as metabolic substrates, which depletes body fat stores
- Increases plasma glucose levels but protects amino acid pools (see later)

Insulin has an important permissive, or facilitatory, role in growth hormone–mediated growth. It enhances the entry of both glucose and amino acids into cells. Growth hormone exerts some of its effects through an intermediary, the somatomedins, or insulin-like growth factors.

Growth hormone secretion is enhanced by various stressful and normal stimuli, including starvation, chronic protein deficiency, hypoglycemia, low plasma levels of free fatty acids, exercise, and the first hours of sleep. Hypothalamic secretion of growth hormone releasing and inhibitory hormones is the primary regulator of growth hormone release.

PROLACTIN

The hypothalamus is the end organ for prolactin secretion. Hypothalamic control of prolactin is unique, in that the normal control of prolactin release is ıypothalamic prolactin inhibitory hormone. Consequently, interruption of the hypothalamo-hypophyseal portal system increases pituitary prolactin release. Prolactin-releasing hormone is important in the suckling reflex (see review, Unit 8).

ANTIDIURETIC HORMONE AND OXYTOCIN

Nerve endings in the *posterior pituitary* secrete oxytocin and antidiuretic hormone (ADH), also known as *vasopressin.* Oxytocin, formed primarily in the paraventricular nucleus of the hypothalamus, promotes uterine contraction during parturition, causing expression of milk ("letdown") following suckling (see Unit 8). ADH is formed primarily in the supraoptic nucleus and is released by increases in plasma osmolarity or by low blood pressure. Stress and trauma can also promote ADH release. The mechanism of ADH control of water and electrolyte balance is discussed in Unit 7.

Thyroid Gland

Thyroid hormone is a conglomerate of three (T_3) or four (T_4) iodinated tyrosine residues. Tri-iodothyronine (T_3) and thyroxine (T_4) together are called thyroid hormone. Thyroid hormone is lipid-soluble, and 99% of thyroid hormone in the plasma is bound to thyroid-binding globulin. Of the two thyroid hormones, T_3 has the most rapid effect on target tissues, requiring 3 days for peak effect; T_4 (the more common) requires 11 days for peak effect.

Thyroid hormone has several functions:

- Increases metabolism, enhancing carbohydrate consumption and increasing the size and density of mitochondria.
- Assists in acclimatization to cold environments by increasing metabolic rate (heat production is a by-product of metabolism)
- Increases DNA translation and transcription
- Increases protein synthesis but also has protein catabolic effects
- Promotes growth and is required for normal growth in children.

Finally, thyroid hormone has a permissive effect to increase other endocrine secretions.

Thyroid hormone is formed in epithelium-lined follicles that contain the glycoprotein thyroglobulin. Thyroglobulin can contain five to six thyroid hormone molecules. Dietary iodine is required for thyroid hormone synthesis. Iodine is oxidized within the follicles, and binds a tyrosine residue (T_1) of thyroglobulin. Iodinated tyrosines are coupled while still part of the thyroglobulin molecule, forming T_3 and T_4. The mature hormone is released by digestion of thyroglobulin, with recycling of unused iodine, T_1, and T_2.

Release of thyroid hormone is regulated by negative feedback by T_4 on thyroid-stimulating hormone (TSH) release at the anterior pituitary. TSH stimulates proteolysis of thyroglobulin, releasing T_3 and T_4. TSH also stimulates iodine uptake by the thyroid for new thyroid hormone synthesis, increasing the activity of thyroid gland cells and increasing thyroid hormone synthesis. TSH release is controlled by the hypothalamic tripeptide thyrotropin-releasing hormone (TRH). Cold exposure is a potent stimulus for TRH release, but the feedback loop for the effect of temperature on TRH is not yet established.

Parathyroid Glands

The endocrine secretion of the parathyroid glands is the polypeptide parathyroid hormone (PTH). A fall in serum calcium levels causes release of PTH: PTH acts on bone, GI tract, and kidneys to increase circulating plasma calcium levels, an action coordinated with vitamin D and calcitonin (see later).

Endocrine Pancreas

The islets of Langerhans of the pancreas secrete three hormones that regulate blood glucose: (1) insulin, (2) glucagon, and (3) somatostatin.

Insulin

Insulin is a small protein derived successively from a preprohormone and a prohormone. Insulin circulates as a free hormone, has a short plasma half-life of about 6 minutes, and is cleared from the plasma primarily by the liver and kidneys. Insulin binds to receptors on the surface of target tissues and enhances glucose transport across the membrane. Insulin decreases blood glucose by enhancing uptake, use, and storage of glucose in hepatic, muscle, and adipose tissues (see later). Insulin enhances amino acid transport into cells; it acts synergistically with growth hormone to promote cell hypertrophy and hyperplasia.

Note that the brain is refractory to insulin and must use glucose for a metabolic substrate. Because the brain glucose transporter has a much higher glucose affinity than the insulin-sensitive transporter, only a severe decline in the blood glucose level can lead to hypoglycemic shock.

Insulin is released after ingestion and absorption of carbohydrates. The initial phase, from release of stored insulin, peaks in 5 minutes. A delayed phase, from synthesis of new insulin, persists until blood glucose returns to fasting levels. The ability of insulin to control plasma glucose levels is the basis of the glucose tolerance test (GTT). In the absence of insulin, fats are used as metabolic substrates. The incomplete oxidation of fatty acids results in the ketoacidosis that is characteristic of untreated diabetes mellitus. The lack of insulin elevates blood glucose, causing an osmotic diuresis (see Unit 7 review). Finally, the lack of insulin promotes protein catabolism and inhibits growth.

Glucagon

Glucagon is an extremely potent hormone that is released when blood glucose levels drop below 90 mg/dl. Glucagon acts on the liver to elevate plasma glucose, an action opposite that of insulin (see later). The second messenger for glucagon is cyclic adenosine monophosphate (cAMP); it allows excessively high glucagon levels to affect other tissues (enhancing cardiac contractility, enhancing bile secretion, and inhibiting gastric acid secretion). Protein ingestion enhances glucagon release as well as insulin release. This simultaneous secretion of insulin and glucagon allow cells to use and store glucose without severely decreasing plasma glucose levels. Glucagon is also released during exercise and helps prevent hypoglycemia despite enhanced glucose use by muscle.

Somatostatin

Somatostatin is a small polypeptide with a short (2-minute) half-life; it has many inhibitory actions. Somatostatin is released after ingestion of a meal and inhibits release of both insulin and glucagon. The net action of somatostatin is to delay nutrient absorption by the GI tract, thus prolonging the duration of intestinal food absorption after a meal.

Adrenal Glands

Adrenal Cortex

Aldosterone. The primary mineralocorticoid secreted by the adrenal cortex is aldosterone. About 50% of aldosterone is free in the plasma; the remainder is bound. Aldosterone is degraded in the liver and is excreted in the urine and feces as a glucuronide or sulfate. Infusion of aldosterone causes a drop in plasma potassium levels by increasing renal excretion of potassium. Plasma potassium concentration is the primary regulator of aldosterone release through a negative feedback control mechanism. Angiotensin II can also promote aldosterone synthesis and release, and adrenocorticotropic hormone (ACTH) has a permissive role in aldosterone production and secretion.

Cortisol. The primary glucocorticoid secreted by the adrenal cortex is cortisol. Following secretion, 94% of cortisol is bound in the plasma to transcortin, a cortisol-binding globulin, and 6% is free. Cortisol is degraded in the liver and is excreted in the urine and feces as a glucuronide or sulfate. Cortisol is a potent metabolic regulatory hormone, increasing plasma glucose and promoting use of alternate metabolic substrates for energy (see later). Cortisol stimulates appetite, which leads to central deposition of fat in some central adipose tissues despite the use of fat from peripheral tissues (see clinical description of Cushing's syndrome). Cortisol's metabolic changes assist the transition to nonglucose support of metabolism in starvation.

Cortisol release is regulated by a hypothalamus-pituitary-adrenal cascade. The hypothalamus secretes corticotropin-releasing hormone (CRH), which is carried by the hypothalamo-hypophyseal portal system to the anterior pituitary gland, where it stimulates ACTH release. ACTH travels in the blood to the adrenal gland, where it promotes conversion of cholesterol to pregnenolone, the rate-limiting step in adrenal glucocorticoid and androgen secretion. Because of a common synthetic pathway, pituitary ACTH also stimulates adrenal androgen production.

ACTH release coincides with the release of other compounds formed from the same pre-prohormone. These include (1) melanocyte-stimulating hormone (which stimulates pigment production in epidermal cells), (2) beta-lipotropin (which may stimulate aldosterone release), and (3) the opiate beta-endorphin.

Cortisol is generally described as a stress hormone. Painful stimuli promote release of CRH from the hypothalamus. Emotional stress generated in the limbic system also promotes hypothalamic release of CRH. Cortisol has significant anti-inflammatory effects, retarding the development and enhancing the resolution of the inflammatory response. Glucocorticoid secretion exhibits a strong diurnal rhythm, found to be highest in the early morning and lowest in the late evening.

Adrenal Medulla

The adrenal medulla secretes the catecholamines epinephrine and norepinephrine, whose actions mimic those of the sympathetic nervous system but have a longer duration. Epinephrine has strong beta-adrenergic effects and is a potent stimulator of heart rate and contractility. Epinephrine has strong metabolic effects and increases metabolic rate by up to 100%. These effects include increasing metabolic substrates in the plasma by lipolysis and glycogenolysis (see later).

Gonads

The sex hormones have important trophic and metabolic effects. The synthetic pathways for estrogens and androgens share many common precursors with each other and with the adrenal cortical steroids. Consequently, sex hormones originate predominantly from the gonads but are secreted in lower amounts from the adrenal glands.

Androgens, primarily testosterone, have a potent anabolic action. Testosterone is controlled by the hypothalamic-pituitary axis, and gonadotropin-releasing hormone (GnRH) and luteinizing hormone (LH) act on the Leydig cells of the testes to promote testosterone synthesis and release. The reproductive significance of testosterone is discussed in Unit 8. A secondary effect of testosterone is to promote protein synthesis as well as the musculoskeletal growth that accompanies puberty.

In the female, LH also stimulates androgen production in the ovarian thecal cells, but the aromatase of the ovarian granulose cells converts the androgens into the estrogen estradiol. The puberty-related increase in musculoskeletal growth and onset of menstruation are a result of increases in the cyclic release of estrogen and progesterone (see Unit 8).

Metabolic Substrates

Plasma Glucose

Glucose is the primary metabolic substrate for the body. The plasma glucose level is normally about 100 mg/dL in both the fed and fasted states. Glucose entry into most cells is insulin-dependent. The notable exception is in the brain; cerebral glucose utilization is independent of insulin and requires a plasma glucose level of only 60 mg/dL—levels below this will disrupt brain function.

Plasma glucose represents the balance between glucose absorption from the diet, movement into and out of storage pools, and utilization by the tissues. Glucose storage pools include glycogen, the glycerol component of fat, and amino acids. Although only insulin acts to decrease plasma glucose levels, the hormones glucagon, cortisol, growth hormone, and epinephrine all can elevate plasma glucose levels. This multiple endocrine control allows protection of one or more glucose storage pools (Fig. U9–6). For example, glucagon mobilizes all storage pools, resulting in increased plasma glucose. Growth hormone prevents gluconeogenesis but increases glucose by the other mechanisms. Cortisol preserves glycogen and fat stores in the center of the body but mobilizes all other glucose pools, including gluconeogenesis. Epinephrine mobilizes fat and glycogen pools.

After a meal, excess plasma glucose is moved into storage, facilitated by insulin. During periods of fasting, glucose is moved from the storage pools, first from glycogen, then from fats, and—if the fast is sufficiently long—from the amino acid pools.

Plasma Amino Acids

Plasma amino acid levels are not controlled by a tight negative feedback mechanism. Ingestion of a protein-rich meal, however, increases both insulin and growth hormone levels. Growth hormone alone enhances cellular uptake of amino acids and preserves amino acid stores (by blocking gluconeogenesis) when insulin is not elevated. When insulin is elevated, the combined action of growth hormone and insulin greatly enhances uptake of amino acids.

Plasma Free Fatty Acids

Free fatty acids are the baseline metabolic substrate and are used unless insulin shifts metabolism to glucose as a metabolic fuel. The heart in particular can oxidize free

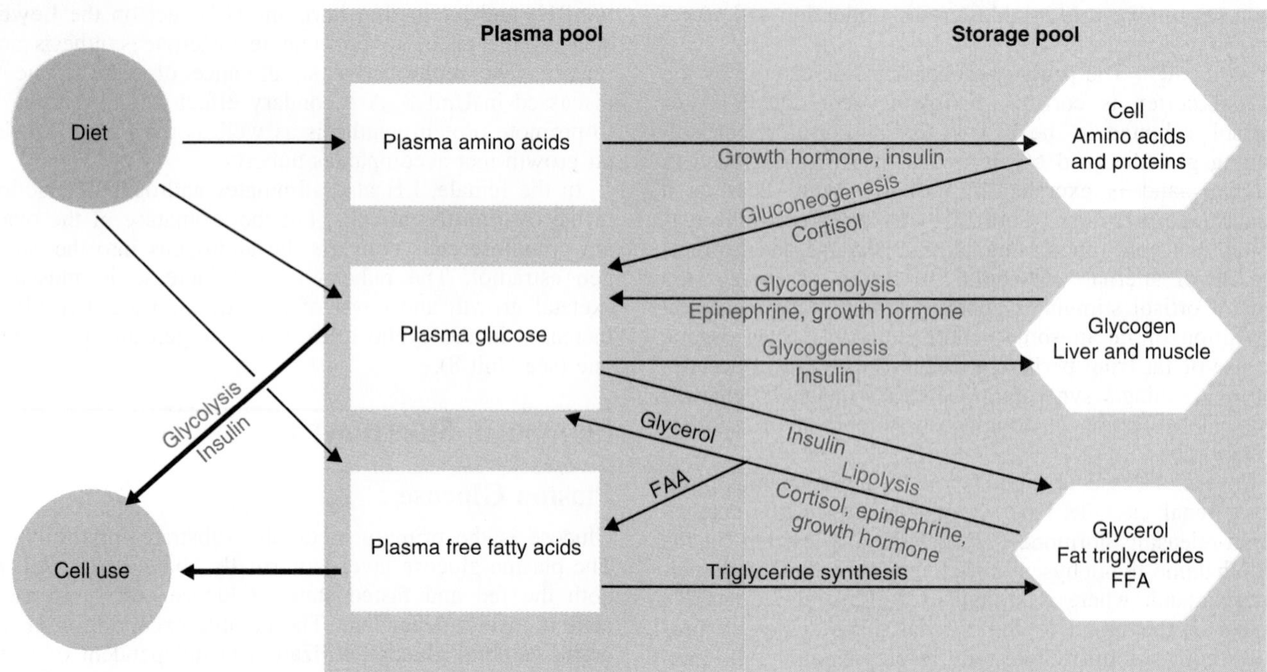

FIGURE U9–6 Regulation of metabolic substrates. Cells consume glucose or fatty acids to support metabolism. Plasma glucose is regulated by multiple endocrine mechanisms, which act primarily on the movement into and out of storage pools. Glucose is stored if the plasma glucose level is above 110 mg/dL; glucose is mobilized from storage pools if the plasma glucose level is below 90 mg/dL. FFA, free fatty acid.

fatty acids and thus is not as dependent on glucose as a metabolic substrate as the remainder of the body is. In the American diet, food is ingested with sufficient frequency that insulin levels are high, and glucose is normally used as the metabolic fuel. When metabolized, fatty acids are incompletely oxidized, however, with ketone bodies produced as a metabolic by-product.

Plasma levels of free fatty acids are not controlled by a tight negative feedback mechanism. A drop in plasma glucose levels, however, causes the release of epinephrine, cortisol, and growth hormone, all of which promote lipolysis. This results in the movement of fatty acids from the storage pool in fat cells into the plasma pool, providing an alternative substrate for metabolism when glucose availability is limited.

Plasma Calcium

The plasma calcium level (Ca^{2+}) is tightly regulated around 9.4 mg/dl, with a normal range of 9 to 10 mg/dl. About 40% of plasma Ca^{2+} is tightly bound to plasma proteins, and an additional 10% is combined in non-ionized salts with citrate and phosphate. About 5 mg/dl (50%) of plasma Ca^{2+} is free.

More than 99% of calcium within the body is stored in bone, most of it combined with phosphate in hydroxyapatite crystals. Regulation of plasma calcium levels involves balancing dietary absorption, renal excretion, and exchange between the plasma and storage areas. PTH and Vitamin D_3 are the major regulators of plasma calcium, with a minor role for the hormone calcitonin.

Infusion of PTH results in elevated plasma calcium levels and decreased plasma phosphate levels. The increase in plasma calcium occurs by enhancing dietary calcium absorption (via vitamin D_3), by decreasing renal calcium excretion, and by mobilizing calcium from the bone storage pools. Plasma calcium is the primary regulator of PTH release. PTH synthesis and release are stimulated by a drop in plasma calcium and helps regulate calcium levels during pregnancy and lactation.

Dietary absorption of calcium requires activated vitamin D. Vitamin D can be absorbed from the diet or synthesized through ultraviolet (sun) light action on 7-dehydrocholesterol. Vitamin D is then converted successively in liver and kidney to 1-25-hydroxcholecalciferol, the active form.

Calcitonin is a polypeptide secreted by the parafollicular C cells of the thyroid gland. While infusion of calcitonin decreases the plasma calcium concentration, its role in regulating plasma calcium levels is minor.

Alterations in plasma calcium levels produce physiologic changes. Hypocalcemia increases neuronal excitability. Motor neurons exhibit spontaneous depolarizations, leading to tetanic muscular contractions. The hand is particularly susceptible, resulting in carpopedal spasm. Hypercalcemia depresses neuronal and muscle activity.

EFFECTS OF AGING

With aging, the functions of the liver, biliary system, and exocrine pancreas all begin to deteriorate. In the liver, the number and size of hepatic cells is reduced, leading to a decreased weight and mass. Fibrotic tissue also increases, leading to a decrease in protein synthesis, liver enzymes, and cholesterol synthesis. The decrease in enzyme activity diminishes the liver's ability to detoxify drugs and increases the risk of toxic levels of a variety of medications in older adults.

The pancreas is also affected by the process of aging, with calcification of the pancreatic vessels, and by changes in the size of the ducts through distention and dilation. These changes lead to decreased production of lipase, resulting in reduced fat absorption and digestion. Older people also may experience a decreased absorption of fat-soluble vitamins and an increase of fat excreted through the feces (steatorrhea).

CONCLUSIONS

Metabolic regulation is a complex body function, involving the gastrointestinal tract, liver, muscle, and fat tissues. The multiple endocrine systems that regulate the availability of metabolic fuels reflect the essential role of glucose and fatty acids in survival. The process is complicated by the fact that the body must cope both with periods of excess nutrients (after a meal) and with prolonged fasting.

BIBLIOGRAPHY

1. Guyton, A. C., & Hall, J. (1996). *Textbook of medical physiology* (9th ed.). Philadelphia: W. B. Saunders.
2. Kacsoh, B. (2000). *Endocrine physiology.* New York: McGraw-Hill.
3. McPhee, S. J., et al. (2000). *Pathophysiology of disease* (3rd ed.) New York: McGraw-Hill.
4. Silverthorn, D. (1998). *Human physiology.* Upper Saddle River, NJ: Prentice-Hall.

CHAPTER 42

Assessment of the Endocrine and Metabolic Systems

Dianne Smolen

Clients with endocrine or metabolic system disorders may have specific complaints such as nausea, diarrhea, or fatigue. These same clients may also have vague, intermittent, generalized manifestations. Because of the different functions of the endocrine glands and the organs of metabolism, there is no single, uniform assessment for clients with endocrine or metabolic disorders. Assessment of clients with such disorders includes a complete health history, physical examination, and diagnostic tests. It is important to perform a complete assessment and analyze the data related to the client's current and past health history.

HISTORY

During the health history interview, help the client place the recalled experiences and manifestations in a time sequence. Linking events and clinical manifestations aids the diagnostic process.

■ BIOGRAPHICAL AND DEMOGRAPHIC DATA

Note biographical and demographic data, such as the client's age, sex, ethnic background, and geographical residence. Some disorders, such as gallbladder disease, diabetes mellitus, and hepatitis, are associated with age or sex as well as where a person lives. For example, as a person ages, fewer hormones and metabolic secretions may be produced or their effect on target organs may diminish.

■ CURRENT HEALTH

Chief Complaint

Thorough investigation of the client's chief complaint is necessary for accurate assessment. Like gastrointestinal manifestations, the manifestations of endocrine and metabolic disorders may be ambiguous with a puzzling origin. Indicate the onset, duration, intensity, and characteristics of manifestations and any alterations in growth patterns, especially changes in weight, height, or hand, foot, or head size.

Symptom Analysis

For purposes of discussion, common manifestations related to the endocrine and metabolic systems are grouped by body system as follows (see Chapter 9):

GASTROINTESTINAL MANIFESTATIONS

- An enlarged, red tongue (*glossitis*)? May be present in clients with diabetes mellitus.
- Weight gain or loss or changes in appetite? These manifestations may be an indication of an endocrine or metabolic disorder. For example, increased eating but loss of weight may indicate hyperthyroidism; gaining weight may suggest hypothyroidism. Excessive appetite (*polyphagia*) may be indicative of diabetes mellitus.
- Excessive thirst (*polydipsia*)? May indicate diabetes mellitus.
- Abdominal pain? Right upper quadrant discomfort suggests gallbladder or liver disorders.
- Nausea or vomiting? Occurs in 70% of clients with pancreatitis.
- Anorexia? Especially prevalent in liver disorders.
- Fatty food intolerance? May be indicative of pancreatic or biliary tract disease.
- Excessive eructation (belching or *aerophagia*)? Suggests gallbladder disease. Heartburn (*pyrosis*)? May be a manifestation of cholecystitis or refluxed acid or bile.
- Disturbed bowel pattern, such as diarrhea (dark-colored, tarry stools)? May be caused by hyperthyroidism or a biliary tract problem.
- Constipation? May indicate hypothyroidism or a biliary disorder. Clay-colored stools or *acholic* (without bilirubin) stools? May occur briefly in viral hepatitis; common in obstructive jaundice.
- Fatty, foul-smelling stools (*steatorrhea*)? May occur with chronic pancreatitis or after gastric surgery; partially the result of rapid gastric emptying, which prevents adequate mixing with pancreatic and biliary secretions.

NEUROLOGIC MANIFESTATIONS

- Weakness? Generalized or localized? May indicate late manifestations of diabetes mellitus.

- Mild depression? May be a manifestation of pancreatic cancer or an endocrine disorder.
- Changes in mental status or mood (increased irritability)? Extreme alterations in consciousness, such as coma, may occur in uncontrolled diabetes mellitus.
- Emotional lability? Alterations in consciousness? These manifestations may indicate liver or endocrine disorders.
- Drowsiness? A change in mental status and neurologic manifestations can signal the development of hepatic encephalopathy or uncontrolled diabetes mellitus.
- Pain? If radiating to the back, it can be a manifestation of a pancreatic, gallbladder, or biliary tract disorder.
- Tremors? If uncontrolled, can indicate hyperthyroidism.
- Loss of sensation, especially in hands or feet? Suggests diabetes mellitus.

GENITOURINARY AND REPRODUCTIVE MANIFESTATIONS

- Dark yellow or tea-colored urine? Indicates impaired excretion of bilirubin caused by hepatocellular disease.
- Frequent urination (*polyuria*)? May be indicative of diabetes mellitus.
- Menstrual cycle irregularities (including amenorrhea)? Loss of libido? Loss or premature development of secondary sex characteristics? Impotence or infertility? These sexual changes are characteristics of endocrine disorders.
- Renal problems? Calcium stone formation may be caused by hyperparathyroidism (because calcium is resorbed from bone).

INTEGUMENTARY MANIFESTATIONS AND CHANGES IN APPEARANCE

- Red, noninflammatory blisters and erosions on dorsum (back) of hands? Commonly demonstrated in clients infected with hepatitis C virus.
- Jaundiced skin? Causes include viral hepatitis, cirrhosis, and obstructive or cholestatic liver disease.
- Unexplained puncture holes? May be the route of entry for hepatitis (type B or C) or other pathogens.
- Spider angiomas? Petechiae? Dilated abdominal veins? May indicate hepatic cirrhosis.
- Skin lesions that do not heal? May indicate pancreatic dysfunction (see Chapter 45).
- Hyperpigmentation or hypopigmentation? Addison's disease, caused by chronic adrenocortical insufficiency, causes excessive pigmentation of skin; areas of hypopigmentation (*vitiligo*) may indicate other endocrine disorders.
- Hard, nonpitting edema? Occurs in adult hypothyroidism (*myxedema*).
- Delayed healing? May indicate diabetes mellitus.
- Changes in hands, head, feet, and face? Acromegaly produces enlargement of the head, hands, and feet and coarsening of facial features. Adrenocortical hyperfunction (Cushing's syndrome)? Is manifested in moon facies, thin extremities, and truncal obesity.
- Growth delayed? Stunted (*dwarfism*)? Excessive (*gigantism*)? Inappropriate (*acromegaly*)? All may indicate a pituitary or other type of endocrine disorder.
- Changes in hair? Distribution, amount, or texture? Excessive hair (*hirsutism*) may indicate ovarian or adrenocortical disorders; loss of pubic and ancillary hair may indicate a pituitary problem; dry, brittle hair may indicate hypothyroidism; and soft, silky hair may indicate hyperthyroidism.

OPHTHALMIC MANIFESTATIONS

- Bulging eyes (*exophthalmos*)? Characteristic of hyperthyroidism.
- Diminished or blurred vision? Visual problems may be caused by diabetes mellitus; visual loss may be caused by a pituitary tumor.

CARDIOVASCULAR MANIFESTATIONS

- Nosebleeds or bruising easily? Hemorrhoids? *Ascites* (fluid accumulation in peritoneal cavity)? Edema of limbs? All may be indicative of a hepatic disorder in which fluid overload results from the liver's improper functioning and metabolism of hormones, such as aldosterone and antidiuretic hormone (ADH).
- Changes in vital signs? Hyperthyroidism may cause elevation of body temperature and pulse rate.
- Hypertension? May be caused by an adrenal tumor (e.g., pheochromocytoma). Insufficient secretion of ADH from the pituitary gland can cause dehydration; oversecretion can cause excessive retention of body water.
- Increased heart rate and flushing? May occur in hyperthyroidism and in pheochromocytoma.
- Kussmaul's respiration (deep, rapid breathing)? A direct result of diabetic ketoacidosis.

OTHER MANIFESTATIONS

- Yellow sclerae? Suggests biliary obstruction.
- Fever? May indicate an acute gallbladder, pancreas, or liver problem.
- Intolerance of alcohol or medications? Fatigue? Malaise? All occur with hepatitis or endocrine disorders.
- Dehydration? May indicate insufficient levels of ADH.
- Bone or joint pain? Hyperparathyroidism may cause calcium to be reabsorbed from bone and contribute to bone pain, fracture, or both. Adrenal insufficiency (Cushing's syndrome) may produce a rapid breakdown of bone.
- Muscle cramps? Tetany? May result from inadequate secretion of parathyroid hormone (PTH).

■ PAST HEALTH HISTORY

Childhood and Infectious Diseases

Ask the client and family members about any episodes of endocrine or metabolic disorders the client may have experienced as a child or an adolescent. For example, did the client have any growth patterns that were different from those of other members of the family? Did these changes in body size occur after physical maturation?

Have there been any changes in head circumference or size of the hands or feet? For instance, has the client needed to buy hats, gloves, rings, or shoes in a larger size?

Ask the client about changes in the amount and distribution of hair, such as increased facial hair (women), decreased hair (men), or changes in pubic or axillary hair (both men and women). Has the client had any episodes of excessive thirst and urination? In addition, ask female clients about their menstrual history, pregnancies, or fertility problems.

Immunization Status

Inquire about the client's immunization status. Did the client receive the routine childhood vaccinations (see Chapter 9)? Were the vaccinations given when the client was an infant or later in life? Was a tetanus shot received recently? Has the client been immunized against hepatitis A or B or ever received post-exposure immunization for hepatitis A?

Major Illnesses, Hospitalizations, and Operations

Ask the client to identify any illnesses or injuries to the head or neck. Is there a history of head trauma, such as a forceful blow? Trauma can lead to hypopituitarism. Has the client been hospitalized for surgery to the head or neck? Does the client have a history of surgery, chemotherapy, or radiation therapy to the head or neck? Ask about diagnosis or treatment for related disorders, such as primary brain or spinal cord tumors, metastatic tumors, meningitis, brain infarctions, diabetes mellitus, diabetes insipidus, hypertension, and goiter.

Have the client describe any past problems with jaundice, hepatitis, abdominal pain, gallbladder disease, anemia, or changes in bowel elimination, such as diarrhea, clay-colored stools, or melena. Has the client ever been hospitalized for any of these disorders or ever had surgery of the liver or gallbladder?

Have diagnostic procedures, such as a gallbladder x-ray study, liver biopsy, or ultrasound examination of the gallbladder ever been performed? Has the client ever received a transfusion of blood or blood products?

Procedures Causing Skin or Membrane Disruption

Has the client had recent blood tests, transfusions of blood products, dental procedures, ear or other body piercing, tattooing, or any intravenous injection with a potentially contaminated needle? Note such procedures in an assessment, because breaks in the skin may be the route of entry for hepatitis virus (type B or C) or other pathogens.

Medications

Ask specifically about the use of hormones and steroids, including name, dose, and duration of use. Does the client have a history of taking anabolic steroids? Ask specifically about medications the client is currently taking or has taken previously, including over-the-counter drugs. Many drugs and chemicals are potentially hepatotoxic, such as alcohol, gold compounds, mercury, phosphorus, anabolic steroids, acetaminophen, isoniazid, halothane, sulfonamides, arsenic, thiazide diuretics, zidovudine (azidothymidine [AZT]), and anticancer drugs, such as methotrexate. Other medications to ask about are oral contraceptives, anesthetic agents, and antipsychotic agents.

Ask about the use of alternative therapies, such as herbal medicines. Herbal medicines used in the treatment of non–insulin-dependent diabetes include aloe vera juice, beans (*Phaseolus* species), bitter gourd, karela (*Momordica charantia*), black tea (*Camellia sinensis*), fenugreek (*Trigonella foenum-graecum*), gumar (*Gymnema sylvestre*), macadamia nut, and Madagascar periwinkle (*Catharanthus roseus*). Effects of these herbs include lowering of blood pressure (fenugreek), a boosting of insulin production (gumar), and increased use of available insulin (black tea).

Kelp (*Fucus vesiculosus*) may help with weight loss in hypothyroid disorders. Milk thistle (*Silybum marianum*) is used for treatment and prophylaxis of chronic hepatotoxicity, inflammatory liver disorders, and certain types of cirrhosis.

Allergies

Ask the client about known allergies to food or medications. Specifically ask about reactions to iodine. Iodine is contained in contrast media used in some diagnostic studies of the metabolic system.

■ FAMILY HEALTH HISTORY

When assessing a client with an endocrine or metabolic disorder, inquire about the family history. A number of endocrine disorders are inherited or tend to run in families. Has any family member had problems similar to those of the client? Disorders to inquire about include growth and development problems, obesity, goiter, hypothyroidism or hyperthyroidism, hypertension, low blood pressure (hypotension), diabetes mellitus, diabetes insipidus, autoimmune diseases (Addison's disease), and problems with the adrenal glands (e.g., pheochromocytoma).

Ask the client whether any family members have had cancer (especially of the bowel, liver, or pancreas), jaundice, bleeding disorders, hepatitis, nutritional deficiencies, alcoholism, obesity, pancreatic disease, or gallbladder disease. A history of these disorders in family members increases the risk of their development in the client.

■ PSYCHOSOCIAL HISTORY

Assessment of the psychosocial history and lifestyle patterns provides data about the client's physical and psychological status. Inquire about the client's occupation, environment, and habits.

Occupation, Geographical Location, and Environment

Because *stress* can increase the severity of disorders such as diabetes mellitus, ask about the client's stress tolerance and coping patterns. Stress can be either *physiologic* (caused by illness) or *emotional*. Ask about job-related stressors, such as amount of time spent on the job both in the work setting and at home. Do strained interpersonal relationships at work contribute to increased stress levels? Does the client have opportunities to retreat from the workplace and to engage in recreational activities?

Ask about the home environment and family interpersonal relationships and obligations. What support systems are available to the client? Does the client report effective current coping strategies? If possible, ask family members to corroborate or to help identify behavior changes.

Ask about the client's occupation and work environment. Are there any factors that are known to cause liver damage? For example, heavy metals such as mercury and lead, anesthetic agents such as nitrous oxide, and chemicals such as carbon tetrachloride and certain pesticides are known hepatotoxins. Does the client engage in activities that increase the risk of exposure to substances that cause hepatitis or pancreatitis? Ask about the following:

- Any close contact with hazardous waste
- Travel in areas where hepatitis or pancreatitis is endemic
- Eating raw or steamed shellfish (oysters, clams, scallops) from polluted water
- Swimming or bathing in polluted water
- Any known contact with hepatitis-infected animals or people
- Ingestion of mushrooms that have not been purchased in a store

Exercise, Nutrition, and Habits

When assessing the client for endocrine or metabolic disorders, also consider other aspects of lifestyle and coping. Ask the client about exercise, food intake, sleep and rest patterns and about the use of alcohol, illicit drugs, or tobacco products. Ask about usual patterns as well as any alteration in patterns. Related to food intake, investigate the following:

- Food preferences
- Daily intake of proteins, carbohydrates, fats, and sodium
- Changes in eating patterns, including onset of changes
- Meal preparation (by whom, style of preparation)
- Recent development of food intolerances

In the case of a chronic condition such as diabetes mellitus, careful control is crucial to prevent complications. Diet and physical activity are important in the management of both type 1 and type 2 diabetes (see Chapter 45). One type, non–insulin-dependent diabetes mellitus, can often be prevented through diet and physical activity. According to *Healthy People 2000*, the goal of the Public Health Service is to "reduce diabetes-related deaths to no more than 34 per 100,000 people (an 11% decrease)."[12] You have an important role in helping clients adjust to chronic conditions such as diabetes mellitus or liver disease by assisting them to adopt health-seeking behaviors related to diet, exercise, and necessary medication.

Carefully explore the client's use of alcohol and other mind-altering substances. Pay attention to alcohol use patterns, because alcoholism often accompanies liver and pancreatic disease causing fatty infiltration of the liver.

Be alert to whether the client provides confusing or conflicting data. Is the client's behavior altered in any way as the assessment proceeds? For example, does the client become angry, silent, or tearful? If significant others are present, do they corroborate the client's account? The client who does not acknowledge a substance abuse problem may not provide reliable information about usage. The client who takes illicit drugs may be unwilling to describe drug use patterns. If you suspect that the client's history is unreliable, ask significant others to provide additional information. (Chapter 24 discusses alcoholism and other drug use.)

■ REVIEW OF SYSTEMS

If an endocrine or metabolic disorder is suspected, a careful review of systems (ROS) is important because endocrine and metabolic disorders can affect multiple systems. During this review, ask about the gastrointestinal, genitourinary, integumentary, cardiovascular, and neurologic systems and mental status (see Chief Complaint and Symptom Analysis). Specifically, inquire about jaundice, pruritus (itching), abdominal swelling indicating edema or ascites (fluid-filled abdomen), dark-colored urine, clay-colored stools, bleeding tendencies (purpura), spider angiomas (spider nevi or telangiectasia), fatigue, excessive thirst, excessive urination, and weight loss or weight gain. Detailed questions for the review of systems may be found in Chapter 9, Box 9–2.

PHYSICAL EXAMINATION

Physical assessment of endocrine or metabolic (liver, biliary, or pancreatic) dysfunction involves careful examination of the entire body and is integrated throughout the interaction with the client. Specifically, the assessment covers general health and nutritional status along with the skin, head, neck, thorax, abdomen, upper and lower extremities, and genitalia. Examine all body systems in a systematic manner from head to toe (see Chapter 10) using inspection, auscultation, percussion, and palpation.

Before the examination, ask the client to point to any painful area; examine that area last. As stated earlier, hepatic or biliary pain is often located in the right upper quadrant (Fig. 42–1). Pain that is dull and difficult to localize or describe may arise from an organ (viscera). Somatic pain is sharp, piercing, and easy to localize, and it arises from nerve endings in the peritoneum.

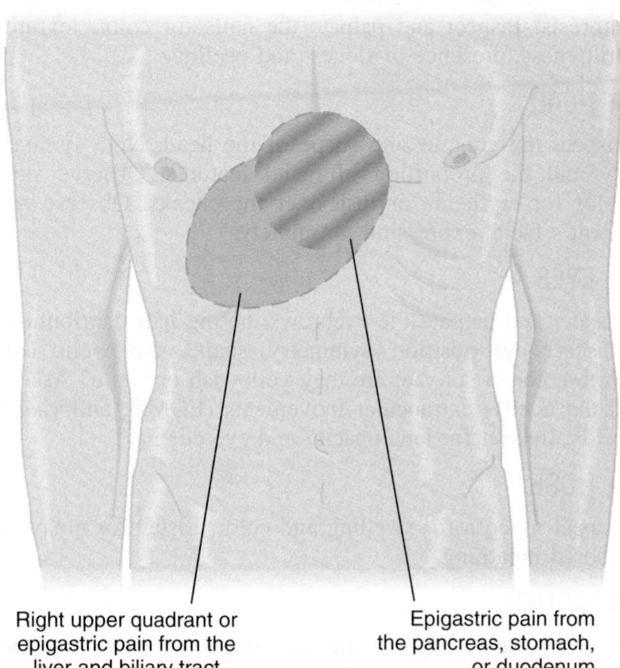

FIGURE 42–1 Location of abdominal pain with hepatic, biliary, or pancreatic disorders.

■ GENERAL APPEARANCE AND NUTRITIONAL STATUS

Begin by assessing the client's general appearance and health status. Is the client alert and responding appropriately to questions? Observe the client's mood, level of consciousness (orientation, alertness), verbal and nonverbal behavior, memory, affect, and speech patterns. Note any anxiety or nervousness, depression, apathy, or anger.

Does the client appear acutely or chronically ill? Question the client's use of alcohol and other substances. Because handwriting deteriorates with diminishing liver function, obtain a handwriting sample for subsequent comparison should the client have progressive hepatocellular damage (see Chapter 47).

Assess nutritional status. Weigh the client, and determine the amount of subcutaneous fat and muscular development. Obesity may accompany gallbladder disease. Ask whether the client has a pattern of right upper quadrant pain after eating certain high-fat foods (e.g., nuts, chocolate). Clients with a history of substance abuse or cirrhosis may be malnourished. Observe the client's state of dress, growth and development, and body size. Chapter 28 describes the assessment of nutrition.

■ VITAL SIGNS

Measure and assess vital signs. Temperature is elevated in hyperthyroidism or may be low-normal or below normal in hypothyroidism. Observe respirations for altered rate and rhythm. Blood pressure alterations include hypotension, hypertension, widening pulse pressure, and orthostatic changes in the pulse rate.

■ INTEGUMENT

Observe hair texture and distribution over body surfaces. Note brittleness or loss of hair *(alopecia)*. Inspect the skin for color, pigmentation, striae, ecchymoses, or mottling. Palpate the skin for texture, thickness, moisture, and diaphoresis. Inspect and palpate the nails for color, texture, brittleness, presence of ridges, and peeling.

■ HEAD

Inspect the contour and shape of the head. Note symmetry and the proportion of facial features. Observe skin color for erythema or rash over the cheeks. Observe the client's facial expression for anxiety.

■ EYES

Inspect and palpate the eyebrows, noting hair distribution. Observe eye position, symmetry, shape, and eyelid lag. Note color of sclerae: are they yellowish or white? Assess visual acuity, extraocular movements (EOMs), and visual fields. Inspect for lens opacity and eye edema.

■ NOSE

Inspect mucosa for swelling and color. Listen for noisy or labored breathing.

■ MOUTH

Note size and shape of the jaw. Inspect the color of the oral mucosa and the condition of the client's teeth. Note malocclusion. Observe tongue size and activity for fasciculations.

■ NECK

Listen to the client's voice for hoarseness or huskiness. Note clarity, pitch, and volume of speech. Ask the client to swallow, and observe for difficulty in swallowing or pain; repeat this maneuver with the client's neck in a hyperextended position. Inspect the neck for symmetry, alignment, thickness, or bulging over the thyroid gland, and examine the midline position of the trachea. Observe for scars related to thyroidectomy, trauma, or other neck surgery. Note presence of hyperpigmentation.

Observe for forceful pulsations over the carotid arteries. Palpate the thyroid gland unless it is noticeably enlarged; vigorous palpation can stimulate release of thyroid hormone, which increases the risk of precipitating a thyroid crisis in a client with thyroid hyperplasia. If the thyroid gland is enlarged, auscultate the lobes for bruits.

The thyroid gland may be palpated by means of an anterior or posterior approach (Fig. 42–2). In both approaches, gently run a finger down the anterior part of the neck, locating the thyroid and cricoid cartilages and the isthmus of the thyroid gland. The isthmus feels soft and compressible compared with the firmer cartilage ring just superior to it. Ask the client to swallow while you palpate the isthmus. It should rise in the neck and should not be enlarged. Figure 42–2 explains the anterior and posterior approaches for palpating the lobes of the thyroid gland. The thyroid gland is normally nonpalpable. If it is palpable, note the texture of the gland because it is usually smooth and firm, without lumps, roughness, hardness, asymmetry, or tenderness (see the Physical Assessment Findings feature).

■ EXTREMITIES

Examine the arms and legs for size, shape, and symmetry, and check their proportionality to the trunk. The distance from the symphysis pubis to the heel is usually about half of the body's total height. Note peripheral edema. Palpate and note peripheral pulse amplitude (see Chapter 10). Assess deep tendon reflexes, and observe their relaxation time (see Chapter 67).

Upper Extremities

Ask the client to extend the hands with palms down; observe for fine tremors and for reddened palms (palmar erythema). Inspect for thenar wasting, Dupuytren's contracture, and nail clubbing (see Chapter 59). Note the size of the client's hands in proportion to the rest of the body. Assess grip strength and muscle strength of the fingers and arms (see Chapter 25).

Lower Extremities

Note the color and distribution of hair. Assess the size of the client's feet in proportion to the rest of the body. Inspect for corns and calluses. Separate the toes, and observe for deformities and skin changes, such as thickening, fissures, and nail thickening. Palpate and note pedal pulses (see Chapter 10). Assess leg muscles for weakness (see Chapter 25).

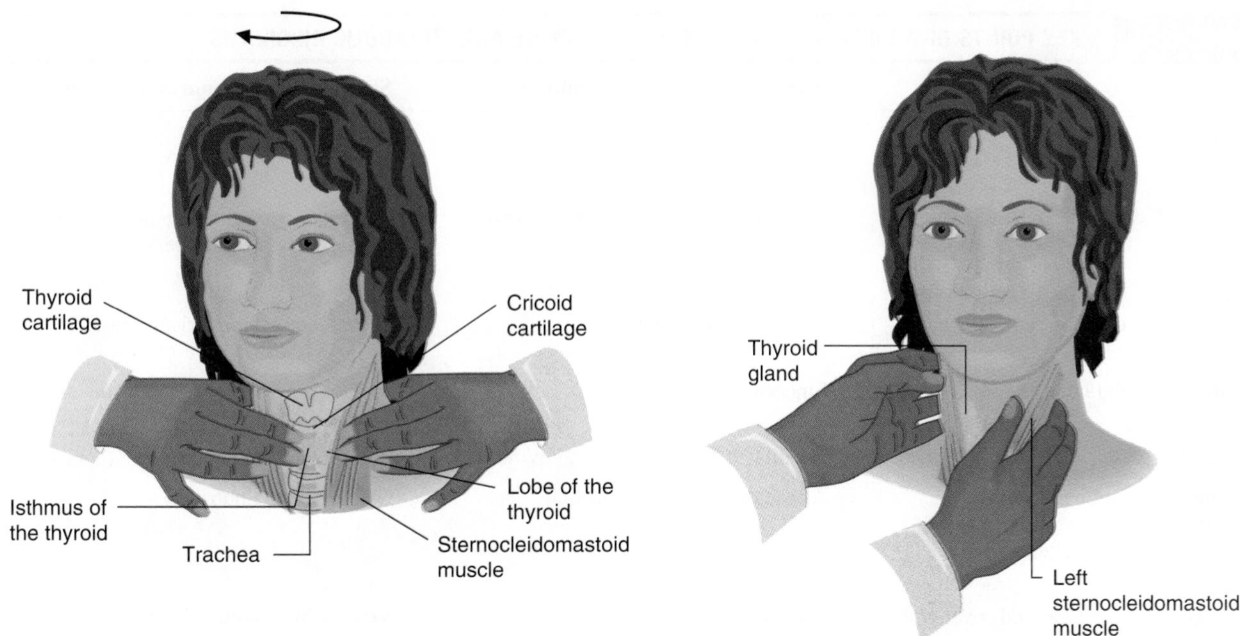

FIGURE 42–2 Palpation of the thyroid. *A*, Posterior approach. Stand behind the client. Ask the client to lower the chin to relax the neck muscles, and tilt the head slightly to the right. To examine the right lobe of the thyroid, use the fingers of your left hand to displace the trachea slightly to the right. This moves the thyroid laterally. You can then palpate between the trachea and the sternocleidomastoid for the right lobe with the fingers of your right hand. Ask the client to swallow while you palpate; doing so causes the gland to rise in the neck. Repeat for the left lobe by reversing your hand placement and positioning the client toward the left. Projection of the thyroid can be enhanced by having the client drink water. *B*, Anterior approach. Stand in front of the client. To palpate the thyroid gland's right lobe, flex the client's head toward the right to relax the neck muscles on that side. Use the fingers of your right hand to displace the trachea slightly to the client's right. Then ask the client to swallow while you palpate the right lobe of the thyroid with the fingers of your left hand. Repeat for the left lobe. You can also assess for thyroid enlargement by palpating deep on each side of the sternocleidomastoid muscle.

THORAX

In males, inspect for gynecomastia (breast enlargement), which can develop because of decreased metabolism of estrogen when the liver is dysfunctional. Auscultate for extra heart sounds, such as a systolic murmur (see Chapter 54).

PHYSICAL ASSESSMENT FINDINGS IN THE HEALTHY ADULT*

Thyroid Gland

Inspection

The thyroid gland is not normally seen on inspection.

Palpation

The gland rises and falls with swallowing. Isthmus at midline, soft. Right lobe slightly larger than the left lobe. Texture rubbery without nodules. Nontender.

Auscultation

No bruits heard over either lobe.

* Findings for the metabolic system are found in Chapter 28 as part of the abdominal assessment.

ABDOMEN

Assessment of the abdomen includes inspection, auscultation, percussion, and palpation. Table 42–1 summarizes the key points of a physical examination for endocrine and metabolic disorders.

Inspection

Note areas of hyperpigmentation, such as in scars or striae. Observe the client for manifestations of pain during light palpation; examine painful areas last. Characteristics of ascites include a distended abdomen with tight and glistening skin, bulging flanks, and prominent abdominal veins. Measure abdominal girth if ascites is present. Ascites may account for recent rapid onset of weight gain with accompanying loss of muscle mass.

Auscultation

Auscultation for possible hepatic or biliary problems is performed by gently placing a warmed stethoscope on the right upper quadrant while the client is supine. Note whether a soft hum is heard during both the systolic and diastolic components of the heartbeat. A *hum* indicates increased collateral circulation between the portal and systemic venous systems, as might occur in hepatic cirrhosis.

TABLE 42-1 KEY POINTS OF A PHYSICAL EXAMINATION: ENDOCRINE AND METABOLIC DISORDERS

Steps	Normal or Common Findings	Significant or Abnormal Findings
Inspection		
Note:		
Color of skin	Same as or lighter than other areas	Redness, cyanosis, jaundice, lesions, ecchymosis, needle marks, or hematomas
Eyes	White sclerae	Sclerae: yellow tint
Symmetry, contour, shape of abdomen	Flat, rounded abdomen	Distended, asymmetrical, masses
Surface of abdomen	Smooth	Tight, shiny; engorged, prominent veins, spider angiomas
Rectal area	No dilated veins (hemorrhoids)	Presence of distended veins (hemorrhoids)
General nutritional state Weigh Observe for ascites	Adequate for height and build	Obesity or malnutrition
Auscultation		
Place stethoscope (warmed) over right upper quadrant. Listen for vascular sounds or friction rubs	No venous hums No friction rubs	Venous hum with both diastolic and systolic components
Percussion		
Abdomen: Note percussion sounds in four quadrants	Tympany over abdomen, bladder, intestines, and aorta, and dull over liver, spleen, pancreas, kidneys, and uterus	Dullness over enlarged organs; indicates need for further assessment for ascites
Liver: Span. Percuss upward from below client's umbilicus on the right midclavicular line (MCL), until dullness is heard. Mark this point. Percuss downward from lung resonance in right MCL to dullness and measure distance between two marks.	Liver span is 6–12 cm. No tenderness	Liver span is greater than 12 cm
Note if tender, soft, or firm, smooth or nodular	Slightly tender, soft, smooth surface	Nodular, more than slightly tender, hard
Spleen: Note size. Percuss downward in left posterior axillary line, beginning with lung resonance until dullness is heard	Dullness between ribs 6 and 10	Dullness extends above sixth rib or covers large area—indicates enlargement
Palpation		
Use palmar surface of extended fingers		
Liver: Palpate lightly on right side and then palpate deeply	No tenderness, pain, masses	Tenderness, rigidity, nodules, enlarged
Spleen: Note: If spleen can be percussed, it is best not to palpate it. Palpate lightly on left side, distal to MCL	No tenderness, pain, masses	Tenderness, rigidity, nodules, enlarged
ADAPTATIONS FOR OLDER ADULTS		
Inspection		
Contour	Sagging and rounded because of loss of muscle tone and accumulation of fat	
Palpation		
Note liver span and borders	Span may be shortened but border more easily palpated	Right upper quadrant or epigastric pain from the liver and biliary tract Epigastric pain from pancreas, stomach, or duodenum

Listen for a *friction rub* (a grating sound heard with respiratory ventilation). A friction rub suggests inflammation of the peritoneal surface of an organ, as from a liver tumor, chlamydial or gonococcal perihepatitis, or recent liver biopsy.

If a systolic *bruit* (swishing sound indicating vascular turbulence) accompanies a hepatic friction rub, carcinoma of the liver is suspected.

Percussion

Percuss the abdomen, especially the liver and spleen. Assess liver size by percussing the span of the liver at the right midclavicular line (RMCL) and the midsternal line (MSL). Begin by percussing in the right midclavicular line either superior or inferior to the estimated borders of the liver. Superiorly, begin at the third intercostal space (ICS) over lung resonance; percuss down the thorax until the sound changes to dull. Mark this level on the skin with a pen. Inferiorly, start over a tympanic area and percuss upward until the sound changes to dull. Also mark this with the pen.

At the midsternal line, percuss upward from above the umbilicus from tympany to dull. Mark where the sound changes. Superiorly, percuss down the sternum until the percussion note changes; mark this too. Measure the distance between each set of marks.

At the right midclavicular line, the liver span ranges from 6 to 12 cm (2½ to 5 inches); at the midsternal line, it ranges from 4 to 8 cm (1½ to 3 inches). The lower border of the liver at the right midclavicular line is usually at the right costal margin, and the upper border is between the fifth and seventh intercostal spaces.

Liver size varies with body size. Measurements larger than the norms indicate liver enlargement. Ask the client to take a deep breath and hold it while you percuss the lower liver border in the right midclavicular line again. With deep inspiration, the pressure of the diaphragm causes the liver to descend lower into the abdomen. The distance of liver descent is marked and measured and ranges from 2 to 3 cm (~1 inch). Use the marked level of liver descent as a guide for later palpation of the liver.

Spleen size may be determined by percussion, particularly if the spleen is enlarged. The spleen is located by percussion as a small area of dullness just posterior to the left midaxillary line (LMAL) between the sixth and 10th ribs. It normally has a span of approximately 7 cm (2½ to 3 inches). If the spleen enlarges, the area of dullness shifts inferiorly below the 10th rib and anteriorly toward or beyond the left anterior axillary line (LAAL).

Percussion is also used to assess for ascites in the abdomen by observing for a *fluid wave*. This infrequently performed maneuver is an advanced physical assessment technique because of the potential difficulty in detecting a fluid wave. A more common method of assessment for ascites is to measure changes in abdominal girth and weight gain over time. Another advanced assessment technique to detect ascites is the *test for shifting dullness,* described in Chapter 32.

The *fluid wave test* is performed while the client is supine. Two nurses participate. One nurse places the edges of the hands on the client's abdominal midline to stabilize the abdominal wall. The second nurse places one hand on one side of the client's abdomen while briskly tapping the opposite side of the abdomen with the other hand. The second nurse feels for the movement of a fluid wave against the palpating hand opposite the side percussed.

Palpation

Use palpation initially to assess for muscle guarding or tenderness. Observe the client for facial grimaces, tensing, or other indications of discomfort. Next, perform deep palpation to evaluate tenderness, indicating possible inflammation. Light and deep palpation techniques are discussed in Chapter 10.

Because the peritoneum is often involved, evaluate for localized peritoneal irritation. Press the abdomen firmly at a point away from any tender area, and quickly remove the examining hand. Severe pain accompanies this maneuver when inflammation is present, indicating *rebound tenderness.*

Perform *liver palpation* standing at the client's right side. Use one of two bimanual techniques:

First technique. Place your left hand under the client's right posterior thorax over the 11th and 12th ribs, and push the thorax upward. Place the right hand below the right costal margin at the previously marked level of liver descent, as determined by percussion. Point your fingers upward toward the costal margin, then gently push up and in as the client takes a deep breath using the abdominal muscles. As the client inhales, feel for the liver's edge to slip over the finger tips as it descends. If the liver's edge is felt, it should feel firm, sharp, smooth, and regular. Palpate at several points medially and laterally to assess the edge along its inferior border.

Second technique. Place the right hand below the right costal margin as described. Superimpose the left hand on the right hand. Perform the remainder of the maneuver as described earlier.

The liver is difficult to palpate in clients who are obese or tense or who have taut abdominal muscles because they are physically fit. Abnormal findings include a hard, nodular feel to the liver and more than minimal tenderness as perceived by the client. If extreme ascites is present, the liver edge is nonpalpable.

Spleen palpation is an advanced physical assessment technique. If percussion has shown that the spleen is enlarged, the nurse does not usually palpate it because of the possibility of rupture. If no enlargement is noted on percussion, perform spleen palpation in a manner similar to that for the liver; however, perform the technique on the left side of the abdomen below the costal margin. Ask the client to turn onto the right side, allowing gravity to bring the spleen forward and down, closer to the abdominal wall. Place your left hand behind the client's left posterior rib cage, and push forward while palpating with the right hand. The spleen is normally nonpalpable. Congestion caused by portal hypertension results in enlargement of the spleen and is a common finding in cirrhosis.

Blunt (fist) percussion is used to determine organ tenderness over the liver. This maneuver is performed after all other abdominal assessment techniques are completed to avoid producing discomfort in the presence of organ tenderness. When assessing for *liver tenderness*, use *only* indirect fist percussion over the costal margin at the right midclavicular line to avoid trauma to the liver. This maneuver is also known as a *liver tap*. For comparison, perform indirect fist percussion over the left costal margin at the midclavicular line (Chapter 10 explains blunt percussion). Tell the client what is going to be done to avoid a reaction of surprise that may be misinterpreted as tenderness. Note the client's reaction to the blows.

Record physical findings for the liver and spleen as part of the abdominal examination. Chapter 28 includes a recording of a normal abdominal physical assessment.

■ GENITALIA AND RECTUM

Observe the pattern of pubic hair distribution, particularly in women. A diamond-shaped (male) pattern is indicative of a masculinizing tumor. Note the size of the testes in male clients and the clitoris in female clients for comparison with expected norms. The remainder of endocrine assessment consists of diagnostic studies, since the only endocrine glands accessible to physical examination are the thyroid and gonads (see Chapter 37).

Inspect the rectal area for dilated veins (hemorrhoids). These may be present in cirrhosis with portal hypertension.

■ MODIFICATIONS FOR OLDER ADULTS

When assessing the older adult client for possible endocrine or metabolic disorders, remember to divide the physical assessment into several parts to avoid fatigue. Allow adequate time for the physical examination so that the information needed is clearly communicated to the client.

When inspecting the abdomen, note the contour and color. A rounded, sagging abdomen is a normal finding because of the tendency for fat to accumulate in the lower abdomen and hips and for the abdominal muscles to weaken. Note any areas of tenderness or discomfort because old age may blunt the manifestations of pain caused by peritoneal inflammation, for example (see Table 42–1).

DIAGNOSTIC TESTS

A client with an endocrine dysfunction may need several general types of diagnostic tests. Blood levels of various hormones specific to the endocrine glands are measured. Some hormones are measured for specific levels; others, such as thyroid hormone, are measured according to how well they combine with plasma proteins or radioactive iodine.

The client may be anxious about the tests and the possible results. In many cases, endocrine disorders have been misdiagnosed for years because of the nonspecific manifestations of the disorders. After the correct diagnosis is made, the client and family may need help coping with ongoing care.

Similarly, a client with a metabolic dysfunction (exocrine pancreas, liver, or biliary tract) frequently requires multiple diagnostic measures. No single laboratory test, radiographic study, or surgical procedure yields sufficient data to confirm a diagnosis or establish the degree of malfunction. Foster a sense of self-worth and understanding in the client during repeated diagnostic procedures. Such a sense promotes cooperation and reduces the fatigue and anxiety that frequently accompany these evaluations.

In the discussion that follows, common diagnostic tests of endocrine function are identified according to specific endocrine organs: pancreas, thyroid, adrenal, and pituitary, after which diagnostic tests involving organs of metabolism (exocrine pancreas, liver, biliary tract, and gallbladder) are discussed.

■ ENDOCRINE FUNCTION STUDIES

Laboratory Studies

A more detailed presentation of laboratory tests for specific endocrine disorders may be found in the chapters on these disorders.

Tests of Pancreatic Function

Diagnostic assessment of pancreatic endocrine function is related to blood glucose levels. Elevated fasting blood glucose is usually the first indication of hyperglycemia. Glycosylated hemoglobin (HbA1c), or glycohemoglobin, is a measure of the average blood glucose over 3 months and can be obtained in the nonfasting state. A more detailed presentation of diagnostic tests related to diabetes appears in Chapter 45.

Tests of Thyroid Function

Several tests are available to assess thyroid function. A brief overview of the most common diagnostic tests follows.

SERUM THYROXINE AND TRIIODOTHYRONINE

Radioimmunoassay can be used to measure serum concentrations of thyroxine (T_4) and triiodothyronine (T_3).

T_4 is transported in the blood largely bound to thyroxine-binding globulin and is an effective indicator of thyroid function; conditions that affect thyroid-binding globulin levels alter the serum T_4 concentration. Hyperthyroidism, viral hepatitis, pregnancy, and oral contraceptives increase serum T_4; hypothyroidism, strenuous exercise, heparin, and lithium decrease serum T_4.

T_3 (like T_4) circulates in the bloodstream, attached to plasma proteins and to erythrocytes. However, T_3 binds far more readily to plasma proteins than to erythrocytes. T_3 binds to erythrocytes only when plasma protein binding sites are limited.

Analysis of T_3 and T_4 concentrations has largely replaced the older technique of estimating basal metabolic rate (BMR). BMR is calculated by measuring the amount of oxygen the body consumes when in a state of complete mental and physical relaxation.

T_3 RESIN UPTAKE

If thyroid function is below normal or if serum protein levels are high, resin uptake of T_3 is depressed. If thyroid function is above normal or serum protein levels are low, resin uptake of T_3 is elevated. T_3 resin uptake is one test used to measure thyroid function but should not be the only one.

RADIOIODINE UPTAKE AND EXCRETION TEST

The body cannot distinguish between radiolabeled ("tagged") iodine and nonradiolabeled iodine. Consequently, the thyroid takes up radioactive iodine (RAIU) and processes it just as it does regular iodine. ^{131}I has been used for measuring thyroid function, but ^{123}I is preferable because it allows the use of a lower radiation dose.[30] Radioiodine is excreted in the urine just as is ordinary iodine. A scintillation scanner is used to measure the amount of radioactive iodine present in the thyroid 24 hours after administration of a radioiodine isotope preparation. The laboratory may measure the client's urine output of radioactive iodine after the test.

Many factors can distort findings. Before the procedure, therefore, question the client about the following, and inform the physician if the client answers "yes" to any of these questions.

- Have you taken any iodine-containing medications within the last 30 days?
- Are you taking estrogens that can cause a false elevation?
- Have you undergone x-ray studies of the gallbladder, ureters, bronchi, fallopian tubes, or heart within the last 10 years?
- Within the last 2 weeks, have you principally eaten seafood? (Seafood is so rich in iodine that ^{131}I uptake can show a falsely low reading.)

SERUM THYROID-STIMULATING HORMONE CONCENTRATION

Measurement of the basal serum thyroid-stimulating hormone (TSH) concentration is useful in the diagnosis of both advanced and subclinical hypothyroidism. In one stage of hypothyroidism, the thyroid gland compensates for a functional abnormality that impairs the ability to synthesize hormones and hypersecretes TSH. In thyrotoxic states, the serum TSH concentration is almost always low or undetectable.

THYROTROPIN-RELEASING HORMONE STIMULATION TEST

Thyrotropin-releasing hormone (TRH) is released from the hypothalamus, and it normally stimulates release of TSH from the pituitary. During the TRH stimulation test, people with thyroid disorders are given TRH intravenously. A rise in TSH levels indicates that the pituitary is functioning normally. TSH levels do not rise in the presence of hyperthyroidism or when the pituitary cells that secrete TSH are diseased.

SERUM CHOLESTEROL

The serum cholesterol level may be elevated in primary hypothyroidism, which may explain why this condition is accompanied by a marked tendency toward atherosclerosis. People with hyperthyroidism usually have a lower serum cholesterol level. Serum cholesterol is not a specific test of thyroid function, however, because its levels are influenced by many factors other than thyroid hormone levels.

ANTITHYROID ANTIBODY TESTS

Many thyroid disorders are presumed to have an autoimmune basis, such as Hashimoto's thyroiditis, some types of myxedema, and Graves' disease (a form of hyperthyroidism). Serologic tests may be performed to determine whether the client's blood contains antithyroid antibodies.

ACHILLES TENDON REFLEXES

The Achilles tendon reflex test measures the amplitude and duration of the ankle jerk with a special instrument, which is used to tap the strong tendon at the back of the heel. Clients with hyperthyroidism may demonstrate a more rapid tendon reflex. Clients with an underactive thyroid gland or diabetes mellitus and pregnant women have slower reflexes and prolonged relaxation times. Chapter 67 covers tendon reflex testing.

Tests of Adrenal Function

Adrenal function tests may be used to evaluate medullary and cortical hormones. Adrenocortical hormones include cortisol (glucocorticoid), aldosterone (mineral corticoid), and small amounts of sex hormones (androgens). Adrenal medullary hormones include epinephrine and norepinephrine (catecholamines).

CORTISOL SUPPRESSION TEST

Cortisol is secreted in a diurnal pattern, and levels are assessed at 8 AM and 8 PM. A cortisol suppression test involves the suppression of pituitary ACTH with dexamethasone. Normally, after administration of dexamethasone, 24-hour levels of ketosteroid in the urine drop by 50%. Dexamethasone can also be given at midnight and serum cortisol then assessed at 8 AM. In clients with increased adrenocortical stimulation, no decrease is seen in ketosteroid production in urine or in serum levels of cortisol.

ALDOSTERONE LEVELS

Plasma levels of aldosterone, angiotensin II, and renin can be measured at any time. Plasma levels of aldosterone can be increased by giving potassium, restricting sodium, or having the client assume an upright position. Plasma levels of aldosterone can be decreased by infusion of saline.

SERUM ADRENOCORTICOTROPIC HORMONE

Serum levels of ACTH can be assessed after infusion of synthetic ACTH. Urine levels of ketosteroid would be expected to rise to 25 mg in 24 hours; plasma levels of cortisol should rise to 10 to 40 μg/dl. Urine levels of ketosteroid can be measured with 24-hour urine specimens. *Ketosteroids* are metabolites of the hormones produced by the adrenal cortex. A preservative is required for the collection bottle. If the client has an indwelling catheter, the urinary drainage bag is emptied frequently and the urine is refrigerated. Collection of 24-hour urine specimens is explained in Chapter 11.

URINARY CATECHOLAMINES

Adrenal medullary function can be assessed through urine levels of catecholamines and their metabolites (vanillylmandelic acid [VMA]). A 24-hour urine sample is collected and assayed. Adrenal medullary secretion can be suppressed by administration of ganglionic blocking agents, which normally decrease the urine levels of catecholamines. In clients with pheochromocytoma (a tumor of the adrenal medulla), ganglionic blocking agents have a negligible effect in controlling blood pressure. An older assessment test for pheochromocytoma, which involved blood pressure manipulation, is rarely performed today.

RADIOGRAPHY

The adrenal cortex can be assessed for tumors by x-ray study, computed tomography (CT), and magnetic resonance imaging (MRI) (see Chapter 11).

Tests of Pituitary Function

RADIOGRAPHY

The structure of the pituitary gland can be assessed by skull x-ray study, CT, or MRI. Tumors of the pituitary may be visualized with these studies (see Chapter 11).

HORMONE ASSAYS

Hormonal disorders caused by malfunction of the pituitary gland can lead to a wide variety of clinical manifestations, depending on which hormone is involved. Growth hormone (GH) and ADH are discussed here.

GROWTH HORMONE LEVELS. GH is secreted in a diurnal pattern, and its level can be assayed. In a determination of basal levels, the blood sample is usually drawn in the morning after the client has had nothing by mouth (*nil per os*, NPO) for 8 to 10 hours. Usual levels for males are less than 5 ng/ml; for females, less than 10 ng/ml. GH can be stimulated by administration of (1) levodopa (500 mg, orally), (2) insulin (0.05 to 0.3 unit/kg, intravenously), or (3) bromocriptine (5 mg, orally). After the stimulus, blood is drawn at intervals for up to 120 minutes. GH levels usually peak 60 minutes after stimulation.

DEHYDRATION TESTS. Absence of ADH leads to diabetes insipidus. A dehydration test is used to confirm the diagnosis of diabetes insipidus. Fluids are withheld long enough to result in stable hourly urinary osmolalities (4 to 18 hours). During this time, the client's vital signs, urine output, and urine specific gravity are assessed hourly. Hypovolemic shock can develop from dehydration. After the third hour of stable urinary osmolality, the client is given vasopressin as 5 units aqueous arginine vasopressin or 1 μg desmopressin by subcutaneous injection or 10 μg desmopressin by nasal spray.[19] A client without diabetes insipidus responds with decreased urine output and increased urine osmolality. A client with diabetes insipidus cannot respond and continues to produce high volumes of dilute urine (low osmolality).

■ METABOLIC FUNCTION STUDIES

Laboratory Studies

The most common laboratory tests for metabolic function (liver, biliary, and exocrine pancreas) include those used to measure levels of serum enzymes, proteins, antigens, antibodies, fats, and bleeding and clotting factors and related urine and stool studies (Table 42–2). Details on hepatitis virus infection are presented in Chapter 47.

Tests of All Metabolic Organ Functions

LIVER, GALLBLADDER, BILIARY TRACT, AND PANCREAS

ULTRASONOGRAPHY. Ultrasonographic examination provides valuable diagnostic information about liver, pancreatic, and biliary tract conditions. The technique is rapid, and little or no preparation is required. Depending on the area to be examined, the client may or may not fast before the procedure. Reassure the client that the test is painless and safe. There are no specific precautions or observations after ultrasonography. See Chapter 11 for a discussion of ultrasonography.

RADIOGRAPHY. Many procedures used to diagnose disorders of the liver, pancreas, and biliary tract involve the use of x-rays. Plain x-ray films of the abdomen may show diaphragm elevation caused by hepatic enlargement or calcification in the abdominal organs. Upper or lower gastrointestinal series using barium contrast medium also provide important information about the accessory organs of digestion (i.e., liver, gallbladder, and pancreas). One such test of the pancreas, hypotonic duodenography, requires insertion of barium sulfate and air into the duodenum via a catheter passed through the client's nose to the duodenum. Spot x-ray films are taken to detect pancreatic and duodenal diseases (i.e., tumor at the head of the pancreas or a stricture caused by chronic pancreatitis).

Radiologic studies with iodinated contrast media permit visualization of tubes and vessels. Before any of these procedures are performed, question the client about known hypersensitivity to iodine (see Chapter 11).

Computed Tomography. CT is used to identify and evaluate liver, biliary tract, gallbladder, and pancreatic disorders. It is useful for distinguishing cysts or tumors and differentiating obstructive from nonobstructive jaundice (Fig. 42–3). The client is instructed to fast, except for water, for 8 to 12 hours before the test. See Chapter 11 for a more detailed discussion of CT.

Angiography. Angiography allows visualization of the hepatic, biliary, and pancreatic arterial vessels after administration of contrast medium. It is used to identify abnormalities of vascular structure and function, observe masses, and note bleeding sites in the pancreas, spleen, and portal system. To inject the contrast medium, the examiner usually introduces a needle into the femoral artery. Next, the needle is exchanged for a catheter, which is then passed into the celiac artery or one of its branches (superior mesenteric or hepatic). After contrast medium injection, rapid sequence filming is done. See Chapter 11 for additional details.

Preprocedure care

Explain the purpose of the examination to the client. The client usually takes nothing by mouth for 6 to 8 hours before the test. Ask the client about any use of medications that might lead to bleeding, such as anticoagulants or nonsteroidal anti-inflammatory drugs (NSAIDs). These medications should be stopped up to a week before the test. Bleeding or clotting tests are usually ordered before the test. Remind the client that it is necessary to lie very still during the examination. Explain that there may be a sensation of pressure during introduction of the catheter. Assess the pulses distal to the insertion site for comparison with pulses afterward.

Postprocedure care

After angiography, assess the needle insertion site for manifestations of bleeding. Clients with liver conditions often have concurrent clotting disorders, which may lead to a hematoma. Assess the pulses below the level of

TABLE 42–2 LABORATORY TESTS OF LIVER, BILIARY, AND PANCREATIC FUNCTION

Measurement	Normal Value*	Procedure	Interpretation
		EXOCRINE PANCREATIC ASSESSMENT	
Serum amylase with isoenzymes	60–160 Somogyi U/dl	Blood drawn 1–2 hr after eating, preferably while no IV solutions are infusing	Pancreatic digestive enzyme released with breakdown of acinar cells; serum levels increase with acute and chronic pancreatitis, obstruction of pancreatic duct, acute alcoholic intoxication, and diabetes mellitus; elevations not directly correlated with severity; decreased with advanced chronic necrosis of liver and chronic alcoholism; amylase test measures both pancreatic and salivary amylase; pancreatic isoamylase is a more specific test
Urine amylase	4–37 U/dl/24 hr	2- or 24-hr urine collection bottle must have a preservative. Specimens collected after initial voiding	Urine levels elevated longer with pancreatitis
Serum lipase	14–280 mU/ml 20–180 IU/L	Blood drawn after client NPO except for water for 8–12 hr	Lipase aids in digesting fats and is increased in acute and chronic pancreatitis, early-stage cancer of pancreas, and obstruction of pancreatic duct; decreased in late cancer of pancreas and hepatitis
Pancreatic function		Oral bentiromide given after overnight fast; urine is collected for 6 hr	Pancreatic chymotrypsin splits bentiromide; para-aminobenzoic acid (PABA), a breakdown product, is excreted in urine; less PABA is excreted with pancreatic insufficiency
		LIVER ASSESSMENT	
Serum bilirubin			
Direct (conjugated)	0.1–0.3 mg/dl	Blood drawn after client NPO after midnight except for water; protect sample from ultraviolet light or sunlight	Direct bilirubin increased with biliary obstruction, causing conjugated fraction to accumulate in plasma
Indirect (unconjugated)	0.2–0.8 mg/dl		Indirect bilirubin increased with excessive erythrocyte hemolysis
Total	0.1–1.2 mg/dl		Total bilirubin measures direct and indirect levels together
Urine bilirubin	0–0.02 mg/dl	Urine collection (urine appears smoky or tea colored); protect from light	Urine bilirubin measures conjugated bilirubin only; increased with biliary obstruction
Urine urobilinogen	Random: 0.3–3.5 mg/dl 24-hr: 0.05–2.5 mg/24 hr	2- or 24-hr afternoon collection placed in brown refrigerated bottle with sodium carbonate preservative	Urine urobilinogen decreased with biliary obstruction or liver damage; increased with erythrocyte hemolysis and certain drugs (e.g., sulfonamides) and liver, toxic, or infectious hepatitis
Fecal urobilinogen	75–275 EU/100 g	Entire stool specimen to laboratory	Fecal urobilinogen decreased with biliary obstruction; increased in erythrocyte hemolysis
Serum cholesterol	150–240 mg/dl <200 mg/dl desired	Blood drawn after low-cholesterol diet for 12 hr	Elevated when excretion blocked by bile duct obstruction, diabetes mellitus, and pancreatitis; may be decreased in chronic liver disease, hyperthyroidism, and adrenal hormone excess (Cushing's syndrome)

Table continues on following page

TABLE 42–2 LABORATORY TESTS OF LIVER, BILIARY, AND PANCREATIC FUNCTION *Continued*

Measurement	Normal Value*	Procedure	Interpretation
Liver enzyme tests†			
Aspartate aminotransferase (AST)	0–35 U/L	Blood drawn without special preparation	Serum AST, ALT, and LDH released from damaged liver, heart, kidney, and muscle cells; prolonged elevation in liver disease may be first indicator of chronic active hepatitis; a rapid drop may signal liver failure
Alanine aminotransferase (ALT)	5–35 U/ml (Frankel)		
Lactate dehydrogenase (LDH) isoenzyme	100–190 IU/L		
Alkaline phosphatase (ALP) and isoenzyme	20–90 U/L at 30° C		Elevated in biliary obstruction; produced by cells lining the biliary tract; this enzyme is also found in bone, intestine, and placenta
Serum 5′-nucleotidase	<17 U/L		Enzyme located mainly in liver and liver disease confirmed if ALP and this enzyme both elevated
Serum γ-glutamyltransferase (GGT)	4–23 IU/L (male) 3–13 IU/L (female)		Enzyme located primarily in liver and kidney; elevation of GGT and ALP significant indication of liver disorders
Leucine aminopeptidase (LAP)	8–22 mU/ml		Elevated in liver disease. LAP frequently ordered with 5′-NT and LAP tests to confirm liver disease
Protein metabolism			
Total protein	6.0–8.2 g/dl	Blood drawn without special preparation	Impaired protein synthesis or utilization caused by chronic liver disease, pancreatic insufficiency (albumin, α- and β-globulins); γ-globulins produced by B lymphocytes, not liver
Serum albumin	3.5–5.0 g/dl		
Serum globulin includes α_1, α_2, β, γ	2.1–4.2 g/dl		
A/G (albumin/globulin) ratio	1.0–2.0 g/dl		Decrease in the ratio may indicate chronic liver disease
Plasma ammonia	15–45 g/dl	Blood drawn after client NPO except for water for 8–12 hr before the test. Blood must be iced and tested immediately	Reduced synthesis of urea from body ammonia in severe hepatocellular damage produces elevated blood ammonia
Hemostatic function			
Prothrombin time (PT)	11–15 sec or 70%–100%	Blood drawn without special preparation	Increase in PT may occur in liver disease. Assesses function of extrinsic pathway in clotting process (factors I, II, V, VII, X). PT prolonged with (1) decreased synthesis of prothrombin because of liver cell damage or (2) decreased vitamin K absorption because of bile duct obstruction. Vitamin K necessary for liver to synthesize prothrombin
Platelets	150,000–400,000 μl (mean = 250,000 μl)		May fall in liver disease (cirrhosis, chronic active hepatitis), anemias, leukemias Elevated in trauma, metastatic carcinoma TB
Metabolism of foreign substances			
Bromsulphalein (BSP) excretion	<5% retention in 1 hr	Control blood specimen (or sample) taken after fasting for 12 hr; BSP given, blood drawn at intervals	Dye retained with diminished hepatocellular ability to remove it from blood and excrete it; test is infrequently used

TABLE 42–2 **LABORATORY TESTS OF LIVER, BILIARY, AND PANCREATIC FUNCTION** *Continued*

Measurement	Normal Value*	Procedure	Interpretation
Antigens and antibodies			
Hepatitis antigens and antibodies	Negative for antigens. Positive or negative for antibodies, depending on history	Blood drawn without special preparation	Antigens indicate hepatitis, antibodies indicate past or present hepatitis or immunization (hepatitis B)
Antimicrobial antibody (AMA)	Negative at 1:5 Positive at >1:160		Test done to differentiate between biliary cirrhosis and other liver diseases
Alpha-fetoprotein (AFP), antigen associated with cancer	<10 ng/ml		AFP is synthesized by fetus but not by healthy adult; AFP level >1000 ng/ml usually indicates hepatocellular carcinoma

*Normal values may differ significantly between laboratories.

†Trends in elevation are of particular importance in predicting the rapidity with which the liver is failing. If levels rise, fall, then rise again, liver failure may be occurring.

A, albumin; AFP, alpha-fetoprotein; ALP, alkaline phosphatase; ALT, alanine aminotransferase; AMA, antimicrobial antibody; AST, aspartate aminotransferase; BSP, Bromsulphalein (sulfobromophthalein sodium); EU = Ehrlich units; G, globulin; GGT, gamma-glutamyltransferase; IV, intravenous; LAP, leucine aminopeptidase; LDH, lactate dehydrogenase; NPO, *nil per os* (nothing by mouth); 5′-NT, 5′-nucleotidase; PABA, para-aminobenzoic acid; PT, prothrombin time; TB, tuberculosis.

Data from Kee, J. L. (1998). *Laboratory and diagnostic tests with nursing implications.* (5th ed.). Stamford, CT: Appleton & Lange.

catheter insertion and compare with the preprocedure baseline findings.

RADIONUCLIDE IMAGING. Radionuclide imaging with technetium 99m dimethylacetanilide (hepato-iminodiacetic acid [HIDA], diethyl-iminodiacetic acid [DIDA], and di-isopropyl-iminodiacetic acid [DISIDA]) involves intravenous infusion of gamma-emitting isotopes. After infusion, a scintillation detector is passed over the abdomen. This procedure is used to investigate biliary obstruction and indicates whether a tumor or abscess is present in the liver, gallbladder, or pancreas. Useful isotopes include colloidal gold (^{198}Au), gallium (^{67}Ga), technetium (^{99}Tc), and selenium (^{75}Se). ^{67}Ga accumulates in inflamed tissue. ^{99}Tc is used to evaluate liver, gallbladder, and biliary tract function. ^{75}Se is useful for identifying pancreatic abnormalities.

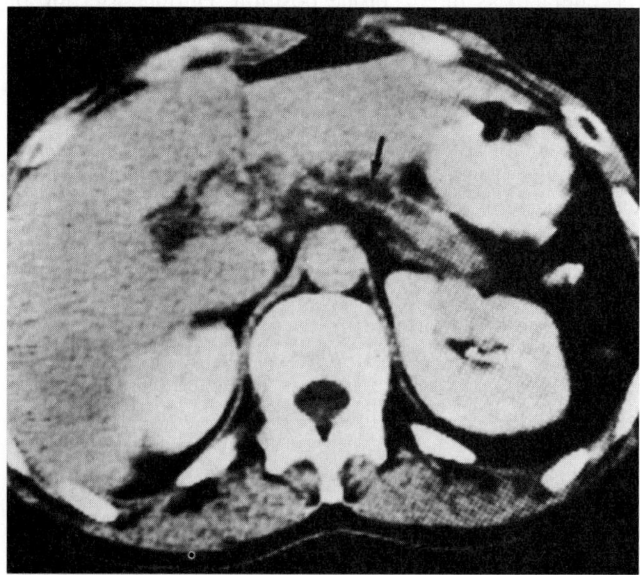

FIGURE 42–3 Computed tomographic scan of chronic pancreatitis. Pancreatic atrophy and a dilated pancreatic duct *(arrow)* are present, but there is no evidence of pancreatic calcification. (From Moss, A. A., et al. [1983]. *Computed tomography of the body.* Philadelphia: W. B. Saunders.)

Tests of Specific Metabolic Organ Functions

LIVER

PERITONEOSCOPY. Insertion of a peritoneoscope through an abdominal stab wound permits direct visualization of the liver and peritoneum. Visualization of structural changes aids in the diagnosis of cirrhosis and cancer. During peritoneoscopy, the examiner may take photographs and perform a biopsy. Peritoneoscopy is relatively safe and simple.

Contraindications include infections of the abdominal cavity, clotting disorders, or intestinal obstruction. In addition, the client must be able to cooperate throughout the procedure. Obesity and ascites interfere with test results.

Preprocedure care

To prepare a client for peritoneoscopy:

- Check that written consent has been obtained.
- Check the laboratory record to make certain the client has normal or adequate clotting factors. If not, inform the physician.

- Check the client and health care record for contraindications to preprocedural medications.
- Inquire whether the client is sensitive to local anesthetics.
- Prepare the skin, and administer preprocedural medication when appropriate.
- Instruct the client to take nothing by mouth and to empty the bowel and bladder just before the procedure begins.
- Provide adequate teaching before and during the actual procedure.
- Explain to the client that it may be difficult to breathe when air is placed in the abdominal cavity.
- Instruct the client to elevate the abdominal wall by holding the breath to protect major organs during needle insertion.

Postprocedure care

When peritoneoscopy includes liver biopsy, bed rest for 24 hours follows the procedure (see discussion of liver biopsy later in this chapter). If biopsy is not performed, the client resumes activity after recovery from the effects of the medication. Complications are uncommon and are more often related to biopsy. Possible complications after peritoneoscopy are pneumothorax, subcutaneous emphysema, air embolism, bile peritonitis, perforation of a hollow organ, and shoulder or abdominal pain.

PORTAL PRESSURE MEASUREMENTS. Measurements of portal pressure and flow help to (1) diagnose portal hypertension, (2) indicate the severity of portal hypertension, and (3) guide decisions about appropriate intervention, which may include surgery. Also, the indirect calculation of sinusoid pressure helps determine the location of an obstruction in the liver and thus identify the underlying disorder. Normal portal pressure is 5 to 10 mm Hg. Portal hypertension is present when the wedged venous pressure is more than 5 mm Hg higher than the inferior vena cava pressure.[8]

The major portal pressure measurements are:

- *Wedged hepatic venous pressure* (WHVP). The portal pressure is obtained indirectly by percutaneous hepatic vein catheterization. The examiner uses either an arm vein or a femoral vein.
- *Umbilical vein catheterization.* This procedure allows direct measurement of portal pressure.
- *Splenic pulp manometry.* During manometry, the examiner places a needle between two of the lower ribs and inserts a manometer into the spleen. Instruct the client to hold the breath during needle insertion and passage.

Preprocedure care

Portal pressure measurements are minor surgical procedures that are performed in the operating room or a special studies laboratory. In many instances, the surgeon may concurrently inject a contrast agent. These measures require standard preoperative and postoperative care (see Chapter 16).

Postprocedure care

Observe for bleeding or pneumothorax. Assess the incision site for hematoma formation. Other nursing care is the same as for the client after liver biopsy (see next).

BIOPSY. Biopsy is the single most valuable diagnostic study because it is often the determining factor for the final diagnosis. It involves removal of a sample of living tissue for analysis. Biopsies may be open or closed procedures.

An *open biopsy* necessitates a general anesthetic and a major abdominal incision. A client may have an open biopsy at the time of a concurrent operative procedure. An advantage of the open biopsy is that the surgeon can observe the entire liver, identify grossly altered tissue, and remove the biopsy specimen for study.

A *closed biopsy*, or percutaneous liver biopsy, is performed to aspirate a core of tissue via needle for histologic study. The biopsy is usually a "blind" procedure (Menghini's technique) performed under local anesthesia using a transpleural or subcostal approach. The primary limitation of Menghini's technique is that the surgeon cannot see where the needle is going. Needle biopsy of the liver is indicated for unexplained hepatomegaly, hepatosplenomegaly, cholestasis (stoppage of bile secretion), persistently abnormal liver function tests, or suspected primary or metastatic liver tumor.

Contraindications to percutaneous liver biopsy are severe thrombocytopenia, local infection of the lung base, prolonged prothrombin time, peritonitis, massive ascites, an uncooperative client, and extrahepatic obstructive jaundice, especially with an enlarged gallbladder. The client with cancer or amyloidosis is at increased risk for postprocedure hemorrhage. If the client is unable to remain still and cooperative during the procedure, the surgeon can accidentally puncture another organ.

Procedure

The liver biopsy procedure may be performed at the bedside, in a procedure room, or in a gastrointestinal unit using a local anesthetic. Sedation and analgesia, such as with diazepam or midazolam, may be given to help allay the client's fears and make the client more comfortable. Place the client either in the supine or left lateral position with the right arm elevated. Less frequently, you may ask the client to assume a prone position. During insertion of the needle, have the client exhale and then hold the breath on expiration for 5 to 10 seconds to avoid puncture of the diaphragm (Fig. 42–4).

When the purpose of liver biopsy is to assess a focal lesion or abnormality, the blind procedure has definite limitations. The chance of inserting the needle into the wrong part of the liver and missing the lesion is great. With the use of concurrent ultrasonography, however, the physician can view the entire procedure and thus guide the needle. Guided biopsy allows better localization of a focal lesion or abnormality.

Fine-needle aspiration biopsy, often performed when a questionable area of the liver is localized, helps to confirm malignancy. This approach is ideal when only a few cells are necessary for cytologic study. The risks of fine-needle aspiration biopsy are far less than those of a guided regular biopsy because the tissue sample is much smaller. This procedure greatly reduces any risk of tumor metastasis along the needle track.

There are few contraindications to the guided regular or fine-needle aspiration biopsy procedures. Clients with impaired coagulation associated with liver disease, however, may not be appropriate candidates for the closed procedure. When biopsy is indicated for these clients, a

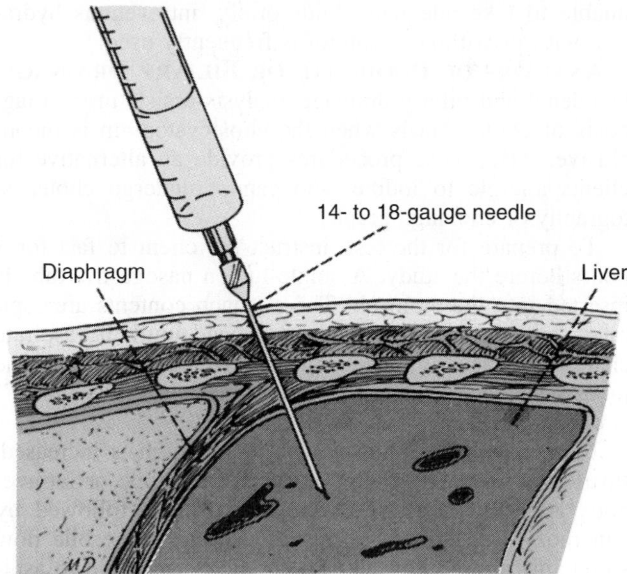

FIGURE 42–4 Percutaneous liver biopsy requires the client's cooperation. The client must be able to lie quietly and hold his or her breath after exhaling.

"plugged" biopsy procedure minimizes the risk of hemorrhage. This procedure allows injection of absorbable gelatin material on withdrawal of the biopsy needle. The gelatin material applies pressure to the bleeding site and closes the potential track. The client must be able to hold the breath for up to 15 seconds.

Preprocedure care

At least 2 weeks before a liver biopsy, the client must refrain from ingesting aspirin, NSAIDs, or anticoagulants. In addition, blood clotting tests (i.e., prothrombin time, bleeding time, partial thromboplastin time, platelet count, and hematocrit) are done beforehand.

Before the procedure is begun, the client fasts for at least 6 hours. Check the client's chart for the coagulation profile results; also check that the client has signed a consent form. Explain the procedure, including its purpose, insertion of an intravenous line during the procedure, and positioning during and after the procedure. When a client is informed about the procedure, the recovery period is smoother and less anxiety-producing than when no information is given. Emotional support is important to decrease apprehension and to help the client feel more in control.

Postprocedure care

After percutaneous liver biopsy, perform the following nursing assessments and interventions:

- Monitor vital signs every 15 minutes for 2 hours, every 30 minutes for 2 hours, and every 60 minutes for 4 hours.
- Assess for tachycardia and decreasing blood pressure, which may indicate hemorrhage.
- Check the puncture site by monitoring the dressing, palpating the surrounding area for crepitus, and observing for hematoma formation.
- Observe for pain in the right upper quadrant of the abdomen caused by a subcapsular accumulation of blood or bile or at the right shoulder as a result of blood on the undersurface of the diaphragm.
- Beginning 2 hours after the procedure, elevate the head of the bed 30 degrees. Two hours later, elevate it to 45 degrees. Maintain the client with bed rest for 24 hours after the procedure. Lying on the right side for the first 1 to 2 hours decreases the risk of hemorrhage and bile leakage.
- Administer postprocedure medications on an individual basis, depending on the client's physical status.
- Give vitamin K if prescribed.
- Assess respiratory status for manifestations of dyspnea.

Inherent risks of the biopsy procedure include hemorrhage and puncture of adjacent organs or structures. Hemorrhage, the most serious complication, may result from penetration of the arterial tree or a distended vein radicle during the first 24 hours after the biopsy procedure. The risk of hemorrhage is increased if vascular channels are distended or if the client breathes during needle insertion into the liver. Puncture of a lung can cause pneumothorax.

A large (14- to 18-gauge) biopsy needle can penetrate a dilated intrahepatic duct in a client with obstructive jaundice. Bile leakage and resultant peritonitis can develop. Bile peritonitis is treated with surgical decompression. Cross-contamination may occur after puncture of an adjacent organ. Clients with potentially effusive conditions (e.g., ascites, chronic lung disease) in addition to liver abnormality are at great risk for cross-contamination.

GALLBLADDER, BILIARY TRACT, AND PANCREAS

ORAL CHOLECYSTOGRAPHY (GALLBLADDER SERIES). Cholecystography is an x-ray test for gallbladder or cystic duct disease. Oral cholecystography (OCG) has been the standard examination for gallstones for almost 50 years but has been largely replaced by ultrasonography. Oral cholecystography is still useful for selecting clients for noninvasive treatment of gallstone disease, such as by lithotripsy or bile acid dissolution therapy. Oral cholecystography is useful in accurate identification of gallstones (90% to 95%)[10] and in assessing the patency of the cystic duct and gallbladder emptying function.

Procedure

During the test, radiography permits visualization of the gallbladder. When contraction of the gallbladder is desirable, the client consumes a high-fat meal during the procedure. After oral cholecystography, some people experience burning on urination because of the presence of the dye in the urine. Forcing fluids decreases this problem.

Poor or no visualization of the gallbladder indicates gallbladder disease, presumably because biliary obstruction prevents passage of the dye. Occasionally, stones can be visualized as shadows within the opaque medium. The test results are accurate only when gastrointestinal and liver function allows absorption and conjugation of the dye.

Preprocedure care

The evening before the examination, the client ingests a radiopaque dye according to the fat content of the evening meal. The client who has a regular or low-fat dinner may receive ipodate sodium. After a high-fat dinner, the client must be given iopanoic acid. These dyes contain iodine. Observe the client for allergic reactions even when the health history reveals no known allergies to iodine. Possible hypersensitive reactions include nausea and vomiting, diarrhea, abdominal pain, rash, and anaphylaxis. If diarrhea develops, the radiopaque dye may not be absorbed, resulting in nonvisualization of the gallbladder.

Conjugation of the dye occurs in the liver. Be aware that these dyes are potentially toxic to the liver and kidneys, especially in clients with pre-existing hepatic or renal failure. After excretion of the opaque medium into the bile, the gallbladder concentrates the contrast medium.

Postprocedure care

The client can eat after the examination. There is no other specific postprocedure care.

CHOLANGIOGRAPHY. Cholangiography or cholangiopancreatography allows visualization of the bile ducts. After administration of an organic iodine dye (iodipamide meglumine), x-ray filming begins. There are four types of cholangiography:

- *Intravenous cholangiography* is used for common bile duct visualization. The radiopaque dye burns intensely upon injection.
- *Percutaneous transhepatic cholangiography* involves injecting the dye directly into the ductal system through the skin via a long, slender needle.
- *Endoscopic retrograde cholangiopancreatography* (ERCP). After a local anesthetic solution is sprayed on the back of the throat, a fiberoptic endoscope is passed through the mouth to the papilla of Vater in the duodenum. The examiner passes a catheter into the common bile duct and, possibly, the pancreatic duct that allows injection of contrast material into pancreatic and biliary systems. The biliary tract and the pancreatic duct are observed for possible strictures, stones, cysts, or tumors.
- T-*tube cholangiography* involves injecting dye into a pre-existing bile drainage tube.

In all four types of cholangiography, failure of the opaque dye to pass through the bile ducts provides evidence of duct obstruction.

Preprocedure care

Explain the procedure to the client and significant others. Check that written consent has been obtained. Ask whether the client has had a history of allergies to iodine or contrast dye. If so, inform the physician. Explain that there may be a flushing sensation when the contrast medium is injected. Food and fluids may be restricted for 8 hours.

Obtain baseline vital signs. Administer sedatives as prescribed.

Postprocedure care

Check vital signs as ordered by the physician. A rising temperature may indicate an infection. Monitor skin color for signs of jaundice, which may indicate a disease process or the result of injury. The client should be monitored for an allergic reaction for 24 hours after the procedure. Warn the client that there may be some discomfort with urination while the dye is excreted. Also, to prevent renal damage, instruct the client to drink ample amounts of fluid after administration of the dye. If the client is unable to take adequate fluids orally, intravenous hydration with or without mannitol is frequently used.

ANALYSIS OF DUODENAL OR BILIARY DRAINAGE. Duodenal and biliary drainage analysis assists in the diagnosis of cholelithiasis when the cholecystogram is inconclusive. Also, these procedures provide an alternative for clients allergic to iodine who cannot undergo cholecystography or cholangiography.

To prepare for the test, instruct the client to fast for 8 hours before the study. A single-lumen nasogastric tube is inserted into the stomach. The stomach contents are aspirated, and the tube is slowly advanced until the aspirate changes to clear, golden, and alkaline. At this point, the tube is in the duodenum and clear golden bile ("A bile") is collected.

Next, the flow of bile into the duodenum is increased. Instillation of magnesium sulfate into the tube or intravenous administration of secretin (sometimes followed by pancreozymin) stimulates bile flow. After these bile flow stimulants are administered, it should be possible to aspirate 30 to 60 ml of concentrated bile ("B bile") from the duodenum. Bile can also be collected through an endoscope.

Collected fluid is sent to the laboratory to be analyzed for volume and bicarbonate, enzyme, and bile content. Disproportions in the bile and pancreatic juice fractions indicate obstruction in the bile or pancreatic duct. The presence of cholesterol crystals indicates lithiasis.

Other Metabolic Function Tests

PARACENTESIS. Paracentesis (peritoneal tap) is used to (1) extract fluid accumulations in the peritoneum (ascites), (2) relieve intra-abdominal tension, which can impair the client's respiratory status, or (3) obtain fluid for culture. After cleaning of the skin and infiltration with a local anesthetic, the physician, using sterile technique, inserts a long aspirating needle with a syringe to collect a fluid specimen. To drain ascitic fluid (if desired), the physician aseptically inserts a trocar through a small stab wound below the umbilicus. This procedure allows fluid (usually several liters) to drain slowly through a catheter into a collection bottle.

Preprocedure care

The nurse actively participates in the procedure, which usually takes place at the bedside. Obtain written permission before the procedure begins, and explain the purpose and steps involved. Ask the client to void immediately before the procedure to decrease the risk of bladder puncture. Have the client sit upright on the edge of the bed with the feet resting on a stool and the back well supported.

Postprocedure care

The major complication of paracentesis is *hypovolemia* and shock secondary to fluid drainage from the peritoneum, the resulting fluid shift from intravascular to interstitial space, and the sudden change in intra-abdominal pressure on the vessels. This fluid shift is exacerbated by hypoalbuminemia.

Assess vital signs and peripheral circulation every few minutes during and immediately after paracentesis. Observe for hypovolemic shock: pallor, tachycardia, decreased blood pressure, oliguria, and dyspnea.

Hepatic encephalopathy, caused by reduced tissue perfusion, is another complication resulting from drainage of ascitic fluid. Because ascitic fluid contains a high concentration of protein, the physician may prescribe albumin infusions for 24 hours after paracentesis to compensate for protein losses. Potassium depletion may also occur after multiple paracentesis procedures. Infection, peritonitis, and bleeding related to vessel trauma occasionally complicate paracentesis.

Carefully assess for abdominal pain after paracentesis. In addition, monitor the puncture site for persistent leakage of ascitic drainage.

CONCLUSIONS

Once you have gained a thorough knowledge of the structure and function of the endocrine and metabolic organs, you must examine the diagnostic assessment of these organs. Systematic assessment of the client with possible disorders of the endocrine and metabolic organs can lead to prompt diagnosis and treatment. You can facilitate the diagnostic process by adequately preparing the client for diagnostic procedures and by assisting with or collecting assessment data.

BIBLIOGRAPHY

1. Banks, P. A. (1998). Acute and chronic pancreatitis. In M. Feldman, B. F. Scharschmidt, & M. H. Sleisenger (Eds.), *Gastrointestinal and liver disease* (Vol. 1, 6th ed.). Philadelphia: W. B. Saunders.
2. Bates, B. (1995). *A guide to physical examination and history taking* (6th ed.). Philadelphia: J. B. Lippincott.
3. Bilhartz, L. E., & Horton, J. D. (1998). Gallstone disease and its complications. In M. Feldman, B. F. Scharschmidt, & M. H. Sleisenger (Eds.), *Gastrointestinal and liver disease* (Vol. 1, 6th ed.). Philadelphia: W. B. Saunders.
4. Birch, C. (1997). Caring for people with endocrine disorders. In J. Luckmann (Ed.), *Saunders manual of nursing care.* Philadelphia: W. B. Saunders.
5. Ebersol, P., & Hess, P. (1998). *Toward healthy aging: Human needs and nursing response* (5th ed.). St. Louis: Mosby–Year Book.
6. Ferri, F. F. (1995). *The care of the medical patient* (3rd ed.). St. Louis: Mosby–Year Book.
7. Friedman, L. S. (1995). Liver, biliary tract, pancreas. In L. M. Tierney, S. J. McPhee, & M. A. Papadakis (Eds.), *Current medical diagnosis and treatment* (34th ed.). Norwalk, CT: Appleton & Lange.
8. Friedman, S. L. (1998). Cirrhosis of the liver and its major sequelae. In J. C. Bennett & F. Plum (Eds.), *Cecil textbook of medicine* (20th ed.). Philadelphia: W. B. Saunders.
9. Ganong, W. F. (1997). *Review of medical physiology* (18th ed.). Norwalk, CT: Appleton & Lange.
10. Greensberger, N. J., & Isselbacher, K. J. (1998). Diseases of the gallbladder and bile ducts. In A. S. Fauci et al. (Eds.), *Harrison's principles of internal medicine* (14th ed., pp. 1725–1736). New York: McGraw-Hill.
11. Guyton, A. C., & Hall, J. E. (1996). *Textbook of medical physiology* (9th ed.). Philadelphia: W. B. Saunders.
12. *Healthy people 2000: National Health Promotion and Disease Prevention Objectives.* (1990). Washington, DC: U.S. Public Health Service.
13. Jarvis, C. (2000). *Physical examination and health assessment* (3rd ed.). Philadelphia: W. B. Saunders.
14. Kee, J. L. (1999). *Laboratory and diagnostic tests with nursing implications* (5th ed.). Stamford, CT: Appleton & Lange.
15. McCance, K., & Heuther, S. (1994). *Pathophysiology: The biological basis for disease in adults and children* (2nd ed.). St. Louis: Mosby–Year Book.
16. Melillo, K. D. (1993). Interpretation of abnormal laboratory values in older adults: Part II. *Journal of Gerontological Nursing, 19*(2), 35–40.
17. Melillo, K. D. (1993). Interpretation of laboratory values in older adults. *Nurse Practitioner, 18*(7), 59–67.
18. Mirowski, G. W. & Berger, T. G. (1998). Oral and cutaneous manifestations of gastrointestinal disease. In M. Feldman, B. F. Scharschmidt, & M. H. Sleisenger (Eds.), *Gastrointestinal and liver disease* (Vol. 1, 6th ed.). Philadelphia: W. B. Saunders.
19. Moses, A. M., & Streeten, D. H. P. (1998). Disorders of the neurohypophysis. In A. S. Fauci et al. (Eds.), *Harrison's principles of internal medicine* (14th ed., pp. 2003–2011). New York: McGraw-Hill.
20. Murray, W. J., & Gabel, T. L. (1998, May). *What about herbal medicine?* Unpublished manuscript, University of Nebraska Medical Center, Omaha.
21. Niedzwick, L., & Stringer, C. (1994). Liver biopsy and nursing intervention. *Gastroenterology Nursing, 17*(1), 17–19.
22. Ober, K. P. (1996). Work-up of endocrine abnormalities. *Hospital Medicine, 32*(10), 15–25.
23. Podolsky, D. K., & Isselbacher, K. J. (1998). Evaluation of liver function. In A. S. Fauci et al. (Eds.), *Harrison's principles of internal medicine* (13th ed., pp. 1663–1667). New York: McGraw-Hill.
24. Price, S., & Wilson, L. (Eds.). (1994). *Pathophysiology* (4th ed.). St. Louis: Mosby–Year Book.
25. Seidel, H. M., et al. (1995). *Mosby's guide to physical examination* (3rd ed.). St. Louis: Mosby–Year Book.
26. Sommers, M. S., & Johnson, S. A. (1997). *Davis's manual of nursing therapeutics for disease and disorders.* Philadelphia: F. A. Davis.
27. Swearingen, P. L. (1994). *Manual of medical-surgical nursing care* (3rd ed., pp. 380–481). St. Louis: Mosby–Year Book.
28. Swearingen, P. L. (1995). *Mosby's medical-surgical nursing* (2nd ed.). St. Louis: Mosby–Year Book.
29. Treseler, K. M. (1995). *Clinical laboratory and diagnostic tests* (3rd ed.). Norwalk, CT: Appleton & Lange.
30. Wartofsky, L. (1998). Diseases of the thyroid. In A. S. Fauci, et al. (Eds.), *Harrison's principles of internal medicine* (14th ed., pp. 2012–2034). New York: McGraw-Hill.
31. Wilson, J., & Foster, D. (1992). *Williams textbook of endocrinology* (8th ed.). Philadelphia: W. B. Saunders.

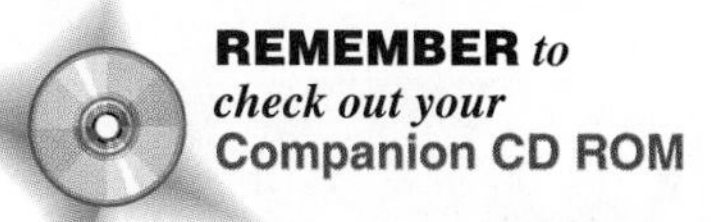

CHAPTER 43

Management of Clients with Thyroid and Parathyroid Disorders

Anne Larson

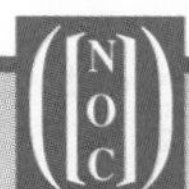

NURSING OUTCOMES CLASSIFICATION (NOC)
for Nursing Diagnoses—Clients with Thyroid and Parathyroid Disorders

Activity Intolerance
Activity Intolerance
Endurance
Energy Conservation
Self-Care: Activities of Daily Living
Altered Nutrition: Less than Body Requirements
Nutritional Status
Nutritional Status: Food and Fluid Intake
Nutritional Status: Nutrient Intake
Altered Nutrition: More than Body Requirements
Nutritional Status: Food and Fluid Intake
Nutritional Status: Nutrient Intake
Weight Control
Altered Urinary Elimination
Knowledge: Disease Process
Symptom Control
Symptom Severity
Urinary Elimination
Constipation
Bowel Elimination
Hydration
Medication Response
Mobility Level
Decreased Cardiac Output
Cardiac Pump Effectiveness
Circulation Status
Tissue Perfusion: Peripheral
Vital Signs Status
Hyperthermia
Thermoregulation
Vital Signs Status
Hypothermia
Thermoregulation
Vital Signs Status
Impaired Social Interaction
Role Performance
Social Interaction Skills
Social Involvement
Risk for Impaired Skin Integrity
Fluid Balance
Immobility Consequences: Physiologic
Nutritional Status
Risk Control
Risk Detection
Thermoregulation
Tissue Integrity: Skin and Mucous Membranes
Tissue Perfusion: Peripheral
Risk for Injury
Knowledge: Personal Safety
Neurological Status
Risk Control
Risk Control: Visual Impairment
Risk Detection
Symptom Control

THYROID DISORDERS

Many terms describe normal and abnormal states of thyroid function. *Euthyroidism* means that the thyroid gland is functioning normally. Like other endocrine disorders, the two primary thyroid disorders are related to increased secretion (*hyperthyroidism*) and decreased secretion (*hypothyroidism*) of the gland's hormones. Such alterations in thyroid hormone (TH) secretion result in increased or decreased rates of metabolic function, heat production, and oxygen consumption. In addition, a third disorder is related to enlargement of the thyroid gland. These enlargements are called *goiters*.

This chapter incorporates material written for the fifth edition by Carol Birch.

GOITER

Enlargement of the thyroid gland may be seen with both hyperthyroidism and hypothyroidism. It generally results from lack of iodine, inflammation, or benign or malignant tumors. Enlargement may also appear in hyperthyroidism, especially Graves' disease, in which the client typically has exophthalmos as well.

Etiology and Risk Factors

There are two major forms of simple goiter: endemic and sporadic.

Endemic goiter is caused principally by nutritional iodine deficiency. It tends to occur in goiter "belts," geographical areas characterized by soil and water that are deficient in iodine. Major goiter belts in the United States are the Midwest, Northwest, and Great Lakes regions. Iodine is readily available in regions with access to salt water and also through consumption of seafood. Hence, goiters are less common in coastal areas.

Endemic goiter typically occurs in fall and winter months and is twice as prevalent in women as in men. Also, because the need for TH is particularly great during growth spurts, pregnancy, and lactation, goiter commonly develops in adolescents, pregnant women, and nursing mothers living in iodine-deficient regions.

Sporadic goiter is not restricted to any geographical area. Major causes include:

- Genetic defects resulting in faulty iodine metabolism
- Ingestion of large amounts of nutritional *goitrogens* (goiter-producing agents that inhibit thyroxine [T_4] production), such as rutabagas, cabbage, soybeans, peanuts, peaches, peas, strawberries, spinach, and radishes, all of which contain goitrogenic glycosides
- Ingestion of medicinal goitrogens, for example, adrenergic antagonists, glucocorticoids, dopamine, methimazole, lithium, iodinated radiographic contrast agents, phenytoin, rifampin, carbamazepine, propylthiouracil (PTU), and thiocarbamides (aminothiazole, tolbutamide)

Health promotion practices include ingestion of iodized salt and avoidance of goitrogens. Health maintenance or restoration interventions include teaching about the use of iodized salt.

Pathophysiology

If a person's diet lacks sufficient iodine or if production of thyroid hormones is suppressed for any other reason, the thyroid enlarges in an attempt to compensate for hormonal deficiency. Under these circumstances, goiter is essentially an adaptation to a deficiency of thyroid hormones. Enlargement of the gland also occurs in response to increased pituitary secretion of thyroid-stimulating hormone (TSH). TSH stimulates the thyroid to secrete more T_4 when blood T_4 levels are low. Eventually, the gland may become so large that it compresses structures in the neck and chest, causing respiratory problems and dysphagia.

Clinical Manifestations

Diagnosis of simple goiter is confirmed by history, clinical findings, and laboratory tests (Fig. 43–1). The client is often euthyroid because the gland enlarges enough to produce normal amounts of T_4. Needle biopsy of the goiter may be indicated to rule out malignancy.

Outcome Management

Medical Management

When enlargement is a compensatory reaction to iodine deficiency and consequent suppression of T_4 secretion, the client can be treated with preparations of iodine and thyroid hormones. Either a strong iodine solution (Lugol's solution) or saturated solution of potassium iodide (SSKI) drops can be administered. Iodine reduces the size and vascularity of the enlarged gland. The availability of iodized salt and thyroid hormones has made replacement therapy with iodine obsolete in the United States.

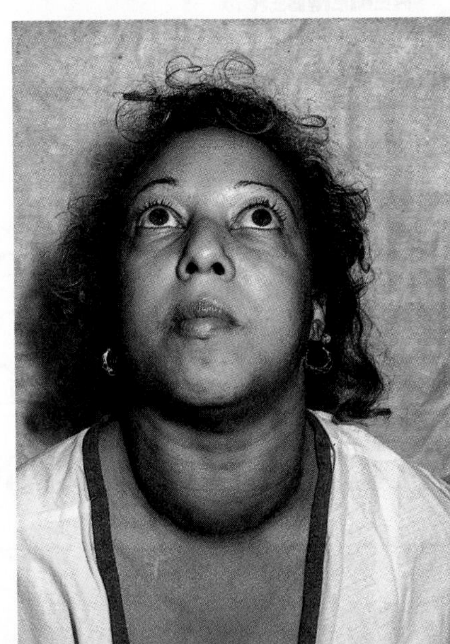

FIGURE 43–1 Massive thyroid enlargement caused by diffuse toxic goiter. *A*, Front view. *B*, Side view. (From Swartz, M. H., [1998]. *Textbook of physical diagnosis* [3rd ed.]. Philadelphia: W. B. Saunders.)

The client's diet should also be higher in iodine. The client may switch to iodized salt. Dietary goitrogens (e.g., turnips, soybeans, rutabagas, and, to a lesser degree, seafood, green leafy vegetables, carrots, and peanuts) should be avoided.

Endemic goiter can be prevented altogether by the use of iodized salt. Adults require at least 50 mg of iodine per day. However, 200 to 300 mg/day is considered the minimum adequate intake needed to prevent goiter. Iodized salt, used in the United States since 1924, contains 1 part iodine to 100,000 parts of salt. Thus, the average person, who ingests about 6.2 g of salt a day, is also taking 474 mg of iodine daily if the salt is iodized.

Many clients do not understand the need for iodized salt as a goiter preventative. Some believe that any additive to food or water is harmful and, therefore, avoid iodized salt. These two problems, along with the fact that many modern foods are processed with cheaper non-iodized salt, contribute to the potential for development of simple goiter. Nurses need to educate the public about the importance of iodized salt.

Surgical Management

Surgery is indicated for a goiter that is very large, does not respond to treatment, or is putting too much pressure on other structures in the neck. Surgery is discussed in detail under Hyperthyroidism.

HYPOTHYROIDISM

Hypothyroidism is a deficiency of TH resulting in slowed body metabolism, decreased heat production, and decreased oxygen consumption by the tissues. The underactivity of the thyroid gland may result from primary thyroid dysfunction or be secondary to anterior pituitary dysfunction.

The term hypothyroidism is not synonymous with m*yxedema* (mucinous edema), a complication of hypothyroidism characterized by a generalized hypometabolic state. *Myxedema coma* is a life-threatening condition in which all body systems are severely compromised by the hypometabolic state.

The frequency of hypothyroidism depends on the population being studied. The incidence of overt hypothyroidism is one to two in 1000 people in community surveys and five to 20 in 1000 clients seeking medical care.

Hypothyroidism affects women more than men (about 4:1). Although hypothyroidism may be congenital (cretinism) and therefore present at birth, the highest incidence is in adults between 30 and 65 years of age. About 95% of all people with hypothyroidism have the *primary* form of the disease. *Central hypothyroidism* resulting from pituitary or hypothalamic disease accounts for fewer than 10% of cases. Myxedema is most commonly identified in postmenopausal, hypothyroid women in their 60s.

Etiology and Risk Factors

Primary hypothyroidism may be caused by:

- Congenital defects of the thyroid (cretinism)
- Defective hormone synthesis
- Iodine deficiency (prenatal and postnatal)
- Antithyroid drugs
- Surgery or treatment with radioactive agents for hyperthyroidism
- Chronic inflammatory (autoimmune) diseases such as Hashimoto's disease, amyloidosis, and sarcoidosis

Hashimoto's disease is the most common type of autoimmune hypothyroidism. In primary hypothyroidism, TH levels are low and TSH levels are elevated, indicating that the pituitary is attempting to stimulate the secretion of thyroid hormones and the thyroid is not responding.

Secondary hypothyroidism develops when there is insufficient stimulation of a normal thyroid gland; consequently, TSH levels are decreased. This condition may start as a malfunction of the pituitary or hypothalamus. It may also be caused by peripheral resistance to TH. When this occurs, both TSH and TH levels are low in the serum.

Tertiary or *central hypothyroidism* can develop if the hypothalamus cannot produce thyroid-releasing hormone (TRH) and subsequently does not stimulate the pituitary to secrete TSH. It may be due to a tumor or other destructive lesion in the hypothalamic region. When this occurs, both TSH and TH levels are again low in the serum.

Subclinical hypothyroidism is defined as hypothyroidism that is diagnosed with an elevated TSH level but a normal to low-normal T_4 level. Manifestations resemble those of mild hypothyroidism with subtle cardiac defects, especially in clients with pre-existing cardiac disease. Subclinical hypothyroidism is found in 20 to 120 of 1000 persons in the community. The causes are the same as those of primary hypothyroidism. Its prevalence increases with age. Low-dose levothyroxine sodium (Synthroid) is effective for relief of manifestations and improvement in cardiac function and lipid profile.

Use of iodized salt and avoidance of goitrogens are health promotion activities. Health restoration practices involve lifelong hormone replacement.

Pathophysiology

The thyroid gland needs iodine to synthesize and secrete thyroid hormones: T_4, triiodothyronine (T_3), and thyrocalcitonin (calcitonin). Production of thyroid hormones depends on secretion of TSH from the anterior pituitary and ingestion of adequate protein and iodine. The hypothalamus regulates the pituitary secretion of TSH via a negative feedback system.

Decreased levels of thyroid hormones lead to overall slowing of the basal metabolic rate. This slowing of all body processes leads to achlorhydria (decreased secretion of hydrochloric acid in the stomach), decreased gastrointestinal tract motility, bradycardia, slowed neurologic functioning, and a decrease in heat production resulting in a decreased basal body temperature.

The most important changes caused by reduced levels of thyroid hormones are those affecting lipid metabolism. The reduction in thyroid hormones causes an increase in serum cholesterol and triglyceride levels and an increase in arteriosclerosis and coronary heart disease in clients with hypothyroidism.

Because thyroid hormones play a role in the production of red blood cells, people with hypothyroidism also show evidence of anemia, with possible vitamin B_{12} and folate deficiency.

Myxedema, a mucinous edema, is caused by accumulation of hydrophilic proteoglycans in the interstitial spaces. The cause of this problem remains unclear.

Clinical Manifestations

The manifestations of hypothyroidism depend on whether it is mild or complicated by myxedema or myxedema coma.

Mild Hypothyroidism

Clients with mild hypothyroidism (the most common form) may be asymptomatic or may experience vague manifestations so ordinary as to escape detection. For example, clients may experience sensitivity to cold, lethargy, dry skin or hair, forgetfulness, depression, and some weight gain (Table 43–1).

The client's physical appearance changes. Often, obesity develops, features become coarse, hair becomes dry and sparse, and the skin feels dry, flaky, and inelastic. In addition, clients with hypothyroidism are sensitive to cold because of a decreased metabolic rate and a decreased basal body temperature. The client's ability to sweat also diminishes. Constipation and fecal impaction related to slowed peristaltic action and lack of normal physical activity are serious problems. Also, there is increased susceptibility to infection.

Vital sign changes may be minimal: the heart rate is normal or slow; blood pressure may be normal, or both systolic and diastolic pressures may be slightly elevated; temperature may be normal to subnormal; and respiratory

TABLE 43–1 MANIFESTATIONS OF HYPOTHYROIDISM AND HYPERTHYROIDISM

System	Hypothyroidism	Hyperthyroidism
Cardiovascular	↓ HR + ↓ SV: ↓ CO ↓ Myocardial O_2 demand ↑ Peripheral vascular resistance Possible hypertension Hyperlipidemia Hypercholesterolemia Distant heart sounds	↑ HR + ↑ SV: ↑ CO ↑ O_2 consumption Systolic BP ↑ 10–15 mm Hg Diastolic BP ↑ 10–15 mm Hg Palpitations Rapid, bounding pulse Possible heart failure, edema
Hematologic	Normocytic, normochromic anemia Macrocytic anemia (pernicious) Easy bruising	No specific changes
Respiratory	Reduced hypoxic drive Hypercapnic ventilatory drive Respiratory muscle weakness Possible CO_2 retention on arterial blood gas tests Dyspnea	↑ Respiratory rate and depth Shortness of breath
Renal	Fluid retention ↓ Urinary output ↑ Total body water Dilutional hyponatremia ↓ Production of erythropoietin	Fluid retention ↓ Output
Gastrointestinal	↓ Peristalsis Anorexia Possible weight gain Constipation ↓ Protein metabolism ↑ Serum lipids Delayed glucose uptake ↓ Glucose absorption	↑ Peristalsis ↑ Appetite Weight loss Diarrhea ↑ Use of adipose and protein stores ↓ Serum lipids ↑ Gastrointestinal secretions Vomiting, abdominal pain
Musculoskeletal	Transient pain Muscle cramps and stiffness Slow movements ↑ Bone density ↓ Bone formation and resorption	Negative nitrogen balance Malnutrition Fatigue Muscle weakness Proximal muscle wasting Incoordination caused by tremors
Integumentary	Dry, coarse, scaly skin Hair that falls out Thick, brittle nails Expressionless face Periorbital edema Thick, puffy skin: face and pretibial areas Cold intolerance	Profuse sweating Moist skin Flushed, warm skin Hair: fine, soft, straight, possible hair loss Heat intolerance
Endocrine	Normal to enlarged thyroid	Thyroid usually enlarged Bruit over thyroid
Neurologic	↓ Deep tendon reflexes Muscle sluggishness Fatigue, somnolence Slow, deliberate speech Apathy, depression, paranoia Impaired short-term memory Lethargy	↑ Deep tendon reflexes Fine tremors Nervousness, restlessness Emotional instability: anxiety, worry, paranoia
Reproductive	Females: menorrhagia, anovulation, irregular menses, decreased libido Males: decreased libido, impotence	Females: amenorrhea, irregular menses, ↓ fertility, ↑ tendency for spontaneous abortion Males: impotence, decreased libido ↓ Sexual development prepuberty
Other	Myxedema	Exophthalmos

BP, blood pressure; CO, cardiac output; CO_2, carbon dioxide; HR, heart rate; O_2, oxygen; SV, stroke volume.

rate and rhythm may be affected by goiter size and degree of respiratory distress.

As the degree of hypothyroidism worsens, the thyroid may enlarge (goiter) in an attempt to produce enough T_4. Typically, clients seek medical advice when the goiter grows large enough to distort the appearance of the neck. They may also experience respiratory distress and dysphagia if the goiter is very large.

MYXEDEMA

Myxedema may develop in clients with undiagnosed or undertreated hypothyroidism who experience stress. Stressors include infection, drugs (phenothiazines, barbiturates, narcotics, anesthetics), respiratory failure, heart failure, cerebral vascular accident, trauma, prolonged exposure to cold, metabolic disturbances, surgery, and seizures.

Myxedema is characterized by a dry, waxy type of swelling with abnormal deposits of mucin in the skin and other tissues. The edema is of the nonpitting type and is common in the pretibial and facial areas (Fig. 43–2).

Myxedema is most commonly diagnosed in hypothyroid women in their 60s. Untreated myxedema has been associated with severe atherosclerosis and has been attributed to the increase in serum cholesterol concentrations, particularity low-density lipoproteins. TH replacement improves these changes.

MYXEDEMA COMA

The major complication of hypothyroidism is myxedema coma, an extremely rare condition with a mortality rate approaching 100%. Myxedema coma is characterized by a drastic decrease in metabolic rate, hypoventilation leading to respiratory acidosis, hypothermia, and hypotension. Complicating conditions include hyponatremia, hypercalcemia, secondary adrenal insufficiency, hypoglycemia, and water intoxication. Myxedema coma may be brought on by stress—as from surgery or infection—or by noncompliance with thyroid treatment.

Diagnostic tests for hypothyroidism confirm the clinical picture of hypometabolism and depressed thyroid activity (Table 43–2). The serum TSH level is elevated in primary hypothyroidism. Radioactive iodide uptake is decreased in hypothyroidism.

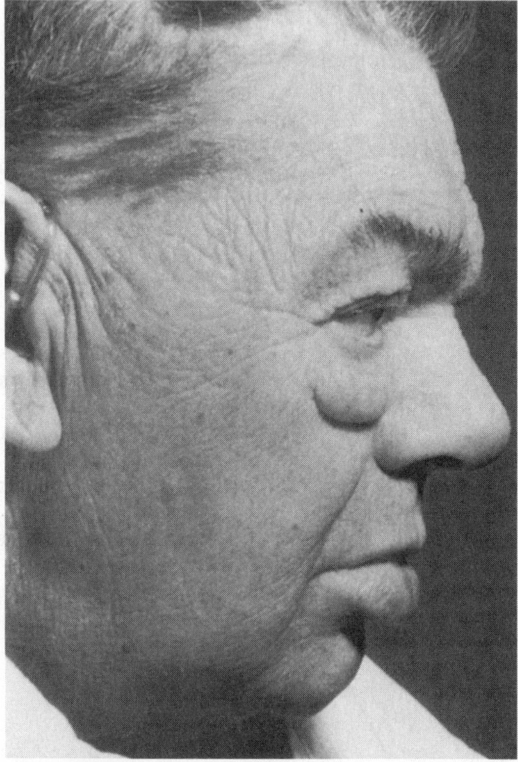

FIGURE 43–2 Typical facial appearance of myxedematous client. (From Jacob, S. W. [1982]. *Structure and function in man* [5th ed.] Philadelphia: W. B. Saunders.)

Clients with myxedema may also have hypercholesterolemia, hyperlipidemia, and proteinemia as a result of T_4 changes in the synthesis, mobilization, and degradation of serum lipids. Elevated lipid levels may contribute to the later development of cardiac problems. Dilutional hyponatremia may develop as a result of the marked impairment of water excretion because of decreased delivery of sodium and volume to the distal renal tubules associated with decreased renal blood flow. Elevated creatine phosphokinase, aspartate aminotransferase, and lactate dehydrogenase may also develop secondary to altered metabolism.

Outcome Management

Hypothyroidism is rarely a primary diagnosis. Usually, the diagnosis is made after the development of another medical problem. Clients with hypothyroidism are typically managed on an outpatient basis with TH replacement. Treatment is an ongoing, lifelong process. Clients with myxedema or myxedema coma are managed as a medical emergency.

Medical Management

MYXEDEMA AND MYXEDEMA COMA

The desired outcome of the medical management of myxedema coma is to reverse the condition to save the client's life. Supportive measures begin immediately and include maintaining a patent airway, giving oxygen, and replacing fluids intravenously. The client is kept warm, and vital signs are closely monitored until the client begins to recover. Vasopressors are used to maintain tissue perfusion.

Levothyroxine sodium is given intravenously with glucose and corticosteroids. When administering TH to a client with myxedema heart disease, assess the client carefully for angina, dyspnea, or orthopnea. The event that precipitated the coma (surgery, infection, noncompliance) must be evaluated and treated as well.

The desired outcomes of the medical management of hypothyroidism are to correct TH deficiency, reverse manifestations, and prevent further cardiac and arterial damage.

CORRECT THYROID HORMONE DEFICIENCY. For hypothyroidism to be reversed permanently, the client must usually take TH for life. Levothyroxine sodium is the principal form of replacement therapy. Dosages vary with age, the severity of the hypothyroidism, general medical condition (particularly cardiovascular disorders), and the client's response to medical treatment at the initiation of TH therapy. Children and older adults receive smaller doses.

Clients who respond to TH therapy receive a maintenance dose of T_4 daily for life. Pharmacologic goitrogens are replaced by drugs that do not interfere with TH function. The drug of choice for thyroid replacement is levothyroxine sodium, which is converted in the body to both T_4 and T_3 (Table 43–3). Desiccated thyroid and liothyronine sodium (Cytomel), once commonly used in replacement therapy, are now used infrequently because of problems with fluctuating plasma levels and side effects.

TABLE 43–2 DIAGNOSTIC TESTS FOR THYROID DISORDERS*

Test	Description	Nursing Notes	Indications
THYROID FUNCTION TESTS			
Thyroid-stimulating hormone (TSH) assay	TSH controls triiodothyronine (T_3) and thyroxine (T_4) release; TSH released from anterior pituitary	None	↑: Hypofunction of thyroid gland; primary hypothyroidism ↓: Pituitary disorders; hyperthyroidism; high dosages of dopamine or corticosteroids
Radioactive iodine uptake	Used to determine the metabolic activity of the thyroid gland by measuring absorption of ^{131}I in thyroid	Client education: radioactive dose is small and harmless Contraindicated in pregnancy Drugs that may elevate results: barbiturates, estrogen, lithium, phenothiazines Seafood may elevate results Drugs that may decrease results: Lugol's solution, saturated solution of potassium iodide (SSKI), antithyroid, cortisone, aspirin, antihistamines 24-hr urine collection begins after oral tracer dose given Thyroid scanned after 24 hr	↑: Hyperthyroidism, thyroiditis, liver cirrhosis; urine: hypothyroidism ↓: Hypothyroidism; urine: hyperthyroidism
Thyroid antibodies	Measures the presence of antibodies produced by body; may cause inflammation and destruction of thyroid gland	Note if client receiving oral contraceptives because they may elevate titers	↑: Thyroiditis
Free thyroxine (FT_4) concentration	FT_4 is metabolically active form of thyroxine	Results may be inaccurate with high estrogen levels or low serum protein levels	↑: Hyperthyroidism ↓: Hypothyroidism
Thyroxine (T_4)	A direct measurement of total amount of T_4 present in blood	Fasting is recommended Note on laboratory slip if client is taking thyroid supplements; levels can be increased by pregnancy or oral contraceptives	↑: Hyperthyroidism Normal–↓: Hypothyroidism
Triiodothyronine (T_3) radioimmunoassay	Measures small amount of potent thyroid hormones; T_3 is active form of thyroid hormone	Same as T_4	↑: Hyperthyroidism, pregnancy, oral contraceptives Normal–↓: Hypothyroidism, hypoprotein conditions
T_3 resin uptake (T_3 RU)	Measures T_3 that is protein bound	None	↑: Hyperthyroidism, low serum protein levels ↓: High serum protein, hypothyroidism
Thyroid-binding globulins (TBGs)	Measures T_4 that is protein bound	None	↑: Hyperthyroidism, low serum protein ↓: High serum protein, hypothyroidism
Thyroid-releasing hormone (TRH)	TRH influences TSH release	None	↑: Hypothyroidism ↓: Hyperthyroidism

TABLE 43–2 DIAGNOSTIC TESTS FOR THYROID DISORDERS* *Continued*

Test	Description	Nursing Notes	Indications
DIAGNOSTIC IMAGING STUDIES			
Thyroid scan	Injection of radioactive isotopes used to identify thyroid gland	No preparation Radioactive iodine taken orally; dose is harmless Scanning done 24 hr later Be aware of contraindications such as potassium iodide, Lugol's solution, seafood intake, thyroid medications	Cold nodules: cancer Hot nodules: benign
Ultrasonography	Identifies presence, size, and location of gland and nodules; differentiates solid tumors from fluid-filled cysts	No preparation necessary Remind clients that they will not be radioactive Provide client education to alleviate anxiety	
Thyroid scan	Injection of radioactive isotopes used to identify thyroid gland	No preparation Radioactive iodine taken orally; dose is harmless Scanning done 24 hr later Be aware of contraindications such as potassium iodide, Lugol's solution, seafood intake, thyroid medications	Cold nodules: cancer Hot nodules: benign
Magnetic resonance imaging	Used to visualize gland size, location, identify abnormalities	Test cannot be done in clients with metal implants (such as pacemakers, arthroplasties, skull plates) Assess for allergy to contrast media Inquire about claustrophobia	
Computed tomography	Identifies location and structure of gland	Client education Noninvasive Contrast media may be used; note allergy history	
OTHER PROCEDURES USED TO DIAGNOSE ENDOCRINE DISORDERS			
Fine-needle aspiration	Provides sample of cells for histologic studies; usually used as thyroid biopsy	Client education for short, relatively pain-free procedure Observe site for swelling and bleeding	Benign or malignant

*The following drugs affect thyroid function test results: amiodarone hydrochloride (HCl) (Cordarone), corticosteroids, cough medicine (with iodine), dopamine HCl (Dopastat, Intropin), estrogens., lithium carbonate (Eskalith, Lithane, Lithobid), phenytoin (Dilantin), salicylates.

Data from Malarkey, L. M., & McMorrow, M. E. (1996). *Nurses' manual of laboratory tests and diagnostic procedures.* Philadelphia: W. B. Saunders.

REVERSE MANIFESTATIONS. Clients with hypothyroidism of long duration notice an improvement in manifestations within 2 to 3 weeks of starting medication; however, hoarseness, anemia, and changes in hair and skin may take many months to resolve.

PREVENT CARDIAC COMPLICATIONS. A client with cardiac complications starts with a small dose of TH. Large doses may precipitate heart failure or myocardial infarction by increasing body metabolism, myocardial oxygen requirements, and, consequently, the workload of the heart.

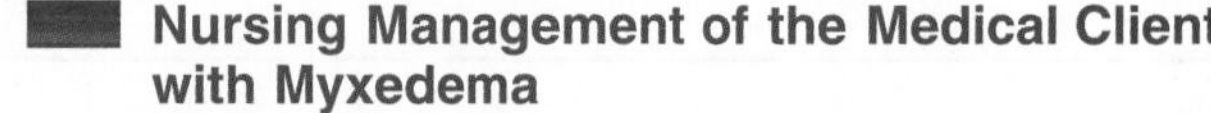

Nursing Management of the Medical Client with Myxedema

ASSESSMENT

Observe the client for the physical manifestations of myxedema, such as periorbital and facial edema, a blank facial expression, a thick tongue, and generalized slowing of all muscle movement. The client's vital signs are also affected and must be monitored closely. The client is hypothermic. Depressed respirations precipitate respiratory acidosis. Alterations in heart rate and blood pressure follow.

TABLE 43–3 NURSING IMPLICATIONS FOR MEDICATIONS USED TO TREAT THYROID DISORDERS

Class	Action	Therapeutic Outcomes	Adverse Outcomes	Dosing
HYPERTHYROID MEDICATIONS (ANTITHYROID DRUGS)				
Propylthiouracil (PTU)	Temporarily inhibits thyroid hormone synthesis	Thyroid hormone level returns to normal; resting heart rate less than 100 beats per minute	Use carefully in combination with any drug that causes agranulocytosis Monitor blood counts for agranulocytosis Observe for signs of hypothyroidism	100–150 mg PO tid Give orally every 8 hr around the clock Urge continued compliance because response is slow
Radioactive iodine (^{131}I)	Antithyroid drug that destroys thyroid tissue; used to treat hyperthyroidism; may be used to treat thyroid cancer	Thyroid hormone level decreases	Monitor for evidence of local irritation from irradiation concentration in the neck	4–10 mCi PO for hyperthyroidism, 50–150 mCi for thyroid cancer Stop all antithyroid medications 1 week before giving ^{131}I Monitor thyroid function closely Give on an empty stomach Institute radiation precautions for body secretions for 3 days after ingestion Tell client to avoid close, prolonged contact with children for 1 week; should also sleep alone for 1 week Client should not resume antithyroid medications for 6 weeks
HYPOTHYROID MEDICATIONS				
Levothyroxine sodium (Synthroid, Levothroid, Levoxine)	Thyroid replacement medication (T_4) used to treat hypothyroidism	Thyroid hormone level returns to normal range; signs and symptoms of decreased thyroid hormones resolve	Watch for adverse effects early in treatment Toxicity may last for weeks with overdose Monitor for improvement of manifestions Serum levels may be decreased when client is also taking aluminum hydroxide antacid Monitor pulse, blood pressure, and thyroid function	Initial low dose daily increased until response to 0.1–0.2 mg/day in hypothyroidism (less in older clients); 0.2–0.5 mg IV in myxedema coma Give a single dose in AM Watch for adverse effects early in treatment Stress need for lifetime replacement Smaller doses required for older clients

DIAGNOSIS, OUTCOMES, INTERVENTIONS

Decreased Cardiac Output. The client with myxedema is susceptible to severe arteriosclerotic heart disease and other cardiac abnormalities, leading to the nursing diagnosis *Decreased Cardiac Output related to sustained bradycardia, resulting in edema and decreased urine output.*

Outcomes. The client will maintain a normal cardiac output and will remain free of heart failure, as evidenced by normal heart rate, evidence of normal perfusion, absence of edema, and urine output of at least ½ ml/kg/hr.

Interventions. As the client proceeds with hormone replacement therapy, the edema and puffiness start to lessen. Continue to monitor the client's intake and output, which will become more balanced. Urinary output should increase significantly during thyroid therapy. Monitor the client's weight daily.

To help prevent further strain on the already overburdened heart, help the client conserve energy. For example, always help the client turn in bed. If any new cardiac manifestations occur, notify the physician immediately. Do not give TH until the physician has reappraised the client's condition.

When administering thyroid preparations, assess the client carefully for manifestations of thyrotoxicosis, such as tachycardia, increased appetite, diarrhea, sweating, agitation, tremor, palpitations, and shortness of breath. If any of these manifestations develop during thyroid therapy, notify the physician at once so that the dosage can be reduced.

Hypothermia. A client with severe myxedema has a very low metabolic rate, leading to an important nursing diagnosis of *Hypothermia related to slowed metabolic rate resulting in subnormal body temperature.*

Outcomes. The client's body temperature will return to normal.

Interventions. Provide the client with a comfortable, warm environment. Remember that hypothyroidism sharply increases sensitivity to cold. If necessary, supply extra clothing and warm blankets. Encourage the client to dress warmly and avoid extreme cold whenever possible. In cases of severe hypothermia, a warming blanket may be necessary.

Risk for Injury: Myxedema Coma. A client with acute hypothyroidism is susceptible to development of myxedema coma, leading to the nursing diagnosis *Risk for Injury: Myxedema coma related to hypersensitivity to anesthetics, sedatives, and narcotics secondary to decreased metabolic rate.*

Outcomes. The client will not receive the usual doses of anesthetics, sedatives, and narcotics so that development of myxedema coma will be prevented and the client will not be injured.

Interventions. The client should not receive sedatives unless it is absolutely necessary. If a sedative or narcotic must be given, administer no more than one-third to one-half the usual dose. Then assess the client carefully for respiratory depression or a decreased level of consciousness.

Risk for Impaired Skin Integrity. A client with myxedema is very susceptible to skin breakdown, leading to the nursing diagnosis *Risk for Impaired Skin Integrity related to edema and dryness secondary to infiltration of fluid into interstitial spaces.*

Outcomes. The client's skin will remain intact, as evidenced by absence of injury and resolution of edema.

Interventions. Monitor the sacrum, coccyx, elbows, scapulae, and other pressure points for redness or tissue breakdown. Remember that edematous tissues are more susceptible to pressure ulcers. Have a strict turning schedule for the client, and use a pressure reduction mattress.

EVALUATION

It is expected that after successful treatment the client will demonstrate no evidence of heart failure, edema, or skin impairment; temperature and urine output will be normal; and there will be no further evidence of myxedema. After the client is out of danger and alert, long-term management begins (see next).

Nursing Management of the Medical Client with Hypothyroidism

ASSESSMENT

Carefully assess the client for manifestations of hypothyroidism. Obtain a careful history; look for evidence of decreased metabolic function, such as weight gain, excessive sleeping, and generalized fatigue. The Critical Monitoring feature on Hypothyroidism lists other manifestations of decreased metabolic functions. Take a thorough diet history, looking particularly at the intake of iodine. Does the client take any goitrogenic substances or reside in a goiter belt?

Ask the client about other medical conditions that might be present, such as a history of hyperthyroidism treated with surgery or radioactive iodine, both of which predispose to hypothyroidism. Does the client use any medication that might lead to hypothyroidism? Lithium, aminoglutethimide, sodium or potassium perchlorate, and cobalt can slow thyroid metabolism.

DIAGNOSIS, OUTCOMES, INTERVENTIONS

Altered Nutrition: More than Body Requirements. The slowed metabolic rate places a hypothyroid client at risk for weight gain, leading to the nursing diagnosis *Altered Nutrition: More than Body Requirements related to a slowed metabolic rate resulting in weight gain.*

Outcomes. The client will return to normal weight, as evidenced by loss of at least 2 pounds weekly.

Interventions. When the client begins taking thyroid medication, the activity level and decreased edema commonly result in a significant initial weight loss without any change in diet. Typically, however, appetite also increases as the medication begins to work. Therefore, teach the client to maintain a low-calorie diet until weight stabilizes at the ideal body weight. The client should gain more energy as the TH level returns to normal, allowing an increase in activity to help in weight loss.

Activity Intolerance. A client with hypothyroidism usually feels fatigued, which commonly leads to the nursing diagnosis *Activity Intolerance related to weakness and*

CRITICAL MONITORING

Hypothyroidism

These manifestations should be monitored in a client who is thought to have a diagnosis of hypothyroidism. Serum laboratory tests confirm the diagnosis:

- Lethargy, depression
- Sensitivity to cold, weight gain; later, an enlarged thyroid
- Dry skin
- Normal to subnormal temperature
- Normal to slow pulse
- Normal respiratory rate unless affected by goiter size
- Normal to slight elevation of blood pressure
- Augmentation of heart failure

apathy secondary to a decreased metabolic rate and resulting in an increased heart rate and shortness of breath with activity.

Outcomes. The client will develop increased tolerance for activity, as evidenced by a return to pre-illness activity levels.

Interventions. While the client still has hypothyroidism, energy levels are decreased and the client tires easily. Usually, the result is a decreased activity level. When TH replacement begins, the client returns to a level of physical and mental activity that should gradually improve with hormone therapy.

Constipation. A client with hypothyroidism has decreased gastrointestinal motility, leading to the nursing diagnosis *Constipation related to decreased peristalsis secondary to slowed metabolic rate and activity intolerance, resulting in decreased frequency of stools and painful defecation.*

Outcomes. The client will experience a return to a normal pre-illness bowel pattern, as evidenced by a bowel movement at least every other day.

Interventions. Implement measures to prevent constipation and fecal impaction. As the hypothyroidism is reversed and cardiac status improves, encourage more activity. Advise the client to drink six to eight glasses of water every day and to eat foods high in fiber, such as fresh fruits, vegetables, and grains. If these measures are ineffective, a stool softener or cathartic may be indicated.

EVALUATION

Once hypothyroidism has been diagnosed and replacement therapy begun, it is expected that the condition will be reversed over 3 to 12 weeks. A maintenance dosage of TH replacement is determined. If reversal of the condition does not continue, the client must be assessed for compliance with the therapeutic regimen.

Self-Care

Hypothyroidism is a lifelong disease that must be managed with the client's full participation. The client should understand the pharmacologic regimen, nutrition, and follow-up required to control the condition.

To promote self-care, focus your teaching on the client's need to understand the manifestations of hyperthyroidism and hypothyroidism, to follow the medication regimen and diet, and to seek medical attention appropriately. Evaluate the client's level of knowledge about the disorder and the importance of taking TH daily for life. Develop and implement a teaching plan based on the client's particular needs. Also, provide a written list (such as the one in the Client Education Guide) of the manifestations of thyroid deficiency or excess. Instruct the client on how to monitor pulse rate. Instruct the client and significant others to telephone the physician if those manifestations develop.

Monitor the client's weight weekly. Physical manifestations of hypothyroidism should decrease over 3 to 12 weeks as TH levels increase. Emphasize the need for iodized salt. Advise the client to drink sufficient fluids, increase physical activity, and eat a high-fiber diet to prevent constipation. Remind the client to have TH levels checked routinely until they stabilize and then at regular intervals to be sure that they remain normal.

Modification for Elderly Clients

Subclinical hypothyroidism refers to a combination of elevated TSH levels, normal T_3 and free thyroxine (FT_4) levels, and no clinical manifestations. Subclinical hypothyroidism occurs in up to 15% of postmenopausal women. The most common causes of are, in order of frequency, autoimmune thyroiditis, Hashimoto's disease, previous thyroid surgery or treatment with radioactive agents, and noncompliance with prescribed T_4 replacements.

CLIENT EDUCATION GUIDE

Thyroid Supplements

The usual initial dosage in adults is 0.025 to 0.1 mg by mouth (PO) per day, increased by 0.05 to 0.1 mg PO every 1 to 4 weeks until the desired response is achieved. The maintenance dose is 0.1 to 0.4 mg/day.

- Take your medication at the same time every day to maintain appropriate levels in your blood. Morning is preferred to prevent insomnia.
- Check your pulse rate, and tell your physician if it is over 100. Side effects may result from your dosage and your sensitivity.
  - Central nervous system effects include nervousness, insomnia, and tremor.
  - Cardiovascular effects may include tachycardia, palpitations, dysrhythmias, angina pectoris, hypertension, and worsening of pre-existing cardiac conditions, such as heart failure.
  - Gastrointestinal effects may include an increase in appetite, nausea, and diarrhea.
  - Other side effects resemble the manifestations of hyperthyroidism: headache, leg cramps, weight loss, heat intolerance, sweating, fever, and menstrual irregularities.
- Do not take a thyroid supplement if you have had a heart attack, thyrotoxicosis, or untreated adrenal insufficiency.
- Use these drugs with caution if you have angina pectoris (chest pain), other cardiovascular disorders, renal insufficiency or failure, or poor circulation.
- Tell your physician right away if you experience angina or manifestations of hyperthyroidism (suggesting overdose or exacerbated or difficult-to-control cardiac disease).
- Notify your other physicians or health care providers that you are taking a thyroid supplement, which will alter your thyroid function test results.
- Thyroid supplements prolong the prothrombin time, a measure of the speed at which your blood clots. Therefore, if you are taking blood thinners, you will need a smaller dose.
- Notify your physician immediately if you are pregnant or plan to become pregnant so that your dose can be adjusted accordingly.

Medical treatment is not indicated for clients who have no manifestations. Clients with generalized complaints may benefit from small doses of T_4, which indicates that their condition was symptomatic rather than subclinical. Remember, a principal hazard in giving T_4 to an elderly client is the development of ischemic heart disease, as evidenced by angina. The response to therapy and serum levels must be observed closely. The client's pulse should be monitored daily.

The difficulty in diagnosing hypothyroidism in older adults is that the manifestations are usually vague and generic to other disease processes. Hypothyroidism must be considered in the differential diagnosis of a variety of conditions affecting older people.

HYPERTHYROIDISM

Hyperthyroidism (excessive secretion of TH) is a highly preventable endocrine disorder. Like most thyroid conditions, it is a disorder predominantly affecting women (in a female-to-male ratio of 4:1), especially women between ages 20 and 40 years.

Etiology and Risk Factors

Hyperthyroidism may be due to overfunctioning of the entire gland or, less commonly, to single or multiple functioning adenomas of thyroid cancer. Overtreatment of myxedema with TH may also result in hyperthyroidism.

The most common form of hyperthyroidism is Graves' disease (toxic, diffuse goiter), which has three principal hallmarks: hyperthyroidism, thyroid gland enlargement (goiter), and exophthalmos (abnormal protrusion of the eyes). Graves' disease is an autoimmune disorder mediated by immunoglobulin G (IgG) antibody that binds to and activates TSH receptors on the surface of the thyroid cells.

Other causes of hyperthyroidism include toxic nodular goiter, toxic adenoma (benign), thyroid carcinoma, subacute and chronic thyroiditis, ingestion of TH, and ingestion of amiodarone hydrochloride for atrial fibrillation. Health maintenance and restoration activities include monitoring TH levels if TH replacement is given, removal of thyroid tumors, and administration of antithyroid medications.

Pathophysiology

Graves' disease may be due to excessive stimulation of the adrenergic nervous system or excessive levels of circulating TH.

Hyperthyroidism is characterized by loss of the normal regulatory controls of TH secretion. Because the action of TH on the body is stimulatory, hypermetabolism results, with increased sympathetic nervous system activity. Excessive amounts of TH stimulate the cardiac system and increase the number of beta-adrenergic receptors, leading to tachycardia and increased cardiac output, stroke volume, adrenergic responsiveness, and peripheral blood flow. Metabolism increases greatly, leading to a negative nitrogen balance, lipid depletion, and a state of nutritional deficiency and weight loss.

Hyperthyroidism also results in altered secretion and metabolism of hypothalamic, pituitary, and gonadal hormones. If hyperthyroidism occurs before puberty, sexual development is delayed in both sexes. After puberty, it results in diminished libido in both men and women. Women also have menstrual irregularities and decreased fertility.

Clinical Manifestations

Because hyperthyroidism is caused by excessive secretion of TH, the clinical picture of Graves' disease is, in many ways, opposite to that of hypothyroidism. Assessment reveals a client who appears extremely agitated and irritable, with a hand tremor at rest. Despite a ravenous appetite, weight loss occurs as a result of the quickened metabolism. Because of the high levels of circulating TH, the client's body processes "speed up." As described in the Critical Monitoring feature called Hyperthyroidism, manifestations include loose bowel movements, heat intolerance, profuse diaphoresis (perspiration), tachycardia, and incoordination related to tremor. The skin becomes warm, smooth, and moist because of accelerated circulation to the tissues. Hair appears thin and soft.

Moreover, the client's emotions are adversely affected by the turbulent activity within the body. Moods may be cyclic, ranging from mild euphoria to extreme hyperactivity to delirium. The excessive hyperactivity in turn leads to extreme fatigue and depression, again followed by episodes of overactivity. As a result of the client's chaotic emotional state, interpersonal relationships may deteriorate, further accentuating the emotional disturbance.

Goiter, the second characteristic of Graves' disease, is due to hyperplasia and hypertrophy of the thyroid cells. The gland may grow to three or four times its normal size. Cellular overgrowth results in the release of excessive amounts of TH into the blood.

Exophthalmos is the third major manifestation of Graves' disease. The cause of the ophthalmologic changes in Graves' disease seems to be autoimmunity against retro-orbital tissues. The client who develops exophthalmos has protruding eyes and a fixed stare caused by accumulation of fluid in the fat pads and muscles that lie behind the eyeballs (Fig. 43–3). Because the eyes are surrounded by unyielding bone, edema forces them forward out of their sockets, producing the typical facies of exophthalmos. In severe cases, clients may be unable to

CRITICAL MONITORING

Hyperthyroidism

These manifestations should be monitored in a client who is thought to have a diagnosis of hyperthyroidism.

- Anxiety, short attention span, irritability
- Heat intolerance, unintentional weight loss
- Warm, moist skin
- Increased temperature
- Increased pulse
- Increased blood pressure
- Fatigue and weakness
- Augmentation of other disorders, such as atrial fibrillation, heart failure, angina pectoris (chest pain), paranoia, and anxiety

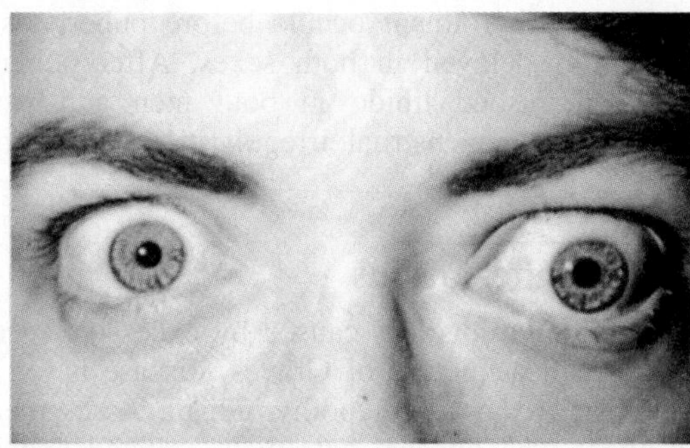

FIGURE 43–3 Extreme exophthalmos in hyperthyroidism. Because the eyes are surrounded by unyielding bone, fluid accumulation in the fat pads and muscles behind the eyeballs causes protruding eyes and a fixed stare in the client with exophthalmos. Without intervention, the client with severe exophthalmos may be unable to close the eyelids and may develop corneal ulceration or infection. Eventually, this can result in total loss of vision. (From Scheie, H. G. [1997]. *Textbook of ophthalmology* [9th ed.] Philadelphia: W. B. Saunders.)

close their eyelids and must have their lids taped shut to protect the eyes. Without intervention, severe exophthalmos can progress to corneal ulceration or infection and loss of vision. In some cases, exophthalmos is not reversed by intervention. It may actually worsen with radioactive iodine therapy.

The diagnosis of Graves' disease is confirmed on the basis of the client's often striking physical appearance (enlarged neck, protruding eyes, agitated expression); the manifestations of agitation, restlessness, and weight loss; and laboratory findings. Serum TH levels are usually all elevated, although they are occasionally within the normal range (so-called euthyroid Graves' disease). Serum cholesterol levels are usually depressed. See Table 43–2 for the usual laboratory findings.

Complications

The three major complications of Graves' disease are exophthalmos, heart disease, and thyroid storm (thyroid crisis, thyrotoxicosis).

EXOPHTHALMOS

Exophthalmos develops as a result of proptosis, lid retraction, muscle swelling, and tissue edema from a prolonged hyperthyroid condition. Manifestations may include a gritty sensation in the eye, photophobia, lacrimation, inflammatory changes, and dyslogia.

Unlike the manifestations of goiter and hyperthyroidism, exophthalmos does not necessarily regress with therapy. Diuretics may alleviate some of the periorbital edema. Glucocorticoids such as prednisone are given in large doses to reduce inflammation of the periorbital tissues. Unfortunately, steroids produce many undesirable side effects, including acute psychoses. Estrogen therapy is occasionally of value in postmenopausal women. Methylcellulose eye drops, 14% four times daily, help reduce eye irritation. Radiation therapy to the retro-orbital tissues may help in severe cases. Surgical decompression of the orbits may be performed when all other measures fail to correct exophthalmos. This procedure may save the client's vision when eye changes are severe.

A number of general nursing interventions also help to reduce eye discomfort and prevent corneal ulceration and infection. Instruct a client with exophthalmos to wear dark eyeglasses. Warn the client to avoid getting dust or dirt in the eyes. If the eyelids cannot be closed easily or at all, have the client wear a sleeping mask (available in drug stores) or lightly tape the eyes shut with nonallergic tape. Elevate the head of the bed at night, and have the client restrict salt intake to relieve edema.

HEART DISEASE

Heart disease poses a serious threat. Tachycardia almost always accompanies thyrotoxicosis, and atrial fibrillation may also appear. Heart failure is found among older clients with long-standing thyrotoxicosis. Propranolol is the drug of choice but is contraindicated if asthma or heart failure is a pre-existing condition. The treatment of these cardiac complications is covered in Unit 12.

THYROID STORM (THYROTOXICOSIS)

Thyroid storm (thyrotoxicosis) is a potentially fatal, acute episode of thyroid overactivity characterized by high fever, severe tachycardia, delirium, dehydration, and extreme irritability. Thanks to modern intervention techniques, this once common problem seldom develops today. Factors that may precipitate a thyroid storm include undiagnosed or untreated hyperthyroidism, infection, thyroid ablation, metabolic catastrophes, surgery, trauma, labor and delivery, myocardial infarction, pulmonary embolus, medication overdosage, or inadequate preparation for thyroid surgery.

A client with thyrotoxicosis may have an increase in clotting factor VIII. Despite this increase, the hyperthyroid client has increased sensitivity to coumarin derivatives because of the accelerated metabolic clearance of the vitamin K–dependent clotting factors. Thyroid storm is a clinical diagnosis; no laboratory tests differentiate hyperthyroidism from thyroid storm in general.

Outcome Management

Medical Management

The desired outcomes of medical management for clients with Graves' disease are to curtail the excessive secretion of TH and to prevent and treat complications. Choice of intervention is based on age, goiter size, and whether other health problems exist. The three major forms of therapy are antithyroid medication, radioiodine therapy, and surgery.

CURTAIL EXCESSIVE SECRETION OF THYROID HORMONE

ANTITHYROID MEDICATION THERAPY. Antithyroid medication is recommended for clients younger than 18 years of age and for pregnant women (see Table 43–3). The major medications used to control hyperthyroidism include iodide, propylthiouracil, and methimazole (Tapazole). Adrenergic blocking agents may be administered as adjunctive therapy.

Propylthiouracil is the most commonly used antithyroid medication. It corrects hyperthyroidism by impairing TH synthesis. With the usual dosage regimen, propylthiouracil ameliorates Graves' disease within 4 to 8 weeks. However, several months may pass before manifestations completely abate. When euthyroid, the client is given a maintenance dose of propylthiouracil, usually three times daily. Although an ideal medication in many ways, propylthiouracil causes significant side effects in about 9% of people who use it.

The most serious toxic effect is agranulocytosis (see Chapter 75). A white blood cell (WBC) count should be obtained before initial administration of the medication. Instruct the client to report a sore throat, fever, or rash immediately so that further WBC tests can be performed and the client's condition evaluated. Less severe adverse reactions include mild allergies (rash and pruritus). Rarely does hepatitis or drug fever develop.

Methimazole blocks the action of TH in the body. Unfortunately, it produces agranulocytosis in a small percentage of people.

Iodine therapy is prescribed for two reasons: (1) to reduce the vascularity of the thyroid gland before subtotal or total thyroidectomy and (2) to treat thyroid storm. Iodine preparations act temporarily to prevent release of TH into the circulation by increasing the amount of TH stored in the gland. The stored TH is eventually released back into the circulation, however, once again producing hyperthyroidism. For this reason, iodine preparations are usually given only for 10 to 14 days before surgery. If iodine is given for a longer period or if it is given alone (not in combination with propylthiouracil), the thyroid gland may "escape" before thyroidectomy. Escape of the thyroid means that the iodine is no longer capable of maintaining TH storage. As a result, TH floods the circulation, and hyperthyroidism becomes more severe than before.

The iodine medication of choice is potassium iodide. Lugol's solution is also used but is more expensive than potassium iodide and tends to inactivate antithyroid preparations in the bowel.

Radioiodine Therapy. Therapy with radioactive iodine (^{131}I) is prescribed mainly for middle-aged and older clients. This intervention offers many advantages: it is economical, is simple to administer, and can be prescribed on an outpatient basis, as described in the accompanying Case Study. Radiotherapy is contraindicated for pregnant women and is rarely used for children.

The rationale behind ^{131}I therapy for Graves' disease is simple. The thyroid gland is unable to distinguish between regular iodine atoms and radioiodine atoms. Consequently, when the client receives a dose of ^{131}I, the thyroid gland picks up the radioiodine and concentrates it just as it would regular iodine. As a result, the cells that concentrate ^{131}I to make T_4 are destroyed by the local irradiation, TH secretion diminishes, and the manifestations of hyperthyroidism and goiter disappear. However, because radioiodine destroys thyroid cells, one of the major possible complications of ^{131}I therapy is hypothyroidism. Therefore, assess for manifestations of hypothyroidism after ^{131}I therapy.

^{131}I is dissolved in water and administered orally. The dosage is determined both by the size of the gland and by the thyroid's uptake of a tracer dose of radioiodine. After receiving the radioiodine, the client may go home unless the dosage is extremely large. In the latter case, the client must be placed in isolation for several days to prevent radioactive contamination.

The manifestations of hyperthyroidism usually subside within 6 to 12 weeks after ^{131}I administration. Because of the delay in achieving a therapeutic response with ^{131}I, concurrent treatment with beta-adrenergic blockers may be desirable. Sometimes resistant clients require a second or, in rare instances, a third dose of radioiodine.

The client who becomes euthyroid still needs regular medical examinations because hypothyroidism may develop several years after radiotherapy. Clients who become hypothyroid require lifelong hormone replacement with thyroid preparations.

Prevent and Treat Complications

Adrenergic Blocking Agents. Adrenergic blocking agents are sometimes given as adjunctive therapy to control the activity of the sympathetic nervous system. There is now evidence that these agents are of great benefit to the "hyperthyroid heart," which has increased sensitivity to catecholamines and an increased number of beta-adrenergic receptor sites. Therefore, these agents help lessen distressing manifestations such as palpitations and tachycardia. Tremor and nervousness may also be alleviated by adrenergic blocking agents. These medications include propranolol and reserpine. Treatment of Graves' hyperthyroidism may involve a long delay (weeks to months) between the start of therapy and substantial improvement or resolution of manifestations.

Dietary Therapy. The client with hyperthyroidism needs a high-calorie, high-protein diet to compensate for the hypermetabolic state. A diet of 4000 to 5000 calories with high protein levels may be necessary to prevent a negative nitrogen balance and weight loss.

Treating Thyroid Storm. Because thyroid storm is an emergency, heroic intervention is needed for control. The high fever is treated with hypothermia blankets; dehydration is reversed with intravenous fluids. Management of thyroid storm involves suppressing hormone release, inhibiting hormone synthesis, blocking conversion of T_4 to the more active T_3, inhibiting the effects of TH on body tissues, and treating the precipitating cause, if known.

Blockade of TH release is usually achieved by oral administration of iodides, such as potassium iodide. Sodium iodide may be given intravenously. Glucocorticoid, dexamethasone, and propylthiouracil are also commonly used oral drugs. Beta-blockers are given to decrease the effects of sympathetic nervous system stimulation and to treat tachycardia.

Nursing Management of the Medical Client

Assessment

Begin your assessment by obtaining a complete history. By asking questions concerning weight, appetite, activity, heat intolerance, and bowel activity, you can assess for the presence of typical manifestations of hyperthyroidism. Also ask about mood alterations. Mood swings, irritability, decreased attention span, and manic behavior may be experienced by the client with hyperthyroidism. Because the client may not be aware of some of the mood changes, consider questioning significant others about changes in the client's behavior.

Hyperthyroidism and Postmenopausal Osteoporosis

Mrs. Gonzales is a 55-year-old Hispanic woman who presents at a free clinic for migrant farm workers. She is dressed in a lightweight sundress and sandals despite outdoor temperatures around 50° F. Mrs. Gonzales complains of pounding in her chest and shortness of breath without exertion. She relates that she has lost 20 pounds in the last 6 weeks even though she has been eating more than usual. A thyroxine (T_4) level determined at the clinic is twice the normal value. The nurse practitioner has arranged for additional outpatient diagnostic studies.

Selected Outpatient Laboratory Values for Mrs. Gonzales

Red blood cells: 3.8 million/mm^3
Hemoglobin, 11.8g/dl
Hematocrit: 35%
White blood cells: 9000/mm^3
Glucose: 90 mg/dl
Thyroxine: 20 mg/dl
Thyroid-stimulating hormone: 0 mIU/ml
^{131}I (radioactive iodine) uptake: 50% in 2 hr without evidence of malignancy
Calcium: 10 mg/dl

Nursing Assessment

Mrs. Gonzales reports that she has worked in the fields all her life. She met her husband in California while they were picking grapes 40 years ago. They have three children, who are married and work in the fields. She does not see them often, however, because they cannot always work in the same area. Mrs. Gonzales was born in Mexico. She speaks fluent Spanish and only a few words of English. She is concerned about how she and her husband will pay for her treatment.

Mrs. Gonzales reports that she went through "the change of life" 14 years ago. She cannot afford hormone replacement therapy. Mrs. Gonzales denies a family history of cancer, heart disease, or diabetes mellitus.

Nursing Physical Examination

Height: 5 ft 5 inches. Weight: 105 lb (47.7 kg)
Vital signs: Blood pressure (BP) 160/94; temperature, pulse, and respirations (TPR) 99.6, 126, 24
Level of consciousness: Awake, alert, restless
Eyes, ears, nose, throat: pupils equal, round, reactive to light and accommodation (PERRLA), increased tears, photophobia, exophthalmos, goiter
Cardiac: Tachycardia, regular rate and rhythm, palpitations
Pulmonary: Lungs clear bilaterally
Abdominal: Soft, nontender, with hyperactive bowel sounds
Genitourinary: Within normal limits
Peripheral pulses: 4/4, with slight pretibial and pedal edema

Initial Outpatient Treatment Plan

Medications: Propranolol (Inderal) 20 mg PO tid
Propylthiouracil (PTU) 100 mg PO tid
Artificial tears or other over-the-counter (OTC) eyedrops as needed; arrange for sample medications if possible)
Diet: As tolerated, no added salt
Activity: As tolerated; monitor heart rate; call if pulse 160 BPM at rest
Other: Call if there is difficulty swallowing or breathing or other signs of enlarging goiter; return to clinic in 2 weeks

On the basis of the diagnostic work-up, Mrs. Gonzales will have radioactive iodine therapy. At her return visit, her T_4 level is within normal limits. She reports that she has not had any more pounding in her chest. Her resting heart rate at the clinic is 84 BPM.

Review of her diet history reveals an average daily intake of about 2000 to 2500 calories consisting largely of tortillas, beans, and the foods currently being harvested in the fields. She reports that she does not drink milk or eat cheese because they cause bloating and diarrhea.

Mrs. Gonzales receives the prescribed dose of radioactive iodine orally and is instructed to return in 30 days for laboratory work and to call if any problems develop.

Discharge and Post-treatment Considerations

1. Average length of stay (LOS): outpatient only
2. Complete post-treatment instruction
3. Coordinate health benefits with department of social services

Questions to Be Considered

1. What influence would Mrs. Gonzales' use of the Spanish language have on her treatment plan? Identify implications for formal nursing education preparation.
2. How might Mrs. Gonzales' care differ from that of a person with health care benefits? Discuss ethical considerations that may affect the allocation of scarce health care resources.
3. Compare and contrast the manifestations of menopause and hyperthyroidism. Discuss the implications for diagnosis and treatment.
4. Discuss the pathophysiology of the relationship between the pituitary gland and the thyroid gland. How is this manifested in Mrs. Gonzales' case?
5. Discuss the management of Mrs. Gonzales' diet before and after radioactive iodine treatment. Include cultural and economic factors in your discussion. In addition, consider the implications of Mrs. Gonzales being postmenopausal and having lactose intolerance.
6. Discuss the nursing implications and client teaching aspects associated with Mrs. Gonzales' prescription medications before radioactive iodine treatment. Identify potential OTC drug contraindications in the pretreatment period. Discuss medication requirements and related client teaching after radioactive iodine treatment.

DIAGNOSIS, OUTCOMES, INTERVENTIONS

Altered Nutrition: Less than Body Requirements. A client with hyperthyroidism is hypermetabolic, leading to the nursing diagnosis *Altered Nutrition: Less than Body Requirements related to accelerated metabolic rate resulting in weight loss and decreased energy levels.*

Outcomes. The client's weight loss will end, as evidenced by an ability to consume sufficient calories to return to ideal body weight.

Interventions. Provide the client with a well-balanced, high-calorie diet. Clients with Graves' disease are usually extremely hungry because of the increased metabolism. Six full meals a day may be needed to satisfy their appetite. Despite unusually large meals, however, clients may lose weight rapidly; they are also usually in a state of negative nitrogen balance. Therefore, encourage the client to eat foods that are nutritious and contain ample amounts of protein, carbohydrates, fats, and minerals. Discourage foods that increase peristalsis and thus result in diarrhea, such as highly seasoned, bulky, or fibrous foods.

The client should be weighed daily, and weight losses of more than 4.4 pounds (2 kg) should be reported. If the client continues to appear malnourished despite an ample diet, supplemental vitamins, particularly vitamin B complex, may be needed.

Activity Intolerance. Another nursing diagnosis related to the client's hypermetabolic state is *Activity Intolerance related to exhaustion secondary to accelerated metabolic rate resulting in inability to perform activity without shortness of breath and significant increases in heart rate.*

Outcomes. The client will engage in a normal level of activity, as evidenced by ability to maintain a proper balance of rest and activity to prevent exhaustion.

Interventions. Provide the client with an environment that is restful both mentally and physically. It is a challenge to help hyperthyroid clients relax. Assign the client to a private room to promote rest and to prevent the client from disturbing others through hyperactivity and restlessness.

Risk for Injury. Many ocular problems can develop in a client with hyperthyroidism. Therefore, an important nursing diagnosis for this client is *Risk for Injury: Corneal ulcerations, infection, and possible blindness related to inability to close the eyelids secondary to exophthalmos.*

Outcomes. The client will not experience corneal ulceration, infection, or blindness, as evidenced by no further development of exophthalmos.

Interventions. Treatment should be started as soon as possible after the diagnosis is made so that exophthalmos—a potentially permanent condition—can be avoided. The client should use artificial tears and eye patches as needed to prevent irritation if exophthalmos has already developed. When treatment has begun, the exophthalmos should not increase; however, it may not diminish quickly or at all.

Hyperthermia. A client with hyperthyroidism is in a hypermetabolic state, leading to the nursing diagnosis *Hyperthermia related to accelerated metabolic rate resulting in fever, diaphoresis, and reported heat intolerance.*

Outcomes. The client will not exhibit hyperthermia, as evidenced by a return to normal body temperature.

Interventions. Tell the client to stay in a cool environment. Use only a lightweight sheet for the top cover, and give the client light, loose pajamas. The client who is diaphoretic may need fresh bed sheets and clothes frequently. Encourage the client not to overexert because doing so raises the body temperature and metabolic rate.

Impaired Social Interaction. A client with hyperthyroidism is hyperactive, possibly leading to the nursing diagnosis *Impaired Social Interaction related to extreme agitation, hyperactivity, and mood swings resulting in inability to relate effectively with others.*

Outcomes. The client will not suffer from impaired social interaction, as evidenced by ability to interact without difficulty and without agitation, hyperactivity, or mood swings.

Interventions. Explain to significant others that any bizarre, difficult behavior is likely to be temporary and should improve steadily with intervention. Maintain a quiet, understanding manner when caring for a client with Graves' disease. Accept the irritation and emotional outbursts as normal expressions of the disease.

Incorporate occupational therapy into care planning. The occupational therapist may be able to provide simple activities designed to distract the client from the disorder (such as putting together a puzzle with large pieces, molding clay, or watching television). For a very restless client, discuss with the physician the need for a sedative such as diazepam (Valium) or possibly an adrenergic blocking agent.

EVALUATION

The client with Graves' disease should recover from the hyperthyroidism without difficulty when the medication regimen has begun.

Surgical Management

THYROIDECTOMY

Surgery for hyperthyroidism has been performed since the early 1880s. Thyroidectomy (removal of the thyroid gland) may be total or partial. *Total* thyroidectomy is performed to remove thyroid cancer. Clients who undergo this operation must take thyroid hormones permanently. *Subtotal* thyroidectomy is performed to correct hyperthyroidism and extreme cases of simple goiter. About five sixths of the gland is removed. Because one sixth of the functioning gland is left intact, hormone replacements may not be necessary.

INDICATIONS AND CONTRAINDICATIONS. Ideally, clients selected are young and free from any condition that makes them poor operative risks (such as diabetes, heart disease, renal disease, or drug allergies).

Preoperative preparation for a subtotal thyroidectomy is extremely important. The client must be euthyroid before the operation, if possible. Preoperative care for a client with Graves' disease includes administration of antithyroid drugs to suppress secretion of thyroid hormones and iodine preparations to reduce the size and vascularity of the organ, thereby diminishing the chance of hemorrhage (see Medical Management). The client should be adequately rested, at optimal weight, and in good health before entering the operating room. Adequate preoperative preparation may take as long as 2 to 3 months.

TABLE 43–4 POSTOPERATIVE ORDERS, RATIONALES, AND ASSOCIATED NURSING INTERVENTIONS AFTER THYROIDECTOMY

Postoperative Order	Rationale	Associated Nursing Interventions
Take vital signs every 15 min until stable; then every hour for next 24 hr.	After thyroidectomy, hemorrhage and respiratory obstruction may develop. Elevated pulse and hypotension indicate hemorrhage and shock. Dyspnea, stridulous respirations, and retraction of neck tissues indicate respiratory obstruction.	Check dressing after checking vital signs. Observe for bleeding at front, sides, and back of neck. Examine back of neck and shoulders for bleeding because blood tends to drain posteriorly. Check dressing for tightness; uncomfortable tautness may indicate bleeding into tissues. Loosen dressing and call surgeon immediately.
Use semi-Fowler position when client conscious unless client is hypotensive. Support head and neck with pillows and sandbags. Ambulation on day 2 as tolerated.	Immobilization of head and neck is essential to prevent flexion and hyperextension of neck with resultant strain on suture line. Semi-Fowler position used for comfort.	Place sandbags on either side of head for immobilization and good alignment. Warn client not to extend or hyperextend neck; reassure client that sandbags will prevent moving head too much. Gently rub back of neck to relieve tension. Support client's head and neck when moving or changing position.
Give fluids by mouth as tolerated. If nausea or vomiting, notify surgeon. Start soft diet on afternoon of day 2.	Give intravenous fluids if nausea or vomiting. Otherwise, start oral fluids as soon as client is fully conscious.	Maintain intake and output record for 2–3 days. Assess for difficulty swallowing. Normally this problem lasts for only 1–2 days postoperatively. Weigh client once a full diet is started; weight lost during early postoperative period should be regained.
Give meperidine (Demerol) or morphine sulfate every 1–2 hr as needed for pain in throat area.	Meperidine and morphine sulfate are both used during early postoperative period to relieve pain and promote rest.	Do not give narcotics if client has respirations below 12/min or respiratory congestion. Consult physician for further orders.
Cough and deep-breathe every hour. Suction mouth and trachea if necessary.	Pooling of mucous secretions in trachea, bronchi, and lungs causes respiratory obstruction with resultant atelectasis and pneumonia. Secretions must be raised to prevent respiratory complications.	Instruct client to cough and deep-breathe as taught during preoperative period. If client cannot raise secretions, gently suction mouth and trachea. Do not oversedate clients with profuse respiratory secretions; given narcotics judiciously.
Have tracheostomy set, endotracheal tube, laryngoscope, and oxygen on hand.	Acute respiratory obstruction due to hemorrhage, edema of glottis, laryngeal nerve damage, or tetany is an emergency. Equipment for establishing an airway and administering oxygen must be available for immediate use.	Continuously assess for manifestations of airway obstruction, such as increasing restlessness, tachycardia, apprehension, cyanosis, stridulous respiration, and retraction of neck tissues. Report any of these manifestations to the surgeon immediately.
Give continuous mist inhalation until chest is clear.	Humidification of air promotes easier breathing and helps to liquefy mucous secretions.	Keep doors closed so that moist air is retained in room.
Take temperature every 4 hr for 24 hr, then routinely.	One of the first manifestations of thyroid storm is elevated temperature.	Carefully assess for manifestations of thyroid storm: elevated temperature, extreme restlessness, agitation, and tachycardia. Report any elevation over 100° F (37.7° C) rectally or 99° F (32.2° C) orally.
Assess client for hypocalcemia and monitor calcium, magnesium, and phosphorus.	Inadvertent removal or devascularization of the parathyroid glands can cause postoperative hypoparathyroidism.	Mild hypocalcemia can be asymptomatic. Severe hypocalcemia can produce circumoral paresthesias, positive Chvostek's or Trousseau's sign. Administer calcium supplements for hypocalcemic levels.

Postoperative orders, rationales, and associated nursing interventions after thyroidectomy are presented in Table 43–4.

COMPLICATIONS. Besides the usual complications of any surgery, which include hemorrhage and infection, the client after thyroidectomy is at risk for thyroid storm, tetany, respiratory obstruction, laryngeal edema, and vocal cord injury. If the client is not euthyroid, the risk of intraoperative or postoperative thyroid storm is greatly increased.

Although uncommon, respiratory obstruction may result from swelling related to the surgical site. Rarely, vocal cord paralysis may result from nerve damage. Hypoparathyroidism may result from inadvertent removal of parathyroid gland tissue. The parathyroid glands lie just behind the lobes of the thyroid and are commonly disturbed and sometimes inadvertently removed during surgery. Careful postoperative monitoring of neurologic irritability and serum calcium levels is performed for this reason.

OUTCOMES. Surgical treatment is effective in most people with Graves' disease. A small percentage remain hyperthyroid, and hypothyroidism develops in some.

Nursing Management of the Surgical Client

ASSESSMENT

Assess the client for typical manifestations of Graves' disease. A hypermetabolic state may be obvious from apparent weight loss, and exophthalmos may be obvious as well. Also, question the client about visual difficulties, fatigue, weakness, tremors, and insomnia, as outlined in the earlier Critical Monitoring feature on Hyperthyroidism.

DIAGNOSIS, OUTCOMES, INTERVENTIONS

Risk for Injury: Thyroid Storm, Hypocalcemia, or Hemorrhage. The client undergoing a thyroidectomy should be euthyroid preoperatively. Thus, an important nursing diagnosis is *Risk for Injury: Thyroid storm, hypocalcemia, or hemorrhage related to surgical procedure and not being in a euthyroid state.*

Outcomes. Thyroid storm, hypocalcemia, or hemorrhage will be prevented or will be detected early and the client protected from injury.

Interventions

Promote Preoperative Euthyroid State. The client must be carefully prepared for a thyroidectomy to avoid complications (such as thyroid storm and hemorrhage). Outcomes of successful preparation for thyroid surgery are as follows:

- The client is euthyroid before entering the operating room. Tests of thyroid function are within normal limits.
- Manifestations of thyrotoxicosis are greatly diminished or absent. The client appears rested and relaxed.
- Weight and nutritional status are normal; any weight lost earlier has been regained.
- Cardiac problems are under control, pulse rate is normal, and preoperative electrocardiograms show no dangerous dysrhythmias.

To help meet these outcomes, antithyroid drugs, iodine preparations, bed rest, a nutritious diet, and supplemental vitamins are prescribed. Cardiac monitoring is maintained. Thorough preparation may take months. When good health has been restored, however, the client can undergo surgery with confidence that the operation will be successful and the manifestations alleviated.

Provide Postoperative Care. The immediate desired outcomes of postoperative care after thyroidectomy are to maintain airway patency, minimize strain on the suture line, relieve discomfort related to the sore throat and tracheal irritation, prevent pooling of respiratory secretions, prevent or relieve complications, and monitor for decreased parathyroid function.

Monitor for Postoperative Complications. Assemble the needed equipment at the bedside before the client returns from surgery. The equipment includes a blood pressure cuff and stethoscope, additional pillows, oxygen, suction equipment, intubation supplies, and a tracheostomy set. Ampules of calcium gluconate should be on hand in the medicine room or on the emergency cart.

As noted earlier, major complications after thyroidectomy may include:

- Respiratory obstruction caused by edema of the glottis, bilateral laryngeal nerve damage, or tracheal compression from hemorrhage
- Hemorrhage
- Weakness and hoarseness of the voice from trauma or damage to one laryngeal nerve
- Hypocalcemia and tetany from accidental removal of one or more parathyroid glands
- Thyroid storm (if the client is not euthyroid preoperatively)

Promote Voice Rest. Temporary hoarseness and voice weakness may occur if there has been unilateral injury to the recurrent laryngeal nerve during surgery. To assess the voice, ask the client's name after full recovery from the anesthesia. Have the client speak every 30 to 60 minutes thereafter, and carefully note any voice changes. If hoarseness or voice weakness is present, reassure the client that the problem will probably subside in a few days. Discourage unnecessary talking to minimize hoarseness.

Monitor and Treat Hypocalcemia. Muscle twitching and hyperirritability of the nervous system may indicate hypocalcemic tetany. Hypocalcemia can develop after thyroidectomy if the parathyroid glands are accidentally removed during surgery. Manifestations may develop 1 to 7 days after surgery. Monitor the client for Chvostek's (facial nerve irritability) and Trousseau's (carpal spasm) signs; report positive responses to the physician immediately. Also, if the client develops numbness and tingling around the mouth, fingertips, or toes; muscle spasms; or twitching, call the physician immediately. Make sure calcium gluconate ampules are available at the bedside and that the client has a patent intravenous line.

EVALUATION

The client should be discharged within several days of surgery without difficulty. The wound should heal within about 6 weeks without infection.

Self-Care

Hyperthyroidism is a chronic disease that must be managed with the client's full participation. When the immediate postoperative period and its dangers have passed, turn your attention to teaching. Several important areas should be included.

NECK EXERCISES. First, teach the client how to support the weight of the head and neck when sitting up in bed. Show the client how to place the hands at the back of the head when flexing the neck or moving. The client will probably be able to perform this maneuver by the first postoperative day.

Second, as the wound heals (about the 2nd to 4th postoperative day), demonstrate range-of-motion exercises to prevent contractures. With the surgeon's permission, teach the client to flex the head forward and laterally, to hyperextend the neck, and to turn the head from side to side. Have the client perform these exercises several times every day.

MEDICATIONS. If a total thyroidectomy has been performed, explain self-administration of thyroid medications (see the Client Education Guide earlier). Teach the client the medication regimen and the need for lifelong replacement therapy.

FOLLOW-UP MONITORING. Make an appointment for the clinic or physician's office after discharge. Serum thyroid levels must be determined to monitor treatment. Emphasize that the client who has had a thyroidectomy must see a physician at least twice yearly to avert possible complications (e.g., hypothyroidism, hypoparathyroidism, or recurrent hyperthyroidism) related to hormonal replacement. TH levels must be measured at regular intervals until the replacement medication is adjusted to a maintenance dose. The client should then see the physician twice a year for examinations.

PROMOTE WOUND HEALING. Teach the client how to care for the incision when it has healed by using lanolin cream to soften the wound and minimize the scar.

Modification for Elderly Clients

Hyperthyroidism in older adults accounts for 10% to 15% of all thyrotoxic clients. Some clients present with typical manifestations of hyperthyroidism, especially when the diagnosis is Graves' disease. However, hyperthyroidism in older people is also notorious for atypical or minimal manifestations. It is often overlooked because the manifestations are not the usual ones.

Indeed, manifestations are commonly attributed to aging. Weight loss, lack of ocular findings, and normal-sized thyroid glands are commonly found on assessment. Many clients actually appear apathetic instead of hyperactive. Cardiovascular abnormalities, such as heart failure, atrial dysrhythmias (usually digoxin resistant), and various degrees of heart block may be caused by hyperthyroidism. If the cardiac condition is pre-existing, it may be exacerbated by hyperthyroidism. Relative lack of tachycardia has been documented; about 40% of elderly clients have heart rates under 100 beats per minute (BPM).

The diagnosis of hyperthyroidism is established by appropriate laboratory tests. It is usual to find elevated T_4 and suppressed TSH levels. Hyperthyroidism in elderly clients is treated with radioactive iodine.

THYROIDITIS

Thyroiditis (inflammation of the thyroid gland) appears in three basic forms:

- Acute suppurative
- Subacute thyroiditis, either granulomatous (painful or de Quervain's thyroiditis) or lymphocytic (silent or painless thyroiditis)
- Chronic thyroiditis, also known as Hashimoto's disease

Etiology and Risk Factors

Acute suppurative thyroiditis is an uncommon inflammatory disease usually caused by bacterial invasion in the form of an abscess of the thyroid gland. *Streptococcus pyogenes, Staphylococcus aureus*, and *Pneumococcus pneumoniae* are the most common etiologic agents. Acute thyroiditis is more common in females. Usually, it affects women between 20 and 40 years of age, although it also occurs in children and older people. Most affected clients have a pre-existing thyroid disorder.

Subacute granulomatous thyroiditis is a self-limiting inflammatory condition. No etiologic agent has been identified, although the condition may be viral in origin and commonly follows a respiratory infection. Autoimmune abnormalities have been described. There also appears to be a genetic predisposition to the development of both subacute granulomatous and lymphocytic thyroiditis. Of people with subacute granulomatous thyroiditis, 80% are women between 40 and 50 years old.

Chronic thyroiditis (Hashimoto's disease) is the most common form of thyroiditis. It is more prevalent in women than men and usually occurs between ages 20 and 50 years. Hashimoto's disease is a long-term inflammatory disorder. It is most commonly caused by autoimmune destruction of the thyroid gland. Genetic predisposition also plays a role in its causation.

Pathophysiology

Acute thyroiditis is a state of acute infection and inflammation. Usually, one lobe of the thyroid is more affected than the other. Follicular destruction, cell infiltration, and colloid depletion occur. Microabscesses form.

Subacute thyroiditis has three phases:

Phase 1: The condition begins with a 3- to 4-week prodromal viral illness. Fever and malaise precede the sudden onset of a tender goiter. The thyroid gland may become two to three times its normal size. Mild hyperthyroidism may be present because of sudden release of thyroid hormones into the circulation as a result of the inflammation and destruction of the thyroid gland.

Phase 2: Mild hypothyroidism develops because of incomplete recovery of the injured gland and exhaustion of stored thyroid hormones. Relapse may occur. Hypothyroidism is rarely permanent.

Phase 3: The recovery phase may begin 2 to 4 months after onset.

Hashimoto's disease is manifested by an enlarged thyroid gland that may produce hypothyroid manifestations if the gland is destroyed by the autoimmune system. A euthyroid state may prevail if the gland is not destroyed.

Clinical Manifestations

Manifestations of acute thyroiditis include abrupt onset of unilateral anterior neck pain with possible radiation to the ear or mandible on the affected side. Fever, diaphoresis, and other manifestations of bacterial toxicity may also be present.

Subacute granulomatous thyroiditis is usually painful, whereas subacute lymphocytic thyroiditis is usually painless. Assessment data may include characteristic anterior, unilateral neck pain that may have an abrupt onset, usually after a respiratory infection or viral episode. Radiation to the ear on the ipsilateral side may occur. There may be manifestations of viral infection, such as myalgia, low-grade fever, lassitude, and sore throat. About 50% of clients present with thyrotoxicosis.

Subacute lymphocytic thyroiditis is characterized by occasional hyperthyroidism and a painless goiter. The goiter is firm, diffuse, and mildly enlarged.

Manifestations of chronic thyroiditis include painless, asymmetrical enlargement of the gland, which causes pressure on the surrounding structures and can lead to dysphagia and respiratory distress. Most clients are euthyroid, about 20% are hypothyroid, and less than 5% are hyperthyroid.

The diagnosis of thyroiditis may be confirmed by evaluation of serum T_3, FT_4, ^{131}I uptake, TSH, erythrocyte sedimentation rate, and thyroid antibodies. See Table 43–5 for the results of these tests. Clients with acute thyroiditis are typically euthyroid according to laboratory tests.

For subacute granulomatous thyroiditis, laboratory findings reveal hyperthyroidism in approximately 50% of clients. With subacute lymphocytic thyroiditis, laboratory diagnosis includes decreased radioactive iodine uptake, elevated T_3 and T_4, and frequently positive thyroid antibodies.

In chronic thyroiditis, immune antibodies are usually positive. Other thyroid function levels may be normal, increased, or decreased.

Outcome Management

Medical Management

Acute thyroiditis usually responds to parenteral antibiotic therapy. Treatment of subacute granulomatous thyroiditis is supportive. Therapy may include salicylates, nonsteroidal anti-inflammatory agents (NSAIDs), and oral glucocorticoids such as prednisone. The desired outcome of treatment in subacute lymphocytic thyroiditis is to provide relief of manifestations of hyperthyroidism with beta-adrenergic blocking agents. Antithyroid medications are not indicated.

The course of Hashimoto's disease varies. Some clients experience spontaneous remission, whereas others remain stable for years. In about one third of cases, hypothyroidism develops from gradual atrophy of the gland. Intervention is intended to reduce the size of the gland and correct any thyroid function abnormalities. Immunologic tests are not useful in monitoring these clients.

Surgical Management

Clients with acute thyroiditis that does not respond to medical treatment may require incision and drainage of the affected gland. Depending on the size of the thyroid area to be incised and concurrent medical problems, the procedure may be done in the physician's office or during a short stay in the hospital. A fine-needle biopsy may be performed to rule out malignancy in chronic thyroiditis.

Nursing Management of the Medical-Surgical Client

Nursing care of a client with thyroiditis is usually supportive until the diagnosis is made. Then, as with other thyroid disorders, care revolves around helping the client learn correct medication administration. If surgery is necessary, care is the same as discussed earlier.

Discharge teaching focuses on ensuring that the client understands the medication and how to take it. Thyroid function is monitored at regular intervals after client discharge for development of hyperthyroidism or hypothyroidism and for testing the effectiveness of medication.

THYROID CANCER

The incidence of thyroid cancer is rising. One reason may be the maturation of people exposed to low-dose radiation early in life. Thyroid cancer accounts for 3 to 4 new cases per 100,000 population per year in the United States and about 1% of cancer deaths. The ratio of females to males is 4:1. Its incidence peaks during the 60s, but it may arise from infancy to old age. Mortality is lowest in the young if the cancer is well differentiated.

Etiology and Risk Factors

Benign adenomas are usually not dangerous, although they occasionally grow large enough to cause respiratory problems by pressing against the trachea. Malignant transformation sometimes occurs, and the benign nodules become cancerous. Also, malignant transformation of benign nodules can apparently follow prolonged stimulation of the thyroid gland by TSH. Other risk factors include genetic predisposition, a family history of thyroid or other endocrine cancer, and a history of thyroid cancer.

TABLE 43–5 DIAGNOSTIC TESTS FOR THYROIDITIS

Test	Acute Thyroiditis	Subacute Thyroiditis	Chronic Hashimoto's or Lymphocytic Thyroiditis
Serum triiodothyronine	Normal–low	↑ at first; ↓ later	↑ or ↓
Free thyroxine	Normal–low	↑ at first; ↓ later	↑ or ↓
Radioactive iodine uptake	Low in about 40%	Low	Low or high-normal
Thyroid-stimulating hormone	↓	↓ at first; ↑ later	↑ or ↓
Erythrocyte sedimentation rate	NA	↑ ↑	NA
Thyroid antibodies	NA	Not detected	↑

NA, not applicable.
Adapted from Luckmann, J. (Ed.) (1997). *Saunders manual of nursing care.* Philadelphia: W. B. Saunders.

Pathophysiology

There are four major types of thyroid cancer:

- Papillary adenocarcinoma
- Follicular adenocarcinoma
- Medullary carcinoma
- Anaplastic carcinoma

These cancers vary in their characteristics, interventions, and prognoses (Table 43–6). Benign adenomas and malignant thyroid tumors constitute the third most common cause of thyroid enlargement, with hypothyroidism and hyperthyroidism being the two most common causes. Like other benign tumors, most thyroid adenomas are usually well encapsulated and, as a result, do not spread or extend into other tissues.

Clinical Manifestations

The major manifestation of thyroid cancer is the appearance of a hard, irregular, painless nodule in an enlarged thyroid gland. The nodule itself is typically solitary, rapidly enlarging, and "cold" (it does not take up radioactive iodine) in contrast to benign adenomas, which may take up radioactive iodine. The examiner can make this determination by giving a tracer dose of ^{131}I and performing a thyroid scan 24 hours later to assess ^{131}I uptake by any nodules. "Hot" nodules absorb more isotope than normal tissue and are usually benign.

If the tumor has metastasized, the lymph nodes are sometimes palpable. In long-standing cases, the client may have respiratory difficulty and dysphagia (difficulty swallowing) resulting from the enlarged thyroid pressing against neck structures. The diagnosis of thyroid cancer is confirmed by fine-needle aspiration biopsy.

Outcome Management

Medical Management

Without prompt, aggressive therapy, a client with thyroid cancer risks death. Chemotherapy, ^{131}I, external radiation, or TSH suppressive therapy may be used for metastasis, as discussed earlier. A client with a benign nodule is likely to undergo long-term suppression therapy with levothyroxine. The desired outcome is to suppress serum TSH without causing hypothyroidism.

TABLE 43–6 TYPES OF THYROID CANCER: INCIDENCE, CHARACTERISTICS, INTERVENTION, AND PROGNOSIS

Type	Incidence	Characteristics	Intervention	Prognosis
Papillary adenocarcinoma	Constitutes 75% of thyroid cancers Affects clients in all age groups	Slow-growing firm tumor Palpable nodule Spreads to regional nodes in about half of cases Radiation-related thyroid cancer with 10- to 20-year latency period	Total or near-total thyroidectomy Others recommend lobectomy and isthmectomy	Excellent if cancer restricted to thyroid gland Lymph node metastasis is common Surgery usually curative
Follicular adenocarcinoma	Constitutes 15% of thyroid cancers Mainly affects clients 50 and older	Slow-growing nodule with about 15% metastasis to regional nodes at diagnosis Associated with radiation, iodine deficiency, edemic goiter, thyrotoxicosis	Total or near-total thyroidectomy Aggressive radioactive iodine therapy for metastases	Good but inferior to that of papillary adenocarcinoma 5-yr survival is 60%–90% Lymph node metastasis is uncommon Distant metastasis is common
Medullary thyroid carcinoma	Constitutes 5%–10% of thyroid cancers Mainly affects clients of all age groups Disease is familial in 20% of all clients	Growth rate is moderate Tends to secrete adrenocorticotropic hormone, serotonin Metastases to surrounding structures at diagnosis in 50% Associated with multiple endocrine neoplasia	Total or near-total thyroidectomy Radioactive iodine to ablate the gland	Lymph node and distant metastases are common 5-yr survival is 70%–80%
Anaplastic carcinoma (nondifferentiated)	Constitutes 5%–15% of thyroid cancers Mainly affects clients between ages 60 and 70	Highly malignant Grows rapidly Local and widespread metastasis within 1 yr	Combination of thyroidectomy, external radiation therapy, chemotherapy, and tracheostomy as needed Aggressive therapy is palliative at best	Grave; mean survival, 6.2 mo; 10-yr survival, 1%

From Baker, K., & Feldman, J. (1993). Thyroid cancer: A review. *Oncology Nursing Forum, 20*(1), 95–104.

Surgical Management

Treatment usually includes removal of all or part of the thyroid. Neck resection may be done for metastases to the neck. (Thyroid surgery has been covered earlier.) As with a thyroidectomy for noncancerous lesions, the major postoperative complications are respiratory distress, recurrent laryngeal damage, hemorrhage, and hypoparathyroidism.

Nursing Management of the Medical-Surgical Client

Nursing care of the client with thyroid cancer is similar to the care of any client undergoing a thyroidectomy. The client also needs the support and teaching that a client with cancer requires. If the client is to have chemotherapy, additional teaching is needed.

If the client has undergone a total thyroidectomy, replacement of thyroid hormones is necessary. Discharge teaching focuses on ensuring that the client understands the medication and how to take it. Home health needs reflect those of any client after thyroidectomy or receiving chemotherapy or radiation therapy. The client should be checked at regular intervals for recurrence, and thyroid function should be monitored.

PARATHYROID DISORDERS

HYPERPARATHYROIDISM

Hyperparathyroidism, a disorder caused by overactivity of one or more of the parathyroid glands, is classified as primary, secondary, or tertiary. It usually occurs in clients older than age 60 and affects women twice as often as men. It is not related to age in clients with renal failure. The overall incidence of hyperparathyroidism is 27 per 100,000.

Etiology and Risk Factors

Primary hyperparathyroidism develops when the normal regulatory relationship between serum calcium levels and parathyroid hormone (PTH) secretion is interrupted. The interruption occurs when an adenoma or hyperplasia of the gland exists without an identifying injury.

Secondary hyperparathyroidism occurs when the glands are hyperplastic because of malfunction of another organ system. It is usually the result of renal failure but may also occur with osteogenesis imperfecta, Paget's disease, multiple myeloma, or carcinoma with bone metastasis.

Tertiary hyperparathyroidism occurs when PTH production is irrepressible (autonomous) in clients with normal or low serum calcium levels.

Pathophysiology

The normal function of PTH is to increase bone resorption, thereby maintaining the proper balance of calcium and phosphorus ions in the blood (see Chapter 42). Excessive circulating PTH leads to bone damage, hypercalcemia, and kidney damage.

PRIMARY HYPERPARATHYROIDISM

The severity of hypercalcemia reflects the quantity of hyperfunctioning parathyroid tissue. Excessive PTH stimulates transport of calcium into the blood from the intestine, kidneys, and bone. Nephrolithiasis is secondary to calcium phosphate kidney stones and deposition of calcium in the soft tissues of the kidney. Pyelonephritis may complicate the nephrolithiasis. Bone resorption related to hypercalcemia may develop.

Myopathy is a common condition characterized by neuropathic atrophy and proximal muscle weakness. Hypercalcemia can stimulate hypergastrinemia, abdominal pain, and peptic ulcer disease. Pancreatitis is also influenced by high calcium levels.

SECONDARY HYPERPARATHYROIDISM

Chronic renal failure and hyperphosphatemia cause secondary hyperparathyroidism. As the glomerular filtration rate (GFR) decreases in chronic renal failure, serum phosphorus levels rise. This increase causes the serum calcium level to fall. PTH secretion is stimulated. This increase decreases renal tubular absorption of phosphorus, causing serum phosphorus levels to return to normal. As the GFR continues to decrease, PTH is secreted in increased amounts in order to decrease tubular reabsorption of phosphorus and maintain serum phosphorus at or close to normal limits.

Clinical Manifestations

Some clients with hyperparathyroidism may be asymptomatic. Others have myriad manifestations arising from the skeletal disease, renal involvement, gastrointestinal tract disorders, and neurologic abnormalities, as outlined in the Critical Monitoring feature Hyperparathyroidism and Hypoparathyroidism and in Figure 43–4.

Manifestations of bone disease range from backache, joint pain, and bone pain to pathologic fractures of the spine, ribs, and long bones. In long-standing cases, assessment reveals deformity and bending of the bones. Osteitis fibrosa with superperiosteal resorption or bone cysts, arthritis, or radiologic osteoporosis may be diagnosed.

Manifestations of renal involvement include polyuria and polydipsia; the appearance of sand, gravel, or stones

CRITICAL MONITORING

Hyperparathyroidism and Hypoparathyroidism

These manifestations should be monitored in a client who is thought to have a diagnosis of hyperparathyroidism or hypoparathyroidism.

Hyperparathyroidism	Hypoparathyroidism
Increased bone resorption	Decreased bone resorption
Elevated serum calcium levels	Depressed serum calcium levels
Depressed serum phosphate levels	Elevated serum phosphate levels
Hypercalciuria and hyperphosphaturia	Hypocalciuria and hypophosphaturia
Decreased neuromuscular irritability	Increased neuromuscular activity, which may progress to tetany

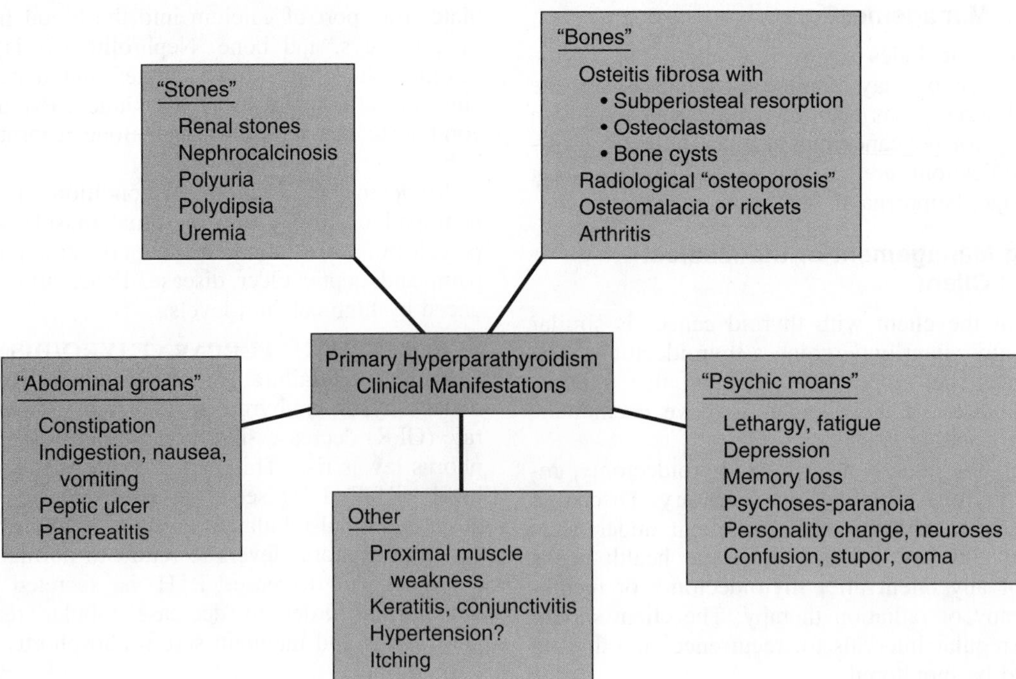

FIGURE 43–4 Clinical manifestations of primary hyperparathyroidism. (Adapted from Strewler, G. J., & Rosenblatt, M. (1995). Mineral metabolism. In P. Felig, J. D. Baxter, & L. A. Frohman [Eds.], *Endocrinology and metabolism* [3rd ed., pp. 1407–1499]. New York: McGraw-Hill.)

(calculi) in the urine; azotemia; and hypertension resulting from renal damage. Without intervention, renal insufficiency may progress to fatal renal hypertension and uremia.

Hypercalcemia produces mainly gastrointestinal manifestations, such as thirst, nausea, anorexia, constipation, ileus, and abdominal pain. Decreased neuromuscular irritability is also common. Often, clients have a history of peptic ulcer or gastrointestinal bleeding. Assessment may also reveal psychiatric manifestations. Listlessness, depression, and paranoia are sometimes associated with high levels of serum calcium. Finally, calcification may form in the eyes, impairing vision.

Major complications include the manifestations associated with hypercalcemia and those associated with treatment, such as dehydration, hypocalcemia, and gastrointestinal problems.

The diagnosis of hyperparathyroidism mainly rests on laboratory and x-ray findings (Table 43–7). Serum calcium levels are elevated, serum phosphate levels are depressed, and both urine calcium and phosphorus levels are high. In addition, alkaline phosphatase is elevated in the 25% of clients who have associated bone disease. Clients with skeletal damage have the following characteristic x-ray findings: diffuse demineralization of bones, bone cysts, subperiosteal bone resorption, and loss of the lamina dura around the teeth. Ultrasonography or magnetic resonance imaging (MRI) may be used for preoperative localization of the parathyroid glands.

Outcome Management

Medical Management

The desired outcomes of the medical treatment of hyperparathyroidism include lowering severely elevated calcium levels and long-term management of hypercalcemia with drugs to increase bone resorption of calcium.

LOWER ELEVATED CALCIUM LEVELS. Serum calcium levels are lowered by hydration and calciuria. Hydration may be achieved with an infusion of normal saline solution. Normal saline is the fluid of choice because it both expands the volume and acts in the kidney to inhibit the resorption of calcium. Furosemide (Lasix), a loop diuretic, may also be used to promote calciuria after rehydration has occurred. Thiazide diuretics are not used because they promote calcium retention in the kidneys. A client with hypercalcemia should have a diet low in calcium and vitamin D.

ANTIRESORPTION AGENTS. Drugs that inhibit bone resorption include plicamycin (Mithracin), gallium nitrate (Ganite), phosphates, and calcitonin (Table 43–8). Plicamycin is a chemotherapeutic drug that is effective in lowering serum calcium levels. The hypocalcemic effect occurs after 24 hours and lasts for about 1 to 2 weeks. The dose is about one-tenth that used for cancer treatment, and the adverse effects are proportionally lower.

Gallium nitrate, a newer drug, is now being used more often because it has even fewer side effects. Glucocorticoids may be used to reduce hypercalcemia by decreasing gastrointestinal absorption of calcium. Etidronate (Didronel) or calcitonin may be used to decrease the release of calcium by bones.

Nursing Management of the Medical Client

ASSESSMENT

There are no obvious manifestations of hyperparathyroidism and the resultant hypercalcemia. Elicit a good history from the client to see whether any risk factors are present. The client may exhibit psychological changes,

TABLE 43–7 DIAGNOSTIC TESTS OF PARATHYROID FUNCTION: PURPOSE, PROCEDURE, NORMAL RANGE, AND INTERPRETATION OF ABNORMAL FINDINGS

Test	Purpose	Procedure	Normal Range	Interpretation of Abnormal Findings	Remarks
Total serum calcium	Measures amount of ionized and nonionized calcium in serum	Venous blood to laboratory	4.8–5.2 mEq/L or 8–11 mg/dl	Elevated in hyperparathyroidism; depressed in hypoparathyroidism, tetany, rickets, nephrosis, and osteomalacia	Normally 50% of total serum calcium is ionized; the amount of ionized calcium available decreases in alkalosis
Qualitative urinary calcium (Sulkowitch test)	Measures roughly amount of calcium in urine; used as quick method for diagnosis if tetany is due to hypoparathyroidism	Collect urine specimen and send to laboratory	Fine white precipitate should form when Sulkowitch reagent is added to urine specimen	Absent or decreased density of precipitate indicates low serum calcium and hypoparathyroidism	Medications that elevate serum calcium levels include vitamin D, parathyroid infection, and dihydrotachysterol
Quantitative urinary calcium (calcium deprivation test)	Measures exact amount of calcium in 24-hr urine specimen	Collect 24-hr urine specimen and send to laboratory	75–175 mg calcium per 24 hr	Elevated in hyperparathyroidism; depressed in hypoparathyroidism	Foods high in calcium include milk, cheese, molasses, turnip greens, and dandelion greens
Serum phosphorus	Measures amount of inorganic phosphorus in serum	Venous blood to laboratory	1.3–1.75 mEq/L (2.5–4.5 mg/dl) in adults	Depressed in hypoparathyroidism, uremia, and alkalosis; elevated in hyperparathyroidism, rickets, and osteomalacia	There is an inverse relationship between serum calcium and serum phosphorus
Serum alkaline phosphatase	Measures amount of alkaline phosphatase in serum; aids in diagnosing bone and liver disorders	Venous blood to laboratory	2.0–5.0 Bodansky units	Elevated in hyperparathyroidism, osteomalacia, rickets, healing fractures, and pregnancy and after ingestion of large amounts of vitamin D	Alkaline phosphatase is an enzyme normally present in small amounts in serum; medications causing false elevations of alkaline phosphatase levels include allopurinol, some androgens, colchicine, erythromycin, methyldopa, some oral contraceptives, procainamide, and tolbutamide
Parathyroid hormone (PTH) radioimmunoassay	Measures level of PTH in serum	Venous blood to laboratory	Depends on serum calcium level	High concentrations indicate hyperparathyroidism	When evaluated in conjunction with serum calcium levels, this is the most specific test for hyperparathyroidism

such as lethargy, drowsiness, memory loss, and emotional lability, all manifestations seen in hypercalcemia.

DIAGNOSIS, OUTCOMES, INTERVENTIONS

Risk for Injury. The client with hyperparathyroidism is at great risk for injury, leading to the nursing diagnosis *Risk for Injury related to demineralization of bones resulting in pathologic fractures.*

Outcomes. The client will remain free from injury, as evidenced by absence of pathologic fractures or hypercalcemia.

Interventions

Prevent Fractures. Protect the client from accidents. If bone involvement exists, pathologic fractures may develop from even small bumps or minor falls. Keep the client's bed in the low position and use the side rails. If the client is weak or has joint or skeletal disease, help with ambulation.

Assist with Activities. If the client suffered from severe osteoporosis or pathologic fractures, some assistance may be required at home. The client may need a visiting nurse to help assess the home situation and to make recommen-

TABLE 43–8 DRUGS USED TO TREAT HYPERCALCEMIA

Class	Action	Therapeutic Outcome	Adverse Outcome	Dosing
Loop diuretic (furosemide)	Promotes renal excretion of calcium	Improved muscle tone and coordination Relief of nausea, vomiting, and anorexia Decreased serum calcium	Monitor intake and output, blood pressure and pulse Watch serum calcium level closely and monitor for numbness, tingling, and other signs of decreased calcium	Up to 100 mg IV Give with 0.9% sodium chloride
Chemotherapeutic agent (plicamycin)	Inhibits bone resorption and lowers serum calcium level	Therapeutic effect in hypercalcemia may not be seen for 24–48 hr and may last 3–15 days Improve muscle tone and coordination Improved appetite and decreased nausea and vomiting	Monitor serum electrolytes, liver enzymes, and BUN and creatinine Monitor platelet count and watch for bleeding Watch for sudden drop in serum calcium; check closely for signs of hypocalcemia	25 mg IV daily for 1–4 days Give antiemetics before administration to reduce nausea
Electrolyte modifier (etidronate disodium)	Decreases release of calcium from bones	Decreased serum calcium May take months for onset of improved muscle tone and coordination and improved appetite	Diarrhea, nausea, bone pain; protect from fractures Elevated serum phosphate; monitor for increased serum phosphate Tell client that onset of therapeutic effect may take several months Monitor renal function	5 mg/kg PO daily as single dose 2 hr before meals, up to dose of 20 mg/kg Do not administer with food or antacids Do not give for more than 6 months continuously; stop, then restart after 3 months
Hormone (calcitonin)	Used in secondary hyperparathyroidism as a phosphate-binding agent and nutritional supplement to the low-phosphate diet; prescribed to decrease acidosis	Decreased serum calcium Improved appetite Improved muscle tone and coordination	Monitor for numbness, tingling, and other signs of hypocalcemia Monitor serum phosphate Warn client about transient facial flushing	4–8 IU/kg SC daily or two to three times a week (salmon) or 0.5 mg two to three times a week (human) or as a nasal spray daily Administer at bedtime to decrease nausea and vomiting Treatment may last for 6 months

BUN, blood urea nitrogen; IV, intravenously; PO, orally; SC, subcutaneously.

dations on how safety might be enhanced. The home should be cleared of articles that can increase the risk of falling, such as throw rugs. The client may also need assistive devices, such as a railing in the bathroom, a bedside commode, or a walker.

Altered Urinary Elimination. The development of urinary lithiasis in clients with hyperparathyroidism may lead to the nursing diagnosis *Altered Urinary Elimination related to renal involvement secondary to hypercalcemia and hyperphosphaturia resulting in urolithiasis, painful urination, hematuria, and spasms.*

Outcomes. The client will resume a normal urinary output, as evidenced by urine production of ½ ml/kg/hr without development of stones.

Interventions

Encourage Fluids. The client should consume at least 3000 ml of fluid a day. Dehydration is dangerous in clients with hyperparathyroidism because it increases the serum calcium level and promotes the formation of renal stones.

Prevent Urolithiasis. Cranberry juice or prune juice may help make the urine more acidic. Acidification helps prevent renal stone formation, because calcium is more soluble in acidic urine than in alkaline urine.

Strain Urine of Stones. If a kidney stone is present, strain all urine to detect gravel and stones. Save any specimens of abnormal urine for the physician to examine and for laboratory analysis. Also, observe the urine for blood and assess the client for renal colic (see Chapter 34).

Altered Nutrition: Less Than Body Requirements. The client is likely to experience nutritional problems, suggesting the nursing diagnosis *Altered Nutrition: Less than Body Requirements related to anorexia and nausea resulting in decreased food intake and weight loss.*

Outcomes. The client will have an adequate intake, as evidenced by absence of nausea and return to or maintenance of ideal body weight.

Interventions. Encourage a low-calcium diet to correct hypercalcemia. Explain that abstaining from milk and milk products may help alleviate some of the distressing gastrointestinal manifestations. A client who has peptic ulcers needs to take antacids or histamine receptor antagonists. Help the client create a diet that is high enough in calories without dairy products. If necessary, have a dietitian see the client to help with meal planning.

Constipation. A client with hyperparathyroidism is susceptible to bowel problems, leading to the nursing diagnosis *Constipation related to adverse effects of hypercalcemia on the gastrointestinal tract resulting in decreased frequency of stools and painful defecation.*

Outcomes. The client will maintain a normal bowel pattern, as evidenced by a daily, soft, formed bowel movement.

Interventions. Work to prevent constipation and fecal impaction resulting from hypercalcemia. Help the client stay as active as the extent of bone disease allows. Increase fluid intake and the amount of fiber in the diet. The client should drink at least six to eight glasses of water a day unless contraindicated. If constipation continues despite these measures, obtain an order for a stool softener or laxative.

EVALUATION

Depending on the cause of the hypercalcemia, medical management may be able to control primary hypercalcemia. If it does not, surgery may be required. If the condition is secondary to renal failure, the management is more chronic in nature.

Surgical Management

PARATHYROIDECTOMY

INDICATIONS. Definitive treatment of primary hyperparathyroidism is surgical removal of the gland or glands causing hypersecretion of PTH. Usually, only the diseased parathyroid glands are resected. If all four glands are hyperplastic, however, three and one-half glands are removed. Fortunately, one half of a parathyroid gland is usually sufficient to maintain normal levels of circulating PTH.

Autotransplantation of the parathyroid glands is a useful modality for the management of certain forms of hyperparathyroidism and radical neck surgery. After partial parathyroidectomy, it is possible to transplant the remaining healthy parathyroid tissue to a safer location, such as the brachioradial muscle of the forearm. Reexploration of the neck in the future may cause laryngeal nerve damage and influence complications of the original surgery. Transplantation procedures take some time to come to full effect. In the meantime, the client must supplement the diet with calcium and vitamin D to prevent hypoparathyroidism and hypocalcemia.

If hyperparathyroidism is surgically treated early in its course, the chance of total recovery is good. Bone pain may disappear within 3 days after removal of parathyroid tissue, and bone lesions may heal completely. Unfortunately, serious renal disease might not be reversible by parathyroid surgery.

COMPLICATIONS. The complications after parathyroidectomy are similar to those following thyroidectomy and rarely occur. Hypocalcemia is a potentially life-threatening complication even if some parathyroid glands are left untouched because edema reduces their function. The client may also experience respiratory distress related to either hemorrhage or recurrent laryngeal nerve damage.

OUTCOMES. The cure rate for primary hyperparathyroidism after surgical removal is greater than 95%. This high success rate is directly related to the experience of the surgeon and adequate exploration of the neck.

Nursing Management of the Surgical Client

ASSESSMENT

The client undergoing surgery may have long-standing hyperparathyroidism and thus should be assessed for complications of the disease. Renal function should be carefully assessed preoperatively.

DIAGNOSIS, OUTCOMES, INTERVENTIONS

Risk for Injury. The client undergoing surgery for hyperparathyroidism is at risk for a number of complications. An important nursing diagnosis is *Risk for Injury related to preoperative drug sensitivities and postoperative complications.*

Outcomes. The client will not suffer injury, as evidenced by the absence of medication reactions preoperatively and by the absence of respiratory distress, hemorrhage, and hypocalcemia postoperatively.

Interventions

Administer Digitalis. If the client is receiving digitalis, administer this medication with extreme caution. Clients with hypercalcemia are hypersensitive to digitalis, and toxic manifestations may develop quickly.

Monitor for Postoperative Complications. During the postoperative period, new problems arise, some of which are the reverse of those found preoperatively. During the immediate postoperative period, nursing care is similar to that after thyroidectomy; that is, assess the client carefully for hemorrhage, airway obstruction, injury to the recurrent laryngeal nerve, and tetany. Also watch for manifestations of hormonal imbalance.

Mild tetany resulting from a drop in the serum calcium level is expected after removal of parathyroid tissue. Typically, the uncomfortable tingling of the hands and around the mouth that follows parathyroid resection is temporary.

If it persists or is severe, however, calcium gluconate is administered intravenously.

Prevent Osteoporosis. Clients with bone disease require additional therapy after surgery. Removal of the parathyroid glands reduces bone resorption, and because bone rebuilding proceeds at a rapid rate, the client may experience the "hungry bones" syndrome. This is characterized by hypocalcemia and severe tetany resulting from the rapid utilization of calcium by the bones.

To prevent low serum calcium levels resulting from bone recalcification, instruct the client to eat foods high in calcium. Tetany is treated with injections of calcium gluconate. To maintain adequate calcium levels, the client usually takes oral calcium preparations for months until the skeletal tissues have been rebuilt. Finally, encourage ambulation as soon as possible after surgery, because weight-bearing speeds the recalcification process.

EVALUATION

If hypercalcemia remains unrelieved by medical management, surgery is usually therapeutic. If a partial parathyroidectomy is unsuccessful, the remaining gland may need to be transplanted to the forearm to reduce absorption of the hormone. This measure usually eliminates the problem. As long as the client is closely observed in the immediate postoperative period, complications of hypocalcemia are usually controllable.

Modification for Elderly Clients

Hyperparathyroidism in older adults is an overlooked disease. It is estimated that 1 of 1000 men and 2 of 1000 women older than 60 years of age experience hyperparathyroidism. This disease often goes undiagnosed in older people because manifestations in the early stages are subtle and attributed to old age, depression, or anxiety. The manifestations intensify as the serum calcium level continues to rise and other physiologic and functional changes occur. Laboratory diagnosis is the same as for a younger client, but treatment may be complicated by medical problems and medication.

HYPOPARATHYROIDISM

Hyposecretion of the parathyroid glands produces the reverse syndrome of hyperparathyroidism. That is, serum calcium levels are abnormally low, serum phosphate levels are abnormally high, and pronounced neuromuscular irritability (tetany) may develop.

Hypoparathyroidism is diagnosed in women more often than men. The incidence is related to thyroid surgery. The incidence of temporary hypoparathyroidism after total thyroidectomy ranges from 6.9% to 25%. The incidence after subtotal thyroidectomy is 1.6% to 9.0%.

Etiology and Risk Factors

The causes of hypoparathyroidism are either *iatrogenic* (treatment-induced) or *idiopathic* (without a specific cause). Iatrogenic causes include accidental removal of the parathyroid glands during thyroidectomy, infarction of the parathyroid glands because of an inadequate blood supply to the glands during surgery, and strangulation of one or more of the glands by postoperative scar tissue. Health maintenance actions include monitoring of PTH, calcium, and phosphorus levels. Calcium supplements are required for life to prevent tetany.

Idiopathic hypoparathyroidism, like Graves' disease and Hashimoto's disease, may be an autoimmune disorder with a genetic basis. It is far less common than the iatrogenic form. *Pseudohypoparathyroidism* (Albright's hereditary osteodystrophy) is an inherited form of hypoparathyroidism involving lack of end-organ responsiveness to PTH.

Pathophysiology

PTH normally acts to increase bone resorption, which maintains proper serum calcium levels. The hormone also regulates phosphate clearance by the renal tubules, thereby maintaining the correct inverse balance between serum calcium and serum phosphate. Consequently, when parathyroid secretion is reduced, bone resorption slows, serum calcium levels fall, and severe neuromuscular irritability develops. Somewhat paradoxically, calcifications form in various organs, such as the eyes and basal ganglia. Also, without sufficient PTH, fewer phosphorus ions are secreted by the distal tubules of the kidney, renal excretion of phosphate falls, and serum phosphate levels rise.

The client may fully recover from the effects of hypoparathyroidism if the condition is diagnosed early, before serious complications begin. Unfortunately, cataracts and brain calcification, once formed, are irreversible.

Clinical Manifestations

The manifestations of hypoparathyroidism result mainly from low serum calcium levels. Manifestations are always more severe in clients with an elevated serum pH (alkalosis) of any cause (such as hyperventilation or ingestion of antacids). They worsen because, when the pH of the blood rises, the amount of ionized calcium drops, although total serum calcium remains the same. With less ionized calcium available to the body, the manifestations resulting from hypocalcemia become more severe until the alkalosis is corrected.

ACUTE HYPOPARATHYROIDISM

Acute hypoparathyroidism is caused by accidental damage to parathyroid tissues during thyroidectomy. It is characterized by greatly increased neuromuscular irritability, which results in tetany. Clients with tetany experience painful muscle spasms, irritability, grimacing, tingling of the fingers, laryngospasm, and dysrhythmias. Assessment also reveals Chvostek's and Trousseau's signs. In some cases, tetany is so severe that a tracheostomy is required to correct acute respiratory obstruction secondary to laryngospasm.

CHRONIC HYPOPARATHYROIDISM

Chronic hypoparathyroidism is usually idiopathic, resulting in lethargy; thin, patchy hair; brittle nails; dry, scaly skin; and personality changes. Ectopic or unexpected calcification may appear in the eyes and basal ganglia. Thus, cataracts and permanent brain damage, accompanied by psychosis or convulsions, may develop. In addition, severe persistent hypocalcemia adversely affects the heart, causing dysrhythmias and eventual cardiac failure.

The diagnosis of hypoparathyroidism is based on the following physical examination findings related to hypocalcemia:

- Presence of Chvostek's sign (spasms of facial muscles after a tap over the facial nerve, signifying facial hyperirritability)
- Presence of Trousseau's sign (spasms of the wrist and hand after compression of the upper arm, as by a blood pressure cuff)
- Hyperactive deep tendon reflexes (DTRs)
- Circumoral paresthesia
- Numbness and tingling of fingers

The diagnosis of hypoparathyroidism also stems from these findings:

- Laboratory findings showing low calcium, low PTH, high phosphorus, decreased urine calcium
- Radiographic studies of the skull or computed tomography (CT) of the head showing areas of calcification
- Ophthalmic examination revealing calcification of the ocular lens, which may lead to cataract formation

Complications

If treatment is not started rapidly in acute hypoparathyroidism, death can result from the respiratory obstruction secondary to tetany and laryngospasms. In chronic hypoparathyroidism, the complications are calcifications in the eye and basal ganglia that can occur if treatment is delayed.

Outcome Management

Medical Management

Acute hypoparathyroidism (with its major manifestation of acute tetany) is a life-threatening disorder. The desired outcomes of emergency care are to elevate serum calcium levels as rapidly as possible, to prevent or treat seizures, and to control laryngeal spasm and consequent respiratory obstruction.

For clients with chronic hypoparathyroidism, the desired outcome of intervention is to restore the serum calcium level to normal concentrations. The calcium level is increased more gradually than in acute hypoparathyroidism.

Elevate Serum Calcium

Calcium Gluconate. In clients with acute hypoparathyroidism, in order to elevate serum calcium levels quickly, the physician prescribes 10% calcium gluconate solution in an intravenous infusion. While administering the calcium gluconate, instruct the client to inhale carbon dioxide by breathing into a paper bag. Carbon dioxide inhalation causes a mild metabolic acidosis, which elevates the amount of ionized calcium in the blood.

Oral Calcium Replacements. When the condition has stabilized and the dangers of tetany have passed, the client is given oral calcium salts to maintain normal serum calcium levels. The desired outcome of therapy for chronic hypoparathyroidism is to keep the client asymptomatic with a serum calcium level of about 8.5 to 9.2 mg/dl. The client is given oral calcium salts (calcium gluconate, calcium lactate, or calcium carbonate).

Vitamin D. The client is given vitamin D in addition to calcium supplements to maintain serum calcium levels. Commercially available forms of vitamin D include ergocalciferol (vitamin D_2) and dihydrotachysterol (Hytakerol). Although ergocalciferol is a more reliable and less expensive drug than dihydrotachysterol or dihydroxycholecalciferol, all three forms of vitamin D are effective in correcting hypocalcemia. They are available as either tablets or oily liquids. Aluminum hydroxide gel (Amphojel) is also prescribed.

Parathyroid Hormone. The ideal treatment of this PTH-deficient condition is replacement of the absent hormone. A pure form of PTH has now been synthesized and is available.

High-Calcium, Low-Phosphate Diet. A client with hypoparathyroidism should receive a diet high in calcium but low in phosphorus. Again, vitamin D is needed to maintain serum calcium levels, and clients should be encouraged to select foods or supplements enriched with vitamin D.

Address Seizures and Laryngeal Spasm

Tetany and laryngeal spasms may occur suddenly and without warning in patients at risk for acute hypoparathyroidism. Calcium gluconate should be readily available at the bedside, and in many cases an order is left to have a tracheotomy tray available at the bedside.

Nursing Management of the Medical Client

Assessment

Carefully assess the client at risk for acute hypoparathyroidism (e.g., the post-thyroidectomy client) for development of hypocalcemia. Question the client about any numbness or tingling around the mouth or in the fingertips or toes. Check for Chvostek's and Trousseau's signs. In addition, assess for any manifestation of respiratory distress secondary to laryngospasm.

In a client with chronic hypoparathyroidism, assess for obvious physical changes, such as dry skin and hair. Also assess for a Parkinson-like syndrome or cataracts. Assess the teeth because pits may encircle them, indicating enamel hypoplasia.

Diagnosis, Outcomes, Interventions

Risk for Injury: Muscle Tetany. A client with hypoparathyroidism is susceptible to hypocalcemia, which can lead to the nursing diagnosis *Risk for Injury: Muscle tetany related to decreased serum calcium levels.*

Outcomes. The client will remain free from injury, as evidenced by a return of calcium levels to normal range, a normal respiratory rate, and blood gases within normal limits.

Interventions

Prevent Respiratory Arrest. When caring for a client with severe hypoparathyroidism, always be prepared for laryngeal spasm and respiratory obstruction. Have an endotracheal tube, laryngoscope, and tracheostomy set available when caring for a client with acute tetany.

Monitor and Prevent Tetany. When a client is at risk for sudden hypocalcemia, as after thyroidectomy, an ampule of intravenous calcium carbonate is usually kept at the bedside for immediate use if necessary. When the intravenous tubing is removed, it is sometimes capped so that rapid venous access is available. Sometimes clients are encouraged to take in a ready source of calcium carbonate, such as Tums.

EVALUATION

If the hypocalcemia is transient after a thyroidectomy, it usually resolves as edema decreases. If it is chronic, the client is usually able to manage the therapeutic regimen with minimal difficulty.

Self-Care

Because hypoparathyroidism can be a chronic condition, the client must be able to provide self-care. Teaching is important for the client with chronic hypoparathyroidism because this client requires lifelong medication and dietary modification.

MEDICATIONS

When teaching the client about take-home medications, make sure the client knows that all forms of vitamin D, except dihydroxycholecalciferol, are slowly assimilated by the body. Therefore, it may take a week or longer for the manifestations to improve.

DIET MODIFICATIONS

Teach the client about a diet high in calcium but low in phosphorus. Remind the client to omit cheese and milk products, which have a high phosphorus content. Explain that calcium supplements may be obtained in either tablet or solution form, depending on preference. Oral calcium administration is usually discontinued when the client responds to vitamin D preparations.

Emphasize the importance of lifelong medical care for the client with chronic hypoparathyroidism. Instruct the client to have serum calcium levels checked by a physician at least three times a year. Normal blood serum calcium levels must be maintained to prevent complications. If hypercalcemia or hypocalcemia develops, the physician will adjust the treatment regimen to correct the imbalance.

CONCLUSIONS

You must make careful assessments of clients with thyroid or parathyroid disorders. These disorders can be controlled and the manifestations reversed if they are discovered in a timely manner and prompt and proper treatment is begun. You are an important resource for these clients, who require considerable education. You are also responsible for closely monitoring any client who needs surgery for either the thyroid or parathyroid gland. The client is particularly vulnerable during this postoperative period, and high-level nursing surveillance and intervention facilitate successful recovery.

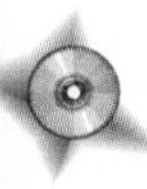

THINKING CRITICALLY

1. **A 64-year-old man comes to the clinic with a 6-month history of progressive fatigue, weakness, and dyspnea. On further questioning, you find that he has had an unintentional weight loss of 30 pounds despite an increased appetite.**

   Your physical examination reveals an alert and oriented man who looks his stated age. He is somewhat anxious. His attention span is short, and you must repeat many questions. His heart rate is 118 BPM; blood pressure, 154/98 mm Hg; temperature, 101 °F; the skin is warm and moist; deep tendon reflexes are hyperactive. What are priorities for care?

Factors to Consider. What additional subjective and objective data should you collect to confirm a diagnosis? What medication might be started after the diagnosis is made?

2. **The client is a woman with a long history of chronic renal failure. She receives dialysis three times a week. She is currently hospitalized for a complicated pneumonia. Upon reviewing her laboratory values, you note that her serum calcium level is 6.8 mg/dl. What are the implications for care?**

Factors to Consider. What is the relationship of calcium metabolism to renal function? What are the dangers associated with this serum calcium level? What treatments should be initiated to treat this and what should be done to prevent recurrence?

3. **A middle-aged woman comes to the clinic with manifestations of weight gain, lethargy, fatigue, and severe constipation. After diagnostic evaluation, the client is given Synthroid, 0.1 mg, for hypothyroidism. What general information should you give the client about hypothyroidism? About the medication?**

Factors to Consider. What should you teach about the expected therapeutic response to this medication? About side effects? How often are blood studies required for the client being treated with thyroid medications?

BIBLIOGRAPHY

1. Angelucci, P. A. (1995). Caring for patients with hypothyroidism. *Nursing, 25*(5), 60–61.
2. Behnia, M. & Gharib, B. (1996). Primary care diagnosis of thyroid disease. *Hospital Practice, 31*(6), *121–134.*
3. Burrow, G. N. (1995). The thyroid: Nodules and neoplasm. In P. Felig, J. D. Baxter, & L. A. Frohman (Eds.), *Endocrinology and metabolism* (3rd ed., pp. 521–549). New York: McGraw-Hill.
4. Corbett, J. V. (1999). *Laboratory tests and diagnostic procedures* (5th ed.). Norwalk, CT: Appleton & Lange.
5. Daylan, C. M. & Daniels, G. H. (1996). Chronic autoimmune thyroiditis. *New England Journal of Medicine, 335*(2), 89–105.
6. DeGroot, L. (Ed.). (1995). *Endocrinology* (3rd ed.). Philadelphia: W. B. Saunders.
7. Dunn, J. (1996). Seven deadly sins in confronting endemic iodine deficiency, and how to avoid them. *Journal of Clinical Endocrinology and Metabolism, 81*(4),1332–1335.
8. Facts and Comparisons Staff. (1999). *Drug facts and comparisons* (2nd ed.). St. Louis: Facts & Comparisons.
9. Fitzpatrick, L., & Arnold, A. (1995). Hypoparathyroidism. In P. Felig, J. D. Baxter, & L. A. Frohman (Eds.), *Endocrinology and metabolism* (3rd ed., pp. 1123–1135). New York: McGraw-Hill.
10. Frohman, L. A. (1995). Diseases of the anterior pituitary. In P. Felig, J. D. Baxter, & L. A. Frohman (Eds.), *Endocrinology and metabolism* (3rd ed., pp. 289–369). New York: McGraw-Hill.

11. Gambert, S. R. (1995). Hyperthyroidism in the elderly. *Clinics in Geriatric Medicine, 11*(2), 181–188.
12. Goldsmith, C. (1999). Clinical snapshot. Hypothyroidism. *American Journal of Nursing, 99*(6), 42–43.
13. Heitman, B., & Irizarry, A. (1995). Hypothyroidism: Common complaints, perplexing diagnosis. *Nurse Practitioner, 20*(3), 54–60.
14. Hubener, J., Arnold, A., & Potts, J. (1995). Hyperparathyroidism. In L. DeGroot (Ed.), *Endocrinology* (3rd ed., pp. 1044–1060). Philadelphia: W. B. Saunders.
15. Jankowski, C. B. (1996). Irradiating the thyroid: How to protect yourself and others. *American Journal of Nursing, 96*(10), 50–54.
16. Kennedy, L. W. & Caro, J. F. (1996). The ABCs of managing hyperthyroidism in the older patient. *Geriatrics, 51*(5), 22–24, 27, 31, 32.
17. Lehne, R. (1998). *Pharmacology for nursing care* (3rd ed.). Philadelphia: W. B. Saunders.
18. Loriaux, G. C. (1996). Endocrine assessment: Red flags for those on the front lines. *Nursing Clinics of North America, 31*(4), 695–714.
19. McKenzie, J. M., & Zakarija, M. (1995). Hyperthyroidism. In L. DeGroot (Ed.), *Endocrinology* (3rd ed., pp. 676–711). Philadelphia: W. B. Saunders.
20. McMorrow, M. E. (1996). Myxedema coma: Do you recognize the clues to this rare complication of hypothyroidism? *American Journal of Nursing, 96*(10), 55.
21. Miller, W. L., & Tyrrell, J. B. (1995). Adrenal cortex. In P. Felig, J. D. Baxter, & L. A. Frohman (Eds.), *Endocrinology and metabolism* (3rd ed., pp. 521–549). New York: McGraw-Hill.
22. Molitch, M. E. (1995). Neuroendocrinology. In P. Felig, J. D. Baxter, & L. A. Frohman (Eds.), *Endocrinology and metabolism* (3rd ed., pp. 221–275). New York: McGraw-Hill.
23. Pagana, K., & Pagana, T. (1997). *Diagnostic testing and nursing implications* (4th ed.). St. Louis: Mosby–Year Book.
24. Robertson, G. (1995). Posterior pituitary. In P. Felig, J. D. Baxter, & L. A. Frohman (Eds.), *Endocrinology and metabolism* (3rd ed., pp. 385–423). New York: McGraw-Hill.
25. Rusterholtz, A. (1996). Interpretation of diagnostic laboratory tests in selected endocrine disorders. *Nursing Clinics of North America, 31*(4), 715–724.
26. Singer, P., et al. (1995). Treatment guidelines for patients with hyperthyroidism and hypothyroidism. *Journal of the American Medical Association, 273*(10), 808–813.
27. Strief, M. M., & Pachucki-Hyde, L. C. (1996). Management of the patient with thyroid disease. *Nursing Clinics of North America, 31*(4), 779–796.
28. Strewler, G. J., & Rosenblatt, M. (1995). Mineral metabolism. In P. Felig, J. D. Baxter, & L. A. Frohman (Eds.), *Endocrinology and metabolism* (3rd ed., pp, 1407–1499). New York: McGraw-Hill.
29. Trivalle, C., et al. (1996). Differences in the signs and symptoms of hyperthyroidism in older and younger patients. *Journal of the American Geriatric Society, 44*(1), 50–53.
30. Tunbridge, W. M. G., & Caldwell, G. (1996). The epidemiology of thyroid diseases. In L. E. Braverman & R. O. Utiger (Eds.), *Werner & Ingbar's the thyroid: A fundamental and clinical text* (7th ed.). Philadelphia: J. B. Lippincott.
31. U.S. Public Health Service. (1996). Put prevention into practice: Thyroid function. *Journal of the American Academy of Nurse Practitioners, 8*(10), 495–496.
32. Utiger, R. (1995). Hypothyroidism. In L. DeGroot (Ed.), *Endocrinology* (3rd ed., pp. 753–768). Philadelphia: W. B. Saunders.
33. Utiger, R. D. (1995). The thyroid: Physiology, thyrotoxicosis, hypothyroidism and the painful thyroid. In P. Felig, J. D. Baxter, & L. A. Frohman (Eds.), *Endocrinology and metabolism* (3rd ed., pp. 435–509). New York: McGraw-Hill.
34. Wartofsky, L. (1995). The thyroid gland. In K. L. Becker, et al. (Eds.), *Principles and practice of endocrinology and metabolism* (2nd ed). Philadelphia: J. B. Lippincott.
35. Young, J. (1999). Actionstat: Thyroid storm. *Nursing, 29*(8), 33.

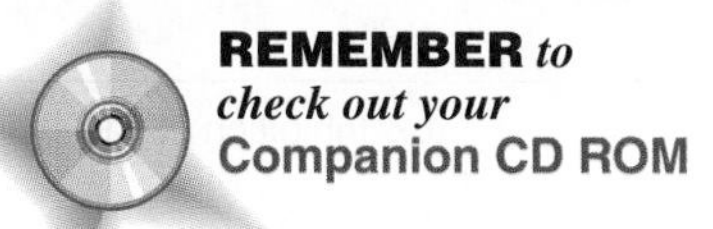

CHAPTER 44

Management of Clients with Adrenal and Pituitary Disorders

Anne Larson

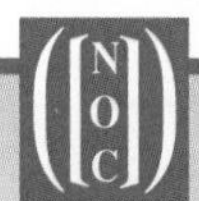

NURSING OUTCOMES CLASSIFICATION (NOC)
for Nursing Diagnoses—Clients with Adrenal and Pituitary Disorders

Activity Intolerance
Activity Tolerance
Endurance
Energy Conservation
Self-Care: Activities of Daily Living (ADL)
Self-Care: Instrumental Activities of Daily Living (IADL)

Altered Thought Processes
Cognitive Ability
Cognitive Orientation
Concentration
Decision-Making
Distorted Thought Control
Identity
Information Processing
Memory
Neurological Status: Consciousness

Knowledge Deficit
Knowledge: Diet
Knowledge: Disease Process
Knowledge: Energy Conservation
Knowledge: Health Behaviors
Knowledge: Health Resources
Knowledge: Illness Care
Knowledge: Infection Control
Knowledge: Medication
Knowledge: Personal Safety
Knowledge: Prescribed Activity
Knowledge: Treatment Procedures
Knowledge: Treatment Regimen

Pain
Comfort Level
Pain Control
Pain: Disruptive Effects
Pain Level

Risk for Impaired Skin Integrity
Immobility Consequences: Physiologic
Nutritional Status
Risk Control
Risk Detection
Tissue Integrity: Skin and Mucous Membranes
Tissue Perfusion: Peripheral
Wound Healing: Primary Intention

Risk for Infection
Immune Status
Knowledge: Infection Control
Nutritional Status
Risk Control
Risk Detection
Tissue Integrity: Skin and Mucous Membranes
Treatment Behavior: Illness or Injury
Wound Healing: Primary Intention

Risk for Injury
Circulation Status
Knowledge: Personal Safety
Neurologic Status
Risk Control
Risk Detection
Safety Behavior: Fall Prevention
Safety Behavior: Home Physical Environment
Safety Behavior: Personal
Safety Status: Physical Injury
Symptom Control
Vital Signs Status

ADRENOCORTICAL DISORDERS

Glandular hypofunction and hyperfunction characterize the major disorders of the adrenal cortex. Underactivity of the adrenal cortex results in a deficiency of glucocorticoids, mineralocorticoids, and adrenal androgens. The person with adrenal hypofunction is a prime candidate for injury, knowledge deficit, and feelings of powerlessness. Overactivity of the adrenal cortex results in excessive production of glucocorticoids, mineralocorticoids, and androgens or estrogens. The person with adrenal hyperfunction needs to focus on preventing injury and infection, acquiring effective coping mechanisms, and learning about the disease process.

ADRENAL INSUFFICIENCY

Hypofunction of the adrenal cortex can originate from a disorder in the adrenal gland itself (primary adrenal insufficiency), or it may result from hypofunction of the pituitary-hypothalamic unit (secondary adrenal insufficiency).

This chapter incorporates material written for the fifth edition by Carol Birch.

PRIMARY ADRENAL INSUFFICIENCY

Commonly known as *Addison's disease,* primary adrenal insufficiency results from idiopathic atrophy or destruction of the adrenal glands by an autoimmune process or other disease. Thomas Addison first described this disorder in 1849.

Etiology and Risk Factors

Primary adrenal insufficiency is caused by hypofunction of the adrenal glands. It is a rare disorder, and its incidence and prevalence in the United States are unknown. An autoimmune process accounts for 75% of primary adrenal insufficiency. It is commonly seen in people with acquired immunodeficiency syndrome (AIDS). Tuberculosis is the cause in about 20% of cases of Addison's disease. Adrenal metastasis from the lung, breast, gastrointestinal tract, melanoma, or lymphoma may also cause primary adrenal insufficiency. Additional causes include bilateral adrenalectomy and hemorrhagic infarction with necrosis of the adrenal gland.

Risk factors for primary adrenal insufficiency include (1) a history of other endocrine disorders, (2) taking glucocorticoids for more than 3 weeks with sudden cessation, (3) taking glucocorticoids more than once every other day, (4) adrenalectomy, and (5) tuberculosis.

Health promotion and health maintenance activities for clients receiving glucocorticoids include instruction on the risks and benefits of this therapy and instruction on the proper means of withdrawing glucocorticoids. Health maintenance activities for those receiving long-term steroid therapy include education about the need for supplemental steroids to prevent acute adrenal insufficiency and having parenteral steroids available for use when the client is unable to take oral steroids. Health restoration activities include ensuring that the client is mindful of the need for follow-up with the physician to monitor steroid levels.

Pathophysiology

Autoimmunity is the most common cause of adrenal insuffciency. Lymphocytic infiltration of the adrenal cortex is the characteristic feature. Addison's disease is frequently accompanied by other immune disorders. Gradual destruction leads to chronic adrenal insufficiency. Continued loss of cortical tissue accompanies a deficiency of mineralocorticoids as well as glucocorticoids. Adrenocortical hypofunction results in decreased levels of mineralocorticoids (aldosterone), glucocorticoids (cortisol), and androgens (Fig. 44–1).

Clinical Manifestations

The onset of Addison's disease is usually insidious. The client experiences mild fatigue, languor, irritability, weight loss, nausea, vomiting, and postural hypotension, usually weeks or months before the diagnosis is confirmed. As the disorder progresses, manifestations intensify. By then, the client has lost more than 90% of both adrenal cortices (Table 44–1).

Diagnosis of Addison's disease depends primarily on

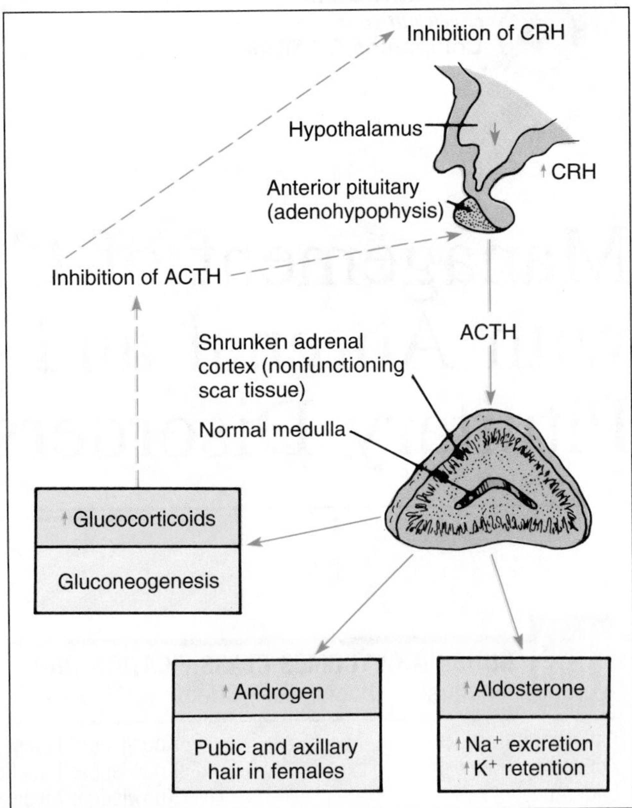

FIGURE 44–1 Effects of Addison's disease. *Dashed arrows* show feedback mechanisms. ACTH, adrenocorticotropic hormone; Na, sodium; K, potassium; CRH, corticotropin-releasing hormone.

blood and urine hormonal assays (Table 44–2). Primary adrenal insufficiency is characterized by a low cortisol production rate and a high plasma adrenocorticotropic hormone (ACTH) concentration.

Other diagnostic tests may be ordered to evaluate the effects of hypofunction of the adrenals on the body: (1) serum electrolytes (especially hyponatremia and hyperkalemia in primary adrenal insufficiency and hyponatremia alone in secondary disease); (2) blood glucose; (3) complete blood count (to assess for anemia); (4) x-ray studies, computed tomography (CT); and (5) magnetic resonance imaging (MRI) of the adrenals and pituitary.

Outcome Management

Addisonian crisis is an emergent condition requiring careful monitoring in the critical care unit. Thereafter, the rate of recovery is client-specific. Normally, Addison's disease can be managed on an outpatient basis if the client is compliant and receives proper self-care instructions.

Medical Management

ADDISONIAN CRISIS

Addisonian crisis, or *acute adrenal insufficiency,* may occur when the client has been under stress without appropriate hormone replacement. Stressors include pregnancy, surgery, infection, states of dehydration or anorexia, fever, and emotional upheaval. Manifestations are related to the degree of hormone deficiency and electrolyte imbal-

TABLE 44–1 ADRENAL HORMONES: FUNCTION AND CONSEQUENCES OF DYSFUNCTION

Hormone	Usual Function	Insufficient State: Addison's Disease	Excess State: Cushing's Syndrome
MINERALOCORTICOIDS			
Aldosterone Stimulated by adrenocorticotropic hormone (ACTH) production Major control is renin-angiotensin system	Promotes retention of Na^+ (and water) in kidney	More than 90% of the adrenal gland is destroyed before the clinical picture of *adrenal insufficiency* emerges Increased excretion of Na^+ and water influences dehydration, hyponatremia, orthostatic hypotension, ↓ urine output, ↓ cardiac output, weight loss, salt craving, acidosis, circulatory collapse, shock	Increased retention of Na^+ and water results in edema, weight gain, hypertension, augmentation of cardiac problems such as left ventricular hypertrophy, congestive heart failure
GLUCOCORTICOIDS			
Cortisol Regulated by ACTH release from anterior pituitary	Promotes gluconeogenesis Maintains plasma glucose level Promotes appetite Causes release of epinephrine from adrenal medulla Assists in adaptation to stress by ↑ gluconeogenesis releasing an anti-inflammatory response; augmenting release of catecholamines (epinephrine, norepinephrine) to increase blood pressure	Decreased gluconeogenesis causes depleted liver glycogen stores manifested by hypoglycemia, weakness, fatigue, anorexia, weight loss, vomiting, mental confusion, emotional disturbances (mild neurosis to depression) Inadequate release of epinephrine produces hypoglycemia, hypotension Lowers resistance to stress and produces a "hyperresponse" to stressors: hypoglycemia, hypotension, hyperthermia	Increased circulating cortisol causes memory loss, poor concentration, depression, euphoria, anxiety, sleep disorders Increased susceptibility to infection and suppression of inflammatory response: vulnerability to infections, poor response to infectious process, poor wound healing
ACTH release controls cortisol secretion	ACTH regulates melanocyte-stimulating hormone (MSH)	Stimulates an increase in MSH: increases skin and mucous membrane pigmentation, especially in fingers, toes, and sun-exposed body parts (skin appears bronzed)	No effect
ANDROGENS			
Regulated by ACTH release from anterior pituitary		Females: oligomenorrhea or amenorrhea, decrease in body hair Males: no manifestations in males because testes produce adequate quantities of sex hormone	Females: acne, thinning of scalp hair, excessive growth of body and facial hair in male pattern (hirsutism), menstrual irregularities, infertility common Males: decreased libido, impotence

ance and include sudden penetrating pain in the back, abdomen, or legs; depressed or changed mentation; volume depletion; hypotension; loss of consciousness; and shock.

CORRECT FLUID AND ELECTROLYTE IMBALANCES. The overall desired outcome of treatment is prevention of the morbidity and mortality associated with the addisonian crisis. Untreated, addisonian crisis is fatal. The cause of the crisis must be determined and treated immediately. Hypotension and electrolyte imbalance need to be corrected quickly. Rapid rehydration is essential. An isotonic solution usually corrects the volume depletion, salt depletion, and hypotension. The client may also need oxygen, vasopressors, or volume expanders. Sodium polystyrene sulfonate (Kayexalate) may be administered orally or as an enema in combination with sorbitol. Kayexalate is a resin that releases sodium ions in exchange for potassium ions.

TABLE 44–2 DIAGNOSTIC TESTS OF ADRENOCORTICAL FUNCTION

Test	Purpose	Nursing Notes	Interpretation
Cortisol level with dexamethasone suppression test	Evaluates function of adrenal cortex	Give dexamethasone before phlebotomy to suppress diurnal formation of adrenocorticotropic hormone (ACTH) Give 1 mg dexamethasone at 11 PM to suppress ACTH formation in time for 8 AM phlebotomy and later at 8 PM; estrogen therapy can falsely increase results	↑ Pituitary tumor, Cushing's syndrome or disease, hyperplasia of adrenal cortex (benign or malignant) ↓ Addison's disease
Cortisol plasma levels	Evaluates function of adrenal cortex	Plasma cortisol levels have diurnal effect: levels higher in AM than PM Fasting prephlebotomy 2 hrs of supine activity are necessary before test because activity increases cortisol level Estrogens increase level Aldactone (spironolactone) can cause false-positives	↑ Pregnancy, recent physical activity, obesity, Cushing's disease or syndrome ↓ Addison's disease
17-Hydroxysteroids (Porter-Silber reaction)	Measures metabolites of glucocorticoids and aldosterone	24-hr urine collection to be kept on ice Many drugs can invalidate results	↑ Cushing's disease or syndrome; ACTH administration; nonadrenal ACTH-producing tumor ↓ Addison's disease or exogenous steroid suppression
Cosyntropin test	Diagnoses adrenal insufficiency with ACTH stimulation	Give ACTH IV; 45 min later, obtain serum cortisol level	↑ Normal ↓ Dysfunction of hypothalamic-pituitary axis Secondary adrenal insufficiency
Computed tomography (CT) or magnetic resonance imaging (MRI) of adrenals	Identifies and locates adrenal glands	No preparation except client education	Small, atrophied glands = autoimmune adrenal insufficiency Bilateral enlarged glands = hemorrhage (with areas of high density), neoplasm
Rapid ACTH stimulation		Give cosyntropin IV; obtain plasma cortisol and aldosterone level at baseline + 30 min	↓ Cortisol and aldosterone = primary adrenal insufficiency
17-Ketosteroids	Measures steroid metabolites from adrenal cortex and testes (does not include testosterone)	24-hr urine test; keep collection cold; may need preservative Many drugs make test invalid	↑ Tumors of adrenal cortex or testes, Cushing's syndrome ↓ Hypofunction of adrenal, or in clients with removal of testes or ovaries

Correct Hypoglycemia. Hypoglycemia must be evaluated and corrected with intravenous (IV) glucose (5% dextrose [D_5] solution IV or IV glucose push bolus).

Replace Steroids. Hydrocortisone at 100 mg is administered as an IV bolus followed by 100 mg IV every 8 hours for 24 hours. The IV hydrocortisone is tapered as the client's status dictates. Oral hydrocortisone is initiated.

Addison's Disease

Addison's disease was once fatal within months. Today, with the availability of synthetic corticosteroids (Table

TABLE 44–2 **DIAGNOSTIC TESTS OF ADRENOCORTICAL FUNCTION** *Continued*

Test	Purpose	Nursing Notes	Interpretation
Aldosterone	Measures mineralocorticoid production	Client to be supine 2 hr before phlebotomy ↑ Aldosterone can cause ↑ extracellular fluid Oral contraceptive, sodium restriction, and potassium may ↑ level	↑ Primary or secondary hyperaldosteronism, severe liver dysfunction ↓ Addison's disease (may be undetectable or ↓ in Addison's)
Urinary cortisol level	Measures cortisol, not metabolites		↑ Adrenal hyperfunction, Cushing's syndrome ↓ Not necessarily adrenal hypofunction
Renin level	Measures renin, an enzyme produced by juxtaglomerular apparatus in response to decreased blood flow to kidneys	Client in supine position Results high in AM Note sodium content in diet on laboratory slip The following medications interfere with results: diuretics, estrogens, oral contraceptives, antihypertensives	↑ Hypertension, upright position with phlebotomy ↓ High-sodium diet
Plasma ACTH or serum corticotropin	Tests anterior pituitary function as it may cause Cushing's syndrome, Addison's disease	Fasting sample Stress may artificially increase results	↑ Cushing's syndrome caused by bilateral adrenal hyperplasia or ectopic ACTH-producing tumors; Addison's disease (primary adrenal insufficiency) caused by adrenal gland failure, surgical removal of adrenals, adrenal suppression with long-term exogenous steroid supply ↓ Secondary adrenal insufficiency caused by hypopituitarism; cushingoid client may have adrenal adenoma as cause of hyperfunction
Captopril test	Rules out renal artery stenosis	Nuclear medicine captopril renal scan done first to evaluate resting glomerular filtration rate (GFR); captopril administered PO; GFR reevaluated after captopril	↓ GFR renal artery stenosis same ↑ GFR after captopril: negative for renal artery stenosis
Corticotropin-releasing hormone (CRH) stimulation	Measures CRH from hypothalamus to pituitary necessary to stimulate ACTH and cortisol release	Give CRH IV; measure plasma ACTH and cortisol at baseline and after 15, 30, and 60 min	↑ ACTH and cortisol indicate primary adrenal insufficiency ↓ ACTH and cortisol indicate pituitary or hypothalamic dysfunction, secondary adrenal insufficiency

44–3), clients with Addison's disease can live normal, active lives, provided they receive adequate glucocorticoid replacement. Use corticosteroids with caution. Table 44–4 shows the adverse consequences of administering corticosteroids in selected disorders. Carefully assess clients for manifestations of hypercortisolism, which can result from excessive long-term cortisol therapy. Most clients receive glucocorticoid and mineralocorticoid replacement.

Osteoporosis is a complication that may develop with excessive use of glucocorticosteroids because the protein matrix in the bones is broken down and therefore

TABLE 44–3 NURSING IMPLICATIONS OF CORTICOSTEROIDS

Class	Action	Therapeutic Outcomes	Adverse Outcomes	Dosing
GLUCOCORTICOIDS				
Long-acting (dexamethasone, Decadron)	Inhibits inflammation Suppresses cell-mediated immune response	Inflammation and allergic responses are reduced	Monitor for infection (use good handwashing) Monitor for hypocalcemia	Take with food or milk Do not stop abruptly
Intermediate-acting (methylprednisolone, Medrol)	Inhibits inflammation Suppresses cell-mediated immune response	Adrenal crisis is averted Muscle strength returns Blood pressure normalizes	Monitor for heartburn Monitor for signs and symptoms of hypercortisolism	Give with food or milk Give as single dose before 9 AM Do not stop abruptly
Short-acting (hydrocortisone, Hydrocortone)	Inhibits inflammation Suppresses cell-mediated immune response	Adrenal crisis is averted Muscle strength returns Blood pressure normalizes	Monitor for heartburn Monitor for signs and symptoms of increased cortical effects, insomnia, mood swings, increased hunger Protect from infection (use good handwashing)	Give oral dose with food or milk Give as single dose before 9 AM Have client wear Medic-Alert bracelet Tell client not to stop drug abruptly
MINERALOCORTICOIDS				
Fludrocortisone (Florinef)	Increases retention of sodium and therefore water	Postural hypotension diminishes	Monitor for edema Monitor for hypokalemia Monitor intake and output Monitor daily weights	Give with food or milk Do not stop abruptly

calcium cannot be retained. Closely observe clients with other medical problems that may be worsened with steroid use.

Nursing Management of the Medical Client

ADDISONIAN CRISIS

ASSESSMENT

Monitor the client's vital signs closely while the disease is being diagnosed. Check the pulse carefully, at least every 4 hours. Take orthostatic blood pressure (BP) readings and pulses. Report drops in BP or orthostatic changes.

As rehydration occurs and electrolyte imbalances are corrected, assess increased physical vitality and emotional well-being. Assess bone prominences for pressure ulcers in immobilized clients. With therapy, listlessness and exhaustion should gradually disappear.

Monitor for exposure to cold and infections. Immediately inform the physician if evidence of infection develops, such as a sore throat or burning on urination. Remember, a client with Addison's disease cannot tolerate stress. Infection imposes additional stress on the body, and cortisol levels need to be higher during infectious illnesses.

Carefully assess for manifestations of sodium and potassium imbalance (see Chapter 13). Obtain daily weights for objective measurement of fluid gain or loss. If steroid replacement therapy is inadequate, sodium loss and potassium retention continue uncorrected. If the steroid dosage is too high, excessive amounts of sodium and water are retained and potassium excretion is high.

TABLE 44–4 CONSEQUENCES OF CORTICOSTEROID USE IN SELECTED DISORDERS*

Disorder	Consequence
Diabetes mellitus	Augments hyperglycemia
Inflammatory bowel disorders	Fluid retention may exacerbate peristalsis
Hypertension	Contributes to fluid retention
Congestive heart failure	Contributes to fluid retention
Renal insufficiency	Worsens fluid retention

*Corticosteroids are contraindicated in clients with viral, fungal, or tubercular infections.

DIAGNOSIS, OUTCOMES, INTERVENTIONS

Risk for Injury: Addisonian Crisis. The client must be diligent in self-care, or the diagnosis may be *Risk for Injury: Addisonian crisis related to adrenal insufficiency.*

Outcomes. The client will not exhibit injury, as evidenced by absence of hypotension, shock, or other manifestations of acute adrenal insufficiency.

Interventions

Monitor for Manifestations of Crisis. Addisonian crisis usually develops over 24 to 48 hours. Closely monitor for sudden profound weakness; severe abdominal, back, and leg pain; hyperpyrexia (although this may be suppressed by steroids) followed by hypothermia; hypotension associated with high cardiac output, normal wedge pressure, and low systemic resistance; coma; renal shutdown; and death.

An adrenal crisis is a medical emergency that must be treated rapidly and vigorously. The three major desired outcomes of intervention are (1) reversal of shock, (2) restoration of blood circulation (the client usually has a deficit of at least 20% of extracellular fluid volume), and (3) replenishment with essential steroids.

Correct Fluid, Electrolyte, Steroid Imbalances. Immediately on admission, 1000 ml of normal saline with water-soluble glucocorticoid (hydrocortisone phosphate or hydrocortisone sodium succinate) added is rapidly infused. The dosage of the prescribed glucocorticoid is gradually reduced. It is administered intramuscularly (IM) or IV every 8 hours on days 1 and 2 of the crisis and gradually reduced thereafter. Hypoglycemia is controlled by a glucose infusion, either an IV bolus or IV drip as part of rehydration. Hyperkalemia is controlled or corrected with Kayexalate. The precipitating event must be corrected. Plasma, oxygen, and vasopressor medications may be indicated.

Throughout the emergency period, monitor BP, administer IV infusion and medications, monitor hourly urine output, report oliguria (a manifestation of shock), and minimize exposure to emotional and physical stress. Observe for manifestations of glucocorticoid overdose and overhydration, such as generalized edema from fluid retention, hypertension, flaccid paralysis from hypokalemia, psychosis, and loss of consciousness. Also evaluate electrolytes for hyperkalemia, hyponatremia, and hypoglycemia, and correlate these findings with the client's manifestations.

With rapid, efficient intervention, addisonian crisis usually resolves within 12 hours. The client's condition stabilizes, and the convalescent period begins. When the client can tolerate food and fluids by mouth, steroid replacement can be administered orally.

Prevent Future Crises. After the immediate crisis is over, help the client avoid further development of adrenal insufficiency. Obtain a medical identification (Medic-Alert) bracelet and an emergency kit before discharge from the hospital. Instruct the client to carry these items at all times. The client's name and diagnosis should appear on the identification bracelet, and a wallet card should state that the client receives daily hydrocortisone and that the medication must be administered by injection in an emergency.

Dexamethasone can be kept in a prepared syringe in an emergency kit with sterile alcohol wipes for cleaning the injection site. The kit should also contain written information about the client's diagnosis, prescribed drugs, dosage schedules, and emergency phone numbers, including the physician's name and phone number.

Adrenal insufficiency is a potentially life-threatening condition, but when properly recognized and treated, it has little or no effect on life span. There are no dietary or activity restrictions.

EVALUATION

The outcome of treatment for addisonian crisis is easily evaluated, usually within 12 hours of treatment. By this time, the client should no longer exhibit any manifestations of addisonian crisis or death would have occurred.

Self-Care

Management of Addison's disease takes place in the community with regular medical follow-up of the client's status. Hence, the focus of management is on self-care. Carefully assess the client's ability to understand and perform self-care. The client needs extensive instruction in self-care activities to achieve independence. Appropriate outcomes for the client with Addison's disease are that the client's weight remains stable, vital signs and cortisol levels remain within normal limits, and the client states that fatigue has decreased.

STEROID REPLACEMENT

The client must learn how to take steroids correctly. Provide the client and significant others with written instructions on self-administration of steroids. (The client and significant others should have demonstrated their ability to prepare and administer injections.) The client needs to know the following information:

- Actions of prescribed hormones (hydrocortisone, fludrocortisone)
- Importance of taking medications daily, without fail, exactly as prescribed
- Principles of self-administration of oral medications (e.g., the client must check the label on the bottle before taking the medication and documenting medications taken and their side effects)
- Manifestations of overdosage and underdosage
- Importance of hydrocortisone self-injection when unable to tolerate oral medication (because of nausea and vomiting) and during times of acute stress (motor vehicle accident, trauma) because the body is unable to provide the needed additional glucocorticoid coverage
- Need for an IM self-injection kit to be available at all times
- Need for a Medic-Alert bracelet showing the diagnosis and the need for cortisol replacement
- Need for the client to call a health care provider if questions arise after discharge from the medical center

Emphasize that the client who takes glucocorticoids must call the physician to obtain a dosage increase when experiencing stressful situations (e.g., emotional upheavals, dental extractions, minor surgery, upper respiratory infections). The general rule is to double the glucocorticoid dosage for up to 1 week, depending on manifestations, and then resume normal dosage. In addition, temporary mineralocorticoid dosage is reduced by 50% to avoid excessive salt retention and hypertension. Encourage the client to consult the physician for dose adjustment. The medication must be administered IM when nausea and vomiting prevent oral administration.

Follow-up Monitoring

Remind clients to keep semiannual appointments with the physician, even when their health is good and self-medication is proceeding smoothly. As with diabetes mellitus, the control of Addison's disease is a lifelong responsibility.

Modification for Elderly Clients

Adrenal diseases are uncommon in older people. The effects of normal aging on the adrenals are unclear. It appears, however, that ACTH and cortisol production remains constant throughout life. Elderly people may be more sensitive to the side effects of steroid therapy because these problems (e.g., osteoporosis, hypertension, diabetes) already exist.

Secondary Adrenal Insufficiency

Secondary adrenal insufficiency results from dysfunction of the hypothalamic-pituitary-adrenal (HPA) axis (Fig. 44–2). The most common cause is chronic treatment with glucocorticoids for nonendocrine uses. Other causes include:

- Hypopituitarism resulting in decreased ACTH secretion by the pituitary gland, which causes decreased secretion of cortisol and androgens by the adrenal gland
- Pituitary tumor or infarction
- Radiation
- Suppression of hypothalamic-pituitary secretion of ACTH related to hypercortisolism caused by either exogenous administration of corticosteroids or oversecretion of corticosteroids by an adrenal tumor (in both cases, the adrenal glands atrophy and become filled with lipids)

Secondary adrenal insufficiency is characterized by low cortisol production and low plasma ACTH. Because circulating levels of corticosteroids remain high, these clients do not experience manifestations of adrenocortical insufficiency unless steroid therapy is discontinued suddenly or the tumor is resected. If corticosteroid therapy is tapered gradually, with the dosage reduced each day, adrenal gland function usually returns to normal.

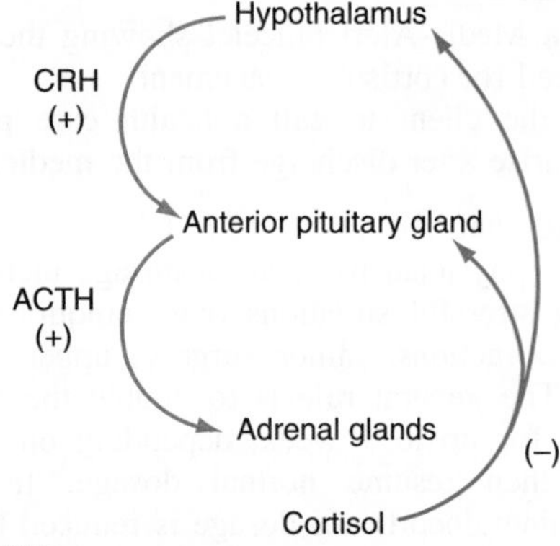

FIGURE 44–2 The hypothalamic-pituitary-adrenal (HPA) axis, demonstrating stimulation and feedback between the hypothalamus, anterior pituitary, and adrenal glands. ACTH, adrenocorticotropic hormone; CRH, corticotropin-releasing hormone.

Assessment reveals that clients with secondary adrenal insufficiency experience cortisol deficiency. Aldosterone continues to be secreted in sufficient amounts. Treatment involves administering glucocorticoids, as in Addison's disease. Mineralocorticoid replacement is unnecessary. Instruct the client to wear an emergency identification bracelet and to carry an emergency kit for hydrocortisone injection in case of an adrenal crisis.

ADRENOCORTICAL HYPERFUNCTION

Hyperfunction of the adrenal cortex can result in excessive production of glucocorticoids, mineralocorticoids, and androgens. Major conditions of adrenocortical hyperfunction are hypercortisolism (glucocorticoid excess) and primary aldosteronism (aldosterone excess).

Hypercortisolism

Hypercortisolism (Cushing's syndrome) was first described by Harvey Cushing in 1932. It results from overactivity of the adrenal gland, with consequent hypersecretion of glucocorticoids. Cushing's syndrome is relatively rare, and its incidence is unknown. It occurs mainly in women ages 20 to 40 years; however, it can occur up to age 60.

Etiology and Risk Factors

Iatrogenic hypercortisolism (resulting from medical interventions) accounts for most cases because of the frequent therapeutic use of high-dose glucocorticoids. Hypersecretion of cortisol can be caused by a cortisol-secreting adrenal tumor or adrenal hyperplasia, resulting from overproduction of ACTH. Adrenal tumors are responsible for about 30% of cases of Cushing's syndromes. Most (85%) are benign, but 15% are malignant. There are two sources of excessive ACTH secretion:

- Pituitary hypersecretion and pituitary tumors, which cause about 70% of cases of Cushing's syndrome. These usually benign tumors are either small basophil adenomas or large chromophobe adenomas. Pituitary hypersecretion of ACTH that results in glucocorticoid excess is called *Cushing's disease.*
- Ectopic secretion of ACTH (or *ectopic ACTH syndrome*). ACTH-secreting tumors located outside the pituitary gland are a rare cause of Cushing's syndrome. Oat cell carcinoma of the lung, pancreatic islet cell carcinoma, and carcinoid tumors of the lung, gut, thymus, and ovary are the tumors that most frequently cause ectopic ACTH syndrome.

Iatrogenic Cushing's syndrome, another form of the disorder, results from exogenous (originating outside the body; e.g., taking supplemental medication) administration of synthetic glucocorticoids in supraphysiologic amounts. Thus, educating clients to avoid unnecessary use of exogenous steroids is an important health promotion activity. Health maintenance activities include (1) educating clients who are at risk for manifestations of Cushing's syndrome; (2) treating clinical manifestations of hypernatremia, hypokalemia, hyperglycemia, and hypertension;

and (3) teaching clients about adrenalectomy and steroid replacement. Health restoration activities include making sure that clients understand the importance of surgery, lifelong steroid replacement, and recognizing disease complications that may have already developed (such as osteoporosis or "buffalo hump," a fat pad on the neck).

Pathophysiology

When Cushing's syndrome develops, the normal function of the glucocorticoids becomes exaggerated and the classic picture of the syndrome emerges (Fig. 44–3). This exaggerated physiologic action of glucocorticoids appears as follows:

- Persistent hyperglycemia (or "steroid diabetes").
- Protein tissue wasting, which results in muscle wasting and weakness; capillary fragility, which results in ecchymosis; and osteoporosis from bone matrix wasting. Osteoporosis can become so severe that even mild trauma can cause fractures. Compression fractures can develop in the osteoporotic spine, leading to kyphosis and loss of height.
- Potassium depletion, leading to hypokalemia, dysrhythmias, muscle weakness, and renal disorders.
- Sodium and water retention, which causes edema and hypertension.
- Hypertension, which eventually predisposes the client to left ventricular hypertrophy, heart failure, and cerebrovascular accidents.
- Abnormal fat distribution (in conjunction with edema), which results in a moon-shaped face, a dorsocervical fat pad on the neck (buffalo hump), and truncal obesity with slender limbs. Also, pink and purple striae appear on the breasts, axillary areas, abdomen, and legs because of thinning of the skin. Striking changes in appearance occur after the development and cure of Cushing's syndrome. Old photographs can be useful in showing changes over time.
- Increased susceptibility to infection and lowered resistance to stress increase vulnerability to microorganisms of all types. Because of suppression of the inflammatory response, people with Cushing's syndrome show few manifestations of infection. They also demonstrate poor wound healing.
- Possible increased production of androgens can cause virilism (masculine characteristics) in women. Manifestations of virilism include acne, thinning of scalp hair, and hirsutism (excessive bodily and facial hair in a male pattern).
- Mental changes include memory loss, poor concentration and cognition, euphoria, and depression. Sometimes a condition called "steroid psychosis" develops. Depression can predispose the client to suicidal thoughts. About 80% of the clients meet the criteria for a major affective disorder: 50% with unipolar depression, 30% with bipolar illness.

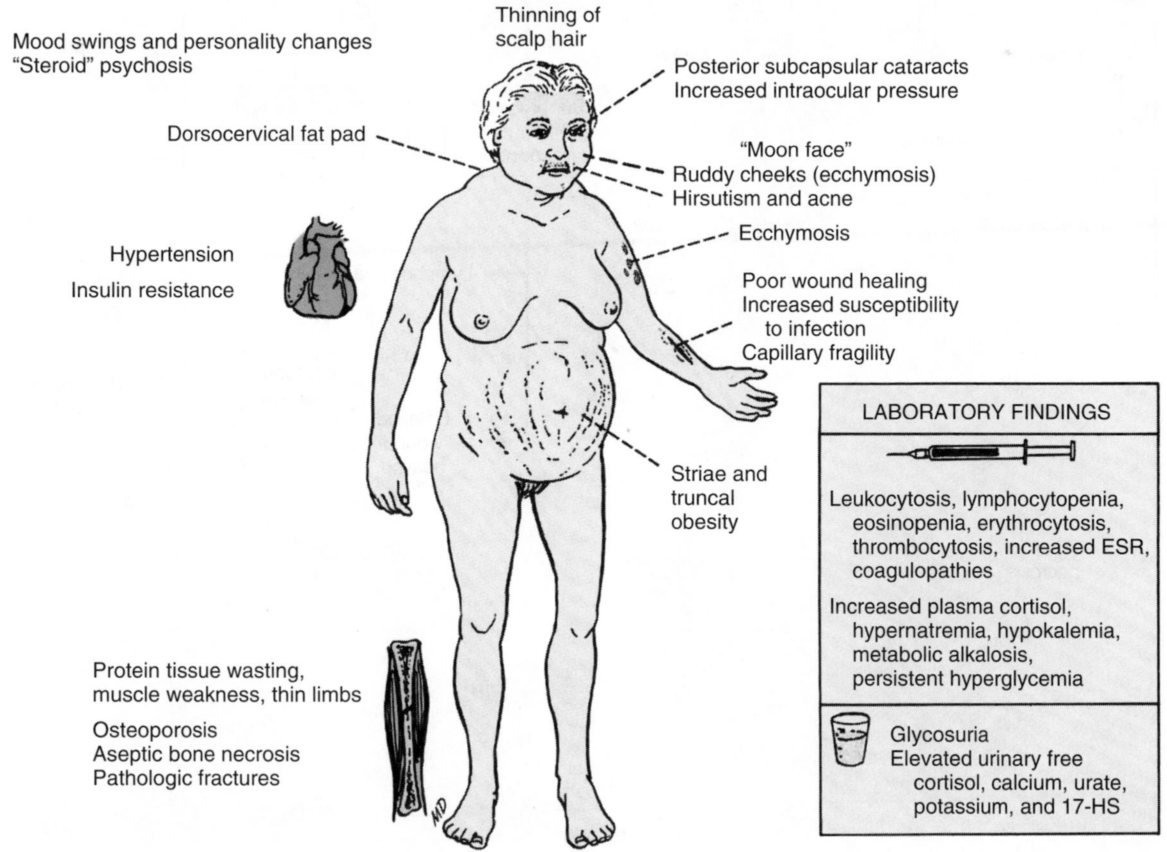

FIGURE 44–3 Assessment data for Cushing's syndrome. *Inset,* Laboratory findings. ESR, erythrocyte sedimentation rate; 17-HS, 17-hydroxysteroid.

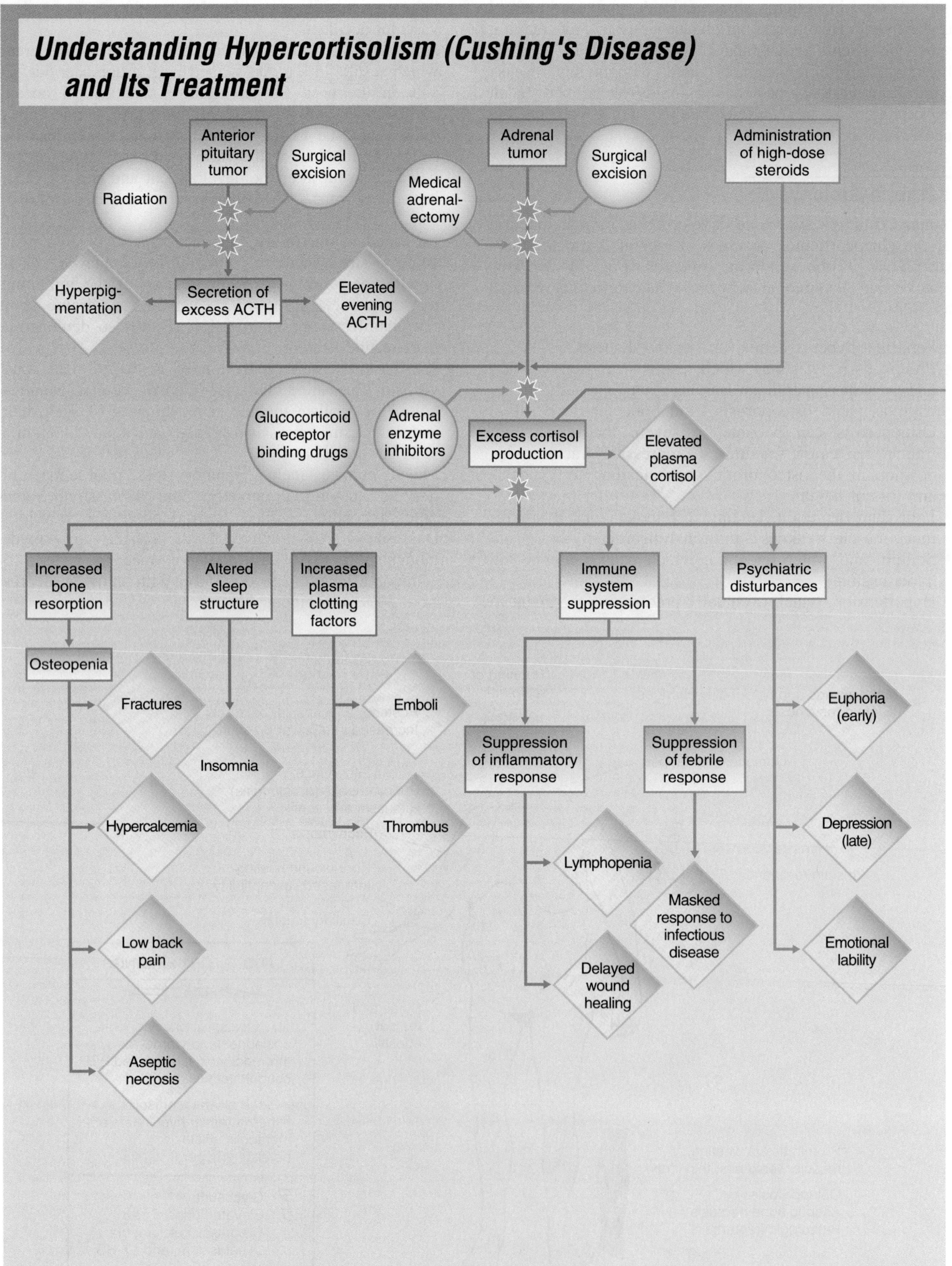

■ ACTH, adrenocorticotropic hormone.

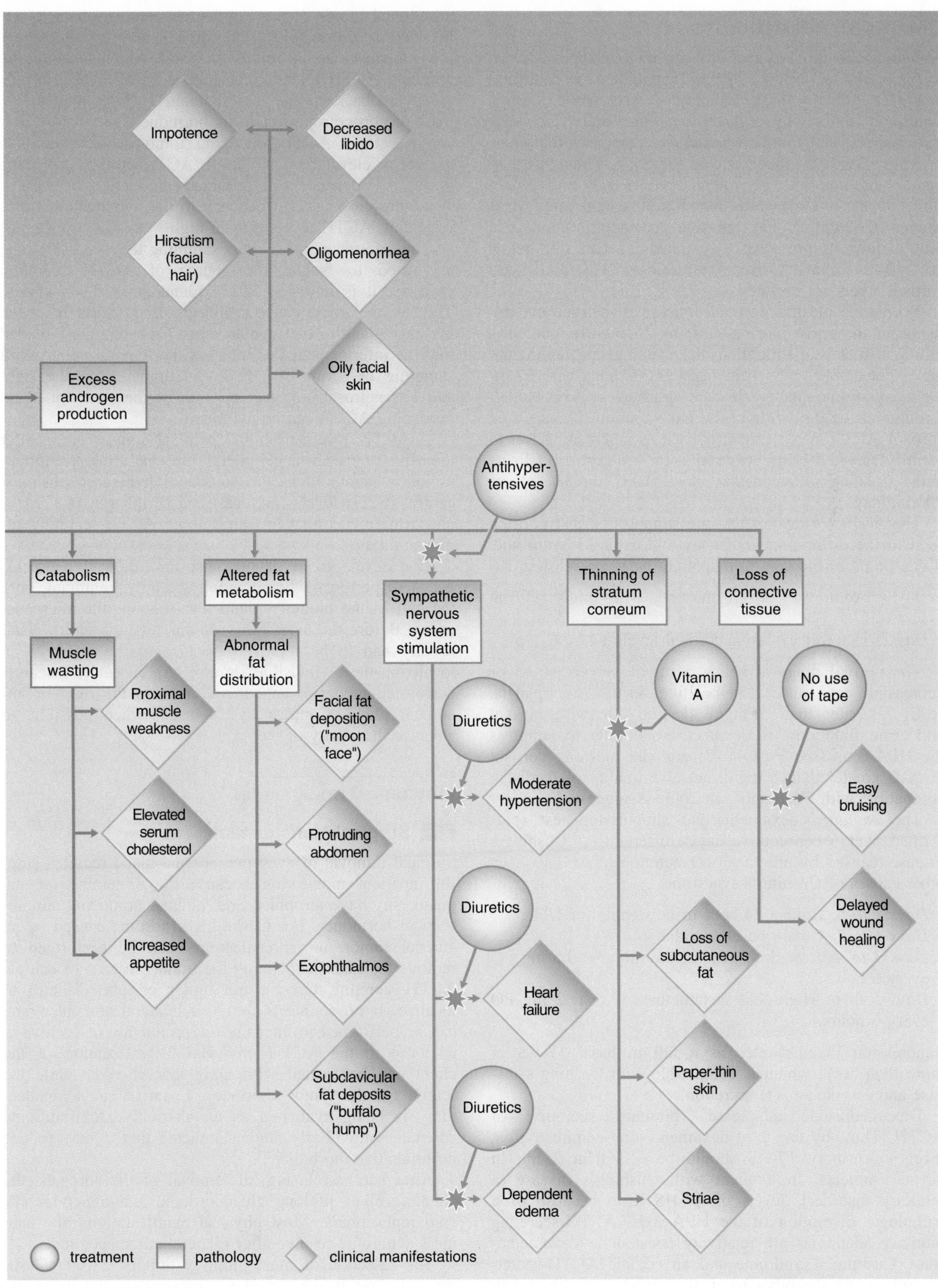
Impotence
Decreased libido
Hirsutism (facial hair)
Oligomenorrhea
Oily facial skin
Excess androgen production
Antihyper-tensives
Catabolism
Altered fat metabolism
Sympathetic nervous system stimulation
Thinning of stratum corneum
Loss of connective tissue
Muscle wasting
Abnormal fat distribution
Vitamin A
No use of tape
Proximal muscle weakness
Facial fat deposition ("moon face")
Diuretics
Moderate hypertension
Easy bruising
Elevated serum cholesterol
Protruding abdomen
Diuretics
Delayed wound healing
Loss of subcutaneous fat
Increased appetite
Exophthalmos
Heart failure
Paper-thin skin
Subclavicular fat deposits ("buffalo hump")
Diuretics
Dependent edema
Striae
treatment
pathology
clinical manifestations

Clinical Manifestations

Although clients have a classic cushingoid appearance, it is important to perform diagnostic studies for confirmation (see Table 44–2). Laboratory tests for Cushing's syndrome reflect hyperglycemia, fluid and electrolyte disturbances, and immunosuppressive responses that characterize excessive glucocorticoid secretion. Thus, in Cushing's syndrome glucose tolerance decreases and glucosuria appears. The white blood cell count often rises above 10,000/mm^3, but the total eosinophil count can drop below 50/mm^3. Also, lymphocytes can fall below 20%. Both urinary 17-hydroxysteroid (17-HS) and blood cortisol levels are elevated.

Normally, plasma cortisol follows a diurnal pattern, rising in the early morning (10 to 25 mg/dl), gradually falling to below 10 mg/dl in the evening, and approaching undetectable levels near midnight. Clients with Cushing's syndrome have elevated plasma cortisol levels throughout the day without diurnal variation. Urinary free cortisol (UFC) measurement is used as a screening test to identify elevated urinary excretion of free cortisol. Clients with Cushing's syndrome have UFC levels above 100 mg/day.

The *overnight* dexamethasone suppression test is often used in the differential diagnosis of Cushing's syndrome. It can be performed on an outpatient basis as follows:

- *Day 1:* Administer dexamethasone, 1 mg orally (PO) at 11 PM.
- *Day 2:* Determine plasma cortisol level at 8 AM.

The normal range is below 5 mg/dl. Severe stress or depression can cause false-positive results (i.e., plasma cortisol greater than 5 mg/dl despite otherwise normal endocrine function). If dexamethasone fails to suppress the HPA axis (see Fig. 44–2) and the morning cortisol level is greater than 5 mg/dl, an abnormality of feedback compatible with Cushing's syndrome is suggested.

The *standard* dexamethasone suppression test (performed over 6 consecutive days) differentiates Cushing's disease (caused by pituitary oversecretion of ACTH) from other causes of Cushing's syndrome:

- *Days 1 to 6:* Collect 24-hour urine sample for UFC.
- *Days 1 to 2:* Obtain baseline value.
- *Days 3 to 4:* Low-dose dexamethasone test: 0.5 mg PO every 6 hours.
- *Days 5 to 6:* High-dose dexamethasone test: 2 mg PO every 6 hours.

Suppression is interpreted as a fall in basal 17-HS of more than 50%, which is compatible with Cushing's disease and ectopic ACTH secretion.

Dexamethasone suppresses pituitary secretion of ACTH. Thus, by day 2 of dexamethasone administration, levels of urinary 17-HS should be less than 2 mg in normal subjects. In a client with Cushing's disease (a pituitary disorder), levels of 17-HS drop because of a pathologic disruption of the HPA axis. ACTH-secreting pituitary adenomas are relatively resistant to dexamethasone. Cushing's syndrome and an ectopic ACTH-secreting tumor, on the other hand, usually do not respond to dexamethasone (i.e., levels of 17-HS do not decrease).

In the plasma ACTH test, low ACTH levels point to an adrenal tumor as the cause of hypercortisolism. Overproduction of cortisol by the adrenal tumor provides negative feedback to the pituitary gland, which responds by reducing ACTH release. The high cortisol level also provides feedback to the hypothalamus, which reduces release of corticotropin-releasing hormone.

An ectopic ACTH-producing tumor usually yields a normal or elevated ACTH level. ACTH production by the tumor is independent of pituitary production of ACTH. Thus, despite negative feedback to the hypothalamic-pituitary unit, ACTH levels remain high.

The inferior petrosal sinus sampling test is a radiologic test used to isolate the source of ACTH secretion (whether it is in the pituitary gland and, if so, where). The left and right petrosal sinuses carry blood from the pituitary gland to the jugular veins. Catheters are threaded into the inferior petrosal sinus via the femoral veins. With sampling of serum ACTH levels drawn from the right and left petrosal sinuses, the side of the pituitary gland producing ACTH can be identified.

If ACTH levels from the petrosal sinuses are greater than this one from a peripheral site (the arm), a pituitary tumor is identified as the source of hypercortisolism. If central ACTH levels (petrosal) and peripheral ACTH levels (arm) are equivalent, an ectopic ACTH-secreting tumor is likely.

The development of this test has allowed neurosurgeons to perform a hemihypophysectomy, removing only the half of the pituitary gland that contains the microadenoma. Before the availability of this test, the entire gland usually had to be removed because of the difficulty in localizing these "invisible" tumors. An adrenal CT scan is performed to detect an adrenal mass in the right or left adrenal gland. Contrast dye is used, when possible, to enhance the clarity of the scan.

Outcome Management

Surgical Management

Surgical removal of even one adrenal gland requires careful inpatient monitoring because the remaining adrenal gland may have atrophied and stopped producing adrenocortical hormones. For Cushing's syndrome caused by an adrenal tumor, an adrenalectomy can be performed to remove the gland containing the tumor. In case of ectopic ACTH-secreting tumors, the tumor can be difficult to localize. If no source is found, a bilateral adrenalectomy can be performed to interrupt the production of cortisol in response to the ACTH produced by the tumor, or the client can be treated with antiglucocorticoids while the search for the tumor continues. Laparoscopic adrenalectomy is being evaluated as an alternative to traditional adrenalectomy. Early studies indicate that it may reduce postoperative morbidity.[27, 31]

After successful surgical removal of the adrenals, the client receives lifelong glucocorticoid and mineralocorticoid replacement. Most physical manifestations of Cushing's syndrome resolve after bilateral adrenalectomy.

The resection of most pituitary tumors causing Cushing's disease is performed via transsphenoidal hypophysectomy (see Chapter 69). Occasionally, large or anatomically complex tumors are excised via a transfrontal approach (see discussion of hypophysectomy). A surgical cure rate of 85% to 90% has been documented. Because the HPA axis has been suppressed, adrenal insufficiency develops postoperatively. The axis takes 12 to 24 months to recover. Replacement steroids are indicated during this time.

Nursing Management of the Surgical Client

PREOPERATIVE CARE

ASSESSMENT

Begin by obtaining a careful history from a client with possible Cushing's syndrome. The client may exhibit the characteristic clinical manifestations identified previously. Support the client during the diagnostic phase of care. At this point, there is often a great deal of uncertainty about the cause of the disorder. Explain to the client why these tests must be performed before treatment can be started.

During the preoperative phase, the client with Cushing's syndrome requires expert nursing assessment and care. The crucial problems of hypertension, edema, possible heart disease, diabetes mellitus, increased susceptibility to infection, decreased resistance to stress, and emotional lability (tendency toward frequent mood changes) or instability must all be assessed and brought under control before surgery.

DIAGNOSIS, OUTCOMES, INTERVENTIONS

Risk for Injury: Fractures, Hypertension, or Diabetes. Until the diagnosis is made and the problem treated, the client is at *Risk for Injury: Fractures, Hypertension, or Diabetes related to osteoporosis, sodium and water retention, or the presence of an insulin antagonist, respectively.*

Outcomes. Injury will not occur, as evidenced by absence of fractures. The client will not have hypertension, hyperglycemia, or diabetes.

Interventions

Prevent Injury. Protect the client from falls and accidents. Clients with Cushing's syndrome have osteoporosis and tend to develop fractures even with mild trauma. Keep the bed in its lowest position, and raise the side rails for protection. Assist clients with ambulation to avoid falls.

Monitor for Hypertension and Diabetes. Monitor vital signs at frequent intervals. Assess the client carefully for evidence of severe hypertension, such as elevated BP, headache, failing vision, irritability, and dyspnea. Check for postural hypotension (but have the client change position slowly to avoid injury from a sudden drop in BP).

Obtain the client's weight daily in a consistent manner. If sodium intake is reduced, edema and weight should diminish. Obtain daily blood glucose levels via finger stick. Positive results may indicate diabetes mellitus (steroid diabetes) caused by the insulin antagonist action of the excessive cortisol.

Knowledge Deficit. A typical nursing diagnosis for the client undergoing surgery to correct adrenocortical excess is *Knowledge Deficit regarding the disease, surgery, and proper diet related to no previous instruction and new diagnosis resulting in anxiety, misinformation, and questions.*

Outcomes. The client will understand the disease, the surgery planned, and the importance of a proper diet, as evidenced by statements of understanding and choice of a proper diet.

Interventions

Explain Disease and Treatment. It is important for clients to understand their condition and the proposed treatment. Give clients an opportunity to ask questions about the treatment, and assess their understanding of it.

Provide Adequate Nutrition. Encourage a diet low in calories, carbohydrates, and sodium but with ample protein and potassium. Such a diet promotes weight loss, reduction of edema and hypertension, control of hypokalemia, and rebuilding of wasted tissue. The client with diabetes mellitus or gastric ulcers requires a special diet.

EVALUATION

It is expected that clients will have minimal complications or have appropriate management of complications before surgery so that they can undergo the adrenalectomy successfully. The client will be able to explain the desired outcome of surgical intervention, possible complications, and related treatment. A glucocorticoid preparation will be given on the morning of surgery to prevent adrenal insufficiency during the procedure.

POSTOPERATIVE CARE

ASSESSMENT

Routine postoperative monitoring of the incision and special assessments for manifestations of shock, addisonian crisis, and renal shutdown are required. Assess the client's ability to perform self-care and to manage the disease for the remainder of his or her life. The client's current level of knowledge must be assessed and a teaching plan carefully developed.

DIAGNOSIS, OUTCOMES, INTERVENTIONS

Risk for Injury. After surgery, the client may have *Risk for Injury related to complications of the surgical procedure.*

Outcomes. Injury will not occur or will be detected early, as evidenced by absence of shock, hemorrhage, infection, or addisonian crisis.

Interventions. On the morning of surgery, administer a glucocorticoid preparation IM or IV as prescribed. A water-soluble cortisol preparation (diluted in an IV infusion) may be given throughout the surgery. Cortisol protects against the development of acute adrenal insufficiency during the adrenalectomy. Even if the surgeon plans to remove only one adrenal gland, temporary glucocorticoid support may be needed until the remaining adrenal gland begins to secrete sufficient cortisol. Because of the excessive secretion of cortisol by the tumorous gland, the healthy gland can atrophy and needs time to readjust.

During the immediate postoperative phase, major desired outcomes are prevention of shock and infection, maintenance of adequate cortisol levels, and control of pain and incisional discomfort. Observe for manifestations of shock related to hemorrhage (hypotension and a rapid, weak pulse). Document vital signs every 15 minutes. Measure urine and record hourly output, observing for oliguria, a manifestation of shock and renal shutdown. Administer IV fluids, pressor amines, and corticosteroids as prescribed.

The manifestations of addisonian crisis resemble those of shock. Closely assess the client for this complication, and administer IV cortisol in high doses until the manifestations subside. The client will require increased amounts of steroids until the remaining adrenal gland returns to a normal level of functioning and the stress associated with the treatment subsides.

Risk for Infection. The client receiving steroid replacement will be at *Risk for Infection related to lowered resistance to stress and compromised immune response.*

Outcomes. Infection will not develop or will be detected early, as evidenced by absence of leukocytosis, fever, and other manifestations of infections.

Interventions. After surgery, encourage the client to cough, turn, and deep-breathe to prevent respiratory infections. Employ meticulous sterile technique with wound care to prevent infection. Paralytic ileus is less common because the flank approach is usually used.

Protect the client from exposure to infectious organisms. Isolate the client from health care personnel and significant others who have contagious disorders. Wash your hands meticulously before contact with the client.

Because glucocorticoids suppress immune and inflammatory reactions, a client with Cushing's syndrome may have only mild manifestations of even a severe infection. The white blood cell count does not show significant elevation in immunosuppressed clients. A slight elevation in body temperature may indicate the presence of a severe infection.

Activity Intolerance. A client receiving steroids may exhibit *Activity Intolerance related to fatigue and muscle weakness from protein wasting, persistent hyperglycemia (and possible diabetes mellitus), and potassium depletion resulting in an inability to maintain a normal activity level without increased heart rate or shortness of breath.*

Outcomes. The client will be able to balance rest and activity.

Interventions. Promote mental and physical rest for the client with Cushing's syndrome. Minimize stress and confusion so that the client can achieve maximal periods of rest.

Risk for Impaired Skin Integrity. A client receiving steroids is at *Risk for Impaired Skin Integrity related to tissue catabolism (thinning of skin), loss of connective tissue, and edema secondary to sodium and water retention.*

Outcomes. The client will maintain intact skin.

Interventions. Monitor the client's skin meticulously for breakdown. The client is extremely susceptible to breakdown from tissue catabolism. Avoid using tape or other irritants that may tear or excoriate the skin.

Altered Thought Processes. The client may exhibit *Altered Thought Processes (memory loss, cognitive impairment, mood swings, euphoria, or depression) related to increased levels of glucocorticoids and ACTH, resulting in an inability to make decisions and remember.*

Outcomes. The client will not have memory loss, cognitive impairment, or mood swings, or these manifestations will be minimized.

Interventions. Anticipate mood swings. Clients may become easily upset by changes in their appearance caused by the disease and may also become alarmed by bizarre feelings and emotions. Reassure clients that appearance and moods should gradually return to normal after treatment unless steroid replacement is necessary. If clients need steroid therapy, some side effects will continue.

EVALUATION

If the surgical management of Cushing's disease is successful, neither injury related to the surgery nor addisonian crisis will develop. If complications do occur, desired outcomes may be related to successful management of the complications, such as control of hemorrhage, prevention of shock, and control of addisonian crisis.

Appropriate outcomes also include the control of side effects of the steroid therapy. Because these cannot be completely avoided, the client's ability to control them is an appropriate area to evaluate. The client should be able to differentiate complications from the side effects of medications.

Medical Management

Usually, a client with primary adrenal hyperplasia is treated surgically as an inpatient. Medical management is reserved for clients with inoperable tumors or metastatic tumors that warrant palliative care (Table 44–5). The outcome, therefore, is related to achieving comfort versus cure. Medical management options include radiation therapy and administration of adrenal blocking agents or ACTH-reducing agents to decrease the effects of the adrenal hyperplasia.

RADIATION THERAPY. Radiation therapy can be used to treat primary pituitary tumors and other ACTH-secreting adenomas. Radiation can be applied to the pituitary gland either internally or externally. Internally, the radiation is applied through a transsphenoidal implant. Radiation must be used with care because of the proximity of the optic nerve. Radiation is not always effective in even palliative treatment of tumors and may destroy normal tissue. For ACTH-secreting adenomas, such as lung tumors, palliation is possible. Radiation therapy is commonly used concurrently with surgical or pharmacologic management to enhance its effectiveness and reduce long-term side effects.

ADRENAL BLOCKING AGENTS. Medications that interfere with ACTH production or adrenal hormone synthesis are available. Mitotane (Lysodren) is a cytotoxic antihormonal agent that inhibits corticosteroid synthesis without destroying cortical cells. Aminoglutethimide (Cytadren) and trilostane (Modrastane) are other cytotoxic agents that block the synthesis of glucocorticoids and adrenal steroids.

ACTH-REDUCING AGENTS. Cyproheptadine (Periactin), bromocriptine, or somatostatin is used to treat hypersecretion caused by pituitary abnormalities and resulting in increased ACTH levels. These agents appear to interfere with ACTH production, thereby reducing the effect on the adrenals.

TABLE 44–5 THERAPIES FOR CUSHING'S SYNDROME, CUSHING'S DISEASE, AND ECTOPIC ACTH SYNDROME

Condition	Responsible Lesion	Therapies	Remarks
Cushing's syndrome	Adrenal tumor (benign or malignant)	Adrenalectomy	Adrenalectomy for benign unilateral tumor; usually curative Bilateral adrenalectomy must be followed by lifelong administration of corticosteroids
	Adrenal carcinoma with widespread metastases	Surgery and chemotherapy (mitotane)	Chemotherapy largely unsuccessful
Cushing's disease	Pituitary tumor (or unidentified lesion) that secretes excessive amounts of ACTH	Microsurgical resection of pituitary adenoma	Pituitary surgery successful in 95% of cases
		Irradiation of pituitary gland	Irradiation successful in 75% of cases; therapeutic effects not apparent for months after initiation of therapy
		Total bilateral adrenalectomy (corrects adrenal hyperplasia caused by excessive ACTH stimulation)	Total bilateral adrenalectomy must be followed by lifelong replacement therapy with glucocorticoid and mineralocorticoid
Ectopic ACTH syndrome	Extra-adrenal malignant tumor	Surgical removal of ectopic malignant tumor; chemotherapy used to control hypercortisolism and promote remission in clients with inoperable cancer	Surgery rarely successful because metastasis usually occurs before diagnosis; chemotherapy purely palliative

ACTH, adrenocorticotropic hormone.

Self-Care

The client with a bilateral adrenalectomy needs to learn self-care, because lifelong glucocorticoid replacement is essential. If only one adrenal gland has been removed, daily cortisol replacement continues until the remaining gland functions normally (usually after 6 to 12 months). Before discharge, the client and significant others need instruction on self-administration of replacement hormones (hydrocortisone). They should successfully demonstrate the injection technique before discharge. The client should also be able to repeat and comply with instructions and to remain free from addisonian crisis or adrenal insufficiency.

Modifications for Elderly Clients

Older clients may exhibit excessive manifestations of Cushing's syndrome because these clients may already have osteoporosis, hypertension, and diabetes. Older clients are also more susceptible to the side effects of steroid replacement therapy.

HYPERALDOSTERONISM

Aldosterone is the most powerful of the mineralocorticoids. Its primary role is to conserve sodium, and it also promotes potassium excretion. The incidence of primary hyperaldosteronism in the hypertensive population is unknown, affecting approximately 1%. It affects women twice as often as men and appears most frequently in the middle-aged.

Etiology and Risk Factors

Primary hyperaldosteronism refers to hypersecretion of aldosterone resulting from an adrenal lesion, which is usually benign. The disease, which produces secondary hypertension, hypokalemia (in most), and hypernatremia, is also known as *Conn's syndrome.*

Secondary hyperaldosteronism results from a variety of conditions that cause overproduction of aldosterone. These conditions include sodium-wasting renal disease, laxative or diuretic abuse, dehydration, cirrhosis with ascites, heart failure, and a decrease in intravascular volume. Hypertension is uncommon.

There are no particular risk factors for primary hyperaldosteronism. Risk factors for secondary hyperaldosteronism include chronic heart failure, cirrhosis with ascites, nephrotic syndrome, and hypertension caused by destructive renal artery disease. Health promotion measures, therefore, are successful treatment and control of the causative disease process. The more successfully these factors are controlled, the less secondary hyperaldosteronism is present.

Pathophysiology

Aldosterone affects tubular reabsorption of sodium and water and excretion of potassium and hydrogen ions in the renal tubular epithelial cells (Fig. 44–4). These effects lead to the development of hypernatremia, hypervolemia, hypokalemia, and metabolic alkalosis. With hypervolemia and hypernatremia, BP increases, often to very high levels, and renin production is suppressed. The hypertension can lead to cerebral infarcts and renal damage.

Secondary hyperaldosteronism is a result of continuous secretion of aldosterone secondary to high levels of angiotensin II, resulting from high plasma renin activity. Decreased renal perfusion of a variety of causes is the underlying mechanism.

Clinical Manifestations

Clients with primary hyperaldosteronism may be asymptomatic, but incidental findings include hypertension, hypernatremia, and hypokalemia. Without intervention, all of the complications of chronic hypertension, such as visual disturbances, heart failure, renal damage, and cerebrovascular accident, may occur. Unfortunately, the renal complications resulting from long-term hypertension tend to be progressive. Therefore, clients with primary hyperaldosteronism need to be identified and treated early in the course of the disease.

Hypokalemia results from excessive urinary excretion of potassium ions. This problem, in turn, causes muscle weakness, paralysis, or cardiac dysrhythmias, because potassium loss reduces normal neuromuscular irritability. In addition, excessive potassium excretion results in polyuria. The large urinary output leads to polydipsia (excessive thirst). Finally, hypokalemia leads to metabolic alkalosis because of shifting of hydrogen ions into the cells in exchange for potassium and exchange of hydrogen ions in the tubular cells for sodium ions from the tubular urine. Metabolic alkalosis causes a decrease in ionized calcium levels, which can result in tetany and respiratory suppression.

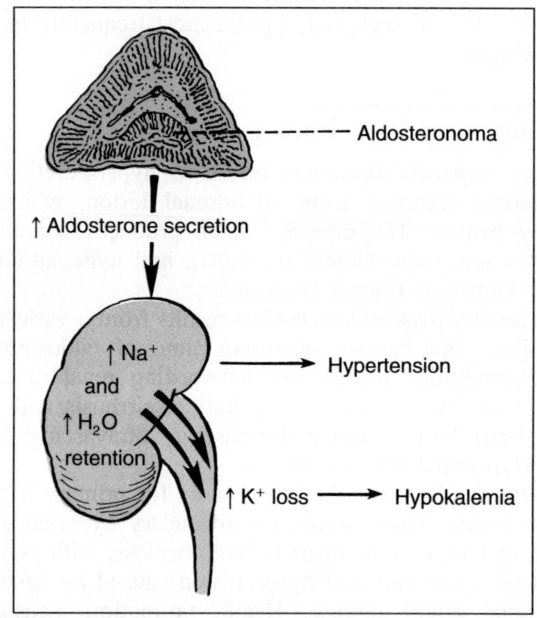

FIGURE 44–4 Effects of primary aldosteronism. Excessive aldosterone secretion causes increased sodium (Na^+) and water (H_2O) retention and increased excretion of potassium (K^+).

Despite sodium retention, clients with hyperaldosteronism rarely develop overt edema. Although extracellular fluid increases moderately, excessive water is normally excreted in the urine with potassium ions. Over time, the kidneys tend to adjust physiologically to excessive secretion of aldosterone, and water excretion reaches an equilibrium with sodium intake. The kidneys' eventual "escape" from the sodium-retaining and water-retaining action of aldosterone is sometimes called the *escape phenomenon.*

The diagnosis of primary hyperaldosteronism is based on low serum potassium levels, alkalosis, and elevated urinary or plasma aldosterone levels with low plasma renin levels (elevated in secondary hyperaldosteronism). In addition, radiographic studies may reveal cardiac hypertrophy resulting from chronic hypertension. Radionuclide scanning techniques using radiolabeled iodocholesterol allow visualization of the tumors.

Outcome Management

Surgical Management

Surgery is the treatment of choice for the client with primary hyperaldosteronism. A unilateral or bilateral adrenalectomy must be performed. A client undergoing a unilateral adrenalectomy may need temporary replacement of glucocorticoids. A client who requires a bilateral adrenalectomy needs permanent replacement (see Addison's Disease). Clients usually receive glucocorticoids preoperatively to prevent adrenal hypofunction. In two thirds of the cases, removal of the aldosterone-secreting tumor completely resolves the hypertension, hypokalemia, and hypernatremia. Most clients have normal BP readings by the third postoperative month.

Nursing Management of the Surgical Client

Help prepare the client for the diagnostic assessment so that the diagnosis of hyperaldosteronism can be achieved rapidly and the treatment performed before permanent damage occurs. Administer prescribed medications, and closely monitor the client for hypertension or renal damage. Preoperative and postoperative management is the same as that described for hypercortisolism.

Discharge planning must include client education about a low-sodium diet, medications, and manifestations of hypokalemia if the client is to be medically treated. The client should also understand the disease process and manifestations.

Medical Management

A client who cannot be treated surgically may receive spironolactone (Aldactone) to increase sodium excretion and to treat the hypertension and hypokalemia. Hypertension may take 4 to 8 weeks to correct. Potassium levels should be carefully monitored for the development of

BOX 44–1 Complications of Spironolactone Administration

Spironolactone is the drug of choice for primary hyperaldosteronism. It effectively lowers blood pressure and improves hypokalemia. The administration of spironolactone is complicated by:

1. Side effects such as gastrointestinal discomfort, impotence, decreased libido, gynecomastia, and menstrual irregularities.
2. Increase in the half-life of digoxin. The client's digoxin dosage may be reduced based on serum levels.
3. Concomitant therapy with salicylates. Salicylates increase renal tubular excretion of canrenone, the major active metabolite of spironolactone, thus decreasing its effectiveness.

hyperkalemia, especially if the client has been receiving potassium supplements or a high-potassium diet (Box 44–1). Amiloride is the drug of choice for clients who cannot tolerate spironolactone.

Nursing Management of the Medical Client

Assess the client's ability to manage the complex therapeutic regimen. Plan and implement a teaching program for self-care.

ADRENOMEDULLARY DISORDERS

Two important tumors occur in the adrenal medulla: *pheochromocytoma,* a tumor that causes hyperactivity of the gland, and *neuroblastoma,* a malignant tumor made up of cells resembling a neuroblast. For a complete description of neuroblastoma, an important tumor in children, consult a pediatric textbook.

PHEOCHROMOCYTOMA

A pheochromocytoma is a catecholamine-secreting tumor of the chromaffin cells of the sympathetic nervous system that is usually found in the adrenal medulla. Pheochromocytomas are rare. In autopsy series, the incidence of pheochromocytoma is 0.1% in clients with diastolic hypertension. The condition is equally common in women and men. Although the disease can occur at any age, it is most common in middle age and rarely occurs after age 60 years.

Etiology and Risk Factors

The cause of pheochromocytomas is unknown. In some cases, they appear to have a familial basis. They often occur together with neuroectodermal diseases and with multiple endocrine neoplasia type IIA. There are no known risk factors for pheochromocytoma.

Pathophysiology

Usually weighing less than 200 g, a pheochromocytoma is composed of chromaffin cells, so named (Latin *affinis, affinitas,* affinity) because these cells stain brownish yellow with chromic salts. In 85% to 95% of cases, pheochromocytomas arise within the adrenal medulla. Occasionally, however, they develop from the chromaffin tissues found in the sympathetic paraganglia. Pheochromocytomas are typically benign; fewer than 10% are malignant. Because of the excessive amounts of epinephrine and norepinephrine they secrete, they can produce severe manifestations and even death (Table 44–6).

Once a pheochromocytoma is diagnosed, certain risk

TABLE 44–6 THE EFFECTS OF EPINEPHRINE AND NOREPINEPHRINE

Epinephrine	Norepinephrine
CARDIOVASCULAR SYSTEM	
Constricts superficial blood vessels; in small doses, dilates muscle, brain, and coronary vessels, thus shunting blood supply to organs; essential for "fight or flight"	Constricts blood vessels (especially peripheral), causing increased peripheral resistance
Raises blood pressure	Raises blood pressure greatly
Increases cardiac output	Decreases cardiac output because of increased peripheral resistance
Increases pulse dramatically	Increases pulse moderately
Constricts spleen, shunting stored red blood cells into general circulation	
Increases coagulability of blood	
RESPIRATORY SYSTEM	
Increases rate and depth of respirations	
Dilates bronchi	
NERVOUS SYSTEM	
Stimulates central nervous system, increasing alertness and producing a feeling of fright, excitation, and impending doom	
Dilates pupils	Dilates pupils
Inhibits gastrointestinal tract	Inhibits gastrointestinal tract
METABOLISM	
Increases nonesterified fatty acid level of blood	Increases nonesterified fatty acid level of blood
Promotes conversion of glycogen to glucose	
Increases body metabolism	Increases body metabolism slightly

Data from DeGroot, L. (Ed.). (1995). *Endocrinology* (3rd ed.). Philadelphia: W. B. Saunders.

factors are known to influence catecholamine release. Catecholamine release occurs with various frequencies and intensities and is called a *paroxysm.* Risk factors that may stimulate a paroxysm include:

- Smoking
- Micturition (voiding reflex)
- Activities that displace abdominal organs, such as bending, exercising, straining, vigorous palpation of the abdomen, and pregnancy
- Certain drugs, such as histamines, anesthetics, atropine, opiates, fentanyl, steroids, and glucagon

Without early intervention, the client is at risk for cerebral hemorrhage and cardiac failure. If a pheochromocytoma is discovered early in its development, it can usually be removed surgically.

Clinical Manifestations

A client with pheochromocytoma may present with manifestations of diabetes mellitus (elevated blood glucose and glucosuria), hypertension (elevated BP, headaches), hyperthyroidism (increased metabolic rate, diaphoresis, agitation, rapid pulse, palpitations, emotional outbursts), and psychoneurosis (emotional instability).

Hypertension is the principal manifestation of pheochromocytoma and can be persistent, fluctuating, intermittent, or paroxysmal (rapid onset and abrupt cessation). Typically, the client has episodes of high BP accompanied by pounding headaches. Other manifestations of sympathetic overactivity include sweating, apprehension, palpitations, nausea, and vomiting. Excessive release of catecholamines also results in excessive conversion of glycogen into glucose in the liver. Consequently, hyperglycemia and glucosuria occur during attacks. Such manifestations can develop spontaneously or may be precipitated by emotional stress, physical exertion, or change in body position.

Acute attacks may be associated with profuse diaphoresis (perspiration), dilated pupils, and cold extremities. Severe hypertension can precipitate a cerebrovascular accident or sudden blindness.

Because pheochromocytoma is curable, early and accurate diagnosis is essential. Current methods of diagnosis include the following:

1. *History and physical examination.* The client may describe symptomatic attacks over weeks, months, or even years. The BP may change with exertion or emotional upset. In long-standing cases, complications of intractable hypertension (such as visual disturbances), manifestations of heart disease (dyspnea, edema), and manifestations of kidney damage (albuminuria, proteinuria, and increased blood urea nitrogen) can coexist.
2. *Chemical tests* of urinary catecholamines and their metabolites (metanephrines and vanillylmandelic acid [VMA]) and of plasma catecholamine concentrations. Assays of catecholamines are performed on single-voided urine specimens, 2- to 4-hour specimens, and 24-hour urine specimens. The normal range of urinary catecholamines is up to 14 mg per 100 ml of urine, with higher levels occurring in clients with pheochromocytoma. Assays of urinary VMA levels are performed only on 24-hour urine specimens. Advise the client to avoid tea, chocolate, vanilla, and all fruits for at least 2 days before urine collection begins, and remind the client not to take any medications for 2 to 3 days before the test. Normally, the amount of VMA is less than 7 mg in 24 hours. Urinary VMA levels increase in clients with pheochromocytoma. Plasma catecholamine concentrations are also determined.
3. *Direct assay* of catecholamines (epinephrine and norepinephrine) in the blood. The normal ranges of catecholamines in the blood are epinephrine, 0.02 to 0.2 mg/L, and norepinephrine, 0.1 to 0.5 mg/L.
4. *X-ray imaging.* Various radiographic techniques, such as CT and MRI, can help confirm and identify adrenomedullary tumor location.
5. *Nonspecific laboratory tests.* In the presence of pheochromocytoma, the basal metabolic rate increases, blood glucose rises to abnormal levels, and glycosuria can occur.

Outcome Management

Surgical Management

ADRENALECTOMY

INDICATIONS. The primary treatment of a pheochromocytoma is surgical removal of one or both adrenal glands, depending on whether the tumor is unilateral or bilateral. The procedure is the same as that described for Cushing's syndrome.

CONTRAINDICATIONS. The presence of complications of pheochromocytoma may make the client a poor surgical risk. Ideally, surgery is performed before complications develop. However, high BP and vascular complications may necessitate treatment before surgery can take place. Alpha-adrenergic blocking agents, such as phentolamine (Regitine), can be used in an IV bolus or IV drip for hypertensive crisis. Oral phenoxybenzamine (Dibenzyline) is used at least 7 days preoperatively to control BP, reduce manifestations, and eliminate paroxysms before surgical removal of the affected gland.

Complications associated with pheochromocytoma that may delay surgery include hypertensive retinopathy, hypertensive nephropathy, myocarditis, increased platelet aggregation, cerebrovascular accident, and heart failure. Death may result from myocardial infarction, cerebrovascular accident, dysrhythmias, irreversible shock, renal failure, or dissecting aortic aneurysm.

COMPLICATIONS. The surgical procedure for pheochromocytoma is not without danger. There are two serious hazards. First, excessive discharge of pressor hormones during induction of anesthesia or manipulation of the tumor can cause extreme rises in BP and cardiac dysrhythmias. Second, after resection of the tumor, BP can fall precipitously.

OUTCOMES. Surgical removal of the pheochromocytoma can be curative in most cases, if the growth is discovered before cardiovascular damage becomes permanent. Some clients may receive less medication at discharge after surgery. Lifelong steroid replacement must be initiated after a bilateral adrenalectomy.

Nursing Management of the Surgical Client

Preoperative Care

Assessment

Assess and control the client's BP preoperatively. Closely monitor the client for the development of stressful episodes before treatment has begun. Evaluate the client's neurologic status in case the client has a stroke because of the extremely elevated BP.

Diagnosis, Outcomes, Interventions

Risk for Injury. The client with a pheochromocytoma is at great risk for injury preoperatively. Write the nursing diagnosis *Risk for Injury related to excessive release of epinephrine and norepinephrine preoperatively.*

Outcomes. Injury will not occur or will be detected early, as evidenced by absence of hypertensive episodes and cardiovascular or cerebral damage.

Interventions. During the preoperative phase, the desired outcome of treatment is preventing attacks of acute paroxysmal hypertension, thereby lowering the risk of further damage to the cardiovascular system. Important nursing interventions include (1) promoting rest and relief from stress; (2) administering prescribed sedatives; (3) providing a diet high in vitamins, minerals, and calories; (4) prohibiting beverages containing caffeine, such as coffee, tea, and colas; and (5) monitoring vital signs. In most cases, the physician prescribes an alpha-adrenergic blocking agent, such as phenoxybenzamine.

Postoperative Care

Assessment

The first 24 to 48 hours after surgery is a critical period demanding vigilant nursing assessment. After surgery, the client should be closely monitored for adrenal insufficiency, hypotension, hemorrhage, and shock. Urine output and BP are assessed hourly.

Diagnosis, Outcomes, Interventions

Risk for Injury. The client is at increased risk for such problems as hypotension postoperatively. Write the nursing diagnosis as *Risk for Injury related to postoperative hypotension, hemorrhage, and shock.*

Outcomes. Injury will not occur or will be detected early, as evidenced by a normotensive state and an absence of hemorrhage, shock, or addisonian crisis.

Interventions

Monitor and Prevent Shock. During the immediate postoperative period, observe for manifestations of shock and hemorrhage. After removal of the tumor, profound shock can develop as catecholamine levels drop. Hypotension can persist for 24 to 48 hours. Hemorrhage can occur because of the high vascularity of the adrenal glands. To prevent postoperative shock, do the following:

1. Give IV fluids as prescribed, such as blood, plasma, dextran, or glucose in water to maintain blood volume.
2. Administer IV pressors as prescribed at a rate sufficient to maintain BP within a safe range. Check BP as often as necessary to titrate the medication.
3. Carefully measure hourly urinary output. If the client voids less than ½ ml/kg/hr, notify the physician. Oliguria can signify impending shock and consequent renal shutdown.
4. Assess the client for manifestations of hemorrhage. Check the dressing every half-hour for bloody drainage. If the client is bleeding internally, an abdominal hematoma can develop, resulting in paralytic ileus or nonmechanical bowel obstruction (see Chapter 33). Manifestations of paralytic ileus include abdominal pain, distention, severe nausea, vomiting, and diminished or absent bowel sounds.
5. If cortical tissue has been resected during surgery, assess the client closely for manifestations of adrenal insufficiency (see Addisonian Crisis). If both adrenal glands have been removed, the client must receive cortisol replacement for life.

Pain. Postoperatively, the client must be monitored for *Pain related to surgery, headache, and other manifestations of pheochromocytoma resulting in verbal reports of pain and guarding behaviors.*

Outcomes. The client will not have pain, as evidenced by the client's statements, normotensive state, and an absence of pained expressions.

Interventions. When administering medication for incisional pain, monitor BP frequently. Although narcotics, particularly meperidine, produce hypotension as a side effect, withholding pain medication can also lead to hypotension (or even hypertension) and severe pain. It is important to control the pain so that the client's level of stress decreases.

Evaluation

It is expected that the client will have no complications postoperatively or that complications that occur will be managed successfully so that the client is discharged within 4 to 5 days postoperatively. Self-care outcomes are evaluated by the client's ability to manage steroid replacement after surgery. Although side effects of steroids cannot be avoided, there are ways to minimize them, and the client's ability to control these and avoid complications can be evaluated.

Self-Care

After a bilateral adrenalectomy, the client must learn self-care measures. When the critical postoperative period is over, most clients experience an uneventful convalescence. A client who will be self-administering corticosteroids needs instruction concerning the administration and side effects (see Addison's Disease).

Modification for Elderly Clients

Damage related to hypertensive episodes associated with the pheochromocytoma tends to affect older clients, whose cardiovascular and cerebrovascular systems may be weak and thus susceptible to damage by elevated BP.

ANTERIOR PITUITARY DISORDERS

Disorders of the pituitary gland occur most frequently in the anterior lobe (Table 44–7; see also Fig. 44–2). Major causes of pituitary disease include functioning tumors, nonfunctioning tumors, pituitary infarction, genetic disor-

TABLE 44–7 PITUITARY HORMONES

Name	Releasing Factor	Target Cells	Response	Increased Level	Decreased Level
ANTERIOR PITUITARY					
GH	GHRH	Bone, muscle	Stimulates growth; promotes active transport of amino acids into cell and influences lipid, CHO, and Ca^{2+} metabolism	Child: gigantism (before epiphyseal closure); child grows very tall Adult: acromegaly (after epiphyseal closure); bones increase in thickness; increase in soft tissue growth	Child: dwarfism Adult: lethargy, increased weight, loss of reproductive function, premature aging
ACTH	CRH	Adrenal cortex	Stimulates adrenal gland secretion of mineralocorticoids and glucocorticoids	Cushing's disease: increased amounts of cortisol and aldosterone	Addison's disease: decreased cortisol and aldosterone, increased MSH
TSH	TRH	Thyroid	Stimulates thyroid to increase secretion of thyroxine (controls rate of most chemical reactions in body)	Goiter; increased BMR; decreased weight; increased cardiac output, HR, and BP; increased cerebration; fine muscle tremors	Reduced thyroid activity; decreased BMR; increased weight; decreased cardiac output, HR, and BP; decreased cerebration; somnolence
Prolactin		Breast	Stimulates breast to lactate	Amenorrhea	Too little milk
FSH	LHRH	Ovaries, testes	Stimulates growth of ovaries and sperm		Late puberty
LH	LHRH	Ovaries, testes	Stimulates growth of follicles and increased secretion of estrogen and progesterone; increases testosterone secretion in the male	Excess testosterone, menstrual cycle disturbance	Amenorrhea; diminished progesterone and testosterone
POSTERIOR PITUITARY					
Oxytocin	Labor, sucking	Uterus, breasts	Stimulates uterus to contract at childbirth; stimulates lactation	Precipitates childbirth, excess milk	Prolonged childbirth, diminished milk
ADH (vasopressin)	Dehydration	Arterioles, distal renal tubule	Vasoconstricts arterioles to increase arterial pressure; increases water reabsorption in distal tubules, stimulates smooth muscle of gastrointestinal tract	Increased BP, decreased urinary output, edema	Diabetes insipidus, dilute urine, increased urinary volume

ACTH, adrenocorticotropic hormone; ADH, antidiuretic hormone; BP, blood pressure; BMR, basal metabolic rate; CHO, carbohydrate; CRH, corticotropin-releasing hormone; FSH, follicle-stimulating hormone; GH, growth hormone; GHRH, growth hormone–releasing hormone; HR, heart rate; LH, luteinizing hormone; LHRH, luteinizing hormone–releasing hormone; MSH, melanocyte-stimulating hormone; TRH, thyrotropin-releasing hormone; TSH, thyroid-stimulating hormone.

Data from DeGroot, L. (Ed.). (1995). *Endocrinology* (3rd ed.). Philadelphia: W. B. Saunders.

ders, and trauma. The three principal pathologic consequences of pituitary disorders are (1) hyperpituitarism, (2) hypopituitarism, and (3) local compression of brain tissue by expanding tumor masses.

HYPERPITUITARISM AND HYPERPROLACTINEMIA

Etiology and Risk Factors

Hyperpituitarism is defined as oversecretion of one or more of the hormones secreted by the pituitary gland. It is caused primarily by a hormone-secreting pituitary tumor, typically a benign adenoma. Syndromes associated with hyperpituitarism are Cushing's syndrome, acromegaly, amenorrhea, galactorrhea, hyperthyroidism, and, rarely, hypergonadism in the male.

Pathophysiology

Prolactin and growth hormone are the hormones most commonly overproduced by adenomas. They lead to hyperprolactinemia and acromegaly (Fig. 44–5), respectively. Increased amounts of growth hormone lead to rapid growth of all body tissues. This increased growth leads to gigantism (Fig. 44–6) if it occurs before closure of the epiphysis and acromegaly if it occurs after epiphyseal closure.

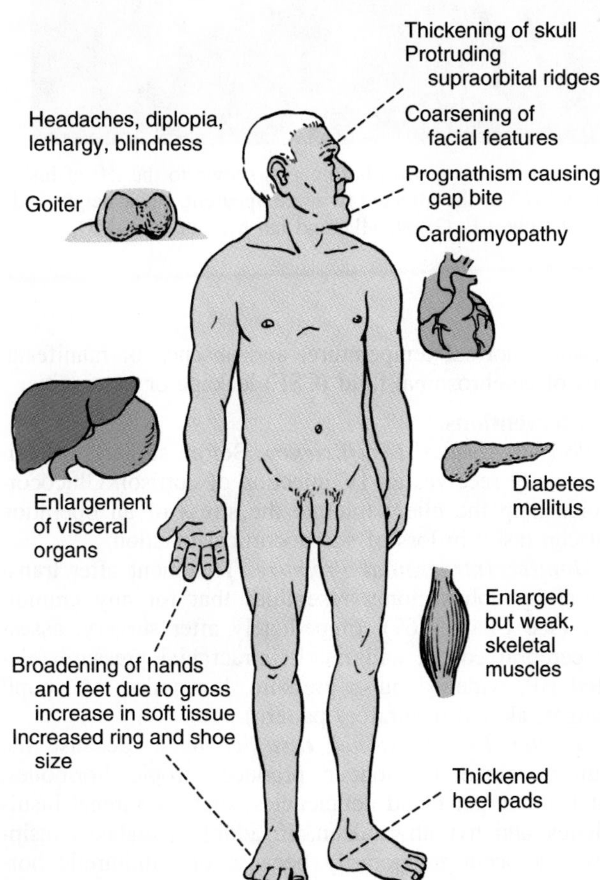

FIGURE 44–5 Assessment data for acromegaly.

Clinical Manifestations

Pituitary tumors produce both systemic and local effects. Systemic effects include excessive or abnormal growth patterns related to overproduction of growth hormone, abnormal milk secretion (galactorrhea), and overstimulation of one or more of the target glands, resulting in release of excessive thyroid, sex, or adrenocortical hormones.

Locally, pituitary tumors produce manifestations because the bony cranium that houses the tumor cannot expand to accommodate a growing mass. Local manifestations include visual field abnormalities resulting from pressure on the optic chiasm, headaches, and somnolence. See Table 44–8 for additional information related to hyperprolactinemia and acromegaly.

Outcome Management

Surgical Management

A client with a pituitary tumor must have the tumor resected. A variety of approaches can be used to remove a pituitary tumor. Usually, a transsphenoidal hypophysectomy is performed (see Chapter 69).

Nursing Management of the Surgical Client

ASSESSMENT

Most clients are frightened by the prospect of having the pituitary gland removed. Provide the client and significant others with emotional support and comfort throughout the preoperative period.

The initial manifestations are vague; therefore, the client may have seen many physicians and may have had multiple examinations and tests while seeking a diagnosis. The client and family may be fearful, skeptical, or relieved with the final diagnosis of pituitary tumor. Assess the client's reaction to the diagnosis, expectations for the surgery, educational needs related to the diagnosis and treatment plan, and available support network after discharge.

Physical assessment includes baseline vital signs and weight as well as neurologic assessment. The client should also have a preoperative eye examination by an ophthalmologist. These findings are essential to establish a baseline for postoperative comparison. To perform the neurologic assessment, check the following:

- Pupil equality and reactivity to light
- Handgrip for strength, equality, and ability to release on command
- Level of consciousness
- Orientation to time, place, person, and location
- Appropriate response to stimuli
- Visual acuity and visual fields

DIAGNOSIS, OUTCOMES, INTERVENTIONS

Knowledge Deficit. Preoperatively, the client must to be taught about the surgery and its implications. A typical nursing diagnosis would be *Knowledge Deficit: Surgery and possible outcomes related to lack of instruction resulting in anxiety, misinformation, and questions.*

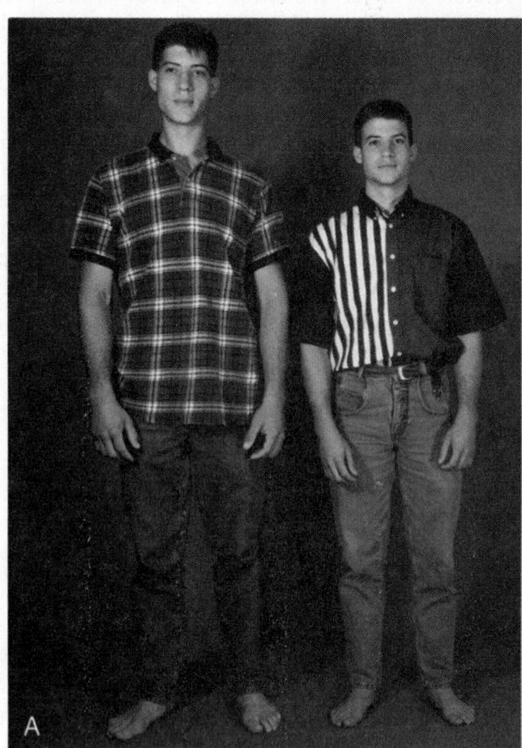

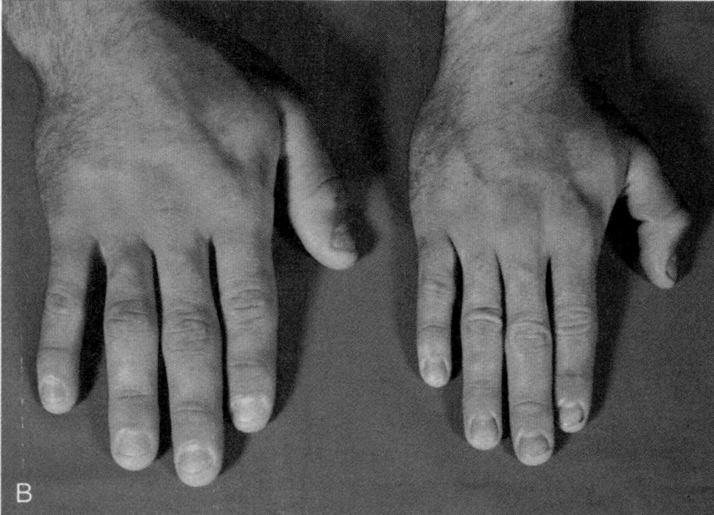

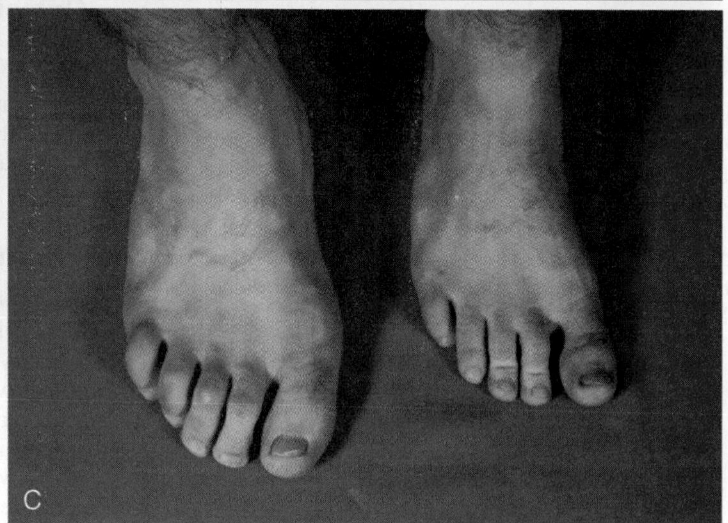

FIGURE 44–6 Primary gigantism. *A,* a 22-year-old man with gigantism due to excess growth hormone is shown to the left of his identical twin. The increased height (*A*), enlarged hand (*B*), and enlarged foot (*C*) of the affected twin are apparent. Their height and features began to diverge at the age of approximately 13 years. (Courtesy of Robert F. Gagel, MD, and Ian McCutcheon, MD, University of Texas M.D. Anderson Cancer Center, Houston, TX.)

Outcomes. The client will understand the planned surgery and possible outcomes as evidenced by his or her statements, questions, and ability to describe the procedure and outcomes.

Interventions. Explain the surgery to the client in detail, along with potential outcomes of surgical treatment. Use drawings of the brain to explain the transsphenoidal approach. Prepare the client for the presence of an indwelling urinary catheter, IV lines, and any other lines or monitors that may be needed after surgery. Tell the client that vital signs will be monitored closely after surgery. Preoperative preparation also includes coaching the client in deep-breathing exercises and assisting in keeping records of intake and output.

Risk for Injury. A typical postoperative nursing diagnosis would be *Risk for Injury related to postoperative complications.*

Outcomes. Injury will not result from surgery as evidenced by absence of addisonian crisis, balanced intake and output, no manifestations of increased intracranial pressure, normal temperature, and absence of manifestations of cerebrospinal fluid (CSF) leakage or meningitis.

Interventions

Prevent Adrenal Insufficiency. Before surgery, the client usually receives an IV injection of cortisol. Glucocorticoids help the client tolerate the stress of an operation that can result in loss of adrenocortical function.

Monitor Intracranial Pressure. Treatment after transfrontal hypophysectomy resembles that for any craniotomy (see Chapter 69). Immediately after surgery, assess for cerebral edema and rising intracranial pressure (elevated BP, widened pulse pressure, low pulse rate, pupil changes, altered respiratory pattern).

Monitor for Hormonal Insufficiencies. Because the pituitary gland no longer produces tropic hormones, watch for target gland deficiencies, such as adrenal insufficiency and hypothyroidism. In addition, diabetes insipidus can occur temporarily because of antidiuretic hormone (ADH, vasopressin) deficiency, as outlined in the accompanying Critical Monitoring feature. This deficiency

TABLE 44–8 **HYPERPROLACTINEMIA AND ACROMEGALY IN HYPERPITUITARISM**

	Hyperprolactinemia	Acromegaly
Hormone secreted	Excessive prolactin (PRL) causes prolactinoma	Excessive growth hormone (GH)
Risk factors	Hyperprolactinemia; estrogen therapy; oral contraceptive use; pregnancy may increase tumor size and dysfunction	None
Etiology	Pregnancy; hypothalamic-pituitary disorders; hypothyroidism; drug ingestion (estrogen or oral contraception)	Anterior pituitary adenoma; abnormal hypothalamic function (rare)
Pathophysiology	PRL-producing tumors deliver excess PRL systemically	GH-producing adenomas deliver excess GH systemically, leading to rapid growth in other body tissues (with exception of the CNS) causing organomegaly; increase in tumor size within confined space can result in destruction of entire pituitary and cause hypopituitarism
Clinical manifestations related to hormone oversecretion	Abnormal lactation (galactorrhea) in nonlactating breast; amenorrhea; decreased vaginal lubrication; decreased libido in men; impotence; depression; anxiety; headache; visual loss	Local overgrowth of bone: skull and mandible; soft tissue overgrowth; lethargy; weight gain; paresthesias; glucose intolerance; coarse facial features; irregular or absent menses; enlargement of hands and feet over 1–10 yr; depression; headache; visual field impairment; osteoarthritis; paresthesias; impotence
Complications related to tumor growth	Headaches; visual disturbances affecting cranial nerves III, IV, VI; hypopituitarism; infertility; decreased bone growth	Hypopituitarism; neoplasms of gastrointestinal tract; increased mortality secondary to cardiovascular atherosclerosis, cerebral atherosclerosis, congestive heart failure, respiratory disease, hypertension, diabetes mellitus
Pharmacologic intervention	Bromocriptine is treatment of choice; bromocriptine can reduce PRL levels in 90% of clients; adverse reactions may contribute to noncompliance: nausea, headaches, dizziness, nasal stuffiness, hypotension, depression	Somatostatin analog octreotide is very effective in reducing GH levels; pharmacologic treatment may cause cholelithiasis; bromocriptine is effective in 60%–80% of clients
Surgical intervention	Transsphenoidal microsurgery; complications: residual tissue may produce elevated hormone levels, visual loss, diabetes insipidus, postoperative infection	Transsphenoidal microsurgery is treatment of choice; complications: same as in hyperprolactinemia
Radiation treatment	May decrease adenoma, but local complications are common because of tissue scarring and impairment of anterior pituitary function (hypopituitarism)	Produces slower decline of GH levels, implying higher morbidity related to atherosclerotic disease, respiratory disease, hypertension, diabetes mellitus, and gastrointestinal cancer; hypopituitarism
Diagnosis	Measurement of GH, ACTH, FSH, LH, PRL, testosterone, gonadotropins; thyroid function tests (T_3, T_4, FT_4, TSH); liver function tests (LDH, CPK, AST, alkaline phosphatase), coagulation studies; kidney function tests (serum creatinine, BUN, 24-hr urine collection for protein, creatinine clearance, GFR); urinalysis; pregnancy testing; CT or MRI for pituitary adenoma localization	Radioimmunoassay or enzyme-linked immunosorbent assay for GH level; serum GH level; insulin-like growth factor; CT scan or MRI for pituitary edema localization; oral GTT may demonstrate hyperglycemia; usually, GTT suppresses normal GH release 1–2 hr after ingestion, but in acromegaly the GH level remains elevated

ACTH, adrenocorticotropic hormone; AST, aspartate aminotransferase; BUN, blood urea nitrogen; CNS, central nervous system; CPK, creatine phosphokinase; CT, computed tomography; FSH, follicle-stimulating hormone; FT_4, free thyroxine; GFR, glomerular filtration rate, GH, growth hormone; GTT, glucose tolerance test; LDH, lactate dehydrogenase; LH, luteinizing hormone; MRI, magnetic resonance imaging; PRL, prolactin; TSH, thyroid-stimulating hormone; T_3, triiodothyronine; T_4, thyroxine.

is related to surgical manipulation. Maintain strict documentation of intake and output. Notify the physician if urine output is above 200 ml/hr with a specific gravity below 1.005.

Monitor for Meningitis. Assess the client carefully for meningitis, a potential complication of surgery. Report any temperature elevation, severe headache, irritability, or nuchal rigidity.

Provide Oral Hygiene. The client who has undergone transsphenoidal hypophysectomy requires frequent oral hygiene with a gauze sponge; the lips should be lubricated with petroleum jelly. The client should not brush the teeth for 2 weeks after surgery.

Monitor for CSF Drainage. The nasal packing is usually removed in 2 to 5 days. After its removal, observe the client for rhinorrhea, which can indicate a CSF leak.

CRITICAL MONITORING

Does Your Client Have an Antidiuretic Hormone (ADH) Imbalance?

	Diabetes Insipidus	Syndrome of Inappropriate Secretion of Antidiuretic Hormone
ADH	↓	↑
Urine output	↑	↓
Urine osmolality	↓	↑
Urine specific gravity	↓	Value insignificant
Serum Na^+	↑	↓
Urine Na^+	↓	↑
Plasma osmolality	↑	↓
Daily weights	↓	Sudden ↑ (without edema)
Mentation changes	Related to electrolyte imbalance and hypotension	Related to degree of hyponatremia

Have the client report frequent postnasal drainage. Collect any serous drainage, and test it for the presence of CSF (see Chapter 67) or send it to the laboratory for analysis. It is possible for the muscle or fat graft to dislodge, causing a CSF leak. Instruct the client to avoid sneezing, coughing, and bending over from the waist to avoid disrupting the graft.

EVALUATION

Appropriate outcomes after a hypophysectomy include the absence of postoperative complications and the client's ability to manage lifetime hormone replacement. If complications occur, appropriate outcomes are that these are controlled without permanent problems.

Self-Care

After a hypophysectomy, the client must take replacement hormones for life. Instruct the client to avoid gastric irritation by taking cortisone with milk, food, or an antacid. Advise the client to notify the physician about gastritis, tarry stools, or frank blood in the stools. Some clients may also require thyroid or sex hormone replacement. In addition, some need vasopressin replacement to treat *diabetes insipidus.* As a result of deficient ADH, clients may experience polyuria (large urine output) and low urine specific gravity readings. Diabetes insipidus is usually transient after surgery but can persist, indicating the need for chronic hormone replacement.

SEXUAL DISTURBANCES

Excess secretion of gonadotropic hormones, such as luteinizing hormone (LH) and follicle-stimulating hormone (FSH), from pituitary tumors can produce sexual precocity in children. Excess prolactin secretion can cause amenorrhea or galactorrhea (excessive flow of milk) in women. Physicians consider surgical removal the treatment of choice for radiologically demonstrable tumors.

Clients with increased prolactin secretion and no radiologic or neurologic evidence of a pituitary tumor often respond to bromocriptine, an ergot-like compound. Clients with prolactinomas can be successfully treated with bromocriptine. A dopamine agonist, bromocriptine inhibits prolactin secretion. Surgery is no longer the treatment of choice in most cases.

HYPOPITUITARISM

In contrast to hyperpituitarism, hypopituitarism is a deficiency of one or more of the hormones produced by the anterior lobe of the pituitary. When both the anterior and posterior lobes fail to secrete hormones, the condition is called *panhypopituitarism.* Hypopituitarism and panhypopituitarism are rare disorders.

Etiology and Risk Factors

The nine most important causes of hypopituitarism are known as the "nine Is":

- Invasion (most common)—pituitary tumors, central nervous system tumors, carotid aneurysm
- Infarction—postpartum necrosis (Sheehan's syndrome), pituitary apoplexy
- Infiltration—sarcoidosis, hemochromatosis
- Injury—head trauma, child abuse
- Immunologic—lymphocytic hypophysitis
- Iatrogenic—surgery, radiation therapy
- Infectious—mycoses, tuberculosis, syphilis
- Idiopathic—familial
- Isolated—deficiency of an anterior pituitary hormone, such as growth hormone, LH, FSH, thyroid-stimulating hormone (TSH), ACTH–lipotropic pituitary hormone (ACTH-LPH), or prolactin

Clinical Manifestations

The pituitary gland has enormous functional reserve; therefore, manifestations of hypopituitarism usually do not appear until 75% of the pituitary has been obliterated by tumor or thrombosis. Manifestations depend on age of onset as well as the hormones that are deficient. The onset of hypopituitarism is usually gradual. The classic course of progressive hypopituitarism is an initial loss of growth hormone and gonadotropin, followed by deficiencies of TSH, then ACTH, and finally prolactin.

Specific disorders resulting from pituitary hyposecretion include:

- *Short stature.* Severely stunted growth results from either a congenital lack of growth hormone or the development of a space-occupying intracranial tumor, meningitis, or brain injury during early childhood.
- *Sexual and reproductive disorders.* Deficiencies of the gonadotropins (LH and FSH) can produce sterility, diminished sex drive, and decreased secondary sex characteristics. Decreased FSH and LH lead to infertility and amenorrhea, diminished spermatogenesis, and testicular atrophy.
- *Hypothyroidism.* Because the synthesis of thyroid hormone depends on TSH, therapeutic ablation or pathologic destruction of the pituitary gland causes hypothyroidism unless the client receives thyroid hormone (see Chapter 43).
- *Secondary adrenocortical insufficiency.* Adrenal insufficiency can follow diminished synthesis of ACTH by the pituitary gland, which, in turn, causes diminished secretion of adrenocortical hormones by the adrenal cortex (see Fig. 44–2).
- *Prolactin deficiency.* This deficiency is indicated by absence of lactation in the postpartum woman.

Diagnosis of growth hormone deficiency rests on the inability of stimulating agents—such as levodopa, arginine, and insulin—to increase plasma growth hormone levels. ACTH levels can be measured to diagnose secondary adrenal insufficiency. Cortisol levels are low in both primary and secondary hypothyroidism; however, when it is a primary deficiency, ACTH levels are high. In a client with secondary hypopituitarism, ACTH levels are low. Low serum thyroid hormone levels, together with low serum TSH levels, establish the diagnosis of hypothyroidism. Sexual and reproductive disorders are diagnosed by low levels of sex steroids and low levels of plasma FSH and LH. Skull x-ray studies may reveal enlargement of the sella turcica, erosion of the sphenoid bone, or calcification of a suprasellar mass. CT or MRI may provide an enhanced view of an x-ray finding.

Outcome Management

Treatment of hypopituitarism involves removal, if possible, of the causative factor (such as a tumor) and permanent replacement of the hormones secreted by the target organs.

Medical Management

Injections of human growth hormone successfully treat growth hormone deficiency. Previously, human growth hormone was scarce and available for only a few clients. Now it is produced by recombinant deoxyribonucleic acid (DNA) technology and is readily available. Medications prescribed to replace hormones include corticosteroids to correct secondary adrenocortical insufficiency, thyroid hormone to treat myxedema, and sex hormones to correct hypogonadism.

Assessment of the client with hypopituitarism focuses on target organs that depend on pituitary secretions (see specific disorders such as Addison's disease and hypothyroidism). Nursing interventions are also directed at problems resulting from deficiency at the target organ. See the appropriate secretions for specific interventions.

Posterior Lobe (Neurohypophyseal) Disorders

Unlike the adenohypophysis, the neurohypophysis is rarely destroyed by disease. Even if the posterior lobe becomes damaged or is surgically destroyed with the anterior lobe, hormonal deficiencies usually do not develop because the hypothalamus continues to synthesize oxytocin and ADH. If the hypothalamus suffers damage, however, deficiencies of oxytocin and ADH develop even if the neurohypophysis is healthy and intact.

The major disorder of the posterior lobe is ADH deficiency, also known as diabetes insipidus (Fig. 44–7). Excessive ADH causes a condition called the *syndrome of inappropriate antidiuretic hormone* (SIADH), which can occur with lung cancer, head injuries, cranial surgery, pituitary tumors, encephalitis, poliomyelitis, and myxedema. Table 44–9 compares diabetes insipidus and SIADH.

Gonadal Disorders

Testicular dysfunction can be primary, a disorder of testicular function, or secondary to a disorder of hypothalamic-pituitary function. Primary testis dysfunction can involve the seminiferous tubules (germ cells or Sertoli's cells), Leydig's cells, or both. Germ cell abnormalities cause infertility by disrupting spermatogenesis. Secondary sexual development and virilization are normal because testosterone production is not interrupted. When Leydig cell function is impaired, testosterone production falls, and virilization is impaired.

Causes of primary hypogonadism include genetic defects, malnutrition, trauma, infection, renal failure, radiation, chemotherapy, and environmental toxins (such as lead or alcohol). The cause, however, is usually unknown. Klinefelter's syndrome, caused by a chromosomal anomaly with a 47,XXY chromosome constitution, is an example of a genetic disorder causing primary testicular failure.

Secondary testicular dysfunction is frequently referred to as *hypogonadotropic hypogonadism* and results from inadequate secretion of gonadotropins. This complication leads to infertility and hypoandrogenism. The extent of LH and FSH deficiency and the age of onset determine clinical manifestations. Prepubertal hypogonadism leads to eunuchoid body proportions (resulting from deficiency in male hormones), small testes, and lack of virilization.

Causes of secondary hypogonadism include hypothalamic or pituitary tumors, trauma, degenerative lesions, and radiation. Kallmann's syndrome, involving a deficiency of gonadotropin-releasing hormone (GRH) production by the hypothalamus, is an example of congenital secondary testicular dysfunction. People with Kallmann's syndrome do not mature normally because of gonadotro-

TABLE 44–9 COMPARISON OF DIABETES INSIPIDUS AND SYNDROME OF INAPPROPRIATE SECRETION OF ANTIDIURETIC HORMONE

	Diabetes Insipidus (DI)	Syndrome of Inappropriate Secretion of Antidiuretic Hormone (SIADH)
Definition	A deficiency of antidiuretic hormone (ADH, vasopressin) results in inability to conserve water	Excessive amounts of ADH secreted from posterior pituitary and other ectopic sources
Incidence	Unknown; DI idiopathic in about 30% of all clients with DI; tumors can be related to 25% of DI cases; head injury accounts for 16%; cranial surgery for 20% of DI cases	Approximately 80% of clients with small cell carcinoma have evidence of impaired ability to excrete water secondary to ectopic production of vasopressin
Etiology	Central CI or neurogenic DI: CNS interruption of anatomic integrity of posterior pituitary; localized or generalized edema from head trauma, vascular lesions, centrally acting drugs, or CNS infections may also cause central DI; ADH synthesis or release is affected; may be transient or permanent Complete DI occurs when there is disruption of hypophyseal tract and a complete absence of ADH Nephrogenic DI: rare hereditary disorder; acquired structural or functional change in kidney occurs; ADH produced normally, but distal and collecting tubules cannot respond Idiopathic DI	Ectopic production of vasopressin by malignancy is most common cause (degree of vasopressin impairment is relative to extent of malignant disease); see Risk factors below
Risk factors	Head injury, neurosurgery, hypothalamic tumors, pituitary tumors, brain infections or inflammation; drugs that inhibit vasopressin release: ethanol, glucocorticoids, adrenergic agents, phenytoin, narcotic antagonists, lithium	Vasopressin overuse (from DI); malignant conditions that may contain ectopic sources of vasopressin-like hormone: bronchogenic carcinoma; lymphoma of duodenum, brain, bladder; pancreatic cancer; prostatic cancer; increased intracranial pressure secondary to infectious processes or brain trauma; infectious processes—viral or bacterial pneumonia; drugs that may stimulate vasopressin release: vincristine, cyclophosphamide, thiazides, phenothiazides, carbamazepine, vinblastine, cisplatin, oxytocin; endocrine disorders: adrenal insufficiency, myxedema, anterior pituitary insufficiency; analgesics; vomiting
Pathophysiology: normally ADH increases kidneys' permeability to water to promote water reabsorption and decrease urine output; ADH is normally released in response to: ↑ serum osmolality and ↓ extracellular volume	With ADH deficiency: permeability of water is diminished resulting in excretion of large volumes of hypotonic fluid Three patterns may develop: (1) transient DI—abrupt onset within first few days after neurosurgery, resolves within several days; (2) permanent DI (prolonged DI)—abrupt and early onset, persists for several weeks or forever, usually occurs after damage to hypothalamus or neurohypophyseal stalk; (3) triphasic DI—immediate postinjury increase in urine volume with decrease in urine osmolality lasting 4–5 days; interphase occurs over next 5–7 days when urine volume decreases to normal and is followed by a permanent phase of polyuria	Key features of ADH excess: (1) water retention, (2) hyponatremia, (3) hypo-osmolality; a continual release of ADH causes water retention from renal tubules and collecting ducts; extracellular fluid volume increases with dilutional hyponatremia; hyponatremia suppresses renin and aldosterone secretions causing a decrease in proximal tubule reabsorption of Na^+
Physical examination	Integumentary: dry, cool skin, dry mucous membranes Cardiovascular: tachycardia Physical manifestations related to specific electrolyte imbalance	Physical manifestations related to hyponatremia: decreased deep tendon reflexes, fatigue, headache, anorexia, nausea, decreased mental status, seizures, coma Physical manifestations related to fluid volume excess: weight gain without edema, jugular venous distention, tachycardia, tachypnea, rales

TABLE 44–9 **COMPARISON OF DIABETES INSIPIDUS AND SYNDROME OF INAPPROPRIATE SECRETION OF ANTIDIURETIC HORMONE** *Continued*

	Diabetes Insipidus (DI)	Syndrome of Inappropriate Secretion of Antidiuretic Hormone (SIADH)
Clinical manifestations	Genitourinary: polyuria—a few liters to 18 L/day; clear urine; urinary frequency; nocturia Gastrointestinal: weight loss; polydipsia (if thirst mechanism intact) Integumentary: dry skin and mucous membranes Neurologic: mentation changes as electrolyte imbalance and hypotension worsen	Related to degree of hyponatremia: confusion, lethargy, irritability, seizures, coma Gastrointestinal: decreased motility with anorexia, nausea, vomiting; abrupt weight gain *without edema* of 5%–10%
Complications	Electrolyte imbalance; hypovolemia; hypotension; shock	Seizures; coma; permanent brain damage; disease processes already in progress may be complicated
Diagnosis	Urine: output—a few liters to 18 L/day; specific gravity 1.005; osmolality <200 mOsm/kg H_2O Plasma osmolality ↑ secondary to hypovolemia and dehydration Serum Na^+ ↑ secondary to hypovolemia and dehydration Serum osmolality >290 mOsm/kg H_2O Serum Na^+ ↓ secondary to volume depletion Water deprivation study: positive results Hypertonic saline test: positive for DI if there is little or no ↑ in plasma ADH levels	Serum Na^+ ↓; urine Na^+ ↑; blood urea nitrogen ↑; serum osmolality ↓; urine osmolality ↑; absence of hypotension, hypovolemia, or edematous states; water load test: positive for SIADH, abnormal water excretion; serum Na^+ remains ↓; serum osmolality remains ↓; urine osmolality remains ↑
Surgical management	Hypophysectomy to remove posterior pituitary tumor	None
Medical management	IV fluids; ADH replacement with DDAVP (desmopressin) IV, SQ, or intranasal; nasal solution bid is drug of choice; onset of action is 1 hr, 6–24 hr duration; Pitressin tannate in oil is given IM; aqueous Pitressin is used for acute, transient form of DI	Hypertonic IV fluids to correct hyponatremia; sodium restriction; diuretics to correct low plasma osmolality; monitor urine electrolyte loss; replace electrolyte loss; demeclocycline to facilitate free water clearance; treat the underlying cause
Nursing management	1. Know which clients are at risk 2. Monitor intake and output 3. Monitor for excessive thirst or urination 4. Assess serum and urine values: ↓ specific gravity, ↓ urine osmolality, ↑ serum osmolality, are early indicators of DI 5. Observe effects of DI on concurrent medical and surgical disorders 6. Client and family teaching	1. Know which clients are at risk 2. Monitor appropriate urine and serum laboratory tests 3. Assess for manifestations of hyponatremia by evaluating neurologic status 4. Monitor daily weights and intake and output 5. Observe for changes in concurrent disorders 6. Administer demeclocycline as ordered to interfere with ADH action; monitor for possible nephrotoxicity 7. Monitor for hypernatremia with fluid overcorrection 8. Client and family teaching
Prognosis	Excellent if there is compliance with vasopressin therapy	Dependent on cause and sodium level and serum osmolality; poor for client with bronchogenic carcinoma; seizures and coma contribute to chronic brain dysfunction

pin deficiency. Midline defects, such as cleft lip or palate, color blindness, anosmia, and ataxia, are common findings in these people.

CONCLUSIONS

Adrenal, pituitary, and gonadal disorders are not common but are extremely complex and diverse. Obtaining a thorough understanding of the adrenal, pituitary, and gonadal anatomy and physiology can help you care for clients with these disorders. Most of these conditions (such as hypopituitarism) are acute and affect many body systems, whereas others become chronic and lead to a wide variety of other problems, such as Addison's disease. Teaching is vital to the care of these clients; understand these conditions so that appropriate teaching plans can be initiated.

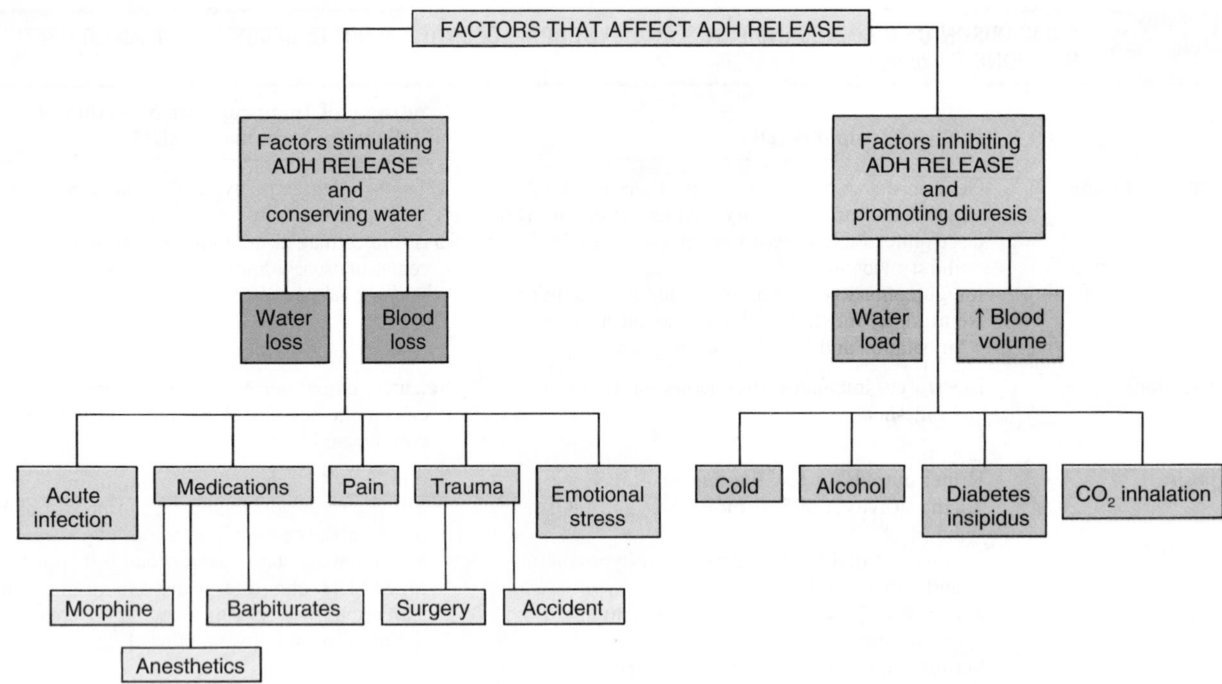

FIGURE 44–7 Factors that stimulate and inhibit the release of antidiuretic hormone (ADH). CO_2, carbon dioxide.

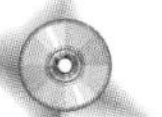

THINKING CRITICALLY

1. **The client is a woman with a 9-year history of Addison's disease. Normally, she takes her prescribed doses of a glucocorticoid (dexamethasone [Decadron]) and a mineralocorticoid (fludrocortisone [Florinef]) without fail. She is 29 years old and is otherwise in good health. The client stayed home from work today because she began to experience nausea, vomiting, diarrhea, and fever with diaphoresis. Because of the nausea and vomiting, she did not take her medications. When her husband returned home at 5:30 PM, he found her unconscious. What events led to the client's unconsciousness? How might missing her medications have affected the client?**

Factors to Consider. What acute disorder do the nausea, vomiting, diarrhea, and fever suggest? How might they affect a person with Addison's disease?

2. **A 50-year-old woman has been taking glucocorticoids for 10 years for asthma. She is admitted to the hospital for sudden onset of severe low back pain. What factors may have contributed to her back pain?**

Factors to Consider. What are the potential long-term effects of oral glucocorticoid therapy? What are their manifestations?

3. **A 23-year-old man is admitted for a head injury related to an automobile accident. While doing your hourly checks, you note that his urine output has been 800 ml since the last check. Over the next 3 hours, the client excretes an additional 3000 ml of very clear urine. His blood pressure has dropped, and urine specific gravity is less than 1.005. What are your priorities for care?**

Factors to Consider. Is the urine output within normal limits? How might his urine output be related to his head injury?

BIBLIOGRAPHY

1. Anonymous. (1998). A quick check of the endocrine system. *Nursing, 28*(7), 32cc12–32cc13.
2. Bianco, C. (1996). Diabetes insipidus: Your role in managing this multifaceted disease. *American Journal of Nursing, 96*(8), 30–31.
3. Birch, C. (1997). Caring for people with endocrine disorders. In J. Luckmann (Ed.). *Saunders manual of nursing care.* Philadelphia: W. B. Saunders.
4. Clayton, L., & Dilley, K. B. (1998). Cushing's syndrome: Here's how to recognize and treat the manifestations of excess corticoids. *American Journal of Nursing, 98*(7), 40–41.
5. Coskeran, P. (1999). Management and treatment of patients with acromegaly. *Nursing Times, 95*(13), 50–52.
6. Cryer, P. (1995). Diseases of the sympathochromaffin system. In P. Felig, J. D. Baxter, & L. A. Frohman (Eds.), *Endocrinology and metabolism* (3rd ed., pp. 713–748). New York: McGraw-Hill.
7. Davies, P. (1996). Caring for patients with diabetes insipidus. *Nursing, 26*(5), 62–63.
8. Davis-Martin, S. (1996). Pearls for practice: Disorders of the adrenal glands. *Journal of the American Academy of Nurse Practitioners, 8*(7), 323–326.
9. DeJong, M. J. (1998). Hyponatremia: A life-threatening complication of the widely used thiazide diuretics. *American Journal of Nursing, 98*(12), 36.
10. Edwards, C. (1995). Primary mineralocorticoid excess syndromes. In L. DeGroot (Ed.), *Endocrinology* (3rd ed., pp. 1775–1803). Philadelphia: W. B. Saunders.
11. Eisenberg, A., & Redick, E. (1999). Caring for a patient after resection of pituitary adenoma. *Critical Care, 29*(12), 32cc1–2, 32cc4–6.
12. Eisenberg, A., & Redick, E. (1998). Preventing complications. Transsphenoidal resection of pituitary adenoma: Using a critical pathway. *Dimensions of Critical Care Nursing, 17*(6), 306–312.
13. Frohman, L. A. (1996). Acromegaly: What constitutes optimal ther-

apy? *Journal of Clinical Endocrinology and Metabolism, 8*(2), 443–445.

14. Go, H., et al. (1995). Laparoscopic adrenalectomy for Cushing's syndrome: Comparison with primary hyperaldosteronism. *Surgery, 117*(1), 11–17.
15. Greenspan, F., & Strewler, G. (Eds.). (1997). Basic and clinical endocrinology (5th ed.). Stamford, CT: Appleton & Lange.
16. Gumowski, J., & Loughran, M. (1996). Diseases of the adrenal gland. *Nursing Clinics of North America, 31*(4), 747–768.
17. Huether, S., & Tomky, D. (1998). Alterations of hormonal regulations. In K. McCance & S. Huether (Eds.), *Pathophysiology: The biologic basis for disease in adults and children* (3rd ed., pp. 656–706). St. Louis: Mosby–Year Book.
18. Jenkins, P. J., et al. (1995). The long term outcome after adrenalectomy and prophylactic pituitary radiotherapy in adrenocorticotropin-dependent Cushing's syndrome. *Journal of Clinical Endocrinology and Metabolism, 80*(1), 165–171.
19. Kee, J., & Hayes, E. (1997). *Pharmacology: A nursing process approach* (2nd ed.). Philadelphia: W. B. Saunders.
20. Keiser, H. (1995). Pheochromocytoma and related tumors. In L. DeGroot (Ed.), *Endocrinology* (3rd ed., pp. 1853–1877). Philadelphia: W. B. Saunders.
21. Loriaux, T. C. (1996). Endocrine assessment: Red flags for those on the front lines. *Nursing Clinics of North America, 31*(4), 695–714.
22. Loriaux, D. L., & McDonald, W. J. (1995). Adrenal insufficiency. In L. DeGroot (Ed.), *Endocrinology* (3rd ed., pp. 1731–1740). Philadelphia: W. B. Saunders.
23. McEwen, D. R. (1995). Transsphenoidal adenomectomy. *AORN Journal, 61*(2), 321–337.
24. Miller, W., & Tyrell, J. B. (1995). The adrenal cortex. In P. Felig, J. D. Baxter, & L. A. Frohman (Eds.), *Endocrinology and metabolism* (pp. 555–711). New York: McGraw-Hill.
25. Molitch, M. (1999). Advances in the management of pituitary tumors. *Endocrinology and Metabolism Clinics of North America, 28*(1), 1–240.
26. Nieman, L., & Cutler, G. B. (1995). Cushing's syndrome. In L. DeGroot (Ed.), *Endocrinology* (3rd ed., pp. 1741–1769). Philadelphia: W. B. Saunders.
27. O'Donnell, M. (1997). Addisonian crisis: Overexertion brought this patient's adrenal insufficiency to light. *American Journal of Nursing, 97*(3), 41.
28. Oekler, W. (1996). Adrenal insufficiency. *New England Journal of Medicine, 335*(16), 1206–1212.
29. Romeo, J. H. (1996). Hyper- and hypofunction in the anterior pituitary. *Nursing Clinics of North America, 31*(4), 769–778.
30. Rusterholtz., A. (1996). Interpretation of diagnostic laboratory tests in selected endocrine disorders. *Nursing Clinics of North America, 31*(4), 715–724.
31. Utiger, R. D. (1997). Treatment and retreatment of Cushing's disease. *New England Journal of Medicine, 336*(3), 215–217.
32. Werbel, S., & Ober, K. P. (1995). Pheochromocytoma. *Medical Clinics of North America, 79*(1), 131–153.
33. Winger, J. M., & Hornick, T. (1996). Age-associated changes in the endocrine system. *Nursing Clinics of North America, 31*(4), 827–844.

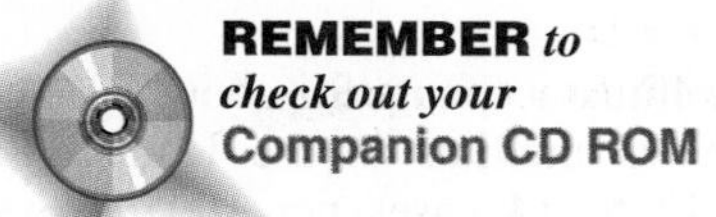

CHAPTER

45

Management of Clients with Diabetes Mellitus

James A. Fain

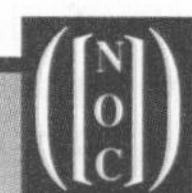

NURSING OUTCOMES CLASSIFICATION (NOC)
for Nursing Diagnoses—Clients with Diabetes Mellitus

Altered Health Maintenance		Risk for Ineffective Management of Therapeutic Regimen (Individuals)
Health Belief: Perceived Resources	Knowledge: Treatment Regimen	Compliance Behavior
Health Promoting Behavior	Participation: Health Care Decisions	Knowledge: Disease Process
Health Seeking Behavior	Psychosocial Adjustment: Life Change	Knowledge: Treatment Regimen
Knowledge: Health Behaviors	Risk Detection	Participation: Health Care Decisions
Knowledge: Health Promotion	Self-Direction of Care	Treatment Behavior: Illness or Injury
Knowledge: Health Resources	Social Support	
	Treatment Behavior: Injury or Illness	

Diabetes mellitus is a chronic systemic disease characterized by either a deficiency of insulin or a decreased ability of the body to use insulin. Diabetes mellitus is sometimes referred to as "high sugars" by both clients and health care providers. The notion of associating sugar with diabetes is appropriate because the passage of large amounts of sugar-laden urine is characteristic of poorly controlled diabetes. However, high levels of blood glucose are only one component of the pathologic process and clinical manifestations associated with diabetes mellitus. Diabetes mellitus can be associated with serious complications, but people with diabetes can take preventive measures to reduce the likelihood of such occurrences.

In 1979, The National Diabetes Data Group[33] (NDDG) developed criteria for the classification and diagnosis of diabetes. In 1997, the Expert Committee on the Diagnosis and Classification of Diabetes Mellitus[23] proposed changes to the original NDDG classification scheme. Such changes were supported by the American Diabetes Association (ADA) and the National Institute of Diabetes and Digestive and Kidney Diseases (NIDDK). Previously, diabetes was classified as either insulin-dependent diabetes mellitus (IDDM) or non–insulin-dependent diabetes mellitus (NIDDM). With the use of insulin therapy commonplace with both types of diabetes, IDDM is now referred to as type 1 diabetes, and NIDDM is referred to as type 2 diabetes. The ADA also recommended using Arabic numerals—type 1 and type 2—rather than Roman numerals in referring to the two types of diabetes.[23]

This chapter incorporates material written for the fifth edition by Carol Birch and Kerry H. Greear.

Type 1 diabetes is characterized by destruction of pancreatic beta cells, usually leading to absolute insulin deficiency. Type 1 diabetes affects 10% of people who have diabetes, and it can develop at any age; usually, however, it is diagnosed before the age of 30 years. The most common form of diabetes, type 2, affects 90% to 95% of people who have diabetes and usually is diagnosed after age 40. Type 2 diabetes is more common among older adults and certain ethnic populations.

Clients who do not have type 1 or type 2 diabetes may nevertheless be classified as having impaired glucose tolerance, also known as *impaired fasting glucose.* This new diagnostic category is defined by fasting glucose levels above 110 mg/dl (milligrams per deciliter), but below 126 mg/dl. These glucose values are higher than the level considered normal but lower than the level diagnostic of diabetes.[23] It is estimated that 11% of the population has impaired fasting glucose.

Diabetes may also result from other disorders or treatments. Genetic defects in the beta cells can lead to the development of diabetes. Several hormones, such as growth hormone, cortisol, glucagon, and epinephrine, antagonize or counteract insulin. Excess amounts of these hormones—as in acromegaly, Cushing's syndrome, glucagonoma, and pheochromocytoma—cause diabetes. In addition, certain drugs, such as glucocorticoids and thiazides, and infections may cause diabetes. Such types of secondary diabetes account for 1% to 2% of all diagnosed cases of diabetes.

Gestational diabetes mellitus is a diagnosis of diabetes mellitus that applies only to women in whom glucose intolerance develops or is first discovered during pregnancy. Gestational diabetes develops in 2% to 5% of all pregnant women but disappears when the pregnancy is over. It occurs more frequently in African Americans, Hispanic Americans, Native Americans, and women with a family history of diabetes, and obesity is also a risk factor. See Box 45–1 for an overview of the types of diabetes mellitus.[19, 21]

Diabetes mellitus is a significant public health concern in the United States. About 16 million people (5.9% of the population) have diabetes, nearly half of whom do not yet know they have it. Some 3.2 million of affected people are 65 years of age or older. Diabetes imposes a heavy economic burden on the United States each year. It is estimated that more than $100 billion in direct and indirect costs (such as disability, work loss, and premature death) are attributed to diabetes mellitus.[13]

Diabetes is the seventh leading cause of death in the United States, with more than 180,000 deaths attributable to the disease in 1995. Even when it does not kill, diabetes can cause major disabilities. For example, diabetes mellitus is the single greatest contributor to the number of cases of blindness in adults, end-stage renal failure, and nontraumatic amputations. Diabetes is the leading cause of new cases of blindness in adults 20 to 74 years of age. It is also the leading cause of end-stage renal disease, accounting for about 40% of new cases. In 1995, about 98,000 people with diabetes underwent dialysis or kidney transplantation. Likewise, more than half of leg amputations are performed among people with diabetes. From 1993 to 1995, about 67,000 amputations were performed each year.[20] The increasing burden of diabetes is alarming, but the good news is that much of the burden of this major public health problem can be prevented by early detection, improved delivery of care, and better education for diabetes self-management.

BOX 45–1 Types of Diabetes Mellitus and Abnormal Glucose Metabolism

Diabetes Mellitus

1. Type 1 diabetes
2. Type 2 diabetes
3. Causes of secondary diabetes
   a. Genetic defects
   b. Diseases of the pancreas (such as pancreatitis, neoplasia, trauma/pancreatectomy)
   c. Endocrinopathies (such as acromegaly, Cushing's syndrome, pheochromocytoma, hyperthyroidism)
   d. Drug/chemical-induced (as from glucocorticoids, thyroid hormone, diazoxide, thiazides, phenytoin sodium [Dilantin], nicotinic acid)
   e. Infections (such as congenital rubella, cytomegalovirus infection)
   f. Genetic syndromes associated with diabetes (such as Down syndrome, Klinefelter's syndrome, Huntington's chorea)
4. Gestational diabetes mellitus

Impaired Glucose Tolerance

1. Impaired fasting glucose

Adapted from American Diabetes Association. (1997). Report of the Expert Committee on the Diagnosis and Classification of Diabetes Mellitus. *Diabetes Care, 20*(7), 1183–1197.

Type 1 diabetes mellitus accounts for about 10% of all known cases of diabetes mellitus in the United States. Annual incidence is 12 to 14 cases per 100,000 people younger than 20 years, with a prevalence of 1 case per 500 people younger than 16 years. It is one of the most common childhood diseases, being three to four times more common than such chronic childhood diseases as cystic fibrosis, juvenile rheumatoid arthritis and leukemia, and 10 times more common than nephrotic syndrome or muscular dystrophy. The incidence of type 1 diabetes mellitus in males is similar to that in females, and the condition is more common in African Americans, Hispanic Americans, Asian Americans, and Native Americans than in whites.[13] Risk factors are less well defined for type 1 diabetes than for type 2 diabetes.

Type 2 diabetes mellitus accounts for about 90% to 95% of all known cases of diabetes mellitus in the United States. About 8 million Americans have this type of diabetes, but an almost equal number of cases are undiagnosed. Type 2 diabetes is present, on average, for about 6.5 years before its clinical identification and treatment. The prevalence is markedly higher in Native Americans, African Americans, and Hispanic Americans, as well as in older and obese people.[13]

Etiology and Risk Factors

TYPE 1 DIABETES MELLITUS

Type 1 diabetes, previously called IDDM or *juvenile-onset diabetes,* is inherited as a heterogeneous, multigenic trait. Identical twins have a risk of 25% to 50% of inheriting the disease, whereas siblings have a 6% risk and offspring a 5% risk. Despite this strong familial influence, 90% of people in whom type 1 diabetes develops do not have a first-degree relative with diabetes. An association also exists between type 1 diabetes and several human leukocyte antigens (HLAs). Environmental factors such as viruses appear to trigger an autoimmune process that destroys beta cells. Islet cell antibodies (ICAs) then appear, increasing in amount over months to years as beta cells are destroyed.[37] Fasting *hyperglycemia* (elevated blood glucose level) occurs when 80% to 90% of beta cell mass has been destroyed.

Identification of ICAs has made it possible to detect type 1 diabetes mellitus in its preclinical stage. Autoantibodies directed against insulin are found in 20% to 60% of clients with type 1 diabetes prior to initiation of exogenous insulin therapy. The combination of large amounts of ICAs, presence of insulin autoantibodies, and decreased first-phase insulin secretion (representing insulin stored in beta cells) can predict the onset of type 1 diabetes mellitus within 5 years.[37]

There are no known health promotion activities to prevent type 1 diabetes mellitus; however, regular exercise and adherence to the prescribed diet may limit the development of complications. Health maintenance activities involve:

- Maintaining blood glucose at levels as normal as possible
- Preventing hypoglycemia and hyperglycemia with stress, illness, or exercise by closely monitoring blood glucose levels and taking early action; performing daily foot care

- Preventing complications of diabetes mellitus by removing or treating coexisting risk factors such as smoking, hypertension, hyperlipidemia, and use of nephrotoxic drugs.

Health restoration actions include:

- Prompt treatment of foot abrasions or infections
- Follow-up visits to assess for complications of diabetes and to reinforce learning needs
- Yearly funduscopic examinations by an ophthalmologist with treatment as needed
- Treatment of coexisting risk factors as described previously

Type 2 Diabetes Mellitus

Type 2 diabetes mellitus, previously called NIDDM or *adult-onset diabetes,* also appears to be a heterogeneous disorder involving both genetic and environmental factors. It is not associated with HLA tissue types, and circulating ICAs are rarely present. Heredity plays a major role in the expression of type 2 diabetes. It is more common in identical twins (58% to 75% incidence) than in the general population. Obesity is also a major risk factor; 85% of all people with type 2 diabetes are obese. It is unclear whether impaired tissue (liver and muscle) sensitivity to insulin or impaired insulin secretion is the primary defect in this type of diabetes.[37] In addition, the prevalence of coronary artery disease in people with type 2 diabetes is twice that in the non-diabetic population, and cardiovascular and total mortality rates are two-fold to three-fold greater than in non-diabetic people.[41]

Cases have been documented of families in which type 2 diabetes is present in all age groups and in which an autosomal dominant inheritance has been established. This form of diabetes is referred to as *maturity-onset diabetes of the young* (MODY).

Health promotion actions for type 2 diabetes mellitus include:

- Eating habits based on the "Food Guide Pyramid" (as noted later on)[40]
- Avoidance of foods high in refined sugars and saturated fats
- Maintaining ideal body weight, starting in childhood
- Exercising regularly
- Returning to pre-pregnancy weight or ideal body weight post partum

Health maintenance activities involve:

- Screening high-risk people, such as those with first-degree relatives who have type 2 diabetes, those who are obese, members of high-risk racial groups, people over age 40 with any other risk factor, people with hypertension or hyperlipidemia, clients with previous impaired glucose tolerance, women with previous gestational diabetes mellitus or those who have had a baby weighing more than 9 pounds, and people with a history of recurrent infections
- Performing periodic assessments to determine the client's learning needs and to assess glycemic control
- Using strategies shown to reduce complications of diabetes by removing or treating coexisting risk factors such as smoking, hypertension, hyperlipidemia, and use of nephrotoxic drugs
- Performing daily foot care
- Preventing hypoglycemia or hyperglycemia by closely monitoring blood glucose levels and taking early action

Health restoration actions include:

- Teach diet and exercise programs to reduce obesity
- Prompt treatment of foot abrasions or infections
- Follow-up visits to assess for complications of diabetes and reinforce learning needs
- Yearly funduscopic examinations by an ophthalmologist with treatment as needed
- Treatment of previously described risk factors
- Control of angina and peripheral vascular disease

Pathophysiology

Type 1 Diabetes Mellitus

The development of type 1 diabetes mellitus can be broken down into five stages:

Stage 1: genetic predisposition
Stage 2: environmental trigger
Stage 3: active autoimmunity
Stage 4: progressive beta cell destruction
Stage 5: overt diabetes mellitus

Type 1 diabetes mellitus does not develop in all people who have a genetic predisposition. Of those in whom gene markers (DR3 or DR4 HLA) indicate risk, diabetes ultimately develops in fewer than 1%. Environmental triggers have long been suspected in type 1 diabetes. Incidence is increased in both spring and fall, and onset is often coincidental with epidemics of various viral diseases. Active autoimmunity is directed against the beta cells of the pancreas and their products. ICAs and insulin antibodies serve to progressively decrease the effective circulating insulin level.

This slow, progressive insult to the beta cells and endogenous insulin molecules can result in an abrupt onset of diabetes. Hyperglycemia can result from acute illness or stress (see the Case Study), which increases insulin demand beyond the reserves of the damaged beta cell mass. When the acute illness or stress resolves, the client may revert to a compensated state of variable duration in which the pancreas once again manages to produce adequate amounts of insulin. This compensated state, referred to as the *honeymoon period,* typically lasts for 3 to 12 months. The process ends when the diminishing beta cell mass cannot produce enough insulin to sustain life. The client then becomes dependent on exogenous insulin (produced outside the body) administration to survive.[32, 37]

Type 2 Diabetes Mellitus

The pathogenesis of type 2 diabetes mellitus differs significantly from that of type 1. A limited beta cell response to hyperglycemia appears to be a major factor in its development. Beta cells chronically exposed to high blood levels of glucose become progressively less efficient when responding to further glucose elevations. This phenomenon, termed *desensitization,* is reversible by normalizing glucose levels. The ratio of *proinsulin* (a precursor to insulin) to insulin secreted also increases.[37]

A second pathophysiologic process in type 2 diabetes mellitus is resistance to the biologic activity of insulin in both the liver and peripheral tissues. This state is known as *insulin resistance.* People with type 2 diabetes have a

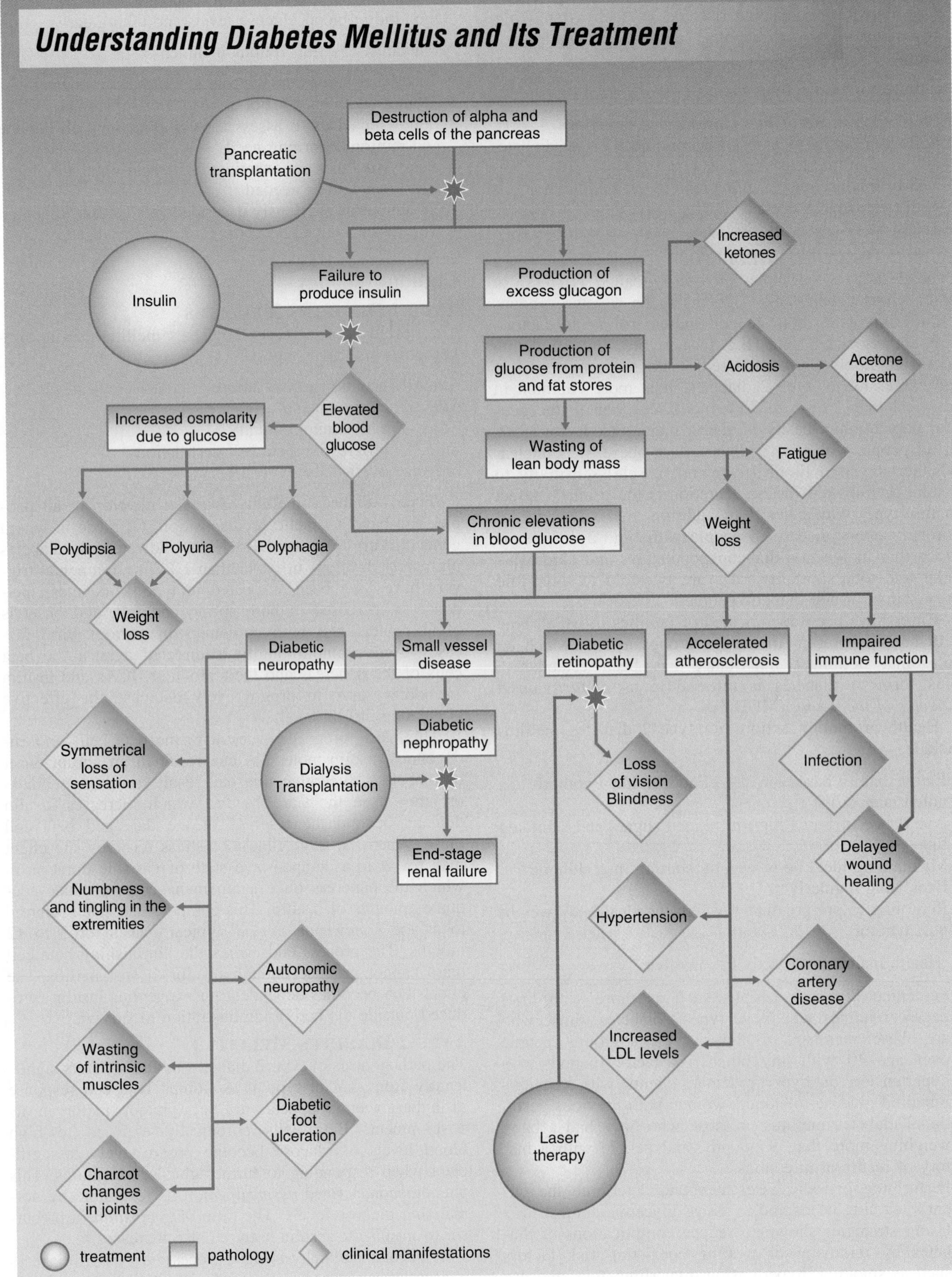
Understanding Diabetes Mellitus and Its Treatment
Pancreatic transplantation
Destruction of alpha and beta cells of the pancreas
Insulin
Failure to produce insulin
Production of excess glucagon
Increased ketones
Production of glucose from protein and fat stores
Acidosis
Acetone breath
Increased osmolarity due to glucose
Elevated blood glucose
Wasting of lean body mass
Fatigue
Polydipsia
Polyuria
Polyphagia
Weight loss
Chronic elevations in blood glucose
Weight loss
Diabetic neuropathy
Small vessel disease
Diabetic retinopathy
Accelerated atherosclerosis
Impaired immune function
Symmetrical loss of sensation
Diabetic nephropathy
Dialysis Transplantation
Loss of vision Blindness
Infection
End-stage renal failure
Delayed wound healing
Numbness and tingling in the extremities
Hypertension
Autonomic neuropathy
Coronary artery disease
Wasting of intrinsic muscles
Increased LDL levels
Diabetic foot ulceration
Laser therapy
Charcot changes in joints
treatment
pathology
clinical manifestations

Diabetes and Pneumonia

Ms. Washington is a 44-year-old black woman who has been sick for the past week. She has been treated with erythromycin (E-Mycin) 500 mg q 6 h and phenylpropanolamine-guaifensin (Entex LA) q 12 h as an outpatient after being seen in the clinic for a persistent cough, loss of voice, chest pain from coughing, fever, chills, and mild nausea without vomiting. She now reports that she has been coughing sputum that is brown to green, with small amounts of red blood present. Ms. Washington is also complaining of left shoulder pain of 3 days' duration, fatigue, sinus pressure, congestion, fullness in the ears, and postnasal drainage. She also reports frequent urination without dysuria or urgency and feeling thirsty all the time.

Her history is significant for gestational diabetes 11 years ago, at which time she administered her own insulin injections. At this time, she is being admitted for failed treatment of pneumonia and control of new-onset diabetes. Consider whether Ms. Washington has type 1 or type 2 diabetes mellitus and the effect of that type of diabetes on her treatment plan and future complications.

Admission Laboratory Values	
RBC count	3.7 million/mm^3
Hb	10.5 g/dl
Hct	31%
WBC count	15,600/mm^3
Neutrophils	81%
BUN	5 mg/dl
Creatinine	0.7 mg/dl
Cholesterol	176 mg/dl
Triglycerides	134 mg/dl
Potassium	5.3 mEq/L
Chloride	96 mEq/L
Sodium	139 mEq/L
Glucose	335 mg/dl

Nursing Admission Assessment

Ms. Washington is a single mother of an 11-year-old son. She works from 6 AM to 2 PM at a fast food restaurant 6 days a week, where she stands at the counter. She reports that the benefits of the job are medical insurance and the free food for herself and discounted food for her son when he stops for breakfast on his way to school. Her father died of diabetes complicated by heart disease, and her mother died of diabetes complicated by stroke. She admits to smoking one pack of cigarettes a day for 20 years and denies use of alcohol. However, she reports drinking 1 gallon of bottled fruit juice daily.

Nursing Physical Examination

Height: 5′7″ Weight: 192 lb (87.3 kg)
Vital signs: BP = 144/94
TPR = 100.8, 78, 18
Level of consciousness: Alert and cooperative

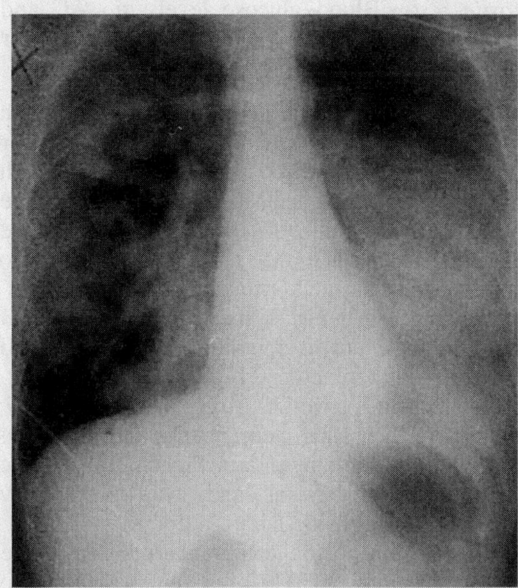

● Ms. Washington's chest x-ray shows thickened bronchioles and left lower-lobe infiltrates. The cardiac silhouette is normal.

EENT: Nasal mucosa unremarkable, yellow-green drainage on pharynx.
Cardiac: Regular rate and rhythm without gallop or murmur
Pulmonary: Decreased breath sounds at bases, with the left greater than the right; wheezes and rhonchi noted at the left lower lobe; increased tactile fremitus
Abdominal: Soft and nontender with active bowel tones
Genitourinary: Reports vaginal itching and white "clumpy" discharge
Peripheral pulses: 3/3, without edema

Initial Treatment Plan

Medications

Cefazolin (Ancef) 1 g IV q 8 h
Triamcinolone acetonide (Kenaject-40) 40 mg IM now
Human insulin (Humulin) NPH 20 U SC AM, 10 U SC PM; sliding-scale insulin AC and HS: Humulin regular SC according to serum glucose level:
<150 mg/dl: 0 units
151–250 mg/dl: 3 units
251–350 mg/dl: 6 units
>350 mg/dl: call physician

Saline flush IV lock bid and after medications

What effect, if any, would the admission medication orders have on Ms. Washington's blood glucose?

Diet: 1200-calorie ADA; develop a sample 24-hour diet plan for Ms. Washington
Activity: As tolerated

Case Study continued on following page

Respiratory treatments: Albuterol (Ventolin) 2.5 mg in 3 ml NS aerosol qid; incentive spirometer q 2 h while awake

Diagnostic tests: Blood glucose levels qid AC and HS; repeat complete blood count, electrolytes, chest x-ray in AM

At 11:00 AM on day 2, Ms. Washington's serum glucose level is 265 mg/dl. How much insulin will she require?

Over the next 3 days, Ms. Washington's blood glucose levels stabilize. Her physician adds 10 U Humulin regular to her routine AM insulin dose and 5 U Humulin regular to her routine PM insulin dose and discontinues the orders for sliding-scale insulin. Metformin (Glucophage) is initiated at 500 mg PO bid with meals. The physician writes an order for the client to continue monitoring blood glucose levels with a glucometer qid. Yesterday, her fluid intake was 1980 ml, and her urinary output was 1575 ml. She remains on her 1200-calorie ADA diet, but says that she would like a hamburger and French fries. Yesterday, the nurse discovered several candy bars in the drawer of Ms. Washington's bedside table.

Ms. Washington no longer complains of sinus pressure or postnasal drainage. Her cough remains productive of small amounts of white, thick sputum. Lung sounds remain diminished, but clear after coughing. She is able to raise her incentive spirometer measurement to 1500 ml. Her antibiotic has been changed to clarithromycin (Biaxin) 500 mg bid with food × 10 days. The physician has also ordered miconazole (Monistat) vaginal cream daily. What instructions would you give Ms. Washington about administration of the vaginal cream?

Most recent laboratory values reveal a potassium of 4.0 mEq/L, chloride of 100 mEq/L, and sodium of 139 mEq/L. Her fasting blood sugar this AM was 95 mg/dl, and the WBC count was 10×10^9/L.

The physician is planning to discharge her tomorrow.

Discharge Criteria

- Average length of stay: 5.5 days without complications; 8.4 days with complications.
- Initiate diabetes instruction for survival, home care, and improved lifestyle. Consider differences in discharge planning between chronic illnesses, such as diabetes, and episodic or acute illnesses, such as sinusitis.
- Complete community referrals. What referrals would you make? Why?

Questions to Be Considered

1. In the progress notes, Ms. Washington's physician reports a shift to the left in her WBC count. What does this mean? Discuss the relationship between diabetes mellitus and susceptibility to infection and response to treatment. What influence do infections exert over control of diabetes mellitus?
2. How would the physician's decision to prescribe mixed-dose insulin and metformin (Glucophage) influence the triangle of control (diet, exercise, pharmacologic agents)? What are the benefits? What are the risks?
3. What influence did her socioeconomic status, race, and heredity have on Ms. Washington's development of diabetes mellitus? What continuing influence will these factors play in her regulation of the diabetes? What effect will her current employment probably have on Ms. Washington's compliance with, and ability to financially afford, diet, foot care, glucose monitoring, and exercise?
4. Describe the pathophysiologic basis for the change in Ms. Washington's potassium levels and her development of polyuria, polydipsia, polyphagia, and weight loss.
5. Ms. Washington's employer telephones the nurses' station and states: "Ms. Washington has informed me that she will be unable to return to work for 10 days. Is this true?" How would you respond? What are the ethical considerations you should make in formulating your response?
6. Ten days after discharge, Ms. Washington complains of fever, nausea, vomiting, and diarrhea. What directions would you give?

AC, at meals; ADA, American Diabetes Association; BP, blood pressure; EENT, eye, ear, nose, throat; Hb, hemoglobin; Hct, hematocrit; IM, intramuscular; NS, normal saline; RBC, red blood cell; SC, subcutaneous; TPR, temperature, pulse, respirations; WBC, white blood cell.

decreased sensitivity to glucose levels, which results in continued hepatic glucose production, even with high plasma glucose levels. This is coupled with an inability of muscle and fat tissues to increase glucose uptake. The mechanism causing peripheral insulin resistance is not clear; however, it appears to occur after insulin binds to a receptor on the cell surface (Fig. 45–1).

Insulin is a building (anabolic) hormone. Without insulin, three major metabolic problems occur: (1) decreased glucose utilization, (2) increased fat mobilization, and (3) increased protein utilization. (See the algorithm called Understanding Diabetes Mellitus and Its Treatment), p. 1152.)

Decreased Glucose Utilization

In diabetes, cells that require insulin as a carrier for glucose can take in only about 25% of the glucose they require for fuel. Nerve tissues, erythrocytes, and the cells of the intestines, liver, and kidney tubules do not require insulin for glucose transport. Skeletal and cardiac muscles and adipose tissues do. Without adequate amounts of insulin, much of the ingested glucose cannot be used.

With inadequate amounts of insulin, blood glucose levels rise. This elevation continues because the liver cannot store glucose as glycogen without sufficient insulin levels. In an attempt to restore balance and return blood glucose levels to normal, the kidney excretes the excess glucose. Glucose appears in the urine (*glucosuria*). Glucose excreted in the urine acts as an osmotic diuretic and causes excretion of increased amounts of water, resulting in fluid volume deficit.[37]

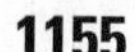

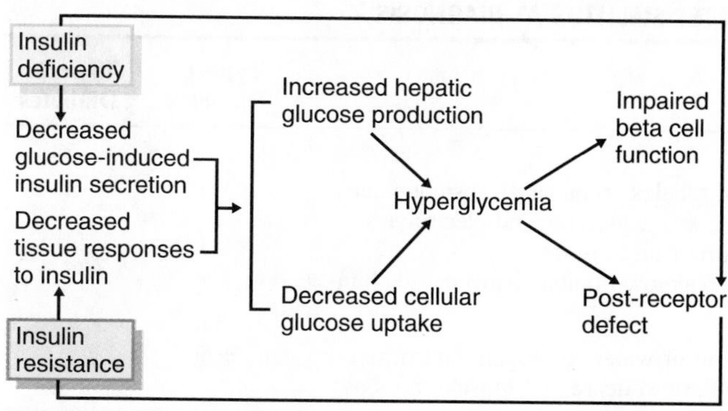

FIGURE 45–1 Relationship between insulin resistance and insulin secretion in type 2 diabetes mellitus. (Modified from American Diabetes Association [1998]. *Medical management of non-insulin dependent (type 2) diabetes* [4th ed., p. 18]. Alexandria, VA: Author.)

Increased Fat Mobilization

In type 1 diabetes and occasionally with severe stress in type 2 diabetes, the body turns to fat stores for energy production when glucose is unavailable. Fat metabolism causes breakdown products called *ketones* to form. Ketones accumulate in the blood and are excreted through the kidneys and lungs. Ketone levels can be measured in the blood and urine; high levels can serve as an indicator of uncontrolled diabetes.

Ketones interfere with the body's acid-base balance by producing hydrogen ions. The pH can fall, and metabolic acidosis (discussed later) can develop. In addition, when ketones are excreted, sodium is also eliminated, resulting in sodium depletion and further acidosis. The excretion of ketones also increases osmotic pressure, leading to increased fluid loss. Also, when fats are the primary source of energy, body lipid levels can rise to five times normal, leading to increased atherosclerosis.[37]

Increased Protein Utilization

Lack of insulin leads to protein wasting. In healthy people, proteins are constantly being broken down and rebuilt. In people with type 1 diabetes, without insulin to stimulate protein synthesis, the balance is altered, which leads to increased catabolism (destruction). Amino acids are converted to glucose in the liver, further elevating glucose levels. If this condition goes untreated, clients with type 1 diabetes appear emaciated. The pathophysiologic processes of diabetes continue, leading to many acute and chronic complications, as discussed later in the chapter.[37, 41]

Clinical Manifestations

Hyperglycemia, the medical term for an elevated blood glucose level, leads to common clinical manifestations associated with diabetes. In type 1 diabetes, the onset is sudden, with diabetic ketoacidosis being the first indication of the disease. In contrast, type 2 diabetes may develop so gradually that some affected people notice few or no manifestations for a number of years. Clients may initially complain of chronic problems, as from peripheral neuropathy (nerve damage in hands and feet). Other times, the diagnosis of type 2 diabetes may be made by a routine laboratory test in clients who have no manifestations.

The classic clinical manifestations of diabetes are increased frequency of urination (*polyuria*), increased thirst and fluid intake (*polydipsia*), and, as the disease progresses, weight loss despite increased hunger and food intake (*polyphagia*). These clinical manifestations are caused by hyperglycemia and the accompanying spillover of excess glucose in the urine. See Tables 45–1 and 45–2 for other common manifestations.

DIAGNOSIS OF DIABETES MELLITUS

Physical examination, medical history, and laboratory tests are employed to evaluate clients with diabetes. Clinical manifestations suggest the presence of diabetes, but laboratory tests are needed to make a definitive diagnosis.

FASTING BLOOD GLUCOSE. Diabetes is diagnosed by measuring blood glucose levels. The fasting blood glucose level is normally less than 110 mg/dl. The diagnosis of diabetes can be made when a client's fasting blood glucose level is above 125 mg/dl. Values between 110 and 125 mg/dl indicate impaired fasting glucose. Critical values in adults are those less than 60 mg/dl or more than 500 mg/dl (see Box 45–2).

A fasting blood glucose sample is drawn when the client has not ingested any nutrients other than water for 8 to 12 hours. This sample generally reflects glucose from hepatic production. If the client is receiving a dextrose IV solution, the results of the test must be analyzed with that variable in mind. In clients who are known to have diabetes, food and insulin are withheld until after the specimen is obtained. The fasting blood glucose gives the best indication of overall glucose homeostasis.

RANDOM BLOOD GLUCOSE. A blood sample for determination of glucose level may be drawn at any time and requires no client preparation. Results should be within normal limits for both non-diabetic and diabetic clients with good control of their blood glucose. Elevated blood glucose levels may occur after meals, after stressful events, if the sample was drawn from above an intravenous (IV) site, or in cases of diabetes. Table 45–3 lists conditions and medications that can cause hyperglycemia or *hypoglycemia* (decreased blood glucose level).

POSTPRANDIAL BLOOD GLUCOSE. Postprandial (after a meal) blood glucose samples are drawn 2 hours after a standard meal and reflect the efficiency of insulin-mediated glucose uptake by peripheral tissues. Normally, blood glucose should return to fasting levels within 2 hours. In older adults, levels are higher, typically rising by 5 to 10 mg/dl per decade after age 50 years because of the normal decline in glucose tolerance associated with aging. Smoking and drinking coffee can lead to falsely elevated values at 2 hours, whereas strenuous exercise can lead to falsely decreased values.

GLYCOSYLATED HEMOGLOBIN. Glucose normally attaches itself to the hemoglobin molecule on a red blood cell. Once attached, it cannot dissociate. Therefore, the higher the blood glucose levels, the higher the levels of glycosylated hemoglobin (HbA_{1C}). The results of this test show the average blood glucose level over the previous 3 months. It is therefore useful in evaluating long-term glycemic control. HbA_{1C} samples can be drawn at any time during the day. Conditions that increase erythrocyte turnover, such as bleeding, pregnancy, or asplenia (absence of

TABLE 45–1 **SELECTED CLINICAL MANIFESTATIONS OF DIABETES MELLITUS AT DIAGNOSIS**

Clinical Manifestation	Pathophysiologic Basis	Type 1 Diabetes	Type 2 Diabetes
Cardinal manifestations			
Polyuria* (frequent urination)	Water not reabsorbed from renal tubules secondary to osmotic activity of glucose; leads to loss of water, glucose, and electrolytes	++	+
Polydipsia* (excessive thirst)	Dehydration secondary to polyuria causes thirst	++	+
Polyphagia* (excessive hunger)	Starvation secondary to tissue breakdown (catabolism) causes hunger	++	+
Weight loss*	Initial loss secondary to depletion of water, glycogen, and triglyceride stores; chronic loss secondary to decreased muscle mass as amino acids are diverted to form glucose and ketone bodies	++	−
Recurrent blurred vision	Secondary to chronic exposure of ocular lens and retina to hyperosmolar fluids	+	++
Pruritus, skin infections, vaginitis	Bacterial and fungal infections of the skin seem to be more common; research conflicting	+	++
Ketonuria	When glucose cannot be used for energy in insulin-dependent cells, fatty acids are used for energy; fatty acids are broken down into ketones in the blood and excreted by the kidneys; in type 2 diabetes, sufficient insulin is present to depress excessive use of fatty acids, but not enough to permit use of glucose	++	−
Weakness and fatigue, dizziness	Decreased plasma volume leads to postural hypotension; potassium loss and protein catabolism contribute to weakness	++	+
Often asymptomatic	The body can "adapt" to a slow rise in blood glucose to a greater extent than it can to a rapid rise	−	++

* Often referred to as *classic manifestations* of diabetes.
+, sometimes seen; ++, usually seen; −, not usually seen.

TABLE 45–2 **DISTINGUISHING FEATURES OF TYPE 1 AND TYPE 2 DIABETES MELLITUS**

Feature	Type 1	Type 2
Synonyms	Insulin-dependent diabetes mellitus (IDDM), juvenile diabetes, labile or brittle diabetes	Non–insulin-dependent diabetes mellitus (NIDDM), adult or maturity-onset diabetes, mild diabetes
Age at onset	Usually occurs before age 30 years, but may occur at any age	Usually occurs after age 30 years, but can occur in children
Incidence	~10%	~90%
Type of onset	Usually abrupt, with rapid onset of hyperglycemia	Insidious, may be asymptomatic or mildly asymptomatic; body adapts to slow onset of hyperglycemia
Endogenous insulin production	Little or none	Below normal, normal, or above normal
Body weight at onset	Ideal body weight or thin	85% of clients are obese; may be of ideal body weight
Ketosis	Prone to ketosis, usually present at onset, frequently present during poor control	Resistant to ketosis, can occur with infection or stress
Manifestations	Polyuria, polydipsia, polyphagia, fatigue	Frequently none, may be mild manifestations of hyperglycemia
Dietary management	Essential	Essential
Exercise management	Essential	Essential
Exogenous insulin administration	Dependent on insulin for survival	20% to 30% of clients may require insulin
Oral hypoglycemic agents	Not effective	Effective
Teaching needs	At diagnosis and ongoing	At diagnosis and ongoing

BOX 45–2 Screening and Diagnosis Guidelines for Diabetes Mellitus

Guidelines for Testing for Diabetes

- Testing for diabetes should be considered in all persons at age 45. If results are normal, test should be repeated at 3-year intervals.
- Testing should be considered at a younger age or performed more often for clients with the following risk factors:
  - Obesity (>120% of desirable body weight or a body mass index above 27 kg/m^2)
  - Diabetes in a first-degree relative
  - Racial predisposition (as in African American, Hispanic, Native American populations)
  - In women, giving birth to a baby weighing more than 9 lb or a history of gestational diabetes
  - Hypertension (blood pressure > 140/90 mm Hg)
  - A high-density lipoprotein level < 35 mg/dl or triglyceride level > 250 mg/dl
  - On previous testing, impaired glucose tolerance or impaired fasting glucose

Guidelines for Diagnosis of Diabetes Mellitus

- Manifestations of diabetes plus random plasma glucose concentration above 200 mg/dl (11.1 mmol/L). *Random* is defined as any time of day without regard to time since last meal. Classic manifestations include polyuria, polydipsia, and unexplained weight loss.

OR

- Fasting plasma glucose level above 126 mg/dl (7.0 mmol/L). Fasting is defined as no caloric intake for at least 8 hours.

OR

- A 2-hour postprandial glucose level above 200 mg/dl during an oral glucose tolerance test. This test should be performed using a glucose load containing the equivalent of 75 g of anhydrous glucose dissolved in water.

Plasma Glucose Values

Fasting plasma glucose	<110 mg/dl	Normal fasting glucose
	110–126 mg/dl	Impaired fasting glucose
	>126 mg/dl	Diagnosis of diabetes
Oral glucose tolerance test, 2 hours after eating	<140 mg/dl	Normal glucose tolerance
	140–200 mg/dl	Impaired glucose intolerance
	>200 mg/dl	Diagnosis of diabetes

Adapted from American Diabetes Association. (1997). Report of the Expert Committee on the Diagnosis and Classification of Diabetes Mellitus. *Diabetes Care, 20*(7), 1183–1197.

the spleen as after splenectomy), will lead to falsely low HbA_{1C} concentrations. High aspirin doses, alcohol ingestion, uremia, elevated hemoglobin levels, and heparin therapy can cause falsely elevated levels of HbA_{1C}. Normal values are 6% to 7%.[24]

GLYCOSYLATED ALBUMIN. Glucose also attaches to proteins, primarily albumin. The concentration of glycosylated albumin (fructosamine) represents the average blood glucose over the previous 7 to 10 days. This measurement is useful when short-term determinations of average blood glucose are desired. The reliability and clinical applicability continue to be evaluated.

CONNECTING PEPTIDE. When the proinsulin produced by pancreatic beta cells is broken apart by an enzyme, two products are formed: insulin and connecting peptide, commonly called *C-peptide.* Because C-peptide and insulin are formed in equal amounts, this test indicates the amount of endogenous insulin production. Clients with type 1 diabetes usually have no or low concentrations of C-peptide. Clients with type 2 diabetes tend to have normal or elevated levels.

ORAL GLUCOSE TOLERANCE TEST. The oral glucose tolerance test is often unnecessary for the diagnosis of diabetes mellitus, especially if the client's fasting blood glucose is above 140 mg/dL. Bed rest, infection, trauma, medications, and stress can alter the test results.

TABLE 45–3 SELECTIVE FACTORS CONTRIBUTING TO HYPOGLYCEMIA AND HYPERGLYCEMIA

Predisposing Factors	Associated Medications
HYPOGLYCEMIA	
Too much insulin	Insulin
Erratic absorption of insulin	Salicylates/NSAIDs
Sudden increase in activity	Sulfonamides
Starvation	Beta-blockers
Alcohol ingestion	Sulfonylureas (oral hypoglycemic agents)
Age >60 years	Allopurinol
Acute illness	Dicumarol
Cerebrovascular accident	Haloperidol
Heart failure	Anticholinergic antagonists
Decreased kidney function	Monoamine oxidase inhibitors
Gastroparesis	
Abnormal liver function	Para-aminobenzoic acid
Hypopituitarism	Dextropropoxyphene
Adrenocortical insufficiency	Clofibrate
	Imipramine
	Histamine H_2-receptor antagonists
HYPERGLYCEMIA	
Inadequate insulin	Diuretics, especially thiazides
Infection	Beta-blockers
Inactivity	Diphenylhydantoin
Obesity	Glucocorticoids
Intravenous dextrose	Lithium
Diabetes	Phenothiazines
Emotional stress	Progestins
Physical stress	Levothyroxine
Liver disease	NSAIDs
Hyperthyroidism	Epinephrine
Lack of oral hypoglycemic agents	Tricyclic antidepressants
Decreased muscle mass	Oral contraceptives
Chronic pancreatitis	Rifampin
	Nicotinic acid
	Isoniazid

NSAID, nonsteroidal anti-inflammatory drug.

This test is not usually recommended in hospitalized clients.

The client needs a diet that offers at least 150 g of carbohydrate per day for 3 days before the test. A sample is drawn to test fasting blood glucose, and the client is given 75 g of glucose in water to drink. Blood samples are taken at intervals afterward (such as at 1 and 2 hours). The client cannot consume any food or fluid other than water between the glucose load ingestion and the end of the test. Diagnosis of diabetes mellitus or impaired glucose tolerance after the glucose tolerance test is dependent on fasting and follow-up glucose levels. The oral glucose load and levels diagnostic of diabetes are different for the pregnant client undergoing testing for gestational diabetes mellitus.[24]

KETONURIA. Urine levels of ketones can be tested by clients, as well as by laboratories, by use of dip-strips. The presence of ketones in the urine (a condition called *ketonuria*) indicates that the body is using fat as a major source of energy, which may result in ketoacidosis. All clients with diabetes should test their urine for ketones during acute illness or stress, when blood glucose levels are consistently elevated, and when they are pregnant or have evidence of ketoacidosis (such as nausea, vomiting, or abdominal pain). The presence of ketones in the urine of a nonfasting client with type 2 diabetes is also a major cause for concern.

PROTEINURIA. A routine urinalysis tests the sample for protein. The presence of protein in the urine (called *proteinuria*) is a manifestation of nephropathy. Testing the urine for microalbuminuria shows early nephropathy, long before it would be evident on routine urinalysis.

SELF-MONITORING OF BLOOD GLUCOSE

The development of devices that enable diabetic clients to monitor their own blood glucose levels has revolutionized diabetes care. These machines use reagent strips or a photometer, or both, and produce a digital readout of blood glucose values. Some have memory chips. Self-monitoring of blood glucose is recommended for all clients with diabetes, but it is required for people with type 1 diabetes, people with type 2 diabetes who need insulin, highly motivated clients with type 2 diabetes, women with gestational diabetes, clients who use insulin pumps, and clients whose diabetes is in poor control. These tests must be performed with extreme care and accuracy, because the results are used to adjust insulin, manage exercise, and monitor dietary management of diabetes. Most devices have a process by which the client can verify accuracy by using control samples. This method of testing is not used to diagnose diabetes, but it is instrumental in managing diabetes.

Self-monitoring of blood glucose levels uses whole blood, whereas laboratories use serum or plasma for glucose determinations. Values obtained with these monitoring methods are not equal. Glucose levels in whole blood are about 12% to 15% lower than those in plasma because glucose is not distributed in hemoglobin. To compare self-monitored levels and laboratory levels of glucose, divide the serum or plasma level by 1.12, which represents the 12% difference between the two. The results of self-monitoring should fall within 15% to 20% of the laboratory results.

Several noninvasive methods of measuring blood glucose levels are being developed and tested. Infrared radiation spectroscopy, polarized light rotation, and the use of minimally invasive devices that analyze interstitial fluid from the skin are some of the methods under active study.

Outcome Management

Medical Management

The desired outcomes with medical management for clients with diabetes include restoring and maintaining blood glucose levels to as near normal as possible by balancing diet, exercise, and the use of oral hypoglycemic agents or insulin.[9, 27, 42] In general, when diabetes is successfully managed, clients avoid the complications of hyperglycemia and hypoglycemia. Unfortunately, complications may develop in some clients with diabetes despite their vigorous efforts to carefully control the disease.[12]

Initial as well as ongoing client education is vital in helping the client manage this chronic condition. Interventions must be individualized to the client's goals, age, lifestyle, nutritional needs, maturation, activity level, occupation, type of diabetes, and ability to independently perform the skills required by the management plan. Incorporation of psychosocial aspects into the overall plan is vital.[16]

REGULATE BLOOD GLUCOSE

Promote Proper Nutrition

Dietary management is an essential component of diabetes care and management. The general goal of dietary management is to help diabetic clients improve metabolic control by making changes in nutrition habits. Specific goals include (1) improving blood glucose and lipid levels, (2) providing consistency in day-to-day food intake (in type 1 diabetes), (3) facilitating weight management (in type 2 diabetes), and (4) providing adequate nutrition for all stages of life and with coexisting medical conditions.[9]

Achieving nutrition-related goals requires a team approach that includes the client. Effective self-management requires an individualized approach, taking into account the client's personal lifestyle and diabetes management goals. A nutritional assessment is used to determine the nutrition prescription on the basis of what the client with diabetes is able and willing to do. Glucose levels (self-monitored), lipid levels, blood pressure, and renal status are all essential aspects of nutrition-related management.

Promote Regular Physical Activity

A program of planned exercise is a crucial part of the treatment plan for a diabetic client. Exercise lowers blood glucose by increasing carbohydrate metabolism, fosters weight reduction and maintenance, increases insulin sensitivity, increases high-density lipoprotein (HDL) levels, decreases triglyceride levels, lowers blood pressure, and reduces stress and tension.[3, 27]

The primary side effect of acute exercise is hypoglycemia (low glucose level). Occasionally, hyperglycemia (elevated glucose level) and ketosis can occur in clients with type 1 diabetes. Hypoglycemia is a significant risk for clients who exercise while taking insulin or oral hypoglycemics. Adjustments are sometimes needed to prevent hypoglycemia in the client taking insulin, because hepatic glucose production is blocked or partially inhibited by exogenous insulin. For example, a reduction in short-acting insulin of 30% to 50% can decrease the risk of hypoglycemia. Clients who use meal planning and exercise alone to control type 2 diabetes are not at risk for hypoglycemia when exercising.

Administer Medications

ORAL ANTIDIABETES AGENTS. Five chemical classes of oral antidiabetes agents are available in the United States for the management of diabetes (Table 45–4):

- Sulfonylureas (oral hypoglycemic agents)
- Meglitinides (oral hypoglycemic agents)
- Biguanides (insulin sensitizers)
- Thiazolidinediones (also insulin sensitizers)
- Alpha-glucosidase inhibitors

Pharmacologic interventions should be considered when the client cannot achieve normal or near-normal plasma glucose levels with nutrition and exercise therapies.[42]

Oral hypoglycemic agents are effective in people with type 2 diabetes after nutrition and exercise therapy have failed. About 35% of clients with type 2 diabetes take oral hypoglycemic agents. The client most likely to respond well to oral antidiabetes agents is one who first has diabetes after age 40, has had diabetes for less than 5 years, is of normal weight or obese, and either has never received insulin or has well-controlled diabetes with less than 40 units of insulin per day. Indications for these agents are (1) random blood glucose levels less than 300 mg/dl, (2) fasting blood glucose level less than 250 mg/dl, (3) and inadequate control after exercise and diet therapies.

INSULIN THERAPY. Clients with type 1 diabetes do not produce enough insulin to sustain life. They depend on exogenous insulin administration on a daily basis. In contrast, clients with type 2 diabetes are not dependent on exogenous insulin for survival. They may need supplemental insulin for adequate glucose control, especially in times of stress or illness.

Insulin Types. Before 1991, insulin was classified by species (beef, pork, and human) and duration of action (short-, intermediate-, and long-acting). Most clients who require insulin therapy now receive human insulin produced by recombinant deoxyribonucleic acid (DNA) technology (Table 45–5).[42] Compared with animal insulins, human insulin peaks more precisely and predictably, has a shorter duration of action, and has reduced antigenicity (ability to produce antigen response), and it does not cause lipoatrophy (loss of subcutaneous fat) or lipodystrophy (fat metabolism disturbance leading to loss of subcutaneous fat) at the injection site.

Insulin works to lower blood glucose by promoting the transport of glucose into cells, and by inhibiting the conversion of glycogen and amino acids to glucose. The type and species of the insulin used, injection technique, site of injection, level of insulin antibodies, and individual client response all can affect the onset, peak, and duration of action of insulin. Insulin injected into the abdomen is absorbed fastest, with less rapid-absorption after injection into the arm and leg, respectively. Insulin inhalers are being developed and may replace the syringes used for insulin injection. The normal secretory pattern of endogenous insulins follows a basal-level secretion, with increased production in response to an incoming carbohydrate load. In clients with type 1 diabetes, the goal is to mimic this increase with injections of exogenous insulin.

Humalog, an insulin analog, was released in 1996. Its action and potency as a hypoglycemic agent are the same as for human regular insulin, but the onset of action is immediate after subcutaneous injection, with a duration of action of about 2 hours. Humalog should be taken immediately before eating. Humalog is approved only for subcutaneous injection or continuous insulin infusion pump use. Humalog provides many benefits in achieving glucose control and may ultimately prevent or delay diabetes-related complications. Remind clients that because Humalog works so quickly, hypoglycemia can develop rapidly if they do not consume adequate calories immediately after injection.

Insulin Dosage. Insulin therapy should be individualized. For a client with newly diagnosed diabetes, a simple regimen with fixed doses may be used at first. The starting dose of insulin is 0.5 unit/kg/day. Two thirds of the dose is commonly given in the morning, one third in the evening. The health care team works to adjust the numbers and timing of injections to smooth out normal patterns. Then the dose can be increased. Algorithms are detailed guidelines to help clients self-adjust the daily insulin dose, based on self-monitored blood glucose levels, food intake, exercise, and departures from normal routine (such as added stress or illness). These guidelines use a prospective (predictive) approach to blood glucose control.[5, 42]

Insulin dosage varies greatly (Fig. 45–2). In determining it, the health care team must consider both the client's requirements and the client's response to the insulin. After initial stabilization, the team helps the client learn how to make adjustments in insulin doses, timing, food intake, and exercise. Unexplained fluctuations in blood glucose often occur. The team needs to help the client feel confident in his or her ability to control the diabetes.

Insulin Pump Therapy. Small portable pumps for the continuous administration of regular insulin are sometimes used (Fig. 45–3). The small pump, worn externally, injects insulin subcutaneously into the abdomen through an indwelling needle site that is usually changed daily. Insulin is normally infused at a low basal rate (a rate that matches the client's basal metabolic needs), with additional infusion of larger amounts (boluses) of insulin before meals.

Insulin pumps commonly improve blood glucose control by means of continuous subcutaneous insulin infusion. However, they do not have a built-in feedback mechanism for monitoring blood glucose levels. To benefit from use of an insulin pump, the client must comply with dietary requirements and usually must deliver the correct premeal bolus of insulin. The client must also monitor blood glucose levels four to six times a day and make decisions about dosages by using problem-solving skills.[1] Complications from use of insulin pumps include infection at the injection site, hypoglycemia from pump malfunction or mistakes in calculating the insulin dosage,

TABLE 45–4 NURSING IMPLICATIONS FOR ORAL ANTIDIABETIC MEDICATIONS

Class with Example Drug	Action(s)	Therapeutic Outcomes	Adverse Outcomes	Dosing
FIRST-GENERATION SULFONYLUREAS				
Chlorpropamide (Diabinese) Includes short-acting, intermediate-acting, and long-acting drugs	Stimulates beta cells of pancreas to secrete insulin Mild diuretic	Control of type 2 diabetes mellitus with blood glucose levels within preset parameters*	Monitor for hypoglycemia and hyperglycemia Monitor for hyponatremia in elderly May cause photosensitivity Monitor for weight gain, gastrointestinal and hematologic defects Increased risk of hyperglycemia with infection, fever, surgery, trauma, injury	Take 1–3 times/day with meals Avoid alcohol as it may result in hypoglycemia Allopurinol, clofibrate, aspirin, anticoagulants, anticonvulsants, beta-blockers may enhance action of drug and lead to hypoglycemia Caffeine, nicotine, glucocorticoids, NSAIDs, oral contraceptives, cough and cold medicines, thiazide diuretics, barbiturates, thyroid hormone, and phenothiazines may decrease action of drug and lead to hyperglycemia Women should avoid if pregnant or breast-feeding
SECOND-GENERATION SULFONYLUREAS				
Glipizide (Glucotrol)	Increases tissue response to insulin (insulin sensitizer); decreases glucose production by liver; stimulates beta cells to secrete insulin Mild diuretic	Control of type 2 diabetes mellitus with blood glucose levels within preset parameters*	Monitor for adverse outcomes similar to those seen with first-generation sulfonylureas	Take 1–2 times/day 30 minutes before breakfast (and evening meal if 2 times/day) Avoid alcohol and medications as described with first-generation sulfonylureas Women should avoid if pregnant or breast-feeding
BIGUANIDES				
Metformin (Glucophage)	Increases tissue response to insulin (insulin sensitizer); decreases hepatic production of glucose; decreases absorption of glucose from small intestine; decreases triglyceride and low-density lipoprotein levels	Control of type 2 diabetes mellitus with blood glucose levels within preset parameters* Decreases amount of insulin needed by type 2 diabetics who use insulin (research shows moderate decrease in insulin needed for type 1 diabetics, but no FDA approval for use in type 1 diabetics)	Monitor for lactic acidosis Hypoglycemia and hyperglycemia not seen because drug does not stimulate beta cells to produce insulin; clients taking other antidiabetic drugs, however, may experience these effects Long-term use results in decreased absorption of amino acids, vitamin B_{12}, folic acid May cause metallic taste at start of therapy	Take 1–3 times/day with or before meals; often given with sulfonylureas or insulin Hold for 24 hours before and after contrast media containing iodine Alcohol, Histamine H_2-receptor antagonists, calcium-channel blockers, and diuretics may increase effect of drug and result in hypoglycemia Avoid in pregnancy, during breast-feeding, in kidney or liver disease Decreases half-life of furosemide

TABLE 45–4 NURSING IMPLICATIONS FOR ORAL ANTIDIABETIC MEDICATIONS *Continued*

Class with Example Drug	Action(s)	Therapeutic Outcomes	Adverse Outcomes	Dosing
ALPHA-GLUCOSIDASE INHIBITORS				
Acarbose (Precose)	Delays digestion of complex carbohydrates and certain sugars, so blunts peak of blood glucose and insulin levels after meals	Control of type 2 diabetes mellitus with blood glucose levels within preset parameters*	Monitor for gastrointestinal effects of flatulence, diarrhea, distension Monitor liver function studies every 3 months Does not cause hypoglycemia, but blood sugar can become so low that client becomes hypoglycemic	Take 3 times/day before meal or with first bite Give with sulfonylurea or metformin, but watch for hypoglycemia Calcium-channel blocker, estrogen, oral contraceptives, thyroid hormone, thiazide diuretics may decrease action of drug and result in hyperglycemia
MEGLITINIDES				
Repaglinide (Prandin)	Stimulates insulin secretion via closing or inhibition of ATP-sensitive K^+ channels in beta cells	Control of type 2 diabetes mellitus with blood glucose levels within preset parameters*	Monitor for hypoglycemia Monitor for hyperglycemia if infection, fever, trauma, or surgery Monitor for upper respiratory infections, which occur more frequently	Take 30 minutes before or with meals 1–3 times/day Given most often with metformin If dose is missed, skip it and take next dose with next meal; skip dose if meal is skipped Calcium-channel blockers, diuretics, beta-blockers, oral contraceptives, estrogen, thyroid hormone may decrease action of drug and result in hyperglycemia
THIAZOLIDINEDIONES				
Rosiglitazone (Avandia)	Increases insulin action at receptors and postreceptor level in hepatic and peripheral tissue (decreases insulin resistance) Decreases triglycerides	Control of type 2 diabetes mellitus with blood glucose levels within preset parameters* Decrease insulin dosage for type 1 and type 2 diabetes if >30 units of insulin/day (dosage may be decreased 10–25%)	Monitor for hypoglycemia in client taking insulin or sulfonylurea	Take once a day before breakfast Avoid cholestyramine because it will decrease drug absorption and lead to hyperglycemia May lead to pregnancy by decreasing effect of oral contraceptives Usually given with sulfonylurea or insulin

* Preset parameters are generally considered to be fasting blood glucose level of 70–130 mg/dl; 2-hour postprandial blood glucose level of <160 mg/dl; glycosylated hemoglobin (HbA_{1C}) of <7.0.
NSAIDs, nonsteroidal anti-inflammatory drugs.

and diabetic ketoacidosis from injecting too little insulin to meet regular or increased metabolic needs.

At the start of insulin pump therapy, the client must be supervised carefully in either an inpatient or an outpatient setting. During this time, the clinician adjusts the pump for basal and bolus doses before meals, according to the client's usual diet and exercise regimen and previous insulin requirements. Researchers are trying to produce an implantable pump that not only administers insulin but also monitors blood glucose levels, much as a normal pancreas does.

INTENSIVE DIABETES THERAPY. In 1983, the NIDDK launched a 10-year, randomized clinical trial to assess the safety and determine the benefits of intensive

TABLE 45–5 TYPES OF HUMAN INSULIN AND COMPARATIVE ACTIONS

Action	Preparation	Appearance	Action (h)*		
			Onset	*Peak*	*Duration*
Short-acting	Humalog (insulin lispro injection)	Clear	Immediate	0.5–1.5	2–4
	Regular	Clear	½–1	2–3	3–6
Intermediate-acting	NPH	Cloudy	2–4	4–10	10–16
	Lente	Cloudy	3–4	4–12	12–18
	Premixed (70% NPH, 30% regular)	Cloudy	½–1	Two peaks: 3–4, 8–12	16–24
Long-acting	Ultralente	Cloudy	6–10	None	18–20

* Absorption rates may vary by 20%–40% from day to day in any one client.

diabetes therapy. The most comprehensive diabetes study ever conducted, it compared the effects of two different treatment methods on the long-term development of diabetes complications—specifically, eye, kidney, and nerve disease.[22]

Twenty-nine medical centers in the United States and Canada enrolled 1441 people in the study; 52% were men and 48% were women. The average age at entry was 27 years. To participate in the study, volunteers had to be 13 to 19 years old; to have had type 1 diabetes for at least 1 year but no more than 15 years; to have no manifestations or only early manifestations of diabetic complications; and to be taking no more than two insulin injections a day. After being invited to participate in the study, clients were randomly assigned to either an intensive treatment group or a conventional treatment group.

Clients in the intensive treatment group learned to adjust their insulin doses to keep their blood glucose levels as close to normal as possible. Treatment included three or more insulin injections a day or the use of an insulin pump, self-monitoring of blood glucose levels four or more times a day, a special diet, an initial hospital stay, and weekly to monthly clinic visits. Clients in the conventional treatment group followed a regimen used by most people with type 1 diabetes: insulin injections once or twice a day, daily self-monitoring of blood glucose, and clinic visits every 3 months. Researchers monitored clients in both groups for signs of diabetic eye disease (retinopathy) as well as kidney (nephropathy) and nerve (neuropathy) disease.

Results of the trial indicated that intensive therapy delayed the onset or slowed the progression of chronic complications of diabetes by 35% to more than 70%. The risk of hypoglycemia was three times higher in the intensive treatment group than in the conventional treatment group. However, the risk of hypoglycemia was believed to be greatly outweighed by the reduction in microvascular and neurologic complications. On the basis of these results, it is recommended that clients with type 1 diabetes receive closely monitored intensive regimens. However, intensive therapy should be implemented with caution in clients who have repeated severe hypoglycemia or an unawareness of hypoglycemia.

With the intensive therapy approach, the client must be willing to monitor blood glucose levels four to six times a day and take three to five insulin injections a day. Throughout the initiating period of intensive therapy, the clinician must assess the client's knowledge of the meal plan, monitoring techniques, management goals, and manifestations of and interventions for hyperglycemia and hypoglycemia. The client also needs to be made aware of the extra financial and emotional burdens of this approach. The family and significant others need to be involved in the teaching process. Finally, the client needs to know that neither protocol is guaranteed to prevent long-term complications.[35]

COMBINATION THERAPY. *Combination therapy* is defined as the use of two or more oral antidiabetes agents or an oral agent combined with insulin. The advantage is that because the various groups of oral agents have different sites and mechanisms of action, they can complement and even augment each other.

In some clients with type 2 diabetes (mostly non-obese clients) in whom sulfonylurea agents alone failed to normalize blood glucose levels, insulin therapy has been required to achieve metabolic control very early in the course of disease. In these clients, daily insulin dosage is markedly higher than in clients with type 1 diabetes. This is attributed to insulin resistance. Because sulfonylurea agents enhance the effect of endogenous insulin by reducing insulin resistance, it has been thought that combining insulin therapy with sulfonylureas may be effective. One prescribed regimen is an injection of an intermediate-acting insulin at bedtime with daytime coverage by a sulfonylurea. This regimen is commonly called BIDS (*b*edtime *i*nsulin with *d*aytime *s*ulfonylurea).[38]

Nursing Management of the Medical Client

Diabetes self-management is the responsibility of clients and their families. The client with diabetes must be empowered to accept self-management and to become the focus of the team approach to treatment. Physiologic treatment of manifestations is neither the means nor the end of responsibility in dealing with a chronic disease like diabetes. Clients require consistent follow-up, updating, and reinforcement. Assessment of the client's level of acceptance of personal responsibility is necessary. This guides the practitioner to appropriate teaching and behavioral techniques to encourage a higher level of acceptance on the client's part.

Because of the multidisciplinary nature of the treatment, a team approach is recommended in managing clients with diabetes. This approach is particularly appropriate for client education when learners must acquire knowledge and skills from a variety of disciplines. Crucial members of the health care team include, whenever possible, a nurse, a dietitian, and a physician as the core members. Depending on need and availability, other members may include a psychologist, a social worker, a pharmacist, an exercise physiologist, and a podiatrist. Team meetings are planned to share information gained from individual client assessments and to develop a plan of action to respond to the client's clinical and educational priorities. The integration of various roles within the team strengthens the communication essential to client self-management.

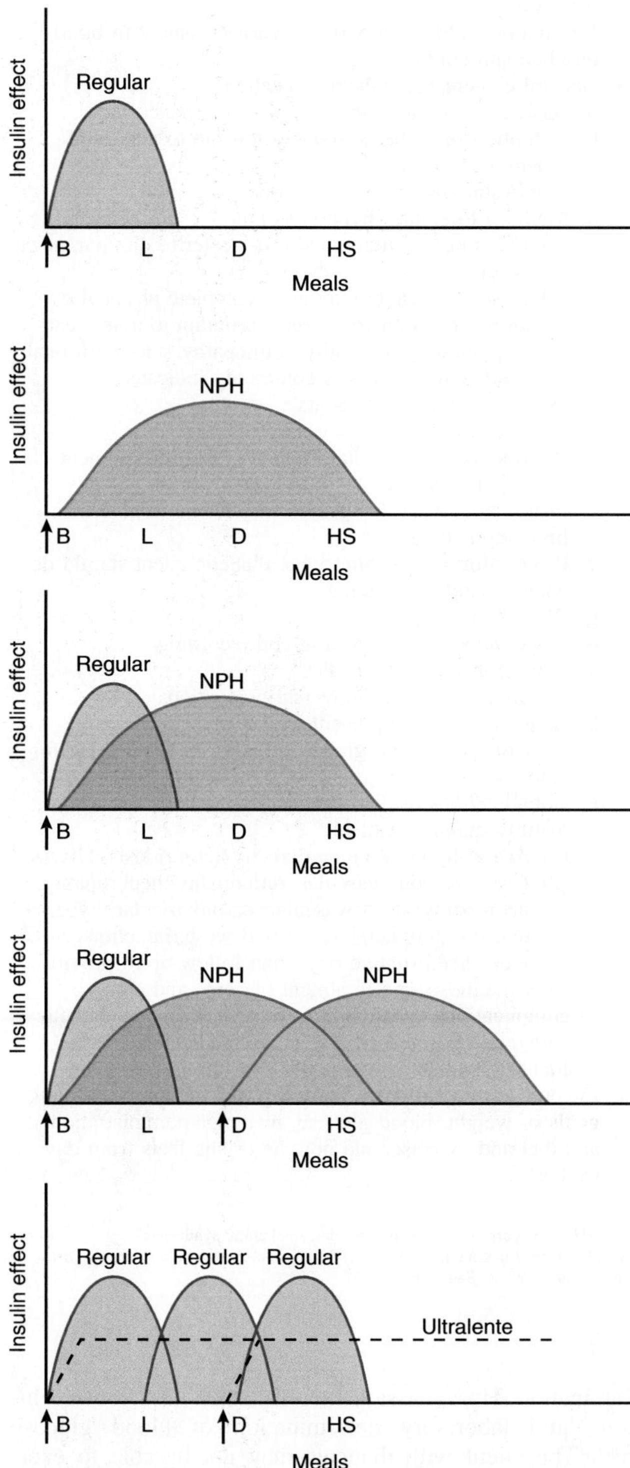

FIGURE 45–2 Insulin regimens. Only a few of a variety of possible regimens are shown here. Some clients require only one injection per day, whereas others may require split mixed doses (such as mixtures of NPH or Ultralente and regular insulin) or several doses of the same type of insulin (such as NPH insulin). Insulin regimens must be individualized for each client. B, breakfast; L, lunch; D, dinner; HS, bedtime.

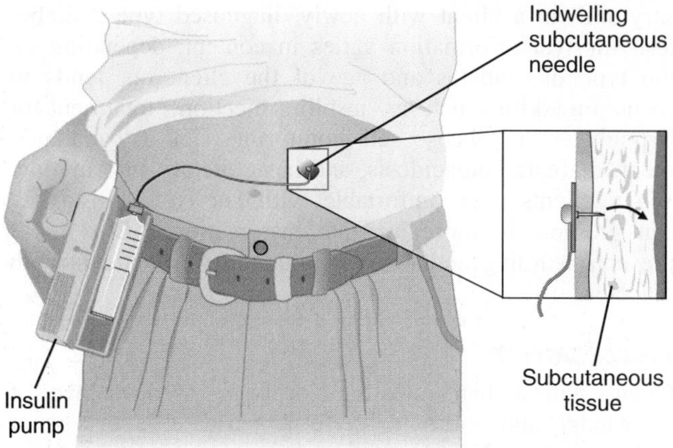

FIGURE 45–3 Insulin pumps are worn externally and connected to an indwelling subcutaneous needle, usually inserted in the abdomen.

There are two approaches to diabetes education[14, 15, 25]:

- The *compliance-based approach* is intended to improve client adherence to the treatment recommendations of health care professionals. It is based on the assumption that health care professionals are diabetes care experts and that in general, clients should comply with their recommendations regarding diabetes self-management.
- In the *empowerment-based approach,* the primary purpose of diabetes education is to prepare clients to make informed decisions about their own diabetes care. This approach assumes that most clients with diabetes are responsible for making important and complex decisions.

Few members of the health care team use one approach all the time to the exclusion of the other approach. Indeed, many health care professionals use some combination of the two approaches based on their own values and understanding of the purposes of education. For example, clients with newly diagnosed diabetes may wish to have the health care team make most of the decisions until they become familiar with the costs and benefits of various options in diabetes self-management.

Survival education includes the crucial information necessary to meet the client's immediate survival needs. These vary widely from client to client. For example, insulin injection is a survival skill for a client with newly diagnosed type 1 diabetes but is unlikely to be a necessary skill in a client with newly diagnosed type 2 diabetes. Survival information varies in content, depending on the type of diabetes and age of the client but tends to focus on skills such as insulin injection, treatment of hypoglycemia, glucose self-monitoring, sick-day management, diabetic ketoacidosis, and basic dietary information. When clients are comfortable with survival skills, they can progress to more in-depth information.[28] Box 45–3 presents learning and teaching guidelines for clients with diabetes.

ASSESSMENT

Clients with diabetes must be closely assessed for level of knowledge and ability to perform self-care. The type of diabetes, clinical status of the client, and plans for treatment are also important assessments. Ask clients if they take any vitamin, mineral, or herbal supplements, whether to decrease blood glucose levels or for other purposes. Chromium and garlic may lower blood glucose and cholesterol levels, and magnesium may increase insulin sensitivity. Blueberries, especially European bilberries, may also decrease blood glucose levels. Niacin may impair glucose tolerance.

DIAGNOSIS, OUTCOMES, INTERVENTIONS

Altered Health Maintenance. The client with diabetes must be able to perform self-care to keep the condition well controlled, leading to the nursing diagnosis *Altered Health Maintenance related to lack of knowledge about diabetes mellitus, lack of knowledge about exercise regimen for diabetes management, and lack of knowledge about dietary management of diabetes mellitus.*

Outcomes. The client will relate the basic pathophysiologic mechanism of diabetes mellitus, explain the need for exercise and diet in the treatment, and list the clinical manifestations of acute and chronic complications. The client will plan an exercise program to maintain blood glucose levels at preset levels and will identify strategies to monitor for and prevent complications associated with exercise.

The client will state the relationship of dietary management to blood glucose control, and will choose foods that meet caloric needs and offer a well-balanced diet. The client will recognize the times at which it is necessary to substitute a food to maintain blood glucose control. The client will discuss with the health care team difficulties seen in compliance with plans for diet, maintain blood glucose levels within preset parameters, and maintain weight within preset parameters.

Interventions

Explain the Pathophysiology of Diabetes. You or a diabetes educator should explain to the client and family the basic pathophysiologic mechanism of diabetes and how the disorder is managed. Sometimes the information is given through classes or by videotape. The client should also receive some form of written information to reinforce the material. Also, the client should be monitored for denial or anger about the diagnosis as part of a coping response.

Plan an Exercise Program. Clients with diabetes must consult the clinician before starting an exercise program. Pre-exercise screening may include a history, physical examination, HbA_{1C} assay, exercise stress test, foot evaluation, and laboratory determination of blood glucose level. The client with diabetes may not be able to exercise intensely to achieve a calculated heart rate because of a pre-existing cardiac condition, advanced age, or joint problems. The client should be helped to choose an exercise regimen and to set reasonable goals, because any increase in activity level is beneficial. Walking is usually well tolerated. Using a stationary bicycle or swimming is possible for clients with foot problems.

BOX 45–3 Learning and Teaching Guidelines for Clients with Diabetes

1. Assess knowledge about diabetes mellitus, correct misinformation
2. Reteach or build on previously learned content to build baseline and confidence
3. General content for diabetic education
   a. Basic anatomy and physiology of the pancreas
   b. Definition of diabetes and relationship to abnormal function of pancreas
   c. Manifestations of hyperglycemia
   d. Methods to control hyperglycemia
      (1) Diet must be individualized—refer to dietitian accordingly
      (2) Exercise—client may need complete physical examination prior to exercise program to assess cardiac status, neuropathy, retinopathy, and nutritional needs (weight loss is commonly indicated)
      (3) Oral antidiabetic agents
      (4) Insulin
      (5) Recognize precipitating factors for development of hyperglycemia
   e. Insulin education: how/when/why/where to give insulin combinations
   f. Basic information about what diabetic client should do when ill and/or traveling
   g. When to call physician
   h. Daily blood glucose testing and recording
   i. Storing insulin and needles
   j. Needle disposal and universal precautions
   k. Using and recycling needles
   l. How to use a blood glucose monitor and test urine for ketones
   m. Complications of diabetes mellitus—definition, cause, manifestations, treatment
      (1) *Acute:* hypoglycemia, diabetic ketoacidosis, HHNS
      (2) *Chronic:* microvascular: retinopathy, nephropathy, neuropathy; macrovascular: cardiovascular, hypertension, peripheral vascular disease, infections
   n. Diabetics need routine physician follow-up to provide early diagnosis and treatment of acute and chronic complications, evaluation of present means of diabetic care, and treatment of coexisting medical disorders
   o. Identify available community and family resources
4. Encourage client to keep written goals and diary outlining goals of weight, blood glucose, medicine administration, and diet and exercise, and how he or she feels from day to day.

HHNS, hyperglycemic, hyperosmolar, nonketotic syndrome.
Adapted from Luckmann, J. (Ed.). (1995). *Saunders manual of nursing care.* Philadelphia: W. B. Saunders.

Clients with diabetes must start any new activity at a well-tolerated intensity level and duration, with gradual (over a period of weeks or months) increases in intensity and duration until preset exercise goals are reached. Exercise should include warm-up and cool-down periods before and after the activity. It is best to exercise at the same time of day, if possible. Because regular exercise is very important, have the client plan an alternative activity in case environmental or other factors make the usual exercise difficult. Unplanned exercise can be dangerous for clients taking insulin or oral hypoglycemic agents. During periods of exercise, the muscles are stimulated to take up glucose. Therefore, blood glucose levels can fall abruptly.[27]

Prevent Complications from Exercise. Clients should make sure they are adequately hydrated before starting exercise. They should eat 15 to 30 g of carbohydrate before exercise if the blood glucose level is less than 100 mg/dl and should carry a carbohydrate snack as well as their diabetes identification. If blood glucose is 100 to 150 mg/dl, the client may exercise and have a snack later. If blood glucose is greater than 250 mg/dl and the client has not just eaten, ketone levels should be checked. Clients with glucose at this level should wait to exercise, because vigorous activity can raise blood glucose levels by releasing stored glycogen. Alcohol and beta-blockers should be avoided because they may increase the risk of hypoglycemia or hyperglycemia.[27]

Plan Nutrition Therapy to Achieve Target Blood Glucose. A balanced nutritional plan is important for all clients, whether or not they have diabetes. Emphasize to the client and family members that they are not eating a "diabetic diet" but, rather, are following a balanced meal plan. Adherence to nutrition principles is one of the most challenging aspects of diabetes management. It requires a team effort. For an effective plan, assessment of the person's present eating patterns, knowledge of a healthy eating plan, and willingness and ability to modify patterns and nutritional needs is vital. Specific nutritional information should include the following[9]:

- Appetite
- Food allergies
- Ethnic and cultural influence on food habits
- Ability to obtain and prepare food (including financial ability)
- Community resources currently used
- Amount and type of physical activity
- Chronic disease requiring dietary modification
- Gastrointestinal disease
- Vitamin, mineral, or food supplements used
- Weight patterns
- Current eating patterns
- Dietary concerns of client
- Dental and oral health
- Medications with nutritional implications

The results of this assessment form a personal profile used to arrive at individualized goals. As a member of the health care team, you must have a knowledge base of both nutritional assessment and appropriate interventions.

Basic nutritional assessment includes anthropometric measures, biochemical tests, physical assessment, and dietary evaluation. No single parameter can measure the client's nutritional status or determine problems or needs. Figure 45–4 shows how assessment fits into the total nutritional plan for the collaborative management of diabetes. After the assessment, individualized goals are determined. Nutritional assessment and the client's understanding that optimal nutrition can lead to reduction of risk factors for chronic health problems and improve overall health constitute the starting point for goal selection.

For example, if the client has type 2 diabetes and is obese, emphasize that nutritional changes can help to lower blood glucose levels, decrease lipid levels, and lower blood pressure as well as help in losing weight. Weight loss also appears to increase insulin sensitivity and to normalize liver glucose production. The client should understand that dietary treatment is the best and initial treatment. If nutritional status does not improve, glucose-lowering medications, insulin, lipid-lowering agents, or antihypertensives may be required.

A standard "diabetic diet" is no longer prescribed for all clients with diabetes; instead, many dietary options exist (Table 45–6). Basically, the client with diabetes should strive to follow the Dietary Guidelines for Americans (the "Food Guide Pyramid") issued by the U.S. Department of Agriculture (USDA) and U.S. Department of Health and Human Services (USDHHS) in 1992 for current recommended nutritional guidelines.[40]

Calories. Caloric restrictions, especially for people with lifelong obesity, may be perceived negatively. Obesity is a complex interaction between genetic and environmental factors. The most successful approach to weight reduction is unclear, but you should understand caloric restriction, regular exercise, behavior modification, and peer and professional support. Moderate caloric reduction is described as a reduction of 250 to 500 calories per day less than usual. Reduction of fat calories may be a good initial modification. Regular exercise (three to five times weekly) enhances weight loss and is a predictor for successful weight maintenance.[9]

Protein. In general, Americans with and without diabetes consume more protein than needed to meet nutritional

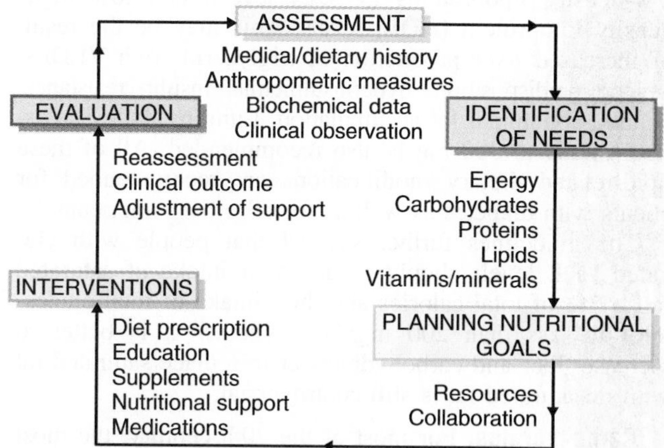

FIGURE 45–4 Assessment as part of the total nutritional plan for the collaborative management of diabetes. (Redrawn from Groth, K. [1995]. Nutritional alterations in critical illness. In L. C. Copstead [Ed.], *Perspectives on pathophysiology* [p. 1124]. Philadelphia: W. B. Saunders.)

TABLE 45–6 CURRENTLY RECOMMENDED NUTRITIONAL GUIDELINES FOR THE CLIENT WITH DIABETES MELLITUS

Calories	Sufficient to achieve and maintain reasonable weight
Protein	Adequate to ensure maintenance of body protein stores; people with diabetes have the same protein requirements as for non-diabetic people; in general 10%–20% of the total daily calories should come from protein (equal to ~0.8 g/kg/day)
Fats	Less than 30% of calories should be from fat, with less than 10% of that from saturated fat sources; if individualized risk factors indicate elevated VLDL and LDL levels, total calories from saturated fat may be reduced to 7%; cholesterol intake should be limited to 300 mg/day or less
Carbohydrates	50% to 60% of total calories should be from carbohydrates; simple and complex sugars do not differ appreciably in their ability to worsen hyperglycemia
Fiber	Clients with diabetes are urged to consume 20–35 g of fiber per day, which is the same as the recommendation for all Americans

LDL, low-density lipoprotein; VLDL, very-low-density lipoprotein.

needs. Protein should be incorporated into the diet through a variety of foods. Very-low-calorie diets are often deficient in protein and may result in accelerated protein breakdown. High protein intake increases renal workload and glomerular filtration rate. Some studies in people with diabetes indicate that lowering protein intake may delay progression of nephropathy. At present, the lower end of the recommended scale for protein intake (about 10% of daily calories) is sufficiently restricted and is recommended for clients with nephropathy. In certain cases, protein requirements vary from the adult recommended daily allowance; this is true for infants, children, adolescents, and pregnant women.[9]

Fat. The USDA national food consumption surveys reveal that most Americans eat too much fat. About 36% of calories in the average adult diet comes from fat, with about 13% from saturated fat. The general recommendation for Americans is to decrease total dietary fat to 30% or less of total calories, with saturated fat decreased to less than 10%. This reduction is consistent with a diet to reduce cardiovascular disease.

Clients with type 2 diabetes often have high triglyceride levels, high low-density lipoprotein (LDL) levels, high very-low-density lipoproteins (VLDL) levels, and low high-density lipoprotein (HDL) levels. This may be the result of increased liver production of triglyceride-rich VLDLs, genetic predisposition, hyperinsulinemia, insulin resistance, or intra-abdominal fat accumulation. Limiting daily cholesterol intake to 300 mg is also recommended. All of these lipid-related dietary modifications are recommended for clients with diabetes as well as for all other Americans.[9]

The guidelines further suggest that people with elevated LDL levels should reduce their intake of saturated fat to 7% of total calories and their intake of total cholesterol to less than 200 mg/day. Whether it is better to increase fiber and carbohydrates or to replace saturated fat with unsaturated fat is still controversial.

Carbohydrates. For most of the 20th century, the most widely held belief about dietary treatment of diabetes was that sugar was to be avoided. Little or no scientific evidence supports this assumption. When fed as a single nutrient, sucrose produces a glycemic response similar to that for bread or pasta. In the United States, the average diet obtains almost half of total carbohydrate intake in the form of simple sugars. Clinical guidelines suggest that 50% to 60% of the diet should consist of carbohydrates, in either simple or complex form. An occasional high-sucrose dessert poses no problem for the client with diabetes when it is accounted for in the day's total caloric and carbohydrate plan. Because some desserts are also high in fat, however, they should be limited.[9]

Working as a team with the client and a nutritionist, make a concrete medical nutrition therapy plan. The following are some helpful questions to ask the client:

- What is your most important goal in managing your diabetes?
- What are some changes you would like to make?
- Of the changes we have talked about, what would you like to work on first?

Team members must remember their roles as providers of information and counselors. Most counseling on nutrition begins with basic overviews of nutrition, diabetes guidelines, and reading of labels. More in-depth counseling on meal planning and calorie counting, for example, can come later. Eating plans vary widely among clients. Consistency within an eating style results in lower levels of glycosylated hemoglobin than does a haphazard eating style.

Diet management for clients with type 1 diabetes. Meals should be adjusted to match insulin action. Breakfast should be eaten within 1 hour after the morning insulin dose and a carbohydrate should be eaten about 3 hours later; lunch should be eaten about 4 to 5 hours after the morning insulin dose. When multiple insulin injections are used, greater flexibility with meal timing is possible.

The following are examples of approaches used successfully to instruct clients with diabetes:

- Handouts available from government sources, such as the USDA's "Food Guide Pyramid"[40] and the USDHHS publication, which uses the four-basic-food-groups approach[39]
- Individualized menus shaped between the client and dietitian
- The exchange system, last revised in 1986, which help with uniform meal planning (available from the ADA

in a simple pamphlet called "Healthy Food Choices," or in an expanded version called "Exchange Lists for Meal Planning")

- Counting components of the diet, such as counting calories and grams of fat
- A point system that utilizes lists of foods with point values and a prescribed number of total points
- The total available glucose system, which looks at foods in terms of their metabolic effects (highly motivated clients who desire flexibility may like this system)

A registered dietitian—preferably a certified diabetes educator—should always be consulted for initial evaluation and teaching of any client with a new diagnosis of diabetes. Each client should receive an individualized meal plan based on ethnic, religious, and cultural background; eating, cooking, and work habits; and food preferences. All clients need to know the dietary basics, which include the following:

- Avoid adding sugar to foods such as coffee and cereal.
- Avoid foods that are sweetened with sugar or honey, such as jellies, jams, cakes, and ice cream.
- Check blood glucose levels regularly.
- Keep periodic appointments with health care providers for evaluation of blood glucose control.
- Be consistent about the amount, distribution, and timing of nutrients.
- Increase the amount of carbohydrate in a meal eaten before sustained exercise.
- Limit intake of saturated fat and cholesterol.

Risk for Ineffective Management of Therapeutic Regimen. A client with diabetes must understand and be able to self-monitor glucose levels and learn self-injection of insulin, leading to the nursing diagnosis of *Risk for Ineffective Management of Therapeutic Regimen (Individuals) related to lack of knowledge and lack of previous experience with testing blood and urine and lack of knowledge and lack of experience with self-injection of insulin.*

Outcomes. The client will state personal goals for urine ketone and blood glucose testing parameters; demonstrate correct techniques for blood glucose testing (including timing), and demonstrate correct technique for urine ketone testing (including timing). The client will test blood glucose at regular times (including during illnesses and when traveling), and will prick the side of the finger, where nerve endings are fewer and more blood is available. The client will test urine for ketones when the glucose level is high (>250 mg/dl) or during illnesses; keep a record of all tests performed and bring this record to regular, scheduled follow-up visits; and store testing materials away from heat, light, and moisture.

The client will state that insulin lowers blood glucose, and will name the type or types of insulin prescribed and the onset, peak, and duration of each. The client will take injections at regular times, 30 to 60 minutes before meals, every day, even when ill. The client will wash hands before preparing insulin injections, demonstrate proper mixing of insulin, and withdraw prescribed dosage using sterile technique.

When taking two types of insulin, the client will withdraw the prescribed dosage of each insulin into one syringe without contaminating either bottle (regular insulin is drawn up first). The client will demonstrate the correct technique of insulin injection, and inject insulin into the same area to ensure consistency in onset, peak, and duration of action. The client will store at least one extra bottle of insulin in the refrigerator, not use insulin past the expiration date, and will purchase insulin syringes before all of the current supply has been used.

The client will wear medical identification (Medic-Alert) bracelet or necklace, or carry a diabetic identification card. The client will state manifestations, describe treatment of hypoglycemia, and will always carry something to treat hypoglycemia.

Interventions

Provide Instruction on Blood Glucose Monitoring. All clients with newly diagnosed diabetes mellitus require teaching about urine and blood glucose monitoring. All clients with diabetes may require review or update of information for self-care. Newer, more accurate blood glucose meters that are easier to use are constantly being made available. Only the basics are covered in this discussion, so you must keep up to date on each meter's advantages and disadvantages.

Many kinds of meters are available. Each client needs to be evaluated so that the proper meter is obtained. The client's ability to calibrate the meter and to visually interpret the digital reading must be considered. Some meters can be connected to a computer, which can convert blood glucose results into bar graphs or other printouts. Glucose meters are available for the visually impaired that give

MANAGEMENT AND DELEGATION

Measuring and Recording Blood Glucose Levels

The measurement and recording of blood glucose levels may be delegated to unlicensed assistive personnel. Delegate the data collection only to those who have demonstrated competency in performing this task. Consider the following issues:

- Initial orientation and demonstration of competence in the performance of blood glucose monitoring, including quality control and equipment management requirements.
- Instruction on the time schedule and frequency to obtain blood glucose levels.
- Proper method of recording and reporting of the blood glucose level.
- Rotation of sites from which to obtain samples in order to minimize patient discomfort.

You are responsible for defining those blood glucose levels that are immediately reportable to you (for example, levels outside the range of 70 to 180 mg/dl). Instruct assistive personnel to report any difficulty in obtaining the sample or concerns the client may raise during the process of obtaining a sample.

Verify the competency of assistive personnel in performing blood glucose level testing during orientation and annually thereafter.

Marsha E. Cloud, BSN, RN, *Clinician II, Surgical Services, University of Virginia Health System, Charlottesville, Virginia*

audio commands for use of the device and announce the blood glucose reading.

In addition to demonstrating the techniques of blood glucose self-monitoring, discuss the normal blood glucose range, goals for good control (individualized for each client), when to test, how to record test results, and what to do for abnormal results. Consult a diabetes educator for assistance in helping the client choose an optimal meter.

Clients can use blood glucose strips if they are unable or unwilling to purchase a meter. Make sure the client is not color blind and can read the results accurately. Compare the client's results with blood glucose meter readings to check for accuracy. With some meters and strips, a 15% difference is seen between capillary blood and venous blood glucose levels. The capillary blood reading is lower. When insulin is being adjusted, make sure to account for this difference. As long as the source of blood is consistent, no adjustment is required.

Both health care agencies and clients need to verify the accuracy of their blood glucose determinations. The Joint Commission on Accreditation of Healthcare Organizations (JCAHO) and other regulating bodies dictate the procedure and frequency for quality control of meters used in health care agencies. The usefulness of many glucose meters is technique-dependent. Because treatment is based on results, correct methods of use must be ensured. Clients can perform a self-test and simultaneously send a blood specimen to the laboratory to compare results. Manufacturers of meters also provide quality-control testing solutions, which clients should be instructed to use routinely (weekly, for example). Quality control of glucose monitors is a constantly changing area; nurses and clients must keep up to date (see Management and Delegation).

Provide Instruction on Urine Testing. Urine testing for glucose is rarely done; however, urine can be tested for ketones (beta-hydroxybutyric acid, acetoacetic acid, and acetone). These substances appear in the urine of clients who are fasting, clients with poorly controlled type 1 diabetes, and clients with type 1 or type 2 diabetes who have a secondary illness. Ketones result from fat metabolism and are therefore present during fasting.[37] In a client with diabetes, however, the presence of ketones may indicate the serious complication of diabetic ketoacidosis (see later).

Provide Instruction on Insulin Administration. When administered correctly, insulin acts as a life-saving medication for the insulin-dependent client. When administered incorrectly, it may cause complications ranging from tissue damage to lethal hypoglycemia (*insulin shock*). To administer insulin properly, the client must be familiar with insulin concentrations, syringes, storage, preparation for injection, and techniques for self-injection, as outlined in the Client Education Guide.[5] Insulin inhalers may someday replace insulin injection syringes.

Insulin concentrations. Insulin is prescribed in units. Thus, pharmaceutical companies prepare types of insulin—such as NPH, regular, or Lente—in 10-ml glass vials that contain 100 units/mL. U-100 insulin contains 100 units of insulin per milliliter. It is the insulin of choice for nearly all clients. Those who require large amounts of insulin may benefit from using U-500 insulin, which contains 500 units of insulin per milliliter and is available in the United States only by prescription.[5, 42]

CLIENT EDUCATION GUIDE

Self-Injection of Insulin

Procedure

1. Wash hands.
2. Clean site with soap and water or 70% isopropyl alcohol (optional).
3. Store insulin vial in original carton to keep clean (or wipe top of insulin vial with 70% isopropyl alcohol).
4. Shake or roll insulin vial in palm of hands to resuspend all but short-acting insulins.
5. Inject an amount of air that is equal to each dose into the bottle—short-acting last. Insulin solution should be clear.
6. Aspirate prescribed amount of short-acting insulin into syringe first, intermediate- or long-acting insulin second.
7. Inspect syringe for air bubbles.
8. Pinch up and hold skinfold and inject at 90-degree angle.
9. If you are thin or have loose skin, inject insulin at 45-degree angle to avoid an intramuscular injection, which is absorbed faster.
10. Routine aspiration is not necessary.
11. Inject insulin.
12. If injection is painful or blood or serum oozes from site, apply pressure for 5 to 10 seconds.

Disposal

State laws require that needles and syringes be disposed of as a single unit in a puncture-resistant container. It is unsafe to recap, bend, or break the needle.

Syringe Reuse

The manufacturer intends that the insulin syringe and needle be disposed after one use. Research demonstrates that most people with diabetes reuse the needle and syringe until the needle becomes dull or bent or comes in contact with any surface other than skin. Most insulins have a bacteriostatic agent in them. If you reuse syringes and needles, recap the needle after each use; reusing may carry increased risk for infection, especially if you have poor personal hygiene, acute concurrent illness, or open wounds on hands. Discuss the practice of reuse with your practitioner before initiating:

- Can you safely recap the needle?
- Can you see clearly enough?
- How is your manual dexterity?
- Do you have a visible tremor?

Store syringes at room temperature. The potential benefit of using alcohol on the needle is unknown. It may remove the silicone coat on the needle and contribute to pain at the puncture site.

Insulin syringes. The most commonly used syringe can deliver a maximum of 100 units of insulin in 1 ml. However, insulin syringes are manufactured with capacities of 0.25, 0.30, 0.50, and 1.0 ml. For smaller prescriptions (50 units, 30 units, or less), smaller syringes are used (Fig. 45–5).[5] A smaller syringe enables a more precise insulin dosage. Two lengths of needles are available: short (8 mm) and long (12.7 mm). Short needles are not recommended for obese clients because of variability of insulin absorption when injected into adipose tissue.

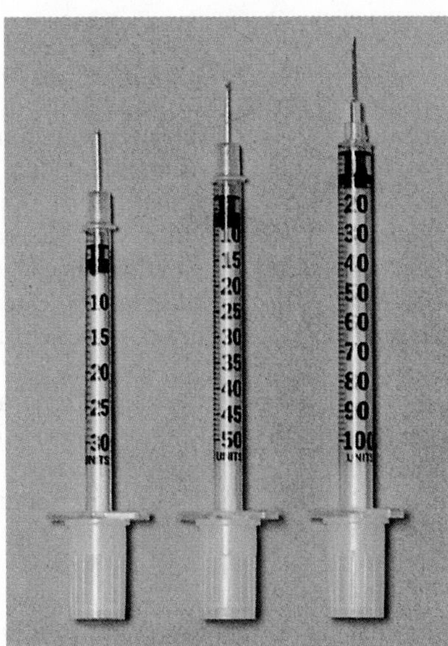

FIGURE 45–5 Examples of the sizes of insulin syringes that are available for precise measurement of insulin doses. (Courtesy of Becton Dickinson Consumer Products, Franklin Lakes, NJ.)

Insulin storage. Vials of insulin not in use should be refrigerated. Avoid temperature extremes of less than 36° F or greater than 86° F. Vials in use may be kept at room temperature. A slight loss of potency may occur after 30 days at room temperature. Humalog, regular insulin cartridges, or prefilled regular insulin pens may be kept unrefrigerated for 28 days. Because of potential variations in temperature, insulin should not be left in a car or checked in airline baggage. Mark the date on the vial when it was initially opened. The client should always have a spare vial on hand.[5, 42]

Insulin preparation and injection. Experts once thought that insulin vials should be rolled between the hands to resuspend the insulin without creating air bubbles. Now they believe that vials containing NPH and Lente suspensions should be agitated vigorously to mix the insulin to deliver consistent insulin concentrations.

To minimize the discomfort of subcutaneous insulin injection, administer the insulin at room temperature. The number of bacteria carried through a small-gauge needle is insufficient for infection to occur, and alcohol preparation is no longer considered necessary. If alcohol is used to clean the site, wait until it has evaporated completely. Have the client try to relax. Penetrate the skin quickly. Do not change the direction of the needle once it has entered the subcutaneous tissue or while it is being withdrawn.[5]

Prefilled syringes. Prefilled syringes are chemically stable for up to 3 weeks when stored vertically, needle upward (so that suspended particles do not clog the needle), in the refrigerator. Self-monitoring of blood glucose levels may need to be performed more frequently to check whether storage of the insulin in prefilled syringes alters its effectiveness in achieving glycemic control. Mixing regular and NPH insulins in one syringe is acceptable and convenient. Premixed, fixed-proportion insulins are available commercially. These insulins are not suitable when daily variations are needed in the dose or when short-acting insulin is required.[42]

Site selection and rotation. Certain sites are best used for insulin injection (Fig. 45–6). Insulin absorption varies from site to site. To avoid possibly dramatic changes in daily insulin absorption, instruct the client to give injections in one area, about an inch apart, until the whole area has been used, before changing to another site. Tell the client to avoid sites above muscles that will be exercised heavily that day, because exercise increases the rate of absorption. The client who is taking two injections daily may use one site for the morning insulin and another site for the evening insulin. Some clinicians instruct their clients to use only the abdomen because of its more even and rapid absorption rate. Emphasize the importance of adhering to a definite injection plan for avoiding tissue damage. Rotate injection sites in one area to decrease the variability of absorption.

Techniques for self-injection. Most clients who take insulin learn to give their own injections (see the Client Education Guide on Self-Injection of Insulin). It is primarily your responsibility to instruct clients with diabetes in the techniques for preparing and injecting insulin. The amount of teaching needed depends on the client's familiarity with insulin and the injection equipment.

Equipment that the client will purchase for home use includes insulin of the type prescribed, absorbent cotton,

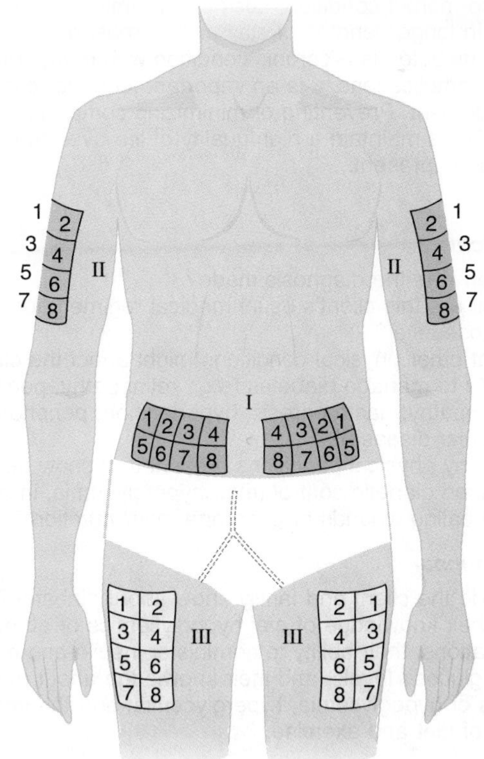

FIGURE 45–6 Sites used for insulin injection. The injection site can affect the onset, peak, and duration of action of the insulin. Insulin injected into the abdomen (area I) is absorbed fastest, followed by insulin injected into the arm (area II) and the leg (area III).

approved syringes with needles, and 70% ethyl or 91% isopropyl alcohol (optional). As noted, alcohol preparation of the injection site is no longer considered necessary, and cleansing of the top of the insulin vial may increase the risk of infection by transferring resident bacteria from fingers to the vial unless gloves are worn. Storing insulin in its original carton or in a container that will keep it clean may be a more practical option.

Although the prospect of daily injections for life is far from pleasant, the client's attitude toward this intervention may be largely influenced by your own attitude. A matter-of-fact approach helps the client understand and accept responsibility for self-care. Schedule a teaching session for self-injection techniques. Some clients find it difficult to inject the needle into their own skin. For these clients, you might select the site and insert the needle. Then, as the first step in self-injection, have the client push in the plunger and remove the needle. As the client gains confidence, self-injecting will be less traumatic. Jet injectors, which are pen-like devices, can be used.

See the Case Management feature for the diabetic client.

EVALUATION

It is expected that clients with type 1 or type 2 diabetes will learn about the disease process and methods of control. If management is successful, complications of diabetes will be avoided as much as possible. For a client with newly diagnosed type 1 diabetes, return demonstration should be expected for all activities with increasing proficiency over time. The client should not be expected to accomplish complete self-care after a single teaching session. The amount of time required varies from client to client. Follow-up visits must be initiated to make sure that the client is following recommendations and has not experienced problems with the therapeutic regimen. Over time, periodic follow-up visits will help you monitor the client's ability to perform self-care and anticipate any potential difficulties.

Self-Care

Before hospital discharge, the client and family must have a basic understanding of diabetes and its management with blood glucose monitoring, insulin injections, foot care, nutrition, and exercise. Because diabetes is a chronic

CASE MANAGEMENT

DIABETES

Although nurses may care for clients with newly diagnosed diabetes, or clients with diabetic ketoacidosis or hypoglycemia, it is much more common for a client to be admitted with another primary problem and with diabetes as a co-morbid condition. Loss of glycemic control may result in longer lengths of stay and increased cost; because diabetes is a chronic condition with many devastating complications, it is an important focus for case management. Preventing or minimizing complications can help clients maintain a high quality of life even though disease is present.

Assess

Physical

- When was the diagnosis made?
- What are this client's usual medical regimen and blood glucose level?
- What other physical conditions might affect the client's ability to manage diabetes (e.g., retinopathy, peripheral neuropathy, gastroparesis, hypertension, peripheral vascular disease)?
- Are any physical conditions present that show decreased diabetic control (e.g., hyperglycemia, infection, nonhealing wounds or gangrene, poor nutrition)?

Educational

What do the client and family know about diabetes? Assess their knowledge of oral hypoglycemics or other medications, their ability to administer insulin and monitor blood glucose levels, and their knowledge about manifestations of hypoglycemia, hyperglycemia, and the importance of diet and exercise.

Advocate

- Allow the client to continue diabetes management as independently as possible (e.g., with self-administration of insulin). Remember, consistent timing of meals and medications is important.
- Be aware of sensory deficits: for instance, during teaching, the client may need large-print materials; special equipment or pain management techniques may be needed to maintain mobility.
- Recognize and discuss the client's feelings related to chronic illness, loss, and changes in lifestyle or family role.

Prevent Readmission

- Make sure that diabetic clients have essential "survival skills," such as how to administer insulin and how to obtain help when necessary.
- Explore financial and practical issues around obtaining medications, equipment and food. Determine whether devices to assist vision-impaired clients to draw up insulin or whether prefilled syringes are needed.
- Stress follow-up with the primary care physician.
- Remind the client to keep records on glucose monitoring, diet, and exercise and to bring them to follow-up visits.
- Know when to refer the client to outpatient diabetic programs, including insurance-sponsored disease management programs.
- Consider home nursing follow-up for clients with newly diagnosed diabetes, clients with changes in management (e.g., from oral medications to insulin injections), and older clients for home nursing follow-up.

Summary

Some new diabetic clients will be started on insulin as outpatients, and newer techniques for delivering insulin via pump are changing management. However, weight reduction and control, smoking cessation, blood pressure and lipid control, infection prevention, and foot care remain important strategies to decrease diabetic complications and to avoid readmissions.

Cheryl Noetscher, RN, MS, *Director of Case Management, Cruse Hospital and Community–General Hospital, Syracuse, New York*

disorder, the client needs time to adapt to as well as to learn about the many changes that are occurring. The client should be encouraged to anticipate a usual day at work, school, or home and should be taught how and when to give insulin, how to monitor blood glucose, and what types of foods to eat.

Clients with diabetes need ongoing monitoring of their self-care ability. Glycosylated hemoglobin (HbA_{1C}) levels are usually checked, as is the client's log of daily glucose levels and insulin. Chronic changes that result from diabetes should also be assessed on an ongoing basis, by checking the client's vision, kidney function, degree of neuropathy, blood pressure, and skin condition. If the client is elderly or debilitated, home nurse visits may be an excellent asset. A referral to a visiting nurse organization or home health care agency should be initiated before discharge.

Modification for Elderly Clients

Diabetes is common among older adults and represents an important health problem for this population. Currently, 6.3 million (19%) of all people over the age of 65 years have diabetes. Many changes that occur with normal aging affect glucose levels. Blood glucose levels increase with age; fasting levels increase by about 1 mg/dl per decade and postprandial values by 6 to 13 mg/dl per decade. It is believed that peripheral receptor sites become less sensitive to insulin with time. A decline also takes place in levels of glucose-regulating hormones (glucagon and epinephrine) and in lean body mass. These changes may be accompanied by decreased physical activity and a poor diet. Elderly people are more susceptible to severe hypoglycemia, which can lead to stroke, myocardial infarction (MI), angina, or seizures. Diminished sensations may mask the manifestations of hyperglycemia. Accompanying changes in liver and kidney function and multi-drug regimens may exacerbate hypoglycemia.

In general, nutritional guidelines for older clients with diabetes are no different than those for older clients without diabetes. However, older people with diabetes are at increased risk for problems that can cause functional limitations, such as:

- Pain
- Urinary incontinence
- Decreased vision (retinopathy, glaucoma, cataracts)
- Decreased proprioception
- Postural hypotension

Impairments in mental status, functional abilities, and sensory function may interfere with the client's ability to understand and follow the treatment plan. In the older client, the risk of acute complications from hypoglycemia may outweigh the benefits of tight glucose control. The older client may enjoy good health and do very well on an individualized treatment plan. A team approach aimed at maximizing health through optimal diet and exercise, may improve the client's quality of life, as well as achieving adequate glucose control.

Surgical Management

Pancreas and Pancreas-Kidney Transplantation

Indications. Some clients with type 1 diabetes are now receiving pancreas transplants. The first pancreas transplant was completed in 1966. Eighty per cent of pancreas transplantation procedures are now done concurrently with kidney transplantation. This is usually because the anti-rejection medication cyclosporine has such severe side effects, including hyperglycemia and nephrotoxicity, that adequate renal function unaffected by nephropathy must be present. The client's own pancreas is left intact (98% of its function is exocrine in nature), and the new pancreas is usually anastomosed (attached) to the iliac artery and vein, through which insulin can enter the systemic pathway. The new pancreas is placed in the lower pelvic cavity, and the duct is connected to the urinary bladder. The exocrine secretions of the new pancreas drain into the bladder and are not absorbed. The surgical procedure generally lasts from 4 to 6 hours. Pancreas-after-kidney transplants and pancreas-only transplants account for the remaining 20% of pancreas transplantation procedures.

There has been renewed interest in the surgical technique of anastomosing the transplanted pancreas to the duodenum to allow for exocrine secretions to be absorbed normally through the gastrointestinal tract. This prevents the dehydration that is common with bladder-drained pancreas transplantation. Research is being conducted on the use of transplanted pancreatic islets rather than the entire pancreas.

Contraindications. Clients with type 1 diabetes must have well-functioning kidneys to receive only a pancreas transplant. If not, the pancreas and kidney must be transplanted simultaneously, or the pancreas must be transplanted following a successful kidney transplant. Other contraindications include problems that make the client unable to withstand the stress of surgery. Clients with type 2 diabetes do not benefit from pancreas transplantation. Type 2 diabetes results from a failure of insulin action, which cannot be improved by adding a pancreas.

Complications. Major complications of pancreas transplantation include vessel thrombosis, rejection, and infection. To help prevent thrombosis, the volume of blood flowing through the pancreas is kept at a high rate for 72 hours. Careful monitoring of laboratory values, fluid and electrolyte status, physical manifestations, and vital sign changes can alert you to possible complications. A sharp and sudden drop in urine amylase levels, rapid increases in serum glucose, gross hematuria (blood in urine), severe pain in the iliac fossa, and tenderness in the graft area are manifestations of vessel thrombosis.

Manifestations of acute and chronic graft rejection include fever, increased serum creatinine and blood urea nitrogen (BUN) levels, weight gain, and graft tenderness. Proteinuria is a primary manifestation of chronic rejection. In addition, fever, decreased urinary amylase levels, increased serum amylase levels, hyperglycemia, and graft tenderness are manifestations of graft rejection. To prevent graft rejection, immunosuppressive therapy with monoclonal antibodies (OKT3) or polyclonal antibody preparations (cyclosporine [Sandimmune], and azathioprine [Imuran] and prednisone) is administered. See Chapter 80 for further discussion of immunosuppressive agents.

Immunosuppressive drugs may be harmful to the transplant recipient. A rise in serum creatinine levels and decreased urine output may be related to the nephrotoxic effects of cyclosporine. Decreased white blood cell counts may be associated with the myelosuppressive effects of azathioprine. Other adverse effects of immunosuppressive agents for which you should monitor are discussed in Chapter 80.

Measures to prevent infection include early removal of invasive lines, adherence to sterile technique with dressing changes and catheter irrigations, pulmonary hygiene measures, and strict hand-washing practices. Antibiotics are used to treat infections.

OUTCOMES. It is expected that the client will recover from the pancreas or pancreas-kidney transplant surgery and will be discharged from the hospital within 7 to 10 days without the need for insulin. Within 3 to 4 months, the client will resume a normal life as long as medication and health care regimens are followed closely. Complications such as rejection and infection will slow postoperative progress. The client's quality of life is improved as a result of freedom from the need for insulin, return to a normal diet, and a less restricted lifestyle. Successful transplantation is indicated by improvement in blood glucose control (levels between 60 and 110 mg/dl) and C-peptide levels.

The survival rate is 91% after transplantation. More than 65% of clients who receive transplants no longer need insulin at 1 year afterward. HLA-DR matching or mismatching affects the results. See Chapter 80 for further discussion of organ transplantation.

Nursing Management of the Surgical Client

Once the client has chosen transplantation as an alternative to medical care and is placed on the recipient waiting list, he or she will need to undergo an extensive physical and psychological evaluation (see Chapter 80). Nursing care focuses on assessing the client's needs for knowledge and information.

The nursing care of the client undergoing a pancreas transplantation procedure is similar to that for any client undergoing major abdominal surgery. Postoperative care is directed not only at caring for the client's postsurgical needs but also at addressing the particular needs of a client who has undergone an organ transplant. Care of the client after organ transplantation is discussed in Chapter 80; renal transplantation is discussed briefly in Chapter 36.

The major focus of care is to monitor for rejection, adverse effects of immunsuppressive agents, infection, and occlusion of vessels. Careful monitoring for changes in vital signs, laboratory values, fluid and electrolyte status, and physical manifestations is important to determine the onset of complications—thrombosis, infection, and rejection. Serum glucose levels will range between 60 and 110 mg/dl, without administration of exogenous insulin. Urine amylase levels will remain constant, with urine pH between 7.0 and 8.5.

Immunosuppressive therapy started before surgery must be continued on a regular schedule postoperatively to prevent rejection of the new pancreas. Nursing implications for immunosuppressive agents to prevent rejection and treat rejection are described in Chapter 80.

You are responsible not only for implementing physical care immediately after transplantation but also for addressing the psychosocial needs of the client and significant others. Keep them informed about the status of the transplanted organ. Allow them to express concerns and ask questions. See Chapter 80 for further discussion of organ transplantation.

Self-Care

The self-care regimen following pancreas or pancreas-kidney transplantation is very complex for the client and significant others. Teach the client and significant others about long-term, ongoing care, which includes frequent follow-up to monitor the status of the new organ(s). Discuss self-care involved in managing medications, diet, physical activity, and manifestations of rejection and infection. Explain why continuing the present medication regimen is important and why the client should never miss a dose. Explain the manifestations of rejection and infection if the client cannot remember, needs a review, or did not receive complete information. See Chapter 80 for additional information related to transplantation.

ACUTE COMPLICATIONS OF DIABETES MELLITUS

HYPERGLYCEMIA AND DIABETIC KETOACIDOSIS

Hyperglycemia results when glucose cannot be transported to the cells because of a lack of insulin. Without available carbohydrates for cellular fuel, the liver converts its glycogen stores back to glucose (glycogenolysis) and increases the biosynthesis of glucose (gluconeogenesis). Unfortunately, however, these responses worsen the situation by raising the blood glucose level even higher.[26, 37]

In type 1 diabetes mellitus, as the need for cellular fuel grows more critical, the body begins to draw on its fat and protein stores for energy. Excessive amounts of fatty acids are mobilized from adipose tissue cells and transported to the liver. The liver, in turn, accelerates the rate at which it produces ketone bodies (ketogenesis) for catabolism by other body tissues, particularly muscle. As fat metabolism increases, the liver may produce too many ketone bodies. Ketone bodies accumulate in the blood (ketosis) and are excreted in the urine (ketonuria). Metabolic acidosis develops from the acidic (pH-lowering) effect of the ketones acetoacetate and beta-hydroxybutyrate. This condition is called *diabetic ketoacidosis.* Severe acidosis may cause the diabetic client to lose consciousness, a condition called *diabetic coma.* Diabetic ketoacidosis always constitutes a medical emergency and requires immediate medical attention.[26, 37]

Diabetic ketoacidosis is the most serious metabolic disturbance in type 1 diabetes and is a common cause of hospital admission. Diabetic ketoacidosis is identified in about 40% of clients with previously undiagnosed diabetes and is responsible for more than 160,000 hospital admissions each year. It occurs most frequently in teenagers and older adults.

Etiology and Risk Factors

Diabetic ketoacidosis is primarily a complication of type 1 diabetes mellitus, although it can also affect clients with type 2 diabetes during periods of extreme stress. A precipitating cause can be identified in 80% of clients. Common causes of diabetic ketoacidosis include:

- Taking too little insulin
- Skipping doses of insulin
- Inability to meet an increased need for insulin created by surgery, trauma, pregnancy, stress, puberty, or infection
- Developing insulin resistance through the presence of insulin antibodies

Pathophysiology

Diabetic ketoacidosis is marked by a relative or absolute lack of insulin. Insulin may be present, but not in sufficient amounts for the increased need for glucose due to the stressors present (such as infection). When the body lacks insulin and cannot use carbohydrates for energy, it resorts to using fats and proteins. Excess production of counterregulatory hormones (glucagon, catecholamines, cortisol, and growth hormones) secondary to stress appears to play an important role in the development of diabetic ketoacidosis. These hormones antagonize the effects of insulin and foster diabetic ketoacidosis by promoting hyperglycemia, osmotic diuresis, lipolysis with secondary hyperlipidemia, and acidosis. Figure 45–7 summarizes the pathophysiologic mechanisms involved. The process of catabolizing fats for fuel gives rise to three pathologic events:

- Ketosis and acidosis
- Dehydration
- Electrolyte and acid-base imbalances[37]

Ketosis

We have already examined the metabolic effect of insufficient insulin on fat metabolism. In diabetic ketoacidosis, buffering of acid by bicarbonate, which is excreted as carbon dioxide and water, fails to compensate for ketosis. Respirations increase in rate and depth (Kussmaul's respirations), and the breath has a "fruity" or acetone-like odor.

The renal system attempts to excrete enough ketone bodies to normalize pH, which leads to osmotic diuresis and hemoconcentration (excessive loss of fluid and electrolytes). Hemoconcentration impedes blood circulation and leads to tissue anoxia and lactic acid production. This rise in lactic acid further acidifies blood pH. The rising tide of ketone bodies eventually overwhelms the body's defenses against hydrogen excess. With its buffer, respiratory, and renal defense systems depleted, the body finally succumbs to its acid overload, and diabetic coma can ensue.

Dehydration

Clients with ketoacidosis lose fluids from several sources. They excrete large amounts of urine in the body's attempt to eliminate excessive glucose and ketones. Second, acidosis can cause severe nausea and vomiting, with further losses of fluid and electrolytes (notably sodium and chloride). Finally, water is lost in the breath as the body attempts to rid itself of excess acetone and carbon dioxide. Typically, clients in diabetic coma lose an amount of water equivalent to 10% of body weight, plus about 40 g of sodium. Severe dehydration resulting from these fluid losses may be followed by hypovolemic shock and lactic acidosis.

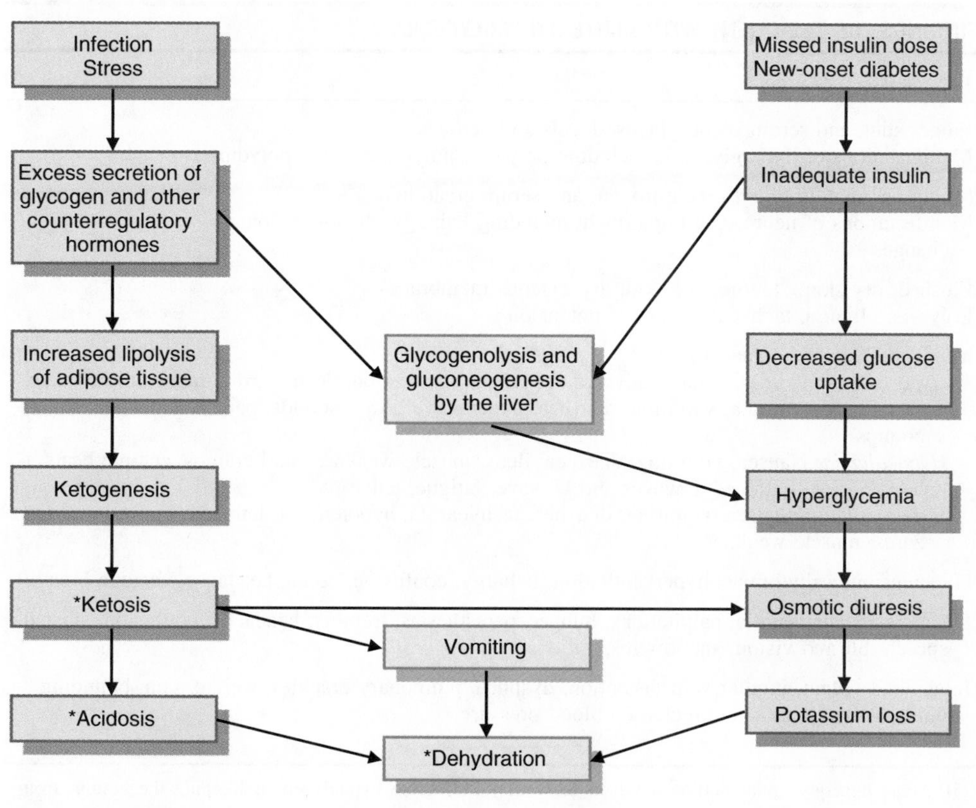

FIGURE 45–7 The pathophysiology of diabetic ketoacidosis. (Adapted from White, N. H., & Henry, D. N. [1996]. Special issues in diabetes management. In D. Haire-Joshu [Ed.], *Management of diabetes mellitus: Perspectives of care across the lifespan* [2nd ed., p. 344]. St. Louis: Mosby–Year Book.)

Electrolyte Imbalance

As the pH of the blood decreases (acidosis), the accumulating hydrogen moves from the extracellular fluid to the intracellular fluid. The movement of hydrogen into the cells promotes the movement of potassium out of the cells into the extracellular fluid, which results in severe intracellular potassium depletion. Initially, the intracellular potassium loss may go unrecognized because serum potassium levels are often normal or elevated. As the resulting osmotic diuresis continues, however, much potassium is excreted in the urine. If the client becomes severely dehydrated, hemoconcentration and oliguria may cause the serum potassium levels to rise still higher. In addition to potassium losses, the client in metabolic acidosis loses excessive amounts of sodium, phosphate, chloride, and bicarbonate in the urine and vomitus.

Clinical Manifestations

Common presenting manifestations of the client in diabetic ketoacidosis are listed in Box 45–4.

BOX 45–4 Common Manifestations of Diabetic Ketoacidosis

- Abdominal pain
- Anorexia
- Dehydration
- Fruity odor of ketones on breath
- Hyperpnea or Kussmaul's respirations
- Hypotension
- Impaired level of consciousness or coma
- Nausea and vomiting
- Polyuria
- Somnolence
- Tachycardia
- Thirst
- Visual disturbances
- Warm, dry skin
- Weakness
- Weight loss

Outcome Management

Medical Management

Assessment priorities for the client with acute hyperglycemia are presented in Table 45–7. Management of diabetic ketoacidosis usually takes place in a hospital setting, with care managed by the physician, nurse, and pharmacist. Dehydration resulting in hypovolemic shock, acute tubular necrosis, and uremia are major causes of death in cases of untreated diabetic ketoacidosis. Diabetic ketoacidosis constitutes an emergency. Rapid medical care and nursing intervention are essential to correct the life-threatening abnormalities. Effective therapy is based on an understanding of metabolic changes that occur during diabetic ketoacidosis. The cornerstone of treatment is the administration of fluids, insulin, and electrolytes.

Management outcomes in diabetic ketoacidosis are rehydration, correction of electrolyte and acid-base imbalances, restoration to a state of carbohydrate catabolism from a state of fat catabolism by providing insulin, and identification and correction of those factors that precipitated the ketoacidosis. The measures to achieve these outcomes must be done with great care. Fully correcting all

TABLE 45–7 ASSESSMENT FINDINGS FOR THE CLIENT WITH ACUTE HYPERGLYCEMIA

Problem	Key Assessments
Hyperglycemia	Finger stick and serum blood glucose levels and ketones Manifestations of hyperglycemia including polyuria, polyphagia, and polydipsia
Hyperosmolality	Serum osmolality, blood urea nitrogen; and serum creatinine Manifestations of neurologic impairment including lethargy, disorientation, and behavioral changes
Dehydration	Flushed, dry skin; "tenting" of skin; dry mucous membranes Polyuria, oliguria, tachycardia, and hypotension
Electrolyte imbalances	Manifestations of imbalances *Hyperkalemia:* Tachycardia, bradycardia, peaked T waves on electrocardiogram, ectopic beats, hypotension, nausea, vomiting, diarrhea, hyperactive bowel sounds, paresthesias, muscle cramps *Hypokalemia:* Nausea, vomiting, diarrhea, ileus, muscle weakness and cramps, ectopic beats, hypotension, flattened T waves and U wave, fatigue, lethargy *Hyponatremia:* Nausea, vomiting, diarrhea, tachycardia, hypotension, lethargy, confusion, seizures, muscle weakness
Metabolic acidosis	Hypotension, arrhythmias, hyperventilation, lethargy, confusion, coma, headache, acetone breath
Hypoglycemia	Diaphoresis, tachycardia, palpitations, hunger, paresthesias, tremors, headache, confusion, slurred speech, blurred vision, shallow respirations
Fluid overload (may develop with insulin treatment for hyperglycemia)	Intake and output, jugular vein distention, dyspnea, pulmonary crackles, weight gain, bounding pulse, edema, confusion, increased blood pressure

Adapted from Reising, D. L. (1995). Acute hyperglycemia: Putting a lid on the crisis; and Acute hypoglycemia: Keeping the bottom from falling out. *Nursing 95, 25*(2), 37, 39, 46.

CRITICAL MONITORING

The Rehydration Process

- The best indication of the degree of dehydration is weight loss, which may be determined if the client's baseline weight is known; loss may be 10% of total body weight.
- Other clinical indices to monitor are tissue turgor, pulse, condition of mucous membranes, level of consciousness, thirst, hematocrit, and positional blood pressure changes (to check for orthostatic hypotension).
- For older adults and clients with heart disease, fluid replacement should be determined according to central venous pressure measurement.
- Too-aggressive fluid replacement (particularly with normal saline) may induce heart failure; frequent auscultation of the lungs is vital.

biochemical abnormalities may take as long as 1 week after the client is able to eat solid food. A comprehensive flow sheet should be kept to record intake and output, body weight, fluids, electrolytes, insulin, and ketones.

REHYDRATE

Intravenous rehydration is required for all clients who are vomiting, are unable to drink, and have acidosis. IV infusions of isotonic or normal saline (0.9% sodium chloride) are started immediately. Usually, the client receives 1000 ml of isotonic solution by the IV route during the first hour (10 to 20 ml/kg), followed by an additional 2000 to 8000 ml of solution over the next 24 hours. Clients with compromised cardiovascular function may require slower IV fluid replacement (see the Critical Monitoring feature and Box 45–5).

A nasogastric tube may be necessary if the client is comatose or is vomiting and likely to aspirate the vomitus. The client's mouth may be dry because of the nasogastric tube and the dehydration. Frequent oral care is important.

Assess bowel sounds frequently for changes. Once the client can tolerate fluids, encourage them. Drinking salted broth is beneficial to replenish needed sodium. Record intake and output accurately. Most clients require a urinary catheter. Because clients with diabetes are susceptible to infection, aseptic catheter care is essential.

REVERSE SHOCK

If the client is in circulatory collapse, the physician may order blood, albumin, or other plasma volume expanders, such as dextran, to be administered alternately with normal saline solution. Also, the client may receive combinations of colloids and saline solution that raise serum levels of both sodium chloride and plasma protein.

RESTORE POTASSIUM BALANCE

Because of the lowered pH in untreated ketoacidosis, potassium leaves the intracellular space, and transient hyperkalemia develops. The total body potassium level is depleted, despite a normal or elevated serum potassium level. Correct potassium replacement requires caution and timely action. Once intervention begins with fluids and insulin, dangerous hypokalemia may develop, manifested by weakness, extreme dyspnea, and even cardiac arrest. Hypokalemia occurs because potassium reenters the cells (along with glucose) after insulin administration and then is excreted in the urine with rehydration and restoration of renal function. General agreement exists on the following points of assessment and intervention:

- Frequently assess and measure urine output. Do not administer potassium to a client with low urine output; dangerous hyperkalemia may develop. Notify the physician promptly if urine output falls dramatically or is less than 0.5 ml/kg per hour.
- Assess the client continuously for evidence of hyperkalemia (bradycardia, cardiac arrest, weakness, flaccid paralysis, oliguria) or hypokalemia (weakness, flaccid paralysis, paralytic ileus, cardiac arrest). Hyperkalemia may be present during the first 4 hours of intervention. Hypokalemia usually develops 4 to 24 hours after the initial intervention.
- Replace potassium carefully following protocols (Box 45–6).
- Plan to begin potassium administration within 1 to 2 hours after starting insulin therapy and after adequate urine output is ensured.
- When the client has recovered sufficiently to resume eating and drinking, give foods and liquids that are high in potassium, such as bananas or orange juice.
- Monitor sodium chloride and phosphate levels. Sodium is replaced by normal saline. Phosphate levels can also vary to the same degree noted for potassium levels. Sometimes the physician will alternate potassium chloride with potassium phosphate in the IV fluid.

CORRECT PH AND ADMINISTER INSULIN

Clients presenting in diabetic ketoacidosis usually have phosphate depletion from a combination of decreased food intake, excessive catabolism, and increased urinary excretion. As with administration of potassium, adminis-

BOX 45–5 Intravenous Fluid Replacement in Diabetic Ketoacidosis*

Hour 1

Provide 15–20 ml/kg of isotonic sodium chloride (0.9%) (normal saline) or full-strength Ringer's lactate (lactated Ringer's solution).

Hour 2

Continue fluid as above at 15 ml/kg. If the client is hypernatremic, in heart failure, or is a child, consider half-strength sodium chloride (0.45% normal saline).

Hour 3

Reduce fluid intake to 7.5 ml/kg in adults. Fluid should be 0.45% normal saline.

Hour 4

Adjust fluid intake to meet clinical need. Consider urine output rate in calculation.

*When blood glucose approaches 250 mg/dl, change fluid to 5% dextrose in half-strength sodium chloride (D_5 0.45% normal saline). Continue intravenous fluids until client can ingest food and drink without vomiting.

Modified from American Diabetes Association. (1998). *Medical management of (type 1) insulin dependent diabetes* (3rd ed.). Alexandria, VA: Author.

BOX 45–6 Potassium Replacement in Diabetic Ketoacidosis

In clients with adequate urine output, lead II of the 12-lead electrocardiogram may be used as a guide for plasma potassium (K^+) concentration. Flattening or inversion of the T wave with U wave and prolongation of the QT interval indicate hypokalemia. Peaking of T waves, loss of P wave, and a disrupted QRS complex indicate hyperkalemia.

Intravenous replacement of potassium is based on plasma K^+ concentration. If K^+ concentration is:

- <3 mEq/L, infuse ≥0.6 mEq/kg/hr
- 3–4 mEq/L, infuse 0.6 mEq/kg/hr
- 4–5 mEq/L, infuse 0.2–0.4 mEq/kg/hr
- 6 mEq/L, withold until K^+ concentration is <6.0 mEq/L

Add K^+ to replacement fluid therapy. If concentration is 20–40 mEq/L and infusion into peripheral vein causes irritation, infuse into central vein.

Recheck plasma K^+ concentration every 2 hours if previous value was <4 or >6 mEq/L.

Adapted from American Diabetes Association. (1998). *Medical management of (type 1) insulin dependent diabetes* (3rd ed.). Alexandria, VA: Author.

tration of insulin enhances movement of phosphate into the cells, which further reduces plasma phosphate concentration. However, administering too much phosphate can induce hypocalcemia. Calcium levels should be checked before phosphate (as potassium phosphate) is given.

Clinicians usually administer sodium bicarbonate only to clients with a blood pH of 7.1 or less. Such replacement therapy partially corrects the metabolic acidosis. As the client's condition improves, normal body mechanisms restore the blood pH to normal.

Low-dosage insulin therapy (5 to 10 units/hour) is ordered for the client in diabetic ketoacidosis. Although the blood glucose concentration is usually sharply elevated in diabetic ketoacidosis, a blood glucose level below 300 mg/dl does not exclude the diagnosis. The client in ketoacidosis may receive an initial IV bolus of regular insulin (0.15 unit/kg) in the emergency department. Before starting an infusion of insulin, ask whether the client has already received insulin that day. Insulin should never be given subcutaneously to someone in diabetic ketoacidosis, because the subcutaneous tissues are dehydrated and poorly perfused as a result of dehydration and hypovolemic shock.

Traditionally, the hyperglycemia associated with diabetic ketoacidosis is treated with an IV bolus of regular insulin. Then an insulin drip should be started. Either 0.9% (normal) saline solution or 0.45% saline may be used, depending on the degree of dehydration and concurrent medical problems. Prepare the last amount of insulin in the smallest IV bag available (e.g., 100 units of regular insulin in 100 ml of IV fluid). This gives a 1:1 ratio of regular insulin to IV fluid. Prime the IV tubing with the IV solution first, and then add the regular insulin, because insulin will adhere to the IV tubing. Label the IV bag clearly with the dose and type of insulin added. The IV regular insulin must be administered very meticulously by a control pump and checked frequently.

After the bolus, infuse insulin at a rate of 0.1 unit/kg/hour. If no improvement in the acidosis occurs within 2 to 4 hours, the infusion rate should be doubled. Severe insulin resistance may be precipitated by severe stress. The glucose level is normalized more quickly than pH.

Blood glucose levels need to be monitored every 30 minutes initially, preferably with a blood glucose meter. Rapid blood glucose test results allow you to adjust the insulin infusion rapidly and correctly. When the blood glucose levels approach 250 mg/dl, the insulin infusion should be reduced and 5% dextrose added to the infusion so that the blood glucose level can be maintained at about 250 mg/dl for the first 12 to 24 hours. Faster correction of hyperglycemia can lead to cerebral edema. Monitor the client's level of consciousness closely to assess for this uncommon complication. Monitor blood glucose levels every 1 to 2 hours after reaching 250 mg/dl until they are stable.

As the client improves, decisions must be made about when to discontinue IV insulin and fluids and begin subcutaneous insulin administration. Normalization of the client's vital signs, correction of acidosis, and ability to take oral fluids are important considerations. Short-acting insulin is usually administered subcutaneously every 4 to 6 hours, with the first dose given 15 to 30 minutes before stopping IV insulin. The initial dose is about 0.2 unit/kg. Subsequent doses are determined by blood glucose levels.

While any metabolic abnormalities are being corrected, the cause of the client's diabetic ketoacidosis must be pursued aggressively. Cultures of urine, throat, sputum, and blood; chest x-ray films; and an electrocardiogram (ECG) may reveal the source of stress. Before discharge of the client from the hospital, the health care team reviews the situation that led to diabetic ketoacidosis and institutes teaching for risk factor reduction.

PREVENT RECURRENCE

Primary prevention of diabetic ketoacidosis is through client education. Preventing diabetic ketoacidosis is the long-term goal of good diabetes management. Clients and their families should understand enough about ketoacidosis to avoid potential causes, to recognize its approach, to slow down or minimize its development, and to seek help fast if it begins to occur. To prevent diabetic ketoacidosis, clients with diabetes should learn to:

- Take insulin in appropriate doses at appropriate times
- Monitor blood glucose frequently, at least before each meal and at bedtime
- Monitor urine ketone levels when blood glucose levels rise above 250 mg/dl
- Schedule regular appointments with a health care provider to review blood glucose levels, weight gains or losses, and general state of health and well-being
- Recognize manifestations of infection—a major cause of diabetic ketoacidosis. The first clinical manifestations of infection (upper respiratory tract, urinary tract, or vaginal infection) should be reported immediately to the health care provider; other stressors, such as family or emotional problems, can also precipitate diabetic ketoacidosis[16]

The client should telephone for assistance if any of the following develop:

- Anorexia, nausea, vomiting, or diarrhea
- Ketonuria persisting for more than 8 hours
- Fever or infection
- Any manifestation of acidosis

Emphasize that the greatest weapons against diabetic ketoacidosis are regular, daily self-monitoring of blood glucose; adherence to the diabetes management program; and early recognition of and intervention in mild ketosis.

HYPERGLYCEMIC, HYPEROSMOLAR, NONKETOTIC SYNDROME

Hyperglycemic, hyperosmolar, nonketotic syndrome (HHNS) is a variant of diabetic ketoacidosis characterized by extreme hyperglycemia (600 to 2000 mg/dl), profound dehydration, mild or undetectable ketonuria, and the absence of acidosis. HHNS most commonly occurs in older clients with type 2 diabetes mellitus (Box 45–7).

Mortality with HHNS is higher than with diabetic ketoacidosis (10% to 40%), primarily because clients typically are older and commonly have significant medical problems. HHNS sometimes occurs in people with undiagnosed diabetes and in known diabetic clients after a long period of uncontrolled hyperglycemia. The precipitating factors for HHNS may be the same as those for diabetic ketoacidosis. There is almost always an identifiable precipitating factor.

The major difference between HHNS and diabetic ketoacidosis is the lack of ketonuria with HHNS. Because some residual ability to secrete insulin remains in type 2 diabetes mellitus, the mobilization of fats for energy usually does not occur. In the absence of adequate insulin, the blood becomes loaded with glucose. Glucose molecules are too large to pass into cells; therefore, osmosis of water occurs from the interstitial spaces and cells to dilute the glucose in the blood. Osmotic diuresis occurs. Eventually, the cells become dehydrated.

The client's fluid intake can initially balance the loss of fluid and glucose through the urine. The imbalance gradually becomes more severe as the client cannot match intake to output. In time, the client becomes obtunded and is unable to respond to thirst. At this point, the process is self-perpetuating.

The four major clinical features of HHNS are:

- Severe hyperglycemia (600 to 2000 mg/dl)
- No or only slight ketosis
- Profound dehydration (10% to 15% loss of body water)
- Hyperosmolality (increased concentration) of plasma and elevated blood urea nitrogen

Typically, the client experiences excessive thirst, altered level of consciousness (coma or confusion), and manifestations of dehydration.

The precipitating event should be determined and corrected as soon as possible, even during resuscitation. HHNS is treated with vigorous fluid replacement and administration of insulin and electrolytes. A common initial intervention is infusion of normal saline solution over a 2-hour period, followed by administration of hypotonic (0.45%) saline solution. As in diabetic IV ketoacidosis, potassium, sodium, chloride, and phosphates are administered.

Insulin is given via an infusion pump, but usually at lower dosages, because the client is producing some insulin. Because of severe dehydration, plasma glucose levels fall rapidly with fluid administration. Dextrose is added to the IV fluid when the blood glucose level reaches about 250 mg/dl, to prevent hypoglycemia. Because many clients who have HHNS are older and have other cardiovascular or renal disorders, fluid volume and electrolyte changes must be carefully assessed, especially if acute or chronic renal failure complicates the course.

As the population ages, an increasing number of clients will experience HHNS and you need to be alert for its manifestations. Before discharge, review the causes of HHNS with the client and family, including insulin injection (if necessary) and blood glucose testing techniques. Help the client understand how serious these acute complications are and how to prevent them in the future.

BOX 45–7 Factors Associated with Hyperglycemic, Hyperosmolar, Nonketotic Syndrome (HHNS)

Therapeutic Agents

- Glucocorticoids
- Diuretics
- Diphenylhydantoin
- Beta-adrenergic blocking agents
- L-Asparaginase
- Immunosuppressive agents
- Chlorpromazine
- Diazoxide

Therapeutic Procedures

- Peritoneal dialysis
- Hemodialysis
- Hyperalimentation
- Surgical stress

Chronic Illness

- Renal disease
- Heart disease
- Hypertension
- Previous stroke
- Alcoholism
- Psychiatric diagnosis
- Loss of thirst

Acute Illness

- Infection
- Gangrene
- Urinary tract infection
- Septicemia
- Burns
- Gastrointestinal bleeding
- Myocardial infarction
- Pancreatitis
- Cerebrovascular accident (stroke)

From American Diabetes Association. (1998). *Medical management of non-insulin dependent (type 2) diabetes* (4th ed.). Alexandria, VA: Author.

HYPOGLYCEMIA

Hypoglycemia (also known as an *insulin reaction* or hypoglycemic reaction) is a common feature of type 1 diabetes mellitus and can also be seen in clients with type 2 diabetes treated with insulin or oral agents. The precise blood glucose level at which clients have manifestations of hypoglycemia varies, but they usually do not occur until the blood glucose level is less than 50 to 60 mg/dl.

Etiology and Risk Factors

Hypoglycemic reactions may result from the following:

- An overdose of insulin or, less commonly, a sulfonylurea
- Omitting a meal or eating less food than usual
- Overexertion without additional carbohydrate compensation
- Nutritional and fluid imbalances caused by nausea and vomiting
- Alcohol intake

Inadvertent or deliberate errors in insulin dose are a frequent cause of hypoglycemia. Other changes in the schedule of meals or insulin administration, vigorous unexpected exercise, or sleeping later than usual in the morning can also cause hypoglycemia. The effects of alcohol, marijuana, or other drugs can mask a client's awareness of hypoglycemia in its earliest stages.

Hypoglycemia can also occur secondary to administration of an oral hypoglycemic agent. Most recorded cases have been in clients receiving chlorpropamide (Diabinese), which has a duration of action of 24 to 72 hours. Clients at risk for hypoglycemia while taking an oral hypoglycemic are over age 60 years, have poor nutritional intake, use alcohol, have hepatic or renal dysfunction, and are receiving multi-drug regimens. The hypoglycemic reactions can be severe and prolonged.

Pathophysiology

Normally, hypoglycemia triggers counterregulatory hormones, primarily glucagon and epinephrine, to promptly increase blood glucose levels by stimulating glucose release from the liver and inhibiting insulin secretion. Under usual conditions, this leads to normoglycemia.

In contrast, clients with type 1 diabetes have abnormalities in this feedback system. Typically, within the first 2 to 5 years of diabetes, the secretion of glucagon becomes deficient. Later, the secretion of epinephrine may become impaired secondary to subclinical neuropathy. The regulation of insulin absorption from subcutaneous fat also becomes impaired.

The combination of these abnormalities makes the client with type 1 diabetes susceptible to frequent development of hypoglycemia. In this respect, hypoglycemic shock is more dangerous than diabetic ketoacidosis. About one in 10 clients with type 1 diabetes suffer one severe reaction per year that requires emergency treatment. Untreated or prolonged hypoglycemia can cause permanent brain damage, memory loss, decreased learning ability, paralysis, and death.

Clinical Manifestations

Hypoglycemic manifestations are generally divided into two major categories (Box 45–8):

BOX 45–8 Manifestations of Hypoglycemia

Adrenergic (increased epinephrine)

- Shakiness
- Irritability
- Nervousness
- Tachycardia, palpitations
- Tremor
- Hunger
- Diaphoresis
- Pallor
- Paresthesias

Neuroglycopenic (decreased glucose to brain)

- Headache
- Mental illness
- Inability to concentrate
- Slurred speech
- Blurred vision
- Confusion
- Irrational behavior
- Lethargy, severe
- Loss of consciousness
- Coma
- Seizure
- Death

1. *Adrenergic* (autonomic) manifestations are associated with rising epinephrine levels and are considered "mild" reactions. Cognitive deficits usually do not occur, and affected people are capable of self-treatment. Diaphoresis, although not mediated via adrenergic nerve endings, is usually grouped with the adrenergic manifestations of hypoglycemia. Adrenergic reactions usually occur during rapid decreases in blood glucose. They have been reported by clients with poorly controlled diabetes when the fall in blood glucose level is rapid, even in the absence of hypoglycemia. These manifestations can also occur during other stressful or anxiety-provoking events. These mild reactions may produce only minimal disruptions of daily activities.
2. *Neuroglycopenic* manifestations are associated with lack of glucose availability to the brain and resultant decrease in cognitive functioning. These reactions typically produce longer-lasting and more severe manifestations than those characteristic of mild reactions. Common manifestations are headache, irritability, drowsiness, weakness, and tremor. The client may need assistance in treatment. Severe hypoglycemic reactions render the client unable to self-treat. The client may be awake and alert, semicomatose, or comatose.

Hypoglycemia can occur at any time of day or night. It seems to occur most commonly during exercise, 8 to 24 hours after strenuous exercise, and in the middle of the night. Severe hypoglycemia seems to occur more often in people who have hypoglycemic unawareness, defective glucose counterregulation, and autonomic neuropathy as well as in clients receiving intensive diabetes therapy.

The period during which the client is most likely to experience an insulin reaction depends on the type of insulin given, the client's response to that type of insulin, and the timing of the insulin injection in relation to food intake. When insulin is given in the morning, short-acting preparations tend to produce reactions before lunch; intermediate-acting insulins, 2 or 3 hours before dinner; and long-acting insulins, between 2:00 AM and breakfast. NPH or Lente insulin injected before dinner (5:00 PM) can cause hypoglycemia around 2:00 AM, when the normal blood glucose level is lowest because of the decrease in metabolism, and again at around 8:00 AM, when the insulin peaks if breakfast is not eaten on time.

Outcome Management

Medical Management

RETURN SERUM GLUCOSE TO NORMAL LEVELS

Management of hypoglycemia depends on the severity of the reaction (Table 45–8). To reverse mild hypoglycemia, 10 to 15 g of simple carbohydrate is given and works quickly to increase blood glucose levels. Reactions that occur during the night should be treated with a carbohydrate followed by a longer-acting mixture of carbohydrate and protein (8 ounces of milk, for example). A blood glucose test (with a glucose meter) should be performed as soon as manifestations begin. If a meter is not available, it is safer to assume and treat hypoglycemia. Blood glucose is retested in 15 to 30 minutes, and treatment is repeated if the level is not over 100 mg/dl. Moderate reactions may need two or more treatments with 10 to 15 g of carbohydrates.

Never force an unconscious or semiconscious client to drink liquids, because fluid may be aspirated into the lungs. The unconscious client with severe hypoglycemia needs glucagon or IV glucose immediately. Family members of clients with diabetes can administer glucagon at home in the event of a serious hypoglycemic reaction. Glucagon, administered intramuscularly or subcutaneously in the amount of 1 mg for adults, may eliminate the need for emergency department intervention. The pharmacy dispenses glucagon in the form of a powder, with the diluent in a separate vial. Instruct family members how and when to mix and inject glucagon, and let them know that the client may experience nausea or vomiting on awakening. Even though glucagon is effective in most clients, its effect is transient and slower than that of dextrose. Hypoglycemia often recurs. Medical assistance is advisable if hypoglycemia recurs, vomiting prevents oral intake, or the client's status does not improve.

A client who experiences severe hypoglycemia in the hospital usually receives 10 to 25 g of IV glucose (as 50% or 25% dextrose) over 1 to 3 minutes. This is followed by an infusion of 5% dextrose at 5 to 10 g/hour until the client is fully recovered and able to eat.

TABLE 45–8 INTERVENTIONS FOR HYPOGLYCEMIA

Clinical Manifestations	Interventions
Mild hypoglycemia	10–15 g of carbohydrate, contained in:
Tremors	4 oz orange juice
Tachycardia	6 oz regular soda
Diaphoresis	6–8 oz 2% milk
Paresthesias	6–8 Life Savers candies
Excessive hunger	1 small (2-oz) tube of cake icing
Pallor	4 tsp granulated sugar
Shakiness	
Moderate hypoglycemia	20–30 g of carbohydrate
Manifestations listed above plus	Glucagon, 1 mg SC or IM
Headache	
Mood swings	
Irritability	
Inability to concentrate	
Drowsiness	
Impaired judgment	
Slurred speech	
Double or blurred vision	
Severe hypoglycemia	50% dextrose, 25 g IV
Disorientation	Glucagon, 1 mg IM or IV
Seizures	
Unconsciousness	

IM, intramuscularly; IV, intravenously; SC, subcutaneously.

PREVENT HYPOGLYCEMIA

Because insulin reactions are so common, clients with newly diagnosed diabetes must understand the following:

- Why hypoglycemia occurs
- When it is most likely to occur
- The early clinical manifestations of hypoglycemia
- The danger of severe or repeated reactions
- The importance of early intervention
- How to prevent insulin reactions

Whenever administration of insulin or an oral hypoglycemic agent begins, the client must be taught to identify clinical manifestations and to manage hypoglycemia. Once a client experiences and then fully recovers from an episode of hypoglycemia, thoroughly reassess the intervention program. In some cases, insulin reactions develop because the client carelessly prepares insulin dosages, fails to eat, or exercises excessively. Explain the dangers of repeated insulin reactions to a client who is careless in maintaining a normoglycemic balance. These dangers include loss of consciousness, trauma caused by falling after losing consciousness, injury from poor decision-making, seizures, loss of brain cells, and eventual death. Emphasize conscientious adherence to the therapeutic program.

In other cases, hypoglycemia develops because the prescribed insulin dosage is too large or the client's dietary intake is too small. Instruct the client to record the time and probable cause of any hypoglycemic episodes on the blood test record. The health care team and the client can then evaluate the record together, making appropriate changes. Teach the client with type 1 diabetes to adjust diet and insulin by monitoring results. Finally, be certain that the client with diabetes obtains a diabetic identification tag or medical identification bracelet or necklace and a diabetic identification card. Sometimes, a client who is experiencing an insulin reaction behaves as if intoxicated or mentally disturbed. By carrying proper identification, the client can avoid being arrested at a time when emergency care is desperately needed. Table 45–9 compares the data and interventions for diabetic ketoacidosis, HHNS, and hypoglycemia.

As in many chronic disorders, the client needs to develop a positive self-concept and a feeling of control. Help the client and significant others understand the complications associated with diabetes. Equally important, help the client develop and maintain self-care skills that meet emotional and social needs as well as physical ones.

OTHER HYPOGLYCEMIC DISORDERS

Other manifestations of altered counterregulatory mechanisms in type 1 diabetes mellitus are (1) hypoglycemic unawareness, (2) hypoglycemia with rebound hyperglycemia (Somogyi effect), and (3) the dawn phenomenon.

■ HYPOGLYCEMIC UNAWARENESS

Hypoglycemic unawareness refers to a syndrome in which people with diabetes are unaware they are hypoglycemic and therefore do not initiate treatment. In the Diabetes Control and Complications Trial, about a third of all episodes of severe hypoglycemia seen in awake, intensively treated clients were not accompanied by manifestations of sufficient severity that clients could effectively prevent neuroglycopenia. In the past, this condition was incorrectly viewed as being rare and associated only with advanced neuropathy.

Repeated episodes of hypoglycemia seem to blunt the hormonal defense mechanisms that prevent it (blunted epinephrine response) and the client's ability to perceive early manifestations. Beta-adrenergic–blocking agents (such as propranolol) can cause hypoglycemic unawareness and blunt adrenergic (epinephrine) effects in clients with diabetes, because these effects are primarily mediated by beta-adrenergic receptors. Therefore, beta-blockers are contraindicated in clients with diabetes.

Clients with hypoglycemic unawareness (absence of manifestations of hypoglycemia when glucose level is below 55 mg/dl) require consultation with an experienced physician. Increasing the frequency of self-monitored blood glucose levels, particularly before driving and after exercise, should be encouraged. Clients may wish to choose a slightly higher blood glucose target before meals and during the night. Self-management education and follow-up must be intensified for these clients. For clients with type 1 diabetes, maintaining good control is as much of a problem during the night as at any other time of day.

■ HYPOGLYCEMIA WITH REBOUND HYPERGLYCEMIA

Hypoglycemia followed by rebound hyperglycemia, known as the *Somogyi effect* or *Somogyi phenomenon,* may complicate diabetes management. This phenomenon was implicated in the past as a common cause of fasting morning hyperglycemia. Studies have found it to be a rare occurrence. It usually results from excessive evening insulin dosing. The pathophysiology involves hypoglycemia, leading to counterregulatory hormone secretion and resultant liver production of glucose. This increase in glucose, along with insulin resistance secondary to increased hormone levels, is thought to contribute to rebound hyperglycemia.

Nocturnal rebound hyperglycemia should be investigated by self-monitoring of blood glucose levels between 2:00 and 4:00 AM and again at 7:00 AM. If early-morning levels are less than 50 to 60 mg/dl and those at 7:00 AM are greater than 180 to 200 mg/dl, rebound hyperglycemia may have occurred. Decreasing the intermediate-acting insulin dose at suppertime, moving the intermediate-acting insulin dose to bedtime, or increasing the size of the bedtime snack should prevent this phenomenon.

■ DAWN PHENOMENON

The dawn phenomenon refers to an early-morning (4 to 8 AM) rise in blood glucose level without preceding nocturnal hypoglycemia. Wearing off of insulin does not appear to be the sole cause of this phenomenon. It has been found in people with both type 1 and type 2 diabetes and probably occurs in people without diabetes. Growth hormone, increased insulin clearance, and diurnal variation in counterregulatory hormone levels seem to play a role.

The key clinical implication of the dawn phenomenon is that attempts to normalize pre-breakfast glucose levels often result in early-morning hypoglycemia. Self-monitoring of blood glucose and education about bedtime snacks, manifestations of nocturnal hypoglycemia, and the importance of avoiding hypoglycemia are vital. Investigation has shown positive effects with the use of Ultralente instead of NPH insulin in the elimination of this phenomenon.

CHRONIC COMPLICATIONS OF DIABETES MELLITUS

Clients with diabetes are living longer, with an increased risk for development of chronic complications (Box 45–9). Chronic complications are the major causes of morbidity and mortality in clients with diabetes. These changes affect many body systems and can be devastating to clients and their families; they affect clients with both type 1 and type 2 diabetes. Complications are classified as one of three types[41]:

- *Macrovascular,* including coronary artery disease, cerebrovascular disease, hypertension, peripheral vascular disease, and infection
- *Microvascular,* including retinopathy and nephropathy
- *Neuropathic,* including sensorimotor and autonomic dysfunction

Sustained increases in glucose levels create an imbalance of substances used for making the matrix between cells. Enzyme systems normally convert glucose to other sugars, such as sorbitol and fructose to lower blood glucose. Sorbitol, fructose, and glucose accumulate in the basement membrane of the cell and between the cells. Intracellular accumulations of sorbitol cause intracellular edema and affect function.

The microcirculation is affected by extracellular accumulation of glucose, sorbitol, and fructose. The thickened basement membrane increases the distance over which

TABLE 45–9 ACUTE COMPLICATIONS OF DIABETES

	Diabetic Ketoacidosis (DKA)	Hyperglycemic, Hyperosmolar, Nonketotic Syndrome (HHNS)	Hypoglycemia
Type of diabetes	Usually type 1; may occur in type 2	Type 2	Type 1 or type 2
Clinical manifestations	Warm/dry skin, nausea, vomiting, flushed appearance, dry mucous membranes, soft eyeballs, Kussmaul's respirations or tachypnea, abdominal pain, impaired consciousness, hypotension, tachycardia, acetone breath, acute weight loss Polyuria (early) Oliguria/anuria (late)	Same as for DKA except Kussmaul's respirations and acetone breath usually not present Alterations in level of consciousness, severe dehydration Nausea and vomiting not present Tachypnea, shallow respirations	Mild reaction: tremors, palpitations, pallor, sweating, hunger Moderate reaction: headache, irritability, drowsiness, weakness, visual disturbances, decreased mental acuity Severe reaction: loss of consciousness, seizures
Precipitating factors	Undiagnosed diabetes Omission of insulin dose Puberty Infection Cardiovascular disorder Other physical or emotional stress, such as pregnancy or surgery Trauma	Undiagnosed diabetes Infection or other stress Medications: phenytoin sodium (Dilantin), thiazide diuretics, steroids, chlorpromazine Dialysis GI bleed Hyperalimentation, myocardial infarction Acute pancreatitis Central nervous system disorders Major burns rehydrated with high volumes of glucose	Delay or omission of meal Insulin overdosage Excessive exercise Improper timing of insulin and food
Onset of manifestations	Slow (hours to days) or quickly	Slow (hours to days)	Rapid (minutes to hours)
Laboratory findings			
Plasma glucose	300–1500 mg/dl	600–2000 mg/dl	60 mg/dl or less
Serum sodium	Normal or decreased	Normal or increased	Normal
Serum potassium	Normal or elevated at first, then decreased	Same as for DKA	Normal
Blood urea nitrogen	Elevated	Elevated	Normal
Serum ketones	Elevated	Absent	Absent
White blood cells	Elevated	Elevated	Normal or elevated
Hematocrit	Elevated	Elevated	Normal
Urine glucose	Elevated	Elevated	Absent
Urine ketones	Elevated	Absent	Absent
Arterial blood gas	Metabolic acidosis with compensatory respiratory alkalosis	Normal (metabolic acidosis of shock is profound and prolonged)	Normal or slight respiratory acidosis
pH	Less than 7.3	Usually normal or slightly decreased	Normal
Osmolality	300–350 mOsm/L	Usually over 350 mOsm/L	Normal
Acute intervention	IV regular insulin IV fluids such as normal saline or half normal saline Potassium when urine output is adequate Sodium bicarbonate, rarely Phosphate, usually Electrocardiogram Correct underlying problem	Correct underlying problem IV regular insulin IV fluids such as normal saline or half normal saline Potassium when urine output is adequate	Mild reaction: 10–15 g of simple carbohydrate Moderate reaction: one or more simple carbohydrate, glucagon may be needed, 0.5–1 mg Severe reaction: glucagon IM or SC, repeat × 1 in 10 minutes prn, may need IV glucose

Table continued on following page

TABLE 45–9 ACUTE COMPLICATIONS OF DIABETES *Continued*

	Diabetic Ketoacidosis (DKA)	Hyperglycemic, Hyperosmolar, Nonketotic Syndrome (HHNS)	Hypoglycemia
Preventive measures	Prompt medical attention when necessary Plan ahead for illness care Frequent SMBG checks during illness or stressful events	Frequent SMBG checks during illness or stressful events Prompt medical attention when necessary	Sleeping late should be planned in advance; if oversleeping >45 min is planned, changes in insulin or food intake may be necessary Have short-acting carbohydrate available when exercising or reduction of insulin dose before exercise Restricting alcohol intake Double-check insulin type and dosage prior to administration
	→→→ Wearing diabetes identification tag or bracelet. Education for self-care. →→→		

GI, Gastrointestinal; IM, intramuscularly; IV, intravenous; SC, subcutaneously; SMBG, self-monitored blood glucose.

nutrients and waste products must travel to and from the cell. As a result, the cells receive inadequate oxygen and nutrition and cannot rid themselves of waste. Unfortunately, the process starts as early as 2 years after the onset of diabetes.

Clinicians often see clients with diabetes in the hospital with an MI, with loss of cognitive or physical function as a result of a cerebrovascular accident, or with a lower limb amputation necessitated by peripheral vascular disease. Prevention of these all-too-common macrovascular health problems should be a major focus of nurses working with clients with diabetes (Table 45–10).

BOX 45–9 Chronic Complications of Diabetes Mellitus

Macrovascular Complications

- Coronary artery disease
- Cerebrovascular disease
- Hypertension
- Peripheral vascular disease
- Infection

Microvascular Complications

- Retinopathy
- Nephropathy

Neuropathic Complications

- Sensorimotor neuropathy
- Autonomic neuropathy
  - Pupillary
  - Cardiovascular
  - Gastrointestinal
  - Genitourinary

Mixed Vascular and Neuropathic Diseases

- Leg and foot ulcers

MACROVASCULAR COMPLICATIONS

Coronary artery disease, cerebrovascular disease, and peripheral vascular disease are more common, tend to occur at an earlier age, and are more extensive and severe in people with diabetes. Macrovascular disease (disease of large arteries) reflects atherosclerosis with deposits of lipids within the inner layer of vessel walls. The risk for development of macrovascular complications is higher in those with type 1 diabetes than with type 2 diabetes.

Macrovascular disease, especially coronary artery disease, is the most common cause of death in diabetic clients, accounting for 40% to 60% of all cases of diabetes-related macrovascular disease. The most common reason for hospitalization in diabetics is for treatment of macrovascular complications. Diabetes not only is an independent risk factor for these complications but also is a major risk factor for hypertension and hyperlipidemia. Typically, very-low-density and low-density lipoproteins are increased and high-density lipoproteins are decreased. The most characteristic lipid abnormality in diabetes is an elevated triglyceride level. Therefore, the influence of diabetes in these diseases is multiplicative, not additive.

Macrovascular disease tends to occur years before the onset of clinical diabetes and to occur in people with impaired glucose tolerance at a rate similar to that in people with type 2 diabetes. This phenomenon, called *syndrome X*, further establishes the need for disease prevention and health promotion.

Health promotion activities include (1) managing obesity and maintaining ideal body weight, (2) exercising, (3) not smoking, and (4) achieving normal blood lipid levels. Health maintenance actions include (1) prompt recognition and treatment of hyperglycemia with exercise, food, and medication; (2) aggressive management of hypertension, including regular blood pressure checks; and (3)

TABLE 45–10 MACROVASCULAR DISEASE IN DIABETES: CLINICAL MANIFESTATIONS, DIAGNOSIS, AND INTERVENTIONS

Clinical Manifestations	Diagnosis	Interventions
CEREBROVASCULAR DISEASE		
Atherothromboembolic infarctions *(transient ischemic attacks and cerebral vascular accidents)* are more severe, have higher mortality rate, have higher recurrence rate	History Manifestations Physical examinations Computed tomography scan Magnetic resonance imaging	Same as for non-diabetics plus: improved glucose control, aspirin, dipyridamole, ticlopidine; ongoing education and support
HEART DISEASE (CORONARY HEART DISEASE)		
Diabetics have a higher incidence of coronary artery changes that influence decreased oxygen and nutrients to myocardium Clients have more *angina* and higher mortality with *myocardial infarction;* manifestations are often "silent" Clients with a history of diabetes mellitus and myocardial infarction have higher incidence of *congestive heart failure, shock,* and *arrhythmias* *Cardiomyopathy* may occur secondary to small vessel infarctions causing myocardial fibrosis and hypertrophy Additional coronary artery disease manifestations: *Exertional weakness, peripheral edema, orthopnea, fatigue* Features such as female gender, which normally protects from premature heart disease, do not pertain to individuals with diabetes	History Manifestations Physical examination Electrocardiogram Cardiac enzymes Cardiac catheterization Stress test Autopsy	Same as for non-diabetics with cerebrovascular disease plus: improved glucose control, exercise, diet Hypertension control: Use of diuretics may worsen hyperglycemia if hypokalemia exists and may adversely affect lipid levels Beta-adrenergic blockers (may cause hypoglycemia), calcium-channel blockers, thrombolytic agents, aspirin, angioplasty, bypass surgery
INFECTION		
Diabetics have a higher incidence of *Pseudomonas external otitis* and *monilial skin infections;* common sites of infection in the diabetic include *urinary tract and skin*	History Manifestations Physical examination Laboratory data: serum—increased WBCs and blood sugar; urine—increased WBCs	Improved glucose control; antibiotics, antifungals as required; follow-up with laboratory data; ongoing client education
PERIPHERAL VASCULAR DISEASE (PVD)		
The incidence of *carotid bruits, intermittent claudication, absent pedal pulses* and *ischemic gangrene* is increased in diabetes mellitus PVD and neuropathy augment the morbidity associated with trauma and infection in the lower extremity	History Manifestations Physical examinations Doppler studies Angiogram Neuropathy identification	Daily foot inspection aimed at prevention and early intervention; meticulous foot care, padded sport socks, well-fitting shoes; weight reduction; smoking cessation; safe exercise programs; ongoing education
HYPERTENSION		
Usually asymptomatic	History Physical examinations Orthostatic blood pressures with pulse recordings Elevated blood pressure readings at 2–3 recordings Urinalysis: 24-h urine collection for protein, creatinine clearance, and GFR Renal angiogram to evaluate for renal artery stenosis from atherosclerotic disease	Eliminate risk factors; educate client on this silent but deadly disease; diet education: low protein, low salt Pharmacologic intervention dependent on blood pressure readings: diuretics, angiotension-converting enzyme inhibitors, calcium-channel blockers, alphablockers

WBC, white blood cell; GFR, glomerular filtration rate.

screening for high-risk clients (such as those with a family history of diabetes). Health restoration activities involve (1) controlling angina, (2) treating peripheral vascular disease, (3) using blood glucose self-monitoring to keep track of manifestations, (4) controlling risk factors for macrovascular disease, (5) stressing medication compliance and follow-up, and (6) working closely with the client.

Some speculate that type 2 diabetes may be one piece of a syndrome caused by insulin resistance. A well-established association has been demonstrated among hyperglycemia, hyperinsulinemia, dyslipidemia, and hypertension, which leads to coronary artery disease and stroke. The acronym CHAOS (*c*oronary artery disease, *h*ypertension, *a*dult-onset diabetes, *o*besity, and *s*tress) has been used to remind health care providers to look at the client's entire risk profile for cardiovascular disease when determining treatment for diabetes.

Successful weight reduction with a balanced diet improves lipid profiles, lessens glucose intolerance, lowers blood pressure, and eliminates obesity; otherwise, successful treatment of macrovascular disease in clients with diabetes parallels that in the non-diabetic population.[2, 9, 12]

■ CORONARY ARTERY DISEASE

Clients with diabetes are two to four times more likely than non-diabetic clients to die of coronary artery disease, and the relative risk factor for cardiovascular disease in women with type 2 diabetes is three to four times greater. Female gender does not protect the diabetic woman from premature macrovascular disease. In many clients with diabetes, macrovascular events or processes such as coronary artery disease are atypical or silent, and they often present as indigestion or unexplained heart failure, dyspnea on exertion, or epigastric pain. Coronary artery disease is common in clients under age 40 years if diabetes is of long duration. Clients with diabetes who have had an MI have an increased chance of complications or of having a second infarction, compared with that in non-diabetic clients who have had an MI. After an MI, diabetic clients also experience a higher incidence of heart failure, shock, and dysrhythmias. It has been suggested that insulin therapy in type 2 diabetes may actually increase the incidence of atherosclerotic disease, because such therapy often leads to weight gain and increased blood pressure.

■ CEREBROVASCULAR DISEASE

Prevention of cerebrovascular disease includes the same strategies as for prevention of coronary artery disease, including (1) control of hypertension, lipid levels, and obesity; (2) smoking cessation; (3) exercise; and (4) good nutritional practices.

Cerebrovascular disease, particularly atherothromboembolic infarctions manifested by transient ischemic attacks and cerebrovascular accidents (CVAs), are more common and severe in diabetes. The incidence is two to three times greater in diabetic clients. The relative risk is higher in females, highest in the fifth and sixth decades of life, and much higher in clients with hypertension. In the United States, the southeastern states are often referred to as the "Stroke Belt" because of the sizable black population in that region with its increased prevalence of hypertension. Many clients presenting with CVA have undiagnosed diabetes. In clients with diabetes, CVAs are more serious and carry higher recurrence and mortality rates, especially with type 2 diabetes.

It is speculated that the increased prevalence of CVA in clients with diabetes may be related to the development of diabetic nephropathy and resultant proteinuria, hypertension, and platelet adhesiveness. Clients who present with CVA and high blood glucose levels have a much poorer prognosis than that in clients with normoglycemia. Ticlopidine, a platelet aggregation inhibitor, may be more effective than aspirin in lowering the risk of cerebral infarction, especially in clients with diabetes. This drug may also cause increased cholesterol levels and neutropenia (decreased neutrophils).

■ HYPERTENSION

A 40% increased rate of hypertension has been noted in the diabetic population. Hypertension is a major risk factor for stroke and nephropathy. Inadequately treated hypertension augments the rate at which nephropathy develops. Individualized pharmacologic treatment for hypertension above 140/90 mm Hg is suggested. Angiotensin-converting enzyme (ACE) inhibitors and calcium-channel blockers are the agents of choice for treatment. Beta-blockers and diuretics may increase glucose tolerance and lipid levels.

■ PERIPHERAL VASCULAR DISEASE

In diabetes, the incidence and prevalence of carotid bruits (abnormal sound or murmur), intermittent claudication, absent pedal (foot) pulses, and ischemic gangrene are increased. More than half of nontraumatic lower limb amputations are associated with diabetic changes such as sensory and autonomic neuropathy, peripheral vascular disease, an increased risk and rate of infection, and poor healing. This chain of events, which may lead to amputation, is illustrated in Figure 45–8.

■ INFECTIONS

Clients with diabetes are susceptible to infections of many types. Once infections occur, they are difficult to treat. Three factors that may contribute to the development of an infection are impaired polymorphonuclear leukocyte function, diabetic neuropathies, and vascular insufficiency. Poor glycemic control augments the importance of these factors. Infected areas heal slowly because the damaged vascular system cannot carry sufficient oxygen, white blood cells, nutrients, and antibodies to the injured site. Infections increase the need for insulin and enhance the possibility of ketoacidosis.[43]

Urinary tract infections are the most common type of infections affecting diabetic clients, particularly women. One factor may be the inhibition of polymorphonuclear leukocyte activity while glucosuria is present. Glucosuria is associated with hyperglycemia. The development of a neurogenic bladder, which results in incomplete emptying and urinary retention, may also contribute to the risk of a urinary tract infection.

Diabetic foot infections are very common. Their occurrence is directly related to the three factors just listed, plus hyperglycemia. Up to 40% of diabetic clients with foot infections may require amputation, and 5% to 10% will die despite amputation of the affected area. With proper education and early intervention, foot infections are usually eliminated in a timely manner. The accompanying Care Plan describes prevention of foot infections.[4] Effective foot care can be the initial break in the chain of events that leads to amputation (see Fig. 45–8 and the Bridge to Home Health Care feature).

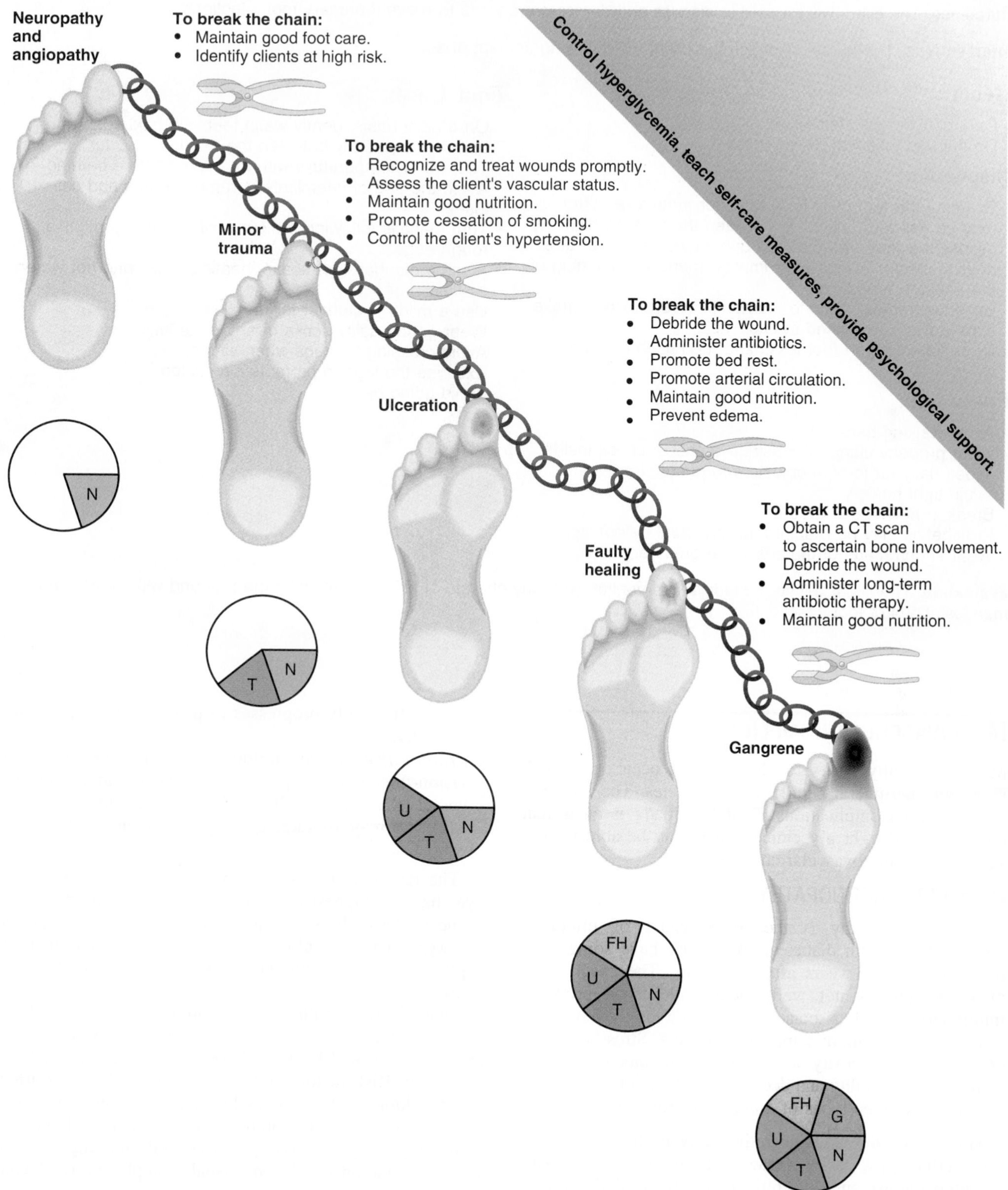
Neuropathy and angiopathy
To break the chain:
• Maintain good foot care.
• Identify clients at high risk.
Control hyperglycemia, teach self-care measures, provide psychological support.
To break the chain:
• Recognize and treat wounds promptly.
• Assess the client's vascular status.
• Maintain good nutrition.
• Promote cessation of smoking.
• Control the client's hypertension.
Minor trauma
To break the chain:
• Debride the wound.
• Administer antibiotics.
• Promote bed rest.
• Promote arterial circulation.
• Maintain good nutrition.
• Prevent edema.
Ulceration
To break the chain:
• Obtain a CT scan to ascertain bone involvement.
• Debride the wound.
• Administer long-term antibiotic therapy.
• Maintain good nutrition.
Faulty healing
Gangrene
N
T
U
FH
G

FIGURE 45–8 Breaking the chain of events that leads to amputation in high-risk clients with diabetes mellitus. High-risk clients (those with neuropathy, vascular disease, structural deformities, abnormal gait, skin or nail deformities, or a history of previous diabetic ulcers or amputations) need frequent monitoring by the health care team. CT, computed tomography. (Adapted from Pecoraro, R. E., & Burgess, E. M. [1992]. Pathways to diabetic limb amputation: Basis for prevention. *Diabetes Spectrum, 5,* 329–334.)

CARE PLAN

■ FOOT INFECTIONS IN THE CLIENT WITH DIABETES MELLITUS

Nursing Diagnosis. Altered Peripheral Tissue Perfusion related to neuropathy and atherosclerosis secondary to diabetes mellitus and lack of knowledge related to diabetic foot care and the prevention of diabetic foot infections

Outcomes. The client will be able to discuss and demonstrate ways to prevent primary foot infections.

Interventions. The nurse will teach the client the following content areas:

General:

- Control hyperglycemia.
- Do not use tobacco.

Inspection:

- Examine the feet daily for any minor trauma (a mirror may be needed), including between the toes. Particularly assess the foot area that has decreased sensation or a healing lesion. Evaluate for improvement or worsening of the affected area.
- Schedule regular visits to the health care provider; make sure feet are examined at each visit.
- Immediately report foot lesions to the health care provider.

Footwear:

- Avoid walking barefoot.
- Wear properly fitting, nonrestrictive shoes; check inside shoes daily for foreign objects, rough areas or wear.
- Avoid tight hosiery.
- Break in new shoes gradually.
- Prosthetics may be required for structural deformities.
- Wear shoes made of materials that breathe.

Foot Care:

- On a daily basis, gently wash feet with mild soap and blot dry (especially between the toes).
- Test water temperature with the elbow before bathing.
- Avoid the use of chemicals to remove corns and calluses.
- Trim toenails following the curve of the toe; gently file rough edges.
- Avoid prolonged foot soaks, heating pads, and hot water bottles.
- Use a mild moisturizer for dry skin.
- Wear good-quality socks of any material.
- Avoid crossing the legs when sitting.
- Exercise the legs to promote circulation.
- Avoid going barefoot.

Evaluation. The client will seek medical intervention with any change of skin integrity with the foot and will remain free of manifestations of foot infections.

MICROVASCULAR COMPLICATIONS

Microangiopathy refers to changes that occur in retinal, renal, and peripheral capillaries in diabetes. The Diabetes Control and Complications Trial has made it clear that consistent and tight glycemic control may be able to prevent or stop microvascular changes.

■ DIABETIC RETINOPATHY

Diabetic retinopathy is the major cause of blindness among clients with diabetes; about 80% have some form of retinopathy 15 years after diagnosis. The exact cause of retinopathy is not well understood but is probably multifactorial and associated with protein glycosylation, ischemia, and hemodynamic mechanisms. Stress from increased blood viscosity is a hemodynamic mechanism that increases permeability and decreases elasticity of capillaries.

There are three types of diabetic retinopathy:

- *Nonproliferative* diabetic retinopathy is the early phase of retinopathy. It is characterized by microaneurysms (outpouching) and intraretinal "dot and blot" hemorrhages. It occurs in most clients with long-term diabetes and in many cases it does not progress or affect visual acuity.
- *Preproliferative* diabetic retinopathy involves further progression of the hemorrhages and decreasing visual acuity. It usually progresses to proliferative diabetic retinopathy.
- *Proliferative* diabetic retinopathy is the final and most vision-threatening type. The weakened and damaged vessels that have proliferated, or formed, in response to ischemia may rupture, causing retinal hemorrhage and exudates.

The retina, which is the most essential structure of the eye, has the highest rate of oxygen consumption of any tissue in the body. Consequently, if the retina is deprived of oxygen-carrying blood secondary to destruction of its capillaries, tissue anoxia (lack of oxygen) develops swiftly.

Diabetic retinopathy is the leading cause of blindness in the United States among adults 20 to 74 years of age and causes from 12,000 to 24,000 new cases of blindness each year. Risk factors under investigation that may affect the development of retinopathy include chronic hyperglycemia, poor glycemic control, disease duration, hypertension, pregnancy, puberty, polyuria, and smoking (see the Client Education Guide on Visual Complications of Diabetes).

Clinical Manifestations

Clinical manifestations of retinopathy typically do not develop until the later stages, when clients have acute vision

BRIDGE TO HOME HEALTH CARE

Diabetic Foot Care

People who have diabetes often develop minor foot problems that progress to major problems, and even amputation. Many foot problems can be prevented or resolved at an early stage. The most important responsibilities of the nurse in diabetic foot care are assessment, education, and direct care measures.

The nurse who initially works with the client in the community needs to do a thorough diabetic assessment that includes evaluation of the client's knowledge, self-care ability, physical status, and needs. Physical assessment of the feet includes:

- Observation of the dermatologic condition, to detect absence of hair, diminished turgor, dry or rough skin, hyperpigmentation, fissures, calluses, ulcers, and lesions or nail problems, such as thickness or discoloration
- Evaluation of the vascular status by checking peripheral pulses, blood return after blanching, and skin temperature, consistency (to rule out edema), and color
- Examination for evidence of orthopedic problems such as hammer toes or bunions
- Evaluation of the neurologic status by testing the deep tendon reflexes and response to pain, vibration, and touch.

Refer the client to a physician if anything abnormal is noted.

Clients who have diabetes must receive very specific education about circulation, self-inspection, protection, and daily foot care. If clients cannot safely perform the necessary tasks independently, it is imperative that other caregivers accept responsibility. Some clients will need a combination of helpers including the home health care nurse, the community health nurse at a foot care clinic, family members, and informal caregivers. Medicare reimbursement for foot care and other home health services is limited. Nurses must advocate for clients and help them obtain the most appropriate and cost-effective services.

Clients who have diabetes need to maximize the circulation of their feet. Teach them to maintain good nutrition and adequate fluid intake. Instruct them not to smoke, cross their legs, or wear restrictive clothing. Demonstrate how to do foot and ankle range-of-motion exercises by writing the alphabet with their feet. Teach them to inspect all areas of their feet daily, looking for open areas, warmth, redness, discharge, formation of calluses or corns, or anything unusual.

Encourage clients to use protective measures, such as (1) always wearing good-fitting, high-quality shoes, (2) avoiding temperature extremes, and (3) seeking immediate medical attention for any injury or problem. Teach daily care of the feet that includes washing with a mild soap; drying thoroughly, especially between the toes; moisturizing feet, except between the toes; and keeping toenails trimmed. If it is necessary to soak feet before trimming toenails, do not soak for longer than 5 to 10 minutes.

Routine foot care performed by nurses in the community may include care of the skin (washing, drying, lubricating, massaging), removal of corns and calluses (shaving to healthy skin with a file or blade), and cutting the toenails. Toenails should be cut straight across or with a slight curve following the shape of the toe and filed smooth to prevent pressure or cutting of adjacent toes.

As with any nursing procedure, appropriate infection control measures should be followed. Cleanse supplies properly, wear gloves and protective eye wear, and dispose of used blades following adequate disposal protocols for sharps.

Debra A. Solomon, RN, MSN, FNP-C, *Clinical Coordinator, Fairview Lakes HomeCaring and Hospice, Chisago City, Minnesota*

problems. Blurred vision is a common manifestation that results from an abnormally high blood glucose level. In addition, seeing floaters or flashing lights may indicate hemorrhage or retinal detachment. Because of a lack of early manifestations, it is important to assess the potential for visual problems in all clients with diabetes, including the date of their last dilated pupil examination.

Outcome Management

Major interventions, particularly in the early phases, include achievement of euglycemia and normalization of blood pressure. When retinopathy threatens vision, outpatient laser therapy (photocoagulation) is usually recommended. It halts or slows the decline in vision in most diabetic clients if it is used before too much damage has occurred. Although extensive photocoagulation usually diminishes peripheral vision and may decrease night vision, its success in preserving good visual acuity makes it worthwhile despite these side effects.

If the extent or location of the damage makes photocoagulation ineffective, or if the vitreous is too scarred or clouded with blood, vision may be improved with a vitrectomy, a surgical procedure that removes the vitreous and replaces it with saline solution. About 70% of clients who have vitrectomies notice an improvement in or stabilization of their sight, and some recover enough to resume reading and driving.

■ NEPHROPATHY

Diabetic nephropathy is the single most common cause of end-stage renal disease (ESRD). About 35% to 45% of clients with type 1 diabetes are found to have nephropathy 15 to 20 years after diagnosis. About 20% of clients with type 2 diabetes are found to have nephropathy 5 to 10 years after diagnosis. A consequence of microangiopathy, nephropathy involves damage to and eventual obliteration of the capillaries that supply the glomeruli of the kidney. This damage leads in turn to a complex of pathologic changes and manifestations (intercapillary glomerulosclerosis, nephrosis, gross albuminuria, and hypertension). Risk factors include poor glycemic control, duration of disease, and hypertension. Some clients now self-check microalbumin levels at home. This test can

CLIENT EDUCATION GUIDE

Visual Complications of Diabetes

- Diabetes can cause diabetic retinopathy, which can lead to vision loss.
- There is a relationship between hyperglycemia and diabetic retinopathy. It is extremely important to normalize blood glucose levels.
- Hypertension can worsen diabetic retinopathy. Its diagnosis and aggressive treatment are important.
- If you have diabetic retinopathy, you should know that isometric exercises raise intraocular pressure and can aggravate proliferative retinopathy.
- An ophthalmologist will be brought in to be part of your diabetes management team. If you have any visual impairments, you can be referred to appropriate organizations for assistance.
- If your vision is blurred while reading, you may have hyperglycemia or macular edema. Floaters may indicate hemorrhage, and flashing lights may indicate retinal detachment. If you experience any of these occurrences, you should report them.
- Early laser photocoagulation therapy can reduce risk of vision loss.

Adapted from American Diabetes Association. (1998). *Medical management of non–insulin dependent (type 2) diabetes mellitus* (4th ed.). Alexandria, VA: Author; and Herman, W. H., & Green, D. A. (1996). Microvascular complications of diabetes. In D. Haire-Joshu (Ed.), *Management of diabetes mellitus: Perspectives of care across the life span* (2nd ed.). St. Louis: Mosby–Year Book.

detect very small quantities of urinary albumin, which can indicate very early renal disease. With worsening of the nephrosis, chronic renal failure ensues. Unless the client can be maintained with hemodialysis or receives a renal transplant, uremia eventually causes death.

Clients with nephropathy monitor their blood glucose levels and blood pressure at home. ACE inhibitors can be used to decrease the microalbuminuria. Hypertension should be treated aggressively, as it can be the catalyst for the progression of nephropathy. Clients with nephropathy are taught to eat a low-protein diet and to avoid nephrotoxic drugs (such as gentamicin). If contrast dye is required for radiographic study, mannitol may be ordered, but the client must drink fluids after the test to clear the dye from the kidneys. Serum creatinine levels should be assessed before the administration of the contrast dye or other nephrotoxic agents.

Like diabetic retinopathy, diabetic nephropathy cannot be cured. However, prompt and adequate interventions for renal and bladder infections can prevent these causes of renal failure. Control of hypertension and tight glycemic control can contribute to a delay in the development of nephropathy or a decrease in its progression. Unsuccessfully treated nephropathy progresses to ESRD. Treatment at this point includes hemodialysis, peritoneal dialysis, or a kidney transplant.

■ NEUROPATHY

Neuropathy is the most common chronic complication of diabetes. Nearly 60% of diabetic clients experience it. Because nerve fibers do not have their own blood supply, they depend on the diffusion of nutrients and oxygen across the membrane. When axons and dendrites are not nourished, their transmission of impulses slows. In addition, sorbitol accumulates in nerve tissue, further diminishing both sensory and motor function. Both temporary and permanent neurologic problems may develop in clients with diabetes during the course of the illness. The neuropathy may be mild (causing minor inconveniences) or so severe that the quality of life is affected. Identified causes of diabetic neuropathy include (1) vascular insufficiency, (2) chronic elevations in blood glucose level, (3) hypertension, and (4) cigarette smoking. Clients may present with mononeuropathy or polyneuropathy and may have sensory or motor impairment, depending on which nerves are involved.

A platelet-derived growth factor, becaplermin (Regranex), that stimulates the body to grow new tissue is being used to promote healing in open wounds associated with lower extremity diabetic neuropathic ulcers that extend into subcutaneous tissue or beyond. The topical agent is applied once daily, spread evenly, and covered with a saline-moistened gauze dressing. After 12 hours, the ulcer is rinsed and re-covered with saline gauze (see Chapter 16).

MONONEUROPATHY

Mononeuropathy, or focal neuropathy, usually involves a single nerve or group of nerves. Mononeuropathies produce sharp, stabbing pains and are usually caused by an infarction of the blood supply. The muscles innervated by nerves affected by focal neuropathies are painful and are at risk for atrophy from disuse. Treatment may include surgical decompression for compression lesions.

POLYNEUROPATHY

Polyneuropathy, or diffuse neuropathy, involves the sensory and autonomic nerves. Sensory neuropathy is the most common type. It is commonly assessed as bilateral, symmetrical, and affecting the lower extremities. The client describes tingling, numbness, burning, and mild to total sensory loss. This complication is a major factor in injuries to the legs.

Treatment includes foot care education to prevent trauma and ulcers. Painful neuropathy may be treated with tricyclic antidepressants, phenytoin, or carbamazepine. Polyneuropathy also may simply resolve spontaneously.

AUTONOMIC NEUROPATHY

Autonomic neuropathy manifests itself in its effect on pupillary, cardiovascular, gastrointestinal, and genitourinary functions.

PUPILLARY. Autonomic neuropathy of the pupil interferes with the pupil's ability to adapt to the dark. Pupil dilation is inadequate. Clients are at risk for accidents when driving at night. The environment should be well lighted at night.

CARDIOVASCULAR. Autonomic neuropathy of the cardiovascular system is evidenced by an abnormal response to exercise. A fixed heart rate may be noted. Orthostatic hypotension may occur, which is dangerous. Resting tachycardia is another possible cardiovascular effect.

GASTROINTESTINAL. Autonomic neuropathy commonly affects the gastrointestinal tract. The client may have dysphagia, abdominal pain, nausea, vomiting, malabsorption, postprandial hypoglycemia, diarrhea, constipation, or fetal incontinence. Gastroparesis (delayed stomach emptying) may give the client the feeling of stomach fullness. This may contribute to anorexia, decreased intake, weight loss, and labile blood glucose levels related to food malabsorption. About 20% to 30% of diabetic clients have gastroparesis, manifestations of which may be alleviated with metoclopramide (Reglan) or cisapride (Propulsid).

Genitourinary. Bladder hypotonicity, or neurogenic bladder, is a common manifestation of autonomic neuropathy. Manifestations may include straining with urination, infrequent urge to urinate with long periods of time between voiding, and a decreased urine stream. Urinary stasis may occur, leading to urinary tract infection. In the male client, autonomic neuropathy can contribute to erectile dysfunction and retrograde ejaculation. Penile injections, implantable devices, or sildenafil (Viagra) may improve function (see Chapter 38 on male reproductive problems). Women with autonomic neuropathy may experience painful intercourse, which estrogen-containing lubricants can resolve (see Chapter 39 on female reproductive problems).

Management of a Diabetic Client Having Surgery

Surgery is a stressful experience for anyone; for a client with diabetes, however, surgery imposes several additional stressors. Surgery interrupts the client's usual therapeutic regimen. The diet must be temporarily changed and the dosage of insulin or oral hypoglycemic agent readjusted. The stress of surgery raises serum glucose levels. The client is susceptible to infection. The surgical incision itself becomes a new potential portal of entry for pathogens. Furthermore, postoperative healing in these clients may be slower than normal.

To offset these problems, clients with diabetes require special interventions, both preoperatively and postoperatively. They may vary, depending on whether the client has type 1 or type 2 diabetes and whether the surgery is elective or performed on an emergency basis.

Preoperative Care

The goal of preoperative care for clients with diabetes is thorough regulation of blood glucose levels before surgery. Clients with type 1 diabetes need to be closely monitored for several days or even weeks before elective surgery to stabilize their condition and, thereby, to decrease surgical risk. If a client with type 1 diabetes and poor glucose control requires emergency surgery, the surgeon must choose between operating on a hypoglycemic or hyperglycemic client and postponing an emergency operation until the diabetes is controlled. In either case, the client needs constant monitoring of vital signs, frequent laboratory and bedside glucose studies, and vigilant nursing intervention.

In contrast, clients with well-controlled type 2 diabetes usually undergo surgery with only slightly more risk than that for the general population. Typically, preoperative preparation for clients with type 1 and type 2 diabetes includes the following:

- Preoperative laboratory tests, including fasting and preprandial blood glucose levels; glycosylated hemoglobin; serum electrolytes, BUN, and serum creatinine; complete blood count; ECG and cardiac enzymes; and chest radiograph
- Early-morning scheduling of surgery so that the client's diet and insulin regimen undergo as little disruption as possible
- Omission of food, water, and oral hypoglycemic agents on the morning of surgery (one long-acting hypoglycemic agent, chlorpropamide, is discontinued 1 to 2 days before surgery because of its long half-life)
- IV infusion of insulin for insulin-dependent or insulin-requiring clients, usually with glucose (5%) to prevent hypoglycemia (if the surgery is relatively minor, such as for cataract removal, the surgeon may order a 5% dextrose solution infusion and half the usual dose of intermediate-acting insulin; the anesthesiologist can monitor blood glucose levels in the operating room)
- A blood glucose determination performed and reported to the physician within 1 hour before the operation to ensure that the client (who has taken nothing by mouth since midnight) will not develop hypoglycemia during surgery

Intraoperative Care

Once the client arrives in surgery, management again depends on the severity of the diabetes and the extent of the surgery. Regular insulin, in a dose based on the client's blood glucose levels and a sliding scale or an insulin protocol, can be given by the IV route. Subcutaneous insulin should not be given intraoperatively because its absorption is affected by body temperature, circulatory blood volumes, and certain anesthetics.

Postoperative Care

After surgery, the goals of postoperative management are to stabilize the client's vital signs, correct fluid and electrolyte imbalances, reestablish control of the diabetes, prevent wound infection, and promote wound healing. The following are important postoperative interventions:

- Administer prescribed IV infusions and regular insulin until the client can take oral nourishment.
- Once the client can tolerate fluids, offer those that contain calories to prevent hypoglycemia. Once the client can eat, make food available. Discuss the client's calorie level with a dietitian to ensure that enough calories are provided for postoperative wound healing.
- Obtain a blood glucose level four to six times daily.
- Resume the client's prescribed preoperative insulin type and dosage once blood glucose control is reestablished, foods are being consumed at adequate levels, and it has been reordered by the physician.
- Observe for evidence of hypoglycemia after surgery, such as a decrease in blood pressure or an increase in heart rate in a client who is still unresponsive from anesthesia.
- Avoid catheterization, if at all possible, to prevent bladder infection.
- Change wound dressings with meticulous sterile technique to prevent wound infection.
- Assess the client's wound and incision frequently for signs of infection. Be alert for abnormal amounts of drainage or foul-smelling drainage.
- Observe for and treat manifestations of skin breakdown,

especially if the client has peripheral vascular disease or neuropathy.

Management of a Sick Diabetic Client

The Client Education Guide presents guidelines for the client to follow during illnesses.

CLIENT EDUCATION GUIDE

Sick Day Management for Diabetes Mellitus*

You should have an individualized plan of care prescribed by the health care team to utilize during illness.

Monitoring is an essential part of diabetes management, but this is even more vital during the stress of illness.

Insulin requirements may be increased secondary to reduced activity and increased secretion of counterregulatory hormones. To prevent diabetic ketoacidosis, you should know the following:

Self-Monitoring of Blood Glucose. It is important to self-monitor blood glucose more frequently during illness, often every 2–4 hours. If premeal blood glucose values stay greater than 250 mg/dl, you should test for urine ketones and contact your health care provider.

Ketones. Urine ketones should be monitored when you feel sick and/or blood glucose is greater than 250 mg/dl. Test for ketones every 2–4 hours.

Insulin. Do not stop taking your insulin, even if you are vomiting and unable to eat. Additional regular insulin may be required, based on self-monitored blood glucose levels.

Nutrition/Fluids. Adequate fluid intake and carbohydrates are essential during illness. Eating 10–15 g of carbohydrate every 1–2 hours and small quantities of fluid every 15–30 minutes is usually sufficient to prevent dehydration and ketoacidosis. Clear broth, tea, and ice chips are usually well tolerated. Examples of foods and beverages containing about 15 g of carbohydrate are as follows:

1 regular whole Popsicle
½ cup applesauce
½ cup regular soft drink
¾ cup ginger ale
½ cup orange or apple juice
1 cup Gatorade
½ cup regular gelatin

Notify your health care provider when you have any of the following problems:

- Illness that persists more than 24 hours
- Severe abdominal pain
- Fever over 100° F, oral
- Persistent diarrhea
- Vomiting with inability to take fluids for more than 4 hours
- Blood glucose levels difficult to control and/or moderate to high levels of ketones in urine
- Shortness of breath or chest pain
- Acute visual loss
- Other unexplained health problems

*Most applicable to clients with type 1 diabetes and those with type 2 diabetes receiving insulin therapy.

CONCLUSIONS

Diabetes mellitus is a chronic disease characterized by abnormalities in carbohydrate, fat, and protein metabolism. The two major categories of diabetes mellitus are type 1 and type 2. Meal planning, exercise, and medication are the main forms of treatment. Acute complications include hyperglycemia with diabetic ketoacidosis and hypoglycemia. Chronic complications are relentlessly progressive and result from multiple changes in small and large vessels. Because diabetes is chronic, nursing management focuses on teaching the client and family how to manage the disorder on a day-to-day basis and how to assess for complications.

THINKING CRITICALLY

1. A client with type 1 diabetes takes 14 units of regular insulin and 32 units of NPH insulin subcutaneously at 7 AM and 5 PM every day. He is now hospitalized for pneumonia and nausea. It is 9:30 AM. On entering his room, you observe the client talking to his plants. What is your priority intervention? How will his confusion be resolved?

Factors to Consider. When does regular insulin peak? What might be the underlying cause of the client's confusion? How might you confirm the presence of hypoglycemia?

2. An older woman with type 1 diabetes calls the clinic and tells the nurse that she has the flu. She tells the nurse that she usually takes Humulin N, 12 units, and Humulin R, 8 units, every morning. She has not taken her insulin this morning because of vomiting, nausea, and an inability to eat. She tells the nurse she lives alone. What telephone advice is appropriate? How often should she monitor her blood glucose levels while she is ill?

Factors to Consider. What learning needs does the client exhibit? When should the insulin be given? Is a clinic visit warranted?

3. The client is a 72-year-old woman who has a 25-year history of type 2 diabetes. She has managed her care adequately over the years; with the advent of home glucose monitoring, her blood glucose levels have been very well controlled. Her main problem is a history of significant hypertension, controlled with a daily antihypertensive. Lately, she finds that small cuts and bruises take longer than usual to heal. What are the chronic complications of diabetes mellitus? What teaching should you consider for this client?

Factors to Consider. What risks does this client face as a result of her long-term diabetic history? How would you approach teaching about complications?

BIBLIOGRAPHY

1. American Diabetes Association. (1998). Continuous subcutaneous insulin infusion (position statement). *Diabetes Care, 21* (suppl. 1), S76.

2. American Diabetes Association (1998). Management of dyslipidemia in adults with diabetes (position statement). *Diabetes Care, 21* (suppl. 1), S36–S39.
3. American Diabetes Association (1998). Diabetes mellitus and exercise (position statement). *Diabetes Care, 21* (suppl. 1), S40–S44.
4. American Diabetes Association (1998). Foot care in clients with diabetes mellitus (position statement). *Diabetes Care, 21* (suppl. 1), S54–S55.
5. American Diabetes Association. (1998). Insulin administration (position statement). *Diabetes Care, 21* (suppl. 1), S72–S75.
6. American Diabetes Association. (1998). Magnesium supplementation in the treatment of diabetes (position statement). *Diabetes Care, 21* (suppl. 1), S80–S81.
7. American Diabetes Association. (1998). *Medical management of insulin-dependent (type 1) diabetes* (3rd ed.). Alexandria, VA: Author.
8. American Diabetes Association. (1998). *Medical management of non–insulin-dependent (type 2) diabetes* (4th ed.). Alexandria, VA: Author.
9. American Diabetes Association. (1998). Nutrition recommendations and principles for people with diabetes mellitus (position statement). *Diabetes Care, 21* (suppl. 1), S32–S35.
10. American Diabetes Association. (1998). Prevention of type 1 diabetes mellitus (position statement). *Diabetes Care, 21* (suppl. 1), S83.
11. American Diabetes Association. (1998). Screening for type 2 diabetes (position statement). *Diabetes Care, 21* (suppl. 1), S20–S22.
12. American Diabetes Association (1998). Standards of medical care for patients with diabetes mellitus (position statement). *Diabetes Care, 21* (suppl. 1), S23–S31.
13. American Diabetes Association. (1998). *Diabetes 1998 vital statistics.* Alexandria, VA: Author.
14. Anderson, R. M. (1995). Client empowerment and the traditional medical model: A case of irreconcilable differences? *Diabetes Care, 18*(3), 412–415.
15. Anderson, R. M., et al. (1995). Patients' empowerment: Results of a randomized clinical trial. *Diabetes Care, 18*(7), 943–949.
16. Auslander, W., & Corn, D. (1996). Environmental influences on diabetes management. Family, health care system, and community contexts. In D. Haire-Joshu (Ed.), *Management of diabetes mellitus: Perspectives of care across the life span* (2nd ed., pp. 513–526). St. Louis: Mosby–Year Book.
17. Beaser, R. S. (1995). Putting DCCT into practice. *Client Care, 29*(6), 15–30.
18. Bergenstal, R., & Rubenstein, A. (1995). Diabetes mellitus therapy. In L. J. De Groot (Ed.), *Endocrinology* (3rd ed., pp. 1482–1505). Philadelphia: W. B. Saunders.
19. Carr, S. R. (1998). Screening for gestational diabetes mellitus: A perspective in 1998. *Diabetes Care, 21* (suppl. 2), B14–B18.
20. Coleman, W. C. (1996). Foot care and lower extremity problems of diabetes mellitus. In D. Haire-Joshu (Ed.), *Management of diabetes mellitus: Perspectives of care across the life span* (2nd ed., pp. 309–332). St. Louis: Mosby–Year Book.
21. Couston, D. R., & Carpenter, M. W. (1998). The diagnosis of gestational diabetes. *Diabetes Care, 21* (suppl. 2), B5–B8.
22. Diabetes Control and Complications Trial Research Group. (1993). The effect of intensive treatment of diabetes on the development and progression of long-term complications in insulin-dependent diabetes mellitus. *New England Journal of Medicine, 329*(14), 977–985.
23. Expert Committee on the Diagnosis and Classification of Diabetes Mellitus. (1997). Report of the Expert Committee on the Diagnosis and Classification of Diabetes Mellitus. *Diabetes Care, 20*(7), 1183–1197.
24. Fajans, S. (1995). Diabetes mellitus: Definition, classification, tests. In L. J. DeGroot (Ed.), *Endocrinology* (3rd ed., pp 1411–1422). Philadelphia: W. B. Saunders.
25. Feste, C., & Anderson, R. M. (1995). Empowerment: From philosophy to practice. *Patient Education and Counseling, 26,* 139–144.
26. Foster, D. W., & McGarry, J. D. (1995). Diabetes mellitus: Acute complications, ketoacidosis, hyperosmolar coma, lactic acidosis. In J. L. DeGroot (Ed.), *Endocrinology* (3rd ed., pp 1506–1521). Philadelphia: W. B. Saunders.
27. Franz, M. (1996). Exercise and diabetes. In D. Haire-Joshu (Ed.), *Management of diabetes mellitus: Perspectives of care across the life span* (3rd ed., pp. 162–201). St. Louis: Mosby–Year Book.
28. Funnell, M. M., & Merritt, J. H. (1996). Diabetes and the older adult. In D. Haire-Joshu (Ed.), *Management of diabetes mellitus: Perspectives of care across the life span* (2nd ed., pp. 755–821). St. Louis: Mosby–Year Book.
29. Guyton, A., & Hall, J. C. D. (1997). *Human physiology and mechanisms of disease* (6th ed.). Philadelphia: W. B. Saunders.
30. Jasper, J. B., & Green, A. J. (1995). The neuropathies of diabetes. In L. J. DeGroot (Ed.), *Endocrinology* (3rd ed., pp. 1536–1568). Philadelphia: W. B. Saunders.
31. Klein, R. (1995). Diabetes mellitus: Late complications: Oculopathy. In L. J. DeGroot (Ed.), *Endocrinology* (3rd ed., pp. 1522–1535). Philadelphia: W. B. Saunders.
32. Lernmark, A. (1995). Insulin dependent (type I) diabetes: Etiology, pathogenesis, and natural history. In J. L. DeGroot (Ed.), *Endocrinology* (3rd ed., pp. 1423–1435). Philadelphia: W. B. Saunders.
33. National Diabetes Data Group. (1979). Classification and diagnosis of diabetes mellitus and other categories of glucose intolerance. *Diabetes, 28,* 1039–1057.
34. Olefsky, J. M. (1995). Diabetes mellitus (type II): Etiology and pathogenesis. In J. L. DeGroot (Ed.), *Endocrinology* (3rd ed., pp. 1436–1463). Philadelphia: W. B. Saunders.
35. Peragallo-Dittko, V. (1996). Tight control: A guide to getting started. *Diabetes Self-Management, 13*(5), 20–24.
36. Powers, M. A. (1996). *Handbook of diabetes nutritional management.* Rockville, MD: Aspen Publishers.
37. Ratner, R. E. (1998). Diabetes disease state: Pathophysiology. In M. M. Funnell, et al. (Eds.), *A core curriculum for diabetes educators* (3rd ed., pp. 167–184). Chicago: American Association of Diabetes Educators.
38. Skyler, J. S. (1997). Insulin theory in type II diabetes. *Postgraduate Medicine, 101,* 85–96.
39. U.S. Department of Agriculture, U.S. Department of Health and Human Services. (1995). *Nutrition and your health: Dietary guidelines for Americans* (4th ed). Hyattsville, MD: USDA Human Nutrition Information Service.
40. U.S. Department of Agriculture (1992). *The Food Guide Pyramid.* Hyattsville, MD: USDA Human Nutrition Information Service.
41. Vinicor, F. (1998). Macrovascular disease. In M. M. Funnell, et al. (Eds.), *A core curriculum for diabetes educators* (3rd ed., pp. 787–809). Chicago: American Association of Diabetes Educators.
42. White, J. R., Campbell, R. K., & Yarborough, P. C. (1998). Pharmacologic therapies. In M. M. Funnell, et al. (Eds.), *A core curriculum for diabetes educators* (3rd ed., pp. 295–360). Chicago: American Association of Diabetes Educators.
43. White, N. H., & Henry, D. N. (1996). Special issues in diabetes management. In D. Haire-Joshu (Ed.), *Management of diabetes mellitus: Perspectives of care across the life span* (2nd ed., pp. 342–404). St. Louis: Mosby–Year Book.

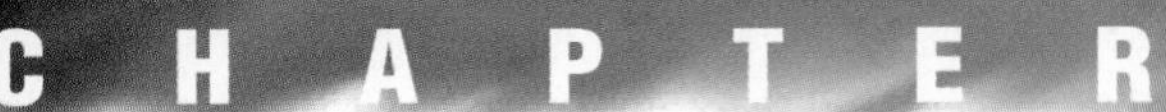

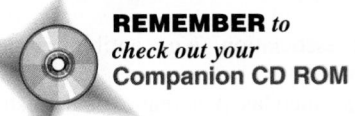

CHAPTER 46

Management of Clients with Exocrine Pancreatic and Biliary Disorders

Dianne Smolen

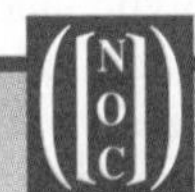

NURSING OUTCOMES CLASSIFICATION (NOC)
for Nursing Diagnoses—Clients with Exocrine Pancreatic and Biliary Disorders

Altered Nutrition: Less Than Body Requirements
Nutritional Status
Nutritional Status: Food and Fluid Intake
Nutritional Status: Nutrient Intake
Altered Oral Mucous Membrane
Oral Health
Tissue Integrity: Skin and Mucous Membrane
Anxiety
Anxiety Control
Coping
Grief Resolution
Psychosocial Adjustment: Life Change
Symptom Control
Effective Management of Therapeutic Regimen: Individual
Adherence Behavior
Compliance Behavior
Family Participation in Professional Care
Knowledge: Treatment Regimen
Participation: Health Care Decisions
Risk Control
Symptom Control
Ineffective Breathing Pattern
Respiratory Status: Airway Patency
Respiratory Status: Ventilation
Vital Signs Status
Knowledge Deficit
Knowledge: Diet
Knowledge: Disease Process
Knowledge: Energy Conservation
Knowledge: Health Behaviors
Knowledge: Health Resources
Knowledge: Illness Care
Knowledge: Medication
Knowledge: Personal Safety
Knowledge: Prescribed Activity
Knowledge: Treatment Procedure(s)
Knowledge: Treatment Regimen
Pain
Comfort Level
Pain Control
Pain: Disruptive Effects
Pain Level
Risk for Fluid Volume Deficit and Electrolyte Imbalance
Bowel Elimination
Cardiac Pump Effectiveness
Electrolyte and Acid/Base Balance
Fluid Balance
Hydration
Knowledge: Disease Process
Knowledge: Health Behaviors
Knowledge: Medication
Knowledge: Treatment Regimen
Nutritional Status: Food and Fluid Intake
Risk Control
Risk Detection
Thermoregulation
Urinary Elimination
Vital Signs Status
Risk for Ineffective Management of Therapeutic Regimen (Individuals)
Compliance Behavior
Knowledge: Disease Process
Knowledge: Treatment Regimen
Participation: Health Care Decisions
Treatment Behavior: Illness or Injury
Risk for Injury
Immune Status
Knowledge: Infection Control
Nutritional Status
Risk Control
Risk Detection
Symptom Control
Treatment Behavior: Illness or Injury
Tissue Integrity: Skin and Mucous Membranes
Vital Signs Status
Wound Healing: Primary Intention

Some disorders of the exocrine pancreas and the biliary tract are acute, and others are chronic. Manifestations may be similar to those of other conditions. The nurse plays an important role in assessing the client's manifestations and in managing the outcomes of medical and surgical treatment.

DISORDERS OF THE EXOCRINE PANCREAS

A client with a pancreatic disorder may have problems with both digestion and utilization of glucose. The relative inaccessibility of the pancreas to direct examination and the nonspecificity of manifestations associated with pancreatic disorders make diagnosis of some conditions difficult. In addition, more than 90% of the pancreas must be damaged before fat and protein digestion problems become apparent.

ACUTE PANCREATITIS

Pancreatitis (inflammation of the pancreas) may be acute or chronic. Acute pancreatitis is an inflammation of the pancreas that may result in autodigestion of the pancreas by its own enzymes. Acute pancreatitis is a fairly common but a potentially lethal inflammatory process associated with edema, various amounts of autodigestion, fat necrosis, and sometimes hemorrhage.

Although the frequency is about 5000 new cases per year in the United States, with a mortality rate of about 10%, the number of clients who have recurrent acute pancreatitis or chronic pancreatitis is not known.[18]

The incidence of pancreatitis varies in different countries and depends on the cause (e.g., alcohol, gallstones, metabolic factors, or drugs). In the United States, acute pancreatitis is related to alcohol consumption more commonly than to gallstones; in England, the opposite is true.

Etiology and Risk Factors

There are many causes of acute pancreatitis, such as alcohol (ethanol) abuse, *cholelithiasis* (gallstones), abdominal trauma, and metabolic factors. The mechanisms by which these conditions trigger pancreatic inflammation have not been identified.

In the United States, alcohol abuse is the major cause of acute pancreatitis, with common bile duct stone disease the second most frequent occurrence. Although the exact cause is not known, acute pancreatitis is thought to result from inappropriate intrapancreatic activation of proteases, which causes autodigestion of the pancreas. Exactly how this occurs is not known. It is thought that alcohol-induced pancreatitis may include a physiochemical alteration of protein that results in plugs that block the small pancreatic ductules. Biliary pancreatitis occurs when a stone migrates through the ampulla of Vater, causing diversion of bile into the pancreatic duct and subsequent bile-induced pancreatic parenchymal injury. Other causes include:

- Hyperlipidemia, which may occur secondary to nephritis, castration, or exogenous estrogen administration, or as hereditary hyperlipidemia
- Hypercalcemia arising as a result of hyperparathyroidism
- Familial cases with no definite mechanism defined
- Pancreatic trauma, such as penetrating or blunt external trauma, intraoperative manipulation, or ampullar manipulation and pancreatic ductal overdistention during endoscopic retrograde cholangiopancreatography (ERCP)
- Pancreatic ischemia during episodes of hypotensive shock, cardiopulmonary bypass, visceral atheroembolism, or vasculitis
- Drugs; although azathioprine and estrogens have been directly linked with the disease, many other drugs are believed to have an association (e.g., antibiotics, anticonvulsants, and diuretics)
- Other general causes, such as pancreatic duct obstruction, obesity, duodenal obstruction, viral infection, carcinoma, scorpion venom, and factors still to be determined

Avoidance of alcohol is the best way to promote health and to reduce the risk of pancreatitis. Limiting or completely stopping ingestion of alcohol may be a health promotion, health maintenance, or health restoration activity, depending on a diagnosis or potential diagnosis of pancreatitis. Other risk factors include cholecystitis, cholelithiasis, hyperlipidemia, hypercalcemia, pancreatic tumor, pancreatic ischemia, obesity, certain medications (estrogens, azathioprine), and any condition that causes pancreatic duct obstruction. Correction of these risk factors, such as cholecystectomy for gallstones, are health maintenance or restoration actions.

Pathophysiology

The etiologic mechanism of pancreatic damage remains unclear. The pathologic changes occurring in the pancreas may be due to premature activation of proteolytic and lipolytic pancreatic enzymes. These enzymes are normally activated in the duodenum. The pancreas normally releases protease in an inactive form. Once protease is in the intestine, the action of intestinal enterokinase converts pancreatic trypsinogen (one of the proteases) into trypsin. In pancreatitis, however, activation of the proteases and lipases occurs before secretion into the intestine. When these enzymes are activated before they are secreted into the intestine, pancreatic tissue damage occurs.

Exactly how the enzymes become active in the pancreas is unknown, but they may be triggered by reflux of bile from the duodenum into the pancreatic duct or by pancreatic duct obstruction. The net effect of this enzymatic activation is autodigestion of the pancreas. Once pancreatic inflammation begins, a vicious circle continues the process of further tissue damage and enzyme activation. As the process becomes chronic, the pancreatic parenchyma is destroyed.

In most clients, acute pancreatitis is a mild disease; in 10% to 15% of clients, however, a severe form of illness develops that leads to a lengthy hospitalization, complications, and significant rates of morbidity and mortality. Such clients present a major medical challenge because they require an intensive care setting, hemodynamic monitoring, and frequent laboratory and radiographic evaluation.

One way to predict the severity of attack and overall prognosis is to use the predictive criteria identified by Ranson in 1974 (Box 46–1):

1. Clients with two or fewer prognostic manifestations generally require only supportive care.
2. Clients with three or four manifestations have a mortality rate of approximately 15%.
3. Clients with five or six prognostic manifestations need intensive care, and the mortality rate reaches 40%.[4]
4. Clients with seven or more manifestations have an even higher mortality rate and truly test the limits of modern medicine.

BOX 46–1 Early Prognostic Manifestations of Acute Pancreatitis

At Admission

Age > 55 years
WBC count > 16,000 cells/mm^3
Blood glucose > 200 mg/dl
Serum LDH > 350 units/L
Serum AST > 250 units/L
Base deficit > 4 mEq/L

Indicators of a Worsening Prognosis in the First 48 Hours

Hematocrit fall > 10 percentage points
BUN elevation > 5 mg/dl
Serum calcium falls to < 8 mg/dl
PaO_2 < 60 mm Hg
Estimated fluid sequestration > 6 L

AST, aspartate aminotransferase; BUN, blood urea nitrogen; LDH, lactic dehydrogenase; PaO_2, partial pressure of arterial oxygen; WBC, white blood cells.

Data from Ranson, J. H. C., et al. (1974) as cited in Friedman, L. S. (1998). Liver, biliary tract, and pancreas. In L. M. Tierney, S. J. McPhee, & M. A. Papadakis (Eds.), *Medical diagnosis and treatment* (37th ed.). Stamford, CT: Appleton & Lange.

Clinical Manifestations

Manifestations in clients presenting with acute pancreatitis are largely the result of activation of proteases and lipases and the resulting autodigestion of the pancreas. Manifestations vary from mild, nonspecific abdominal pain to profound shock with coma and death. The predominant clinical feature is abdominal pain caused by edematous distention of the pancreatic capsule, local peritonitis due to enzyme release into the peritoneum, ductal spasm, or pancreatic autodigestion stimulated by increased enzyme secretion when eating.

Pain normally begins in the midepigastrium and achieves maximal intensity several hours later. In most clients, an extreme epigastric or umbilical pain radiates to the back. In clients with alcohol-associated pancreatitis, pain often begins 12 to 48 hours after an episode of inebriation. Clients with gallstone-associated pancreatitis typically experience pain after a large meal. Nausea and vomiting are frequently present because pain stimulates the vomiting center and gastric and intestinal hypomotility.

Physical examination reveals a distressed, anxious client with abdominal distention and tenderness and with fever caused by paralytic ileus of the small bowel due to localized peritonitis. Severe hemorrhagic pancreatitis may produce two distinctive manifestations: (1) *Turner's sign* (bluish discoloration of the left flank) and (2) *Cullen's sign* (bluish discoloration of the periumbilical area). These manifestations, which occur in fewer than 3% of cases, are the result of tissue catabolism and blood-stained retroperitoneal fluid, respectively. Jaundice, caused by common bile duct obstruction by pancreatic edema, may be present in clients with gallstone-associated pancreatitis but otherwise is uncommon in the initial phase of the disease.

Clients with severe pancreatitis may exhibit severe circulatory complications, such as hypotension; pallor; cool, clammy skin; hypovolemia; hypoperfusion; obtundation; and shock. Shock is not unusual; it may result from:

- Hypovolemia secondary to loss of blood and plasma proteins into the retroperitoneal space
- Increased formation and release of kinins, which cause vasodilation and increased vascular permeability
- Systemic effects of proteolytic and lipolytic enzymes released into the circulation

As many as one third of clients have evidence of left pleural effusion or left hemidiaphragmatic elevation.

Other clinical findings include subcutaneous fat necrosis and cerebral abnormalities, such as belligerence, confusion, psychosis, and coma, that are caused by hyperosmolality, hypoperfusion and hypoxia, cerebral fat embolism, or disseminated intravascular coagulopathy. Transient hyperglycemia is found in 50% of clients, probably as a result of damage to the islets. All of the hormonal (endocrine) functions of the pancreas may be disrupted from tissue damage, and diabetes may develop secondary to the disease. Hypocalcemia occurs in up to 30% of clients, since calcium may be deposited in areas of necrosis and undigested intestinal fat traps calcium in feces.

Serum amylase analysis is the most widely used test for the diagnosis of pancreatitis. In most cases, hyperamylasemia is seen within 24 hours of the onset of manifestations and resolves within 7 to 14 days. Persistent hyperamylasemia may indicate the development of complications.

The measurement of urinary amylase appears to be a sensitive index of pancreatitis. Some support the use of the amylase-creatinine clearance ratio in the diagnosis. Unfortunately, acute pancreatitis may occur with a normal amylase-creatinine clearance ratio.

The serum lipase value is one of the most specific indicators of acute pancreatitis because lipase is solely of pancreatic origin. The duration of hyperlipasemia often exceeds that of hyperamylasemia. However, hyperlipasemia may also be seen in perforated peptic ulcer, acute cholecystitis (inflammation of the gallbladder wall), intestinal ischemia, hereditary hyperlipidemia–associated pancreatitis, or alcohol-induced pancreatitis. Additionally, a white blood cell (WBC) count above 10,000 cells/mm^3 is common; hyperglycemia, mild azotemia, abnormal liver function tests, and hypocalcemia may also be present.

Chest film findings may show left basilar atelectasis, elevated left hemidiaphragm, and left pleural effusion. Abdominal films may reveal nonspecific abnormalities, such as (1) the presence of air in the duodenal loop, indicating duodenal ileus; (2) the "sentinel loop" sign, representing a dilated proximal jejunal loop; (3) the colon "cutoff" sign, indicating distention of the transverse colon; (4) gallstones; or (5) pancreatic calcifications.

Nearly all acute pancreatitis clients have some abnormality on a computed tomography (CT) scan. Pancreatic changes include parenchymal enlargement, edema, or necrosis. A CT scan is also helpful in identifying other structural changes, such as pancreatic pseudocyst, abscess, or phlegmon. A magnetic resonance imaging (MRI) study reveals the same information as CT. Scans with radio pharmaceuticals such as ^{99}mTc-labeled (technetium) *N*-substituted iminodiacetic acids (HIDA, DIDA, DISIDA) may be useful in acute pancreatitis to evaluate the gallbladder and biliary tree.

Although ERCP has no role in the standard diagnostic evaluation of most clients with acute pancreatitis, it has proved helpful in some clients with recurrent pancreatitis by identifying correctable abnormalities (e.g., duct abnormalities).

Prognosis

The mortality rate for severe acute pancreatitis—more than three Ranson criteria (see Box 46–1)—is high, especially when cardiovascular, renal, or hepatic impairment is present or when pancreatic necrosis develops. Recurrences of acute pancreatitis are common in clients with alcoholic pancreatitis.

Outcome Management

Medical Management

REDUCE PAIN

Pain is usually treated with narcotic analgesics, meperidine being the drug of choice. Morphine is contraindicated because it may cause spasm of the sphincter of Oddi, which may then potentiate ongoing pancreatic parenchymal injury.

MAINTAIN VOLUME STATUS, ELECTROLYTE BALANCE, AND NUTRITIONAL STATUS

Acute pancreatitis is commonly associated with fluid loss due to emesis. Fluids can accumulate in the bowel secondary to ileus or in the peripancreatic region because of edema. Management of the client involves replacing lost body fluids, correcting hypovolemia, and restoring electrolyte balance. Normally, the success of fluid and electrolyte restoration is monitored by assessment of heart rate, blood pressure, and urinary output. In clients with pre-existing cardiac, pulmonary, or renal disease or in those with severe pancreatitis, invasive monitoring, including urinary catheterization, central venous pressure monitoring, or monitoring cardiac output and filling via a Swan-Ganz catheter, is indicated. Clients with severe hemorrhagic pancreatitis may require transfusions of blood or clotting factors to correct coagulation problems.

Clients with acute pancreatitis commonly have a variety of electrolyte abnormalities. Clients with severe and persistent vomiting may require saline solutions containing potassium chloride. Serum calcium levels may be depressed secondary to hypoalbuminemia. Mild hyperglycemia is usually corrected with fluid volume replacement, but marked hyperglycemia or glycosuria calls for careful insulin administration.

Treatment may involve attempts to suppress pancreatic exocrine function. Therapy to decrease these enzymes may include nasogastric suction or administration of histamine (H_2)-receptor antagonists, antacids, anticholinergics, glucagon, calcitonin, somatostatin, and proglumide.

Pancreatitis may also be associated with nutritional problems when the client has been allowed nothing by mouth (NPO; *nil per os*), has nausea and vomiting, or has undergone nasogastric suction. Nutritional problems are detailed later in this chapter.

MAINTAIN PANCREATIC REST

Pancreatic rest involves withholding food and liquids by mouth initially, because food ingestion increases pancreatic secretion, which may increase inflammation and pain. No food or fluids should be given orally until the client is largely free of pain and has bowel sounds. Clear liquids are then given, and gradual advancement to a regular low-fat diet is prescribed, guided by the client's tolerance and by the absence of pain. Caution must be taken, because premature return to oral intake has been associated with development of pancreatic abscess and reactivation of inflammation.

Clients with moderate to severe pancreatitis need to be supported nutritionally by total parenteral nutrition (TPN). Administration of a carbohydrate and amino-acid solution along with lipids as a source of calories may be necessary.

TREAT COMPLICATIONS

Complications of pancreatitis include *pancreatic* disorders (e.g., pancreatic abscess, infected necrosis), which may warrant surgery, or *nonpancreatic* disorders (e.g., colonic or bile obstruction or metabolic, renal, or pulmonary disorders). Clients with pulmonary or respiratory complications may require supportive measures, such as endotracheal intubation and positive pressure ventilation.

OTHER MEASURES

Antibiotics are not routinely administered because they are without proven benefit; they are generally reserved for documented infections. Calcium gluconate must be given intravenously if there is evidence of hypocalcemia with tetany. The role of somatostatin in severe acute pancreatitis is unknown, but octreotide and histamine H_2 blocker therapy are thought to be of no benefit.

It may be necessary to perform peritoneal dialysis to rid the peritoneum of potentially toxic compounds commonly found in exudate from acute pancreatitis. Histamine, vasoactive kinins, elastase, prostaglandins, phospholipase A, trypsin, and chymotrypsin may mediate adverse systemic effects, such as hypotension, pulmonary failure, hepatic failure, and altered vascular permeability. This form of therapy is usually reserved for clients who show early clinical deterioration in spite of maximal intensive care support.

Nursing Management of the Medical Client

ASSESSMENT

Until a confirmed diagnosis is made, concentrate on preparing clients for diagnostic procedures and on assessing and treating manifestations of disease (see earlier). Assess the location, severity, and character of the pain as well as the onset, duration, and precipitating or relieving factors. Evaluate the client's response to pain and the therapies used to relieve discomfort. Much of your role focuses on educating the client and significant others about procedures and their rationales.

DIAGNOSIS, OUTCOMES, INTERVENTIONS

Pain. A common nursing diagnosis for the client with pancreatitis is *Pain related to inflammation of the pancreas and surrounding tissue, biliary tract disease, obstruction of pancreatic ducts, and interruption of the blood supply.*

Outcomes. The client will demonstrate an absence of or a decrease in pain, as evidenced by verbalizing this fact and resting quietly.

Interventions

Administer Pain Medications. Administer pain medications in a timely manner. Meperidine is the drug of choice because opiate narcotics may stimulate spasm of the ducts and increase pain. Other drugs may be ordered (e.g., anticholinergics, histamine-receptor antagonists) to quiet the pancreas and to decrease enzyme secretion.

Promote Pancreatic Rest. Keeping the client on NPO status (taking nothing by mouth) not only rests the gastrointestinal tract but also decreases pancreatic stimulation and pain. Allowing no oral alimentation and using a nasogastric (NG) tube suction decrease gastrin release from the stomach and prevent gastric contents from entering the duodenum. Nasogastric suctioning removes hydrochloric acid (a powerful stimulant to the release of pancreatic enzymes) and helps to decrease distention, thereby promoting comfort. Check the system frequently to ensure that nasogastric suction is functioning properly. According to some studies, however, nasogastric suction offers only a mild to moderate advantage in the treatment of severe acute pancreatitis and should be considered elective rather than mandatory.

Provide Comfort Measures. Nonpharmacologic measures are often helpful in relieving pain, relaxing the client, and enhancing the effects of narcotics. Correct positioning (particularly a side-lying, knee-chest position with a pillow pressed against the abdomen or a sitting position with the trunk flexed), back rubs, relaxation techniques, and a quiet environment all help to promote comfort and rest.

Risk for Fluid Volume Deficit and Electrolyte Imbalance. A possible complication of acute pancreatitis is *Risk for Fluid Volume Deficit and Electrolyte Imbalance related to vomiting, nasogastric suctioning, NPO status, shifting of body fluids, fever, and diaphoresis.*

Outcomes. The client will remain normovolemic and maintain electrolyte levels within normal limits.

Interventions. Monitor vital signs for changes in pulse and blood pressure (fluid volume changes) and respiration (acid-base imbalance). If necessary, use hemodynamic monitoring to check for changes in fluid and electrolyte status. Electrocardiographic (ECG) findings of cardiac rhythm changes may be the first indication of electrolyte imbalance.

Check laboratory values for significant changes, and observe for physical manifestations of hyperglycemia, hypocalcemia, and hypokalemia. Monitor the client's response to fluid administration and blood products by monitoring intake and output and assessing for edema, adventitious lung sounds, skin turgor, and mucous membrane alterations. Report significant changes promptly because these clients are at increased risk.

Altered Nutrition: Less Than Body Requirements. Pancreatitis leads to many gastrointestinal manifestations making *Altered Nutrition: Less Than Body Requirements related to nausea and vomiting, NPO status, and nasogastric suctioning* a common nursing diagnosis for this client.

Outcomes. The client will maintain adequate nutritional status, as evidenced by maintaining normal body weight, keeping blood glucose within normal limits, and showing no evidence of muscle wasting.

Interventions. Depending on the severity of illness, these clients may be kept on NPO status for an extended length of time. When extended fasting is necessary, nutrition is provided through hyperalimentation and lipids (see Chapter 29). Assess the overall nutritional status of the client by checking daily weights, tissue integrity, and the presence of adequate body fat and muscle mass.

Clients with acute pancreatitis are allowed an oral diet when all abdominal pain and tenderness have resolved; however, if oral intake is resumed too soon, reexacerbation of manifestations may occur. Therefore, monitor the client's response to oral intake carefully, and begin intake slowly with liquids before the client progresses to a normal diet. It may be necessary to administer antispasmodics, anticholinergics, histamine-receptor antagonists, and antacids to reduce gastric and pancreatic secretions.

If the pancreas has been severely damaged, it may be necessary to give replacement pancreatic enzymes to replace the enzyme deficit and aid digestion. Monitor the effects of these drugs.

Ineffective Breathing Pattern. The client with acute pancreatitis has the potential for development of many problems. One appropriate nursing diagnosis is *Ineffective Breathing Pattern related to abdominal distention or ascites, pain, or respiratory complications.*

Outcomes. The client will maintain an effective breathing pattern, as evidenced by a respiratory rate within normal limits, relaxed respiratory effort, absence of cyanosis, and clear lungs.

Interventions. Assess the client's respirations for rate and effort. Your assessment should include lung auscultation for decreased lung sounds (potential for atelectasis), rales or rhonchi (potential for pneumonia and pleural effusion), and cyanosis. Many times, these clients have been given a prescription of bed rest, which precludes the need for prophylactic nursing interventions of pulmonary hygiene (e.g., turning, coughing, deep breathing, and incentive spirometry). Keeping the client comfortable with analgesics enhances full inspiration and normal breathing patterns. Positioning, such as placing the client in the semi-Fowler or a side-lying position, may facilitate normal respiration.

Anxiety. Because of the uncertainty of the disease and the possibility of recurrence, an appropriate nursing diagnosis is *Anxiety related to change in health status, change in environment, fear of pain returning, and alcohol abuse withdrawal.*

Outcomes. The client will express and demonstrate decreasing manifestations of anxiety, as evidenced by calmly discussing his or her apprehension, stating that anxiety and fear are decreasing, admitting that alcohol is a problem and seeking help with abstinence, and displaying behavior associated with relaxation (e.g., resting quietly).

Interventions. Assess the client's level of anxiety by listening and observing. Reassure the client, and acknowledge that the unknown is frightening. Explain procedures that may cause anxiety for the client. Because clients who are in pain or who have acute anxiety may have a shortened attention span, keep instructions simple and direct. Allow significant others to remain with the client when appropriate for added reassurance and comfort.

The client must be encouraged to face the problem that alcohol is causing if it is the source of the pancreatitis. Spend time with the client to encourage him or her to talk about the problem. Recommend groups such as Alcoholics Anonymous, and encourage the client to join such a program. Discuss supportive services available as necessary with the client and significant others.

EVALUATION

Within a few days of treatment, the client is expected to experience less pain and to gradually resume eating and drinking. For more severe cases, the client must remain on NPO status and rest the pancreas for a much longer time. If this occurs, the client will require TPN to maintain adequate nutrition.

Surgical Management

INDICATIONS. Operative intervention is indicated in four specific circumstances:

- Uncertainty of diagnosis
- Treatment of pancreatic necrosis and pancreatic abscess
- Correction of associated biliary tract disease
- Progressive clinical deterioration despite optimal supportive care

If clients with severe pancreatitis do not respond to medical management, operative intervention may be indicated to debride necrosis or, again, to exclude other possible diagnoses as causative factors.

If it is necessary to facilitate drainage of a pancreatic abscess, a laparotomy with sump drainage is usually required. It is usually necessary to resect necrotic tissue because undrained pancreatic abscesses are associated with a high mortality rate.

If the client has extensive disease of the entire gland, a subtotal pancreatectomy may be performed. The operation involves attaching a small remnant of the remaining head of the pancreas to the duodenum. A more extensive procedure, Whipple's operation (pancreaticoduodenectomy), may be necessary if the pancreatitis is confined to the head of the pancreas. In this instance, the distal third of the stomach, the duodenum, common bile duct, gallbladder, and head of the pancreas are removed.

Because it may be difficult to identify acute pancreatitis, exploratory laparotomy may be indicated to eliminate processes such as perforated viscus or acute mesenteric ischemia. If uncomplicated acute pancreatitis is present, no manipulation is needed and the surgery is terminated. In presumed gallstone-associated pancreatitis, cholecystectomy and intraoperative cholangiography are favored. In clients with severe hemorrhagic pancreatitis with necrosis, debridement of necrotic tissue is performed and retroperitoneal drainage is established.

Treatment of pancreatic abscess combines antibiotic therapy and surgical drainage. Operative debridement is necessary to remove the thick, debris-filled, paste-like collections of infected necrotic material.

CONTRAINDICATIONS. In the past, biliary tract surgery for gallstone-associated pancreatitis was deferred for up to 8 weeks; however, up to 50% of clients awaiting elective surgery experienced a recurrence of pancreatitis. Today most surgeons proceed with surgery as soon as the initial manifestations of pancreatitis resolve.

COMPLICATIONS. Ileus, abdominal distention, and vomiting are possible postoperative complications and require nasogastric suction if they occur. A serious complication of acute pancreatitis is adult respiratory distress syndrome (ARDS), which can occur within 3 to 7 days of the onset of pancreatitis and after the administration of large volumes of fluid and colloids given to sustain blood pressure and adequate urine output. The Critical Monitoring feature presents the findings mandating early intervention in ARDS secondary to acute pancreatitis.

OUTCOMES. Clients are expected to recover from the surgical procedure and not experience postoperative complications. Once bowel sounds have returned approximately 3 days after surgery, the nasogastric tube is discontinued. If tube removal is tolerated and pain is relieved, the client will begin liquids within the next 24 to 72 hours. The client is discharged once a low-fat diet is tolerated.

Nursing Management of the Surgical Client

PREOPERATIVE CARE

Preparing a client for pancreatic surgery requires the usual preoperative care. In addition, close monitoring of WBC count, hematocrit, serum electrolytes, serum calcium, serum creatinine, blood urea nitrogen (BUN), aspartate aminotransferase (AST), lactic dehydrogenase (LDH), and arterial blood gases (ABGs) is essential. Other measures may be necessary, depending on the severity of the client's illness, such as insertion of a nasogastric tube, continued replacement of fluids, monitoring of central venous pressure, and blood culture results.

Preoperative nursing management of the client with acute pancreatitis is similar to that described under Nurs-

CRITICAL MONITORING

Manifestations of Adult Respiratory Distress Syndrome Secondary to Acute Pancreatitis

Acute respiratory distress: tachypnea, dyspnea, accessory muscle breathing, and cyanosis
Fever and dry cough that develop over a short time period
Fine crackles heard throughout lung fields on auscultation
Possible confusion and agitation
Hypoxemia with partial pressure of oxygen (Po_2) < 50 mm Hg
Early—hypocapnia and respiratory alkalosis
Late—hypercapnia and respiratory acidosis

ing Management of the Medical Client. Pay special attention to the nutritional status of the client as well as to the breathing pattern, fluid volume and electrolyte levels, control of pain, and possible complications as the client is prepared for surgery. The client will require preoperative teaching about the procedure and what to expect postoperatively (see Chapter 15). Encourage clients to ask questions about their condition, treatment, and progress.

Postoperative Care

Assessment

After pancreatic surgery, you should:

1. Have a clear idea of the surgical procedure performed, its purpose, steps, and dangers.
2. Be aware of the location and purpose of each drain inserted during surgery. If there are multiple drains, especially external drains, assess each for proper function.
3. Continually assess tubes or drains that are in place for decompression. If a T tube or internal stent becomes nonfunctional, alert the surgeon immediately to prevent leakage at the internal insertion site. Leakage may lead to peritonitis or fistula formation. Assess for placement, location (internal or external), and proper function and patency of the drains. If the drains do not appear to be functioning, notify the physician immediately.

After pancreatic excision, it is important to know how much pancreatic tissue was removed. When there is a decrease in endocrine tissue, control of blood glucose with insulin and diet becomes necessary. Exocrine loss does not pose immediate postoperative problems but does necessitate lifelong enzyme replacement when oral ingestion is resumed. Assess the functional ability of remaining pancreatic tissue after excision of the pancreas, determining both endocrine and exocrine functioning and its long-term implications. If the client has lost all endocrine function, insulin administration will be necessary (see Chapter 45). Continue to monitor the client for manifestations of hypoglycemia and hyperglycemia.

With the loss of exocrine function, replacement of pancreatic enzyme function with medications such as pancrelipase (Pancrease) becomes necessary. When the client begins to eat, watch for the development of diarrhea and steatorrhea (fatty stools), which indicate that insufficient pancreatic enzymes are present.

Diagnosis, Outcomes, Interventions

See the nursing diagnoses discussed under Nursing Management of the Medical Client with acute pancreatitis relating to pain, fluid and electrolyte balance, anxiety, ineffective breathing pattern, and nutrition. All are applicable in the postoperative situation. In addition, the following nursing diagnoses are specifically related to the postoperative period.

Risk for Ineffective Management of Therapeutic Regimen (Individuals). After pancreatectomy, the client will have many and complex learning needs, leading to the nursing diagnosis *Risk for Ineffective Management of Therapeutic Regimen (Individuals) related to care, postoperative nutritional needs, diabetic care, and pancreatic enzyme replacement.*

Outcomes. The client will understand discharge instructions, as evidenced by the ability to describe and demonstrate appropriate wound care, diet, proper diabetes care, and correct administration and side effects of the medication regimen.

Interventions. Assess the knowledge of the client and significant others before providing appropriate learning guidelines before discharge. Provide instructions for wound care. The client will require changes in diet necessitated by diabetes. Provide guidelines for nutritional needs and an appropriate low-fat diet.

Provide the client with important information concerning diabetes, including information about hyperglycemia (polyuria, polydipsia, and polyphagia) and hypoglycemia (see Chapter 45). Explain medication (pancreatic enzymes), including action, side effects, and when to notify the physician.

Effective Management of Therapeutic Regimen: Individual. If the client has an alcohol problem, there will be a need to control it and other potential problems associated with the disease, leading to the nursing diagnosis *Effective Management of Therapeutic Regimen: Individual related to alcohol abuse, surgical procedure, severity of the pancreatitis, and need for follow-up care.*

Outcomes. The client will discuss strategies to address the progression or complications of alcoholism and pancreatitis that challenge his or her continued successful management.

Interventions. The client with loss of pancreatic endocrine function requires extensive education regarding diabetes and its care (see Chapter 45). All clients require instruction on good nutrition to maintain adequate output. The client will need to understand and to follow a nutritious low-fat diet.

Avoidance of alcohol is another area of postoperative education. Explain the problems that alcohol is creating and the importance of stopping drinking before irreversible damage is done.

Evaluation

If there are no complications, the client can be discharged about a week after surgery. Hence, a visiting nurse may visit the client after discharge to assess the client's ability to follow the postoperative regimen. The client will need to be seen at regular intervals to ensure compliance.

The client's ability to abstain from alcohol should be carefully assessed and further counseling provided, if needed. In the short term, the client should recover from acute pancreatitis without complications. Long-term recovery, however, often depends on the client's willingness and ability to alter one's lifestyle.

Self-Care

Because of the complex nature of pancreatitis and the importance of the client's understanding in lowering the risk of recurrence, clients must become knowledgeable about the causes of the disease, treatment, possible complications, and home health care.

Before discharge to the home, ask the client and significant others to verbalize home health care needs related to the diet; medications, including indications, dosage, frequency, and side effects; and the manifestations of recurrence.

MEDICATIONS

Prepare clients for discharge by assessing their level of understanding and their learning needs. Discuss the medication regimen with the client, including its purpose, dosage, frequency, and possible side effects. Explain that an insulin supplement may be required because of pancreatic damage. Begin your teaching as soon as possible to ensure that the client and significant others are fully prepared to cope with glucose monitoring, diet, and insulin administration (see Chapter 45).

DIET MODIFICATIONS

Instruct the client about dietary restrictions, such as avoiding alcohol, tea, coffee, spicy foods, and heavy meals, which stimulate pancreatic secretions and produce attacks of pancreatitis. Clients should understand the benefit of eating small, frequent meals high in protein, low in fat, and moderate to high in carbohydrate.

TEACH MANIFESTATIONS OF RECURRENCE

Ensure that the client is aware of the manifestations of recurrence of pancreatitis and the importance of reporting these manifestations immediately. These manifestations include steatorrhea; severe back or epigastric pain; persistent gastritis, nausea, and vomiting; weight loss; elevated temperature; and evidence of hyperglycemia. If the client has had surgery, routine postoperative teaching (see Chapter 15) and education about care of drains, if still in place, will be needed.

CHRONIC PANCREATITIS

Chronic pancreatitis is a progressive, inflammatory, destructive disease of the pancreas. The incidence in the United States is approximately 4 in 100,000.

Pathophysiology

Chronic pancreatitis involves progressive fibrosis and degeneration of the pancreas. Characteristically, the pancreas is progressively destroyed by repeated flares of usually mild attacks of pancreatitis. After repeated attacks of acute pancreatitis, this inflammatory process results in scarring and calcification of pancreatic tissue. The damage is irreversible, affecting both endocrine and exocrine pancreatic functions.

In the United States and in other industrial countries, chronic alcoholism is the most frequent cause of chronic calcifying pancreatitis. In up to 25% of American adults, chronic pancreatitis is of unknown or idiopathic cause; it may also be hereditary. A gene for hereditary pancreatitis, transmitted as an autosomal dominant trait with variable penetrance, has been identified on chromosome 7. Protein malnutrition is a cause in other parts of the world. Other causes include untreated hyperparathyroidism, congenital anomalies, and pancreatic trauma.

Clinical Manifestations

In chronic pancreatitis, as in acute pancreatitis, dull pain alternates with severe pain, vomiting, constipation, fever, and jaundice. The client may experience some pain relief by sitting in bed with the knees flexed and pressing a pillow to the abdomen. The client generally experiences more pain when supine. Attacks may last only a few days or as long as 2 weeks.

Because food may worsen the pain, the client usually reduces food intake, resulting in weight loss. Reduction in digestive enzyme secretion eventually causes malnutrition and contributes to the weight loss. Ultimately, because of involvement of islet tissue, hyperglycemia develops with manifestations of diabetes. Insulin-dependent diabetes mellitus occurs in up to one third of clients.

The client also suffers from (1) abdominal distention with flatus and cramps and (2) frequent passage of foul fatty stools (steatorrhea). Thus, the clinical group of manifestations that serves as a classic presentation of chronic pancreatitis is abdominal pain, weight loss, diabetes, and steatorrhea. Additionally, many clients present with a history of narcotic analgesic abuse in an effort to control pain. Pain or digestive disturbance may motivate a person with chronic pancreatitis to seek help.

Because clients with chronic pancreatitis have a reduced amount of functioning tissue, pancreatic enzyme analysis may be normal. Blood studies may reveal a mild leukocytosis. Glycosuria may be present. X-ray studies may show reduced bowel motility, calcifications, and adhesions. Both ultrasonography and the more expensive CT study provide useful diagnostic data. Angiography indicates vascular changes. Cholangiography and cholecystography show biliary alterations, which may be either a cause or a consequence of the pancreatic disorder.

Outcome Management

Medical Management

RELIEVE PAIN

The control of pain can be a major problem and is generally the sole indication for surgical intervention. Attempts to control pain pharmacologically should begin with non-narcotic analgesics and should progress to narcotic analgesics, if needed. For alcohol-related pancreatitis, total abstinence from alcohol is imperative and sometimes successful in itself for pain relief. A low-fat diet should be prescribed and may reduce painful stimulation of pancreatitis enzyme secretion.

Steatorrhea may be treated with pancreatic supplements selected for their high lipase activity. Concurrent administration of sodium bicarbonate H_2-receptor antagonists (e.g., ranitidine) or a proton pump inhibitor (e.g., omeprazole) may decrease the inactivation of lipase by acid and thereby may further decrease steatorrhea.

TREATMENT OF ENDOCRINE INSUFFICIENCY

Exogenous insulin therapy may be necessary because of destruction of islet tissue.

TREATMENT OF EXOCRINE INSUFFICIENCY

Exocrine insufficiency is treated with exogenous pancreatic enzyme therapy. This therapy may include lipase, trypsin, or H_2-receptor antagonists.

Surgical Management

The three major goals of surgical intervention for chronic pancreatitis are to:

1. Correct the primary tract disease (ampullar procedure)
2. Relieve ductal obstruction (ductal drainage)
3. Alleviate pain (ablative procedure)

Several surgical approaches are available. The major operations are depicted in Figure 46–1.

Endoscopic or surgical drainage is indicated for pseudocysts that cause manifestations. Pancreatic ascites or pancreaticopleural fistulae resulting from a disrupted pancreatic duct can be managed by endoscopic placement of a stent across the disrupted duct. Breaking up stones (calculi) in the pancreatic duct by lithotripsy and endoscopic removal of stones from the duct at ERCP or placement of a stent across pancreatic duct strictures may relieve pain. For clients with chronic pain and nondilated ducts, a percutaneous celiac plexus nerve block may be ordered, although results are often disappointing.

The prognosis for the client with chronic pancreatitis is good if acute attacks decrease in frequency. Replacement therapy for chronic fat indigestion permits a fairly normal life. If the client continues to drink alcohol, the prognosis is poor. Repeated attacks eventually cause death from shock or renal failure.

PANCREATIC PSEUDOCYSTS

Pancreatic pseudocysts are localized collections of pancreatic secretions (high concentrations of amylase, lipase, and trypsin) in a cystic structure usually adjacent to the pancreas rather than within the parenchyma. Pseudocysts account for up to 75% of all cystic lesions of the pancreas. They develop in up to 10% of clients after an attack of acute alcoholic pancreatitis, but they may be associated with acute pancreatitis of other causes, chronic pancreatitis, trauma, and pancreatic neoplasm.

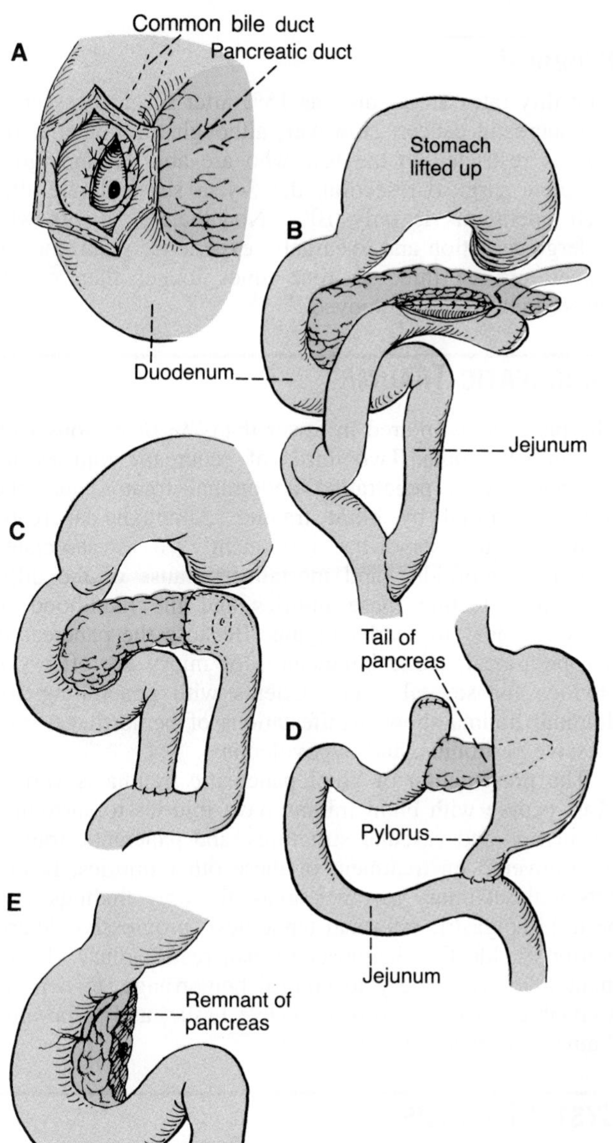

A. **Sphincteroplasty (ampullary)**
Indicated for stenosis of sphincter of Oddi with dilation of pancreatic duct. This procedure has limited application in pancreatitis, and its use is decreasing.

B. **Side-to-side pancreaticojejunostomy (ductal drainage)**
Indicated when gross dilation of pancreatic ducts is associated with septa and calculi. The most successful procedure, with rates of 60% to 90%.

C. **Caudal pancreaticojejunostomy (ductal drainage)**
Indicated for the uncommon cases of isolated proximal pancreatic ductal stenosis not involving the ampulla.

D. **Pancreaticoduodenal resection (ablative) (with preservation of pylorus) (Whipple procedure)**
Indicated when major changes are confined to head of pancreas. Preservation of pylorus avoids usual sequelae of gastric resection.

E. **Subtotal pancreatectomy (ablative)**
Indicated when other operations fail and when ducts are unsuitable for decompression. Because metabolic sequelae are significant, this procedure is declining in popularity.

FIGURE 46–1 Surgical procedures for chronic pancreatitis and pancreatic cancer.

The most common clinical picture of a client with pancreatic pseudocyst involves abdominal pain, early satiety, nausea, and vomiting. Less common manifestations include pruritus, jaundice, sepsis, and hemorrhage. Essentially, diagnosis of pseudocyst is made through the same assessment as that used for pancreatitis.

Treatment is based on the presence or absence of manifestations, the client's age, and the size of the cyst. Cysts smaller than 6 cm in diameter often resolve spontaneously. Clients with such cysts are followed up with frequent ultrasound studies to determine whether the cyst is decreasing in size. Clients with persistent manifestations or pseudocyst-related complications, such as infection, require operative intervention. Erosion of an inflammatory process into a blood vessel can result in a major hemorrhage into the cyst.

Surgical procedures include internal drainage of the pseudocyst (cystojejunostomy, cystogastrostomy, and cystoduodenostomy), pancreatic resection, distal pancreatectomy, and, least often, percutaneous or endoscopic drainage.

PANCREATIC CANCER

Cancer is the most common neoplasm affecting the pancreas. About 75% of cancers occur in the head, and 25% are in the body and tail of the pancreas. Pancreatic cancer is the fifth most common cause of death from cancer, exceeded only by lung, colorectal, breast, and prostate cancer. Of clients with pancreatic cancer, 90% die within the first year of diagnosis. Cancer of the pancreas is more common in blacks than in whites, in smokers, and in men. It appears to be linked to diabetes mellitus, use of alcohol, history of previous pancreatitis, smoking, and ingestion of a high-fat diet and organic chemicals, such as coke, coal gas, and benzidine. Health promotion actions include avoidance of risk factors and pancreatitis. Health maintenance and health restoration activities are limited because of the poor prognosis associated with pancreatic cancer.

Duct cell adenocarcinoma accounts for more than 90% of cell types of malignant pancreatic exocrine tumors. Less common types of pancreatic exocrine cancer include cystadenocarcinoma and acinar cell carcinoma. Periampullary adenocarcinomas originate in the region of the ampulla of Vater. Clients typically present with jaundice, significant unexplained weight loss, and abdominal pain. Many clients are managed operatively by either resection (~30%) or palliative therapy to relieve manifestations such as jaundice.[11]

Carcinomas of the tail and body of the pancreas usually present with significant weight loss and abdominal pain. Because of their location, these tumors generally grow to a large size before manifestations occur and the diagnosis is made. Therefore, the resectability rate is low (<7%), and the prognosis is poor (a 5- to 6-month mean survival). The response to chemotherapy (fluorouracil) has been disappointing.

Cystadenocarcinoma of the pancreas is most frequently seen in women between ages 40 and 60 years, and it accounts for fewer than 2% of all pancreatic exocrine neoplasms. Acinar cell carcinoma of the pancreas is very rare, showing no sex predominance. Surgical treatment is the same as that used for ductal adenocarcinoma.

Outcome Management

Medical Management

Medical treatment for pancreatic cancer includes radiation therapy (e.g., high-dose external beam, interstitial seed of iodine 125 or iridium 192, brachytherapy, and intraoperative radiation therapy) and drugs (e.g., 5-fluorouracil alone or with radiation therapy and nitrosourea, mitomycin-C, and doxorubicin). A newer chemotherapeutic agent with success is gemcitabine (Gemzar), which inhibits the movement of cells from the G1 to the S phase of the cell cycle.

Surgical Management

Surgical treatment is Whipple's operation, which involves a pancreaticoduodenectomy with removal of the distal third of the stomach, pancreaticojejunostomy, gastrojejunostomy, and choledochojejunostomy (see Fig. 46–1). The nursing care for these clients is similar to that for Nursing Management of the Surgical Client with acute pancreatitis.

Prognosis

Mortality rates are as high as 15% after surgical resection of pancreatic cancer. However, although the potential for cure is restricted to the few who are able to undergo a complete surgical resection, the 5-year survival rate after such operations is only 10%. Nonetheless, clients who undergo resection and eventually experience recurrence of cancer survive three to four times longer than clients whose tumor is not removed.[11]

PANCREATIC TRAUMA

The pancreas is injured in fewer than 2% of persons with abdominal trauma. Two thirds of pancreatic injuries are associated with penetrating abdominal trauma, and the rest are caused by blunt trauma. Although pancreatic trauma occurs somewhat infrequently, it is associated with high morbidity and mortality because of the difficulty in detecting these injuries and the likelihood of massive injury to nearby organs. Because the pancreas is retroperitoneal, clinical indicators of injury are often not obvious for several hours. Clients with penetrating abdominal trauma show manifestations of hemorrhage, progressive peritonitis, and hypovolemia.

The presentation of blunt pancreatic trauma is varied. Most people with blunt trauma have injuries to surrounding organs and vascular structures, and pancreatic trauma is discovered on treatment of these other injuries. In clients without injury to other areas, the only findings may be mild epigastric pain and tenderness; progressive deterioration yields the diagnosis of pancreatic injury. Treatment involves surgery to control hemorrhage, to debride nonviable tissue, to preserve viable tissue, and to provide drainage of pancreatic secretions.

CYSTIC FIBROSIS

Cystic fibrosis (CF) is a hereditary, chronic disease characterized by abnormal secretions of the exocrine glands.

It is genetically transmitted as an autosomal recessive trait. Approximately 4% to 5% of the population are carriers, and the incidence in the United States is about 1 in every 1600 to 2000 births in whites. CF is diagnosed and managed in childhood, but improvements in care have allowed many clients to survive into adulthood.

Pulmonary complications are the most physically visible. Clients have obvious respiratory compromise, with frequent bronchopneumonia and chronic bronchitis. Some improvements in the management of infants and children with CF have led to a greater number of adults with CF. Typically, these adults have a small stature and appear somewhat emaciated. They are barrel-chested and have clubbed fingers. Because the digestive problems encountered with CF are generally managed with diet and oral administration of pancreatic enzymes and fat-soluble vitamins, clients are hospitalized for treatment of respiratory complications rather than for intestinal problems.

In addition to pulmonary problems, clients experience impaired pancreatic exocrine function because of decreased lipase released into the bowel. The result is malabsorption of lipids with blockage of the pancreatic ducts by thick mucus. Pancreatic degeneration, fibrosis, and atrophy of tissues follow, with eventual development of fatty infiltration and loss of function. The intestines have thick, viscous mucus, which may cause a thick mass within the bowel. The lack of pancreatic enzymes causes steatorrhea.

The current trend is to hospitalize the client routinely for thorough pulmonary hygiene with a full course of intravenous (IV) antibiotics, with emphasis on antifungal agents, and respiratory therapy.

Nursing management of the client with CF focuses on two major nursing diagnoses: (1) *Ineffective Airway Clearance* and (2) *Altered Nutrition: Less than Body Requirements*. Interventions for clients with CF include:

- Prophylactic pulmonary support (expectorants, postural drainage, antibiotics)
- Administration of pancreatic enzymes
- A high-protein, high-calorie, high-salt, low-fat diet
- Replacement of fat-soluble vitamins

BILIARY TRACT DISORDERS

Disorders of the gallbladder and ducts are extremely common. In the United States alone, biliary tract disorders account for more than 500,000 hospitalizations annually. Disorders include gallstones, inflammatory conditions, infections, tumors, and congenital malformations.

The two most common conditions are gallstones and associated cholecystitis (inflammation of the gallbladder). Approximately 98% of clients who present with symptomatic gallbladder disease have gallstones. Malignancies and congenital anomalies of the biliary tract are relatively uncommon.

Before beginning this discussion, note the list of terms (Table 46–1) used in association with these conditions.

TABLE 46–1 BILIARY TRACT TERMINOLOGY

Term	Definition
Chole-	Pertaining to bile
Cholang-	Pertaining to bile ducts
Cholangiography	X-ray study of bile ducts
Cholangitis	Inflammation of bile duct
Cholecyst-	Pertaining to gallbladder
Cholecystectomy	Removal of gallbladder
Cholecystitis	Inflammation of gallbladder
Cholecystography	X-ray study of gallbladder
Cholecystostomy	Incision and drainage of gallbladder
Choledocho-	Pertaining to common bile duct
Choledocholithiasis	Stones in common bile duct
Choledochostomy	Exploration of common bile duct
Cholelith-	Pertaining to gallstones
Cholelithiasis	Presence of gallstones
Cholescintigraphy	Radionuclide imaging of biliary system

CHOLELITHIASIS (GALLSTONES)

Approximately 20 million people in the United States have gallstones, and almost 475,000 cholecystectomies are performed every year. The incidence of gallstones increases with age, as do the risks associated with cholelithiasis. In the United States, more than 10% of men and 20% of women have gallstones by age 65 years. Women account for nearly 70% of those treated for gallstones, although the mortality rate may be higher in men. Twice as many white Americans as black Americans are affected, and although gallstones are less common in black people, cholelithiasis attributable to hemolysis occurs in more than one third of people with sickle cell anemia.

The prevalence of gallstones is much the same in Europe and Australia. Clients with diabetes mellitus, obesity, Crohn's disease, and those with cirrhosis show an increased incidence.

Most of our present knowledge of cholesterol gallstones comes from the study of Pima Native American women in south-central Arizona, in whom the occurrence is 75% over age 25 years. Pigment stones are dominant in Asians and in African Americans.

Etiology and Risk Factors

Gallstones are crystalline structures formed by concretion (hardening) or accretion (adherence of particles, accumulation) of normal or abnormal bile constituents. According to various theories, there are four possible explanations for stone formation.

First, bile may undergo a change in composition. Studies of subjects with cholesterol gallstones indicate that their bile is supersaturated with cholesterol but deficient in bile salts. The cholesterol saturation of bile seems to increase with age. Changes in bile composition, however, do not completely explain why gallstones form.

Second, gallbladder stasis may lead to bile stasis. Bile stasis may (1) change the composition of bile, (2) supersaturate bile with cholesterol, and (3) precipitate some bile constituents. Gallbladder stasis may result from decreased contractility and emptying of the gallbladder and spasm of the sphincter of Oddi. Circumstances in which gallbladder stasis occurs (e.g., TPN; low-fat, weight-reduction diets; spinal cord injury, pregnancy) are associated with a high rate of gallstone formation. More specifically, TPN without oral intake for longer than 1 month is associated with gallbladder sludge formation and cholelithiasis. Delayed emptying of the gallbladder may correlate with hormonal factors. In pregnant women, there is an increase in the female sex hormone estrogen. Estrogen increases dietary uptake of cholesterol and increases biliary cholesterol secretion. This may explain why gallstones seem to be associated with pregnancy.

Third, infection may predispose a person to stone formation. Inflammatory debris can form a *nidus* (point of origin) for stone growth. The related tissue injury may alter the composition of bile by increasing the reabsorption of bile salts and lecithin. Certain organisms may also play a part in stone formation by altering the composition of bile. For example, *Escherichia coli* increases the amount of bilirubin available for pigment stones and *Streptococcus faecalis* reduces bile salts.

Fourth, genetics and demography may affect stone formation, as shown by the higher prevalence in Pima and Chippewa Native Americans, Northern Europeans, and South Americans than in Asians.

Health promotion activities to minimize gallstone formation include maintaining a low-fat diet, maintaining ideal body weight, and limiting the number of pregnancies. Clients receiving TPN for longer than 1 month should be monitored closely as health maintenance and restoration actions.

Pathophysiology

Gallstone formation involves several factors:

1. Bile must become supersaturated with cholesterol or calcium.
2. The solute must precipitate from solution as solid crystals.
3. Crystals must come together and fuse to form stones.

Gallstones are generally of three types: (1) cholesterol, (2) pigment, and (3) mixed. Because the incidence of a pure stone formation is rare, stones are generally classified by the predominant substance.

Cholesterol stones are the most common type; the incidence increases with age, and the prevalence is higher in women. Stones are usually smooth and whitish yellow to tan.

Pigment stones are present in about 30% of people with cholelithiasis in the United States. In these people, bile contains an excess of unconjugated bilirubin. Pigment stones may be black (associated with hemolysis and cirrhosis) or earthy calcium bilirubinate (associated with infection in the biliary system).

Mixed stones may be a combination of cholesterol and pigment stones or either of these with some other substance. Calcium carbonate, phosphates, bile salts, and palmitate make up the more common minor constituents.

Most gallstones are formed in the gallbladder, but they may also form in the common duct or hepatic ducts of the liver. The actual incidence is not known, however, because some stones do not cause manifestations and they pass through the ducts into the bowel unnoticed.

The pathologic findings are best interpreted from the clinical manifestations of the disease, which may be acute or chronic. Once a client becomes symptomatic, treatment and follow-up are essential to prevent progression to a more severe, and sometimes fatal, complication of gallbladder disease. About one third of these complications are due to free perforation, which occurs when a gangrenous area becomes necrotic and bile breaks into the peritoneal cavity. The mortality rate is about 20% for peritonitis with systemic distribution of pepsin.

Pericholecystic abscess accounts for 50% of the complications and is the least severe, with a mortality rate of approximately 15%. Abscess formation occurs while the perforation is walled off by omentum or an adjacent organ (e.g., colon, stomach, or duodenum). Much less frequently, in about 15% of clients, a fistula occurs when the gallbladder becomes attached to a portion of the gastrointestinal tract and perforates it. The duodenum, followed by the colon, is the most common site for this event.

Occasionally, a stone is discharged into the small intestine. If the stone is large enough, it can obstruct the narrow terminal ileum, causing gallstone ileus.

Clinical Manifestations

Manifestations of biliary tract disorders are similar to those of several other conditions. Box 46–2 lists some of the more common diseases that must be differentiated from acute and chronic cholecystitis.

Fewer than half of people with gallstones report any

BOX 46–2 Disorders with Manifestations Similar to Those of Chronic and Acute Cholecystitis

Chronic Cholecystitis

Angina pectoris
Chronic pancreatitis
Esophagitis
Hiatal hernia
Peptic ulcer
Pyelonephritis
Spastic colitis

Acute Cholecystitis

Acute appendicitis
Acute hepatitis
Acute myocardial infarction
Acute pancreatitis
Acute pyelonephritis
Intercostal neuritis
Intestinal obstruction
Perforated ulcer
Pleurisy
Renal calculus
Right lower lobe pneumonia

distress, because gallstones cause no manifestations unless complications develop. The most specific and characteristic manifestation of gallstone disease is pain or biliary colic, which is caused by spasm of the biliary ducts as they try to dislodge the stones. This pain usually follows the temporary obstruction of the gallbladder outlet. Characteristically, the pain starts in the upper midline area. It may radiate around to the back and right shoulder blade, although some clients complain that it passes straight through to the back and substernal areas. The client is often restless, changing positions frequently to relieve the intensity of the pain. Pain may persist for only a few hours or several days, and the interval between attacks is variable.

If the stone is blocking the cystic duct, manifestations of acute cholecystitis (see Acute Cholecystitis) may occur. If the stone lodges in the common duct, gallstones may be complicated by *cholangitis* (inflammation of the bile duct) and pancreatitis. *Jaundice* appears only when common duct obstruction is present.

Nausea and vomiting may occur; occasionally, self-induced vomiting alleviates the manifestations. Assessment may further reveal a history of flatulence, bloating, epigastric pain, belching, intolerance for fatty foods, and vague upper abdominal sensations. Occasionally, clients who have these problems still have them after cholecystectomy.

Assessment of these clients becomes important, in that manifestations of biliary colic and coronary artery disease are remarkably similar. Considering the prevalence of both of these problems, accurate diagnosis is essential. Many times, the diagnosis is based on the manifestations alone. Physical findings are present only during an attack with pain, pain being the cardinal manifestation. The right upper quadrant or epigastric area is tender to palpation with voluntary muscle guarding, but manifestations of peritonitis are absent. The gallbladder is not palpable, and the temperature is normal.

Blood test results are unremarkable. For confirmation of the presence of gallstones, an abdominal ultrasound study is very accurate and has advantages over oral cholecystography. Radionuclide scanning (HIDA, DIDA, or DISIDA) after administration of ^{99}mTc (technetium) is an accurate test for confirming acute cholecystitis. Other tests may include CT, cholescintigraphy, cholangiography, and, rarely, biliary drainage analysis.

The current trend is to use ERCP and endoscopic retrograde catheterization of the gallbladder (ERCG) in diagnosis, especially for common duct stones (see Chapter 42). Biliary ultrasonography (cholecystosonography) may be the initial study because it is accurate and safe, does not expose the client to ionizing radiation, and can be performed without preparation.

Outcome Management

Medical Management

Reduce Pain

Pain may arise from contraction of the gallbladder during transient obstruction of the cystic duct by gallstones. Administration of parenteral analgesics, usually meperidine (Demerol), may be administered intramuscularly (IM) on a schedule or as needed for pain. Antacids are given to neutralize gastric hyperacidity and to reduce associated pain, and antiemetics are given to minimize nausea and vomiting. Antibiotics are administered to reduce the likelihood of infection. Nitroglycerin may reduce biliary colic as well.

Monitor Fluid and Electrolyte Balance

During an acute attack of biliary colic, the client remains on NPO status, with IV fluids administered to maintain hydration. The client may lose fluids if a nasogastric tube has been inserted for symptomatic relief of vomiting or if pancreatitis is a probable diagnosis.

The diet progresses according to the client's tolerance. The client is advised to avoid foods that precipitate biliary colic. Instructions may include avoiding a fatty meal or a large meal after fasting.

Nonsurgical Approaches to Eradicate Stones

Endoscopy. Retrograde endoscopy for stone removal is an important nonsurgical alternative. To remove a gallstone from the common bile duct, the physician passes an endoscope orally into the duodenum, then passes a wire snare into the common bile duct through the ampulla of Vater, securing and removing the obstructing stone (Fig. 46–2). The physician may choose to enlarge the ampulla of Vater by endoscopic papillotomy to allow passage of stones. If stones remain in the common bile duct after cholecystectomy and a T tube is still in place, the physician may pass a stone-retrieving basket or other device through the T tube tract to remove the stone.

Gallstone Dissolution (Cholesterol-Dissolving Agents). The use of oral administration of agents for dissolving cholesterol gallstones is an important nonsurgical intervention. Chenodeoxycholic acid (CDCA), or chenodiol, is not widely used because of its tendency to produce dose-related diarrhea. However, ursodeoxycholic acid, or ursodiol (UDCA) has become popular because it is effective and produces no side effects. Both drugs act to reduce the amount of cholesterol in bile; however, each drug uses a different mechanism. Oral chenodiol is contraindicated in clients with liver disease and in women of childbearing years because of its hepatotoxic effects on the developing fetus. The two drugs, administered together, appear to produce a slightly better effect than when used individually. Diarrhea does not occur when the two drugs are combined.

Extracorporeal Shock Wave Lithotripsy. Extracorporeal shock wave lithotripsy (ESWL) may be used as an ambulatory treatment in some instances. The client should have symptomatic cholelithiasis with fewer than four stones, each smaller than 3 cm in diameter, and no history of liver or pancreatic disease. Contraindications to the procedure are the presence of common duct stones, recent acute cholecystitis, cholangitis, and pancreatitis.

Up to 1500 shock waves are directed at the stones until they are crushed during the hour-long procedure. The minute particles are then able to travel through the biliary ductal system to be excreted via the intestine (Fig. 46–3). IV conscious sedation with fentanyl citrate (Alfenta) or midazolam hydrochloride (Versed) may be used

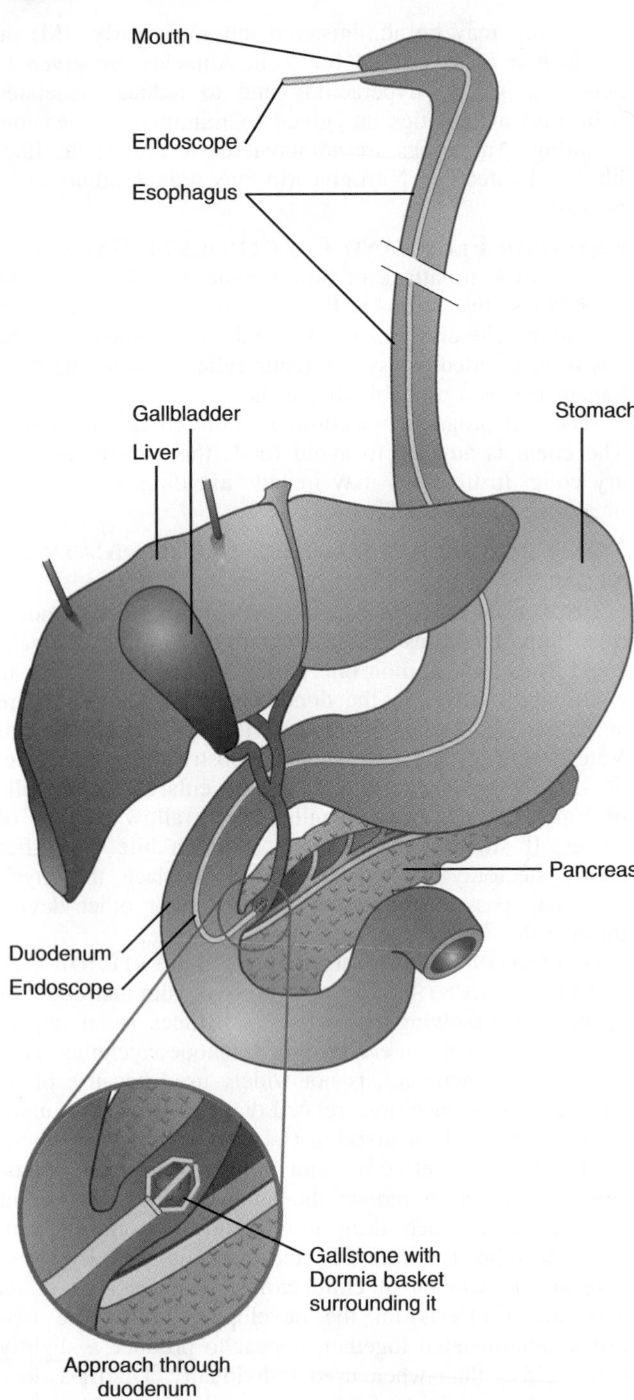

FIGURE 46–2 Cholendoscopic removal of gallstones.

to minimize the mild discomfort that some clients experience while expelling the tiny stone fragments.

After lithotripsy, minor complications may include ecchymosis over the area of entry of the shock waves, gross or microscopic hematuria because of the proximity of the right kidney, and biliary pain when large fragments pass through the cystic duct. About 50% of clients experience a recurrence of gallstones within 5 years of lithotripsy.[6]

MONITOR FOR COMPLICATIONS

Monitoring for complications of gallstone disease includes observing, most commonly, for development of manifestations of biliary colic. Conditions such as bile duct obstruction, cholangitis, pancreatitis, acute calculus, and cholecystitis may occur and cause manifestations consistent with gallbladder disease and subsequent sepsis and death. People with diabetes mellitus and gallstones appear to be somewhat more susceptible to complications of sepsis.

Because the gallbladder is left in place in all interventions except cholecystectomy, recurrence of stones is likely. Investigation continues on long-term prevention of the recurrence of gallstones.

Nursing Management of the Medical Client

ASSESSMENT

If the client is being admitted for evaluation and treatment of manifestations, your assessment should focus on collecting subjective and objective data and noting the client's response to medications. Assess the client's manifestations carefully to help determine the diagnosis. Check vital signs at regular intervals to document inflammation associated with stones. Also assess the client's knowledge of the diagnostic process. Closely monitor the client for manifestations of obstruction from the gallstones.

DIAGNOSIS, OUTCOMES, INTERVENTIONS

Pain. Because one of the major manifestations of the disease is pain, *Pain related to biliary spasms* is the major nursing diagnosis.

Outcomes. The client will demonstrate absence of or a decrease in pain, as evidenced by the client's verbalizing that pain is absent or decreased and that he or she is resting quietly.

Interventions

Administer Pain Medications. Administer pain medication as ordered; document and note the client's response to the medication. Encourage the client to verbalize the effectiveness of the medication by describing whether the pain is absent or decreased. Meperidine is the drug most frequently ordered. Morphine is contraindicated because it may increase spasm of the sphincter of Oddi. Nitroglycerin may be ordered sublingually (under the tongue) to relax smooth muscle and, thereby, to decrease colic.

Provide Comfort Measures. Other comforting measures may be helpful. Providing a quiet environment and using relaxation techniques, such as a back rub, or comfortable positioning may promote rest and enhance the effects of the analgesics.

Risk for Fluid Volume Deficit and Electrolyte Imbalance. Because of the associated gastrointestinal manifestations, write the nursing diagnosis as *Risk for Fluid Volume Deficit and Electrolyte Imbalance related to vomiting and nasogastric suctioning.*

Outcomes. The client will maintain adequate hydration and electrolyte balance, as evidenced by normal skin turgor, moist oral mucous membranes, adequate urinary output, and no manifestations of electrolyte imbalance.

Interventions

Insert a Nasogastric Tube. If the client continues vomiting, obtain an order for a nasogastric (NG) tube with a suction attachment to relieve distention and vomit-

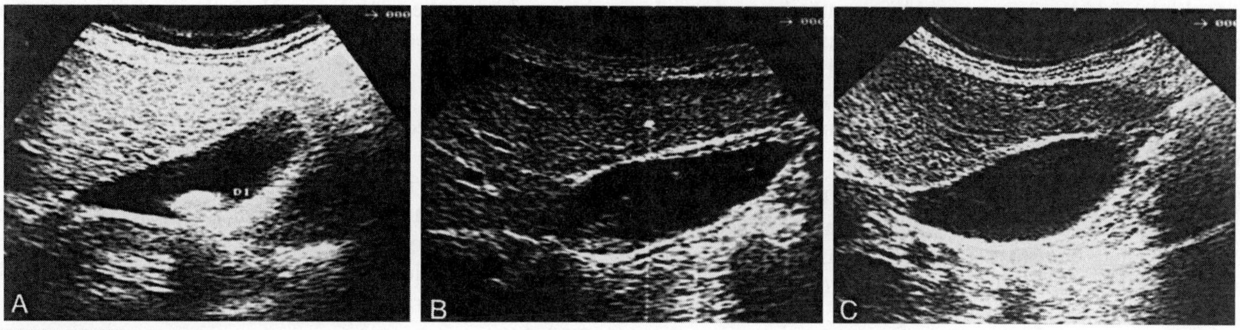

FIGURE 46–3 Ultrasonogram of the gallbladder with a single stone before *(A),* 1 day after *(B),* and 6 weeks after *(C)* extracorporeal shock-wave lithotripsy (ESWL). At day 1 after treatment, multiple small fragments are visible that had disappeared 6 weeks after ESWL and adjuvant bile acid dissolution therapy. (From Paumgartner G. [1998]. Nonsurgical management of gallstone disease. In M. Feldman, B. F. Scharschmidt, & M. H. Sleisenger [Eds.], *Sleisinger and Fordtran's gastrointestinal and liver disease* [Vol. 1, 6th ed., p. 989]. Philadelphia: W. B. Saunders.)

ing. Suction also removes the gastric juices that stimulate cholecystokinin, which in turn causes painful contractions of the gallbladder. NG suction is usually maintained on a low intermittent setting when a single-lumen tube (e.g., Levine) is used or on a low continuous setting when a double-lumen (e.g., Salem Sump) tube is used.

Administer IV Fluids and Electrolytes. Assess and document intake, output, and electrolyte laboratory values, communicating discrepancies to the physician. Assess the client for manifestations of dehydration, such as dry mucous membranes, poor skin turgor, and urinary output less than ½ ml/kg/hr.

Risk for Injury. The client undergoing endoscopic retrograde stone removal is assigned the nursing diagnosis *Risk for Injury related to medication during the procedure and possible introduction of bacteria into common bile duct.*

Outcomes. The client will remain free from injury and infection following endoscopic retrograde stone removal, as evidenced by the airway remaining patent without aspiration and absence of manifestations of infection, such as elevated temperature.

Interventions. For the client undergoing endoscopic retrograde papillotomy or stone removal, a local anesthetic solution is sprayed on the back of the throat. This intervention facilitates the passing of the endoscope. After the endoscopic papillotomy, carefully check for the return of the gag reflex before allowing oral intake. If the client receives sedation, raise the side rails on the bed for protection and keep the call light within reach. Antibiotics are often administered during the procedure to minimize the risk of infection from introduction of bacteria from the intestine into the common bile duct.

EVALUATION

Most clients recover from acute cholecystitis in a few days without complications. Once the biliary system is allowed to rest, inflammation decreases and recovery progresses. Clients should be monitored for the development of chronic cholecystitis.

Self-Care

The client and significant others will need to learn about the suggested therapeutic regimen, diet changes, indications for drugs and their side effects, dosage, and administration instructions, and ways to prevent recurrence. Clients who undergo gallstone dissolution most frequently receive UDCA. Chenodeoxycholic acid (CDCA) administration may result in mild to moderate elevation in liver function test values and serum cholesterol levels. In addition, clients receiving CDCA may experience disabling diarrhea.

MEDICATIONS

After assessing the level of understanding and learning needs, educate the client about the purpose of oral dissolution therapy, expected responses, and possible untoward reactions. Because oral dissolution medication must be taken over a long period of time, help the client devise ways to remember to take the medication daily. For example, a pillbox that is divided into the days of the week clearly indicates whether the client has missed a dose.

The client who is being treated medically may be sent home with oral analgesics or other medications for comfort as well as with an oral dissolution agent. Be sure that the client and significant others can relate all necessary information to the nurse before discharge.

DIET MODIFICATIONS

Diet instructions may be necessary if ingestion of food precipitated the attack; that is, if a fatty food caused the biliary colic, inform the client about the need for a low-fat diet.

PREVENT RECURRENCE

Advise the client about what to do should another attack occur. The client has probably been encouraged by the physician to consider elective cholecystectomy or other surgical intervention before gallbladder disease progresses further. Provide written material on gallbladder disease at this time to aid the client in understanding and decision-making.

Surgical Management

Whether to operate on a client with asymptomatic cholelithiasis ("silent gallstones") is an area for debate. The potential for serious complications (e.g., acute cholecystitis, choledocholithiasis, sepsis) can pose a significant risk. Older people and clients with insulin-dependent diabetes have a high incidence of gallstones. Because such people are at high risk during acute biliary attacks and emergency procedures, surgeons may recommend that they undergo elective cholecystectomy to avoid later emergency surgery. Other procedures that may be performed include percutaneous cholecystolithotomy and laparoscopic cholecystectomy.

Percutaneous Cholecystolithotomy

With a percutaneous cholecystolithotomy, surgeons extract stones using cystoscopes, stone baskets, and instruments designed for nephrolithotomy. Stones too large to be extracted manually can be fragmented by means of a lithotriptor or laser fiber. General anesthesia is not necessary for this procedure.

The use of percutaneous insertion of a contact dissolution agent is now being investigated. In this procedure, a catheter is inserted into the gallbladder through the skin and methyl *tert*-butyl ether (MTBE) is instilled directly into the gallbladder to dissolve cholesterol gallstones. When small amounts are infused and withdrawn four to six times per minute, stones dissolve in 1 to 3 days. Early results have been excellent.

Laparoscopic Cholecystectomy

Indications. Laparoscopic cholecystectomy has become the treatment of choice for symptomatic gallbladder disease. The procedure is suitable for most clients, even those with acute cholecystitis, because there is minimal trauma to the abdominal wall. This makes it possible for clients to go home within 24 hours after the procedure and return to work within a few days instead of a few weeks, as is the case with a cholecystectomy.

With the client under general anesthesia, carbon dioxide is used to create pneumoperitoneum through a needle inserted near the umbilicus. Near the umbilicus, an endoscope is inserted through a small incision to view the gallbladder and to determine the feasibility of success associated with this procedure. Three other small incisions are created: one for grasping the gallbladder, one for suction and irrigation, and one for dissection instruments and applying clips (Fig. 46–4).

Contraindications. Laparoscopic cholecystectomy is contraindicated if stones are known to exist in the common bile duct. Laparoscopic cholecystectomy does not allow exploration or removal of stones from the common duct.

Complications. Possible complications of surgery or anesthesia include damage to the biliary tract and hemorrhage. However, the advantages of small scars and a short hospital stay have influenced surgeons to opt for this procedure more often. Clients who undergo this procedure are at less risk because they are ambulatory sooner and usually require only oral analgesia. Because of the carbon dioxide pressing on the diaphragm, nausea, vomiting, and shoulder pain are more frequent if the client's head and torso are elevated too soon after surgery.

Outcomes. Most clients are discharged the day of surgery or the day after. In most cases, they can resume normal activities and return to work after 3 to 4 days.

Cholecystectomy

Indications. A cholecystectomy consists of excising the gallbladder from the posterior liver wall and ligating the cystic duct, vein, and artery. The surgeon usually approaches the gallbladder through a right upper paramedian or upper midline incision. If necessary, the common duct may be explored through this incision. When stones

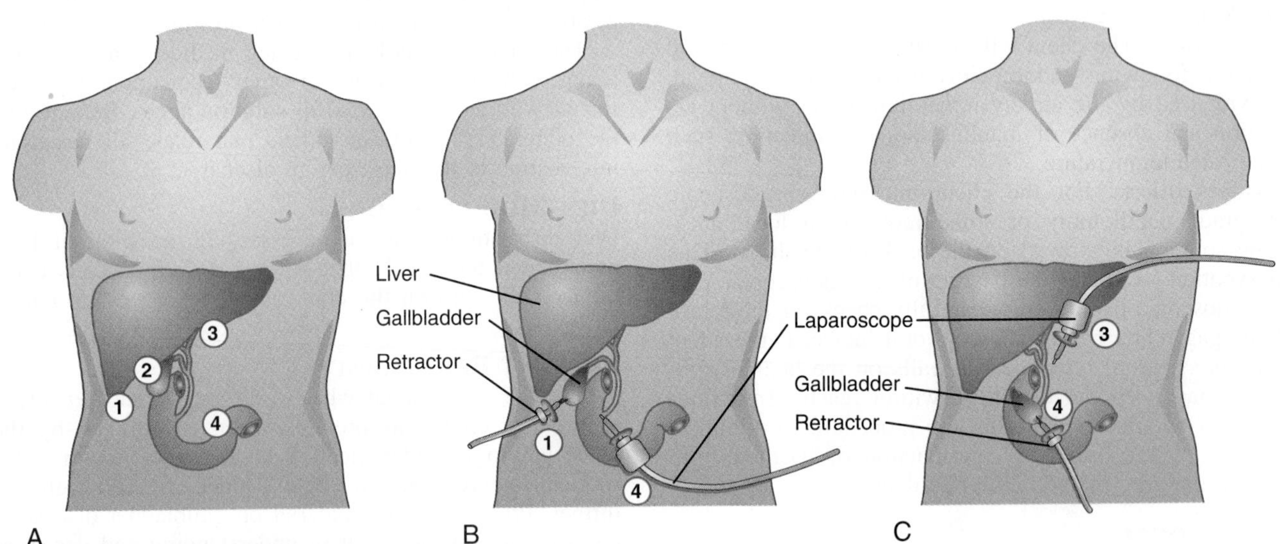

FIGURE 46–4 Laparoscopic cholecystectomy.

A, Standard sites of four ports used in laparoscopic cholecystectomy. 1, The lateral port is used to retract the gallbladder. 2, The subcostal port is used to retract the gallbladder. 3, The superior midline port is used to insert the laparoscope later in the procedure while the gallbladder is being withdrawn from the umbilical port. 4, The umbilical port is most often used to insert the laparoscope for most of the procedure and then is used to withdraw the gallbladder after the laparoscope is moved to the superior midline port.

B, Preparing the gallbladder for removal by ligating it from attachments (e.g., cystic duct, artery, vein). 1, The gallbladder is retracted through the lateral port. 4, A laparoscope is inserted through the umbilical port to visualize the gallbladder.

C, Removal of the gallbladder. 3, Laparoscope through the superior midline port. 4, Removal of the gallbladder through the umbilical port.

are suspected in the common duct, operative cholangiography may be performed (if it has not been ordered preoperatively). The surgeon may dilate the common duct if it is not already dilated as a result of a pathologic process. Dilation facilitates stone removal. The surgeon passes a thin instrument into the duct to collect the stones, either whole or after crushing them.

After exploring the common duct, the surgeon usually inserts a T tube to ensure adequate bile drainage during duct healing (*choledochostomy*). The T tube also provides a route for postoperative cholangiography or stone dissolution, when appropriate (Fig. 46–5).

A conventional open cholecystectomy is indicated when a laparoscopic cholecystectomy does not allow for retrieval of a stone in the common bile duct and when the client's physique does not allow access to the gallbladder. Occasionally, when a person is very obese, the gallbladder is not retrievable via laparoscopic instruments. Further, a surgeon may have difficulty accessing the gallbladder in an adult with a small frame and may need to perform the conventional open cholecystectomy.

CONTRAINDICATIONS. A client's physical condition may not be able to withstand the stress of surgery, including loss of fluid, electrolytes, and anesthesia. Cholecystotomy, incision and drainage of the gallbladder, may be performed as an alternative procedure.

COMPLICATIONS. After cholecystectomy, monitor the client for the usual postoperative complications, such as hemorrhage, pneumonia, thrombophlebitis, urinary retention, and ileus. The risk of bile leakage into the abdominal cavity is more applicable to surgeries involving the gallbladder. With hemorrhage and bile leakage, the client feels severe pain and tenderness in the right upper quadrant, abdominal girth increases, bile or blood may leak from the wound, blood pressure drops, and tachycardia develops.

OUTCOMES. Cholecystectomy results in immediate cessation of pain in most clients and prevents development of complications such as acute cholecystitis, choledocholithiasis, and cholangitis. Persistence of manifestations after removal of the gallbladder indicates (1) a possible misdiagnosis or functional bowel disorder, such as esophagitis, peptic ulceration, pancreatitis, or irritable bowel syndrome; (2) a technical error; (3) a retained or recurrent common bile duct stone; or (4) spasm of the sphincter of Oddi. Clients must be hospitalized for about 3 days before dismissal. They may be sent home with a T tube in place for 1 to 2 weeks.

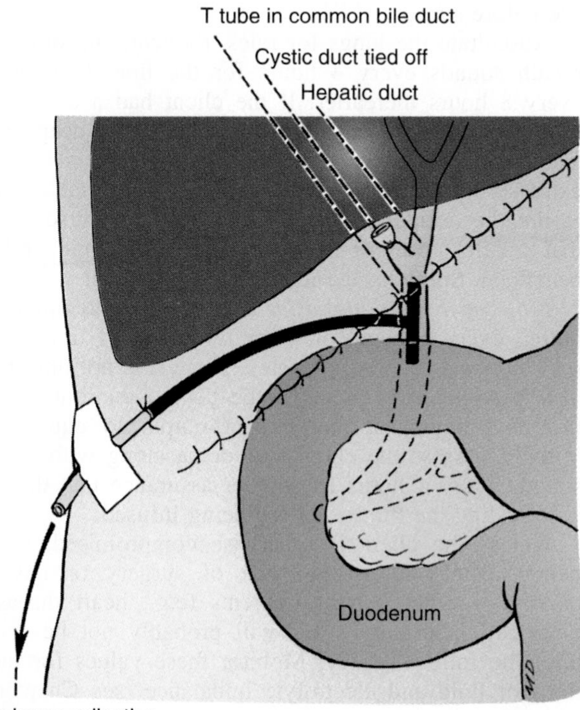

FIGURE 46–5 Placement of a T tube. The surgeon ties off the cystic duct and sutures the T tube to the common bile duct with the short arms of the T tube toward the hepatic duct and duodenum. The long arm of the T tube exits the body near the incision site. Skin suture and tape secure placement.

Nursing Management of the Surgical Client

PREOPERATIVE CARE

Preoperative care of the client facing gallbladder or biliary surgery is the same as that described in Chapter 15. In addition, preparation involves careful monitoring for early clinical findings that may indicate the onset of complications from infection or obstruction. For laparoscopic cholecystectomy, preoperative preparation involves the same measures taken for other clients going to surgery. They include (1) NPO status after midnight, (2) skin preparation (i.e., showering with bacterial soap, such as Safeguard, Dial, Hibiclens), (3) occasionally an enema to reduce colon mass and to reduce the chance of incontinence contaminating the operative field, and (4) sometimes an antibiotic.

ASSESSMENT

Generally, surgical management of cholelithiasis is elective and is not performed in an emergency situation unless obstruction has occurred. Consequently, although the client is typically knowledgeable about the procedure and the rationale for it, assess client concerning knowledge of preoperative and postoperative care.

DIAGNOSIS, OUTCOMES, INTERVENTIONS

Knowledge Deficit. The preoperative client may not be completely knowledgeable about surgical procedures, particularly gallbladder surgery. The diagnosis, therefore, can be *Knowledge Deficit related to gallbladder surgery and recovery.*

Outcomes. The client will indicate an understanding of the procedure, as evidenced by ability to verbalize information regarding it; will demonstrate an ability to carry out coughing, deep breathing, and leg exercises; and will have knowledge regarding the immediate postoperative course.

Interventions. Reinforce information given to the client about the surgical procedure. Determine the level of understanding and the learning needs of the client and significant others. Provide material, if available, that can be read or viewed at the client's own pace. Give verbal instructions and a demonstration to ensure that the client can perform postoperative exercises (turning, coughing, deep-breathing, and wound splinting) properly and can understand their importance.

Clients also need some knowledge of what to expect postoperatively, such as IV fluids, T tube placement and drainage, and pain control and activity). Studies have shown that preoperative client education significantly reduces the risk for development of postoperative complications.

Anxiety. Because of the surgery and associated stress, a nursing diagnosis appropriate to these clients is *Anxiety related to the procedure and outcome.*

Outcomes. The client will express and demonstrate feelings of comfort and show decreasing manifestations of anxiety, as evidenced by calmly discussing his or her apprehension, affirming that anxiety is decreasing, and ventilating feelings regarding the surgical procedure and diagnosis.

Interventions. Assess the client's level of anxiety by listening and observing. Reassure the client and acknowledge that the unknown is frightening. Thoroughly explain those topics that may frighten the client, such as diagnostic or preparatory procedures. Allow significant others to stay with the client as appropriate.

POSTOPERATIVE CARE

Respiratory status is carefully monitored after surgery of the gallbladder or biliary tract because of the potential for development of atelectasis and pneumonia. Closely monitor drainage from all biliary tubes and drainage from the incision site, for amount, character, and color. Carefully assess cardiovascular status and manifestations of hemorrhage or shock. Hemorrhage, although rare, may occur if an inflamed gallbladder has adhered to the liver.

Analgesia for pain management is important and should be given on a regular basis to promote comfort and rest as well as to enhance the individual's ability to cough and deep breathe.

Maintain hydration and fluid balance IV until the client is no longer on NPO status and can receive fluids orally. When the client is allowed oral intake, the amount of fluid and food should be sufficient and well balanced enough to maintain renal function and body weight (minimal loss of weight). Clients are generally allowed to progress to a regular diet, with fat content included as tolerated.

ASSESSMENT

Postoperative assessment of the client is important; it includes careful monitoring of vital signs, breath and bowel sounds, and general level of responsiveness to check for complications such as hemorrhage, respiratory problems, or infection. In addition, intake is monitored to reflect renal function and output carefully measured including wound drainage, vomiting, or nasogastric suctioning.

Assess the client's incision for redness or swelling. Monitor the level of pain as well as the location, severity, and the effectiveness of any interventions.

After a laparoscopic cholecystectomy, referred pain to the shoulder is a common postoperative pain pattern. Shoulder pain occurs because of the carbon dioxide that has not been released or absorbed by the body. Carbon dioxide causes irritation of the phrenic nerve and diaphragm and may decrease respiratory excursion.

DIAGNOSIS, OUTCOMES, INTERVENTIONS

Risk for Injury. The postoperative client is at risk for the development of many complications leading to the nursing diagnosis *Risk for Injury related to postoperative complications of hemorrhage, infection, fluid and electrolyte imbalance, pulmonary changes (atelectasis, pneumonia), urinary retention, ileus, and decreased gastrointestinal motility.*

Outcomes. The client will receive appropriate assessments and interventions for early detection and prevention of injury from postoperative complications, as evidenced by stable vital signs; normal pulmonary function; normal gastrointestinal function; laboratory values within normal limits; normal urinary function, which returns within 6 to 8 hours postoperatively; an intact incision that does not exhibit redness, odor, or purulent drainage; and no manifestations of thrombus or embolus.

Interventions

Assess Postoperatively. Take routine postoperative vital signs, and assess for manifestations of shock, such as cyanosis; diaphoresis; cold, clammy skin; decreased blood pressure; and increased pulse. As vital signs are checked, check dressings and drainage tubes at the same time for unusual amounts of bleeding or drainage. If any of the aforementioned manifestations or changes occur, check vital signs frequently and notify the physician.

Prevent Pneumonia. The client should change position at least every 2 hours. While the client is awake for turning, help him or her to cough and deep breathe. Some hospitals use devices such as incentive spirometry to encourage lung expansion and spontaneous coughing. When these devices are used, it is helpful to demonstrate their use before surgery.

Auscultate the lungs for rales, rhonchi, and diminished breath sounds every 4 hours for the first 24 hours and every 8 hours thereafter. If the client had a cholecystectomy, it will be even more difficult to take deep breaths and cough because of the location of the incision. Take extra care to ensure that the client is comfortable enough to breathe normally. Many physicians and nurses believe that smaller doses of narcotics given more frequently are beneficial. Splinting the incision helps as well.

Monitor Fluids and Electrolytes. Measure intake and output every 4 hours or more frequently if ordered. Assess amounts for discrepancies. Since it is not unusual for new postoperative clients to be behind on fluids for the first few hours, do not expect output to equal intake initially. Assess the client for edema along with the lung sounds every 4 hours as another assurance that the client is tolerating the fluids that are being infused.

Unless the client is otherwise compromised, such as being acutely ill at the time of surgery or having a history of other health problems (e.g., heart disease or diabetes), laboratory work will probably not be ordered until the following day. Monitor these values for indications of fluid and electrolyte imbalance (see Chapters 12 and 13).

Monitor Urinary Output. Generally, the client can void within 6 to 8 hours after surgery; if not, assess the bladder for distention. The client may not to be able to void because of pain, discomfort, and position, or absence of feeling the need to void because of the effects of anesthesia and narcotics. The client may need to be catheterized to empty the bladder initially.

Maintain Nasogastric Tube. Occasionally, after gallbladder surgery, the client may return with a nasogastric tube attached to suction. Check the tube frequently to ensure that it is patent and that placement is correct for adequate drainage. A plugged or displaced tube not only causes distention, nausea, and vomiting but also may place undue stress on the surgical site. Auscultate bowel sounds every 8 hours to note return of normal bowel activity. Depending on the surgery, the client may or may not be allowed oral intake before bowel sounds return.

Offer oral care at least every 2 hours while the client is on NPO status. This may consist of rinsing the mouth with water, using mouthwash, swabbing with a moist swab, or assisting the client with brushing the teeth. Assess the oral mucous membranes at least every 8 hours for integrity, color, and moistness. While the client is taking nothing orally, it may be helpful to place a wet washcloth over the lips to humidify the air. Offering ice chips or sips of liquid as soon as allowed also provides much relief.

Advance Diet as Tolerated. For the more involved surgical procedure, such as a cholecystectomy, clients are usually not allowed a normal diet until they have begun to pass flatus and until bowel sounds are heard. After the client is allowed to have fluids or food, continue to assess the client for abdominal distention and normal bowel sounds to ensure that the intake is being tolerated. Early activity also helps the return of intestinal motility, so the client should be encouraged to begin progression of regular activities as soon as possible.

Prevent Infection. If the nurse is to change the dressings, the incision should be checked simultaneously for redness, swelling, drainage characteristics and amounts, and odor. If drains are present, such as a T tube, observe the drainage for its characteristics and amount. Check the client's temperature at least every 4 hours or more frequently if necessary. Keep the dressing and incision clean and dry because moisture enhances bacterial growth. Subjective complaints of increased pain may be the first manifestation that an infectious process is taking place. This is why it is important to document the location, type, and amount of pain routinely so that comparison can be made and a significant change in condition noted immediately. Many times it is your assessment that alerts the physician and facilitates the diagnosis of infection.

Pain. The client may have problems with postoperative pain. Therefore, the following nursing diagnosis, *Pain related to surgical procedure and incision,* is applicable.

Outcomes. The client will feel relief of pain, as evidenced by resting comfortably and quietly; blood pressure and heart rate will be within normal limits, and the client will be able to tolerate postoperative exercises and activities.

Interventions. Assess and document the level, location, and type of pain as well as the client's response to pain medication. You may need to intervene and obtain new medication orders if the medication ordered is ineffective. It may be necessary to administer medication to coincide with activity to keep the client active. Nonpharmacologic measures are helpful as well. Providing a quiet environment (even limiting visitors, if necessary), changing the client's position, and rubbing the client's back all are important in relaxing the client and in enhancing the effects of the pain medication. Assist the client in splinting the incision, and instruct the client on the best way to get out of bed and to lie down.

EVALUATION

The client should heal without difficulty and may be discharged within about 3 to 4 days after cholecystectomy. The client will be able to resume normal activities in 4 to 6 weeks. After laparoscopic cholecystectomy, the client is usually discharged the day of or day after surgery and can return to normal activities within 3 to 4 days.

Self-Care

Because the client will be faced with early discharge from the health care setting, the client should be able to verbalize and accurately demonstrate home health care needs and skills, for example, (1) identifying manifestations of infection; (2) demonstrating wound care; (3) naming medications, their purpose, side effects, and administration instructions; and (4) stating activity and dietary restrictions.

Teach the client about home health care as soon after surgery as possible to assess the client's learning potential and learning needs. Instruction should include wound care, dressing changes with a return demonstration, and assessing for manifestations of infection.

TEACH MANIFESTATIONS TO REPORT

Be sure the client is knowledgeable about which manifestations should be reported to the physician and how to contact the physician. Advise the client to report fever, chills, nausea and vomiting, jaundice, dark-colored urine, pale-colored stools, and pruritus. If the client is discharged with a drain or T tube in place, he or she should know the purpose of the tube, how to secure it, how to empty it, what amounts of drainage can be expected, and abnormal characteristics of drainage.

DIET AND ACTIVITY MODIFICATIONS

Explain and reinforce activity and dietary restrictions thoroughly. Advise that heavy lifting (>10 pounds) or strenuous work or sports for as long as prescribed by the physician should be avoided. Instruct and question the client as to the medications he or she is being discharged with, the possible adverse effects, and the dosage and frequencies of the medications. Explain that a low-fat (to be increased gradually), a high-carbohydrate, high-protein diet is needed and that alcohol should be avoided to minimize the risk of pancreatic involvement.

Modifications for Elderly Clients

In older clients, gallstones do not necessarily cause pain, fever, or jaundice. Mental confusion, shakiness, and an elevated alkaline phosphatase may be the only manifestations of gallstones in the elderly population. Nonsurgical decompression techniques may be preferred in high-risk older clients.

When the older client undergoes a cholecystectomy, he or she is at greater risk for injury related to anesthesia, pain medications, and sometimes the response to the trauma of surgery. Postoperative care should be modified to prevent injury. Especially in the immediate postoperative period, the side rails should be up, the bed in low position, and the call light within easy reach.

Depending on the client's response to anesthesia and pain medication, frequent reorientation to the environment and circumstances may be necessary. Remind the older client how to summon help and why it is important to not get up alone. Be sure that all IV lines and drainage tubes are secure to prevent the client from inadvertently disconnecting them.

In particular, be alert to the fact that older people tend to become confused after surgery, especially at night. You may need to take precautions by having a physician order soft wrist or vest restraints or a device such as a bed check machine, which is placed under the client and sounds an alarm if it senses weight is no longer on it.

ACUTE CHOLECYSTITIS

Acute cholecystitis refers to acute inflammation of the gallbladder wall. There is an increased incidence of cholecystitis in clients who are overweight, especially those with a sedentary lifestyle. Certain ethnic groups, including Chinese, Jewish, and Italians, have a higher rate of the disease.

Etiology and Risk Factors

Cholecystitis is associated with gallstones and obstruction of the cystic duct by a stone in 90% of cases.[4] Obstruction of a cystic duct by a stone is the usual cause of acute cholecystitis. In 5% to 10% of clients, however, calculi obstructing the cystic duct are not found during surgery (*acalculous cholecystitis*, or cholecystitis without stones). In more than 50% of such cases, an underlying cause of the inflammation is not found.[6] Hepatic *Helicobacter* bacteria have been implicated in cholecystitis.

The major preventable risk factors are sedentary lifestyle and obesity. If the client increases his or her level of activity and maintains a low-fat diet, the risk of cholecystitis can be reduced. Encourage clients to engage in exercise and to follow healthy dietary habits.

Pathophysiology

Acute calculous cholecystitis, which appears to be caused by obstruction of the cystic duct, in turn causes distention of the gallbladder. Subsequently, (1) venous and lymphatic drainage is impaired, (2) proliferation of bacteria occurs, (3) localized cellular irritation or infiltration, or both, take place, and (4) areas of ischemia may develop. The inflamed gallbladder wall is edematous and thickened, may have areas of gangrene, or necrosis may be present. The term *empyema* describes a gallbladder that contains pus, which is the equivalent of an intra-abdominal abscess and may be associated with severe sepsis. Recurrent episodes of acute cholecystitis cause fibrosis of the wall of the gallbladder.

Complications of untreated acute cholecystitis are usually associated with septic complications. Others are consequences of ischemia, inflammation, adhesions, and gangrene: perforation, pericholecystic abscess, and fistula.

Acalculous cholecystitis (cholecystitis without stones) is far less common than cholecystitis due to gallstones. It apparently can be triggered by (1) multiple blood transfusions, (2) gram-negative bacterial sepsis, or (3) tissue damage after burns, trauma, or extensive surgery. Other possible contributing factors include hyperalimentation, prolonged fasting, hypotension, anesthesia, narcotic analgesics, and mechanical ventilation with positive end-expiratory pressure. Clients with diabetes mellitus and systemic arteritis are also susceptible.

Clinical Manifestations

Inflammation of the gallbladder may be acute or chronic. The most common and reliable finding on physical examination is tenderness in the right upper quadrant, epigastrium, or both. Although clients with chronic and acute cholecystitis may complain of the same type of pain, the distinguishing factor is the severity and persistence of the pain. Chronic cholecystitis rarely lasts more than a few hours, whereas acute cholecystitis may last several days.

Pain in acute cholecystitis may be located in the epigastric, subscapular, or right upper quadrant regions. Sometimes the pain is referred to the right scapula. The pain usually starts suddenly, increases steadily, and reaches a peak in about 30 minutes. Abdominal examination may reveal a tender abdomen with right upper quadrant guarding. Murphy's sign may be elicited when the client is asked to take a deep breath. About 60% to 70% of clients with acute cholecystitis have experienced biliary colic episodes in the past from ductal spasm when a stone moves from the gallbladder into ducts causing waves of pain (biliary colic).

In addition to pain, the following problems may be revealed in clients with acute cholecystitis:

1. Nausea and vomiting occur in 60% to 70% of clients as a result of impulses transmitted to the vomiting center from distention of bile ducts.
2. Approximately 80% of clients have an elevated temperature from the response to inflammation, but this may be absent in older clients, immunocompromised clients, and clients receiving steroidal therapy.
3. Mild jaundice occurs in only 10% of cases.
4. Right upper quadrant tenderness, fever, and leukocytosis suggest acute cholecystitis, particularly if other assessment data support this diagnosis.

The diagnostic examination for acute cholecystitis includes the following:

1. Biliary ultrasonography is often the initial diagnostic procedure. Sonographic findings consistent with acute cholecystitis include (a) cholelithiasis, (b) focal tenderness over the gallbladder (sonographic Murphy's sign), (c) thickening of the gallbladder wall (>3 mm), and (d) distention of the gallbladder lumen (>5 cm).
2. Aminotransferase, alkaline phosphatase, and bromsulfophthalein values may be slightly abnormal.
3. An abdominal x-ray study occasionally reveals the enlarged gallbladder. In 15% of cases, the gallstones contain enough calcium to be visible on film.

4. Radionuclide imaging (cholescintigraphy) can provide additional information (when the diagnosis is clinically obscure) by pinpointing cystic duct obstruction. Confirmation is based on nonvisualization of the gallbladder.
5. The WBC count is elevated in 85% of clients, with the exception of the elderly and those receiving steroid therapy.

Outcome Management

Medical Management

Clients thought to have acute cholecystitis may need to be hospitalized, and initial management should include administration of antibiotics effective against organisms found in the bile in approximately 80% of the cases. These organisms include both gram-positive and gram-negative aerobes and anaerobes: *E. coli, Klebsiella aerogenes, S. faecalis, Clostridium welchii, Proteus* species, *Enterobacter* species, *Helicobacter* species, and anaerobic streptococci.

Antibiotics that are effective given singly include ampicillin, cephalosporins, or aminoglycosides. A combination of these drugs may be more effective in clients with diabetes mellitus or with debilitated conditions. Further medical management is the same as for symptomatic cholelithiasis (see Cholelithiasis).

Nursing Management of the Medical Client

Assessment becomes extremely important because several other disease entities may produce the same manifestations (see Box 46–2). Collect subjective and objective data, and note the client's response to medications.

Nursing care is the same as for medical management of cholelithiasis except for the certainty that these clients will receive a course of antibiotics. Observe the client for the development of complications, which may include increased pain in the right upper quadrant or jaundice (from an obstruction) and decreased or absent bowel sounds (from peritonitis). For additional information on nursing management, see Nursing Management of the Medical Client under Cholelithiasis.

Surgical Management

Once the diagnosis of acute cholecystitis is made, the decision for early or delayed cholecystectomy depends on the risk factors. Delayed surgery is usually the correct decision in those clients who have unstable angina, significant carotid artery disease, congestive heart failure, cirrhosis, and other conditions that would increase their risk.

Cholecystectomy for the client with acute cholecystitis is more difficult than elective surgery because of the distended, inflamed gallbladder. Usually, the gallbladder must be decompressed first to allow complete visualization of all surrounding structures and to avoid injury to the extrahepatic bile ducts.

Cholecystotomy (surgical drainage of the gallbladder) is usually performed only when cholecystectomy is too dangerous, given all the risk factors. Although the procedure relieves the obstruction, the cure depends on the ability of the client's immune system to resolve the inflammatory process. Treatment of complications of cholecystotomy is usually cholecystectomy. See Nursing Management of the Surgical Client under Cholelithiasis.

Acute Acalculous Cholecystitis

Acute acalculous cholecystitis (without stones) accounts for approximately 4% to 8% of all cases of acute cholecystitis. Although data are inconclusive, this condition is said to be increasing. It tends to occur after or in association with other conditions, especially major trauma, burns, or surgery. Other pre-existing conditions include the postpartum period after a prolonged childbirth, bacterial sepsis, and debilitating systemic diseases, such as cardiovascular disease, tuberculosis, and sarcoidosis. However, no apparent precipitating factor is present in as many as 50% of the clients.

The pathologic process does not differ from that of the calculous type, although the incidence of gangrene and perforation is higher. It is debatable whether this is an inherent feature of the disease or the result of delayed diagnosis.

Recognition of the disease may be delayed when the client cannot communicate well because of concomitant disease or post-traumatic or postoperative states. The manifestations are the same as those of acute calculous cholecystitis—pain in the right upper quadrant, epigastrium, or both, and vomiting. However, although pain is the cardinal manifestation in the calculous type, it may be obscured or absent in acalculous cholecystitis because of narcotic administration, decreased level of consciousness, or abdominal pain from an incision or from another disease process. Significant physical findings are the same as those in acute calculous cholecystitis, and the same diagnostic procedures are used.

The standard treatment is emergency cholecystectomy because of the increased risk of gangrene and perforation.

Chronic Cholecystitis

Chronic cholecystitis sometimes arises as a sequela to acute cholecystitis. Typically, however, it develops independently of acute cholecystitis. In addition, it is almost always associated with gallstones. Chronic cholecystitis principally affects middle-aged and older obese women. The female-to-male ratio is 3 : 1.

Assessment data for chronic cholecystitis are similar to those of acute cholecystitis with certain exceptions. In chronic states, (1) the pain is less severe, (2) the temperature is not as high, and (3) the leukocyte count is lower. Vague manifestations of indigestion, epigastric pain, fat intolerance, heartburn, and flatulence accompany chronic cholecystitis. The client has usually experienced these manifestations for a long time as well as repeated attacks (mild or severe) of acute cholecystitis. Eventually, fibrous tissues begin to replace the normal muscle and mucosal tissues of the gallbladder. As a consequence, the gallbladder loses its ability to concentrate bile.

Diagnosis depends largely on ultrasonography, and other diagnostic procedures provide supplementary information. Diagnostic findings include (1) cholelithiasis, (2) gallbladder wall thickening (>3 mm), and (3) delayed visualization or nonvisualization of the gallbladder on radionuclide scanning. Scarring from chronic inflammation may partially or completely obstruct the cystic duct and thus account for this delay in visualization or nonvisualization. It may be difficult to differentiate chronic cholecystitis from other disorders. Conditions that produce manifestations similar to the manifestations of cholecystitis (acute and chronic) are listed in Box 46–2. The diagnostic process serves to rule out these conditions.

Conservative interventions include (1) a low-fat diet, (2) weight reduction, and (3) administration of anticholinergics, sedatives, and antacids. When medical intervention is ineffective, cholecystectomy may be the treatment of choice. About 90% of clients obtain relief of manifestations after cholecystectomy. Of the gallbladders removed, 95% contain stones.

CHOLEDOCHOLITHIASIS AND CHOLANGITIS

Choledocholithiasis is defined as stones in the common duct. Common bile duct calculi can arise from the gallbladder or hepatic ducts. Thus, common duct stones can occur in the absence of a gallbladder and are classified as *primary*. *Cholangitis* is inflammation of the bile duct.

Common duct stones are found in 10% to 15% of clients with cholelithiasis. The incidence increases with age and the frequency of gallstones in the elderly population may be as high as 50%.[3] Frequently, inflammation or bacteria are present, and cholangitis may develop.

Etiology and Risk Factors

The cause is essentially the same as for cholelithiasis. This condition is sometimes combined with a narrowing of the papilla, which traps stones. The risk factor for choledocholithiasis is that a small stone may pass from the gallbladder and lodge in the common bile duct.

Pathophysiology

The pathophysiology is essentially the same as for cholelithiasis. Most bile duct stones are cholesterol or mixed stones. They form in the gallbladder and move into the biliary tree through the cystic duct.

Clinical Manifestations

Common duct calculi may be asymptomatic or cause biliary colic, bile duct obstruction, cholangitis, or pancreatitis. Early manifestations of choledocholithiasis are not easily distinguished from gallbladder colic or acute cholecystitis. Pain may be mild or severe and cannot be differentiated from gallbladder pain. Jaundice is intermittent if obstruction is intermittent but may be progressive if the stone becomes impacted in the cystic duct or bile duct.

Chills and fever, frequently recurring attacks of right upper quadrant severe pain, a history of jaundice, and mild elevation of serum bilirubin are manifestations of *cholangitis*. The WBC count is normal except when cholangitis is present. It is characteristic, however, to see an elevation of serum bilirubin and alkaline phosphatase levels, which result from obstruction. The serum amylase level should always be determined to determine the presence of secondary pancreatitis.

Infrequently, manifestations of cholangitis are accompanied by shock and confusion, coma, or other central nervous system manifestations. These manifestations signal the presence of *acute toxic cholangitis*, a condition in which infected bile or pus is under pressure within the duct system. Emergency decompression of the duct system is necessary to prevent death.

To determine the diagnosis, ultrasonography, CT scan, and radionuclide imaging may be performed. Although they are not reliable for the detection of common duct stones, they can detect common duct dilation. Endoscopic retrograde cholangiography is indicated for clients with bile duct obstruction (as indicated by persistent jaundice) or bile duct dilation on ultrasonography. It allows visualization and endoscopic sphincterotomy when indicated.

Outcome Management

Medical Management

Medical management of pain is based on its severity and frequency and is similar to medical management described for cholelithiasis. Management of inflammation involves antibiotic therapy when cholangitis is present.

Surgical Management

INDICATIONS. Indications for surgical management of common duct calculi may include emergency intervention, which is rare unless severe ascending cholangitis is present. Usually, however, surgical management in some form is necessary for symptomatic choledocholithiasis.

Treatment includes hospitalization, treatment of infection, and removal of stones. The removal of stones may be accomplished surgically in clients with an intact gallbladder by cholecystectomy and choledochotomy. As many as 20% of clients undergoing cholecystectomy will prove to have common bile duct stones in addition to stones in the gallbladder. With the development and refinement of laparoscopic cholecystectomy, the management of common bile duct stones in the presence of gallstones is becoming more easily defined. To remove common bile duct stones, preoperative ERCP with endoscopic papillotomy and stone extraction is the preferred approach. Postoperative ERCP may also be done if necessary. As laparoscopic cholecystectomy becomes more perfected as a technique, the need for preoperative ERCP is expected to decrease.

Common duct stones in a client who has previously had a cholecystectomy is best treated by endoscopic sphincterotomy. The surgeon opens the sphincter of Oddi and allows passage of gallstones up to 1 cm. The success rate is approximately 90%. Extracorporeal shock wave lithotripsy is used when stones are too large to extract via the endoscopic approach. Success can be achieved in 70% to 85% of these complicated cases. Most common duct stones are found and removed at the time of cholecystectomy.

Liver function should be thoroughly evaluated preoperatively by measuring the prothrombin time. If results are abnormal, function should be restored to normal with administration of vitamin K. Antimicrobial agents (e.g., mezlocillin IV along with either metronidazole or gentamicin IV) should be given.

Another procedure, *choledochostomy*, consists of opening the common duct surgically, removing stones, and inserting a T tube for drainage. Choledochostomy may be performed in conjunction with cholecystectomy. Otherwise, cholecystectomy may be necessary at a later date.

Postoperative antibiotics are not usually given after biliary tract surgery unless specimens of the bile obtained for culture during the surgery are positive for organisms.

Contraindications. Contraindications to surgical management of choledocholithiasis include elderly clients and those who are poor surgical risks.

Complications. Surgical traumas or the presence of stones may result in ductal edema after choledochostomy. Inserting a T tube prevents bile from spilling into the peritoneal cavity and maintains patency of the duct (see Fig. 46–5). T tubes may be attached to continuous gravity drainage or to collapsible bags in the dressing site.

Avoid tension on long tubing and obstruction by kinking. Carefully measure drainage from the T tube. The tube usually drains 300 to 500 ml in the first 24 hours. This amount decreases to less than 200 ml after 3 to 4 days. Record the volume and color of the drainage. To prevent excessive loss of bile, place the drainage bag for the T tube at the level of the abdomen rather than hanging the bag below the bed. At this height, bile flows into the bag only when pressure is high in the biliary tree.

Excessive T tube drainage may indicate obstruction. Occasionally, it signals development of a biliary fistula. Excessive bile losses may necessitate recycling the client's bile drainage. The bile may be returned to the client through a nasogastric tube or orally in fruit juice.

Thick bile or bile containing blood clots may prevent drainage or cause inadequate amounts of drainage from the T tube. Without intervention, bile may begin to leak from the choledochotomy site instead of through the T tube. To prevent this problem, the physician may decide to irrigate the tube with sterile saline.

On rare occasions, tube dislodgment causes failure of the T tube to drain. The tube may dislodge from the common duct when the client moves from a supine to a sitting position. This complication may result from excessive tension during T tube insertion in surgery.

After a few days, the T tube will probably be clamped during meals to aid fat digestion.

The tube remains in place for about 10 days. A T tube cholangiogram should be done on or about the seventh or eighth postoperative day to assess for bile duct obstruction. When the T tube cholangiogram indicates absence of obstruction, the surgeon may decide to remove the T tube. If a retained stone is discovered during cholangiography, the client may go home with the T tube in place. The surgeon may remove the stone through the T tube tract with a catheter at a later time.

Outcomes. When stones are extracted, the client is likely to experience a reduction in pain and a general increase in well-being and quality of life. Encourage the client to increase his or her level of activity and maintain a low-fat diet to reduce the risk of forming additional future stones.

Nursing Management of the Surgical Client

Nursing management is the same as for the client with a cholecystectomy.

Sclerosing Cholangitis

Sclerosing cholangitis is an uncommon, inflammatory disease of the bile ducts that causes fibrosis and thickening of their walls and multiple short, concentric strictures. The disease is progressive and gradually causes cirrhosis, portal hypertension, and death from hepatic failure. It may also predispose the client to the development of cholangiocarcinoma. Some cases are associated with inflammatory bowel disease, especially ulcerative colitis. Sclerosing cholangitis and papillary stenosis are important complications of acquired immunodeficiency syndrome (AIDS). In addition, cytomegalovirus and cryptosporidium are observed frequently in such clients, indicating that these organisms may be involved in causing primary sclerosing cholangitis.

The cause has been linked to altered immunity, toxins, and infectious agents. Clients often have the hepatocompatible antigen HLA-B, suggesting that genetic factors may play a role. The disease is most common in men 20 to 40 years of age. The male-to-female ratio is 3:2.

Usually, clients present with fatigue, anorexia, weight loss, jaundice, and pruritus. They sometimes complain of vague upper abdominal pain. The diagnosis is usually made by endoscopic retrograde cholangiography, clinical findings, and liver biopsy.

Medical management consists of corticosteroids and broad-spectrum antimicrobial therapy when cholangitis is a recurrent problem. Immunosuppressants, bile acid-binding agents, colchicine, and penicillamine have been used with inconsistent and unpredictable results. These agents do not alter the slow, progressive course of the disease. Ursodiol, which improves primary biliary cirrhosis, is now being evaluated in the treatment of sclerosing cholangitis. Cholestyramine may help control the pruritus.

The success of surgical intervention is limited by the progressive nature of the disease and the recurrent cholangitis. Surgery is generally limited to procedures to open the ducts. Cholecystectomy should not be performed unless there is definite evidence of cholecystitis or cholelithiasis. Although surgical therapy may be life-saving in some circumstances, it has to be considered palliative in the overall context of the disease. The definitive management of these clients is liver transplantation, which is the procedure of choice. Survival rates with transplantation are 85% at 3 years.[10]

Carcinoma of the Gallbladder

Although cancer of the gallbladder is the most common malignant lesion of the biliary tract, it accounts for only 5% of all cancers at the time of autopsy. Most cancers of the gallbladder develop in conjunction with stones rather than polyps. Of all clients with this malignancy, 91% are over age 50 and the incidence in women is four times that of men. However, the incidence of bile duct cancer is predominant in men. Native Americans, Hispanics, northeastern Europeans, Israelis, and Japanese immigrants to the United States are at greatest risk for cancer of the gallbladder. At least 70% of these clients have gallstones. Adenocarcinoma accounts for 82% of all cases.

The clinical presentation differs according to stage of the disease. There is no distinct pattern because the manifestations depend on the site of the lesion, its extent, and the presence or absence of pre-existing biliary manifestations. Usually, however, the clinical manifestations are unrelenting right upper quadrant pain, weight loss, jaundice, and a palpable right upper quadrant mass.

At this point, treatment modalities and their effectiveness are widely debated. Treatment varies from radical resection, to palliative relief of duct obstruction, to chemotherapy or radiation. None of the treatments have been found to increase survival.

The prognosis for cancer of the gallbladder is poor. About 88% of clients die within the first year, and only about 5% are alive at 5 years. Trials of radiation and chemotherapy in clients with primary gallbladder cancer have been disappointing. The long-term survivors are generally those in whom the diagnosis of cancer had not been made prior to cholecystectomy and was determined by pathologic study.

CONCLUSIONS

Biliary and exocrine pancreatic disorders are common but are extremely complex and diverse. Some of these conditions are treated without further difficulty, such as cholecystitis, whereas others can become chronic and lead to a wide variety of other problems, such as pancreatitis. Teaching is vital to the care of these clients, and the nurse must understand these conditions to initiate appropriate teaching plans.

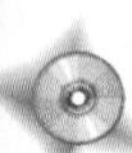

THINKING CRITICALLY

1. **You are assigned to care for a 35-year-old writer who has been admitted with severe upper abdominal pain radiating to his back and recurrent vomiting. This is his second admission for pancreatitis. He admits to drinking 1 pint of whiskey daily on the weekends and having several drinks nightly on weekdays. His alcohol intake has been greater in the past. Laboratory data include an amylase level of 750 units/L (normal 25 to 125 units); lipase, is 5.6 units/ml (normal, 10 to 140 units); aspartate aminotransferase (AST), 150 units/L (normal, 5 to 40 units) and alanine aminotransferase (ALT), 60 units (normal, 1 to 45 units). How do you feel about caring for this client?**

Factors to Consider. Are you comfortable with the client's lifestyle? Do the biochemical studies support a diagnosis of pancreatitis? What do you need to consider if he complains of pain? What should you do if you discover he is allergic to meperidine? Should a nasogastric tube be inserted?

2. **A 45-year-old woman is admitted to the hospital complaining of colicky pain in the right upper abdominal quadrant. She states that the pain is worse when she eats fried foods. She also states that she has vomited on several occasions and it seems to relieve her manifestations. What are your priorities in assessing and caring for the client?**

Factors to Consider. What types of diagnostic procedures should be scheduled? Why is an accurate assessment of the clinical manifestations important? What indications warrant insertion of a nasogastric tube?

3. **A 70-year-old woman comes to the emergency department with complaints of recurrent episodes of epigastric pain during the past 9 months. Chills, fever, and jaundice have occurred for the first time and have persisted for 4 days. Her white blood cell count is normal. Serum bilirubin and alkaline phosphatase values are elevated. There is no history of alcoholism, blood transfusions, or hepatitis. The client takes no medications except an occasional "Bufferin for my arthritis." Her past medical history is unremarkable except for a cholecystectomy 10 years ago after an episode of cholecystitis. What are the priorities for care?**

Factors to Consider. What are the client's clinical manifestations? Would surgical treatment alleviate the problem? What might cause stricture of the bile ducts?

BIBLIOGRAPHY

1. Andreoli, R. E., et al. (1996). *Cecil essentials of medicine* (4th ed.). Philadelphia: W. B. Saunders.
2. Copstead, L. C., & Banasik, J. L. (2000). *Pathophysiology: Biological and behavioral perspectives* (2nd ed.). Philadelphia: W. B. Saunders.
3. Frey, C. F. (1993). Management of necrotizing pancreatitis. *Western Journal of Medicine, 159,* 675–680.
4. Friedman, L. S. (1998). Liver, biliary tract, and pancreas. In L. M. Tierney, S. J. McPhee, & M. A. Papadakis (Eds.), *Medical diagnosis and treatment* (37th ed.). Stamford, CT: Appleton & Lange.
5. Greenberger, N. J., Toskes, P.P., & Isselbacher, K. J. (1998). Acute and chronic pancreatitis. In A. S. Fauci, E. Braunwald, K. J. Isselbacher, et al. (Eds.), *Harrison's principles of internal medicine* (14th ed.). New York: McGraw-Hill.
6. Greenberger, N. J., & Isselbacher, K. J. (1998). Diseases of the gallbladder and bile ducts. In A. S. Fauci, E. Braunwald, K. J. Isselbacher, et al. (Eds.), *Harrison's principles of internal medicine* (14th ed.). New York: McGraw-Hill.
7. Guyton, A. C., & Hall, J. E. (1996). *Textbook of medical physiology* (9th ed.). Philadelphia: W. B. Saunders.
8. Hansen, M. (1998). *Pathophysiology: Foundations of disease and clinical intervention.* Philadelphia: W. B. Saunders.
9. Malka, D., et al. (1998). Chronic obstructive pancreatitis due to a pancreatic cyst in a patient with autosomal dominant polycystic kidney disease. *Gut, 42*(1), 131–134.
10. McCance, K. L., & Heuther, S. E. (1998). *Pathophysiology: The biologic basis for disease in adults and children* (3nd ed.). St. Louis: Mosby–Year Book.
11. Mayer, R. J. (1998). Pancreatic cancer. In A. S. Fauci, E. Braunwald, K. J. Isselbacher, et al. (Eds.), *Harrison's principles of internal medicine* (14th ed.). New York: McGraw-Hill.
12. Mergener, K., & Baille, J. (1997). Chronic pancreatitis. *Lancet, 350*(9088), 1379–1385.
13. Noone, J. (1995). Acute pancreatitis: An Orem approach to nursing assessment and care. *Critical Care Nurse, 15*(4), 27–37.
14. Price, T. F., Payne, R. L., & Oberleitner, M. G. (1996). Familial pancreatic cancer in South Louisiana. *Cancer Nursing, 19*(4), 275–282.
15. Soergel, K. H. (1996). Pancreatitis. In J. C. Bennett, & F. Plum. (Eds.), *Cecil textbook of medicine* (20th ed.). Philadelphia: W. B. Saunders.

16. Stabile, B. E. (1998). Laparoscopic cholecystectomy-associated bile duct injuries. *Western Journal of Medicine*, *168*(1), 40–41.
17. Stephens, C. D. (1998). Gemcitabine: A new approach to treating pancreatic cancer. *Oncology Nursing Forum, 25*(1), 87–93.
18. Toskes, P. P., & Greenberger, N. J. (1998). Approach to the patient with pancreatic disease. In A. S. Fauci, E. Braunwald, K. J. Isselbacher, et al. (Eds.), *Harrison's principles of internal medicine* (14th ed.). New York: McGraw-Hill.
19. Vaona, B., et al. (1997). Food intake of patients with chronic pancreatitis after onset of the disease. *American Journal of Clinical Nutrition*, *65*(30), 851–854.
20. Warsaw, A. L., et al. (1998). Middle segment pancreatectomy: A novel technique for conserving pancreatic tissue. *Archives of Surgery, 133*(3), 327–331.
21. Woodward, J., & Colagiovanni, L. (1998). Feed the patient, fool the pancreas. *Nursing Times, 94*(8), 65–67.

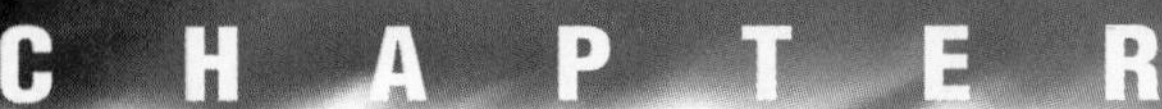

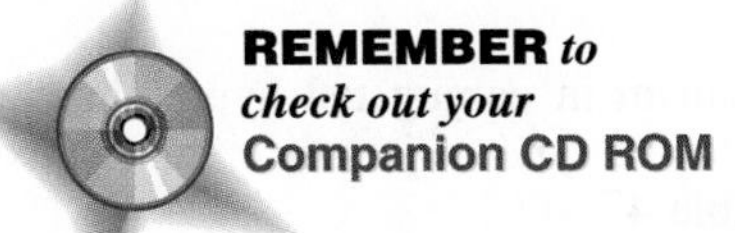

CHAPTER 47

Management of Clients with Hepatic Disorders

Dianne Smolen

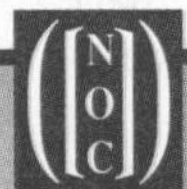

NURSING OUTCOMES CLASSIFICATION (NOC) for Nursing Diagnoses—Clients with Hepatic Disorders

Activity Intolerance
Activity Tolerance
Endurance
Energy Conservation
Self-Care: Activities of Daily Living (ADL)
Self-Care: Instrumental Activities of Daily Living (IADL)
Acute Confusion
Cognitive Ability
Distorted Thought Control
Information Processing
Memory
Neurologic Status: Consciousness
Altered Health Maintenance
Health Belief: Perceived Resources
Health-Promoting Behavior
Health-Seeking Behavior
Knowledge: Health Behaviors
Knowledge: Health Promotion
Knowledge: Health Resources
Knowledge: Treatment Regimen
Psychosocial Adjustment: Life Change
Risk Detection
Self-Direction of Care
Social Support
Treatment Behavior: Illness or Injury
Altered Nutrition: Less Than Body Requirements
Nutritional Status
Nutritional Status: Food and Fluid Intake
Nutritional Status: Nutrient Intake
Weight Control
Altered Protection
Abuse Protection
Immunization Behavior
Infection Status
Altered Tissue Perfusion
Tissue Perfusion: Cardiac
Tissue Perfusion: Pulmonary
Vital Signs Status
Anxiety
Anxiety Control
Coping
Social Interaction Skills
Body Image Disturbance
Body Image
Grief Resolution
Psychosocial Adjustment: Life Change
Self-Esteem
Fatigue
Activity Tolerance
Endurance
Energy Conservation
Nutritional Status: Energy
Psychomotor Energy
Fluid Volume Deficit
Electrolyte and Acid-Base Balance
Fluid Balance
Hydration
Nutritional Status: Food and Fluid Intake
Fluid Volume Excess
Electrolyte and Acid-Base Balance
Fluid Balance
Hydration
Impaired Skin Integrity
Immobility Consequences, Physiologic
Nutritional Status
Risk Control
Tissue Perfusion: Peripheral
Tissue Integrity: Skin and Mucous Membranes
Wound Healing: Primary Intention
Wound Healing: Secondary Intention
Ineffective Breathing Pattern
Respiratory Status: Airway Patency
Respiratory Status: Ventilation
Vital Signs Status
Risk for Impaired Gas Exchange
Electrolyte and Acid-Base Balance
Respiratory Status: Gas Exchange
Respiratory Status: Ventilation
Tissue Perfusion: Pulmonary
Vital Signs Status
Risk for Ineffective Management of Therapeutic Regimen: Families
Family Functioning
Family Participation in Professional Care
Risk for Ineffective Management of Therapeutic Regimen: Individuals
Compliance Behavior
Knowledge: Treatment Regimen
Participation: Health Care Decisions
Treatment Behavior: Illness or Injury
Risk for Injury
Knowledge: Personal Safety
Neurologic Status
Risk Control
Risk Detection
Safety Behavior: Fall Prevention
Safety Status: Physical Injury
Symptom Control

The liver plays a central role in many essential physiologic processes. It is the primary organ of lipid synthesis, and it detoxifies endogenous and exogenous substances such as hormones, drugs, and poisons. When the normal physiologic processes are altered, numerous hepatic and extrahepatic manifestations of liver disease appear. These manifestations offer the initial clue to liver disease, regardless of the cause.

This chapter describes the clinical features of liver diseases, medical and surgical management, and measures the nurse can take to assist clients with such nursing diagnoses as *Impaired Skin Integrity, Fluid Volume Ex-*

cess, Fatigue, and *Altered Nutrition: Less than Body Requirements.*

JAUNDICE

Jaundice, or icterus, is the yellow pigmentation of the sclerae, skin, and deeper tissues caused by excessive accumulation of bile pigments in the blood. It is a common manifestation of a variety of liver and biliary diseases and serves as a starting point for evaluating many of these disorders. Bilirubin (bile pigment), a product of red blood cell (RBC) breakdown, is deposited in the skin and excreted in the urine when present in the blood in excessive amounts (hyperbilirubinemia). This characteristic makes jaundice a valuable indicator of a variety of disorders involving either hemolysis or biliary obstruction. When there is an obstruction blocking the flow of bile into the intestine, jaundiced clients also may have clay-colored stools owing to lack of bilirubin and its metabolites in the intestine.

Bilirubin is formed from the breakdown of hemoglobin from RBCs by macrophages. This unconjugated bilirubin measured as ("indirect bilirubin") is not water-soluble, cannot be filtered in the kidney, and thus is not excreted in the urine. Normally, the unconjugated bilirubin returns to the liver via the bloodstream and is conjugated with glucuronic acid to form conjugated bilirubin (measured as "direct bilirubin"), which is water-soluble. The conjugated bilirubin travels to the gallbladder and eventually to the intestines. In the bowel, bacterial action converts bilirubin to urobilinogen. A small amount of urobilinogen is absorbed into the bloodstream to be returned to the liver or excreted in the urine.

Etiology and Risk Factors

The cause of jaundice may be described according to the location of the pathologic change. Jaundice may occur because of a problem (1) outside the liver (resulting in unconjugated hyperbilirubinemia, in which the accumulated bilirubin is predominantly of the unconjugated type) or (2) in the liver or biliary tract (resulting in conjugated hyperbilirubinemia, with predominantly conjugated bilirubin). When the problem is in the liver or biliary tract, the cause may be hereditary cholestatic syndromes, hepatocellular dysfunction, or biliary obstruction.

Pathophysiology

The underlying pathophysiologic mechanism in jaundice relates to whether the jaundice results from accumulation of predominantly unconjugated or conjugated bilirubin in the serum.

UNCONJUGATED HYPERBILIRUBINEMIA

Unconjugated hyperbilirubinemia may result from overproduction of bilirubin due to hemolysis, to impaired hepatic uptake of bilirubin caused by certain drugs, or to impaired conjugation of bilirubin by glucuronide, as in Gilbert's syndrome, Crigler-Najjar syndrome, or drug reactions.

CONJUGATED HYPERBILIRUBINEMIA

Conjugated hyperbilirubinemia may result from impaired excretion of bilirubin from the liver due to hepatocellular disease, drugs, sepsis, hereditary disorders such as Dubin-Johnson syndrome, or extrahepatic biliary obstruction. The pathologic mechanism in conjugated hyperbilirubinemia varies according to the type of jaundice (mechanisms are summarized in Table 47–1).

Hereditary Cholestatic Syndromes

Jaundice related to hereditary cholestatic syndromes or intrahepatic cholestasis (stagnation of bile in liver or bile ducts) results from faulty excretion of bilirubin conjugates, as in conditions such as Dubin-Johnson syndrome or Rotor's syndrome.

Hepatocellular Disease

Hepatocellular jaundice is due to defective uptake, conjugation, or transport of bilirubin by the liver. Liver cell dysfunction or necrosis caused by hepatitis, for example, or defective bile transport in the bile canal and small bile duct can cause hyperbilirubinemia. Unknown channels absorb the pooled bile components into the bloodstream. Although "obstructive jaundice" usually refers to jaundice caused by an obstruction such as a stone, hepatic cellular damage can also result in obstruction sufficient to cause jaundice.

Biliary Obstruction

Biliary obstruction, the cause of obstructive jaundice, results from impaired bilirubin transport and excretion in the biliary system. In this case, the problem arises from obstruction of an extrahepatic bile duct by gallstones.

Clinical Manifestations

Manifestations of jaundice include yellow sclerae, yellowish-orange skin, clay-colored feces, tea-colored urine, pruritus (itching), fatigue, and anorexia. Table 47–1 presents reference values for the laboratory diagnostic tests used to identify the underlying cause and type of jaundice. The following diagnostic test results are consistent with jaundice:

Abnormality	*Reason/Result*
Increased levels of conjugated serum bilirubin (direct bilirubin >0.4 mg/dl)	Bile excretion is blocked
Increased levels of unconjugated serum bilirubin (indirect bilirubin >0.8 mg/dl)	Liver damage with impaired conjugation of bilirubin; increased hemolysis of red blood cells
Bilirubin in urine	Liver damage or biliary obstruction of conjugated bilirubin
Increased urinary excretion of urobilinogen (>4 mg/24 hr)	Liver's ability to absorb urobilinogen from portal vein is impaired
Reduced fecal excretion of urobilinogen (<40 mg/24 hr)	Urobilinogen does not reach intestine
Increased alkaline phosphatase and cholesterol serum levels	Normal excretion of alkaline phosphatase and cholesterol into bile cannot occur owing to liver cell damage
In extreme cases of liver failure, an unusually low cholesterol level	Liver cannot synthesize cholesterol
Increased levels of serum bile salts	Bile salts are deposited in the skin, causing pruritus
Prolonged prothrombin time (>40 seconds)	Absorption of vitamin K is reduced

TABLE 47–1 TYPES OF JAUNDICE (ICTERUS)

Type of Jaundice	Causes	Assessment	Laboratory Test Results: Reference Values*									
			Conjugated (Direct) Bilirubin (0.1–0.3 mg/dl)	*Unconjugated (Indirect) Bilirubin (0.2–0.8 mg/dl)*	*Total Bilirubin (0.1–1.0 mg/dl)*	*Urinary Bilirubin (0)*	*Urinary Urobilinogen (0–4 mg/day)*	*Fecal Urobilinogen (40–280 mg/day)*	*AST (5–40 U/L)*	*ALT (5–35 U/L)*	*PTT (30–40 sec)*	*PT (12–15 sec)*
Unconjugated hyperbilirubinemia	Increased bilirubin production (hemolytic anemias, hemolytic reactions, hematoma infarction) Impaired bilirubin uptake and storage (post-hepatitis or with Gilbert's syndrome, Crigler-Najjar syndrome, drug reactions) Defective albumin binding	Liver function usually normal; compensates for ↑ bilirubin by ↑ metabolism of bilirubin Weakness or abdominal or back pain may occur with acute, mild jaundice	Normal	↑	↑	None	↑	↑	Normal	Normal	Normal	Normal
▪ Hereditary cholestatic syndrome	Faulty excretion of bilirubin conjugates; Dubin-Johnson syndrome	May be asymptomatic May have pruritus, light-colored stools, occasional malaise	↑	↑	↑	↓	↓	↓	↑	↑	Prolonged	Prolonged
▪ Hepatocellular disease	Liver's inability to conjugate or transport bilirubin to canaliculi for excretion due to hepatitis, liver congestion, cirrhosis, metastatic cancer, prolonged use of medications metabolized by liver, etc.	Liver may be enlarged Abdomen may be tender May have bruising or bleeding due to vitamin K malabsorption†	↑	↑	↑	↑	⇅	↓	↑	↑	Prolonged	Prolonged

Table continued on following page

TABLE 47–1 TYPES OF JAUNDICE (ICTERUS) *Continued*

Type of Jaundice	Causes	Assessment	Laboratory Test Results: Reference Values*									
			Conjugated (Direct) Bilirubin (0.1–0.3 mg/dl)	*Unconjugated (Indirect) Bilirubin (0.2–0.8 mg/dl)*	*Total Bilirubin (0.1–1.0 mg/dl)*	*Urinary Bilirubin (0)*	*Urinary Urobilinogen (0–4 mg/day)*	*Fecal Urobilinogen (40–280 mg/day)*	*AST (5–40 U/L)*	*ALT (5–35 U/L)*	*PTT (30–40 sec)*	*PT (12–15 sec)*
▪ Biliary obstruction	Blocked flow of bile into duodenum due to inflammation, scar tissue, stones, or tumors in liver, biliary, or pancreatic system	↑ Level of unconjugated bilirubin if liver cell function is diminished May have bruising or bleeding due to vitamin K malabsorption (bile is necessary for vitamin K absorption)† Abdomen may be tender Stools are clay-colored (bile gives stool its dark color) Urine is brown to foamy (conjugated bilirubin is excreted in urine)	↑	Normal or ↑	↑	↑	↓	Absent or ↓	Normal or slightly ↑	Normal or slightly ↑	Prolonged	Prolonged

ALT, alanine aminotransferase; AST, aspartate aminotransferase; PTT, partial thromboplastin time; PT, prothrombin time; U, units.

*Reference values vary among laboratories.

†Parenteral vitamin K will improve prothrombin time only if jaundice is due to posthepatic cause.

Modified from Friedman, L. S. (1998). Liver, biliary tract, and pancreas. In L. M. Tierney, (Eds.), *Medical diagnosis and treatment manual* (37 ed., pp. 628–630). Stamford, CT: Appleton & Lange.

Outcome Management

Medical Management

DETERMINE CAUSE OF JAUNDICE

An early goal in managing jaundice is to determine which category of disease explains the client's jaundice. The clinical evaluation is an important element in this determination. It includes a carefully documented health history, physical examination, basic tests of liver function, and a complete blood count (CBC). Additional tests, such as imaging studies, serologic tests, and laboratory pathologic evaluation, may be required.

The health history should focus on specific manifestations, including presence and character of pain, fever or other manifestations of active inflammation, and changes in appetite, weight, and bowel habits. The clinical evaluation should focus on features of the client's illness that point to hereditary cholestatic syndromes, hepatocellular disease, or biliary obstruction.

REDUCE PRURITUS AND MAINTAIN SKIN INTEGRITY

Pruritus, caused by an accumulation of bile salts in the skin, results from obstructed biliary excretion. Some clients experience only mild itching; others suffer such extreme itching that they tear at their skin or scratch during sleep. If skin lesions develop and become infected, antibiotics may be ordered.

Oral cholestyramine resin provides some relief by binding bile salts in the intestine so that they can be excreted. Antihistamines and phenobarbital (which enhances bile flow) may also relieve itching.

Nursing Management of the Medical Client

ASSESSMENT

The client should be observed closely for development of jaundice. Often, the first manifestation the client notices is a change in taste, manifested as a distaste for a food or drink the client previously liked, such as coffee. Pruritus is another early manifestation of incipient jaundice. Check the sclerae daily for the development of yellow coloration.

DIAGNOSIS, OUTCOMES, INTERVENTIONS

Impaired Skin Integrity. The most common nursing diagnosis for the client with jaundice is *Impaired Skin Integrity related to pruritus.*

Outcomes. The client's itching will be controlled, as evidenced by the client's statements of relief, decreased dryness of skin, and a decrease in scratching by the client.

Interventions. Administer antihistamines and phenobarbital as prescribed to relieve the itching. For clients with extreme itching, administer oral cholestyramine resin to bind with bile salts in the intestine so that they can be excreted. Suggest other interventions, including tepid water or emollient baths, avoidance of alkaline soap, and frequent application of lotions. Encourage the client to wear loose, soft clothing. Provide soft bed linens (cotton is best), and change soiled linens as soon as possible. Keep the room cool.

Body Image Disturbance. Clients with jaundice often experience problems associated with the nursing diagnosis *Body Image Disturbance related to yellowing of skin and sclerae.*

Outcomes. Clients will cope with body image disturbance, as evidenced by clients not isolating themselves, verbalizing and demonstrating acceptance of appearance (grooming, dress, posture, eating patterns, and self-presentation), and initiating or reestablishing support systems.

Interventions. Reassure the client that the discoloration is usually temporary. Assist the client in personal hygiene as needed, and promote activity as tolerated. Encourage clients to express their feelings about their self-image.

Altered Health Maintenance. Clients with jaundice may lack understanding of the condition, leading to the nursing diagnosis *Altered Health Maintenance related to lack of knowledge of jaundice.*

Outcomes. The client will understand the cause of jaundice, as evidenced by the client's statements and ability to define the illness.

Interventions. Clients often wonder why they have jaundice, how long the condition will last, and how to cope with the problem. Encourage clients with jaundice to ask questions about their health, treatment, and progress.

EVALUATION

Jaundice should resolve with treatment of the underlying condition. It usually begins to disappear within 4 to 6 weeks. The return of normal stool and urine color is an indication of resolution. As the jaundice lessens, the client's appetite and body image improve and the pruritus subsides.

Surgical Management

Surgical exploration of the common bile duct (choledochostomy) enables the diagnostician to differentiate choledocholithiasis (stone in the common bile duct) from tumor. If carcinoma (usually of the head of the pancreas) is discovered during exploration, the surgeon may perform a palliative anastomosis of the gallbladder to the jejunum to bypass the common bile duct. Chapter 46 describes surgical management of the client undergoing a choledochostomy.

HEPATITIS

Simply stated, hepatitis is inflammation of the liver. This inflammation may be caused by viruses, toxins, or chemicals (including drugs). Jaundice usually develops, and the liver is tender. Other manifestations depend on the causative agent and the degree of organ disruption. There are several types of hepatitis, such as viral, toxic, chronic, and alcoholic.

VIRAL HEPATITIS

The development of serologic tests has made it possible to identify a growing number of specific viruses that cause hepatitis. The most common of these are hepatitis A virus, hepatitis B virus, hepatitis C virus, hepatitis D virus (delta agent), and hepatitis E virus—which cause hepatitis A through E, respectively. A sixth agent, hepatitis G virus, has been discovered, but its role in acute viral hepatitis has not been established. Although the manifestations of infection are similar in hepatitis A through E plus G, these conditions differ in incubation period, mode of transmission, and severity (Table 47–2). As noted in

TABLE 47–2 COMPARISON OF SIX TYPES OF VIRAL HEPATITIS

Factor	Hepatitis A	Hepatitis B	Hepatitis C	Hepatitis D (Delta Hepatitis)	Hepatitis E	Hepatitis G
Occurrence	Endemic in areas of poor sanitation Common in fall and early winter	Worldwide, especially in drug addicts, homosexuals, people exposed to blood and blood products Occurs all year	Posttransfusion, those working around blood and blood products IV drug users Occurs all year	Hepatitis D virus causes hepatitis only in association with hepatitis B virus and only in presence of HBsAg Endemic in Mediterranean	Parts of Asia, Africa, and Mexico where there is poor sanitation	Associated with chronic viremia lasting 10 years
Incubation period	5–45 days Mean 25 days	30–180 days Mean 60–90 days	15–160 days Mean 50 days	Same as for hepatitis B	14–60 days Mean 40 days	—
Risk factors/high-risk groups	Close personal contact or by handling feces-contaminated wastes Poor sanitation	Health care workers in contact with body secretions, blood, and blood products Hemodialysis and posttransfusion clients Homosexually active males and drug abusers	Similar to that for hepatitis B	Same as for hepatitis B	Traveling or living in areas where incidence is high	Heath care workers in hemodialysis, IV drug users, hemodialysis clients, chronic hepatitis B or C clients
Transmission	Infected feces, fecal-oral route May be airborne if copious secretions Shellfish from contaminated water No carrier state	Parenteral, sexual contact, and fecal-oral route Carrier state	Contact with blood and body fluids Source of infection uncertain in many clients Carrier state	Coinfects with hepatitis B, close personal contact Carrier state	Fecal-oral route, food- or water-borne No carrier state	Percutaneous
Severity	Mortality low Rarely causes fulminating hepatic failure	More serious, may be fatal Mortality rate 10%–20%	Can lead to chronic hepatitis	Similar to hepatitis B More severe if occurs with chronic active hepatitis B	Illness self-limiting Mortality rate in pregnant women 10%–20%	Does not appear to cause liver disease
Diagnostic tests	Anti-HAV–IgM–positive in acute hepatitis; IgG-positive after infection	HBsAg or anti-HBc–IgM, HBeAg	Anti-HCV or anti-HDV Recombinant immunoblot assay	HDAg-positive HDV RNA in serum	Anti-HEV	Anti-HGV
Prophylaxis and active or passive immunity	Hygiene Immune globulin (passive) Inactivated hepatitis A vaccine (active)	Hygiene, avoidance of risk factors HBIG (passive) Recombinant hepatitis B vaccine (active)	Hygiene Immune globulin (passive)	Hygiene Hepatitis B vaccine (active)	Hygiene, sanitation No immunity	Hygiene

anti-HAV, antibody to hepatitis A virus; anti-HBc–IgM, antibody to hepatitis B–IgM; HBeAg, hepatitis Be antigen; anti-HCV, antibody to hepatitis C virus; anti-HEV, antibody to hepatitis E virus; HBsAg, hepatitis B surface antigen; anti-HGV, antibody to hepatitis G virus; HBIG, hepatitis B immune globulin; IV, intravenous.

Modified from Friedman, L. S. (1998). Liver, biliary tract, and pancreas. In L. M. Tierney, S. J. McPhee & M. A. Papadakis (Eds.). *Medical diagnosis and treatment* (37th ed). Stamford, CT: Appleton & Lange.

the Etiology and Risk Factors section, various other viruses can also cause viral hepatitis.

Viral hepatitis occurs worldwide. It is a reportable disease in the United States, with approximately 50,000 cases reported annually to the Centers for Disease Control and Prevention (CDC). Because viral hepatitis is often asymptomatic, it is likely that many cases remain undiagnosed.[12]

Hepatitis A

Hepatitis A is endemic (prevalent) in some areas of the world, especially areas with poor sanitation. However, epidemics also occur in countries with good sanitation.

Hepatitis B

Hepatitis B occurs worldwide, even in remote areas. The incidence of hepatitis B increases in areas of high population density and poor hygiene.

Hepatitis C

Hepatitis C accounts for over 90% of cases of post-transfusion hepatitis and many sporadic cases of hepatitis. Only 4% of cases of hepatitis are caused by the hepatitis C virus; intravenous (IV) drug use accounts for half of these.[10]

Hepatitis D

Hepatitis D virus (delta agent) is always found with hepatitis B virus. The hepatitis D virus is endemic in some areas, such as in the Mediterranean countries, where up to 80% of hepatitis B carriers may be superinfected with hepatitis D.[10]

Hepatitis E

Hepatitis E virus is a ribonucleic acid (RNA) virus distinct from hepatitis A virus and the enteroviruses. This agent is a water-borne virus and has been associated with hepatitis outbreaks in India, Burma, Afghanistan, Algeria, and Mexico.

Hepatitis G

The agent of hepatitis G is a flavivirus that spreads through contact with blood transfusions, contaminated needles, and body fluids.

Etiology and Risk Factors

Agents that may cause viral hepatitis include hepatitis A–E and G viruses, rubella virus, varicella virus, retroviruses, yellow fever virus, adenoviruses, and Marburg virus. Epstein-Barr virus (which causes infectious mononucleosis), cytomegalovirus, and herpes simplex virus are other possible causes of viral hepatitis, especially in immunocompromised people.

Hepatitis A. Hepatitis A, also known as infectious hepatitis, is caused by an RNA virus of the enterovirus family. Causes of epidemics include infected water, milk, and food, especially raw shellfish from contaminated waters.

People who work with animals imported from areas where hepatitis A is endemic are at increased risk, as are people who eat raw or steamed shellfish. In the general population, children under 15 years of age are at most risk.

Hepatitis A is transmitted primarily by the fecal-oral route. It spreads from person to person by close contact or by the handling of feces-contaminated articles. Because the infected client's feces contain the virus before the onset of manifestations, other household members are at risk for infection. In addition, hepatitis A may spread in institutions such as day care centers, prisons, or facilities for developmentally disabled people. Spread of the disease is enhanced by crowding and poor sanitation.

Hepatitis B. Health care workers are at high risk for acquiring hepatitis B because of their close contact with the blood of carriers. Clients who have had multiple blood transfusions or dialysis are also vulnerable. Other high-risk populations are homosexual men, morticians, people who undergo tattooing, and IV drug users.

The major sources of hepatitis B are carriers and clients in the acute phase of the infection. Contact with the serum of an infected person is the major mode of transmission. The virus also may be transmitted by other body fluids such as saliva and semen. Hepatitis B virus can survive on environmental surfaces for at least a week.

Hepatitis C. Hepatitis C is transmitted parenterally through the blood, by personal contact, and possibly by the fecal-oral route. In contrast to hepatitis A, but like hepatitis B, hepatitis C may be spread by carriers. Because hepatitis C is also parenterally transmitted, the risk factors are similar to those for hepatitis B.

Hepatitis D. Hepatitis D is transmitted only through blood contact and is thus seen most commonly in clients exposed to blood and blood products, such as IV drug users and people with hemophilia. The risk factors for hepatitis D are the same as for hepatitis B.

Hepatitis E. The hepatitis E virus is a water-borne virus. This form of hepatitis primarily affects young adults. It has a short incubation, and there is no evidence that it becomes chronic. The risk factors for hepatitis E include travel to countries that have a high incidence of hepatitis E and consuming food or water contaminated with the virus.

Hepatitis G. Hepatitis G is spread through contact with blood, blood products, and body fluids. Risk factors are the same as those for hepatitis B and hepatitis C.

Prevention

To a great extent, viral hepatitis can be prevented by proper controls within the home, community, and health care facility setting. Table 47–2 describes each disease and contains information on prophylaxis for the hepatitides.

Hepatitis A

Personal Hygiene. Because transmission of hepatitis A (and possibly hepatitis C) is by the fecal-oral route, good personal hygiene is important. Strict isolation of clients is not necessary, but hand-washing after a bowel movement is required. Food handlers must wash their hands thoroughly. In some facilities, transmission of the disease occurs because residents are unable to properly perform self-care, including hygiene measures. Care providers must supervise hand-washing by ambulatory residents. Personnel in day care centers need to wash their hands carefully after changing diapers.

Water Supply. Treatment of municipal water supplies prevents transmission of hepatitis A. Private water supplies can be sources of contamination, and polluted fishing waters pose a threat. Shellfish that come from such waters are a major source of hepatitis A.

Restaurants. It is important for local health authorities to inspect eating establishments consistently and thoroughly. Serologic screening of food handlers for hepatitis A reduces its transmission. Because the disease can be transmitted via food, a person with active hepatitis A should not work in food services.

Animal Care. Isolating newly imported animals for a 2-month period would reduce the incidence of hepatitis A among people who handle them. If isolation is impossible, these people need to wear protective clothing and use good hand-washing technique. If the risk of contamination is high, some physicians prescribe prophylactic standard immune globulin (see later under prevention of hepatitis A).

Active Immunization. An inactivated hepatitis A vaccine (Havrix) is available commercially. It is recommended for children and adults who travel, work, or live in countries or communities with a high rate of hepatitis A and for people with chronic liver disease, homosexual men, and IV drug users. Children older than 2 years and adolescents receive two doses given 1 month apart, followed by a booster dose 6 to 12 months after the first two doses. Adults receive an initial dose followed by a booster 6 to 12 months later. All injections are intramuscular. Adverse effects include headache, abdominal pain, diarrhea, syncope, fever, fatigue, jaundice, and local soreness.[19]

Passive Immunization. Physicians may prescribe standard immune globulin. Adverse effects of intramuscular injection include pain, tenderness, and at times hematoma formation. Administration of immune globulin (gamma globulin [Gammar]) is helpful prophylaxis both before and after exposure. Immune globulin is administered intramuscularly after exposure but not after the development of clinical manifestations. Clients who live in or visit high-risk areas can be protected for up to 3 months by immune globulin. The earlier in the incubation period that the prophylactic immune globulin is given, the greater the protection.

Hepatitis B

Control of Blood, Blood Products, and Skin-Piercing Instruments. Because hepatitis B is transmitted by the serum of infected people, all blood, blood products, and instruments that pierce the skin and contact the vascular system are potential sources of contamination. Some donor-related precautions that reduce the incidence of hepatitis B are the following:

- Screening of donors' blood for hepatitis B virus surface antigen (HBsAg), antibody to hepatitis B core antigen (anti-HBc), antibody to HbsAg (anti-HBs), hepatitis B, antigen (HbcAg), and hepatitis B virus deoxyribonucleic acid (DNA) (HBVDNA)[10]
- Use of volunteer rather than paid donors
- Registration of carriers
- Sharing of accurate records between institutions
- Testing of all pregnant women for HBsAg

It is possible to reduce the transfusion recipient's exposure to hepatitis B by using blood products only when necessary, using only the necessary amount of blood or blood products, cross-checking laboratory data to reduce errors of reported results, avoiding commercially obtained blood, and encouraging clients who are having elective surgery to donate their own blood (autologous transfusions).

Many health care facilities use disposable equipment, especially needles and syringes, to reduce hepatitis transmission. Nondisposable equipment must be sterilized. All health care workers, of course, must follow CDC standard precautions.

Personal Hygiene. Good personal hygiene reduces transmission. Clients with hepatitis B and hepatitis B carriers should not share razors, toothbrushes, washcloths, cigarettes, or other personal items.

Active Immunization. Hepatitis B vaccine may provide active immunization before exposure to hepatitis B virus. The injection is best given into the deltoid muscle. Hepatitis B vaccine is given in three doses. The first and second doses must be separated by at least 1 month. The third dose is administered at least 4 months after the initial dose. Adverse reactions include headache, fever, nausea, vomiting, abdominal cramps, local soreness, redness, and swelling. Authorities strongly recommend this killed virus vaccine for all people. Hepatitis B vaccine is now included in the routine vaccination schedule for children (see Chapter 17). It is also recommended for adolescents and adults not previously immunized with the hepatitis B vaccine.

The hepatitis B vaccine is highly recommended for all people in high-risk categories for hepatitis B, including not only health care workers but also dialysis clients and attending personnel, clients requiring repeated transfusions, spouses of HBsAg-positive clients, people who have multiple sex partners (especially homosexual men), prison workers, and handlers of primates. It may be used in conjunction with the preparation *hepatitis B immune globulin* (HBIG) after documented exposure to hepatitis B.

Passive Immunization. Standard immune globulin may contain antibodies against hepatitis B. However, HBIG contains much higher levels of antibody. HBIG is given within 24 hours of exposure to hepatitis B or as soon as possible after exposure. Physicians may prescribe HBIG for prophylaxis after percutaneous exposure to blood that contains HBsAg.

Hepatitis C

Transmission of hepatitis C is similar to that of hepatitis B. Many of the same measures are useful in its prevention, although available evidence suggests that hepatitis C is less readily transmitted through sexual and household contacts than is hepatitis B. Physicians may prescribe standard immune globulin for passive immunization after exposure to hepatitis C. However, the role of this intervention as a preventive measure remains unclear; at present, immune globulin is not officially recommended for prophylaxis. There is no vaccine for active immunization against hepatitis C.

Hepatitis D

Because hepatitis D must coexist with hepatitis B, the hepatitis B vaccine can help prevent hepatitis D also. The precautions that help prevent hepatitis B also are useful in preventing delta hepatitis.

Hepatitis E

Because the hepatitis E virus is water-borne and infection occurs by the fecal-oral route in various parts of the world, attention to matters of personal hygiene and sanitation helps prevent the spread of this form of hepatitis, as it does with hepatitis A and hepatitis B.

Hepatitis G

Hepatitis G virus (HGV) is spread through contact with blood, blood products, and body fluids. HGV has been detected in 50% of IV drug users, 20% of people with hemophilia, and 15% of clients with chronic hepatitis B or C.

Pathophysiology

The pathophysiologic features in viral hepatitis are similar regardless of the cause. Hepatocytes undergo pathologic changes induced by the body's immune response to the virus. Inflammation of the liver with areas of necrosis occurs, and the resultant damage leads to impairment of function. The degree of functional impairment depends on the amount of hepatocellular damage. The endoplasmic reticulum—responsible for protein and steroid synthesis, glucuronide conjugation, and detoxification—is the first cellular organelle (a specialized part of a cell that performs a definite function) to undergo change, and liver functions that depend on these processes are altered. Kupffer cells (fixed phagocytic cells found in sinusoids of liver) increase in size and number. Vascular and ductular tissues undergo inflammatory changes. Healing of the damaged hepatic tissue generally occurs in 3 to 4 months.

Some complications of hepatitis occur, though rarely. (See Complications of Hepatitis below.)

Hepatitis A

Antibodies to hepatitis A virus (anti-HAV) appear early in the course of the illness. Both immunoglobulin M (IgM) and immunoglobulin G (IgG) anti-HAV are detectable in the serum soon after the onset of illness. IgM anti-HAV titers peak during the first week of the disease and usually disappear within 3 to 6 months. Detection of IgM anti-HAV is a valid test for demonstrating acute hepatitis. IgG anti-HAV peak titers occur 1 month after onset of the disease but may stay elevated for years; this finding is therefore an indicator of past infection.

Hepatitis B

The hepatitis B virus is a DNA virus that has an inner core and a surface envelope. The body forms antibodies to the viral antigens HBcAg and HBsAg. The presence of HBsAg in the blood denotes (1) a previous or resolving infection with hepatitis B, (2) a continuing, chronic infection, or (3) immunization with immunoglobulin or hepatitis B vaccine.

Hepatitis C

The hepatitis C virus is a single-stranded RNA virus with properties similar to those of the hepatitis B and hepatitis D viruses. Hepatitis C virus is thought to be a pathogenic factor in conditions such as glomerulonephritis and autoimmune thyroiditis.

Hepatitis D

Hepatitis D virus is a small defective RNA virus that causes hepatitis only in hepatitis B virus infection, and specifically only in the presence of HBsAg. Hepatitis D virus requires the helper function of hepatitis B virus for its replication and expression. Hepatitis D virus can either infect a person simultaneously with hepatitis B virus (*co-infection*) or infect a person already infected with hepatitis B virus (*superinfection*).

Hepatitis E

The hepatitis E virus alters hepatocellular function in almost the same way as for the other types of hepatitis viruses. It causes necrosis and liver cell damage.

Hepatitis G

Hepatitis G virus, like hepatitis C virus, is a blood-borne RNA virus. Current data indicate that a large portion of clients infected with hepatitis G are also infected with hepatitis C. Hepatitis G virus does not alter the severity of hepatitis C, nor is it associated with acute or chronic liver injury, although the latter finding requires continued study.

Clinical Manifestations

Clients with viral hepatitis all experience liver inflammation and other pathologic changes that are similar. Hepatitis B, hepatitis C, and hepatitis D are usually the most severe, although they may be asymptomatic in some clients. The onset of manifestations ranges from abrupt to insidious, according to the incubation period and the degree of infectivity.

Manifestations of viral hepatitis are systemic and vary from client to client. Manifestations occurring during the earlier (prodromal) phase may include jaundice, lethargy, irritability, myalgia, arthralgia, anorexia, nausea, vomiting, abdominal pain (caused by stretching of Glisson's capsule surrounding the liver due to inflammation), diarrhea or constipation, fever, and other flu-like manifestations. Fever is caused by the release of pyrogens in the inflammatory process. Fatigue and malaise are the result of reduced energy metabolism by the liver. Pruritus (itching), the result of bile salt accumulation in the skin, is typically mild and transient and may be more intense at its onset and termination. Jaundice, caused by impaired excretion of conjugated bilirubin, may or may not be present; when it is, it is first seen in the sclerae of the eyes and mucous membranes.

Anicteric (without jaundice) hepatitis may or may not precede jaundice. Children with hepatitis are usually anicteric. Adults often note the appearance of darker urine (the color of tea or mahogany) and clay-colored stools a few days before clinical jaundice develops. The darker urine is from the presence of urobilinogen, which is excreted through the kidneys instead of the bowel as normally occurs. The other manifestations often abate when jaundice appears, but they also may worsen.

If irritability and drowsiness become severe, assess for the possibility of hepatic encephalopathy. Deterioration of handwriting is an early manifestation of hepatic encephalopathy; thus, at each shift ask clients to write their name and observe their writing closely for changes. *Asterixis*, an abnormal muscle tremor sometimes called "liver flap," may accompany encephalopathy. This manifestation is easily elicited by applying a blood pressure cuff on the upper arm and noting whether the tremor is present when the cuff is released. Mild depression is not uncommon because of (1) the nature of the illness (weakness, jaundice, itching, and nausea), (2) its long duration and the expense of treatment, (3) the need for confinement, and (4) forgetfulness and the inability to concentrate on completion of activities of daily living (ADL).

Bleeding tendencies may develop either from reduced prothrombin synthesis by injured hepatic cells or from reduced absorption of the fat-soluble vitamin K due to reduced levels of bile in the intestines. Anemia may occur because of the decreased life span of erythrocytes

(RBCs). Erythrocyte destruction results from liver enzyme alterations. A transient hyperglycemia sometimes develops, and a client with diabetes may need to increase insulin dosage at this time.

The liver is larger than normal in hepatitis and is tender to palpation. Some people with viral hepatitis have spider angiomas, palmar erythema, and gynecomastia, which disappear during the recovery period. A small percentage (5% to 15%) of clients experience splenomegaly or enlargement of the posterior cervical lymph nodes. Occasionally, hepatitis B is accompanied by arthralgias, rash, vasculitis, or glomerulonephritis.

Occasionally, cholestatic viral hepatitis syndrome may develop. This uncommon disease process resembles mechanical obstruction; it is difficult to differentiate cholestatic viral hepatitis from biliary tract obstruction due to gallstones, strictures, and tumors.

The cause and pathophysiology of this hepatitis variant are unclear. Cholestatic viral hepatitis syndrome causes jaundice, itching, and the typical flu-like and gastrointestinal problems of hepatitis, but the manifestations often last longer and are more severe. Serum bilirubin reaches levels of 10 to 15 mg/dl. Diagnostic studies reveal elevations of serum lipoproteins, globulins, cholesterol, and alkaline phosphatase. Rarely, the liver progressively enlarges.

Fulminant viral hepatitis may develop. This life-threatening form resembles acute liver failure with manifestations of encephalopathy (increased excitability, insomnia, somnolence, and impaired mentation). The liver rapidly decreases in size. Other problems include gastrointestinal bleeding, disseminated intravascular coagulation (DIC), fever with leukocytosis and neutrophilia, hepatorenal problems of oliguria and azotemia, edema and ascites, hypotension, respiratory failure, hypoglycemia, bacterial infection of the respiratory or urinary tract or both, and thrombocytopenia and coagulopathy. The prognosis is poor, and death may occur before jaundice appears. Liver transplantation may be performed to save the client's life.

Presence of hepatitis B surface antigen (HBsAg) in the blood usually indicates that the person is infectious. Another antigen, HBeAg, is often associated with progression of acute hepatitis to chronic hepatitis and indicates a highly infectious state.

Levels of serum aminotransferases first rise and then begin to fall as bilirubin starts to increase. Levels that rise, peak, drop, and then rise again indicate severe liver damage and a poor prognosis. Jaundice may not be clinically recognizable until levels are about 3 mg/dl. Bilirubin that rises above 20 mg/dl and remains elevated for a long period may indicate severe liver necrosis, which has a poor prognosis. Mild prolongation of the prothrombin time sometimes occurs. The gamma globulin fraction and alkaline phosphatase are elevated in some clients. If hepatitis B is responsible, detection of HBsAg is possible before the level of aspartate aminotransferase (AST) (formerly serum glutamic-oxaloacetic transaminase [SGOT]) rises.

Prognosis

By 8 to 10 weeks, nearly all clients with acute viral hepatitis demonstrate normal results on liver function tests. However, the clinical course, morbidity, and mortality of viral hepatitis may vary considerably. In most cases, clients recover in 3 to 16 weeks, with abnormal results on liver function testing for a longer time. Most clients recover completely. The mortality rate is less than 1%, with the rate reportedly being higher in older people.[7]

Outcome Management

Medical Management

The acute manifestations of hepatitis generally subside over 2 to 3 weeks. Complete clinical and laboratory recovery occurs in hepatitis A by 9 weeks and in hepatitis B and hepatitis C by 16 weeks. Severe complications develop in fewer than 1% of clients with hepatitis. Clients who have severe nausea and vomiting and have difficulty maintaining normal fluid balance need to be hospitalized if there is progressive deterioration.

Reduce Fatigue

Rest is advisable in proportion to the severity of manifestations. Bed rest is usually not necessary but is recommended on an as-needed basis during the initial prodromal, anicteric phase of the disease, when the infection is most active and there is decreased metabolism by the liver. Return to normal activity during the convalescent period should be gradual. If pruritus (itching) disturbs rest, cholestyramine, antihistamines, emollients, and lipid creams may be prescribed.

Maintain Nutritional and Fluid Balance

No specific dietary measures are indicated, but most clients find a low-fat, high-carbohydrate diet more easily digested and more palatable. During the most severe phase of the illness, when there are changes in the stomach or bowel, anorexia and nausea may be so extreme that oral intake of any kind is greatly reduced. In such cases, IV administration of 10% glucose is indicated. As the client's manifestations abate and appetite improves, food and fluid intake may be resumed as tolerated. All alcoholic beverages should be avoided.

Reduce Effects of Hepatitis

Few medications are available for treating vital hepatitis. Antibiotics are not prescribed. Antiemetics control nausea and vomiting, but phenothiazines should not be used because they are biotransformed in the liver and are therefore potentially toxic. Parenteral vitamin K may be given to clients with prolonged prothrombin time. Antihistamines may provide relief of pruritus but may cause sedation.

Steroids. Corticosteroids are not necessary in uncomplicated cases of acute viral hepatitis, and authorities have questioned their use. Although they may reduce serum aminotransferase and bilirubin levels, they have no effect on liver necrosis or regeneration.

Estrogens. Estrogens can raise serum bilirubin levels. Therefore, clinicians need to consider the advisability of oral contraceptive use during acute viral hepatitis.

Bile Acid Sequestrants. The administration of bile acid sequestrants cholestyramine (Questran) or colestipol (Colestid) can relieve pruritus associated with elevated levels of bile acids that may result from severe cholestatic liver disease. Both drugs bind bile acids in the gastrointestinal tract forming an insoluble complex that is excreted in the feces. The result of this action is increased clearance of cholesterol.

IMMUNE GLOBULIN. Immune globulin, although not used to treat viral hepatitis, does provide prophylaxis for family and friends. If given early, standard immune globulin (a preparation of proteins capable of acting as antibodies, formerly termed "immune serum globulin") can prevent hepatitis A or mitigate the severity of manifestations. The hepatitis A virus does not remain in the blood long; therefore, there is no healthy carrier state for hepatitis A as there is for hepatitis B.

VACCINES. Vaccines are available to promote immunity to hepatitis A and hepatitis B. In addition to immune globulin, they may be administered prophylactically in persons exposed to infected clients.

MEDICATIONS TO AVOID. Clinicians administer very few medications to clients with hepatitis. Medications such as chlorpromazine, aspirin, acetaminophen, and a variety of sedatives are given as infrequently as possible because of their hepatotoxic properties.

COMPLICATIONS OF HEPATITIS

Persons with viral hepatitis typically recover completely from the illness in 3 to 16 weeks. Clients who are otherwise healthy usually recover from hepatitis A without major sequelae. Although hepatitis A is associated with a low mortality rate, very rarely fulminant hepatitis may result. The fulminant form, resembling acute liver failure, also occurs with infection due to other hepatitis viruses. Clients with hepatitis B tend to experience more complications. One in 10 persons develops chronic active hepatitis as a result of hepatitis B, often leading to destruction of the liver. Cirrhosis may follow a severe case of hepatitis B or chronic active hepatitis. Primary hepatocellular carcinoma is a potential complication of chronic hepatitis. Other possible complications of hepatitis include chronic persistent hepatitis, chronic carrier state, and aplastic anemia.

FULMINANT HEPATITIS

Fulminant hepatitis (massive hepatic necrosis) is rare and is primarily seen in hepatitis B and hepatitis D as well as in hepatitis E and hepatitis A. Fulminant hepatitis causes severe illness and is fatal in 1% to 2% of all cases and in up to 20% of cases occurring in pregnant women. Fulminant hepatitis involves a progression of manifestations that include jaundice, hepatic encephalopathy, and ascites. The mortality rate varies with age but approaches 90% to 100%, especially in people over 60 years of age.

CHRONIC HEPATITIS

Chronic hepatitis exists when liver inflammation continues beyond a period of 3 to 6 months. This disease may take the form of *chronic persistent hepatitis* (CPH) or *chronic active hepatitis* (CAH). Both CPH and CAH may follow hepatitis B or hepatitis C. Biopsy findings in CPH and CAH are compared in Figure 47–1.

■ CHRONIC PERSISTENT HEPATITIS

CPH is the most common form of chronic hepatitis. Most clients have no manifestations, although some may report fatigue, anorexia, and abdominal pain. Recurrent episodes are not acute in nature, and extrahepatic involvement seldom occurs. The clinical course is benign; fibrotic liver and cirrhosis develop only rarely. Clients with CPH generally have an excellent prognosis.

■ CHRONIC ACTIVE HEPATITIS

CAH is demonstrated by elevation of serum transaminase levels for more than 6 months. It is a complication of hepatitis B and hepatitis C. A more severe illness is caused by CAH than by CPH. CAH leads to hepatic inflammation, hepatic necrosis, and progressive fibrosis, with accompanying manifestations of chronic liver disease such as splenomegaly and spider angiomas. Affected clients are also at risk for hepatocellular carcinoma.

In most instances, CAH results from an autoimmune response or from hepatitis B virus infection with or without superimposed hepatitis D virus infection. Autoimmune CAH is more common in women, whereas hepatitis B CAH is more common in men. The pathogenesis in hepatitis B CAH also indicates an autoimmune response,

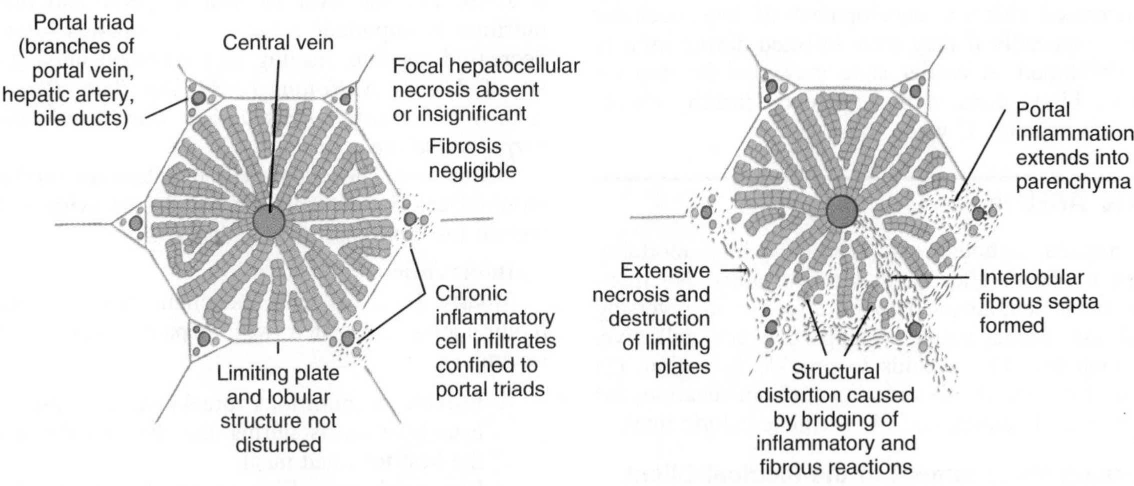

FIGURE 47–1 Comparison of biopsy findings in hepatitis. Inflammation is confined to portal triads in chronic *persistent* hepatitis but extends into the parenchyma in chronic *active* hepatitis.

with low-level anti-HBc IgM present in 70% of the clients.

Cytomegalovirus infection during an immunosuppressed state is another viral cause. CAH may also follow acute hepatitis C or post-transfusion hepatitis. When CAH presents in adolescents, it may arise from Wilson's disease, a hereditary disorder. In addition, methyldopa, dantrolene, nitrofurantoin, and isoniazid may cause inflammatory changes consistent with CAH. Discontinuing the medication usually resolves the inflammatory process.

The onset of CAH is gradual. Some clients report the manifestations of acute viral hepatitis, cirrhosis, or extrahepatic problems. Clients come to the acute care setting primarily for liver biopsy and the identification of extrahepatic sequelae, such as thyroiditis, hemolytic anemia, amenorrhea, arthritis, urticaria, or glomerulonephritis.

Treatment of CAH varies. In the past, steroids, with or without azathioprine (Imuran), were often prescribed for treatment of idiopathic CAH. These drugs often reduced manifestations, improved laboratory test results, suppressed the inflammatory response viewed on biopsy, and lowered the short-term and long-term morbidity and mortality. More recently, a combination of two antiviral drugs for treatment of chronic hepatitis C was introduced. A series of ribavirin (Rebetron) capsules and interferon alfacon-1 (Infergen) injections for 6 months has proved very effective in reducing the virus to undetectable levels in about one half of clients who received this treatment.

Clients receiving treatment for CAH require close follow-up. They need periodic liver testing, monitoring for possible side effects of drug treatments, and liver biopsy every 6 months to 1 year. Clients with untreated CAH have a high mortality rate. Death results from hepatic failure, bleeding varices, hepatic encephalopathy, or primary hepatocellular carcinoma. Liver transplantation is a consideration for clients with end-stage liver disease that can no longer be managed medically.

Chronic Carrier State

A carrier state is possible in clients who demonstrate persistent HBsAg without clinically evident disease but who are able to transmit the disease. Carriers of HBsAg are at increased risk for development of hepatocellular carcinoma, especially if they were infected during infancy or early childhood. A carrier state may also develop for hepatitis C; blood donated by apparently healthy clients may transmit hepatitis C when transfused.

Aplastic Anemia

Aplastic anemia, although rare, carries a high mortality rate when it occurs after acute viral hepatitis. No treatment has been demonstrated to be effective in reversing this condition. Management is supportive and palliative. Therapy includes (1) IV fluids to provide hydration, (2) correction of electrolyte abnormalities, (3) medications for relief of pain and nausea, and (4) adequate caloric intake.

Nursing Management of the Medical Client

Assessment

To determine the type of hepatitis present, always begin by questioning the client about possible exposure to risk factors. Ask about common manifestations, especially jaundice, and about manifestations of disease progression, such as hepatic encephalopathy (see Hepatic Encephalopathy under Cirrhosis, later on). Assess results of liver function studies, and monitor them to ascertain progression of the disease. Also assess the client's and family's ability to provide home and self-care. Their understanding of the disease and its implications is vital to its successful management in the home setting.

Diagnosis, Outcomes, Interventions

Fatigue. The client with hepatitis has tremendous metabolic demands, leading to the nursing diagnosis *Fatigue related to decreased metabolic energy production secondary to liver dysfunction.*

Outcomes. The client will convey reduced fatigue and heightened energy, as evidenced by compliance with activity restrictions and a gradual increase in activity to the pre-illness level.

Interventions. Fatigue associated with hepatitis may interfere with ADL. Most clients experience the greatest fatigue during the *anicteric phase* (before jaundice occurs) and begin to feel stronger during the icteric phase. Fatigue may persist, however, even after the jaundice clears. Clients with severe jaundice may suffer pruritus (see Jaundice for nursing interventions for *Impaired Skin Integrity related to pruritus*). During the period of severe fatigue, advise the client to rest in bed. Most clients who feel capable of being up and around can do so without harm if they rest after meals and do not engage in any activity to the point of becoming overly tired. Because prolonged bed rest itself can lead to weakness, a reasonable activity level is more conducive to recovery than enforced bed rest.

Encourage ADL such as exercise of bathroom privileges, performance of personal hygiene measures, and self-feeding unless they cause excessive fatigue. Advise the client to plan rest periods while jaundice is present, especially after meals. Clients who engage in excessive activity too early in the recovery phase sometimes experience a relapse, potentially leading to liver failure.

Altered Nutrition: Less Than Body Requirements. For the liver to heal properly and regenerate, nutrition is important. Clients with hepatitis often have a decreased appetite, leading to a common nursing diagnosis of *Altered Nutrition: Less Than Body Requirements related to anorexia, nausea, bile stasis, and altered absorption and metabolism.*

Outcomes. The client will maintain an intake of the required calories to maintain weight, as evidenced by no weight loss and possible weight gain.

Interventions

Modify Diet. To help the client meet the nutritional requirements associated with hepatitis, perform the following:

1. Provide a nutritious breakfast. Because anorexia usually worsens during the day, breakfast may be the best-tolerated meal.
2. Encourage the client to avoid fatty foods, which can induce nausea.
3. Include the optimal amount of protein and carbohydrates to allow recovery of injured liver cells with-

out overfeeding. If the client has no problem with protein metabolism, a normal intake is helpful for tissue repair. However, clients with very severe hepatitis who are at risk for development of hepatic encephalopathy require a diet low in protein (to prevent the buildup of ammonia in the blood from incomplete clearing of protein metabolic wastes). Alterations in fat metabolism differ according to the degree of interruption of bile production and excretion.

4. Suggest multiple small meals. This approach allows the client with anorexia to ingest a diet of 2500 to 3000 calories more comfortably. Also, candy, juice, sweetened tea, and carbonated drinks can supply calories when nausea is a problem.

Avoid Alcohol. Remind the client to avoid alcohol, which is an extremely hepatotoxic agent.

Provide Vitamin Supplements. Explain that vitamin supplements are not generally necessary in uncomplicated hepatitis if the diet is adequate in nutrients. Vitamin K supplements, as ordered, may be administered if the prothrombin time is longer than normal.

Relieve Nausea and Vomiting. Clients who experience severe nausea and vomiting may obtain relief with antiemetics. However, before administering these medications, review their effect on liver function. Phenothiazines such as prochlorperazine (Compazine) are usually contraindicated. If the client cannot tolerate any oral intake, provide IV nutrition.

Anxiety. It is often difficult to predict the outcome of hepatitis; therefore, the nursing diagnosis *Anxiety related to uncertainty of the effects of hepatitis* is a common one.

Outcomes. The client will experience a decrease in anxiety, as evidenced by the ability to discuss his or her feelings about the disease.

Interventions. Encourage clients with hepatitis to express their feelings concerning the following:

- The illness
- The duration and cost of the illness
- Alterations in home life and in financial status (especially for the parent of young children or for the sole family earner)
- The effect of the illness on future health problems
- The possibility of death in clients who are very ill

Suggest psychosocial and financial counseling for the client who is disturbed. Increase the client's knowledge and understanding of the illness by teaching the facts about the illness and its management. Increased knowledge can reduce anxiety.

Altered Health Maintenance. In order for the client and family members to manage hepatitis at home, the nursing diagnosis of *Altered Health Maintenance related to cause of disease, modes of transmission, and its course* must be addressed.

Outcomes. The client will understand the disease and its treatment, as evidenced by the client's ability to state the causes of the disease and the rationales for treatment.

Interventions

Provide Client Teaching. Teaching for the client with hepatitis varies with the causative agent. Teach the client how to prevent recurrence and spread. Instruct the client to return to former activity levels slowly in order to avoid a relapse. Provide clear instructions concerning diet.

Administer Medications. Administer medications and provide supportive management. Discontinue any medications that may be causing inflammatory changes. Clients who cannot tolerate large doses of steroids may benefit from azathioprine and smaller steroid doses. Clinicians generally do not recommend steroid therapy for subclinical CAH, especially in older adults.

Promote Rest. Encourage bed rest during the active phase of the disease. The client usually remains at home to convalesce. There may be periods of remission during which liver necrosis continues. Discuss with the client the need for help at home after discharge (such as with housework or shopping), because limits on activity will still have to be maintained. The client will need to see a physician at regular intervals after discharge to ensure that the liver is healing and no further damage has occurred.

EVALUATION

Because the clinical course of acute viral hepatitis varies considerably from client to client, the nurse must assess outcomes carefully to determine whether they have been met. Recovery without permanent liver damage is expected to occur within 1 to 4 months. Permanent damage may result if the therapeutic regimen is not followed.

Self-Care

Most clients recover from acute viral hepatitis, do not require hospitalization, and are appropriately managed at home. However, clinical and biochemical relapses may occur before full recovery. In addition, complications of acute viral hepatitis may develop, necessitating careful monitoring, especially in older clients.

AVOID HEPATOTOXINS

There is no specific ongoing pharmacologic management of clients recovering from acute viral hepatitis. Advise the client to avoid alcohol and medications such as aspirin, acetaminophen, and sedatives because of their hepatotoxicity.

PROMOTE NUTRITION

Encourage clients to continue eating a well-balanced, nutritional diet. A low-fat, high-carbohydrate diet is generally tolerated best. A well-balanced diet promotes liver healing, leading to improved tolerance for activity.

PROVIDE CLIENT TEACHING

One of the primary areas to cover in teaching the client and family members is how to avoid reinfection or possible spread of the infection to others. Caution the client and significant other to avoid sexual activity until there is no longer a chance of disease transmission (generally after liver function tests have returned to normal), and to check with the physician before resuming sexual relations.

PROMOTE REST

Help the client understand the need for adequate rest so that the liver can heal on its own. The client needs to be active enough to prevent complications of immobility but not so active as to risk relapse. The client is also expected to resume pre-hepatitis activities and to remain free from complications.

PREVENT INFECTION AND REINFECTION
Teach the client to avoid reinfection or possible spread of the infection to other family members. You may recommend vaccination for hepatitis A and B to promote health maintenance.

TOXIC HEPATITIS

Toxins and drugs may produce a wide variety of pathologic lesions in the liver. Some agents may cause toxic hepatitis, whereas others produce necrosis, cholestasis, or neoplasms. The extent and type of hepatitis produced by the toxin depends on the degree of exposure, the chemical properties of the hepatotoxin, and the genetic make-up of the individual. Most commonly, the causative agent is a toxic metabolite formed by the drug-metabolizing enzymes within the liver. Table 47–3 lists some hepatotoxic agents. Liver necrosis occurs within 2 or 3 days after acute exposure to a dose-related hepatotoxin. However, several weeks may pass before manifestations of idiosyncratic reactions appear. People experiencing either type of hepatotoxicity demonstrate abnormal results on liver function testing.

People who are repeatedly exposed to hepatotoxins in minimal amounts but over long periods of time may develop chronic hepatitis or cirrhosis. Clients experiencing a hypersensitivity reaction may demonstrate eosinophilia, fever, arthralgia, and sometimes xanthomatosis (an excessive accumulation of lipids brought about by faulty lipid metabolism).

Nursing intervention begins with obtaining a detailed drug history and information about past exposure and the response to a suspected agent. Ensure removal of the causative agent and adequate rest, promote alleviation of side effects (e.g., with cholestyramine for pruritus), and provide a high-calorie diet with fats and protein as tolerated. Restrict protein intake if there is evidence of impending hepatic encephalopathy. Steroids have not proved of value in treatment of drug-induced liver disease, although they may suppress the manifestations caused by the reaction of the toxic agent.

Renal failure sometimes appears as a complication of toxic hepatitis. Assessment and interventions for renal failure are discussed in Chapter 36.

ALCOHOLIC HEPATITIS

Alcoholic hepatitis may be acute or chronic. It is caused by parenchymal necrosis resulting from heavy alcohol ingestion. Although sometimes reversible, this condition is the most frequent cause of cirrhosis. This fact is important because cirrhosis of the liver is a common cause of death among adults in the United States.

Clinical manifestations of alcoholic hepatitis usually develop after a bout of heavy drinking. Assessment reveals anorexia, nausea, abdominal pain, splenomegaly, hepatomegaly, jaundice, ascites, fever, and encephalopathy. Laboratory studies typically show anemia, leukocytosis, and an elevated serum bilirubin. Liver biopsy reveals fatty hepatic tissue. Hepatitis due to excessive alcohol intake carries a poor prognosis, particularly if the client continues to ingest alcohol.

TABLE 47–3 SUBSTANCES KNOWN TO BE HEPATOTOXIC

Type of Hepatotoxicity	Type of Liver Alteration: *Hepatitis*	*Cholestasis*
Dose-related	Acetaminophen	Oxymetholone
	Amanita phalloides (mushroom)	
	Aspirin	
	Benzene	
	Carbon tetrachloride	
	Chloroform	
	Methotrexate	
	Phosphorus	
	Tetracyclines	
	Vitamin A	
Idiosyncratic	Halothane	Allopurinol
	Isoniazid	Anabolic steroids
	Methyldopa	Carbamazepine
	Nitrofurantoin	Chlordiazepoxide
	Oxacillin	Chlorpromazine
	Phenytoin	Chlorpropamide
	Quinidine	Diazepam
	Streptomycin	Erythromycin estolate
	Sulfasalazine	Flurazepam
	Sulfanilamides	Oral contraceptives
	Sulfonamides	Propylthiouracil
	Other sulfa drugs	Thiazides
	Valproic acid	

Data from Di Marin, A. J. (1994). Gastrointestinal diseases. In A. R. Myers (Ed.), *Medicine* (2nd ed.; pp. 225–226). Philadelphia: JB Lippincott.

Nursing interventions include providing a high-vitamin, high-carbohydrate diet and administration of folic acid and thiamine supplements and administration of parenteral fluids as ordered. Administration of liquid formulas may be useful in increasing caloric intake. Steroids sometimes have a beneficial effect, although their use remains controversial.

CIRRHOSIS

Cirrhosis of the liver is a chronic, progressive disease characterized by widespread fibrosis (scarring) and nodule formation. Cirrhosis occurs when the normal flow of blood, bile, and hepatic metabolites is altered by fibrosis and changes in the hepatocytes, bile ductules, vascular channels, and reticular cells.

There are four major types of cirrhosis:

- Alcoholic (historically called "Laënnec's cirrhosis" or micronodular or portal)
- Postnecrotic (macronodular or toxin-induced)
- Biliary
- Cardiac

The types are compared in Table 47–4. The two major clinical problems in cirrhosis are (1) decreased liver func-

TABLE 47–4 COMPARISON OF POSTNECROTIC, BILIARY, CARDIAC, AND ALCOHOLIC CIRRHOSIS

Definition	Etiology	Pathology	Assessment Data	Diagnosis and Prognosis	Intervention(s)
POSTNECROTIC (MACRONODULAR) CIRRHOSIS					
Most common worldwide form Massive loss of liver cells, with irregular patterns of regenerating cells	Postacute viral (types B and C) hepatitis Postintoxication with industrial chemicals Some infections and metabolic disorders	Liver small and nodular	As in alcoholic cirrhosis except less muscle wasting and more jaundice	Needle biopsy of liver establishes pathologic processes Within 5 years 75% die of complications ↑ serum aminotransferases ↑ gamma globulins	Treat complications as needed
BILIARY CIRRHOSIS					
Bile flow is decreased with concurrent cell damage to hepatocytes around bile ductules	*Primary* Chronic stasis of bile in intrahepatic ducts Cause unknown Autoimmune process implicated *Secondary* Obstruction of bile ducts outside of liver	Early-stage biopsy reveals inflammatory process with necrosis of cells and ducts Hepatocytes are lost and scar tissue remains End stage similar to postnecrotic type	Generalized pruritus Dark urine Pale stools Jaundice Impaired bile flow Steatorrhea ↓ absorption of fat-soluble vitamins Elevated serum lipids ↑ cholesterol deposits in subcutaneous tissues Signs of portal hypertension	Elevated serum bilirubin levels *Early:* 3–10 mg/100 ml *Late:* >50 mg/100 ml High elevations of alkaline phosphatase ↑ gamma globulins ↑ blood lipids Presence of lipoprotein X ↑ serum bile salts Hypoprothrombinemia ↑ antimitochondrial antibody in primary cases ↑ serum copper in primary cases	*Primary* Treatment is symptomatic, e.g., high-calorie diet, lower intake of fats by 30–40 g/day if problems develop Cholestyramine for pruritus Supplement of fat-soluble vitamins *Secondary* Treatment to relieve mechanical obstruction
CARDIAC CIRRHOSIS					
Chronic liver disease associated with severe right-sided long-term heart failure (fairly rare)	Atrioventricular valve disease Prolonged constrictive pericarditis Decompensated cor pulmonale	*Early* Dark-colored liver enlarged by blood and edema fluid *Late* Liver capsule thickens and nodular scarring occurs	Slight jaundice, enlarged liver, and ascites in person with severe cardiac impairment over 10-year span RUQ pain during acute congestion Cachexia Fluid retention Circulatory problems	↑ conjugated bilirubin in serum ↑ sulfobromophthalein ↓ albumin in serum ↑ serum aminotransferases ↑ alkaline phosphatase Liver biopsy *Prognosis* Depends on course of cardiac disease	Cause of chronic heart failure is treated if possible
ALCOHOLIC CIRRHOSIS					
Alcoholic cirrhosis (Laënnec's, micronodular) Small nodules form as a result of persistence of some offending agent	Associated with alcohol abuse	Scarring and collagen tissue deposits Regenerating nodules are very small Normal lobular structure is destroyed	May produce no symptoms for long periods Onset of symptoms may be insidious or abrupt *Early:* Weakness, fatigue, weight loss *Later:* Anorexia, nausea, and vomiting Abdominal pain Ascites Menstrual irregularities Impotence Enlarged breasts in men Hematemesis Spider angiomas	Liver biopsy; history of alcohol abuse; high AST; high bilirubin (slight); anemia Prognosis depends on presence of complications and continued abuse of alcohol	Correction of vitamin and mineral deficiencies if any (e.g., folate, thiamine, pyridoxine, vitamin K, and minerals [magnesium and phosphate]); treat complications as needed (e.g., ferrous sulfate for anemia, IV vasopressin for esophageal varices, reduce or withhold dietary protein for hepatic encephalopathy or vitamin K for hemorrhagic tendency)

AST, aspartate aminotransferase; IV, intravenous; RUQ, right upper quadrant.

Data from Friedman, L. S. (1995). Liver, biliary tract and pancreas. In L. M. Tierney et al. (Eds.), *Medical diagnosis and treatment manual* (pp. 568–571). Norwalk, CT: Appleton & Lange; and Friedman, L. S. (1996). Cirrhosis of the liver and its major sequelae. In J. C. Bennett & F. Plum (Eds.), *Cecil textbook of medicine* (20th ed.). Philadelphia: W. B. Saunders.

tion and (2) portal hypertension. The latter problem develops in severe cirrhosis.

Cirrhosis is the 11th leading cause of death in the United States, with an age-adjusted mortality rate of 10.4 deaths per 100,000 population. Of those deaths, 45% were alcohol-related.[10] Men are more likely than women to have alcoholic (Laënnec's) cirrhosis. Worldwide, postnecrotic cirrhosis is the most common form; it is also more common in women. Mortality is higher from all types of cirrhosis in men and nonwhites.

Etiology and Risk Factors

The causes of cirrhosis have not been clearly identified, although the relationship between cirrhosis and excessive alcohol ingestion is well established. Countries with the highest incidence of cirrhosis have the greatest per capita consumption of alcohol. Genetic predisposition with a familial tendency, as well as a hypersensitivity to alcohol, is seen in alcoholic cirrhosis.

The primary risk factor for cirrhosis is alcohol ingestion, especially in the absence of proper nutrition. Any client with a family history of alcoholism should avoid alcohol because of the increased risk. Hence, cessation of alcohol consumption may be a health promotion, health maintenance, or health restoration activity. The amount of alcohol consumed daily appears to be a more important factor than the pattern of drinking (binge versus daily) or the type of alcoholic beverage consumed. If the client is in a poor nutritional state, the likelihood of damage is greater and the damage is more severe. Viral hepatitis is the primary risk factor for postnecrotic cirrhosis, which makes prevention of hepatitis through vaccination and good hygiene the most important health promotion activity.

Other risk factors for cirrhosis of the liver are biliary cirrhosis with intrahepatic cholestasis or obstruction of bile ducts; use of drugs (such as acetaminophen, methotrexate, or isoniazid); hepatic congestion from severe right-sided heart failure; constrictive pericarditis; valvular disease; $alpha_1$-antitrypsin deficiency; infiltrative disease (such as amyloidosis, glycogen storage diseases, or hemochromatosis); Wilson's disease; and nutritional deficits related to jejunal bypass.

Pathophysiology

Cirrhosis is the final stage in many types of liver insults. The cirrhotic liver usually has a nodular consistency, with bands of fibrosis (scar tissue) and small areas of regenerating tissue. There is extensive destruction of hepatocytes. This alteration in the architecture of the liver alters flow in the vascular and lymphatic systems and bile duct channels. Periodic exacerbations are marked by bile stasis, precipitating jaundice.

Portal vein hypertension develops in severe cirrhosis. The portal vein receives blood from the intestines and spleen. Thus, an increase of pressure in the portal vein causes (1) a retrograde increase in pressure resistance and enlargement of the esophageal, umbilical, and superior rectus veins, which may result in bleeding varices; (2) ascites (the result of osmotic or hydrostatic shifts leading to fluid accumulation in the peritoneum); and (3) incomplete clearing of protein metabolic wastes, with a resultant increase in ammonia, thus leading to hepatic encephalopathy.

Continuation of the process as a result of unknown causes or of alcohol abuse usually results in death from hepatic encephalopathy, bacterial (gram-negative) infection, peritonitis (bacterial), hepatoma (liver tumor), or complications of portal hypertension. See the algorithm on page 1236 for a summary of pathophysiologic changes, clinical manifestations, and treatment of cirrhosis.

Clinical Manifestations

Manifestations of cirrhosis diminish if the process is arrested at an early stage. Cirrhosis is a disease that initially progresses slowly. Thus, people with cirrhosis often discover the condition incidentally when seeking health care for other problems. In the early stages of cirrhosis, findings include hepatomegaly (enlarged liver), vascular changes, and abnormal results of laboratory tests. Palpation reveals a firm (scarred), lumpy (nodular), usually enlarged liver (although the liver becomes hard and shrunken in late cirrhosis).

In advanced cirrhosis, assessment reveals the following severe complications with their physiologic bases: ascites caused by malnutrition, portal hypertension, hypoalbuminemia, and hyperaldosteronism. Gastrointestinal bleeding arises from esophageal varices (swollen veins), hypoprothrombinemia, thrombocytopenia, and portal hypertension and often results in encephalopathy. Splenomegaly (enlargement of the spleen) indicates severe portal hypertension. Anemia, leukopenia, or thrombocytopenia may result from splenomegaly. Portal hypertension may cause prominent abdominal wall veins and internal hemorrhoids. Infections may be present as a result of an enlarged, overactive spleen, causing leukopenia. In addition, the bacteria that remain in the portal venous blood bypass the liver and are not removed by Kupffer cells and hence may cause infection. Ammonia no longer removed by the liver accumulates to levels toxic to the brain, resulting in encephalopathy. Renal failure occurs with rapidly failing hepatic function. Laboratory determinations reveal impaired hepatocellular function: elevated serum levels of liver enzymes (AST, alanine aminotransferase [ALT], and lactate dehydrogenase [LDH]), hypoalbuminemia, anemia, and prolonged prothrombin time. Liver biopsy allows for definitive diagnosis and demonstrates the associated pathologic changes.

Outcome Management

Medical Management

Monitor for Complications

Ascites, bleeding esophageal varices, and hepatic encephalopathy are discussed in depth later in this chapter. They are the most feared complications of cirrhosis. Renal failure (hepatorenal syndrome) and infection also are deadly. Family members and the client are taught manifestations of progressive liver failure. The family members should know what manifestations they need to report to the physician and when to seek immediate assistance, such as when variceal bleeding or a decrease in the level of consciousness occurs. Clients with encephalopathy may need extensive home care.

Maximize Liver Function

Although cirrhosis is a progressive, degenerative disorder, steps are taken to minimize the risk of trauma and maximize regeneration, thereby slowing the course of the disease and prolonging life. A nutritious diet is recommended for clients with cirrhosis. The diet should be palatable, with adequate calories and protein (75 to 100 g/day) unless hepatic encephalopathy is present, in which case protein is limited. A list of foods to be included in the diet is given to the client and family. Fat intake need not be restricted. If there is edema or fluid retention, restrict sodium and fluids. If the client is receiving a thiazide diuretic, the diet should be high in potassium. The B vitamins and fat-soluble vitamins (vitamins A, D, E, and K) are commonly given to clients with alcoholic cirrhosis. Adequate rest also is important to maximize regeneration of the liver. In postnecrotic or posthepatic cirrhosis, the clinician may prescribe corticosteroids to reduce manifestations of cirrhosis and improve liver function. Other medications may be used to treat the complications.

Treat the Underlying Causes

It is important that exposure to hepatotoxins be eliminated, that use of alcohol be avoided, and that biliary obstruction be removed. Medications that should be avoided (listed in Table 47–5) are specified to the client. The client should be encouraged to seek help (e.g., from Alcoholics Anonymous) with alcohol abstinence.

Prevent Infection

Prevention of infection is accomplished by adequate rest, appropriate diet, and avoidance of hepatotoxic substances (alcoholic beverages, and medications and chemicals toxic to the liver). Before the discovery of antibiotics, infection was the major cause of mortality in cirrhosis.

TABLE 47–5 CIRRHOSIS AND DRUG-INDUCED LIVER FAILURE

Drugs to Restrict or Avoid	Rationale
Acetaminophen	Can cause fatal liver damage
Phenobarbital, phenytoin, chlorpromazine (Thorazine)	Stimulates liver's major drug-metabolizing system; when liver diseased or damaged, drugs may not be metabolized properly and toxicity may occur; may also cause alteration in sensory perception and thought processes related to hepatic encephalopathy
Morphine, paraldehyde, codeine	Can cause spasms and pressure in the biliary tract, thus increasing discomfort
Alcohol	Stimulates liver's major drug metabolizing system; can damage liver further

Nursing Management of the Medical Client

Assessment

Because the manifestations of cirrhosis are sometimes vague and nonspecific, the client may not be aware of the disease early in its course. Assess the client closely for the presence of early manifestations, such as hepatomegaly, and carefully check the laboratory data for any indication of cirrhosis. As the disease progresses, assess for manifestations of complications of cirrhosis, such as ascites, portal hypertension, or hepatic encephalopathy. These are discussed later in the chapter.

When a client with cirrhosis is hospitalized, use laboratory data and the client's physical and psychosocial assessment data to guide care planning. See the Case Study on cirrhosis for further information about these tests. Also, assess the client and family members for their knowledge of the important aspects of self-care.

Diagnosis, Outcomes, Interventions

Altered Tissue Perfusion. Because of the increased risk of bleeding in the client with cirrhosis, the nursing diagnosis *Altered Tissue Perfusion related to bleeding tendencies and varices that may hemorrhage* is common.

Outcomes. Hemorrhage will be prevented, as evidenced by absence of bleeding, normal vital signs, and urine output of at least 0.5 ml/kg/hr.

Interventions

Monitor for Hemorrhage. Monitor the client for bleeding gums, purpura, melena, hematuria, and hematemesis. Check vital signs as ordered to assess for signs of shock. In addition, monitor urine output. Report volume that is less than 0.5 ml/kg/hr.

Prevent Hemorrhage. Protect the client from physical injury from falls or abrasions, and give injections only when absolutely necessary, using only small-gauge needles. Be sure to apply gentle pressure after an injection, but do not rub the site because this might cause bruising.

Provide Client Teaching. Instruct the client to avoid vigorous nose-blowing and straining with bowel movements. Sometimes stool softeners may be ordered to prevent straining with rupture of varices. Antidiarrheal agents may be administered to control diarrhea. If bleeding gums are noted, advise the client to use a soft toothbrush and to refrain from flossing until the bleeding has ceased.

Altered Nutrition: Less Than Body Requirements. In order for the liver to regenerate, the client must have adequate levels of vital nutrients; otherwise, the unmet requirements lead to the nursing diagnosis *Altered Nutrition: Less Than Body Requirements related to anorexia, impaired liver function, decreased absorption of fat-soluble vitamins, and diarrhea.*

Outcomes. The client will take in adequate nutrition, as evidenced by no weight loss and no manifestations of malnutrition.

Interventions

Modify Diet. The diet should provide ample protein to rebuild tissue but not enough protein to precipitate hepatic encephalopathy. The diet should supply sufficient carbohydrates to maintain weight and to spare protein

Text continued on page 1239

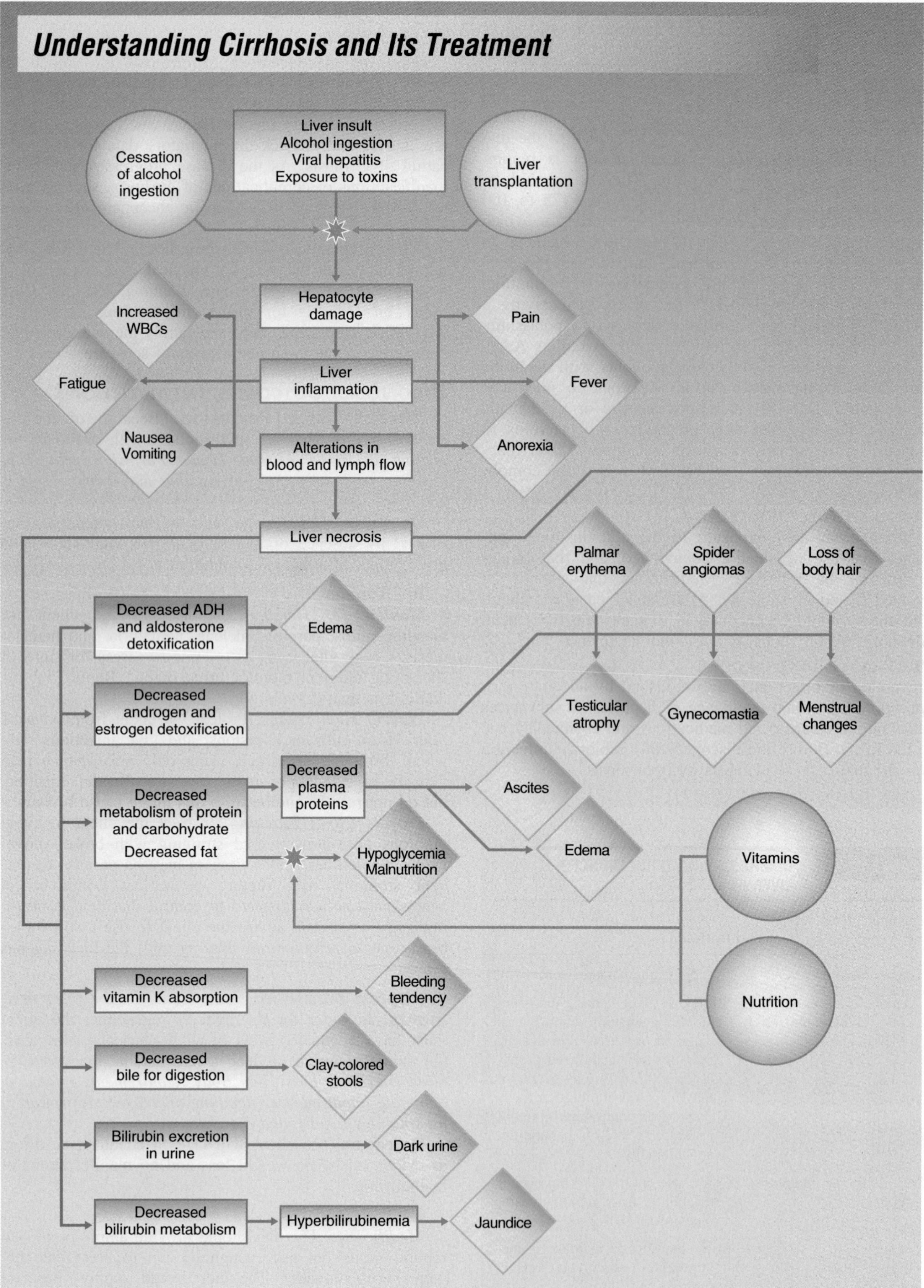
Understanding Cirrhosis and Its Treatment
Cessation of alcohol ingestion
Liver insult
Alcohol ingestion
Viral hepatitis
Exposure to toxins
Liver transplantation
Hepatocyte damage
Increased WBCs
Fatigue
Nausea
Vomiting
Liver inflammation
Pain
Fever
Anorexia
Alterations in blood and lymph flow
Liver necrosis
Palmar erythema
Spider angiomas
Loss of body hair
Decreased ADH and aldosterone detoxification
Edema
Decreased androgen and estrogen detoxification
Testicular atrophy
Gynecomastia
Menstrual changes
Decreased metabolism of protein and carbohydrate
Decreased fat
Decreased plasma proteins
Ascites
Edema
Hypoglycemia
Malnutrition
Vitamins
Nutrition
Decreased vitamin K absorption
Bleeding tendency
Decreased bile for digestion
Clay-colored stools
Bilirubin excretion in urine
Dark urine
Decreased bilirubin metabolism
Hyperbilirubinemia
Jaundice

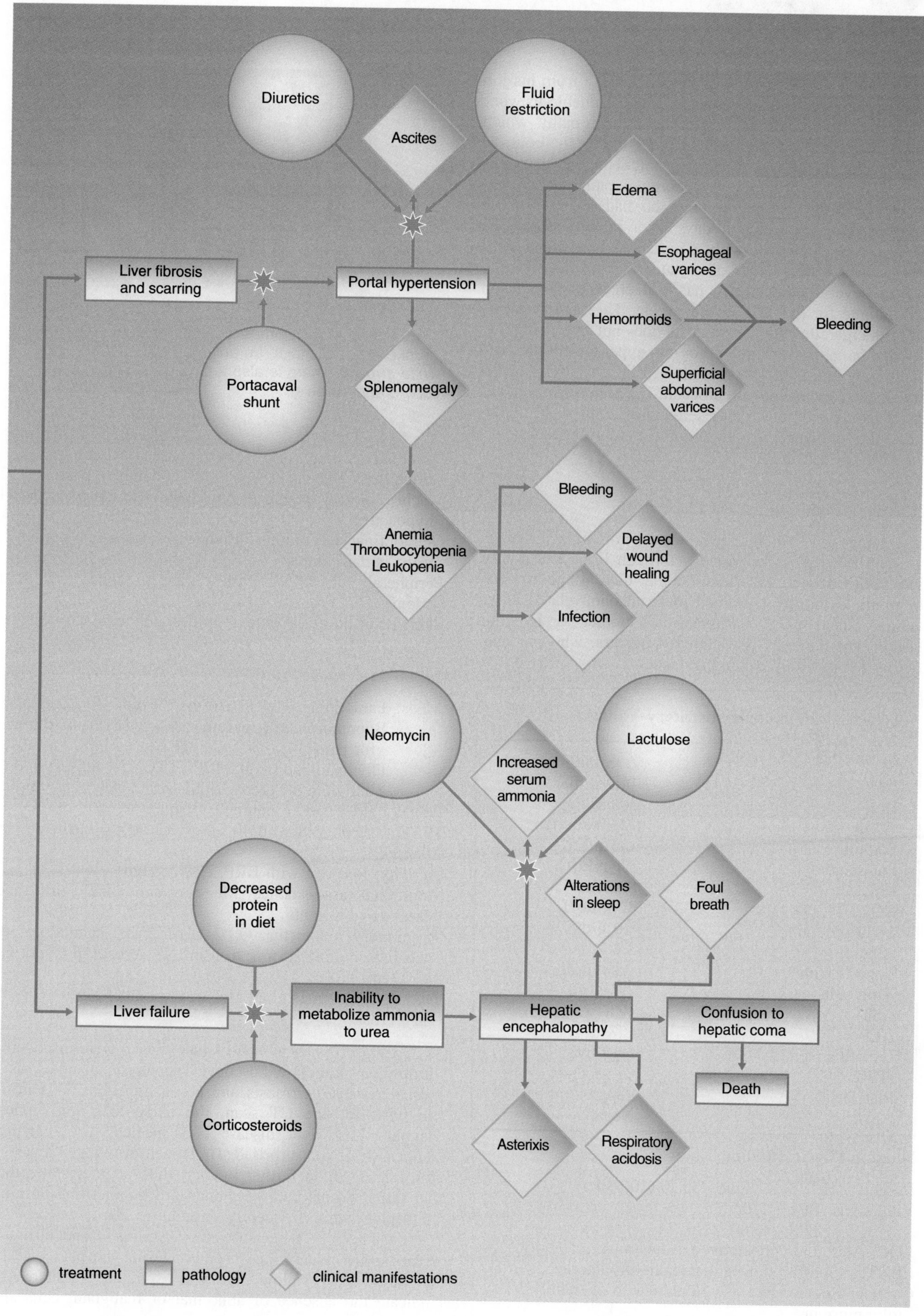
Diuretics
Ascites
Fluid restriction
Edema
Liver fibrosis and scarring
Portal hypertension
Esophageal varices
Hemorrhoids
Bleeding
Superficial abdominal varices
Portacaval shunt
Splenomegaly
Anemia
Thrombocytopenia
Leukopenia
Bleeding
Delayed wound healing
Infection
Neomycin
Increased serum ammonia
Lactulose
Decreased protein in diet
Alterations in sleep
Foul breath
Liver failure
Inability to metabolize ammonia to urea
Hepatic encephalopathy
Confusion to hepatic coma
Death
Corticosteroids
Asterixis
Respiratory acidosis
treatment
pathology
clinical manifestations

Cirrhosis

Mr. James is a 53-year-old man on disability from his job as a warehouse forklift driver. He became unable to work after developing idiopathic peripheral neuropathy which resulted in frequent falls and inability to run the controls of the forklift. He uses a cane to ambulate. Mr. James is being admitted with severe abdominal pain and coffee-grounds emesis. He reports that he had been vomiting bright red blood in the 2 days prior to admission. His abdomen is distended, with a measured abdominal girth of 52 inches. Mr. James also states that he has recently gained several pounds and has had shortness of breath and fatigue for the past several weeks. He reports that he smokes cigarettes but says that he does not use alcohol.

Mr. James is scheduled for an upper gastrointestinal endoscopy and paracentesis followed by a CT scan of the abdomen. Review the preprocedure preparations and client teaching required for these diagnostic tests. Also consider the influence of the preprocedure preparations on the order of scheduling these procedures.

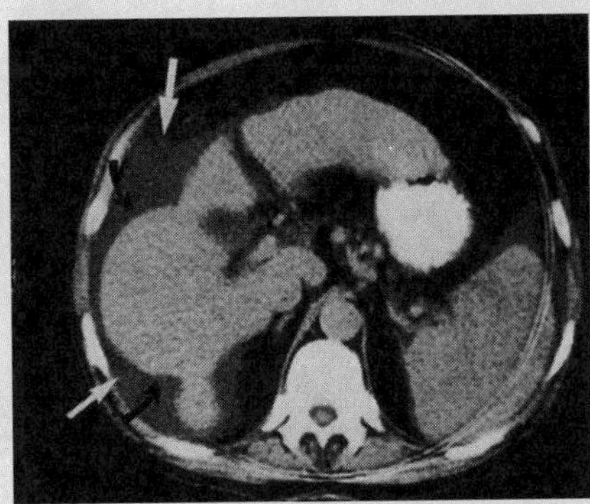

● A CT scan of Mr. James' abdomen revealed a shrunken, cirrhotic liver, an enlarged spleen, and ascites *(white arrows)*. There is also a large regenerating nodule *(curved dark arrows)*.

Nursing Admission Assessment

Mr. James lives in his own home with his wife of 32 years. His wife works Monday through Friday as a cook in a public school. Mr. James' father died at age 50 years of multiple injuries sustained in an alcohol-related motor vehicle accident. His 75-year-old mother is in good health. The Jameses have three daughters, who are married and live within driving distance.

Selected Admission Laboratory Values	
RBC	2.78 million/mm³
Hb	11.0 g/dl
Hct	30.6%
WBC	12,300/mm³
Sodium	133 mEq/L
Potassium	3.1 mEq/L
Chloride	89 mEq/L
CO_2	32 mEq/L
Total protein	5.0 g/dl
Albumin	2.1 g/dl
Total bilirubin	1.5 mg/dl
Ammonia	79 μg/dl
AST	47 U/L
ALP	178 U/L
Hepatitis panel	Negative
aPTT	62 seconds
Platelets	184,000/mm³
ANA	Negative

Nursing Physical Examination

Height: 5′10″ Weight: 235 lb (106.8 kg)
Vital signs: BP = 110/75
TPR = 100.3, 95, 25
LOC: Alert and cooperative
EENT: Moon-faced; sclerae are slightly icteric
Cardiac: Regular rate and rhythm with a grade I/VI systolic murmur
Pulmonary: Slight crackles in the bases bilaterally
Abdominal: Distended and taut; abdominal girth = 52 inches; fluid wave noted; bowel sounds high-pitched and hypoactive
Genitourinary: Voiding infrequently in small amounts; urine is dark amber
Peripheral pulses: 3/3 with pitting pretibial and pedal edema
Skin: Bruising noted on extremities and abdomen

Initial Treatment Plan

Meds: Famotidine (Pepcid) 20 mg IV bid
Buprenorphine (Buprenex) 0.3 mg IV q 4–6 h prn for pain
Phytonadione (AquaMEPHYTON) 2 mg IM qod
Multivitamin preparation with folate and biotin (M.V.I.-12) 1 ampule IV qd
IV: D_5 and 0.5 NS with 40 mEq KCl at 100 ml/hr
Diet: NPO
Activity: Bed rest with BRP, elevate HOB
Additional assessments: Measure abdominal girth and I&O daily weights
Respiratory treatments: O_2 2 L per nasal cannula, albuterol (Ventolin) 2.5 mg in 3 ml NS aerosol qid, spot O_2 oximetry qd
Diagnostic tests: Hb and Hct q 4 h; call if Hb <10 g/dl, aPTT daily

Oozing esophageal varices (see figure) were discovered during Mr. James' endoscopy. The physician notes, as a probable cause, cirrhosis and portal hypertension. During the visit for the CT scan, the nurse tells Mr. James' daughter that liver disease is suspected. The daughter replies, "I'm not surprised. He's been drinking like a fish for years." Upon further inquiry, the daughter states that her father drinks both beer and hard liquor from morning until night while frequently skipping meals.

Mr. James' CT scan reveals a shrunken and cirrhotic liver, splenomegaly, and ascites. During the paracentesis, 60 ml of clear yellow fluid was aspirated. Initial results indicate the absence of abnormal or malignant cells and bacteria. Following diagnostic examinations, the physician discontinues the buprenorphine and orders acetaminophen (Tylenol) 650 mg q 4 h prn. Consider the rationale for this change.

In addition, the physician orders bumetanide (Bumex) 1 mg IV bid. A one-time dose of salt-poor albumin 25 g IV is also ordered. Consider the rationale of using these medications for treatment of ascites. Which of these orders should be implemented first? Why?

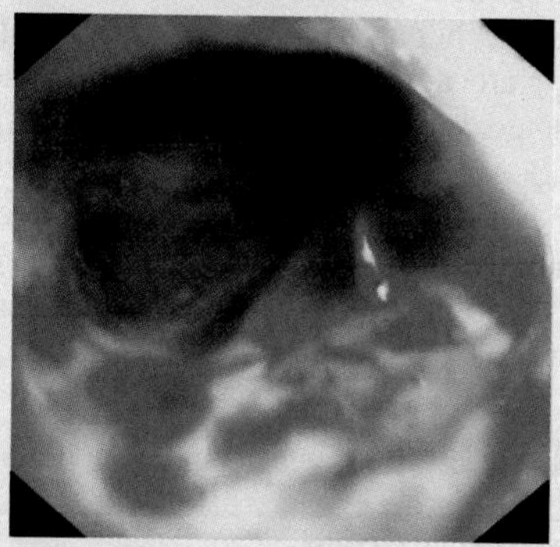

● Oozing varix. (Courtesy of Martin Sears, Internal Medicine and Diagnostic Problems, Fremont, NE.)

Mr. James' hemoglobin level remains stable, and no further bleeding is noted. He is started on an all-cooked, high-carbohydrate, moderate-protein (60–70 g/day) and low-sodium (1–2 g/day) diet. He is to limit his intake of fluids to 1500 ml/day. The intravenous and intramuscular vitamin K preparations are discontinued. Vitamin K (phytonadione) 5 mg PO twice a week and a daily supplement of B vitamins are added to his medication orders. The famotidine is changed from the intravenous route to the oral route of administration. Lansoprazole (Prevacid) 15 mg PO every AM, 30 minutes before breakfast, is added. The bumetanide IV order is discontinued and replaced with an order for spironolactone (Aldactone) 25 mg bid and potassium (K-Dur) 20 mEq/day. Docusate (Colace) 100 mg/day is also ordered. Discharge is planned for tomorrow morning.

Discharge Criteria

Average length of stay (LOS): 6.6 days

Initiate teaching of client and significant others about diet, medications, drug and alcohol incompatibilities, fluid restriction, and need to report of bleeding and changes in mental status.

Complete community referrals for client and significant others.

What referrals would you make? Why?

Questions to Be Considered

1. Discuss the pathophysiologic changes that have led to Mr. James' ascites, peripheral edema, weight gain, bruising, and esophageal varices.
2. Discuss what further changes in Mr. James' diet and medications might be needed if certain laboratory values suggest progression of the disease process (e.g., serum ammonia levels, bleeding studies, liver enzymes, serum protein, bilirubin, etc.).
3. Mr. James' family decides to confront him about his alcohol consumption. Discuss the nurse's role in supporting the family's decision. Consider the ethical ramifications of your decision.
4. If Mr. James continues to abstain from alcohol, he is at risk of developing delirium tremens (DTs). What are the manifestations of this syndrome, and what treatments are indicated?
5. What is Mr. James' prognosis? Would he be eligible for a liver transplant? What factors would influence the transplant team's decision?
6. Had Mr. James' bleeding not been controlled, what medical and nursing interventions would have been indicated? Consider both medical and surgical management.

Abbreviations: ALP, alkaline phosphatase; ANA, antinuclear antibodies; aPTT, activated partial thromboplastin time; AST, aspartate aminotransferase; BP, blood pressure; BRP, bathroom privileges; CO_2, carbon dioxide; CT, computed tomography; D_5, 5% dextrose; EENT, eye-ear-nose-throat; Hb, hemoglobin; Hct, hematocrit; HOB, head of bed; IM, intramuscularly; I&O, intake and output; IV, intravenously; KCl, potassium chloride; L, liter; LOC, level of consciousness; LOS, length of stay; Meds, medications; NPO, *nil per os* (nothing by mouth); NS, normal saline; O_2, oxygen; PO, *per os* (orally); prn, as needed; qd, once daily; RBC, red blood cell(s); TPR, temperature/pulse/respirations; WBC, white blood cell(s).

stores. Fat restriction is not necessary. Total daily calories should range between 2000 and 3000. Place the client on daily weight, intake and output, and calorie counts to assess fluid and nutritional balance.

Closely monitor the laboratory and nutritional panels for manifestations of improvement or further deterioration. If ammonia levels rise (normal levels are 70 to 200 mg/dl in whole blood and 56 to 150 mg/dl in plasma), foods high in protein may be restricted.

If the client has ascites or edema, sodium and fluids should be restricted in the diet. Small, frequent meals make it easier for clients with anorexia to eat enough food. Adequate rest and a stable environmental temperature should be ensured to allow optimal use of calories. Administer prescribed medications such as antacids, antiemetics, antidiarrheals, or cathartics to decrease gastric distress, but avoid antiemetics such as phenothiazines.

Provide Vitamin Supplements. The physician usually prescribes a maintenance multivitamin preparation or, in severe malnutrition, therapeutic levels of vitamins. Also, vitamins A, D, E, and K are supplied if fat absorption is adequate. The client with severe malabsorption may require IV vitamins with calcium gluconate supplementation. Encourage family or friends to provide desirable foods as permitted.

Activity Intolerance. The client with cirrhosis often experiences severe fatigue, leading to the nursing diagnosis *Activity Intolerance related to bed rest, fatigue, lack of energy, and altered respiratory function secondary to ascites.*

Outcomes. The client will maintain a balance between rest and activity, as evidenced by the absence of fatigue and problems associated with immobility.

Interventions. Clinicians often prescribe rest for clients with cirrhosis, but how much rest is necessary is debated. During periods of acute malfunction, rest reduces metabolic demands on the liver and increases circulation. Long-term planning should include counseling the client to rest frequently and to avoid unnecessary fatigue.

Risk for Injury. Because the liver is in a very precarious state, intake of alcohol or other hepatotoxins should cease immediately. Otherwise, the nursing diagnosis *Risk for Injury related to continued intake of hepatotoxins* becomes appropriate.

Outcomes. The client will not suffer injury from continued intake of hepatotoxins as evidenced by cessation of drinking and avoidance of medications that may cause further damage.

Interventions. Ensure that all known hepatotoxic medications (including alcohol) are removed from therapeutic regimens, and that dosages of all drugs thought to be metabolized by the liver have been lowered. Avoid administration of sedatives and opiates.

Altered Protection. Because of portal hypertension and decreased filtering capability of the liver, the nursing diagnosis *Altered Protection related to alcohol abuse and inadequate nutrition* may be appropriate.

Outcomes. The client will not experience systemic infection or spontaneous bacterial peritonitis with ascites.

Interventions. Clients with cirrhosis may experience spontaneous bacterial peritonitis with ascites. Mortality is high when this occurs. Your role as nurse is to monitor for manifestations of infection and to administer antibiotics as prescribed. Antibiotics may be required to control intestinal flora that aggravate encephalopathy.

Altered Health Maintenance. The client with cirrhosis must become involved in self-care if the treatment is to be successful. Therefore, *Altered Health Maintenance related to lack of knowledge of the disease and long-term treatment is an important nursing diagnosis.*

Outcomes. The client with cirrhosis will understand the disease and the implications of long-term management, as evidenced by the client's statements.

Interventions. Provide the client and significant others with information to manage care at home. Clients with cirrhosis will live longer if they get adequate rest, abstain from alcohol, and eat nutritious meals.

Encourage clients with a history of alcohol abuse to seek assistance from support groups such as AA to stop drinking. Even if cirrhotic changes have begun in the liver, it is vital for the client to stop drinking before irreparable damage occurs. See Chapter 24 for further information on alcoholism.

EVALUATION

The outcome in cirrhosis depends on the client's ability to stop intake of alcohol, or any other substances toxic to the liver, early enough to prevent irreparable liver damage. If biliary obstruction is the cause of the cirrhosis, the client must seek further medical or surgical treatment. Once extensive damage has occurred, the client will not recover and the disease will progress with manifestations of liver failure.

Self-Care

Clients with cirrhosis are managed at home unless they encounter complications or are in the end stage of the disease process. Hence, it is important to teach them how to maintain adequate nutrition, to alternate rest and activity, and to avoid hepatotoxic substances. Refer the client to the appropriate agency or support group for assistance with alcohol cessation such as AA, Al-Anon, or Al-Ateen. Provide referrals to community nursing support agencies as needed. If the client is exposed to hepatotoxic agents in the workplace, suggest that the client try to change jobs. Emphasize that regular check-ups and blood tests to follow the progress of the disease are needed.

COMPLICATIONS OF CIRRHOSIS

PORTAL HYPERTENSION

Portal hypertension exists when there is a persistent increase in blood pressure in the portal venous system occurring as a result of increased resistance to or obstruction of blood flow through the portal venous system into the liver.

Etiology and Risk Factors

Most cases of portal hypertension in the United States are associated with cirrhosis. The portal vein is likely to be obstructed by a thrombus; a tumor is the next most common cause. Box 47–1 lists factors that may cause portal hypertension.

Pathophysiology

The normal blood flow to and from the liver depends on proper functioning of the portal vein (70% of inflow), the hepatic artery (30% of inflow), and the hepatic veins (outflow). Disease processes that damage the liver or its

BOX 47–1 Factors in the Pathogenesis of Cirrhotic Portal Hypertension

1. *Presinusoidal obstruction*
   a. Outside liver
      (1) Portal vein thrombosis
   b. Within liver
      (1) Schistosomiasis
2. *Postsinusoidal obstruction*
   a. Distal to liver
      (1) Budd-Chiari syndrome
      (2) Right-sided heart failure
   b. Within liver
      (1) Veno-occlusive disease
3. *Increased inflow beyond vessel capacity*
   a. Arterial–portal venous fistulas
   b. Splenomegaly

Adapted from Friedman, S. L. (1996). Cirrhosis of the liver and its major sequelae. In J. C. Bennett & F. Plum (Eds), *Cecil textbook of medicine* (20th ed.). Philadelphia: W. B. Saunders.

major vessels or alter the flow of blood through these structures are responsible for the development of portal hypertension. Portal hypertension may result either from increased blood flow in the portal vein or from an increased resistance to flow within the portal venous system.

The most common cause of portal hypertension is cirrhosis. The pathophysiologic mechanism in cirrhosis is increased resistance, which is intrahepatic and primarily sinusoidal. Portal hypertension may also arise from presinusoidal obstruction, either outside the liver (as in portal vein thrombosis) or within it (as in schistosomiasis). In addition, lesions leading to portal hypertension may be postsinusoidal, either within the liver (as in veno-occlusive disease) or distal to it (as in Budd-Chiari syndrome or right-sided heart failure). Rarely, portal hypertension can occur in the normal liver from markedly increased inflow beyond the capacity of the compliant portal vessels to absorb. Arterial–portal venous fistulas and massive splenomegaly due to infection or neoplasm are examples of causes of this type of portal hypertension. The degree of liver dysfunction varies with the causative process, the duration of the process, and individual client characteristics.

Normal portal venous blood pressure is 5 to 10 mm Hg. Portal hypertension exists when the pressure rises 5 mm Hg higher than the inferior vena cava pressure. Collateral vessels develop in an effort to equalize pressures between the two venous systems. The spleen and other organs that empty into the portal venous system also begin to undergo the effects of congestion.

Clinical Manifestations

In clients with portal hypertension, assessment reveals a network of slightly tortuous epigastric vessels that branch off the area of the umbilicus and lead toward the sternum and ribs (caput medusae); an enlarged, palpable spleen; internal hemorrhoids; bruits, which may be heard over the upper abdomen; and ascites, which typically appears when there is concurrent liver disease.

Direct measurement of portal venous blood pressure is possible only during laparotomy. The diagnosis of portal hypertension often relies on indirect measurements of portal pressure—obtained at liver scanning, splenoportography, abdominal angiography, or liver biopsy—and on other laboratory data (see Chapter 42). Radiography and endoscopy procedures may be used to differentiate variceal hemorrhage from other types of gastrointestinal bleeding.

Outcome Management

Medical Management

One of the most serious disabling complications of portal hypertension is dilatation of the superior rectal veins, abdominal wall veins, and esophagogastric veins. With conditions such as cirrhosis, portal venous blood pressure increases, causing esophageal veins to swell and distend. These swollen, dilated veins are called *varices*. Several factors can contribute to the rupturing of varices (Fig. 47–2): increased portal venous blood pressure, increased intrathoracic pressure (coughing and straining at stools), irritation by food or alcohol, and erosion by gastric juices. The veins of the stomach and esophagus are most subject to rupture; when rupture occurs, it constitutes a medical emergency.

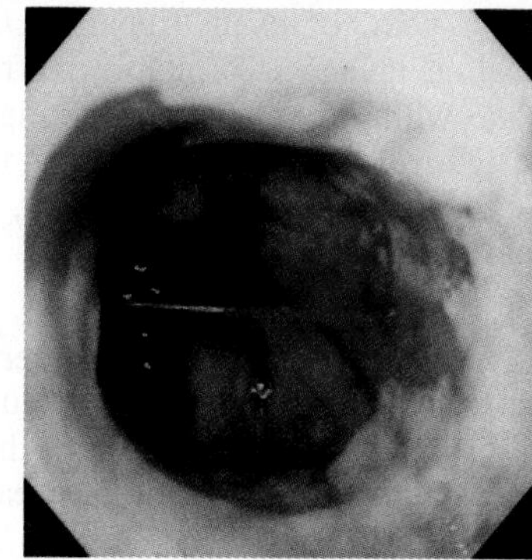

FIGURE 47–2 A bleeding esophageal varix. (Courtesy of Martin Sears, M.D., Internal Medicine and Diagnostic Problems, Fremont, NE.)

Another mechanism that leads to hemorrhage involves the spleen. The splenic vein merges with the superior mesenteric vein to form the portal vein. When pressure increases in the portal venous system, damage to the spleen occurs. Damage to the spleen is not proportional to the increase in portal venous blood pressure. As the spleen enlarges, it destroys blood cells, especially platelets, which increases the risk of hemorrhage and anemia.

Hepatic encephalopathy is an extremely dangerous complication of portal hypertension. This problem usually arises following a period of bleeding into the gastrointestinal tract. Digestion of this blood takes place in the intestines. Because blood is a protein, this process increases ammonia in the gut and bloodstream. In turn, the excessive ammonia disturbs brain function. The Critical Monitoring feature lists assessment findings that mandate early intervention in esophageal bleeding secondary to portal hypertension. Hepatic encephalopathy is discussed later in this chapter.

Death often follows rupture of esophageal varices if the hemorrhage is not immediately controlled. To stop hemorrhage, health practitioners perform emergency measures: administration of vasopressin, balloon tamponade, injection sclerotherapy, endoscopic electrocautery, direct ligation of the bleeding varices, transhepatic embolization

CRITICAL MONITORING

Esophageal Bleeding Secondary to Portal Hypertension

Blood pressure ≤ 90/60 mm Hg
Heart rate ≥ 100 BPM
Cool, clammy skin
Distal pulses <2+ on a 0–4+ scale
Slowed capillary refill (>2 seconds)
Diminished orientation to person, place, and time
Restlessness

of the left gastric vein, or even urgent portacaval shunt surgery. Cold saline lavage is probably ineffective but is occasionally done while the client is awaiting transport to surgery or the gastrointestinal laboratory. Fluids, especially volume expanders and blood products, are administered to maintain volume.

Control Hemorrhage

Sclerotherapy. To perform sclerotherapy, the operator passes an endoscope into the esophagus and injects a sclerosing agent (e.g., morrhuate sodium) that flows into the varices. The sclerosing agent initially causes inflammation of the vein wall and then fibrosis. The operator may give repeated injections over a period of weeks until the varices are no longer prominent.

Transjugular Intrahepatic Portosystemic Shunt. For years, surgical decompression procedures were used to lower portal pressure in clients with bleeding esophageal varices. However, survival rates in clients with hepatitis were not improved with portal vein–systemic (portosystemic) shunt surgery. Decompression can now be accomplished without surgery through the percutaneous placement of a portosystemic shunt, called a transjugular intrahepatic portosystemic shunt (TIPS). With the use of fluoroscopy, an expandable metal stent is used to keep open a parenchymal tract created between the hepatic vein and the intrahepatic portion of the portal vein. Physiologically, the TIPS is similar to a side-to-side surgical shunt. Placement is successful in more than 90% of the clients and bleeding is controlled in 90 to 95% of clients.

Vasopressin. When varices rupture, IV vasopressin is routinely administered to stop variceal bleeding. Administration of vasopressin achieves temporary lowering of portal pressure. These agents reduce portal venous blood flow by constricting afferent arterioles. Direct infusion of vasopressin into the superior mesenteric artery is most effective. Serious side effects include hypothermia, myocardial and gastrointestinal tract ischemia, and acute renal failure. It is therefore contraindicated in clients with a recent myocardial infarction. Vasopressin may be given in conjunction with nitroglycerin, which is administered intravenously, sublingually, or by patch to minimize vasoconstrictive side effects. Alternatively, somatostatin is at least as effective as vasopressin. Drug therapy may stop bleeding, but it has no effect on survival.

Beta-Adrenergic–Blocking Agents. The effectiveness of beta-adrenergic–blocking agents (e.g., propranolol [Inderal], metoprolol [Lopressor] or nadolol [Corgard]) in the management of acute variceal bleeding is limited, because they reduce the heart rate (and hence the blood pressure) and mask the early manifestations of hypoglycemia. However, studies suggest that such therapy has been effective in preventing a first episode of variceal bleeding or subsequent episodes after an initial bleed.

Balloon Tamponade. Applying pressure to ruptured varices via balloon tamponade may stop the hemorrhage. For this intervention, the clinician inserts a Sengstaken-Blakemore or Minnesota tube into the stomach and inflates the esophageal and gastric balloons (Fig. 47–3). The pressure of the esophageal balloon against the varices may stop the bleeding. It is important to release this pressure periodically to prevent tissue necrosis. The esophageal balloon is not left inflated for more than 24 hours. Also, it is important to remove secretions and saliva that accumulate above the balloon to prevent aspiration. The Minnesota tube has an additional port for aspiration of secretions above the esophageal balloon. Ensure that the gastric balloon is inflated to prevent migration of the tube. You should also have scissors at the bedside in order to be able to remove the tube in an emergency. Complications of balloon tamponade may occur in 15% or more of clients and include aspiration pneumonitis as well as esophageal rupture. This intervention is performed less frequently today now that other treatment is available.

Nursing Management of the Medical Client

Assessment

The major assessment for you to make is for the presence of hemorrhage. The other important aspect of assessment is to check for indicators of the client's clinical status after any intervention to treat the hemorrhage, such as in assessing tube function after placement of a Sengstaken-Blakemore or Minnesota tube. Monitor the client's vital signs continuously for any significant changes.

Diagnosis, Outcomes, Interventions

Altered Tissue Perfusion. With rupture of varices, the nursing diagnosis that must be addressed immediately is *Altered Tissue Perfusion related to portal hypertension and rupture and hemorrhage of esophageal varices.*

Outcomes. Hemorrhage will be controlled, as evidenced by the return of vital signs to normal and no further bleeding.

Interventions. The client can learn activities to help reduce the risk of rupture of esophageal varices.

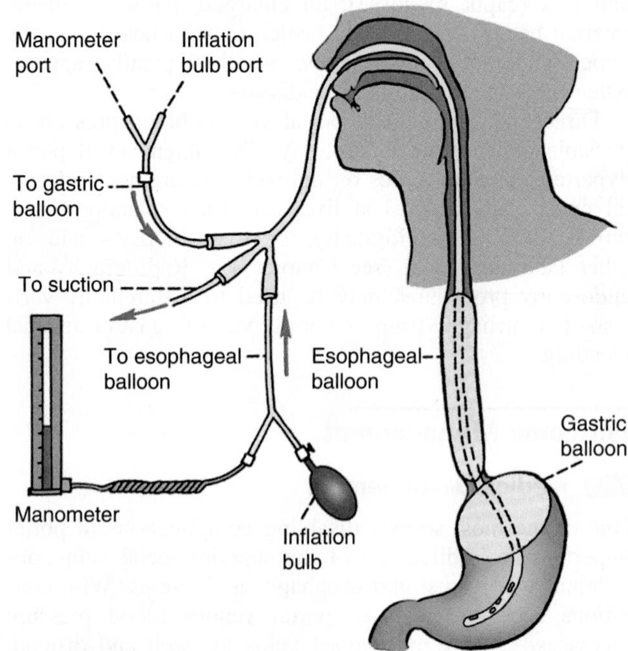

FIGURE 47–3 A Sengstaken-Blakemore tube may be used to control ruptured esophageal varices, a potential complication of portal hypertension.

Prevent Hemorrhage. The nurse should instruct the client as follows:

- Avoid straining maneuvers that increase intra-abdominal or intrathoracic pressure.
- Avoid rough foods, which may traumatize the esophagus, and spicy foods, which may irritate the esophageal mucosa.
- Develop an emergency plan in case severe esophageal varices should rupture. Include in this plan a list of all emergency telephone numbers. Discuss the plan with both the client and family members.

Monitor for Hemorrhage. If hemorrhage from ruptured varices occurs, monitor blood pressure, pulse, respiration, and urine output continuously, and assist with interventions to restore circulating blood volume. Monitor vital signs closely throughout this period. This is a critical time for nursing intervention and can be a very stressful time for the client, family members, and nurse. Further information on the assessment and treatment of shock and hemorrhage can be found in Chapter 81.

Risk for Impaired Gas Exchange. The client with ruptured varices is prone to many problems. A major potential problem is addressed in the nursing diagnosis *Risk for Impaired Gas Exchange related to decreased oxygen supply secondary to aspiration pneumonitis or obstruction occurring after balloon tamponade with the Sengstaken-Blakemore tube.*

Outcomes. The client will not suffer injury related to the Sengstaken-Blakemore tube, as evidenced by no respiratory distress, absence of aspiration, and absence of esophageal ischemia.

Interventions

Prevent Esophageal Necrosis. The pressure of the esophageal balloon on the esophagus not only stops hemorrhage but also may cause esophageal necrosis. As noted earlier, you must release the pressure on the esophagus periodically to prevent tissue damage. Consult the physician on how often to release balloon pressure, because practices vary widely.

Prevent Aspiration Pneumonia. Aspiration pneumonia is another complication of balloon tamponade. The inflated balloon in the esophagus prevents saliva and secretions from reaching the stomach. Ascertain whether the tube used for tamponade has a suction port above the esophageal balloon. If not, insert a nasogastric tube to the upper balloon level or perform suctioning frequently to remove accumulating fluid.

Prevent Nares Erosion. Tubes inserted through the nose may cause erosion of the nares, especially if traction is applied to the tamponading tube (practices differ). To prevent this complication, clean and lubricate the external nares. Provide padding if necessary.

Prevent Airway Obstruction. Airway obstruction, another complication of balloon tamponade, occurs when the gastric balloon deflates or breaks and traction on the tube pulls the esophageal balloon up into the oropharynx. Keep scissors at the bedside. If this emergency arises, cut the tube and pull it out to restore airway patency. To prevent airway obstruction, label each port of the tube to prevent accidental deflation of the gastric balloon.

Acute Confusion. Because of the potential buildup of ammonia, the client with bleeding varices is likely to have the nursing diagnosis *Acute Confusion related to portosystemic encephalopathy and hepatic coma occurring in conjunction with gastrointestinal bleeding and accumulation of ammonia.*

Outcomes. The client will be oriented to person, place, and time. Serum ammonia levels will not increase, and level of consciousness will not decrease.

Interventions

Monitor Level of Consciousness. Assess the client's level of consciousness and orientation on a regular basis (after performing a baseline assessment). Ask clients to write their name each day, and assess for writing deterioration and possible rising ammonia levels. Also assess the client regularly for the development of asterixis (liver flap or flapping tremor). Monitor for evidence of gastrointestinal bleeding, including melena or hematemesis, because bleeding can precipitate hepatic coma. Report the bleeding promptly to the physician.

Protect from Injury. Protect the client from injury by keeping the side rails up and the bed in the lowest position. Assist the client with ambulation as needed. Use caution when administering sedatives, antihistamines, and other agents that affect the central nervous system (CNS).

EVALUATION

Although the acute episode of bleeding from esophageal varices can usually be controlled, the development of varices is a sign of deterioration of the liver and increasing portal hypertension. The client will need careful and continued follow-up to prevent recurrence or further complications.

Surgical Management

PORTOSYSTEMIC SHUNT

Several surgical procedures can be used to reduce the danger of hemorrhage from varices caused by portal hypertension. These procedures involve anastomosing the high-pressure portal venous system to the low-pressure systemic venous system. This creates a portosystemic shunt.

Surgical creation of a portosystemic shunt reduces portal hypertension by sending portal venous blood directly into the inferior vena cava, bypassing the liver. Other vessels may be altered, depending on the type of shunt selected. Such a procedure lowers portal venous blood pressure, thus decreasing the risk of rupture of esophageal varices. Figure 47–4 illustrates some of the many possible portosystemic (portal vein–vena cava) shunt procedures.

Overall, clients who require portosystemic shunts are poor surgical candidates because of their suboptimal nutritional status, increased risk of infection, and deteriorating liver function. The role of portosystemic shunt surgery in the management of bleeding esophageal varices after initial medical control of bleeding is uncertain.

INDICATIONS. Although surgical shunting reduces the risk of recurrent hemorrhage, the overall mortality of clients undergoing such surgery is comparable with that of

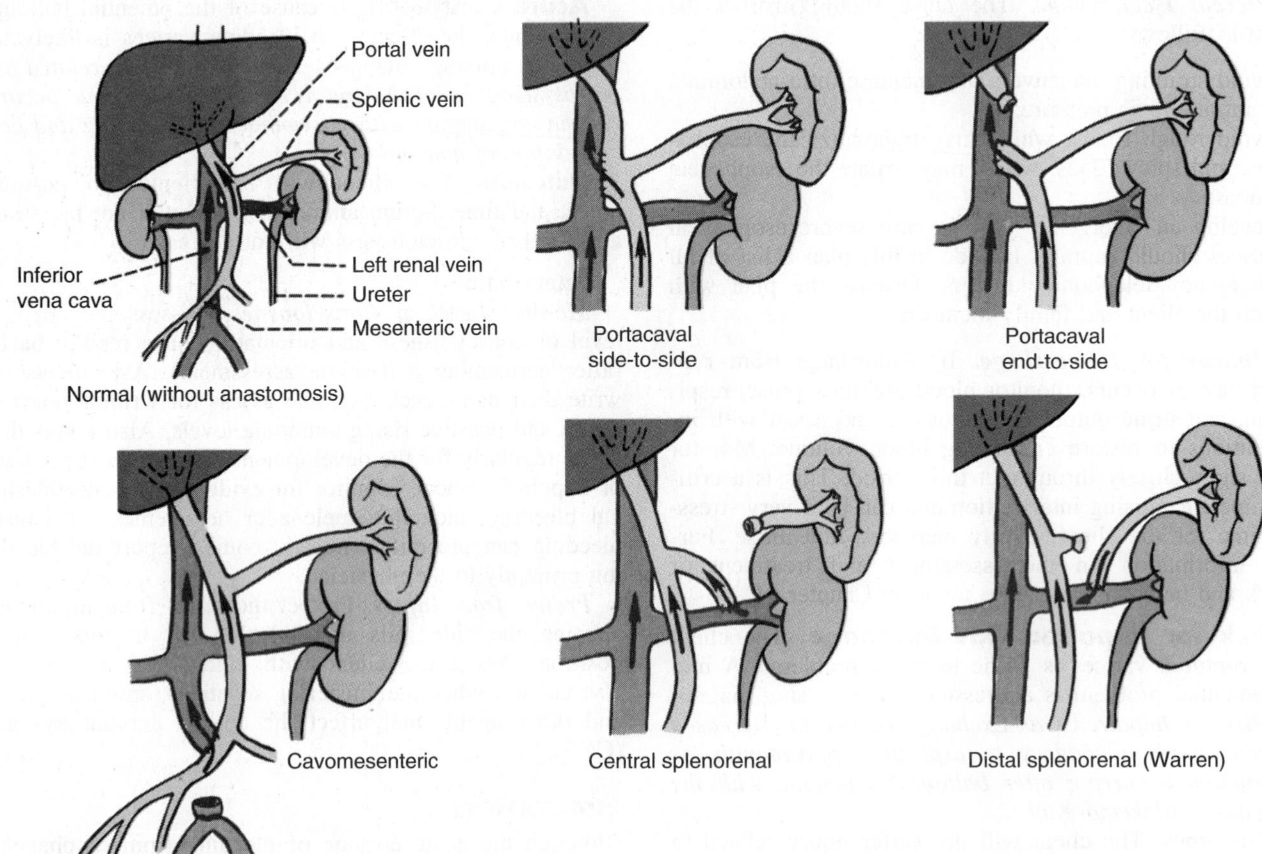

FIGURE 47–4 Some types of portacaval or portosystemic shunt procedures used to reduce portal hypertension.

clients managed medically. The similarity of outcomes is related to the increased incidence of encephalopathy in surgically managed clients when the shunted blood is not cleared of toxic substances, and to the higher incidence of death from progressive liver failure with their increased longevity. For these reasons, surgical creation of a portosystemic shunt is reserved for clients who have not responded to other treatment, and who, despite periodic endoscopic sclerotherapy, continue to bleed.

CONTRAINDICATION. The main contraindication to portosystemic shunt procedures is poor general health, so that the client is not able to withstand the trauma, blood and fluid loss, and anesthesia of surgery.

COMPLICATIONS. Major complications after a shunt procedure are bacteremia and DIC, heart failure, shunt clotting, and hepatic encephalopathy. Clients must he monitored closely to detect the onset of these complications, and corrective measures implemented quickly if they arise.

OUTCOMES. Clients who undergo portosystemic shunt procedures require surgery because other methods of controlling bleeding have been unsuccessful. The goal of these procedures is (1) to reduce portal venous blood flow enough to prevent variceal hemorrhage, (2) to preserve enough blood inflow to the liver to prevent hepatic encephalopathy and hepatic failure, and (3) to increase client comfort (the shunting is a palliative procedure).

Nursing Management of the Surgical Client

PREOPERATIVE CARE

Preoperative management of the client undergoing a portosystemic shunt procedure includes an appraisal of the client's general physical condition and readiness for surgery along with assessment of the client's neurologic, respiratory, and renal systems to establish a baseline. Blood and urine may be examined for the presence of infectious organisms and an arterial blood gas analysis may be performed to assess general respiratory function.

Blood clotting mechanisms are analyzed, as well as the client's fluid and electrolyte status and levels of ammonia, protein, bilirubin, and liver enzymes. If the client has an inappropriate level of any one of these substances, measures are taken to correct the problem. If the hemoglobin and hematocrit are low, the client may receive a blood transfusion. The client's general nutritional status is important, and protein hydrolysates are administered by total parenteral nutrition (TPN) if indicated.

POSTOPERATIVE CARE

ASSESSMENT

After portosystemic shunt surgery, assess the client's respiratory, renal, and hemodynamic status. In addition, observe the client and inspect the operative site carefully for any manifestations of shunt clotting, such as pain, distention, or nausea. Assess the client after portosystemic shunt surgery by monitoring for the following:

- Presence of hemorrhage, hypovolemia, and oliguria
- Fluid and electrolyte imbalance (dilutional hyponatremia, ascites)
- Respiratory rate and rhythm (rales, atelectasis, labored breathing, pneumonia)
- Hypoalbuminemia
- Hypoglycemia
- Manifestations of infection (fever, increased white blood cells [WBCs])
- Pain levels
- Mental status (alertness)

DIAGNOSIS, OUTCOMES, INTERVENTIONS

Nursing diagnoses associated with care of the client after portosystemic shunt surgery include *Altered Tissue Perfusion, Impaired Gas Exchange,* and *Acute Confusion* (see Nursing Management of the Medical Client). In addition, *Fluid Volume Excess* is a pertinent nursing diagnosis for the client undergoing portosystemic shunt surgery.

Fluid Volume Excess. The client who has undergone portosystemic shunt surgery often retains excess fluid, leading to the nursing diagnosis *Fluid Volume Excess related to retention of fluids secondary to portal hypertension, liver failure, and hemodilution of blood related to the new portosystemic shunt.*

Outcomes. A normovolemic state will be maintained, as evidenced by a stable or decreasing abdominal girth and a regular respiratory rate and rhythm.

Interventions

Assess for Fluid Volume Excess. Assess the client for retention of fluid, which is likely to occur because of hemodynamic fluid shifts. Measure abdominal girth to obtain a baseline, and then recheck daily or every shift, as appropriate, to detect development of ascites. Also, monitor weight and intake and output. Output should not be less than intake. Assess for the presence of edema and document its degree, from 1+ (barely noticeable) to 4+ (deep and pitting). Be sure to check for clinical indicators of pulmonary edema, including dyspnea and orthopnea. See that appropriate pulmonary and respiratory therapy is initiated if the client has any respiratory involvement.

Monitor and Treat Postprocedure Complications. Assess the client for hepatic encephalopathy. If portal hypertension is due to liver disease, carefully monitor for postoperative hemorrhage, because bleeding tendencies often arise from liver cell malfunction. Assess cardiovascular function carefully, because the shunt increases venous return to the heart, thus increasing the workload of the heart and placing the client at risk for heart failure.

After surgery, carefully monitor laboratory data, including hemoglobin, hematocrit, prothrombin time, ammonia level, blood urea nitrogen (BUN) level, bilirubin level, blood gas concentrations, and fluid and electrolyte levels. If the hemoglobin and hematocrit are below normal, you may need to administer a blood transfusion. However, many times the low hematocrit and hemoglobin levels occur because of hemodilution that results after the shunt is completed. If clotting time (prothrombin time) is not within normal limits, administer vitamin K. If the client is having difficulty breathing because of ascites, it is doubly important after surgery to implement measures that improve respirations (turning, coughing, and deep-breathing; respiratory treatments; and maintaining any chest drainage system). Other areas in which you may need to intervene for clients who have undergone portosystemic shunt surgery include the following:

- Administering IV fluids plus blood or volume expanders such as dextran and maintaining line patency and prescribed flow rates
- Monitoring blood and urine values and noting any manifestations of infection (such as increased WBCs and elevated erythrocyte sedimentation rate)
- Eliminating medications that sedate, depress the CNS, or are known hepatotoxins (e.g., acetaminophen)
- Maintaining nutrition: while client is receiving nothing by mouth, i.e., is on *nil per os* (NPO) status, usually for several days postoperatively, administer TPN; when food intake begins, protein intake may be limited and increased slowly if BUN and ammonia levels and mental status remain within normal limits
- Maintaining sterile technique when changing dressing(s)
- Maintaining patency if a gastrointestinal tube is in place
- Assisting the client and family to cope with postoperative discomfort and with issues pertinent to chronic liver disease and its sequelae

When emergency shunt surgery is performed, there may be little time to complete preoperative teaching of appropriate information to the client and significant others. Present careful explanations postoperatively to compensate for the lack of preoperative teaching.

EVALUATION

Although shunt procedures may decrease the bleeding, the long-term prognosis for the client is poor. Severe encephalopathy often develops, followed by coma and death.

ASCITES

Etiology and Risk Factors

Ascites is the accumulation of fluid in the peritoneal cavity that results from the interaction of several pathophysiologic changes. Portal hypertension, lowered plasma colloidal osmotic pressure, and sodium retention all contribute to this condition. Disease processes that lead to these events include cirrhosis of the liver, right-sided heart failure, tuberculous peritonitis, cancer, and complications of pancreatitis.

Pathophysiology

Any process that blocks the flow of blood through the liver sinusoids to the hepatic veins and vena cava causes an increase in hydrostatic pressure in the portal venous system. Most commonly, this problem develops in cirrhosis of the liver or right-sided heart failure. As portal pressure increases, plasma leaks directly from the liver capsule and the congested portal vein into the peritoneal cavity. Congestion of lymph channels occurs, leading to the leakage of more plasma into the peritoneal cavity. Loss of plasma proteins into ascitic fluid from the portal venous system reduces oncotic pressure in the vascular compartment. Reduction in oncotic pressure limits the vascular system's ability to hold onto or collect water.

In addition, hepatocellular damage reduces the liver's ability to synthesize normal amounts of albumin. Decreased albumin synthesis leads to hypoalbuminemia, which is exacerbated by leakage of protein into the peritoneal cavity. The circulating blood volume decreases from loss of colloid osmotic pressure. The secretion of aldosterone increases to stimulate the kidneys to retain sodium and water. As a result of hepatocellular damage, the liver is unable to inactivate aldosterone. Thus, sodium and water retention continue. More fluid is held, and the volume of ascitic fluid grows.

Clinical Manifestations

Ascitic fluid typically produces abdominal distention, bulging flanks, and a downward-protruding umbilicus. Figure 47–5 depicts a client with ascites. Although large accumulations of ascitic fluid are obvious, small or moderate amounts may be more difficult to detect.

Diagnostic tests to confirm the presence of ascites include paracentesis, abdominal x-ray studies, ultrasonography, and computed tomography (CT) scan. These tests may locate fluid in the peritoneal cavity. Paracentesis provides samples of fluid for analysis. Findings help determine the underlying cause of the ascites; for example, the finding of malignant cells may indicate a tumor.

Outcome Management

Medical Management

Correct Fluid and Electrolyte Imbalance

Fluid and electrolyte balance is corrected by improving renal sodium excretion and restricting sodium and water intake. This involves discontinuing medications that inhibit prostaglandin synthesis and thus impair renal sodium excretion (e.g., aspirin, ibuprofen, indomethacin).

Paracentesis. Repeated large-volume paracentesis, in combination with IV administration of albumin to maintain plasma volume, is used to manage clients with ascites resulting from cirrhosis. However, repeated removal of fluid, protein, and electrolytes from the body causes severe disturbances in homeostasis. It is becoming more common to remove the least amount of fluid, such as 100 ml, sufficient to relieve manifestations such as shortness of breath. Clients must be monitored for rupture of the umbilicus.

Albumin. The physician may prescribe IV administration of albumin to replace each liter of ascitic fluid removed.

Diet Modifications. The diet is low in sodium with restriction of fluids. Protein intake is moderate unless the client has manifestations of hepatic encephalopathy.

Promote Effective Breathing Pattern

Edema in the form of ascites, besides compressing the liver and thus affecting its function, may also cause shallow breathing and impaired gas exchange, resulting in respiratory compromise. When ascites is present, potassium-sparing diuretics (e.g., spironolactone) are prescribed. Oxygen may be prescribed, and arterial blood gas analysis and pulse oximetry may be ordered. Semi-Fowler or high Fowler position, as well as daily or every-shift measurement of abdominal girth, is often prescribed.

Maintain Skin Integrity

When edema is present in liver disease, the client is at increased risk for development of skin impairment and possibly infected skin lesions. If jaundice is present, tepid water or emollient baths may be ordered, along with use of non-alkaline soaps and application of emollient lotions. If antihistamines are prescribed, observe for excessive sedation.

Nursing Management of the Medical Client

Assessment

Some simple assessments to perform at the bedside are the following:

- Percussion of the abdomen; if the client has ascites, the sound will be dull
- Measurement of circumference (abdominal girth)

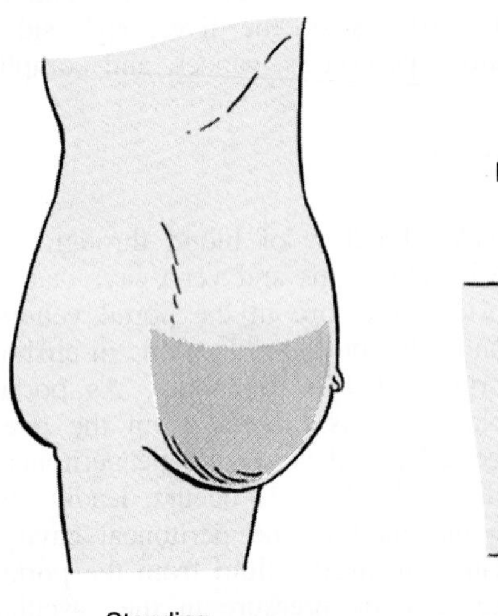

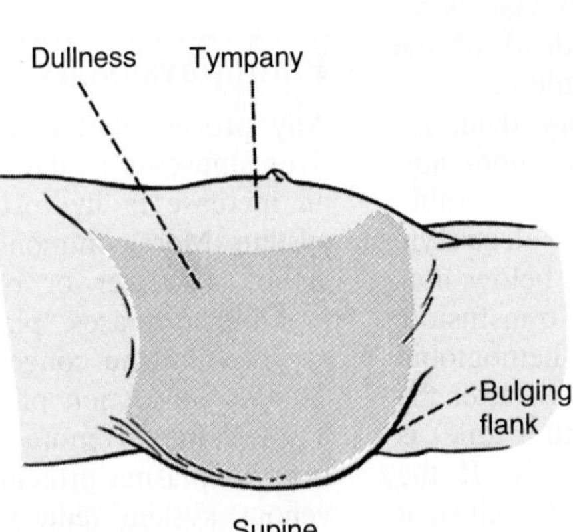

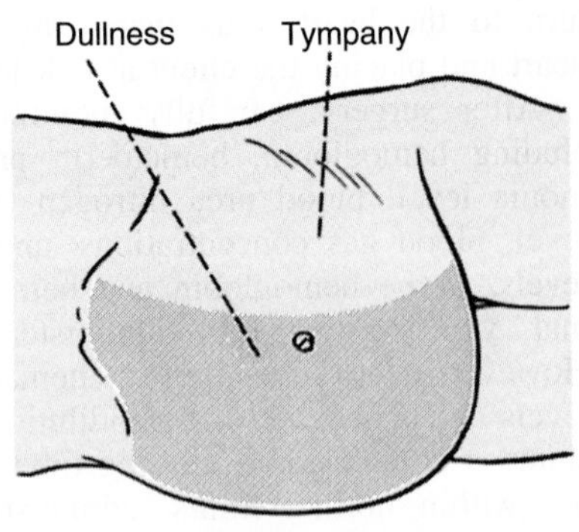

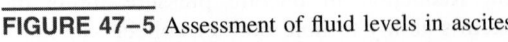

FIGURE 47–5 Assessment of fluid levels in ascites.

- Turning the client laterally and percussing the abdomen (see Fig. 47–5). Because ascitic fluid flows to the lowest point in the abdomen, it will move downward when the client turns; this causes a shift in the area where dullness is heard
- Tapping the abdomen to elicit a fluid wave

Assess the amount of distress caused by the ascites. Ask whether the fluid is interfering with sleeping, eating, and breathing. Assess for the presence of a hydrothorax or misplaced point of maximal impact (PMI). See the Care Plan on Management of the Client with Hepatic Failure.

DIAGNOSIS, OUTCOMES, INTERVENTIONS

Fluid Volume Excess and Fluid Volume Deficit. The client with ascites has a combination of volume problems leading to the nursing diagnoses *Fluid Volume Excess* and *Fluid Volume Deficit related to fluid shifts secondary to portal hypertension, hypoalbuminemia, and hyperaldosteronism.*

Outcomes. A normal balance of fluid between the intracellular and extracellular spaces will be maintained, as evidenced by absence of hypovolemia, normal serum albumin, decreased abdominal girth, and normal blood pressure.

Interventions

Restrict Fluids. The client's fluid restriction must be strictly followed. Give medications with meals, if possible, so that mealtime fluids can be used for taking medications.

Monitor Intake and Output. Measure abdominal girth daily (sometimes twice a day), and weigh the client daily. Monitor intake and output daily. Output should be equal to or exceed intake.

Administer Albumin and Diuretics. Administer albumin and diuretics as ordered. Give the albumin first to pull fluid back into the blood vessels. Give the diuretics second to promote excretion of the extra fluid. Assess the client for electrolyte imbalance and heart failure.

Avoid Hepatotoxins. Avoid adminstering aspirin and nonsteroidal anti-inflammatory drugs (NSAIDs), because they inhibit prostaglandin synthesis and, as noted previously, impair sodium excretion by the kidney.

Monitor after Paracentesis. Monitor the client closely after a paracentesis procedure. Check vital signs frequently to ensure that the client has tolerated the procedure well, and check the dressing carefully to ensure that excessive amounts of fluid are not lost. Sometimes a pouch is placed to collect leaking fluid. If too much fluid is lost, the physician may suture the site closed to prevent excess loss.

Ineffective Breathing Pattern. Ascites leads to many other problems. *Ineffective Breathing Pattern related to increased intra-abdominal pressure on the diaphragm* is a common nursing diagnosis in clients with ascites.

Outcomes. The client will not experience an ineffective breathing pattern, as evidenced by the absence of shortness of breath and the presence of normal respiratory excursion.

Interventions. Position the client in the high Fowler position to facilitate breathing, and monitor respiratory status for the development of atelectasis or pneumonia. Ask the client to cough and take a deep breath hourly to maintain adequate respiratory function. The client may need to use an incentive spirometer or receive ultrasound treatments if the cough does not loosen and bring up respiratory secretions.

Risk for Impaired Skin Integrity. In clients with ascites, severe edema as well as other problems may develop, leading to the nursing diagnosis *Risk for Impaired Skin Integrity related to immobility, edema, and pressure from the abdomen.*

Outcomes. The client will maintain skin integrity.

Interventions. Turn the client frequently, providing adequate support for the distended abdomen. If the client is on bed rest, recommend a specialty mattress used to prevent skin breakdown. Inspect the client's skin carefully daily, and apply lotions and creams as necessary. Keep the skin cool, and change soiled bed linens as soon as possible.

Altered Health Maintenance. Once the acute problems associated with ascites are controlled, the client and family members are faced with long-term control of the problem, often leading to the nursing diagnosis *Altered Health Maintenance related to lack of knowledge about ascites, treatment, and self-care.*

Outcomes. The client will understand ascites, its treatment, and self-care after discharge, as evidenced by the client's statements, compliance with the treatment regimen, and abstinence from alcohol.

Interventions. Help the client to understand ascites, its treatment, and self-care needs after discharge. Discuss the causes of ascites with the client, making sure that the client understands ways to slow the recurrence. Ensure that the client understands the need for dietary modifications, fluid restrictions, and home health care measures. Help the client to understand that all alcohol intake must be stopped. Refer the client to AA and other support groups for assistance with abstinence if necessary.

EVALUATION

The client's ascites may be controlled to an extent, but once cirrhosis is advanced, it is difficult to control. The optimal outcome is that the client will stop drinking, thereby preventing further liver damage.

Surgical Management

PERITONEOVENOUS SHUNT

The client with refractory and disabling chronic ascites may obtain relief from the insertion of a peritoneovenous (LeVeen or Denver) shunt.

INDICATIONS. Insertion of a peritoneovenous shunt may be indicated for clients whose ascites is not responding to medical management. As Figure 47–6 shows, a properly functioning shunt moves fluid from the peritoneal (abdominal) cavity into the superior vena cava. Resolution of ascites may be dramatic after implantation of a peritoneovenous shunt. The shunt contains a one-way valve that prevents back-flow of ascitic fluid.

CONTRAINDICATION. The main contraindication to placement of a peritoneovenous shunt is a state of health too poor for the client to withstand the trauma of surgery.

COMPLICATIONS. Complications of shunt implantation include infection, hemodilution, DIC, heart failure, and shunt clotting. For additional information, see the earlier discussion of surgical management of portal hypertension.

MANAGEMENT OF THE CLIENT WITH HEPATIC FAILURE

Nursing Diagnosis. Activity Intolerance related to fatigue, anemia from poor nutrition and bleeding, ascites, dyspnea from pressure of ascites on diaphragm, muscle wasting.

Outcomes. Client will feel rested, with fewer complaints of fatigue and increased tolerance for activity.

Interventions	Rationales
1. Alternate rest and activity.	1. Conserves energy and reduces demands on liver.
2. Monitor hemoglobin and hematocrit.	2. Allows detection of gastrointestinal bleeding.
3. Assist with activities of daily living (ADL).	3. Conserves energy and reduces demands on liver.
4. Administer iron supplements or blood transfusions as ordered to treat anemia.	4. Increases activity tolerance.
5. Assist with measures to decrease edema and ascites (see Fluid Volume Excess below).	5. Increases lung capacity.

Evaluation. Within a day after paracentesis or shunting surgery, the client will have decreased volume of ascitic fluid, tolerate activity better, perform more ADL, and experience less dyspnea and tachycardia. If ascitic fluid reaccumulates after paracentesis, the activity intolerance will return. Continued improvement will be seen after various shunting procedures. Blood transfusions will immediately improve hemoglobin and hematocrit levels, while iron replacement therapy will take longer to be effective.

Nursing Diagnosis. Altered Nutrition: Less than Body Requirements related to impaired utilization and storage of nutrients, increased pressure on stomach and intestines, feeling full, anorexia, nausea, loss of nutrients from vomiting.

Outcomes. Client will maintain or increase body weight to ideal weight and will consume adequate nutrients.

Interventions	Rationales
1. Weigh daily.	1. Monitors weight loss or gain
2. Provide oral hygiene before meals.	2. Improves taste of food.
3. Administer antiemetics as ordered.	3. Relieves nausea and vomiting.
4. Provide small, frequent meals.	4. Prevents feeling of fullness and ensures adequate nutritional intake.
5. Determine food preferences and assist in selection of those that contain low or no protein and/or low salt, as ordered.	5. Allows preferred foods, when possible, to encourage nutrition.
6. Prevent constipation.	6. Reduces abdominal pressure.

Evaluation. With interventions, the client will maintain weight (not fluid) or begin to gain weight by consuming adequate nutrients and following diet restrictions.

Nursing Diagnosis. Altered Protection related to decreased filtering of bacteria by liver and impaired synthesis of clotting factors.

Outcomes. Client will remain free of infection and will have no bruising or hemorrhage.

Interventions	Rationales
1. Monitor for manifestations of hemorrhage.	1. Decreased synthesis of clotting factors can lead to hemorrhage.
2. Provide assistance with ambulation and ADL.	2. Minimizes risk of trauma and injury.
3. Use small-gauge needles for injections and apply prolonged pressure after injection.	3. Minimizes risk of bleeding into tissues.
4. Recommend soft-bristle toothbrush.	4. Reduces injury to oral tissues.
5. Teach to avoid vigorous blowing of nose or straining at stool.	5. Reduces risk of hemorrhage.
6. Administer vitamin K as ordered.	6. Necessary for synthesis of clotting factors.
7. Follow infection control procedures.	7. Minimizes risk of infection.
8. Monitor for manifestations of infection (temperature, leukopenia).	8. Promotes identification and treatment of infection.

Evaluation. If interventions are successful, the client will not experience hemorrhage or infection.

Nursing Diagnosis. Confusion related to portal systemic encephalopathy occurring in conjunction with gastrointestinal bleeding and accumulation of ammonia in the bloodstream.

Outcomes. Client will be oriented to person, place, and time. Serum ammonia levels will not increase, and level of consciousness will not decrease.

Interventions	Rationales
1. Monitor for manifestations of encephalopathy such as disorientation, changes in handwriting or speech, or coma.	1. Liver is unable to convert ammonia to urea for excretion.
2. Encourage fluids (unless restricted).	2. Promotes excretion of ammonia and urea.
3. Give laxatives and enemas.	3. Decreases serum ammonia.
4. Provide low-protein diet.	4. Reduces generation of ammonia, which is a by-product of protein metabolism.

5. Limit activity.
6. Treat gastrointestinal bleeding as ordered.

5. Reduces generation of ammonia, a by-product of metabolism.
6. Reduces generation of ammonia, a by-product of bacterial action on blood.

Evaluation. Within 1 or 2 days of treatment, the client's serum ammonia levels will decrease and the client will become oriented to person, place, and time.

Nursing Diagnosis. Body Image Disturbance related to yellowing of skin and sclerae (jaundice), ascites, and edema.

Outcomes. Client will cope with body image disturbance; avoid isolation, and initiate or reestablish support systems.

Interventions

1. Assess client's response to changes in body.
2. Promote accepting and nonjudgmental attitude.
3. Listen and encourage ventilation of feelings.
4. Suggest clothing colors and options and make-up suggestions.

Rationales

1. Determines extent of body image disturbance.
2. Respects client's sensitivity to body image changes.
3. Helps client feel valued.
4. Enhances self-esteem.

Evaluation. Within 1 to 2 days of beginning treatment, some of the body changes will be corrected. Jaundice usually resolves in about 3 weeks. The volume of ascitic and edematous fluid can be reduced in a few days. Some degree of ascites and muscle wasting is irreversible, and the client will learn to accept the altered body image. In addition, it is expected that the client will maintain or establish new interpersonal relationships and activities.

Nursing Diagnosis. Fluid Volume Excess related to retention of fluids secondary to decreased serum albumin, increased sodium and water, portal hypertension, and possible shunting procedures causing hemodilution of blood.

Outcomes. Client will maintain a normovolemic state and adequate respirations and will have a decreased abdominal girth.

Interventions

1. Follow sodium and fluid restrictions.
2. Administer diuretics as ordered.
3. Weigh daily.
4. Measure abdominal girth every day or shift.
5. Monitor intake and output.
6. Monitor electrolytes, hemoglobin, and hematocrit.
7. Implement measures to prevent skin breakdown (see Impaired Skin Integrity below).
8. Administer albumin as ordered.
9. Assist with paracentesis procedure.

Rationales

1. Helps decrease ascites and edema.
2. Promotes excretion of fluid.
3. Evaluates treatment measures.
4. Evaluates treatment measures.
5. Evaluates treatment measures.
6. Diuretics may cause electrolyte imbalances; shunting may cause hemodilution.
7. Edema causes skin to break down faster.
8. Albumin pulls fluid into blood vessels, where the action of diuretics can remove the excess fluid.
9. Paracentesis removes a liter or more of fluid.

Evaluation. If some liver function is restored, the client will produce more albumin to promote return of fluid into blood vessels. Administration of albumin and diuretics will promote diuresis within hours, but repeated administration may be necessary because their effect is temporary. Paracentesis is a temporary solution; ascitic fluid will accumulate again if albumin levels remain low and portal hypertension is untreated.

Nursing Diagnosis. Ineffective Breathing Pattern related to pressure on diaphragm and reduced lung capacity secondary to ascites.

Outcomes. Client will breathe with minimal difficulty; there will be no manifestations of hypoxia.

Interventions

1. Place the client in the semi-Fowler or Fowler position with arms supported with pillows.
2. Assess for manifestations such as crackles or increased respirations.
3. Administer oxygen as needed.

Rationales

1. Relieves pressure on diaphragm.
2. Identifies fluid in lungs.
3. Improves gas exchange.

Evaluation. Treatment of ascites will enable the client to breathe with minimal difficulty.

Nursing Diagnosis. Impaired Skin Integrity related to pruritus (itching), edema, ascites, decreased mobility.

Outcomes. Client will maintain skin integrity and obtain relief from pruritus.

Interventions

1. Limit bathing to every 2–3 days, with sponge baths in between.
2. Use warm (95–100° F) rather than hot water.

Rationales

1. Keeps skin moist and minimizes itching.
2. Cool water minimizes vasodilation and itching.

Care Plan continued on following page

continued

3. Avoid alkaline soaps.	3. Soaps dry skin.
4. Apply emollients (mineral oil, lanolin, baby oil).	4. Emollients reduce evaporation and keep skin moist.
5. Use cool, light cotton clothing, which promotes evaporation.	5. Minimizes irritation and itching.
6. Keep clothing and bedding dry.	6. Minimizes itching.
7. Keep the environment cool (65–70° F).	7. Minimizes vasodilation and itching.
8. Avoid activities that promote sweating.	8. Minimizes vasodilation and itching.
9. Keep nails short and smooth.	9. Prevents breaking skin integrity when scratching.
10. Administer cholestyramine as ordered.	10. Combines with bile salts and promotes intestinal elimination to decrease itching.
11. Administer diphenhydramine hydrochloride (Benadryl) at night.	11. Antihistamine that has antipruritic and sedative effect; itching is worse at night.
12. Encourage diversional activities.	12. Decreases perception of itching and improves coping.
13. Encourage the client to avoid trauma.	13. May have impaired clotting activity, which will result in bruises with trauma.
14. Monitor manifestations.	14. Observes for changes that suggest improvement or worsening of condition.
15. Restrict sodium intake.	15. Prevents additional fluid retention.
16. Restrict fluids as ordered.	16. Reduces fluid retention.
17. Administer prescribed diuretics.	17. Reduces fluid retention and promotes diuresis.
18. Monitor intake and output.	18. Assesses renal function and fluid retention.
19. Weigh daily.	19. Assesses fluid retention.
20. Reposition every 2 hours.	20. Relieves pressure over bony prominences.
21. Use special mattress such as alternating air mattress or eggcrate mattress.	21. Reduces likelihood of skin breakdown.

Evaluation. After jaundice resolves in about 3 weeks, the client will have relief from pruritus, be able to sleep without interruption, and maintain skin integrity.

Nursing Management of the Surgical Client

Pre-and postoperative management of a client with ascites is similar to that of a client who has undergone surgery for portal hypertension and esophageal varices. See the discussion of nursing care of the client with surgical treatment of a hepatic problem.

HEPATIC ENCEPHALOPATHY

Etiology and Risk Factors

Hepatic encephalopathy constitutes a spectrum of CNS disturbances. These disturbances may appear in conjunction with severe liver injury or liver failure or after porto-

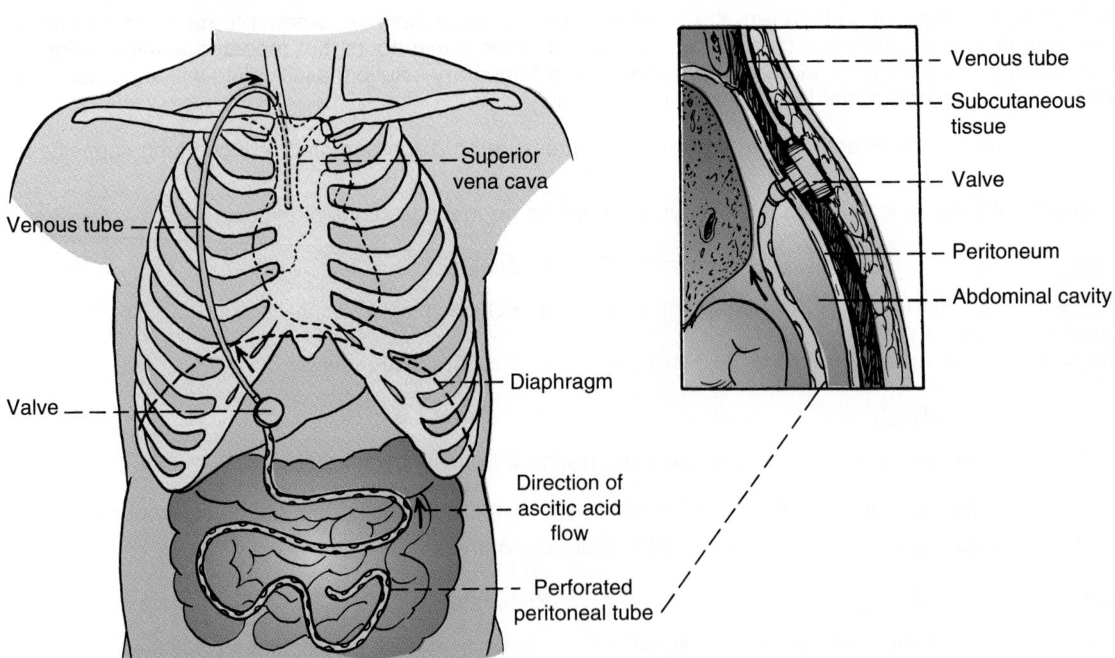

FIGURE 47–6 LeVeen peritoneovenous shunt for chronic ascites moves fluid from the peritoneal (abdominal) cavity into the superior vena cava.

BOX 47–2 Hepatic Encephalopathy: Causes or Precipitating Factors

- Decrease in hepatocellular function
- Hypoxia
- Infection
- Diuretics (produce hypokalemia, alkalosis, and hypovolemia)
- Depressants: (produce phenobarbital, narcotics, tranquilizers, and sedatives)
- Gastrointestinal bleeding
- Medications containing ammonium or amino compounds
- Paracentesis
- Increased protein intake
- Constipation
- Dehydration
- Hypokalemia
- Portosystemic and portacaval shunts

systemic shunt surgery. The cause of this disorder is the liver's inability to metabolize ammonia to form urea, so that it can be excreted. Ammonia is a CNS depressant. Changes during the initial stages of hepatic encephalopathy include reduced mental alertness, confusion, and restlessness. Loss of consciousness, seizures, and irreversible coma occur in the terminal stage.

Pathophysiology

The specific cause of hepatic encephalopathy is unknown, but it is characterized by elevations of ammonia levels in the blood and cerebrospinal fluid (CSF). Ammonia is produced in the gastrointestinal tract when protein is broken down by bacteria, by the liver, and, in lesser amounts, by gastric juices and peripheral tissue metabolism. The kidneys are another source of ammonia in the presence of hypokalemia. More recently implicated as a cause of encephalopathy are false neurotransmitters, elevated levels of mercaptans (organic chemicals that contain the sulfhydryl radical, formed when the oxygen of an alcohol molecule is replaced by sulfur), and fatty acids.

Normally, the liver converts ammonia into glutamine, which is stored in the liver and is later converted to urea and excreted through the kidneys. Blood ammonia rises when the liver cells are unable to perform this conversion. Failure of the liver to perform this function may be due to liver cell damage and necrosis. It also may result from the shunting of blood from the portal venous system directly into the systemic venous circulation (bypassing the liver). In either case, as blood ammonia levels rise, many unusual compounds begin to form. Some of these (e.g., octopamine) apparently act as false neurotransmitters in the CNS. Ammonia also is a CNS toxin, affecting glial and nerve cells; it leads to altered CNS metabolism and function.

Any process that increases protein in the intestine, such as increased dietary protein or gastrointestinal bleeding, causes elevated blood ammonia levels and possible manifestations of hepatic encephalopathy in clients with hepatocellular failure or who have undergone portosystemic shunt surgery (Box 47–2).

Clinical Manifestations

The manifestations of hepatic encephalopathy are primarily neurologic and range from mild mental confusion to deep coma. The neurologic changes occur with cerebral accumulation of ammonia or gastrointestinal bleeding. Hepatic encephalopathy impairs memory, attention, concentration, and rate of response. Sleep pattern reversal often occurs, with the client awake at night and sleepy during the day. Handwriting and speech show significant changes as intellectual deterioration occurs. Asterixis may be present. In some clients with hepatic encephalopathy, hyperventilation with respiratory alkalosis develops because high ammonia levels stimulate the respiratory center. The presence of methylmercaptan causes a characteristic odor on the breath called *fetor hepaticus.*

As the client's condition deteriorates, characteristic delta waves appear on the electroencephalogram (EEG). As the syndrome progresses, the client's level of consciousness slowly diminishes, and confusion becomes more severe. However, the level of CNS depression commonly fluctuates. Coma may eventually ensue, which deepens until there is no pain response and the reflexes, including the corneal reflex, are completely absent. Box 47–3 lists the stages of hepatic encephalopathy.

Laboratory results show elevated blood ammonia and CSF glutamine. Although these findings help to confirm the diagnosis of encephalopathy, they are not specific to it. Monitor serum ammonia levels, electrolytes, blood gases, and hepatic function test results (bilirubin, albumin, prothrombin, and enzymes) throughout the course. These

BOX 47–3 Stages of Hepatic Encephalopathy

Stage 1

Fatigue
Restlessness
Irritability
Decreased intellectual performance
Decreased attention span
Diminished short-term memory
Personality changes
Sleep pattern reversal

Stage 2

Deterioration in handwriting
Asterixis
Drowsiness
Confusion
Lethargy
Fetor hepaticus

Stage 3

Severe confusion
Inability to follow commands
Deep somnolence, but arousable

Stage 4

Coma
Unresponsive to painful stimuli
Possible decorticate or decerebrate posturing

findings help determine the degree of imbalance and the extent of hepatic injury (see Chapter 42).

Prognosis

Although intervention usually alleviates hepatic encephalopathy, the client may succumb to circulatory or respiratory complications, infection, or delirium and convulsions. Mortality is high among clients who progress into coma with hepatic failure. Health practitioners often use dramatic measures to reduce toxic levels of ammonia in the blood. Such measures include hemodialysis and exchange transfusions, which involve removal and replacement of approximately 80% of the client's blood. A liver transplant may be performed in cases of fulminant liver failure.

Outcome Management

Medical Management

IDENTIFY AND TREAT PRECIPITATING CAUSES

Factors that may precipitate or severely aggravate hepatic encephalopathy in clients with severe liver disease include gastrointestinal bleeding, increased dietary protein, constipation, infection, CNS-depressant drugs (e.g., opiates, benzodiazepines), and dehydration. Gastrointestinal bleeding and increased protein intake may lead to increased bacterial formation of nitrogenous compounds that induce encephalopathy. The use of CNS-depressant drugs should be avoided in these clients.

Protein may be totally eliminated from the diet, with an intake of only fruit juices and IV fluids, although this radical restriction leads to catabolism of the client's own protein stores. The usual protein restriction is 20 to 40 g/day. The client with chronic hepatic encephalopathy may need to adjust to a long-term, low-protein diet (50 to 60 g/day), which can be difficult. Vegetable and dairy protein may be better tolerated than meats. These proteins contain fewer ammonia-forming amino acids than those in meat. A diet high in vegetables and dairy products also helps prevent constipation, thus further reducing ammonia production.

REDUCE NITROGENOUS WASTE (AMMONIA) IN BLOOD AND BACTERIA IN COLON

Neomycin and lactulose are given to reduce bacteria in the intestinal tract. Because it is not absorbed into the circulation, neomycin exerts a powerful effect on the intestinal bacteria that are responsible for ammonia production. Undesirable side effects result from the depletion of intestinal flora (e.g., diarrhea, vitamin K deficiency). Also, because neomycin is nephrotoxic, its use must be avoided in clients with renal insufficiency. Lactulose, which helps decrease blood ammonia levels by reducing absorption of ammonia, is given to clients to produce two to four stools a day. Antibiotics are administered to inhibit growth of gastrointestinal bacteria, and oral magnesium sulfate or enemas are given after hemorrhage to clean out the intestines.

MAINTAIN FLUID VOLUME BALANCE

With the accumulation of fluid in the abdominal area (ascites), bleeding, and decreased fluid intake, the client may experience a fluid volume deficit. This deficit, along with electrolyte imbalances that may occur, should be corrected. IV fluids are administered, with the quantity and rate of administration carefully monitored.

Nursing Management of the Medical Client

ASSESSMENT

When working with a client susceptible to hepatic encephalopathy, use interviewing and assessment techniques to evaluate psychophysiologic status. For example, has the client's normally neat handwriting become sloppy and difficult to read? Is speech slow and slurred? Observe the client for personality changes with labile feeling states, and elicit liver flap or flapping tremor (asterixis) by asking the client to dorsiflex the hand with the rest of the arm resting on the bed. (In asterixis, the hand cannot be held steady.)

The nurse who is with the client over time is often the best person to assess a change in level of mental functioning. Early detection of a depressed or confused level of consciousness greatly improves the client's chances of recovery. To make nursing progress notes relevant, describe behavior vividly and objectively, as in "States pigeons are pecking at his bedclothes," rather than offering interpretations that may have a different meaning for each reader, such as "Seems more confused." As the client progresses into coma, make ongoing neurologic checks to determine the level of consciousness. See Unit 15 for neurologic assessment of comatose clients.

DIAGNOSIS, OUTCOMES, INTERVENTIONS

Risk for Ineffective Management of Therapeutic Regimen: Individuals and Risk for Ineffective Management of Therapeutic Regimen: Families. The client and family members are vital players in the control of encephalopathy. Thus, the nursing diagnoses *Risk for Ineffective Management of Therapeutic Regimen: Individuals,* and *Risk for Ineffective Management of Therapeutic Regimen: Families, related to reduction in protein in the diet and long-term pharmacologic intervention with neomycin* are common with hepatic encephalopathy.

Outcomes. The client will understand and comply with the reduction of protein in the diet and long-term pharmacologic intervention with neomycin, as evidenced by the client's following a low-protein diet and stating reasons why neomycin should be taken.

Interventions

Promote Low-Protein Diet. It is important that the client understand the importance of the reduced protein diet in order to have the motivation to remain on this diet.

Monitor for Gastrointestinal Hemorrhage. In addition to ensuring a low-protein diet, assess for manifestations of gastrointestinal bleeding, checking for bright red blood in the stool or for black, tarry stools. As previously noted, bleeding results in protein accumulation in the gastrointestinal tract, which exacerbates hepatic encephalopathy. To reverse the progression of manifestations, constipation must be prevented. Administer cathartics and enemas to hasten the exit of protein material from the intestine.

Encourage Bowel Cleansing. The client may need to learn to manage diarrhea, a possible side effect related to the laxative action of lactulose or neomycin sulfate. Intervention in severe hepatic encephalopathy commonly combines neomycin therapy with protein restriction and bowel cleansing. Administer the prescribed maintenance doses of neomycin and provide a low-protein diet for clients with chronic hepatic encephalopathy. In addition, administer oral lactulose, a combination of galactose and fructose that passes through the intestine unchanged, to decrease ammonia by trapping ammonium ions and allowing their evacuation from the bowel. As noted earlier, the appropriate lactulose dosage causes two to four soft stool evacuations daily. If severe diarrhea occurs, the dosage is reduced to prevent further electrolyte imbalance.

Fluid Volume Deficit. The client often has difficulties with fluid volume, leading to the nursing diagnosis *Fluid Volume Deficit related to bleeding, decreased intake, and ascites.*

Outcomes. The client will maintain a balanced fluid volume, as evidenced by normal blood pressure, absence of edema, absence of ascites, and balanced intake and output.

Interventions. Hypovolemia often precipitates hepatic encephalopathy by reducing hepatocellular perfusion. Fluid balance must be achieved, maintained, and monitored to prevent further hepatic injury and reduced renal perfusion. Deliver IV fluids evenly over time. Monitor vital signs frequently. If necessary, measure urine output hourly.

Electrolyte and acid-base disturbances such as hypokalemia and alkalosis may precipitate hepatic encephalopathy or may develop during its course. Laboratory tests indicate which replacement therapy is necessary.

Risk for Injury. Because of the multitude of problems faced by the client with encephalopathy, the nursing diagnosis *Risk for Injury related to loss of protective mechanisms secondary to hepatic coma* is common.

Outcomes. Injury or complications of immobility will be prevented or will be identified early, as evidenced by the absence of problems related to immobility.

Interventions. Hepatic coma may create a multitude of problems for the client with encephalopathy.

Prevent Hypoxemia. Hypoxemia may precipitate hepatic encephalopathy by damaging the hepatic cell. To prevent and treat hypoxemia, attend to respiratory interventions (e.g., maintain a patent airway).

Prevent Infection. Concurrent infection, with accumulation of protein from tissue catabolism, necessitates rapid intervention. The client is particularly vulnerable to nosocomial (hospital-acquired) infections. Wash your hands thoroughly, and take other measures to prevent cross-contamination.

Prevent Ammonia Toxicity and Hypokalemia. Be alert to possible harmful accumulations of ammonia due to diuretic therapy. Hypokalemia from the use of diuretics contributes to hepatic encephalopathy by increasing ammonia production in the kidney.

Avoid Sedation. Agents with CNS-depressant effects may precipitate coma, and their use should thus be avoided. If agitation occurs in early encephalopathy, administer agents that are excreted partially through the kidney, instead of the liver (e.g., phenobarbital). *Administer phenobarbital with caution!* Know which narcotics, tranquilizers, and sedatives are biotransformed by the liver; they are often contraindicated in clients with decreased hepatic function.

Prevent Complications of Immobility. The immobile client who lacks protective reflexes (blink or gag reflex) is vulnerable to numerous complications. Preventing complications requires intensive nursing intervention. Measures for intervention are discussed further in Chapter 68 on the care of the client in a coma. Prevent pneumonia and skin breakdown by turning the client frequently and promoting lung aeration.

As the body accumulates metabolic substances, physiologic disturbances develop that may produce a state of agitation. Therefore, protect the client from self-injury, for example, by lowering the bed and padding the side rails. See Chapter 68 for further discussion of the comatose client and the client with neurologic disturbances.

EVALUATION

The prognosis for the client with hepatic encephalopathy is poor. Generally, the best outcome that can be hoped for is maintenance with slowed deterioration.

Self-Care

As the acute stages of cirrhosis subside, the ongoing care of the client continues. If the care plan includes discharge from the hospital, provide extensive discharge teaching for the client with cirrhosis who has experienced complications. Family members and significant others need to know how to reduce the incidence of complications from cirrhosis. Review the potential complications with the caregivers as well as how to prevent and treat them.

MEDICATIONS

Review all medications, along with scheduled times of administration and their intended and adverse side effects. Potential medications include lactulose, diuretics, and vitamin supplements.

DIET MODIFICATIONS

Explain the importance of a well-balanced, nutritional diet to the client, with specific information about limitations on dietary protein, sodium, and water. Teach family members and significant others about the need to encourage eating and still maintain food intake within prescribed limits.

HOME MODIFICATIONS

Teach that the client's home may need to be altered to adjust for limitations in mobility. Safety precautions should be taken to help prevent injury to the client. The client's bedroom should be near the bathroom if the client is receiving diuretics.

FOLLOW-UP ASSESSMENTS

The client's status should be followed closely. Be sure that the client's caregivers are aware of any changes that require immediate medical attention. They should also know that diagnostic testing at regular intervals is continued to monitor the status of the liver.

FATTY LIVER (HEPATIC STENOSIS)

Lipid infiltration may lead to hepatic stenosis, or "fatty liver," one of the more common metabolic diseases of the liver. This pathologic process causes liver enlargement and increased firmness and may result in decreased function. Liver biopsy establishes the diagnosis. Laboratory studies reveal that triglyceride is the major lipid involved, but small amounts of cholesterol and phospholipid also may have infiltrated the liver.

Major causes of lipid infiltration include chronic alcoholism, protein malnutrition in early life, diabetes mellitus, obesity, Cushing's syndrome (natural or induced), jejunoileal bypass, prolonged IV hyperalimentation, chronic illnesses that involve impaired nutrition or malabsorption, some hepatotoxins (carbon tetrachloride and DDT [dichlorodiphenyltrichloroethane]), and Reye's syndrome in children.

The manifestations of fatty liver are related to the degree of fat infiltration, the amount of time fat has been accumulating, and the underlying cause. Clients with moderate to severe lipid infiltration are frequently asymptomatic. However, clients with massive infiltration experience anorexia, abdominal pain, and sometimes jaundice. Laboratory studies demonstrate elevated serum alkaline phosphatase and bilirubin levels.

Recovery begins after the source of the problem is removed and metabolic balance and adequate nutrition are restored. Residual damage, if it occurs, usually follows persistent fatty infiltration and chronic alcoholism. Fat embolization may occur and can cause death.

Nursing intervention for clients with fatty infiltration of the liver includes the following:

- Directing attention to correction of the cause (abstinence from alcohol, control of diabetes, weight loss, or correction of the intestinal absorptive defect)
- Preparing the client for diagnostic procedures
- Giving emotional support by allowing verbalization of concerns and fears
- Giving supportive physical care including adequate nutritional intake
- Designing teaching guidelines that promote proper diet and prevent a recurrence

LIVER NEOPLASMS

Tumors of the liver are either primary or metastatic. Primary liver tumors may arise from hepatocytes, connective tissue, blood vessels, or bile ducts. These tumors are either benign or malignant (Fig. 47–7). Figure 47–8 presents a classification of the primary liver neoplasms. Metastatic malignant tumors arise from the gastrointestinal tract (particularly the colon), the breasts, and the lungs.

BENIGN HEPATIC TUMORS

Hepatic adenomas are benign tumors of the liver occurring most commonly in women in their 20s and 30s. Nearly 90% of cases are associated with oral contraceptive use. The fact that the tumors occur more commonly in women, especially women who take oral contraceptives, suggests a hormonal influence in their pathogenesis.

Although these tumors are classified as benign, they are nevertheless dangerous because of their vascularity. A benign adenoma may rupture, with consequent hemorrhage. Diagnosis is made by a combination of tests including sonography, CT scanning, selective hepatic arteriography, and radionuclide scanning. Liver biopsy is not warranted because the tumors are hypervascular.

Intervention for benign adenoma depends on its cause. Discontinuation of oral contraceptives or androgens, when a tumor appears to be hormone-dependent, may correct the condition. Otherwise, treatment may include surgical excision of the involved liver segment. If acute hemorrhage calls for surgery, the surgeon may perform a hepatic lobectomy. Benign hepatic tumors are associated with an excellent prognosis if they can be removed surgically before they rupture and cause death from hemorrhage.

MALIGNANT HEPATIC TUMORS

PRIMARY HEPATOCELLULAR CANCER

Primary hepatocellular cancer (malignant hepatoma) is one of the most common tumors worldwide. It is four times more common in men than in women. About 15,300 new cases of liver cancer were expected in the United States in 2000, which represents a 71% increase from the mid-1970s.[1, 2] Etiologic factors that may contribute to hepatoma are hepatitis B, hepatitis C, cirrhosis,

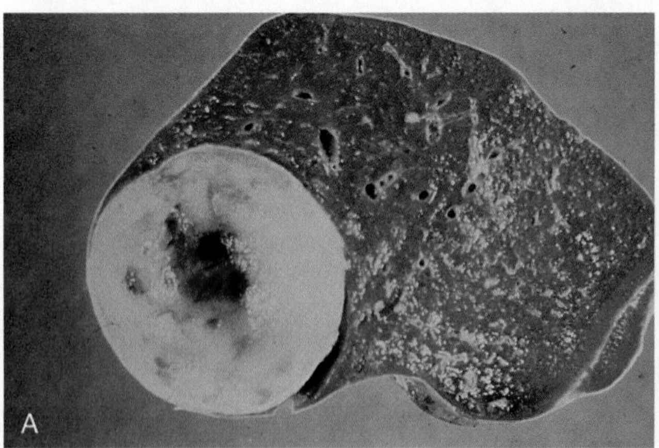

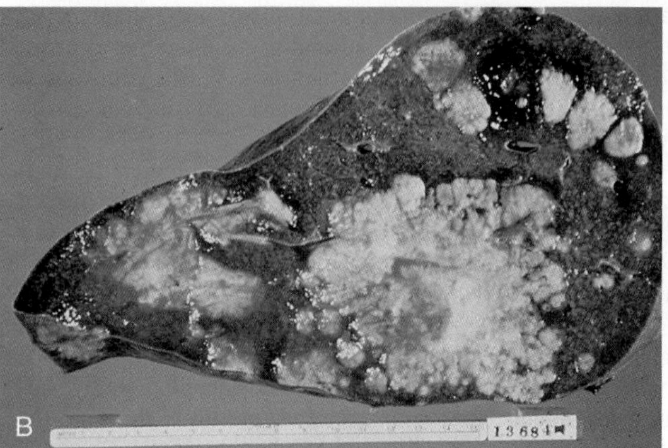

FIGURE 47–7 Benign liver tumor *(A)* and metastatic malignant liver tumor *(B)*.

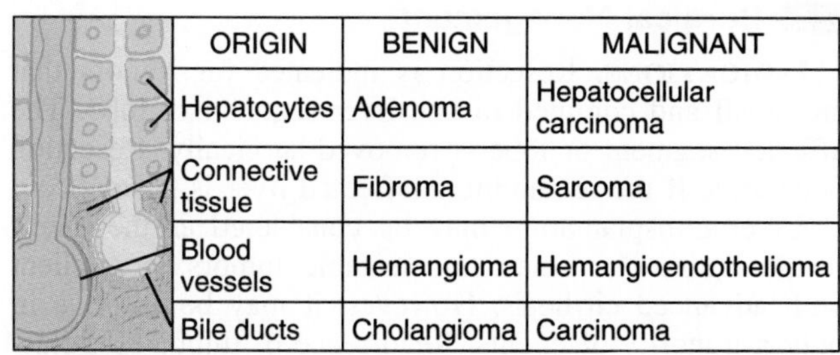

ORIGIN	BENIGN	MALIGNANT
Hepatocytes	Adenoma	Hepatocellular carcinoma
Connective tissue	Fibroma	Sarcoma
Blood vessels	Hemangioma	Hemangioendothelioma
Bile ducts	Cholangioma	Carcinoma

FIGURE 47–8 Classification of primary liver neoplasms.

chronic liver disease, hemochromatosis, ingestion of certain mycotoxins (aflatoxins), anabolic steroid use, and long-term androgen therapy. Primary hepatocellular carcinoma is the main cause of death from cancer in many areas of the world, including sub-Saharan Africa and parts of Asia.

After the diagnosis of liver cancer and if intervention fails to terminate the neoplastic process, the client usually dies of hepatic failure within 3 to 6 months. Surgical resection of the tumor is the only method of cure and may be attempted if the tumor is confined to one lobe. Many clients, however, do not have a resectable tumor because of underlying cirrhosis and involvement of both lobes.

METASTATIC HEPATIC CANCERS

The liver is one of the common sites of metastasis for all cancers. In the United States, metastatic cancers of the liver are 20 times more common than primary liver tumors.

Etiology and Risk Factors

The liver is a common site of metastasis because of the liver's high rate of blood flow, its size, and portal venous drainage from the major abdominal organs. Tumors of the gastrointestinal tract, lung, and breast metastasize to the liver more frequently than do tumors of the prostate or thyroid.

Pathophysiology

Metastatic cancers spread to the liver in three ways: by direct extension from adjacent organs (stomach and gallbladder), via the hepatic arterial system, or via the portal venous system. Also, as a result of cell migration, the surface of the liver may become seeded with metastatic cells.

Clinical Manifestations

Clients with primary (benign and malignant) and secondary (metastatic) tumors often present with similar manifestations. Early indicators of liver neoplasm are usually vague. Many clients with metastatic malignancy of the liver present with the following three types of manifestations:

- Manifestations that are specific only to the primary tumor, hepatic involvement being discovered incidentally in the course of a diagnostic evaluation
- Nonspecific manifestations of anorexia, diaphoresis, fever, weight loss, and weakness
- Manifestations of active liver disease, such as abdominal pain, ascites, and hepatomegaly

Diagnostic studies and physical examination may reveal the following: elevated alkaline phosphatase, hepatomegaly, a liver mass, a friction rub or bruit over the liver, angiographic evidence of neoplasm hypoproteinemia, blood-tinged ascitic fluid, decreased liver function, and reversal of the albumin-globulin (A/G) ratio. The A/G ratio is a calculation of the distribution of two major protein fractions, albumin and globulin. The value of the A/G ratio is >1.0, albumin divided by globulin ($A \div G$). A high ratio is considered insignificant. However, a low ratio occurs in liver and renal diseases.

Some clients also may have metabolic derangements such as in polycythemia, blood glucose disorders, and high levels of calcium. Other clients may present with marked leukocytosis and anemia. Jaundice occurs more often when a bile duct is the site of a primary tumor or when the tumor mass obstructs a major outflow duct. Other manifestations may be present, depending on the concurrent pathologic condition. At times, the tumor process causes elevation of the diaphragm and some respiratory problems.

Although neoplasms of the liver create numerous clinical manifestations, many pathologic features may not appear until the tumors have grown quite large. Malignant tumor cells may have replaced as much as 90% of normal liver tissue before liver insufficiency becomes clinically evident.

In primary hepatocellular cancers, diagnostic tests often reveal high levels of alpha-fetoprotein (AFP). This substance is sometimes present in clients who have metastatic tumors, but levels rarely reach those found in clients with primary tumors.

A diagnosis of liver cancer is suggested by an elevated serum alkaline phosphatase level and by abnormal findings on ultrasonography, CT, liver scanning, or magnetic resonance imaging (MRI). Cytologic examination of aspirated fluid can also be used to establish the diagnosis.

Liver biopsy is very helpful in establishing the diagnosis. The route of access may be percutaneous, direct via laparotomy, or through a peritoneoscope. Each method has its limitations. Percutaneous procedures may cause seeding of tumor cells along the biopsy needle pathway as it is withdrawn. Laparotomy requires anesthesia, which may be too dangerous. Peritoneoscopy may be impossible if there are extensive adhesions. Because all of these biopsy procedures require internal membrane puncture, be sure the client has an acceptable prothrombin time (PT) because of the risk of hemorrhage if the time is too prolonged.

Prognosis

Because hepatic tumors may be far advanced before clinical manifestations or laboratory data indicate their presence, and because severe liver disease (e.g., cirrhosis) frequently coexists, liver cancer carries a poor prognosis. In the United States, median survival from the time of diagnosis is about 6 months.

Outcome Management

Medical Management

Relief of Manifestations and Promotion of Palliation

As noted previously, treatment of liver cancer is aimed at relieving manifestations and supporting the client physically and emotionally. The treatment options for medical management include chemotherapy, radiation therapy, and other approaches such as cryoablation.

Chemotherapy. Regional perfusion of the liver with infusions given directly into the hepatic artery to relieve pain or slow tumor growth may be useful and may produce fewer side effects than those incurred with systemic chemotherapy. Various chemotherapeutic agents have been used singly or in combination with other agents infused into the hepatic artery, or have been given by regional infusion with other agents given systemically.

During surgery, the surgeon may implant a chemotherapy infusion pump. Such pumps, filled percutaneously, deliver medication continuously into the hepatic artery. With metastatic growths, the oncologist may prescribe systemic chemotherapy to reduce tumor size and pain.

Chemotherapeutic agents used to induce regression of primary and metastatic tumors of the liver include 5-fluorouracil (5-FU) and doxorubicin. (Adriamycin) for single-dose therapy and 5-FU with carmustine (BCNU), semustine (methyl CCNU), or streptozocin for combination therapy.

Radiation Therapy. Radiation therapy has produced disappointing results. Irradiation of liver tumors may provide temporary pain relief but does not promote survival.

Other Approaches. Some of the other approaches that have been used for treatment of primary hepatic tumor include alcohol ablation via ultrasound-guided percutaneous injection, ultrasound-guided cryoablation, and gene therapy with retroviral vectors containing genes that express cytotoxic agents. Biliary drainage achieved percutaneously or through an internal stent placed surgically helps increase the passage of bile into the duodenum, decreasing jaundice and discomfort.

Nursing Management of the Medical Client

Nursing diagnoses and interventions for clients with liver neoplasms vary according to the amount of liver dysfunction and the treatment modalities. Plan to assess the client for metabolic malfunctions, pain, bleeding problems, ascites, edema, inability to biotransform endogenous and exogenous (drug) wastes, hypoproteinemia, jaundice, and endocrine complications.

Take time to prepare the client in the diagnostic stage for the various procedures, and assess carefully for post-procedure complications. If pain is a problem, administer medication at the prescribed time and dosage. In addition, assist the client and family members to gain knowledge about the condition and offer support necessary for them to cope with the uncertainty and fear associated with cancer. See Chapters 18 and 19 for detailed discussions of nursing care of clients with malignant tumors. See also the Care Plan on Management of the Client with Hepatic Failure.

Surgical Management

Indications. Resection is indicated for tumors that are small and confined to one liver segment or lobe. The affected segment or lobe is removed surgically. Resection is curative if the remaining unaffected liver is normal.

Liver transplantation may be considered as the therapeutic option for small unresectable tumors in a client with advanced cirrhosis. However, it may be curative in only a minority of clients. Recurrence of tumor or metastasis after transplantation has limited its usefulness.

Contraindications. The client may not be able to withstand the stress of surgery. An additional contraindication to surgery is the presence of liver disease too extensive for surgery to be beneficial.

Complications. Tumor rupture, gastrointestinal hemorrhage from varices, progressive cachexia, and hepatic failure are the primary complications of hepatic tumors. Management of the client with these complications is supportive and palliative and will vary according to the client's overall condition, degree of liver impairment, and extent of surgery.

Outcomes. Prognosis is poor. Most clients with hepatic carcinoma have a median survival time of 3 to 6 months.

Nursing Management of the Surgical Client

Nursing management of the client preoperatively and postoperatively includes many responsibilities. See the discussion of nursing management of the client who has undergone surgery for complications of portal hypertension, earlier in the chapter.

LIVER TRANSPLANTATION

Surgical Management

Liver transplantation is now considered a feasible form of intervention for a variety of end-stage liver diseases. The number of liver transplants has continued to grow each year. In 1995, more than 3700 people in the United States received liver transplants. The demand for livers for transplantation continues to outpace availability. As many as 6000 clients in the United States remain on a donor liver waiting list.

The duration of the surgical procedure is generally 8 hours but can be from 6 to 18 hours. The surgery may be *orthotopic,* involving removal of the diseased liver and insertion of the donor liver. Anastomoses of the vena cava, portal vein, hepatic artery, and bile duct are performed. In the *heterotopic* approach, the diseased liver is left in and the transplanted liver is inserted alongside. Orthotopic surgery is by far the more common of the two. Because excessive bleeding may occur, large amounts of blood, blood products, and volume expanders are needed.

Indications. The most appropriate candidates for liver transplant are people who, in the absence of contraindications, have severe, irreversible liver disease for which alternative medical or surgical treatments have not been successful or are not available. Ideally, transplantation should be considered in clients with end-stage liver disease who are experiencing life-threatening complications of liver dysfunction, whose quality of life has increasingly deteriorated, or who are predicted to experience neurologic effects of liver damage. If the surgery is performed sufficiently early, contraindications and extrahepatic deterioration are less likely.[12]

Some of the most common conditions warranting transplantation are as follows:

- Primary and secondary biliary cirrhosis (adult)
- Hepatitis—chronic with cirrhosis, chronic viral or fulminant (usually adult)
- Primary sclerosing cholangitis (adult)
- Biliary atresia (pediatric)
- $Alpha_1$-antitrypsin deficiency (usually pediatric)
- Confined hepatic malignancy (adult or pediatric)
- Wilson's disease
- Budd-Chiari syndrome (hepatic vein obstruction)
- Alcoholic cirrhosis

Choosing clients with alcoholic cirrhosis, chronic viral hepatitis, and primary hepatocellular malignancies as liver transplant recipients may be questionable. Clients with any one of these conditions are considered to be high-risk surgical candidates, but liver transplantation may be offered to carefully selected individuals. The alcoholic client, for example, must be willing to adhere to certain guidelines such as abstinence and a substance abuse treatment program in order to be eligible for the procedure. The client must be psychologically stable and have good support systems for the complex postoperative course.

CONTRAINDICATIONS. Contraindications include (1) life-threatening systemic diseases; (2) uncontrolled extrahepatic bacterial or fungal infections; (3) pre-existing advanced cardiovascular or pulmonary disease; (4) multiple, uncorrectable, life-threatening congenital anomalies; (5) metastatic malignancy; (6) active alcoholism or drug abuse; (7) cholangiocarcinoma; and (8) human immunodeficiency virus (HIV) infection. See Chapter 80 for other contraindications to transplantation.

COMPLICATIONS. Postoperative complications can be *hepatic* and *nonhepatic.* They may include cardiovascular and pulmonary problems as well as infection, rejection, hemorrhage, atelectasis, failure of anastomosis, and acute renal failure. Rejection occurs most commonly between postoperative days 4 and 10. Manifestations of acute rejection include fever, tachycardia, right upper quadrant or flank pain, and increasing jaundice. Drugs including azathioprine, cyclosporine, FK506, OKT3, and steroids such as prednisone and methylprednisolone are used to stop or prevent rejection; otherwise, liver function rapidly deteriorates. Chapter 80 describes management of clients undergoing transplantation.

OUTCOMES. It is expected that the client will recover from the liver transplant surgery, be discharged from the hospital in 1 week, and within 3 to 4 months be able to resume a normal life as long as medication and health care regimens are followed closely. Complications such as rejection and infection will slow the progress of affected clients.

The survival rate after liver transplantation has improved steadily since 1983, approximately 70% in the early 1980s to 80% to 90% in the mid-1990s. The 5-year survival rate is about 60%. Survival rate is higher and quality of life better after transplantation in people who had less hepatic damage before surgery and in those who had fewer extrahepatic manifestations.

Nursing Management of the Surgical Client

PREOPERATIVE CARE

Once the client has chosen transplantation as an alternative to care and is placed on the recipient waiting list, an extensive physical and psychological evaluation is required (see Chapter 80). The client must undergo a variety of tests, including blood analysis, hepatic angiogram, abdominal CT scan, chest and hip x-ray studies, electrocardiogram (ECG), bone density studies, and nutritional assessment. The client may also have the opportunity to meet the transplant team. Matching donor and recipient organ size and blood and tissue type are important considerations in donor selection.

Focus on assessing the client's needs in relation to the amount of knowledge and information he or she has. Ascertain how the client and family members are coping with the situation. In addition, the needs dictated by the extent of organ failure will guide care. The specific nursing care needs of clients during the waiting period for a liver transplant depend on the degree of end-stage liver disease.

POSTOPERATIVE CARE

The major focus of care is to monitor for rejection, infection, and occlusion of vessels. Immunosuppressive therapy, which is started before surgery, must be continued on a regular schedule postoperatively to prevent rejection of the new liver. The client requires constant monitoring of respiratory, cardiovascular, neurologic, and hemodynamic status. Liver function is monitored through assessment of serum transaminases (ALT, AST), bilirubin, albumin, and clotting factors. Monitor fluid and electrolyte status, serum glucose, and pH. Clients are always somewhat fluid-overloaded from receiving extensive volumes of blood products during the long surgical procedure. This overload can lead to pulmonary edema and heart failure. Serum potassium will be decreased as a result of transplantation, and serum glucose will be increased. The serum pH will be normal to acidic.

Monitor wound drains and bile drains for patency, and note bile characteristics (amount, color, consistency). Obstruction of wound drains causes increased intra-abdominal pressure from accumulation of ascitic fluid and blood. Obstruction of bile flow can cause damage to the liver and biliary system.

Assess the needs of family members and significant others, who may have traveled long distances from home and may be feeling powerless, stressed, and anxious. Much of the care and many of the nursing diagnoses for a client who undergoes liver transplantation are the same as for a client after any other type of surgery. See Chapter 80 for care of the client after transplantation.

LIVER ABSCESS

A liver abscess is a localized collection of pus and organisms within the parenchyma of the liver. Liver abscess usually develops in association with one of the following three conditions:

- *Bacterial cholangitis,* which results from obstruction of the bile ducts by stone or stricture
- *Portal vein bacteremia,* which may develop following bowel inflammation or organ perforation
- *Amebiasis* (infestation with amebae from tropical or subtropical areas)

Other predisposing factors are diabetes mellitus, infected hepatic cysts, metastatic liver tumors with secondary infection, and diverticulitis.

The client commonly reports right upper quadrant pain and abdominal and right shoulder pain. Assessment may also reveal liver enlargement, tenderness, nausea, vomiting, weight loss, anorexia, fever, and diaphoresis. Sometimes a right pleural effusion may develop. The liver's proximity to the base of the right lung contributes to this process.

Liver scanning is extremely valuable in diagnosis. Other useful diagnostic modalities include ultrasonography, CT, and arteriography. Laboratory data reflect slight to marked elevations of aminotransferases, alkaline phosphatase, and bilirubin. High levels indicate the presence of concurrent obstruction. Blood culture yields positive results in some cases.

Intervention in hepatic abscess consists of (1) percutaneous drainage of the abscess with antimicrobial therapy, (2) surgical drainage of large abscesses with postoperative antimicrobial therapy, or (3) antimicrobial therapy without drainage for a few months. Abscesses due to amebic infestation (such as by *Entamoeba histolytica*) call for treatment with metronidazole (Flagyl) or chloroquine phosphate (Aralen phosphate) instead of broad-spectrum antibiotics. Early diagnosis and therapy for uncomplicated amebic liver abscess result in less than 1% mortality.

When caring for the client with liver abscess, assess vital signs regularly. High temperature and rapid pulse may indicate the presence of general sepsis, a likely complication. Encourage movement, coughing, and deep breathing to prevent or limit pulmonary complications related to hepatic abscess. Increase the client's fluid intake and provide skin care in the event of hyperpyrexia. Dispose of feces carefully, and wash your hands to prevent transmission of amebic infestations.

HEMOCHROMATOSIS

Hemochromatosis is an uncommon disorder of iron metabolism that is often associated with portal hypertension and hepatomegaly. It affects men more often than women. *Primary* hemochromatosis, a recessive inherited metabolic defect, causes increased iron absorption from the gastrointestinal tract. *Secondary* hemochromatosis is caused by alcoholism, excessive dietary intake of iron, or conditions in which repeated blood transfusions have been required, such as chronic anemias.

Total body iron in most clients ranges from 2 to 5 g. Clients with hemochromatosis often have levels of 20 g or higher. The excess iron travels to parenchymal cells, where it is deposited as ferritin (form in which iron is stored in the liver) or hemosiderin (an iron-containing pigment derived from hemoglobin breakdown and one way iron is stored until needed for hemoglobin synthesis). The liver and pancreas are most at risk for iron deposition and its untoward effects. The heart, spleen, kidney, and skin undergo less damage. As these organs become fibrotic in response to iron deposition, loss of function occurs. As a result, the more common problems associated with hemochromatosis include diabetes, enlarged liver, cirrhosis, cardiac disease, increased skin pigmentation, and arthritis. Pseudogout, a form of arthritis in which calcium phosphate crystals accumulate in large joints, is also associated with hemochromatosis. It is often the arthritis that prompts clients to seek medical attention.

Diagnosis depends on the presence of (1) elevated plasma iron levels (>150 mg/ml), (2) more than 60% saturation of iron-binding protein (transferrin), and (3) manifestations of specific organ dysfunction. Liver biopsy provides the definitive diagnosis.

Intervention involves phlebotomy (a surgical opening of a vein to withdraw blood) performed on a biweekly or weekly basis over a 1- or 2-year period (2 ml of blood = 1 mg of iron). Once the excess iron has been removed from the body, two or three maintenance phlebotomies per year keep the level of body iron normal. If hemochromatosis is diagnosed before cirrhosis develops, phlebotomy can reverse or prevent all of the manifestations except arthropathy and hepatocellular carcinoma. Desferrioxamine mesylate, a chelating agent, also facilitates the removal of iron from the body.

AMYLOIDOSIS

Amyloid is a proteinaceous, starch-like substance that can infiltrate the liver and other organs. Accumulation of amyloid deposits causes tissues to cease functioning. Clinicians classify amyloidosis according to the type of protein that forms the amyloid deposits. In the most common form of amyloidosis (*primary*), light-chain amyloid formed from immunoglobins is deposited. This abnormal protein material causes the most damage to tissues of cardiac, smooth muscle, skin, kidney, and liver origin. However, light-chain amyloid can accumulate in every organ or system except the CNS.

Amyloidosis due to deposition of protein A is associated with chronic inflammation in conditions such as tuberculosis, rheumatoid arthritis, osteomyelitis, and bronchiectasis. Tissues most disturbed by this type of amyloidosis include those of the spleen, kidney, and liver. Although many organs may be affected, the liver incurs the greatest damage. Assessment reveals that hepatomegaly is the most noticeable effect of this pathologic process. Liver function remains relatively unaffected. Clinical jaundice rarely appears. Liver biopsy provides excellent diagnostic data, but there is a high incidence of post-biopsy hemorrhage or liver rupture.

Chemotherapy may be prescribed to provide symptomatic relief of inflammation and pain for the client with light-chain amyloidosis.

CONGENITAL CONDITIONS

Three congenital conditions affecting the liver are Wilson's disease, Caroli's syndrome, and congenital hepatic fibrosis.

Wilson's Disease

Wilson's disease leads to an accumulation of copper in the tissue of the liver, brain, and kidney. The primary manifestations of this disorder are abnormal liver function and neurologic changes. Hepatic manifestations may occur from early childhood to adulthood. This disease is usually chronic but also may be acute. The acute form is often fatal unless transplantation can be performed. One of the hallmarks of this disease is the presence of Kayser-Fleischer rings encircling the corneas. These greenish-yellow–pigmented rings are due to copper deposits. Copper deposits also can be seen on liver biopsy. Penicillamine is the drug of choice to treat this problem.

Caroli's Syndrome

Caroli's syndrome is characterized by dilated bile ducts and cyst formations. The condition may be localized or widespread. Clinical manifestations usually present soon after birth, but the syndrome may not be diagnosed until early adulthood. Fever and bacterial cholangitis are usually the two manifestations that lead to diagnosis. Other manifestations may include right upper quadrant pain and jaundice, both of which may be caused by obstruction of the biliary tract by one or more cysts or stones. Treatment consists of antibiotics, external biliary drainage, or even liver transplantation.

Congenital Hepatic Fibrosis

Congenital hepatic fibrosis is characterized by portal hypertension caused by portal vein fibrosis. It usually presents as upper gastrointestinal bleeding from gastric or esophageal varices. Treatment ranges from blood transfusions and sclerotherapy to portacaval shunting.

LIVER TRAUMA

Liver injury usually results from a penetrating injury or blunt trauma. Either may lead to laceration and hemorrhage. Penetrating injuries are usually knife or missile (gunshot) wounds. A knife wound generally is superficial and leaves a sharp clear edge, whereas missile wounds cause perforations through the liver tissue, that is, the entrance and exit points. The greater the velocity of the missile, the greater the damage. Often, a close-range missile injury is fatal because of the large amount of damage. Blunt trauma (e.g., from a steering wheel or a fall) can have various effects, ranging from small hematomas that remain under the liver capsule to large, star-like lacerations from severe impact forces.

Management of liver injuries consists of control of the hemorrhage, debridement, and drainage. Surgical resection of liver lobes may be necessary, but more often the major goal of surgical intervention is to control hemorrhage. Monitor victims of trauma carefully for falling blood pressure and tachycardia, which may indicate hemorrhage. The problem is more difficult when the liver's blood vessels or bile ducts are damaged as well. Later complications include bile peritonitis and abscess formation.

CONCLUSIONS

Hepatic disorders are complex and difficult for all involved. You should have a thorough understanding of the liver and its functions to care for these clients. Many hepatic disorders are the result of the client's lifestyle, further complicating an already difficult problem. The nurse must therefore consider both the physiologic and psychosocial problems associated with many hepatic disorders. Helping the client make appropriate lifestyle changes is an important nursing function.

THINKING CRITICALLY

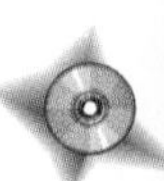

1. **A 37-year-old man is admitted to the hospital with a 10-day history of anorexia, fatigue, malaise, low-grade fever, dark urine, and upper abdominal discomfort. There is no history of jaundice, IV drug use, or blood transfusions. He is homosexual. Alcohol intake consists of several mixed drinks nightly and wine with dinner. Findings on physical examination include temperature of 99.6° F, jaundice, blood pressure of 150/80 mm Hg, and no spider nevi. The liver measures 12 cm in the midclavicular line and is moderately tender. The spleen is not palpable. Initial laboratory data: total bilirubin, 6.8 mg/dl (normal, 0.2 to 1.2 mg/dl); alkaline phosphatase, 240 units (U)/L (normal, 20 to 90 U/L); AST, 980 U/L (normal, 5 to 40); ALT, 1200 U/L (normal, 5 to 35 U/L). The WBC count is 5600/mm^3, with a normal differential count. What are the priorities for care in this situation? What interventions might be used?**

Factors to Consider. Without further data, what would appear to be the major organ systems involved? What additional information do you, as his nurse, think it is necessary to obtain? If you are caring for this client and you inadvertently sustain a needle-stick from a syringe used to give an injection to this client, what action would you take?

2. **A 48-year-old man arrives in the emergency department. He felt well until 2 hours previously, when he became nauseated and subsequently vomited a large amount of red blood and clots. He reports a long history of heavy alcohol use and cigarette smoking. He takes no medications. Laboratory data: hemoglobin, 9.6 g/dl; hematocrit, 28.4%; platelet count, 92,000/mm^3; prothrombin time, 16.5 seconds (normal, 11 to 15); alkaline phosphatase, 120 U/L (normal, 20 to 90); AST, 265 U/L; ALT, 112 U/L. What is likely to be a major underlying cause of this client's problem? Is it reversible? Can further damage be stopped? With the client vomiting blood, what should your priority interventions be?**

Factors to Consider. What gastrointestinal disorders can be manifested in people who consume large quantities of alcohol? What risks does the client face in the present situation?

3. Your client is a 68-year-old man with cirrhosis. He is admitted for treatment of ascites and acute upper right abdominal pain. His abdomen is very large, and the ascitic fluid shifts from side to side whenever he moves. Diagnostic studies reveal that the cause of his pain is cholelithiasis, and surgery is scheduled. What are the client's priority needs on admission? What complications might he face following surgery?

Factors to Consider. What are the clinical manifestations of cirrhosis? Is the client with cirrhosis a good candidate for abdominal surgery?

BIBLIOGRAPHY

1. Alexander, I. M. (1998). Viral hepatitis: Primary care diagnosis and management. *American Journal of Primary Care Health, 23*(10), 13–20.
2. American Cancer Society. (2000). *Cancer facts and figures.* Atlanta: Author.
3. Bass, N. M. (1996). Toxic and drug-induced liver disease. In J. C. Bennett & F. Plum (Eds.), *Cecil textbook of medicine* (20th ed., pp. 772–776). Philadelphia: W. B. Saunders.
4. Burke, W., et al. (1998). Hereditary hemochromatosis. *Journal of the American Medical Association, 280*(2), 172–178.
5. Caregaro, L., et al. (1996). Malnutrition in alcoholic and virus-related cirrhosis. *American Journal of Clinical Nutrition, 63*(4), 602–609.
6. Chappell, S. M. (1997). Anxiety in liver transplant patients. *MEDSURG Nursing, 6*(2), 98–103.
7. Dienstag, J. (1998). Liver transplantation. In A. S. Fauci, et al. (Eds.), *Harrison's principles of internal medicine* (14th ed.). New York: McGraw-Hill.
8. Feldman, M., Scharschmidt, B.F., & Sleisenger, M. H. (Eds.) (1998). *Sleisenger and Fordtran's gastrointestinal and liver disease: Pathophysiology, diagnosis, management* (6th ed., pp. 1721–1725). Philadelphia: W. B. Saunders.
9. Friedman, L. S. (1996). Cirrhosis of the liver and its major sequelae. In J. C. Bennett & F. Plum (Eds.), *Cecil textbook of medicine* (20th ed., pp. 788–796). Philadelphia: W. B. Saunders.
10. Friedman, L. S. (1998). Liver, biliary tract, and pancreas. In L. M. Tierney, S. J. McPhee, & M. A. Papadakis (Eds.), *Current medical diagnosis and treatment 1998* (37th ed., pp. 628–665). Stamford, CT: Appleton & Lange.
11. Gubby, L. (1998). Assessment of quality of life and related stressors following liver transplantation. *Journal of Transplant Coordination, 8*(2), 113–118.
12. Hansen, M. (1998). *Pathophysiology: Foundations of disease and clinical intervention.* Philadelphia: W. B. Saunders.
13. Isselbacher, K. J., & Dienstag, J. L. (1998). Tumors of the liver and biliary tract. In A. S. Fauci, et al. (Eds.), *Harrison's principles of internal medicine* (14th ed., pp. 578–581). New York: McGraw-Hill.
14. Jonsen, E., Athlin, E., & Suhr, O. (1998). Familial amyloidotic patients' experience of the disease and liver transplantation. *Journal of Advanced Nursing, 27,* 52–58.
15. Kaplan, L. M., & Isselbacher, K. J. (1998). Jaundice. In A. S. Fauci, et al. (Eds.), *Harrison's principles of internal medicine* (14th ed., pp. 249–254). New York: McGraw-Hill.
16. Kelvin, J. F., & Scagliola, J. (1998). Metastases involving the gastrointestinal system. *Seminars in Oncology Nursing, 14*(3), 87–98.
17. King, R. (1997). Hepatitis C: Past, present and future issues. *Advances for Nurse Practitioners, 5*(3), 51–56.
18. Lee, W. M. (1997). Hepatitis B virus infection. *New England Journal of Medicine, 337*(24), 1733–1745.
19. Lerner-Durjava, L. (1998). Nurse's guide to immunizations. *Nursing 98, 28*(7), 10–12.
20. LoBiondio-Wood, G., et al. (1997). Impact of liver transplantation on quality of life: A longitudinal perspective. *Applied Nursing Research,* 10(1), 27–32.
21. Maddrey, W. C. (1996). Parasitic, bacterial, fungal, and granulomatous liver disease. In J. C. Bennett & F. Plum (Eds.), *Cecil textbook of medicine* (20th ed.). Philadelphia: W. B. Saunders.
22. Marx, J. F. (1998). A, B, C, D, E, and G: Understanding the varieties of viral hepatitis. *Nursing 98, 28*(7), 43–49.
23. McEwen, D. R. (1996). Management of alcoholic cirrhosis of the liver. *AORN Journal, 64*(2), 209–220.
24. Moyer, L. A., & Mast, E. E. (1998). Hepatitis A through E. *Journal of Intravenous Nursing, 21*(5), 286–290.
25. Ockner, R. K. (1996). Chronic hepatitis. In J. C. Bennett & F. Plum (Eds.), *Cecil textbook of medicine* (20th ed., pp. 776–781). Philadelphia: W. B. Saunders.
26. Podolsky, D. K., & Isselbacher, K. J. (1998). Major complications of cirrhosis. In A. S. Fauci, (Eds.), *Harrison's principles of internal medicine* (14th ed.). New York: McGraw-Hill.
27. Reed, S. L. (1998). Amebiasis and infection with free-living amebas. In A. S. Fauci, et al. (Eds.), *Harrison's principles of internal medicine* (14th ed., pp. 1176–1180). NY: McGraw Hill.
28. Sabiston, D. C., Jr. (1997). *Textbook of surgery: The biologic basis of modern surgical practice* (15th ed.). Philadelphia: W. B. Saunders.
29. Schaffner, W. (1998). The bright spot: Immunizations in 1998. *Patient Care, 32*(13), 123–126, 135–138, 141–144.
30. Scharschmidt, B. F. (1996). Acute and chronic hepatic failure and hepatic encephalopathy. In J. C. Bennett & F. Plum (Eds.), *Cecil textbook of medicine* (20th ed., pp. 797–800). Philadelphia: W. B. Saunders.
31. Scharschmidt, B. F. (1996). Hepatic tumors. In J. C. Bennett & F. Plum (Eds.), *Cecil textbook of medicine* (20th ed., pp. 802–805). Philadelphia: W. B. Saunders.
32. Scharschmidt, B. F. (1996). Bilirubin metabolism and hyperbilirubinemia. In J. C. Bennett & F. Plum (Eds.), *Cecil textbook of medicine* (20th ed., pp. 755–759). Philadelphia: W. B. Saunders.
33. Thanassi, W. T. (1998). Topics in primary care medicine: Immunization for international travelers. *Western Journal of Medicine, 168*(3), 197–202.
34. Wong, J. C., et al. (1998). Pretreatment evaluation of chronic hepatitis C: Risks, benefits, costs. *JAMA, 280*(24), 2088–2093.
35. Zakim, D., & Boyer, T. D. (1996). *Hepatology: A textbook of liver disease* (3rd ed.). Philadelphia: W. B. Saunders.
36. Zollo, A. J. (1997). *Medical secrets.* Philadelphia: Hanley & Belfus, Inc.
37. Zollo, A. J. (1998). Infectious diseases in the United States: A snapshot. *Patient Care, 32*(13), 188–194.
38. Zollo, A. (1998). Understanding hepatitis C. *Patient Care Nurse Practitioner, 1*(8), 32.

UNIT 10

Integumentary Disorders

Anatomy and Physiology Review

The Integumentary System

Robert G. Carroll

The integument, or skin makes up 15% to 20% of body weight. Intact skin is the body's primary defense system. It protects us from invasion by organisms, helps regulate body temperature, manufactures vitamins, and provides our external appearance. Skin has three primary layers (i.e., (*epidermis,* or outer layer; the *dermis,* or inner layer; and the *hypodermis,* or subcutaneous layer) as well as epidermal appendages (i.e., eccrine glands, apocrine glands, sebaceous glands, hair follicles, and nails).

The skin is the most prominent organ containing *epithelium,* which is composed of cells that provide a continuous barrier between the body contents and the outside environment. Epithelial cells also cover the gastrointestinal (GI) tract, pulmonary airways and alveoli, renal tubules and the urinary system, and the ducts that empty onto the surface of the skin (lumen) of the GI and respiratory systems. Epithelial cells allow selective transport of ions, nutrients, and metabolic wastes and have a permeability to water that is partially regulated. Epithelial cells are joined to each other through tight junctions and express different populations of protein transporters on the apical side (generally facing a lumen) and the basolateral (facing the blood, or serosal) side. The functional significance of epithelial transport is covered in the GI and renal chapters (see Units 6 and 7).

STRUCTURE OF THE INTEGUMENTARY SYSTEM

EPIDERMIS

The epidermis is the thin, stratified outer skin layer that is in direct contact with the external environment (Fig. U10–1). The thickness of the epidermis ranges from 0.04 mm on the eyelids to 1.6 mm on the palms and soles. *Desmosomes* (points of intercellular attachment that are vital for cell-to-cell adhesion) are found in the epidermis. *Keratinocytes,* the principal cells of the epidermis, produce *keratin* in a complex process. The cells begin in the basal cell layer and change constantly, moving upward through the epidermis. On the surface, they are sloughed off or lost by abrasion. Thus, the epidermis constantly regenerates itself, providing a tough keratinized barrier.

Skin color reflects both the production of pigment granules *(melanin)* by melanocytes and, in light-skinned people, the presence of blood *(hemoglobin).* Skin color reflects a combination of four basic colors:

- Exogenously formed carotenoids (yellow)
- Melanin (brown)
- Oxygenated hemoglobin in arterioles and capillaries (red)
- Reduced hemoglobin in venules (blue)

Melanin plays the largest role in skin color; it is produced in the epidermis and in corresponding layers of the hair follicle. Although melanin is not produced in the dermis, it can be deposited in the dermis from the epidermis through various processes (such as inflammation).

Melanosomes are granules in melanocytes that synthesize melanin. Skin color differences result from the size and quantity of melanosomes as well as from the rate of melanin production. In natives of equatorial Africa, there is an increase in the size and number of melanosomes (not melanocytes) as well as increased melanin production. The melanosomes are large, discrete, and dispersed. In natives of northern Europe, the melanosomes are small and aggregated, producing less melanin. Sun exposure initially increases the size and functional activity of both melanocytes and melanosomes. With chronic sun exposure, there is an increase in concentration of melanocytes as well as in size and functional activity. The presence of melanin limits the penetration of sun rays into the skin and protects against sunburn and development of ultraviolet light–induced skin carcinomas.

Epidermal Appendages

Epidermal appendages are downgrowths of epidermis into the dermis and consist of eccrine glands, apocrine units, sebaceous glands, hair, and nails.

GLANDS

Eccrine glands produce sweat and play an important role in thermoregulation. They are found throughout the skin except on the vermilion border (junction of the pink area of the lip with the surrounding skin), the ears, nail bed, glans penis, and labia minora. They are more numerous on the palms, soles, forehead, and axillae. Sweat is similar to plasma but is more dilute. Eccrine gland secretion is stimulated by heat as well as by exercise and emotional stress. Eccrine glands exit the body independently of the hair shaft (see Fig. U10–1).

Apocrine glands occur primarily in the axillae, breast areolae, anogenital area, ear canals, and eyelids. In lower-order animals, apocrine secretions function as sexual attractants (pheromones), and the apocrine secretion musk is used as a perfume base. The role, if any, in humans is not established. Mediated by adrenergic innervation, apocrine glands secrete a milky substance that becomes odoriferous when altered by skin surface bacteria. These glands do not function until puberty, and they require a high output of sex hormone for activity.

Sebaceous glands are found throughout the skin except on the palms and soles and are most abundant on the face, scalp, upper back, and chest. They are associated with hair follicles that open onto the skin surface, where *sebum* (a mixture of sebaceous gland-produced lipids and epidermal cell-derived lipids) is released. Sebum has a lubricating function and bactericidal activity. Androgen is responsible for sebaceous gland development. In utero

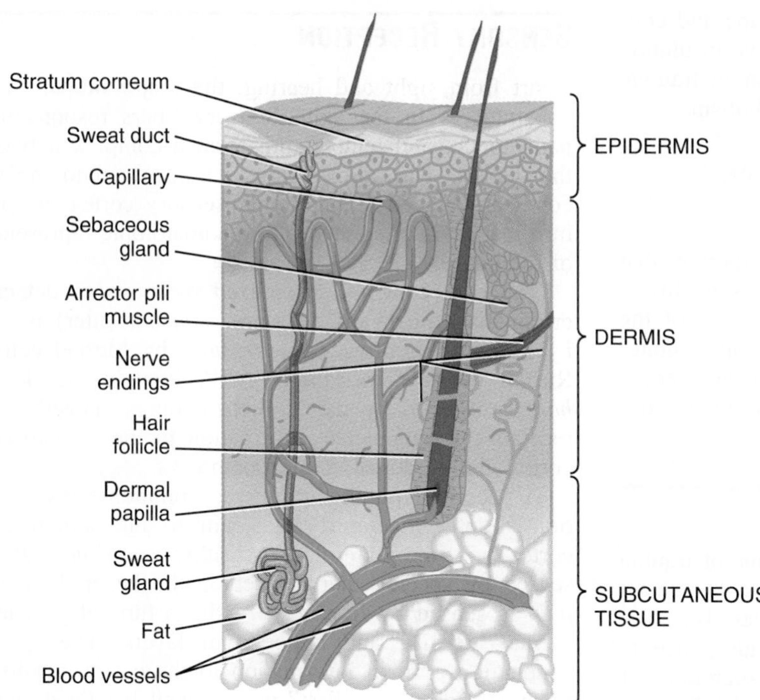

FIGURE U10–1 Structure of the skin.

androgen causes neonatal acne; after puberty, sebum production can cause acne in adolescents.

Hair and Nails

Hair is a nonviable protein end-product found on all skin surfaces except the palms and soles. Each hair follicle functions as an independent unit and goes through intermittent stages of development. Hair develops from the mitotic activity of the hair bulb. The rate of hair growth varies in different parts of the body. In a typical adult scalp, 85% to 90% of hairs are in an *anagen* (growth) phase. The remainder are in a *telogen* (rest) phase. About 50 to 100 hairs are lost each day. As a rule, the growing phase of hair on the eyebrows, trunk, and extremities does not exceed 6 months. Its resting phase is 3 to 4 months.

Hair form (straight or curly) depends on the shape of the hair in cross-section. Straight hair has a round cross-section; curly hair has an oval or ribbon-like cross-section. Curved follicles also affect the curliness of hair. Melanocytes in the bulb determine hair color. Hair follicles usually occur with sebaceous glands, and together they form a pilosebaceous unit. *Arrector pili* muscles of the dermis attach to hair follicles and elevate the hairs when body temperature falls, producing "goose bumps."

Nails are horny scales of epidermis. The nail matrix is the source of specialized, nonkeratinized cells. They differentiate into keratinized cells, which make up the nail protein. The matrix for nail formation is located in the proximal nail bed. It grows forward from the nail fold to cover the nail bed. Fingernails grow about 0.1 mm/day; complete reproduction takes 100 to 150 days. Toenails grow one third as fast as fingernails do. A damaged nail matrix, which may result from trauma or aggressive manicuring, produces a distorted nail. Nails are also sensitive to physiologic changes; for instance, they grow more slowly in cold weather and during periods of illness.

Nails and hair consist of keratinized and, therefore, "dead" cells. The ingestion of gelatin has not been shown to increase nail growth or strength.

Dermis

The dermis, a dense layer of tissue beneath the epidermis, gives the skin most of its substance and structure. It varies from 1 to 4 mm in thickness and is thickest over the back. The dermis contains fibroblasts, macrophages, mast cells, and lymphocytes, which promote wound healing. The skin's lymphatic, vascular, and nerve supplies, which maintain equilibrium in the skin, are in the dermis.

The dermis is divided into two parts: papillary and reticular. The papillary dermis, which contains increased amounts of collagen, blood vessels, sweat glands, and elastin, is in contact with the epidermis. The *reticular* dermis also contains collagen but with increased amounts of mature elastic tissue. The dermis houses many specialized cells, blood vessels, and nerves.

The epidermis and dermis meet at the *dermoepidermal junction.* This area contains wave-like projections from the dermis called *papillae,* which correspond to reciprocal structures in the epidermis. The *subepidermal basement membrane zone* is a semipermeable filter that permits fluid exchange of components such as nutrients, metabolites, and waste products.

Hypodermis

The *subcutaneous layer* is a specialized layer of connective tissue. It is sometimes called the *adipose layer* because of its fat content. This layer is absent in some sites such as the eyelids, scrotum, areola, and tibia. Age, heredity, and many other factors influence the thickness of the subcutaneous layer. Subcutaneous fat is generally thickest on the back and buttocks, giving shape and contour over the bone. This layer functions as insulation from extremes of hot and cold, as a cushion to trauma, and as a source of energy and hormone metabolism.

FUNCTION OF THE INTEGUMENTARY SYSTEM

The skin is a morphologically complex structure that serves several functions essential to life. The skin differs anatomically and physiologically in various areas of the body. Functions of the skin include protection, maintenance of homeostasis, thermoregulation, sensory reception, vitamin synthesis, and processing of antigenic substances.

PROTECTION

The skin protects the body against many forms of trauma (e.g., mechanical, thermal, chemical, radiant). The intact tough epidermal layer is a mechanical barrier. Bacteria, foreign matter, other organisms, and chemicals penetrate it with difficulty. The oily and slightly acid secretions of its sebaceous glands protect the body further by limiting the growth of many organisms. The thickened skin of the palms and soles provides additional covering to absorb the constant use of or trauma to these areas.

HOMEOSTASIS

Skin forms a barrier that prevents excessive loss of water and electrolytes from the internal environment and also prevents the subcutaneous tissues from drying out. The effectiveness of this impermeable membrane is readily recognized when one observes the extreme loss of fluids that occurs with damage to the skin, as with burns and other injuries. Insensible loss of water and electrolytes occurs only through pores in this effective barrier.

THERMOREGULATION

The skin, under normal conditions, adjusts heat loss to balance metabolic heat production. The rate of heat loss depends primarily on the surface temperature of the skin, which is in turn a function of the skin's blood flow. The blood flow of the skin varies in response to changes in the body's core temperature and to changes in temperature of the external environment. Generally, the vessels dilate during warm temperatures and constrict during cold. The hypothalamus is partly responsible for regulating skin blood flow, particularly to the extremities, the face, ears, and the tip of the nose. Maintenance of the thermal balance allows the internal temperature of the body to remain at approximately 37° C (98.6° F).

Under severe heat stress, increased cutaneous blood flow is inadequate to dissipate the thermal load. Eccrine glands produce sweat, and cooling is enhanced by fluid evaporation from the skin. Eccrine gland innervation is unique, in that these sympathetic cholinergic nerves use acetylcholine (rather than norepinephrine) as the neurotransmitter. Sweating contributes significantly to the body's capacity for thermoregulation.

SENSORY RECEPTION

Apart from sight and hearing, the major human sensory apparatus is in the skin. Sensory fibers responsible for pain, touch, and temperature form a complex network in the dermis. This information is transmitted to the spinal cord and relayed to the somatosensory cortex, where the information is integrated into a somatotopic representation of the body.

The skin contains specialized receptors to detect discriminative touch and pressure. *Touch* (flutter) is sensed by Meissner's corpuscles; *pressure,* by Merkel cells and Ruffini endings; *vibration,* by Pacinian corpuscles; and *hair movement,* by hair follicle endings. Together these receptors communicate information to the somatosensory cortex via the dorsal column pathways.

A second grouping of nerves communicates information about temperature and pain to the somatosensory cortex via the anterolateral pathways. *Temperature* is sensed by specific thermoreceptors in the epidermis, and *pain* is sensed by free nerve endings throughout the epidermal, dermal, and hypodermal layers. The speed of conduction of pain information to the cortex results in a functional division. "Fast" pain is well localized, and has a short latency. "Slow" pain is more diffuse, has a longer latency, and is more difficult to endure.

The density of receptors determines the sensitivity of the skin. For example, two-point discrimination is most acute on the skin of the fingers and face, where the highest density of touch receptors occurs. In contrast, the skin on the back has a low density of touch receptors and the ability to localize touch is therefore reduced.

VITAMIN D PRODUCTION

The epidermis is involved in synthesis of vitamin D. In the presence of sunlight or ultraviolet radiation, a sterol found on the malpighian cells is converted to form cholecalciferol (vitamin D_3). Vitamin D_3 assists in the absorption of calcium and phosphate from ingested foods.

PROCESSING OF ANTIGENIC SUBSTANCES

Langerhans cells are scattered among the keratinocytes located primarily in the epidermis; however, they can also be seen in the dermis. These cells originate in the bone marrow and migrate to the epidermis. Langerhans cells play a role in the cell-mediated immune responses of the skin through antigen presentation.

Cells in both the epidermis and dermis of the skin are important in the immune function. Skin is now recognized not only as a physical barrier but also as a participant in immunologically mediated defense against various antigens. These specialized cells include Langerhans cells and keratinocytes located in the epidermis and lymphocytes located in the dermis. An antigen entering immunologically competent skin is likely to encounter a coordinated response of Langerhans and T cells to neutralize its effect. An antigen entering diseased skin can induce and elicit immune responses. These reactions may be involved in the pathogenesis of many inflammatory skin diseases.

Dermatologic Care

As the largest and most visible organ of the body, the skin plays a major role in our physical and mental health and protects us from an array of natural and man-made attacks. Yet, the skin is rarely taken as seriously as other organ systems, such as the heart and the lung. In both outpatient and inpatient practice settings, as a nurse you have a unique opportunity to affect a client's dermatologic care. You can teach clients to appreciate the skin's important role and to recognize that some skin conditions are indeed life-threatening. For example, forecasts have indicated that by the year 2000, as many as 1 in 75 Americans would be afflicted by malignant melanoma, an often fatal skin cancer. In the United States today, one person dies every hour from skin cancer. Also, burn injuries continue, despite advances in fireproofing homes and clothes. Pressure ulcers, a serious alteration in skin integrity, poses a growing concern as the elderly population increases and may result in 60,000 deaths per year.

Appearance and Self-Esteem

Skin is integral to self-image and self-esteem. Each client's unique appearance is established through the skin. The skin was once thought to reflect the normal "aging process" and how that aging process affected the genetic skin types we inherit. We now know that skin type more likely reflects the cumulative amount of sun exposure over a lifetime. It is hoped that with education, untanned skin will once again be viewed as attractive and healthy. Cosmetic surgery should not be considered a procedure for vanity but a procedure to enhance self-esteem.

Today's society has a long-standing prejudice that needs to be dispelled regarding impaired skin. Historically, skin diseases were perceived as divine punishment for being spiritually and physically "unclean." Subtle punishment for skin diseases still exists because of ignorance. For example, a woman with atopic dermatitis may sit isolated and shunned in a waiting room because others view eczematous lesions as contagious. A waitress may be encouraged to work in the back of the kitchen so that customers will not notice the healed burn scars on her hands and body. Vitiligo, loss of pigment in the skin, is sometimes mislabeled "white leprosy," and so on. Clients who have visible chronic skin problems often withdraw from social situations and have altered interpersonal relationships and increased social isolation. When these clients seek professional care for skin problems, psychosocial as well as physical concerns need to be met.

Another function of skin, hair, and nails is to provide an outward appearance or *cosmetic adornment.* The appearance of our skin, hair, and nails is crucial to our psychosocial well-being and can affect our experiences positively or negatively. Skin disorders are often a major cause of a morbidity because we live in a beauty-conscious society. Health care providers must be acutely aware of the role of the skin in a person's self-esteem and ability to function in relationships.

Effects of Aging

The skin undergoes numerous changes that a person can see and feel throughout the life span. Many of these changes are natural, unchangeable, and harmless. Some may be bothersome or painful and are treated until there is an acceptable resolution or acceptance of the condition. Other skin changes may go unnoticed or not be bothersome because they are slow-growing, such as senile keratosis. Table U10–1 lists some age-associated changes.

Adolescence

During puberty, hormone secretion stimulates the maturation of hair follicles, sebaceous glands, and apocrine and eccrine units in certain body areas. Hair follicles on the face (males), pubic region, and axillae activate to produce coarse terminal hairs. Normal changes may bother teen-

TABLE U10–1 COMMON SKIN CHANGES ASSOCIATED WITH AGING

Skin Change	Description
ADOLESCENCE	
Folliculitis	Hair follicle inflammation
Acne	Inflammation of pilosebaceous follicle
Increased perspiration	Response to heat, emotional stress, exercise
Apocrine secretion	Related to sex hormone activity
Skin irritation	Often caused by overuse of over-the-counter skin products
Pigmented nevi	Benign cluster melanocyte-like cells
ADULTHOOD	
Melasma	Blotchy hyperpigmentation
Alopecia	Baldness (hormonal and genetic factors)
Excessive facial or body hair	Androgen-related problem in women
Actinic keratosis	Slightly raised, red papules (premalignant)
Sebaceous cyst	Enclosed cyst in dermis (potentially infectious)
Acrochordon	Small, flesh-colored papule
OLDER ADULTHOOD	
Xerosis	Dry skin (decreased natural oils and sweat)
Wrinkling	Natural change affected by many factors (e.g., loss of elasticity and subcutaneous fat, sun exposure, gravity, cigarette smoking)
Skin tears	Epidermal thinning; seen most in clients using oral corticosteroids
Senile lentigenes	Black or brown flat lesions ("liver spots")
Seborrheic keratosis	Harmless raised black or brown spots or wart-like growths
Cherry angiomas	Dilated blood vessels that form loops

agers, but caution adolescents about the potential for irritating the skin with excessive use of over-the-counter products.

New nevi can appear after adolescence. At any age, raised, pigmented lesions that bleed or change in color or size should be assessed by a physician to determine whether they require only minor care or removal because of early malignant changes.

Adulthood

Temporary *hormonal changes* account for some adult skin changes. Pregnancy and birth control pills may alter hormonal status and thus change skin structures that are hormonally linked. Pregnancy may cause changes in hair growth patterns and a temporary thinning of hair after pregnancy.

Heredity and exposure to environmental factors, such as sun, tobacco, alcohol, and chemicals, play a major role in many of the skin changes that occur in adults. Some lesions (i.e., seborrheic keratosis and acrochordons) may be removed for cosmetic reasons, if desired, or if physically irritating. Actinic keratoses (because of their premalignant status) and sebaceous cysts (because of their infectious potential) need to be assessed and may be removed.

Older Adulthood

The skin of older people reflects the cumulative influence of environmental insults, decreased circulation, and diminished function of various skin structures. As the stratum corneum becomes thinner, the skin reacts more readily to minor changes in humidity, temperature, and other irritants. The skin also becomes more transparent. Hair loss is often noticeable on the trunk, pubic area, axillae, and limbs. Loss of pigment causes gray hair. Nails become brittle and may yellow or thicken. Skin may be leathery from overexposure to ultraviolet light. There is no known treatment for past overexposure; protection from ultraviolet light is the only preventive measure.

CONCLUSIONS

The skin is the largest and most visible organ of the body. Anatomically, the skin is divided into (1) the epidermis (outer layer), (2) the dermis (inner layer), and (3) the hypodermis (subcutaneous layer). The skin serves many functions. It is the first line of defense against many forms of trauma. Skin maintains body temperature, prevents water loss, and provides sensations of touch, temperature, and pain. Skin also produces vitamin D and recognizes antigens. Finally, healthy skin is aesthetically pleasing.

BIBLIOGRAPHY

1. Arndt, K. A., et al. (1996). *Cutaneous medicine and surgery.* Philadelphia: W. B. Saunders.
2. Freedburg, I., et al. (Ed.). (1998). *Fitzpatricks' dermatology in general medicine.* New York: McGraw-Hill.
4. Pogue, S. (1995). Vitamin D synthesis in the elderly. *Dermatology Nursing, 1*(2), 103–105.
5. Silverthorn, D. (1998). *Human physiology.* Upper Saddle River, NJ: Prentice Hall.

CHAPTER 48

Assessment of the Integumentary System

Noreen Heer Nicol

A thorough health history assists in diagnosis of integumentary disorders, such as occupationally related contact dermatitis, or in revealing psychosocial aspects of disease processes. The medication history is important because side effects of certain medications can cause skin changes. The physical examination can confirm integumentary disorders as well as reveal disorders that the client may have omitted during the history.

HISTORY

The history includes questions about the current manifestations, past health history (including medications and allergies), family health history, psychosocial history (including occupational and travel history), and a review of systems.

■ CURRENT HEALTH

Chief Complaint

The most common problems related to the integument are itching (pruritus), dryness, rashes, lesions, ecchymoses (small hemorrhagic patches), lumps, and masses. Ask about changes in the skin, hair, and nails that may be related to the chief complaint. Sample questions that elicit pertinent information related to the presenting dermatologic problem are listed in Table 48–1.

Symptom Analysis

Conduct a symptom analysis, including the factors noted in Table 48–1. Sexual history may also be important if the differential diagnosis includes a sexually transmitted disease (STD) (see Chapter 37).

■ PAST HEALTH HISTORY

Various systemic diseases are characterized by cutaneous manifestations. Does the client have other systemic disorders relevant to the skin (i.e., immunologic, endocrine, collagen, vascular, renal, or hepatic conditions)? Ask about recent exposure to ticks, other insects, or infectious or childhood diseases, and find out about the vaccination status. Previous trauma and surgical intervention may explain unusual lesions or their location. A history of past allergic reactions to foods or medications is important for avoiding inadvertent reaction through readministration.

Medications

Note prescription and over-the-counter medications that the client is currently taking or has recently finished. Sensitivity to antibiotics or other drugs in the form of a drug rash may not occur until the end of a routine course of therapy. Photosensitizing drugs (e.g., phenothiazides, tetracyclines, diuretics, sulfonamides) may cause a sunburn-like rash in areas of sun exposure. Topical preparations may include preservatives or active ingredients that are known sensitizers. The most commonly encountered are neomycin, benzocaine, and diphenhydramine hydrochloride. Oral corticosteroids (e.g., prednisone), if used at high doses or routinely, can cause acne breakouts, thinning of skin, stretch marks, and many other systemic side effects.

Ask about self-treatment with herbal remedies. Aloe vera (*A. barbadensis, A. ferox, A. africana, A. spicata)* is used for relief of eczema and psoriasis, and to promote wound healing. Chamomile (*Matricaria recutita, Chamaemelum nobile)*, comfrey (*Symphytum officinale*), evening primrose (*Oenothera biennis*), and gotu kola (*Centella asiatica*) have similar uses.

Allergies

Ask the client about allergies to medications and foods. Does the ingestion of certain foods cause itching, burning, or eruption of rashes? Fresh fruits that have been treated with pesticides or preservatives may also be problematic, as may prepared foods containing preservatives.

There is a difference between allergy and irritation. *Allergy* is an immunologic response that happens consistently with exposure. *Irritation* can occur unpredictably. Inquire about substances that may cause local skin irritation or lesions on direct contact, such as textiles or metals. Wool is irritating to most people. Jewelry containing nickel may cause skin discoloration, irritation, rash, or other problems in people who are sensitive to this metal.

TABLE 48–1 **DERMATOLOGIC ASSESSMENT HISTORY: SAMPLE QUESTIONS**

Information Needed	Questions
Chief complaint	"Please tell me what brings you here today."
Definition of problem (onset, location)	"Tell me more about the problem. Where did it start? Have you noticed this problem before?"
Duration	"When did it start? Does it come and go? Has it changed? Has it become better or worse?"
Accompanying manifestations	"Did you have any feelings—such as fatigue, nausea, skin tightness, skin burning—before this problem started? Does it itch?"
Evolution of lesion or eruption	"How does it feel now? Are you experiencing any discomfort? Do you feel tenderness, tightness? Does clothing irritate your skin? Do you have any problems sleeping? Does it limit any of your activities? Has it interfered with your normal daily routine?"
Aggravating and relieving factors	"Have you noticed whether the problem worsens after any of these activities: eating particular foods? Using cosmetics? Using soaps? Wearing clothing? Do changes in temperature or climate affect the problem? Does it worsen or improve with changes in season? Are you more comfortable when warm or when cool?"
Medical intervention	"Did you see a physician about this? Were you told what the problem was? Was any treatment recommended? Did it help?"
Self-treatment	"What have you tried to do on your own to get relief? What did you use? What over-the-counter medications or home remedies have you tried? What do you do yourself that helps the problem?"
Compliance and treatment factors	"How often were you able to apply or take prescribed medication? Were you able to complete prescribed treatment? How did you use the medication? (e.g., How did you apply it? How did you take it? For how long? Why did you stop?)"

■ FAMILY HEALTH HISTORY

A family health history helps determine genetic predisposition to skin disorders as well as predisposition to parasitic or other conditions related to the family's lifestyle and living environment. Many dermatologic disorders or systemic disorders with a dermatologic presentation are passed on genetically. Genetically transmitted dermatologic conditions include alopecia (loss of patches of hair), ichthyosis (thickened, scaly skin), atopic dermatitis, and psoriasis. Systemic diseases with dermatologic manifestations include diabetes mellitus, blood dyscrasia, and collagen-vascular diseases (e.g., lupus erythematosus). Other diseases, such as scabies, are likely to be passed on to family members because of close and frequent exposure.

■ PSYCHOSOCIAL HISTORY

Psychosocial factors that influence dermatologic disorders often play a large role, particularly in long-term and chronic processes. Skin disease can greatly affect lifestyle and self-image. Cultural and familial influences in caring for a particular disorder may conflict with prescribed therapies. Misconceptions about skin problems (e.g., acne lesions can be scrubbed away) need to be determined and corrected. Visually or physically disabling chronic skin diseases have been associated with chronic unemployment, poor mental health, and even suicide. Assess the sexual history, which can help alert to or explain the presence of tissue trauma or lesions caused by STDs (see Chapter 37).

Do not overlook socioeconomic factors. Compliance with outlined therapies and return for follow-up care are influenced by social expectations and ability to pay for medications or treatments. When recommending therapies or medications, consider the impact on the client's day-to-day routine as well as the type of prescription insurance plan. Many topical therapies—whether or not they are covered by insurance—are expensive, and expense is a factor that affects compliance.

Occupation and Travel

Occupational history is important because a large number of skin problems are caused or worsened by exposure to irritants and chemicals in the home and work environment. Learn what substances the client comes in contact with and to what extent. For example, chronic flaring of hand eczema may be caused by use of certain glues and glazes in a hobby project, total body rash by chemical mists penetrating nonprotective gear at the work site, or hand rash by latex glove allergies.[14, 19]

The travel history can be helpful, especially if it includes hiking or exposure to outdoor agents that result in dermatologic disorders, such as poison ivy, poison sumac, or poison oak or Lyme disease.

Habits

Inquire about the client's habits. Determine the frequency of hygiene practices, the products used (e.g., soaps, lotions, abrasives), and whether cosmetics are used. Record the products used, including brand names. Inquire whether there have been any changes in clothing or bedding, and discuss how these items are cleaned. Review the client's diet history for intake of sufficient nutrients, such as water, protein, dietary fat, and vitamins A, D, E, and C. Also, ask about exercise and sleep patterns, which affect circulation, nourishment, and repair of the skin.

Does the client engage in recreational activities that involve prolonged exposure to the sun, unusual cold, or other conditions that may damage the integument? For example, does the client visit tanning salons? More than 1 million persons use tanning salons each day, and federal regulation of salons is limited. Advise clients that exposure leads to premature aging, increased risk of skin cancer, risk of corneal burns if eye guards are not worn, exacerbation of photosensitivity disorders, and increased development of lentigines ("liver spots").[18]

REVIEW OF SYSTEMS

Obtain a complete history of the skin. Specifically, ask about past problems with unusual itching, dryness, lesions, rashes, lumps, ecchymoses, and masses. Has the client had problems with moles or other lesions, especially if they have undergone changes in size, shape, or color? A more complete list of questions for the review of systems appears in Chapter 9, Box 9–2.

PHYSICAL EXAMINATION

Examine the skin as thoroughly as any other body organ. This procedure cannot be done properly in the hall or at a quick glance, which the dermatologist or the nurse is often requested to do. Use inspection, palpation, and olfaction to assess hair, nails, and skin. Effective assessment requires knowledge, awareness, and practice in describing skin of individuals of all ages and different lifestyles and in recognizing normal and abnormal skin changes. The Physical Assessment Findings in the Healthy Adult feature describes normal conditions of the integumentary system.

PHYSICAL ASSESSMENT FINDINGS IN THE HEALTHY ADULT

Integumentary System

Inspection

Skin. Even skin tones, darker on exposed areas of face, neck, arms, and lower legs; lighter on trunk and back. Small tan freckles scattered over face and arms. Scars, striae absent.

Hair and Scalp. Hair evenly distributed over scalp. Clean, without nits or lice. No dandruff, scaling, or scalp lesions. Axillae and legs probably shaved; pubic hair distributed as inverted triangle from symphysis pubis to perineum (female). Pubic hair distributed in diamond pattern from below umbilicus to perineum (male).

Nails. Regular, smooth, oval shape. Pink nail beds. Cuticles manicured, clean. Nail bed angle 160 degrees (no clubbing).

Palpation

Skin. Warm, well hydrated, smooth, elastic, nontender. No lesions, masses, or lumps.

Hair and Scalp. Hair non-oily, even textured, resilient. Scalp smooth, intact, nontender.

Nails. Firm without tenderness or bogginess. Rapid blanch response.

TERMINOLOGY

The terms used in dermatology have been referred to as a "foreign language" and have been known to inhibit use of the correct terminology for skin disorders by health care providers. Use of standard terminology often leads to differential diagnosis. This section clarifies some commonly used dermatologic terms and should assist the reader in recognizing and describing skin disorders. Table 48–2 is a glossary of commonly used dermatologic terms.

TYPES OF LESIONS

Examination and making the correct diagnosis of skin disorders depend on identifying skin lesions or changes. Two major types of lesions are distinguished: *primary* and *secondary* lesions.

The primary lesion is the first lesion to appear on the skin and has a visually recognizable structure. Figure 48–1 depicts 10 primary lesions: macule, papule, plaque, nodule, tumor, wheal, vesicle, bulla, cyst, and pustule. Frequently, the health care provider does not see a primary lesion and must depend on the client's description of "how it looked when it first appeared."

When a primary lesion undergoes changes, it becomes a secondary lesion. These alterations, brought about by the client or by the client's environment, often occur in the epidermal layer. The changes may result from many factors, including scratching, rubbing, medication, natural disease progression, or processes of involution and healing. Figure 48–2 presents nine secondary lesions: scale, crust, erosion, deep ulcer, scar, lichenification, excoriation, fissure, and atrophy.

EXAMINATION ENVIRONMENT

The best setting for conducting a dermatologic assessment is a well-lit, private room with moderate temperature and neutral, white, or cream-colored walls. Excessive warmth can produce changes in skin color (e.g., redness) by causing vasodilation. Colored walls can affect normal skin hue (color). For a complete examination, ask the client to undress and provide a gown. Explain that all skin surfaces will be examined. Avoid unnecessary exposure during the examination. Have warm hands to avoid stimulation of the skin and to add to the overall comfort of the client.

DEPTH OF EXAMINATION

The examination is systematic and as complete as appropriate. A total-body skin examination involves assessment of the hair, scalp, nails, mucous membranes, and skin, including the axillae, areas in skinfolds, external genitalia, webs between toes and fingers, palms of hands, and soles of feet. Begin at the head, and proceed to the toes. General changes can alter total-body skin color (e.g., jaundice, cyanosis, pallor), thickness, turgor, temperature, and vascularity (e.g., purpura, petechiae). General findings can suggest systemic disease and may require complete physical examination and appropriate evaluation. The diagnosis of skin disorders is accomplished by careful observation and evaluation of individual lesions. This discussion is limited to assessment of hair, scalp, nails, and skin lesions.

Table 48–2 GLOSSARY OF DERMATOLOGIC TERMS

Term	Definition
Actinic	Pertaining to ultraviolet light (UVL)
Amelanotic	Without pigment
Circinate (pronounced *sir-sin-ate*)	Circular
Circumscribed	Limited to a certain area by sharply defined border
Coalesce	To merge one with another
Comedo	Plug in a skin duct containing keratin (open, blackhead; closed, whitehead)
Cytotoxic	Toxic to cells
Dermatome	Area of skin supplied by a single dorsal nerve root
Dermatophyte	Fungus that enters the skin's surface, causing infection
Desquamation	Scaling, peeling of epidermis
Discoid	Coin-like
Eczematous	General term for disease process characterized by scaling, weeping, crusting, and inflammation
Erythema	Redness
Exacerbation	Worsening of disease state
Exfoliative	Shedding of skin in fairly large quantities
Folliculitis	Hair follicle inflammation
Guttate	Small, water drop–sized lesions, usually widespread
Hives	Spontaneously occurring wheals
Hyperkeratosis	Thickening of stratum corneum, usually from repeated pressure or friction
Hyperpigmentation	Increased or excessive skin pigmentation (melanin) causing an area of skin to be darker than surrounding areas
Hypopigmentation	Decreased pigmentation
Indurated	Hard (tissue)
Intertrigo	Irritation of body areas with opposing skinfolds that are subject to friction
Lesion	Detectable change from normal skin structure
Maceration	Tissue softening or disintegration from excessive moisture
Milia	Small, white papules
Perioral	Around the mouth
Periungual	Under the nail plate
Pigmentation	Degree of skin or mucous membrane color
Plantar	Pertaining to sole of the foot
Polymorphic	Existing in many forms
Pruritus	Itching
Punctate	Pinpoint or dot-shaped
Sclerosis	Hardening or induration of skin
Sebum	Lipid excretion produced by sebaceous glands
Tautness	Degree of skin tightness
Texture	Tactile or visual skin characteristics (e.g., coarseness, dryness)
Ultraviolet light (UVL)	Electromagnetic radiation from the sun (wavelengths 4–400 nm)
Urticaria	Wheals (hives)
Verruca	Lesion characterized by surface roughness (e.g., wart)
Wheal	Lesion found in hives

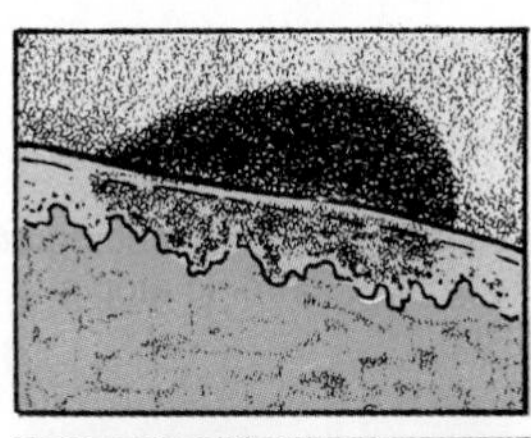

MACULE: Skin color change without elevation, i.e., flat (e.g., freckles or petechia). Described as a "patch" if greater than 1 cm (e.g., vitiligo).

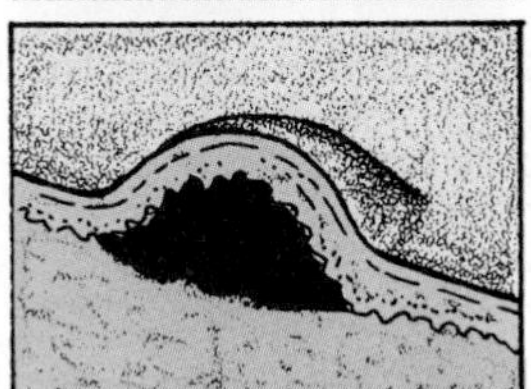

PAPULE: Elevated, solid lesion of less than 1 cm, varying in color (e.g., warts or elevated nevus).

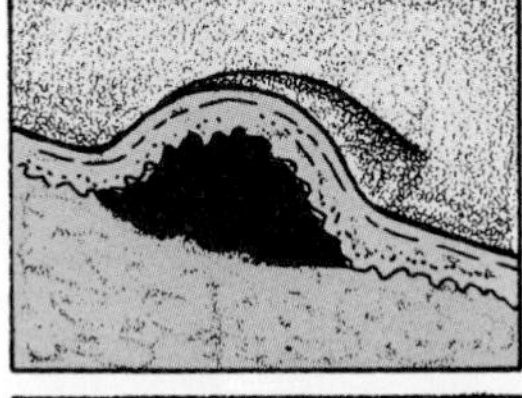

PLAQUE: Raised, flat lesion formed from merging papules or nodules.

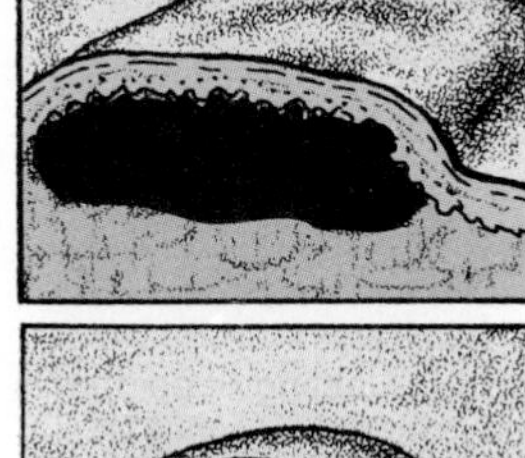

NODULE: Larger than a papule. Raised solid lesion extending deeper into the dermis.

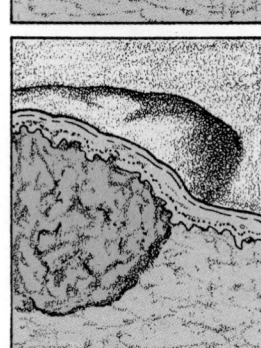

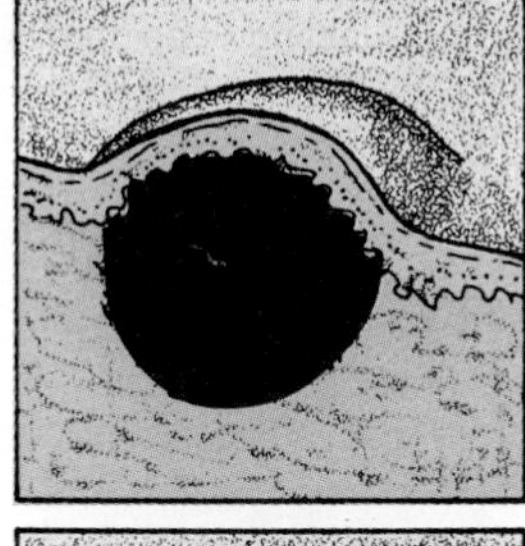

TUMOR: Larger than a nodule. Elevated firm lesion that may or may not be easily demarcated.

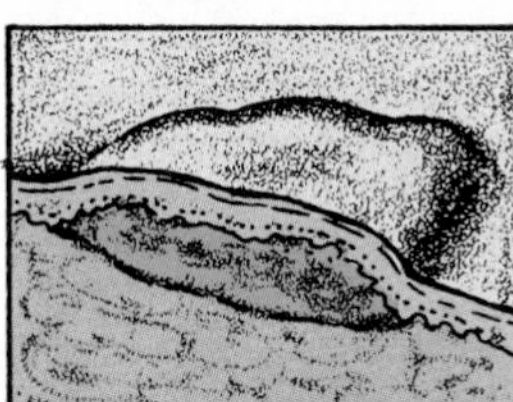

WHEAL (hive): Fleeting skin elevation that is irregularly shaped because of edema (e.g., mosquito bite or urticaria).

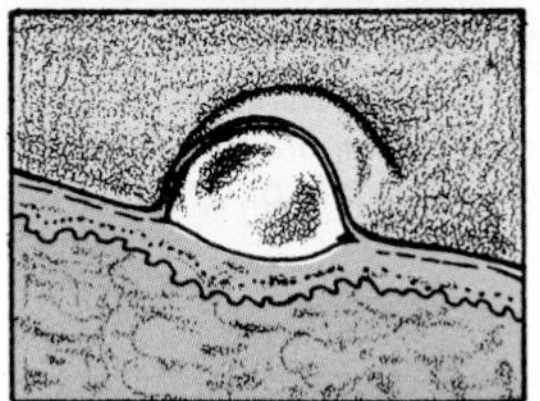

VESICLE (blister): Elevated, sharply defined lesion containing serous fluid. Usually less than 1 cm (e.g., blister, chickenpox, or herpes simplex).

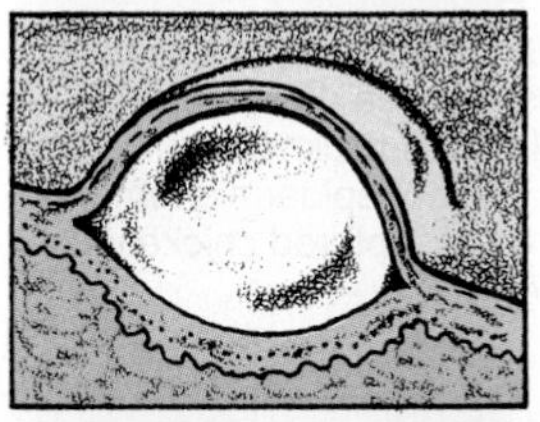

BULLA (plural, *bullae*): Large, elevated, fluid-filled lesion greater than 1 cm (e.g., second-degree burn).

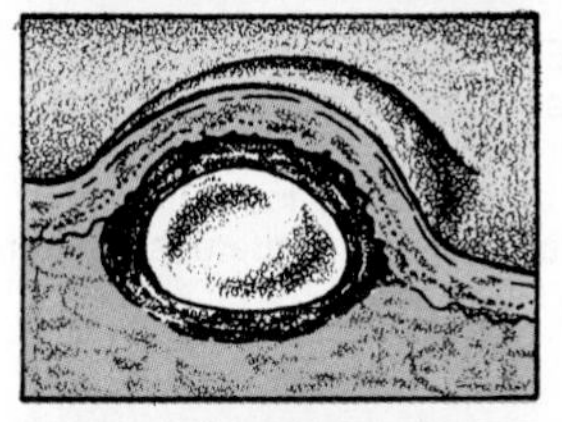

CYST: Elevated, thick-walled lesion containing fluid or semisolid matter.

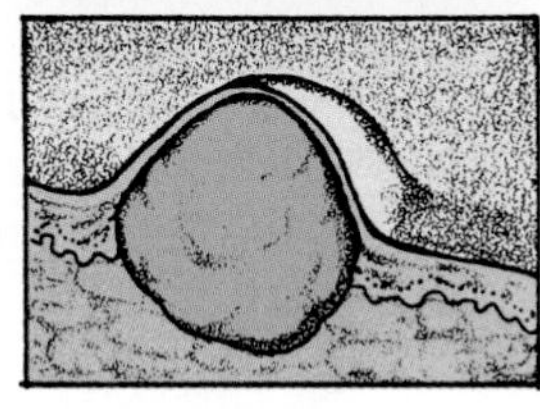

PUSTULE: Elevated lesion less than 1 cm containing purulent material. Lesions larger than 1 cm are described as boils, abscesses, or furuncles (e.g., acne, or impetigo).

FIGURE 48–1 Primary lesions: visually recognizable structural changes in the skin that have specific characteristics.

Although you may examine the client's integument over the complete body surface at one time, this is usually not done in the screening examination. Instead, integument assessment is integrated as each body region is examined. For the purpose of discussion, however, assessment of the integument is presented as a separate body system. Significant or abnormal findings are commonly reported as part of each regional assessment rather than separately.

■ INSPECTION AND PALPATION

Hair and Scalp

Examine *hair distribution* patterns for symmetry and distribution according to age and sexual development. Fine hair covers much of the body and is the same color as scalp hair. Increased distribution occurs normally in the axillae and pubic area. Having excess body hair is known as *hirsutism.*

Inspect the hair and scalp under good light. Wear gloves if you suspect lesions or infestation with lice. Inspect and palpate the hair for distribution, thickness, texture, lubrication, and signs of infestation or infection. Because natural hair color varies greatly, ask the client whether hair dye is used, as it alters texture. Hair should be resilient and distributed evenly over the scalp. Individual hair shafts can range from thin and fine to thick and coarse; the shape of hair fibers can be straight, curly, or wavy. Texture and lubrication are affected by the type of hair care products used (e.g., harsh shampoo, curling irons, or hair dryers) as well as by a protein-deficient diet or health problems, such as febrile illness, all of which tend to leave hair dry and brittle. Hair loss or thinning *(alopecia)* can result from genetic predisposition to bald-

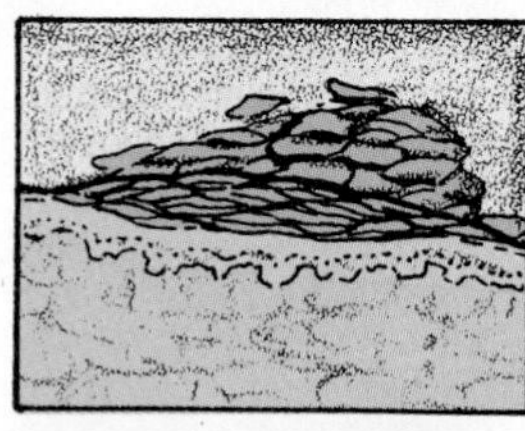

SCALE: Dried fragments of sloughed epidermal cells, irregular in shape and size and white, tan, yellow, or silver in color (e.g., dandruff, dry skin, or psoriasis).

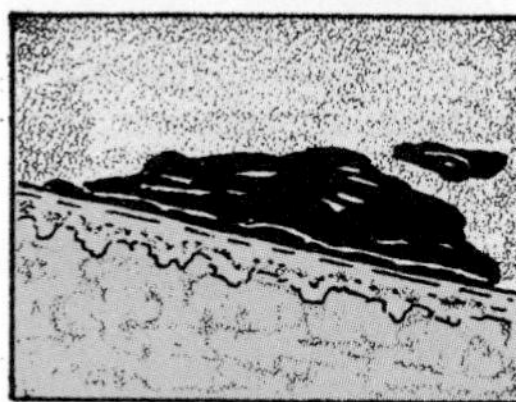

CRUST: Dried serum, sebum, blood, or pus on skin surface producing a temporary barrier to the environment (e.g., impetigo).

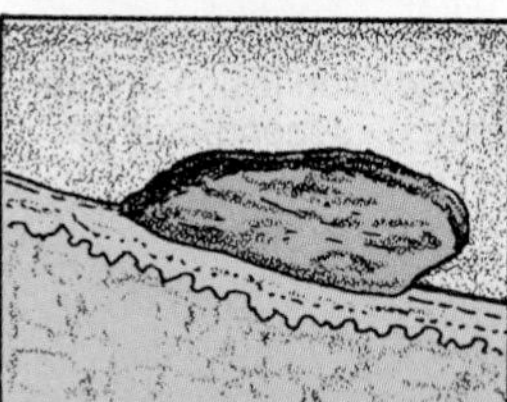

EROSION: A moist, demarcated, depressed area due to loss of partial- or full-thickness epidermis. Basal layer of epidermis remains intact (e.g., ruptured chickenpox vesicle).

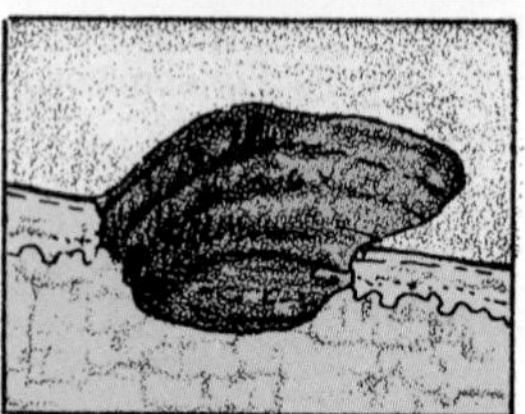

ULCER: Irregularly shaped, exudative, depressed lesion in which entire epidermis and upper layer of dermis are lost. Results from trauma and tissue destruction (e.g., stasis ulcer).

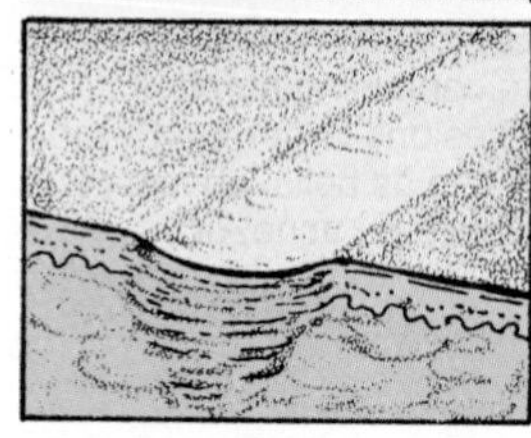

SCAR: Mark left on skin after healing. Replacement of destroyed tissue by fibrous tissue.

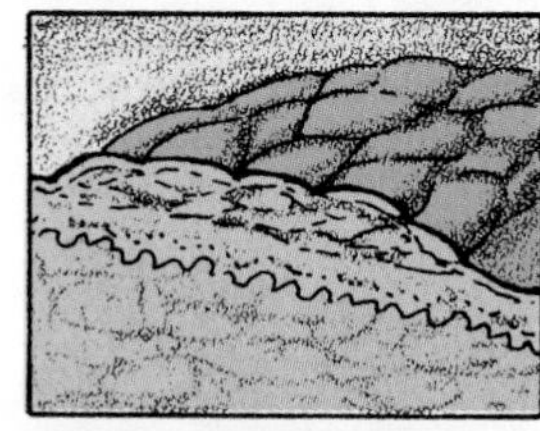

LICHENIFICATION: Epidermal thickening resulting in elevated plaque with accentuated skin markings. Usually results from repeated injury through rubbing or scratching (e.g., chronic atopic dermatitis).

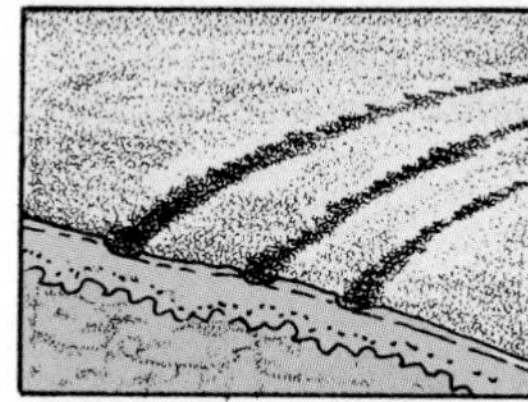

EXCORIATION: Superficial, linear abrasion of epidermis. Visible sign of itching caused by rubbing or scratching (e.g., atopic dermatitis).

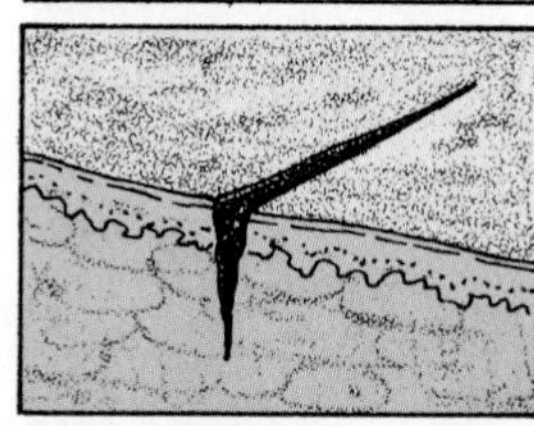

FISSURE: Deep linear split through epidermis into dermis (e.g., tinea pedis).

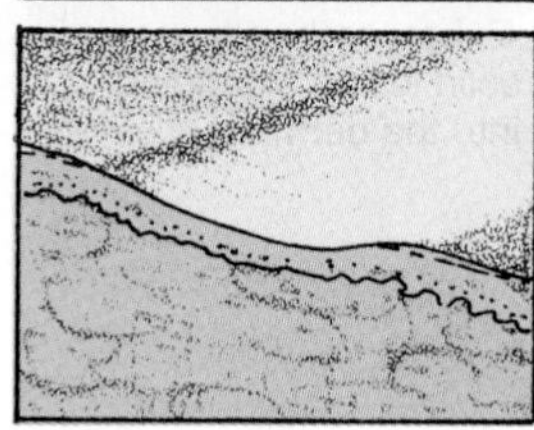

ATROPHY: Wasting of epidermis in which skin appears thin and transparent, or of dermis in which there is a depressed area (e.g., arterial insufficiency).

FIGURE 48–2 Secondary lesions: primary lesions that have changed because of the natural progression of the lesion or because of physical change (e.g., scratching, irritation, or secondary infection).

ness or a health problem, such as recent chemotherapy or a thyroid disorder.

Inspect and palpate the *scalp* for lesions, excoriations (from scratching), lumps, or bruises, which should be absent. Examine hair shafts for the presence of nits, which are the eggs of the human head louse *(Pediculus humanus capitis)* and appear as particles of oval dandruff. Adult lice often bite the scalp behind the ears and along the back of the neck, which results in pustular lesions. It may be difficult to see adult lice on the scalp; they are very small (1 to 2 mm) and have gray-white bodies.

If you see lesions, describe them and ask the client about recent trauma or injury to the head. If the client has not already provided information during the health history interview, conduct a symptom analysis.

Nails

Inspect the client's nails for color, shape, texture, integrity, and thickness (Table 48–3). The nails reflect the client's overall health, indicating nutrition and respiratory status.

Color and Shape

The nail plate is usually transparent and colorless and, when viewed from the side, has a convex shape. The vascular bed underlying the nail plate gives the nail its color. The color is pink in white clients and darker in dark-skinned clients. A hemoglobin deficiency is seen in the nail bed as pallor, and decreased arterial circulation appears as cyanosis.

Perform a *blanch test* by palpating the nail beds to assess capillary refill. Press the nail bed firmly for 5 seconds, then quickly release while observing the rate of color return to the nail bed. Color should return within 3 to 5 seconds in healthy individuals. Document results of the blanch test as "rapid" or "sluggish" capillary refill. When palpated, the nail bed feels firm with no softness (i.e., bogginess) or tenderness.

Texture

Texture should be smooth; healthy nails are of uniform thickness with no signs of dryness, softness, brittleness, splitting, peeling, ridges, or pitting. The *angle* formed between the nail plate and posterior nailfold is approximately

TABLE 48–3 ASSESSING THE NAILS

Assessment Finding	Description	Causes
Normal nail	Nail shape is convex, and nail plate angle is approximately 160°	
Beau's line	Horizontal depression in nail plate; depressions can occur singly or in multiples	Nail growth is disturbed temporarily; related to systemic illness (e.g., infection) or direct injury to the nail root
Splinter hemorrhages	Linear (vertical) red or brown streaks in the nail bed	Minor trauma to the nail bed; subacute bacterial endocarditis; trichinosis
Paronychia	Inflammation of the skinfold at the nail margin	Trauma; skin infection at the nail base
Spoon shape	Nail shape is concave as the nail curves upward from the nail bed	Use of strong detergents; iron deficiency anemia; syphilis
Clubbing	Increased angle between nail plate and nail base	Long-standing hypoxia

160 degrees without separation (see Table 48–3). Changes in nail shape and nail bed angle can indicate health problems. Clubbing of the nails refers to an increase of more than 160 degrees in the angle between the nail plate and nail base. The base of a clubbed nail is spongy and soft on palpation. These changes result from hypoxia (diminished tissue oxygenation). Nail clubbing commonly occurs in clients with congenital heart defects or chronic lung disease.

INTEGRITY

The tissue surrounding the nail should appear intact without signs of inflammation, jagged edges (hangnail), or dryness. Inferior or lateral nailfold inflammation is a sign of paronychia (i.e., nailfold infection). If these abnormalities are noted, ask the client about nail care habits such as biting or cutting cuticles.

THICKNESS

While examining the fingers and toes, you may note common abnormalities such as calluses or corns. A *callus* is a flat, painless thickening of a circumscribed area of skin. Calluses usually occur on the hands and feet. A *corn* is a horny induration and thickening of the skin caused by friction and pressure and is often painful.

Skin

Color

Assess overall skin color during the health history interview. Conduct a more thorough assessment as you proceed through the remainder of the physical examination. Observe the client's face and visible skin surfaces for color tones, which should be congruent with the stated race. Abnormal findings include pallor (paleness), a flushed or ruddy complexion, cyanosis (blue cast), jaundice (yellow cast), and areas of irregular pigmentation. Normal variation occurs from one region of the body to another, particularly in areas protected from the sun and exposure by clothing; these areas are lighter. Overall color should be uniform. Skin tone may range over a variety of colors including light ivory to deep brown or blue-black, yellow to olive, or light pink to dark, ruddy pink.

Areas that are less pigmented reveal abnormal findings more readily than more heavily pigmented surfaces. For example, *pallor* is best seen in the buccal (mouth) mucosa, especially in clients with dark skin. *Cyanosis* is evident more readily in less pigmented areas, such as the nail beds, lips, and palms. *Jaundice* sharply contrasts with the white of the sclera, especially in dark-skinned clients who have more carotene deposits. Jaundice is best assessed in dark-skinned clients by inspecting color changes in the hard palate.

Examine local areas of color change closely. *Hyperpigmentation* describes areas of increased pigmentation; *hypopigmentation* describes areas of decreased pigmentation. Skin color also results from the circulation; an increased blood supply may lead to the redness of inflammation *(rubor)*, whereas extreme pallor may be a result of anemia or impeded arterial circulation to the area.

Moisture

Moisture refers to the skin's hydration level in terms of both wetness and oiliness. Overall skin moisture in healthy individuals can be described as well hydrated. Skin moisture often reflects ambient temperature and humidity levels. Moistness usually occurs in intertriginous areas (where skin touches skin), such as the axillae and groin. Skin that feels overly moist and cool (i.e., clammy) or overly dry, scaling, or cracked is abnormal.

Temperature

Assess temperature with the dorsum of the hand. The skin should feel uniformly warm because it reflects circulation. Compare areas of hypothermia or hyperthermia with the same areas on the opposite side. See Figure 48–3.

Texture

Palpate *texture* by stroking the skin lightly with the fingertips. The skin should feel smooth, soft, and resilient. There should be no areas of lumps or unusual thickening or thinning (atrophy).

Turgor

Turgor, a reflection of the skin's elasticity and hydration status, is measured by the time needed for the skin and underlying tissue to return to their original contour after being "pinched up." Lightly pinch the skin over the forearm between the thumb and index finger, then release it.

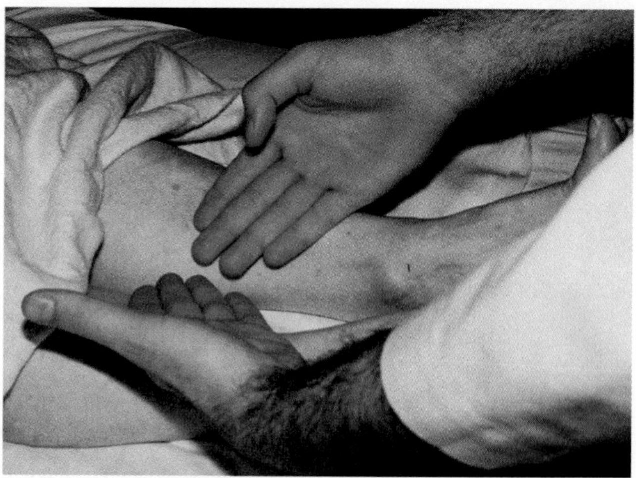

FIGURE 48–3 Assessing skin temperature. (Courtesy of Mary Sieggreen.)

If the skin remains elevated (i.e., tented) for more than 3 seconds, turgor is decreased. Skin with normal turgor is mobile and elastic and should return to baseline contour within 3 seconds. Turgor decreases with age as the skin loses elasticity. Assessment of turgor is discussed in Chapter 10.

Edema

Palpate for *edema* (fluid retention), particularly if areas of taut, shiny skin are noted. Edema refers to a collection of fluid in underlying tissues that separate the skin's surface from pigmented and vascular layers, which results in a blanched appearance. It is an abnormal finding. Palpate edematous areas for consistency, temperature, shape (i.e., extent), tenderness, and mobility. Assess and describe edematous areas using the technique described in Chapter 51. Areas examined for edema include those over the sacrum (especially in bedridden clients), the feet, the ankles, and the shins (over the tibia).

Tenderness

Tenderness is an abnormal finding and is elicited with palpation. No areas of tenderness should be found in a healthy, uninjured client.

Odor

The skin should be free of pungent odors. Odors, when noted, are usually present in the axillae and skinfolds or in open wounds and are related to the presence of bacteria on the skin, inadequate hygiene, or infection. Assess odor in open wounds after cleansing the wound, since odor can be related to the drainage itself or to the type of dressing used (e.g., hydrocolloid).

Lesions

Inspect the skin for detectable lesions. Assess and describe lesions in an orderly fashion: location, distribution, size, arrangement, color, configuration, secondary changes, and presence of drainage. Palpate skin lesions to determine the characteristics of contour (e.g., flat, raised, or depressed), size (using a measuring device), consistency (e.g., firm, soft), mobility, and tenderness. Lesions can be mobile or immobile (fixed to underlying tissue). Photographing lesions of concern is an excellent way to document changes over time.

LOCATION, DISTRIBUTION, AND SIZE. *Location* is described in reference to anatomic landmarks. Measure the lesions for *size* to help classify their type (e.g., macule, papule). If multiple lesions are present, the *distribution pattern* can be helpful in determining the diagnosis. Note the extent of the lesions. Lesions can be (1) localized (confined to a specific area), (2) regional, or (3) generalized (present over a large surface). Compare sides bilaterally to determine whether lesions are symmetrical or asymmetrical. Another commonly noted distribution is on sun-exposed areas. Certain diseases feature a classic lesion distribution; for example, lesions of herpes zoster follow along a nerve root dermatome. Table 48–4 presents common configurations and distributions. Figure 48–4 depicts the locations of common skin disorders found during physical examination.

ARRANGEMENT. The *arrangement* refers to the pattern of nearby lesions. Two of the typical patterns are "linear" and "satellite," which can also be helpful in confirming diagnosis. Linear lesions appear in a straight line (e.g., in scabies). Satellite lesions appear as small peripheral lesions around a central larger lesion (e.g., in diaper candidiasis).

COLOR. Skin lesions are found in a wide variety of colors; they may be skin-colored, brown, red, yellow, tan, or blue. Color can be influenced by many factors, including the client's normal skin hue, which may make accurate description difficult. Slight color changes can best be assessed in areas having the least amount of natural pigmentation and those with superficial capillary beds (i.e., buccal membrane of the mouth, mucosa, lips, nail beds,

TABLE 48–4 TERMINOLOGY FOR SKIN LESION CONFIGURATION AND DISTRIBUTION

	Description
CONFIGURATION*	
Annular	Ring-shaped
Iris	Concentric rings, "bull's eyes"
Gyrate	Spiral-shaped
Linear	Forming a line
Nummular	Coin-like
Polymorphous	Occurring in several forms
Punctate	Marked by points or dots
Serpiginous	Snake-like
DISTRIBUTION†	
Solitary	Single lesion
Satellite	Single lesion occurring in close proximity to but separate from a large group of lesions
Grouped	Clustered
Confluent	Merged together
Diffuse	Widely distributed
Discrete	Separate from other lesions
Generalized	Diffusely distributed
Localized	Limited, clearly defined
Symmetrical	Bilaterally distributed
Asymmetrical	Unilaterally distributed
Zosteriform	Band-like distribution of lesions along a dermatome

*Position of lesions relative to other lesions.
†Grouping, or pattern, of lesions over entire skin surface.

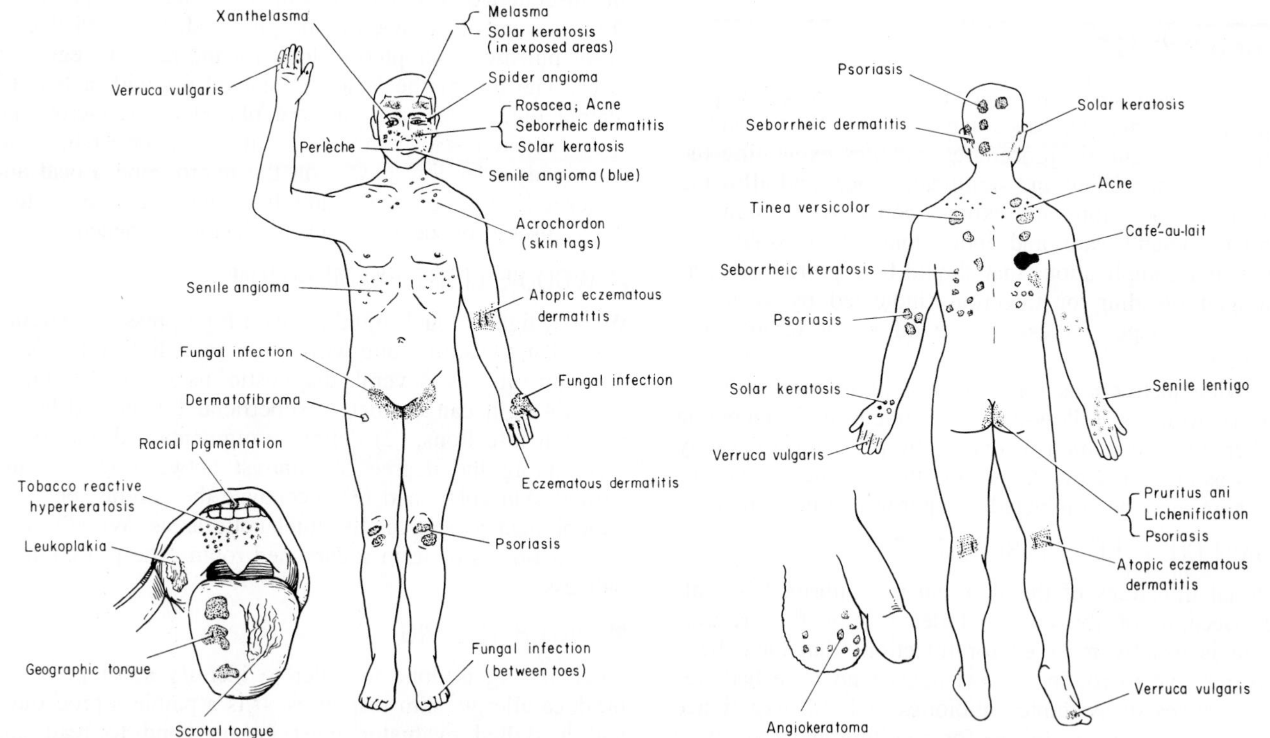

FIGURE 48–4 Common disorders encountered during physical examinaton of the skin. (From Fitzpatrick, T. B., et al. [1993]. *Dermatology in general medicine* [4th ed]. New York: McGraw-Hill.)

ocular conjunctiva, palms, and soles). These areas are especially important in assessing darkly pigmented skin.

CONFIGURATION. The term configuration refers to the shape or the outline of the lesion. Most lesions are circular. The term *nummular* is used for a circular lesion that is the size of a large coin (i.e., nummular eczema). *Annular* describes lesions with an active ring-shaped border and some central clearing (e.g., granuloma annulare). Table 48–4 shows other configurations that may be found during assessment.

■ SKIN SELF-EXAMINATION

Although it is crucial that all health care providers learn to perform an accurate and complete assessment of the skin, it is more important to teach every individual how to do a skin self-examination. Routine self-examination greatly lowers individual risk for severe skin disorders, such as skin cancer. Teach clients to examine their entire bodies to look for any changes in the skin or their moles or skin lesions. See the Client Education Guide in Chapter 49.

Danger signals to look for are the *ABCDs* of melanoma:

A = *Asymmetry*: one half unlike the other half;
B = *Border*: irregular, scalloped, or poorly circumscribed border;
C = *Color*: varied from one area to another, shades of two colors, or changing colors;
D = *Diameter*: larger than 6 mm as a rule (diameter of a No. 2 pencil eraser).

Also see the Physical Assessment Findings in the Healthy Adult feature in this chapter. Encourage clients to visit their health care provider for further evaluation of any suspicious-looking lesions.

DIAGNOSTIC TESTS

Before a diagnostic skin procedure (or treatment), perform an assessment and document findings. Nursing intervention for diagnostic procedures includes explaining the procedure to the client and significant others and allowing them to ask questions and express concerns. Explain appropriate wound care and indications of possible side effects and complications that should be reported, such as prolonged bleeding or infection (indicated by swelling, redness, drainage, increased discomfort, or temperature elevation).

Provide instructions (preferably written) for follow-up care as well as follow-up appointment and telephone number. Documentation of diagnostic procedures (exactly what was done and by whom) and the specific location of the lesion must be completed by appropriate personnel.

■ SKIN CULTURE AND SENSITIVITY

Bacterial infections of the skin can be confirmed by culture. Because of the cost and delay in getting results, culture is usually reserved for infections that have been nonresponsive to routine care. Clients who have had frequent courses of systemic antibiotics and still experience skin infections are candidates for a culture and sensitivity test to determine which antibiotic is indicated for treatment.

■ POTASSIUM HYDROXIDE EXAMINATION AND FUNGAL CULTURE

Fungal infection of skin, hair, or nails may be confirmed by microscopic identification or culture of scrapings from the area or both. Any area of scaly dermatitis may be scraped for this test. Typical sites are the scalp, intertriginous areas (between the toes, axillae, groin, under or between the breasts, abdominal folds), and the nailfold.

Fine scales from the edge of the site are scraped with a No. 15 scalpel blade or the edge of a glass slide onto a second glass slide. A drop of 10% to 20% potassium hydroxide is added to the scale, and a coverslip is placed over the specimen. Gentle pressure is applied to the coverslip to flatten the scales. The slide may be gently heated to dissolve the keratin or the cells more quickly. The scrapings are examined under the microscope. For a culture, scrapings from a suspicious lesion are implanted in the appropriate culture medium. For a nail culture, an altered, dystrophic nail is snipped and implanted in the medium. Debris from the nail's subungual area is less suitable for culture.

■ TZANCK'S SMEAR

Tzanck's smear is used for microscopic assessment of fluids and cells from vesicles or bullae. The presence of multinucleated giant cells establishes a diagnosis of viral infection, such as herpes simplex or herpes zoster infection. An intact, recently evolved vesicle's top is removed, and its base is scraped with a scalpel or small curet. The debris is smeared onto a labeled slide and sent for cytologic assessment.

■ SCABIES SCRAPING

The most difficult part of the test for scabies is selecting an unscratched lesion from which to take the specimen. Often several areas need to be prepared. When visible, a linear burrow is sampled to look for the mite, its eggs, or feces. The top of the lesion is shaved off with a No. 15 scalpel blade. The shavings are placed on a microscope slide, covered with immersion oil and a coverslip, and examined under low power on the microscope. Local anesthesia is not necessary, and fine bleeding is expected. Some discomfort occurs when the lesion is opened.

■ WOOD'S LIGHT EXAMINATION

Wood's light ("black light") uses a high-pressure mercury lamp that transmits long-wave ultraviolet light (UVA), or 360 nm; it has several diagnostic uses. For example, Wood's light can (1) detect superficial fungal and bacterial skin infections, (2) delineate pigmentary disorders by highlighting the degree of contrast between lesions and normal skin color, and (3) accentuate the contrast between hypopigmented and totally amelanotic areas. Wood's light examination is done in a darkened room. The procedure is painless.

■ PATCH TESTING

Patch testing is done in order to identify substances that produce allergic skin responses. It is a painless procedure, and a skilled evaluator must be on hand to read and interpret the results. Patch testing is often done to differentiate between an *irritant* contact dermatitis and an *aller-*

gic contact dermatitis. Small amounts of various substances or allergens are applied to the skin using a commercially prepared tape containing the allergens, or allergens are placed on aluminum discs on a special tape. The client and significant others need to understand that whereas potential allergic substances (allergens) can produce inflammatory skin reactions, compounds of low concentration are used to prevent possible excessive irritation.

Patch testing should not be performed if acute dermatitis is present; the potential allergen may worsen the dermatitis.

The tape must be worn for 48 hours without disturbing the patches; then it is removed. Interpretations are made at 48, 72, and 96 hours and sometimes at 1 week. An eczematous response at the test site with erythema, papules, or small vesicles indicates a positive reaction and confirms an allergic contact sensitivity to the substance on the disc.

■ BIOPSY

Skin biopsy refers to removal of a skin tissue specimen for histologic (cellular microscopic) assessment. There are three types: shave, dermal punch, and surgical excision. In all three procedures, local anesthesia is used. Small-gauge (26- to 30-gauge) needles are recommended to limit trauma to the skin.

Depending on the size and location of the biopsy specimen and the skill of the practitioner, the procedure is usually quick and almost painless. The most common source of pain is the initial administration of local anesthetic. The specimen is placed in a preservative such as formalin solution, properly identified, and sent for pathologic assessment. Use clean or sterile technique, as appropriate, to dress or cover the biopsy site.

PROCEDURES

SHAVE BIOPSY

A shave biopsy is performed to obtain tissue for analysis from possibly malignant epidermal growths except potential melanoma (Fig. 48–5*A*). After skin cleaning and infiltration of local anesthesia, tissue is removed with a lateral motion by use of a scalpel with a No. 15 blade. Alternatively, a specimen can be obtained by snipping with curved tissue scissors. Tissue removed includes the epidermis and upper portions of the dermal layers.

Hemostasis of the biopsy site is obtained by applying pressure, by using ferric subsulfate (Monsel's solution) or aluminum chloride solution, or by instituting electrodesiccation (cautery).

PUNCH BIOPSY

For a dermal punch biopsy, a circular instrument with a sharp cutting edge is used to remove a specimen of skin

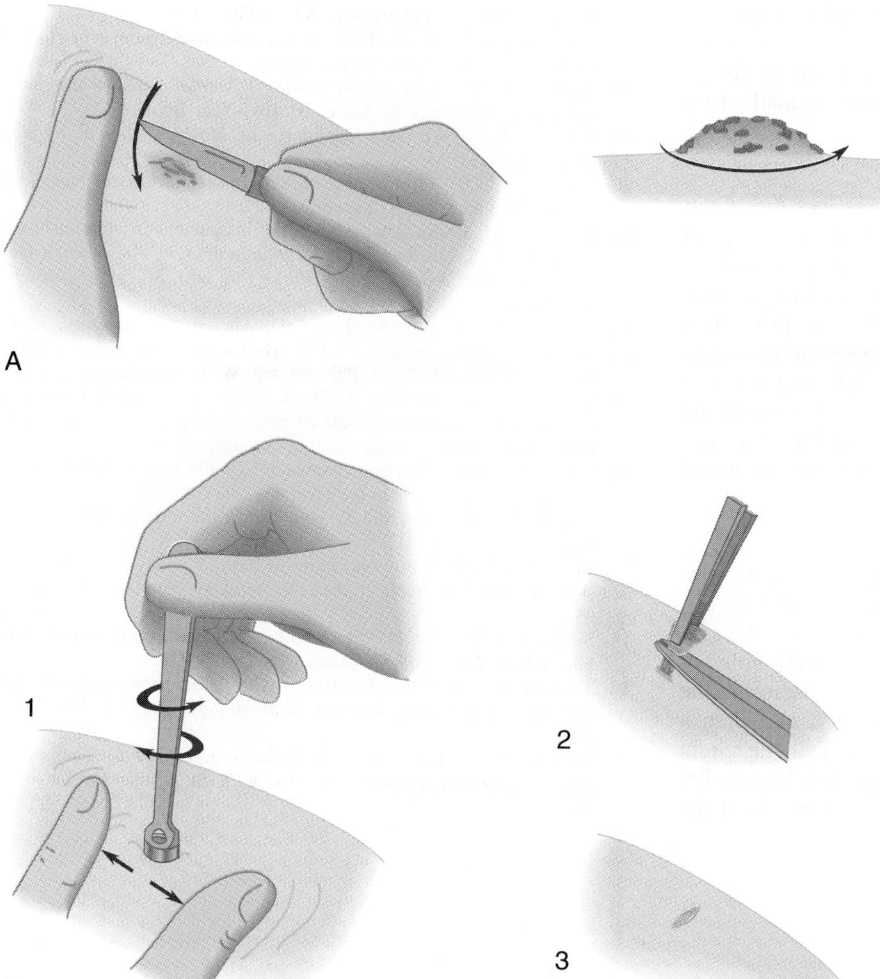

FIGURE 48–5 Skin biopsies. *A, Shave* biopsy. A tissue specimen is obtained by use of a scalpel (No. 15 blade) in a horizontal-lateral motion. *B, Punch* biopsy. A tissue specimen is obtained with the instrument pressed down firmly on the skin. The specimen is freed from surrounding tissue by a rotary back-and-forth cutting motion. The specimen base is severed with tissue scissors.

that includes epidermal, dermal, and subcutaneous tissue. This method is used to obtain a biopsy specimen of a well-developed, mature lesion (Fig. 48–5*B*). An appropriate-sized punch is chosen (from 2 to 6 mm). The skin site is cleaned, and a local anesthetic is injected. Skin surrounding the lesion is stretched taut, and the punch is pressed firmly downward into the skin site. The instrument is rotated back and forth in a cutting motion that frees the specimen from surrounding tissue. The specimen is then gently grasped with a tissue forceps or needle, and its base is severed with scissors or a scalpel blade.

Depending on the size of the specimen, hemostasis can be achieved with pressure or application of Monsel's solution or aluminum chloride solution. The oval defect may be closed with a 4-0 or 5-0 silk or nylon suture to produce a linear scar. Sutures are removed after about 7 to 14 days (with facial biopsies, 3 to 5 days).

SURGICAL EXCISION BIOPSY

The surgical excision biopsy is used (1) when it is necessary to excise a lesion completely (e.g., when full skin thickness is needed), (2) when a lesion's borders are indistinct from surrounding skin, or (3) when there is a recurrent or aggressive cancer, such as malignant melanoma. The site is cleansed, the excisional lines are marked with a gentian violet pen, and local anesthetic is administered. The lesion is excised with a scalpel by means of a variety of surgical techniques; a commonly used technique is an elliptical incision.

Hemostasis is achieved with pressure and ligation (suturing closed) of superficial vessels. The incision is closed with sutures. The suture site is rinsed with saline-dampened gauze. A pressure dressing of sterile nonadhering gauze is applied and taped in place.

PREPROCEDURE CARE

Depending on the size of the excision, instruct the client to avoid the use of aspirin and products containing aspirin for 48 hours before the biopsy to avoid a prolonged postprocedure bleeding time. If the client is taking anticoagulants (e.g., heparin or warfarin), notify the physician. Review the client's medical history for systemic disorders such as liver malfunction, which affects clotting time. If the client has a history of cardiac valve replacement, be sure that prophylactic antibiotics are prescribed. The client should eat a light meal before the procedure to avoid syncope (fainting).

POSTPROCEDURE CARE

After the procedure, cover the majority of biopsy sites with an antibiotic ointment and a clean bandage or dry dressing unless ordered otherwise. Many nonadhesive types of dressings are available and may be preferable for clients who have fragile or sensitive skin. Remind the client that follow-up assessment is necessary, and plan a follow-up appointment for suture removal. Tell the client how and when biopsy results will be reported. Remember that individuals have different levels of anxiety about the biopsy results, depending on the anticipated possible outcome (e.g., melanoma versus wart).

CONCLUSIONS

Although the skin is the largest organ in the body, it is often taken for granted. The skin protects us from the sun and many dangerous elements and helps fight diseases and infections. The top layers of healthy skin have the ability to regenerate and repair themselves every 3 to 4 weeks. Skin must be handled with care to maintain its many functions.

BIBLIOGRAPHY

1. Arnold, H. L., Odom, R. B., & James, W. D. (1990). *Andrew's diseases of the skin* (8th ed.). Philadelphia: W. B. Saunders.
2. Bates, B. (1995). *A guide to physical examination* (6th ed.). Philadelphia: J. B. Lippincott.
3. Burrage, R., et al. (1991). Physical assessment. An overview with sections on the skin, eye, ear, nose and neck. In W. Chenitz, et al. (Eds.), *Clinical gerontological nursing*. Philadelphia: W. B. Saunders.
4. Callen, J. P. (1995). *Current practice in dermatology*. Philadelphia: W. B. Saunders.
5. Dellasega, C., & Burgunder, C. (1991). Perioperative nursing care for the elderly surgical patient. *Todays OR Nurse, 13*(6), 12–17.
6. Dermatology Nurses' Association. (1998). *Dermatology nursing essentials: A core curriculum*. Pitman, NJ: Anthony J. Jannetti.
7. Fitzpatrick, T. B., & Eisen, T. B. (1992). *Dermatology in general medicine* (4th ed.). Hightstown, NJ: McGraw-Hill.
8. Fitzpatrick, T. B., et al. (1997). *Color atlas and synopsis of clinical dermatology*. New York: McGraw-Hill.
9. Habif, T. (1996). *Clinical dermatology: A color guide to diagnosis and therapy* (3rd ed.). St. Louis: Mosby–Year Book.
10. Hill, M. J. (1994). Skin disorders. In *Mosby's clinical nursing series*. St. Louis: Mosby–Year Book.
11. Jarvis, C. (2000). *Physical examination and health assessment* (3rd ed.). Philadelphia: W. B. Saunders.
12. Nicol, N. H. (1998). Alteration in the integument in children. In J. McCance & S. Huetner (Eds.), *Pathophysiology: The biologic basics for disease in adults and children* (3rd ed.). St. Louis: Mosby–Year Book.
13. Nicol, N. H., & Hill, M. J. (1994). Altered skin integrity. In R. Foster, M. Hunsberger, & C. Betz (Eds.), *Family-centered nursing care of children* (2nd ed.). Philadelphia: W. B. Saunders.
14. Nicol, N. H., Ruszkowski, A. M., & Moore, J. A. (1995, February). Contact dermatitis and the role of patch testing in its diagnosis and management. *Dermatology Nursing, Supplement*, 5–10.
15. Pogue, S. (1992). Nursing assessment of the elderly for dermatologic procedures. *Dermatology Nursing, 4*(1), 15–23.
16. Pogue, S. (1995). Vitamin D synthesis in the elderly. *Dermatology Nursing, 7*(2), 103–105.
17. Rudy, S. (1991). From conception to birth: The development of the skin and nursing implications. *Dermatology Nursing, 3*(6), 381–392.
18. Sinni-McKeehen, B. (1995). Health effects and regulation of tanning salons. *Dermatology Nursing, 7*(5), 307–312.
19. Truscott, W., & Roley, L. (1995). Glove-associated reactions: Addressing an increasing concern. *Dermatology Nursing, 7*(5), 283–292.
20. Weston, W. L., Lane, A. T., & Morelli, J. G. (1996). *Color textbook of pediatric dermatology* (2nd ed.). St. Louis: Mosby–Year Book.

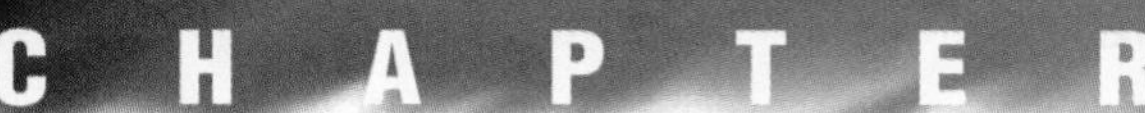

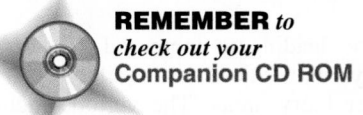

CHAPTER 49

Management of Clients with Integumentary Disorders

Noreen Heer Nicol
Joyce M. Black

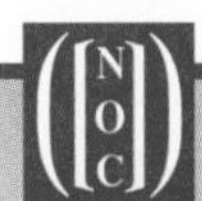

NURSING OUTCOMES CLASSIFICATION (NOC)
for Nursing Diagnoses—Clients with Integumentary Disorders

Altered Tissue Perfusion: Peripheral
Sensory Function: Cutaneous
Tissue Perfusion: Peripheral
Anxiety
Aggression Control
Anxiety Control
Coping
Impulse Control
Self-Mutilation Restraint
Social Interaction Skills
Body Image Disturbances
Body Image
Grief Resolution
Psychosocial Adjustment: Life Change
Self-Esteem
Chronic Low Self-Esteem
Self-Esteem
Fear
Fear Control
Impaired Skin Integrity
Tissue Integrity: Skin and Mucous Membranes
Wound Healing: Primary Intention
Wound Healing: Secondary Intention
Pain
Comfort Level
Pain Control
Pain: Disruptive Effects
Pain Level
Risk for Infection
Immobility Consequences: Physiologic
Immune Status
Immunization Behavior
Knowledge: Infection Control
Risk Control
Risk Detection
Risk for Impaired Skin Integrity
Immobility Consequences: Physiologic
Nutritional Status
Nutritional Status: Biochemical Measures
Physical Aging Status
Risk Detection
Tissue Integrity: Skin and Mucous Membranes
Wound Healing: Primary Intention
Wound Healing: Secondary Intention
Sleep Pattern Disturbance
Anxiety Control
Rest
Sleep
Well-Being
Ineffective Management of Therapeutic Regimen: Individual
Compliance Behavior
Knowledge Treatment Regimen
Participation: Health Care Decisions
Treatment Behavior: Illness and Injury

The skin is the largest and most visible organ of the body. Thus, disorders of the skin offer the nurse an opportunity to provide care that makes a noticeable and rewarding difference to clients. Five primary dermatologic therapies—topical medications, wound dressings, soaks and wet wraps, skin lubricants, and ultraviolet light (UVL) therapy—are reviewed in this chapter. These therapies are the most common interventions provided by nurses for a variety of dermatologic conditions.

TOPICAL MEDICATIONS

■ TOPICAL THERAPY

The skin's large surface area allows the absorption, penetration, and permeation of topically applied preparations. The factors that determine how well these processes occur include the client's age, the size of the affected region, the condition of the stratum corneum, the cutaneous blood supply, and the medication vehicle (the word *vehicle* is used here to mean the substance containing the medication or the form in which the medication is delivered).

Topical therapy can be used to:

- Restore hydration
- Alleviate clinical manifestations
- Reduce inflammation
- Protect the skin
- Reduce scale and callus
- Clean and debride
- Eradicate causative organisms

Topical medications are chosen both for the action of the active ingredients (which are delivered directly to the skin surface) and for the vehicle. Topical medications have many different actions and cover a large spectrum of drug categories, including anti-infective, corticosteroid, and antipruritic (Table 49–1).

■ TOPICAL VEHICLES

Examples of various topical medication vehicles (Table 49–2) are ointments, creams, gels, aerosols, lotions, solutions, and powders. Ointments are more occlusive and therefore provide better delivery of the medication by preventing water loss from the skin. However, in some cases, especially under conditions of excessive heat or humidity, this occlusion may result in increased itching or skin infection; in such cases, creams may be better tolerated. Although creams spread more easily than ointments, they are less occlusive, leading to increased skin drying in some people. Sprays and lotions are available for use on the scalp and other hairy areas. The various ingredients used to formulate the different bases may be irritating to the skin, and care must be taken in recommending any product.

Both the active ingredient and the vehicle must be appropriate for the condition being treated. For acute dermatosis (i.e., weeping, blistering lesions), an aqueous (water-based) compound provides a drying effect. A greasy vehicle has the opposite effect; it promotes lubrication and occlusion and helps treat the dryness and scaling caused by chronic dermatosis. Differences in skin permeability also influence the effectiveness of topical medications. For example, absorption is increased in inflamed skin. Depending on the medication and the specific condition, topical medication may be applied to localized lesions or to larger skin

TABLE 49–1 NURSING IMPLICATIONS FOR MEDICATIONS USED TO TREAT SKIN DISORDERS

Class (Example)	Assessing Therapeutic Responses	Assessing Adverse Responses	Nursing Implications
Corticosteroids Triamcinolone (Kenalog)	Inflamed areas should become less red, painful, and swollen	Assess for thinning of skin and delayed healing	Apply evenly over skin Use with caution in clients with systemic bacterial, fungal, or viral infections May be applied to hydrated skin to increase penetration
Antipruritics *Wet Dressings* Potassium permanganate 1:4000–1:16,000) Aluminum acetate Burow's solution (1:10–1:40) Boric acid (1 tbsp in 1 L of water) Normal saline (2 tsp salt in 1 L of water) Magnesium sulfate (8 tsp in 1 L of water)	Pruritic areas should become less "itchy," and evidence of scratching should decrease	Assess for allergy or contact sensitivity to substances	Use in bathtub for full body immersion or on dressings for local use Use caution in tub bathing; solutions are slippery Protect linens from stains when wet dressings are used
Topical Lotions Calamine lotion			Apply frequently unless solution contains anesthetic agents; then apply as directed
Anti-infectives Bacitracin and polymyxin B (Polysporin)	Reduce or eliminate bacterial infection	Superinfection Allergic reaction	Remove adherent crust before applying Apply 1–4 times/day
Nystatin (Mycostatin)	Reduce or eliminate fungal infection	Nausea, vomiting, diarrhea	Requires twice-daily application for 2–3 wk
Lindane (Kwell)	Eradicate scabies and pediculosis	Vomiting, restlessness, ataxia, seizures Observe for reinfestation	Treat webs of fingers and toes Avoid eyes Full course of treatment must be completed
Benzoyl peroxide	Decreased number of anaerobic bacteria and free fatty acids in sebaceous follicles	Extreme dryness, redness, or scaling	Apply once or twice daily after washing Apply sparingly Improvement should occur in 2 weeks

TABLE 49–2 TOPICAL MEDICATION VEHICLES

Category	Examples	Action	Use	Nursing Implications
Powders	Talc, cornstarch	Leaves a film of powder May absorb fluid	Intertriginous dermatitis	Dry surface before applying to prevent caking; reapply often
Lotions				
Suspension-based	Calamine lotion	Leaves a thin film of powder as water evaporates	Pruritus	Shake lotions well before applying Observe for overdrying of skin Apply in long, even strokes along direction of hair growth
Solutions	Salicylic acid	Leaves a film of powder as alcohol base evaporates	Warts, acne	Shake well before applying; observe for skin overdrying and drying and tightness of skin due to alcohol Apply as for suspension
Aerosols	Triamcinolone acetonide aerosol	Leaves a thin film after alcohol evaporates	Pruritus, when direct application is painful	Shake well before applying; prevent inhalation by turning client's face to the side
Gels	Fluocinonide gel	Promotes drying of the skin	Eczema Pruritic rash	Observe for skin drying; avoid application to open skin areas
Creams	Hydrocortisone cream Eucerin	Leaves medication on skin after evaporation	Pruritus Eczema	Apply in thin layer along direction of hair growth Use during daytime Reapply often because perspiration or drainage may remove preparation
Ointments	Hydrocortisone ointment			
Water-in-oil	—	Lubricates skin	Xerosis Dermatitis	Removable with soap and water
Absorbent	Aquaphor	Lubricates skin	Xerosis, dermatitis	Difficult to remove; may feel greasy
Water-repellent	Petrolatum	Promotes absorption of water and medication	Xerosis, dermatitis	Retains heat, difficult to remove; observe for maceration; avoid use in hair-bearing areas

surfaces. When increased absorption of the medication is needed, topical medication may be prescribed for application under an occlusive dressing (Table 49–3). Ointments, creams, and gels have greatly increased absorption if they are applied to skin that is wet.

■ TOPICAL CORTICOSTEROIDS

Corticosteroids are among the most commonly used topical medications for treatment of a variety of dermatologic conditions. Corticosteroids can also be injected directly

TABLE 49–3 OCCLUSIVE DRESSINGS FOR INCREASED ABSORPTION OF MEDICATION

Purpose/Desired Effect	Nursing Implications
Produces airtight barrier, usually with plastic film Enhances absorption of topically applied medication (e.g., corticosteroids, keratolytics) by preventing evaporation Increases stratum corneum rehydration Softens hyperkeratotic areas by moisture retention	Clean skin site of debris and "old" medication before applying prescribed topical medication Apply topical medication while skin is still damp Apply plastic film (e.g., Saran wrap) snugly Use plastic bags for feet, polyethylene gloves for hands, plastic shower cap for scalp Press air out; seal borders with paper tape Leave dressing intact for 2–12 hr (as prescribed); then remove and gently cleanse the site Observe and document complications—maceration, oozing, signs of secondary fungal or bacterial infection, folliculitis With prolonged use in conjunction with topical corticosteroids, striae, nonhealing ulcerations, telangiectases, erythema, and skin atrophy may develop

into the lesion or given systemically. Attempts to diagnose the condition before any corticosteroid use are important because the effects of the medication can mask or change the clinical manifestations. Topical corticosteroids reduce inflammation by relieving itching, by reducing blood flow via vasoconstriction, which reduces redness of the skin from capillary dilation (erythema), and by interfering with the action of inflammatory cells.

A large selection of topical steroids, ranging in potency from low to high, is available today. Low-potency topical steroids are now available in over-the-counter (OTC) formulations (e.g., hydrocortisone, 0.5% or 1.0%) and in prescription strength (e.g., desonide, alclometasone). Generally, low-potency steroids are safe to use for longer periods of time and even on thin-skinned areas like the face, groin, or axilla. Prolonged use should still be monitored. Medium-potency (e.g., triamcinolone, fluocinolone) to high-potency (e.g., halcinonide, fluocinonide) corticosteroids should be used with caution and for short periods of time and not on the face, groin, or axilla. High-potency or superhigh-potency (e.g., betamethasone dipropionate, clobestasol) steroids should be reserved for use on very acute or resistant dermatoses (e.g., contact dermatitis) or areas with thick plaque such as in psoriasis.

Clients should know the strength of the topical steroid they are taking and its potential side effects. The lowest-potency corticosteroid that is effective should be used. Side effects are more likely with prolonged use of medium-potency to high-potency topical corticosteroids. The most common side effect is skin atrophy, which presents as thin, shiny skin with increased prominence of blood vessels, telangiectases, easy bruising, and striae.

Clients must clearly understand how, when, and where to use topical steroids. Properly applying the medication evenly and sparingly once or twice daily to the affected areas can eliminate many potential problems. It is rarely helpful to apply the topical corticosteroid more than twice a day. More frequent application increases the chance of side effects, makes the therapy more costly, and does not usually increase effectiveness. As the skin disorder resolves, the frequency of use may be changed or a less potent topical corticosteroid prescribed. The condition can recur if treatment is stopped abruptly. When the skin disease disappears or comes under good control, a tar preparation, moisturizer, or other topical preparation may be substituted for the topical steroid.

WOUND DRESSINGS

Application of wound dressings allows control of the affected skin's environment and remains important in the treatment of wounds, ulcers, and recalcitrant dermatitis. Historically, the primary role of wound dressings has been protection. Today, the role of dressings is to create an environment that promotes healing (see Table 49–3). Dressings limit the exposure of injured skin to dirt, mechanical trauma, and irritants. Ulcers and denuded skin heal more quickly when kept damp by an occlusive or semi-occlusive dressing because regenerating epithelium migrates more easily across a moist surface. These wounds are also less painful when kept damp, and absorption of topical medications is enhanced.

The clinician is challenged to understand the properties of the hundreds of wound care dressings on the market. Wound dressing materials include film, hydrocolloid, hydrogel, foam, alginates, and gauze, among others (see Table 49–3).

■ UNNA BOOT

The Unna boot, a dressing designed to be removed only by medical personnel at a later clinical visit, can be extremely useful for treatment of stasis ulcers in clients who have venous insufficiency or in whom there is a concern about compliance, scratching, or even self-injury. The Unna boot is a fixed, protective dressing applied to the foot and ankle that stimulates granulation tissue and restores epithelial growth. It is made from dressing materials impregnated with zinc oxide paste, glycerin, and gelatin, which harden into a cast-like "boot" after application. The "boot" protects the skin from mechanical injury, promoting venous return.

Before application, the damaged skin surface is gently irrigated with warm saline to remove previous medication and debris. The damaged skin area is then measured and assessed. Prescribed topical agents (i.e., antibiotic ointments) may be applied. Next, starting at the dorsum of the foot, the dressing is applied. It is wrapped obliquely over the heel and up the calf. The greatest pressure is applied at the ankle and over the lower third of the leg. The boot ends just below the popliteal space. A layer of tube gauze is applied over the dressing. For additional support, an elastic bandage is secured appropriately with tape. The Unna boot is usually removed weekly so that damaged skin can be assessed and normal skin cleaned.

Ideally, with all wound dressings, the area of damaged skin decreases, granulation tissue forms, and signs of inflammation are reduced. Treatment may continue for weeks until improvement occurs. Instruct the client and family numbers to keep the dressing intact and to notify the primary health care provider if there is excessive drainage or localized pain (signs of infection). Routine follow-up examination is very important in wound care.

SOAKS AND WET WRAPS

Soaks serve several purposes. Moisture softens dry epidermis, which aids in removal of crusts. Removal of cellular skin debris promotes healing and improves absorption of topical medication. The risk of infection is reduced by removal of necrotic tissue and occlusive crusts. Cooling also results from the gradual evaporation of water and has an anti-inflammatory effect, thus relieving itching (pruritus).

Soaks can be accomplished by either soaking the affected area or bathing for 15 to 20 minutes in warm—not hot—tap water. The agent added to the soaks is the least important aspect of this therapy. Addition of substances such as colloidal oatmeal (Aveeno) or starch to the bath water may be soothing for some people but does nothing to increase water absorption. Coal tar preparations (Balnetar, T/Derm) have an anti-inflammatory effect and can be helpful in some eczematous and psoriatic conditions. Aluminum acetate (Burow solution), aluminum sulfate and calcium acetate (Domeboro), and povidone-iodine (Betadine) are also effective antibacterial substances; however, they have drying effects. Bath oils are not recommended because they give the client a false sense of lubrication and make the bathtub very slippery.

After bathing, clients should remove excess water by gently patting the skin with a soft towel. Then they should immediately apply the recommended occlusive substance. Immediate application of this substance to damp skin is the most important detail, because if the occlusive barrier is not provided within 3 to 5 minutes, evaporation begins to occur.

Wet wraps used immediately after soaking and occlusion can optimize hydration and topical therapy; this also promotes cooling of the skin. Wet wraps and occlusion can be applied in various ways. The location and severity of lesions often determine the choices. Total-body wet wraps can be accomplished by putting on wet pajamas or wet long underwear followed by dry pajamas or a dry or plastic sweat suit. The hands and feet can be covered with wet tube socks or wet cotton gloves followed by dry tube socks. Any extremity or the trunk can be covered with wet rolled (e.g., Kerlix) gauze and occluded with elastic bandages or by pieces of tube sock, wet followed by dry. The face can be wrapped with two layers of wet Kerlix gauze, followed by two layers of dry Kerlix gauze held in place with elasticized netting or other tubular dressings; holes are cut out for the eyes, nose, and mouth (Fig. 49–1). If the dressing becomes dry, it should be rewetted before removal because debridement by the wet-to-dry method produces tissue damage and pain. Gentle debridement usually still occurs if dressings are removed when damp.

SKIN LUBRICANTS

Agents to hydrate the skin play an important role in many xerotic, pruritic, and inflammatory skin disorders. Measures to prevent skin dryness include elimination of irritating or drying compounds, which may include *soaps* and *solvents,* and use of *cleansing agents* and *moisturizers.* Moisturizers may be classified as follows:

1. *Occlusive* preparations are extremely effective when applied to damp skin because they prevent evaporative water loss and replace oils in the stratum corneum. The primary means of correcting dryness is to add water to the skin by bathing and then apply an occlusive substance to retain the absorbed water. To seal in the water, use occlusives such as white petrolatum (Vaseline) or petrolatum with mineral oil and wool wax alcohol (Aquaphor ointment). Occlusives are greasy and may be cosmetically unacceptable to some people.
2. *Emollients* contain fatty acids, oil, and other agents that soften and soothe the skin. There are many emollients available in the form of creams and lotions. Creams contain less water than lotions and therefore evaporate less quickly and provide more skin hydration. Clients often prefer these cosmetically pleasing products because they can be rubbed into the skin without leaving a greasy residue. Although the chemicals in these lotions provide benefit, the water loss continues. Lotions and creams may be irritating and drying because of the evaporative property of water and the substances used as preservatives, solubilizers, and fragrances.
3. If emollient products are not successful, more potent agents may be necessary. *Humectants* are substances such as urea (Aquacare 10%, Carmol 20% to 40%) that attract and hold water, which results in transepidermal water migration, and they have a concentration-dependent desquamation action. Ammonium lactate (Lactydrin) is also an effective keratolytic which moisturizes and thickens the stratum corneum. The alpha-hydroxy acids (AHAs) have become extremely popular and effective additives; these hold moisture and reduce the rough scale that creates the sensation of dryness. The AHAs are naturally derived organic acids and include citric acid, glycolic acid, malic acid, and tartaric acid. Many of the AHAs have been used for years; the industry has invested in reformulating and promoting these products. Also popular with clients are additives such as aloe, vitamin E, jojoba, elastin, and collagen; however, no scientific evidence has shown that these substances have special, intrinsic properties beyond their minimal lubricating effects. Clients should be taught the basic principles of hydration and moisturization to avoid spending unnecessarily high prices for any needed products.

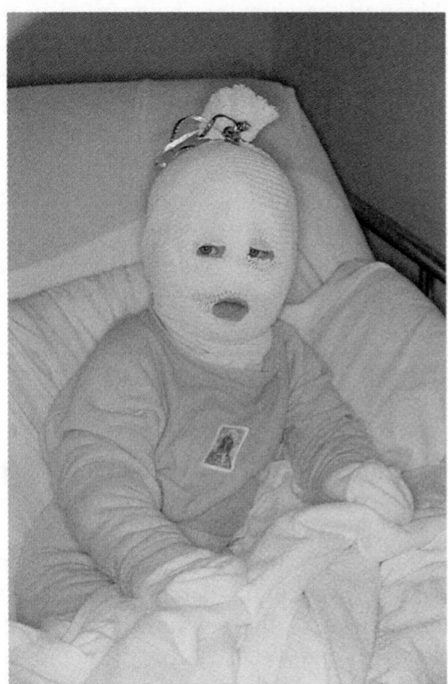

FIGURE 49–1 Wet wraps applied to the entire body.

ULTRAVIOLET LIGHT THERAPY

Artificially reproduced forms of ultraviolet light (UVL) are used therapeutically with topical or systemic photosensitizing drugs to cause desquamation (shedding or peeling of the epidermis). UVL also temporarily suppresses mitosis of the basal cell layer by inhibiting deoxyribonucleic acid (DNA) mitosis. Ultraviolet A (UVA) light and ultraviolet B (UVB) light are used to treat diseases responsive to UVL, such as psoriasis, vitiligo, cutaneous T-cell lymphoma, uremic pruritus, and chronic eczematous eruptions. At present, three treatment modalities involve UVL: (1) UVA; (2) UVB, in the Goeckerman or modified Goeckerman regimen; and (3) photochemotherapy, or PUVA (psoralen plus UVA). Many of these regimens are given two or three times a week initially, and the frequency is then decreased to two to four times per month.

Obtain a complete history and physical examination in every client before initiation of any UVL therapy. Record the highlights of the client's history; take care to include the complete medication history, because the client may be taking one or more of the many photosensitizing drugs (e.g., thiazide diuretics, tetracyclines). Ask clients specifically about previous herpes simplex infections, which can be stimulated by UVL. Pre-treatment assessment includes identifying solar energy–induced skin malignancies, cataracts, or lupus erythematosus and any additional photosensitive skin changes. Clients with a history of basal cell or squamous cell epithelioma are at risk for additional neoplastic changes with this treatment. Thus, potential benefit is weighed against potential risk.

A complete ophthalmologic examination before treatment begins is important and should be performed yearly during long-term treatment. A history of cataract formation is a potential contraindication to PUVA therapy. Clients who exhibit early cataract changes need extra photoprotective measures (e.g., the complete occlusion provided by goggles or PUVA glasses) and more frequent ophthalmologic assessments (every 3 to 6 months). The skin changes of lupus erythematosus are worsened by sun exposure, and phototherapy is thus contraindicated. Before therapy is initiated, an antinuclear antibody (ANA) test should rule out this condition when suspected.

Be aware that because treatments to the face and genitalia add to the cumulative effects of UVL, minimal exposure is indicated. Periodic assessments must be done throughout the course of therapy for signs of actinic damage (e.g., severe wrinkling, "tissue paper" transparency) or cutaneous malignancy. After completion of therapy, clients must be observed for potential side effects including dry skin, pruritus, and potential delayed (36 to 48 hours after exposure) phototoxic reaction (erythema, vesicles, and pain). All phototherapy should be administered by qualified and well-trained dermatologic personnel. Use of home UVL equipment and tanning salons should be considered only when the client has no access to qualified dermatologic personnel. Numerous risks are associated with home and salon therapy.

■ ULTRAVIOLET B THERAPY

UVB therapy requires no oral medications and is usually the first-line UVL therapy used before progression to PUVA. Types of UVB therapy include (1) plain UVB treatment, (2) UVB with topical tar and topical anthralin, the *Ingram method,* and (3) UVB with topical tar, referred to as the Goeckerman treatment or regimen.

One of the most common types of UVB therapy is the *Goeckerman regimen* and variants of it. The photosensitizing, keratoplastic, and antipruritic properties of topical tar preparations are used in conjunction with UVL in UVB wavelengths. This method is often used to treat psoriasis vulgaris and atopic dermatitis. The regimen includes a therapeutic tar emulsion bath, followed by an application of topical tar medication (e.g., crude coal tar in petrolatum). Several hours later, a specific dose of UVL is administered to the skin surface. If the skin condition is severe, hospitalization or daily care in an ambulatory or day care setting may be necessary for this treatment. Outpatient phototherapy, combined with treatment baths and tar applications at home, can be helpful for clients with less severe involvement.

■ PHOTOCHEMOTHERAPY

Photochemotherapy (PUVA) combines oral or topical 8-methoxypsoralen with UVA. PUVA is used to treat severe, unresponsive forms of psoriaris, atopic dermatitis, cutaneous T-cell lymphoma, and alopecia areata or vitiligo. The potent systemic photosensitizing medications used in PUVA increase skin sensitivity to long-wave UVL (UVA). In conjunction with exposure to artificially reproduced forms of UVA light, these medications induce repigmentation (melanin production) in vitiligo and have an antimitotic effect in psoriasis and cutaneous T-cell lymphoma.

Dosage is determined by body weight. The medication is taken orally with food to minimize nausea 1 to 2 hours before UVL irradiation. Topical medication is used to treat localized sites and for clients in whom systemic administration is contraindicated (such as clients with liver or renal disease).

The skin must be protected from ambient UVL irradiation before and for 8 hours after taking the photosensitizing medication. The client should (1) wear protective clothing, such as long sleeves, (2) apply sunscreen to exposed skin, (3) minimize natural skin exposure, and (4) wear dark green or brown plastic sunglasses that can screen both UVA and UVB to protect the eyes for 48 hours after taking the medication.

■ COMBINATION THERAPIES

Many combination therapies are being used in phototherapy units across the United States. These include PUVA with various topical medications, PUVA with retinoid therapy (RE-PUVA), PUVA with methotrexate, PUVA with cyclosporine, PUVA with UVB therapy, UVB therapy with retinoids, and UVB with methotrexate. The purpose of combination therapy is to accelerate clearing of lesions and to reduce the total cumulative dose of UVL. These therapies should be administered according to protocol and by highly qualified dermatologic personnel.

PSYCHOSOCIAL ASPECTS OF SKIN DISORDERS

Anger, frustration, and anxiety are commonly experienced by clients with skin disorders, which often exacerbates the condition. Clients with skin disease are more likely to respond to stress, frustration, embarrassment, or any emotionally upsetting event with itching and scratching. Excitability and arousal of the central nervous system from an emotional upset can intensify the vasomotor and sweat responses in the skin, leading to the *itch-scratch-itch cy-*

cle (see Pruritus). In some instances, scratching is used as an expression of anger, because typically it will get an immediate response from those nearby. The added dimension of family hostility, rejection, and guilt can damage the family structure.

Learning about the acute or chronic nature of the given disorder, the exacerbating factors, and the management measures that can control it is important for both the client and family members. Maintaining a healthy outlook is important. Counseling and other psychosocial interventions are often helpful in dealing with the frustrations of skin disease, especially for adolescents and young adults, who may consider the lesions disfiguring.

The educational needs of people affected by skin disease are vast. Health care providers need to consistently provide information that includes detailed skin care plans, general disease information, and availability of client-oriented support organizations as well as updates on encouraging research results. Clients tend to forget or confuse the important skin care recommendations without written instructions. Clearly outlining the skin care recommendations orally and in writing is essential for good outcomes.

The accompanying Client Education Guide provides information about skin self-examination. Nurses play the major role in providing this important aspect of care. Adequate time and client teaching materials are needed to provide education effectively. Be resourceful in obtaining or writing educational materials and instruction sheets. Client education pamphlets are available through a variety of sources, including the many dermatologically oriented client support groups and professional dermatology agencies such as the Dermatology Nurses' Association and the American Academy of Dermatology.

CLIENT EDUCATION GUIDE

Skin Self-Examination

You will need a bright light; a full-length mirror; a hand mirror; two chairs or stools; a blow dryer; body maps; and a pencil.

A. Examine your face—especially the nose, lips, mouth, and ears—front and back. Use one or both mirrors to get a clear view.
B. Thoroughly inspect your scalp, using a blow dryer and mirror to expose each section to view. Get a friend or family member to help, if you can.
C. Check your hands carefully: palms and backs, between the fingers, and under the fingernails. Continue up the wrists to examine both the front and back of your forearms.
D. Standing in front of the full-length mirror, begin at the elbows and scan all sides of your upper arms. Do not forget the underarms.
E. Next, focus on the neck, chest, and torso. Women should lift breasts to view the underside.
F. With your back to the full-length mirror, use the hand mirror to inspect the back of your neck, shoulders, upper back, and any part of the back of your upper arms you could not view previously.
G. Still using both mirrors, scan your lower back, buttocks, and backs of both legs.
H. Sit down; prop each leg in turn on the other stool or chair. Use the hand mirror to examine the genitals. Check front and sides of both legs, thigh to shin; ankles; and tops of feet, between toes, and under toenails. Examine soles of the feet and the heels.

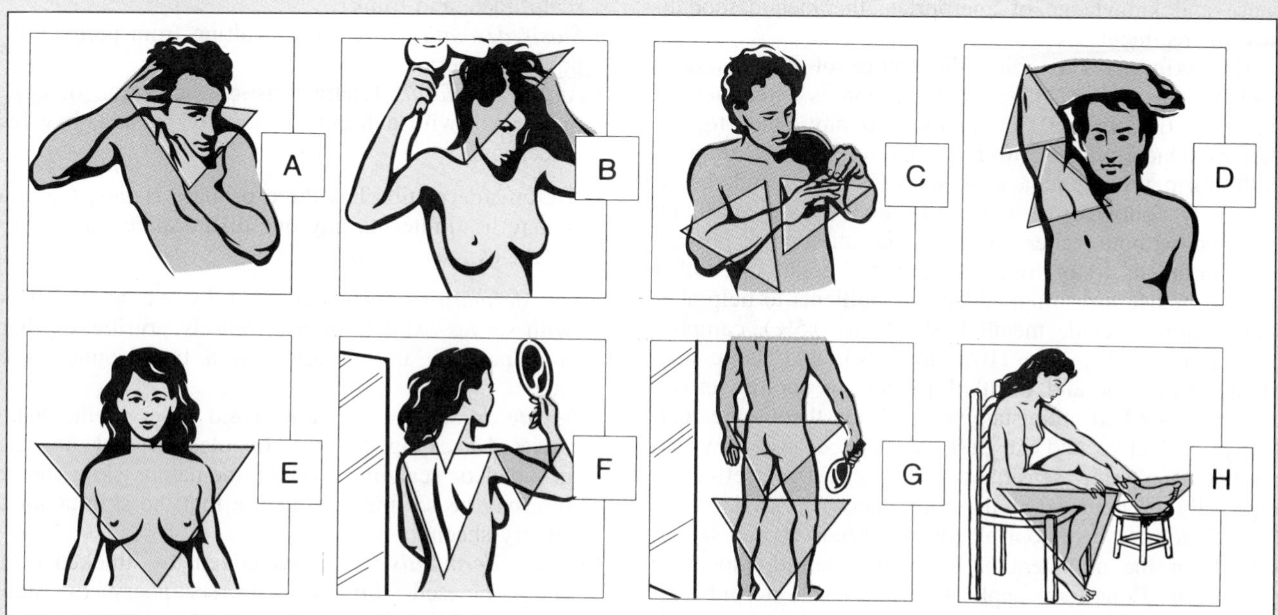

From The Skin Cancer Foundation (1992). *Skin cancer. If you can spot it, you can stop it.* New York: Author.

COMMON SKIN DISORDERS

PRURITUS

Pruritus (itching), one of the most common manifestations of skin problems, is a symptom, not a disease. It has been defined as an unpleasant skin sensation, resulting in a strong desire to scratch, localized to or generalized over a body area. Pruritus can lead to damage if scratching injures the skin's protective barrier, with possible resultant infection and scarring. Relieving this symptom, especially for chronically ill clients, is a nursing challenge because of its common occurrence and the major effect it may have on quality of life.

Pruritus can be a secondary clinical manifestation of conditions ranging from dry skin to cancer. Systemic diseases that can cause generalized and severe pruritus include chickenpox, liver failure, diabetes mellitus, uremia, drug hypersensitivity reaction, intestinal parasites, leukemia, and lymphoma.

Stimulation of itching can be initiated by almost any chemical or physical substance, especially if skin is damaged. Once the itch sensation is established, the client has an almost uncontrollable urge to scratch. Scratching leads to further skin damage and increased inflammation. Pruritus therefore worsens, and the urge to scratch is also intensified. Thus, the itch-scratch-itch cycle develops. To minimize skin trauma caused by scratching, clients should keep fingernails short.

The client usually volunteers subjective reports of the degree and location of itching. Listen carefully to the client's description of the severity and location of pruritus, and seek information about how pruritus interferes with activities of daily living. Objective signs include excoriations and other secondary skin changes such as lichenification. Document all assessment findings.

Appropriate management of itching requires a complete assessment that attempts to discover the underlying cause and knowledge of appropriate therapeutic modalities for treatment.

Dry skin may be either the source of pruritus or a contributing factor, and good hydration is often helpful (see Xerotic Eczema), in addition to any other topical therapy. One bath or shower per day for 15 to 20 minutes with warm water and a mild soap is recommended, immediately followed by the application of an emollient, with or without other topical medications, to prevent evaporation of water from the hydrated epidermis. Other topical medications often added to emollients to help alleviate itching include menthol (0.25% to 0.5%), camphor (0.25% to 0.5%), urea (10% to 20%), and lactic acid (12%). Camphor and menthol produce a cooling effect. Topically applied antihistamines and anesthetics are relatively ineffective and are best avoided because they can be potent allergic sensitizers. The sensitizing effect is especially pronounced if these products are used on inflamed skin. Use of topical corticosteroids should be reserved for the treatment of a specific steroid-responsive dermatosis. Long-term application of topical steroids, especially on skin not affected with an eczematous condition, may result in thinning of the skin, striae, telangiectases, and easy bruising.

Systemic antihistaminic agents are most helpful in disorders in which histamine is the principal mediator but may be of benefit through a sedative or even placebo effect. A trial of a histamine$_1$ (H_1) blocker (hydroxyzine, diphenhydramine, chlorpheniramine) is appropriate either on a regular schedule or as indicated for itching. Tricyclic antidepressants (TCAs) (doxepin HCl, amitriptyline HCl) have a high binding capacity for H_1 receptors and may be helpful in clients who would benefit from their antidepressant as well as antipruritic effect.

Older clients may have difficulty in following through with frequent bathing or showering because of decreased mobility. In such clients, when hydration cannot precede the application of moisturizers, more frequent application and use of more hydrating products may be needed. In addition, elderly people may have difficulty applying the needed topical agents properly, and assistive personnel may be required to ensure proper therapy. Antihistaminics should be administered carefully, with use of small doses initially, because many older people have a very low tolerance of these agents and may experience severe drowsiness, especially at the initiation of therapy.

ECZEMATOUS DISORDERS

Eczema is not a specific disease. *Dermatitis* and eczema are terms that may be used interchangeably to describe a group of disorders with a characteristic clinical appearance. Some examples of eczema or dermatitis are:

- *Allergic contact dermatitis* (eruptions from allergy to poison ivy, sumac, or oak or a proven allergen)
- *Irritant dermatitis* (eruption from direct contact with irritating substances such as cosmetics, chemicals, dyes, or detergents)
- *Nummular eczema* (appearance of coin-shaped, oozing, crusting patches)
- *Seborrheic dermatitis* (yellowish pink scaling of the scalp, face, and trunk)
- *Stasis dermatitis* (eruption resulting from peripheral venous disorders)
- *Atopic dermatitis* (characteristic distribution of eczema in persons with a family history of asthma, hay fever, or eczema)

Eczema/dermatitis has three primary stages; the condition may be limited to any one of the three stages, or the three stages may coexist.

Acute dermatitis is characterized by extensive erosions with serous exudate or by intensely pruritic, erythematous papules and vesicles on a background of erythema.

Subacute dermatitis is characterized by erythematous, excoriated, scaling papules or plaques that are either grouped or scattered over erythematous skin; the scaling may be so fine and diffuse that the skin acquires a silvery sheen.

Chronic dermatitis is characterized by thickened skin and increased skin marking secondary to rubbing and scratching (lichenification); excoriated papules, fibrotic papules, and nodules (prurigo nodularis); and postinflammatory hyperpigmentation and hypopigmentation.

ATOPIC DERMATITIS

Atopic dermatitis is a common, chronic, relapsing, pruritic type of eczema. The word "atopic" refers to a group of three associated allergic disorders: asthma, allergic rhinitis (hay fever), and atopic dermatitis.

Etiology

According to several studies, 75% to 80% of clients with atopic dermatitis have a personal or family history of asthma, hay fever, eczema, or food allergies. Atopic dermatitis is a common disorder, affecting 10% to 20% of children in the United States. The cause is unknown.

Pathophysiology

It is clear that an immune dysfunction exists in clients with atopic dermatitis, but whether the dysfunction is the cause or the effect of the disorder is still unclear. Altered $CD4^+$ T-helper cells produce interleukins which stimulate IgE. Mast cells release histamine and tumor necrosis factor (TNF). Compared with normal skin, the dry skin of atopic dermatitis has reduced water-binding capacity, higher rate of transepidermal water loss, and decreased water content.[73] Water loss leads to further drying and cracking of the skin, which leads to more itching. Rubbing and scratching of itchy skin are responsible for many of the changes seen in the skin.

Clinical Manifestations

Atopic dermatitis begins in many clients during infancy. The dermatitis is usually of acute onset, with a red, oozing, crusting rash. Over time, the skin tends to show the chronic form of dermatitis, with thickened dry texture, brownish-gray color, and scales. The rash tends to become localized to the large folds of the extremities as the client becomes older (Fig. 49–2). It is found mainly on elbow bends, the backs of the knees, the neck, the eyelids, and the backs of the hands and feet. Hand and foot dermatitis becomes a significant problem in some adults.

Pruritus is the major clinical manifestation of atopic

ALTERNATIVE THERAPY

Integumentary Disorders

The management of skin disorders is often difficult. Nutritional and herbal approaches to the treatment of skin problems have been shown to be effective for some disorders, often with fewer side effects than with conventional methods.

In a general article on atopic dermatitis, commonly known as eczema, naturopathic physician Michael Murray touches on a number of possible causes and treatments of this chronic condition.[4] He cites evidence that food allergies may be the culprit, at least in some people. Commonly, milk, eggs, and peanuts may be the offending foods. Food allergy tests using a small sample of blood, such as the enzyme-linked immunosorbent assay (ELISA) and immunoglobulin E (IgE) and IgG tests, are now available. These tests expose the blood sample to food antigens to determine reactivity to foods. Controversial but of interest, breast-feeding of infants may be preventive for atopic dermatitis and allergies in general. Breast-fed infants who developed eczema due to food allergy experienced relief of manifestations when the mothers refrained from eating specific foods.

Another nutritional issue is the ratio of omega-3 to omega-6 fatty acids in the diet. This ratio appears to be lower in people who have eczema. Supplementation with fish and/or flaxseed oils or consumption of coldwater fish may therefore be of benefit in the treatment of eczema.

Chinese herbs have long been used in Asian countries for the treatment of skin diseases. A landmark study done in England showed the effectiveness of Chinese herbs in treating atopic dermatitis.[5] This study was undertaken after dermatologists were impressed by the results seen in their patients who were also under the care of a Chinese herbalist. Participants in the study who received the active herbal formula reported decreases in the number of lesions and itching as well as improved sleep.

A traditional Australian plant remedy, tea tree oil (from *Melaleuca alternifolia*), has been shown to be effective in the treatment of acne.[1] In a single-blind, randomized study, topical tea tree oil was compared with topical benzoyl peroxide (both in a 5% solution). Although both treatments produced significant improvement after three months of daily application, the frequency of side effects such as dryness, burning, and skin redness was 44% with the tea tree oil and 79% with benzoyl peroxide.

A topical mixture of the essential plant oils of thyme, rosemary, lavender, and cedarwood, in a carrier of jojoba and grapeseed oils, was found to have significant effect in the treatment of alopecia areata.[3] This treatment was called "aromatherapy" in the study because such oils are commonly used in aromatherapy, but topical use of the preparation might be better regarded as a medicinal herbal application. Forty-four per cent of the subjects in the essential oil treatment group improved, compared with 15% of those in the placebo group.

In a 1998 published report from Taiwan,[2] acupuncture was stated to be effective in the treatment of urticaria (hives). Although the authors noted a lack of controlled studies in this area, they proposed that the improvement frequently observed clinically with use of this modality warrants consideration of acupuncture in the treatment of both acute and chronic urticaria.

References

1. Bassett, I. B., Pannowitz, D. L., & Barnetson, R. St. C. (1990). A comparative study of tea-tree oil versus benzoyl peroxide in the treatment of acne. *Medical Journal of Australia, 153,* 455–458.
2. Chen, C. J., & Yu, H. S. (1998). Acupuncture treatment of urticaria. *Archives of Dermatology, 134,* 1397–1399.
3. Hay, I. C., Jamieson, S. R. N., & Ormerod, A. D. (1998). Randomized trial of aromatherapy: Successful treatment for alopecia areata. *Archives of Dermatology, 134,* 1349–1352.
4. Murray, M. T. (1999). Atopic dermatitis (eczema). *Natural Medicine Journal, 2*(4), 1–6.
5. Sheehan, M. P., et al. (1998). Efficacy of traditional Chinese herbal therapy in adult atopic dermatitis. *Lancet, 340,* 13–17.

James Higgy Lerner, RN, LAc, *Private practice of acupuncture, traditional Oriental medicine, and feedback*

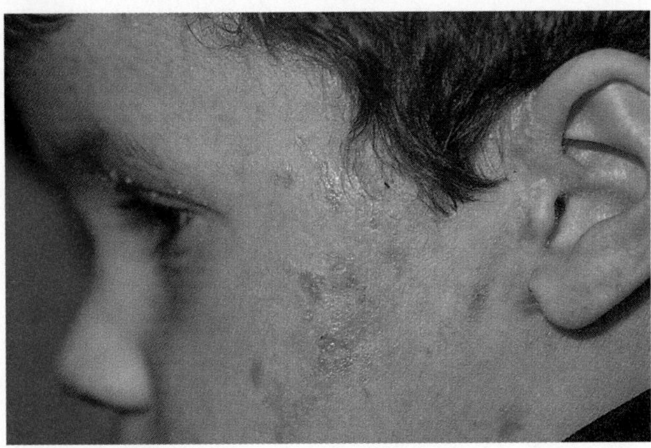

FIGURE 49–2 Atopic dermatitis. Intense pruritus leading to scratching and open lesions.

dermatitis and causes the greatest morbidity. The condition may be mild and self-limiting, or it may be intense, provoking scratching that results in severely excoriated lesions, infection, and scarring.

Complications

Clients with atopic dermatitis tend to experience viral, bacterial, and fungal skin infections. It is not clear whether these cutaneous infections arise secondary to a disruption of normal barrier function or are due to reduced local immunity. The most common viral infection is herpes simplex, which tends to spread locally or become generalized. Honey-colored crusting, extensive serous weeping, folliculitis, pyoderma, and furunculosis indicate bacterial infection, usually secondary to *Staphylococcus aureus* in clients with atopic dermatitis. Clients with atopic dermatitis are frequently heavily colonized with *S. aureus.* Superficial fungal infections may also appear more frequently.

Outcome Management

The goal of therapy is to break the inflammatory cycle that causes excess drying and cracking as well as the itching and scratching.[34] The health care team's understanding of each client's disease pattern and the discovery and reduction of exacerbating factors are crucial to effective management of this chronic disorder.

Medical Management

Lubricate the Skin

Hydration is the key to management but is often difficult to achieve. Management begins with daily skin care that hydrates and lubricates the skin. Soaks followed by application of occlusive substances are usually prescribed (see Soaks and Wet Wraps).

Remove Allergens

Allergens, food, aeroallergens, and emotional stresses may be inciting factors in this disorder. Clients should avoid exposure to substances for which there is a positive result on allergy testing and which are suspected to precipitate dermatitis. Stringent restrictions on lifestyle and activities are unjustified. Air conditioning may help reduce aeroallergen exposure at home and in the workplace. It is important to identify and eliminate triggers that cause the atopic dermatitis to flare. Many of these triggering factors are the same irritants that contribute to generalized pruritus (see Pruritus).

Dietary management of atopic dermatitis has continued to be controversial. Food allergies in the causation of atopic dermatitis seem to be more significant in certain populations of young children and infants. The most common allergens appear to be eggs, cow's milk, soy, wheat, nuts, and fish. Known allergens are avoided. People with food allergies must be taught to read labels. Care must be taken to avoid malnutrition when any type of restrictive diet is used.

Occlusives, emollients, topical corticosteroids, and tar preparations all can be employed in various combinations to control atopic dermatitis. The use of topical steroids is an important component of therapy for eczema (see Topical Corticosteroids). These preparations are best absorbed into hydrated skin or by using wet wraps and occlusion. Topical agents containing chemicals or drugs with the potential to cause skin eruptions are avoided.

Systemic medications may include antibiotics and antihistaminics. The use of a systemic corticosteroid is rarely warranted in atopic dermatitis. Some clients view the systemic use of steroids as a "quick cure" and find these agents much easier to use than hydration and topical therapy. Systemic corticosteroids should be avoided in this chronic, non–life-threatening disorder. Although there may be dramatic improvement with their use, the recurrence of dermatitis after their discontinuation is equally dramatic. The side effects of long-term systemic steroid use are both unpleasant and dangerous.

If a short-term course of oral steroid therapy is given, it is important to taper the dosage as the drug is discontinued. Intensified skin care should also be instituted during the taper to suppress flaring of the dermatitis.

Various therapeutic approaches are becoming available. Results are promising with the use of the new immune response modifier tacrolimus for therapy of moderate to severe atopic dermatitis as well as with the use of cyclosporine and other experimental modalities. Clients with severe, recalcitrant disease should be made aware of research advances and encouraged to participate in trials, when possible, to give them a sense of hope.

Nursing Management of the Medical Client

Assess the client with atopic dermatitis for bathing habits, use of moisturizers, medication regimen, exposure to known allergens, environmental exposure, and history of skin eruptions. Nursing management of the client with atopic dermatitis is presented in the accompanying Care Plan.

Modifications for Elderly Clients

Dermatitis is a common skin disorder in the elderly population. It may be caused by venous insufficiency, allergens, irritants, or underlying malignancy such as leukemia or lymphoma. Because older adults often take many medications, the potential for dermatitis from drug-drug interactions is increased. The fragility of the skin as a result of the flattened epidermal-dermal junction and loss of dermis should be considered in planning any form of treatment.

THE CLIENT WITH ATOPIC DERMATITIS

Nursing Diagnosis. Impaired Skin Integrity related to skin dryness

Outcomes. The client will maintain skin that has good hydration and reduced inflammation, as evidenced by:

- Verbalizing increased skin comfort
- Decreased flaking and scaling
- Decreased redness
- Decreased excoriations from scratching
- Healing of previous areas of breakdown

Interventions	Rationales
1. Bathe the client at least once every day, soaking for 15 to 20 minutes. Immediately upon leaving the bath, apply an appropriate emollient or prescribed topical agent. Bathe more often when clinical manifestations increase.	1. Soaking saturates the stratum corneum. Application of an occlusive moisturizer 2 to 4 minutes after the bath is critical for preventing evaporation of water from the hydrated epidermis.
2. Use warm water.	2. Hot water causes vasodilation, which may increase pruritus.
3. Use superfatted soaps (e.g., Dove or Basis) or soaps for sensitive skin (e.g., Oil of Olay, Eucerin, Neutrogena, Vanicream, Aveeno, Oilatum, Cetaphil). Avoid bubble baths.	3. The use of drying soap may compound the problem. Superfatted soaps are less alkaline and less drying to the skin. "Sensitive skin" formulas are usually fragrance-free.
4. Apply occlusive topical emollient (e.g., Aquaphor ointment, cream (Eucerin) or lotion, Vanicream, Cetaphil cream or lotion) or prescribed topical preparation two or three times per day.	4. Ointments and creams seal in water and thereby hydrate the skin. The particular emollient selected depends mostly on client preference and whether the ingredients in the base are irritants.

Evaluation. Outcomes should be met in 48 to 96 hours, depending on severity of eczema, frequency of baths, and adequate application of appropriate occlusive topical agent. Evaluate skin as often as possible.

Collaborative Problem. Alteration in Comfort related to pruritus

Outcomes. The client will experience a decrease in pruritus, as evidenced by:

- Decrease in observed and reported scratching
- Decreased excoriations from scratching
- Decreased restlessness during sleep
- Verbalizing increased skin comfort

Interventions	Rationales
1. Explain the itching symptom as it relates to cause (i.e., dryness of the skin) and the principles of the selected therapy (i.e., hydration) and the itch-scratch-itch cycle.	1. Understanding the physiologic or psychological process and principles of itching and its treatment increases cooperation.
2. Wash all new clothes before wearing for removal of formaldehyde and other chemicals, and avoid use of fabric softeners.	2. Pruritus is often precipitated by irritant or allergic effects of certain chemicals or components of fabric softeners.
3. Change to a milder detergent, and add a second rinse cycle to ensure removal of soap.	3. Residual laundry detergent in clothing may be irritating. The actual laundry soap that is used is not the key; rather, all soap is rinsed out so that an irritant effect is avoided.
4. Wear open-weave, loose-fitting, cotton-blend clothing. Avoid overdressing, rough or wool fabrics, and tightly woven fabrics.	4. Light cotton-blend clothing allows air circulation and minimizes perspiration, which intensifies itching.
5. Work and sleep in comfortable surroundings with a fairly constant temperature (68° to 75° F) and humidity level (45% to 55%). Air conditioning in the home, particularly the bedroom, may be beneficial.	5. Extremes of temperature cause pruritus frequently secondary to vasodilation and increased cutaneous blood flow. In addition to providing a cooler environment, air conditioning decreases aeroallergen exposure.
6. Keep fingernails short, smooth, and clean.	6. Trimmed nails prevent damage and infection to the skin.
7. Appropriate use of oral antihistamines may reduce itching to some degree.	7. Histamine is one of the best-known itch mediators. The sedating antihistaminics also provide relief through tranquilizing effects.
8. Use sunscreen on a regular basis.	8. Sunburn may cause flare of dermatitis.
9. Immediately after swimming, take a shower or bath, washing with a mild soap from head to toe, and then apply an appropriate moisturizer.	9. Residual chlorine or bromine on the skin after swimming in a pool may be irritating.

Care Plan continued on following page

Evaluation. Outcomes may not be achieved for days or weeks after eczema has been brought under control. Itching can become a learned behavioral response brought on by many factors, which may need to be modified through counseling, oral medications, and maintenance of good skin care.

Nursing Diagnosis. Risk for Infection related to skin excoriation or decreased resistance to cutaneous viral, fungal, and staphylococcal organisms

Outcomes. The client will be free of infectious lesions, as evidenced by absence of pustules, exudate, or crusting.

Interventions	Rationales
1. Explain to the client the signs of infection, and be sure the client understands that the presence of these signs indicates need for medical intervention.	1. Infections are a potentially serious complication of disorders of open skin.
2. Ensure that the client understands the importance of not self-treating with leftover medication at home.	2. Leftover medications may be outdated and may be inappropriate treatment. Medications can become contaminated, leading to infection, or may lose their potency.
3. Emphasize the importance of taking the antibiotic on schedule over the entire course.	3. The entire course of medication will completely eradicate the infectious organism.

Evaluation. Outcomes are usually achieved with 7 to 10 days of oral antibiotic therapy. However, some clients require an extended course for complete clearing. Evaluation should be done no later than at 7 days after initiation of therapy.

Nursing Diagnosis. Body Image Disturbance related to skin lesions and/or response of significant others to appearance

Outcomes. The client will exhibit a positive self-concept, as evidenced by engaging in social activities, expressing feelings of importance and self-worth, and enjoying interpersonal interactions.

Interventions	Rationales
1. Encourage the client to teach others that eczema is not contagious unless the lesions are severely infected.	1. Eczema can be mistaken for impetigo or as an indication of uncleanliness, causing social isolation.
2. Encourage the client and significant others to share feelings with one another and professional counselors, as needed, regarding the client's appearance and the chronic nature of eczema.	2. Unidentified fears and concerns may hinder interpersonal relationships.
3. Reinforce the client's sense of identity and personal competence. Encourage self-management of eczema and the understanding that controlling scratching will greatly reduce lesions.	3. Allowing the client to determine the need for various treatment modalities, such as when to initiate wet wraps or minor alterations in topical therapy, promotes a positive self-concept.

Evaluation. Outcomes are totally dependent on the degree of negative self-concept, chronicity of this process, and the degree to which eczema can be controlled. Depending on the age and motivation of the client, outcomes can be reached in weeks, months, years, or—unfortunately for a small few—never. Professional intervention should be facilitated early.

XEROTIC ECZEMA

Xerotic (dry) skin is dehydrated. Xerotic eczema may present as erythematous, scaling, and finely cracked skin. Xerosis occurs in patches and may involve any skin surface. It is common in the elderly population. If xerosis is severe, the skin is tight, itchy, and painful. Water loss causes xerotic chapping. The problem may be accentuated by use of drying skin cleansers, soaps, disinfectants, and solvents and infrequent use of moisturizers. Environmental factors play a large role, especially those that increase water loss in the stratum corneum. Any factors that decrease the relative humidity exacerbate this condition, such as cold or dry winter air, especially in artificially heated rooms.

Management includes hydration and moisturizing the skin plus avoiding irritating factors. Teaching the client correct daily skin care is essential to treating this condition. See the earlier discussion on soaks and wet wraps and skin lubricants.

STASIS DERMATITIS

Stasis dermatitis is characterized by the development of areas of very dry skin and sometimes shallow ulcers on the lower legs, primarily as a result of venous insufficiency. The process of dermatitis begins with edema of the leg due to slowed venous return. The client commonly has a history of varicose veins or deep vein thrombosis. As the venous stasis continues, the tissue becomes hypoxic from stagnant blood supply. As the blood pools, hemoglobin is released from the red blood cell and is deposited in the tissues, causing brown stains on the skin. Fluids escape into the interstitial space, and edema develops. This poorly nourished tissue begins to undergo necrosis.

Clinical manifestations include itching, a feeling of heaviness in the legs, brown-stained skin, and open shallow lesions (Fig. 49–3). Dilated veins may be obvious. The lesions are very slow to heal because of the lack of oxygenated blood.

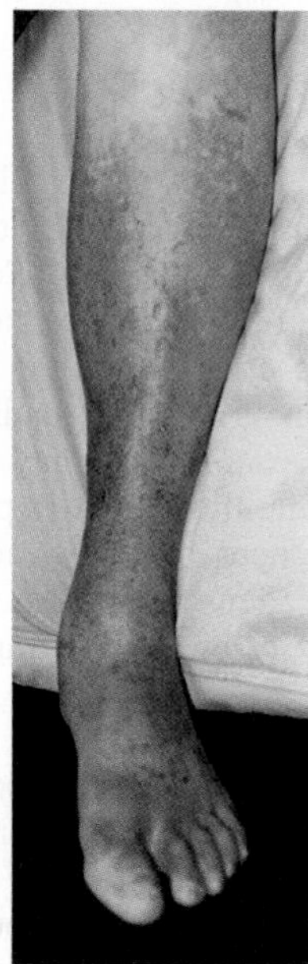

FIGURE 49–3 Stasis dermatitis. Note the dark, stained, shiny skin on the leg as well as the absence of hair.

Improvement of venous return in the legs is needed. This can be accomplished with leg elevation, wearing support hose or elastic wraps daily, and refraining from crossing the legs. Clients should be instructed to raise the legs periodically during the day, especially if their occupation requires standing still for long periods of time (e.g., cashier). Walking instead of standing or performing calf exercises while standing is encouraged to increase circulation. In addition, it is beneficial to raise the foot of the bed with two-by-four blocks or books.

Stasis ulcers are treated with moisture-retentive dressings and gradient pressure wraps. Unna boots can be used. Skin grafts may be required to heal large ulcers.

■ CONTACT DERMATITIS

Contact dermatitis is an inflammatory response of the skin to chemical or physical allergens. *Irritant contact dermatitis* is due to exposure to a chemical or physical irritant (cleaning product, fragrance, or topical skin care product), not to an immune-mediated response. Clinical manifestations range from mild erythema to vesicles to ulceration (Fig. 49–4).

Allergic contact dermatitis is a delayed hypersensitivity reaction resulting from contact with an allergen. This reaction is an immune-mediated response by previously sensitized lymphocytes to a specific allergen. Common examples are poison ivy, nickel sensitivity, and formaldehyde allergy. Clinical manifestations begin at the site of exposure with itching, stinging, erythema, and edema, which may extend to involve more distant sites. Manifestations may develop within an hour of contact or as late as 7 to 14 days after contact. With even brief contact of the irritant with the skin, an allergic response is possible. For example, contact with poison ivy may have happened quickly and the evident irritant washed off. However, areas of dermatitis may continue to appear for many days following the initial exposure.

Management begins with identification of the causative agent. First, question the client about recent exposure to chemicals, metals, and the like. Patch testing is done to attempt to determine the specific agent. Pain and itching may be controlled with topical medication or wet dressings (see earlier). Antihistaminic agents and topical or systemic steroids may be required. Each patch in a standardized test panel (T.R.U.E. test [thin-layer, rapid-use epicutaneous test]) contains a substance that is known to be a common cause of allergic contact dermatitis. When these tests elicit a positive reaction, much can be done to teach the client about what to avoid (see Chapter 48).

■ INTERTRIGO

Intertrigo is a superficial inflammatory dermatitis that occurs between two apposed (touching) skin surfaces. Adequate ventilation, friction, heat, and moisture buildup result in erythema and maceration, itching, and burning. Erosions and fissures with erythema and secondary bacterial or *Candida albicans* infection may occur. Whenever candidiasis is present, a careful evaluation is indicated. In an otherwise healthy person, candidiasis is a self-limiting disease that responds well to topical antifungal therapy; however, it can be the presenting sign of underlying systemic disease affecting the endocrine system (e.g., diabetes) or the immune system (e.g., immunodeficiency syndromes). Intertrigo is common in hot, humid weather in neck creases, axillae, antecubital fossae, the perineum, finger and toe webs, and abdominal skinfolds and beneath the breasts, particularly in obese clients. One of the most common causes of intertrigo is contamination with body fluids, as occurs in urinary incontinence.

The treatment of intertrigo is to eliminate maceration by promoting drying and to aerate the body skinfolds. For mobile clients, review environmental changes that promote drying of the body folds, such as wearing loose-fitting cotton-blend clothing or periodic removal of clothing to dry off. Instruct clients to avoid tight-fitting clothing such as jeans and activities that promote sweating. Care recommendations are very dependent on the degree of involvement and the overall condition of the skin. If the skin is still intact, recommendations include washing the area gently with tap water twice daily and

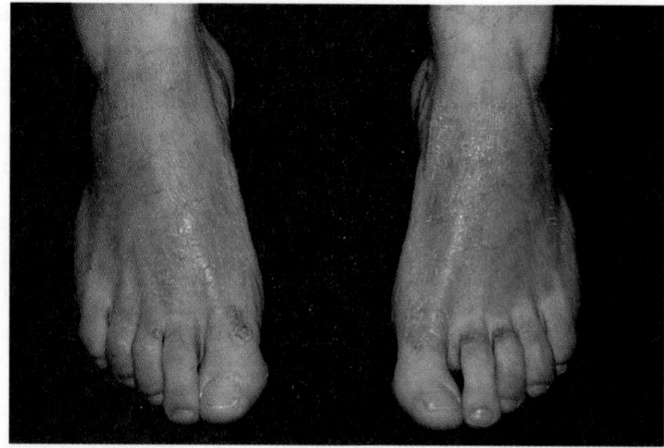

FIGURE 49–4 Contact dermatitis. Note the distinct line of erythema.

then rinsing and drying the area, followed by liberal application of a talc-containing powder or a cellulose-containing powder (e.g., Zeasorb) for extra absorption. Never use cornstarch because it encourages *C. albicans* overgrowth.

If inflammation is present, a low-potency topical corticosteroid in a nonocclusive vehicle (e.g., hydrocortisone 1.0% or 2.5% cream or lotion) or a combination steroid-antibiotic-antifungal agent (Vytone 1%) may initially be helpful, but long-term use should be avoided. Apply cool, wet soaks with tap water or Burows solution three to four times daily for removal of exudate if secondary infection is present. Applying folded gauze or clean cotton handkerchiefs in skinfolds promotes healing by keeping skin surfaces apart.

PSORIASIS VULGARIS

Psoriasis vulgaris is a chronic, recurrent, erythematous, inflammatory disorder involving keratin synthesis. Pruritus can be severe. Psoriasis occurs in both genders, usually commencing in early adulthood. The Latin *vulgaris* (from *vulgus* "the public") means "common." The cause of psoriasis vulgaris is unknown. However, alterations in cyclic nucleotides and possible immunologic abnormalities have been noted. Genetic predisposition is also possible.

Pathophysiology

Rapidly proliferating epidermal cells which do not mature form small, scaly patches of skin that develop into erythematous, dry, scaling patches of various sizes. The course of psoriasis vulgaris is prolonged and unpredictable. Anxiety and stress often precede flares. Exacerbations and remissions are common. The condition usually recurs at intervals and lasts for increasingly longer periods. Spontaneous clearing is uncommon. Clients with psoriasis have greater than normal numbers of staphylococci in colonized plaques. Psoriatic clients who are seropositive for human immunodeficiency virus (HIV) are at high risk of HIV infection from self-inoculation.

Clinical Manifestations

Psoriatic patches are covered with silvery white scales. The eruptions (usually in a symmetrical distribution) commonly occur on the scalp, elbows, knees, and sacral regions (Fig. 49–5). Lesions may develop at the site of a previous injury, which is known as Koebner's phenomenon. A generalized eruption may occur with severe psoriasis vulgaris. In a rare form of psoriasis, known as pustular psoriasis, generalized, sterile cutaneous pustules are produced. Severe systemic involvement can be fatal. About 15% to 20% of clients with psoriasis have psoriatic arthritis, which primarily affects the distal joints and may be deforming. Nail dystrophies and pitting occur in about 30% to 50% of clients.

Outcome Management

The goals of medical management of psoriasis are to control the rate of epidermal cell turnover and to monitor for complications of therapy.

Medical Management

REDUCE RATE OF EPIDERMAL CELL TURNOVER

Mild psoriasis may be treated locally with natural sunlight or topical therapy, including tar preparations and topical corticosteroids (see Topical Corticosteroids) or intralesional corticosteroids. Injecting small, dilute amounts of corticosteroids (e.g., triamcinolone acetonide) into or just beneath a lesion gives a high drug concentration at the injection site. Keratolytic agents (e.g., salicylic acid) may remove scale and allow greater penetration of topical agents. Anthralin reduces mitotic action in the cell and is an effective topical agent for treatment of psoriasis with widespread discrete lesions consisting primarily of thick plaques.

Scalp care in psoriasis consists of removing scales and treating inflammation. Tar shampoos with keratolytic agents, followed by topical corticosteroid lotions, are useful. Use of steroids under occlusion (under dressings) is often necessary to enhance percutaneous absorption; on the scalp, a plastic shower cap can be used for this purpose. There is no consistently effective treatment of psoriatic involvement of the nails. Usually, the scalp and nails improve with remission of psoriasis on the body surface.

Antimetabolites (e.g., methotrexate) in small doses are useful for inhibiting deoxyribonucleic acid (DNA) synthesis. Methotrexate is a folic acid antagonist used to treat psoriasis that is unresponsive to all topical therapies; it is reserved for the most severe cases.

Systemic treatment is sometimes prescribed for widespread psoriasis. The vitamin A derivative etretinate (Tegison) has been shown to be useful in pustular and erythrodermic psoriasis but less so in chronic plaque-type psoriasis. The mode of action may involve the correction of abnormal polyamine metabolism or leukocyte migration.

MONITOR FOR COMPLICATIONS

Potential localized side effects of corticosteroids include atrophy, hypopigmentation, infection, and, rarely, ulceration. The side effects of etretinate are similar to those of the oral retinoid isotretinoin (see Acne Vulgaris later). Because of the teratogenicity of the drug and its extremely long half-life, its use in women of childbearing age is contraindicated. Widespread involvement may require whole-body irradiation with UVL (see earlier).

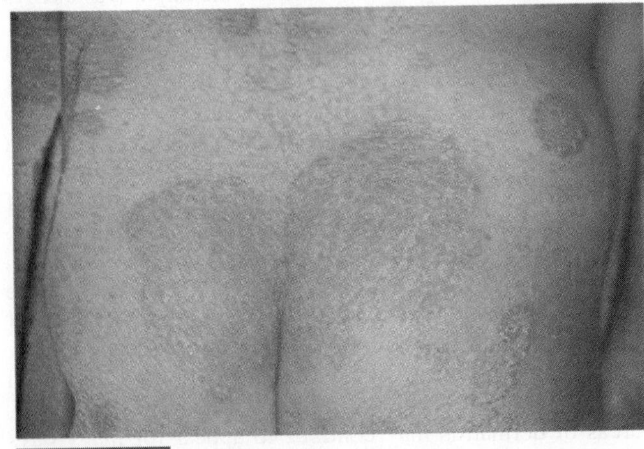

FIGURE 49–5 Plaque psoriasis of the buttocks.

Methotrexate is potentially toxic to the renal, hepatic, and hematopoietic systems. Thus, baseline assessment (e.g., blood chemistry, complete blood count, liver biopsy) is important before this medication is started. During treatment, periodic assessments are needed, including re-biopsy of the liver. If any serious side effects develop, such as bone marrow depression (decreased white blood cell count and platelet count) or gastrointestinal tract bleeding, treatment is discontinued. To limit potential liver damage, advise the client not to consume alcohol throughout therapy. Because methotrexate may cause chromosomal abnormalities, effective birth control methods are important for both women and men before and during treatment. Nausea, the most common side effect, can be limited by taking methotrexate with food or with prophylactic antiemetics.

Nursing Management of the Medical Client

Although the physician orders the medical regimen for the client, the nurse and the physician collaborate in the ongoing assessment of the client's response to treatment and the development of new lesions.

There are various methods of application of topical medications. With all methods, it is important to apply medication only to the affected lesions, avoiding contact with normal surrounding skin. The client should wash the hands immediately after application. The medication must be left on for the prescribed period of time and then removed by showering or bathing.

Anthralin products have the potential to stain fabric, hair, skin, nails, furniture, and bathroom fixtures. To avoid excessive staining, it is recommended that the medication be carefully applied and that as much medication as possible be removed with a tissue or a previously stained towel before bathing.

Self-Care

Your role in client self-care centers on teaching the client about the UVL treatments and medications. Assist the client in coping with an altered self-concept. The appearance of skin lesions may make the client feel "dirty" or untouchable. In addition, the smell of the tar preparations and the stain may add to the psychological reaction. Because open lesions are at high risk for secondary infection, the client should be taught to keep the creams or ointments on and to keep the area clean and dry.

To keep psoriasis in remission, the client needs to control the causative factors. Adequate rest, nutrition, and exercise promote health. Stress should be minimized, and illness and infection should be treated early.

ACNE VULGARIS

Acne is a common, self-limiting, multifactorial disorder. One in four clients affected has disease of sufficient severity for them to seek professional treatment. Potential facial disfigurement is a major concern. Acne requires active treatment for control until it spontaneously resolves.

Etiology

The exact cause of acne is unknown. The principal etiologic factors are abnormal keratinization of the follicular epithelium, excessive sebum production, proliferation of *Propionibacterium acnes,* and inflammation secondary to the action of extracellular inflammatory products produced by *P. acnes.* There is no scientific evidence that consumption of chocolate, nuts, or fatty foods affects acne. It is important to take time to dispel this popular misconception about foods, because frequently guilt related to "eating the wrong foods" causes major family confrontations. However, exacerbations coinciding with the menstrual cycle result from hormonal activity. Heat, humidity, and excessive perspiration also have a role in worsening of acne.

Clinical Manifestations

The types of acne lesions are comedones (open and closed), pustules, papules, and nodules (Fig. 49–6). A closed *comedone,* or whitehead, is a noninflamed lesion that develops as the follicle enlarges, with retention of horny cells. Open comedones, or blackheads, result from the continuing accumulation of horny cells and sebum, which dilate the follicles. Inflammation does not usually occur in comedones unless they are self-manipulated. *Pustules* and *papules* result as the inflammatory process progresses. With papules, the level of involvement of the dermis is deeper than it is with pustules. *Nodules* result from total disintegration of a comedone with subsequent collapse of the follicle. Nodules are the hallmark of serious acne, and deep scarring may result. Aggressive management is always indicated with nodular acne.

Outcome Management

Medical Management

Treatment depends on the severity of acne. There is no convincing evidence that dietary management, use of abrasive scrubs, or oral vitamin A has any beneficial effects on the management of acne. Some people with acne may notice an improvement in the summer months as a result of additional UVL exposure. Clients should be instructed to use products labeled noncomedogenic and cosmetics that are water-based, because contact with oily or oil-based products is known to exacerbate acne.

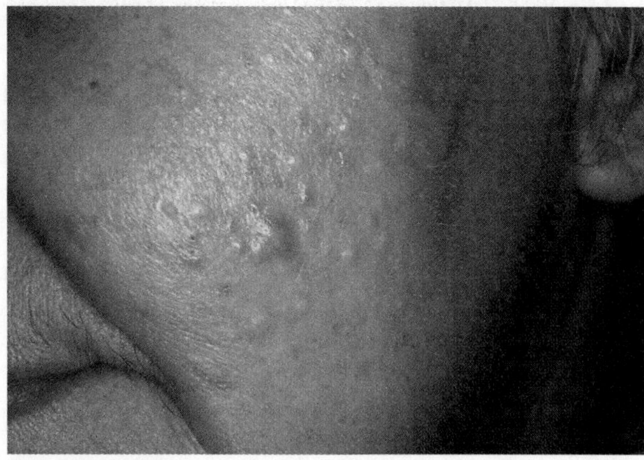

FIGURE 49–6 Acne. (From Cullen, J. P., et al. [1993]. *Color atlas of dermatology.* Philadelphia: W. B. Saunders.)

To prevent scarring, it is important to suppress inflammation. See Table 49–1 for a listing of acne medications. Benzoyl peroxide (a component of Desquam, Benzagel, Persa-Gel, Panoxyl) in 5% and 10% concentrations has a potent antimicrobial effect. The agent reduces the size and number of comedones present and may inhibit sebum secretion. Topical antibiotics (clindamycin and erythromycin) are also used. Topical retinoid products such as tretinoin (Retin-A, Avita) and adapalene (Differin) are two of the most effective comedolytic agents, used alone or in combination with benzoyl peroxide. The irritant effects sometimes limit the usefulness of these agents. Clients should receive written instructions regarding use of topical retinoids.

With failure of response to topical agents, the addition of oral antibiotics (tetracycline or erythromycin) should be considered. Tetracycline or erythromycin administered over an extended period (e.g., several months) suppresses *P. acnes* and decreases inflammation. However, long-term administration of systemic antibiotics can lead to monilial vaginitis and gastrointestinal disorders, and clients should be informed how to monitor for these problems and what interventions to use. Improvement may not be apparent for 4 to 6 weeks.

Hormone therapy may be indicated for severe cystic acne. Medication containing estrogens suppresses sebaceous gland activity. Estrogenic therapy requires treatment through a minimum of three to four menstrual cycles.

In severe cystic acne resistant to standard management, isotretinoin (Accutane) is used to inhibit inflammation. Dosage is determined by body weight. The drug is taken in divided daily doses for several months. Isotretinoin produces many side effects, necessitating frequent follow-up visits and laboratory evaluations. Adverse effects include elevated triglycerides, skin dryness, cheilitis (lip inflammation), and eye discomfort (i.e., dryness, burning). Isotretinoin is a teratogen; thus, women of childbearing age should use an effective contraceptive for at least 1 month before starting this medication and should have a pregnancy screening test 2 weeks before treatment. This drug should not be used in women without strict and adequate contraception throughout the course of therapy and for a determined period after therapy. Reinforce the fact that close medical follow-up is needed and that dry skin and cheilitis can be controlled by use of emollients and lip balms. Vitamin A supplements are stopped during this treatment.

Explain the mechanism of acne and the treatment plan, and set therapeutic goals. The client should understand that improvement is not usually seen for 4 to 8 weeks and that therapy is usually required for months to years to achieve control. Assess the client's skin care practices. Reinforce compliance with topical or systemic therapy regimens and appropriate skin-cleansing methods, with special emphasis on gentle washing technique and use of appropriate topical agents. Note areas of self-induced skin damage, and emphasize to the client the importance of refraining from squeezing, pricking, or picking at lesions.

■ ACNE ROSACEA

Acne rosacea is a chronic inflammatory eruption characterized by erythema, papules, pustules, and telangiectases. It occurs on the face, especially the cheeks and over the bridge of the nose. Unlike with acne vulgaris, comedones are generally not seen. The onset is insidious, usually between 30 and 50 years of age, and women are affected more frequently than men. It is more common in fair-skinned people with a history of easy facial flushing. Precipitating factors that appear to make the flushing worse include tea, coffee, alcohol (especially wine), caffeine-containing products, sunlight, extremes of hot and cold, spicy foods, and emotional stress.

Sebaceous hyperplasia of the nose (rhinophyma) often develops after many years of chronic acne rosacea. This condition results from chronic inflammation with an increase in the amount of connective tissue and may be mistaken for an indication of excessive alcohol consumption. Ocular changes such as eyelid inflammation and conjunctivitis may occur.

Outcome Management

Avoidance of the stimuli that trigger acne rosacea may be sufficient for management of mild forms of the disorder. Instruct clients to avoid factors that provoke facial vasodilation, such as caffeine, excessive sunlight, alcohol (especially wine), temperature extremes, hot liquids, and spicy foods. Systemic antibiotics used to be the mainstay of therapy. Antibiotics are given in small, usually tapered doses for long periods. Remind the client that improvement with systemic antibiotics occurs gradually.

Topical metronidazole (MetroGel) is the drug of choice for treatment of acne rosacea. A thin layer is applied twice daily with usually only minimal problems of dryness or burning. Relapse is common in clients who discontinue therapy.

SKIN TEARS

Skin tears are wounds resulting from the separation of epidermis from the underlying connective tissue, creating a flap. The most common sites for skin tears, in order of frequency, are the forearm, hand, elbow, and upper arm.

Etiology

Most often, the actual cause of the skin tear is unknown. When known, causes typically are trauma such as falls and injury from wheelchair handles or brakes or injury that incurred during transfer to a chair. Even though the actual skin damage is minor, families and residents are disturbed by presence of skin tears, perceiving the injury as resulting from abuse. Skin tears are most common in older adults as a result of a thinning of the epidermis, a flattening of the dermal-epidermal junction, and reduced adhesion of the dermis to the epidermis.[28]

Outcome Management

Before choosing a dressing, determine whether the edges of the tear can be approximated or the flap can be replaced to cover the wound. Gently irrigate excess blood from the site with normal saline. If possible, replace the flap to approximate the wound edges, and affix the edges to the skin with wound closure strips (Steri-Strips). Protect the site from further damage and drying by applying rolled gauze. Do not apply tape to the skin, and do not cover the wound with a transparent dressing.

For tears with small to moderate losses of epidermal tissue, irrigate the wound as described earlier. Replace any flaps of epidermis, and secure as noted. Cover the open wound with nonocclusive, moisture-retentive dressing, such as petrolatum-impregnated gauze or opaque foam dressing. Past management techniques for this type of wound included the use of transparent film dressings. Although these dressings appear to provide needed skin protection, they have important drawbacks such as maceration of tissue related to the increased heat and moisture and the additional skin trauma incurred upon removal.

For tears with complete loss of epidermal tissue, use the same technique for cleansing as described previously, cover the wound with opaque foam dressing or petrolatum (Vaseline)-impregnated gauze, and wrap with rolled gauze to secure.

Prevention is important. Use protective gloves on the client's hands and soft armrests on wheelchairs, and train caregivers for proper transfer techniques (e.g., use of transfer belts). Less frequent bathing and use of emollient soap also help to prevent skin dryness. Daily assessment by unlicensed assistive personnel is critical to identify lesions early (see Management and Delegation).

PRESSURE ULCERS

A pressure ulcer is any lesion on the skin caused by unrelieved pressure resulting in damage to underlying tissue. Pressure ulcers occur commonly in areas subject to high pressure from body weight on bony prominences. Pressure ulcers have also been called "bed sores" and "decubitus ulcers." The word *decubitus* comes from the Latin *decumbere,* to lie down. The ulcers were so named because they are common in bedridden clients.

Etiology and Risk Factors

Pressure ulcers develop when soft tissue (skin, subcutaneous tissue, and muscle) are compressed between a bony prominence and a firm surface for a prolonged period of time. Therefore, immobility is a major risk factor. In bedridden or chair-bound clients, infrequent turning and repositioning or lack of padding between surfaces that touch (e.g., knees) is a common cause. The length of time of exposure to pressure before skin breakdown varies among clients; in very debilitated clients, permanent tissue damage can result in less than 2 hours. Cognitive or sensory impairments also increase risk because the client cannot recognize the need to turn or move.

Protein-calorie malnutrition is a major risk factor. Malnourished clients have poor skin integrity, and their skin

MANAGEMENT AND DELEGATION

Skin Inspection

Unlicensed assistive personnel frequently are in the position to observe the skin of clients as they assist with various activities of daily living and provide assistance with personal hygiene. Be sure to fully delineate their role in identifying and reporting skin abnormalities. Reportable findings are listed as follows.

- *Bruising or a change in skin color.* Ecchymosis, erythema, jaundice, and pallor may indicate a serious disease process or acute tissue injury. Identification of these changes in skin color by unlicensed assistive personnel should be immediately reported to you for thorough assessment and intervention. Redness overlying bony structures may indicate prolonged or undue pressure. Unlicensed assistive personnel should ensure pressure relief by assisting the client with frequent position changes.
- *Lumps.* Assess any skin lesion or growth in further detail.
- *Dry, scaling, or cracked skin.* Dry skin may indicate dehydration or other integumentary disorders. You may delegate the application of over-the-counter lotions to unlicensed assistive personnel if the skin is not broken. Some clients may need specific lubricants or medications prescribed by a physician; therefore, have any findings of dry skin reported to you.
- *Skin that feels excessively moist and cool or excessively warm.* It is appropriate for unlicensed assistive personnel to cover clients with extra bedding if they feel cool or to offer cool compresses for warm skin (see Chapter 27). Localized areas of warmth may indicate underlying processes that need your prompt attention. Clearly communicate that any of these findings should be immediately reported to you for prompt assessment and intervention.
- *Any break in the skin with drainage or bleeding.* You may delegate the application of sterile gauze to the surface of the skin to unlicensed assistive personnel for the purpose of containing drainage (see Chapter 15). Skin tears should be treated with nonsticky dressings. Assess such skin abnormalities promptly after identification by unlicensed assistive personnel.
- *Taught and/or shiny skin.* This finding may indicate fluid shifting from the intravascular space. Such skin is prone to breakdown and infection. Employ proactive measures to prevent any undue pressure or damage to the skin. Assess the area carefully, and report any unknown disorders or significant change to a physician. Elevate the area to decrease swelling.
- *Client complaints of itching or tenderness:* Instruct unlicensed assistive personnel identifying such client complaints to communicate these findings to you promptly. Assess the client for potential allergic reaction, an underlying tissue pathologic process, or the need for additional analgesics.
- *Rashes.* New rashes or other skin eruptions sometimes suggest allergic reactions. Instruct that such findings be reported to you promptly.

Remember, you are ultimately responsible for thorough, ongoing assessment and evaluation of integument.

Kimberly Elgin, BSN, RN, *Clinician III, Clinical Manager, Surgical Services, University of Virginia Health System, Charlottesville, Virginia*

is damaged easily. In addition, incontinence, friction, and skin shearing can also lead to breakdown.

The reported incidence (number of new cases per year) of pressure ulcers in acute care facilities ranges from 2.7% to 29.5%. The prevalence (number of cases at one point in time) in acute care settings ranges from 3.5% to 29.5%. Several populations are at increased risk. Quadriplegic clients, older adults with femoral fractures, and clients in critical care facilities have the highest risk. Prevention of pressure ulcers begins with identifying the client at risk. Risk factors for alteration in skin integrity can be determined by assessing sensory perception, moisture, activity, mobility, nutrition, friction, and shear.

Pathophysiology

Continuous pressure on soft tissues between bony prominences and hard surfaces compresses capillaries and occludes blood flow. If the pressure is relieved, a brief period of rebound capillary dilation (called reactive hyperemia) occurs, and there is no tissue damage. If pressure is not relieved, microthrombi form in capillaries and completely occlude blood flow. A blister may form initially if there has been damage only to superficial tissues. Damage to underlying tissues creates a necrotic area of tissue. The necrotic tissue undergoes the process of inflammation as the body tries to get rid of it and ready the tissue for healing.

Healing occurs through secondary intention. Granulation tissue fills the base of the wound. Contraction of the ulcer edges closes the wound. Eventually, epithelial cells cover the wound. Stage III and IV pressure ulcers often require debridement and surgery to close the wound. Scar tissue predominates in ulcers healed without surgery.

Clinical Manifestations

The clinical manifestations of pressure ulcers have been described in four stages (Fig. 49–7). Ulcers most commonly occur on the sacrum, heel, greater trochanter (Fig. 49–8), and ischial tuberosities. The ulcer may or may not be covered with devitalized tissue, which can be yellow, white, brown, or black. Ulcers covered with devitalized tissue cannot be staged accurately until it is excised.

With pressure ulcers, few additional diagnostic assessments are required. Sometimes osteomyelitis is present in deep wounds. Bone scans are used for confirming this problem. If malnutrition is suspected as a cause, serum protein, albumin, or prealbumin levels may be monitored.

Outcome Management

Medical Management

Management of the client with a pressure ulcer begins with a complete history and physical examination. There are many causes of delayed wound healing, and delayed healing of pressure ulcers may be the result of other health problems. The goal of medical management is to heal the wound by relieving the pressure over the lesion or decreasing tissue load, cleaning and dressing the wound, and improving nutrition. In addition, the ulcer is monitored for healing, and the client is monitored for complications.

MANAGE TISSUE LOAD

The term *tissue load* refers to the distribution of pressure, friction, and shear on the tissues. Interventions are designed to decrease tissue load and thereby decrease pressure. Special low-pressure beds may be required for clients with multiple pressure ulcers. Heels should be elevated from the bed by placing pillows under the calf or using pressure reduction boots.

PROVIDE ULCER CARE

Moist, devitalized tissue supports bacterial growth. Therefore, devitalized tissue must be removed from the ulcer. Several forms of debridement can be used depending on the client's goals and needs for healing. *Sharp debridement* is the use of a scalpel to excise devitalized tissue (eschar). This technique works best for a thick, adherent eschar. *Mechanical debridement* is the use of wet-to-dry dressings, hydrotherapy, wound irrigation, and dextranomers to soften and remove devitalized tissues. *Enzymatic debridement* is the use of topical debriding agents, such as collagenase, to remove necrotic tissues. Finally, *autolytic debridement* involves the use of synthetic dressings to cover an ulcer, allowing enzymes in the wound bed to digest the devitalized tissues. This form of debridement is the slowest and is usually reserved for clients who cannot tolerate the other forms. Heel ulcers are not debrided unless they are clearly infected. All forms of debridement (except autolytic) are painful; the client should be given analgesics before beginning.

MONITOR HEALING

If the ulcer does not heal within 2 weeks despite adequate nutrition, pressure reduction, daily cleaning, and use of appropriate dressings, the ulcer may be infected. An infected pressure ulcer looks like any other infected wound, with foul-smelling drainage, increasing size, increasing pain in the wound, and fever or elevation in white blood cell count. Older clients do not invariably demonstrate all of the signs of infection and are at risk for development of confusion; therefore, vigilance in assessing the ulcer for changes is critical. If infection is suspected, a 2-week trial of topical antibiotics is considered. Swab cultures are not appropriate for diagnosis of infection in the ulcer. All pressure ulcers are colonized (covered with surface bacteria), and a swab culture will grow only organisms that colonize the surface. Use a quantitative culture for suspected infection. Systemic antibiotics are used when the infection cannot be controlled locally or for systemic infection (manifested by fever or positive blood cultures).

Many conditions are associated with delays in healing. Diabetes, paralysis, and arterial diseases require close assessment because of increased risk of infection. Urine and bowel incontinence lead to skin excoriation and can contaminate open wounds.

IMPROVE NUTRITION

The association of malnutrition with pressure ulcer formation and delayed healing is quite clear. In fact, many clinicians believe that pressure ulcers are a specific indicator of malnutrition. If the client's serum albumin concentration is less than 3.5 g/dl, if the total lymphocyte count is less than 1800/mm^3, or if the client is not eating or is at a body weight that is less than 80% of ideal, consider nutritional supplementation. If the client has no

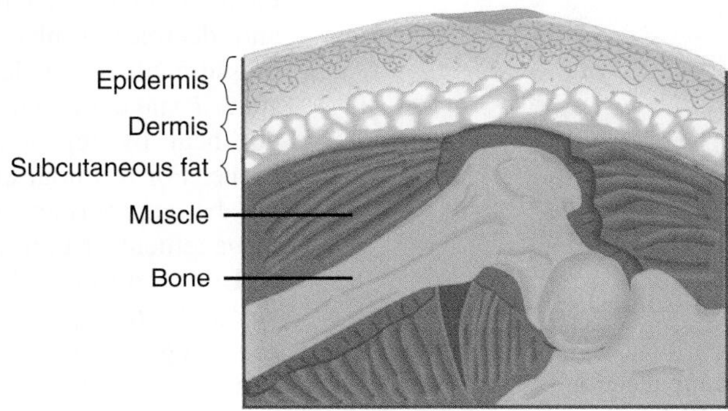
Stage I
Epidermis
Dermis
Subcutaneous fat
Muscle
Bone
Non-blanching erythema of intact skin; the heralding lesion of skin ulceration

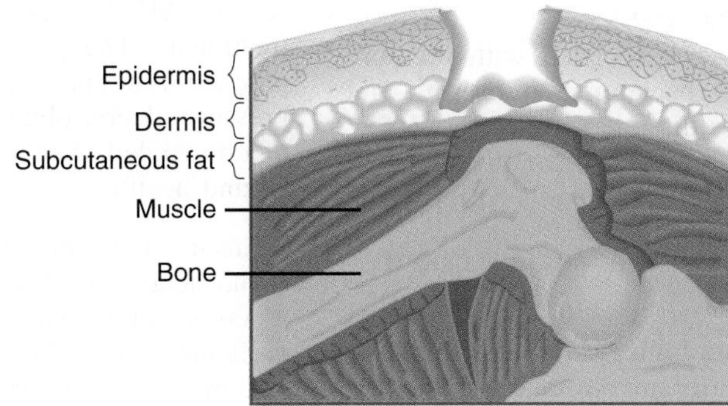
Stage II
Epidermis
Dermis
Subcutaneous fat
Muscle
Bone
Partial-thickness skin loss involving epidermis and/or dermis. The ulcer is superficial and presents clinically as an abrasion, blister, or shallow crater.

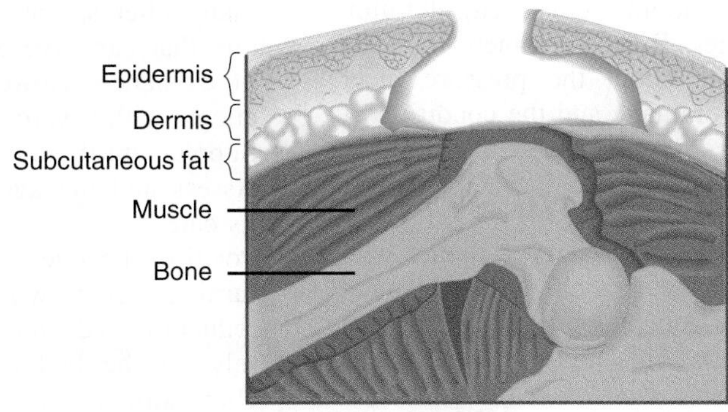
Stage III
Epidermis
Dermis
Subcutaneous fat
Muscle
Bone
Full-thickness skin loss involving damage or necrosis of subcutaneous tissue, which may extend down to, but not through, the underlying fascia. The ulcer presents clinically as a deep crater with or without undermining of adjacent tissue.

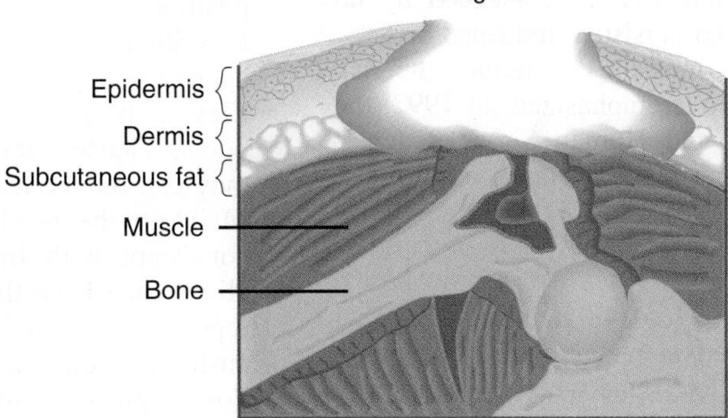
Stage IV
Epidermis
Dermis
Subcutaneous fat
Muscle
Bone
Full-thickness skin loss with extensive destruction, tissue necrosis, or damage to muscle, bone, or supporting structures (e.g., tendon, joint capsule, etc.)

FIGURE 49–7 Stages of pressure ulcers.

gastrointestinal disorders, feed oral supplements, or give tube feeding. Some clinicians use the phrase "if the gut works, use it" to summarize this recommendation. If the client has gastrointestinal problems, consider total parenteral nutrition. These more aggressive forms of feeding must be compatible with the client's wishes. Monitor nutritional status (as described previously) every 3 months. Body weight should be assessed every 1 to 4 weeks.

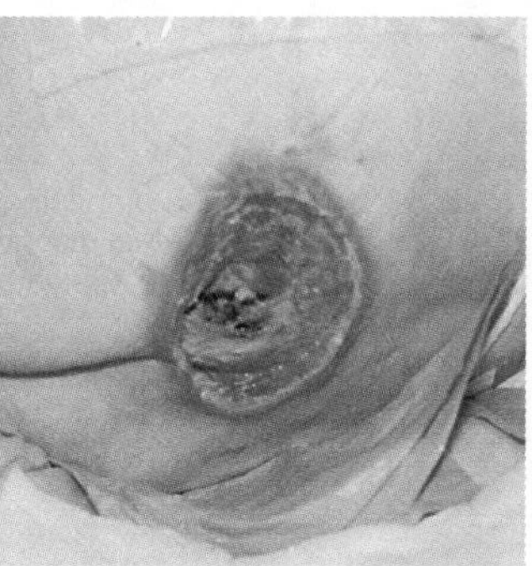

FIGURE 49–8 A stage IV pressure ulcer on the sacrum. The center of the ulcer contains necrotic tissue.

MONITOR FOR COMPLICATIONS

Many complications have been associated with pressure ulcers, including osteomyelitis, bacteremia and sepsis, and cellulitis. Amyloidosis, endocarditis, heterotopic bone formation, septic arthritis, and formation of a fistula from the ulcer to the perineum are rare but have been reported.

Nursing Management of the Medical Client

ASSESSMENT

The assessment of the client at high risk for development of pressure ulcers should identify any specific risk factors. The Braden Scale (Fig. 49–9) is an assessment tool that evaluates risk. This scale has been developed to assist the nurse in predicting which clients are at greatest risk. Assess laboratory data on hemoglobin, hematocrit, albumin, total protein, and lymphocytes. Risk assessment must be ongoing. Note objective data about the pressure ulcer (i.e., size, depth, or stage of drainage and the condition of periulcer tissue).

DIAGNOSIS, OUTCOMES, INTERVENTION

Risk for Impaired Skin Integrity. Clients who score between 12 and 16 on the Braden risk assessment scale are considered at risk for pressure ulcers. Scores below 12 indicate a high risk. This nursing diagnosis is written as *Risk for Impaired Skin Integrity related to malnutrition and unrelieved pressure.*

Outcomes. The client will experience a reduction in the risk of impairment of skin integrity, as evidenced by no actual tissue breakdown and no persistent reddened areas.

Interventions. Preventive measures to reduce the risk of pressure ulcers cannot be overemphasized. In 1992, the U.S. Department of Health and Human Services developed guidelines for prediction and prevention of pressure ulcers in adults[9] (Box 49–1).

EVALUATION

Outcomes should be met in 24 to 48 hours. Recall that skin integrity can be impaired in just 2 hours. Therefore, several hours are needed to determine whether skin injury occurred prior to risk reduction measures.

Impaired Skin Integrity. Use this diagnosis to describe an actual pressure ulcer. State the diagnosis as *Impaired Skin Integrity related to pressure ulcer secondary to prolonged immobility, malnutrition, and unrelieved pressure.*

Outcomes. The client will experience healing of the ulcer, as evidenced by development of granulation tissue and decreasing ulcer size. Do not use lower stages of pressure ulcers to describe healing. For example, do not state a stage IV will heal to a stage III. The body does not heal by regeneration of tissue but, rather, by scar tissue. For terminal clients, outcomes such as healing may not be appropriate. For these clients, outcomes of pain management or comfort may be more appropriate.

Interventions. Consistency in the nursing care provided is an important aspect of interventions directed at achieving wound healing. It is important to develop scientific protocols in ulcer care and to use them consistently. It is also important to give one protocol time to work before changing to another.

In 1994, the Agency for Health Care Policy and Research (AHCPR) established guidelines for pressure ulcer treatment.[8] The guidelines are summarized here. If your practice routinely involves nursing care of clients with pressure ulcers, obtaining the actual AHCPR document is recommended. See also Chapter 16 for information on wound healing.

- Ensure adequate dietary intake to prevent malnutrition and delayed healing.
- Assess nutritional status at least every 3 months in clients at risk for malnutrition, such as those in long-term care facilities. Clients in acute care settings need nutritional assessment weekly.
- Provide oral supplementation, tube feeding, or hyperalimentation to achieve positive nitrogen balance. For many clients, the decision not to eat is an important one that can give a sense of control over some aspect of existence. However, pressure ulcers cannot heal in clients with severe malnutrition.
- Supplement the diet with vitamins and minerals.
- Assess and manage pain associated with the ulcer and its care.
- Position the client to stay off the ulcer. If there is no turning surface without a pressure ulcer, use a pressure reduction bed and continue to turn the client. Do not rely on the bed exclusively to move the client. The client still needs to be repositioned. You cannot assess the skin if you cannot see it.
- Use positioning devices to hold the client in various positions. Do not use doughnut-type devices. Establish a written turning schedule, and post it according to agency policy.
- Elevate heels off the bed by using pillows or foam boots. Fleece heel covers do not relieve pressure, but they can reduce friction.
- Maintain the head of the bed at the lowest elevation consistent with the client's medical condition. If the client must have the head elevated to prevent aspiration, reposition into a 30-degree lateral position. Use a seat cushion in the chair, and assess for sacral ulcers daily. For dyspneic clients, position erect and assess for sacral and ischial ulcers daily.
- Use support surfaces for clients with multiple ulcers and for those who are not able to keep off the ulcer surface. Begin with a dynamic surface or mattress overlay. Progress to low-air-loss beds or air-fluidized beds (Fig. 49–10) if the ulcer does not heal.

RISK PREDICTORS FOR SKIN BREAKDOWN

Patient's Name__________ Evaluator's Name__________

SENSORY PERCEPTION ability to respond to discomfort	1. **Completely limited:** Unresponsive to painful stimuli, either because of state of unconsciousness or severe sensory impairment, which limits ability to feel pain over most of body surface	2. **Very limited:** Responds only to painful stimuli (but not verbal commands) by opening eyes or flexing extremities. Cannot communicate discomfort verbally, OR has a sensory impairment which limits the ability to feel pain or discomfort over one half of body surface	3. **Slightly limited:** Responds to verbal commands by opening eyes and obeying some commands, but cannot always communicate discomfort or need to be turned, OR has some sensory impairment which limits ability to feel pain or discomfort in one or two extremities.	4. **No impairment:** Responds to verbal commands by obeying. Can communicate needs accurately. Has no sensory deficit which would limit ability to feel pain or discomfort
MOISTURE degree to which skin is exposed to moisture	1. **Very Moist:** Skin is kept moist almost constantly by perspiration and urine. Dampness is detected every time patient is moved or turned. Linen must be changed more than one time each shift	2. **Occasionally Moist:** Skin is frequently, but not always kept moist, linen must be changed two to three times every 24 hours	3. **Rarely Moist:** Skin is rarely moist more than three to four times a week, but linen does require changing at that time	4. **Never Moist:** Perspiration and incontinence are never a problem linen changed at routine intervals only
ACTIVITY degree of physical activity	1. **Bedfast:** Confined to bed	2. **Chairfast:** Ability to walk severely impaired or nonexistent and must be assisted into chair or wheelchair. Is confined to chair or wheelchair when not in bed	3. **Walks occasionally:** Walks occasionally during day, but for very short distances, with or without assistance. Spends majority of each shift in bed or chair	4. **Walks frequently:** Walks a moderate distance at least once every 1 to 2 hours during waking hours
MOBILITY ability to change and control body position	1. **Completely Immobile:** Unable to make even slight changes in position without assistance	2. **Very limited:** Makes occasional slight changes in position without help but unable to make frequent or significant changes in position independently	3. **Slightly limited:** Makes frequent though slight changes in position without assistance but unable to make or maintain major changes in position independently	4. **No limitations:** Makes major and frequent changes in position without assistance
NUTRITION usual food intake pattern	1. **Very Poor:** Never eats a complete meal. Rarely eats more than 1/3 of any food offered. Intake of protein is negligible. Takes even fluids poorly. Does not take a liquid dietary supplement, OR is NPO and/or maintained on clear liquids or IV for more than 5 days	2. **Probably Inadequate:** Rarely eats a complete meal and generally eats only about one half of any food offered. Protein intake is poor. Occasionally will take a liquid dietary supplement, OR receiving less than optimum amount of liquid diet or tube feeding	3. **Adequate:** Eats over half of most meals. Eats moderate amount of protein source one to two times daily. Occasionally will refuse a meal. Will usually take a dietary supplement if offered OR is on a tube feeding or TPN regimen which probably meets most of nutritional needs	4. **Excellent:** Eats most of every meal. Never refuses a meal. Frequently eats between meals. Does not require a dietary supplementation
FRICTION AND SHEAR	1. **Problem:** Requires moderate to maximum assistance in moving. Complete lifting without sliding against sheets is impossible. Frequently slides down in bed or chair, requiring frequent repositioning with maximum assistance. Either spasticity, contractures or agitation leads to almost constant friction	2. **Potential Problem:** Moves feebly Independently or requires minimum assistance. Skin probably slides against bedsheets or chair to some extent when movement occurs. Maintains relatively good position in chair or bed most of time but occasionally slides down	3. **No Apparent Problem:** Moves in bed and in chair independently and has sufficient muscle strength to lift up completely during move. Maintains good position in bed or chair at all times	

Key: 16, minimum risk; 13–14, moderate risk; 12 or less, high risk;
NPO, nothing by mouth; IV, intravenously; TPN, total parenteral nutrition.

FIGURE 49–9 The Braden Scale for evaluation of risk of pressure ulcers. (Courtesy of Barbara Braden and Nancy Bergstrom. Copyright 1988.)

BOX 49–1 Prevention of Pressure Ulcers

- Perform a systematic skin inspection for all clients at risk at least once a day, with particular attention paid to the bony prominences.
- Document results of skin inspection.
- Cleanse the skin at the time of soiling and at routine intervals. The frequency of skin cleaning should be individualized according to need and client preference.
- Avoid hot water; use a mild cleaning agent that minimizes irritation and dryness of the skin. During the cleaning process, take care to minimize the force and friction applied to the skin.
- Minimize environmental factors leading to skin drying, such as low humidity (<40%) and exposure to cold. Treat dry skin with moisturizers.
- Avoid massage over bony prominences, which may be harmful.
- Minimize skin exposure to moisture from incontinence, perspiration, or wound drainage. When these sources of moisture cannot be controlled, apply underpads or briefs that are made of materials that absorb moisture and present a quick-drying surface to the skin. Topical agents that act as barriers to moisture can also be used.
- Minimize skin injury due to friction and shear forces through proper positioning, transferring, and turning techniques. In addition, help reduce friction injuries by the use of lubricants (e.g., cornstarch and creams), protective films (e.g., transparent film dressings and skin sealants), protective dressings (e.g., hydrocolloids), and protective padding.
- When apparently well-nourished clients do not have an adequate dietary intake of protein or calories, caregivers should first attempt to discover the factors compromising intake and offer support with eating. Other nutritional supplements or support may be needed. If dietary intake remains inadequate and if consistent with overall goals of therapy, consider more aggressive nutritional intervention (enteral or parenteral feedings).
- For nutritionally compromised clients, implement a plan of nutritional support or supplementation that meets individual needs and is consistent with the overall goals of therapy.
- If the potential exists for improving the client's mobility and activity status, institute rehabilitation efforts if these measures are consistent with the overall goals of therapy. Maintaining current activity level, mobility, and range of motion is an appropriate goal for most clients.
- Use a written schedule for systematically turning and repositioning the client.
- For clients in bed, use pillows to keep bony prominences (such as knees or ankles) from direct contact with one another.
- For clients in bed who are completely immobile, the care plan should include the use of devices that totally relieve pressure on the heels, most commonly by raising the heels off the bed. Do not use doughnut-type devices; they tend to cause pressure ulcers, not prevent them.
- When the side-lying position is used in bed, avoid positioning the client directly on the trochanter.
- Maintain the head of the bed at the lowest degree of elevation consistent with medical conditions and other restrictions. Limit the amount of time during which the head of the bed is elevated.
- Use a lifting device (trapeze, bed linen) to move, rather than drag, clients in bed who cannot assist during transfers and position changes.
- Place at risk clients on a pressure-reducing device, such as a foam, static air, alternating air, or water mattress.
- Ensure that any person at risk for a pressure ulcer avoids uninterrupted sitting in chair or wheelchair. The client should be repositioned, with appropriate shifts of the points under pressure, at least every hour. Teach clients who are able to shift their weight every 15 minutes.
- For chair-bound clients, select a pressure-reducing device, such as one made of foam, air, or a combination of these. Do not use a doughnut-type device.
- When positioning chair-bound clients, consider postural alignment, distribution of weight, balance and stability, and pressure relief.
- Provide a written plan for the use of positioning devices and schedules to help chair-bound clients.

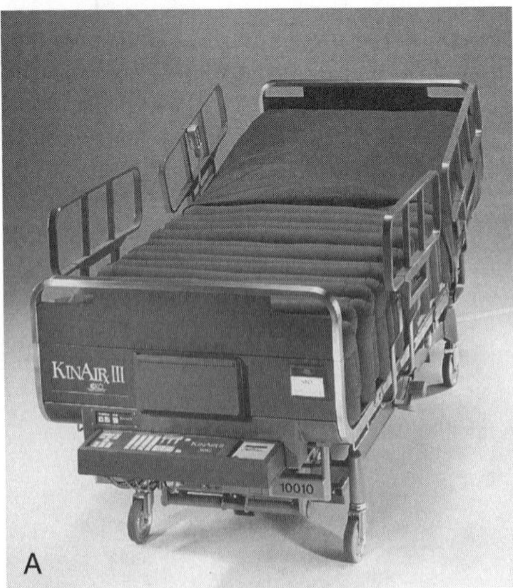

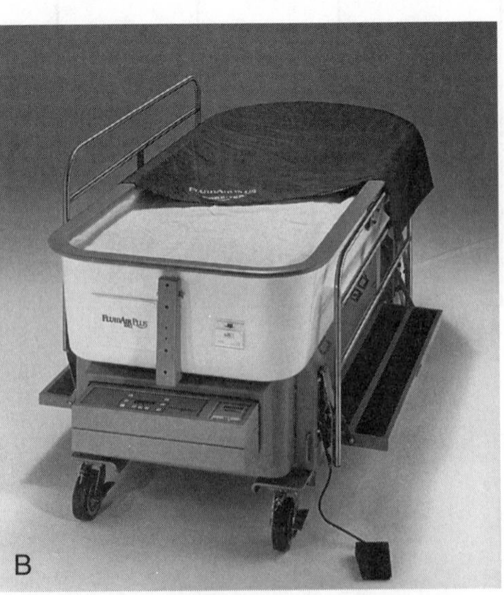

FIGURE 49–10 Pressure reduction surfaces. *A,* KinAir beds provide controlled air suspension to redistribute body weight away from bony prominences. *B,* FluidAir beds use air flow and bead fluidization. Both of these beds are covered with Gore-Tex fabric, which resists tearing. This fabric is also waterproof and acts as a barrier against bacteria. (Courtesy of Kinetic Concepts, Inc., San Antonio, TX.)

- Check for bottoming out beneath the mattress (Fig. 49–11). Place your hand between the mattress and the bed. If you feel less than an inch between the client's body and the mattress surface, the support is not adequate.
- Prevent moisture from coming in contact with the client's skin.
- Use support cushions for the wheelchair-bound client or for any client who prefers to sit.
- Teach wheelchair-bound clients to reposition themselves every 15 minutes.
- Debride the ulcer of devitalized tissue. Medicate for pain before debriding the ulcer.
- Clean the wound with normal saline. Avoid antiseptics on the wound bed.
- Use irrigation to clean the wound. Safe pressure ranges from 4 to 15 pounds per square inch. A 35-ml syringe with a 19-gauge angiocatheter is a good device for irrigation.
- Once the ulcer is free of devitalized tissue, apply dressings that keep the wound bed moist and the surrounding skin dry. Do not use occlusive dressings on ulcers that may be infected.
- Follow body substance isolation precautions; use clean gloves and clean dressings for wound care.

Reducing the risk of pressure ulcer development and identifying early signs of pressure ulcers are frequently delegated to unlicensed personnel (see the Management and Delegation feature). Case managers often assist in managing care between facilities. When preparing for discharge to home, case managers assist with advocating and preventing readmission (see the Case Management feature).

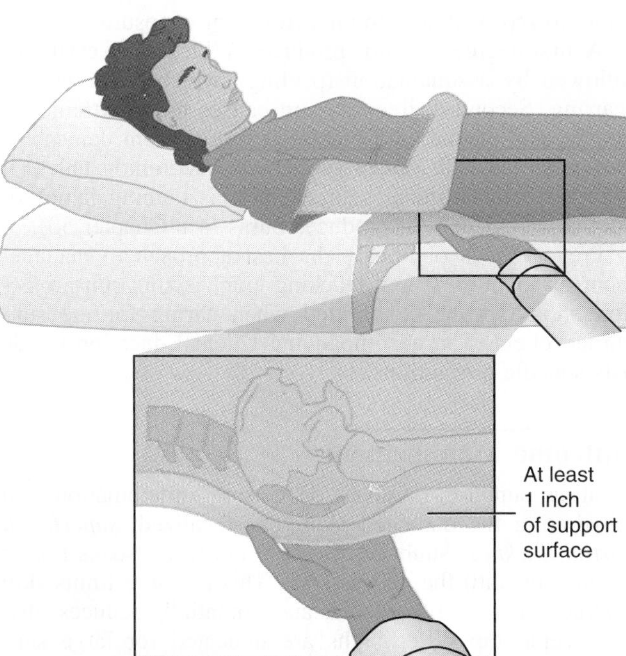

FIGURE 49–11 Assessment of pressure relief ("bottoming out"). Slide your hand (palm up and fingers flat) under the support surface, just under the pressure point. Do not flex your fingers. With adequate support, there will be at least 1 inch of uncompressed support surface between your hand and the client's body. (Modified from Gaymar Industries, Inc., Orchard Park, NY.)

EVALUATION

As the wound heals, assess the degree of outcome attainment every 3 to 4 days. Allow 2 weeks before changing the plan of care, unless the ulcer is deteriorating.

Self-Care

The clients at high risk for development of pressure ulcers should be referred to a home health agency before discharge from the acute care facility so that devices to reduce pressure can be obtained for home use. The family and the client need to understand the importance of frequent turning. A client who is wheelchair-bound and has arm function should be taught to lift the body, using the arms, off the chair twice every hour for repositioning. A client who is incontinent needs to wear protective pads to absorb the urine or stool and should be assessed often. The U.S. Department of Health and Human Services has developed a "patient guide" for preventing and treating pressure ulcers.[8, 9]

If the client is going home with an unhealed ulcer, the client and one or more family members must be taught

MANAGEMENT AND DELEGATION

Care of Clients with Pressure Ulcers

When working with unlicensed assistive personnel in the care of clients with pressure ulcers, help them to keep the following points in mind:

- Report any areas of skin redness that do not disappear after pressure relief.
- Report any development of foul odor or drainage from pressure ulcers.
- Reposition the client *at least* every 2 hours. Even a small shift in the client's body weight may be sufficient, but it must be done every 2 hours at a minimum.
- *Do not position the client on the ulcer.* If an ulcer is on the client's trunk, use a dynamic or overlay mattress. However, the use of these support surfaces does not eliminate the need for turning.
- If the client is wheelchair-bound, ensure that the padding provides adequate pressure relief by checking for "bottoming out."
- Keep all pressure off the client's heels. Use small pillows or foam padding to prevent direct contact.
- Keep the head of the bed at the lowest elevation to reduce shear and friction on the skin of the client's lower back.
- Keep the client's skin dry.

Be aware that even though you have delegated the skin care of these clients, you are still accountable for their skin condition. Assess the entire skin surface every day. Ask for help in turning the client so that you can see the client's heels and sacrum. Use an assessment guide such as the Braden Scale to determine the risk of further ulceration.

Donna W. Markey, MSN, RN, ACNP-CS, *Clinician IV, Surgical Services, University of Virginia Health System, Charlottesville, Virginia*

CASE MANAGEMENT

The Client with Impaired Skin Integrity

Impaired skin integrity, caused by breakdown, stasis, or iatrogenic conditions, is responsible for the expenditure of millions of health care dollars per year. When skin integrity is compromised, long lengths of stay and time-consuming, complex treatments are the result. The human costs—in terms of pain and suffering, infection, surgical procedures (amputation, debridement, grafting), and death—are even more staggering. Case management calls for primary prevention of skin breakdown and meticulous care and client education when skin integrity is impaired.

Advocate

It is much easier to prevent skin breakdown than to heal it after it occurs. Turning or ambulation schedules as well as good nutrition and hydration are often neglected in place of more complex nursing interventions, but they are just as important. When skin breakdown is present, be sensitive to the client's privacy needs and embarrassment resulting from the site of the problem or from the necessity of several caregivers to assist with treatment. Manage pain, allowing time for the analgesic to take effect before performing treatments or applying dressings. Sometimes skin breakdown occurs when clients can no longer care for themselves or do not realize the care needed. Help to realistically assess the client's needs after discharge from the facility, including the ability to return home.

Prevent Readmission

During hospitalization, the client may have benefited from use of a special low-pressure mattress or bed, special wound dressings, or ambulation and turning schedules. Surgical debridement or grafting may have facilitated wound healing. The fragile tissue can easily be damaged if conditions causing skin breakdown are able to reoccur.

Special beds, mattresses, or other equipment, such as a lifting device, may be useful as the client returns home. Make referrals for these devices (e.g., air-fluidized bed) and home nursing visits, aide support, physical therapy, and meal services as appropriate. Make sure that caregivers can manage the expected treatments and know how to use body mechanics and lifting devices.

Emphasize nutrition and hydration, and teach tube feeding or total parenteral nutrition techniques. Make sure that the client and caregivers are aware of hygiene and care for incontinence and know how to summon emergency assistance.

Cheryl Noetscher, RN, MS, *Director of Case Management, Crouse Hospital and Community–General Hospital, Syracuse, New York*

wound care, wound assessment, and in some cases the administration of intravenous (IV) antibiotics. Teach these interventions before the day of discharge, so that return demonstrations can be used to evaluate learning. In addition, procurement of equipment is often necessary, which takes time. Community nurses need to be involved early in the planning for the discharge of the client with an ulcer. The Bridge to Home Health Care describes ways to help the client and family manage pressure ulcers.

Surgical Management

Surgical repair is frequently performed on stage III and stage IV ulcers (see Fig. 49–7), on ulcers over 2 cm in diameter, and in clients who can tolerate surgery. In stage III ulcers, undamaged tissue near the wound is rotated to cover the ulcer. In stage IV ulcers, musculocutaneous flaps are often used (see later).

PRECANCEROUS CHANGES IN THE SKIN

Precursors to cancer of the skin include damage from recurrent skin trauma and various skin lesions. In order to understand the role of prevention of skin cancer, these precursor conditions are discussed first.

■ SUNBURN

Pathophysiology

Sunburn is an acute inflammatory skin response that occurs as a reaction to excessive exposure to sunlight. Dermatopathologic changes include the production of epidermal cells that exhibit cytoplasmic and nuclear changes. These changes are cumulative over the life span and lead to an increased incidence of skin cancer. *Photodamage* refers to repeated skin trauma from sun exposure.

A first-degree sunburn produces mild, tender erythema followed by desquamation (peeling), which heals without scarring. Second-degree sunburn causes more extreme erythema and edema, and blistering results from damage to the epidermal cells. Deep sunburn is uncommon unless it is induced by artificial sources such as tanning lamps or booths. Deep sunburn produces burns (see Chapter 50).

Prevention is obviously the best approach to management of sunburn. Client teaching emphasizing sun protection should never be omitted when caring for the sunburned client. The accompanying Client Education Guide lists specific precautions.

Outcome Management

Treating sunburn involves decreasing inflammation and rehydrating the damaged skin. For localized, *superficial, partial-thickness* sunburn, use cool tap water soaks for 20 minutes or until the skin is cool. This measure limits skin destruction, prevents edema, and potentially reduces blisters. Tepid tap water baths are indicated for large sunburned areas. After a bath or soak, apply water-based emollients, preferably refrigerated for an additional cooling effect. Emollients should also be applied throughout the day to soothe the skin and relieve dryness. Lotions or foams containing camphor and menthol (e.g., Sarna) can also be beneficial. Avoid the use of OTC remedies containing local anesthetics—such as benzocaine, dibucaine

BRIDGE TO HOME HEALTH CARE

Managing Pressure Ulcers

For the client with pressure ulcers, a smooth transition from hospital to home care requires planning, preparation, and communication. For example, it may take a home health nurse several days to obtain special wound care supplies or pressure relief devices not ordinarily stocked by the home health agency. If a pressure relief bed or mattress overlay is required, the agency then contacts a durable medical equipment company and arranges delivery at a predetermined time. To facilitate the transition from hospital care, the home health agency should be notified of the referral before the client's discharge from the hospital and should receive specific instructions per physician orders for wound cleansing, dressing materials, and frequency of dressing changes. In addition, sending a day's supplies home with the client helps to minimize disruption in the wound treatment regimen.

Clients who are eligible for Medicare and have stage IV or draining, infected pressure ulcers may initially require daily skilled nursing visits. However, as the infection is treated and drainage subsides, the frequency of skilled nursing visits is usually decreased and the family member or informal caregiver is taught to perform the dressing change. Caregivers should participate in or at least observe dressing change procedures in the hospital, and should receive information about turning and other aspects of care. The earlier the caregiver is introduced to prevention and treatment goals, the faster the client can reach the desired clinical outcome. Hospital nurses can significantly enhance the continuity of care by coordinating educational efforts with the home health agency. The home health nurse should obtain copies of any teaching materials distributed in the hospital. Older adults are often fearful of leaving the security of an inpatient setting; therefore, reinforcing familiar teaching materials and wound care procedures helps to ensure a more seamless transition from inpatient to outpatient management.

Maintaining equipment and supplies is more difficult in the home than in inpatient settings. Estimate the needed amount of skin and wound care supplies, and arrange for delivery in a timely manner. Establish an intercommunication sheet in the home that flags a change in wound care orders for other members of the health care team. Leave specific directions for product use, especially when more than one product is being used. *Normal saline* can be made by using the following recipe: mix 8 teaspoons of salt in 1 gallon of bottled or boiled water. Do not use water from an outdoor well.

Adapting the home environment to meet the needs of the client and family members or other caregivers requires creativity and skill. Note the conditions under which the client spends prolonged periods of time. Any firm, unyielding surface can contribute to development of a pressure ulcer in unusual body areas. Sitting on ridged, corded edges of chairs or stools or a firm toilet seat for extended periods can restrict blood flow, leading to pressure ulcer development.

The limitations of older clients and their older caregivers pose additional changes. For example, it may not be possible for a debilitated client to be turned as often as needed during the night to relieve pressure over bony prominences. Frequent turning schedules usually result in increased anxiety and sleep deprivation for older caregivers. Accurately assessing the client's risk category and using an effective pressure-relieving mattress overlay can help to reduce the physical demands for caregivers and increase the possibility that the client can receive needed care and remain at home.

Janice Z. Cuzzell, MA, RN, *Vice-President, Island Health Care, Inc., Savannah, Georgia*

(Nupercaine), or lidocaine (Xylocaine)—because they are rarely effective and have the potential to induce contact sensitivity.

For *partial-thickness* sunburn, apply continuous cool, normal saline soaks or soaking baths to reduce oozing and edema. Aspirate very large blisters, and apply sterile dressings. Avoid debridement unless there is evidence of secondary bacterial infection. Silver sulfadiazine may be prescribed.

Prostaglandin inhibitors (nonsteroidal anti-inflammatory drugs [NSAIDs]) may be used to reduce erythema and inflammation in adults. Topical corticosteroids may be prescribed to be used sparingly in nonocclusive vehicles (i.e., lotion, spray, gel) for their vasoconstrictive effects. Systemic corticosteroids are prescribed only for clients with very extensive, painful burns, but their use has declined because they seem to offer little efficacy when given in a reasonable dose range.

■ ACTINIC KERATOSIS

Actinic keratosis, the most common epithelial precancerous lesion in white people, is caused by sun exposure. It affects nearly 100% of older white adults. There is a small but definite risk of malignant degeneration and subsequent metastatic potential in neglected lesions.

Actinic keratosis most frequently occurs in areas of chronic, usually high-intensity sun exposure including the face, the tops of the ears, the back of the neck, the forearms, and the backs of the hands.

The clinical appearance of actinic keratoses can be quite varied. The typical lesion is an irregularly shaped, flat, slightly erythematous macule or papule with indistinct borders and an overlying hard keratotic scale or horn. In some cases, the erythema or the horn may be absent. This scale can be periodically shed or peeled off, but then it regrows. The lesion varies in size from a pinhead to several centimeters across and is often more easily palpated than observed. Single lesions may be seen, but more often they appear in groups on a background of sun-damaged skin.

Outcome Management

The goals of medical management are to eradicate the lesion and to educate the client how to reduce risk and recognize early skin changes.

CLIENT EDUCATION GUIDE

Simple Guidelines to Help Protect You from the Damaging Rays of the Sun

1. Minimize sun exposure during the hours of 10 AM to 2 PM (11 AM to 3 PM Daylight Saving Time), when the sun is strongest. Try to plan your outdoor activities for the early morning or late afternoon.
2. Wear a hat, long-sleeved shirt, and long pants when out in the sun. Choose tightly woven materials for greater protection from the sun's rays.
3. Apply a sunscreen before every exposure to the sun and reapply frequently and liberally—at least every 2 hours—as long as you stay in the sun. The sunscreen should always be reapplied after swimming or perspiring heavily, because products differ in degree of water resistance. Sunscreens with an SPF (sun protection factor) of 15 or more printed on the label are recommended.
4. Use a sunscreen during high-altitude activities such as mountain climbing and skiing. At high altitudes, where there is less atmosphere to absorb the sun's rays, your risk of burning is greater. The sun is also stronger near the equator, where the sun's rays strike the earth most directly.
5. Do not forget to use your sunscreen on overcast days. The sun's rays are as damaging to your skin on cloudy, hazy days as they are on sunny days.
6. If you are at high risk for skin cancer (if you work outdoors, are fair-skinned, or have already had skin cancer), apply sunscreen daily.
7. Photosensitivity—an increased sensitivity to sun exposure—is a possible side effect of certain medications, drugs and cosmetics, and birth control pills. Consult your physician or pharmacist before going out in the sun if you are using any such products. You may need to take extra precautions.
8. If you develop an allergic reaction to your sunscreen, change sunscreens. One of the many products on the market today should be right for you.
9. Beware of reflective surfaces! Sand, snow, concrete, and water can reflect more than half of the sun's rays onto your skin. Sitting in the shade does not guarantee protection from sunburn.
10. Avoid tanning parlors. The ultraviolet light emitted by tanning booths causes sunburn and premature aging and increases your risk of developing skin cancer.
11. Keep young children out of the sun. Begin using sunscreens on children at 6 months of age, and then allow sun exposure with moderation.
12. Teach children sun protection early. Sun damage occurs with each unprotected sun exposure and accumulates over the course of a lifetime.

From The Skin Cancer Foundation, New York.

ERADICATE THE LESION

Topical application of 5-fluorouracil (5-FU) (Efudex), a topical antimetabolite, is at present one of the best approaches to treatment of widespread actinic damage, with multiple lesions. The advantage of 5-FU is that large areas of widespread disease can be treated at the same time. Use of 5-FU not only removes the majority of premalignant and superficial malignant lesions that can be seen but also uncovers and destroys clinically undetectable lesions of this type. However, the major disadvantage is the therapeutic inflammatory response that often accompanies successful treatment. This response sequence is erythema usually followed by vesiculation, erosion, ulcerations, necrosis, and epithelialization.

The medication should be applied twice daily with a gloved hand, carefully avoiding eyes, nose, mouth, and scrotum. A porous gauze dressing may be applied over the medication for cosmetic reasons without increase in reaction. However, occlusive dressing should be avoided because of increased inflammatory response. Medication should be continued until the inflammatory response reaches the erosion, necrosis, and ulceration stage, at which time the medication should be stopped. The usual duration of therapy is 2 to 4 weeks; by then, the client may experience extreme discomfort requiring pain medication. At the time 5-FU is stopped, topical corticosteroid creams may be applied to reduce inflammation and provide the client with additional pain relief. Complete healing of the lesions may not be evident for 1 to 2 months after cessation of therapy.

Surgical Management

CRYOTHERAPY

Cryotherapy using liquid nitrogen is the most common treatment for single lesions or for small numbers of actinic keratoses. Liquid nitrogen is usually applied with a cotton-tipped applicator or spraying device (Fig. 49–12*A*). No local anesthetic is required but the freezing process is associated with a small amount of discomfort, which may linger afterward. Intermittent application of a warm, damp wash cloth to the site may bring relief. Freezing frequently results in inflammation with blister formation, and blister care should be reviewed with the client. Care must be taken to avoid overfreezing the site, which may result in scarring. Cryotherapy is cost-effective and easy to perform and has minimal side effects.

ELECTRODESICCATION AND CURETTAGE

Electrodesiccation produces superficial destruction through generation of radiofreqency waves that cause a very hot spark to arc onto the lesion. The procedure is usually done using local anesthesia (Fig. 49–12*B*). The tissue is destroyed by mechanical disruption of cells and heat. The tissue is removed by scraping or scooping with a loop-shaped instrument called a curet (Fig. 49–12*C*). This method provides tissue for histologic diagnosis if needed. The curetted areas usually heal quickly with adequate wound care. The wound site should be kept moist with a nonsensitizing topical antibiotic ointment such as bacitracin.

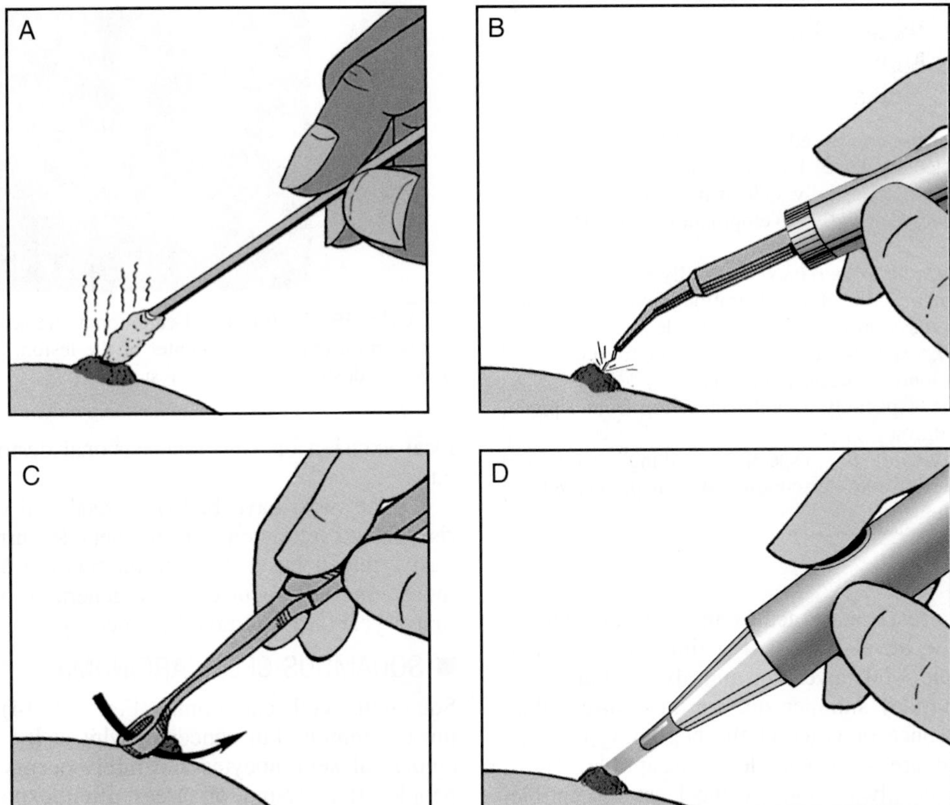

FIGURE 49–12 Methods for destroying skin lesions. *A,* Cryotherapy. Liquid nitrogen is applied with a saturated cotton-tipped applicator directly to the lesion or sprayed on. This causes tissue destruction by freezing. *B,* Electrodesiccation. Tissue is destroyed by heat from an electrical current; note the gloved hand. *C,* Curettage. A curet (cutting instrument) removes tissue by scraping or scooping; note gloved hand. *D,* The laser removes tissue by vaporizing it.

Laser Excision

Laser uses light energy to vaporize lesions (Fig. 49–12*D*). Depending upon the wave length of the light, various portions of the cell are heated. Tissue is not available for histologic examination. Local anesthesia is used.

Shave or Excisional Biopsy

Shave (excisional) biopsy is indicated for lesions that are large or have other characteristics of a cutaneous malignancy (induration, erythema, erosion). It is often difficult to distinguish a large actinic keratosis from a squamous cell carcinoma without histologic diagnosis. Biopsy should also be done on lesions that persist after adequate treatment with 5-FU. Local anesthesia is used for the biopsy procedure and allows electrodesiccation to be done painlessly after biopsy. Excisional biopsy requires primary closure of the site and may be a more extensive procedure than the lesion warrants; however, it ensures removal of the entire growth (see Chapter 48, Fig. 48–4).

Skin Cancer

Skin cancer is the most common cancer in the United States, and the number of new skin cancers and the number of skin cancer deaths are increasing at alarming rates. Skin cancer is a malignant condition caused by uncontrolled growth and spread of abnormal cells in a specific layer of the skin. The several different kinds of skin cancer are distinguished by the types of cells involved. The three most common types are (1) basal cell carcinoma, (2) squamous cell carcinoma, and (3) malignant melanoma. More than 90% of all skin cancers fall into the first two classifications. Both basal cell carcinoma and squamous cell carcinoma are slow-growing tumors with a cure rate of 95% or greater after early treatment.

Etiology and Risk Factors

The cause of skin cancer is well known. Prolonged or intermittent, repeated exposure to UVL radiation from the sun, especially when it results in sunburn and blistering, plays a key role in the induction of skin cancer, especially malignant melanoma. The majority of all non-melanoma skin cancers occur on parts of the body unprotected by clothing (face, neck, forearms, and backs of hands) and in people who have received considerable exposure to sunlight. All people are at risk of skin cancer regardless of skin tone and hair color; however, some are at much greater risk than others. In general, people with red, blond, or light brown hair with light complexions or freckles, many of Celtic or Scandinavian origin, are most susceptible; blacks and Asians are least susceptible.

All clients should be taught to look for new moles or lesions and to evaluate them for danger signs of cancer. Danger signals in moles (pigmented nevi) are presented in Box 49–2. Suspicious lesions should be examined by a physician.

BOX 49–2 Danger Signals Suggestive of Malignant Transformation of Moles

- *Change in color,* especially red, white, and blue; sudden darkening; mottled shades of brown or black
- *Change in diameter,* especially sudden increase
- *Change in outline,* especially development of irregular margins
- *Change in surface characteristics,* especially scaliness, erosion, oozing, crusting, bleeding, ulceration, development of a mushrooming mass on the surface of the lesion
- *Change in consistency,* especially softening or friability
- *Change in symptoms,* especially pruritus
- *Change in shape,* especially irregular elevation from a previously flat condition
- *Change in surrounding skin,* especially "leaking" of pigment from the lesion into surrounding skin or pigmented "satellite" lesions

The pattern of reaction to acute sun exposure can be correlated with the development of actinic keratosis and skin cancer. People who never tan and always burn after 1 to 2 hours of midday summer sun are most susceptible. People who burn once or twice at the beginning of summer and then tan are somewhat less susceptible. Those who never burn and always tan are the least susceptible. The most severely affected people usually have a history of long-term occupational (farmers, construction workers, surveyors, sailors) or recreational (swimmers, skiers, surfers, sunbathers) sun exposure.

Clinical Manifestations

■ BASAL CELL CARCINOMA

Basal cell carcinoma, the most common form of skin cancer, is a malignant epithelial tumor of the skin that arises from the basal cells in the epidermis. The tumor is usually painless and slow-growing, generally appearing on sun-exposed skin of the face, ears, head, neck, or hands. Occasionally, basal cell carcinoma may appear on the trunk, especially the upper back and chest. The majority of cases are caused by chronic overexposure to UVL radiation, and only a few cases can be linked to arsenic, burns, scars, exposure to radiation, or genetic predisposition. Clinical and histologic findings are used to identify the tumor.

The most common clinical presentation of basal cell carcinoma is the nodular lesion (Fig. 49–13). This is a dome-shaped papule with a well-defined border having a classic "pearly" texture. Basal cell carcinoma has this flesh-colored "pearly" or shiny appearance because it does not keratinize. Telangiectatic vessels frequently overlie the lesion. As the lesion enlarges, the center may flatten or ulcerate; however, the border is still raised, giving a "rolled-edge" appearance.

Although basal cell carcinomas almost never metastasize, they can be locally destructive and invasive through tissue. This is particularly true on the face, where a lesion can invade deep structures with resultant loss of an eye or ear or the nose. If untreated, the tumor can invade through bone and brain. If the tumor is identified and treated early, local excision or even nonexcisional destruction is usually curative.

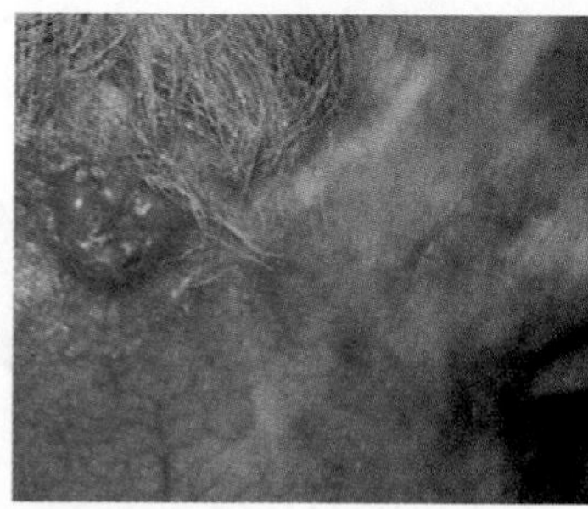

FIGURE 49–13 Basal cell carcinoma characterized by rolled edges and a crater in the center of the lesion. Scars are from previous destruction of skin lesions.

Clients who have had one basal cell carcinoma are at risk for development of another. Recurrences of previously treated basal cell carcinomas are also possible but more unusual; recurrence is generally noted within the first 2 years after removal or therapy.

■ SQUAMOUS CELL CARCINOMA

Squamous cell carcinoma (Fig. 49–14) is the second most common skin cancer in whites. It is a tumor of the epidermal keratinocytes and rarely occurs in dark-skinned people. It is found on areas often exposed to the sun, typically the rim of the ear, the face, the lips and mouth, and the backs of the hands.

Squamous cell carcinoma is more difficult to characterize than basal cell carcinoma. The tumor is poorly marginated; the edge often blends into surrounding sun-damaged skin. Squamous cell carcinoma may present as an ulcer, a flat red area, a cutaneous horn, an indurated plaque, or a hyperkeratotic papule or nodule. Often it presents as a red- to skin-colored papule surmounted by varying amounts of scale.

The lesions grow more rapidly than does basal cell carcinoma. These tumors are potentially dangerous because they may infiltrate surrounding structures and metastasize to lymph nodes, with a fatal outcome.

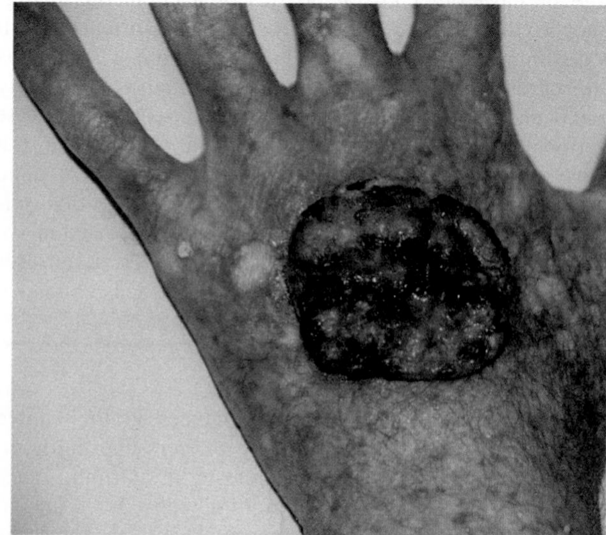

FIGURE 49–14 Squamous cell carcinoma on the hand.

MALIGNANT MELANOMA

Malignant melanoma (Figs. 49–15 and 49–16) is a cancer of melanocytes; it is the deadliest form of skin cancer. The incidence of and death rate from melanoma are rising worldwide. In countries populated with fair-skinned white people, the incidence of melanoma and the mortality rate have risen by 7% to 15% per year, more than doubling during the 1990s. Whites have 10 times the incidence of blacks.

Exposure to UVL continues to be one of the most important causes of malignant melanoma. However, melanoma can appear anywhere on the body, not just on sun-exposed areas. Most malignant melanomas appear to be associated with the intensity rather than the duration of sunlight exposure, in contrast to basal cell and squamous cell carcinomas. Melanoma tends to be observed more often in whites who have had a history of blistering sunburns or a family history of melanoma or atypical moles. The suspicion of melanoma is based on history as well as the clinical appearance.

Clinical Manifestations

The cardinal clinical manifestation of melanoma is a change in a skin lesion observed over a period of months. If a lesion grows so fast that it doubles in size in 10 days, it is usually an inflammation. If a lesion changes so slowly that neither the client nor family is sure of a change, it is usually benign. Changes that may signal melanoma include doubling size in 3 to 8 months, change in diameter, bleeding, itching, ulceration, a change in color, or development of a palpable lymph node.

Melanomas usually have the following features: (1) various shades of brown, black, or blue within one lesion, (2) an irregular raised surface, (3) an irregular perimeter, (4) ulceration of the surface, and (5) crusting. Four types of melanoma are presented in Table 49–4. The tumor can metastasize, usually to the brain, lungs, bones, liver, and skin, and is ultimately fatal. The prognosis with melanoma has become more predictable. Clinically, metastatic melanoma is universally fatal. Prognosis and mortality for melanoma that is not clinically metastatic at presentation depend on the depth of the lesion at the time of excision.

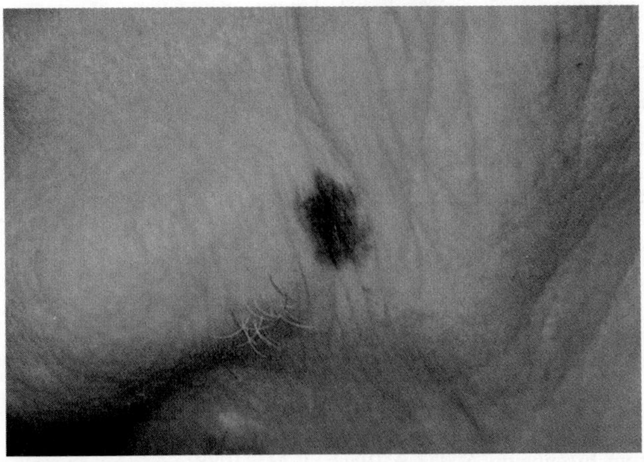

FIGURE 49–15 Superficial spreading melanoma.

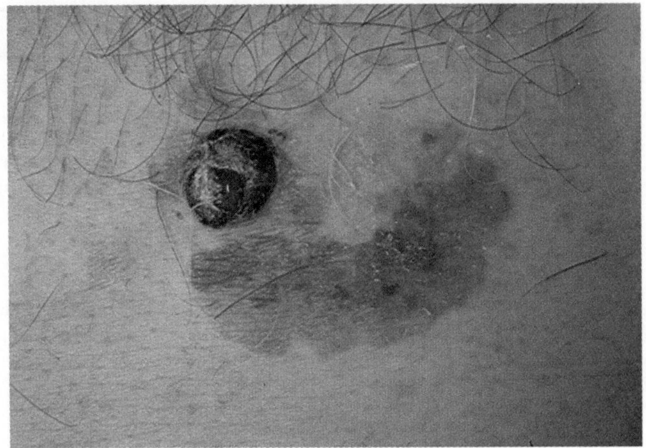

FIGURE 49–16 Nodular melanoma.

The more superficial or "thin" the tumor, the better the prognosis.

Outcome Management

Medical Management

Medical management begins with a high level of suspicion for any type of skin cancer but specifically for melanoma. The need for early detection cannot be overemphasized. Any indication, whether it is a confirmed risk factor or a suspicious lesion, is adequate reason for referral. The most exciting medical development in the treatment of melanoma is the creation and testing of therapeutic vaccines. A variety of vaccines targeting melanoma cell antigens are in the clinical trial phase.

Surgical Management

Treatment of all skin cancers requires removal of the lesion. The margins of the resected specimen must be free of tumor to a specified distance (depending on the type of skin cancer) to guarantee full removal.

A special surgical technique primarily used for the removal of skin malignancies such as basal cell carcinoma and squamous cell carcinoma is *Mohs' surgery,* which is also indicated for primary lesions in areas in which preservation of normal skin is necessary (e.g., eyelids, pinna, nasolabial folds). The technique involves a series of excisions with careful microscopic tissue assessment to "map" the presence or absence of malignant cells within each specimen. The procedure may be lengthy. After all tumor tissue is removed, the wound is closed with sutures or with a flap or allowed to close by secondary intention.

Basal cell carcinomas and squamous cell carcinomas can also be excised and the surgical wound closed primarily (with skin edges sewn together) or with a skin flap. The advantage of this technique is that it requires much less time, and the scar is controllable as a fine line. The tumor is completely excised with adequate margins of tumor-free tissue. If there is doubt about adequacy of margins, the specimen is sent for pathologic diagnosis (by frozen section technique).

TABLE 49–4 TYPES OF MELANOMA

Tumor Type	General Information	Clinical Manifestations
Superficial spreading melanoma (SSM)	The most common form of melanoma; slowly changing lesion with more rapid growth just before diagnosis	Deeply pigmented area contained within a brown nevus (freckle); usually flat and asymmetrical; as lesion grows, color changes may occur, ranging from jet black to dark blue to pale gray or white; looks lacy; lesions may have areas of no color; usually 2 cm wide
Nodular melanoma (NM)	Second most common form of melanoma; more aggressive tumor than SSM, with shorter clinical onset time	Common on the trunk, head, and neck; usually 1–2 cm in diameter; frequently begin in normal skin, rather than in a pre-existing lesion; dark and more uniform in color; may resemble a blood blister or hemangioma; dome-shaped with sharp borders
Lentigo maligna melanoma (LMM)	Fairly uncommon tumor; typically appears on the face of white women; usually has been present for long period of time (5–15 yr)	Generally a large, flat lesion that looks like a stain on the skin; typically tan with various shades of brown; metastasis less common
Acral lentiginous melanoma (ALM)	Commonly occurs on palms and soles; more common in dark-skinned people; usually occurs in older adults; may evolve over a few months to years	Large lesion, about 3 cm in diameter; resembles LMM (a tan or brown flat lesion on the palm or sole); can be misdiagnosed as a corn; ulceration is common; likely to metastasize

The treatment of malignant melanoma is wide local excision. Surgical excision begins with biopsy to determine the stage of the cancer. Biopsies are performed whenever a benign nature of the lesion is uncertain. Excisional biopsy is the removal of the lesion and a narrow margin of normal-appearing tissue. This tissue is examined, and the melanoma is staged (Fig. 49–17).

Surgeons differ on the timing of the definitive surgery. Some surgeons excise the lesion after frozen section examination while the client is still on the operating table.

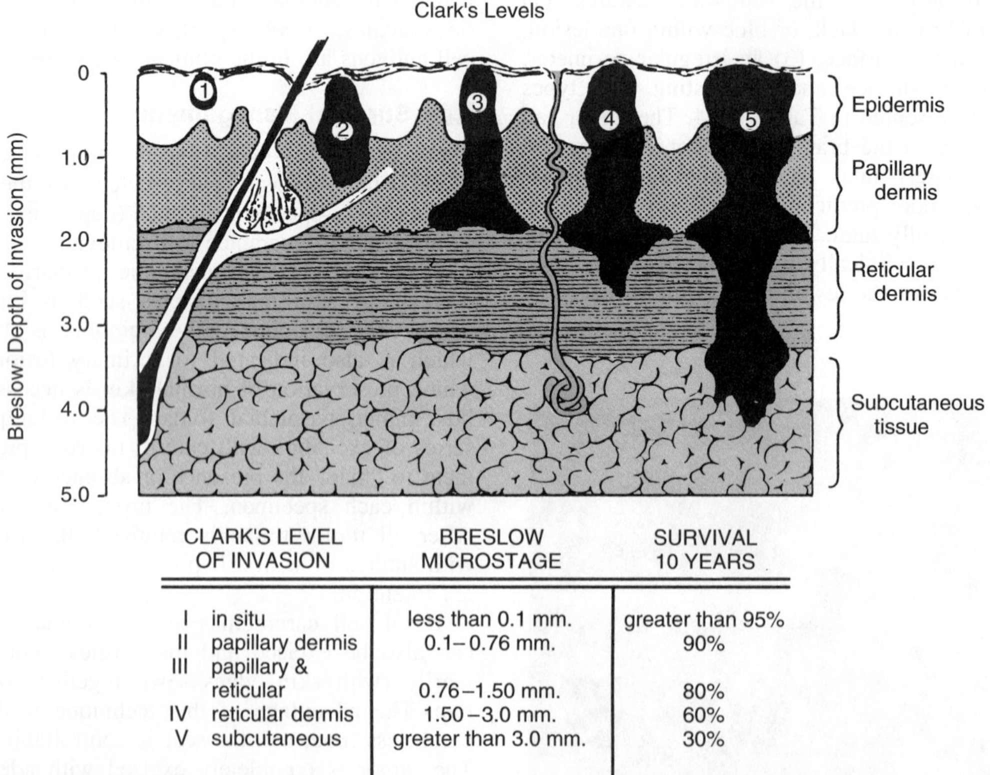

CLARK'S LEVEL OF INVASION	BRESLOW MICROSTAGE	SURVIVAL 10 YEARS
I in situ	less than 0.1 mm.	greater than 95%
II papillary dermis	0.1–0.76 mm.	90%
III papillary & reticular	0.76–1.50 mm.	80%
IV reticular dermis	1.50–3.0 mm.	60%
V subcutaneous	greater than 3.0 mm.	30%

FIGURE 49–17 The combination of Clark's level of invasion and Breslow's depth of invasion allows prediction of 10-year survival in melanoma. (From Eisenbaum, S. L., & Black, J. M. [1988]. Melanoma. *Plastic Surgical Nursing, 8,* 42–47.)

Other surgeons wait for the results of permanent section pathologic diagnosis and then proceed with definitive treatment. The final excision is usually completed within 1 week of biopsy. Although there is a theoretical risk of tumor spread during biopsy, there is no convincing evidence that waiting 1 to even 6 weeks after biopsy jeopardizes the outcome. In fact, sometimes the delay gives the client time to prepare for surgery, both physically and psychologically.

The tumor is excised with a 1- to 3-cm margin of normal-appearing tissue. The margin width is based on the type of melanoma. The surgical wound is closed either primarily or with grafts or flaps.

Most clients with metastatic melanoma live less than 1 year. There is no cure today for metastatic melanoma, but some of the new developments in clinical trials may change currently accepted treatments. A treatment plan is formulated on the basis of several factors: site of the tumor, number of metastases, rate of tumor growth, previous treatments, response to treatment, and the age, general health, and desires of the client. Some treatments include surgery to remove metastatic lesions, radiation therapy, chemotherapy, and local hyperthermia. Of course, the client can opt for no further treatment.

■ CUTANEOUS T-CELL LYMPHOMA (MYCOSIS FUNGOIDES)

Cutaneous T-cell lymphoma (CTCL), or mycosis fungoides, is a malignant disease involving the T helper cells. Malignant T cells in the blood migrate to the skin, where they have an affinity for the epidermis. The malignant cells continue to grow and change, eventually moving into the dermis. The cause is not known, and the course is unpredictable, varying with the type of presentation.

The three distinct clinical presentations are patch, plaque, and tumor. Clinical manifestations include eversion of the eyelids and hyperkeratosis of the palms and soles, often with fissuring. Finally, the plaques form tumors that ultimately ulcerate. Tumors can also develop spontaneously in previously unaffected areas, and eventual visceral or organ involvement ensues. This disease is often described as a slow-growing but highly disfiguring debilitating cancer. Clients often feel desperate by the time diagnosis is confirmed, which adds to the psychological difficulties. The tumor presentation carries the worst prognosis, with a survival period of 3 years or less.

CTCL is extremely difficult to diagnose and is often misdiagnosed. In its early stages, CTCL can clinically mimic eczematous processes. The initial erythematous papules resemble those in other eczematous conditions, including psoriasis and atopic dermatitis. The original eruptions of CTCL may be either transitory or of prolonged duration and sometimes are pruritic.

Outcome Management

Control of pruritus is essential at all stages and is accomplished by rehydration of the skin, various dry skin therapies (see Xerotic Eczema), topical corticosteroids, and PUVA therapy (see Ultraviolet Light Therapy). Prevention of secondary infections is important. Nitrogen mustard and other chemotherapy agents are administered topically. Daily application of chemotherapeutic agents often constitutes the initial treatment. Photophoresis, a treatment involving the removal of small amounts of blood that is irradiated and then returned to the body, is used frequently in more advanced stages. Total-body electron beam therapy with or without adjuvant chemotherapy is an aggressive approach often used.

The primary systemic drug was formerly intravenous methotrexate. With advances in treatment, newer drugs have replaced methotrexate: one is denileukin diftitox (Ontak) used primarily in the treatment of persistent or recurrent CTCL. This agent has produced sustained regression of the tumors, in some cases for longer than 2 years. Unfortunately, fatalities remain extremely high in this disease as a result of progression to systemic involvement.

■ KAPOSI'S SARCOMA

Kaposi's sarcoma is a vascular malignancy that presents as a skin disorder. It has a long history. Kaposi's sarcoma used to be a skin disease seen predominantly in 50- to 60-year-old men in Central or Eastern Europe. It was also seen, although less frequently, in blacks and the immunosuppressed (e.g., renal transplant recipients). In the past two decades, Kaposi's sarcoma has been seen more often in clients with acquired immunodeficiency syndrome (AIDS).

Etiology and Risk Factors

The cause of Kaposi's sarcoma is not known, although infection with HIV and herpesvirus have been suggested as cofactors in its development. It is considered to be due to a failure in the immune system, perhaps as a result of frequent or overwhelming infections. The lesions begin in the mid-dermis and extend upward into the epidermis.

The client history must include specific details of the sexual history when lesions of this type are present. All known risk factors for AIDS should be identified, such as homosexual activity, intravenous (IV) drug use, and multiple sexual partners.

Clinical Manifestations

The lesions of Kaposi's sarcoma begin as red, dark blue, or purple macules on the lower legs that coalesce into larger plaques (Fig. 49–18). These large plaques frequently ulcerate or open and drain. The lesions spread by metastasis through the upper body and then to the face and oral mucosa. Lesions of the lymph nodes, gastrointestinal tract, and lungs develop in about 75% of clients. Clients also report pain and itching in the lesions; as Kaposi's sarcoma progresses, the legs become edematous.

The diagnosis of Kaposi's sarcoma is confirmed by skin biopsy. A high index of suspicion should exist for those clients with immunosuppression.

Outcome Management

Local lesions can be excised or treated with intralesional chemotherapy. Systemic lesions are treated with a combination of interferon-alpha, cytotoxic agents, and radiation therapy. In general, response to treatment is poor. A complete discussion of AIDS may be found in Chapter 79.

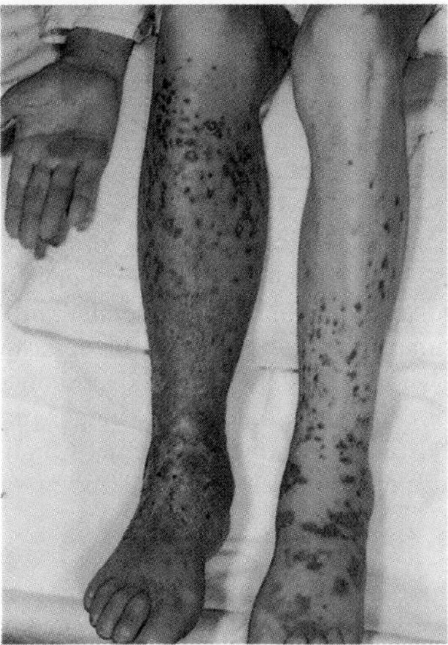

FIGURE 49–18 Kaposi's sarcoma.

Nursing interventions include obtaining informed consent for HIV testing and addressing the client's questions and concerns. Client education should include guidelines for safe sex and giving clients the addresses and telephone numbers of appropriate local and national resource groups.

BULLOUS DISORDERS: PEMPHIGUS

Pemphigus is a chronic disorder that results in the development of blisters (*bullae*). It is fairly uncommon in the general population, but the incidence is increased in Jewish and Mediterranean peoples. There are several types: pemphigus vulgaris, pemphigus foliaceus, and pemphigus erythematosus. This discussion focuses on pemphigus vulgaris, the most common type.

Pemphigus is an autoimmune disease caused by circulating immunoglobulin G (IgG) autoantibodies. These autoantibodies react with the intracellular cement—the substance that holds epidermal cells together. The reaction causes intraepidermal bulla (blister) formation and acantholysis (loss of cohesion between epidermal cells).

Clinical manifestations include flaccid bullae that rupture easily, emitting a foul-smelling drainage and leaving crusted, denuded skin. Nikolsky's sign is the result when the epidermis can be rubbed off by slight friction or injury; this sign is a hallmark of pemphigus. Even slight pressure on an intact blister may cause it to spread to adjacent skin. The lesions are common on the face, back, chest, groin, and umbilicus.

Outcome Management

Management includes large doses of steroids and immunosuppressives. Plasmapheresis has been of some benefit in the treatment of pemphigus. If a large proportion of the skin is denuded, management is similar to that for a burn-injured client. The client is at increased risk for infection, fluid and electrolyte imbalance, and stress response complications (i.e., stress ulcers, body system failure). In addition, nursing management focuses on self-concept and pain management. Potassium permanganate baths may be used to reduce the risk of infection, control the odor of the drainage, and ease the pain.

INFECTIOUS DISORDERS

Several organisms lead to skin infections and infestations. Common skin infections are described in Table 49–5. A few are discussed in detail here.

■ ERYSIPELAS AND CELLULITIS

Erysipelas is an acute, superficial, rapidly spreading inflammation of the dermis and lymphatics. The usual causative agent is beta-hemolytic group A streptococci. The organism enters tissue via an abrasion, bite, trauma, or wound. Fever and leukocytosis (elevated white blood cell count) are present. The initial lesion is small, elevated, and bright red. The involved area spreads peripherally to become a plaque with sharp, indurated borders. Lesions are most common on the face and extremities. Recurrence in the same area is common, possibly because of underlying lymphatic obstruction.

Cellulitis is a skin infection extending into the deeper dermis and subcutaneous fat that results in deep, red erythema without sharp borders that spreads widely through tissue spaces (see Fig. 49–19). The skin is erythematous, edematous, tender, and sometimes nodular. *Streptococcus pyogenes* is the usual cause of this infection; however, other pathogens may be responsible. Lymphangitis may occur; if cellulitis is untreated, gangrene, metastatic abscesses, and sepsis result.

At increased risk for erysipelas and cellulitis are older adults and clients with lowered resistance from diabetes, malnutrition, steroid therapy, or the presence of wounds or ulcers. Other predisposing factors include the presence of edema and of other cutaneous inflammation or wounds (e.g., tinea, eczema, burns, trauma). There is a tendency for recurrence, especially at sites of lymphatic obstruction.

Erysipelas and cellulitis are treated by either oral or IV antibiotics that are effective against both streptococci and *Staphylococcus aureus.* Before antibiotics are administered, a wound specimen for culture and sensitivity testing should be obtained, although culture rarely yields the causative organism. Soaks may reduce edema and inflammation. The enzymes that facilitate a rapid spread of infection also seem to produce other significant manifestations such as high fever, tachycardia, confusion, and hypotension; appropriate interventions should be undertaken if these occur. Monitor the client's temperature and administer prescribed antipyretic medication. Prevent cross-contamination by teaching the client proper hand-washing technique and careful handling of soiled linen, clothing, dressings, and so forth. Universal precautions should be used as appropriate. Close follow-up evaluation is necessary.

■ HERPES ZOSTER (SHINGLES)

Herpes zoster (Fig. 49–20), or shingles, is an infection caused by the reactivation of the varicella virus in clients who have had chickenpox. Although zoster is much less

TABLE 49–5 COMMON SKIN INFECTIONS AND INFESTATIONS

Disease with Causative Organism	Clinical Manifestations	Management
PARASITIC		
Scabies: *Sarcoptes scabiei*	Multiple straight or wavy thread-like lines beneath the skin, itching	Application of a scabicide with re-treatment in 1 wk to kill residual eggs. All clothing and linen should be washed and dried in hot cycles or dry cleaned.
Lice: *Pediculus humanus, Phthirus pubis*	Intense itching; scratch marks may be evident	Application of pediculicides. For *head lice,* the shampoo should be worked into dry hair until it is saturated. A fine-toothed comb should be used to remove dead lice and nits. Brushes and combs should be washed in pediculicide also. For *body lice,* a pediculicide lotion is applied to involved body areas. Clothing should be washed and dried in hot cycles or dry cleaned. Other items can be stored in plastic bags for 30–35 days. Family members, close contacts, and sexual partners should be treated, too.
BACTERIAL		
Impetigo: group A streptococci, staphylococci	Pruritic vesicle or pustule that breaks and leaves a thick honey-colored crust	Antibiotics given until culture results available include erythromycin or dicloxacillin. Mupirocin preferable to oral antibiotics when lesions limited to small, localized area. Teach control of contagion; infection is contagious as long as skin lesions are present. Thorough hand-washing, separate laundry for client's linens, separate washing of client's dishes.
Folliculitis, furuncles, carbuncles: *Staphylococcus aureus*	White pustules on forehead, chest, upper back, neck, thighs, groin, and axillae; furuncles are deeper inflamed nodules; carbuncles are interconnected furuncles and often rupture, expelling purulent, foul-smelling thick drainage	Localized folliculitis is treated with warm compresses, gentle washing, and topical antibiotics. Furuncles are treated as for folliculitis with incision and drainage (I&D) to avoid rupture. Carbuncles are treated with systemic antibiotics and I&D. Instruct client to use disposable razors to avoid reinfection. Reduce spread of infection by careful hand-washing and separate laundry of linens.
FUNGAL		
Candidiasis: *Candida albicans*	Appearance depends on location; in the *mouth,* infection is called thrush and appears as white plaques with an underlying red base with fissures on corners of the mouth; *skin* lesions are pruritic, red, and moist with eroded scales, commonly found in the axilla and gluteal, perianal, and interdigital folds; *vaginal* thrush causes intense itching and a cheesy drainage	Eliminate or control predisposing factors such as antibiotics (which alter the flora), malnutrition, diabetes, immunosuppression, pregnancy, or use of birth control pills. Use topical antifungal powders and creams. Keep the skin dry, the environment cool.
Tinea: variety of dermatophytes (tinea corporis, on body; tinea capitis, on scalp; tinea cruris, jock itch; tinea pedis, athlete's foot)	Tinea corporis: round red macules and papules with scales—lesions have advancing borders and healing centers; tinea capitis: patchy hair loss, inflammation, scales, and folliculitis; tinea cruris: red lesions with raised borders; tinea pedis: scaling, maceration, pain, and vesicles	Infection is controlled with antifungal solutions and creams. Acute lesions may require wet dressings, keratolytic agents, or both to remove the scales. Client is taught to reduce risk by thoroughly drying after a bath or shower, wearing absorbent underwear and socks, applying talc to intertriginous areas, and wearing open shoes during warm weather.

Table continued on following page

TABLE 49–5 COMMON SKIN INFECTIONS AND INFESTATIONS *Continued*

Disease with Causative Organism	Clinical Manifestations	Management
VIRAL		
Herpes simplex: herpes simplex virus	Vesicles preceded by sensation of itching or burning; clear exudate from vesicles, followed by crusting; common to the nose, lips, cheeks, ears, and genitalia	No cure is available. Treatment includes pain relief and topical anesthetics. Acyclovir, an antiviral drug, may decrease viral shedding and hasten healing. Avoiding the sun and using sunscreens reduce recurrent lesions on the lips. Reduce contagiousness by frequent hand-washing, not picking at lesions, avoiding sexual intercourse and kissing while lesions are active, and not sharing lipsticks. Try to identify (and avoid or control) personal triggers for lesions.
Warts: human papillomavirus	Rough, fresh, or gray-colored skin protrusion	Numerous therapies, some with over-the-counter medication. May require electrodesiccation or cryosurgery. Intralesional injections of cytotoxic drugs may also be used. No treatment also an acceptable option.

communicable than varicella, people who have not had chickenpox are at risk after exposure to a person with herpes zoster. An increased incidence of herpes zoster is seen in clients with lymphoma, leukemia, or AIDS, probably because of their decreased immunologic response.

Diagnostic tests may not be necessary because of the specific characteristics of herpes zoster; however, a Tzanck test demonstrates multinucleated giant cells (see Chapter 48), and a viral culture also is helpful.

Clinical Manifestations

The primary lesion of zoster is a vesicle. The classic presentation is grouped vesicles on an erythematous base along a dermatome. The vesicles appear 1 to 2 days after onset of pain and itching at the site. Occasionally, only papules appear and not vesicles. Because they follow nerve pathways, the lesions do not cross the body's midline; however, rarely, the nerves of both sides may be involved. Herpes zoster lesions evolve into ulcers on the superficial mucous membrane.

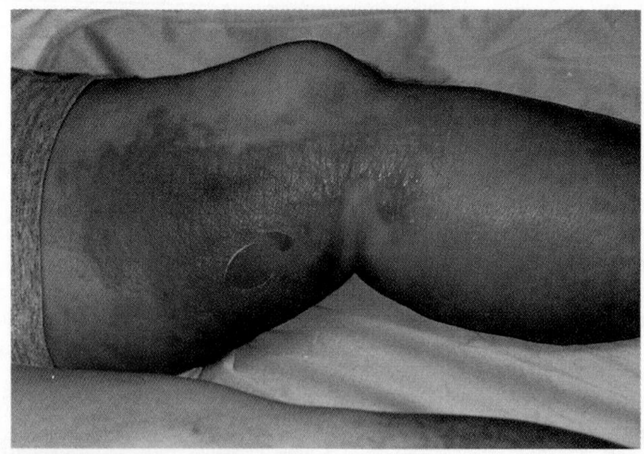

FIGURE 49–19 Cellulitis in a client with long-standing diabetes and stasis dermatitis.

The eruption generally clears in about 2 weeks, unless the period between the pain and the eruption is longer than 2 days. In such cases, a prolonged convalescence may be expected. Residual pain, called postherpetic neuralgia, and itching are the major complications with herpes zoster. The pain may be constant or intermittent and may range from light burning to a deep visceral sensation. The duration of the pain can be weeks or months to years. Unfortunately, in older clients, the pain generally lasts months to years. Another potential complication is loss of sight when herpes zoster involves the facial or acoustic nerve. Involvement of the ophthalmic branch of the facial nerve requires close medical attention to avoid ocular damage.

Outcome Management

Treatment for herpes zoster is administration of antiviral medications such as acyclovir (Zovirax), given in large doses orally or smaller doses intravenously five times daily. Newer antiviral agents (Valtrex) have more convenient dosing schedules. Antivirals, when started early in the course of the disease, reduce acute pain and also accelerate healing of the lesions. Studies now suggest that early oral antiviral therapy may assist in reducing postherpetic neuralgia. Analgesics and sedatives are prescribed for pain relief.

Topical therapy is primarily symptomatic: applications of cool compresses, use of cooling antipruritic preparations (see Table 49–1), and measures to prevent secondary infection. If pain is present, the client's normal pain tolerance and current pain level must be assessed. Systemic analgesics are usually required, and occasionally narcotics; however, in chronic pain, use of these agents raises the possibility of addiction. Assess the effectiveness and side effects of prescribed analgesics. Because postherpetic neuralgia can last a long time, the client and significant others need continued intervention and support. Chronic pain management may include the use of tricyclic antidepressants, phenothiazines, and other

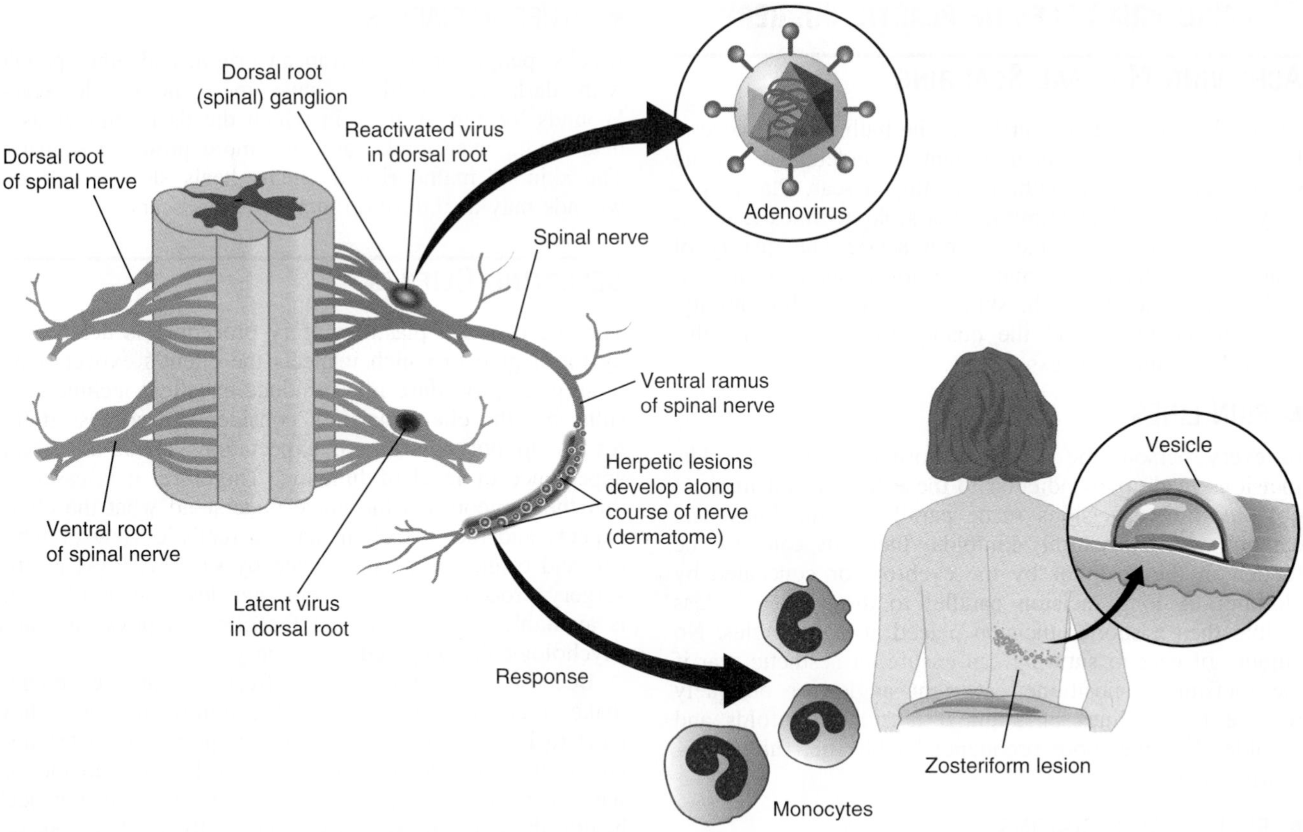

FIGURE 49–20 Pathophysiology of herpes zoster. The dormant herpes virus is reactivated causing vesicular lesions along the dermatome.

local physical modalities such as electrical stimulating units.

PLASTIC SURGERY AND OTHER COSMETIC/RESTORATIVE PROCEDURES

Plastic surgery is the surgical subspecialty that concentrates on the restoration of function and form to body structures damaged by trauma, transformed by the aging process, changed by disease processes (such as skin cancer), or malformed as a result of congenital defects. Plastic surgery can be divided into two major areas: (1) aesthetic (cosmetic) and (2) reconstructive.

Aesthetic plastic surgery improves physical features that are already within "normal" range. It is performed for changes that result from aging, to alter inherited features, or because of a client's personal desire. Clients seeking aesthetic surgery are so dissatisfied with the appearance of one or more body parts that they are willing to undergo surgery. Because aesthetic surgery is considered "cosmetic," it is not covered by insurance; clients pay out of pocket. Most clients are enthusiastic and happy because the surgery is a culmination of a personal desire that they may have held for a long time. In contrast, other clients may or may not have social support for their decision. The client may feel vain, embarrassed, or guilty about taking health care away from "people who really need it." Become sensitive to these feelings in the client, and be comfortable with a person's normal desires to feel good about the way he or she looks.

Reconstructive surgery attempts to restore a more normal appearance or function in a person who has an abnormal body part or in whom a body part is missing. The abnormality may be a result of injury or disease, it may be congenital, or it may be the cause of other medical problems. People undergoing reconstructive surgery are typically motivated to try to gain increased function of body parts and to improve their appearance. Although they may hope that plastic surgery will make them "normal," they usually know this may be unrealistic. Such clients are often struggling with diverse emotions: hope for a future without disease recurrence, eagerness to see final surgical results, anxiety over the surgery itself and impending postoperative pain, and weariness of the illness. The client having reconstructive surgery does have the advantage of social approval. Inasmuch as such a client is seen as a victim, society, as represented by either individuals or institutions, often provides treatment or makes appeals for payment of the operations.

Because of the significant impact of plastic surgery procedures on body image and self-esteem, psychological care is imperative. Plastic surgery is not only an operation on the skin; it reaches into the psyche of the person undergoing the surgery.

BASIC PRINCIPLES OF PLASTIC SURGERY

ACHIEVING MINIMAL SCARRING

Minimal postoperative scarring is the hallmark of successful plastic surgery. It is important to understand that no surgery can be done without creating a scar. Plastic surgery is conducted to minimize scars, so at times it seems that surgery can be done without scars. The quality of scarring is affected by many variables, such as the client's age, general health, skin type, and healing ability. Surgical technique and the quality of wound care also affect the healing process.

■ SKIN LINES

In every person, the skin has normal lines and folds. Incisions made perpendicular to these lines result in more obvious scars. Incisions made parallel to the lines heal camouflaged by natural skinfolds. Incisions can also be hidden in the scalp or by the eyebrow or concealed by clothing. A long incision parallel to these lines is less visible than a shorter incision placed at right angles. No amount of care in suturing can ensure an aesthetic scar if the incision is positioned at right angles or obliquely relative to the lines of minimal tension. Skinfolds and wrinkles become more pronounced with age, further obscuring incision lines.

■ ELLIPTICAL INCISIONS

When excising a lesion, the surgeon designs the incision lines to be longer than the lesion (Fig. 49–21). The resulting defect is elliptical, and the skin edges can be approximated easily. When the defect is round, tissues bunch at the ends of the incision, resulting in "dog ears."

■ SUTURING TECHNIQUES

To heal with minimal scarring, the edges of the skin incision must be approximated precisely, without undue tension. Each suture puncture represents a miniature wound, and scar tissue forms at the site of each puncture. Suture lines must be kept clean; otherwise, stitch abscesses may develop, increasing scarring. Sutures removed within 7 days leave no discernible suture marks or "tracks." Unfortunately, the skin on some areas of the body (e.g., the back) is thick and slower to heal, so that sutures must remain in place for a longer period of time. It is difficult to achieve fine scarring in these areas.

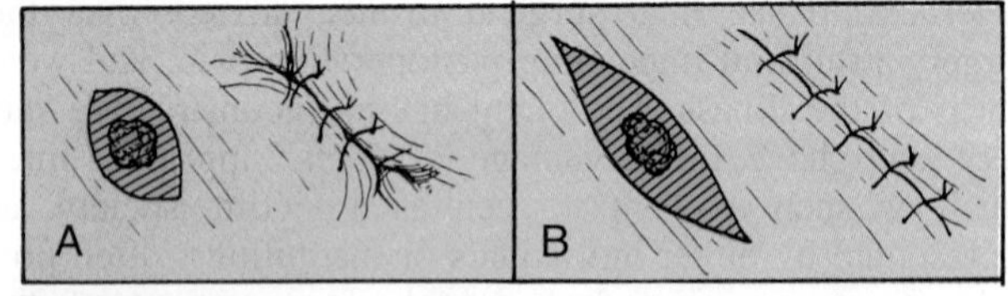

FIGURE 49–21 Elliptical excisions are used to reduce the scar. The *shaded area* shows the area of tissue removed with each lesion. *A,* If the ellipse is too short, puckers ("dog ears") form at the ends of the incision. This creates an unsightly scar. *B,* The correct length of elliptical incision for minimal scarring. (Redrawn from Grabb, W., & Smith, J. [1979]. *Plastic surgery* [3rd ed]. Boston: Little, Brown.)

■ OTHER VARIABLES

Blacks, people of Mediterranean origin, and other people with dark skin tend to have more noticeable scars. Wounds located in areas in which the tissue moves as it heals (e.g., over joints) are also more prone to scarring. The skin of malnourished clients heals slowly, and the wounds may also develop more obvious scars.

SELECTING CLIENTS

The success of a plastic surgery procedure is determined by the degree to which it meets the client's expectations. A surgical procedure may produce excellent technical results, but the client may not consider it a success if the results do not conform to expectations about a specific appearance or level of function. Therefore, it is essential that the surgeon and the nurse understand what the client expects and that the client have a realistic view of what can and cannot be accomplished by surgery. Most plastic surgery procedures are not emergencies, and ample time is available to ascertain that the client is physically and psychologically prepared for surgery.

Because most procedures affect appearance, clients make a considerable emotional commitment when they elect to have plastic surgery. It is important to determine client characteristics that may indicate lack of satisfaction with a result. In addition to being in good physical health, the client must be psychologically healthy. Assessing the client's motivation is essential. Plastic surgery neither cures a person's underlying emotional problems nor alleviates major stress. An external change does not make a happy, well-adjusted person out of a person who is unhappy, poorly adjusted, or excessively stressed. Clients who expect plastic surgery to do so are poor candidates for plastic surgery. Nurses help to identify appropriate candidates for surgery. In most situations, the client feels that the physician is too busy and talks more openly to the nurse about the desires for the surgical outcome.[27]

■ UNDERSTANDING MOTIVATIONS FOR SURGERY

The desire to be attractive or beautiful is present in people of all cultures, but the perception of what is attractive varies. Adorning the body with paints or scars dates from ancient times to the present (e.g., lipstick, nail polish, tattoos). Some people decorate the body by wearing objects in their noses, ear lobes, or lips. Western society pressures people to continue to look young (perhaps by exercise) and to combat the normal physical changes of aging (perhaps by plastic surgery). For many years, people were limited to highlighting their positive features with make-up and clothing.

The importance of physical appearance varies from person to person; however, it is an integral part of the sense of self. The desire to want to physically resemble one's peers reasonably closely—for instance, to have acceptably "normal" facial features—is a normal desire. Clients' physical aspects are consistent with their idea of who they are as people. Trauma, disease states, congenital deformities, or multi-stage reconstruction procedures can result in alterations in appearance that have an impact on self-esteem and body image. Physical appearance carries significant meaning to overall quality of life for both men and women and should be considered throughout all phases of treatment.

A significant portion of any deformity rests in the client's perception of the abnormality. Perceptions develop in part from body image. Body image describes a person's perception of his or her body—how the person *thinks* he or she looks, rather than an objective assessment of the person's characteristics. Body image is a factor in determining self-image, self-concept, and self-esteem. People with a positive body image display more confidence and interact more easily with others. Body image changes continually, depending on individual expectations and feedback from others.

A person with a physical deformity, real or perceived, can have a severely damaged body image. Even the usual processes of aging can be detrimental to body image. A self-perception of "getting old" can impair self-confidence, affect behavior, and interfere with interactions in society. Body image is an important factor in the nursing assessment of the client having plastic surgery.

The client's ability to cope with a temporary or permanent or a perceived or actual disfigurement is also assessed. Assess the client's coping mechanisms. Some coping mechanisms may be effective; others may be ineffective. Men may have more difficulty expressing their feelings about their appearance than that typically noted in women. Listen to the client, be alert for positive and negative self-statements, and note the degree of anxiety and fear. Evaluate the client's willingness or unwillingness to touch or look at involved body areas and the client's comfort with being near other people.

Techniques for working with clients who have alterations in body image are presented in Box 49–3.

DETERMINING REALISTIC EXPECTATIONS

A client who understands what is and what is not a possible surgical outcome is said to have realistic expectations. Determining a client's expectations is a crucial first step before any surgery is performed. Most clients with conditions requiring plastic surgery have some degree of deformity. The deformity can be *actual,* that is, objectively observable by others (e.g., a missing breast or a deviated septum), or it can be *perceived*—that is, the client is aware of the deformity, but it may not be noticeable to other people (e.g., fine facial wrinkling indicative of aging). It is important to clearly understand what the client sees and wants changed.

Clients with realistic expectations understand that facial rejuvenating surgery cannot stop the clock. A face lift (rhytidectomy) cannot make a 65-year-old woman look like a 40-year-old. Realistic expectations are the realization that appearance will be improved, but aging continues.

Obviously, a face lift cannot get an unfaithful spouse to return home. Expectations can be very private and may be hidden from the physician and the nurse during interviews. Clients with documented or suspected psychiatric illness may or may not be candidates for plastic surgery. A consultation with the psychiatrist or psychologist who

BOX 49–3 Supporting the Client Who Has a Changed Body Image

Many clients undergoing plastic surgery experience some form of body image alteration. Clients may experience body image changes before surgery due to disease or injury. They may also have problems after surgery from edema, bruising, or less than desired results. Try to anticipate these problems and work with the client as soon as possible to facilitate needed adjustments. You may want to work with the nursing diagnosis of *Risk for Body Image Disturbance* or *Self-Esteem Disturbance related to perceived or actual disfigurement and changes in self-concept.* The expected outcome must be tailored to the client but may include improved self-image with incorporation of the changed body part into the body image, as evidenced by effective coping and appropriate use of defense mechanisms; verbalizing feelings comfortably and appropriately; expressing satisfaction with the changed body image; having the ability to openly verbalize feelings; making positive statements about self; having a normal level of anxiety and normal fears; comfortably looking at self in mirror and/or touching the deformed body area, healed surgical site, or other scars; being able to be with others comfortably; and having no indications of depression.

Some interventions that you may find effective with clients who are experiencing body image disturbances include the following:

- Continue to assess apparent self-concept, coping methods, defense mechanisms, degree of anxiety, and fears frequently.
- Assist the client to explore and express feelings; do not use phrases such as "I know how you feel." These empty phrases build barriers to communication, whereas statements such as "you are angry" or "you seem depressed," for example, identify the feeling.
- Be sensitive to the client's feelings and needs.
- Acknowledge the client's feelings.
- Present reality; building false hope is detrimental (reality need not be brutal, however).
- Healing is unpredictable; refer questions about healing to the surgeon.
- Do not force the client to view or touch himself or herself; gently assist the client to look at and touch the deformity or healed surgical site (help incorporate it into the client's self-concept and body image).
- Encourage the client to begin meeting in public to begin desensitization to the reactions of others, such as by taking walks in halls; desensitization begins in safe environments and proceeds to new situations, prepare the client for stares and remarks.
- Discuss others' reaction to the client; support grief reactions.
- If the client has a facial deformity, prepare visitors and family members before they see the client.
- Look for vocal expression or hand gestures in cases of facial disfigurement; facial expression may be limited in clients with extensive facial scars or skin grafts.
- Refer the client and family to local support groups, such as About Face.
- Assist the client with techniques to camouflage scars; licensed aestheticians can assist with make-up choices and techniques.

is providing treatment for the client is necessary before any operation is undertaken.

The realistic client understands that plastic surgery does not occur as depicted in films: the bandages do not come off the next day, leaving the client perfectly healed and changed into a new person. Bruising can last for 2 weeks, and swelling can persist for 6 months.

Realistic clients understand that some scarring is inevitable, but that the scars are to be hidden in normal skinfolds and will therefore be less noticeable. Help clients to understand that any incision results in the formation of scar tissue. It is essential that the client have a realistic expectation of the location and extent of scarring that will result from the surgical procedure. Remind the client that a scar matures over a long period of time. Some scars take as long as several years to achieve their final appearance.

Explain that postoperative activities must be curtailed temporarily. Clients who are very athletic and refuse to remain inactive during healing and workaholics who refuse to take time off from work, present potential management problems. Preoperative teaching includes helping the client develop realistic postoperative expectations. Explain how the surgery will affect usual routines. Thorough planning ensures minimum disruption in routines. Preoperative teaching must include information about restrictions on activity, the location and extent of scars, and the clinical manifestations of possible complications. Including family members in the teaching process promotes an effective support system for the client.

The ideal candidate would have support from relatives and significant others. Family members may react negatively, regarding the surgery as a waste of time, a waste of money, or an expression of vanity, creating unnecessary stress during surgery. With short hospital stays, the family has taken over the caregiver role by providing postoperative care, which was in the past provided by nurses. The client may feel hesitant to rely on nonsupportive family members or may fear a negative postoperative result. You have the unique opportunity to serve as the facilitator of positive interaction between the family and the client.

Finally, the ideal candidate for surgery is healthy. Disorders such as hypertension and diabetes increase risk, but they do not prevent the client from having surgery. Alcohol and tobacco use should be stopped before surgery is undertaken. Nutritional impairments are identified and corrected before surgery. Other diagnostic assessments vary with specific procedures or with specific preexisting medical problems.

■ DOCUMENTATION THROUGH PHOTOGRAPHY

Photographs are used extensively in plastic surgery. Document the client's condition before any surgical intervention. Once changes have been made in appearance, it is very difficult to remember the details of the original appearance; photographic documentation provides an accurate record.

In office settings, nurses commonly photograph the client before and after surgery. By protecting the client's privacy and explaining the importance of photographic documentation, you can make a photography session much less uncomfortable and embarrassing. The client must give written permission for photographs to be taken, especially if they are to be used for teaching purposes in addition to documentation for the medical record. Specific and standardized positions are used. Consistent positioning is crucial for comparison of preoperative and postoperative views.

FACIAL REJUVENATING SURGERY

In childhood, skin is very elastic and is supported at maximum distention by adipose tissue ("baby fat"). During aging, the skin loses elasticity and the subcutaneous fat diminishes and changes character. Skinfolds and wrinkles become increasingly noticeable. The tissue around the eyes and jaw line sags, producing a drooping, tired, weary, or worried expression. The rate of skin change varies among people. Weight loss, sun exposure, genetic tendencies, and alcohol and tobacco use affect the speed and character of the changes.

Habitual exposure to the sun leads to several alterations in the skin. Many of the cutaneous changes once attributed to normal aging are in large measure due to chronic exposure to sunlight. Skin exposed to sunlight (natural sun and sun lamps) develops a chronic state of inflammation, which in its final stages leads to disintegration of the support matrix of elastin and collagen.

RHYTIDECTOMY (FACE LIFT)

A rhytidectomy *(face lift)* consists of removal of the larger skin wrinkles and folds from the face and neck. The ideal candidate for the procedure has large wrinkles or sagging facial skin. Fine circumoral wrinkles cannot be removed with a face lift. Physical manifestations of aging occur throughout the body but are most obvious to others on the face. Rhytidectomy may restore a more youthful appearance to the face (perhaps from 5 to 10 years younger) by removing wrinkled skin from the forehead and around the eyes and mouth (Fig. 49–22). Rhytidectomy does not result in removal of all of the wrinkles of the face. Clients may require acid peeling for fine wrinkles (see following).

Rhytidectomy is usually performed on an outpatient basis with the client under general anesthesia, or using local anesthesia with intravenous (IV) sedation. Incisions are made from the temple along the ear and out into the hair-bearing scalp behind the ear (Fig. 49–23). Through the incisions, excess facial skin is undermined and pulled back toward the ear. *Undermining* is a surgical technique in which the skin is separated from underlying structures. Most clients elect to have additional procedures done, such as tightening of the underlying fascia or facial suction lipectomy. Further adjuncts to face lift include brow lift, blepharoplasty (eyelid revision), mentoplasty (chin revision), and, occasionally, rhinoplasty (nose revision). On completion of the operation, facial compression dressings are applied.

Nursing Management

Postoperatively, the client is placed in the Fowler position to reduce the risk of edema. Cold compresses can also be used to reduce swelling and bleeding. Suction drains are used to eliminate dead space and remove wound drainage.

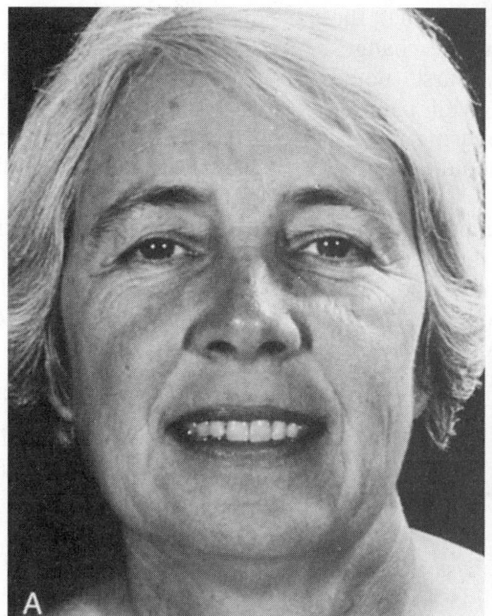

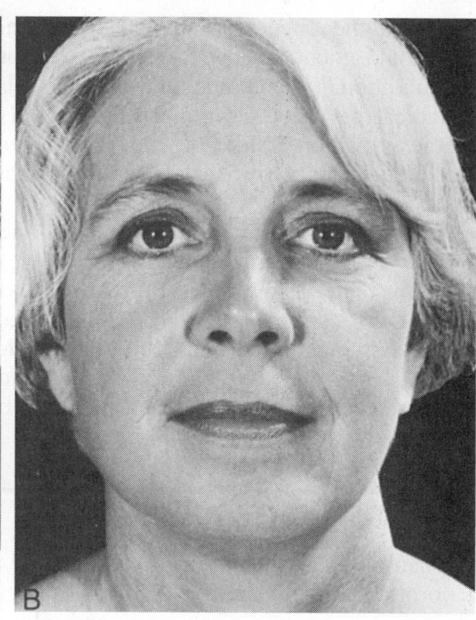

FIGURE 49–22 Before (*A*) and after (*B*) a face lift (rhytidectomy) and blepharoplasty.

Drains are removed in 24 to 48 hours, when drainage has subsided. Facial movement (talking and chewing) should be limited. Localized increases in blood pressure should be avoided by keeping the head elevated; any prescribed antihypertensive medications should also be resumed. Coughing also increases blood pressure and should be avoided (by not operating on clients with colds) or treated if it occurs after surgery.

Use antiemetics to reduce nausea and vomiting. Vomiting increases blood pressure and the risk of bleeding. Pain is minimal and can usually be managed with oral analgesics.

Complications

Complications associated with a face lift include hematoma, hair and skin loss, and nerve injury. Hematomas are caused by the resumption of bleeding in small vessels after the wound is closed. Large hematomas can cause tissue necrosis and must be surgically removed. Hematoma formation occurs most often in people who smoke or have pre-existing hypertension. Postoperative nausea and vomiting can also increase bleeding and hematoma formation. Hair loss is presumably due to altered circulation to hair follicles. The hair almost always grows back. Skin loss occasionally develops behind the ear, perhaps as a result of swelling or hematoma. Such a wound is allowed to heal by secondary intention and does not result in a very large scar. Nerve damage causing facial paralysis is a rare but devastating complication. Occasionally, facial paralysis results from nerve compression by a suture. When facial paralysis is observed, immediate surgical exploration to correct the problem and to prevent permanent damage is necessary.

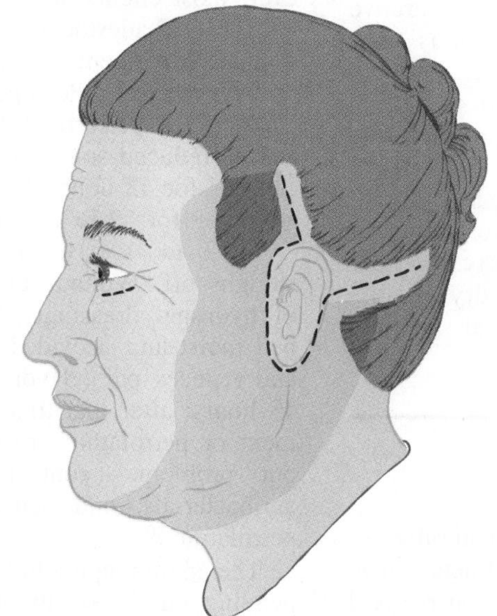

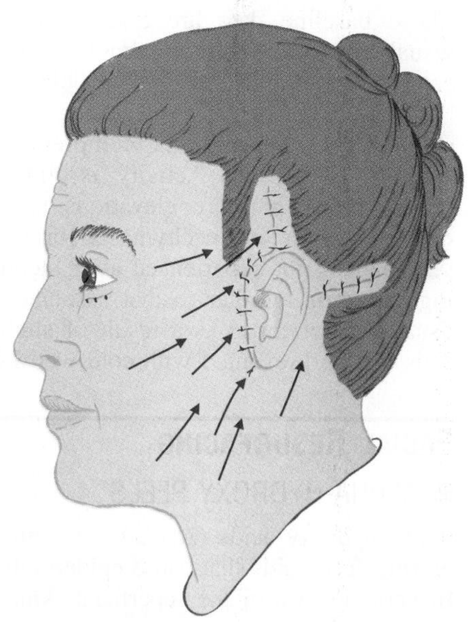

FIGURE 49–23 Face lift (rhytidectomy) and blepharoplasty. Face lifts enable removal of large wrinkles and folds of skin from the face and neck. *A,* Area in pink shows amount of tissue that is undermined (lifted from the fascial connection) and moved during a face lift. For the face lift, the incision lines go around the ear and into the hair-bearing scalp; other incisions may also be used. Note also the incision line beneath the eyelid for the blepharoplasty, which enables removal of excess eyelid tissue. *B,* The postoperative near-final result, with tightened facial skin and neck folds.

Assess the client for complications, and instruct the family and client in how to recognize reportable changes in condition. Hematoma development is first noted as increasing facial asymmetry associated with pain or tightness on one side of the face. Increasing drainage and changes in facial sensation should also be reported.

Teach the client to keep the head of the bed elevated for 1 week to minimize edema and to rest the face for 1 week to achieve fine scars (minimize talking, and limit chewing by eating a soft diet). The surgeon usually removes dressings the morning after rhytidectomy. The face and hair may then be gently washed. Dandruff shampoo is avoided. Creams or cosmetics should not be applied to the suture line until healing is complete.

BLEPHAROPLASTY

Blepharoplasty is the surgical removal of excess skin and periorbital fat from the upper or lower eyelid. The aging process causes a loss of elasticity and relaxation of eyelid skin. Excess eyelid tissue in young and middle-aged people may be an inherited characteristic, may reflect an allergic reaction, or may be the result of cardiovascular or thyroid disease. Complete medical assessment is essential to rule out physical causes of excess eyelid skin. Most blepharoplasties are considered aesthetic operations, but if eyelid tissue obstructs vision, blepharoplasty is medically indicated.

Blepharoplasty is usually performed on an outpatient basis. General or local anesthesia with sedation can be used. Wide elliptical incisions are made on the upper eyelids. The excised wedge of excess tissue is lifted off, and herniated fat is removed. A lower-lid blepharoplasty incision is placed ⅛ inch below the edge of the eyelid.

Rapid, uneventful recovery is typical. Blepharoplasty can be performed alone or with rhytidectomy (face lift). Complications from blepharoplasty are rare.

Assess preoperative near and distant vision in each eye by asking the person to read from a book and from something in the distance while one eye is covered. These baseline data are crucial to assess postoperative visual changes. An ophthalmologic examination is indicated before surgery if vision problems are noted.

After blepharoplasty, the head is elevated to reduce edema. Iced normal saline compresses are applied to the eyes as prescribed. Activity is limited for 1 week to reduce blood pressure elevations that often lead to increased edema and ecchymosis (bruising). Normally, severe pain is not experienced after blepharoplasty. An itching sensation, similar to that associated with dry eyes, is usually experienced as a result of slight corneal swelling. This can be prevented with cold wet dressings.

FACIAL RESURFACING

■ ALPHA-HYDROXY PEELS

Alpha-hydroxy acids (AHAs) are a group of naturally occurring fruit acids that cause epidermolysis and detachment of keratinocytes of the superficial skin. AHAs can be used to remove acne scars, keratoses, warts, and superficial layers of skin. The best candidates for AHA peels are thin-skinned women with a fair complexion and fine facial wrinkling. Trained nurses perform the peel procedure.

The skin is prepared for the peel with a 2-week skin care regimen consisting of a facial wash and application of daytime treatment lotion and nighttime cream. The actual peel begins with the application of a pre-peel solution. Skin that will not be peeled is protected. For the peel, a thin layer of acid is applied to the face for a few minutes, and then it is neutralized. Care after the peel includes application of skin moisturizers, gentle cleansing, use of sunscreen, and avoidance of abrasive agents.

■ TRICHLOROACETIC ACID PEELS

Trichloroacetic acid (TCA) is generally used when a medium-depth peel is required. TCA is indicated for clients with moderate actinic damage or for clients with pigment changes.

The skin is prepared with a 2-week regimen of tretinoin (Retin-A) or glycolic acid in combination with a bleaching agent. If clients are taking estrogen, they should stop its use for 2 weeks before the peel. The choice of skin preparation can affect the depth of the peel. TCA is applied to the face for a few minutes until the skin "frosts." TCA does not need to be neutralized. Care after the peel includes application of skin moisturizers, use of hydrocortisone to reduce edema and erythema, gentle cleansing, and use of sunscreen. The client often resumes the pre-peel skin regimen after the peel. Hyperpigmentation is the most common complication.

■ LASER RESURFACING

Laser treatment of skin wrinkles is becoming the preferred method of facial resurfacing. The wound produced is shallow because the energy is absorbed very superficially. An ultra-pulse laser is used.

Laser irradiation is quite painful. Some clients can tolerate the procedure with anesthesia provided by local sedation or through the use of topical anesthetics such as eutectic mixture of local anesthetic (EMLA). The cream is applied 1 to 2 hours before the procedure and covered with an occlusive wrap (cellophane works well). However, most clients need nerve blocks and local infiltration with a local anesthetic agent.

Laser treatments result in skin injury similar to a second-degree burn. Postoperative edema is significant, especially if the periorbital area has been treated. The edema can be reduced somewhat with ice packs and oral corticosteroids for 48 hours. Some clients also experience a burn sensation for 12 to 18 hours after treatment.

In 2 to 4 days, the residual tissue separates and sloughs off. Wound care after that time usually consists of hydrogel dressings. These dressings keep the wound bed moist and occluded, which promotes epithelialization and reduces pain. Hydrogel dressings are used for about 48 hours; after that time, thin layers of antibacterial ointment or petrolatum are applied. Neither product is without problems—contact dermatitis can develop from antibacterials, and acne-like lesions can develop from petrolatum.[40]

The skin reepithelializes in about 5 to 10 days, depending on the depth of the injury. Varying degrees of erythema can remain, but clients can effectively cover the erythema with make-up that has a green foundation color.

Milia can form and may require tretinoin or they can be manually expressed. Sun-blocking agents are a must, as hyperpigmentation can develop.

■ DERMABRASION

Dermabrasion is a process of sanding the surface layers of skin on cheeks and forehead with an electric rotating brush to smooth out pitting and surface blemishes. This operation is the preferred treatment for depressed acne scars and other deep scars. Local anesthesia with sedation is used. The abraded surfaces are covered with antibiotic ointment and gauze. After removal of the gauze, the facial skin weeps serous fluid for 5 to 7 days. Once the weeping stops and new skin has appeared, the client can apply make-up to camouflage the redness. The redness fades over the following 6 weeks.

■ COLLAGEN INJECTION

Collagen is sometimes injected to fill in small wrinkles or depressed blemishes in the skin. The client's reaction to collagen is tested before treatment, because some people experience induration (hard, raised area) and swelling at the injection site. Clients with autoimmune disorders are not candidates for collagen injection.

After collagen injections, the face should not be washed and face cream or make-up should not be applied for 3 to 4 hours. Normal skin care can then continue. Exposure to strong sunlight, alcohol consumption, and excessive exercise can cause mild swelling and should be avoided as prescribed (e.g., for a week).

RHINOPLASTY

Rhinoplasty is the surgical correction of nasal deformities. This procedure is frequently performed as an outpatient procedure using either local anesthesia and sedation or general anesthesia. Incisions are made inside the nose. The surgical plan is individualized and may include reshaping the bony dorsum of the nose, the tip of the nose, and/or the cartilage along the nares (nostrils). The nasal bones may be fractured to achieve the desired result. After surgery, the inside of the nose may be packed and an external splint applied.

Preoperative nursing care focuses on teaching the client to breathe through the mouth after surgery and to not touch the nose. Postoperatively, assess for bleeding. While the client is sleepy from the anesthesia, excessive swallowing may be the only sign of bleeding. Examine the back of the throat with a flashlight to look for blood. Some bleeding is normal down the back of the throat and on the nasal packs and dressings. The nurse promptly reports excessive bleeding to the surgeon. The head of the bed is kept elevated to control postoperative edema. Nasal packing can be very uncomfortable. Pain management is important and can usually be achieved with oral analgesics (e.g., codeine, acetaminophen). Aspirin is avoided for 1 week before and 3 weeks after surgery. Postoperative care is discussed in the Client Education Guide.

CLIENT EDUCATION GUIDE

Postoperative Care After Rhinoplasty

After the procedure, follow these instructions:

1. Sleep with the head of the bed elevated for 1 week.
2. Do not remove the external splints or nasal packing.
3. Do not blow the nose. Sneeze only through an open mouth.
4. Continue a soft diet for 2 days.
5. After nasal packs are removed, avoid decongestant nasal sprays because they cause vasoconstriction and decrease the blood supply needed for healing.
6. After nasal packs and splints are removed, the nose will remain swollen and bruised for a while. Wait 12 months before judging the final results of the procedure.

BODY-CONTOURING SURGERY (LIPECTOMY)

Body-contouring surgical procedures (lipectomy) remove excess fatty tissue, skin folds, or subcutaneous fat from various body parts, including the abdomen, thighs, arms, and buttocks. Generally, obesity is best treated by diet and exercise before any body-contouring surgery is performed. In exceptional cases, the client may become highly motivated to follow a weight-reducing diet *after* such surgery. In still other cases, despite an appropriate diet and exercise regimen, there may be no reduction in the size of fat deposits in certain areas of the body. Fat distribution is based on sex, heredity, and corticosteroid use. It is generally accepted that rapid growth of fat cells occurs during childhood. It is also accepted that few new fat cells are made during adult life. Fat cells deposited during childhood are very resistant and their number does not dwindle during dieting. Surgical removal then becomes an option. As with all surgery, careful preoperative assessment is necessary to determine whether the client's expectations are realistic.

SUCTION-ASSISTED LIPECTOMY

Suction-assisted lipectomy, or liposuction, is a technique used (1) to aspirate fatty tissue from areas of the body resistant to diet and exercise (lipodystrophy), (2) to contour flaps, and (3) to remove lipomas (benign fatty tumors). It is also used adjunctively with other plastic surgery procedures to create better contour and to enhance the aesthetic result.

A blunt, hollow cannula is inserted through a very small incision (Fig. 49–24). The cannula, attached to a powerful suction machine, is passed back and forth through the subcutaneous tissue, sucking up adipose tissue and creating a series of tunnels. The blunt tip pushes aside nerves and blood vessels. Precise surgical technique avoids ridges and dimpling on the surface as fatty tissue is suctioned away. Compression dressings or elastic compression garments may be used to help collapse the tunnels, thereby preventing fluid collection (hematoma and seroma); to maintain the desired body contour; and to promote healing. Tumescent technique involves the additional use of large volumes of dilute lidocaine and epinephrine. These medications promote vasoconstriction to minimize bleeding and provide postoperative analgesia. Ultrasonic lipectomy is the use of ultrasound to ease the removal of fat.[1, 2]

Complications of liposuction include hematoma, skin necrosis, infection, and undesirable scars or skin dimpling. If large volumes of fat were removed, the client can also develop hypovolemia. Pulmonary embolism has also been reported.

After liposuction, assess the client for hypovolemia and electrolyte imbalance (manifested by syncope, dizziness, and abnormal blood values). If drains are used, monitor the quantity and quality of drainage. Ice is effective in managing postoperative pain. Dressings usually remain in place for at least 24 hours. Nurses must ensure that dressings remain smooth and uniform; otherwise, contour irregularities can result. Sometimes the client wears a compression garment for several weeks postoperatively.

Clients may gradually resume normal activity except for strenuous exercise. It may be 4 to 6 weeks before the client works up to the preoperative level of exercise. Resuming activity too rapidly may result in soreness and swelling. Bruising is common after liposuction and may take weeks to disappear completely.

Many clients expect the results of liposuction to be immediate. Usually up to 6 months is required for final results to be apparent after edema subsides and subcutaneous tissue heals. Reinforce that results may not be apparent for 6 months following surgery. This period of time is required for complete resolution of edema and reconnection of soft tissues.

ABDOMINOPLASTY

Abdominoplasty is the removal of excess abdominal skin and fat and the repair and tightening of separated abdominal muscles. An incision is made across the lower abdomen, and tissue is undermined to the costal margin. The excess skin and fatty tissue are excised and recontoured. The umbilical stalk is detached and reattached once the overlying skin is in its proper position.

During abdominoplasty, the surgeon repairs diastasis (lateral separation of the rectus abdominis muscles) and/or umbilical hernia. Indications for abdominoplasty include abdominal skin flaccidity (e.g., after multiple pregnancies or major weight loss) and marked striae from pregnancy. An indwelling urinary catheter and surgical drains are inserted, and sequential compression devices are applied at the end of the surgical procedure.

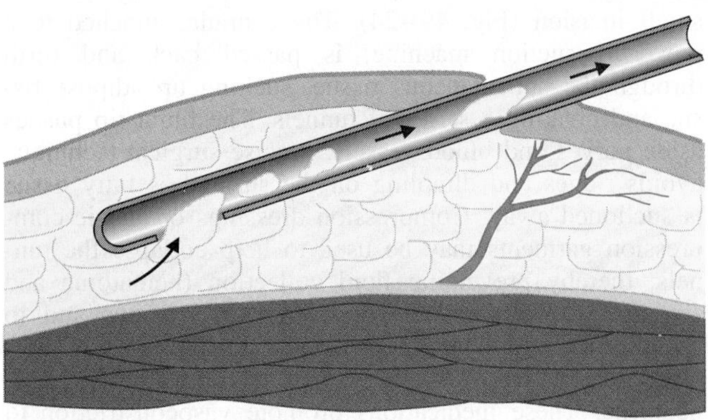

FIGURE 49–24 Suction-assisted lipectomy. To prevent extraction of subdermal fat, the surgeon directs the opening of the suction cannula toward the muscle fascia.

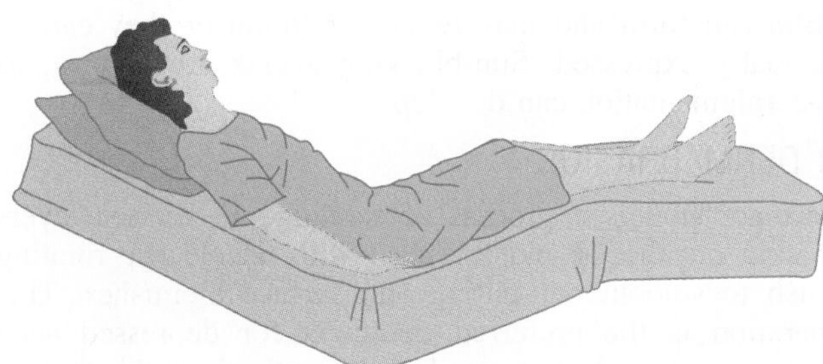

FIGURE 49–25 Position the client after abdominoplasty in a modified semi-Fowler position, with the knees bent, to reduce strain on the incision line.

Preoperative nursing care includes informing the client that drains and a urinary catheter will be in place after surgery, that a blood transfusion may be required, and that an IV infusion is continued until a diet is tolerated. After surgery, inspect the incision line for signs of pallor and/or lack of capillary refill. The operative site can swell, with resulting impairment of capillary blood supply. Smoking is prohibited, because nicotine further restricts blood flow to the skin. Tension on the suture line must be minimized; therefore, the client must lie in a contouring position (Fig. 49–25).

The client also needs to walk in a "hunched-over" position until the swelling decreases and abdominal skin relaxes. Teach the client postoperative pain management techniques. Abdominoplasty is an abdominal operation and produces significant postoperative discomfort. Adequate analgesia and other pain-relieving measures are essential. Reinforce to unlicensed personnel that these clients require usual postoperative care (see the Management and Delegation feature).

PANNICULECTOMY

In people who have experienced major weight loss, excess loose skin and subcutaneous tissue may develop over

MANAGEMENT AND DELEGATION

Care of Clients Recovering from Plastic Surgery

When unlicensed assistive personnel are caring for clients after plastic surgery, reinforce the need for adequate pain management and routine postoperative care. It is not uncommon for these clients to feel uncomfortable about asking for pain medications and for nursing assistance. Some people have the notion that surgery "for vanity" should hurt a little. This is a dangerous philosophy and should not be condoned. Any incision hurts, and these clients do not differ in their need for pain control. Likewise, routine vital signs, pulmonary care, monitoring intake and output, and encouraging ambulation are routine aspects of postoperative nursing care. Withholding care is not an acceptable manner of providing care.

Donna W. Markey, MSN, RN, ACNP-CS, *Clinician IV, Surgical Services, University of Virginia Health System, Charlottesville, Virginia*

the abdomen, thighs, and arms. This tissue may hang in large folds, and laxity is greater in older people who have lost skin elasticity. Panniculectomy, the removal of excess folds of tissue, usually requires more than one operation. The surgery is lengthy, and there is risk of major blood loss. As much as 10 pounds of redundant tissue has been surgically removed during one of these operations.

Clearly, this operation is not for the cure of the client's obesity, but it can offer some positive gains in self-esteem and reduction in health-related problems.

Postoperative care is usually focused on reducing stress on the long suture lines. For example, place the client in the Fowler position after abdominal panniculectomy. Monitor the suture lines closely for signs of non-healing. Fatty tissue is poorly perfused, and the client may have pre-existing diet-induced malnutrition. During the healing phase, the client needs to consume adequate amounts of protein and carbohydrate to heal.

RECONSTRUCTIVE PLASTIC SURGERY

One of the greatest challenges in plastic surgery is the reconstruction of deformities. In planning reconstruction, it is important to consider the following questions:

- *What tissue is missing?* Is bone, muscle, subcutaneous tissue, or skin missing? If only skin is missing (e.g., burns), skin grafts are used for reconstruction. People with large pressure sores may be missing muscle, subcutaneous tissue, and skin, and a rotation flap containing all of these tissues may be used to repair the defect. Facial trauma may result in loss of bone as well as of other tissues, and vascularized bone may be used in reconstruction.
- *Where is tissue available?* Some small defects have adequate tissue for repair nearby. This is ideal, because the tissue can be lifted from its base and rotated into the defect. Nearby tissue has the same color, thickness, and hair-bearing tendencies, contributing to a more natural appearance. If the tissue needed is not nearby, it may be moved from its location and attached to the defect by microscopic anastomosis (i.e., suturing small vessels and nerves with the aid of a microscope). Reconstruction with this technique is called *free flap reconstruction.*
- *What deficit might result from moving donor tissue?* Obviously, a person does not want a larger defect in the donor site than in the area being reconstructed! For example, a toe is often used to reconstruct a missing finger, but it is unlikely that a person would give up a finger to rebuild a toe.
- *What is the simplest method to achieve the desired results?* The simplest method to close any wound is simple suturing. More complex methods are used if adequate tissue is not available for primary closure or if a greater defect would result from simple suturing (e.g., a defect on the cheek could be closed by suturing, but this approach might pull the eyelid down into ectropion as it healed). Another method of closing a wound is to use a flap of nearby tissue and to rotate it onto the wound, maintaining the flap's own blood supply. Skin grafting is the third choice for reconstruction. The most complex form of wound closure is the free flap of skin, subcutaneous tissue, and, as indicated, muscle or bone.

RECONSTRUCTIVE MODALITIES

■ SKIN GRAFTS

A graft is tissue (e.g., skin, bone, nerve, or vessel) that is harvested without a blood supply from a donor site. It is transferred to a recipient site, where it develops a new blood supply. For the tissue to remain viable, or to *take,* a healthy vascular supply must be present at the recipient site.

Skin grafts are used extensively to resurface exposed surfaces. The grafts vary in thickness from very thin split-thickness skin grafts (STSGs), which contain epidermis and a very thin layer of dermis, to full-thickness grafts (FTSGs), which contain epidermis and all of the dermis. Thinner grafts are more likely to contract during healing, but they are also more likely to develop adequate blood supply. FTSGs are used in areas in which contraction would limit function, such as on the hand or over joints. FTSGs leave a full-thickness defect in the donor site that must be closed, either primarily or with an STSG.

Skin grafts can be expanded to cover a greater surface area by use of meshing techniques. Meshing the graft, achieved by cutting small slits in it, allows the skin to be expanded (like an accordion). Meshed skin grafts are used when there is little uninjured skin to use as a donor site (e.g., a major burn).

BANKING SKIN

Skin grafts can be removed or harvested during one surgical procedure and stored for application later, when a wound is clean or when an earlier graft has failed. Banked skin is folded in a dermis-to-dermis fashion, to preserve moisture, and then wrapped in moist saline gauze. The gauze with skin is placed into a dressing impregnated with ointment (such as petrolatum gauze); this is put into a bottle, which creates an airtight environment. Banked skin can be stored at 4° C for 10 to 21 days. Later, the skin graft can be placed on the wound without the need for another operation.

SKIN GRAFT SURVIVAL

A skin graft requires enough blood in its recipient site for survival. Capillary buds must revascularize the graft before the cells die. Blood supply that supports the growth of granulation tissue is usually adequate to support a skin graft. Good contact between the graft and the recipient bed is also critical. A thin fibrin network develops almost immediately after placement and serves as a temporary glue of sorts to hold the graft in place. Skin grafts require about 7 to 10 days to adhere and longer to mature.

Several factors reduce contact and thereby reduce skin graft survival. Collections of fluid between the graft and bed, improper tension on the graft, and movement of the graft on the bed are three common problems that lead to graft failure. Blood, serum, and purulent material may separate the graft from the bed. This collection prevents revascularization of the graft. A hematoma only 0.5 mm in diameter delays the time for revascularization by 12 hours. A 5-mm-thick hematoma delays revascularization by 120 hours. At body temperature, the skin graft cannot survive for the additional time, and necrosis begins.

Proper tension on the skin graft is crucial once the skin graft has been sutured in place. If tension is insufficient, wrinkles develop that will never revascularize because they are not in contact with the recipient bed. If the skin graft is too tight, it is stretched like a drumhead above the recesses of the wound, where the blood supply exists.

Movement between the graft and the bed shears capillary buds from the bed, which prevents revascularization. When skin grafts are applied to extremities, the adjacent joints are splinted to prevent movement. Tie-over dressings are commonly used to prevent the graft from moving.

HEALED SKIN GRAFTS

Skin grafts tend to carry their natural color. Grafts from the clavicle are a blush (pink) shade, whereas grafts from below the clavicle take on a yellow or brownish hue. Sweat gland, hair-bearing, and sebaceous features occur only in thick STSGs and FTSGs. Nerves regenerate from the edges of the graft, and in the absence of dense scarring, sensation parallels that of nearby skin. If the skin graft regains sensation, it is fairly durable. Grafted skin will usually grow in a manner parallel to that of the rest of the body.

Meshed skin grafts heal with a pebbled appearance. Therefore, they are only used on body areas normally covered by clothing.

Nursing Management

Skin graft recipient sites are covered with dressings, which should not be altered for at least 72 hours. Assess the site, and document pain, bleeding through the dressings, and adjacent skin color and temperature.

The donor site is usually covered with a hydrophilic dressing, such as hydrocolloid gel. Because clients have more pain in the donor site than in the grafted site, it is important to keep the open area covered.

It is imperative to keep a skin-grafted extremity elevated. If the graft is on the chest or back, be certain that it is anchored well and that the client is positioned off the grafted site. Avoid moving the grafted part. After the dressings are removed, continue to assess the skin graft for healing. The skin graft should become pink throughout (a graft with viability assured by a healthy pink color is called a *take*). Blisters (small blebs of serum) can also shear the skin graft from the underlying wound.

Document the presence of blisters and report this finding to the surgeon. Blisters under a skin graft sometimes need to be drained. When prescribed, this is accomplished by inserting a small (25-gauge) sterile needle into the blister and letting the fluid run out onto a sterile dressing or a cotton-tipped applicator. Rolling fluid to the edges of the skin graft is not advised, because it shears the graft from the capillaries in the bed en route. A standing order (as needed [prn]) may be given for this intervention. Large accumulations may require surgical removal.

FLAPS

Flaps are areas of tissue raised from one area of the body without being completely detached, so that the blood supply is intact; the flap is transferred (e.g., by rotation) to adjacent areas. Flaps of tissue can also be transferred to distant areas, where a blood supply is reestablished; these are called *free flaps* and are discussed later on. Local flaps are rotated or advanced to reconstruct an adjacent defect (see Fig. 49–26). An important consideration with the use of flaps is the preservation of the nutrient blood vessels. The tissue attachment containing these vessels is sometimes called the *pedicle,* because in the past, flaps were moved from site to site with a visible portion of tissue that "carried" the flap to the recipient site. This style of flap can be seen in the deltopectoral flaps used to repair neck resection tissue loss. Flaps are also used to cover extensive wounds from pressure ulcers and long-standing defects from osteomyelitis.

The skin of the flap, after transfer, maintains its original color and texture. This is why skin from the head and neck is used to reconstruct facial defects. If, for example, abdominal skin were used for facial reconstruction, it would be bulky and would increase in size if the patient gained weight, because the graft would respond just as if it were still in the abdomen.

Hair growth and sebaceous secretion remain the same as they were in the donor area. Sensation and sweating are lost immediately after transfer and usually return sometime between 6 weeks and 3 years later. These functions reappear as superficial nerves regrow into the tissues; therefore, the sensation and sweating capacity match those of recipient site tissues.

MUSCULOCUTANEOUS FLAPS

Flaps comprising both muscle and skin are called *musculocutaneous flaps.* They are commonly used to fill in defects where muscle is missing or where muscle can provide ample blood flow to heal osteomyelitis. These flaps are named by the muscle of origin. For example, large trochanteric pressure ulcers can be repaired with tensor fasciae latae flaps, named for the tensor fasciae latae muscle of the lateral thigh. Intrathoracic muscle flaps used for chest wall reconstruction include serratus anterior, latissimus dorsi, and pectoralis muscles.

Tissue defects of the leg can also be managed with muscle flaps and skin grafting or with musculocutaneous flaps. Attempts are made to salvage all extremities unless nerve or vascular damage is irreparable, in which case amputation is preferred. It is common to treat less severe tissue loss in compound lower leg fractures with local rotation muscle flaps if possible. The use of these flaps has been overshadowed in recent years by the excitement over microvascular techniques, but definite indications exist for use of these local muscle flaps.

Care of the client after a flap reconstruction centers on maintaining perfusion and reducing tissue injury to the flap. You may choose to design your nursing care under the nursing diagnosis of *Risk for Altered Peripheral Tissue Perfusion related to tissue transfer.*

The outcome is that the client will maintain adequate peripheral tissue perfusion, as evidenced by usual color of skin, no pallor or cyanosis, warm and dry skin, blanching (capillary refill) in 3 to 5 seconds, no edema or blebs, intact incisions, and controllable pain.

The flap is monitored for color, capillary refill, and dermal bleeding. Look for pallor, coolness, decreased capillary refill, or dark dermal blood on lancing (see the Critical Monitoring feature) (lancing may not be allowed in some settings). It takes a fair amount of experience in clinical assessment of flaps to predict early flap demise using these subjective methods. Findings can vary because of oxygen content of the blood, capillary dilation, blood flow, and skin pigmentation. Therefore, in complex flaps, temperature and Doppler monitors are used to mon-

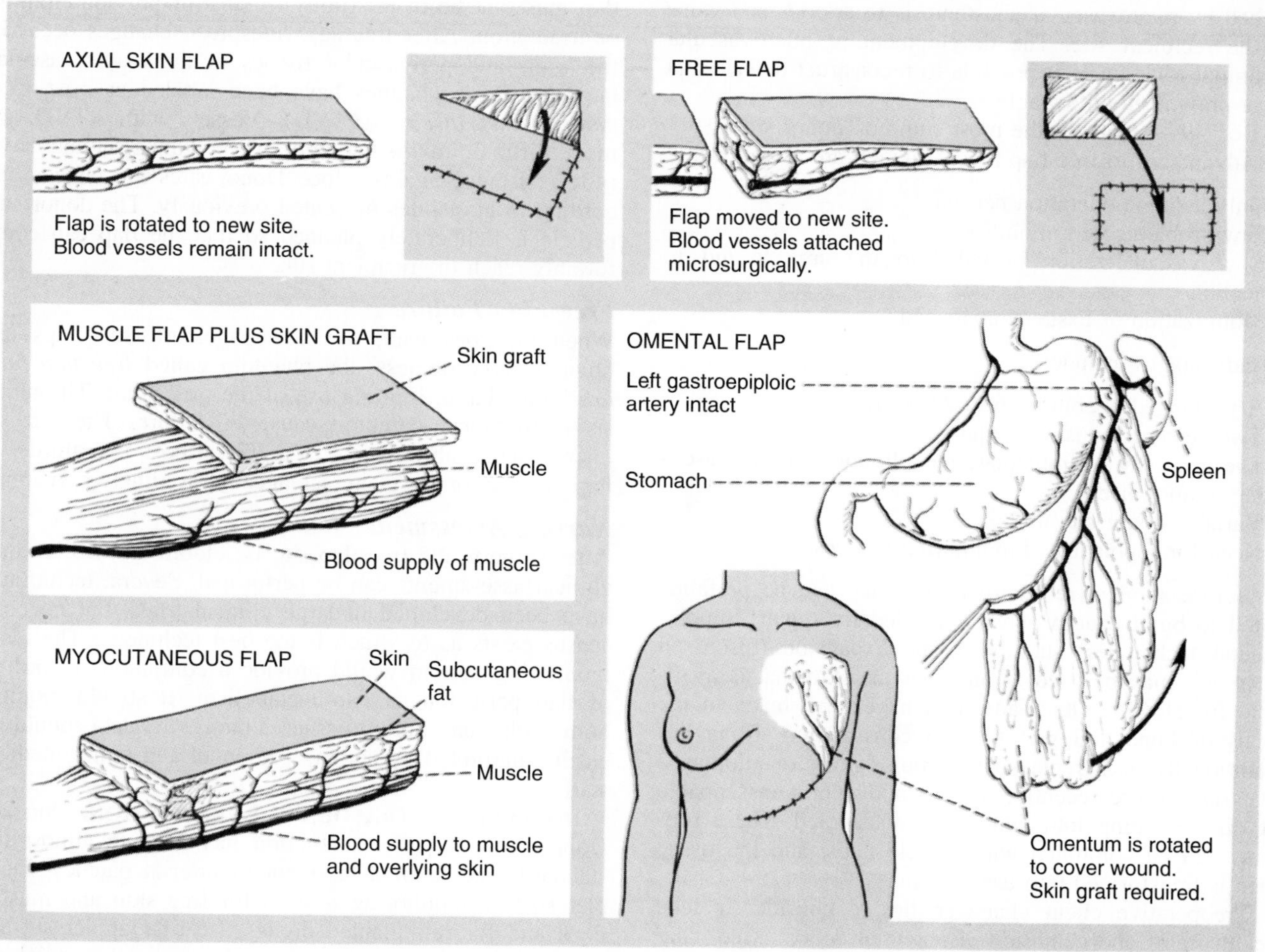

FIGURE 49–26 Common flaps.

itor circulation. The extremity is usually elevated to improve venous return as long as elevation does not interfere with arterial flow.

Protecting the blood supply to a flap is a primary nursing responsibility. Nursing interventions are designed to avoid factors that can jeopardize blood flow. Position the client so that the flap is relaxed and elevated. Gravity promotes edema and venous congestion, both of which impede blood flow. Interventions to increase venous return include elevating the involved body part and applying elastic stockings or wraps as prescribed. Tension on the flap can stretch or kink the feeding blood vessels, reducing the flow of blood to the tissues. A blood clot can restrict blood flow. The first sign of compromised blood flow is pallor.

Know the location of the pedicle that carries blood vessels to the flap. Most of the time the pedicle is buried, and little can be done to harm it. Some exceptions exist, though. When skin flaps are used, such as the deltopectoral flap, the pedicle is visible. Tracheostomy ties should not be tied tightly around the flap; otherwise, circulation to the distal portions will be compromised. When the breast is reconstructed after mastectomy with a latissimus dorsi flap, the pedicle is located in the ipsilateral axilla. The client cannot lie on the ipsilateral side.

Hydrate the client well, if prescribed, to help perfuse the flap. Maintain any postoperative splints to prevent tension on vessels. Limit the use of caffeine by the client and prohibit the use of nicotine by the client and by visitors.

Problems due to impaired arterial supply are apparent early after surgery. Altered perfusion due to venous obstruction may not be evident for a few hours.

FREE FLAPS

Free flaps are harvested from one area of the body to reconstruct a defect in a distant area. The donor tissue (skin, muscle, bone, or a combination of these) is detached from its blood supply at the donor site and reat-

> **CRITICAL MONITORING**
>
> **Musculocutaneous Reconstruction**
>
> Report the following findings immediately:
>
> - Development of coolness in the flap
> - Development of duskiness or pallor in the flap
> - Slowing of capillary refill in the flap
> - Loss of pulses (palpable or detected by Doppler) in the flap
> - Increasing pain in the flap

tached by microvascular anastomosis to arteries and veins at the recipient site. The development of microvascular techniques has made it possible to reconstruct defects that were previously untreatable.

Box 49–4 includes the most common donor sites.

Advantages to free flap reconstruction are as follows:

- Only a single operation needed
- Few problems with mobility
- New vascularization provided to the area to aid in healing
- Mobilization of tissues maximized

Disadvantages include:

- A prolonged operation (6 to 24 hours)
- Two separate incisions required
- The necessity of immediate reexploration of any vascular compromise
- Variable donor site mobility
- Need for sophisticated monitoring devices

Before surgical reconstruction, a flap can be prefabricated to build exactly what is needed for repair. Supplemental techniques, such as tissue expansion (discussed later on), may be used to augment the skin that is available for closure. Other advances have been made in the areas of bone and soft tissue reconstruction. Bone has traditionally been replaced with bone grafts or alloplastic materials. More recently, osteoinductive proteins capable of differentiating into bone were discovered. These proteins can be combined with muscle flaps, and the tissue then is transformed into useful bone.

Preoperative client characteristics to consider include health status and condition of potential donor tissue. Diabetes and cardiovascular, renal, and pulmonary disease do not present absolute contraindications, but these diseases do increase risk of flap failure. The vessels used for a flap must not be in proximity to sites of previous trauma or irradiation. After trauma, widespread changes occur in the walls and perivascular tissues of the major vascular bundles. These changes have been labeled as *post-traumatic vessel disease* (PTVD). Vessels with PTVD are more difficult to dissect, are easily damaged, and have little resistance against clots. Donor sites are chosen according to guidelines presented previously. The donor site pedicle is deliberately planned so that the flap can comfortably reach the recipient site.

BOX 49–4 Common Donor Sites for Free Flaps

- *Temporalis fascia,* a thin conforming flap, is used to cover the dorsum of the foot or hand.
- *Radial forearm,* a flap of skin and fascia, can be used for reconstruction of intraoral and extraoral defects; it can be combined with portions of the radius if bony reconstruction is needed.
- *Lateral forearm,* a flap of skin and fascia, is used to cover body areas that demand thicker skin, such as weight-bearing surfaces.
- *Omentum,* the fatty drape over the anterior abdomen, can be transplanted into spaces that require pliability, such as the frontal sinuses or chest wounds.
- *Latissimus dorsi,* a large flap muscle with a skin segment, has a long pedicle and is useful for large bulky defects; it is the "workhorse" of flap reconstruction and is common for facial, chest, and breast reconstruction.
- *Rectus abdominis,* midline abdominal muscle and skin, has a long pedicle and is used for defects that require bulk.
- *Gracilis,* a skin and muscle flap with a short pedicle, is used to reconstruct defects of the distal tibia, ankle, and heel, and for facial reanimation.
- *Serratus anterior,* an easily sculpted flap, provides bulk and protects lower extremity defects.

Free Flap Failure

When all goes well, the advantages of free flaps are obvious. Nevertheless, the phantom called *free flap failure* looms large, limiting use of the procedure. Thrombosis is the most common cause of failure. The rate of microvascular thrombosis is 3.7%; almost two thirds of flaps with thrombosis are salvageable by timely revisions.

Nursing Assessment

After surgery, the free flap site is seldom dressed, so that clinical assessments can be performed. Several techniques have been developed in large clinical trials, but no consensus exists as to which is the best technique. The ideal monitoring system would provide a continuous recording of flap perfusion or flap metabolism. It should monitor both visible and buried tissues. Finally, the data should be easily interpreted by nursing personnel and junior medical staff.

DOPPLER ULTRASOUND EXAMINATION. Surface Doppler ultrasound examination has become almost the standard method of assessment of arterial patency. Doppler surface monitoring is used for free skin and muscle flaps and for reimplanted digits. Use of Doppler surface monitoring has some limitations, however. The axial artery must be located superficially, and sometimes venous obstruction still produces an arterial "hum." If venous obstruction is suspected, compression of the flap will produce a louder "hum." Implanted Doppler probes are also available and are in use in some centers.

TRANSCUTANEOUS OXYGEN DETERMINATION. Determination of tissue oxygen tension ($PtCO_2$) constitutes the simplest technique for monitoring perfusion. Absolute $PtCO_2$ greater than 20 mm Hg seems to suggest adequate perfusion. Sudden falls of $PtCO_2$ below 20 mm Hg that do not respond to the administration of oxygen suggest arterial occlusion. As in other forms of monitoring, trends in data, rather than absolute values, should be monitored. Implantable probes have been developed for oxygen monitoring also.

TISSUE PH. Measurement of tissue pH has been shown to be a more reliable index of perfusion than tissue oxygen. Arterial occlusion produces a rapid fall in tissue pH (0.66 pH unit per hour in laboratory animals, compared with a fall of only 0.27 pH unit per hour with venous occlusion).

PULSE OXIMETRY. Pulse oximetry is a good monitor for viability of digital free flaps or reimplanted digits. Digits remain viable if the oxygen saturation remains above 95%. Loss of pulsatile flow is indicative of arterial occlusion; a decrease in saturation to 85% indicates venous obstruction.

MUSCLE CONTRACTILITY. Ischemic muscles lose their contractility, and free muscle transfers can therefore be monitored by the continuing ability of the muscle to contract in response to electrical stimulation. Nerve stimulators are used to irritate the nerve every 15 minutes, and the response is recorded. A decrease in amplitude of the evoked potential is indicative of ischemia.

PHOTOPLETHYSMOGRAPHY. Photoplethysmography is commonly used to monitor several types of free flaps, because it is noninvasive and reliable. Infrared light from a light-emitting diode penetrates about 3 mm below the surface of the skin. Some of the light is reflected back to a photoelectric cell. Pulsatile changes in flow alter the proportion of light reflected back. Waveforms are monitored for changes. The waveforms can also be transmitted by telephone to remote stations for interpretation.

CLINICAL ASSESSMENT. Postoperative monitoring of free flaps used to be based solely on clinical assessment, which relied heavily on the experience of the nurse. In the 1990s, the monitors just described were used. It is interesting to note that some surgeons have abandoned external monitoring devices and are once more relying solely on the nurse's judgment. Most centers use a flow sheet to document color, texture, and temperature of the flap, as well as Doppler pulses and drainage from wound drains. Other postoperative care includes maintaining adequate hydration, keeping the client warm, managing pain, and allowing only the appropriate activities. Clients may express some concern with the decision to salvage a body part and/or may fear that the flap will fail and amputation will be required. The nurse needs to be supportive of the decision for surgery and allow time for expression of fears.

Long-Term Results

The ability to obtain soft-tissue coverage and limb salvage of a massively traumatized lower limb approaches 95%. A true measure of the adequacy of reconstruction, however, is whether the client can use the limb. A study was completed to examine the functional outcomes of 70 leg salvage procedures. The functional demands on the lower limb are great and include strength, stability, motion, and balance. Functional analysis of tibial shaft injuries revealed marked limb shortening and decreased ambulation and mobility. Most clients require some sort of ambulatory-assist devices. Clients requiring free flaps or foot resurfacing did not have limb shortening, and all of them could wear shoes.

■ IMPLANTS

Implant material can be used to augment or replace tissue in all parts of the body. Facial structures (including the nose, chin, ears, orbital floor, and malar complex), breasts, bones and joints, and genitalia are often augmented or reconstructed with implant material. Polymers such as medical-grade silicone are used most frequently in plastic surgical procedures. Silicone prostheses can be very soft (breast prostheses), flexible (finger and toe joints), or rigid (bones and joints). Stainless steel, cobalt-chromium alloy (Vitallium), and titanium plates, screws, and wire are used to approximate, replace, and stabilize bone fragments (Fig. 49–27). Injectable collagen can be used to fill out skin depressions and fine wrinkles. Material for implants must be biocompatible and not rejected by body tissues. It must not cause severe foreign body reaction or infection. Implants must be noncarcinogenic, nontoxic, nonallergenic, and sterile.

Postoperatively, assessment and intervention focus on preventing displacement of the implant, ensuring adequate blood flow to the operative site, and preventing infection. Infection is a serious complication that can necessitate removal of the implant. Changes in temperature and local changes (e.g., drainage, increasing edema, hyperemia, increasing skin temperature) may indicate a developing infection or implant rejection. Excellent wound care is imperative. Teach the client to recognize the clinical manifestations of infection so that treatment can be initiated quickly. Implants themselves are not painful, but the surgical procedure causes mild to moderate pain. Pain not relieved with analgesics must be investigated.

■ SKIN EXPANSION

Skin expansion is a technique used to increase the amount of local tissue available to reconstruct a defect. An inflatable silicone balloon is placed under the skin or muscle flap adjacent to a defect. The expander is inflated sequentially over several weeks or months to stretch the overlying tissue. When tissue is sufficient to resurface the adjacent defect, the balloon is removed and the flap is contoured (shaped) and advanced to cover the defect.

The process of skin expansion involves an extended period of time, commitment, and significant, although temporary, disfigurement. It is essential that the client be motivated, well prepared for the experience, and able to comply with the treatment regimen. The client must be able to make additional trips to the physician's office where the expander will be inflated under sterile conditions. Each expander has an injection site into which a sterile needle is inserted percutaneously. Saline is injected slowly until the tissue is very tight over the expander.

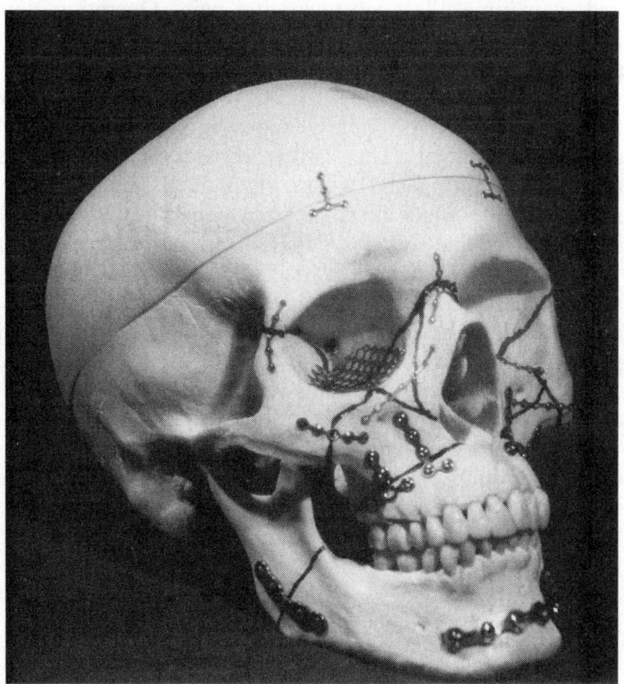

FIGURE 49–27 Titanium plates and screws used to treat facial fractures.

Sometimes a small amount of saline needs to be withdrawn to reduce discomfort. The tightness may be uncomfortable for several hours, but it subsides as the tissue begins to expand.

Teach the client to keep the incision and the injection site clean and dry to prevent infection. Make sure that the client understands that pressure on the expander compromises blood flow and can cause tissue breakdown. Infection may require that the expander be removed altogether. If dehiscence of the incision line occurs, exposing the expander, the treatment need not necessarily be aborted. Fluid can be removed from the expander to relieve the tension. When the incision has healed sufficiently, expansion can begin again.

In most cases, the client can camouflage the expander with clothing. The clothing must be loose so that no pressure is placed on the expander. Advise the client to sleep in a position that protects the expander from pressure. When the expander is placed in an exposed area, such as the neck or scalp, the client must be able to cope with the temporary physical inconvenience and insult to body image.

Nurses are instrumental in assisting the client in disguising the deformity caused by the expander. For example, when one breast is being expanded before reconstruction, the other breast will not match in size or shape. Assist the client in padding the other side of the bra to reduce obvious asymmetry.

■ LASERS

The laser (*l*ight *a*mplification by *s*timulated *e*mission of *r*adiation) is a coagulating, vaporizing, and cutting instrument. A precise beam of laser light is directed onto tissue. The light is converted into heat energy that is absorbed by the cells. The heat vaporizes the cells. The advantages of laser surgery include precision and accuracy of cell destruction, reduced bleeding and swelling, and, sometimes, less postoperative pain. Operating time may be longer, but tissue damage is less, and the postoperative infection rate is lower.

Laser light can be of different colors and wavelengths. Each is absorbed differently depending on cell pigment and water content. The carbon dioxide (CO_2) laser is primarily a cutting and vaporizing tool. Its energy is absorbed by the water in cells, so it penetrates tissue only superficially. The CO_2 laser is used primarily to excise or vaporize lesions such as warts, keloids, and vascular lesions. Argon, copper vapor, and pulsed-dye laser energy are preferentially absorbed by hemoglobin and are used primarily for coagulation. These types of lasers are used to treat birthmarks (e.g., port-wine stain), superficial vascular lesions, and pigmented lesions.

Laser energy generates intense heat, and clients experience a burning sensation or a pin-prick sensation. The tissue reaction can be similar to that of a second-degree burn with blistering. Ointment applied to the affected area for 2 to 4 weeks keeps the tissue moist until healing is complete. It is also essential that the area treated with laser energy be protected from sun exposure for several weeks.

Laser treatment to remove large pigmented lesions may require many operations. A single application may address only a small portion of the lesion, and the results are appreciated slowly as the site heals. Clients must be prepared for the length of time required and the inconvenience of multiple procedures.

REPAIR OF TRAUMATIC INJURIES

FACIAL INJURIES

Injuries to the face are a common result of automobile accidents and physical violence. Although they may be serious, facial injuries are seldom fatal. Proper management helps to avoid sensory impairment and permanent disability and can minimize disfigurement.

■ LACERATIONS

Facial lacerations can range from very small injuries (0.50 cm) that can be repaired using local anesthesia to extensive lacerations with soft tissue injury that require repair with the client under general anesthesia. Before closure, wounds are cleansed of debris and devitalized tissue.

Facial lacerations and facial soft tissue injuries are usually distressing to the injured client and family. Although it is important to remain optimistic about the outcome and reduce anxiety, it is also essential to provide accurate information. Explain that a scar forms with any injury. Scar revision can be performed later.

Excellent wound care, including cleansing and applying prescribed topical antibiotics, promotes the healing of facial abrasions and lacerations. A client who is receiving nothing by mouth (i.e., is on *nil per os* [NPO] status) and has dried blood in the mouth needs frequent oral care. If oral tissue contains sutures, the mouth is simply rinsed with saline. Oral care *must* be performed, however. With severe facial trauma, soft toothbrushes suffice for oral care. Use of oral irrigation devices (e.g., Water Pik) may further damage such injuries and is usually contraindicated. The nurse takes measures to prevent aspiration during oral care.

Teach the client and family members to keep facial incision lines clean and to apply a prescribed topical antibiotic. Skin incisions must not get wet (e.g., in the shower), because moisture allows bacteria to enter the wound along the sutures. Infected incisions tend to produce more scar tissue. (Wound care is also discussed in Chapter 16.)

■ FACIAL FRACTURES

Fractures can occur in the individual bones of the face: the nasal bones, orbit, malar prominence, mandible, or maxilla. Le Fort fractures are facial fractures with specific patterns (Fig. 49–28); they are classified as follows:

Le Fort I: transverse fracture of the alveolar process separating the upper dental arch from the maxilla
Le Fort II: fracture of the midface, maxilla, and orbits
Le Fort III: fracture of the orbits that leads to craniofacial dissociation

The client with facial fractures has often been involved in an automobile accident or an assault or has suffered a sports injury. Pain, improper bite (malocclusion), swelling, bruising, diplopia (double vision), facial asymmetry,

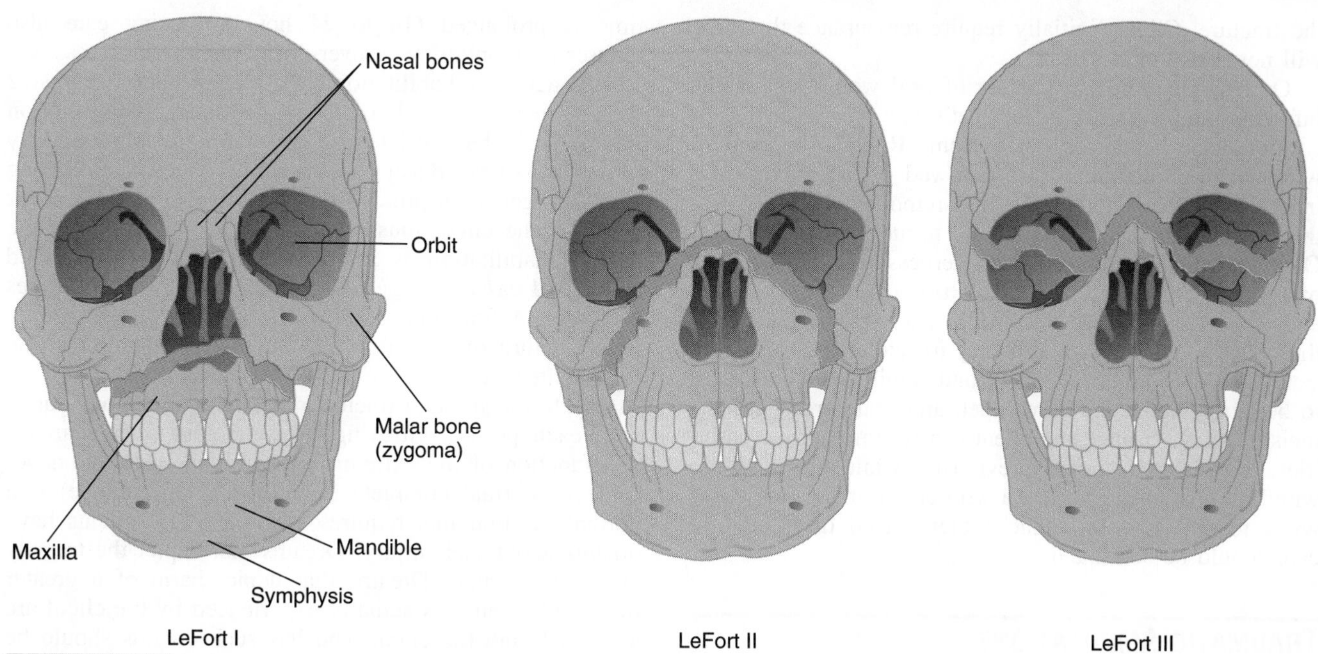

FIGURE 49–28 Le Fort fractures.

enophthalmos (sunken eye), and exophthalmos (bulging eye) are clinical manifestations of facial fractures. Diagnostic assessment includes x-ray studies. Life-threatening problems (e.g., airway obstruction, hemorrhage, or cervical spine injury) that may accompany facial trauma must be managed immediately. Repair of facial fractures can be delayed for up to 3 weeks and still achieve good results.

Like all fractures, facial fractures must be reduced, stabilized, and immobilized to ensure proper healing. Methods vary according to the location of the fractures. Nasal fractures are reduced and then splinted or stabilized with nasal packing and immobilized with an external nasal splint, which usually remains in place for at least 1 week.

Fractures of the mandible and maxilla and Le Fort fractures can be reduced and stabilized with intermaxillary fixation (wiring the upper and lower jaws together in occlusion) using arch bars. The jaws usually remain wired for 4 to 6 weeks. When small plates and screws are used to stabilize bone fragments, intermaxillary fixation may not be necessary.

Blowout fractures of the orbit can involve trapping of orbital structures between bone fragments, which may result in diplopia or enophthalmos. The integrity of the orbital floor is reestablished surgically, and the fracture fragments are stabilized with wire or small plates and screws. Implant material or bone graft may be used to complete the reconstruction. Malar (cheekbone) fractures may produce facial asymmetry. These fractures may also be stabilized with wire or small plates with screws. Malar implants may be necessary to reestablish facial symmetry.

Assesses airway patency and breath sounds every 2 hours (more often if bleeding is present). Suction equipment is present at the bedside. Teach the client to breathe through the nose. Trying to open the mouth may dislocate the fracture. When the client has intermaxillary wiring, wire cutters should be in the client's possession at all times. If airway problems develop that cannot be managed with suction, the wires should be cut. The nurse and the client need to be informed about which wires should be cut. Two wires are usually present on each side of the mouth, and they are the only wires that attach the top and bottom teeth. Do not try to cut off the bands attached to the teeth.

Facial edema and ecchymoses may be present. The head of the bed is elevated. Artificial tears may be needed if the client's ability to blink is decreased as a result of swelling, injury, or nerve damage.

Assess the client for diplopia and blurred vision. When these disorders are present, the nurse assists the client during ambulation to prevent injury.

The client continues a liquified diet until the wires are removed. Without adequate nutrition, clients can lose 10 to 20 pounds during convalescence. Instruct the client how to "blenderize" food and to maintain an adequate balance of carbohydrates, fat, protein, and calories. Milkshakes can be made with a wide variety of foods. High-calorie food supplements can augment the regular diet, and liquid multivitamins may be useful. Alcoholic and carbonated beverages can cause nausea and can fizz and foam in the back of the throat, leading to airway problems; they are to be avoided.

Assess the client for clear rhinorrhea or otorrhea. Rhinorrhea or otorrhea may indicate leaking cerebrospinal fluid (CSF), which must be reported to the physician. With CSF leakage, the potential exists for development of meningitis. To assess for rhinorrhea or otorrhea, inspect the bed linens; CSF dries in concentric, halo-like rings and does not crust.

Initially, you and the client must establish a means of communication. Although talking is possible through clenched teeth, hand signals or writing may be most effective initially. Trying to open the mouth may dislocate the fracture. Clients initially require reassurance that they will not choke or suffocate.

Oral hygiene aids in healing of oral wounds, prevents infection and destruction of teeth and gums, increases comfort, and enhances self-esteem. Rinsing the mouth with water or a mouthwash followed by use of an oral irrigation device on low pressure removes particles from the front of the mouth while the tissues are still tender. Once the initial swelling and tenderness subside, the teeth must be brushed and the mouth rinsed after every meal and at bedtime. Pieces of paraffin wax can be placed on the open ends of the wires if they irritate buccal surfaces.

Before discharge, the client and family members need to be taught about the wires, diet, and oral care. Once the incisions have healed, the client can resume normal activities. However, as noted previously, while the jaws are wired, the client must carry a wire cutter and know which wires to cut. A well-balanced blenderized diet and oral care should be continued.

TRAUMATIC AMPUTATIONS

Immediate care of a person who has sustained a traumatic amputation, like that of any other injured person, focuses on life-saving activities (see Chapter 82). Hemorrhage is controlled with direct pressure on the bleeding points. Tourniquets and cautery are not used because they may damage surrounding tissue, so that reimplantation becomes impossible. All amputated parts, including small pieces of tissue, are sent to the health care facility with the injured person. As soon as possible, these parts are (1) rinsed with sterile normal saline, (2) wrapped in sterile wet gauze, (3) sealed in a watertight bag, and (4) placed on ice. Cooling the amputated part reduces metabolism, increasing the time the part can survive without blood. For example, an amputated finger can survive for 18 hours if effectively cooled. Although the part is rinsed with normal saline, it is never stored in normal saline or on dry ice, or frozen, which causes extensive cellular damage.

Reimplantation surgery is performed using a regional block or with the client under general anesthesia. An operating microscope guides the surgical reattachment of arteries, veins, tendons, and nerves. With severe injuries, such an operation may take 12 to 18 hours. After surgery, incisions are dressed, the extremity is immobilized with casts or splints, and the entire extremity is elevated.

After reimplantation, the client requires careful, frequent nursing assessment (every 15 minutes) including documentation of the reimplanted part's color, temperature, and capillary refill. Arterial or venous blood flow in the reimplanted part may become blocked; if the problem is not immediately corrected surgically, the part will die. Toes and fingertips are usually left uncovered for assessment. Doppler assessments help monitor pulses in the part. Temperature probes are often placed on the extremity. The surgeon usually states the ideal temperature range for reimplantations. A temperature decrease of 2° C or more in an hour or a decline to 32° C (89.6° F) demands immediate attention and is promptly reported to the surgeon. Aspirin is usually prescribed to reduce blood-clotting tendencies. A temperature of 34° to 36° C (93.2° to 96.5° F) is considered excellent for a reimplanted finger. Because anesthesia time is prolonged (18 to 24 hours), nursing care also focuses on monitoring recovery from anesthesia.

An active rehabilitation program usually begins 2 weeks after injury and continues for months. Joint motion initially may be restricted by pins through joints and by bulky dressings. Because peripheral nerves take a long time to regenerate, protective sensation may be absent for months. The client must be careful to avoid injuring the part. Rehabilitation is accomplished through prescribed active and passive range-of-motion exercises several times each day. A final indication of the success of reimplantation is return of sensory and motor nerve function in the reimplanted part.

Psychosocial adjustment after reimplantation varies with each person. Grieving over the loss of appearance and function of the extremity (the reimplanted part never achieves normal complete function and appearance) is a normal reaction that requires support. Many clients have dreams about their injury. Dreams that depict the tragedy again are normal. Dreams that depict harm of a greater magnitude than was actually experienced by the client are abnormal, and the client who has such dreams should be counseled by a psychologist. Praise and encouragement during rehabilitation are very helpful.[4]

Teach the client to avoid activities and substances that cause vasoconstriction (which precipitates necrosis) for 2 weeks after surgery (e.g., tobacco, nicotine, cocaine, amphetamines). Exposure to air conditioning is also harmful. Advise the client to avoid cold and chilling (such as by wearing extra clothing and having the car prewarmed before entering to prevent vasoconstriction).

NAIL DISORDERS

Disorders of the nail can indicate any of several dermatologic processes. Potential causes include an infection of the nail (e.g, paronychia), a fungal infection of the nail (e.g., onychomycosis), a dermatologic disease with prominent nail changes (e.g., psoriasis), or pigmentary abnormalities of the nail (as in melanoma).

Unguis incarnatus (ingrown nail) is one of the most common nail conditions and is caused by improper nail trimming and by wearing tight or ill-fitting shoes. It primarily involves the great toe. A painful, warm inflammatory reaction results from excessive lateral growth of the nail into the nailfold. The nail acts as a foreign body, promoting granulation tissue. Decrease inflammation with warm soaks for 20 minutes several times a day. If the problem is minor, lifting the lateral portion of the nail by inserting a cotton wick prevents contact with the nailfold. Sometimes, the involved segment of the nailfold needs to be excised.

Paronychia, or infection around the nail, is characterized by red, shiny skin often associated with painful swelling. These infections frequently result from trauma, picking at the nail, or disorders such as dermatitis. Often these sites become secondarily infected with bacteria or fungi, which later involve the nail. As with ingrown toenail, warm soaks three or more times a day may reduce pressure and pain; however, incision and drainage of inflamed sites is frequently required. Samples for appropriate cultures of the purulent material and the nail should be obtained.

Onychomycosis refers to any fungal infection of the nail, whether due to dermatophytes or candidiasis. Prescribed topical or systemic antibiotic or antifungal therapy, with emphasis for compliance is important. Unfortunately, even with good compliance, recurrence of fungal infections in nails is frequent.

Clients should understand the importance of reducing trauma and irritation to involved nails by (1) trimming nails straight across to reduce further trauma, (2) avoiding overmanicuring or self-induced trauma, (3) limiting harsh chemical irritants such as abrasive cleansers and drying nail products, and (4) keeping the nails dry.

CONCLUSIONS

Skin disorders range from those that are a mere nuisance (such as dry skin) to life-threatening disorders (such as melanoma). Nurses frequently manage skin disorders independently; therefore, a thorough knowledge of the use of topical medications and therapies is crucial. Because much of the needed skin care is provided by the client or a family member, the nurse must use excellent teaching skills to convey the necessary self-care information.

THINKING CRITICALLY

1. You are caring for an older woman who has had a stroke that left her with residual paralysis on the left side. She also has a pressure ulcer on the left trochanter, in part because she lies on her left side all the time. While caring for her on Monday, you convince her to sit in a chair and to lie on her right side. When you care for her again on Thursday, the ulcer is twice as large and deeper. She refuses to turn to the right and says: "I like lying on my left side." What can you do to help this client?

Factors to Consider. What pressure reduction methods should be instituted? Is there any harm in lying on a pressure ulcer? Why might she be at increased risk because of malnutrition?

2. The client is a 72-year-old white man who had undergone a wide excisional biopsy on his forearm to rule out squamous cell carcinoma. The next day the client calls the office complaining of pain at the surgery site. What additional questions need to be asked? What potential interventions might be necessary?

Factors to Consider. What clinical manifestations would indicate an infection is present? Is age a factor in wound healing?

3. The client is an otherwise healthy 41-year-old woman who presented to the clinic with a week-long history of intensely itchy, erythematous red lesions under her breasts. The rash appears to be spreading, and the centers of some of the lesions are seen to contain tiny pustules. In addition, the woman complains of a 12-pound weight loss over the past 6 months despite always feeling hungry and thirsty. She denies any medical problems and reports that she does not currently take systemic or topical medications.

Factors to Consider. What is the common cause of intertriginous dermatitis? What diagnostic study can determine the cause of the problem? What endocrine disorder is suggested by the history of skin rash, thirst, and weight loss?

BIBLIOGRAPHY

1. Ablaza, V., Jones, M. R., & Gingrass, M. K. (1998). Ultrasound assisted lipoplasty: Part 1. An overview for nurses. *Plastic Surgical Nursing, 18*(1), 25–32.
2. Ablaza, V., Jones, M. R., & Gingrass, M. K. (1998). Ultrasound assisted lipoplasty: Part 2. Clinical management. *Plastic Surgical Nursing, 18*(1), 16–25.
3. American Society of Reconstructive Surgical Nurses. (1996). *Core curriculum for plastic and reconstructive surgical nurses* (2nd ed). Pitman, NJ: Author.
4. Anderson, K., & Maksud, D. (1994). Psychological adjustments to reconstructive surgery. *Nursing Clinics of North America, 29*(4), 711–724.
5. Anderson, L. G., & Leroux, C. (1996). Routine surgery, routine patients? Never. *Plastic Surgical Nursing, 16*(1), 41–42.
6. Anderson, S. V. (1998). Laser resurfacing: A survey of pre- and post-procedural care. *Plastic Surgical Nursing, 18*(4), 229–234.
7. Bergstrom, N., & Braden, B. (1987). The Braden scale for predicting pressure sore risk. *Nursing Research, 36*(4), 205–210.
8. Bergstrom, N., et al. (1994). *Treatment of pressure ulcers: Clinical practice guideline No. 15.* Rockville, MD: U.S. Department of Health and Human Services, Public Health Service, Agency for Health Care Policy and Research. AHCPR Pub. No. 95-0652.
9. Bergstrom, N., et al. (1992). *Pressure ulcers in adults: prediction and prevention.* Rockville, MD: U.S. Department of Health and Human Services, Public Health Service, Agency for Health Care Policy and Research. AHCPR Publ. No. 95-0050.
10. Black, J. (1996). Surgical options for wound healing. *Critical Care Nursing Clinics, 8*(2), 169–182.
11. Black, S. (1995). Venous stasis ulcers: A review. *Ostomy/Wound Management, 41*(8), 20–32.
12. Bondville, J. (1994). Pain-free harvesting of skin grafts with EMLA. *Plastic Surgical Nursing, 14*(4), 231–233.
13. Bueller, H. A., & Bernhard, J. D. (1998). Review of pruritus therapy. *Dermatology Nursing, 10*(2), 101–107.
14. Burris, L. M., & Roenigk, H. (1997). Chemical peel as a treatment for skin damage from excessive sun exposure. *Dermatology Nursing, 9*(2), 99–104.
15. Camisa, C., & Warner, M. (1998). Treatment of pemphigus. *Dermatology Nursing, 10*(2), 115–118, 123–131.
16. Clamon, J., & Netscher, D. (1994). General principles of flap reconstruction: Goals for aesthetic and functional outcomes. *Plastic Surgical Nursing, 14*(1), 9–14.
17. Dermatology Nurses' Association. (1996). *Phototherapy administration guidelines for nurse phototherapists and phototechnicians.* Pitman, NJ: Author.
18. Fitzpatrick, T. B. (1996). *Dermatology in general medicine* (5th ed). New York: McGraw-Hill.
19. Formica, K., & Alster, T. S. (1998). Complications for cutaneous laser resurfacing: A nursing guide. *Dermatology Nursing, 10*(5), 353–356.
20. Frankel, E. (1995). Psoriasis. *Journal of the American Academy of Nurse Practitioners, 7*(5), 237–240.
21. Fraser, M., Goldstein, A., & Tucker, M. (1997). The genetics of melanoma. *Seminars in Oncology Nursing, 13*(2), 108–114.
22. Gregory, R. (1997). Laser blepharoplasty. *Plastic Surgical Nursing, 17*(3), 129–133, 151–153.
23. Hinojosa, R. (1995). Postoperative nausea and vomiting: How nurses can help. *Plastic Surgical Nursing, 15*(2), 85–88.
24. Hinojosa, R. (1996). Anxiety of elective surgical patients' family members: Relationship between anxiety levels, family characteristics. *Plastic Surgical Nursing, 16*(1), 43–45.
25. Licata, A. G. (1998). High-dose adjuvant interferon therapy for melanoma. *Dermatology Nursing, 10*(5), 334–336.

26. Lusis, S. (1994). Nursing management of the elderly surgical patient. *Plastic Surgical Nursing, 14*(3), 139–146.
27. Maksud, D., & Cogwell-Anderson, R. (1995). Psychological dimensions of aesthetic surgery: Essentials for nurses. *Plastic Surgical Nursing, 15*(3), 137–144.
28. Malone, M., et al. (1991). The epidemiology of skin tears in the institutionalized elderly. *Journal of the American Geriatric Society, 39,* 591–595.
29. McClelland, P. (1997). New treatment options for psoriasis. *Dermatology Nursing, 9*(5), 295–306.
30. McClelland, P., et al. (1997). Psoralen photochemotherapy. *Dermatology Nursing, 9*(6), 403–417.
31. Mendez-Eastman, S. (1998). Negative pressure wound therapy. *Plastic Surgical Nursing, 18*(1), 27–29, 32–37.
32. Morgan, P., et al. (1997). UVB therapy: dermatology nursing considerations. *Dermatology Nursing, 9*(5), 309–321.
33. Morton, D., & Barth, A. (1996). Vaccine therapy for malignant melanoma. *CA: A Cancer Journal for Clinicians, 46*(4), 225–244.
34. Nicol, N. H., & Boguniewicz, M. (1999). Understanding and treating atopic dermatitis. *Nurse Practitioner Forum 10(2),* 48–55.
35. Nicol, N. H., Ruszkowski, A., & Moore, J. A. (1995, February). Contact dermatitis and the role of patch testing in its diagnosis and management. *Dermatology Nursing* (Suppl.), 5–10.
36. Payne, R., & Martin, M. (1990). The epidemiology and management of skin tears in older adults. *Ostomy/Wound Management, 26,* 26–27.
37. Pochi, P. E., et al. (1991). Report on the Consensus Conference on Acne Classification. *Journal of the American Academy of Dermatology, 24*(3), 495–500.
38. Salisbury, C. C., & Kaye, B. (1998). Complications of rhytidectomy. *Plastic Surgical Nursing, 18*(2), 71–77, 89.
39. Sams, V. M., & Lynch, P. (1990). *Principles and practice of dermatology.* New York: Churchill Livingstone.
40. Seckel, B. R., & Watson, L. (1997). Complications of laser resurfacing. *Plastic Surgical Nursing, 17*(3), 138–143, 151–153, 161.
41. Smith, P., Black, J., & Black, S. (1999). Infected pressure ulcers in the long-term care facility. *Infection Control and Hospital Epidemiology, 20*(5), 358–361.
42. Spencer, K. W. (1994). Selection and preoperative preparation of plastic surgery patients. *Nursing Clinics of North America, 29*(4), 697–710.
43. Springer, R. (1996). Rhytidectomy: From consultation to recovery. *Plastic Surgical Nursing, 16*(1), 27–30.
44. Springer, R. (1996). Liposuction: An overview. *Plastic Surgical Nursing, 16*(4), 215–224.
45. Strohl, R. A. (1998). Cutaneous manifestations of malignant disease. *Dermatology Nursing, 10*(1), 23–25.
46. Taylor, C. R. (1998). Photosensitivity: Classification, diagnosis, and treatment. *Dermatology Nursing, 10*(5), 323–330.
47. Urist, M. (1996). Surgical management of primary cutaneous melanoma. *CA: A Cancer Journal for Clinicians, 46*(4), 217–224.

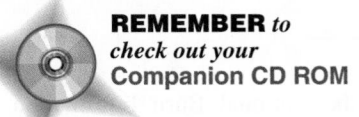

CHAPTER 50

Management of Clients with Burn Injury

Pamela Cornwell

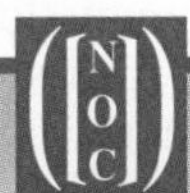

NURSING OUTCOMES CLASSIFICATION (NOC) for Nursing Diagnoses—Clients with Burns

Altered Nutrition: Less Than Body Requirements
Nutritional Status
Nutritional Status: Food and Fluid Intake
Nutritional Status: Nutrient Intake
Altered Tissue Perfusion: Peripheral
Sensory Function: Cutaneous
Tissue Integrity: Skin and Mucous Membranes
Tissue Perfusion: Peripheral
Altered Tissue Perfusion: Renal
Electrolyte and Acid-Base Balance
Fluid Balance
Hydration
Urinary Elimination
Vital Signs Status
Fluid Volume Deficit
Electrolyte and Acid-Base Balance
Fluid Balance
Hydration
Nutritional Status: Food and Fluid Intake
Hypothermia
Thermoregulation
Impaired Gas Exchange
Electrolyte and Acid-Base Balance
Respiratory Status Gas Exchange
Respiratory Status: Ventilation
Tissue Perfusion: Pulmonary
Impaired Physical Mobility
Ambulation: Walking
Ambulation: Wheelchair
Body Positioning: Self-Initiated
Joint Movement: Active
Mobility Level
Transfer Performance
Impaired Skin Integrity
Tissue Integrity: Skin and Mucous Membranes
Wound Healing: Primary Intention
Wound Healing: Secondary Intention
Impaired Tissue Integrity
Tissue Integrity: Skin and Mucous Membranes
Ineffective Airway Clearance
Aspiration Control
Respiratory Status: Airway Patency
Respiratory Status: Gas Exchange
Respiratory Status: Ventilation
Ineffective Family Coping: Compromised
Family Coping
Family Normalization
Knowledge Deficit
Knowledge: Health Resources
Knowledge: Illness Care
Knowledge: Infection Control
Knowledge: Medication
Knowledge: Personal Safety
Knowledge: Prescribed Activity
Knowledge: Treatment Procedures
Knowledge: Treatment Regimen
Pain
Comfort Level
Pain Control
Pain: Disruptive Effects
Pain Level
Risk for Infection
Immobility Consequences: Physiologic
Immune Status
Knowledge: Infection Control
Treatment Behavior: Illness or Injury
Self-Esteem Disturbance
Self-Esteem
Body Image
Hope
Mood Equilibrium

Injuries that result from direct contact with or exposure to any thermal, chemical, or radiation source are termed *burns.* Burn injuries occur when energy from a heat source is transferred to the tissues of the body. The depth of injury is related to the temperature and the duration of exposure or contact.

Burn care has improved in recent decades, resulting in a lower mortality rate for victims of burn injuries.[2, 71] Dedicated burn centers have been established in which multidisciplinary burn team members work together to care for the burn client and family. Advances in prehospital and inpatient care have contributed to survival. However, despite these advances, many people are still injured and die each year from burns. In the United States, 1.2 million people suffer burn injuries each year, resulting in 60,000 hospitalizations and 6000 deaths annually.[60]

Etiology

Burn injuries are categorized according to the mechanism of injury.

Thermal Burns

Thermal burns are caused by exposure to or contact with flame, hot liquids, semiliquids (e.g., steam), semisolids (e.g., tar), or hot objects. Specific examples of thermal burns are those sustained in residential fires, explosive automobile accidents, scald injuries, clothing ignition, and ignition of poorly stored flammable liquids.

Chemical Burns

Chemical burns are caused by tissue contact with strong acids, alkalis, or organic compounds. The concentration, volume, and type of chemical, as well as the duration of contact, determine the severity of a chemical injury. Chemical burns can result from contact with certain household cleaning agents and various chemicals used in industry, agriculture, and the military. Between 33,000 and 63,000 chemicals in use today have been recognized as hazardous and capable of causing chemical injuries.[77] Chemical injuries to the eyes and inhalation of chemical fumes are particularly serious.

Electrical Burns

Electrical burn injuries are caused by heat that is generated by the electrical energy as it passes through the body.[26] Electrical injuries can result from contact with exposed or faulty electrical wiring or high-voltage power lines. People struck by lightning also sustain electrical injury.

The extent of injury is influenced by the duration of contact, the intensity of the current (voltage), the type of current (direct or alternating), the pathway of the current, and the resistance of the tissues as the electrical current passes through the body. Contact with electrical current of greater than 40 volts is potentially dangerous; however, current of greater than 1000 volts is considered to be high-voltage current and is associated with extensive tissue damage.[23]

Radiation Burns

Radiation burns are the least common type of burn injury and are caused by exposure to a radioactive source. These types of injuries have been associated with nuclear radiation accidents, the use of ionizing radiation in industry, and therapeutic irradiation. Sunburn, from prolonged exposure to ultraviolet rays (solar radiation), is also considered to be a type of radiation burn.

The amount of radioactive energy received after exposure depends on the distance the person is from the source of the radiation, the strength of the radiation source, the duration of exposure, the extent of body surface area exposed, and the amount of shielding between the source and the person. An acute localized radiation injury appears similar to a cutaneous thermal injury and is characterized by skin erythema, edema, and pain. In contrast, whole-body radiation exposure causes systemic symptoms (radiation sickness) that are dose-dependent.[52]

Inhalation Injury

Exposure to asphyxiants and smoke commonly occurs with flame injuries, particularly if the victim was trapped in an enclosed, smoke-filled space (e.g., in a residential fire). Victims who die at the scene of the fire usually do so as a result of hypoxia and carbon monoxide poisoning.[18]

The pulmonary pathophysiologic changes that occur with inhalation injury are multifactorial and relate to the severity and type of smoke or gases inhaled. Exposure to asphyxiants, smoke poisoning, and direct thermal (heat) injury to lung tissue constitute the three facets of an inhalation injury. However, not all of these injury components may be present in the client suffering from an inhalation injury.[14, 70]

Risk Factors

Data collected from the National Burn Information Exchange reveal that 75% of all burn injuries result from the actions of the victim, with many of these injuries occurring in the home environment. Most at risk to suffer serious burn injuries are young children, older adults, and people with mental or physical limitations.[8]

Contact with scalding liquids is the leading cause of burn injury.[18] Toddlers (children 2 to 4 years of age) suffer more scald injuries than any other age group. Scald injuries are frequently the result of mishaps in the performance of everyday tasks such as bathing and cooking. Overturned coffeepots, cooking pans spilling hot liquid and grease, overheated foods, liquids cooked in microwave ovens, and hot tap water have been identified as specific causes.[68] In an effort to reduce the incidence of scald injuries the Consumer Products Safety Commission and Underwriters Laboratory has recommended that the maximum temperature on the thermostats of hot water heaters be lowered and that a warning label identifying the potential for injury be affixed to hot water heaters. Legislation requiring public buildings to lower water temperature to 120° F (48.8° C) has proved successful in reducing scald injuries.[59] In addition, a thermostatic control system (anti-scald device) has been developed that, when installed at the faucet or shower head, shuts off the flow of water when the temperature rises above a predetermined temperature, typically 119° F (48.3° C).

Direct contact with flame in the young adult (17 to 25 years of age) is the second leading cause of burn injury.[18] Frequently seen flame injuries in this category are burns to the hands and face that result from an explosion of flammable liquid, known as flash burns. Actions such as using gasoline to start or accelerate a fire and priming a carburetor on an automobile or boat can result in flash explosions.

Clothing ignition during routine meal preparation has also been cited as a leading cause of burn injury, particularly in the elderly population.[68] Synthetic fabrics are especially dangerous, as they melt and adhere to the skin, causing prolonged contact with the heat. Another age group at risk for clothing ignition is the pediatric population. During the early 1970s, the fatality rate among young children burned from ignition of sleepwear was significant. In 1975 it was mandated that children's sleepwear, sizes 0 to 6X, pass a standard flame test. This action significantly lowered mortality associated with children's clothing ignition.[65] The mandate for sleepwear to pass a flame test has since been repealed, and testing will no longer be required. This decision may add significantly to the risk of serious burn injury in the young. See Box 50–1 for burn injury prevention in the home.

Structural fires account for only 5% of burn-related hospital admissions; however, they are responsible for the greatest number of burn-related deaths.[18] Approximately 30% of all burn-related deaths are a result of structural fires,[14] seemingly from the associated smoke inhalation.[16, 70] Ignition from cigarettes is the nation's largest single cause of all fire deaths.[5, 9] Approximately 10% of residential fire deaths are caused by children playing with matches or other ignition sources.[59] Additionally, faulty chimneys, flue vents, fixed heating units, fireplaces, central heating

BOX 50–1 Residential Burn Injury Prevention Recommendations

In the kitchen:

- Turn pot handles toward the back of the stove.
- Purchase a stove with controls on the front or side to reduce the likelihood of clothing ignition as one reaches across the hot elements.
- Place a screen around any heating appliance to function as a barrier.

In the home:

- Adjust the thermostat setting on the water heater to produce a temperature no higher than 120° F (48.8° C).
- Install water temperature–regulating valves (anti-scald device) that obstruct the flow of water when the water temperature exceeds a preset level.

systems, wood-burning stoves, ignition of wood-shingled roofs, as well as human error, all have been implicated.

Of primary importance in reducing injuries and deaths from residential fires is the presence of a working smoke detector and fire extinguisher. It has been estimated that the risk of dying in a residential fire is reduced 50% when an operating smoke detector is in place.[5]

Pathophysiology

The pathophysiologic changes that occur following a cutaneous burn injury depend on the extent or size of the burn. For smaller burns, the body's response to injury is localized to the burned area. However, with more extensive burns (i.e., involving 25% or more of the total body surface area [TBSA]), the body's response to injury is systemic and proportional to the extent of the injury.[64] The clinical manifestations of burn trauma evolve in dramatic fashion over the postinjury clinical course. Extensive burn injuries affect all major systems of the body. The systemic response to burn injury is typically biphasic, characterized by early hypofunction followed later by hyperfunction of each of the organ systems.

Direct Injury to the Skin

With direct injury to the skin, heat from an external source is conducted to the skin, where it denatures (devitalizes) the cells. The amount of damage is dependent upon the length of exposure to the heat and the temperature. At sustained temperatures of 40° to 44° C (104° F to 111.2° F), various cellular enzyme systems and cellular systems fail. The sodium-potassium pump fails, which leads to cellular edema. As the temperature rises to 44° C, cell necrosis occurs. In addition, free radicals are produced, increasing cell damage. The processes of cellular damage continue until the heat source is withdrawn and cooling processes return the cell temperature to a tolerable range.

Protein destruction occurs in tissues destroyed by heat. The directly damaged skin is coagulated and fully destroyed. This area of burned tissue is called the *zone of coagulation* (Fig. 50–1) and represents the area of direct heat injury. In surrounding skin, which has been exposed to heat, the tissue is edematous and has impaired blood flow. This middle zone is called the *zone of stasis* and consists of skin that initially is viable but may also eventually die from ischemia. The outer ring of tissue injury is called the *zone of hyperemia* and consists of tissue that is inflamed and vasodilated.

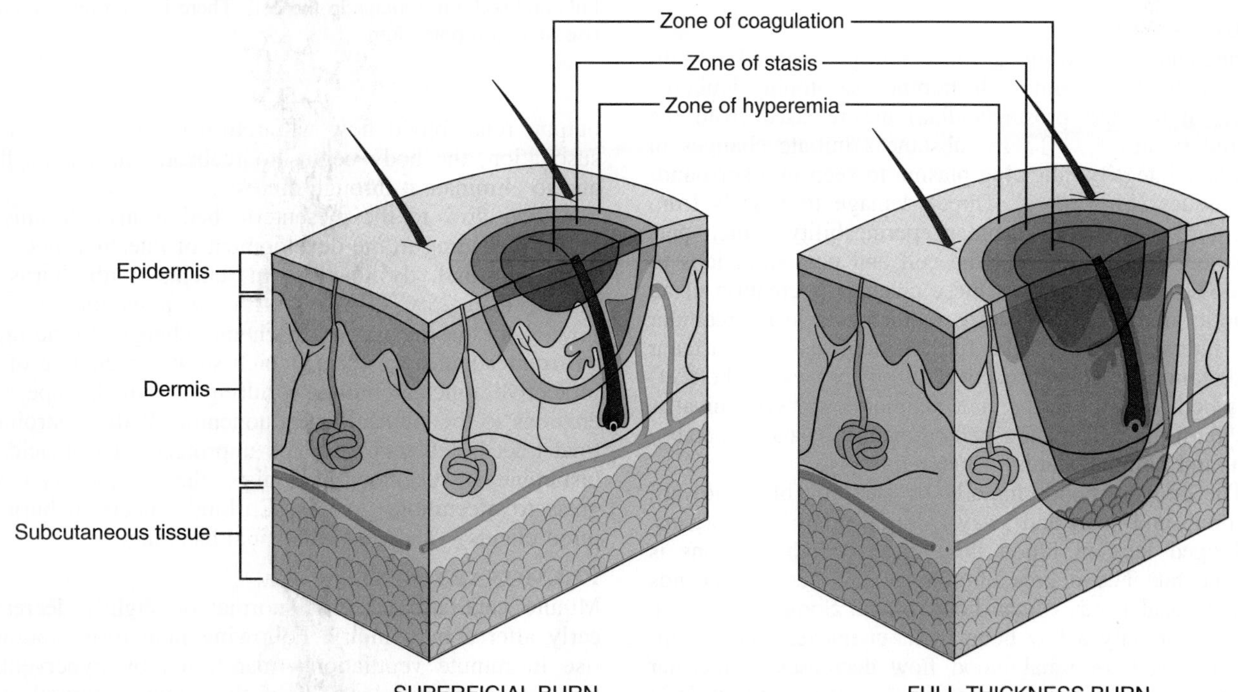

FIGURE 50–1 Zone of tissue injury. The zone of coagulation is the center of the burn wound and represents actual tissue damage. The zone of stasis is the surrounding area and represents areas of potential tissue loss. The outer ring is the zone of hyperemia and is unburned tissue that is inflamed.

Some types of burn create unique patterns of injury. In electrical injuries, heat is generated as the electricity travels through the body, resulting in internal tissue damage.[29] The concept of "the tip of the iceberg" is helpful to understand these injuries. For instance, only a very small percentage of total injury from an electrical burn can be seen from the body's surface. Cutaneous burn injuries may appear negligible, but muscle and soft tissue damage may be extensive, particularly with high-voltage electrical injuries. The voltage, type of current (direct or alternating), contact site, and duration of contact are important considerations because they may affect morbidity. Electricity seeks ground as it exits the body; en route, it creates heat and may pass though vital organs. Alternating current (AC) is more dangerous than direct current (DC). AC is often associated with cardiopulmonary arrest, ventricular fibrillation, tetanic muscle contractions, and long bone or vertebral compression fracture. The risk of acute renal failure is noteworthy in clients following an electrical injury. Hemoglobin, released from heat-damaged erythrocytes together with myoglobin, the protein that supplies muscles with oxygen, is released in significant quantities into the blood stream after deep burn injuries involving muscle damage. These substances pass through the glomeruli and are excreted in urine. However, these materials may precipitate and obstruct the renal tubules, causing renal damage unless a brisk urine output is maintained.[64] In addition, victims of electrical injuries may have fallen from the point of electrical contact and sustained associated injuries. Cataract formation is also associated with high-voltage electrical injury, especially in cases in which contact points are on the head or neck. In chemical burns, systemic toxic effects may result from cutaneous absorption of the offending agent. Organ failure and even death have resulted from prolonged contact with and absorption of different chemicals.

Fluid Shifts

Immediately following a burn injury, vasoactive substances (catecholamines, histamine, serotonin, leukotrienes, kinins, and prostaglandins) are released from the injured tissues.[34, 60] These substances initiate changes in capillary integrity, allowing plasma to seep into surrounding tissues (Fig. 50–2). Direct damage to vessels from heat further increases capillary permeability, which permits sodium ions to enter the cell and potassium ions to exit. The overall effect of these changes is creation of an osmotic gradient, which leads to increases in intercellular and interstitial fluid and further depletes intravascular fluid volumes. The vasoactive substances exert their effects both locally (in the area of injury) and systemically. The burn-injured client's hemodynamic balance, metabolism, and immune status are altered.

The body responds initially by shunting blood toward the brain and heart and away from all other body organs. Prolonged lack of blood flow to these other organs is detrimental. The degree of damage that results depends on the basal needs of the body organ. Some organs can survive for only a few hours without nutrient blood supply. The lack of renal blood flow decreases glomerular filtration rate, leading to oliguria (low urine output).[64] If fluid resuscitation is delayed or inadequate, hypovolemia progresses, and acute renal failure may occur. However, with adequate fluid resuscitation and a rise in cardiac output, renal blood flow will return to normal. After resuscitation, the body begins to reabsorb the edema fluid and to eliminate it through diuresis.

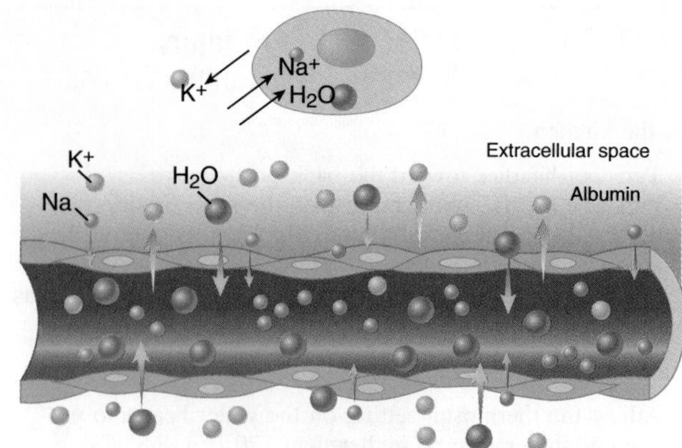

Fluid and electrolyte shift during burn shock

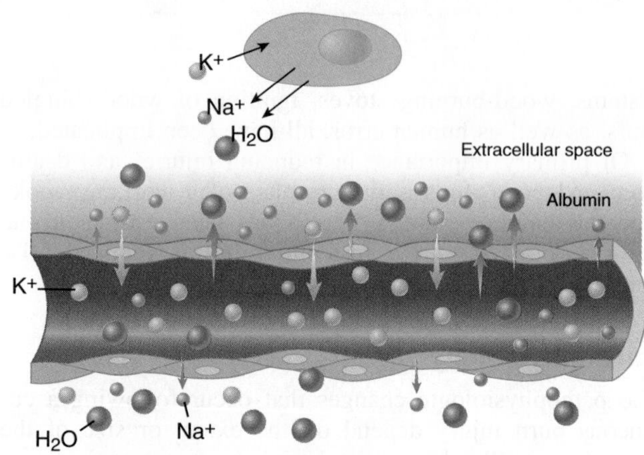

Fluid and electrolyte shift after burn shock

FIGURE 50–2 Changes in capillary permeability allow plasma to seep into interstitial spaces. In addition, the sodium pump fails and sodium remains in the cell. There is a corresponding rise in serum potassium.

Blood flow to the mesenteric bed is also diminished initially, leading to the development of intestinal ileus and gastrointestinal dysfunction in clients with burns of greater than 25% TBSA.[59] With the reduction in blood flow to the gastric mucosa, ischemic changes to the upper gastrointestinal tract occur, which slows production of the protective mucous lining, resulting in small, superficial erosions to the stomach and duodenum. If the gastrointestinal tract is left untreated and unprotected by antacids or histamine H_2-receptor antagonists, the erosions can progress to ulcerations—called Curling's ulcers in burn injured clients—and gastrointestinal bleeding.

Pulmonary System

Minute ventilation is often normal or slightly decreased early after a burn injury. Following fluid resuscitation, a rise in minute ventilation—manifested by hyperventilation—may occur especially if the client is fearful, anxious, or in pain. This hyperventilation is the result of an increase in both respiratory rate and tidal volume and appears to be the result of the hypermetabolism that is seen after burn injury. It typically peaks in the second postinjury week and then gradually returns to normal as the burn wound heals or is closed by grafting.[59]

Pulmonary vascular resistance may increase slightly, and lung compliance may decrease. The changes in lung compliance cause a proportionate increase in the work of breathing; however, these changes are typically small, and in the absence of any pulmonary parenchymal (tissue) damage, they require no specialized treatment.

INHALATION INJURY. Exposure to asphyxiants is the most common cause of early mortality from inhalation injury.[18] Carbon monoxide (CO), a common asphyxiant, is produced when organic substances (e.g., wood or coal) burn. It is a colorless, odorless, and tasteless gas that has an affinity for the body's hemoglobin that is 200 times greater than that of oxygen. With inhalation of CO, the oxygen molecules are displaced, and CO binds to hemoglobin to form carboxyhemoglobin (COHb). Tissue hypoxia occurs from an overall decrease in the blood's oxygen-delivering capability.

Direct heat injury to the upper airway results from inhalation of the air heated by fire. The heat immediately produces injury to the airway, which results in edema, erythema, and ulceration. Thermal burns to the lower airways of the pulmonary system are rare because of the protective reflex closure of the glottis and the ability of the respiratory tract to exchange heat effectively. However, thermal burns to the lower airways can occur with the inhalation of steam or explosive gases or with aspiration of scalding liquids.

Smoke poisoning results from the inhalation of the by-products of combustion: noxious chemicals and particulate matter. The pulmonary response includes a localized inflammatory reaction, a decrease in bronchial ciliary action, and a decrease in alveolar surfactant. Mucosal edema occurs in the smaller airways. After several hours, sloughing of the tracheobronchial epithelium may occur, and hemorrhagic tracheobronchitis may develop. Adult respiratory distress syndrome may follow.[18]

MYOCARDIAL DEPRESSION

Some research investigators have suggested that a myocardial depressant factor exists and circulates in the early postinjury period. More recently, a combination of inflammatory mediators and hormones has been suggested as the cause of myocardial depression occurring after the injury.[6]

ALTERED SKIN INTEGRITY

The burn wound itself exhibits pathophysiologic changes caused by disruption of the skin and alterations to the tissue beneath the surface. The skin, nerve endings, sweat glands, and hair follicles injured by burn lose normal functioning. Most important, the skin's barrier function is lost. Intact skin normally keeps bacteria from entering the body and body fluids from seeping out, controls evaporation, and maintains body warmth. With destruction of the skin in burn injury, mechanisms for maintaining normal body temperature can be altered, the risk of infection from invasion of bacteria increases, and evaporative water loss increases.[31] Depending upon the depth of the injury, nerve endings either become exposed, resulting in pain and discomfort until wound closure, or are damaged, leaving the innervated area insensate, with potential for permanent impairment of ability to sense touch, pressure, and pain.

IMMUNOSUPPRESSION

Immune system function is depressed following burn injury. Depression of lymphocyte activity, a decrease in immunoglobulin production, suppression of complement activity, and an alteration in neutrophil and macrophage functioning are evident following extensive burn injuries.[53] In addition, the burn injury disrupts the body's primary barrier to infection, the skin. Together these changes result in an increased risk of infection and life-threatening sepsis.

PSYCHOLOGICAL RESPONSE

Numerous psychological and emotional responses to burn injuries have been identified, ranging from fear to psychosis.[7] A victim's response is influenced by age, personality, cultural and ethnic background, the extent and location of the injury, and the resulting impact on body image. In addition, separation from family and friends during hospitalization and the change in the client's normal role and responsibilities affect the reaction to burn trauma. Four stages in the psychosocial response to burn trauma have been described: (1) impact, (2) retreat or withdrawal, (3) acknowledgment, and (4) the reconstructive period.[37]

Clinical Manifestations

DEGREE OF INJURY

Depending on the skin layers damaged, burn wounds are termed either partial-thickness burns or full-thickness burns. Burn wounds are also classified as first-, second-, third-, or fourth-degree burns. Partial-thickness burns involve injury to the epidermis and portions of the dermis (Fig. 50–3). *First-degree* partial-thickness burns are superficial and painful and appear red. They heal on their own by epidermal cell regeneration within about 3 to 7 days. Sunburn is a good example of a first-degree partial-thickness burn. *Second-degree* partial-thickness burns appear wet or blistered and are extremely painful but can heal on their own (that is, without skin grafting) if they are small and do not become infected.

Third-degree full-thickness burns are characterized by damage throughout the dermis (Figs. 50–4 and 50–5). A

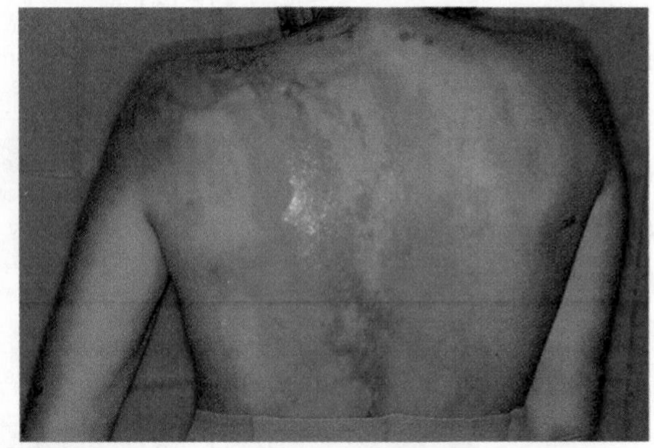

FIGURE 50–3 Partial-thickness burn injury (second-degree burn).

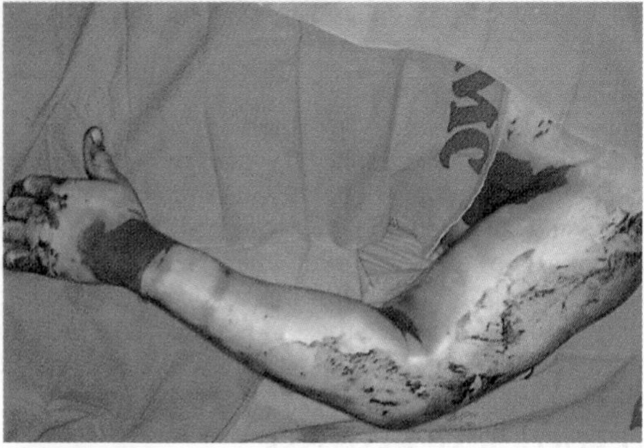

FIGURE 50–4 Full-thickness burn injury (third-degree burn).

full-thickness burn appears dry and may be black, brown, white, or ivory. The denatured skin is called eschar (pronounced "ĕs-car"). The burned tissue is painless as a result of damage to the nerve endings; however, the surrounding skin is painful. Unless the area is very small (the size of a half-dollar), the full-thickness burn must be skin-grafted to heal. The appearance of the burn relative to the depth of injury is described in Figure 50–6.

Fourth-degree full-thickness burns involve skin, fat, muscle, and sometimes bone. The skin appears charred or may be completely burned away. Areas of a fourth-degree burn require extensive surgical debridement and grafting. Amputations are common in these deep injuries.

In addition to altered physical appearance, the loss of skin leads to other problems. Hypothermia results from loss of body heat through the burn wound and is characterized by a core body temperature below 98.6° F. Hypothermia is extremely harmful because it leads to shiver-

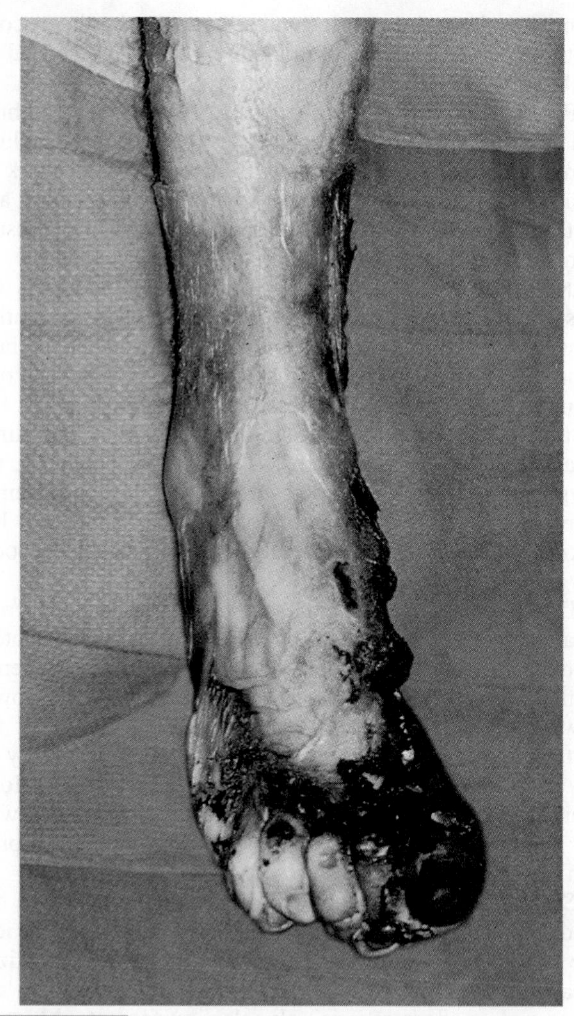

FIGURE 50–5 Full-thickness burn injury (fourth-degree burn).

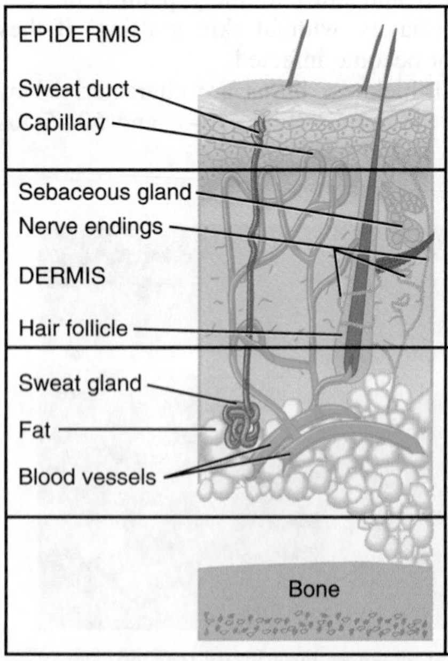

Skin layer	Burn type	Degree	WOUND APPEARANCE	WOUND SENSATION	COURSE OF HEALING
EPIDERMIS; Sweat duct; Capillary	PARTIAL-THICKNESS BURN	1st-degree	Epidermis remains intact and without blisters. Erythema; skin blanches with pressure.	Painful	Discomfort lasts 48–72 hours. Desquamation in 3–7 days
Sebaceous gland; Nerve endings; DERMIS; Hair follicle	PARTIAL-THICKNESS BURN	2nd-degree	Wet, shiny, weeping surface. Blisters. Wound blanches with pressure.	Painful. Very sensitive to touch, air currents	Superficial partial-thickness burn heals in < 21 days. Deep partial-thickness burn requires > 21 days for healing. Healing rates vary with burn depth and presence/absence of infection.
Sweat gland; Fat; Blood vessels	FULL-THICKNESS BURN	3rd-degree	Color variable (i.e., deep red, white, black, brown). Surface dry. Thrombosed vessels visible. No blanching	Insensate (↓ pinprick sensation)	Autografting required for healing
Bone	FULL-THICKNESS BURN	4th-degree	Color variable. Charring visible in deepest areas. Extremity movement limited	Insensate	Amputation of extremities likely. Autografting required for healing

FIGURE 50–6 Burn injury classification according to depth of injury.

ing, which in turn increases oxygen consumption and caloric demands.

The evaporative water loss through the burn contributes to the client's diminished fluid volume and compromised hydration status. Evaporative losses not compensated for by fluid replacement will be evidenced by a low blood pressure, decreased urine output, dry mucous membranes, and poor skin turgor.

FLUID AND ELECTROLYTE IMBALANCE

Hyponatremia, hypernatremia, and hyperkalemia are common electrolyte abnormalities that affect the burn-injured client at different points in the recovery process. Extensive burns (greater than 25% TBSA) result in generalized body edema affecting both burned and nonburned tissues and in a decrease in circulating intravascular blood volume (Fig. 50–7).[18, 60, 65] Hematocrit levels are elevated in the first 24 hours after injury, demonstrating hemoconcentration from the loss of intravascular fluid. In addition, evaporative fluid losses through the burn wound are 4 to 20 times greater than normal and remain elevated until complete wound closure is obtained. The result is a decrease in organ perfusion. If the intravascular space is not replenished with intravenous (IV) fluids, hypovolemic (burn) shock and, ultimately, death ensue for the victim of an extensive burn.[2, 18, 20, 34, 46, 74]

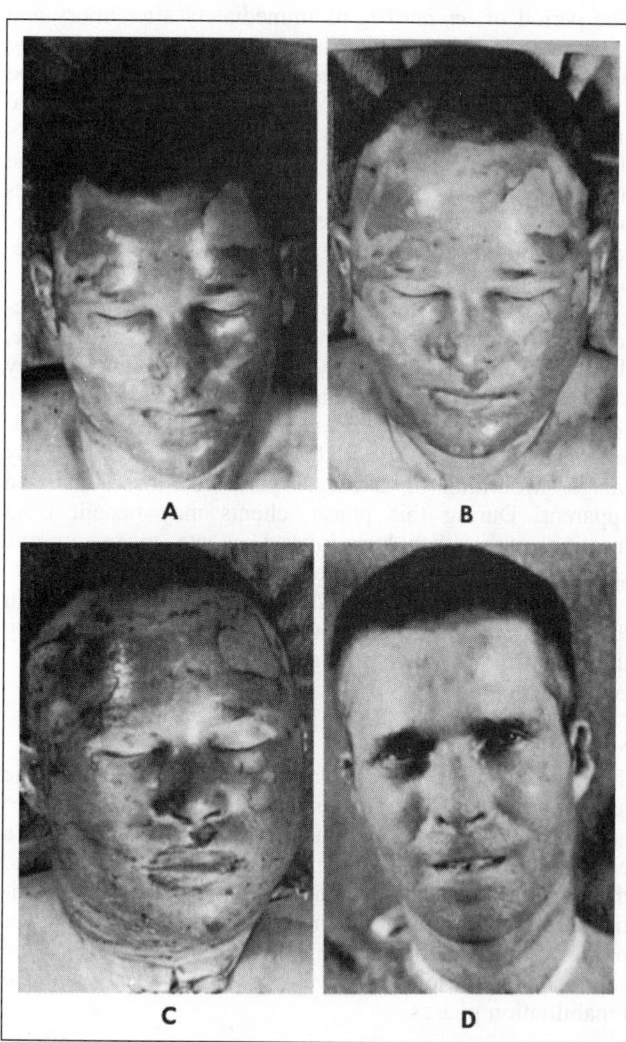

FIGURE 50–7 Edema formation after a burn injury to the face and neck. Edema worsens over the first 24 to 48 hours after burn injury. *A,* At 3 hours after burn. *B,* At 8 hours after the burn. *C,* At 24 hours after burn, when edema has typically maximized. *D,* Complete healing after 40 days. (From Artz, C. P., et al. [1979]. *Burns: A team approach.* Philadelphia: W. B. Saunders.)

TABLE 50–1 CLINICAL MANIFESTATIONS OF CARBON MONOXIDE (CO) POISONING

CO Level (%)	Clinical Manifestations
5–10	Impaired visual acuity
11–20	Flushing, headache
21–30	Nausea, impaired dexterity
31–40	Vomiting, dizziness, syncope
41–50	Tachypnea, tachycardia
>50	Coma, death

Adapted from Cioffi, W. G., & Rue, L. W. (1991). Diagnosis and treatment of inhalation injuries. *Critical Care Clinics of North America, 3*(2), 195.

Urine output for the adult client receiving insufficient fluid replacement following a major burn injury will diminish to less than 0.5 ml/kg of body weight. Physical findings of the urine sample will demonstrate dehydration, characterized by dark amber, concentrated urine and elevated specific gravity. Laboratory tests reveal elevated blood urea nitrogen (BUN) levels until the client has been adequately hydrated.

Manifestations of decreased gastrointestinal motility following major burn injuries include the absence of bowel sounds, stool, or flatus; nausea and vomiting; and abdominal distention. After adequate fluid resuscitation, gastrointestinal motility returns, signaled by a return of hunger/appetite, bowel sounds, flatus, and stool production.

At approximately 18 to 36 hours after burn injury, capillary membrane integrity begins to be restored. The initial rise in hematocrit seen early after injury falls to below normal by the third or fourth day after injury owing to red blood cell loss and damage incurred at the time of injury. Over the ensuing days and weeks, the body begins to reabsorb the edema fluid, and the excess fluid is excreted via diuresis (see Fig. 50–7).

ALTERATIONS IN RESPIRATION

The client may exhibit tachypnea following the burn injury. Arterial blood gas analysis may demonstrate a relatively normal arterial partial pressure of oxygen (PaO_2), with oxygen saturation lower than expected relative to the PO_2. Diagnosis is made by measuring the COHb level in the blood. The clinical manifestations of acute CO poisoning are directly related to the level of COHb saturation and relative degree of tissue hypoxia (Table 50–1). The onset of clinical manifestations will typically not occur until COHb levels reach 15%. Initial signs and symptoms are related to decreased cerebral tissue oxygenation and are neurologic in nature. The neurologic problems caused by CO exposure can lead to progressive and permanent cerebral dysfunction.

Thermal burns to the upper airways (mouth, nasopharynx, and larynx) characteristically appear erythematous and edematous, with mucosal blisters or ulcerations. Increasing mucosal edema can lead to upper airway obstruction, typically between the first 24 and 48 hours after injury. Clinical manifestations, including stridor, dyspnea, increased work of breathing, and eventually cyanosis, may be noted when critical narrowing of the airway is present.[14, 38, 57]

Physical findings on admission indicative of smoke exposure include soot on the face and nares, facial burns, soot in the sputum, coughing, and wheezing. The manifestations of tracheobronchitis typically do not present until 24 to 48 hours after injury. Early signs consist of bronchospasm evidenced as wheezing and bronchorrhea. Lung compliance is decreased, causing an increased work of breathing. Impaired clearance of secretions accentuates the problem. Normally, ventilation and perfusion are matched by equal volumes of air and blood on the alveolar-capillary level. The client with smoke inhalation exhibits pathophysiologic changes that reduce alveolar ventilation, causing a ventilation-perfusion (V-Q) mismatch, which in turn impairs gas exchange.[19, 42]

Decreased Cardiac Output

Following a major burn injury, heart rate and peripheral vascular resistance increase in response to the release of catecholamines and to the relative hypovolemia, but initial cardiac output falls (hypofunction).[10] At approximately 24 hours after burn injury in clients receiving adequate fluid resuscitation, cardiac output returns to normal and then increases (2 to 2.5 times normal) to meet the hypermetabolic needs of the body (hyperfunction). This change in cardiac output occurs even before circulating intravascular volume levels are restored to normal. Arterial blood pressure is normal or slightly elevated unless severe hypovolemia exists. The decreased cardiac output seen initially after burn injury is evidenced by a decreased blood pressure, decreased urine output, weak peripheral pulses, and if monitored via a pulmonary artery catheter, a cardiac output below 4 L/min, cardiac index of less than 2.5 L/min, and systemic vascular resistance of less than 900 dyne-sec/cm.[5, 18]

Pain Responses

The client experiences substantial pain as a result of the burn wound and exposed nerve endings from lack of skin integrity.[42, 43] Burn victims typically describe two types of pain resulting from their injury: background pain and procedural pain. Background pain is experienced when the client is at rest or engages in non–procedure-related activities, such as shifting position in bed, or with chest or abdominal wall movements that occur with deep breathing or coughing. Background pain is described as continuous in nature and low in intensity, typically lasting for the duration of the clinical course.[17] Procedural pain is experienced during the performance of therapeutic measures commonly used in burn care. Nearly 52% of clients report moderate to severe pain during burn wound debridement.[19] Procedural pain is described as acute and high in intensity. Clinical responses to pain may include an increase in blood pressure, heart rate, and respiratory rate and dilated pupils, rigid muscle tone, and guarded positioning.

Altered Level of Consciousness

Rarely do burn-injured clients suffer neurologic damage. The client with a major burn injury is most often awake and alert on admission to the hospital. If agitation develops in the immediate postinjury period, the client may be suffering from hypoxemia or hypovolemia and needs further assessment for identifying the origin of these changes. When an alteration in level of consciousness is present, it is most often related to neurologic trauma (e.g., fall, motor vehicle accident), impaired perfusion to the brain, hypoxemia (as from a closed-space fire), inhalation injury (as from exposure to asphyxiates or other toxic materials from the fire), electrical burn injury, or the effects of drugs present in the body at the time of injury.

Clients with associated head trauma may have scalp lacerations, swelling, tenderness, or ecchymosis. Level of consciousness may fluctuate between intervals of lucidity followed by rapid deterioration. Pupils may be of unequal size. Neurologic manifestations may include headache, dizziness, memory loss, confusion or loss of consciousness, disorientation, visual changes, hallucinations, combativeness, and coma.

Psychological Alterations

The period of *impact* begins immediately after injury and is characterized by shock, disbelief, and feelings of being overwhelmed. The client and family members may be aware of what is happening but may be coping with the situation poorly. During this period, families of critically ill clients have a need for assurance, proximity to the injured person, and information. Specifically, families want to know how the client is being treated, specific facts about the client's progress, and why certain procedures are being done.

Retreat is characterized by repression, withdrawal, denial, and suppression. Although seemingly destructive, these coping strategies may be protective in that they allow the client to maintain an intact psyche.

The third phase, *acknowledgment,* begins when the client accepts the injury and the resultant change in body image. Mourning of actual or perceived losses may be apparent. During this phase, clients may benefit from meeting with other burn-injured clients in one-on-one contact or group support meetings.

The final phase, the *reconstructive period,* begins when the client and family accept the limitations imposed by the injury and begin to plan realistically for the future.

Outcome Management

The burn client undergoes a wide range of physiologic and metabolic changes in response to the burn injury. To accomplish the best outcomes, it is essential to have a clear understanding of the pathophysiologic process and the necessary treatment modifications needed over the entire course of burn treatment. Three distinct periods or phases of treatment can be defined in the care of the seriously burned client: the emergent, the acute, and the rehabilitation phases.

Emergent Phase

The emergent phase of burn injury consists of the time between the initial injury and 36 to 48 hours after injury. This phase ends when fluid resuscitation is complete.

During this phase, life-threatening airway and breathing problems are of major concern. It is also characterized by the development of hypovolemia which results as capillaries leak fluid from the intravascular spaces into the interstitial spaces, causing edema. Although the fluid remains in the body, it is unable to contribute to maintaining adequate circulation, because it is no longer in the vascular space. The burn itself, except for initial assessment of severity and depth and, in certain cases, a procedure (escharotomy) performed to restore perfusion to areas exhibiting circulatory compromise, is of less immediate concern. The adequacy of initial treatment of pulmonary and circulatory abnormalities sets the stage for subsequent management. Any early management error will lead to a dramatic increase in morbidity and mortality during the subsequent injury phases.

Management of the burn client begins at the scene of the accident. The first step should be removing the victim from the area of immediate danger, followed by stopping the burning process. Basic life support measures should be implemented during transport of the client to the hospital.

Medical Management in the Emergent Phase of Burn Injury

ASSESS BURN SEVERITY

The American Burn Association has published a severity classification schedule for burn injuries (see Table 50–2). These guidelines are intended to assist the clinician in determining injury severity for the burn client. This classification schedule separates injuries into major, moderate, and minor categories. Clients with major burns are usually transferred to a specialized burn care facility after local emergency treatment has been provided. Clients with moderate burns can usually be managed on an inpatient basis at the receiving hospital. Clients with minor burns usually receive initial care in the emergency department and are then discharged for follow-up care on an outpatient basis.

The severity of a burn injury is classified according to the risk of mortality and the risk of cosmetic or functional disability.[3] Several factors influence injury severity.

BURN DEPTH. The deeper the burn wound, the more serious the injury. Deep partial-thickness and full-thickness burns are more likely to become infected, have more profound systemic effects, and are more frequently associated with contractures.

BURN SIZE. The size of a burn (percentage of injured skin, excluding first-degree burns) is determined by one of two techniques: (1) the rule of 9s and (2) an age-specific burn diagram or chart.[45, 61] Burn size is expressed as a percentage of TBSA. The *rule of 9s* was introduced in the late 1940s as a quick assessment tool for estimating burn size. The basis of the rule is that the body is divided into anatomic sections, each of which represents 9%, or a multiple of 9%, of the TBSA (Fig. 50–8). This method is easy and requires no diagrams to determine the percentage of TBSA injured. Therefore, it is frequently used in emergency departments, where initial triage occurs. A *burn diagram* charts the percentages for body segments according to age and provides a more accurate estimate of burn size (Fig. 50–9). It should be noted that the extent of burn injury is most accurate after initial debridement and should therefore be verified again at that time.

BURN LOCATION. With burns of the head, neck, and chest, associated pulmonary complications are frequent. When burns involve the face, associated injuries often include corneal abrasions. Burns of the ears are prone to auricular chondritis and are susceptible to infection and further loss of tissue. Management of burns of the hands and joints often requires intense physical and occupational therapy, with the potential for major loss of work time and for permanent physical and vocational disability. Burns involving the perineal area are prone to infection owing to autocontamination by urine and feces. Circumferential burns of extremities may produce a tourniquet-like effect, leading to distal vascular compromise. Circumferential thorax burns may lead to inadequate chest wall expansion and pulmonary insufficiency.

AGE. The client's age affects the severity and outcome of the burn. Mortality rates are higher for children younger than 4 years, particularly in newborns and infants up to 1 year of age, and for clients older than 65 years.[5, 18, 68] High mortality and morbidity rates in the older burn-injured client result from the combination of age-related functional impairments (slower reaction time, impaired judgment, and decreased mobility), living alone, environmental hazards, and significant preburn morbidity. Compounding this vulnerability to burn injury is the thinning of the skin and atrophy of skin appendages that occur with aging.

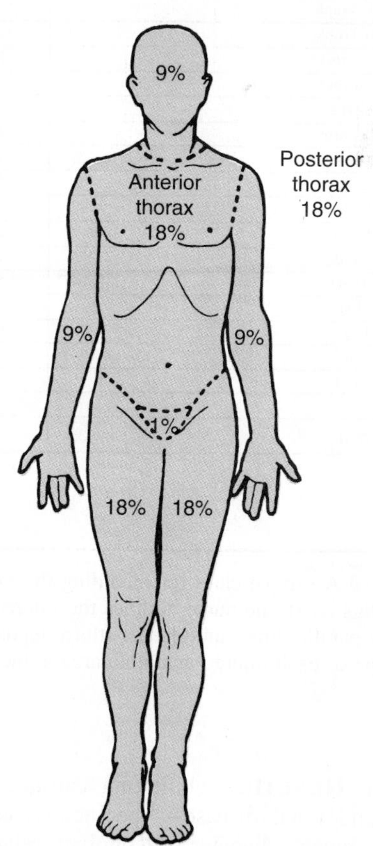

FIGURE 50–8 The rule of 9s provides a quick method for estimating the extent of a burn injury in the adult.

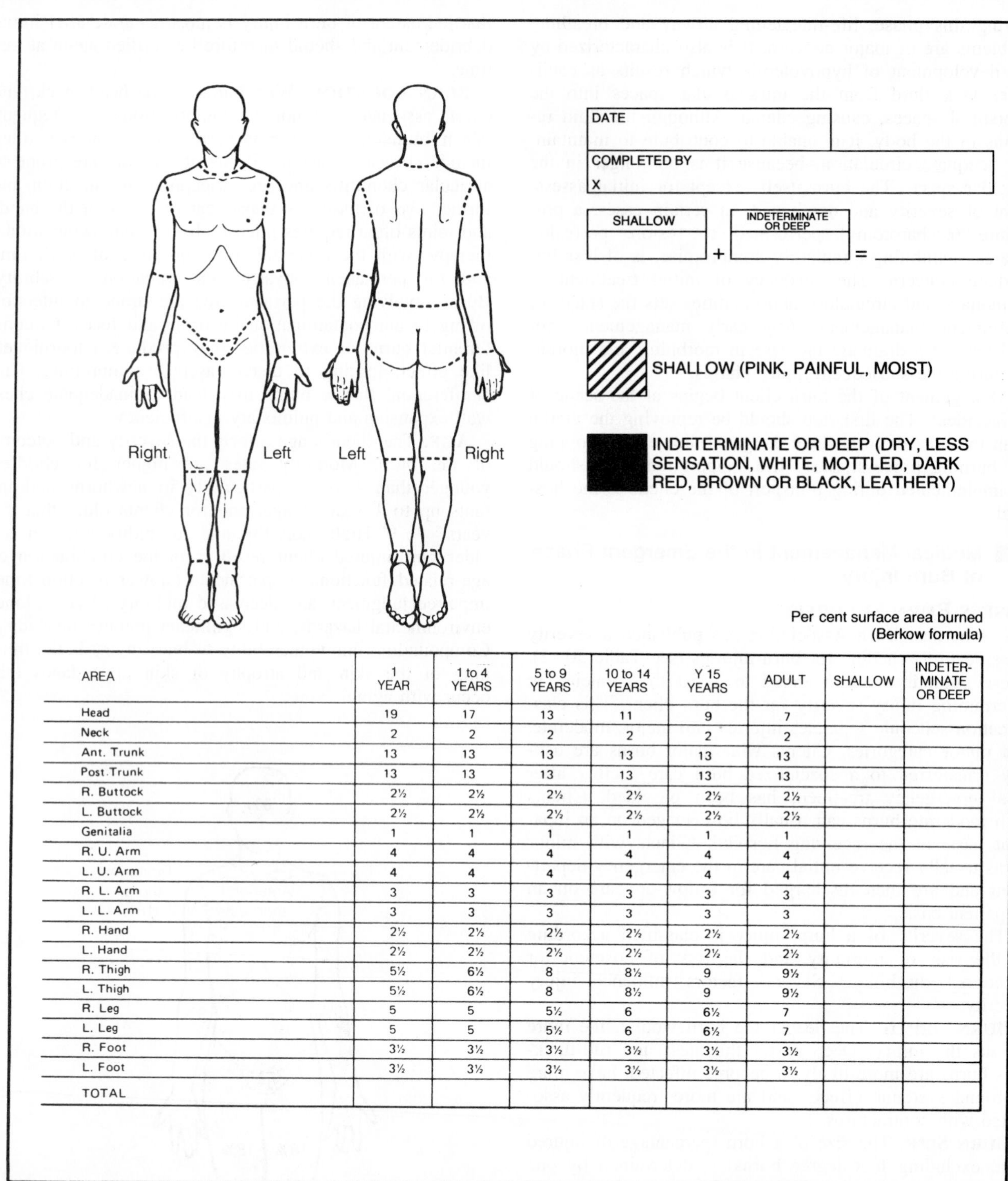

AREA	1 YEAR	1 to 4 YEARS	5 to 9 YEARS	10 to 14 YEARS	Y 15 YEARS	ADULT	SHALLOW	INDETER-MINATE OR DEEP
Head	19	17	13	11	9	7		
Neck	2	2	2	2	2	2		
Ant. Trunk	13	13	13	13	13	13		
Post.Trunk	13	13	13	13	13	13		
R. Buttock	2½	2½	2½	2½	2½	2½		
L. Buttock	2½	2½	2½	2½	2½	2½		
Genitalia	1	1	1	1	1	1		
R. U. Arm	4	4	4	4	4	4		
L. U. Arm	4	4	4	4	4	4		
R. L. Arm	3	3	3	3	3	3		
L. L. Arm	3	3	3	3	3	3		
R. Hand	2½	2½	2½	2½	2½	2½		
L. Hand	2½	2½	2½	2½	2½	2½		
R. Thigh	5½	6½	8	8½	9	9½		
L. Thigh	5½	6½	8	8½	9	9½		
R. Leg	5	5	5½	6	6½	7		
L. Leg	5	5	5½	6	6½	7		
R. Foot	3½	3½	3½	3½	3½	3½		
L. Foot	3½	3½	3½	3½	3½	3½		
TOTAL								

FIGURE 50–9 A sample chart for recording the extent and depth of a burn injury using the Berkow formula. To estimate burn extent using this chart, the nurse outlines the injured areas, excluding first-degree burns. Shallow (second-degree) burns are designated by parallel lines, and deeper (third-degree and fourth-degree) burns are designated by shading in the appropriate areas. The percentage of each injured anatomic area is then estimated using the age-specific table. Total body surface area burn is then calculated.

General Health. Debilitating cardiac, pulmonary, endocrine, and renal disease—specifically, cardiopulmonary insufficiency, diabetes, alcoholism-related disease, and renal failure—have been observed to influence the client's response to injury and treatment.[58] The mortality rate for clients with pre-existing cardiac disorders is 3.5 to 4 times higher than that for burn-injured clients without cardiac disorders. Alcoholic clients with burn injury have a threefold increase in mortality rate over that of nonalcoholic clients with burns. In addition, alcoholic clients who survive their burn injury have longer hospital stays and more complications. The increased morbidity among clients with burn injury who are alcoholics may be related to impaired immune function. Obese clients with burn injury are also at increased risk owing to cardiopulmonary complications.

MECHANISM OF INJURY. The mechanism of injury is another factor used to determine the severity of injury. In general, special attention to this aspect of the injury is required for any electrical or chemical burn injury or any burn associated with inhalation injury. The client, people at the scene of the injury, and emergency medical personnel may have important information that could help in determining the severity of the burn. Useful information includes the time of injury, the level of the client's consciousness at the scene, whether the injury occurred in an enclosed or open space, the presence of associated trauma, and the specific mechanism of injury. If the victim has suffered a chemical burn, knowledge of the offending agent, its concentration, the duration of exposure, and whether irrigation was initiated at the scene is useful. For victims of electrical injuries, knowledge of the electrical source, type of current, and the current voltage is useful in determining the extent of the injury. Information concerning the client's past medical history as well as his or her general health should be obtained. Specifically, information regarding cardiac, pulmonary, endocrine, or renal disease should be obtained because it may have implications for treatment. Known allergies should also be identified, as should any current medication regimen.

TREAT MINOR BURNS

Care of the client with minor burn injuries is frequently provided on an ambulatory or outpatient basis. In making the decision about whether to manage a client as an outpatient, the seriousness of the injury must first be assessed. As outlined in Table 50–2, a minor burn injury in the adult is generally considered to be less than 15% TBSA in clients younger than 40 years of age or 10% TBSA in clients older than 40 years, without a risk of cosmetic or functional impairment or disability.[3] In addition, the client's or caregiver's ability to perform wound care in the home environment must be considered. Medical care of the minor burn includes wound evaluation and initial care, tetanus immunization, and pain management. While providing initial wound care, the nurse is responsible for teaching home wound care and the clinical manifestations of infection that necessitate further medical care. Other teaching needs include the need to perform active range of motion (ROM) exercises to maintain normal joint function and to decrease edema formation. The need for any follow-up evaluations or treatments should be confirmed with the client at this time.

TREAT MAJOR BURNS

The medical goals for burn care depend on the phase of care. Initial goals are saving life, maintaining and protecting the airway, and restoring hemodynamic stability. Later goals are replacement of missing skin, promoting healing, and assessing and correcting complications.

MONITOR AIRWAY AND BREATHING. The adequacy of the airway and breathing should take prime importance during the emergent phase of burn injury.[11, 21, 30, 39, 45, 54] The oropharynx should be inspected for evidence of erythema, blisters, or ulcerations, and the need for endotracheal intubation should be considered. If inhalation injury is suspected, administration of 100% oxygen via a tight-fitting facemask continues until COHb levels fall below 15%.[18] Hyperbaric oxygen is also considered with any exposure to CO. If breathing appears to be compromised by tight circumferential trunk burns, bilateral escharotomies of the trunk may be necessary to relieve ventilatory compromise.

PREVENT BURN SHOCK. In adults with burn injuries affecting more than 15% TBSA, IV fluid resuscitation is generally required.[2, 46] Two peripheral large-bore IV lines placed through nonburned skin, proximal to any extremity burns, is recommended. IV lines may be placed through burned skin if necessary; however, these lines should be secured with a suture. For clients with extensive burns or limited peripheral IV access sites, cannulation of a central vein (subclavian, internal or external jugular, or femoral) by a physician may be necessary.

TABLE 50–2 AMERICAN BURN ASSOCIATION SEVERITY CLASSIFICATION FOR BURN INJURIES

MAJOR BURN INJURY
25% TBSA burn in adults <40 yr of age 20% TBSA burn in adults >40 yr of age 20% TBSA burn in children <10 yr of age
or
Burns involving the face, eyes, ears, hands, feet, and perineum likely to result in functional or cosmetic disability
or
High-voltage electrical burn injury
or
All burn injuries with concomitant inhalation injury or major trauma
MODERATE BURN INJURY
15%–25% TBSA burn in adults <40 yr of age 10%–20% TBSA burn in adults >40 yr of age 10%–20% TBSA burn in children <10 yr of age
with
Less than 10% TBSA full-thickness burn without cosmetic or functional risk to the face, eyes, ears, hands, feet, or perineum
MINOR BURN INJURY
<15% TBSA burn in adults <40 yr of age <10% TBSA burn in adults >40 yr of age <10% TBSA burn in children <10 yr of age
with
<2% TBSA full-thickness burn and no cosmetic or functional risk to the face, eyes, ears, hands, feet, or perineum

TBSA, total body surface area.

Adapted from American Burn Association. (1984). Guidelines for service standards and severity classification in the treatment of burn injury. *American College of Surgeons Bulletin, 69*(10), 24–28.

Fluid resuscitation is used to minimize the deleterious effects of the fluid shifts. The goal of fluid resuscitation is to maintain vital organ perfusion while avoiding the complication of inadequate or excessive fluids. Several formulas used to calculate fluid requirements are listed in Table 50–3. In the calculation of fluid infusion rates, the time of injury, not the time at which fluid resuscitation was initiated, serves as time zero. Thus, if a burned client is delayed 2 hours in reaching an emergency department, those 2 hours must be considered in any calculation of needed fluid.

Although each formula is different, fluid management during the first 24 hours after burn injury generally includes the infusion of balanced salt solution, typically lactated Ringer's solution. The exact amount of fluid is based on the client's weight and the extent of injury. Other factors to be considered include the presence of an inhalation injury, a delay in initiation of resuscitation, and deep tissue damage. These factors tend to increase the amount of IV fluid required for adequate resuscitation above the calculated amount.[18] With the exception of the Evans and Brooke formulas, colloid-containing solutions are not given during this period because of the changes in capillary integrity that allow leakage of protein-rich fluid (e.g., albumin) into the interstitial space, resulting in the formation of additional edematous fluid. During the second 24 hours after burn injury, colloid-containing solutions are administered, along with 5% dextrose and water in varying amounts. It is important to remember that all resuscitation formulas are only guides and that fluid resuscitation volumes should be adjusted according to the client's physiologic response. Adequacy of fluid resuscitation is based upon urine output when hemodynamic monitoring is not used.[20] An indwelling urethral catheter connected to a closed drainage system should be placed to measure hourly urine production and to guide IV fluid replacement.

Vital signs are used to provide a baseline of information as well as additional data for determining the adequacy of fluid resuscitation. Baseline laboratory studies should include blood glucose, BUN, serum creatinine, serum electrolytes, and hematocrit levels. Arterial blood gas and COHb levels should also be obtained, particularly if an inhalation injury is suspected. A chest x-ray film should be obtained for all clients with extensive burns or inhalation injury. Other laboratory tests in addition to the radiographic study should be performed in all clients with associated trauma, as indicated. Depending on the circumstance of the injury, an alcohol and/or drug screen may be appropriate. Continuous electrocardiographic (ECG) monitoring should be initiated in all clients with major burn injuries, particularly those who have suffered a high-voltage electrical injury or who have a history of cardiac ischemia.

Prevent Aspiration. Many burn centers advocate the placement of a nasogastric tube for management of unresponsive clients and clients with burns of 20% to 25% TBSA or more, to prevent emesis and reduce the risk of aspiration. Gastrointestinal dysfunction results from the intestinal ileus that develops almost universally in clients during the early post–burn injury period.[54] All oral fluids should be restricted at this time.

TABLE 50–3 FLUID RESUSCITATION FORMULAS USED IN BURN CARE

	First 24 Hours			Second 24 Hours		
Formula Name	*Electrolyte-Containing Solution*	*Colloid-Containing Solution*	*Dextrose in Water*	*Electrolyte-Containing Solution*	*Colloid-Containing Solution*	*Dextrose in Water*
Evans	Normal saline 1 ml/kg/% burn	1 ml/kg/% burn	2000 ml	½ of first 24-hr requirement	½ of first 24-hr requirement	2000 ml
Brooke	Lactated Ringer's 1.5 ml/kg/% burn	0.5 ml/kg/% burn	2000 ml	½–¾ of first 24-hr requirement	½–¾ of first 24-hr requirement	2000 ml
Modified Brooke	Lactated Ringer's 2 ml/kg/% burn	None	None	None	0.3–0.5 ml/kg/% burn	Titrate to maintain urine output
Parkland	Lactated Ringer's 4 ml/kg/% burn	None	None	None	0.3–0.5 ml/kg/% burn	Titrate to maintain urine output
Hypertonic saline solution	Fluid containing 250 mEq of sodium/L to maintain hourly urine output of 70 ml in adults	None	None	Same solution to maintain hourly urine output of 30 ml in adults	None	None

Adapted from Rue, L. W., & Cioffi, W. G., Jr. (1991). Resuscitation of thermally injured patients. *Critical Care Nursing Clinics of North America 3*(2), 185; and Wachtel, T. L., & Fortune, J. B. (1983). Fluid resuscitation for burn shock. In T. L. Wachtel et al. (Eds.), *Current topics in burn care* (p. 44). Rockville, MD: Aspen Publishers.

Minimize Pain. Pain management for the patient with a moderate or major burn is achieved through the administration of IV narcotic agents, typically morphine sulfate. In the adult, small doses are given and repeated in 5- to 10-minute intervals until pain appears to be under control. The intramuscular and subcutaneous routes are *not* used during this phase because absorption from the soft tissues is unreliable during the emergent period, when peripheral perfusion is sporadic. The oral route for pain medication administration is not used owing to the likelihood of gastrointestinal dysfunction.

Clients presenting to emergency departments with minor burn injuries often are initially given small doses of IV narcotics (e.g., morphine sulfate). Oral analgesic agents are then prescribed for outpatient use.

Wound Care

Stop the Burning Process. All burn wound care begins at the scene of the injury. Flame and scald burns should be cooled by submerging small burns in cool water until the sensation of burning stops. Major burn victims should have an initial "wet down" at the scene to stop the burning process, but not be submerged in water. Smoldering clothing should be carefully removed, and the client should be covered with a blanket to preserve body heat. Ideally, treatment of chemical burn wounds also begins at the scene of the injury. All clothing should be promptly removed; any chemical powder should be brushed off the skin. Wet chemical burns should be irrigated continuously with copious amounts of water,[13] for at least 20 minutes. Neutralizing agents are not recommended because the neutralizing reaction causes heat, which results in further tissue damage.

For chemical eye injuries, irrigate the eyes with a gentle stream of normal saline, flushing both the injured eye and the conjunctiva. It is recommended to irrigate the eyes from the inner canthus outward, to avoid washing any chemicals down the tear duct or toward the other eye.

Electrical burn care also includes stopping the burning process. It is important to remember to shut off any power source before approaching the victim. Early care is directed at assessment of the entire person, owing to the potential path of the electricity through the body (e.g., dysrhythmias, fractures).

Immediate Care. If transfer to a burn center will be accomplished within 12 hours of injury, wound care should consist of covering the wound with sterile towels and placing clean dry sheets and blankets over the client. Unless transport time to the receiving medical facility is prolonged, debridement and application of topical antimicrobial agents are unnecessary. Definitive wound care begins following inpatient admission to the hospital.[30]

Wound care for burns consists of cleansing, debridement, removal of any damaging agents (e.g., chemicals, tar), and application of an appropriate topical agent and a dressing. Burn wounds should be washed with a mild soap and rinsed thoroughly with warm water.[4] Loose, nonviable tissue should be carefully trimmed away, and any hair should be shaved to within a 1-inch margin around the burn wound.[12]

The removal of tar or asphalt is easily accomplished with the use of a citrus-petroleum product such as Medisol (Orange-Sol, Inc. Chandler, Ariz.) or with mineral oil and a petroleum-based antibiotic ointment such as bacitracin or polymyxin-neomycin-bacitracin (Neosporin).

Clients with minor burns are generally taught wound care and discharged home with instructions to continue wound care twice daily and return to the outpatient clinic or their private physician for follow-up assessment and care.

Prevent Tetanus. Burns, even minor ones, are tetanus-prone wounds. The current protocol for tetanus immunization in clients with minor burns is the same as in clients with any other type of trauma.[54] Clients who have been previously immunized against tetanus, but not within the past 5 years, should receive a tetanus toxoid booster. For clients who have not been immunized, tetanus immune globulin (a passive immunizing agent) and the first of a series of active immunizations with tetanus toxoid should be administered.

Prevent Tissue Ischemia

Circumferential burns of the extremities may compromise circulation in the affected limb.[31] Elevating injured extremities above the level of the heart and active exercise help to reduce dependent edema formation. However, circulatory compromise may still occur. Therefore, frequent assessment of distal extremity perfusion is necessary. Doppler flowmeter assessment of the palmar arch vessels (for the upper extremity) and the posterior tibial artery (for the lower extremity) provides the most precise indication of peripheral perfusion and should be performed regularly during the resuscitation period. The absence of flow or the progressive diminution of the Doppler flowmeter signal intensity is an indication that perfusion is impaired.

An escharotomy is the appropriate treatment for circulatory compromise due to constricting, circumferential burns.[18, 49] A midlateral or midmedial incision of the involved extremity is made from the most proximal to the most distal extent of the full-thickness burn. The depth of the incision is limited to the eschar. It is generally performed at the bedside without local or general anesthesia, because full-thickness burns are insensate. However, viable tissue beneath the escharotomy may bleed if cut, and then the client may feel pain. Bleeding can be controlled with pressure, suture ligation, or electrocautery. Pain control is achieved with IV narcotic administration. After escharotomy, the burn wound can be dressed with topical antimicrobial creams and gauze dressings.

If adequate tissue perfusion does not return following escharotomy, a fasciotomy may be necessary. This procedure, in which the fascia is incised, is performed in the operating room with the client under general anesthesia. A fasciotomy is usually necessary only in injuries caused by high-voltage electricity or those with concomitant crush injury (Fig. 50–10).

Transport to a Burn Facility

Consideration of transfer to a specialized burn care facility is appropriate for all clients with major burn injuries (see Table 50–2). Prompt contact with the receiving burn center is important to facilitate a smooth transfer. All copies of medical records, which should include all fluids and medications given, hourly urine output values, and vital signs, must accompany the client.[20] The client's burn

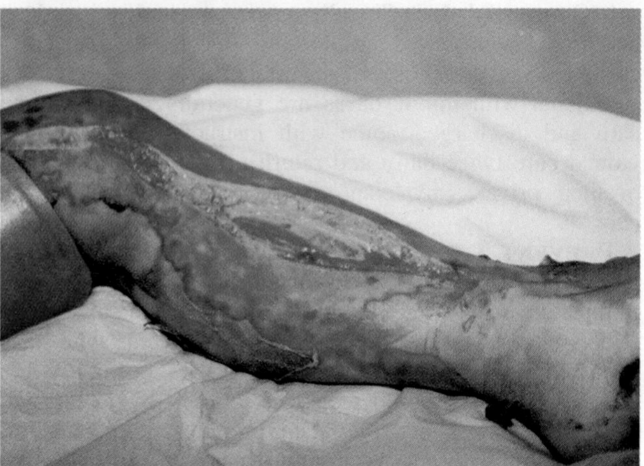

FIGURE 50–10 Escharotomy. Incision is made through the constricting burn eschar to permit expansion of the underlying subcutaneous tissues as edema forms.

wounds should simply be covered with a sterile sheet and blankets. The burn center will perform a complete assessment of the wounds; therefore, it is best if topical care has not been initiated.

Nursing Management of the Medical Client in the Emergent Phase of Burn Care

ASSESSMENT

Because the body's immediate physiologic responses to burn injury can either be life-threatening or lead to significant morbidity, prudent nursing assessment during the emergent phase of burn injury is crucial.

DIAGNOSIS, OUTCOMES, INTERVENTIONS

Impaired Gas Exchange. Effective gas exchange may become impaired when clients have experienced smoke inhalation because of tracheobronchial swelling, the presence of carbonaceous debris in the airway, or CO poisoning.

Outcomes. Adequate gas exchange will be evidenced by a PaO_2 of greater than 90 mm Hg; oxygen saturation (SaO_2) of greater than 95%, arterial partial pressure of carbon dioxide ($PaCO_2$) of 35 to 45 mm Hg; respiratory rate of 16 to 24 breaths/min with a normal pattern and depth; and clear bilateral breath sounds.

Interventions. The client must be frequently assessed for signs of respiratory distress such as restlessness, confusion, labored breathing, tachypnea, dyspnea, diminished or adventitious breath sounds, tachycardia, decrease in PaO_2 and SaO_2, and cyanosis. Monitor SaO_2 continuously in clients with major burns during the emergent phase of burn injury. Draw and monitor arterial blood gas and COHb levels per physician order. Report changes in the client's condition immediately.

Instruct the client on the use of the incentive spirometer to encourage deep breathing every 2 hours. Elevate the head of the bed to facilitate lung expansion and to reduce facial edema.

Ineffective Airway Clearance. Because of the occurrence of airway epidermal sloughing, increase in secretions, inflammation and swelling of the nasopharyngeal mucous membranes from smoke irritation, and depressed ciliary action from inhalation injury, the client becomes at risk for ineffective airway clearance.

Outcomes. Clients will have an effective airway clearance, as evidenced by clear bilateral breath sounds, clear to white pulmonary secretions, effective mobilization of pulmonary secretions, and unlabored respiration with a respiratory rate of 16 to 24 breaths/min.

Interventions. A thorough pulmonary assessment should be performed every 1 to 2 hours during the first 24 hours after injury, and every 2 to 4 hours the second 24 hours after injury, evaluating breath sounds, rate and depth of respirations, and level of consciousness. Be alert to a declining respiratory status as evidenced by crackles, rhonchi, stridor, labored breathing, dyspnea, tachypnea, restlessness, or a decreasing level of consciousness. Report significant findings promptly. Have the client turn, cough, and deep-breathe every 1 to 2 hours for 24 hours and then every 2 to 4 hours. Place an oral suctioning device within the client's reach for independent use. Perform endotracheal or nasotracheal suction as needed. Assess and document the character and amount of secretions.

Fluid Volume Deficit. The client with a major burn injury is at risk for hypovolemia, most significantly during the first 36 hours after burn injury. The fluid volume deficit is directly related to the increased capillary leakage and fluid shift from the intravascular to the interstitial space after the burn insult.

Outcomes. The client will have improved fluid balance, as evidenced by a urine output of 0.5 to 1.0 ml/kg/hr, clear sensorium, pulse rate less than 120 beats per minute (BPM), absence of dysrhythmias, adequate amplitude of peripheral pulses (2+ or better) and blood pressure within the expected range for age and medical history.

Interventions. Assess the client for signs of hypovolemia every hour for 36 hours, including tachycardia, decreased blood pressure, decreased amplitude of peripheral pulses, urine output of less than 0.5 ml/kg/hr, thirst, and dry mucous membranes. Report significant findings.

Carefully monitor and document intake and output, administering fluid therapy as prescribed; titrate the infusion every hour to maintain urine output between 0.5 and 1.0 ml/kg/hr. Large volumes of fluid may be required to produce adequate urine volumes.

Monitor serum electrolyte and hematocrit values. Hyponatremia, hyperkalemia, and elevated hematocrit levels are common findings during the emergent phase. As the circulation is restored, levels should return to normal values.

Altered Tissue Perfusion: Renal. Clients who have suffered deep burn and tissue injury, such as in electrical injury or crush injuries, and those in whom adequate fluid resuscitation has not been achieved are at risk for renal failure. Myoglobin and hemoglobin released from the damaged muscles and red blood cells that precipitate in the renal tubules can create acute tubular necrosis.

Outcomes. The client with evidence of deep tissue injury will maintain a urinary output of 75 to 100 ml/hr, or 1 ml/kg/hr, or higher, until the pigment load has decreased.

Interventions. Monitor and document hourly output and urine color. A dark brown or red color is indicative of the presence of hemochromagens. Send urine samples for myoglobin or hemoglobin assay per physician order to provide quantitative information for documentation of the client's condition. Ensure that the catheter is patent, as the tubing may become plugged with hemochromagens. Administer IV fluids per physician orders. Hemochromagens must be flushed from the body; therefore, the rate of fluid administration is based on maintaining an hourly urine output of 1 ml/kg/hr or greater.

Altered Tissue Perfusion: Peripheral. The client may exhibit altered peripheral tissue perfusion as a result of constricting circumferential burns.

Outcomes. The client will have adequate peripheral perfusion, as evidenced by the presence of pulses on palpation or Doppler flowmeter assessment, capillary refill time for unburned skin of less than 2 seconds, absence of numbness or tingling, and absence of increased pain with active ROM exercises.

Interventions. Remove all constricting jewelry and clothing, because constricting items may compromise circulation as edema formation ensues. Limit the use of the blood pressure cuff on the affected extremity, as the cuff can reduce arterial inflow and venous return. Elevate the burned extremity above the level of the heart to promote venous return and to prevent excessive dependent edema formation.

Monitor arterial pulses by palpation or with the use of an ultrasonic flow detector (Doppler flowmeter) hourly for up to 72 hours after burn injury. Pulses will diminish with circulation impairments. Assess capillary refill of unburned skin on the affected extremity; capillary refill will be prolonged with impaired circulation. Encourage ROM exercises, and assess the level of pain associated with efforts. Increasing pain with movement is a result of tissue ischemia. When pain is not present, increased movement of the affected area will promote venous return and assist in decreasing edema.

If tissue perfusion is threatened, anticipate and prepare the client for an escharotomy. Once the underlying tissue edema has exceeded the expansion ability of the burned skin, an escharotomy will be needed to restore perfusion. After the procedure is complete, recheck for restoration of circulation by assessing pulses, color, movement, and sensation of the affected extremity. Anticipate some bleeding after escharotomy, as the tissue beneath the eschar bleeds. Bleeding can be controlled by electrocautery or suturing by the physician. Continue to observe and assess the extremity after the procedure.

Risk for Infection. The burn-injured client faces an increased risk for infection related to inadequate primary and secondary defenses resulting from traumatized tissue, bacterial proliferation in burn wounds, and an immunocompromised status.

Outcomes. The client will remain free from significant burn wound microbial invasion, as evidenced by quantitative wound cultures containing less than 100,000 colony-forming units (CFUs)/g. In addition, core body temperature will be maintained between 99.6° and 101.0° F (37.5° C to 38.3° C); there will be no swelling, redness, or purulence present at IV line insertion sites; and results of blood, urine, and sputum cultures will be negative.

Interventions. Tetanus prophylaxis should be administered per physician order, as the anaerobic environment beneath eschar is ideal for tetanus organism growth. Intramuscular or IV antibiotic therapy is not used because the area of potential infection is avascular and would not be reached by antibiotics. Antimicrobial agents are used to deter the growth of bacteria on the surface of the wound.

It is essential to maintain infection control techniques at all times during the client's hospitalization to prevent cross-contamination. Ensure aseptic technique when administering care to burned areas and performing invasive techniques. Enforce strict hand-washing, and instruct family members or significant others on infection control measures.

When wound care is performed, it is important to debride the wound of loose, nonviable tissue, which serves as a medium for bacterial growth. Hair within and around a wound should be shaved (with the exception of eyebrows and eyelashes), as hair is contaminated and also prevents adherence of the burn cream. Apply a topical therapeutic agent (an antimicrobial) and loose gauze dressings.

Impaired Physical Mobility. The client's mobility during the emergent phase of burn injury is impaired by tissue edema, pain, and dressings.

Outcomes. The outcomes related to physical mobility are measured throughout the hospitalization and recovery process. The long-term outcome goal is return of the client to maximum independence in performance of activities of daily living (ADL) with minimum disability and disfigurement. Although this outcome will be demonstrated long after the emergent phase, it is important to initiate care on the day of admission and to follow through continually throughout hospitalization.

Interventions. Encourage the client to participate in self-care and ROM exercises at the earliest time possible. The time of the emergency department visit is not too soon to help motivate the client and to overcome fear and dependence related to the injury. Additionally, during early postinjury fluid shifts, increasing movement helps to improve circulation and decrease edema. Consult with occupational and physical therapists for initial assessment and follow-up care throughout the hospitalization.

Ineffective Family Coping: Compromised. Because of the urgent and critical nature of the injury, the client and family are at risk for ineffective coping skills.

Outcomes. Family members and significant others will have accurate information about the immediate status of the client, as evidenced by their ability to verbalize an understanding of the client's injury and treatment goals. Support services will be provided as needed.

Interventions. It is important to prepare family members or significant others for their first visit with the client after injury. Provide a simple explanation of procedures and equipment, communicate the extent of the burn, and describe changes in the client's appearance. For impending client transfer, provide family members or significant others with support services to assist with travel arrangements. Providing support at this time will help to reduce their anxiety during the client's transfer. Families of clients remaining in the facility should be provided with information that meets their basic needs (e.g., information about lodging, location of cafeteria, parking).

ACUTE PHASE

The acute phase of recovery following a major burn begins when the patient is hemodynamically stable, capillary integrity is restored, and diuresis has begun. This is generally 48 to 72 hours after the time of injury. Many of the same principles of care outlined for the emergent phase apply to the acute phase; however, more emphasis is placed on restorative therapies. The acute phase continues until wound closure is achieved.

Medical Management in the Acute Phase of Burn Injury

PREVENT INFECTION

Infection control is a major component of burn management. An infection control policy is necessary for managing burn-injured clients to control the transmission of microorganisms that can lead to infection or colonization.[23, 75] Universal precautions should be followed in caring for all clients with burn injuries; however, specific infection control practices and isolation techniques exist for all burn centers. These practices include the use of gloves, caps, masks, shoe covers, scrub clothes, and plastic aprons. Strict hand-washing is stressed to reduce the incidence of cross-contamination between clients and is the single most important means of preventing the spread of infection. Staff and visitors are generally prevented from client contact if they have any skin, gastrointestinal, or respiratory tract infections. See Box 50–2 for basic infection control strategies. All visitors as well as health-care providers from other departments should be oriented to established infection control practices before their first contact with the burn-injured client.

PROVIDE METABOLIC SUPPORT

Maintenance of adequate nutrition during the acute phase of burn care is essential in promoting wound healing and preventing infection.[36, 78] Basal metabolic rates may be 40% to 100% higher than normal levels, depending on the extent, of the burn. This response is thought to be the result of a resetting of the homeostatic "thermostat" of the hypothalamic-pituitary-adrenal axis, leading to an increase in heat production. Metabolic rates decrease as wound coverage is achieved.

BOX 50–2 Basic Principles of Infection Control

1. Thorough hand-washing should be done before and after each contact with the burn-injured client.
2. Protective garb (aprons or gowns) should be donned before each contact and promptly discarded after leaving the bedside or room.
3. Gloves should be changed when they become contaminated with secretions or fluids from one anatomic site before contact with another site.
4. Equipment, materials, and surfaces are considered contaminated for the individual client and should be properly decontaminated before use with another client.

From Weber, J. M., & Tompkins, D. M. (1993). Improving survival: Infection control and burns. *AACN Clinical Issues in Critical Care Nursing 4*(2), 418–419.

TABLE 50–4 ENERGY CALCULATION FORMULAS USED FOR THE BURN-INJURED ADULT

Formula/Author Name	Formula for Daily Caloric Expenditure Estimate
Curreri	(25 kcal/kg body weight) + (40 kcal × % TBSA burn)
Modified Harris-Benedict	RMR × activity factor × injury factor
U.S. Army Institute of Surgical Research	[Age- and gender-specific BMR × (0.89142 + 0.01335 × % TBSA burn) × m^2 × 24 × activity factor]

TBSA, total body surface area; RMR, resting metabolic rate; BMR, basal metabolic rate.

Aggressive nutritional support is required to meet the increased energy requirements necessary to promote healing and to prevent the untoward effects of catabolism.[22, 62] Several different formulas (Table 50–4) are currently used to estimate energy requirements by factoring different indices: weight, gender, age, extent of burn, and amount of activity. Additional support is generally indicated for the burn-injured client with any of the following: 30% or greater TBSA burn, clinical course requiring multiple operations, need for mechanical ventilatory support, compromised mental status, and poor preinjury nutritional state. Methods for delivering nutritional support include oral intake, enteral tube feedings, peripheral parenteral nutrition, and total parenteral nutrition, which may be used alone or in combination. The preferred feeding route is oral or enteral[44]; however, the decision of how to best meet the client's nutritional needs should be individualized. Typically, parenteral nutrition is reserved for clients with a prolonged ileus or for those in whom enteral feedings fail to meet nutritional needs.[27]

MINIMIZE PAIN

Pain continues to be a significant problem throughout the client's hospitalization. During the acute phase of injury, an attempt is made to find the right combination of medications and interventions to minimize the discomfort and pain associated with the injury. As in the emergent phase, the most common approach to pain control is with the use of pharmacologic agents. However, in addition to the narcotics used during the emergent phase, other modalities may be utilized during the acute phase of burn injury to help alleviate the client's pain. Patient-controlled analgesia devices, inhalation analgesics such as nitrous oxide, oral analgesic "pain cocktails," and narcotic agonist-antagonist agents may be beneficial during the acute phase of burn injury.[32, 42] Nonsteroidal anti-inflammatory agents (NSAIDs) are also prescribed for the treatment of mild to moderate pain. When NSAIDs are used, extra precautions must be taken to prevent gastric ulceration.

Nonpharmacologic modalities used to treat burn-related

pain include hypnosis, guided imagery, art and play therapy, relaxation techniques, distraction, biofeedback, and music therapy. These modalities have been found to be effective in decreasing anxiety, thereby decreasing the perception of pain. They are often used as adjunctive therapies to the pharmacologic treatment of burn pain.[43]

PROVIDE WOUND CARE

Care of the burn wound is ultimately aimed at promoting wound healing. Daily wound care involves cleansing, debridement of eschar (devitalized tissue), and dressing of the wound.[12]

WOUND CLEANSING. The practice of hydrotherapy remains a mainstay of burn treatment plans for cleansing the wounds.[66] This is accomplished by immersion, showering, or spraying (Fig. 50–11). A hydrotherapy session of 30 minutes or less is optimal for clients with acute burns. Longer time periods may increase sodium loss (water is hypotonic) through the burn wound and may promote heat loss, pain, and stress. During hydrotherapy, the wounds are gently washed using any one of a variety of solutions. Care should be taken to minimize bleeding and to maintain body temperature during this procedure. To prevent cross contamination between clients, single-use plastic hydrotherapy tub liners are available. Clients excluded from hydrotherapy are generally those who are hemodynamically unstable and those with new skin grafts. If hydrotherapy is not used, wounds are washed and rinsed while the client is in bed, before the application of antimicrobial agents.

DEBRIDEMENT. Burn wound debridement involves the removal of the eschar. This serves to promote wound healing by preventing bacterial proliferation in and under the eschar.[75] Debridement of the burn wound is accomplished through mechanical, enzymatic, or surgical means.

Mechanical debridement can be accomplished with careful use of scissors and forceps to lift and trim away loose eschar. Hydrotherapy softens and loosens eschar so that it is more easily removed. Wet-to-dry dressing changes are another effective means of mechanical debridement. Coarse gauze dressings are saturated with a prescribed solution, wrung out until the dressing is slightly moist, and applied to the wound. The dressing is left in place to dry. Typically 6 to 8 hours later the gauze is carefully removed from the wound, mechanically lifting drainage, exudate, and loose necrotic tissue that has dried on to the gauze. Mechanical debridement of the burn wound can be extremely painful; therefore, effective pain management is paramount.

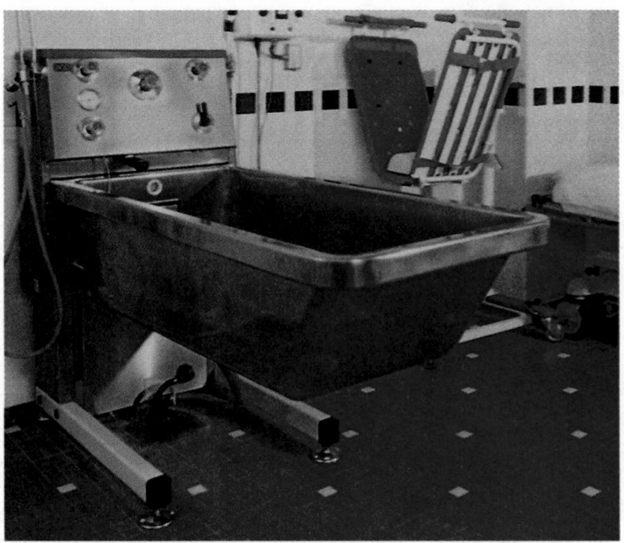

FIGURE 50–11 A low-boy whirlpool tank is used for immersion hydrotherapy treatment of burn wounds. (Courtesy of Shriners Hospitals for Children of Northern California.)

Enzymatic debridement involves the application of commercially prepared proteolytic and fibrinolytic topical enzymes to the burn wound, which facilitates eschar removal. These agents require a moist environment to be effective and are applied directly to the burn wound. Enzymatic debridement is not widely practiced, as several serious side effects are associated with use of these agents.[47] As the enzyme digests necrotic tissue, it also opens up thrombosed blood vessels. This causes some oozing of blood from the blood vessels and creates a site for bacteria to enter the bloodstream. Bacteremia, pain, and bleeding can occur; therefore, if enzymatic debridement is used, the client should be assessed for complications continuously throughout the course of treatment. The use of enzymatic debridement agents is contraindicated for wounds communicating with major body cavities, and for wounds with exposed nerves or nervous tissue.

Surgical debridement of the burn wound involves excision of the eschar and coverage of the wound. Early surgical excision begins during the first week after injury, once the client is hemodynamically stable. Advantages of early excision include early mobilization, reduction of pain (which is otherwise experienced with repeated dressing changes), early wound closure (which reduces the potential for wound infection), and reduced length of hospitalization.[33, 76] A disadvantage of early excision is the risk of excising viable tissue that may heal with time.

Two techniques of surgical debridement are currently used.[50] In *tangential* excision, very thin layers of eschar are sequentially shaved until viable tissue is reached. *Fascial* excision involves removing the burn tissue and underlying fat down to fascia. This technique is frequently used for debridement of very deep burns.

TOPICAL ANTIMICROBIAL TREATMENT. Deep partial-thickness or full-thickness burn wounds are treated initially with topical antimicrobial agents.[73] These agents are applied once or twice daily following cleansing, debridement, and inspection of the wound. The nurse assesses for eschar separation, the presence of granulation tissue or reepithelialization, and signs of infection. The most commonly used topical antimicrobial agents are listed in Table 50–5. Although no single agent is used universally, many burn centers choose silver sulfadiazine cream as the initial topical agent.[31]

Burn wounds are treated using either an open or a closed dressing technique. For the *open method,* the antimicrobial cream is applied with a gloved hand (Fig. 50–12) and the wound is left open to the air without gauze dressings. The cream is reapplied as needed, although formal reapplication is necessary every 12 hours in keeping with the duration of activity of the agent. The

TABLE 50–5 TOPICAL ANTIMICROBIAL AGENTS USED IN BURN CARE

Agent	Antimicrobial Spectrum	Application	Side Effects	Nursing Considerations
WATER-BASED CREAMS				
1% silver sulfadiazine	Broad spectrum; effective against some fungi and yeast	2× daily, 1/16-inch thickness Gauze dressing not required	Transient leukopenia typically appearing after 2 or 3 days of treatment Macular rash	Do not store in warm environment (e.g., warm client room)
Mafenide acetate	Broad spectrum; little antifungal activity	2× daily, 1/16-inch thickness Gauze dressing not required	Hyperchloremic metabolic acidosis from bicarbonate diuresis due to the inhibition of carbonic anhydrase Pain/burning sensation on application to superficial burns Maculopapular rash	Assess for side effects Assess adequacy of pain management; if pain and discomfort continue, consider other topical treatments Use cautiously in clients with acute renal failure
SOLUTIONS				
5% mafenide acetate	Broad spectrum	Gauze dressing required, moistened with solution for application to the wound	Pain on application Pruritus Rash Fungal colonization	Assess for side effects Assess adequacy of pain management
0.5% silver nitrate	Broad spectrum; effective against *Candida* species	Multiple layers of gauze dressing required, moistened with solution for application to the wound	Hyponatremia Hypochloremia Hypokalemia Hypocalcemia	Check serum electrolytes daily Penetrates eschar poorly Remoisten dressings every 2 hours to avoid wound desiccation Protect the environment; stains everything a blackish-brown color
PETROLEUM-BASED OINTMENTS				
Polymyxin B	Gram-negative organisms	Apply as needed in a thin layer; gauze dressing not used unless clothing protection is needed	Hypersensitivity (rash)	Assess for side effects
Neomycin sulfate	Predominantly gram-negative organisms		Overgrowth of nonsusceptible organisms including fungi	
Bacitracin	Predominantly gram-positive organisms			

advantages of the open method include increased visualization of the wound, greater freedom for mobility and joint motion, and simplicity in wound care. The disadvantages include an increased chance of hypothermia from exposure.

In the *closed method* of wound care, gauze dressing is impregnated with antimicrobial cream and applied to the wound. To prevent circulatory compromise in extremity burns, the gauze should be wrapped from the most distal portion of the extremity in a proximal direction. The advantages of the closed method are decreases in evaporative fluid and heat loss from the wound surface. In addition, gauze dressings may aid in debridement. The disadvantages of gauze dressings are mobility limitations and a potential decrease in effectiveness of ROM exercises. Wound assessment is also limited to the times at which dressing changes are performed.

Temporary wound coverings (skin substitutes) are frequently used as a kind of wound "dressing." Table 50–6 outlines the most common biologic, biosynthetic, and synthetic wound coverings available. These products are temporary wound coverings, and each has specific indications.[25, 63, 67] The character of the wound (depth of injury, amount of exudate, location of the wound on the body, and phase of recovery) and treatment goals are considered in choosing the most appropriate wound covering.

MAXIMIZE FUNCTION. Maintenance of optimal physical functioning in the client with a burn injury is a challenge for the entire team. Nurses work closely with occupational and physical therapists to identify the reha-

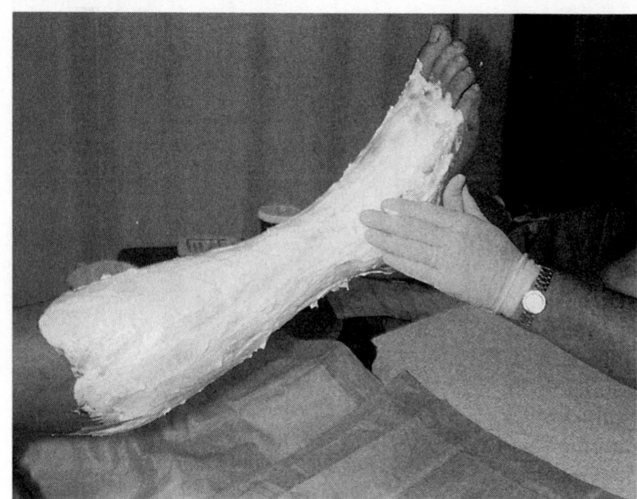

FIGURE 50–12 Silver sulfadiazine, a common antimicrobial cream used in burn care, is applied to the burn wound using a sterile, gloved hand. (Courtesy of the University of Washington Burn Center, Harborview Medical Center, Seattle.)

bilitative needs of the burn-injured client. An individualized program of splinting, positioning, exercise, ambulation, performance of ADL, and pressure therapy should be implemented in the acute phase of recovery to maximize functional recovery and cosmetic outcome. Therapeutic goals at this stage in recovery are to prevent early contracture formation and to maintain soft tissue length.

Wound contracture and hypertrophic scarring are two major problems for the burn-injured client.[72] Wound contractures are typically more severe with extensive burns. Areas seemingly predisposed to contracture are the hands, head and neck, and axilla.[71] Measures used to prevent and treat wound contractures include therapeutic positioning, ROM exercises, splinting, and client/family education.

Table 50–7 lists corrective and therapeutic techniques for positioning clients with specific areas of burn injury during periods of inactivity or immobilization. Allowing the burn-injured client to assume a position of comfort most often contributes to contracture formation. Therefore, proper positioning, both in and out of bed, should be maintained for the burn-injured client. These techniques place affected body parts in positions that are in opposition to positions of potential contracture or deformity. The natural tendency with healing and immobility is for muscles and joints to contract into a shortened, flexed position. Thus, for example, to reduce the risk of neck contractures, the use of pillows—which place the neck in flexion—is not allowed.

Active ROM exercises are prescribed early in the acute phase of recovery to promote resolution of edema and to maintain strength and joint function. In addition, ADL can be effective in maintaining function and ROM. Ambulation also maintains strength and ROM of the lower extremities and should begin as soon as the client is physiologically stable. Passive ROM and stretching exercises should be included as part of the daily treatment plan if the client is unable to perform active ROM exercises.

Splints are used to maintain proper joint position and to prevent or correct contractures.[28] Two types of splints are frequently used. A *static splint* immobilizes the joint. Static splints do not replace exercise and are frequently applied for periods of immobilization or during sleeping hours or are used for clients who cannot maintain proper positioning. In contrast, *dynamic splints* exercise the affected joint. Care must be taken to ensure that all splints fit properly and do not apply excessive pressure, which may lead to further tissue or nerve damage.[73]

PROVIDE PSYCHOLOGICAL SUPPORT

The longest period of adjustment occurs during the acute phase. The burn-injured adult may demonstrate a variety of emotional and psychological responses. Anxiety and fearfulness related to potential disfigurement and perceived changes in role and identity plague the client during this time period. Depression, withdrawal, and regression may result.[7]

The client may begin discussing the burn injury or accident, recounting significant events and searching for the meaning of what has happened.[1] Allowing the expression of these worries and validating that they are "normal" are essential in providing support. Staff members need to actively listen and to allow the client to talk about the accident. Detailed and repetitious recounting of the injury is useful in desensitizing clients to the horror of what has happened and in decreasing nightmares.[7]

Clients who have little information about specific treatment procedures, potential associated discomfort or pain, and available resources or options for pain management typically react with anxiety and a heightened pain response. Providing the client with information about what will occur during a particular procedure or what is expected over the course of recovery is a concept known as providing preparatory information. This technique is a psychologically based method that has proved successful in reducing pain and anxiety during certain procedures.[1, 7] To enhance the client's sense of personal control, teaching should include education about various coping mechanisms and the use of nonpharmacologic methods for pain control.

Involving clients in their own care helps them to feel some control over the situation at hand. Clients can be encouraged to participate in wound care (e.g., bathing, simple debridement, dressing application) and physical therapy (e.g., active versus passive ROM exercises, application of splints and pressure garments). These interventions have been found to be effective in supporting the client's psychological needs.[43]

Nursing Management of the Medical Patient in the Acute Phase of Burn Injury

Impaired Gas Exchange. Note that the consequences of smoke inhalation may not be fully appreciated until the acute phase of burn care. The decreased ciliary action in the airways leads to a high risk for infection (which usually is not manifested until day 3 or 4 after the burn injury); that is demonstrated first by tracheobronchitis and followed by bronchopneumonia.

Outcomes. The client will have improved gas exchange, as evidenced by unlabored respirations, a respiratory rate of 16 to 24 breaths/min, PaO_2 of greater than 90

TABLE 50–6 TEMPORARY WOUND COVERINGS USED IN BURN CARE

Category/Examples	Description	Indications	Nursing Considerations
Biologic			
Amnion	Amniotic membranes collected from human placentas	To protect partial-thickness burns To protect granulation tissue prior to autograft application	Cover dressing is changed every 48 hours with amnion
Allograft homograft	Donated human cadaver skin harvested within 24 hours after death	To debride exudative wounds To cover excised wounds and test for receptivity prior to autograft application To cover and protect meshed autografts	Observe for wound exudate and signs of infection that may be indicative of a wound infection beneath the allograft/xenograft
Xenograft heterograft	Porcine skin is harvested after slaughter, then cryopreserved or lyophilized for storage	To promote healing of clean, superficial partial-thickness wounds	Xenograft over granulation tissue is changed every 2–5 days For superficial wounds, ensure that the wound is clean and well rinsed; apply xenograft with slight overlapping of edges to allow for shrinkage; trim away xenograft when skin beneath it has healed
Biosynthetic			
Biobrane (Bertek Pharmaceuticals, Morgantown, WV)	Nylon fabric bonded to a silicone rubber membrane containing collagenous porcine peptides	Donor site dressing Protective cover over meshed autografts To promote healing of clean superficial partial-thickness wounds	Secure to the surrounding intact skin by staples, skin closure strips, tape, or sutures and then wrap with a gauze dressing; this outer dressing can be removed by 48 hours to check for adherence of the Biobrane; once adherence has occurred, the tape, sutures, and staples can be removed; the Biobrane can then be left exposed to the air New and healing donor sites of the legs require support during ambulation; the figure eight elastic (Ace) bandage wrapping technique is recommended to minimize trauma to newly formed capillaries Assess for infection beneath the fabric and at wound periphery
Integra (Integra Life Sciences, Plainsboro, NJ)	Bilaminate substitute composed of collagen (dermal analog) and a Silastic covering (epidermal analog) The dermal analog is allowed to incorporate into the wound, becoming permanent	For application to excised wounds	The Silastic portion is removed after 2–3 days, providing a wound bed for placement of a very thin split-thickness skin graft Assess for infection Protect the site from mechanical shearing forces
Calcium alginates (Curasorb, Kendall Co, Mansfield, MA; Kalginate, DeRoyal Textiles, Camden, SC)	Dressing material derived from brown seaweeds (alginate) and calcium/sodium salts	Donor site dressing To promote healing of superficial partial-thickness wounds (contraindicated in full-thickness wounds)	To apply, irrigate wound with a physiologic solution, apply calcium alginate dressing to the wound, cover with an absorptive dressing The entire dressing should be changed when the outer dressing is saturated with drainage
Transparent films (Bioclusive, Johnson & Johnson, Arlington, TX; Op-Site, Smith & Nephew, Memphis, TN)	Hypoallergenic film dressing that is occlusive, waterproof, and permeable to moisture vapor	Donor site dressing To promote healing of clean, small, superficial partial-thickness wounds	Use a margin of intact skin around the entire wound or donor site to adequately secure the dressing Assess for pooling exudate; if significant exudate forms that threatens the integrity of the closed dressing, drain the exudate aseptically with a small gauge needle and syringe; seal hole with a film patch
Non-adhering gauze (Aquaphor gauze, Beiersdorf Inc. Norwalk, CT; Xeroform gauze, Sherwood Medical, St. Louis)	Fine-mesh gauze impregnated with ointment	Donor site dressing To cover meshed autografts To cover fragile, newly healed epithelium	Dressing material over donor site should remain intact until healed beneath (10–14 days) New and healing donor sites of the legs require support during ambulation; the figure eight (Ace) wrapping technique is recommended to minimize trauma to newly formed capillaries

TABLE 50–7 THERAPEUTIC POSITIONING FOR THE BURN-INJURED CLIENT

Burned Area	Therapeutic Position	Positioning Techniques
Neck		
Anterior	Extension	No pillow Small towel roll beneath shoulders to promote neck extension
Circumferential	Neutral toward extension	No pillow
Posterior or asymmetrical	Neutral	No pillow
Shoulder/axilla	Arm abduction to 90–110 degrees	Splinting Arms positioned away from the body and supported on arm troughs
Elbow	Arm extension	Elbow splint Elbows positioned in extension with slight bend at the elbow (no more than 10 degrees of elbow flexion) Arms supported on arm troughs with the forearm in slight pronation
Hand		
Wrist	Wrist extension	Hand splint
MCP	MCP flexion at 90 degrees	Hand splint
PIP/DIP	PIP/DIP extension	Hand splint
Thumb	Thumb abduction	Hand splint with thumb abduction
Finger web spaces	Finger abduction	Web spacers of foam, silicone products, or custom-fitted pressure garments to decrease webbing formation
Hip	Hip extension	Supine with the head of bed flat and legs extended Trochanter roll to maintain neutral hip rotation (toes should be pointing toward the ceiling) Prone positioning
Knee	Knee extension	Supine with knees extended (toes should be pointing toward the ceiling) Prone positioning with feet extended over the end of the mattress Sitting in chair with legs extended and elevated Knee splint
Ankle	Neutral	Padded footboard Ankle positioning devices (avoid heel cord tightening)—provide heel protection to prevent pressure sore development

MCP, metacarpal interphalangeal joint(s); PIP/DIP, proximal/distal interphalangeal joint(s).

mm Hg, $PaCO_2$ of 35 to 45 mm Hg, SaO_2 greater than 95%, and clear bilateral breath sounds.

Interventions. Interventions continue unchanged from the emergent phase of injury. Comprehensive respiratory assessment and preventive pulmonary toilet should be performed every 2 hours.

Ineffective Airway Clearance. Upper airway and facial edema caused by heat-induced tissue and mucosal damage begins to resolve between 2 and 4 days after injury with superficial burns. Full-thickness injuries, however, resolve more slowly, making ineffective airway clearance a problem that may last well into the acute phase of treatment.

Outcomes. The client will have effective airway clearance, as evidenced by clear bilateral breath sounds, clear to white pulmonary secretions, effective mobilization of pulmonary secretions, and unlabored breathing.

Interventions. Continue interventions begun in the emergent phase of treatment. Pulmonary toilet including turning/coughing/deep breathing, use of an incentive spirometer every 2 to 4 hours while the client is awake, and endotracheal suctioning as needed will facilitate clearance of secretions and sputum. Leave an oral suctioning device within the client's reach for independent use.

Hypothermia. Clients remain at risk for loss of body heat through burn injuries until wound closure is complete. During dressing changes, clients are especially at risk for becoming hypothermic.

Outcomes. The client will maintain a core body temperature between 99.6° and 101.0° F (37.5° and 38.3° C).

Interventions. To help prevent the loss of heat from open wounds that occurs as a result of evaporation, limit hydrotherapy treatment sessions to 30 minutes or less with water temperatures of 98° to 102° F (36.6° C to 38.8° C). Cover the client with sterile sheets after the hydrotherapy session, exposing only limited areas of body surface during topical agent–dressing application. Provide heat lamps or heat shields and increase the ambient temperature in the treatment room and/or in the client's room if the client exhibits subnormal temperatures.

Risk for Infection. During the acute phase of injury, infection remains an ongoing risk owing to inadequate primary and secondary defenses secondary to traumatized tissue, bacterial proliferation in the burn wound, presence of invasive lines or urinary catheters, and an immunocompromised status.[24]

Outcomes. The client will have no significant burn wound microbial invasion, as evidenced by quantitative wound cultures containing less than 100,000 CFUs/g. In addition, the client will maintain core body temperature at 99.6° to 101° F; will demonstrate evidence of no swelling, redness, or purulence at invasive line insertion sites; and will have negative results on blood, urine, and sputum cultures.

Interventions. Continue to follow infection control policy for burn-injured clients in an effort to prevent cross-contamination. Assess for clinical signs of infection in the burn wound: discoloration of wounds (e.g., brown, black, or hemorrhagic); drainage; odor; delayed healing; or spongy eschar. As in the emergent phase, provide meticulous wound care in an aseptic fashion, cleaning and rinsing the wound, and debriding loose nonviable tissue to discourage bacterial growth. Apply a topical antimicrobial agent to the wound to decrease the risk for local wound infection. Continue to shave or cut body hair around wound margins until wound closure.

Observe for clinical indicators of sepsis: headache, chills, anorexia, nausea, changes in vital signs, hyperglycemia and glycosuria, paralytic ileus, and confusion, restlessness, or hallucinations. Assess for signs of infection at the catheter insertion site. Obtain cultures per physician order, and administer antibiotics and antipyretics as prescribed.

Impaired Tissue Integrity. Remember that stress ulcers can occur at any time after a burn injury. The assessment and preventive treatment started in the emergent phase of injury should continue until wound coverage is completed.[40]

Outcomes. The client will exhibit no signs of gastrointestinal bleeding and will maintain gastric pH above 5.

Interventions. Monitor and document gastric pH values and heme content every 2 hours while the client's nasogastric tube is in place. Administer antacids and/or H_2 blockers per physician order to reduce the gastric acid content, as high acid levels may lead to bleeding. Monitor stools for occult blood.

Altered Nutrition: Less Than Body Requirements. The burn-injured client must maintain adequate protein and caloric intake to meet metabolic demands for wound healing.

Outcomes. The client will have adequate nutrition, as evidenced by maintenance of 85% to 90% of preburn weight and healing of burn wounds, donor sites, and skin grafts.

Interventions. Caloric needs are based upon preburn weight. Obtain a daily weight to assess whether caloric needs are being met and to provide documentation for staff to follow trends. Assess eating habits and patterns, and identify food preferences and food allergies. Order meals high in calories and proteins. Encourage family members or significant others to bring favorite foods from home. Provide nutritious supplements between meals.

Document daily caloric intake, and consult with the dietitian to perform a nutritional assessment. Consider other methods to meet caloric needs such as tube feeding or total parenteral feeding, as oral feeding may not provide adequate calories for healing.

Performing oral hygiene during each nursing shift and as needed helps to prevent stomatitis and enhance appetite. Provide an a esthetically pleasing environment, which is conducive to eating. Schedule treatments to provide for uninterrupted meal times. Allow a period of rest before meal times if the client has endured a painful procedure or treatment, because pain will decrease appetite.

Pain. The client can be expected to experience a significant amount of pain during the acute burn phase. The pain experienced during this phase of recovery is directly associated with the burn wound and donor sites, wound care procedures, and ROM exercises.

Outcomes. The client will verbalize a level of acceptable pain control.

Interventions. Continue to frequently assess for pain, and administer appropriate narcotic and anxiolytics. Time the administration of medications so that the client receives the benefit of the drug's peak performance during painful procedures, and evaluate the effectiveness of interventions as initiated during the emergent burn phase.

During the acute phase, nonpharmacologic interventions should be initiated to enhance medication effects and to assist in controlling pain. Explore the benefits of relaxation techniques, guided imagery, music therapy, distraction, and biofeedback.

Impaired Physical Mobility. Impaired physical mobility during the acute phase of burn treatment is related to pain, the presence of dressings and splints, surgical procedures, and wound contractures.

Outcomes. The client will maintain soft tissue length, as evidenced by maintaining ROM without signs of early contracture formation.

Interventions. The main interventions during the acute phase of injury are splinting, positioning, and ROM exercises. Collaboration with physical and occupational therapists is essential for guidance in an individualized program for each client.

Optimal positioning of the client involves continuing use of anticontracture positions. Maintaining burned areas in a position of physiologic function by either splinting or positioning will help to prevent or reduce contracture development.

Encourage the client to participate in ADL, to ambulate, and to spend time sitting up in a chair. These activities will not only improve mobility but also assist in moving the client toward independence.

Self-Esteem Disturbance. During the acute burn phase, the client recognizes the extent of injury and realizes that his or her body is changed forever. Depression, grief, fear, and anxiety confront the client.

Outcomes. The client will acknowledge body changes and demonstrate movement toward incorporating these changes into the self-concept. The client will not exhibit maladaptive responses such as severe depression.

Interventions. The client should be expected to experience emotional lability in progress through recovery. Staff members should provide an accepting atmosphere for the client, although the client should be assisted to exercise control over any destructive behaviors. Family members or significant others should be involved in care as much as possible to demonstrate continued support for the client. Staff members should be available to provide information about the appearance of burns and grafts and to explain changes that can be expected over time (up to 1 year). Providing information helps to reduce misconceptions and can give hope that the painful procedures can produce good results.

Ineffective Family Coping Skills. Recognize that families often imagine that the survival of the family unit is threatened following a member's injury. Normal coping mechanisms become overwhelmed.

Outcomes. Family members will demonstrate coping strategies, as evidenced by verbalizing realistic expectations for client outcomes, expressing knowledge of the goals of treatment regimen, interacting appropriately with the client, and demonstrating decreased emotional stress.

Interventions. Once beyond the emergent phase, it will be important to provide the family members or significant others with information about what to expect for the burn-injured client in the future. It is helpful to provide families with daily updates regarding changes in the client's condition. This assists in maintaining realistic perceptions of the client's progress. Assist the family in finding ways to nurture the client and to participate in some aspects of care. These measures not only assure the client of the family's love and acceptance but also allow family members or significant others to regain some feelings of control. It may also be useful to introduce the family members to the local burn support group. Burn survivors and their families can provide emotional support and validation and also can reinforce the concept that it is possible to survive burns and live acceptable happy lives.

Surgical Management in the Acute Phase of Burn Injury

Definitive wound care for full-thickness burns is accomplished by *autografting,* the surgical removal of a superficial layer of the client's own unburned skin, which is subsequently grafted to the excised or clean and granulating burn wound. Because the epidermis is split (in layers) rather than taken in full, these grafts are referred to as *split-thickness grafts.* This procedure is performed in the operating room while the client is under general anesthesia. Autografts can be applied either as a *sheet* (*sheet graft*) or in a meshed form (*meshed graft*).

A sheet autograft is applied to the excised wound bed without alteration in its integrity. Sheet autografts are frequently used to graft burns in visible areas.

In contrast, a meshed autograft contains many little slits that allow for expansion of the donor skin. Meshing permits coverage of larger areas of irregularly shaped wounds and allows for drainage from a bleeding wound bed. When healed, the meshed pattern of the autograft remains visible. Therefore, meshed grafts are used on hidden body areas. When a thicker layer of skin is removed, consisting of the epidermis and the dermis, this is referred to as a *full-thickness graft.* For all autografts, the area of the body from which the skin was removed is referred to as the donor site (Fig. 50–13).

Graft adherence is dependent on the formation of a fibrin bond between the recipient bed and the graft.[50] There are no vascular connections between the graft and the wound bed immediately after surgery. The graft is held in place only by weak fibrin bonds and is nourished by the diffusion of serum from the wound bed. The graft begins to stabilize after 3 days as a fibrovascular and collagen network form and provide durability to the graft. A bleeding wound bed, hematoma formation, or shearing of the graft will disrupt formation of this bond between graft and bed. Care must be taken during the postoperative period to assess for bleeding, remove accumulated serum beneath sheet grafts (as described next in the discussion on nursing management of the surgical client), and prevent unwanted movement and shearing of autografts.[49]

Various types of dressings are used to cover donor sites, depending on the size, location, and condition of adjacent skin or tissue.[35] However, despite the differences in dressings, the donor site wound requires the same meticulous care as for other partial-thickness wounds, to expedite healing and prevent infection. If the donor site becomes infected, the dressing should be gently removed or soaked off. The wound can then be thoroughly cleansed and an antimicrobial agent applied. Once the donor site has healed, lubricating lotions can be applied to soften the area and reduce itching. Donor sites can be reused after they are healed.

Cultured *epithelial autografting* is a technique for closure of massive burn wounds.[49, 51] The process of autolo-

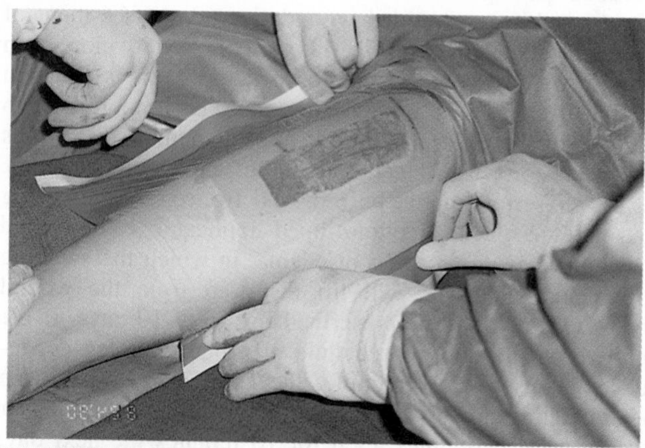

FIGURE 50–13 Harvesting donor skin from the lateral portion of the client's thigh.

gous epithelial cell growth begins with taking a full-thickness skin specimen from an uninjured body site. This specimen is sent to a specialized laboratory for culture and growth. Typically, in 3 to 4 weeks, several sheets of cultured epithelial autografts are ready for application. In the operating room, the cultured epithelial autograft sheets are carefully applied to an excised and non-bleeding wound bed and are secured in place with staples. Dressings are applied and moistened with an antibiotic solution shown to be nontoxic to the cultured epithelial autografts.

Reports demonstrating the success of cultured epithelial autografts in the treatment of massive burn wounds have been limited. Both early and late cultured epithelial autograft loss due to mechanical shearing, nutritional imbalance, infection, or an autoimmune response have been reported.[69]

Nursing Management of the Surgical Client in the Acute Phase of Burn Injury

PREOPERATIVE CARE

Routine care of clients undergoing surgery is discussed in Chapter 15. Specific preoperative care of the client scheduled for debridement includes providing information about areas to be debrided and plans for pain control. Debridement cases are usually considered contaminated in the operating room and are often done at the end of the surgical list; therefore, clients may wait for many hours before undergoing the scheduled procedure. Specific orders for medications to be given or withheld, and the time to begin *nil per os* (NPO) (i.e., nothing by month) status should be obtained.

Before skin grafting, clients need information on the type of skin graft to be used, the location of the donor site, the postoperative plans for pain control, and the need for immobility and elevation of the graft site. Fears over scarring should be addressed; in general, scarring cannot be predicted because scar tissue requires a full year to mature. Both debridement and grafting can be multiple procedures, and clients may become anxious over repeated surgical procedures. Severe anxiety should be communicated to the surgeon and anesthesia personnel.

POSTOPERATIVE CARE

Routine postoperative care is discussed in Chapter 15. Care specific to debrided wounds includes assessment of bleeding and pain control. Many clients report more pain in donor sites (owing to exposed nerve endings) than in recipient sites. Skin-grafted sites must be immobilized to promote adherence of the graft to the wound bed. Various techniques are used, including suture, tape, and dressings. Blebs of serum should be removed from graft sites using a small needle and cotton-tipped applicator. Skin-grafted sites are elevated to prevent edema, in which the swelling of edematous tissue will lift the graft from the wound bed. Bed rest may be prescribed for up to 10 days. If the graft is on the legs, a schedule of progressive leg dependency is used. For example, the client can position the legs hanging down ("dangling") while sitting in a chair or walking for 5 minutes, then for 10 minutes the next day, and so on. The graft site is inspected for rubor and edema after each episode.

REHABILITATION PHASE

The rehabilitation phase of recovery represents the final phase of burn care and encompasses the time from wound closure to discharge and beyond. In order for the best outcomes to be achieved, caregivers must understand the consequences of burn injury, and treatment for rehabilitation must begin from the day of injury. Rehabilitation should overlap the acute care phase and last well beyond the acute inpatient hospitalization. Ultimately, a burn rehabilitation program is designed for maximal functional and emotional recovery. Measures to promote wound healing, to prevent or minimize deformities and hypertrophic scarring, to increase physical strength and function, to promote emotional support, and to provide education are a part of the ongoing rehabilitation phase.

See the Bridge to Home Health Care: Managing After Burns.

Medical Management in the Rehabilitation Phase of Burn Injury

MINIMIZE FUNCTIONAL LOSS

Early wound excision helps to minimize short-term and long-term functional loss by removing the nonpliable eschar and eliminating wound pain.[49] A skin graft, although more elastic than eschar, still does not have normal elasticity, and wound stiffness will still be present, which must be counterbalanced with aggressive therapy and splinting.

Exercise, splinting, and positioning continue through all phases of burn injury; however, it is during this phase that the importance of these efforts becomes paramount. These measures are crucial to the client's progression to optimal functional independence.[73]

Hypertrophic scarring, which results from an overabundant deposition of collagen in the healed burn wound, can be minimized with the use of massage and pressure therapy.[56] Constant pressure applied to healing burn wounds has been found to reduce the scarring process. Several commercially available products provide the constant, even pressure required. Although hypertrophic scarring usually does not peak until several months after the injury, it is important to plan ahead before the onset of loss of function. By the rehabilitation phase of injury, the client should be measured for custom-fitted anti–burn scar support garments for any area that did not heal within 3 weeks of injury[56] (Fig. 50–14).

PROVIDE PSYCHOSOCIAL SUPPORT

In this, the last phase of burn injury, during which the wounds are almost healed and specific plans are made for hospital discharge, the client must face numerous issues and overcome many concerns.[55] Self-image issues, pain, physical limitations, and fear of rejection represent only a few of the issues the client must deal with as discharge nears.[7] During this time, it is important to maintain good communication with the client. It is beneficial to the client for the staff to encourage independence and carry the message that survivors can find ways to achieve whatever goals they set for themselves. Pain control and anxiety prevention continue to require assessment and medical management as needed.[41] Psychosocial assistance for the client and family members or significant others should carry through from admission to discharge.

BRIDGE TO HOME HEALTH CARE

Managing After Burns

When admitting the burn-injured client to home health services, remember that each case is unique and involves detailed treatment instructions. Include the client's and family members' responses to the client's discharge from the hospital and to the client's being home in the nursing assessment. If clients require assistance with activities of daily living (ADL), they will need a primary caregiver to provide both emotional support and direct care. This person is a critical member of the health care delivery team.

Work with the client and the primary caregiver to set up a place in the home for dressing changes and storage of needed dressing materials that limits the possibility of contamination. This area should be comfortable and relaxing and off-limits to family pets. If possible, select a room that clients do not use for other activities, especially sleeping, so that they do not associate these activities with pain from dressing changes. The dressing materials and an up-to-date wound care plan can be neatly organized and stored in a sealed plastic box or plastic bag. Supplies should be ordered on a weekly basis in quantities that can be used for one dressing change. In some agencies, prepackaged wound care kits provide an excellent method of infection control and reduce the amount of waste significantly.

Although dressing changes and physical therapy can be painful experiences for the client, both are essential for recovery. Identify ways to decrease the pain or the length of time for which pain will occur. Work with the physical therapist, the client, and the family to determine the best schedule for these activities. Consider scheduling joint visits if this would improve the care given to the client. Instruct a family member to give prescribed pain medications 1 hour before the scheduled dressing change to provide the best relief for the client. While changing dressings, use soft music or relaxation techniques, and involve the client and family as much as possible. These strategies offer a sense of control and can decrease the client's perception of pain.

Unless mechanical debridement of the wound is necessary, the dressings should not stick to the wound bed. Avoid removing dried-on dressings because they cause unnecessary pain. If the dressings are sticking, soak them off with normal saline, or after obtaining the physician's approval, remove them in the shower. Collaborate with the primary physician or a wound care nurse to obtain an appropriate moisture-retentive dressing, to reduce or eliminate pain with dressing changes.

Rehabilitation of people who have suffered burn injury involves more than dressing changes and physical therapy. It is also important to consider the psychological stress of the initial injury, scarring, and surgical procedures and other treatments as well as the financial burden from loss of work time and the lengthy recovery period. Evaluate the need of the client and family members for referrals to local agencies that offer social, counseling, financial, and spiritual services as well as support groups. Such services may be essential in order for clients and their families to cope with the traumatic life event that a major burn injury with its sequelae represents.

Roxanne Rivard, RN, BSN, CWOCN, *Enterostomal Therapy Nurse, Fairview Lakes HomeCaring and Hospice, Chisago City, Minnesota*

Nursing Management of the Medical Client in the Rehabilitation Phase of Burn Injury

Impaired Physical Mobility. During the rehabilitation phase of burn injury, the client's physical mobility and ability to provide self-care are impaired by the presence of dressings, pain, scarring, contracture, and muscle atrophy.

Outcomes. The client will have improved physical mobility, as evidenced by maximum independence in performance of ADL, with minimum disability and disfigurement.

Interventions. The physical and occupational therapy consultations initiated in the early phases of burn injury are especially important for continued treatment in the rehabilitation phase as the client works toward functional independence. Typically, the therapist provides an individualized rehabilitation schedule as well as needed assistive devices for the client.

Motivate the client to participate in self-care activity such as brushing teeth and self-feeding, as this increased activity will not only improve mobility but also lessen dependence. Provide assistive devices furnished by therapy consultants to assist the client with any limitations. Expect tasks to take longer when the client works independently. Allow adequate time for the client to complete the undertaking. Self-confidence will be gained with independent functioning regardless of the time spent.

Encourage active ROM every 2 to 4 hours while the client is awake unless contraindicated because of a recent grafting procedure. Increased activity prevents muscle atrophy, tendon adherence, joint stiffness, and capsular tightness. Help the client to ambulate, to promote muscle strength and cardiopulmonary reserve. Provide passive exercise and stretching if the client is unable to actively participate (e.g., if the client is comatose or paralyzed).

Wrap donor sites on both burned and unburned legs with elastic bandage wraps (Ace bandages), using a figure-eight technique, before placing the limbs in a dependent position. The support will decrease capillary venous stasis, which impairs wound healing. Explain the rationale for activities to the client and family members, as understanding improves compliance. Avoid the position of comfort, and maintain burned areas in the position of physiologic function, within the client's limit of endurance. Continue to follow the splinting and positioning regimen recommended in the therapy consultation.

Pain. Pain experienced during the rehabilitation phase of burn injury is typically associated with wound care and therapeutic activity, particularly ROM exercises.

Outcomes. The client will have an acceptable level of comfort, as evidenced by verbalizing relief or control of pain or discomfort and actively participating in care.

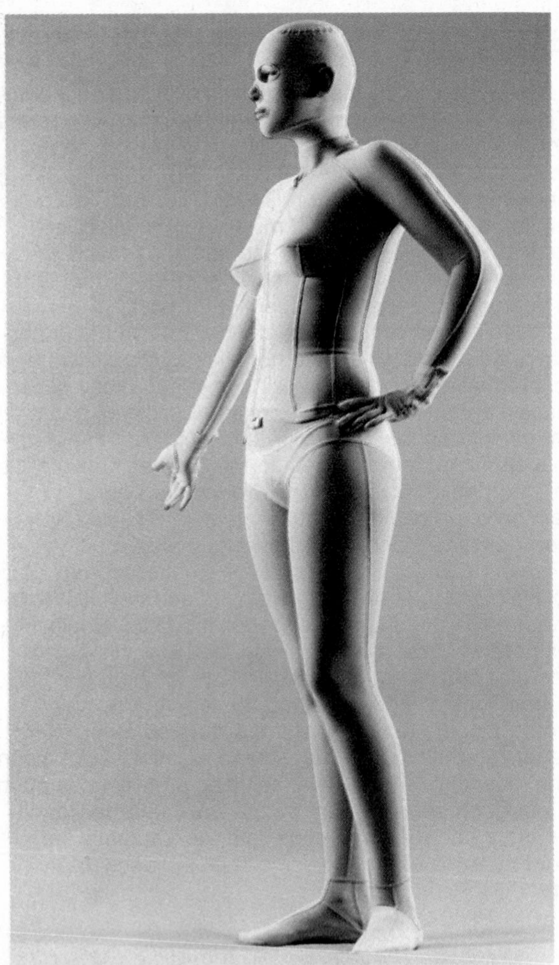

FIGURE 50–14 The model is wearing custom-fitted anti-scar support garment. When worn 23 hours a day, this garment is effective in providing pressure over healing burn wounds. Pressure therapy helps to minimize the development of hypertrophic scarring. (Courtesy of Medical Z Corporation, San Antonio.)

Interventions. Formulate a plan for controlling the client's pain based on an assessment of the client's response to pain and documentation of previous successful treatment regimens. As in the earlier phases of injury, allow adequate time for the onset of the medication for maximum benefits of the medication (5 to 10 minutes for the IV route; 45 minutes for the oral route). Nonpharmacologic methods of pain control, such as relaxation techniques, music therapy, guided imagery, distraction, and hypnosis, may improve the client's comfort, even if such methods were not successful in early phases of injury. As described earlier, effective communication assists in decreasing the client's anxiety. In preparation for impending discharge, the client should at some point during the rehabilitation phase progress to analgesia given only by the oral route.

Self-Esteem Disturbance. The client is at risk for self-esteem disturbances related to threatened or actual change in body image, physical loss, and loss of role responsibilities.

Outcomes. The client will develop improved self-esteem, as evidenced by making social contact with others outside the immediate family, developing effective coping mechanisms throughout the stages of recovery, and verbalizing feelings about self-concept.

Interventions. Allowing time for two-way communication with the client is especially important during this phase of injury. Provide an atmosphere of acceptance as the client tries various coping strategies to deal with the injury. Provide honest and accurate information about the client's projected appearance in an effort to reduce misconceptions that he or she may have.

Assess the need for limit-setting for maladaptive behavior. Consult with burn team members to establish such limits and to formulate a treatment plan for such behaviors; explain limit-setting to family members or significant others and assist them to maintain the same limits. Promote the client's self-confidence by providing information about the progress made, and support the client's role in care and treatment, providing encouragement and positive reinforcement.

Encourage family members to interact with the client, as this encouragement facilitates societal reintegration. During this phase of recovery, encourage the client to interact with others outside the facility. Use of a family day pass during this time is useful. Help to prepare the client for social interaction after discharge by discussing potential situations and how the client might deal with them. Such preparation provides rehearsal of events and reduces anxiety.

Impaired Skin Integrity. The expectation is that by the time the client reaches the rehabilitation phase of burn injury, the majority of wounds will be either healed or grafted. The new skin over areas of donor site, graft, and healed burn is characteristically very thin, with disrupted oil glands. The skin therefore is fragile; it becomes very dry and shears or cracks easily; and it is prone to infection.

Outcomes. The client will have intact skin with no evidence of infection, breakdown, or blistering.

Interventions. Daily wound and skin care should continue throughout hospitalization. Clean burned areas, grafts, and donor sites daily with a mild soap (without fragrance) and water. Rinse thoroughly to remove the soap. After cleaning, the healed skin should be lubricated with a nonirritating, alcohol-free moisturizer. Itching associated with dry skin can be minimized with application of the moisturizer at least 3 times a day. Avoid any shearing of tissue with dressings, clothing, or splints.

Knowledge Deficit. The burn-injured client or a family member or significant other must have knowledge of important treatment modalities that need continuation after discharge from the hospital.

Outcomes. The client or a family member or significant other will verbalize knowledge and demonstrate techniques that facilitate continued wound healing and limb mobility.

Interventions. Demonstrate and discuss the following skin care interventions with the client and appropriate family member or significant other: daily skin and wound care and dressing instructions if any; lubrication of grafts, donor sites, and healed burn wounds using an alcohol-free skin moisturizer at least 3 times daily; wearing pressure dressings or garments for 23 hours daily; and complete avoidance of direct sunlight for 1 year after injury owing to increased sensitivity to ultraviolet rays.

Review current medications and the dosage, precautions, and potential side effects. Discuss nutritional needs and the benefits of diets with adequate protein and calories.

Provide information on support groups or peers and counseling as needed for adjustment to life outside the hospital setting. Stress the need for follow-up care, and provide appointment dates and times if these have been established.

CONCLUSIONS

Nursing care of the burn-injured client is both complex and challenging. The psychological and physical trauma sustained following a burn injury can be devastating for both the victim and family members or significant others. Having a thorough understanding of the pathophysiologic changes that occur after a burn, knowing what to expect clinically as a result of the injury, and becoming familiar with the standards of care will guide nursing care to promote positive patient outcomes. As a key member of the burn team, you are responsible for an individualized plan of care that reflects the client's changing needs during progression through the different phases of recovery. Priority issues and care change as the client moves from the critical emergent phase into and, ultimately, through the rehabilitation period.

THINKING CRITICALLY

1. **You are working on the night shift in your hospital's burn center and receive a call that a client is in transport via ambulance to your unit. He will be a direct admission and bypass the emergency department. The telephone report reveals that the client was found unconscious on the floor of the bedroom. He is covered with soot and has obvious burns on his face, arms and torso. An intravenous line of lactated Ringer's solution was started and is running wide open. Oxygen is being administered via face mask. On admission, the client is received lying in the supine position on a gurney. He is restless, confused, and combative. He appears anxious and in pain. The eyebrows, eyelashes and hair are singed. There is soot in the nares and mouth and on the tongue. His voice is raspy, and he is coughing up thick black sputum. Breath sounds with scattered crackles; oxygen saturation, 75%. Face mask is in place but was disconnected from oxygen tank while the client was being moved onto the burn center gurney.**

   Heart rate is 142 BPM, with sinus tachycardia. Respiratory rate is 40 breaths/min and labored. Blood pressure is 144/88; temperature is 35° C. Bowel sounds are absent. There is thick, white leathery eschar on the chest, neck, left and right arm, and hands. The skin of the face and back are pink, moist, and blistered. The body from the waist to the feet is unburned. An IV line is infusing the LR right saphenous vein. Weight, 85 kg. What priorities should be set for the client's care? What interventions should be undertaken?

Factors to Consider. What is the client's respiratory status? Do the physical examination and history provided by the ambulance crew give you any clues to his respiratory status? What should you consider when administering pain medication or anxiolytics to this client? What is the client's fluid volume status? How will you monitor adequate fluid resuscitation?

2. **It is now 7 days after the injury, and the client has just returned to the unit after receiving grafts on the chest, neck, bilateral arms, hands, and axillae. Donor skin was taken circumferentially from both thighs. What assessments should you perform? What interventions should be undertaken?**

Factors to Consider. What factors disrupt graft adherence? What can you do to help prevent contracture formation?

3. **It is now 2 months since the client was injured, and the team begins to discuss discharge plans. The client tells you that he does not want to go home and does not want to talk any more about discharge. What can you do to help the client?**

Factors to Consider. What concerns might a burn survivor face upon discharge from the hospital? What professional resources might be helpful in addressing this situation? What lay resources might be helpful?

REFERENCES

1. Adcock, R., Boeve, S., & Patterson, D. (1998). Psychological and emotional recovery. In G. J. Carrougher (Ed.), *Burn care and therapy* (pp. 329–347). St. Louis: Mosby–Year Book.
2. Ahrns, K. S., & Harkins, D. R. (1999). Initial resuscitation after burn injury: Therapies, strategies, and controversies. *AACN Clinical Issues in Critical Care Nursing, 10*(1), 46–60.
3. American Burn Association. (1984). Guidelines for service standards and severity classification in the treatment of burn injuries. *Bulletin of the American College of Surgeons, 69*(10), 24–28.
4. Atkinson, A. (1998). Nursing burn wounds on general wards. *Nursing Standard, 12*(1), 58–65.
5. Barillo, D. J., & Goode, R. (1996). Fire fatality study: Demographics of fire victims. *Burns, 22*(2), 85–88.
6. Barton, R. G., & Saffle, J. R. (1997). Resuscitation of thermally injured patients with oxygen transport criteria as goals of therapy. *Journal of Burn Care and Rehabilitation, 18*(1), 1–9.
7. Blakeney, P., & Meyer, W. (1996). Psychosocial recovery of burned patients and reintegration into society. In D. N. Herndon (Ed.), *Total burn care* (pp. 556–563). London: W. B. Saunders.
8. Brigham, P. A., & McLoughlin, E. (1996). Burn incidence and medical care in the United States: Estimates, trends, and data sources. *Journal of Burn Care and Rehabilitation, 17*(2), 95–107.
9. Brigham, P. A., & McGuire, A. (1995). Progress towards a safe cigarette. *Journal of Public Health Policy, 16*(4), 433–439.
10. Carleton, S. C., Tomassoni, A. J., & Alexander, J. K. (1995). The cardiovascular effects of environmental traumas. Cardiac problems associated with burns. *Cardiology Clinics, 13*(2), 257–262.
11. Carrougher, G. J. (1999). Inhalation injury. *AACN Clinical Issues in Critical Care Nursing, 10*(1), 367–376.
12. Carrougher, G. J. (1998). Burn wound assessment and topical treatment. In G. J. Carrougher (Ed.), *Burn care and therapy* (pp. 133–159). St. Louis: Mosby–Year Book.
13. Cartotto, R. C., et al. (1996). Chemical burns. *Canadian Journal of Surgery, 39*(3), 205–220.

14. Cioffi, W. G. (1998) Inhalation injury. In G. J. Carrougher (Ed.), *Burn care and therapy* (pp. 35–59). St. Louis: Mosby–Year Book.
15. Cusick, J. M., & Grant, E. J. (1997). Children's sleepwear: Realization of the Consumer Product Safety Commission's flammability standards. *Journal of Burn Care and Rehabilitation, 18*(5), 469–474.
16. Darling, G. E., et al. (1996). Pulmonary complications in inhalation injuries with associated cutaneous burn. *Journal of Trauma Injury, 40*(1), 83–89.
17. Davis, S. T., & Sheely-Adolphson, P. (1997). Psychosocial interventions: Pharmacologic and psychologic modalities. *Nursing Clinics of North America, 32*(2), 331–340.
18. Demling, R. H. (1998). *Burn trauma*. New York: Thieme.
19. Everett, J. J. (1994). Pain assessment from patients with burns and their nurses. *Journal of Burn Care and Rehabilitation, 15*(2), 194–198.
20. Gordon, M., & Goodwin, C. (1997). Initial assessment, management and stabilization. *Nursing Clinics of North America, 32*(2), 237–248.
21. Gordon, M., & Winfree, J. (1998). Fluid resuscitation after a major burn. In G. J. Carrougher (Ed.), *Burn care and therapy* (pp. 107–126). St. Louis: Mosby–Year Book.
22. Gottschlich, M., & Jenkins, M. (1998). Metabolic consequences and nutritional needs. In G. J. Carrougher (Ed.), *Burn care and therapy* (pp. 213–226). St. Louis: Mosby–Year Book.
23. Greenfield, E., & McManus, A. (1997). Infectious complications. Prevention strategies for their control. *Nursing Clinics of North America, 32*(2), 297–308.
24. Harris, B., & Gelfand, J. (1995). The immune response to trauma. *Seminars in Pediatric Surgery, 4*(2), 77–81.
25. Hansbrough, J., & Franco, E. (1998). Skin replacements. *Clinics in Plastic Surgery, 25*(3), 407–423.
26. Heimbach, D., Mann, R., & Engrav, L. (1996). Evolution of the burn wound. Management decisions. In D. N. Herndon (Ed.), *Total burn care* (pp. 81–97). London: W. B. Saunders.
27. Hildreth, M., & Gottschlich, M. (1996). Nutritional support of the burned patient. In D. N. Herndon (Ed.), *Total burn care* (pp. 237–245). London: W. B. Saunders.
28. Hurren, J. S. (1995). Rehabilitation of the burned patient: James Laing memorial essay for 1993. *Burns, 21*(2), 116–126.
29. Jain, S., & Bandi, V. (1999). Electrical and lightning injuries. *Critical Care Clinics, 15*(2), 319–329.
30. Jordan, B., & Barillo, D. (1998). Prehospital care and transport. In G. J. Carrougher (Ed.), *Burn care and therapy* (pp. 61–88). St. Louis: Mosby–Year Book.
31. Jordan, B., & Harrington, D. (1997). Management of the burn wound. *Nursing Clinics of North America, 32*(2), 251–270.
32. Kealey, G. P. (1995). Pharmacologic management of background pain in burn victims. *Journal of Burn Care and Rehabilitation, 16*(3), 358–362.
33. Kirn, D S., & Luce, E. A. (1997). Early excision and grafting versus conservative management of burns in the elderly. *Plastic and Reconstructive Surgery, 9*, 1013–1017.
34. Kramer, G., & Nguyen, T. (1996). Pathophysiology of burn shock and burn edema. In D. N. Herndon (Ed.), *Total burn care* (pp. 44–52). London: W. B. Saunders.
35. Ladin, D. (1998). Understanding dressings. *Clinics in Plastic Surgery, 25*(3), 433–440.
36. LeBoucher, J., & Cynober, L. (1997). Protein metabolism and therapy in burn injury. *Annals of Nutrition and Metabolism*, 41, 69–82.
37. Lee, J. (1970). Emotional reactions to trauma. *Nursing Clinics of North America, 5*(4), 577–587.
38. Lee-Chiong, T. (1999). Smoke inhalation injury. When to suspect and how to treat. *Postgraduate Medicine, 105*(2), 55–62.
39. Lim, J., Rehmar, S., & Elmore, P. (1998). Rapid response: Care of burn victims. *AAOHN Journal, 46*(4), 169–178.
40. Linares, H. A. (1996). The burn problem: A pathologist's perspective. In D. N. Herndon (Ed.), *Total burn care* (p. 372). London: W. B. Saunders.
41. Malenfant, A., et al. (1998). Tactile, thermal and pain sensibility in burned patients with and without chronic pain and paresthesia problems. *Pain, 77*, 241–251.
42. Marvin, J. (1998). Management of pain and anxiety. In G. J. Carrougher (Ed.), *Burn care and therapy* (pp. 167–179). St. Louis: Mosby–Year Book.
43. Marvin, J., et al. (1996). Pain response and pain control. In D. N. Herndon (Ed.), *Total burn care* (pp. 529–544). London: W. B. Saunders.
44. Mayes, T. (1997). Enteral nutrition for the burnpatient. *Nutrition in Clinical Practice, 12*(1), S43–S45.
45. Mlcak, R., Dimick, A., & Micak, G. (1996). Prehospital management, transport and emergency care. In D. N. Herndon (Ed.), *Total burn care* (pp. 33–43). London: W. B. Saunders.
46. Monafo, W. (1996). Initial management of burns. *New England Journal of Medicine, 335*(21), 1581–1586.
47. Monafo, W. (1996). Wound care. In D. N. Herndon (Ed.), *Total burn care* (pp. 88–97). London: W. B. Saunders.
48. Moritz, A. R. (1945). The effect of inhaled heat on the air passages and lung: An experimental investigation. *American Journal of Pathology, 21*(2), 311–332.
49. Mozingo, D. (1998). Surgical management. In G. J. Carrougher (Ed.), *Burn care and therapy* (pp. 233–246). St. Louis: Mosby–Year Book.
50. Muller, M., et al. (1996). Modern treatment of a burn wound. In D. N. Herndon (Ed.), *Total Burn Care* (pp. 136–147). London: W. B. Saunders.
51. Munster, A. (1996). Cultured skin for massive burns. *Ann Surg, 224*(3), 372–377.
52. Nenot, J. C. (1990) Medical and surgical management for localized radiation burns. *Journal of Radiation Biology, 57*(4), 783–795.
53. Nguyen, T., et al. (1995). Current treatment of severely burned patients. *Annals of Surgery, 223*(1), 14–25.
54. Oman, K., & Reilly, E. (1998), Initial assessment and care in the emergency department. In G. J. Carrougher (Ed.), *Burn care and therapy* (pp. 89–101). St. Louis: Mosby–Year Book.
55. Partridge, J., & Robinson, E. (1995). Psychologic and social aspects of burns. *Burns, 21*(6), 453–457. Patino, O., et al. (1998) Massage in hypertrophic scars. *Journal of Burn Care and Rehabilitation, 20*(3), 268–271.
56. Pessina, M., & Ellis, S. (1997). Rehabilitation. *Nursing Clinics of North America, 32*(2), 365–373.
57. Pruitt, B., & Cioffi, W. (1995). Diagnosis and treatment of smoke inhalation. *Journal of Intensive Care Medicine, 10*(3), 117–127.
58. Pruitt, B., & Goodwin, C. (1995). Thermal injury. In J. H. Davis & G. F. Sheldon (Eds.), *Clinical surgery*. St. Louis: Mosby–Year Book.
59. Pruitt, B., & Mason, A. (1996). Epidemiological, demographic and outcome characteristics of burn injury. In D. N. Herndon (Ed.), *Total burn care* (pp. 5–15). London: W. B. Saunders.
60. Ramzy, P., Barret. J., & Herndon, D. (1999). Thermal injury. *Critical Care Clinics, 15*(2), 333–352.
61. Richard, R. (1998). Assessment and diagnosis of burn wounds. *Advances in Wound Care, 12*(9), 468–471.
62. Rodriguez, D. (1996). Nutrition in patients with severe burns: State of the art. *Journal of Burn Care and Rehabilitation, 17*(1), 62–70.
63. Rose, J. K., et al. (1997). Allograft is superior to topical antimicrobial therapy in the treatment of partial-thickness scald burns in children. *Journal of Burn Care and Rehabilitation, 18*(4), 338–341.
64. Rutan, R. (1998). Physiologic response to cutaneous burn injury. In G. J. Carrougher (Ed.), *Burn care and therapy* (pp. 1–28). St. Louis: Mosby–Year Book.
65. Sakurai, H., Traber, L., & Traber, D. (1998). Altered systemic organ blood flow after combined injury with burn and smoke inhalation. *Shock, 3*(5), 369–374.
66. Shankowsky, H. A., Callioux, L. S., & Tredget, E. E. (1994). North America survey of hydrotherapy in modern burn care. *Journal of Burn Care and Rehabilitation, 15*(2), 143–146.
67. Smith, D. (1995). Use of Biobrane in wound management. *Journal of Burn Care and Rehabilitation, 16*(3), 317–320.
68. Thompkins, R. M., & Carrougher, G. J. (1998). Burn prevention. In G. J. Carrougher (Ed.), *Burn care and therapy* (pp. 497–522). St. Louis: Mosby–Year Book.
69. Tompkins, R., and Burke, J. (1996). Alternative wound coverings. In D. N. Herndon (Ed.), *Total burn care* (pp. 164–183). London: W. B. Saunders.
70. Traber, D., & Polland, V. (1996). Pathophysiology of inhalation injury. In D. N. Herndon (Ed.), *Total burn care* (pp. 175–183). London: W. B. Saunders.
71. Ward, C. G. (1998). What's new in burns? *Journal of the American College of Surgery, 186*(2), 123–126.
72. Ward, R. S (1998). Physical rehabilitation. In G. J. Carrougher (Ed.), *Burn care and therapy* (pp. 293–320). St. Louis: Mosby–Year Book.

73. Ward, R. S., & Saffle, J. R. (1995). Topical agents in burn and wound care. *Physical Therapy, 75*(6), 526–538.
74. Warden, G. D. (1996). Fluid resuscitation and early management. In D. N. Herndon (Ed.), *Total burn care* (pp. 53–60). London: W. B. Saunders.
75. Weber, J. (1998). Epidemiology of infections and strategies for control. In G. J. Carrougher (Ed.), *Burn care and therapy* (pp. 185–206). St. Louis: Mosby–Year Book.
76. Williams, W., & Phillips, L. (1996). Pathophysioiogy of the burn wound. In D. N. Herndon (Ed.), *Total burn care* (pp. 63–70). London: W. B. Saunders.
77. Winfree, J., & Barillo, D. (1997). Nonthermal injuries. *Nursing Clinics of North America, 32*(2), 275–294.
78. Wolfe, R. (1996). Metabolic responses to burn injury: Nutritional implications. In D. N. Herndon (Ed.), *Total burn care* (pp. 217–222). London: W. B. Saunders.

UNIT 11

Circulatory Disorders

Anatomy and Physiology Review
The Circulatory System
Robert G. Carroll

The vascular system is a vast network of vessels through which blood circulates in the body. The major functions of the cardiovascular system—delivery of nutrients to tissues and removal of metabolic wastes—are accomplished in the capillaries. Blood leaving the ventricles is distributed through arteries and arterioles, in progressively smaller branches to the capillaries (a *divergent* pattern, like a river to a delta). Blood leaving the capillaries follows progressively larger venules and veins on its way back to the atria (a *convergent* pattern, like tributaries flowing into a river).

The anatomic arrangement of blood vessels allows regulation of blood flow at the individual tissue level, so that blood flow delivery can be proportional to the tissue's metabolic needs. Because the volume of blood flowing from the arteries to the capillaries is a major determinant of blood pressure, the blood pressure control systems also include control of arteriolar diameter by the sympathetic nervous system and circulating hormones.

STRUCTURES OF THE VASCULAR SYSTEM

Two series of blood vessels—the systemic and the pulmonary circulations—distribute blood to the capillaries and return blood to the heart. Blood exiting the left ventricle enters the *systemic circulation,* passing progressively through the aorta, arteries, arterioles, capillaries, venules, veins, and finally the vena cava before entering the right atrium (Fig. U11–1). For the *pulmonary circulation,* blood flows from the right ventricle into the pulmonary artery, then passes through arterioles, pulmonary capillaries, and venules, before returning to the pulmonary vein and the left atrium.

GENERAL BLOOD VESSEL STRUCTURE

The anatomic division of blood vessels into arteries, arterioles, capillaries, venules, and veins is based on the presence of up to three histologic layers (Fig. U11–2).

1. The *tunica intima* (innermost layer) consists of endothelial cells that separate the blood from the extravascular spaces. The tightness of the junctions between the endothelial cells varies among tissues. For example, the very tight junctions of cerebral capillaries restrict movement of some drugs to brain cells (the blood-brain barrier). In contrast, the endothelial cell holes and relatively loose junctions in the liver and spleen allow easy transit between the blood and tissue spaces in those organs. The endothelium generates substances such as endothelial-derived relaxing factor (EDRF, or nitric oxide), allowing nitroglycerin, friction, and stress to cause vasodilation. Damage to the endothelium may allow blood to enter the middle layer of a blood vessel, creating an aneurysm.
2. The *tunica media* (middle layer) consists of elastic connective tissue and smooth muscle cells. Particularly in the aorta and large arteries, the elastic tissue contributes to the shape of the arterial pressure pulse. The amount of smooth muscle contraction regulates the diameter of the vessel and causes a change in blood flow and blood pressure. Smooth muscle is normally partially contracted because of sympathetic nerve activity. Smooth muscle contraction can also be regulated by circulating hormones and (in the smaller vessels) by tissue metabolic factors.
3. The *tunica adventitia* (outermost layer) consists of a relatively thin layer of connective tissue providing shape for the blood vessels. This layer also houses the vasa vasorum, the small arteries and veins that provide nutrients to the cells of the blood vessel.

VASCULAR SEGMENTS

Arteries

Arteries, particularly the aorta, have an extensive elastic tissue layer that accounts for the difference between arterial pressure (120/80 mm Hg) and left ventricular pressure (120/10 mm Hg). The elastic tissue stretches during ventricular ejection, storing energy. When the aortic valve closes and ventricular ejection stops, recoil of the elastic tissue slows the fall of arterial pressure during the interval until the next period of ventricular ejection. The efficiency of the elastic tissue decreases with age and with atherosclerosis, contributing to the rise in systolic arterial blood pressure usually seen in older adults.

Arterioles (5 to 100 μm in diameter) contain a high proportion of vascular smooth muscle. The degree of contraction of this muscle is regulated by background activity of the autonomic nervous system, primarily the sympathetic nerves. In addition, circulating hormones such as epinephrine, norepinephrine, and angiotensin can also cause smooth muscle contraction.

Capillary Beds

Capillary beds include the small arterioles and venules, and the vessels connecting them (see *Inset,* Fig. U11–1). The smooth muscle of these small arterioles is contracted by sympathetic nerves, but local factors become increasingly important as the diameter of the vessel decreases. The *precapillary sphincters* (the last band of smooth muscle before the capillaries) respond only to local factors. Blood passes from the arterioles into capillaries (5 to 10 μm in diameter). The capillary diameter approaches that

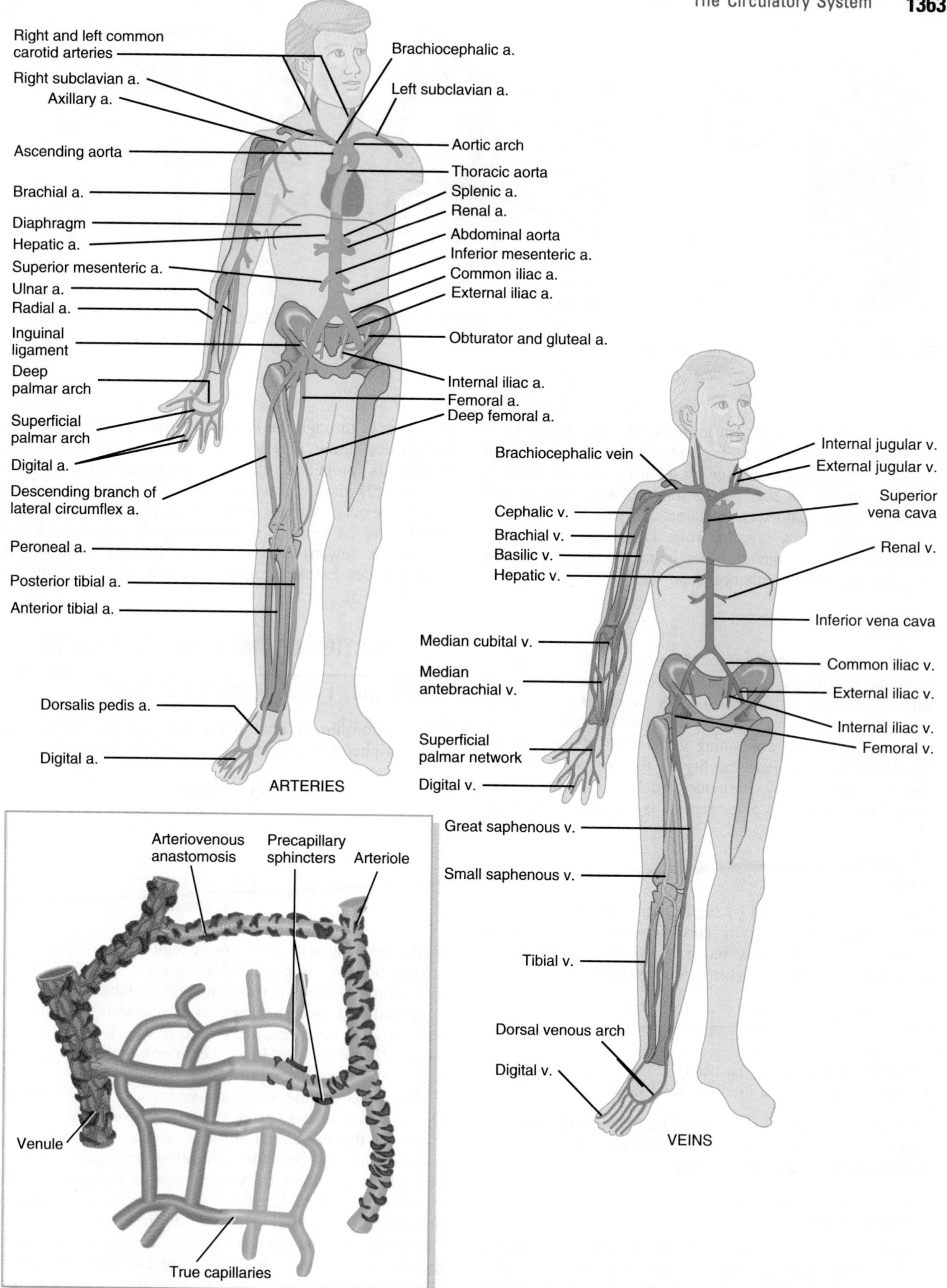
Right and left common carotid arteries
Right subclavian a.
Axillary a.
Ascending aorta
Brachial a.
Diaphragm
Hepatic a.
Superior mesenteric a.
Ulnar a.
Radial a.
Inguinal ligament
Deep palmar arch
Superficial palmar arch
Digital a.
Descending branch of lateral circumflex a.
Peroneal a.
Posterior tibial a.
Anterior tibial a.
Dorsalis pedis a.
Digital a.
Brachiocephalic a.
Left subclavian a.
Aortic arch
Thoracic aorta
Splenic a.
Renal a.
Abdominal aorta
Inferior mesenteric a.
Common iliac a.
External iliac a.
Obturator and gluteal a.
Internal iliac a.
Femoral a.
Deep femoral a.
ARTERIES
Brachiocephalic vein
Internal jugular v.
External jugular v.
Superior vena cava
Cephalic v.
Brachial v.
Basilic v.
Hepatic v.
Renal v.
Inferior vena cava
Median cubital v.
Median antebrachial v.
Common iliac v.
External iliac v.
Internal iliac v.
Femoral v.
Superficial palmar network
Digital v.
Great saphenous v.
Small saphenous v.
Tibial v.
Dorsal venous arch
Digital v.
VEINS
Arteriovenous anastomosis
Precapillary sphincters
Arteriole
Venule
True capillaries

FIGURE U11–1 Major systemic arteries and veins. *Inset,* Capillary network.

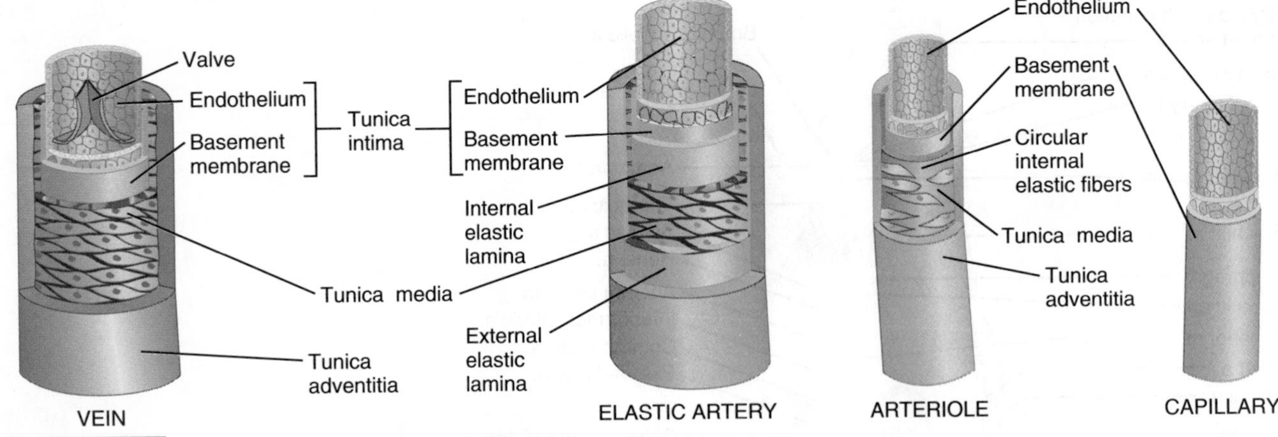

FIGURE U11–2 Structure of blood vessels.

of the red blood cell (7 μm in diameter). Capillaries have only a tunica intima (see Fig. U11–2), and the small wall thickness facilitates exchange by diffusion. In tissues such as the skin, blood also passes through *metarterioles* (10 to 100 μm in diameter). Metarterioles are not exchange vessels but serve a separate role. Decreased blood flow through cutaneous metarterioles helps the body conserve heat; increased flow enhances heat loss.

Venules

Venules (10 to 100 μm in diameter) collect drainage from the capillaries in a convergent flow pattern. Venule smooth muscle is innervated by sympathetic nerves. Along with the veins, venules serve as capacitance (volume storage) areas, containing up to 75% of the circulating blood volume. Permeability of the postcapillary venules is regulated by hormones such as histamine and bradykinin. Note that angiogenesis is initiated in the venules.

Veins

Veins are characterized by high volume and low pressure. Sympathetic nerve activity constricts the smooth muscle of the veins and helps move blood toward the heart. Blood flow toward the heart is also assisted by:

- A drop in intrathoracic pressure during respiration
- Extravascular compression of veins in exercising skeletal muscle,
- Gravity (for veins in the head)
- Valves that insure a unidirectional flow

Damage to venous valves can cause swellings, such as varicose veins, and lack of leg muscle movement can lead to venous stasis and clotting.

Lymphatics

Lymphatics are a network of endothelial tubes that merge to form two large systems that enter the vena cava. Terminal lymphatics lack tight junctions, allowing large proteins (and metastasizing cancer cells) to enter the circulatory system through the lymphatic system. In the GI tract, lymphatics allow digested fats to enter the circulation. Lymph is propelled by (1) massaging from adjacent muscle, (2) tissue pressure, and (3) contraction of the lymph vessels. Valves ensure that the flow of lymph, which over 24 hours is a volume equal to the total blood volume, is toward the vena cava. Lymph is filtered in lymph nodes before progressing back to the circulation (Fig. U11–3).

FUNCTION OF THE VASCULAR SYSTEM

PRESSURE, FLOW, AND RESISTANCE

The relationship of arterial pressure, cardiac output, and total peripheral resistance is shown by the equation

$$Q = \Delta P/R$$

or

$$\text{flow} = \frac{\text{pressure gradient}}{\text{resistance}}$$

In the body, arterial *pressure* is regulated. A decrease in arterial pressure is corrected by a reflex increase in cardiac output and an increase in total peripheral resistance, both mediated by an increase in sympathetic nervous system activity. For a capillary bed, however, *flow* is regulated. If flow is too low, the arteriole dilates and the decrease in resistance allows flow to increase.

Resistance in the vascular system can be affected by (1) the radius of the vessel, (2) fluid viscosity, and (3) the length of the vessel. Of these, vessel radius is the most powerful mechanism for controlling resistance and the one that is physiologically important. If the radius of the vessel decreases to ½ of the starting value, resistance to flow increases 16-fold. The body utilizes vascular smooth muscle to alter the diameter of arteries and arterioles and, therefore, to regulate both pressure and flow. Occasionally, changes in blood viscosity can alter resistance, particularly when the hematocrit is increased (polycythemia)

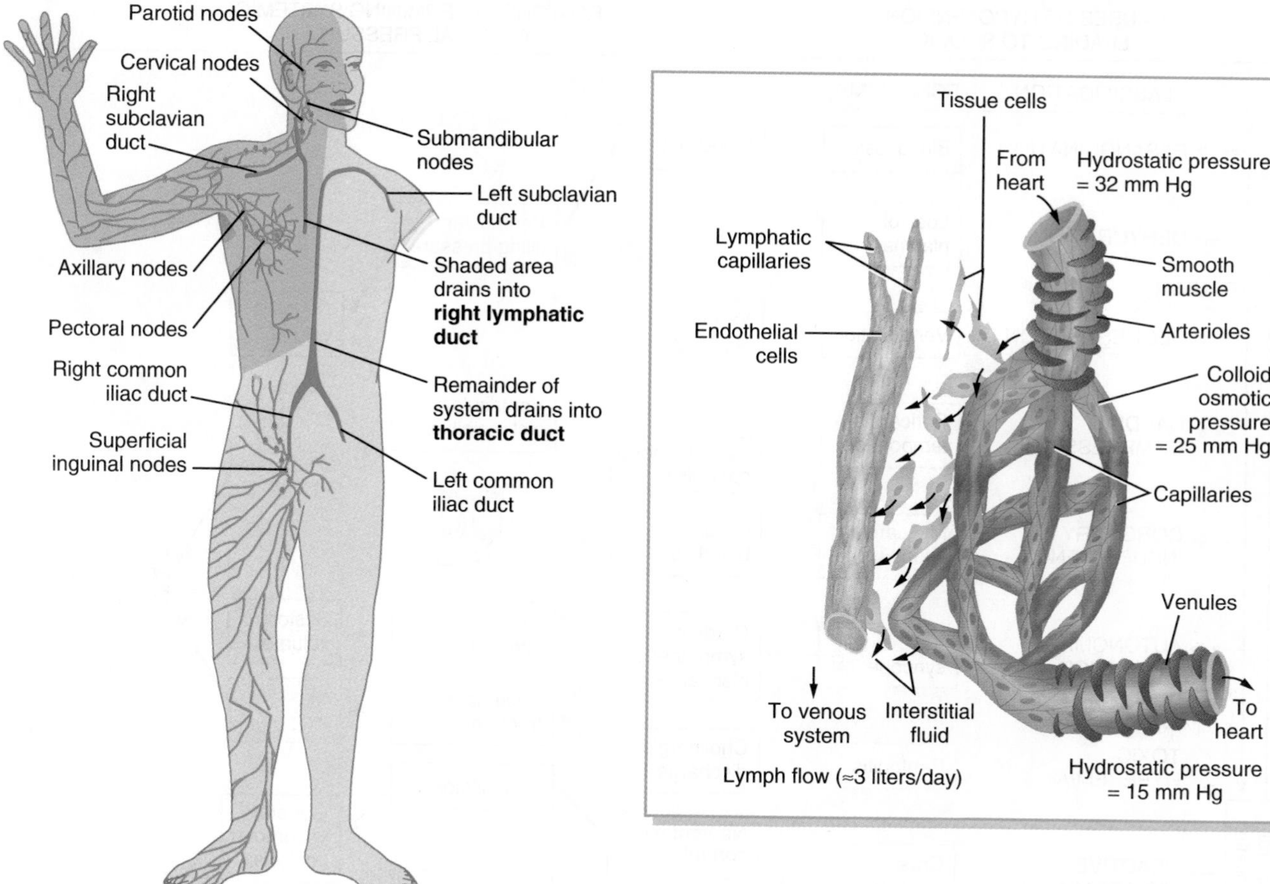

FIGURE U11–3 Major lymphatic vessels and drainage. *Inset,* Fluid exchange at the capillary bed. The primary driving force to move fluids from the capillary is *hydrostatic pressure.* The primary pulling force to bring fluids back into the vessel is *colloid osmotic pressure* from the proteins in the capillary fluids (e.g., albumin). The hydrostatic pressure at the arterial end of the capillary is 32 mm Hg. As the fluid moves through the capillary, the pressure falls. Because proteins do not move across the capillary endothelium, colloid osmotic pressure is constant at 25 mm Hg. Thus, at the arterial end the hydrostatic pressure is greater than the colloid osmotic pressure, and fluids then move into interstitial spaces. The opposite is true at the venous end where pressure falls to 15 mm Hg. The hydrostatic pressure is lower than the colloid osmotic pressure, and fluids thus return to the capillary. There is a net loss of fluids out of the capillary (~3 L/day). This fluid is absorbed by the lymphatic system and is returned to circulation at the lymphatic duct.

or decreased (anemia). Resistance increases as viscosity increases and decreases as viscosity decreases.

Capillary Exchange

Exchange of nutrients and wastes between the blood and the tissues is the primary purpose of the cardiovascular system. The movement of nutrients from the blood to the tissue and removal of metabolic wastes are driven by diffusion, filtration, and pinocytosis.

Diffusion

Diffusion is quantitatively the most important process. The rate of diffusion is enhanced by (1) increasing the surface area available for exchange, (2) increasing the concentration gradient, and (3) decreasing the distance that a compound must travel. In tissues such as exercising skeletal muscle, an increase in the number of perfused capillaries enhances the delivery of nutrients to the tissues.

Filtration

Fluid movement across the capillary depends on the balance of the hydrostatic pressure gradient (which favors filtration) and the oncotic pressure gradient from plasma proteins (which favors reabsorption) (Fig. U11–4). The net force favors filtration at the arteriolar end of the capillary bed, and reabsorption at the venular end of the capillary bed. In most capillary beds, the volume filtered is slightly greater than the volume absorbed, and the excess fluid is removed from the tissue spaces by the lymph vessels. *Edema* (accumulation of fluid in the tissue spaces) occurs because of (1) increased filtration, (2) decreased reabsorption, or (3) impaired lymph drainage.

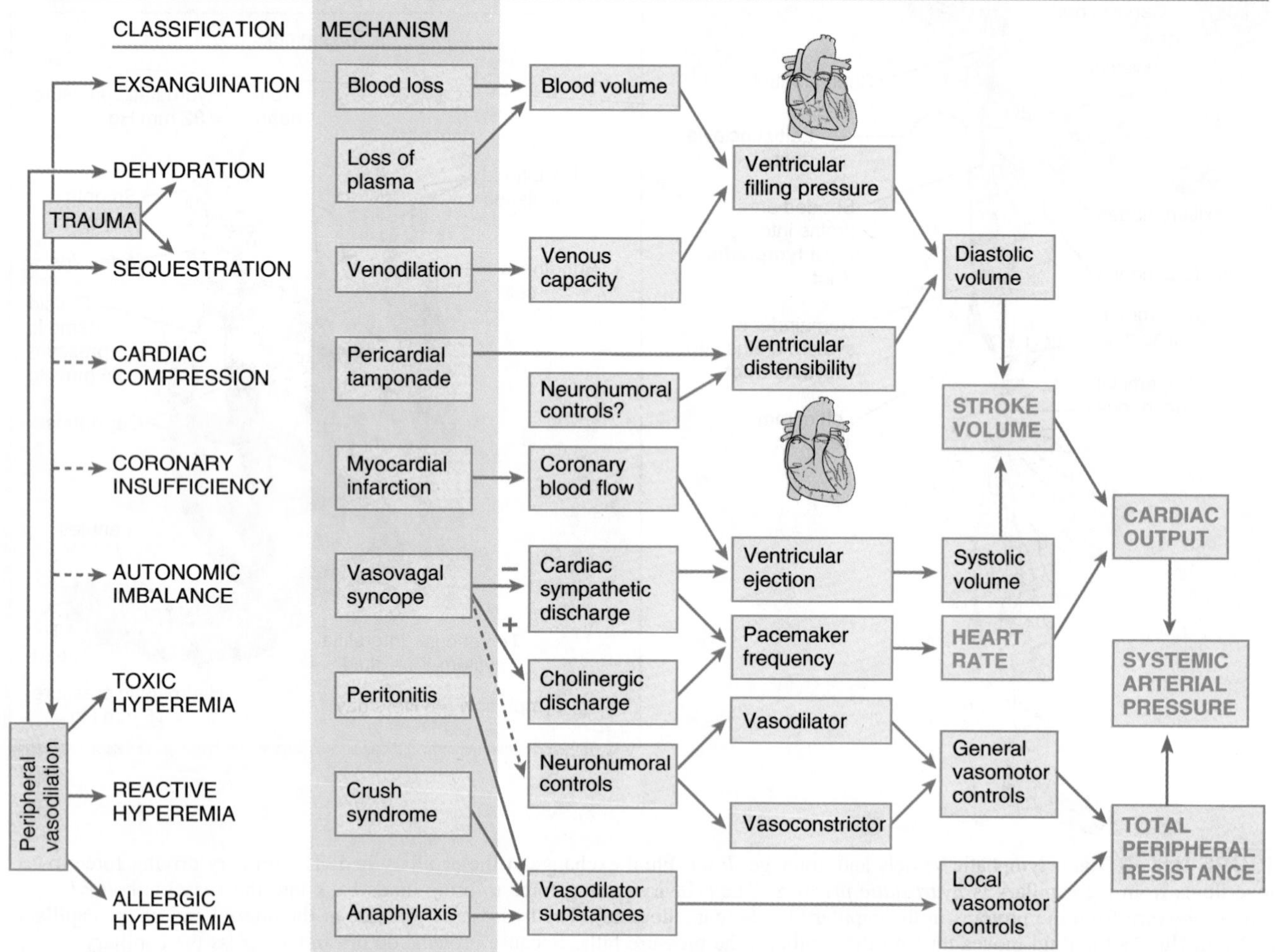

FIGURE U11–4 Control of arterial pressure. Arterial blood pressure is controlled by several factors. *Right,* Blood pressure is controlled by two major factors: cardiac output and total peripheral vascular resistance. Cardiac output is also a function of two factors: stroke volume and heart rate. Reading the diagram from the right, you will find the factors that govern each step. Each bifurcation represents possible compensatory mechanisms. *Far left,* Disorders that can lead to shock. These factors are extremes of the various control mechanisms. (Modified from Rushmer, R. F. [1976]. Cardiovascular dynamics [p. 207]. Philadelphia: W. B. Saunders.)

Pinocytosis

Pinocytosis is the movement of vesicles, especially from outside the cell to inside the cell. Pinocytosis is thought to be important only as a route for large proteins to cross the capillary wall.

Cardiovascular Control

Much like the power and water supply systems in a city, the distribution of blood flow in the body depends on a sufficient driving pressure (arterial pressure), allowing the end users (capillary beds) to determine how much of the resource to utilize. Cardiovascular control is best described in terms of (1) regulation of arterial pressure and (2) local regulation of tissue blood flow.

■ REGULATION OF ARTERIAL PRESSURE

The normal arterial pressure is maintained by a negative feedback mechanism called the *baroreceptor reflex.* Pressure-sensitive nerve endings in the aortic arch and carotid sinus monitor arterial pressure. This information is transmitted to the cardiovascular centers of the medulla, where it is integrated with other sensory information. The cardiovascular centers then adjust the activity of the sympathetic and parasympathetic nervous systems. Parasympathetic nerves help slow the heart rate; sympathetic nerves can increase heart rate, increase cardiac contractility, constrict the veins (to decrease venous capacity, thus increasing venous return), and constrict the arterioles (to increase total peripheral resistance and, therefore, arterial pressure). The relationships among all of these events in controlling arterial pressure are shown in Figure U11–4. Thus, a decrease in blood pressure activates the sympathetic nervous system, increasing cardiac output (heart rate, venoconstriction for venous return, and cardiac contractility) and increasing peripheral resistance to trap blood within the arteries.

Baroreceptor control of blood pressure is augmented by volume-sensitive receptors in the low-pressure atria and veins, which control renal fluid balance, and endocrine vasoconstrictor agents such as angiotensin II, antidiuretic hormone (ADH), and norepinephrine. Chronic regulation of blood pressure depends on the volume of blood in the system and, ultimately, is tied to renal regulation of body fluid balance.

■ LOCAL REGULATION OF BLOOD FLOW

If arterial pressure is sufficient, tissues can regulate their blood flow to match their metabolic needs. If blood flow is inadequate, metabolites such as carbon dioxide, adenosine, potassium, and acids accumulate, acting as vasodilators of the arteriolar smooth muscle only of that local area. The resulting increase in blood flow washes out the metabolites and diminishes the vasodilator stimulus. This control system allows tissue blood flow to increase as tissue metabolic activity increases and accounts for the period of increased blood flow that follows a period of occlusion. In the long term, inadequate blood flow to a tissue can cause the growth of new capillaries, again matching blood flow to the tissue's metabolic needs. Blood flow to tissues such as the brain and myocardium is dominated by local control.

At the other extreme of regulation, cutaneous blood flow responds primarily to neural control. Because skin blood flow is tied to thermoregulation rather than nutrition, metabolic control is poorly developed. Other vascular beds, such as the kidney and the splanchnic circulation, respond both to sympathetic control and to local control. During increased sympathetic activity, blood flow to these tissues is decreased and is shunted to the brain and the myocardium.

CARDIOVASCULAR ADJUSTMENT TO EXERCISE

Cardiovascular control must balance the need for a steady arterial blood pressure against the ability to respond to a physiologic challenge. Exercise, which increases skeletal muscle consumption of oxygen and other nutrients, requires a marked increase in both cardiac output and skeletal muscle blood flow. The increase in cardiac output results from a cerebral cortical stimulation of the medullary cardiovascular center and activation of the sympathetic nervous system. The increased cardiac output requires an increased venous return, accomplished both by the vasodilation of the skeletal muscle beds and by a sympathetic-mediated venoconstriction. In rhythmic activity such as running, compression of the veins by the contracting skeletal muscle along with the negative intrathoracic pressure from breathing assists the flow of blood toward the heart.

The increased cardiac output is preferentially directed to the exercising muscles (including the heart). Local factors in the exercising muscles cause a vasodilation of those vascular beds. The sympathetic activity constricts the arteriolar smooth muscle of the nonexercising vascular beds, such as the gastrointestinal tract, the kidney, and the nonworking muscles. Cerebral blood flow remains unchanged because that vascular bed is regulated primarily by local control. Cutaneous blood flow may be diminished initially but increases as the heat generated by the exercising muscles raises body core temperature, and cutaneous vasodilation helps to cool the body.

CONCLUSIONS

The vascular system is a series of vessels that transport blood to the capillary exchange vessels. In the capillaries, nutrients pass to the tissues and wastes pass into the blood for transport to excretory organs. Blood pressure regulation by the baroreceptor reflex ensures that arterial pressure remains sufficient to propel blood toward the tissues. Tissue blood flow is controlled by the metabolic needs of the tissues, and it increases when tissue metabolism increases.

BIBLIOGRAPHY

1. Berne, R., and Levy, M. (1998). *Physiology (4th ed.)*. St. Louis: Mosby–Year Book.
2. Gartner, L., and Kiatt, J. (1997). *Color textbook of histology*. Philadelphia: W. B. Saunders.
3. Guyton, A., and Hall, J. (1996). *Textbook of medical physiology (9th ed.)*. Philadelphia: W. B. Saunders.
4. Silverthorn, D. (1998). *Human physiology*. Saddle River, NJ: Prentice Hall.

CHAPTER 51

Assessment of the Vascular System

Mary Sieggreen

Peripheral vascular disease is common among elderly and diabetic clients. It is characterized by disturbances of blood flow through the peripheral vessels. These disturbances eventually damage tissues as a result of ischemia, excessive accumulation of waste and fluid, or both. Damage can be due to any disorder that narrows, obstructs, or injures blood vessels, thus impeding blood flow. Without intervention, damage may progress to the point of tissue or organ death. Assessment of the peripheral vascular system includes data collection through the health history, physical examination, and diagnostic tests when indicated.

HISTORY

When assessing the client, note risk factors for atherosclerosis (see Chapter 52), diabetes (see Chapter 45), and cardiac (see Chapters 55 and 58) as well as arterial, venous (see Chapter 53), and lymphatic disorders. Some clients are reluctant to mention what they believe to be minor symptoms. Consequently, perform a careful assessment, ask specific questions skillfully, and be alert for information that may indicate early manifestations of insidious conditions.

■ BIOGRAPHICAL AND DEMOGRAPHIC DATA

Biographical data include the client's age. Atherosclerosis (hardening of the arteries) is more prevalent in older people. Venous disease, although also more prevalent in the elderly, may be identified in younger people. Ask about occupation, and clarify whether the occupation increases the risk for vascular disease. If the client is retired, ask about the previous employment history.

■ CURRENT HEALTH

Ask about frequency and duration of clinical manifestations that may indicate a vascular disorder. The following section describes the typical chief complaints of clients who have arterial and venous disorders.

Chief Complaint

ARTERIAL DISORDERS

In arterial insufficiency of the lower extremities, the chief complaint is often cramping leg pain in the calf muscles during ambulation that disappears with 1 to 2 minutes of rest. The pain is called *intermittent claudication.* The pain occurs in the muscle group distal to the diseased artery (see Chapter 53).

Intermittent claudication results from inadequate tissue oxygenation (*ischemia*) due to arterial stenosis, usually secondary to atherosclerosis. It is a pathologic process similar to angina. Claudication is predictable and reproducible; this means that (1) the client can walk the same distance each time before pain occurs and (2) the pain occurs each time that this distance is walked.

As an artery becomes more stenosed, the pain may become more severe. When clients report distal forefoot burning, numbness or tingling, pain at rest, or pain that awakens them during the night (*rest pain*), urgent attention is needed. This pain is related to arterial disease and exacerbated by decreased cardiac output during sleep. The relative leg elevation while in a supine position decreases blood flow through stenosed arteries. Pain is relieved when the client stands because gravity pulls the blood toward the feet. Even during non-sleep hours, elevation of the legs decreases blood flow and increases pain. Clients may report that they sleep upright with the legs dependent (below heart level) to control pain.

Ask about precipitating factors, duration and persistence of the discomfort, the manner of its onset, and associated manifestations. Document the activity required to cause pain. The extent of disease involvement can be gauged by the distance the client is able to walk without pain, or *claudication distance.* For example, one client may be able to walk only one block before experiencing pain, whereas another may be able to walk six blocks.

Disorders of the aorta and iliac vessels can lead to impotence. If a male client has aortoiliac disease, ask about problems with penile erection. Sexuality may be a sensitive issue; ask questions carefully to elicit areas of concern or problems (see Chapters 9 and 37).

VENOUS DISORDERS

Chronic venous disease has an insidious onset. Many clients do not recall any precipitating event. There may be a positive family history for venous disease, a job history involving many hours of standing in one place, or multiple pregnancies. Obesity may be a factor. In contrast to the pain in arterial disorders, pain in chronic venous disease has a slow onset and is not associated with exercise or rest. Clients may also have varicose veins and a history of phlebitis. In these clients, the leg veins have been subjected to increased pressure and return of venous blood has been obstructed. Vein walls are compliant and distend with increased pressure. Valves become incompetent because the distended wall prevents the valve leaflets from meeting each other when they close. An *incompetent vein* allows the column of blood to flow backward, increasing the hydrostatic pressure in the venous end of the capillary. This increase in pressure against the vein wall moves fluid from the intravascular to the interstitial space, causing edema. As the process continues, blood flow slows and tissues become hypoxic (lacking in oxygen). The client may report a feeling of heaviness in the legs or nighttime cramping. Exercise and elevation generally relieve the discomfort and swelling because venous return of blood is improved.

In more severe forms of chronic venous disorders, lower extremity edema may be the initial complaint. Edema worsens toward the end of the day and diminishes after nighttime leg elevation. Pitting edema (see discussion of edema) may be seen at first, but as the edema becomes more chronic, tissue sclerosis develops and the tissue becomes more difficult to compress.

Initial skin changes noted with chronic venous disorders may include erythema (redness), followed in the late stages by lipodermatosclerosis (brawny, thick, darkly pigmented skin). The skin becomes dry and flaky, which leads to itching and scratching. Continued irritation results in stasis dermatitis, and the skin eventually ulcerates. Ulcers develop in the lower third of the leg, most commonly above the medial malleolus, where venous pressure is highest and there are more perforator veins than elsewhere in the leg. Chronic venous edema and sclerotic subcutaneous tissue may compress the lymph vessels.

Lymphatic disorders also lead to edema. If the lymphatic obstruction is prolonged, edematous tissue becomes fibrotic and almost impossible to compress. Chapter 74 describes the assessment of the lymphatic system.

Symptom Analysis

Vascular disease may be arterial, venous, or lymphatic. Table 51–1 compares the clinical manifestations of arterial and venous disorders in the lower extremities.

The client who has venous disease may report chronic aching pain in the legs when they are in a dependent position. Chronic venous insufficiency produces the following manifestations:

- Edema
- Dependent cyanosis
- Brown discoloration of the skin at the ankle
- Ulcers
- Pruritus

Skin temperature remains normal or slightly elevated and pulses are present, although they may be difficult to palpate through the edema.

Chronic arterial insufficiency produces the following manifestations:

- Decrease or absence of arterial pulses
- Thin, shiny, hairless skin
- Thick, ridged toenails
- Cool skin temperature
- Pain with ambulation (claudication)
- Pain with leg elevation, or at night (rest pain)

The skin is pale when the legs are elevated above heart level and dusky red after they are placed in a dependent position (*dependent rubor*). Edema is not usually present in pure arterial insufficiency. There may be ulcers from trauma, over pressure points, or on the tips of toes.

PAST HEALTH HISTORY

Note any history of vascular impairment. Inquire about changes that indicate vasospastic disorders, such as changes in color or temperature of digits. Ask specifically whether the client has a history of hypertension, diabetes, stroke, transient ischemic attacks (TIAs), changes in vision, pain in legs during activity, leg cramps, phlebitis, venous or arterial blood clots, pulmonary emboli, edema, varicose veins, leg ulcers, or extremities that are cold,

TABLE 51–1 CLINICAL MANIFESTATIONS IN LOWER EXTREMITY DISORDERS

Manifestation	Arterial Disorder	Venous Disorder
Pain	Intermittent claudication. Rest pain may be present, or pain may worsen with elevation	Aching, heaviness Exercise and elevation decrease pain Nocturnal cramping Heaviness in the legs at the end of day
Skin	Absence of hair in chronic condition. Thin, shiny skin Thick toenails if fungal infection present	Brown discoloration Normal toenails
Color	Pale with dependent rubor	Brown discoloration. Dependent cyanosis
Temperature	Cool	No change, or may be warmer than unaffected areas
Sensation	Decreased; tingling, numbness may be present	Pruritus may be present
Pulses	Decreased to absent	Present, but may be difficult to palpate if edema is present
Edema	May be present but usually absent	Present, worse at end of day, improved with elevation
Muscle mass	Reduced in chronic disease	Unaffected in pure venous disease
Ulcers	Small, painful ulcers on pressure points, points of trauma, between toes, or distal most point, especially lateral malleolus and toes	Broad, shallow, slightly painful ulcers of the ankle and lower leg. Surrounding skin is brown, fibrotic

pale, or blue. Question any previous history of frostbite, which increases risk of vasospasm. Visual changes and TIAs may indicate carotid artery disease. Ask about any past medical tests, operations, or treatments involving the vascular system and about any previous treatment for diabetes mellitus, collagen disorders, or hypertension.

In addition, note medications that the client takes, including over-the-counter drugs and herbal remedies. Some medications increase risk for vascular disorders (e.g., birth control pills.

Herbal remedies used to self-treat peripheral vascular disorders include those for hypertension, varicose veins, atherosclerosis, and vascular spasm. Herbs with antihypertensive action include garlic (*Allium sativum*), hawthorn (*Crataegus oxyacantha*), kudzu (*Pueraria lobata*), nettle (*Urtica dioica*), onion (*Allium cepa*), purslane (*Portulaca oleracea*), reishi mushroom (*Ganoderma lucidum*), and valerian (*Valeriana officinalis*). Garlic is also thought to be preventive for atherosclerosis. *Ginkgo biloba* is used for varicose veins, obliterative arterial disease of the lower extremities, and intermittent claudication. Horse chestnut (*Aesculus hippocastanum*) is used for varicose veins and phlebitis, and valerian is used as an antispasmodic. Antihypertensive spices include basil, black pepper, fennel, and tarragon.

Note allergies, especially to iodine. Iodine is found in contrast agents used in diagnostic testing for vascular disorders.

■ FAMILY HEALTH HISTORY

The family health history helps to determine risk factors and provides clues about reported and observed manifestations. Note any family history of diabetes, hypertension, coronary artery disease, collagen diseases, and peripheral vascular disease.

■ PSYCHOSOCIAL HISTORY

Record the occupational history. If the client's occupation is unfamiliar to you, ask questions about the number of hours spent in various positions or activities (e.g., standing, prolonged sitting, walking, using vibrating machinery). In addition, some occupations involve contact with chemicals or are associated with cold or wet environments; note these also.

Find out whether or not the client smokes or has ever used any tobacco products. Ask about the use of prescription and over-the-counter nicotine products. Nicotine in any form is a potent vasoconstrictor.

Determine the client's nutrient and fluid intake (see Chapters 12 and 28). Ask about the usual intake of protein and calories. Also ask about sodium, cholesterol, and fat intake.

Assess the client's activity, rest, and sleep habits. Assess the extent to which clinical manifestations interfere with activities of daily living. Obtaining information about the frequency and duration of manifestations, precipitating activities, and their influence on daily life enables determination of disease severity. Assessment of the client's stress level, emotional state, and coping mechanisms (including the use of tobacco products, alcohol, or recreational drugs) is important.

Remain sensitive to the emotional effect of peripheral vascular disorders. Clients who have visible lesions may be embarrassed. Clients may have concern about the inability to perform self-care and about changes in role and sexual performance. Fear of amputation or functional loss may be significant.

■ REVIEW OF SYSTEMS

Review each body system as it relates to peripheral vascular disorders. Inquire about headaches, dizziness, TIAs, stroke, visual disturbances, hypertension, diabetes, pulmonary emboli, phlebitis, blood clots, leg pain or cramps, varicose veins, leg or foot ulcers, and cold hands or feet. Also see Chapter 9 for additional information about the review of systems.

PHYSICAL EXAMINATION

Physical examination of the vascular system involves inspection, palpation, and auscultation. Before starting the physical examination, prepare the environment. Natural lighting is the best because it allows assessment of subtleties in skin color. Warm the room to minimize cutaneous vasoconstriction. A quiet room is helpful for auscultating the low-pitched sounds commonly found in blood vessels. Clients who are free of vascular disorders display characteristics such as those described in the feature Physical Assessment in the Healthy Adult.

■ INSPECTION

Observe the extremities, noting skin color, hair distribution, nail beds and capillary refill, presence of muscle atrophy or edema, venous pattern, and ulcers. These are reviewed in detail next. Compare one side with the other. Begin with the head and upper extremities, and proceed toward the legs and feet.

Skin Color

A range of normal skin color is noted among people. Localized areas of cyanosis, rubor, or pallor are easily

PHYSICAL ASSESSMENT FINDINGS IN THE HEALTHY ADULT

Peripheral Vascular System

Inspection

Extremities of even contour, without edema. Even hair distribution; symmetrical venous pattern. Varicosities, skin lesions, and ulcers absent. Capillaries refill in less than 3 seconds on blanching.

Palpation

Extremities warm and dry without areas of localized heat or tenderness. Pulses (temporal, carotid, brachial, radial, ulnar, femoral, popliteal, posterior tibial, dorsalis pedis) are bilaterally equal and regular. No aneurysmal dilation of aorta.

Auscultation

Blood pressures equal in the upper extremities. Orthostatic hypotension absent. No bruits.

noticed in a person with fair skin (Fig. 51–1) but are more difficult to see in a person with darker skin tones (Fig. 51–2). For all clients, changes in skin color are best assessed by comparison with the contralateral limb. Ischemic pallor may be detected by comparing the palms of the hands, the soles of the feet, or the nail beds. Clients with arterial disorders may have pale extremities and cyanotic (blue-tinged) or red extremities with venous disorders.

Hair Distribution

Lack of hair growth may indicate chronically inadequate circulation to an area. This sign must be correlated with other signs of arterial insufficiency. It is not a valid indicator of acute arterial insufficiency.

Capillary Refill

Capillary refill time is an evaluation of peripheral perfusion and cardiac output. This assessment is usually completed while pulses are assessed. Depress the nail bed or the pad of the toe or finger until it blanches (becomes pale) (Fig. 51–3). Release pressure on the blanched area, and note the length of time for usual skin color to return. Capillaries usually refill in a fraction of a second, but "normal" times range up to 3 seconds for color return. With diminished blood flow, the return to the baseline color is delayed and a refill time of more than 3 seconds is sometimes called "sluggish." Note whether the room in which you are conducting the test is cold, because external temperatures can delay capillary refill.

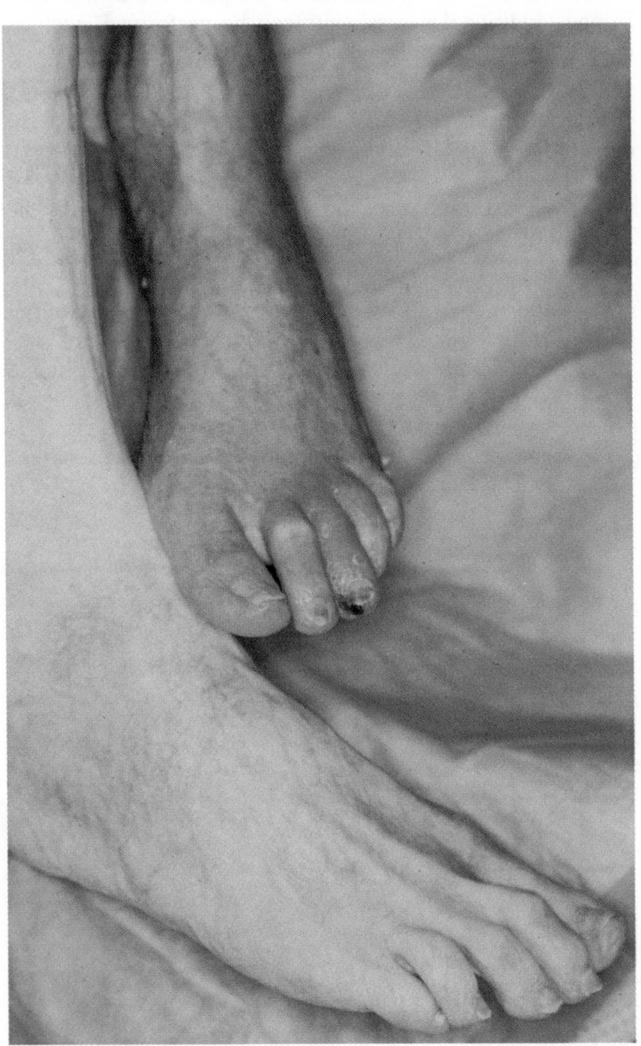

FIGURE 51–1 Dependent rubor is noted as a ruddy color in severe arterial insufficiency in this white client's left leg just minutes before amputation. (Note area of ulceration and necrosis on the third toe.)

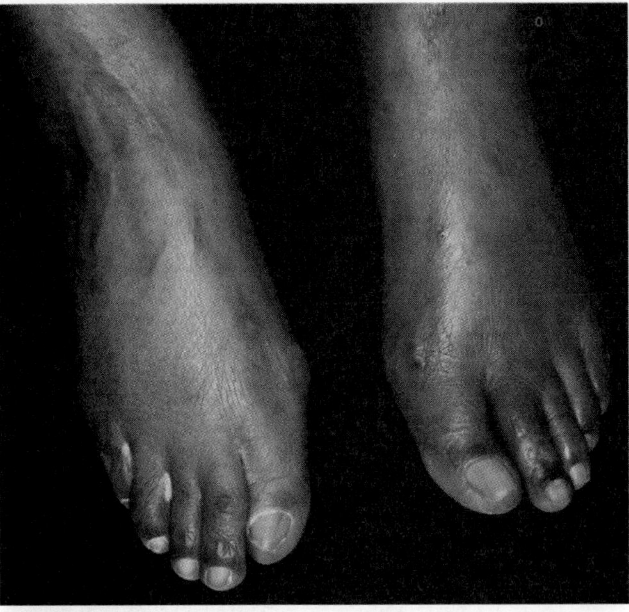

FIGURE 51–2 Dependent rubor in dark skin in the client's left foot has a reddish hue when compared to the unaffected right foot.

Muscle Atrophy

There can be many reasons for muscle atrophy in an extremity. If atrophy is noted, it may represent longstanding arterial insufficiency. Measure the muscle circumference, and compare it with that of the muscle on the opposite side.

Edema

To assess edema of the leg, push with your thumb on the skin over the client's foot or tibia for 5 seconds. If the skin is edematous, an indentation or pit will remain (thus the term *pitting edema*). Edema is often graded; however, scales used to grade edema are not universal. Because there is no established standard, it is most accurate to describe the edema as *present* or *absent, pitting* or *nonpitting* (Fig. 51–4).

Edema resulting from cardiac disease is generally bilateral and occurs in dependent areas (in the legs of a client who is ambulatory and the sacrum of a client who is bedridden). Unilateral edema is usually caused by oc-

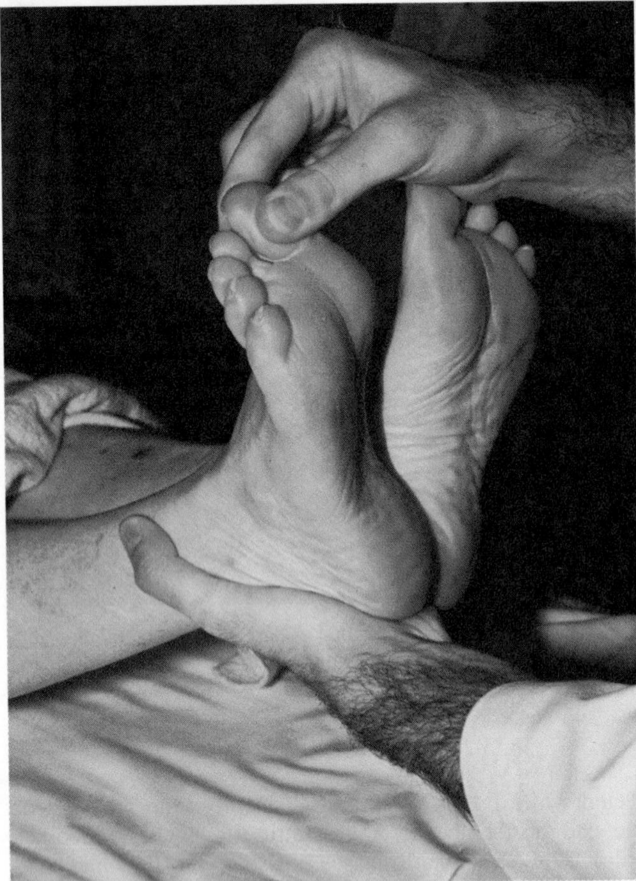

FIGURE 51–3 Determine capillary refill time by compressing the great toe and then releasing pressure. Count the number of seconds required for color to return to the skin.

clusion of a deep vein. Long-standing edema destroys the structure of the skin and the subcutaneous tissue and is easily recognized from its fibrotic appearance and firm texture.

Venous Pattern

Varicosities may indicate superficial or deep venous insufficiency. Note the presence, location, and distribution of *telangiectasias,* or "spider veins."

Ulcers

Note the presence of skin lesions or scar tissue (indicating healed ulcers); fissures of the feet and ulcers of the ankles and heels may be signs of arterial insufficiency. Tissue necrosis (see Fig. 51–1) and gangrene may be present with severe arterial disease. Examine between the toes for moist ulcers penetrating into the web spaces (Fig. 51–5).

Note the presence of other lesions, such as *angiomas* (benign tumors of blood and lymph vessels) and *petechiae* (small, purplish spots on the skin from several causes, including hemorrhage).

Additional Inspections

If arterial or venous disease is suspected but not confirmed, additional assessments can be performed, such as elevation pallor and Trendelenburg's test.

ELEVATION PALLOR

If arterial insufficiency is suspected, perform the test for elevation pallor. Because leg elevation can cause pain, perform this test only when needed. Note the degree of pallor at rest, and use the test only to determine the severity of ischemia. Perform the test as follows:

1. Elevate the legs 30 cm (12 inches) (Fig. 51–6). Pallor occurring within 60 seconds indicates arterial insufficiency.
2. Have the client dangle the legs from the side of the bed or examination table. Normally, the color returns within 10 seconds. Severe arterial insufficiency causes an exaggerated color change of dependent rubor.

FIGURE 51–4 To assess peripheral edema, press a finger into the skin over the client's tibia. Note the presence, depth, and persistence of any resulting depression. Use descriptive terms to record your findings.

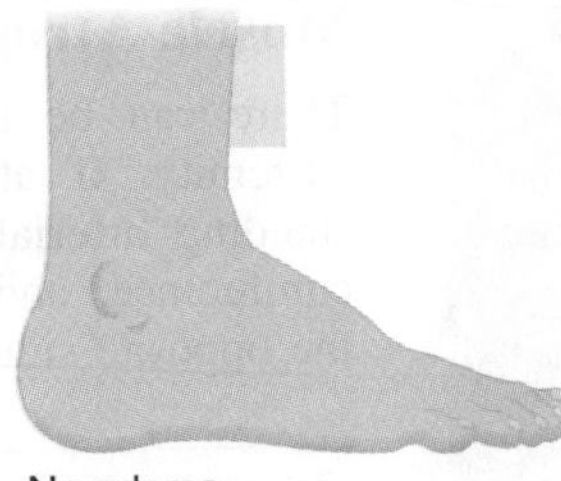

No edema

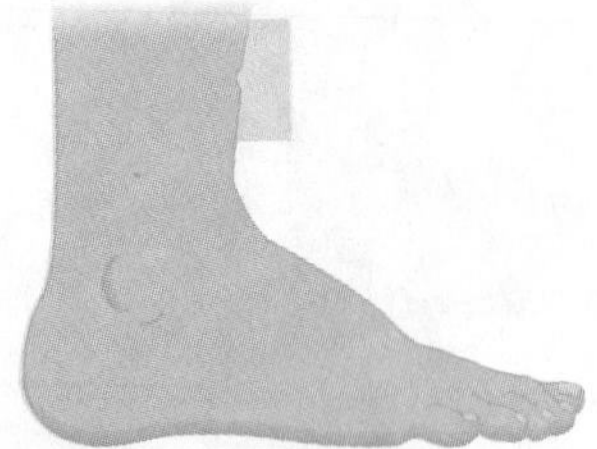

A barely detectable depression accompanied by normal foot and leg contours

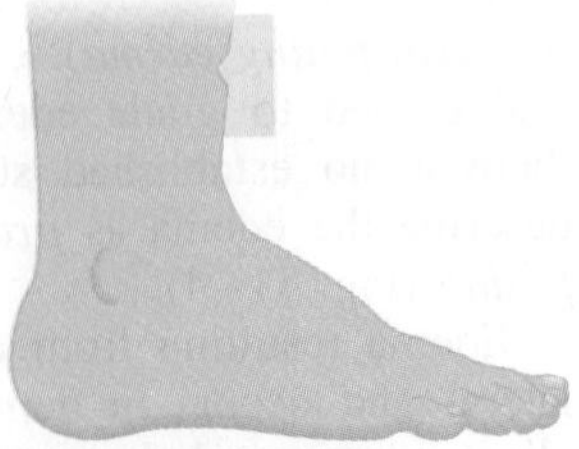

A deeper depression (less than 5 mm) accompanied by normal foot and leg contours

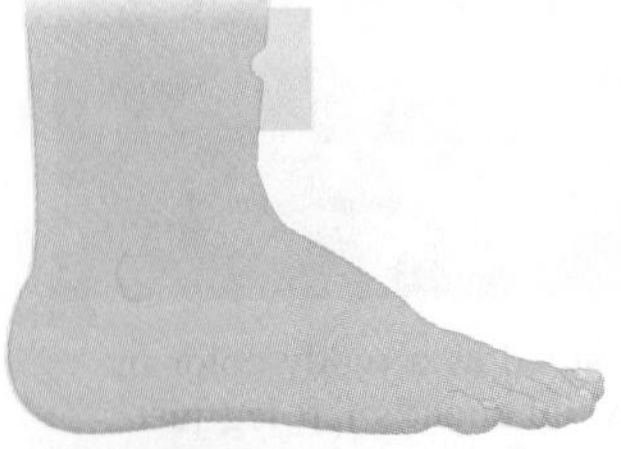

A deep depression (5 to 10 mm) accompanied by foot and leg swelling

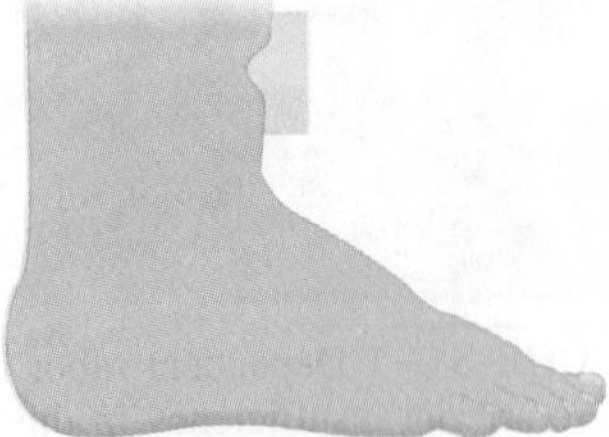

An even deeper depression (more than 1 cm) accompanied by severe foot and leg swelling

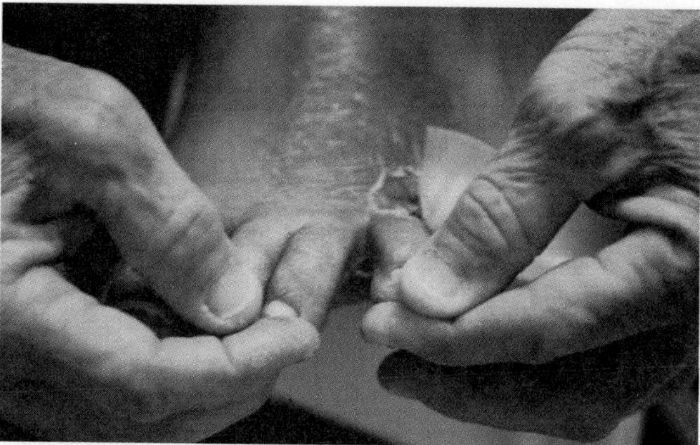

FIGURE 51–5 Carefully examine the web spaces for ulcers or maceration when assessing the foot.

TRENDELENBURG'S TEST

Intended to help detect abnormal venous filling time, Trendelenburg's test reveals valvular incompetence of the deep veins. Superficial varicose veins are easy to recognize. They appear as dilated, tortuous (twisted) veins. This test helps confirm leg vein valve competence. This noninvasive assessment maneuver may be performed by nurses who possess advanced assessment skills, as follows:

1. Have client lie down with the leg elevated until the veins empty.
2. Apply a tourniquet at midthigh snugly enough to occlude the superficial veins.
3. With the tourniquet in place, help the client stand.
4. Note the time required for the veins to fill from below. Veins usually fill in about 30 seconds.
5. After 60 seconds, release the tourniquet. Normally, when the tourniquet is released, no further blood fills the veins. Additional blood flowing into the vein from above indicates that a valve is incompetent and has allowed back-flow of blood.

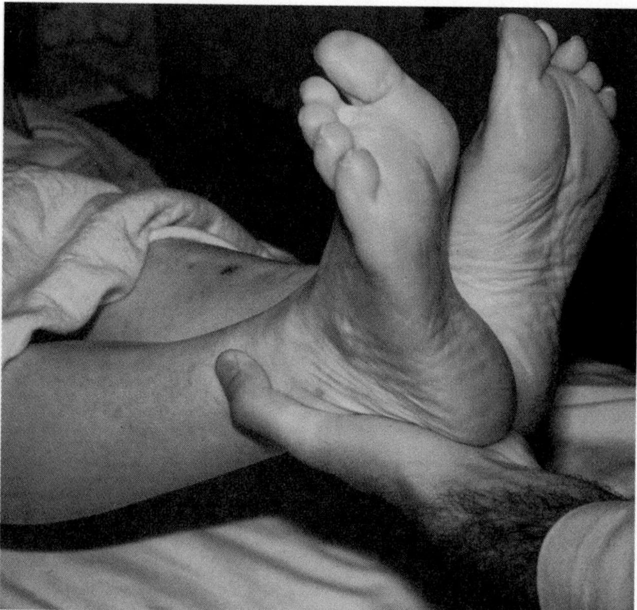

FIGURE 51–6 Assess for elevation pallor if arterial insufficiency is suspected.

PALPATION

Temperature

Palpate the arms and legs with the dorsal surface of your hand, and note the temperature (see Chapter 48, Fig. 48–3). Temperature should be similar in both contralateral limbs. Vasoconstriction produces cold, pale skin. Bilateral vasoconstriction may be caused by smoking, environmental temperature, anxiety, or generalized arterial disease. Unilateral or localized arterial vasoconstriction indicates arterial disease. Venous disorders may cause an increase in local skin temperature.

Pulses

Palpate pulses by placing the first three fingers of your dominant hand along the length of the selected artery. Apply gentle pressure against the artery, followed by a gradual release. Palpate temporal, carotid, brachial, radial, and ulnar pulses (upper extremities), and femoral, popliteal, posterior tibial, and dorsalis pedis pulses (lower extremities), as shown in Figure 51–7. Palpate pulses bilaterally and simultaneously, except for the carotid pulse (Fig. 51–8). Palpate carotid pulses separately to avoid stimulation of the carotid sinus, which may produce bradycardia or sinus arrest. Assess the ulnar pulse during Allen's test, as described later.

Palpate the abdominal aortic pulse by placing the palm of your hand over the upper abdomen just beneath the sternum while the client is supine. Use gentle pressure to push the abdomen downward. When you feel the aortic pulse, cup your fingers and thumb together to determine the width of the aorta (Fig. 51–9). You can use both hands if the client is large. When using both hands, place the lateral side of your right hand just left of the midline of the abdomen. Palpate using gentle pressure on the side of the aorta. Then place your left hand to the right of the abdominal midline. Estimate the width of the aorta as it pulsates toward your hands. In very obese clients, you may not be able to feel the aorta.

Always note the rhythm, amplitude, and symmetry of pulses. Compare peripheral pulses on the two sides for rate, rhythm, and quality. There are no standard numerical grades or rating scales for pulses. It is most accurate to describe the pulse as *palpable* (or present), *diminished* (weak), *absent,* or *aneurysmal* (easily palpable, bounding).

Note whether a pulse feels unequal on the two sides. The dorsalis pedis pulse is congenitally absent in approximately 10% to 17% of the normal adult population. The posterior tibial pulse is absent congenitally in 9% of the black adult population of the United States. In the elderly, dorsalis pedis and posterior tibial pulses may be more difficult to palpate. If they are found, mark the site with a pen to facilitate later examinations. Clients who have arterial grafts may have palpable pulses along the length of the graft.

If there is any question about the presence of a specific pulse, position your hand below the pulse you are seeking; then attempt to palpate the client's pulse again. This position will reduce the chance of mistaking your pulse for that of the client by establishing the difference between the two pulses.

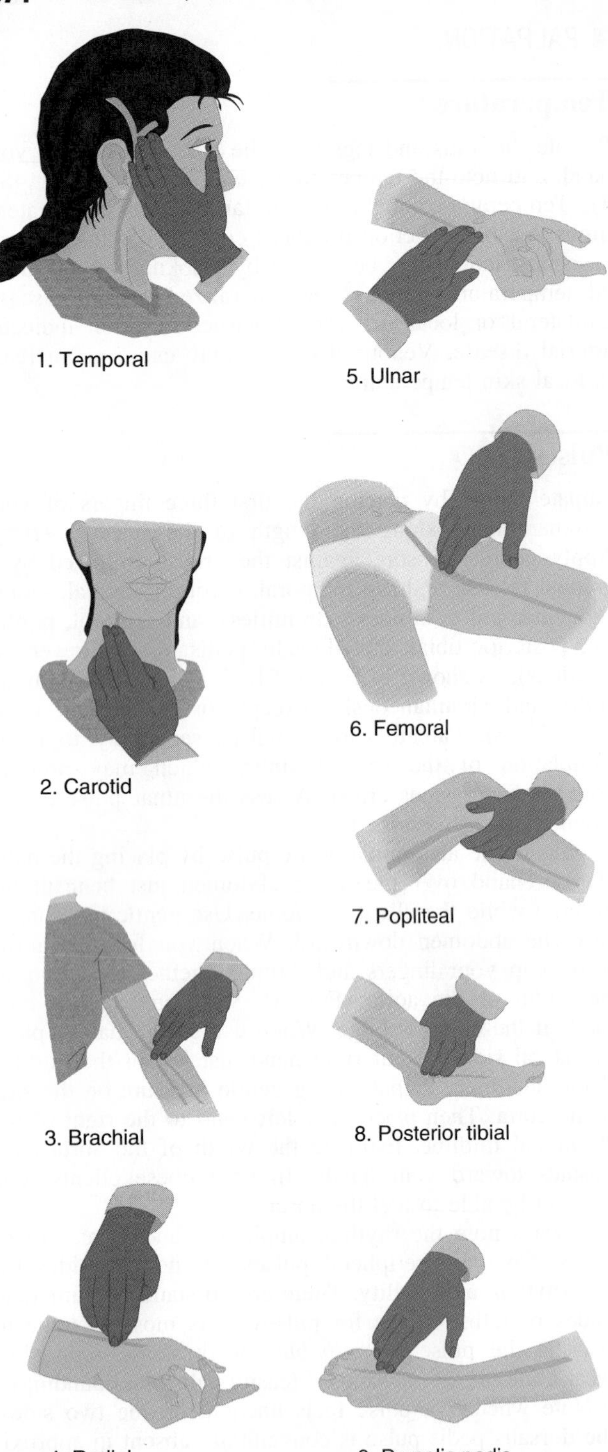

FIGURE 51–7 Assess pulses bilaterally from head to toe, comparing one side to the other for amplitude, rhythm, and symmetry. To prevent possible carotid sinus massage, do not palpate carotid pulses simultaneously. The carotid sinus is nerve tissue, located in the wall of the carotid artery, that helps regulate blood pressure. Massaging over this area may cause sinus bradycardia or syncope.

Allen's Test

Blood flow to the hand is supplied by both the ulnar and the radial arteries, which join at the volar arch in the palm. Allen's test is used to assess the patency of the radial and ulnar arteries distal to the wrist. It is commonly performed before arterial blood samples are drawn for analysis (see Chapter 14) or before an arterial line is inserted (see Chapter 55). Perform Allen's test as follows:

1. Ask the client to make a tight fist while you compress the radial and ulnar arteries.
2. Have the client open the hand, which should be pale and mottled.
3. Release the pressure on the radial artery while continuing to compress the ulnar artery. If the client's hand regains full color within about 6 seconds, the radial artery has normal patency.
4. Repeat steps 1 to 3, this time releasing the pressure on the ulnar artery to assess its patency.

If the client's hand remains pale during either portion of the test, the artery being tested may be occluded. Allen's test is shown in Chapter 59, Figure 59–14.

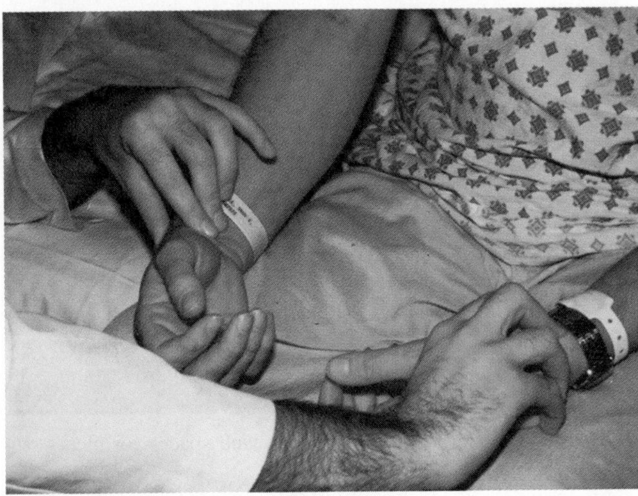

FIGURE 51–8 Palpating radial pulses.

Homans' Sign

The test for Homans' sign involves gently compressing the gastrocnemius muscle of the calf and asking the client whether this maneuver causes pain or tenderness. The test

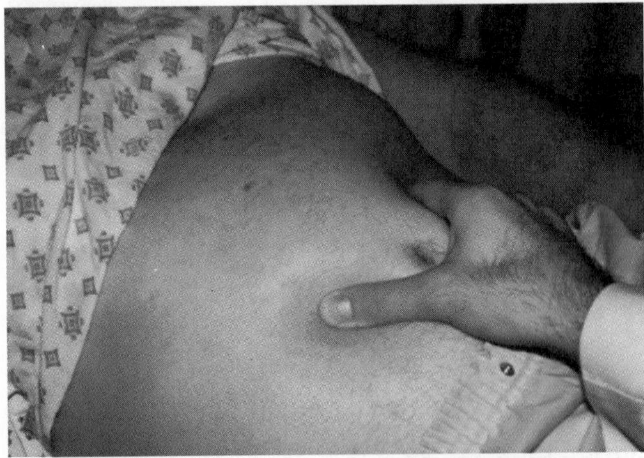

FIGURE 51–9 Palpate the abdomen for aortic aneurysm.

can also be performed by quickly dorsiflexing the foot (pointing the toes downward); calf pain that occurs with this maneuver is a positive finding of Homans' sign.

Homans' sign is unreliable, however. Studies indicate that only about 35% of people with deep venous thrombosis (DVT) have a positive response to Homans' test. Superficial phlebitis, Achilles' tendinitis, and plantar muscle injury can also elicit a positive Homans' sign. Therefore, 50% of the people who display a positive response to Homans' test do not have DVT. Doppler studies (see later discussion) are more accurate and should be used to confirm the diagnosis.

■ AUSCULTATION

Limb Blood Pressure

The measurement of arterial blood pressure is the most commonly performed noninvasive test of cardiac and vascular function. It may be the best single indicator of arterial perfusion. Arterial stenosis or occlusion produces regional hypotension. Arterial blood pressure is measured with a sphygmomanometer and a properly fitting cuff. For an accurate reading, place the cuff on the client's arm at the level of the heart; it should be wide enough to transmit pressure to the center of the arm and long enough to encircle the arm firmly. Auscultate the blood pressure in both arms. A few points' difference between readings is normal. A difference of 20 mm Hg between extremity readings may indicate aortic dissection or subclavian artery stenosis. Document asymmetrical readings. All subsequent blood pressure measurements should be performed on the arm with the higher reading. Measure blood pressure while the client is in supine, sitting, and standing positions when possible, and document the position of the client and the site used for each reading. Note *orthostatic* (positional) changes in blood pressure.

Auscultate over the carotid artery, aorta, and renal, femoral, and popliteal arteries to assess for the presence of bruits. A *bruit* is a "whooshing" sound that may be soft or loud; it results from turbulent blood flow from vessel wall irregularities. The presence of a bruit indicates some arterial narrowing. These arterial sounds are best heard with the bell of the stethoscope.

DIAGNOSTIC TESTS

■ NONINVASIVE VASCULAR LABORATORY TECHNIQUES

Noninvasive diagnostic techniques have assumed an increasingly important role in the management of vascular disorders. Noninvasive diagnostic tests provide reliable, objective data that can be used to evaluate the extent of vascular disease. Variables include blood flow velocity, blood flow abnormality, and some measure of functional limitations.

Doppler Ultrasonography

Hand-held Doppler ultrasonographic instruments permit assessment of arterial disease through (1) evaluation of audible arterial signals or (2) measurement of limb blood pressures (Fig. 51–10). Doppler ultrasonography is simple and inexpensive, but the technique may not detect minor disease, and it is less accurate than duplex scanning (see later). There is no special client preparation for this test.

Brightness-mode (*B-mode*) ultrasound refers to the creation of a two-dimensional image from ultrasound waves. It can be used to assess a vessel's size and compressibility, flow patterns, the presence or absence of thrombus, and valve function.

Ankle-Brachial Index

The ankle-brachial index (ABI) is a commonly used parameter for overall evaluation of extremity status. There is no special preparation for this test.

The client assumes a supine position, and a regular arm blood pressure cuff is applied to the leg above the malleolus. Doppler probes are used to identify the systolic end-point at both the dorsalis pedis and the posterior tibial sites (see Fig. 51–7). The higher of the two pressures is used as the indication of ankle blood pressure status. This number is then divided by the higher of the two brachial systolic artery pressures by means of the following formula:

$$\text{Ankle-brachial index} = \frac{\text{higher systolic ankle pressure}}{\text{higher systolic brachial pressure}}$$

A systolic ankle pressure of 60 mm Hg with a systolic brachial pressure of 120 mm Hg yields an ABI of 0.5. In normal circulation, ankle pressure is the same as or higher than the brachial pressure. Thus, an ABI of 1 or more is considered a normal finding; the client with an ABI of 0.5 to 0.8 typically experiences claudication, and the client with an ABI of 0.4 or less typically experiences rest pain.

In the presence of diabetes, the ABI is artificially elevated because of calcification, which prevents vessel wall compression. A toe-brachial index (TBI) is more reliable in clients who have diabetes (see Fig. 51–10).

Ultrasonic Duplex Scanning

Ultrasonic duplex scanners are used to (1) localize vascular obstruction, (2) evaluate the degree of stenosis, and (3) determine the presence or absence of vascular reflux (backward flow). This anatomic and physiologic test eval-

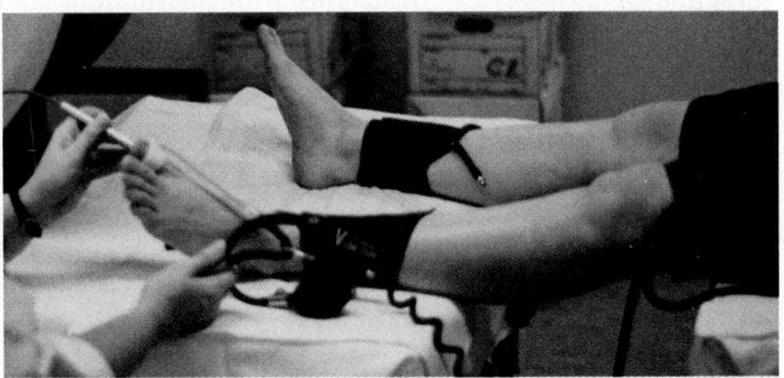

FIGURE 51–10 A Doppler probe is used to check toe pressures in the client with diabetes. Ankle pressures may be erroneously high because of calcification in the vessel wall.

uates the hemodynamic effects of arterial lesions. It is also the most sensitive and specific noninvasive modality for detecting DVT. Both an ultrasound image of the vessel and a Doppler audible signal and waveform are provided. The visual ultrasound data allow more specific localization of stenosis than simple pressure or waveform techniques. No special client preparation is required.

Air Plethysmography

Air plethysmography (APG) uses a pneumatic plethysmograph to measure volume changes in the legs. Venous reflux, venous obstruction, calf muscle pump function, and venous volume can be measured. A large cuff is applied to the client's calf, and a known volume of air is instilled to calibrate the cuff. Venous volume, ejection fraction, and residual volume fractions are then measured.

Impedance Plethysmography

Impedance plethysmography (IPG) and photoplethysmography (PPG) are also used to measure venous blood volume changes in the extremities. During the procedure, electrodes from a plethysmograph are applied to a limb along with a pressure cuff. As pressure is increased, electrical resistance is increased; thus, the quality of venous blood flow is demonstrated.

Inform the client about the purpose of the procedure. Explain that a technique similar to blood pressure measurement will be used. The client must be able to assume a supine position with the involved extremity elevated above the level of the heart.

Exercise Testing

Exercise or stress testing provides an objective measurement of the severity of intermittent claudication. It suggests the extent to which intermittent claudication interferes with the client's lifestyle. The most commonly used method for stress testing is the *treadmill exercise test.* This test is similar to that used for clients who have had a myocardial infarction, except that walking speed is usually 1.5 to 2 miles per hour (mph) with a grade elevation of 10% to 20% and a time limit of 5 minutes. A client who can walk 5 minutes is considered mildly symptomatic; a walking time of 1 minute represents severe disease.

Performance on the treadmill test is also gauged by measurement of ankle systolic pressure. In asymptomatic clients, the time required for return to pre-exercise ankle pressure is usually less than 3 minutes with a drop from baseline of 20% or less. In clients with intermittent claudication, recovery time is longer; ankle pressure is usually less than 50 mm Hg, and may be unrecordable during recovery.

The client undergoing stress testing should wear loose-fitting clothes and comfortable walking shoes. Explain the procedure so that the client knows what to expect. Inform the client that exercise will be stopped at the maximal level of exertion or when clinical manifestations become disabling.

Computed Tomography

Computed tomography (CT) provides a cross-section of vessel walls and other structures. CT scans can be used in the diagnosis of abdominal aortic aneurysms and postoperative complications, such as graft infection, graft occlusion, hemorrhage, and abscess. Chapter 11 covers client preparation during CT.

Magnetic Resonance Imaging

Magnetic resonance imaging (MRI) is used to detect tissue changes, such as tumors, aneurysms, and DVT, in the pelvic iliac veins and leg veins (see Chapter 11). Blood flow in an extremity is evaluated, with the limb to be examined placed in a cradle-like support in a flow cylinder.

In the future, MRI techniques likely will supply much of the information that today is available only with invasive angiography. Although MRI does not require ionizing radiation or injection into the arterial system, the expense and time necessary limit its use for routine screening and follow-up.

Magnetic Resonance Angiography

Magnetic resonance angiography (MRA) uses magnetic imaging techniques to access blood vessels. The advantage of this technique is that the images are not obscured by bone, bowel gas, fat, or vascular calcification. The vessel anatomy is displayed as a three-dimensional angiogram. MRA can be used to measure blood flow volume and blood viscosity. It is a noninvasive modality. The disadvantages are its limited availability, its cost, and the need for the client to hold still during the procedure. MRA cannot be used for people who have cardiac pacemakers or intracranial aneurysm clips.

■ INVASIVE TECHNIQUES

Angiography

Contrast angiography is the most invasive of the diagnostic procedures for arterial disorders and poses the greatest risk for the client. It is frequently performed before a vascular operation and can be used intraoperatively to evaluate the results of an operation.

Procedure

The procedure involves injecting a contrast agent into the arterial system and performing radiographic studies. Angiography is performed in an interventional laboratory or a special procedures room in the radiology department. The procedure is performed under sterile conditions. Local anesthesia is given at the injection site, and a catheter is placed percutaneously. After injection of a contrast agent through the catheter, fluoroscopy may be performed. Serial pictures of the dye movement are taken by cameras positioned over the study field (see Chapter 11).

Preprocedure Care

Explain the procedure, and obtain an informed consent. The client is given nothing by mouth (NPO) for 2 to 6 hours before the procedure. A mild sedative may be used.

Postprocedure Care

Nursing care after angiography usually involves routine postprocedural orders, including the following:

1. Frequent assessment of vital signs and neurologic function and distal pulse checks, with particular attention to the extremity that has been punctured.
2. Assessment of the puncture site for hematoma (bruising) and of the appearance of the extremity distal to the puncture site.
3. Bed rest for 6 to 8 hours, with the punctured extremity kept in straight alignment if the transfemoral approach was used. Use of the transaxillary approach does not require postprocedure bed rest.
4. Continuous intravenous (IV) hydration for 6 to 8 hours to assist with contrast excretion. Encourage oral fluid intake.
5. Assessment of blood urea nitrogen (BUN) and creatinine levels the next day.
6. Resumption of preprocedure diet and medications. If the client was receiving heparin, its administration may not be resumed until sealing of the puncture site has been confirmed.

Also assess motor and sensory function, especially if the client has undergone catheter insertion at the axillary site. Bleeding can compress the brachial plexus, resulting in permanent neurologic deficits. Report changes in neurologic function of the upper extremity immediately because they require emergency attention from the physician.

Pain at the injection site is fairly common and can usually be managed with mild analgesics. Severe pain or pain distal to the puncture site requires further assessment of peripheral pulses, neurovascular assessment, and palpation for masses, which may indicate a hematoma. Notify the physician of abnormal assessment data.

Complications of angiography, in addition to allergic reaction to the contrast medium, include thrombi, vessel wall perforation, emboli, renal failure, and pseudoaneurysm. *Pseudoaneurysm* is a significant complication and may extend the inpatient stay. A pseudoaneurysm is caused by blood leaking outside the vessel wall but within a contained area adjacent to the artery. There is a persistent communication between the artery and the fluid mass. Pseudoaneurysms generally result from arterial trauma (after arterial puncture). They provide a site for potential infection, can be a source of emboli, or may cause intravascular thrombosis. Pseudoaneurysms can become enlarged, compress an adjacent structure, and even rupture, although rupture is rare.

Venography

Venography, performed in a manner similar to that for angiography, is used to examine the venous system. Venograms can be used to detect DVT and other abnormalities, such as incompetent valves. This diagnostic test is performed less frequently than in the past. Newer, noninvasive vascular laboratory studies pose less risk, are more accurate, and provide functional information.

Procedure

For an *ascending* venogram, dye is injected into a vein in the foot to record patency of the veins. A *descending* venogram involves injecting a contrast agent into the femoral vein at the groin to evaluate vein reflux and valve incompetence.

Preprocedure Care

Document the presence and quality of peripheral pulses before the procedure. The client is usually given clear liquids for 3 to 4 hours before the procedure to help maintain adequate hydration. (See the earlier discussion of angiography and Chapter 11 for information about client preparation, informed consent, and use of contrast medium.)

Postprocedure Care

After the procedure, a pressure dressing is placed on the injection site. The client should remain at bed rest for 2 hours after the procedure if the femoral vein was punctured. Monitor pulses distal to the site for the next 4 to 6 hours. Continue IV fluids for 8 to 24 hours after the procedure to help promote dye excretion. Assess fluid balance: observe for signs of fluid overload (also see Chapter 12). When the client returns to the nursing unit, monitor vital signs, palpate pulses, and observe the insertion site frequently for bleeding or hematoma formation.

Vascular Endoscopy (Angioscopy)

Vascular endoscopy permits imaging of intra-arterial disease with the use of fiberoptic technology. Images are in color and in three dimensions. Equipment consists of a flexible fiberoptic angioscope, a light source, an irrigation system, a camera, a video recorder, and a monitor. The major advantage of angioscopy is the internal visualization of the vessel lumen. This enables identification of thrombus (blood clot), plaque, hemorrhage, ulceration, or embolus (clot that has broken off from a thrombus and lodged in a more distal artery). Angioscopes can be used to remove debris from vessels and to check the integrity of an anastomosis (suture line that connects a vessel grafted to a native vessel) from within a vessel. They may also be used to remove venous valves in preparation for use of the vein as a bypass graft.

Complications of vascular endoscopy are rare but may include intimal damage, vessel spasm, thrombosis or embolism, perforation, fluid overload, and infection. Postprocedure care is similar to that for clients who have undergone angiography.

Intravascular Ultrasonography

Intravascular ultrasonography provides information about the atherosclerotic intima beneath the luminal surface. It can thus determine the thickness of the arterial wall and can distinguish thrombus and calcium from vascular tissue, allowing more exact removal of lesions. One current limiting factor is the need for specialized interpretation of the scans.

CONCLUSIONS

Vascular assessment requires inspection, palpation, and auscultation skills. Knowledge of anatomy is critical for correct performance of assessments. Diagnostic modalities can range from simple noninvasive tests to complex, sophisticated, invasive technology. A clear understanding of the indications for diagnostic tests and interpretation of the findings assists the clinical decision-making.

BIBLIOGRAPHY

1. Baker, J. D. (1991). Assessment of peripheral arterial occlusive disease. *Critical Care Nursing Clinics of North America, 3*(3), 493–498.
2. Barnes, R. W. (1991). Noninvasive diagnostic assessment of peripheral vascular disease. *Circulation, 83*(suppl. I), I-20–I-27.
3. Bright, L. D., & Georgi, S. (1992). Peripheral vascular disease: Is it arterial or venous? *American Journal of Nursing, 92*(9), 34–43.
4. Fahey, V. (1999). *Vascular nursing* (3rd ed.). Philadelphia: W. B. Saunders.
5. Herbert, L. M. (1997). *Caring for the vascular patient.* New York: Churchill Livingstone.
6. Kerstein, M. D., & White, J. V. (1995). *Alternatives to open vascular surgery.* Philadelpia: J. B. Lippincott.
7. Moore, W. S. (Ed). (1998). *Vascular surgery: A comprehensive review.* Philadelphia: W. B. Saunders.
8. Rutherford, R. B. (Ed). (2000). *Vascular surgery* (5th ed.). Philadelphia: W. B. Saunders.
9. Sloan, H., & Wills, E. M. (1999). Ankle-brachial index: Calculating your patient's vascular risks. *Nursing, 99*(10), 58–59.

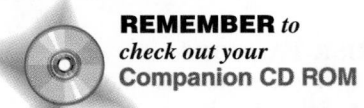

CHAPTER 52

Clients with Hypertensive Disorders: Promoting Positive Outcomes

Jean Elizabeth DeMartinis

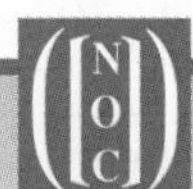

NURSING OUTCOMES CLASSIFICATION (NOC)
for Nursing Diagnoses—Clients with Hypertensive Disorders

Altered Health Maintenance
Health Belief: Perceived Resources
Health-Promoting Behavior
Health-Seeking Behavior
Knowledge: Health Behaviors
Knowledge: Health Promotion
Knowledge: Health Resources
Participation: Health Care Decisions
Psychosocial Adjustment: Life Changes
Risk Detection
Self-Direction of Care
Social Support
Treatment Behavior: Illness or injury

Altered Nutrition: More than Body Requirements
Nutritional Status: Food and Fluid Intake
Nutritional Status: Nutrient Intake
Weight Control

Ineffective Management of Therapeutic Regimen (Individual)
Compliance Behavior
Knowledge: Treatment Regimen
Participation: Health Care Decisions

Noncompliance
Adherence Behavior
Compliance Behavior
Symptom Control
Treatment Behavior: Illness or Injury

Pain
Comfort Level
Pain Control

HYPERTENSION

Arterial hypertension, simply put, is high blood pressure. It is defined as a persistent elevation of the systolic blood pressure at a level of 140 mm Hg or higher and of diastolic pressure at a level of 90 mm Hg or higher. The National Institute of Health's Sixth Report of the Joint National Committee on Detection, Evaluation, and Treatment of High Blood Pressure (JNC VI) and the Centers for Disease Control and Prevention (CDC) publications *Healthy People 2000* and *Healthy People 2010* have documented the advances made over the last few decades regarding prevention, detection, and treatment of hypertension.[16, 25] Members of the public have become more knowledgeable about high blood pressure, are more likely to visit a health care provider for hypertension, and are more likely to follow medical advice. The use of increasingly effective antihypertensive agents has also dramatically reduced the mortality rate associated with hypertension. The percentage of people receiving treatment for their hypertension has increased from 31% to 55%, and of those with controlled hypertension, from 10% to 29%. Ultimately, the combined effects of these measures have contributed to a 60% decline in stroke and a 53% decline in coronary artery disease mortality.[13] These impressive gains have been seen across all age groups, in both men and women, and in special populations.

However, the JNC VI and *Healthy People 2010* reports also document some disturbing current trends. After years of decline, the mortality rates for coronary heart disease and stroke leveled off and have begun to rise again. Hypertension prevalence is on the rise, and control rates are decreasing. Arterial hypertension affects approximately 50 million persons—1 in 4—in the United States, with the highest rates of occurrence among the elderly, African Americans, less educated, and poorer people. It is estimated that only 25% of all people with hypertension have blood pressure controlled at a target level below 140/90 mm Hg. Lack of client compliance and providers' continued ignorance of the need to prescribe and manage holistic treatment protocols are cited as the two major factors that have contributed to this abysmal decline in improvement in client outcomes toward identification and control of their hypertension.[9, 11, 16, 25]

Coronary events such as a "heart attack" are still the most common result of hypertension.[30] Increased blood pressure level is related to increased severity of atherosclerosis, stroke, nephropathy, peripheral vascular disease, aortic aneurysms, and heart failure. Nearly all people with heart failure have antecedent hypertension. If hypertension is left untreated, nearly half of hypertensive clients will die of heart disease, a third will die of stroke, and the remaining 10% to 15% will die of renal failure.[16] Hypertension is also a "silent factor" in the etiology of many deaths attributed to stroke or heart attacks.[25, 26]

These disturbing trends indicate the need for renewed vigor in the battle against hypertension.[23] Hypertension-related morbidity and mortality will not decrease until providers appreciate the need for changes in existing treatment protocols that support a comprehensive holistic management plan, and that are based on quantifiable client outcomes. The *Healthy People 2000/2010* guidelines are prevention-focused, and the JNC VI guidelines are also now primarily prevention-focused and strongly recommend the use of nonpharmaceutical as well as pharmaceutical measures to prevent and treat hypertension.[16, 25] Nurses are faced with a profound urgency to enhance public and professional education toward this end and to translate the results of research into improved practice.[30] An ambitious, but nevertheless feasible, goal is the diagnosis and treatment of hypertension in all affected people in the United States.

Types of Hypertensive Disease, Etiology, and Severity

Hypertension is characterized by type, cause, and severity (Box 52–1).[2, 10–12, 17, 23, 24] People with hypertensive disease have either combined systolic and diastolic elevations in pressure or isolated systolic pressure elevation alone. The blood pressure remains elevated and continues to rise over time because of a persistent and progressive increase in peripheral arterial resistance. The persistent rise in arterial resistance is due to inappropriate renal retention of salt and water and/or abnormalities of or within the vessel wall. The severity of the condition directly relates to the number and magnitude of risk factors present, the length of time for which these risk factors have been present, and the presence of accompanying disease states.

Epidemiology and Risk Factors

Primary *(essential)* hypertension constitutes more than 90% of all cases of hypertension. Fewer than 5% to 8% of adult hypertensive clients have secondary hypertension. However, hypertension, regardless of type, results from an array of genetic and environmental factors. The following text discusses the major nonmodifiable and modifiable risk factors that contribute to the development of hypertension. There is necessarily some overlap between categories.[2, 10, 12, 16, 24]

Secondary hypertension is an elevation in blood pressure from an identifiable disease, such as renal failure. *Malignant* hypertension, or persistent severe hypertension, is a sustained elevation in blood pressure combined with end-organ damage.

Nonmodifiable Risk Factors

Family History. Hypertension is thought to be polygenic and multifactorial—that is, in any person with a family history of hypertension, several genes may interact with each other and the environment to cause the blood pressure to elevate over time. The genetic predisposition that makes certain families more susceptible to hypertension may be related to an elevation in intracellular sodium levels and to lowered potassium-to-sodium ratios. This is found more often in blacks. Clients with parents who have hypertension are at greater risk for hypertension at a younger age.

Age. Primary hypertension typically appears between the ages of 30 and 50 years. The incidence of hypertension increases with age; 50% to 60% of clients older than 60 years have a blood pressure over 140/90 mm Hg.

BOX 52–1 Types of Hypertension

Primary hypertension—also known as *essential* or idiopathic hypertension. The etiology is a multifactorial, with no identifiable cause, but several interacting homeostatic forces are generally involved concomitantly. Most cases of combined systolic and diastolic elevation fall into this category. Severity of sequelae increases as the blood pressure, both systolic and diastolic, increases.

Secondary hypertension—results from an identifiable cause. Various specific disease states or problems are responsible for the elevation in blood pressure (see Box 52–2), and underlying causes may be correctable. Therefore, it is important to isolate the root of the problem so that the most appropriate treatment regimen can be prescribed. Severity depends on underlying causes, personal and environmental factors, and duration of concurrent disease states.

"White coat hypertension"—defined as hypertension in people who are actually normotensive except when their blood pressure is measured by a health care professional. An intermittent vasovagal response accounts for the transient elevation in blood pressure. Differentiation between this diagnosis and essential or secondary hypertension is crucial so that the latter can be treated effectively. Treating this false hypertension produces significant hypotension and severe deleterious sequelae. However, the converse is also true; essential or secondary hypertension disguised as "white coat" hypertension and left undiagnosed and untreated can have ominous consequences over time.

Isolated systolic hypertension (ISH)—occurs when the systolic blood pressure is 140 mm Hg or higher but the diastolic blood pressure remains less than 90 mm Hg. It is thought to emerge because of increased cardiac output or atherosclerosis-induced changes in blood vessel compliance or both in older adults. The likelihood of development of ISH increases with advancing age, as does the severity of ISN.

Malignant hypertension—persistent *severe* hypertension characterized by a diastolic blood pressure above 110 to 120 mm Hg. It results when hypertension is left untreated or is unresponsive to treatment and becomes a truly severe emergency condition as the pressure continues to rise unchecked.

However, epidemiologic studies have shown a poorer prognosis in clients whose hypertension began at a young age. Isolated systolic hypertension occurs primarily in people older than 50 years, with almost 24% of all people affected by age 80 years. Among older adults, systolic blood pressure readings are a better predictor of possible future events such as coronary heart disease, stroke, heart failure, and renal disease than are diastolic blood pressure readings.

GENDER. The overall incidence of hypertension is higher in men than in women until about age 55 years. Between the ages of 55 and 74 years, the risk in men and that in women are almost equal; then, after age 74 years, women are at greater risk. Men are also at greater risk for cardiovascular morbidity and mortality. The reasons are not clear.

ETHNICITY. Mortality statistics indicate that the death rate for adults with hypertension is lowest for white women at 4.7%; white men have the next lowest rate at 6.3%, and black men have the next lowest at 22.5%; the death rate is highest for black women at 29.3%. The reason for the increased prevalence of hypertension among blacks is unclear, but the increase has been attributed to lower renin levels, greater sensitivity to vasopressin, higher salt intake, and greater environmental stress.

MODIFIABLE RISK FACTORS

STRESS. Because stress is a matter of perception, people's interpretations of events are what create most stressors and stress responses. Environmental factors or events, personality characteristics, and physiologic phenomena may either cause or set the stage for the mobilization of the stress response. Stressors such as noise, infection, inflammation, pain, decreased oxygen supply, heat, cold, trauma, prolonged exertion, responses to life events, obesity, old age, drugs, disease, surgery, and medical treatment can elicit the stress response. These noxious stimuli are perceived by a person as a threat or capable of causing harm, and subsequently a psychophysiologic "fight-or-flight" response is initiated in the body.

Stress increases peripheral vascular resistance and cardiac output and stimulates sympathetic nervous system activity. Over time, hypertension can develop. Chronic stress, when unable to be stopped, will aggravate existing physical and emotional instability, further exacerbating the response. Should stress arousal be excessive or prolonged, target organ dysfunction or disease will result. A report from the American Institute of Stress estimates that 60% to 90% of all primary care visits involve stress-related complaints.[3]

OBESITY. Obesity, especially in the upper body (giving an "apple" shape), with increased amounts of fat about the midriff, waist, and abdomen, is associated with subsequent development of hypertension. However, people who are overweight but who carry most of their excess weight in the buttocks, hips, and thighs (giving a "pear" shape) are at far less risk for development of hypertension secondary to increased weight alone.

NUTRIENTS. Sodium consumption can be an important factor in the development of essential hypertension. A high-salt diet may induce excessive release of natriuretic hormone, which may indirectly increase blood pressure. Sodium loading also stimulates vasopressor mechanisms within the central nervous system (CNS). Studies also show that low dietary intake of calcium, potassium, and magnesium can contribute to the development of hypertension.

SUBSTANCE ABUSE. Cigarette smoking, heavy alcohol consumption, and some illicit drug use all are risk factors for hypertension. The nicotine in cigarette smoke and drugs such as cocaine cause an immediate rise in blood pressure that is dose-dependent; however, *habitual* use of these substances has been implicated in increased incidence of hypertension over time. The incidence of hypertension is also higher among people who drink more than 3 ounces of ethanol per day. The impact of caffeine is controversial. Caffeine raises blood pressure acutely but does not have sustained effects.

Pathophysiology

PRIMARY (ESSENTIAL) HYPERTENSION

The exact pathologic underpinnings of primary hypertension remain to be established. Any factor producing an alteration in peripheral vascular resistance, heart rate, or stroke volume affects systemic arterial blood pressure. Four control systems play a major role in maintaining blood pressure[12]: (1) the arterial baroreceptor and chemoreceptors system, (2) regulation of body fluid volume, (3) the renin-angiotensin system, and (4) vascular autoregulation. Hypotheses derived to explain the onset of primary hypertension in people at risk propose that a defect or malfunction must exist in some or all of these systems. Probably no single defect causes essential hypertension in all affected people.

Arterial baroreceptors and chemoreceptors work reflexively to control blood pressure (Fig. 52–1). Baroreceptors, major stretch receptors, are found in the carotid sinus, aorta, and wall of the left ventricle. They monitor the level of arterial pressure and counteract rises through vasodilatation and slowing of the heart rate via the vagus nerve. Chemoreceptors, located in the medulla and carotid and aortic bodies, are sensitive to changes in concentrations of oxygen, carbon dioxide, and hydrogen ions (pH) in the blood. A decrease in arterial oxygen concentration or pH causes a reflexive rise in pressure, whereas an increase in carbon dioxide concentration causes a decrease in blood pressure. The major reflex response is to changes in oxygen saturation, and effects of changes in pH and carbon dioxide are minor.

The role of the arterial baroreceptors and chemoreceptors in hypertension is not well understood. The stretch receptors may become desensitized because they must continue to "reset" as prolonged, sustained increases in pressure continue. Chemoreceptor autoregulation may be altered as blood volume rises, and sympathetic overstimulation becomes apparent.

Changes in fluid volume affect systemic arterial pressure. Thus, an abnormality in the transport of sodium in the renal tubules may cause essential hypertension. When sodium and water are in excess, total blood volume increases, thereby increasing blood pressure. In functional kidneys, a rise in pressure leads to diuresis. Pathologic changes that alter the pressure threshold at which kidneys excrete salt and water alter systemic blood pressure. In addition, the overproduction of sodium-retaining hormones has been implicated in hypertension.

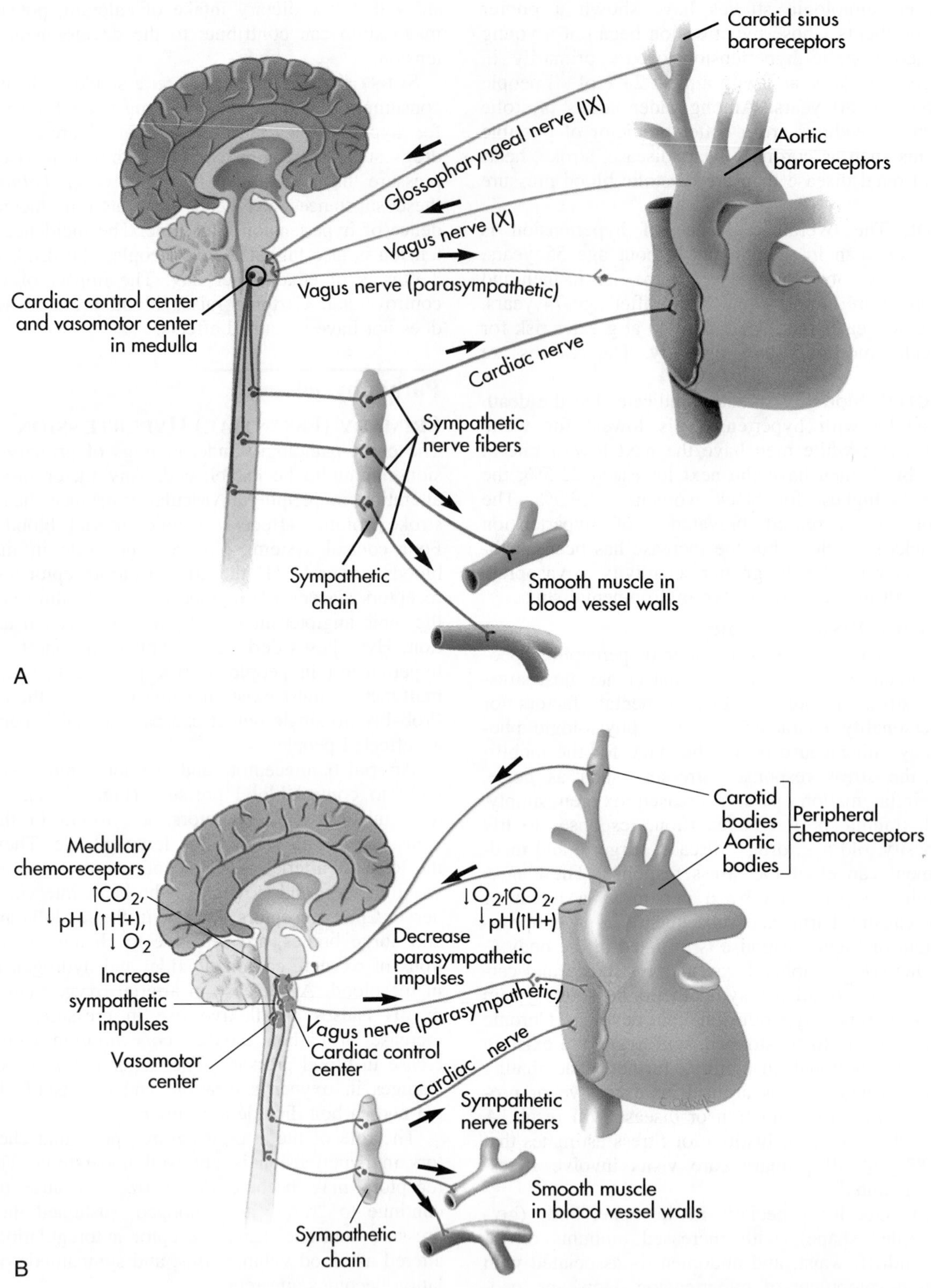

FIGURE 52–1 Baroreceptor and chemoreceptor reflex control of blood pressure. *A,* Baroreceptor reflexes. Baroreceptors located in the carotid sinuses and aortic arch detect changes in blood pressure. The heart rate can be decreased by the parasympathetic system; the heart rate and stroke volume can be increased by the sympathetic system. The sympathetic system also can constrict or dilate blood vessels. *B,* Chemoreceptor reflexes. Chemoreceptors located in the medulla oblongata and in the carotid and aortic bodies detect changes in blood oxygen, carbon dioxide, or pH. In response, the vasomotor center can cause vasoconstriction or dilation of blood vessels by the sympathetic system, and the cardioregulatory center can cause changes in the pumping activity of the heart through the parasympathetic and sympathetic systems. (From Seeley, R. R., Stephens, T. D., & Tate, P. [1995]. *Anatomy and physiology* [3rd ed.]. St. Louis: Mosby–Year Book.)

Renin and angiotensin play a role in blood pressure regulation. Renin is an enzyme produced by the kidney that catalyzes a plasma protein substrate to split off angiotensin I, which is removed by a converting enzyme to the lung to form angiotensin II and then angiotensin III (Fig. 52–2). Angiotensin II and III act as vasoconstrictors and also stimulate aldosterone release. With increased sympathetic nervous system activity, angiotensin II and III also seem to inhibit sodium excretion, which results in elevated blood pressure. Increased renin secretion has been investigated as a cause of increased peripheral vascular resistance in primary hypertension. Hypertension may also develop from deficiencies in vasodilator substances, such as prostaglandins, from congenital abnormalities in resistance vessels (arterioles), or from defects in neuroendocrine secretion.

SECONDARY HYPERTENSION

Many renal, vascular, neurologic, endocrine, and drug- and food-induced problems that directly or indirectly negatively affect the kidneys can result in serious insult to these organs that interferes with sodium excretion, renal perfusion, or the renin-angiotensin-aldosterone mechanism, leading to an elevation in blood pressure over time (Box 52–2).

Chronic renal disease, mainly chronic glomerulonephritis and renal artery stenosis, is the most common cause of secondary hypertension. Also, the adrenal glands cause secondary hypertension as a result of primary excesses of aldosterone, cortisol, and catecholamines. Primary aldosteronism usually arises from solitary benign adenomas of the adrenal cortex that release excess aldosterone. Excess aldosterone causes renal retention of sodium and water, expands blood volume, and elevates blood pressure. Pheochromocytoma, a small tumor of the adrenal medulla, can cause dramatic hypertension because of the release of excessive amounts of epinephrine and norepinephrine. Other adrenocortical problems can result in excess production of cortisol (Cushing's syndrome). Clients with Cushing's syndrome have an 80% risk for development of hypertension. Cortisol increases blood pressure by increasing renal sodium retention, angiotensin II levels, and vascular reactivity to norepinephrine. Chronic stress induces prolonged elevated blood levels of catecholamines, certain hormones, and cortisol.

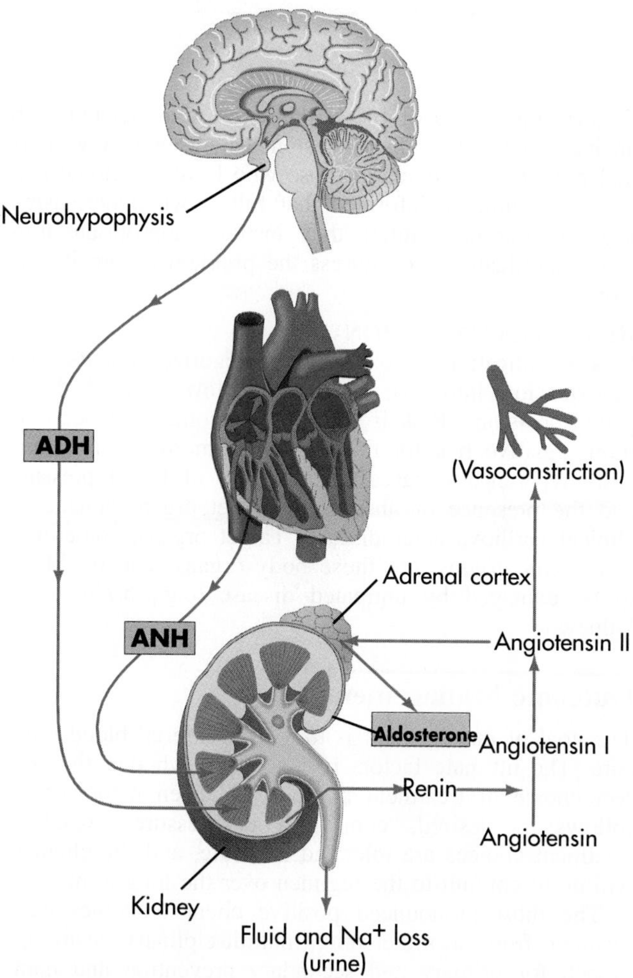

FIGURE 52–2 Renin-angiotensin-aldosterone regulation of blood pressure. (From Thibodeau, G. A., Patton, K. T. (1999). *Anatomy and physiology: A student survival guide*. St. Louis: Mosby.

VESSEL CHANGES

Early in the course of development of hypertension, there may be no obvious pathologic changes in the blood vessels and organs other than intermittent elevations of blood pressure (*labile* hypertension). Slowly, widespread pathologic changes take place in both the large and small blood vessels and in the heart, kidneys, and brain.[12]

The large vessels, such as the aorta, coronary arteries, basilar artery to the brain, and peripheral vessels in the limbs, become sclerotic, tortuous, and weak. Their lumina narrow, with resultant decreased blood flow to the heart, brain, and lower extremities. As the damage continues, large vessels may become occluded or may hemorrhage, causing infarction of the tissue supplied by the vessel that has suddenly been robbed of its blood supply.

Small vessel damage, equally dangerous, causes structural changes in the heart, kidneys, and brain. Elevated diastolic blood pressure damages the intimal lining of the small vessels. Because of intimal damage, fibrin accumulates in the vessels, local edema develops, and intravascular clotting may occur. The net results of these changes are (1) a decreased blood supply to the tissues of the heart, brain, kidneys, and retina; (2) progressive functional impairment of these organs; and (3) finally, as a consequence of the chronic ischemia, infarction of the tissue supplied by these vessels, originating in much the same way as with occlusion of the large vessels.

Clinical Manifestations

In the early stages of development of hypertension, there are no clinical manifestations overt to clients or practitioners. Eventually, the blood pressure will rise, but early on, no clinical manifestations are present to alert the client of the problem. If elevated blood pressure is not caught during a routine screening, clients are still unaware that they have an elevated pressure and therefore do not seek health care for diagnosis of the cause and management of the condition. If the condition is left un-

BOX 52–2 Causes of Secondary Hypertension

Renal disorders

Renal parenchymal disease
- Acute glomerulonephritis
- Chronic nephritis
- Polycystic disease
- Connective tissue diseases
- Diabetic nephropathy
- Hydronephrosis

Renal artery stenosis
Renin-producing tumors

Endocrine disorders

Acromegaly
Hypothyroidism
Hyperthyroidism
Adrenal disorders
- Cortical
  - Cushing's syndrome
  - Primary aldosteronism
- Medullary
  - Pancreatitis
  - Pheochromocytoma

Neurologic disorders

Increased intracranial pressure
- Brain tumor
- Encephalitis

Sleep apnea
Autonomic dysreflexia

Medications

Oral contraceptives
Glucocorticoids
Mineralocorticoids
Cyclosporine
Erythropoietin
Monoamine oxidase (MAO) inhibitors
Tricyclic antidepressants
Cocaine use
Amphetamine use

Tyramine-containing foods

Aged cheeses (especially cheddar)
Chicken liver
Yeast extract
Beer, wine

Acute stress

Psychogenic hyperventilation
Hypoglycemia
Burns
Alcohol withdrawal

Vascular disorders

Arteriosclerosis
Coarctation of the aorta
Sickle cell crisis
Increased intravascular volume

Pregnancy-induced hypertension

diagnosed, the blood pressure will continue to rise, clinical manifestations will become apparent, and clients will eventually report to a provider's office with complaints of persistent headaches, fatigue, dizziness, palpitations, flushing, blurred or double vision, or epistaxis.[11, 16, 18, 23, 24]

Assessment of the client with hypertension involves the following three main objectives:

- To determine the extent of target organ involvement
- To ascertain the presence of other cardiovascular risk factors
- To identify the type of hypertension (primary or secondary)

Clinicians can obtain information relevant to these areas from the history, physical examination, and laboratory studies (Box 52–3).[21] The diagnosis of hypertension is made when, after the seated client has been allowed to rest for at least 5 minutes, the average of two or more readings separated by at least 2 minutes is 140 mm Hg or higher for the systolic blood pressure and 90 mm Hg or higher for the diastolic pressure. Follow-up examinations are scheduled to diagnose or rule out the presence of hypertension (see Table 52–1), unless first-visit measurement averages fall into either stage 2 or stage 3 or the client is in risk group C (see later). In such cases, the client is diagnosed with hypertension on the basis of the first-visit measurements, and a temporary management plan is implemented to bring the blood pressure down immediately or in a short time. However, careful differentiation of primary from secondary causes of the high blood pressure must precede any long-term management plan.

Hypertension is classified into stages 1 through 3 according to the blood pressure readings (see Table 52–2). It is important to identify "high-normal" values as well, because this range of blood pressures is associated with an increased risk of hypertension. Clients with high-normal pressures, particularly those who have additional risk factors, should be informed that full-blown hypertension may be imminent unless they institute appropriate lifestyle modifications to address the problem before it gets worse.

RISK STRATIFICATION

Risk stratification (Table 52–3) categorizes clients with hypertension into risk groups to allow optimal therapeutic decisions. Risk is based on outcome evidence outlining relative risk for morbidity and mortality in clients with hypertension based on the level of blood pressure and the presence or absence of target organ damage or clinical cardiovascular disease. Target organs, sometimes called *end organs,* are those body organs that are likely to be damaged by untreated disease (e.g., brain, eyes, kidneys).

Outcome Management

The goal of management is to control arterial blood pressure. The ultimate factors in evaluating whether the correct choice of treatment regimen has been made are as follows: the desired, "control" blood pressure is reached, treatment choices are tolerated and safe, and the client is willing to commit to the regimen over the long term.

The most pronounced positive client outcomes have resulted from a systematic, multidisciplinary team approach for primary and secondary prevention and management of hypertension using diverse qualified health care professionals.[11, 24–26, 29, 30] Multidisciplinary teams can provide the most comprehensive, cost-effective care of clients with a multitude of prevention and management

BOX 52–3 Assessment of the Client with Hypertension

History

Note the following points when interviewing the hypertensive client:

- Family history of hypertension, diabetes mellitus, cardiovascular disease, hyperlipidemia, or renal disease, smoking, stress, obesity, or sedentary lifestyle
- Previous documentation of high blood pressure, including age at onset, level of elevation, and currently prescribed medical regimen
- History of all prescribed and over-the-counter medications and the client's exact compliance with taking the medications—*Note:* Medications that may either raise blood pressure or interfere with the effectiveness of antihypertensive medications include oral contraceptives, steroids, nonsteroidal anti-inflammatory drugs, nasal decongestants, appetite suppressants, cyclosporine, tricyclic antidepressants, monoamine oxidase inhibitors, and erythropoietin
- History of any disease or trauma to target organs
- Results and side effects of previous antihypertensive therapy
- Clinical manifestations of cardiovascular disorders, such as angina, dyspnea, or claudication
- History of or recent weight gain, exercise activities, sodium intake, fat intake, alcohol use, and smoking
- Psychosocial and environmental factors (e.g., emotional stress, cultural food practices, economic status) that may influence blood pressure control

Physical Examination

Physical assessment should include accurate determination of blood pressure as well as evaluation of target organs.

- Vital signs and weight
- Blood pressure—because blood pressure is variable and can be affected by multiple factors, it should be measured so that readings are representative of the client's usual level; the following techniques are strongly recommended:
  - The client should be seated with the arm bared, supported, and positioned at heart level. The client should not have smoked tobacco or ingested caffeine within the previous 30 minutes.
  - Measurement should begin after at least 5 minutes of quiet rest. The client's back should be supported, and both feet should be flat on the floor with the legs uncrossed. The client should not speak while the blood pressure is being monitored.
  - Use of the appropriate cuff size will ensure an accurate measurement. The rubber bladder should encircle at least 80% of the limb being measured. The bladder's width should be one-third to one-half the circumference of the limb. Several sizes of cuffs (e.g., child, adult, large adult) should be available.
- Measurements should be taken with a mercury sphygmomanometer, a recently calibrated aneroid manometer, or a validated electronic device.
- Postural blood pressures should be measured and recorded according to position and arm used, including lying, sitting, and standing measurements from both arms.
  - Both systolic and diastolic blood pressures should be recorded. The disappearance of sound (phase V) should be used for the diastolic reading.
  - Two or more readings should be averaged. If the first two readings differ by more than 5 mm Hg, additional readings should be obtained.
- Funduscopic examination for retinal arteriolar narrowing, hemorrhages, exudates, and papilledema
- Examination of the neck for distended veins, carotid bruits, and enlarged thyroid
- Auscultation of the heart for increased heart rate, dysrhythmias, enlargement, precordial impulses, murmurs, and S3 and S4 heart sounds
- Examination of the abdomen for bruits, aortic dilation, and enlarged kidneys
- Examination of extremities for diminished or absent peripheral pulses, edema, and bilateral inequality of pulses
- Neurologic evaluation for signs of cerebral thrombosis or hemorrhage

Laboratory Studies

Studies used in the routine evaluation of hypertension include a complete blood count, urinalysis, determinations of serum potassium and sodium levels, fasting blood glucose level, serum cholesterol level, blood urea nitrogen and serum creatinine levels, electrocardiogram, and chest radiography. These tests provide useful information in determining the severity of vascular disease, the extent of target organ damage, and the possible causes of hypertension. Clients with potential for secondary hypertension may need more extensive studies.

needs, including those related to the prevention, diagnosis, and management of hypertension.

Long-term compliance/adherence has emerged as the most essential element in reducing morbidity and mortality associated with hypertension.[9] However, poor compliance with or adherence to antihypertensive therapy persists as one of the most frustrating blocks to effective therapeutic management. More than two thirds of clients with hypertension do not have adequate control of their blood pressure because of poor compliance or adherence. The reasons vary; the client may choose not to have the initial prescription filled, may successfully initiate therapy only to abandon it after a few weeks or months, or may comply with only part of the regimen and thus fail to achieve optimal control.

NORMALIZING ARTERIAL PRESSURE

The outcome goal of prevention and management of hypertension is to restore the elevated blood pressure to as normal a level as possible using lifestyle modification alone or in combination with drug therapy in order to prevent morbidity and mortality associated with the sequelae of hypertension. The objective is to achieve and maintain arterial blood pressure below 140/90 mm Hg, or

TABLE 52–1 FOLLOW-UP CRITERIA FOR FIRST-OCCASION MEASUREMENT OF BLOOD PRESSURE

Initial Screening Blood Pressure (mm Hg)*		
Systolic	*Diastolic*	**Follow-up Recommended†**
<130	<85	Recheck in 2 yr
130–139	85–89	Recheck in 1 yr‡
140–159	90–99	Confirm within 2 mo‡
160–179	100–109	Evaluate or refer to care within 1 mo
≥180	≥110	Evaluate or refer to care immediately or within 1 wk, depending on clinical situation

*If the systolic and diastolic categories are different, follow recommendation for the shorter follow-up time.

†The scheduling of follow-up visits should be modified by reliable information about past blood pressure, other cardiovascular risk factors, or target organ disease.

‡Encourage lifestyle modifications.

From the Joint National Committee. (1997). The sixth report of the Joint National Committee on the Detection, Evaluation, and Treatment of Hypertension. *Archives of Internal Medicine, 157,* 2418.

TABLE 52–2 CLASSIFICATION OF BLOOD PRESSURE IN ADULTS 18 YEARS OF AGE AND OLDER*

	Blood Pressure (mm Hg)	
Category	*Systolic*	*Diastolic*
Normal	<130	<85
High-normal	130–139	85–89
Hypertension		
Stage 1: mild	140–159	90–99
Stage 2: moderate	160–179	100–109
Stage 3: severe	≥180	≥110

*Not taking antihypertensive medications and not acutely ill. When systolic and diastolic pressures fall into different categories, the higher category should be selected to classify the client's blood pressure status. For example, 170/96 would be classified as stage 2, and 178/112 would be classified as stage 3.

From the Joint National Committee. (1997). The sixth report of the Joint National Committee on the Detection, Evaluation, and Treatment of Hypertension. *Archives of Internal Medicine, 157,* 2417.

as near to that goal as possible, while controlling modifiable risk factors for cardiovascular disease.[11, 16, 25, 26, 30]

Lifestyle Modifications

Strong research evidence has conclusively illustrated that lifestyle modifications are effective in lowering blood pressure and reducing cardiovascular risk factors at little overall cost and with minimal risk. Lifestyle modifications are widely advocated to prevent high blood pressure. They are suggested as definitive therapy for some clients, at least for the first 6 to 12 months after initial diagnosis.

Lifestyle modification is also strongly encouraged as adjunctive therapy for all clients with hypertension who are also receiving pharmacologic therapy. Positive adjustments in lifestyle alone may completely normalize the blood pressure for an extended period of time or indefinitely. When lifestyle management alone is not entirely successful in normalizing pressure, continued healthy lifestyle practices can reduce the number and dosage of antihypertensive medications needed to manage the condition.

Weight Reduction

Excess body weight, exhibited by a body mass index (BMI)—weight in kilograms divided by height in meters squared—of 27 or greater, correlates closely with elevated blood pressure. Also, excess body fat accumulated in the torso with a waist circumference of 34 inches or greater for women and 39 inches or more for men has

TABLE 52–3 RISK STRATIFICATION AND TREATMENT IN CLIENTS WITH HIGH BLOOD PRESSURE

	Treatment*		
Blood Pressure	*Risk Group A No Risk Factors, No TOD/CCD*	*Risk Group B At Least 1 Risk Factor, Not Including Diabetes; No TOD/CCD*	*Risk Group C TOD/CCD ± Diabetes, ± Other Risk Factors*
High-normal: 130–139/85–89	Lifestyle modification	Lifestyle modification	Drug therapy†
Stage 1: 140–159/90–99	Lifestyle modification (up to 12 mo)	Lifestyle modification‡ (up to 6 mo)	Drug therapy
Stages 2 and 3: ≥160/≥100	Drug therapy	Drug therapy	Drug therapy

*Lifestyle modification should be adjunctive therapy in all clients receiving pharmacologic therapy.

†For clients with heart failure, renal insufficiency, or diabetes.

‡For clients with multiple risk factors, clinicians should consider drug therapy as initial treatment plus lifestyle modifications.

TOD/CCD, target organ disease/clinicial cardiovascular disease.

Modified from the Joint National Committee. (1997). The sixth report of the Joint National Committee on the Detection, Evaluation, and Treatment of Hypertension. *Archives of Internal Medicine, 157,* 2419.

also been associated with increased risk for hypertension. For many people with hypertension whose body weight is more than 10% over ideal, weight reduction of as little as 10 pounds can lower blood pressure. Weight reduction also enhances effectiveness of antihypertensive medications. Therefore, reassess the client's blood pressure during weight loss, and make appropriate changes in pharmacologic interventions as needed.

Sodium Restriction

An estimated 40% of people with hypertension are sodium-sensitive. A moderate restriction of sodium intake to 2.3 g of sodium, or 6 g of salt, can be used to lower blood pressure in some cases of stage I hypertension. The amount of medication otherwise needed may be decreased if sodium intake is lowered. In addition, this moderate sodium restriction may reduce the degree of potassium depletion that often accompanies diuretic therapy.

Dietary Fat Modification

Modification of dietary intake of fat by decreasing the fraction of saturated fat and increasing that of polyunsaturated fat has little, if any, effect on decreasing blood pressure but can decrease the cholesterol level significantly. Because dyslipidemia is a major risk factor in the development of coronary artery disease, diet therapy aimed at reducing lipids is an important adjunct to any total dietary regimen. In addition to the usual recommendations for sensible eating following the Food Pyramid (see Chapter 3), the Dietary Approaches to Stop Hypertension (DASH) diet (Table 52–4) which is rich in fruits, vegetables, nuts, and low-fat dairy foods with reduced saturated and total fats, should be recommended for clients who need a more structured, fat-limited, dietary intervention.

Exercise

A regular program of aerobic exercise adequate to achieve at least a moderate level of physical fitness facilitates cardiovascular conditioning and can aid the obese hypertensive client in weight reduction and reduce the risk for cardiovascular disease and all-cause mortality. Blood pressure can be reduced with moderate-intensity (as low as 40% to 60% of maximum oxygen consumption) physical activity, such as a brisk walk (about 2.5 to 3 miles per hour) for 30 to 45 minutes most days of the week.

Weight training using *light* weights is a positive addition to any exercise regimen. However, lifting *heavy* weights may be harmful, because blood pressure rises, sometimes to very high levels, with the vasovagal response that occurs during an intense isometric muscle contraction. Advise hypertensive clients to initiate exercise programs gradually, slowly increasing intensity and duration of activity as the body adjusts and becomes more conditioned with ongoing professional surveillance.

Alcohol Restriction

The consumption of more than 1 ounce of alcohol per day is associated with a higher prevalence of hypertension, poor adherence to antihypertensive therapy, and, occasionally, refractory hypertension. Carefully assess alcohol intake. Advise clients who do drink to do so in moderation (i.e., no more than 1 ounce of ethanol per day for men and 0.5 ounce for women). There is 1 ounce (30 ml) of ethanol in 2 ounces (60 ml) of 100-proof whiskey, in 10 ounces (300 ml) of wine, or in 24 ounces (720 ml) of beer.

Caffeine Restriction

Although acute ingestion of caffeine may raise blood pressure, chronic moderate caffeine ingestion appears to have no significant effect on blood pressure. Therefore, caffeine restriction is not necessary unless cardiac response or other excessive sensitivity to caffeine is present.

Relaxation Techniques

A variety of relaxation therapies, including transcendental meditation, yoga, biofeedback, progressive muscle relaxation, and psychotherapy, reduce blood pressure in hypertensive clients at least transiently. Although each modality has its advocates, none has been conclusively shown to be either practical for the majority of hypertensive clients or effective in maintaining a significant long-term effect.[3, 20]

Smoking Cessation

Although smoking has not been statistically linked to the development of hypertension, nicotine definitely increases heart rate and produces peripheral vasoconstriction, which does raise arterial blood pressure for a short time during smoking and afterward. Smoking cessation is strongly recommended, however, to reduce the client's risk for cancer, pulmonary disease, and cardiovascular disease. Smokers appear to have a higher frequency of malignant hypertension and subarachnoid hemorrhage. In addition, risk reduction brought about by antihypertensive therapy may not be as great in smokers as in nonsmokers.

Potassium Supplementation

The high ratio of sodium to potassium in the modern diet has been held responsible for the development of hypertension. However, even though potassium supplements may lower blood pressure, they are too costly and potentially too hazardous for routine use. A reduction in consumption of high-sodium, low-potassium processed foods with an increase in consumption of low-sodium, high-potassium natural foods may be all that is needed for maximum benefits.

Pharmacologic Intervention

Considerable debate continues regarding the appropriate time and circumstances for the initiation of pharmacologic management of hypertension. Although antihypertensive agents are known to be effective in decreasing cardiovascular morbidity and mortality associated with hypertension, clinicians sometimes question whether the benefit of immediate initiation of medication therapy, particularly in mildly hypertensive clients, outweighs the risks in terms of untoward effects of the drugs and other inconveniences. Other clinicians prefer to recommend lifestyle modification, as indicated in the previous section, and to add drug therapy as needed.

In any event, once a decision has been made to use pharmacologic intervention, any one of several drugs can be used.[6, 8, 11, 14, 15, 19, 24, 28, 30] Table 52–5 outlines the major antihypertensive agents.

Antihypertensive medications can be classified into the following categories: diuretics, alpha- and beta-adrenergic antagonists, $alpha_2$-agonists, vasodilators, calcium antago-

Text continued on page 1391

TABLE 52–4 *D*IETARY *A*PPROACHES TO *S*TOP *H*YPERTENSION (DASH) DIET

The DASH eating plan shown below is based on 2000 calories a day. Depending on your caloric needs your number of daily servings in a food group may vary from those listed. This eating plan is from the "Dietary Approaches to Stop Hypertension" (DASH) clinical study supported by the National Institutes of Health. The DASH combination diet lowered blood pressure and so may help prevent and control high blood pressure.

Food Group	Daily Servings (No.)	Serving Size	Examples	Significance of Each Food Group to DASH Diet Pattern
Grains and grain products	7–8	1 slice bread; ½ cup dry cereal; ½ cup cooked rice, pasta, or cereal*	Whole wheat breads, English muffin, pita bread, bagel, cereals and fiber, grits, oatmeal	Major source of energy and fiber
Vegetables	4–5	1 cup raw, leafy vegetable; ½ cup cooked vegetable; 6 oz vegetable juice	Tomatoes, potatoes, carrots, peas, squash, broccoli, turnip greens, collards, kale, spinach, artichokes, beans, sweet potatoes	Rich sources of potassium, magnesium, and fiber
Fruits	4–5	6 oz fruit juice, 1 medium fruit; ¼ cup dried fruit; ½ cup fresh, frozen, or canned fruit	Apricots, bananas, dates, grapes, oranges, orange juice, grapefruit, grapefruit juice, mangoes, melons, peaches, pineapples, prunes, raisins, strawberries, tangerines	Important sources of potassium, magnesium, and fiber
Low fat or nonfat dairy foods	2–3	8 oz milk; 1 cup yogurt; 1.5 oz cheese	Skim or 1% milk, skim or low-fat buttermilk, nonfat or low-fat yogurt, part skim mozzarella cheese, nonfat cheese	Major sources of calcium and protein
Meats, poultry, fish	2 or less	3 oz cooked meats, poultry, or fish	Select only lean; trim away visible fats; broil, roast, or boil, instead of frying; remove skin from poultry	Rich sources of protein and magnesium
Nuts, seeds, and legumes	4–5/wk	1.5 oz or ⅓ cup nuts; ½ oz or 2 tbsp seeds; ½ cup cooked dry beans	Almonds, filberts, mixed nuts, peanuts, walnuts, sunflower seeds, kidney beans, lentils and peas	Rich sources of energy, magnesium, potassium, protein, and fiber
Fats and oils†	2–3	1 tsp soft margarine; 1 tbsp low-fat mayonnaise; 2 tbsp light salad dressing; 1 tsp vegetable oil	Soft margarine, low-fat mayonnaise, light salad dressing Vegetable oil (such as olive, corn, canola, or safflower)	Besides considering the fats added to foods, choose foods that contain less fats
Sweets	5/wk	1 tbsp sugar; 1 tbsp jelly or jam; ½ oz jelly beans; 8 oz lemonade	Maple syrup, sugar, jelly, jam, fruit-flavored gelatin, jelly beans, hard candy, fruit punch, sorbet ices	Sweets should be low in fat

*Serving sizes vary between ½ and 1¼ cups. Check the nutrition label.

†Fat content changes per serving size of fats and oil, for example, 1 tbsp regular salad dressing equals 1 serving. 1 tbsp low-fat dressing equals ½ serving. 1 tbsp fat-free dressing equals zero servings.

Modified from Kolasa, K. M. (1999). Dietary Approaches to Stop Hypertension (DASH) in clinical practice: A primary care experience. *Clinical Cardiology, 22*(7 suppl), III-16–22.

TABLE 52–5 **MEDICATIONS USED TO TREAT HYPERTENSION**

Drug Class with Example(s)	Action	Therapeutic Outcome	Adverse Outcomes	Dose
Thiazide and Related Diuretics Hydrochlorothiazide (HydroDIURIL)	Promote renal excretion of water, sodium, potassium, and hydrogen	Lower BP, diuresis, weight loss Generally a first-line agent	Hypotension, dehydration, hypokalemia	12.5–50 mg/d daily to twice daily Administer in AM These drugs potentiate other antihypertensive medications; monitor BP closely
Loop Diuretics Bumetanide (Bumex) Furosemide (Lasix)	Inhibits absorption of sodium and chloride from ascending loop of Henle, causing excretion of water, sodium, potassium, chloride, magnesium, and calcium	Lower BP, reduce edema First-line agent in clients with renal failure	Hypotension, dehydration, hypokalemia Drugs decrease effect of antidiabetic agents	Lasix: 20–40 mg q 6–8 h initially Bumex: 0.5–4 mg Maintenance dose given daily or twice daily Administer last dose in early evening Monitor BP and positional BP, daily weight, I&O Closely monitor potassium levels
Potassium-Sparing Diuretics Amiloride hydrochloride (Midamor) Spironolactone (Aldactone)	Competes with aldosterone for receptor sites in distal renal tubules, increasing sodium and chloride excretion	Management of edema associated with hyperaldosteronism Weak diuretics	Hyperkalemia, dehydration, impotence	Daily to twice-daily dosing Amiloride: 5–10 mg daily Spironolactone: 25–100 mg
Selective Beta Blocker Metoprolol (Lopressor)	Selective inhibitor of $beta_1$-adrenergic receptors; no effect on $beta_2$ receptors	Decreased BP, decreased heart rate May be less effective in treating black clients and the elderly	Hypoglycemia in diabetics, with masking of clinical manifestations except for diaphoresis, dizziness, fatigue	50–300 mg bid Monitor I&O, BP, daily weight
Nonselective Beta Blocker Propranolol (Inderal)	Nonselective inhibitor of $beta_1$- and $beta_2$-adrenergic receptors	Decreased BP, decreased heart rate, decreased myocardial oxygen demand	Bronchial constriction Hypoglycemia in diabetics (as for metoprolol above), dizziness, fatigue, insomnia	Daily to twice-daily dosing 40–480 mg/day Monitor I&O, BP, daily weight Avoid using in clients with asthma
Peripheral-Acting Adrenergic Antagonist Guanadrel (Hylorel)	Deplete the brain and peripheral nerve tissues of norepinephrine, decreasing peripheral vascular resistance	Decreased heart rate and standing BP	Depression, weight gain, bradycardia, postural hypotension (due to loss of norepinephrine) GI upset	Daily or twice-daily dosing 10–75 mg/day Often used in combination with other diuretics or beta-blockers Concurrent use of digitalis or quinidine may potentiate dysrhythmias
Centrally Acting $Alpha_2$ Agonists Clonidine (Catapres) Methydopa (Aldomet)	Suppress sympathetic nervous system Action potentiated by alcohol, sedatives, propranolol	Decreased BP Bradycardia	Xerostomia, dizziness, headache, fatigue, GI disturbances	Clonidine 0.1 mg bid Methyldopa 250 mg bid–tid Used only for severe hypertension or renin-dependent hypertension Monitor BP closely Monitor for bradycardia Chewing gum or hard candy may relieve dry mouth

Table continued on following page

TABLE 52–5 MEDICATIONS USED TO TREAT HYPERTENSION *Continued*

Drug Class with Example(s)	Action	Therapeutic Outcome	Adverse Outcomes	Dose
Calcium Channel Blockers Diltiazem (Cardizem SR or CD) Verapamil (Calan SR) Nifedipine (Procardia XL)	Blocks entry of calcium into smooth muscle channels in arterioles Used for cardioprotective effects with angina, atrial fibrillation, diabetes	Vasodilation Decreased peripheral vascular resistance Reduce heart rate, slow ventricular conduction, depress contractility	Hypotension Bradycardia from heart block Nocturia	Daily dosing Diltiazem 120–360 mg/day or bid Verapamil 80–120 mg tid **Short-acting forms, particularly nifedipine, should no longer be used because of increased risk of MI and mortality after MI**
Angiotensin-Converting Enzyme (ACE) Inhibitors Captopril (Capoten) Enalapril (Vasotec) Fosinopril (Monopril)	Inhibit the conversion of angiotensin I to angiotensin II, thereby preventing release of renin	Reduces peripheral vascular resistance without changing cardiac output	Digitalis toxicity Hyperkalemia Ticklish, dry cough Renal damage	5–40 mg (qid to tid) Do not administer with antacids Monitor potassium levels, urine protein, leukocyte counts
Alpha$_1$-Receptor Blockers Doxazosin (Cardura) Prazosin (Minipress)	Competitively inhibits postsynaptic receptors	Vasodilation, decreased peripheral vascular resistance	Orthostatic hypotension, with loss of consciousness especially with first dose	Given 1–4 times daily Doxazosin: 1 mg up to qid Prazosin: 2–30 mg bid–tid Monitor BP closely Titrate dose based on standing BP Teach clients to move slowly to prevent orthostasis
Alpha/Beta-Blocker Labetalol (Normodyne)	Same as for alpha/beta-blockers	Same as for alpha/beta-blockers	Same as for alpha/beta-blockers	May be more effective in black clients than a beta-blocker alone
Vasodilator Hydralazine (Apresoline)	Direct vasodilation of arterioles, no effect on veins	Decreased peripheral vascular resistance	Orthostatic hypotension, palpitations, tachycardia, flushing, headache	10–70 mg 4 times daily Monitor positional BP closely, especially when drug given IV Headache responds to acetaminophen and ice compresses

BP, blood pressure; GI, gastrointestinal; I&O, intake and output (fluid); MI, myocardial infarction.

nists, and angiotensin-converting enzyme (ACE) inhibitors. If therapy is chosen carefully, more than half of mild hypertension cases can be controlled with a single drug, and more than 90% should be controlled with no more than two drugs. Cultural aspects of antihypertensive medications are discussed in the Diversity in Health Care feature.

Provider Responsibilities

Stepped-Care Therapy

The goal of antihypertensive therapy is to control blood pressure with a minimum of side effects. The stepped-care approach is prescribed as treatment for hypertension (Box 52–4). Prevention-based healthy lifestyle change with the addition of pharmacologic therapy as indicated is the preferred treatment regimen. An individualized approach to prescription of lifestyle management and drug therapy is used, taking into consideration demographic concerns, concomitant diseases or therapies, and the client's perceived quality of life within the confines of the treatment regimen.

If more than one drug is necessary, several combination therapies have proved effective. For example, the combination of a diuretic with a beta-adrenergic blocker or other adrenergic inhibitor has been effective in both blacks and whites, in contrast to the responses to the individual drugs, whereas blacks respond less well to

DIVERSITY IN HEALTH CARE

Ethnopharmacology and Hypertension

Ethnopharmacology

How medications are metabolized varies not only in relation to a person's age, gender, body composition, and size but also with ethnicity[3]; these factors, therefore, must be considered in any treatment regimen. The variation in metabolism is called drug polymorphism and is influenced by several ethnicity-related factors. In this regard, Kudzma[3] has identified environmental, cultural, and genetic factors.

Environmental factors affect the assimilation and half-life of a medication and include diet, smoking, and alcohol use. Cultural factors include (1) values and beliefs, which can influence adherence to a medication regimen, (2) reporting or nonreporting of manifestations, and (3) use of herbal and homeopathic remedies. Some people may doubt the need for medication when manifestations ease or disappear, and some may be unwilling to accept the use of particular routes of medication. In addition, religious beliefs may dictate fasting periods, which may affect medication absorption.[5]

Genetic factors determine medication metabolism in terms of genetic polymorphism, because each person's inherited genes affect liver metabolism. Some people are slow or poor metabolizers, whereas others are rapid or extensive metabolizers. An estimated 9% of whites and 32% of Asians are slow metabolizers.[5] In rapid metabolizers, a drug is more efficient but may sometimes be metabolized so quickly that full benefit is not realized. In slow metabolizers, a drug is less effective and greater drug toxicity may be experienced.[3] The speed of metabolism is an important issue in determining the appropriate dose of medication for a client and has been examined in some studies of ethnic groups, although more studies across a variety of groups need to be done.

Hypertension

Hypertension, as well as some other related conditions such as stroke, has been connected to cultural, economic, social, and political factors that have had a negative impact upon the health of African Americans in large urban areas.[4] Davis and Curley[1] have described African Americans as having the poorest health of all ethnic groups in the United States, as measured by certain indicators. Giger and Davidhizar[2] note that the incidence of hypertension has been reported to be significantly higher in African Americans than in white Americans. In addition, the age at onset of hypertension is younger and the level of severity is higher.

Because the incidence of hypertension is higher among blacks than among whites, many studies have been conducted to investigate the effectiveness of commonly prescribed medications among blacks. What has not yet been clearly determined is whether genetics, the pathophysiology of hypertension, or some other factor is responsible for the results. Kudzma[3] reported that most of the major classes of antihypertensive drugs—diuretic agents, angiotensin-converting enzyme (ACE) inhibitors, beta-blockers, and calcium-channel blockers—are found to be effective in blacks. However, if only one drug is used, blacks appear to respond better to diuretics than to ACE inhibitors or beta-blockers. Also, lower doses are required for some drugs in blacks than in whites.

In general, become aware that drug metabolism differs across ethnic groups for a variety of reasons and that certain medications may be more effective for some groups than for others. In addition to considering the differences that may occur in treatment response, consider the many factors that may have contributed to certain conditions occurring in higher frequencies in some groups. Such factors include diet, socioeconomic status, habits, beliefs and norms, and access to and acceptability of preventive care. Try to improve the health outcomes of clients by monitoring their responses to medication, communicating pertinent information to physicians, and assisting clients in modifying the impact of the multiple factors, both internal and external, affecting them.

References

1. Davis, C. M., & Curley, C. M. (1999). Disparities of health in African Americans. *Nursing Clinics of North America, 34*(2), 345–357.
2. Giger, J. N., & Davidhizar, R. E. (1999). *Transcultural nursing: Assessment and intervention* (3rd ed.). St. Louis: Mosby.
3. Kudzma, E. C. (1999). Culturally competent drug administration. *American Journal of Nursing, 99*(8), 46–51.
4. Leininger, M. (1995). *Transcultural nursing: Concepts, theories, research and practices.* New York: McGraw-Hill.
5. Pavlovich-Davis, S. (1999). Drug of choice? Medicinal effects vary widely, depending on ethnicity and culture. *Nursing Spectrum,* Oct. 4, 18–19.

Sandra Sharma, PhD, ARNP, CS, *James A. Haley Veterans Hospital, Tampa, Florida*

BOX 52–4 Stepped-Care Approach to Management of Hypertension

Step 1: Implement lifestyle modifications.
Weight reduction
Moderation of alcohol intake
Regular aerobic physical activity
Reduction of sodium intake with maintenance of adequate intake of potassium, calcium, and magnesium
Decreased intake of saturated fats and cholesterol
Smoking cessation

If there is inadequate blood pressure control, move to step 2.

Step 2: Continue lifestyle modifications and make initial pharmacologic selection; diuretics or beta-blockers are recommended because of studies that demonstrate reduced morbidity and mortality. If co-morbid conditions exist, evidence supports the use of other drugs as first-line therapy.

- Start with lowest therapeutic dose of a long-acting drug given once daily, then titrate dose.
- Low-dose combination drugs may be appropriate.

If there is inadequate blood pressure control, move to step 3.

Step 3: Increase drug dose.
OR
Substitute another drug if no response or side effects become apparent.
OR
Add second drug from a different class or a diuretic if not already used, particularly if there is an inadequate response but initial drug well tolerated and at maximum dose.

If there is inadequate blood pressure control, move to step 4.

Step 4: Add second or third drug if not already prescribed; continue to add medications from other classes; consider referral to a hypertensive specialist.

From the Joint National Committee. (1997). The sixth report of the Joint National Committee on the Detection, Evaluation, and Treatment of Hypertension. *Archives of Internal Medicine, 157,* 2430.

beta-adrenergic blockers alone or as first-line treatment. The combination of a diuretic with an ACE inhibitor or a calcium-channel blocker has additive effects on blood pressure.

Finally, combination drugs can be less expensive than the individual drugs, and the need for only one drug may improve compliance in a client who does not like "taking so many pills."

Follow-up Care: Step-Down Therapy

Reducing the number and amounts of antihypertensive medications should be considered once a client's blood pressure has been controlled effectively for at least 1 year. Medication dosages must be decreased slowly and progressively until the lowest effective dosages are reached and maintained. Step-down methods are most often successful in clients who are also participating in healthy lifestyle change interventions. Lifestyle change habits should be established and can be regulated to provide the most appropriate and practical regimen for each client. Regular follow-up evaluation is essential if drug therapy has been completely stopped, because blood pressure can rise again over time, especially if positive lifestyle change practices have been neglected or also stopped.

Nursing Management

ASSESSMENT

The many sequelae of untreated hypertension can be prevented, or the severity of such problems reduced, if hypertension is well managed. Client education and understanding are crucial to successful management.

Ineffective Management of Therapeutic Regimen (Individual). Use the nursing diagnosis *Ineffective Management of Therapeutic Regimen (Individual)* to identify the learning needs of the newly diagnosed hypertensive client. The diagnosis can be written *Risk for Ineffective Management of Therapeutic Regimen (Individual) related to a new diagnosis, no previous learning about the disease process, potential consequences, the rationale for intervention, and proper administration of prescribed medications.*

Outcomes. The client and significant others will demonstrate knowledge required for self-care, as evidenced by (1) describing hypertension and its associated risk factors; (2) discussing the importance of lifelong medical follow-up; (3) listing the prescribed medications, including drug name, rationale for use, dosage, frequency, potential side effects, and measures to minimize side effects; and (4) demonstrating proper blood pressure measurement technique for home blood pressure monitoring.

Interventions. Because of the chronicity of hypertension and its dangerous complications, clients with hypertension need clear, practical, and realistic learning guidelines. Guidelines should include information concerning hypertension and its management. Use written materials with clear illustrations for teaching the client with newly diagnosed hypertension about the condition. Teach the client to measure blood pressure at home at least once a week and to record the findings in a diary.

Inform clients of their blood pressure reading, and advise them of the need for periodic remeasurement. When working with most clients, the examiner should refer to hypertension as *high blood pressure* to help avoid confusion associated with the term *hypertension.* Many clients unfamiliar with medical terms may believe that hypertension denotes a state of being "hypertense"—that is, being worried or agitated. For these clients, the term *high blood pressure* more accurately conveys the nature of the health problem.

Altered Nutrition: More Than Body Requirements. Dietary adjustments can reduce the severity of hypertension and in some cases reduce the need for medication. Client teaching about and assessment of needed changes constitute an important aspect of nursing care. Write the diagnosis as *Altered Nutrition: More Than Body Requirements related to high sodium, fat, and total calorie intake.*

Outcomes. The client will demonstrate knowledge of and adherence to the nutritional regimen, as evidenced by describing specific dietary modifications including sodium, fat, and calorie restrictions and their rationales (see the three Client Education Guides to these topics), by reduction in levels of urine sodium and blood cholesterol, and by losing weight.

Interventions. The two most important aspects of dietary intervention for hypertension are weight reduction (for overweight clients) and mild to moderate sodium restriction. Therefore, advise the client with hypertension to eat a diet low in salt, calories, cholesterol, and saturated fat. Discuss the prescribed diet with the household members who prepare food. If possible, enlist the aid of a dietitian to provide detailed dietary instructions. Before dietary intervention begins, assess the client's patterns of food intake, lifestyle, food preferences, and ethnic, social, cultural, and financial influences. A highly individualized approach to dietary counseling is crucial to compliance and adherence.

Restrict Sodium. Sodium is a hidden ingredient in many processed foods, beverages (including water from certain sources), and over-the-counter drugs (particularly antacids, cough remedies, and laxatives). It cannot be seen and is often not tasted. The average adult daily intake of salt is 5 to 15 g, but the therapeutic effects of sodium reduction on blood pressure do not occur until salt intake is reduced to equal to or below 6 g/day. Low-salt diets can be very difficult to adhere to, at least initially. Reassure the client that dietary adherence becomes easier as the palate adjusts to decreased salt over a period of several weeks to months. After the client becomes fully accustomed to the low-salt diet, unsalted foods usually cease to taste bland. The Client Education Guide on low-salt diets presents guidelines for teaching clients about sodium reduction.

Reduce Fat and Cholesterol. Hypertension and high serum cholesterol (>250 mg/dl) are linked as risk factors in the development of coronary artery disease. The level of serum cholesterol is partly determined by the consumption of cholesterol, saturated and polyunsaturated fats, and total calories. Cholesterol is contained in animal fats and dairy products. Saturated fats occur predominantly in animal fats and tropical oils (e.g., coconut and palm oils). Unsaturated fats predominate in most plant-derived fats. Polyunsaturated fats occur predominantly in vegetable and seed oils. A diet low in saturated fats and high in polyunsaturated fats is beneficial in reducing blood pressure. (See DASH diet, Table 52–4.) The Client Education Guide on low-fat, low-cholesterol diets also provides guidelines for teaching clients about fat and cholesterol reduction.

Reduce Calories and Weight. Not all clients with hypertension need to lose weight. As discussed previously, only people with a BMI of greater than 27 should consider the need to lose weight. Ideally, the rate of weight loss should be no more than 0.5 kg (about a pound) a week. Advise the average adult with hypertension to reduce caloric intake by at least 250 calories per day. Caution the client to avoid over-the-counter appetite suppressants because these preparations often contain sympathomimetic agents, which elevate blood pressure. The Client Education Guide on calorie-restricted diets provides advice on regulating caloric intake.

Altered Health Maintenance. Exercise is like dietary management: A regular exercise program can lower blood pressure in hypertensive clients. This diagnosis can be written as *Altered Health Maintenance related to a lack of regular exercise regimen.*

Outcomes. The client will begin and maintain an appropriate exercise program, as evidenced by self-report, demonstration of ability to monitor heart rate during exercise, sensation of reduced physical and emotional stress, and reduced blood pressure.

CLIENT EDUCATION GUIDE

Low-Fat, Low-Cholesterol Diet

Client Instructions

Avoid foods high in saturated fats and cholesterol:

Use margarine and vegetable oils instead of butter.
Avoid gravies, creams, and cheese sauces.
Avoid fried foods; instead, eat broiled, baked, or boiled foods
Use skim or low-fat milk and milk products.
Choose lean cuts of meat. Trim off all visible fat. Remove all poultry skin.
Use a wire rack when roasting, broiling, or baking meats so that the fat can drip off.
Keep in mind that poultry, fish, and veal have a relatively low fat content. Chicken and turkey breasts are the leanest poultry available. Avoid duck and goose. Haddock, cod, and water-packed tuna are the leanest fish available.
Use pans with a nonstick coating when cooking to reduce the need for oil or shortening.
Prepare meat stews, soups, and gravies in advance and chill them until the fat hardens. Then skim off the fat.
Eat no more than three egg yolks per week. Egg whites are low in cholesterol, as are many egg substitutes.
Limit your intake of organ meats and shellfish.

CLIENT EDUCATION GUIDE

Low-Sodium Diet

Client Instructions

Avoid foods high in sodium:

Read labels of foods carefully for "sodium," "Na^+," "salt," "NaCl," "bicarbonate of soda," and "MSG" because these are all sources of sodium. If these words appear in the first four to five ingredients listed on the package, avoid the food item.
Avoid common commercial preparations that are high in sodium, including baking powder, baking soda, monosodium glutamate, meat tenderizer, and soy sauce.
Avoid canned, boxed, and some frozen foods to which sodium has been added. (Frozen fruits and vegetables are okay.)
Avoid canned, smoked, pickled, or cured meat and fish products. (Canned tuna in water is okay.) Pickled or preserved vegetables always contain salt.
Be aware that not all dietetic foods are sodium-free; read the labels before purchasing and using.
In restaurants, choose foods that are baked, broiled, boiled, or roasted and without salted gravies or juices. Avoid soups and salted or cheesy dressings. Carry your own salt substitute if desired. Be aware that "fast foods" also tend to be high in sodium.

CLIENT EDUCATION GUIDE

Calorie-Restriction Diet

Client Instructions

To regulate your caloric intake:

Never eat when you are doing something else, such as watching television or reading. Chew properly and slowly, and always sit down to eat.

Begin each meal with raw vegetables or salad.

Do not eat more than one slice of bread at a time. Except for a piece of toast with breakfast or a sandwich at lunch, do not eat bread with meals. Do not put butter or margarine on bread.

Stop eating when you feel not quite full. (A feeling of satiety will usually occur about 20 minutes after eating.)

Never wait until you are very hungry before you eat. Eat low-calorie, between-meal snacks if necessary.

Eat something before going to parties. Avoid high-calorie party snacks such as potato and corn chips and peanuts, almonds, and other nuts.

Drink only low-calorie beverages, such as coffee or tea (decaffeinated). Avoid adding sugar to them, although nonfat milk may be added. Do not quench your thirst with milk; use water.

Drink one to two glasses of water before drinking an alcoholic beverage. Alcoholic beverages are high in calories (7 kcal/ml).

Avoid sugar; use artificial sweeteners instead.

To appease an irresistible urge to eat something sweet, take ⅕ teaspoon of sugar or a tiny bite from a chewy candy. Leave the sugar on your tongue for as long as possible. Doing this even up to six times a day will provide fewer calories than a piece of cake or several cookies.

Intervention. Exercise programs can heighten the client's sense of well-being, provide an outlet for emotional tensions, and raise the levels of high-density lipoproteins (HDLs) relative to total blood cholesterol. Elevated HDL levels are associated with a decreased risk of cardiovascular morbidity and mortality. Instruct the client, however, to avoid heavy weight-lifting, isometric exercises, and other activities inappropriate to the client's physical limitations. A modest but consistent exercise program provides greater benefits than those obtainable with spurts of strenuous activity mixed with periods of inactivity. A gradually increasing program of aerobic activity such as walking, jogging, or swimming can thus be recommended.

Current recommendations include aerobic exercise of an intensity aimed at maintaining 45% to 75% of maximal heart rate for 20 to 30 minutes, three times a week, depending on age and the coexistence of other co-morbid conditions. Maximal heart rate is calculated by subtracting the client's age from 220. Before advising and initiating an exercise prescription for your client, a qualified specialist must conduct a careful performance evaluation.

Risk for Noncompliance. Many aspects of hypertension management set the stage for noncompliance. Several factors related to specific drug use, including side effects, interference with lifestyle, cost, and inconvenience of physician visits and taking prescribed medications, play an important role in noncompliance. Assess the reasons for noncompliance, and then state the diagnosis as *Risk for Noncompliance related to a lack of understanding about the seriousness of high blood pressure, cost of therapy, side effects of medications, complexity of management,* or *multiple changes in lifestyle.*

Outcomes. The client will actively participate in creating a treatment plan, describing the underlying causes of hypertension and self-care strategies, adhering to scheduled follow-up appointments, describing the actions and side effects of current medications, and expressing commitment to and self-responsibility for controlling hypertension.

Intervention. The greatest problem in the management of chronic hypertension involves the client's lack of adherence to nonpharmacologic and pharmacologic interventions. An estimated 40% to 60% of clients with hypertension fail to comply with prescribed therapy. There are several reasons why hypertensive clients do not follow prescribed regimens:

1. The asymptomatic nature of the disease tends to minimize the perceived seriousness of the problem and importance of intervention.
2. Therapeutic regimens often demand difficult lifestyle changes, such as low-sodium diets, weight loss, and smoking cessation.
3. Many hypertensive agents produce annoying side effects, and clients who require antihypertensive medication may consider the intervention worse than the disease.
4. The high cost of medications and the inconvenience of obtaining health care also contribute to noncompliance.

Nursing interventions for promoting compliance with the antihypertensive treatment regimen include individualizing care, ensuring adequate follow-up, communicating often with the client, and teaching the client and family. Compliance usually improves dramatically when the client understands the causative factors underlying hypertension as well as the consequences of inadequate intervention and health maintenance.

EVALUATION

Medications can bring blood pressure down quickly. The remainder of interventions, such as stress management, exercise, and smoking cessation, are more difficult to implement and maintain. Expect the client to struggle with compliance with all of the necessary changes. Ask specific questions in a nonjudgmental manner. As needed, recommend involvement in various self-help groups, such as smoking cessation groups.

Modifications for Elderly Clients

Hypertension is one of the most prevalent cardiovascular diseases among older adults, and because of their advanced age, these clients are more likely to suffer from end organ damage secondary to chronically elevated pressure.[10, 22] Blood pressure readings in older adults show greater variability from one measurement to the next than seen in younger clients; therefore, the diagnosis is made after several readings. Recent research findings indicate a need to treat hypertension in elderly people, regardless of whether both the systolic *and* diastolic pressures are involved or there is evidence of only isolated systolic hypertension. Older adults are more likely to experience adverse reactions to antihypertensive drugs and are monitored closely for evidence of such reactions; they are given detailed advice on the specifics of their medication regimens; and the clinical course of the disease is carefully followed.

The ultimate goal of antihypertensive therapy in older adults is not to try to lower the pressure to "normal" values but, rather, to lower the pressure gradually to a level sufficient to eliminate target organ damage and to minimize the risk of hypoperfusion. "Start low and go slow" is the principle followed for prescribing medications to the older adult. Too rapid a reduction in blood pressure in elderly clients, particularly those with chronic hypertension, may produce cerebral hypoperfusion manifested by decreased mental status, weakness, and dizziness. These changes may appear at measured blood pressures still above the upper limit of normal.

HYPERTENSIVE CRISES: URGENCY VERSUS EMERGENCY[11, 16, 18, 22, 25]

Elevated blood pressure alone, in the absence of clinical manifestations or new or progressive target organ damage, rarely requires *emergency* therapy. In most cases, the hypertensive crisis really constitutes a hypertensive *urgency,* in which severe elevation in blood pressure has been reached but there is mild or no acute target organ damage. Hypertensive urgencies include cases in which it is desirable to reduce blood pressure within a few hours to 24 hours.

However, *malignant hypertension,* a seldom-used term today, constitutes a true medical emergency and is currently referred to as *persistent severe hypertension.* The seriousness of the crisis correlates not so much with the level of blood pressure elevation as with the extent of target organ damage. Without treatment, persistent severe hypertension results in a 90% mortality rate within 1 year secondary to renal or heart failure, cerebrovascular accident, myocardial infarction, or aortic dissection. The most common cause of persistent severe hypertension is untreated hypertension. Other causes include eclampsia, dissecting aortic aneurysm, pyelonephritis, sudden catecholamine release (as from a pheochromocytoma), drug or toxic substance ingestion or exposure, and food and drug interactions (e.g., between a monoamine oxidase inhibitor [MAO] and aged cheese).

Clinical manifestations include those of hypertensive encephalopathy evidenced by restlessness, changes in level of consciousness (e.g., confusion, somnolence, lethargy, memory defects, coma, seizures), blurred vision, dizziness, headache, nausea, and vomiting. Assessment may also reveal renal insufficiency, proteinuria, hematuria, urinary sediment casts, hemolytic anemia, left ventricular failure, and pulmonary edema. Severe headache may be occipital or anterior in location, is steady and throbbing in quality, and is often worse in the morning. Visual blurring, reduced visual acuity, and even blindness can occur. Acute renal failure, rapid vascular deterioration, and stroke can also develop.

Outcome Management

True hypertensive emergencies are uncommon but do occur occasionally; in such cases, immediate blood pressure reduction is imperative to prevent or limit target organ damage. The usual initial treatment is parenteral administration of appropriate pharmacologic agents in an emergency department or an intensive care unit. Conversely, hypertensive urgencies can be managed in a hospital or clinic setting with *oral* doses of drugs with relatively fast onset of action. Oral and parenteral drugs currently used for hypertensive urgencies and emergencies are listed in Table 52–6. Although sublingual administration of nifedipine had been widely used for this purpose, it is no longer considered appropriate therapy because of several reports of severe adverse effects from its use.

The initial goal of therapy in hypertensive crisis is to reduce mean arterial pressure by no more than 25% within the first minutes to 2 hours. Then reduction in blood pressure toward 160/100 mm Hg is accomplished over the next 2 to 6 hours. Blood pressure is monitored frequently (every 5 to 15 minutes depending on the drug and route of administration used), and medications are titrated to manage the course of blood pressure reduction. It is essential to avoid excessive falls in blood pressure, which can precipitate renal, cerebral, or coronary ischemia. Consequently, restoration of normal blood pressure must be done slowly and with care. Once the client is out of immediate danger, oral medications are adjusted while vital signs are monitored continuously, and changes in drug therapy regimens are made if necessary.

COMMUNITY SCREENING AND SELF-CARE

Public Health Initiative

Research showing the importance of normalized blood pressure for clients' optimum health led to the introduction by the National Heart, Lung and Blood Institute (NHLBI) of the National High Blood Pressure Education Program (NHBPEP) in 1972.[25] The NHBPEP is the first large-scale public outreach and education campaign to reduce high blood pressure. Its promotion of the detection, treatment, and control of high blood pressure has been credited with influencing the dramatic increase in the public's understanding of hypertension and its role in heart attacks and strokes.

However, the prevention and treatment of hypertension continues to represent a major public health concern for the United States.[16, 25] Prevention of hypertension and early discovery of new cases depend on a broader national public health effort. With guidance from the *Healthy People 2000/2010* initiatives, this national effort has begun. In addition to the diligent work of the NHBPEP, government support is increasing, and nationwide attention and assistance from business and industry, labor organizations, health care institutions, voluntary associations, and local communities are also on the rise. Revised goals of the national public health plan are as follows:

- To prevent the rise of blood pressure with age
- To decrease the existing prevalence of hypertension
- To increase hypertension awareness and detection
- To improve control of hypertension
- To reduce cardiovascular risks

TABLE 52–6 PHARMACOLOGIC TREATMENT FOR HYPERTENSIVE URGENCIES AND EMERGENCIES

Drug Class with Example(s) and Dosage	Monitoring*	Comments/Nursing Considerations
HYPERTENSIVE URGENCIES		
ACE Inhibitors		
Captopril (Capoten)—first-line agent 25 mg PO; may repeat in 30 min Enalapril (Vasotec)—second-line agent 5 mg PO, may repeat in 30 min	BP should be checked at 15-min intervals over first hour, at 30-min intervals over second hour, then hourly	Very effective first-line therapy in hypertensive *urgency* with diastolic BP >110 mm Hg when client has no end-organ problems and oral treatment over several hours is indicated.
Centrally Acting Alpha$_2$ Agonist		
Clonidine (Catapres) 0.1–0.2 mg loading dose, followed by 0.1 mg every 20 min to 1 h up to 0.7–0.8 mg total	Monitor level of consciousness BP should be checked at 15-min intervals over first hour, at 30-min intervals over second hour, and then hourly	Effective second-line treatment of hypertensive urgency. Sedation is a common side effect. After 8 h, clonidine dosing may begin again if necessary.
Adrenergic Inhibitor		
Labetalol is the most commonly used agent in this group—see under Hypertensive Emergencies for discussion Oral dose determined per client situation.	BP should be checked at 15-min intervals over first hour, at 30-min intervals over second hour, and then hourly	Effective second-line treatment of hypertensive urgency. Be particularly watchful for the development of heart block—adrenergic blockade of normal cardiac conduction.
Calcium Antagonists/Calcium Channel Blockers		
Diltiazem (Cardizem) and verapamil (Calan) are drugs of choice in this category but are currently used cautiously; therapy must be completely individualized	Monitor pulse closely BP should be checked at 15-min intervals over first hour, at 30-min intervals over second hour, and then hourly	May be effective and efficient choice if BP elevation is secondary to a tachyarrhythmia. Be particularly watchful for the development of heart block—adrenergic blockade of normal cardiac conduction. Sublingual nifedipine or any fast-acting form of nifedipine is now **contraindicated** in the treatment of hypertensive emergency.
HYPERTENSIVE EMERGENCIES		
(Drugs listed in order of rapidity of action, with most rapid listed first)		
Vasodilators		
Sodium nitroprusside (Nipride) 0.25–10 μg/kg/min as IV infusion† (maximal dose for 10 min only) Fenoldopam mesylate 0.1–0.3 μg/kg/min IV infusion Nitroglycerin 5–100 μg/min as IV infusion Nicardipine hydrochloride 5–15 mg/h IV Hydralazine hydrochloride 10–20 mg IV 10–50 mg IM Enalaprilat 1.25–5 mg q 6 h IV	For all of these drugs: careful and continuous monitoring of IV lines and blood pressure is essential Monitor for too rapid a fall in BP or increase in pulse Monitor for side effects; most cause GI disturbance in varying degrees such as nausea/vomiting, tachycardia, headache, flushing, sweating—all secondary to increased vasodilation IV use of these drugs restricted to hospital emergency room and intensive care settings; drug titration continued until normotensive status prevails and persists	Nipride, fenoldopam, and nicardipine are most commonly used in hypertensive emergencies, with certain precautions to indicate which drug to use in a given situation. Nitroglycerin is drug of choice when coronary ischemia is also present (may use with extreme caution in combination with sodium nitroprusside). Enalaprilat may be most effective with acute left ventricular failure; however, it must be avoided in acute myocardial infarction.
Adrenergic Inhibitors		
Esmolol hydrochloride 250–500 μg/kg/min for 1 min, then 50–100 μg/kg/min for 4 min; may repeat sequence Phentolamine 5–15 mg IV Labetalol hydrochloride 20–80 mg IV bolus q 10 min 0.5–2.0 mg/min IV infusion	In addition to foregoing outcome and monitoring considerations, be particularly watchful for development of heart block—adrenergic blockade of normal cardiac conduction	Labetalol is the only one of this group that is commonly used for most hypertensive emergencies, except in acute heart failure. All of these drugs may be used in combination with vasodilators to increase effectiveness. Esmolol and phentolamine are reserved for specific underlying causes of increased blood pressure (i.e., aortic dissection and catecholamine excess, respectively).

*See Table 52–5 for drug actions and therapeutic outcomes.
ACE: angiotensin-converting enzyme; BP, blood pressure.

- To increase the recognition of the importance of controlled isolated systolic hypertension
- To improve recognition of the importance of the persistence and damage from high-normal blood pressures
- To reduce ethnic, socioeconomic, and regional variations in hypertension
- To improve opportunities for treatment
- To enhance community programs

Managed Care and Community Screening

Because high blood pressure is very common, its management requires a major commitment from clinicians and managed care organizations. Managed care programs offer the opportunity for a coordinated systematic, multifactorial, multidisciplinary approach to care. Nurse-managed clinics offer attractive opportunities to improve adherence and outcomes.

Hypertensive clients usually find out about their condition through incidental screening in health care facilities or through organized community screening in public settings (e.g., shopping malls, schools, the workplace). Nurses are actively involved in both approaches. About 80% of Americans come into contact with some aspect of the health care system at least once a year (e.g., in a health care provider's office, clinic, or hospital). Each encounter with the health care system presents an opportunity for incidental blood pressure screening. Blood pressure measurement should be a routine procedure at every initial encounter with a health care practitioner and annually thereafter.

Organized community screening programs help assess the remaining 20% of Americans not in contact with any part of the health care system.[29] Such programs identify not only clients with untreated hypertension but also those who have discontinued intervention or whose hypertension is not adequately controlled by current intervention. In addition, screening programs provide an opportunity to educate the public. It is particularly important to screen members of high-risk "target groups," such as black and elderly populations. Community services need to keep target groups in mind when choosing the setting for blood pressure screenings. Practitioners who take blood pressure readings need to inform clients in writing of their blood pressure and its significance and, if necessary, the importance of follow-up evaluation. Culturally and linguistically appropriate counseling by health care providers is important to those efforts.

Self-Measurement of Blood Pressure

Measurement of blood pressure outside a health care provider's office can provide valuable information for initial evaluation and subsequent follow-up of people with hypertension. Most drug, medical supply, and grocery stores provide standardized blood pressure monitors that their customers can use at no cost. These monitoring stations are generally located near the pharmacy or medical supplies department. Such stores also usually carry a variety of self-measurement blood pressure devices for home use. Choosing a monitoring device may be confusing for some people; however, several models of accurate and appropriate electronic or aneroid-type sphygmomanometers are available. Most insurance packages cover the cost of a home blood pressure unit, and these devices are generally easy to use.

Manual and electronic arm and wrist cuffs are the most accurate. Finger monitors are available but have proved inaccurate in standardized testing. Periodically, the accuracy of the instrument used in the home should be checked by comparing home readings with those obtained in the health care provider's office, at a "health fair," or in a community nursing clinic.

SYNCOPE

Syncope (fainting) is defined as generalized muscle weakness and inability to stand erect accompanied by loss of consciousness. It is a good measure of cardiovascular status because it may indicate decreased cardiac output, fluid volume deficits, or defects in cerebral tissue perfusion.

Syncope is a common occurrence when a person tries to stand after being bedridden for a time. This form of syncope, called *postural hypotension,* can be seen in clients attempting to ambulate the first few times after surgery, in clients who have been on prolonged bed rest, and clients who have dysrhythmias. When a person quickly moves to a standing position, blood normally pools in the lower legs. The arterial pressure receptors in the aortic arch detect the fall in cardiac output that occurs with the lack of venous return, and they increase sympathetic tone to compress arterioles to improve venous return.[5] If the sympathetic response is not adequate or is blocked by medication, the person becomes dizzy because of the decreased cerebral perfusion. All medications taken to reduce blood pressure have the potential to cause orthostatic hypotension or postural hypotension—some more than others, such as potent diuretics, alpha$_1$-receptor blockers, and vasodilators.

When a client reports dizziness or is at risk of syncope because of medication use or prolonged bed rest, assess fluid volume status and check the pulse for irregularities. If syncope develops, it can usually be managed by having the client move slowly to a sitting position and rest a moment before standing. If the client becomes dizzy, instruct him or her to breathe deeply and to keep both eyes open. Syncope should resolve within moments. If it is prolonged, place the client supine, use leg exercises to improve venous return, and wait until the blood pressure returns to a normotensive state. Confused clients who do not wait for syncope to resolve before walking are at risk for falls. Bed alarms may be needed.

CONCLUSIONS

New coalitions between health care providers and individual communities are forming to focus on the prevention and management of hypertension throughout all stages of life. Support from the community and greater use of technology such as the Internet will play an increasingly greater role in promoting long-term adherence to lifestyle and pharmacologic regimens. Achieving long-term control of blood pressure risk factors requires that the same interest and attention given to initial evaluation and treatment decisions also be given to long-term management issues.

THINKING CRITICALLY

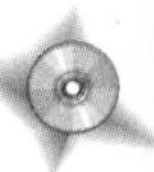

A 50-year-old obese black man presents to your clinic with persistent elevated blood pressure. He has

had hypertension for 7 months. Despite attempts at lifestyle management, his blood pressure continued to rise. He was started on a regimen of antihypertensive medication 1 month ago. He has returned to the clinic today for a follow-up visit. His blood pressure is higher than it was initially. What might explain his continued elevated blood pressure?

Factors to Consider. What other history and physical examination data should you obtain in order to more effectively analyze this case? When and how long should lifestyle modifications alone be encouraged? How long does it take for various medications to be effective? What diseases worsen hypertension? What psychosocial factors affect compliance with or adherence to a treatment regimen? What modifications in the pharmacologic treatment plan, if any, would be most appropriate at this time?

BIBLIOGRAPHY

1. Patient education. Understanding hypertension. (1999). *Nurse Practitioner: American Journal of Primary Health Care, 24*(5), 38.
2. Ambler, S. K., & Brown, R. D. (1999). Genetic determinants of blood pressure regulation. *Journal of Cardiovascular Nursing, 13*(4), 59–77.
3. Benson, H., & Friedman, R. (1996). Harnessing the power of the placebo effect and renaming it "remembered wellness." *Annual Review of Medicine, 47,* 193–199.
4. Bushnell, K. L., & Smith, L. A. (1998). Hypertension clinical outcomes in a nurse practitioner managed care setting. *Seminars in Nursing Management, 6*(3), 155–160.
5. Engstrom, J. W., & Aminoff, M. J. (1997). Evaluation and treatment of orthostatic hypotension. *American Family Physician, 56,* 1378–1384.
6. Fagan, T. C. (1995). Calcium antagonists and mortality: Another case of the need for clinical judgment. *Archives of Internal Medicine, 155,* 2145.
7. Kolasa, K. M. (1999). Dietary Approaches to Stop Hypertension (DASH) in clinical practice: A primary care experience. *Clinical Cardiology, 22*(7 suppl.), III16–III22.
8. Kuncl, N., & Nelson, K. M. (1997). Antihypertensive drugs: Balancing risks and benefits. *Nursing, 27*(8), 46–49.
9. Kyngas, H., & Lahdenpera, T. (1999). Compliance of patients with hypertension and associated factors. *Journal of Advanced Nursing, 29*(4), 832–839.
10. Lever, A. F., & Ramsey, L. E. (1995). Treatment of hypertension in the elderly. *Current Science, 13,* 571–579.
11. Mancia, G., & Grassi, G. (1998). Antihypertensive treatment: Past, present and future. *Journal of Hypertension, Supplement, 16*(1), S1–S7.
12. McCance, K. L. (1998). Structure and function of the cardiovascular and lymphatic systems. In K. L. McCance & S. E. Huether (Eds.), *Pathophysiology: The biologic basis for disease in adults and children* (pp. 968–1023). St. Louis: Mosby–Year Book.
13. McPaul, K. (1999). New hypertension guidelines: Commentary. *AAOHN Journal, 47*(3), 114–116.
14. Michels, K. B., et al. (1998). Prospective study of calcium-channel blocker use, cardiovascular disease, and total mortality among hypertensive women. The Nurses' Health Study. *Circulation, 97,* 1540–1548.
15. Moser, M. (1998). Why are physicians not prescribing diuretics more frequently in the management of hypertension? *Journal of the American Medical Association, 279*(22), 1813–1816.
16. National High Blood Pressure Education Program, National Institutes of Health, National Heart, Lung and Blood Institute. (1997). *The Sixth Report of the Joint National Committee on Detection, Evaluation, and Treatment of High Blood Pressure* (NIH Publication No. 98-4080). Bethesda, MD: U.S. Government Printing Office.
17. Pinkowish, M. D. (1995). What is white-coat hypertension? *Patient Care, 23*(2), 15.
18. Porsche, R. (1995). Hypertension: Diagnosis, acute antihypertension therapy, and long-term management. *AACN Clinical Issues, 6,* 515–525.
19. Psaty, B. M., et al. (1997). Health outcomes associated with antihypertensive therapies used as first-line agents. A systematic review and meta-analysis. *Journal of the American Medical Association, 277,* 739–745.
20. Schneider, R. H., et al. (1995). A randomized controlled trial of stress reduction for hypertension in older African Americans. *Hypertension, 26,* 820–827.
21. Seidel, H. M., et al. (1999). *Mosby's guide to physical examination* (4th ed.). St. Louis: Mosby.
22. Sullivan, J. A. (1998). Hypertension in the elderly: Don't treat too quickly! *Journal of Emergency Nursing, 24*(1), 20–26.
23. Tobin, L. J. (1999). Evaluating mild to moderate hypertension. *Nurse Practitioner, 24*(5), 22, 25–26, 29–30.
24. Uphold, C. R., & Graham, M. V. (1998). *Clinical guidelines in family practice* (3rd ed.). Gainesville, FL: Barmarrae Books.
25. U.S. Department of Health and Human Services. (2000). *Healthy People 2010: National health promotion and disease prevention objectives.* Washington, DC: Public Health Service.
26. U.S. Department of Health and Human Services. (1995). *Clinical practice guideline number 17: Cardiac rehabilitation.* (AHCPR Pub. No. 96-0672). Rockville, MD: Author.
27. Van Wissen, K., Litchfield, M., Maling, T. (1998). Living with high blood pressure. *Journal of Advanced Nursing, 27*(3), 567–574.
28. Vantrimpont, P., et al. (1997). Additive beneficial effects of beta-blockers to angiotensin-converting enzyme inhibitors in the Survival and Ventricular Enlargement (SAVE) study. *Journal of American College of Cardiology, 29,* 229–236.
29. Wang, C., & Abbott, L. J. (1998). Development of a community-based diabetes and hypertension preventive program. *Public Health Nursing, 15*(6), 406–414.
30. Weber, M. (1999). Guidelines for assessing outcomes of antihypertensive treatment. *American Journal of Cardiology, 84*(2A), 2K–4K.

CHAPTER 53

Management of Clients with Vascular Disorders

Janice D. Nunnelee

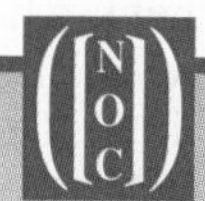

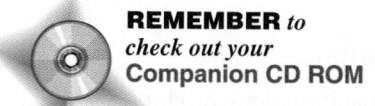

NURSING OUTCOMES CLASSIFICATION (NOC)
for Nursing Diagnoses—Clients with Vascular Disorders

Altered Tissue Perfusion
Pain Level
Tissue Perfusion: Cardiac
Tissue Perfusion: Pulmonary
Vital Signs Status

Anxiety
Anxiety Control
Coping

Delayed Surgical Recovery
Endurance
Infection Status
Self-Care: Activities of Daily Living (ADL)
Wound Healing: Primary Intention
Wound Healing: Secondary Intention

Health Seeking Behaviors
Adherence Behaviors
Health Beliefs
Health Promoting Behavior
Health Seeking Behavior
Knowledge: Health Promotion
Knowledge: Health Resources

Impaired Gas Exchange
Electrolyte and Acid-Base Balance
Respiratory Status: Gas Exchange
Respiratory Status: Ventilation
Tissue Perfusion: Pulmonary

Impaired Physical Mobility
Ambulation: Walking
Body Positioning: Self-Initiated
Immobility Consequences: Physiologic
Mobility Level
Transfer Performance

Knowledge Deficit
Knowledge Deficit: Disease Process
Knowledge Deficit: Health Behaviors
Knowledge Deficit: Health Resources
Knowledge: Medication
Knowledge Deficit: Illness
Knowledge: Prescribed Activity
Knowledge Deficit: Treatment Procedure(s)
Knowledge: Treatment Regimen

Pain
Comfort Level
Pain Control
Pain: Disruptive Effects
Pain Level

Risk for Activity Intolerance
Coping
Health Beliefs: Perceived Control
Mood Equilibrium
Nutritional Status: Energy
Symptom Control
Symptom Severity

Risk for Fluid Volume Deficit
Bowel Elimination
Electrolyte and Acid-Base Balance
Fluid Balance
Hydration
Nutritional Status: Food and Fluid Intake
Urinary Elimination

Risk for Impaired Skin Integrity
Immobility Consequences: Physiologic
Nutritional Status
Physical Aging Status
Risk Control
Risk Detection
Tissue Integrity: Skin and Mucous Membranes
Tissue Perfusion: Peripheral

PERIPHERAL ARTERY DISORDERS

Peripheral vascular disease encompasses three systems: the arterial, the venous, and the lymphatic. Peripheral arterial occlusive disorders involve narrowing of the arterial lumen or damage to the endothelial lining. Narrowing can be partial (stenosis) or complete (occlusion). The clinical manifestations and management may differ, depending on the client's needs and the degree of occlusion. Additionally, the manifestations of chronic disease differ considerably from those of acute arterial disease.

Etiology and Risk Factors

Peripheral arterial occlusive diseases are caused primarily by atherosclerosis. Other causes include embolism, thrombosis, trauma, vasospasm, inflammation, and autoimmunity. Obesity is a risk factor for arterial disorders. The cause of some disorders remains unknown. Most of the pathologic changes that occur in peripheral arterial occlusive disease are caused by atherosclerosis. Atherosclerosis is considered in detail in Chapter 56.

Pathophysiology

The peripheral arterial system delivers oxygen-rich blood to the peripheral vascular beds. Any alteration in blood flow disrupts the balance between oxygen supply and demand. Prolonged reduction in blood flow or the presence of large areas of decreased perfusion initiates vasodilation and promotes the development of collateral arterial pathways and utilization of anaerobic pathways for oxygen demands to be met. These compensatory mechanisms are designed to bring in new blood supplies but are limited in effectiveness. Vasodilation has a limited effect because arteries that are deprived of oxygen quickly become maximally dilated. Collateral vessels needed to improve blood supply develop slowly over time. Cellular anaerobic metabolism tries to meet the basic requirements, but the waste products of lactic acid and pyruvic acid build up quickly, are extremely toxic, and are excreted slowly. Significant increases in these two acids can lead to acidosis.

As the compensatory mechanisms prove inadequate to meet peripheral arterial needs, and without other intervention, the eventual result is pain. The pain is analogous to anginal pain and is called *intermittent claudication,* which occurs when a muscle is forced to contract without an adequate blood supply to meet the metabolic needs of exercise. It is a specific manifestation of peripheral arterial disease and results from muscular hypoxia and metabolite accumulation. Any muscle can claudicate, including muscles in the arms, legs, jaw, or anywhere that decreased arterial supply exists. This section primarily focuses on lower extremity disease.

The physiologic effect of any given stenosis is variable because it is determined not only by the degree of narrowing but also by the number of collateral vessels that have developed. The lower limbs are more susceptible to arterial occlusive disorders and atherosclerosis than the upper limbs because of the natural collateral system in the upper extremities. The most common locations of stenosis supplying a lower extremity are the aortoiliac bifurcation and the femoral bifurcation (Fig. 53–1). In general, stenoses occur at bifurcations in arteries.

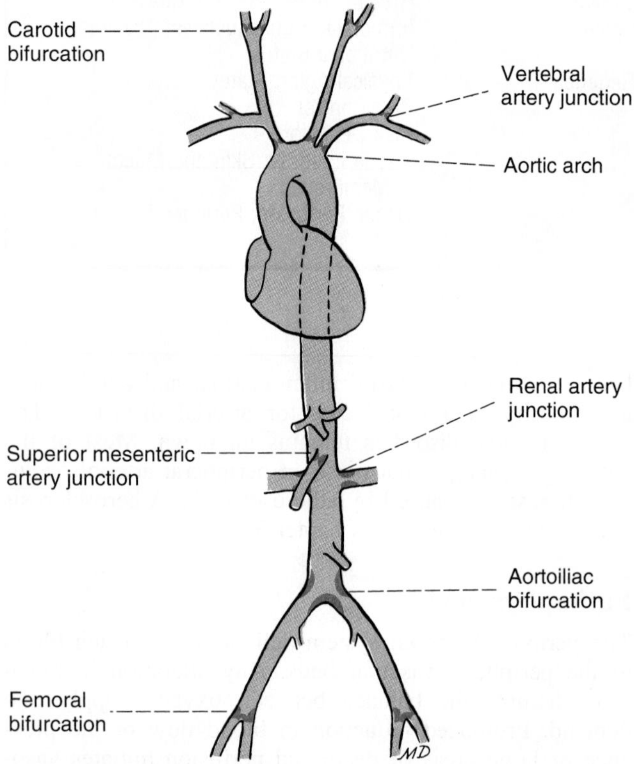

FIGURE 53–1 Major sites of peripheral atherosclerotic occlusive disease.

Clinical Manifestations

The most important manifestations of chronic arterial occlusive disease are *intermittent claudication* and *rest pain.* The client typically complains of pain described as tightening pressure in the calves or buttocks or a sharp, cramp-like or burning sensation that occurs during walking and disappears with rest. The pain is reproducible and not positional. It always occurs in a muscle distal to the stenosis or occlusion.

Intermittent claudication is influenced by the speed and incline of the walk, conditions that increase the demand for oxygen by muscles of the legs. The more rapid the speed or the greater the incline, the faster claudication occurs. The client's exercise tolerance generally decreases over time; episodes of claudication occur with less exertion. Claudication response is constant, reproducible, and not positional. *Reproducible* means that the client who walks the same distance at the same speed and incline has manifestations at the same distance each time. The client who cannot walk the length of a house because of leg pain one day but can walk indefinitely the next day does not have intermittent claudication.

Another hallmark of chronic arterial insufficiency is a dusky, purplish discoloration of the foot and leg when the foot is placed in a dependent position. This *dependent rubor* changes to white pallor when the leg is elevated.

Clinical manifestations of chronic arterial occlusion may not appear for 20 to 40 years. Claudication, usually insidious in onset, generally occurs in men, although the incidence rises in women after menopause. Usually, claudication strikes males in their 50s or 60s. Nearly half of clients who experience claudication also have associated severe coronary artery disease.

As the disease progresses, clinical manifestations become more severe. The development of pain at rest, usually occurring at night when the client lies supine, indicates limb-threatening disease. Usually described as a dull, deep pain in the toes or forefoot, this sensation awakens clients from sleep and may cause them to hang the foot over the side of the bed or to get up and walk around for relief. Clients may start to sleep in a chair with their legs dependent. Placing the leg in a dependent position provides increased gravitation supply of blood. This often results in a moderate degree of lower extremity edema. The affected foot usually demonstrates dependent rubor.

Manifestations of cutaneous arterial insufficiency are nonspecific. Their presence in combination with claudication, however, indicates advanced disease. Skin and subcutaneous tissues require little blood flow for maintenance of normal nutrition. Coldness of feet is an unreliable sign, but a sudden onset of coldness suggests acute arterial insufficiency or occlusion. Other objective data associated with arterial insufficiency include weak or absent peripheral pulses, dependent rubor and pallor with elevation, hypertrophied toenails, tissue atrophy, ulceration, and gangrene (Fig. 53–2). Paresthesias with exertion indicate ischemia of the peripheral nerves because of the phenomenon of *arterial steal.* This phenomenon occurs as arterioles of the muscles are maximally dilated because of hypoxia. To meet muscular metabolic needs, these arterioles steal from cutaneous and peripheral nerve vessels,

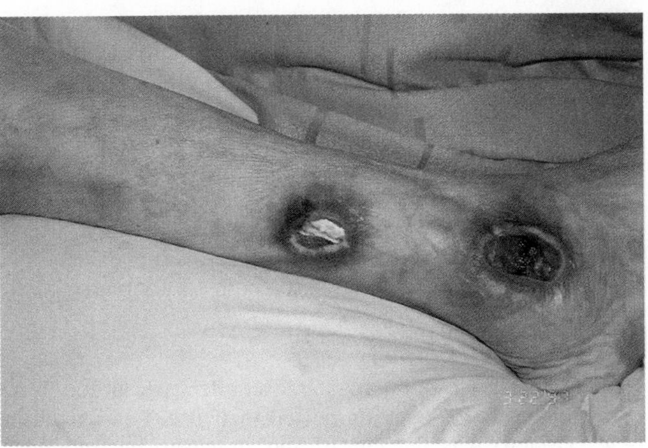

FIGURE 53–2 Arterial ulcers of the lateral malleolus and distal lateral portion of the leg. Note round, smooth shape.

which results in coldness and a "pins and needles" sensation.

Lower extremity pain may also appear in several other disorders unrelated to arterial disease. Other conditions that cause a similar type of pain include arthritis, lumbar disc protrusion, neuritis, and muscle cramps. However, the pain of other conditions is not consistent or replicable. The pain of arthritis, disc protrusion, and neuritis may also be positional.

Aortoiliac disorders are a form of chronic arterial occlusive disease characterized by aortoiliac stenosis and occlusion. These disorders result in clinical manifestations in the legs (Fig. 53–3). Assessment reveals hip, thigh, and buttock claudication with absent or diminished femoral and distal pulses. In males, impotence is also part of the syndrome known as Leriche's syndrome. Dependent rubor is common when aortoiliac and femoropopliteal disorders are combined.

A femoropopliteal disorder refers to an occlusion in the chief arteries of the proximal leg or thigh. The most common manifestation of superficial femoral artery and popliteal disease is calf claudication, which may improve, stay the same, or potentially progress to rest pain. Popliteal artery disease and stenosis in the anterior or posterior tibial artery results in claudication in the distal leg and foot.

Diagnostic evaluation of the lower extremity includes both noninvasive and invasive techniques. Techniques range from simple measurement of ankle/brachial index (ABI) to the use of magnetic resonance imaging (MRI) to measure arterial blood flow. Recording of an ABI provides information at the bedside. Segmental Doppler systolic blood pressure and pulse waveform analysis provide more objective information about the level and severity of occlusive disease. Treadmill examination, a form of lower extremity stress testing, measures the fall of arterial pressure with ambulation and the rapidity with which it returns to baseline. Color flow imaging visualizes the blood flow in the vessels and records pressures within the vessel. It is possible that imaging may replace arteriography in the future.

Arteriography is the definitive examination when surgery is being considered. It reveals the lumen of the blood vessels. It is not a measurement of actual blood flow, as the noninvasive assessment is, but instead shows the outline of the contrast media within the lumen. Because of the contrast media, there are many potential complications. Computed tomography (CT) angiography, sometimes called spiral CT, is in its infancy but may replace conventional angiography.

Outcome Management

The goals of management are to reduce the risk of progressive arterial disease, promote arterial flow, and reverse the disease that is present. Important outcomes include improving the quality of life if no other intervention is possible. Specialists in the field exist in both the medical and advanced nursing practice realm. Medical management is appropriate for clients with intermittent claudication and non-limb-threatening ischemia. Additionally, medical management may be the only course of action in the client with multiple morbidities who is a poor surgical risk.

Medical Management

RISK REDUCTION

WEIGHT REDUCTION. Clients are advised and counseled to reduce body weight by following a low-fat, low-

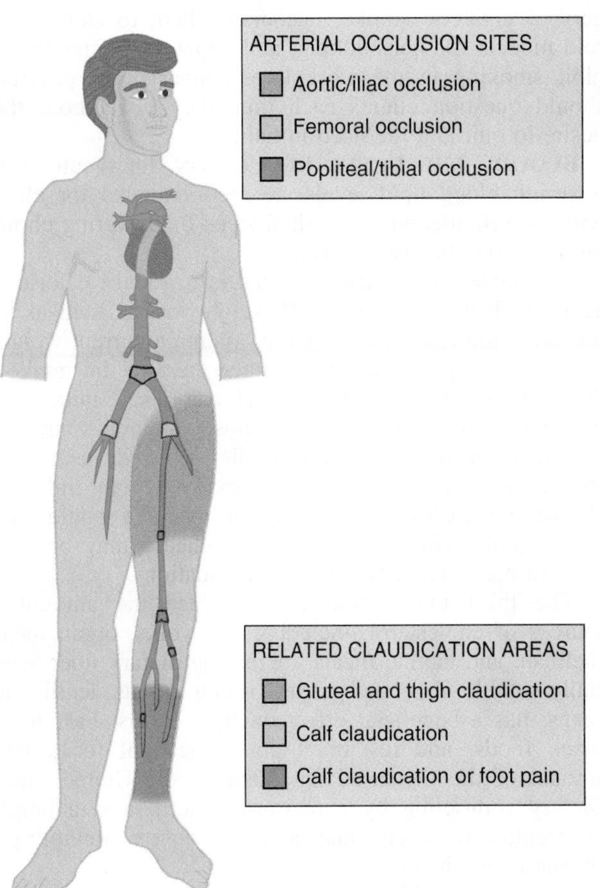

FIGURE 53–3 Occlusion of the arterial system at any given location leads to a specific portion of claudication in distal tissues.

cholesterol diet containing more fruits and vegetables. There is no evidence that any special diet alters the course of atherosclerosis once it has appeared. Small studies claim that rigid diets reverse atherosclerosis, but no major body of data exists to support this hypothesis.

EXERCISE. A prescribed moderate program of exercise and rest helps increase collateral circulation and improve conditioning. Several studies have shown that clients involved in an exercise program generally feel better and can slowly improve their walking distance. Clients are instructed to walk every day, provided that no skin ulcerations are present. The exercise program should begin judiciously and progress gradually until the client has substantially lengthened walking distances. For obese and chronically ill clients, an exercise program should be (1) individually tailored to the client's abilities, goals, interests, and resources and (2) written with specific instructions.[20] Most clients can significantly increase their walking distance, and many can avoid surgery if they exercise regularly and stop smoking.

SMOKING CESSATION. Cigarette smoking influences vascular disability. Nicotine is a potent vasoconstrictor. Clients who stop smoking improve their treadmill walking distance. Smoking cessation is extremely difficult, because nicotine is a highly addictive chemical. Social support, especially of friends and family members, seems to be an important factor in assisting smokers to quit. Pharmacologic measures may be instituted by the primary care provider if necessary. Educate clients about the dangers of cigarette smoke, encourage them to stop, act as role models for nonsmoking, and support policies to prohibit smoking in the workplace. Primary care providers should question clients each time they visit about their desire to quit and the need to quit.

BLOOD LIPID LEVEL REDUCTION. Interventions for lowering blood lipid levels are recommended for clients with hyperlipidemia. The initial steps for lowering cholesterol involve dietary intervention.

For obese clients, the first goal is to reduce calories to achieve ideal body weight. If weight loss is seen as improbable, the client should try to maintain current weight.

The next major step is to reduce the total fat intake in the diet to 30% or less of total calories. Saturated fat intake should be reduced. The most common sources of saturated fat in the American diet are red meat, fried foods, and dairy products, especially whole milk and cheese. Increasing the quantity of fish and poultry and changing to skim milk and nonfat cheese may be sufficient to meet saturated fat recommendations.

The third major goal is to reduce the amount of sources of cholesterol, including egg yolks, organ meats, shellfish, and animal meats. Increasing dietary fiber, especially soluble fiber, such as that found in oats, lentils, and beans, has a beneficial effect on lipid levels. Fast foods, snack foods, and restaurant dining account for a large amount of the increased fat intake in the United States. Dietary counseling by a registered dietitian is a helpful intervention for clients and families who are attempting to change eating habits.

Pharmacologic intervention may be needed for clients with high levels of hyperlipidemia and for those whose dietary changes have been less than successful. The major drug groups include nicotinic acid, fibrin acid derivatives, bile acid resins, meglutol (hydroxymethylglutaryl), coenzyme A (CoA) reductase inhibitors, and probucol. These medications have varying degrees of effectiveness, and each produces important side effects. Guidelines have changed over the past few years, with intervention encouraged when the low-density lipoproteins (LDLs) reach 160 in a client with no risk factors and 130 (with levels of 100 recommended) in diabetic clients or when clients have two or more risk factors. Controversy exists over treatment in younger clients with high LDLs or triglycerides.

PROMOTE ARTERIAL FLOW

Vasodilators were popular in the remote past, although no convincing studies ever supported their use. Pentoxifylline (e.g., Trental) was introduced and shown to be somewhat effective in increasing walking distance in combination with conditioning exercise. Pentoxifylline is reported to reduce blood viscosity and enhance oxygen delivery to the muscle of the affected limb. The major side effect is gastrointestinal upset, which may be avoided by taking the medication with meals. A new drug, cilostazol (Pletal), helps to increase walking distance with or without exercise. Ongoing trials will give evidence to its efficacy.

In severe cases of arterial insufficiency, the physician may order that the reverse Trendelenburg position be used. The head of the client's bed should be elevated on 6-inch blocks (either constructed, or use steady books such as encyclopedias) so that blood from the heart flows more easily, via gravity, to the extremities when the client sleeps or rests.

Nursing Management of the Medical Client

ASSESSMENT

The history should include an account of arterial problems, surgery, medications, and ulcerations. Because of the chronic nature of the problem, a psychosocial assessment is warranted. Feelings of powerlessness may exist. Some clients are not aware of chest pain, shortness of breath, or fatigue because their attention is focused on leg discomfort. Question them carefully about these discomforts. Medical or surgical intervention may reduce pain and thus improve walking ability.

The physical examination should include peripheral pulses, ABI, assessment of quality of arterial flow with a hand-held Doppler, notations of skin color, assessment of skin integrity (including the presence of ulcers, darkened areas of skin, tinea pedis, thickened nails), capillary refill ($\leq$3 seconds is normal), and the presence of venous filling when the foot is dependent.

DIAGNOSIS, OUTCOMES, INTERVENTIONS

Altered Tissue Perfusion. The ideal nursing diagnosis for clients with arterial disorders is *Altered Peripheral Tissue Perfusion.* Write the diagnosis as *Altered Peripheral Tissue Perfusion related to interruption of blood flow secondary to arterial occlusion.*

Outcomes. The client will maintain adequate peripheral tissue perfusion in affected extremities, as evidenced by warm, dry skin with normal peripheral pulse, color, temperature, motor and sensory function, and capillary filling.

Interventions

Promote Arterial Flow. For safe positioning of a client with peripheral vascular disease, first learn whether the disorder is arterial or venous in nature. Because blood flows to dependent parts of the body (i.e., parts lower than the heart), position clients with arterial disease so that blood flows toward the legs and feet. In milder cases, clients can benefit from sitting for periods of time with their feet flat on the floor. If the reverse Trendelenburg position is used, assess for dependent edema. Remind clients with arterial insufficiency to avoid raising their feet above heart level unless the physician has specifically prescribed this as an exercise. Authorities vary in their opinion as to the best position for enhancing arterial flow to the feet.

Prevent Vasoconstriction. Explain the dangers of smoking to the client who uses tobacco. Encourage the client to stop smoking completely. The client who realizes that smoking literally threatens life and limbs may develop sufficient motivation to quit. Help the client locate therapy groups or biofeedback training. Do not recommend the use of nicotine patches. Patches provide continuous administration of nicotine and can cause continuous vasospasm.

Encourage the client to avoid stressful situations and to try to relax, both mentally and physically. Counseling services may be indicated for nervous, high-strung clients. Offer information regarding stress reduction classes. Remember to involve significant others.

Prevent the client from becoming chilled. Clients should wear protective clothing in layers during cold weather, warm cars before entering them, and follow winter driving precautions.

Risk for Impaired Skin Integrity. Because of altered peripheral tissue perfusion, the client is at risk of arterial ulceration and skin infection. Write the diagnosis as *Risk for Impaired Skin Integrity related to decreased peripheral circulation.* If the client has an arterial ulcer, this diagnosis can still be used for the remaining intact skin.

Outcomes. The client will maintain intact skin surfaces, with healed skin surfaces, freedom from signs of infection, and signs of wound healing.

Interventions. Prevent injury to the extremities, particularly the feet. Excellent foot care should be an integral part of the daily routine of clients with peripheral vascular disorders, because prevention is easier to initiate and maintain than is correction (see the Client Education Guide on foot care).

CLIENT EDUCATION GUIDE

Foot Care

Client Instructions

Daily Hygiene

Do not soak your feet; use mild soap and a washcloth to clean them.
Dry well between your toes.
Check water temperature with a bath thermometer or your elbow, not your toes, to prevent burns; 32.2° to 35° C (90° to 95° F) is safe.
Gently rub corns or calluses. Avoid cutting, digging, or using harsh commercial products.

Daily Inspection and Lubrication

Use good lighting.
Put on your glasses or contacts, if you wear them.
Promptly report ulcerations, redness, calluses, blisters, or cracking of the skin on the feet or thickening of the nails to the physician.
Rub soothing lotions or lanolin on your hands, feet, legs, and arms to prevent dryness.
Do not use lotion on sores or between your toes.
Do not use perfumed lotions.
Dust your feet lightly with cornstarch if they sweat.

Care of Toenails

Use clippers, not scissors or razor blades.
Cut straight across the nail.
Do not perform "bathroom surgery."
If your eyesight is poor or if you are unable to reach your toes, find qualified assistance.
Place lamb's wool between overlapping toes.

Proper Footwear

Never go barefoot, not even at the beach or at home.
Avoid high heels and shoes with pointed toes.
Make sure nothing is in your shoes before putting them on your feet.
Avoid tight socks and shoes.
Wear cotton socks for absorbency. Change your socks daily.
Alternate several pairs of comfortable, firm, well-made shoes during the week.
Avoid shoes that cause your feet to perspire (for example, canvas shoes and rubber boots).
Make sure that your shoes and slippers fit well and are sturdy enough to prevent foot injury.

Safety

Avoid sunburn.
Avoid scratching insect bites on your legs to prevent creating open lesions.
Do not use heating pads.
Wear adequate foot protection on cold days.
Turn on the lights before entering a dark hallway or room.
Avoid sitting with your legs crossed.
Use a cane or walker, if indicated.
When in doubt, ask for help. Have telephone numbers of people who can assist you at hand.

Activity

Walking is good, but get your physician's permission before beginning a regular program.
Do not walk if you have open ulcerations.
Walk until pain begins, stop and rest, then begin again.
Elevate your feet if they swell.
Find a nurse and a physician who will get to know you and your foot problems and will take the time to talk with you when you need help.

Pain. Intermittent claudication is caused by ischemia. The diagnosis can be written *Pain related to inadequate arterial blood supply to the legs.*

Outcomes. The client will experience increased comfort, as evidenced by self-report and demonstrated knowledge of pain relief measures, both pharmacologic and nonpharmacologic.

Interventions. The pain of ischemia is usually chronic, continuous, and difficult to relieve. Arterial leg ulcers are exquisitely painful. Because of pain, clients with arterial disorders are often depressed and irritable. Pain limits their activities, disturbs their sleep, saps their energy, and has a demoralizing emotional effect. Thus, pain must be relieved if the client is to rest and improve.

Help clients assess and plan ways of correcting the position of their beds at home. The head of the bed can be elevated to promote blood flow to the legs. Remind the client with arterial insufficiency to:

- Avoid standing in one position for more than a few minutes
- Avoid crossing the legs at the knees
- Seek the most comfortable position
- Watch for and report edema

Any measure that increases circulation to the extremities helps alleviate ischemic pain. Although pain also can be subdued by analgesics, interventions that augment circulation are best. For more information on pain control, see Chapter 23. When strong analgesics such as morphine are necessary around the clock, the client may require amputation. Amputation can improve the quality of life by diminishing pain and improving mobility with a prosthesis.

Risk for Activity Intolerance. The client's pain (intermittent claudication) may greatly deter activity. This common diagnosis is written as *Risk for Activity Intolerance related to leg pain after walking.*

Outcomes. The client will develop appropriate levels of activity free from pain and excess fatigue, as evidenced by normal vital signs, absence of pain, and verbalized understanding of the benefits of gradual increase in activity and exercise.

Interventions. When assisting the client with a walking program, assert that *pain* should be the guide for the amount of activity to be undertaken. Intermittent claudication signals that the muscles and tissues of the legs are not receiving enough oxygen. Before the client begins a walking program, take a careful history and perform a physical assessment. Establish a cardiopulmonary profile, and carefully examine the client's feet and legs to locate open ulcerations or anatomic deformities. The client should have sturdy shoes to prevent foot trauma.

Although exercise helps most clients with vascular disorders, some clients must not exercise, such as clients with leg ulcers, pain at rest, cellulitis, deep vein thrombosis (DVT, unless the client is receiving low-molecular-weight heparin), or gangrene. Exercise and activity increase the metabolic needs of tissues and, consequently, tissue requirements for oxygenated blood. Thus, clients with tissue breakdown or necrosis must remain for a period on complete bed rest. Even minimal activity raises the oxygen requirements of the tissues above those that damaged arteries can provide.

Knowledge Deficit. The nursing diagnosis *Knowledge Deficit* can be used as a guide to teaching the client about a walking program. State the diagnosis as *Knowledge Deficit related to walking program as evidenced by no previous experience.*

Outcomes. The client will follow a progressive walking program.

Interventions. Remind clients that at first it may be painful to walk any distance and they may need to stop frequently to rest. They should walk through the pain as much as possible without causing undue distress. Encourage them to walk in enclosed shopping malls in the winter for safety from falls on icy pavement and to avoid vasoconstriction from the cold outdoors. In the summer, malls help to avoid heat exhaustion or stress on other comorbidities. It is important to emphasize that small increments of exercise increase are not dramatic but are evidence of improvement. Even improvements that enable clients to shop in the grocery store is a cause for celebration.

Health-Seeking Behaviors. Health-conscious clients may request information about self-improvement and interventions to reduce the severity of manifestations. Write the diagnosis as *Health Seeking Behaviors related to lack of knowledge about the role of exercise, weight reduction, and smoking cessation in management of arterial disease.*

Outcomes. The client will begin and maintain the chosen health promotion program, as evidenced by demonstrated knowledge of the specific activities of the program, regular evaluation of goals against performance, and verbalized feelings of increased well-being.

Interventions. Instruct the client in areas of concern or interest (see the nonpharmacologic intervention methods described earlier). Refer the client to groups in the community if available. The client with intermittent claudication caused by arterial disease should be routinely reexamined at least every 3 months for progression of the disease. Use the information in the Alternative Therapies feature to teach clients about other treatments.

EVALUATION

Arterial disorders are chronic, and you should not expect to see reversal of the problems. Write outcomes that allow for time and client adjustments.

Modifications for Elderly Clients

Age-related changes and impairments of physiologic function concomitant with arterial disease affect the nursing diagnoses of *Activity Intolerance* (possibly increased), *Altered Peripheral Tissue Perfusion* (possibly reduced), and *Pain.* Recognition of pain may be complicated by physical or cognitive impairments, ongoing drug therapy, and psychosocial factors (e.g., depression or social isolation). Additionally, sight reduction and flexibility limitations may prevent or decrease self-care. Diminished sight may increase risks for falls or other injury, which may be disastrous in the client with impaired circulation.

Surgical Management

ENDOVASCULAR INTERVENTIONS

Endovascular interventional therapies use angioscopy, intraluminal ultrasonography, balloon angioplasty, laser,

ALTERNATIVE THERAPY

Vascular Disorders

A number of natural therapies may be useful in the treatment of vascular problems. During the 1940s and 1950s, researchers found that vitamin E can be useful in the treatment of intermittent claudication, with a number of randomized, double-blind trials supporting the use of vitamin E. Dosages from the most successful studies were 400 to 800 mg/day, with effects becoming apparent generally after 3 months. However, recent studies indicate doses above 400 mg/day increase the risk of intracranial bleeding, especially if used with aspirin. Interestingly, vitamin E use "was associated with marked decreases in the rate of leg amputation and even overall mortality, in addition to decreasing claudication."[2] No further trials of vitamin E in treating intermittent claudication have been conducted since the 1970s, perhaps because of the resistance in the medical community to nutritional, nonpharmaceutical therapies.

A number of herbs have been studied for their circulatory effects. Ginkgo biloba has been found minimally effective for intermittent claudication as well as for decreased cerebral circulation leading to reduced function. Manifestations can include decreased memory, vertigo, tinnitus, and mood swings with anxiety.[4] One study of ginkgo use in clients with mild to moderate cognitive impairment found improvements in a number of parameters as well as significant decreases in diastolic blood pressure in those receiving a low (40 mg three times a day) daily dose of ginkgo.[5] Optimal dosage may need to be determined by further research.

In the treatment of chronic venous insufficiency, horse-chestnut seed extract (HCSE, *Aesculus hippocastanum*) may be superior to placebo, equivalent to a reference medication, and therapeutically equivalent to compression stocking therapy.[3] German health authorities have approved HCSE for the treatment of chronic venous insufficiency as well as for pain and heaviness in the legs and varicose veins. Gastrointestinal side effects may occur but are uncommon.[4]

Garlic has been studied for its effects on arteriosclerosis and lipids with varying results. The amount of fresh garlic a person would need to eat for a therapeutic dosage is quite high and likely to cause gastric upset. Garlic preparations vary widely in terms of their active constituents. In one study of garlic powder versus a placebo in people with advanced plaque buildup in the arteries beneficial effects were noted from the powder. All subjects had at least one additional risk factor for heart disease, such as hypertension, diabetes, or a smoking history. Whereas subjects on placebo experienced an increase of plaque volume over 48 months, those taking garlic experienced plaque reductions.[1]

Caution must be exercised and clients taking anticoagulants should be advised regarding the use of certain vitamins and herbs, including garlic, ginkgo, and vitamin E. Although natural, these substances can obviously have potent therapeutic activity. This may in part be due to anticoagulant effects, which may potentiate the action of blood-thinning drugs. Health practitioners should be aware of the use of such substances so that any interactions can be monitored safely. Not enough controlled research is available to make definite predictions.

References

1. Kosielny, J. et al. (1999). The antiatherosclerotic effect of Allium sativum. *Atherosclerosis, 144,* 237–249.
2. Goodwin, J. S., & Tangum, M. R. (1998). Battling quackery: Attitudes about micronutrient supplements in American academic medicine. *Archives of Internal Medicine, 158,* 2187–2191.
3. Pittler, M. H., & Ernst, E. (1998). Horse-chestnut seed extract for chronic venous insufficiency: A criteria-based systematic review. *Archives of Dermatology, 134,* 1356–1360.
4. Tyler, V. E. (1994). *Herbs of choice: The therapeutic use of phytomedicinals.* Binghamton, NY: Pharmaceutical Products Press.
5. Winther, K. (1998). Effects of ginkgo biloba extract on cognitive function and blood pressure in elderly subjects. *Current Therapeutic Research, 59,* 881–888.

James Higgy Lerner, RN, LAc, *Private practice of acupuncture, traditional Oriental medicine, and biofeedback*

mechanical atherectomy, thrombolytic therapy, and stents to treat vascular disorders. The goal is to operate from within the artery to remove partial or total blockages. Most of the procedures can be performed in the radiology department or in cardiac catheterization laboratories. Benefits of endovascular interventions include use of a small puncture wound for access rather than a long incision and minimal postoperative care. Complications from long-duration (>3 hours) general anesthetics are reduced and the client is quickly ambulatory. Obvious cost reduction occurs.

Percutaneous Transluminal Angioplasty. Percutaneous transluminal angioplasty (PTA), or balloon angioplasty, is a procedure in which a catheter with a distal inflatable balloon is used to dilate stenotic vessels mechanically. Angioplasty stretches the artery, thereby enlarging the lumen. Observation of a segment of an arterial wall that has undergone PTA reveals rupture of the plaque at its thinnest place, stretching of the artery wall away from the plaque, and rupture of the media with the lumen of the artery being maintained by the adventitia. The enlarged vessel's new dimensions are maintained by the hydrostatic pressure of the increased luminal blood flow.

Preprocedural Care

Assess and document peripheral pulse quality. Use a pen to mark the location of pulses on the foot to guide later assessments. Note color, skin temperature of the feet, and level of rest pain. Document the location and characteristics of any open lesions. Teach clients about the procedure and any sensations they will feel.

PTA has been used successfully, in varying degrees, for the treatment of hemodynamically significant stenoses in the coronary, aortic, iliac, femoral, popliteal, tibial, mesenteric, and renal circulations as well as for stenoses in arteriovenous dialysis shunts. Current practice also is to place a stent in the area that was treated with angioplasty to reduce the recurrence of stenosis. Several types of stents have been developed, including flexible, rigid, balloon-expandable, and self-expanding varieties. After a stent has been in place for about 8 months, it becomes covered by a thin neointimal layer. After the procedure, clients are given aspirin to reduce the risk of occlusion.

Complications of balloon angioplasty include bleeding, hematoma and thrombus formation at the insertion site, perforation, and dissection of the artery. Reocclusion that occurs over a longer period of time is caused by accelerated cell growth of the intima (intimal hyperplasia), which occurs in response to injury to the vessel.

Postprocedural Care

Nursing care is similar to that for routine diagnostic arteriography (Chapter 11). Major concerns are acute reocclusion and bleeding. Clients are given heparin as an anticoagulant during the procedure; thus, the arterial puncture site requires frequent assessment for swelling, bleeding, ecchymosis, or hematoma formation. Peripheral pulses are usually assessed every 15 to 30 minutes during the first hour following the procedure, then hourly for the next 4 to 8 hours. Report clinical manifestations of circulatory compromise immediately (e.g., sudden change in limb color or temperature, increasing muscle discomfort, pain at rest, and motor or sensory paresthesias). Long-term aspirin administration is prescribed after angioplasty to prevent occlusion.

Thrombolytic Therapy. Thrombolytic therapy is an important aspect of management of extensive venous or arterial thrombosis. Streptokinase and urokinase are used to treat acute arterial emboli and arterial graft occlusion. Contraindications to therapy include surgery within the past 10 days (e.g., arteriogram, lumbar puncture, paracentesis), recent trauma (e.g., cardiopulmonary resuscitation), renal or liver biopsy, and pregnancy. Renal function must be adequate because of the amount of contrast material given during thrombolytic therapy.

Thrombolytic agents are administered through a peripheral vein or through an intra-arterial catheter. A test dose is given; if it is determined to be safe, it is followed by a loading dose and then by continuous infusion. The agents have a half-life of 16 to 18 minutes. Activated partial thromboplastin times (aPTT), fibrinogen levels, or both may be monitored to be certain that the thrombolytic system has been activated. Major adverse reactions include hemorrhage, allergic reactions, and fever.

Nursing management is related to the stage of fibrinolytic therapy: preinfusion, intrainfusion, and postinfusion. Prior to infusion, the client is monitored closely (usually in intensive care). Baseline values are obtained for aPTT, prothrombin time (PT), thrombin time, platelet count, hematocrit, and white blood cell (WBC) count. Because of the risk of hemorrhage, if data reveal a bleeding disorder, the physician is notified. A history of recent streptococcal infection may diminish the drug's effects. Baseline pulses and assessments are performed in each extremity with Doppler ultrasonography if needed.

During infusion, vital signs, pulses, skin color, movement, and sensation are assessed frequently. Assess for clinical manifestations of bleeding and hematoma formation. If bleeding occurs apply direct pressure, stop the infusion, and notify the physician. Bleeding is usually from the gastrointestinal or genitourinary tract or is intramuscular, intracerebral, or retroperitoneal. Intracerebral bleeding presents as pain in the head or neck, changes in cognition, or loss of motor function. Retroperitoneal bleeding presents as back or flank pain.

No intramuscular injections are given for 24 hours after infusion, and any medications that have bleeding as a side effect are used with caution. There is also a chance that a partially lysed thrombus will embolize. After infusion, pressure is continued on the puncture site. The involved extremity is positioned in straight alignment to facilitate perfusion. The client's leg remains immobile. Heparin therapy in low doses is also begun. Streptokinase is administered from glass bottles because it is inactivated by plastic containers. Administration is regulated by a volume-control pump.

Arterial Bypass

Arterial obstruction can be reconstructed with bypass operations. Clients are selected for surgery after a careful history and physical and diagnostic assessments, including arteriography. Arteriography provides a necessary road map to indicate the level of obstruction, because it is essential to reconstruct the arterial inflow to the legs before correcting the outflow. This process prevents newly placed bypass grafts from becoming thrombosed because of inadequate blood supply to the graft. During the operation, the surgeon assesses inflow, and a distal site is chosen for outflow after it is ascertained that inflow to the femoral system is adequate.

Improvements in vascular surgery have provided outstanding examples of long-term limb salvage in clients who in the past would have required amputation. Revascularization should be the first option considered in clients with critical limb ischemia. This recommendation is based on observations that previous revascularization does not raise the level of amputation, mortality rates for amputation are at least as high as those for arterial bypass, and there is no difference in cost between amputation and successful bypass surgery.

Various locations along the arterial system can be reconstructed as follows. Femoral artery bypass grafting or axillofemoral reconstruction (Fig. 53–4) is used if the aortoiliac segment is obstructed. The operative mortality rate is 1%. The patency rates of aortofemoral grafts are 80% to 90% at 5 years.

Axillofemoral grafting is reserved for clients who have increased operative risk, usually because of their cardiopulmonary status or the presence of intra-abdominal infection. The graft begins at the axillary artery and travels subcutaneously along the lateral chest wall to the femoral artery. It may then be combined with a femorofemoral graft to revascularize both extremities. Axillofemoral grafts have a higher incidence of occlusion than aortofemoral grafts and carry a mortality rate of 4% to 5%, but the necessary anesthesia time is greatly reduced. The patency rates are 60% to 70% at 5 years, in part because thrombi are easily removed from axillofemoral grafts.

The femoral artery can be bypassed with grafts anastomosed (surgically connected) to any one of three lower leg arteries (posterior tibial, anterior tibial, or peroneal artery). The success of bypass grafts of the legs depends largely on what material is used for grafting. The client's own saphenous vein remains the most successful grafting material used today. Seventy-five per cent of saphenous vein grafts are patent after 5 years; in contrast, only 12%

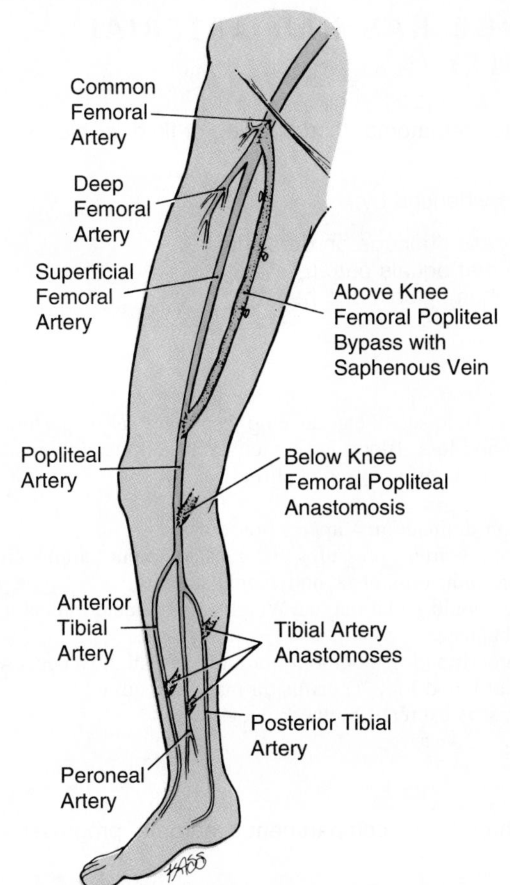

FIGURE 53–4 Femoral artery bypass grafts. The anastomosis can be to any one of three tibial arteries. (From Fahey, V. A. [1994]. *Vascular nursing.* Philadelphia: W. B. Saunders.)

of synthetic material (polytetrafluoroethylene [PTFE]) is patent after the same length of time. (Gore-Tex is a common brand name for PTFE.) Unfortunately, the client's own saphenous vein is not always large enough or long enough for the surgery, or it may have been removed during another operation. In these cases, PTFE is used. In situ grafts can also be used for reconstruction. In situ grafting permits the client's own vein to be used for a bypass of the artery. A section of vein is anastomosed proximally and distally, and the valves are disabled. The vein then acts as an artery.

Anticoagulant medications (e.g., heparin) are used in clients who have had previously thrombosed femoral bypass grafts. Low-molecular-weight heparin may be safer, with fewer bleeding side effects and rare occurrences of heparin-induced thrombocytopenia. It is also possible to treat some clients with fibrinolytics; however, these agents are seldom used immediately after surgery because of the potential for bleeding. Three drugs—streptokinase, urokinase, and tissue plasminogen activator (TPA)—are in current clinical use. All three drugs convert the client's plasminogen to the active molecule plasmin, which instigates fibrinolysis. The client is eventually given warfarin sodium based on the International Normalized Ratio (INR). Dextran is sometimes used to improve blood flow in the microcirculation but is only recommended in complex cases. Medications that decrease platelet aggregation (aspirin, clopidogrel [Plavix] are also used to increase the length of graft patency. Some authors recommend the use of anticoagulants in clients who have never had an occluded graft, including clients with poor outflow, complicated procedures, or a small-caliber graft. Broad-spectrum antibiotics are used before and after surgery.

Nursing Management of the Surgical Client

Preoperative Care

Preoperatively, obtain baseline vital signs and document the character of peripheral pulses, comparing one side with the other. Know exactly which pulses are palpable and which pulses can be assessed only with Doppler. Mark with ink the sites where peripheral pulses can be palpated to assist with postoperative assessment.

Before surgery, it is common to begin administration of intravenous (IV) fluids, insert a urinary catheter, and weigh the client. Just before surgery, arterial and central venous pressure (CVP) lines may be inserted. In addition, broad-spectrum antibiotics normally are prescribed for 48 hours preoperatively. All infections (e.g., tooth abscesses, urinary tract and respiratory infections) must be resolved, especially if the surgeon plans to use a synthetic graft. Adequate circulating blood volume must be maintained to permit good perfusion throughout the period of arterial repair.

As with any preoperative assessment, perform careful cardiac and pulmonary evaluations. Even though the incision for a femoral artery bypass is peripheral and major complications are infrequent, the client probably has other manifestations of atherosclerosis (such as heart and kidney disease) that may complicate the surgery. If the operation is not an emergency, malnutrition can be reversed and open wounds can be cleaned. The client should have a complete medical evaluation, and hypertension should be controlled. If the blood pressure is outside normal parameters, or well above the client's normal value, report it to the surgeon or anesthesia department.

The client and family are taught the various procedures involved and are offered psychological support. First assess the client's readiness and desire to learn about the surgery. The importance of maintaining the medication routine is to be stressed with appropriate guidance from the physician or anesthesia department.

Postoperative Care

The client is placed on bed rest for the evening after surgery, with the leg flat in bed. The leg is wrapped with light dressings or a vascular boot. Boots are commonly used in clients who had a loss of sensation prior to surgery or who are at risk for pressure ulcers. Elastic wraps are not used if vein grafts have been used for reconstruction. Leg swelling is common after revascularization resulting from the reperfusion of ischemic muscles and surgical dissection around lymphatic drainage systems in the leg. If edema worsens when the client's leg is dependent, elastic wraps can be used. Edema usually resolves within 4 to 8 weeks, especially with ambulation.

Oxygen saturation monitors may also be used to measure tissue perfusion. Daily aspirin is usually required after surgery. Incisions are carefully monitored for clinical manifestations of infection. The Care Plan describes the remainder of nursing care of the client after bypass surgery.

C A R E P L A N

POSTOPERATIVE CARE OF THE CLIENT WHO HAS HAD ARTERIAL BYPASS SURGERY OF THE LOWER EXTREMITY

Nursing Diagnosis. Risk for Fluid Volume Deficit related to hemorrhage, hematoma, third spacing of fluid, or diuresis from contrast given during angiography

Outcomes. The client will maintain adequate vascular fluid volume, as evidenced by:

- Hemodynamic stability
- Urine output ≥30 ml/hr
- Warm, dry skin
- Being alert, awake
- No excess drainage on dressings
- Intake that equals output
- Stable hemoglobin and hematocrit

Interventions	Rationales
1. Observe the client for an increase in pulse, decrease in blood pressure, anxiety, restlessness, pallor, cyanosis, thirst, oliguria, clammy skin, venous collapse, and decreasing level of consciousness.	1. Hemorrhagic shock can develop from surgical or postoperative blood loss. Blood is shunted from peripheral stores because of the effect of epinephrine.
2. Check the client's dressings for excessive drainage.	2. Incision drainage first appears on dressings.
3. Assess the client's pulmonary artery pressures and cardiac output if parameters are available.	3. Pulmonary artery pressures and cardiac output parameters are reliable indicators of hemodynamic stability.
4. Check the client's daily weights; monitor intake and output closely.	4. Intake should equal output. Weight is a reliable indicator of fluid balance.
5. Check hematocrit and hemoglobin values and notify the physician if they are abnormal.	5. Hematocrit and hemoglobin normally fall slightly because of surgical blood loss. Transfusion may be required.
6. Check the client's creatinine level after angiography.	6. Contrast is excreted by the kidneys.

Evaluation. This outcome should be attainable within 24 hours.

Nursing Diagnosis. Risk for Altered Tissue Perfusion related to graft thrombosis, compartment syndrome, progressive arterial disease, or inadequate anticoagulation

Outcomes. The client will maintain adequate tissue perfusion to the lower extremities, as evidenced by full pedal pulses, intact sensory and motor function, and minimal swelling.

Interventions	Rationales
1. Check the client's pedal pulses every hour for 24 hours, then every shift, unless otherwise ordered. Obtain Doppler pressures per doctor's orders.	1. Pedal pulses indicate graft patency.
2. Check the sensory and motor function of the client's extremities.	2. Compartment syndrome may develop because of bleeding.
3. Check the client's leg for hematoma or severe swelling.	3. Severe swelling may impede the flow through the graft.
4. Monitor creatine phosphokinase levels when appropriate.	4. Enzymes are released from ischemic muscle.
5. Observe for a change in color and the presence of red blood cells in the client's urine.	5. These manifestations may be caused by a release of myoglobin secondary to muscle ischemia.
6. Avoid raising the knee section of the gatch bed and placing pillows under the client's knees.	6. Pressure may increase the risk of thrombosis.

Evaluation. Outcomes related to tissue perfusion should be met within 48 hours.

Nursing Diagnosis. Risk for Impaired Skin Integrity related to altered circulation, altered nutritional state, infection, and multiple surgical procedures

Outcomes. The client will maintain adequate skin integrity.

Interventions	Rationales
1. Inspect the client's lower extremities on daily basis.	1. Early detection of ulceration will improve the chances of healing
2. Provide proper skin care using lanolin-based creams.	2. Soft skin does not crack open.
3. Protect the client's lower extremities from trauma.	3. Tissue perfusion is decreased and injured sites heal poorly.
4. Use sheepskin, a bed cradle, or heel protectors when appropriate.	4. These devices are used to protect the skin from breakdown.
5. Check the sensory and motor function of the client's extremities.	5. Compartment syndrome may develop because of bleeding or edema.
6. Avoid using tape on the skin below the client's knee.	6. Tape burns from tape removal may be slow to heal.

Interventions	Rationales
1. Monitor the client's nutritional status and albumin level. Obtain a dietitian's consultation, if necessary.	1. Malnutrition is the most common cause of delayed healing.
2. Observe strict aseptic technique during dressing changes.	2. Aseptic technique reduces risk of infection.
3. Monitor the client for low-grade fever, elevated white blood cell count, any drainage from the wound, and graft exposure at each shift.	3. These are clinical manifestations of wound infection.
4. If ordered, apply Ace bandages below the knee to the affected extremity when the client is out of bed.	4. Edema, although normal after surgery, can inhibit wound healing.
5. Instruct client to inspect feet and incisions daily. (See Foot Care Guide.)	5. Circulation to the legs and feet is impaired from arteriosclerosis. Daily assessment and proper care can lead to early intervention.
6. Assess for presence of footdrop.	6. Nerve injury due to ischemia can lead to footdrop.

Evaluation. Expect the wound to heal slowly over 10 days if arteriosclerosis is extensive.

Nursing Diagnosis. Impaired Physical Mobility related to a surgical procedure, pain, or nerve injury secondary to ischemia

Outcomes. The client will maintain intact motor function, avoid potential complications of immobility, and demonstrate use of adaptive devices to increase mobility.

Interventions	Rationales
1. Assess the causative factors for immobility and the client's range of motion and ability to ambulate.	1. Mobility can be facilitated once the cause is known.
2. Encourage progressive ambulation and range of motion while the client is in bed.	2. These activities promote venous return and muscle strength.
3. Request a physical therapy consult when appropriate.	3. Assistive devices may be necessary for ambulation.
4. Encourage independence in the client's activities of daily living.	4. Independence improves both physical and psychological recovery

Evaluation. Outcomes related to mobility may require several days, depending on initial physical status.

Nursing Diagnosis. Pain related to surgical incision

Outcomes. The client verbalizes and demonstrates an increased level of comfort.

Interventions	Rationales
1. Assess the client's level of pain: type, duration, and location.	1. This assessment provides baseline data to evaluate the effectiveness of treatment.
2. Provide comfort measures and means of distraction.	2. Distraction is a nonpharmacologic method of pain management.
3. Medicate with prescribed analgesics as needed.	3. Adequate pain management promotes healing.
4. Evaluate the effectiveness of pain medication after each administration.	4. This evaluation allows the adequacy of analgesics to be determined.

Evaluation. Acute pain should subside over 48 to 72 hours.

Adapted from Fahey, V. A. (1994). *Vascular nursing.* Philadelphia, W. B. Saunders.

COMPLICATIONS

Bleeding may develop along the suture line and can indicate a disruption in the suture line, pseudoaneurysm formation, or a slipped ligature (suture). For these problems, additional surgery is required. Reclotting of the graft is also possible. Peripheral tissue perfusion is monitored, and noninvasive follow-up studies are performed to assess patency.

Infection is not a common complication after bypass surgery, but it can occur, especially when synthetic grafting material is used. Because infection in a synthetic graft necessitates its removal, infection often results in the loss of a limb. Poorly nourished clients appear to be at highest risk for infection and delayed healing.

Compartment syndrome may also develop from swelling around the fascial compartments of the leg. In addition to loss of sensation and function, muscle cells can die and release myoglobin, which can cause acute tubular necrosis in the kidney. The manifestations of compartment syndrome include pain out of proportion to the surgery, a tense swollen leg and pain with muscle stretching, and decreased sensation. A change involving any of these manifestations or change in the color of the urine to rusty brown should be reported immediately.

Self-Care

Most clients are discharged home. Because activity was limited by claudication before surgery, the client needs to begin regular permissible exercise, including climbing stairs and going out of doors. Explain that swelling of the operative leg is normal. Elastic wraps can be used when the client is ambulating, but they should not be worn continuously.

AMPUTATION

Amputation is the oldest operation, existing before recorded history. Early amputations were done as punishment for crime. Today's amputations are used to treat injuries, cancer, overwhelming limb gangrene, and limb-threatening arterial disease or rest pain. Amputation is common, with nearly 2 million people in the United States having undergone the procedure. Unlike many other forms of surgery, such as removal of a body organ, amputation is followed by a replacement with a prosthetic device that can restore a reasonable degree of function. However, the surgical loss is visible, and therefore amputation has an emotional component that does not exist in the same manner following removal of many other body organs.

For many years, amputation was performed with an apology and often a sense of failure. More recently, there has been increasing media attention featuring amputees who have "overcome their handicap" and are back in mainstream society. There are organizations of amputee skiers, golfers, and runners. Publicity has removed much of the old stigma.

Clients with peripheral vascular disease are the most frequent candidates for amputation of the lower extremities. Diabetes mellitus is a major cause of arterial occlusion and has been associated with more than 55% of major amputations in clients with lower extremity occlusive disease. Traumatic injuries are also a common cause of amputation, especially in younger clients.

PREOPERATIVE ASSESSMENT

Usual preoperative assessment is performed (see Chapter 15). In addition, a rehabilitation team designs an individualized care plan focusing on the whole client rather than on a diseased or missing limb. Before amputation, the surgeon and rehabilitative team should consider the client's physical condition and attitude toward amputation and the type and level of amputation required.

PHYSICAL CONDITION. The following physical conditions may predicate the rehabilitation potential of clients: age, ability to become ambulatory or remain ambulatory, comprehension level, willingness to participate in a rehabilitation program, and pre-existing conditions (e.g., chronic and progressive mental deterioration, advancing neurologic problems, chronic obstructive pulmonary disease, or cardiac disease with heart failure or angina). Ideally, clients should attain independent function with the use of a prosthesis.

TYPE OF AMPUTATION PERFORMED. There are two types of amputation procedures: the *open,* or guillotine, amputation and the *closed,* or "flap," amputation. The major indication for guillotine amputation is infection. In open amputation, the surgeon does not close the stump with a skin flap immediately but leaves it open, allowing the wound to drain freely. Antibiotics are used. Once the infection is completely eradicated, the client undergoes another operation for stump closure.

During a "flap" amputation, the surgeon closes or covers the stump with a flap of skin sutured over the end of the stump. This type of amputation is performed when there is no evidence of infection and, consequently, no need for open drainage. However, the surgeon may insert small drains (e.g., Jackson-Pratt drain) to promote wound healing.

LEVEL OF AMPUTATION REQUIRED. The level of amputation for any extremity should be as distal as possible (Fig. 53–5). Arteriography is used to guide the decision about the level of amputation. Clients with below-knee amputations (even bilateral) more successfully achieve independent function with a prosthesis than do those with above-knee amputations.

CLIENT'S GENERAL ATTITUDE TOWARD AMPUTATION. Attitude toward amputation depends, to a large degree, on the client's age and maturity. Young clients may resist amputation, even though it might greatly improve function. For some, the thought of amputation dramatically conflicts with their ideal self-image. Conversely, some clients who suffer from the pain of chronic ischemia may welcome amputation. These clients are more concerned with removing the source of their pain than with altering their body image or function.

Diagnostic assessments include the usual preoperative blood studies and x-rays. In addition, arteriography may be done to determine the level of blood flow in the extremity. Doppler studies are used to measure blood flow velocity, and transcutaneous tissue oxygen levels may also be measured (see Chapter 51). These studies assist with determining the level of amputation most likely to heal.

PREOPERATIVE CARE

ASSESSMENT

Perform the usual preoperative assessments (see Chapter 15). In addition, assess the peripheral vascular system thoroughly, palpate pulses, and assess the skin temperature, sensation, and capillary refill in both extremities to serve as a baseline for comparison. If the nails have hypertrophied, assess the skin of the toe as a measure of capillary refill. If the client is diabetic, assess blood glucose levels and follow orders for sliding scale insulin to maintain normal glycemic levels.

DIAGNOSIS, OUTCOMES, INTERVENTIONS

Anxiety. Clients may fear amputation because it destroys a familiar body image, imposes physical and social limitations, and temporarily upsets their personal lifestyle. Such fears and anxiety must be resolved preoperatively to ensure successful postoperative recovery. Depending on the reason for the amputation, fear may lead the client to experience anticipatory grief. State this nursing diagnosis as *Anxiety related to impending loss of limb, change in mobility, pain, changes in body image, fear about feelings after amputation.* Other nursing diagnoses may also be appropriate, such as *Ineffective Individual Coping, Self Esteem Disturbance,* or *Body Image Disturbance.*

Outcomes. The client will openly discuss feelings and express reduced anxiety before surgery.

Interventions. Establish open, honest communication. Allow free expression of fears and negative feelings about the loss of a limb. Ask significant others how they feel about the amputation and how they perceive the

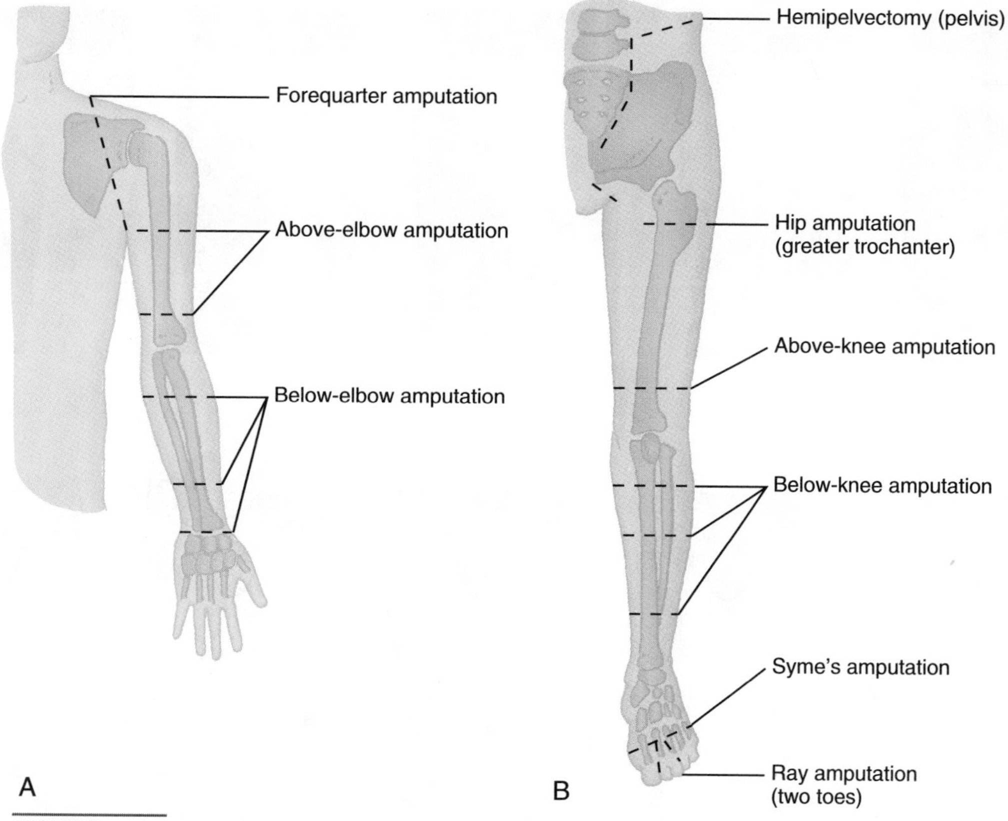

FIGURE 53–5 Common sites of amputation: *A,* upper extremity; *B,* lower extremity.

client to be responding. The social worker or psychologist may need to be involved if the client is responding poorly.

The client may also be anxious about unknown consequences and sensations after the amputation. Provide and reinforce information. Most clients feel less anxious when they know what to expect on awakening from surgery. Prepare the client for *phantom limb sensation* (see later discussion). Most clients with new amputations experience the peculiar sensation that their missing limb is still present. This phantom limb sensation may or may not be painful.

Delayed Surgical Recovery. For clients who require amputation on an emergent basis, the usual preoperative care to stabilize health conditions cannot occur. The need for emergent surgery can create a risk for delayed recovery. State this nursing diagnosis as *Delayed Surgical Recovery related to pre-existing health conditions.*

Outcomes. The risk for delayed surgical recovery will be minimized.

Interventions. Clients with diabetes mellitus are a high-risk surgical group and require careful preoperative assessment of their metabolic status. Blood glucose is normalized with blood testing four times a day and sliding scale insulin. Clients with ulcerated legs or osteomyelitis may be treated with wound packing, antibiotics, and leg elevation with bed rest. Malnourished clients are nourished with foods high in protein or tube-feeding. They also may benefit from vitamin and mineral supplements. Severely anemic clients may require iron preparations and blood transfusions. Dehydrated clients should receive preoperative IV fluids to restore fluid balance.

Pain. The client may experience very severe to moderate pain before surgery. The nursing diagnosis of *Pain related to ischemia of the limb* is used.

Outcomes. The client will be comfortable, as evidenced by statements of reduced pain, use of unchanging doses of narcotics (e.g., pain is controlled without increasing dosage), ability to move about comfortably, and ability to sleep or rest.

Interventions. Administer prescribed analgesics as necessary to relieve pain. Intervene with supportive measures. For example, use footboards and cradles to avoid pressure on injured or ischemic limbs. Keep ischemic limbs warm with wraps.

Knowledge Deficit. The diagnosis can be written as *Knowledge deficit related to expectations after surgery.*

Outcomes. The client will express an understanding of the usual postoperative regimens.

Interventions. Clients want to know what to expect after surgery and what will be expected of them by health care professionals. Emphasize that the client is the most important member of the rehabilitation team. To achieve independence, teach the client about

- Exercising legs and arms several times a day
- Strictly limiting weight-bearing (for leg amputations) until instructed otherwise
- Learning the intricacies of stump and prosthesis care
- Mastering the use of the prosthesis.

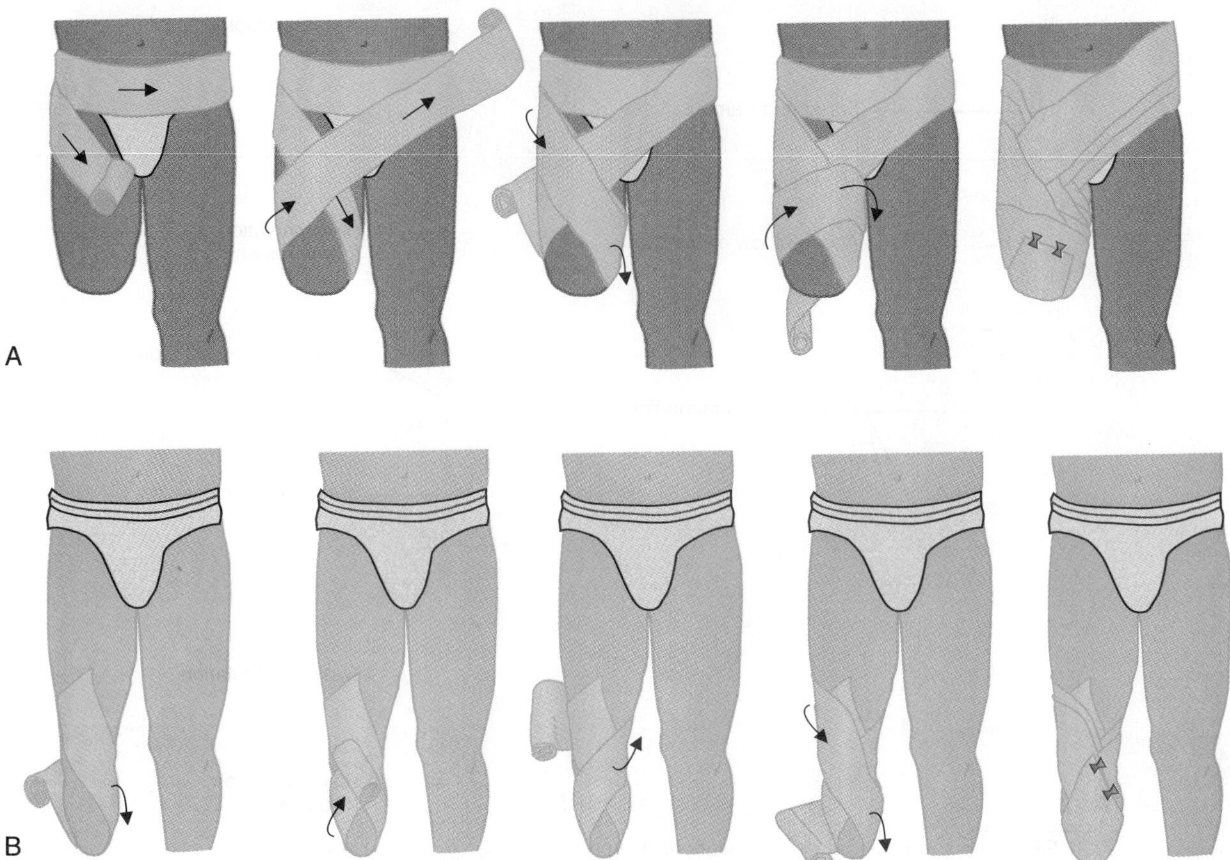

FIGURE 53–6 Common methods of stump wrapping. *A,* For an above-knee stump, two bandages are required. *B,* For a below-knee stump, one bandage is usually sufficient.

Postoperative Care

After the operation is completed, the surgeon applies a dressing on the incision (such as silk or Telfa bandage) and places a small amount of fluffed gauze over the end of the stump. A rigid dressing (usually a cast) is applied, distributing pressure evenly over the end of the stump. The cast protects the stump from injury and reduces swelling by gently compressing the tissues. The socket of the distal end of the cast connects to a pylon, an adjustable rigid support, the proximal end of which attaches to the below-knee socket or to the knee unit of an above-knee prosthesis. The distal end connects to a foot-ankle assembly. The rigid dressing is usually changed three to four times before application of a permanent prosthesis. Cast changes are necessary because the stump tends to shrink as it heals and, consequently, is no longer adequately compressed by the original cast.

Edema is controlled by elevating the stump for the first 24 hours after surgery. The stump then is placed flat on the bed to reduce hip contracture. Edema is also controlled by stump wrapping techniques. In below-knee amputations, the knee is immobilized to eliminate joint flexion. A trapeze and frame are attached over the bed to assist the client to develop upper arm and shoulder strength.

Phantom Limb Sensation

Phantom sensations are feelings that the amputated part is still present. Although these sensations are often referred to as *phantom pain,* not all of the sensations are painful. The client may describe sensations of warmth, cold, itching, or pain, especially in amputated fingers or toes. Phantom sensations are caused by intact peripheral nerves proximal to the amputation site that carried messages between the brain and the now amputated part. These sensations are normal, and the client should be prepared for them. Phantom sensations often are felt immediately after surgery and gradually decrease over the next 2 years.

Phantom pain is a form of central pain. The client reports actual pain that is usually burning, cramping, squeezing, or shooting in nature. Phantom pain is less well understood than phantom sensations and may occur in a large percentage of clients. Although it is thought to be caused by a combination of physiologic and psychological components, no research has identified a link between phantom pain and any clinical psychological disorder. Phantom pain occurs most often in clients who have had pain in the limb before the amputation. Interventions that may reduce phantom pain include range-of-motion exercises, visual imaging, and other interventions for chronic pain (see Chapter 23).

Rehabilitation

Fit the Prosthesis. For clients with a below-knee amputation, the patellar tendon–bearing limb prosthesis is the most common choice. The interior of the prosthesis contacts all surfaces of the stump, and weight-bearing is on several areas. Clients with an above knee amputation are fitted with either a quadrilateral socket or an ischial containment prosthesis. Weight is borne on the ischial tuberosity and soft tissues of the proximal stump, respectively.

Prostheses for the upper extremity consist of a hook or hand device, a harness to supply force to the hand, and a socket for attachment. The client coping with an upper extremity amputation must be highly motivated to master the prosthesis and to achieve independence. For successful rehabilitation, the client must integrate the prosthetic arm and hand into the total body image.

Cosmetic prostheses are primarily used to enhance self-esteem and to make reentry into society minus a limb more tolerable for clients who are not candidates for a functioning prosthesis. Because the construction of cosmetic prostheses does not allow weight-bearing, caution the client never to attempt transfers or ambulation with a cosmetic prosthesis.

Immediate prosthetic fitting is not always possible. However, anyone with a new amputation who can walk should receive a temporary prosthesis as soon as possible after surgery. When a conventional delayed prosthesis fitting is anticipated, the client returns from surgery with the stump dressed and covered with elastic bandages or stump socks (Fig. 53–6). When the sutures are removed 2 to 3 weeks after surgery, the surgeon or prosthetist fits the client with a provisional temporary prosthesis made of plaster of Paris or plastic. A permanent prosthesis is fitted once the stump is healed and molded (Fig. 53–7).

Provide Gait Training. Physical mobility is compromised for the client who has just experienced an amputation. Amputating a limb displaces the center of gravity, normally located just below the umbilicus. A client coping with an amputation must relearn balance because the prosthesis, however similar, is not an exact replica in weight and movement of the lost limb. Adapting to a change in the center of gravity occurs slowly but progressively until the conscious effort of maintaining balance comes under unconscious control. Physically, the client increases strength and endurance with regularly scheduled exercise, controls weight-bearing until the wound completely heals, and practices ambulating with the new prosthesis until a skillful, automatic gait is developed. Physi-

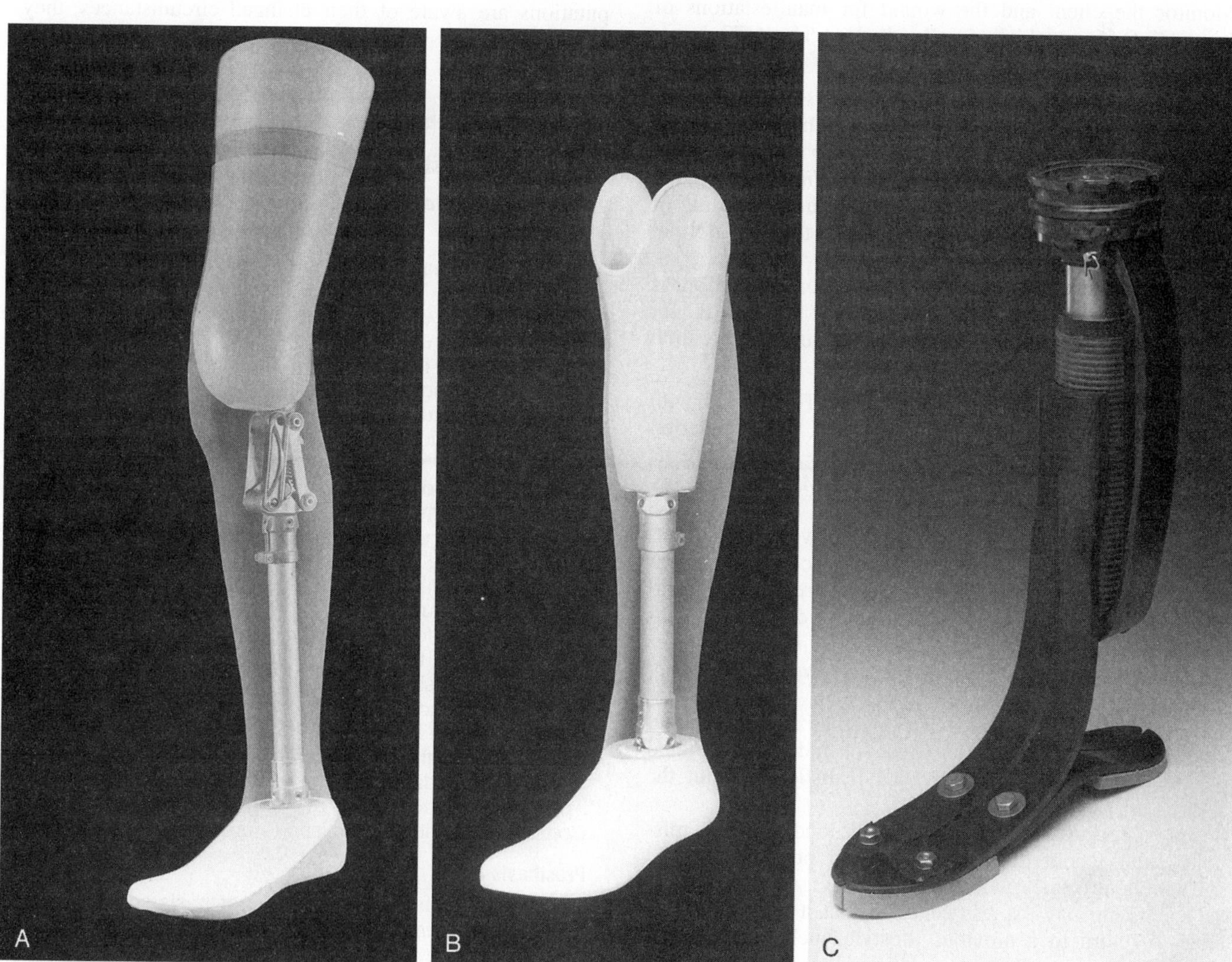

FIGURE 53–7 Permanent lower-extremity prostheses. *A,* Above-knee prosthesis. *B,* Below-knee prosthesis. *C,* Flex-foot prosthesis, which connects to the distal end of the pylon of an above-knee or below-knee prosthesis and provides increased flexibility for people who want to be more active than they are able to be with a traditional foot-ankle assembly. (*A* and *B,* Courtesy of Otto Bock Orthopedic Industry, Inc., Minneapolis. *C,* Courtesy of Flex Foot, Inc., Mission Viejo, CA.)

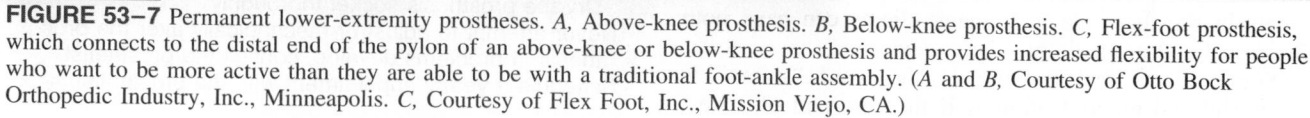

cal therapists usually work with the client twice daily for strengthening and gait training.

When the prosthesis is not worn (e.g., during the night), turning also requires a readaptation in body balance. Consequently, the client may need assistance while turning until the new center of gravity is comfortable.

DIAGNOSIS, OUTCOMES, INTERVENTIONS

After an amputation, the usual postoperative care is given. Look for bleeding or oozing. Outline the drainage, including the time on the temporary prosthesis or soft dressing. If drains are placed in the wound, carefully monitor the amount and type of drainage.

Postoperative management of acute pain is essential. Acute surgical pain management is similar to other postoperative techniques. To prevent increased pain, handle the stump carefully when assessing the site or drainage beneath the stump or dressings.

Because of pre-existing conditions such as diabetes, open infected wounds, and decreased perfusion, the client remains at high risk for infection. Broad-spectrum antibiotics are usually prescribed for several days after surgery until there is an indication that the wound is healing. Monitor the client and the wound for manifestations of wound infection, which usually develop about 72 hours after surgery.

Pain. Following amputation, phantom limb sensation is often present. State this diagnosis as either *Pain related to phantom sensation in amputated limb* or *Anxiety related to phantom sensation in amputated limb.*

Outcomes. The client will express an understanding of the sensations present and recognize that they are normal and usually diminish in time.

Interventions. Emphasize that phantom sensation is usual and, more important, subsides in time. It is not helpful to correct clients by telling them that the limb cannot be hurting because it is absent.

Ineffective Individual Coping. For clients with some chronic disorders, such as diabetes, the amputation may signal further losses in their battle. These clients may express anger openly or covertly. Many clients express depression after amputation. Clients may cry easily, eat little, sleep poorly or sleep more, or avoid interactions with others. Depression is a common reaction to the fear that they will never walk again, and therefore early ambulation is therapeutic. State the nursing diagnosis as *Ineffective Individual Coping related to a reaction or response to change in body image, or fear over loss of independence.*

Outcomes. The client openly verbalizes fears about changes in body image and loss of independence and begins to speak optimistically and realistically about the future.

Interventions. Listen to the client, and confront misconceptions about the rehabilitation. If possible, arrange for the client to meet with an amputee.

The client may express concerns that it will be impossible to return to a previous lifestyle, including job, leisure activities, or intimate relationships. With advancements in prosthetic devices, many clients can have both functional and aesthetic prosthetic devices.

Some clients feel the use of the word "stump" is distasteful and report feeling as if they are part of a tree. Use of other terms may be controversial, however, if such words encourage or support denial of the problem. Some rehabilitation specialists use the term "residual limb" instead.

Knowledge Deficit. Clients require information and time to learn all the new information about the care of the stump and the prosthesis. Use the nursing diagnosis *Knowledge deficit related to gait training, care of the stump, and care of the prosthesis.*

Outcomes. The client will express and demonstrate ability to don and doff the prosthesis and to inspect the stump for abrasions.

Interventions. The Client Education Guide: Stump and Prosthesis Care suggests ways for clients with a lower limb amputation to care for their stump and prosthesis in the health care facility or at home.

Self-Care

When making discharge plans for the client with a new amputation (and probably a prosthesis), consider the client's ambulatory level and the tasks with which the client may need help. Frequently, by the time clients with amputations are aware of their changed circumstances, they

CLIENT EDUCATION GUIDE

Stump and Prosthesis Care

Client Instructions

Stump Care

Inspect the stump daily for redness, blistering, or abrasions.

Use a mirror to examine all sides and aspects of the stump. Skin breakdown on the stump is extremely serious because it interferes with prosthesis training and may prolong hospitalization and recovery. If you have diabetes mellitus, you are particularly susceptible to skin complications, because changes in sensation may obliterate your awareness of stump pain.

Perform meticulous daily hygiene. Wash the stump with a mild soap, then carefully rinse and dry it. Apply nothing to the stump after it is bathed. Alcohol dries and cracks the skin, whereas oils and creams soften the skin too much for safe prosthesis use.

Wear woolen stump socks over the stump for cleanliness and comfort. Wash woolen socks in cool water and mild soap to prevent shrinkage. To prevent stretching, wash socks gently. Dry stump socks flat on a towel. Replace torn socks; mending creates wrinkles that irritate the skin.

Put on the prosthesis immediately when arising and keep it on all day (once the wound has healed completely) to reduce stump swelling.

Continue prescribed exercises to prevent weakness.

Prosthesis Care

Remove sweat and dirt from the prosthesis socket daily by wiping the inside of the socket with a damp soapy cloth. To remove the soap, use a clean damp cloth. Dry the prosthesis socket thoroughly.

Never attempt to adjust or mechanically alter the prosthesis. If problems develop, consult the prosthetist.

Schedule a yearly appointment with the prosthetist.

are at home, alone, and without the informed and professional advice that can prepare them for their altered lives. Schedule home visits from community health care nurses until such clients have adjusted to their new situation and feel reasonably comfortable and confident in their ability to provide self-care.

TRAUMATIC AMPUTATION

Not all amputations are planned. Some clients suffer traumatic loss of a limb due to farm machinery accidents, chain saw accidents, and automobile accidents. Sometimes the amputated limb can be replanted because usually both the client and the limb were healthy up to the time of injury. It is important to properly store and transport the amputated limb prior to replantation. The limb should be wrapped in a cloth and placed in a plastic bag and then on ice. The limb or digit should not come in contact with ice or water to prevent direct tissue damage. No promises should be made to the client about the ability to successfully replant an amputated limb prior to an evaluation by the replantation surgery team. People whose limbs are amputated because of trauma have not had time before surgery to grieve the loss or adjust to their perceived alterations in body image. They may express sadness or anger or may show a strong determination not to let the amputation alter their ability to function.

Outcomes after replantation vary with the complexity of repair required and the amount of tissue replanted. Months of rehabilitation are required, and the peripheral nerve repairs itself very slowly.

ACUTE ARTERIAL OCCLUSION

Etiology and Pathophysiology

Acute occlusion of a limb's main artery may be caused by trauma, embolism, or thrombosis and may occur in a healthy or diseased artery; about 90% occur in the lower limbs. In arterial embolism, the wall of the artery is often healthy; the obstruction in the artery arises most frequently from a thrombus within the heart. Causes include atrial fibrillation, myocardial infarction, prosthetic heart valves, and rheumatic heart disease. Sometimes portions of a blood clot, such as platelet emboli that form at points of turbulence and then lodge at a bifurcation, can initiate a thrombus. Atheromatous emboli sometimes block small arteries. In the lower extremity, more than half the emboli lodge in either the superficial femoral or the popliteal artery. Other noncardiac sources of emboli are laminated clots in an abdominal aortic aneurysm or peripheral aneurysm, and up to 20% are from an unidentified source. Most of these emboli lodge in the lower extremities, and about 15% travel to the arms. Arterial thrombosis is usually superimposed on atherosclerosis and consequently develops in a damaged vessel. However, coagulopathy from heparin-induced thrombocytopenia, inherited coagulation disorders, disseminated intravascular coagulation, or polycythemia vera may also occur.

The circulatory changes that follow arterial occlusion and that predict the outcome are complex and depend on various factors. Acute occlusion produces a fall in mean and pulse pressures in the distal arteries and a decrease in tissue perfusion and oxygenation. In a normal artery, blood flow is restored by collateral channels; with acute emboli, collateral vessels have not had time to develop.

It is important to differentiate between *arterial thrombosis* and *arterial embolism.* Acute arterial thrombosis is usually caused by arterial obstruction from a blood clot that forms in an artery that has been damaged by atherosclerosis. Arterial thrombosis may also develop in an arterial aneurysm, especially an aneurysm that has formed in the popliteal artery. Arterial emboli form in the terminal end of an artery and lead to distinct areas of necrotic tissue.

Clinical Manifestations

The classic manifestations of acute ischemia caused by peripheral thrombus or embolism, which are known as the *six P's,* are shown in Box 53–1. Muscle necrosis may start as early as 2 to 3 hours after occlusion. Paresthesias indicate advanced damage. Complete paralysis with stiffness of muscles and joints (rigor mortis) indicates irreversible damage. The leg must be amputated to prevent systemic reaction to the products of massive muscle destruction and systemic sepsis.

Outcome Management

Surgery is required to correct arterial embolism. Arterial emboli can be removed by an embolectomy.

Surgery for thrombosis usually involves an arterial reconstructive procedure for revascularization of the leg. If the decision is made to remove the occluding embolus or thrombus, surgery should be performed as quickly as possible, generally with the client under local anesthesia. If hours have elapsed since the occlusion occurred, the viability of the limb determines whether embolectomy should be attempted.

If surgery is not performed immediately, anticoagulants are used to reduce the risk of further occlusion. Heparin is usually continued for a minimum of 2 to 7 days, after which a change to an oral anticoagulant may be made. The prevailing practice is to treat all clients who have a definite source of embolism and who have satisfactorily recovered from the acute episode of occlusion with long-term anticoagulant therapy. Fibrinolytic agents may also be used to dissolve a thrombus or embolus (see Chapter 58).

While decisions about surgery are being made, put the

BOX 53–1 Clinical Manifestations of Acute Arterial Occlusion: The Six *P*'s

1. *P*ain or loss of sensory nerves secondary to ischemia
2. *P*ulselessness
3. *P*oikilothermia (coldness)
4. *P*allor caused by empty superficial veins and no capillary filling; pallor can progress to a mottled, cyanotic, cadaverous, cold leg
5. *P*aresthesias and loss of position sense; the client cannot detect pressure or sense a pinprick; the client cannot tell whether toes are flexed or extended
6. *P*aralysis

client to bed in a comfortable, warm room. Protect the limb from pressure and other trauma, and keep it at room temperature, neither warm nor chilled. The best position for the limb is level or slightly dependent.

ARTERIAL ULCERS

Areas of an ischemic foot subjected to local pressure or minor trauma may undergo skin breakdown. The usual sites of arterial ulcers are the medial and lateral metatarsal heads and the tip of the heel. The ulcers are very painful, which distinguishes them from venous stasis ulcers. Arterial ulcers also have a sharp edge and a pale base and often are surrounded by atrophic tissue (see Fig. 53–7). In contrast, venous stasis ulcers are irregular and have a red healthy base (see later).

Once an ulcer develops, it tends to heal poorly if at all (especially in diabetic clients). Without adequate blood flow, the damaged tissues do not receive needed oxygen, nutrients, antibodies, and leukocytes, and the process of tissue damage continues. Eventually, the client may be forced to undergo limb amputation.

Although skin grafting may ultimately be required to cover the site of arterial ischemic leg ulcers (once the ulcerated area is free from infection and granulation tissue is evident), intervention for the skin lesion does not cure the underlying disease. For most ulcers, revascularization is required for healing. Arterial bypass surgery improves circulation when the client has an aortoiliac or femoropopliteal occlusion. For this surgery to be successful, however, the arteries in the leg must be healthy enough to carry sufficient blood to the foot once the block has been removed or bypassed.

General intervention involves keeping the area of ulceration clean and free from pressure and irritation. Bed rest reduces the oxygen needs of the impaired tissues. Whirlpool treatments provide debridement. If surgical debridement is necessary, a qualified health care provider should perform this procedure. After revascularization, if the ulcer bed is clean and granulating, healing is enhanced with damp normal saline dressings or a moist occlusive dressing, such as DuoDerm.

ANEURYSMS

An aneurysm is a permanent localized dilation (50% increase in size) of an artery. Once formed, an aneurysm tends to enlarge gradually; this, along with the thrombus that develops within the aneurysm, leads to the usual complications: rupture, pressure on surrounding structures, thrombosis, and distal embolization. Atherosclerotic aneurysms occur about 10 times more often in men than in women and, for the most part, after age 50 years. There is a hereditary tendency for abdominal aortic aneurysms, with a 25% increase in the rate among first-degree relatives (male).

The most common cause of arterial aneurysms is atherosclerosis. Less common causes include congenital defects of the arterial wall (e.g., Marfan's syndrome), trauma (both blunt and penetrating types), infection (including syphilis), polyarteritis, and hereditary abnormalities of connective tissue. Hypertension seems to enhance aneurysm formation.

A combination of factors, such as "wear and tear," impaired nutrition, and inherited elastin insufficiency, results in weakening of the arterial wall over time, which leads to tortuosity (twisted), dilation, and aneurysm formation in atherosclerotic arteries. The most common sites of arteriosclerotic aneurysms are the thoracic and abdominal aorta, the iliac arteries, and the femoral and popliteal arteries.

■ CLASSIFICATION

Aneurysms may be classified according to the following characteristics:

1. *Location.* Aneurysms are designated as being either *venous* or *arterial.* They are also described according to the specific vessel in which they develop (e.g., aortic, iliac artery) and, more precisely, the exact area of the vessel that they affect (e.g., thoracic aorta, abdominal aorta).
2. *Etiology.* Aneurysms can be classified according to the cause, such as atherosclerotic aneurysm, mycotic aneurysm (caused by bacterial infection), anastomotic graft aneurysm, or syphilitic (luetic) aneurysm.
3. *Gross Appearance.* Classification of aneurysms is sometimes based on their shape, anatomic features, and size. *Fusiform* aneurysms are localized, rather uniform dilations of an artery; the term *saccular* is used to describe an outpouching of an artery at a point at which the medial coat is thinned (Fig. 53–8). A *dissecting* aneurysm occurs as the hematoma in the arterial wall forms a localized enlargement of the involved artery, separating the layers of the arterial wall. A dissecting aneurysm may be either acute or chronic. A *pseudoaneurysm,* or false aneurysm, results from the development of a sac around a hematoma that maintains a communication with the lumen of an artery whose wall has been ruptured or penetrated.

■ ABDOMINAL AORTIC ANEURYSMS

Abdominal aortic aneurysms (Fig. 53–9*A*) occur about four times more often than thoracic aneurysms. The natural course of an untreated abdominal aortic aneurysm is to expand and rupture. The aorta is under greater stress than the rest of the arterial system because of its large diameter and its exposure to high pressure during each systolic ejection of blood. Abdominal aneurysms may extend into the iliac arteries. When the aneurysm reaches about 5 cm in diameter, it can usually be palpated, except in the obese client. An abdominal aneurysm measuring 6 cm or more in diameter has a 20% chance of rupturing in 1 year.

Most abdominal aneurysms are asymptomatic; discovery is usually made on physical or x-ray examination of the abdomen or lower spine for other reasons. Smaller aneurysms and aneurysms in obese clients may be more difficult to confirm. The most common clinical manifestation is the client's awareness of a pulsating mass in the abdomen, with or without pain, followed by abdominal pain and back pain. Groin pain and flank pain may be experienced because of increasing pressure on other structures. Sometimes mottling of the extremities or distal em-

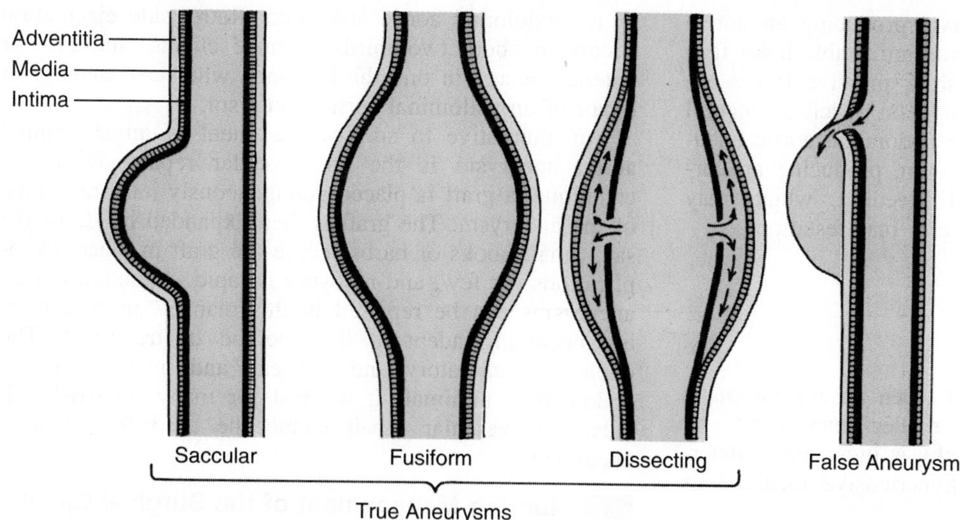

FIGURE 53–8 Classification of aneurysms. In a true aneurysm, layers of the vessel wall dilate in one of the following ways: *saccular,* a unilateral outpouching; *fusiform,* a bilateral outpouching; or *dissecting,* a bilateral outpouching in which layers of the vessel wall separate, with creation of a cavity. In a false aneurysm, the wall ruptures, and a blood clot is retained in an outpouching of tissue, or there is a connection between a vein and an artery which does not close.

boli in the feet can alert the clinician to a source in the abdomen.

Ultrasonography and CT are the most accurate diagnostic tools. Abdominal aortography is not essential for making the diagnosis but helps identify circulatory anomalies important at the time of resection. Therefore, angiography is not performed until surgery is contemplated.

The most frequent complication is rupture, which occurs most often in aneurysms 5 cm or more in diameter. The abdominal aneurysm may rupture in the following body areas:

- Into the peritoneal cavity (usually with fatal results)
- Into the mesentery
- Behind the peritoneum (the most common type of rupture with the best prognosis)
- Into the inferior vena cava (resulting in shock and heart failure from massive arteriovenous fistula)
- Into the duodenum or rectum (causing severe gastrointestinal hemorrhage)

Ruptured abdominal aortic aneurysm presents with a triad of manifestations, including:

- Abdominal pain combined with intense back and flank pain and possible scrotal pain
- A pulsating abdominal mass or a rigid abdomen from the hemorrhage
- Shock, with systolic blood pressure below 100 mm Hg and apical pulse rate greater than 100 per minute

Other manifestations include syncope; ecchymosis in the flank and perianal area; severe sudden pain in the abdomen, paravertebral area, or flank; lightheadedness; and nausea with sudden hypotension. In addition, the red blood cell (RBC) count falls and the WBC count rises. These are also the signs of a ruptured postoperative abdominal bypass graft.

After the initial retroperitoneal rupture, the blood may be walled off in the retroperitoneal space, or tamponaded, for a period. If the ruptured abdominal aortic aneurysm can be identified during this phase, the client has a much greater chance of survival. Once the aorta ruptures anteriorly into the peritoneal cavity, death is almost certain because there are no structures in the abdomen to wall off the bleeding, such as the retroperitoneal space. Rupture occurring more than an hour away from medical care severely decreases the chances of survival.

Surgery is the only intervention for clients with ruptured abdominal aortic aneurysm. New surgical and grafting techniques and faster methods for transport (e.g., helicopters) now permit rapid resection of ruptured abdominal aortic aneurysm and sometimes save the client's life. Even with new advances in surgery, the operative mortality rate for repair of ruptured abdominal aneurysm may be as high as 35%.

About 4% of all ruptured abdominal aortic aneurysms

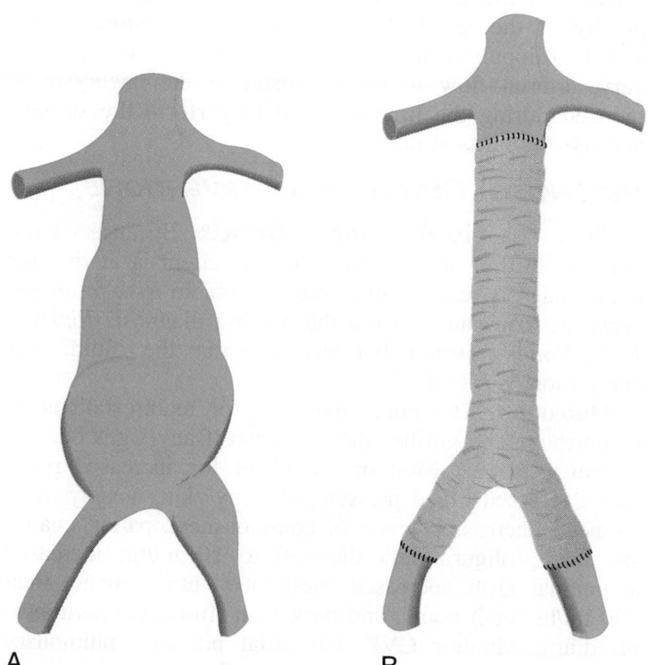

FIGURE 53–9 *A,* An abdominal aortic aneurysm. *B,* A bifurcated synthetic graft in place.

rupture into the inferior vena cava, producing an aortocaval fistula. Manifestations include intractable heart failure because of the right-to-left shift, massive lower extremity edema, acute abdominal pain, ascites, pleural effusions, and hepatomegaly. The abdominal aortic aneurysm may rupture into the duodenum, producing an aortoenteric fistula. Gastrointestinal bleeding, which may progress to shock, is the beginning of manifestations.

Outcome Management

Medical Management

Surgery is usually not performed when an asymptomatic abdominal aortic aneurysm is smaller than 4 to 5 cm. Every 6 months, an ultrasonography is indicated to determine any change in size. Antihypertensive medications are usually prescribed if indicated.

Surgical Management

Surgical management of an aneurysm may be performed as either an emergency or an elective procedure. Elective resection and graft replacement carry a surgical mortality of less than 5%; emergency surgical treatment after the aneurysm has ruptured is associated with a much higher mortality rate.

The surgical technique involves exposing the aneurysm, applying clamps just above and below the aneurysm, opening the aneurysm, and placing a polyester (Dacron) graft within the aneurysm. The aneurysm sac is then wrapped around the graft to protect it (see Fig. 53–9*B*). Excision of an abdominal aneurysm is done through a midline incision that extends from the xiphoid process to the symphysis pubis.

Abdominal aortic aneurysm repair is considered a major operation, and many specific postoperative complications can develop. Complications after abdominal aortic aneurysm repair are generally caused by underlying coronary artery disease and chronic obstructive pulmonary disease (COPD). These conditions decrease the excretion of the anesthetic, increase the risk of postoperative atelectasis, and decrease the client's tolerance of hemodynamic changes from blood loss and fluid shifts.

One of the most serious complications is acute myocardial infarction. To reduce the risk of this complication, many clients undergo coronary artery bypass grafting (CABG) before aneurysm repair.

Prerenal failure can develop for several reasons. The kidney can sustain ischemia from decreased aortic blood flow, decreased cardiac output, emboli, inadequate hydration, or the need for clamps on the aorta above the renal arteries during surgery.

Emboli can also develop and lodge in the arteries of the lower extremities or mesentery. Clinical manifestations include those of acute occlusion in the leg. Bowel necrosis is exhibited as fever, leukocytosis, ileus, diarrhea, and abdominal pain.

The spinal cord can also become ischemic, resulting in paraplegia, rectal and urinary incontinence, or loss of pain and temperature sensation. Spinal cord ischemia tends to occur more commonly when an abdominal aortic aneurysm has ruptured.

Changes in sexual function may also occur after repair of an abdominal aortic aneurysm. Retrograde ejaculation occurs in about two thirds of male clients, and loss of potency occurs in one third of men who have undergone repair of an abdominal aortic aneurysm.

An alternative to surgical treatment of an abdominal aortic aneurysm is the endovascular repair. With this technique, a graft is placed percutaneously into the lumen of the aneurysm. The graft is then expanded inside of the sac. Small hooks or barbs secure the graft in place. Complications are few, and recovery is rapid. Although not all aneurysms can be repaired in this manner, more centers are becoming adept at this method of treatment. The client is ambulatory and can eat, and invasion of the abdomen is minimal. It is ideal for many poor-risk clients. Endovascular repair cannot be used for ruptured aneurysms.

Nursing Management of the Surgical Client

PREOPERATIVE CARE

Abdominal aortic surgery is major surgery and lasts approximately 4 hours. During the hours under anesthesia, the client is at high risk for pulmonary and cardiac complications. Preoperative assessment must include detection of concurrent coronary artery disease and cerebrovascular disease. Assess all peripheral pulses for baseline comparison postoperatively. If dissection or rupture occurs, the client may receive IV fluids (often in large volumes) for maintenance of tissue perfusion.

For endovascular repair, the procedure is much shorter. Standard evaluation must occur because the potential for an open repair of the aneurysm still exists.

POSTOPERATIVE CARE

ASSESSMENT

A very comprehensive postoperative assessment of the client after open surgical repair of an abdominal aortic aneurysm is essential. Potential complications are many, because of the seriousness of the problem and the complexity of the repair. Even though extracorporeal perfusion (cardiopulmonary bypass) is not needed for the surgery, arterial flow to tissues distal to the aneurysm is reduced during the time required to perform the surgery because the aorta is clamped.

DIAGNOSIS, OUTCOMES, INTERVENTIONS

Risk for Fluid Volume Deficit. Because of the risk of bleeding at the graft site, the client is at risk for hemorrhage. Use the collaborative problem *Risk for Hemorrhage.* You can also use the nursing diagnosis *Risk for Fluid Volume Deficit,* but recognize that the "fluid" that can be lost is blood.

Outcomes. The nurse monitors for manifestations of hemorrhage and notifies the physician if any signs occur.

Interventions. Monitor the client for increased pulse rate, decreased blood pressure, clammy skin, anxiety, restlessness, decreasing levels of consciousness, pallor, cyanosis, thirst, oliguria less than 30 to 50 ml/hr, increased abdominal girth, increased chest tube output greater than 100 ml/hr for 3 hours, and back pain (from retroperitoneal bleeding). Monitor CVP, left atrial pressure, pulmonary artery pressure, and pulmonary capillary wedge pressure (PCWP) continuously. Assess for changes indicating hypovolemia. Report any of these manifestations immediately.

Impaired Gas Exchange. The large abdominal incision impairs deep inspiration and usually reduces effective coughing. Write the diagnosis as *Impaired Gas Exchange related to ineffective cough secondary to pain from large incision.*

Outcomes. The client will demonstrate improved gas exchange, as evidenced by oxygen saturation or PaO_2 greater than 95%, increasing effectiveness in coughing, and clearing of lung sounds.

Interventions. Monitor settings on the ventilator to ensure that the client is adequately oxygenated. Assess lung sounds every 1 to 2 hours, and report any adventitious sounds. Monitor oxygen saturation continuously, and report any desaturation. After extubation, assist with coughing by using incentive spirometry, provide splinting pillows before coughing, encourage ambulation, and provide adequate analgesia to promote coughing with severe pain.

Altered Tissue Perfusion. During the operation, the aorta is clamped to stop bleeding while the graft is placed. During that time, peripheral tissues are not perfused. The graft site can also become occluded with thrombus. In addition, the client often has pre-existing arterial disease. Write the diagnosis as *Altered Peripheral Tissue Perfusion related to temporary decrease in blood supply.*

Outcomes. The client will maintain adequate tissue perfusion, as evidenced by pedal pulses, warm feet, capillary refill of less than 5 seconds, absence of numbness or tingling, and dorsiflexion and plantiflexion of both feet equally.

Interventions. Assess dorsalis pedis and posterior tibial pulses every hour for 24 hours. Report changes in pulse quality or absent pulses; assess with Doppler imaging if needed. Assess dorsiflexion and plantiflexion and sensation (needles and pins sensation) every hour for 24 hours. Inspect lower extremities for mottling, cyanosis, coolness, or numbness every 4 hours.

Pain. Abdominal aortic aneurysm repair necessitates a long incision. Write this common postoperative diagnosis as *Pain related to surgical incision.*

Outcomes. The client will experience increased comfort, as evidenced by self-report of decreasing levels of pain, use of decreasing amounts of narcotic analgesics for pain control, and ambulating and coughing without extreme pain.

Ischemia of the Bowel. Extensive aortic procedures that involve clamping the mesenteric vessels can result in ischemic colitis. In addition, the inferior mesenteric artery can embolize. The lack of blood supply may lead to ischemia and ileus. This diagnosis is a collaborative problem.

Outcomes. The nurse will monitor the client for abdominal distention, diarrhea, severe abdominal pain, sudden elevations in WBC count, and bowel sounds.

Interventions. Maintain accurate intake and output, and analyze data hourly for 24 hours. Notify the physician if output falls below 30 to 50 ml/hr. Assess urine specific gravity and daily weight. Monitor blood urea nitrogen (BUN) and creatinine levels. Assess bowel sounds every 4 hours. The client should have nothing by mouth. Provide oral care every 2 to 4 hours. Provide routine nasogastric (NG) tube care, and assess nares for tissue impairment. Perform guaiac tests of NG drainage every 4 hours or if bleeding is suspected (i.e., drainage has dark, coffee-ground appearance or is bright red).

Self-Care

Most clients who require abdominal aortic aneurysm repair have significant degrees of arterial disease. Many of the postoperative instructions should address care of clients with arterial disorders (see earlier). Review all medications to be used to be certain that the client understands their purpose, scheduling, and side effects. Explain incision care and manifestations of infection.

The client should ambulate as tolerated, including climbing stairs and walking outdoors. If leg swelling develops, the leg should be wrapped in elastic bandages or support stockings should be used. Activities that involve lifting heavy objects, usually more than 15 to 20 pounds, are not permitted for 6 to 12 weeks postoperatively. Activities that involve pushing, pulling, or straining may also be restricted. Driving may also be restricted because of postoperative weakness and decreased response time.

Clients can resume sexual activity as soon as they can walk without shortness of breath (e.g., two flights of stairs), usually in 4 to 6 weeks. The risk of impotence in male clients should be discussed before discharge. Causes vary from pre-existing aortoiliac disease or diabetes to side effects from aortic cross-clamping. Referral may be appropriate if the client is amenable.

AORTIC DISSECTION

Aortic dissection, the longitudinal splitting of the medial (muscular) layer of the aorta by blood flowing through it, is the most common catastrophe involving the aorta. Dissection occurs following a tear in the intima, or inner lining, of the aorta, which allows blood to dissect between it and the medial layer. As the dissection progresses, blood flow through the arterial branches of the aorta becomes blocked and blood flow to the organs served by these branches is reduced. Aortic dissections occur more often in men between ages 50 and 70 years, most of whom are hypertensive. Aortic dissections differ from *aneurysms,* in that a false lumen is formed by separation of the intima from the medial layers of the aorta. An aneurysm is a dilation of the entire aortic wall.

Etiology and Classification

The exact cause of dissection is not known. The medial layer of the aorta can become necrotic and thereby lose strength. Marfan's syndrome (a hereditary condition of connective tissue that predisposes it to aneurysm formation) is associated with a high incidence of dissection. Blunt trauma to the chest wall, such as impact on the steering wheel during a car accident, can also lead to tearing of the aorta.

Dissections are classified by the anatomic location and time of occurrence:

- Type I—the most common and most lethal form—starts above the aortic valve and extends to the iliac bifurcation, traversing the entire aorta.

- Type II is confined to the ascending aorta and proximal transverse arch and is most often seen in conjunction with Marfan's syndrome.
- Type III dissections begin just distal to the left subclavian artery and extend to the iliac bifurcation; they carry the best prognosis and are usually treated medically.

Dissections are also classified as *acute* (occurring during the preceding 2 weeks) and chronic (persisting more than 2 weeks). If dissections are untreated, 50% of clients die within the first 48 hours, 60% to 70% within the first week, and 90% within 3 months after dissection.

Clinical Manifestations

Abrupt, excruciating pain is the most common presenting manifestation in clients with aortic dissection. Clients describe the pain as "ripping" or knife-like tearing sensations that radiate to the back, abdomen, extremities, or anterior part of the chest. Hypertension is a common finding, although the client looks "shocky," is sweating profusely, is severely apprehensive, and has diminished peripheral pulses. Other manifestations of decreased perfusion include unequal pulses, different blood pressures in the arms, paraplegia or hemiplegia, decreased urine output or hematuria, mental status changes, and chest pain. A murmur of aortic regurgitation can be heard if the dissection proceeds proximally.

Chest x-ray studies reveal a widened mediastinum and sometimes fractured ribs. Echocardiography can be used to determine the size, shape, and location of the tear. Laboratory tests during emergency settings are usually not helpful except for hemoglobin and hematocrit assays to calculate blood loss and transfusion needs. If the client's condition is stable, aortography can be used to determine the extent of the dissection.

Complications

Cardiac tamponade can develop in the presence of dissection of the ascending aortic arch. This life-threatening complication occurs when blood escapes from the area of dissection into the pericardial sac. Clients have pulsus paradoxus, muffled heart sounds, narrowed pulse pressure, and distended neck veins. Pulsus paradoxus occurs when beats are weaker in amplitude during inspiration and are stronger with expiration. Blood pressure readings decrease more than 10 mm Hg during inspiration and increase with expiration.

Because the dissection decreases blood supply to many vital organs, ischemic changes in many organs can occur. The spinal cord, kidneys, and abdominal organs are most commonly affected. Ischemia of the spinal cord can lead to manifestations ranging from weakness to paralysis. Renal ischemia can lead to oliguria. Ileus is the most common sign of decreased bowel perfusion.

Management

Emergency management is directed at lowering the blood pressure to decrease the force of the blood tearing the aorta. Potent vasodilators, such as trimethaphan and nitroprusside, are used to quickly reduce blood pressure. Beta-blockers can also be used to decrease myocardial contractility.

If the client's condition is stable, the goals are to reduce pain, initiate blood transfusion (as needed), and manage heart failure (as needed). Pain levels are used as a guide for needed treatment. Pain subsides when the dissection stabilizes.

Surgery is warranted for clients whose condition is unstable, who have severe heart failure, who have a leaking aneurysm, or whose arteries to major organs are occluded. During surgery, the torn area is resected and repaired with synthetic graft materials. The operation is similar to that for repair of an abdominal aortic aneurysm.

Nursing care is directed at reducing blood pressure. The client is kept on bed rest in a semi-Fowler position. Unnecessary environmental stresses (e.g., noise) should be minimized. Narcotics are administered to reduce pain; tranquilizers may also be needed. If the client is receiving potent antihypertensive agents, monitor blood pressure continuously with an arterial line. Usually, the desired parameters for blood pressure are maintained by titrating the vasodilators. Observe the client often for signs of further tearing or rupture. Monitor peripheral pulses, level of anxiety, level of pain, and pulse pressure, and check for pulsus paradoxus.

If the client is being managed medically, explain the need for antihypertensive agents and beta-blocker drugs. The client and family should understand that if pain recurs, they should return immediately to the emergency room.

■ THORACIC AORTIC ANEURYSMS

Aneurysms of the thoracic aorta appear most often in hypertensive men between ages 40 and 70 years. The aneurysms can develop in any portion of the aorta (ascending, transverse, or descending) and are the most common aneurysms to dissect. The thoracic aorta is relatively out of the reach of physical examinations unless the aorta becomes large enough to be palpable above the clavicle. Therefore, the aneurysm is usually asymptomatic early. If the mass presses on other structures in the chest, various manifestations develop. Respiratory manifestations are a result of compression of the trachea or bronchus and can include cough, dyspnea, and hemoptysis. Respiratory arrest can develop, and pressure on the recurrent laryngeal nerve can lead to hoarseness. Dysphagia can result from pressure on the esophagus. Swelling of upper extremity and head can ensue from superior vena cava obstruction. Aortic valve insufficiency can occur if the aneurysm is located in the ascending aorta. The aneurysm can be seen on a chest x-ray and an angiogram.

The client with a ruptured aneurysm reports intense chest pain; hemoglobin is decreased, and hemodynamic instability develops. The pain is described as a ripping sensation up or down the aorta and is more intense when the client lies supine. The pain is usually substernal but may be noted in the back, lower back, shoulders, or abdomen. Increased pain intensity usually indicates rapid enlargement or imminent rupture and is a sign of extreme peril. Unless fortuitous tamponade develops in local tissue, death ensues rapidly. Surgical repair and postoperative management are the same as that for abdominal aortic aneurysm.

RAYNAUD'S SYNDROME

Raynaud's syndrome, a condition in which the small arteries and arterioles constrict in response to various stimuli, can be classified as *vasospastic* or *obstructive.* Manifestations of vasospastic Raynaud's syndrome can be induced by cold, nicotine, caffeine, and stress. Obstructive Raynaud's syndrome is often found in association with autoimmune disorders such as systemic lupus erythematosus, scleroderma, or rheumatoid arthritis.

Raynaud's syndrome may be a benign primary disorder (formerly, *Raynaud's disease*) or secondary to another disease or underlying cause (formerly, *Raynaud's phenomenon*). Manifestations of both types are the same.

Clinical Manifestations

Raynaud's syndrome causes classic color changes in the hands. Exposure to causative stimuli leads to spasm of the digital arteries, which results in pallor. The resulting tissue hypoxia causes the arteries to dilate slightly. Because the fingers carry mainly deoxygenated hemoglobin, they look cyanotic (bluish). Finally, rubor (redness) develops when arterial spasms stop completely.

Criteria for the diagnosis of primary Raynaud's disease include

- Manifestations for at least 2 years
- Intermittent attacks of pallor or cyanosis of the digits from exposure to cold or emotional stimuli
- Bilateral or symmetrical involvement
- No evidence of occlusive disease in the digital arteries or of any systemic disease that might be the cause of the changes
- Gangrene, which (when it occurs) is limited to the skin of the tips of the digits

Noninvasive blood flow studies to determine finger pressures both pre-cold and post-cold challenges may be necessary. Occasionally, the presence of vasospasm during examination makes the use of cold challenge unnecessary.

Outcome Management

Conservative measures are helpful for most clients. These measures include keeping hands and feet warm and dry, protecting all parts of the body from cold exposure to prevent reflex sympathetic vasoconstriction of the digits, and cessation of tobacco use. Biofeedback has helped some clients.

Medication is used when the vasospastic attacks interfere with the client's ability to work or to perform activities of daily living. Medications are used to induce smooth muscle relaxation, to relieve spasm, and to increase arterial flow. Calcium antagonists, such as nifedipine and verapamil, are the drugs of choice because they can decrease the frequency, duration, and intensity of vasospastic attacks. Other categories of drugs used in treatment include alpha-adrenergic receptor blockers and agents that interfere with sympathetic nerve activity (sympatholytic drugs). Medications may be necessary only during the winter months. People who rarely go out in the cold weather may take medications prophylactically 1 to 2 hours before exposure to cold.

Because the manifestations of Raynaud's syndrome may be alarming, reassure the client that the condition is unlikely to lead to a serious disability. Advise the client to stay warm by wearing wool gloves and turtleneck sweaters, turning up the thermostat at home if necessary, and staying out of drafts. Advise the client to warm up a cold car before driving. Body core heating is important to prevent chilling and the shunting of blood from the extremities to the trunk. Encourage clients to limit their intake of caffeine or chocolate. They must stop smoking to control the disease. Stress can also bring on vasospasm, and stress management workshops and biofeedback programs may prove beneficial. Teach the client about any prescribed medications.

THROMBOANGIITIS OBLITERANS (BUERGER'S DISEASE)

Thromboangiitis obliterans is a vasculitis of small and medium-sized veins and arteries in the extremities of young adults. The disease process starts distally and progresses cephalad, involving both upper and lower extremities. The cause remains unknown. The most commonly affected clients are young men who smoke heavily. Many clients have a hypersensitivity reaction to intradermal injection of tobacco products. Therefore, the probable etiologic mechanism is an exaggerated autoimmune reaction.

Clinical Manifestations

Pain is the outstanding clinical manifestation. Digital ulcerations and pain may result from ischemia. The pain may be accompanied by manifestations of ischemia, such as color or temperature changes in the fingers. Cold sensitivity, with color changes and pain, may be another early manifestation. Various types of lower extremity paresthesias may occur. Claudication-type pain is common with pain in the arch of the foot. Pulsations in the posterior tibial and dorsalis pedis arteries are weak or absent. In advanced cases, the extremities may be abnormally red or cyanotic, particularly when they are dependent.

Ulceration and gangrene are common complications and may occur early in the course of the disease. These lesions can appear spontaneously from migratory superficial thrombophlebitis but can also occur after trauma. Gangrene usually occurs in one extremity at a time. Edema of the legs is fairly common in advanced cases. Changes may appear in the nails and skin, and segmental thrombophlebitis affects the smaller veins in about 40% of clients.

Outcome Management

The goals of management include arresting progress of the disease, producing vasodilation, relieving pain, and providing emotional support.

The primary diagnostic study is leg arteriography. Biopsy may also be in order; inflammatory lesions are usually noted.

The need for smoking cessation must be clearly and unequivocally conveyed to the client and family. Provide information about programs to promote abstinence from tobacco. Because of vasoconstriction, teach the client to avoid exposure to cold.

For clients with rest pain and ischemic lesions, adequate pain control is essential. Vasodilation by calcium-channel blockers may be helpful in a few cases. Regional sympathetic ganglionectomy also produces vasodilation and may be recommended. In the past, it was the only method of treatment but is rarely used today. Ulcerations need wound care to facilitate healing. Amputation should be deferred until conservative interventions have failed. Thromboangiitis is usually not life-threatening; however, it does result in disability from pain and amputation.

■ PERIPHERAL ANEURYSMS

Peripheral aneurysms are found more commonly in the lower extremities than in the upper extremities, most commonly in the popliteal space. Popliteal aneurysms cause ischemic manifestations in the lower limbs, and pulses are easily palpable. Although the client may be aware of an enlarged area behind the knee, discomfort is seldom present. Peripheral aneurysm is differentiated from other swellings by the presence of expansile pulsation. Thrombosis may occur and may result in severe ischemia with gangrene and loss of the limb. Popliteal artery aneurysms may also become entrapped, with marked flexion of the knee, or may embolize to the feet.

Bypass operations are the only satisfactory intervention for aneurysms of the popliteal artery and must be performed before emboli develop. Results are excellent in uncomplicated cases.

SUBCLAVIAN STEAL SYNDROME

Subclavian steal syndrome produces arm ischemia arising from subclavian artery blockage. The arm is perfused from the vertebral artery as blood is taken from the brain to supply the arm. The most prevalent physical finding is a significant difference in blood pressure of the right and left arms (20 mm Hg or more). Other manifestations include dizziness and syncope when the arm is exercised. Arm paresthesias and bruit in the supraclavicular fossa are present. The client may not be symptomatic, and no intervention is necessary.

Intervention is surgical, by carotid-subclavian bypass, transluminal dilation of the subclavian artery, or endarterectomy of the subclavian artery.

THORACIC OUTLET SYNDROMES

Thoracic outlet syndromes are a group of disorders that produce symptoms affecting the neck, shoulder, and upper extremities by compression or mechanical irritation of the brachial plexus, subclavian artery, or subclavian vein as these structures pass through the thoracic outlet.

Aching or throbbing pain and paresthesias of the neck and upper limb are the most prominent clinical manifestations. In more than half of the clients, the manifestations appear to follow a hyperextension injury to the neck or upper back. Intervention is usually nonsurgical and involves physical therapy. The syndrome has sometimes been treated by surgical removal of the first rib, but this intervention is controversial.

Arterial thoracic outlet syndromes result from chronic compression of the subclavian artery. This leads to the formation of intimal and mural thrombus and, eventually, to peripheral embolization. Arterial thoracic outlet syndrome is more serious because it frequently results in severe ischemia of the upper extremity. Diagnosis is made by arteriography; treatment involves surgical excision of the anatomic abnormality and removal of the emboli.

Venous thoracic outlet syndrome is caused by external compression of the axillosubclavian vein that results in thrombosis. The primary symptoms are sudden swelling, pain, and cyanosis of the upper extremity. Management is conservative and may involve arm elevation and anticoagulation, thrombectomy, or thrombolytic therapy.

VENOUS DISORDERS

Venous disorders can be *acute* (e.g., thromboembolism) and *chronic.* Chronic venous disorders can be further separated into varicose vein formation and chronic venous insufficiency. Acute venous disorders are discussed first.

ACUTE VENOUS DISORDERS

Acute venous disorders are caused by thrombus (clot) formation, which obstructs venous flow. Blockage may occur in the superficial veins, the deep veins, or both.

Superficial thrombophlebitis is usually an easily diagnosed condition and may be iatrogenic, resulting from IV catheters or instillation of caustic chemicals. Deep vein thrombosis (DVT) is thrombophlebitis of the deep veins. DVT is a common disorder, affecting more women than men and adults more than children. It is particularly common among hospitalized clients. Around one third of clients older than 40 years who have had either major surgery or an acute myocardial infarction have DVT, and clients with cancer or a family history of clotting disorders are at high risk.

Etiology and Risk Factors

Thrombus formation is usually attributed to Virchow's triad: (1) venous stasis, (2) hypercoagulability, and (3) injury to the venous wall. At least two of the three preceding conditions must be present for thrombus formation.

Venous stasis is usually caused by immobilization or absence of the calf muscle pump. Other etiologic factors are age over 40 years, surgery, immobility, prolonged travel, stroke, obesity, pregnancy, paralysis, and heart disease, such as heart failure, myocardial infarction, or cardiomyopathy.

Hypercoagulability often accompanies malignant neoplasms (especially visceral and ovarian tumors). Dehydration and blood dyscrasias may raise the platelet count, decrease fibrinolysis, increase the clotting factors, or increase blood viscosity. Oral contraceptives and hematologic disorders may also increase blood coagulability.

Conditions that may cause vein wall trauma are IV injections, fractures and dislocations, severe blows to an area, chemical injury from sclerosing agents, contrast x-rays, certain antibiotics (such as chlortetracycline), and thromboangiitis obliterans (Buerger's disease). The resulting damage to the vein wall attracts platelets, and blood debris accumulates. Platelets do not stick to an intact endothelium. This injury, in combination with low blood flow and a hypercoagulable state, results in thrombus formation.

There are many risk factors for the development of venous thrombosis (Box 53–2). Untreated immobile clients with DVT are at lower risk for pulmonary embolism than clients who are ambulatory. Thus, the risk of pulmonary embolism is often underestimated after hospital discharge in clients who have "low-risk" surgery. Presumably, hospitalized clients are treated prophylactically with antiembolism stockings and anticoagulants. Clients discharged to their homes seldom receive this prophylaxis.

Pathophysiology

Usually, venous return is aided by the calf muscle pump. When the legs are inactive or the pump is ineffective, blood pools by gravity in the veins (Fig. 53–10). Thrombus development is a local process. It begins by platelet adherence to the endothelium. Several factors promote platelet aggregation, including thrombin, fibrin, activated factor X, and catecholamines. In addition, where the platelets adhere to collagen, adenosine diphosphate (ADP) is released. ADP is also released from the damaged tissues and disrupted platelets. ADP produces platelet aggregation that results in a platelet plug.

Deep vein thrombi vary from 1 mm in diameter to long tubular masses filling main veins. Small thrombi are found commonly in the pocket of deep vein valves. As thrombi become larger in diameter and length, they obstruct the veins. The resulting inflammatory process can destroy the valves of the veins; thus, venous insufficiency and postphlebitic syndrome are initiated.

Newly formed thrombi may become pulmonary emboli. Probably 24 to 48 hours after formation, thrombi undergo lysis or become organized and adhere to the vessel wall. Lysis diminishes the risk of embolization.

BOX 53–2 Common Conditions Associated with Venous Thrombosis and Thromboembolism

- Age above 40 years
- Surgery requiring more than 30 minutes of general, spinal, or epidural anesthesia
- Venous stasis (bed rest, prolonged travel, stroke)
- Previous deep vein thrombosis
- Cardiac disease (heart failure, myocardial infarction, cardiomyopathy)
- Pregnancy
- Trauma, especially of the lower extremities
- Estrogen therapy or oral contraceptives
- Malignancy
- Obesity
- Family history of clotting disorders

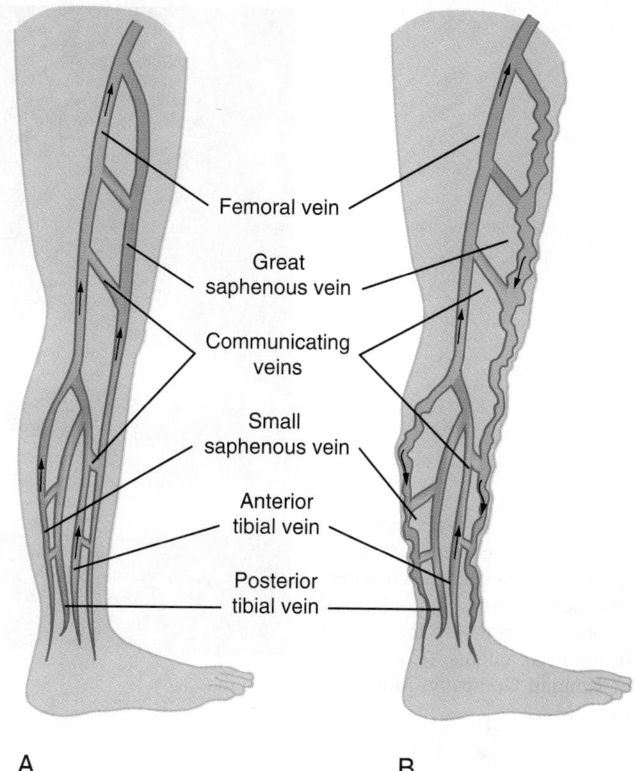

FIGURE 53–10 Venous return from the legs. *A,* Normal flow. *B,* Varicosities and retrograde venous flow.

If a thrombus occludes a major vein (e.g., femoral, vena cava, axillary), venous pressure and volume rise distally. Conversely, if a thrombus occludes a deep small vein (e.g., tibial, popliteal), collateral venous channels usually relieve the increased venous pressure and volume.

Pulmonary emboli, most of which start as thrombi in the large deep veins of the legs, are an acute and potentially lethal complication of DVT. Pulmonary embolism is discussed in Chapter 61.

Prevention

Prevention is geared toward reversing the three risk factors by promoting venous stasis, treating hypercoagulability, and reducing risk of injury to the venous wall.

Venous stasis is improved by any activity that causes the leg muscles to contract. Passive or active contraction, such as leg exercises and ambulation, promote venous return. Passive leg muscle contraction occurs by using sequential intermittent pneumatic compression (IPC) devices (Fig. 53–11). Use of these devices is initiated at the time of many operations and continues until the client is ambulatory. The leggings or boots are attached by polyethylene tubing to an electric pump attached to the foot of the bed. Air is pumped sequentially into three chambers (ankle, calf, and thigh) at a pressure of 45 to 60 mm Hg for 15 to 20 seconds. The compression is followed by deflation and a 45-second resting period. IPC is clinically effective in reducing the incidence of DVT and is also a good alternative for clients who cannot tolerate any anticoagulation therapy. These devices should not be used in clients with known DVT. Other

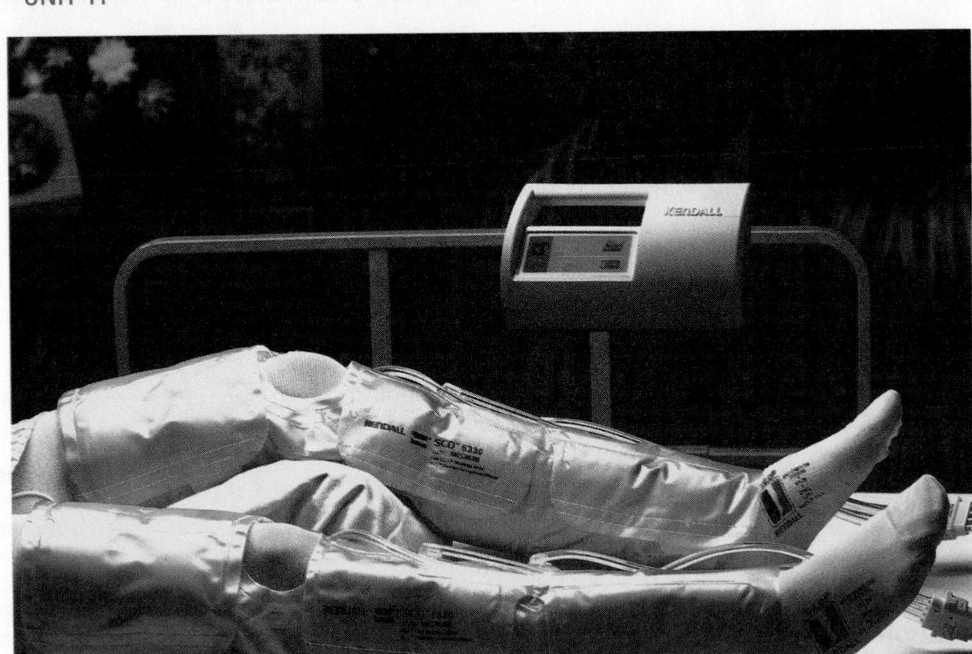

FIGURE 53–11 Pneumatic compression devices, such as the Kendall sequential compression device, are commonly used to prevent deep vein thrombosis in high-risk clients. (Courtesy of Kendall Company, Mansfield, MA.)

methods of promoting venous return include elevating the foot of the bed, applying compression stockings, using motorized foot devices, and providing passive range-of-motion exercises. Encouraging postoperative deep-breathing exercises promotes thoracic pull that is due to negative thoracic pressure on venous stores in the legs.

Pharmacologic prevention directed at reducing the hypercoagulability includes warfarin, platelet antiaggregation agents (aspirin being the most common), heparin, and dextran. Other methods to reduce coagulation include preventing the venous blood from pooling. Avoid using pillows under the client's knees postoperatively. Teach the client to avoid sitting or standing in one position for prolonged periods.

Measures to prevent injury to the vein wall include the avoidance of infiltration during intravenous therapy, pressure on the calf veins during prolonged surgery, and trauma to veins in procedures requiring prolonged positioning (delivery, colonoscopy). In addition, access ports should be used in clients requiring multiple IV sticks.

Clinical Manifestations

Clinical manifestations of superficial thrombophlebitis include redness (rubor), induration (tumor), warmth (calor), and tenderness (dolor) along a cord following the course of the involved vein. Discomfort may be relieved by application of heat. Activity should be encouraged, and a supportive wrap or stocking should be applied.

The clinical manifestations of DVT are less distinctive; about 50% of clients are asymptomatic. The most common clinical manifestation is unilateral swelling distal to the site. Other clinical manifestations include pain, redness or warmth of the leg, dilated veins, and low-grade fever. Unfortunately, the first clinical manifestation may be pulmonary embolism. Clients may have thrombi in both legs even though the manifestations are unilateral, but this is more common in the client with cancer.

Homans' sign—discomfort in the upper calf during forced dorsiflexion of the foot—is commonly assessed during physical examination. Unfortunately, it is not reliable. It is present in fewer than a third of clients with documented DVT. In addition, more than 50% of clients with a positive Homans sign do not have venous thrombosis.

Venous duplex scanning has become the primary diagnostic test of DVT because it allows visualization of the vein, which provides an extremely reliable diagnosis of venous thrombus. Venography, previously the gold standard of diagnosis, results in exposure to contrast and is seldom used.

The Doppler ultrasonographic flowmeter determines blood flow in the larger blood vessels and the patency of vessels. Reliability of the test is directly related to the skill of the examiner; its accuracy is affected by an inability to detect partially or totally occluded veins, inaccessibility of deep pelvic and thigh veins, and inability to distinguish collateral circulation from that in native veins.

The D-dimer test is being used more frequently in evaluation of DVT. The D-dimer is a product of fibrin degradation and is indicative of fibrinolysis that occurs with thrombosis. The use of the D-dimer, a risk assessment score, and duplex imaging appear to be excellent at predicting and diagnosing DVT in asymptomatic people.

Plethysmography of the venous system is seldom used; however, these studies may be found in client records. In the past, the test was performed by recording volume changes in a limb during venous filling and emptying. Impedance plethysmography measures maximal venous filling capacity by applying a pneumatic cuff at thigh level and then recording the rate of venous emptying after cuff release.

Outcome Management

Medical Management

The goals of medical management are to detect the thrombus early, prevent extension or embolization of the thrombus, and prevent further thrombus formation.

Superficial thrombophlebitis can be managed with local measures, such as warm packs and elevation of the extremity. Ambulation is encouraged. Sometimes anti-inflammatory medications are required. Encourage clients to be seen in follow-up, because an extension of a superficial phlebitis can result in DVT.

ANTICOAGULATION

Anticoagulant therapy is based on the premise that the initiation or extension of thrombi can be prevented by inhibiting the synthesis of clotting factors or by accelerating their inactivation.

HEPARIN. Heparin is the drug of choice for the treatment of thromboembolic disease. Unfractionated heparin prevents the activation of clotting factor IX and inhibits the action of thrombin in forming fibrin threads. The primary anticoagulant effect is from the binding on antithrombin III. Heparin has a 4-hour half-life and, in the event of bleeding, is stopped immediately. The specific antidote to heparin is protamine sulfate, which neutralizes the effects of heparin immediately and lasts for 2 hours. Unfortunately, an excessive dose of protamine may actually prolong clotting.

Heparin is contraindicated in any conditions of bleeding or disorders that increase the risk of bleeding, including severe hypertension, cerebrovascular hemorrhage, active gastrointestinal ulceration, recent neurosurgery, and overt bleeding from the gastrointestinal, genitourinary, or respiratory tract.

Low-molecular-weight (LMW) heparin is a variant of heparin. Its primary action is from inactivation of factor Xa; advantages include decreased bleeding complications, subcutaneous (not IV) route, no need for laboratory testing, and ability of the client to be ambulatory. The anticoagulants heparin and warfarin do not induce thrombolysis, but they effectively prevent clot extension. The use of LMW heparin allows the client to ambulate, to go home, and to treat the DVT with an injectable medication. LMW heparin therapy is still followed by 3 to 6 months of warfarin therapy.

WARFARIN. Warfarin (Coumadin) inhibits hepatic synthesis of the vitamin K–dependent clotting factors. The effect of the warfarin is determined by measurement of the INR. The therapeutic level for DVT is an International Normalized Ratio (INR) of 2.0 to 3.0. The antidote for the warfarin derivatives is vitamin K (Mephyton). The warfarin derivatives require 24 to 48 hours to eliminate the vitamin K–dependent factors. Therefore, anticoagulation can include both medications. Heparin, which is fast-acting, is used initially with warfarin and discontinued when the warfarin begins to take effect. Anticoagulation therapy is usually continued about 3 to 6 months after an acute venous thrombosis and after pulmonary embolism.

FIBRINOLYTIC AGENTS. Fibrinolytic medications (e.g., streptokinase and urokinase) dissolve thrombi by stimulating the conversion of plasminogen to plasmin, an enzyme that decomposes fibrin (see Chapter 58).

Nursing Management of the Medical Client

Goals of nursing management are to prevent existing thrombi from becoming emboli and to prevent new thrombi from forming. Nurses also closely monitor the effect of anticoagulant medications.

ELEVATE THE CLIENT'S LEGS

Elevation of the legs above the level of the heart facilitates blood flow by the force of gravity. The increase of blood flow prevents venous stasis and the formation of new thrombi. Elevation of the legs also decreases venous pressure, which in turn relieves edema and pain. Elevate the foot of the bed 6 inches (Trendelenburg's position), with a slight knee bend to prevent popliteal pressure. The veins of the legs should be level with the right atrium. The head of the bed may be raised to facilitate eating and bathing.

Various forms of elastic support are used to promote venous return. Elastic bandages are advantageous for clients with large or misshapen legs. Apply elastic wraps snugly from toe to groin. Include the heel with wrapping. Rewrap the legs every 4 to 8 hours. If compression stockings are prescribed, they must be fitted correctly and removed for a short time every day.

RELIEVE DISCOMFORT

Elevation of the extremity and application of warm packs usually relieve discomfort. Some clients need a mild sedative or analgesic.

MONITOR ANTICOAGULANT THERAPY

Most physicians use an algorithm to adjust the dose of heparin based on the client's partial thromboplastin time (PTT) levels. Blood is sampled every 4 to 8 hours for PTT or INR, and the dose is adjusted accordingly. Use of warfarin therapy requires that PT or INR be monitored on a regular basis. LMW heparin therapy requires no testing. When invasive studies are necessary (e.g., arterial blood gas analyses), apply pressure for 30 minutes to the puncture site.

Bleeding can occur in any client receiving anticoagulation therapy. Observe the client observed for the following:

- Bleeding, evidenced by pink-tinged or frank blood in the urine, tarry or frank blood in the stool, and bleeding after brushing the teeth
- Subcutaneous bruising
- Flank pain

MONITOR THE CLIENT FOR DEVELOPMENT OF PULMONARY EMBOLISM

Pulmonary embolism is an acute and potentially lethal complication of DVT. Chest pain is the most common clinical manifestation of pulmonary embolism, but it is not diagnostic of the condition. The pain most often associated with pulmonary embolism is pleuritic. Pleuritic pain is caused by an inflammatory reaction of the lung parenchyma or by pulmonary infarction or ischemia caused by obstruction of small pulmonary arterial branches. Pleuritic chest pain is typically sudden in onset and is worsened by breathing.

Hemoptysis occurs in about 30% of clients. The presence of hemoptysis indicates that pulmonary infarction or atelectasis has produced alveolar hemorrhage. Other clinical manifestations may include cough, diaphoresis, dyspnea, and apprehension. Because of the seriousness of pulmonary embolism, promptly notify the physician of these clinical manifestations. Document the lack of manifestations of pulmonary embolism in the medical record to provide evidence of monitoring for the condition. Pulmonary embolism is discussed in Chapter 61.

Surgical Management

Surgical treatment of thrombophlebitis is directed against pulmonary embolism by filtering blood flow from the lower extremities and pelvis through a filter inserted into the inferior vena cava. In the past the direct removal of venous thrombi was recommended; now this procedure is rarely performed because of the high incidence of recurrent postoperative thrombosis. Excision of the pulmonary emboli from the lung can also be performed, but this procedure is also rare.

VENA CAVA FILTERS (UMBRELLA)

A filter is inserted in the vena cava to trap large emboli. Devices include those that look like umbrellas and those that are a complex web of threads (bird's nest) to stop the emboli. The surgeon can insert these devices, using local anesthesia, by threading the device through the femoral or jugular vein. Indications for surgery include the presence of a large thrombus or the presence of "showers" of emboli. A rare complication of this technique is the migration of the filter into the iliac vein, renal vein, right atrium, right ventricle, or pulmonary artery. Another complication includes complete obstruction of the filter. This results in back pain and swelling of the lower extremities.

Self-Care

Prevention is key in DVT. Therefore, teach clients about the risk factors of DVT and how to avoid them. Continue to explain medications being taken, actions, doses, timing, adverse effects, and the importance of monitoring coagulation status. Begin teaching on the first day of heparinization, and discuss the need for anticoagulants. Clients need to know who to contact and how to reach a health care provider in the event that problems develop. Inform the client about the monitoring required while they are receiving anticoagulants. Some clients may be apprehensive about being up and about while they have DVT, when past practice has been recommend bed rest. Reassure clients about the change in practice.

CHRONIC VENOUS DISORDERS

■ VARICOSE VEINS

Varicose veins are permanently distended and develop because of the loss of valvular competence. Faulty valves elevate venous pressure, causing distention and tortuosity of the superficial veins. The greater and lesser saphenous veins and perforator veins in the ankle are common sites of varicosities.

Primary varicose veins often result from a congenital or familial predisposition that leads to loss of elasticity of the vein wall. *Secondary* varicosities occur when trauma, obstruction, DVT, or inflammation causes damage to valves.

Varicose veins affect many adults 24 million Americans. Prevalence increases with age and peaks in people between their 40s and 50s. Varicose veins are more common in women; however, the sex ratio decreases with advancing age and almost disappears in clients older than 70 years. Prolonged standing has been implicated as a cause, but epidemiologic studies have not demonstrated an association between standing at work and an increased incidence of varicose veins.

Clients often complain of aching, a feeling of heaviness, itching, moderate swelling, and, frequently, the unsightly appearance of their legs. Severity of discomfort is difficult to assess and does not seem related to the size of varicosities. A superficial inflammation may occasionally develop along the path of the varicose vein. To assess for varicose veins, carefully examine both of the client's legs in good lighting. Varicosities appear as dilated, tortuous skin veins (Fig. 53–12).

Outcome Management

Medical Management

In the early stages of varicosity, the goals are to reduce venous pooling, prevent complications, and improve comfort levels. The simplest form of treatment is the applica-

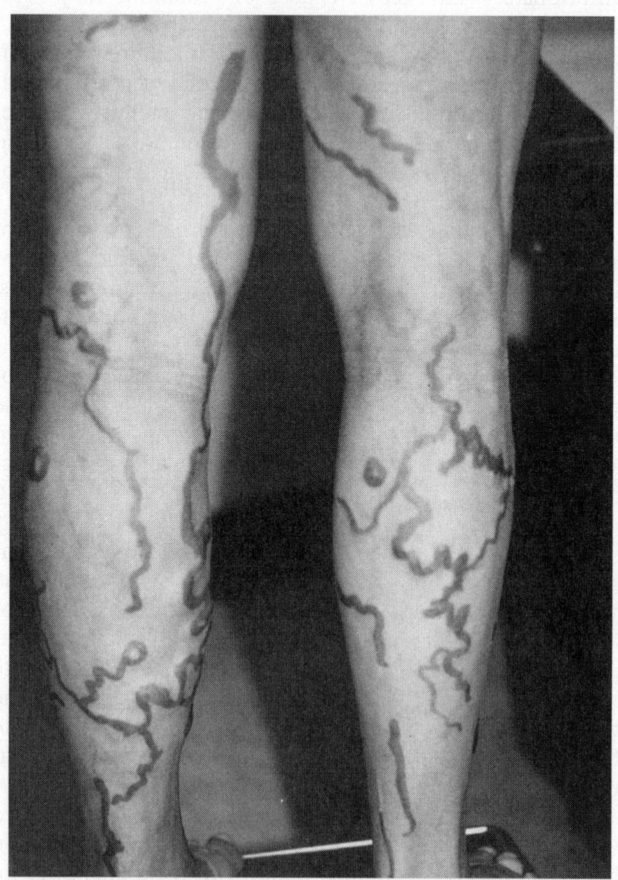

FIGURE 53–12 Varicose veins marked with a pen on the legs. Note the tortuous pattern.

tion of below-knee compression stockings or elastic wraps. These stockings are designed to exert the greatest amount of pressure over the ankle. Teach the client to avoid standing still in one position for extended periods.

Surgical Management

SCLEROTHERAPY

Sclerotherapy is the injection of an agent into the varicose vein that damages the vein and endothelium, causing an aseptic thrombosis that closes the vein. Application of pressure causes the vein walls to grow together. Sclerotherapy is usually performed for cosmetic reasons but may also relieve the discomfort of both short segments of varicosities and spider veins. It is most effective in closing small, residual varicosities after surgical intervention for varicose veins. (Sclerotherapy is contraindicated before such surgery, because it makes vein stripping more difficult.) Within minutes after injection, elastic compression and active walking should commence. Elastic support is worn for 1 to 3 weeks, morning to night.

VEIN LIGATION AND STRIPPING

Surgical management of varicose veins consists of ligation (tying off) of the greater saphenous vein with its tributaries at the saphenofemoral junction, combined with removal of the saphenous vein (stripping) and ligation of incompetent perforator veins. Removal of the vein is performed through multiple, short incisions. An incision is made at the ankle over the saphenous vein, and a nylon wire is threaded up the vein to the groin. The wire is brought out through the groin and capped, and the wire and vein are then pulled out through the ankle incision. If the perforator veins alone are ligated, ligation may be done through multiple, small endoscopic incisions.

Elastic compression bandages are applied from foot to groin. The client is rarely hospitalized overnight. Complications are infrequent and include bleeding, infection, and nerve damage. Hemorrhage most commonly occurs at the surgical wound site in the groin. Bleeding comes primarily from the stripped canal. The risk of serious bleeding can be decreased by carefully wrapping the leg from foot to groin and by applying compression, especially to the upper thigh and groin. Some discoloration with bruising along the stripped tract is normal. Saphenous nerve damage may occur. In the distal third of the leg, the saphenous nerve runs close to the saphenous vein. Thus, the risk of nerve injury increases when the distal part of the vein is involved. DVT, embolism, and infection are rare following varicose vein surgery, especially if postoperative precautions (e.g., bandaging, movement, exercise) are taken.

Some clients only require tying off of the junction of the saphenous and the femoral vein at the groin. This involves one short incision, often local anesthesia, and no hospital stay. Postoperative care is the same.

Nursing Management of the Surgical Client

Provide routine postoperative assessment and care. Specific care includes maintaining firm elastic pressure over the whole limb, reducing the risk of thrombophlebitis by promoting regular movement and exercise of the legs, and improving venous return by elevating the foot of the bed 6 to 9 inches so that the legs are above the heart level when the client is in bed. The client ambulates for short periods, starting immediately after surgery. Clients should walk rather than stand or sit. After ambulation, elevate the client's legs again.

CHRONIC VENOUS INSUFFICIENCY

Chronic venous insufficiency, a group of disorders resulting from faulty venous valves, is also known as *postphlebitic syndrome.* It follows most severe cases of DVT but may take as long as 5 to 10 years to develop; however, about 20% of clients with chronic venous insufficiency have no history of DVT.

Within 5 years of a known DVT, almost 50% of clients develop chronic induration and stasis dermatitis, and 20% suffer from venous stasis ulcer. Therefore, clients with a history of DVT must be monitored periodically for life. Alert these clients to observe for the slightest skin changes. Once the skin is broken and a venous ulcer develops, the client faces a frustrating chronic problem. Venous stasis ulcers do not heal well.

Chronic venous insufficiency results from dysfunctional valves that reduce venous return, which thus increases venous pressure and causes venous stasis. Skin ulcerations also occur. Because existing valves are destroyed, venous blood flow is bidirectional, resulting in inefficient venous outflow. The net effect of this change is that the weight of the venous blood column from the right atrium is transmitted along the full length of the veins. Very high venous pressure is exerted at the ankle, and the venules become the final pathway for the highest venous pressure. It is hypothesized that the abnormal capillaries lead to extravasation of RBCs, activation of endothelial cells, and WBC trapping. The end result is capillary thrombosis.

Chronic venous insufficiency is marked by chronically swollen limbs; thick, coarse, brownish skin around the ankles (the "gaiter" area); venous stasis ulceration; and itchy, scaly skin (Fig. 53–13).

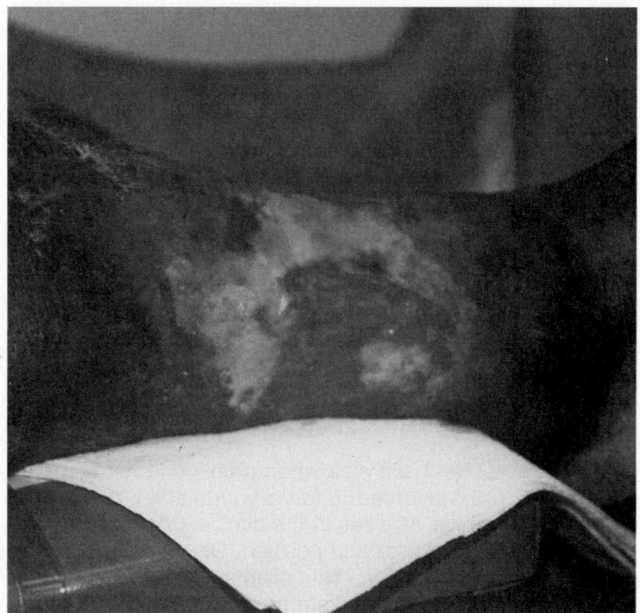

FIGURE 53–13 Severe post-phlebitic syndrome with liposclerosis and scars from healed ulcers.

Management

Goals of management are to increase venous blood return and to decrease venous pressure. Antigravity measures increase blood return to the heart and include elevating the client's legs above the heart level and avoiding prolonged standing or sitting. Advise the client to avoid:

- Crossing the legs
- Sitting in chairs that are too high to allow the feet to touch the floor or that are too deep (and press on the popliteal area)
- Wearing garters or tightly rolled socks or stockings
- Garments that exert pressure above the legs (e.g., tight girdles)

Encourage the client to sleep with the foot of the bed elevated 6 inches. At least one third of every 24 hours should be spent with the feet and legs elevated above the heart.

The Bridge to Home Health Care feature describes how increased venous pressure on the tissues of the leg can be counteracted by the compression of elastic support hose. Ideally, this support should just balance the increased venous pressure. Thus, hose should be fitted individually to the client's legs. Measurements of the ankle and calf circumference and from 1 inch below the knee or 1 inch below the groin to the bottom of the foot are usually taken. Measure after the client has been recumbent and leg edema is minimal. Stockings that extend above the knee often bind the popliteal space and act as a tourniquet, especially when the knee is bent. Knee-length elastic stockings are preferable. Elastic wraps are often preferable for clients who have periods of leg swelling. Apply the elastic wrap using a graded technique, placing more tension on the lower leg. The problem with elastic wraps is that most of them only maintain their elastic properties for a few washings, and clients tend to use them long past their effective compression. Additionally, wraps often are not used properly and do not exert adequate compression. See the Alternative Therapy chart earlier for information about nontraditional therapies.

After thrombosis of a deep calf vein, clients should wear elastic support for at least 3 to 6 months and probably for life. Elastic support compresses the superficial veins when the client walks, and blood flow in the larger veins is increased while venous pressure is kept to a minimum. Standing and sitting are not allowed for long periods during the acute phase because they increase the hydrostatic pressure in the capillaries, which pro-

BRIDGE TO HOME HEALTH CARE

Managing Peripheral Vascular Disease

Many clients who are referred to home health agencies or clinics that serve older people have peripheral vascular disease. Consider what you can do to help clients prevent further complications through assessment and evaluation, blood pressure monitoring, health education, and reporting changes in your clients' status to their physicians.

Assessment

Inspect clients for temperature variations; color changes in the skin; dorsal and ankle foot pulses; extremity size comparisons; shiny, taunt, hairless, or blistered skin; diminished toenail growth and color change; pain with palpation, dependent position, or weight-bearing; and skin breakdown and ulcerations. As part of the assessment, measure the calves, ankles, and feet correctly, as the involved areas of edema indicate. Use a monofilament (thin plastic filament) test for sensation and dorsiflexion and plantiflexion of the great toe (proprioception), especially for diabetic clients. The loss of touch sensation may require special foot protection. The loss of proprioception of the foot (position perception) indicates the need to discourage or stop driving. For many clients, this news is very traumatic. You may want to discuss this safety recommendation with a family member or significant other. Be prepared to problem-solve transportation alternatives.

Use the correct cuff size when monitoring the blood pressure. You may need to travel with a child, adult, and large cuff or have all sizes in the clinics. For consistency, document the cuff size and position. Discuss the benefits of self-monitoring devices with clients. Because clients may have decreased hand strength or arthritis, they may have difficulty pumping the bulb of a partially automatic cuff. Fully automatic, one-button devices are reasonably accurate and may be better options. When your clients have checkups, suggest that they take their blood pressure equipment along and compare their readings with those obtained at the clinic. Instruct them to record and share their list of self-recorded measurements with you and their physician, a strategy that is helpful for blood pressure management.

Education

Health education is an essential component of the care you provide. It is important for clients to avoid smoking, wearing constrictive clothing, and applying excessive heat to their extremities. Clients need information about elevating their legs and performing daily foot hygiene. They may be able to reduce lower extremity edema by wearing properly fitted antiembolic hose or compression socks (Siguaris or TEDS); home health clients need physicians' orders. Before ready-made compression socks are bought, measure the heel to knee or heel to thigh and the largest calf circumference; the cost ranges from $8 to $15. Before purchasing custom-ordered antiembolic socks, clients need a prescription and are measured by a supply company; these socks cost up to several hundred dollars. Clients need to exercise caution when using compression socks. Most ready-made ones lose significant compression after 6 to 12 months and need to be replaced. When possible, use the "open toe" design to prevent excess pressure on the toes, especially with diabetic clients. The nylon content in these socks causes moisture retention and leads to skin maceration in clients who have poor circulation. The socks should not be worn around the clock.

Deborah S. Bjerstedt, RNCS, MSN, FNP, *Family Nurse Practitioner, Allina Medical Clinic-Shoreview, St. Paul, Minnesota*

motes edema. Encourage walking and exercises in bed to decrease venous pressure and to promote blood flow.

■ VENOUS STASIS ULCERATION

Venous stasis ulceration is the end stage of chronic venous insufficiency. Prolonged venous pressure prevents nutrient blood flow, depriving cells of needed oxygen, glucose, and other substances. Skin of the lower legs ulcerates (*stasis ulcer*) because it occurs as a result of stasis of blood and is characteristically located in the malleolar area (Fig. 53–14).

Outcome Management

Management of venous stasis ulceration includes leg elevation, wound care, moist dressings, and support stockings. Gravity is the major enemy of venous stasis disease. Clients should rest with their legs elevated 6 inches. Regular walking is encouraged.

When ulcers are present, specimens are often obtained for culture for clients with painful, odorous, or weeping wounds to rule out infection. Antibiotics may be required to treat infection or cellulitis. Local wound care is essential by a health care provider familiar with the disease process. For some ulcers, debridement of eschar is necessary; for others, protection is needed. Techniques of wound care are addressed in Chapter 17.

Hydrocolloid dressings are used to protect new epithelium. Protect granulation tissue with wet-to-moist saline dressings, petroleum jelly (Vaseline) gauze, or moist occlusive dressings. Almost all ointments, creams, powders, and local antibiotics are harmful to healing tissue. They contribute to skin sensitivity problems, which complicate healing. To clean the ulcer, use sterile normal saline. The surrounding skin is probably dry and scaly. Gently clean the area and apply a lanolin-containing lotion (e.g., Eucerin, Alpha-Keri) every day. Avoid lotions containing alcohol and perfumes because they dry and irritate the skin. Solutions such as povidone-iodine (Betadine) are often used to control infection, but any solution other than normal saline retards healing.

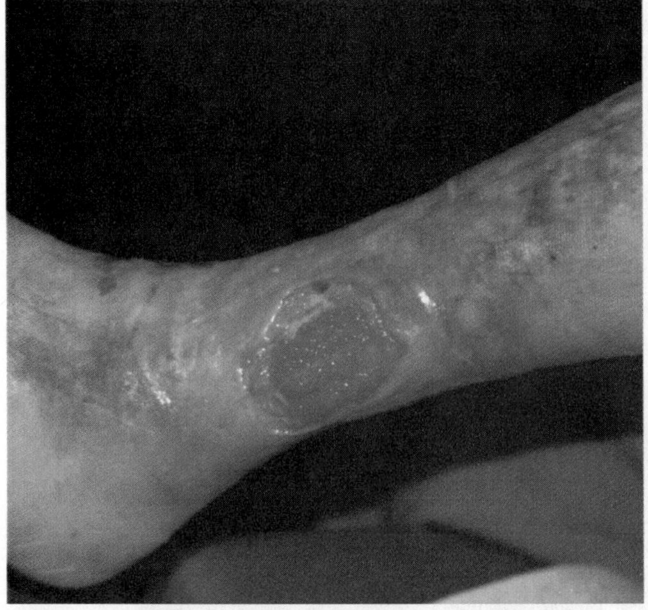

FIGURE 53–14 Venous stasis ulcers usually develop in the lower outer leg, appear irregular, and have a beefy-red base.

No topical treatment is adequate without compression. Stockings are the easiest to apply, but soiling may be a problem. In addition, stockings do not fit abnormally shaped legs or those clients with dressings over the ulcer. Elastic wraps may provide one alternative because they can be adjusted for size. Elastic wraps must be wrapped with the most tension at the foot and ankle and rewrapped twice daily.

An *Unna boot* is a popular form of bandage impregnated with calamine, zinc oxide, and glycerin. When wrapped snugly around the leg, it provides excellent compression during ambulation and applies minimal pressure during limb elevation. An Unna boot is a permeable dressing that can be applied directly over skin ulcers, thereby allowing drainage of exudate. It creates a moist and warm interface between the ulcerated skin and the bandage. It can be changed on a weekly or biweekly basis, which clients wear without interruption, and thereby improves compliance. The Unna boot has been shown to achieve healing rates of 70%.

Disadvantages include allergy, skin irritation, discomfort, difficulty in bathing, and pain while one is changing the boot.

Skin grafting is rarely necessary to achieve healing. Surgery to remove incompetent varicose veins or incompetent perforator veins may also be necessary.

LYMPHATIC DISORDERS

LYMPHEDEMA

Lymphedema is swelling caused by impaired transcapillary fluid transport and transportation of lymph. Failure of lymph transport allows the plasma proteins in the interstitial fluid to accumulate. The increase in interstitial colloid osmotic pressure encourages fluid accumulation. The osmotic pressure is reduced by drawing water into interstitial areas. In addition, as the lymph channels dilate, valves become incompetent. The fluid seeks new pathways through the tissues, which causes inflammation, lymphatic thrombosis, and, eventually, fibrosis. Lymphedemas are best classified into primary and secondary forms.

Primary lymphedema may be classified according to age at onset: congenital (present at birth), praecox (before age 35), or tarda (after age 35). Congenital and familial lymphedema is also called Milroy's disease. It is inherited as an autosomal dominant trait.

Secondary lymphedema occurs because of some damage or obstruction to the lymph system by another disease process or by a procedure: trauma, neoplasms (primary or metastatic), filariasis, inflammation, surgical excision, or high doses of radiation. Postoperative lymphedema is usually seen after surgical excision of axillary, inguinal, or iliac nodes. These operations are usually performed as a prophylactic or therapeutic treatment for metastatic tumor. For example, lymphedema of the arm is encountered after mastectomy (see Fig. 53–15*A*) Radiation in moderate amounts does not appear to damage the lymph vessels. However, heavy radiation for a particularly resistant tumor usually leads to lymphatic obstruction.

Of the primary forms, lymphedema praecox encompasses the largest group of clients; it peaks in the teenage years and is more common in females than in males. The edema usually appears spontaneously and without known cause (Fig. 53–15*B*).

Filariasis, caused by the filarial nematode *Wuchereria bancrofti* (and others), is one of the most common diseases in undeveloped nations; it is transmitted by mosquitoes from human to human. The living embryos (microfilariae) of the adult worms are found in the bloodstream. The larvae migrate to the lymphatics, where they mature into adult worms. Adult worms in the lymph nodes and lymphatics lead to obstruction, lymphedema, and elephantiasis.

Lymphedema secondary to neoplasms in the lymph nodes is common. The malignant disease may be primary (lymphoma or Hodgkin's disease) or metastatic from another site.

Clinical Manifestations

Primary lymphedema presents as bilateral mild edema of ankles and legs in women at puberty or shortly after puberty, unilateral edema of the entire leg in men and women (see Fig. 53–14), or bilateral edema present at birth or early age. The skin of clients with congenital lymphedema contains vesicles (blisters) filled with lymph. A dull, heavy sensation is present, but actual pain is absent. Elevation of the limb and rest in bed cause a reduction but not disappearance of the sensation. Smooth skin becomes roughened; the edema is nonpitting. Acute lymphangitis and cellulitis are infrequent. Ulceration of the skin does not occur. However, the limb becomes greatly enlarged, uncomfortable, and unsightly (Fig. 53–16). Lymphedema can be diagnosed with isotopic lymphography, lymphangiography, and phlebography.

Outcome Management

There is no known cure for lymphedema once the swelling appears. The goal of treatment is to remove as much fluid as possible from the affected extremity and to maintain a normal appearance.

Physical therapy for arm or leg lymphedema involves mechanical or manual squeezing of the tissue in order to press the stagnant lymphatic fluid to the proximal part of the limb. This is followed by specific active and passive exercises to transport the lymph farther into the lymphatic system and finally into the bloodstream. Many pneumatic pumping devices for intermittent compression are available. Diuretics may also be prescribed. Elastic stockings or sleeves are used to maintain the effects of the pneumatic pump.

To reduce the swelling, the extremity is elevated above the right atrium. Pneumatic pumps may be used to reduce the extremity size. If pumps are used, teach the client how to apply the device, the frequency of application, and the reasons for its use. When stockings are used, ascertain that the stockings fit and do not gather behind the knee. Activity such as walking, rather than sitting or standing, should be promoted. For bedridden clients, teach bed exercises to promote venous and lymphatic return and to maintain muscle strength.

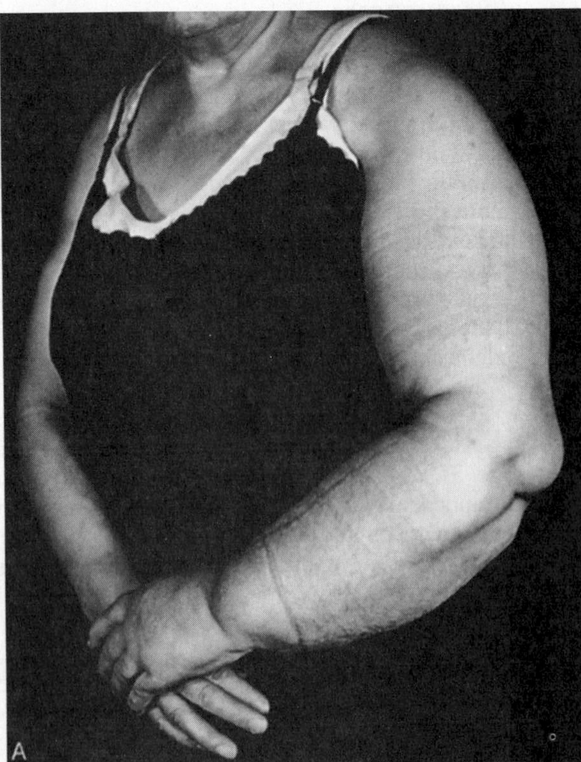

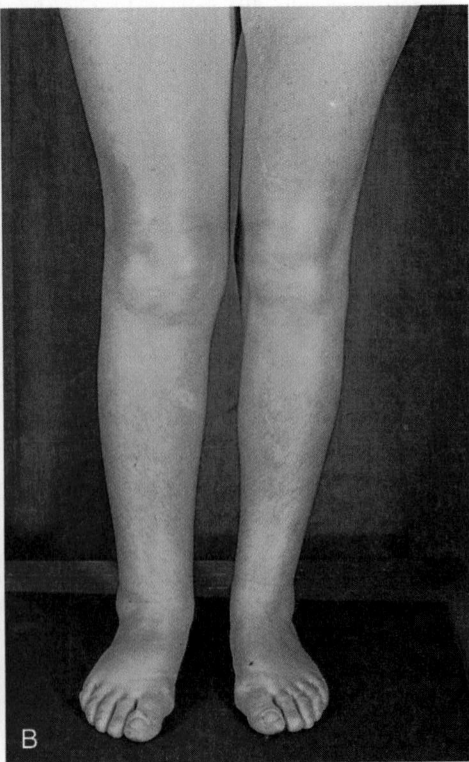

FIGURE 53–15 Types of lymphedema. *A,* Secondary lymphedema of the arm following mastectomy. *B,* Primary lymphedema.

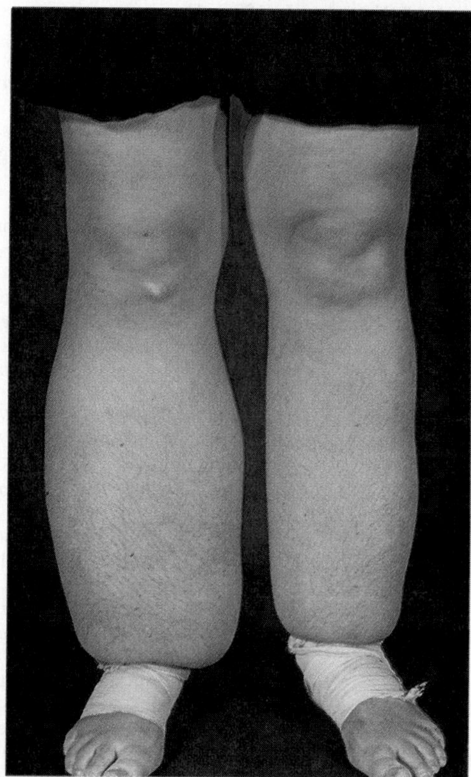

FIGURE 53–16 Severe lymphedema. The client's feet were bandaged so that shoes could be worn.

The client with lymphedema is at high risk for infection. The affected extremity is monitored for clinical manifestations of infection such as redness, warmth, and pain. Meticulous skin care is given to the extremity using mild soaps and lotions. Nails are kept trimmed.

Clients with lymphedema may suffer from disturbances in self-concept because of the visibility of their deformity. Encourage the client to discuss these feelings and help the client understand that such feelings are normal. Variations in clothing style may be suggested to disguise the deformity. When caring for clients with lymph disorders, remember that these clients must cope with difficult, chronic diseases. Take time to give emotional support to the client and the family. Emphasize the possible need for lifelong follow-up.

When lymphedematous limbs are massively swollen to the point that compression devices or stockings are no longer beneficial, surgery may be required. The most common surgical procedure for lymphedema is excision, in which all skin, subcutaneous tissue, and deep fascia in the leg are removed. The leg is covered with skin grafts. Scarring is evident, and the cosmetic appearance may not be acceptable to all clients. Another form of surgery, removal of the bulk of edematous tissues, is not curative, but the final appearance may be more acceptable.

CONCLUSIONS

Clients with vascular diseases can challenge a broad range of the nurse's capability and skill, from monitoring a client with rupture of an abdominal aortic aneurysm in an intensive care unit, to performing and teaching meticulous foot care, to educating and counseling a client to make significant lifestyle changes. Vascular diseases involve a broad spectrum of arterial, venous, and lymphatic problems.

Nursing care for clients with arterial disorders centers on promoting circulation and adequate tissue perfusion, protecting against skin breakdown and injury, managing pain, and encouraging positive lifestyle changes. Limb amputation requires particularly sensitive assessment, teaching, and counseling skills.

Nursing care for clients with venous disorders focuses on monitoring therapeutic regimens such as thrombolytic therapy, controlling and preventing thrombus formation, and promoting circulation by increasing venous blood return and decreasing venous pressure. Nursing care for lymphedema is palliative. The unique nursing care needs of clients with vascular disorders along with the exploding knowledge base that nurses need to command led to the growth of vascular nursing as a recognized area of specialty practice. The Society for Vascular Nursing was founded in 1982 and is an international organization with the *Journal of Vascular Nursing* as its scientific voice.

THINKING CRITICALLY

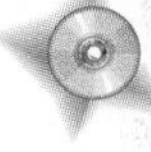

1. A male client is admitted to the hospital for the care of leg ulcers. He is homeless and usually wanders the streets, sleeping on external heating grates in the sidewalk. He has large, irregularly shaped ulcers covered with thick, yellow, devitalized tissue. The ulcers are weeping, and his stockings have adhered to the ulcers. What type of ulcers are present? What type of wound care does he need? How can he continue to do wound care after discharge?

Factors to Consider. How would you distinguish arterial from venous ulcers? Is it important to remove the devitalized tissue? If so, how? How does the client's lifestyle influence his recovery?

2. A middle-aged man enters the emergency department with complaints of a painful leg. The pain began about 3 hours earlier after he noted a very rapid heartbeat. You note that his leg and foot are cold and white. What may have happened? What other factors need to be addressed in relation to to his leg? What are the possible treatments available? What might his post-hospital instructions include?

Factors to Consider. How do you determine the acuteness of the tissue insult? What are the potential outcomes if you delay treatment? What might be the source of emboli, and how can this be assessed?

BIBLIOGRAPHY

1. Adams, S. (1999). Evaluation and conservative management of chronic lower extremity arterial disease. *Clinical Excellence for Nurse Practitioners, 3*(2), 88–96.
2. Anderson, L. (1999). Ischemic venous thrombosis: Its hidden agenda. *Journal of Vascular Nursing, 17*(1), 1–5.

3. Aster, R. (1995). Heparin induced thrombocytopenia and thrombosis. *New England Journal of Medicine, 332,* 1330–1335.
4. Blebea, J., et al. (1999). Deep venous thrombosis after percutaneous insertion of vena caval filters. *Journal of Vascular Surgery, 30*(5), 821–829.
5. Bradbury, A., et al. (1994). Recurrent varicose veins: Assessment of the sapheno-femoral junction. *British Journal of Surgery, 1,* 373–375.
6. Braun, C., Colucci, A., & Patterson, R. (1999). Components of an optimal exercise program for the treatment of clients with claudication. *Journal of Vascular Nursing, 17*(2), 32–36.
7. Clagget, G., & Krupski, W. (1995). Antithrombotic therapy in peripheral arterial occlusive disease. *Chest, 108*(4), 431S–443S.
8. Defraigne, J., Vazquez, C., & Limet, R. (1999). Systematic review of randomized controlled trials of aspirin and oral anticoagulants in the prevention of graft occlusion and ischemic events after infrainguinal bypass. *Journal of Vascular Surgery, 30*(4), 701–709.
9. Ekers, M., & Hirsch, A. (1999). Vascular medicine and vascular rehabilitation. In V. Fahey (Ed.), *Vascular nursing* (3rd ed., pp. 188–211). Philadelphia: W. B. Saunders.
10. Executive Committee, Nicolaides, A. (chair), American Venous Forum. (1996). Classification and grading of chronic venous disease in the lower limbs: A consensus statement. In P. Gloviczki & J. S. T. Yao (Eds.), *Handbook of venous disorders* (pp. 652–660). London: Springer-Verlag.
11. Fahey, V. (1995). Heparin induced thrombocytopenia. *Journal of Vascular Nursing, 13,* 112–116.
12. Gardner, A., & Poehlman, E. (1995). Exercise rehabilitation programs for the treatment of claudication pain: A meta-analysis. *Journal of the American Medical Association, 274*(12), 975–980.

12a. Gardner, A. W. (1996). The effect of cigarette smoking on exercise capacity in clients with intermittent claudication. *Vascular Medicine, 1*(3), 181–186.

13. Gross, K. (1999). Ultrasonographic diagnosis and guided compression repair of fenoral artery pseudoaneurysm: An update for the vascular nurse. *Journal of Vascular Nursing, 17*(3), 59–64.
14. Haraldur, B., et al. Iliofemoral deep venous thrombosis: Safety and efficacy outcome during 5 years of catheter directed thrombolytic therapy. *Journal of Vascular and Interventional Radiology, 8,* 405–418.
15. Hirsch, A., et al. (1997). The role of tobacco cessation, anti-platelet and lipid lowering therapies in the treatment of peripheral arterial disease. *Vascular Medicine, 2,* 243–251.
16. Johnson, M. (1997). Treatment and prevention of varicose veins. *Journal of Vascular Nursing, 15*(3), 97–103.
17. Katzenschlager, R., et al. (1995). Incidence of pseudoaneurysm after diagnostic and therapeutic angiography. *Radiology, 195,* 463–466.
18. Kowallak, D., & DePalma, R. (1999). A new approach to an old and vexing problem: Subfascial endoscopic perforator surgery. *Journal of Vascular Nursing, 17*(3), 65–70.
19. Kramer, S. (1999). Effect of providone-iodine on wound healing: A review. *Journal of Vascular Nursing, 17*(1), 17–23.
20. Kurgan, A., & Nunnelee, J. (1995). Upper extremity venous thrombosis. *Journal of Vascular Nursing, 13*(1), 21–23.
21. Lawrence, P., et al. (1999). The epidemiology of surgically repaired aneurysms in the United States. *Journal of Vascular Surgery, 30*(4), 632–640.
22. Lennox, A., et al. (1999). Combination of a clinical risk assessment score and rapid whole blood D-dimer testing in the diagnosis of deep vein thrombosis in symptomatic clients. *Journal of Vascular Surgery, 30*(5), 794–804.
23. Lensing, A., et al. (1995). Treatment of deep venous thrombosis with low molecular weight heparins—a meta-analysis. *Archives of Internal Medicine, 155,* 601–607.
24. Liem, T., & Silver, D. (1997). Options for anticoagulation. In A. Whittimore, D. Bandyk, & J. Cronnenwett (Eds.), *Advances in vascular surgery* (pp. 201–221.) St. Louis: Mosby–Year Book.
25. Lombardo, K. (1997). Endovascular grafting of abdominal aortic aneurysms. *Journal of Vascular Nursing, 15*(3), 83–87.
26. Moore, W., & Rutherford, R. (1996). Transfemoral endovascular repair of abdominal aortic aneurysm: Results of the North American EVT phase 1 trial. *Journal of Vascular Surgery, 23,* 543–553.
27. Nunnelee, J. (1997). Low molecular weight heparin. *Journal of Vascular Nursing, 15,* 94–96.
28. Nunnelee, J. (1999). Medications used in vascular clients. In V. Fahey (Ed.), *Vascular nursing (3rd ed.,* pp. 159–174). Philadelphia: W. B. Saunders.
29. Nunnelee, J., & Kurgan, A. (1993). Interruption of the inferior vena cava for venous thromboembolic disease. *Journal of Vascular Nursing, 11*(3), 80–82.
30. Racelis, M. (1995). Vascular medicine: An alternative approach to arterial disease. *Journal of Vascular Nursing, 13*(3), 69–74.
31. Regensteiner, J., Steiner, J., & Hiatt, W. (1996). Exercise training improves functional status in clients with peripheral arterial disease. *Journal of Vascular Surgery, 23,* 104–115.
32. Sasso, C., et al. (1999). Vascular procedures. In L. Morgan & J. Nunnelee (Eds.), *Core curriculum for radiologic nursing* (pp. 319–368). Oak Brook, IL: American Radiological Nurses Association.
33. Schaefer, A. (1996). Low molecular weight heparin: An opportunity for home treatment of venous thrombosis. *New England Journal of Medicine, 334,* 724–725.
34. Sutton, K., et al. (1999). Contrast media. In L. Morgan & J. Nunnelee (Eds.), *Core curriculum for radiologic nursing* (pp. 5–56). Oak Brook, IL: American Radiological Nurses Association.
35. Twardowski, P., & Green, D. (1999). Thrombotic disorders in vascular clients. In V. Fahey (Ed.), *Vascular nursing (3rd ed.,* pp. 175–187). Philadelphia W. B. Saunders.
36. Weitz, J., et al. (1996). Diagnosis and treatment of chronic arterial insufficiency of the lower extremities: A critical review. *Circulation, 94*(11), 3026–3049.
37. Zheng, Z., et al. (1997). Associations of ankle-brachial index with clinical coronary heart disease, stroke and preclinical carotid and popliteal atherosclerosis: The Atherosclerosis Risk in Communities (ARIC) Study. *Atherosclerosis, 131*(1) 115–125.

UNIT 12

Cardiac Disorders

Anatomy and Physiology Review: *The Heart*

Robert G. Carroll

The human heart, through rhythmic contraction, provides the pressure necessary to propel blood through the body. Blood flow is essential to deliver nutrients to the tissues of the body and to transport metabolic wastes, including heat, to removal sites. Presence of an arterial pulse, caused by the beating of the heart, is appropriately designated as a vital sign.

The heart weighs about 300 g and is located within the mediastinum; it is cone-shaped and tilted forward and to the left. Because of its orientation during fetal development, the apex of the heart (tip of the cone) is at its bottom and lies left of the midline. The base is at the top, where the great vessels enter the heart, and lies posterior to the sternum. The heart consists of four chambers: two smaller atria at the top (the base) of the heart, and two larger ventricles at the apex. A band of fibrous tissue separates the atria from the ventricles and seats the four cardiac valves. A muscular septum separates the right from left atrium, and the right from left ventricle. Table U12–1 describes the basic structures and their functions.

Functionally, the heart is actually two pumps working simultaneously (Fig. U12–1). The right atrium and right ventricle generate the pressure to propel the oxygen-poor blood through the pulmonic circulation; the left atrium and left ventricle propel oxygen-rich blood to the remainder of the body through the systemic circulation. At rest, each side of the heart pumps approximately 5000 ml (5 liters) of blood per minute *(cardiac output)*. This is accomplished by a contraction frequency *(heart rate)* of 72 beats per minute (BPM), with each contraction ejecting a volume of 70 ml *(stroke volume)* into the arterial system. Cardiac output can increase five-fold during exercise as a result of increases in both heart rate and stroke volume.

TABLE U12–1 THE HEART: ITS STRUCTURE AND FUNCTIONS

Structure	Function
Pericardium	Two-layered sac that encases and protects the heart
Atrium	Upper, receiving chambers of the heart
Right atrium	Receives deoxygenated systemic blood via superior and inferior vena cava; blood passes to right ventricle
Left atrium	Receives oxygenated blood from the lungs. Blood passes to the left ventricle.
Ventricles	Lower, pumping chambers of the heart
Right ventricle	Receives blood from atrium via the tricuspid valve; pumps it to the pulmonary circulation
Left ventricle	Receives blood from atrium via the bicuspid (mitral) valve; pumps it to the systemic circulation
Cardiac valves	Prevent backflow of blood
Tricuspid and bicuspid (mitral) valves	Prevent backflow from right ventricle to right atrium and from left ventricle to left atrium, respectively
Semilunar valves	Prevent backflow from pulmonary artery to right ventricle *(pulmonic semilunar)* and from aorta to left ventricle *(aortic semilunar)*
Coronary arteries (common pattern)	Provide blood supply to the heart
Right coronary artery	Perfuses right atrium, right ventricle, inferior portion of the left ventricle and posterior septal wall, SA node, and AV node
Left coronary artery:	
Left anterior descending artery	Supplies blood to anterior wall of left ventricle, anterior ventricular septum, and apex of left ventricle
Circumflex artery	Provides blood to left atrium, lateral and posterior surfaces of left ventricle, occasionally the posterior interventricular septum; also, sometimes supplies SA and AV nodes
SA node	"Pacemaker" node, initiates heartbeat by generating an electrical impulse
AV node	Normal pathway for impulses originating in the atria to be conducted to ventricles; can be a secondary pacemaker
Bundle of His, bundle branches, Purkinje's fibers	Rapidly transmit cardiac action potentials to enable synchronous contraction of ventricles

AV, atrioventricular; SA, sinoatrial.

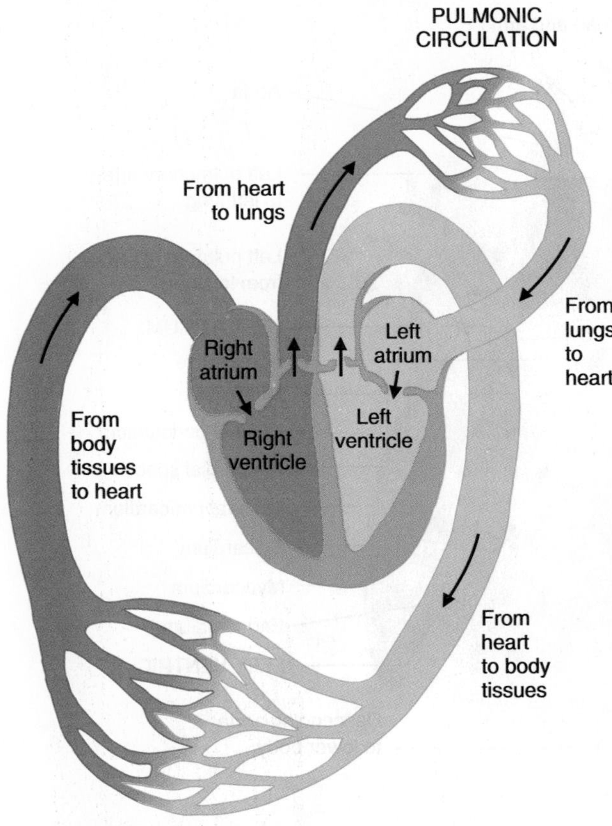

FIGURE U12–1 Functions of the heart. In the peripheral capillaries, blood oxygen is exchanged for carbon dioxide. The deoxygenated blood returns to the right atrium and right ventricle to be pumped into the lungs, where carbon dioxide is exchanged for oxygen. Oxygenated blood from the lungs enters the left atrium and left ventricle of the heart to be pumped once again into the systemic circulation.

STRUCTURE OF THE HEART

LAYERS OF THE HEART

The heart consists of three distinct layers of tissue: endocardium, myocardium, and epicardium (Fig. U12–2, *inset*). The *endocardium* (innermost layer) consists of thin endothelial tissue lining the inner chambers and the heart valves. The *myocardium* (middle layer) consists of striated muscle fibers forming interlaced bundles and is the actual contracting muscle of the heart. The *epicardium* or *visceral pericardium* covers the outer surface of the heart. It closely adheres to the heart and to the first several centimeters of the pulmonary artery and aorta.

The visceral pericardium is encased by the *parietal pericardium,* a tough, loose-fitting, fibrous outer membrane that is attached anteriorly to the lower half of the sternum, posteriorly to the thoracic vertebrae, and inferiorly to the diaphragm. Between the visceral pericardium and the parietal pericardium is the *pericardial space,* which holds 5 to 20 ml of pericardial fluid. This fluid lubricates the pericardial surfaces as they slide over each other when the heart beats. Excessive fluid accumulation in the pericardial space can diminish the filling of the ventricles *(cardiac tamponade).*

CHAMBERS OF THE HEART

The heart consists of four chambers: two upper collecting chambers *(atria)* and two lower pumping chambers *(ventricles)* (see Fig. U12–2). Muscular walls *(septa)* separate the chambers of the right side from those of the left side. The *right atrium* receives deoxygenated blood from the body. The blood moves to the *right ventricle,* which pumps it to the lungs against low resistance. The *left atrium* receives oxygenated blood from the lungs. The blood flows into the *left ventricle* (the heart's largest, most muscular chamber), which pumps it against high resistance into the systemic circulation.

CARDIAC VALVES

The cardiac valves are delicate, flexible structures that consist of endothelium covered by fibrous tissue. They permit only unidirectional blood flow through the heart. The valves open and close passively, depending on pressure gradients in the cardiac chambers (Fig. U12–3). "Leaky" valves that do not seal when closed are called *regurgitant* or *insufficient.* "Stiff" valves that cannot open completely are called *stenotic.*

Cardiac valves are of two types: (1) atrioventricular (AV) and (2) semilunar (see Table U12–1). *Atrioventricular valves* lie between the atria and ventricles. The *tricuspid valve,* on the right side, is composed of three leaflets. The *mitral (bicuspid)* valve, on the left, is composed of two. Attached to the edges of the AV valves are strong, fibrous filaments called *chordae tendineae,* which arise from papillary muscles on the ventricular walls. The papillary muscles and chordae tendineae work together to prevent the AV valves from bulging back into the atria during ventricular contraction (systole).

The *semilunar valves* consist of three cup-like cusps that open during ventricular contraction and close to prevent backflow of blood into the ventricles during relaxation (diastole). Unlike the AV valves, the semilunar valves open during ventricular contraction The *pulmonic semilunar valve* (right ventricle to pulmonary artery) and the *aortic semilunar valve* (left ventricle to aorta) do not have papillary muscles.

CARDIAC BLOOD SUPPLY

The heart muscle requires a rich oxygen supply to meet its own metabolic needs. The *coronary arteries* (right and left) branch off the aorta just above the aortic valve, encircle the heart, and penetrate the myocardium (Fig. U12–4). Coronary vessel distribution can vary greatly, but the pattern described in Table U12–1 is the most common.

Contraction of the muscle of the left ventricle generates enough extravascular pressure to occlude the coronary blood vessels and prevent blood flow to the muscle of the heart during ventricular systole. Thus, 75% of the coronary artery blood flow occurs during diastole, when the heart is relaxed and resistance is low.[1] For adequate blood flow through the coronary arteries, the diastolic blood pressure must be at least 60 mm Hg. Coronary blood flow increases with increased heart work load (i.e.,

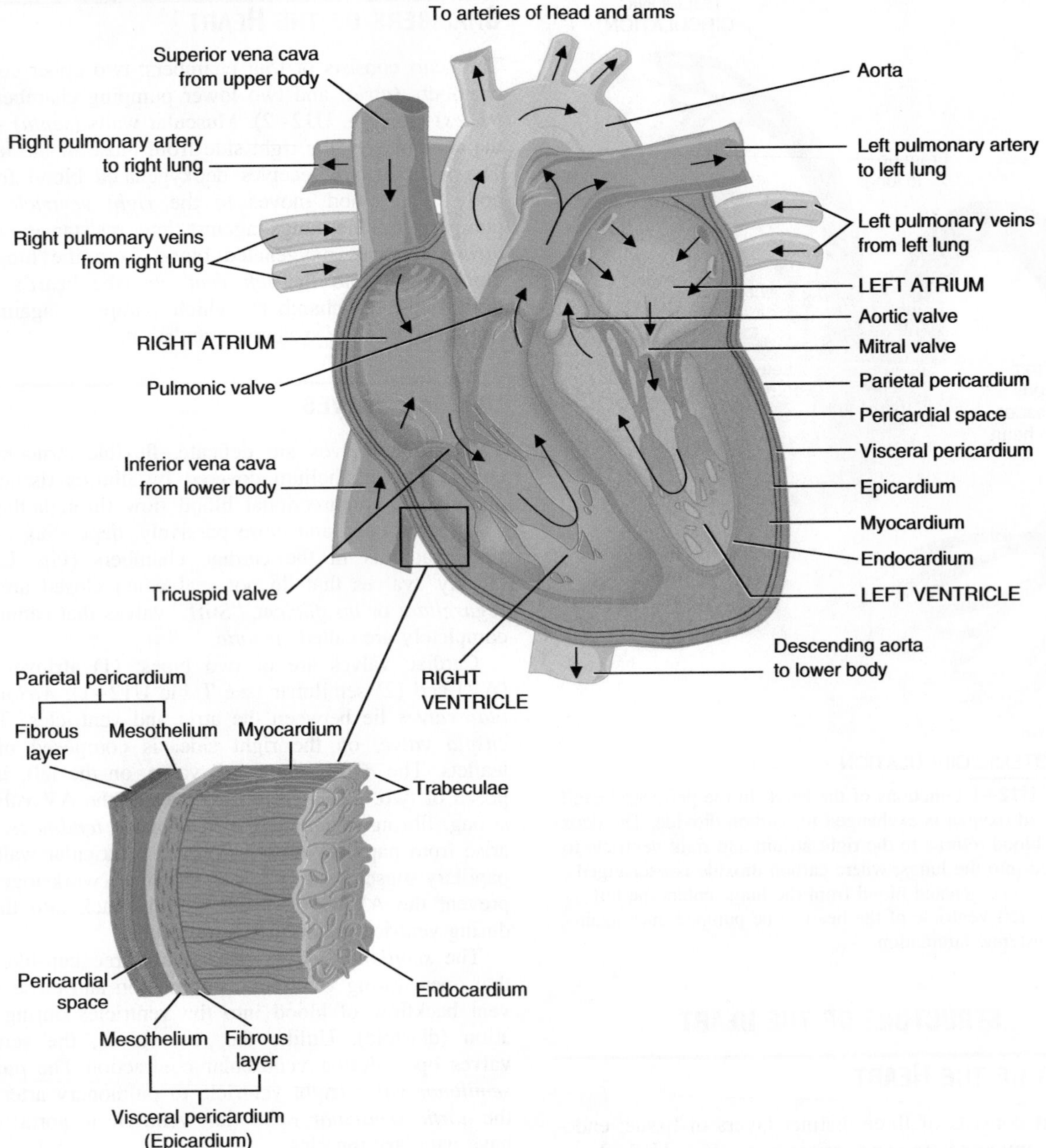

FIGURE U12–2 Structure of the heart and circulation of blood through the heart. Blood entering the left atrium from the right and left pulmonary veins flows into the left ventricle. The left ventricle pumps blood into the systemic circulation through the aorta. From the systemic circulation, blood returns to the right atrium through the superior and inferior venae cavae. From there, the right ventricle pumps blood into the lungs through the right and left pulmonary arteries. *Inset,* The pericardium and layers of the heart.

exercise). The coronary veins return blood from most of the myocardium to the coronary sinus of the right atrium. Some areas, particularly on the right side of the heart, drain directly into the cardiac chambers.

FUNCTIONS OF THE HEART

ELECTROPHYSIOLOGIC PROPERTIES

The electrophysiologic properties of cardiac muscle regulate the heart rate and rhythm. These properties include excitability, automaticity, contractility, refractoriness, and conductivity.

Excitability

The ability of cardiac muscle cells to depolarize in response to a stimulus—*excitability*—is influenced by hormones, electrolytes, nutrition, oxygen supply, medications, infection, and autonomic nerve activity.

In myocardial cells, as in other types of muscle and neurons, differences in intracellular and extracellular ion concentrations create electrical and concentration gradients for ionic movement across the semipermeable cell membrane. At rest, the inside of a myocardial cell is more negative than the outside. This *resting membrane potential* results primarily from the differences in concen-

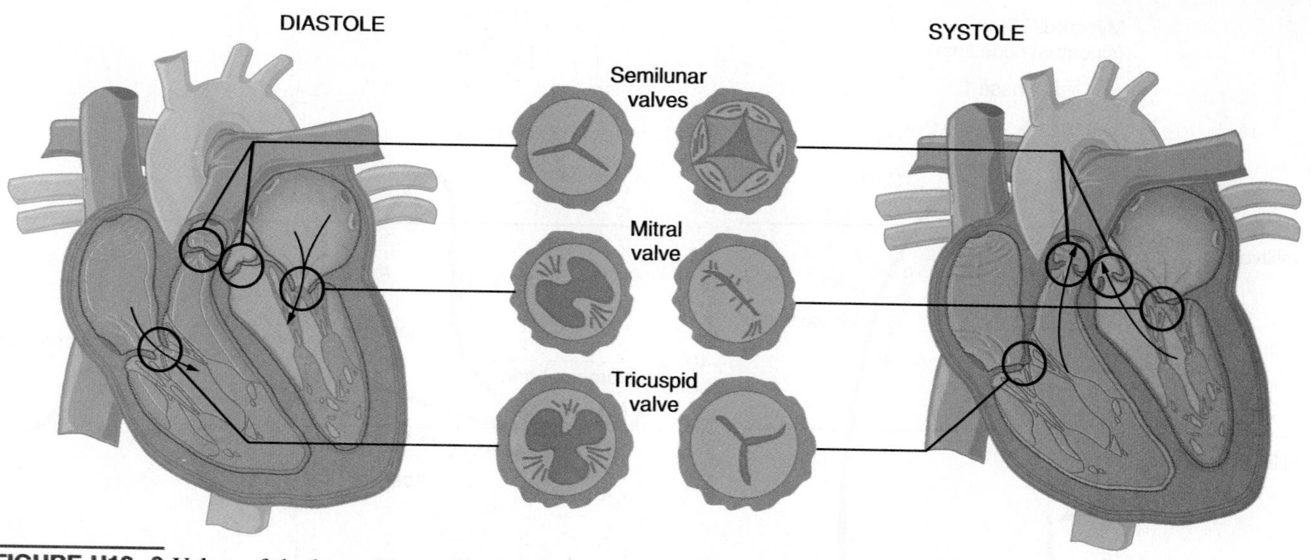

FIGURE U12–3 Valves of the heart. The semilunar, mitral, and tricuspid valves are shown as they appear during diastole, or ventricular filling *(left)* and during systole, or ventricular emptying *(right)*.

trations of potassium (K^+) and sodium (Na^+). Although both ions are present on either side of the cell membrane, potassium has a greater intracellular concentration and sodium has a greater extracellular concentration. Selective channels can increase membrane permeability for specific ions, allowing the ion to move down the electrochemical gradient and to alter the resting membrane potential.

When the cardiac cell is stimulated to a certain threshold, a sequence of ion permeability changes cause a dramatic change in the transmembrane potential, this is known as an *action potential* (Fig. U12–5*A*). The action potential consists of depolarization and repolarization phases. The electrocardiogram (ECG) reflects currents generated by the depolarization and repolarization of regions of the heart.

Depolarization is caused by an increase in cell membrane permeability to sodium. The cell returns to its resting (relaxed) state during *repolarization.* Sodium permeability drops sharply, and potassium permeability in-

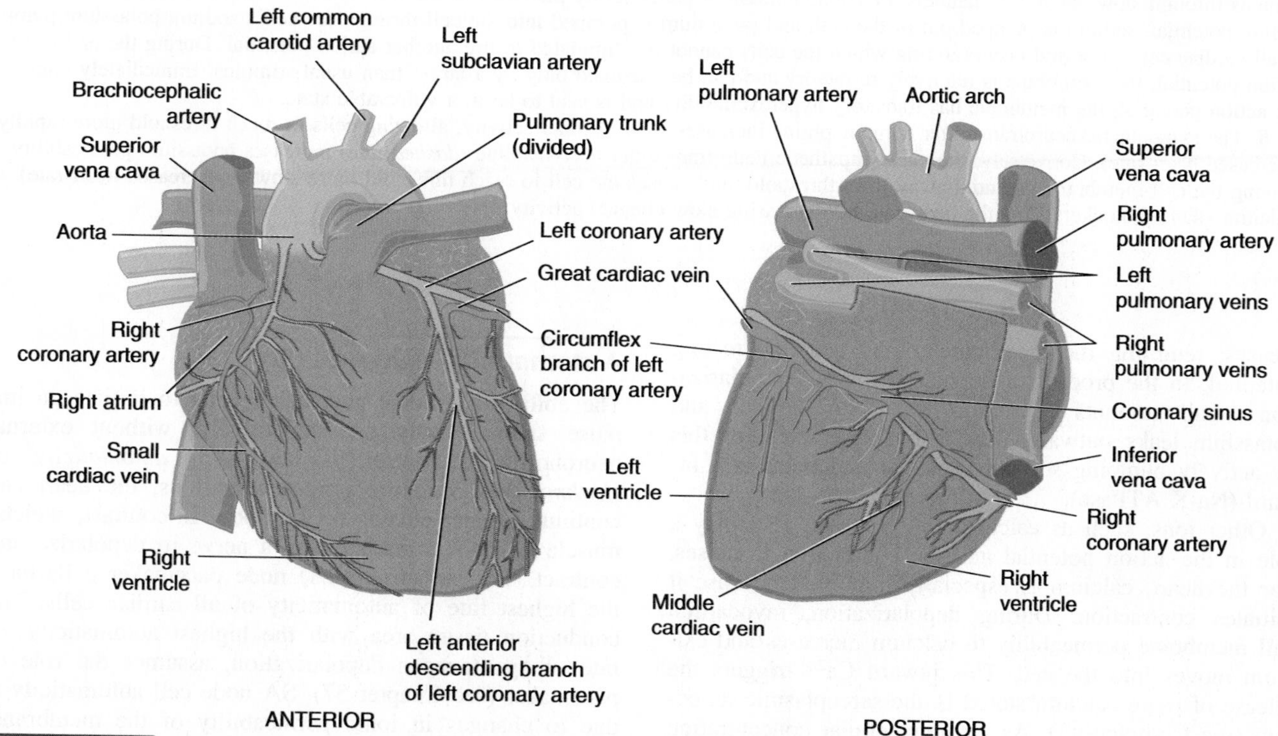

FIGURE U12–4 The coronary arteries. The right and left coronary arteries branch off the aorta just above the aortic valve; they normally supply the myocardium with oxygenated blood.

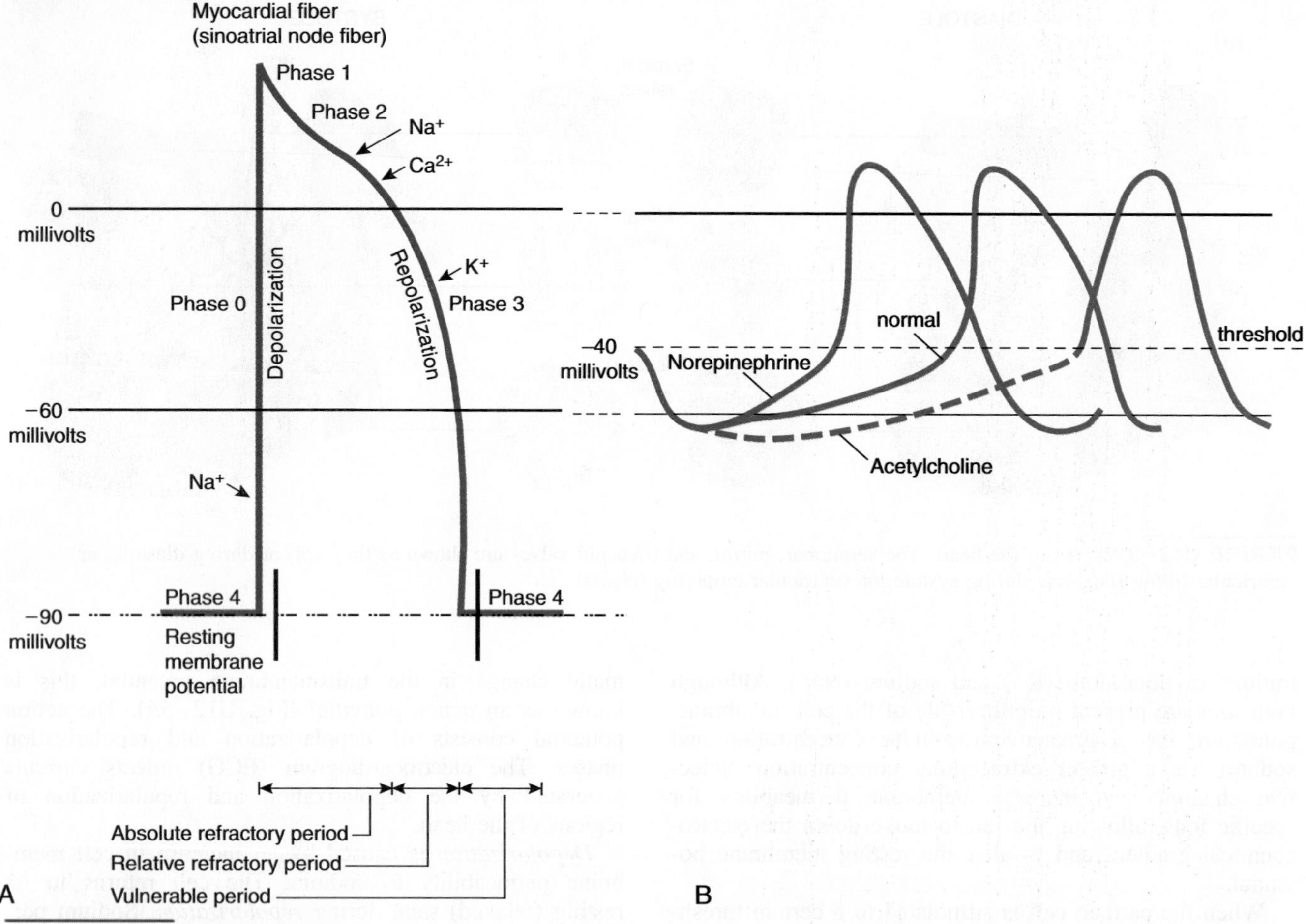

FIGURE U12–5 Action potential.

A, The action potential of cardiac cells has five phases: *Phase 0:* Sodium permeability increases through fast sodium channels, and cell depolarization (contraction) begins. *Phase 1:* The fast sodium channels close. *Phase 2:* Some sodium and calcium permeability remains through slow Na^+/Ca^{2+} channels. *Phase 3:* Potassium permeability increases in the cell. *Phase 4:* The cell returns to its resting potential, sodium is pumped out of the cell, and potassium is pumped into the cell through the cell's sodium-potassium pump. In all cardiac cells, a period occurs during which the cells cannot be stimulated to fire another action potential. During the end of the action potential, the membrane is relatively refractory and can be reexcited only by a larger than usual stimulus. Immediately after the action potential, the membrane has transitory hyperexcitability and is said to be in a vulnerable state.

B, The sympathetic neurotransmitter norepinephrine increases slow channel activity, allowing cells to reach threshold more rapidly (increased heart rate). Conversely, the parasympathetic neurotransmitter acetylcholine *(dashed line)* increases potassium permeability, moving the cell membrane potential away from threshold, and causes the cell to reach threshold more slowly (decreased heart rate). Calcium channel blockers slow the heart rate by decreasing slow channel activity.

creases, returning the membrane to the negative resting potential. In the process of depolarization and repolarization, small amounts of sodium leak into the cell and potassium leaks outward. The cell compensates for this by actively pumping sodium back out and potassium inward (Na-K ATPase).

Other ions, such as calcium and chloride, also play a role in the action potential and the contraction it causes. For the heart, calcium is especially important because it initiates contraction. During depolarization, myocardial cell membrane permeability to calcium increases and calcium moves into the cell. This inward Ca^{2+} triggers the release of more calcium stored in the sarcoplasmic reticulum (see Contractility). As the intracellular concentration of calcium increases, calcium reacts with contractile elements and myocardial muscle fibers contract.

Automaticity (Rhythmicity)

The ability of cardiac pacemaker cells to initiate an impulse spontaneously and repetitively, without external neurohormonal control, is known as *automaticity,* or *rhythmicity.* Given the proper conditions, the heart can continue to beat outside of the body. In contrast, skeletal muscle must be stimulated by a nerve to depolarize and contract. The sinoatrial (SA) node pacemaker cells have the highest rate of automaticity of all cardiac cells. The conduction tissue area with the highest automaticity, or rate of spontaneous depolarization, assumes the role of pacemaker (see Chapter 57). SA node cell automaticity is due to changes in ionic permeability of the membrane. Even at rest, a decreasing potassium permeability and increasing slow channel permeability (for Na^+ and Ca^{2+}

ions) move the cell membrane potential more positively towards threshold voltage. When threshold is reached, the cell initiates an action potential. Norepinephrine and acetylcholine cause heart rate to increase and decrease, respectively (Fig. U12–5*B*). The rate of spontaneous depolarization can also be affected by other hormones, body temperature, drugs, and disease.

Contractility

The heart muscle is composed of long, narrow cells or fibers. Cardiac muscle fibers, like striated skeletal muscle, contain myofibrils, Z bands, sarcomeres, sarcolemmas, sarcoplasm, and sarcoplasmic reticulum. Contraction results from the same sliding filament mechanism described for skeletal muscle (see Unit 5 review).

The action potential initiates the muscle contraction by releasing calcium through the T tubules of the cell membrane. The calcium reaches the sarcoplasmic reticulum, causing additional calcium release. The intracellular calcium diffuses to myofibrils, where it binds with troponin. When the actin filaments become activated by calcium, the heads of the cross-bridges from the myosin filaments immediately become attracted to the active sites of the actin. Contraction then occurs by power stroke repetition. After contraction, free calcium ions are actively pumped back into the sarcoplasmic reticulum, and muscle relaxation begins.

One important difference between cardiac and skeletal muscle is that cardiac muscle needs extracellular calcium. All of the calcium involved in skeletal muscle comes from the sarcoplasmic reticulum. In cardiac muscle, however, extracellular calcium enters through the T tubules and triggers release of more calcium from the sarcoplasmic reticulum. Because of this, calcium channel blockers can alter contraction of the heart, but not the contraction of skeletal muscle.

Refractoriness

Refractoriness is the heart's inability to respond to a new stimulus while still in a state of depolarization from an earlier stimulus. Refractoriness develops when the sodium channels of the cardiac cell membrane become inactivated and unexcitable during an action potential. Thus, the heart muscle does not respond to restimulation, preventing the possibility of tetanic contractions that are seen in skeletal muscle.

Refractoriness occurs in two periods (see Fig. U12–5*A*). The *absolute refractory period* occurs during depolarization and the first part of repolarization. During this period, cardiac cells do not respond to any stimuli, however strong. The *relative refractory period* occurs in the final stages of repolarization; refractoriness diminishes and a stronger-than-normal stimulus can excite the heart muscle to contract. At the end of the refractory period, there is a transient hyperexcitability *(vulnerable period).* The sodium channels are reset and the cardiac cells can again conduct action potentials.

Normally, the ventricles have an absolute refractory period of 0.25 to 0.3 seconds, which approximates the duration of the action potential. The relative refractory period for the ventricles lasts about 0.05 seconds. The atria have a refractory period of about 0.15 seconds, and they can therefore contract rhythmically much more quickly than the ventricles. The duration of the action potential and the refractory period are not fixed, however; both can shorten as heart rate increases.

Conductivity

Conductivity is the ability of heart muscle fibers to propagate electrical impulses along and across cell membranes. The heart muscle must conduct the action potential from its origin throughout the heart both rapidly and smoothly so that the atria and ventricles contract as a unit. Intercalated disks join adjacent myocardial cells, allowing the action potential to travel over the entire muscle mass (Fig. U12–6). However, the fibrous band of tissue that separates the atria and ventricles lacks intercalated disks. Thus, the atria are isolated electrically from the ventricles except for the only normal conduction pathway, the atrioventricular node. The conduction system consists of the following major parts:

- Sinoatrial (SA) node
- AV node
- Bundle of His and bundle branches
- Purkinje fibers

The *SA node,* or *pacemaker,* is located at the junction of the superior vena cava and right atrium. Under normal circumstances, the SA node initiates electrical impulses (heartbeats) approximately 60 to 100 times per minute but it can adjust its rate. Three internodal and one interatrial tract carry the wave of depolarization through the right atrium to the AV node and to the left atrium, respectively.[2] The sympathetic and parasympathetic nervous systems regulate the SA node. Any myocardial tissue that generates impulses at a higher rate than the SA node can become an abnormal pacemaker.

The (AV) node, or *AV junction,* is located in the lower aspect of the atrial septum. The AV node can be a secondary cardiac pacemaker, but it normally receives electrical impulses from the SA node and is the only pathway for conducting impulses from the atria to the ventricles. Within the AV node, the impulse is delayed 0.07 second while the atria contract. This delay enables atrial contraction to be completed before the ventricles contract.

The common *bundle of His* in the interventricular septum is relatively short, branching into right and left segments. The *right bundle branch* (RBB) courses down the right side of the interventricular septum. The *left bundle branch* (LBB) bifurcates into anterior and posterior fascicles, both of which extend into the left ventricle. The right and left bundle branches terminate in Purkinje fibers.

Purkinje fibers are a diffuse network of conducting strands beneath the ventricular endocardium; they rapidly spread the wave of depolarization through the ventricles. Activation of the ventricles begins in the septum and then moves from the apex of the heart upward. Within the ventricular walls, depolarization proceeds from endocardium to epicardium. Repolarization occurs in each cell and does not involve the conduction system. Repolarization occurs in reverse order, so that the last cells to depolarize are the first to repolarize. The action potentials of Purkinje fibers have the longest duration, and their

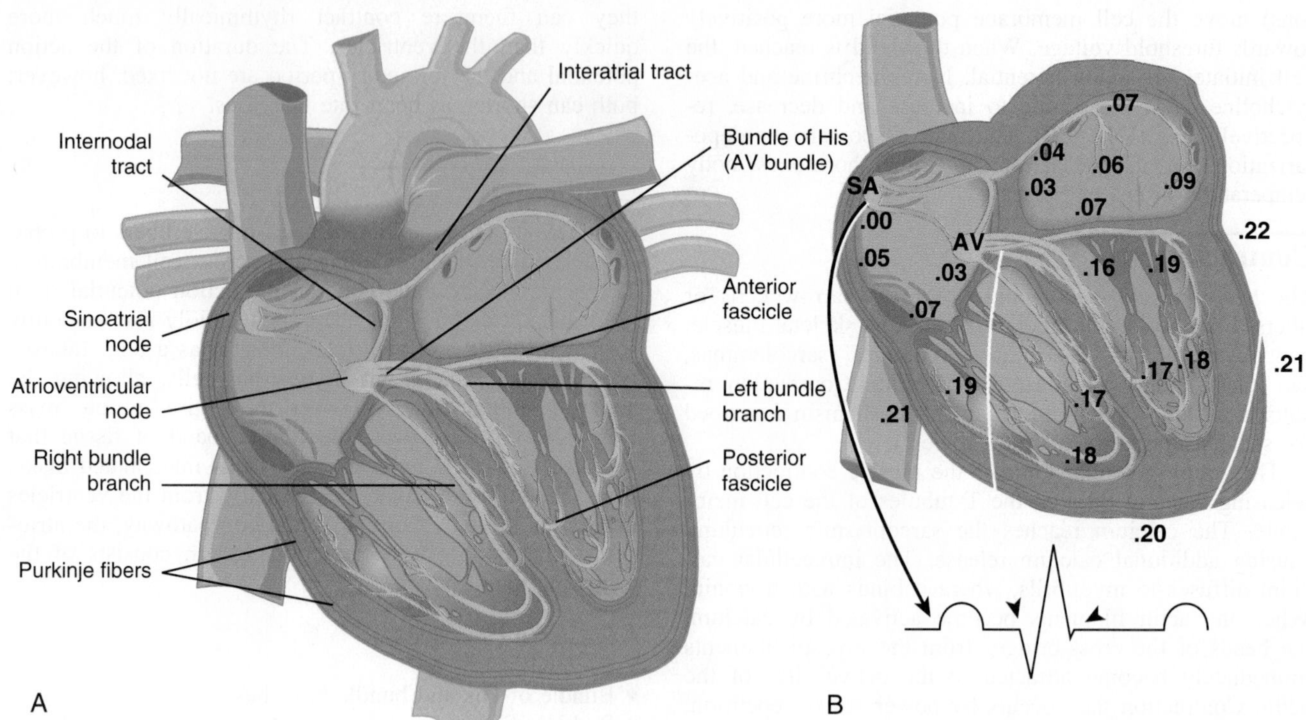

FIGURE U12–6 *A,* The cardiac conduction system. *B,* Transmission of the cardiac impulse through the heart, showing the time of appearance (in fractions of a second) of the impulse in different parts of the heart. (*B,* After Guyton, A. C., & Hall, J. E. [1996]. *Textbook of medical physiology* [9th ed.]. Philadelphia: W. B. Saunders).

repolarization is occasionally seen as a U wave of the ECG.

CARDIAC CYCLE

One cardiac cycle (Fig. U12–7) is equivalent to one complete heartbeat. The sequence of events in the cardiac cycle is divided into two parts: ventricular *systole* (contraction) and ventricular *diastole* (relaxation). The cardiac cycle normally begins with the spontaneous depolarization of the pacemaker cells of the SA node and ends following the filling of the relaxed ventricles.

Atrial Systole

Depolarization of the SA node spreads through the atria, both cell to cell and using the internodal and interatrial pathways. Depolarization of the atrial cells (P wave of the ECG) allows calcium entry, followed by contraction and pressure generation (a wave of the venous pressure tracing). Contraction of the atria propels a small amount of blood into the ventricles.

Ventricular Systole

Following a delay at the AV node, the wave of depolarization enters the ventricles, where it is rapidly spread by the bundle branches and Purkinje fibers (QRS complex of the ECG). Following depolarization, calcium enters, initiating contraction of the ventricle. In the *isovolumic contraction phase,* the ventricles begin to contract, closing the AV valves and building up pressure within the ventricles. As the AV valves close, the first heart sound (S_1) is heard. Because the aortic and pulmonic valves remain closed at this point, no blood leaves the ventricle. The *ejection phase* begins when pressure in the ventricles exceeds the aortic and pulmonic pressures. The semilunar valves open, and the ventricles pump blood into the systemic and pulmonary circulations.

Ventricular Diastole

In early diastole, as the ventricles begin to relax, aortic and pulmonic pressures exceed ventricular pressures, and the semilunar valves close. The valve closure causes the second heart sound (S_2). The AV valves remain closed, and no blood moves in or out of the ventricles. This is called *isovolumic relaxation.* As the ventricles continue to relax, pressure in the ventricles falls below that of the atria, the AV valves open, allowing blood which has been pooling in the atria to flow into the ventricles *(ventricular filling).* When the ventricles have filled passively, the cardiac cycle is ready to begin again.

Extra Heart Sounds

The ventricular wall must expand to accommodate rapid ventricular filling. If ventricular wall compliance is decreased (as in heart failure or valvular regurgitation), structures within the ventricular wall vibrate and a third heart sound (S_3) may be heard. An S_3 heart sound may be a normal finding in people younger than age 30 years. During the last phase of ventricular diastole, atrial contraction (atrial systole or atrial kick) occurs, contributing 5% to 30% more blood volume to the ventricles.

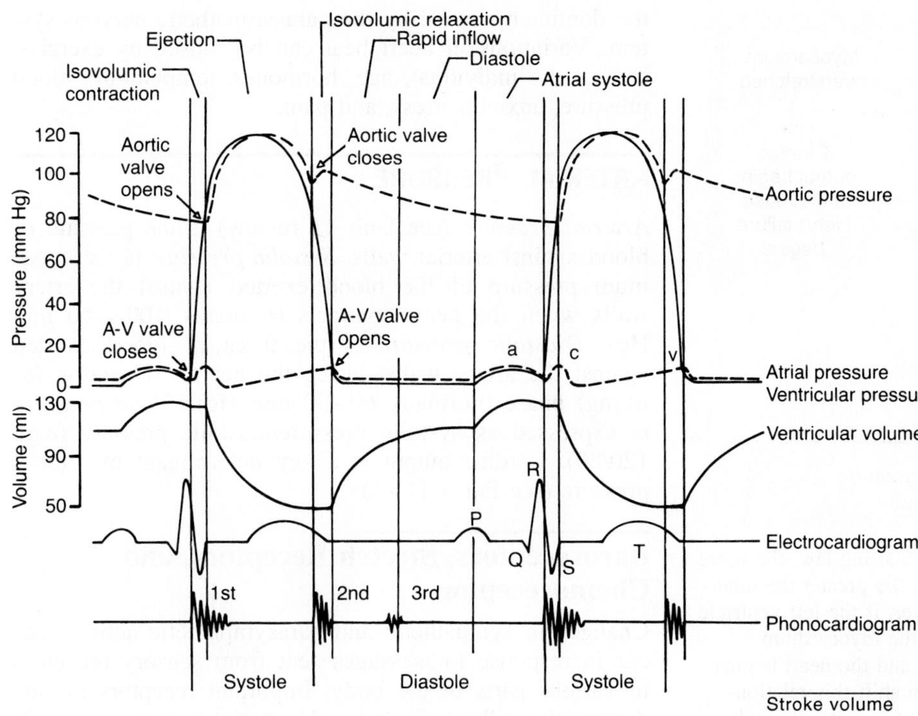

FIGURE U12–7 Changes that occur during the cardiac cycle in left atrial pressure, left ventricular pressure, aortic pressure, ventricular volume, the electrocardiogram, and the phonocardiogram. (From Guyton, A. C., & Hall, J. E. [1996]. *Textbook of medical physiology* [9th ed.]. Philadelphia: W. B. Saunders.)

A fourth heart sound (S_4) may be heard on atrial systole if resistance to active ventricular filling is present. This is not a normal finding. It may be a result of hypertrophy, disease, or injury of the ventricular wall.

CARDIAC OUTPUT AND CARDIAC INDEX

Cardiac output (CO) is the volume of blood ejected per minute by rhythmic ventricular contraction. At the end of ventricular diastole (and atrial kick), each ventricle contains approximately 140 ml of blood (end-diastolic volume [EDV]). Normally, during systole, the heart ejects approximately half of its EDV. The volume ejected with each contraction (heartbeat) of the ventricle is the stroke volume. Cardiac output can be calculated as

$$CO = [EDV - ESV] \times HR$$

where ESV is the end-systolic volume and HR is the heart rate.

Cardiac output averages between 4 and 8 L/min in adults. For a normal 150-pound (70-kg) adult at rest, cardiac output is 5 to 6 L/min. Adjustments in either stroke volume or heart rate can compensate for fluctuations in the other, or both can rise or fall.

Cardiac output is commonly measured by thermodilution with the use of a pulmonary artery (Swan-Ganz) catheter. Several other approaches can also be used, such as obtaining heart rate from an ECG and stroke volume through ventricular imaging techniques.

Clinicians compute the *cardiac index* (CI) from the cardiac output to compensate for individual differences in body size:

$$CI = \frac{\text{cardiac output}}{\text{body surface area}}$$

The normal cardiac index is 2.5 to 4.0 L/min/m².

Stroke volume has a major influence on cardiac output and is determined by (1) preload, (2) afterload, and (3) the contractile state of the heart.

Preload

Preload is the myocardial fiber length of the left ventricle at end diastole. It is determined by the EDV. The Frank-Starling law of the heart states that the greater the resting myocardial fiber length, or stretch, the greater its force of contraction. Preload therefore increases when increased EDV (e.g., from increased venous return) subjects myocardial fibers to greater stretch. The ventricles respond with a greater force of contraction, producing a larger stroke volume and increased cardiac output. This phenomenon, however, has limits (Fig. U12–8), such as the greatly distended ventricles characteristic of heart failure.[3]

Afterload

Afterload is the resistance to left ventricular ejection. More specifically, it is the amount of pressure required by the left ventricle to open the aortic valve during systole and to eject blood. Afterload directly relates to arterial blood pressure and the characteristics of the valves.[6] If arterial blood pressure is high, the heart must work harder to pump blood into the circulation. Stroke volume is inversely related to afterload. For example, if afterload increases because of peripheral vasoconstriction (which increases arterial blood pressure), myocardial fiber shortening is reduced and ejections are less effective. Then the ventricles cannot eject a normal stroke volume.

Contractile State

The contractile *(inotropic)* state refers to the vigor of contraction generated by the myocardium regardless of its

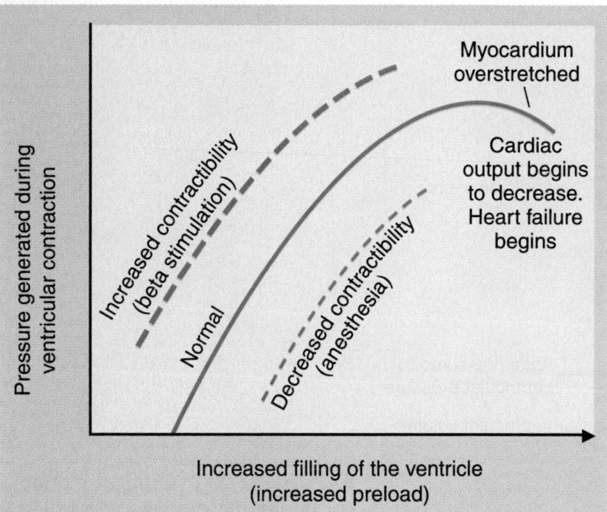

FIGURE U12–8 According to the Frank-Starling law, the more the left ventricle fills with blood (preload), the greater the quantity of blood ejected into the aorta. However, if the left ventricle fills to such an extent that it overdistends the myocardium *(arrow),* cardiac output begins to decrease and the heart begins to fail. Agents that change contractility can shift this relationship. Norepinephrine increases contractility (+ inotrope) and improves cardiac performance; anesthesia decreases contractility (− inotrope) and impairs cardiac performance.

blood volume (preload). Unlike skeletal muscle, the myocardium can alter contractile velocity and, therefore, force. The rate of cross-bridge cycling in the myocardium is calcium-dependent, and agents that increase intracellular calcium thus increase contractile force. For example, sympathetic stimulation increases myocardial contractility and ventricular pressure, thereby ejecting blood more rapidly and increasing stroke volume. Metabolic abnormalities (e.g., hypoxemia) and metabolic acidosis decrease myocardial contractility, therefore reducing stroke volume (see Fig. U12–8).

Cardiac Pressures

With the use of a pulmonary artery pressure (Swan-Ganz) catheter, pressures in the right atrium, right ventricle, and pulmonary artery can be measured. Inflation of a balloon at the catheter tip allows measurement of pulmonary capillary wedge pressure (PCWP), an estimate of left atrial pressure. Assuming normal aortic valve function, arterial systolic pressure reflects left ventricular systolic pressure. These pressures are useful in determining factors that characterize cardiac performance, such as preload, afterload, volume, filling pressures, and resistance. Normal cardiac pressures are shown in Figure U12–9.

HEART RATE

The normal heart rate is 60 to 100 BPM. *Sinus tachycardia* is a rate of more than 100 BPM; *sinus bradycardia* is a rate of fewer than 60 BPM. (The *sinus* in these terms indicates that the impulse arose in the sinoatrial node, the normal pacemaker region of the heart.) The intrinsic heart rate is 90 BPM. At rest, the heart rate of 70 BPM reflects the dominant control by the parasympathetic nervous system. Variations in heart beat can be caused by exercise, size of the individual, age, hormones, temperature, blood pressure, anxiety, stress, and pain.

ARTERIAL PRESSURE

Arterial pressure (see Unit 11 review) is the pressure of blood against arterial walls. *Systolic pressure* is the maximum pressure of the blood exerted against the artery walls when the heart contracts (normally 100–140 mm Hg). *Diastolic pressure* is the force of blood exerted against the artery walls during the heart's relaxation (or filling) phase (normally 60–90 mm Hg). *Blood pressure* is expressed as systolic pressure/diastolic pressure (e.g., 120/80). Cardiac output is a key determinant of arterial pressure (see Fig. U11–5).

Baroreceptors, Stretch Receptors, and Chemoreceptors

Changes in sympathetic and parasympathetic activity occur in response to messages sent from sensory receptors in various parts of the body. Important receptors in cardiovascular reflexes include: (1) arterial baroreceptors, (2) stretch-sensitive cardiopulmonary receptors of the atria and veins, and (3) chemoreceptors.

Baroreceptors (pressoreceptors) are stretch-sensitive nerve endings affected by changes in arterial blood pressure. They are located in the walls of the aortic arch and carotid sinuses. Increases in arterial pressure stimulate baroreceptors (Fig. U12–10), which send impulses to the medulla oblongata, resulting in heart rate and arterial pressure decreases (the vagal response). When arterial pressure decreases, baroreceptors receive less stretch and thus send fewer impulses to the medulla oblongata. Then sympathetic-mediated increase in heart rate and vasoconstriction occurs.

Cardiopulmonary stretch receptors are located in terminal sections of the vena cava and the atria. These receptors respond to length changes, which reflect circulatory volume status. When blood pressure decreases in the vena cava and the right atrium (e.g., hypovolemia), stretch receptors send fewer impulses than usual to the central nervous system (CNS). This process results in a sympathetic response, particularly to the kidney, to enhance salt and water retention. These changes also stimulate release of antidiuretic hormone (ADH) from the posterior pituitary. Hypervolemia produces the opposite effects.

Chemoreceptors, found in the aortic arch and carotid bodies, are primarily sensitive to increased carbon dioxide and decreased arterial pH (acidemia) and secondarily sensitive to hypoxemia. When these changes occur, chemoreceptors transmit impulses to the CNS to increase heart rate.

THE AUTONOMIC NERVOUS SYSTEM AND THE HEART

The autonomic nervous system (ANS) is the effector limb of the baroreceptor reflex, and plays an important role in regulating:

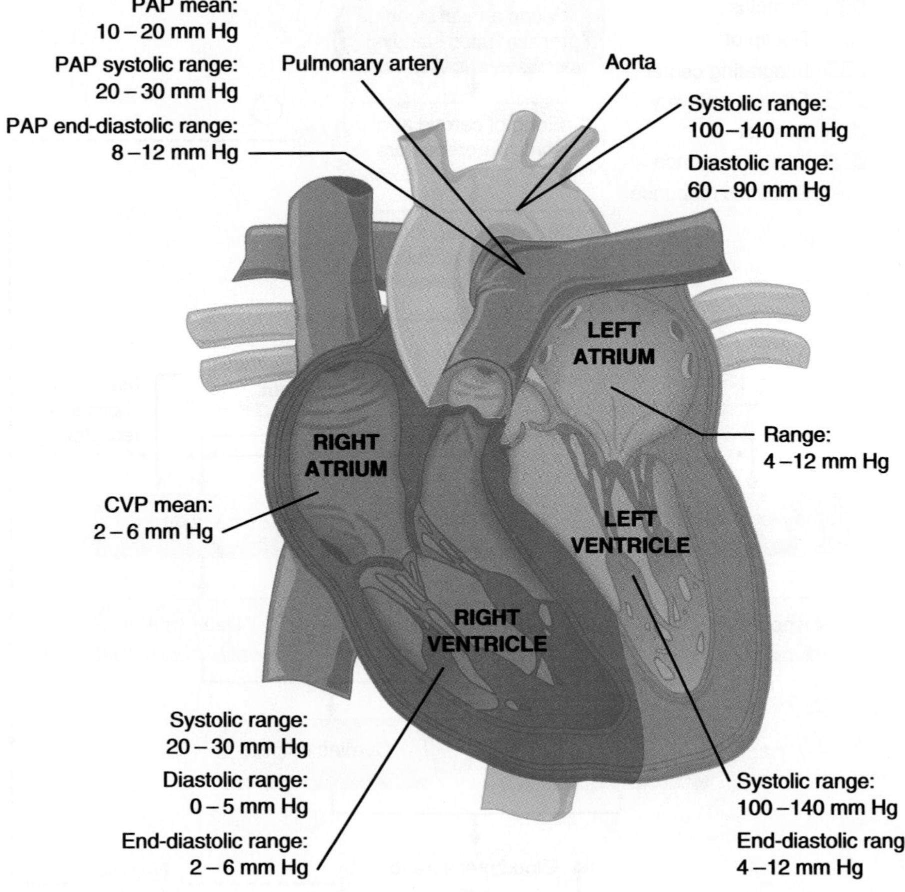

FIGURE U12–9 Normal pressures in the cardiac chambers and associated major blood vessels. CVP, central venous pressure; PAP, pulmonary artery pressure.

- Heart rate (chronotropic effect)
- Myocardial contractility (inotropic effect)
- Conduction velocity at the AV node
- Peripheral vascular resistance (arteriole constriction and dilation)
- Venous return (venule and vein constriction and dilation)

The two subdivisions of the autonomic nervous system (sympathetic and parasympathetic) generally exert opposing influences and balance their activities to promote cardiovascular adaptation to internal and external demands. Autonomic nervous system responses are involuntary.

Parasympathetic nerves arise from the dorsal motor nucleus of the vagus nerve, located in the medulla oblongata. They innervate the SA node atria, AV node, and to a lesser extent the ventricles and Purkinje system. When stimulated, parasympathetic nerve endings release the neurotransmitter acetylcholine, which produces inhibitory effects by binding to muscarinic receptors. Parasympathetic stimulation decreases the rate of SA node firing, thus lowering heart rate; atrial conductivity lessens as well.

Sympathetic nerve fibers originate between the first and fifth thoracic vertebrae and terminate in all areas of the heart. With stimulation, the nerve endings release the neurotransmitter norepinephrine and produce the following effects: (1) increased heart rate, (2) increased conduction speed through the AV node, (3) increased atrial and ventricular contractility, and (4) peripheral vasoconstriction, by bending to adrenergic receptors, activation of G proteins, and opening of ionic channels.

The sympathetic nervous system influences adrenal activity. The adrenal medulla responds to stimulation by secreting catecholamines (norepinephrine and epinephrine) into the circulation. Norepinephrine and epinephrine interact with adrenergic receptors found within cell membranes of the heart and blood vessels. The response to stimulation depends on the type and location of adrenergic receptors involved. The five types of receptors follow:

1. *Alpha$_1$-adrenergic receptors* are located in peripheral arteries and veins. When stimulated, alpha receptors produce a dramatic vasoconstrictive response.
2. *Alpha$_2$-adrenergic receptors* are located in several tissues. Their actions include contraction of some vascular smooth muscle, inhibition of lipolysis, inhibition of neurotransmission, and promotion of platelet aggregation.
3. *Beta$_1$-adrenergic receptors* are predominantly located in the heart. When stimulated, beta$_1$ receptors cause an increase in heart rate, AV node conduction, and myocardial contractility. This may result in increased cardiac output and blood pressure.
4. *Beta$_2$-adrenergic receptors* are found in the arterial and bronchial walls. Stimulation of beta$_2$ receptors causes smooth muscles to dilate, producing vasodilation of arterial vessels and bronchodilation.

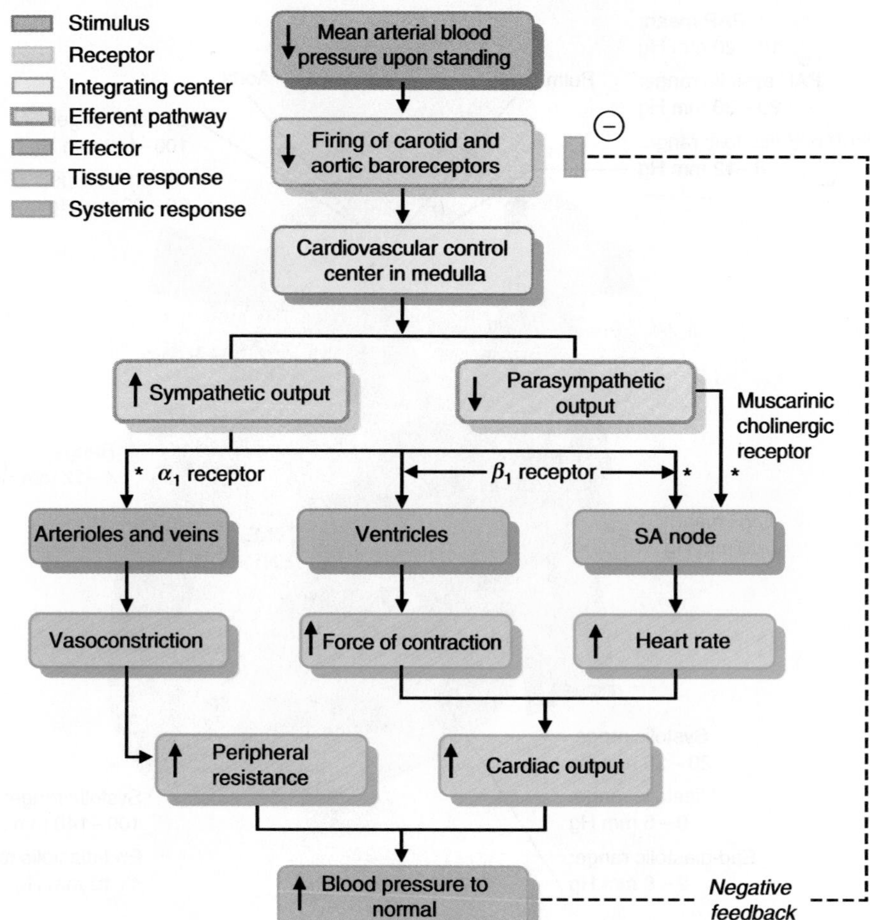

FIGURE U12–10 Baroreceptor control of cardiac function. Baroreceptors sense changes in blood pressure and stimulate either a sympathetic nervous system response to constrict peripheral blood vessels or the parasympathetic system to relax blood vessels. These actions maintain blood pressure at a steady state. SA, sinoatrial. (Modified from Silverthorn D. *Human physiology,* 1988. Upper Saddle River, NJ: Prentice Hall.)

5. *Beta$_3$-adrenergic receptors* are found in adipose tissue, where they promote lipolysis. Indirectly, this may assist cardiac performance because the myocardium can utilize fatty acids as metabolic fuels. Currently, no direct cardiac role for beta$_3$ adrenoreceptors has been identified.

Hormonal and Other Influences

In addition to epinephrine and norepinephrine from the adrenal medulla, several other hormones regulate cardiac output indirectly by controlling body fluid volume (and thus venous pressure and venous return). The most important hormones include ADH and the renin-angiotensin-aldosterone mechanism.

Other factors also influence cardiac activity and blood pressure. For example, cerebral cortical input from anger, fear, pain, or excitement can augment the effects of the sympathetic nervous system.

EFFECTS OF AGING

At birth, the neonate ventricles are of equal size. However, the vascular changes associated with birth lead to a decrease in pulmonary vascular resistance and pressure and an increase in systemic vascular resistance and pressure. During childhood, the greater work of the left ventricle to eject its cardiac output into the high pressure systemic circulation causes a hypertrophy of the left ventricular muscle, which is characteristic of the adult heart. The heart muscle also undergoes changes with further aging that lead to dilation of the cardiac chambers and lessening of contractility. This has little effect on stroke volume, but it reduces cardiac reserve. Coronary arteries become thickened and rigid. These changes decrease the ability of the heart to respond to additional demands and increase the likelihood of coronary artery disease. Heart valves may thicken and become incompetent, resulting in a systolic ejection murmur.

CONCLUSIONS

Although the heart can be viewed simply as a pump, this remarkable, durable organ is much more than that. The heart is a continuously beating organ that never rests. It moves blood throughout the body to oxygenate cells for energy. It propels blood through its four chambers in one direction, from right to left. Left ventricular contraction moves blood into the arteries under high pressure. This pressure propels blood through the systemic circulation.

Heart disease remains the major cause of death and involves disorders both of structure and of function of the heart. These disorders are studied in the following chapters.

BIBLIOGRAPHY

1. Ahrens, T., & Taylor, L. (1992). *Hemodynamic waveform analysis.* Philadelphia: W. B. Saunders.
2. Berne, R. M., & Levy, M. N. (1998). *Physiology* (4th ed.). St. Louis: Mosby–Year Book.
3. Braunwald, E., et al. (Ed.). (1992). Normal and abnormal circulatory function. In *Heart disease: A textbook of cardiovascular medicine* (4th ed.). Philadelphia: W. B. Saunders.
4. Guyton, A. C., & Hall, J. E. (1996). *Textbook of medical physiology* (9th ed.). Philadelphia: W. B. Saunders.
5. Hurst, J. W. (1990). *The heart.* New York: McGraw-Hill.
6. Hurst, J. W., et al. (1988). *Atlas of the heart.* New York: McGraw-Hill.
7. Jarvis, C. (1999). *Physical examination and health assessment* (3rd ed.). Philadelphia: W. B. Saunders.
8. Silverthorn, D. (1998). *Human physiology.* Upper Saddle River, NJ: Prentice Hall.

Bibliography

1. Alspach, J., & Taylor, L. (1992). *Hemodynamic waveform analysis.* Philadelphia: W. B. Saunders.
2. Berne, R. M., & Levy, M. N. (1988). *Physiology* (4th ed.). St. Louis: Mosby–Year Book.
3. Braunwald, E., et al. (Ed.) (1992). Normal and abnormal circulatory function. In *Heart disease: A textbook of cardiovascular medicine* (4th ed.). Philadelphia: W. B. Saunders.
4. Guyton, A. C., & Hall, J. E. (1996). *Textbook of medical physiology* (9th ed.). Philadelphia: W. B. Saunders.
5. Hurst, J. W. (1990). *The heart.* New York: McGraw-Hill.
6. Hurst, J. W., et al. (1988). *Atlas of the heart.* New York: McGraw-Hill.
7. Jarvis, C. (1996). *Physical examination and health assessment* (2nd ed.). Philadelphia: W. B. Saunders.
8. Silverthorn, D. (1998). *Human physiology.* Upper Saddle River, NJ: Prentice Hall.

CHAPTER

54

Assessment of the Cardiac System

Kathleen Popelka

Cardiovascular disease (CVD) is the leading cause of illness and death in the United States, affecting more than one in five people. According to the National Center for Health Statistics (NCHS), if all forms of major CVD were eliminated, life expectancy would rise by almost 10 years. About one sixth of those who die of CVD are younger than 65 years of age.[3] CVD is not just a "man's disease." More than 52.6% of deaths in women are due to CVD. CVD has claimed the lives of more women than men (47.4%) since 1984—more than half a million women every year, or more than the next 16 causes of death combined.[3, 20] The gap between male and female CVD-related death widens as women approach menopause, lose the protective effect of estrogen, and have a continuously rising risk of heart disease and stroke with age.

The prevalence and complications of CVD have significant implications for nurses to utilize physical assessment skills. Assessment of the cardiovascular system incorporates data from history-taking, relating the information to the physical examination and diagnostic tests, and correlating it with the underlying pathophysiology.

HISTORY

The history of CVD is inseparable from the client's total health history. Important information may be overlooked unless previous illnesses, manifestations, habits, lifestyle, socioeconomic considerations, and family history are examined. Table 54–1 summarizes common risk factors for CVD. Significant cardiovascular data are obtained by assessment of the following areas.

■ RISK FACTOR ANALYSIS

During the interview, be alert for data indicating the presence of CVD. Note whether the client has ever had an illness or problem related to the heart or blood vessels, such as an enlarged heart, heart murmur, rheumatic heart, heart attack, or heart failure. When reviewing the demographic data, ask whether the client has not been accepted for the armed services or sports, not passed an insurance examination, or had a high rating on an insurance examination.

While conducting the symptom analysis and review of systems, note statements about the following: chest discomfort or pain; shortness of breath on exertion or while sleeping; ankle swelling; dizzy spells; fainting spells; palpitations or rapid heartbeats; unexplained fatigue; coughing at night; coughing up blood; and cramps or pain in the calves, thighs, or hips while walking that is relieved by rest.

Must the client sleep on more than one pillow to breathe comfortably at night? Does the client need to arise several times during the night to urinate? Does the client have tender or swollen calves or varicose veins? These questions screen for the presence of heart disease that is producing physiologic impairment.[11, 36] With the exclusion of chest pain and palpitations, the manifestations are all traceable to the secondary effects of heart disease on other organs, particularly the lungs, brain, kidneys, and blood vessels.

Tailor questions to the client, depending on the manifestations, prior illnesses, physical findings, and other information gathered in order to help determine possible causes. Of all the CVDs tracked by the American Heart Association (AHA), the following are considered to be major[3, 4]:

- Ischemic (coronary) heart disease (CHD)
- Hypertensive disease
- Rheumatic fever or rheumatic heart disease
- Cerebrovascular disease (stroke)

Classification of the functional severity of illness is also important. Although there is a rough correlation between severity of heart disease, manifestations, and client limitations, the pathophysiologic impairment does not always correlate closely with the manifestations. This lack of correlation is sometimes true even with far advanced heart disease. Diagnostic studies and the client's actual capacities and limitations warrant further investigation.

Ask about current activities and limitations. Do any activities bring on shortness of breath (SOB), chest discomfort, fatigue, or dizziness? How far can the client walk, run, and climb steps? Can the client complete housework, mow the lawn, participate in sports, shop, do a full day's work, or have sexual intercourse?[11, 36]

Evaluation of previous treatments, medications, and surgical and nonsurgical interventions provides a foundation for further therapeutic regimens. Ascertain whether the client understood and followed previously prescribed medical regimens. Clients are often said not to respond to therapy when, in reality, they do not take the medications

TABLE 54–1 **RISK FACTOR ANALYSIS FOR CARDIOVASCULAR DISEASE**

Risk Factor	High Risk	Highest Risk
Sex and age	Women after menopause	Men older than 60
Family history of high blood pressure	Two blood relatives	Three or more blood relatives
Family history of heart attack	One relative, before age 60	Two relatives, before age 60
Family history of diabetes	One or more relatives with type 1 diabetes	One or more relatives with type 2 diabetes
Blood pressure† (degree of control somewhat modifiable)	Systolic: 160–200 mm Hg Diastolic: 90–110 mm Hg	Systolic: >200 mm Hg Diastolic: >110 mm Hg
Diabetes† (degree of control somewhat modifiable)	Type 1 diabetes uncontrolled or type 2 diabetes controlled	Type 2 diabetes uncontrolled
Weight*	30%–40% overweight	50% or more overweight
Cholesterol level†	240–280	Over 280
Serum triglycerides, fasting†	400–1000	Over 1000
Percentage of fat in diet†	30%–50%	Over 50%
Frequency of recreational exercise*	Minimal	No activity
Frequency of occupational exercise*	Minimal	Sedentary occupation
Cigarette smoking*	20–40 a day	Over 40 a day
Stress at home*	High	Extremely high
Stress at work†	High	Extremely high
Behavior pattern (especially men)†	Type A	Type A
Use of oral contraceptives (women)†	Younger than 40 and use oral contraceptives	Older than 40 and use oral contraceptives
Air pollution†	Moderate	High
Sleep patterns*	More than 8 hr sleep a night	4–6 hr sleep a night

*Modifiable risk factors.
†Possibly modifiable risk factors.

correctly. Diets are commonly not adhered to as prescribed. Confusion about the use, frequency, and amount of different medications or the expense is the cause of noncompliance and of the lack of expected improvement. Question the client's understanding of the illness so that appropriate education can be initiated, corrected, or reinforced.

■ BIOGRAPHICAL AND DEMOGRAPHIC DATA

Biographical and demographic data include name, age, sex, place of birth, race, marital status, occupation, and ethnic background. Alterations in health status may have caused changes in occupation and status within the family as the provider. There are known transcultural considerations regarding heart disease and stroke among culturally diverse individuals. Mortality from heart disease for Native Americans is twice as high as that for all Americans. Black men are nearly twice as likely to die from stroke as white men. Among American adults age 20 and older, the estimated prevalence of coronary heart disease is 7.2% for the general population, 7.5% for non-Hispanic whites, 6.9% for non-Hispanic blacks, and 5.6% for Mexican Americans.[3, 40]

■ CURRENT HEALTH

Documenting the progression of the first manifestations to the current complaints or problems helps organize the history and reveals the sequence of events that led the client to seek help.

Chief Complaint

Inquire about the chief complaint or complaints to establish priorities for intervention and to evaluate how well the client understands the presenting condition. Common clinical manifestations of CVD are listed in Box 54–1.[20, 36] There may be more than one major manifestation. When this occurs, assess them in order of importance.

Symptom Analysis

Conduct a symptom analysis to evaluate and clarify the chief complaint. Chapter 9 describes symptom analysis. Following are the more common cardiac manifestations.

CHEST PAIN

Chest pain is one of the most important manifestations of cardiac disease. It may result from pulmonary, intestinal, gallbladder, and musculoskeletal disorders. *Angina pectoris* is the true symptom of coronary artery disease (CAD). Angina is caused by myocardium ischemia (hypoxia), an imbalance of oxygen supply and demand as the coronary arteries support myocardial tissue. Because chest pain is caused by a number of conditions, it is highly variable. Evaluate chest pain and its cause with a careful symptom analysis. Table 54–2 compares selected cardiac, pulmo-

BOX 54–1 Important Manifestations of Cardiac Disease

- Chest pain
- Irregularities of heart rhythm—palpitations
- Respiratory manifestations—dyspnea
- Syncope
- Fatigue
- Weight gain, dependent edema
- Cyanosis
- Hemoptysis

TABLE 54–2 DIFFERENTIAL ASSESSMENT OF CHEST PAIN

Condition	Location	Quality	Quantity	Timing	Aggravating and Relieving Factors	Associated Manifestations
Angina pectoris	Substernal or retrosternal region; radiates to neck, jaw, epigastrium, shoulders, arms (especially left)	Pressure, burning, squeezing, tight heaviness, indigestion	Moderate to severe	<10 min	Aggravated by exertion, cold, stress, or after meals; relieved by rest or nitroglycerin; atypical (Prinzmetal's) angina may be unrelated to activity and caused by coronary artery spasm	Sinus tachycadia, bradycardia, S_4, paradoxical split S_2 during pain episode
Coronary insufficiency	Same as angina	Same as angina	Increasingly severe	>10 min	Same as angina, with gradually decreasing tolerance for exertion	Same as angina
Myocardial infarction	Precordial, substernal; may radiate like angina	Heaviness, crushing pressure, burning, constriction	Severe, sometimes mild (in 30% of clients)	Sudden onset; lasting longer than 15 min	Unrelieved	Dyspnea, sweating, weakness, nausea, vomiting, severe anxiety
Pericarditis	Usually begins over sternum and may radiate to neck and down left upper extremity	Sharp, stabbing, knife-like	Moderate to severe	Lasts many hours to days	Aggravated by deep breathing, rotating chest or supine position; relieved by sitting up and leaning forward	Fever, infection, pericardial friction rub, syncope, dyspnea, orthopnea
Dissecting aortic aneurysm	Anterior chest; radiates to thoracic area of back; may be abdominal; pain shifts in chest	Tearing	Excruciating, tearing, knife-like	Sudden onset, lasts for hours	Unrelated to anything	Lower blood pressure in one arm, absent pulses, CVA, dyspnea, murmur of aortic insufficiency, pulsus paradoxus, stridor; myocardial infarction can occur
Mitral valve prolapse syndrome	Usually not substernal; sometimes radiates to the left arm, back, jaw	Stabbing, sharp, sticky quality, "kick"	Variable; generally mild but can become severe	Sudden, recurrent	Not related to exertion, not relieved by nitroglycerin or rest	Variable palpitations, dysrhythmias, dizziness, syncope, dyspnea, late systolic or pansystolic murmur
Pulmonary embolism (many pulmonary emboli do not produce chest pain)	Substernal, "anginal"	Deep, crushing; if pulmonary infection, may be pleuritic	Can be absent, mild, or severe	Sudden onset; lasts minutes to <1 hr	May be aggravated by breathing	Fever, tachypnea, tachycardia, hypotension, elevated jugular venous pressure, right ventricular lift, accentuated pulmonary valve (P_2) sound during S_2, occasional murmur of tricuspid insufficiency and right ventricular S_4; with infarction usually in the presence of heart failure; crackles, pleural rub, hemoptysis, clinical phlebitis present in minority of cases

Table continued on following page

TABLE 54–2 DIFFERENTIAL ASSESSMENT OF CHEST PAIN *Continued*

Condition	Location	Quality	Quantity	Timing	Aggravating and Relieving Factors	Associated Manifestations
Spontaneous pneumothorax	Unilateral	Sharp, well localized, stabbing	Moderate, severe	Sudden onset; lasts many hours	Painful breathing	Dyspnea, shock, tension pneumothorax
Pneumonia with pleurisy	Localized over area of consolidation	Sharp, grabbing aching	Variable	Sudden	Painful breathing	Dyspnea, cough, fever, hemoptysis, crackles, occasional pleural rub
Gastrointestinal disorders (esophageal reflux)	Lower substernal area, epigastric, right or left upper quadrant	Burning, colic-like aching, tightness, pressure	Moderate to severe	Waves, continuous radiation	Precipitated by recumbency, large meals, alcohol ingestion	Nausea, regurgitation, food intolerance, melena, hematemesis, jaundice
Musculoskeletal disorders	Variable	Aching	Variable	Short or long duration Prolonged period of time	History of muscle exertion, viral illness	Tender to pressure or movement
Neurologic disorders (herpes zoster)	Dermatomal in distribution	Aching constant burning, pins and needles, sharp	Moderate, severe	Unassociated with external events	Aggravated by systemic stress	Pain before rash, vesicles
Psychogenic states (depression, self-gain, or attention-seeking)	Usually localized to a point	Vague, burning, diffuse	Mild to moderate, disabling	Varies; usually very brief	Situational anger, depression, anxiety	Sighing, chest wall tenderness, fatigue, dyspnea, anorexia

CVA, cerebrovascular accident; P_2, pulmonic second sound; S_2, second heart sound; S_4, fourth heart sound.
Modified from Andreoli, K., et al. (1987). *Comprehensive cardiac care* (6th ed., pp. 54–55). St. Louis: Mosby–Year Book; Seller, R. H. (1996). *Differential diagnosis of common complaints* (3rd ed., pp. 57–68). Philadelphia: W. B. Saunders; and Hill, B., & Geraci, S. A. (1998). A diagnostic approach to chest pain based on history and ancillary evaluation. *Nurse Practitioner, 23*(2), 20–45.

nary, gastrointestinal, musculoskeletal, neurologic, and anxiety-related conditions in relation to chest pain.[20, 32, 36] Table 54–3 compares gender differences in manifestations associated with angina.[34]

TIMING. Note the time the pain begins and ends to determine the duration of discomfort. Several intermittent small episodes of chest pain are not considered as one long period of pain. Generally, the pain of myocardial infarction lasts longer than 30 minutes or until intervention is begun. Conversely, angina is usually relieved within 5 to 15 minutes by rest, with or without the use of vasodilator drugs such as nitroglycerin. Angina pectoris rarely lasts less than 1 minute or more than 15 minutes in the absence of myocardial infarction or persistent dysrhythmias (abnormal heart rhythms).[2]

QUALITY. Chest pain may be described as a "strange feeling," indigestion, a dull heavy pressure, burning, crushing, constricting, aching, stabbing, or tightness. Angina pectoris characteristically has a crescendo (gradually increasing) pattern at onset. Pain described as "shooting" or "stabbing" and reaching maximum intensity virtually instantaneously is often not angina but musculoskeletal or neural in origin.[2]

QUANTITY. To better quantify chest pain, ask the client to use a scale of 1 (least severe) to 10 (most severe). This recorded scale can then be used to compare future episodes of chest pain. For example, the client may report 10/10 for pain on admission and then report 3/10 for pain after administration of a vasodilating medication.

LOCATION. The site of discomfort provides additional information for determining its cause. Anginal pain is ordinarily retrosternal, felt slightly to the left of the midline or partly under the sternum. The chest pain of myocardial ischemia tends to radiate bilaterally across the chest into the arms, left greater than right, and into the neck and lower jaw. Occasionally, radiation to the back or occiput is noted. Chest pain may be diffuse, localized, or so minor that clients dismiss true ischemic pain or possible infarction. Painless or atypical presentation of myocardial infarction occurs in up to 30% of clients, particularly in diabetic and older clients.[2]

PRECIPITATING OR AGGRAVATING FACTORS. The pain may be associated with certain factors or conditions. Emotional or sexual excitement, temperature extremes, exertion, deep sleep, position changes, deep breathing, straining during bowel movements, or eating may trigger the onset of chest pain.

RELIEVING FACTORS. Anginal pain may be relieved by rest, nitroglycerin, oxygen, and a change in position. Chest pain that is not relieved by these interventions and lasts 20 minutes or longer highly suggests myocardial infarction.[2]

ASSOCIATED MANIFESTIONS. Ask the client whether other manifestations accompany the onset of chest pain, for example, anxiousness, shortness of breath, nausea, vomiting, diaphoresis (perspiration), vertigo, palpitations, or a feeling of impending doom. Pain associated with transmural Q-wave infarction is usually more severe and longer lasting than angina and is often associated with nausea, vomiting, and diaphoresis. Myocardial infarction is frequently accompanied by symptoms of sustained left ventricular dysfunction (*dyspnea* [labored breathing] and *orthopnea* [difficult breathing except in an upright position]) and evidence of autonomic nervous system hyperactivity (tachycardia, diaphoresis, bradycardia).[2]

TABLE 54–3 GENDER DIFFERENCES IN MANIFESTATIONS ASSOCIATED WITH ANGINA

Rank in Frequency	Among Women	Among Men
1	Fatigue	Rest pain
2	Rest pain	Fatigue
3	Weakness	Shortness of breath
4	Shortness of breath	Weakness
5	Dizziness	Arm pain
6	Arm pain	Dizziness
7	Nausea	Sweating
8	Back pain	Neck pain
9	Lost of appetite	Nausea
10	Neck pain	Heartburn
11	Sweating	Palpitations
12	Heartburn	Throat pain
13	PND	Back pain
14	Palpitations	Loss of appetite
15	Jaw pain	Jaw pain
16	Throat pain	PND
17	Toothache	Toothache

PND, paroxysmal nocturnal dyspepsia.

From Penque, S., et al. (1998). Women and coronary artery disease: Relationship between descriptors of signs and symptoms and diagnostic and treatment course. *American Journal of Critical Care, 7*(3), 175–182.

IRREGULARITIES OF HEART RHYTHM—PALPITATIONS

The word "palpitation" is derived from the Latin *palpitare*, "to throb." *Palpitations* are uncomfortable sensations in the chest associated with a wide range of dysrhythmias (Box 54–2). They are common and do not necessarily indicate serious heart disease. A palpitation is a sensation of rapid heartbeats, skipping, irregularity, thumping, or pounding and may be accompanied by anxiousness.

Tachycardia (rapid heart rate), increased force of myocardial contraction (as can occur with ingestion of caffeine or with emotional or physical stress), or premature ventricular beats may cause palpitations. Any condition in which there is an increased stroke volume, as in aortic regurgitation, may be associated with a sensation of forceful contraction.

The onset and termination of palpitations are often abrupt. Question the client about (1) medications; (2) the frequency of palpitations, precipitating factors, and aggravating or relieving factors; and (3) any manifestations such as dizziness or shortness of breath associated with the onset of the palpitations. See Box 54–2 for common causes of palpitations.[2, 32]

RESPIRATORY MANIFESTATIONS—DYSPNEA

Dyspnea is defined as shortness of breath or labored breathing. Like chest pain, this common manifestation affects clients with cardiac and pulmonary disorders. *Acute dyspnea* may occur with a fever, exposure to high altitude, acute pulmonary edema, hyperventilation, anemia, pneumonia, pneumothorax, pulmonary emboli, and

BOX 54–2 Common Causes of Palpitations

Dysrhythmias

1. Bradyarrhythmias
   a. Heart block
   b. Sinus arrest
2. Extrasystoles
   a. Premature atrial contractions (PACs)
   b. Premature nodal contractions
   c. Premature ventricular contractions (PVCs)
3. Tachyarrhythmias
   a. Atrial fibrillation
   b. Atrial flutter
   c. Multifocal atrial tachycardia
   d. Paroxysmal supraventricular tachycardia
   e. Ventricular tachycardia

Other

1. Anemia
2. Anxiety states
3. Caffeine
4. Drugs
   a. Antidepressants
   b. Bronchodilators
   c. Digitalis
5. Fever
6. Hyperthyroidism
7. Hypoglycemia
8. Perimenopausal
9. Pheochromocytoma
10. Smoking
11. Thyrotoxicosis

airway obstruction. *Chronic dyspnea* also may occur in clients experiencing anxiety, depression, left ventricular heart failure, pulmonary disease, pleural effusion, asthma, obesity, poor physical fitness, and various psychosomatic conditions.

Although dyspnea can develop in any form of heart disease, it usually occurs with cardiac enlargement and other pathologic, cardiovascular, structural, and physiologic changes. Dyspnea develops when the left ventricle fails to function and the lungs become congested with fluid.[2]

There are several forms of dyspnea: exertional dyspnea, orthopnea, and paroxysmal nocturnal dyspnea.

EXERTIONAL DYSPNEA. This is the most common form of cardiac-related dyspnea. Also known as *dyspnea on exertion* (DOE),[2] it occurs during mild to moderate exercise or activity and disappears with rest. If severe, exertional dyspnea can greatly limit activity tolerance. Ask the client to describe the degree of activity that typically precipitates the onset of dyspnea, for example, walking up one flight of stairs or walking to the mailbox. Noncardiac conditions such as obesity, poor physical conditioning, anemia, asthma, and obstructions of the nasal passages may also lead to dyspnea after mild exercise.

ORTHOPNEA. Orthopnea (difficult breathing) results from an increase in hydrostatic pressure in the lungs when the person is lying flat and is relieved when the person assumes an upright or semivertical position. It consists of a cough and dyspnea in clients with left ventricular failure or mitral valve disease. Clients with orthopnea need to use two or more pillows when lying down. Clients with severe obstructive lung disease, especially acute asthma, also cannot lie flat comfortably.

Ask clients what actions they take to facilitate breathing. Do they sit up in a chair or dangle their feet at the bedside? What position do they sleep in? How many pillows do they sleep with? Record the degree of head elevation required to breathe. Orthopnea usually indicates a more serious compromise of the cardiovascular system than does exertional dyspnea.[2]

PAROXYSMAL NOCTURNAL DYSPNEA. Paroxysmal nocturnal dyspnea (PND) is dyspnea during sleep that awakens the sleeper with a "terrifying breathing attack." It commonly occurs 2 to 3 hours after the person goes to bed and is relieved when the person assumes an upright position. The dyspnea usually does not recur after the client goes back to sleep. Episodes can be mild, or they can be severe with wheezing, coughing, gasping, and apprehension. Some episodes associated with severe left ventricular failure progress to pulmonary edema.[2]

SYNCOPE

Syncope, or fainting, is a transient loss of consciousness related to inadequate cerebral perfusion. Certain cardiac disorders, especially cardiac dysrhythmias (irregular heart rhythms), can precipitate a sudden decrease in cardiac output. Valvular disorders may also lead to an adverse change in circulatory hemodynamics and cause syncope or vertigo. Clients who are susceptible to syncopal episodes (e.g., those with Stokes-Adams syndrome) should wear Medic-Alert bracelets to inform emergency health care providers.[2]

FATIGUE

Easy fatigability on mild exertion is a frequent problem for clients experiencing cardiac disease; it is a common manifestation of decreased cardiac output. Progressive deterioration of activity tolerance results from the heart's inability to pump an effective volume of blood to meet the varying metabolic demands of the body. Fatigue, however, is not specific for cardiac problems. The most common causes of fatigue are anemia, anxiety, chronic diseases, depression, and thyroid dysfunction.

WEIGHT GAIN AND DEPENDENT EDEMA

As the heart fails, or the blood volume expands, fluid accumulates. A client may notice weight gain, shortness of breath, swelling of the lower extremities, or a combination of these. An increase in body weight of 3 pounds or more within 24 hours results from fluid rather than body mass changes. Body weight is a sensitive indicator of water and sodium retention and increases even before edema occurs. The client with heart failure has symmetrical edema of the lower extremities that worsens as the day progresses. Daily weight measurement is important for clients with cardiac problems. Changes in weight should be reported to the health care provider.[2]

OTHER ASSOCIATED MANIFESTATIONS

Cyanosis is a subtle bluish discoloration. Cyanosis from birth is associated with congenital heart lesions. *Differential cyanosis* is related to a right-to-left shunt through a patent ductus arteriosus (PDA). In right-to-left shunting resulting from pulmonary hypertension, blood in the pulmonary artery crosses the PDA, which is located below the carotid and left subclavian arteries; deoxygenated blood is pumped to the lower extremity, producing cyanosis in only that location. *Peripheral cyanosis* is due to increased oxygen extraction in states of low cardiac output and is seen in cooler areas of the body such as the nail beds and the outer surfaces of the lips.

Clubbing of the fingernails is seen in association with significant cardiopulmonary disease.[2]

Hemoptysis refers to coughing up of blood. A careful description of hemoptysis is essential because it can include clots of blood as well as blood-tinged sputum. Recurrent episodes of hemoptysis may result from mitral stenosis and pulmonary causes.[2]

■ PAST HEALTH HISTORY

Ask the client about the following areas.

Childhood and Infectious Diseases

In addition to the usual information about common childhood diseases and immunizations, ask about the client's experiences with rheumatic fever, scarlet fever, and severe streptococcal infections. These conditions are associated with structural mitral valve disease. Investigate known or corrected congenital anomalies (e.g, atrial or ventricular septal defect, persistent PDA, tetralogy of Fallot, Eisenmenger's syndrome).[2, 12, 38]

Immunizations

Clients with chronic conditions, such as cardiovascular disorders, should be vaccinated yearly against influenza. Indications for the pneumococcal polysaccharide vaccine are similar to those for the influenza vaccine. Revaccination is recommended every 6 to 10 years.[21]

Major Illnesses and Hospitalizations

Note conditions that influence the client's current cardiovascular performance, that is, diabetes mellitus, chronic obstructive lung disease, kidney disease, anemia, hypertension, stroke, gout, thrombophlebitis (vein inflammation associated with thrombus formation), collagen diseases, and bleeding disorders. Explore previous hospitalizations, surgical procedures, obstetric history, and outpatient interventions. Inquire about previous cardiovascular diagnostic studies, such as an electrocardiogram (ECG), exercise stress test, and echocardiogram. The results of such studies provide baseline data for comparative analysis when later studies are performed.[12, 38]

Medications

Evaluate the use of prescription medications, over-the-counter medications, herbs, and recreational drugs. Whenever possible, use brand names or simple descriptors instead of generic names. For example, ask clients whether they are currently taking "water pills," "heart pills," or "blood pressure" medications.

Numerous medications can affect the cardiovascular system. Ask specifically about the use of antihypertensives, diuretics, vasodilators (nitroglycerin), cardiotonic drugs (digoxin), anticoagulants, bronchodilators, contraceptives, and steroids. Noncardiac medications can have profound secondary effects on cardiovascular performance. For example, tricyclic antidepressants and other psychotropic medications can potentiate dysrhythmias. Oral contraceptives increase the incidence of thrombophlebitis. Steroid use increases fluid retention and may cause hypertension. Various antineoplastic agents may be cardiotoxic, causing dysrhythmias and cardiomyopathy.

Discuss the use of recreational drugs. Cocaine toxicity is a major threat to the cardiovascular system. The systemic sympathomimetic effects of cocaine result in a "fight-or-flight" reaction that increases heart rate, contractility, blood glucose levels, and peripheral vasoconstriction. Cocaine can potentiate the effects of circulating catecholamines (epinephrine and norepinephrine), resulting in sudden death.

Finally, discuss the use of over-the-counter drugs such as aspirin, cold remedies, and vitamins. Note the dose and times of administration. Ask about use of herbal remedies. Herbs are used for cardiac disorders such as angina, dysrhythmias, and heart disease and for related disorders such as high blood pressure (BP) and peripheral vascular disease.[16, 42]

Antianginal herbs include angelica (*Angelica archangelica*), bilberry (*Vaccinium myrtillus*), evening primrose (*Oenothera biennis*), flaxseed (*Linum usitatissimum*), garlic (*Allium sativum*), ginger (*Zingiber officinale*), hawthorn (*Crataegus*), khella (*Ammi majus*), kudzu (*Pueraria lobata*), onion (*Allium cepa*), purslane (*Portulaca oleracea*), Sichuan lovage (*Ligusticum chuanxiong*), and willow (*Salix*). Some of these herbs are anticoagulants (e.g., evening primrose, garlic, Sichuan lovage, willow). Others are vasodilators (e.g., bilberry, hawthorn, khella, kudzu). Some have calcium-channel blocking action (e.g., angelica). Hawthorne, garlic, bilberry, evening primrose, and flaxseed can lower BP and cholesterol levels. Antioxidants include ginger and purslane.

Herbs known to have antidysrhythmic action include angelica, astragalus (*Astragalus*), barberry (*Berberis vulgaris*), canola (*Brassica*), cinchona (*Cinchona*), ginkgo (*Gingko biloba*), hawthorn, horehound (*Marrubium vulgare*), khella, motherwort (*Leonurus cardiaca*), purslane, reishi (*Ganoderma lucidum*), Scotch broom (*Cytisus scoparius*), and valerian (*Valeriana officinalis*).

Other herbs used for heart disease include chicory (*Cichorium intybus*), grape (*Vitis vinifera*), olive (*Olea europaea*), peanut (*Arachis hypogaea*), pigweed (*Amaranthus*), and rosemary (*Rosmarinus officinalis*). Chicory has digitalis-like properties. Red grape and olive products protect against heart attack. Pigweed is high in omega-3 fatty acids, preventing blood clots that can trigger a heart attack. Peanut and rosemary are antioxidants.

In addition to the types and names of the medications the client takes, ask how many pills and how often they are taken. Is the client currently taking these medications? Clients with cardiac disease occasionally stop taking prescribed medications because they (1) are taking too many pills, (2) are experiencing unwanted side effects, (3) believe that the problem has resolved, or (4) worry about the cost. A client may neglect to take prescribed diuretics because "it makes me go to the bathroom all the time." Clients receiving antihypertensive medications may stop taking them when their BP reaches a normal range because they perceive that the problem has resolved. Careful questioning can identify areas for client teaching.

Review for substance abuse including cigarette smoking and using alcohol or street drugs. Determine the pack-year history (number of cigarette packs smoked per day multiplied by the number of years smoked) of tobacco abuse and the history of alcohol consumption and dependence. If the client is not smoking currently, does he or she use a nicotine inhalation system or a nicotine transdermal product or chew nicotine gum or smokeless tobacco? All nicotine products have a vasoconstrictive effect on the heart and vessels.

Allergies

Note and describe any environmental, food, or drug allergies. Clearly document the manifestations of an allergic reaction, such as rashes, itching, or anaphylaxis (a sudden severe allergic reaction).

■ FAMILY HEALTH HISTORY

Ask about prolonged contact with a communicable disease or the effect of a family member's illness on the client. Specifically, inquire about a family history of heart disease, high BP, stroke, diabetes, or kidney disease. A detailed health history of the client's family can provide insight into possible genetic, environmental, and lifestyle conditions contributing to a cardiac condition. Note nonmodifiable cardiac risk factors such as heredity, age, sex, and race.

Genetic factors contribute to four traits that increase the incidence of atherosclerosis: hypertension, dyslipidemia, diabetes, and obesity. Modifiable risk factors, when corrected, significantly reduce the likelihood of a cardiac event. Modifying risk factors includes reducing stress, losing weight, reducing cholesterol levels, stopping tobacco abuse, and becoming more physically active.[3–6, 10, 17, 33, 35]

■ PSYCHOSOCIAL HISTORY

The psychosocial history includes data on lifestyle, household members, marital status, children, relationships with significant others, education, military service, religious beliefs (in relation to perceptions of health and treatment), the living environment, employment, and hobbies. Note data that help identify support systems and coping mechanisms. Psychosocial data provide information about risk factors for the development of CVD (see Chapter 58). Background information can be used to formulate a plan to assist the client in making necessary lifestyle adaptations to promote health and lessen disease.

Occupation

Inquire about all occupations the client has had and the duration of each. The present occupation may be relevant to the significance of the disease; that is, coronary artery disease or dysrhythmias may be incompatible with continuing a career as an airline pilot or truck driver. The amount of perceived job-related stress may need to be evaluated; stress is a modifiable risk factor for CVD.

Geographical Location

Where one lives is significantly related to death caused by cardiac events. The American Heart Association categorizes age-adjusted death rates for total CVD, coronary heart disease, and stroke by state. See Box 54–3.

Environment

Ask the client about the following:

- The home, such as safety issues, type of dwelling (number of steps), state of repair, exits for fire, heating and cooling adequacy
- Mode of transportation
- Access to public transportation
- The neighborhood, in regard to noise, pollution, and violence
- Access to family and friends, grocery store, a pharmacy, laundry, church, and health care facilities

After a stroke or with deteriorating cardiac function and output, a client may need assistance or environmental adjustments to live safely and fully and meet daily needs.

Exercise

Ask about the type and amount of exercise routinely engaged in during an average week before and after the

BOX 54–3 Death Rates from Total Cardiovascular Disease, United States (2000)

Rate	State
300.7 to 339.4	Alaska, Arizona, Colorado, Hawaii, Idaho, Massachusetts, Minnesota, Montana, New Mexico, Oregon, Utah, Washington, Wyoming
345.2 to 366.7	California, Connecticut, Florida, Iowa, Kansas, Maine, Nebraska, New Hampshire, North Dakota, Rhode Island, South Dakota, Vermont, Wisconsin
368.3 to 409.8	Delaware, District of Columbia, Illinois, Maryland, Michigan, Nevada, New Jersey, North Carolina, Ohio, Pennsylvania, Texas, Virginia
411.4 to 480.0	Alabama, Arkansas, Georgia, Indiana, Kentucky, Louisiana, Mississippi, Missouri, New York, Oklahoma, South Carolina, Tennessee, West Virginia

Total cardiovascular diseases are defined here as ICD/9 390–459.

Source: National Center for Health Statistics (NCHS) compressed mortality file for the years 1994 to 1996. Age adjustments are based on the 2000 standards.

onset of current manifestations. Research confirms that a sedentary lifestyle potentiates the lethality of myocardial infarction, and it is considered a significant risk factor in the development of coronary artery disease.

Effective, routine *aerobic* exercise is thought to lower the likelihood of a coronary event. Aerobic exercise includes such activities as swimming, jogging, brisk walking, bicycling, and rowing.

To be beneficial, aerobic exercise should raise the heart rate from 50% to 100% of baseline (depending on age and prior physical conditioning) for at least 30 minutes three to five times a week. Along with general body conditioning, this form of exercise increases the heart's efficiency in using oxygen. Advise clients who are older than 40 years of age or who have a history of CVD to consult their physician before beginning an exercise program.[2, 3, 9]

Nutrition

Assess excess or deficit caloric intake and the client's approximate intake of foods high in sodium, cholesterol, saturated fat, and caffeine. Although these are common components of the average American diet, they have been linked to the development of atherosclerosis and hypertensive disease. Elevated serum cholesterol levels are associated with coronary artery disease. This correlation diminishes with age but still remains. Elevated serum triglyceride levels are positively related to the development of coronary artery disease, especially in women.

Examine not only daily food habits but also attitudes toward food and resistance to therapeutic alterations in diet. Cultural beliefs and economic status greatly affect food choices. Consider these factors before recommending dietary changes. Identify and include the primary food purchaser and preparer in dietary instruction.[2, 6, 10, 17, 24, 35]

Results from the Dietary Approaches to Stop Hypertension (DASH) study have established that a diet high in fruits, vegetables, and low-fat dairy products and low in cholesterol and total and saturated fat reduces BP significantly. These changes occurred in the absence of weight loss or fluid restriction. A subgroup analysis of that study suggested that although all groups benefited significantly in terms of systolic BP reduction, two subgroups gained the most from adopting these dietary changes in daily life.[37] The DASH diet resulted in (1) lower systolic BP in African Americans than in whites (6.8 versus 3.0 mm Hg) and (2) an even lower systolic BP in clients with hypertension than in those with high-normal BP (11.4 versus 3.4 mm Hg).[37]

Habits

If the client smokes, inquire about the duration of the smoking habit and the number of cigarettes smoked daily. Cigarette smoking increases the risk of coronary artery disease and worsens hypertension. Nicotine, a major ingredient in cigarettes, causes peripheral vasoconstriction, increasing resistance to left ventricular emptying and thus increasing the myocardial workload. Smoking increases the mortality rate of middle-aged clients with coronary artery disease and greatly potentiates the development of peripheral vascular disease. The death rate for coronary heart disease is 70% higher in cigarette smokers than in nonsmokers. Clients who stop smoking will, after several years, have a death rate from heart attack almost as low as that of people who never smoked.[3, 4]

Evidence that caffeine and alcohol ingestion increases the risk of atherosclerosis is inconclusive. Nevertheless, caffeine is a stimulant that, in excessive amounts, can increase heart rate and BP and contribute to palpitations, both of which can raise the myocardial workload and precipitate angina pectoris, heart failure, and some dysrhythmias. Therefore, assess caffeine intake and caution those with known heart disease to limit caffeine intake to the equivalent of two 8-oz cups of coffee per day.

Researchers state that only excessive alcohol intake has deleterious effects on the cardiovascular system and its performance. An intake of 100 g of pure (100%) alcohol may slightly increase BP and heart rate. This amount is approximately equal to three beers or one mixed drink. Alcoholism, in contrast, has been associated with the development of hypertension and damage to the heart muscle, leading to congestive cardiomyopathy. Ask about the client's approximate daily and weekly alcohol consumption (see Chapter 2). Keep in mind that the alcoholic client may lie about the type and amount consumed.

■ REVIEW OF SYSTEMS

Ask about past problems involving the cardiovascular system, including chest pain, palpitations, fatigue, edema, shortness of breath, orthopnea, wheezing, fainting (syncope), weight gain, heart murmurs, hypertension, paroxysmal nocturnal dyspnea, and history of rheumatic fever.

Cardiovascular problems also affect the pulmonary, renal, and neurologic systems. Ask about productive cough, decreased urination, dark or concentrated urine, edema of the legs, dizzy spells, and memory loss. Detailed questions for the review of systems may be found in Chapter 9, Box 9–2.

PHYSICAL EXAMINATION

The cardiac physical examination includes the following:

- A general inspection
- Assessment of BP, arterial pulses, and jugular venous pulse
- Percussion, palpation, and auscultation of the heart
- Evaluation for edema

The client is supine. Stand at the client's right side. The head of the bed or examination table may be elevated slightly for comfort. Proceed in logical fashion from head to foot. Necessary equipment includes a stethoscope with diaphragm and bell, a penlight, ruler, and an applicator stick. Ensure a woman's privacy by keeping her breasts draped. The female left breast overrides part of the area examined in a cardiac examination. Gently displace the breast upward, or ask the woman to hold it out of the way.[12, 37] See the accompanying Physical Assessment Findings in the Healthy Adult feature.

■ GENERAL APPEARANCE

Begin with inspection. Much may be learned through simple observation. Look at the client and consider the following:

PHYSICAL ASSESSMENT FINDINGS IN THE HEALTHY ADULT

Cardiovascular System

Inspection

Skin color even; capillary refill less than 3 seconds. Thorax symmetrical, without visible lifts or point of maximal impulse (PMI). Jugular venous distention absent with client at 45-degree angle. Lower extremity superficial vessels without tortuosity upon standing.

Palpation

Skin warm. PMI palpable in fifth intercostal space at left midclavicular line, approximately 1 cm in diameter. Forceful thrusts, heaves, and pulsations absent. No palpable thrills. Abdominal aorta pulsations slightly palpable over epigastrium without lateral radiation. Carotid and peripheral pulses equal and readily palpable bilaterally. Evidence of unimpeded arterial flow and venous return to upper and lower extremities. No edema evident.

Percussion

Right heart border not discerned.

Auscultation

S_1 and S_2 heard without splitting. Apical rate, 72 BPM, regular. Murmurs and extra heart sounds absent.

- Does the client lie quietly, or is there restlessness or continual moving about?
- Can the client lie flat, or is only an upright, erect position tolerated?
- Does the facial expression reflect pain or obvious signs of respiratory distress?
- Are there signs of significant cyanosis or pallor?
- Can the client answer questions without dyspnea during the interview?

■ LEVEL OF CONSCIOUSNESS

Note the client's general *level of consciousness* (LOC). The level of consciousness reflects the adequacy of cerebral perfusion and oxygenation. Also assess whether the client manifests appropriate behavior for the surroundings:

- What is the client's affect?
- Are there obvious signs of anxiety, fear, depression, or anger?
- How does the client react to those in the immediate vicinity, including significant others?

Assessment of general appearance and level of consciousness provides an initial composite picture of the client and indicates the level of comfort and distress.

■ HEAD, NECK, NAILS, AND SKIN

When examining the head, pay particular attention to the eyes, ear lobes, lips, and buccal mucosa. Examine the eyes for *arcus senilis* (a light gray ring around the iris, possibly caused by cholesterol deposits) and *xanthelasma* (yellow raised plaques around the eyelids resulting from lipid deposits). Both findings are common in elderly clients but may indicate a predisposition to atherosclerosis.

Observe the skin and mucous membranes for abnormalities such as central or peripheral *cyanosis*. The presence of a bluish tinge or duskiness is indicative of central cyanosis, indicating poor arterial circulation. Central cyanosis indicates serious heart or lung disease in which hemoglobin is not fully saturated with oxygen. Peripheral cyanosis, seen in lips, ear lobes, and nail beds, suggests peripheral vasoconstriction.

Assess *capillary refill* (circulation) by putting slight pressure on a nail bed until it blanches (see Chapter 59). Quickly release the pressure. When circulation is adequate, nail color returns to baseline in less than 2 seconds. Always check capillary refill before using pulse oximetry; if capillary refill is abnormal, pulse oximetry findings are inaccurate.

Check fingers for *clubbing*, in which the distal tips of the fingers become bulbous and the angle between the base of the nail and the skin next to the cuticle increases from the normal 160 to 180 degrees or more (see Chapter 59). In addition, the nails feel soft and spongy. Finger clubbing is associated with pulmonary and cardiovascular disease. Splinter hemorrhages of the nail are classically associated with subacute bacterial endocarditis.

Assess *skin turgor* (elasticity) by lifting a fold of skin over the sternum or lower arms and releasing it (see Chapter 48). Normal skin immediately returns to the baseline position, but skin with decreased turgor stays pinched (tenting) for up to 30 seconds. Decreased skin turgor occurs with dehydration, volume depletion, rapid weight loss, and advanced age. The temperature of the skin may reflect cardiac disease. Severe anemia, beriberi, and thyrotoxicosis tend to make the skin warmer; intermittent claudication (leg pain related to peripheral vascular disease) is associated with coolness of the lower extremity compared with the upper extremity.[2, 12, 30, 38]

■ EDEMA

Edema occurs in right-sided heart failure when the excess intravascular volume begins to increase capillary hydrostatic pressure and force fluid into the interstitium.

Inspect dependent areas for edema. In the mobile client, edema is best seen in the feet, ankles, and lower legs. In the chair-ridden or bedridden client, edema may be palpated over the sacrum, abdomen, or scapula. Assess the severity of edema by pressing a thumb or finger carefully into the area. A depression that does not rapidly resume its original contour is noted as orthostatic, or pitting, edema. Because there is a wide discrepancy in edema grading scales, record the actual amount of time in seconds for the indentation to resolve (see Chapter 51).[2, 12, 38]

■ BLOOD PRESSURE

Measure BP in both arms initially to rule out dissecting aortic aneurysm, coarctation of the aorta, vascular obstruction, vascular outlet syndromes, and errors in measurement. If the arms are inaccessible, obtain pressures from the thighs and popliteal arteries or the calves and posterior tibial arteries. When pressures are difficult to auscultate, systolic pressures can be determined through palpation or by Doppler ultrasonography.

When recording measurements, note both systolic and diastolic pressures, for example, 120/70. The muffling of

Korotkoff's sounds may also be included and recorded as 120/80/70. The American Heart Association recommends recording the point at which the sound disappears (fifth Korotkoff sound) as the diastolic pressure in adults. Also, record the arm in which the measurement was taken and the client's position at the time of the reading.

Postural Blood Pressure

Perform a postural BP reading when an extracellular volume depletion or decreased vascular tone is suspected. Note the client's position at the time of the reading (Fig. 54–1).

Paradoxical Blood Pressure (Pulsus Paradoxus)

Pulsus paradoxus is an abnormal fall in systolic BP of more than 10 mm Hg during inspiration. It is frequently found in clients with pericardial tamponade, constrictive pericarditis (inflammation of the pericardial sac), and pulmonary hypertension.

Use a sphygmomanometer and stethoscope to assess for a paradoxical pulse over the brachial artery. Instruct the client to breathe normally. Inflate the cuff 20 mm Hg above the systolic BP. Slowly deflate the cuff (1 to 2 mm Hg/sec), and listen for Korotkoff's sounds to appear only during expiration. (Sounds are first heard during expiration and then during inspiration.) Continue deflating the cuff until Korotkoff's sounds are heard equally well during inspiration and expiration.

The paradoxical pressure is the difference between the BP when the sounds are first heard during expiration and the BP when the sounds are heard on both expiration and inspiration. Normally, this difference is less than 10 mm Hg. If the client is breathing normally and the systolic difference is greater than 10 mm Hg, cardiac compression, such as cardiac tamponade, may be present.

■ PULSE

Pulse characteristics can vary. If the pulse is irregular, assess for a pulse deficit by taking apical and radial pulses simultaneously, noting differences in rate. Peripheral pulse assessment is discussed in Chapter 51.

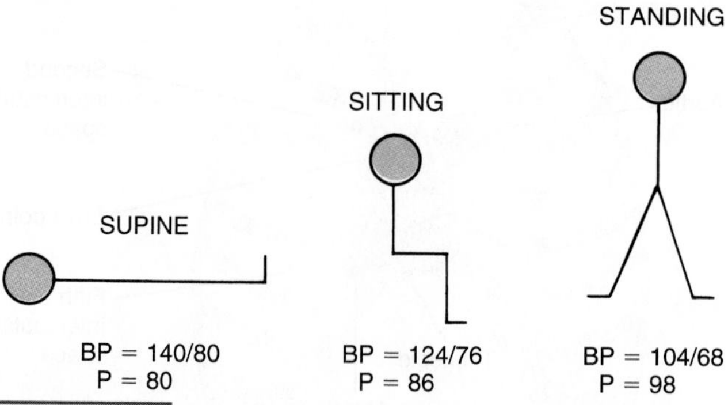

FIGURE 54–1 Recording postural blood pressure (BP). After measuring the client's BP and pulse in the supine position, leave the BP cuff in place and help the client sit. Then measure the BP within 15 to 30 seconds. Help the client stand, and measure again. Postural hypotension is indicated by a BP drop of more than 10 to 15 mm Hg systolic pressure and more than 10 mm Hg diastolic pressure. Postural hypotension is typically accompanied by a 10% to 20% increase in heart rate (pulse).

■ RESPIRATIONS

Note the rate, rhythm, depth, and quality of the breathing pattern. Variations in the respiratory rate and character may indicate heart failure or pulmonary edema. Auscultate the lungs for the presence of crackles, rhonchi (dry rattling), or other abnormal breath sounds (see Chapter 59). Severe left ventricular failure may produce pulmonary congestion and resultant frothy sputum with deep respiratory efforts.

■ HEAD AND NECK

Neck Veins

Neck vein distention can be used to estimate *central venous pressure* (CVP). The amount of distention reflects pressure and volume changes in the right atrium. The internal jugular veins, although more difficult to detect than the external jugular veins, are more reliable indicators of CVP. The external jugular vein engorges easily with only slight provocation, for example, by holding the breath, twisting the neck, and being constricted by clothing (except in weight lifters, football players, and professional speakers and singers, who have overdeveloped neck muscle tendons). The vessels are prominent and visible but soft and compressible.

A relaxed supine position with the head of the bed inclined between 15 and 30 degrees maximizes jugular vein prominence. Clients who have greatly increased right atrial pressure may require head elevation from 45 to 90 degrees. Support the client's head with a small pillow and avoid sharp neck flexion. Turn the client's head slightly away from you. Loosen or remove clothing that compresses the neck or upper thorax. Tangential (oblique) lighting enhances the veins' appearance. Observe both sides of the neck. The internal jugular vein lies deep to the sternocleidomastoid muscle and runs parallel along its length to the jaw and ear lobe (Fig. 54–2). Identify the pulsations of the internal jugular. Use the external jugular vein if the internal jugular is not visible.

Note the highest point at which the internal jugular pulses can be seen (the *meniscus*). The *sternal angle* (manubrial joint) is a reference point to measure the height of venous pulsation, approximately 4 to 5 cm above the center of the right atrium. Use a centimeter ruler to measure the vertical distance between the sternal angle and the point of highest venous pulsations. See Figure 54–3.

The value is usually less than 3 or 4 cm above the sternal angle when the head of the bed is elevated 30 to 40 degrees. Higher values indicate increased right atrial or right ventricular pressure, as seen in right ventricular failure, tricuspid regurgitation, and pericardial tamponade. Flat jugular veins in a supine client suggest extracellular volume depletion. Unilateral distention may indicate vessel obstruction on that side.

The timing and amplitude of the jugular vein pulsations may also be assessed to evaluate right-sided heart function, tricuspid valve performance, and the presence of certain dysrhythmias.[12, 30, 38]

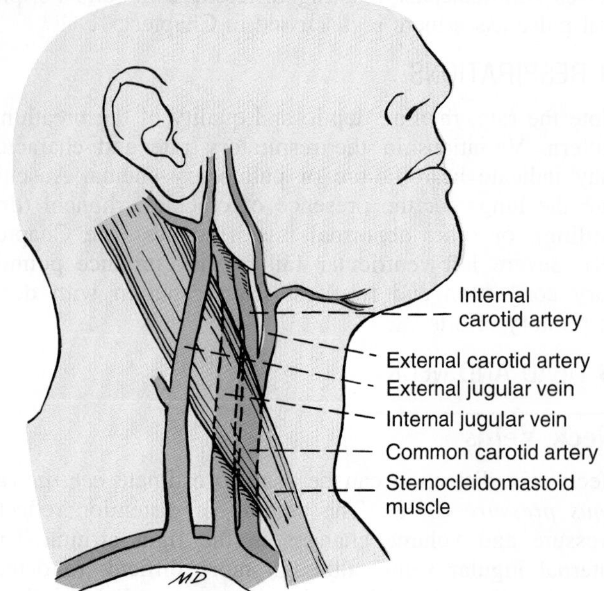

FIGURE 54–2 Location of the internal jugular vein.

Carotid Arteries

Carotid artery examination indicates the adequacy of stroke volume and the patency of the arteries. Using your finger tips, gently palpate the carotid arteries one side at a time. Check and compare the rate, rhythm, and amplitude of the pulses. Note whether a *bruit* (a blowing sound) is present by listening with the diaphragm of a stethoscope over the arteries while the client holds the breath. Tracheal breath sounds are heard while respiration is ongoing. A bruit generally indicates that the carotid artery has narrowed. Bruits typically result from atherosclerosis or radiation of sounds from an aortic valve murmur.

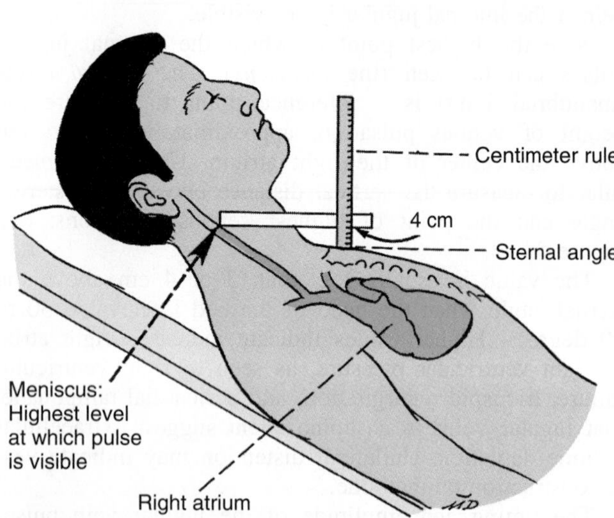

FIGURE 54–3 Estimation of jugular vein measurement to assess central venous pressure.

■ CHEST

Precordium

Perform inspection and palpation of the precordium together to determine the presence of normal and abnormal pulsations. Ideally, the client should be supine with the chest exposed. The left lateral position allows the heart to move closer to the chest wall, accentuating precordial movements and certain heart sounds. Good lighting and a warm, quiet environment are essential. Stand at the client's right side and observe the anterior chest for size, shape, symmetry of movement, and any evident pulsations. Record the location of pulsation in relation to the intercostal space and the midclavicular line. Confirm your observation with palpation. When palpating, use the fingers and palm of the hand.

The *point of maximum intensity* (PMI) or apical impulse is usually seen at the apex. The PMI is associated with left ventricular contraction and should appear at the fifth intercostal space medial to the left midclavicular line. It may be prominent in thin people and obscured in those who are obese or have large breasts. When palpated, the PMI is a single, faint, instantaneous tap beneath the fingers, no more than 2 cm in diameter. The left lateral recumbent position may enhance locating the PMI, but its position is displaced. With left ventricular enlargement and aneurysm, the PMI is more diffuse, sustained, and displaced downward and to the left of the midclavicular line.

Right ventricular enlargement can produce an abnormal pulsation that may be seen as a sustained thrust along the left sternal border. Termed *"heaves" or "lifts,"* these pulsations may be found with various disorders, such as valvular disease and pulmonary hypertension. *Thrills* represent turbulent blood flow through the heart, especially across abnormal heart valves. Use the heel or ulnar surface of the hand to palpate over each of the five cardiac landmarks (Fig. 54–4). Thrills are perceived as a rushing

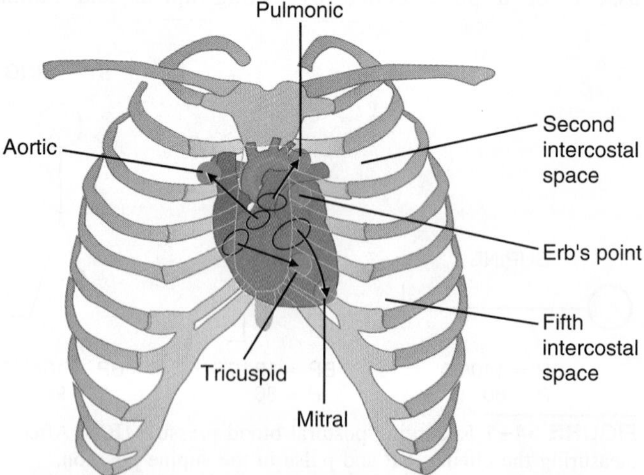

FIGURE 54–4 Precordial locations for cardiac palpation and auscultation of heart sounds. Closure of mitral and tricuspid valves produces the S_1 heart sound; closure of pulmonic and aortic (semilunar) valves produces the S_2 heart sound.

vibration, much like feeling the throat of a purring cat. Thrills are associated with significant heart murmurs. They may also be palpated over partially obstructed blood vessels.[12, 30, 38]

Heart Sounds

Auscultation of the precordium yields valuable information about normal or abnormal heart rate and rhythm, ventricular filling, and blood flow across heart valves. Assessment of heart sounds is a sophisticated skill, requiring study of heart sound characteristics and extensive clinical practice. To become skilled, you must be thoroughly familiar with normal cardiac sounds. With practice and experience, you will be able to detect abnormal heart sounds.

Discerning abnormal heart sounds is difficult even for skilled practitioners under ideal circumstances. The sensitivity of the human ear falls sharply when the frequency of sound vibrations is below 1000 Hz. Most cardiac murmurs and sounds are below that frequency. A reliable stethoscope is a must. Use the bell to hear low-pitched sounds and the diaphragm to hear high-pitched sounds. Always warm the chestpiece before placing it on the client's skin.

The environment is key to successful auscultation. The surroundings should be warm and quiet. An exposed chest is ideal, but prevent shivering, which can greatly distort heart sound transmission. Instruct the client to breathe through the nose while supine. The left lateral position may facilitate auscultation. An upright position, leaning forward and holding the breath after exhalation, helps when assessing early diastolic murmurs and pericardial friction rubs.

Always use a systematic approach when evaluating heart sounds. Methods vary. Develop your own routine to ensure a thorough assessment each time you perform cardiac auscultation.

Examination of heart sounds may progress from the base (right second intercostal space) of the heart to the apex or from the apex to the base. Whichever approach you use, pay special attention to each of the precordial locations diagrammed in Figure 54–4. Each area corresponds to a specific valvular outflow tract. Concentrate on one component of the cardiac cycle at a time, that is, the first heart sound (S_1), then the second heart sound (S_2), and so on. It is difficult to assess everything at one time. As many as three or four abnormalities may occur simultaneously. Listen to several complete cardiac cycles at each of the five precordial areas. Listen carefully, noting the quality (crisp or muffled), intensity (loud or soft), rhythm (irregular or regular), and presence of extra sounds (murmurs, gallops, rubs, or clicks). Repeat this process using the bell over each of the precordial areas.[7, 12, 30, 38]

NORMAL HEART SOUNDS

The *first heart sound (S_1)* is linked to closure of the mitral and tricuspid valves (atrioventricular [AV] valves). It marks the onset of systole (ventricular contraction). It is heard best with the diaphragm at the apex (the mitral valve area) and left lower sternal border (the tricuspid valve area). S_1 results from abrupt closure of the AV valves, which causes some blood turbulence and vibration of structures within the ventricles. This vibration is transmitted across the chest wall as a heart sound. Phonetically, if both heart sounds are appreciated as "lub-dup," S_1 is "lub." Although closure of both mitral and tricuspid valves is heard as a single sound, the mitral valve closes a fraction of a second earlier.

The intensity of S_1 may vary in certain pathologic conditions. Diseased and stiffened AV valves (as seen in rheumatic heart disease) may augment S_1; rhythms of asynchrony between the atria and ventricles (as in atrial fibrillation and AV block) cause varying intensity of S_1. If you are not sure which sound is S_1, check the carotid artery for a pulsation or look for the upstroke of the R wave in the QRS complex (described later) on the ECG monitor.

The *second heart sound (S_2)* is related to closure of the pulmonic and aortic (semilunar) valves and is heard best with the diaphragm at the aortic area. Phonetically, it is the "dup" of the heart sounds. It signifies the end of systole and the onset of diastole (ventricular filling). At the base of the heart, normal S_2 is always louder than S_1, whereas both sounds are usually of nearly equal intensity at the left sternal border over Erb's point. Usually, S_1 is the louder of the two sounds at the apex and occurs just after or along with the carotid pulse.

Knowing the usual quality of sounds that occur over the precordium can help you to distinguish between S_1 and S_2 during rapid heart rates. Simultaneous palpation of the carotid pulse during auscultation also helps discriminate sounds. Carotid pulsation occurs with systole or S_1. Figure 54–5 shows the relationship of heart sounds to events during the cardiac cycle.

Physiologic (normal) *splitting of S_2* occurs during inspiration. Normal splitting results from delayed closure of the pulmonic valve. During S_2, both the aortic and pulmonic components of S_2 (A_2 and P_2) can be heard. Inspiration creates negative pressure within the thoracic cavity, "pulling" blood from the periphery into the right side of the heart. Because of this transient augmentation of venous return, right ventricular volume increases and emptying is delayed, delaying pulmonic valve closure. The "split-second heart sound" is best heard over the pulmonic and mitral areas. The two components of S_2 occur so close together that the pause between them produces a phonetic gap similar to the "pl" sound in the word "split." If a split S_2 is heard when the client is sitting or during expiration, it usually indicates right ventricular failure or other cardiac disease.[2, 7]

ABNORMAL HEART SOUNDS

Many abnormal heart sounds may indicate a serious heart disorder or change in cardiac function. You may not be able to label each abnormality, but with a thorough understanding of the normal sounds, you should be able to recognize various abnormal sounds and refer the problem to the physician.

PATHOLOGIC SPLITTING OF S_2

A wide splitting of S_2 may be heard during both inspiration and expiration, with an increase during inspiration. This form of splitting occurs in right bundle branch block and is related to delay in depolarization of the right ventricle and late closure of the pulmonic valve. Fixed split-

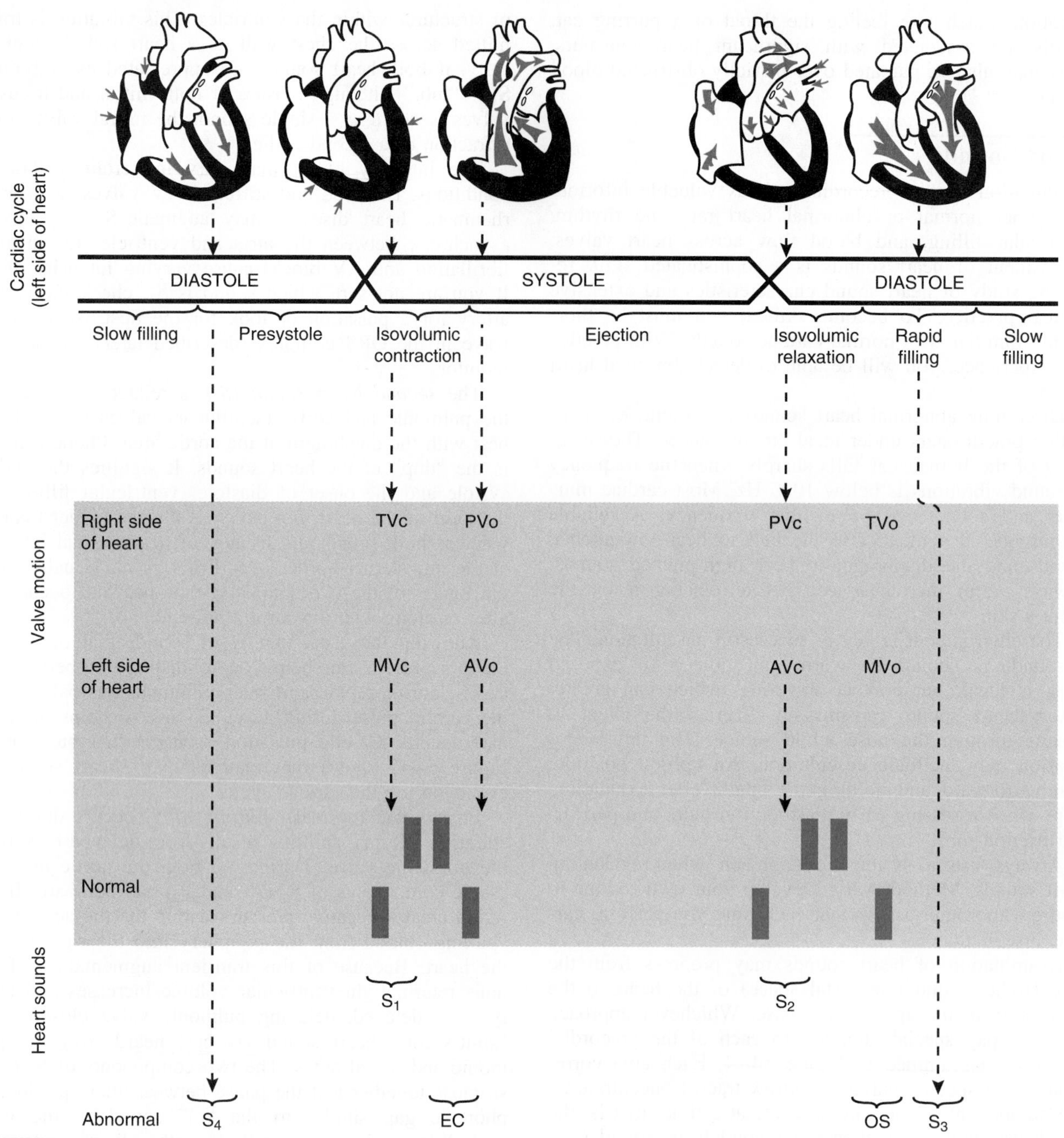

FIGURE 54–5 Relationship of heart sounds to events during the cardiac cycle. Understanding heart sounds is facilitated when they are correlated with cardiac cycle events and valvular movements. MVc, mitral valve closing; TVc, tricuspid valve closing; PVo, pulmonic valve opening; AVo, aortic valve opening; AVc, aortic valve closing; PVc, pulmonic valve closing; TVo, tricuspid valve opening; MVo, mitral valve opening; EC, ejection click; OS, opening snap.

ting is the hallmark of atrial septal defect. This form of S_2 split is continuous and does not vary with respirations. Fixed splitting occurs because the emptying of the right ventricle is prolonged. Paradoxical splitting results from a delay in closure of the aortic valve because of aortic stenosis, left bundle branch block, or patent ductus arteriosus. In paradoxical splitting, the S_2 split is heard during expiration rather than inspiration.[2, 7]

GALLOPS

Diastolic filling sounds or *gallops* (S_3 and S_4) occur during the two phases of ventricular filling. Sudden changes of inflow volume cause vibrations of the valves and ventricular supporting structures, producing low-pitched sounds that occur either early (S_3) or late (S_4) in diastole. Such sounds can originate in either side of the heart. These extra heart sounds create a triplet rhythm, acoustically mimicking a horse's gallop. For that reason, the term "gallop" is often used to denote these heart sounds.

A gallop sound that occurs in early diastole, during passive, rapid filling of the ventricles, is known as the *third heart sound (S_3)*. It is heard best with the bell at the apex and with the client in the left lateral recumbent position. An S_3 immediately follows S_2 and is a dull, low-pitched sound. An S_3 gallop is considered a normal finding in children and young adults. In adults older than 30 years of age, an S_3 is considered characteristic of left ventricular dysfunction.[2, 7]

Clinical conditions associated with an S_3 gallop are those that precipitate heart failure, such as myocardial infarction and valvular incompetence. Third heart sounds arising in the left ventricle are best heard at the apex, with the client on the left side. Right ventricular gallops are best detected along the left sternal border, with the client supine.

A *fourth heart sound,* or *S_4 gallop*, occurs in the later stage of diastole, during atrial contraction and active filling of the ventricles. This soft, low-pitched sound is heard immediately before S_1 and is also referred to as an atrial gallop. An atrial gallop is found most commonly in disorders involving increased stiffness of the ventricle, such as ventricular hypertrophy, ischemia, and fibrosis. These conditions are often associated with elevated diastolic ventricular pressures and a vigorous atrial contraction. The ventricles become resistant to filling, and the structures within the ventricles vibrate in response to the added blood input during the "atrial kick."

The presence of S_4 may result from myocardial infarction (transient S_4), hypertension, hypertrophy, fibrosis, cardiomyopathy, cor pulmonale, aortic stenosis, or pulmonic stenosis. S_4 is never heard in the absence of atrial contraction (i.e., atrial fibrillation). S_4 is heard best with the bell of the stethoscope at the apex, with the client in the supine, left lateral position.[2, 7]

QUADRUPLE RHYTHM

At times a quadruple rhythm is noted when both S_3 and S_4 are audible. Clients with this unusual heart sound often have tachycardia, which causes the diastolic filling sounds to fuse, forming a *summation gallop* that may be louder than S_1 or S_2. It can be heard best at the apex and resembles the sound of a galloping horse.

CLICKS

Clicks are extracardiac sounds that can be heard any time during the cardiac cycle in clients with aortic stenosis, valve prolapse, or prosthetic valves. There are three basic types of clicks[2, 7]:

1. *Click.* A *simple click* occurs during systole and is usually caused by a prolapsed mitral valve.
2. *Ejection sound.* An *ejection click* is a high-pitched sound heard in systole. It can be associated with either opening of the semilunar valves or prolapse (inversion) of the mitral valve. Ejection clicks heard during early systole usually result from sudden tensing of the aortic or pulmonic root at the peak of systolic ejection. They are often the result of high ventricular pressure generated in order to open a rigid, calcified aortic valve. Middle to late systolic clicks are more likely to be due to a benign form of mitral insufficiency (regurgitation). When a billowing mitral valve allows prolapse of the leaflets into the left atrium, a click can be heard as the chordae tendineae act as a tether and prohibit further leaflet excursion into the atria.
3. *Opening snap.* Valves normally open silently, but when they become calcified or rigid from disease, greater pressure is required to force them open. When they do "pop" open, they produce a characteristic sound. Opening snaps occur with the opening of a stenotic mitral and (rarely) tricuspid valve. The resulting sound is brief, high-pitched, and of a snapping quality. It is heard early in diastole at the apex using a diaphragm.

PERICARDIAL FRICTION RUB

A pericardial friction rub is produced by inflammation of the pericardial sac (pericarditis). The roughened parietal and visceral layers of the pericardium rub against each other during cardiac motion. The sound has three components corresponding to cardiac activity: ventricular systole, ventricular diastole, and atrial systole.

A pericardial friction rub is best detected with the diaphragm at the apex and along the left sternal border. It may be accentuated when a person leans forward or lies prone and exhales. Friction rubs produce a sound that is described as "to and fro," scratchy, grating, rasping, and much like "squeaky leather." Friction rubs may be present during the first week after myocardial infarction or after open heart surgery. Differentiate a pericardial friction rub from a pleural friction rub by noting the timing of the rub in relation to breathing. Pleural friction rubs are heard during inspiration. Pericardial friction rubs are heard throughout the respiratory cycle.

MURMURS

Murmurs are heard as a consequence of turbulent blood flow through the heart and large vessels. Turbulent blood flow produces vibrations in the heart and great vessels that can be detected as a blowing or swooshing sound. Murmurs are caused by (1) increased rate or velocity of blood flow, (2) abnormal forward or backward flow across stenosed or incompetent valves, (3) flow into a dilated chamber, or (4) flow through an abnormal passage between heart chambers. Bruits are due to turbulence in vessels. Murmurs are best heard with the bell of the stethoscope when the client is in the left lateral recumbent position. Table 54–4 describes the characteristics of murmurs. Box 54–4 gives the scale for grading the loudness of murmurs.

Systolic murmurs, also called "benign" murmurs, are often caused by vigorous myocardial contraction or strong blood flow. They are common in children, adults younger than 50 years of age, and pregnant women. All diastolic murmurs are pathologic and are produced by mitral and tricuspid valve stenosis or aortic or pulmonic insufficiency.[2, 7, 12, 29, 38] Table 54–5 presents a comparison of selected heart murmurs.

Lungs

Because the cardiovascular and respiratory systems are intimately related, assessment of the cardiovascular system must include evaluation of the respiratory system. The respiratory assessment is covered in Chapter 59. Common respiratory findings related to CVD are as follows.

TACHYPNEA

Tachypnea, or rapid respirations, is often associated with pain and anxiety accompanying myocardial ischemic pain. Tachypnea is also a common compensatory mechanism in heart failure and pulmonary edema.

TABLE 54–4 CHARACTERISTICS OF MURMURS

Characteristic	Description
Location	Area where the murmur is best heard
Pitch	Classified as either high or low; describe quality as musical, harsh, blowing, or buzzing
Timing	Refers to whether the murmur occurs in systole or diastole. Systolic murmurs, unlike diastolic murmurs, are harmless
Place and duration	When the murmur occurs during the cardiac cycle: early, middle, or late. Holosystolic or pansystolic murmurs are heard during the entire systolic phase. An ejection murmur is best heard during midsystole
Loudness	Graded on a six-point scale from I (barely audible) to VI (audible without stethoscope)
Quality	A murmur's sound pattern. A *crescendo* starts low and grows louder; a *decrescendo* starts loud and gets softer; a *crescendo-decrescendo* starts softly, becomes loud, and then becomes soft again; *a plateau* is a consistent sound
Radiation	Sound migration to other parts of the body; for example, aortic murmurs often radiate to the carotid arteries, and mitral murmurs radiate to the axilla
Variations	Changes that occur with movement or interruption of normal respirations

From Alexander, R. W., et al. (Eds.). (1998). *Hurst's the heart* (9th ed.). New York: McGraw-Hill, and O'Hanlon-Nickols, T. (1997). The adult cardiovascular system. *American Journal of Nursing, 97*(12), 34–40.

CRACKLES

Crackles frequently signal left ventricular failure and usually occur just after the onset of an S_3 gallop. As pulmonary capillary pressure rises because of the backward pressure of left ventricular failure, fluid shifts into the intra-alveolar spaces and crackles can be auscultated. Crackles may also result from atelectasis (incomplete lung expansion) related to limited chest wall excursion during prolonged bed rest, chest splinting from pain, and the effects of sedatives and narcotics. Crackles are high-pitched, noncontinuous sounds. Crackles are best heard at the lung bases (because of gravitational effects on the fluid) during late inspiration.[2]

BLOOD-TINGED SPUTUM

Pink, frothy sputum may indicate acute pulmonary edema. This manifestation accompanies diffuse pulmonary crackles and denotes serious left ventricular failure. Frank hemoptysis may be associated with pulmonary embolus. A cough frequently occurs with hemoptysis.

CHEYNE-STOKES RESPIRATIONS

Cheyne-Stokes respirations are characterized by abnormal periods of deep breathing alternating with periods of apnea. They are a common finding in heart failure, anemia, and brain damage (from anoxic encephalopathy).

BOX 54–4 Grading of Heart Murmurs

Grade I	Faint; heard after listener has "tuned in"
Grade II	Faint murmur heard immediately
Grade III	Moderately loud, with accompanying thrill
Grade IV	Loud
Grade V	Very loud; heard only with the stethoscope
Grade VI	Very loud; heard without the stethoscope

■ ABDOMEN

Examination of the abdomen provides information regarding cardiac competence. Findings, however, are of less value than those of other examinations discussed in this section. Abdominal assessment is described in Chapters 28 and 42.

Inspection and Palpation

Inspection may reveal abdominal distention. Palpation may confirm the presence of *ascites* (fluid accumulation in the peritoneal cavity) and an enlarged liver. Both of these findings indicate liver failure, which can be a sequela (result) of chronic right ventricular failure. In addition, you may elicit a hepatojugular reflex in the client with right ventricular distention.

After assessing for jugular vein distention, apply mild pressure with one hand over the liver for 1 minute. An increase in jugular vein distention during and immediately after liver compression indicates chronically elevated right ventricular pressure.

Auscultation

Auscultation can yield the following clues about cardiovascular function. Decreased bowel tones may accompany potassium (K^+) depletion. Potassium depletion can complicate chronic diuretic use without sufficient potassium replacement. Increased bowel tones, indicative of hypermotility, may result from laxative use or may be a side effect of certain antiarrhythmic agents (such as quinidine). Loud bruits, heard with the bell just over or above the umbilicus, may indicate an aortic obstruction or aortic aneurysm (the latter can be detected by a palpable abdominal pulsation). Bruits heard over the upper midline or toward the back typically arise from renal arterial stenosis.

TABLE 54–5 HEART MURMURS

Type of Heart Sound	Origin	Preferred Method of Auscultation
Systolic murmurs Ejection type 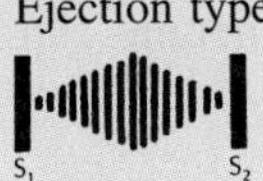	Systolic ejection murmurs are associated with forward blood flow during ventricular contraction across stenotic aortic or pulmonic valves	Use the stethoscope diaphragm. Ejection murmurs are typically of medium pitch and harsh quality and may be associated with early ejection click. Aortic ejection murmurs are best heard over aortic valve and radiate into the neck, down left sternal border, and occasionally to apex. May be accompanied by decreased S_2. Pulmonic ejection murmurs are heard best over pulmonic valve, and radiate toward left shoulder and left neck vessels. May be accompanied by a wide split S_2
Pansystolic regurgitant murmurs 	Pansystolic murmurs occur when blood regurgitates through incompetent mitral and tricuspid valves (AV valves) or ventricular septal defect as pressures rise during systole and blood seeks chambers of lower pressure. Damage to valve leaflets, papillary muscles, and chordae tendineae results in mitral valve insufficiency (blood regurgitates from left ventricle to left atrium) and tricuspid valve insufficiency (blood regurgitates from right ventricle to right atrium). Ventricular septal defect results in blood regurgitation from left ventricle to right ventricle	All regurgitant murmurs are high-pitched, and those of AV valve incompetence have blowing quality. Mitral regurgitant murmurs are heard at apex, radiate into left axilla, and may be accompanied by ejection click and signs of left ventricular failure. Tricuspid regurgitant murmurs are heard loudest over the tricuspid area and radiate into the sternum. Ventricular septal defects are usually loud, harsh, and heard best over left sternal border in fourth, fifth, and sixth intercostal spaces and radiate over the precordium but not the axilla
Early systolic murmurs 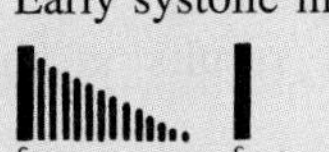	Early systolic (innocent) murmurs are associated with high cardiac outputs, as blood flow velocity is increased across normal semilunar valves. Causes include anemia, tachycardia, thyrotoxicosis, and fever. Murmur disappears with correction of underlying condition. Normal variant in children	These are best heard with bell over base of heart or along lower left sternal border. Are usually no greater than grade II, are of medium pitch, and have blowing quality. Intensity may increase during inspiration with client in left recumbent position or with increased heart rates
Late systolic murmurs 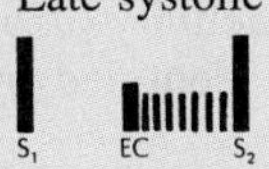	These imply mild mitral regurgitation as mitral valve balloons into left atrium late in ventricular systole	Best heard with diaphragm of stethoscope over apex and are often preceded by mid-systolic or late systolic ejection click
Diastolic murmurs Early diastolic murmur S_1 S_2 S_1	These (decrescendo murmurs) are usually caused by semilunar valve insufficiency, with regurgitation due to valvular deformity or dilation of valvular ring. Are heard immediately after S_2 and then diminish in intensity as pressure in aorta or pulmonary artery falls and ventricles fill	Heard best with diaphragm at base of heart while the client leans forward in deep expiration. Are high-pitched and blowing and radiate down left sternal border, perhaps to apex or down right sternal border. Accompanying signs of heart failure may be present
Diastolic filling rumbles S_1 S_2 S_1	Caused as blood flows across stenotic AV valves (more often mitral). May also occur during augmented blood flow across normal AV valves. Murmur has two phases, becoming louder as the blood flow from the atrium to ventricle increases with passive ventricular filling just after AV valve opening and again during atrial contraction (presystole)	With the bell, this murmur is heard over only a small area at and just medial to the apex. Exercise and a left lateral position of the client increase the intensity of the sound. It is a low-pitched, rumbling sound often accompanied by an augmented S_1 and an opening snap

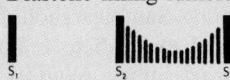

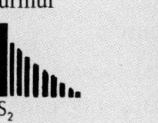

AV, atrioventricular.

Modified from Huang, S. L., et al. (1989). *Coronary care nursing* (2nd ed., p. 19). Philadelphia: W. B. Saunders; and Alexander, R. W., et al. (Eds.). (1998). *Hurst's the heart* (9th ed.) New York: McGraw-Hill.

Diagnostic Tests

The four most common types of diagnostic procedures used in the diagnosis of CVD are:

- Laboratory tests
- Graphic procedures (e.g., ECG)
- Radiographic (x-ray) studies
- Hemodynamic studies

Nursing responsibilities in diagnostic testing include the following:

- Explaining the purpose and the procedure and answering any questions
- Witnessing signing of the consent form
- Scheduling the test
- Providing any necessary preliminary care (e.g., adjustments in medications and special diets)
- Promoting maximal emotional and physical comfort

After the procedure, review instructions for home care, returning to work, and general aftercare.

LABORATORY TESTS

Laboratory test data are used to (1) diagnose a variety of cardiovascular ailments (e.g., myocardial infarction), (2) screen people considered at risk for CVD, (3) determine baseline values, (4) identify concurrent disorders (e.g., diabetes mellitus, electrolyte imbalance) that may affect treatment, and (5) evaluate the effectiveness of intervention. Tests that are more commonly used to determine cardiovascular function and disease are discussed here.[31]

Prepare the client for the laboratory test by explaining the procedure. Determine whether the client should fast or refrain from intake of a particular substance before blood is drawn; if so, provide clear instructions. Determination of therapeutic levels of specific medications may require documenting the last time the drug was taken by the client to correlate with the laboratory value. Ask whether the client is taking any blood thinners such as warfarin sodium (Coumadin), which would require a longer time and pressure over the venipuncture site.

Handle blood samples carefully. Gently invert laboratory tubes to prevent clotting of specimens for a complete blood count (CBC). Avoid vigorous handling of specimens, which may lead to hemolysis and falsely elevated levels of intracellular ions, such as potassium and magnesium. Apply pressure to the puncture site until bleeding stops. Assess the site for hematoma formation.

Complete Blood Cell Count

The *red blood cell (RBC) count* or *erythrocyte count* is usually decreased in rheumatic fever and infective endocarditis. The count is usually increased in heart diseases characterized by inadequate tissue oxygenation, for example, right-to-left congenital shunts and heart conditions accompanied by obstructive lung disease.

Measuring the packed cell volume, or *hematocrit*, is the easiest way to ascertain the concentration of red blood cells in the blood. An elevated hematocrit can result from obstructive lung disease and conditions of vascular volume depletion with hemoconcentration (e.g., hypovolemic shock and excessive diuresis). Decreases in hematocrit and hemoglobin indicate anemia, which is commonly caused by hemorrhage, hemolysis (from prosthetic valves), and chronic disease states. Clients with anemia have a significant reduction in red blood cell mass and a decrease in oxygen-carrying capacity. Anemia can be manifest as angina or exacerbate heart failure and produce heart murmurs.

The *white blood cell (WBC) count* is elevated in infectious and inflammatory diseases of the heart (e.g., infective endocarditis and pericarditis). It is also elevated after myocardial infarction because large numbers of WBCs are necessary to dispose of the necrotic tissue resulting from the infarction.

Cardiac Enzymes

Enzymes are special proteins that catalyze chemical reactions in living cells. Cardiac enzymes are present in high concentrations in myocardial tissue. Tissue damage causes release of enzymes from their intracellular storage areas. For example, myocardial infarction causes cellular anoxia, which alters membrane permeability and causes spillage of enzymes into the surrounding tissue. This leakage of enzymes can be detected by rising plasma levels.

Myoglobin is a useful marker of myocardial necrosis that is rapidly released from the circulation within 1 to 2 hours of infarction. Its release allows very early detection, but its short half-life makes it less useful in clients who present several hours after onset. Measurement of myoglobin levels is not recommended if there is evidence of muscle damage, trauma, or renal failure because of the greater potential for false-positive test results in these circumstances.[28]

The enzymes most commonly used to detect myocardial infarction are *creatine kinase* (CK) and *lactic acid dehydrogenase* (LDH). Serum elevations of these two enzymes occur in sequence after myocardial insult. Because these enzymes are also found in other organs and tissues (e.g., skeletal muscle and liver), cardiac specificity must be determined by measuring isoenzyme activity. *Isoenzymes* are various forms of CK and LDH, identified by a process known as electrophoresis.

There are three isoenzymes of CK:

- CK-MM (skeletal muscle)
- CK-MB (myocardial muscle)
- CK-BB (brain)

Elevated CK-MB indicates myocardial damage. Plasma MB is significantly elevated within 6 to 8 hours of the onset of manifestations of myocardial infarction, maximal levels are reached between 14 and 36 hours, and levels return to normal after 48 to 72 hours. Samples should be taken immediately on admission and every 6 to 8 hours for the first 24 hours. Diagnosis of injury requires no fewer than two samples separated by at least 4 hours.

Of the five isoenzymes for LDH (numbered 1 to 5), only LDH_1 and LDH_2 are cardiac-specific. If the serum concentration of LDH_1 is higher than the concentration of LDH_2, the pattern is said to have "flipped," signifying myocardial necrosis. Eighty per cent of clients have elevations in LDH within 48 hours after myocardial infarction.

The use of *troponin* has led to increased specificity in the detection of myocardial infarction. Troponin has three components: I, C, and T. Troponin I modulates the contractile state, troponin C binds calcium, and troponin T binds I and C. Although troponin is present in all striated muscle, troponin components in cardiac muscle have different amino acid sequences. Therefore, antibodies against cardiac troponins I and T are very specific. Elevated levels of troponin I are as sensitive as CK-MB for the detection of myocardial injury. They correlate highly with the development of new areas of regional dysfunction determined by echocardiography and correlate in a linear fashion with the development of complications. Troponins are useful for diagnosis after 4 to 6 hours have elapsed. Once present, troponin I persists for 4 to 7 days.[15, 19, 28]

Because of their higher specificity for myocardial injury, troponins can be used to exclude myocardial infarction when CK-MB may be falsely positive, as in athletes, clients with skeletal trauma, and after direct-current (DC) cardioversion, or when CK totals may be high and MB missed, as in the postoperative state.

As well as indicating myocardial damage, elevations in serum cardiac enzymes can reveal the timing of the acute cardiac event (see Chapter 58).

Blood Coagulation Tests

Blood coagulation tests are used to examine the ability of blood to clot. Evaluate coagulation tests such as *prothrombin time* and *partial thromboplastin time* in people with a greater tendency to form thrombi (e.g., clients with atrial fibrillation, infective endocarditis, or prosthetic valves). Research has shown an increase in coagulation factors during and after a myocardial infarction. Therefore, the client is at greater risk for thrombophlebitis and extension of clots in the coronary artery. Chapter 74 discusses coagulation tests in detail.

Serum Lipids

Serum lipids play a major role in the development of atherosclerosis. They are composed of fatty substances that are insoluble in water. These lipids are derived from fats in the diet or synthesized in the liver. The lipid profile shows serum cholesterol, triglyceride, and lipoprotein levels and is used to assess the risk for development of coronary artery disease. Serum lipids are discussed in Chapter 51.

Serum Electrolytes

Fluid and electrolyte regulation may be affected by cardiovascular disorders. Electrolyte balance is also altered by certain medications. Chapters 12 and 13 describe fluids and electrolytes.

POTASSIUM. The serum potassium level decreases as a result of diuretic therapy, vomiting, diarrhea, and alkalosis. *Hypokalemia* (abnormally low potassium) increases cardiac electrical instability, the occurrence of ventricular dysrhythmias, and the risk of digitalis toxicity. A characteristic change on the ECG is a U wave. A high serum potassium level is usually associated with kidney and endocrine disorders. *Hyperkalemia* can lead to a tall T wave on the ECG, asystole, and ventricular dysrhythmias.

SODIUM. The serum sodium level reflects water balance and may decrease (i.e., *hyponatremia*, indicating water excess) with heart failure, stress, excessive intravenous (IV) infusion of hypotonic fluids, and vomiting. Extensive use of diuretics and severely restricted sodium intake also lower serum sodium.

CALCIUM. The serum calcium level decreases as a result of multiple transfusions of citrated blood, renal failure, alkalosis, and laxative and antacid abuse (phosphate excess). *Hypocalcemia* can lead to serious ventricular dysrhythmias, a prolonged QT interval, and cardiac arrest. *Hypercalcemia* occurs with thiazide diuretic use, acidosis, adrenal insufficiency, immobility, and vitamin D excess. Hypercalcemia shortens the QT interval and causes AV block, tachycardia, bradycardia, digitalis hypersensitivity, and cardiac arrest.

MAGNESIUM. Magnesium helps regulate intracellular metabolism, activates essential enzymes, and aids in the transport of sodium and potassium across the cell membrane. It plays a vital role in neuromuscular excitability.

Hypomagnesemia may result from prolonged use of diuretics, malnutrition, chronic alcoholism, severe diarrhea, and dehydration. Manifestations include mental apathy, facial tics, leg cramps, respiratory depression, and severe cardiac dysrhythmias, including ventricular tachycardia and fibrillation. *Hypermagnesemia* may develop in the client with chronic renal failure. Manifestations include profound muscle weakness, hyporeflexia, hypotension, and bradycardia with a prolonged PR interval and wide QRS complex.

PHOSPHORUS. Most extracellular phosphorus is present in the bone with calcium (85% of the body's total phosphorus). A small amount of phosphorus is found in intracellular fluid. There it helps regulate energy formation (adenosine triphosphate [ATP]) and maintain acid-base balance and neuromuscular excitability. Phosphate levels are inversely related to calcium levels as the kidneys retain or excrete one or the other. Interpret the two levels together.

Hypophosphatemia may result from hyperparathyroidism, diabetic ketoacidosis, prolonged use of IV dextrose infusions, or renal tubular acidosis. Manifestations of hypophosphatemia include bleeding, decreased WBC levels, muscular weakness (including respiratory muscles), and nausea and vomiting.

Hyperphosphatemia usually occurs in clients with chronic renal failure or skeletal disease (including healing fractures) and those undergoing chemotherapy. Manifestations are similar to those of hypocalcemia, with muscle tetany being the most common finding.

Blood Urea Nitrogen

Blood urea nitrogen (BUN) is an indicator of renal function, specifically the ability of the kidney to excrete urea and protein. It is elevated in kidney diseases, during water and saline depletion, and cardiac disorders that adversely affect renal circulation, for example, heart failure and cardiogenic shock.

Blood Glucose

Diabetes mellitus is a major risk factor for the development of atherosclerosis. In addition, the stress of an acute cardiac event can greatly elevate blood glucose, causing unstable *hyperglycemia* in clients with latent diabetes mellitus. For these reasons, blood glucose is routinely assessed in all clients with acute cardiovascular disorders.

■ ELECTROCARDIOGRAM

PROCEDURE

The ECG is an essential tool in evaluating the heart rhythm. Electrocardiography detects and amplifies the very small electrical potential changes between different points on the surface of the body as the myocardial cells depolarize and repolarize, causing the heart to contract. The same electrical impulses spread outward from the heart to the skin, where they can be detected by electrodes attached to the skin. The ECG displays the electrical action of the heart.

There are several types of ECGs: continuous monitoring, 12-lead, signal-averaged, and Holter monitored ECGs. Analysis of ECG waveforms allows identification of disorders of cardiac rate, rhythm, or conduction.

Electrocardiography is a common noninvasive test. It is performed for clients older than 40 years of age before surgery to detect any unknown heart disease and is frequently used for clients with known or suspected heart disease.

PREPROCEDURE CARE

Prepare the client for a 12-lead ECG or continuous monitoring. Explain that the test helps evaluate the heart's function by recording its electrical activity. The steps required for ECG monitoring are (1) attaching the electrodes to the client's skin, (2) connecting the electrodes to the monitor by a cable, and (3) adjusting the monitor to obtain a readable ECG. During the procedure, advise the client to lie still, breathe normally, and refrain from talking. Record the client's age, height, and weight, and note any cardiac medications being taken.[2]

POSTPROCEDURE CARE

After the procedure, disconnect the equipment. If using conductive gel, wipe the gel from the client's skin. If using conductive stickers, remove them unless serial ECG readings are to be done. If serial ECGs are ordered, leave the stickers in place to ensure consistent lead placement.

CONTINUOUS ELECTROCARDIOGRAM MONITORING

For the client who is undergoing continuous ECG monitoring, adjust the monitor by setting the alarms for desired high and low rates. Reassure the client that the equipment does not cause electrical shock or hurt. Clients receiving telemetry are monitored continuously with radiofrequency waves rather than by direct cable attachment. They can get up and move about their rooms or walk in the halls while their heart rhythm is monitored.

Attaching the Electrodes

Electrodes detect electrical impulses from the heart on the skin. Unless the signal is detected accurately, ECG monitoring has little value. The most common electrodes are disc-type or floating electrodes, which are separated from the skin by a spacer filled with conductive gel. The gel improves the signal by reducing local electrical interference on the skin. An adhesive ring surrounds the gel. Peel the paper backing off the pad and apply the electrode to the skin. Three electrodes are required for continuous ECG monitoring. Two of these detect the heart's activity; the third is an electrical ground.

Attach the electrodes to the lead wires before applying them to the chest wall. This process makes it unnecessary to apply pressure to the electrode, which could hurt the client and squeeze the gel outward, reducing contact.

Thorough skin preparation improves impulse conduction. Clean the areas where electrodes are to be applied. Wipe the skin with alcohol, and allow it to air-dry before applying the electrodes. If the client has a great deal of chest hair, clip the hair to improve contact.

Position the electrodes on the chest wall by selecting locations that will provide the clearest ECG waveforms. Two common positions are (1) the conventional position and (2) the modified chest lead position (Fig. 54–6). The lead II waveform (shown) is the most common rhythm strip lead. MCL_1 (shown), V_1, and V_6 are more helpful for detecting dysrhythmia. When close monitoring of ST

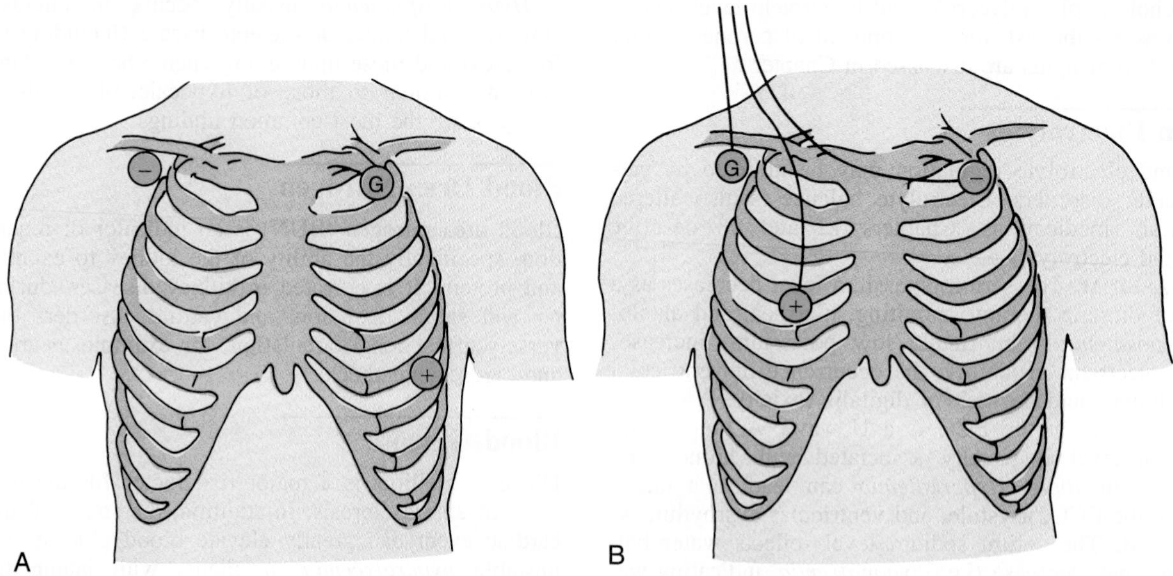

FIGURE 54–6 Common positions for continuous monitoring lead placement. Use lead II *(A)* or lead V_1 *(B)*. (From Phillips, R. E., & Feeney M. K. [1990]. *The cardiac rhythms. A systematic approach to interpretation* [3rd ed.]. Philadelphia: W. B. Saunders.).

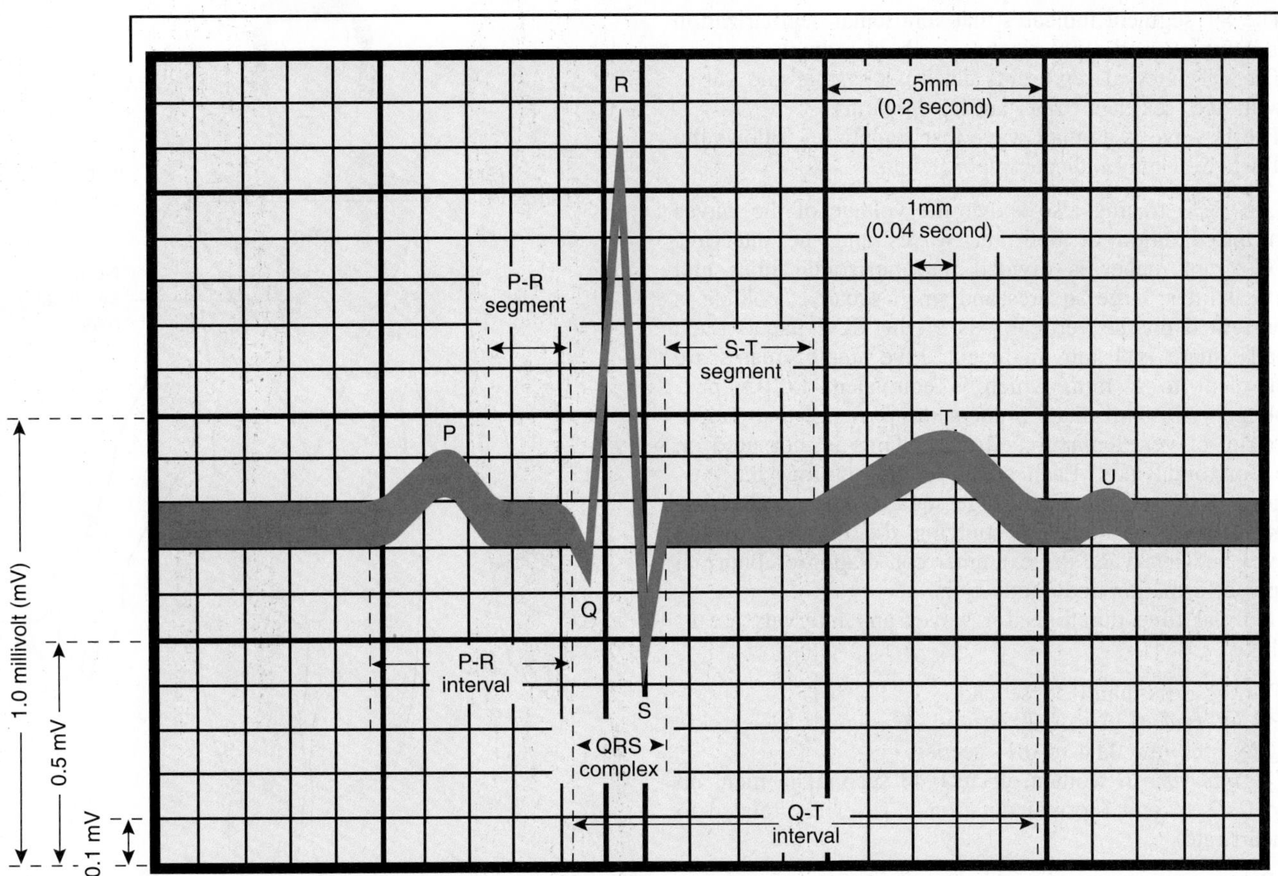

FIGURE 54–7 Normal electrocardiographic (ECG) pattern. The P wave represents depolarization of the atria to the ventricles. The QRS complex represents depolarization of the ventricles, and the T wave represents repolarization of the ventricles. The small U wave is sometimes seen following the T wave. Time and voltage lines of ECG paper: *vertically,* 1 mm = 0.1 mV; 5 mm = 0.5 mV; 10 mm = 1.0 mV; *horizontally,* one small box = 0.04 second; five small boxes = 0.20 second; 25 small boxes = 1 second.

segments is essential, such as after cardiac bypass surgery, thrombolytic therapy, or coronary angioplasty, the lead most closely associated with the area of involved heart muscle should be monitored. Change electrodes if the tracing is unclear, the electrodes become dry, or skin contact is lost. Electrodes should be routinely changed every 48 hours to avoid skin irritation and to ensure that electrode gel is sufficient for clear conduction.

Connecting the Monitor

The electrodes are connected to the monitor by lead wires, which are 12 to 18 inches long. One end snaps onto the electrode, and the other end is attached to a cable that is connected to the monitor. The cable has a receptacle for the attachment of each wire. The receptacle and lead wires are color coded to facilitate connection.

Adjusting the Monitor

The ECG pattern should be clear and distinct. If the pattern is not clear, recheck the first steps. Monitor adjustments depend on the brand of monitor in use. Refer to the operating instructions for assistance.

Setting the Alarms

Set alarm limits appropriately to signal any acute changes. Many monitors have default alarm settings. Verify these for each client. If there are no default settings or institutional standards, alarm limits should be set approximately 20 beats above and below the client's typical heart rate.

At times, false alarms may occur because of poor electrode contact or client movement. Occasionally, you may find that the alarm limits have been set far apart (e.g., 40 to 180 beats per minute [BPM]) or, worse, that the alarms have been turned off completely. This practice defeats the purpose of the alarm system and should never be adopted.

Electrocardiogram Tracings

When continuous ECG monitoring is used, assess the heart rhythm hourly. Log rhythm strips into the medical record routinely as well as when dysrhythmias are noted. Dysrhythmias are discussed in Chapter 57.

The impulse waves, recorded by the ECG machine on graph paper, are arbitrarily designated by the letters P, Q, R, S, and T. The QRS letters are generally referred to as the QRS complex. Figure 54–7 depicts the typical ECG pattern formed by these waves.

The components of the ECG are defined as follows:

- The P wave represents depolarization of the atria.
- The PR interval represents the time it takes for the impulse to spread from the atria to the ventricles.
- The QRS complex represents depolarization of the ventricles.

- The T wave represents repolarization of the ventricles.
- The ST segment indicates that ventricular depolarization is complete and repolarization is about to begin.
- The QT interval represents electrical systole and varies with age, sex, heart rate, and medications.
- The U wave is a small wave that sometimes follows the T wave. It may indicate hypokalemia.

An ECG tracing also shows the voltage of the waves and the duration of both the waves and the intervals. ECG graph paper is divided into horizontal lines and vertical lines, large squares and small squares. Voltage is represented on the vertical axis of the ECG paper. Each small square is 1 mm in height. Five small squares are equivalent to 5 mm, which is equivalent to 0.5 mV. Voltage yields information about the presence and degree of atrial or ventricular hypertrophy. Time is measured on the horizontal axis. Each small square signifies the passage of 0.04 second. Each large square indicates the passage of 0.20 second. By studying the duration of the waves and intervals, the examiner can diagnose abnormal impulse formation and conduction.

Normal time durations for waves and intervals are as follows:

- *P wave:* less than 0.11 second
- *PR interval:* 0.12 to 0.20 second (average, 0.16 second)
- *QRS complex:* 0.04 to 0.11 second
- *QT interval:* in women, up to 0.43 second; in men, up to 0.42 second (normal duration is inversely related to heart rate)

Because of its normal variation in configuration, more must be said about the QRS complex. The Q wave is always the first downward (negative) deflection of the complex. The R wave is always the first upward (positive) deflection. If there is a negative deflection (below the baseline) after an R wave, it is labeled an S wave. In most instances, a Q wave is not obvious on the ECG of the normal heart. The QRS complex may appear as a mostly positive or mostly negative deflection, depending on the recording electrode used.

Electrocardiogram Variations

The 12-Lead Electrocardiogram

Indications for a 12-lead ECG are listed in Box 54–5.

The standard ECG has a 12-lead system, offering 12 points of reference for recording the electrical activity of the heart. The 12-lead ECG can be conceptualized as 12 different views of the heart, looking in both horizontal and vertical planes. The standard 12-lead ECG has six *limb* leads (used to view the heart in a frontal or vertical plane) and six *precordial* leads (used to view the heart in a horizontal plane).

BOX 54–5 Indications for a 12-Lead Electrocardiogram

Dysrhythmias
Chest pain
Myocardial infarction
Heart rate determination
Chamber dilation or hypertrophy
Preoperative assessment
Pericarditis
Effect of medications (especially cardiac)
Effect of systemic disease on the heart (i.e., renal or pulmonary disease)
Effect of electrolyte disturbances (especially potassium)

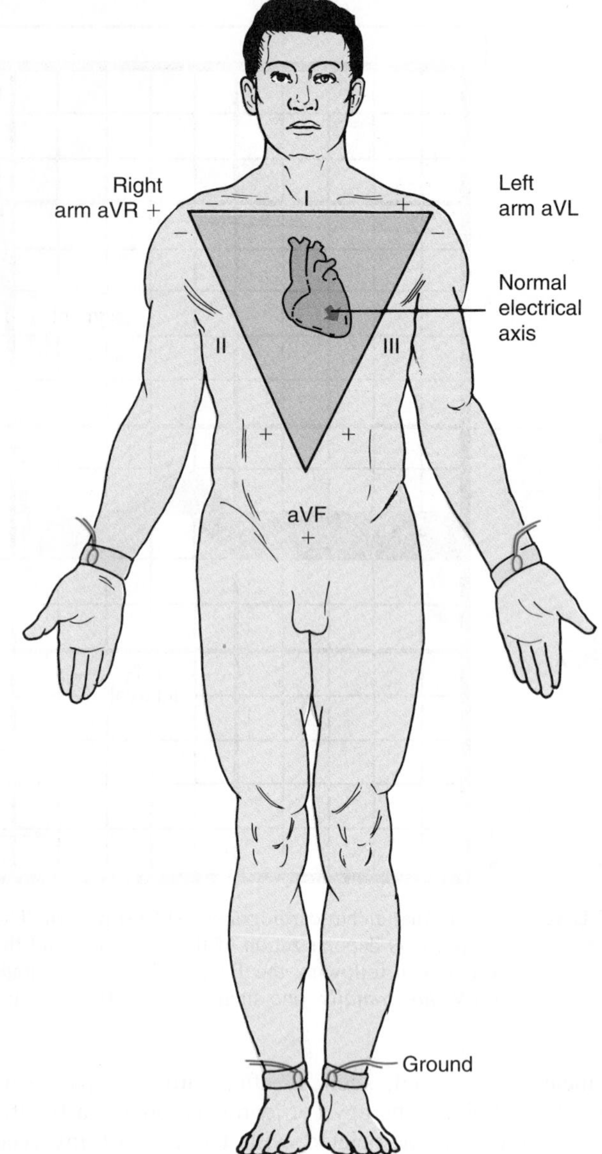

FIGURE 54–8 Standard positions for electrocardiogram leads. Bipolar limb leads are I, II, and III (Einthoven's triangle). Augmented unipolar limb leads: aVR (right arm), aVL (left arm), and aVF (left leg).

The limb leads are composed of three *bipolar* leads (leads I, II, and III) and three *unipolar* leads (leads aVR, aVL, and aVF). The bipolar leads have two electrodes and measure the difference in electrical potential flowing through the heart between two extremities. The unipolar leads compare the electrical potential of a positive electrode, placed on one limb, and a negative pole within a central terminal that averages the potential of the other two limb leads.

Standard bipolar limb leads are called I, II, and III (Fig. 54–8):

- *Lead I* measures the difference in electrical potential between the left arm and right arm.
- *Lead II* measures the difference in potential between the left leg and right arm.
- *Lead III* measures the difference in potential between the left leg and left arm.

Augmented unipolar limb leads are as follows (see Fig. 54–8):

- aVR measures electrical potential between the center of the heart and the right arm.
- aVL measures electrical potential between the center of the heart and the left arm.
- aVF measures electrical potential between the center of the heart and the left leg.

The precordial leads (V_1, V_2, V_3, V_4, V_5, and V_6) provide six views of the heart from the anterior and left lateral vantage points. These unipolar leads compare the electrical potential between a positive electrode (in the six different chest locations) and a central, negative terminal that represents an average potential of the three standard limb leads (Fig. 54–9).

Together, the 12 leads permit multidirectional examination of the electrical events in the heart. The location of pathologic change within the heart, which alters electrical activity, can be pinpointed. Table 54–6 correlates the area of infarct with expected ECG changes and coronary artery lesion location. Views from the different leads are oriented to various surfaces of the myocardium:

- Leads I, aVL, V_5, and V_6 record electrical events occurring on the lateral surface of the left ventricle.
- Leads II, III, and aVF record electrical events occurring on the inferior surface of the left ventricle.
- Leads V_1 and V_2 record electrical events occurring on the surface of the right ventricle and anterior surface of the left ventricle.
- Leads V_3 and V_4 record electrical events occurring within the septal region of the left ventricle.

The placement of 12-lead electrodes is shown in Figures 54–8 and 54–9. Unbroken contact must be made

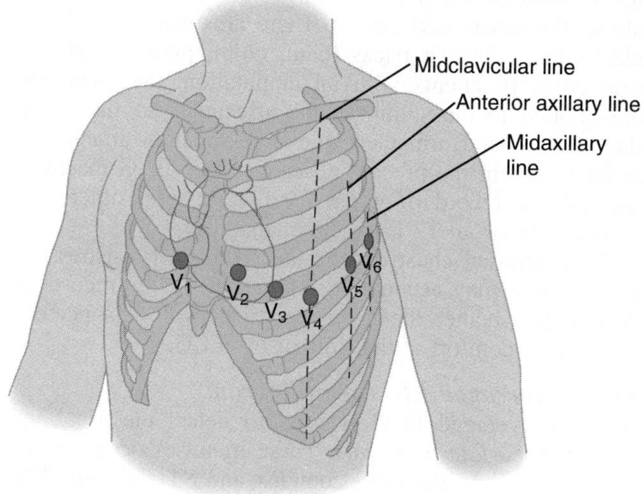

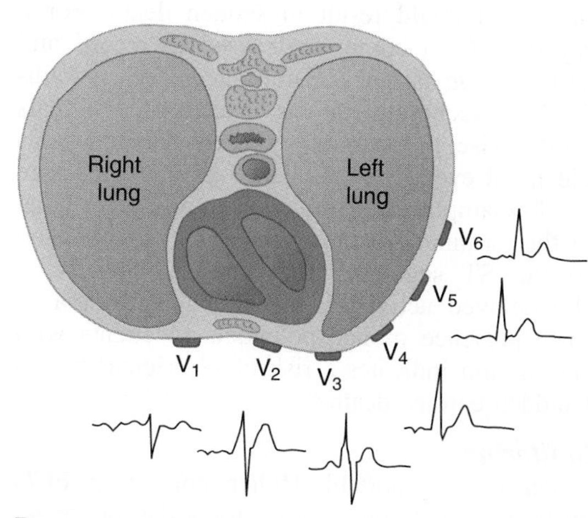

FIGURE 54–9 Placement of the chest (V) leads. *A*, Precordial (chest) lead placement. *B*, Normal electrocardiographic findings with corresponding chest leads to cross-section at the fourth rib level.

TABLE 54–6 CORONARY ARTERY LESION LOCATION, AREA OF INFARCT, AND ELECTROCARDIOGRAPHIC (ECG) CHANGES

Coronary Artery	Area of Infarct	ECG Leads	Dysrhythmias
LAD	Anterior	V_{2-4}	RBBB, LAH, Mobitz type II, CHB
	Septal	V_{1-2}	
	Anteroseptal	V_{1-4}	
Circumflex	Lateral	I, aVL	Ventricular and possibly SA and AV node conduction disturbances
	Anterolateral	I, aVL, V_{5-6}	
	Inferolateral	aVF, II, III, V_{5-6}	
	Posterior	Reciprocal, V_{1-3}	
RCA	Inferior	II, III, aVF	SA node, AV node, and His bundle conduction disturbances
	Right ventricle	II, III, aVF, V_{4-6R}	

AV, atrioventricular, CHB, complete heart block; LAD, left anterior descending, LAH, left anterior hemiblock; RBBB, right bundle branch block; RCA, right coronary artery; SA, sinoatrial.

From Alspach, J. G. (Ed.) (1992). *Instructor's resource manual for the AACN core curriculum for critical care nursing*. Philadelphia: W. B. Saunders.

between the skin and the electrodes. To facilitate contact, the electrodes are placed firmly on the flat surface just above the wrists and ankles. There are many varieties of electrodes: adhesive back, foam, cloth, plastic, and suction cups. In clients with an amputation, the electrodes are applied to the stump of the affected extremity. Note that the leg and arm electrodes must remain attached in order to obtain the precordial leads. Some ECG machines are able to record only one lead at a time; others can record 3, 6, or all 12 leads simultaneously.

Note unusual chest deformities, respiratory distress, or tremors that may account for alterations in the recording. Also note whether the client experiences angina pectoris or chest discomfort at the time of the ECG.

Signal-Averaged Electrocardiogram

A signal-averaged ECG is used to detect electrical impulses called *late potentials*. These impulses occur during diastole late into the QRS complex and ST segment. This noninvasive test may be done at the bedside and is used to determine whether the client is susceptible to ventricular tachycardia that could result in sudden death. For a signal-averaged ECG, a computer is used to record and process low-level signals that are not detected by a traditional ECG. This technique allows detection of signals that might otherwise be masked by noise that conceals the small electrical events of the heart. Late potentials are multiphasic, low-amplitude, high-frequency spikes that appear after the terminal portion of the QRS complex and extend into the ST segment. They are thought to be generated by delayed activation in an abnormal area of the heart. The presence of late potentials in clients with normal sinus rhythm indicates a risk of ventricular tachycardia and sudden cardiac death.[2]

Holter Monitoring

When the client wears a portable Holter monitor, an ECG tracing may be recorded continuously for a day or longer on an outpatient basis, whereas a standard ECG is obtained in a relatively short time. Thus, Holter monitoring is used to detect dysrhythmias that may not appear on a routine ECG but occur when the client is ambulating at home or work. Holter monitoring is also useful in evaluating the effectiveness of antiarrhythmic or pacemaker therapy.[2] The monitoring system records at preset time intervals and when it senses an unusual event.

To prepare the client, place two to three electrodes on the chest and attach them to the telemetry unit. This unit is not much larger than a beeper and is worn in a sling about the chest or waist. Encourage the client to go about the usual daily activities and keep a written account of these activities along with any manifestations that develop. These data are used to document transient dysrhythmias and correlate the client's perceived symptoms with the underlying rhythm.

EXERCISE ELECTROCARDIOGRAM (STRESS TESTING)

PROCEDURE

Exercise testing defines the body's reaction to measured increases in acute exercise. Changes in heart rate, BP, respirations, and perceived level of exertion provide data for quantitative estimation of cardiovascular conditioning and function. The exercise testing may be used in conjunction with myocardial radionuclide testing. Regardless of the technique used, the optimal exercise testing protocol lasts 6 to 12 minutes and is adjusted to the type of client being tested. The advantages of the exercise test are that it is easily performed, relatively inexpensive, and completely noninvasive.

Exercise testing may consist of single or multiple stages. A single-stage test is one in which the exercise workload is constant throughout. Multiple-stage testing involves increasing the exercise workload in increments until a desired point is reached. The incremental increases in workload may occur every 1 to 5 minutes. The duration of testing varies with the type of test being used and the client's tolerance.

There are two major modes of exercise used for stress testing:

1. *Bicycle ergometry* involves a device equipped with a wheel operated by pedals that can be adjusted to increase the resistance to pedaling (multistage testing). It can be used for arm cranking, foot pedaling, or both. Advantages are that this mode of exercise is relatively inexpensive and the equipment is portable. However, frequent recalibration is required and localized muscle group fatigue is often induced.
2. *Treadmill testing* is the most common mode of stress testing, especially when used in conjunction with thallium 201 imaging. The treadmill is a motorized device that has an adjustable conveyor belt able to reach speeds of 1 to 10 miles per hour. The conveyor belt can be adjusted from a horizontal position to a 20% gradient, allowing the client to walk or run on slopes of different angles.[2, 11]

PREPROCEDURE CARE

Before stress testing, inform the client of the purposes and risks of exercise testing and obtain a signed consent. Instruct the client not to eat or smoke for 2 to 3 hours before the test and to dress appropriately for exercise. No strenuous physical efforts should be made for at least 12 hours before testing. Most clients are allowed to take their usual medications; the physician orders otherwise.

Brief history-taking and physical examination are performed. Obtain a baseline resting ECG immediately before testing. A standing ECG and BP should be recorded to determine vasoregulatory abnormalities, particularly ST-segment depression. Prepare the skin for electrode placement as previously described. Secure electrodes to the chest with tape or a belt. Drape lead wires, cable, and BP cuff to allow maximal freedom of movement. See the Client Education Guide for further client instructions. During the exercise test, the client's BP (taken with an automatically inflating cuff) and ECG are closely monitored by a physician or appropriately trained person.

During the procedure, perform the following:

- Obtain baseline BP, heart rate, and rhythm strip.
- Observe the ECG monitor constantly for changes.
- Record the client's BP, heart rate, rhythm strip, and activity level and time at specified intervals.
- Monitor the client for chest pain, dysrhythmias, ST-segment changes, unexpected changes in BP, or other cardiac manifestations (extreme dyspnea, claudication, vertigo).

CLIENT EDUCATION GUIDE

Stress Testing

- Get sufficient rest the night before the test.
- Avoid eating a heavy meal just before the test, although it is advisable to eat a light meal 1 to 2 hours before the test.
- Avoid smoking, alcohol, and beverages containing caffeine during the day of testing.
- Wear nonconstrictive, comfortable clothing and rubber-soled, supportive shoes during testing. Only a loose-fitting, front-buttoning shirt (or blouse) should be worn. (Women should wear a brassiere.)
- Continue all usual medications unless specified otherwise by the physician. (An inquiry about this should be made to the physician.)
- After the test, rest and keep the physician informed of any lingering manifestations of cardiovascular distress (i.e., chest pain, shortness of breath, or dizziness).
- Avoid taking a hot shower for 1 to 2 hours after the test because it may potentiate hypotension, resulting in a fainting episode. If bathing is desired, use only tepid water.

A multilead monitoring system is most often used to provide maximal views of the heart wall. The examiner makes frequent observations throughout testing for untoward manifestations related to impaired cardiovascular performance. These include chest pain, ventricular dysrhythmia, extreme dyspnea, claudication (leg pain), vertigo, and a sudden drop in BP. Reasons for terminating the test are as follows:

1. Chest pain or fatigue
2. Greatly increased heart rate (age-related):
    a. 20 to 29 years: 170 BPM
    b. 30 to 39 years: 160 BPM
    c. 40 to 49 years: 150 BPM
    d. 50 to 59 years: 140 BPM
    e. 60 to 69 years: 130 BPM
3. Untoward manifestations of myocardial ischemia or heart failure
4. Failure of systolic BP to rise or a drop in BP (below resting levels)
5. Sudden development of bradycardia
6. Serious cardiac dysrhythmia
7. Severe hypertension
8. Severe dyspnea
9. ST-segment depression (greater than 2 to 4 mm)
10. Sudden loss of coordination (cerebral ischemia)

Because these manifestations occur with some frequency, an emergency cart containing cardiac drugs and resuscitation equipment is kept close at hand at all times. Clients rarely die because of this procedure, but some may need assistance with resuscitation from dysrhythmias.

A positive exercise test is one that must be terminated before the predicted maximal (or submaximal) limits have been achieved because of manifestations of cardiovascular intolerance. Generally, the earlier these manifestations appear, the more serious the disease. Alterations in the ST segment and T wave on the ECG during exercise and recovery are often considered diagnostic of coronary artery disease because these alterations reflect an imbalance between myocardial oxygen demand and supply. There is, however, controversy about what extent of ST-segment change constitutes an abnormal response to exercise. The most widely held position is that the stress test is positive when the configuration and magnitude of the ST segment fulfill any of the following criteria:

- A 1-mm flat (horizontal) ST-segment depression lasting for 0.08 second
- A 1-mm downsloping ST-segment depression lasting for 0.08 second (this has the highest predictive value)
- A 1.5- to 2.0-mm upsloping ST-segment depression lasting for 0.08 second (this characteristic alone does not constitute a positive response)

Although the exercise test is helpful as an adjunct diagnostic study for coronary artery disease, it can produce false-positive findings in some cases, especially in women. In some people, ST-segment alterations may occur during exercise even though coronary artery disease is not present. Hyperventilation, certain drugs, and electrolyte imbalances can produce false-positive readings. For this reason, a diagnosis cannot be based on exercise findings alone.

False-negative findings also occur, although with less frequency. Medications such as beta-blocking agents and nitrates can produce false-negative results. Another limitation of the study is that it is absolutely contraindicated for clients with various cardiovascular and noncardiac conditions. See Box 54–6 for contraindications to exercise testing.

Become familiar with the stress testing procedure to provide clear teaching guidelines to clients scheduled for exercise testing. Many clients have misconceptions and unnecessary fears. Although not painful, the procedure can produce great fatigue. Warn the client that this test

BOX 54–6 Contraindications to Exercise Testing

Acute Cardiovascular Disease

Acute myocardial infarction (usually avoided in clients less than 2 weeks after infarction)

Unstable angina pectoris
Heart failure
Pericarditis
Myocarditis
Endocarditis
Life-threatening dysrhythmias
Thrombophlebitis
Recent systemic embolism
Dissecting or enlarging aneurysm

Others

Severe diseases restricting mobility
Renal failure
Severe pulmonary disruptions
Orthopedic disorders affecting the spine or lower extremities
Neurologic impairment (e.g., stroke or paralysis)
Systemic infection
Left ventricular outflow obstruction (aortic stenosis, hypertension, or hypertrophic cardiomyopathy)

may trigger chest pain and dyspnea. Along with this warning, explain that the procedure is performed in a controlled environment under close nursing and medical attention. It is essential that the client arrive for the exercise testing appointment relaxed and well rested. Teaching guidelines for stress testing appear in the Client Education Guide.

Postprocedure Care

After the procedure, assist the client to a chair, cart, or bed for recovery. Periodically monitor the client's BP, heart rate, and rhythm strip for a least 15 minutes after test completion or until the ECG returns to baseline.

■ ELECTROPHYSIOLOGIC STUDIES

The electrophysiologic study is an invasive method of recording intracardiac electrical activity. It is used to (1) shed light on the mechanisms of dysrhythmias, (2) differentiate between supraventricular and ventricular dysrhythmias, (3) evaluate sinoatrial (SA) or AV node dysfunction, (4) determine the need for a pacemaker, and (5) evaluate the effect of antiarrhythmic agents used to prevent the occurrence of tachycardias.

An electrophysiologic catheter has four electrodes at the distal tip that record or stimulate (pace). Under fluoroscopy, the catheter is threaded into the heart via the femoral, basilic, or subclavian vein. The catheter sites selected depend on the purpose of the examination. One catheter is placed at the bundle of His just beneath the AV node as a point of reference. An additional catheter is introduced high in the right atrium. If Wolff-Parkinson-White syndrome is suspected, a catheter may be placed in the coronary sinus. A catheter may also be placed in the right ventricle. During mapping of ventricular tachycardia, a catheter may be introduced into the left ventricle via an artery.

The purpose of the procedure is to reproduce any dysrhythmia so that its origin may be isolated. Ventricular tachycardia is induced by using programmed stimulation to fire an impulse at different times during the cardiac electrical cycle. If dysrhythmia is induced, the client's BP and hemodynamic responses are observed. It is possible to record simultaneously arterial pressure, surface ECGs, and ECGs from intracavitary catheters. The morphology and rate of the induced tachycardia are compared with those of the client's spontaneous ventricular tachycardia. Ventricular tachycardia is often terminated by rapid ventricular decremental pacing. If the tachycardia cannot be stimulated, IV isoproterenol may be infused to simulate stress or exercise, which may produce the tachycardia.

Antiarrhythmic drugs may be administered during the study to evaluate their effect. After the initial antiarrhythmic has been given, induction of ventricular tachycardia is attempted. If ventricular tachycardia is induced, the dosage may be increased or other drugs administered. The electrophysiologic studies are repeated in several days to determine the effectiveness of antiarrhythmic drug therapy.

Frequently, when the irritable focus has been identified (e.g., accessory pathway or bundle of His), ablation (destruction) may be performed. Ablation of the irritable focus may be accomplished by the use of radiofrequency waves, direct current, ethyl alcohol, or cryosurgery. Radiofrequency ablation is the most popular method because its effect may be localized, with less damage to surrounding tissue.

Preprocedure and Postprocedure Care

Preprocedure and postprocedure nursing care of the client undergoing electrophysiologic studies is similar to that of the client undergoing cardiac catheterization. Because these studies attempt, under controlled circumstances, to induce potentially lethal dysrhythmias, it is imperative that emergency drugs, equipment, and a defibrillator be immediately accessible.

■ CARDIAC DIAGNOSTIC IMAGING

X-ray studies, magnetic resonance imaging (MRI), ultrasonography, and radioisotopes are discussed in Chapter 11. Use of these diagnostic tools to evaluate the heart is discussed next. See Chapter 11 for the preprocedure care and postprocedure care for each of these diagnostic examinations.

Chest X-ray Studies

Posteroanterior, lateral, and oblique chest x-ray films help to determine the size, silhouette, and position of the heart. For the acutely ill client, a portable anteroposterior x-ray study is performed at the bedside. Specific pathologic changes of the heart are difficult to determine with x-ray examination, but anatomic changes in the heart and pulmonary sequelae of various cardiac conditions can be seen. Assessed on x-ray film are valvular and pericardial calcifications; pulmonary congestion (from heart failure); pericardial effusion; and placement of central lines, endotracheal tubes, hemodynamic monitoring devices, and intra-aortic balloon catheters.

Magnetic Resonance Imaging

Although MRI is one of the most expensive noninvasive diagnostic options, a variety of information may be obtained in a single image. MRI provides the best information on chamber size, wall motion, valvular function, and great vessel blood flow. MRI is commonly used for examination of the aorta and detection of tumors or masses, cardiomyopathies, and pericardial disease. MRI can show the heart beating and the blood flowing in any direction. All standard quantitative functional indices can be obtained from a MRI study with the exception of transstenotic gradients.

Information obtained from MRI includes the following:

- Normal morphology and structural changes
- Wall thickness, chamber volumes, valve areas, vessel cross-sections, and extent, location, and size of lesions
- Global and regional biventricular function, including ejection fraction, stroke volume, and cardiac output
- Blood flow quantifications within vessels over the cardiac cycle
- Tissue characterization of paracardiac and intracardiac masses, pericardial effusions, and myocardial infarction

Positron Emission Tomography

The positron emission tomographic (PET) scanner is a diagnostic imaging tool that allows visualization of regional physiologic function and biochemical changes that often separate normal from diseased myocardium. Cellular metabolic information is obtained by mapping regional myocardial glucose metabolism. Combining information from the perfusion and metabolism images provides a thorough assessment of regional cardiac viability. For further discussion of PET, see Chapter 11.

The scanning procedure takes about 2 to 3 hours. An IV radiopharmaceutical, [^{13}N]-ammonia, is administered and a 20-minute blood flow image is begun. An IV injection of glucose follows. Localization of glucose in the myocardium takes about 40 minutes. Final uptake of the tracer is proportional to the glucose metabolic activity of myocardial cells and provides an excellent indication of regional tissue viability.

The following are clinical indications for PET scanner use:

- Detection of coronary artery disease
- Assessment of myocardial viability
- Assessment of progression of coronary artery stenosis
- Documentation of collateral coronary circulation
- Differentiation of ischemia from dilated cardiomyopathy

The terms "match" and "mismatch" describe the relationship between the perfusion and metabolism studies. A perfusion study showing poor blood flow and a metabolic study showing decreased glucose uptake of necrotic tissue are described as a *match.* A perfusion study that shows poor blood flow and a metabolic study that shows only stunned viable myocardium that has survived the initial insult are described as a *mismatch.*

Echocardiography

Echocardiography, a noninvasive diagnostic procedure based on the principles of ultrasonography, is used to evaluate structural and functional changes in a wide variety of heart ailments.

An echocardiogram is obtained by placing a transducer on several areas of the chest wall. Bursts of ultrasound waves are directed at the part of the heart under investigation. The echocardiogram records the structure and motion of that area in relation to its distance from the anterior chest wall (Fig. 54–10). An ECG is recorded simultaneously on the graph. Two-dimensional echocardiography generates a continuous picture of the beating heart. These images are recorded on videotape for analysis.

Echocardiograms are used to help assess and diagnose pericardial effusion, cardiomyopathy, valvular disorders (including prosthetic valves), cardiac shunts, myocardial ischemia, chamber size, left ventricular function, ventricular aneurysms, and cardiac tumors (atrial myxoma). In addition, they are useful during heart biopsies because the physician can view the heart on a monitor while taking tissue samples.

Transesophageal Echocardiography

Procedure

Transesophageal echocardiography (TEE) yields a higher quality picture of the heart than does regular echocardiography. It is especially useful for clients who have thickened lung tissue or thick chest walls or who are obese. The procedure may also be used intraoperatively, where conventional echocardiography is ineffective. Dobutamine stress testing is now being used in combination with TEE to evaluate clients with suspected coronary artery disease and to evaluate left ventricular wall motion.

This combination test involves inserting a flexible endoscope equipped with an ultrasonic transducer tip into the esophagus of a sedated client, administering dobutamine to mimic the effects of exercise (by increasing myocardial oxygen demand through stimulation of $beta_1$ receptors), and recording ultrasonic images of the heart's response. Because the probe is placed behind the heart, it allows the left atrium to be viewed. TEE allows clearer visualization of the heart and its structures and is most useful in diagnosis of cardiac masses, prosthetic valve function, aneurysm, and posterior effusions. The procedure lasts approximately 15 minutes to 1 hour.[1, 2, 14]

Preprocedure Care

Explain the procedure to the client. Obtain an informed consent. Assure the client that sedation will be used. The client should receive nothing by mouth for 6 to 8 hours before the procedure.

During the procedure, do the following. Administer sedation and topical anesthetic as ordered. If the client has a nasogastric tube in place, remove it before the esophageal scope is inserted. If dobutamine is used, the nurse is responsible for calculating the dose according to

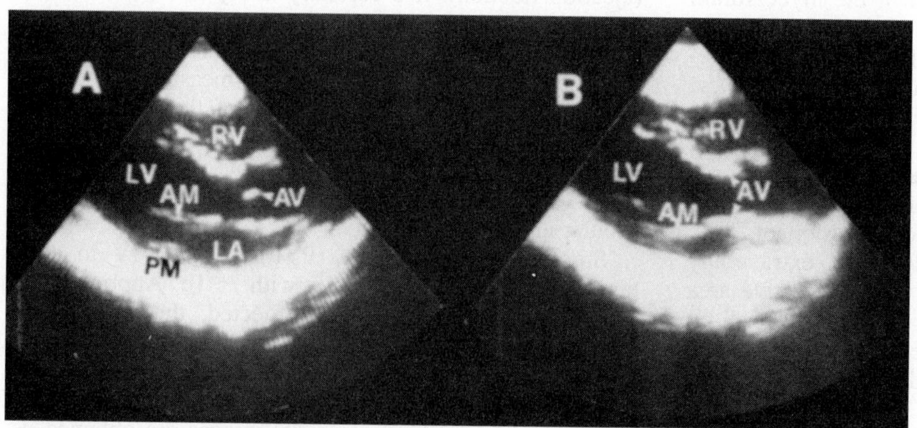

FIGURE 54–10 Long-axis, cross-sectional echocardiographic images of the left ventricle (LV), right ventricle (RV), mitral valve, aortic valve, and left atrium (LA) during diastole *(A)* and systole *(B).* During diastole, the anterior (AM) and posterior (PM) mitral leaflets are apart and the aortic valve leaflets (AV) come together as a single echo in the midportion of the aorta *(A).* With systole *(B)* the mitral leaflets come together and the aortic valve leaflets separate. (From Braunwald, E. [1992]. *Heart disease* [4th ed., p. 67]. Philadelphia: W. B. Saunders.)

the client's weight. To imitate the effects of increasing physical activity, the dose is slowly increased from a baseline infusion of 2.5 to 5 μg/kg/min and thereafter increased in increments of 5 to 10 μg/kg/min up to a maximum of 40 μg/kg/min. Each dose is infused for 5 minutes; images are captured during the final 2 minutes of the infusion. Monitor the client's vital signs, ECG, respiratory status, and pulse oximetry throughout the procedure.

POSTPROCEDURE CARE

After the procedure, closely monitor vital signs for 30 minutes and record the ECG every 10 minutes. Keep the client fasting until the gag reflex is fully restored. Instruct the client that there may be mild throat discomfort for a day or two and to report significant discomfort or hemoptysis to the physician immediately. Because of the sedation, advise the client not to drive or operate machinery for 24 hours.

Phonocardiography

Phonograms are recordings of audible vibrations from the heart and great vessels. Phonograms are used to assist in determining the timing of cardiac sounds and murmurs. Microphones are placed under elastic straps, usually at the base and apex of the heart. No preparation is required for this assessment.

Myocardial Scintigraphy

Myocardial function, motion, and perfusion may be studied by a method called scintigraphy, which involves IV injection of a radioactive isotope. As the isotope is absorbed by the blood cells of the heart muscle, photons are emitted. These photons are detected by an external gamma camera, which produces a radionuclide image. Because these nuclear imaging techniques are relatively noninvasive, they are frequently used diagnostic tools.

THALLIUM 201 SCINTIGRAPHY

Thallium 201 is the most widely used isotope for myocardial perfusion because of its short half-life (73 hours) and low total body radiation dose. Thallium 201 is a radioactive analog of potassium that is easily extracted by smooth skeletal and cardiac muscle fibers that have the potassium active transport system. Eighty-eight per cent of blood-borne ^{201}Tl is taken up on its first pass through the heart. The amount of ^{201}Tl found in the myocardium after an IV injection depends on the regional myocardial perfusion and the efficiency of cellular extraction. Regional perfusion is dependent on coronary artery patency. Areas of the myocardium that receive less blood flow also receive less thallium.

A high concentration of ^{201}Tl is present in well-perfused cells, and a lower concentration remains in the blood, setting up a concentration gradient for diffusion of ^{201}Tl. Infarcted or scarred myocardium does not extract any ^{201}Tl and shows up as "cold spots." If the defective area is ischemic, the cold spots fill in or become "warm" on the delayed images. Infarcts continue to appear cold with little or no perfusion of ^{201}Tl either during a stress test or with delayed images.

The perfusion scanning is performed with a special camera that is capable of showing the source of emitted low-energy photons on a screen. Each photon detected by the camera is recorded on film and a computer screen over a half-hour period. The computer refines and enhances the images and then provides quantitative information about the myocardial walls.

Thallium 201 imaging can be performed before or after an exercise ECG study or as a resting study only. Ischemic myocardium may be detected by a resting ^{201}Tl study. Two sets of images are taken 3 hours apart and compared. The ^{201}Tl stress test begins with a graded exercise protocol on a treadmill. The client receives a slow IV infusion of normal saline. The ECG is monitored continuously. About 1 minute before the peak of the stress test, ^{201}Tl is injected intravenously. The client should exercise for the last minute to ensure ^{201}Tl distribution to the heart during 85% maximum stress. The client then cools down and reclines on an examination table for the perfusion scan. Continuous imaging in a 180-degree arc over the chest is performed. The client then waits for 3 hours and returns for repeated films. Before the delayed images are obtained, the client receives additional ^{201}Tl by IV injection. The two sets of images are then carefully compared.

DIPYRIDAMOLE THALLIUM 201 TEST

This test may be used as an alternative to standard treadmill exercise when the client is not able to achieve a vigorous level of exercise. Dipyridamole serves as a pharmacologic stress agent. It is given IV to dilate the coronary arteries, which would normally dilate during the stress of exercise. Arteries that are narrowed as a result of coronary artery disease do not expand as much as normal arteries. Infusion of dipyridamole for 5 minutes is followed by injection of ^{201}Tl. Thallium 201 travels easily through normal arteries that have dilated and travels less freely through narrowed arteries. At 7 minutes, images are taken.

Any form of caffeine as well as medications for asthma, such as theophylline or aminophylline, should be omitted before this test. Aminophylline is an antagonist of dipyridamole and may be given slowly IV to reverse any adverse side effects.

TECHNETIUM 99m VENTRICULOGRAPHY (MULTIPLE GATED ACQUISITION SCANNING)

This test is used to study the motion of the left ventricular wall and measure the ventricle's ability to eject blood (ejection fraction). If a coronary artery is narrowed, causing ischemia, the segment of the myocardium it serves exhibits diminished wall motion or contractility. In addition, hemodynamic changes may be measured by observing the actual filling and emptying of the cardiac chambers. Changes in cardiac output as well as ejection fraction may be obtained. Multiple gated acquisition (MUGA) scans represent the blood pool within the ventricular and atrial chambers.

Stannous pyrophosphate (PYP) is given IV to allow tagging of the red blood cells with ^{99m}Tc. Approximately 20 minutes after the PYP is injected, the ^{99m}Tc is injected. A heart monitor is then attached, and images are begun.

MUGA scans use counts from any one of a number of consecutive beats. Multiple serial images are obtained using a gamma camera. The cardiac cycle is broken into intervals, with counts taken during these intervals for a number of beats. These counts are stored and then displayed in a weighted average picture.

If a stress study is to be performed, the client is put on a bicycle ergometer with a gamma camera positioned to project the right and left blood pools. The ECG is monitored continuously. Images are obtained at rest and during each stage of exercise.

First-Pass Cardiac Study

Procedure

During a first-pass study, a single IV injection of ^{99m}Tc is administered and traced as it passes through the heart. Only the initial pass of the ^{99m}Tc through the cardiac chambers is recorded. Ejection fraction and information about ventricular wall motion are obtained. A first-pass study may be performed during exercise or rest.

Preprocedure Care

Before the procedure, ask female clients if they are or may be pregnant because these studies involve radiation exposure (although minimal). Explain the purpose of the procedure, and tell the client what to expect during the procedure. Explain that electrodes will be placed on the chest and an IV line will be inserted for administration of the radioisotope. Generally, total exposure to radiation during these scans is less than or equal to that of one chest x-ray study.

Instruct the client to wear walking shoes if exercise on the treadmill or bicycle is anticipated. Follow the diet protocol of the institution. Some tests may require fasting. A light meal is preferred if the scan is to be performed during exercise as it prevents nausea and stomach cramping during exercise and allows better uptake of the radioisotope. Instruct the client to avoid alcohol and smoking on the day of the procedure.

Check the physician's orders for omission of any medications. Usually, beta-blockers, calcium-channel blockers, and xanthines are prohibited before the procedure. Ensure that the client signs a consent form. During the procedure, ask the client to notify the nurse or technologist of any chest pain (ischemia).

Postprocedure Care

After the procedure, again ask the client to report any chest pain. If the client must return for follow-up scanning, instruct the client to rest between studies.

Cardiac Catheterization

This complex procedure involves insertion of a catheter into the heart and surrounding vessels to obtain detailed information about the structure and performance of the heart, the valves, and the circulatory system. Specifically, cardiac catheterization is performed to:

- Confirm a diagnosis of heart disease and determine the extent to which the disease has affected the structure and function of the heart
- Determine congenital abnormalities
- Obtain a clear picture of cardiac anatomy before heart surgery
- Obtain pressures within the heart chambers and the great vessels (aorta and pulmonary artery [PA])
- Measure blood oxygen concentration, tension, and saturation within the heart chambers
- Determine cardiac output
- Perform angiography for better coronary artery visualization
- Obtain endocardial biopsy specimens
- Allow infusion of fibrinolytic agents directly into an occluded coronary artery in an attempt to restore coronary blood flow

Cardiac catheterization is usually performed in the controlled environment of a cardiac catheterization laboratory. Typically, only one side of the heart is catheterized, although it is sometimes necessary to insert the catheter into both sides of the heart. See Chapter 11 for discussions of the preprocedure and postprocedure nursing care and possible complications after cardiac catheterization.[1, 2, 39]

Right-Sided Catheterization

For right-sided cardiac catheterization, the physician inserts a sterile, radiopaque catheter through the antecubital or femoral vein. Under fluoroscopic guidance, the catheter is advanced slowly to the right atrium and right ventricle and is finally wedged in a small branch of the PA. The ECG is continuously monitored during the procedure. Premature ventricular contractions may occur as the catheter is being passed through the ventricles. The client may experience fluttering sensations or palpitations as the catheter passes through the heart. If they occur frequently, cardiac output falls and the physician may need to withdraw the catheter temporarily or order administration of lidocaine (an antiarrhythmic).

Left-Sided Catheterization

This procedure is far more difficult to perform than right-sided catheterization. There are two major methods of catheter introduction. (1) The catheter can be passed retrograde (backward) from the brachial or femoral artery into the aorta and then to the left ventricle. (2) Rarely during right-sided catheterization, the middle or lower third of the atrial septum is punctured and the catheter is passed transseptally into the left atrium.

As the catheter is passed through the venous or arterial system and into various heart chambers, the desired studies are performed. The catheter has several end or side holes that allow blood withdrawal for oxygen analysis from the various cardiac chambers. Pressures can be obtained by attaching the catheter to a transducer with its connecting amplifier and recording device. Radiopaque contrast materials and indicator solutions can be injected via the catheter into the left ventricle to examine the mitral valve, the left ventricular outflow tract, wall motion and thickness, left ventricular end-diastolic volume, and ejection fraction.[7] The client may experience pain when contrast material is injected and the dye replaces blood flowing through the arteries. The lack of oxygenated blood causes regional cardiac hypoxia.

Angiography

Angiocardiography involves IV injection of contrast material into the heart during cardiac catheterization. Immediately after the injection, a series of x-ray films are taken that reveal the course of the contrast material as it circulates through the heart, lungs, and great vessels. (See Chapter 11, Fig. 11–7.)

Cineangiography is a technique in which moving pictures are taken during cardiac catheterization. The examiner can view the film at both rapid and slow speeds, permitting detailed and unlimited review of the study.

Coronary angiography involves injection of contrast material directly into the coronary arteries (via the coronary ostia) during cardiac catheterization. Table 54–7 outlines the various forms of angiocardiography. See Chapter 11 for preprocedure and postprocedure nursing care.

■ HEMODYNAMIC STUDIES

Hemodynamic status is assessed with four parameters: CVP, PA pressure, cardiac output, and intra-arterial pressure. Each parameter is obtained through an invasive procedure. Critical care nurses perform all of these studies routinely at the bedside. Hemodynamic studies provide a wealth of information reflecting the earliest changes in the circulatory system that are not yet clinically detectable.

Hemodynamic pressure monitoring provides information about blood volume, fluid balance, and how well the heart is pumping. Current technology allows measurement of right atrial pressure (CVP), PA pressures during systole and diastole (reflecting right and left ventricular pressures), and pulmonary capillary wedge pressure (PCWP) (an indirect indicator of left ventricular pressure).

The Pulmonary Artery Catheter

Development of the balloon-tipped, flow-directed catheter has enabled continuous direct monitoring of PA pressure (see Bridge to Critical Care).

The PA catheter has four lumina. The proximal lumen terminates in the right atrium, allowing CVP measurement, fluid infusion, and venous access for blood samples. The distal lumen terminates in the PA and measures PA systolic pressure, PA diastolic pressure, PA mean pressure, and PCWP. A small, third lumen is used for inflation and deflation of the balloon. The fourth lumen is the thermistor port and permits measurement of cardiac output. In addition, some catheters have a fifth port for infusion of fluids and capabilities for cardiac pacing and measuring oxygen saturation of the blood.

TABLE 54–7 MAJOR TYPES OF ANGIOCARDIOGRAPHY

Angiocardiography Procedure	Method Employed
Right-sided angiocardiography	Contrast medium is injected into the right heart chambers and pulmonary artery by means of a catheter threaded up a vein and into the heart during cardiac catheterization
Left-sided angiocardiography	Contrast medium is injected into the left side of the heart through a transvenous catheter passed through the atrial septum during cardiac catheterization or via a catheter passed retrograde through an artery into the left heart
Selective coronary artery angiocardiography	Contrast medium is injected directly into the ostium of each coronary artery via a catheter that is placed retrograde through an artery into the aorta

INSERTING THE CATHETER

Insertion of a PA catheter involves risk for the client. The potential complications are PA infarction, pulmonary embolism, injury to the heart valves, and injury to the myocardium. In addition, while the catheter is in place, the heart valves are unable to close completely.

PA monitoring must be carried out in a critical care unit under careful scrutiny of an experienced nursing staff. Before insertion of the catheter, explain to the client that (1) the procedure may be uncomfortable but not painful, and (2) a local anesthetic will be given at the catheter insertion site. Support of the critically ill client at this time helps promote cooperation and lessen anxiety.

The physician inserts the PA flow-directed catheter at the bedside via percutaneous puncture of the brachial, subclavian, jugular, or femoral vein using sterile technique. The catheter is connected to a transducer and a fluid-filled pressure monitoring system. Pressure levels and fluctuations are monitored both graphically and by numerical display.

The inflated balloon follows the direction of blood flow through the right ventricle into the PA, where it finally wedges in the right or left branch of the PA. Clinicians can follow the path of the balloon by observing waveforms and pressure readings on the monitor (see Bridge to Critical Care).

When wedged, the catheter is "pointing" indirectly at the left end-diastolic pressure. Therefore, PCWP is the most accurate, although indirect, indicator of left ventricular end-diastolic pressure or left ventricular *preload* available at the bedside. The normal PCWP is 8 to 13 mm Hg. Elevations of PCWP (greater than 18 to 20 mm Hg) indicate increased left ventricular pressure, as seen in left ventricular failure, and may coincide with the onset of pulmonary congestion. Pressures climbing to more than 30 mm Hg generally herald the onset of pulmonary edema. Conversely, low PCWP suggests insufficient volume and pressure in the left ventricle, as seen in hypovolemic shock. Pressure changes commonly related to various cardiac conditions are shown in the Bridge to Critical Care.

Central Venous Pressure

Central venous pressure is the pressure within the superior vena cava. It reflects the pressure under which the blood is returned to the superior vena cava and right atrium. CVP is determined by vascular tone, blood volume, and the ability of the right side of the heart to receive and pump blood. When the tricuspid valve is open at the end of diastole, the atrium and ventricle are, in effect, one chamber. At this time, the CVP is equal to the pressure in the right ventricle and indicates right ven-

BRIDGE TO CRITICAL CARE

Swan-Ganz Monitoring

Positioning the Swan-Ganz Catheter

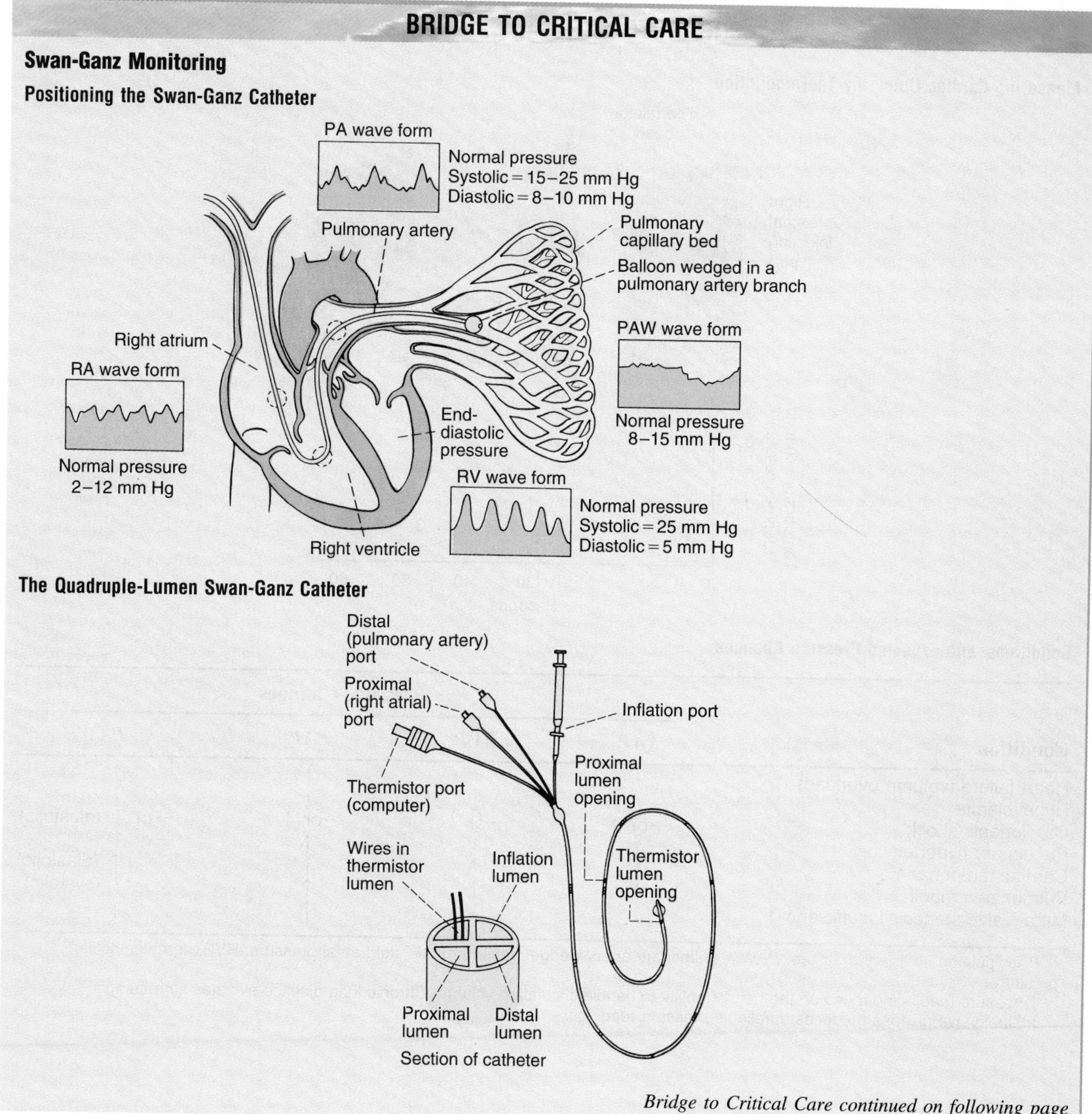

Bridge to Critical Care continued on following page

tricular function (Table 54–8). CVP can also be seen as a measurement of preload on the right side of the heart. Preload is the amount of blood presented to the heart or when the ventricle is full before the next ejection. Preload is the right ventricular end-diastolic pressure. (Preload is also discussed in Chapter 55.)

CVP can be measured with a central venous line placed in the superior vena cava or a balloon flotation catheter in the PA. Normal CVP pressure is 2 to 12 mm Hg. A drop in CVP pressure indicates a decrease in circulating volume, which may result from fluid imbalance, hemorrhage, or severe vasodilation and pooling of blood in the extremities with limited venous return. A rise in CVP indicates an increase in blood volume because of a sudden shift in fluid balance, excessive IV fluid infusion, renal failure, or sodium and water retention.

Accurate CVP measurement requires a baseline for the transducer position. The zero point on the transducer needs to be at the level of the right atrium. The right atrium is located at the midaxillary line at the fourth intercostal space when measured while the client is supine with the head of the bed elevated to no more than 45 degrees for the most accurate reading.

During measurement of CVP, the client should be relaxed. Straining, coughing, or any other activity that increases intrathoracic pressure can cause falsely high measurements. When measuring the CVP of a client with a

BRIDGE TO CRITICAL CARE *Continued*

Measuring Cardiac Output by Thermodilution

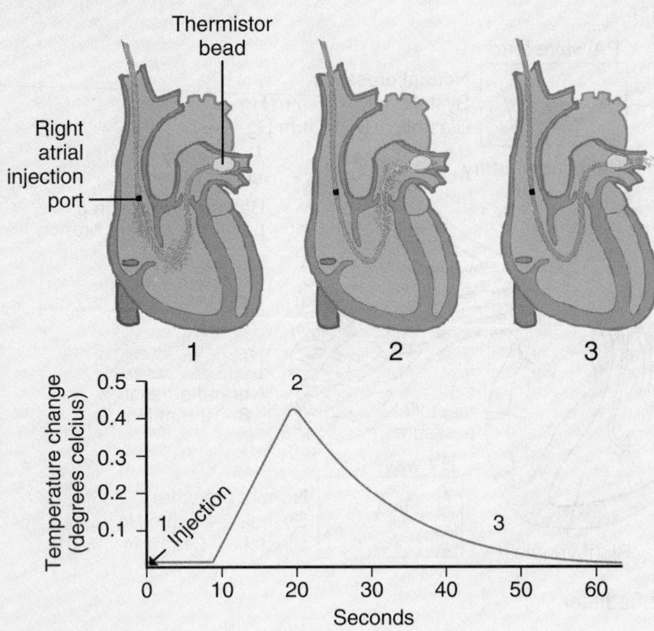

Conditions with Expected Pressure Changes

Condition	RAP	RVP	PAP	PAWP
	Pressure Changes			
Heart failure (volume overload)	↑	↑	↑	↑
Hypovolemia	↓	↓	↓	↓
Cardiogenic shock*	—or ↑	—or ↑	—or ↑	—or ↑ (diastolic)
Pulmonary hypertension	↑	↑	↑	—or ↑
Cardiac tamponade	↑	↑	↑	↑ (diastolic)
Pulmonary emboli	↑	↑	↑	↑ (systolic)
Mitral valve stenosis/insufficiency†	↑	↑	↑	↑

PAP, pulmonary artery pressure; PAWP, pulmonary artery wedge pressure; RAP, right atrial pressure; RVP, right ventricular pressure.

* Pressure readings depend on the heart's ability to handle circulating volume. Chronic lung disease elevates all readings.

† Mitral valve disease produces unreliable pressure readings.

TABLE 54–8 INDICATIONS FOR CENTRAL VENOUS PRESSURE (CVP) AND HOW THEY MAY AFFECT THE READINGS

To Assess	↑ CVP (>11 cm H_2O)	↓ CVP (<3 cm H_2O)
Right-sided heart hemodynamics	Right heart failure (including chronic heart failure, LVF) Constrictive pericarditis Cardiac tamponade Valvular stenosis Pulmonary hypertension	Early LVF
Blood volume	↑ Circulating volume	↓ Circulating volume
Vascular tone	Vasoconstriction Hypertension	Vasodilation, peripheral pooling Septic shock

LVF, left ventricular failure.

Modified from Huang, S. H., et al. (1989). *Coronary care nursing* (2nd ed., p. 101). Philadelphia: W. B. Saunders.

ventilator, take the readings at the point of end expiration for greatest accuracy.

Check the connections between the catheter and the attachments frequently to ensure that they are secure (in order to prevent air embolism). Change the dressing at the insertion site according to health care facility policy to prevent infection. In order to maintain patency of the system, a small amount of fluid is delivered under pressure at a constant rate of flow. This fluid may or may not be heparinized. Complications of the procedure include pneumothorax, phlebitis, air emboli, pulmonary emboli, fluid overload, dysrhythmia, sepsis, and microelectric shock.

Pulmonary Artery Pressure

The CVP is unsatisfactory for determining the status of left-sided heart function, especially in critically ill people, for example, those who are immediately recovering from cardiac surgery, have experienced myocardial infarction, have cardiomyopathy, or are in cardiogenic shock. Significant changes can occur in the left side of the heart and not be reflected for some time in the right side of the heart. Failure to detect such changes can lead to delayed or inappropriate intervention.

During diastole, blood flows freely from the PA through the pulmonary capillaries, left atrium, and open mitral valve to the left ventricle. Therefore, the pressure in the left ventricle at the end of diastole approximates the diastolic pressure in the PA, pulmonary capillaries, and left atrium.

Starling's principle indicates that the heart muscle contracts most effectively when under slight stretch. PA pressure measurements can assist in determining whether the ventricle is understretched (in need of fluids), overstretched (in need or diuretics), or appropriately stretched (at maximal function).

Cardiac Output Measurement

As detailed in the anatomy and physiology feature for the cardiac system, cardiac output is the amount of blood pumped out of the left ventricle into the arterial system every minute. That is, cardiac output is equal to the stroke volume (volume of blood pumped out with each beat) multiplied by the heart rate. If the stroke volume of the left ventricle is between 50 and 90 ml (average, 70 ml) and the heart rate is 80 BPM, the normal cardiac output of the left ventricle is approximately 4 to 8 L/min. Table 54–9 lists the conditions that change cardiac output. The cardiac output of the right ventricle is considered equal to that of the left because the right ventricle, although not as muscular as the left ventricle, pumps against less resistance.

TABLE 54–9 CONDITIONS THAT CAUSE A CHANGE IN CARDIAC OUTPUT

Conditions That Decrease Cardiac Output	Conditions That Increase Cardiac Output
Acute heart failure	Hypoxia
Pericarditis with effusion	Hyperthyroidism
Old age	Excitement
Arterial hemorrhage	Exercise
Standing motionless, which decreases venous return to the heart	Food intake
Myxedema	Oral and intravenous fluid intake
Shock	Early stage of septic shock
Valvular heart disease	Pregnancy
Myocardial ischemia	
Dysrhythmias	
Paroxysmal atrial tachycardia (PAT)	
Atrial fibrillation	
Heart block	
Ventricular tachycardia	
Heat stroke	

Intra-arterial Pressure Monitoring

PROCEDURE

Systemic intra-arterial monitoring is a common method for obtaining BP measurements in the acutely ill client. This method provides continuous detection of arterial BP via an indwelling catheter. It is of greatest benefit for clients whose cuff BP measurements are undetectable or unreliable, such as those with low cardiac output, fluctuating hemodynamic status, and excessive peripheral vasoconstriction. Note that intra-arterial pressure readings are at least 10 mm Hg higher than cuff BP readings. The intra-arterial line simplifies obtaining blood samples for arterial blood gas and blood studies, minimizing the need for arterial or venous punctures. Major complications of intra-arterial monitoring include hemorrhage caused by loose connections of the monitoring system, hematoma at the insertion site, infection (local or systemic), and embolization of the artery that supplies the distal portion of the cannulated extremity.

The physician introduces a short, nonreactive polytetrafluoroethylene (Teflon) catheter into an artery (radial, brachial, axillary, femoral, or dorsalis pedis) using sterile technique.

PREPROCEDURE CARE

Informed consent is required. Before catheter insertion, the adequacy of circulation in the selected extremity must be assessed. If the radial artery is chosen as the site for insertion, blood flow to the hand is evaluated with an Allen test to determine ulnar artery patency. Allen's test is described in Chapter 59. If ulnar artery obstruction is suspected, cannulation of the radial artery should not be attempted.

Besides accurate monitoring and recording of arterial pressure, nursing responsibilities focus on preventing complications of arterial cannulation. Do the following: Check all connections frequently to ensure that they remain tight and secure. Evaluate the cannulated extremity for neurovascular function every 2 hours. Assess color, temperature, capillary filling, and sensation distal to the site of cannulation. Check the insertion site for redness or signs of infection daily, and change dressing per institutional policy.

POSTPROCEDURE CARE

After removal of the arterial cannula, maintain firm constant pressure for 5 to 15 minutes over the site of the artery to prevent hematoma formation. Secure a pressure dressing over the site for 12 hours. Monitor for infection (increased redness, warmth, tenderness, and induration at the catheter insertion site, elevated temperature) and neurovascular compromise (pain, paresthesia [abnormal touch sensation], decreased pulse quality, pallor, coolness). Report these complications immediately to the physician.

CONCLUSIONS

Cardiovascular assessment can range from taking blood presssure to monitoring hemodynamic parameters. Learning how to perform adult cardiac assessment takes time and perseverance. Abnormal heart sounds are harder to interpret than normal heart sounds; be persistent and practice frequently. Even though invasive diagnostic tests are more prevalent, you need to be able to evaluate accurately the client's history, BP, and physical assessment. These data are just as important as the results of invasive studies if the nurse continues to assess the client effectively, provide primary preventive care, and monitor treatment. Assessment skills and nursing interventions can make a significant difference in the client's quality of life by preventing complications and improving outcomes.

BIBLIOGRAPHY

1. Aiello, S. (1997). Radiologic workup for angina. *American Journal of Nursing, 97*(12), 50.
2. Alexander, R. W., et al. (Eds.). (1998). *Hurst's the heart* (9th ed.). New York: McGraw-Hill.
3. American Heart Association. (1998). *Heart and stroke: Statistical update*. Dallas: Author.
4. American Heart Association. (1998). *HeartStyle*. Dallas: Author.
5. Arnold, E. (1997). The stress connection: Women and coronary artery disease. *Critical Care Nursing Clinics of North America, 9*(4), 565–575.
6. Carney, R. M., et al. (1998). New CAD risk factors: How useful? *Patient Care, 32*(11), 134–165.
7. Cheitlin, M., et al. (1998). The art of auscultation. *Patient Care, 32*(23), 35–48.
8. Colbath, J. D. (1997). Holistic health options for women. *Critical Care Nursing Clinics of North America, 9*(4), 589–599.
9. Cox, M. H., & DiNubile, N. A. (1997). Exercise for coronary artery disease: A cornerstone of comprehensive treatment. *Physician and Sportsmedicine, 25*(12), 27–35.
10. Eckel, R. H., & Krauss, R. M. (1998). American Heart Association call to action: Obesity is a major risk factor for coronary heart disease. *Circulation, 97*(21), 2099–2100.
11. Ellestad, M. H. (1997). Is the standard exercise ECG test obsolete? *Internal Medicine, 18*(11), 33–45.
12. Epstein, O., et al. (1997). *Clinical examination* (2nd ed.). Philadelphia: Mosby–Year Book.
13. Evanoski, C. A. M. (1997). Myocardial infarction: The number one killer of women. *Critical Care Nursing Clinics of North America, 9*(4), 489–496.
14. Frizzell, J. (1997). Transesophageal echocardiography. *American Journal of Nursing, 97*(9), 17–18.
15. Gasperetti, C. M. (1997). Recent development in the rapid diagnosis of acute chest pain syndromes. *Veterans Health System Journal, 2*(5), 51–55.
16. Glisson, J., et al. (1999). Review, critique, and guidelines for the use of herbs and homeopathy. *Nurse Practitioner, 24*(4), 44–67.
17. Hahn, R. A., et al. (1998). Cardiovascular risk factors and preventive practices among adults—United States, 1994: A behavioral risk factor atlas. *Morbidity and Mortality Weekly Report, 47*(SS–5), 35–69.
18. Halm, M. A., & Penque, S. (1999). Heart disease in women. *American Journal of Nursing, 99*(4), 26–31.
19. Hamm, C., et al. (1997). Emergency room triage of patients with acute chest pain by means of rapid testing for cardiac troponin T or troponin I. *New England Journal of Medicine, 337*(23), 1648–1688.
20. Hill, B., & Geraci, S. A. (1998). A diagnostic approach to chest pain based on history and ancillary evaluation. *Nurse Practitioner, 23*(4), 20–45.
21. Immunization Action Coalition. (August 1999). *Summary of recommendations for adult immunization*. St. Paul, MN: Author.
22. Jadin, R. L., & Margolis, K. (1998). Coronary artery disease in women: How customary expectations can interfere with interpretation of test results. *PostGraduate Medicine, 103*(3), 71–84.
23. JNC VI guidelines: Hypertension treatment shifts to total CV risk. (1997). American Heart Association 70th scientific sessions. *Geriatrics, 52*(12), 52–58.
24. Laurienzo, J. M. (1997). Detection of coronary artery disease in women. *Critical Care Nursing Clinics of North America, 9*(4), 469–475.
25. Meyer, N. (1999). Using physiologic and pharmacologic stress testing in the evaluation of coronary artery disease. *Nurse Practitioner, 24*(4), 70–82.
26. Miller, D. B. (1997). Secondary prevention for ischemic heart disease: Relative numbers needed to treat with different therapies. *Archives of Internal Medicine, 157*(18), 2045–2052.

26a. Miracle, V. A., & Sims, J. M. (1999). Making sense of the 12-lead ECG. *Nursing, 29*(7), 34–39.

27. Montes, P. (1997). Managing outpatient cardiac catheterization. *American Journal of Nursing, 97*(8), 34–37.
28. Murphy, M. J., & Berding, C. B. (1999). Use of measurements of myoglobin and cardiac troponins in the diagnosis of acute myocardial infarction. *Critical Care Nurse, 19*(1), 58–66.
29. Norman, E. M. (1997). Combining dobutamine stress testing and TEE. *American Journal of Nursing, 97*(7), 16HH and 16MM.
30. O'Hanlon-Nickols, T. (1997). The adult cardiovascular system. *American Journal of Nursing, 97*(12), 34–40.
31. Pagana, J. D., & Pagana, T. J. (1998). *Mosbys manual of diagnostic and laboratory tests*. St. Louis: Mosby.
32. Paul, S. (1997). Arrhythmias in women. *Critical Care Nursing Clinics of North America, 9*(4), 545–553.
33. Pennington, J. C., Tecce, M. A., & Segal, B. L. (1997). Heart protection: Controlling risk factors for cardiovascular disease. *Geriatrics, 52*(12), 40–50.
34. Penque, S., et al. (1998). Women and coronary artery disease: Relationship between descriptors of signs and symptoms and diagnostic and treatment course. *American Journal of Critical Care, 7*(3), 175–182.
35. Pinkowish, M. D. (1998). New CAD risk factors: Interesting, but how useful? *Patient Care, 32*(11), 134–165.
36. Seller, R. H. (1996). *Differential diagnosis of common complaints* (3rd ed.). Philadelphia: W. B. Saunders.

36a. Siomka, A. J. (2000). Demystifying cardiac markers. *American Journal of Nursing, 100*(1), 36–40.

37. Svetkey, L. P., et al. (1999). Effects of dietary patterns on blood pressure: Subgroup analysis of the Dietary Approaches to Stop Hypertension (DASH) randomized clinical trial. *Archives of Internal Medicine, 159*(3), 285–293.
38. Swartz, M. H. (1998). *Textbook of physical diagnosis: History and physical* (3rd ed.). Philadelphia: W. B. Saunders.
39. Tremko, L. A. (1997). Understanding diagnostic cardiac catheterization. *American Journal of Nursing, 97*(2), 16K–16R.
40. Trends in ischemic heart disease death rates for black and whites—United States, 1981–1995. (1998). *Morbidity and Mortality Weekly Report, 47*(44), 945–949.
41. Wingate, S. (1997). Cardiovascular anatomy and physiology in the female. *Critical Care Nursing Clinics of North America, 9*(4), 447–452.
42. Youngkin, E. Q., & Israel, D. S. (1996). A review and critique of common herbal alterative therapies. *Nurse Practitioner, 21*(10), 39–62.

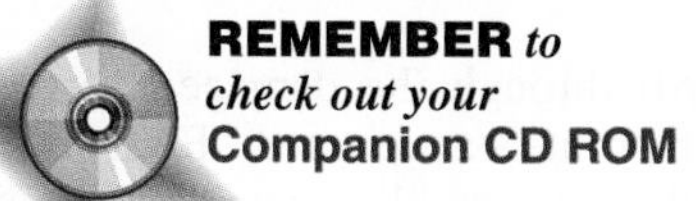

CHAPTER 55

Management of Clients with Structural Cardiac Disorders

Barbara B. Ott

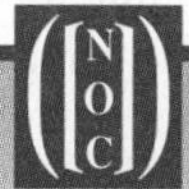

NURSING OUTCOMES CLASSIFICATION (NOC)
for Nursing Diagnoses—Clients with Structural Cardiac Disorders

Activity Intolerance
Activity Tolerance
Endurance
Energy Conservation
Altered Nutrition: Less Than Body Requirements
Nutritional Status: Food and Fluid Intake
Decreased Cardiac Output
Cardiac Pump Effectiveness
Circulation Status
Tissue Perfusion: Abdominal Organs
Tissue Perfusion: Peripheral
Vital Signs Status
Impaired Gas Exchange
Respiratory Status: Ventilation
Tissue Perfusion: Pulmonary
Vital Signs Status
Impaired Physical Mobility
Ambulation: Walking
Joint Movement: Active
Mobility Level
Pain
Comfort Level
Pain Control
Pain: Disruptive Effects
Risk for Altered Tissue Perfusion: Cerebral
Neurological Status: Consciousness
Tissue Perfusion: Cerebral
Risk for Ineffective Airway Clearance
Aspiration Control
Respiratory Status: Airway Patency
Respiratory Status: Ventilation
Risk for Ineffective Management of Therapeutic Regimen: Individuals
Compliance Behavior
Participation: Health Care Decisions
Risk for Infection
Immune Status
Tissue Integrity: Skin and Mucous Membranes

Adequate tissue perfusion is essential to good health. Many disorders of the heart can cause inadequate tissue perfusion. Specifically, disorders that affect the structure of the heart may decrease the heart's pumping ability and thus may result in inadequate tissue perfusion.

INFECTIOUS DISORDERS

Bacteria and other microbes are found in abundance in our environment. The heart can become infected by these microbes, a process that prompts an inflammatory response. Involvement of the heart can be lethal during the acute stage or lead to structural damage.

RHEUMATIC FEVER

Rheumatic fever is a diffuse inflammatory disease. It is a delayed response to an infection by group A beta-hemolytic streptococci. Although this infection remains common, the incidence of rheumatic fever has declined dramatically to about 2 per 100,000 people in the United States. This decline is due to an emphasis on prevention. The incidence in developing countries is about 100 per 100,000 people.[7]

Etiology and Risk Factors

Rheumatic fever develops in only a relatively small percentage of people (3%), even after a virulent bout of streptococcal infection; there is, therefore, some evidence of host predisposition. Genetic links are less advanced and less widely performed than for other diseases such as cancer.[13] Once rheumatic fever is acquired, the person becomes more susceptible than the general population to recurrent infection. Poor hygiene, crowding, and poverty are risk factors for acute rheumatic fever. If appropriate antibiotic therapy for group A beta-hemolytic streptococcal infection is given within the first 9 days, rheumatic fever can usually be prevented.[7]

Prevention is the best treatment. The most effective measures against rheumatic fever are probably socioeconomic. In the affluent neighborhoods of Western cities, where there is spacious housing with no crowding, the incidence of rheumatic fever is low. Identification of high-risk persons is also important. Nurses can help to identify mitral valve prolapse (see later) early to prevent valvular disease. Nurses in community settings can identify those with beta-hemolytic streptococcal infections and refer clients for appropriate diagnosis and medical management.

Pathophysiology

Rheumatic fever initiates a diffuse, proliferative, and exudative inflammatory process. In rheumatic fever, the heart, joints, subcutaneous tissue, central nervous system (CNS), and skin are affected. Although the cellular disease process is not clear, the mechanism is probably an abnormal humoral and cell-mediated response to streptococcal cell membrane antigens. These antigens bind to receptors on the heart, other tissues, and joints, which begins the autoimmune response. The inflammatory process often produces permanent and severe heart damage.

Rheumatic fever produces *carditis* (inflammation of the heart). Carditis affects the pericardium, epicardium, myocardium, and endocardium. There may be Aschoff's bodies, minuscule nodules with localized fibrin deposits surrounded by areas of necrosis in the myocardium, which are due to the inflammation of rheumatic fever. Endocardial inflammation causes swelling of the valve leaflets, which leads to valve dysfunction and murmurs. Small bacterial vegetations form on the valve tissues. Rough eroded areas of the valves attract platelets, which adhere and form platelet-fibrin clumps that eventually cause scarring and shortening of the valve. The valves lose their elasticity, and cardiac function is impaired.

First, the damaged valve may become stenosed. This increases the cardiac workload, because higher pressure must be generated to propel blood through the narrow valve. Second, the valve leaflets may become so short that they cannot close securely. As a result, blood regurgitates (leaks backward) through the damaged valve into the chamber from which it was ejected. Both valvular stenosis and regurgitation eventually cause heart failure from the high workload (Table 55–1).

Complications of rheumatic fever include valvular disorders, cardiomegaly, and heart failure. These complications may be fatal.

Clinical Manifestations

The clinical manifestations of rheumatic fever are related to the inflammatory response and include fever, weakness, malaise, weight loss, anorexia, arthritis, carditis, subcutaneous nodules, erythema marginatum, chorea, abdominal pain.

Fever, with a temperature of 38° C (100.4° F) or higher, alternates with normal temperature. Weakness, malaise, weight loss, and anorexia probably develop as a result of fever, pain, and the general debilitation associated with serious illness.

Arthritis, a prominent finding, is painful and migratory. It most often affects the larger joints, such as the ankles, knees, elbows, shoulders, and wrists. The arthritis may or may not be symmetrical. If the client takes aspirin early in the course of the disease, arthritis manifestations may not be as apparent. Joint manifestations may last hours or days.

Carditis, one of the most common manifestations of rheumatic fever, is the most destructive consequence of this disease. Characteristics include a significant murmur, cardiomegaly, pericarditis that produces a significant friction rub, and heart failure. Chest pain due to pericardial inflammation may be present. Sometimes there is myocardial involvement that produces atrioventricular (AV) conduction defects or atrial fibrillation.

Subcutaneous nodules are small, painless, firm nodules that adhere loosely to the tendon sheaths, especially in knees, knuckles, and elbows. They are usually evident

TABLE 55–1 EFFECTS OF RHEUMATIC FEVER ON THE MYOCARDIUM, ENDOCARDIUM, AND PERICARDIUM

Condition	Characteristic Lesion	Cause of Lesion	Significance of Pathophysiologic Involvement
Rheumatic myocarditis	Aschoff's bodies (minute nodules in connective tissue around small arteries in myocardium)	Formed by leukocytes that mass in inflamed tissues	Nodules may eventually become fibrotic. Damage from fibrosis may eventually damage arteries in myocardium. Myocarditis may cause temporary loss in contractile power of heart. Permanent damage rarely results.
Rheumatic endocarditis	Tiny vegetations resembling little beads form along line of closure of valve leaflets (primarily mitral and aortic valves)	Probably result from inflammation, ulceration, and erosion of valve leaflets	Progressive fibrosis, scarring, and calcification of valve leaflets result in valvular incompetence and stenosis
Pericarditis	Nonspecific lesions	Result from diffuse, nonspecific fibrinous or serofibrinous inflammatory reaction	May cause pericardial friction rub; usually no serious sequelae.

only during the first week or so and, generally, only in children.

Erythema marginatum is an unusual rash seen primarily on the trunk. The lesions are crescent-shaped and have clear centers. The rash is transitory and may change in appearance in minutes or hours.

Chorea, a CNS disorder, is manifested by sudden, irregular, aimless, involuntary movements. Chorea disappears without treatment and produces no permanent sequelae.

Abdominal pain, a common clinical manifestation, varies in site and severity. The pain may be related to engorgement of the liver.

No single diagnostic feature identifies rheumatic fever. Many of the common clinical manifestations are associated with other disorders as well as rheumatic fever. The Jones criteria were developed to assist in diagnosis (Box 55–1). The clinical manifestations of rheumatic fever may last 3 months.

A positive throat culture for group A beta-hemolytic streptococci can help to confirm the diagnosis. An elevated white blood cell (WBC) count, erythrocyte sedimentation rate (ESR), and C-reactive protein may indicate inflammation.

Outcome Management

Medical Management

The goals of medical management include (1) eradicating infection, (2) maximizing cardiac output, and (3) promoting comfort.

BOX 55–1 Guidelines for the Diagnosis of Initial Attack of Rheumatic Fever (Jones Criteria)*

Major Manifestations

1. Carditis
2. Polyarthritis
3. Chorea
4. Erythema marginatum
5. Subcutaneous nodules

Minor Manifestations

1. Clinical findings
   a. Arthralgia
   b. Fever
2. Laboratory findings
   a. Elevated acute phase reactants
      (1) Erythrocyte sedimentation rate
      (2) C-reactive protein
   b. Prolonged P-R interval

Supporting Evidence of Antecedent Group A Streptococcal Infection

1. Positive throat culture or rapid streptococcal antigen test
2. Elevated or rising streptococcal antibody titer

*If supported by evidence of preceding group A streptococcal infection, the presence of two major manifestations, or of one major and two minor manifestations, a high probability of acute rheumatic fever is indicated.

Modified from Diagnosis of Rheumatic Fever—Special Writing Group (1992). *Journal of the American Medical Association, 268*(15), 2069–2073.

ERADICATE INFECTION

The first priority is to eradicate the streptococcal infection. Usually this can be accomplished with oral administration of penicillin. For penicillin-allergic clients, the physician usually prescribes erythromycin.

The client typically takes prophylactic agents for rheumatic fever for 5 years after the initial attack. After 5 years, recurrences are rare. Clients who have had rheumatic fever remain vulnerable to bacterial endocarditis. Therefore, in addition to the antibiotics they take to prevent rheumatic fever recurrence, they must be referred for evaluation for possible prophylactic medications before and after any surgical procedure or dental work. Specific evaluation for prophylaxis medication must be individualized according to recommendations by the American Heart Association.[6]

Careful monitoring for side effects of multiple cardiac drugs that may be prescribed for clients with valvular disease is essential.

MAXIMIZE CARDIAC OUTPUT

Corticosteroids are used to treat carditis, especially if heart failure is evident. If heart failure develops, treatment, including cardiac glycosides and diuretics, is effective.

PROMOTE COMFORT

Clients with arthritic manifestations obtain clinical relief with salicylates; however, because these drugs can result in a misdiagnosis, a firm diagnosis should be in place before administration of salicylates. Bed rest is usually prescribed to reduce cardiac effort until evidence of inflammation has subsided. For clients with rheumatic valvular heart disease, bacterial endocarditis prophylaxis may be necessary (see Infective Endocarditis).

Nursing Management of the Medical Client

ASSESSMENT

Nursing assessment involves gathering baseline and ongoing subjective and objective data. Assess vital signs to reveal the presence of fever, tachycardia, and stability of blood pressure. Vital signs are also used as a measure of activity tolerance. Auscultate heart sounds for presence of a friction rub, and palpate peripheral pulses. A baseline electrocardiogram (ECG) is documented. Assess baseline nutritional and hydration data.

Assess psychosocial data on the client's feelings regarding restrictions of activity, support systems, coping strategies, level of discomfort, and knowledge (the client's and family's) concerning the nature of, and intervention for, rheumatic fever.

DIAGNOSIS, OUTCOMES, INTERVENTIONS

Activity Intolerance. A reduced cardiac reserve and enforced bed rest can quickly lead to activity intolerance. The nursing diagnosis statement would be *Activity Intolerance related to reduced cardiac reserve and enforced bed rest.*

Outcomes. The client will progress toward an optimal level of physical activity tolerance, based on underlying cardiovascular status and psychosocial readiness, as evidenced by ability to (1) pace activity, (2) verbalize improvement in fatigue, (3) express acceptance of any imposed activity restrictions, and (4) steadily increase activity level to include climbing one flight of stairs without chest pain or without ECG changes, while the heart rate remains under 90 BPM (beats per minute).

Interventions. Bed rest is important in the acute phase, because it reduces myocardial oxygen demand, and usually continues until the following criteria are met:

- Temperature remains normal without use of salicylates
- Resting pulse remains under 100 BPM
- ECG tracings show no signs of myocardial damage
- ESR returns to normal
- Pericardial friction rub is not present

Once ambulatory, the client must still be careful not to overdo. Assess the client's stamina and response to exercise to gauge the degree of gradual activity progression. Assess vital signs before and after exercise. After 3 to 5 minutes of rest, reassess vital signs. The client should reduce or discontinue activity if chest pain, vertigo, dyspnea, confusion, a drop in blood pressure, or an irregular pulse develops. The length of activity restriction depends on whether carditis develops and the extent of permanent heart damage. Restrictions may extend for months. In severe cases of rheumatic carditis, clients may be forced to undergo restrictions on a permanent basis. Encourage a gradual increase in activity within the limits of the client's condition.

The client experiencing chorea requires sedatives, bed rest, and protection from self-injury. A carefully planned and supervised activity schedule should be maintained and evaluated.

Pain. The inflammatory response in the joints can lead to pain. The nursing diagnosis statement would be *Pain related to the inflammatory response in the joints.*

Outcomes. The client will experience increased comfort, as evidenced by (1) reports of restful sleep and reduced discomfort, (2) expression of joint pain relief, (3) reduced use of pain medications, and (4) a relaxed body posture and calm facial expression.

Interventions. Obtain a clear description of the pain or discomfort. Identify the source of greatest discomfort as a focus for intervention. Administer analgesics as needed. Balance rest and activity according to the degree of pain and activity tolerance. Other pain interventions are discussed in Chapter 23.

Altered Nutrition: Less Than Body Requirements. Hypermetabolism seen with fever and inflammation and other factors in rheumatic fever can lead to protein calorie malnutrition. This diagnosis is stated as *Altered nutrition: Less Than Body Requirements, related to fever, inflammation, anorexia, and fatigue.*

Outcomes. The client will maintain or restore adequate nutritional balance, as evidenced by (1) resumption of body weight before the illness or no further weight loss, (2) consumption of 75% or more of each meal served, (3) normal serum albumin or prealbumin, and (4) a positive nitrogen balance.

Interventions. A high-protein, high-carbohydrate diet helps maintain adequate nutrition in the presence of fever and infection. Hypermetabolic states (fever and infection) can induce a catabolic state, thus delaying healing. Vitamin and mineral supplements may also benefit the client. Oral hygiene every 4 hours, small attractive meal servings, and foods that are not overly rich, sweet, or greasy stimulate the appetite. Adequate fluid intake prevents dehydration resulting from fever. If the client shows signs of severe carditis or heart failure, sodium and fluids must be restricted. Daily weights can serve as an indication of nutritional and fluid status.

Risk for Ineffective Management of Therapeutic Regimen (Individuals). Following rheumatic fever, the client must follow a lifelong regimen to reduce risk of rheumatic heart disease. This diagnosis is stated as *Risk for Ineffective Management of Therapeutic Regimen (Individuals) related to a need for lifelong therapy.*

Outcomes. The client and family will demonstrate adequate knowledge of rheumatic fever and its cause, course, and therapy, as evidenced by the ability to accurately describe the causes and process of rheumatic fever, its clinical manifestations, its prevention, and the rationale for prescribed interventions.

Interventions. Today, streptococcal infections do not have to develop into rheumatic fever if the client seeks immediate assessment and begins antibiotics. Clients who have recovered from an episode of rheumatic fever may avoid subsequent attacks by taking prophylactic doses of antibiotics and observing good health practices. Because repeated attacks may lead to serious heart disease and permanent cardiac disability, it is important to emphasize means of avoiding subsequent attacks.

Instruct the client how to reduce exposure to streptococcal infection as follows:

1. Take good care of teeth and gums, and obtain prompt dental care for cavities and gingivitis. Prophylactic medication may be needed before invasive dental procedures, and individualized evaluation for prophylaxis medication is needed.[6]
2. Avoid people who have an upper respiratory infection or who have had a recent streptococcal infection.
3. Notify the physician if any of the manifestations of streptococcal sore throat (pharyngitis) develop. It is extremely important to begin antibiotic therapy promptly for any infection. The clinical manifestations include fever (102° to 104° F), chills, sore throat, and enlarged, painful lymph nodes. Advise clients who have had rheumatic fever that they must guard against infections for the rest of their lives to avoid development of heart disease.

EVALUATION

Rheumatic fever is treated over 10 days. Expect activity tolerance to improve once fever and pain are controlled. Altered nutrition may require more than 2 weeks to show improvement, depending on the severity of anorexia and the fever.

INFECTIVE ENDOCARDITIS

Endocarditis is an inflammatory process of the endocardium, especially the valves. This disorder was once lethal, but morbidity and mortality have been greatly reduced with the use of antibiotics and advanced diagnostic procedures.

In the past, many different terms and classifications were used to describe infective endocarditis. You may still see these terms used or find them in old medical records. Some are defined here.

- *Subacute bacterial endocarditis* (SBE): develops gradually over several weeks or months; usually caused by organisms of low virulence, such as *Streptococcus viridans,* which has a limited ability to infect other tissues
- *Acute bacterial endocarditis:* develops over days or weeks with an erratic course and earlier development of complications; commonly caused by *Staphylococcus aureus,* which is capable of infecting other body tissues
- *Native valve endocarditis:* an infection of a previously normal or damaged valve
- *Prosthetic valve endocarditis:* an infection of a prosthetic valve
- *Nonbacterial thrombotic endocarditis:* caused by sterile thrombotic lesions (often aggregates of platelets), which may develop in people with cancer or other chronic diseases

Changes in the population at risk are altering the classic picture of endocarditis. The incidence is continuing to rise. Each year, about 15,000 to 20,000 new cases are appearing. Infective endocarditis is now the fourth leading cause of life-threatening infectious disease syndromes.[3] The median age of clients has increased from 30 to 40 years in the early antibiotic era to 47 to 64 years in recent decades.[12] Fewer clients are being seen with the classic physical signs of advanced endocarditis, such as Osler's nodes, finger clubbing, or Roth's spots (see Clinical Manifestations). The proportion of cases due to streptococci has fallen slightly. The proportion of cases caused by gram-negative bacilli, fungi, and other unusual microbes is increasing.

The changes are traced to several notable alterations in the population. The increased incidence of endocarditis caused by yeasts and fungi is attributable to the increased number of persons with valve prostheses, to the increased number of persons using intravenous (IV) drugs, and rising use of long-term antimicrobial therapy or immunosuppression.

The decreased incidence of rheumatic fever results in a lower incidence of endocarditis, whereas the number of children surviving congenital heart disease results in an increased incidence. The growing elderly population also leads to an increase in the number of endocarditis episodes.

Etiology and Risk Factors

Common infecting organisms include staphylococci (*S. aureus, S. faecalis, S. epidermidis*), streptococci, *Escherichia coli*, gram-negative organisms (*Klebsiella, Pseudomonas, Serratia marcescens*) and fungi (*Candida, Aspergillus*). These organisms enter the body through the oral cavity after dental procedures, mouth or tooth abscesses, oral irrigations, or oral irritations from dental floss or bridgework. The upper respiratory tract is another port of entry following surgery, intubations, or infections. Direct exposure of the bloodstream to organisms can occur with prolonged IV catheters, hemodialysis catheters, and IV drug use. Procedures involving the gastrointestinal and genitourinary tracts (e.g., barium enemas, sigmoidoscopy, colonoscopy, percutaneous liver biopsy, catheterization, urethrotomy, prostatectomy, cystoscopy) have been associated with infective endocarditis.

Reproductive conditions have also been linked (e.g., delivery of a newborn, abortion, intrauterine devices, pelvic inflammatory diseases). Defective heart valves causing changes in blood flow and pressures encourage the proliferation of vegetations. Open heart surgery to replace damaged valves increases the risk of endocarditis. Fortunately, coronary artery bypass grafting (CABG), one of the most frequently performed surgical procedures in the United States, carries a low risk of infective endocarditis because the endocardium is not invaded during the operation.

Circulating microorganisms in the bloodstream attach to the endocardial surface and multiply. Usually the multiplication of these organisms requires a rough or abnormal endocardium. IV drug abusers may be injecting particulate matter into the bloodstream, with damage to the previously normal endocardium that allows the organism to adhere, thereby initiating acute bacterial endocarditis.

Pathophysiology

Microorganisms enter the bloodstream in many ways. Once the colonization process begins on the endothelium, replication occurs and bacterial colonies form within layers of platelets and fibrin. As the colonies become entangled within the tight layers of fibrin and platelets, the colony becomes less and less vulnerable to the body's defense mechanisms. The bacteria stimulate the humoral immune system to produce nonspecific antibodies, but the bacteria are protected by the fibrin-platelet aggregation. It is not uncommon for these vegetations to form clots that travel to other organs, forming abscesses. The vegetations can severely damage heart valves by perforating and deforming the valve leaflets (Fig. 55–1). Extensions of the

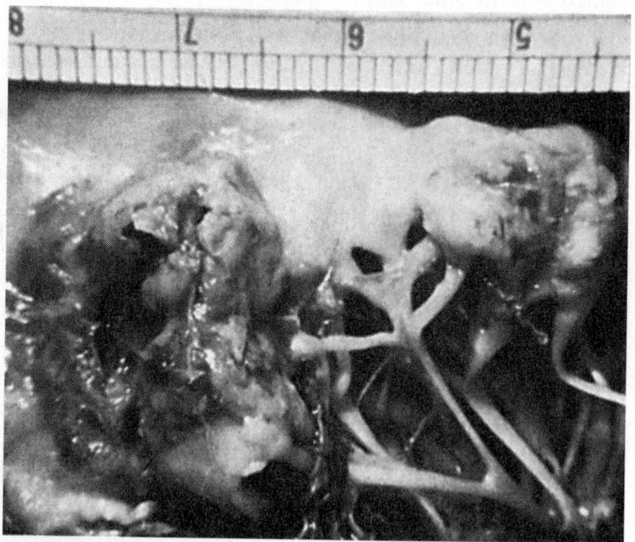

FIGURE 55–1 Vegetations of the heart valves resulting from infective endocarditis. Large vegetations were present on the leaflets of the mitral valve. (From Braunwald, E. [1992]. *Heart disease: A textbook of cardiovascular medicine* [4th ed.] Philadelphia: W. B. Saunders.)

bacteria may invade the aorta or pericardium. The amount of damage depends on the type and virulence of the organisms causing the infection.

There are many possible complications. Heart failure may develop as a result of structural valvular damage. Arterial emboli can occur from the vegetation. Systemic embolization occurs in 30% of clients with left-sided infective endocarditis. Common infarction sites are the kidney, spleen, and brain. Pulmonary embolus is associated with right-sided infective endocarditis. Emboli can also travel to the brain and produce myriad manifestations. Occasionally, immune complex glomerulonephritis will develop. Renal function usually returns to normal after the infection has been controlled.

Clinical Manifestations

Clinical manifestations of infective endocarditis include those related to the infectious process, embolization, and the immune response.

Clinical manifestations related to the infection include fever, chills alternating with sweats, malaise, weakness, anorexia, weight loss, pallor, backache, and splenomegaly.[24] Clients may report feeling as if they have the flu with headaches and musculoskeletal aching. In acute infection, clients appear very ill. Fever, chills, and prostration are so severe that hospital admission is usually necessary within a few days.

Cardiac murmurs eventually develop, but they may be absent in the early stages of infection. In clients with preexisting valvular disease, new murmurs may be heard. Heart failure may develop suddenly in either acute or subacute endocarditis. Mechanical complications include perforation of a valve leaflet, rupture of one of the chordae tendineae, or development of a functional stenosis from obstruction of blood flow by large vegetations.

Embolization occurs in about 30% of clients with infective carditis. Clinical manifestations related to embolization can occur in any part of the body. They are presented here in order from head to toe:

- Stroke, transient ischemic attacks, aphasia, or ataxia
- Loss of vision from embolization to the brain or retinal artery
- Petechiae on the neck, conjunctiva, chest, abdomen and mouth
- Roth's spots—a white or yellow center surrounded by a bright-red, irregular halo seen by ophthalmoscope
- Myocardial infarction, which may develop as a result of coronary artery embolism
- Pulmonary embolus
- Splinter hemorrhages, which look like tiny splinters under the nail
- Osler's nodes—painful, erythematous, pea-sized nodules on tips of the fingers and toes resulting from inflammation around a small, infected embolus
- Finger clubbing, although less common today, may occur in clients with long-standing infective endocarditis; pathogenesis remains unclear
- Janeway's lesions—flat, small, nontender red spots on the palms of the hands and the soles of the feet
- Evidence of an immunologic reaction to infection, including arthralgia, proteinuria, hematuria, casts, and acidosis

Because the clinical manifestations of endocarditis are numerous and often nonspecific, several modalities are employed for differential medical diagnosis. Blood cultures for bacteria, fungus, and yeast are the most important diagnostic tests. Blood cultures should be obtained for all clients with both fever and heart murmur. ECGs should be done on admission to the hospital and repeated during the hospital stay. Although a negative ECG does not rule out endocarditis, transesophageal echocardiography can be useful in arriving at a diagnosis. A chest x-ray study is useful in identifying early heart failure. A complete blood count (CBC) and other routine diagnostic procedures are also helpful.

Outcome Management

Medical Management

The chief aims of management are to eradicate the infecting organism and to treat complications. The advent of antimicrobial therapy has changed this infection from one that was almost always fatal to one that is rarely fatal. The choice of antibiotic depends on the organism involved. Penicillin and streptomycin are commonly used. Therapy is usually administered by the IV route and continued for 4 to 6 weeks. Drug administration is usually begun in the hospital but is occasionally continued at home with extensive discharge planning and education.

Occasionally, after the infection is under control (negative blood cultures, absence of fever, and normal WBC count), it may be necessary for the client to undergo heart valve replacement for reversal of newly developed heart failure. Complications that could have developed as a result of the infecting organism warrant careful evaluation.

Nursing Management of the Medical Client

Nursing assessment focuses on gathering data about the client's hemodynamic stability (particularly the presence of a new heart murmur and embolic complications), level of comfort, coping ability, support from significant others, and potential for self-care.

Administer IV antibiotics as prescribed. Antibiotics relieve much discomfort within a few days. Treat fever, when present, with rest, cooling measures, forced fluids, and sometimes salicylates. As with most infectious processes, encourage the client to eat a nutritious diet, drink sufficient fluids, and rest mentally and physically.

The client may need to be hospitalized for 2 to 6 weeks if home care is not an option. Do not enforce complete bed rest unless fever or signs of heart damage develop. Auscultate the heart every 8 hours for heart murmurs. Assess for rapid pulse, easy fatigability, dyspnea, restlessness, signs of heart failure, and embolic manifestations. Document these manifestations if they occur, and report them to the physician.

When the client's condition improves, plan and implement a progressive activity schedule and a teaching plan (see the Client Education Guide: Infective Carditis) As activity increases, monitor the client's physical response to exercise. For example, assess blood pressure, heart rate, diaphoresis, vertigo, and weakness.

CLIENT EDUCATION GUIDE

Infective Endocarditis

1. Continue taking your intravenous antibiotics with the help of a family member after you leave the hospital.
2. Follow your doctor's advice about gradually resuming activities. A month of convalescence at home is typical.
3. Tell your physician and dentist about having had infective endocarditis. If you are going to have surgery or extensive dental work, be sure you take a full course of antibiotics first.
4. Floss every day, and brush with a soft toothbrush. Consult your dentist before using water-jet cleaning devices because these devices may cause gums to bleed and may put you at risk for infection.
5. Monitor yourself for manifestations of infective endocarditis. Take your temperature every day for the next month; and keep a record of your readings. Report any fever, chills, malaise, loss of appetite, weight loss, or increased fatigue to your physician.

Self-Care

The trend toward early hospital discharge has changed the course of treatment for clients with infective endocarditis. IV therapy may now be routinely given in the home. Clients who are alert, cooperative, and reasonably stable and who want to return home may be allowed to do so. Typically, the nurse, pharmacist, and physician teach the techniques of self-administered IV antibiotics. Before discharge, the client must demonstrate the knowledge and technique required. The physician's office or home health care nurses often monitor the client's progress.

Home IV antibiotic therapy offers many benefits. It is less costly than hospital care, motivates clients to become active participants in their own care, reestablishes a more normal lifestyle, and promotes a sense of control that aids in psychosocial and physiologic recovery. To be effective, this program calls for exceptional communication and cooperation between health care team members and the client.

MYOCARDITIS

Myocarditis is an inflammation of the myocardial wall. It can be caused by almost any bacterial, viral, or parasitic organism as well as by radiation, toxic agents such as lead, and drugs such as lithium and cocaine. Myocarditis affects people of all ages and may be acute or chronic. An immunodeficient person is at greater risk for myocarditis. Frequently, the inflammation is not limited to the myocardium but extends to the pericardium, with production of an associated pericarditis. The incidence is not possible to ascertain[17] and varies with the client's age and with various etiologic agents.

Etiology

In the United States, most cases of myocarditis are due to viral infections. Viruses associated with this disorder include coxsackieviruses A and B, mumps, influenza virus serotypes A and B, rubella virus, measles virus, adenoviruses, echoviruses, cytomegalovirus, and Epstein-Barr virus.

Other causes include bacterial infections from diphtheria, typhoid fever, staphylococci, pneumococci, tetanus, and tuberculosis. Myocarditis can also be caused by hypersensitivity immune reactions seen with acute rheumatic fever and postcardiotomy syndrome, toxins and chemicals such as alcohol, large doses of radiation therapy to the chest for the treatment of malignancy, and parasitic infections, including Chagas' disease and toxoplasmosis.

Pathophysiology

Myocardial damage from acute myocarditis is usually the result of the direct invasion or the toxic effects of the microorganism in cardiac myocytes. This can cause an alteration in cellular energy systems and cellular damage. Endomyocardial biopsies are used in diagnosis of the viral infection.[17]

Usually, myocarditis involves both ventricles. If myocardial contractility is impaired, ventricular diastolic pressures and volumes may be elevated in order to maintain stroke volume. Disruptions leading to cardiac dysrhythmias can decrease cardiac output.

Clinical Manifestations

Clinical manifestations vary widely, and there may be no clinical manifestations at all. The health history may reveal a recent upper respiratory infection, a viral pharyngitis, or tonsillitis. The most frequent manifestations, however, are fatigue, dyspnea, palpitations, and chest pain. The client often experiences chest pain as a mild continuous pressure or soreness in the chest. Thus, the chest pain of myocarditis can be distinguished from the effort-induced pain of angina pectoris. Tachycardia, if present, may be disproportionate to the degree of fever, exertion, or illness. Dysrhythmias can also occur, sometimes producing a fatal circulatory collapse. There may be a pericardial friction rub if the client has pericarditis.

In most cases, myocarditis is self-limiting and uncomplicated. If myocardial involvement becomes extensive or prolonged, myofibril degeneration can produce heart failure, with pulmonary congestion, dyspnea, neck vein distention, peripheral edema, and cardiomegaly. Recurrent myocarditis can produce cardiomyopathy. Possible complications include heart failure, dilated cardiomyopathy, and sudden death from lethal dysrhythmias or rupture of a myocardial aneurysm.

The chest x-ray may show an enlarged cardiac silhouette due to ventricular enlargement or pericardial effusion. Blood tests may show a moderate leukocytosis and elevated cardiac enzymes. Echocardiography is helpful in determining heart chamber size and ventricular functioning. Gallium scan shows regional wall abnormalities, dilated ventricles, and hypokinesis of the left ventricle. ECG abnormalities and elevated serum levels of cardiac enzymes are helpful in the diagnosis. The ECG may show a bundle branch block or complete AV heart block, ST-segment elevation, or T-wave flattening.

Outcome Management

Clients with acute myocarditis are usually admitted to the hospital for observation. Clients with pericardial effusion, dysrhythmias, heart failure, or hypotension are usually admitted to the intensive care unit (ICU). Medical management begins with specific therapy for the underlying infection. Bed rest is suggested to decrease cardiac work. Supplemental oxygen may be prescribed for clients with low cardiac output or dysrhythmias. Immunosuppressive therapy had been previously considered helpful, but new research does not support this therapy.[11, 27] Antipyretic agents are helpful for the fever and its hemodynamic effects, which result in increased myocardial workload. Clients who remain at home may use Holter monitoring, which provides continuous surveillance of the client's heart rhythm.

The outlook for clients with myocarditis is generally good. Although most clients recover rapidly, some have recurrent or chronic myocarditis and some become very ill and die.

Nursing management for the client experiencing myocarditis is essentially the same as that provided to clients with infective endocarditis and rheumatic fever. Review those sections within this chapter.

Teaching begins when acute manifestations have subsided and the client has demonstrated physical and emotional readiness. Teach clients how to monitor their pulse rate and rhythm. Instruct them to report any sudden changes in heart rate, rhythm, or palpitations immediately. Encourage family members to take cardiopulmonary resuscitation (CPR) training, which can be obtained from such groups as the local fire department, the American Red Cross, or the American Heart Association. Educating family members about CPR can enhance their sense of preparedness for an emergency.

Because the myocardial infectious process resolves slowly and late complications can occur, advise clients to continue self-monitoring and to schedule clinical follow-up appointments, even after apparent recovery.

The potential of lethal dysrhythmias may frighten the client and significant others. The client who is experiencing extreme anxiety, fear, and ineffective coping may manifest insomnia, tearfulness, somatic complaints, inability to problem-solve, and agitation. Determine with the client (and family) the specific focus of anxiety. Clarify any misconceptions that arise. Speak slowly and calmly, and focus on the present situation, giving feedback about current reality. Encourage the use of relaxation techniques to help allay stress. Schedule activities around periods of undisturbed sleep.

PERICARDITIS

Pericarditis may be either acute or chronic (*recurrent*). It is not known why pericarditis may be an acute illness in some clients and recurrent in others. Chronic pericarditis (*constrictive* pericarditis) is present when a fibrotic, thickened, and adherent pericardium restricts diastolic filling of the heart. This process eventually results in cardiac failure.

■ ACUTE PERICARDITIS

Pathophysiology

Acute pericarditis is a syndrome resulting from inflammation of the parietal and visceral pericardium. Because of the proximity of the pericardium to the pleura, lungs, sternum, diaphragm, and myocardium, pericarditis may be a consequence of a number of inflammatory or infectious processes (Box 55–2). Acute pericarditis is usually viral (idiopathic) in origin.

Agents or processes causing pericardial inflammation create an exudate of fibrin, WBCs, and endothelial cells. The exudate covers the pericardium and causes further inflammation of the surrounding pleura and tissues. The fibrinous exudate may localize to one region of the heart or may be generalized. Acute pericarditis may be either *dry* (fibrinous) or *exudative*. Under normal conditions, the pericardial sac contains about 50 ml of clear, serous-like fluid. Volumes from 100 to 3000 ml of serofibrinous exudate can accumulate with pericarditis. The exudate accumulates in the pericardial sac, causing cardiac tamponade that restricts cardiac filling and emptying. Without prompt treatment, shock and death can result from decreased cardiac output.

Dry pericarditis can occur after a common viral infection, myocardial infarction, tuberculosis, bacteremia, or renal failure. Delicate adhesions form within the pericardial space along with serous fibrin deposition, hemorrhage, and calcification. Adhesions may eventually obliterate the pericardial sac. Inflammation of the pericardium frequently penetrates the myocardium to some degree, which produces myopericarditis.

Clinical Manifestations

The most characteristic subjective clinical manifestation of pericarditis is chest pain. The nature of this pain varies with the client. Sometimes the pain is similar to that of

BOX 55–2 Causes of Pericarditis

Infections
- Viral: coxsackie, influenza
- Bacterial: tuberculosis, staphylococcus, streptococcus, meningococcus, pneumococcus
- Parasitic
- Fungal

Myocardial injury
- Myocardial infarction (Dressler's syndrome)
- Cardiac trauma: blunt or penetrating
- Post cardiac surgery
- Hypersensitivity

Collagen diseases
- Rheumatic fever
- Scleroderma
- Systemic lupus erythematosus
- Rheumatoid arthritis

Drug reaction
- Procainamide
- Methysergide
- Hydralazine

Radiation therapy
Cobalt therapy
Metabolic disorders
- Uremia
- Myxedema

Chronic anemia
Neoplasm: lymphoma
Aortic dissection

myocardial infarction; at other times, it mimics the pain of pleurisy. The pain is exacerbated with respiration and rotating the trunk but usually does not radiate to the arms. Sitting up often relieves the pain.

Pericardial *friction rub* is a classic objective manifestation of acute pericarditis. The rub is produced by inflamed, roughened pericardial layers that create friction as their surfaces rub together during heart movement. Auscultation over the precordium reveals a scratchy, leathery, or creaky sound that is heard anywhere over the precordium but most frequently at the third intercostal space left of the sternal border. The rub is best heard with the diaphragm of the stethoscope and with the client holding his or her breath. In some clients, the sound is best heard with the client sitting up. Pericardial friction rubs vary in intensity from hour to hour and from day to day.

Fever is another common finding in clients with pericarditis. The temperature may rise to 39.4° C (103° F). Chills, malaise, joint pain, anorexia, nausea, and weight loss accompany the fever. Dyspnea and chest pain can potentiate anxiety. An increase in heart rate usually corresponds to the degree of fever and anxiety.

The ECG may indicate bradycardia or atrial fibrillation. The ECG frequently shows a decrease in the amplitude of the QRS complex and changes in the ST-segment elevation in leads I, II, aVF, and V_4 to V_6 and inversion of the T wave.[15] Laboratory studies show an elevated ESR and may show an elevated WBC count. Cardiac enzymes are usually normal but may be elevated.

Outcome Management

When the cause of acute pericarditis is known, treatment of the cause can be planned accordingly. If no causal agent is known, symptomatic intervention for acute dry pericarditis is provided. Pain and fever, usually self-limited, may be eased by aspirin given in maximally tolerated doses. The physician may prescribe a nonsteroidal anti-inflammatory drug (NSAID). Stronger analgesia, such as morphine sulfate, may be necessary if chest pain becomes severe.

If acute pericarditis is present after a myocardial infarction, reassure the client that the pain experienced with pericarditis is not to be associated with another infarction. If the client becomes anxious, thinking that this pain might be that of another infarction, oxygen demand increases and myocardial ischemia may develop.

The focus of nursing care related to pericarditis is the same as that described for the other inflammatory cardiac diseases discussed in this chapter. Nursing assessment of the client with pericarditis also includes scrutiny for the presence of pericardial tamponade (pulsus paradoxus, distended neck veins). Vigilant assessment is necessary. Provide reassurance concerning the temporary nature of the disease.

■ ACUTE PERICARDITIS WITH EFFUSION

Acute pericarditis with effusion results when fluid accumulates within the pericardial sac. Rapid or excessive fluid accumulations may compress the heart and reduce ventricular filling and cardiac output. When fluid accumulates slowly, the fibrous pericardium is better able to stretch and accommodate its presence. Clients can tolerate 1 to 2 L of fluid without an increase in intrapericardial pressure if accumulation is slow. However, the normal unstretched pericardial sac can accommodate the rapid addition of only 80 to 200 ml of fluid without a decrease in cardiac output.

Pericardial effusion may be asymptomatic. If dry pericarditis precedes the condition, the friction rub may disappear. Fever may develop. Heart sounds may be muffled because the pericardial fluid accumulates between the stethoscope and the heart valves and chambers quieting the heart sounds.

Pulsus paradoxus can be present. If the client has normal breathing and a systolic difference of greater than 10 mm Hg, evaluation for cardiac compression and possibly cardiac tamponade should be performed.[15]

Echocardiography is the most accurate technique for evaluating pericardial effusion.[15] The test is sensitive enough to detect as little as 20 ml of pericardial fluid. Pericardiocentesis is not indicated unless there is evidence of cardiac compression caused by cardiac tamponade (see next). If pericardial effusion is present, an enlarged cardiac silhouette is seen on the chest radiograph.

Care of the client with pericardial effusion is similar to the plan of intervention for dry pericarditis. Bed rest, analgesia, and proper positioning can help alleviate symptoms. Psychological support is very important.

■ CHRONIC CONSTRICTIVE PERICARDITIS

Chronic constrictive pericarditis is a chronic inflammatory condition in which the pericardium changes into a thick, fibrous band of tissue. This tissue encircles, encases, and compresses the heart, preventing proper ventricular filling and emptying. Cardiac failure eventually results from this slow compression.

This condition usually begins with an episode of acute pericarditis characterized by fibrin deposition, often with pericardial effusion. In most cases, the visceral and parietal layers become completely fused. The heavily fibrosed pericardium restricts diastolic filling in all chambers and decreases systolic ejection.

Clinical manifestations include right ventricular failure first, followed by decreased cardiac output manifesting as fatigue on exertion, dyspnea, leg edema, ascites, low pulse pressure, distended neck veins, and delayed capillary refill time.[18]

Constrictive pericarditis is a progressive disease without spontaneous reversal of manifestations. Relatively few clients survive for many years with minor symptoms. Most of these clients become progressively more disabled over time.

Treatment is both surgical and medical. Medical treatment includes digitalis, diuretics, and sodium restriction to relieve manifestations of right ventricular failure. Surgical intervention involves the excision of the damaged pericardium (pericardiectomy) and should be performed early in the course of the disease.

■ CARDIAC TAMPONADE

Cardiac tamponade is a life-threatening complication caused by accumulation of fluid in the pericardium. This fluid, which can be blood, pus, or air in the pericardial sac, accumulates fast enough and in sufficient quantity to compress the heart and restrict blood flow in and out of the ventricles. *This is a cardiac emergency!*

Large or rapidly accumulating effusions raise the intrapericardial pressure to a point at which venous blood cannot flow into the heart, which decreases ventricular filling. As a result, venous pressure rises and cardiac output and arterial blood pressure fall. A narrowing pulse pressure signals cardiac tamponade. The heart attempts to compensate by beating rapidly (tachycardia), but tachycardia cannot sustain cardiac output for very long. Prompt intervention is necessary to prevent shock and death.

In the client with cardiac tamponade, assessment reveals hypotension, tachycardia, jugular venous distention, cyanosis of lips and nails, dyspnea, muffled heart sounds, diaphoresis, and paradoxical pulse (a decrease in systolic arterial pulsation exceeding 10 mm Hg, during inspiration). The client may be comfortable and quiet one minute and then very restless with a feeling of impending doom. Clients may panic when fluid accumulates rapidly. Slowly developing tamponade is characterized by manifestations resembling those of heart failure: nonspecific ECG changes, decreased voltage, and visualization of fluid in the pericardial sac on echocardiogram (see Critical Monitoring: Cardiac Tamponade).

Immediate intervention is required. The emergency intervention of choice is pericardiocentesis, a procedure in which fluid or air is aspirated from the pericardial sac (Fig. 55–2). This procedure relieves pressure on the heart, thereby improving cardiac function and perhaps saving the client's life. Pericardiocentesis is now performed with a soft catheter, which is resulting in fewer cardiac lacerations.[15]

CARDIOMYOPATHY

Cardiomyopathy (Fig. 55–3) is a heart muscle disorder of unknown cause (idiopathic). The three major classes are:

- Dilated (congestive)
- Hypertrophic (also called hypertrophic subaortic stenosis)
- Restrictive

> **CRITICAL MONITORING**
>
> **Cardiac Tamponade**
>
> Report the following manifestations of cardiac tamponade immediately!
>
> Elevated venous pressure (increased central venous pressure)
> Distended neck veins
> Kussmaul's sign (distended neck veins on inspiration)
> Hypotension
> Narrowed pulse pressure
> Tachycardia
> Dyspnea
> Restlessness, anxiety
> Cyanosis of lips and nails
> Diaphoresis
> Muffled heart sounds
> Pulsus paradoxus
> Decreased friction rub
> Decreased QRS voltage and electrical alternans

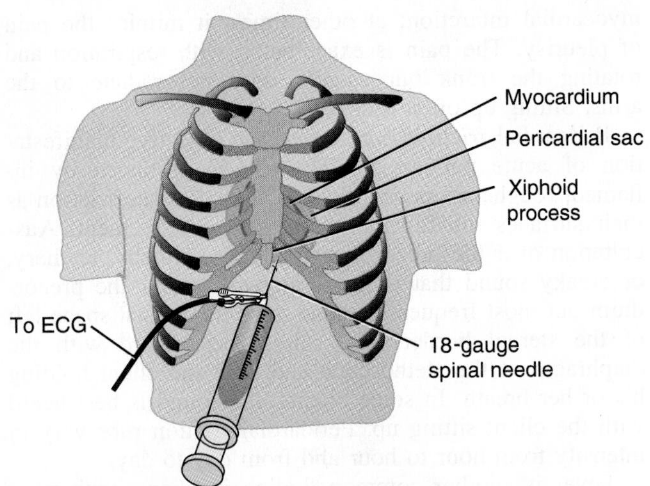

FIGURE 55–2 Pericardiocentesis. ECG, electrocardiogram.

Four conditions seem to increase the risk for its development:

- Chronic ingestion of excessive amounts of alcohol
- Pregnancy
- Systemic hypertension
- Various infections

Table 55–2 compares diagnostic data for the three types of idiopathic cardiomyopathy. These forms of cardiomyopathy are described separately.

■ DILATED CARDIOMYOPATHY

Pathophysiology

Dilated (congestive) cardiomyopathy is the most common form. Usually, both the left and right ventricles dilate, the myocardial fibers degenerate, and fibrotic tissue replaces viable tissue. Severe dilation of the heart occurs, but reduced contractility results in decreased stroke volume, low cardiac output, and a compensatory increase in heart rate. These changes eventually lead to heart failure accompanied by lethal ventricular dysrhythmias. The combined problem of ventricular dilation and ineffective myocardial contractility also increases the risk of blood pooling within the heart and subsequent clot formation. Many clients (75%) with idiopathic dilated cardiomyopathy die within 5 years after the onset of manifestations.[27]

Some forms of dilated cardiomyopathy are idiopathic. Other etiologic mechanisms include viral myocarditis, infections, metabolic problems, toxins, pregnancy, neuromuscular disorders, connective tissue disorders and genetic predisposition (20% of cases). Dilated cardiomyopathy associated with pregnancy can disappear. There may be spontaneous rapid improvement in some women and early fatality in others.

Clinical Manifestations

Clinical manifestations usually develop gradually. Fatigue and weakness are common. Chest pain may be present and may be associated with ischemic heart disease. Right-

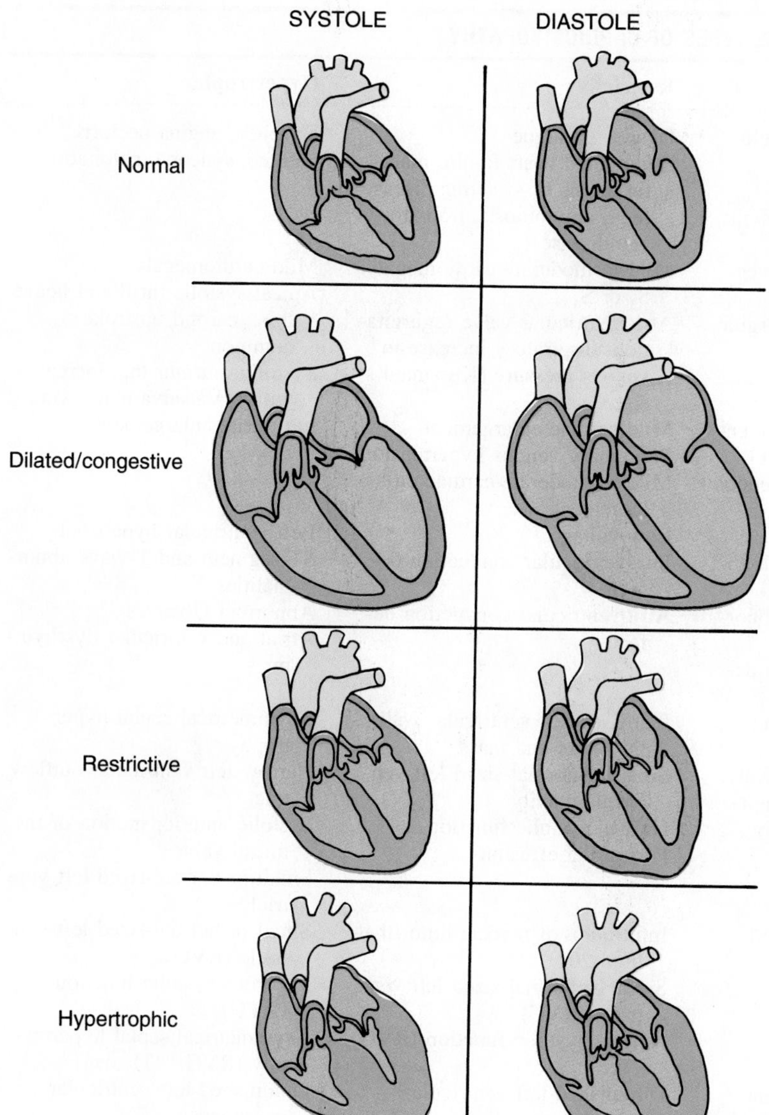

FIGURE 55–3 The three types of cardiomyopathy.

sided heart failure is a late and ominous sign. Systemic blood pressure is usually normal or low. Heart failure develops steadily and is seen as dyspnea, orthopnea, tachycardia, palpitations, peripheral edema, enlargement of jugular veins, and liver engorgement.

An S_4 gallop often precedes the development of heart failure, and an S_3 gallop generally occurs with heart failure. If the heart rate is rapid, both S_4 and S_3 may fuse to form a summation gallop sound. There may be a systolic murmur of mitral or tricuspid insufficiency, because ventricular dilation prevents sufficient closure of those valves. Gallop sounds and regurgitant murmurs may be intensified by an isometric hand grip exercise because of the increase it causes on systemic vascular resistance. Pulmonary crackles become audible as failure progresses.

Diagnostic tests, including ECG, cardiac biopsy, echocardiography, chest x-ray, and blood chemistries, are useful for diagnosis. ECG findings include sinus tachycardia, ventricular dysrhythmias, ST-segment changes, and left bundle branch block.

Outcome Management

Treatment is similar to that for heart failure. Inotropic agents are used to enhance myocardial contractility and to unload the heart. Nitroglycerin as a vasodilator can be used to decrease preload and afterload. Diuretics and sodium-restricted diets are used to decrease pulmonary congestion and to reduce fluid overload. Anticoagulants may help prevent clots and emboli. Antidysrhythmic agents may help suppress ventricular irritability. In appropriate candidates, the implantation of the automatic internal cardiac defibrillator may be used to prevent sudden cardiac death[27] (see Chapter 57).

Rest improves cardiac function and reduces heart size. Most clients experience severe activity intolerance during the later stages of the disease, which automatically limits their activities. However, during the earlier stages, most clients find it difficult to accept rigidly imposed restrictions on activity. Clients should avoid poorly tolerated activities. Advise clients that physical and emotional stress exacerbate the disease. Because alcohol depresses

TABLE 55–2 DIAGNOSTIC DATA FOR THE THREE TYPES OF CARDIOMYOPATHY

	Dilated	Restrictive	Hypertrophic
Manifestations	Heart failure, particularly left-sided Fatigue and weakness Systemic or pulmonary emboli	Dyspnea, fatigue Right-sided heart failure manifestations of systemic disease (e.g., amyloidosis, iron storage disease)	Dyspnea, angina pectoris Fatigue, syncope, palpitations
Physical examination	Moderate to severe cardiomegaly: S_3 and S_4 Atrioventricular valve regurgitation, especially mitral	Mild to moderate cardiomegaly: S_3 or S_4 Atrioventricular valve regurgitation; inspiratory increase in venous pressure (Kussmaul's sign)	Mild cardiomegaly Apical systolic thrill and heave; brisk carotid upstroke S_4 common Systolic murmur that increases with a Valsalva maneuver
Chest x-ray	Moderate-to-marked cardiac enlargement, especially left ventricular pulmonary venous hypertension	Mild cardiac enlargement Pulmonary venous hypertension Mild to moderate cardiac enlargement	Left atrial enlargement
Electrocardiogram	Sinus tachycardia Atrial and ventricular dysrhythmias ST-segment and T-wave abnormalities Intraventricular conduction defects	Low voltage Intraventricular conduction defects Atrioventricular conduction defects	Left ventricular hypertrophy ST-segment and T-wave abnormalities Abnormal Q waves Atrial and ventricular dysrhythmias
Echocardiogram	Left ventricular dilation and dysfunction Abnormal diastolic mitral valve motion secondary to abnormal compliance and filling pressures	Increased left ventricular wall thickness and mass Small or normal-sized left ventricular cavity Normal systolic function Pericardial effusion	Asymmetrical septal hypertrophy Narrow left ventricular outflow tract Systolic anterior motion of the mitral valve Small or normal-sized left ventricle
Radionuclide studies	Left ventricular dilation and dysfunction (RVG)	Infiltration of myocardium (thallium 201 scan) Small or normal-sized left ventricle (RVG) Normal systolic function (RVG)	Small or normal-sized left ventricle (RVG) Vigorous systolic function (RVG) Asymmetrical septal hypertrophy (RVG ^{201}Tl scan)
Cardiac catheterization	Left ventricular enlargement and dysfunction Mitral/tricuspid regurgitation Elevated left-sided and often right-sided filling pressures Diminished cardiac output	Diminished left ventricular compliance Square root sign in ventricular pressure recordings Preserved systolic function Elevated left-sided and right-sided filling pressures	Diminished left ventricular compliance Mitral regurgitation Vigorous systolic function Dynamic left ventricular outflow gradient

RVG, radionuclide ventriculogram.
From Braunwald, E. (1997). *Heart disease: A textbook of cardiovascular medicine* (5th ed.). Philadelphia: W. B. Saunders.

myocardial contractility, the client should abstain from drinking alcoholic beverages.

Only transplantation and specific vasodilator therapy (hydralazine plus nitrates) have resulted in prolonged life.[27] Heart transplantation shows a 5-year survival of greater than 70% in appropriately selected clients.[27]

HYPERTROPHIC CARDIOMYOPATHY

Pathophysiology

Hypertrophic cardiomyopathy (sometimes called *asymmetrical septal hypertrophy)* is disproportionate thickening of the interventricular septum, compared with the free wall of the ventricle. This overgrowth leads to wall rigidity and thereby increases resistance to blood flow from the left atrium. There is also obstruction of left ventricular outflow. Although this disease is also known as idiopathic hypertrophic subaortic stenosis, many clients do not have the obstructive or stenotic component of the disease. Therefore, it is more accurate to use the term *hypertrophic cardiomyopathy* to describe this disease.

Hypertrophic cardiomyopathy appears to be a genetically transmitted disease (~50% of cases). It can also be idiopathic, caused by hypertension or hypoparathyroidism. It appears most often in young adults, both men and women.

In its severest form, the left ventricular wall reaches tremendous dimensions and encroaches on the left ventricular chamber, which becomes small and elongated. Septal hypertrophy may obstruct the left ventricular outflow tract during systole. Frequently, there is diastolic dysfunction in the form of stiffness of the left ventricle during diastolic filling. This stiffness raises left ventricular end-diastolic pressure, which eventually results in elevation of left atrial, pulmonary venous, and pulmonary capillary pressures.

Clinical Manifestations

Clients with hypertrophic cardiomyopathy most commonly present with clinical manifestations in late adolescence or early adulthood, but clinical manifestations may appear at any age. Many clients with hypertrophic cardiomyopathy are asymptomatic and can lead long lives. Interestingly, they often have relatives with incapacitating manifestations of the disease. Sadly, sudden death is frequently the first clinical manifestation of the disease in asymptomatic clients. Sudden death appears more often in younger clients and, if the presence of the disease is known, may be avoided by elimination of strenuous exercise.

The most common manifestation is dyspnea. Dyspnea is due to the high pulmonary pressures produced by the elevated left ventricular end-diastolic pressure. Angina pectoris, fatigue, and syncope are also common clinical manifestations. Cardiac dysrhythmias are frequently present. Palpitations, paroxysmal nocturnal dyspnea, and frank heart failure are less common. Many clients complain of dizzy spells. Exertion tends to worsen most manifestations.

Physical examination may be normal in asymptomatic clients. The appearance of a fourth heart sound may be the only sign of the disease. An increase in the intensity of the heart murmur usually suggests progression of the condition. ECG, chest film, echocardiogram, and radionuclide scanning are very useful in the diagnosis.[27]

Management

The goals of intervention for hypertrophic cardiomyopathy are to reduce ventricular contractility and to relieve left ventricular outflow obstruction. Beta-adrenergic blocking agents, such as propranolol, and calcium channel blockers provide the mainstay of medical intervention. These medications reduce myocardial contractility. With decreased vigor of ventricular contraction, outflow obstruction diminishes. Beta-adrenergic blockade also reduces the heart rate (which further reduces myocardial workload) and prevents dysrhythmias.

Medications that decrease preload (e.g., nitrates, diuretics, morphine) and that increase contractility (e.g., isoproterenol, dopamine, digitalis) are to be avoided. Anticoagulants are used if the client is in atrial fibrillation. The client is at risk for endocarditis and should follow the prophylactic care for that condition.

RESTRICTIVE CARDIOMYOPATHY

Pathophysiology

Restrictive cardiomyopathy, the least common form, is characterized by excessively rigid ventricular walls. This rigidity impairs filling during diastole; however, contractility with systole is usually normal. Any infiltrative process of the heart that results in fibrosis and thickening can cause restrictive cardiomyopathy. The most frequently associated disease is amyloidosis (deposition of eosinophilic fibrous protein in the heart). Other disorders include glycogen storage disease, hemochromatosis, and sarcoidosis.

Fibrotic infiltrations into the myocardium, endocardium, and subendocardium cause the ventricles to lose their ability to stretch. Filling pressures increase, and cardiac output falls. Eventually, cardiac failure and mild ventricular hypertrophy occur.

Restrictive cardiomyopathy causes decreased cardiac output. As cardiac output falls and intraventricular pressures rise, manifestations of heart failure appear. The earliest manifestations may include exercise intolerance, fatigue, and shortness of breath, followed by neck vein distention, peripheral edema, and ascites. In severe or end-stage disease, the clinical manifestations of restrictive cardiomyopathy are indistinguishable from those of chronic constrictive pericarditis (see preceding discussion of pericarditis). Cardiac murmurs are usually minimal or absent. The manifestations progress rapidly producing a high mortality.[27]

Outcome Management

At present there are no specific interventions for restrictive cardiomyopathy. Intervention aims at diminishing heart failure. A pacemaker, diuretics, vasodilators, and salt restriction may help accomplish this goal.[27] Digitalis may help in some forms of restrictive cardiomyopathy.

Death attributable to dysrhythmia may occur suddenly, or a more progressive course may be followed by eventual, intractable heart failure. The prognosis largely depends on the underlying cause. Unfortunately, intervention rarely brings about long-term improvement.

Surgical Management for Cardiomyopathy

Surgical intervention for hypertrophic cardiomyopathy may become necessary if medical management is ineffective. Several surgical procedures have been developed to reduce the outflow gradient. The most popular surgical treatment involves an incision into the ventricular septum with or without resection of part of the septum.

The excision of fibrotic endocardium is successful in a limited number of clients with restrictive cardiomyopathy. Recent advances in surgical treatment have shown some success. Surgery has been effective for some dysrhythmias. Cardiac transplantation is becoming increasingly common for the treatment of dilated cardiomyopathy. Valve replacement may also be required, but it is not commonly performed.

Nursing Management

The management of the client with cardiomyopathy is outlined in the Care Plan. In addition, clients who are acutely or chronically ill with cardiomyopathy require strong psychosocial support. The uncertain and serious consequences of the disease create fear and anxiety. The chronic nature of the disorder can deplete coping resources, leaving those afflicted with feelings of helpless-

C A R E   P L A N

THE CLIENT WITH CARDIOMYOPATHY

Collaborative Problem. Risk for Heart Failure related to mechanical dysfunction of the heart

Outcomes. Monitor the client for the following clinical manifestations of heart failure:

- Peripheral edema
- Pulmonary edema
- Decreased renal perfusion
- Decreased CO
- Diaphoresis
- Dyspnea, orthopnea
- Anxiety
- Frothy, pink sputum

Interventions	Rationales
1. Assess the client every 4 to 8 hours for: • Neck vein distention • Peripheral edema • Altered lung sounds • Dyspnea or orthopnea • Tachycardia • Hypotension • Confusion • Urine output > 30 ml/hr	1. These assessments can help detect early signs of heart failure; as the heart muscle fails to pump effectively, falling cardiac output stimulates the adrenergic system and the renin-angiotensin-aldosterone system. These changes lead to tachycardia and oliguria. Increased preload and afterload lead to neck and vein distention, peripheral edema, altered lung sounds, dyspnea, and orthopnea. Hypoxia may lead to confusion.
2. Monitor BUN, bilirubin, liver enzymes, and creatinine.	2. Laboratory results can indicate liver congestion.
3. Monitor fluid balance every 8 to 24 hours, and record daily weights.	3. Clients are given potent diuretics to reduce pulmonary and peripheral edema. Accurate assessment of fluid balance and weight assist in determining effectiveness of treatment.

Evaluation. Heart failure will remain an active problem. Some clients will show improvement after diuresis. Others may have such severe cardiomyopathy that the goal is to have no further deterioration.

Nursing Diagnosis. Decreased Cardiac Output related to alterations in cardiac structure and function

Outcomes. The client will demonstrate improved cardiac output, as evidenced by:

- Clear lung sounds
- Vital signs WNL
- Warm, dry skin
- Normal sinus rhythm
- Absence of S_3 or S_4
- Urine output > 30 ml/hr
- Decreased peripheral edema, neck vein distention, and ascites

Interventions	Rationales
1. Monitor for clinical manifestations of decreasing CO.	1. Early detection of decreasing CO improves treatment options.
2. Encourage bed rest during acute phase; limit self-care.	2. Rest decreases oxygen consumption and demand on myocardium.
3. Avoid Valsalva's maneuver (with hypertrophic cardiomyopathy).	3. Valsalva's maneuver impedes venous return and impairs outflow.
4. Observe and record dysrhythmias every 4 to 8 hours.	4. Dysrhythmias may further impair CO.
5. Monitor intake and output every 1 to 8 hours.	5. Fluid retention may occur with decreased CO and CHF.
6. Restrict IV and oral fluids as ordered.	6. This restriction decreases the amount of circulating fluids.
7. Administer unloading and inotropic agents.	7. These agents are used to improve ejection, reduce preload, and improve contractility.
8. Administer calcium antagonists as ordered.	8. These agents are used to decrease LV outflow obstruction and to increase LV compliance to improve ventricular filling.
9. In hypertrophic cardiomyopathy, avoid nitrates, beta-adrenergic agents, and cardiac glycosides.	9. These agents increase contractility and increase obstruction.
10. Hemodynamic monitoring: monitor arterial pressure, RAP, PAP, PCWP, CO/I every 2 to 4 hours as indicated.	10. These monitor the degree of heart failure and the response to therapy.

Evaluation. Like heart failure, decreased cardiac output will remain an active problem. Degree of outcome attainment varies greatly.

CARE PLAN

continued

Nursing Diagnosis. Activity intolerance related to mechanical dysfunction of the heart and decreased cardiac reserve.

Outcomes. The client will show an improved activity tolerance, as evidenced by:

- Demonstrating a progression of activity appropriate to the disorder
- Showing a willingness to combine rest and activity
- Demonstrating minimal change in pulse or BP during activities
- Having pulse, respirations, and BP return to normal range within 3 minutes of the activity
- Accepting any imposed restrictions

Interventions	Rationales
1. Assess the tolerance to activities in bed before ambulating	1. This assessment provides a baseline to plan activity.
2. During activity, monitor pulse, respiration, color, and ECG.	2. Changes in vital signs, skin color, and ECG are evidence of orthostatic changes and the ability of the diseased myocardium to meet oxygen demand with exercise.
3. Discontinue activity if chest pain, dyspnea, cyanosis, dizziness, hypotension, sustained tachycardia, or dysrhythmias develop.	3. These manifestations are evidence of myocardial hypoxia.
4. Monitor pulse, respirations, and BP 3 minutes after activity.	4. These measures aid in evaluating tolerance of activity.
5. Explore which sedentary activities client may enjoy.	5. Sedentary activities may provide diversion if activity is not permitted; sedentary activities do not place a demand on the diseased myocardium.

Evaluation. If the cardiomyopathy is severe, plan to achieve only small increments in activity tolerance. This problem will remain active, since the condition is not curable.

BP, blood pressure; BUN, blood urea nitrogen; CO, cardiac output; CO/I, cardiac output/cardiac index; ECG, electrocardiogram; IV, intravenous; LV, left ventricular; PAP, pulmonary artery pressure; PCWP, pulmonary capillary wedge pressure; RAP, right atrial pressure; WNL, within normal limits.

ness and hopelessness. As physical capabilities diminish, feelings of inadequacy, frustration, and poor self-esteem grow. Clients may become irritable, angry, withdrawn, or dependent.

Even though the prognosis is often poor, you can help clients who suffer from this debilitating disorder to maintain hope and dignity. Encouragement, a caring touch, a listening ear, and attainable goals can promote a high quality of life. Create an environment in which clients can openly express concerns and acknowledge fears. Acceptance, empathy, and kindness can help clients with cardiomyopathies adopt more successful coping strategies.

Self-Care

With hypertrophic cardiomyopathy, syncope or sudden death may follow physical exertion. Therefore, warn the client with hypertrophic cardiomyopathy to avoid strenuous physical exercise such as running or active competitive sports. In addition, encourage household members to learn CPR. Although chest pain often accompanies this disease, nitroglycerin can worsen obstruction. Instead, clinicians treat chest pain with reduced activity and beta-blocking agents.

Hypertrophic cardiomyopathy predisposes the client to the risk of infective endocarditis. Advise clients with this cardiomyopathy to check with their physician about taking prophylactic antibiotics before and after dental and surgical procedures as American Heart Association Guidelines have changed.[6]

All clients with cardiomyopathy need clear, honest education concerning the disease and its cause and intervention. Both you and the client must be watchful for untoward effects of therapy. Clients with restrictive cardiomyopathy are especially vulnerable to the toxic effects of digitalis (see Chapter 56).

VALVULAR HEART DISEASE

Valvular dysfunction occurs when the heart valves cannot fully open or fully close. A stenosed valve may impede the flow of blood from one chamber to the next; an insufficient (incompetent) valve may allow blood to regurgitate (flow backward) (Fig. 55–4). The aortic and mitral valves become dysfunctional more often than the pulmonary and tricuspid valves. This change occurs because the left side of the heart is a system of higher pressures; the right side of the heart is exposed to the lower pressures in the pulmonary circulation.

Valvular heart disease remains fairly common in the United States even though the incidence is steadily decreasing as the incidence of rheumatic fever decreases. Mitral valve prolapse syndrome is one of the most common cardiac abnormalities; as much as 5% of the population is affected, with women affected more than men.[16]

MITRAL VALVE DISEASE

Disorders of the mitral valve obstruct the flow of blood from the atrium to the ventricle (stenosis) or allow blood to leak back from ventricle to atrium (regurgitation). *Mitral stenosis* is a block in blood flow resulting from an abnormality of the mitral valve leaflets that prevents proper opening of the valve during diastole. This disorder

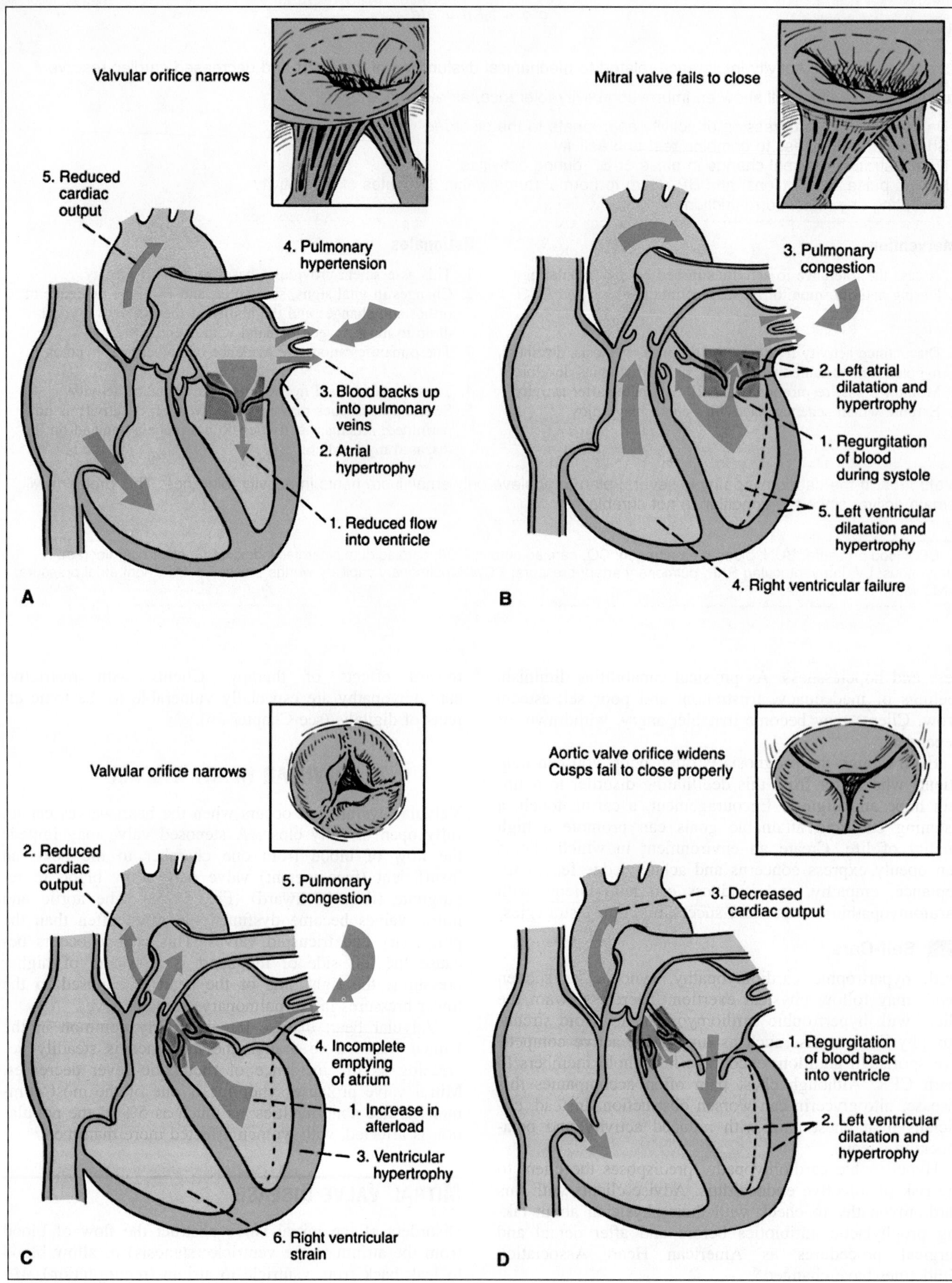

FIGURE 55–4 Dysfunctions of the cardiac valves. *A*, Mitral stenosis. *B*, Mitral regurgitation. *C*, Aortic stenosis. *D*, Aortic regurgitation.

causes overwork for the left atrium. *Mitral regurgitation* occurs when blood from the left ventricle is ejected back into the left atrium during systole because of abnormalities in the mitral valve. This disorder results in overwork for the left atrium and left ventricle. Regurgitation of the mitral valve sometimes occurs with mitral stenosis.

In *mitral valve prolapse* (see later), one or both of the valve leaflets bulge into the left atrium during ventricular systole. Various names have been given to the disorder: late apical systolic murmur, Barlow's syndrome, and floppy mitral valve syndrome. Usually a benign disorder, it may progress to a stage of pronounced regurgitation and ventricular dilation. Although it is often an isolated abnormality, this syndrome is associated with a number of other conditions, such as endocarditis, myocarditis, atherosclerosis, systemic lupus erythematosus, muscular dystrophy, acromegaly, and cardiac sarcoidosis. In addition, there may be a genetic component.

Etiology and Risk Factors

Factors leading to the development of acquired valvular disease include acute rheumatic fever, infectious endocarditis, and connective tissue abnormalities. Rheumatic heart disease, the most common cause of valvular heart disease, is preventable. Community health nurses working in health care centers or schools can often detect people with beta-hemolytic streptococcal infections (the precursor to rheumatic heart disease). Refer these clients for appropriate diagnosis and intervention.

Pathophysiology

Acquired valvular dysfunction is usually caused by inflammation of the endocardium due to acute rheumatic fever or infectious endocarditis. The inflammation causes the valve leaflets and chordae tendineae to become fibrous. The chordae tendineae shorten, which narrows the outflow tract.

In the client with valvular stenosis, the valve orifice narrows, and the valve leaflets (cusps) may become fused or thickened in such a way that the valve cannot open freely. With valvular insufficiency, scarring and retraction of the valve leaflets result in incomplete closure. Either problem increases the heart workload. Valvular stenosis subjects the chamber behind the stenotic valve to greater stress (e.g., the left ventricle in aortic stenosis). This is because the heart must generate more pressure to force blood through the narrowed opening. In the client with valvular insufficiency, the chambers in front and behind the valve are taxed.

For a time, the heart may be able to compensate for the additional strain through dilation and eventual hypertrophy. If valvular damage worsens, however, without intervention the heart eventually fails.

MITRAL STENOSIS

As the valves become calcified and immobile, the valvular orifice narrows, which prevents normal passage of blood from the left atrium to the left ventricle. The valve orifice normally is 4 to 6 cm². When the orifice is mildly stenosed, it is reduced to 2 cm². This mild stenosis allows blood to flow from the left atrium to the left ventricle only if increased pressure is generated.

The obstruction of blood flow across the mitral valve during diastolic filling creates a pressure gradient between the left atrium and the left ventricle of approximately 20 mm Hg in critical stenosis.[4] Therefore, the pressure in the left atrium is elevated to approximately 25 mm Hg. The elevated left atrial pressure, in turn, raises the pulmonary venous and pulmonary capillary pressures. The left atrium hypertrophies to accommodate the increase in pressure and volume, and the right ventricle hypertrophies because of the chronic pulmonary hypertension. Right ventricular failure can result, and inadequate filling of the left ventricle (preload) can result in reduced cardiac output[4] (Fig. 55–4*A*).

MITRAL REGURGITATION

Mitral regurgitation occurs during systole. During the systole, much pressure is generated within the left ventricle. The blood in the left ventricle is ejected forward into the aorta and also backward into the left atrium through the mitral valve that is not completely closed. The backward flow of blood causes left atrial and left ventricular enlargement. The left atrium responds to the large volume of blood it is receiving during systole, causing dilation and hypertrophy. The left ventricle responds to the large amount of blood lost to the left atrium by pumping harder to preserve cardiac output. This causes hypertrophy of the left ventricle and, eventually, left ventricular failure (Fig. 55–4*B*).

Over time, the increase in blood to the left atrium causes a rise in left atrial pressure. This pressure is reflected backward into the pulmonary venous and arterial system. With continued high pressures, right-sided heart failure can develop.

MITRAL VALVE PROLAPSE

In the client with mitral valve prolapse, the anterior and posterior cusps of the mitral valve billow upward into the atrium during systolic contraction (Fig. 55–5). The chordae tendineae can be lengthened, which allows the valve cusps to stretch upward. The cusps may be enlarged and thickened. If blood leaks backward into the atrium during systole, mitral regurgitation is present.

Clinical Manifestations

The clinical manifestations of valvular heart disease may appear gradually or suddenly.

MITRAL STENOSIS

On auscultation, a loud first heart sound and then an opening snap that ushers in a low-pitched, rumbling diastolic murmur is heard. The opening snap is best heard at the apex with the diaphragm of the stethoscope. The diastolic murmur is best heard at the apex using the bell of the stethoscope while the client is in a left lateral recumbent position.

Atrial fibrillation is a common finding in clients with mitral stenosis. During episodes of atrial fibrillation, the pulse becomes irregular and faint and the blood pressure often drops. In some cases of mitral stenosis, systemic embolization is present. Ineffective atrial contractions allow some stagnation of blood in the left atrium and encourage the formation of mural thrombi. These thrombi easily break away and travel as emboli throughout the arterial system, causing tissue infarction.

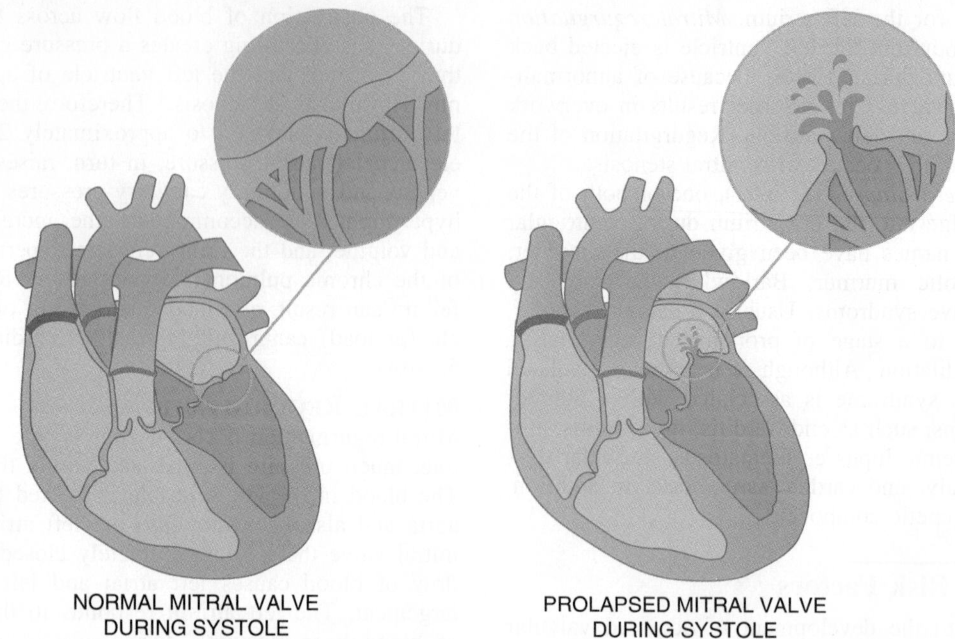

FIGURE 55–5 Mitral valve prolapse. The main figure shows a normal mitral valve; the *inset* shows a prolapsed mitral valve. Prolapse permits the valve leaflets to billow back into the atrium during left ventricular systole. The billowing causes the leaflets to part slightly, permitting regurgitation of blood into the atrium.

Mitral Regurgitation

Clients with mitral regurgitation may be asymptomatic, but if cardiac output falls, manifestations will develop. When cardiac output falls, fatigue and dyspnea are the first manifestations. Clinical manifestations gradually increase to include orthopnea, paroxysmal nocturnal dyspnea, and peripheral edema. Pulmonary manifestations are less severe than in mitral stenosis because changes in the mean pulmonary capillary pressure are less exaggerated. However, when the right side of the heart is affected, the manifestations are the same as in mitral stenosis.

Auscultation reveals a blowing, high-pitched systolic murmur with radiation to the left axilla, heard best at the apex. The first heart sound may be diminished, and often a splitting of the second sound will be heard. Severe regurgitation is associated with a third heart sound (S_3).

Vital signs are usually normal unless mitral regurgitation is severe. Atrial fibrillation is common in clients with this condition; however, emboli and hemoptysis occur far less often than in mitral stenosis.

Mitral Valve Prolapse

It is not uncommon for many clients with mitral valve prolapse to be completely asymptomatic. In a healthy client, a physical examination may reveal a regurgitant murmur or a midsystolic click on auscultation. Manifestations, if present, may include tachycardia, lightheadedness, syncope, fatigue, weakness, dyspnea, chest discomfort, anxiety, and palpitations related to dysrhythmias.[4] Manifestations may be vague. Minimal morbidity and mortality are associated with mitral valve prolapse. Clinically, clients have no physical limitations.

Various diagnostic assessments are used to detect valvular lesions or structural heart changes. These studies include echocardiography, chest radiography, stress tests and cardiac catheterization.[4]

Outcome Management

The goals of medical management are to maintain cardiac output and activity tolerance. When cardiac output falls or the client is unable to tolerate simple activities, the valve can be surgically replaced.

Mitral Stenosis

Improvement of manifestations may be achieved with oral diuretics and a sodium-restricted diet. Digitalis is useful in clients with atrial fibrillation for slowing the ventricular heart rate. Beta-blockers may decrease the heart rate and, therefore, increase exercise tolerance. Anticoagulants are helpful in these clients. A client with untreated mitral stenosis can progress from having mild disability to severe disability in about 3 years.[4]

Mitral Regurgitation

The client should restrict physical activities that produce fatigue and dyspnea. Reducing sodium intake and promoting sodium excretion with diuretics can lessen the work of the heart. Nitrates, digitalis and angiotensin-converting enzyme (ACE) inhibitors have brought about hemodynamic improvement and symptomatic relief in clients with chronic mitral regurgitation.[4]

Mitral Valve Prolapse

Treatment of mitral valve prolapse depends on the manifestations. Beta-blockers are helpful in relieving syncope, palpitations, and chest pain. For preventing infective endocarditis, the client may receive antibiotics prophylactically before any invasive procedures.

Aortic Valve Disease

Aortic valve disease is far less common than mitral valve disease but often occurs in conjunction with mitral valve disease. Aortic stenosis obstructs the forward flow of blood during systole from the left ventricle into the aorta and systemic circulation. This obstruction to flow creates a resistance to ejection and increased pressure in the left ventricle. *Aortic regurgitation* (aortic insufficiency) allows blood to leak back from the aorta into the left ventricle. During systole, blood that is ejected into the aorta reenters the left ventricle. To maintain normal pressures, the left ventricle hypertrophies. Both aortic stenosis and regurgitation overwork the left ventricle.

Etiology and Risk Factors

Aortic stenosis can be caused by several congenital defects of the aortic valve and by two degenerative processes: (1) calcification of the valve in older adults and (2) retraction and stiffening of the valve from rheumatic fever. As the population in the United States ages, the incidence of aortic stenosis from calcification has been rising.[4]

Aortic regurgitation is most often a result of infectious disorders such as rheumatic fever, syphilis, and infective endocarditis. Connective tissue disorders can also lead to aortic regurgitation.

Pathophysiology

Aortic Stenosis

In the client with aortic stenosis, the orifice of the aortic valve becomes narrowed, which causes a decrease in the blood flow from the left ventricle into the aorta. The pressure within the left ventricle rises as the blood is ejected through the narrowed opening. A pressure gradient develops between the left ventricle and the aorta. The elevated pressure in the left ventricle during systole causes the ventricle to hypertrophy. Dilation of the left ventricle occurs over time when there is a deterioration of the contractility of the hypertrophied muscle. Eventually, dilation and hypertrophy of the left ventricle are unable to maintain adequate cardiac output, resulting in elevated left ventricular end-diastolic pressure, decreased cardiac output, and increased pulmonary hypertension (Fig. 55–4*C*).

Aortic Regurgitation

Aortic regurgitation is a diastolic event in which blood that is propelled forward into the aorta regurgitates back into the left ventricle through an incompetent valve. This causes abnormal filling and a volume overload of the left ventricle. The magnitude of the overload depends on the severity of the incompetence. However, a small incompetent area can result in significant aortic regurgitation over time.

Because the left ventricle receives blood from both the atrium and the systemic circulation, aortic regurgitation gradually increases left ventricular end-diastolic volume. Left ventricular stroke volume is increased to produce an effective forward-moving volume into the systemic circulation. There is a compensatory dilation of the left ventricle but minimal increase in left ventricular end-diastolic pressure.[4] The compensatory mechanisms of dilation and hypertrophy help to maintain an adequate cardiac output. As the condition progresses and the contractile state of the myocardium declines, however, cardiac output falls (Fig. 55–5*D*).

Clinical Manifestations

Aortic Stenosis

Clinical manifestations of aortic stenosis tend to occur gradually and late in the course of the disease. There is usually a long latent period in which the client is asymptomatic. Manifestations begin to appear as the obstruction and ventricular pressure increase to critical levels. Angina pectoris (chest pain) is a frequent finding in approximately 60% of clients. The character of the angina is similar to that in clients with coronary artery disease, and pain is commonly brought on by exertion and relieved by rest. Myocardial oxygen consumption is higher in clients with aortic stenosis because of the hypertrophy of the left ventricle, and this probably accounts for the angina.

Syncope, another common clinical manifestation, also occurs during exertion because of a fixed cardiac output and an increased demand.[4] Syncope at rest may be due to dysrhythmias. Exertional dyspnea, paroxysmal nocturnal dyspnea, and pulmonary edema occur with increasing pulmonary venous hypertension attributable to left ventricular failure. In severe aortic stenosis, additional manifestations may include palpitations, fatigue, and visual disturbances.

On auscultation, the systolic murmur may be associated with a diminished second heart sound and an early ejection click. A systolic thrill is present over the aortic areas.

Aortic Regurgitation

Clients with chronic severe aortic regurgitation may be asymptomatic for a long time. During this time, the left ventricle gradually enlarges. Clients may complain of an uncomfortable awareness of the heartbeat and palpitations. These manifestations are due to the large left ventricular stroke volume with rapid diastolic runoff. This is also apparent with prominent pulsations in the neck and even head-bobbing with each heartbeat. Sinus tachycardia or premature ventricular contractions may make palpitations more pronounced.

On physical examination, systolic blood pressure may be due to the large stroke volume and a decreased diastolic blood pressure due to the regurgitation and distal runoff. Carotid artery pulsations may be exaggerated. The arterial pulse pressure widens, and palpable pulse amplitude increases. This may be noted as a sudden sharp pulse, followed by a swift collapse of the diastolic pulse (Corrigan's or water-hammer pulse). Auscultation reveals a soft, high-pitched, blowing decrescendo diastolic murmur heard best at the second right intercostal space and radiating to the left sternal border.

Outcome Management

Medical Management

The goals of medical management are to maintain or improve cardiac function and activity tolerance. When the client reaches maximum benefit from medications, surgery may be warranted.

Aortic Stenosis

Noninvasive assessment of clients with Doppler echocardiography should be performed. Advise clients with known or suspected critical obstruction of the aortic valve to avoid vigorous physical activity. Clients with mild obstruction may continue exercise if it is tolerated.

Prophylactic antibiotics may be given on an individual basis for invasive medical or dental procedures for prevention of infective endocarditis. Digitalis and diuretics that are usually used for ventricular failure must be used with caution.[4] Beta-blockers are not usually ordered because they can depress myocardial function and induce left ventricular failure. Cardiac dysrhythmias should be treated pharmacologically.

AORTIC REGURGITATION

Medical intervention for aortic regurgitation is the same as for aortic stenosis: relief of manifestations of heart failure and prevention of infection in the already deformed aortic cusps.

TRICUSPID VALVE DISEASE

Tricuspid stenosis, or *regurgitation*, usually develops from rheumatic fever or in combination with other structural disorders of the heart.[4] Because the tricuspid valve is on the right side of the heart, the major hemodynamic alterations are decreased cardiac output and increased right atrial pressure. The inability of the right atrium to propel blood across the stenosed valve may account for these changes. With *tricuspid regurgitation*, although pressure in the right atrium is elevated, it is due to regurgitation of the blood volume in the right ventricle back into the right atrium during systole.

Clinical manifestations of tricuspid stenosis are dyspnea and fatigue, pulsations in the neck, and peripheral edema. Physical assessment reveals prominent waves in the neck veins as the atrium vigorously contracts against the stenotic valve. A diastolic murmur is heard best along the left lower sternal border. The murmur increases with inspiration. The ECG reveals tall, tented P waves in leads II, III, and aV. Tricuspid insufficiency causes hepatic congestion and peripheral edema. Often atrial fibrillation is present, and jugular waves are evident. The murmur is holosystolic along the left sternal border.

Tricuspid stenosis usually responds well to diuretics and digitalis therapy. If the leaflets are severely stenotic, surgery may be required.

PULMONIC VALVE DISEASE

Abnormalities of the *pulmonic valve* are usually congenital defects. Few lesions develop after birth. Pulmonary hypertension, caused by mitral stenosis, pulmonary emboli, or chronic lung disease, can precipitate functional pulmonary regurgitation. Pulmonic stenosis and regurgitation lead to a decrease in cardiac output because blood does not reach the left side of the heart in adequate supply for metabolic demands. Pulmonic regurgitation may lead to dyspnea and fatigue. The murmur is a high-pitched diastolic blow along the left sternal border. There are no significant changes in the ECG.

Pulmonic stenosis causes similar clinical manifestations, but the murmur is often a crescendo-decrescendo type. Right-sided heart failure can also develop.

Intervention focuses on ameliorating the underlying cause and right-sided heart failure.

Outcome Management

Nursing Management of the Medical Client

Nursing assessment should address the type, severity, and progress of the valvular disorder; presence of fatigue; clinical manifestations of heart failure; heart rhythm (including ECG); vital signs; auscultation and palpation of the heart; the client's support systems; and the degree of knowledge that the client and family have concerning the nature of and intervention in the disorder.

The main focus of nursing intervention in valvular heart disease is to help the client maintain a normal cardiac output, thereby preventing manifestations of heart failure, venous congestion, and inadequate tissue perfusion. To evaluate the effectiveness of therapeutic interventions, perform ongoing hemodynamic assessment. Monitor vital signs closely every 1 to 4 hours. A decrease in cardiac output is manifested in a compensatory rise in heart rate, a drop in blood pressure, or a decrease in urinary output. Carefully auscultate the chest every 4 hours to identify the presence of abnormal breath sounds (crackles, rhonchi) or heart gallops (S_3, S_4).

Self-Care

Clients with valvular heart disease require lifelong management. With a sincere desire to understand and accept each client's response to chronic illness, you can help these clients adapt to difficult lifestyle changes and achieve a positive sense of well-being.

Clients may find it difficult to cope physically and psychosocially after hospital discharge. The chronicity of valvular heart disease and its potential complications can create an atmosphere of uncertainty, fear, and frustration. Take time to help the client identify support people, personal strengths, and coping strategies. Assess how the client handles frustration or anger and which activities are particularly relaxing. Address the client's fears and misconceptions. In some instances, counseling referrals may help. Stress the importance of follow-up physical examinations and intervention.

Before discharge, prepare detailed teaching material for the client and family concerning the therapeutic regimen, the disease process, factors contributing to manifestations, and the rationale for intervention. Give information concerning prescribed medications. Medications frequently prescribed include digoxin, quinidine, diuretics, beta-blockers, potassium supplements, anticoagulants, and sometimes prophylactic antibiotics. Explain their rationale, dosages, side effects, and special considerations in their use.

Review exercise prescriptions with the client. Clients with aortic stenosis often require activity restrictions. The client should demonstrate ability to pace activity, verbalize improvement in fatigue, and accept activity restrictions.

Address dietary restrictions, and plan interdisciplinary follow-up. Make sure the client knows whom to call when questions arise.

Surgical Management

When conservative medical intervention fails to improve hemodynamic status in valvular disorders, surgical intervention is indicated. Mitral valve repair is becoming more common because it carries relatively few complications, good long-term survival, and low hospital mortality.[24] Additionally, long-term anticoagulant therapy is not needed.[14]

Surgical intervention should be considered for aortic stenosis when the pressure gradient is greater than 50 mm Hg or the valve orifice is less than 0.8 cm^2. The prognosis for clients with symptomatic aortic stenosis is poor without surgical intervention. The incidence of sudden death rises once myocardial failure develops. Surgical replacement of the incompetent valve provides the only effective long-term intervention for aortic regurgitation. A high percentage of clients with aortic regurgitation and aortic stenosis show striking clinical improvement with valve replacement.[4]

CONGENITAL DISORDERS

Congenital heart disorders result from faulty development of cardiac structures in utero. Congenital disorders include septal defects, vessel stenosis, abnormally positioned vessels, and patency of the ductus arteriosus. Advances in the medical and surgical treatment of people with congenital heart disease have assisted an ever-growing number of clients to survive into adulthood. As this number grows, medical and nursing support has grown also.

With today's available treatments, about 85% of children with congenital heart disease will survive into adulthood.[8] Therefore, we can expect to see more adults with congenital defects in the future.[19] Each congenital defect brings its own morbidity and mortality statistics; in general, however, people with the less complex defects will have a longer survival than those with more complex defects (the course for such defects is still uncertain).

Operations may be palliative or corrective. Most adult clients today underwent their surgical procedures many years ago during the developmental phase of these interventions. Their course would probably be quite different from that followed today. Many refinements in surgical techniques continue to be developed so that clinical outcomes vary significantly.

Many people with a congenital heart defect have remained asymptomatic; others have had varying levels of functional ability. Clients may have both residual problems (those not corrected or improved at the time of the surgical repair) and sequelae (results of the surgery).[19] Common lifelong problems include the risk of infective endocarditis in clients with artificial valves or with suture repair of an atrial septal defect. It is not uncommon for a client with a repaired coarctation of the aorta to find that the aorta has gradually become narrowed again. In such cases, hypertension may develop. Clients who as children underwent repair for cyanotic defects tend to experience sequelae and complications in adulthood.[19] There may be some degree of exercise intolerance that can be better managed after proper stress testing.

Dysrhythmias frequently present a lifelong complication. Clients who have had intraventricular repairs may present with ventricular dysrhythmias or complete heart block. A 24-hour Holter monitor and stress testing may help evaluate the client's tolerance for activity.

Many people who have had surgical procedures as infants and children had to have repeated operations as they "outgrew" their repairs or prosthetic devices. Our growing geriatric population also may be experiencing unknown late consequences of congenital heart disease or surgical repair. It is important to encourage these people to participate in long-term follow-up.

Your role as a nurse who is caring for the adult with congenital heart disease varies with the setting. However, you play an integral role in helping these clients achieve optimal health and functioning. Nursing assessment, intervention, education, and follow-up are directed toward improving functional levels, managing medications, psychosocial adjustment, and preventing complications.

CARDIAC SURGERY

Cardiac surgery is performed when the probability of survival with a useful life is greater with surgical treatment than with nonsurgical treatment. The first heart surgery, performed in 1923 by Cutler and Levine,[43] was a repair of a stenosed mitral valve. Since that time, heart surgery has been revolutionized by the development of open heart techniques that allow surgeons to visualize the heart directly while they explore, cut, repair, and sew. Further advances include minimally invasive open heart surgery. These improved operating conditions have enabled today's surgeons to replace diseased valves with prosthetic valves, to repair severe congenital lesions, and to perform heart transplantation procedures. Today, under ideal conditions, the hospital mortality rate associated with cardiac surgery should be approaching zero. However, reporting the results of cardiac surgery by hospital mortality alone (as is frequently done in the popular press) is not sufficient. The preoperative condition of the client's heart and other body systems greatly influences the results of cardiac surgery. The identification of incremental risk factors should continue to improve results.

TYPES OF HEART SURGERY

There are three types of cardiac surgery:

1. *Reparative* procedures are likely to produce cure or excellent and prolonged improvement. Examples: closure of a patent ductus arteriosus, atrial septal defect, and ventricular septal defect; repair of mitral stenosis; and simple repair of tetralogy of Fallot.
2. *Reconstructive* procedures are more complex. They are not always curative, and reoperation may be needed. Examples: coronary artery bypass grafting (CABG) and reconstruction of an incompetent mitral, tricuspid, or aortic valve.
3. *Substitutional* procedures are not usually curative because of the preoperative condition of the client. Examples: valve replacement, cardiac replacement by transplantation, ventricular replacement or assistance, and cardiac replacement by mechanical devices.

■ VALVULAR SURGERY

The repair or replacement of cardiac valves with acquired stenosis or incompetence is not considered curative, but the results are generally good and long-lasting. Cure is usually unattainable because of the preoperative condition of the heart or other body systems. Indications for surgery include the following:

1. Progressive impairment of cardiac function due to scarring and thickening of the valve with either impaired narrowing of the valvular opening (stenosis), or incomplete closure (insufficiency, regurgitation)
2. Gradual enlargement of the heart with manifestations of decreased activity, shortness of breath, and heart failure.
3. Surgical therapy for mitral valve stenosis, which can include valve repair. Valve repair can be accomplished if the preoperative assessment indicates that the valve is pliable. If the valve is not pliable, valve replacement is necessary. In clients with mitral regurgitation, valve reconstruction or annuloplasty may be done. This may include the use of a flexible ring that is sewn into the valve for stabilization. Aortic stenosis may be surgically treated with valve replacement or balloon aortic valvuloplasty. In the valvuloplasty procedure, a catheter with a balloon is used to dilate the valve orifice (Fig. 55–6). Surgery for the client with aortic regurgitation is not always the treatment of choice but may be considered.

Artificial cardiac valves are continuing to show improvements in design, safety, function, and durability. Mechanical and tissue prosthetic valves are available. The type of valve prosthesis used is based on a number of considerations. The surgeon primarily considers (1) the client's tolerance of anticoagulation and (2) the durability of the valve.

Clients with mechanical valves require continuous anticoagulation therapy for the remainder of their lives. Therefore, if the client has a preoperative history of bleeding or noncompliance with pharmacologic regimens, the surgeon may decide to use a tissue valve. The overall advantages and disadvantages of tissue and mechanical valves are almost equal. Mechanical valves are very durable, but anticoagulant therapy is necesssary; no anticoagulation therapy is needed for tissue valves, but they are less durable. Some physicians recommend mechanical valves in clients younger than 65 or 70 years of age and tissue valves in clients 70 years or older.[4] Artificial valves are shown in Figure 55–7.

Potential complications of heart valves include a risk of thrombus formation, especially in mechanical valves. Newer types of heart valves have shown reduced rates of thrombosis. Most clients require long-term anticoagulation therapy. The major drawback with tissue valves is durability. The leaflets of these valves may degenerate or calcify or may develop structural abnormalities. Mitral valves tend to fail usually because of the higher stress on the valve. The rate of tissue valve failure is 2% to 5% for the first 6 years, with the rate accelerating thereafter. Almost every client with a tissue valve will require replacement eventually.[4]

Management of the client after heart surgery is discussed later in this section.

■ HEART TRANSPLANTATION

Cardiac transplantation is now a standard and effective treatment for clients with end-stage cardiac disease. Formerly, widespread application of heart transplantation depended on the development of improved immunosuppressive therapy. The use of cyclosporine has resulted in superior results. Later favorable results resulted from the rapidly accumulating experience.

In 1998, 2389 hearts were transplanted in the United States. The number of clients who died while on the waiting list was 773, and 4167 clients remained on the list at the end of 1998.[25] As of 1999, 85% of heart transplant clients survived 1 year and 76% survived 3 years.[25] Heart transplant recipients who die following the

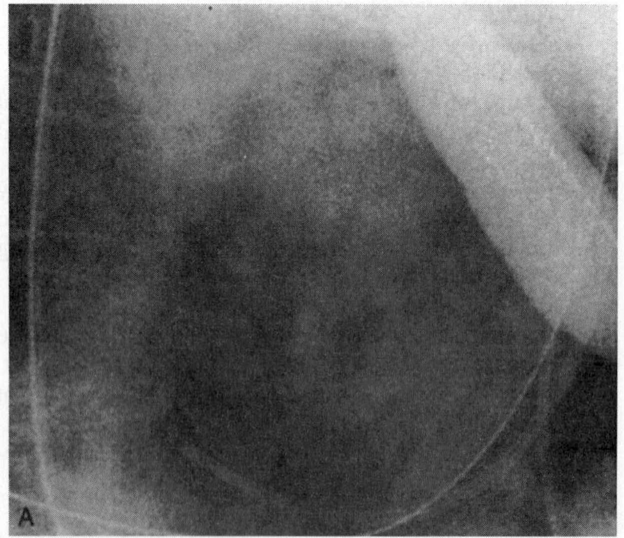

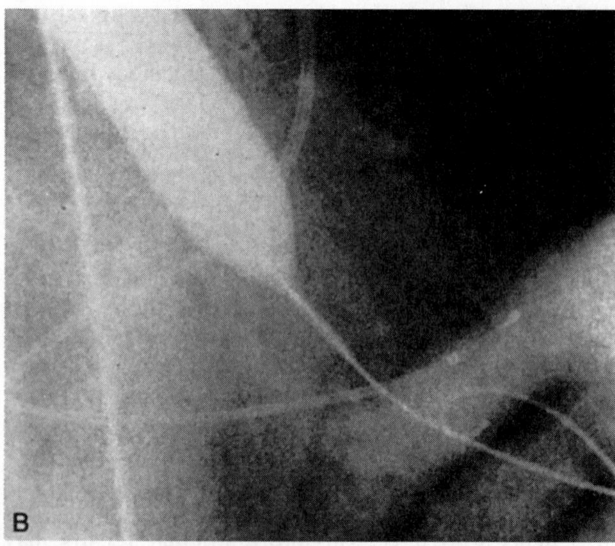

FIGURE 55–6 Valvuloplasty. *A*, The valvuloplasty balloon is inflated across the aortic valve. Note the indentation ("waist") in the balloon. *B*, The valvuloplasty balloon inflated across the aortic valve after dilation. Note the disappearance of the indentation seen in *A*. (From Barden, C., et al. [1990]. Balloon aortic valvuloplasty: Nursing care implications. *Critical Care Nurse, 10*[6], 26.)

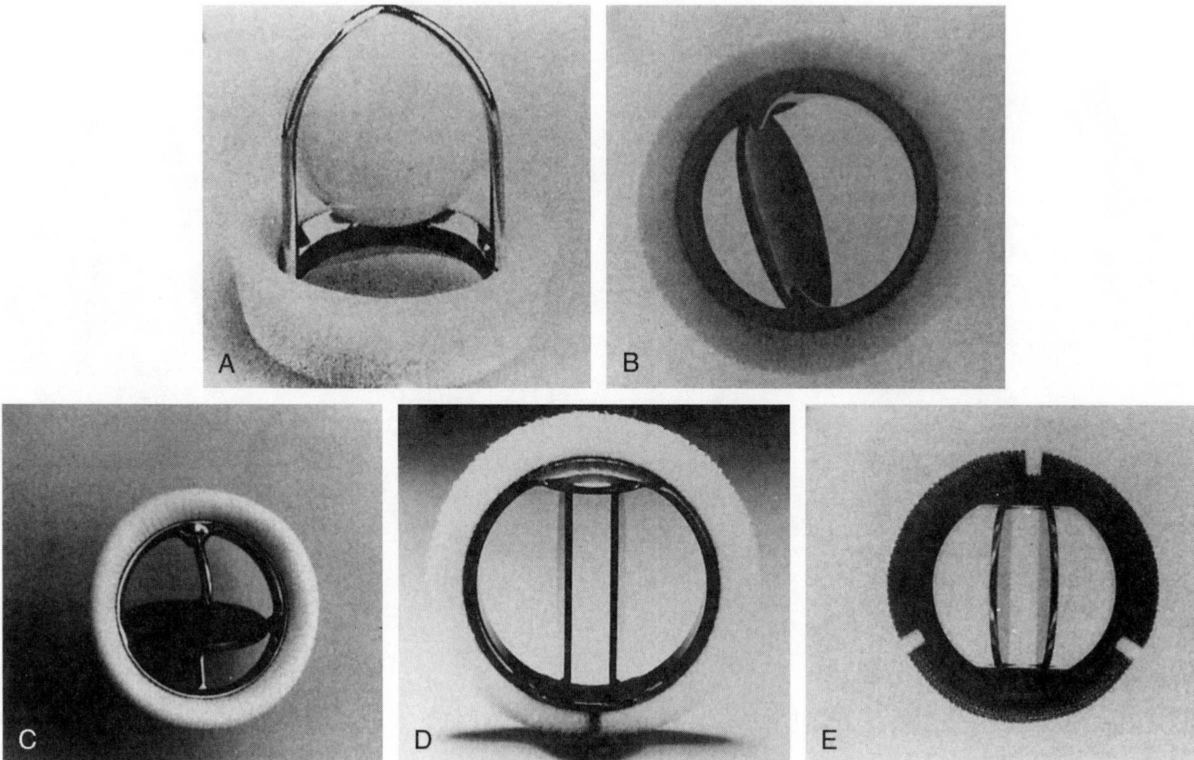

FIGURE 55–7 Prosthetic heart valves. *A*, Starr-Edwards cage and ball valve with a cloth sewing ring and bare struts. *B*, Omniscience valve. *C*, Medtronic-Hall valve. *D*, St. Jude valve. *E*, Carbomedics bileaflet valve. (From Braunwald, E. [1997]. *Heart disease: A textbook of cardiovascular medicine* [5th ed., p. 1062]. Philadelphia: W. B. Saunders.)

procedure usually do so within the first 30 days postoperatively. Clients at greatest risk are those who deteriorate rapidly before the transplant procedure. Infection, cardiac failure, or rejection is usually the cause of death.

Potential candidates must be evaluated and screened. Their cardiac status is evaluated to determine the need for the heart transplant. The candidates are also evaluated for underlying conditions that predispose to an unfavorable outcome. Selection criteria for heart transplantation are shown in Box 55–3.

The current *orthotopic* technique retains a large portion of the right and left atrium in the recipient and implants the donor heart to the atria (Fig. 55–8). Cardiopulmonary bypass is used during the operation (see later). Temporary pacemaker wires and chest drainage catheters are inserted.

Another type of procedure, the *heterotopic* technique, is performed only rarely. The donor heart is placed parallel to the recipient's heart (Fig. 55–9). The right side of the client's heart can continue to function while the dysfunctional left side of the heart is bypassed.

Recognition and treatment of rejection are the most difficult tasks in heart transplantation. The most reliable technique for assessing organ rejection is the endomyocardial biopsy, which enables identification of the diffuse interstitial infiltrate associated with rejection.

Drug therapy is adjusted to give the maximum amount of immunosuppression with the minimum amount of side effects. This is a very individualistic regimen. There is a higher risk of acute rejection soon after transplantation that decreases dramatically after 3 months. Immunosuppression treatment relies on several drugs: cyclosporine, prednisone, methylprednisolone, and azathioprine (Table 55–3). Even with this intensive regimen, 84% of heart transplant recipients experience at least one episode of rejection during the first 3 months.

For these rejection episodes, pulse therapy with methylprednisolone is used. High doses are given for 3 consecutive days, then gradually reduced over the next 2 weeks. Because of the side effects of increased steroid therapy, the client must be monitored carefully for infec-

BOX 55–3 Selection Criteria for Heart Transplantation

- End-stage heart disease
- Current medical management is unsuccessful
- New York Heart Association class III or IV
- Prognosis of less than 1 year to live
- Under 65 years of age
- Nonsmoker
- No drug or alcohol abuse
- Client is well motivated and will follow postoperative instructions and medications
- No underlying condition that would limit survival:
  - Systemic infection
  - Irreversible hepatic insufficiency
  - Irreversible renal insufficiency
  - Cancer
  - Active peptic ulcer
  - Recent pulmonary embolus
  - Irreversible pulmonary insufficiency

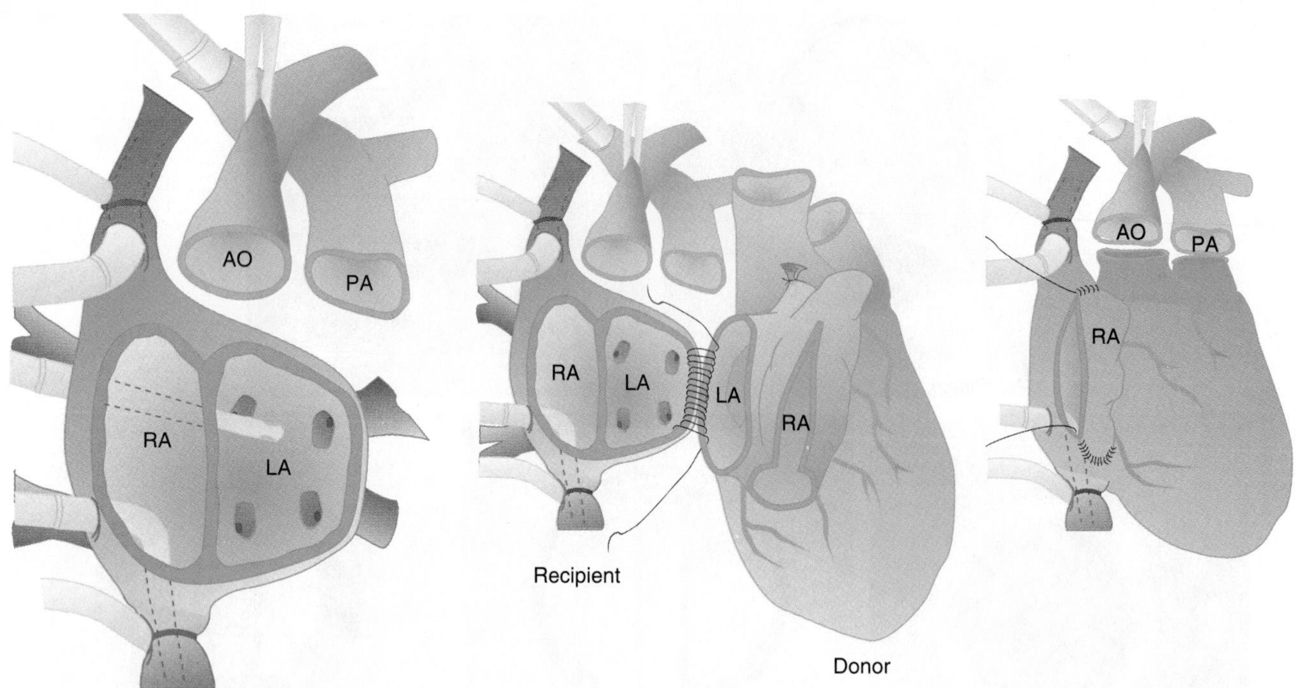

FIGURE 55–8 Orthotopic technique of heart transplantation. AO, aorta; PA, pulmonary artery; RA, right atrium; LA, left atrium.

tions. If the steroid therapy has not been successful in reversing the rejection, other, more aggressive therapy is begun. Equine antithymocyte globulin or OKT3 monoclonal antibody therapy may be used. Some clients have persistent recurrent rejection episodes, which may be treated with total lymphoid irradiation. In the long term, survival and rehabilitation can be expected in most recipients.

■ ASSISTED CIRCULATION AND MECHANICAL HEARTS

Cardiac failure leads to multisystem organ failure if it is not reversed. Sometimes, despite maximal therapy, the failing heart cannot adequately respond to therapy. If, for various reasons, cardiac transplantation is not an immediate option, other therapies are sought. It is in these cases that assisted circulation devices or mechanical hearts seem to be the only option (see Intra-aortic balloon counterpulsation). Other modalities being used in practice include ventricular assist devices, implantable left ventricular assist systems, and orthotopic biventricular replacement prostheses (artificial hearts). Many of these devices offer a bridge to transplantation when the client's heart is failing and a donor heart is not readily available. These devices can maintain a client until transplantation can be performed. The total artificial heart is available only as a bridge to transplantation. Research is continuing on a device that will be suitable for long-term outpatient use.[20]

■ OPEN HEART SURGERY

Cardiopulmonary bypass is used during cardiac surgery to divert the client's unoxygenated blood and to return reoxygenated blood to the client's circulation. This technique, called extracorporeal circulation (ECC), is accomplished with a pump oxygenator (heart-lung machine). Diversion of the client's blood allows the surgeon to visualize the heart directly during the operation. The pump oxygenator, more than any other device, has made sophisticated open heart surgery possible (Fig. 55–10). It is used to:

- Divert circulation from the heart and lungs, providing the surgeon with a bloodless operative field
- Perform all gas exchange functions for the body while the client's cardiopulmonary system is at rest
- Filter, rewarm, or cool the blood

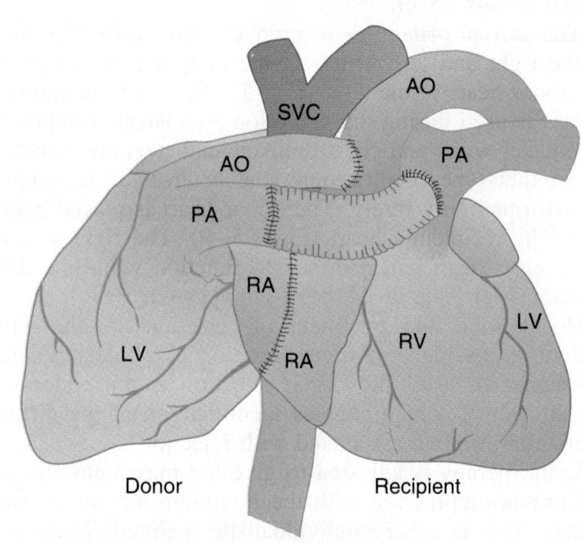

FIGURE 55–9 Heterotopic technique of heart transplantation. AO, aorta; PA, pulmonary artery; RA, right atrium; RV, right ventricle; LV, left ventricle; SVC, superior vena cava.

TABLE 55–3 IMMUNOSUPPRESSIVE PROTOCOL FOR HEART TRANSPLANTATION

Medication	Early Postoperative	Late Postoperative
Cyclosporine	6–10 mg/kg/day PO* *or* 0.5–2 mg/kg/day IV	3–6 mg/kg/day PO
or		
Tacrolimus	0.15–0.30 mg/kg/day PO	0.15–0.30 mg/kg/day PO
Methyprednisolone	500 mg IV after cardiopulmonary bypass	125 mg q 8 hr × 3 doses
Prednisone	1 mg/kg/day PO tapered to 0.4 mg/kg	0.1–0.2 mg/kg/day PO
Azathioprine	2 mg/kg/day PO†	1–2 mg/kg/day PO

* Not given if preoperative serum creatinine is greater than 1.5 mg/dl, given IV instead.
† Not given if white blood cell count is below 4000 mm².
PO, orally.
From Braunwald, E. (1997). *Heart disease: A textbook of cardiovascular medicine* (5th ed.). Philadelphia: W. B. Saunders.

- Circulate oxygenated, filtered blood back into the arterial system

Although the pump oxygenator is considered safe, there are some risks; for instance, the pump can crush and destroy blood cells, sludging of cells can lead to thrombus formation, or air emboli can form. Other complications related to ECC are shock, hemorrhage, fluid overload, hemolysis, and kidney or lung damage.

Outcome Management

Medical Management Before Cardiac Surgery

Preoperative laboratory tests include urine tests and blood electrolyte, enzyme, and coagulation studies. Important diagnostic studies that provide valuable information about cardiac status include the ECG, echocardiogram, vectorcardiogram, chest x-ray films, and cardiac catheterization.

Any physiologic imbalance or problem in cardiac or respiratory status is corrected when possible by means of rest, diet, medication, or other appropriate therapy. Physiologic baselines should be established for postoperative comparison of vital signs, weight, and laboratory values.

Preparation for surgery in general is discussed in Chapter 15. For the client undergoing the stress of heart surgery, special preparation and instruction are needed.

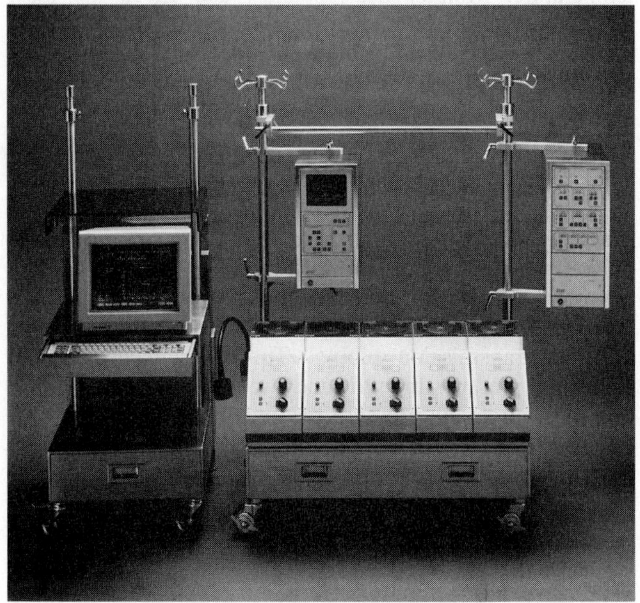

FIGURE 55–10 Stöckert heart-lung bypass machine with a computer-aided perfusion system—a type of pump-oxygenator, or heart-lung bypass machine. Machines like this are used during open heart surgery to circulate oxygenated blood while the heart is unable to pump. (Courtesy of Sorin Biomedical, Irvine, CA.)

ASSESSMENT

The client undergoing heart surgery has probably experienced cardiopulmonary clinical manifestations for months or years. Data to collect during the initial assessment include the following:

- The primary cardiovascular problem requiring surgical correction and its duration
- The purpose of the surgery and the risk involved stated in the client's own words
- Past cardiopulmonary illnesses that may predispose the client to postoperative complications (e.g., bacterial endocarditis, pulmonary embolus, allergy, abnormal bleeding)
- The degree of cardiac impairment (e.g., does the client have manifestations when at rest or only during exertion?)
- The types of medications, herbal or natural substances, and interventions that the client has received or is currently receiving (e.g., digitalis, quinidine, oxygen)

Note the client's psychological readiness for surgery and his or her reaction to the need for heart surgery. The client may initially experience shock and grief over the impending surgery. Chief concerns may be helplessness and fear of disability or death.

The psychological preparation of the cardiac surgery client is very important. Many hospitals throughout the United States have extensive preoperative education programs that greatly reduce client and family anxiety. Such a program should include a thorough explanation of the preoperative, intraoperative, and postoperative procedures. Also helpful is the introduction of the client to involved health care team members and the health care facility environment. Box 55–4 provides a list of topics for education. Your institution probably has written material for you to use.

Allow clients to tell you in their own words about their heart problem and the surgery. Correct any misconceptions, using pictures and a model of the heart. Clients tend to ask the greatest number of questions about what will happen to them in the recovery room and intensive care unit (ICU).

BOX 55-4 Guidelines to Preparing the Client Undergoing Cardiac Surgery

Plan teaching well in advance of the surgical date, if possible. By the time of surgery, the client should be prepared by the following:

1. Describe the surgical procedure:
   a. All steps, including heart-lung machine
   b. Review of anatomy and physiology of heart and valves
   c. Brief definition of unfamiliar technical terms
   d. Length of time in surgery and approximate time of first visit by family
   e. Giving the client pictures of the heart and involved valve for future reference
2. Describe the intensive care unit (ICU) environment and monitoring equipment:
   a. Cardiac monitor and alarm
   b. Endotracheal (ET) tube and projected length of time with ET tube in place
   c. Mechanical ventilator and alarm
   d. Suctioning procedure
   e. Arterial line and automatic blood pressure cuff
   f. Any limitation on visits from family
   g. Chest tubes or mediastinal tubes
   h. Nasogastric tube and length of NPO (nothing by mouth) status
   i. Urinary catheter
   j. High noise level in ICU
   k. Multiple intravenous lines and fluids
3. Describe preoperative preparation:
   a. Showering with antimicrobial soap
   b. Shaving of chest, abdomen, neck, and groin
   c. Special cardiac studies: echocardiogram, electrocardiogram, cardiac catheterization
4. Describe comfort measures:
   a. Pain relief
   b. Turning, range-of-motion exercises
   c. Out of bed next morning
   d. Medication for sleep, if needed

Explain that they will awaken from anesthesia with a chest tube in place. Discuss the ventilator that will assist the client's breathing for the first 8 to 24 hours. Remind clients that during this time they will be unable to talk. Explain that an IV line for fluid or blood will be inserted in an arm and that various equipment that continuously monitors vital signs will be attached to their skin.

Answer questions concerning the necessity of using blood products. Use these facts to respond to concerns about transfusion. Blood transfusions postoperatively are used only as needed; blood is screened carefully, and there is little risk of contracting acquired immunodeficiency syndrome (AIDS). Family members can be screened for possible donation of blood. Emphasize that although the client will experience pain, the pain will be swiftly relieved by medication and comfort measures.

Finally, explain that the client will be awakened frequently in the ICU for vital nursing assessments and interventions. Give examples of scheduled activities: vital signs every 15 minutes; temperature every 2 hours; frequent turning, coughing, and deep breathing; blood drawn for tests every morning.

Clients also need information concerning discharge from the ICU and health care facility. Explain the average length of stay in the ICU, the room to which the client will return from the ICU, the average length of stay in the health care facility, and the diet and activities permitted once the client returns home. Be general in the discussion. Remember, many unforeseen events can arise and greatly alter the postoperative course.

Give verbal and written information concerning health care facility services, rules, and regulations; visiting hours; the chaplain's name and visiting hours (if appropriate); and names of clinical nurse-specialists and other health care professionals who can be contacted for information.

Most clients benefit from a tour of the recovery room and ICU. If they are not physically able to participate in a tour, audiovisual material is helpful.

Familiarize the client with the equipment that will be used in the ICU (e.g., chest drainage tubes, oxygen apparatus, ventilators, cardiac monitors, IV setups). Reassure the client that lights and alarm noises are part of the critical care environment and are not indicators that something is wrong.

Nursing Care Before Cardiac Surgery

Preparation the evening before and the day of surgery is essentially the same as the preparation of clients for any thoracic surgery (see Chapter 62). The client may take several showers with an antimicrobial soap; skin preparation (shaving) for a thoracotomy is performed in the operating room. If the surgeon plans a CABG, the legs may also be prepared in the operating room (see Chapter 15).

Nursing Management After Cardiac Surgery

ASSESSMENT

The most reliable measures of cardiovascular function and tissue perfusion are the vital signs, including arterial blood pressure, pulses, venous and left heart filling pressures, and temperature. Monitor heart sounds, and check the ECG continuously as appropriate. Stabilization of vital signs after heart surgery usually indicates adequate cardiovascular function. Conversely, severe deviations indicate a complication such as hemorrhage, shock, cardiac tamponade, or infection. The normal ranges for each vital sign after cardiac surgery and the meaning of deviations follow.

ARTERIAL BLOOD PRESSURE. For an accurate blood pressure reading postoperatively, an 18- or 20-gauge polytetrafluoroethylene (Teflon) catheter is inserted into an artery (usually the radial artery) and attached to a strain-gauge transducer via stiff connecting tubing called pressure transmission tubing. This is connected to an electronic pressure monitor and oscilloscope. The monitor provides numerical pressure readings and produces a continuous tracing of the arterial pressure wave form (see Bridge to Critical Care). The arterial line is usually irrigated (continuously or at intervals) with heparinized water or saline. The arterial line is sometimes used as a route for obtaining blood for laboratory studies.

Most pressure monitors are able to monitor the pulmonary artery, arterial pressures, and ECG tracing simultaneously. This capability assists in determining the possible effect of surgery on hemodynamic status and cardiac output and demonstrates the effect of a dysrhythmia or change in body temperature on cardiac output.

In general, the physician will request that the blood pressure be maintained between 20 mm Hg above and 20 mm Hg below the baseline blood pressure. Frequently, this is a mean arterial pressure of 70 mm Hg or above. After mitral and aortic valve surgery, clients may tolerate a low systolic blood pressure of 90 mm Hg without difficulty. After coronary artery surgery, clients may not tolerate systolic blood pressure drops of more than 10 mm Hg below preoperative baseline because the myocardium may not be adequately perfused. Maintaining a sufficient diastolic blood pressure is also important because the myocardium receives 70% of its blood supply during this phase of the cardiac cycle. Careful assessment and monitoring of the client's hemodynamic status are essential.

Hypertension is also dangerous in a client who has undergone a CABG procedure because high blood pressure may cause the new graft to break loose or leak. Vasoactive medications (e.g., vasodilators such as nifedipine, nitroprusside, phentolamine, labetalol) can be used to improve cardiac function.

PULSES. Check radial pulse for rate, rhythm, and volume. A rapid radial pulse may indicate dysrhythmia, shock, fear, fever, hypoxia, heart failure, or hemorrhage. A slow radial pulse may indicate heart block or severe anoxia. Check the apical radial pulse for a pulse deficit, which may indicate atrial fibrillation, a frequent complication of mitral stenosis.

Assess peripheral pulses. Absence of pedal pulses may indicate the presence of peripheral emboli blocking a blood vessel in the extremity. Report this finding immediately to the surgeon. If pulses are absent, assess all pulses in the extremity and check the lower extremities for coldness, pallor, or cyanosis.

VENOUS AND LEFT-HEART FILLING PRESSURES. The central venous and pulmonary artery pressures are usually monitored postoperatively. A pressure higher than normal may be acceptable after open heart surgery, because a heart that has been diseased and then subjected to surgical trauma is weak and needs a higher filling pressure to strengthen the force of myocardial contraction and to maintain an adequate cardiac output. Therefore, the surgeon usually specifies values for venous and pulmonary artery pressures that address this problem.

If a pulmonary artery catheter is in place, a pulmonary artery wedge pressure (PAWP) can be obtained and cardiac output measured by the thermodilution method. The PAWP is a reflection of the left atrial filling pressure. (See Bridge to Critical Care, Chapter 57, which covers the Swan-Ganz catheter and these measurements.)

Causes of abnormally elevated central venous pressure (CVP) and left heart filling pressure include hypervolemia and ineffective myocardial contractions. Abnormally decreased CVP and left heart filling pressure result from hypovolemia.

BODY TEMPERATURE. Initially, the client has a low temperature of 35° to 36° C (95° to 96.8° F) because of hypothermia induced during surgery. With careful warming in a heating blanket, the client's temperature may become normal within 4 hours. Be aware that the blood pressure may drop as body temperature rises as a result of vasodilation.

The temperature may rise 1° to 1.5° C (2° or 3° F) above normal during the first or second day postoperatively and may remain elevated for 3 to 4 days. Treat this elevation with acetaminophen suppositories as prescribed and with minimal bed covering. For persistent elevations, apply ice bags or use a hypothermia blanket if prescribed.

Report abnormal findings, such as an elevated temperature to 38.5° C (101° F) or higher or an elevation that persists for more than 4 or 5 days. Abnormal temperature elevation may result from infection, dehydration, hemolysis due to transfusion reaction, or atelectasis. The untoward effects of the elevated temperature include increased metabolic demands (which increase the work of the heart), dehydration, and hypovolemia.

Abnormally low temperatures ranging from 34.4° C (94° F) to 36° C (96.8° F) result from shock or cardiac decompensation. The physician may order a warming blanket to increase temperature. Rectal, oral, or tympanic temperature readings are the most accurate.

RESPIRATIONS. To assess respiratory function, prevent respiratory complications, and provide appropriate intervention, closely monitor the rate and depth of respirations, the presence of dyspnea, and the presence of wheezing.

Make certain the ventilator is set at a rate that adequately ventilates the client and delivers an appropriate tidal volume and oxygen percentage. A conscious client may initiate respirations in addition to those delivered by the ventilator (usually the assist light will come on). Adjust the rate, tidal volume, and oxygen level to ensure adequate ventilation of the lungs and oxygenation of the blood. Adjustments are usually determined by arterial blood gas (ABG) analysis and the assessments by the physician and the nurse.

Assessment of depth of respiration may reveal shallow respirations, which may be due to pain. Give a narcotic if vital signs are stable.

Assessment of dyspnea may reveal that the client is "fighting" the ventilator (breathing against instead of with the machine), which can lead to inadequate ventilation. The client may feel short of breath. Airway obstruction (possibly due to excessive secretions), pain, fear, anoxia, acidosis, hemorrhage, and improper placement of the tube may cause difficulty in breathing and must be investigated immediately. The physician usually orders ABG studies and a chest film. The ventilator settings may need adjustment, and the client may require sedation (see Bridge to Critical Care for ventilators, Chapter 63). While the client is on the ventilator, make sure the ventilator alarms are functioning. Never turn off the alarms, not even during suctioning.

Wheezing results from pulmonary edema, bronchospasm, or airway obstruction. It may be treated with bronchodilators.

Assess the amount of pulmonary secretion. Is it copious or scant?

Assess the color of sputum. Sputum is normally white and translucent. Yellow suggests infection and represents the presence of WBCs. Green represents old retained secretions with the breakdown of WBCs. Green and foul-smelling secretions usually suggest *Pseudomonas* infection. Red denotes fresh blood. Streaking with red suggests upper airway or tracheal bleeding. Brown represents old blood residue.

Assess for accompanying signs of retained secretions, such as apprehension, perspiration, rapid pulse, dyspnea, cyanosis, and gurgling respirations.

Assessment of respiration in the pre-extubation period involves drawing blood for ABG analysis and obtaining respiratory values, including inspiratory effort and tidal volume. The client is ready for extubation if these values are within normal limits.

Respiratory assessment in the postextubation period begins with careful assessment of clinical manifestations of respiratory distress. Check the rate, depth, and character of respirations frequently. Note the client's skin color and vital signs; changes may indicate inadequate ventilation and the need for reintubation. Perform ABG analysis to determine whether the client is breathing adequately after extubation.

HEART SOUNDS. For the first 2 days postoperatively, assess heart sounds at least every 4 hours. Pericardial rubs are commonly caused by the irritation and inflammation from surgery. A new murmur may indicate valve problems. Notify the physician if one develops. A gallop probably indicates hypervolemia. See discussion of cardiovascular assessment in Chapter 54.

ELECTROCARDIOGRAM TRACINGS. Monitor the electrical activity of the client's heart continuously for at least 3 or 4 days after surgery. Observe carefully for abnormal ECG tracings; heart block, ventricular tachycardia, and atrial fibrillation commonly complicate open heart surgery. The physician requests 12-lead ECGs preoperatively, immediately postoperatively, and before discharge to observe for signs of perioperative infarction.

Most dysrhythmias can be treated effectively with antidysrhythmic medications. Clients with certain life-threatening dysrhythmias require defibrillation or cardioversion (see Chapter 57).

During surgery, the surgeon may implant atrial or ventricular pacing wires. These small wires lead from the myocardium through the chest wall. They can be connected to an external pacemaker and are used to treat bradycardia or heart block. These wires should always be insulated. When connecting them to a pacemaker, wear rubber gloves. Microshocks to these wires may result in atrial or ventricular fibrillation. Atrial pacing wires can also be connected to the chest leads of an ECG machine for differential diagnosis of atrial dysrhythmias.

CHEST DRAINAGE. The surgeon inserts chest tubes to drain air and fluid from the pleural cavity, thereby allowing the lungs to respond after surgery. Chest tubes that drain the pericardial sac are called *mediastinal tubes.*

Measure and observe chest drainage by collecting drainage in a calibrated cylinder (most hospitals use disposable chest drainage setups that are clearly calibrated). Measure findings and record hourly. Up to 100 ml of drainage may be lost during the first hour postoperatively as a result of reexpansion of the lungs, which forces drainage through the chest tube. Approximately 500 ml of drainage occurs over the first 24 hours. Large gushes of drainage are sometimes expelled when the client coughs or turns. Usually dark red during the early postoperative phase, the drainage gradually becomes more serous as time passes. Chest tubes are described in Chapter 62.

Bloody mediastinal drainage that is collected from the chest tubes can be transfused back into the client *(autotransfusion).* This transfused blood has the advantage of not originating at the blood bank. There is reduced risk of infection or disease to the client and less cost when the client's own blood is used. The bloody drainage is infused via filtered IV tubing. Some manufacturers produce disposable chest drainage systems that have this autotransfusion capability.

FLUID BALANCE. Carefully measure and record intake and output. Obtain daily weights to determine accurately whether the client is retaining fluids within tissues or losing excessive fluid rapidly. Significant fluctuations in weight act as a guide to fluid replacement.

RENAL FUNCTION. Measure urine volume hourly for the first 8 to 12 hours after surgery. The client almost always has an indwelling urinary catheter. Normal urine output is greater than 30 ml/hr except during the night, when it is lower. Urine may be bloody as a result of hemolysis of erythrocytes during ECC.

Assess the urine 24-hour specific gravity. The normal value is 1.015 to 1.020. Specific gravity may rise because of oliguria or the presence of red blood cells. Lowered specific gravity results from overhydration or inability of kidney tubules to filter waste products.

ELECTROLYTE BALANCE. Daily electrolyte studies are performed to determine blood levels of sodium, potassium, and chloride. The physician replaces electrolytes parenterally if the values are deficient. If diuretics are given to reduce volume overload, monitor potassium closely and replace as prescribed. The heart may be particularly sensitive to hypokalemia (low potassium level) soon after surgery. Obtain hematocrit, hemoglobin, and prothrombin time daily to determine extent of blood loss or hemorrhage, and check ABG values daily to determine the pH and partial pressures of arterial carbon dioxide ($PaCO_2$) and oxygen (PaO_2) (see Chapter 14).

NEUROLOGIC RESPONSE. After heart surgery, carefully observe the client's level of consciousness, pupil size and reaction, orientation, and ability to move extremities.

The client should awaken within 1 to 2 hours after surgery. Not awakening may result from embolization of air, calcium, fat, or thrombotic particles to the brain. Slow return to consciousness (over 2 to 4 days) may result from a diffuse neurologic deficit due to poor cerebral capillary perfusion during ECC.

Check pupils hourly during the early postoperative period for size, equality in size, and reaction to light. Pupils dilate when blood contains excess carbon dioxide.

Disorientation and restlessness may indicate anoxia or embolization to the brain. Also, fatigue or fear can produce mental confusion.

Hemiplegia (inability to move an extremity) or extreme weakness of an extremity may indicate embolization to the motor area of the brain.

After cardiac surgery, clients may become disoriented, delusional, and psychotic. Severe depression is not uncommon. Causes of confusion, hallucinations, and psychotic behavior include:

- Isolation in the ICU
- Sensory deprivation
- Lack of rest and sleep over an extended period

- Fear and anxiety
- An impersonal environment if care providers are preoccupied with monitors and machines
- Desynchronization of circadian rhythm (ICUs are active and well lighted 24 hours a day).

Causes of postoperative depression include fatigue and debility after surgery along with resumption of responsibilities.[53]

Diagnosis, Outcomes, Intervention

Risk for Decreased Cardiac Output. Heart failure, metabolic acidosis, weakening of the left ventricle, dysrhythmias, and cardiac tamponade can decrease cardiac output. State this diagnosis as *Risk for Decreased Cardiac Output related to (appropriate cause).*

Outcomes. The client will have improved cardiovascular function, as evidenced by adequate tissue perfusion, stabilization of vital signs, clear lung sounds on auscultation, stable body weight, adequate urine output (30 ml/hr or greater), no reported or observed dyspnea or orthopnea, regular heart sounds without S_3 or S_4, and decreased or absent peripheral edema (blood pressure within 20 mm Hg of baseline values).

Interventions. Interventions for a failing heart muscle often involve administration of inotropic agents (e.g., dopamine, dobutamine), which increase cardiac contractility. Administer inotropic agents cautiously because they also increase the work of the heart and its need for oxygen.

Complications resulting from persistent hypotension are cerebral ischemia, renal shutdown, myocardial infarction, and shock. To correct these complications, the surgeon may use a mechanical device to support the failing heart if medications are unsuccessful.

The intra-aortic balloon pump (IABP) is a counterpulsation device that supports the failing heart by increasing coronary artery perfusion during diastole and reducing afterload. It consists of a sausage-shaped balloon catheter that is passed through the femoral artery and positioned in the descending thoracic aorta just distal to the subclavian artery. The catheter is attached to a power console that inflates and deflates the balloon in time with the heart.

The balloon is inflated during diastole; blood is pushed back into the aorta, and coronary artery perfusion is improved.

The balloon is deflated during systole; resistance is decreased, and the workload of the heart is thus reduced (see Bridge to Critical Care). The timing of the balloon inflations and deflations is critical. A nurse educated in the use of the balloon pump is assigned to care for the client. Monitoring the effects of the pumping on the client's vital signs requires special skills.

Risk for Ineffective Airway Clearance. Retained secretions are common after open heart surgery. State the diagnosis as *Risk for Ineffective Airway Clearance related to retained secretions.* Also consider using the diagnosis of *Impaired Gas Exchange* if the client has marginal levels of oxygen saturation.

Outcomes. The client will exhibit improved airway clearance, as evidenced by clear lung sounds, afebrile state, strong nonproductive cough, and ABG values within normal limits.

Interventions. Turn and suction the intubated client frequently. Monitor the client's response to suctioning, noting changes in heart rhythm, restlessness, or pallor. Suctioning is seldom indicated routinely and is done when the secretions can be heard in the endotracheal tube. Today, most clients are extubated within hours of surgery. Skilled nursing care to promote pulmonary hygiene is crucial. Help the nonintubated client to turn, take deep breaths, and cough every 1 to 2 hours; suction the trachea if the temperature rises to above 38.5° C (101° F) and the client is coughing ineffectively.

After the endotracheal tube is removed, the client can wear a high-humidity oxygen mask to aid in loosening secretions; chest physiotherapy may also be used. In rare cases, bronchoscopy may be indicated for removal of secretions. Complications of retained secretions include atelectasis, pneumonia, and subsequent inadequate oxygenation of the tissues. Monitor oxygen saturation continuously.

Risk for Hemorrhage. State the collaborative problem as *Hemorrhage related to surgical trauma or slipped ligature (suture).*

Outcomes. Collaborative problems are monitored only by the nurse. Therefore, the expected outcome addresses your actions, not the client's goals. The nurse will monitor the client for amounts of drainage that exceed 2 ml/kg of body weight per hour or a sustained period of bleeding through the chest tube.

Interventions. If bleeding is noted, notify the physician because the client may need to be returned to the operating room for repair of the bleeding sites. Replace blood by transfusion as prescribed. The chest drainage may be autotransfused back into the client from the chest drainage system through an IV line. The use of blood transfusions has decreased dramatically since the onset of human immunodeficiency virus (HIV) infection. However, sometimes it is necessary to replace blood lost during surgery. If the client's hematocrit is adequate, albumin or high-molecular-weight plasma expanders, such as hetastarch, may be prescribed in place of blood.

Risk for Cardiac Tamponade. Occlusion in the pericardial drainage system can lead to cardiac tamponade. State this collaborative problem as *Risk for Cardiac Tamponade related to occlusion of the pericardial drainage system.*

Outcomes. The nurse will monitor the client for sudden cessation of chest drainage with an increase in venous pressure, pulsus paradoxus, dyspnea, oliguria, distant or inaudible heart sounds, or lowered left atrial pressure.

Interventions. Gently milk the chest tube to express clots that may be blocking drainage. Do not pull vigorously on the tube or strip the tube by creating negative pressure in it. If clots cannot be removed by gentle milking of the tube, the physician may need to declot the tube using a long catheter with an inflatable balloon on the end. The client may need to be returned to the operating room or may need a pericardial tap for removal of fluid.

Risk for Renal Failure. State this collaborative problem as *Risk for Renal Failure related to* (add specific risk). Hypovolemia, decreased cardiac output, or hemolysis of erythrocytes during cardiopulmonary bypass can result in acute renal failure.

Outcomes. The nurse will monitor the client's urinary output, expecting output greater than 30 ml/hr. Also mon-

BRIDGE TO CRITICAL CARE

Intra-aortic Balloon Pumping–Counterpulsation Device

When the left ventricle fails to support adequate circulation and perfusion, an intra-aortic balloon pumping (IABP) device can be used to augment coronary artery filling and decrease left ventricular workload. A polyethylene balloon is inserted via the femoral artery into the descending thoracic aorta distal to the left subclavian artery and connected to an external pneumatic pumping system. The pump inflates the balloon with helium or carbon dioxide during diastole, and deflates it during systole. The inflation-deflation cycle is triggered by the client's ECG, specifically by the R wave, which signals the beginning of systole. Balloon inflation during diastole augments coronary artery filling. Systolic balloon deflation decreases afterload.

IABP inflating at end of systole (dicrotic notch)
Blood pressure waves

BPM, beats per minute; ECG, electrocardiogram.

The IABP device is used in clients with cardiogenic shock, septic shock, acute anterior myocardial infarction (MI), complications following MI, angioplasty with MI, ventricular dysrhythmias with ischemia, left ventricular failure, unstable angina refractory to medications, and low cardiac output after surgery.

Guidelines for Management

1. Select an ECG lead that optimizes the R wave.
2. Time the IABP device using an arterial waveform.
3. Monitor perfusion in the extremity with IABP.
4. Monitor perfusion in arms (catheter can occlude subclavian artery)
5. Monitor arterial pressures (which should improve).
6. Monitor urine output (the catheter can occlude the renal artery).
7. Keep the affected limb straight to prevent dislodgment of the catheter.
8. Monitor for balloon rupture and misplacement (loss of augmentation, wrinkled appearance in safety chamber, blood in tubing).
9. Monitor for bleeding resulting from anticoagulant use.
10. Monitor for aortic dissection (acute back, retroperitoneal, testicular or chest pain, decreased pulses, variations in blood pressure between arms, decreased cardiac output, tachycardia, decreased filling pressures, decreased hemoglobin, decreased hematocrit).
11. Monitor skin integrity on the sacrum, the coccyx and the heels.
12. Do not elevate the head of the bed above 15 degrees.
13. Clarify or reinforce the client's and family's understanding of the IABP device.

Complications

Dissection of the femoral or iliac artery or aorta
Bleeding
Plaque dislodgment, which can cause embolization
Balloon rupture
Arterial occlusion with limb ischemia or neuropathy
Mechanical destruction of red blood cells
Inability to wean from the IABP device
Hematoma at the insertion site
Mesenteric/renal ischemia (catheter too low)
Arm ischemia (catheter too high)

Weaning

The ratio of IABP-assisted beats to unassisted beats is decreased from 1:1 to 1:2 based on the following parameters:

- Heart rate < 110 BPM
- No dysrhythmias
- Mean arterial pressure > 70 mm Hg without vasopressors
- Pulmonary arterial wedge pressure < 18 mm Hg
- Cardiac index > 2.5
- Capillary refill > 3 sec
- Urine output > 0.5 ml/kg/min
- SvO_2 between 70% and 80%

itor laboratory values for blood urea nitrogen (BUN), creatinine, and potassium.

Interventions. A client with decreased urine output may be treated with extra fluids (sometimes called a *fluid challenge*) if dehydration is the probable etiologic factor. Other interventions may include correcting shock or low output failure and administering a diuretic (e.g., furosemide) via the IV route. If renal failure occurs, peritoneal dialysis or hemodialysis should be instituted.

During the course of surgery, the client typically receives 3 to 4 L of extra fluid. Often this fluid accumulates as edema and does not greatly increase the vascular volume. However, this additional fluid does place the client at high risk for circulatory overload. For this reason, IV fluids are administered judiciously for the first 3 days postoperatively to prevent overwork of the heart. Typically, 500 to 700 ml/m^2 body surface over 24 hours, including oral intake (normal surface area is 1.5–2.0 m^2), is given. Administer sodium-containing fluids cautiously to prevent circulatory overload and heart failure.

Risk for Paralytic Ileus. Sympathetic responses leading to shunting of blood from the gastrointestinal tract during surgery, side effects of anesthesia and narcotics, and immobility lead to paralytic ileus. State this collaborative problem as *Risk for Paralytic Ileus related to (appropriate cause* [all may apply in this case]).

Outcomes. The nurse will monitor the client for clinical manifestations of ileus, as evidenced by hypoactive or absent bowel sounds, abdominal distention, nausea, vomiting, lack of appetite, and no passing of flatus.

Interventions. Give sips of water 4 hours after extubation if the client is fully responsive and not nauseated. The client may have clear liquids next, followed by solid foods. Watch for signs of abdominal distention and paralytic ileus (see Chapter 15). If either condition develops, stop oral fluids and notify the physician.

Risk for Pain. Sternal and leg incisions cause intense pain after surgery. Express this common diagnosis as *Risk for Pain related to sternal and leg incision.*

Outcomes. The client will experience increased comfort, as evidenced by normal heart rate, absence of restlessness, normal respiratory rate, verbalization of increased comfort, decreasing use of narcotics, and periods of rest.

Interventions. Give narcotic analgesics for pain postoperatively as ordered. Avoid overmedicating a client who is recovering from hypothermia because narcotic metabolism is slowed and the medication may not be excreted. Attempt to relieve the pain and restlessness with comfort measures before administering a narcotic. Most clients have more pain in the legs than in the sternum.

Risk for Altered Tissue Perfusion. The surgical procedure, hemodynamic stability, electrolyte imbalances, hypoxia, medications, and several other potential problems can lead to impaired cerebral circulation. Use this nursing diagnosis early after surgery. Later, if confusion develops, use *Risk for Injury or Acute Confusion* as the best diagnosis.

Outcomes. The client will demonstrate adequate cerebral tissue perfusion, as evidenced by continuous progress toward an alert level of consciousness.

Interventions. To prevent mental confusion, undue fear, anxiety, and tension, always address the client by name and introduce yourself by name. Take an interest in the client. Do not ignore the client while working with monitors and equipment. Place a calendar and clock at the bedside to orient the client to date and time of day. Position the cardiac monitor so that it is out of the client's view. Many clients become nervous watching their own heart action.

Schedule the day so that periods of nursing intervention alternate with periods of rest and relaxation. Encourage the client to freely discuss fears and anxieties. Prepare significant others for changes in the client's sensorium after surgery. Before visiting times, warn visitors if the client is hallucinating or is severely depressed so that they know what to expect. Explain all interventions to the client, and allow time for questions.

Risk for Impaired Physical Mobility. Prolonged bed rest after surgery and a weakened condition before surgery lead to impaired physical mobility. State this diagnosis as *Impaired Physical Mobility related to prolonged bed rest or weakened condition before surgery (or both).*

Outcomes. The client will demonstrate postoperative mobility, as evidenced by having mobility that is equal to or greater than preoperative mobility.

Interventions. Prolonged periods of bed rest after heart surgery (or any surgery) may cause weakness, pooling of respiratory secretions, atelectasis, thrombophlebitis, osteoporosis, urinary retention, renal calculi, and a negative nitrogen balance. Planned activity is the most important single factor in preventing the complications of bed rest. The type and amount of activity allowed for each client depend on the type of surgery and the client's general postoperative condition.

If the client is hemodynamically stable, turn him or her from side to side at intervals for pressure relief. Perform passive exercises and leg flexion every 2 hours to prevent thrombosis of lower extremities.

The day after surgery, the client usually dangles the legs over the side of the bed for a short period. That evening or on postoperative day 2, the client usually sits in a chair for a brief time. On day 3 to 5, the client begins to ambulate in the room and up and down the hallway. By day 8 to 10, the client is usually fully ambulatory. Cardiac monitors are used to evaluate the client's response to increasing activity.

It usually takes 8 to 10 weeks for clients to fully regain strength after surgery. On discharge home, the client gradually increases activity until moderate walks and climbing stairs do not cause undue fatigue. The client usually returns to work 2 months after surgery.

Risk for Transplant Rejection. Recall that the body's normal response to foreign protein is to recognize and destroy it. Rejection of the transplanted heart is a common concern. State this collaborative problem as *Risk for Transplant Rejection related to immune response after surgery.*

Outcomes. The nurse will monitor the client for clinical manifestations of rejection, as evidenced by decreases in oxygenation, fever, malaise, anxiety, and infiltrates on chest film.

Interventions. Rejection and infection are the most common complications of cardiac transplantation. The prevention of rejection with immunosuppression is continually being examined (see immunosuppressive protocol, Table 55–3). Cyclosporine has been helpful in preventing rejection, but it is toxic. Renal failure, hypertension, liver toxic effects, and neurologic disturbances are not uncommon.

Risk for Infection. The loss of primary defenses and use of immunosuppressive agents in transplant recipients makes these clients excellent candidates for infection. State this common nursing diagnosis as *Risk for Infection related to loss of primary defenses (skin incision) and use of immunosuppression.*

Outcomes. The client will be free from clinical manifestations of infection, as evidenced by remaining afebrile and having WBC levels within normal limits, no malaise, and no abnormal heart sounds.

Interventions. Infection remains the major cause of death in the early postoperative period as well as a major cause of death after 1 year in heart transplant recipients. Clients are treated prophylactically with antibiotics. Nonhealing sternal wounds are treated promptly. Myocutaneous flaps may be required (see Chapter 49).

EVALUATION

Clients who have open heart surgery for coronary bypass may have a leg incision from a saphenous vein graft. These long incisions can be slow to heal, in part due to decreased peripheral circulation. Delayed leg wound healing is a common problem. Wounds are usually cleaned twice daily with povidone-iodine and redressed.

The degree of expected outcome attainment should be examined frequently. Some of the problems discussed in the care of the client after heart surgery require prompt treatment (e.g., dysrhythmias); others can be evaluated over longer periods of time.

Self-Care

At home, the client's activity level will continue to increase. It takes approximately 6 weeks postoperatively for the sternum to heal. During that time, advise the client to lift nothing heavier than 5 pounds. Also, the client must refrain from driving, which may strain the incision. As the client gets into and out of bed or a chair, the arms should not bear weight; the arms are used only for balance. Teach the client and significant others to inspect the incision daily. Care of the incision may include swabbing with povidone-iodine and applying dry dressings over oozing areas.

In some cities, exercise rehabilitation programs have been developed for clients who have had heart attacks or heart surgery. These programs involve supervised, closely monitored exercise sessions and teaching. It is important for the partner or significant other to understand how much activity is desired, since many partners who mean well allow the client to assume a "sick role" once home and ultimately delay healing and recovery. See Bridge to Home Health Care.

BRIDGE TO HOME HEALTH CARE

Recovery After Heart Surgery

Following cardiac surgery, your role as a nurse is to assess for the early onset of complications; teach clients, their families, and their informal caregivers to identify problems; and evaluate recovery progress during each visit. It is also important that you encourage clients to reduce their risks and adopt a healthier lifestyle in relation to smoking, hypertension, hyperlipidemia, inactivity, and stress.

Cardiac dysrhythmias, such as atrial fibrillation, often occur after surgery and can be identified during your nursing assessment by a portable electrocardiogram (ECG) monitor. Auscultate heart tones to assess for a pericardial rub; it may not be present until 2 weeks after surgery and can be safely managed with anti-inflammatory medications. Instruct clients to weigh themselves daily and to report gains of 2 pounds in 24 hours or 5 pounds in a week. Such weight gain may indicate heart failure.

Assess pulmonary status to detect early evidence of pneumonia. Evaluate incentive spirometry measurements; decreasing lung volumes indicate early pneumonia or an enlarging pleural effusion. Instruct clients to use their incentive spirometers a minimum of 10 times each day until presurgical lung volume returns. Typically, the goal is to increase lung volume by 200 ml every other day.

Incisions remain red and tender for 2 to 3 weeks but should not demonstrate discolored drainage, increased edema, or heat at the site. Instruct clients to take a daily shower, pat their incisions dry, and keep them open to air unless drainage occurs. If you remove staples or sutures, apply Steri-strips over the incisions. If the Steri-strips do not fall off in the shower, they can be removed within 2 weeks.

Even though clients usually have a poor appetite for the first 4 to 6 weeks after surgery, they need to eat a diet that promotes healing; the diet should be 300 to 500 kilocalories (kcal) above their basal metabolic rate. Clients, their family members, and informal caregivers are often concerned about limiting fats during the recovery period. However, anorexic clients need to limit only sodium and caffeine until their incisions heal. Encourage a high fiber intake to prevent constipation. Most clients will be ready to begin the American Heart Association Step 2 diet 3 to 4 weeks after surgery.

Urge clients to take their prescribed pain medication to promote comfort, to enable them to perform their deep-breathing exercises, and to foster restful sleep. Clients should use several pillows to obtain a comfortable position and to minimize pain. Women should wear a supportive brassiere to decrease sternal stress. Instruct clients to use stretching and range-of-motion exercises to reduce left shoulder discomfort, which results from positioning during surgery. Transient postoperative depression is common. Instruct clients that the "blues" may occur between 2 and 6 weeks after hospital discharge and should subside in a few weeks.

Typical recovery instructions include increasing low level activity, such as walking, by 2 minutes each day until the client is able to tolerate 20 minutes of sustained activity. Clients are instructed not to lift anything heavier than 5 pounds, and driving is generally restricted for 1 month per physician's order. Clients, young and old, want to know when they can safely resume sexual relations. When the client can tolerate climbing two flights of stairs, sexual activity is safe. Clients are instructed to assume passive positions that will not stress the sternum for the first few months after surgery.

Ann K. Frantz, RN, BSN, *Independent Health Care Consultant, Pontiac, Michigan*

Low-sodium and low-cholesterol diets are often prescribed for clients after cardiac surgery. For the client to be able to comply with dietary instruction, the diet must be carefully planned (see Chapter 56).

Teach the client or significant other to check the pulse daily for rate and regularity and to call the physician if the resting heart rate rises by more than 20 beats per minute or a new irregularity is present. The client can also use heart rate to monitor responses to exercise. Authorities usually recommend a rise of not more than 20 BPM for the immediate postoperative period.

Make sure the client knows how and when to schedule follow-up appointments. Instruct the client to report the following to the primary health care provider:

- Manifestations of infection, including fever, and increased redness, tenderness, or swelling of incisions
- Palpitations, tachycardia, or irregular pulse (if normally regular)
- Dizziness or increased fatigue
- Sudden weight gain or peripheral edema
- Shortness of breath

Modifications for Elderly Clients

Older clients commonly have many other disorders that interfere with or delay their ability to respond to the hemodynamic changes of surgery and recovery. The elderly client is also at risk for skin breakdown and renal impairment. Fluids must be closely titrated because of the possibility of a pre-existent heart disorder.

CONCLUSIONS

The client with a cardiac disorder frequently has activity intolerance, decreased cardiac output, and ineffective coping due to the seriousness of the disorder. Nurses must be skilled in the physical and psychosocial aspects of disease when providing care.

THINKING CRITICALLY

1. **A 45-year-old man arrives in the emergency department after an automobile accident. Initially, he does not complain about himself, but then he is more concerned about his daughter, who was injured in the accident. Neither the child nor the client were wearing seat belts when their car was struck from behind. While sitting at his daughter's bedside in the emergency department, the client becomes more and more anxious; his respiratory rate increases, and he becomes restless. The vital signs reveal a blood pressure of 88/72, pulse of 118, and respirations of 28. What other assessments are needed to rule out cardiac tamponade? What intervention will relieve pressure on the heart and improve cardiac function?**

Factors to Consider. What are the clinical manifestations of cardiac tamponade? How is cardiac output affected by cardiac tamponade?

2. **The client is a 60-year-old man with dilated cardiomyopathy. His prognosis is very poor. He is able to tolerate only minimal amounts of activity: using the bedside commode, feeding himself, and shaving himself in bed. Today, he continues to be short of breath but seems particularly withdrawn. Repeated physical assessment to identify cardiovascular status shows no change in assessment findings. He continues to take his medications at the proper dosages. His physician thinks these medications are at their maximal levels. Repeated psychosocial assessment would show that the client is withdrawn because he is anxious that he will become physically worse, hospitalized, and placed on a ventilator again. He does not wish to be placed on a ventilator. He was terrified the last time and sees no purpose in just prolonging his dying. What nursing actions might help your client?**

Factors to Consider. What are the clinical manifestations of cardiomyopathy? What are the psychological considerations for the client's care?

3. **A 52-year-old man with a lengthy history of mitral valve prolapse is recovering from kidney transplantation surgery. This is his fourth postoperative day, and he and his spouse are asking questions about care at home. What priorities for client education should be established?**

Factors to Consider. What complication is associated with mitral valve prolapse? How does the medication regimen following transplantation surgery further place the client at risk?

BIBLIOGRAPHY

1. Alexander, R. W., Schlant, R. C., & Fuster, V. (1998). *Hurst's the heart* (9th ed.). New York: McGraw-Hill.
2. Bates, B. (1995). *A guide to physical examination and history taking.* Philadelphia: J. B. Lippincott.
3. Bayer, A.S., et al. (1998). AHA Scientific Statement: Diagnosis and management of infective endocarditis and its complications. *Circulation, 98,* 2936–2948.
4. Braunwald, E. (1997). Valvular heart disease. In E. Braunwald (Ed.), *Heart disease* (pp. 1007–1076). Philadelphia: W. B. Saunders.
5. Carpenito, L. J. (1995). *Nursing diagnosis.* Philadelphia: J. B. Lippincott.
6. Dajani, A.S. (1997). Prevention of bacterial endocarditis: Recommendations by the American Heart Association. *Journal of the American Medical Association, 277*(22), 1794–1801.
7. Dajani, A. S. (1997). Rheumatic fever. In E. Braunwald (Ed.), *Heart disease* (pp. 1769–1775). Philadelphia: W. B. Saunders.
8. Findlow, D., & Doyle, E. (1997). Congenital heart disease in adults. *British Journal of Anesthesia, 78,* 416–430.
9. Futterman, L. G., & Lemberg, L. (1995). New indications for dual chamber pacing: Hypertrophic and dilated cardiomyopathy. *American Journal of Critical Care, 4*(1), 82–87.
10. Halm, M. A. (1996). Acute gastrointestinal complications after cardiac surgery. *American Journal of Critical Care, 5*(2), 109–117.
11. Kawai, C. (1999). From myocarditis to cardiomyopathy: Mechanisms of inflammation and cell death. *Circulation, 99*(8), 1091–1100.
12. Karchmer, A. W. (1997). Infective endocarditis. In E. Braunwald (Ed.), *Heart disease* (pp. 1077–1104). Philadelphia: W. B. Saunders.
13. Lashley, F. R. (1999). Genetic testing, screening, and counseling issues in cardiovascular disease. *Journal of Cardiovascular Nursing, 13*(4), 110–126.

14. Lawrie, G. M. (1998). Mitral valve repair vs. replacement. *Cardiology Clinics, 16*(3), 437–448.
15. Lorell, B. H. (1997). Pericardial Diseases. In E. Braunwald (Ed.), *Heart disease* (pp. 1478–1534). Philadelphia: W. B. Saunders.
16. McLachlan, J., Reddy, P., & Ratts, T. E. (1998). Mitral valve prolapse: A common diagnosis in women. *Journal of the Louisiana State Medical Society, 150,* 92–96.
17. Micevski, V. (1999). The use of molecular technologies for the detection of enteroviral ribonucleic acid in myocarditis. *Journal of Cardiovascular Nursing, 13*(4), 78–90.
18. Myers, R. B.,& Spodick, D. H. (1999). Constrictive pericarditis: Clinical and pathophysiologic characteristics. *American Heart Journal, 138,* 219–232.
19. Perloff, J. K. (1997). Congenital heart disease in adults. In E. Braunwald (Ed.), *Heart disease* (pp. 963–987). Philadelphia: W. B. Saunders.
20. Richenbacher, W. E., & Pierce, W. S. (1997). Assisted circulation and the mechanical heart. In E. Braunwald (Ed.), *Heart disease* (pp. 534–547). Philadelphia: W. B. Saunders.
21. Riddle, M. M., Dunstan, J. L., & Castanis, J. L. (1996). A rapid recovery program for cardiac surgery patients. *American Journal of Critical Care, 5*(2), 152–159.
22. Simpson, T., & Lee, E. R. (1996). Individual factors that influence sleep after cardiac surgery. *American Journal of Critical Care, 5*(3), 182–189.
23. Simpson, T., Lee, E. R., & Cameron, C. (1996). Patients' perceptions of environmental factors that disturb sleep after cardiac surgery. *American Journal of Critical Care, 5*(3), 173–181.
24. Sparacino, P. A. (1999). Cardiac infections: Medical and surgical therapies. *Journal of Cardiovascular Nursing, 13*(2), 49–65.
25. United Network of Organ Sharing (1999). Transplant patient data source. Available: *http://www.unos.org*
26. Wakowski, C. A., & Bierman, P. Q. (1995). Dual chamber pacing in patients with hypertrophic obstructive cardiomyopathy: A case study. *American Journal of Critical Care, 4*(2), 165–168.
27. Wynne, J., & Braunwald, E. (1997). The cardiomyopathies and myocarditides. In E. Braunwald (Ed.), *Heart disease* (pp. 1404–1463). Philadelphia: W. B. Saunders.

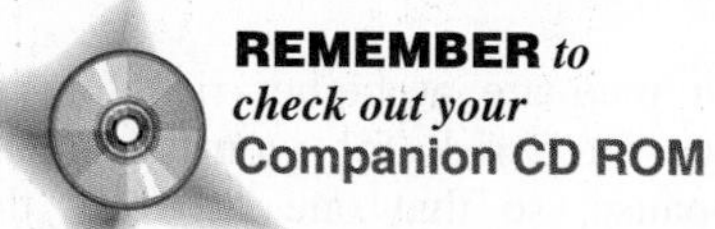

CHAPTER

56

Management of Clients with Functional Cardiac Disorders

Peggy Gerard
Janice Tazbir

NURSING OUTCOMES CLASSIFICATION (NOC)
for Nursing Diagnoses—Clients with Functional Cardiac Disorders

Altered Tissue Perfusion
Sensory Function: Cutaneous
Tissue Perfusion: Peripheral
Tissue Perfusion: Pulmonary
Decreased Cardiac Output
Cardiac Pump Effectiveness
Circulation Status
Tissue Perfusion: Abdominal Organs
Vital Signs Status
Fluid Volume Excess
Electrolyte and Acid/Base Balance
Fluid Balance
Hydration
Impaired Gas Exchange
Electrolyte and Acid/Base Balance
Respiratory Status: Ventilation
Risk for Activity Intolerance
Activity Tolerance
Endurance
Energy Conservation
Self-Care: Activities of Daily Living
Self-Care: Instrumental Activities of Daily Living
Risk for Anxiety
Anxiety Control
Coping
Risk for Impaired Skin Integrity
Tissue Integrity: Skin and Mucous Membranes

Normal functioning of the heart is based on a balance between oxygen supply and oxygen demand. In order to function as an effective pump, the heart muscle must be adequately supplied with blood from the coronary arteries. In *coronary heart disease* (CHD), atherosclerosis develops in the coronary arteries, causing them to become narrowed or blocked. When a coronary artery is narrowed or blocked, blood flow to the area of the heart supplied by that artery is reduced. If the remaining blood flow is inadequate to meet the oxygen demand of the heart, the area may become ischemic and injured and myocardial infarction (MI) may result. In addition, the heart may fail to pump sufficient blood supply to the other organs and tissues in the body. Over time, changes resulting from CHD may lead to the development of chronic heart failure.

The term coronary heart disease, also called *coronary artery disease* or *ischemic heart disease,* refers to diseases of the heart that result from a decrease in blood supply to the heart muscle. This chapter reviews the risk factors, etiology, pathophysiology, clinical manifestations, and medical and nursing intervention for two major disorders of cardiac function: CHD and heart failure. The related conditions of angina pectoris and MI are discussed in Chapter 58.

CORONARY HEART DISEASE

CHD is the single largest killer of men and women in the United States and currently affects more than 12 million people.[7] Although these numbers seem high, the death rate from coronary heart disease decreased 24.2% from 1986 to 1996. Contributing to this decline in the death rate are factors such as improved technology for diagnosis and treatment, use of thrombolytic drugs in acute MI, improved interventional therapies and surgical techniques, and modification of risk factors in populations at risk.

Etiology and Risk Factors

CHD results from the development of obliterative atherosclerotic lesions within the coronary arteries that narrow or obstruct these vessels. Atherosclerosis is a disorder of lipid metabolism and underlies most causes of cardiovascular disease and death.

Although CHD claims more lives each year than any other disease, its causes are poorly understood. Clinical evidence suggests that many factors contribute to the onset of atherosclerosis. Risk factors that precipitate CHD can be presented in two categories: major risk factors and contributing risk factors (Box 56–1). Major risk factors are those that are significantly associated with the development of CHD. Contributing risk factors are those that are associated with the risk of cardiovascular disease but whose significance and prevalence have not been determined.

The more risk factors a person has, the greater the risk of CHD. Although risk factors influence the development of CHD in all people, the importance of selected risk factors may vary by gender and race. Overall, risk factors are found more frequently in lower socioeconomic and educational groups.[49] Although a few risk factors cannot be changed, a person may reduce the risk of CHD by controlling risk factors that can be modified by lifestyle or medication.

MAJOR NONMODIFIABLE RISK FACTORS

Heredity (Including Race)

Children whose parents had heart disease are at higher risk for CHD. This increased risk is related to genetic factors that contribute to four risk factors that increase the incidence of CHD:

- Hypertension
- Dyslipidemia
- Diabetes
- Obesity

For people ages 35 to 74 years, the age-adjusted death rate from CHD for African American women is 72% higher than that for white women. The prevalence of CHD is lowest among Mexican Americans.[6]

Increasing Age

Age influences both the risk and the severity of CHD. Symptomatic CHD appears predominantly in people older than 40 years of age, and four out of five people who die of CHD are age 65 years or older. However, angina and MI can occur in a person's 30s and even in one's 20s. At older ages, women who have heart attacks are twice as likely as men to die of the heart attack.[6]

Gender

CHD is the number one killer of both men and women. In 1996, mortality from CHD was almost equal for men and women. Although men are at higher risk for heart attacks at younger ages, the risk for women increases significantly at menopause, so that one of every three women in the United States 65 years of age and older has CHD.

Women who take oral contraceptives and who smoke or have high blood pressure are at greater risk for CHD. Women with an early menopause are also at higher risk than are women with a normal or late menopause.[6, 49]

Two lifestyle changes during the past two decades may be responsible for the increased incidence of CHD among women. More women (many with full responsibility for the household and children) have entered the work force, and more women have begun to smoke tobacco at an earlier age.

BOX 56–1 Risk Factors for Coronary Heart Disease

Nonmodifiable Major Risk Factors

- Heredity, including race
- Age
- Gender

Modifiable Major Risk Factors

- Cigarette smoking
- Hypertension
- Elevated serum cholesterol
- Diabetes mellitus
- Physical inactivity
- Obesity

Contributing Risk Factors

- Stress
- Homocysteine level

MAJOR MODIFIABLE RISK FACTORS

Smoking, hypertension, elevated serum cholesterol levels, physical inactivity, obesity, and diabetes mellitus constitute the other major risk factors. Their effect on CHD can be modified or reduced by treatment.

Smoking

Smokers are two times more likely to have a heart attack and to die from it than nonsmokers. Recent evidence suggests that nonsmokers who are exposed to second-hand tobacco smoke at home or work may also have a higher mortality rate from CHD. Smoking triples the risk of heart attack in women and doubles the risk of heart attack in men. Clients who smoke have two to four times the risk of sudden cardiac death.[6, 49]

Although the means by which smoking causes CHD remains unknown, the three substances thought to increase the prevalence of CHD are tar, nicotine, and carbon monoxide. Tar contains hydrocarbons and other carcinogenic substances. Nicotine increases the release of epinephrine and norepinephrine, which results in peripheral vasoconstriction, elevated blood pressure and heart rate, greater oxygen consumption, and increased likelihood of dysrhythmias. In addition, nicotine activates platelets and stimulates smooth muscle cell proliferation in the arterial walls. Carbon monoxide reduces the amount of blood available to the intima of the vessel wall and increases the permeability of the endothelium. Clients who quit smoking lose their increased risk in 3 to 5 years.[49]

Hypertension

High blood pressure afflicts nearly 50 million American adults and children. It increases the workload of the heart, thus causing the heart to enlarge and weaken over time. As blood pressure increases, the risk of a serious cardiovascular event also escalates. When hypertension is combined with other risk factors, such as obesity, smoking, high cholesterol levels, and diabetes, the risk of heart attack or stroke increases significantly.

Compared with whites, African Americans have hypertension at an earlier age and it is more severe at any age. Consequently, the rate of heart disease in African Americans is 1.5 times greater than that of whites. Although hypertension cannot always be prevented, it should be treated to lower the risk of CHD and premature death.[6, 7]

Elevated Serum Cholesterol Levels

The risk of CHD increases as blood cholesterol levels increase. The risk increases further when other risk factors are present. In adults, total cholesterol levels of 240 mg/dl are classified as "high" and levels ranging from 200 to 239 mg/dl are classified as "borderline-high." At young and middle ages, men have higher cholesterol levels. In women, cholesterol levels continue to increase up to about age 70.[49]

Cholesterol, a sterol found in animal tissue, circulates in the blood in combination with triglycerides and protein-bound phospholipids. This complex is called a *lipoprotein.* There are four basic groups of lipoproteins, all produced in the intestinal wall. Elevation of lipoproteins is called *hyperlipoproteinemia.* Elevation of lipids, a component of lipoproteins, is called *hyperlipidemia.* Lipoproteins and their functions are as follows:

- Chylomicrons primarily transport dietary triglycerides and cholesterol.
- Very-low-density lipoproteins (VLDLs) mainly transport triglycerides synthesized by the liver.
- Low-density lipoproteins (LDLs) have the highest concentration of cholesterol and transport endogenous cholesterol to body cells.
- High-density lipoproteins (HDLs) have the lowest concentration of cholesterol and transport endogenous cholesterol to body cells.

Recent investigations have documented how the presence of lipoproteins may predispose the body to CHD. People with high levels of HDL in proportion to LDL are at less risk for CHD than people with a low HDL:LDL ratio. High concentrations of HDL seem to protect against the development of CHD. Experts believe that the cholesterol in HDL, in contrast to that in LDL, does not become incorporated into the fatty plaques that develop in the lining of the artery wall.

The ratio of total cholesterol to HDL or of LDL to HDL is the best test for predicting the risk of CHD. Exercise and low-fat, low-cholesterol diets increase the amount of HDL in the blood. Current recommendations[21] for cholesterol and lipoproteins are:

- Total blood cholesterol < 200 mg/dl
- LDL < 160 if fewer than two other risk factors (<130 mg/dl if two or more risk factors)
- HDL > 35 mg/dl

Triglycerides are not an independent risk factor in men, but their significance in women is unknown. However, the combination of a high triglyceride level and a low HDL level seems to be a more important predictor of CHD in women than in men. The Consensus Panel Statement from the American Heart Association (AHA) recommends that triglyceride levels be below 200 mg/dl.[21]

In the average American diet, approximately 45% of the total calories come from fat. This level exeeds that recommended in the *AHA Step 1 Diet.* Dietary fat comes in many forms and disguises. A high intake of cholesterol and saturated fats is associated with the development of CHD, whereas a proportional intake of polyunsaturated and monounsaturated fats is linked with lower risk. The AHA Step 1 Diet contains no more than 30% of calories from fat, 55% from carbohydrate (at least half of which should be complex), and 15% from protein. When fat intake does not exceed 30% of total calories, the expected rise in triglycerides from a high carbohydrate diet is minimal. Saturated fats should account for no more than 10% of caloric intake.[7, 21]

Physical Inactivity

Twenty-five per cent of adults in the United States report no leisure-time physical activity even though regular aerobic exercise is important in preventing heart and blood vessel disease. The Framingham Study demonstrated an inverse relationship between exercise and the risk of CHD. Those who exercise reduce their risk of CHD because they have (1) higher HDL levels; (2) lower LDL cholesterol, triglyceride, and blood glucose levels; (3) greater insulin sensitivity; (4) lower blood pressure; and (5) lower body mass index.[9]

Obesity

Obesity places an extra burden on the heart, requiring the muscle to work harder to pump enough blood to support added tissue mass. In addition, obesity increases one's risk for CHD because it is often associated with elevated serum cholesterol and triglyceride levels, high blood pressure, and diabetes.

Distribution of body fat is also important. In older women, a waist-to-hip ratio of 0.8 or higher is one of the major risk factors for CHD. People can lower their heart disease risk by losing as little as 10 to 20 pounds.[6] However, an alternating pattern of weight gain and weight loss is associated with an increased risk for CHD.[49]

Diabetes

Diabetes frequently appears in middle-aged, overweight people. A fasting blood glucose level of more than 126 mg/dl or a routine blood glucose level of 180 mg/dl and glucosuria signals the presence of diabetes and represents an increased risk for CHD. Diabetes leads to early atherosclerosis and in women increases the risk of CHD by three-fold to seven-fold.[49]

Contributing Risk Factors

Response to Stress

A person's response to stress may contribute to the development of CHD. Some researchers have reported a relationship between CHD risk and stress levels, health behaviors, and socioeconomic status. Stress appears to increase CHD risk through its effect on major risk factors. For example, people may respond to stress by overeating or by starting or increasing smoking. Stress is also associated with elevated blood pressure. Although stress is unavoidable in modern life, an excessive response to stress can be a health hazard. Significant stressors include major changes in residence, occupation, or socioeconomic status.

Homocysteine Levels

Researchers have reported that elevated levels of plasma homocysteine (an amino acid produced by the body) are associated with an increased risk of CHD. However, scientists do not know whether homocysteine directly or indirectly increases CHD risk because homocysteine levels are related to renal function, smoking, fibrinogen, and C-reactive protein. Elevated homocysteine levels can be reduced by treatment with folic acid, vitamin B_6, and vitamin B_{12}. Experts currently recommend that homocysteine levels be measured in people with a history of premature CHD, cerebrovascular accident, or both in the absence of other risk factors.[9]

Menopause

The incidence of CHD markedly increases among women after menopause. Before menopause, estrogen is thought to protect against CHD risk by raising HDL and lowering LDL levels. Epidemiologic studies have shown that the loss of natural estrogen as women age may be associated with increases in total and LDL cholesterol and a gradually increasing CHD risk. If menopause is caused by surgical removal of the uterus and ovaries, the risks of CHD and MI rise.

Estrogen replacement therapy (ERT) is currently recommended for women without a confirmed diagnosis of CHD who are not at high risk for breast cancer or thromboembolism. A large number of studies suggest that ERT substantially decreases the risk of coronary events and is associated with increases in HDL and decreases in LDL and fibrinogen levels.

Evidence regarding the role of ERT for women with diagnosed CHD is conflicting. Observational studies indicate that ERT is beneficial for women with diagnosed CHD; however, recent results from a large multicenter clinical trial show an increase in cardiovascular events after 1 year of treatment with estrogen and progesterone therapy but a decrease in cardiovascular events in years 4 and 5.[26] Additional research is being conducted in this area.[34]

Pathophysiology

There are three layers in the arterial wall:

1. The *intima,* a single layer of cells on the inner surface of the artery, normally provides an impermeable barrier to proteins in the blood.
2. The *media* (middle layer) is made up almost entirely of smooth muscle cells.
3. The *adventitia* consists mainly of smooth muscle cells, fibroblasts, and loose connective tissue.

Atherosclerosis primarily affects the intima of the arterial wall and normally takes years to develop. When clinical manifestations develop, atherosclerosis is usually well advanced.

Pathogenesis of Atherosclerosis

In the 1950s, pathologists proposed that atherosclerosis progressed through three developmental stages: the fatty streak, the fibrous plaque, and the complicated lesion. This classification system was commonly used until the late 1990's. In 1995, the AHA published a report that reclassified atherosclerosis into five phases, including six progressive types of lesions (Table 56–1).[46] *Phase I* is present in most people 30 years of age and younger and is characterized by lesions of types I through III that do not appreciably thicken the arterial wall or narrow the arterial lumen. Lesion types I and II, also called *early lesions,* occur primarily in infants and children but also may be present in adults.

Type I lesions are microscopic, occur most often near branches in the arteries, and consist of adaptive thickening of the smooth muscle and lipid-filled macrophages, called foam cells. Type I lesions progress and mature into *type II* lesions that consist of fatty streaks containing intracellular lipid droplets, clusters of foam cells, and smooth muscle cells.[16, 17]

Type III lesions, known as *intermediate* lesions, develop during one's 20s. These lesions appear as raised fatty streaks in which extracellular connective tissue, fibrils, and lipid deposits surround the smooth muscle cells. Type III lesions are also referred to as "pre-atheromas" because they form the bridge between early and advanced lesions. In phase I, the progression of lesions is predictable, characteristic, and uniform.[17, 46]

Phase II, characterized by type IV and V lesions, represents the development of vulnerable plaques that contain pools of extracellular lipids. The *type IV* lesion, also called an *atheroma,* is characterized by further changes in the intimal structure caused by the accumulation of large amounts of extracellular lipids and fibrous tissue localized into a lipid core. The lipid core thickens the artery wall but often does not narrow the lumen of the artery. The periphery of type IV lesions is vulnerable to rupture, which may lead to rapid progression to more severe lesions.

When new fibrous connective tissue forms a thin protective cap over the atheroma, the lesion is classified as *type V.* These lesions are further subdivided into types Va, Vb, and Vc. *Type Va* lesions contain irregularly stacked multiple layers of lipid cores separated by thick layers of fibrous connective tissue. These lesions may rapidly progress to a *type VI* lesion or may continue to develop into stenotic plaques that may eventually occlude the entire lumen of the artery.[16] A type V lesion that contains calcium in the lipid core and other parts of the lesion is referred to as type *Vb.* The absence of a lipid core, with minimal lipid deposition in other parts of the lesion, is characteristic of a type *Vc* lesion. Type Vc lesions are often seen in arteries in the legs.[17, 46]

Phase III is marked by the acute disruption of type IV and V lesions that causes thrombus formation and the development of a type VI lesion (*complicated*). If thrombus formation during phase III does not limit the flow of blood through the artery, these events are often asymptomatic. The net result of phase III is a rapid increase in plaque size that may result in stable angina. However, if the thrombus reduces or significantly blocks flow through the artery (*phase IV*), an acute coronary syndrome such as unstable angina, MI, or sudden cardiac death often results (see Chapter 58). Type VI lesions are characterized by a core containing extracellular lipids, tissue factor, collagen, platelets, thrombin, and fibrin. These lesions may also be associated with disruption of the plaque surface, hematoma or hemorrhage into the plaque, and thrombosis.[17, 46]

Phase V follows a phase III or IV event and occurs when the thrombus over the disrupted plaque begins to calcify (type Vb lesion) or fibrose (type Vc lesion), forming a chronic stenotic lesion. The phase V lesion often contains organizing thrombus from several earlier episodes of plaque disruption, ulceration, hemorrhage, and organization. As the phase V lesion progresses, it occludes a greater portion of the arterial lumen and eventually may lead to total occlusion. Phase V lesions are associated with chronic stable angina and are often accompanied by the development of collateral circulation.[17, 46]

Collateral circulation is the presence of more than one artery supplying a muscle. There is normally some collateral circulation in the coronary arteries, especially in

TABLE 56–1 PROGRESSION OF ATHEROSCLEROSIS, CLINICAL MANIFESTATIONS, AND ASSOCIATED LESIONS

Phase of Coronary Heart Disease	Type and Characteristics	Earliest Onset	Clinical Manifestation	Illustration
Phase I	*Type I (initial lesion)* Isolated macrophage foam cells Intimal thickening located near bifurcations of artery	Infancy and childhood	Clinically silent	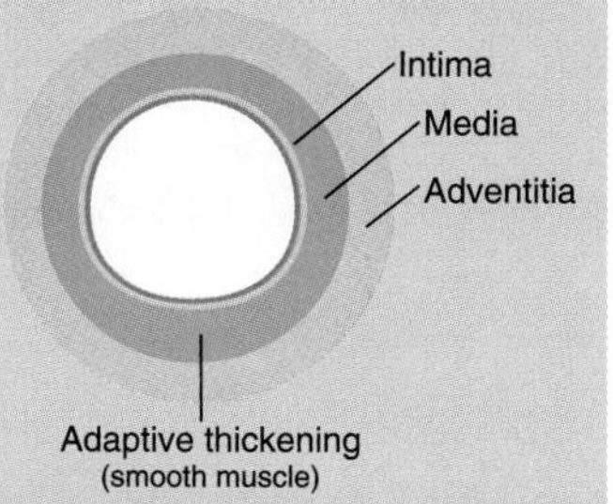 Intima Media Adventitia Adaptive thickening (smooth muscle)
	Type II (fatty streak) No decrease in lumen Flat, fatty streaks Lipid accumulation with clusters of macrophage foam cells	Infancy and childhood	Clinically silent	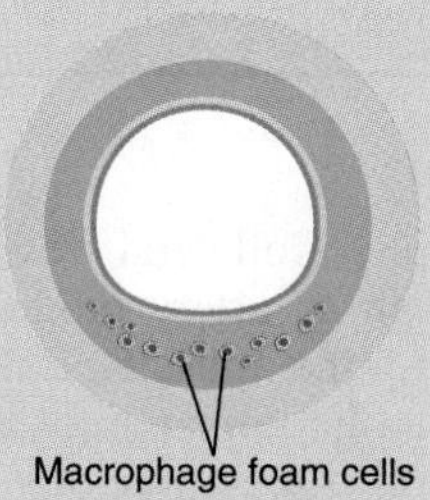 Macrophage foam cells
	Type III (preatheroma) Raised fatty streaks Lipid-filled foam cells and smooth muscle cells	From third decade on	Clinically silent	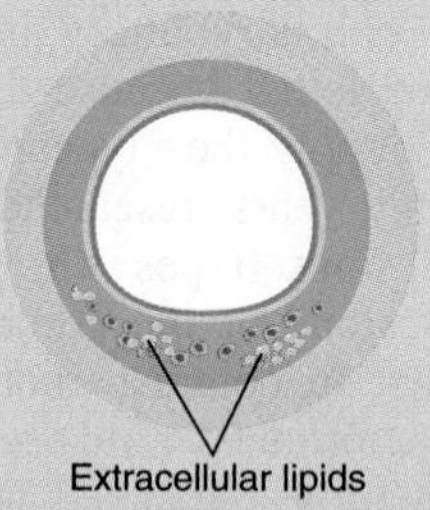 Extracellular lipids
Phase II	*Type IV (atheroma)* Disturbed intimal structure with extracellular lipid and fibrous tissue in core Small to moderate decreases in lumen	From third decade on	Clinically silent	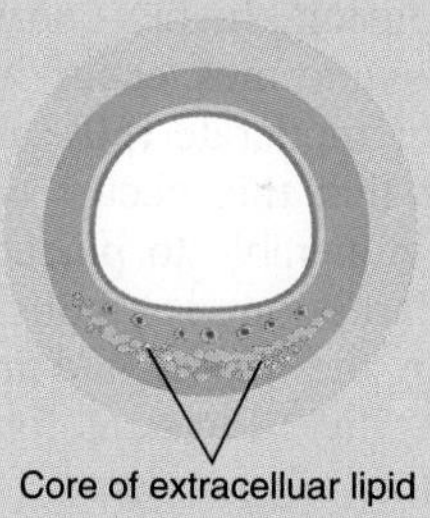 Core of extracelluar lipid
	Type Va (fibroatheroma) Lipid core with fibrotic layer Multiple lipid cores and fibrotic layers	From fourth decade on	Va is usually clinically silent, whereas Vb may be associated with chronic stable angina	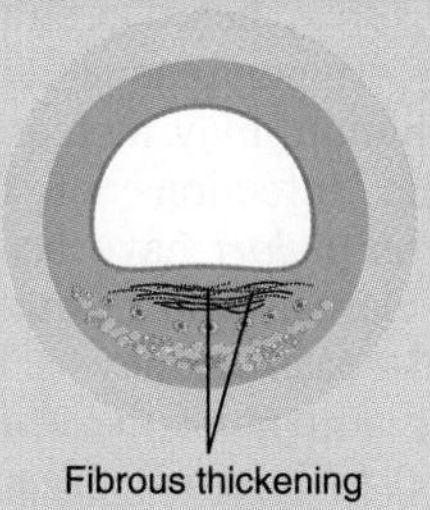 Fibrous thickening
Phase III	*Type VI (complicated lesion)* Plaque rupture Mural thrombus with partial occlusion of lumen	From fourth decade on	Angina pectoris that is due to partial occlusion of vessel	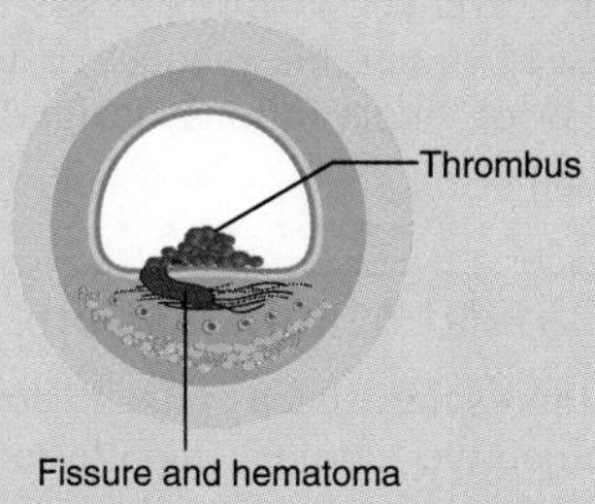 Thrombus
Phase IV	*Type VI lesion* Same as above except greater degree of occlusion	From fourth decade on	Acute syndromes, unstable angina, myocardial infarction, sudden death	Fissure and hematoma

Table continued on following page

TABLE 56–1 PROGRESSION OF ATHEROSCLEROSIS, CLINICAL MANIFESTATIONS, AND ASSOCIATED LESIONS *Continued*

Phase of Coronary Heart Disease	Type and Characteristics	Earliest Onset	Clinical Manifestation	Illustration
Phase V	*Type Vb-c* Complicated plaques from phase III become calcified (Vb) or fibrotic (Vc)	From fourth decade on	Stable angina	Organized thrombus covered over by fibrous or calcified tissue

older people. Collateral vessels develop when the blood flow through an artery progressively decreases and causes ischemia to the muscle. Extra blood vessels develop to meet metabolic demands of the muscle. The development of collateral circulation takes time. Therefore, an occlusion of a coronary artery in a younger person is more likely to be lethal because there are no collateral arteries present to supply the myocardium with blood.

For many years, researchers thought that the more obstructive lesions (types Vb and Vc) were responsible for most occlusions of the coronary arteries and acute coronary events. In contrast, more recent studies suggest that lesions that produce mild stenosis (types IV and Va) are more frequently associated with rapid progression to coronary occlusion. In fact, nearly 60% to 70% of all acute coronary syndromes occur in arteries with mild (<50% stenosis) or moderate (50% to 70% stenosis) occlusion. It is thought that this occurs because less occlusive lesions are more vulnerable to plaque rupture and thrombosis.[44, 54] Plaque disruption is thought to result from external stresses on the vessel and internal changes that increase plaque fragility. Physical forces that exert external pressure on the atherosclerotic plaques such as blood and pulse pressures, heart contraction, vasospasm, and shear stress may trigger plaque rupture.[54] Internal factors, such as inflammation, may increase plaque vulnerability.

Systemic infections of *Chlamydia pneumoniae* and *Helicobacter pylori* have been linked to the development of atherosclerosis and are thought to contribute to plaque instability because they activate the inflammatory response. Treatment of these infections with antibiotics has been found to improve the prognosis after an acute coronary event.[22, 23] Researchers are investigating methods to detect vulnerable plaques and are evaluating the effectiveness of interventions designed to stabilize atherosclerotic plaques.

Clinical Manifestations

Atherosclerosis by itself does not necessarily produce subjective clinical manifestations. For manifestations to develop, there must be a critical deficit in the blood supply to the heart in proportion to the demands for oxygen and nutrients. In other words, a supply-and-demand imbalance must exist. When atherosclerosis progresses slowly, the collateral circulation that develops generally can meet the heart's demands. Thus, whether manifestations of CHD develop depends on the total blood supply to the myocardium (by way of the coronary arteries and collateral circulation) and not solely on the condition of the coronary arteries.

Rapid progression of atherosclerotic lesions (type VI) may cause ischemia and may result in the development of acute coronary syndromes of unstable angina, MI, and sudden cardiac death. Slow progression of atherosclerotic lesions (types Vb and Vc) is associated with stable coronary artery disease and the clinical manifestation of chronic stable angina. These lesions usually cause ischemia during periods when myocardial oxygen demand increases.[17] Angina, MI, and sudden cardiac death are discussed in Chapter 58.

Techniques to determine the extent of CHD and identify the affected vessels include the electrocardiogram (ECG), B-mode ultrasonography, Doppler flow studies, intravascular ultrasound, electron-beam computed tomography, and thallium, sestamibi, or echocardiographic stress tests (see Chapter 58).[46]

Outcome Management

Medical Management

The primary goals that guide the medical management of a client with CHD are reducing and controlling risk factors and restoring blood supply to the myocardium.

Reduce Risk Factors

Prevention, rather than treatment, is the goal with regard to CHD. Modification of risk factors can significantly improve prognosis even after an acute coronary event.[17] Recent findings indicate that risk factor reduction may limit and even prevent the progression of CHD by increasing the stability of atherosclerotic plaques, decreasing thrombogenicity, and limiting external stress on the vessel. Consensus Panel Statements, revised in 1999, outline recommendations for primary prevention of CHD as well as comprehensive risk reduction for clients with diagnosed CHD.[6] For people without diagnosed CHD, the goal of medical treatment is to prevent the development of risk factors and clinical disease. Cessation of cigarette smoking, participating in regular exercise, and controlling blood pressure, diabetes, cholesterol levels, and weight can reduce the risk of CHD.[6]

Primary and secondary prevention goals are in place for all of the major risk factors. Ideally, primary prevention should begin with promoting healthy lifestyles in children. Primary care should include family-oriented risk factor education, review of family history, and risk factor modification. For clients with diagnosed CHD, the goals of prevention are to (1) reduce the incidence of subsequent coronary events, (2) decrease the need for treatments such as angioplasty and coronary artery bypass graft (CABG) surgery, (3) extend overall survival, and (4) improve quality of life.

People should stop smoking and avoid contact with secondary smoke. Health professionals should provide counseling, nicotine replacement, and referrals to smoking cessation programs for clients who smoke. Blood pressure should be measured at least every 2 years in adults, and clients should be encouraged to control blood pressure by maintaining ideal weight, exercising regularly, moderating alcohol intake, and following a moderately low sodium diet. Blood pressure should be below 140/90 (<130/85 for those with heart failure, diabetes, or renal insufficiency). Antihypertensive therapy should begin if blood pressure exceeds 140/90 after 6 months of lifestyle modification or if the initial blood pressure exceeds 160/100 (130/85 mm Hg for those with heart failure, diabetes, or renal insufficiency).[6, 9]

Total, LDL, and HDL cholesterol should be measured annually for adults older than 20 years of age. Primary prevention goals for cholesterol management are as follows:

- LDL < 160 mg/dl if no or one risk factor
- LDL < 130 mg/dl if two or more risk factors
- HDL > 35 mg/dl
- Triglycerides < 200 mg/dl

Secondary prevention goals for cholesterol management are:

- LDL < 100 mg/dl
- HDL > 35 mg/dl
- Triglycerides < 200 mg/dl

The AHA Step 1 Diet should be recommended for clients not meeting primary prevention goals, and the Step 2 Diet should be recommended for those with CHD who do not meet recommended goals. In addition, drug therapy is recommended for clients who do not meet recommended goals for cholesterol management.[9, 20, 28]

During routine physical examinations, health professionals should determine the client's activity level and participation in exercise. Clients should be encouraged to exercise three to four times weekly for 30 to 60 minutes and to increase their physical activity in daily life. An exercise test may be needed to guide an exercise prescription for clients with confirmed CHD.[6, 9]

Clients should be encouraged to maintain ideal body weight as indicated by a body mass index (BMI) between 21 and 25 kg/m^2 and a waist circumference less than 40 inches in men and 36 inches in women. Height, weight, BMI, and waist-to-hip ratio should be measured at each visit. People with BMIs and waist circumferences higher than those recommended should be counseled regarding weight management and physical activity.[6, 9]

Fasting blood glucose should be maintained near normal levels in clients with diabetes mellitus. Hypoglycemic therapy should be used to achieve normal fasting plasma glucose, as indicated by hemoglobin A_{1c} (HbA_{1c}). Other risk factors should be treated aggressively.[6, 9]

ERT should be considered for all postmenopausal women without diagnosed CHD, particularly if they have multiple risk factors. However, the decision regarding therapy should be made by considering the risks for breast cancer, gallbladder disease, thromboembolic disease, and endometrial cancer.[6, 49] It has been reported that estrogen-progesterone therapy increases cardiovascular events in women with diagnosed CHD during the first year of treatment but decreases events in the fourth and fifth years. Consequently, initiating estrogen and progesterone therapy for women with confirmed CHD is not recommended. For women with CHD who have already been receiving ERT for more than 1 year, continuing therapy is recommended until the results of additional research are known.[34]

Additional management strategies are recommended for clients with diagnosed CHD. These include the use of antiplatelet therapies such as acetylsalicylic acid (aspirin), heparin, and low-molecular-weight heparin if not contraindicated.[6, 17] Aspirin reduces the risk of fatal or nonfatal MI by 71% during the acute phase, by 60% at 3 months, and by 52% at 2 years.[17] Adjunctive therapies, such as angiotensin-converting enzyme (ACE) inhibitors, beta-blockers, and nitrates, are also recommended.[6, 9, 17]

Glycoprotein IIb/IIIa receptor antagonists are the most recent pharmacologic treatment for secondary prevention of CHD. These drugs prevent platelet aggregation in acute coronary syndromes, and when combined with aspirin, they decrease the incidence of recurrent cardiac events.[17] The therapeutic effects, adverse responses, and nursing implications of pharmacologic agents used in the primary prevention of CHD are outlined in Table 56–2.

RESTORE BLOOD SUPPLY

For some clients, even aggressive management of risk factors fails to prevent coronary occlusion. Various techniques have been developed to open the vessels and restore blood flow through the coronary arteries. Collectively, these procedures—coronary angioplasty, intracoronary stent placement, and laser atherectomy—are called *interventional cardiology*.[12, 15]

Percutaneous Transluminal Coronary Angioplasty

Percutaneous transluminal coronary angioplasty (PTCA) is a technique in which a balloon-tipped catheter is inserted into a leg artery and threaded under x-ray guidance into a blocked coronary artery. The balloon is inflated several times to reshape the lumen by stretching it and flattening the atherosclerotic plaque against the arterial wall, thus opening the artery (Fig. 56–1). In 1996, more than 482,000 PTCA procedures were performed in the United States. The success rate (defined as >20% reduction in stenosis) was reported as 82%. PTCA is less invasive and less expensive than open heart surgery and therefore is an attractive alternative.[7]

Guidelines for selection of clients for PTCA are rap-

TABLE 56–2 PREVENTIVE PHARMACOTHERAPY IN CORONARY HEART DISEASE

	Assessing Therapeutic Responses	Assessing Adverse Responses	Nursing Implications
Antiplatelet-aggregating agents			
Acetylsalicylic acid (ASA)	ASA blocks prostaglandin synthesis action, which prevents formation of the platelet-aggregrating substance thromboxane A_2. The therapeutic response would be the absence or slowed formation of coronary artery disease.	Clients may experience heartburn, stomach pains, nausea and vomiting, rash, weakness, hemolytic anemia, and gastrointestinal (GI) ulceration. Overdose symptoms include tinnitus, headache, dizziness, confusion, and metabolic acidosis.	▪ Avoid use in clients with severe liver or renal disease. ▪ Monitor serum concentrations, renal function, hearing changes, skin inflammation, and abnormal bleeding. ▪ Administer with food or large quantities of water to decrease GI upset. ▪ Instruct clients to avoid concurrent use of over-the-counter products that contain ASA.
Antilipemic agents			
Simvastatin	It inhibits an enzyme, 3-hydroxy-3-methylglutaryl coenzyme A reductase, which is responsible for catalyzing an early step in the synthesis of cholesterol. Total cholesterol and low-density lipoprotein levels will decline.	Clients may experience headache, dizziness, abdominal cramps, constipation, diarrhea, flatus, heartburn, and rashes.	▪ Monitor plasma triglycerides, cholesterol, and liver function tests. ▪ Instruct clients to report any unexplained muscle pain or weakness. ▪ Administer with food. ▪ Advise clients that medication should be used along with diet restrictions.

Data from Armstrong, L. L. (Ed.). *The University of Chicago formulary of accepted drugs.* Hudson, OH: Lexi-Comp, Inc., 1998.

idly changing. Clients with no or mild manifestations to clients with unstable angina may be suitable candidates. PTCA may also be successful in single-vessel or multiple-vessel disease. However, balloon angioplasty is most successful in men who are younger than age 70 and have normal pumping ability; no more than two blocked arteries; and no history of diabetes, MI, or coronary artery bypass surgery.[12] One study indicated that clients with "type A" behavior, specifically hostility, carry an increased risk of restenosis after PTCA.[19] In addition to PTCA, new therapeutic devices for coronary application continue to evolve as alternatives to bypass surgery.

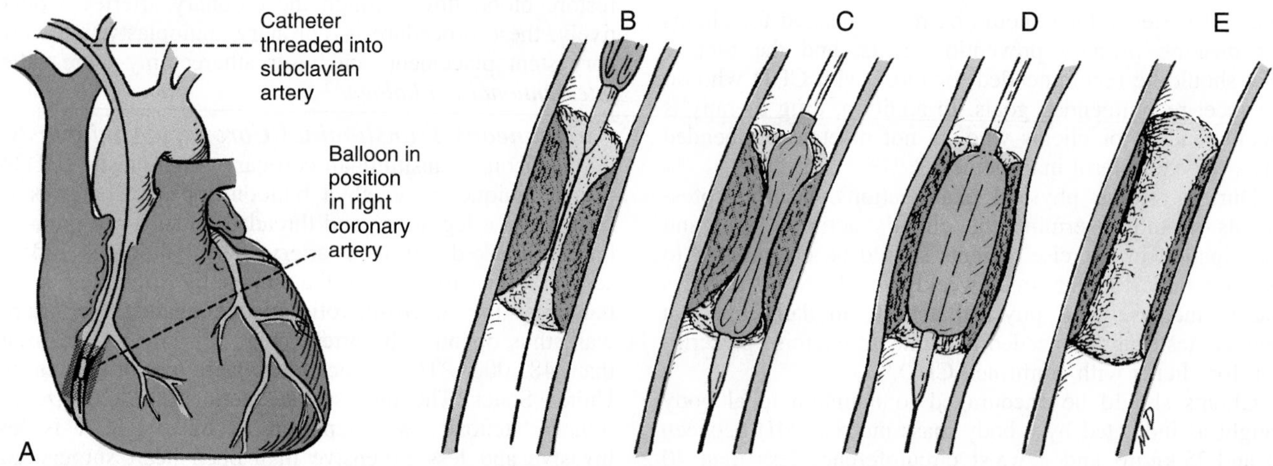

FIGURE 56–1 Percutaneous transluminal coronary angioplasty (PTCA). *A,* A balloon-tipped catheter positioned in a blocked artery. *B,* The balloon is centered. *C,* The balloon expands to compress the blockage (*D*). *E,* The artery is restored to its original diameter.

Directional Coronary Atherectomy

Atherectomy was designed to overcome two of the most significant complications of PTCA: restenosis and abrupt closure of the coronary artery.[15, 42] Restenosis occurs in 25% to 50% of clients within 2 to 6 months after PTCA, whereas abrupt closure resulting from plaque fracture, coronary artery dissection, localized thrombus, or coronary artery spasm occurs in 2% to 6% of clients after PTCA. Directional coronary atherectomy (DCA) reduces coronary stenosis by excising and removing atheromatous plaque. The DCA cutter consists of a catheter that contains a rigid cylindrical housing with a central rotating blade (Fig. 56–2). The blade shaves off the atherosclerotic material and deposits it in the nose cone of the housing for later histopathologic study. Because the spinning of the cutter can cause vibrations that irritate the vessel wall and cause coronary vasospasm, calcium-channel blockers are usually given before the procedure.[15]

DCA is very appropriate for lesions in medium to large coronary arteries located in the proximal or middle portions of the vessel. It is not recommended for use with tortuous vessels, distal lesions, or heavily calcified lesions. The large size of the catheter (10 or 11F) limits the usefulness of DCA in treating women. The use of DCA has decreased because of the increasing use of stents and reports that the results are not comparable to those of PTCA.[12] Complications of DCA include embolus formation, acute vessel occlusion, vessel perforation, and arterial spasm. After DCA, clients are given enteric-coated aspirin to prevent thrombosis.

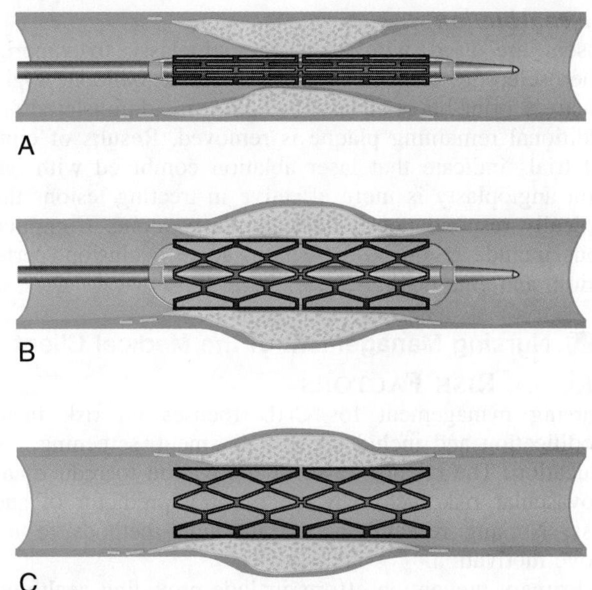

FIGURE 56–3 Placement of a coronary artery stent. *A,* The stent is positioned at the site of the lesion. *B,* The balloon is inflated, expanding the stent. The balloon is then deflated and removed. *C,* The implanted stent is left in place.

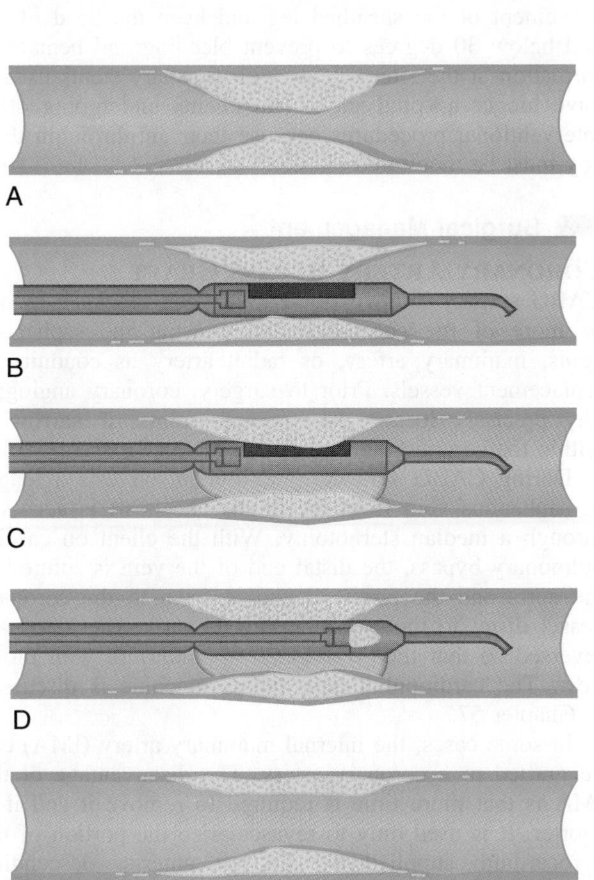

FIGURE 56–2 Atherectomy. *A,* Lesion. *B,* The catheter is advanced through the artery so that the cutting device is positioned over the lesion. *C,* The balloon on the device is inflated to stabilize the catheter. *D,* The cutting portion of the catheter is advanced, slicing away the lesion and trapping it in the cylindrical housing. The balloon is then deflated, and the catheter is removed. *E,* Result of the procedure.

Intracoronary Stents

Intracoronary stents were originally designed to reduce restenosis and abrupt closure of coronary vessels resulting from complications of coronary angioplasty. They are now used instead of PTCA to eliminate the risk of acute closure and to improve long-term patency.[15] There are several different stent designs, but most are balloon-expandable or self-expandable tubes that, when placed in a coronary artery, act as a mechanical scaffold to reopen the blocked artery (Fig. 56–3). Coronary stents are made of numerous materials, ranging from stainless steel to bioabsorbable compounds.

The procedure for placing a stent is similar to that for PTCA. Once the coronary lesion is identified by angiography, the balloon catheter bearing the stent is inserted into the coronary artery and the stent is positioned at the site of the occlusion. A major concern related to stent placement is the prevention of acute thrombosis, especially during the first several weeks after the procedure. During the initial recovery period, clients receive an antiplatelet, such as ticlopidine, and an anticoagulant. To prevent thrombosis, clients must take antiplatelet inhibitors over the long term. If anticoagulation is continued after discharge, clients are usually given warfarin for 6 weeks after the procedure. Long-term anticoagulation therapy is required only when optimal stent expansion is not achieved or when the resulting lumen diameter is less than 3 mm.[15] Complications include stent occlusion, bleeding secondary to anticoagulation, and coronary artery dissection.[12, 15]

Laser Ablation

Lasers are used with balloon angioplasty to vaporize atherosclerotic plaque. After the initial balloon angioplasty, a brief burst of laser radiation is administered and additional remaining plaque is removed. Results of clinical trials indicate that laser ablation combined with balloon angioplasty is more effective in treating lesions that typically respond poorly to angioplasty alone. Complications include coronary dissection, acute occlusion, perforation, and embolism.[12, 15]

Nursing Management of the Medical Client

Reduce Risk Factors

Nursing management for CHD focuses on risk factor modification and includes risk assessment, screening, and education. The client's level of motivation to reduce cardiovascular risk factors is the primary predictor of success. Nursing researchers are studying methods to improve motivation.

Primary prevention efforts include providing health education on reducing risk factors for CHD. Encourage clients to reduce their risk by lowering dietary intake of fats and cholesterol, exercising, controlling diabetes and hypertension, keeping body weight near ideal levels, and ceasing smoking. The risk and incidence of CHD are so high that many clients are doing these activities on an ongoing basis. Reinforce these behaviors. Participate in risk factor screening for children and adults, and maintain a high index of suspicion for clients at increased risk for CHD. Teach stress reduction techniques, such as progressive muscle relaxation and guided imagery. Instruct postmenopausal women to discuss the need for estrogen replacement therapy (ERT) with their physician. Monitor blood pressure control in clients with diagnosed hypertension, and monitor HbA_{1c} levels in diabetic clients.

Nursing interventions for clients with diagnosed CHD include assessing their CHD risk and explaining diagnostic tests, when to seek treatment, clinical manifestations of complications, and the actions, dosages, and side effects of prescribed medications. Assess cardiovascular risk factors, and provide individualized education on risk reduction. Emphasize the importance of adopting risk-reduction behaviors and participating in cardiac rehabilitation to prevent recurrence or progression of CHD. Teach clients the clinical manifestations of angina and MI. Monitor therapeutic drug levels as appropriate. Emphasize the importance of keeping follow-up appointments with health care practitioners. Most important, instruct clients to seek prompt medical attention if symptoms of CHD return.

Many clients use forms of alternative therapies for self-treatment of heart disease. See the Alternative Therapy feature.

Restore Blood Supply

Before interventional procedures, the client is usually given an antiplatelet medication, such as aspirin. The client is also given an anticoagulant (heparin) to prevent occlusion and calcium-channel blockers or nitrates to reduce coronary spasm during the procedure. After the procedure, the client may continue with this drug regimen to prevent reocclusion or arterial spasms.[15, 24]

The client's blood is also typed and crossmatched in the event that emergency CABG surgery is needed. A consent form is signed for the interventional procedure and surgery, if required, for spasm, perforation of the artery, or acute occlusion. Following interventional procedures, monitor the client for changes in vital signs, especially the quality and rhythm of pulse, and in the ECG. Report any indication of coronary ischemia to the physician. ST-segment monitoring is frequently used to detect ischemia. If the client complains of chest pain, obtain a 12-lead ECG immediately. Force fluids, orally or intravenously, to assist the body in excreting contrast, which causes diuresis and may cause acute tubular necrosis. Monitor the puncture site for hematoma, and palpate pulses to assess peripheral perfusion. Complications include bleeding and hematoma formation at the puncture site, acute MI resulting from perforation of an artery, refractory spasm, or occlusion. The physician may order bed rest for longer periods for clients undergoing stent placement and DCA because of the larger sheaths used to dilate the vessels in these procedures.

Nursing considerations specific to the care of the client with a coronary stent include close monitoring of anticoagulation status and ongoing assessment for bleeding. Until the sheath is removed, instruct the client to limit movement of the sheathed leg and keep the head of the bed below 30 degrees to prevent bleeding and hematoma formation at the site. Clients with coronary stents usually have longer hospital stays than clients undergoing other interventional procedures because their antithrombin therapy must be monitored closely.[47, 48]

Surgical Management

Coronary Artery Bypass Graft

CABG surgery involves the bypass of a blockage in one or more of the coronary arteries using the saphenous veins, mammary artery, or radial artery as conduits or replacement vessels. Prior to surgery, coronary angiography precisely locates lesions and points of narrowing within the coronary arteries.

During CABG surgery, the surgeon harvests a length of saphenous vein from the thigh. The heart is accessed through a median sternotomy. With the client on cardiopulmonary bypass, the distal end of the vein is sutured to the aorta and the proximal end is sewn to the coronary vessel distal to the blockage (Fig. 56–4). The veins are reversed so that their valves do not interfere with blood flow. The cardiopulmonary bypass machine is discussed in Chapter 57.

In some cases, the internal mammary artery (IMA) can be grafted to a coronary artery. The disadvantage of the IMA is that more time is required to remove it and it is shorter. It is used only to revascularize the portion of the myocardium supplied by the left anterior descending (LAD) artery. An advantage is that IMA grafts have a greater chance of remaining patent. Radial arteries have been used as an alternative to saphenous vein conduits and show excellent short-term and long-term patency rates.[52]

A new approach to CABG surgery, called minimally invasive direct CABG (MIDCABG) surgery, is being per-

ALTERNATIVE THERAPY

Cardiac Disorders

Cardiovascular disease has been shown to be largely related to lifestyle habits such as exercise, diet, and smoking. Unfortunately, although many people are aware of the importance of these factors, they are often ignored. New research continues to elucidate the effects of often simple lifestyle changes that can help prevent cardiac problems. An examination of fiber intake and coronary heart disease (CHD) among women in the Nurses' Health Study, a very large cohort study of female nurses followed for 10 years, found that high fiber intake from cereal sources reduced the risk of CHD.[11] Another study, looking again at the Nurses' Health Study as well as men in the Health Professionals' Follow-up Study, found a protective benefit from consumption of fruit and vegetables, particularly green leafy and cruciferous vegetables and citrus fruit and juice, for ischemic stroke.[3] The former study examined a cohort of nearly 70,000; the latter examined 113,000 people.

An intensive program of lifestyle changes pioneered by Dean Ornish has been shown to lead to regression of coronary atherosclerosis.[8] The lifestyle changes included a vegetarian diet limited to 10% fat intake, aerobic exercise, stress management, smoking cessation, and group psychosocial activity. Although some have debated the results achieved and whether other lifestyle modifications might be as successful, there is little doubt that lifestyle changes can be not only preventive but also therapeutic in managing clients with heart disease.[2, 4, 7]

CoEnzyme Q10 (CoQ10), or ubiquinone, is synthesized in all human cells and is also present in many foods. First isolated in 1957, CoQ10 was later produced in large quantities, and many studies demonstrated its therapeutic benefits in the treatment of heart problems.[9] CoQ10 has been helpful in treating angina, heart failure, and dysrhythmias and in preventing problems following heart surgery. It is thought that a deficiency of CoQ10 may be a factor in the development of heart disease in certain people. Certain medications may lower CoQ10 levels. Many cardiologists are now aware of the research on CoQ10, and laboratory tests are available to monitor its levels. CoQ10 has the potential to be an important adjunct in the treatment of a number of heart problems.

The nutrients magnesium, thiamine (vitamin B_1), and carnitine have all been found to have potentially positive effects in the management of heart failure. Interestingly, drugs such as diuretics, commonly used in treating heart failure, may lead to depletion of nutrients such as magnesium and thiamine. Many older adults, especially those on poorer diets, may have thiamine and other nutritional deficiencies that could have an impact on cardiovascular health.[5]

The leaves, berries, and flowering tops of the herb hawthorn *(Crataegus monogyna)* have been traditionally used for heart problems. Although hawthorn may improve cardiac output, decrease angina, and lower cholesterol,[6] the German Commission E has only approved the leaf with flowers for treatment of decreased cardiac output in patients with stage II of the New York Heart Association's classification for 1994.[1] Tyler[10] comments that although hawthorn is "devoid of side effects," it may be difficult to obtain adequate quality preparations of it, and he questions the wisdom of self-treatment for problems as serious as cardiac ones.

References

1. Blumenthal, M. (Ed.). (1998). *The complete German Commission E monographs: Therapeutic guide to herbal medicines.* Austin, TX: American Botanical Council.
2. Herbert, P. N. (1999). Effect of lifestyle changes on coronary heart disease. [Letter]. *Journal of the American Medical Association, 282,* 130.
3. Joshipura, K. J., et al. (1999). Fruit and vegetable intake in relation to risk of ischemic stroke. *Journal of the American Medical Association, 282,* 1233–1239.
4. Lear, S. A. (1999). Effect of lifestyle changes on coronary heart disease. [Letter]. *Journal of the American Medical Association, 282,* 131.
5. Murray, M. T. (1997). Natural support for congestive heart failure. *American Journal of Natural Medicine, 4*(5), 14–17.
6. Murray, M. T. (1999). Important considerations in angina. *Natural Medicine Journal, 2*(2), 1–8.
7. Miller, M. (1999). Effect of lifestyle changes on coronary heart disease. [Letter]. *Journal of the American Medical Association, 282,* 130.
8. Ornish, D. et al. (1998). Intensive lifestyle changes for reversal of coronary heart disease. *Journal of the American Medical Association, 280,* 2001–2007.
9. Sinatra, S. T. (1999). CoEnzyme Q10: A cardiologist's commentary. *Natural Medicine Journal 2*(2), 9–15.
10. Tyler, V. E. (1994). *Herbs of choice.* Binghamton, NY: Pharmaceutical Products Press.
11. Wolk, A., et al. (1998). Long-term intake of dietary fiber and decreased risk of coronary heart disease among women. *Journal of the American Medical Association, 281,* 1998–2000.

James Higgy Lerner, RN, LAc, *Private practice of acupuncture, traditional Oriental medicine, and biofeedback*

formed in many institutions. MIDCABG surgery is a less invasive approach for clients who need revascularization of the anterior coronary arteries. The internal mammary arteries are used as conduits, and the client does not have to be placed on cardiopulmonary bypass. MIDCABG surgery is less costly than traditional CABG surgery and is associated with fewer postoperative complications.[32]

Surgical methods only ease the manifestations. Surgery cannot halt the process of atherosclerosis, although it may prolong life in some cases. The surgical management of CHD in women is being studied. Data from several studies have reported that, compared with men, women have higher operative mortality rates, lower rates of graft patency, less frequent use of arterial conduits for grafting, more frequent reoperations, increased incidence of perioperative infarction and heart failure, and less long-term symptomatic relief.[49] However, a report from the Bypass Angioplasty Revascularization Investigation found better outcomes for women than men in nonemergent situations.[27] Scientists are continuing to conduct research in this area.

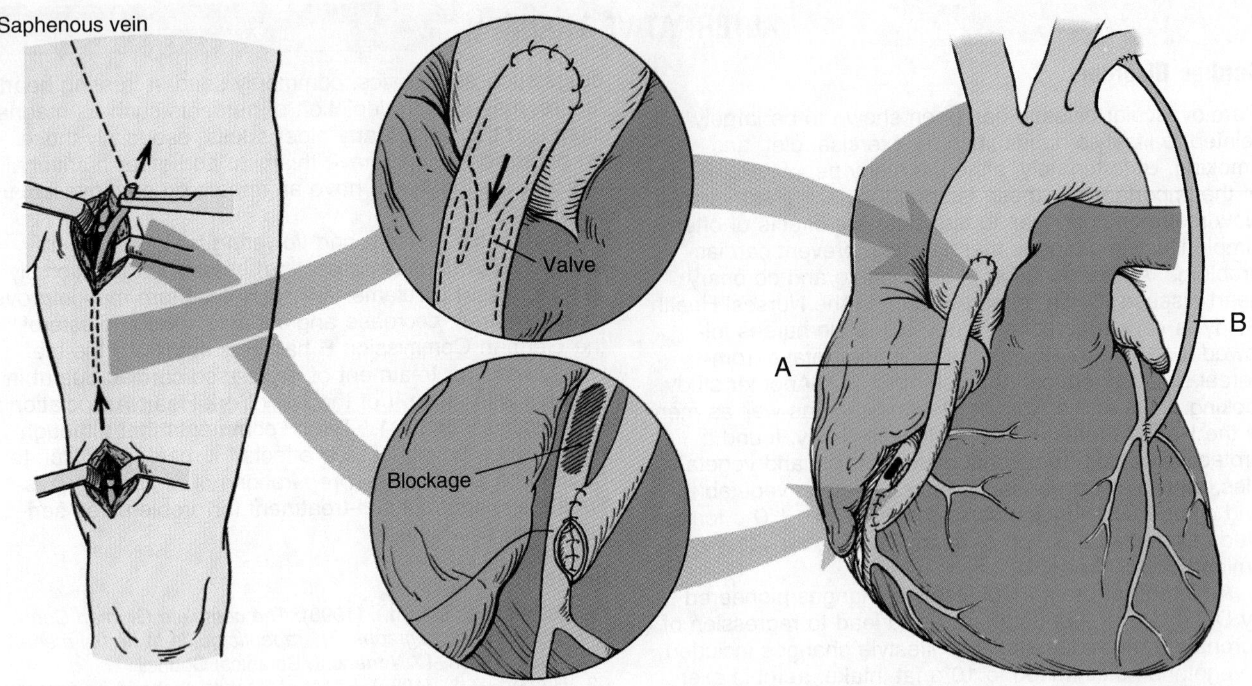

FIGURE 56–4 Coronary artery bypass grafting (CABG). *A,* A section of saphenous vein is harvested from the leg and anastomosed (upside down, because of its directional valves) to a coronary artery to bypass an area of occlusion on the right coronary artery. *B,* Bypass of the left coronary artery with mammary artery.

Possible complications of CABG surgery include:

- Postoperative bleeding
- Wound infection and dehiscence
- Intraoperative stroke
- MI
- Blood clots
- Multiple organ system failure
- Death

The development of calcium-channel blockers and nonsurgical interventions such as PTCA, atherectomy, and stents have reduced the number of CABG surgical procedures being performed. Survival rates in CABG have not been significantly better than survival rates of medically treated clients. CABG nevertheless remains a common procedure, and because it can reduce angina in 80% to 90% of clients who do not respond to medical management, it will continue as an important intervention in the management of CHD. Benefits from CABG surgery also include prolongation of life, increased exercise tolerance, reduced need for medication, and ability to resume former activities.

Transmyocardial Revascularization

A new procedure that is still experimental shows promise for clients with widespread atherosclerosis involving vessels that are too small and numerous for replacement or balloon catheterization. In transmyocardial revascularization (TMR), a high-powered laser is used to open up channels in the heart through a relatively small chest incision by punching holes in a fraction of a second in the beating heart. The laser beam is applied between heartbeats when the ventricle is filled with blood. The laser creates from 15 to 40 1-mm channels through the myocardium into the distal two thirds of the left ventricle.

The exact mechanism by which TMR works has not been established. However, scientists believe that the "controlled trauma" caused by creating the channels promotes vascular growth or angiogenesis. TMR should be used only for the most severely debilitated clients who are not helped by PTCA or CABG surgery. The procedure is estimated to cost $15,000, slightly more than angioplasty but much less than CABG. Sustained improvement has been seen up to 27 months after the operation.[4, 11]

Modifications for Elderly Clients

More than half of all CABG procedures are performed on people older than 65 years of age, and 71% of them on men.[7] Older clients have a postoperative recovery similar to that for younger clients, but the pace is slower and they typically remain hospitalized an average of 2 to 4 days longer. They also have a higher mortality rate.

Postoperative complications that are more prevalent in older clients include dysrhythmias related to aged sinoatrial node cells, drug toxicity associated with impaired hepatic and renal perfusion, multiple drug interactions, and decreased physical stamina. These complications contribute to a 15-day mean length of hospital stay for clients older than age 80.

During the first and second weeks after discharge, depression, fatigue, incisional chest discomfort, dyspnea, and anorexia are common. By the fourth to fifth weeks, elderly clients report improved mood, comfort, and appetite. At 1 year, almost all (93%) are pleased with the outcome and improved quality of life.

Nursing Management of the Surgical Client

Many hospitals have initiated rapid recovery programs for cardiac surgery clients that reduce the hospital stay to 4 days. With rapid recovery programs, most of the client's recovery takes place in the home, with the client and family assuming primary responsibility for many aspects of care. Discharge planning begins at the time of admission, activity progression in the postoperative period is accelerated, and client and family education continues on a daily basis throughout hospitalization. Many hospitals have developed clinical pathways for CABG. Use the clinical pathway for your client to assist you in planning your clients' care (see Guide to Clinical Pathway: Coronary Bypass Grafting, p. 1529). In addition, a three-phase program of activity is implemented (see discussion that follows).

Phase I (In-Hospital) Rehabilitation Programs

Most CABG clients participate in cardiac rehabilitation following surgery. Phase I begins immediately after the client returns from surgery. The goals of phase I inpatient rehabilitation are as follows:

- To prevent the negative effects of prolonged bed rest
- To assess the client's physiologic response to exercise
- To manage the psychosocial issues related to recovery from CABG surgery
- To educate the client and family concerning recovery and the adoption of risk reduction behaviors

While in the intensive care unit, the client is turned every 2 hours during the first several hours after surgery. Once extubated, the client gets up in a chair and ambulates in the room. After transfer to the intermediate care unit, the client continues to walk three or four times a day, increasing the distance walked each time.

Assess the client's blood pressure, heart rate, ECG, and oxygen saturation before, during, and after activity. Systolic blood pressure should not increase more than 20 mm Hg or decrease more than 10 to 15 mm Hg after exercise. Heart rate should not increase more than 20 beats per minute (BPM) above resting, and no significant dysrhythmias should occur. Activity levels will be reduced if clients have adverse physiologic responses (e.g., tachycardia, dysrhythmias, pain) to exercise. Clients are seated for all meals. Research has demonstrated that early mobilization improves cardiac function and benefits the client psychologically.[5]

Education for a healthier lifestyle is an important part of each phase of cardiac rehabilitation. The emphasis in phase I is on the identification and modification of reversible risk factors to prevent further deleterious cardiac events.

Self-Care

Before hospital discharge, instruct the client and family (or significant other) about medication actions and side effects, dietary restrictions, physical activity restrictions and progression, and wound care. Because it is not always possible to anticipate all of the problems clients may encounter the first few days at home, instruct the client whom to call when there is an emergency or when there are questions or concerns. If possible, introduce the client to the home health nurse who will be supervising home care. Following discharge, the home health care nurse provides additional education and counseling and assesses the client for complications.[32, 47, 53] In addition, instruct the client on how to assess response to exercise and activity.[40, 41]

Before discharge, a low-level symptom-limited exercise test may be performed to evaluate the client's ability to perform activities of daily living (ADL) and exercise. The test results are used to prescribe a safe and effective exercise program for the first few weeks at home and serve as a basis for the initial exercise prescription in phase II.[5]

Phase II (Outpatient Exercise Training) Rehabilitation Programs

Outpatient (phase II) exercise training usually takes place in a facility that provides continuous ECG monitoring, emergency equipment, and medically supervised exercise. Outpatient treatment usually begins 10 to 14 days after discharge and requires physician referral. The goals of phase II are as follows:

- To restore clients to a desirable exercise capacity appropriate to their health status, lifestyle, and occupation
- To provide additional education and support to the client and family for adoption of risk-reduction behaviors
- To meet the psychosocial needs of clients and families, restore confidence, and minimize anxiety and depression
- To promote early identification of medical problems through close observation and monitoring of clients during exercise
- To assist clients in returning to occupational and leisure activities

Exercise therapy is conducted three times weekly for 2 to 3 months. The duration of the aerobic exercise session ranges from 20 to 40 minutes at an intensity of 70% to 85% of the baseline exercise heart rate. During each exercise session, blood pressure, heart rate, respiratory rate, and ECG are monitored before, during, and after exercise. Activity levels are increased gradually, based on the client's response. A nutritionist may counsel clients about proper diet, and a psychologist or social worker may counsel clients on stress management and adoption of other risk prevention behaviors.

At the end of the program, clients are given a symptom-limited exercise test and are reevaluated. Decisions regarding progression to a phase III or home program are based on the client's results of the stress test, ability to self-monitor his or her response to exercise, the client's stability, and psychological or emotional status. Periodic evaluations are scheduled so that activity progression and cardiopulmonary function can be assessed.[5, 50]

Phase III (Community) Rehabilitation Programs

Phase III programs are conducted in community settings, such as a "Y" or a health club. The goals of phase III are as follows:

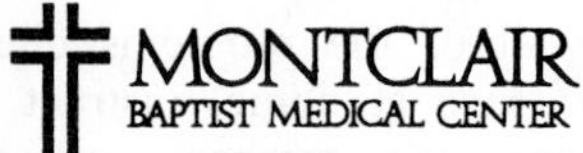

MONTCLAIR BAPTIST MEDICAL CENTER

CABG/VALVE CAREMAP

(Addressograph)

PRE-OP	Date:	INITIAL Met	INITIAL Not Met
General Safety:	Fall Precautions Bed Rails Up x 2 Bed in Preventive Mode		
Activity	As ordered.		
	Goal:		
Dietary: Consult Date/Time Completed ______	NPO after midnight		
	Goal: %		
Respiratory: Consult Date/Time Completed ______	Spirometry teaching per respiratory therapy/nurse.		
	Goal: SaO_2 > 90%. **Goal:** Performs correct Incentive Spirometry technique **Goal:** Clear, patent airway		
Rehab: Consult Date/Time Completed ______	**Goal:**		
Discharge Planning: Consult Date/Time Completed ______	Assess support system for post-hospital stay and notify social services if not adequate.		
	Goal: Adequate support system.		
Nursing: Consult Date/Time Completed ______	Vital signs as ordered. B/P in both arms, height, actual weight, and SaO2 recorded on front of chart. Pre-op teaching by floor nurse and/or CCU nurse. Give patient/caregiver cardiac packet for "Open Heart Surgery Patient". Patient/Caregiver to review "Open Heart Surgery" video on patient education channel. Telemetry. Call MD if SaO2 < 90%. Do not continue Coumadin, Ticlid, Persantine, Plavix, or ______. Notify cardiologist, attending M.D., surgeon and surgeon's/physician's assistant of admission/surgery as appropriate. Request and obtain old records immediately and send old chart to surgery with patient. Antimicrobial scrub for a total of two (1 HS and 1 AM). Shave with electric surgical razor. Obtain appropriate Operative and Blood permits. Encourage patient/cargiver to verbalize and ask questions. Consult Pastoral Care. If emergency, beep on-call chaplain.		
	Goal: Patient/Caregiver verbalizes understanding of pre-op teaching. **Goal:** No symptomatic dysrhythmias.		
Tests:	Labwork (If labwork done within 14 days, call lab to obtain results and do not repeat). CBC, S7, PT (only obtain PT if patient on Coumadin). EKG (if done within 3 months, call for report). CXR (If age > 70 or re-operation and not done within 6 months). Type and screen 2 units packed red cells. If patient is re-operation or HCT < 35, type and crossmatch 2 units of packed red cells.		
	Goal: Blood work WNL.		

G-99-5179-2PG REV. 11/15/99

- To maintain and, if possible, increase exercise capacity
- To institute long-term follow-up of risk-reduction behavior change
- To encourage clients to take responsibility for continuing lifestyle changes

Exercise consists of walking, jogging, weight training, and recreational games. Clients are usually not monitored while exercising, although some facilities obtain exercise ECGs on a monthly basis. Clients are responsible for monitoring their own heart rate response to exercise, although blood pressure can be taken by program personnel if indicated.[5, 50]

HOME EXERCISE REHABILITATION PROGRAMS

For CABG clients, a home exercise program is usually prescribed in conjunction with or in place of the outpatient program. Clients are given detailed exercise instruc-

GUIDE TO CLINICAL PATHWAY

Coronary Bypass Grafting

Immediately following coronary bypass grafting (CABG) the client is in the intensive care unit (ICU). The focus of care in the ICU includes monitoring and treating hemodynamic instability and assessing respiratory status. Stays in the ICU have become very short, and many clients who were healthy before surgery are treated on "fast-track" programs to decrease their length of stay. This full care map projects a 5-day stay, with 1 day in the ICU.

Because postoperative fluid shifts increase pulmonary fluid accumulation and chest incisions create pain with deep breathing, the risk of pneumonia is great. The care map includes many interventions to promote lung aeration. Respiratory therapists assist with monitoring and care, including the use of percussion to loosen thick secretions. Use pillows to splint the incision. Ambulation is an important aspect of recovery; be certain that the client ambulates three times the second day after surgery. Administer medications as ordered for pain prior to ambulation, and monitor the client closely for dysrhythmias and desaturation during ambulation.

Many intravenous lines and tubes are discontinued on day 2. Before pulling the lines or tubes, be sure that the parameters needed (such as minimal chest tube output) are within established standards. On day 3, pacer wires are removed. In most facilities, a nurse must be certified to pull pacer wires.

Care of leg incisions varies by surgeon. Most clients report more pain in the leg than in the chest. Be prepared to explain that this is common and does not mean anything is wrong.

Discharge teaching begins on day 2. This information is an important component of full recovery. Many clients and their spouses are fearful of "doing something wrong" on discharge, and clients have been allowed to become dependent rather than independent. Work with the client and educate the family on the advantages and importance of activity to promote recovery.

The CareMap is reprinted with permission from Baptist Health System.

The CareMap shown is an excerpt of one that covers the Preoperative phase through phase III.

Helen Andrews, BSN, RN, *Care Manager, Alegent Health Bergan Mercy Medical Center, Omaha, Nebraska,* and **Linda R. Haddick, MSN, RN,** *Clinical Nurse Specialist, Alegent Health Home Care & Hospice, Omaha, Nebraska*

tions and are told to keep a log of heart rates, perceived exertion rates, exercise parameters, and any problems that may occur during the home program. Cardiac rehabilitation staff members or the client's physician should analyze the data and adjust the home exercise program if necessary. Once clients reach their optimal level of functional capacity, they are instructed to continue to exercise at least three times weekly so that cardiopulmonary exercise capacity can be maintained.[50]

HEART FAILURE

Despite aggressive medical and surgical treatment, CHD may eventually lead to the development of heart failure. Heart failure is a significant cardiac functional disorder that can result in reduced oxygen delivery to the body's organs and tissues. Heart failure affects approximately 4.8 million people in the United States, with 465,000 new cases diagnosed each year. In contrast to decreases in mortality rates associated with other cardiovascular diseases, the incidence of heart failure and the mortality associated with it have increased steadily since 1975.[7] Annually, about 250,000 clients die from direct or indirect consequences of heart failure, and the number of deaths that are due to heart failure has increased six-fold over the past 40 years.[7, 35]

Heart failure can affect both women and men, although it occurs more often in men, with a poorer prognosis.[38] There are also racial differences; at all ages, death rates are higher in African Americans than in non-Hispanic whites. Heart failure is primarily a disease of older adults, affecting 6% to 10% of those over 65 years of age. It is also the leading cause of hospitalization in older people.[7]

Heart failure is a physiologic state in which the heart cannot pump enough blood to meet the metabolic needs of the body (determined as oxygen consumption). Heart failure results from changes in systolic or diastolic function of the left ventricle. The heart fails when, because of intrinsic disease or structural defects, it cannot handle a normal blood volume or, in the absence of disease, cannot tolerate a sudden expansion in blood volume (e.g., during exercise). Heart failure is not a disease itself; instead, the term refers to a clinical syndrome characterized by manifestations of volume overload, inadequate tissue perfusion, and poor exercise tolerance. Whatever the cause, pump failure results in hypoperfusion of tissue, followed by pulmonary and systemic venous congestion. Because heart failure causes vascular congestion, it is often called *congestive heart failure,* although most cardiac specialists no longer use this term. Other terms used to denote heart failure include *cardiac decompensation, cardiac insufficiency,* and *ventricular failure.*[30]

Etiology and Risk Factors

The performance of the heart depends on four essential components:

- Contractility (inotropic state) of the muscle
- Preload (amount of blood in the ventricle at the end of diastole)
- Afterload (the pressure against which the left ventricle ejects)
- Heart rate

Table 56–3 defines the terms commonly used to describe cardiac function. Adverse changes in these determinants of myocardial performance ultimately cause the heart to fail. CHD is the primary cause of heart failure in two thirds of clients with decreased ventricular dysfunction.

TABLE 56–3 TERMS USED TO DESCRIBE CARDIAC FUNCTION

Term	Function
Afterload	Force that the ventricle must develop during systole in order to eject the stroke volume
Cardiac output	Stroke volume × heart rate
Inotropic state	A measure of contractility
Preload	Stretch of myocardial fibers at end-diastole
Stroke volume	The amount of blood ejected from the ventricle with each contraction

However, heart failure may also be caused by other disorders. The causes of heart failure can be divided into three subgroups[38]:

- Abnormal loading conditions
- Abnormal muscle function
- Conditions or diseases that limit ventricular filling

Abnormal Loading Conditions

Abnormal loading is associated with any condition that increases either the pressure or the volume load of the ventricle. The effect of increasing volume on the ventricle can be explained by the analogy that the heart muscle is like a stretched rubber band. When the rubber band is stretched, it contracts with more force. The heart muscle does the same. Venous return stretches the heart and improves contractility. When the rubber band is overstretched, it becomes limp and cannot contract. Likewise, when the heart is overloaded with blood, excessive stretch and decreased contraction occur. Overload develops because blood does not leave the ventricles during contraction. Therefore, cardiac workload increases in an effort to move blood.

Preload refers to the stretch of the ventricular myocardial fibers just before ventricular contraction. The load or stretch placed on the ventricular fibers corresponds to the end-diastolic ventricular volume and pressure. Preload is determined by the condition of the heart valves (especially the mitral valve), blood volume, ventricular wall compliance, and venous tone.

Table 56–4 lists conditions that increase preload. Increased preload usually increases contractility (more stretch on the rubber band) and stretch because of filling pressures from venous return and previous volume. Stretch and filling pressures may rise beyond the capabilities of the normally compliant heart. This increased preload lessens the force and efficiency of ventricular contraction. Cardiac output decreases. Under the strain of this load, the heart will fail.

Increased pressure load in the ventricle is related to *afterload,* the amount of tension the heart must generate to overcome systemic pressure and to allow adequate ventricular emptying. Thus, afterload indicates how hard the heart must pump to force blood into circulation. The tone of systemic arterioles, the elasticity of the aorta and large arteries, the size and thickness of the ventricle, the presence of aortic stenosis, and the viscosity of the blood all determine afterload. High peripheral vascular resistance and high blood pressure force the ventricle to work harder to eject blood (see Table 56–4). Subjected to prolonged high pressures, the ventricle eventually fails.[90]

Abnormal Muscle Function

Certain conditions interfere directly with myocardial contractility and affect the inherent contractility of cardiac muscle:

- MI
- Myocarditis, an inflammation of the myocardium associated with viral, bacterial, fungal, or parasitic diseases or toxic chemical injury
- Cardiomyopathy
- Ventricular aneurysm

Such disorders impair the contractile function of the myocardial fibrils, which reduces ventricular emptying and stroke volume.[38]

After an MI, some of the heart muscle is replaced by noncontracting scar tissue and the ventricles pump less efficiently. Some degree of heart failure, either chronic or transient, appears in more than half of clients after MI. Other conditions that affect the intrinsic condition of the heart muscle are listed in Table 56–4.

TABLE 56–4 ETIOLOGY OF HEART FAILURE

Abnormal Loading Conditions	Abnormal Muscle Function	Limited Ventricular Filling
Conditions that increase preload		
Regurgitation of mitral or tricuspid valve	Myocardial infarction	Mitral or tricuspid stenosis
Hypervolemia	Myocarditis	Cardiac tamponade
Congenital defects (left-to-right shunts)	Cardiomyopathy	Constrictive pericarditis
Ventricular septal defect	Ventricular aneurysm	Hypertrophic obstructive cardiomyopathy
Atrial septal defect	Long-term alcohol consumption	
Patent ductus arteriosus	Coronary heart disease	
	Metabolic heart disease	
	Endocrine heart disease	
Conditions that increase afterload		
Hypertension, pulmonary or systemic		
Aortic or pulmonic stenosis		
High peripheral vascular resistance		

LIMITED VENTRICULAR FILLING. Certain conditions externally compress the heart, thereby limiting ventricular filling and myocardial contractility. Disorders that greatly restrict cardiac chamber filling and myocardial fiber stretch include *constrictive pericarditis,* an inflammatory and fibrotic process of the pericardial sac; and *cardiac tamponade,* which involves the accumulation of fluid or blood within the pericardial sac. Because the pericardium encloses all four heart chambers, compression of the heart both decreases diastolic relaxation, thereby elevating diastolic pressure, and hampers forward blood flow through the heart.[38] Other conditions that limit ventricular filling are listed in Table 56–4.

Some clients have pre-existing mild to moderate heart disease with no evidence of heart failure. In these clients, adequate cardiac output depends on functional compensatory mechanisms. When the heart undergoes undue stress, these compensatory mechanisms may prove inadequate and the heart fails. Careful assessment helps identify precipitating causes of the great increase in cardiac workload. Recognition of these factors allows prompt treatment and long-term prevention.[30] Precipitating factors are described next.

CONDITIONS THAT PRECIPITATE HEART FAILURE

Heart failure can be precipitated by conditions that increase cardiac and systemic oxygen demand, reduce the ability of the heart to contract, or increase the workload of the heart. Conditions that increase demand for oxygen delivery include physical or emotional stress, dysrhythmias (most notably tachycardia), infections, anemia, thyroid disorders, pregnancy, and Paget's disease. Thiamine deficiency can precipitate heart failure because it reduces myocardial contractility, causing tachycardia and ventricular dilation. Chronic pulmonary disease and volume overload can precipitate heart failure because they increase the workload of the heart.

Pathophysiology

The healthy heart can meet the demands for oxygen delivery through the use of cardiac reserve. Cardiac reserve is the heart's ability to increase output in response to stress. The normal heart can increase its output up to five times the resting level. The failing heart, even at rest, however, is pumping near its capacity and thus has lost much of its reserve. The compromised heart has a limited ability to respond to the body's needs for increased output in situations of stress.

When cardiac output is not sufficient to meet the metabolic needs of the body, compensatory mechanisms, including neurohormonal responses, become activated. These mechanisms initially help improve contraction and maintain integrity of the circulation but, if continued, lead to abnormal cardiac growth and reconfiguration (remodeling) of the heart. The compensatory responses to a decrease in cardiac output are ventricular dilation, increased sympathetic nervous system stimulation, and activation of the renin-angiotensin system.

VENTRICULAR DILATION

Ventricular dilation refers to lengthening of the muscle fibers that increases the volume in the heart chambers. Dilation causes an increase in preload and thus cardiac output, because a stretched muscle contracts more forcefully (Starling's law). However, dilation has limits as a compensatory mechanism. Muscle fibers, if stretched beyond a certain point, become ineffective. Second, a dilated heart requires more oxygen. Thus, the dilated heart with a normal coronary blood flow can suffer from a lack of oxygen. Hypoxia of the heart further decreases the muscle's ability to contract.[35]

INCREASED SYMPATHETIC NERVOUS SYSTEM STIMULATION

Sympathetic activity produces venous and arteriolar constriction, tachycardia, and increased myocardial contractility, all of which work to increase cardiac output and improve delivery of oxygen and nutrients to tissues. However, this compensatory effect occurs at the cost of increasing peripheral vascular resistance (afterload) and myocardial workload. In addition, sympathetic stimulation reduces renal blood flow and stimulates the renin-angiotensin system.[35, 38]

STIMULATION OF THE RENIN-ANGIOTENSIN SYSTEM

When blood flow through the renal artery is decreased, the baroreceptor reflex is stimulated and renin is released into the bloodstream. Renin interacts with angiotensinogen to produce angiotensin I. When angiotensin I comes into contact with ACE, it is converted to angiotensin II, a potent vasoconstrictor. Angiotensin II increases arterial vasoconstriction, promotes release of norepinephrine from sympathetic nerve endings, and stimulates the adrenal medulla to secrete aldosterone, which enhances sodium and water absorption. Stimulation of the renin-angiotensin system causes plasma volume to expand and preload to increase.

Cardiac compensation exists when the initial compensatory mechanisms of ventricular dilation, sympathetic nervous system stimulation, and renin-angiotensin system stimulation succeed in maintaining an adequate cardiac output and oxygen delivery to the tissues in the presence of pathologic changes. Once cardiac output is restored, the body produces counterregulatory substances that restore cardiovascular homeostasis. If underlying pathologic changes are not corrected, prolonged activation of the compensatory mechanisms eventually leads to changes in the function of the myocardial cell and overexpression of the neurohormones. These processes are responsible for the transition from compensated to decompensated heart failure. At this point, manifestations of heart failure develop because the heart cannot maintain adequate circulation.[3, 35, 38]

When compensatory mechanisms fail, the amount of blood remaining in the left ventricle at the end of diastole increases. This increase in residual blood in turn decreases the ventricle's capacity to receive blood from the left atrium. The left atrium, having to work harder to eject blood, dilates and hypertrophies. It is unable to receive the full amount of incoming blood from the pulmonary veins, and left atrial pressure increases. This leads to pulmonary edema (Fig. 56–5).

The right ventricle, because of the increased pressure in the pulmonary vascular system, must now dilate and hypertrophy in order to meet its increased workload. It

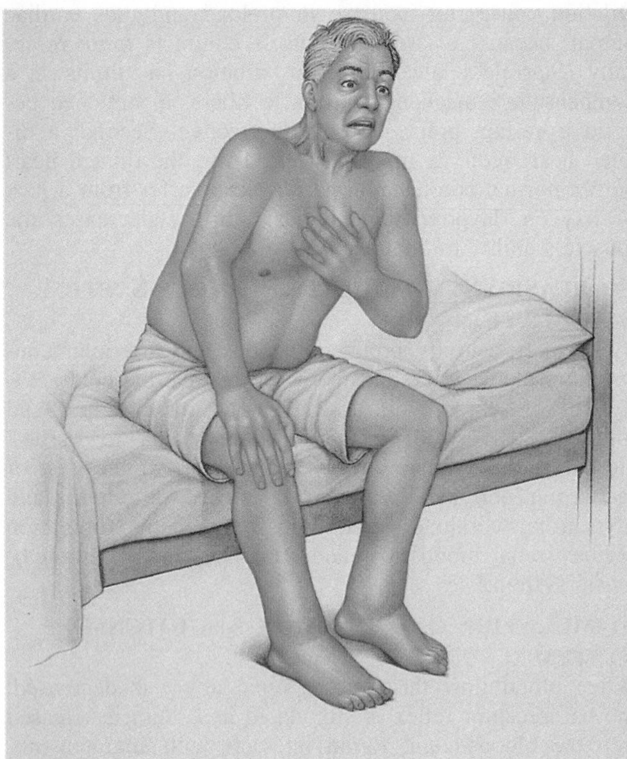

FIGURE 56–5 Appearance of a client with both right-sided and left-sided heart failure. (From *Mayo Clinic Health Letter* (1997), *15*:1–3. Mayo Foundation for Medical Education and Research, Rochester, MN. By permission of Mayo Foundation.)

too eventually fails. Engorgement of the venous system then extends backward to produce congestion in the gastrointestinal tract, liver, viscera, kidneys, legs, and sacrum, with edema as the main manifestation. Right ventricular failure (RVF) results. RVF usually follows left ventricular failure (LVF), although occasionally it may develop independently.

Decompensated Heart Failure

Remodeling

Several structural changes, known as remodeling, occur in the ventricle during decompensated heart failure. Remodeling is thought to result from hypertrophy of the myocardial cells and sustained activation of the neurohormonal compensatory systems. Recall that one of the initial compensatory responses to a decrease in cardiac output is dilation of the ventricle. This dilation increases cardiac output but also increases wall stress in the ventricle. To reduce wall stress, the myocardial cells hypertrophy, resulting in a thickening of the ventricular wall. According to Laplace's law, an increase in wall thickness reduces wall stress.

When used over time, these compensatory responses produce changes in the structure, function, and gene expression of the myocardial cell. Changes in the myocardial cells eventually increase failure by reducing myocardial contractility, increasing ventricular wall stress, and increasing oxygen demand. In addition to increasing myocardial dysfunction, the genetically abnormal myocytes die prematurely and at an accelerated rate through the process of apoptosis (programmed cell death). Apoptosis affects cells scattered throughout the myocardium and causes a further reduction in cardiac function.[2, 35, 38]

Sustained Neurohormonal Activation

Remodeling changes continue to increase wall stress and further stimulate neurohormonal activity. Long-term sympathetic activation exerts a direct toxic effect on the heart that promotes myocyte hypertrophy and apoptosis. Prolonged activation of the renin-angiotensin system also stimulates myocyte hypertrophy and myocardial fibrosis. This creates a self-perpetuating cycle of cell death and further hypertrophy.[2, 35, 38]

Clinical Manifestations

The manifestations of heart failure depend on the specific ventricle involved, the precipitating causes of failure, the degree of impairment, the rate of progression, the duration of the failure, and the client's underlying condition. Manifestations of pulmonary congestion and edema dominate the clinical picture of LVF. RVF is associated with signs of abdominal organ distention and peripheral edema.[30] Heart failure has been classified into several stages based on a client's functional ability and clinical manifestations (Box 56–2).

Types of Heart Failure

Heart failure may be categorized as (1) LVF versus RVF, (2) backward versus forward, and (3) high-output versus low-output.[3]

Left Ventricular Versus Right Ventricular Failure

The theory of LVF versus RVF is based on the fact that fluid accumulates behind the chamber that fails first.

BOX 56–2 New York Heart Association Classification of Cardiovascular Disability

Class I

No limitation on physical activity. Ordinary physical activity does not cause undue fatigue, palpitation, dyspnea, or anginal pain.

Class II

Slight limitation of physical activity. Comfortable at rest, but ordinary physical activity results in fatigue, palpitation, dyspnea, or anginal pain.

Class III

Marked limitation of physical activity. Comfortable at rest, but less than ordinary physical activity causes fatigue, palpitation, dyspnea, or anginal pain.

Class IV

Unable to carry on any physical activity without discomfort. Symptoms of cardiac insufficiency or of the anginal syndrome may be present even at rest. If any physical activity is undertaken, discomfort is increased.

From Konstam, M., et al. (1994). *Heart failure: Evaluation and care of patients with left-ventricular systolic dysfunction. Clinical practice guideline No. 11* (AHCPR Pub. No. 94-0612). Rockville, MD: Agency for Health Care Policy and Research, Public Health Service, U.S. Department of Health and Human Services.

However, because the circulatory system is a closed circuit, impairments of one ventricle commonly progress to failure of the other. This is referred to as *ventricular interdependence.* Figure 56–6 depicts clinical manifestations that differentiate LVF from RVF.

Left Ventricular Failure

LVF causes either pulmonary congestion or a disturbance in the respiratory control mechanisms. These problems in turn precipitate respiratory distress. The degree of distress varies with the client's position, activity, and level of stress.

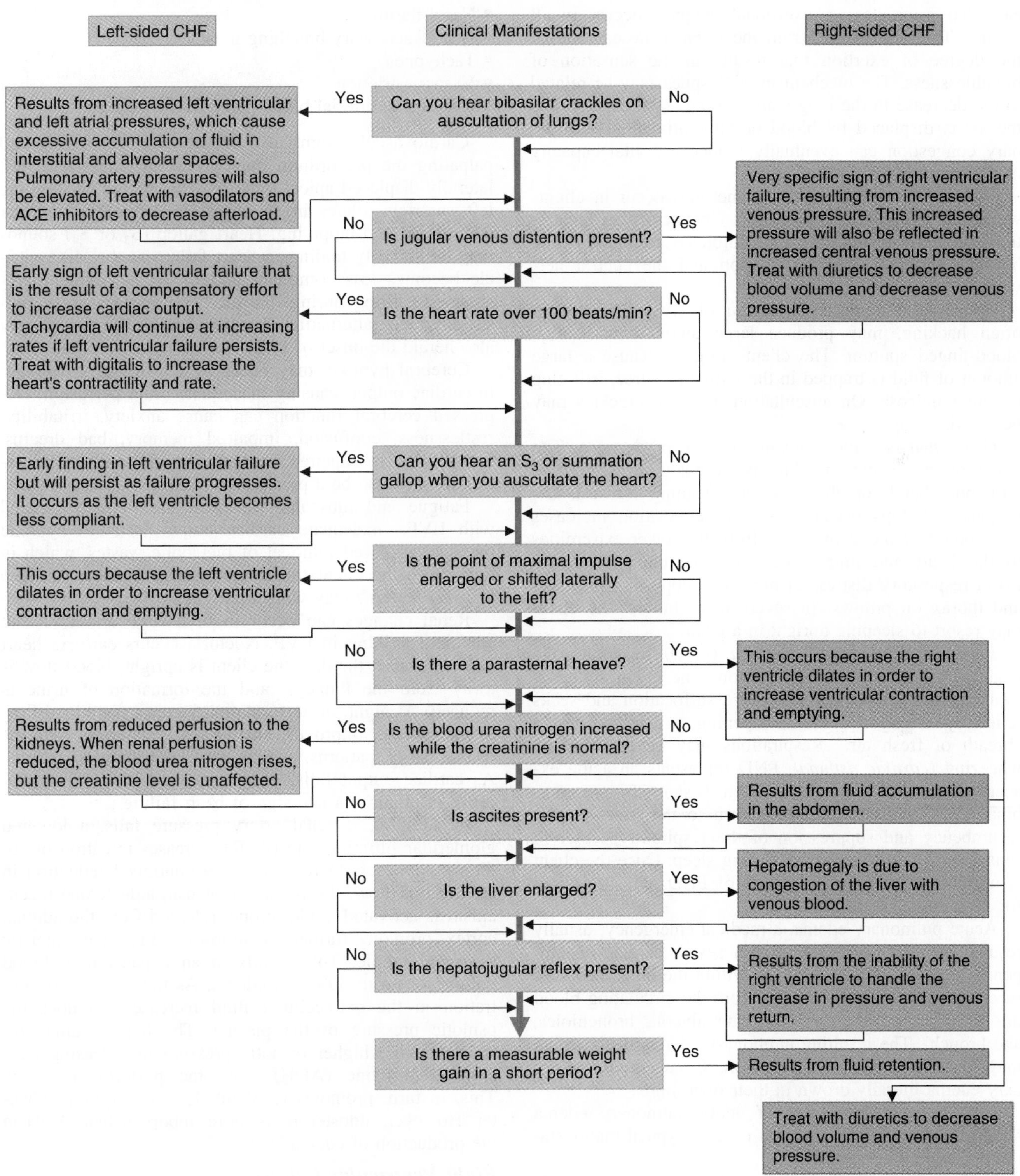

FIGURE 56–6 Clinical manifestations of left-sided and right-sided heart failure. CHF, congestive heart failure.

Dyspnea (difficult breathing) is a subjective problem and does not always correlate with the extent of heart failure. Because breathing is usually effortless at rest, the feeling of breathlessness can mean anything from an awareness of breathing to extreme distress. An apprehensive client with only moderate ventricular failure may be more aware of dyspnea than a client with advanced disease. To some degree, exertional dyspnea occurs in all clients. Therefore, elicit from the client a description of the degree of exertion that results in the sensation of breathlessness. The mechanism of dyspnea may be related to the decrease in the lung's air volume (vital capacity) as the air is displaced by blood or interstitial fluid. Pulmonary congestion can eventually reduce the vital capacity of the lungs to 1500 ml or less.

Cheyne-Stokes respirations sometimes occur in clients with severe forms of heart failure. Cheyne-Stokes respirations probably result from the prolonged circulation time between the pulmonary circulation and the central nervous system (CNS).

Cough is a common symptom of LVF. The cough, often hacking, may produce large amounts of frothy, blood-tinged sputum. The client coughs because a large amount of fluid is trapped in the pulmonary tree, irritating the lung mucosa. On auscultation, bilateral crackles may be heard.

Orthopnea is a more advanced stage of dyspnea. The client often assumes a "three-point position," sitting up with both hands on the knees and leaning forward. Orthopnea develops because the supine position increases the amount of blood returning from the lower extremities to the heart and lungs (preload). The client learns to avoid respiratory distress at night by supporting the head and thorax on pillows. In severe heart failure, the client may resort to sleeping upright in a chair.

Paroxysmal nocturnal dyspnea (PND) resembles the frightening sensation of suffocation. The client suddenly awakens with the feeling of severe suffocation and seeks relief by sitting upright or opening a window for a "breath of fresh air." Respirations may be labored and wheezing (*cardiac asthma*). PND represents an acute exacerbation of pulmonary congestion. It stems from a combination of increased venous return to the lungs during recumbency and suppression of the respiratory center to sensory input from the lungs during sleep. Once the client is upright, relief from the attack of PND may not occur for 30 minutes or longer.

Acute pulmonary edema, a medical emergency, usually results from LVF. In clients with severe cardiac decompensation, the capillary pressure within the lungs becomes so elevated that fluid is pushed from the circulating blood into the interstitium, then into the alveoli, bronchioles, and bronchi. The resulting pulmonary edema, if untreated, may cause death from suffocation. Clients with pulmonary edema literally drown in their own fluids.

The dramatic symptoms of acute pulmonary edema terrify the client and significant others. Typical manifestations include the following:

- Severe dyspnea
- Orthopnea
- Pallor
- Tachycardia
- Expectoration of large amounts of frothy, blood-tinged sputum
- Fear
- Wheezing
- Sweating
- Bubbling respirations
- Cyanosis
- Nasal flaring
- Use of accessory breathing muscles
- Tachypnea
- Vasoconstriction
- Hypoxia in arterial blood gas (ABG) findings

Cardiovascular signs also denote LVF. Inspecting and palpating the precordium may reveal an enlarged or left laterally displaced apical impulse. This occurs because the left ventricle dilates in an effort to augment ventricular contraction and emptying. Heart gallop (S_3 or S_4) sounds may be an early finding in heart failure as the left ventricle becomes less compliant and its walls vibrate in response to filling during diastole. The appearance of pulsus alternans (alternating strong and weak heartbeats) may also herald the onset of LVF.

Cerebral hypoxia may occur as a result of a decrease in cardiac output, causing inadequate brain perfusion. Depressed cerebral function can cause anxiety, irritability, restlessness, confusion, impaired memory, bad dreams, and insomnia. Impaired ventilation with resultant hypercapnia may also be a precipitant.

Fatigue and muscular weakness are often associated with LVF. Inadequate cardiac output leads to hypoxic tissue and slowed removal of metabolic wastes, which in turn cause the client to tire easily. Disturbances in sleep and rest patterns may worsen fatigue.

Renal changes can occur in both RVF and LVF but are more striking in LVF. Nocturia occurs early in heart failure. During the day, the client is upright, blood flow is away from the kidneys, and the formation of urine is reduced. At night, urine formation increases as blood flow to the kidneys improves. Nocturia may interfere with effective sleep patterns, which may contribute to fatigue. As cardiac output falls, decreased renal blood flow may result in oliguria, a late sign of heart failure.

In addition, if renal artery pressure falls, a lowered glomerular filtration rate (GFR) increases retention of sodium and water. In response to a continued reduction in renal blood flow, the renin-angiotensin-aldosterone mechanism is activated. Aldosterone, released from the adrenal cortex, promotes further retention of sodium and water by the renal tubule. This results in an expansion in blood volume of up to 30% and edema. As the sodium concentration in the extracellular fluid increases, so does the osmotic pressure of the plasma. The hypothalamus responds to the higher osmotic pressure by releasing antidiuretic hormone (ADH) from the posterior pituitary. This, in turn, promotes renal tubular reabsorption of water. However, aldosterone is more important than ADH in the production of edema.[30, 35]

Right Ventricular Failure

When right ventricle functioning decreases, peripheral edema and venous congestion of the organs develop. Liver enlargement (hepatomegaly) and abdominal pain occur as the liver becomes congested with venous blood.

If this occurs rapidly, stretching of the capsule surrounding the liver causes severe discomfort. The client may notice either a constant aching or a sharp pain in the right upper quadrant. In chronic heart failure, abdominal tenderness generally disappears.

In severe RVF, the lobules of the liver may become so congested with venous blood that they become anoxic. Anoxia leads to necrosis of the lobules. In long-standing heart failure, these necrotic areas may become fibrotic and then sclerotic. As a result, a condition called *cardiac cirrhosis* develops, manifested by ascites and jaundice.

In chronic heart failure, the increased workload of the heart and the extreme work of breathing increase the metabolic demands of the body. Anorexia, nausea, and bloating develop secondary to venous congestion of the gastrointestinal tract. The combination of increased metabolic needs and decreased caloric intake results in a marked wasting of tissue mass and cardiac cachexia.[35] Anorexia and nausea may also result from digitalis toxicity. This is a common problem because digitalis is usually prescribed for heart failure.[31]

Dependent edema is one of the early signs of RVF. Venous congestion in the peripheral vascular beds causes increased hydrostatic capillary pressure. Capillary hydrostatic pressure overwhelms the opposing pressure of plasma proteins, and fluid shifts out of the capillary beds and into the interstitial spaces, with resultant pitting edema. Edema is usually symmetrical and occurs in the dependent parts of the body, where venous pressure is highest. In ambulatory clients, edema begins in the feet and ankles and moves up the lower legs. It is most noticeable at the end of the day and often subsides after a night's rest. In the recumbent client, pitting edema may develop in the presacral area and, as it worsens, progress to the genital region and medial thighs. Concurrent jugular vein distention differentiates the edema of heart failure from that of lymphatic obstruction, cirrhosis, and hypoproteinemia.

Anasarca, a late sign in heart failure, is substantial and generalized edema. It can involve the upper extremities, genital area, and thoracic and abdominal walls. Cyanosis of the nail beds appears as venous congestion reduces peripheral blood flow.

Clients with heart failure often feel anxious, frightened, and depressed. Almost all clients realize that the heart is a vital organ and that when the heart begins to fail, health also fails. As the course of the disease progresses and manifestations worsen, the client may have an overwhelming fear of permanent disability and death. Clients express their fears in varying ways: nightmares, insomnia, acute anxiety, depression, or withdrawal from reality.

Backward Versus Forward Failure

The clinical presentation of heart failure arises from inadequate cardiac output, the pooling of blood behind the failing chamber, or both. *Backward* failure focuses on the ventricle's inability to eject completely, which increases ventricular filling pressures, causing venous and pulmonary congestion. *Forward* failure is a problem of inadequate perfusion. It results when reduced contractility produces a decrease in stroke volume and cardiac output. As cardiac output falls, blood flow to vital organs and peripheral tissues diminishes. This causes mental confusion, muscular weakness, and renal retention of sodium and water. Each of these types of failure is usually present to some degree in the client with heart failure.[3, 35]

High-Output Versus Low-Output Failure

High-output failure occurs when the heart, despite normal-output to high-output levels, is simply not able to meet the accelerated needs of the body. Causes include sepsis, Paget's disease, beriberi, anemia, thyrotoxicosis, arteriovenous fistula, and pregnancy.

Low-output failure occurs in most forms of heart disease, resulting in hypoperfusion of tissue cells. The underlying disorder is related not to increased metabolic needs of the tissues but to poor ventricular pumping action and a low cardiac output.

Acute Versus Chronic Heart Failure

The onset of heart failure may be *acute,* as when a client experiences an MI, or *gradual,* as in chronic heart failure. In chronic heart failure, there is a progression of compensatory events: a decrease in contractility, neurohormonal activation, increased preload and afterload, and finally cardiac remodeling.[3]

Diagnostic Findings

The diagnosis of heart failure rests primarily on presenting manifestations and pertinent data from the client's health history. Diagnostic studies assist in determining the underlying cause and the degree of heart failure. Such studies include an echocardiogram, chest x-ray, and ECG.[37]

The most useful diagnostic test is a two-dimensional (2-D) echocardiogram coupled with Doppler flow studies.[3] It provides information about cardiac chamber size and ventricular function and aids in assessing myocardial, valvular, congenital, endocardial, and pericardial heart disease. It allows the clinician to determine whether the dysfunction is systolic or diastolic.

In LVF, chest x-ray often depicts an enlarged cardiac silhouette, pulmonary and venous congestion, and interstitial edema. Interstitial edema on x-ray produces images called Kerley's B lines. Pleural effusions may develop and generally reflect biventricular failure.

ABG analysis is performed. Early heart failure with pulmonary edema may lead to respiratory alkalosis that is due to hyperventilation. As the disorder progresses and oxygenation becomes more impaired, acidosis develops. Pulse oximetry values show decreased oxygen levels.

Liver enzymes may reflect the degree of liver failure. Elevated blood urea nitrogen (BUN) and creatinine levels reflect decreased renal perfusion.

An ECG may give clues to the cause of LVF. Abnormalities in the ECG arise from the underlying cardiac disorder and from therapeutic agents. It may demonstrate evidence of a prior MI, dysrhythmias, or left ventricular dysfunction.

Outcome Management

Medical Management

When clients experience acute heart failure, the body compensates in many ways. The short-term effects from these compensatory mechanisms are beneficial and directed toward restoration of normal cardiac output. If cardiac output continues to fall, however, these same compensatory mechanisms become counterproductive and lead to progressive deterioration in cardiac function.

The use of various drugs is typically the mode of therapy for the treatment of heart failure. However, mechanical devices may provide respite for the heart in acute failure. The most common devices are venoarterial bypass (see later) and counterpulsation (see Chapter 57). The goals of the management are to improve ventricular pump performance, reduce myocardial workload, and prevent further heart failure by affecting the process of cardiac remodeling.

Improve Ventricular Pump Performance

Oxygen

Administer oxygen in high concentrations by mask or cannula to relieve hypoxia and dyspnea and to improve oxygen–carbon dioxide exchange. For hypoxemia, the physician may order a partial rebreather mask with a flow rate of 8 to 10 L/min to deliver oxygen concentrations of 40% to 70%. A non-rebreathing mask can achieve higher oxygen concentrations. If these methods do not raise the arterial oxygen tension (PaO_2) above 60 mm Hg, the client may need intubation and ventilatory management. Intubation provides a route for removing secretions from the bronchi. If severe bronchospasm or bronchoconstriction occurs, bronchodilators are given. Monitor the client's heart rhythm because some bronchodilators also stimulate the myocardium and may lead to dysrhythmias.

Digoxin

Digoxin exerts a direct and beneficial effect on myocardial contraction in the failing heart. Improved cardiac output enhances kidney perfusion, which may create a mild diuresis of sodium and water. For a more complete discussion on digitalis, see Box 56–3.

Digoxin does not appear to have an effect on long-term mortality in clients with heart failure.[3] It is for clients who remain symptomatic despite ACE inhibitor and beta-blocker therapy. It is very effective in heart failure associated with low cardiac output caused by ischemic, rheumatic, hypertensive, or congenital heart disease. Digoxin therapy may also be initiated to control the ventricular response in atrial fibrillation, the most common dysrhythmia in heart failure. Digoxin is not given for heart failure associated with high cardiac output states, such as anemia and thyrotoxicosis. Digoxin is contraindicated in constrictive pericarditis or cardiac tamponade and should be used with caution in acute MI because it increases myocardial oxygen demand.

When administering digoxin, assess for signs of digoxin toxicity. Digoxin levels can become elevated as a result of medication interactions. The most common medications that increase digoxin levels are quinidine, verapamil, and amiodarone. Digoxin dosage may need to be reduced if the client is taking any of these medications.[29] Clients at risk for the toxic effects of digoxin are older people and those with advanced heart disease, severe dysrhythmias, or acute MI.

Digoxin toxicity occurs in approximately one in five clients and may present with systemic or cardiac manifestations (Box 56–3). Digoxin toxicity is more prevalent when the serum concentration is equal to or greater than 2 μg/L, serum potassium is less than 3 mEq/L, or serum magnesium is low. If any of these manifestations are present, notify the physician, withhold digoxin, and initiate interventions to abate the undesirable symptoms.

Digoxin toxicity may be a life-threatening condition. Carefully follow the guidelines in Box 56–3 to prevent toxicity.

Inotropes

Inotropic agents such as dopamine, dobutamine, and amrinone may be ordered for clients with severe low-output heart failure. These medications facilitate myocardial contractility and enhance stroke volume. Dopamine is a naturally occurring catecholamine with alpha-adrenergic, beta-adrenergic, and dopaminergic activity.

Dopamine, when given in small doses (<4 μg/kg/min), stimulates the dopaminergic receptors in the renal, mesenteric, cerebral, and coronary vascular beds, which causes vasodilatation. The primary result is an increase in renal blood flow, GFR, and sodium excretion. The alpha-adrenergic and beta-adrenergic receptors in the vasculature and myocardium are affected by moderate doses of dopamine (4 to 8 μg/kg/min). The results are increases in heart rate, stroke volume, and cardiac output. Alpha-adrenergic effects, such as intense vasoconstriction, dominate when dopamine is given in doses larger than 10 μg/kg/min.[48] Although dopamine may improve cardiac output, it may do so at the expense of the myocardium and renal blood flow. Tachycardia may increase myocardial oxygen demands and decrease myocardial oxygen supply, which may prove costly to the already ischemic myocardium.

Another inotropic agent, dobutamine, is a synthetic derivative of dopamine that produces strong beta-stimulatory effects within the myocardium; it increases heart rate, atrioventricular (AV) conduction, and myocardial contractility. Dobutamine is capable of increasing cardiac output without increasing myocardial oxygen demands or reducing coronary blood flow.

Amrinone is also used to increase cardiac output in severe heart failure. In addition to the positive inotropic effects, amrinone increases renal blood flow and GFR.

Reduce Myocardial Workload

Positioning the Client

The client is placed in a high Fowler position or chair to reduce pulmonary venous congestion and to relieve the dyspnea. The legs are maintained in a dependent position as much as possible. Even though the legs are edematous, they should not be elevated. Elevating the legs increases venous return rapidly.

Reducing Preload

Diuretic therapy plays an integral part in the successful management of heart failure in clients with a predisposition for fluid retention. Diuretics enhance renal excretion of sodium and water, which reduces circulating blood volume, diminishes preload, and lessens systemic and pulmonary congestion. Table 56–5 describes the characteristics of a commonly used diuretic.

BOX 56-3 Cardiac Glycoside—Digoxin

Actions and Therapeutic Responses

Action: increases ventricular contractility (positive inotropic effect), increases ventricular emptying, slows conduction of impulses through the atrioventricular (AV) node and Purkinje's fibers, increases AV nodal refractory period, augments stroke volume, and increases cardiac output.

Therapeutic responses: slows heart rate and increases cardiac output.

Administration Guidelines and Rationales

Guidelines	*Rationales*
1. Always take the client's apical pulse for 1 full minute before administration.	1. Apical pulse for a full minute is the most reliable method for obtaining an accurate pulse rate.
2. Withhold digoxin if heart rate is below 60 or newly irregular.	2. Bradycardia or dysrhythmias may be indicative of digoxin toxicity.
3. Check most recent digoxin and electrolyte levels before administration.	3. The digoxin level must be below or within therapeutic range before administering. Hypokalemia increases myocardial sensitivity to digoxin.
4. Intravenous (IV) administration must be given over 5 minutes.	4. Rapid IV administration may potentiate side effects.
5. Serum levels should be drawn at least 4 hours after an IV dose and 6 hours after an oral dose.	5. To obtain accurate results in levels, they should be drawn after peak effect.

Pharmacokinetics

Onset: oral 1–2 hours, IV 5–30 minutes
Duration: 3–4 days in both forms
Peak effect: oral 2–8 hours, IV 1–4 hours
Absorption: upper small intestine

Excretion: renal
Half-life: 38–48 hours
Therapeutic plasma levels: 0.8–2.0 ng/ml
Toxic plasma levels: above 2.4 ng/ml

Drugs That May Increase or Decrease Serum Digitalis Concentrations

Increase	*Decrease*
Amiodarone	Antacids
Cyclosporine	Cholestyramine
Diltiazem	Colestipol
Diuretics	Kaolin-pectin
Erythromycin	Metoclopramide
Propantheline	Neomycin
Quinidine/quinine	P-aminosalicylic acid
Spironolactone	Rifampin
Tetracycline	Sulfasalazine
Verapamil	
Captopril	

Assessing Adverse Responses

The client may exhibit nausea, vomiting, abdominal pain, diarrhea, anorexia, sinus bradycardia, AV or sinoatrial (SA) block, dysrhythmias, drowsiness, fatigue, headache, lethargy, blurred vision, halos, green or yellow vision, or diplopia.

Evidence of Digoxin Toxicity

Digoxin toxicity is manifested by a wide array of signs and symptoms and is often difficult to differentiate from effects of cardiac disease. Nausea and vomiting are the most common early indicators of toxicity. Other signs include anorexia, diarrhea, abdominal discomfort, headache, weakness, visual disturbances, and confusion. Cardiac signs include ventricular tachycardia, premature ventricular contractions, bradycardia, AV block, ST depression, PR prolongation, and atrial and ventricular fibrillation.

Treatment of Toxicity

Discontinue digoxin administration. Digoxin immune Fab is administered intravenously. Each 40 mg binds approximately 0.6 mg of digoxin. Digoxin immune Fab causes hypokalemia; therefore, serum potassium levels must be obtained and replaced appropriately.

Data from Armstrong, L. L. (Ed.). *The University of Chicago Hospitals Formulary of Accepted Drugs.* Hudson, OH: Lexi-Comp, Inc., 1998.

TABLE 56–5 NURSING IMPLICATIONS FOR MEDICATIONS USED IN HEART FAILURE

Class (Example)	Assessing Therapeutic Responses	Assessing Adverse Responses	Nursing Implications
DECREASES MYOCARDIAL WORKLOAD			
Diuretic (furosemide)	The urine output should increase. The reduction in circulating volume decreases central venous pressures, pulmonary congestion, and peripheral edema. It may also decrease systemic blood pressure.	Clients may experience orthostatic hypotension, hypokalemia, electrolyte imbalance, blurred vision, headache, loss of appetite, hearing loss, and stomach cramps and pain.	Monitor electrolytes, intake and output, weight, blood pressure, and renal function. Intravenous (IV) administration should not exceed 0.5 mg/kg/min, and hearing loss is possible with high doses. Teach clients to rise slowly to avoid orthostatic hypotension.
Venous vasodilator (nitroglycerin)	Reducing peripheral resistance decreases blood pressure, and the reduction in preload may decrease the heart rate and pulmonary congestion. Vasodilatation of coronary vessels should keep clients free of anginal pain.	Clients may experience flushing, weakness, headache, postural hypotension, dizziness, and reflex tachycardia.	Monitor clients for hypotension. Ointment and patches should be rotated daily, and clients may need a nitrate-free interval to avoid tolerance. Avoid getting ointment on fingers. IV nitroglycerin should be in glass bottles with tubing specific for nitroglycerin. If a client is receiving continuous IV nitroglycerin, the blood pressure and heart rate should be continually monitored.
Vein and arteriole dilator (sodium nitroprusside)	The peripheral vasodilatation decreases the blood pressure. Decrease in afterload increases cardiac output by enhancing contractility.	Clients may experience hypotension, sweating, palpitations, restlessness, headache, nausea, and vomiting. Cyanide toxicity is possible in clients with decreased liver function, and thiocyanate toxicity is possible in clients with decreased kidney function or anyone who has prolonged use of nitroprusside. Signs of thiocyanate toxicity include psychoses, blurred vision, tinnitus, and seizures. Signs of cyanide toxicity include metabolic acidosis, tachycardia, decreased pulse and reflexes, and coma.	Solution must be mixed with 5% dextrose in water (D_5W) and wrapped with opaque material to protect it from light. Blue color indicates almost complete degradation to cyanide. Constant blood pressure and heart rate monitoring is necessary. Monitor acid/base status, as acidosis can be the earliest indicator of cyanide toxicity. Monitor thiocyanate levels if infusion is for more than 3 days or the dose is more than 4 mg/kg/min.
Angiotensin-converting enzyme (ACE) inhibitor (captopril)	The decrease in afterload increases cardiac output by enhancing contractility. The neurohormonal effects include inhibition of ACE and vasodilatation and a decrease in systemic blood pressure.	Clients may experience oliguria, chest pain, palpitations, insomnia, dizziness, fatigue, nausea, vomiting, maculopapular rash, and cough.	Monitor blood pressure. Administer 1 hour before meals. Two weeks of therapy may be necessary before the full therapeutic effect is achieved. May increase blood urea nitrogen, creatinine, liver enzymes, and potassium levels. If given concurrently with digoxin, it may cause an increase in digoxin levels.

Beta-adrenergic antagonist (atenolol)	The effects of blockade of beta-adrenergic receptors are seen clinically by decreased heart rate, blood pressure, and cardiac output. The neurohormonal response inhibits the sympathetic nervous system that causes vasodilatation and decreasing automaticity in the heart. Clinically, this decreases blood pressure and the heart rate and the incidence of dysrhythmias.	Clients may experience brochoconstriction, severe bradycardia, or hypotension. They may also experience atrioventricular conduction abnormalities, dizziness, confusion, constipation or diarrhea, and vomiting. Male clients may experience impotence.	Clients must be instructed not to stop taking medication abruptly because they may experience angina. The drug should not be given in clients with a history of bronchospastic pulmonary disease. If the client is diabetic, it may potentiate hypoglycemia. The nurse must monitor the heart rate, rhythm, and blood pressure frequently and assess pulmonary status for bronchoconstriction.
INCREASES PUMP PERFORMANCE			
Cardiac glycoside (digoxin)	The increased contractility increases cardiac output. Suppression of the atrioventricular node decreases the heart rate.	The client may experience nausea, vomiting, abdominal pain, diarrhea, anorexia, bradycardia, dysrhythmias, drowsiness, fatigue, and visual disturbances. Digoxin toxicity is a potentially fatal condition that must be assessed for whenever a client is on digoxin therapy.	Always take apical pulse for 1 minute and hold if the rate is under 60 or if the pulse is newly irregular. The most recent digoxin and electrolyte levels must be assessed prior to administration. IV doses should be given over 5 minutes. Serum levels should be drawn no sooner than 4 hours after an IV dose and 6 hours after an oral dose.
Inotrope (dobutamine)	The enhanced myocardial contractility increases cardiac output and may increase the heart rate and blood pressure.	Clients may experience anginal pain, increased heart rate, palpitations, premature ventricular beats, paresthesia, headache, nausea, and vomiting. Extravasation should be avoided; if present, treat with phentolamine.	Monitor the electrocardiogram and blood pressure continuously. Observe for hypertension and tachycardia. Use a central line for administration if possible. Observe the IV site frequently.
Inotrope (dopamine)	The enhanced myocardial contractility increases the systolic blood pressure, heart rate, and cardiac output. Improved circulation to renal vascular beds results in increased urine output in low to moderate doses.	The client may experience palpitations, cardiac dysrhythmias, tachycardia, vasoconstriction, or hypotension. Estravasation should be avoided; if present, treat with phentolamine.	Continuous monitoring of the blood pressure and heart rate is necessary. In higher doses, observe for decreases in urine output, cool extremities, and decreased pulses. The IV site must be monitored frequently to avoid extravasation. Central lines are preferred, especially in clients with occlusive vascular disease or diabetic endarteritis. The hemodynamic effects are dose dependent.

Data from Armstrong, L. L. (Ed.). *The University of Chicago Hospitals Formulary of Accepted Drugs.* Hudson, OH: Lexi-Comp, Inc., 1998.

Although they are effective, diuretics should be administered cautiously because of their side effect profile. Diuretics can produce mild to severe electrolyte imbalance. Hypokalemia, a particularly dangerous problem, potentiates digitalis toxicity and can cause myocardial weakness and cardiac dysrhythmias. Moreover, vigorous diuresis may produce hypovolemia and hypotension, jeopardizing cardiac output.

Reducing Afterload

Vasodilating agents have become an increasingly important intervention in clients with heart failure. Vasodilators vary in their mechanisms of action, which include:

- Direct dilation of veins
- Dilation of arterioles
- Combined action on veins and arterioles
- Inhibition of ACE

Closely assess the client receiving vasodilators, which can cause a rapid fall in blood pressure.

Venous dilators relax venous smooth muscle and increase the capacity of the systemic venous bed; blood is "trapped" in the veins, and venous return to the heart is decreased. This increased venous capacity reduces preload. Examples include nitroglycerin and isosorbide dinitrate.

Arteriolar dilators reduce systemic arteriolar tone, which decreases peripheral vascular resistance and afterload. Reduction in afterload reduces the left ventricular workload and increases cardiac output. Improved renal perfusion may initiate diuresis. Hydralazine is the most commonly used arterial dilator. Note that hydralazine may precipitate reflex tachycardia.

Combined venous and arteriolar dilators decrease both preload and afterload. Sodium nitroprusside helps manage severe heart failure. A potent vasodilator, sodium nitroprusside relaxes the smooth muscles of both veins and arterioles. It does not directly affect the heart muscle or heart rate.

ACE inhibitors suppress the renin-angiotensin-aldosterone system, blocking production of the potent vasoconstrictor angiotensin II. This results in an increase in renal blood flow and a decrease in renal vascular resistance, which enhances diuresis. They also lessen the effect of neurohormonal influences in heart failure. ACE inhibitors reduce remodeling changes in the hearts of animals and can increase client survival. One ACE inhibitor, captopril, improves hemodynamic status. All clients with left systolic heart failure should receive ACE inhibitors unless they cannot tolerate the drugs.

Beta-adrenergic antagonists (beta-blockers) are now used in clients with heart failure because they inhibit the effects of the sympathetic nervous system. They have been shown to increase clinical improvement[14] and to decrease mortality. These findings are apparent when clients are concurrently receiving ACE inhibitory therapy, suggesting that the combination of two agents that have inhibitory effects on two neurohormonal systems may have an additive effect.[3]

VENTRICULAR ASSIST DEVICES. For the past few decades, when conventional therapy such as medications and the intra-aortic balloon pump (IABP) became ineffective, there was little hope for the client with heart failure. Advances continue to be made in perfecting methods of mechanical ventricular support. The goal of mechanical circulatory support is to decompress the hypokinetic ventricle, decrease myocardial workload, reduce oxygen demands, and maintain adequate systemic perfusion to sustain end-organ function. In the client with heart failure, the two most common options are ventricular assist devices (VADs) as a bridge to transplantation and as permanent support.[43] VADs have the capability to support circulation, either partially or totally, until the heart recovers or is replaced. Devices may be right ventricular, left ventricular, or biventricular VADs. Complications of any VAD include bleeding, hemolysis, thromboembolism, infection, and multiorgan failure.[8, 26]

Traditionally, nonpulsatile pumps have been used as VADs. Difficulties with these devices include end-organ dysfunction, thromboembolic complications, and the need for full anticoagulation. Their use in clients with heart failure is diminishing because better technology is available. These pumps can be used for a relatively short period of approximately 10 days.

Pulsatile pumps are the newest, most advanced forms of mechanical support. Pulsatile flow decreases the amount of hemolysis, decreases thromboembolic episodes, and allows better perfusion to organs. They allow extended use with minimal anticoagulation.

External pulsatile VADs are utilized as a bridge to transplantation. They offer both short-term and long-term support. Cardiopulmonary bypass is not required for insertion. If the client is stable, they allow for mobility. Thromboembolism is the major concern with the external pulsatile devices.

Implantable VADs are currently approved as permanent devices to bridge over to transplantation. They were designed with larger clients in mind because these clients often have to wait the longest for a transplantation. The greatest advantage of the device is that it allows mobility for the client. It reduces the risk of infection, prevents muscle disuse, and prevents other systemic complications, such as pneumonia. Cardiopulmonary bypass is required to insert these devices. They are also more costly than the external pulsatile VADs.

Total artificial hearts provide complete control of the cardiovascular system and allow total mobility. Their use is limited in smaller people, because the device may not fit the client's small body. Complications include infection, thromboembolism, and the possibility of mechanical failure. Initially, total artificial hearts were limited to people awaiting transplantation. Currently, these devices are being used when there are contraindications to transplantation, such as advanced age.[39]

Extracorporeal membrane oxygenation (ECMO) systems are widely used for short-term hemodynamic stabilization. These devices remove blood from the inferior vena cava to a centrifugal pump that pumps the blood to an oxygenator. The oxygenated blood is returned to the client via the femoral artery. Long-term use (>48 hours) does not promote recovery. In addition, bleeding is a concern because anticoagulation therapy is needed.

As the number of people who require cardiac transplantation increases and the options for mechanical assist devices grow, the nurse needs to become more aware of these devices for clients with end-stage heart disease. Traditionally, clients were cared for in the intensive care unit (ICU), but today a critical care environment is not needed, except for those on ECMO, once the client is stabilized.

Reduce Fluid Retention

Controlling sodium and water retention improves cardiac performance. Sodium restrictions are placed on the diet to prevent, control, or eliminate edema. Diets with 2 to 4 g of sodium are usually prescribed (Table 56–6).

From the use of some loop diuretics, potassium is lost via the kidneys, which can lead to dysrhythmias and electrolyte imbalances. Hypokalemia sensitizes the myocardium to digitalis and therefore predisposes the client to digitalis toxicity. Potassium supplements and adequate dietary potassium are important.

It is usually not necessary to restrict fluid intake in clients with mild or moderate heart failure. In more advanced cases, however, it is beneficial to limit water to 1000 ml/day (1 L/day). The reason is that excessive water intake tends to dilute the amount of sodium in body fluids and may produce a low-salt syndrome (*hyponatremia*). Hyponatremia is characterized by lethargy and weakness; it results more often from the combination of a restricted sodium diet, increased sodium loss during diuresis, and excessive water intake.

Reduce Stress and Risk of Injury

In addition to improving ventricular pump performance and reducing myocardial workload, the client also needs to reduce physical and emotional stress. Sometimes clinicians overlook rest as an intervention to diminish the workload of the heart. The proper use of rest as the initial step in management offers many benefits. Rest can promote diuresis, slow the heart rate, and relieve dyspnea, all of which allow more conservative use of pharmacologic agents (e.g., ACE inhibitors, diuretics, beta-blockers).

Whether the physician prescribes complete, modified bed rest depends on the seriousness of the client's condition. The physician may prescribe a mild sedative or small doses of barbiturates and tranquilizers to promote rest and overcome problems of restlessness, insomnia, and anxiety.

The client may also be at risk for injury because of immobility. The client should be confined to bed only long enough to regain cardiac reserve but not so long as to promote complications of immobility. Give the client confined to bed rest specific guidelines to prevent the harmful effects of immobility. Clients should perform passive leg exercises several times daily to prevent venous stasis, which may lead to the formation of venous thrombi and pulmonary emboli. The physician may also initiate anticoagulant therapy to prevent these potentially deadly complications.[29]

Nursing Management of the Medical Client

The goals of nursing management for the client with heart failure are to:

- Monitor for reduced cardiac output
- Maintain adequate fluid balance
- Reduce myocardial workload
- Assess response to medical therapies
- Educate the client about self-care following discharge (see Bridge to Home Health Care, p. 1546)

Use Figure 56–6 to help differentiate right-sided from left-sided failure. Consider the psychosocial effect of heart failure on the client and family. Nursing diagnoses that may apply to the client with heart failure are discussed in the Care Plan.

TABLE 56–6 SODIUM CONTENT OF SELECTED FOODS

FOODS LOW IN SODIUM	
Dairy products	Skim milk, eggs, cottage cheese, cream cheese, ice cream
Meats*	Turkey, chicken, veal, lamb, liver, fresh fish, tuna packed in water (meats should be unprocessed)
Fruits and vegetables*	Any fresh or frozen food in this group
Beverages	Any juice (except tomato or V8 brand vegetable), coffee, tea, bottled water
Breads	Some breads and cereals
Seasonings	Garlic, onion, bay leaf, pepper, dill, nutmeg, rosemary, allspice, thyme, sage, caraway, cinnamon, almond and vanilla extract, fresh dried herbs
Fats	Margarine, oils, shortening, unsalted salad dressings
Desserts	Sherbet, fruit ice, gelatin, fruit drinks
Miscellaneous	Unbuttered, unsalted popcorn; unsalted nuts; vinegar
FOODS HIGH IN SODIUM	
Milk and dairy products	Aged, hard cheese; pasteurized, processed cheese; buttermilk
Meats	Sausage, frankfurters, ham, bacon, corned beef; all smoked, pickled, or cured meats; canned meats, salami, most luncheon meats, beef jerky; frozen "TV" dinners
Fruits and vegetables	Pickled or canned fruits and vegetables, olives, sauerkraut, pickles
Breads and cereals	Salted crackers, macaroni and cheese, pretzels, rye rolls, pizza, commercial pancake mixes
Beverages	Tomato juice, V8 vegetable juice, beef broth, bouillon
Fats	Commercial salad dressings, dips and party spreads, peanut butter
Seasonings	Garlic, celery, or onion salt; Accent, monosodium glutamate (MSG), meat tenderizer, soy sauce, ketchup, steak sauce, mustard, canned soup
Desserts	Fruit pies, doughnuts, cakes, commercial puddings
Miscellaneous	Baking soda, baking powder, salted popcorn, salted nuts, potato chips

* Food sources high in potassium.

Text continued on page 1546

THE CLIENT WITH HEART FAILURE

Nursing Diagnosis. Decreased Cardiac Output related to heart failure or dsyrhythmias or both.

Outcomes. The client will have an increase in cardiac output, as evidenced by regular cardiac rhythm, heart rate, blood pressure, respirations, and urine output within normal limits.

Interventions	Rationales
1. Assess blood pressure for hypotension or hypertension and respiratory rate for tachypnea q 1 hr (more or less frequently, depending on the client's stability).	1. Hypotension may indicate decreased cardiac output and may lead to a decrease in coronary artery perfusion. Hypertension may be caused by chronic vasoconstriction or may indicate fear or anxiety, and increased respiratoryl rate may indicate fatigue or increased pulmonary congestion.
2. Assess heart rate and rhythm q 1 hr for tachycardia or the presence of dysrhythmias.	2. Tachycardia can increase myocardial and oxygen demands and may be a compensatory mechanism related to the decreased cardiac output (increased heart rate to compensate for decrease in stroke volume). Ventricular enlargement decreases conduction of cardiac impulses and may lead to dysrhythmias. Dysrhythmias further compromise cardiac output by reducing ventricular filling time and myocardial contractility and by increasing myocardial oxygen demands. Common dysrhythmias include premature atrial contractions (PACs), premature ventricular contractions (PVCs), and paroxysmal atrial tachycardia (PAT). Ventricular dysrhythmias must be watched for because they can increase the chance of sudden death.
3. Document rhythm strips q 8 hr and if dysrhythmias occur. Measure and note rate, QRS, PR, and QT intervals and ST segment with each strip and note any deviations from baseline.	3. Documentation of rhythm confirms rhythm and gives a baseline for changes. Changes in the ST segment may indicate myocardial ischemia, which may be present because of decreased coronary artery perfusion.
4. Report dysrhythmias to the physician.	4. Dysrhythmias can decrease cardiac output and may lead to life-threatening dysrhythmias.
5. Auscultate heart rate q 2 hr for changes in heart sounds such as murmurs, S_3, or S_4.	5. Delayed filling time, incomplete ejection, and structural changes within the heart and fluid overload may cause abnormal heart sounds detected by auscultation. S_3 may indicate a noncompliant or stiff ventricle, and S_4 may indicate a weak, overdistended ventricle.
6. Monitor lung sounds q 2 hr for advantageous sounds such as crackles and for the presence of coughing.	6. Increased ventricular pressures are transmitted back to the pulmonary circulation, increasing pulmonary capillary hydrostatic pressure and exceeding oncotic pressure fluid moves within the alveolar septum, and are evidenced by the auscultation of crackles, increased shortness of breath, and sputum production. This indicates a further decrease in cardiac output and the possibility of the development of pulmonary edema. Coughing can be caused by the increased fluid in the lungs or by angiotensin-converting enzyme (ACE) inhibitors.
7. Monitor intake and output (I & O) and assess findings q 8 hr and as required (PRN). Note color and amount of urine q 2 hr and PRN.	7. If intake exceeds output, the patient is at risk for fluid overload and may not be able to clear fluids because of a decompensating heart. Dark, concentrated urine and oliguria may reflect a decrease in renal perfusion. Diuresis is expected in clients receiving diuretic therapy.
8. Assess for changes in mental status.	8. Change in mental status may indicate decreased cerebral perfusion or hypoxia.
9. Assess peripheral pulses for strength and quality and for pulsus alternans.	9. Decreased strength of peripheral pulses is often found in clients with decreased cardiac output, and a further decrease in pulses from baseline may indicate further cardiac failure. Pulsus alternans may be detected and indicates severe heart failure.
10. Administer prescribed medications and evaluate responses.	10. Prescribed medications are utilized to increase contractility and decrease preload or afterload, and their responses must be evaluated. Therapeutic levels must be monitored. Clients need to be monitored for potential side effects.
11. Encourage physical and psychological rest.	11. Increased physical or mental strain can increase myocardial and oxygen demands.
12. Encourage clients to eat small meals and rest afterward.	12. Larger meals increase myocardial workload and may cause vagal stimulation, which may lead to bradycardia.

Evaluation. Client's vital signs will be within normal parameters, and urine output will be normal.

Nursing Diagnosis. Fluid Volume Excess related to reduced glomerular filtration, decreased cardiac output, increased antidiuretic hormone (ADH) production, and sodium and water retention.

Outcomes. The client will demonstrate adequate fluid balance, as evidenced by output equal to or exceeding intake, clearing breath sounds, and decreasing edema.

Interventions	Rationales
1. Monitor I & O q 4 hr (more or less frequently depending on clients status).	1. I & O balance reflects fluid status.
2. Weigh clients daily.	2. Body weight is a sensitive indicator of fluid balance, and an increase indicates fluid volume excess.
3. Assess for presence of peripheral edema.	3. Heart failure causes venous congestion, resulting in increased capillary pressure. When hydrostatic pressure exceeds interstitial pressure, fluids leak out of the capillaries and present as edema in the legs, sacrum, and scrotum.
4. Assess for jugular vein distention, hepatomegaly, and abdominal pain.	4. Elevated volumes in the venae cavae occur as right atrium preload increase from inadequate emptying from right atrium and are transmitted to the jugular vein and present as distention; they can also be the cause of hepatomegaly, splenomegaly, and abdominal pain.
5. Low-sodium diet or fluid restriction.	5. Decreased systemic blood pressure can trigger renin, leading to a cascade of events that ends with stimulation of aldosterone, which causes increased renal tubular absorption of sodium. Low-sodium diet helps prevent increased sodium retention, which decreases water retention. Fluid restriction may be utilized to decrease fluid intake, hence decreasing fluid volume excess.
6. Auscultate breath sounds q 2 hr and PRN for the presence of crackles and monitor for sputum production.	6. When increased pulmonary capillary hydrostatic pressure exceeds oncotic pressure, fluid moves within the alveolar septum and is evidenced by the auscultation of crackles. Frothy, pink-tinged sputum is an indicator the client is developing the life-threatening complication of pulmonary edema.
7. Administer diuretic therapy as ordered and evaluate effectiveness of the therapy.	7. Diuretics are commonly prescribed to promote the diuresis of accumulated fluid. The nurse should expect an increase in urine output after the client receives diuretic therapy

Evaluation. The client has clear breath sounds, decrease in weight, equal or increased output in relationship to intake, and decreased peripheral edema.

Nursing Diagnosis. Impaired Gas Exchange related to fluid in alveoli.

Outcomes. The client will have improved gas exchange, as evidenced by decreased dyspnea, no cyanosis, normal arterial blood gases, and a decrease in pulmonary congestion upon auscultation.

Interventions	Rationales
1. Auscultate breath sounds q 2 hr.	1. Auscultation of crackles may indicate pulmonary congestion.
2. Encourage the client to turn, cough, and deep-breathe q 2 hr.	2. This will help facilitate oxygen delivery and clear the airways.
3. Administer oxygen if ordered.	3. Oxygen therapy will improve oxygenation by increasing the amount of oxygen available for delivery.
4. Assess respiratory rate and rhythm q 2 hr and PRN.	4. Increased respiratory rate indicates difficulty with oxygenation, and a decreased respiratory rate may indicate impending respiratory failure.
5. Assess for cyanosis q 4 hr and PRN.	5. Circumoral cyanosis or cyanosis to the finger tips or end of nose indicates hypoxia from lack of oxygen in peripheral tissues.

Care Plan continued on following page

6. Position the client to facilitate breathing and observe for paroxysmal nocturnal dyspnea.	6. Fowler position and orthopneic positioning facilitate diaphragmatic excursion. Paroxysmal nocturnal dyspnea may occur because as the client assumes a supine position, venous return to the heart is increased. This increase in return increases preload and will increase pulmonary capillary hydrostatic pressure and lead to pulmonary alveolar edema.
7. Monitor pulse oximetry.	7. A low SaO_2 reflects hypoxia.
8. Obtain arterial blood gases if ordered.	8. Arterial blood gases indicate whether the patient has hypoxia, acidosis, or both.
9. Administer diuretic therapy as ordered, and monitor for effectiveness.	9. Diuretics promote fluid loss in the alveoli as well as systemically.

Evaluation. The client has clear breath sounds, normal arterial blood gases, and saturation. Respiratory rate is normal.

Nursing Diagnosis. Altered Tissue Perfusion related to decreased cardiac output.

Outcomes. The client will have adequate tissue perfusion as evidenced by warm dry skin, peripheral pulses, and adequate urine output.

Intervention	Rationales
1. Note color and temperature of the skin q 4 hr.	1. Cool, pale skin is indicative of decreased peripheral tissue perfusion.
2. Monitor peripheral pulses q 4 hr.	2. Decreased pulses are indicative of decreased tissue perfusion from vasoconstriction of the vessels.
3. Provide a warm environment.	3. A warm environment promotes vasodilatation, which decreases preload and promotes tissue perfusion.
4. Encourage active range of motion.	4. Range of motion helps decrease venous pooling and promotes tissue perfusion.
5. Monitor urine output q 4 hr.	5. Decreased perfusion to the kidneys may result in oliguria.

Evaluation. The client has warm skin, adequate peripheral pulses, and normal urine output.

Nursing Diagnosis. Risk for Activity Intolerance related to decreased cardiac output.

Outcomes. The client will have improved levels of activity without dyspnea.

Interventions	Rationales
1. Space nursing activities.	1. Clustering activities increases myocardial demand and may cause extreme fatigue.
2. Schedule rest periods.	2. Rest periods help alleviate fatigue and decrease myocardial workload.
3. Monitor the client's response to activities.	3. Dyspnea, tachycardia, angina, diaphoresis, dysrhythmias, and hypotension are all indicative that the activity required more myocardial demand than the body was able to compensate for. Assess vital signs before and after an activity. The time it requires for the vital signs to return to baseline indicates the degree of cardiac deconditioning.
4. Increase activity as ordered or according to the rehabilitation nurse's direction.	4. Gradually and appropriately increasing physical activity may help the client gain cardiac conditioning and improve activity tolerance.
5. Instruct the client to avoid activities that increase cardiac workload.	5. Activities such as stair climbing, working with arms above the head, or sustained arm movement may cause extreme fatigue and demand more cardiac output than the body can supply.

Evaluation. The client will perform spaced activities without dyspnea and will gradually increase activity tolerance.

Nursing Diagnosis. Risk for Impaired Skin Integrity related to decreased tissue perfusion and activities.

Outcomes. The client will maintain intact skin.

Interventions

1. Reposition the client q 2 hr.
2. Provide a therapeutic mattress or bed while client is in bed.
3. Assess the skin, especially bony prominences, for redness, each shift, and as needed. Utilize protective devices if redness is noted.
4. Assist the client with morning care.

Rationales

1. Changing position frequently deters the formation of pressure ulcers by decreasing the amount of time of pressure on any given area.
2. Pressure reduction mattresses and beds are available to decrease the pressure on the sacrum when the client is in bed.
3. Redness is indicative of increased pressure to an area and is the first sign of breakdown. Risk areas include the sacrum, coccyx, heels, elbows, and back of the head.
4. Clients may have difficulty providing themselves with adequate skin care, and the nurse must ensure the skin is clean and has proper moisture.

Evaluation. The client has intact skin.

Nursing Diagnosis. Risk for anxiety related to decreased cardiac output, hypoxia, diagnosis of heart failure, and fear of death or debilitation.

Outcomes. The client will not exhibit signs of anxiety and will be able to express concerns.

Interventions

1. Provide a calm environment.
2. Explain in advance all procedures and routine regimens.
3. Encourage the client to ask questions.
4. Provide emotional support to clients and their significant others.
5. Encourage the client to utilize additional support systems.

Rationales

1. A calm environment decreases additional anxiety.
2. By providing information in advance, the client will not feel anxious about the routine care provided.
3. By encouraging the client to ask questions, the nurse is providing an open forum for discussion with the client.
4. Allowing clients and their support systems to vent fears and anxiety, the nurse assists them in decreasing anxiety.
5. Additional support people such as religious leaders, social workers, counselors, and clinical nurse specialists may increase the client's support system and decrease anxiety.

Evaluation: The client is calm, without apparent anxiety.

BRIDGE TO HOME HEALTH CARE

Managing Heart Failure

One third of all clients hospitalized for heart failure are readmitted within 90 days of discharge. Problems with self-monitoring techniques, medication, and diet are the primary reasons. Home health and outpatient care nurses can make a positive difference in readmission rates through nursing interventions.

Review clients' cardiovascular history, disease etiology, and medical management plan to guide your assessment. Auscultate the heart and lungs during each visit, and look for signs of fluid accumulation. Measure blood pressure with both the client sitting and standing. If blood pressure decreases significantly and the client experiences lightheadedness or dizziness, it may be necessary to adjust diuretic or vasoactive medications. Worsening cardiac status or drug toxicities can cause changes in pulse rate or rhythm.

Clients may experience unique manifestations such as fullness in their ears, increased urination at night, and chest heaviness. The client, family members, and informal caregivers need to be educated about the correlation between manifestations and clinical status. Evaluate changes in the prevalence and severity of manifestations. The assessment can include measuring intake and output, abdominal girth and lower extremities, and weight. Instruct clients to call you or their physicians if they lose or gain 2 to 3 pounds in 1 day or 5 to 7 pounds in 1 week. When manifestations are noted and cardiac decompensation is detected early, heart failure can be managed successfully in non-institutional, outpatient settings.

Use various techniques to help clients manage their medications. Write the medication schedule clearly, and suggest reminder systems such as pill boxes. Examine all pill bottles for the drug name, strength, expiration date, and available refills. Review brand versus generic labeling to minimize confusion and prevent drug administration errors. Simplify dosing frequencies; by limiting doses to twice a day (bid), three times a day (tid), or four times a day (qid), medication administration can be associated with daily routines such as meals and bedtime. Flexible dose times can promote drug tolerance and increase accurate administration. Discourage the use of over-the-counter medications because of the potential for drug interactions.

Limiting sodium intake to 2000 mg a day can help prevent fluid retention. Rarely do clients need to restrict fluid intake to less than 2000 ml/day. Evaluate the client's appetite, meal frequency, portion sizes, and food preferences, and provide appropriate health education. If possible, open cupboards and the refrigerator to gain insight into the client's eating patterns. Suggest a food diary to accurately assess intake. Teach clients, family members, and informal caregivers how to distinguish the sodium content of foods by reading food labels.

Because a client's functional status is often severely impaired, explain energy-conservation techniques before initiating limited mobility and aerobic routines. Even the most severely affected client may benefit from chair exercises, done while in a sitting position. Instruct clients to keep an activity log to demonstrate their progress toward activity goals. Clients should perceive their activities as only somewhat hard to do and should not participate in activities that worsen their manifestations or produce fatigue.

Clients who have chronic illnesses, including heart failure, often have feelings of depression. Consider whether clients need psychosocial and financial assistance. Antidepressant medications benefit some clients and improve their sense of well-being.

Cynthia A. Bolin, RN, *Program Coordinator, Congestive Heart Failure Management Center, St. Luke's Hospital, St. Louis, Missouri*

Surgical Management for Heart Failure

HEART TRANSPLANTATION

When the heart is irreversibly damaged and no longer functions adequately and when the client is at risk of dying, cardiac transplantation and the use of an artificial heart to assist or replace the failing heart are measures of last resort. With the development of cyclosporine, and more recently FK-506 and mycophenolate mofetil, and with improvements in the procurement and preservation of donor hearts, cardiac transplantation has become an accepted therapeutic procedure. One-year survival rates after transplantation are greater than 85%. Although transplantation may not be appropriate for all clients, it may be the only option available to some. Heart transplantation is discussed in Chapter 57.

CARDIOMYOPLASTY

For clients with low cardiac output who are not candidates for cardiac transplantation, a procedure called *cardiomyoplasty* may support the failing heart. Initially developed in 1985, this procedure involves wrapping the latissimus dorsi muscle around the heart and electrostimulating it in synchrony with ventricular systole.

Immediate postoperative care is similar to that of any cardiac surgery client. Continuous cardiac and hemodynamic monitoring is initiated. Inotropic and vasopressor agents are administered to maintain cardiac output until the pulse generator is activated (within 2 to 3 weeks). Because the muscle flap obliterates the left upper lobe and can reduce vital capacity by as much as 20%, aggressive pulmonary hygiene and judicious pain management are essential to prevent atelectasis or pneumonia. In addition, an upper extremity exercise regimen is prescribed.

Modifications for Elderly Clients

Heart failure is becoming increasingly a disorder of the very old. Cardiac decompensation can be triggered by seemingly minor illnesses and dietary indiscretions.[45] Medications commonly used by older people may have an impact on heart performance even though they pose little risk of interaction with cardiovascular medications. Nonsteroidal anti-inflammatory drugs (NSAIDs) tend to worsen heart disease because they promote sodium retention; tricyclic antidepressants (TCAs) and neuroleptic

CASE MANAGEMENT

Heart Failure

Heart failure is one of the most prevalent chronic diseases in the United States, causing millions of dollars of health care resources to be spent on hospitalizations and frequent readmissions. Without management and follow-up, clients tend to be readmitted repeatedly as they become more debilitated. Many case management programs have been initiated in an attempt to break the cycle of constant readmission. Through programs involving assessment, education, rehabilitation, and follow-up, clients have been able to have fewer manifestations and to return to a higher level of function. Moreover, scarce health care resources have been saved.

Assess

- What are the underlying causes of the heart failure (coronary artery disease, acute myocardial infarction, hypertension, valvular disease, cardiomyopathy, congenital heart disease, infections, dysrhythmias)?
- Are there co-morbid diseases that might worsen the condition (e.g., diabetes mellitus, renal disease, chronic obstructive pulmonary disease)?
- What are the warning manifestations for this client when an episode of heart failure is beginning?
- What did the client experience before this admission or readmission (shortness of breath, weight gain, cough, chest pain, fatigue, lower extremity or abdominal edema)?
- What does this client know about preventing an episode of heart failure, and what is your assessment of the client's ability to follow the care plan after discharge?

Advocate

A diagnosis of heart failure may be frightening; clients may think that "failure" means that the heart is not beating or that they will die. Carefully explain what "heart failure" means in terms the client can understand. Discuss care needs openly and honestly. This client may need assistance in making decisions regarding increased care or changes in residence. Caregivers, especially spouses, may need respite or assistance, but may be reluctant to ask for help.

Be alert for cognitive impairments or decreased mental function due to low oxygen saturation levels. Most clients take multiple medications, necessitating accurate administration and considerable cost. Does the client have financial concerns, or will lack of finances prevent obtaining medications?

Do environmental or safety issues in the home make it difficult for the client to manage, such as entry stairways or upstairs bedrooms? Be alert for manifestations of anxiety and stress in work or home situations that may exacerbate heart failure, and review safety measures if home oxygen therapy is to be used.

Prevent Readmission

Make sure that clients know about each medication they will be taking; help to create a schedule for them to follow at home.

Emphasize the need to manage hypertension and lipid levels. Discuss diet, sodium restrictions and weight gain. Clients may not be aware of the high sodium content in canned or prepared foods; in fact, they may use these products because of their easier preparation.

Find out if a scale is available at home; teach taking daily weights at the same time each day and how to keep a weight record.

Review the need for rest periods (sitting with legs elevated) and for some exercise. Evaluate the need for cardiac rehabilitation, referral for smoking cessation, or home care services.

Investigate the availability of telephone or home visitation follow-up through area hospitals or community or insurer disease management programs.

Finally, make sure the client knows about the manifestations needing immediate physician intervention, the need for follow-up visits with the primary physician, and how to obtain emergency assistance.

Cheryl Noetscher, RN, MS, *Director of Case Management, Crouse Hospital and Community–General Hospital, Syracuse, New York*

agents lead to orthostatic hypotension. Conversely, cardiac performance can affect the medication's action. The development of RVF can markedly increase the prothrombin time and thereby increase the action of anticoagulants.[45] See the Case Management feature on heart failure.

CONCLUSIONS

Disorders of cardiac function are the leading causes of death in the industrialized world. It is imperative that you fully understand the care of clients with heart disease to improve the outcomes and quality of life and to reduce morbidity and mortality. CHD is the precursor to several problems. Your role is to educate the client about risk reduction. Heart failure is a frequent end-point of cardiac disease. It is important to maximize cardiac output and reduce system demands on the heart.

THINKING CRITICALLY

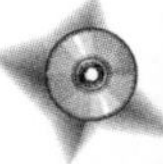

1. **Your client is a 67-year-old man with newly diagnosed insulin-dependent diabetes in end-stage heart failure. The client was recently released from the hospital. You are to begin intravenous dobutamine therapy during this initial home visit. What assessment should be made prior to initiating dobutamine therapy? What other assessment interventions might be done?**

Factors to Consider. How does heart failure respond to the administration of dobutamine? What teaching or learning needs might be assessed in the client?

2. **A 70-year-old man is scheduled for a coronary artery bypass graft. What postoperative complications are most prevalent in older adults?**

Factors to Consider. How is CABG surgery accomplished? Why is CABG surgery a popular option?

BIBLIOGRAPHY

1. Abou-Awdi, N. L., & Samuels, W. L. (1995). Transmyocardial laser revascularization. *Seminars in Perioperative Nursing, 4,* 173–176.
2. Albert, N. (1994). Laser angioplasty and intracoronary stents: Going beyond the balloon. *AACN Clinical Issues in Critical Care Nursing, 5,* 15–20.
3. Albert, N. (1999). Heart failure: The physiologic basis for current therapeutic concepts. *Critical Care Nurse, 19*(suppl. 6), 2–13.
4. Allen, B., et al. (1999). Comparison of transmyocardial revascularization with medical therapy in patients with refractory angina. *New England Journal of Medicine, 341,* 1029–1036.
5. American Association of Cardiovascular and Pulmonary Rehabilitation. (1995). *Guidelines for cardiac rehabilitation programs.* Champaign, IL: Human Kinetics.
6. American Heart Association. (1999). *Scientific statement on prevention of cardiovascular diseases.* Dallas: Author.
7. American Heart Association. (1998). *1999 heart and stroke statistical update.* Dallas: Author.
8. Aregenziano, M., et al. (1997). The influence of infection on survival and successful transplantation in patients with left ventricular assist devices. *Journal of Heart and Lung Transplantation, 16,* 822–831.
9. Assmann, G., et al. (1999). Coronary heart disease: Reducing the risk. *Arteriosclerosis, Thrombosis, and Vascular Biology, 19,* 1819–1824.
10. Baig, M. K., et al. (1998). The pathophysiology of advanced heart failure. *Heart and Lung, 28,* 87–97.
11. Ballard, J. C., Wood, L. L., & Lansing, A. M. (1997). Transmyocardial revascularization: Criteria for selecting patients, treatment, and nursing care. *Critical Care Nurse, 17,* 42–49.
12. Bittl, J. A., & Thomas, P. (1996). Beyond the balloon. *Harvard Health Letter, 21,* 4.
13. Cheng, J. W. M., & Rovera, N. G. (1998). Infection and atherosclerosis: Focus on cytomegalovirus and *Chlamydia pneumoniae. Annals of Pharmacotherapy, 32,* 1310–1315.
14. Cohn, J., et al. (1997). The U.S. carvedilol heart failure study: Safety and efficacy of carvedilol in severe heart failure. *Journal of Cardiac Failure, 3,* 173–179.
15. Davis, C., et al. (1997). Vascular complications of coronary interventions. *Heart and Lung, 26,* 118.
16. Doering, L. V. (1999). Pathophysiology of acute coronary syndromes leading to acute myocardial infarction. *Journal of Cardiovascular Nursing, 13*(3), 1–20.
17. Fischer, A., Gutstein, D. E., & Fuster, V. (1999). Thrombosis and coagulation abnormalities in the acute coronary syndromes. *Cardiology Clinics, 17,* 283–294.
18. Futterman, L. G., & Lemberg, L. (1999). The use of antioxidants in retarding atherosclerosis: Fact or fiction. *American Journal of Critical Care, 8,* 130–133.
19. Goodman, M., et al. (1996). Hostility predicts restenosis after percutaneous transluminal coronary angioplasty. *Mayo Clinic Proceedings, 71,* 729–734.
20. Gotto, A. M. (1998). Assessing the benefits of lipid-lowering therapy. *American Journal of Cardiology, 82,* 2m–4m.
21. Grundy, S. M., et al. (1997). Guide to primary prevention of cardiovascular disease: A statement for healthcare professionals from the Task Force on Risk Reduction. *Circulation, 95,* 2329–2331.
22. Gurfinkel, E., et al. (1997). Randomized trial of roxithromycin in non–Q-wave coronary syndromes: ROXIS pilot study. *Lancet, 2,* 404–407.
23. Gutstein, D. E., & Fuster, V. (1998). Pathophysiologic bases for adjunctive therapies in the treatment and secondary prevention of acute myocardial infarction. *Clinical Cardiology, 21,* 161–168.
24. Homes, L. M., & Hollabaugh, S. K. (1997). Using continuous quality improvement process to improve the care of patients after angioplasty. *Critical Care Nurse, 17,* 56–65.
25. Horvath, K. A., et al. (1996). Transmyocardial laser revascularization: Operative techniques and clinical results at two years. *Journal of Thoracic and Cardiovascular Surgery, 111*(15), 1047–1053.
26. Hulley, S., et al., Heart and Estrogen/Progestin Replacement Study (HERS) Research Group. (1998). Randomized trial of estrogen plus progestin for secondary prevention of coronary heart disease in postmenopausal women. *Journal of the American Medical Association, 280,* 605–613.
27. Jacobs, A. K., et al. (1998). Better outcome for women compared with men undergoing coronary revascularization: A report from the Bypass Angioplasty Revascularization Investigation (BARI). *Circulation, 98,* 1279–1285.
28. Keller, K. B., & Lemberg, L. (1998). Therapy for hyperlipidemia when it is the only risk factor: Fact or fiction? *American Journal of Critical Care, 7,* 395–397.
29. Kinney, M. R. (1995). Assessment of quality of life in recovery settings. *Journal of Cardiovascular Nursing, 10,* 88–96.
30. Konstam, M., et al. (1994). *Heart failure: Evaluation and care of patients with left ventricular systolic dysfunction. Clinical practice guideline No. 11* (AHCPR Pub. No. 94-0612). Rockville, MD: Agency for Health Care Policy and Research, Public Health Service, U.S. Department of Health and Human Services.
31. Michael, K., & Parnell, K. J. (1998). Innovations in the pharmacologic management of heart failure. *AACN Clinical Issues, 9,* 172–191.
32. Mizell, J. L., Maglish, B. L., & Matheny, R. G. (1997). Minimally invasive direct coronary artery bypass graft surgery. *Critical Care Nurse, 17,* 46–55.
33. Moore, S. M. (1995). A comparison of women's and men's symptoms during home recovery after coronary artery bypass surgery. *Heart and Lung, 24,* 495–501.
34. Mosca, L., et al. (1999). Guide to preventive cardiology for women. *Circulation, 99,* 2480–2484.
35. Moser, D. K. (1998). Pathophysiology of heart failure update: The role of neurohormonal activation on the progression of heart failure. *AACN Clinical Issues, 9,* 157–171.
36. Packer, M. (1997). End of the oldest controversy in medicine: Are we ready to conclude the debate on digitalis? *New England Journal of Medicine, 336,* 575–576.
37. Packer, M., & Cohn, J. N. (1999). Consensus recommendations for the management of chronic heart failure. *American Journal of Cardiology, 83,* 1A–38A.
38. Piano, M., Bondmass, M., & Schwertz, D. (1998). The molecular and cellular pathophysiology of heart failure. *Heart and Lung, 27,* 3–19.
39. Poirier, V. (1997). The heartmate left ventricular assist system: Worldwide clinical results. *European Journal of Cardio-Thoracic Surgery, 11,* 539–544.
40. Redeker, N. S., et al. (1995). Women's patterns of activity over 6 months after coronary artery bypass surgery. *Heart and Lung, 24,* 502–511.
41. Riddle, M. M., Dunston, J. L., & Castanes, J. L. (1996). A rapid recovery program for cardiac surgery patients. *American Journal of Critical Care, 5,* 152–159.
42. Saatvedt, K., Dragsundm, M., & Nordstrandt, K. (1996). Transmyocardial laser revascularization and coronary artery bypass grafting. *Annals of Thoracic Surgery, 62*(1), 323–324.
43. Scherr, K., Jensen, L., & Koshal, A. (1999). Mechanical circulation as a bridge to cardiac transplantation: Toward the 21st century. *American Journal of Critical Care, 8,* 324–335.
44. Shah, P. K. (1996). Pathophysiology of plaque rupture and the concept of plaque stabilization. *Cardiology Clinics, 14*(1), 17–28.
45. Stanley, M. (1997). Current trends in the clinical management of an old enemy: Congestive heart failure in the elderly. *AACN Clinical Issues, 8,* 616–626.
46. Stary, H. C., et al. (1995). A definition of advanced types of atherosclerotic lesions and a histological classification of atherosclerosis. *Circulation, 92,* 1355–1374.
47. Strimike, C. L. (1995). Caring for a patient with an intracoronary stent. *American Journal of Nursing, 95,* 40–45.
48. Sulzbach, L. M., Hazard-Munro, B., & Hirshfield, J. (1995). A randomized clinical trial of the effect of bed position after PTCA. *American Journal of Critical Care, 4,* 221–226.
49. Wenger, N. K. (1998). Addressing coronary heart disease risk in women. *Cleveland Clinic Journal of Medicine, 65,* 464–469.
50. Wenger, N. K. (1999). Women, myocardial infarction, and coronary revascularization. *Cardiology in Review, 7,* 117–120.
51. Wenger, N. K., et al. (1995). *Cardiac rehabilitation as secondary prevention. Clinical practice guideline: Quick reference guide for clinicians, No. 17* (AHCPR Pub No. 96-0672). Rockville, MD:

Agency for Health Care Policy and Research, and the National Heart, Lung, and Blood Institute, Public Health Service, U.S. Department of Health and Human Services.

52. Wolff, C. A., Scott, C., & Banks, T. A. (1997). The radial artery: An exciting alternative conduit in coronary artery bypass surgery. *Critical Care Nurse, 17,* 34–39.

53. Zevola, D. R., et al. (1997). Clinical pathways and coronary artery bypass surgery. *Critical Care Nurse, 17,* 20–33.

54. Zhou, J., et al. (1999). Plaque pathology and coronary thrombosis in the pathogenesis of acute coronary syndromes. *Scandinavian Journal of Clinical and Laboratory Investigation, 59*(suppl. 230), 3–11.

CHAPTER

REMEMBER *to check out your* Companion CD ROM

57 Management of Clients with Dysrhythmias

Maribeth Guzzo

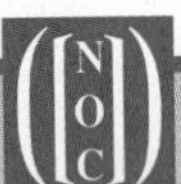

NURSING OUTCOMES CLASSIFICATION (NOC)
for Nursing Diagnoses—Clients with Dysrhythmias

Anxiety
Anxiety Control
Coping

Decreased Cardiac Output
Circulation Status
Vital Signs Status

The heart is endowed with a specialized system for generating rhythmic electrical impulses and for conducting these impulses rapidly throughout the heart to cause contraction of the heart muscle. When this system functions normally, the atria contract about one-sixth of a second ahead of the ventricles. This orderly electrical activity must precede contraction to provide adequate cardiac output for perfusion of all body organs and tissues.

The rhythmical and conduction systems of the heart are susceptible to damage by heart disease, especially by ischemia of the heart tissues resulting from decreased coronary artery blood flow. The consequence is often a bizarre heart rhythm or abnormal sequence of contraction through the heart chambers. The abnormal rhythms, called *dysrhythmias* (or arrhythmias), can severely decrease the heart's ability to pump effectively, even to the extent of causing death.

Before reading about dysrhythmias, you may want to review the electrical conduction system of the heart in the Unit 12 review and/or the electrocardiogram (ECG) in Chapter 54.

A *normal sinus rhythm* is a heart rhythm that begins in the sinoatrial (SA) node, is between 60 and 100 beats per minute (BPM), and has normal intervals and no aberrant or ectopic beats (Fig. 57–1). Characteristics of normal sinus rhythm are shown in Table 57–1.

DYSRHYTHMIAS

Dysrhythmias (abnormal heart rhythms) are common in people with cardiac disorders but also occur in people with normal hearts. Dysrhythmias are often detected because of associated manifestations of dizziness, palpitations, and syncope. Abnormalities in conduction are dangerous because of reduced cardiac output, which can lead to impaired cerebral perfusion. The most serious complication of a dysrhythmia is sudden death.[1, 9] Since seconds can literally make the difference between life and death for the person who is experiencing a serious dysrhythmia, evaluating responsiveness, quickly activating the emergency medical service (EMS), and initiating cardiopulmonary resuscitation (CPR) can determine the outcome.

Etiology and Risk Factors

Dysrhythmias result from disturbances in three major mechanisms: (1) automaticity, (2) conduction, and (3) problems with reentry of impulses.[6, 8, 32]

DISTURBANCES IN AUTOMATICITY

The term *automaticity* is used to describe alterations in the normal heart rates produced by various pacemaker cells in the myocardium. Recall that the SA node is the pacemaker of the heart because it possesses the highest level of automaticity. It normally produces a rhythm of 60 to 100 BPM. The SA node is regulated by the nervous system through the vagus nerve. Sympathetic stimulation increases the rate of firing; lack of sympathetic stimulation or vagal stimulation (which is parasympathetic) decreases the rate.

If the SA node fails to initiate an impulse, every other muscle cell in the myocardium can start the impulse. This fail-safe mechanism is crucial during heart disease. Latent pacemaker cells in the atrioventricular (AV) junction usually assume the role of pacemaker of the heart but at a slower rate (40 to 60 BPM). Such a pacemaker is called an "escape" pacemaker. If the AV junction cannot take over as the pacemaker because of disease, an escape pacemaker in the electrical conduction system below the AV junction (i.e., in the bundle branches or Purkinje

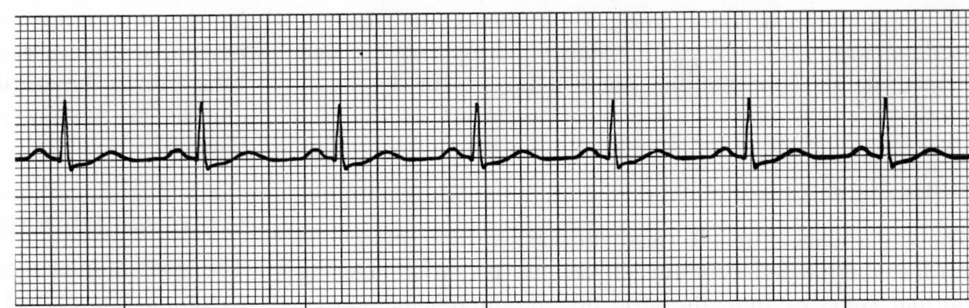

FIGURE 57–1 Normal sinus rhythm as seen on an electrocardiogram (ECG) strip. Note the regular R-R interval, a rate of 80 beats per minute, and a P-R interval of 0.16 second.

fibers) may take over at a still lower rate (<40 BPM). In general, the farther the escape pacemaker is from the SA node, the slower it generates electrical impulses.

These impulses can also occur prematurely—before the SA node would normally fire again. Premature impulses occur when the heart is ischemic, as with coronary artery disease. Myocardial infarction (MI) or heart failure is characterized by areas of calcification along different points in the heart as a normal variant or by irritation of the AV node, Purkinje system, or myocardium from drugs, nicotine, or caffeine.

Under a variety of circumstances, cardiac cells in any part of the heart, whether they are latent pacemaker cells or nonpacemaker myocardial cells, may take on the role of a pacemaker and start generating extraneous electrical impulses. When impulses begin from other sites, the sites are called "ectopic" pacemakers. For instance, if the SA node fails to fire, other sites in the atria can fire. If the atria do not initiate a beat, it can begin in the AV node; if the AV node does not initiate a beat, one can start in the ventricles. When an ectopic pacemaker initiates a beat, the appearance of the ECG differs from the way it looks with a normal sinus rhythm beat.

Each of these areas of myocardium (atria, AV node, ventricles) has its own intrinsic rate:

- Sinus node, 60 to 100 BPM
- Atria, 60 to 100 BPM
- AV node, 40 to 60 BPM
- Ventricles, 20 to 40 BPM

Latent pacemaker cells can also fire at increased rates beyond their inherent rate. When rates exceed these values, the rhythm is called "accelerated" and classified as a problem of "altered automaticity." For example, an accelerated junctional tachycardia can develop with a rate higher than 60 BPM (the inherent AV node rate). Abnormal automaticity is commonly caused by ischemia, hyperkalemia, hypocalcemia, hypoxia, increased catecholamine levels, digitalis toxicity, and administration of atropine. A rhythm faster than the intrinsic rate is called *tachycardia*. A rhythm slower than the intrinsic rate is called *bradycardia*. Therefore, sinus bradycardia is identified as a heart rate below 60 BPM and sinus tachycardia is defined as a heart rate above 100 BPM.

Disturbances in Conduction

Conduction is the speed the impulse travels through the sinus node, AV node, and Purkinje fibers. Conduction may be either too rapid or too slow. Blocks that slow or stop an impulse can occur anywhere along the pathway. Blocks can result from ischemia of the tissues, scarring of conduction pathways, compression of the AV bundle by scar tissue, inflammation of the AV node, extreme vagal stimulation of the heart, electrolyte imbalances, increased atrial preload, digitalis toxicity, beta-blocking agents, impaired cellular metabolism, MI (especially inferior), and valvular surgery.

Blocks result in ECG changes in appearance. Because the blocked impulse needs more time to travel to its destination, the wave is wider than normal. Disturbances in conduction can also lead to decreased cardiac output and life-threatening dysrhythmias.

Reentry of Impulses

Reentry is the activation of muscle for a second time by the same impulse. The waves of electrical impulse are not extinguished but persist because of a combination of slow conduction and blocks. Therefore, the conduction system is delayed or blocked (or both) in one or more segments while being transmitted normally through the rest of this system.

The problem occurs when some cells have been repolarized sufficiently so that they can prematurely depolarize again, producing ectopic beats and rhythms. Hyperkalemia and myocardial ischemia are the two most common causes of delay or block in the conduction system responsible for the reentry mechanism. The reentry mechanism can result in atrial fibrillation (AFib) and ventricular fibrillation (VFib).

Risk Factors

Understanding which client populations are at risk for development of abnormal heart rhythms can be useful in preventing and correcting these abnormalities. Myocardial

TABLE 57–1 CHARACTERISTICS OF NORMAL SINUS RHYTHMS

Rhythm	Regular, P–P intervals and R–R intervals may vary as much as 3 mm and still be considered regular
Rate	60–100 beats per minute
P waves	One P Wave preceding each QRS complex
P–R interval	0.12–0.20 second, consistent with each complex
QRS complex	0.04–0.10 second, consistent with each complex
Q–T interval	<0.40 second

ischemia, hypoxia, autonomic nervous system imbalances, lactic acidosis, electrolyte imbalances, drug toxicity, and hemodynamic abnormalities are risk factors for dysrhythmias.

Pathophysiology

The significance of all dysrhythmias is their effect on cardiac output and cerebral or vascular perfusion. During normal sinus rhythm, the atria fill and stretch the ventricles with about 30% more blood. This process is called the *atrial kick.* The extra stretch improves contractility of the ventricles and thereby increases cardiac output. When the impulse starts in the AV node or in the ventricles, atrial and ventricular contraction are no longer coordinated. Atrial kick is lost and cardiac output falls. For example, during contractions initiated in the ventricle the impulse begins in the ventricle and travels backward up the heart. As a result, the atria fill the ventricles while they are contracting or even afterward. Obviously, the efficiency of the heart as a pump is restricted during dysrhythmias and the clinical manifestations noted are due to changes in cardiac output.

Clinical Manifestations

The reduced cardiac output leads to clinical manifestations of dysrhythmias: palpitations, dizziness or syncope, pallor, diaphoresis, altered mentation (restlessness and agitation to lethargy and coma), hypotension, sluggish capillary refill, swelling of the extremities, and diminished urinary output. Palpitations, dizziness, and syncope are the clinical manifestations that are most effectively evaluated by ambulatory ECG monitoring. The client wears a portable ECG monitor and manually records (writes down) worrisome manifestations, and the correlation of manifestations to the heart rhythm can then be assessed. Shortness of breath, chest pain, and fatigue may also be caused by dysrhythmias. However, these manifestations are probably caused by other factors, such as myocardial ischemia and heart failure.

Depending upon the type of dysrhythmia, physical assessment findings may reveal (1) a heart rate below 50 or above 140 BPM; (2) an extremely irregular heart rhythm or pulse; (3) a first heart sound that varies in intensity; (4) sudden appearance of heart failure, shock, and angina pectoris; and (5) a slow, regular heart rate that does not change with activity or medications such as atropine or epinephrine.

Diagnostic findings include ECG abnormalities. The key to dysrhythmia interpretation is the analysis of the form and interrelations of the P wave, the P-R interval, and the QRS complex. The ECG should be analyzed with respect to its rate, rhythm, and site of the dominant pacemaker as well as the configuration of the P and QRS waves. Remember, any ECG findings should be correlated with clinical observations of the client; that is, "treat the client, not the monitor."

You will find it necessary to develop a method of analyzing ECG strips that allows you to consistently identify the rhythm demonstrated. The analysis of rhythms is one of two types: sight reading or paper analysis. Sight readers analyze ECGs by looking at the whole rhythm. Much experience and continual, regular viewing of rhythm strips are required for this technique, which is of little use to the beginner. Health care providers with less experience need to develop a method of ECG analysis (Box 57–1).

Outcome Management

The goal of management is to control or ablate the dysrhythmia and reduce potential complications from it. The specific management of dysrhythmias depends on the type and on the client's response to it. All dysrhythmias can reduce cardiac output, which can cause a client to have no manifestations or to have many. Rhythm disturbances resulting in syncope, near-syncope, or sudden death warrant further evaluation. Ventricular dysrhythmias can be life-threatening, demanding immediate treatment. This chapter reviews dysrhythmias and their management, progressing from problems arising (1) in the atria, (2) in the AV junction, and (3) in the ventricles.

ATRIAL DYSRHYTHMIAS

DISTURBANCES IN AUTOMATICITY

SINUS TACHYCARDIA

Sinus tachycardia is characterized by a rapid, regular rhythm at a rate of 100 to 180 BPM with a normal P wave and QRS complex (Fig. 57–2*A*). It often occurs in response to an increase in sympathetic stimulation or decreased vagal (parasympathetic) stimulation. Causes include the following:

- Fever
- Emotional and physical stress
- Heart failure
- Fluid volume loss
- Hyperthyroidism
- Hypercalcemia
- Medications, including, atropine, nitrates, epinephrine, and isoproterenol
- Caffeine
- Nicotine
- Exercise

Most clients do not experience clinical manifestations except for occasional palpitations. However, the clinical manifestations depend on the heart rate and its effect on cardiac output. Between these quick beats, there is little time for ventricular filling and atrial contraction. Clients with underlying heart disease may not tolerate the increased myocardial workload and reduced coronary artery filling time that accompanies the increased heart rate. These clients may experience hypotension and angina pectoris (chest pain).

Management focuses on alleviating the underlying cause and reducing further demands on the heart. Medications such as digitalis, beta-adrenergic blocking agents (e.g., propranolol), and calcium channel blockers may be prescribed.[1, 23, 32] Bed rest is ordered to reduce metabolic demand. Oxygen may be prescribed to supply the myocardium adequately.

BOX 57–1 Electrocardiographic Interpretation of Dysrhythmias

There are seven basic steps to assist you in the identification of dysrhythmias. The electrocardiogram (ECG) should be studied in an *orderly* fashion as follows:

Step 1

Calculate the heart rate. The simplest method for obtaining the rate is to count the number of R waves in a 6-inch strip of the ECG tracing (which equals 6 seconds). Multiply this sum by 10 to get the rate per minute (BPM). Because the ECG paper is marked into 3-inch intervals (at the top margin), the approximate heart rate can be rapidly calculated.

Another method is to count the number of large squares between R waves. Find an R wave crossing a large square. Count the number of large squares until the next R wave. The approximate heart rate is

1 large square = 300 BPM
2 large squares = 150 BPM
3 large squares = 100 BPM
4 large squares = 75 BPM
5 large squares = 60 BPM
6 large squares = 50 BPM
7 large squares = 43 BPM
8 large squares = 37 BPM
9 large squares = 33 BPM
10 large squares = 30 BPM

Step 2

Measure the regularity (rhythm) of the R waves (ventricular rhythm). This can be done by gross observation or actual measurement of the intervals (R-R).

If the R waves occur at regular intervals (variance <0.12 second between beats), the ventricular rhythm is normal. When there are differences in R-R intervals (>0.12 second), the ventricular rhythm is said to be irregular. The division of ventricular rhythm into regular and irregular categories assists in identifying the mechanism of many dysrhythmias.

Note atrial regularity and measure the atrial rate. Measure the regularity (rhythm) of the P waves (P-P). Use the above method, but calculate the distance between the same point on two consecutive P waves.

Step 3

Examine the P waves. If P waves are present and precede each QRS complex, the heartbeat originates in the sinus node and a sinus rhythm exists. The absence of P waves or an abnormality in their position with respect to the QRS complex indicates that the impulse started outside the sinoatrial node and that an ectopic pacemaker is in command.

Step 4

Measure the P-R interval. Normally, this interval should be between 0.12 and 0.20 second. Prolongation or reduction of this interval beyond these limits indicates a defect in the conduction system between the atria and the ventricles.

Step 5

Measure the duration of the QRS complex. If the width between the onset of the Q wave and the completion of the S wave is greater than 0.12 second (three fine lines on the paper), an intraventricular conduction defect exists.

Step 6

Examine the ST segment. Normally, this segment is isoelectric, meaning it is neither elevated nor depressed because the positive and negative forces are equally balanced during this period. Elevation or depression of the ST segment indicates an abnormality in the onset of recovery of the ventricular muscle, usually because of injury (e.g., acute myocardial infarction).

Step 7

Examine the T wave. Normally, the T wave is upright and one-third the height of the QRS complex. Any condition that interferes with normal repolarization (e.g., myocardial ischemia) may cause the T waves to invert. An abnormally high serum potassium level causes the T wave to become very tall—sometimes the height of the QRS complex.

SINUS BRADYCARDIA

Sinus bradycardia occurs when the SA node fires at a rate of less than 60 times per minute. The P wave and QRS complex are normal (Fig. 57–2*B*). Sinus bradycardia may result from the following:

- Increased vagal (parasympathetic) tone, as occurs with Valsalva's maneuver (e.g., straining while moving bowels)
- Drugs (especially digitalis, propranolol, or verapamil)
- MI (most often inferior MI)
- Hyperkalemia
- Various diseases, such as hypothyroidism, myxedema, and obstructive jaundice

In some people, sinus bradycardia can be a normal condition. Athletes often have sinus bradycardia because their heart is an effective pump with a greater than normal stroke volume. Because cardiac output is the product of stroke volume and heart rate, the heart rate decreases, yet cardiac output is adequate.

Clients may be asymptomatic; when manifestations do develop, it is because cardiac output is decreased. Fatigue, hypotension, lightheadedness, syncope, shortness of breath, decreased level of consciousness, pulmonary congestion, or heart failure may develop. The slowed rate of SA discharge may allow junctional or ventricular pacemakers to take over, thereby producing ectopic beats.

The aim of management is to correct the underlying cause of sinus bradycardia, and the goal of intervention is to increase the heart rate just enough to relieve manifestations but not enough to cause tachycardia. The intervention sequence for treating symptomatic bradycardia is atropine, transcutaneous pacing if available, dopamine, epinephrine, and isoproterenol or insertion of a temporary transvenous pacemaker.[1, 23, 32]

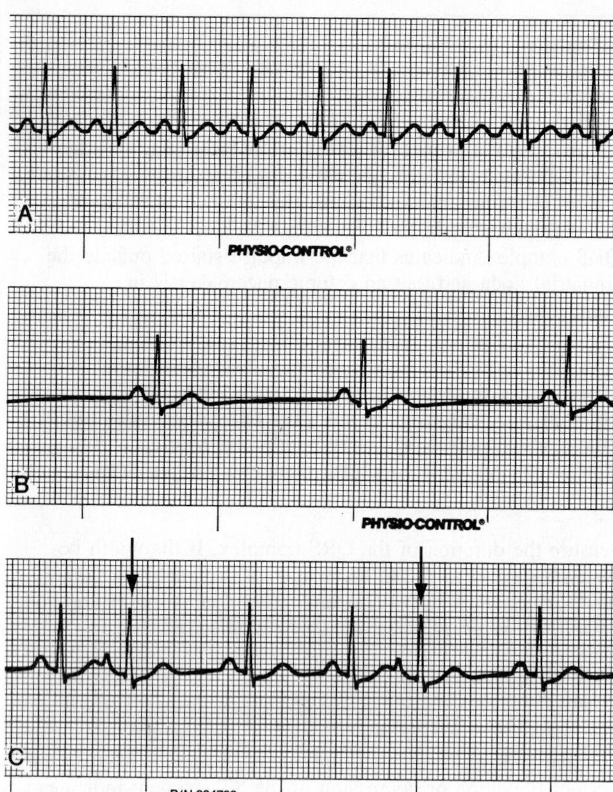

FIGURE 57–2 Atrial dysrhythmias. *A*, Sinus tachycardia—regular R-R interval, rate 125 beats per minute (BPM); P-R interval, 0.16 second. *B*, Sinus bradycardia—regular R-R interval, rate 40 BPM; P-R interval, 0.16. *C*, Premature atrial contractions. The second and fifth beat are premature atrial contractions (PACs). Note the difference in appearance of the P wave and the shortened R-R interval.

Sinus Dysrhythmia

Sinus dysrhythmia is characterized by phasic changes in the automaticity of the SA node, which cause it to fire at varying speeds. The heart rate generally ranges between 60 and 100 BPM. The ECG shows a normal P wave, P-R interval, and QRS complex; the only abnormality is an irregular P-P interval.

Sinus dysrhythmia may develop from alterations in vagal tone and in response to delayed atrial filling with inhalation. During inspiration, venous return to the right atrium is delayed because of increased intrathoracic pressure. In quiet respiration, the heart rate can decrease about 5%; with deep respiration, the rate can decrease up to 30%.

Clients with sinus dysrhythmia do not usually require intervention other than alleviation of the underlying cause. Cardiac output is not affected.

Premature Atrial Contractions

Premature atrial contractions (PACs) are early beats arising from ectopic atrial foci, interrupting the normal rhythm. Commonly resulting from enhanced automaticity of the atrial muscle, PACs occur in both normal and diseased hearts. PACs are associated with valvular disease and atrial chamber enlargement; they may also be seen with stress, fatigue, alcohol, smoking, coronary artery disease (CAD), cardiac ischemia, heart failure, cardioactive medications (digitalis, quinidine, procainamide), pulmonary congestion, and pulmonary hypertension. Frequent PACs may mark the onset of AFib or heart failure or may reflect electrolyte imbalances.

In clients with PACs, P waves are premature and differ from the normal sinus P wave in appearance, size, or shape (Fig. 57–2*C*). Premature beats from any ectopic focus can be palpated as skipped or irregular beats. The client who experiences numerous PACs may note palpitations, or "missed beats." PACs are usually benign; however, if the client has increasing numbers of "skipped beats" or feels palpitations often, the problem should be evaluated. Intervention usually focuses on correcting the underlying cause and may include administration of quinidine or procainamide.

DISTURBANCES IN CONDUCTION

Sinoatrial Node Conduction Defects

Under certain circumstances, the impulse from the SA node is either (1) not generated in the SA node *(SA arrest)* or (2) not conducted from the SA node *(sinus exit block)*. Causes of SA node conduction abnormalities include the following:

- Conditions that increase vagal tone
- Coronary artery disease
- MI
- Digitalis and calcium channel blocker toxicity
- Hypertensive disease
- Tissue hypoxia
- Scarring of intra-atrial pathways
- Electrolyte imbalances

During *SA arrest*, neither the atria nor the ventricles are stimulated, resulting in a pause in the rhythm. An entire PQRST complex will be missing for one or more cycles. After the pause of sinus arrest, a new pacemaker focus assumes the pacing responsibility. The new pacer paces the heart at its inherent rate, which is usually slower than the original SA node rate. The new pacer site is often another atrial focus, but the junction or ventricle can also assume pacing responsibility.

During *sinus exit block*, there is a conduction delay between the sinus node and the atrial muscle. Unlike the rhythm in SA arrest, the rhythm of SA node discharge in sinus exist block remains constant and uninterrupted. The ECG characteristically displays a normal sinus rhythm that is interrupted intermittently by pauses. This creates a pattern of pauses that, when measured, are multiples of the underlying P-P interval. Sinus arrest differs from SA exit block, in that the SA node at times does not fire at all. The result is the occurrence of pauses that are longer and not a multiple of the underlying P-P interval. These pauses are also frequently terminated by escape ectopic beats. Sinus arrest often is associated with a more serious prognosis.

The client usually remains asymptomatic, depending on the duration and frequency of the pauses; however, lengthy pauses can cause lightheadedness or syncope. Intervention is unnecessary unless the client becomes symptomatic and exhibits manifestations of decreased cardiac output. An irregular pulse can be palpated or auscultated. Clinicians can only infer impulse formation within the SA node from the appearance of P waves, which reflect atrial depolarization.

Intervention may include administration of a vagolytic (atropine) or a sympathomimetic (isoproterenol) agent to increase the rate of SA node firing. If pharmacologic measures fail, a pacemaker may be required. Finally, the physician must determine and treat the underlying cause of the dysrhythmia.[1, 23, 32]

REENTRY OF IMPULSES

PAROXYSMAL ATRIAL TACHYCARDIA

Paroxysmal atrial tachycardia (PAT) is the sudden onset and sudden termination of a rapid firing from an ectopic atrial pacemaker (Fig. 57–3*A*). PAT is due to the reentry phenomenon. This process allows (1) the atrial impulses to travel down less refractory conduction pathways to the bundle of His and (2) retrograde conduction through previously refractory parallel fibers. A circular circuit for rapid repetitive depolarizations results from these events.

PAT occasionally appears in clients with a normal heart but most commonly develops in clients with cardiac disease. Common cardiac problems precipitating PAT include the following:

- MI
- Cardiomyopathy
- Extreme emotions
- Caffeine ingestion
- Fatigue
- Smoking
- Excessive alcohol intake

Less common causes include rheumatic heart disease, valvular disease, pulmonary emboli, cor pulmonale, thyrotoxicosis, digitalis toxicity (PAT with block), and cardiac surgery.

Clinicians identify PAT by three or more consecutive atrial ectopic beats occurring at a rate greater than 150 BPM alternating with normal sinus rhythm. The P waves are usually upright, narrow, and peaked in lead II. At faster atrial rates, the P waves may become lost in the preceding T wave. The P-R intervals may be normal. However, rapid atrial rates may overcome the conduction limits of the AV node, causing varying degrees of AV block. Atrial tachycardia with 2:1 block (i.e., two P waves for every QRS complex) most often results from digitalis toxicity. The QRS complexes are usually normal, although aberrant ventricular conduction may occur at

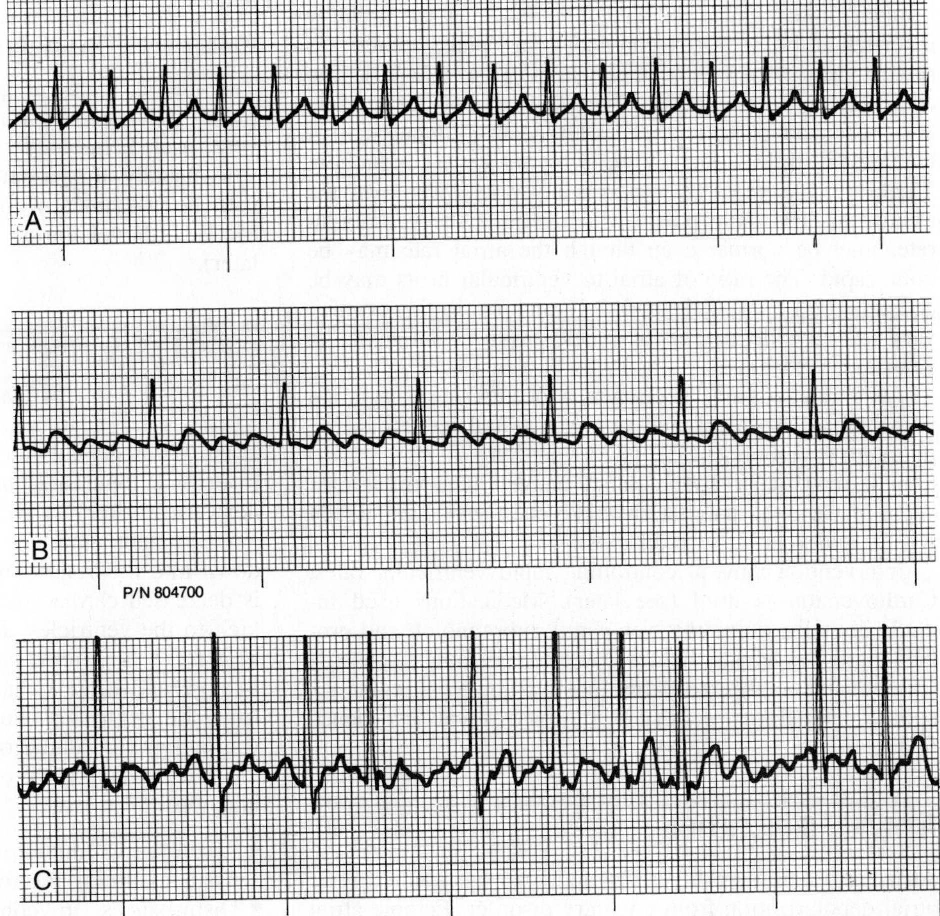

FIGURE 57–3 *A*, Paroxysmal atrial tachycardia (PAT). The rate is rapid, about 175 beats per minute (BPM). The P wave is not distinguishable, but the QRS complex is narrow, indicating that the impulse began above the atrioventricular node. *B*, Atrial flutter. Note the saw-toothed appearance of the P waves. There are three P waves for every QRS complex, indicating a 3:1 block. Atrial rate is 75 BPM. *C*, Atrial fibrillation is identifiable by a chaotic P wave, not one clear P wave, and an irregular R-R interval.

very rapid atrial rates or when a conduction defect exists within the ventricle.

PAT decreases ventricular filling time and mean arterial pressure and also increases myocardial oxygen demand. Clients may report palpitations and lightheadedness.

Management varies with the severity of manifestations. Clients with extremely rapid heart rates or significant underlying cardiovascular disease may experience syncope and heart failure. In such instances, heart rate must be immediately reduced. Any maneuver that stimulates the vagus nerve can successfully terminate PAT or increase AV block. The vagus nerve can be stimulated by carotid sinus massage and Valsalva's maneuver (bearing down). Useful pharmacologic agents include adenosine, verapamil, and beta-blockers. Sedatives may also be used to reduce sympathetic stimulation. The physician may also employ cardioversion (see later) as an effective means of terminating PAT if medications and vagal stimulation are not effective.

Ablation procedures that destroy a part of the reentrant path are being more widely used (see later). Such procedures can result in a long-term cure in selected clients.[1, 6, 21, 23, 32]

ATRIAL FLUTTER

Atrial flutter is a dysrhythmia arising in an ectopic pacemaker or the site of a rapid reentry circuit in the atria, characterized by rapid "saw-toothed" atrial wave formations and usually by a slower, regular ventricular response. Atrial flutter differs from PAT, in that it produces a much more rapid atrial rate. The P waves are actually inverted or bidirectional, producing a "picket fence" or saw-toothed pattern of "flutter waves" (Fig. 57–3*B*). The atrial rate generally ranges from 220 to 350 BPM. The AV node cannot conduct all of the atrial impulses that bombard it; that is, the AV node blocks a 1:1 conduction. Therefore, the ventricular rate is always slower than the atrial rate. Thus, the pulse, which reflects the ventricular rate, may be normal even though the atrial rate may be quite rapid. The ratio of atrial to ventricular beats may be constant (2:1, 3:1, 4:1, and 7:1, and so forth) or may vary. A variable degree of block produces an irregular ventricular rhythm.

Atrial flutter most commonly occurs in association with organic diseases such as CAD, mitral valve disease, pulmonary embolus (PE), and hyperthyroidism. In addition, it may occur after cardiac surgery. The client may sense occasional palpitations and chest pain, especially when rapid ventricular rates exist.

Intervention aims at controlling rapid ventricular rates. Cardioversion is used (see later). Medications used include digitalis, quinidine, verapamil, propranolol, and procainamide, especially if cardioversion is not successful. Carotid sinus massage helps to slow the ventricular response temporarily so that flutter waves can be identified.[1, 23, 32]

ATRIAL FIBRILLATION

Atrial fibrillation (AFib) is characterized by rapid, chaotic atrial depolarization from a reentry disorder. Ectopic atrial foci produce impulses between 400 and 700 BPM. At extremely rapid rates, however, the entire atrium may not be able to recover from one depolarization wave before the next begins. This results in mechanical and electrical disorganization of the atria. As with atrial flutter, the AV node is bombarded with more impulses than it can conduct. Most of these impulses are blocked; however, as a result of the erratic atrial impulses, there is a very irregular ventricular rhythm. The ventricular rate ranges from 160 to 180 BPM.

Examination of the ECG reveals erratic or no identifiable P waves and underlying ventricular rhythm that appears to be irregular and undulating (Fig. 57–3*C*). Because of atrial disorganization, there is no "atrial kick." This loss of additional blood volume can decrease cardiac output by as much as 20% to 30%. With increasing ventricular rates, cardiac output falls even further and may result in angina pectoris, heart failure, and shock.

AFib may be associated with sick sinus syndrome, hypoxia, increased atrial pressure, pericarditis, and many other conditions. Clients may be asymptomatic, or they may note an irregular pulse and palpitations. The client may have a pulse deficit between apical and radial pulses.

Mural thrombi formation can severely complicate the condition. Blood pools in the "quivering" atria because of lack of adequate contraction of atrial muscle. This blood can clot, which increases the potential for cerebral and pulmonary vascular emboli. Most clients with sudden onset of AFib are given heparin as an anticoagulant to reduce risk of stroke and PE until the impulses are controlled.

Outcome Management

The initial treatment goal is to control the rate of impulses with administration of drugs such as diltiazem, verapamil, beta-blockers, or digoxin. Chemical cardioversion, usually after a period of anticoagulation therapy, can then be attempted with procainamide or quinidine. Electrical cardioversion is the third therapeutic option (see later).

ATRIOVENTRICULAR JUNCTIONAL DYSRHYTHMIAS

If the SA node fails to fire and an impulse is not initiated in other ectopic sites in the atria, the AV junction is the next pacemaker for the heart. An impulse begins in the junction and simultaneously spreads up to the atria and down into the ventricles. During junctional rhythms, there is decreased cardiac output resulting from a lack of atrial kick to the ventricles. Junctional rhythms are not dependable for a long-term cardiac pacemaker because the rate is slow and more irritable ectopic foci may fire, such as from the ventricles. Consider junctional rhythms to be a warning or forerunner of more serious dysrhythmias.

Two major types of dysrhythmias arise in the AV junction:

- Disturbances in automaticity, with the AV junctional tissue assuming the role of the pacemaker
- Disturbances in conduction, with the AV junction

blocking impulses journeying from the atria to the ventricles

Both types of dysrhythmias may result from ischemia or trauma in the area of the AV junction (i.e., after MI or cardiac surgery). Digitalis toxicity, quinidine toxicity, and hyperkalemia may also cause junctional dysrhythmias.

Junctional rhythms produce abnormal upward direction of impulse (e.g., in lead II the P waves are inverted), because the impulse is traveling through the atria in a direction opposite to that found in normal sinus rhythm. Also, the P-R interval shortens to less than 0.12 second. The impulse may spread through the atria at the same time that the ventricles are being activated by the AV junction. In this instance, the P wave would be buried in the QRS complex and not observed on the ECG. Also, the atria may contract after the ventricles. In this case, the P wave would follow the QRS complex. The QRS complex is normal if ventricular conduction is normal.

DISTURBANCES IN AUTOMATICITY

The major junctional dysrhythmias caused by changes in automaticity are (1) premature junctional contractions (PJCs), (2) junctional escape rhythm, and (3) junctional tachycardias. As with PACs, an ectopic focus in the AV junctional tissue may develop increased automaticity and discharge prematurely, initiating depolarization of the heart.

PREMATURE JUNCTIONAL CONTRACTIONS

A PJC is the single, early firing of a junctional ectopic focus (Fig. 57–4). PJCs are slower as a result of lower intrinsic rates. Usually, clients can tolerate junctional rhythms, although clients with severe forms of cardiac disease may not because of decreased cardiac output.

PAROXYSMAL JUNCTIONAL TACHYCARDIA

A junctional rhythm with a rate that exceeds 60 BPM is termed a *junctional tachycardia.* It usually stops and starts abruptly, thereby acquiring the name *paroxysmal junctional tachycardia,* or PJT. The usual rate is 140 to 220 BPM.

Causes of PJT include metabolic imbalances and increased sympathetic stimulation. Rapid ventricular rates can lead to left ventricular failure resulting from increased myocardial oxygen demand and decreased blood supply. PJT that cannot be distinguished from PAT on the ECG is called *supraventricular tachycardia* (SVT).

Management of rapid junctional rhythms begins with vagal stimulation such as carotid sinus massage. If clinical manifestations develop, treatment consists of pharmacologic agents and cardioversion. Common medications include propranolol, quinidine, and digitalis. Evaluation of digitalis intoxication and potassium levels may also be indicated.[1, 32]

DISTURBANCES IN CONDUCTION

AV block comprises the second group of disturbances arising in the area of the AV junction. Impulses passing through the AV junction are blocked to varying degrees. Therefore, the conduction of impulses from the atria to the ventricles slows or stops entirely, depending on the degree of the AV block. Normally the impulse coming from the SA node is delayed at the AV junction for less than 0.20 second before traveling on to the bundle of His. If the AV junction has been damaged by ischemia, rheumatic fever, or drug toxicity, impulses are delayed or completely blocked at the AV junction for abnormally long periods of time.

FIRST-DEGREE ATRIOVENTRICULAR BLOCK

First-degree AV block is a delay in passage of the impulse from atria to ventricles. This delay usually occurs at the level of the AV node. The rhythm is regular, and each P wave is followed by a QRS complex; however, the P-R interval is prolonged beyond the normal 0.20 second. The P-R interval usually remains constant (Fig. 57–5*A*). This characteristic is an important differentiation between first-degree AV block and the other AV blocks. This block is often associated with CAD, increased vagal tone, and congenital anomalies and may also result from digitalis administration.

First-degree AV block, existing alone as the only abnormal feature of a client's ECG, produces no clinical manifestations and requires no intervention. If the block is a result of digitalis, the medication may be discontinued. Because first-degree AV block can progress to a higher-degree AV block, the client requires observation and ECG monitoring.[1, 32]

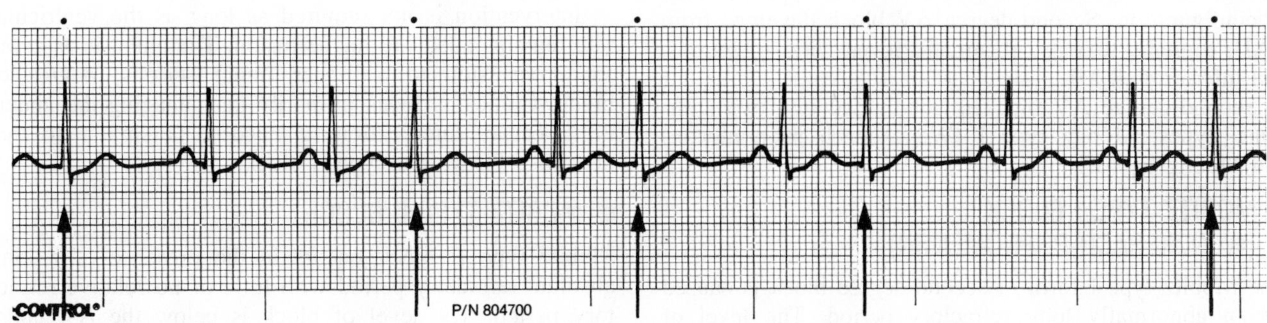

FIGURE 57–4 A premature junctional contraction. The beats marked with *arrows* are premature junctional contractions. Note the absence of a P wave but otherwise normal deflection, indicating that the impulse was initiated above the ventricles.

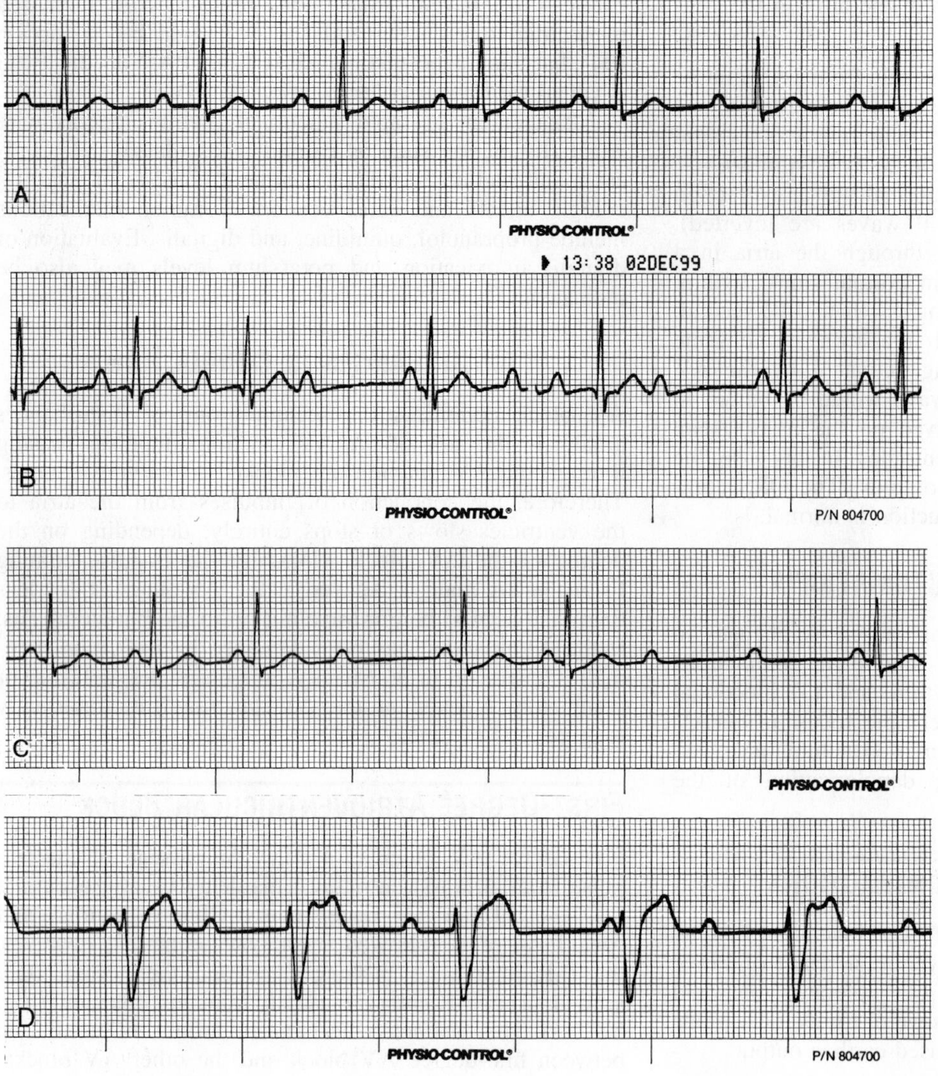

FIGURE 57–5 Junctional dysrhythmias. *A*, First-degree atrioventricular (AV) block. *B*, Second-degree AV block (Mobitz type I, Wenckebach phenomenon; note the regularly occurring P waves and the increasing P-R intervals). *C*, Second-degree AV block (Mobitz type II). *D*, Third-degree AV block (note variable P-R interval and lack of association of the P wave with the QRS complex).

SECOND-DEGREE ATRIOVENTRICULAR BLOCK

In a client with second-degree AV block, a more serious form of conduction delay in the heart, some impulses are conducted and others are blocked. Second-degree block results in intermittently dropped QRS complexes. Atrial depolarization continues without disturbance, and normal-appearing P waves occur at regular intervals. Second-degree AV block does not usually affect conduction through the ventricles, and QRS complexes appear normal in configuration. Second-degree AV block develops from CAD, digitalis toxicity, rheumatic fever, viral infections, and inferior wall MI.

Second-degree AV block is subdivided into two additional types: Mobitz type I (Wenckebach phenomenon) and Mobitz type II.

■ MOBITZ TYPE I BLOCK (WENCKEBACH PHENOMENON)

The Mobitz type I form of second-degree block is caused by an abnormally long refractory period. The level of block occurs at the AV node. On the ECG, the P-R interval gradually lengthens until a P wave is not conducted (Fig. 57–5*B*). This is the mildest form of second-degree heart block. This dysrhythmia is due to increased vagal tone, digoxin administration or congenital anomalies.

Mobitz type I does not usually result in clinical manifestations because the ventricular rate is adequate; however, the client may have an irregular pulse. Vertigo, weakness, or other signs of low cardiac output may be experienced if the ventricular rate drops precipitously.

Intervention is not required as long as the ventricular rate remains adequate for perfusion. The client is assessed for progression to a higher (more serious) degree of block. Clinicians focus primarily on managing the underlying cause. Intervention, if needed, is similar to that described for Mobitz type II block.[1, 23, 32]

■ MOBITZ TYPE II BLOCK

Mobitz type II block occurs in the presence of a long absolute refractory period with little or no relative refractory period. The level of block is below the AV node, usually a consequence of a block within the His bundle system. The P waves are normal and are followed by normal QRS complexes at regular intervals, until suddenly a QRS complex is dropped (Fig. 57–5*C*). Mobitz type II blocks result from ischemia, digitalis, or quinidine toxicity or from anterior wall MI.

Mobitz type II, a more serious condition than Mobitz type I, may progress to third-degree AV block, especially in clients with an anterior wall MI. Clients with second-degree AV block require close ECG monitoring for possible progression to complete heart block.

Interventions include (1) administration of atropine and isoproterenol (which speed the rate of impulse conduction), (2) insertion of a temporary or permanent pacemaker, and (3) withholding cardiac depressant drugs (e.g., digitalis). Second-degree block, which occurs after MI, particularly an inferior MI, may be reversible as the injury of ischemia heals.[1, 23, 32]

THIRD-DEGREE ATRIOVENTRICULAR BLOCK

Third-degree AV block is the complete absence of conduction of the electrical impulses due to a block in the AV node, bundle of His, or bundle branches. Third-degree heart block is sometimes called *AV dissociation*, because the two halves of the heart are working independently of each other. The atria are paced by the SA node, but because the message is blocked, the ventricles are being paced by a ventricular ectopic pacemaker (Fig. 57–5*D*). The atrial rate is always equal to or faster than the ventricular in complete heart block. The ventricular rate is typically 40 to 60 BPM.

Other features of the ECG in third-degree heart block include (1) regular P-P intervals, (2) regular R-R intervals, (3) an absence of meaningful or consistent P-R intervals, and (4) normal-appearing P waves. The greatest danger inherent in third-degree AV block is ventricular standstill or asystole, characterized by the Stokes-Adams attack. If a focus in the ventricles does not initiate a heartbeat, asystole leads to immediate loss of consciousness and even death.

Third-degree AV block results from a variety of causes, including:

- Fibrotic or degenerative changes in the conduction system
- MI (especially anterior wall MI)
- Congenital anomalies
- Cardiac surgery
- Myocarditis
- Viral infections of the conduction system
- Drug toxicity (digitalis, beta blockers, calcium channel blockers)
- Trauma
- Cardiomyopathy
- Lyme disease

The slow ventricular rate leads to decreased cardiac output and circulatory impairment. Clients may experience hypotension, angina pectoris, and heart failure.

The major interventions in complete heart block are atropine, transcutaneous pacing, catecholamine infusions (dopamine or epinephrine), and transvenous pacemaker. If asystole develops, CPR is used until a pacemaker can be inserted. Isoproterenol is rarely indicated.[1, 23, 32]

DISTURBANCES IN CONDUCTION

BUNDLE BRANCH BLOCK

Bundle branch block indicates that conduction is impaired in one of the bundle branches (distal to the bundle of His) and thus the ventricles do not depolarize simultaneously. The abnormal conduction pathway through the ventricles is causing a wide or notched QRS complex. The defect may result from:

- Myocardial fibrosis
- Chronic CAD
- MI
- Cardiomyopathies
- Inflammation
- Pulmonary embolism
- Severe left ventricular hypertrophy
- Congenital anomalies

These disturbances of conduction through the ventricles result in either a right bundle branch block (RBBB) or a left bundle branch block (LBBB). Because of its association with left ventricular disease, LBBB carries a worse prognosis. The left bundle branch is composed of anterior and posterior fascicles (small bundles) of which one or both may be involved.

There is no specific intervention for this conduction defect. However, if RBBB exists along with block in one of the fascicles of the left bundle, the one remaining fascicle represents the only conduction pathway to the ventricles. Therefore, in this situation a pacemaker is required.[1, 31, 32]

VENTRICULAR DYSRHYTHMIAS

Ventricular dysrhythmias arise below the level of the AV junction. Like dysrhythmias in the atria or junction, dysrhythmias in the ventricles are caused by abnormalities of automaticity or conduction. Ventricular dysrhythmias are generally more serious and life-threatening than atrial or junctional dysrhythmias, because ventricular dysrhythmias more commonly develop in association with intrinsic heart disease. Also, ventricular dysrhythmias usually cause greater hemodynamic compromise (e.g., hypotension, heart failure, and shock). The independent contraction of the ventricles results in a reduced stroke volume and, therefore, a reduced cardiac output. Rapid ventricular rates prevent optimal filling of the ventricular chambers and reduce stroke volume even further. At rates of less than 40 contractions per minute, cardiac output is simply not sufficient to support the body's vital functions.

The ECG tracing of a client with ventricular dysrhythmias reveals wide and bizarre QRS complexes. Normally, impulses traverse the ventricles via the shortest, most efficient route. This normal pathway results in a narrow QRS complex. When an impulse originates in the ventricles, however, the impulse follows an abnormal pathway through the ventricular muscle tissue. This abnormality appears as a wide (>0.12 second) complex on the ECG.

DISTURBANCES IN AUTOMATICITY

Dysrhythmias due to problems in automaticity are characterized by ectopic impulses, which result from either myocardial irritability or the phenomenon of reentry. The four ventricular dysrhythmias due to automaticity are:

- Premature ventricular contractions (PVCs)
- Ventricular fibrillation (VFib)
- Ventricular tachycardia (VT)
- Torsades de pointes

PREMATURE VENTRICULAR CONTRACTIONS

PVCs, also called ventricular premature beats, are the most common of all dysrhythmias other than those of the sinus node. They are usually caused by the firing of an irritable pacemaker in the ventricle. PVCs result from enhanced ventricular automaticity or reentry. Factors promoting PVCs include:

- Myocardial hypoxia
- Hypokalemia
- Hypocalcemia
- Acidosis
- Alcohol
- Caffeine
- Nicotine
- CAD
- Heart failure
- Toxic agents (e.g., digitalis, tricyclic antidepressants)
- Exercise
- Hypermetabolic states
- Intracardiac catheters

PVCs produce easily recognized ECG changes. They occur earlier than the expected beat of the underlying rhythm and are usually followed by a compensatory pause. On the ECG, an unusually wide and bizarre QRS appears, interrupting the underlying rhythm (Fig. 57–6*A*).

Isolated PVCs are usually not treated. If the client becomes symptomatic because of decreased cardiac output, lidocaine or any of the other class I antidysrhythmics can be given to treat PVCs. In clients with acute MI, the development of PVCs indicates that the myocardium is ischemic; in such instances, ectopic foci become irritated and fire more often.

PVCs are dangerous when they are:

- Frequent (>6/min)
- Coupled with normal beats (bigeminy)
- Multiform (Fig. 57–6*B*)
- In pairs after every third beat (trigeminy) (Fig. 57–6*C*)
- A result of acute MI
- On the T wave (Fig. 57–6*D*)

Clinicians refer to "falling on the T wave" as the *R-on-T phenomenon*. The downward slope of the T wave is the most vulnerable period of the cardiac cycle. If the heart is stimulated at this time, it often cannot respond to the stimulus in an organized fashion because the muscle fibers are in various stages of repolarization. Therefore, PVCs that occur during this vulnerable period can precipitate the more life-threatening dysrhythmias of ventricular tachycardia (VTach) (Fig. 57–6*E*) and VFib.

Outcome Management

Management of dangerous PVCs involves administration of antidysrhythmic agents that have myocardial depressant actions. In acute situations, the clinician may administer class I and class II antidysrhythmic agents intravenously (IV), followed by a continuous IV drip. Table 57–2 describes a variety of antidysrhythmic agents.[1, 15, 17, 20, 22, 23, 32]

Nursing Management of the Medical Client

Assessment

Assess the client for clinical manifestations of decreased cardiac output. Monitor the ECG continuously for patterns of PVCs that indicate further deterioration (e.g., PVCs moving closer to the preceding T wave).

DIAGNOSIS, PLANNING, INTERVENTIONS

Decreased Cardiac Output. Dysrhythmias often lead to decreased ventricular filling due to rapid rate or from not being coordinated to allow for atrial kick. Express this common nursing diagnosis as *Decreased Cardiac Output related to decreased ventricular filling time secondary to (name the rhythm).*

Outcomes. The client will have an adequate cardiac output, as evidenced by (1) return of normal heart rate, rhythm, palpable pulse, and blood pressure to baseline levels; (2) return of level of consciousness to baseline value; (3) warm and dry skin; (4) clear lung sounds; (4) absence of S_3 or S_4; (5) absence of dysrhythmias; and (6) adequate urine output.

Interventions. Monitor heart rate and rhythm and vital signs continuously, aided by the computer when needed. Assess skin temperature, lung sounds, heart sounds, and peripheral pulses every 2 to 4 hours. Monitor laboratory studies, especially if an MI is suspected. Give antidysrhythmic medications according to orders. Use blood levels as a guide to dosage. Many medications, especially antidysrhythmics, can rise to toxic levels, especially if the client has a pre-existing liver, renal, or electrolyte disorder.

Maintain a quiet atmosphere, and administer analgesics to control pain. Stimulation can lead to increased levels of catecholamine release and may trigger tachycardias and increased oxygen demand.

Apply oxygen with nasal prongs to supplement serum levels. Hypoxia can lead to further myocardial ischemia and dysrhythmias.

If life-threatening dysrhythmias develop, many nurses are trained to use defibrillation for the client. Other emergency interventions include CPR, various medications, and preparation of the client for a transcutaneous or permanent pacemaker.

Anxiety. The risk of death from sudden onset of life-threatening dysrhythmias weighs heavily on most clients. Express this nursing diagnosis as *Anxiety related to fear about unknown outcome.*

Outcomes. The client will experience a reduced level of anxiety, as evidenced by (1) a report of feeling less anxious and not voicing feelings of helplessness or hopelessness, (2) increased ability to sleep and rest, (3) return of heart rate to baseline level, and (4) reduction of dyspnea.

Interventions. Identify the client's anxiety and assist the client in discussing sources of fear. Clarify miscon-

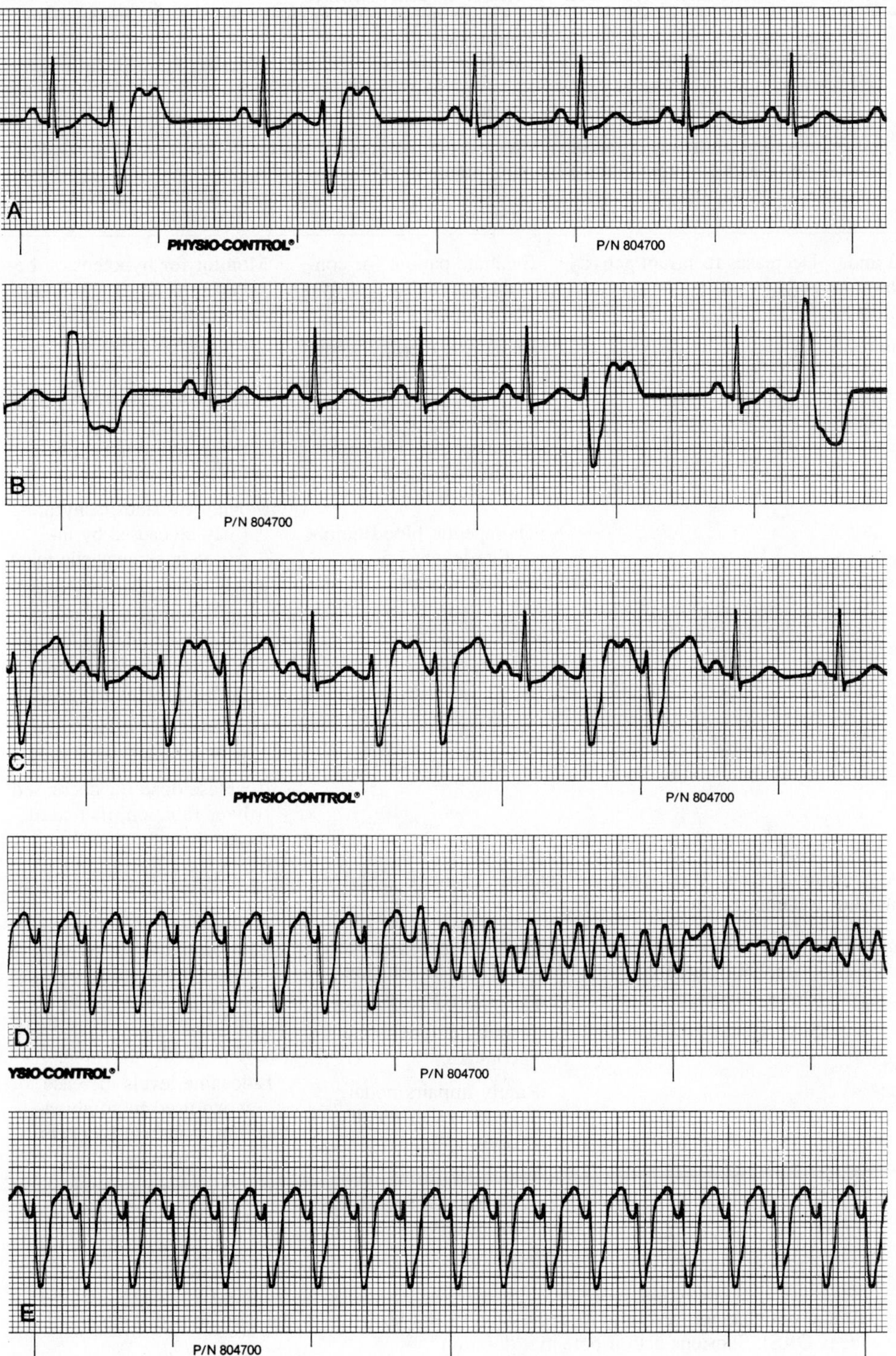

FIGURE 57–6 Ventricular dysrhythmias. *A*, Beats 2 and 4 are unifocal premature ventricular contractions (PVCs). *B*, Multifocal PVCs. *C*, Paired PVDs. *D*, R-on-T phenomenon, leading to ventricular fibrillation. *E*, Ventricular tachycardia.

ceptions. Commonly, the client or a member of the family has had a heart condition and the client's ability to cope may be directly influenced by that experience.

Explain the equipment present in the room. Most rooms are stocked with several types of equipment, and its presence does not always indicate the severity of the client's condition.

Remain with the client and tell the client and family what is happening now and what will be happening (e.g., blood will be drawn soon).

Finally, explore the usual coping methods with the client. Positive coping methods are usually supported; discuss maladaptive coping mechanisms, and suggest substitutions. For example, smoking may be a common coping mechanism, but it is not permitted with cardiac disorders or in most hospitals. Therefore, if smoking is the client's coping mechanism when stressed, a substitute would need to be found, such as nicotine patches or chewing gum. Be aware that these patches actually can increase the levels of nicotine because they provide constant levels of the drug. Light smokers require less nicotine. Adjust the dose of the patch, beginning with the lowest levels.

TABLE 57–2 NURSING IMPLICATIONS FOR MEDICATIONS USED TO TREAT DYSRHYTHMIAS

Prototype	Actions	Evaluation of Therapeutic Effect	Evaluation of Adverse Effects	Nursing Considerations
CLASS I ANTIDYSRHYTHMICS				
Drugs with local anesthetic effects and membrane-stabilizing properties. Affect stroke velocity of phase 0. They are subdivided based on the magnitude of effects on phase 0, action potential duration, and effective refractory period				
Type IA: Slowing of phase 0 upstroke (fast sodium channel). Prolongs action potential. Lengthens effective refractory period.				
Quinidine	Inhibits peripheral and myocardial alpha-adrenegic receptors Inhibits muscarinic receptors and causes a reflex increase in sympathetic tone Slows conduction Increases effective refractory period	Decreases reentrant activity Decreases ventricular and atrial dysrhythmias Decreases ventricular response to AFib and WPW	Evaluate patient for conduction delay and dysrhythmias Readdress therapy when: QRS widens >50%; QRS widens >20% with IVCD: QRS duration > 140 msecs and prolonged QT > 500 msecs Therapeutic blood quinidine levels 2.5 −5.0 mg/ml	Monitor for hypotension because of alpha-adrenergic inhibition (especially with IV administration, although rarely used) Monitor for pro-dysrhythmic effects; measure Q–T interval and duration of QRS complex Monitor for sinus tachycardia (may be caused by increase in sympathetic tone) Watch for drug interactions: increased digoxin levels, increases anticoagulation for clients receiving warfarin (Coumadin) May cause GI upset; give with meals Decrease dose for decreased liver function, increased age
Type IB: Effects similar to type IA. Slowing of phase 0 upstroke (fast sodium channel). Shortens action potential duration. Class IB agents act selectively on diseased or ischemic tissues.				
Lidocaine (Xylocaine)	Blocks fast sodium channel Shortens action potential Acts selectively on diseased or ischemic tissue	Suppression of dysrhythmia associated with cardiac surgery Suppression of VT	Half-life increases with >24 hour infusion Usually not associated with hemodynamic changes Rarely impairs nodal functions or conduction Watch for drowsiness, numbness, speech disturbances	After initial IV dose, drug is distributed rapidly and must be followed by an infusion to maintain therapeutic blood level Lidocaine levels increase when used in combination with beta-blockers and cimetidine Decreased dose for clients with liver disease Decreased dose for elderly clients
Type IC: Powerful inhibition of the fast sodium channel, resulting in depression of the upstroke of the cardiac action potential. Inhibits His-Purkinje conduction (widens QRS). Shortens action potential duration.				
Propafenone (Rhythmol)	Blocks fast inward sodium channel Increases P–R and QRS intervals No effect on Q–T interval Mild beta-blocking properties Mild calcium channel–blocking properties	Suppression of ventricular tachyarrhythmias Suppression of SVT (including WPW) Suppression of AFib and atrial flutter	P–R/QRS prolongation Conduction block SA node inhibition Negative inotrope may exacerbate heart failure	Not used for clients with structural heart disease Drug interactions include increased serum digoxin levels and increased anticoagulation when taken with Coumadin Monitor for adverse effects when used in combination with other conduction-blocking drugs

Table continued on following page

TABLE 57–2 NURSING IMPLICATIONS FOR MEDICATIONS USED TO TREAT DYSRHYTHMIAS *Continued*

Prototype	Actions	Evaluation of Therapeutic Effect	Evaluation of Adverse Effects	Nursing Considerations
CLASS II ANTIDYSRHYTHMICS				
Beta-adrenergic blocking agents. General myocardial depressants for both supraventricular and ventricular rhythm disturbances.				
Metoprolol (Lopressor)	Blocks sympathetic stimulation at the sinus node Reduced automaticity in Purkinje fibers	Suppression of inappropriate sinus tachycardia, paroxysmal atrial tachycardia, ventricular dysrhythmias and dysrhythmias of increased beta-adrenergic activity	Relatively safe Watch for bradycardia Can cause bronchospasm; contraindicated in bronchial asthma, bronchospasm, and COPD	Not recommended for clients with conduction defects Contraindicated in bronchial asthma
CLASS III ANTIDYSRHYTHMICS				
Act by lengthening action potential duration. Lengthen effective refractory period.				
Sotalol (Betapace)	Lengthens action potential duration Prolonged atrial and ventricular refractory periods Inhibits conduction along bypass tracts Mixed class II and III agent	Used for treatment of life threatening arrhythmia	May lengthen Q–T interval Q–T interval should not exceed 500 msec	Monitor vital signs and ECG closely Monitor Q–T interval Avoid inpatients with conduction defects
CLASS IV ANTIDYSRHYTHMICS				
Calcium-channel blockers				
Verapamil (Calan)	Blocks slow calcium channel; has slight nonspecific sympathetic depressant effect Increases relative refractory period through AV node Interferes with reentry of impulses at AV node	Used in controlling rapid ventricular response in AFib and atrial flutter Used for suppression of AV nodal reentry tachycardia	Hypotension, syncope, peripheral edema, constipation, bradycardia, AV blocks; may precipitate or worsen heart failure Watch P–R interval	Monitor vital signs and heart rhythm Monitor lung sounds and liver function tests Administer with food Monitor blood pressure and P–R interval
UNCLASSIFIED ANTIDYSRHYTHMICS				
Digoxin	Decreases AV node conduction to control ventricular response to AFib		Increases irritability and automaticity of ectopic sites in atria and ventricles	Given as rapid IV bolus to convert PSVT to NSR
Adenosine (Adenocard)	An endogenous nucleoside; decreases AV node conduction; interrupts AV reentry pathways			

AFib, atrial fibrillation; AV, atrioventricular; ECG, electrocardiogram; GI, gastrointestinal; IV, intravenous; IVCD, intraventricular conduction delay; NSR, normal sinus rhythm; PSVT, paroxysmal supraventricular tachycardia; PVCs, premature ventricular contractions; SA, sinoatrial; SVT, supraventricular tachycardia; VT, ventricular tachycardia; WPW, Wolff-Parkinson-White syndrome.

From Ophie, L. H., & Marcus, F. I. (1997). Antiarrhythmic drugs. In L. H. Ophie (Ed.), *Drugs for the heart* (4th ed.). Philadelphia: W. B. Saunders; and Zipes, D. P. (1997). Management of cardiac arrhythmias: Pharmacological, electrical and surgical techniques. In E. Braunwald (Ed.), *Heart disease* (5th ed.). Philadelphia: W. B. Saunders.

Data from Katzung, B. G. (1992). *Basic and clinical pharmacology* (5th ed.). Norwalk, CT: Appleton & Lange; Koda-Kimble, M. A., et al. (1992). *Handbook of applied therapeutics* (2nd ed.). Vancouver, WA: Applied Therapeutics.

EVALUATION

The degree of expected outcome attainment is assessed hourly (or more often) if the client has life-threatening dysrhythmias. Dysrhythmias are treated promptly and usually stop quickly once treatment is begun. Clients with recalcitrant dysrhythmias may require several medications. Anxiety can sometimes abate quickly but usually requires several days. Some clients remain anxious for their entire hospital stay.

VENTRICULAR FIBRILLATION

Ventricular fibrillation (VFib) is a life-threatening dysrhythmia characterized by extremely rapid, erratic impulse formation and conduction. This lethal dysrhythmia causes abrupt cessation of effective cardiac output. It usually results from severe myocardial damage, hypothermia, R-on-T phenomenon, hypoxia, contact with high-voltage electricity, electrolyte imbalance, or toxicity from quinidine, procainamide, or digitalis.

The ECG tracing displays bizarre, fibrillatory wave patterns, and it is impossible to identify P waves, QRS complexes, or T waves (Fig. 57–7*A*). VFib may be either coarse or fine. Untreated, the deflections become smaller and eventually all ventricular activity ceases. Death results within minutes without immediate intervention (i.e., defibrillation, CPR, and medications).

When VFib appears, the clinician must immediately initiate CPR until the defibrillator is engaged. Defibrillate up to three times if needed. Defibrillation can be performed by nurses who have advanced training (see Defib-

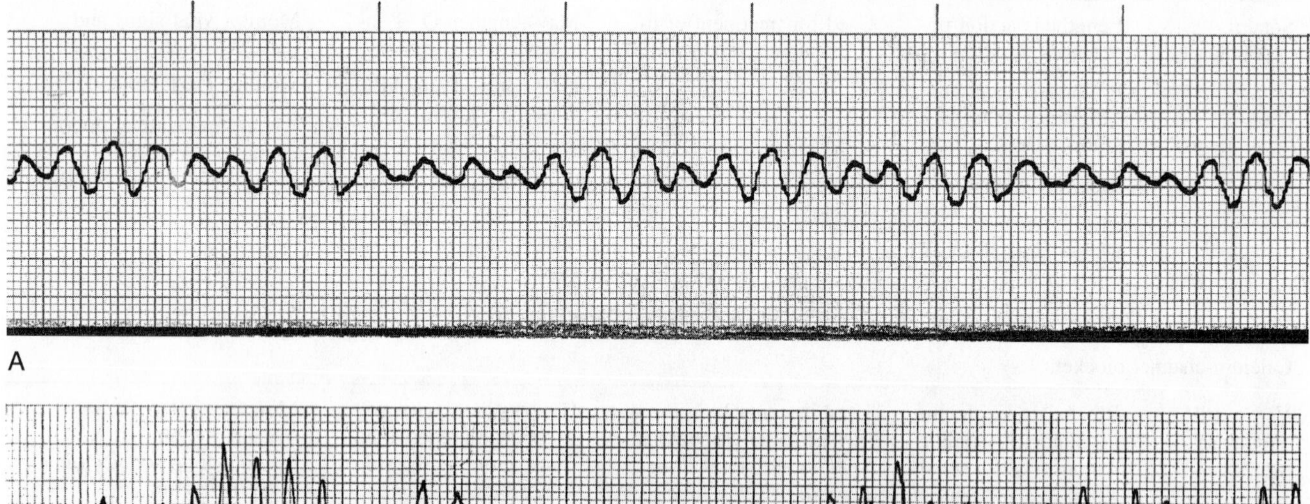

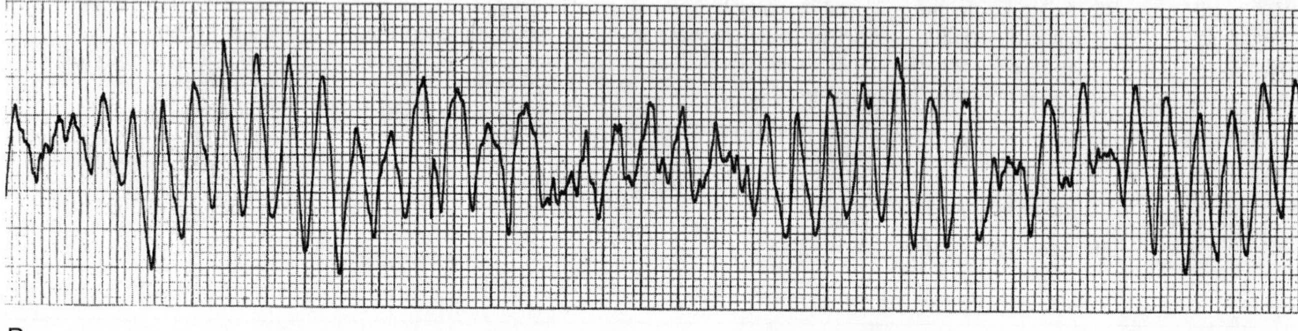

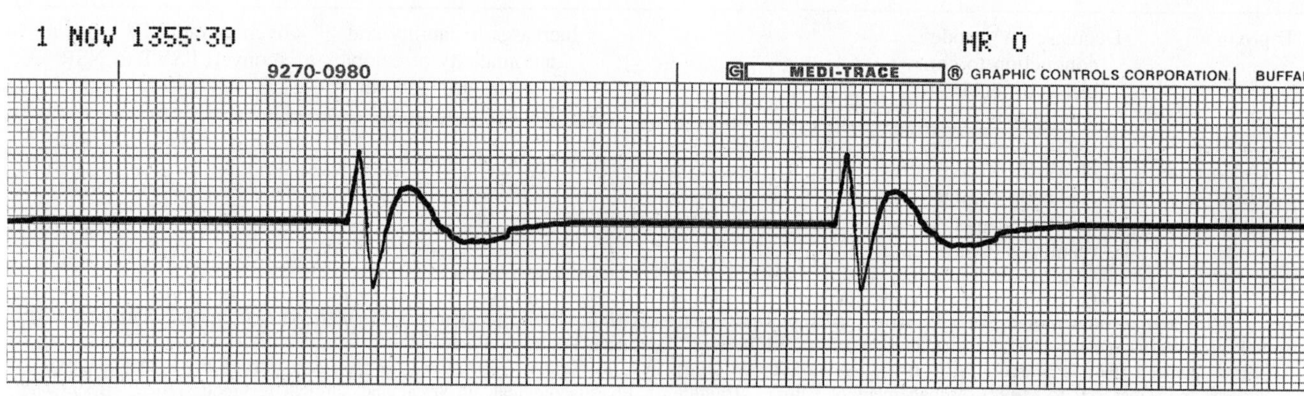

FIGURE 57–7 *A*, Coarse ventricular fibrillation. *B*, Torsades de pointes. *C*, Ventricular asystole in a dying heart. (*B*, From Phillips, R. E., & Feeney, M. K. [1990]. *The cardiac rhythms: A systematic approach to interpretation.* [3rd ed., p. 393]. Philadelphia: W. B. Saunders.)

rillation later). A standard pattern of energy and current is used. Defibrillation begins with 200 joules (J); if not successful, it is advanced to 300 J, then to 360 J. With persistent VFib, epinephrine is given and the clinician defibrillates at 360 J. Other medications are alternated with defibrillation (lidocaine, bretylium, magnesium sulfate, sodium bicarbonate), depending on the client's cardiac rhythm and electrolyte and acid-base balance.[1, 23, 32]

VENTRICULAR ASYSTOLE

Ventricular asystole (cardiac standstill) represents the total absence of ventricular electrical activity (Fig. 57–7*C*). The client has no palpable pulse (no cardiac output), and a rhythm is absent if the client is monitored. The occurrence of sudden ventricular asystole in a conscious person results in faintness, followed within seconds by loss of consciousness, seizures, and apnea. If the dysrhythmia remains untreated, death ensues. Ventricular asystole must be treated immediately.

Cardiac standstill can occur as a primary event, or it may follow VFib or pulseless electrical activity. Asystole can occur also in clients with complete heart block (CHB) in whom there is no escape pacemaker. Possible causes include:

- Hypoxia
- Hyperkalemia and hypokalemia
- Pre-existing acidosis
- Drug overdose
- Hypothermia

The treatment of choice consists of CPR, epinephrine, atropine, transcutaneous pacing, and correction of the cause.[1, 23, 32]

PULSELESS ELECTRICAL ACTIVITY

Pulseless electrical activity represents the presence of some electrical activity in the heart, as seen on the monitor, other than VFib or VT; however, a pulse cannot be detected by palpation of any artery. Common causes include cardiac tamponade, massive pulmonary embolus, tension pneumothorax, and severe hypovolemia.

Rapid searching for the cause is imperative. Until the cause is located, CPR is initiated and fluid volume is restored.

REENTRY OF IMPULSES

VENTRICULAR TACHYCARDIA

Ventricular tachycardia (VTach or VT) is a life-threatening dysrhythmia that occurs when an irritable ectopic focus in the ventricles takes over as the pacemaker. It occurs in the presence of significant cardiac disease, such as in clients with CAD, cardiomyopathy, mitral valve prolapse, heart failure, acute MI with hypoxia and acidosis, and digitalis toxicity.

VT is characterized by rapidly occurring series of PVCs (three or more) with no normal beats in between (Fig. 57–12*E*). P waves are absent, and the P-R interval is absent. The QRS complex is wide (>0.12 second) and bizarre. The ventricular rate ranges between 100 and 220 BPM, usually 130 to 170 BPM. The ventricular rhythm is slightly irregular. VT produces a very low cardiac output that can quickly lead to cerebral and myocardial ischemia. At any time, VT can develop into VFib. Clients with VT commonly express that they are experiencing feelings of impending death.

Sustained but hemodynamically stable VT is initially treated with antidysrhythmics (i.e., lidocaine, procainamide, or bretylium). Cardioversion may be required for conversion to sinus rhythm. VT that causes loss of consciousness must be terminated immediately with defibrillation. The physician may also order IV antidysrhythmic agents, usually lidocaine. Another drug gaining favor is magnesium sulfate, particularly if the client has low magnesium levels.[1, 19, 23, 32]

TORSADES DE POINTES

Torsades de pointes is a form of VT in which the QRS complexes appear to be constantly changing. Delayed repolarization of the ventricle is revealed as a prolonged Q-T interval and a broad flat T wave in the preceding sinus rhythm. The rhythm is regular or irregular with a ventricular rate of 150 to 300 BPM (Fig. 57–7*B*). The QRS complex is wide and bizarre.

Torsades de pointes is usually a result of drug toxicity (procainamide, quinidine, disopyramide) or electrolyte imbalances (hypokalemia or hypomagnesemia). Clinical manifestations begin with palpitations and syncope. This rhythm often precedes VFib and sudden death.

Torsades de pointes is treated only if the Q-T interval is prolonged with temporary overdrive ventricular or atrial pacing. Discontinuation of offending agents is also crucial. IV magnesium sulfate is considered the treatment of choice.[1, 19, 32]

PRE-EXCITATION SYNDROMES

Pre-excitation syndromes occur when part or all of the ventricle is reentered by a depolarization wave traveling down a congenital or acquired accessory conducting pathway between the atrium and ventricle.

An accessory pathway is abnormal conductile tissue connecting the atria and ventricle. Normally, the AV node is the only connection between the atria and ventricles and controls (blocks) rapid atrial rates that prevent rapid ventricular rates (e.g., AFib). When accessory pathways are present, there is nothing to block rapid atrial rates, and ventricular rates soar.

There are several types of disorders in this category, of which *Wolff-Parkinson-White syndrome* (WPW) appears most frequently. In clients with WPW, sudden attacks of very rapid supraventricular dysrhythmias suddenly develop. Most adults with WPW have normal hearts, but if the tachydysrhythmias occur persistently, myocardial fatigue and ventricular failure may result.

Clients with WPW do not require intervention unless they experience recurring tachydysrhythmias. In this instance, the physician may elect to use vagotonic maneuvers, cardioversion, adenosine, amiodarone (Cordarone), esmolol administration, or chemical, mechanical, or radiofrequency ablation. Ablation is an interventional procedure that destroys the accessory pathway.

Outcome Management

Medical Management of Life-Threatening Dysrhythmias

The goal of management is to immediately stop the dysrhythmia and restore normal sinus rhythm. Remember, because there is inadequate or no perfusion of blood during these dysrhythmias, CPR is performed. Finally, the cause of the dysrhythmia is identified and treated.

Life-threatening dysrhythmias can often be effectively managed with exogenously delivered currents of electricity. The most crucial element for survival after cardiac arrest is the time interval from collapse to care, especially defibrillation. With each passing minute, the chances of survival decline as much as 10%. Electrical intervention can (1) abruptly stop the heart's erratic electrical discharge or (2) resume the flow of electrical current where there is none. Methods of electrical therapy include defibrillation and cardioversion.

DEFIBRILLATION

The use of defibrillation delivers an electrical current (shock) of preset voltage to the heart through paddles placed on the chest wall (closed chest procedure). This current causes the entire myocardium to depolarize completely at the moment of shock, thus producing transient asystole and allowing the heart's intrinsic pacemakers to regain control. The amount of energy required to produce this effect is largely determined by the client's transthoracic impedance, or resistance to current flow. Because of this factor, the amount of energy that reaches the heart is less than the amount that the defibrillator is charged to deliver.[1, 15, 18]

The procedure is associated with potential hazards, particularly myocardial damage. The higher the amount of energy or frequency of the shocks, the greater the risk of injury. Advances in the equipment now allow measurement of transthoracic impedance. Once impedance is determined, the defibrillator automatically selects the amount of current needed that can restore rhythm and cardiac output. It is expected this mode of defibrillation will reduce the risk of complications.[1, 32]

The degree of transthoracic resistance depends on several variables:

1. *Energy level.* The higher the energy level selected, the more current follows.
2. *Number and frequency of shocks.* The more shocks administered and the shorter the time interval between them, the lower the transthoracic resistance.
3. *Ventilation phase.* Resistance is lower when shocks are delivered during exhalation, when there is less air (and therefore less diameter) in the lungs.
4. *Paddle size.* The larger the paddle, the lower the resistance.
5. *Chest size.* The smaller the distance between the defibrillator electrodes once they are in place, the lower the resistance.
6. *Paddle-skin interface material.* Conductive material between the skin and paddles reduces transthoracic impedance.
7. *Paddle pressure.* Applying firm pressure increases contact between the skin and the paddles, helping to overcome transthoracic resistance. Exert about 25 pounds of pressure on each paddle.
8. *Paddle placement.* Place one paddle on the upper chest, to the right of the sternum; place the other on the lower left chest, to the left of the nipple, with the center of the paddle in the midaxillary line.

If the client has a permanent pacemaker or an internal cardiac defibrillator, place the paddles at least 5 inches away from the generator to avoid damaging it. If a temporary pacing system is in use, disconnect the pacing lead from the pulse generator immediately before defibrillation and reconnect it after the shock.[1, 5, 7, 10, 11, 18]

Most defibrillators can be used to perform either *synchronized* cardioversion or *unsynchronized* cardioversion (commonly called defibrillation). Defibrillation is always indicated in VFib and is also used in VT when the client is unconscious and pulseless. Specially trained nurses, emergency medical technicians, and physicians perform this procedure in acute settings.

CARE BEFORE DEFIBRILLATION. Immediately before defibrillation, assess the client's responsiveness and do the following:

1. If the client is not responsive, activate the EMS system.
2. Call for the defibrillator.
3. Assess the client's airway, breathing, and circulation (ABCs). Open the airway. Look, listen, and feel.
4. If the client is not breathing, give two slow breaths.
5. Assess the client's circulation; if there is no pulse, start CPR.
6. Perform CPR until the defibrillator is in place.
7. Check the ECG to verify the presence of VFib or pulseless VT.
8. Check leads for any loose connections.
9. Remove any nitroglycerin patch.

On confirmation of the emergency, the code alarm is given over the health care facility intercom system or to their pagers to summon the emergency team (e.g., "Code 99, Dr. Blue"). In the meantime, CPR measures are started by the first person on the scene. The clinician turns on the defibrillator and sets it at 200 J. In the presence of VFib, the synchronous mode must not be used. Start an IV line, as needed, for administration of resuscitation medications. Intubation is completed with oxygen supplementation.

CARE DURING DEFIBRILLATION. When VFib develops, clinicians must attempt defibrillation at the earliest opportunity. The paddles are lubricated with electrode paste or conducting pads to enhance conduction and prevent burning of the skin. The paste should not extend beyond the paddles, and the paddles must lie flat against the body in order to avoid burns. The clinician places the paddles firmly against the chest. A transverse (anterolateral) position for paddle placement is used. One paddle is placed at the second intercostal space, at the right of the sternum, and the other paddle is positioned at the fifth intercostal space on the anterior axillary line (Fig. 57–8).

To ensure safe defibrillation, people who perform defibrillation must always announce when they are about to shock. The phrase "One. I'm clear. Two. You're clear. Three. All clear." is recommended. Because electricity is carried along metal devices and the client, all personnel, including the clinician administering the shock, must stand back from the bed. Open chest defibrillation occurs when electrical current is applied directly to the heart.

CARE AFTER DEFIBRILLATION. The clinician immediately assesses the ECG and pulse after defibrillation. If the first countershock is unsuccessful, immediate debrillation must be performed again at a higher energy level (300 and 360 J). Defibrillation may be applied up to three times (200, 300, 360 J), if needed, for persistent VFib or pulseless VT. Defibrillators are frequently equipped with paddles that can monitor the ECG, even immediately after defibrillation. Therefore, if the paddles are left in place after the shock has been delivered, the cardiac response can be quickly evaluated.

CPR should be continued if the three defibrillations have not been successful. A member of the health care team administers appropriate medications again before the next defibrillation attempt. A successful response is indicated by cessation of fibrillation, restoration of sinus rhythm, and palpation of a regular pulse. After successful defibrillation, continuous ECG monitoring is required. The client's vital signs and neurologic status must also be continuously assessed.

For clients with a pacemaker or an automatic implantable cardioverter-defibrillator (AICD), a programmer-analyzer should be available to examine the system for damage and erroneous reprogramming after defibrillation. Continue to monitor for pacemaker malfunction for at least the next 24 hours.

In documenting the outcome of defibrillation, record the following points:

- Preprocedure rhythm
- Times and voltage of shocks delivered
- Postdefibrillation rhythm pattern
- Names, times of administration, and doses of administered medications
- Other hemodynamic data available before, during, and after defibrillation

TERMINATION OF RESUSCITATION. Generally, if an organized rhythm and pulse have not returned, the Advanced Cardiac Life Support team leader can cease efforts to resuscitate clients from confirmed and persistent asystole when the client has received successful endotracheal intubation, successful IV access, suitable basic CPR, and all rhythm-appropriate medications. Always consider any pre-existing problems that may make the client less responsive to defibrillation (acidosis, hypokalemia, hyperkalemia, hypoxia, hypovolemia), and treat them appropriately. In many cases, clients may have other, noncardiac, disorders that make resuscitation attempts futile.

The 1996 American Heart Association guidelines for emergency cardiac care do not state a specific time limit beyond which rescuers can never have a successful resuscitation. Cardiac arrests in special situations such as hypothermia, electrocution, and drug overdose present ex-

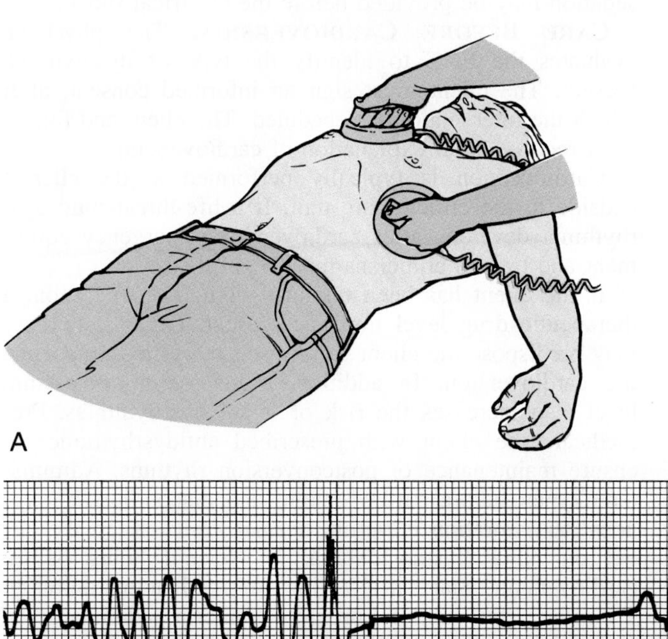

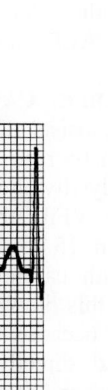

FIGURE 57–8 *A*, Anterolateral paddle placement for external countershock. External paddles are placed at the second right intercostal space and at the anterior axillary line in the fifth left intercostal space. *B*, Ventricular fibrillation converted to normal sinus rhythm.

ceptions to any rules. Special situations call for common sense and clinical judgment.[1, 23, 32]

Television portrayal of defibrillation and CPR contributes to many misconceptions about these treatments. One article discusses whether the information on television provides accurate information.[9] Three television shows were viewed (*ER, Chicago Hope,* and *Rescue 911*). The cause of the cardiac arrest, the demographics of the client, the underlying illness, and the outcomes were recorded. A total of 97 episodes of the three shows were reviewed. Of the 60 clients who received CPR, 46 (77%) survived the immediate cardiac arrest. Survival rates for CPR on these television programs are much higher than the highest rates reported in the literature. Most people resuscitated were children, teenagers, and young adults. In the hospital, cardiac arrest is most common in older adults. On television, most cardiac arrests have been caused by trauma; in reality, most cardiac arrests are due to heart disease. During the same episodes, 37 people died. In only eight of the situations in which people died was there any discussion about the use of CPR or reference to do-not-resuscitate orders.

Clients participate in discussions about their health care today more than ever before. Many people have few resources from which to hear about acute care. Consequently, images in the media strongly shape the public's belief about medical care, illness, and death. The portrayal of CPR and death on three popular programs has been misleading. Misrepresentation of CPR on television may lead people to misinterpret the outcomes seen there as real life. Nurses need to be able to clarify misconceptions.

OTHER FORMS OF DEFIBRILLATION

AUTOMATED EXTERNAL DEFIBRILLATOR. An automated external defibrillator (AED) delivers electrical shocks to a client after it identifies VT or VFib. The device is attached to the client with adhesive sternal-apex pads on flexible cables, which allows "hands-free" defibrillation, a feature available with conventional defibrillation as well. AEDs also have an internal microprocessor-based detection system that analyzes the rhythm for the characteristics of VFib or VT. When VFib or VT is present, the AED "advises" the operator to deliver a shock.

AEDs are "automated," in the sense that the device—not the operator—analyzes the rhythm and determines the presence of VFib or VT.[1, 5] The most common cause of unconsciousness in an adult is VFib. Defibrillation is the only effective treatment. AEDs are thus common in emergency response units.

AUTOMATIC IMPLANTABLE CARDIOVERTER-DEFIBRILLATOR. The AICD consists of a pulse generator and a sensor that continuously monitors heart rhythm. When the device detects a dysrhythmia, it automatically delivers a countershock. For VFib, the AICD gives an electrical countershock within 15 to 20 seconds. It can also detect and treat VT with cardioversion. Compared with external defibrillation, this implanted system does not require as much energy because less energy is lost when the impulse is applied directly to the heart. In addition, a back-up pacemaker helps to control the rhythm.

The AICD is implanted surgically into a pouch into the abdominal wall through a thoracotomy incision or transvenously for two types of conditions[1, 5, 32]:

- Survival of one or more episodes of sudden cardiac death resulting from VT or VFib
- Recurrent, refractory, life-threatening ventricular dysrhythmias that can develop into VT or VFib, or both, despite antidysrhythmic therapy

Clients who require AICDs have a great deal of anxiety. Anxiety can develop from past episodes of near death as well as from feelings of not ever being able to die. Other clients may fear that the AICD will not be able to reverse the dysrhythmia. Be sensitive to these thoughts, and facilitate their discussion.[1, 5, 7, 10, 13, 18]

CARDIOVERSION

Cardioversion, most often an elective procedure, involves the use of a synchronized direct current (DC) electrical countershock that depolarizes all the cells simultaneously, allowing the SA node to resume the pacemaker role. The electrical discharge is synchronized with or triggered by the client's QRS complex for avoidance of accidental discharge during the repolarization phase when the ventricle is vulnerable to the development of VFib. A QRS complex must be present for successful conversion of the dysrhythmia.

Low voltages (50 to 100 J) are tried initially. If the attempt is unsuccessful, cardioversion using larger voltages can be repeated. Only specially trained physicians can perform this procedure.[1, 23, 32]

Cardioversion is used to treat SVT, AFib, and atrial flutter that is resistant to medication, and VT in an unstable patient. The unstable client may be hypotensive or dyspneic, may be experiencing chest pain, or may have evidence of heart failure, MI, or ischemia. Analgesia or sedation may be provided before the electrical shock.

CARE BEFORE CARDIOVERSION. The physician evaluates the ECG to identify the type of dysrhythmia present. The client must sign an informed consent, after which the intervention is scheduled. The client and family must receive a full explanation of cardioversion.

Cardioversion is typically performed at the client's bedside in the critical care unit. If a life-threatening dysrhythmia develops after cardioversion, emergency equipment and trained clinicians must be in the room.

If the client has been taking a digitalis preparation, a therapeutic drug level must be present. Digitalis toxicity may predispose the client to ventricular dysrhythmias during cardioversion. In addition, a low serum potassium level also increases the risk of lethal dysrhythmias. Premedicate the client with prescribed antidysrhythmics to ensure maintenance of postconversion rhythms. Administer oxygen before cardioversion, and discontinue if oxygenation saturation is within normal limits. Keep the client on NPO (fasting) status for several hours before cardioversion. Start an IV line for medication delivery. To reduce fear and to promote amnesia, administer an antianxiety medication IV as prescribed.

CARE DURING CARDIOVERSION. The physician performs the following steps:

1. Sets the machine within a range of 50 to 200 J (more or less, depending on the underlying impedances).

2. Turns the synchronizer switch to "on" to deliver the shock during the QRS complex, not on the down-slope of the T wave.
3. Lubricates the paddles and places them exactly as described for defibrillation.
4. Calls for all health care personnel to stand back from the bed.
5. While standing back from the bed, depresses and holds the buttons on the paddles until the shock is delivered.

Newer equipment for cardioversion includes adhesive skin paddles attached to the client's chest and back.

CARE AFTER CARDIOVERSION. Clinicians immediately assess the ECG and pulse after the procedure. In some cases, VFib or VT occurs, an event demanding emergency action. Monitor the client's ECG rhythm and vital signs continuously for at least 2 hours, and carefully assess for rhythm changes and complications. A successful response to cardioversion resolves the dysrhythmia and restores normal sinus rhythm. With a good response and no complications, the client may be discharged later that day when fully awake and able to eat.

SUPPRESSING IRRITABLE FOCI

Improving Myocardial Oxygen

Oxygen is an essential component of dysrhythmia management, especially for dysrhythmias that result from irritable foci in an ischemic myocardium. These include PVCs and other ventricular dysrhythmias. Oxygen should be given to all clients at risk of ventricular dysrhythmias, such as those with chest pain or hypoxemia or during cardiac arrest.

Antidysrhythmic Therapy

Do not attempt to memorize Table 57–2; rather, commit a few drugs to memory (atropine, lidocaine, epinephrine, verapamil, and procainamide). These medications may be administered orally or by continuous IV infusion. You must be diligent in monitoring for the intended effect and side effects of the medication.

ABLATING CONDUCTION PATHWAYS

A variety of procedures can be used to treat dysrhythmias when use of medications are unsuccessful in bringing about conversion of the abnormal rhythm to a normal rhythm. Interventions include (1) chemical and mechanical ablation and (2) radiofrequency of the abnormal pathway. These procedures involve risk to normal conduction tissue, and a pacemaker may be needed either temporarily or permanently.[5, 21, 32]

CHEMICAL ABLATION. Alcohol or phenol is inserted into involved areas of the myocardium through an angioplasty catheter. Test injections with saline or lidocaine are given to determine whether the dysrhythmia ceases before the final injection. Postprocedural care is the same as that for angioplasty.

MECHANICAL ABLATION. The abnormal pathway is surgically removed or treated with a cryoprobe to interrupt its effect on heart rhythms. SVT, AFib, atrial flutter, and WPW syndrome may be treated with this method when the client does not respond to medication. Before the procedure, the myocardium is mapped to determine whether other forms of surgery (e.g., coronary bypass grafting, valve replacement) may correct the dysrhythmia. Mapping also isolates the area to be treated. The procedure may be performed through open-heart or closed-heart methods.

Postprocedure care and recovery are similar to those following cardiac catheterization.

RADIOFREQUENCY ABLATION. Radiofrequency catheter ablation (RFA) is used primarily for SVT associated with WPW or AV nodal reentry, although it has also been used successfully to treat refractory VT. A steerable pacing catheter directs low-power, high-frequency current to a localized accessory pathway and necroses a small portion of the heart. When this current is applied, the temperature of the contact tissue rises, water is driven out, and coagulation necrosis results. The amount of tissue injury depends on the amount of energy delivered (5 to 50 watts), the length of time it is delivered (10 to 90 seconds), and the resistance at the end of the catheter. RFA produces lesions that are smaller and more controllable than DC catheter ablation lesions.

The major advantage of RFA is the high rate of success (99% at some centers) and low morbidity. RFA is more successful than conventional medical therapies or DC ablation but equal in success to surgical treatment.

Although RFA is a relatively safe procedure, some complications can occur:

- Cardiac tamponade (1%)
- Deep vein thrombosis (1%)
- Trauma to vessel (1%)
- Transient ischemic attack or stroke (0.5%)
- Perforation of AV leaflet (extremely rare)
- Hematoma at introducer site (common)
- Unintentional AV block requiring pacemaker implantation (up to 10%)

Postprocedure nursing care and recovery are similar to those following cardiac catheterization. Specific nursing responsibilities include (1) preprocedure education of client and family, (2) interventions to reduce anxiety before and during the RFA procedure, (3) monitoring of vital signs and lower extremity perfusion during and after the procedure, and (4) discharge instructions. Clients are usually discharged within 24 hours after RFA and are instructed to gradually resume normal activities but to avoid strenuous activities for 7 to 10 days. ECGs are obtained routinely at 1, 3, 6, and 9 months after RFA. Aspirin, 325 mg, is prescribed for 14 days after RFA to prevent clot formation and platelet aggregation at the ablation site.[5, 32]

Surgical Management

RESTORING IMPULSE GENERATION

Pacemakers

Pacemakers provide an artificial SA node or Purkinje system. Pacemakers can be *permanent* or *temporary*.

An artificial pacemaker is indicated if the conduction system fails to transmit impulses from the sinus node to the ventricles, to generate an impulse spontaneously, or to maintain primary control of the pacing function of the heart. Many conditions may affect the ability of the heart's conduction system to function normally, creating

BOX 57–2 Conditions That May Necessitate a Pacemaker

- Ablation
- Acute myocardial infarction
- Autonomic nervous system failure
- Cardiac surgery
- Drug toxicity (antidysrhythmics)
- Electrolyte imbalance
- Myocardial ischemia

circumstances that warrant pacing (Box 57–2). Pacemakers can be used temporarily or prophylactically until the condition underlying the disturbance resolves. Pacemakers also can be used on a permanent basis if the client's condition persists despite adequate therapy.

An artificial pacemaker is intended to provide a physiologic back-up for the heart during failure of the conduction system to depolarize the myocardium and maintain adequate cardiac output. When cardiac output is diminished because of lack of depolarization of the ventricles, artificial pacing can provide the necessary stimulus directly to the atria or ventricles, or both, to bring about contraction. If cardiac output is compromised because an ectopic pacemaker is causing the ventricles to depolarize and contract at a rate that does not promote adequate ventricular filling, artificial pacing competes with the ectopic pacemaker to assume the primary pacing function of the heart.

Pacemaker Design

An artificial pacemaker provides an external source of energy for impulse formation and delivery, and stimulation of myocardial tissue. Whereas numerous pacemaker models are available, each with unique capabilities, every pacemaker consists of a pulse generator with circuitry, the lead, and the electrode system.

The pulse generator is essentially the pacemaker's power source. It houses the electronic circuitry responsible for sending out appropriately timed signals and for sensing cardiac activity. The output circuit controls the current pulse delivery rate, pulse duration, and refractory period. The sensing circuit is responsible for identifying and analyzing any spontaneous intrinsic electrical activity and responding appropriately.

The pulse generator can be external or internal. The external unit is designed for temporary pacing, primarily for support of transient dysrhythmias that impair cardiac output.

The unit is the size of a small transistor radio and operates by dry-cell batteries (Fig. 57–9). There are dials for adjustment of power, rate of discharge, and mode. The pulse generator can also be permanently implanted. The surgeon places the permanent pulse generator into a small tunnel burrowed within the subcutaneous tissue below the right (Fig. 57–10) or left clavicle or in the abdominal cavity. The pulse generator is a small—about the size of a stethoscope head—hermetically sealed (to prevent exposure to body fluids) lithium battery. Most of the new generators can be reprogrammed after insertion, as needed.

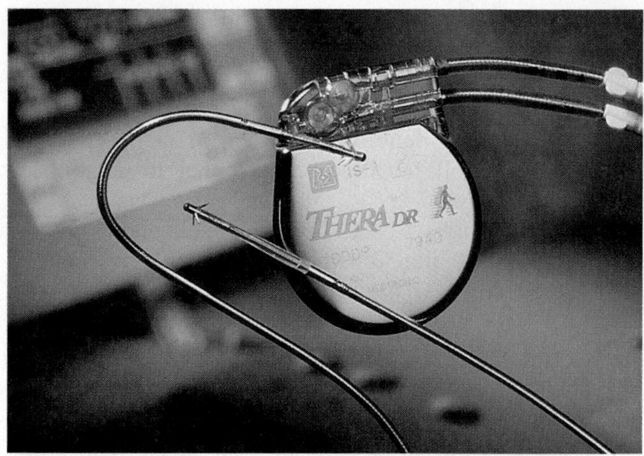

FIGURE 57–9 A permanent pacemaker (pulse generator). (Courtesy of Medtronic, Inc., Minneapolis, MN.)

The lead delivers the electrical impulse from the pulse generator to the myocardium. The leads consist of flexible conductive wires enclosed by insulating material. The electrode is the end of the lead that delivers the impulse directly to the myocardial wall. It is usually made of platinum-iridium, a highly conductive material that also deters the adherence of platelets. This system not only delivers electrical impulses but also relays information about spontaneous intracardiac signals back to the sensing circuit within the pulse generator.

Electrodes can be *unipolar* or *bipolar*. Unipolar designs incorporate the cardiac electrode as the negative

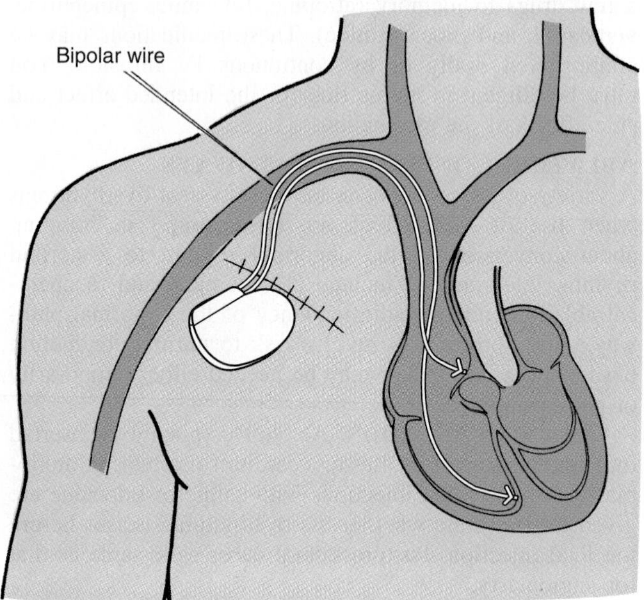

FIGURE 57–10 Transvenous temporary endocardial pacing is routine for most cardiac surgical procedures. This can be established by insertion of electrode wires through a vein (subclavian or internal jugular) and into the right atrium or right ventricle. Temporary pacing wires can also be advaned through pulmonary artery catheters. (From Thelan, L. A., et al. [1998]. *Critical care nursing* [3rd ed.]. St. Louis: Mosby–Year Book.)

terminal of the electrical circuit with the metallic shell or second wire of the impulse generator as the positive electrode. Bipolar systems use two wires, each ending in an electrode a short distance apart.

Single-chamber pacemakers pace either the ventricles or atria; *dual-chamber* pacemakers pace both the ventricles and atria.

Pacemaker Methods

Impulses can be delivered to myocardial tissue by three major modes of artificial pacing: external, epicardial, and endocardial.

External (Transcutaneous) Pacing. The heart is stimulated through large gelled electrode pads placed anteriorly and posteriorly and connected to an external transcutaneous pacemaker. Transcutaneous pacing is the treatment of choice in emergency cardiac care because it can be started quickly while a temporary transvenous pacemaker is being inserted or as prophylaxis against dysrhythmias. It is also the least invasive pacing technique. Because no vascular puncture is needed for electrode placement, transcutaneous pacing is preferred in clients who are receiving anticoagulation therapy or who may require thrombolytic therapy.

Because the anterior electrode is placed to the left of the sternum and centered close to the point of maximal impulse (PMI), excessive chest hair must be clipped or

TABLE 57–3 PACEMAKER MALFUNCTIONS AND NURSING INTERVENTIONS

Problem	Possible Cause	Nursing Interventions*
FAILURE TO PACE PROPERLY		
Intermittent or complete absence of pacing artifact Rapid, inappropriate firing of pacemaker (pacemaker-mediated tachycardia)	Battery failure A break or loose connection anywhere along the system Pulse generator failure Circuitry failure "Oversensing" or "undersensing" by the pacemaker	Replace pulse generator Replace battery unit Check and tighten all connections between pulse generator and leads Reduce or increase sensitivity threshold of pacemaker unit Assess client's tolerance of pacemaker failure; have emergency drugs on hand; perform CPR as indicated
FAILURE TO CAPTURE		
Pacing artifact present but is not followed by a QRS complex or P wave	Increased pacing threshold. Can be related to electrolyte imbalance, ischemia, drug toxicity, perforation, or excessive fibrosis of tissue at electrode site Lead displacement due to migration, or idle manipulation of pulse generator ("twiddler's syndrome")	Increase voltage by 1–2 mA (temporary pacemaker) Increase amplitude of pacemaker output/pulse width Reposition client to either side in attempt to improve contact of electrode with endocardium; in temporary pacemaker, try moving arm if lead wire is inserted in antecubital area Obtain chest film to determine pacemaker position Have emergency drugs on hand; initiate CPR if necessary
FAILURE TO SENSE		
Pacing artifact present despite the presence of QRS complexes and P waves A competitive rhythm may develop	Sensitivity threshold set too low Intrinsic beats are of too-low voltage and go undetected by pacemaker's sensing mechanism Dislodged or fractured lead Circuitry failure Electromagnetic interference	Increase sensitivity threshold on pulse generator Reposition client If client's intrinsic rhythm or rate is adequate, turn off pacemaker Increase pacing rate to overdrive client's intrinsic heart rate Give antidysrhythmics to decrease ectopy Notify physician Obtain chest x-ray to determine electrode placement
OVERSENSING		
Results from the inappropriate sensing of extraneous electrical signals or myopotentials (which should be ignored)	Sensitivity threshold set too high T wave sensing myopotentials Electromagnetic interference Two leads touching	Decrease sensitivity threshold Correct conditions that produce large T waves

* For all problems, document malfunction by an electrocardiogram. If pacemaker is programmable, have reprogramming machine available. Monitor client's tolerance to pacemaker malfunction (vital signs, chest pain).

CPR, cardiopulmonary resuscitation.

Modified from Huang, S. H., et al. (1989). *Coronary care nursing* (2nd ed.). Philadelphia: W. B. Saunders; and Thelan, L. A. et al. *Critical care nursing* (3rd ed.). St. Louis: Mosby–Year Book.

shaved to ensure good contact, or alternative pacing electrode positions must be used. The pacing device is usually activated at a rate of 80 BPM. Electrical capture is characterized by widening of the QRS complex and broadening of the T wave. Many clients feel extreme discomfort with each paced beat; this is a significant limitation to transcutaneous pacing.

Narcotic analgesia and sedation may be given to clients who are conscious or who regain consciousness to reduce discomfort and anxiety. Additional complications of external transcutaneous pacing can include skin burns, muscle twitching, psychological reactions, failure to "capture" (inability of the impulse to initiate a contraction), and failure to "sense" (inability of the pacemaker to sense intrinsic electrical activity) (Table 57–3).

EPICARDIAL (TRANSTHORACIC) PACING. With this method of artificial pacing, the electrical energy travels from an external pulse generator through the thoracic musculature directly to the epicardial surface of the heart via lead wires. Epicardial pacing is most commonly used during and immediately after open-heart surgery because there is direct access to the epicardium at this time. Some occasional complications may include lead dislodgment, microshock, cardiac tamponade, infection, psychological reactions, failure to capture, and failure to sense.

ENDOCARDIAL (TRANSVENOUS) PACING. Endocardial pacing is the most common mode of pacing the heart in emergency situations. The surgeon inserts the pacing electrode via the transvenous route (via the antecubital, femoral, jugular, or subclavian vein) and then threads the electrode into the right atrium or right ventricle so that it comes into direct contact with the endocardium. This procedure can be done at the bedside under fluoroscopic control or in a cardiovascular laboratory.

Major drawbacks include thrombophlebitis, infection at the insertion site, sepsis from unsterile technique, increased chance of lead displacement as the client changes position, and the discomfort of having the extremity nearest the insertion site immobilized (Fig. 57–11). Other additional complications occasionally seen are pacer-induced dysrhythmias, hiccups, abdominal twitching, myocardial irritability, perforation of chamber or septum, failure to capture, and failure to sense.

Temporary Pacing

Temporary pacing may be used in emergent or elective situations that require limited, short-term pacing (<2 weeks). The pulse generator is external. Temporary pacemakers can be applied transcutaneously and can be inserted transthoracically or, more commonly, transvenously.

Although the principles of cardiac pacing are the same for temporary and permanent pacemakers, each type presents distinct issues for nurses to assess and to teach to the client and family. Clients with a temporary pacemaker need the following:

- An explanation about the pacemaker
- Monitoring for response to the pacemaker
- Maintenance of electrical safety
- Monitoring for pacing parameters (sensing, capturing, threshold)
- Protection against injury and infection

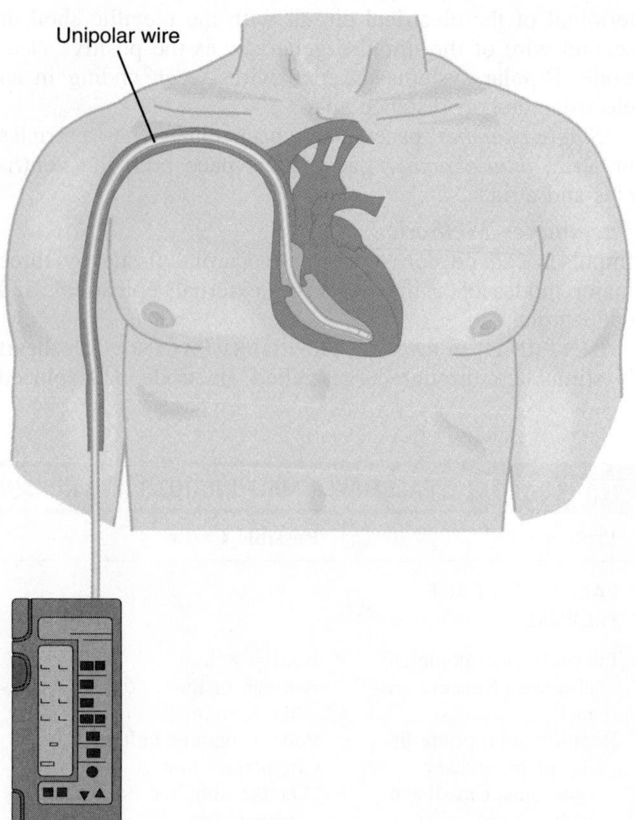

FIGURE 57–11 A temporary endocardial pacemaker.

Before the procedure, explain the purpose of the temporary pacemaker to the client and family. Ensure that a permit for the procedure has been signed and that all questions have been answered. Necessary equipment is gathered, and the external generator is checked (battery and sense and pace modes). Assess the client's vital signs, and obtain a rhythm strip.

During the procedure, monitor the client's ECG and vital signs continuously. Large P waves are seen as the catheter passes through the atrium, and larger QRS complexes are seen in the ventricles. Set and maintain the stimulus and sensitivity settings according to the physician's orders. Tape or suture the electrode at the insertion site.

After the procedure, assess vital signs routinely along with heart rhythm and emotional reactions to the procedure and pacing. Secure and check all connections. Monitor battery and control settings. Clean and dress the incision site according to protocols. Keep the generator dry and protect the controls from mishandling. The client must be protected from electrical microshocks and electromagnetic interference. Wear rubber gloves when exposed wires are handled. Check electrical equipment for adequate grounding. Limit motion of the extremity at the insertion site. Stabilize arm, catheter, and pacemaker to an arm board and avoid movement of the arm above shoulder level. Do not lift the client from under the arm. If the leg is the insertion site, limit its motion, especially hip flexion and outward rotation.

In addition to protecting the client from injury, monitor pacemaker function. Document the location and

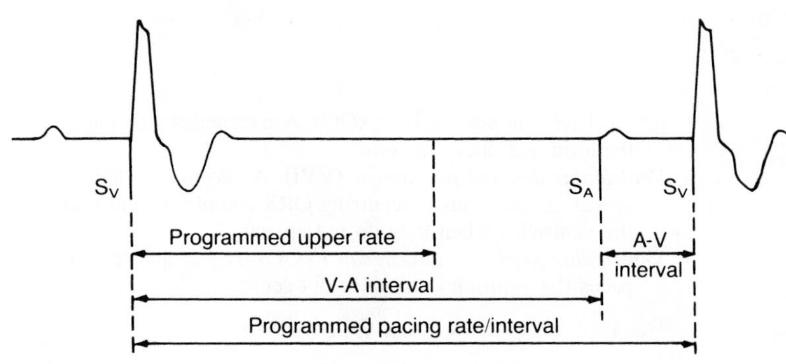

FIGURE 57–12 Pacing intervals. The atrioventricular (A-V, delay) interval can be thought of as an artificial P-R interval. The programmed pacing rate, or interval, is also called the ventriculoventricular (V-V) interval. Ventricular pacing occurs if intrinsic ventricular activity does not occur within the V-V interval. (From *Symbiotics series: Selecting the DDD patient* [1984]. Minneapolis: Medtronic.)

type of pacing lead. Note the pacing mode, stimulus threshold, sensitivity setting, pacing rate and intervals, and intrinsic rhythm. Pacing intervals are shown in Figure 57–12.

Permanent Pacing

Permanent pacing is indicated for chronic or recurrent dysrhythmias that are severe, unresponsive to antiarrhythmic medication, and caused by AV block or sinus node malfunction. The need for permanent pacemakers is confirmed through ECGs, electrophysiology studies, and Holter monitoring. Indications for permanent pacemakers have been grouped into three classes. Class I criteria are identified in Box 57–3.[31, 32]

Clinical manifestations that are directly attributable to the slow heart rate include transient dizziness, lightheadedness, near syncope or frank syncope as manifestations of transient cerebral ischemia, and more generalized manifestations such as marked exercise intolerance or frank heart failure.[12, 31, 32]

BOX 57–3 Clinical Conditions That Warrant Permanent Pacemakers (Class I Criteria)

A. Complete heart block (permanent or intermittent), associated with the following complications:
   1. Symptomatic bradycardia
   2. Left ventricular heart failure
   3. Ectopic rhythms that suppress the automaticity of escape pacemakers and result in symptomatic bradycardia
   4. Documented periods of asystole greater than 3 seconds or any escape rate less than 40 beats per minute in a symptom-free client
   5. Confusional states that clear with temporary pacing
   6. Post-AV (atrioventricular) junctional ablation
B. Second-degree AV block, permanent or intermittent, with symptomatic bradycardia
C. Atrial fibrillation, atrial flutter, supraventricular tachycardia with complete heart block or advanced AV block, bradycardia (the bradycardia must be unrelated to digitalis or drugs known to impair AV conduction)

From Zaim, B, Zaim, S., & Kutalek, S. (1994). Indications for use of permanent cardiac pacemakers. *Heart Disease and Stroke, 3,* 71–76.

Pacemaker Modes

There are two basic kinds of pacemakers:

1. *Fixed-rate* (non-demand or asynchronous). Fixed-rate pacemakers are designed to fire constantly as a preset rate without regard to the electrical activity of the client's heart. This mode of pacing is appropriate in the absence of any electrical activity (asystole) but is dangerous in the presence of an intrinsic rhythm because of the potential of the pacemaker to fire during the vulnerable period of repolarization and initiate lethal ventricular dysrhythmias.
2. *Demand* pacemakers contain a device that senses the heart's electrical activity and fires at a present rate only when the heart's electrical activity drops below a predetermined rate level (Fig. 57–13).

In addition to a variety of capabilities, permanent pacemakers now have special programmable and antitachyarrhythmic functions that are quite complex. In order to communicate all the functions of the individual pacemakers, international codes were developed. Pacemakers are identified with a five-digit letter code. Although the last two letters contain pertinent information, commonly a pacemaker is referred to only by its first three letters (Box 57–4).

Pacemaker Function

Because there are many types of pacemakers with more than 250 programs, the general functions are discussed first. A simple demand pacing system works in the following manner. The cardiac cycle normally begins with the client's own beat. The pacemaker's sensor senses

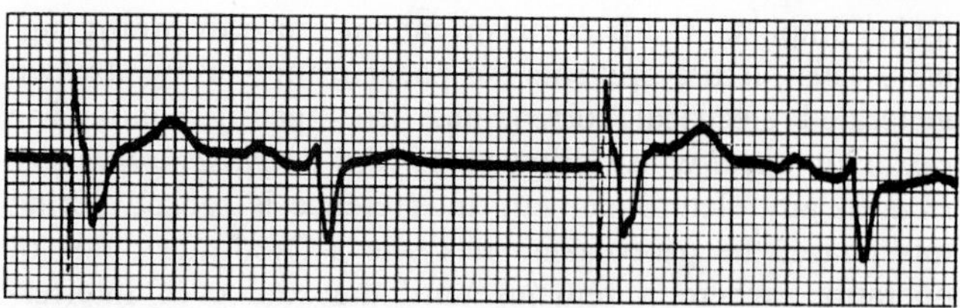

FIGURE 57–13 Demand pacing. The pacemaker initiates an electrical impulse when the sinus node fails to pace the heart. (From Phillips, R. E., & Feeney, M. K. [1990]. *The cardiac rhythms: A systematic approach to interpretation* [3rd ed.]. Philadelphia: W. B. Saunders.)

BOX 57–4 Classification System for Pacemakers

First Letter: Chamber-Paced

Indicates which chamber(s) of the heart will be stimulated.

V = Ventricle
A = Atrium
D = Dual-chamber (both atria and ventricles stimulated)

Second Letter: Chamber-Sensed

Indicates the chamber(s) of the heart in which the lead is capable of recognizing intrinsic electrical activity.

V = Ventricle
A = Atrium
D = Dual-chamber (sensing capabilities in atria and ventricles)
O = No sensing capability

Third Letter: Mode of Response

Indicates how the pacemaker will act based on the information it senses.

T = Triggered (may have energy output triggered)
I = Inhibited (pacing output inhibited by intrinsic activity)
D = Dual-chamber (may be either inhibiting or triggering of both chambers)

Fourth Letter: Programmable Functions

Indicates ability to change function once the pacemaker has been implanted.

P = Programmable for one or two functions
M = Multiprogrammable ability to change functions other than the rate or output

Fifth Letter: Tachyarrhythmic Functions

Indicates specific methods of interrupting tachyarrhythmias.

B = Bursts of pacing
N = Normal rate competition
S = Scanning

Examples

Pacing Modes Within Single-Chamber Pacemakers

Atrial demand pacemaker (AAI). A pacemaker that senses spontaneously occurring P waves and paces the atria when they do not appear.

Atrial fixed-rate pacemaker (AOO). A pacemaker that paces the atria and does not sense.

Ventricular demand pacemaker (VVI). A pacemaker that senses spontaneously occurring QRS complexes and paces the ventricles when they do not appear.

Ventricular fixed-rate pacemaker (VOO). A pacemaker that paces the ventricles and does not sense.

Pacing Modes Within Dual-Chamber Pacemakers

Atrial synchronous ventricular pacemaker (VDD). A pacemaker that senses spontaneously occurring P waves and QRS complexes and paces the ventricles when QRS complexes fail to appear after spontaneously occurring P waves, as in complete atrioventricular (AV) block. In this type of pacemaker, the pacing of ventricles is synchronized with the P waves, so that the ventricular contractions follow the atrial contractions in a normal sequence. A major benefit is that it permits the heart rate to vary, and AV synchrony occurs, depending on the physiologic demands of the body. A built-in safety mechanism causes ventricular depolarizations to occur at a fixed rate should atrial rates become too fast.

AV synchronous pacemaker (VAT). A pacemaker that has ventricular pacing, atrial sensing, and triggered response to sensing. The ventricular pacing stimulus will fire at a set time after sensing of a spontaneous atrial depolarization.

AV sequential pacemaker (DVI). A pacemaker that senses spontaneously occurring QRS complexes and paces both the atria and ventricles (the atria first, followed by the ventricles after a short delay) when QRS complexes do not appear.

AV sequential fixed-rate pacemaker (DOO). A pacemaker that paces both the atria and ventricles, but does not sense.

Optimal sequential pacemaker (DDD). A pacemaker that senses spontaneously occurring P waves and QRS complexes and (1) paces the atria when P waves fail to appear, as in sick sinus syndrome, and (2) paces the ventricles when QRS complexes fail to appear after spontaneously occurring or paced P waves. In this type of pacemaker, like the VDD pacemaker, the pacing of ventricles is synchronized with the P waves, so that the ventricular contractions follow the atrial contractions in a normal sequence.

whether the intrinsic beat has occurred; if not, the pacer sends out an impulse to begin myocardial depolarization through a pulse generator. The impulse generator is said to "capture" the myocardium and thereby maintain heart rhythm.

For a predetermined amount of time after the pacemaker impulse, the pacemaker cannot sense incoming signals. This feature prevents the pacer from sensing its own generated electrical current and from acting again. The *refractory period* is followed by the *noise-sampling period*. If any electromagnetic interference is sensed during this phase, the pacemaker goes into a fixed-rate mode of operation, where it remains until the source of interference is removed. At the end of the noise-sampling period, the *alert period* begins and the cycle starts over again. If a PVC or PAC occurs during the alert period, the pacemaker can sense it and start its cycle over again without emitting any impulse.

Electrocardiography of Paced Beats

The ECG appearance of a paced rhythm differs from that of a normal sinus rhythm. A pacing artifact is seen. With atrial pacing, a P wave follows the artifact but may be hidden in some leads. Examination of leads II and V_1 is best for deciding whether a P wave follows a pacer spike. The QRS complex appears normal with atrial pacing; the impulse travels through usual conduction systems.

The ECG with ventricular pacing shows an abnormal QRS complex because the impulse begins in the ventricle. With right ventricular endocardial pacing, a pseudo-LBBB ECG wave is created. If the left ventricle is paced, a pseudo-RBBB is created.

Assess the ECG strip for pacer spikes followed by the expected appearance of a P wave or QRS complex. Spikes not followed by depolarization waves or paced beats that appear too early or too late may signal pacemaker failure.

Pacemaker Failure

Malfunctions can occur in the pacemaker's sensor or pulse generator. Complications associated with the components of the pacemaker system itself (see Table 57–3) may include:

1. *Failure to sense*—an inability of the sensor to detect the client's intrinsic beats; as a result, the pacemaker sends out impulses too early (Fig. 57–14*A*). The failure may be due to improper position of the catheter, tip or lead dislodgment, battery failure, the sensitivity set too low, or a fractured wire in the catheter.
2. *Failure to pace*—a malfunction of the pulse generator. The ECG shows an absence of any impulse (Fig. 57–14*B*). Component failure to discharge (pace) can be due to battery failure, lead dislodgment, fracture of the lead wire inside the catheter, disconnections between catheter and generator, or a sensing malfunction.
3. *Failure to capture*—a disorder in the pacemaker electrodes; the impulse does not generate depolarization (Fig. 57–14*C*). This complication can result from low voltage, battery failure, faulty connections between the pulse generator and catheter, improper position of the catheter, catheter wire fracture, fibrosis at the catheter tip, or a catheter fracture.

Clinical manifestations associated with pacemaker malfunctioning include syncope, bradycardia or tachycardia, and palpitations. When these manifestations occur, the malfunctioning leads or pacemaker must be replaced.

Teach the client and family how to care for the pacemaker and the precautions to follow (see Client Education Guide).[11, 32, 34]

Nursing Management of Clients with Pacemakers

ASSESSMENT

Assess the client for *subjective* clinical manifestations of dysrhythmias and alterations in cardiac output. These include palpitations, syncope, fatigue, shortness of breath, chest pain, or skipped beats felt in the chest. The client may also feel anxiety about the heart disorder and may manifest nervousness, fear, sleeplessness, uncertainty, or hopelessness. *Objective* clinical manifestations may include diaphoresis, pallor or cyanosis, variations in radial and apical pulses such as bradycardia or tachycardia, rhythm changes, hypotension, crackles, and decreased mental acuity. The client may be fearful of being left alone. Monitoring is begun, and the heart rhythm is observed continuously by a nurse, a computer, and an ECG technician. Rhythm strips are examined at least every shift.

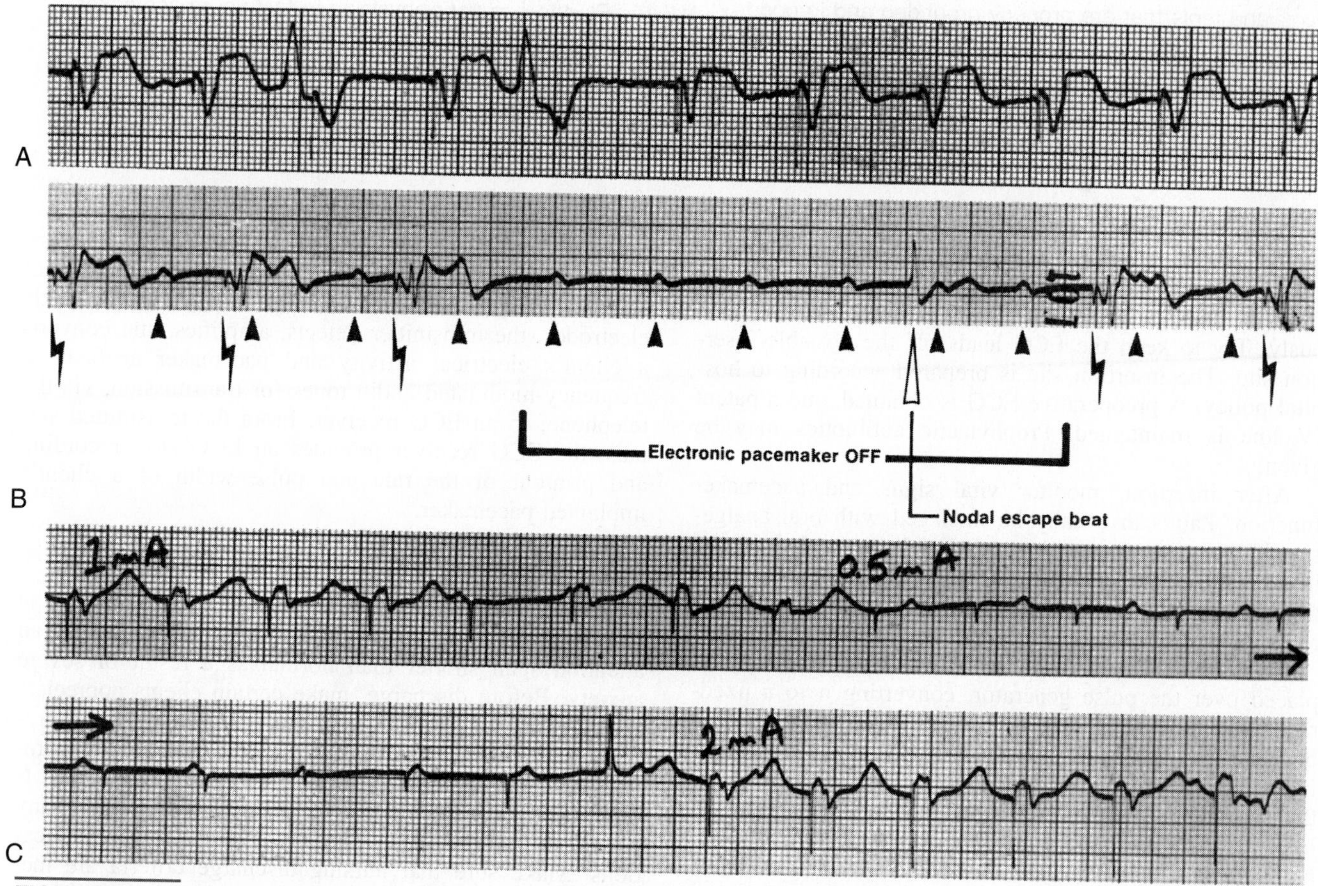

FIGURE 57–14 Pacemaker failures. *A*, Failure to sense. *B*, Failure to pace. *C*, Failure to capture. (From Phillips, R. E., & Feeney, M. K. [1990]. *The cardiac rhythms: A systematic approach to interpretation* [3rd ed.]. Philadelphia: W. B. Saunders.)

CLIENT EDUCATION GUIDE

The Client with a Permanent Pacemaker

Wound Care

1. Assess your wound daily.
2. Report any signs of inflammation (fever, redness, tenderness, discharge, or warmth) to the physician.
3. Avoid constrictive clothing (e.g., tight brassiere straps), which puts excessive pressure on the wound and the pulse generator.
4. Avoid extensive "toying" with the pulse generator, because this may cause pacemaker malfunction and local skin inflammation.

Pacemaker Management

1. Take your pulse daily in your wrist or on your neck. You will be taught how to do this before leaving the hospital.
2. Notify the physician if your pulse is slower than the set rate; also report sensations of feeling your heart "racing," beating irregularly, or of dizziness.
3. Avoid being near areas with high voltage, magnetic force fields, or radiation; this can cause pacemaker problems.
4. Avoid being near large running motors (gas or electric) and standing near high-tension wires, power plants, radio transmitters, large industrial magnets, and arc welding machines. Riding in a car is safe, but do not bring the pacemaker to within 6 to 12 inches of the distributor coil of a running engine.
5. You can continue to safely operate most appliances and tools that are properly grounded and in good repair, including microwave ovens, televisions, video recorders, AM and FM radios, electric blankets, lawn mowers, leaf blowers, and cars.
6. You can safely operate the following office and light industrial equipment that is properly grounded and in good repair, such as electric typewriters, copying machines, and personal computers.
7. An airport's metal detector may be triggered by the pacemaker's metal casing and the programming magnet. Mention your pacemaker to security guards. The metal detector itself does not harm the pacemaker.
8. At all times, carry a pacemaker identity card (including programming information—pacemaker manufacturer, emergency phone numbers). Wear a medical alert bracelet.
9. Avoid activity that might damage the pulse generator, such as playing football and firing a rifle with the butt end against the affected shoulder.
10. Some stores sell antitheft devices that may affect pacemaker function. If you suddenly become dizzy, move away from the area and notify the store clerk about the pacemaker.
11. If radiation therapy has been prescribed to the area in which the pulse generator was implanted, the pulse generator must be relocated.
12. Do not lift more than 5 to 10 pounds (equivalent to a full grocery sack or a gallon of milk) for the first 6 weeks after surgery. Do not move your arms and shoulders vigorously for the first 6 weeks. Normal activities (including sexual activity) can be resumed in 6 weeks.
13. Discuss with the nurse the purpose, dose, schedule, and possible side effects of prescribed medications. Consult your written information sheets to reinforce learning.
14. Plan to see your physician to test your pacemaker. Your cardiologist will periodically reevaluate pacemaker function and can reprogram it if needed. You may also be able to check your pacemaker by telephone. If this is possible, you will receive instructions.

Explain the purpose of the pacemaker and the experience of having a pacemaker inserted to the client and family. Most permanent pacemakers are inserted transvenously. Try to keep the ECG leads off the possible insertion site. The insertion site is prepared according to hospital policy. A preoperative ECG is obtained, and a patent IV line is maintained. Prophylactic antibiotics may be given.

After insertion, monitor vital signs and pacemaker function. Pain can usually be managed with oral analgesics if the transvenous approach has been used. Initially, instruct the client to avoid excessive extension or abduction of the arm on the operative side. Perform passive range-of-motion exercises on the arm.

Obtain paced and nonpaced ECGs. A magnet may be placed over the pulse generator, converting it to a fixed-rate pacing mode, so that the client's intrinsic rhythm can be determined. The location of the pacemaker electrodes is determined by x-ray. The model and serial numbers of the pulse generator and leads along with the date of implantation and programmed functions of the initial implant are recorded.

Transtelephonic Pacemaker Monitoring

Special telephone monitoring of the client's ECG may be done from time to time on an outpatient basis. Telephone ECG systems are designed for follow-up monitoring of clients with pacemakers. Via finger tip, wrist, or ankle electrodes, the transmitter detects, amplifies, and converts a client's electrical activity and pacemaker artifacts to frequency-modulated audio tones for transmission, via the telephone, to an ECG receiver. From the transmitted signals, the ECG receiver provides an ECG strip recording and printout of the rate and pulse width of a client's implanted pacemaker.

Self-Care

It may be necessary to teach about the nature of the disorder several times, because the client may have an attention span shorter than normal as a result of severe anxiety. Before discharge, make certain clients appreciate the importance of taking antidysrhythmic agents as prescribed. Include details concerning medication administration, dosage, and side effects in the discharge plan. If discharged too early and in an unstable condition, many clients risk further exacerbations or additional complications. Make sure that nursing discharge criteria are met and documented.

Clients who have experienced cardiac dysrhythmias

while at a health care facility may be apprehensive about leaving the facility. Those who have experienced innocuous dysrhythmias may need only calm reassurance and an explanation of the cause of their disorder. Clients with recurring life-threatening dysrhythmias, such as VT, require comprehensive and specialized attention. These clients may have experienced many frightening events in the course of their hospitalization.

When a client is at risk for development of a life-threatening dysrhythmia, ascertain whether the client's housemates and significant others know how to perform CPR. Refer them to community agencies that provide CPR training (e.g., the American Heart Association, the American Red Cross, local fire department, local hospital).

Sometimes clients with serious, chronic, or potential dysrhythmias use portable telemetry units for self-monitoring at home after discharge. This allows resumption of daily activities while providing continuous 24-hour surveillance of cardiac rhythm. Nurses are often responsible for instructing clients in the use of these units. Ask the client to keep a diary of daily activities so that clinicians can correlate factors in the client's life that may be contributing to the development of dysrhythmias.

Finally, instruct clients concerning the importance of regular medical follow-up. Advise them to keep regular appointments with their physician after discharge. Explain to the client and significant others how to obtain emergency medical attention if necessary.

Living under the constant threat of sudden death provokes anxiety, depression, and, occasionally, dependent behavior. In some cases, psychological counseling may bolster coping resources. Recommend community and private counseling services for the client and significant others.

CONCLUSIONS

Common dysrhythmias usually do not interfere with everyday activities. In fact, most people with dysrhythmias lead a productive and relatively normal life. Clients need to follow a prescribed medical regimen, to take medications as directed, to report any manifestations and side effects, and to become aware of the importance of continued medical care.

THINKING CRITICALLY

1. You are walking with a client in the hospital. He is recovering from an MI. A dysrhythmia develops. What assessments should you perform? What care does the client need?

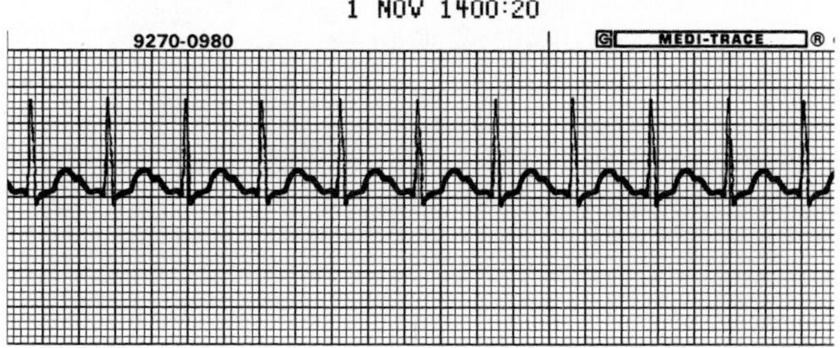

ECG Strip.

Factors to Consider. What is the usual heart rhythm response to activity? How can you assess if your client is tolerating this rhythm? How should the client be returned to his room?

2. An 82-year-old woman is brought to the emergency department by her son after losing consciousness and hitting her head upon falling. She is now awake and states that she has been having periods of dizziness and blackouts for the past few weeks. During your physical examination, you notice what appears to be a pacemaker device implanted under her left clavicle. What additional assessments should you make? What information should you obtain about the pacemaker?

Factors to Consider. What might have happened to the pacemaker during the fall? Could a faulty pacemaker be responsible for the loss of consciousness?

BIBLIOGRAPHY

1. American Heart Association. (1996). *Handbook of emergency cardiac care for health care providers 1996*. Dallas: Author.
2. American Heart Association. (1999). *Heart and stroke facts*. Dallas: Author.
3. Aronow, W. S. (1995). Treatment of ventricular arrhythmias in older adults. *Journal of the American Geriatrics Society 43*(6), 688–695.
4. Brown, D. L. (1998). *Cardiac intensive care*. Philadelphia: W. B. Saunders.
5. Bubien, R., et al. (1993). What you need to know about radiofrequency ablation. *American Journal of Nursing, 93*(7), 30–36.
6. Bush, D. E. (1994). Permanent cardiac pacemakers in the elderly. *Journal of the American Geriatrics Society, 42*(3), 326–334.
7. Conover, M. B. (1996). *Understanding electrocardiography* (7th ed.). St. Louis: Mosby–Year Book.
8. Collins, M. A. (1994). When your patient has an implantable cardioverter defibrillator. *American Journal of Nursing, 94*(3), 34–39.
9. Diem, S., Lantos, J., & Tukley, J. (1996). Cardiopulmonary resuscitation on television: Miracles or misinformation. *New England Journal of Medicine 334*(12), 1578–1582.
10. Dunn, F. G. (1990). Prevention of sudden cardiac death. *Cardiovascular Clinics, 20*(3), 95–109.
11. Frye, R. L., et al. (1984). Guidelines for permanent cardiac pacemaker implantation: A report of the Joint American College of Cardiology/American Heart Association Task Force of the Assessment of Cardiovascular Procedures. *Circulation, 70,* 331A–337A.
12. Hasemeier, C. S. (1996). Permanent pacemaker. *American Journal of Nursing, 96*(2), 30–31.
13. Hayes, D. L. (1992). The next 5 years in cardiac pacemakers: A preview. *Mayo Clinic Proceedings, 67*(4), 379–384.
14. Higgins, C. A. (1990). The AICD: A teaching plan for patients and families. *Critical Care Nurse, 10*(6), 69–74.
15. Kater, K. M., et al. (1992). Corralling atrial fibrillation with "maze" surgery. *American Journal of Nursing, 92*(7), 34–38.
16. Karnes, N. (1995). Adenosine: A quick fix for PSVT—paroxysmal supraventricular tachycardia. *Nursing 25*(7), 55–56.
17. King, K. B. (1994). Preparing patients and families for health care procedures. *Heart Disease and Stroke, 3*(2), 95–97.
18. Massie, B. M., & Amidon T. A. (1997). Disturbances in rate and rhythm. In L. M. Tierney, et al. (Eds.), *Current medical diagnosis and treatment* (36th ed.). Stamford, CT: Appleton and Lange.
19. Massie, B. M., & Amidon, T. A. (1997). Conduction disturbances. In L. M. Tierney, et al. (Eds.), *Current medical diagnosis and treatment* (36th ed.). Stamford, CT: Appleton and Lange.
20. Nattel, S. (1995). Newer developments in the management of atrial fibrillation. *American Heart Journal 130*(5), 1094–1106.
21. Moser, S. A., Crawford, D., & Thomas, A. (1993). Updated care guidelines for patients with automatic implantable cardioverter defibrillators. *Critical Care Nurse, 13*(4), 62–71.

22. Ophie, L. H, & Marcus, F. I. (1997). Antiarrhythmic drugs. In L. H. Ophie (Ed.)., *Drugs for the heart* (4th ed.). Philadelphia: W. B. Saunders.
23. Petrosky-Pacini, A. J. (1996). The automatic implantable cardioverter defibrillator in home care. *Home Healthcare Nurse 14*(4), 238–243.
24. Porter, L. A. (1995). Drug profiles: Maximizing therapeutic effectiveness. *Journal of Cardiovascular Nursing, 10*(1), 64–72.
25. Porterfield, L. M., Porterfield, J. G., & Collins, S. W. (1993). The cutting edge in arrhythmias. *Critical Care Nurse, 13*(suppl. 6), 8–9.
26. Rakel, R. E. (1992). *Conn's current therapy*. Philadelphia: W. B. Saunders.
27. Saver, C. L. (1994). Decoding the ACLS algorithms. *American Journal of Nursing, 94*(1), 26–36.
28. Schron, E. B., et al. (1996). Relation of sociodemographic, clinical, and quality of life variables to adherence in the cardiac arrhythmia suppression trial. *Cardiovascular Nursing, 32*(2), 1–5.
29. Simons, L. H., Cunningham, S., & Catanzaro, M. (1992). Emotional responses and experiences of wives of men who survive a sudden cardiac death event. *Cardiovascular Nursing, 28*(2), 17–21.
30. Sims, J. M., & Miracle, V. (1997). Ventricular tachycardia. *Nursing 97, 21*(11), 47.
31. Sirles, A. T., & Selleck, C. S. (1989). Cardiac disease and the family: Impact, assessment, and implications. *Journal of Cardiovascular Nursing, 3*(2), 23–32.
32. Sommers, M. S. (1992). Preventing complications of CPR. *Medical-Surgical Nursing Quarterly, 1*(1), 44–54.
33. Sommers, M. S. (1992). The near-death experience after cardiopulmonary arrest. *Medical-Surgical Nursing Quarterly, 1*(1), 55–62.
34. Stuart, J. V., & Sheehan, A. M. (1991). Permanent pacemakers: The nurse's role in patient education and follow-up care. *Journal of Cardiovascular Nursing, 5*(3), 32–43.
35. Thelan, L. A., et al. (1998). Temporary pacemakers. In L. A. Thelan, et al. (Eds.), *Critical care nursing: Diagnosis and management* (3rd ed.). St. Louis: Mosby–Year Book.
36. Thelan, L. A., et al. (1998). Implantable cardioverter defibrillator. In L. A. Thelan, et al. (Eds.), *Critical care nursing: Diagnosis and management* (3rd ed.). St. Louis: Mosby–Year Book.
37. Whalley, D. W., Wendt, D. J. & Grant, A. O. (1995). Basic concepts in cellular cardiac electrophysiology: II. Block of ion channels by antiarrhythmic drugs. *Pacing and Clinical Electrophysiology, 18,* 1686–1703.
38. Zaim, B., Zaim, S., & Kutalek, S. P. (1994). Indications for use of permanent cardiac pacemakers. *Heart Disease and Stroke, 3*(2), 71–76.
39. Zipes, D. P. (1997). Management of cardiac arrhythmias: Pharmacological, electrical, and surgical techniques. In E. Braunwald (Ed.), *Heart disease* (5th ed.). Philadelphia: W. B. Saunders.
40. Zipes, D. P. (1997). Specific arrhythmias: Diagnosis and treatment. In E. Braunwald (Ed.), *Heart disease* (5th ed.). Philadelphia: W. B. Saunders.

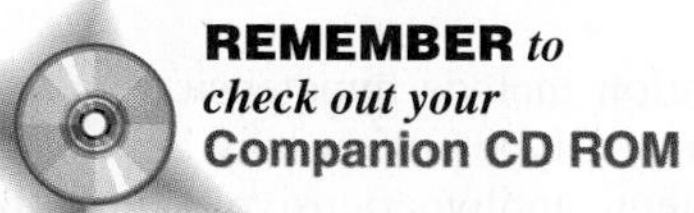

CHAPTER 58

Management of Clients with Myocardial Infarction

Janice Tazbir
Peggy Gerard

NURSING OUTCOMES CLASSIFICATION (NOC)
for Nursing Diagnoses—Clients with Myocardial Infarction

Altered Health Maintenance
Health Promoting Behavior
Health Seeking Behavior
Knowledge: Health Behaviors
Participation: Health Care Decisions
Psychosocial Adjustment: Life Change
Self-Direction of Care

Altered Tissue Perfusion (Cardiopulmonary)
Pain Level
Tissue Perfusion: Cardiac

Anxiety and Fear
Anxiety Control
Coping
Fear Control

Decreased Cardiac Output
Cardiac Pump Effectiveness
Circulation Status
Vital Signs Status

Fluid Volume Excess
Electrolyte and Acid-Base Balance
Fluid Balance
Hydration

Impaired Gas Exchange
Electrolyte and Acid-Base Balance
Respiratory Status: Ventilation

Pain
Comfort Level
Pain Control
Pain: Disruptive Effects
Pain Level

Powerlessness
Depression Control
Depression Level
Health Beliefs: Perceived Ability to Perform
Health Beliefs: Perceived Control
Health Beliefs: Perceived Resources

Risk for Activity Intolerance
Cardiac Pump Effectiveness
Circulation Status
Energy Conservation
Knowledge: Prescribed Activity

Risk for Constipation
Bowel Elimination
Mobility Level
Nutritional Status: Food and Fluid Intake

Risk for Impaired Skin Integrity
Immobility Consequences: Physiologic
Tissue Integrity: Skin and Mucous Membranes
Tissue Perfusion: Peripheral

Risk for Injury
Risk Control

The heart requires a balance between oxygen supply and oxygen demand in order to function properly. The integrity of the coronary arteries is an important determinant of oxygen supply to the heart muscle. Any disorder that reduces the lumen of an artery may cause a decrease in blood flow and oxygen delivery to heart muscle and may result in the acute coronary syndromes of angina, myocardial infarction (MI), and sudden cardiac death. Coronary heart disease (CHD) is the primary underlying cause of these syndromes and is the single largest killer of American men and women.[2]

The clinical syndromes associated with CHD are familiar to most Americans. Almost every day, the news media covers a story on a celebrity who has suffered from or was treated for chest pain, heart attack, or cardiac arrest. Turn on any television hospital drama and you will see someone seeking treatment for an episode of chest pain. Many of us also have had personal experience with CHD through the illness of a relative or close friend.

Acute coronary syndromes are responsible for more than 250,000 deaths annually and result from a progressive atherosclerotic process that culminates in rupture of atherosclerotic plaques and thrombus formation.[2] This chapter reviews the risk factors, pathophysiology, clinical manifestations, and medical and nursing interventions for the acute coronary syndromes of angina pectoris (a type of chest pain) and MI.

ANGINA PECTORIS

As vessels become lined with atherosclerotic plaques, plaques may be disrupted and thrombi may form, leading to clinical manifestations of inadequate blood supply in the tissues supplied by these vessels. Problems such as stroke, claudication, and angina develop. Stroke is described in Chapter 70 and claudication is discussed in Chapter 53.

Angina pectoris is chest pain resulting from myocardial ischemia (inadequate blood supply to the myocardium).[29] It is a common manifestation of CHD and affects about 6,200,000 Americans—2,300,000 men and 3,900,000 women. According to the Framingham Heart Study, approximately 350,000 new cases of angina occur each year.[2] Angina can also occur in clients with normal coronary arteries, but it is less common. Clients with aortic stenosis, hypertension, and hypertrophic cardiomyopathy can have angina pectoris.

Etiology and Risk Factors

Angina pectoris is associated with atherosclerotic lesions and is a manifestation of CHD (see Chapter 56). Angina can be caused either by chronic or acute blockage of a coronary artery or by coronary artery spasm. Chronic blockages are associated with fixed calcified (type Vb) or fibrotic (type Vc) atherosclerotic lesions that occlude more than 75% of the vessel lumen.[8]

When fixed blockages are present in the coronary arteries, conditions that increase myocardial oxygen demand (e.g., physical exertion, emotion, exposure to cold) may precipitate episodes of angina. Because the severely stenosed arteries cannot deliver enough oxygen to meet the increased demand, ischemia results.[31, 36] In contrast, acute blockage of a coronary artery results from rupture or disruption of vulnerable atherosclerotic plaques that cause platelet aggregation and thrombus formation (see etiology of MI).[2] Acute blockages are associated with unstable angina and MI.

Primary prevention is through the lifelong commitment to reducing the risk factors of CHD (see Chapter 56). Secondary prevention is through recognition and early treatment of anginal attacks. Tertiary prevention is resolution of angina before myocardial damage occurs.

Pathophysiology

The coronary arteries normally supply the myocardium with blood to meet its metabolic needs during varying workloads. The coronary vessels are usually efficient and perfuse the myocardium during diastole. When the heart needs more blood, the vessels dilate. As the vessels become lined and eventually occluded with atherosclerotic plaques and thrombi, the vessels can no longer dilate properly.

Myocardial ischemia develops if the blood supply through the coronary vessels or oxygen content of the blood is not adequate to meet metabolic demands. Disorders of the coronary vessels, the circulation, or the blood may lead to deficits in supply.

Disorders of the coronary vessels include atherosclerosis, arterial spasm, and coronary arteritis. Atherosclerosis increases resistance to flow. Arterial spasm also increases resistance. Coronary *arteritis* is inflammation of the coronary arteries caused by infection or autoimmune disease.

Disorders of circulation include hypotension and aortic stenosis and insufficiency. Hypotension may be a result of spinal anesthesia, potent antihypertensive drugs, blood loss, or other factors that result in decreased blood return to the heart. Aortic valve stenosis or insufficiency results in decreased filling pressure of the coronary arteries.

Blood disorders include anemia, hypoxemia, and polycythemia. Anemia and hypoxemia result in decreased oxygen flow to the myocardium. Polycythemia increases blood viscosity, which slows blood flow through the coronary arteries.

The opposite of supply is demand, and increased demands can be placed on the heart. Conditions that increase demands on the myocardium are those that increase cardiac output or increase myocardial need for oxygen (see Box 58–1).

Myocardial ischemia occurs when either supply or demand is altered. In some people, the coronary arteries can supply adequate blood when the person is at rest; when the person attempts activity or is taxed in some other manner, however, angina develops. Myocardial cells become ischemic within 10 seconds of coronary artery occlusion. After several minutes of ischemia, the pumping function of the heart is reduced. The reduction in pump-

BOX 58–1 Factors Influencing Myocardial Supply and Demand

Factors That Decrease Supply

Coronary Vessel Disorders

Atherosclerosis
Arterial spasm
Coronary arteritis

Circulation Disorders

Hypotension
Aortic stenosis
Aortic insufficiency

Blood Disorders

Anemia
Hypoxemia
Polycythemia

Factors That Increase Demand

Increased Cardiac Output

Exercise
Emotion
Digestion of a large meal
Anemia
Hyperthyroidism

Increased Myocardial Need for Oxygen

Damaged myocardium
Myocardial hypertrophy
Aortic stenosis
Aortic insufficiency
Diastolic hypertension
Thyrotoxicosis
Strong emotions
Heavy exertion

ing deprives the ischemic cells of needed oxygen and glucose. The cells convert to anaerobic metabolism, which leaves lactic acid as a waste product. As lactic acid accumulates, pain develops. Angina pectoris is transient, lasting for only 3 to 5 minutes. If blood flow is restored, no permanent myocardial damage occurs.

Clinical Manifestations

Characteristics of Angina

Angina pectoris produces transient paroxysmal attacks of substernal or precordial pain with the following characteristics:

Onset. Angina can develop quickly or slowly. Some clients ignore the chest pain, thinking that it will go away or that it is indigestion. Ask what the client was doing when the pain began.

Location. Nearly 90% of clients experience the pain as retrosternal or slightly to the left of the sternum.

Radiation. The pain usually radiates to the left shoulder and upper arm and may then travel down the inner aspect of the left arm to the elbow, wrist, and fourth and fifth fingers. The pain may also radiate to the right shoulder, neck, jaw, or epigastric region. On occasion, the pain may be felt only in the area of radiation and not in the chest. Rarely is the pain localized to any one single small area over the precordium.

Duration. Angina usually lasts less than 5 minutes. However, attacks precipitated by a heavy meal or extreme anger may last 15 to 20 minutes.

Sensation. Clients describe the pain of angina as squeezing, burning, pressing, choking, aching, or bursting pressure. The client often says the pain feels like gas, heartburn, or indigestion. Clients do not describe anginal pain as sharp or knife-like.

Severity. The pain of angina is usually mild or moderate in severity. Rarely is the pain described as severe.

Associated characteristics. Other manifestations that may accompany the pain include dyspnea, pallor, sweating, faintness, palpitations, dizziness, and digestive disturbances.

Atypical presentation. Women and older adults may have atypical presentations of CHD that are equivalent to angina. In women, CHD may be manifested as epigastric pain, dyspnea, or back pain, whereas the elderly frequently experience dyspnea, fatique, or syncope.[3]

Relieving/aggravating factors. Angina is aggravated by continued activity, and most anginal attacks quickly subside with the administration of nitroglycerin and rest. The typical "exertion–pain, rest–relief" pattern is the major clue to the diagnosis of angina pectoris.

Treatment. Has the client treated the pain with nitroglycerin? Did it work? Angina should subside after nitroglycerin use.

Patterns of Angina

Classic angina pectoris can be subdivided into the following basic patterns:

Stable angina. Stable angina is paroxysmal chest pain or discomfort triggered by a predictable degree of exertion (e.g., walking 20 feet) or emotion. Characteristically a stable pattern of onset, duration, severity, and relieving factors is present.[10, 13]

Unstable angina. Unstable angina (preinfarction angina, crescendo angina, or intermittent coronary syndrome) is paroxysmal chest pain triggered by an unpredictable degree of exertion or emotion, which may occur at night. Unstable angina attacks characteristically increase in number, duration, and severity over time. Once unstable angina is diagnosed, the client must receive immediate medical attention.[10, 34]

Variant angina. Variant angina (*Prinzmetal's angina*) is chest discomfort similar to classic angina but of longer duration; it may occur while the client is at rest. These attacks tend to happen in the early hours of the day. Variant angina may result from coronary artery spasm and may be associated with elevation of the ST segment on the electrocardiogram (ECG).

Nocturnal angina. Nocturnal angina is possibly associated with rapid eye movement (REM) sleep during dreaming.

Angina decubitus. Angina decubitus is paroxysmal chest pain that occurs when the client reclines and lessens when the client sits or stands up.

Intractable angina. Intractable angina is chronic incapacitating angina that is unresponsive to intervention.

Post-infarction angina. Pain occurs occurs after MI, when residual ischemia may cause episodes of angina.

Diagnostic Tests

The following modalities are described in Chapter 54.

Electrocardiography. The ECG tracings remain normal in 25% to 30% of clients with angina pectoris. An ECG taken in the presence of pain may document transient ischemic attacks with ST-segment elevation or depression. An ECG taken during an episode of pain also suggests coronary artery involvement and the extent of cardiac muscle affected by the ischemic event.[34]

Exercise Electrocardiography. During a *stress test,* the client exercises on a treadmill or stationary bicycle until reaching 85% of maximal heart rate. ECG or vital sign changes may indicate ischemia.[34]

Radioisotope Imaging. Various nuclear imaging techniques are used to evaluate myocardial muscle. Regions of poor perfusion or ischemia appear as areas of diminished or absent activity (cold spots).

Electron-Beam (Ultrafast) Computed Tomography. This promising noninvasive method enables detection of the amount of calcium in coronary arteries. Because calcification occurs with atherosclerotic plaque formation, measurement of coronary calcium may reflect the extent of coronary atherosclerosis. High coronary calcium values have been associated with obstructive coronary disease.

Coronary Angiography. Angiography provides the most accurate information about the patency of the coronary arteries and allows visualization of the artery and any partial or complete blockages.

Outcome Management

The aims of therapy in the treatment of angina are to alleviate manifestations and to prevent the progression of

CHD. The ultimate goal is to reduce the risk of MI and death. This goal is accomplished through (1) pharmacologic intervention, (2) education and counseling regarding the most effective way to control or eliminate known cardiovascular risk factors, and, (3) in some instances, revascularization through interventional cardiology or coronary artery bypass graft (CABG) surgery. Smoking cessation reduces the risk of coronary heart disease by 37%; a 10% reduction in cholesterol lowers the risk of CHD by 20%; and a 6-mm reduction in diastolic blood pressure lowers the risk of CHD by 10%.[2] The American Heart Association (AHA) recommends that people with angina control their modifiable risk factors and seek prompt treatment for episodes of chest pain.

Clients with chronic stable angina (CSA) are usually managed effectively with risk factor reduction and pharmacologic therapy. Revascularization through interventional cardiology procedures or CABG surgery is reserved for these clients with triple-vessel or left main coronary artery disease, with left ventricular dysfunction, or whose manifestations are not adequately controlled by pharmacologic therapy. Revascularization is used most often for clients with unstable angina or MI. Interventional cardiology procedures and CABG are discussed in Chapters 55 and 56.

Medical Management

Medical management of clients with angina pectoris focuses on two goals: (1) relief of the acute attack and (2) prevention of further attacks to reduce the risk of MI.

The diagnosis of angina pectoris is confirmed by history and various tests. Obtain a complete history of the pain and its pattern. Encourage clients to describe the pain in their own words. Record a complete analysis of manifestions. This description provides a baseline that can be used in ongoing care.

Most physical findings are transient. The client exhibits pallor or has cold, clammy skin. Tachycardia and hypertension may be recorded. Pulsus alternans (the force of each beat varies) may be present at the onset of ischemic attacks. On auscultation, an S_3 or S_4 gallop or a paradoxical split of S_2 may be noted. If mitral regurgitation is present because of ischemia of the papillary muscle, a murmur can be heard.

Relieve Acute Attack

The primary goal of pharmacologic treatment of angina is to balance myocardial oxygen supply and demand by altering the various components of the process, thereby increasing oxygen supply to the myocardium or reducing myocardial oxygen demand. The components of myocardial oxygen consumption that can be pharmacologically treated are (1) blood pressure, (2) heart rate, (3) contractility, and (4) left ventricular volume. Drugs used in the treatment of angina and associated nursing implications are listed in Table 58–1.

The major types of medications used to treat the acute attack in angina pectoris are as follows:

1. *Opiate analgesics* are used to relieve acute pain.
2. *Vasodilators* help reduce acute pain and prevent further attacks by widening the diameter of coronary arteries and increasing the supply of oxygen to the myocardium. *Nitroglycerin,* a *short-acting* nitrate, has been the treatment of choice against anginal attacks since 1867. Administered sublingually, per tablet, or via translingual spray, nitroglycerin helps relieve anginal pain within 1 to 2 minutes. *Long-acting* nitrates help maintain coronary artery vasodilation, thereby promoting greater flow of blood and oxygen to the heart muscle.
3. *Beta-adrenergic blockers* help reduce the workload of the heart, decrease myocardial oxygen demand, and may decrease the number of anginal attacks.
4. *Calcium-channel blockers* are used to dilate coronary arteries, thereby increasing oxygen supply to the myocardium.
5. *Antiplatelet* agents inhibit platelet aggregation and reduce coagulability, thus preventing clot formation.

Prevent Further Attacks

Education and counseling regarding modification of risk factors are necessary to reduce the progression of CHD andto prevent further attacks. Recommendations should follow the guidelines established by the AHA for primary and secondary prevention of CHD. Specific recommendations for risk factor modification are described in Chapter 56.

Nursing Management of the Medical Client

Relieve Acute Attack

In addition to documenting the clinical manifestations of angina, ascertain how long the client has had angina, whether risk factors for CHD are present, and the client's emotional reaction to chest pain. Start cardiac monitoring, obtain a 12-lead ECG, and control ongoing angina. Until the angina is controlled and coronary blood flow is reestablished, the client is at risk for myocardial damage from myocardial ischemia. If the client reports angina, assess the pain and ask the client whether the pain is the same as experienced in the past. Note new characteristics or increased pain.

Give sublingual nitroglycerin tablets or spray as prescribed. Because nitroglycerin causes vasodilation and hypotension, monitor blood pressure. If the pain is not relieved after three nitroglycerin tablets, each taken 5 minutes apart, or after morphine, notify the physician. In addition, an environment that provides rest and security as well as allays fear and anxiety helps reduce pain.

Prevent Further Attacks Through Self-Care

The client must be knowledgeable about the care of episodes of angina and how to reduce the risk factors that exacerbate the process. Use the following information as needed to help clients control risk factors for angina pectoris.

1. Educate the client to avoid activities or habits that precipitate angina (eating large meals, drinking coffee, smoking, exercising too strenuously, going out in cold weather, being exposed to excessive stress). If an attack begins, the client should stop the activity and sit down. An antianginal medication (e.g., nitroglycerin) should be taken. One pill can be

TABLE 58–1 NURSING IMPLICATIONS FOR MEDICATIONS USED TO TREAT ANGINA PECTORIS

Class	Example	Assessment of Therapeutic Responses	Assessment of Adverse Responses	Nursing Implications
Vasodilators	Nitroglycerin	Dilates coronary arteries, improves collateral blood flow, and decreases cardiac oxygen demands. Clinically, a decrease in chest pain, resolving ST segments, is observed.	The client may experience flushing, weakness, headache, postural hypotension, dizziness, and reflex tachycardia.	Monitor client for chest pain and hypotension. IV nitroglycerin should be in non-PVC sets, and blood pressure and heart rate should be continuously monitored. Titrate IV 5 μg/min every 3–5 minutes until pain subsides. Because tablets are inactivated by light, heat, air, and moisture, store in tight-fitting amber glass containers. Nitroglycerin tablets may be taken 5 minutes apart. If pain is not resolved after three tablets, contact physician immediately.
Beta-adrenergic blocking agents	Atenolol	The effects of blockade of beta-adrenergic receptors and the neurohormonal response that inhibits the sympathetic nervous system are seen clinically by a decreased heart rate, and the vasodilatation decreases blood pressure. It also decreases the automaticity, decreasing heart rate and the incidence of dysrhythmias. Over the long term, the client experiences less mortality and less incidence of heart failure.*	The client may experience bronchoconstriction, severe bradycardia, or hypotension. The client may also experience A-V conduction abnormalities, dizziness, confusion, constipation or diarrhea, and vomiting. Male clients may experience impotence.	Do not give to clients with a history of bronchospastic pulmonary disease. If the client has diabetes, it may potentiate hypoglycemia. Monitor the heart rate and blood pressure frequently. Assess pulmonary status for bronchoconstriction.
ACE inhibitor	Captopril	The decrease in afterload increases cardiac output by enhancing contractility. The neurohormonal effects may cause vasodilatation and a decrease in systemic blood pressure. Long-term effects include a decrease in mortality and decrease in the incidence of heart failure.*	The client may experience hypotension, oliguria, palpitations, insomnia, dizziness, fatigue, nausea, vomiting, maculopapular rash, and cough.	Monitor blood pressure closely. Full therapeutic effect may take weeks to achieve. May increase BUN, creatinine, liver enzymes, and potassium levels.

Table continued on following page

TABLE 58–1 NURSING IMPLICATIONS FOR MEDICATIONS USED TO TREAT ANGINA PECTORIS *Continued*

Class	Example	Assessment of Therapeutic Responses	Assessment of Adverse Responses	Nursing Implications
Opiate analgesics	Morphine	Binds with opiate receptors in the CNS causing inhibition of ascending pain pathways altering the perception of pain. Decreases afterload by vasodilatation and may decrease blood pressure.	The client may experience respiratory depression, hypotension, bradycardia, drowsiness, constipation, pruritus, and weakness.	Monitor heart rate, blood pressure, and respiratory status frequently. Naloxone is the antidote for overdose and should be available when giving morphine IV.
Antiplatelet aggregating agent	Acetylsalicylic acid (ASA)	ASA blocks prostaglandin synthesis action, which prevents formation of the platelet aggregating substance thromboxane A_2. Clinically, this limits the formation or progression of a thrombus and decreases mortality.†	The client may experience heartburn, stomach pains, nausea and vomiting, rash, weakness, hemolytic anemia, and gastrointestinal ulceration. Overdose symptoms include tinnitus, headache, dizziness, confusion, and metabolic acidosis.	Avoid use in clients with severe renal or liver disease. Monitor serum concentrations, renal function, hearing changes, skin inflammation, and for abnormal bleeding. Administer with food or large quantities of water to decrease gastrointestinal upset. Instruct the client to avoid concurrent use of over-the-counter products that contain ASA.
Calcium-channel blockers	Diltiazem	Inhibits influx of calcium ion through the cell membrane, resulting in a relaxation of coronary vasculature smooth muscle and coronary vasodilation, decreasing anginal pains.	Clients may experience hypotension, dysrhythmias, syncope, Stevens-Johnson syndrome, and weakness.	Monitor heart rate for dysrhythmias and blood pressure for hypotension. May increase liver enzymes. Use in MI is investigational for non–Q wave MIs.

ACE, angiotensin-converting enzymes; A-V, atrioventricular; BUN, blood urea nitrogen; IV, intravenous; MI, myocardine infarction; CNS, central nervous system; PVC, premature ventricular contraction.

*See Moser D., et al. (1999, October). The role of the critical care nurse in preventing heart failure after acute myocardial infarction. *Critical Care Nurse Supplement,* 11–15.

†See Feldman, M., & Cryer, B. (1999). Aspirin absorption rates and platelet inhibition times with 325-mg buffered aspirin tablets (chewed or swallowed intact) and with buffered aspirin solution. *American Journal of Cardiology, 84,* 404–409.

taken sublingually three times in 5-minute intervals. If the pain does not subside, worsens, or radiates, the client should be taken or driven to an emergency department. Stress this point, because if the client is experiencing an MI, the sooner the treatment is initiated, the lower the mortality rate.[18]

2. Explain the importance of daily management of hypertension. Advise the client to take daily medication even if no clinical manifestations are evident (see also Chapter 53).
3. Encourage and help plan a regular program of daily exercise to promote improved coronary circulation and weight management.
4. Instruct clients who smoke to quit smoking at once. Smoking cigarettes raises carboxyhemoglobin levels in the blood, which reduces the amount of oxygen available to the myocardium. Clients with angina pectoris exposed for 2 hours to cigarette smoke demonstrate elevations in carboxyhemoglobin concentration, decreased exercise time, increased heart rate, and elevated blood pressure. Advise clients to avoid "passive smoking" (i.e., being with a smoker or in a smoke-filled room).
5. Urge overweight clients to lose excess weight. Encourage them to eat small meals, avoid high-calorie and high-cholesterol diets, abstain from gas-forming foods, and rest for short periods after meals. In addition, recommend a high-fiber diet, which not only may prevent constipation and other intestinal tract ailments but also may decrease the number and severity of anginal attacks. Diets high in fiber may also help lower serum cholesterol and triglyceride levels. CHD is less common among clients with a high intake of dietary fiber than in those with a low intake. High-fiber diets can also decrease hypertension.
6. Help the client who leads an active, hectic life to adjust activities to a level below that which precipitates anginal attacks. Encourage brief rest periods throughout the working day, an early bedtime, and longer or more frequent vacations. Advise clients who are anxious and nervous to consider counseling. Relaxation techniques may also be used.

ACUTE MYOCARDIAL INFARCTION

Acute MI, also known as a heart attack, coronary occlusion, or simply a "coronary," is a life-threatening condition characterized by the formation of localized necrotic areas within the myocardium. MI usually follows the sudden occlusion of a coronary artery and the abrupt cessation of blood and oxygen flow to the heart muscle. Because the heart muscle must function continuously, blockage of blood to the muscle and the development of necrotic areas can be lethal.

Every year about 1.1 million Americans have MIs. Indeed, MI is the leading cause of death in America and is responsible for an estimated 500,000 deaths each year. During an MI, men are more likely than women to die before they reach the hospital, whereas women have higher in-hospital mortality than men.[2, 7, 25] This difference may result from differences in treatment for men and women. In one study, women with MI received aspirin, beta-blocking drugs, coronary thrombolysis, and acute cardiac catherization, percutaneous transluminal coronary angioplasty (PTCA), or CABG surgery less often than did men with MI.[40] About 250,000 people a year die before they reach the hospital. Studies indicate that half of all MI victims wait more than 2 hours before getting help.[45] On the basis of data from the Framingham study, about 45% of all MIs occur in people under age 65 years and 5% occur in those under age 40. Four out of five people who die of MI are 65 years of age or older.[2]

Etiology and Risk Factors

The most common cause of MI is complete or nearly complete occlusion of a coronary artery, usually precipitated by rupture of a vulnerable atherosclerotic plaque and subsequent thrombus formation. Plaque rupture can be precipitated by both internal and external factors.

Internal factors include plaque characteristics, such as the size and consistency of the lipid core and the thickness of the fibrous cap as well as conditions to which it is exposed, such as coagulation status and degree of arterial vasoconstriction. Vulnerable plaques most frequently occur in areas with less than 70% stenosis and are characterized by an eccentric shape with an irregular border; a large, thin lipid core; and a thin, fibrous cap.[8, 28]

External factors result from actions of the client or from external conditions that affect the client. Strenuous physical activity and severe emotional stress, such as anger, increase sympathetic activity that in turn increases hemodynamic stress that may lead to plaque rupture. At the same time, sympathetic activity increases myocardial oxygen demand. Scientists have reported that external factors, such as exposure to cold and time of day, also affect plaque rupture. Acute coronary events occur more frequently with exposure to cold and during the morning hours. Researchers hypothesize that the sudden increases in sympathetic activity associated with these factors may contribute to plaque rupture.[8, 27]

Regardless of the cause, rupture of the atherosclerotic plaque results in (1) exposure of the plaque's lipid-rich core to flowing blood, (2) seepage of blood into the plaque, causing it to expand, (3) triggering of thrombus formation, and (4) partial or complete occlusion of the coronary artery. *Unstable angina* is associated with short-term partial occlusion of a coronary artery, whereas MI results from significant or complete occlusion of a coronary artery that lasts more than 1 hour.[8, 35] When blood flow ceases abruptly, the myocardial tissue supplied by that artery dies. Coronary artery spasm can also cause acute occlusion. The risk factors that predispose a client to a heart attack are the same as for all forms of CHD (see Chapter 56).

Pathophysiology

MI can be considered the end-point of CHD. Unlike the temporary ischemia that occurs with angina, prolonged unrelieved ischemia causes irreversible damage to the

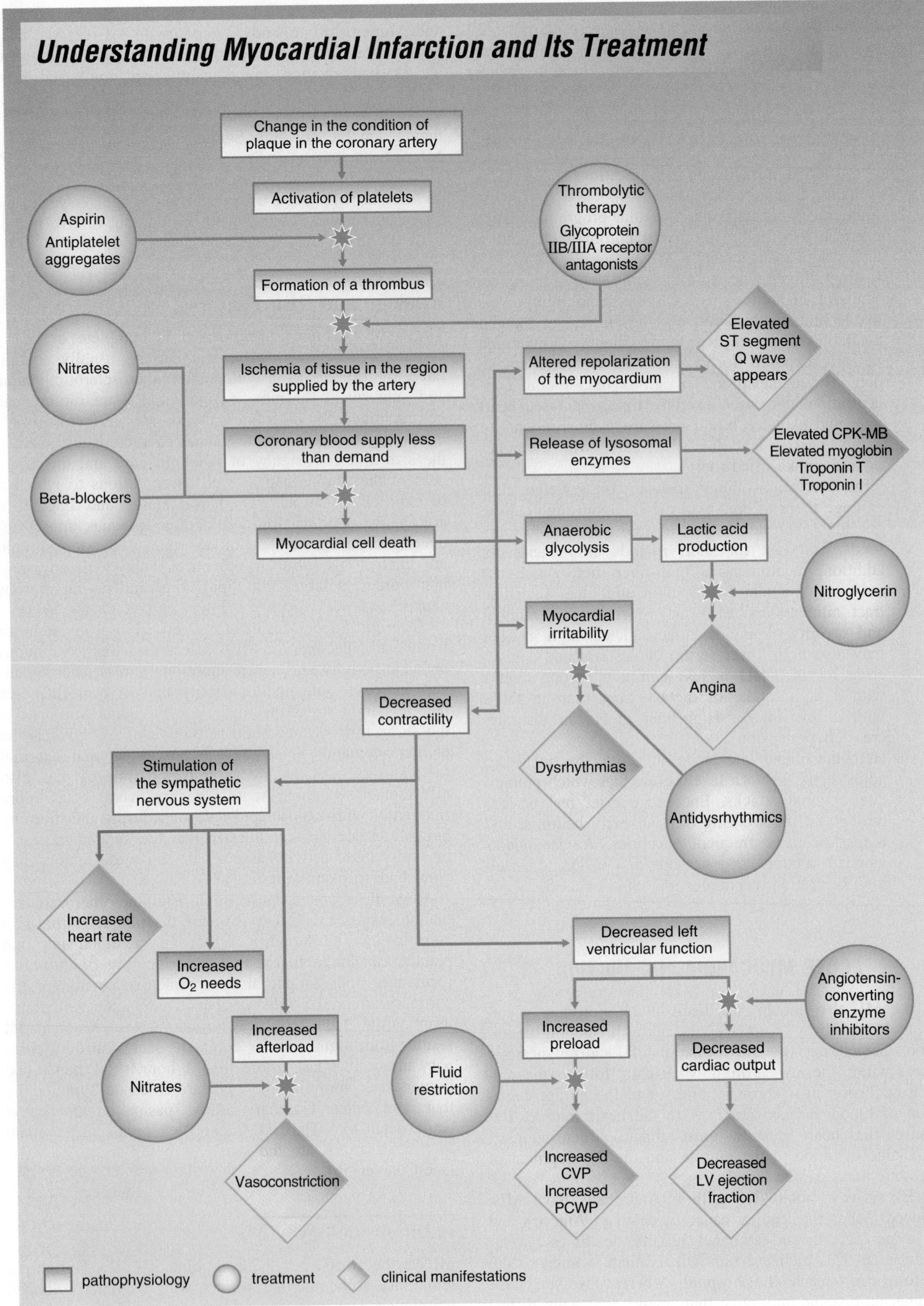
Understanding Myocardial Infarction and Its Treatment
Change in the condition of plaque in the coronary artery
Activation of platelets
Aspirin
Antiplatelet aggregates
Thrombolytic therapy
Glycoprotein IIB/IIIA receptor antagonists
Formation of a thrombus
Nitrates
Elevated ST segment Q wave appears
Ischemia of tissue in the region supplied by the artery
Altered repolarization of the myocardium
Coronary blood supply less than demand
Release of lysosomal enzymes
Elevated CPK-MB Elevated myoglobin Troponin T Troponin I
Beta-blockers
Myocardial cell death
Anaerobic glycolysis
Lactic acid production
Nitroglycerin
Myocardial irritability
Angina
Decreased contractility
Dysrhythmias
Stimulation of the sympathetic nervous system
Antidysrhythmics
Increased heart rate
Increased O2 needs
Decreased left ventricular function
Angiotensin-converting enzyme inhibitors
Increased afterload
Increased preload
Decreased cardiac output
Nitrates
Fluid restriction
Vasoconstriction
Increased CVP Increased PCWP
Decreased LV ejection fraction
pathophysiology
treatment
clinical manifestations

myocardium. Cardiac cells can withstand ischemia for about 20 minutes before they die. Because the myocardium is metabolically active, signs of ischemia can be seen within 8 to 10 seconds of decreased blood flow. When the heart does not receive blood and oxygen, it converts to *anaerobic metabolism,* creating less adenosine triphosphate (ATP) and more lactic acid as a by-product. Myocardial cells are very sensitive to changes in pH and become less functional. Acidosis causes the myocardium to become more vulnerable to the effects of the lysosomal enzymes within the cell. Acidosis leads to conduction system disorders, and dysrhythmias develop. Contractility is also reduced, decreasing the heart's ability to pump. As the myocardial cells necrose, intracellular enzymes are introduced into the bloodstream, where they can be detected by laboratory tests.

Figure 58–1 illustrates the depth of various types of infarctions in the wall of the ventricle. Cellular necrosis occurs in one layer of myocardial tissue in subendocardial, intramural, and subepicardial infarctions. In a transmural infarction, cellular necrosis is present in all three layers of myocardial tissue. The infarct site is called the *zone of infarction and necrosis.* Around it is a zone of hypoxic injury. This zone can return to normal but may also become necrotic if blood flow is not restored. The outermost zone is called the *zone of ischemia;* damage to this area is reversible.

Transmural infarctions cause changes in the architecture of the left ventricle, called "remodeling," which can result in acute or chronic heart failure. Within the first few hours of an MI, the necrotic area stretches in a process called "infarct expansion." This expansion may continue for up to 6 weeks after an MI and is accompanied by progressive thinning and lengthening of infarcted and noninfarcted areas. This remodeling results in left ventricular dsyfunction and produces increases in ventricular volumes and pressures. Remodeling may continue for years after an MI and may result in chronic heart failure (see Chapter 56).[8]

The most common site of MI is the *anterior wall* of the left ventricle near the apex, resulting from thrombosis of the descending branch of the left coronary artery (Fig. 58–2). Other common sites are (1) the *posterior wall* of the left ventricle near the base and behind the posterior cusp of the mitral valve and (2) the *inferior (diaphragmatic) surface* of the heart. Infarction of the posterior left ventricle results from occlusion of the right coronary artery or circumflex branch of the left coronary artery. An inferior infarction occurs when the right coronary artery is occluded. In nearly 25% of inferior wall MIs, the right ventricle is the site of infarction. Atrial infarctions develop less than 5% of the time. See Understanding Myocardial Infarction and Its Treatment.

Clinical Manifestations

The clinical manifestations associated with MI result from ischemia of the heart muscle and the decrease in function and acidosis associated with it. The major clinical manifestation of MI is chest pain (Fig. 58–3), which is similar to angina pectoris but more severe and unrelieved by nitroglycerin. The pain may radiate to the neck, jaw, shoulder, back, or left arm. The pain also may present near the epigastrium, simulating indigestion. MI may also be associated with less common clinical manifestations, including:

- Atypical chest, stomach, back, or abdominal pain
- Nausea or dizziness
- Shortness of breath and difficulty breathing
- Unexplained anxiety, weakness, or fatigue
- Palpitations, cold sweat, or paleness

Women experiencing MI frequently present with one or more of the less common clinical manifestations.[17]

ELECTROCARDIOGRAPHY

When blood flow to the heart is decreased, ischemia and necrosis of the heart muscle occur. These conditions are reflected in altered Q wave, ST segment, and T wave on the ECG. The Q-wave change is significant; normally, the Q wave is very small or absent. Ischemic tissue produces an elevation in the ST segment and a peaked T wave or inversion of the T wave. Through the course of an MI, changes occur first in the ST segment, then the T wave, and finally the Q wave. As the myocardium heals, the ST segment and T waves return to normal but the Q-wave changes persist (Fig. 58–4).[34]

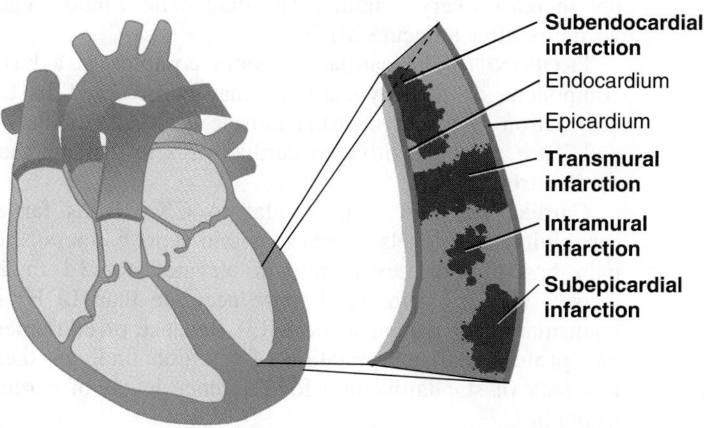

FIGURE 58–1 Depth of infarction in the wall of the ventricle. Subendocardial, intramural, and subepicardial injuries are only in one layer. Transmural infarction extends through all three layers.

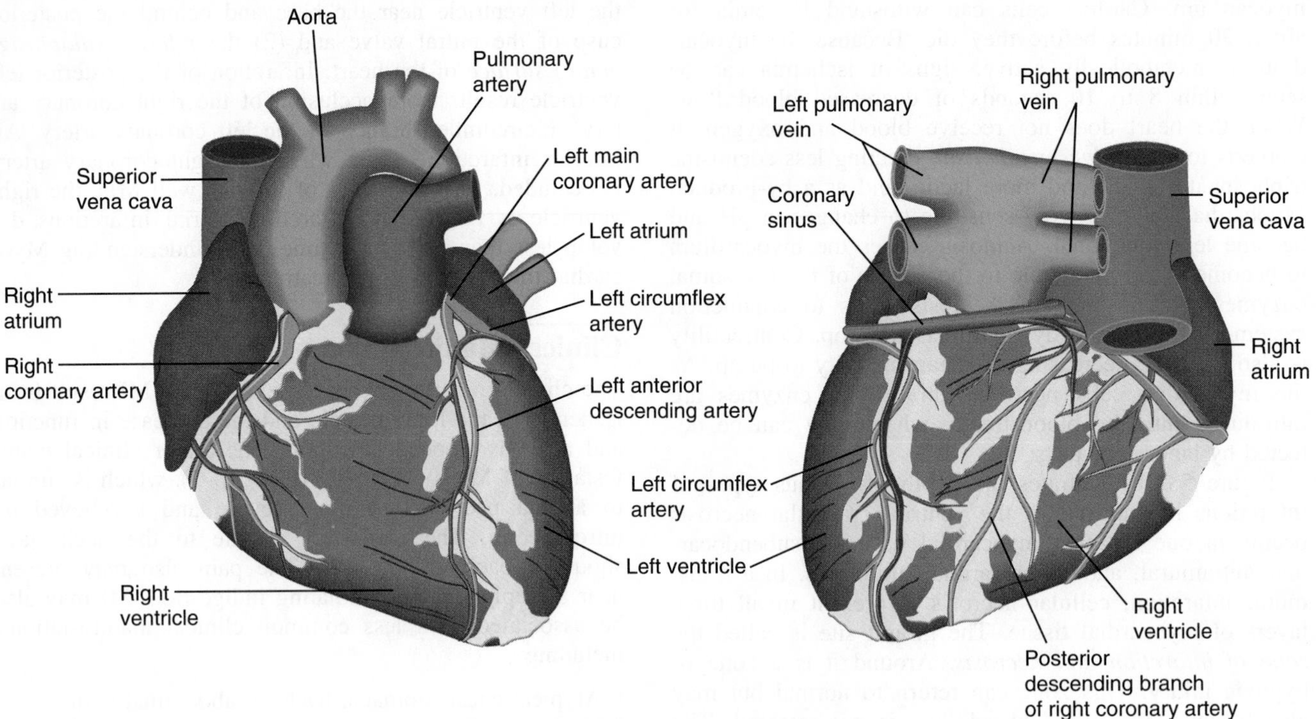

FIGURE 58–2 Areas of the myocardium affected by arterial insufficiency of specific coronary arteries.

Laboratory Tests

Laboratory findings include elevated levels of serum creatine kinase (CK)–MB isoenzyme, myoglobin, cardiac troponin T, and cardiac troponin I. Historically, elevations in lactate dehydrogenase (LDH) M1 isoenzyme, serum aspartate transaminase (AST), and leukocytosis (increased leukocytes), and erythrocyte sedimentation rate (ESR) have aided in the diagnosis of acute MI.

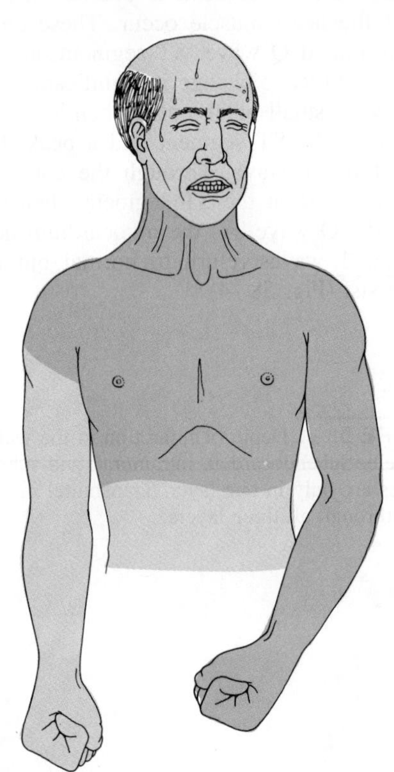

FIGURE 58–3 Possible extent of pain resulting from a myocardial infarction.

CK-MB. Serum levels of CK-MB (an isoenzyme of CK found primarily in cardiac muscle) increase 3 to 6 hours after the onset of chest pain, peak in 12 to 18 hours, and return to normal levels in 3 to 4 days.

Myoglobin. Myoglobin is a heme protein found in striated muscle fibers. Myoglobin is rapidly released when myocardial muscle tissue is damaged. Because of the rapid release, it can be detected within 2 hours after an acute MI. Although many other factors can raise the serum myoglobin level, (strenuous exercise, heavy ethanol use), myoglobin is a highly sensitive indicator of acute MI if serum levels double when a second sample is drawn within 2 hours of the first. Conversely, it is reliable to exclude the diagnosis of acute MI if the levels do not increase every 2 hours. The diagnostic window ends 24 hours after an acute MI.[22]

Troponin. The cardiac troponin complex is a basic component of the myocardium that is involved in the contraction of the myocardial muscle. Cardiac troponin T and I are more sensitive to cardiac muscle damage than cardiac troponin C.

Cardiac *troponin T* is similar to CK-MB as far as sensitivity, and levels increase within 3 to 6 hours after pain has started. Levels remain elevated for 14 to 21 days.[16] This is useful (and more accurate than LDH) in confirmation of distant acute MI.[16] Because of equipment and professional interpretation of research findings, there is a lack of standardization for reference levels of cardiac troponin C.[22]

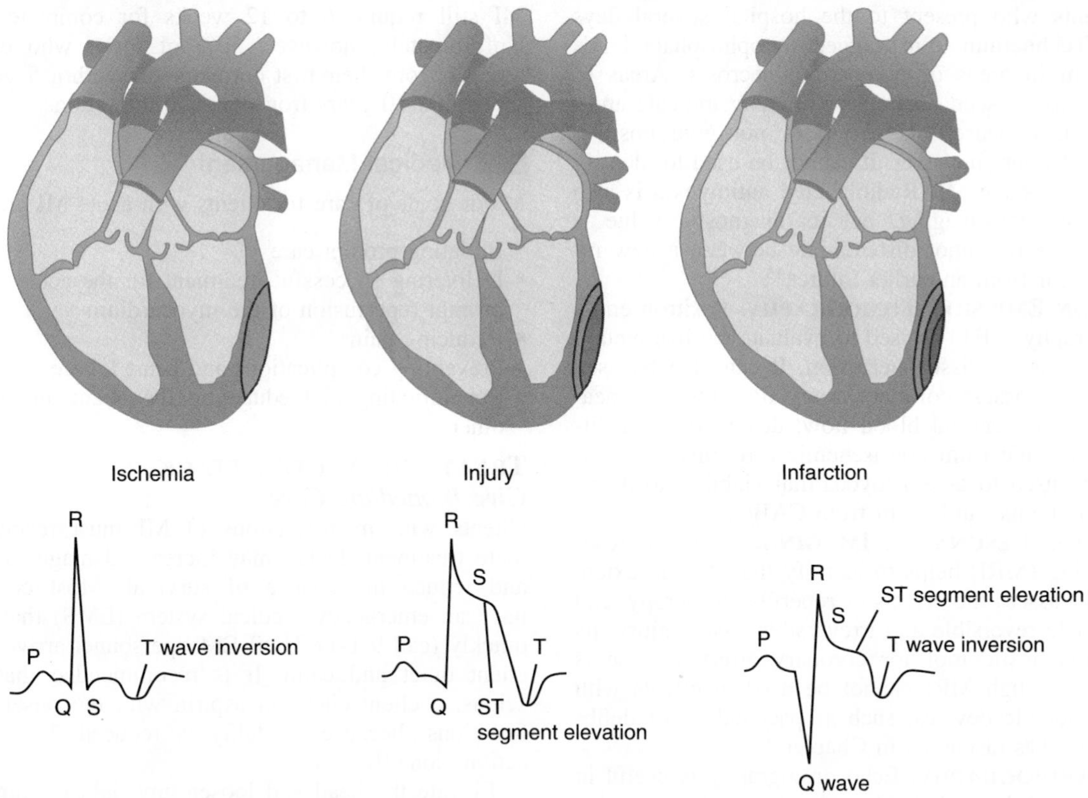

FIGURE 58–4 Zones of hypoxic injury, zone of infarction, and zone of necrosis and the electrocardiographic patterns accompanying these changes during myocardial infarction.

Cardiac *troponin I* levels rise 7 to 14 hours after an acute MI. It is a very specific and sensitive indicator of acute MI and is not affected by any other disease or injury except cardiac muscle.[22] Like cardiac troponin C, it lacks a standardization for reference. Elevation persists for 5 to 7 days.

LDH. The LDH_1 subunit is plentiful in heart muscle and is released into the serum when myocardial damage occurs. Serum levels of LDH elevate 14 to 24 hours after onset of myocardial damage, peak within 48 to 72 hours, and slowly return to normal over the next 7 to 14 days. Figure 58–5 illustrates the pattern of enzyme changes after MI.

AST. Serum levels of AST rise within several hours after the onset of chest pain, peak within 12 to 18 hours, and return to normal within 3 to 4 days.

LEUKOCYTOSIS. Leukocytosis (10,000 to 20,000 mm^3) appears on the second day after an MI and disappears in 1 week.

IMAGING STUDIES

Radionuclide imaging studies provide information on the presence of coronary artery disease as well as the location of ischemic and infarcted tissue. Cardiac imaging studies have been used to provide information for triage decisions and the management of clients who present to the emergency department with acute chest pain.[33]

When a client experiences acute chest pain, perfusion imaging with agents such as thallium, sestamibi, and teboroxime can be used to identify ischemic and infarcted tissue. Perfusion imaging is sometimes called "cold spot" imaging because the radioisotope in the bloodstream is not taken up by ischemic or infarcted tissue.

Infarct, or "hot spot" imaging, is useful in confirming

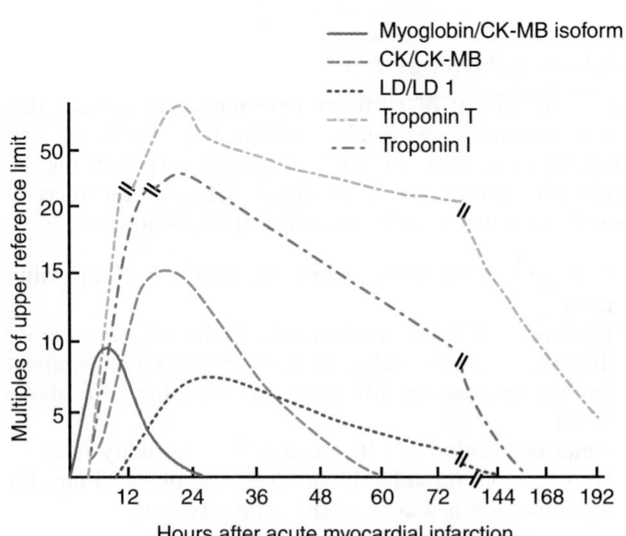

FIGURE 58–5 Isoenzyme alterations in acute myocardial infarction. (From Wong, S. S. [1996.] Strategic ultilization of cardiac markers for the diagnosis of acute myocardial infarction. *Annals of Clinical Laboratory Science, 26,* 301—312. Copyright 1996 by the Institute for Clinical Science, Inc.)

MI in clients who present to the hospital several days after MI. Technetium 99m–tagged pyrophosphate binds with calcium in areas of myocardial necrosis. Areas of uptake (hot spots) seen on nuclear imaging indicate areas of infarction. Because this test does not give positive results for 24 hours however, it cannot be used to identify an acute, early-stage MI. Radiolabeled antimyosin is also used for hot spot imaging, but its diagnostic value is limited because it cannot differentiate between a new infarct and a scar from an earlier infarct.[15]

POSITRON EMISSION TOMOGRAPHY. Positron emission tomography (PET) is used to evaluate cardiac metabolism and to assess tissue perfusion. It can also be used to detect CHD, assess coronary artery flow reserve, measure absolute myocardial blood flow, detect MI, and differentiate ischemic from non-ischemic cardiomyopathy. It may also be used to assess myocardial viability to determine which clients can benefit from CABG.

MAGNETIC RESONANCE IMAGING. Magnetic resonance imaging (MRI) helps to identify the site and extent of an MI, to assess the effects of reperfusion therapy, and to differentiate reversible and irreversible tissue injury. Its use as a diagnostic tool for coronary artery disease is increasing, although MRI cannot be used in clients with implanted metallic devices, such as pacemakers or defibrillators.[37] MRI is discussed in Chapter 11.

ECHOCARDIOGRAPHY. Echocardiography is useful in assessing the ability of the heart walls to contract and relax. The transducer is placed on the chest, and images are relayed to a monitor screen. Wall motion is abnormal in ischemic or infarcted areas.[5]

TRANSESOPHAGEAL ECHOCARDIOGRAPHY. Transesophageal echocardiography (TEE) is an imaging technique in which the transducer is placed against the wall of the esophagus. The image of the myocardium is clearer when the esophageal site is used because no air is between the transducer and the heart. This technique is particularly useful for viewing the posterior wall of the heart.[5]

Outcome Management

Since the advent of coronary care units and devices that aid in promptly recognizing and treating life-threatening dysrhythmias, 70% to 80% of people experiencing an acute MI survive the initial attack. Chances for survival greatly diminish with the presence of the following:

- Old age (clients 80 years or older have a 60% mortality rate)
- Evidence of other cardiovascular disease, respiratory disease, or uncontrolled diabetes mellitus (concomitant angina or previous MI carries a mortality rate above 30%)
- Anterior location of MI (about a 30% mortality rate)
- Hypotension (systolic blood pressure of <55 mm Hg on admission betokens a 60% mortality rate)

Deaths generally result from severe dysrhythmias, cardiogenic shock, heart failure, rupture of the heart, and recurrent MI.

Clients fortunate enough to avoid complications after MI still require 6 to 12 weeks for complete recovery. Unfortunately, however, 50% of those who completely recover from their first coronary die within 5 years; 75% die within 10 years from massive infarctions.

Medical Management

Major goals of care for clients with acute MI are:

- Initiating prompt care
- Delivering successful treatment for the acute attack and prompt reperfusion of the myocardium
- Reducing pain
- Preventing complications and heart failure
- Rehabilitating and educating the client and significant others

TREAT THE ACUTE ATTACK

Give Immediate Care

Clients with manifestations of MI must receive immediate treatment. Delay may increase damage to the heart and reduce the chance of survival. Most communities have an emergency medical system (EMS) that responds quickly (call 9-1-1). Until EMS personnel arrive, keep the client quiet and calm. It is recommended that, if conscious, a client chew an aspirin with the onset of manifestations, because mortality is reduced 23% with this action alone.[11]

Elevate the head and loosen any tight clothing around the neck. Once EMS workers arrive, the client is assessed and transported quickly to an emergency department. The client is given oxygen; an intravenous (IV) line is inserted, and the client is connected to a heart monitor. Clients who become unconscious before reaching the emergency department may require cardiopulmonary resuscitation (CPR).

Many people who experience manifestations of MI delay calling for help because they misinterpret what they are sensing. Their expectations of what an acute MI should "feel like" and their experience are not the same.[44] Many studies have documented an average client delay time that exceeded 7 hours.[44] In women, this delay may even be longer.[40] Community education to "call first, call fast" is important.

The client experiencing an acute MI needs immediate admission to a hospital with a coronary care unit if possible. The first 24 hours after an MI is the time of highest risk for sudden death. There is a significant benefit if treatment is administered within the first 12 hours of onset of manifestations.[18] The first 6 hours after the onset of pain is the crucial time frame for salvage of the myocardium. Because of this, efforts have been made to decrease the time for initial treatment. In 1994, the National Heart Attack Alert Program recommended that all emergency departments treat acute MI clients within 30 minutes of presenting to the hospital. The mnemonic *4D*'s (*d*oor, *d*ata, *d*ecision, and *d*rug), along with treatment algorithms, has been adopted by many emergency departments to treat those with acute MI.

Reduce Pain

Upon admission, the client who complains of chest pain is admitted to the emergency department, given oxygen therapy, and placed on ECG monitoring. An IV line is placed, serum cardiac markers are drawn, and a 12-lead ECG is undertaken. Pain control is a priority, usually with IV morphine. Continued pain is a manifestation of myocardial ischemia. Pain also stimulates the autonomic nervous system and increases preload, which in turn increases myocardial oxygen demand. Oxygen is used to treat tissue hypoxia. Because dysrhythmias are common, ECG monitoring is essential and antidysrhythmic medications should be at hand. A two-dimensional echocardiogram and full exercise stress test may be performed in the emergency department to aid in ruling in or ruling out an acute MI.

Improve Perfusion

The general principles of pharmacologic treatment of acute MI consist of anti-ischemic and antithrombotic therapies.[39] The actions, side effects, and nursing implications of drugs used to treat acute MI are described in Table 58–2. Anti-ischemic therapy usually consists of beta blockade and IV nitroglycerin.

Antithrombotic therapy and the combination of different antithrombotic agents are being studied widely. Antithrombotic therapy is usually initiated with the administration of an aspirin if the client has not taken one before reaching the emergency department. Heparin therapy is the next step.

Clinicians treat acute MI with medications that lyse (dissolve) the clot that forms part of the blockage of the coronary artery. Thrombolytic therapy includes streptokinase, urokinase, tissue-type plasminogen activator (t-PA), anisoylated plasminogen-streptokinase activator complex (anistreplase, APSAC), alteplase, urokinase plasminogen activator, and the newest, reteplase. For best efficacy, thrombolytic agents must be given within 6 hours, (preferably 3 hours) after the onset of chest pain. The choice of thrombolytic agent is not as important as the speed with which it is given.[18] After the thrombolytic agent is administered, IV heparin or a glycoprotein IIB/IIIA is usually continued. All of these thrombolytic agents can be given intravenously. See Understanding Myocardial Infarction and Its Treatment (p. 1586).

Not all clients with MI are suitable candidates for thrombolytic therapy. History of recent cerebral vascular accident, surgery, pregnancy or use of anticoagulants would contraindicate thrombolytic therapy. Complications of thrombolytics include bleeding, allergic reactions, and stroke. Successful reperfusion of the coronary arteries is evidenced by (1) return of ECG changes to normal; (2) relief of chest pain; (3) presence of reperfusion dysrhythmias, usually sudden onset of frequent premature ventricular contractions (PVCs) or short runs of PVCs; and (4) a rapid, early peak of the CK-MB isoenzyme ("washout"). If reperfusion is not attained or if the client is not a candidate for thrombolytic therapy, then primary angioplasty, stenting, or CABG may be performed. Interventional cardiology procedures and bypass surgery are discussed in Chapter 56.

Antidysrhythmic agents are initiated. Some clinicians begin angiotensin-converting enzyme (ACE) inhibitors within 72 hours of onset because ventricular remodeling starts at that time.[21] Stool softeners are used to relieve constipation and to lower the risk of bradycardia from straining that stimulates the vagus nerve.

Monitor for Complications

The possibility of death from complications always accompanies an acute MI. Thus, prime collaborative goals include the prevention of life-threatening complications or at least recognition of them.

DYSRHYTHMIAS. Dysrhythmias are the major cause of death after an MI (40% to 50% of deaths). Ectopic rhythms arise in or near the borders of intensely ischemic and damaged myocardial tissues. Damaged myocardium may also interfere with the conduction system, causing dissociation of the atria and ventricles (*heart block*). Supraventricular tachycardia (SVT) sometimes occurs as a result of heart failure. Spontaneous or pharmacologic reperfusion of a previously ischemic area may also precipitate ventricular dysrhythmias.

Provide continuous cardiac monitoring and frequent counts of PVCs (many monitoring systems count continuously). Notify the physician if more than six PVCs occur per minute and the client is symptomatic (e.g., hypotension, chest pain). For *dysrhythmias*, provide prompt intervention per protocol or orders. For new-onset, symptomatic *ventricular ectopy* (runs, couplets, salvos), administer lidocaine per order. For *ventricular tachycardia,* administer lidocaine, procainamide, or bretylium or provide elective cardioversion. For *ventricular fibrillation,* provide immediate defibrillation. For *SVT,* administer a vagal maneuver, adenosine, verapamil, or lidocaine, and provide elective cardioversion. For *heart block,* administer atropine or isoproterenol (with caution) and use a temporary pacemaker.[26] Dysrhythmias are discussed in Chapter 57.

CARDIOGENIC SHOCK. Cardiogenic shock accounts for only 9% of deaths from MI, but an estimated 80% of clients who develop shock die from it. Causes include decreased (1) myocardial contraction with diminished cardiac output, (2) undetected dysrhythmias, and (3) sepsis.

Clinical manifestations include systolic blood pressure significantly below the client's normal range; diaphoresis; rapid pulse; restlessness; cold, clammy skin; and grayish skin color.

Shock can be prevented with rapid relief of pain and sufficient IV fluids to prevent circulatory collapse. It is also vital to identify dysrhythmias rapidly.

Administer vasopressors (norepinephrine, dopamine, dobutamine, metaraminol [Aramine]) as prescribed, to raise blood pressure by increasing peripheral resistance. In other cases, vasodilators (nitroprusside) promote better blood flow in the microcirculation. Positive inotropic agents (dobutamine, epinephrine, isoproterenol) increase cardiac contractility and cardiac output and improve tissue perfusion. Administer oxygen therapy and antidysrhythmic agents as prescribed, and continuously monitor arterial and pulmonary artery pressures.[26] Chapter 81 explains shock in detail.

HEART FAILURE AND PULMONARY EDEMA. The most common cause of in-hospital death in clients with cardiac disorders is heart failure. Heart failure disables

TABLE 58–2 NURSING IMPLICATIONS FOR ANTITHROMBOTIC MEDICATIONS USED TO TREAT ACUTE MYOCARDIAL INFARCTION

Class	Example	Assessment of Therapeutic Responses	Assessment of Adverse Responses	Nursing Implications
Antiplatelet aggregrating agent	Acetylsalicylic acid (ASA)	ASA blocks prostaglandin synthesis action, which prevents formation of the platelet aggregating substance thromboxane A_2. Clinically, this limits formation or progression of a thrombus and decreases mortality.*	The client may experience heartburn, stomach pains, nausea and vomiting, rash, weakness, hemolytic anemia, and GI ulceration. Overdose manifestations include tinnitus, headache, dizziness, confusion, and metabolic acidosis.	Avoid use in clients with severe renal or liver disease. Monitor serum concentrations, renal function, hearing changes, skin inflammation, and for abnormal bleeding. Administer with food or large quantities of water to decrease GI upset. Instruct client to avoid concurrent use of over-the-counter products containing ASA.
Indirect thrombin inhibitor	Heparin	Heparin increases ability of antithrombin to inactivate circulating thrombin, limiting formation or progression of a thrombus. Clinically, this is seen as a more patent coronary vessel, with resolving ST segments, decreased angina, and lower mortality.†	The client is at risk for bleeding. Monitor for manifestations of occult and overt bleeding. The client may also experience rash or urticaria. Once medication is discontinued, the client is at risk for "rebound" ischemia.	Assess client for manifestations of bleeding or bruising. Monitor ST segments. Monitor aPTT levels during therapy. Protamine sulfate is the antidote for heparin. Many drugs can increase the risk of bleeding if used concurrently with heparin.
Glycoprotein IIB/IIIA receptor antagonists	Abciximab	After atherosclerotic plaque ruptures, platelets attach. Glycoprotein receptor agonists do not allow platelet to become activated, which does not allow fibrinogen to attach to platelet. These actions do not allow further platelet aggregation. Clinically, this is depicted as a more patent coronary vessel, with a decrease in chest pain, resolving ST segments, and a lower mortality.†‡§	Severe bleeding may occur, which rapid transfusion of platelets reverses. Ventricular dysrhythmias, pulmonary emboli, hypotension, and bradycardia may occur.	Assess the client for manifestations of occult and overt bleeding. Monitor platelets while the client is on therapy. Monitor ST segments and chest pain.
Thrombolytic agents	Reteplase	By converting plasminogen to plasmin, the fibrin strands that hold thrombus together are broken down, hence destroying the thrombus. Clinically, this is seen as a decrease in angina, resolving ST segments, and decreased mortality. Long-term effects include preserved ventricular function and reduced incidence of heart failure.†	Clients may experience bleeding, ventricular fibrillation, reperfusion dysrhythmias, and cardiac arrest.	Client must be on cardiac monitor during infusion. Anticipate dysrhythmias, and have appropriate medications on hand. Observe for bleeding. Assess for reduction of chest pain and resolving ST segment elevation. Clients are not candidates for therapy if they have had recent surgery, CVA, or GI bleeding or are currently receiving warfarin or are pregnant. Start treatment as soon as possible for best results.¶

aPTT, activated partial thromboplastin time; CVA, cerebrovascular accident; GI, gastrointestinal.

*See Feldman, M., & Cryer, B. (1999). Aspirin absorption rates and platelet inhibition times with 325-mg buffered aspirin tablets (chewed or swallowed intact) and with buffered aspirin solution. *American Journal of Cardiology, 84,* 404–409.

†See Dracup, K., & Cannon, C. (1999). Combination treatment strategies for management of acute myocardial infarction. *Critical Care Nurse Supplement,* 1–17.

‡See Gensini, G., Comeglio, M., & Falai, M. (1999). Advances in antithrombotic therapy of acute myocardial infarction. *American Heart Journal, 138*(2), S171–S176.

§See Verheugt, F. (1999). What an interventional cardiologist should know about the pharmacological treatment of acute myocardial infarction. *Seminars in Interventional Cardiology, 4,* 17–20.

¶See Kosnik, L. (1999, October). Treatment protocols and pathways: Improving the process of care. *Critical Care Nurse Supplement,* 3–7.

CASE MANAGEMENT

Acute Myocardial Infarction

Clients who have had an acute myocardial infarction (MI) have experienced a serious, life-threatening event. Case management involves prevention of complications, education regarding current treatment plans and rehabilitation, and lifestyle modification. Ideally, modifiable risk factors for coronary artery disease (smoking, hypertension, high cholesterol levels, sedentary lifestyle) should be reduced before MI occurs. The client with an uncomplicated MI usually has a 4-day length of stay with interventions such as angioplasty or stenting during the same admission. The needs of each client vary according to the type, extent, and prognosis as well as age, comorbidities, and plans for intervention.

Assess

- What type of MI has been sustained?
- What should you expect based on the pathophysiology involved (e.g., dysrhythmia, conduction disturbances)?
- Has this client had a previous MI; was there a particular precipitating cause?
- Is unstable angina (pain) part of the clinical picture?
- What other diagnoses might worsen or make it difficult to control this condition (hypertension, heart failure, anemia, diabetes, hyperthyroidism, cardiomyopathy, emotional distress)?
- What were the presenting manifestations, and how long did the client wait before seeking assistance?
- What is the client's pain level? Has pain been relieved?

Advocate

Even if the client has had angina in the past, having a heart attack is an unexpected event that causes anxiety and fear. Being connected to various monitoring devices with warning alarms, being in a special unit with unknown schedules or procedures, and having to make decisions about unfamiliar tests or treatments all contribute to feelings of powerlessness and anxiety. What is routine for the nurse is not routine for the client.

Try to explain tests and procedures thoroughly to the client and family members. Many hospitals have developed educational materials or clinical pathways that may assist. Address difficult questions, such as advanced directives and wishes for resuscitation.

If an emergency occurs, try to remain calm and focused on the situation. Be honest with family members and clients. As recovery progresses, clients may have questions about resuming work or sexual activity. Work with the client and physician to obtain answers and alleviate fear.

Prevent Readmission

As you administer medication, start teaching the name, purpose, and side effects of each medication. If nitroglycerin is prescribed, explain correct use (including prophylactic administration) and storage.

Discuss the factors that caused the need for hospital admission and how the client might prevent future problems by modifying lifestyle or diet; be aware of ethnic or cultural preferences.

Consider appropriate referrals for home care, cardiac rehabilitation or exercise programs, smoking cessation, nutritional counseling, and emergency response systems.

Make sure the client knows how to obtain emergency help, when to call the physician, and the time and date of the first follow-up appointment.

Encourage family members to learn cardiopulmonary resuscitation and to become aware of their own cardiovascular risks.

Investigate support groups and other community resources available through specific institutions, insurers, or the American Heart Association.

Cheryl Noetscher, RN, MS, *Director of Case Management, Crouse Hospital and Community–General Hospital, Syracuse, New York*

20% of clients who experience an MI and is responsible for one third of deaths after an MI.

Heart failure may develop at the onset of the infarction or may occur weeks later. Clinical manifestations include dyspnea, orthopnea, weight gain, edema, enlarged tender liver, distended neck veins, and crackles. It is managed by correcting the underlying cause, relieving clinical manifestations, and enhancing cardiac pump performance.[23, 24, 30] Heart failure is discussed in Chapter 56. The Case Study presents a scenario involving cardiogenic shock, tachycardia, and heart failure.

PULMONARY EMBOLISM. Pulmonary embolism (PE) may develop secondary to phlebitis of the leg or pelvic veins (venous thrombosis) or from atrial flutter or fibrillation. PE occurs in 10% to 20% of clients at some point, during either the acute attack or convalescence. PE is discussed in Chapter 62.

RECURRENT MYOCARDIAL INFARCTION. Within 6 years after an initial MI, 21% of men and 33% of women may experience recurrent MI.[2] Possible causes include overexertion, embolization, and further thrombotic occlusion of a coronary artery by an atheroma. The clinical manifestation is the return of angina. Management is the same as for acute MI.

COMPLICATIONS CAUSED BY MYOCARDIAL NECROSIS. Complications that are due to necrosis of the myocardium include ventricular aneurysm, rupture of the heart (*myocardial rupture*), ventricular septal defect (VSD), and ruptured papillary muscle. These complications are infrequent but serious, usually occurring about 5 to 7 days after MI.[19] Weak, friable necrotic myocardial tissue increases vulnerability to these complications (Fig. 58–6).

Text continued on page 1596

Cardiogenic Shock, Tachycardia, and Heart Failure

Mr. Borg is a 70-year-old retired African American man who was admitted to the ED after arriving by rescue squad. According to his wife, he had been vomiting and experiencing progressive weakness earlier in the day. When the rescue squad arrived at his home, he was in supraventricular tachycardia with a rate over 180 BPM. The squad administered adenosine (Adenocard) 6 mg IV, followed by an additional 12 mg 3 minutes later.

Mr. Borg denied the presence of chest pain or shortness of breath upon admission to the ED. He was cyanotic with no palpable blood pressure and a regular heart rate of 160 BPM. A bolus of diltiazem (Cardizem) 10 mg was administered IV push and normal sinus rhythm was briefly restored. When supraventricular tachycardia returned, a diltiazem drip was initiated. Blood gases drawn in the ED showed a pH of 7.3 and a $PaCO_2$ of 55 mm Hg. Mr. Borg was transferred to the ICU with the diltiazem drip and oxygen at 4 L per nasal cannula.

In the ICU, Mr. Borg's hypotension and tachycardia persisted and a low-dose dopamine drip was initiated at 2 μg/kg/min. Mr. Borg became more hypotensive, tachycardic, and hypoxic. He was then intubated and placed on a ventilator with 100% oxygen. A Swan-Ganz catheter was placed, and his initial PAWP was 30 mm Hg. Furosemide (Lasix) 80 mg and procainamide (Pronestyl) 500 mg IV bolus were administered. A 2 mg/min IV drip of procainamide was continued, and the diltiazem drip was discontinued.

The next morning, Mr. Borg was no longer acidotic, with a pH of 7.36. His heart rate was 140 BPM, and systolic BP was around 100 mm Hg while he was receiving 9 μg/kg/min of dopamine. The ECG revealed that the distal two thirds of the left ventricle was akinetic. Admission and follow-up CPK levels were within normal limits, which indicates that Mr. Borg had an extensive anterior myocardial infarction at an earlier date. Mr. Borg is scheduled to have a right and left heart catheterization at 1:00 PM today. Given his condition, he is not considered a candidate for percutaneous transluminal coronary angiography at this time.

Selected Laboratory Values	
RBC	4.08 million/mm^3
Hb	14.2 g/dl
Hct	41.7%
WBC	20,500/mm^3
Sodium	135 mEq/L
Potassium	3.3 mEq/L
Chloride	94 mEq/L
Cholesterol	264 mg/dl
Triglycerides	334 mg/dl

Nursing Admission Assessment

Mr. Borg is a former mail carrier who retired 10 years ago. He and his wife recently celebrated their 50th wedding anniversary. Their two sons live in cities 1500 miles away, and they will be flying in to visit their father as soon as possible. His wife reports that he stopped smoking 20 years ago and continues to drink two to four alcoholic beverages per day. He has gained 40 pounds during the past 10 years. His wife is concerned that he eats and drinks too much and that he spends most of the day sitting in front of the television. Mr. Borg's wife also reports that he has been taking benazepril (Lotensin) 10 mg/day.

Nursing Physical Examination

Height: 5′11″ Weight: 210 pounds (95.45 kg)
Vital signs: BP = 90/40; TPR = 101, 135, 20

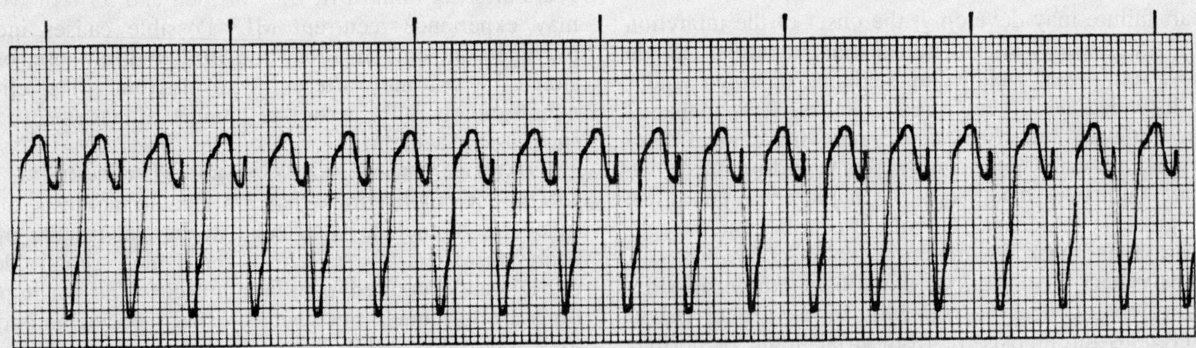

When the rescue squad arrived at Mr. Borg's home, he was in supraventricular tachycardia, with a rate of more than 180 BPM.

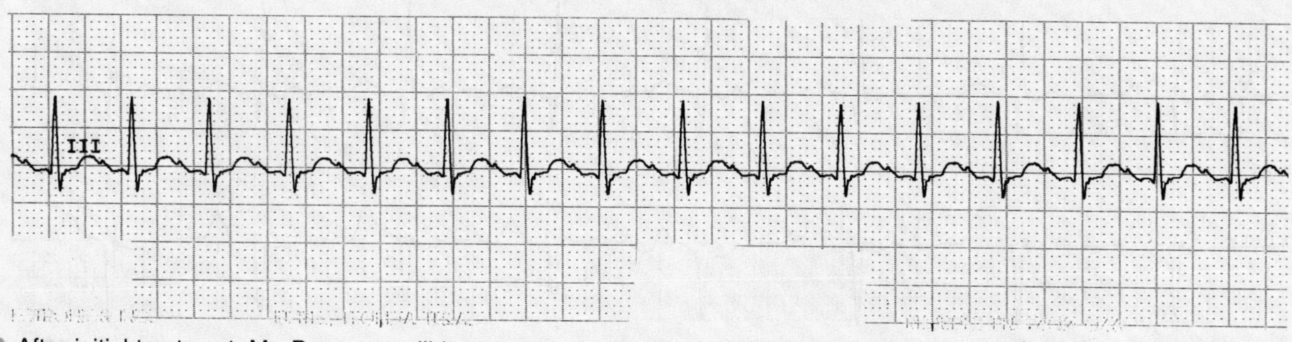

After initial treatment, Mr. Borg was still in supraventricular tachycardia, but his heart rate had dropped to 140 BPM.

LOC: Sedated and intubated
EENT: Within normal limits
Cardiac: S_1, S_2 audible without murmur, questionable S_3 regular rate, unable to assess neck vein distention
Pulmonary: Rhonchi present throughout lungs with fine basilar rales bilaterally
Abdominal: Within normal limits
Genitourinary: Foley catheter in place draining clear yellow urine.
Peripheral pulses: 1/1 with 1+ pitting edema which extends to midcalf

Current Treatment Plan

Meds: Dopamine 1600 mg in 500 ml D_5W; titrate to keep systolic BP >90 mm Hg
Furosemide 40 mg IV tid
Potassium 40 mEq in 100 ml D_5W over 4 hr bid
Thiamine 100 mg IM qd
MVI 1 ampule IV qd
Methylprednisolone (Solu-Medrol) 100 mg IV q 8 hr
Ceftriaxone (Rocephin) 1 g q 12 hr IV
Saline lock as needed for medications, flush bid, prn
Diet: NPO
Activity: Bed rest
Respiratory treatments: 70% FIO_2, IMV = 10, tidal volume = 750 ml with 5 cm PEEP
Diagnostic tests: Repeat chest x-ray, ECG, CBC, metabolic profile, cardiac enzymes this AM

The results of the cardiac catheterization reveal 100% occlusion of the left coronary artery and severe diffuse disease of the left anterior descending coronary artery. The physicians have determined that the client is a poor surgical risk and plan to treat him medically. Mr. Borg has interpreted this as an indication that his problem is temporary and states, "You can't keep a good man down."

Over the next several days, Mr. Borg's BP stabilizes and he is weaned from the dopamine. Furosemide is changed to an oral dose, and potassium dosage is reduced to 10 mEq PO tid. IV procainamide is discontinued after oral procainamide (Procan SR) is initiated at 250 mg bid. Mr. Borg is given digitalis and will be maintained on digoxin 0.25 mg qd. His resting heart rate has been approximately 70 BPM. A nitroglycerin (Nitro-Dur) patch is ordered daily to be applied in the morning and removed at bedtime. Mr. Borg is also extubated and placed on a no-added-salt, low-fat diet. He is to begin a cardiac rehabilitation program. The physician is planning to discharge him tomorrow after a recovery treadmill test.

Discharge Criteria

Average length of stay: 5.4 days
Cardiac rehabilitation initiated and follow-up appointments scheduled (includes diet, exercise, stress management, and medication teaching)

Questions to Be Considered

1. Compare and contrast left versus right ventricular, backward versus forward, and high-output versus low-output heart failure. Given the information provided, how would you categorize Mr. Borg's heart failure?
2. Compare and contrast the effects of Mr. Borg's cardiac medications: dopamine, diltiazem, adenosine, procainamide, digoxin, nitroglycerin. Why are the furosemide and potassium ordered?
3. What ramifications does Mr. Borg's lifestyle have on the success of his cardiac rehabilitation program? How might a home health nurse facilitate Mrs. Borg's participation in his rehabilitation program?
4. Eight weeks after discharge, Mr. Borg asks the cardiac rehabilitation nurse if new lights have been installed because "they all have a yellow ring round them and the edges are fuzzy." Upon further investigation the nurse determines that Mr. Borg has also had a decreased appetite, intermittent nausea and vomiting, and decreased ability to complete his entire exercise protocol. What should the nurse suspect? What recommendations should she make?
5. Six months after discharge, the physician resumes Mr. Borg's medication orders for benazepril 10 mg PO qd. Describe the pharmacodynamics of this drug and how it compares with furosemide.

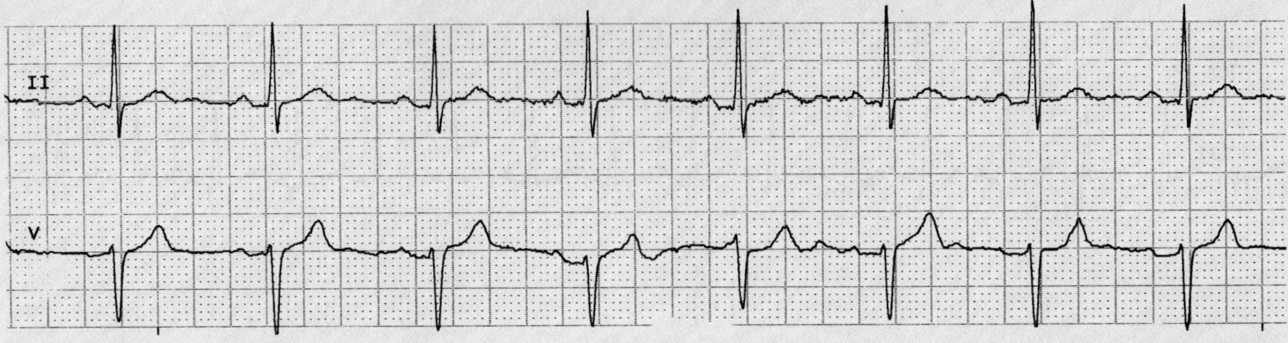

After several days of treatment, Mr. Borg is in normal sinus rhythm, with a resting heart rate of approximately 70 BPM.

ABG, arterial blood gas; BP, blood pressure; BPM, beats per minute; CBC, complete blood count; CPK, creatine phosphokinase; D_5W, 5% dextrose in water; ECG, electrocardiogram; ED, emergency department; EENT, eyes-ears-nose-throat; Hb, hemoglobin; Hct, hematocrit; ICU, intensive care unit; IMV, intermittent mechanical ventilation; IV, intravenous; LOC, loss of consciousness; PEEP, positive end-expiratory pressure; PAWP, pulmonary artery wedge pressure; PO, by mouth; RBC, red blood cell; TPR, temperature, pulse, respirations; WBC, white blood cell.

Manifestations of heart failure develop with ventricular aneurysm, rupture of the ventricular septum, and rupture of the papillary muscle. Manifestations of severe mitral insufficiency often develop when the papillary muscle of the left ventricle ruptures. Ventricular dysrhythmias (e.g., frequent PVCs and ventricular tachycardia) occur often in the presence of a ventricular aneurysm (the necrotic tissue is very irritable). Manifestations of cardiac tamponade develop with rupture of the heart.

The goal of treatment is to decrease the workload of the heart and increase the oxygen supply to keep the area of infarction and necrotic tissue as small as possible.

Surgery is performed to (1) excise the ventricular aneurysm, (2) replace the mitral valve if the papillary muscle is ruptured, or (3) repair the VSD. Pericardiocentesis and immediate surgery help relieve cardiac tamponade that occurs after rupture of the heart.

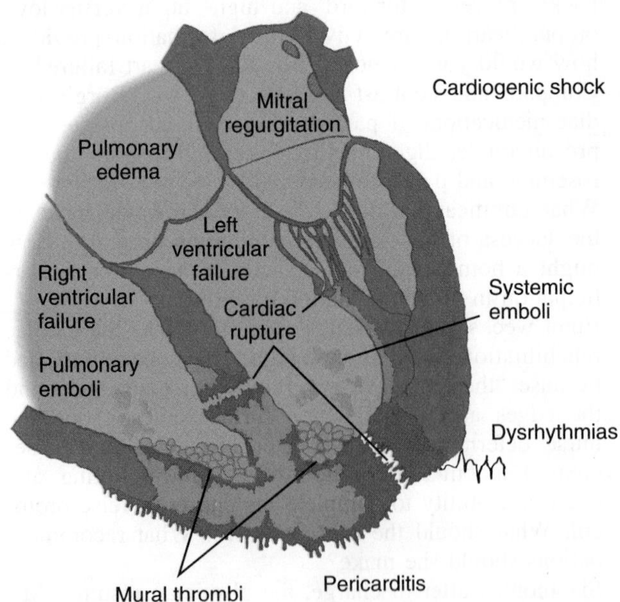

FIGURE 58–6 Major complications of acute myocardial infarction. (From O'Rourke, R. A. [1982]. The bedside diagnosis of the complications of myocardial infarction. In R. S. Eliot [Ed.], *Cardiac emergencies.* Mount Kisco, NY: Futura Publishing.)

PERICARDITIS. Up to 28% of clients with an acute transmural MI develop early pericarditis (within 2 to 4 days). The inflamed area of the infarction rubs against the pericardial surface and causes it to lose its lubricating fluid. A pericardial friction rub can be auscultated across the precordium. The client complains that chest pain is worse with movement, deep inspiration, and cough. The pain of pericarditis is relieved by sitting up and leaning forward.

Frequent assessment may lead to early identification and intervention. Relieve pain with analgesics, such as acetaminophen, nonsteroidal anti-inflammatory drugs (NSAIDs), or other anti-inflammatory agents. Reduce the client's anxiety by differentiating the pain of pericarditis from the pain of MI.

DRESSLER'S SYNDROME (LATE PERICARDITIS). Dressler's syndrome, a form of pericarditis, can occur as late as 6 weeks to months after an MI. Although the etiologic agent is unknown, an autoimmune cause is suggested. The client usually presents with a fever lasting 1 week or longer, pericardial chest pain, pericardial friction rub, and occasionally pleuritis with pleural effusions. This is a self-limiting phenomenon, and no prevention is known. Treatment includes aspirin, prednisone, and narcotic analgesics for pain. Anticoagulation therapy may precipitate cardiac tamponade and should be avoided in these clients.

REHABILITATION AND EDUCATION

Strengthen the Myocardium

A successful rehabilitation program begins the moment the client enters the coronary care unit for emergency care and continues for months and even years after discharge from the health care facility.[1] The overall goal of rehabilitation is to help the client live as full, vital, and productive a life as possible while remaining within the limits of the heart's ability to respond to increases in activity and stress. Six important subgoals of the rehabilitation process are as follows:

- Developing a program of progressive physical activity
- Educating the client and significant others about the cause, prevention, and treatment of CHD
- Helping the client accept the limitations imposed by illness

- Aiding the client in adjusting to changes in occupational goals
- Lessening the exposure to risk factors
- Changing the psychosocial factors adversely affecting recovery from CHD.[42, 43]

Cardiac rehabilitation is a comprehensive, long-term program that involves periodic medical evaluation, prescribed exercises, and education and counseling about cardiac risk factor modification.[42] Cardiac rehabilitation is a multifactorial program that begins when the client is still hospitalized and continues throughout recovery. Cardiac rehabilitation consists of four phases[1]:

- Phase 1 (inpatient)
- Phase II (immediate outpatient)
- Phase III (intermediate outpatient)
- Phase IV (maintenance outpatient)

Phase I (Inpatient)

Phase I begins with admission to the coronary care unit. After an MI, clients usually remain on bed rest for less than 24 hours unless complications such as heart failure or dysrhythmias develop. Although the myocardium must rest, bed rest puts the client at risk for hypovolemia, hypoxemia, muscle atrophy, and pulmonary embolus. Thus, the client must avoid both invalidism and reckless overexertion.

Provide complete bed rest for the first day or so with use of a bedside commode for bowel movements. Most clients receive a 2-g sodium diet. If the client is nauseated, provide a clear liquid diet until nausea subsides. A coronary care nurse or physiotherapist should start passive exercises. As the client regains strength, have the client sit for brief periods on the side of the bed and dangle the feet. Allow the client to ambulate to a bedside chair for 15 to 20 minutes after the first day if dangling has been tolerated. When the client is transferred from the coronary care unit to an intermediate or regular unit, bathroom privileges and self-care activities are encouraged. Wireless heart monitoring (telemetry) may continue. Allow brief walks in the hall with supervision. The length and duration of these walks are increased progressively, working up to 5 to 10 minutes according to the client's endurance.[6]

The client loses 10% to 15% of skeletal muscle and contractile strength within the first week of bed rest and 20% to 25% after 3 weeks of bed rest. The client must increase activities gradually to avoid overtaxing the heart as it pumps oxygenated blood to the muscles. The metabolic equivalent test (MET) provides one way of measuring the amount of oxygen needed to perform an activity:

$$1 \text{ MET} = 3.5 \text{ ml } O_2/\text{kg/min}$$

One MET is about equivalent to the oxygen uptake a client requires when resting. Early mobilization activities after an acute MI should not exceed 1 to 2 METs, as from shaving, washing, and self-feeding. (Later activities can increase to 10 or 11 METs, such as cycling or running.)

With each activity level increase, monitor the heart rate, blood pressure, and fatigue level, adjusting the client's activity level accordingly. During early activities, the heart rate should not rise more than 25% above resting level. Blood pressure must not rise more than 25 mm Hg above normal.[1]

Help the client avoid fatigue. Dyspnea, chest pain, tachycardia, and a sense of exhaustion warn that the client is attempting to do too much. Instruct the client regarding these warning signs of overexertion.

During phase I, client education should include cardiac anatomy and physiology risk factors and management of CHD, behavioral counseling, and home activities.

Phase II (Immediate Outpatient)

If no complications arise, the physician discharges the client to the home by the end of the second week. Nearly 50% of clients after an acute MI have an uncomplicated hospital course without evidence of angina, heart failure, or major dysrhythmias. There is a growing trend toward early discharge of clients with uncomplicated MI. A team at one health care facility discharges post-MI clients at the end of the 4th day but allows clients to go home early only if the household has adequate help and is conducive to rest. Such clients are followed up carefully by trained nurse-clinicians who visit the home and supervise physiologic status, exercise, and diet every other day. Researchers hope that earlier discharge after MI reduces depression as well as hospital expenses. The Bridge to Home Health Care provides suggestions for helping the client to adjust to convalescence at home.

Resuming sexual activity may be one of the most difficult aspects of returning to normal life after an MI. One study reports that more than 50% of a group of women had fear of resuming sexual activity after MI (44% of their partners reported similar concerns). Sexual intercourse may resume 4 to 8 weeks after MI if the physician agrees. The client should be able to climb two flights of stairs before resuming sexual activity. Caution clients not to eat or drink alcoholic beverages immediately before intercourse. Taking nitroglycerin before intercourse may help prevent exertional angina.[20, 32]

Advise the client to stop smoking. Encourage frequent walks, but warn against strenuous activities, such as shoveling snow. The walking program aims for a goal of 2 miles in less than 60 minutes.

A monitored group program may help the client achieve the best possible physical conditioning. These programs typically last from 10 to 12 weeks and are implemented in a supervised setting. They offer various training devices, such as treadmills, stationary bicycles, and rowing machines, to facilitate fitness. During phase II, the client performs large-muscle exercises for at least 20 to 30 minutes three or four times a week. In addition, clients are trained in warm-up and stretching exercises.[1, 6, 42] During the sessions, cardiac rehabilitation staff monitor cardiac rhythm, heart rate, and blood pressure before exercise, at peak exercise, and during recovery. Clients also report their level of perceived exertion several times during the exercise session.

Some clients may be able to return to work at the end of 8 or 9 weeks if they remain asymptomatic. Clients with less physically strenuous jobs can sometimes resume a full-time schedule, but manual laborers may have to work part time or find less taxing work. Occupational evaluations can be done to assess cardiac impairment in relation to job requirements and client skills.[41]

Between the 8th and 10th weeks, the client requires a complete physical examination, including ECG, exercise stress tests, lipid analysis, and chest x-ray study. Clini-

BRIDGE TO HOME HEALTH CARE

Heart-Healthy Living After a Myocardial Infarction

The role of the home health nurse is to help clients who had a myocardial infarction (MI) adjust to their lifestyle by teaching healthy heart living. Focus your teaching on areas that will help clients become responsible for self-care. Assume that you need to repeat health education that was provided in the hospital during the acute MI episode. When stress is high, clients usually recall little of what was taught.

Instruct the client and significant other or family member to monitor for clinical manifestations that may indicate extensions and recurrences of the MI. Clients need to report indigestion, shortness of breath, increased edema, and palpitations. Learning when to call the physician or nurse for these physical problems is very important.

Determine what your clients know about their medications. Knowing what the medication is called, its function, the schedule for taking it, and its side effects is required for client safety. Generally, multiple medications are prescribed, and you need to give the client written instructions and information about each medication. Many pharmacists provide a computer printout of medications and interactions for the client to keep. Medication planners that have compartments for various times of day allow the client to prefill medications for a week at a time and may prevent errors.

The convalescence period for the client and family creates anxiety about daily activities. Instruct the client to avoid prolonged baths or showers to prevent vasodilation. Use tepid water and a stool or bath chair in the shower. Encourage the use of energy-conservation techniques, such as keeping the arms at waist level and getting enough rest to prevent fatigue. Routine household activities and mild recreational activities, such as playing golf, are usually permitted.

Climbing more than two flights of stairs and lifting more than 20 pounds are restricted. If clients do not ask about resuming sexual relations, consider introducing the topic. They may be too timid to consult their physicians about this subject.

An appropriate unsupervised exercise is a prescribed indoor walking program. Exercising after a heavy meal or during mild illness is contraindicated. Instruct the client to begin each exercise session with a warm-up period that may last as long as 15 minutes and to end the session with a cool-down period. Walking should be constant and should last long enough to increase blood flow to the muscles.

The client or caregiver should have an emergency plan that includes having someone available to drive if a ride is needed and someone in the home who knows basic cardiopulmonary resuscitation (CPR). A personal emergency response system may be appropriate for clients who live alone. Some emergency response systems are worn around the neck, and the push of a button summons medical assistance. Caregiver stress, communication problems, and fear of the unknown are valid concerns. Community resources and additional information can be obtained by calling the American Heart Association's toll-free number, 800-242-8721.

Pamela Singh, RN-CS, MSN, FNP, *Family Nurse Practitioner, San Diego, California*

cians must correct pre-existing health problems that might have contributed to the development of CHD (e.g., hypertension, anemia, hyperthyroidism).

Recovery after an MI may be lengthy and difficult. The client may have undergone surgery or may have been managed medically. In either case, a serious threat to integrity has occurred. Initially after an MI, clients attempt to prove that they are not seriously ill. Coping strategies include denial and minimization. Some clients conceal the recurrence of chest pain. As recovery continues, clients begin to comprehend that a heart attack has really occurred, to understand why it happened, and to consider its impact on the future. Clients begin the process of life adjustment to find a lifestyle that can be tolerated and maintained while preserving a sense of self-worth. Several strategies are used to regain self-control, such as gauging progress, seeking reassurance, learning about health, and being cautious. Eventually, clients come to terms with the fact that they will not be living life to the fullest. Clients learn to accept limitations and to refocus on other aspects of life. Some clients are unable to adjust. Sometimes clients find that they have had too many setbacks and are powerless to make changes or gain control. The education and counseling that accompany a structured cardiac rehabilitation program can help to improve psychological well-being, social adjustment, and functioning.[41]

Phase III (Intermediate Outpatient)

The extended outpatient phase of cardiac rehabilitation lasts from 4 to 6 months. Exercise sessions continue to be supervised, and clients are taught how to monitor their exercise intensity by taking their pulse or, if in a walking program, by counting the number of steps they take in a 15-second interval. Clients with dysrhythmias are monitored more closely, and intermittent rhythm strips may be taken. For clients who prefer to exercise at home, clinicians trained in cardiac rehabilitation can provide detailed, written instructions for a long-term exercise program. Various methods are used to determine the appropriate exercise routines. Periodic evaluation is necessary to assess the client's endurance and tolerance to the prescribed exercise program.

Phase IV (Maintenance Outpatient)

Phase IV, the final phase of cardiac rehabilitation, usually takes place in the home or community and is unsupervised. The client maintains a program of regular exercise and other lifestyle modifications to modify cardiac risk. Clients should undergo an exercise testing and risk factor assessment annually.[6]

Nursing Management of the Medical Client

The goals of nursing management after an MI are as follows:

Text continued on page 1605

C A R E P L A N

THE CLIENT WITH A MYOCARDIAL INFARCTION

Nursing Diagnosis. Pain related to myocardial ischemia resulting from coronary artery occlusion with loss or restriction of blood flow to an area of the myocardium and necrosis of the myocardium.

Outcomes. The client will experience improved comfort in the chest, as evidenced by a decrease in the rating of the chest pain, the ability to rest and sleep comfortably, less need for analgesia or nitroglycerin, and reduced tension.

Interventions	Rationales
1. Assess the characteristics of chest pain, including location, duration, quality, intensity, presence of radiation, precipitating and alleviating factors, and associated manifestations. Have the client rate pain on a scale of 0 to 10, and document findings in nurses' notes.	1. Pain is an indication of myocardial ischemia. Assisting the client in quantifying pain may differentiate pre-existing and current pain patterns as well as identify complications. Usually a scale of 0 to 10 is used, 10 being the worst pain and 0 being none.
2. Assess respirations, blood pressure, and heart rate with each episode of chest pain.	2. Respirations may be increased as a result of pain and associated anxiety. Release of stress-induced catecholamines increases heart rate and blood pressure.
3. Obtain a 12-lead electrocardiogram (ECG) on admission, then each time chest pain recurs for evidence of further infarction.	3. Serial ECGs and stat ECGs record changes that can give evidence of further cardiac damage and location of myocardial ischemia.
4. Monitor the response to drug therapy. Notify the physician if pain does not abate within 15 to 20 minutes.	4. Pain control is a priority because it indicates ischemia.
5. Provide care in a calm, efficient manner that will reassure the client and minimize anxiety. Stay with the client until discomfort is relieved.	5. External stimuli may worsen anxiety and cardiac strain and limit coping abilities.
6. Limit visitors as the client requests.	6. Limiting visitors prevents overstimulation and promotes rest.
7. Administer morphine as ordered.	7. Morphine is an opiate analgesic and alters the client's perception of pain and reduces preload time vasoconstriction.
8. Administer nitrates as ordered.	8. Nitrates relax the smooth muscles of coronary blood vessels, decreasing ischemia and hence decreasing pain.

Evaluation. The client should be pain-free within 15 to 20 minutes after administration of drug therapy. The client will verbalize relief of pain and will not exhibit associated manifestations of pain.

Nursing Diagnosis. Altered Tissue Perfusion (cardiopulmonary) related to thrombus in coronary artery, resulting in altered blood flow to myocardial tissue.

Outcomes. The client will demonstrate improved cardiac tissue perfusion, as evidenced by a decrease in the rating of pain and resolving ST segments.

Interventions	Rationales
1. Keep the client on bed rest with a quiet environment.	1. Stress activates the sympathetic nervous system and increases myocardial oxygen needs.
2. Administer oxygen as ordered.	2. Oxygen increases myocardial supply of oxygen.
3. Administer thrombolytics as ordered.	3. Thrombolytic therapy can break apart the thrombus and increase myocardial tissue perfusion.
4. Monitor ST segments.	4. ST segment elevation indicates myocardial tissue injury; ST segment depression indicates decreased myocardial perfusion.

Evaluation. The client will have a decrease in pain and a normal ST segment.

Collaborative Problem. Dysrhythmias related to electrical instability or irritability secondary to ischemia or infarcted tissue, as evidenced by an increase or decrease in heart rate, change in rhythm, and dysrhythmias.

Outcomes. The client will have no dysrhythmias, as evidenced by normal sinus rhythm or return to the client's own baseline rhythm.

Interventions	Rationales
1. Teach the client and family about the need for continuous monitoring. Keep alarms on and limits set at all times.	1. Continued monitoring keeps staff aware of myocardial changes. Family anxiety is decreased.
2. Assess the apical heart rate. Auscultate for change in heart sounds (murmurs, rub, S_3, and S_4).	2. The apical heart rate suggests early cardiac decompensation and potential loss of cardiac output.
3. Document the rhythm strip every shift and prn (as needed) if dysrhythmias occur. Measure the pulse rate, QRS, PR, and QT segments with each strip. Note and report any deviations from the client's baseline values.	3. Dysrhythmias are the most common complication after a myocardial infarction (MI).

Interventions	Rationales
4. Report six or more multifocal premature ventricular contractions (PVCs) per minute to the physician.	4. Multifocal PVCs indicate ventricular irritability, which decreases cardiac output and may lead to life-threatening dysrhythmias.
5. Give antidysrhythmic agents as ordered.	5. Antidysrhythmic drugs reduce myocardial irritability.
6. Monitor the effects of antidysrhythmic agents.	6. The desired results are increased diastolic threshold potential and decreased action potential duration.
7. Monitor serum potassium levels.	7. Altered potassium levels can affect cardiac rhythms.
8. Maintain a patent intravenous (IV) line or heparin lock at all times.	8. This measure is for emergency administration of IV cardiac medications.
9. Monitor ST segments, and document changes.	9. ST depression indicates myocardial ischemia, and ST elevation indicates injury; either may precipitate dysrhythmias.

Evaluation. Within 24 hours of admission, the client's cardiac rhythm will remain stable and the client will exhibit no manifestations of rhythm disturbance.

Nursing Diagnosis. Decreased Cardiac Output related to negative inotropic changes in the heart secondary to myocardial ischemia, injury, or infarction, as evidenced by change in the level of consciousness, weakness, dizziness, loss of peripheral pulses, abnormal heart sounds, hemodynamic compromise, and cardiopulmonary arrest.

Outcomes. The client will have improved cardiac output, as evidenced by normal cardiac rate, rhythm, and hemodynamic parameters, dysrhythmias controlled or absent; and absence of angina.

Interventions	Rationales
Assess for and document the following as evidence of myocardial dysfunction with decreasing cardiac output:	
1. Mental status—be alert to restlessness and decreased responsiveness.	1. Cerebral perfusion is directly related to cardiac output and aortic perfusion pressure and is influenced by hypoxia and electrolyte and acid-base variations.
2. Lung sounds—monitor for crackles and rhonchi.	2. Crackles may develop, reflecting pulmonary congestion related to alterations in myocardial function.
3. Blood pressure—monitor for hypertension or hypotension.	3. Hypotension related to hypoperfusion, vagal stimulation, dysrhythmias, or ventricular dysfunction may occur; it may be related to pain, anxiety, catecholamine release, or preexisting vascular problems.
4. Heart sounds—note the presence of gallop, murmur, and increased or decreased heart rate.	4. Bradycardia may be present because of vagal stimulation or conduction disturbances related to the area of myocardial injury. Tachycardia may be a compensatory mechanism related to decreased cardiac output. A gallop may be related to fluid volume overload or heart failure, and a murmur may be present if a ruptured chordae tendineae occurred.
5. Urinary output—be alert to output less than 30 ml/hr.	5. Urinary output less than 30 ml/hr may reflect reduced renal perfusion and glomerular filtration as a result of reduced cardiac output.
6. Peripheral perfusion—monitor for pallor, mottling, cyanosis, coolness, diaphoresis, and peripheral pulses.	6. Decreased peripheral pulses may indicate a decrease in cardiac output.
7. Monitor arterial blood gas (ABG) levels.	7. Acidosis may cause dysrhythmias and depressed cardiac function.
8. If a pulmonary artery catheter is used, record hemodynamic parameters every 2 to 4 hours and as required (prn). Be alert to pulmonary capillary wedge pressure (PCWP) >18 mm Hg, cardiac output <4 L/min, and cardiac index <2.5 L/min.	8. A PCWP above 18 may indicate fluid volume overload or heart failure. A cardiac output below 4 and a cardiac index of below 2.5 indicate heart failure or decrease in cardiac output. Use hemodynamic monitoring to assess drug therapy and for prevention or early detection of complications of MI (i.e., extension, heart failure, cardiogenic shock).
9. Maintain hemodynamic stability by monitoring the effects of beta-blockers and inotropic agents.	9. Assess the effect of drug therapy on myocardial contractility and function.
10. Monitor and assess angina for type severity and duration.	10. Angina indicates myocardial ischemia, which may decrease cardiac output.

Evaluation. Within 2 to 3 days of admission, the client will have normal hemodynamic pressures, normal vital signs, clear breath sounds, no shortness of breath, normal ABG values. Normal sinus rhythm with rate between 60 to 100 beats/min (BPM).

Nursing Diagnosis. Impaired Gas Exchange related to decreased cardiac output, as evidenced by cyanosis, impaired capillary refill, reduced arterial oxygen tension (PaO_2), and dyspnea.

Outcomes. The client will demonstrate improved gas exchange, as evidenced by absence of cyanosis, brisk cap refill, absence of dyspnea, and ABG levels within normal limits.

Interventions	Rationales
1. Administer oxygen as ordered; maintain continuous oximetry.	1. Increases amount of oxygen available for myocardial uptake; oximetry measures peripheral oxygen saturation.
2. Monitor ABGs as ordered.	2. The presence of hypoxia indicates a need for supplemental oxygen. Monitoring provides data on the adequacy of tissue perfusion and oxygenation.
3. Continue to assess the client's skin, capillary refill, and level of consciousness every 2 to 4 hours and prn.	3. Cyanosis (circumoral or at extremities) indicates hypoxia. Capillary refill >3 seconds indicates poor perfusion and possibly hypoxia.
4. Assess respiratory status for dyspnea and crackles.	4. Dyspnea may indicate inadequate oxygenation, and the presence of crackles may impair gas exchange because of decreased exchange of oxygen and carbon dioxide through fluid in alveoli.
5. Prepare for intubation and mechanical ventilation if hypoxia increases.	5. With increasing hypoxia, mechanical ventilation may be necessary to oxygenate the client adequately.

Evaluation. Within 2 to 3 days of admission, client's breath sounds will be clear, and ABG values will be within normal limits.

Nursing Diagnosis. Risk for Injury related to coagulopathies associated with thrombolytic therapy.

Outcomes. The client will maintain hemostasis; if bleeding does occur, it will be recognized and treated at once.

Interventions	Rationales
1. Obtain coagulation studies as ordered.	1. Coagulation studies can help determine the tendency to bleed.
2. Monitor invasive line sites for active bleeding.	2. Thrombolytic therapy disrupts the normal coagulation process, and bleeding may occur at any invasive site.
3. Inspect all body fluids for presence of blood.	3. Internal bleeding may be manifested through body fluids.
4. Hold pressure on any discontinued lines 15 minutes; if arterial, hold for 30 minutes.	4. It takes longer to achieve hemostasis at catheter sites.
5. Observe neurologic status.	5. A change in neurologic status may indicate intracranial bleeding.
6. Avoid intramuscular (IM) injections.	6. IM injections may cause bleeding.
7. Assess for back or flank pain.	7. Flank or back pain may suggest retroperitoneal bleeding.
8. Keep an IV line patent.	8. In case of active bleeding, a patent line must be maintained to transfuse blood products.
9. Maintain an active type and crossmatch on the client.	9. If the client requires blood or blood products, an active type and crossmatch help eliminate any delay in treatment.

Evaluation. The client will be free from overt or occult bleeding.

Nursing Diagnosis. Powerlessness related to the hospital environment and anticipated lifestyle changes, as evidenced by verbalized "feelings of doom," crying, and anger.

Outcomes. The client will regain a sense of "control," as evidenced by feeling able to express feelings of powerlessness over the present situation and future outcomes.

Interventions	Rationales
1. Provide opportunities for the client to express feelings about oneself and the illness.	1. These opportunities create a supportive climate and send the message that caregivers are willing to help.
2. Explore reality perceptions, and clarify if necessary.	2. Listening to the client's feelings and words can help the client acquire a more hopeful outlook.
3. Eliminate the unpredictability of events by allowing adequate preparation for tests and procedures.	3. Information helps the client and family feel more hopeful and be more willing to participate in care.
4. Reinforce the client's right to ask questions.	4. Maintain a supportive climate to let the client feel free to ask questions or have information repeated.
5. Allow choices when possible.	5. Self-care allows the client to feel independent.
6. Provide positive reinforcement for increased involvement in self-care.	6. When clients participate in planning for care, they are more likely to feel a sense of control and to follow through with actions.
7. Help the client identify strengths and areas of control.	7. Self-confidence and security come with a sense of control; foster full client participation.

Evaluation. Within 24 hours of admission, client will verbalize a feeling of control over the situation and will actively participate in decisions regarding care.

Nursing Diagnosis. Anxiety and Fear related to hospital admission and fear of death, as evidenced by client and family appearing restless, hostile, or withdrawn; client and family verbalize fatalism or act extremely emotional as if in the grieving process.

Outcomes. The client will have reduced feelings of anxiety and fear, as evidenced by demonstrating appropriate range of feelings and initial signs of effective coping (participating in the treatment regimen) being able to rest, and asking fewer questions.

Interventions	Rationales
1. Limit nursing personnel; provide continuity of care.	1. Continuity of care promotes security and development of rapport with and trust of health care providers.
2. Allow and encourage the client and family to ask questions; do not avoid questions. Bring up common concerns.	2. Accurate information about the situation reduces fear, strengthens the client-nurse relationship, and assists the client and family to face the situation realistically.
3. Allow the client and family to verbalize fears.	3. Sharing information elicits support and comfort and can relieve tension and unexpressed worries.
4. Stress that frequent assessments are routine and do not necessarily imply a deteriorating condition.	4. The client may feel reassured after learning that frequent assessments may prevent development of more serious complications.
5. Repeat information as necessary because of the reduced attention span of the client and family.	5. The client's attention span is short, and time perception may be altered. Anxiety decreases learning and attention.
6. Provide a comfortable, quiet environment for the client and family.	6. A comfortable environment enhances coping mechanisms and reduces myocardial workload and oxygen consumption.

Evaluation. Within 2 days of admission, client will exhibit signs of effective coping and progression through stages of recovery.

Nursing Diagnosis. Risk for Constipation related to bed rest, pain medications, and NPO (nothing by mouth) or soft diet, as evidenced by subjective feeling of fullness, abdominal cramping, painful defecation, and palpable impaction.

Outcomes. The client will have improved bowel elimination, as evidenced by eliminating a stool without straining or having a vasovagal response (bradycardia).

Interventions	Rationales
1. Ensure that the client has adequate bulk in diet and adequate fluid intake (without violating fluid restrictions).	1. Bulk and fluid within the colon prevent straining.
2. Monitor the effectiveness of softeners or laxatives. Instruct the client on prevention of straining and avoiding the Valsalva (vasovagal) maneuver.	2. Stool softeners decrease the myocardial workload of straining. The Valsalva maneuver causes bradycardia, decreasing cardiac output.
3. Encourage the client to use a bedside commode rather than a bedpan.	3. Use of bedpans necessitates more straining and increases the vasovagal response.

Evaluation. Within 2 to 3 days of admission, client will have normal bowel function.

Nursing Diagnosis. Altered Health Maintenance related to MI and implications for lifestyle changes.

Outcomes. The client and family will learn about the medical regimen and lifestyle changes, as evidenced by verbalizing an understanding of a heart attack and the necessary lifestyle changes regarding diet, medications, stress reduction, quitting smoking, and cholesterol, weight, and blood pressure reduction.

Interventions	Rationales
1. Explain the following, providing both oral and written instructions: anatomy and functions of heart muscle, coronary arteries, and atherosclerotic process; definition of a "heart attack"; healing process of the heart; and role of collateral circulation.	1. Use of multiple learning methods enhances retention of material; information helps the client understand the underlying problems of overall heart functions.
2. Assist the client with identifying personal risk factors.	2. Risk factor identification is the first step before changes can be implemented.
3. Assist the client in devising a plan for risk factor modification (e.g., diet; smoking cessation; cholesterol, stress, and blood pressure reduction).	3. This information is helpful in providing opportunity for the client to identify risk factors, assume control, and participate in a treatment regimen.
4. Provide guidelines for a diet low in cholesterol and saturated fat. Arrange for dietary consultation before hospital discharge.	4. Consultation with other health professionals enhances client learning from others. Guidelines developed with the client and family before discharge help once they are home.

5. Teach the client and family about medications that will be taken after hospital discharge (name, purpose, dosage, schedule, precautions, potential side effects).	5. The more clients understand the medical regimen and potential side effects, the more adept they will be in monitoring for them.
6. Discuss post-MI activity progression; arrange for a cardiac rehabilitation consultation.	6. Continued follow-up will let clients know how they are doing; outpatient cardiac rehabilitation supports and assists clients in the lifestyle changes necessary for a healthy recovery and life.
7. Utilize other professionals to collaborate in the care of the client.	7. Dietitians can assist in diet education; social services can identify assistance in the area; cardiac rehabilitation personnel can assist in exercise regimens; clergy can assist in coping strategies; and support groups can assist in social support.

Evaluation. Within 2 days of admission, the client and family will be able to verbalize understanding of heart attack and identify personal risk factors and necessary lifestyle changes.

Nursing Diagnosis. Risk for Activity Intolerance related to an imbalance between oxygen supply and demand, as evidenced by weakness, fatigue, change in vital signs, dysrhythmias, dyspnea, pallor, and diaphoresis.

Outcomes. The client will have improved activity tolerance, as evidenced by participating in desired activities, meeting activities of daily living (ADL), reduced fatigue and weakness, vital signs within normal limits during activity, absence of cyanosis, diaphoresis, and pain.

Interventions	Rationales
1. Monitor vital signs before and immediately after activity and 3 minutes later.	1. Data are provided about the client's response to increased activity. Vital signs should return to baseline levels in 3 minutes. If blood pressure decreases and heart rate increases, cardiac decompensation is suggested and activity should be decreased. The development of chest pain or dyspnea may indicate a need for an alteration in exercise regimen or medication.
2. Monitor for tachycardia, dysrhythmias, dyspnea, diaphoresis, weakness, fatigue, or pallor after activity.	2. These indicators of myocardial oxygen deprivation may call for decreased activity, changes in medications, or use of supplemental oxygen.
3. Encourage verbalization of feelings or concerns regarding fatigue or limitations.	3. Knowing limitations prevents exertion and increasing myocardial workload.
4. Provide assistance with self-care activities, and provide frequent rest periods, especially after meals.	4. Large meals may increase myocardial workload and cause vagal stimulation, with resultant bradycardia or ectopic beats; caffeine, a cardiac stimulant, increases heart rate.
5. Increase activity per cardiac rehabilitation nurse and physician orders.	5. Gradual increase in activity increases strength and prevents overexertion, enhances collateral circulation, and restores a normal lifestyle as far as possible.

Evaluation. Within 3 to 4 days of admission, the client will progress normally through steps of phase I cardiac rehabilitation without manifestations of exercise intolerance.

Collaborative Problem. Risk for Heart Failure related to disease process, as evidenced by tachycardia, hypotension or hypertension, S_3 or S_4 heart sounds, dysrhythmias, ECG changes, decreased urine output, decreased peripheral pulses, cool ashen skin, diaphoresis, crackles, jugular vein distention, edema, and chest pain.

Outcomes. The nurse will monitor for clinical manifestations of heart failure by assessing cardiac rate, rhythm, hemodynamic parameters, skin perfusion, renal perfusion, and CNS perfusion.

Interventions	Rationales
1. Auscultate the apical pulse.	1. Atrial (S_3) or ventricular (S_4) gallop rhythms are common and reflect tissue noncompliance or distention of chambers.
2. Assess heart rate and rhythm.	2. Sinus tachycardia, paroxysmal atrial contractions, paroxysmal atrial tachycardia, multifocal atrial tachycardia, and PVCs are commonly seen with heart failure.
3. Document dysrhythmias, if present, as necessary.	3. Dysrhythmias reduce ventricular filling time, decrease myocardial contractility, and increase myocardial oxygen demands, which further compromises cardiac output.
4. Note lung sounds every 2 to 4 hours and as needed.	4. Crackles may develop; ineffective cardiac output causes an increase in venous congestion that transcends to the pulmonary vasculature and leaks into the alveolar tissue, resulting in congestion.
5. Palpate peripheral pulses every 2 to 4 hours and as necessary.	5. Pulses may be weak, thready, or difficult to obtain when cardiac output is decreased.

6. Monitor blood pressure every 2 to 4 hours and as needed.	6. Hypotension related to hypoperfusion, vagal stimulation, or ventricular dysfunction may occur. Hypertension may be related to pain, anxiety, catecholamine release, or pre-existing vascular problems.
7. Inspect skin for pallor, cyanosis, and diaphoresis every 2 to 4 hours and as needed.	7. Pallor is associated with vasoconstriction, reduced cardiac output, and anemia. Cyanosis may develop during severe episodes of pulmonary edema. Dependent areas are often blue or mottled with increased venous congestion.
8. Monitor urine output, noting changes or decreasing output and dark or concentrated urine, every 2 to 4 hours and as needed.	8. Urinary output below 20 ml/hr may reflect reduced renal perfusion and glomerular filtration as a result of reduced cardiac output.
9. Assess for chest pain.	9. Chest pain may indicate inadequate cardiac perfusion related to the hypertrophied myocardium.
10. Assess for peripheral edema.	10. In heart failure, especially right-sided, the inability to pump venous blood back to the heart results in venous pooling, increased pressure in the vascular space that leaks in the interstitium and presents as peripheral edema.
11. Assess changes in sensorium.	11. Cerebral perfusion is directly related to cardiac output, and mentation may be a sensitive indicator of deterioration.
12. Provide frequent rest periods.	12. Physical rest decreases the production of catecholamines, which raises heart rate, myocardial oxygen demand, and blood pressure.
13. Instruct the client on avoidance of activities that increase cardiac workload.	13. Avoidance of activities provides an opportunity for myocardial recovery and decreases workload and myocardial oxygen consumption.
14. Provide a bedside commode. Avoid the Valsalva maneuver.	14. The Valsalva maneuver causes bradycardia and temporarily decreases cardiac output.
15. Elevate the client's legs and avoid pressure under the knees. Permit increase in activity as tolerated.	15. This position enhances venous return, reduces dependent swelling, decreases venous stasis, and may reduce the incidence of thrombus and embolus formation.
16. Administer medications as ordered.	16. ACE inhibitors and beta blockade help reduce the incidence of heart failure after MI in clinical trials.[38]

Evaluation. The client will not manifest heart failure after an MI.

Nursing Diagnosis. Fluid Volume Excess related to reduced glomerular filtration rate (GFR), decreased cardiac output, increased antidiuretic hormone (ADH) production, and sodium and water retention, as evidenced by orthopnea, S_3 heart sound, oliguria, edema, jugular neck vein distention, increased weight, increased blood presssure, respiratory distress, and abnormal breath sounds.

Outcomes. The client's fluid volume balance will be adequate, as evidenced by balanced intake and output (I&O), clear or clearing breath sounds, vital signs within normal limits, stable weight, and absence of edema.

Interventions	Rationales
1. Monitor I&O (especially note color, specific gravity, and amount) every 2 to 4 hours, and as needed, and 24-hour totals.	1. Intake greater than output may indicate fluid volume excess. If client receives diuretic therapy, an increase in output is expected.
2. Maintain chair or bed rest in the semi-Fowler position.	2. This position promotes diuresis by recumbency-induced increased GFR and reduced ADH hormone production.
3. Involve the client and family in fluid schedules, especially if there are restrictions, and provide frequent oral care.	3. Involving the client in the therapy regimen may enhance a sense of control and fosters cooperation with restrictions.
4. Weigh the client daily.	4. Daily weights can show the increase or decrease in congestion and edema in response to therapy. A gain of 5 pounds represents about 2 L of fluid.
5. Assess for jugular neck vein distention, edema, peripheral pulses, and presence of anasarca.	5. Excessive fluid retention may be demonstrated by venous engorgement and edema formation. Peripheral edema often begins in the feet and ascends upward as heart failure worsens.
6. Auscultate breath sounds. Note adventitious sounds, and monitor for dyspnea or tachypnea.	6. These manifestations of pulmonary congestion reflect increased vascular volume and pulmonary hypertension or worsening of heart failure.
7. Monitor for sudden extreme shortness of breath and feelings of panic.	7. These are manifestations of extreme pulmonary capillary hypertension (pulmonary edema).
8. Palpate for hepatomegaly. Note complaints of right upper quadrant pain or tenderness.	8. Advancing heart failure leads to venous congestion, which results in liver engorgement and altered liver function (i.e., impaired drug metabolism, prolonged drug half-life).
9. Note increased lethargy, hypotension, and muscle cramping.	9. These are manifestations of hypokalemia and hyponatremia that may occur because of fluid shifts and diuretic therapy.

10. Evaluate the effectiveness of diuretics and potassium supplements.	10. Fluid shifts and use of diuretics can alter electrolytes, especially potassium and chloride, which affects cardiac rhythm and contractility.
11. Assess the need for dietary consultation as needed.	11. Restrictions of foods high in sodium may be necessary. The client may need to eat foods enriched with potassium when taking loop diuretics.

Evaluation. Within 3 days of admission, the client's fluid volume will be normal. I&O will be balanced, breath sounds will be clear, vital signs will be normal, and weight will be stable, with no signs of peripheral or central edema.

Nursing Diagnosis. Risk for Impaired Skin Integrity related to bed rest, edema, and decreased tissue perfusion, as evidenced by reddened areas and the presence of areas of breakdown.

Outcomes. The client will have intact skin integrity, as evidenced by an absence of reddened areas and no areas of breakdown.

Interventions	Rationales
1. Inspect the client's skin; note bone prominences, edema, altered circulation, pigmentation, obesity, and emaciation.	1. Altered skin color in isolated areas suggests damage caused by pressure or decreased circulation.
2. Assist with active or passive range-of-motion (ROM) exercises.	2. ROM exercises enhance venous return. Isometric exercises may adversely affect cardiac output by increasing myocardial work and oxygen consumption.
3. Reposition the client every 2 hours in a bed or chair.	3. Repositioning increases circulation and reduces the time that weight deprives any one area of blood flow.
4. Provide pressure-reducing devices, sheepskin, or elbow and heel protectors if needed.	4. These devices reduce pressure to bone prominences and improve skin integrity.
5. Assess and provide special air or flotation beds for clients at high risk for pressure ulcers.	5. These beds reduce pressure to skin and may improve circulation.

Evaluation. Within 2 to 3 days of admission, the client will have intact skin integrity and will have no reddened areas or skin breakdown.

- Recognize and treat cardiac ischemia
- Administer thrombolytic therapy as ordered, and observe for complications
- Recognize and treat potentially life-threatening dysrhythmias
- Monitor for complications of reduced cardiac output
- Maintain a therapeutic critical care environment
- Identify the psychosocial impact of MI on the client and family
- Educate the client in lifestyle changes and rehabilitation

Nursing diagnoses or collaborative problems that may apply to the client after acute MI are discussed in the Care Plan. Case managers are assigned to these clients to coordinate their care (see Case Management feature).

CONCLUSIONS

CHD is a progressive occlusive disorder that commonly results in reduced coronary blood flow. This reduction is manifested clinically by angina and MI. MI, permanent damage to the myocardium, may be the first indicator of how serious the heart disease is. Your responsibilities in the care of these clients are to educate them about the warning signs of MI, to monitor their response to therapy, to prevent complications, and to promote rehabilitation.

THINKING CRITICALLY

1. **Mrs. Polk, a 62-year-old housewife who cares for her two grandchildren, is admitted to the emergency department with complaints of chest pain. She is diaphoretic and pale and reports pain "under my left breast that pushes to my back." She rates the pain an 8 on a scale of 1 to 10. Her ECG shows a depressed ST segment. She is placed on oxygen therapy, and an IV line is inserted. Cardiac serum markers are drawn and sent to the laboratory. Her vital signs are temperature 36.9° C, apical pulse 110, and blood pressure 108/68.**

Factors to Consider. What additional testing is necessary to rule in or role out an acute MI? What other information from Mrs. Polk's history might aid in the diagnosis?

2. **The physician immediately orders reteplase, a thrombolytic agent, for Mrs. Polk.**

Factors to Consider. What information must be obtained from Mrs. Polk to safely initiate thrombolytic therapy?

3. **You administer the thrombolytic therapy as ordered. Mrs. Polk states her pain is now a 1 on a scale of 1 to 10. ST segments are resolving, and she is no longer diaphoretic.**

Factors to Consider. What effects from the thrombolytic therapy appear to be occurring? Which side effects of the therapy should you be anticipating?

4. **A client with long-standing coronary artery disease experiences severe chest pain unrelieved by**

nitroglycerin. He is admitted with an acute MI to the coronary care unit. What are the priorities on admission? What medical treatment may be instituted in the first hours following the infarction?

Factors to Consider. What time frame is considered most crucial to the salvage of myocardial muscle? What care is given to the newly admitted client?

BIBLIOGRAPHY

1. American Association of Cardiovascular and Pulmonary Rehabilitation. (1995). *Guidelines for cardiac rehabilitation programs.* Champaign, IL: Human Kinetics.
2. American Heart Association. (1998). *1999 Heart and stroke statistical update.* Dallas: Author.
3. Beattie, S. (1999). Management of chronic stable angina. *Nurse Practitioner, 24*(5), 44, 49, 53, 56, 59–61.
4. Braunwald, E., et al. (1994). *Unstable angina: Diagnosis and management. Clinical practice guideline No. 10* (AHCPR Pub. No. 94-0602). Rockville, MD: Agency for Health Care Policy and Research and the National Heart, Lung, and Blood Institute, Public Health Service, U.S. Department of Health and Human Services.
5. Colon, P., et al. (1998). Utility of stress echocardiography in the triage of patients with atypical chest pain from the emergency department. *American Journal of Cardiology, 82,* 1282–1284.
6. Cox, M. H. (1997). Exercise for coronary artery disease. *Physician and Sports Medicine, 25*(12), 27–32.
7. Dempsey, S. J., Dracup, K., & Moser, D. K. (1995). Women's decision to seek care for symptoms of acute myocardial infarction. *Heart and Lung, 24,* 444.
8. Doering, L. V. (1999). Pathophysiology of acute coronary syndromes leading to acute myocardial infarction. *Journal of Cardiovascular Nursing, 13*(3), 1–20.
9. Dracup, K., & Cannon, C. (1999, April). Combination treatment strategies for management of acute myocardial infarction. *Critical Care Nurse Supplement,* 1–17.
10. Fallon, E. M., & Roques, J. (1997). Acute chest pain. *AACN Clinical Issues, 8,* 382–397.
11. Feldman, M., & Cryer, B. (1999). Aspirin absorption rates and platelet inhibition times with 325-mg buffered aspirin tablets (chewed or swallowed intact) and with buffered aspirin solution. *American Journal of Cardiology, 84,* 404–409.
12. Gensini, G., Comeglio, M., & Falai, M. (1999). Advances in antithrombotic therapy of acute myocardial infarction. *American Heart Journal, 138*(2), S171–S176.
13. Gersh, B. J., Braunwald, E., & Rutherford, J. D. (1997). Chronic coronary artery disease. In E. Brunwald (Ed.), *Heart disease: A textbook of cardiovascular medicine.* Philadelphia: W. B. Saunders.
14. Goodwin, M., et al. (1999). Early extubation and early activity after open heart surgery. *Critical Care Nurse 19*(5), 18–26.
15. Hudak, C. M., Gallo, B. M., & Lohr, P. G. (1998). *Critical care nursing* (7th ed.). Philadelphia: Lippincott-Raven.
16. Hudson, M., et al. (1999). Cardiac markers: Point of care testing. *Clinica Chimica Acta, 28*(4), 223–237.
17. Jensen, L., & King, K. M. (1997). Women and heart disease: The issues. *Critical Care Nurse, 17*(2), 45–52.
18. Kosnik, L. (1999, October). Treatment protocols and pathways: Improving the process of care. *Critical Care Nurse Supplement,* 3–7.
19. Kuhn, F. E., & Gersch, B. J. (1996). Mechanical complications of acute myocardial infarction. In V. Fuster, R. Ross, & E. J. Topol (Eds.), *Atherosclerosis and coronary artery disease* (Vol. 2). Philadelphia: Lippincott-Raven.

19a. Lee, T. H., & Goldman, L. (2000). Evaluation of the patient with acute chest pain. *New England Journal of Medicine, 342*(16), 1187–1193.

20. McCauley, K. M. (1995). Assessing social support in patients with cardiac disease. *Journal of Cardiovascular Nursing, 10,* 73–80.
21. Moser, D., et al. (1999, October). The role of the critical care nurse in preventing heart failure after acute myocardial infarction. *Critical Care Nurse Supplement,* 11–15.
22. Murphy, M., & Berding, C. (1999). Use of myoglobins and cardiac troponins in the diagnosis of acute myocardial infarction. *Critical Care Nurse, 19*(1), 58–65.
23. O'Connor, C. M., Gattis, W. A., & Swedberg, K. (1999). Current and novel pharmacologic approaches in advanced heart failure. *Heart and Lung, 28,* 227–239.
24. Rich, M. W. (1999). Heart failure disease management: A critical review. *Journal of Cardiac Failure, 5*(1), 64–75.
25. Riegel, B., & Gocka, I. (1995). Gender differences in adjustment to acute myocardial infarction. *Heart and Lung, 24,* 457.
26. Ryan, T. J., et al. (1996). ACC/AHA guidelines for the management of patients with acute myocardial infarction: A report of the American College of Cardiology/American Heart Association Task Force on practice guidelines (Committee on Management of Acute Myocardial Infarction). *Journal of the American College of Cardiology, 28,* 1328–1428.
27. Sayer, J. W., et al. (1997). Attenuation or absence of circadian and seasonal rhythms of acute myocardial infarction. *Heart, 77,* 325–329.
28. Shah, P. K. (1996). Pathophysiology of plaque rupture and the concept of plaque stabilization. *Cardiology Clinics, 14,* 17–28.
29. Skillings, J. (1998). Atherosclerosis. *Lippincott's Primary Care Practice, 2*(5), 437–451.
30. Soran, O., Schneider, V. M., & Feldman, A. M. (1999). Basic therapy for congestive heart failure: Current practice, new prospects. *Journal of Critical Illness, 14*(2), 78–89.
31. Stary, H. C., et al. (1995). A definition of advanced types of atherosclerotic lesions and a histological classification of atherosclerosis. *Circulation, 92,* 1355–1374.
32. Steinke, E. F., & Patterson, P. (1995). Sexual counseling of MI patients by cardiac nurses. *Journal of Cardiovascular Nursing, 10,* 81–87.
33. Tatum, J., et al. (1997). Comprehensive strategy for the evaluation and triage of the chest pain patient. *Annals of Emergency Medicine, 29,* 116–23.
34. Thelan, L. A., et al. (1998). *Critical care nursing: Diagnosis and management* (3rd ed.). St. Louis: Mosby–Year Book.
35. Theroux, P., & Fuster, V. (1998). Acute coronary syndromes: Unstable angina and non-Q-wave myocardial infarction. *Circulation, 97,* 1195–1206.
36. Tofler, G. H. (1997). Triggering and the pathophysiology of acute coronary syndromes. *American Heart Journal, 134,* S55–S61.
37. van derWall, E. E., et al. (1995). Magnetic resonance imaging in coronary artery disease. *Circulation, 92,* 2723–2739.
38. Vantrimpont, P., et al. (1997). Additive beneficial effects of beta-blockers to angiotensin-converting enzyme inhibitors in the survival and ventricular enlargement (SAVE) study. *Journal of the American College of Cardiology, 29,* 229–236.
39. Verheugt, F. (1999). What an interventional cardiologist should know about the pharmacological treatment of acute myocardial infarction. *Seminars in Interventional Cardiology, 4,* 17–20.
40. Wenger, N. K. (1999). Women, myocardial infarction, and coronary revascularization. *Cardiology in Review, 7,* 117–120.
41. Wenger, N. K. (1997). Cardiac rehabilitation: Implications of the AHCPR guideline. *Hospital Medicine, 33*(4), 31–38.
42. Wenger, N. K., et al. (1995). *Cardiac rehabilitation as secondary prevention. Clinical practice guideline: Quick reference guide for clinicians. No. 17.* Rockville, MD: Agency for Health Care Policy and Research and the National Heart, Lung, and Blood Institute, Public Health Service, U.S. Department of Health and Human Services.
43. Wu, C. Y. (1995). Assessment of postdischarge concerns of coronary artery bypass graft patients. *Journal of Cardiovascular Nursing, 10,* 1–7.
44. Zerwic, J. (1998). Symptoms of acute myocardial infarction: Expectations of a community sample. *Heart and Lung, 27,* 75–81.
45. Zerwic, J. (1999). Patient delay in seeking treatment for acute myocardial infarction symptoms. *Journal of Cardiovascular Nursing, 13,* 21–32.

The Implantable Cardioverter-Defibrillator and Quality of Life

QUESTIONS

How does implantation of a cardioverter-defibrillator affect a recipient's and the family's quality of life (QOL)?

What are their concerns and fears?

CITATION

Gallagher, R. D., McKinley, S., Mangan, B., et al. (1997). The impact of the implantable cardioverter defibrillator on quality of life. *American Journal of Critical Care, 6,* 16–24.

STUDIES

Eighteen studies examined QOL after insertion of an implantable cardioverter defibrillator (ICD). Published between 1993 and 1995, the studies were identified in the critical care, nursing, medical, and technical literature. The method used to identify the studies included in the review was not specified. A total of 489 recipients (average age, 57 years) participated.

Summary of Findings

Overall, recipients felt that the ICD maintained or improved their QOL,[2, 9, 16, 18] and most indicated they had resumed their normal activities.[2, 12, 20] A majority reported having successfully incorporated the device into their body image over time.[13, 18, 20] In one study, QOL initially declined but returned to the preimplant level by 1 year.[13] Despite overall success, ICDs do cause problems and life changes for clients and their families.

Psychological Issues

Fear

Seventeen per cent to 47% of clients reported pain when a shock was dispensed[2, 16]; in one study, the pain was perceived by most people as being moderate (5 to 7 level on a 10-point Visual Analogue Scale).[2, 6] Descriptions of the shock varied from "like a spark plug" to "a bolt of lightning."[6, 16]

Reported rates of fear vary greatly, from 85% to 12.5%, with most subjects experiencing fear after a shock.[3, 6, 12, 16] Forty-three per cent of recipients reported being afraid that the shocks would not be successful,[12, 16] whereas others feared battery failure.[3, 6] In one study, 88% of recipients reported general nervousness after a shock and felt a need to talk about the experience.[6] The unpredictability of shocks and the possibility of loss of consciousness contribute to their fear.[10, 15]

Many recipients responded to this lack of predictability by attributing the shock to a specific activity (e.g., bending), and then by changing their normal behavior in an effort to prevent further shocks.[6, 19] A small study found that seven of 17 recipients reduced or totally abstained from sexual activity because of fear of shocks.[3] Syncope was unpredictable in these clients; even the absence of earlier syncope did not predict the absence of loss of consciousness during subsequent shocks.[10]

Anxiety

Recipients of ICDs reported higher levels of anxiety than the general population, but the source of the anxiety remains unclear. The anxiety might be due to the presence of the device, but it also might be due to the experience of receiving a shock, the anticipation of being shocked, malfunction of the device, [1, 3, 12, 16] or a residual effect from prior sudden cardiac arrest or ventricular tachycardia experience.[13] Since the ICD is to prevent adverse results of arrest or dysrhythmia, one might argue that recipients should have lower levels of anxiety; indeed, several studies have shown this effect.[16, 20] In one of these studies, 78% of the recipients reported reduced or no anxiety, some even viewed the device as a source of security and a life extender.[16]

It is unclear whether recipients who receive more shocks are more anxious than those who receive fewer shocks.[6, 9, 12] Generally, older people were less anxious than younger people.[12] Body image was a problem for 35% of recipients experiencing shocks[3, 16]; depression, global stress, confusion, and anger were also present.[4, 5, 16, 209]

Psychiatric Disorders

A retrospective study of 20 recipients and their families found that six of the patients had a transient psychiatric disorder (such as adjustment problems or panic attacks), four had major psychiatric disorders, and 9 of the families felt distressed.[14] These incidents are comparable to those found in other groups with chronic medical problems. Like anxiety, these disorders may be related to the presence of cardiac disease with all its implications or to prior experiences of sudden cardiac arrest.

Coping Strategies

Coping strategies of recipients and their families vary widely. Overall, optimism, denial, and confrontation are frequently reported,[4, 5, 11] although evasion is frequently used to cope with physical stresses.[11] Whether coping by recipients and family members improves or declines over the first year is not clear.[4, 13]

Spouses and families tend to be overprotective[18] and to be more concerned about the effects of the ICD and shock experiences on the family than recipients are.[18] Both recipients and families appear to have difficulty seeking and obtaining social support even though they feel a need for it.[4, 11]

Physical Function

Many recipients found that their ability to perform normal physical activities did not return to previous levels.[4, 11, 12, 16, 18] Difficulty sleeping and reduced energy were the most frequently reported limitations.[4, 11, 12, 16, 19] Many of the findings have been contradictory. For example, one study found that only 14% of recipients reported a limited QOL, but 47% of recipients reported an inability to return to an active life.[12] Also, in interpreting the findings regarding physical functioning, remember that many of the recipients have other cardiac conditions; one study reported a 68% incidence of cardiac disease and a 36% incidence of low cardiac output.[17]

Driving has been a controversial issue. About 6% of drivers have received shocks while driving, sometimes with associated syncope, but no accidents resulted.[8]

The Implantable Cardioverter-Defibrillator and Quality of Life *Continued*

Intellectual Function

In a small (n = 15) but comprehensive study of neurocognitive changes, confusion and low global cognitive functioning were often present at the time of implantation, although they returned almost to normal by 1 year.[4] However, memory and construction of thoughts were below normal at implantation and improved only slightly during the recovery year. These findings are limited in credibility by the fact that only 65% of the people contacted participated in the study, and poor coping was given as the main reason for nonparticipation; this suggests that recipients with more severe problems might not have been represented in the data. In another small study, decreased attention span and memory loss were reported.[18]

Work and Social Function

Given the recipients' problems with physical and intellectual activities, it is logical to expect that work and social functioning also would be disrupted after implantation. However, the findings are contradictory; the disparate findings may be the result of the different populations studied, improved technology over the years, or the research methods used.

Of two studies examining social activities after implantation, one noted reduced social interaction (i.e., found more social isolation),[16] whereas the other showed a decrease in social isolation.[19] Several studies have documented a decrease in employment, but estimates range from 38% to 66%.[2, 7, 12, 13, 16] Preexisting cardiac conditions, voluntary retirement, nearing or reaching retirement age, and a history of sudden cardiac arrest all contributed to the decision to stop working.

Driving is an important issue for recipients. Approximately 92% of recipients have continued to drive even though some of them had been advised not to do so.[8] Several subsequent studies have examined the safety of driving and the advice currently given to ICD recipients (see update).[21–24]

Updated, Annotated Study Reports, 1995–1999

Chevalier, P., et al. (1996). Improved appraisal of the quality of life in patients with automatic implantable cardioverter defibrillator. *Psychotherapy and Psychosomatics, 65,* 49–56.

This French study examined the impact of shock delivery on QOL as well as social, psychological, and physical well-being in ICD recipients. Slightly fewer than half the 32 recipients reported a good or very good physical tolerance of the ICD, whereas 75% reported a good or very good psychological tolerance. Better control of cardiac health was reported by 59%, and 82% felt more secure after receiving an ICD. QOL scores were negatively correlated with anxiety and depression, whereas occurrence of shocks had no influence on psychological well-being. Recipients with a psychiatric diagnosis had less favorable psychosocial and QOL outcomes. The single most important factor leading to negative psychosocial outcomes was low physical tolerance of the device itself, although the current miniaturization of devices might diminish this effect.

Dubin, A. M., Batsford, W. P., Lewis, R. J., and Rosenfeld, L. E. (1996). Quality-of-life in patients receiving implantable cardioverter defibrillators at or before age 40. *Pacing and Clinical Electrophysiology, 19,* 1555–1559.

Sixteen recipients 40 years of age or younger who had an ICD in place for an average of 3 years previously completed a functional health questionnaire; 63% were employed, with most holding the same job before and after ICD placement. Four of the nine women became pregnant after implantation, and all delivered healthy infants. All recipients considered their health good to excellent, with 38% reporting improved health since ICD placement. Moderate physical activities were freely performed by 68% of them. Of the recipients, 75% felt that the ICD interfered with social interactions and 50% were concerned about its effect on sexual relationships.

Jung, W., and Luderitz, B. (1996). Quality of life and driving in recipients of the implantable cardioverter-defibrillator. *American Journal of Cardiology, 78*(suppl 5A), 51–56.

Of the European cardiologists who responded to the survey, 67% recommended temporary abstinence from driving for 3 to 18 months (average 9 ± 4 months) after ICD insertion. Despite medical advice not to drive, most recipients resumed driving within 12 months. However, only two experienced ICD shocks while driving—and no motor vehicle accidents resulted. It was concluded that risk of causing an accident varies considerably, depending on the original reason for the implant as well as the nature of the shock experiences of the recipient during the first 6 months after implantation.

Pinski, S. L., and Fahy, G. J. (1999). Implantable cardioverter-defibrillators. *American Journal of Medicine, 106,* 446–458.

This review article summarizes a broad range of findings from randomized clinical trials. The authors conclude that the studies examining QOL show unchanged or improved QOL after implantation. Most recipients perceive ICD shocks as quite uncomfortable, comparing them with a jolt from an electric socket or a kick in the chest. A small proportion (<15%) lose consciousness as a result of the lag between dysrhythmia and the corrective shock. Serious adjustment difficulties do occur, albeit in a small number of recipients.

A survey of American physicians over a 12-year period revealed that the driving fatality and injury rates for persons with ICDs were significantly lower than in the general population. The American Heart Association has advised that recipients with ICDs inserted for sustained, fast, ventricular dysrhythmias refrain from driving for 6 months after implantation and for 6 months after each subsequent shock.

Rosenqvist, M., Beyer, T., Block, M., den Dulk, K., Minten, J., & Lindemans, F. (1998). Adverse events with transvenous implantable cardioverter-defibrillators: A prospective multicenter study. *Circulation, 98,* 663–670.

The Implantable Cardioverter-Defibrillator and Quality of Life *Continued*

Adverse events associated with one ICD model were classified and their incidences reported; 778 European patients were observed for an average of 4 months after implantation. In total, 356 adverse events were observed in 259 recipients. Of the recipients, 50% experienced an adverse event within the first year after ICD implantation. The most frequently observed severe events included (1) inappropriate detection of dysrhythmia, (2) wound or pocket problems, and (3) lead or ICD dislodgment. The impact of adverse events on QOL was not examined, although clearly there is an association.

Limitations/Reservations. When applying the studies' findings, take into account the caveat that the experiences of older people are represented to a greater extent than the experiences of younger people who are now receiving ICDs. Remember, many of the studies in the review were conducted with 30 or fewer participants.

Research-Based Practice

From the evidence presented, it is clear that ICDs relieve recipients of worries about life-threatening dysrhythmias. Yet they also introduce new concerns, and restraints on how recipients live. The rate of occurrence of an adverse event, be it serious or mild, in the first year after implantation is high enough (50%) to contribute to anxiety at the least and to major adjustment disorders at the worst. These problems and responses highlight the need for educational or supportive interventions that cover the first year. Given the levels of problems and psychological stresses, many recipients might benefit from having access via telephone at all times to a nurse who can advise or reassure them.

Education of recipients and their families must carefully balance the possibility of problems with the benefits to be gained. Counseling in how to deal with problems at both emotional and practical problem-solving levels should be provided. Recipients should be encouraged to discuss problems with the nurse who will be seeing them over the long term. When discussing driving, take into account what driving means to the recipient in terms of practical and self-image ramifications. Counseling regarding driving should follow the guidelines provided by the American Heart Association.

The findings enable us to identify recipients who are at risk for poor adjustment to the ICD, namely those who:

- Had experienced sudden cardiac arrest or symptomatic ventricular tachycardia
- Have experienced loss of consciousness with a dysrhythmia-cardioversion event
- Have other serious cardiac disease (e.g., heart failure)
- Have a history of a psychiatric disorder
- Experience an adverse event

These recipients are in particular need of ongoing support.

Cited References

1. Badger, J., & Morris, P. (1989). Observations of a support group for automatic implantable cardioverter-defibrillator recipients and their spouses. *Heart and Lung, 18,* 238–243.
2. Bainger, E., & Fernsler, J. (1995). Perceived quality of life before and after implantation of an internal cardioverter defibrillator. *American Journal of Critical Care, 4,* 36–43.
3. Cooper, D., et al. (1986). The impact of automatic implantable cardioverter defibrillator on quality of life. *Clinical Progress in Electrophysiologic Pacing, 4,* 306–309.
4. Dougherty, C. (1994). Longitudinal recovery following sudden cardiac arrest and internal cardioverter defibrillator implantation: survivors and their families. *American Journal of Critical Care, 3,* 145–154.
5. Dougherty, C. (1995). Psychological reactions and family adjustment in shock versus nonshock groups after implantation of cardioverter defibrillator. *Heart and Lung, 24,* 281–291.
6. Dunbar, S., Warner, C., & Purcell, J. (1993). Internal cardioverter defibrillator device discharge: Experiences of patients and family members. *Heart and Lung, 22,* 494–501.
7. Kalbfleisch, K., et al. (1989). Reemployment following implantation of the automatic cardioverter defibrillator. *American Journal of Cardiology, 64,* 199–202.
8. Keelan, E., et al. (1995). Driving habits and experiences of patients with implantable cardioverter-defibrillators (Abstract). *Journal of the American College of Cardiology, 25*(pt II, suppl A), 145A.
9. Keren, R., Aaron, D., & Veltri, E. (1991). Anxiety and depression in patients with life-threatening ventricular arrhythmias: Impact of the implantable cardioverter-defibrillator. *PACE Pacing and Clinical Electrophysiology, 14,* 181–186.
10. Kou, W., et al. (1991). Incidence of loss of consciousness during automatic implantable cardioverter-defibrillator shocks. *Annals of Internal Medicine, 115,* 942–945.
11. Kuiper, R., & Nyamathi, A. (1991). Stressors and coping strategies of patients with automatic implantable cardioverter defibrillators. *Journal of Cardiovascular Nursing, 5,* 65–76.
12. Luderitz, B., et al. (1993). Patient acceptance of the implantable cardioverter defibrillator in ventricular tachyarrhythmias. *PACE Pacing and Clinical Electrophysiology, 16,* 1815–1821.
13. May, C., et al. (1995). The impact of the implantable cardioverter defibrillator on quality-of-life. *PACE Pacing and Clinical Electrophysiology 18,* 1411–1418.
14. Morris, P., et al. (1991). Psychiatric morbidity following implantation of the automatic implantable cardioverter defibrillator. *Psychosomatics, 32,* 58–64.
15. Porterfield, J., et al. (1991). A prospective study utilizing a trans-telephonic electrocardiographic transmission program to manage patients in the first several months post-ICD implant. *PACE Pacing and Clinical Electrophysiology, 14,* 308–311.
16. Pycha, C., et al. (1990). Patient and spouse acceptance and adaptation to cardioverter-defibrillators. *Cleveland Clinic Journal of Medicine, 57,* 441–444.
17. Saksena, S., et al. (1992). Long-term multicenter experience with a second-generation implantable pacemaker-defibrillator in patients with malignant ventricular arrhythmias. *Journal of the American College of Cardiology, 19,* 490–499.
18. Sneed, N., & Finch, N. (1992). Experiences of patients and significant others with automatic cardioverter defibrillators after discharge from the hospital. *Progress in Cardiovascular Nursing, 7,* 20–24.
19. Vitale, M. B., & Funk, M. (1995). Quality of life in younger persons with an implantable cardioverter defibrillator. *Dimensions of Critical Care Nursing, 14,* 100–111.
20. Vlay, S., et al. (1989). Anxiety and anger in patients with ventricular tachyarrhythmias: Responses after automatic internal cardioverter defibrillator implantation. *PACE Pacing and Clinical Electrophysiology, 12,* 366–372.

The Implantable Cardioverter-Defibrillator and Quality of Life *Continued*

Added References

21. Chevalier, P., et al. (1996). Improved appraisal of the quality of life in patients with automatic implantable cardioverter defibrillator. *Psychotherapy and Psychosomatics, 65,* 49–56.
22. Jung, A., & Luderitz, B. (1996). Quality of life and driving in recipients of the implantable cardioverter-defibrillator. *American Journal of Cardiology, 78*(suppl. 5A), 51–56.
23. Pinski, S. L., & Fahy, G. J. (1999). Implantable cardioverter-defibrillators. *American Journal of Medicine, 106,* 446–458.
24. Rosenqvist, M., et al. (1998). Adverse events with transvenous implantable cardioverter-defibrillators: A prospective multicenter study. *Circulation, 98,* 663–670.

Sarah Jo Brown, PhD, RN, *Principal and Consultant, Practice-Research Integrations, Norwich, Vermont*

UNIT 13

Oxygenation Disorders

Anatomy and Physiology Review

The Respiratory System

Robert G. Carroll

Our body needs a constant supply of oxygen to support metabolism. The respiratory system brings oxygen through the airways of the lung into the alveoli, where it diffuses into the blood for transport to the tissues. This process is so vital that difficulty in breathing is experienced as a threat to life itself. Whether death is a real possibility or not, people with respiratory disorders are often very anxious and fearful that they may die, perhaps agonizingly.

The respiratory system also has other essential functions:

1. Expels carbon dioxide (CO_2), a metabolic waste product that is transported from the tissues to the lungs for elimination.
2. Filters and humidifies air that enters the lungs.
3. Traps particulate matter in the mucus of the airways and propels it toward the mouth for elimination by coughing or swallowing.

An active immune system helps prevent the entry of inhaled pathogens.

Respiratory control is tied most closely to arterial blood and brain CO_2 levels as well as to arterial blood oxygen levels. Respiration is also controlled by higher cortical centers. For example, an increase in ventilation accompanies exercise and keeps arterial blood gases within the normal range.

Respiratory problems are widespread. Acute disorders range from minor inconveniences (colds or flu) to more life-threatening problems (asthma, some types of pneumonia, and chest trauma). Chronic disabling conditions include *chronic airflow limitation* (also called chronic obstructive pulmonary disease, or COPD), and certain restrictive lung diseases. Chronic respiratory problems affect many people, often causing them to make radical lifestyle changes, such as retiring from work earlier than they wish.

Respiratory problems are associated with many causes: allergies, occupational factors, genetic factors, smoking and tobacco use, infection, neuromuscular disorders, chest abnormalities, trauma, pleural conditions, and pulmonary vascular abnormalities. The most significant factor in chronic respiratory illness and lung cancer is cigarette smoking.

STRUCTURE OF THE RESPIRATORY SYSTEM

UPPER AIRWAYS

The airways are the regions through which air passes on its way to the exchange areas of the lungs. The upper airways consist of the nasal cavities, pharynx, and larynx.

Nasal Cavity

The nose is formed from both bone and cartilage. The nasal bone forms the bridge, and the remainder of the nose is composed of cartilage and connective tissue (Fig. U13–1). Each opening of the nose on the face (*nostrils* or *nares*) leads to a cavity *(vestibule)*. The vestibule is lined anteriorly with skin and hair that filter foreign objects and prevent them from being inhaled. The posterior vestibule is lined with a mucous membrane, composed of columnar epithelial cells, and goblet cells that secrete mucus. The mucous membrane extends throughout the airways, and cilia (hair-like projections) propel mucus to the pharynx for elimination by swallowing or coughing. The portion of mucous membrane that is located at the top of the nasal cavity, just beneath the cribriform plate of the ethmoid bone, is specialized *(olfactory)* epithelium, which provides the sense of smell. Because the olfactory epithelium does not lie along the usual path of air movement, smell is enhanced by sniffing.

Along the sides of the vestibule are *turbinates,* mucous membrane-covered projections that contain a very rich blood supply from the internal and external carotid arteries. They warm and humidify inspired air.

Paranasal sinuses, open areas within the skull, are named for the bones in which they lie—frontal, ethmoid, sphenoid, and maxillary. Passageways from the paranasal sinuses drain into the nasal cavities. The nasolacrimal ducts, which drain tears from the surface of the eyes, also drain into the nasal cavity.

The mouth is considered part of the upper airway but only because it can be used to deliver air to the lungs when the nose is obstructed or when high volumes of air are needed, such as during exercise. The mouth does not perform the nasal functions efficiently, especially those of warming, humidifying, and filtering air.

Pharynx

The pharynx is a funnel-shaped tube that extends from the nose to the larynx. It can be divided into three sections.

The *nasopharynx* is located above the margin of the soft palate and receives air from the nasal cavity. From the ear, the eustachian tubes open into the nasopharynx. The pharyngeal tonsils (called *adenoids* when enlarged) are located on the posterior wall of the nasopharynx.

The *oropharynx* serves both respiration and digestion. It receives air from the nasopharynx and food from the oral cavity. Palatine (faucial) tonsils are located along the sides of the posterior mouth, and the lingual tonsils are located at the base of the tongue.

The *laryngopharynx (hypopharynx),* located below the base of the tongue, is the most inferior portion of the pharynx. It connects to the larynx and serves both respiration and digestion.

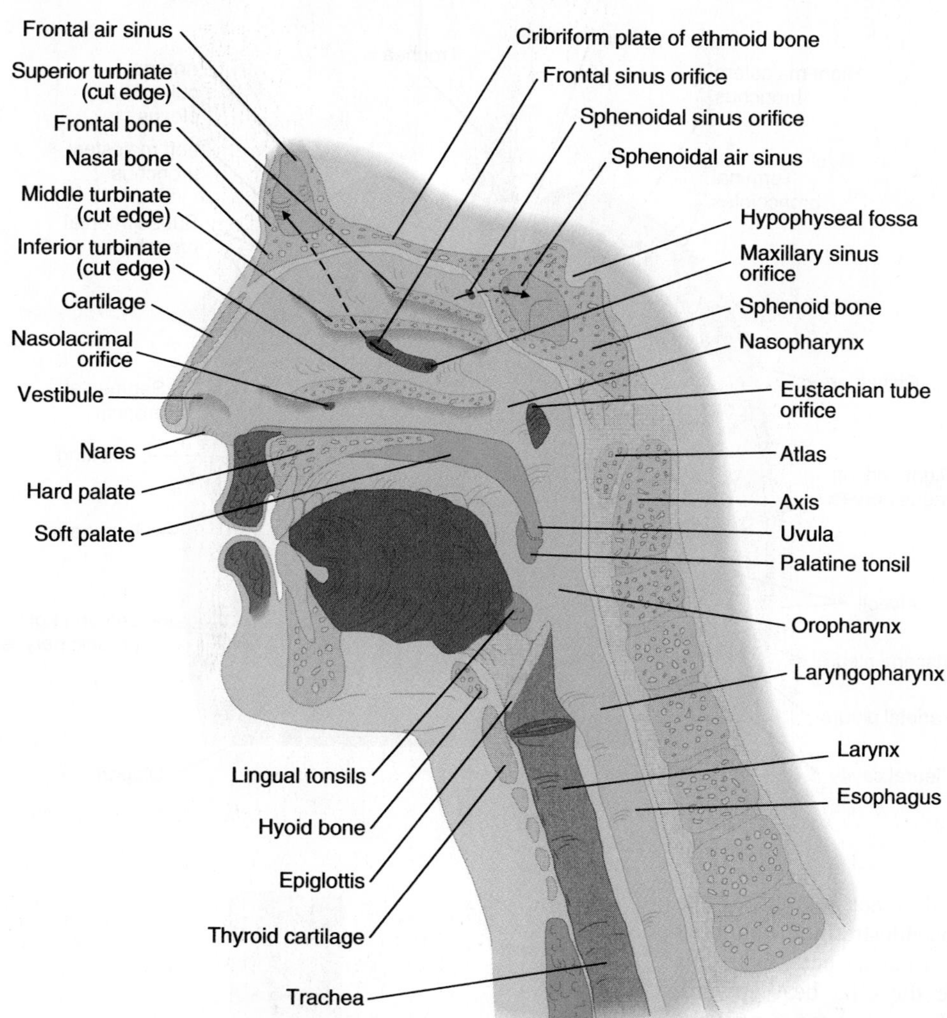

FIGURE U13–1 Structures of the upper airway.

Larynx

The larynx is commonly called the *voice box.* It connects the upper (pharynx) and lower (trachea) airways. The larynx lies just anterior to the upper esophagus. Nine cartilages form the larnyx: three large unpaired cartilages (epiglottis, thyroid, cricoid) and three smaller paired cartilages (arytenoid, corniculate, cuneiform). The cartilages are attached to the hyoid bone above and below the trachea by muscles and ligaments, all of which prevent the larynx from collapse during inspiration and swallowing.

The larynx consists of the endolarynx and a surrounding triangle-shaped bone and cartilage. The endolarynx is formed by two paired folds of tissue, forming the false and the true vocal cords. The slit between the vocal cords forms the *glottis.* The *epiglottis,* a leaf-shaped structure immediately posterior to the base of the tongue, lies above the larynx. When food or liquids are swallowed, the epiglottis closes over the larynx, protecting the lower airways from aspiration.

The thyroid cartilage protrudes in front of the larynx, forming the "Adam's apple." The cricoid cartilage lies just below the thyroid cartilage and is the anatomic site for an artificial opening into the trachea (tracheostomy, or cricothyroidotomy). The internal portion of the larynx is composed of muscles that assist with swallowing, speaking, and respiration and that contribute to the pitch of the voice. The blood supply to the larynx is through the branches of the thyroid arteries. The nerve supply is through the recurrent laryngeal and superior laryngeal nerves.

Lower Airways

The lower airway or tracheobronchial tree is composed of the trachea, right and left mainstem bronchi, segmental bronchi, subsegmental bronchi, and terminal bronchioles (Fig. U13–2). Smooth muscle, wound in overlapping clockwise and counterclockwise helical bands, is found in all of these structures. This arrangement allows contraction of the smooth muscle to decrease the diameter of the airways, increasing the resistance to air flow. This muscle is subject to spasm in many airway disorders. The lower airways continue to warm, humidify, and filter inspired air en route to the lungs.

Trachea

The trachea (windpipe) extends from the larynx to the level of the seventh thoracic vertebrae, where it divides into two main *(primary)* bronchi. The point at which the trachea divides is called the *carina.* The trachea is a flexible, muscular, 12-cm long air passage with C-shaped

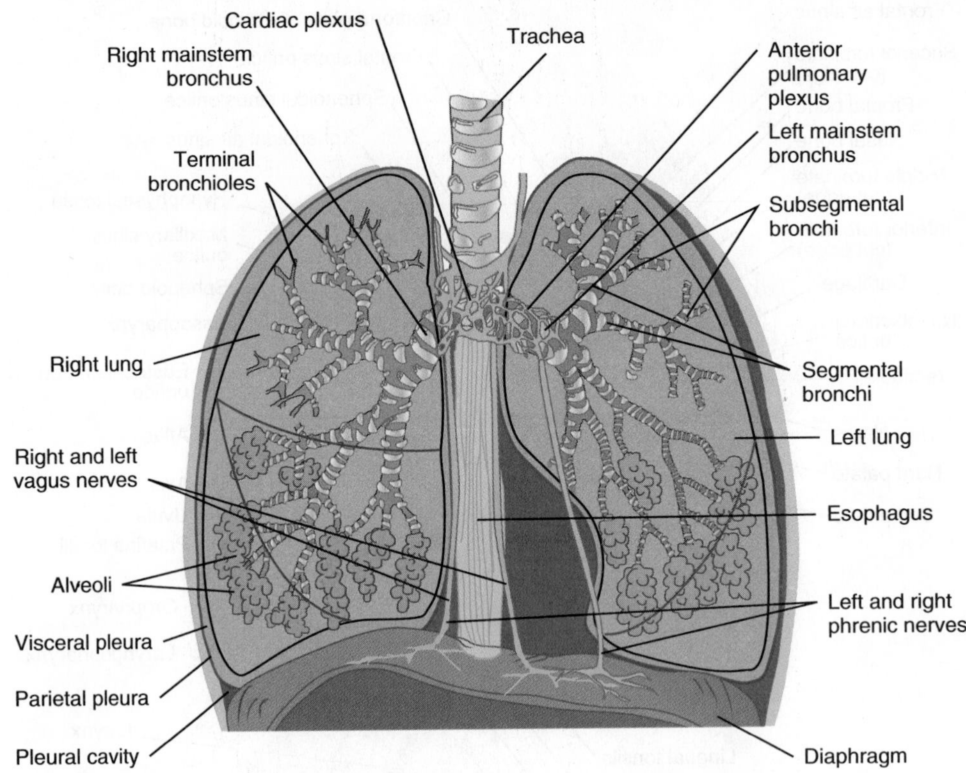

FIGURE U13–2 Structures of the lower airways.

cartilaginous rings. Along with all other regions of the lower airways it is lined with pseudostratified columnar epithelium that contains goblet (mucus-secreting) cells and cilia (Fig. U13–3). Because the cilia beat upward, they tend to carry foreign particles and excessive mucus away from the lungs to the pharynx. (No cilia are present in the alveoli.)

Bronchi and Bronchioles

The right mainstem bronchus is shorter and wider, extending more vertically downward, than the left mainstem bronchus. Thus, foreign bodies are more likely to lodge here than in the left mainstem bronchus. The *segmental* and *subsegmental bronchi* are subdivisions of the main bronchi and spread in an inverted, tree-like formation through each lung. Cartilage surrounds the airway in the bronchi, but the bronchioles (the final pathway to the alveoli) contain no cartilage and thus can collapse and trap air during active exhalation.

The *terminal bronchioles* are the last airways of the conducting system. The area from the nose to the terminal bronchioles does not exchange gas and functions as *anatomic dead space.* The lack of gas exchange means that the first air out of the mouth during exhalation resembles room air, but the last air out (end-tidal air) resembles alveolar air.

LUNGS AND ALVEOLI

Lungs

The lungs lie within the thoracic cavity on either side of the heart (see Fig. U13–2). They are cone-shaped, with

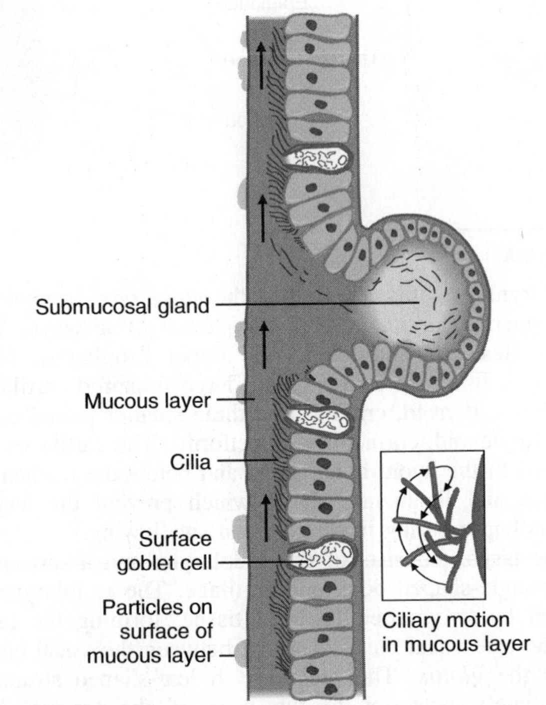

FIGURE U13–3 The mucociliary blanket is an important respiratory defense mechanism. Mucus is secreted by surface goblet cells. About 100 ml of mucus is normally secreted each day by the submucosal glands. Mucus covers the epithelial lining of the tracheobronchial tree in two layers—the watery solution layer close to the mucosal surface and the thicker gel layer. The cilia (hair-like projections) beat in an upward direction toward the upper airway. Particulate matter is trapped on the mucous layer and moved upward by the cilia. Debris-laden mucus is then either swallowed or expectorated as sputum.

the apex above the first rib and the base resting on the diaphragm. Each lung is divided into superior and inferior lobes by an oblique fissure. The right lung is further divided by a horizontal fissure, which bounds a middle lobe. The right lung, therefore, has three lobes; the left lobe has only two. In addition to these five lobes, which are visible externally, each lung can be subdivided into about 10 smaller units *(bronchopulmonary segments).* Each segment represents the portion of the lung that is supplied by a specific tertiary bronchus. These segments are important surgically, because a diseased segment can be resected without the need to remove the entire lobe or lung. The two lungs are separated by a space (the *mediastinum*), where the heart, aorta, vena cava, pulmonary vessels, esophagus, part of the trachea and bronchi, and the thymus gland are located.

The lungs contain gas, blood, thin alveolar walls, and support structures. The alveolar walls contain elastic and collagen fibers; these form a three-dimensional, basket-like structure that allows the lung to inflate in all directions. These fibers are capable of stretching when a pulling force is exerted on them from outside of the body or when they are inflated from within. The elastic recoil helps return the lungs to their resting volume.

Branches of the pulmonary artery provide most of the blood supply to the lungs. The blood is oxygen-poor, but oxygen is supplied by inspired air. The trachea and bronchioles, which are not part of the oxygen exchange surface, receive oxygen-rich blood from branches of the aorta.

Lung Volumes

The lungs of an average 19-year-old man have a total capacity of about 5900 ml. However, a person cannot exhale all the air from the lungs, and about 1200 ml of air always remains, no matter how forceful the expiration. This remaining volume *(residual volume)* prevents the collapse of the lung structures during expiration. The volume of air that moves in and out with each breath is called the *tidal volume.* During quiet breathing, tidal volume is about 500 ml. When we take a deep breath, the lung is more fully expanded. The amount of extra air inhaled, beyond the tidal volume, is called the *inspiratory reserve volume;* the extra air that can be exhaled after a normal breath is called the *expiratory reserve volume.*

Lung volumes are often combined into capacities:

- *Total lung capacity* (all four volumes)
- *Vital capacity* (all volumes except residual volume), which is the amount we can ventilate
- *Functional reserve capacity* (expiratory reserve plus residual volumes)
- *Inspiratory capacity* (tidal volume plus inspiratory reserve volume)

These volumes and capacities are frequently altered by disease. Lung volumes as measured by spirometry are shown in Figure U13–4. (Pulmonary function tests are described in Chapter 39.)

Alveoli

The lung parenchyma, which consists of millions of alveolar units, is the working area of the lung tissue. At birth, we have about 24 million alveoli; by age 8 years, we have 300 million. The total working alveolar surface area is approximately 750 to 860 square feet. The blood supply flowing toward the alveoli comes from the right ventricle of the heart.

The entire alveolar unit (respiratory zone) is made up of respiratory bronchioles, alveolar ducts, and alveolar sacs (Fig. U13–5). The alveolar walls are extremely thin, with an almost solid network of interconnecting capillaries. Because of the extensiveness of the capillary system, the flow of blood in the alveolar wall has been described as a "sheet" of flowing blood.

Oxygen and CO_2 are exchanged through a respiratory membrane, about 0.2 mm thick (Fig. U13–6). The average diameter of the pulmonary capillary is only about 5 μm, but red blood cells (7 μm in diameter) must squeeze through, actually touching the capillary wall. Thus, the distance across which oxygen and CO_2 must diffuse is greatly reduced. Thickening of the respiratory membrane

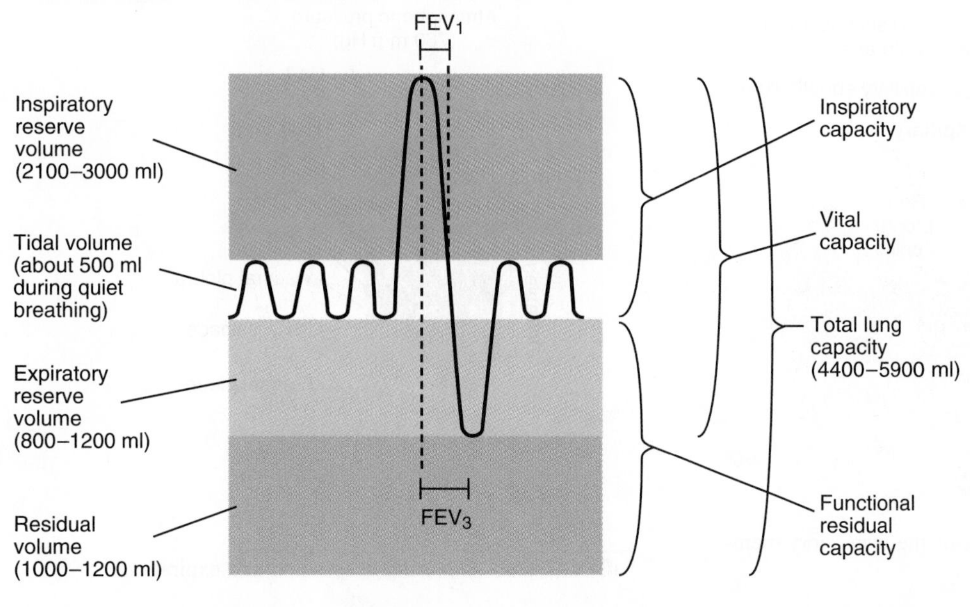

FIGURE U13–4 Lung volumes and capacities as measured by spirometry. The four volumes of the lungs are combined to form four capacities.

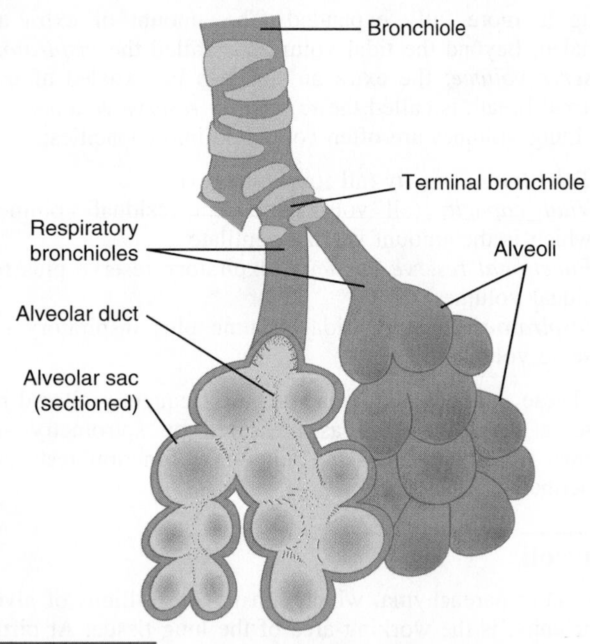

FIGURE U13–5 Gas exchange occurs in the respiratory zone, which consists of the respiratory bronchioles, alveolar ducts, and alveolar sacs.

(e.g., with pulmonary edema or fibrosis) may interfere with normal exchange of gases.

The alveolus comprises two cell types: *Type I pneumocytes,* which line the alveolus, are thin and incapable of reproduction but are effective in gas exchange. *Type II pneumocytes* are cuboidal and do not exchange oxygen and CO_2 well. They produce surfactant and are important in lung injury and repair. They differentiate into type I cells; oxygenation is impaired during the transition from type II to type I cells.

THORAX

The bony thorax provides protection for the lungs, heart, and great vessels. The outer shell of the thorax is made up of 12 pairs of ribs. The ribs connect posteriorly to the transverse processes of the thoracic vertebrae of the spine. Anteriorly, the first seven pairs of ribs are attached to the sternum by cartilage. The 8th, 9th, and 10th ribs *(false ribs)* are attached to each other by costal cartilage. The 11th and 12th ribs *(floating ribs)* allow full chest expansion because they are not attached in any way to the sternum.

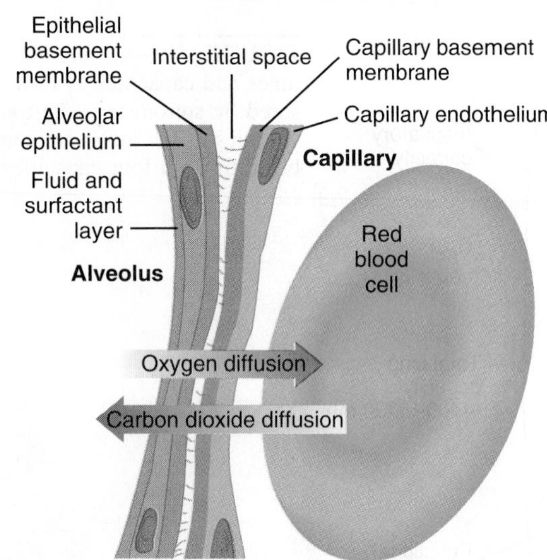

FIGURE U13–6 The ultrastructure of the respiratory membrane, where oxygen is exchanged.

DIAPHRAGM

Breathing is accomplished by skeletal muscle alteration of the thoracic space. The diaphragm is the primary muscle of breathing, and serves as the lower boundary of the thorax (Fig. U13–7). The diaphragm is dome-shaped in the relaxed position, with central muscular attachments to the xiphoid process of the sternum and the lower ribs. Contraction of the diaphragm pulls the muscle downward, increasing the thoracic space and inflating the lungs. The diaphragm's nerve supply (phrenic nerve) comes through

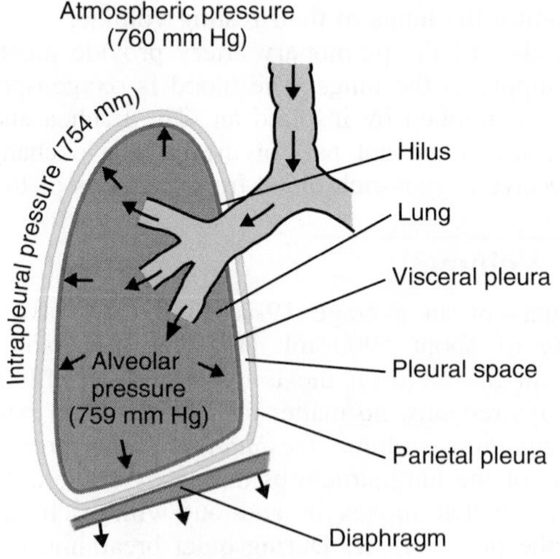

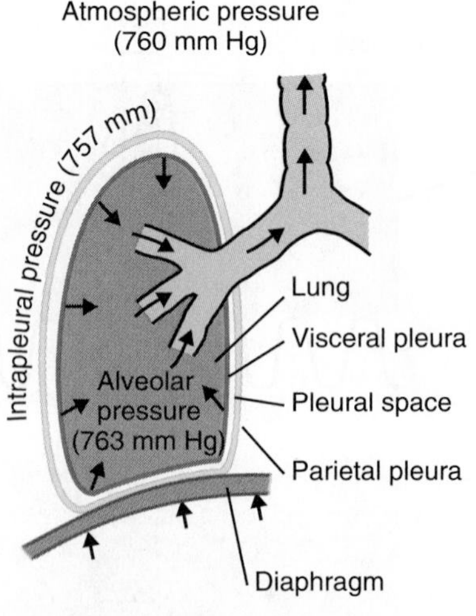

FIGURE U13–7 Normal inspiration and expiration.

the spinal cord at the level of the third cervical vertebra. Thus, spinal injuries at C3 or above can impair ventilation.

PLEURAE

The pleurae are serous membranes that enclose the lung in a double-walled sac. The *visceral* pleura covers the lung and the fissures between the lobes of the lung. The *parietal* pleura covers the inside of each hemithorax, the mediastinum, and the top of the diaphragm; it joins the visceral pleura at the *hilus* (a notch in the medial surface of the lung, where the mainstem bronchi, pulmonary blood vessels, and nerves enter the lung).

Normally, no space exists between the pleurae; the *pleural space* is a potential space between the two layers of pleura. A thin film (only a few milliliters) of serous fluid acts as a lubricant in the potential space. The fluid also causes the moist pleural membranes to adhere, creating a pulling force that helps to hold the lungs in an expanded position. The action of the pleurae is analogous to coupling two sheets of glass with a thin film of water. It is extremely difficult to separate the sheets of glass at right angles, yet they readily slide along each other. Because of the nature of this coupling, the movement of the lungs closely follows the movement of the thorax. If air or increased amounts of serous fluid, blood, or pus accumulates in the thoracic space, the lungs are compressed and respiratory difficulties follow. These conditions constitute *pneumothorax* (air in the pleural space) or *hemothorax* (blood in the pleural space).

FUNCTION OF THE RESPIRATORY SYSTEM

The respiratory system enhances gas exchange. Inspiration brings oxygen-rich air into the alveoli. The upper and lower airways filter and humidify inspired air. Gas exchange between the air and the blood occurs in the alveolus. Oxygen diffuses into the blood, and CO_2 diffuses from the blood into the alveolar air. The CO_2-enriched air is removed from the body during expiration. The large number and large surface area of alveoli are necessary to meet both resting and exercise gas exchange requirements.

The thorax and diaphragm alter pressures in the thorax to drive air movement. The movement of air depends on pressure gradients between the atmosphere and the air in the lungs, with air flowing from regions of higher pressure to regions of lower pressure. On inspiration, the dome of the diaphragm flattens and the rib cage lifts. As thoracic and lung volumes increase, alveolar pressure decreases and air moves into the lungs.

Airway resistance also affects air movement and is affected primarily by the diameter of the airways. Decreasing the diameter by half results in a 16-fold increase in airway resistance. Thus, a decreased diameter of the airways due to bronchial muscle contraction or to secretions in the airways increases resistance and decreases the rate of air flow. This is a common finding in obstructive airway diseases such as asthma.

During quiet breathing, expiration is usually passive, that is, does not require the use of muscles. The chest wall, in contrast to the lungs, tends to recoil outward. The opposing forces of lung and chest wall create a subatmospheric (negative) force of about −5 cm of water in the intrapleural space at the end of quiet exhalation. Exhalation is also a result of elastic recoil of the lungs.

VENTILATION

Ventilation, the movement of air in and out of the lungs, involves three forces: (1) compliance properties of the lung and the thorax (chest wall), (2) surface tension, and (3) the muscular efforts of inspiratory muscles.

Compliance

Compliance refers to the ease with which the lung expands and indicates the relationship between the volume and the pressure of the lungs. The lungs are elastic structures that tend to recoil to a volume slightly less than *residual volume* (the volume of gas remaining in the lungs after a full exhalation). The force required to distend the lungs is the difference between the alveolar pressure and the intrapleural pressure. Diseases that cause fibrosis of the lungs result in "stiff" lungs with low compliance; stiff lungs require high inspiratory pressures to achieve a set volume of gas. In contrast, diseases such as emphysema that damage the elastic structure of the alveolar walls result in "floppy" lungs with greater compliance. Relatively low pressures can achieve the same volume of air during inspiration, but passive exhalation is impaired.

Surface Tension

Changes in the surface tension of the liquid film lining the alveoli also affect compliance by changing resistance. *Surface tension,* the result of the air-liquid interface at each alveolus, restricts alveolar expansion on inspiration and aids alveolar collapse on expiration. Surfactant produced by type II cells in the alveolar lining lowers surface tension and thus increases compliance and aids ventilation. A deficiency of surfactant results in stiff lungs. Premature babies lacking surfactant may suffer infant respiratory distress syndrome (IRDS), or hyaline membrane disease.

Muscular Effort

Ventilation also requires muscular effort. For inspiration to occur, the pressure within the lungs (alveolar pressure) must be less than atmospheric pressure. Contraction of the diaphragm and the external intercostal muscles enlarges the size of the thorax. The external intercostal muscles pull the ribs upward and forward, thus increasing the transverse and anteroposterior diameter. Two accessory muscles of inspiration—the scalene and sternocleidomastoid muscles—elevate the first and second ribs during inspiration to enlarge the upper thorax and stabilize the chest wall. The sternocleidomastoid muscle elevates the sternum. The expanding thorax creates a more negative intrapleural pressure, which expands the lungs. When the alveolar pressure becomes lower than the atmospheric pressure, air flows into the lungs.

During exhalation, the inspiratory muscles relax. The elastic recoil of the lung tissue, increases alveolar pressure above atmospheric pressure and causes air to move out of the lungs. Air flow stops when the recoil pressure of the lungs balances the muscular and elastic forces of the chest (see Fig. U13–7).

Although expiration is usually passive, forced expiration and coughing employ accessory muscles to decrease the size of the thoracic space and cause expiration. Contraction of the abdominal muscles forces the diaphragm upward to its dome-shaped position. Contraction of the internal intercostal muscles pulls the ribs inward, thus decreasing the anteroposterior diameter of the chest wall.

Work of Breathing

Respiratory muscle contraction represents a significant metabolic load. Tidal volume and respiratory rate are adjusted to minimize the workload on the body. For example, clients with obstructive lung disease use slower but deeper breaths to maintain appropriate alveolar ventilation. Clients with restrictive lung disease use frequent, shallow breaths to maintain alveolar ventilation.

RESPIRATORY CONTROL

Human metabolism is not one of steady state. The oxygen needs of the tissues change with changing metabolic demands. Respiratory control mechanisms match the elimination of CO_2 and supply of oxygen to the metabolic needs. The lungs have no intrinsic control of themselves; instead, they are controlled by the central nervous system (CNS).

CENTRAL NERVOUS SYSTEM CONTROL. The medulla has several levels of respiratory centers. The dorsal respiratory group primarily provides for inspiration. The ventral respiratory group is normally quiet unless increased ventilation is needed or if active exhalation is performed. The pons has an apneustic center, which contains both expiratory and inspiratory neurons. The upper pons contains the pneumotaxic center, which fine-tunes breathing. For example, the pneumotaxic center allows for talking and breathing.

Output from the respiratory neurons, located in the medulla, descends via the ventral and lateral columns of the spinal cord to phrenic motor neurons of the diaphragm and intercostal motor neurons of the intercostal muscles. The result is rhythmic respiratory movements.

The cortex also allows voluntary control of breathing (holding our breath or altering the rate or depth of breathing).

REFLEX CONTROL. The cough reflex is a neural reflex stimulated by mechanical stimuli (Table U13–1). Inhaled irritants and mucus (mechanical stimuli) excite rapidly adapting pulmonary stretch receptors concentrated in the region of the carina and the large bronchi. The stimulation of the receptors results in high-velocity expiratory gas flow (cough).

PERIPHERAL CONTROL. Peripheral control of respiration is due to the sensing of partial pressure of oxygen (PO_2) and of partial pressure of CO_2 (PCO_2) in the blood. In the blood, CO_2 is an acid. An increase in PCO_2 causes acidosis, or a fall in pH. Receptors that are responsive to changes in oxygen, CO_2, and pH are located in the brain and in structures adjacent to blood vessels. Arterial blood oxygen and CO_2 pressures are sensed by receptors in the carotid body and the aortic body. The carotid body receptors are located close to the carotid sinus, and the aortic bodies are located near the aortic arch. Chemoreceptors are also located on the brain side of the blood-brain barrier. These receptors respond only to PCO_2 (or pH). An elevated PCO_2 in arterial blood is the normal stimulus to increase ventilation. Low levels of partial pressure of oxygen in arterial blood ($PaCO_2$) can stimulate ventilation, but only when PO_2 drops below 70 mm Hg. There is a powerful synergism between these respiratory stimuli, with the greatest ventilatory drive caused by a simultaneous increase in PCO_2 and decrease in PO_2.

GAS EXCHANGE AND TRANSPORT

The exchange of gases occurs between air and blood in the respiratory membrane. Respiration is the exchange of oxygen and CO_2 at the alveolar-capillary level *(external respiration)* and at the tissue-cellular level *(internal respiration)*. During respiration, body tissues are supplied with oxygen for metabolism and CO_2 is released.

In the earth's atmosphere, air contains 20.84% oxygen, 78.62% nitrogen, 0.04% CO_2, and 0.50% water vapor. Each gas exerts a pressure *(partial pressure)* as if it were the only gas present. The sum of the partial pressures is the *barometric pressure.* When a liquid is exposed to a gas, gas enters the liquid in proportion to the individual pressures. PO_2 in the alveoli is about 104 mm Hg, and PCO_2 is about 40 mm Hg. Venous blood has a PO_2 of 40 mm Hg and a PCO_2 of about 45 mm Hg. These differences in concentration result in the movement of oxygen into the pulmonary capillary bloodstream and of CO_2 out of the pulmonary capillary bed into the alveoli (Fig. U13–8).

TABLE U13–1 PHYSIOLOGIC ELEMENTS OF A COUGH

Deep inspiration	Inhaled volume of air must be sufficient to increase lung volume, to increase diameter of bronchi and bronchioles, and to move mucus up and out of airways
Inspiratory pause	Pause (inspiratory pause) allows a buildup and distribution of air and pressure distal to mucus
Closed glottis	Intact muscles and nerves supplying larynx required; allows development of high intrapleural pressures, resulting in a high air flow velocity to propel mucus out of airway
Abdominal muscles	Increase intra-abdominal pressure, which forces diaphragm upward to increase intrapleural pressure against closed glottis
Open glottis	After intrapleural pressures increase, glottis opens suddenly to allow a high velocity of air to leave lungs; flow rates may be as high as 300 L/min
Mucus is expelled	Expulsion due to high velocity of air leaving airway

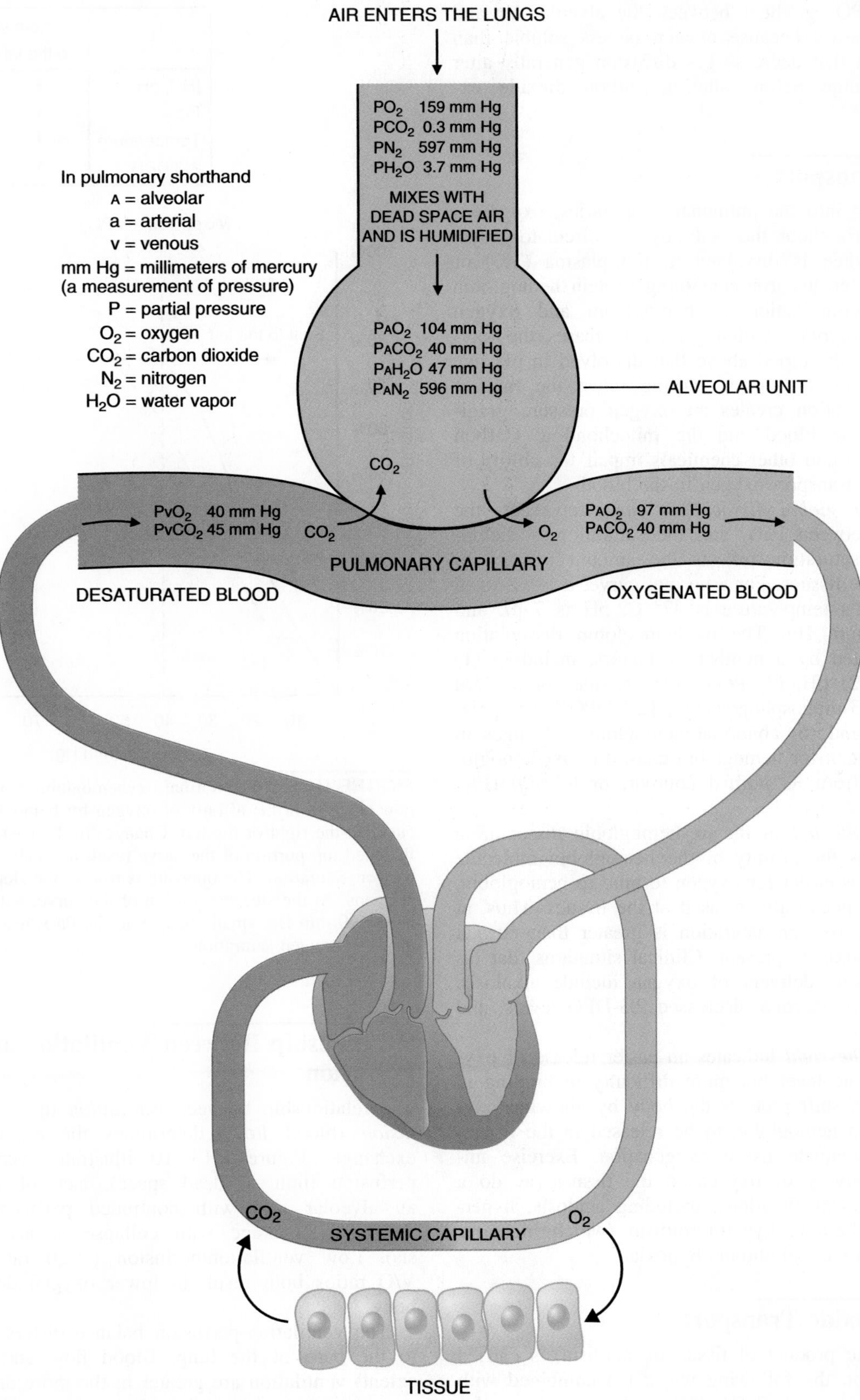

FIGURE U13–8 Partial pressures of gases during normal respiration.

The high PO_2 gradient between the alveolar air and blood is necessary because oxygen is less soluble than CO_2. Diseases that decrease gas diffusion generally alter oxygen exchange before altering carbon dioxide exchange.

Oxygen Transport

After diffusing into the pulmonary capillaries, oxygen is transported throughout the body by the circulatory system. The oxygen is dissolved in the plasma (3%) or bound in the ferrous iron-containing protein hemoglobin (97%). The combination of hemoglobin and oxygen forms *oxyhemoglobin,* which greatly increases the oxygen content of the blood above that dissolved in plasma. Tissues take up oxygen at varying rates; the rate of oxygen consumption creates an oxygen pressure gradient between the blood and the mitochondria. Carbon monoxide (CO) and other chemicals impair the ability of hemoglobin to transport oxygen in the blood.

The *oxyhemoglobin dissociation curve* represents the relationship between PaO_2 and the saturation of hemoglobin. This saturation reflects the amount of oxygen available to the tissues. For a normal curve, it is assumed that the client's temperature is 37° C, pH is 7.40, and PCO_2 is 40 mm Hg. The oxyhemoglobin dissociation curve is affected by a number of factors, including (1) temperature, (2) pH, (3) PCO_2, (4) enzymes in the red blood cell (2,3-diphosphoglycerate [2,3-DPG]), (5) presence of CO, and (6) abnormal hemoglobin. Changes in affinity of oxygen for hemoglobin cause the oxyhemoglobin to move from its normal contour, or to *shift* (Fig. U13–9).

A *shift to the left* of the oxyhemoglobin dissociation curve increases the affinity of the hemoglobin molecule for oxygen. It is easier for oxygen to bind to hemoglobin, but oxygen is not easily released at the tissues. Thus, at any PO_2 level, oxygen saturation is greater than normal but tissue hypoxia is present. Clinical situations that diminish the tissue delivery of oxygen include alkalosis, hypocapnia, hypothermia, decreased 2,3-DPG levels, and CO poisoning.

A *shift to the right* indicates an easier release of oxygen at the tissue level but more difficulty in binding in the lungs. This shift protects the body by allowing oxygen attached to hemoglobin to be released in the tissues to maintain adequate tissue oxygenation. Exercise improves the delivery of oxygen to the tissues, as do a number of clinical situations, including acidosis, hypercapnia, hyperthermia, hyperthyroidism (which increases 2,3-DPG), anemia, and chronic hypoxia.

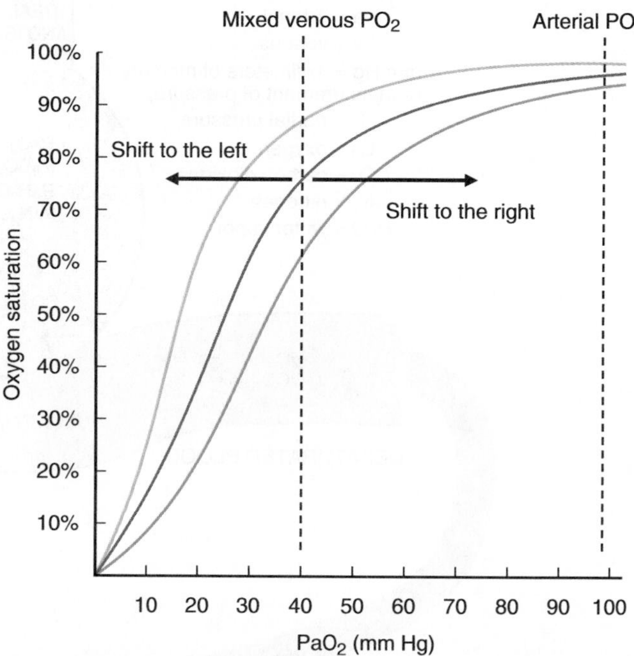

	Factors shifting curve...	
	To the left	To the right
$[H^+]$, pH	↑	↓
PCO_2	↓	↑
Temperature	↓	↑
2,3 DPG	↓	↑

FIGURE U13–9 The normal oxyhemoglobin wave, showing how changes in the affinity of oxygen for hemoglobin shift the curve to the right or the left. Changes in the PaO_2 at the flattened top portion of the curve result in small changes in oxygen saturation. The opposite is true as the slope of the curve steepens. At the steepest portion of the curve, with the PaO_2 below 60 mm Hg, small changes in the PaO_2 result in large drops in oxygen saturation.

Carbon Dioxide Transport

CO_2, the waste product of tissue metabolism, is carried by the blood in the following ways: (1) combined with water as carbonic acid (70%), (2) coupled with hemoglobin (23%), or (3) dissolved in plasma (7%). Red blood cells contain the enzyme carbonic anhydrase, which rapidly breaks down CO_2 into hydrogen ions and bicarbonate ions. When venous blood enters the lungs for gas exchange, this reaction reverses, forming CO_2, which is then exhaled.

Relationship Between Ventilation and Perfusion

The relationship between *ventilation* (air flow) and *perfusion* (blood flow) determines the efficiency of gas exchange. Figure U13–10 illustrates ventilation with perfusion (unit of dead space), lack of ventilation of an alveolar unit with continued perfusion (a shunt), and total blockage with collapse of alveoli (atelectasis). Low ventilation/perfusion (V/Q) ratios and high V/Q ratios both result in lower oxygen delivery to the body.

The ventilation-perfusion balance differs from the top to the base of the lung. Blood flow and (to a lesser extent) ventilation are greater in the more dependent lung segments at the base of the lung. Consequently, the base of the lung has the lowest V/Q ratio, and the apex of the lung has the highest V/Q ratio.

The V/Q balance is controlled at both the airway and vascular levels. Hypoxia, resulting from underventilation of an alveolar region, causes vasoconstriction, which redirects blood to well-ventilated alveoli. CO_2 in the

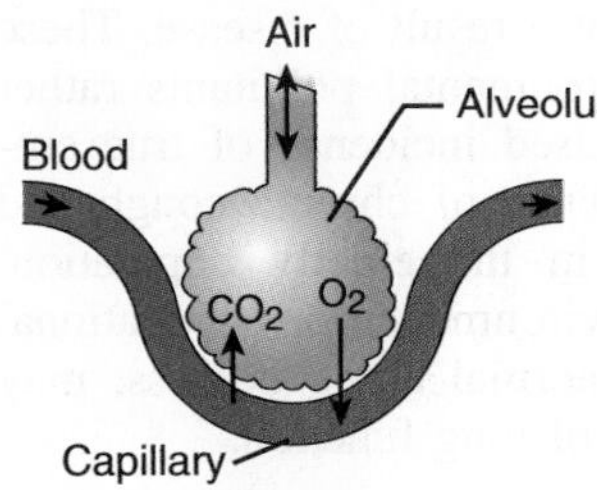

NORMAL
A normally functioning alveolus and normal pulmonary capillary flow. Ventilation and perfusion match.

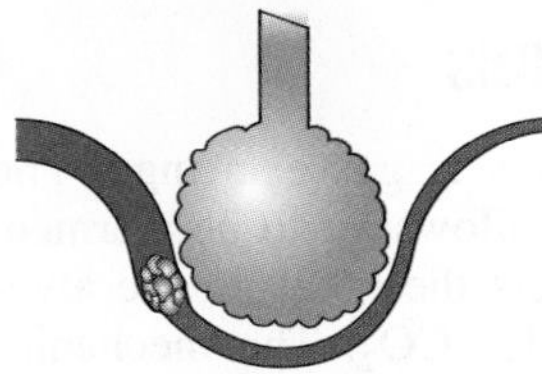

DEAD SPACE UNIT
When there is ventilation without perfusion, a dead space unit exists. Example: Pulmonary embolus preventing blood flow through the pulmonary capillary

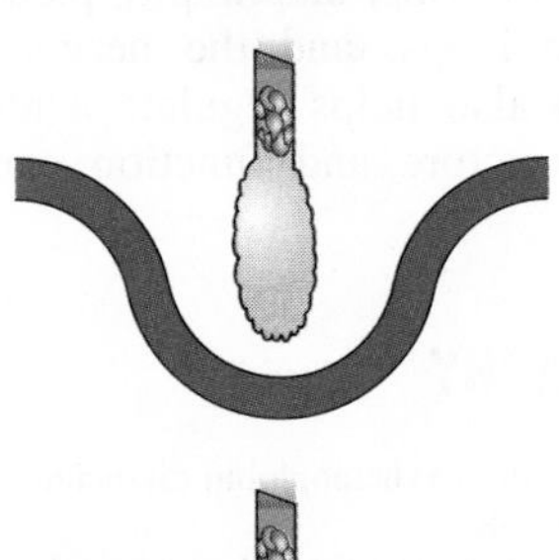

SHUNT UNIT
When there is no ventilation to an alveolar unit but perfusion continues, a shunt unit exists, and unoxygenated blood continues to circulate. Examples: atelectasis, pneumonia. The alveoli collapse.

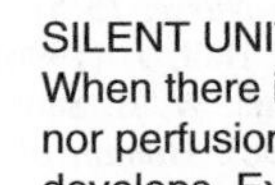

SILENT UNIT
When there is neither ventilation nor perfusion, a silent unit develops. Example: Pulmonary embolus combined with ARDS (adult respiratory distress syndrome). The alveoli collapse.

FIGURE U13–10 Relationships between ventilation (air flow) and perfusion (blood flow).

airways dilates the airway smooth muscle. Poorly perfused alveoli have low CO_2 levels, and the resultant airway constriction directs ventilation to better-perfused alveoli.

Regulation of Acid-Base Balance

The lungs, through gas exchange, have a key role in regulating the acid-base balance of the body. Pulmonary disorders that change the CO_2 level in the blood cause either respiratory acidemia or respiratory alkalemia. Insufficient ventilation causes *hypercapnia,* a respiratory acidemia caused by retention of excessive amounts of CO_2. Hyperventilation, conversely, causes *hypocapnia,* a respiratory alkalemia due to the low amounts of CO_2 in the blood.

The effectiveness of ventilation is best measured by the P_{CO_2} in the arterial blood (Pa_{CO_2}). Because the respiratory system is normally set to maintain a Pa_{CO_2} between 35 and 45 mm Hg at sea level, a Pa_{CO_2} above this range represents *hypoventilation.* Anesthetic agents, sedatives, and narcotics all tend to increase the resting Pa_{CO_2}. (Acid-base balance is detailed in Chapter 14.)

Reaction to Injury

The elaborate defense mechanisms of the lungs involve clearance mechanisms, defense by the respiratory epithelium, and immunologic responses in the lungs. Any injury to the lung affects the barrier between the atmosphere and the bloodstream. This barrier, which lies within the alveolar septum, is made up of epithelial (types I and II pneumocytes) and vascular endothelial cells. Injury resulting from airborne or blood-borne agents may increase vascular permeability and cause pulmonary edema. Inflammatory cells (e.g., neutrophils) arrive soon after acute injury. Then the proportion of lymphocytes, monocytes, and macrophages increases.

The basic lung repair processes include lymphatic drainage of excess fluid and phagocytic removal of protein and debris. This action generally restores lung function and structure. More severe injury requires endothelial and epithelial cell regeneration and proliferation of interstitial cells (fibroblasts). Type II cells that are generated for defense eventually differentiate into thin type I cells, which permit gas exchange. The lung's ability to recreate alveolar septa determines the degree to which normal lung function and structure are restored.

Defense by Clearance Mechanisms

The *upper airways* filter particles. Because the nose has a larger surface-volume ratio and a much more tortuous pathway for airflow than the mouth, particle deposition and conditioning of the air are more efficient when we breathe through the nose. Larger particles ($>$10 mm) are generally trapped; smaller particles ($<$1 mm) may readily enter the lower airways.

There are four clearance mechanisms of the lower airways and alveoli:

- Cough (first five to eight bronchial generations)
- Mucociliary system (to terminal bronchioles)
- Macrophages (alveoli and respiratory bronchioles)
- Lymphatics (alveoli and interstitium)

The cough, an automatic protective reflex used to clear the trachea, occurs most rapidly in the clearing process (see Table U13–1). If the swallowing reflex is delayed or absent, a cough may be stimulated to avoid aspiration of particles into the lower airways.

Defense by the Respiratory Epithelium

Unlike the upper and lower airways, the alveoli lack a mucous layer to trap foreign particles and cilia to propel them to the pharynx for elimination. The alveolar lining is made up of flat, membranous pneumocytes (type I cells) and rounded granular (type II) cells. The type II cells are resistant to injury and cover most of the alveolar surface after exposure to infectious agents. Alveolar macrophages, derived from blood monocytes that migrate into the lungs, are also found over the surface of the alveoli. Alveolar macrophages are active phagocytes that remove dead cells and protein and that synthesize and secrete substances that regulate the immune system. They leave the lung by the mucociliary system or the lymphatic system.

Defense by Immunologic Mechanisms

The systemic immune system responds to the lung during inflammatory processes by mobilizing blood neutrophils and monocytes. Recruited thymus-dependent (T) and thymus-independent (B) lymphocytes contribute to local cell-mediated immune reactions and the production of specific antibodies within the alveoli. Cell-mediated immunity is a key determinant in resistance to organisms such as *Mycobacterium tuberculosis* and *Pneumocystis carinii.* Immune mechanisms are generally a host defense function. However, hypersensitivity immune reactions lead to tissue injury and are responsible for clinical conditions such as asthma, granuloma formation, and lung transplant rejection. (Chapter 76 describes types I, II, III, and IV hypersensitivity reactions.)

EFFECTS OF AGING

Most of the changes that occur with aging affect the lower airway. Movement of cilia in the upper airway slows and becomes less effective. This change predisposes older clients to a greater number of respiratory infections.

Lung structure also changes with age. The lungs become rounder as a result of increased anteroposterior diameter, circumference, area, and height of the lung. The proportion of the lung formed by alveolar duct air increases, and alveolar air decreases. Loss of alveolar wall tissue and its elastic tissue fibers is seen. The result is a deterioration of lung function.

The air spaces enlarge, although this is not referred to as emphysema because it is not a result of disease. These changes may be due to environmental pollutants rather than to aging alone. An increased incidence of true emphysema and a greater prevalence of chronic cough and sputum production are seen in the elderly population. These findings suggest that environmental or occupational pollutants, in addition to the normal aging process, may be a component in the decline of lung function.

CONCLUSIONS

The primary function of the lungs is gas exchange. The physical structure of the airways allows air to be warmed, filtered, and humidified as it enters the body. In the alveolar sacs, oxygen is exchanged for CO_2. The mechanics of breathing are coordinated by the ribs, diaphragm, pleural space, elastic recoil of the lungs, and the nervous system. The respiratory system also helps regulate acid-base balance. Alterations in structure and function can result in various disorders.

BIBLIOGRAPHY

1. Dickson, S. L. (1995). Understanding the oxyhemoglobin dissociation curve. *Critical Care Nurse, 15*(5), 54–58.
2. Guyton, A. C., and Hall, J. (1996). *Textbook of medical physiology* (9th ed.). Philadelphia: W. B. Saunders.
3. Silverthorn, D. (1998). *Human physiology.* Upper Saddle River, NJ: Prentice-Hall.
4. West, J. (1995). *Respiratory physiology: The essentials* (5th ed.). Baltimore: Williams & Wilkins.
5. West, J. (1997). *Pulmonary pathophysiology: The essentials* (5th ed.). Baltimore: Williams & Wilkins.

CHAPTER

59

Assessment of the Respiratory System

Amy Verst

GENERAL RESPIRATORY ASSESSMENT

Nurses caring for clients experiencing respiratory disorders perform and interpret a variety of assessment procedures. This chapter discusses the physical assessment and diagnostic procedures for clients who have respiratory disorders. The assessment data are used to plan client care.

HISTORY

A respiratory history contains information about a client's present condition and previous respiratory problems. Interview the client and family, and focus on the clinical manifestations of the chief complaint, events leading up to the current condition, past health history, family history, and psychosocial history.

The detail and time taken for a respiratory history depend on the client's condition (e.g., acute, chronic, or emergent). State questions simply using short, easy to understand sentences. When necessary, reword questions to clarify statements the client seems not to understand. Ask questions in the context of the client's daily activities, for instance, Are you able to carry the groceries in from the car? Are you able to make your bed, vacuum the house, bathe yourself, or dress yourself without stopping to rest and catch your breath?

■ BIOGRAPHICAL AND DEMOGRAPHIC DATA

Begin the history by obtaining biographical data. Include the client's name, age, sex, and living situation.

Demographic data are usually recorded on an agency assessment form. Note the client's biologic age and compare it with the client's appearance. Does the client look his or her stated age? Disorders such as lung cancer and chronic lung disorders often make the client appear older. The living situation, whether it be alone, with children, or with significant others, is important in planning for discharge.

■ CURRENT HEALTH

Chief Complaint

The chief complaint helps to establish priorities for intervention and to assess the client's level of understanding of the current condition. Common respiratory complaints include dyspnea (difficulty breathing), cough, sputum production, hemoptysis (blood-stained sputum), wheezing, stridor (a high-pitched respiratory sound), and chest pain. Focus on the manifestations, and prioritize questions to elicit a symptom analysis (see Chapter 9).

In emergency or acute situations, simple questions are all that may be asked until the client is stable and comfortable. Whenever possible, ask significant others for further details.

Take as extensive a respiratory history as the client's condition allows. Detailed questioning provides valuable clues to (1) the client's manifestations, (2) the client's degree of existing respiratory dysfunction, (3) the client's and family's understanding of the condition and its management, and (4) the family's support system and ability to cope with the manifestations and management of the condition on an ongoing basis.

Dyspnea

Dyspnea (difficulty breathing) is one of the most common manifestations experienced by clients with pulmonary and cardiac disorders. It is a subjective symptom and a reflection of the client's assessment of the degree of work of breathing for a given task or effort. Clients may define dyspnea as shortness of breath, suffocation, tightness, being winded, or being breathless.

The assessment of dyspnea involves several aspects. The subjective nature of dyspnea makes it difficult to quantify objectively. Several methods are used to assess accurately the level of dyspnea experienced by a client. The Visual Analogue Scale (Fig. 59–1) is used to quantify breathlessness in response to particular questions. It is easy to understand, and the amount of dyspnea during various activities can be assessed. The Modified Borg Category Ratio Scale (Table 59–1) is used to rate the intensity of dyspnea. It is simple, and results have been reproduced in several populations.

The Pulmonary Functional Status and Dyspnea Questionnaire (PFSDQ) is used to quantify dyspnea and changes in activity with dyspnea. This instrument was developed and initially tested in a hospital-based pulmonary rehabilitation program.[9]

In addition to subjective assessment, conduct a symptom analysis to document the characteristics of the dysp-

FIGURE 59–1 The Visual Analogue Scale of dyspnea. Although the scale can be in the form of either a vertical or a horizontal line, the most commonly used scale consists of a 100-mm horizontal line, like the one shown here.

How short of breath are you right now?

None ———————————————————— Extremely Severe

nea. Assess all of the characteristics because there are many respiratory and nonrespiratory causes.

COUGH

Detail the many aspects of the client's *cough* by conducting a symptom analysis. Note when and how the cough began (suddenly or gradually) and how long it has been present. Determine the frequency of the cough and the time of day when the cough is better or worse (early morning, late afternoon, nighttime). Use the client's own words to describe the cough. A cough may be described as hacking, dry, hoarse, congested, barking, wheezy, or bubbling.

Determine which medications or treatments the client has used for the cough (e.g., antitussives, codeine, inhalers, nebulizers, rest, sitting up). Find out what precautions are used to prevent the spread of infection (if present). Use the opportunity to remind the person about good hand-washing, proper disposal of soiled tissues, and completion of a full course of antibiotics (if prescribed).

Coughing may lead to stress incontinence; you may want to ask female clients about this embarrassing problem. The incontinence should clear when the coughing subsides; protective padding may be helpful.

SPUTUM PRODUCTION

Sputum is the substance expelled by coughing or clearing the throat. The tracheobronchial tree normally produces about 3 ounces of mucus a day as part of the normal cleaning mechanism; however, sputum production with coughing is not normal. Question the client about sputum color (clear, yellow, green, rusty, bloody), odor, quality (watery, stringy, frothy, thick), and quantity (teaspoon, tablespoon, cup). Document changes in color, odor, quality, or quantity in the client's medical record. Ascertain whether sputum is produced only after the client is lying in a certain position. The amount of sputum produced is increased in several disorders; for instance, clients with bronchitis may expectorate several cups of sputum daily.

Sputum may be a secretion from the oral or nasopharyngeal area or sinuses rather than from the tracheobronchial tree. For example, draining sinuses may provoke a productive cough.

TABLE 59–1 THE MODIFIED BORG CATEGORY-RATIO SCALE FOR ASSESSMENT OF DYSPNEA

Score	Intensity
0	Nothing at all
0.5	Very, very slight
1	Very slight
2	Slight
3	Moderate
4	Somewhat severe
5	Severe
6	
7	Very severe
8	
9	Very, very severe
10	Maximal

Modified from Burden, J., et al. (1982). The perception of breathlessness. *American Review of Respiratory Diseases, 126,* 825–828.

HEMOPTYSIS

Hemoptysis refers to blood expectorated from the mouth in the form of gross (visible to the naked eye) blood, frankly bloody sputum, or blood-tinged sputum. Attempt to identify the source of the blood—lungs, nosebleed, or stomach. Blood from the lungs is usually bright red because blood in the lungs stimulates an immediate cough reflex. If the blood remains in the lungs for any period of time, it may turn dark red or brown. Ask the client whether the hemoptysis occurred as a result of forceful coughing. Also, obtain an estimate of the amount of blood expectorated (teaspoon, tablespoon, cup).

Pulmonary causes of hemoptysis include chronic bronchitis, bronchiectasis, pulmonary tuberculosis, cystic fibrosis, upper airway necrotizing granulomas, pulmonary embolism, pneumonia, lung cancer, and lung abscesses. Cardiovascular abnormalities, anticoagulants, and immunosuppressive drugs that cause parenchymal (lung tissue) bleeding may also cause hemoptysis.

WHEEZING

Wheezing sounds are produced when air passes through partially obstructed or narrowed airways on inspiration or expiration. *Wheezing* may be audible or may be heard only with a stethoscope. The client may not complain of wheezing but may complain of chest tightness or chest discomfort instead. Ask the client to identify when the wheezing occurs and whether it resolves spontaneously or whether medication (such as inhaled bronchodilators) is required for relief. Not all wheezing is caused by asthma. Wheezing can be caused by mucosal edema, airway secretions, collapsed airways resulting from loss of elastic tissue, and foreign objects or tumors partially obstructing air flow.

STRIDOR

Stridor is the name given to high-pitched sounds produced when air passes through a partially obstructed or narrowed upper airway on inspiration. Stridor is associated with respiratory distress and can be life-threatening because the airway is compromised. Several conditions can lead to stridor: epiglottitis, sleep apnea (cessation of breathing), heart failure, and aspiration. Inquire about changes in voice character, hoarseness, difficulty swallowing, sleep-related disorders such as insomnia, degree of snoring, hypersomnolence (excessive sleepiness) in the morning, early morning headaches, weight gain, fluid retention, apnea, and restlessness.

CHEST PAIN

Chest pain may be associated with pulmonary and cardiac problems, and distinguishing between the two is important. Conduct a complete symptom analysis for any chest pain. *Angina pectoris* (from Latin, pain of the chest) may be associated with decreased blood flow to the heart and is a potentially life-threatening problem.

Determine the location, duration, and intensity of the chest pain to provide early clues to the cause. Coughing and pleuritic infections can cause chest pain. Pleuritic chest pain is commonly a sharp, stabbing pain that occurs at one site on the chest wall and increases with chest wall movement or deep breathing. Retrosternal (behind the sternum) pain is usually burning, constant, and aching. Pain can also originate in the bony and cartilaginous parts of the thorax.

The characteristics of angina pectoris and other chest pains differ from each other. Cardiac chest pain is usually described as an aching, heavy, squeezing sensation with pressure or tightness in the substernal area. Angina pectoris can also radiate into the neck or arms (see Chapter 54, Table 54–2, for comparison of types of chest pain). Ask the client what brings on the pain (activity, coughing, movement) and what relieves the pain (nitroglycerin, splinting the chest wall, heat).

Symptom Analysis

To obtain a complete history of the respiratory system, assess the characteristics of any clinical manifestation. Assessment of these characteristics leads to a comprehensive symptom analysis. When the client describes a specific respiratory manifestation, assess the following factors.

SETTING

In what setting does the symptom occur most often? The *setting* refers to the time and place or particular situation—physical setting and psychological environment—in which the client experiences the complaint. For example, the client may cough in the morning after smoking a cigarette or may complain of respiratory distress at work.

TIMING

Timing encompasses both onset (the gradual or sudden appearance of the symptom) and the period (days, weeks, months) during which the problem has occurred. Ask the client whether there is a specific time of day when the problem occurs most frequently, for example, the morning cough or shortness of breath associated with lying flat at night.

CLIENT'S PERCEPTION

Phrase the *client's perception* in the client's own words. Note any unique properties of the complaint. Use a direct quotation to document the client's complaint. For example, client reports a "catch" in the left posterior chest with deep breaths.

QUANTITY AND QUALITY

Describe the *quantity and quality* of the problem in common language. Ask the client to report the amount, size, number, and extent of the chief complaint. Especially with sputum production, ask the client to estimate how much sputum is produced a day—a cup, a tablespoon, or teaspoon. Avoid using terms such as "a little" or "a lot," which have different meanings among clients and health care providers. Often a scale of 1 to 10, with 1 being the least and 10 the most, is used to describe pain or distress.

In an assessment of a cough, the cough may be described as tight, loose, dry, hacking, or congested. Have clients describe the characteristics of their cough in their own words.

LOCATION

Note the *location* of the manifestation. Ask the client to identify its exact location. Location is especially important when the complaint is chest pain because it is essential to determine whether the pain is cardiac or respiratory in origin.

AGGRAVATING AND RELIEVING FACTORS

The *aggravating* and *relieving factors* precipitate, worsen, or alleviate a symptom. Environmental allergens, such as dog or cat dander, dust mites, mold, and pollen, are often described as aggravating factors. Sitting up or lying down may relieve or exacerbate the symptom. Medication may also worsen or relieve the symptom.

ASSOCIATED MANIFESTATIONS

Associated manifestations occur in conjunction with the chief complaint. Examples include chills, fever, night sweats, anorexia, weight loss, excessive fatigue, anxiety, and hoarseness. You may be able to recognize that chills and fever commonly accompany infectious lung disorders, whereas anorexia and weight loss can occur in clients with disorders that result in dyspnea.

■ PAST HEALTH HISTORY

Examine the past health history of the client and family members for data related to the upper and lower respiratory systems (the upper respiratory history and physical examination are discussed later). These systems are common sources of both acute and chronic health problems. Assess clients with chronic conditions for changes in their ongoing respiratory manifestations (e.g., cough, dyspnea, sputum production, or wheezes) because these changes provide clues to the cause of the new problem. Include questions about the following areas.

Childhood and Infectious Diseases

In addition to obtaining data regarding common childhood diseases and vaccinations, ask the client about the occurrence of tuberculosis, bronchitis, influenza, asthma, and pneumonia and the frequency of lower respiratory infections after upper respiratory infection. Determine the existence of congenital problems, such as cystic fibrosis and premature birth history. These problems are associated with respiratory complications, such as obstructive and restrictive pulmonary disease.

Immunizations

Inquire about vaccination against pneumonia (polyvalent pneumococcal vaccine [Pneumovax]) and influenza. Ask the client to list the dates of these vaccinations. Pneumovax provides lifelong immunity against pneumococcal pneumonia, whereas "flu shots" must be received annually in the fall of the year.

Major Illnesses and Hospitalizations

Ask the client about previous hospitalizations or treatment for respiratory problems. Determine dates of illnesses or hospitalization, the specific respiratory problem, medical treatment (including surgery, use of a ventilator, and inhalation treatments or oxygen therapy), and the present status of the problem.

Has a chest x-ray film been taken? When? Have other pulmonary diagnostic tests been performed? These test results can provide baseline data for the evaluation of the current problem. Inquire about previous injuries to the mouth, nose, throat, or chest (such as blunt trauma, fractured ribs, or pneumothorax).

Medications

Obtain detailed information regarding both prescribed and over-the-counter medications, including herbal remedies, because many products affect the respiratory system. The client may have taken antibiotics for respiratory infections, bronchodilators, or steroids. Specify the route of administration (pill, liquid, or inhalation). Many respiratory medications are inhaled through a metered-dose inhaler (MDI) or mini-nebulizer. If an MDI is used, the client may use a spacer to disperse the medication properly. Ask the client to demonstrate the use of the MDI and spacer.

Herbal medicines for respiratory problems include remedies for nasal discharge and congestion, cough, sore throat, fever and headache, and immunostimulant effects. *Ephedra* (*E. sinica, E. vulgaris*) is a stimulant and is illegal in some areas. Expectorants include anise (*Pimpinella anisum*), coltsfoot (*Tussilago farfara*), and horehound (*Marrubium vulgare*). Coltsfoot and horehound are also believed to have antitussive action.

Sore throat remedies include mint (*Mentha piperita* [peppermint], *Mentha spicata*, [spearmint]) and slippery elm (*Ulmus rubra*). Remedies for the fever and headache that may accompany colds and influenza include boneset (*Eupatorium perfoliatum*), feverfew (*Tanacetum parthenium*), and white willow (*Salix purpurea, Salix fragilis, Salix daphnoides*).

Stimulants of the immune system, believed to help ward off colds and flu, include *Echinacea* (*E. angustifolia, E. pallida, E. purpurea*) and goldenseal (*Hydrastis canadensis*).

Allergies

Question the client about a history of allergies and timing of manifestations to help identify a possible allergic basis for the condition. Ask about precipitating and aggravating factors, such as foods, medications, pollens, smoke, fumes, dust, and animal dander. Sources of molds that may cause allergic manifestations include the water reservoir of a furnace humidifier, air conditioners, and plant soil.

Ask the client to describe the allergic manifestations experienced (e.g., chest tightness, wheezing, cough, rhinitis, watery eyes, scratchy throat) and their severity. Determine the age at which allergies first occurred and whether they have become progressively more severe.

Has the client been tested for allergies? When? Are medications (including allergy shots) taken prophylactically or on an as-needed basis to provide symptomatic relief?

FAMILY HEALTH HISTORY

Question the client about the family history of respiratory diseases. Identify blood relatives (in regard to *genetically transmitted* diseases) and family members (in regard to *infectious* conditions) who have had asthma, cystic fibrosis, emphysema or chronic obstructive pulmonary disease (COPD), lung cancer, respiratory infections, tuberculosis, or allergies. List the age and cause of death of each deceased family member.

Do any household members smoke cigarettes, pipes or cigars? Secondary inhalation of smoke often precipitates or worsens respiratory manifestations.

PSYCHOSOCIAL HISTORY

Respiratory status is affected by numerous factors that may lead to acute problems or that may affect the client's coping with chronic problems such as COPD. Areas to be assessed are described next.

Occupation

Identify any environmental agents that may contribute to the client's condition. Ask specifically about the work environment and hobbies. Focus on exposure to dust, asbestos, beryllium, silica, and other toxins or pollutants. Farmers are exposed to airborne particles that may be inhaled, such as grain dust, fertilizers, and animal dander. Hobbies may involve chemicals, heat, dust, and airborne particles from grinding, soldering, or welding.

Geographical Location

Ask about recent travel to areas where respiratory diseases are prevalent, such as Asia (tuberculosis), the Ohio River valley (histoplasmosis), or the San Joaquin valley (valley fever). Polluted city air has also been related to increasing incidence and severity of asthma.

Environment

Ask about the client's living conditions. How many people are in the household? Crowded living conditions increase risk of exposure to infectious respiratory diseases such as tuberculosis and cold viruses. Recent exposure to continuous air conditioning in a hotel or motel setting may be related to legionnaires' disease.

Assess for environmental hazards such as stairs or poor air circulation. A client with a chronic respiratory condition may have difficulty climbing stairs or breathing unfiltered air.

Habits

Inquire about any history of smoking tobacco products. Calculate the pack-years, which helps quantify the smoking history, as follows:

$$\text{years of smoking} \times \text{packs smoked per day} = \text{pack-years}$$

Smoking has been associated with decreased ciliary function of the lungs, increased mucus production, and the development of lung cancer. Ask the client about the use of smokeless tobacco (such as snuff, chewing tobacco) and smoking nontobacco substances (such as marijuana and clove cigarettes).

Ask about alcohol use. Ciliary action is slowed by alcohol, which reduces mucus clearance from the lungs. Heavy alcohol ingestion depresses the cough reflex and increases risk of aspiration. Clients who use and abuse recreational drugs are at risk for drug overdose and respiratory failure. Sharing needles increases the risk of human immunodeficiency virus (HIV) infection and the development of acquired immunodeficiency syndrome (AIDS) and opportunistic infections such as *Pneumocystis carinii.*

Exercise

Clients who are active may describe the onset of coughing and wheezing during exercise. These clients need to be further evaluated for exercise-induced asthma before continuing workouts. Clients with chronic respiratory conditions often do not have the lung capacity to sustain even mild forms of exercise and subsequently become dyspneic. Has tolerance for activity decreased or remained stable? Ask the client to describe typical activities, such as walking, light housekeeping chores, or grocery shopping, that are tolerated or, conversely, that result in shortness of breath.

Nutrition

Maintaining a nutritious diet is important for clients with chronic respiratory disease, which can result in decreased lung capacity and greater workload for the lungs and cardiovascular system. The added workload increases caloric expenditure, and weight loss may occur. Clients may become anorectic because of the effects of medications and fatigue. The client may not have enough energy to consume the needed calories to maintain body weight. Ask the client to recall intake for the last 24 hours. Assess the amount of protein, kilocalories, and sodium intake (see Chapter 28).

■ REVIEW OF SYSTEMS

Ask the client to describe other manifestations associated with the respiratory system. In addition to cough, dyspnea, sputum production, hemoptysis, wheezing, stridor, and chest pain, include breathlessness, fever, hoarseness, night sweats, anorexia, weight loss, and dependent edema. Upper respiratory manifestations include colds, nasal discharge, postnasal drip, sinus pain and swelling, epistaxis (nosebleed), and sinus headaches.

Hypoxia may precipitate subtle neurologic alterations, such as restlessness, fatigue, disorientation, and personality changes. Tachycardia usually accompanies respiratory problems as the body attempts to compensate for decreased oxygen delivery. Stomach upset, nausea, and vomiting can result from accumulation of excess mucus swallowed from draining sinuses. Anorexia and weight loss are seen in many chronic respiratory conditions. Detailed questions for the review of systems may be found in Chapter 9, Box 9–2.

PHYSICAL EXAMINATION

Physical examination follows the health history. Use the techniques of inspection, palpation, percussion, and auscultation. Successful examination requires that you be familiar with the anatomic landmarks of the posterior, lateral, and anterior thorax (Fig. 59–2). Use these landmarks to locate and visualize the underlying structures, particularly the lobes of the lungs, the heart, and major vessels. Compare the findings on one side of the thorax with those on the other side. Palpation, percussion, and auscultation proceed in a back-and-forth or side-to-side manner so that you continually evaluate findings by using the opposite side as the standard for comparison.

Note the condition and color (pale, red, blue) of the client's skin throughout the examination of the thorax, and record abnormalities. Assess respiratory rate, depth, and rhythm, if not assessed previously with the vital signs, during inspection of the thorax (see Chapter 10). Assess the client's level of consciousness and orientation throughout the examination to determine adequate gas exchange. See the Physical Assessment Findings in the Healthy Adult feature for expected respiratory findings.

■ INSPECTION

The physical examination begins during the history-taking stage as you observe the client and the client's response to questions. Note manifestations of respiratory distress at this time: position of comfort, tachypnea (rapid, shallow breathing), gasping, grunting, central cyanosis, open mouth, flared nostrils, dyspnea, color of facial skin and lips, and use of accessory muscles. Note the *inspiratory-to-expiratory (I:E) ratio.* Because the normal length of expiration is twice that of inspiration, the normal ratio is 2:1.

Observe the client's speech pattern. How many words or sentences can be said before another breath is taken? Clients who are short of breath may be able to say only three or four words before taking another breath. During the physical examination, the client should be bare to the waist while privacy and warmth are maintained. Inspection and palpation, often performed together, are discussed separately.

Head and Neck

Begin inspection with observation of the head and neck for any gross abnormalities that would interfere with respiration. Note the odor of the breath and whether sputum is present. Note nasal flaring, breathing with pursed lips, or cyanosis of the mucous membranes. Record the use of accessory muscles, such as flexion of the sternocleidomastoid muscle.

Chest

CHEST WALL CONFIGURATION

Continue inspection by observing the chest wall configuration. Observe chest size and contour, and note the *anteroposterior* (AP) diameter. Calculate the ratio of the AP diameter to the transverse diameter. The transverse diameter is generally twice the AP diameter (Fig. 59–3*A*).

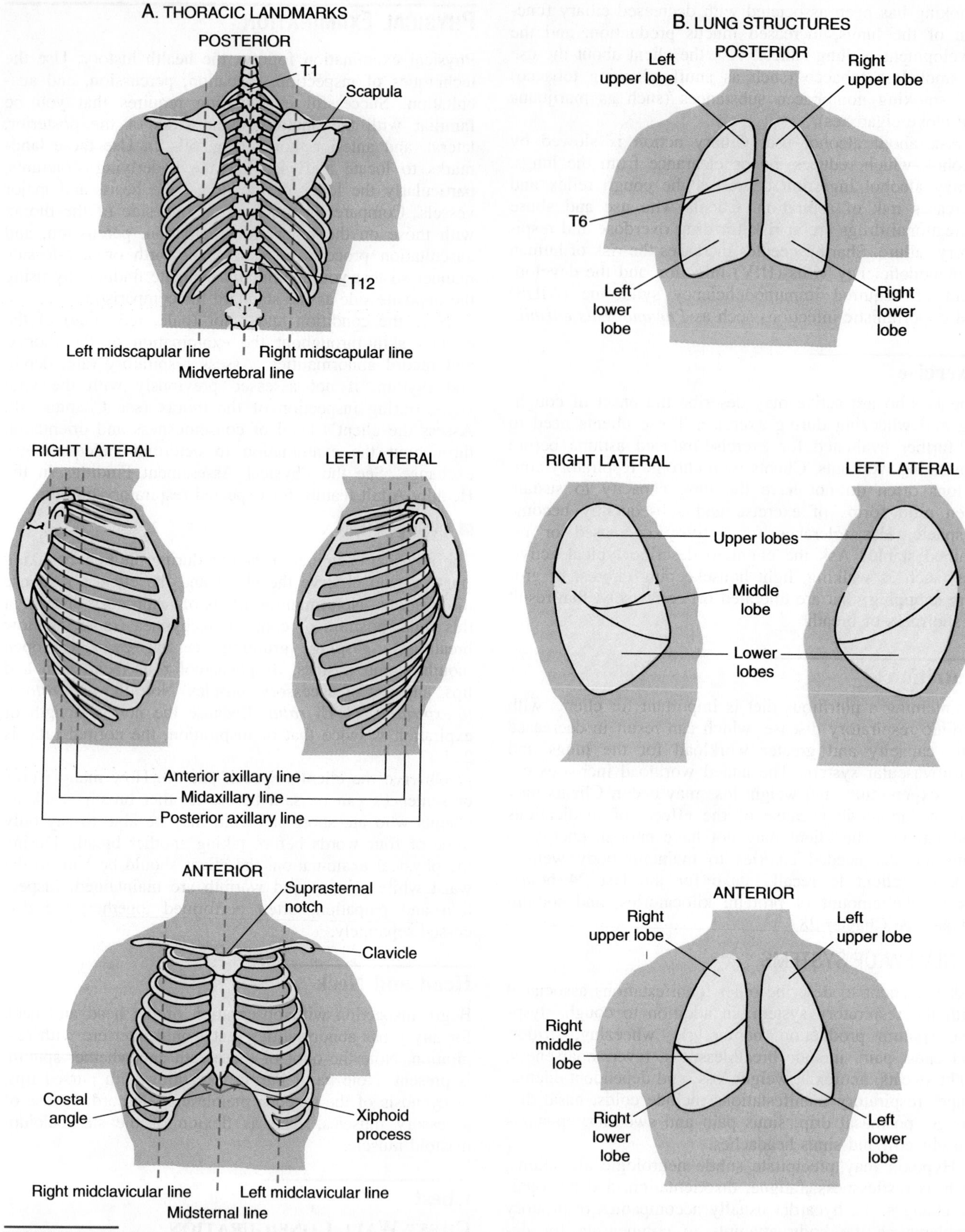

A. THORACIC LANDMARKS

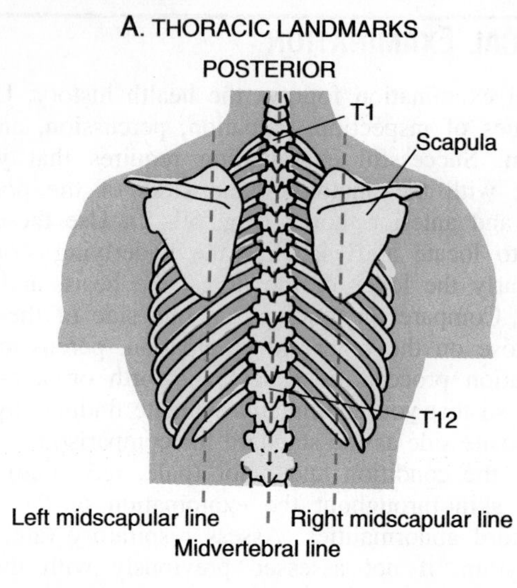

B. LUNG STRUCTURES

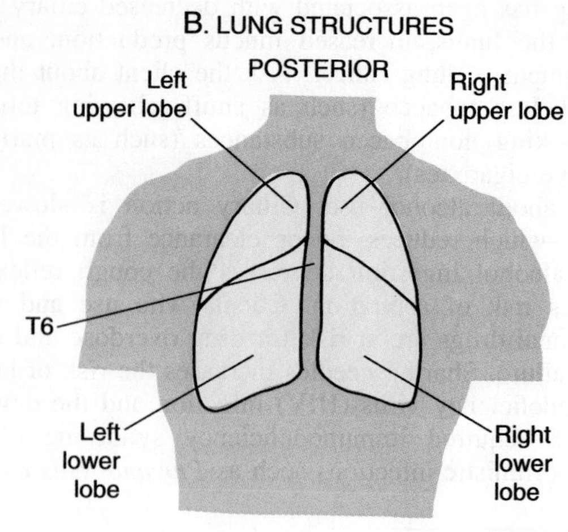

RIGHT LATERAL

LEFT LATERAL

Anterior axillary line

Midaxillary line

Posterior axillary line

RIGHT LATERAL

LEFT LATERAL

Upper lobes

Middle lobe

Lower lobes

ANTERIOR

Suprasternal notch

Clavicle

Costal angle

Xiphoid process

Right midclavicular line

Left midclavicular line

Midsternal line

ANTERIOR

Right upper lobe

Left upper lobe

Right middle lobe

Right lower lobe

Left lower lobe

FIGURE 59–2 Thoracic landmarks and underlying lung structures. During chest examination, it is important to document in a universally understood manner the location of unusual or abnormal findings. Use the terminology of thoracic landmarks and lung structure to do so.

PHYSICAL ASSESSMENT FINDINGS IN THE HEALTHY ADULT

Respiratory System

Inspection

Nose. Nose straight, without flaring or discharge; nares patent; mucosa pink and moist; septum midline, without masses or perforation

Sinuses. Transilluminate

Thorax. Even color; regular, even contour; respirations quiet, unlabored, of even depth, and without retractions, bulges, masses, or use of accessory muscles; anteroposterior-transverse diameter ratio 1:2

Digits. Clubbing absent; nail beds pink; immediate capillary refill on blanching

Palpation

Nose. Nontender, without masses or lesions

Sinuses. Nontender, without swelling or bogginess

Trachea. Midline and mobile without crepitus

Thorax. Chest wall symmetrical, smooth, without lumps, masses, tenderness, or crepitus; thoracic excursion symmetrical; tactile fremitus present

Percussion

Sinuses. Nontender

Thorax and Lungs. Resonant throughout peripheral lung fields; cardiac dullness; diaphragmatic excursion ranges from 3 to 6 cm for each hemidiaphragm, with the right side slightly higher than the left

Auscultation

Thorax and Lungs. Vesicular sounds throughout peripheral lung fields; bronchovesicular sounds over the area of tracheal bifurcation, both anteriorly and posteriorly; bronchial sounds over the trachea anteriorly; adventitious sounds absent; vocal resonance absent

BARREL CHEST. Barrel chest is present when the AP diameter is increased and equals the transverse diameter (Fig. 59–3*B*). It is a characteristic finding in clients with chronic disorders that interfere with ventilation (e.g., emphysema).

PIGEON CHEST. Pigeon chest (pectus carinatum) is the opposite of funnel chest. The sternum juts forward and increases the AP diameter (Fig. 59–3*C*). Congenital atrial or ventricular septal defects are the most common cause of pigeon chest, but rickets, Marfan's syndrome, and severe primary kyphoscoliosis may contribute to pigeon chest.

FUNNEL CHEST. Funnel chest (pectus excavatum) is a deformity in which the sternum is depressed and the organs that lie below it are compressed (Fig. 59–3*D*). In severe cases, the sternum may actually touch the spinal column. In most cases, however, pectus excavatum is clinically insignificant. Some causes of funnel chest, including Marfan's syndrome and congenital connective tissue disorders, may be serious.

THORACIC KYPHOSCOLIOSIS. Thoracic kyphoscoliosis is an accentuation of the normal thoracic curve (Fig. 59–3*E*). The client takes on a hunched-over or hunchback appearance. Causes include congenital defect, osteoporosis secondary to aging, spinal tuberculosis, rheumatoid arthritis, and poor posture over a long period of time. The underlying lungs are distorted, which can make interpretation of lung findings difficult.

CHEST MOVEMENT

Observe chest movement during respiration. Normal respiratory rate is 12 to 22 breaths per minute. Note the amplitude, or depth of expansion, and rhythm. Abdominal breathing is more apparent in men, whereas women use their thoracic muscles. Note the use of accessory muscles, retractions, symmetry, and any paradoxical movements.

Fingers and Toes

Examination of the fingers and toes may reveal *clubbing,* which may be present in clients with pulmonary fibrosis, lung cancer, or bronchiectasis. Clubbing occurs as a compensatory measure in chronic hypoxia. The physiologic cause of clubbing has not yet been identified, although some hypotheses have been proposed. The body develops collateral circulation around an area of impaired circulation to provide more oxygen to that area. With clubbing, the nail bed loses its normal angle of 160 degrees between the nail plate and the finger, and the angle increases to 180 degrees. The base of the nail bed may feel spongy and soft. With advanced clubbing, the finger takes on a bulbous or spoon-like appearance. Assess early clubbing by using the Schamroth technique (Fig. 59–4).

Note the color of the nail beds to assess the status of peripheral tissue oxygenation. Nail beds should be pink, without cyanosis or a dusky blue color. Quickly and gently compress (between thumb and index finger) and release several of the client's nail beds on each extremity. Continuously observe for the *blanch response* and *capillary refill.* With compression, the nail bed becomes pale as capillary blood is squeezed from the tissue. Upon release of the pressure, oxygenated arterial blood fills the capillary bed. Normal capillary refill occurs within 3 seconds; a refill time longer than 3 seconds indicates delayed capillary refill.

■ PALPATION

Palpation is the use of the hands to feel various structures on and below the surface of the body. The technique of palpation is described in Chapter 10.

Trachea

Gently place the thumb of the palpating hand on one side of the trachea and the remaining fingers on the other side. Move the trachea gently from side to side along its length while palpating for masses, *crepitus* (air in the subcutaneous tissues), or deviation from the midline. The trachea is usually slightly movable and quickly returns to the midline position after displacement. A chest mass, goiter, or an acute chest injury may displace the trachea.

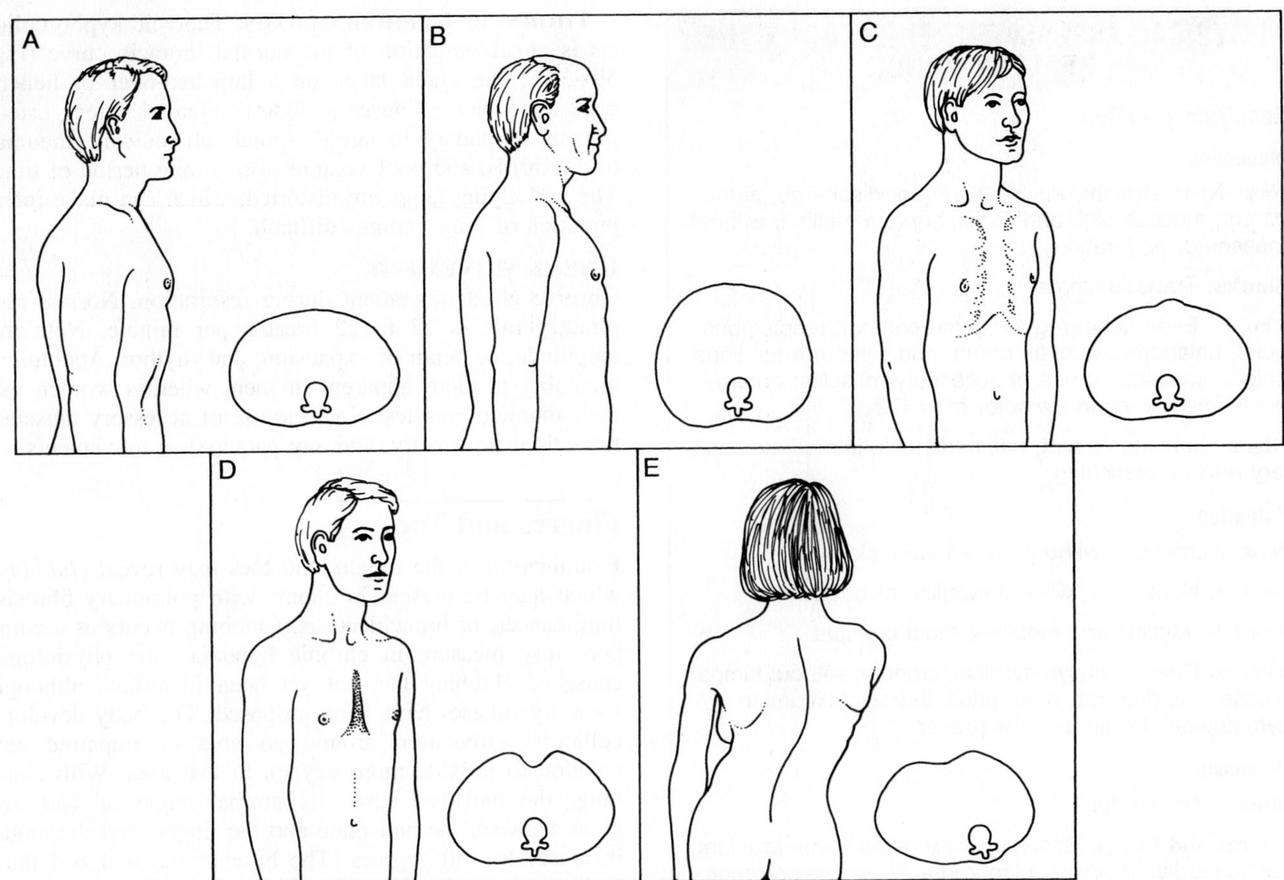

FIGURE 59–3 Chest deformities. *A,* Normal adult, for comparison. The ratio of anteroposterior diameter to transverse diameter can be seen here as 1 : 2. *B,* Barrel chest. The anteroposterior-transverse diameter ratio is 1 : 1. *C,* Pigeon chest (pectus carinatum). *D,* Funnel chest (pectus excavatum). *E,* Thoracic kyphoscoliosis.

Chest Wall

Palpate the chest wall, holding the heel or ulnar aspect of your hand against the client's chest. During palpation, continue the investigation of abnormalities found on inspection. Palpation combined with inspection is particularly effective in assessing whether the movements, or thoracic excursion of the chest during inspiration and expiration, are symmetrical and equal in amplitude. During palpation, assess for crepitus, defects or tenderness of

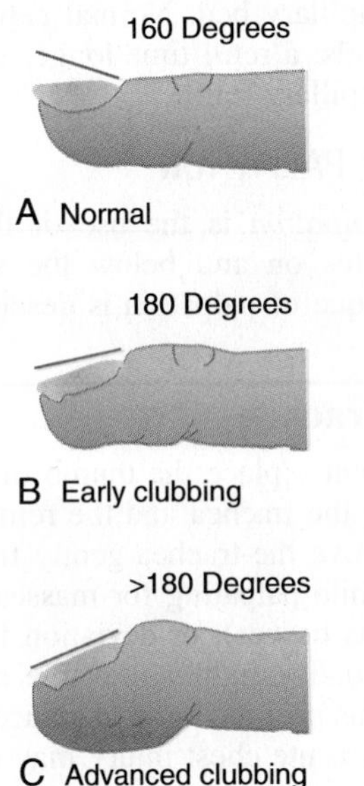

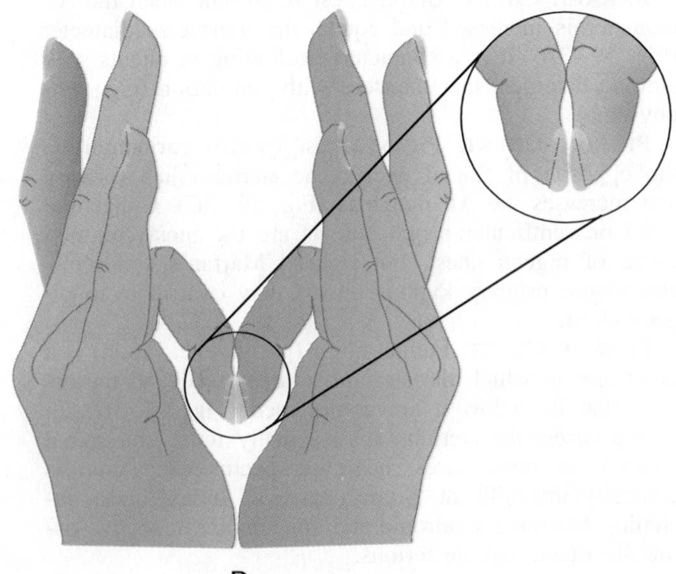

FIGURE 59–4 Clubbing. *A,* A normal digit, with an angle of 160 degrees. *B,* A flattened angle between the nail and the skin, exceeding 180 degrees. *C,* Advanced clubbing, with a rounded nail. *D,* Assess clubbing with the use of the Schamroth technique. Instruct the client to place the nails of the fourth (ring) fingers together while extending the other fingers and to hold the hands up. A diamond-shaped space between the nails is a normal finding and indicates the absence of clubbing.

the chest wall, muscle tone, edema, and tactile *fremitus* (the vibration of air movement through the chest wall while the client is speaking).

Thoracic Excursion

For the evaluation of thoracic excursion, the client sits upright. Place your hands on the client's posterior chest wall (Fig. 59–5). The thumbs oppose each other on either side of the spine, and the fingers face upward and out like butterfly wings. As the client inhales, your hands should move up and out symmetrically. Any asymmetry suggests a disease process in that region.

Tactile Fremitus

Palpate the posterior chest wall while the client says words that produce relatively intense vibrations (e.g., "ninety-nine"). The vibrations are transmitted from the larynx via the airways and can be palpated on the chest wall (Fig. 59–6). Compare the intensity of vibrations on both sides for symmetry. Stronger vibrations are felt over areas where there is consolidation of the underlying lung (e.g., pneumonia). Decreased tactile fremitus is usually associated with abnormalities that move the lung farther from the chest wall, such as pleural effusion and pneumothorax.

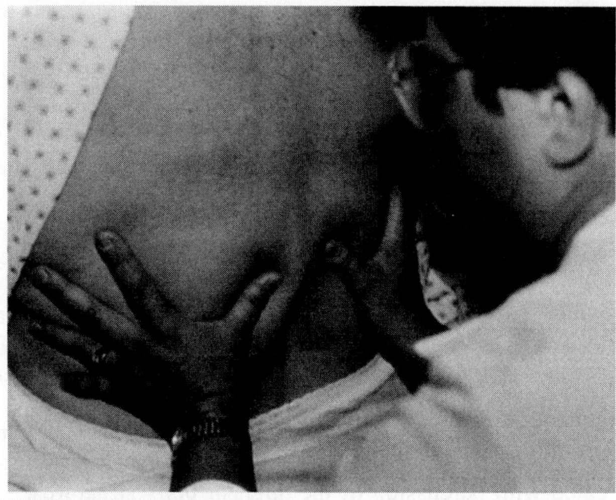

FIGURE 59–5 Assessment of thoracic excursion to determine the degree and symmetry of chest movement.

■ PERCUSSION

Percussion is an assessment technique of producing sounds by tapping on the chest wall with the hand (see Chapter 10). Tapping on the chest wall between the ribs

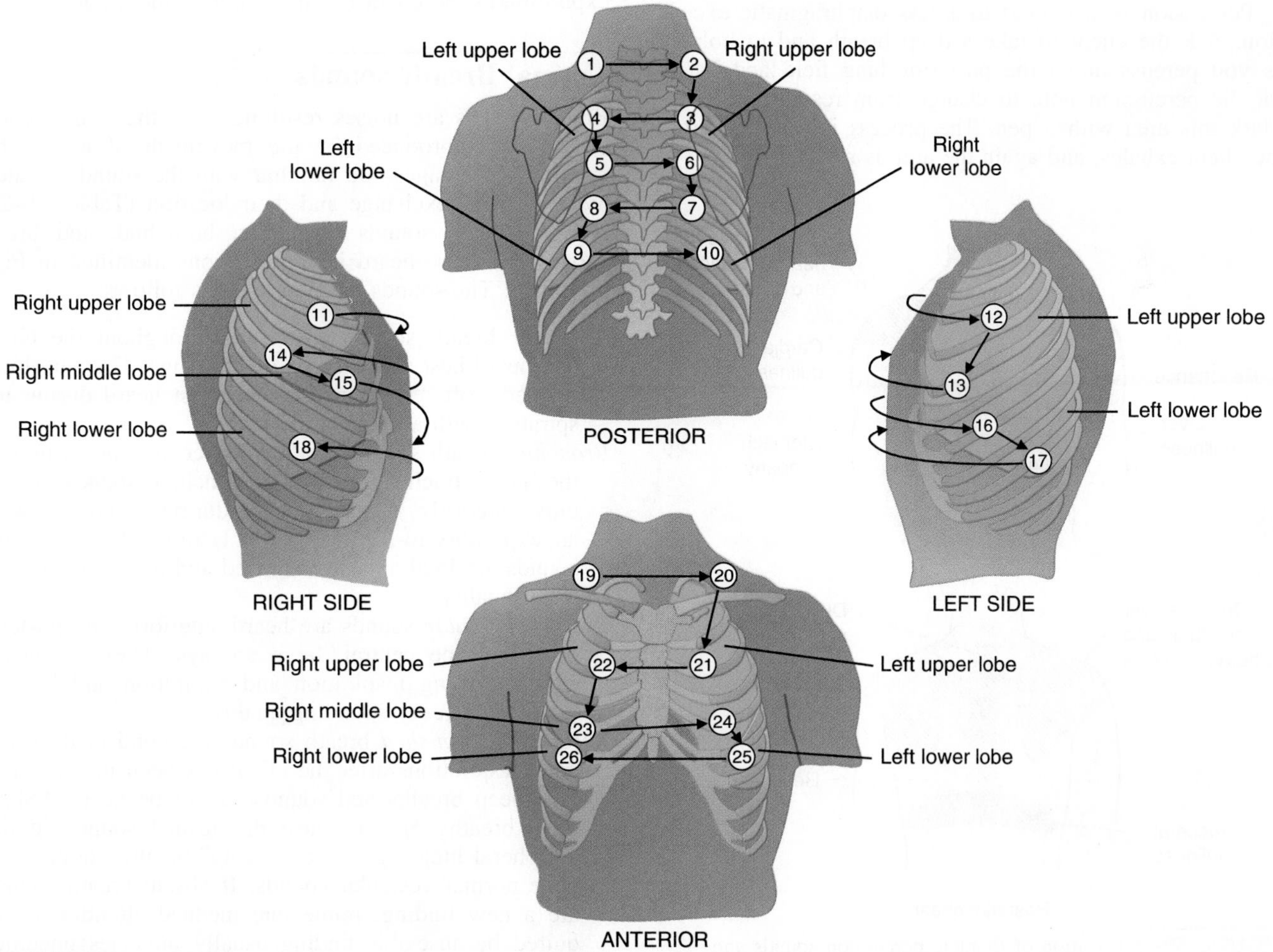

FIGURE 59–6 Sequence of palpation, percussion, and auscultation of the thorax (posterior, lateral, and anterior).

produces various sounds that are described in relation to their acoustic properties:

- *Resonant* sounds are low-pitched, hollow sounds heard over normal lung tissue.
- *Hyperresonant* sounds indicate an increased amount of air in the lungs or pleural space. These sounds are louder and lower-pitched than resonant sounds. Hyperresonant sounds are produced by emphysema and pneumothorax; they are normally heard in children and in very thin adults.
- *Dull* sounds occur over dense lung tissue, such as a tumor or a consolidation. These sounds are thud-like, medium-pitched. They are normally heard over the liver and heart.
- *Flat* notes are soft and high-pitched; they result from percussion over airless tissue. This sound can be replicated with percussion of the thigh or bony structures.
- *Tympanic* notes are high, hollow, drum-like sounds heard with percussion over the stomach, a large tension pneumothorax, or a large air-filled chamber (such as the empty stomach).

Figure 59–7 illustrates the location of percussion sounds of the chest.

Begin percussion at the apices and proceed to the bases, moving from the posterior to the lateral and then to the anterior areas (see Fig. 59–6). The posterior chest is best percussed with the client in an upright position and with arms crossed to separate the scapulae.

Percussion is also used to assess diaphragmatic excursion. Ask the client to take a deep breath and to hold it as you percuss down the posterior lung field and listen for the percussion note to change from resonant to dull. Mark this area with a pen. The process is repeated after the client exhales, and again the area is marked.

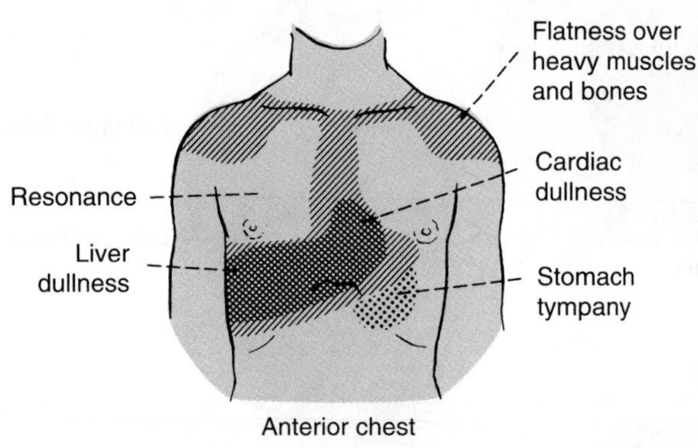

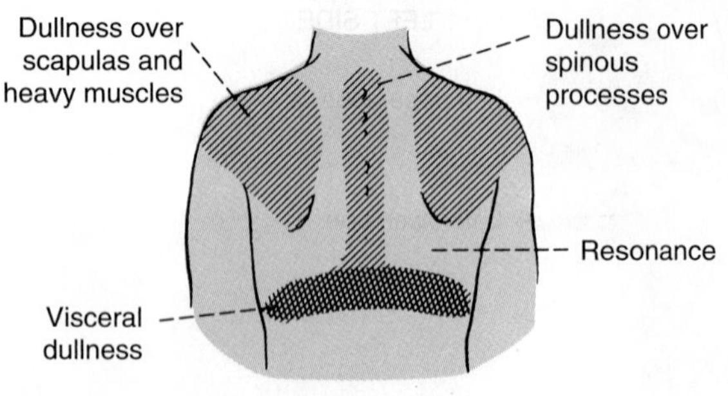

FIGURE 59–7 Location of thoracic percussion sounds and their associated structures.

Assess both right and left sides. The distance between the two marks should be 3 to 6 cm; smaller spans are found in females and larger spans in males. The marks on the right are slightly higher because of the presence of the liver. A client with an elevated diaphragm related to a pathologic process has decreased diaphragmatic excursion.

If the client has lung disease in the lower lobes (e.g., consolidation or pleural fluid), the same dull percussion note is heard. When abnormalities are found, other diagnostic tests should be used to assess the problem fully.

■ AUSCULTATION

Auscultation involves listening to chest sounds with a stethoscope. By listening to the lungs while the client breathes through an open mouth, you can assess:

- The character of the breath sounds
- The presence of adventitious sounds (described later)
- The character of the spoken and whispered voice

Figure 59–6 identifies a sequence for auscultation with comparison of sounds from right to left.

Listen to all areas of the lungs over a bare chest; do not listen to lungs over sheets, gowns, or shirts. The sounds heard may be from the movement of fabric beneath the stethoscope. At each position, listen at the diaphragm for a full respiratory cycle of inspiration and expiration as the client breathes through the mouth.

Normal Breath Sounds

Breath sounds are noises resulting from the transmission of vibrations produced by the movement of air in the respiratory passages. Be familiar with the sounds created by normal air exchange and their location (Table 59–2). Normal breath sounds (vesicular, bronchial, and bronchovesicular) are heard in the locations identified in Figure 59–8. The sounds are described as follows:

Vesicular breath sounds are heard throughout the chest and heard best in the bases of the lungs. They are low-pitched, soft, "swishing" sounds best heard during inspiration with an I:E ratio of 5:2.

Bronchial breath sounds are heard over the manubrium in the large tracheal airways. Bronchial sounds, heard only anteriorly, are best heard during expiration with an expiratory-to-inspiratory (E:I) ratio of 2:1. These sounds are loud and high-pitched and have a hollow or harsh quality.

Bronchovesicular sounds are heard anteriorly and posteriorly over the central, large airways. They are heard equally during inspiration and expiration and have a tubular or breezy-sounding quality.

Absent or *diminished* breath sounds are confirmed during deep respirations after the client has been instructed to take deep breaths and sounds cannot be heard. "Shallow" breaths may produce diminished sounds in the peripheral lung regions, but "deep" breaths should produce normal vesicular sounds. If absent breath sounds are a new finding, immediate medical attention is required because this finding usually indicates pneumothorax or other respiratory emergency.

TABLE 59–2 CHARACTERISTICS OF NORMAL BREATH SOUNDS

	Pitch	Amplitude	Duration	Quality	Normal Location
Bronchial (tracheal)	High	Loud	Inspiration < expiration	Harsh, hollow, tubular	Trachea and larynx
Bronchovesicular	Moderate	Moderate	Inspiration = expiration	Mixed	Over major bronchi where fewer alveoli are located: posterior, between scapulae, especially on the right; anterior, around the upper sternum in the first and second intercostal spaces
Vesicular	Low	Soft	Inspiration > expiration	Rustling, like the sound of the wind in the trees	Over peripheral lung fields where air flows through smaller bronchioles and alveoli

From Jarvis, C. (1996). *Physical examination and health assessment* (2nd ed.) Philadelphia: W. B. Saunders.

Adventitious Breath Sounds

Adventitious sounds (Table 59–3) are abnormal sounds superimposed on normal breath sounds. The current American Thoracic Society nomenclature for adventitious sounds is used throughout this chapter. Adventitious sounds include (1) crackles, (2) rhonchi, (3) wheezes, and (4) pleural friction rubs.

CRACKLES

Crackles (formerly called *rales*) are audible when there is a sudden opening of small airways that contain fluid. The sound of a crackle can be reproduced by rubbing a lock of hair between the thumb and finger close to the ear. Crackles are usually heard during inspiration and do not clear with a cough. Crackles can be found in clients with pulmonary edema, pulmonary fibrosis, or pneumonia.

RHONCHI

Rhonchi (also called "gurgles") occur as the result of air passing through fluid-filled, narrow passages. Diseases in which there is excess mucus production, such as pneumonia, bronchitis, or bronchiectasis, are associated with rhonchi. Rhonchi are usually heard on expiration and may clear with a cough.

WHEEZES

A wheeze is a continuous musical or hissing noise that results from the passage of air through a narrowed airway. Wheezes are heard during inspiration or expiration or both. Severe wheezes are audible without a stethoscope. Wheezing is commonly associated with asthma and its bronchoconstriction and edema, but foreign bodies can also cause airway narrowing and wheezing.

PLEURAL FRICTION RUBS

Pleural friction rubs are the result of pleural inflammation often associated with pleurisy, pneumonia, or pleural infarct. A rub is described as a creaking, grating noise similar to that made by two pieces of leather rubbing together. A rub is audible on inspiration and expiration over the area of the inflammation. Chest wall splinting can be associated with a pleural friction rub.

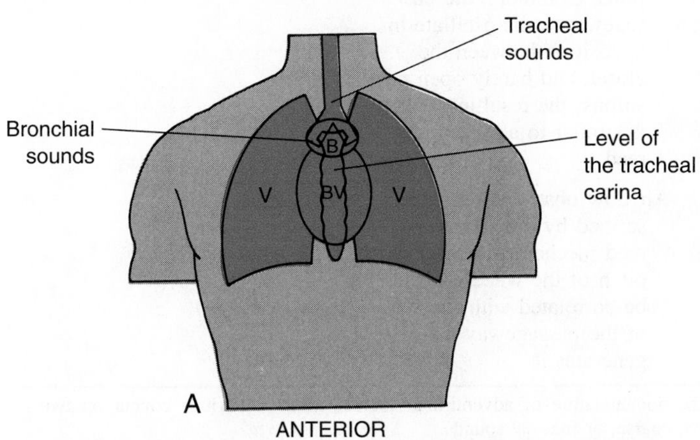

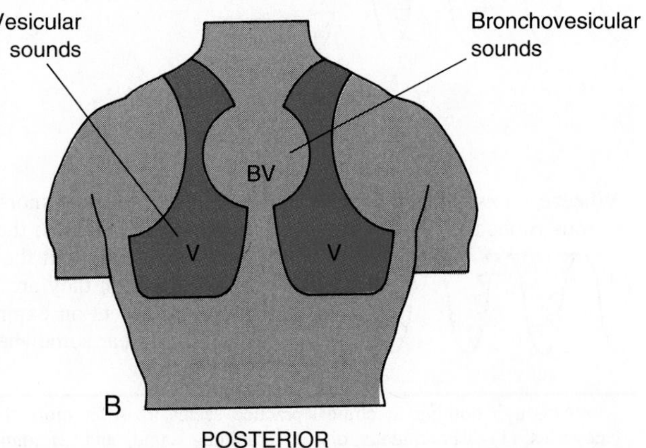

FIGURE 59–8 *A* and *B*, Location of normal breath sounds.

TABLE 59–3 ADVENTITIOUS BREATH SOUNDS

Sound*	Description	Mechanism	Clinical Example
DISCONTINUOUS SOUNDS			
Crackles—fine (rales, crepitations) Inspiration Expiration	Discontinuous, high-pitched, short crackling, popping sounds heard during inspiration that are not cleared by coughing; this sound can be simulated by rolling a strand of hair between the fingers near the ear, or by moistening thumb and index finger and separating them near the ear	Inhaled air collides with previously deflated airways; airways suddenly pop open, creating a crackling sound as gas pressures between the two compartments equalize	*Late inspiratory crackles* occur with restrictive disease: pneumonia, heart failure, and interstitial fibrosis *Early inspiratory crackles* occur with obstructive disease: chronic bronchitis, asthma, and emphysema
Crackles—coarse (coarse rales)	Loud, low-pitched, bubbling and gurgling sounds that start in early inspiration and may be present in expiration; may decrease somewhat by suctioning or coughing but will reappear shortly; sound like opening a self-fastening tape (Velcro) fastener	Inhaled air collides with secretions in the trachea and large bronchi	Pulmonary edema, pneumonia, pulmonary fibrosis, and in the terminally ill who have a depressed cough reflex
Atelectatic crackles (atelectatic rales)	Sound like fine crackles, but do not last and are not pathologic; disappear after the first few breaths; heard in axillae and bases (usually dependent) of lungs	When sections of alveoli are not fully aerated, they deflate and accumulate secretions; crackles are heard when these sections reexpand with a few deep breaths	In aging adults, bedridden people, or in people just aroused from sleep
Pleural friction rub	A very superficial sound that is coarse and low-pitched; it has a grating quality as if two pieces of leather are being rubbed together; sounds just like crackles, but *close* to the ear; sounds louder if the stethoscope is pushed harder onto the chest wall; sound is inspiratory and expiratory	Caused when pleurae become inflamed and lose their normal lubricating fluid; their opposing roughened pleural surfaces rub together during respiration; heard best in the anterolateral wall where there is greatest lung mobility	Pleuritis, accompanied by pain with breathing (rub disappears after a few days if pleural fluid accumulates and separates pleurae)
CONTINUOUS SOUNDS			
Wheeze—high-pitched (sibilant rhonchi)	High-pitched, musical squeaking sounds that predominate in expiration but may occur in both expiration and inspiration	Air squeezed or compressed through passageways narrowed almost to closure by collapsing, swelling, secretions, or tumors; the passageway walls oscillate in apposition between the closed and barely open positions; the resulting sound is similar to a vibrating reed	Obstructive lung disease such as asthma or emphysema
Wheeze—low-pitched (sonorous rhonchi)	Low-pitched, musical snoring, moaning sounds; they are heard throughout the cycle, although they are more prominent on expiration; may clear somewhat by coughing	Air flow obstruction as described by the vibrating reed mechanism above; the pitch of the wheeze cannot be correlated with the size of the passageway that generates it	Bronchitis

*Although nothing in clinical practice seems to differ more than the nomenclature of adventitious sounds, most authorities concur on two categories: (1) discontinuous, discrete crackling sounds and (2) continuous, coarse, or musical sounds.

Modified from Jarvis, C. (1996). *Physical examination and health assessment* (2nd ed.). Philadelphia: W. B. Saunders.

Voice Sounds

Assess voice sounds (vocal resonance) by auscultation if tactile fremitus is abnormal. Auscultation while the client speaks normally reveals muffled and indistinct sounds. The sound is louder medially over the larger airways and softens toward the periphery. Consolidation results in *bronchophony* or increased resonance, so that when the client says "ninety-nine," it is heard clearly.

If bronchophony is present, assess for egophony next. *Egophony* involves a change in the sound of the letter *e* to that of the letter *a*, indicating consolidation. The sound also has a nasal or bleating quality.

A third voice test for consolidation is *whispered pectoriloquy.* Ask the client to whisper "one-two-three." If the words are distinct, the abnormal finding of whispered pectoriloquy is present. Consolidation enhances the transmission of sound vibrations and results from lung tumors, pneumonia, or pulmonary fibrosis.

ASSESSMENT OF THE NOSE, PHARYNX, AND SINUSES

HISTORY

Upper respiratory problems can occur alone or progress to lower respiratory complications, such as viral infections.

■ CURRENT HEALTH

Chief Complaint

The client may present with a current complaint of nosebleeds (epistaxis); sinus infection; hay fever; postnasal drip; rhinitis; sneezing; or nasal, facial, or referred ear pain. Obstruction by engorged mucous membranes or nasal polyps may occlude the upper airway. Loss of or a decreased sense of smell may accompany manifestations of the common cold and allergies or may signal a more serious neurologic problem.

Inquire whether the client has experienced these manifestations previously and, if so, when and how often. Ask the client to describe self-treatment measures, such as nasal sprays, decongestants, antihistamines, and other over-the-counter and herbal cold and allergy medications. For example, an herbal remedy for hay fever is nettle (*Urtica dioica*). See the earlier discussion of herbal remedies.

Symptom Analysis

Perform a complete symptom analysis to determine the nature of the problem, including onset, duration, and severity.

AGGRAVATING AND RELIEVING FACTORS

Ask the client about factors that alleviate or worsen the manifestations, such as increased humidity, sitting upright, lying supine, weather and seasonal changes, or allergies. Nasal and sinus problems may be allergy-related and provoked by pollen, fumes, smoke, animal dander, or dust particles. Nosebleeds may increase during the winter months if mucous membranes are dry because of insufficient humidity.

ASSOCIATED MANIFESTATIONS

A foul taste in the mouth, unpleasant breath odor (halitosis), nasal obstruction, and facial pain (particularly over the frontal and maxillary sinuses) may accompany sinusitis. Chronic sinusitis may be accompanied by headache or facial pain present on awakening and diminishing during the day (because the sinuses drain when the client sits or stands).

■ PAST HEALTH HISTORY

Ask about past problems with frequent colds, sinus infections, nasal stuffiness, or trauma (fracture). Explore episodes of epistaxis for cause (e.g., hypertension), frequency, and treatment (e.g., cauterization or nasal packing).

PHYSICAL EXAMINATION

Inspect and palpate the client's nose and sinuses. The structures assessed include the external nose, vestibule, nasal mucosa, septum, turbinates, nasal canals, and sinuses. Function of the first cranial nerve (olfactory) is usually not tested unless a deficit in the sense of smell is reported or suspected.

■ NOSE

External Nose

Inspect and palpate the external nose for deviations from normal alignment, symmetry, color, discharge, nasal flaring, lesions, and tenderness. Normal findings are listed. The skin color over the nose is the same as that of the facial skin. Alignment is straight and symmetrical without deviation from the midline. Discharge from the nares (nostrils) should be absent, and the nares should not flare (spread) with respirations. The client is able to breathe quietly through the nose rather than breathe through the mouth. Masses, lesions, and tenderness are absent.

Check the nasal canals for patency by asking the client to occlude one naris with a finger and to breathe through the open naris while closing the mouth. Repeat this for the opposite naris. The client should be able to breathe without difficulty through both nares. Ask the client to tip the head back, and inspect the outer nares for crusting, bleeding, or dryness, which should be absent.

Internal Nose

Next, inspect the vestibules with a penlight while the client's head is tipped back. Normal findings include coarse hairs, a clear passage without discharge, and a midline septum. Further examination of the internal nose requires use of a nasal speculum and is not conducted unless indicated. If a detailed examination of the internal nose is performed, either attach a nasal speculum tip to the otoscope head or use a metal nasal speculum (Fig. 59–9) and penlight for illumination. While the client tips the head back, gently insert the speculum into one naris, taking care not to scrape the mucosa. Inspect one naris at a time.

Hold the speculum correctly, and insert the blades gently about ½ inch into the nostril. Gain additional control of the speculum by resting the index finger of the dominant hand on the side of the client's nose. Steady the client's head with the nondominant hand. Open the blades gently and vertically, avoiding pressure on the septum and turbinates. Slowly move the head to inspect all areas

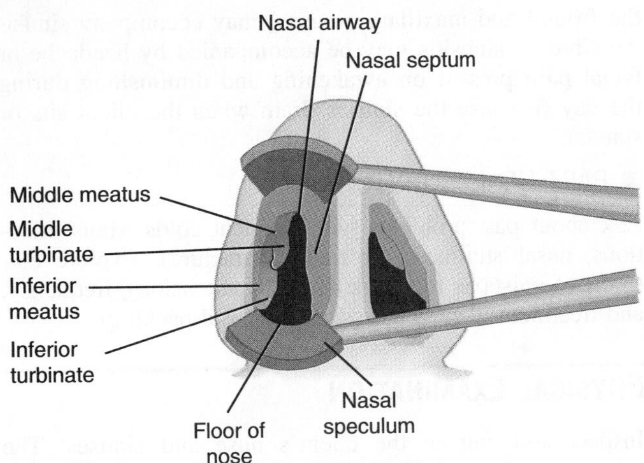

FIGURE 59–9 Internal inspection of the nose with a nasal speculum.

of the nasal chamber. Observe the condition of the mucous membrane (e.g., pallor, redness, swelling). Normally, the mucosa is moist and dark pink without sign of inflammation, pallor, or a blue color. Presence of discharge is abnormal. The septum divides the nasal cavity into halves without deviation, masses, perforation, or exudate. The turbinates are the same color as the mucosa and should be free of exudate, swelling, or inflammation (only the inferior and part of the middle turbinate are visible; the superior is not). Look for polyps and other masses. Observe mucous plugs for color, consistency, amount, and odor.

Inspection may be hampered by nasal congestion. It may be necessary to shrink the nasal mucosa with a topical vasoconstrictor (e.g., phenylephrine hydrochloride) for adequate inspection. When the agent is instilled into the nose, ask the client to say *e* and hold the sound. Use of this technique raises the posterior tongue, occludes the upper airway, and prevents the fluid from running into the pharynx.

NASOPHARYNX

The nasopharynx is best examined with a mirror while the tongue is depressed with a tongue blade or pulled forward and grasped with a gauze sponge. Prevent fogging of the mirror by warming it before putting it into the mouth. Hold the mirror to one side of the uvula, and focus light on it. A small part of the nasopharynx can be observed with a nasal speculum. Specialists may use a nasopharyngoscope to examine the nasopharynx.

PARANASAL SINUSES

Assess the paranasal sinuses by (1) inspecting and palpating the soft overlying tissues, (2) observing any nasal secretions (it is possible to determine which sinus is infected according to where discharge appears), and (3) transilluminating the maxillary and frontal sinuses. Palpate and percuss the frontal and maxillary sinuses to assess for swelling and tenderness, which are normally absent.

Palpate the frontal sinuses simultaneously by placing the thumbs above the eyes, just under the bony ridge of the orbits, and apply gentle pressure. Palpate the maxillary sinuses by using either the index and third fingers or thumbs to press gently on each side of the nose just under the zygomatic bones. Use direct percussion over the eyebrows for the frontal sinuses and on either side of the nose below the eyes in line with the pupils for the maxillary sinuses.

Transillumination is a technique used to assess the sinuses further if tenderness is present. Either a penlight or the otoscope handle fitted with a transilluminator head (see Chapter 10) is used. Darken the room. Place the light against the orbital bones immediately below the eyebrows and direct upward. Shield the light source with one hand. Normally, a reddish glow appears above the frontal sinus area. Lack of illumination may indicate sinus congestion and purulent fluid accumulation. Assess the maxillary sinuses by placing the light beneath the center of the eyes and the zygomatic bones and directing it down and in toward the roof of the mouth. Ask the client to open the mouth. A glow should appear on the hard palate on the side being illuminated. For a more complete assessment of sinus conditions, radiologic studies may be done. Air, normally present in the sinuses, appears as a dark area on a developed film.

SMELL

The senses of taste and smell are closely related. Many conditions affect taste and smell, such as viral infections, normal aging, head injuries, and local obstruction. Some medications can affect smell and taste, such as metronidazole, local anesthetics, clofibrate, some antibiotics, some antineoplastics, allopurinol, phenylbutazone, levodopa, codeine, morphine, carbamazepine, lithium, and trifluoperazine. Smell impairment may be (1) *hyposmia* (decrease in smell sensitivity) or (2) *anosmia* (bilateral and complete absence of smell sensitivity).

Assess smell by having the client identify various odors. Various substances are placed in individual test tubes (covered to eliminate visual cues). Test each nostril separately; have the client sniff the tubes (first with the eyes closed and then with the eyes open). Document whether the client can (1) perceive each odor and (2) identify each odor accurately.

Smell is perceived mainly via the olfactory nerves, although some smell is perceived via the trigeminal nerves. Trigeminal irritants are perceived even by clients with anosmia. (Therefore, a client who claims not to smell trigeminal irritants may be experiencing a conversion hysterical loss of smell rather than hyposmia or anosmia.) A client with a tracheostomy may not be able to smell because of limited upper airway movement. Olfactory stimulants and trigeminal stimulants commonly used to assess smell are listed in Box 59–1. See Chapter 67 for further discussion of smell assessment.

BOX 59–1 Substances Used in Assessing Smell

Olfactory stimulants	Trigeminal stimulants
Coffee (instant powder)	Ammonia
Phenylethyl alcohol	Acetone
Almond oil	Menthol
Peppermint	Distilled water
Musk	

DIAGNOSTIC TESTS

Diagnostic procedures augment the assessment of clients with respiratory disorders. To clarify which diagnostic test is used when and for what purpose, the tests are discussed here in the framework of what is being evaluated: functional status, anatomy, or specimens. The diagnostic test may be used for any or all of these reasons. This listing is limited to the most commonly used diagnostic tests.

■ TESTS TO EVALUATE RESPIRATORY FUNCTION

The diagnostic tests used to evaluate the functional status of the pulmonary system include:

- Pulmonary function tests
- Pulse oximetry
- Capnography
- Arterial blood gas (ABG) analysis
- Ventilation-perfusion studies

Pulmonary Function Tests

Pulmonary function tests (PFTs) provide information about respiratory function by measuring lung volumes, lung mechanics, and diffusion capabilities of the lungs (Table 59–4). PFTs performed in a pulmonary function laboratory can measure respiratory volumes and capacities. PFTs done outside a laboratory are modified to include ventilation tests of forced expiratory volume, vital capacity, and maximal voluntary ventilation measures. A measure of expiratory flow obtained with a hand-held device is called a *peak flow*. Many clients with asthma use a peak flowmeter (Fig. 59–10) at home to monitor changes in their condition and responses to treatment.

Education about the purpose, procedure, and implications of the test is performed by the nurse and reinforced by the examiner. Explicit instructions for each maneuver are given during the testing. Instruct clients that it is normal to feel short of breath after the test. Clients should not smoke or use a bronchodilator 6 hours before undergoing a PFT.

FORCED SPIROMETRY

The flow and volume capacities of the lungs are measured with forced spirometry. The volume of air inhaled and exhaled is plotted against time during a series of ventilatory maneuvers. Flow volume loops are created as visual patterns. Normal loop spirograms and spirogram patterns with obstructive and restrictive disorders are shown in Figure 59–11. Table 59–4 defines maneuvers used to test lung mechanics.

LUNG VOLUME DETERMINATION

Lung volume is measured by a gas dilution technique or body plethysmography. The two most commonly used gas dilution methods are (1) the *open-circuit* nitrogen method and (2) the *closed-circuit* helium method. These tests are most often used to measure functional residual capacity (FRC).

In the open-circuit method, all exhaled gas is collected while the client breathes pure oxygen. Measurement of the total amount of nitrogen washed out from the lungs permits calculation of the volume of gas present in the lungs at the beginning of the maneuver. The open-circuit method also allows assessment of the uniformity of ventilation in the lungs.

When helium is used to test the lungs in the closed-circuit method, the client inhales a mixture of air with a known concentration of helium. Helium does not significantly diffuse into the pulmonary bed. The helium diffuses throughout the air in the breathing box and lungs. The client exhales and is disconnected from the box. Changes in helium concentration in the box are computed to determine total lung volume.

The body plethysmograph, or *body box* (Fig. 59–12), is a device used to measure lung volumes. The lung volume changes seen with obstructive and restrictive lung disorders are shown in Table 59–5. While sitting in the airtight box, the client is instructed to perform a panting maneuver. Changes in the box pressure reflect changes in thoracic volume. Clients who cannot pant, who cannot tolerate closed spaces, or who have equipment that would interfere with the procedure cannot be tested by this method.

DIFFUSION CAPACITY

Studies of the lung diffusing capacity (DL) or carbon monoxide lung diffusion capacity [DL_{CO}]) measure gas transfer of carbon monoxide (CO) across the alveolar capillary membrane. The DL indicates the ease with which CO diffuses across the alveolar capillary membrane and binds with hemoglobin. (Hemoglobin has 250 times greater affinity for CO than for oxygen.) With normal hemoglobin and normal ventilatory function, the only limiting factor to diffusion of CO is the alveolar capillary membrane. The test involves inhaling room air mixed with 0.3% CO and 10% helium.

In many diseases, such as sarcoidosis, systemic lupus erythematosus, and emphysema, the alveolar membrane is thickened and oxygen transfer and diffusion are impaired, resulting in a decrease in DL. An increased DL is found with exercise, polycythemia, and hypervolemia.

Instruct the client to exhale forcefully, then inhale quickly, and hold the breath for 10 seconds and exhale. A sample of the exhaled air is collected for analysis.

Pulse Oximetry

PROCEDURE

Pulse oximetry is a safe and simple method of assessing oxygenation. It has the advantage that the data are obtained noninvasively and continuously. Previously, oxygenation was most commonly assessed by use of ABG determinations. Pulse oximetry was originally used in surgery but has been extended to most acute care settings. In fact, it is so common that it has been called the "fifth vital sign."

The pulse oximeter (Fig. 59–13) passes a beam of light through the tissue, and a sensor attached to the finger tip, toe, or ear lobe measures the amount of light absorbed by the oxygen-saturated hemoglobin. The oximeter then gives a reading of the percentage of hemoglobin that is saturated with oxygen (SaO_2). SaO_2 is closely correlated with the saturations obtained from the pulse oximeter if it is above 70%. Table 59–6 provides a quick guide for comparison of SaO_2 and partial pressure of arterial oxygen (PaO_2).

TABLE 59–4 PULMONARY FUNCTION TEST (PFT) COMPONENTS

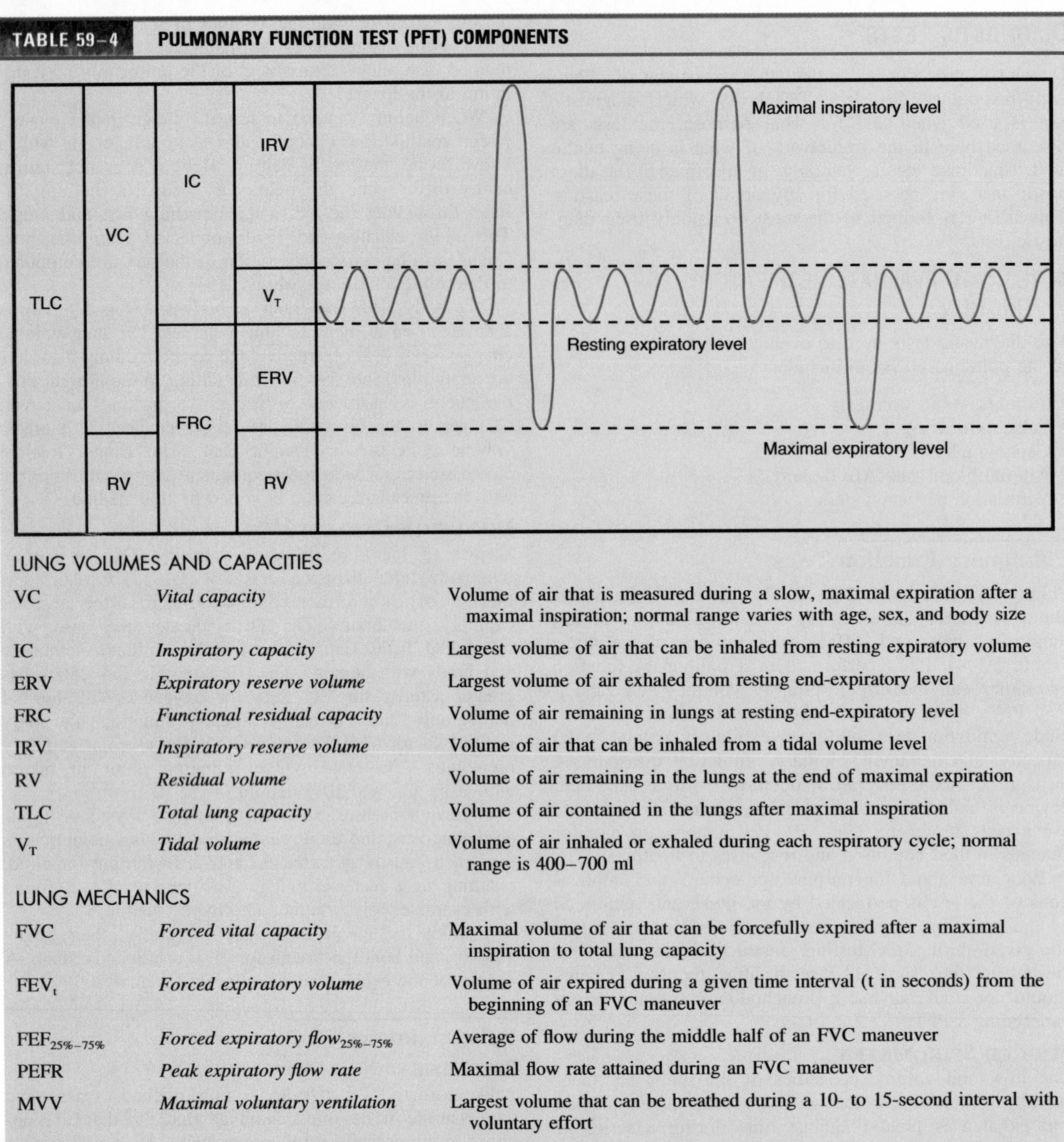

LUNG VOLUMES AND CAPACITIES		
VC	*Vital capacity*	Volume of air that is measured during a slow, maximal expiration after a maximal inspiration; normal range varies with age, sex, and body size
IC	*Inspiratory capacity*	Largest volume of air that can be inhaled from resting expiratory volume
ERV	*Expiratory reserve volume*	Largest volume of air exhaled from resting end-expiratory level
FRC	*Functional residual capacity*	Volume of air remaining in lungs at resting end-expiratory level
IRV	*Inspiratory reserve volume*	Volume of air that can be inhaled from a tidal volume level
RV	*Residual volume*	Volume of air remaining in the lungs at the end of maximal expiration
TLC	*Total lung capacity*	Volume of air contained in the lungs after maximal inspiration
V_T	*Tidal volume*	Volume of air inhaled or exhaled during each respiratory cycle; normal range is 400–700 ml
LUNG MECHANICS		
FVC	*Forced vital capacity*	Maximal volume of air that can be forcefully expired after a maximal inspiration to total lung capacity
FEV_t	*Forced expiratory volume*	Volume of air expired during a given time interval (t in seconds) from the beginning of an FVC maneuver
$FEF_{25\%-75\%}$	*Forced expiratory flow*$_{25\%-75\%}$	Average of flow during the middle half of an FVC maneuver
PEFR	*Peak expiratory flow rate*	Maximal flow rate attained during an FVC maneuver
MVV	*Maximal voluntary ventilation*	Largest volume that can be breathed during a 10- to 15-second interval with voluntary effort
MIP	*Maximal inspiratory pressure*	Greatest negative or subatmospheric pressure that can be generated during inspiration against an occluded airway
MEP	*Maximal expiratory pressure*	Highest positive pressure that can be generated during a forceful expiratory effort against an occluded airway

Limitations of pulse oximetry are still present despite the advancement of the technology. Motion at the sensor site changes light absorption. The motion mimics the pulsatile motion of blood, and because the detector cannot distinguish between movement of blood and movement of the finger, results can be inaccurate. Hypotension, hypothermia, and vasoconstriction reduce arterial blood flow to the sensor; keeping the finger warm may help with this problem. There are also sensors for the nose that can be used to improve accuracy. The sensor should not be placed distal to blood pressure cuffs, pressure dressings, arterial lines, or invasive catheters and should not be taped to the client's finger.

Readings for clients with severe right-sided heart failure and those with high levels of positive end-expiratory pressure (PEEP) may be inaccurate because of the creation

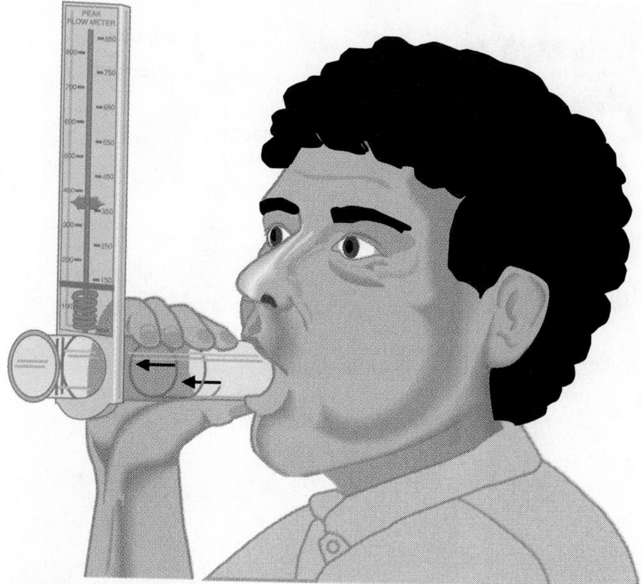

FIGURE 59–10 Use of a peak flowmeter to measure peak expiratory flow volume. The client stands and exhales into the mouthpiece. Normal peak flow values for adults are based on age, sex, height, and underlying lung disorder. Normal values range from 300 to 700 L/min but are best assessed when compared against a client's baseline values.

of pulsatile venous blood. Dark nail polish (especially blue, green, black, and brown-red) may interfere with accuracy. Red nail polish and artificial nails do not affect accuracy. Hyperbilirubinemia can also lead to false results.

Continue to assess the whole client, not just the oxygen saturation monitor. If values fall below preset norms (usually 90%), instruct the client to breathe deeply (if appropriate). Sometimes the amount of inspired oxygen is increased (titrated) to keep oxygen saturation above 90%. If the probe comes off the client's finger, the monitor usually indicates that the probe is off. Seldom is a loose probe the cause for readings of low levels of oxygen saturation.

Preprocedure Care

Tell the client about the need for the monitor. The test is noninvasive and painless. Explain that an infrared light probe will be attached to a finger, toe, or ear lobe. The client should avoid moving the sensor because movement disrupts the sensor and results in false readings.

Capnography

Procedure

Capnography, another noninvasive procedure, is used to measure exhaled carbon dioxide (CO_2) concentrations of

LOOP SPIROGRAM PATTERNS AND EXPLANATION

NORMAL PATTERN

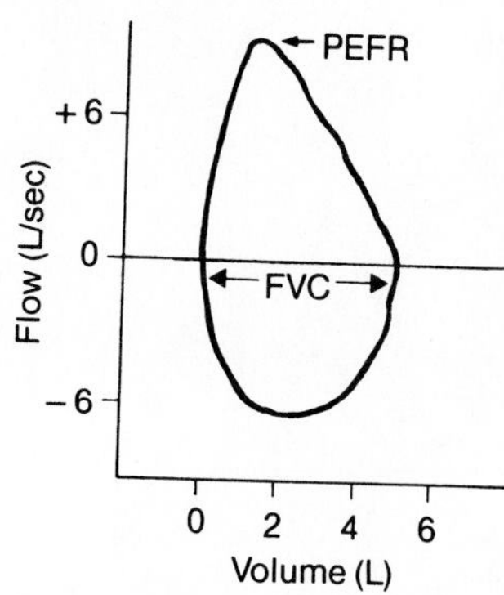

The expiratory curve shows a straight line decrease in flow after peak flow (PEFR). The inspiratory curve has a normal rounded pattern.

OBSTRUCTIVE PATTERN

Minimal-mild

Scooping

Mild-moderate

↓$FEF_{50\%}$

The expiratory curve shows scooping at low lung volumes (minimal to mild obstruction). As obstruction increases, the scooping becomes more marked and is accompanied by a decreased $FEF_{50\%}$ (mild to moderate obstruction).

Severe (e.g., emphysema)

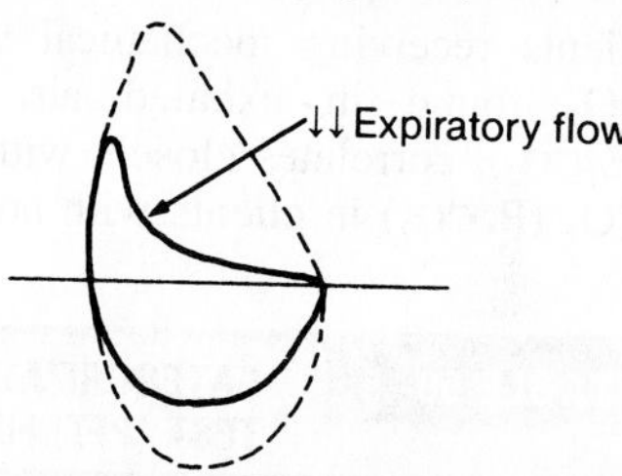

The expiratory curve shows a sudden decrease in PEFR in an "index finger" pattern, followed by a nearly horizontal line.

The inspiratory curve is normal, except for absolute decreases in flow rates.

RESTRICTIVE PATTERN

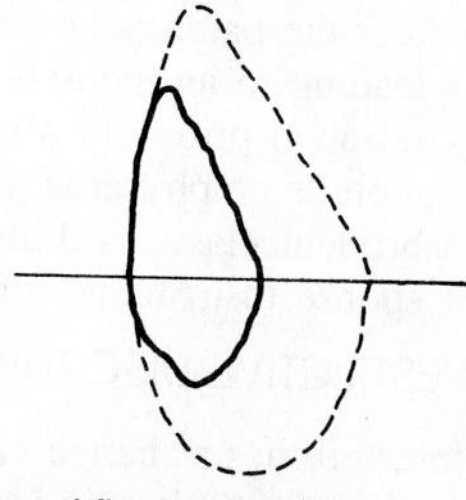

The entire loop resembles a miniature normal flow-volume loop. The FVC is markedly reduced. The expiratory curve shows a straight line decrease in flow with decreasing lung volumes. Peak flow rates may be normal, increased, or decreased, depending on the degree of respiratory impairment.

*The dotted lines represent the boundaries of the normal flow-volume loop.

FIGURE 59–11 A normal flow volume loop pattern and patterns for obstructive and restrictive lung disease. (From Kersten, L. D., et al. [1989]. *Respiratory nursing* [p. 382]. Philadelphia: W. B. Saunders.)

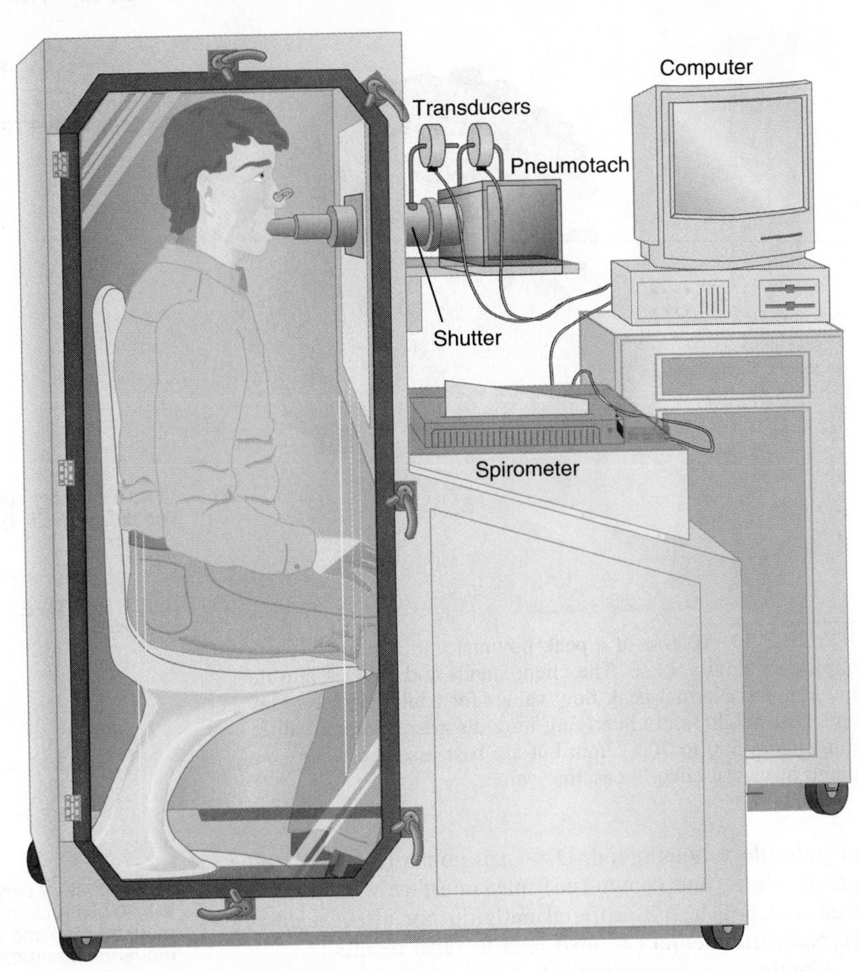

FIGURE 59–12 The volume plethysmograph—the "body box."

clients receiving mechanical ventilation. The amount of CO_2 found in exhaled air, end-tidal carbon dioxide (E_TCO_2), correlates closely with partial pressure of arterial CO_2 ($PaCO_2$) in clients with normal respiratory, cardiovascular, and metabolic function. The normal $PaCO_2$-E_TCO_2 gradient is approximately 5 mm Hg. As the $PaCO_2$ increases with hypoventilation or decreases with hyperventilation, associated changes are noted in E_TCO_2.

TABLE 59–5 CATEGORIZATION OF OBSTRUCTIVE AND RESTRICTIVE PULMONARY DISORDERS AND PULMONARY FUNCTION TEST (PFT) FINDINGS

	PFT Findings					
	VC	FEV_1	FEV_t/VC	FRC	TLC	RV
OBSTRUCTIVE DISORDERS						
Affect the patency or elasticity of the airways, leading to an increase in airway resistance; expiration is primarily affected. Obstructive disorders include emphysema, chronic bronchitis, asthma, bronchiectasis, and airway inflammation in response to irritants, infections, or allergies.	↓	↓	↓	↑	↑	↑
RESTRICTIVE DISORDERS						
Interfere in or change chest wall or lung parenchyma; inspiration is primarily affected. Restrictive disorders include kyphoscoliosis, pulmonary fibrosis, neuromuscular diseases and disorders, chest wall trauma, congenital chest wall changes, and tumors.	Normal or ↓	Slightly ↓	or Normal ↑	↓	↓	↓

FEV, forced expiratory volume in a unit of time; FRC, functional residual volume; RV, residual volume; TLC, total lung capacity; VC, vital capacity.

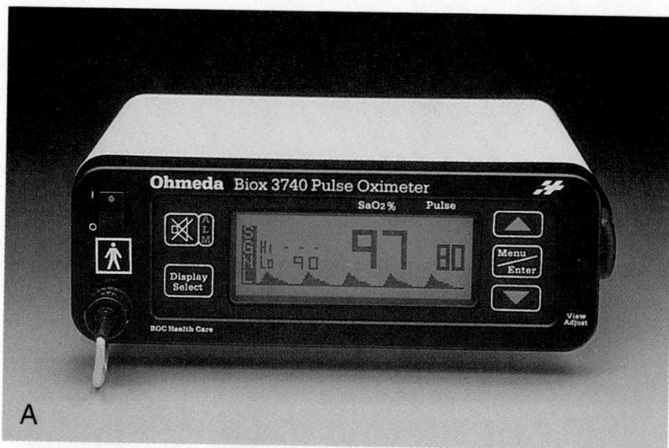

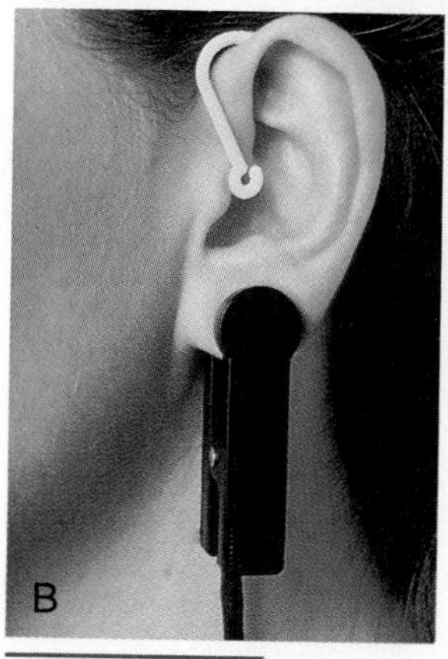

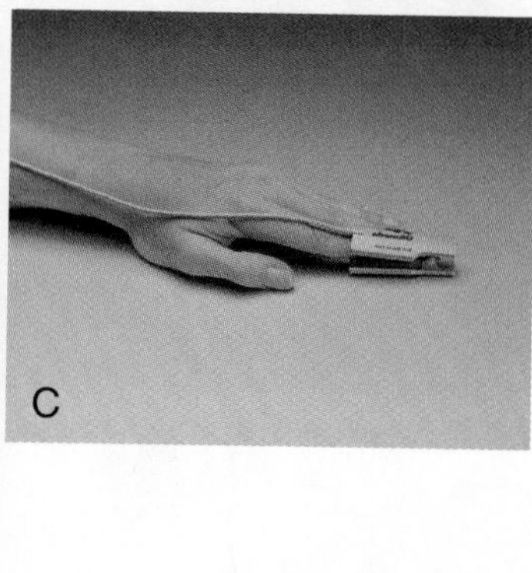

FIGURE 59–13 Oximetry. *A,* Noninvasive monitoring of oxygen saturation (SaO_2) is performed with a pulse oximeter. This unit has an ear probe and a finger probe. The ear probe *(B)* is used during measurements of SaO_2 while the client is exercising. The finger probe *(C)* is most frequently used for stationary measurement. (Courtesy of Ohmeda, Boulder, CO.)

Capnography requires continuous sampling of exhaled air.

Preprocedure Care

Explain the purpose of this test to the client. The test is noninvasive and painless. Clients who require capnography already have an endotracheal tube or tracheostomy tube in place for mechanical ventilation or airway management. A sensor is attached to the endotracheal tube or tracheostomy tube to measure E_TCO_2.

Arterial Blood Gas Analysis

ABG analysis (see Chapter 14) involves the use of arterial, rather than venous, blood to measure PaO_2, $PaCO_2$, and pH directly. Other data, such as bicarbonate (HCO_3^-) and SaO_2, are calculated. ABG analysis is an excellent diagnostic tool. PaO_2 reflects the efficiency of gas exchange, whereas $PaCO_2$ reflects the effectiveness of alveolar ventilation. The acid-base status of the body (see Chapter 14) is indicated by the pH of arterial blood. ABG analysis is essential for the assessment of clients who are acutely ill with pulmonary and nonpulmonary disorders, who require an artificial airway, who are dependent on mechanical ventilation, or who are experiencing chronic respiratory disease.

TABLE 59–6 COMPARING OXYGEN SATURATION TO PARTIAL PRESSURE OF ARTERIAL OXYGEN (PaO_2)

Oxygen Saturation (%)	PaO_2 (mm Hg)	Client Status
50	25	Life-threatening hypoxemia
75	40	Moderate hypoxemia
90	55	Mild hypoxemia

Procedure

A sample of arterial blood is obtained by arterial puncture. A sterile needle (connected to a heparinized syringe) is inserted into one of the superficial arteries (i.e., radial, brachial, or femoral) (Fig. 59–14). Arterial blood is differentiated from venous blood by its bright red color. The radial artery is most commonly used because it is readily accessible, is easily palpated, and is associated with fewer complications. Low complication rates are related to ease of access and presence of collateral circulation via the ulnar artery. Send the sample to the laboratory immediately on ice. For serial ABG analyses or ongoing respiratory monitoring, multiple punctures may be avoided by using an arterial line (i.e., a sterile cannula inserted into one of the arteries).

A systematic approach to ABG interpretation, in conjunction with the client's overall status, can lead to the identification of potentially life-threatening abnormalities. First, assess the client's oxygenation status. Acid-base interpretation then follows to evaluate imbalances. Include the following steps in the ABG analysis: PaO_2, pH, $PaCO_2$, HCO_3^-, the presence and degree of compensation, and identification of the primary disorder.

The physician or other clinician skilled in arterial puncture collects the blood sample. In most hospitals, physicians are the only personnel allowed to draw from the femoral artery; nurses and respiratory therapists with special training can take radial or brachial samples.

Preprocedure Care

Educate the client about the procedure and the need for the test. Explain that the needle-stick will be painful for a moment and that it is necessary to hold very still during the procedure to avoid inadvertent injury to the nerves, vessels, or tendons. After the test is completed, tell the client that pressure must be held at the puncture site for 5 to 10 minutes and it may be uncomfortable.

An Allen test must be completed before the procedure is initiated (see Fig. 59–14*A–C*). Before the sample is drawn, treat the site with a disinfectant and allow to dry. Position the area to facilitate the puncture. Help the client remain calm during the test by explaining what is happening. If the client is anxious about the test or other problems and is hyperventilating, the results of the test may be altered. The amount of blood needed for the sample varies from laboratory to laboratory but may be as small as 0.5 ml or as large as 10 ml.

Postprocedure Care

After the sample is drawn, apply continuous pressure to the site for 5 minutes for radial and brachial sites and 10 minutes for femoral sites. Pressure bandages are com-

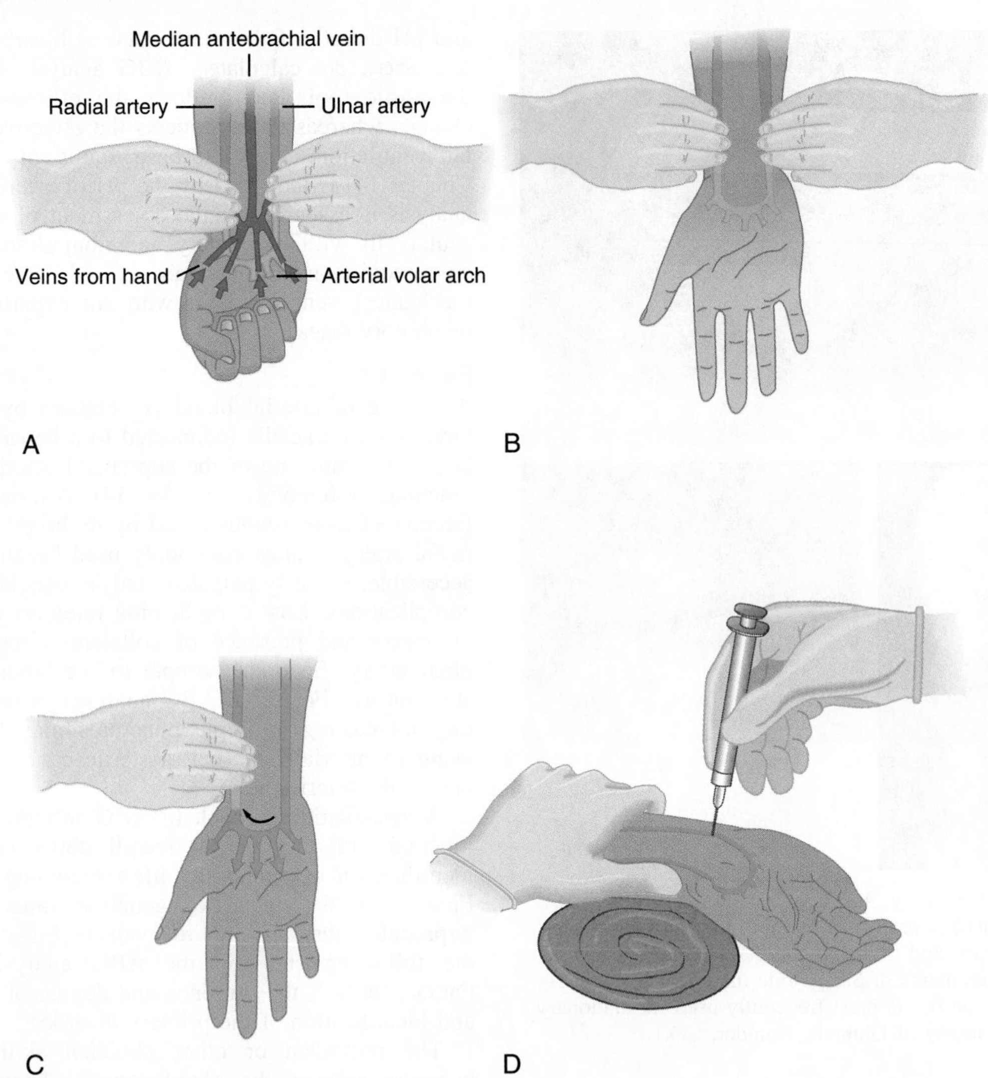

FIGURE 59–14 Obtaining a sample of arterial blood by arterial puncture. First, perform Allen's test, a quick assessment of collateral circulation in the hand. This test is essential before radial artery puncture. *A,* Occlude both the radial and the ulnar arteries with your fingers. Ask the client to close the hand into a fist. *B,* When the client opens the hand with the arteries still occluded, the hand is pale. *C,* When you release either the radial or the ulnar artery, the client's hand should become pink because of collateral circulation. Assess the patency of each of the two arteries in this way, one at a time. *D,* If collateral circulation is adequate, you can draw arterial blood from the radial artery with a heparinized needle and syringe, as shown.

monly used. If the client has a tendency to bleed or is receiving anticoagulant medication, pressure is needed for a longer period.

When interpreting the results, note whether the client is receiving oxygen; record the amount and source of oxygen on the laboratory request form. The results are evaluated in light of the oxygen needed. For example, if the PaO_2 is 85 mm Hg with 50% oxygen, the client has a more significant problem with oxygen transport than a client whose PaO_2 is 85 mm Hg with room air (21% oxygen).

Complications of arterial sampling include bleeding or hematoma formation at the site and injury to the artery and surrounding structures. Report any of these signs to the physician.

Ventilation-Perfusion Lung Scan

Ventilation-perfusion (V/Q) scanning is used to assess lung ventilation and lung perfusion. V/Q scans are valuable in identifying pulmonary embolism, pulmonary infarction, emphysema, fibrosis, and bronchiectasis. Quantitative perfusion scans may be helpful in preoperative assessment of clients undergoing surgical resection of thoracic malignancy.

Procedure

The scan consists of two parts, which may be done together or separately: (1) assessment of the distribution of ventilation (ventilation scan) and (2) assessment of the pulmonary vasculature (perfusion scan).

Ventilation Scan. Radioactive gas is inhaled and produces an image of the areas where ventilation is occurring. Assessment of the pattern of deposition of radioactive gas in the alveoli is also possible.

Ventilation images are compared with the pictures taken during the perfusion scan. The same amount of radioactivity should be discernible on both ventilation and perfusion pictures. If there are areas in which there is ventilation but little or no perfusion, a pulmonary embolus is suspected (Fig. 59–15). Further assessment may be needed. If there is doubt about the cause of impaired perfusion, pulmonary angiography may be needed.

Perfusion Scan. Radiologic material (non–iodine-based) is injected intravenously and carried into the pulmonary vasculature. Decreased blood flow to any part of the lungs is revealed as a decrease in the amount of radioactivity shown on either the x-ray film with use of a rectilinear scanner or on Polaroid film with use of a gamma or scintillation camera. Scanning is done in both the anterior and posterior views.

PREPROCEDURE CARE

Explain the procedure to the client. The test is painless except for local discomfort when radiologic material is injected for the perfusion scan. The client will hear clicking noises during the scan, but the noise is not loud. If the client has dyspnea while lying down, reassure the client that sitting up is possible during the procedure. Radiation exposure is minimal. The client may remain dressed with all metal items removed. The procedure takes 30 to 60 minutes to complete.

■ TESTS TO EVALUATE ANATOMIC STRUCTURES

Diagnostic tests used to evaluate anatomic structures include:

- Radiographic imaging
- Radionuclide studies
- Endoscopy
- Alveolar lavage

Chest X-ray Studies

Chest x-ray studies provide information about the chest that may not be available through other assessment means and may be able to graphically illustrate the cause of respiratory dysfunction. Chest films may reveal abnormalities when there are no physical manifestations of pulmonary disease.

Chest films show the bony structures (e.g., ribs, sternum, clavicles, scapulae, and upper portion of the humerus). The vertebral column is visible vertically through the middle of the thorax. The two hemidiaphragms normally appear rounded, smooth, and sharply defined, with

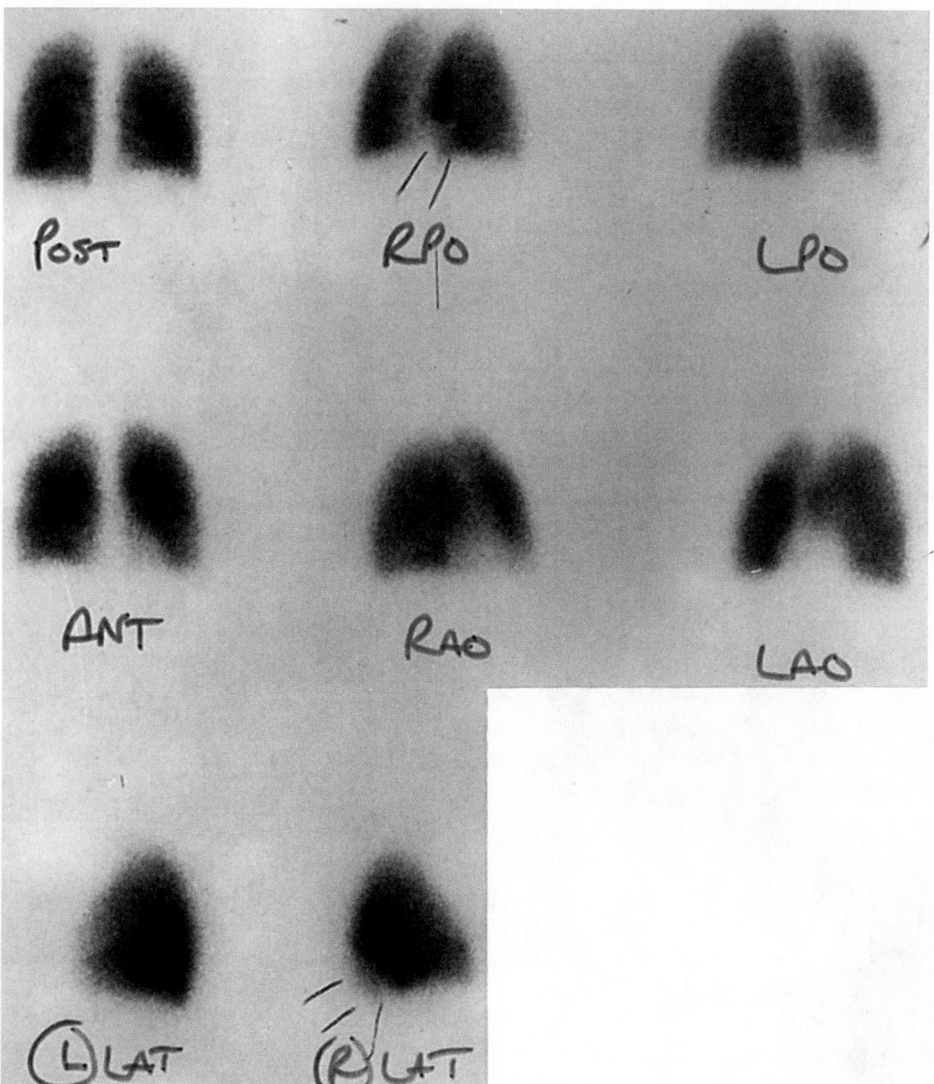

FIGURE 59–15 A ventilation-perfusion scan with technetium 99m. This upright radionuclide pulmonary perfusion study indicates a perfusion deficit of the right posterior basilar segment of the lung, suggesting a pulmonary embolism or pneumonia. This client then underwent a pulmonary venogram (see Chapter 61) that documented the presence of pulmonary embolism.

the right hemidiaphragm slightly higher than the left. The junction of the rib cage and the diaphragm, called the costophrenic angle, is normally clearly visible and angled. Heart tissue is dense and appears white but less intensely white than bone. The heart shadow is normally clearly outlined, extends primarily onto the left side of the thorax, and occupies no more than one third of the chest width. Close observation shows the trachea in the upper middle chest almost superimposed above the cervical and thoracic vertebrae. The trachea bifurcates at the level of the fourth thoracic vertebra into the right and left mainstem bronchi. The pulmonary blood vessels, bronchi, and lymph nodes are located in the hilum on both the right and left sides of the midthorax. Lung tissue appears black on x-ray film. Vascular lung structures are visible as white, thin, wispy strings fanning out from the hilum (Fig. 59–16).

Chest x-ray studies may be performed:

- As part of a routine screening procedure
- When pulmonary disease is suspected
- To monitor the status of respiratory disorders and abnormalities (e.g., pleural effusion, atelectasis, and tubercular lesions)
- To confirm endotracheal or tracheostomy tube placement
- After traumatic chest injury
- In any other situation in which radiographic information helps in the management of a respiratory problem

PROCEDURE

Routine adult chest x-ray studies are performed with the client standing or sitting facing the x-ray film, with the chest and shoulders in direct contact with the film cassette. Several positions are possible.

Posteroanterior View. The client's shoulders are rotated forward to pull the scapulae away from the lung field. The x-ray beam penetrates from the back, for the posteroanterior (PA) position. The radiograph is usually taken on full inspiration, which causes the diaphragm to move downward. Radiographs taken on expiration are sometimes requested in order to demonstrate the degree of diaphragm movement or to assist in the assessment and diagnosis of pneumothorax.

Anteroposterior View. For clients who cannot be transported to the radiology department, portable chest radiography may be performed. These radiographs are usually taken with the film placed behind the client and the x-ray beam entering from the front of the chest—the AP position. Because the x-ray beam enters from the front, the heart appears larger than it really is and larger than on a PA view.

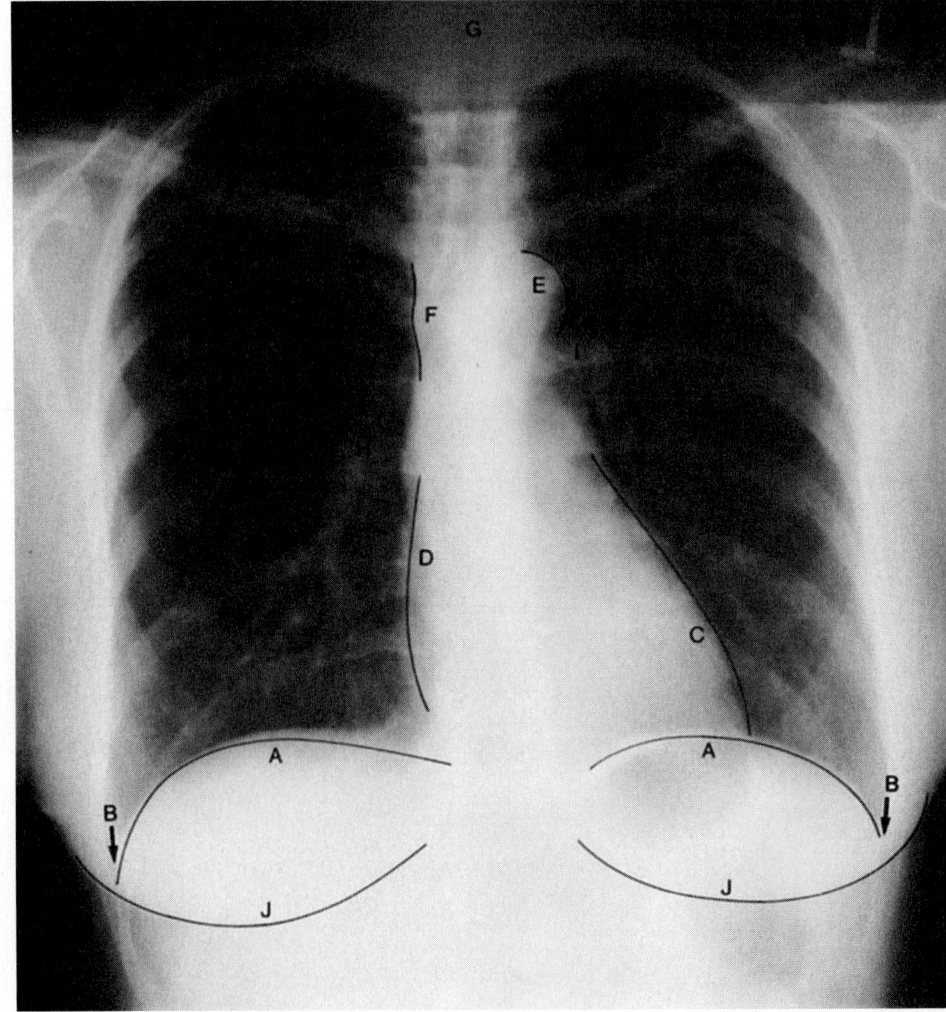

FIGURE 59–16 A normal chest x-ray film taken from the posteroanterior view. The backward "L" in the upper right corner is placed on the film to indicate the left side of the client's chest. A, diaphragm: B, costophrenic angle; C, left ventricle; D, right atrium; E, aortic arch; F, superior vena cava; G, trachea; H, right bronchus; I, left bronchus; J, breast shadows.

Lateral View. The lateral view usually accompanies a standard PA view. It is taken from the right or left side of the chest. The arms are raised above the head, and the side of the chest is placed against the film. The lateral view allows better visualization of the heart and the dome of the diaphragm. In conjunction with a PA film, a lateral radiograph gives a three-dimensional view, allowing more specific identification of the location of an abnormality.

Lateral Decubitus View. The lateral decubitus (from the Latin, lying down) position may be used when it is necessary to determine whether opaque areas on the pleura are due to solid or liquid media. The client lies on the right or left side, depending on which side of the chest is being assessed. In a left lateral decubitus position, the client lies on the left side.

Oblique View. The oblique position is used to visualize behind and around underlying structures. The shoulders are rotated to either the right or left of the film. By turning the client, the examiner can shift the angle at which the x-ray beam passes through the chest. In a right oblique position, the right side is closest to the film. The view may be taken from an anterior or posterior position.

Lordotic View. The lordotic position, consisting of a forward curve of the lumbar spine, is useful if clearer visualization of the upper lung fields is needed. The angle of the cathode x-ray tube is lowered and the beam directed at an upward angle. This angle results in removal of the clavicles and first and second ribs from the field of vision.

PREPROCEDURE CARE

Instruct the client about the need for radiologic testing. The test is painless, and exposure to radiation is minimal. The client must remove all jewelry and underclothes and put on a gown. Assess the client's pregnancy status; pregnant women should not be exposed to radiation. All gonads should be shielded during the study. The test takes 5 to 10 minutes to complete.

Ultrasonography

Ultrasonic waves (sound waves too high in frequency for a human ear to detect) are used diagnostically to assess various body structures. Ultrasonography may be used in conjunction with other pulmonary diagnostic procedures, such as thoracentesis and pleural biopsy, to assess fluid or fibrotic abnormalities. Ultrasonography is especially helpful and accurate in detecting the amount and location of 50 ml or less of pleural fluid. In comparison, positive detection by chest radiography requires at least 500 ml of liquid. If the technique is used in combination with thoracentesis, the ultrasonographer can determine the best location for needle placement as well as the depth of the fluid. This approach facilitates obtaining an adequate amount of fluid for laboratory analysis without unnecessary puncturing and probing.

The client may remain dressed or put on a gown (see Chapter 11 for client preparation needed for ultrasonography). The test takes 15 to 30 minutes to complete.

Fluoroscopy

Fluoroscopy makes it possible for the chest and intrathoracic structures to be observed while they function dynamically (see Chapter 11). Fluoroscopy is not used routinely; rather, it is used when continuous observation of the thorax is an advantage (e.g., observing transbronchial passage of biopsy forceps during bronchoscopy). Other uses for fluoroscopy include:

- Observing the diaphragm during inspiration and expiration
- Detecting mediastinal movement during deep breathing
- Assessing the heart, blood vessels, and related structures
- Identifying esophageal abnormalities
- Detecting mediastinal masses

Instruct the client about the need for this test. The test is painless. Sometimes a radiopaque (non–iodine-based) contrast agent is administered intravenously to help distinguish the structures being assessed. The client must remove all jewelry and underclothes and put on a gown. The test takes 30 to 45 minutes to complete. Exposure to radiation is minimal, but pregnant women should not be exposed to fluoroscopy.

Images obtained by fluoroscopy are not as clear and definitive as those obtained on a standard chest film. If abnormalities are discovered, still photographs and cinefluorography may be used to obtain a permanent record. Cinefluorographs are motion pictures that allow more leisurely study and restudy of the area photographed without exposure of radiology personnel or clients to unnecessary radiation.

Computed Tomography

Computed tomography (CT) provides more sophisticated tomography than is possible with conventional x-ray equipment (see Chapter 11).

CT scans are particularly helpful in identifying peripheral (e.g., pleural) or mediastinal disorders. Special techniques can be used to view pulmonary nodules. Thin cuts of CT scans are used in diagnosing interstitial lung disorders such as pulmonary fibrosis and bronchiectasis.

Magnetic Resonance Imaging

Magnetic resonance imaging (MRI) employs magnetic fields rather than radiation to create images of body structures. MRI is used in much the same way as CT. MRI is more definitive than CT because it creates more detailed images of anatomic structures. See Chapter 11 for a detailed discussion of MRI and client preparation.

Gallium Scans

Gallium scanning is usually done 24 to 48 hours after intravenous injection of radioactive gallium citrate. Many organs take up radioactive gallium, as do some tumors and areas of inflammation. A gallium scan might be used to distinguish embolism from pneumonitis as the cause of an infiltrate on a chest radiograph. Gallium has an affinity for areas of inflammation, such as those associated with pneumonia; however, there is little inflammation with a nonseptic pulmonary embolism. Therefore, gallium accumulates around pneumonitis but not around a pulmonary embolism. The usefulness of gallium scanning in clinical pulmonary assessment is limited.

Educate the client about the test. The test is painless except for local pain at the injection site. Gallium is not iodine-based and produces no side effects. The client returns for serial scans at 24, 48, or 72 hours. Scanning is performed with the client supine. The client may remain dressed but must remove all metal objects. The scan takes 45 to 60 minutes to complete.

Bronchoscopy

PROCEDURE

Bronchoscopy involves passage of a lighted bronchoscope into the bronchial tree (Fig. 59–17). It may be performed with rigid steel or flexible fiberoptic instruments. Bronchoscopy may be performed for diagnostic or therapeutic purposes. Diagnostic purposes include:

- Examination of tissue
- Further evaluation of a tumor for potential surgical resection
- Collection of tissue specimens for diagnosis
- Evaluation of bleeding sites

Therapeutic bronchoscopy is used to:

- Remove foreign bodies
- Remove thick, viscous secretions
- Treat postoperative atelectasis
- Destroy and remove lesions

PREPROCEDURE CARE

Explain the procedure to the client and family, and obtain informed consent. Instruct the client not to eat or drink anything 6 hours before the test. Explain that the throat may be sore after bronchoscopy and there will be some initial difficulty in swallowing. Before sedation, the client should remove dentures, contact lenses, and other prostheses. The client undresses and puts on a gown. Local anesthesia and intravenous sedation are used to suppress cough and to relieve anxiety. A topical anesthetic agent is also sprayed into the back of the throat. The test takes 30 to 45 minutes to complete.

During the procedure, the client lies supine with the head hyperextended. Monitor vital signs, talk to and reassure the client, and assist the physician as necessary.

POSTPROCEDURE CARE

After the procedure, monitor vital signs according to agency protocol. Observe the client for signs of respiratory distress, including dyspnea, changes in respiratory rate, use of accessory muscles, and changes in or absent lung sounds. Expectorated secretions are inspected for evidence of hemoptysis. Nothing is given by mouth until the cough and swallow reflexes have returned, usually in 1 to 2 hours. When the client can swallow, feeding may begin with ice chips and small sips of water.

Lung sounds are monitored for 24 hours. Development of asymmetrical or adventitious sounds should be reported to the physician. Pneumothorax has been noted after bronchoscopy.

Alveolar Lavage

Sterile saline can be injected during bronchoscopy to wash tissues. The saline is aspirated and examined for

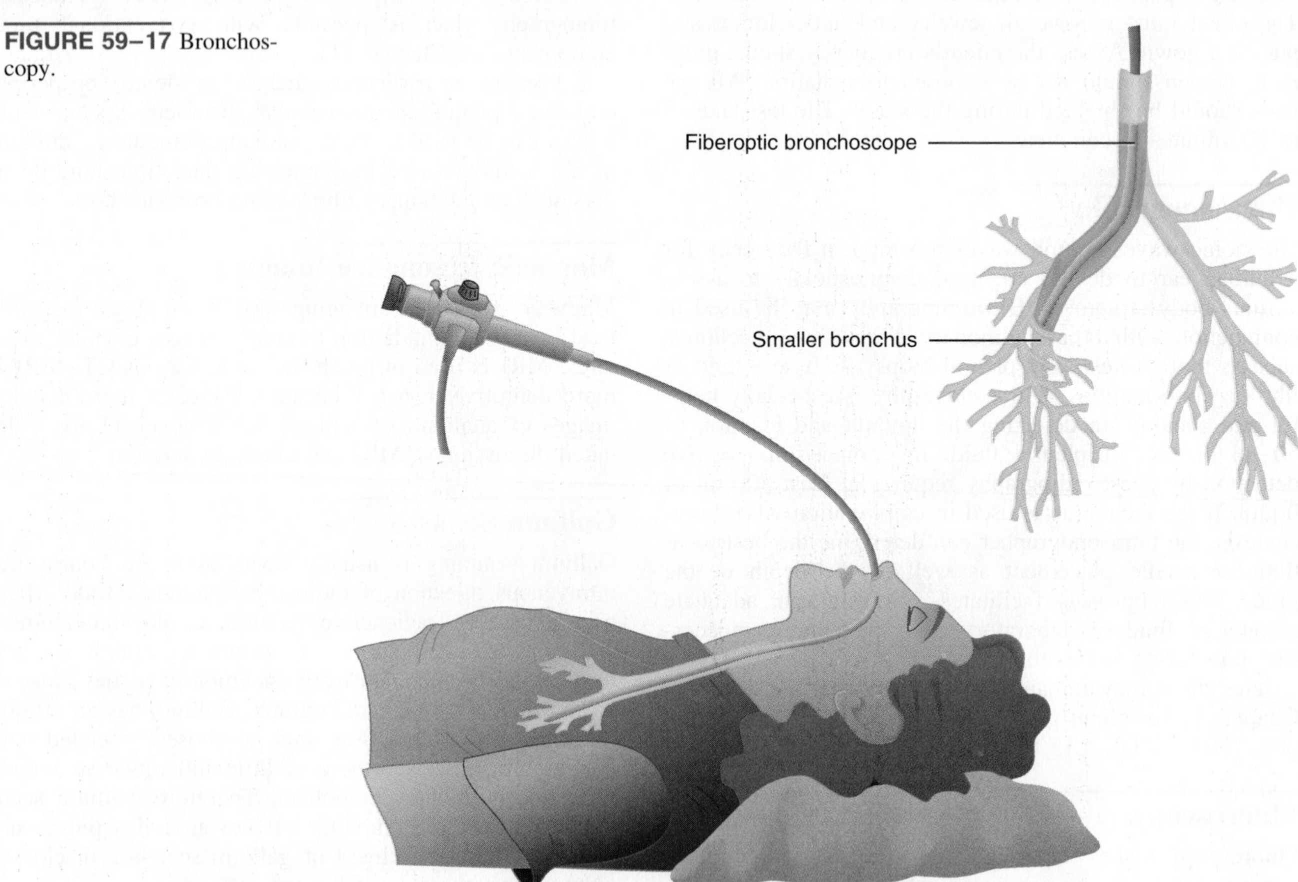

FIGURE 59–17 Bronchoscopy.

atypical cells. Alveolar lavage may be used in the diagnosis of interstitial lung disease, sarcoidosis, hypersensitivity pneumonitis, and *P. carinii* pneumonia. No additional client preparation is needed because this procedure is done during bronchoscopy.

Endoscopic Thoracotomy

Endoscopic thoracotomy is a diagnostic procedure that is an alternative to open-lung biopsy and thoracotomy for pleural surface disorders.

PROCEDURE

Typically, three small incisions are made into the middle chest wall. A scope attached to a camera and video projector is inserted through the first incision to inspect tissue, and tissues are manipulated and biopsy specimens obtained through the other incisions. A chest tube is inserted to promote lung reexpansion. Advantages of the procedure include reduced anesthesia time, less pain, and shortened hospital stay. In addition, biopsy specimens may be obtained from the lower lobes, which is not routinely done during open-lung biopsy procedures.

PREPROCEDURE CARE

Instruct the client about the need for this test, and obtain a signed informed consent form. Endoscopic thoracotomy is a surgical procedure, and general anesthesia is administered (see Chapter 15 for a discussion of the needs of the surgical patient). Explain that a chest tube will be in place and that it will be necessary to perform coughing and deep-breathing exercises.

Pulmonary Angiography

Sometimes the vascular structure of the thorax must be assessed. Angiography and other procedures designed to examine specific vascular structures (i.e., aortography for the aorta) all use similar techniques.

Pulmonary angiography may be done to detect the following:

- Congenital abnormalities of the pulmonary vascular tree
- Abnormalities of the pulmonary venous circulation
- Acquired diseases of the pulmonary arterial and venous circulation (e.g., primary pulmonary arterial hypertension)
- Destructive effects of emphysema
- Potential benefits of resection for bronchogenic carcinoma
- Peripheral pulmonary lesions
- Extent of thromboembolism in the lungs

PROCEDURE

Contrast medium is injected into the vascular system through an indwelling catheter. During pulmonary angiography, the catheter may be inserted either peripherally or directly into the main pulmonary artery or one of its branches. The contrast agent is injected while cinefluorographs or still photographs are taken. (Pulmonary angiography is discussed in Chapter 61.)

Instruct the client about the need for this test, and obtain informed consent. The test is painless and does not involve exposure to radiation. Further preprocedure and postprocedure care of the client is as for angiography (see Chapter 11).

■ SPECIMEN RECOVERY AND ANALYSIS

The following procedures are used for recovery and analysis of pulmonary specimens:

- Sputum collection
- Thoracentesis
- Biopsy

Sputum Collection

Normally, the goblet cells produce 100 ml of mucus a day, but an infectious process can lead to excessive production of mucus (commonly called *sputum*). Assessment of sputum for bacteria, fungus, or cellular elements guides the treatment of an underlying infection.

PROCEDURE

Inspect the sputum for color, quantity, quality, presence of blood, food particles, or other unusual contents. If possible, sputum should be collected before antimicrobial treatment is begun.

Acid-fast smear and culture specimens are collected in the morning, at which time sputum is more plentiful and concentrated because of pooling through the night. Sputum can be collected by (1) the direct method, (2) the indirect method, or (3) gastric lavage.

PREPROCEDURE CARE

Explain the need for and purpose of this test to the client. When a specimen is obtained by the direct method, the client brushes the teeth to reduce contamination and then coughs into a sputum specimen container. Encourage the client to cough, not spit, in order to obtain sputum. Inhaling nebulized saline or water can be used to thin the sputum to facilitate expectoration.

Indirect techniques for obtaining sputum consist of a sterile suction catheter with an attached sputum trap. Sputum can also be obtained by transtracheal aspiration. A puncture is made with a needle through the cricothyroid membrane into the trachea, and sputum is aspirated.

Although gastric lavage is not a common technique for obtaining sputum, it can be used for uncooperative or extremely ill clients. Lavage is based on the assumption that sputum is swallowed during sleep and sometimes after coughing. A nasogastric tube is inserted by appropriate technique. Gastric juice is aspirated with a syringe and sent to the laboratory. The tube is then removed.

The collected sputum is analyzed for Gram's stain, culture, and sensitivity study. Gram's stain is used to classify bacteria as gram-positive or gram-negative and, along with the sputum culture, provides guidelines for appropriate antimicrobial therapy. After the Gram stain, the sputum is incubated for 24 hours or longer on the appropriate culture medium and studied by a microbiologist. Obtaining a specimen for the culture allows further identification of the infecting organism. When the organism is identified, its sensitivity to antibiotic treatment is tested and an appropriate antibiotic is prescribed.

Identification of organisms that cause tuberculosis and similar diseases (acid-fast bacilli) requires tests other than Gram's stain, culture, and sensitivity study.

Regardless of the technique used to obtain the specimen, note the color, consistency, odor, and amount of sputum obtained.

Nose and Throat Cultures

Bacteria in the nose and throat can be identified by culture during assessment of the upper airway. Some bacteria are normally present (e.g., streptococci, staphylococci, pneumococci, *Haemophilus influenzae,* and *Klebsiella pneumoniae*). Other organisms are abnormal (e.g., those causing diphtheria or tuberculosis).

Swab the nose and throat using a sterile cotton swab. Place the swab in a sterile culture tube. Some laboratories require the swab to be suspended in a tube containing 2 ml of fluid to keep air in the tube moist and prevent evaporation and drying of the specimen. Because the fluid is not a culture medium, the swab should not touch the fluid. If Loeffler's medium is used in the tube (i.e., if diphtheria is suspected), the medium should touch the swab. When culture tubes without fluid are used, take the specimen to the laboratory immediately, where the swab is streaked across a culture plate.

Thoracentesis

Procedure

Thoracentesis is performed to drain fluid or air found in the pleural space. Therapeutic thoracentesis removes an accumulation of pleural fluid or air that has caused lung compression and respiratory distress. When the main goal is to determine the cause of an infection or empyema, diagnostic thoracentesis is performed. The fluid collected is sent to the laboratory for assessment of specific gravity, glucose, protein, and pH; culture; sensitivity study; and cytologic evaluation. The color and consistency of the pleural fluid are also documented.

Preprocedure Care

Obtain informed consent, and instruct the client about the procedure and the need for it. The client must sit upright while leaning over the tray table (Fig. 59–18*A*). In the upright position, pleural fluid accumulates in the base of the thorax. Alternatively, place the client in a recumbent position with the arm resting under the head. Insertion of the needle is painful. Explain the importance of holding still during the procedure. Sudden movement may force the needle through the pleural space and injure the visceral pleura or lung parenchyma. State that you will help to hold the client, and provide reassurance. The test takes 5 to 15 minutes to complete.

During the procedure, assist the physician; monitor vital signs; and observe for dyspnea, complaints of difficulty breathing, nausea, or pain.

Postprocedure Care

After the procedure, the client is usually turned onto the unaffected side for 1 hour to facilitate lung expansion. Assess vital signs according to the facility's policy. Carefully assess the respiratory rate and character and breath sounds. Tachypnea, dyspnea, cyanosis, retractions, or diminished breath sounds, which may indicate pneumothorax, should be reported to the physician.

Record the amount of fluid withdrawn as fluid output. Chest films may be obtained to evaluate the degree of lung reexpansion or pneumothorax. Subcutaneous emphysema may follow this procedure, because air in the pleu-

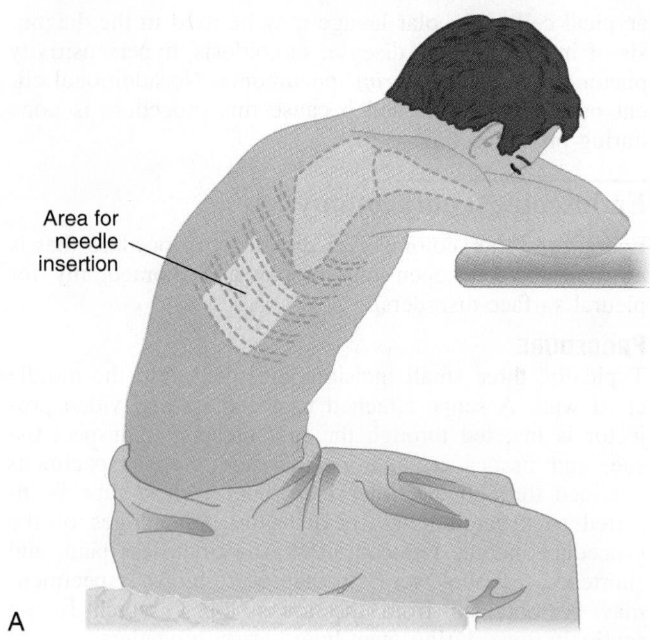

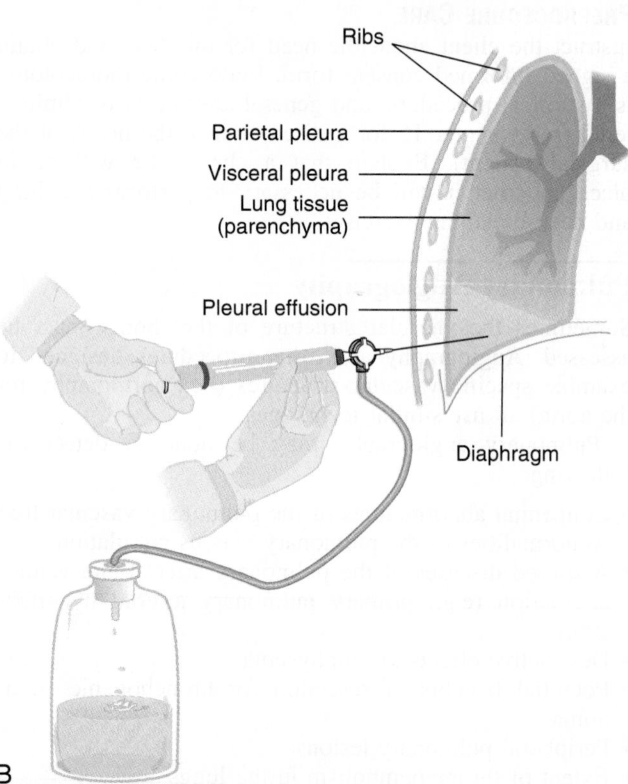

FIGURE 59–18 Thoracentesis. *A,* Correct position of the client for the procedure. The arms are raised and crossed. The head rests on the folded arms. This position allows the chest wall to be pulled outward in an expanded position. If an institutional overbed table is not available, you may leave the client's arms down, but position them toward the client's hips or cross them in front of the chest. *B,* Usual site for insertion of a thoracentesis needle for a right-sided effusion. The actual site varies, depending on the location and volume of the effusion. The needle is kept as far away from the diaphragm as possible but is inserted close to the base of the effusion so that gravity can help with drainage.

ral cavity leaks into subcutaneous tissues. The tissues feel like lumpy paper and crackle when palpated (crepitus). Usually, subcutaneous emphysema causes no problem unless it is increasing and constricting vital organs (e.g., trachea). Clients often need reassurance about this disorder.

If the client has pleural effusion related to a malignancy, cytotoxic medications may be inserted into the pleural space after thoracentesis. Some of these agents burn; with others, the client must roll about in order to have the medication coat the entire pleural space. Review the interventions used with the various medications.

Biopsy

Biopsy specimens may be taken from various respiratory tissues for examination. As mentioned previously, specimens from tracheobronchial structures may be obtained during bronchoscopy. Biopsy specimens of scalene and mediastinal nodes may be obtained (with local anesthesia) for pathologic study, culture, or cytologic assessment.

Pleural Biopsy

Procedure

Pleural biopsies may be performed surgically through a small thoracotomy incision or during thoracentesis with the use of a Cope needle. Needle biopsy is a relatively safe, simple diagnostic procedure that can help determine the cause of pleural effusions. The needle removes a small fragment of parietal pleura, which is used for microscopic cellular examination and culture. If bacteriologic studies are needed, the biopsy specimen should be obtained before chemotherapy is begun.

Preprocedure Care

Obtain informed consent, and instruct the client about the need for and purpose of the test. Preparation and positioning of a client for pleural biopsy are similar to those for thoracentesis. The test is painful, and the client must hold still. Assist and reassure the client. The test takes 15 to 30 minutes to complete.

Postprocedure Care

Rare complications include temporary pain associated with intercostal nerve injury, pneumothorax, and hemothorax. After the biopsy procedure, observe for indications of complications (e.g., dyspnea, pallor, diaphoresis, excessive pain). A pneumothorax associated with needle biopsy may develop. Chest tubes and chest drainage equipment must be available. Follow-up chest x-ray studies are usually done after the procedure. Development of hemothorax is indicated by a substantial increase in fluid in the pleural space and requires immediate thoracentesis.

Lung Biopsy

As with pleural biopsy, lung biopsy may be done by surgical exposure of the lung (open-lung biopsy) with or without endoscopy using a needle designed to remove a core of lung tissue. The tissue is examined for abnormal cellular structure and bacteria. Lung biopsies are most often performed to identify pulmonary tumors or parenchymal changes (e.g., sarcoidosis).

Procedure

Needle puncture (aspiration) biopsy of chest lesions is done with fluoroscopy. After a lesion is identified on a chest film and localized by fluoroscopy, topical anesthesia is administered and the needle is inserted through the chest wall into the lung tissue and lesion. A small sample of cells is aspirated for microscopic study, and the needle is withdrawn. Aspiration biopsy may enable definitive diagnosis of malignant neoplasms, granulomas, or other nonmalignant growths. Possible complications of needle aspiration lung biopsy are hemoptysis, hemothorax, and pneumothorax.

Postprocedure Care

After the procedure, examine any sputum closely for evidence of blood. Observe for respiratory distress (may indicate pneumothorax). Monitor the client's vital signs, breath sounds, skin color, and temperature.

CONCLUSIONS

Respiratory assessment begins with obtaining a thorough client history. One of the most essential aspects of history-taking is determining the degree of dyspnea and the impact it has on activities of daily living. Note the client's smoking history and occupational risks because they are common risk factors for respiratory disorders. The chest is inspected for obvious deformity and shape. Percussion, palpation, and auscultation assist in locating areas of possible fluid accumulation or consolidation that interfere with breathing.

Chest x-ray studies, bronchoscopy, pulmonary function tests, and ABG analysis are common diagnostic assessments. Educate the client about the diagnostic modalities, and monitor for potential complications after the study.

BIBLIOGRAPHY

1. Bates, B., et al. (1998). *A guide to physical assessment and history taking* (7th ed.). Philadelphia: J. B. Lippincott.
2. Burton, G., Hodgkin, J., & Ward, J. (1997). *Respiratory care: A guide to clinical practice.* Philadelphia: J. B. Lippincott.
3. Gift, A. G., & Narsavage, G. (1998). Validity of the numeric rating scale as a measure of dyspnea. *American Journal of Critical Care, 7*(3), 200–204.
4. Gift, A. G., & Nield, M. D. (1991). Dyspnea: A case for nursing diagnosis status. *Nursing Diagnosis, 2*(2), 66–71.
5. Govette, L. A. (1994). Back to basics: Interpreting chest x-ray films. *Journal of the American Academy of Physician Assistants, 7*(3), 205–207.
6. Guyton, A. C. (1996). *Textbook of medical physiology* (9th ed.). Philadelphia: W. B. Saunders.

6a. Horne, C., & Derrico, D. (1999). Mastering ABGS: The art of arterial blood gas measurement. *American Journal of Nursing, 99*(8), 26–33.

7. Jarvis, C. (2000). (3rd ed.). *Physical examination and health assessment.* Philadelphia: W. B. Saunders.
8. Kelly-Heidenthal, P., & O'Connor, M. (1994). Nursing assessment of portable AP chest x-rays. *Dimensions of Critical Care Nursing, 13*(3), 127–132.
9. Lareau, S., et al. (1998). Development and testing of the modified version of the Pulmonary Functional Status and Dyspnea Questionnaire (PFSDQ). *Heart and Lung Journal of Critical Care, 27*(3), 159–168.
10. Malley, W. (1990). *Clinical blood gases: Application and noninvasive alternates.* Philadelphia: W. B. Saunders.
11. McCord, M., & Cronin-Stubbs, D. (1992). Operationalizing dyspnea: Focus on measurement. *Heart and Lung, 21*(2), 167.
12. Murray, J. F., & Nadel, J. A. (1994). *The textbook of respiratory medicine* (2nd ed.). Philadelphia: W. B. Saunders.

13. O'Hanlon-Nichols, T. (1998). Basic assessment series: The adult pulmonary system. *American Journal of Nursing, 98*(2), 39–45.
14. Owen, A. (1998). Respiratory assessment revisited. *Nursing, 28*(4), 48–49.
15. Pierson, D., & Kacmarek, R. (1999). *Foundations of respiratory care.* New York: McGraw-Hill.
16. Ripamonti, C., & Bruera, E. (1997). Dyspnea: Pathophysiology and assessment. *Journal of Pain and Symptom Management, 13*(4), 220–232.
17. Ruppel, G. (1994). *Manual of pulmonary function testing* (5th ed.). St. Louis: Mosby–Year Book.
18. Shapiro, B. A., et al. (1991). *Clinical application of respiratory care* (4th ed.). St. Louis: Mosby–Year Book.
19. Shapiro, B. A., et al. (1994). *Clinical application of blood gases* (5th ed.). St. Louis: Mosby–Year Book.
20. Shortall, S. P., & Perkins, L. A. (1999). Interpreting the ins and outs of pulmonary function tests. *Nursing, 29*(12), 41–47.
21. Speck, D., et al. (1993). *Respiratory control: Central peripheral mechanisms.* Lexington, KY: University of Kentucky.
22. Von Rueden, K. T. (1990). Noninvasive assessment of gas exchange in the critically ill. *AACN Clinical Issues in Critical Care Nursing, 1*(2), 239-247.
23. West, J. B. (1995). *Respiratory physiology* (5th ed.). Baltimore: Williams & Wilkins.
24. Wong, F. W. H. (1999). A new approach to ABG interpretation. *American Journal of Nursing, 99*(8), 34–36.

www.wbsaunders.com/SIMON/Black/medsurg

REMEMBER *to check out your* **Companion CD ROM**

CHAPTER 60

Management of Clients with Upper Airway Disorders

Linda K. Clarke

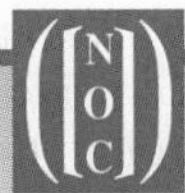

NURSING OUTCOMES CLASSIFICATION (NOC) for Nursing Diagnoses—Clients with Upper Airway Disorders

Altered Nutrition: Less Than Body Requirements
Nutritional Status: Food and Fluid Intake
Anxiety and Fear
Anxiety Control
Coping
Fear Control
Social Interaction Skills
Impaired Verbal Communication
Communication Ability
Communication Ability: Expressive Ability
Ineffective Airway Clearance
Aspiration Control
Respiratory Status: Airway Patency
Risk for Aspiration
Respiratory Status: Gas Exchange
Risk Control
Risk Detection
Risk for Constipation
Hydration
Mobility Level
Nutritional Status: Food and Fluid Intake
Risk Control
Risk Detection
Risk for Impaired Gas Exchange
Respiratory Status: Gas Exchange
Vital Signs Status
Risk for Ineffective Management of Therapeutic Regimen (Families)
Family Functioning
Family Participation in Professional Care
Risk for Ineffective Management of Therapeutic Regimen (Individuals)
Compliance Behavior
Knowledge: Treatment Regimen
Risk for Infection
Immobility Consequences: Physiologic
Knowledge: Infection Control
Nutritional Status
Risk Control
Risk Detection
Tissue Integrity: Skin and Mucous Membranes
Wound Healing

The initial complaint for clients with disorders of the upper airway is a problem with breathing. Obstructions to nasal breathing are observed in clients with nasal polyps, deviated nasal septum, or nasal fractures. After surgical interventions, nasal breathing continues to be compromised because of postoperative edema. Laryngeal disorders may also result in breathing problems. Tumors of the larynx create obstruction to air entering the trachea, as well as to air being exhaled. Vocal cord paralysis and laryngospasm may also affect the passage of air through the larynx and vocal cords. Clients with epistaxis and sinusitis exhibit nasal bleeding and drainage, respectively, and may have fever and pain. Inflammation associated with these problems results in obstruction to breathing. Surgical intervention and nasal packing further exacerbate breathing problems.

METHODS OF CONTROLLING THE AIRWAY

Airway obstruction can be prevented or treated with many modalities. Antihistamine treatment is discussed in Chapter 76. Intubation to support ventilation and oxygenation is discussed in Chapter 63. This chapter begins with tracheostomy because it is a common method of airway management in hospitalized clients.

TRACHEOSTOMY

A *tracheotomy* is a surgical incision into the trachea through overlying skin and muscles for airway management. A *tracheostomy* is the surgical creation of a stoma, or opening, into the trachea through the overlying skin (Fig. 60–1). These terms are often used interchangeably. For simplicity, the term "tracheostomy" is used here.

Tracheostomy can be performed as an emergency procedure or as an elective procedure, depending on the indication. A tracheostomy provides the best route for long-term airway maintenance. Because of the many indications for this procedure, it is discussed at the beginning of this chapter rather than under a particular disorder. Indications for tracheostomy include:

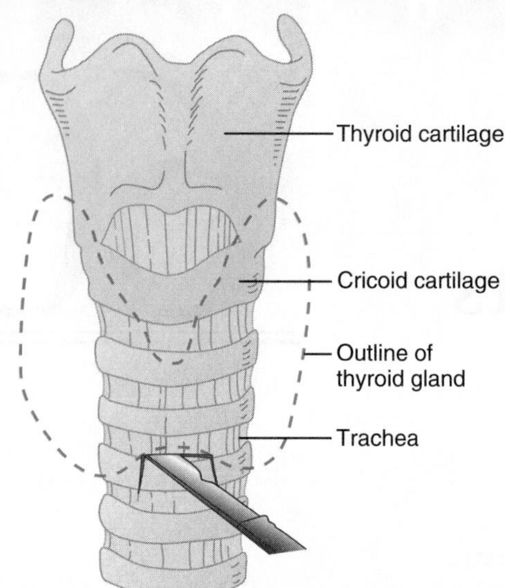

FIGURE 60–1 Incision for a tracheostomy is made through the fibrous tissue above the third tracheal cartilage. Two small vertical incisions create a flap that can be closed later.

- Relief of acute or chronic upper airway obstruction
- Access for continuous mechanical ventilation
- Prevention of aspiration pneumonia
- Promotion of pulmonary hygiene
- Bilateral vocal cord paralysis
- Prolonged endotracheal tube insertion resulting in erosion or pain

A tracheostomy is by far the most satisfactory artificial airway. It bypasses the upper airway and glottis, making stabilization, suction, and the attachment of respiratory equipment much easier than with other types of artificial airways. The client can eat and, with some adjustments, talk.

■ TRACHEOSTOMY TUBES

The tracheostomy opening is fitted with a tube to maintain airway patency. Tracheostomy tubes vary in their composition, number of separate parts, shape, and size. Tracheostomy tubes are chosen specifically for each client. Incorrectly fitted tubes can precipitate permanent or life-threatening damage.

The diameter of a tracheostomy tube should be smaller than the trachea so that it will lie comfortably within the tracheal lumen. Air should be able to pass between the outer wall of the tracheostomy tube and the tracheal mucosa. Although there is no standard tracheostomy tube sizing system, all packages indicate the inner and outer diameters in millimeters.

The length and curve of a tracheostomy tube are important. Tracheostomy tubes may be long (e.g., Hollinger tube, Shiley single-cannula tube) or short. They may be angled, the angle ranging from 50 to 90 degrees. Short to moderately short tubes with an angle of about 60 degrees are most often used. A tube must be long enough to avoid dislodgment into paratracheal tissue when the client coughs or turns the head. The lower end of a tracheostomy tube should be located above the carina. The tube's curve must allow the tip to be in a straight line with the trachea, rather than pressing on the anterior or posterior tracheal wall.

Tracheostomy tubes may be cuffed or uncuffed. An inflated cuff permits mechanical ventilation and protects the lower airway by creating a seal between the upper and lower airways (Box 60–1). Tracheostomy cuffs do not hold the tube in place.

Tracheostomy tubes are made of various substances, such as nonreactive plastic, stainless steel, sterling silver, or silicone. Plastic tubes are disposable and used for only one person. Metal tubes may be reused after being sterilized.

Universal Tracheostomy Tube

The most common tube is a universal, or standard, tracheostomy tube (Fig. 60–2) having three parts: (1) outer cannula with cuff, flange, and pilot tube; (2) inner cannula; and (3) obturator. The parts fit together as one unit and may not be interchanged with other units. Therefore, all three parts of each individual set are kept together.

The outer cannula fits in the tracheostomy stoma to keep it open. The outer cannula has a flange or neckplate that fits flush with the neck and has holes on each side to attach the securing tapes or ties. A tracheostomy tube must be secured in place to prevent accidental extubation, excessive motion, or misalignment. Cloth tape or commercially available self-fastening (Velcro) ties may be used.

The obturator is placed into the outer tube before insertion. Its rounded tip smooths the end of the cannula and facilitates nontraumatic insertion of the tube into the stoma. The obturator is removed immediately after insertion, to open the tube. Place the obturator in a plastic wrapper and tape it to the head of the client's bed in a conspicuous place. If the tracheostomy tube is accidentally displaced, the obturator can be immediately placed into the outer cannula for quick reinsertion.

Once the obturator is removed, the inner cannula is placed into the outer cannula. Lock it into place to prevent accidental removal (e.g., when the client coughs). Frequent removal and cleaning of the inner cannula maintain airway patency. At the distal end, most inner cannulas have a standard 15-mm adapter that fits respiratory therapy and anesthesiology equipment.

Single-Cannula Tracheostomy Tube

A single-cannula tracheostomy tube is slightly longer than a standard, double-cannula tube. Because it does not have an inner cannula that can be cleaned to eliminate secretions, a single-cannula tube should not be used in clients with excessive secretions or difficulty clearing secretions. Clients in whom a single-cannula tube is used must have continuous supplemental humidification to prevent obstruction by accumulated secretions. The longer single-cannula tube is used in the client with a thick neck or with an altered airway in whom a standard tracheostomy tube would be too short.

Fenestrated Tracheostomy Tube

A fenestrated tracheostomy tube has one large opening (Latin, *fenestra*), or several small ones, on the curvature of the posterior wall of the outer cannula. Fenestrated tubes have an inner cannula and may be cuffed or cuffless. When the inner cannula is removed, the fenestration permits air to flow through both the upper airway and the

BOX 60–1 Inflation and Deflation of Tracheostomy Tube Cuff*

Inflation (Minimal Leak Technique)

Objective

Inflate the cuff with the minimum volume of air required to adequately seal the trachea during positive-pressure ventilation and to prevent aspiration of foreign material while exerting the lowest possible cuff–to–tracheal wall pressure.

Intervention

1. Withdraw all residual air from the cuff.
2. Place 6 cc of air in a syringe.
3. Place the diaphragm of a stethoscope over the client's neck in the area of the tracheostomy tube cuff.
4. On inhalation, slowly inject air through the one-way valve into the pilot line in 1-cc increments.
5. Auscultate the neck area over the cuff.
6. Apply positive pressure to the tracheostomy tube with a manual self-inflating bag. An audible air leak can be heard via the stethoscope unless the cuff is inflated.
7. Continue slowly injecting air until the air leak is no longer present during inhalation.
8. When a leak is no longer auscultated, withdraw a small amount of air from the cuff until a very small leak is heard. This is called a *minimal leak.*
9. Note the amount of air necessary to achieve the minimal leak. This is the *minimal occluding volume* (MOV).
10. Once minimal leak is attained, measure the cuff pressure with a manometer.
11. Routinely measure and document cuff pressures.

Deflation

Objective

Allow air to flow around the tracheostomy tube, to permit phonation and to provide an opportunity to blow secretions above the cuff into the oropharynx, where they can be removed by suctioning.

Intervention

Routinely deflating the cuff is not necessary provided that safe cuff inflation and cuff pressure measurements are performed.

1. Remove the ventilator assembly (if present), and attach a self-inflating bag to the 15-mm adapter on the inner cannula.
2. Hyperoxygenate, hyperinflate, and suction the trachea to remove secretions below the cuff. Remove secretions above the cuff by gently applying suction deep into the oropharynx.
3. Insert an empty syringe into the one-way valve, and pull back on the plunger to remove the air in the cuff. At the same time, apply positive pressure with the manual self-inflating bag. This maneuver blows secretions lying directly above the cuff into the mouth, to prevent secretions accumulated above the cuff from draining into the trachea and lower airway.
4. Suction the oropharynx again.
5. If the person is ventilator-dependent, remember that with the cuff "down" or deflated, a portion of ventilation volume will not reach the lungs. Air will escape through the upper airway, which may compromise the person's respiratory status. This volume loss creates an audible leak. Phonation is possible during the exhalation phase of ventilation.

* The same procedure is used for inflation and deflation of endotracheal tube cuffs.

tracheostomy opening. This permits speech and more effective coughing. This tube may be used while a client is being weaned from a tracheostomy and for a client in whom use of the tracheostomy is expected to be prolonged. When the inner cannula is in place, the fenestration is closed, and the tube functions as a universal tracheostomy tube. For weaning a mechanically ventilated client, remove the inner cannula and deflate the cuff to allow the client to breathe through the fenestrae and around the tube.

TRACHEOSTOMY SPEAKING VALVES

For a "talking tracheostomy," a one-way valve in a plastic T-piece is attached to the 15-mm end of the inner cannula of a universal tracheostomy tube. This modification permits talking without the need to plug the tracheostomy tube. The one-way valve allows air (and the aerosol of supplemental humidification and oxygen) to flow into the arm of the T-piece during inspiration. On exhalation, the one-way valve closes, directing air from the lungs up through the vocal cords and upper airway. Phonation and effective coughing are facilitated by this normal passage of air.

A talking tracheostomy is *never* used unless there is enough room around the tracheostomy tube to permit sufficient air flow for breathing. *Always deflate* a cuffed tracheostomy tube before the client uses the talking tracheostomy adapter. Cuff inflation prevents exhalation, potentially causing suffocation.

COMMUNITRACH TUBE

The Communitrach tube allows speech by coordination of phonation efforts. Ventilation and phonation are separated because of different air sources. With this device, an air flow tube (that looks like a second pilot tube) runs outside the pilot (main) tube and opens just above the cuff. There is a port at the distal end of the air flow tube. When the port is occluded by a finger and compressed air or oxygen is directed through the air flow tube, a current of air is generated up through the vocal cords. With practice, the client learns to use this air flow for speech, although the "voice" produced in this way does not sound normal. Mucosal irritation may develop from the forced flow of air or oxygen into the upper airway.

TRACHEOSTOMY BUTTON

Use of a tracheostomy button is sometimes indicated during weaning as an intermediate measure between using a standard tracheostomy tube and extubation. A button is a short, straight tracheostomy tube that fits into the stoma of a tracheostomy but is not deep enough to enter the tracheal lumen. It has a removable cap with a one-way flap inside that permits inhalation but not exhalation. Exhalation occurs through the normal upper airway. When the cap is on, the client can talk.

A button cannot be used with a ventilator. It replaces a standard tracheostomy tube for people with retained secretions who do not require ventilatory assistance. A button creates less airway resistance than that produced by a

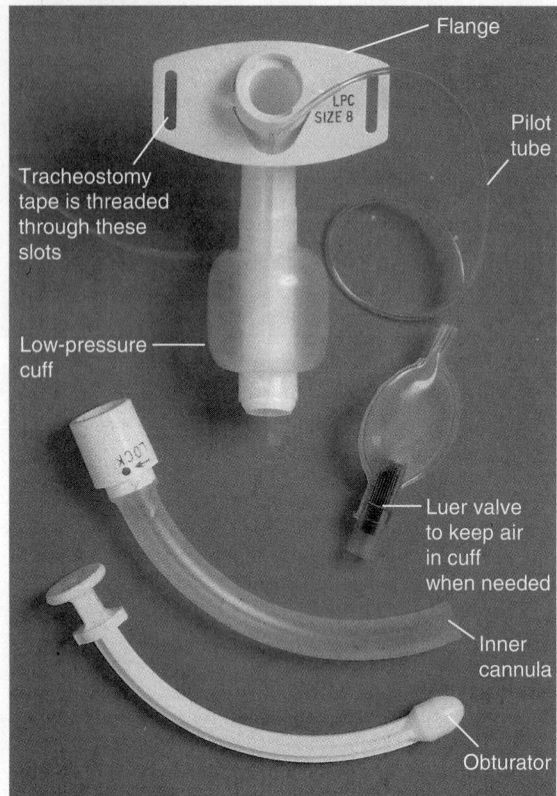

FIGURE 60–2 Parts of a tracheostomy tube. (Courtesy of Shiley, Inc., Irvine, CA.)

plugged standard tracheostomy tube; hence, breathing is easier. Artificial humidification of inspired air is necessary with a button (as with any tracheostomy tube), because the natural airway is bypassed.

Permanent Tracheostomy

Most clients with a permanent tracheostomy use a universal cuffless tracheostomy tube or an Olympic tracheostomy button. For appearance's sake, many people prefer a low-profile inner cannula. This design does not incorporate a 15-mm adapter. Instead, the inner cannula fits into the outer cannula and lies flush with the neck. If the client has had a total laryngectomy, the cut end of the trachea is sutured to the skin, creating a permanent stoma. Once the stoma is healed, most laryngectomy clients do not need a tube.

Metal Tracheostomy Tube

Metal tracheostomy tubes are made of sterling silver or stainless steel. The most popular type is the Jackson tracheostomy tube. Metal tubes are cuffless and most often used in clients who have a permanent tracheostomy or laryngectomy. The inner cannula locks together with the outer cannula. Because metal tubes do not have a standard 15-mm adapter, rapid adaptation to respiratory or anesthesia equipment is impossible unless a specific adapter is available. The Hollinger tube is also made of metal and is similar to the Jackson tube.

■ POTENTIAL PROBLEMS ASSOCIATED WITH TRACHEOSTOMY TUBES AND CUFFS

Most tracheostomy tube cuffs are designed to exert a low pressure against the tracheal wall. These cuffs are easily distensible, so that they accept a high volume of air without generating excessive force (i.e., high-volume, low-pressure cuffs). Low cuff pressure is necessary to prevent damage to the tracheal mucosa. The volume of air in the cuff determines the pressure exerted on the tracheal mucosa. Cuff pressures should not exceed 20 cm H_2O. With pressures above 42 cm H_2O, circulation to the tracheal mucosa is impaired, resulting in ischemia and necrosis. This is because the normal pressure within tracheal arteries is 42 cm H_2O. In the veins and lymphatic vessels the normal pressures are 24 cm H_2O and 7 cm H_2O, respectively.

Tracheal damage from cuff pressure is a frequent complication of intubation. Cuffed tubes can cause tracheal damage in as few as 3 to 5 days.

Tracheal Wall Necrosis

Necrosis of the tracheal wall can lead to the formation of an abnormal opening between the posterior trachea and the esophagus. This problem is called *tracheoesophageal fistula.* The fistula allows air to escape into the stomach, causing distention. It also promotes aspiration of gastric contents. Fistulae most often develop when a cuffed tube is used in conjunction with a standard nasogastric (NG) tube. Use of small-lumen NG tubes can decrease the risk of fistula. Necrosis of the anterior trachea can lead to the rare but life-threatening complication of hemorrhage due to erosion into the innominate artery. This complication is manifested as the bleeding in and around or from the tracheostomy or by pulsation of the tracheostomy tube. Immediate intervention is mandatory because the client can exsanguinate.

When long-term tracheostomy is required, uncuffed tracheostomy tubes are usually used unless the client is at high risk of aspiration. Some clients who require long-term mechanical ventilation can tolerate uncuffed tracheostomy tubes. Tidal volumes and respiratory rates may be adjusted on the ventilator to produce satisfactory ventilation and arterial blood gas (ABG) concentrations while eliminating the risks associated with the use of tracheostomy tube cuffs.

Tracheal Dilation

Prolonged intubation can lead to dilation of the trachea from the cuff. This complication should be suspected when increasing amounts of air are needed to seal the cuff, or when bulging of the tracheal wall is seen on x-ray films.

Tracheal Stenosis

Tracheal stenosis is narrowing of the trachea and may be noted 1 week to 2 years after intubation. It results from scar formation in the inflamed trachea. The severity of stenosis can be prevented by choosing the right size of tube, maintaining adequate cuff pressure, keeping intubation time short, preventing infection, and reducing movement of the tube.

Airway Obstruction

The flow of air through a tracheostomy tube may become occluded for several reasons. The tracheostomy tube may be misaligned so that its opening lies against the tracheal wall, preventing air flow. Cuff overinflation causes the cuff to herniate over the tip of the tube, obstructing air flow. Without adequate airway care, the inner cannula can become occluded with dried secretions or excessive bronchial secretions.

INFECTION

Tracheostomies increase the risk of bronchopulmonary infection because they (1) bypass upper airway protective mechanisms (i.e., filtering, warming, and humidifying) and (2) decrease mucociliary transport and coughing, thus increasing retained secretions. Stoma site infection may occur as well. Nosocomial infection is also a potential problem. The lower airway (below the larynx) is normally sterile. Therefore, all solutions and equipment entering the trachea must be sterile. Organisms (e.g., *Pseudomonas aeruginosa* and other gram-negative bacteria) grow readily in respiratory equipment, which can then contaminate the lower airway. In addition, some bacteria may colonize a tracheostomy without causing infection.

Recommendations for changing tracheostomy tubes vary. Most physicians and health care facilities have established protocols. Some facilities direct that tracheostomy tubes be changed as often as every week, whereas others allow longer periods between tube changes. Ideally, the tube should be changed at least every 6 to 8 weeks, or more frequently if the person is at risk of recurrent tracheobronchial infections. Each client has a unique set of circumstances that dictate the frequency of tracheostomy tube changes.

ACCIDENTAL DECANNULATION

A tracheostomy tube that is not properly secured may be accidentally dislodged from the stoma. Because most new tracheostomy tubes are sutured in place, decannulation is rare, but it is serious nonetheless. Decannulation may occur while the ties are being changed. Manipulation of a tracheostomy tube or suctioning often produces vigorous coughing, which can expel the tube from the stoma unless the tube is held firmly. With accidental extubation, if the stoma is less than 4 days old, it may close, because a tract is not yet formed.

If extubation occurs, call for help immediately. Maintain ventilation and oxygenation by bag and mask. If ventilation is impossible, you must reinsert the tube. To do so, deflate the cuff, remove the tube's inner cannula, insert the obturator in the outer cannula, elevate the person's shoulders with a pillow, and gently hyperextend the neck. You may need to use tracheal dilators (spreaders) to hold the stoma open. Insert the outer cannula with obturator into the client's neck, and immediately remove the obturator. Auscultate for breath sounds. If breath sounds are present, insert the inner cannula and reconnect it to oxygen and ventilation equipment. If the tracheostomy tube cannot be reinserted in 1 minute, (call a code) for respiratory arrest. Unless the client is breathing adequately, an emergency cricothyroidotomy will be necessary (see Chapter 82).

If accidental decannulation occurs once a tract has formed following a tracheostomy, the same procedure is used, but reinsertion of the tube is generally easier. If bleeding occurs or the airway is obstructed, use emergency measures, as indicated earlier.

SUBCUTANEOUS EMPHYSEMA

Subcutaneous emphysema develops when air escapes from the tracheostomy incision into the tissues, dissects fascial planes under the skin, and accumulates around the face, neck, and upper chest. These areas appear puffy, and slight finger pressure produces a crackling sound and sensation. Generally this is not a serious condition; the air is eventually absorbed.

WEANING, REMOVAL, AND RESCUE BREATHING

■ WEANING FROM A TRACHEOSTOMY TUBE

When continuous mechanical ventilation becomes unnecessary, weaning from a tracheostomy tube begins by deflating the cuff to determine the client's ability to manage secretions without aspirating them. A smaller, uncuffed tube may be inserted to ensure adequate ventilation around the tube. The tube is then plugged briefly to assess the client's ability to breathe through the upper airway. The time is gradually lengthened according to the client's respiratory status, general medical condition, and confidence. Eventually, the tracheostomy tube can be removed. The weaning process takes a variable length of time (typically 2 to 5 days) depending on the client's ability to breathe through the upper airway. If the tracheal opening is still needed for some intervention, an uncuffed tube, a fenestrated tube, or a tracheal button may be used.

Plugging a tracheostomy tube is usually done by inserting a tracheostomy plug (decannulation stopper) into the opening of the outer cannula. This closes off the tracheostomy, and air flow and respiration occur normally, through the nose and mouth. *When a cuffed tracheostomy tube is plugged, the cuff must be deflated.* If the cuff remains inflated, ventilation cannot occur, and respiratory arrest could result.

Explain the process to the client and family. Naturally, most clients are anxious about weaning because they fear they may not be able to breathe. Constant, supportive observation during weaning is necessary. Encourage the client to begin to think about breathing through the nose again. This breathing is a strange sensation for people who have used a tracheostomy tube for a long time. Explain ways to facilitate optimal respiration and to maintain control of breathing (e.g., inhale slowly and completely through the nose; avoid holding the breath).

ABG analysis and measurement of spontaneous respiratory mechanics (respiratory rate, tidal volume, vital capacity, inspiratory effort, expiratory effort) are important assessments during weaning. Oximetry and other noninvasive assessment modes may also be used once baseline ABG values are established.

During weaning from tracheostomy, assess for indications of respiratory distress or ventilation impairment. Clinical manifestations of problems may include the following:

- Abnormal respiratory rate and pattern
- Use of accessory muscles to assist breathing
- Abnormal pulse and blood pressure
- Abnormal skin and mucous membrane color
- Abnormal ABG levels or oxygen saturation

Remove the tracheostomy plug immediately if any sign of respiratory distress or ventilation impairment appears. Also assess the client's quality of phonation and ability to deep-breathe and cough effectively. If oxygen has been administered via the tracheostomy, administer it at the prescribed rate of flow using nasal prongs.

■ REMOVING A TRACHEOSTOMY TUBE

A tracheostomy tube is removed after resumption of normal respirations as indicated by the client's ability to breathe comfortably with the tracheostomy plugged, as well as to cough and raise secretions, and normal ABG values or oxygen saturation. Gradually increase the length of plugging sessions until the client is comfortable and confident with the tube plugged continuously for at least 24 hours.

After a tracheostomy tube is removed, place a dry sterile dressing over the stoma. Initially, every 8 hours, clean the skin around the stoma; remove mucus with hydrogen peroxide; rinse the area with normal saline; and apply a fresh, dry dressing over the healing stoma. Document the condition of the stoma and the surrounding skin. If either appears irritated or infected, notify the physician. Topical antibiotic ointment may be prescribed. A tracheostomy stoma closes gradually (over a period of several days). As long as the stoma is open, an air leak is present. Instruct the client to place clean fingers firmly over the dressing to facilitate normal speech and coughing.

After extubation, ongoing assessment of respiratory function is necessary. Some complications of tracheostomy, such as tracheal stenosis, can appear months after tracheostomy tube removal.

■ PERFORMING RESCUE BREATHING

Emergency rescue breathing in the mouth-to-neck mode (i.e., mouth to tracheostomy or mouth to stoma) may be necessary if a client who has a tracheostomy or laryngectomy experiences respiratory depression or respiratory arrest. If a tracheostomy tube is in place, provide ventilation by attaching a manual self-inflating bag to the standard 15-mm adapter on the inner cannula. Some volume is lost from an uncuffed tube. Adequate ventilation can often be compensated for by altering the usual method of manual inflation (e.g., compress the bag more forcefully and quickly). If the tracheostomy tube is cuffed, inflate the cuff and maintain ventilation at the correct rate—that is, 12 to 16 breaths per minute for an adult. If inflation of the cuff impedes ventilation, immediately deflate the cuff, and attempt to compensate for volume loss by compressing the bag more forcefully or quickly. If ventilation continues to be impaired or prevented and you determine the cause is a malfunction in the tube, remove the tube immediately and provide mouth-to-stoma ventilation. Keep the client's nose and mouth closed during mouth-to-stoma rescue breathing to prevent air from escaping through the upper airway.

Nursing Management of the Client with a Tracheostomy

PREOPERATIVE CARE

For clients who are to undergo elective tracheostomy, reinforce education provided by the physician. You may delegate some respiratory assistance tasks to other staff members, as discussed in the Management and Delegation feature, Assisting with Respiratory Care. The client's understanding of the tracheostomy tube may be enhanced by looking at anatomic diagrams and by handling a tracheostomy tube. The postoperative changes in ability to speak and eat should be explained. If the tracheostomy is expected to be permanent, information about living a productive life with modifications in clothing can be provided. A visit by a client with a permanent tracheostomy may be desirable.

When an emergency tracheostomy is needed, precious seconds may be all the time available for teaching. The client may be anxious or even unconscious. Education is often provided to the family in lieu of the client.

POSTOPERATIVE CARE

ASSESSMENT

After tracheostomy, frequent assessment is required, including monitoring vital signs; assessing amount, color, and consistency of secretions; and observing for indications of shock, hemorrhage, respiratory insufficiency, or complications related to the client's general condition or the surgical intervention.

DIAGNOSIS, OUTCOMES, INTERVENTIONS

Ineffective Airway Clearance. Numerous factors can lead to ineffective airway clearance in clients with tracheostomy—for example, dehydration, fever, anesthesia, anticholinergic drugs, sedatives, and immobility.

Outcomes. The client will have an effective airway clearance, as evidenced by no retained secretions, clear (or clearing) lung sounds, and no fever.

Interventions. Promote airway clearance and pulmonary aeration by changing the client's position frequently, providing humidification and hydration, using sedatives cautiously, and performing frequent hyperinflation and suctioning to promote lung expansion and reduce the risks of atelectasis, pulmonary infection, and ineffective gas exchange. Hyperinflation creates an "artificial sigh," improving lung aeration and facilitating removal of tracheobronchial secretions by enhancing the cough effort. When the client's condition is stabilized sufficiently, coughing may be enhanced by having the client place a finger over the tracheostomy tube opening while attempting to cough. It is important that the client wash the hands before doing this. Have the person cough into paper tissues and dispose of them carefully.

Perform Suctioning. When a cuffed tracheostomy tube is used, secretions collect above the cuff. It is difficult to remove such secretions by oropharyngeal suctioning. However, the secretions can be "blown" into the mouth by simultaneously deflating the cuff and giving a deep manual inflation. The client may also be instructed to cough during cuff deflation to expel accumulated secretions through the tracheostomy tube. If the client is unable to produce an effective cough, suction the tracheostomy tube during deflation to prevent aspiration of secretions into the lower airway.

Suction the airway as needed. The use of careful technique reduces mucosal trauma, which can lead to tracheal infection. Mucosal trauma is indicated by tracheal irritation, tracheitis, and bloody tracheal secretions. If tracheal secretions are thick and not easily removed, instill 3 to 5 ml of sterile normal saline into the trachea; the saline reduces viscosity of secretions for easier removal and acts to mechanically stimulate the cough reflex. Instill the saline directly into the tracheostomy tube during inha-

MANAGEMENT AND DELEGATION

Assisting with Respiratory Care

Assisting with respiratory care is one of the more controversial areas involving the use of assistive personnel. Opinions differ widely on the role of assistive personnel in caring for clients who need respiratory care. The performance of suctioning in particular is central to this debate. Your clinical facility should provide you with clear guidelines about the role of assistive personnel in this aspect of care.

The following aspects of respiratory care are commonly delegated to unlicensed assistive personnel:

- Setting up of oxygen delivery equipment and suction equipment
- Stocking routine respiratory care supplies at the bedside
- Assisting clients with the use of an incentive spirometer (after client instruction from a nurse or respiratory care clinician)
- Assisting clients with coughing and deep-breathing (after client instruction from a nurse or a respiratory care clinician)
- Performing tracheostomy care
- Measuring peripheral oxygen saturation (Spo_2)

Controversial aspects of respiratory care less commonly delegated to unlicensed assistive personnel are as follows:

- Suctioning via an artificial airway
- Performance of chest physiotherapy to promote the loosening of secretions

Before the delegation of any aspect of respiratory care, consider the following:

- What is the client's respiratory status? Complete a thorough respiratory assessment.
- What is the indication for respiratory care? Is the client's condition stable? A client with acute respiratory compromise should receive your full attention and care; the care of such a client should not be delegated.
- Is your client on oxygen therapy? Oxygen is a type of medication for your client. All guidelines that pertain to medications also apply to oxygen. You may delegate the setup of oxygen delivery equipment to assistive personnel. However, you are responsible to verify that the ordered amount (dose) of oxygen is actually being delivered to the client.
- Has the client been instructed in the use of the incentive spirometer or coughing and deep-breathing exercises? Does the client need reinforcement or reinstruction? Reinforcement can be provided by assistive personnel; education and instruction should always be provided by a registered nurse or a respiratory care clinician.
- Does the client have a *new* artificial airway, such as an oral airway, nasotracheal or endotracheal tube, or tracheostomy? Have you assessed the client during suctioning? How has the client tolerated suctioning previously? Well-tolerated suctioning via an existing artificial airway may be delegated to a skilled assistant, if this is consistent with training and institutional policy.
- Does this client have a new or long-term tracheostomy? A new tracheostomy should always be managed by a registered nurse. The tracheostomy tube that has been placed through a new surgical incision should be evaluated as for any other fresh postoperative site.
- Have the client and family members managed this tracheostomy at home? This is an opportunity to evaluate their sterile technique, to provide reinforcement, and to review instructions with the client and family. After doing so, you may choose to delegate suctioning for this client to assistive personnel.
- Are the assistive personnel aware that suctioning and care of artificial airways are sterile procedures? The sterile technique of assistive personnel should be evaluated intermittently.

Findings that are immediately reportable to you, the Registered Nurse, should be described for the assistive personnel. These include any change or difficulty that the caregiver or the client experiences during the provision of care, changes in the respiratory rate or pattern, and changes in the consistency, color, and quantity of respiratory secretions.

Donna W. Markey, MSN, RN, ACNP-CS, *Clinician IV, Surgical Services, University of Virginia Health System, Charlottesville, Virginia*

lation. If the client is unable to cough, suction the airway through the tracheostomy tube. Refer to the Management and Delegation feature, Assisting with Respiratory Care, before delegating activities to unlicensed assistive personnel.

Provide Tracheostomy Care. Tracheostomy care is detailed elsewhere in fundamentals textbooks. Reinsertion of the clean inner cannula is shown in Figure 60–3.

Provide Adequate Hydration. The normal hydrating mechanisms of the upper airway are bypassed by a tracheostomy. Hydration can be provided by an oral, parenteral, or inhalation route. Inhalation techniques include increasing the humidity of room air with a room humidifier and administering aerosols with dry gases such as oxygen.

If humidification is insufficient, the body tries to make up the deficit by taking fluid from body water. The result is inspissated (very thick) mucus, which can compromise airway patency and increases the risk of secretion pooling and subsequent infection. Dried mucus also occludes air passages and leads to atelectasis, pneumonia, and potentially severe gas exchange abnormalities.

Prevent Tube Movement. Secure a tracheostomy tube properly. If the tube tapes for this purpose require knotting, tie a square knot. Avoid placing the knot over the client's carotid artery or spine. Make sure the tapes are not too tight (i.e., allow room for two fingers to slide comfortably under the tape). Inspect the skin under the securing tape for skin irritation. In clients in whom a tracheostomy is required for prolonged periods, the use of fastening devices such as padded straps with self-adhesive fasteners promotes comfort. Secure the tube in midline tracheal alignment. Support ventilator and aerosol tubing to prevent pulling on the tracheostomy tube.

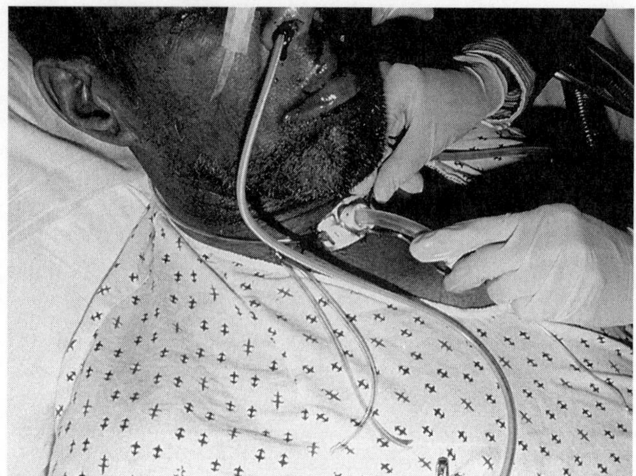

FIGURE 60–3 Reinserting a cleaned inner cannula.

Be careful not to disconnect tubing when turning the client.

Risk for Impaired Gas Exchange. After tracheostomy, impaired gas exchange may occur because of various factors. Factors affecting oxygen delivery include:

- Aspiration of blood, oral secretions, or gastric contents
- Restricted lung expansion from immobility
- Excessive tracheobronchial secretions
- Inability to cough and deep-breathe
- Pre-existing medical conditions (e.g., obesity, fever, inadequate hydration, pneumonia, tracheal injury such as from burns)

Factors affecting the removal of carbon dioxide include (1) the use of sedatives or anesthetic agents, (2) deteriorating level of consciousness, and (3) any other condition potentially affecting ventilatory efficiency and leading to hypoventilation and retention of carbon dioxide.

Outcomes. The client will have adequate gas exchange, as evidenced by maintaining oxygen saturation at greater than 90% (or ABG values within normal limits) and having no manifestations of respiratory distress.

Interventions. Assessment of gas exchange by ABG analysis is important immediately after tracheostomy and whenever there is a change in the client's condition or a change in treatment. Noninvasive monitoring such as pulse oximetry is appropriate once baseline values are established by ABG analysis. Remember, if shock or hypotension exists, or if peripheral vasoconstrictive drugs are used, data obtained by transcutaneous monitoring will be incorrect because of vasoconstriction.

Do not allow smoking in the room of a person who has a tracheostomy. Do not use aerosol spray cans (e.g., room deodorizers) near the person. Do not shake bedding or create dust clouds. Be careful when shaving or tending the person's hair that whiskers or hair does not fall into the trachea. Cover the tracheostomy with a thin cloth towel during shaving.

Risk for Infection. The tracheostomy bypasses normal upper airway protective mechanisms. The client also has an incision. Both areas can become infected.

Outcomes. The client will exhibit no indications of infection, as evidenced by the absence of fever and also a clean and dry tracheostomy site, healing incisions, and clear sputum.

Interventions. Use aseptic technique when working with the tracheostomy. Careful hand-washing, appropriate use of gloves, use of sterile supplies and solutions, and changing and decontaminating respiratory equipment every 24 hours are essential. Create a "loop" in the aerosol or ventilator tubing assembly; that is, let the tube loop down to catch condensate. Drain water and condensate in the tubing away from the tracheostomy into a receptacle.

Clean and inspect the skin around the stoma and the stoma itself. Observe for indications of irritation, inflammation, skin breakdown, and purulent drainage. If skin or stomal infection does occur, a topical antibacterial ointment may be prescribed.

Tracheostomy dressings (Fig. 60–4) are often used, especially in the early postoperative stage. Damp blood- and mucus-soaked dressings constitute a perfect medium for the growth of microorganisms. These conditions promote tissue irritation and breakdown. Change dressings whenever they are soiled or damp. Using hydrogen peroxide and cotton-tipped applicators, carefully clean the skin each time the dressing is changed. Rinse with normal saline and dry the area. Do not use plastic-backed or waterproof dressings. Moisture, secretions, and blood may seep behind the dressings, which hold warmth and moisture in. Skin then becomes irritated and macerated.

Risk for Aspiration. The presence of a tracheostomy increases the risk of aspiration because the tubes tether the larynx, preventing normal upward movement of the larynx and closure by the epiglottis on swallowing.

Outcomes. The client will exhibit no evidence of aspiration—that is, will have clear lung sounds, no fever, and no choking on swallowing.

Interventions. Intravenous fluids are usually given during the first 24 hours after tracheostomy. Then, if the client is alert and swallowing and if gag mechanisms are intact, oral intake of fluid and food may be attempted.

If a cuffed endotracheal tube was used before the tracheostomy, assess for the presence of tracheoesophageal fistula before permitting oral feedings. To assess for fistula, give the client a "test swallow" of water (at room temperature and colored blue with food coloring) before giving fluid or food. Severe coughing or blue fluid suctioned from the tracheostomy tube may indicate aspiration or a fistula. In either case, withhold oral food and fluid, and continue feeding by NG tube or other methods.

A client in whom normal swallowing is not expected to return for some time, or in whom the swallowing mechanism is permanently impaired (e.g., after a cerebrovascular accident), requires gastrostomy feedings or a permanent feeding tube (see Chapter 29). Tube-feedings may cause reflux, and the nutritive substance may be aspirated into the trachea. Before administering tube-feedings, inflate the cuff of the tracheostomy tube. Leave it inflated for at least 1 hour after feeding. Suction above the cuff before deflating it to remove any tube-feeding material.

When feeding a client with a tracheostomy, have the client sit upright. Often, food and fluids with semisolid consistency (e.g., pudding) are easier to swallow than water. Tipping the chin toward the chest narrows the

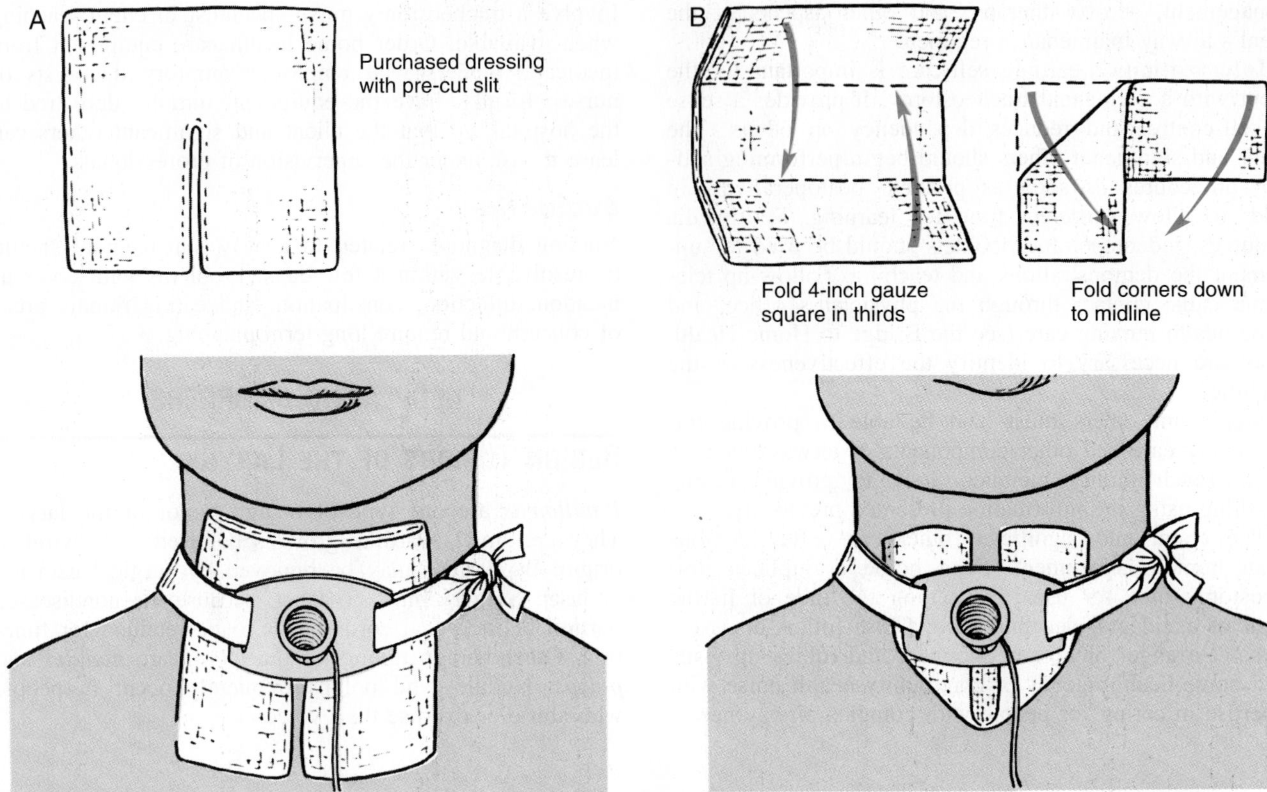

FIGURE 60–4 Tracheostomy dressings. If there is significant bleeding or tracheal secretions, cleaning the skin and changing the dressing frequently may prevent infection and skin breakdown. *A,* Manufactured dressing with a precut slit has no fine threads that could unravel and enter the stoma. Place the dressing around the tracheostomy tube with the slit downward, as shown, or upward. *B,* A 4 × 4 gauze pad is folded and placed under the tracheostomy tube. There should not be any cut edges that might unravel.

airway and helps food enter the esophagus. Overinflation of the cuff causes swallowing difficulty. If oral fluid intake is limited, continue intravenous fluids.

Impaired Verbal Communication. Because the vocal cords are bypassed by the tracheostomy tube, the client cannot talk. The nursing diagnosis of *Impaired Verbal Communication* may need to be combined with the diagnosis of *Fear* or *Anxiety* if the client feels afraid of not being able to summon help.

Outcomes. The client will have a satisfactory method of communicating with the nursing staff, as evidenced by being able to summon help and have needs met.

Interventions. Make sure the client can always reach an emergency call system to summon help. Do not use an intercom system because the client cannot talk. Be sure all staff members know this. Make a written list of common needs, words, and phrases that the client can point to (e.g., "I want to pass urine"; "I am thirsty"; "I have pain") to communicate needs. Provide paper and pencil or a picture communication board to facilitate communication. When possible, assess the client's reading ability preoperatively and select appropriate communication tools to be used postoperatively.

Risk for Constipation. When the glottis and vocal cords are bypassed (as with tracheostomy), the client cannot perform a Valsalva maneuver. This deficit impairs the person's ability to defecate.

Outcomes. The client will have regular bowel movements (according to a usual schedule).

Interventions. Assess for most recent bowel movement. Elimination is a frequently overlooked area of client care. Use prescribed stool softeners, laxatives, and even enemas or suppositories as necessary.

Anxiety and Fear. Anxiety and fear are due to various factors affecting the client with a tracheostomy—for example, inability to talk, fear of suffocating, anxiety about diagnosis, or fear that the tracheostomy tube will come out.

Outcomes. The client will have decreasing manifestations of anxiety and fear, as evidenced by a pulse rate within normal limits, a calm facial expression, the ability to communicate, and no expressed fears.

Interventions. Frequent observation is essential. Your presence and skilled nursing care are reassuring. Be certain to allow the client adequate time to communicate needs and concerns. Assist the family in reassuring the client that nurses are present and that the client is not alone.

Risk for Ineffective Management of Therapeutic Regimen (Individuals) and Risk for Ineffective Management of Therapeutic Regimen (Families). The client and family members need a lot of new information about permanent or long-term tracheostomy care.

Outcomes. Before discharge from the health care facility, the client and significant others will be confident in performing tracheostomy care, suctioning, and preoxygenation and the use of safety measures, emergency airway management, aerosol therapy, and other aspects of the client's airway maintenance regimen.

Interventions. Learning self-care is important for the client with a permanent tracheostomy. It provides a sense of self-control and reduces dependency on others. The client and significant others should begin performing self-care procedures as soon as possible postoperatively in order to allow sufficient time for learning. Multimedia resources, videotape, and booklets should be used to supplement the demonstrations and teaching. Follow-up telephone calls, contact through the physician's office, and home health nursing care (see the Bridge to Home Health Care) are necessary to identify the effectiveness of the teaching.

Significant others must also be able to provide tracheostomy care and other components of airway management. Teach family members how to provide rescue breathing using the information presented previously.

The client and significant others are often anxious about home management. Send home a duplicate tracheostomy tube for use in changing the tube or in the event of accidental decannulation. Close follow-up is essential. Arrange for home equipment and follow-up visits by a home health agency or community health nurse with expertise in caring for people with complex airway needs. Involve a tracheostomy nurse specialist in client teaching when available. Order home health care equipment from medical suppliers who employ respiratory therapists or nurses. Ideally, have the equipment initially delivered to the hospital, so that the client and significant others can learn its use under the supervision of professionals.

Evaluation

Nursing diagnoses related to airway management should be resolvable within a few days. Problems with communication, infection, constipation, and eating remain areas of concern and require long-term planning.

NEOPLASTIC DISORDERS

BENIGN TUMORS OF THE LARYNX

Papillomas are one type of benign tumor of the larynx. They are small, wartlike growths believed to be viral in origin. Papillomas may be removed by surgical excision or laser. Surgery must be exact, because the nondiseased portion of the vocal cords needs to be retained for function. Other benign tumors of the larynx are *nodules* and *polyps.* Nodules and polyps frequently occur in people who abuse or overuse their voice.

BRIDGE TO HOME HEALTH CARE

Living with a Tracheostomy

Common indications for discharging clients to home health care with tracheostomy tubes include the following:

- Long-term ventilatory support
- Inability to clear secretions
- Presence of a tumor that obstructs breathing
- Swelling from extensive neck surgery
- Vocal cord paralysis

Plastic or metal tracheostomy tubes are appropriate for long-term situations. Metal tubes can be disinfected and reused and are therefore cost-effective for home health care clients. However, metal tubes cannot be used for the client who is dependent on a ventilator because they lack the adapter that attaches to the ventilator tubing.

Daily tracheostomy care at home consists of skin care around the tube, cleaning the inner cannula, and suctioning. The home health nurse needs to teach these procedures to the client, family member, or informal caregiver. Use a clean wash cloth and mild soap and water to cleanse the skin around the tracheostomy tube. Keep the skin clean and dry to avoid skin maceration and potential skin breakdown. Keep a dry, lint-free dressing around the tube. Using a skin barrier after cleansing can help to prevent skin irritation. Remove and clean the inner cannula of the tracheostomy tube once per day or more often, depending upon mucus buildup. Wash inner cannulas in hot soapy water, and then disinfect them by boiling in water or soaking in alcohol or in hydrogen peroxide.

Excess secretions are common in clients with tracheostomy tubes for several reasons: (1) presence of the tube as a foreign body, (2) increased secretions due to respiratory illness, and (3) prevention of the normal process by which mucus is carried to the oropharynx and swallowed. Therefore, it is necessary to teach the process of suctioning. Ideally, family members and informal caregivers should learn to assess the need for suctioning by auscultating the client's lungs for "gurgles" with a stethoscope or by listening for signs of excess mucus. Do not encourage oversuctioning; it can irritate the mucosa. In some cases, clients may be able to cough up secretions on their own, or at least into the tracheostomy tube, which can then be suctioned. The caregiver must never apply suction when the suction catheter is inserted and must never apply suction for more than 10 seconds to avoid deoxygenating the client.

The entire tracheostomy tube is usually changed at least once a month. This procedure may be performed by the home health nurse or taught to a willing and capable client, family member, or informal caregiver. When this procedure is performed for the first time, it must be done in the physician's office or an outpatient setting. There is a risk of bleeding, and the client's response to the procedure is unknown. Once tolerance to the tube change is established, the procedure can be performed regularly in the home. It is best to remove and replace the tracheostomy tube with the client in an upright rather than a supine position, to decrease the sensation of choking and the risk of aspiration. An extra tracheostomy tube in a smaller size should be kept in the home in the event that the home health nurse or the client is unable to replace it with the existing size. It is not uncommon for the tracheostomy stoma to narrow over time.

Lisa A. Gorski, RN, MS, *Clinical Nurse Specialist, Covenant Home Health and Hospice, Milwaukee, Wisconsin*

CANCER OF THE LARYNX

Cancer of the larynx accounts for 2% to 3% of all malignancies. Care of the client with cancer of the larynx presents a unique challenge to the nurse because of the cosmetic and functional deformities commonly resulting from the disorder and its treatment. Benign and early malignant tumors may be treated with limited surgery, and the client recovers with little functional loss. Advanced tumors require extensive treatment, including surgery, radiation treatments, and chemotherapy. When a total laryngectomy is required, postoperatively the client is unable to speak, breathe through the nose or mouth, or eat normally. In addition, the defect left by the operation and its reconstruction may cause a significant deformity, necessitating further surgery to restore appearance.

Laryngeal cancer is classified and treated by its anatomic site. Cancer of the larynx (voice box) may occur on the glottis (true vocal cords), the supraglottic structures (above the vocal cords), or the subglottic structures (below the vocal cords) (Box 60–2).

There are an estimated 10,600 new cases of laryngeal cancer each year, most occurring in men. However, the incidence of cancer of the larynx in women is increasing.[14] If untreated, cancer of the larynx is inevitably fatal; 90% of untreated people die within 3 years. Like other cancers, however, it is potentially curable if discovered early enough.

Etiology and Risk Factors

The primary etiologic agent in laryngeal cancer is cigarette smoking. Three of four clients who develop laryngeal cancer have smoked or currently smoke. Alcohol appears to act synergistically with tobacco to increase the risk of developing a malignant tumor in the upper airway. Additional risk factors include occupational exposure to asbestos, wood dust, mustard gas, and petroleum products and the inhalation of other noxious fumes. Chronic laryngitis and voice abuse may also contribute to the disorder. Research now points to a link between tobacco exposure and mutation of the *p53* gene in squamous cell carcinoma of the head and neck.[28]

Pathophysiology

Squamous cell carcinoma is the most common malignant tumor of the larynx, arising from the membrane lining the respiratory tract. Metastasis from cancer of the glottis is unusual because of the sparse lymphatic drainage from the vocal cords. Cancer elsewhere in the larynx spreads more quickly because there are abundant lymphatic vessels. Metastatic disease often may be palpated as neck masses. Distant metastasis may occur in the lungs. Patterns of spread of head and neck cancer are shown in Figure 60–5.

Clinical Manifestations

The earliest clinical warning signs of laryngeal cancer (Box 60–3) are dependent on the location of the tumor. In general, hoarseness that lasts longer than 2 weeks should be evaluated. Hoarseness occurs when the tumor invades muscle and cartilage surrounding the larynx, causing fixation of the vocal cords. Unfortunately, most clients wait before seeking a diagnosis for chronic hoarseness.

Tumors on the glottis prevent glottic closure during speech, which causes hoarseness or a voice change. Supraglottic tumors may cause pain in the throat (especially with swallowing), aspiration during swallowing, a sensation of a foreign body in the throat, neck masses, or pain radiating to the ear by way of the glossopharyngeal and vagus nerves. Subglottic tumors have no early manifestations; clinical evidence does not appear until the lesion grows to obstruct the airway.[30]

Diagnostic Findings

The diagnosis of laryngeal cancer is made by visual examination of the larynx using direct or indirect laryngoscopy. The nasopharynx and posterior soft palate are inspected indirectly with a small mirror or an instrument resembling a telescope. While the mirror is inserted, slight pressure is applied to the tongue, and the client is instructed to say "a" and then "e," which elevates the soft palate (Fig. 60–6*A*). The instrument should not touch the tongue, or the client will gag. The nasopharynx is then inspected for drainage, bleeding, ulceration, or masses. Direct visualization of the larynx may be accomplished with use of several different instruments; most devices used are lighted endoscopes. The client is instructed to protrude the tongue, and the examiner *gently* holds the tongue with a gauze sponge and pulls it forward. A laryngeal mirror or telescopic endoscope is inserted into the oropharynx; again, contact with the tongue is avoided. The client is instructed to breathe in and out rapidly through the mouth, or to "pant like a puppy." Panting decreases the gagging sensation caused by the examination. During quiet respiration, the base of the tongue, epiglottis, and vocal cords are examined for signs of infection or tumor (Fig. 60–6*B*). The client is instructed to vocalize a high-pitched *eee* to approximate (close) the vocal cords. The examiner observes the movement of the cords, the color of the mucous membranes, and the presence of any lesions. If the client is unable to cooperate as described, the examination may be performed with a fiberoptic endoscope inserted through the nose.

Before any definitive treatment for tumor is initiated, a panendoscopy and biopsy should be performed to determine the exact location, size, and extent of the primary tumor. Computed tomography (CT) or magnetic resonance imaging (MRI) is used to assist with this process. Laboratory analysis includes a complete blood count, determination of serum electrolytes including calcium, and kidney and liver function tests. These data help to determine the physiologic readiness of the client for surgery. Because the airway will be altered after surgery, the client requires a thorough pulmonary assessment with ABG analysis for identification of any pre-existing pulmonary disorders that would interfere with breathing. Clients who are to undergo partial laryngectomy must have an adequate pulmonary reserve in order to produce an effective cough postoperatively. The operation is associated with an increased risk of aspiration, and the client must be able to cough to rid the airway of aspirated secretions.

BOX 60–2 Clinical Manifestations of Laryngeal Cancer

Area	Manifestations
Glottic Tumor 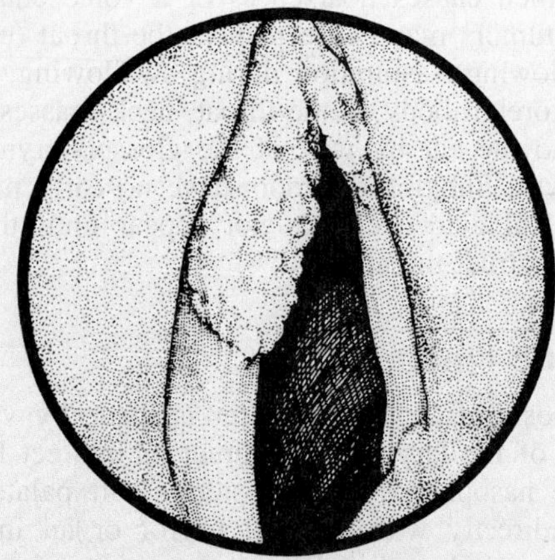 True glottic tumors interfere with normal closure and vibration of the vocal cords	*Early:* voice change, hoarseness, hemoptysis *Late:* dyspnea, respiratory obstruction, dysphagia, weight loss, pain *Metastasize:* through regional lymph nodes (rare except in superior or inferior tumors)
Supraglottic Tumor 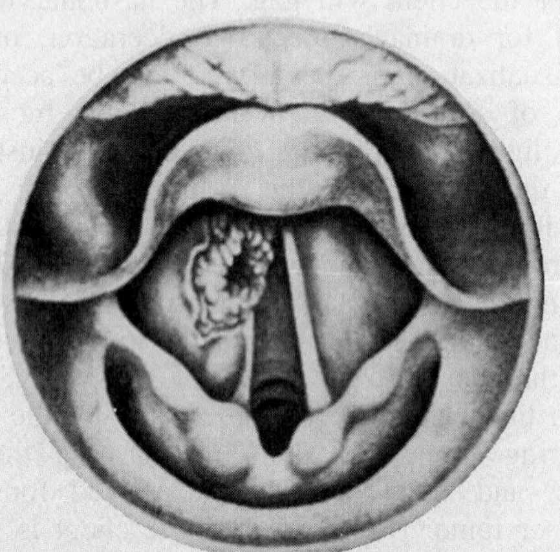 Carcinoma of the false cord partially hiding the true cord	*Early:* aspiration on swallowing (especially liquids), persistent unilateral sore throat, foreign-body sensation, dysphagia, weight loss, neck mass, hemoptysis (expectoration of blood) *Late:* dyspnea, pain in the throat or referred to the ear
Subglottic Tumor 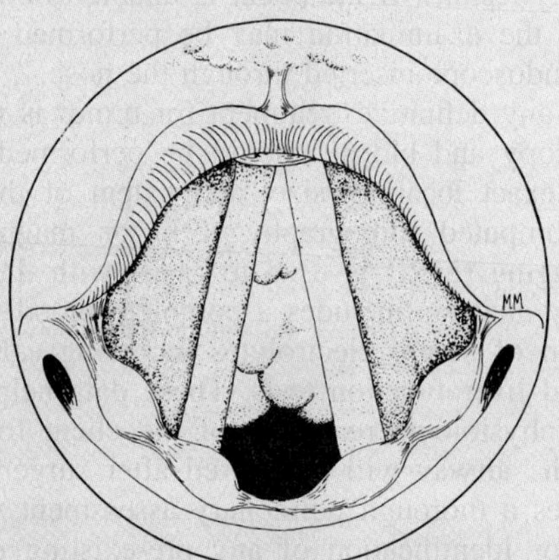 Subglottic polyp; this type of polyp can be single and smooth or lobulated as shown	*Early:* None *Late:* dyspnea, airway obstruction, dysphagia, weight loss, hemoptysis

Top and bottom figures from DeWeese, D. F., & Saunders, W. H. (1982). *Textbook of otolaryngology* (6th ed.). St. Louis: Mosby–Year Book; middle figure from Del Regato, J. A., et al. (1985). *Ackerman and Del Regato's cancer* (6th ed.). St. Louis: Mosby–Year Book.

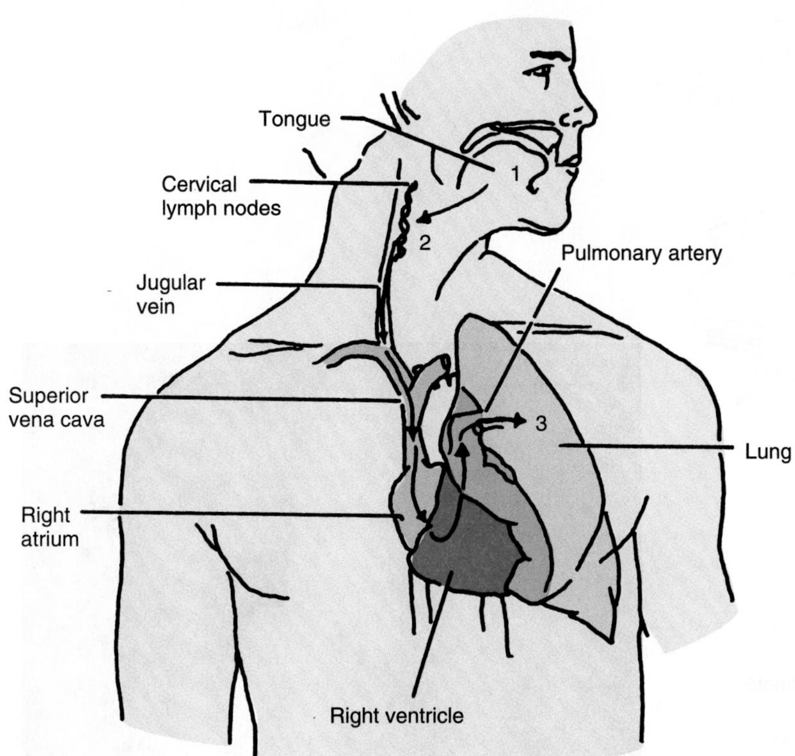

FIGURE 60–5 Pattern of spread of head and neck cancer. (From Black, J. [1991]. Reconstructive surgery in the elderly. *Plastic Surgical Nursing, 11,* 157.)

Finally, for ascertaining possible tumor spread or other primary tumors, a chest radiography and barium swallow study or esophagography are performed.

Once the tumor has been identified and a biopsy performed, the tumor can be staged. Staging has important implications for treatment choice and outcome. It is essential to determine the extent of the primary tumor in order to select the most appropriate intervention. Staging is accomplished by (1) measuring the size of the primary tumor, (2) determining the presence of enlarged lymphatic nodes, and (3) determining the presence of distant metastasis. This system of staging is called the TNM (tumor-node-metastasis) classification system (see Chapter 19).

Outcome Management

Medical Management

TUMOR ABLATION

The goal of client care is ablation of the tumor, with sparing of undiseased tissue when possible. The choice of treatment for glottic cancer depends on the degree of tumor involvement. If the tumor is limited to the true vocal cord, without causing limitation of the cord's movement, radiation therapy is usually the best treatment, with cure rates of 85% to 95%. The radiation dose depends on the size and location of the tumor; it is usually a minimum dose of 5500 to 6000 cGy (*gray* is a more accurate unit than *rad*) over 5 to 7 weeks. During radiation therapy, the client needs to be assessed for signs of destruction of normal tissue, ability to eat, airway distress, and other side effects. The complications of radiation therapy to the larynx include skin irritation, xerostomia, mucositis, laryngeal edema, and delayed healing. Radiation therapy is discussed fully in Chapter 19.

Supraglottic tumors may be treated with radiation therapy or a partial laryngectomy, with or without lymph node dissection. Subglottic tumors are usually more advanced carcinomas in which the tumor has spread to surrounding tissues. Metastasis is common. Treatment requires a total laryngectomy with or without radical neck dissection on the same or both sides of the tumor. (See later discussion.) The operative site may require reconstruction with pectoralis myocutaneous flaps (see Chapter 49).

Chemotherapy alone is not considered to be curative in treating head and neck cancers. However, it may be administered preoperatively to reduce tumor size, postoperatively to reduce the risk of metastasis, or as palliative treatment. Evidence now exists that larynx preservation may be possible with induction chemotherapy followed by radiation. Chemotherapy is generally not effective in advanced laryngeal cancer, but it may have the ability to control the development of new primary tumors through a process called chemoprevention.

Clients with laryngeal tumors often present in a compromised nutritional state due to dysphagia and weight

BOX 60–3 Clinical Warning Signs of Laryngeal Cancer

- Change in voice quality
- A lump anywhere in the neck or body
- Persistent cough, sore throat, or earache
- Hemoptysis
- Sores within the throat that do not heal
- Difficulty in swallowing or breathing

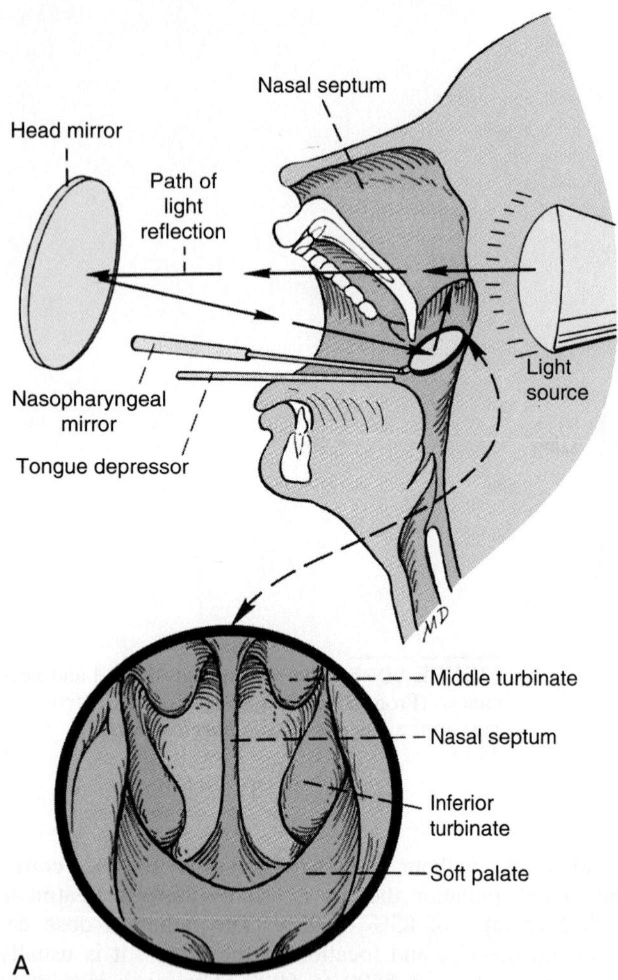

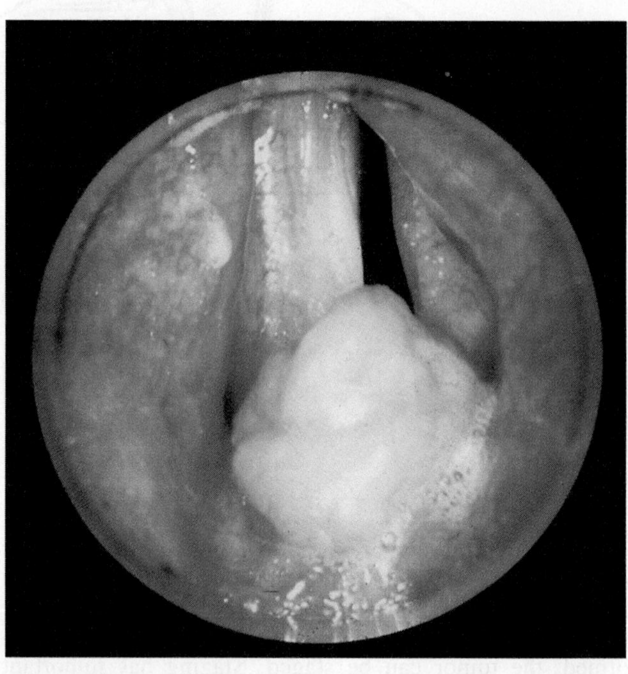

FIGURE 60–6 Laryngoscopy. *A,* Indirect laryngoscopy enables assessment of the pharynx and buccal cavity and some visualization of the larynx. (Laryngeal structure and function are best assessed by direct visualization, such as with flexible or rigid laryngoscopy or flexible fiberoptic bronchoscopy.) A head mirror, tongue depressor, light source, and small examining mirror are used in the indirect method. The mirror is positioned behind the soft palate after the tongue is depressed. To visualize the larynx, gently grasp the tongue with a gauze sponge and pull it forward. Place the mirror against the soft palate in front of the uvula, and move it gently until the cords are visualized. Have the client vocalize the high-pitched sound *eee,* which causes the larynx to move. The larynx is assessed for symmetrical cord motion. *B,* Large granular cell tumor of the true vocal cord, as seen during laryngoscopy. (From Wenig, B. M. [1993]. *Atlas of head and neck pathology.* Philadelphia: W. B. Saunders.)

loss. In addition, surgery, radiation therapy, and chemotherapy can directly affect oropharyngeal structures and impair swallowing. Nutritional intervention should begin before treatment to prevent malnutrition, thereby improving the overall prognosis.

Nursing Management of the Medical Client

The client undergoing radiation therapy for laryngeal cancer should be taught about the procedure and how to assess for and manage any expected problems at home. Written material is usually best, so that the client and family can refer to it as needed. Skin care for the irradiated site should include the use of prescribed creams and sunscreens, which are "patted" onto the skin; avoiding extremes of temperature; avoiding rough or tight garments; and avoiding rubbing or scratching the area.

Surgical Management

The goals of surgical intervention for laryngeal cancer are to (1) remove the cancer, (2) maintain adequate physiologic function of the airway, and (3) achieve a personally acceptable physical appearance. Many clients require tracheostomy for airway management (see earlier discussion). Most clients with advanced laryngeal cancer also have malnutrition from obstruction to swallowing by the tumor, as well as from the effects of the cancer. Before surgery, supplemental nutrition may be provided by NG tube-feedings or gastrostomy feedings. If long-term difficulty in swallowing is anticipated, a gastrostomy tube may be inserted at the time of surgery.

Laser Surgery

Small tumors can often be eradicated with the use of laser. Laser surgery for vocal cord tumors can preserve much of the normal glottis, leaving the client with a usable voice. Sometimes laser surgery is combined with radiation therapy.

Partial Laryngectomy

For cancer involving one true vocal cord, or one cord plus a portion of the other, a partial laryngectomy is

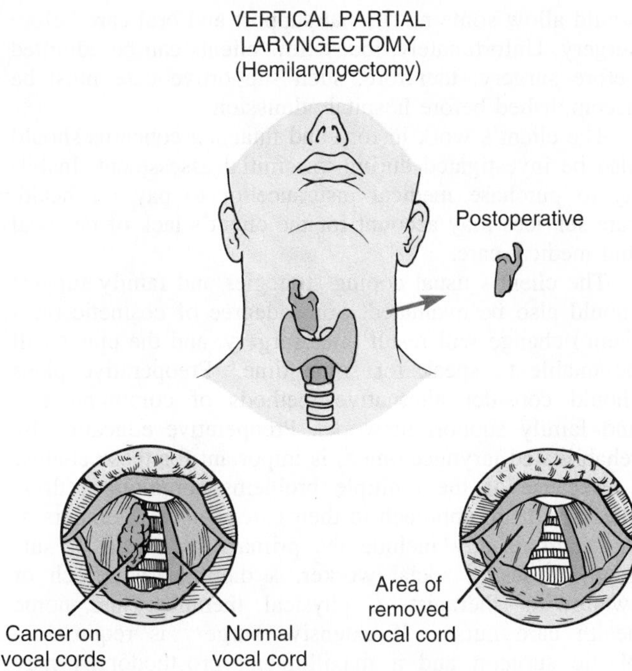

FIGURE 60–7 Technique of partial laryngectomy.

feasible. This procedure is also called a vertical partial laryngectomy and involves the removal of half or more of the larynx (Fig. 60–7). A horizontal neck incision is made, and the diseased portion of the vocal cord is removed. Sometimes up to a third of the contralateral cord is also removed. This operation is generally well tolerated, and the client has only mild difficulty swallowing and an altered but adequate voice.

Another form of partial laryngectomy is the supraglottic laryngectomy. This procedure is performed for cancer of the supraglottis. The surgeon removes the superior portion of the larynx from the false vocal cords to the epiglottis and may also remove a portion of the base of the tongue. Lymph node dissection also may be performed. Because the true vocal cords are preserved, voice quality is maintained. The major postoperative problem is risk of aspiration, because the epiglottis, which normally closes over and protects the larynx, has been removed. The airway is managed with a tracheostomy after surgery; when the edema subsides in surrounding tissues, the tracheostomy tube can usually be removed and the stoma allowed to heal. The client then needs to be taught how to swallow to avoid aspiration.

For selected, confined transglottic carcinomas, a supracricoid partial laryngectomy may be indicated. This conservative procedure preserves functional speech and swallowing without a permanent tracheostomy.[34]

Total Laryngectomy

For large glottic tumors with fixation of the vocal cords, a total laryngectomy is required. The larynx is the connection of the pharynx (upper airway) and the trachea (lower airway) (Fig. 60–8*A*). When the larynx is removed, a permanent opening is made by suturing the trachea to the neck. The esophagus remains attached to the pharynx (Fig. 60–8*B*). Because no air can enter the nose, the client loses the sense of smell. The biggest problem for the client after laryngectomy is loss of voice. The client should be made aware that without surgery, the voice quality will worsen as the tumor enlarges, but in any case the loss of voice constitutes a serious psychological issue. Because the trachea and esophagus are permanently separated by surgery, there is no risk of aspira-

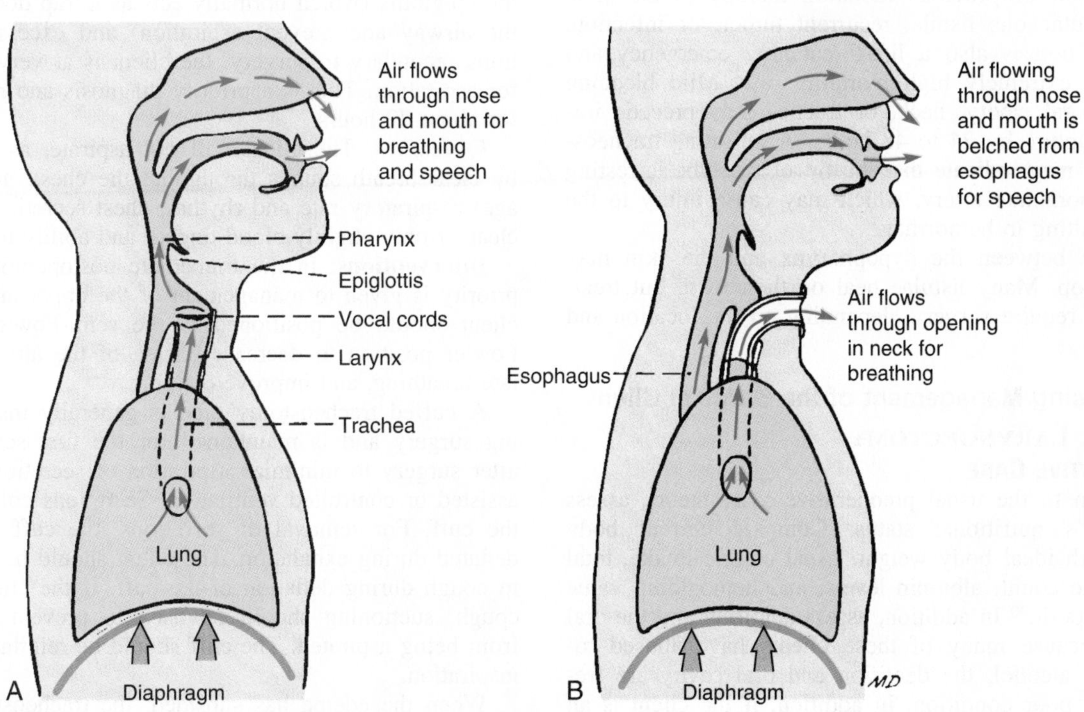

FIGURE 60–8 *A,* Before laryngectomy, air flow is through the nose and mouth. *B,* After surgical removal of the larynx, a new opening must be made for air passage. The trachea and esophagus are separated.

tion unless a fistula forms from the trachea to the esophagus. Besides this, the potential complications of the total laryngectomy are the same as for the partial laryngectomy (see earlier discussion).

Cervical Lymph Node Dissection

Metastasis to the cervical lymph nodes is common with tumors of the upper aerodigestive tract. Surgical management of laryngeal tumors often includes neck dissection. Radical neck dissection (also called en bloc) involves the removal of lymphatic drainage channels and nodes, the sternocleidomastoid muscle, the spinal accessory nerve, the jugular vein, and tissue in the submandibular area. A modified radical neck dissection spares the spinal accessory nerve, and a selective neck dissection removes only the lymph nodes within the area of anticipated spread.[28, 30]

Complications

Possible complications after laryngeal surgery are airway obstruction, hemorrhage, carotid artery rupture, and fistula formation. Airway obstruction is due to edema in the surgical site, bleeding into the airway, or loss of airway from a plugged tracheostomy tube. Airway obstruction constitutes an emergency and requires immediate intervention for restoration of the airway.

Hemorrhage is usually the result of inadequate hemostasis during surgery. Some blood-tinged sputum is expected in the tracheal secretions for the first 48 hours, but frank bleeding from the tracheotomy site or tube is a sign of hemorrhage and must be reported to the physician immediately. Also assess the client for other signs of bleeding such as evident hematoma or unilateral swelling, tachycardia, hypotension, and changes in respiratory patterns.

Carotid artery rupture is usually a late complication and is related to poor condition of the neck tissue. It may be the result of previous radiation therapy to the area, pharyngocutaneous fistula, recurrent tumor, or infection. This condition is also a life-threatening emergency and carries an extremely high mortality rate. Mild bleeding from the oral cavity, neck, or trachea may precede impending rupture by 24 to 48 hours. A pulsating tracheostomy tube may indicate that the tip of the tube is resting on the innominate artery, which may cause injury to the artery resulting in hemorrhage.

Fistulae between the hypopharynx and the skin may also develop. Many fistulae heal on their own, but treatment may require surgery, depending on the location and size.

Nursing Management of the Surgical Client

Partial Laryngectomy

Preoperative Care

In addition to the usual preoperative assessments, assess the client's nutritional status. Compare current body weight with ideal body weight, usual caloric intake, total lymphocyte count, albumin levels, and hemoglobin value and hematocrit.[30] In addition, assess dentition and the oral cavity. Because many of these clients have abused tobacco and alcohol, the dentition and oral cavity are frequently in poor condition. In addition, if the client is an active alcoholic, plans should consider support through the period of alcohol withdrawal. The ideal plan of care would allow some nutritional support and oral care before surgery. Unfortunately, today, few clients can be admitted before surgery; therefore, such supportive care must be accomplished before hospital admission.

The client's work history and financial concerns should also be investigated during this initial assessment. Inability to purchase medical insurance or to pay for health care services may account for the client's lack of personal and medical care.

The client's usual coping strategies and family support should also be evaluated. Some degree of cosmetic (aesthetic) change will result after surgery, and the client will be unable to speak for some time.[6] Preoperative plans should consider alternative methods of communication and family support networks. Preoperative education by rehabilitated laryngectomees is important for these clients.

Because of the multiple problems common in these clients, a team approach to their care is used. Members of the team usually include the primary physician or surgeon, nurses, a social worker, a dietitian, a speech or swallowing therapist, a physical therapist, and home health care nurses. If extensive surgery is required, a plastic surgeon and a maxillofacial prosthodontist may also care for the client during reconstruction.

Postoperative Care

Assessment

In addition to the routine postoperative assessments, after a partial laryngectomy the client needs to undergo careful assessment of the airway, lung sounds, and position of the tracheostomy tube, as well as checking for potential complications related to the surgical procedure and the tracheostomy tube (see earlier discussion).

Diagnosis, Outcomes, Interventions

Risk for Aspiration. Because of the removal of the epiglottis (which normally acts as a trap door to close the airway and prevent aspiration) and excessive secretions secondary to surgery, the client is at very high risk for aspiration. This is a priority diagnosis and remains so for about 72 hours.

Outcomes. The client will not aspirate, as evidenced by clear breath sounds throughout the chest, normal (for age) respiratory rate and rhythm, chest secretions that are clear or only slightly blood-tinged, and ability to cough.

Interventions. In the immediate postoperative period, priority is given to management of the upper airway. The client should be positioned in the semi-Fowler to high Fowler position to decrease edema of the airway, facilitate breathing, and improve comfort.

A cuffed tracheostomy tube is generally inserted during surgery and is maintained for the first several days after surgery to minimize aspiration of secretions and for assisted or controlled ventilation. Secretions collect above the cuff. For removal of secretions, the cuff should be deflated during exhalation. The client should be instructed to cough during deflation of the cuff. If the client cannot cough, suctioning should be used to prevent secretions from being aspirated. The cuff should be reinflated during inspiration.

When the edema has subsided, the tracheostomy tube may be removed. The decannulation process is slow and begins with observation of the client for aspiration, as follows. The cuff of the tube is deflated, and the client is observed for the ability to swallow saliva and other secretions without coughing or requiring additional suctioning. If increased secretions are present through and around the tracheostomy tube, aspiration is occurring and the cuff should be reinflated. If no aspiration is occurring, the tracheostomy tube can be replaced with a smaller, uncuffed tube. If the uncuffed tube is tolerated without aspiration, the tube is capped (plugged) to determine the client's ability to breathe through the upper airway. If the client can breathe through the upper airway for 24 hours, the tracheostomy tube is removed, and the stoma is taped closed and covered with an occlusive dressing[2, 29] (Fig. 60–9).

Ineffective Airway Clearance. The physical alteration in the airway and the presence of a tracheostomy tube interfere with normal movement of mucus up and out of the bronchial tree. In addition, as a result of prior smoking, the cilia have become ineffective. *Ineffective Airway Clearance* is also a priority nursing diagnosis for several days.

Outcomes. The client will have improved airway clearance, as evidenced by effortless, quiet respirations at baseline rate and clear breath sounds.

Interventions. The client may have copious secretions because of the presence of the tracheostomy tube, a history of chronic obstructive lung disease, and aspiration. There may also be oral secretions that cannot be swallowed. Oral secretions accumulate because of the disruption of normal airflow, and swallowing may be impaired as a result of surgery. In the alert and conscious client, coughing and deep-breathing will mobilize and eliminate many of these secretions. However, in the client who has undergone head and neck surgery and is just emerging from anesthesia, these measures may not be possible. Suctioning of the trachea will be needed for the first 24 to 48 hours after surgery. The frequency of suctioning depends on the client's needs, but suctioning every hour or more often is common for the first 24 hours. Sterile technique must be used to avoid introducing microorganisms into the tracheobronchial tree in a client with impaired immune defenses due to malignancy and surgery. (Suctioning techniques can be found in fundamentals of nursing textbooks.)

The inner cannula of the tracheostomy tube should be cleaned as often as necessary to provide a clear airway. In the immediate postoperative phase, the inner cannula is cleaned after suctioning. Once the client is ambulatory and can handle secretions safely, the cannula can be cleaned three times a day and as necessary.

Chest physiotherapy, ultrasonic nebulization, and aerosol administration of bronchodilators and mucolytics into deeper parts of the respiratory tract for sputum induction are recommended to prevent pulmonary complications.

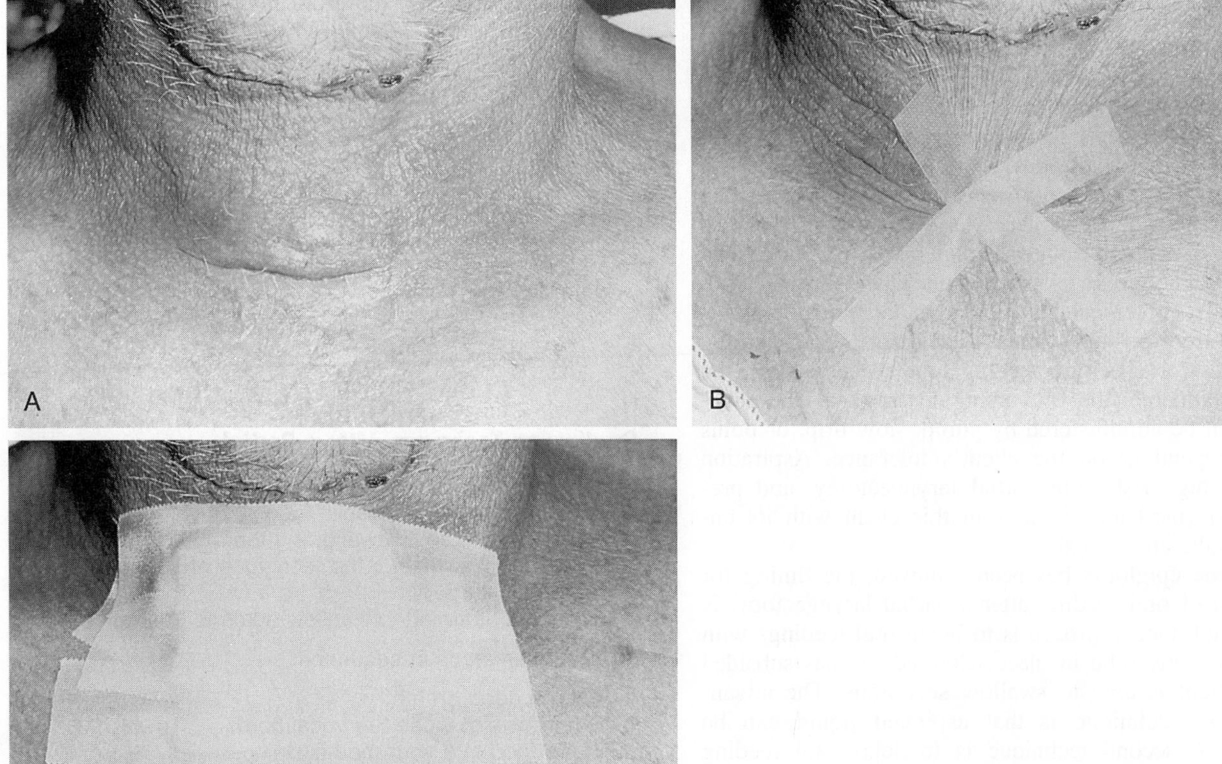

FIGURE 60–9 *A,* Closing stoma after decannulation. The skin is cleaned with hydrogen peroxide and protected with tincture of benzoin. *B,* The skin edges are pulled together and taped in an X. *C,* An occlusive dressing is applied.

These treatments are performed every 4 hours for the first few days after surgery and then usually decreased to four times a day once the client can ambulate.[30]

Risk for Impaired Gas Exchange. Like other postoperative clients, clients with neck surgery have a high risk for atelectasis related to low tidal volume breathing secondary to pain, sedation, and increased mucus production.

Outcomes. The client will have adequate oxygenation, as evidenced by pulse oximetry values above 90%, ABG values within normal limits (that take into consideration any pre-existing lung disorders, such as emphysema), no air hunger, and clear lung sounds.

Interventions. Oxygenation is assessed through ABG analysis or pulse oximetry and the fraction of inspired oxygen (FiO_2) may be adjusted. If the client has pre-existent chronic air flow limitations, oxygen may have to be delivered at lower percentages or not at all. Compressed air with high humidity may be substituted in such cases.

Altered Nutrition: Less Than Body Requirements. A combination of the pre-existing malignancy and swallowing difficulties sets the stage for malnutrition. In addition, concomitant lung disorders and alcoholism, which are common in this population, increase the tendency for malnutrition.

Outcomes. The client will have an improved nutritional status, as evidenced by maintaining baseline body weight or losing less than 5 pounds; consuming adequate fluid, protein, fat, and carbohydrate each 24 hours; swallowing without aspirating or choking; and hemoglobin, hematocrit, albumin, and total lymphocyte values remaining within normal limits.

Interventions. Immediately after surgery, typically an NG tube is inserted for removal of gastric secretions until postoperative ileus subsides. If long-term difficulty in swallowing is anticipated, a gastrostomy tube may be inserted at the time of surgery. Assess for bowel sounds, passage of flatus, and hunger as signs of returning gastrointestinal function. In some clients, tube-feeding with commercial supplements is indicated. Continually ascertain the correct position of the tube before each feeding. (Techniques for checking feeding tube placement can be found in fundamentals of nursing textbooks.) The tube-feeding can be administered by pump, slow drip, or bolus feeding, depending on the client's tolerance. Aspiration remains a high risk with partial laryngectomy, and precautions to guard the client from this event with its untoward results are critical.

When the epiglottis has been removed, the timing for resumption of oral feeding after a partial laryngectomy is controversial. One approach is to begin oral feedings with the tracheostomy tube in place when edema has subsided and the client is able to swallow secretions. The advantage of this technique is that aspirated liquid can be suctioned. A second technique is to delay oral feeding until the client has been decannulated and the stoma has healed. The advantage of this technique is that with a closed stoma, the client is able to increase intrathoracic pressure and remove any aspirated material through an effective cough.

Whenever the client eats, eating should begin with a nonpourable pureed diet; liquids are reserved until swallowing has been relearned. The accompanying Client Education Guide describes one technique for swallowing after a partial laryngectomy. Once swallowing can be accomplished without aspiration, carbonated beverages may be added. Thin liquids should be withheld until the risk of aspiration is minimal.[2, 29, 30]

Risk for Infection. The loss of primary defenses of the skin and delayed healing due to pre-existing malignancy and malnutrition make *Risk for Infection* a common nursing diagnosis.

Outcomes. The client will have no clinical manifestations of wound infection, as evidenced by continued approximation of incisional edges; decrease in the amount of wound drainage; absence of purulent drainage; absence of redness, swelling, tenderness, or warmth beyond the suture lines; absence of fever; and a white blood cell count within normal limits.

Interventions. During surgery, a wound drain is placed into the surrounding tissues of the neck and attached to constant suction. A commonly used device for collecting the drainage is a closed wound drainage system (Hemovac) container, which is attached to the client's gown to prevent accidental dislodgment. Using universal precautions, assess the amount and color of the drainage every 4 hours for the first 24 hours. Assess the wound for signs of hematoma or seroma formation by noting whether the amount of drainage is increasing or if there is a change in the color or consistency of the drainage. Also assess the color of the surgical incisions. If the amount of drainage is decreasing, the drain may be removed by the physician. Dressings are placed over the drain puncture sites on the skin. Small to moderate amounts of serosanguineous drainage should be expected for another 48 to 72 hours.

The suture lines should be cleaned at least twice daily with hydrogen peroxide followed by a water or saline rinse. A thin film of antibiotic ointment may be applied to the suture line to prevent crusting of secretions and promote healing.

CLIENT EDUCATION GUIDE

Swallowing Technique After a Partial Laryngectomy

- Begin with soft or semisolid foods.
- Stay with a nurse or swallowing therapist during meals until you master the technique of swallowing without choking.
- Be patient; learning to swallow again is frustrating.

Follow these steps in sequence:

1. Take a deep breath.
2. Bear down to close the vocal cords.
3. Place food into your mouth.
4. Swallow.
5. Cough to rid the closed cord of accumulated food particles.
6. Swallow.
7. Cough.
8. Breathe.

EVALUATION

Expect the problems with airway management to resolve within a few days. Infection, apart from atelectasis, will not arise for about 72 hours. Nutritional problems and problems with healing may require several weeks to resolve.

Self-Care

The client who has undergone partial laryngectomy may be discharged from the hospital before completion of wound healing. If upper airway edema has not subsided, the client is discharged with a temporary tracheostomy. The client and significant others should understand and demonstrate proper care of the tube, including inner cannula care, technique for insertion of the entire tube in case of accidental decannulation, suctioning, humidification techniques, and emergency resuscitation measures.

Once decannulation has been performed, the stoma must be cleansed and an occlusive dressing applied at least once a day (see Fig. 60–9). Additional wound care includes cleaning the incision area with hydrogen peroxide and water and applying an antibiotic ointment. All instructions given to the client should be in writing, with additional teaching materials used as available. Ongoing assessment for healing, recurrent tumor, or a new tumor is required.

TOTAL LARYNGECTOMY

The nursing management of the client after a total laryngectomy is the same as the care given to a client with a partial laryngectomy, except for feeding and teaching about permanent stoma care. Clients who have a total laryngectomy will have a permanent tracheostomy and need to learn how to speak using alternative methods.

NUTRITION. Immediately after surgery, the client's nutrition is supplemented with NG tube-feedings. The client remains on tube-feedings until edema has subsided and suture line healing has occurred. When the client can swallow secretions, oral feedings can begin. The diet usually begins with liquid or semisoft foods and progresses as healing occurs.

COMMUNICATION. For the first few days after surgery, the client should communicate by writing. If the client is very fatigued, requests such as "I need something for pain" may be expressed by using a communication board so that the client can just point to the statement. Even though the client cannot speak, conversation should still include the client's input through nodding and pointing and not be directed only to others such as the family. Avoiding conversation with the client because of difficulty in communication is demeaning to the client and leads to frustration.

ARTIFICIAL LARYNX. An artificial larynx may be used as early as 3 to 4 days after surgery. These battery-operated speech devices are held alongside the neck or can be adapted with a plastic tube that is inserted in the mouth. The air inside the mouth is vibrated, and the client articulates as usual (Fig. 60–10). The speech quality is monotone and mechanical-sounding but intelligible.[4, 29]

ESOPHAGEAL SPEECH. Esophageal speech is a technique that requires the client to swallow and hold air in the upper esophagus. By controlling the flow of air, the client can pronounce as many as 6 to 10 words before stopping to reswallow more air. The voice is deep but is loud and effective once the technique is mastered.

TRACHEOESOPHAGEAL PUNCTURE. Tracheoesophageal puncture (TEP) is a surgical technique that also restores speech (Fig. 60–11). A small puncture is made into the upper tracheostoma to the cervical esophagus for creation of a fistula. After the fistula tract has healed, a small one-way valve, or voice prosthesis, is inserted. By occlusion of the prosthesis, air can be shunted into the esophagus and used to produce speech. The TEP may be done concurrently with a total laryngectomy or as a secondary procedure after healing and radiation therapy. These devices require maintenance; therefore, only clients who are highly motivated, are able to perform self-care, and have good manual dexterity are eligible for this procedure. Care of the TEP surgical wound is presented in the accompanying Client Education Guide (see p. 1671).

Self-Care

Clients should be discharged with an extra tracheostomy tube to allow daily changes at home (Fig. 60–12). To provide supplemental humidification, normal saline may be instilled into the stoma several times each day to stimulate coughing, moisten the mucosa, and loosen dried secretions and crusts. Use of a bedside humidifier or vaporizer also aids in humidifying the inspired air. A stoma bib or covering should be worn to warm and filter inspired air and to prevent foreign bodies from entering the stoma. These coverings can be purchased, or the client may improvise by using a scarf, necktie, or turtleneck shirt.[4, 30, 31]

The client must be encouraged to continue speech therapy as begun in the hospital. The techniques to restore speech require much time for mastery; the client is seen by a speech therapist after dismissal from the hospital. Community support groups for clients after laryngectomy—the Lost Cord Club and the International Association of Laryngectomees—offer needed reassurance. Much patience is required by the client and family while the client is relearning to speak. The process is time-consuming and frustrating, and progress may sometimes be slow. Encourage the family to give the client enough time to formulate the words and not speak for the client.

Once the incision has completely healed, the tracheostomy tube is no longer required (Fig. 60–13). This process varies but usually takes about 6 to 8 weeks. Occasionally, the tube may be required at night, if the stoma is small or the client does not get adequate air exchange during sleep. Once the tracheostomy tube has been removed, the client can disguise the stoma with clothing and begin to regain a sense of normalcy.

Tub baths or showers are permitted, but the client must use caution to prevent introduction of water into the stoma. Commercial stoma shower covers are available, and the water spray should be aimed at midchest. Water sports are prohibited. If the client fishes, a life preserver must be worn at all times on the boat.

The client should wear a medical alert bracelet or carry an emergency wallet card to identify the fact that resuscitation cannot be performed through the mouth. Information about obtaining these forms of identification is available from the American Cancer Society. The use of mouth-to-stoma rescue breathing is imperative when re-

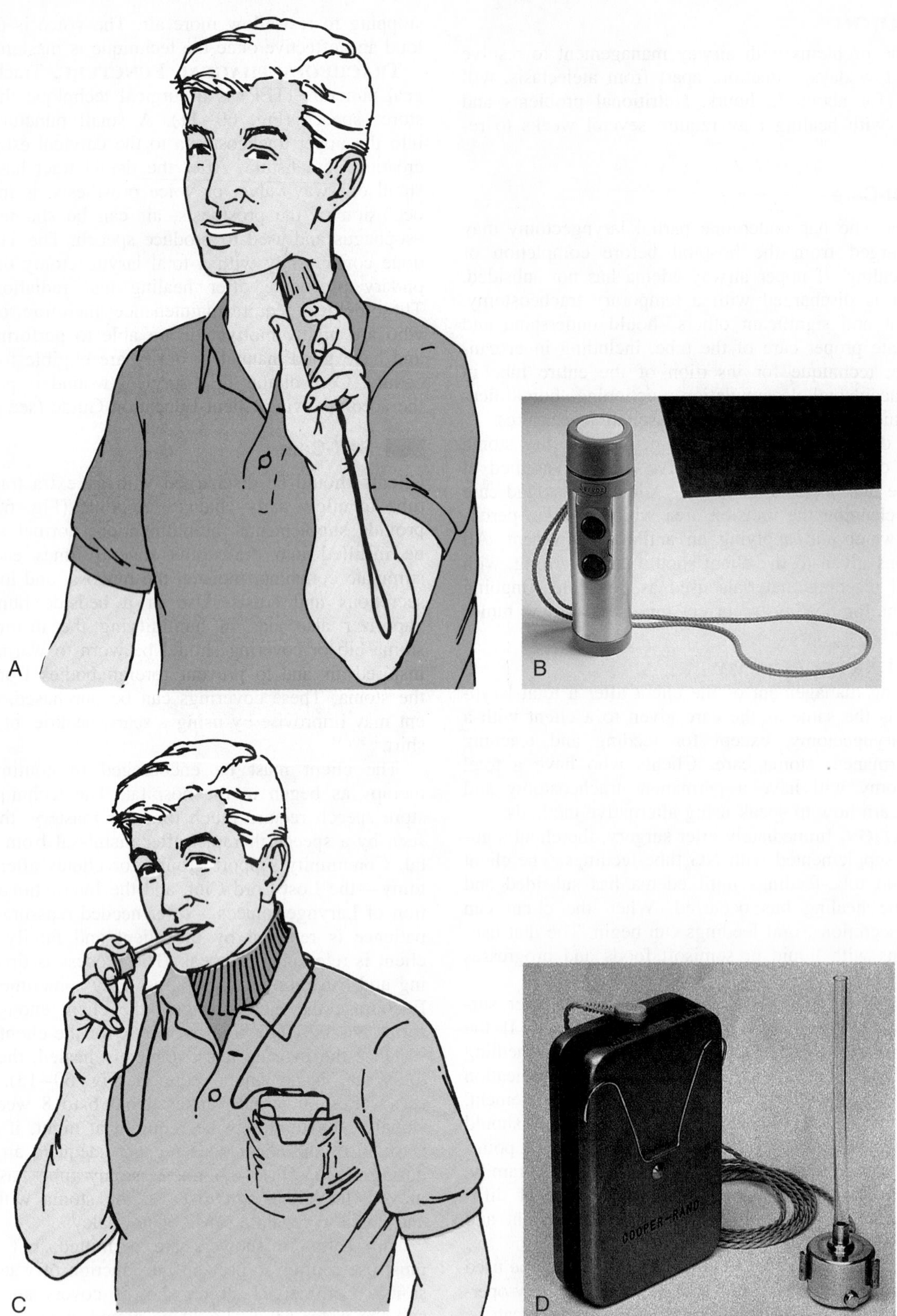

FIGURE 60–10 *A* and *B*, Artificial larynx. This hand-held, battery-powered speech aid is placed against the neck. *A*, When the artificial larynx is activated, it creates a vibration that is transmitted to the neck and into the mouth. Words silently formed by the mouth become sounds from the vibrations emitted by the device. Any type of artificial larynx requires muscle and tongue control and hand strength; usually, such a device is not used until immediate postoperative neck tenderness has subsided. (*B*, Courtesy of Servox Electrolarynx Manufacturing by Siemans Hearing Instruments, Inc., Union, NJ.) *C* and *D*, Electronic speech aid (Cooper Rand) allows the client to adjust tone, pitch, and volume. An oral connector permits speech without the necessity of placing the device against the neck. This is an advantage immediately after surgery, when the neck is too sensitive for a neck-vibrating device. (*D*, Courtesy of Luminaud, Inc., Mentor, OH.)

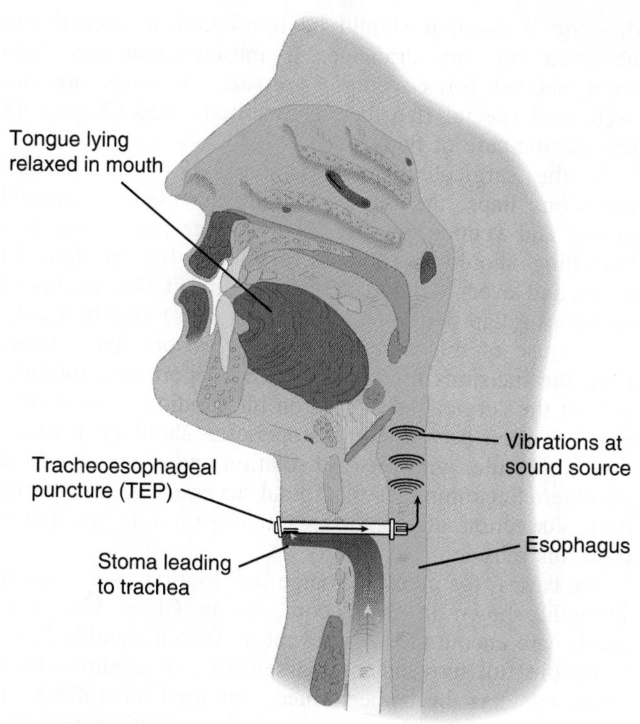

FIGURE 60–11 Tracheoesophageal puncture for voice rehabilitation after laryngectomy. A prosthesis is inserted into a fistula created in the neck. The prosthesis has a one-way valve that permits air to pass into the esophagus but prevents accidental aspiration. To speak, the client occludes the prosthesis with a finger or attachment. Exhaled air is then shunted through the prosthesis, where it vibrates, and exits the mouth as a spoken word.

suscitation is needed in these clients. Family members should be directed to a community program that teaches mouth-to-stoma resuscitation. For additional security, a wireless "beeper" or automatic response monitoring device can be useful.[8]

The client may require a nutritional plan for the first few weeks at home. The dietitian should work with the client and family to determine the consistency of food easiest to swallow as well as the kinds of foods required to obtain needed protein and calories.

It is essential that the client not smoke so that lung function is preserved and the formation of other aerodigestive tract tumors is prevented. For some clients after laryngectomy, the process of smoking cessation seems pointless. Some clients continue to smoke by inhaling the cigarette smoke through the stoma. The attitude is one of "Why quit now? What else could happen to me?" Use extra support and encouragement with the client, remembering to be an advocate of the client's choice as well as providing assurance that the quality of life after smoking cessation improves.

Follow-up care is important to assess the healing process, to evaluate coping mechanisms, and to examine the client for possible metastasis or new tumors. The client should be taught to report any of the following signs or symptoms to the physician:

- A lump anywhere in the neck or body
- Persistent cough, sore throat, or earache
- Hemoptysis
- Sores around the stoma or within the trachea that do not heal
- Difficulty swallowing or breathing

CLIENT EDUCATION GUIDE

Care of a Tracheoesophageal Puncture Wound

1. A 10 Fr., 12 Fr., or 14 Fr. red rubber catheter is inserted into the puncture site to maintain the opening until a tract has formed (Fig. A).
2. Tie a knot at the end of the catheter to prevent the back-flow of gastric secretions onto your chest.
3. Tape the catheter securely to your chest.
4. If the catheter comes out and cannot be reinserted, contact your physician or speech therapist immediately.
5. Once the voice prosthesis is able to be inserted, clean your neck and stoma. Using the inserter, place the prosthesis into the fistula.
6. Tape the prosthesis to the skin of your neck (Fig. B).
7. To use the prosthesis, take a breath, cover your stoma with your thumb, and speak. The air from your lungs will pass through the prosthesis and vibrate the walls of the throat. The mouth is used for producing the words.
8. If food or fluid leaks around the prosthesis, it may need to be replaced.

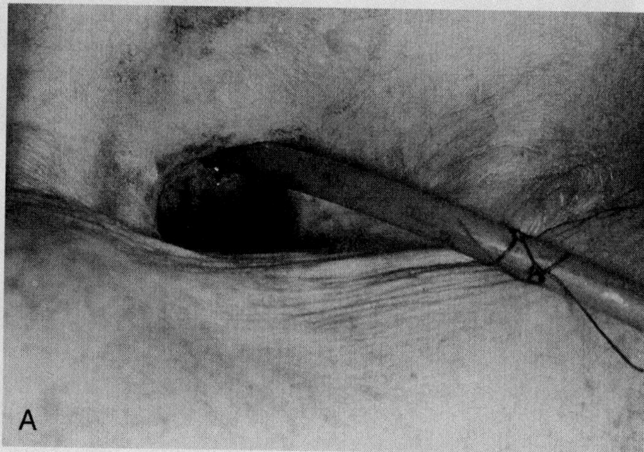

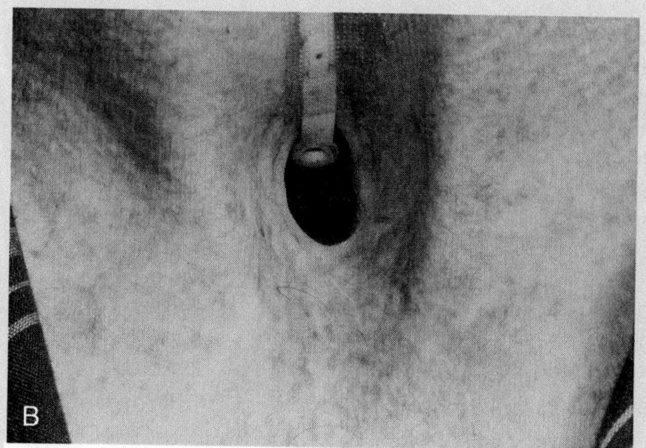

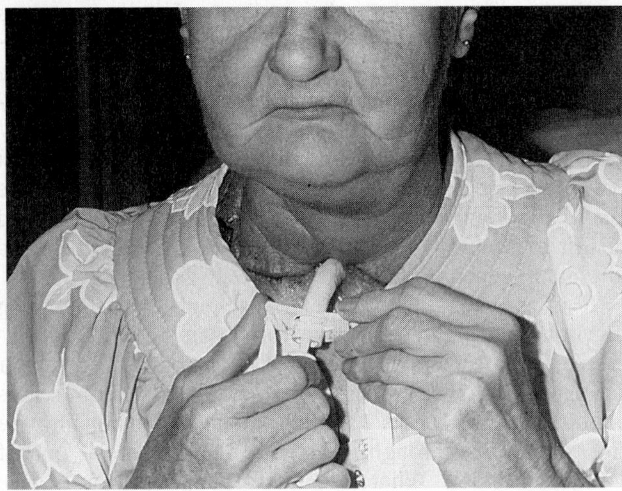

FIGURE 60–12 Insertion of a laryngectomy tube into a permanent tracheostoma. The obturator or guide is inserted into the outer cannula. After the tube is lubricated with water-soluble ointment, the client takes a deep breath and the lubricated tube is inserted. The obturator is removed, and the tube is tied in place.

NECK DISSECTION

PREOPERATIVE CARE

Before surgery, the client's understanding of the plans for surgery should be assessed. Determine what the surgeon has told the client and how much information has been retained or lost because of anxiety. In addition, address the fears the client has about the diagnosis of cancer and fears of deformity after surgery. Assist the client to understand the anatomic and physiologic alterations that will occur as a result of radical surgery. Explain to the client and family what to expect after surgery (e.g., placement in the intensive care unit, tracheostomy, drainage tubes) and review postoperative care (e.g., communication techniques to be used if a tracheostomy is to be placed).

The client's support systems and degree of coping should be assessed. If the client is an alcoholic, the use of alcohol may be the usual coping tool. Because alcohol will not be available, assess the other coping mechanisms available to the client, and encourage the client to use them. Sources may include friends and family. Identify new support systems, if needed, such as interaction with people who have had the same surgery or diagnosis.

POSTOPERATIVE CARE

After surgery, the usual postoperative assessments are performed, with special attention given to the airway. Airway patency can be lost as a result of edema of the neck or bleeding within the area. Assess the client for signs of airway edema or bleeding. Auscultate lung sounds every 2 hours for the first 24 hours. Report signs of airway obstruction immediately.

Place the client in a semi-Fowler position to minimize postoperative edema. Monitor neck drainage for volume and color. Sanguineous or serosanguineous drainage is expected for the first 72 hours after surgery. Once drainage has stopped, the wound drains are removed.

Pressure dressings may be used in the immediate postoperative period, depending on physician preference. If a dressing is used, it should be reinforced as needed and observed for any drainage. If musculocutaneous flaps were needed for coverage, pressure dressings are not used, and special flap care is required. (See Chapter 49 for specific care of flaps.)

If the surgical defect was repaired with musculocutaneous flaps, the flap should be assessed for arterial inflow and venous outflow. Flap temperature, color, and blanching should be noted every hour for the first 24 hours and every 4 hours after that time. Other means of monitoring flap perfusion (Doppler signals) may be used.

Because of the disruption of the sensory nerve fibers from the incisions used, most clients report only minimal pain at the surgical site. If an en bloc radical neck dissection has been performed, postoperative shoulder dysfunction is the rule, with forward rotation and dropping of the shoulder. Sectioning of the spinal accessory nerve during neck dissection also interrupts innervation to the upper trapezius muscle.

Exercises to increase range of motion and muscle strength, shown in the accompanying Client Education Guide, are encouraged to prevent a "frozen shoulder" and to restore full movement. If a selective or modified neck dissection has been performed, minimal alterations in range of motion and muscle strength are anticipated. Encourage use of exercise to prevent permanent disability.[3, 25]

Self-Care

After neck dissection, caution clients about the potential for injury to neck tissue due to lack of sensation. The use of a heating pad or exposure to temperature extremes may result in tissue injury (burns, frostbite) in a client who cannot feel these temperatures. Clients who have a tracheostomy need specific instructions for its management. Explain ongoing evaluations and follow-up.

HEMORRHAGIC, INFECTIOUS, AND INFLAMMATORY DISORDERS

EPISTAXIS

Epistaxis (nosebleed) may result from irritation, trauma, infection, foreign bodies, or tumors. In addition, epistaxis

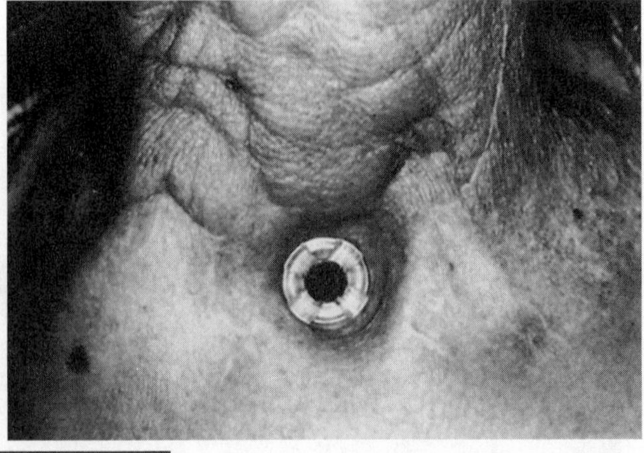

FIGURE 60–13 Healed tracheostomy incision.

CLIENT EDUCATION GUIDE

Exercises After Radical Neck Surgery

Step 1: Begin by gently moving your head from side to side, tipping your ear toward your shoulder on the same side, and moving your chin toward your chest.

Step 2: To exercise your shoulders using the hand on the nonaffected side, lean on or hold onto a low table or chair. Bend your body slightly at the waist and

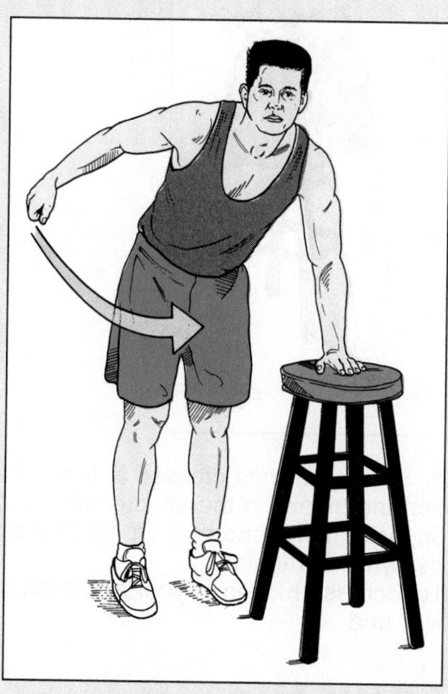

a. Swing your shoulder and arm from left to right

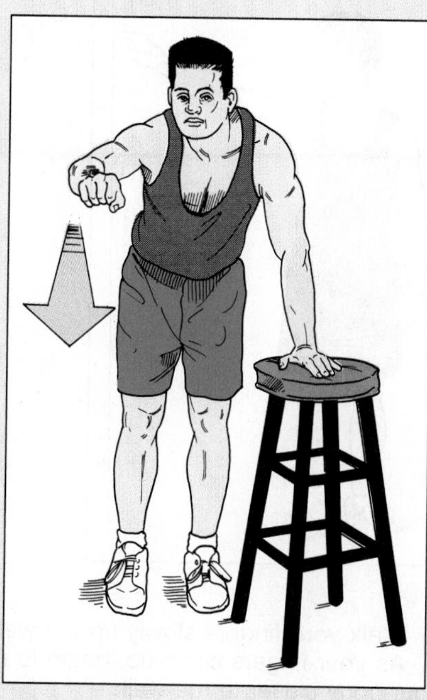

b. Swing your shoulder and arm from front to back.

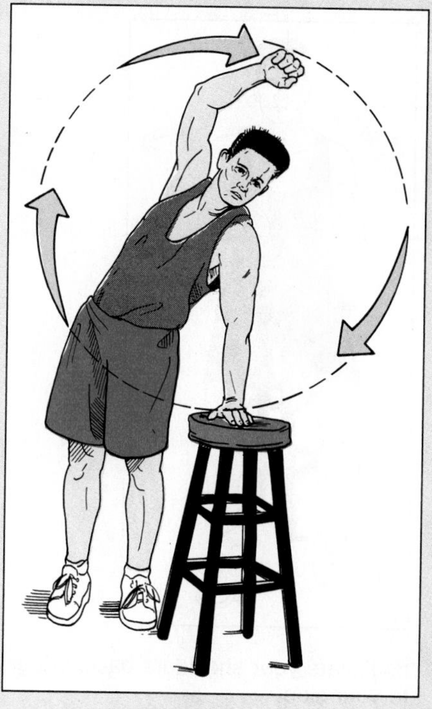

c. Swing your shoulder and arm in a wide circle, gradually bringing your arm all the way over your head.

Step 3: To strengthen your neck muscles, sit on a stool and

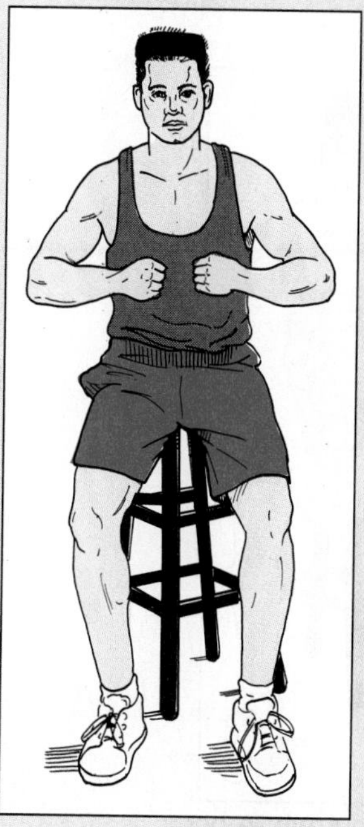

a. Place your hands in front of you with your elbows at right angles, sticking out from your body.

Guide continued on following page

CLIENT EDUCATION GUIDE *Continued*

Exercises After Radical Neck Surgery

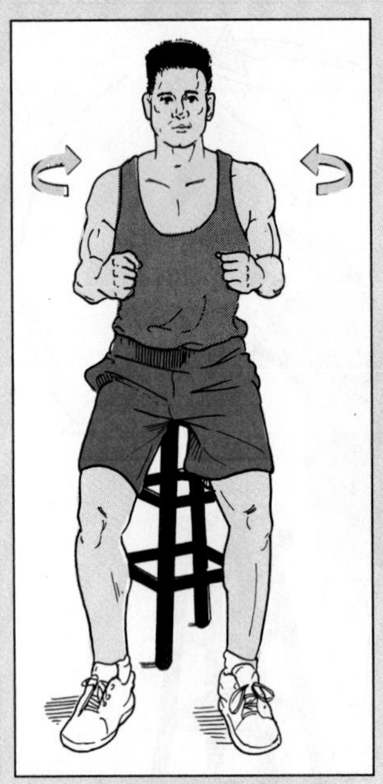

b. Rotate your shoulders back, bringing elbows to your side.

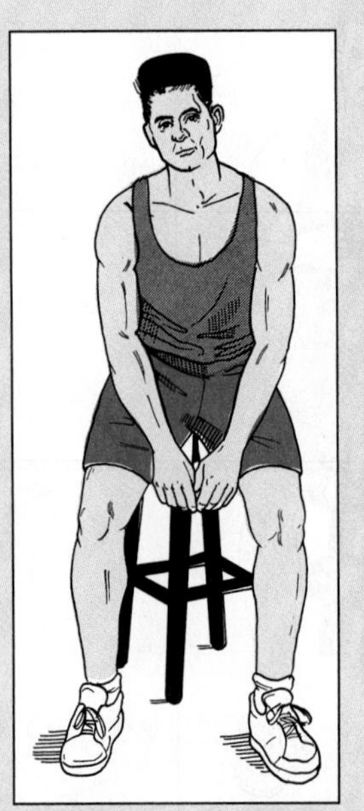

c. Relax your whole body.

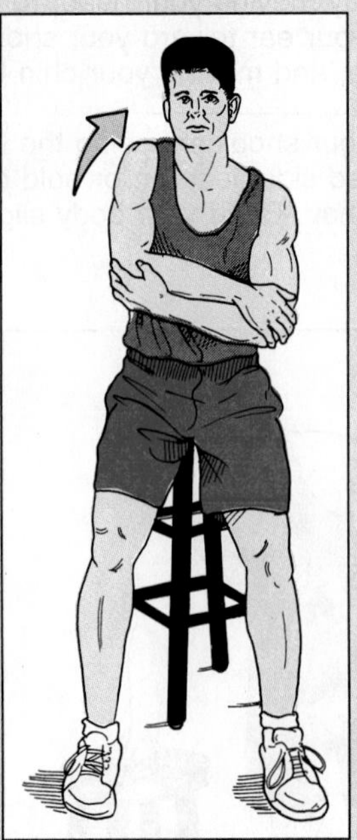

d. With your arms crossed in front of you, support the elbow on the affected side with your opposite hand, and help lift the arm and shoulder while shrugging.

Step 4: To increase motion in your shoulder, stand at a wall and

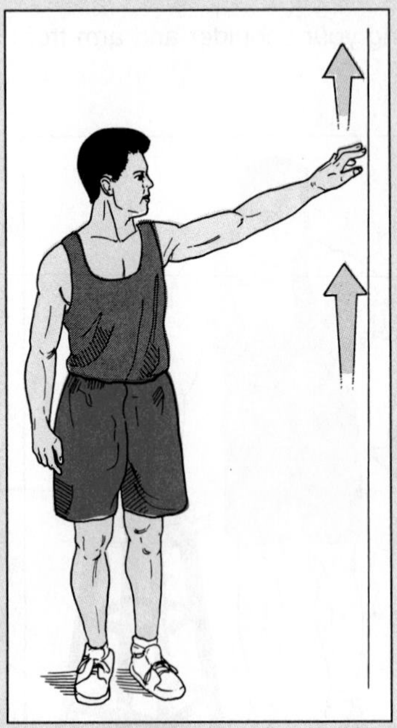

a. Walk your fingers slowly up the wall.
b. As your fingers climb up, begin to move your body closer to the wall.
c. Continue until your arm is high above your head and shoulder.

CLIENT EDUCATION GUIDE *Continued*

Exercises After Radical Neck Surgery

Step 5: To gain shoulder and upper arm strength, attach a hook to a wall or door. Hang a short rope knotted at each end over the hook. Under the hook, place a straight-backed chair or stool. It would be helpful to do this exercise before a mirror.

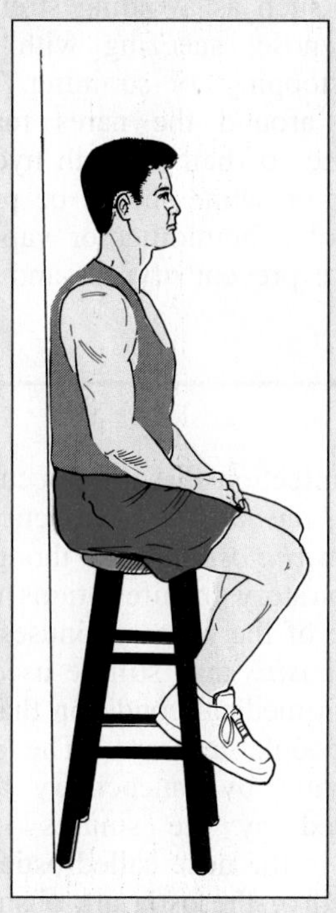

a. Sit straight, with your back against the wall.

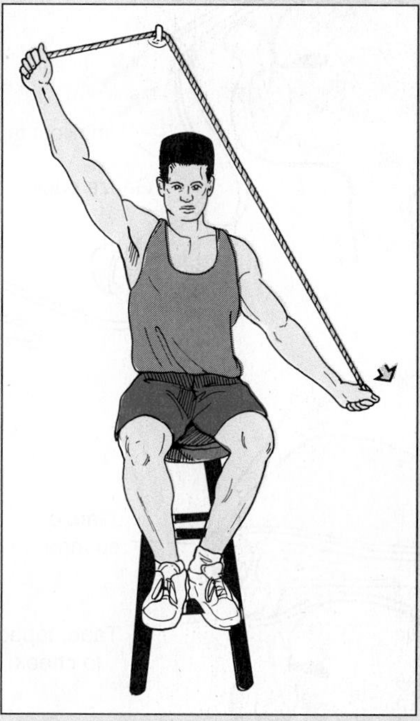

b. Pull one arm and shoulder up with the rope by bringing the other arm and shoulder down. Repeat with the other arm. It is important in this exercise not to bend your body. Keep the motion in the shoulder.

may also be the result of systemic disease (e.g., atherosclerosis, hypertension, blood dyscrasias) or systemic treatment (e.g., chemotherapy or anticoagulants).

Outcome Management

Medical Management

Ninety per cent of nosebleeds are anterior, most occurring in children and young adults. Anterior epistaxis is initially treated by assisting the client to a sitting position. Apply pressure by pinching the anterior portion of the nose for a minimum of 5 to 10 minutes. This maneuver is often successful because the most common source of epistaxis is the anterior part of the septum in an area known as Kisselbach's plexus, a venous plexus vulnerable to trauma. In addition, the application of ice compresses to produce vasoconstriction may also reduce bleeding. If more definitive treatment is necessary, anterior epistaxis can usually be controlled by cauterization of the bleeding vessel with applications of silver nitrate. If these measures do not stop the bleeding, nasal packing may be inserted unilaterally or bilaterally. Antibacterial ointment such as bacitracin or polymyxin B–neomycin (Neosporin) is applied to half-inch gauze, which is then gently but firmly inserted into the anterior nasal cavities to apply pressure to the bleeding vessels. The use of petrolatum gauze packing should be avoided, because it has no antimicrobial properties, and a malodorous discharge may develop within 1 to 2 days of insertion. Nasal packing should remain in place for a minimum of 48 to 72 hours.[9, 30]

Ten per cent of nosebleeds are posterior, usually occurring in older adults. For clients with posterior epistaxis, a *posterior plug* may be necessary in addition to the anterior nasal packing (Fig. 60–14). Insertion of a posterior plug is very uncomfortable, and a mild analgesic may be required to reduce anxiety and discomfort. A small, red rubber catheter is passed through the nose into the oropharynx and mouth. A gauze pack is tied to the catheter, and the catheter is withdrawn; this moves the pack into proper placement in the nasopharynx and posterior nose to apply pressure. The nasal cavity is packed with half-inch gauze, and the strings from the posterior pack are tied around a rolled gauze or bolus to maintain its position outside the nasal vestibule. The ties from the oral cavity are taped to the client's face to prevent loosening or dislodgment of the plug. A nasal balloon may be substituted for the traditional nasal pack. When the balloon is inflated with normal saline, pressure is applied to the lateral nasal wall.[26]

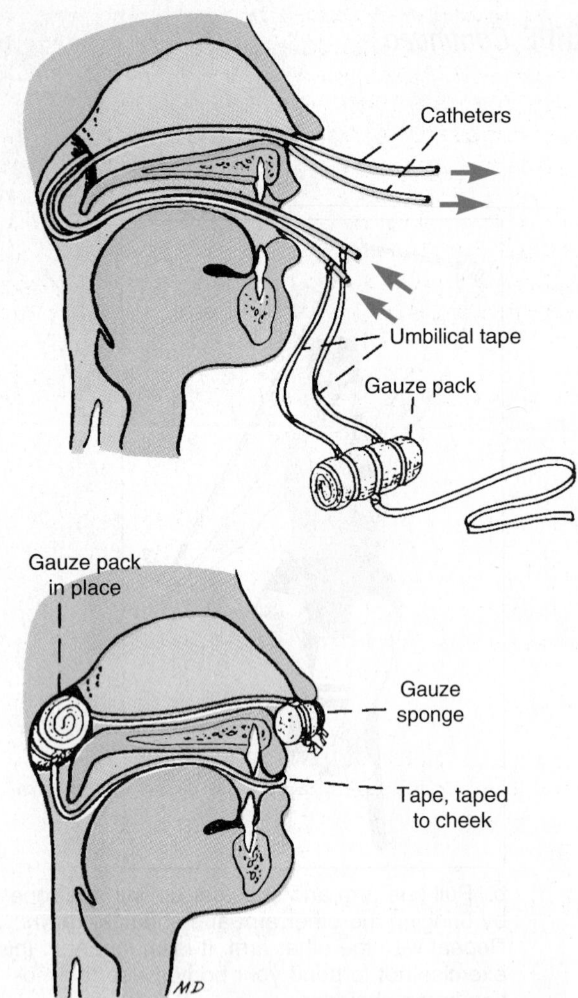

FIGURE 60–14 Instillation of a posterior nasal pack (plug), typically used in an emergency.

Nursing Management of the Medical Client

Clients with a posterior plug and anterior nasal packing are admitted to the hospital and monitored closely for hypoxia. General comfort measures, such as humidification, the use of a drip pad to collect bloody drainage and mucus, and application of water-soluble ointment around the nares to provide lubrication, help to alleviate the discomfort. Monitor the client closely for any signs of airway obstruction and bleeding from the anterior or posterior nares. Inspect the oral cavity for the presence of blood, soft palate necrosis, and proper placement of the posterior plug. If the posterior plug is visible, notify the physician for readjustment of the packing. Posterior nasal packs remain in place for 5 days.[9, 30] Prophylactic antibiotics are used to prevent toxic shock syndrome and sinusitis.

Surgical Management

If anterior and posterior packs fail to control epistaxis, internal maxillary or ethmoidal surgical *artery ligation* may be required. An incision is made in the gum line above the incisor on the affected side, and the maxillary sinus is entered. The artery that supplies the area of bleeding is identified, and a metal clip or suture is used to ligate the artery.

Nursing Management of the Surgical Client

The nasal packing inserted to control epistaxis remains in place for a minimum of 24 hours, during which time the client must be observed for additional bleeding, evidence of hypertension or hypotension, and infection. Upon discharge, the client is instructed to minimize activity for approximately 10 days, such as avoiding strenuous exercise; not blowing the nose; sneezing with the mouth open; and not lifting, stooping, or straining. The use of water-soluble ointment around the nares may provide comfort, and mouth rinses of half-strength hydrogen peroxide mixed with water or saline should be provided for oral hygiene. The use of a humidifier or vaporizer adds supplemental moisture to prevent dryness and crusting of secretions.

SINUSITIS

Sinusitis is a common infection that may occur in any of the paranasal sinuses. *Pansinusitis* is infection of more than one sinus. The term *rhinosinusitis* is thought to more accurately describe respiratory manifestations referable to an inflammatory disease of the nose or sinuses. However, the terms *rhinitis* and *sinusitis* may still be used.

Sinusitis is a common medical condition that affects an estimated 35 million people a year.[12] The sinuses are protected against infection by mucociliary action. The normal mucus produced by the sinuses is removed through small openings in the nose called ostia. When the ciliary action is impaired or the ostia are obstructed, mucus can accumulate in the sinus, which may then become infected. Blockage of the ostia may be due to a deviated nasal septum, bony abnormalities, congenital malformations, infections, or allergy.

A medical diagnosis of sinusitis is suggested by the client's clinical manifestations and confirmed by x-ray findings. Fever and chills along with headaches and facial pain exacerbated with bending, pain or numbness in the upper teeth, and a purulent or discolored nasal discharge may be present. Sinus radiographs or CT scans may show opacification of the sinus, thickened mucous membranes, and an air-fluid level (due to accumulation of secretions in the sinus), all indicative of sinusitis.

Outcome Management

Medical Management

Medical management of sinusitis includes (1) use of the appropriate antibiotic to manage the bacterial infection, (2) decongestants to reduce nasal edema, (3) corticosteroid nasal sprays to reduce mucosal inflammation, and (4) humidification by use of normal saline solution irrigations or a vaporizer or humidifier to prevent nasal crusting and to moisten secretions.

Antral irrigation or sinus lavage may be performed in clients who are not responding to treatment or who have increased purulent exudate in the maxillary sinus. Antral irrigation is performed with the use of a local anesthetic. A trocar (a sharp metal instrument) is inserted through the ostium in the lateral wall of the nose into the sinus. Prepare the client for the procedure with thorough explanations of the anesthetic procedure, the sensation of passage of the trocar through the ostium, and feelings of pressure. Normal saline solution is then injected through the cannula to rinse the sinus of purulent exudate. The client is placed in a sitting position, leaning slightly forward with the mouth open to allow drainage of the irrigating solution through the nose and mouth. A specimen of the exudate may be obtained for culture to determine the causative organism for prescription of an appropriate antibiotic.[30]

Surgical Management

Functional Endoscopic Sinus Surgery

If nonoperative measures fail, functional endoscopic sinus surgery (FESS) may be necessary. The major objective of FESS is the reestablishment of sinus ventilation and mucociliary clearance.[13] FEES is usually performed as an outpatient surgical procedure using local anesthesia (with or without conscious sedation) or with the patient under general anesthesia. Small fiberoptic endoscopes are passed through the nasal cavity and into the sinuses to allow direct visualization of the sinuses in order to remove diseased tissue and to enlarge sinus ostia (Fig. 60–15). A more popular method of performing FESS is with the use of small, powered instruments offering precision and safety in the surgical approach.[13]

Possible complications of FESS include nasal bleeding, pain, scar formation, and rarely, cerebrospinal fluid leak and blindness resulting from intraorbital hematoma formation or direct injury to the optic nerve. After FESS, nasal packing may be inserted to minimize nasal bleeding. Packing is removed within a few hours of the surgical procedure.

Caldwell-Luc Procedure

The Caldwell-Luc procedure is another surgical procedure performed for the management of chronic maxillary sinusitis. An incision is made into the gingival buccal sulcus above the lateral incisor teeth with the patient under general anesthesia, or local anesthesia may be used. Through this opening, the diseased mucous membrane is removed. In addition, an opening between the maxillary sinus and lateral nasal wall (nasal antral window) may be created to increase aeration of the sinus and to permit drainage into the nasal cavity.

After the procedure, the maxillary sinus and anterior nasal cavity are packed with half-inch gauze. Because of the packing, nasal breathing is obstructed. The oral cavity must be frequently evaluated for the presence of blood or packing that may have become dislodged, obstructing the pharynx. If packing is present in the pharynx, the visible portion may be held with a hemostat and cut with scissors. Be certain that the hemostat is holding the trimmed gauze; otherwise, it may be aspirated.[9, 29]

External Sphenoethmoidectomy

External sphenoethmoidectomy is a surgical procedure performed to remove diseased mucosa from the sphenoidal or ethmoidal sinus. A small incision is made over the ethmoidal sinus on the lateral nasal bridge, and the diseased mucosa is removed. Nasal and ethmoidal packing is then inserted. An eye pressure patch is usually applied to decrease periorbital edema.[30]

Nursing Management of the Surgical Client

After sinus surgery, observe the client for profuse nasal bleeding, respiratory distress, ecchymosis, and orbital and facial edema for the first 24 hours postoperatively. Apply ice compresses to the nose and cheek to minimize edema and control bleeding. Place the client in a semi-Fowler to

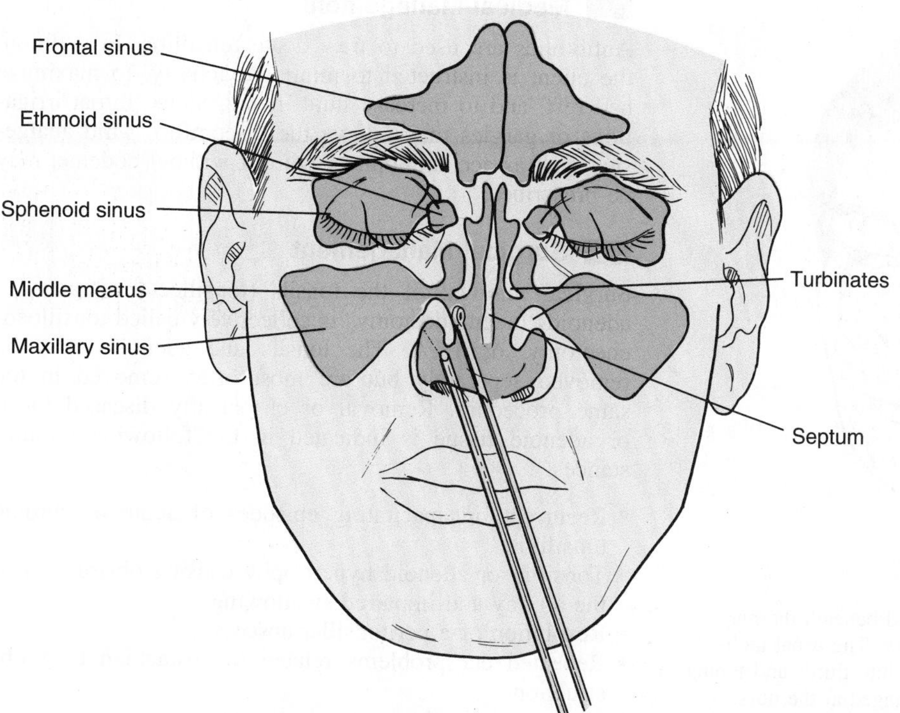

FIGURE 60–15 Functional endoscopic surgery. The middle meatus is the site to which most of the sinuses drain; if it is plugged, drainage is obstructed. With an endoscope, the sinuses can be seen and obstructions removed.

high Fowler position for 24 to 48 hours after surgery to minimize postoperative edema. The nasal packing is generally removed the morning after surgery; however, antral packing may remain in place for 36 to 72 hours. Give mild analgesics to the client to minimize discomfort postoperatively and before removal of the packing.

Instruct clients to increase fluid intake, which maximizes the water content of secretions. Although there may be some pain, a mild analgesic is usually all that is required. Minor nasal bleeding is expected for 24 to 48 hours after surgery. Use of a drip pad under the nose may eliminate the need for constant wiping (Fig. 60–16). Instruct clients to avoid blowing the nose for 7 to 10 days after surgery; tell them to sniff backward or spit, not blow. Teach the client to sneeze only with the mouth open. Nasal saline sprays may be started 3 to 5 days after surgery to moisten the nasal mucosa. Explain that the client is to engage in minimal physical exercise and to avoid strenuous activity, lifting, and straining for approximately 2 weeks. After FESS, the client needs to return to the physician's office for removal of crusts and debris and examination of the nose.

After a Caldwell-Luc procedure, the client may have temporary numbness of the upper teeth caused by interruption of sensory nerves from the mucosal incision. This abnormality may persist for several weeks.[9, 11, 30, 31]

PHARYNGITIS

Pharyngitis is inflammation of the pharynx and may be viral, bacterial, or fungal in origin. Beta-hemolytic streptococci are the most common infecting organisms. A culture of the pharyngeal mucosa is sometimes indicated before treatment is started. Clients may complain of a sore throat, difficulty in swallowing, fever, malaise, and cough and have an elevated white blood cell count. Treatment of pharyngitis depends on the causative agent. Both viral pharyngitis and bacterial pharyngitis are contagious by droplet spread. Good hand-washing technique is essential, and the use of a mask may prevent spread. Antibiotics are used to treat the bacterial pharyngitis; antifungal agents are used to treat fungal infections; and use of comfort measures is required for viral types. Bed rest, fluids, warm saline irrigations or gargles, analgesics, and antipyretics are recommended until the clinical manifestations are alleviated.

Chronic pharyngitis (chronic pharyngeal inflammation) is most common in people who habitually use tobacco and alcohol, have a chronic cough, are employed or live in dusty environments, or use their voices excessively. Clinical manifestations vary according to the degree of irritation and inflammation.

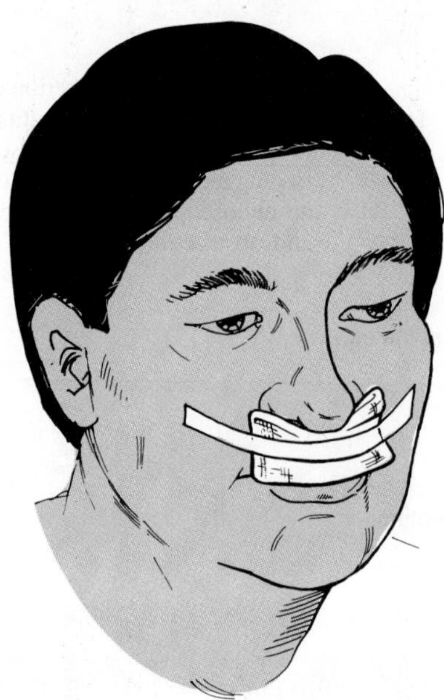

FIGURE 60–16 A nasal drip pad is taped beneath the nares to absorb drainage after nasal or sinus surgery. The usual technique consists of folding 4 × 4 dressings into thirds and taping them in place. These dressings can be changed at the nurse's discretion.

ACUTE TONSILLITIS

Tonsillitis is an infection of the tonsils. *Streptococcus* is the most common infecting organism, although tonsillitis can be caused by *Haemophilus influenzae* and other organisms.

The client with tonsillitis reports throat pain, difficulty in swallowing, otalgia (referred pain to the ear), and generalized malaise. Examination discloses an acutely inflamed mucous membrane around the tonsillar area with or without the presence of purulent exudate. In some clients, lymphadenopathy of the cervical lymph nodes may also be present.

Complications from streptococcal tonsillitis include pneumonia, nephritis, osteomyelitis, and rheumatic fever. Acute tonsillitis may become chronic. Acute otitis media, acute rhinitis, acute sinusitis, and peritonsillar abscess or other deep neck abscesses may also develop.

Medical Management

Antibiotics are used to treat acute tonsillitis. In addition, the client is instructed to minimize activity, to maximize bed rest, and to increase fluid intake. Saline throat irrigations or gargles may relieve the discomfort. Mild analgesics such as acetaminophen, with or without codeine, may be prescribed.

Surgical Management

Surgical removal of the tonsils (tonsillectomy) and the adenoids (adenoidectomy) is collectively called tonsilloadenectomy, or T&A. The tonsils and adenoids may be removed separately but are most often removed in the same procedure. Removal of chronically diseased tonsil or adenoid tissue is indicated in the following circumstances:

- Recurrent, incapacitating episodes of acute or chronic tonsillitis
- Tonsillar or adenoid hypertrophy causing obstruction of the airway and impaired swallowing
- Resolution of a peritonsillar abscess
- Repeated ear problems related to eustachian tube obstruction
- Sinus complications

T&A is most often done in children. Tonsillectomy may also be indicated for a carrier of diphtheria, because tonsils may "seed" the body with infectious organisms. Adults with recurrent sore throat, ear pain, or hearing dysfunction, or who snore because of hypertrophied adenoid or tonsillar tissue, may also benefit from this procedure. Although T&A is not as routine as in the past, it is indicated in clients who have repeated episodes of infection. T&A is performed as an outpatient procedure or as a same-day surgery procedure. Tonsillectomy may be performed with the use of either general or local anesthesia, although general anesthesia is more commonly used. Surgical intervention is contraindicated during an acute infection, that is, upper respiratory infection. Other contraindications to T&A include hematologic disorders such as hemophilia, aplastic anemia, purpura, and leukemia.

Nursing Management of the Surgical Client

After tonsillectomy, place the client in a lateral decubitus position until awake and alert. This position provides for drainage of blood and other secretions through the nose and mouth. Gently inspect the oropharynx and mouth for fresh blood frequently during the first several hours postoperatively. Monitor vital signs closely. Hemorrhage is the most serious complication after tonsillectomy and is most often seen during the first 12 to 24 hours. If postoperative hemorrhage occurs, resuturing or cauterization of the bleeding vessel is mandatory.

The client should begin taking oral feedings once recovery from anesthesia is complete. Encourage cool fluids, and introduce appropriate foods to provide a soft, bland diet, as tolerated. Highly seasoned foods, as well as any food the client finds difficult to swallow, should be avoided.

Pain in the first 7 to 10 postoperative days is common after tonsillectomy. Most clients report generalized throat pain as well as otalgia. Mild analgesics such as acetaminophen with or without codeine may be required to alleviate pain. Increased swallowing of fluids also helps to minimize discomfort. Aspirin is contraindicated because of the risk of bleeding associated with its use.

Encourage clients to seek immediate medical attention if bleeding occurs after hospital discharge. Delayed bleeding may occur once the healing membrane separates from the underlying tissue (7 to 10 days postoperatively). The surgical site is usually well healed in 14 to 21 days, and the client should have little difficulty after this time.[30, 31]

CHRONIC TONSILLITIS

The most frequent manifestation of chronic tonsillitis is recurrent sore throat. Between episodes of acute tonsillitis, the throat remains uncomfortable. The tonsils are often enlarged, and if they are infected, a sharp line may be seen between the color of the buccal mucosa and that of the tonsillar pillar. The most reliable indication of chronic tonsillitis is the expression of purulent material from the tonsillar crypts with a wooden tongue blade. Once chronic tonsillitis is diagnosed, surgical removal is recommended. Surgery is contraindicated during acute tonsillar infection, although tonsillectomy may be performed in a client with acute peritonsillar abscess.

PERITONSILLAR ABSCESS (QUINSY)

Peritonsillar abscess (quinsy) may arise from acute streptococcal or staphylococcal tonsillitis. The tissue between the tonsils and the fascia covering the superior constrictor muscles becomes infected, causing extensive swelling of the soft palate and the pharyngeal wall. The uvula may be pushed to one side, and up to half of the pharyngeal opening may be occluded. Pus formation in the fascial space pushes the tonsil forward toward the midline of the throat.

Peritonsillar abscess is typically manifested several days after the onset of acute tonsillitis. As the tonsillitis-related problems begin to resolve, increasing pain develops on one side of the throat and ear. Inflammation and edema create a partial obstruction to swallowing. Often, the client keeps the mouth partially open to allow drooling, rather than attempting painful swallowing. The voice takes on a characteristic "hot potato" or muffled sound. Thick secretions are raised with difficulty.

A peritonsillar abscess may rupture spontaneously. If spontaneous rupture does not occur, surgical intervention may be necessary. With the client in a sitting position (to allow expectoration of pus and blood), an incision is made and the abscess drained.

Topical anesthetic throat sprays, analgesic agents, hot saline throat irrigations (at temperatures of 40.5° to 43.3° C [105° to 110° F]), saline or alkaline mouthwashes or gargles, and ice collars may be used to make the throat more comfortable. Cool and room-temperature fluids are tolerated best. Ingestion of cool to warm soft foods may also be possible. High-dose antibiotics are often prescribed early to avoid the need for incision and drainage. It takes at least 1 month for the infection of a peritonsillar abscess to subside. Usually, a tonsillectomy is performed following resolution of the abscess and infection, to prevent recurrence. However, a "quinsy tonsillectomy" may be performed during the acute infection.[19, 30, 31]

RHINITIS

Rhinitis, or rhinosinusitis, is inflammation of the nasal mucosa. The classic manifestations of rhinitis are increased nasal drainage, nasal congestion, and paroxysmal sneezing. Normally, nasal drainage is composed of clear mucus. If the infection spreads to the sinuses, however, drainage may become yellow or green. Rhinitis may be classified as acute, allergic, vasomotor, or drug-related (rhinitis medicamentosa).

Acute rhinitis is also known as the common cold, or coryza. Acute rhinitis may be bacterial or viral in origin; it is treated symptomatically. Acute rhinitis usually lasts 5 to 7 days, with or without treatment. Common interventions for acute rhinitis are symptomatic and include supplemental humidification, decongestants to reduce the edema of the nasal mucosa, increased fluids to prevent dehydration, and analgesics to relieve the generalized myalgia. Sometimes antibiotics are given to prevent a secondary infection by bacteria.

Allergic rhinitis occurs most often as a seasonal disorder. In addition to obstruction to nasal breathing, the client may also experience irritation of other mucous membranes (e.g., the conjunctiva, causing tearing and edema of the eyelids). Treatment is symptomatic. A complete allergy evaluation may be required to determine the offending allergen. Most clients are placed on a desensitization program and instructed to avoid the antigen (substance that causes the allergic reaction); treatment is with antihistamines, steroids, or mast cell–stabilizing sprays.[18]

Vasomotor rhinitis causes the same manifestations as those of acute and allergic rhinitis but has no known cause. Clients with vasomotor rhinitis in whom results of culture and allergy evaluation are negative are given symptomatic treatment. If medications have been prescribed for the treatment of rhinitis (especially nasal sprays), the client must be taught the use of medications, including side effects and possible interactions with other medications.

Rhinitis medicamentosa is caused by abuse or overuse of topical nasal decongestant sprays or intranasal cocaine. These substances initially cause vasoconstriction. When used frequently, however, the initial decongestion is followed by severe mucosal edema. The edema is self-treated with more medication, and the rhinitis becomes cyclic. Management of rhinitis medicamentosa consists of avoidance of the causative agent and evaluation and treatment of the original problem.[30, 31]

LARYNGITIS

Laryngitis may be caused by an inflammatory process or vocal abuse. The laryngeal membrane is continuous with the lining of the upper respiratory tract, and infections in other areas of the nose and throat may include the larynx. Edema of the vocal cords caused by the chronic irritation of an upper respiratory tract infection inhibits the normal mobility of the vocal cords, which causes an abnormal sound.

Laryngitis may also be the result of gastroesophageal reflux disorder (GERD). In this syndrome, the cardiac sphincter between the stomach and the esophagus relaxes, and gastric acid is allowed to enter the esophagus. Reflux of gastric secretions, especially during sleep, may result in the aspiration of gastric secretions into the larynx, causing a chemical irritation or burning of the mucous membrane lining the larynx.[18, 25, 30] Clients with gastroesophageal reflux may complain of hoarseness from the chemical irritation of the gastric acid on the vocal cords, increased mucus production from the body's natural tendency to protect the irritated membrane, foreign body sensation, or sore throat. Chronic cough and asthma may also be associated symptoms of GERD.

Hoarseness is a common manifestation of disorders of the larynx and may be caused by inflammation of the vocal cords, abnormal movements of the vocal cords, or a benign or malignant tumor of the vocal cords. All of these problems interfere with normal mobility of the vocal cords, which produces a change in sound. Abnormal voice may also be the result of vocal abuse. Screaming, shouting, and loud speaking over a period of time may produce edema of the vocal cords and the formation of nodules or polyps—outpouchings of inflamed mucous membranes.

The treatment of laryngitis is aimed at the causative factors. If inflammatory laryngitis is suspected, the inflammation should be treated. Antibiotics may be used if a bacterial infection is suspected. In severe cases, systemic steroids (e.g., methylprednisolone [Medrol]) may be prescribed to reduce inflammation and edema. Supplemental humidification may add increased moisture to liquify secretions, and mucolytic agents may be prescribed to thin and mobilize mucus. The client with laryngitis may also be placed on voice rest to allow the edema of the vocal cords to subside without added strain. Caution the client to avoid whispering, which also causes excessive vocal cord strain.

Gastroesophageal reflux is initially treated symptomatically. The client is instructed to elevate the head of the bed to minimize reflux; to avoid eating or drinking for 2 to 3 hours before going to sleep; to avoid caffeine, alcohol, and tobacco, which are known to increase gastric secretions; and to use antacids and hydrogen inhibitors (famotidine [Pepcid], ranitidine [Zantac], omeprazole [Prilosec]) to neutralize and decrease acid production.[7, 30, 31]

Chronic laryngitis may stem from repeated infections, allergy, chronic irritant exposure, long-term voice abuse, or reflux esophagitis of acidic gastric contents. Chronic laryngitis is manifested as a tickling sensation in the throat, voice huskiness, and painful or difficult phonation. Management involves correction or removal of the irritation, in addition to measures to increase comfort. Long-term voice retraining may be necessary if improper use or overuse of the voice is the main cause of chronic laryngitis. This retraining includes (1) learning to use the voice without straining and (2) forming and projecting words to use the diaphragm without shouting.[30, 31]

DIPHTHERIA

Diphtheria is an acute, communicable disease caused by *Corynebacterium diphtheriae.* The incidence of diphtheria has declined in the United States as a result of required vaccination. Diphtheria is a highly contagious disease that is spread easily in populations with poor hygiene, crowding, and limited access to medical care.

Humans are the only natural reservoir for *C. diphtheriae.* This organism colonizes the mucosal surface of the nasopharynx and multiplies. The bacteria release a toxin that causes the tissues to necrose, forming a tough pseudomembrane covering the tonsils and pharyngeal walls. This membrane is difficult to dislodge and causes bleeding if removed. Systemic toxins can damage distal sites such as the heart, nerves, and kidneys.

Diphtheria is spread by aerosolization of the pathogen (droplet infection), and when objects used by diphtheria-infected people, such as eating utensils, towels, or handkerchiefs, are used by others. Healthy people, as well as clients recovering from the disease, may harbor the organism in the throat for 2 to 4 weeks.

The clinical manifestations can range from a single, localized lesion without systemic manifestations to those of a rapidly progressive fatal illness.

The two types of diphtheria are tonsillar and pharyngeal. *Tonsillar* diphtheria is seldom life-threatening, although it can progress rapidly to more fatal forms. A low-grade fever, fatigue, headache, and sore throat are common manifestations.

Pharyngeal diphtheria is the more serious form of diphtheria, especially when a membrane covers the larynx or bronchus. The client is gravely ill, with a weak pulse, restlessness, and confusion. Fever may or may not be present. Because of the location of the membrane, the airway is often obstructed, and the client exhibits stridor and cyanosis. The neck may also be swollen and warm.

Diphtheria is diagnosed by culture of the material with the enzyme-linked immunosorbent assay (ELISA) or the Elek test (toxigenicity test). Gram staining or fluorescent antibody staining may also be performed; these tests yield results more quickly. Although cultures are used to identify the organism, treatment begins immediately, before definitive results have been obtained. Treatment consists of antitoxin administration.

To prevent transmission of the disease, the client is placed in strict isolation. Contacts need to be identified, screened, immunized, and treated. Specimens from all contacts should be obtained for culture. People vaccinated 5 or more years previously should receive a booster dose. People who were never immunized should be given vaccine and antibiotics. During antitoxin administration, observe the client for anaphylaxis; epinephrine is kept at the bedside.[23]

Nursing management focuses on management of the airway obstruction. Suction equipment and a tracheotomy tray should be kept at the bedside. Oxygen is administered. Clients experience pain, especially with swallowing. In addition to analgesia, pain can be reduced by limiting the diet to liquids and soft foods. Throat irrigation and fluids may also help control pain.

OBSTRUCTIONS OF THE UPPER AIRWAY

ACUTE LARYNGEAL EDEMA

Acute laryngeal edema may be associated with inflammation, injury, or anaphylaxis. This condition is manifested by hoarseness and dramatic shortness of breath of acute onset. Dyspnea progresses rapidly, and unless a patent airway is established, respiratory arrest occurs. Endotracheal intubation may be very difficult because the larynx is edematous and is likely to bleed. Emergency tracheostomy may be required. If anaphylaxis is the precipitating cause, subcutaneous epinephrine 1:1000 is given. Intravenous corticosteroids are also used.[5]

CHRONIC LARYNGEAL EDEMA

Chronic laryngeal edema may occur when lymph drainage is obstructed, as with infection or tumor or after radiation therapy. If the edema is significant, an artificial airway may be required (either a tracheostomy or an endotracheal tube). The choice of route depends on the severity of the edema.

LARYNGOSPASM

Laryngospasm (spasm of the laryngeal muscles) may occur (1) after administration of some general anesthetic agents, (2) after repeated and traumatic attempts at endotracheal intubation, (3) as a response to some inhaled agents and foreign material, such as industrial fumes, dusts, and chemicals, and (4) from hypocalcemia.

Management is directed at reestablishing the airway as quickly and efficiently as possible. Administer 100% oxygen until the airway is fully reestablished and the larynx relaxes and spasms stop. Titrate FiO_2 according to ABG or pulse oximetry values. If the laryngospasm persists, paralysis with neuromuscular blocking agents, such as succinylcholine, may be required to allow intubation until the spasm subsides. Manual or mechanical ventilation is then necessary until the effects of the paralyzing agent have worn off. Occasionally, emergency cricothyroidotomy or tracheotomy may be necessary and should not be delayed.

LARYNGEAL PARALYSIS

Laryngeal paralysis may be the result of neck surgery, peripheral disorders, central nervous system (CNS) disorders, tumor, or viral infections or may be of unknown cause. One of the most common causes of laryngeal paralysis is trauma to the recurrent laryngeal nerve during thyroidectomy. Other causes of laryngeal paralysis are aortic aneurysm; mitral stenosis; thoracic surgery; thyroid gland carcinoma; neck injuries; tuberculosis; tumors of the bronchi, lungs, and mediastinum; metallic poisons (e.g., lead); and infection (e.g., diphtheria). CNS disorders that may lead to laryngeal paralysis include cerebrovascular accident (stroke) and myasthenia gravis. Bilateral laryngeal paralysis is rare, and when it occurs, the client usually exhibits difficulty in breathing or stridor.

With unilateral vocal cord paralysis (in which only one vocal cord is affected), the airway is usually not impaired and the primary manifestation is hoarseness. The client may have a breathy quality of the voice. Aspiration of food or saliva may occur until the normal, moving cord compensates by approximating the paralyzed cord (bringing the cords together). The client must be observed for manifestations of aspiration such as coughing upon swallowing, ineffective cough, decreased breath sounds, and crackles, rhonchi, or wheezes. The client with bilateral vocal cord paralysis can have a near-normal voice if the vocal cords are paralyzed in the adducted position. However, the major concern is airway compromise, especially on exertion. Dyspnea, intercostal muscle retraction, and stridor may occur with activity or upper airway infections.[29, 30]

If the paralyzed cords are bilaterally adducted, an emergency tracheotomy may be required. Surgery, such as arytenoidectomy, in which one or both arytenoid cartilages are removed and the vocal cords are held in an open position, may be used to open the glottis.

Injection of absorbable sponge (Gelfoam), as a temporary measure, or of polytetrafluoroethylene (Teflon), for permanent correction, may be used if the client with unilateral vocal cord paralysis exhibits signs of aspiration or requires strength or projection of the voice. The injected material is placed into the paralyzed cord to add bulk, to allow better approximation with the functioning cord.

Type I thyroplasty is recommended for permanent unilateral vocal cord paralysis. For this procedure, a window is made in the thyroid cartilage through an external incision, and a stent is inserted to move the paralyzed vocal cord into a midline position. The client may show signs of airway edema from both the injection and the thyroplasty and should be observed for respiratory distress.

LARYNGEAL INJURY

Laryngeal injury most often results from trauma during a motor vehicle accident, when the driver's neck strikes the steering wheel. Other causes include inhalation of hot gases and aspiration of caustic liquids. If complete airway obstruction does not occur, carefully assess for post-traumatic edema, which may lead to complete obstruction. Few outward signs may be present. It is often easy to overlook potential problems in the neck structures while focusing on other, possibly more dramatic injuries. Observe for increased dyspnea, intercostal muscle retraction, neck swelling, laryngeal tenderness, dysphagia, stridor, inability to speak, and change in respiration patterns.

The thyroid cartilage may be fractured. This problem leads to soft tissue and laryngeal edema as well as hematoma formation. If airway obstruction occurs, tracheostomy may be necessary. Indications of a fractured thyroid cartilage include (1) a tender, swollen ecchymotic neck; (2) stridor; (3) cyanosis in some cases; and (4) subcutaneous emphysema in some cases.

Damage to the larynx above the cricoid cartilage may lead to tracheal stenosis. The cricoid cartilage forms the only complete circle of cartilage in the upper airway, and it maintains the open lumen of the upper end of the airway.

CHRONIC AIRWAY OBSTRUCTION

NASAL POLYPS

Nasal polyps are outpouchings of mucous membrane lining the nose or paranasal sinuses and may occur as solitary or multiple lesions. Polyps may be exacerbated by allergic symptoms, although they are not caused by allergies.[9] Most people who have symptomatic polyps seek medical attention for obstruction to nasal breathing.

The medical management of clients with nasal polyps is symptomatic. Attempts are made to reduce the size of the polyps by eliminating or treating the causative factor (i.e., allergy). In many clients, surgery is needed to remove nasal polyps in order to restore nasal breathing before allergy treatment. Nasal polypectomy (removal of nasal polyps) can be done in the physician's office or in the operating room. Nasal polypectomy is usually performed with use of a local anesthetic. The anesthetic (commonly lidocaine with epinephrine) eliminates discomfort while also producing vasoconstriction to minimize bleeding during the procedure. A snarelike instrument is used to remove the polyps. The bleeding sites are cauterized, and intranasal packing is inserted. Intranasal splints can be used to prevent formation of adhesions. The nasal packing is maintained for several hours to minimize the possibility of postoperative bleeding and is generally removed before discharge of the client from the health care facility.

Because of the presence of nasal packing and edema, clients need to breathe through the mouth for the first 24 to 48 hours. The use of humidification, frequent mouth care, and increasing oral fluids help to minimize the dryness and oropharyngeal discomfort. Inspect the oral cavity frequently to evaluate the effectiveness of these measures. Clients with polyps frequently also have asthma (when combined with aspirin allergy, this is called "triad disease"). Asthmatic symptoms may be exacerbated after surgery.[9]

The client is placed in a semi-Fowler to high Fowler position after surgery to minimize edema. In addition, continuous use of ice compresses is recommended for the first 48 hours to reduce edema and to control bleeding. With the proper application of nasal packing at the time of surgery and the use of ice compresses in the immediate postoperative period, nasal bleeding should be minimal. However, the client should be assessed for changes in vital signs and the oropharynx inspected for the presence of blood. Because the nasal packing absorbs anterior bleeding, it is essential to observe the client for posterior nasal bleeding. Manifestations of active posterior bleeding include frequent swallowing and the presence of blood in the throat.

Most clients experience only minimal discomfort after a nasal polypectomy. Mild analgesics may be given for any postoperative discomfort. The use of aspirin and aspirin-containing products should be avoided because of their anticoagulant effects. Instruct the client not to blow the nose and to refrain from sneezing if possible. When the stimulus to sneeze cannot be overcome, the client should sneeze through an open mouth.[30, 31]

DEVIATED NASAL SEPTUM AND NASAL FRACTURE

The nasal septum (the dividing structure of the nose) is usually straight and separates the nose into two equal chambers. After trauma, the septum may become deviated, creating asymmetrical breathing passages. For some clients, the deviation may cause an obstruction to nasal breathing, dryness of the nasal mucosa leading to bleeding, and occasionally a cosmetic deformity. A deviated nasal septum changes the velocity of air, altering normal nasal activity resulting in dryness, crusting, nasal bleeding, and changes in the membranes lining the nose.

If a nasal fracture occurs, immediate medical management is advised. Within several hours of nasal injury, severe edema may occur, which causes difficulty in reducing the fracture. Immediately after the injury, ice should be applied. A simple nasal fracture may be reduced in an emergency facility with use of local anesthesia. If immediate reduction of the nasal fracture is not possible, it is advisable to wait several days until edema subsides but before healing begins.

For correction of a deviated nasal septum, reconstruction of a cosmetic deformity of the nose, and reduction of a nasal fracture, the principles of surgical management are similar. All three procedures are usually performed with use of local anesthesia combined with mild sedation. Because of the vasoconstrictor properties of local anesthetics, these agents reduce bleeding during and immediately after surgery. Surgery to correct a deviated nasal septum is known as a nasal septoplasty and consists of making an incision on either side of the septum, elevating the mucous membrane, and straightening or removing the offending portion of the cartilage. If a cosmetic deformity is also of concern or if the deformity interferes with septal reconstruction, a rhinoplasty (reconstruction of the external nose) may be done in conjunction with the nasal septoplasty or as a separate procedure. (See also Chapter 49.)

After these three procedures, intranasal packing and internal splints may be used to maintain the position of the septum, to control bleeding, and to prevent hematoma formation. If the patient has undergone rhinoplasty or reduction of a nasal fracture, an external splint and a small dressing may also be applied. Postoperative care is directed at airway management, control of edema and hemorrhage, and pain relief. Because of the presence of bilateral nasal packing, clients require the same care as discussed for the client who has undergone nasal polypectomy.

CONCLUSIONS

Disorders of the upper airway range from a simple cold to cancer of the larynx. This chapter presents care of clients most commonly hospitalized with upper airway disorders. Nursing management ranges from assessment of life-threatening airway obstruction to teaching techniques that reduce the spread of infection.

THINKING CRITICALLY

1. **The client has a temporary tracheostomy after undergoing a supraglottic laryngectomy. On the second postoperative day, the client indicates to you that he is having trouble breathing. How should you evaluate the client and eliminate the problem?**

Factors to Consider. What principles are used as the basis of tracheostomy care? How does evaluation of pulse oximetry contribute to decision-making for care?

2. **You walk into the room of a client who underwent total laryngectomy 12 hours ago. The client is complaining of severe nausea but has not vomited. What are the client's risks following this type of surgery? How should you respond to the present problem?**

Factors to Consider. What risks are inherent in the occurrence of tracheal interruption? How well can the client communicate with you at this time?

3. **You enter the room of a client in whom a nosebleed has developed. Bright red blood is seeping continuously from the nares, and the client states that it feels like some blood is going down the back of his throat. What is the priority intervention? What are the implications if the bleeding continues?**

Factors to Consider. What are the causes of epistaxis? What are the psychological effects of a nosebleed?

BIBLIOGRAPHY

1. Brennan, J. A., et al. (1995). Association between cigarette smoking and mutation of the *p53* gene in squamous-cell carcinoma of the head and neck. *New England Journal of Medicine, 332,* 712–717.
2. Bryce, J. C. (1995). Aspiration: Causes, consequences and prevention. *ORL—Head and Neck Nursing, 13*(2), 14–20.
3. Byers, R. M., & Roberts, D. B. (1998). The selective neck dissection for upper aerodigestive tract carcinoma: Indications and results. In K. T. Robbins (Ed.), *Advances in head and neck oncology* (pp. 37–45). San Diego: Singular Publishing Group.
4. Clarke, L. C. (1998). Rehabilitation for the head and neck cancer patient. *Oncology, 12*(1), 81–94.
5. Cyr, M. H., Hickey, M. M., & Higgins, T. S. (1998). Tracheal, esophageal conditions and care. In L. L. Harris & M. B. Huntoon (Eds.), *Core curriculum for otorhinolaryngology and head-neck nursing* (pp. 246–271). New Smyrna Beach, FL: Society of Otorhinolaryngology and Head-Neck Nurses.
6. Dropkin, M. J. (1997). Coping with disfigurement/dysfunction and length of hospital stay after head and neck cancer surgery. *ORL—Head and Neck Nursing, 15*(1), 22–26.
7. Goldsmith, C. (1998). Gastroesophageal reflux disease. *American Journal of Nursing, 98*(9), 44–45.
8. Haynes, V. (1996). Caring for the laryngectomy patient. *American Journal of Nursing, 96*(5), 161–164.
9. Higgins, T. S., et al. (1998). Nasal cavity, paranasal sinuses, nasopharynx conditions and care. In L. L. Harris & M. B. Huntoon (Eds.), *Core curriculum for otorhinolaryngology and head-neck nursing* (pp. 169–206). New Smyrna Beach, FL: Society of Otorhinolaryngology and Head-Neck Nurses.
10. Kim, M. J., McFarland, G. K., & McLane, A. M. (1993). *Pocket guide to nursing diagnosis.* St. Louis: Mosby–Year Book.
11. Krouse, H. J., Krouse, J. H., & Christmas, D. A. (1997). Endoscopic sinus surgery in otorhinolaryngology nursing using powered instrumentation. *ORL—Head and Neck Nursing, 15*(2), 22–25.
12. Krouse, J. H. (1999). Introduction to sinus disease: I. Anatomy and physiology. *ORL—Head and Neck Nursing, 17*(2), 7–12.
13. Krouse, J. H., & Krouse, H. J. (1999). Introduction to sinus disease: II. Diagnosis and treatment. *ORL—Head and Neck Nursing, 17*(3), 6–16.
14. Landis, S. H., et al. (1999). Cancer statistics, 1999. *CA: A Cancer Journal for Clinicians, 49*(1), 8–31.
15. Leder, S. B., & Blom, E. D. (1998). Tracheoesophageal voice prosthesis fitting and training. In E. D. Blom, M. I. Singer, & R. C. Hamaker (Eds.), *Tracheoesophageal voice restoration following total laryngectomy* (pp. 57–65). San Diego: Singular Publishing Group.
16. Lockhart, J., & Bryce, J. (1993). Restoring speech with tracheoesophageal puncture. *Nursing 93, 23*(1), 10–13.
17. Lockhart, J., Troff, J., & Artim, L. (1992). Total laryngectomy and radical neck dissection. *AORN Journal, 55*(2), 458–479.
18. Mabry, C. S., & Mabry, R. L. (1996). Making the diagnosis of allergy. *ORL—Head and Neck Nursing, 14*(1), 13–14.
19. McCall, M. (1993). It killed George: Managing the peritonsillar abscess patient effectively. *ORL—Head and Neck Nursing, 11*(1), 10–13.
20. McKenna, M. (1999). Postoperative tonsillectomy/adenoidectomy hemorrhage: A retrospective chart review. *ORL—Head and Neck Nursing, 17*(3), 18–21.
21. Minasian, A., & Dwyer, J. T. (1998). Nutritional implications of dental and swallowing issues in head and neck cancer. *Oncology, 12*(8), 1155–1169.
22. Mood, D. W. (1997). Cancers of the head and neck. In C. Varricchio (Ed.), *A cancer source book for nurses* (7th ed., pp. 271–283). Atlanta: American Cancer Society.
23. Postma, G. N., & Koufman, J. A. (1998). Laryngitis. In B. J. Bailey & K. H. Calhoun (Eds.), *Head and neck surgery—otolaryngology* (2nd ed., Vol. 1, pp. 731–739). Philadelphia: Lippincott-Raven.
24. Repasky, T. M. (1995). Epiglottitis. *American Journal of Nursing, 95*(9), 52.
25. Robbins, K. T. (1998). Targeted cisplatin chemotherapy for advanced head and neck cancer. In K. T. Robbins (Ed.), *Advances in head and neck oncology* (pp. 59–71). San Diego: Singular Publishing Group.
26. Santos, P. M., & Lepore, M. L. (1998). Epistaxis. In B. J. Bailey & K. H. Calhoun (Eds.), *Head and neck surgery—otolaryngology* (2nd ed., Vol. 1, pp. 513–530). Philadelphia: Lippincott-Raven.

27. Seay, S. J., & Gay, S. L. (1997). Problem in tracheostomy patient care: Recognizing the patient with a displaced tracheostomy tube. *ORL—Head and Neck Nursing, 15*(2), 10–11.

28. Sigler, B. A. (1995). Nursing care for head and neck tumor patients. In S. E. Thawley & W. R. Panje (Eds.), *Comprehensive management of head and neck tumors* (pp. 79–100). Philadelphia: W. B. Saunders.

29. Sigler, B. A. (1998). Nursing management of the patient with a tracheostomy. In E. N. Myers, J. T. Johnson, & T. Murray (Eds.), *Tracheotomy—airway management, communication, and swallowing* (pp. 57–65). San Diego: Singular Publishing Group.

30. Sigler, B. A., & Schuring, L. T. (1993). *Ear, nose and throat disorders.* St. Louis: Mosby–Year Book.

31. Society of Otorhinolaryngology and Head and Neck Nurses. (1996). *Guidelines for otorhinolaryngology and head and neck nursing practice.* New Smyrna Beach, FL: Author.

32. Thibodeau, G. A., & Patton, K. T. (1993). *Anatomy and physiology* (2nd ed.). St. Louis: Mosby–Year Book.

33. Weilitz, P. B., & Dettenmeier, P. A. (1994). Back to basics: Testing your knowledge of tracheostomy tubes. *American Journal of Nursing, 94*(2), 46–50.

34. Weinstein, G. S., & Laccoureye, O. (1998). Supracricoid partial laryngectomy. In K. T. Robbins (Ed.), *Advances in head and neck oncology* (pp. 83–98). San Diego: Singular Publishing Group.

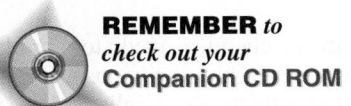

CHAPTER 61

Management of Clients with Lower Airway and Pulmonary Vessel Disorders

Sherill Nones Cronin
Kim Miracle

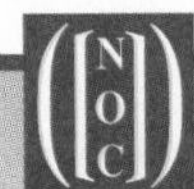

NURSING OUTCOMES CLASSIFICATION (NOC)
for Nursing Diagnoses—Clients with Lower Airway and Pulmonary Vessel Disorders

Activity Intolerance
Activity Tolerance
Altered Nutrition: Less Than Body Requirements
Nutritional Status
Nutritional Status: Food and Fluid Intake
Anxiety
Anxiety Control
Coping
Impaired Gas Exchange
Respiratory Status: Gas Exchange
Respiratory Status: Ventilation
Ineffective Airway Clearance
Respiratory Status: Airway Patency
Respiratory Status: Gas Exchange
Respiratory Status: Ventilation
Ineffective Breathing Pattern
Respiratory Status: Ventilation
Anxiety Control
Asthma Control
Ineffective Individual Coping
Coping
Information Processing
Role Performance
Social Support
Knowledge Deficit
Knowledge: Disease Process
Knowledge: Health Behaviors
Knowledge: Medication
Knowledge: Treatment Regimen

A distinguishing feature of lower airway and pulmonary vessel disorders is the presence of dyspnea. *Dyspnea* (shortness of breath) is a subjective experience that results when air flow, oxygen exchange, or both are impaired. The sensation of uncomfortable breathing can be as distressing as pain and may lead to severe functional disability. The intensity and frequency of dyspnea as well as its association with specific activities must be assessed to develop realistic expectations of treatment outcomes. Because the experience of dyspnea is associated with much anxiety, nursing interventions to relieve this manifestation are essential to the care of clients with conditions of the lower airways and pulmonary vessels.

DISORDERS OF THE LOWER AIRWAYS

ASTHMA

Asthma is a disorder of the bronchial airways characterized by periods of reversible bronchospasm (spasms of prolonged contraction of the airway). Asthma is often called "reactive airway disease." This complex disorder involves biochemical, immunologic, endocrine, infectious, autonomic, and psychological factors. Asthma affects about 5% to 10% of the United States population, making it the most common chronic disease in children and adults. Mortality and morbidity rates from the disease have risen since the mid-1980s, despite a concomitant rise in general knowledge about the disease.[3]

Etiology and Risk Factors

Asthma occurs in families, which suggests that it is an inherited disorder. Apparently, environmental factors (e.g., viral infection, allergens, and pollutants) interact with inherited factors to produce disease. Other inciting factors can include excitatory states (stress, laughing, crying), exercise, changes in temperature, and strong odors. Asthma also is a component of *triad* disease: asthma, nasal polyps, and allergy to aspirin.

Pathophysiology

Asthma involves a chronic inflammatory process that produces mucosal edema, mucus secretion, and airway inflammation. When people with asthma are exposed to extrinsic allergens and irritants (e.g., dust, pollen, smoke, mold, medications, foods, respiratory infections), their airways become inflamed, producing shortness of breath, chest tightness, and wheezing. Initial clinical manifestations, termed *early-phase reaction,* develop immediately and last about an hour.

When a client comes in contact with an allergen, immunoglobulin E (IgE) is produced by B lymphocytes. IgE antibodies attach to mast cells and basophils in the bronchial walls. As shown in the Pathophysiology and Treatment algorithm, the mast cell empties, releasing chemical mediators of inflammation, such as histamine, bradykinin, prostaglandins, and slow-reacting substance of anaphylaxis (SRS-A). The substances induce capillary dilation, leading to edema of the airway in an attempt to dilute the allergen and wash it away. They also induce airway constriction in an attempt to close the airway to prevent inhalation of more allergen.

About half of all asthma clients also experience a *delayed (late-phase) reaction.* Although clinical manifestations are the same as in early phase, they do not begin until 4 to 8 hours after exposure and may last for hours or days.

In both phases, release of chemical mediators produces the airway response. In the late-phase response, however, the mediators attract other inflammatory cells and create a self-sustaining cycle of obstruction and inflammation. This chronic inflammation produces hyperresponsiveness of the airways. This hyperresponsiveness causes subsequent episodes in response not only to specific antigens but also to stimuli, such as physical exertion and breathing cold air. Clinical manifestations may occur with increasing frequency and severity.

Both alpha-adrenergic and beta-adrenergic receptors of the sympathetic nervous system are found in the bronchi. Stimulation of alpha-adrenergic receptors causes bronchoconstriction; conversely, stimulation of beta-adrenergic receptors causes bronchodilation. Cyclic adenosine monophosphate (cAMP) balances the two receptors. Some theories suggest that asthma may be a result of lack of beta-adrenergic stimulation.

Clinical Manifestations

During asthma attacks, clients are dyspneic and have marked respiratory effort. Manifestations of marked respiratory effort include nasal flaring, pursed-lip breathing,

CASE MANAGEMENT

Chronic Obstructive Pulmonary Disease

Chronic obstructive pulmonary disease (COPD) accounts for a high volume of inpatient admissions. Treatment of a COPD exacerbation may be attempted on an outpatient basis, with the administration of nebulized bronchodilators and intravenous steroids in an emergency department or observation unit. Clients who cannot be stabilized or who may have multiple problems are admitted for longer-duration therapy. Case management for these clients involves discovery of underlying risks, education, and health promotion to prevent constant readmission.

Assess

- What manifestations is this client experiencing on admission?
- Are there specific triggers or times when manifestations occur (e.g., stressful situations, environmental factors)?
- What medications does this client take?
- Is the client using the metered-dose inhaler correctly?
- What is the impact of this illness on activities of daily living, family roles, and ability to work or attend school?
- What other co-morbid conditions or practices might worsen this client's respiratory status (e.g., heart failure, cor pulmonale, pneumonia, smoking)?
- Has this client had recent or frequent hospital admissions?

Advocate

Give clients who experience difficulty breathing extra reassurance and attention.

Alleviate their fear and anxiety by anticipating needs and checking frequently to assure them that you are monitoring their condition and are available to assist them.

Ensure that they understand correct sequencing of medications (e.g., bronchodilator before steroid use); also correct use of metered-dose inhalers, spacers, or other equipment as well as cleaning (to prevent oral thrush).

Discuss home oxygen safety, especially if the client is still smoking. Discourage continued tobacco use and offer resources to assist with smoking cessation.

Help to plan a schedule that includes rest periods and smaller, more frequent meals.

Prevent Readmission

Wean the client from oxygen, if possible, and test oxygen saturation levels during activity as well as at rest. If oxygen will be needed at home, make appropriate referrals. For some clients, especially those with asthma, monitoring peak flow levels is recommended, and a meter should be obtained. Ensure that the client is knowledgeable about medications and how to handle dyspneic episodes correctly.

Discuss prevention of infection, including appropriate flu and pneumonia immunization, disposal of secretions, hand-washing, and care of respiratory equipment. Stress the need for hydration and good nutrition.

Make referrals for nursing care, pulmonary rehabilitation, or smoking cessation programs. The client must also know about planned follow-up, when to call the physician, and how to get emergency assistance.

Encourage participation in community support groups and disease management programs through hospitals, insurer groups, and the American Lung Association.

Cheryl Noetscher, RN, MS, *Director of Case Management, Crouse Hospital and Community–General Hospital, Syracuse, New York*

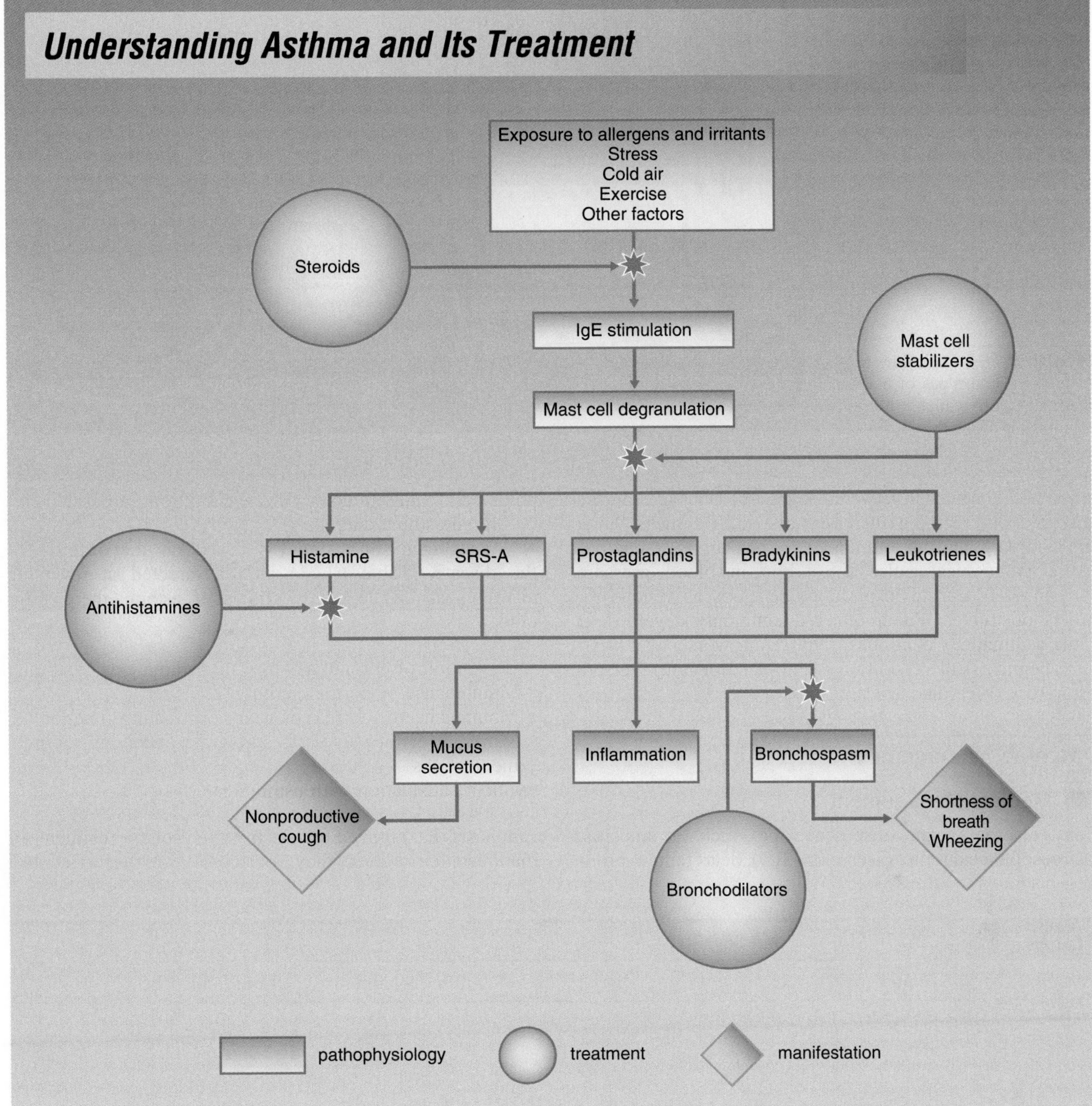

and use of accessory muscles. Cyanosis is a late development.

Auscultation of breath sounds usually reveals wheezing, especially during expiration. The inability to auscultate wheezing in an asthmatic client with acute respiratory distress may be an ominous sign. It may indicate that the small airways are too constricted to allow any air flow. The client may require immediate, aggressive medical intervention. In addition, bronchospasm may lead to almost continuous coughing in an attempt to clear the airway.

The diagnosis of asthma is based on clinical manifestations, spirometry results, and response to treatment. Spirometry reveals decreased peak expiratory flow rate (PEFR), forced expiratory volume timed (FEV_1), and forced vital capacity (FVC). Functional residual capacity (FRC), total lung capacity (TLC), and residual volume (RV) are increased because air is trapped within the lungs. A 12% improvement in forced expiratory volume in 1 second (FEV_1) after inhaled administration of a beta-agonist bronchodilator implies a reversible air flow obstruction, that is, by definition, asthma. Figure 61–1 shows peak flowmeters for monitoring air flow.

Baseline assessment of pulmonary status also may include pulse oximetry and arterial blood gas (ABG) analysis. Pulse oximetry usually reveals low oxygen saturation. ABGs often show some degree of hypoxemia, with elevated partial pressures of arterial carbon dioxide ($Pa{CO_2}$) in severe cases.

Status asthmaticus is a severe, life-threatening complication of asthma. It is an acute episode of bronchospasm

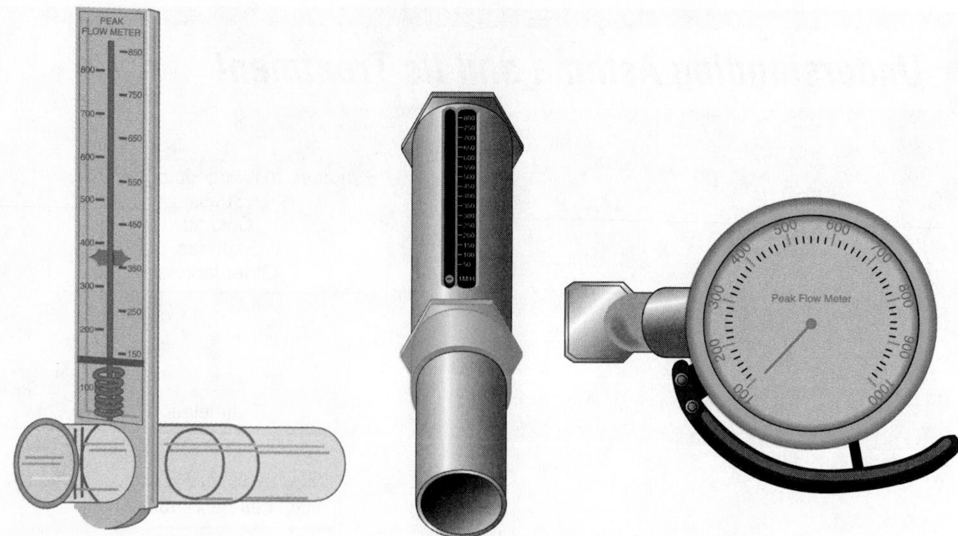

FIGURE 61–1 Peak flowmeters. Several types of portable meters are available for self-monitoring of air flow.

that tends to intensify. With severe bronchospasm, the workload of breathing increases five to 10 times, which can lead to acute cor pulmonale. When air is trapped, a severe paradoxical pulse (i.e., drop in blood pressure >10 mm Hg during inspiration) develops as venous return is obstructed. Pneumothorax commonly develops. If status asthmaticus continues, hypoxemia worsens and acidosis begins. If the condition is untreated or not reversed, respiratory or cardiac arrest ensues.

Outcome Management

Medical Management

Many disorders can cause wheezing, such as sinusitis, gastroesophageal reflux disease (GERD), heart failure, bronchitis, and lung tumors. These conditions are ruled out before an asthma diagnosis is given.

Management of asthma is based on the severity of the disease (Table 61–1) and is directed at reversing airway spasm. The general goals of asthma therapy include:

- Prevention of chronic asthma and asthma exacerbations
- Maintenance of normal activity levels
- Maintenance of normal or near-normal lung function
- Minimal or no side effects while receiving optimal medications
- Client satisfaction with asthma care[19]

Emphasis has moved away from episodic treatment of manifestations after they occur to long-term control

TABLE 61–1 CLASSIFYING ASTHMA SEVERITY

	Symptoms	Nighttime Symptoms	Lung Function
STEP 4 Severe Persistent	Continual symptoms Limited physical activity Frequent exacerbations	Frequent	FEV_1 or PEF ≤ 60% predicted PEF variability >30%
STEP 3 Moderate Persistent	Daily symptoms Daily use of inhaled short-acting $beta_2$ agonist Exacerbations affect activity Exacerbations ≥2 times a week; may last days	>1 time a week	FEV_1 or PEF > 60% to <80% predicted PEF variability >30%
STEP 2 Mild Persistent	Symptoms >2 times a week but <1 time a day Exacerbations may affect activity	>2 times a month	FEV_1 or PEF ≥ 80% predicted PEF variability 20%–30%
STEP 1 Mild Intermittent	Symptoms ≤2 times a week Asymptomatic and normal PEF between exacerbations Exacerbations brief (from a few hours to a few days); intensity may vary	≤2 times a month	FEV_1 or PEF ≥ 80% predicted PEF variability <20%

FEV_1, forced expiratory volume in 1 second; PEF, peak expiratory flow.

From National Institutes of Health. (1997). *Guidelines for the diagnosis and management of asthma.* NIH Pub. No. 97-4051. Washington, DC: Author.

through inhaled corticosteroids to prevent asthma whenever possible.

Reverse Airway Spasm

A severe asthma episode may constitute a medical emergency. Medical intervention for such episodes is aimed primarily at:

- Maintaining a patent airway by relieving bronchospasm and clearing excess or retained secretions
- Maintaining effective gas exchange
- Preventing complications, such as acute respiratory failure and status asthmaticus

Emergency management of the client begins with inhaled beta$_2$ agonists. Beta$_2$ agonists stimulate the beta-adrenergic receptors and dilate the airways. If the spasm does not abate (i.e., if FEV_1 remains $<50\%$ of predicted), nebulized atropine sulfate or intravenous (IV) steroids may be given. Atropine is an anticholinergic that blocks the effect of the parasympathetic system. When the vagus nerve is stimulated, bronchial smooth muscle tone increases. If these treatments do not reverse the clinical manifestations, the client usually is admitted to the hospital for further treatment. If the client has an acute asthma attack and no medications are nearby, the attack sometimes can be lessened by *pursed-lip breathing,* which increases pressure in the airways so that they remain open and so that trapped air can be exhaled more easily.

Supplemental oxygen is indicated if partial pressure of arterial oxygen (PaO_2) levels decrease to less than 60 mm Hg. Monitor the client closely for clinical manifestations of increasing anxiety, increased work of breathing, and indications of tiring. Endotracheal intubation and mechanical ventilation may be necessary. Sedation, and in rare cases administration of paralytic agents, may be necessary to blunt the client's respiratory effort and to prevent further air trapping and pressure increases. Status asthmaticus is treated with aggressive use of IV corticosteroids and frequent administration of inhaled beta-adrenergic medications to avoid intubation and mechanical ventilation.

Control Inflammation

Mucosal inflammation is controlled through the use of inhaled corticosteroids. Steroids prevent the mast cell from emptying, reducing the edema and spasm.

Leukotriene inhibitors and mast cell stabilizers are included in special circumstances. Leukotriene inhibitors are thought to be important mediators in the pathogenesis of asthma. Zafirlukast (Accolate) and zileuton (Zyflo) are two such drugs that have been approved for prophylaxis and treatment of mild to moderate asthma. Mast cell stabilizers, such as cromolyn (Nasalcrom, Intal) and nedocromil (Tilade), suppress the release of bronchoconstrictive substances during antigen-antibody reactions.

Nursing Management

Assessment

Initially, assess the client for clinical manifestations of airway distress. If present, they constitute an emergency that must be managed before a detailed history of the disease is obtained. The Critical Monitoring feature lists manifestations of acute airway distress.

Asking clients to rate dyspnea on a scale of 0 to 10 is an easy and effective measure of present dyspnea and may help you monitor and evaluate dyspnea in clinic and home care settings: "On a scale of 0 to 10, indicate how much shortness of breath you are having right now, with 0 meaning no shortness of breath and 10 meaning shortness of breath as bad as can be."

Determine known medication allergies so that allergenic medications can be avoided during treatment. Ascertain whether the client has a history of cardiac disease because beta$_2$ agonists can produce tachycardia and stress a diseased heart.

Once the acute episode is controlled, explore the history of the client's asthma. Assist the client to determine whether there is a pattern to the manifestations. These data may help identify a trigger that precipitates the asthmatic manifestations. If an extrinsic trigger can be identified, it may be possible to reduce or eliminate it. For example, if the client is allergic to mold, common sources of mold can be avoided. Ask about current medications. Some clients are inadvertently given medications that may induce bronchospasms. For example, a noncardioselective beta-blocker, such as propranolol (Inderal), prescribed for hypertension may cause bronchospasm.

Within the psychosocial domain, ask about the client's ability to manage the asthma and his or her general adaptation to the illness. Denial of the illness can interfere with early treatment. Determine whether the client feels control over the illness and feels capable of managing it. Clients who have this feeling of control show better compliance with treatments. Determine whether the client is experiencing an increased number of stressors. A stressful lifestyle may exacerbate asthma.

Assess the attitude of the family. The family can be a great source of support and can assist the client in recognizing early manifestations. In contrast, an unsupportive family may contribute to denial or may be an additional source of stress to the client. Involve the Case Manager (see the Case Management feature).

The client with a new diagnosis of asthma may be asked to assess the home and work environment for likely triggers of the clinical manifestations. In addition, skin testing for allergy may be performed. The presence of

CRITICAL MONITORING

Asthma

Notify the physician if the client still has the following manifestations after treatment for asthma:

- Increased anxiety
- Increased respiratory rate and effort
- Wheezing, both inspiratory and expiratory
- Almost continuous, nonproductive cough
- Nasal flaring as respiratory distress increases
- Lips pursed while exhaling
- Use of accessory muscles of breathing
- Increasing tachycardia (tachycardia is a normal response to beta-adrenergic drugs)
- Paradoxical pulse as bronchospasm worsens
- Cyanosis and central nervous system depression as late findings

pets that shed hair or dander, cigarette smoke, or occupational exposure to other allergens may require some lifestyle changes. In many cases, the pets can remain in the house but cannot sleep with the asthmatic client. Encourage clients to stop smoking, and teach clients and others about the dangers of second-hand smoke. Elimination of irritants is generally performed in a reasonable fashion, such as removing exposure to one allergen at a time. Potential improvements in a client's manifestations that might result from a major lifestyle change, such as job change or loss of a pet, may be quickly offset by the stress felt from such a change.

DIAGNOSIS, OUTCOMES, INTERVENTIONS

Ineffective Breathing Pattern. Because of airway spasm and edema, the client cannot move air in and out of the lungs as needed to maintain adequate tissue oxygenation. The correct nursing diagnosis would be *Ineffective Breathing Pattern related to impaired exhalation and anxiety.* Anxiety with dyspnea is another cause of breathing pattern problems.

Outcomes. The client will have improved breathing patterns, as evidenced by (1) a decreasing respiratory rate to within normal limits; (2) decreased dyspnea, less nasal flaring, and reduced use of accessory muscles; (3) decreased signs of anxiety; (4) a return of ABG levels to normal limits; (5) oxygen saturation greater than 95%; and (6) vital capacity measurements within normal limits or greater than 40% of those predicted.

Interventions. Assess the client frequently, observing respiratory rate and depth. Assess the breathing pattern for shortness of breath, pursed-lip breathing, nasal flaring, sternal and intercostal retractions, or a prolonged expiratory phase. During an acute asthma attack, these assessments may be conducted continuously.

Place the client in the Fowler position, and give oxygen as ordered. Monitor ABGs and oxygen saturation levels to determine the effectiveness of treatments. Compare pulmonary function test results with normal levels. The degree of dysfunction assists you in planning client activity.

Ineffective Airway Clearance. The excessive production of mucus and spasm in the airway makes it difficult to keep the airway patent. The nursing diagnosis *Ineffective Airway Clearance related to increased production of secretions and bronchospasm* is appropriate.

Outcomes. The client will have effective airway clearance, as evidenced by (1) decreased inspiratory and expiratory wheezing; (2) decreased rhonchi; and (3) decreasing dry, nonproductive cough.

Interventions. If the airway is compromised, the client may require suctioning. Some clients experience asthma episodes as a result of pulmonary infection. Monitor the color and consistency of the sputum, and assist the client to cough effectively. Encourage oral fluids to thin the secretions and to replace fluids lost through rapid respiration. The humidity in the room may be increased slightly. If chest secretions are thick and difficult to expectorate, the client may benefit from postural drainage, lung percussion and vibration, expectorants, and frequent position changes. Give frequent oral care, every 2 to 4 hours, to remove the taste of the secretions.

Impaired Gas Exchange. When air is trapped within alveoli, they are eventually drained of oxygen and the client can become hypoxic. The nursing diagnosis is *Impaired Gas Exchange related to air trapping.*

Outcomes. The client will have adequate gas exchange, as evidenced by (1) decreased inspiratory and expiratory wheezing; (2) decreased rhonchi; (3) $Pa{O_2}$ greater than 60 mm Hg; (4) $Pa{CO_2}$ equal to or less than 45 mm Hg, (5) pH of 7.35 to 7.45; (6) usual skin color (no cyanosis); and (7) decreasing dry, nonproductive cough.

Interventions. Assess lung sounds every hour during acute episodes to determine the adequacy of gas exchange. Assess skin and mucous membrane color for cyanosis. Cyanosis is a late manifestation of hypoxia and an indication of serious gas exchange problems. Monitor pulse oximetry for oxygen saturation levels. Administer oxygen as ordered.

Refer to the Care Plan for the client with chronic obstructive pulmonary disease (COPD) when working with clients with diagnoses of *Activity Intolerance, Anxiety, Altered Nutrition,* or *Sleep Pattern Disturbance.*

EVALUATION

Generally, asthma episodes can be reversed quickly if there is no underlying problem, such as infection. Expect the client to be hospitalized only briefly; plan a coordinated approach to assessment and follow-up.

Self-Care

The approach to pharmacologic therapy often is referred to as *step care,* meaning that the medications ordered and the frequency of administration are adjusted according to the severity of the client's asthma. Asthma medications are categorized into two major classes: (1) *long-term–control* medications, used to achieve and maintain control of persistent asthma, and (2) *quick-relief* medications, used to treat acute air flow obstruction and its accompanying manifestations. The most effective long-term–control medications are those that reduce inflammation, with inhaled steroids being the most potent. Quick-relief medications include short-acting inhaled $beta_2$ agonists and oral steroids (Table 61–2).

For clients who respond poorly to inhaled agents, theophylline and aminophylline are used sometimes. These medications are regarded as weak bronchodilators with wide variations in their rates of metabolism and a high potential for toxicity, however, and their use is declining. Theophylline levels must be monitored to evaluate effectiveness and possible toxicity.

Figure 61–2 depicts a stepwise approach for managing asthma in adults. All clients with asthma require a short-acting inhaled $beta_2$ agonist as needed for acute manifestations. Clients with mild, moderate, or severe persistent asthma require daily long-term–control medications. The preferred treatment strategy is to start with more intensive therapy to achieve rapid control, then "step down" to the minimum therapy needed for maintenance.

Changes in the treatment plan may be needed as asthma severity and control vary over time. Follow-up visits every 1 to 6 months are recommended to monitor the disease and to maintain control. The presence of one or more indicators of poor control (i.e., awakening at night with dyspnea or coughing, increased use of short-

TABLE 61–2 MEDICATIONS USED IN TREATMENT OF CHRONIC OBSTRUCTIVE PULMONARY DISEASE

Drug Class/ Medication	Action	Expected Outcomes	Adverse Effects	Dosing
Steroids Beclomethasone (Vanceril) (inhaled) Methylprednisolone (Solu-Medrol) (injectable) Prednisone (Deltasone) (oral)	Reduce inflammation and inflammatory response in bronchial walls by suppressing action of WBCs and immune system	Long-term prevention of manifestations; suppression, control, and reversal of inflammation; reduced dyspnea, improved FEV_1	Hypertension, heart failure, peptic ulcer, dysphoria, hyperglycemia, cough, oral thrush, fragile skin, adrenal suppression in high doses	Rinse mouth after inhalation Administer oral forms with food Taper dose to withdraw
Beta$_2$ agonists Albuterol sulfate (Proventil) (inhaled)	Relax smooth muscles in bronchial tree by acting on beta$_2$ receptors	Prevention of nighttime manifestations and episodes brought on by exercise; increased mucociliary clearance; improved FEV_1	Tachycardia, skeletal muscle tremors, hypokalemia; GI upset, nausea	Monitor blood pressure and pulse rate Monitor potassium levels Shake inhaler well before using; hold breath 10 seconds after inhalation
Leukotriene inhibitors Zafirlukast (Accolate) (oral)	Block leukotriene (a mediater of inflammation)	Long-term control and prevention of manifestations	Inhibits metabolism of warfarin (Coumadin), nausea	Monitor prothrombin times Small frequent meals and good mouth care may reduce any nausea
Methylxanthines Theophylline (Theo-Dur) (oral) Aminophylline (parenteral)	Bronchodilator by increasing tissue concentrations of cyclic AMP	Long-term control of manifestations; increased myocardial contractility and mucociliary clearance; improved FEV_1	Gastric upset, tachycardia, nausea and vomiting (possible toxicity), nervousness, diuresis	Monitor blood levels Many drug interactions possible Charcoal-broiled foods reduce half-life by 50%
Anticholinergics Ipratropium (Atrovent) (inhaled)	Blocks action of acetylcholine at parasympathetic sites in bronchial smooth muscle	Relief of acute symptoms; bronchodilation; decreased mucus secretions; improved FEV_1	Dry mouth, nervousness, dizziness, fatigue, headache	Shake canister well Monitor liquid intake Provide thorough oral care Contraindicated in clients with BPH or glaucoma Assess appropriate use of inhaler or nebulizer Hold breath 10 seconds after inhalation

AMP, adenosine monophosphate; BPH, benign prostatic hypertrophy; FEV_1, forced expiratory volume in 1 second; GI, gastrointestinal.

acting inhaled beta$_2$ agonists, urgent care visits) may suggest a need to "step up" therapy. Before increasing medications, however, consider other possible reasons for poor control (Table 61–3).

Nebulized medications can be difficult to learn how to use. The client must coordinate inhalation with compression of the metered-dose inhaler canister (Fig. 61–3). The Client Education Guide provides directions for using an inhaler. Observe the client's use of the nebulizer to ascertain whether the medication is entering the airway.

Through appropriate use of the peak flowmeter and medications, clients with asthma should be able to anticipate most exacerbations and enhance their quality of life. Many clients can manage their asthma effectively with a thorough action plan to guide their decisions. An action plan for asthma is presented in Figure 61–4.

CHRONIC OBSTRUCTIVE PULMONARY DISEASE

Also known as *chronic obstructive lung disease,* COPD refers to several disorders that affect the movement of air in and out of the lungs. Although the most important of these—obstructive bronchitis, emphysema, and asthma—may occur in a pure form, they most commonly coexist, with overlapping clinical manifestations. The term *COPD*

Stepwise Approach for Managing Asthma in Adults and Children Over 5 Years Old: Treatment

Long-Term Control

Preferred treatments are in bold print.

Step 4 Severe Persistent

Daily medications:
- **Anti-inflammatory: inhaled steroid (high dose)** AND
- Long-acting bronchodilator: either **long-acting inhaled beta$_2$-agonist** (adult: 2 puffs q 12 hours; child: 1-2 puffs q 12 hours), sustained-release theophylline, or long-acting beta$_2$-agonist tablets AND
- Steroid tablets or syrup long term; make repeated attempts to reduce systemic steroid and maintain control with high-dose inhaled steroid.

Step 3 Moderate Persistent

Daily medication:
- Either
  —**Anti-inflammatory: inhaled steroid (medium dose)**

OR

—**Inhaled steroid (low-to-medium dose)** and add a long-acting bronchodilator, especially for nighttime symptoms: either **long-acting inhaled beta$_2$-agonist** (adult: 2 puffs q 12 hours; child: 1-2 puffs q 12 hours), sustained-release theophylline, or long-acting beta$_2$-agonist tablets.
- If needed
  —Anti-inflammatory: **inhaled steroids (medium-to-high dose)**
  AND
  —Long-acting bronchodilator, especially for nighttime symptoms; either **long-acting inhaled beta$_2$-agonist**, sustained-release theophylline, or long-acting beta$_2$-agonist tablets.

Step 2 Mild Persistent

Daily medication:
- **Anti-inflammatory:** either **inhaled steroid (low dose)** or **cromolyn** (adult: 2-4 puffs tid-qid; child: 1-2 puffs tid-qid) **or nedocromil** (adult: 2-4 puffs bid-qid; child: 1-2 puffs bid-qid) (children usually begin with a trial of cromolyn or nedocromil).
- Sustained-release theophylline to serum concentration of 5-15 mcg/mL is an alternative, but not preferred, therapy. Zafirlukast or zileuton may also be considered for those ≥12 years old, although their position in therapy is not fully established.

Step 1 Mild Intermittent

- No daily medication needed.

Quick-Relief

All Patients

Short-acting bronchodilator: **inhaled beta$_2$-agonist** (2-4 puffs) as needed for symptoms. Intensity of treatment will depend on severity of exacerbation.

NOTES:
- *The stepwise approach presents general guidelines to assist clinical decision-making. Asthma is highly variable; clinicians should tailor medication plans to the needs of individual patients.*
- **Gain control** as quickly as possible. Either start with aggressive therapy (e.g., *add* a course of oral steroids or a higher dose of inhaled steroids to the therapy that corresponds to the patient's initial step of severity); or start at the step that corresponds to the patient's initial severity and step up treatment, if necessary.
- **Step down:** Review treatment every 1 to 6 months. Gradually decrease treatment to the least medication necessary to maintain control.
- **Step up:** If control is not maintained, consider step up. Inadequate control is indicated by increased use of short-acting beta$_2$-agonists and in: step 1 when patient uses a short-acting beta$_2$-agonist more than two times a week; steps 2 and 3 when patient uses short-acting beta$_2$-agonist on a daily basis or more than three to four times in 1 day. But before stepping up: Review patient inhaler technique, compliance, and environmental control (avoidance of allergens or other precipitant factors).
- A course of oral steroids may be needed at any time and at any step.
- Patients with exercise-induced bronchospasm should take two to four puffs of an inhaled beta$_2$-agonist 5 to 60 minutes before exercise.
- Referral to an asthma specialist for consultation or comanagement is *recommended* if there is difficulty maintaining control or if the patient requires step 4 care. Referral may be *considered* for step 3 care.

FIGURE 61–2 Stepwise approach for managing asthma in adults. (From National Institutes of Health. [1997]. *Practical guide for the diagnosis and management of asthma.* NIH Pub. No. 97-4053. Washington, DC: Author.)

commonly is used, but some pulmonologists think that it is not completely accurate and the term *chronic air flow limitation* may be used in its place.

COPD may occur as a result of increased airway resistance secondary to bronchial mucosal edema or smooth muscle contraction. It may also be a result of decreased elastic recoil, as seen in emphysema. Elastic recoil, similar to the recoil of a stretched rubber band, is the force used to passively deflate the lung. Decreased elastic recoil results in a decreased driving force to empty the lung.

COPD is a widespread disorder, affecting more than 14 million Americans. COPD now ranks as the fourth

TABLE 61–3 POSSIBLE REASONS FOR POOR ASTHMA CONTROL—"ICE"

*I*nhaler technique	Check client's technique
*C*ompliance	Ask when and how much medication the client is taking
*E*nvironment	Ask client whether something in the environment has changed
Also consider	
Alternative diagnosis	Assess client for presence of concomitant upper respiratory disease or alternative diagnosis

From National Institutes of Health. (1997). *Practical guide for the diagnosis and management of asthma.* NIH Pub. No. 97-4053. Washington, DC: Author.

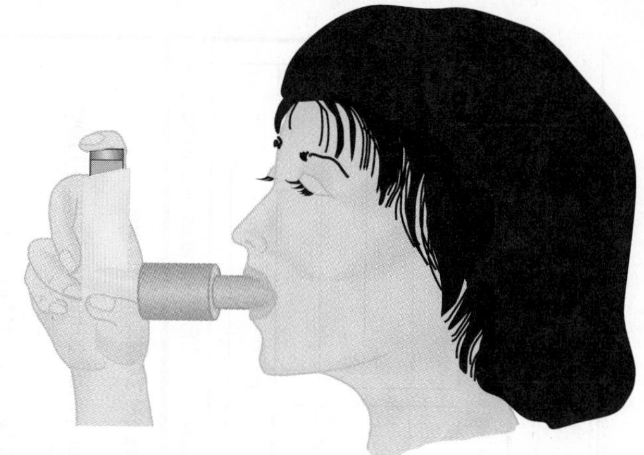

FIGURE 61–3 A client using a metered-dose inhaler with a spacer.

leading cause of death in the United States. The overall cost of caring for clients with COPD has been estimated at $40 billion annually, with $1.6 billion for long-term oxygen therapy alone.[27]

Etiology and Risk Factors

The specific causes of COPD are not clearly understood. The effects of numerous irritants found in cigarette smoke (i.e., stimulation of excess mucus production and coughing, destruction of ciliary function, and inflammation and damage of bronchiolar and alveolar walls), however, make smoking the leading risk factor for COPD development. Chronic respiratory infections, including sinusitis, contribute to development of COPD, as does the aging process. Heredity and genetic predisposition also appear to have a role.

Pathophysiology

COPD is a combination of chronic obstructive bronchitis, emphysema, and asthma. The pathophysiology of bron-

CLIENT EDUCATION GUIDE

Asthma

Client Instructions

Asthma may be triggered by pollen, dust, animal dander, molds, smoke, or other allergens. Learn what triggers your asthma and minimize your exposure to it.

Monitor the pollution index and pollen counts. Limit outdoor activities when these indicators are high.

Take all medications as prescribed by your physician. If you are taking both a bronchodilator and a steroid via inhaler, take the bronchodilator first to open the airways.

Use these directions for using an inhaler:

- Remove the cap and shake the inhaler well.
- Hold the canister upright with your index finger on the top and your thumb on the bottom.
- Breathe out through your mouth.
- Place the mouthpiece 1 to 2 inches away from your opened mouth (unless using a spacer).
- Begin with a slow, deep breath. As you breathe in, press the canister down with your finger to give yourself one puff of medication.
- Hold your breath in for at least 5 to 10 seconds.
- Slowly breathe out, holding your lips tight (pursed).
- If your physician has prescribed more than one puff, wait 1 minute between puffs to let the medication open up the upper airway. That way the next puff can reach lower into your lungs.

Pursed-lip breathing, progressive muscle relaxation, and tripod positioning (i.e., leaning on your arms positioned in front of you) may improve your breathing during asthma episodes.

Unless your physician has told you to limit fluids, drink 8 to 10 glasses of water every day. Water helps to thin your sputum so that you can cough it up more easily.

Some forms of asthma may be triggered by exercise. Discuss an exercise plan with your physician before starting.

Keep track of your peak flows. Often they fall about 1 day before an asthma attack.

Follow these directions on how to use a peak flowmeter:

- Attach the mouthpiece and set the pointer to zero (0).
- Stand up and take a deep breath.
- Put the mouthpiece in your mouth, and close your lips tightly around it.
- Blow into the mouthpiece as hard and as fast as you can.
- Record the value and reset the meter.
- Repeat the procedure for a total of three readings.
- Record the highest value on your record sheet.

Call your physician if you experience any of the following manifestations:

- Wheezing and shortness of breath, even though you are taking your medications as prescribed
- Fever, muscle aches, chest pain, or thickening of sputum
- Sputum color changes to yellow, green, gray, or red (bloody)
- Problems that may be related to your medications (e.g., rash, itching, swelling, or trouble breathing)

ASTHMA ACTION PLAN FOR ______________ Doctor's Name ______________ Date ______________

Doctor's Phone Number ______________ Hospital/Emergency Room Phone Number ______________

GREEN ZONE: Doing Well

- No cough, wheeze, chest tightness, or shortness of breath during the day or night
- Can do usual activities

And, if a peak flow meter is used,
Peak flow: more than ______________
(80% or more of my best peak flow)

My best peak flow is: ______________

Take These Long-Term-Control Medicines Each Day (include an anti-inflammatory)

Medicine	How much to take	When to take it

Before exercise ❑ ______________ ❑ 2 or ❑ 4 puffs 5 to 60 minutes before exercise

YELLOW ZONE: Asthma Is Getting Worse

- Cough, wheeze, chest tightness, or shortness of breath, or
- Waking at night due to asthma, or
- Can do some, but not all, usual activities

-Or-

Peak flow: ______ to ______
(50% - 80% of my best peak flow)

FIRST → **Add: Quick-Relief Medicine – and keep taking your GREEN ZONE medicine**

______________ (short-acting $beta_2$-agonist) ❑ 2 or ❑ 4 puffs, every 20 minutes for up to 1 hour
❑ Nebulizer, once

SECOND → **If your symptoms (and peak flow, if used) *return to GREEN ZONE* after 1 hour of above treatment:**

❑ Take the quick-relief medicine every 4 hours for 1 to 2 days.
❑ Double the dose of your inhaled steroid for ______ (7-10) days.

-Or-

If your symptoms (and peak flow, if used) *do not return to GREEN ZONE* after 1 hour of above treatment:

❑ Take: ______________ (short-acting $beta_2$-agonist) ❑ 2 or ❑ 4 puffs or ❑ Nebulizer

❑ Add: ______________ (oral steroid) ______ mg. per day For ______ (3-10) days

❑ Call the doctor ❑ before/ ❑ within ______ hours after taking the oral steroid.

RED ZONE: Medical Alert!

- Very short of breath, or
- Quick-relief medicines have not helped, or
- Cannot do usual activities, or
- Symptoms are same or get worse after 24 hours in Yellow Zone

-Or-

Peak flow: less than ______
(50% of my best peak flow)

Take this medicine:

❑ ______________ (short-acting $beta_2$-agonist) ❑ 4 or ❑ 6 puffs or ❑ Nebulizer

❑ ______________ (oral steroid) ______ mg.

Then call your doctor *NOW*. Go to the hospital or call for an ambulance if:

- You are still in the red zone after 15 minutes AND
- You have not reached your doctor.

DANGER SIGNS

- **Trouble walking and talking due to shortness of breath**
- **Lips or fingernails are blue**

→

- **Take ❑ 4 or ❑ 6 puffs of your quick-relief medicine *AND***
- **Go to the hospital or call for an ambulance (______________) *NOW!***

FIGURE 61–4 Asthma action plan. (From National Institutes of Health. [1997]. *Practical guide for the diagnosis and management of asthma.* NIH Pub. No. 97-4053. Washington, DC: Author.)

chitis and emphysema is presented here (see pathophysiology of asthma earlier).

CHRONIC OBSTRUCTIVE BRONCHITIS

Inflammation of the bronchi (chronic obstructive bronchitis) causes increased mucus production and chronic cough. In contrast to those of acute bronchitis, the clinical manifestations of chronic bronchitis continue for at least 3 months of the year for 2 consecutive years. Additionally, if the client has a decreased FEV_1/FVC ratio of less than 75% and chronic bronchitis, the client is said to have chronic *obstructive* bronchitis, indicating that the client has obstructive lung disease combined with chronic cough. Chronic bronchitis is characterized by:

- An increase in the size and number of submucous glands in the large bronchi, which increases mucus production
- An increased number of goblet cells, which also secrete mucus
- Impaired ciliary function, which reduces mucus clearance

The lung's mucociliary defenses are impaired, and there is increased susceptibility to infection. When infection occurs, mucus production is greater and the bronchial walls become inflamed and thickened. Chronic bronchitis initially affects only the larger bronchi, but eventually all airways are involved. The thick mucus and inflamed bronchi obstruct airways, especially during expiration. The airways collapse, and air is trapped in the distal portion of the lung. This obstruction leads to reduced alveolar ventilation. An abnormal ventilation-perfusion ($\dot{V}/\dot{Q}$) ratio develops, with a corresponding fall in PaO_2. Impaired ventilation may also result in increased levels of $PaCO_2$. As compensation for the hypoxemia, polycythemia (overproduction of erythrocytes) occurs.

EMPHYSEMA

Emphysema is a disorder in which the alveolar walls are destroyed. This destruction leads to permanent overdistention of the air spaces. Air passages are obstructed as a result of these changes, rather than from mucus production, as in chronic bronchitis. Although the precise cause of emphysema is unknown, research has shown that the enzymes protease and elastase can attack and destroy the connective tissue of the lungs. Emphysema may result from a breakdown in the lung's normal defense mechanisms ($alpha_1$-antitrypsin [AAT]) against these enzymes. Difficult expiration in emphysema is the result of destruction of the walls (septa) between the alveoli, partial airway collapse, and loss of elastic recoil. As the alveoli and septa collapse, pockets of air form between the alveolar spaces (blebs) and within the lung parenchyma (bullae). This process leads to increased ventilatory dead space from areas that do not participate in gas or blood exchange. The work of breathing is increased because there is less functional lung tissue to exchange oxygen and carbon dioxide. Emphysema causes destruction of the pulmonary capillaries, decreasing oxygen perfusion and ventilation further.

There are three types of emphysema (Fig. 61–5): centrilobar, panlobar, and paraseptal.

Centrilobular (or *centriacinar*) *emphysema,* the most common type, produces destruction in the bronchioles, usually in the upper lung regions. Inflammation develops in the bronchioles, but usually the alveolar sac remains intact. *Panlobular emphysema* affects both the bronchioles and the alveoli and most commonly involves the

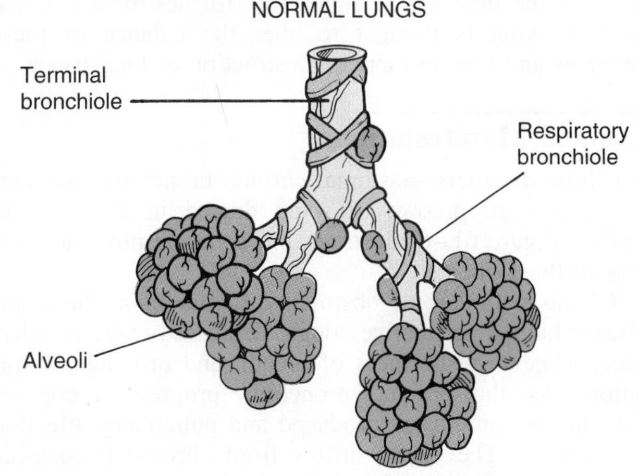

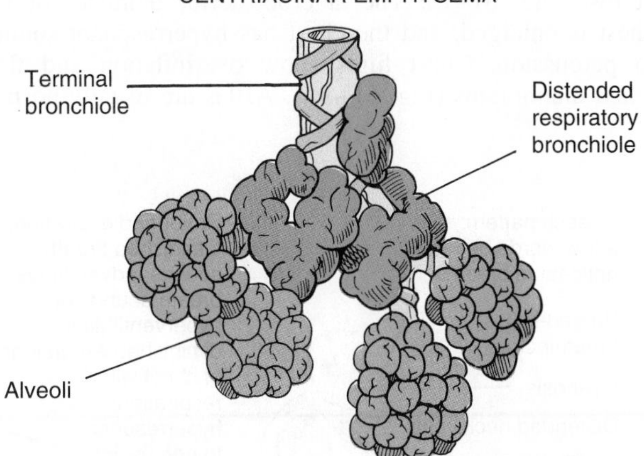

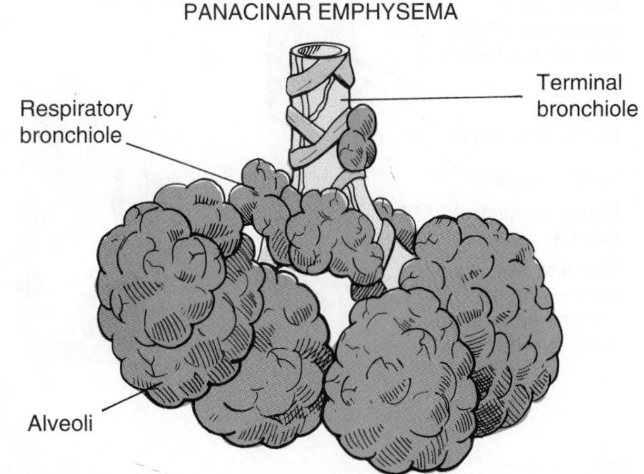

FIGURE 61–5 Two types of emphysema.

lower lung. These forms of emphysema occur most often in smokers.

Paraseptal (or *panacinar*) *emphysema* destroys the alveoli in the lower lobes of the lungs, resulting in isolated blebs along the lung periphery. It is believed to be the likely cause of spontaneous pneumothorax. Paraseptal emphysema occurs in the elderly and in clients with an inherited deficiency of AAT. Normally, AAT inhibits the action of enzymes that break down proteins. Clients without AAT are at increased risk for COPD because the walls of the lung are at higher risk for destruction. Cigarette smoking is thought to alter the balance of these enzymes and thus to increase destruction of lung tissue.

Clinical Manifestations

All three disorders—asthma, chronic bronchitis, and emphysema—are present to some degree in clients with COPD. Figure 61–6 illustrates the common physical findings in these clients.

Clients with chronic obstructive bronchitis as the major disease have a productive cough, decreased exercise tolerance, wheezing, shortness of breath, and prolonged expiration. As the chronic bronchitis progresses, copious amounts of sputum are produced and pulmonary infection is common. The client suffers from chronic hypoxemia and hypercapnia (Fig. 61–7).

Clients who have primary emphysema have progressive dyspnea on exertion that eventually becomes dyspnea at rest (Fig. 61–8). The anteroposterior diameter of the chest is enlarged, and the chest has hyperresonant sounds to percussion. Chest films show overinflation and flattened diaphragms (Fig. 61–9*A*). ABGs are usually normal until later stages. Table 61–4 contrasts common findings in chronic bronchitis and emphysema.

Complications

Respiratory infections commonly develop in clients with COPD. This situation is a result of alterations in the normal respiratory defense mechanisms and decreased immune resistance. Because respiratory status already is compromised, infection frequently leads to acute respiratory failure and is a common reason for hospitalization (see Chapter 63).

Spontaneous pneumothorax may develop from rupture of an emphysematous bleb. This rupture results in a closed pneumothorax and requires insertion of a chest tube for reexpansion of the lung (see Chapter 62).

Similar to asthma, chronic obstructive bronchitis and emphysema may worsen at night. Clients often report sleep-onset dyspnea and frequent or early-morning awakenings. During sleep, there is a decrease in the muscle tone and activity of the respiratory muscles. This decreased tone leads to hypoventilation, an increase in resistance of the airways, and $\dot{V}/\dot{Q}$ mismatch. Eventually, the client becomes hypoxemic.

Outcome Management

Medical Management

The treatment goals for the client with COPD are to improve ventilation, to facilitate the removal of bronchial secretions, to prevent complications, to slow the progression of clinical manifestations, and to promote health

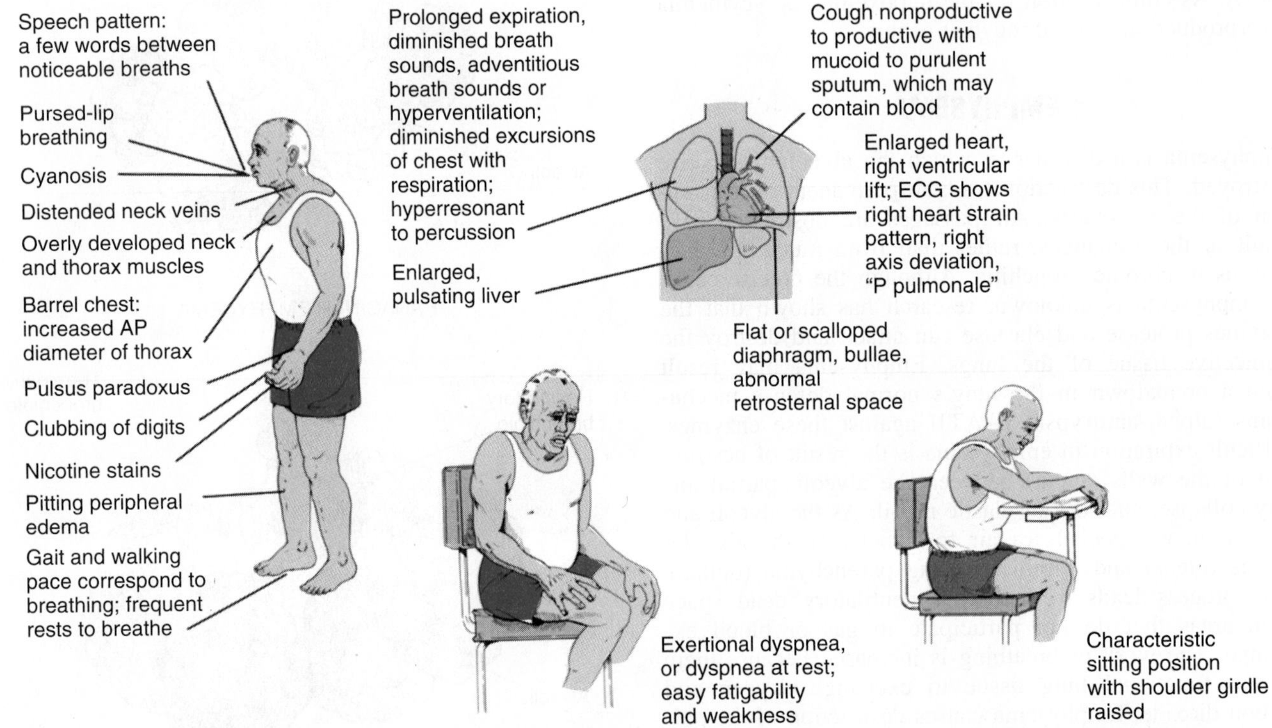

FIGURE 61–6 Typical assessment findings in chronic obstructive pulmonary disease (COPD). AP, anterior-posterior; ECG, electrocardiogram.

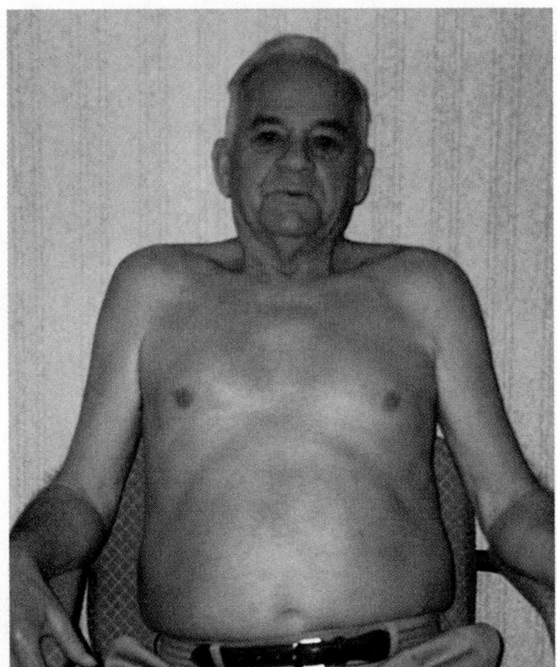

FIGURE 61–7 A client with chronic obstructive bronchitis. Note the stocky build and the presence of pursed-lip breathing and barrel chest. The slight gynecomastia is a side effect of corticosteroid therapy. The client's shoulders are raised because of shortness of breath and increased work of breathing.

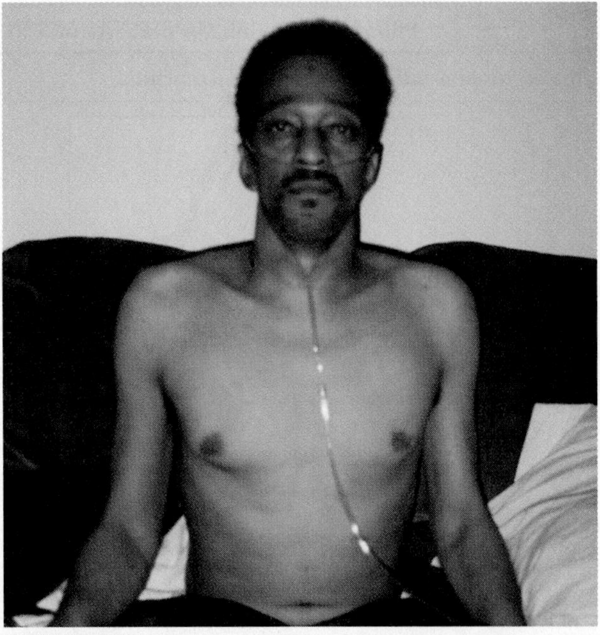

FIGURE 61–8 A client with emphysema. Note the thin appearance and the presence of continuous oxygen therapy. The use of accessory muscles of respiration (neck and shoulder muscles) reflects the client's shortness of breath and increased work of breathing necessary to increase minute ventilation and to maintain adequate arterial blood gas values.

maintenance and client management of the disease. At times, the client may receive continuous mechanical ventilation for adequate oxygenation. Ventilator-dependent clients with COPD may be managed in critical care, although some centers have non–critical care areas for clients on ventilators.

IMPROVE VENTILATION

Bronchodilators and steroids are also used in the treatment of COPD (see Table 61–2). As with asthma, they are used to stop the reversible portion of airway spasm. Narcotics, tranquilizers, and sedatives are used with caution because they depress the respiratory center. The fu-

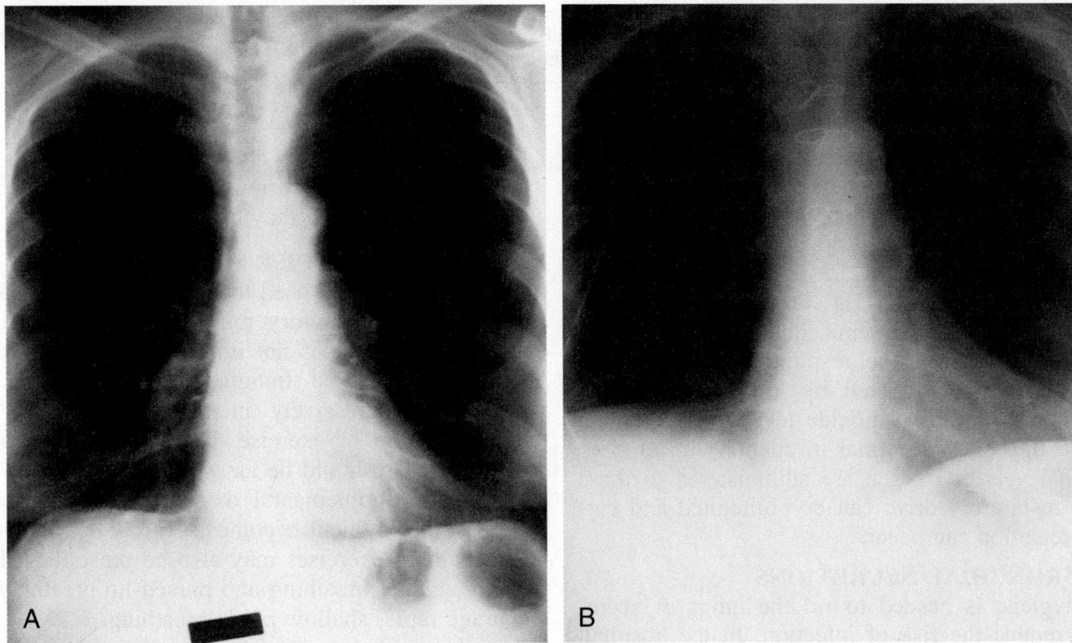

FIGURE 61–9 *A,* Preoperative chest x-ray of a client with emphysema. Note the flattened diaphragm and the laterally hyperexpanded chest walls. *B,* Postoperative chest x-ray after lung volume reduction surgery. The right side of the diaphragm is rounded and no longer flattened by emphysematous lung tissue. (From Allen, G. [1996]. Surgical treatment of emphysema using bovine pericardium strips. *AORN Journal, 63*(2), 373–388.)

TABLE 61–4 PRIMARY CLINICAL MANIFESTATIONS IN CHRONIC BRONCHITIS AND EMPHYSEMA

Clinical Manifestations	Chronic Bronchitis	Emphysema
Onset of symptoms	Age 40–50 yr	Age 50–75 yr
Physical appearance	Stocky build with no history of weight loss; use of accessory muscles to breathe in late stages; cyanotic; barrel chest	Cachectic appearance with history of major weight loss; tachypnea and use of accessory muscles to breathe, even in early stages; pink skin color
Chief complaint	Persistent cough and copious sputum production	Persistent shortness of breath with progressive exertional dyspnea
Clinical course	Variable, with exacerbations usually related to respiratory infection	Progressive deterioration
ABGs	Decreased PaO_2, increased $PaCO_2$	PaO_2 normal or slightly decreased; $PaCO_2$ low or normal until end stage
Pulmonary function	Small airways affected early (reduced $FEF_{25\%-75\%}$); FEV_1 reduced later as airway damage progresses; normal to variable diffusion capacity	Reduced $FEF_{25\%-75\%}$ and FEV_1; reduced diffusion capacity because of destruction of alveoli
Associated findings	Frequent episodes of cor pulmonale with dependent edema (especially in late stage); elevated hematocrit	No history of cor pulmonale until very late stage; no edema; on auscultation, diminished breath sounds even with deep breathing

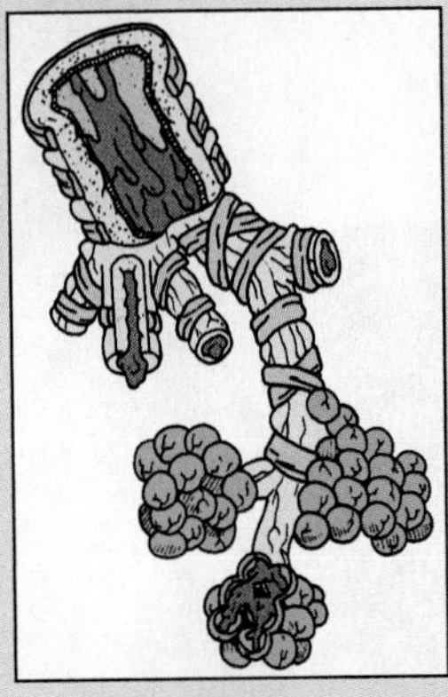

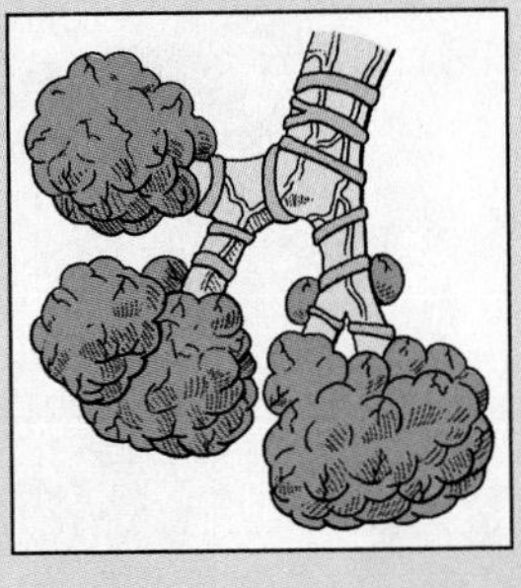

ABGs, arterial blood gases; $FEF_{25\%-75\%}$, forced expiratory flow, midexpiratory phase; FEV_1, forced expiratory volume in 1 second; $PaCO_2$, partial pressure of arterial carbon dioxide; PaO_2, partial pressure of arterial oxygen.

ture looks promising for the treatment of early emphysema with AAT replacement therapy.

Oxygen is used when the client has severe exertional or resting hypoxemia (PaO_2 < 40 mm Hg). Oxygen (1 to 3 L) by nasal cannula may be required to raise the PaO_2 to no less than 60 mm Hg. Oxygen is used cautiously in clients with emphysema, however. Because of long-standing hypercapnia, the respiratory drive in emphysematous clients is triggered by low oxygen levels rather than increased carbon dioxide levels. The drive to breathe is the opposite of normal in clients with emphysema. If high levels of oxygen are administered to these clients, their respiratory drive can be obliterated and carbon dioxide retention can occur.

Remove Bronchial Secretions

Pulmonary hygiene is needed to rid the lungs of secretions and to reduce the risk of infection. In the hospital, the client may be treated with nebulized bronchodilators and positive-pressure air flow or positive end-expiratory pressure devices to increase the caliber of the airways. Postural drainage and chest physiotherapy may be prescribed to move the secretions from the small to the large airways, from which they can be expelled.

Promote Exercise

Aerobic exercise is used to enhance cardiovascular fitness and to train respiratory muscles to function more effectively. Exercise does not improve lung function. Respiratory muscles can be strengthened even when the lungs are diseased. Progressively increased walking is the most common form of exercise. Before a walking program is begun, ABGs should be assessed and compared with resting levels. Supplemental oxygen should be used during exercise if the client becomes severely hypoxemic.

Breathing exercises may also be prescribed. Encourage diaphragmatic breathing and pursed-lip breathing, and discourage rapid, shallow *panic* breathing.

Control Complications

Edema and cor pulmonale are treated with diuretics and digitalis. Phlebotomy may be used to reduce blood volume in clients with marked elevations in hematocrit (>60%). Phlebotomy also reduces cardiac workload.

IMPROVE GENERAL HEALTH

The most effective way to slow disease progression is for the client to stop smoking. Exposure to known allergens should be minimized. All clients with COPD should avoid high altitudes, and supplemental oxygen may be required for air travel. No specific climate has been shown to alter the course of the disorder.

Adequate nutrition is essential to maintain respiratory muscle strength. Malnutrition is common and contributes to decreased respiratory muscle strength and reduced diaphragmatic mass. Consult a clinical dietitian to assist clients in modifying their diet to meet their caloric needs. Clients with COPD often have difficulty eating because of dyspnea. Offer the client frequent small meals, rather than large meals. When the client must be tube-fed, understand that substrate metabolism also may affect lung function. Macronutrients are metabolized to produce carbon dioxide and water. The ratio of carbon dioxide produced to oxygen consumed is the respiratory quotient (RQ). The RQ of carbohydrate oxidation is 1.0, and the RQ of fat oxidation is 0.7. Excess carbohydrate leads to increased production of carbon dioxide and can lead to respiratory distress. Enteral formulas are designed for pulmonary disease and provide more calories from fat. It is equally important not to overfeed the client with carbohydrates.

Adjust oxygen delivery devices so that the mouth is not obstructed but oxygen is delivered through the nose during eating. Calculate the liter flow of the nasal cannula when converting from a mask style (see formulas in Table 61–5). For example, if a client is using a Venturi oxygen mask at 28%, he or she would receive the same amount of oxygen on 2 L by nasal cannula.

Nursing Management of the Medical Client

ASSESSMENT

The nursing history can ascertain whether the client's clinical manifestations are primarily those of chronic bronchitis, emphysema, or asthma. Determine the client's ability to recognize manifestations that require further care. For example, if a client says, "I knew I was developing an infection and went to the doctor," the statement indicates an understanding of the disorder. In contrast, if a client does not fully understand the reasons for hospitalization, educate the client about COPD. A review of past medical history helps determine whether the client has other disorders, such as heart disease, that may affect treatment.

Complete a physical examination with an emphasis on the respiratory and cardiac system. Note the degree of dyspnea, decreased breath sounds, and clinical manifestations of heart failure. Evaluate mental status because confusion and restlessness may be early indicators of increasing hypoxia and hypercapnia.

Consider the impact of stressors that may have led to exacerbations of COPD. Possible factors include the progressive illness itself, marital or other family problems, and financial concerns. Review the client's usual coping strategies. Determine whether these strategies are working now; if not, why not? Support systems, such as friends and family, also are important components of psychosocial stability. Determine the reliability of the client's support system.

The psychosocial impact of COPD is significant. Clients commonly have feelings of loss of control over their bodies and their social environment. These responses leave the client socially isolated and depressed. A Canadian study found that clients with poor adjustment to COPD used more health care dollars for disease management.[16] Psychosocial intervention is important.

A thorough history may need to be delayed until the client is able to breathe comfortably, or it may be taken over short periods of time or obtained through the family. Likewise, the physical examination should not tire the client.

DIAGNOSIS, OUTCOMES, INTERVENTION

Common nursing diagnoses and interventions for the client with COPD are listed in the Care Plan for the client with COPD. Because COPD is very common, many institutions use care maps to guide care. (See the feature on care maps.)

Evaluation

Dyspnea will be slow to improve. Expect several days for the client to return to baseline levels.

Clients with COPD often continue to deteriorate despite medical care. It is difficult to cope with failing health that limits activity and employment. As much as possible, encourage the client to live an active life with

TABLE 61–5 CONVERTING LOW-FLOW TO HIGH-FLOW OXYGEN SYSTEMS*

100% Oxygen Flow Rate (L)	FiO_2 (%)
NASAL CANNULA OR CATHETER	
1	24
2	28
3	32
4	36
5	40
6	44
OXYGEN MASK	
5–6	40
6–7	50
7–8	60
MASK WITH A RESERVOIR BAG	
6	60
7	70
8	80
9	90
10	100

* A normal ventilatory pattern is assumed.
FiO_2, fraction of inspired oxygen.

GUIDE TO CLINICAL PATHWAY

Chronic Obstructive Pulmonary Disease

The client hospitalized with acute exacerbation of chronic obstructive pulmonary disease may have increasing dyspnea because of a chest cold or pneumonia. This care map shows a 5-day length of stay with the major focus on the interventions directed at restoring a balance between energy demands for oxygen (activity) and ability to maintain oxygenation (dyspnea).

By day 2 of the care map, the client's underlying problem (such as pneumonia) has been diagnosed and is being treated. It is expected that once the problem is treated, the client can be weaned from the oxygen levels needed while the presenting problem was acute. Carefully assess the degree of dyspnea, pulse oximetry levels, and amount of oxygen needed. Level of activity progresses while you closely monitor the client's ability to tolerate it. If the client is too dyspneic to eat, ask a dietitian to see the client. Foods that are calorie-dense and do not create carbon dioxide are important changes that can be made in the diet.

By day 3, nebulized bronchodilators are changed to metered-dose inhalers. Validate that the client understands and uses these devices correctly. Intravenous corticosteroids (used to decrease the inflammation) are changed to an oral route. Oral steroids are ulcerogenic and given with meals. Shortness of breath is not expected on day 3. Assessment changes to watch for include bronchospasm, which might occur while activity increases.

On day 4, the client's understanding of self-care is validated. Many of these treatments may have been used previously by the client. Record the client's ability to use equipment safely.

The CareMap is reprinted with permission from Baptist Health System. The CareMap shown is an excerpt of one that covers emergency department admission through day of discharge.

Helen Andrews, BSN, RN, *Care Manager, Alegent Health Bergan Mercy Medical Center, Omaha, Nebraska,* and **Linda R. Haddick, MSN, RN,** *Clinical Nurse Specialist, Alegent Health Home Care & Hospice, Omaha, Nebraska*

daily exercise. The support of significant others is essential.

Surgical Management

Surgery is relatively uncommon in the treatment of COPD. At times, bullectomy (removal of large bullae, which compress the lung and add to dead space) may benefit clients with recurrent spontaneous pneumothorax.

LUNG VOLUME REDUCTION SURGERY

Advances have been made with lung volume reduction surgery (LVRS). Portions of diffusely emphysematous lungs are removed to help restore more normal chest wall configuration and to improve respiratory mechanics and functional capacity (see Fig. 61–9). LVRS also improves quality of life in selected patients. More data are needed regarding the procedure and its long-term effects, however, and multicenter studies are under way.[7]

Candidates for LVRS include people with severely limited pulmonary function (FEV $<$ 30% of normal), maximally flattened diaphragm on radiograph with maximal overdistention of lung volume and evidence of bullae, significant impairment in activities of daily living, and for whom medical management is no longer effective. Before surgery, clients should have stopped smoking for at least 6 months and must complete a 6- to 12-week pulmonary rehabilitation program.[23]

LVRS may be performed via a median sternotomy or thoracotomy. Bovine pericardium strips can be used to reinforce staple lines of resected lung tissue. This technique reduces the problem of air leaks, common in earlier LVRS procedures. Another approach to this intervention is video-assisted thoracoscopy, which avoids a large thoracic incision and may reduce postoperative respiratory complications.[20]

Nursing Care of the Surgical Client

After surgery, monitor closely the client's ABG values. Chest assessment and radiograph help determine whether the lungs are expanding. Assess the chest tubes for air leaks and drainage. Intensive pulmonary toilet is essential. Repeated coughing and deep breathing help prevent pulmonary complications. Many clients have chest physiotherapy every 4 hours and nebulized aerosol treatments. Clients usually ambulate soon after surgery, sometimes the same day as the operation. Manage pain aggressively to promote activity and pulmonary hygiene.

After discharge, the client is assessed for adequate ventilation and tissue oxygenation (with pulse oximetry) and progressive wound healing. Pulmonary treatments may continue until lung sounds are clear. The client is weaned from oxygen and placed into a formal pulmonary rehabilitation program.

Modifications for Elderly Clients

COPD is the second most significant disorder of people in the middle to late adult years. The elderly client frequently has other problems that influence the treatment of COPD. For example, the client may have decreased exercise tolerance, impaired nutrition, or a long-standing habit of smoking that retards rehabilitation. Also consider the possibility of drug-drug interactions in elderly clients.

The older adult has special requirements when chronic conditions are exacerbated (see the Case Management feature in Chapter 72).

Self-Care

Pulmonary rehabilitation is designed to reduce the toll of pulmonary disease for the client and the health care system. The goals of pulmonary rehabilitation are to relieve clinical manifestations, to maximize functional level, and to educate patients to manage their disease process successfully and to maintain an active and independent lifestyle.[27] Clients are taught how to administer medications, what side effects to look for and how to manage them, and the safe and correct use of oxygen. Lower body exercise (walking, cycling) is commonly prescribed. Upper body exercise is also used in some cases.

To facilitate self-care and adherence, the client and significant others need thorough information about the

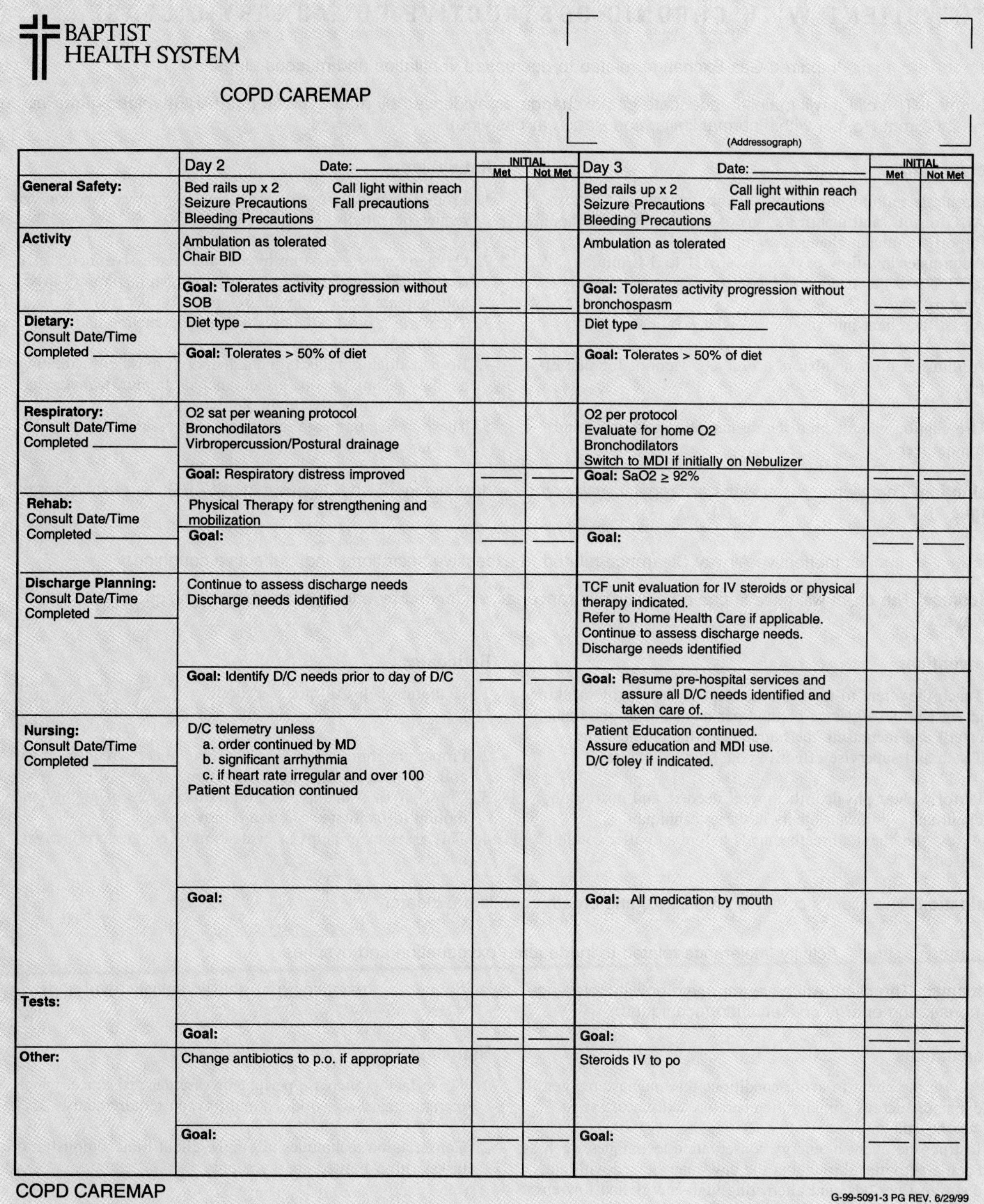

BAPTIST HEALTH SYSTEM

COPD CAREMAP

(Addressograph)

	Day 2 Date: ______	INITIAL Met	INITIAL Not Met	Day 3 Date: ______	INITIAL Met	INITIAL Not Met
General Safety:	Bed rails up x 2 Seizure Precautions Bleeding Precautions Call light within reach Fall precautions			Bed rails up x 2 Seizure Precautions Bleeding Precautions Call light within reach Fall precautions		
Activity	Ambulation as tolerated Chair BID			Ambulation as tolerated		
	Goal: Tolerates activity progression without SOB			**Goal:** Tolerates activity progression without bronchospasm		
Dietary: Consult Date/Time Completed ______	Diet type ______			Diet type ______		
	Goal: Tolerates > 50% of diet			**Goal:** Tolerates > 50% of diet		
Respiratory: Consult Date/Time Completed ______	O2 sat per weaning protocol Bronchodilators Virbropercussion/Postural drainage			O2 per protocol Evaluate for home O2 Bronchodilators Switch to MDI if initially on Nebulizer		
	Goal: Respiratory distress improved			**Goal:** SaO2 $\geq$ 92%		
Rehab: Consult Date/Time Completed ______	Physical Therapy for strengthening and mobilization					
	Goal:			**Goal:**		
Discharge Planning: Consult Date/Time Completed ______	Continue to assess discharge needs Discharge needs identified			TCF unit evaluation for IV steroids or physical therapy indicated. Refer to Home Health Care if applicable. Continue to assess discharge needs. Discharge needs identified		
	Goal: Identify D/C needs prior to day of D/C			**Goal:** Resume pre-hospital services and assure all D/C needs identified and taken care of.		
Nursing: Consult Date/Time Completed ______	D/C telemetry unless a. order continued by MD b. significant arrhythmia c. if heart rate irregular and over 100 Patient Education continued			Patient Education continued. Assure education and MDI use. D/C foley if indicated.		
	Goal:			**Goal:** All medication by mouth		
Tests:						
	Goal:			**Goal:**		
Other:	Change antibiotics to p.o. if appropriate			Steroids IV to po		
	Goal:			**Goal:**		

COPD CAREMAP

G-99-5091-3 PG REV. 6/29/99

disease process. Review the signs of impending respiratory problems (e.g., increased confusion or drowsiness), respiratory infection, and right-sided heart failure (e.g., peripheral edema, distended neck veins) so that prompt intervention can be obtained should these complications develop. The need for routine respiratory follow-up should also be discussed. In your teaching, include a discussion of the hazards of infection and ways to decrease personal risk (i.e., avoid crowds during the flu and colds season, clean respiratory equipment well, obtain pneumococcal and flu vaccines yearly). Review the need for lifestyle modifications.

Text continued on page 1705

C A R E P L A N

THE CLIENT WITH CHRONIC OBSTRUCTIVE PULMONARY DISEASE

Nursing Diagnosis. Impaired Gas Exchange related to decreased ventilation and mucous plugs.

Outcomes. The client will maintain adequate gas exchange as evidenced by arterial blood gas (ABG) values (i.e., Pao_2 of at least 60 mm Hg, pH within normal limits, and $Paco_2$ at baseline).

Interventions	Rationales
1. Regularly monitor the client's respiratory rate and pattern, ABG results, and manifestations of hypoxia or hypercapnia. Report significant changes promptly.	1. Prompt recognition of deteriorating respiratory function can reduce potentially lethal outcomes.
2. Administer low-flow oxygen therapy (1 to 3 L/min on 24% to 31% Fio_2) as needed via nasal prongs or a high-flow Venturi mask.	2. Oxygen corrects existing hypoxemia. Excessive increases in oxygen (55% to 70% Fio_2) may diminish respiratory drive and increase carbon dioxide retention further.
3. Assist the client into the high-Fowler position.	3. The upright position allows full lung excursion and enhances air exchange.
4. Administer bronchodilators if ordered. Monitor for side effects.	4. Bronchodilators relax bronchial smooth muscle, facilitating air flow. Common side effects include tremor, tachycardia, and other cardiac dysrhythmias.
5. Use caution when administering narcotics, sedatives, and tranquilizers.	5. These medications are respiratory depressants and can impair ventilation further.

Evaluation. The client's respirations are regular, unlabored, and between 12 and 20 per minute. ABGs are within normal range.

Nursing Diagnosis. Ineffective Airway Clearance related to excessive secretions and ineffective coughing.

Outcomes. The client will have improved airway clearance, as evidenced by effective coughing techniques and patent airways.

Interventions	Rationales
1. Teach the client to maintain adequate hydration by drinking at least 8 to 10 glasses of fluid per day (if not contraindicated) and increasing the humidity of the ambient air.	1. Hydration helps to thin secretions.
2. Teach and supervise effective coughing techniques.	2. Proper coughing techniques conserve energy, reduce airway collapse, and lessen client frustration.
3. Perform chest physical therapy, if needed, and instruct the client and significant others in these techniques.	3. Chest physical therapy techniques use forces of gravity and motion to facilitate secretion removal.
4. Assess the client's breath sounds before and after coughing episodes.	4. This assessment helps in evaluation of coughing effectiveness.

Evaluation. The client's cough is productive, and breath sounds are clearer.

Nursing Diagnosis. Activity Intolerance related to inadequate oxygenation and dyspnea.

Outcomes. The client will have improved activity tolerance, as evidenced by maintaining a realistic activity level and demonstrating energy conservation techniques.

Interventions	Rationales
1. Advise the client to avoid conditions that increase oxygen demand, such as smoking, temperature extremes, excess weight, and stress.	1. These factors increase peripheral vascular resistance, which increases cardiac workload and oxygen requirements.
2. Instruct the client in energy conservation techniques, such as pacing activities throughout the day, interspersed with adequate rest periods, and alternating high-energy and low-energy tasks.	2. Conservation techniques allow the client to accomplish more tasks with a limited energy supply.
3. Assist the client in scheduling a gradual increase in daily activities and exercise.	3. Gradual increases in physical activity improve respiratory and cardiac conditioning, thus improving activity tolerance.
4. Teach the client to use pursed-lip and diaphragmatic breathing techniques during activities.	4. Breathing retraining ensures maximal use of available respiratory function. Pursed-lip breathing leaves positive end-expiratory pressure in the lungs and helps keep airways open.
5. Schedule active exercise after respiratory therapy or medication (e.g., bronchodilator in metered-dose inhaler).	5. Lung function is maximized during peak periods of treatment and drug effect.
6. Maintain supplemental oxygen therapy as needed.	6. Supplemental oxygen helps alleviate exercise-induced hypoxemia, thus improving activity tolerance.

7. Assess the client for signs of a negative response to activity (e.g., significant change in respiratory rate, failure of pulse to return to near resting rate within 3 minutes of activity, changes in mental status).

7. Significant changes in respiratory, cardiac, or circulatory status signal activity intolerance.

Evaluation. The client performs activities of daily living and other activities with no significant deterioration in respiratory status.

Nursing Diagnosis. Anxiety related to acute breathing difficulties and fear of suffocation.

Outcomes. The client will express an increase in psychological comfort and demonstrate use of effective coping mechanisms.

Interventions	Rationales
1. Remain with the client during acute episodes of breathing difficulty, and provide care in a calm, reassuring manner.	1. Reassures the client that competent help is available if needed. Anxiety can be contagious; remain calm.
2. Provide a quiet, calm environment.	2. Reduction of external stimuli helps promote relaxation.
3. During acute episodes, open doors and curtains and limit the number of people and unnecessary equipment in the room.	3. Environmental changes may lessen the client's perceptions of suffocation.
4. Encourage the use of breathing retraining and relaxation techniques.	4. A feeling of self-control and success in facilitating breathing helps reduce anxiety.
5. Give sedatives and tranquilizers with extreme caution. Nonpharmaceutical methods of anxiety reduction are more useful.	5. Oversedation may cause respiratory depression.

Evaluation. The client's anxiety is decreased; the client demonstrates use of relaxation techniques and appears rested.

Nursing Diagnosis. Altered Nutrition: Less Than Body Requirements related to reduced appetite, decreased energy level, and dyspnea.

Outcomes. The client will maintain body weight within normal limits for gender and body build, and hemoglobin and albumin levels will be within normal ranges.

Interventions	Rationales
1. Assist the client with mouth care before meals and as needed.	1. Coughing and sputum production may impair appetite. Mouth-breathing dries mucous membranes.
2. Advise the client to eat small, frequent meals (e.g., six meals a day) that are high in protein and calories.	2. Large meals may create an excessive feeling of fullness that may make breathing uncomfortable and difficult. High protein and calorie levels are needed to maintain nutritional status in light of the increased work of breathing.
3. Advise the client to avoid gas-producing foods, such as beans and cabbage.	3. Gas-forming foods may cause abdominal bloating and distention and thus impair ventilation.
4. Instruct the client in the use of high-calorie liquid supplements if indicated.	4. Liquid supplements provide high-calorie concentrations in a relatively small volume.
5. Advise hypoxemic clients to use oxygen via nasal cannula during meals.	5. Adequate oxygenation increases the energy available for eating.
6. Suggest methods to make meal preparation more convenient (e.g., Meals on Wheels program).	6. Reducing the energy expenditure of preparation maximizes the energy available for eating.
7. Monitor the client's food intake, weight, and serum hemoglobin and albumin levels.	7. Changes in body weight reflect the degree of nutrition or malnutrition. Hemoglobin and albumin levels reflect protein intake.

Evaluation. The client maintains normal body weight and blood protein levels.

Nursing Diagnosis. Sleep Pattern Disturbance related to dyspnea and external stimuli.

Outcomes. The client will report feeling adequately rested.

Interventions	Rationales
1. Promote relaxation by providing a darkened, quiet environment; ensuring adequate room ventilation; and following bedtime routines.	1. The hospital environment can interfere with relaxation and sleep. Using established bedtime rituals increases relaxation.
2. Schedule care activities to allow periods of uninterrupted sleep.	2. For most people, completing four to five complete sleep cycles (60 to 90 minutes) per night promotes a feeling of being rested.

Care Plan continued on following page

3. Instruct the client in measures to promote sleep;

a. Plan physical exercise during the day and passive, nonstimulating activities in the evening.	a. Activity increases the need for sleep and contributes to a feeling of tiredness.
b. Avoid stimulants, such as caffeine.	b. Stimulants increase metabolism and inhibit relaxation.
c. Maintain a consistent bedtime and a regular bedtime routine.	c. Consistency promotes relaxation and prevents disruptions of the biologic clock.
d. Eat a high-protein snack before bedtime.	d. Protein digestion produces tryptophan, an amino acid that has a sedative effect.
e. Use relaxation techniques (e.g., meditation, massage, warm bath, warm beverage).	e. Sleep is difficult unless the client is relaxed.
f. If the client awakens during the night, suggest a quiet, diverting activity, such as reading, in another room.	f. Frustration over being awake deters sleep efforts further. The bedroom should be associated mentally with sleep to enhance future sleep promotion.
g. If dyspnea is severe, a recliner chair or hospital bed may be more comfortable than a regular bed.	g. The upright position facilitates ventilation.

Evaluation. The client gets at least 4 to 5 hours of uninterrupted sleep per night and reports feeling rested.

Nursing Diagnosis. Altered Family Processes related to chronic illness of a family member.

Outcomes. The family will verbalize their feelings, participate in the care of the ill family member, and seek external resources as needed.

Interventions	Rationales
1. Plan interventions considering the client and significant other as the unit of care. Encourage participation in the planning process.	1. COPD affects not only the client experiencing the condition but also the client's significant others.
2. Assess family communication patterns, and intervene if they are ineffective. Family counseling may be needed.	2. Effective communication helps each member to understand his or her own and others' feelings. Counseling may facilitate healthy interaction.
3. Encourage as wide a social support network as feasible.	3. The use of a wide support group prevents a few family members from being overloaded with responsibility.
4. Encourage the client and family to seek support from other sources (e.g., self-help groups and support groups, such as the Better Breathers clubs sponsored by the American Lung Association).	4. Clients may benefit from opportunities to share common experiences and to learn from others in similar situations.
5. Provide the family with anticipatory guidance as the client's COPD progresses.	5. Knowing what to expect facilitates family adjustment.

Evaluation. The client's family copes effectively with the stress of the client's illness, communicates openly, and supports the client.

Nursing Diagnosis. Sexual Dysfunction related to dyspnea, reduced energy, and changes in relationships.

Outcomes. The client will report increased satisfaction with sexual function.

Interventions	Rationales
1. Provide an opportunity for the client to discuss concerns.	1. Many people are embarrassed or reluctant to talk about their sexual concerns.
2. Suggest measures that may facilitate sexual activity (e.g., alternative positions, use of bronchodilator therapy before beginning sexual activity).	2. Such measures can reduce physical exertion and maximize available oxygen levels.
3. Encourage the client and partner to consider alternative forms of sexual expression (e.g., hugging, cuddling, stroking, kissing).	3. Alternative methods require less energy expenditure compared with intercourse.
4. Recommend a professional sex therapist if appropriate.	4. Talking with a skilled professional may assist client with constructive problem-solving.

Evaluation. The client discusses concerns and verbalizes more satisfaction with sexual relations.

Clients with end-stage lung disease experience significant, intensely distressing manifestations. Whether care is provided in the home or an extended-care facility, the focus is on minimizing these manifestations and making the client as comfortable as possible (see Bridge to Home Health Care).

TRACHEOBRONCHITIS

Acute tracheobronchitis is an inflammation of the mucous membranes of the trachea and the bronchial tree. This disorder commonly follows viral infections of the upper respiratory tract. It may also result from inhalation of noxious or irritating gases and particulate matter (including cigarette smoke), bacterial pneumonia, overvigorous tracheobronchial suctioning, and harsh paroxysms of coughing.

Manifestations include a raw burning pain over the upper anterior chest wall over the midsternum. Pain is increased with exposure to cold environments, cigarette smoke, cough, and tracheobronchial suctioning. In addition, the client may have a cough that progresses from dry to productive as the irritation increases. Fever, headache, and malaise may be present. Observe for cough-related syncope. Lightheadedness or fainting may occur with forceful coughing spells. Fainting is caused by prolonged elevation of intrapulmonary pressure during the compressive phase of a cough. The increased pressure impairs venous return to the thorax, causing a decrease in cardiac output.

Outcome Management

Treatment is focused on the cause of the cough. Cough suppressants are rarely effective. Antibiotics, bronchodilators, corticosteroids (inhaled and systemic), and anticholinergics are the primary treatments. Sinusitis is a common accompanying finding as well as a cause of tracheobronchitis.

Priority nursing goals include relief of pain and elimination of the tracheal irritation. Strongly advise the client to stop smoking. Whenever possible, eliminate other irritating gases or substances from the environment. Promote airway clearance by encouraging effective coughing, increased fluid intake, changing positions, and increasing inspired humidity. Inspired humidity may be increased through the use of aerosols. Advise clients to avoid cold air and to cover the mouth and nose before going outdoors.

BRONCHIECTASIS

Bronchiectasis, an extreme form of bronchitis, causes permanent, abnormal dilation and distortion of bronchi and bronchioles. It develops when bronchial walls are weak-

BRIDGE TO HOME HEALTH CARE

Conserving Oxygen with Chronic Obstructive Pulmonary Disease

Clients with chronic obstructive pulmonary disease (COPD) are challenged to make the most of their lives, given their available oxygen.

Usually, home health nurses are primarily responsible for monitoring manifestations; reviewing and reinforcing previously taught oxygen-conservation techniques; giving further instructions; and determining whether referrals to registered dietitians and occupational, physical, or respiratory therapists are needed. Evaluate what your clients already know, and proceed from there. Be certain that your clients understand the importance of using pursed-lip breathing, abdominal breathing, and metered-dose inhalers consistently and correctly. Have them demonstrate their technique.

Help your clients develop an oxygen-conservation plan that allows them to participate in activities that are most important to them. Ask them to keep a simple diary and to record their usual behavior during a 1- or 2-day period that includes all waking hours. When you analyze the diary, identify your clients' priorities. Help them relate specific activity to feelings of dyspnea during the day. In this way, you can teach specific oxygen-conservation techniques and pacing of activities to meet their priorities. To increase comfort, have your clients schedule the use of inhalers before activities and keep them within easy reach.

Encourage clients who are concerned about adequate oxygen for sexual activity to assume passive positions and to allow their partner to be more active. If winded, clients should use massage and other relaxation techniques as part of foreplay.

Adequate nutrition is essential to clients who have COPD; they may be malnourished because of respiratory muscle wasting. The diet may be high in protein and calories and low in carbohydrates. Answer your clients' questions, and determine whether they are willing or able to purchase, prepare, and eat the foods that were suggested. Encourage easy food preparation to prevent fatigue. Use foods that are prepackaged or can be heated in the microwave. Consider home-delivered meals. Use liquid food supplements to increase protein and calories; many brands are available, including some that are specially formulated for people who have pulmonary problems.

Encourage clients to rest just before eating and to follow these suggestions. Eat in a relaxed and quiet area. Small, frequent meals are best. Schedule meals early in the day if fatigue increases as the day continues. Snack frequently. Schedule inhalers after meals because inhalers can taint the taste of food and make it more difficult to achieve adequate nutrition.

Clients who have COPD often feel isolated because of their decreased ability to leave their homes. Suggest that they and their families join local support groups where they can share their experiences and feelings about the disease and learn new techniques to improve their quality of life. Many hospitals sponsor groups. Another valuable resource is the American Lung Association, which has local offices throughout the United States; call for information about prevention and the latest developments in treatment.

Rebecca M. Dudley, RN, *Staff Nurse, Fairview Lakes HomeCaring and Hospice, Chisago City, Minnesota*

ened by chronic inflammatory changes in the bronchial mucosa and occurs most often after recurrent inflammatory conditions. Any condition producing a narrowing of the lumen of the bronchioles, however, may result in bronchiectasis, including tuberculosis, adenoviral infections, and pneumonia.

Some forms of bronchiectasis are congenital and are associated with cystic fibrosis, sinusitis, dextrocardia (heart located on right side), and alterations in ciliary activity (Kartagener's syndrome). Bronchiectasis is usually localized to a lung lobe or segment rather than generalized throughout the lungs. At times, however, persistent, nonresolving infection may cause the disorder to spread to other parts of the same lung.

Diagnosis may be confirmed by chest radiograph, bronchogram, or computed tomography (CT) scan.

Manifestations vary according to the etiologic agent. The main manifestations are cough and purulent sputum production in large quantities. Fever, hemoptysis, nasal stuffiness, and drainage from sinusitis also are common. The client may complain of fatigue and weakness. Clubbing of the fingers may be found on physical assessment.

Outcome Management

Management of bronchiectasis is the same as for COPD. Most clients are managed medically to prevent progression of the disorder and to control clinical manifestations. Antibiotics, chest physical therapy, hydration, bronchodilators, and oxygen commonly are prescribed. Severe cases may be treated by surgical resection if the pathologic process is well localized in one lobe or two adjacent lobes and when no contraindications to surgery exist.

DISORDERS OF THE PULMONARY VASCULATURE

PULMONARY EMBOLISM

Pulmonary embolism (PE) is an occlusion of a portion of the pulmonary blood vessels by an embolus. An embolus is a clot or other plug (thrombus) that is carried by the bloodstream from its point of origin to a smaller blood vessel, where it obstructs circulation. Depending on its size, an embolus can be lethal. It is estimated that, in the United States, more than 250,000 people are hospitalized annually for venous thromboembolism. For those with a PE, the mortality rate is approximately 15%.[11]

Etiology and Risk Factors

Virtually all PEs develop from thrombi (clots), most of which originate in the deep calf, femoral, popliteal, or iliac veins. Other sources of emboli include tumors, air, fat, bone marrow, amniotic fluid, septic thrombi, and vegetations on heart valves that develop with endocarditis.

Major operations, especially hip, knee, abdominal, and extensive pelvic procedures, predispose the client to thrombus formation because of the reduced flow of blood through the pelvis. Preventive measures, such as early ambulation, frequent leg exercises, sequential compression stockings, and low-dose heparin prophylaxis, are essential.

Pathophysiology

When emboli travel to the lungs, they lodge in the pulmonary vasculature. The size and number of emboli determine the location. Blood flow is obstructed, leading to decreased perfusion of the section of lung supplied by the vessel. The client continues to ventilate the lung portion, but because the tissue is not perfused, a $\dot{V}/\dot{Q}$ mismatch occurs, resulting in hypoxemia.

If an embolus lodges in a large pulmonary vessel, it increases proximal pulmonary vascular resistance, causes atelectasis, and eventually reduces cardiac output. If the embolus is in a smaller vessel, less dramatic clinical manifestations follow but perfusion is still altered.

The arterioles constrict because of platelet degranulation, accompanied by a release of histamine, serotonin, catecholamines, and prostaglandins. The chemical agents result in bronchial and pulmonary artery constriction. This vasoconstriction probably plays a major role in the hemodynamic instability that follows PE.

PE can lead to right-sided heart failure. Once the clot lodges, affected blood vessels in the lung collapse. This collapse increases the pressure in the pulmonary vasculature. The increased pressure increases the workload of the right side of the heart, leading to failure. Massive PE of the pulmonary artery can also result in cardiopulmonary collapse from lack of perfusion and resulting hypoxia and acidosis.

Clinical Manifestations

The clinical manifestations of PE are nonspecific and, in some clients, may not appear until late in the event. The most common manifestations of PE are tachypnea, dyspnea, anxiety, and chest pain. Because these clinical manifestations are similar to those seen with myocardial infarction and other cardiovascular illnesses, overdiagnosis is as likely as underdiagnosis. Extensive differential diagnosis often is required. The pain usually experienced with PE is pleuritic in nature, caused by an inflammatory reaction of the lung parenchyma or by pulmonary infarction or ischemia, caused by obstruction of small pulmonary arterial branches. Typical pleuritic chest pain is sudden in onset and exacerbated by breathing. The client is usually dyspneic, especially if the embolus has occluded major arteries or major portions of lung tissue. Apprehension, cough, diaphoresis, syncope, and hemoptysis may occur. The presence of hemoptysis indicates that the infarction or areas of atelectasis have produced alveolar damage.

Respirations typically increase. Crackles, an accentuated second heart sound, tachycardia, and fever may also develop. Less common findings include heart gallops, edema, heart murmur, and cyanosis.

Diagnostic Findings

When PE is suspected, the optimal strategy for diagnosis is an integrated approach that includes a thorough history and physical examination, supplemented by selective diagnostic tests. ABG analysis indicates arterial hypoxemia (low PaO_2) and hypocapnia (low $PaCO_2$) in massive PE. There may be a severe respiratory alkalosis. Lactate dehydrogenase (LDH) isoenzymes show an increase in LDH_3

if there is lung tissue injury. A chest radiograph may help to rule out other pulmonary diagnoses.

The best noninvasive diagnostic test for PE is the $\dot{V}/\dot{Q}$ lung scan. A radioisotope lung scan is performed by IV injection of particles of human serum albumin that have been labeled with iodine 131 or technetium 99m. These particles are trapped in the pulmonary microvasculature and are distributed according to pulmonary flow. Both lungs are scanned with a scintillation counter, and the amount of radioactivity counted gives an indication of obstruction to flow. A lung scan can be seen in Chapter 59.

An alternative to lung scanning is spiral CT scan of the chest. This approach is particularly effective for identifying PE in the proximal pulmonary vascular tree.

Pulmonary angiography remains the definitive means of diagnosis of PE (Fig. 61–10). A radiopaque contrast agent is injected into the right atrium and pulmonary artery via a catheter threaded through a peripheral vein. Visualization of any filling defects of the heart and right pulmonary artery is achieved by taking sequential radiographs. Because of the invasive nature of the test, pulmonary angiography typically is reserved for cases in which there is a high index of clinical suspicion despite nondiagnostic findings on other tests.

Outcome Management

Medical Care

Successful management of PE depends on prompt recognition of the condition and immediate treatment. Goals are to stabilize the cardiopulmonary system and reduce the threat of a further PE with anticoagulation therapy. For some clients, the clot can be lysed.

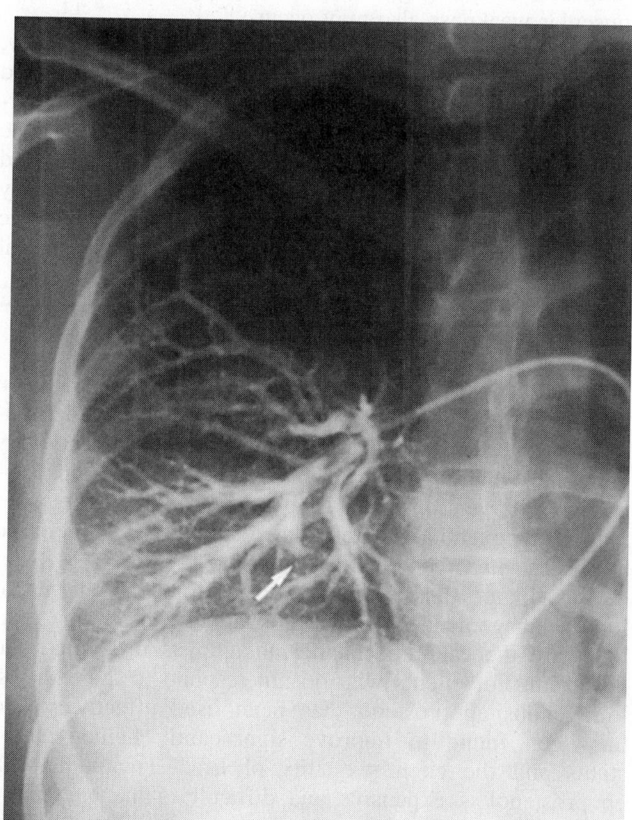

FIGURE 61–10 Angiogram showing a pulmonary embolus (*arrow*).

Stabilizing the Cardiopulmonary System

Maintenance of cardiopulmonary stability is the first priority. Cardiopulmonary support varies with the client's manifestations. Sometimes hypoxemia can be reversed with low-flow oxygen by nasal cannula. Other clients may require endotracheal intubation to maintain PaO_2 greater than 60 mm Hg. Hypotension is treated with fluids. If fluids do not raise the preload (right ventricular end-diastolic pressure) enough to raise blood pressure, inotropic agents may be required. Acidosis, which has a powerful vasoconstricting effect, is corrected with bicarbonate.

Anticoagulant Therapy

Typically, anticoagulation begins with IV standard (unfractionated) heparin sodium to reduce the risk of further clots and to prevent extension of existing clots. Anticoagulants do not break up existing clots. Clinical trials have shown that subcutaneously administered low-molecular-weight heparin is as safe and effective as standard heparin in the treatment of hemodynamically stable clients with PE. Anticoagulants are administered until a therapeutic partial thromboplastin time (PTT) is achieved. In general, the initial target International Normalized Ratio should be 2.5 to 3.0. Administration of sodium warfarin is begun about 3 to 5 days before heparin is stopped to provide a transition to oral anticoagulation. Because the half-life of warfarin is long, about 2 to 3 days is required to achieve adequate anticoagulation. Clients are maintained on warfarin for 3 to 6 months.

Fibrinolytic Therapy

The effectiveness of fibrinolytic therapy in the management of a massive PE is not clear, but it may be useful in clients who are hemodynamically unstable. Thrombolytic agents lyse the clots and restore right-sided heart function; however, some clinicians have found that although the clot dissolves, the mortality rate is not improved.

Nursing Management of the Medical Client

Monitor the client closely for hypoxemia and respiratory compromise, and assess vital signs and lung sounds frequently. Monitor ABG values, and monitor the client for manifestations of right-sided heart failure. Auscultate heart sounds frequently, assessing for murmurs or extra heart sounds. Check for peripheral edema, distended neck veins, and liver engorgement.

To facilitate breathing, elevate the head of the bed and apply oxygen per physician's orders. Because the usual cause of a PE is thrombus from the lower legs, elevate the legs with caution to avoid severe flexure of the hips. Such flexure would slow blood flow and increase the risk of new thrombi.

The client typically experiences fear with the sudden onset of severe chest pain and inability to breathe. Anxiety, restlessness, and apprehension are common. Emotional support can reduce anxiety and lessen dyspnea. Stay with the client and give calm (yet efficient) nursing care.

Analgesics are given as needed to reduce pain and anxiety. Morphine is the most common agent. Anxiety and pain increase oxygen demand and dyspnea. Administer oral care with soft brushes or rinses while oxygen is in use, especially if the client breathes through the mouth.

Once anticoagulation is achieved, watch for manifestations of excess anticoagulation, such as blood in the urine, in the stool, or along the gums or teeth; subcutaneous bruising; or flank pain. When invasive studies, such as ABGs, are necessary, apply pressure to the puncture site for at least 10 minutes. The client is discharged with oral anticoagulation therapy. Instruct the client about side effects, the importance of follow-up to monitor prothrombin times, and precautions to prevent bleeding. Review methods to reduce thrombophlebitis, if that was the likely cause of the embolus (see Chapter 53).

Surgical Management

Surgical interventions that may be used in treatment of PE include (1) vena cava interruption with the insertion of a filter (Fig. 61–11) and (2) pulmonary embolectomy. The Greenfield filter, a basket-like cone of wires bent to look like an umbrella, is the filter most commonly used. The surgeon inserts the filter by threading it up the veins in the leg or neck until it reaches the vena cava at the level of the renal arteries. The filter allows blood flow while trapping emboli.

Embolectomy is used in clients with significant hemodynamic instability caused by the embolus, especially those with unstable circulation and contraindications to thrombolytic therapy. An embolectomy involves surgical removal of emboli from the pulmonary arteries by either a thoracotomy or an embolectomy catheter. Newly developed catheters use high-velocity jets of saline to draw the thrombus toward the catheter tip and pulverize it.[11]

PULMONARY HYPERTENSION

Pulmonary hypertension is defined as a prolonged elevation of the mean pulmonary artery pressure (PAP) above 25 mm Hg at rest (normal, 10 to 20 mm Hg) or above 30 mm Hg during exercise (normal, 20 to 30 mm Hg). Severe forms of pulmonary hypertension are classified as either *secondary* or *idiopathic (primary)*. Secondary pulmonary hypertension is usually associated with underlying heart or lung disease (e.g., PE, venocclusive disease, COPD). The cause of the idiopathic form is, by definition, unclear. It occurs most often in young adults between the ages of 30 and 40 years. Women are affected more often than men.[29] The condition is progressive, leading to right-sided heart failure and severe dyspnea.

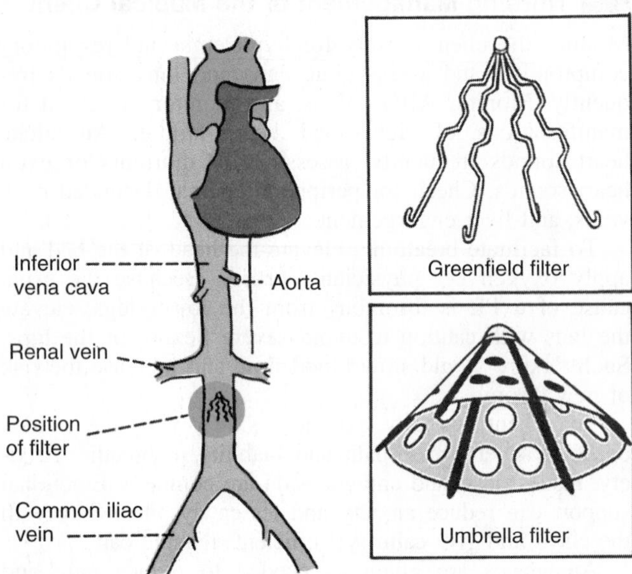

FIGURE 61–11 Inferior vena cava filters, such as the Greenfield and umbrella filters, prevent emboli from traveling to the lung.

Etiology

The pulmonary circulation is generally a low-pressure, low-resistance system. Increased cardiac output in a healthy person, as with exercise, causes minimal elevations in PAP because of the large pulmonary vascular reserve. When pulmonary vasoconstriction is present, however, pressure elevation occurs because the pulmonary vasculature cannot accommodate increased blood flow.

Mild forms of pulmonary hypertension are normally caused by pulmonary vasoconstriction resulting from chronic hypoxia, acidosis, or both. Administration of oxygen, correction of acid-base imbalance, and use of vasodilating medications in selected cases generally return PAP to normal, either completely or partially.

Clinical Manifestations

Clients with mild pulmonary hypertension may be relatively asymptomatic. In moderate to severe forms, the main (and occasionally only) manifestation is dyspnea. Fatigue, syncope, angina-like chest pain, palpitations, and muscular weakness also may occur.

Chest x-ray study shows right ventricular hypertrophy, enlarged pulmonary arteries, prominent hilar vessels, and normal or reduced intrapulmonary vascular markings. Cardiac catheterization provides the most valuable diagnostic measurements. Typical findings include elevated PAP and increased arteriovenous oxygen differences accompanied by normal systemic blood pressure and normal to low cardiac output. Pulmonary wedge pressures (PWPs) remain normal because left ventricular function is typically unchanged.

Outcome Management

The overall prognosis in severe pulmonary hypertension is poor. There is no known cure for the disorder, although treatment of the underlying cause of secondary pulmonary hypertension may slow its progression. Supportive intervention with supplemental oxygen helps to reduce hypoxemia, whereas anticoagulants may be used to prevent thromboembolic events.

Vasodilator therapy is the cornerstone of pharmacologic management. First-line vasodilators used for treatment are the calcium channel antagonists nifedipine and diltiazem. For clients who do not respond to these drugs, intravenous epoprostenol has been used effectively and has been found to improve significantly hemodynamic status and the client's quality of life.[5] Treatment with epoprostenol is expensive and difficult to manage, however, because it requires long-term, continuous central infusion. Some clients with severe pulmonary hypertension may undergo heart-lung transplantation, although data regarding long-term effectiveness are not yet available. Interventions appropriate for underlying diseases and preparation for diagnostic procedures are incorporated into nursing care.

CONCLUSIONS

Lower airway disorders include asthma, chronic air flow limitations, and inflammations of the airways. Nursing care centers on reversal of any airway spasms and education of the client on how to live with the disorder and to reduce the risk of future problems. PE is a potentially life-threatening disorder that usually can be managed effectively with prompt recognition.

THINKING CRITICALLY

1. **A 52-year-old woman is being treated at the neighborhood health clinic for chronic bronchitis. Her husband of 30 years smoked two to three packs of cigarettes a day. The client never smoked. During this exacerbation, she presents with shortness of breath; wheezing; a deep, throaty, productive cough when she tries to talk; and fatigue. Her blood pressure is 180/90 mm Hg, pulse is 90 beats per minute, respirations are 28 per minute and labored, and temperature is 99.4° F. She tells you that she tried to shovel the driveway on this cold winter day and did not wear a scarf over her mouth as she usually does. She further states that her inhalers did not seem to help her. She is taking a diuretic for hypertension, with blood pressure controlled at about 160/86 mm Hg. What is your priority nursing action? What teaching is appropriate at this time?**

Factors to Consider. What are the clinical manifestations of chronic obstructive emphysema? What nursing assessments are in order?

2. **An elderly client is recovering from pelvic surgery. Because of a previous cerebrovascular accident, she is hemiplegic. She has been on bed rest since the surgery. While the nursing assistant is giving her a bath, she notices the client grimacing as if in pain. The client responds to her question by pointing to her chest and nodding when asked if the pain is severe. The nursing assistant notifies you that the client is in distress. What is the priority assessment?**

Factors to Consider. What complications of surgery and resulting bed rest might pose a risk for this client? How would you compare and contrast the clinical manifestations for pneumonia and pulmonary embolus?

3. **You enter the room of the client from Question 2 and discover that she is apprehensive. She is trying to hold her breath because it hurts to breathe. She is sweating, and there is frothy sputum on her lips. What nursing interventions are appropriate? What treatment might be ordered?**

Factors to Consider. What are the clinical manifestations of a pulmonary embolus? What diagnostic studies may be ordered?

BIBLIOGRAPHY

1. Allen, G. (1996). Surgical treatment of emphysema using bovine pericardium strips. *AORN Journal, 63*(2), 373–388.
2. Bennett, J., & Plum, F. (1996). *Cecil textbook of medicine* (20th ed.). Philadelphia: W. B. Saunders.
3. Bone, R. C. (1996). Goals of asthma management: A step-care approach. *Chest, 109*(4), 1056–1065.
4. Burns, S. M., & Lawson, C. (1999). Pharmacological and ventilatory management of acute asthma exacerbations. *Critical Care Nurse, 19*(4), 39–53.
5. Cheever, K. H., Kitzes, B., & Genthner, D. (1999). Epoprostenol therapy for primary pulmonary hypertension. *Critical Care Nurse, 19*(4), 20–27.
6. Couser, J. I., et al. (1995). Pulmonary rehabilitation improves exercise capacity in older elderly patients with COPD. *Chest, 107*(3), 730–734.
7. Faul, J. L., et al. (1999). Quality of life and lung volume reduction surgery. *American Journal of Critical Care, 8*(6), 359–396.
8. Ferraro, J. (1996). Here's the result of poor treatment for lung infections. *RN, 59*(11), 54–56.
9. Gift, A. G. (1995). Application in research: Issues in asthma self-management. *Perspectives in Respiratory Nursing, 6*(4), 5–6.
10. Gift, A. G., & Narsavage, G. (1998). Validity of the numeric rating scale as a measure of dyspnea. *American Journal of Critical Care, 7,* 200–204.
11. Goldhaber, S. Z. (1998). Medical progress: Pulmonary embolism. *New England Journal of Medicine, 339*(2), 93–104.
12. Graling, P., Hetrick, V., & Kiernan, P. (1996). Bilateral lung volume reduction surgery. *AORN Journal, 63*(2), 389–404.
13. Heslop, A., & Shannon, C. (1995). Assisting patients living with long-term oxygen therapy. *British Journal of Nursing, 4*(19), 1123–1128.
14. Janssen, W. (1996). Treatment for emphysema: An overview of lung volume reduction surgery. *Perspectives in Respiratory Nursing, 7*(1), 1–5.
15. Leidy, N. K. (1995). Functional performance in people with chronic obstructive pulmonary disease. *Image, 27*(1), 23–35.
16. Lewis, D., & Bell, S. K. (1995). Pulmonary rehabilitation, psychological adjustment, and use of healthcare services. *Rehabilitation Nursing, 20*(2), 102–107.
17. Madison, J. M., & Irwin, R. S. (1998). Chronic obstructive pulmonary disease. *Lancet, 352*(9126), 467–473.
18. McKinney, B. (1995). Under new management: Asthma and the elderly. *Journal of Gerontological Nursing, 21*(11), 39–45.
19. National Institutes of Health. (1997). *Guidelines for the diagnosis and management of asthma.* NIH Pub. No. 97-4051. Washington, DC: Author.
20. Newsome, E. A., & Ott, B. B. (1997). Lung volume reduction: Surgical treatment for emphysema. *American Journal of Critical Care, 6*(6), 423–429.
21. Pfister, S. M. (1995). Home oxygen therapy: Indications, administration, recertification, and patient education. *Nurse Practitioner, 20*(7), 44–56.
22. Reid, W. D., & Samrai, B. (1995). Respiratory muscle training for patients with chronic obstructive pulmonary disease. *Physical Therapy, 75*(11), 996–1005.
23. Schedel, E. M., & Connolly, M. A. (1999). Lung volume reduction surgery: New hope for emphysema patients. *Dimensions of Critical Care Nursing, 18*(1), 28–34.
24. Scherer, Y., Schmieder, L., & Shimmel, S. (1995). Outpatient instruction for individuals with COPD. *Perspectives in Respiratory Nursing, 6*(3), 1–8.
25. Shelmerdine, L. (1995). Occupational asthma: Assessing the risk. *Nursing Standard, 10*(4), 25–28.
26. Tarpy, S. P., & Celli, B. R. (1995). Current concepts: Long-term oxygen therapy. *New England Journal of Medicine, 333*(11), 710–714.
27. Tiep, B. L. (1997). Disease management of COPD with pulmonary rehabilitation. *Chest, 112*(6), 1630–1656.
28. Verderber, A., Gallagher, K., & Severino, R. (1995). The effect of nursing interventions on transcutaneous oxygen and carbon dioxide tensions. *Western Journal of Nursing Research, 17*(1), 76–90.
29. Wallace, L. S. (1998). Pulmonary hypertension: A deadly threat. *RN, 61*(10), 48–54.

CHAPTER 62

REMEMBER to check out your Companion CD ROM

Management of Clients with Parenchymal and Pleural Disorders

Nancy York

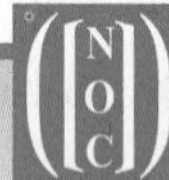

NURSING OUTCOMES CLASSIFICATION (NOC)
for Nursing Diagnoses—Clients with Parenchymal and Pleural Disorders

Activity Intolerance
Activity Tolerance
Endurance
Altered Nutrition: Less Than Body Requirements
Nutritional Status
Nutritional Status: Food and Fluid Intake
Altered Oral Mucous Membrane
Tissue Integrity: Skin and Mucous Membrane
Anxiety
Anxiety Control
Coping
Impaired Gas Exchange
Respiratory Status: Gas Exchange
Respiratory Status: Ventilation
Ineffective Airway Clearance
Aspiration Control
Respiratory Status: Airway Patency
Ineffective Breathing Pattern
Respiratory Status: Airway Patency
Respiratory Status: Ventilation
Ineffective Individual Coping
Coping
Information Processing
Role Performance
Social Support
Knowledge Deficit
Knowledge: Disease Process
Knowledge: Health Behaviors
Knowledge: Medication
Knowledge: Treatment Regimen
Pain
Comfort Level
Pain: Disruptive Effects
Sleep Pattern Disturbance
Anxiety Control
Rest
Sleep

The parenchyma of any organ, in this case the lung, is the tissue essential for the function of the organ. This chapter reviews disorders of the lung parenchyma, such as pneumonia, tuberculosis, cystic fibrosis, and cancer.

ATELECTASIS

Atelectasis is the collapse of lung tissue at any structural level (e.g., segmental, basilar, lobar, or microscopic). It develops when there is interference with the natural forces that promote lung expansion. Such interference may result from a reduction in lung distention forces, localized airway obstruction, insufficient pulmonary surfactant, or increased elastic recoil. Examples of each of these causes are given in Box 62–1. Atelectasis is particularly common after surgery, especially upper abdominal or thoracic procedures. Clients who are elderly, obese, or bedridden or have a history of smoking are also susceptible to atelectasis.

Atelectasis may be diagnosed through physical examination, although generally, it is initially detected on chest x-ray. Some clients are asymptomatic. If significant hypoxemia (low level of oxygen in the blood) is present, however, dyspnea (difficult or labored breathing), tachypnea (rapid breathing), tachycardia (rapid heartbeat), and cyanosis (bluish discoloration of skin and mucous membranes) may occur. Chest auscultation may reveal bronchial or diminished breath sounds and crackles over the involved area. Fever of less than 101° F is common. However, elderly people with atelectasis typically do not exhibit a fever.

If atelectasis is severe, physical assessment findings include the following:

- A tracheal shift toward the side of the atelectasis
- A decrease in tactile fremitus over the affected lung area
- A dull percussion note over the atelectatic region
- Decreased chest movement on the involved side

None of these signs is specific for atelectasis, and the entire clinical picture must always be considered.

One of the primary goals of nursing intervention is to prevent atelectasis in the high-risk client. Frequent position changes and early ambulation help promote drainage of all lung segments. Deep-breathing and effective coughing enhance lung expansion and prevent airway obstruc-

BOX 62–1 Causes of Atelectasis

Reduction in Lung Distention Forces

Pleural space encroachment (e.g., pneumothorax, pleural effusion, pleural tumor)
Chest wall disorders (e.g., scoliosis, flail chest)
Impaired diaphragmatic movement (e.g., ascites, obesity)
Central nervous system dysfunction (e.g., coma, neuromuscular disorders, oversedation)

Localized Airway Obstruction

Mucus plugging
Foreign body aspiration
Bronchiectasis

Insufficient Pulmonary Surfactant

Respiratory distress syndrome
Inhalation anesthesia
High concentrations of oxygen (oxygen toxicity)
Lung contusion
Aspiration of gastric contents
Smoke inhalation

Increased Elastic Recoil

Interstitial fibrosis (e.g., silicosis, radiation pneumonitis)

tion. Incentive spirometry is an excellent means of encouraging a client to deep-breathe.

If atelectasis develops, treatment is directed toward the underlying cause. If the client becomes hypoxic, oxygen should be administered as prescribed (e.g., per cannula, 1 to 4 L/min). More aggressive measures to maintain airway patency, such as postural drainage, chest physiotherapy, and tracheal suctioning, may also be ordered. If an airway obstruction is causing atelectasis, bronchoscopy may be used to remove the material.

INFECTIOUS DISORDERS

INFLUENZA

The term "flu" is often used inappropriately to describe many clinical manifestations and disorders. *Influenza* actually refers to an acute viral infection of the respiratory tract.

Influenza usually occurs seasonally in epidemic form. People most at risk are very young children, the elderly, people living in institutional settings, people with chronic diseases, and health care personnel.

The first flu virus was identified in the 1930s. Since then, influenza viruses have been identified as types A, B, and C. Type A is the most prevalent and is associated with the most serious epidemics. Type B outbreaks also can reach epidemic levels, but the disease produced is generally milder than that caused by type A. Type C viruses have never been connected with a large epidemic.

Clinical manifestations of influenza include fever, myalgias (muscular pain), and cough. Influenza predisposes to complications such as viral bronchitis or pneumonia, bacterial pneumonia, and superinfections (infections that occur during the course of antimicrobial therapy).

Influenza differs from a common cold primarily in its sudden onset and widespread occurrence within the population.

Chest findings are usually negative unless pneumonia results. Conversely, colds have a slow onset of manifestations, usually do not cause fever, have malaise as a major manifestation, and commonly cause nasal manifestations.

Outcome Management

Intervention for influenza is based on manifestations as they arise (i.e., supportive measures to relieve fever, myalgia, and cough). In 1999, two new anti-influenza drugs (zanamivir and oseltamivir) were developed that appear to be extremely effective in preventing massive multiplication of the virus. They must be administered within 24 hours of onset. Rimantadine can be used to treat influenza type A in adults, but it has no effect on type B infections. When taken within 48 hours after the onset of illness, rimantadine reduces the duration of fever and other manifestations and allows clients to return to their daily routines more quickly. These drugs do not, however, replace the need for immunization.

Influenza is a communicable disease spread by droplet infection. Prevent the spread of this infection by encouraging clients with influenza to remain at home, practice frequent hand-washing, and cover the nose and mouth when sneezing or coughing.

Encourage clients at risk for influenza to obtain an annual immunization before the start of the "flu season" each winter. Vaccination controls influenza for many high-risk clients. However, clients who are allergic to eggs or have a history of Guillain-Barré syndrome should not receive an influenza immunization.

PNEUMONIA

Pneumonia (pneumonitis) is an inflammatory process in lung parenchyma usually associated with a marked increase in interstitial and alveolar fluid. Advances in antibiotic therapy have led to the widespread perception that pneumonia is no longer a major health problem in the United States. However, pneumonia and influenza are currently the sixth most common cause of death for all ages and one of the most common causes in the elderly. Among all nosocomial infections, pneumonia is the second most common but has the highest mortality.[8, 22]

Etiology and Risk Factors

There are many causes of pneumonia, including bacteria, viruses, mycoplasmas, fungal agents, and protozoa (Table 62–1). Pneumonia may also result from aspiration of food, fluids, or vomitus or from inhalation of toxic or caustic chemicals, smoke, dusts, or gases. Pneumonia may complicate immobility and chronic illnesses. It often follows influenza.

Major risk factors for pneumonia include (1) advanced age, (2) a history of smoking, (3) upper respiratory infection, (4) tracheal intubation, (5) prolonged immobility, (6) immunosuppressive therapy, (7) a nonfunctional immune system, (8) malnutrition, (9) dehydration, and (10) chronic disease states, such as diabetes, heart disease,

TABLE 62–1 ASSESSMENT AND TREATMENT OF PNEUMONIA

Common Name	Clinical Manifestations	Management
Pneumococcal pneumonia (caused by *Streptococcus pneumoniae*)	Sudden onset with a single shaking chill, high fever, stabbing-pleuritic chest pain, malaise, weakness, occasional vomiting, tachypnea, dyspnea, and elevated WBC count Single or multiple lobar consolidation on the chest x-ray Cough productive of rusty brown or blood-streaked purulent sputum that turns yellow and mucoid	Primary: penicillinase-resistant penicillin, doxycycline, levofloxacin Alternative: azithromycin or clarithromycin, second- or third-generation cephalosporin Prevention: Vaccine available
Staphylococcal pneumonia (caused by *Staphylococcus aureus*)	Sudden onset with fever, multiple chills, pleuritic pain, dyspnea, rales, decreased breath sounds, elevated WBC count, and exaggerated cough productive of purulent golden-yellow or blood-streaked sputum Chest x-ray may show patchy infiltrates, empyema, abscesses, and pneumothorax Disease may start with headache, cough, and myalgia	Primary: penicillin, cephalosporin; vancomycin for non–penicillinase-producing organism; penicillinase-resistant penicillin if organism produces penicillinase; vancomycin if organism is methicillin resistant
Influenzal pneumonia (caused by *Haemophilus influenzae*)	Similar to those of pneumococcal pneumonia Cough productive of apple- or lime-green purulent sputum, which may be blood-tinged	Primary: cefuroxime, chloramphenicol, ampicillin
Gram-negative bacterial pneumonia (most commonly caused by *Klebsiella pneumoniae*)	Sudden onset with high fever, multiple chills, pleuritic pain, dyspnea, cyanosis, and elevated WBC count Lobar consolidation and cavitation on chest x-ray Cough productive of red sputum resembling currant jelly (mucoid, sticky, and difficult to expectorate)	Primary: aminoglycosides, third-generation cephalosporins, TMP-SMZ, extended-spectrum penicillin, ciprofloxacin
Anaerobic bacterial pneumonia, hypostatic pneumonia (caused by normal oral flora)	Insidious onset with low-grade fever, dyspnea, crackles, cyanosis, hypertension, tachycardia, and elevated WBC count Patchy infiltrates in dependent lung segments on chest x-ray Cough productive of purulent greenish-yellow, foul-smelling sputum	Primary: third-generation cephalosporins (such as cefotaxime) or penicillin G Alternative: cefoxitin, clindamycin, or chloramphenicol
Legionnaires' disease (caused by *Legionella pneumophila*)	Prodrome of 24–48 hours with fever, headache, and malaise followed by high fever with pulse-temperature dissociation, dyspnea, hypoxia, pleuritic pain, nausea, vomiting, diarrhea, confusion, and elevated WBC count Single or multilobar consolidation and small pleural effusions on chest x-ray Dry cough productive of scant mucoid or blood-tinged sputum	Primary: erythromycin Alternative: TMP-SMZ, fluoroquinolone, levofloxacin
Mycoplasma pneumonia (caused by *Mycoplasma* microorganisms)	Insidious onset with slowly rising fever, headache, myalgia, malaise, and normal WBC count Pulmonary infiltrate—sometimes extensive—on chest x-ray Cough productive of scant mucoid sputum Client may show only minimal signs and symptoms	Primary: tetracycline Alternative: erythromycin, ciprofloxacin
Viral pneumonia (caused by influenza A virus)	Prodrome with headache and myalgia followed by high fever, dyspnea, normal breath sounds with occasional wheezing and crackles, and normal or slightly elevated WBC count Diffuse, patchy infiltrates on chest x-ray Dry cough with initial mucoid sputum that later turns purulent Cough may be unproductive	Antiviral agents, symptomatic treatment

TABLE 62–1 ASSESSMENT AND TREATMENT OF PNEUMONIA *Continued*

Common Name	Clinical Manifestations	Management
Fungal pneumonia (caused by histoplasmosis, blastomycosis, coccidioidomycosis, aspergillosis, candidiasis)	Usually asymptomatic When manifestations occur, they range from brief periods of malaise to severe, life-threatening illness Typical illness resembles influenza	Amphotericin B and other oral imidazoles (ketoconazole, fluconazole)
Parasitic pneumonia (caused by protozoa, nematodes, platyhelminths); common organism is *Pneumocystis carinii*	Clients who have *P. carinii* pneumonia are invariably immunocompromised (HIV) Cough, dyspnea, pleuritic chest pain, fever and night sweats, crackles	Diamidines, folate antagonists (TMP-SMZ), and other agents (clindamycin)

HIV, human immunodeficiency virus; TMP-SMZ, trimethoprim-sulfamethoxazole; WBC, white blood cell.

chronic lung disease, renal disease, and cancer. Additional risk factors are exposure to air pollution, altered consciousness (from alcoholism, drug overdose, general anesthesia, or a seizure disorder), inhalation of noxious substances, aspiration of foreign or gastric material, and residence in institutional settings where transmission of the disease is more likely.

Pathophysiology

The feature common to all types of pneumonia is an inflammatory pulmonary response to the offending organism or agent. The defense mechanisms of the lungs lose effectiveness and allow organisms to penetrate the sterile lower respiratory tract, where inflammation develops. Disruption of the mechanical defenses of cough and ciliary motility leads to colonization of the lungs and subsequent infection. Inflamed and fluid-filled alveolar sacs cannot exchange oxygen and carbon dioxide effectively. Alveolar exudate tends to consolidate, so it is increasingly difficult to expectorate. Bacterial pneumonia may be associated with significant ventilation-perfusion mismatch as the infection grows.

Clinical Manifestations

The onset of all pneumonias is generally marked by any or all of the following manifestations: fever, chills, sweats, pleuritic chest pain, cough, sputum production, hemoptysis, dyspnea, headache, and fatigue. Elderly clients may present not with fever or respiratory manifestations but with altered mental status and dehydration.

Chest auscultation reveals bronchial breath sounds over areas of *consolidation* (dense white areas on the chest film). Consolidated lung tissue transmits bronchial sound waves to outer lung fields. Crackling sounds (from fluid in interstitial and alveolar areas) and whispered *pectoriloquy* (transmission of the sound of whispered words through the chest wall) may be heard over affected areas. Tactile fremitus is usually increased over areas of pneumonia, whereas percussion sounds are dulled. Unequal chest wall expansion may occur during inspiration if a large area of lung tissue is involved; this is due to decreased distensibility in the affected area. Table 62–1 lists the clinical manifestations of specific types of pneumonia.

Definitive diagnosis is usually determined through sputum culture analysis and sensitivity or serologic testing. At times, fiberoptic bronchoscopy or transcutaneous needle aspiration or biopsy may be necessary for confirmation. Additional diagnostic testing may consist of (1) skin tests, if tuberculosis or coccidioidomycosis is suspected, (2) blood and urine cultures to assess systemic spread, and (3) transcutaneous oxygen level analysis or arterial blood gas (ABG) measurements to assess the need for supplemental oxygen.

Chest x-ray examination provides information about the location and extent of pneumonia. As already mentioned, on a chest film, areas of pneumonia appear as consolidation.

Pneumonia may involve one or more lobe segments of the lungs (*segmental pneumonia*), one or more entire lobes (*lobar pneumonia*) (Fig. 62–1*A*), or lobes in both lungs (*bilateral pneumonia*). On the basis of location and radiologic appearance, pneumonias may be classified as bronchopneumonia, interstitial pneumonia, alveolar pneumonia, or necrotizing pneumonia. *Bronchopneumonia* (bronchial pneumonia) (Fig. 62–1*B*) involves the terminal bronchioles and alveoli. *Interstitial (reticular) pneumonia* involves inflammatory responses within lung tissue surrounding the air spaces or vascular structures rather than the air passages themselves. In *alveolar,* or *acinar, pneumonia*, there is fluid accumulation in a lung's distal air spaces. *Necrotizing pneumonia* causes the death of a portion of lung tissue surrounded by viable tissue; x-ray examination may reveal cavity formation at the site of necrosis. Necrotic lung tissue, which does not heal, constitutes a permanent loss of functioning parenchyma.

Outcome Management

Medical Management

Treatment of pneumonia should include specific antibiotic therapy, respiratory support as needed, nutritional support, and fluid and electrolyte management. Initial drug therapy

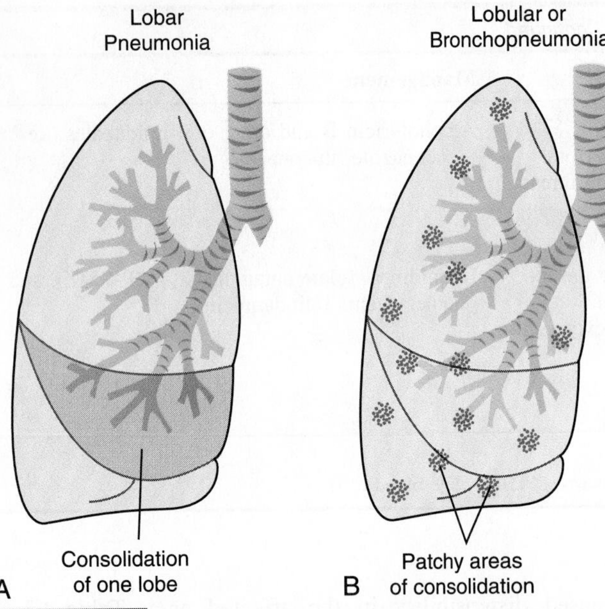

FIGURE 62–1 Two types of pneumonia. *A*, Lobar pneumonia with consolidation in one lobe of one lung. *B*, Lobular or bronchopneumonia with patchy consolidation throughout lobes of one or both lungs.

should consist of broad-spectrum antibiotics until the specific organism has been identified (see Table 62–1). Oxygen should be administered as ordered, and bronchodilator medications, postural drainage, chest physiotherapy, and tracheal suctioning may be used to maintain airway patency.

Nursing Management of the Medical Client

ASSESSMENT

The nursing history should explore the following areas with the client in whom pneumonia is suspected or confirmed:

- Contact with other clients experiencing similar manifestations (suggests viral or mycoplasmal pneumonia)
- Factors suggesting the presence of noninfectious diseases that produce manifestations similar to those of pneumonia (e.g., pulmonary embolism, allergic reaction to drugs or other substances, neoplasm)
- Presence of tuberculosis or contact with others who have active tuberculosis
- Presence and character of any chest pain
- Presence and character of cough and sputum production

Perform respiratory assessment every 4 hours, including determination of the rate and character of respirations, auscultation of breath sounds, and assessment of skin and nail beds to determine the severity of hypoxia. In addition to the physical examination, transcutaneous oxygen level analysis or ABG measurements may be used to evaluate the need for oxygen support.

DIAGNOSIS, PLANNING, INTERVENTIONS

Nursing diagnoses common to pneumonia are described here. Other applicable nursing diagnoses are: *Fluid Volume Deficit related to fever, diaphoresis, and mouth breathing; Altered Nutrition: Less Than Body Requirements related to dyspnea; Pain related to frequent coughing;* and *Altered Oral Mucous Membrane related to mouth breathing and frequent cough.*

Ineffective Airway Clearance. The inflammation and increased secretions seen with pneumonia make it difficult to maintain a patent airway. An appropriate nursing diagnosis is *Ineffective Airway Clearance related to excessive secretions and weak cough.*

Outcomes. The client will maintain effective airway clearance, as evidenced by keeping a patent airway and effectively clearing secretions.

Interventions. Take measures to promote airway patency, such as increasing fluid intake, teaching and encouraging effective coughing and deep-breathing techniques, and frequent turning. Clients with an altered level of consciousness should be turned at least every 2 hours and should be placed in side-lying positions, unless contraindicated, to prevent aspiration. Administer bronchodilating medications, if prescribed. If indicated, more aggressive measures to maintain airway patency may be required (e.g., chest physiotherapy, suctioning, artificial airway).

Ineffective Breathing Pattern. Many clients experience compensatory tachypnea because of an inability to meet metabolic demands. This occurs because affected alveoli cannot effectively exchange oxygen and carbon dioxide. Higher respiratory rates can also develop as a result of chest pain and increased body temperature. An appropriate nursing diagnosis is *Ineffective Breathing Pattern related to tachypnea.*

Outcomes. The client will have improved breathing patterns, as evidenced by (1) a respiratory rate within normal limits, (2) adequate chest expansion, (3) clear breath sounds, and (4) decreased dyspnea.

Intervention. Position the client for comfort and to facilitate breathing (e.g., raise the head of the bed 45 degrees). Teach the client how to splint the chest wall with a pillow for comfort during coughing and about the use of incentive spirometry. Administer prescribed cough suppressants and analgesics; be cautious, however, because narcotics may depress respirations more than desired. Routinely monitor respiratory rate and transcutaneous oxygen levels, auscultate the chest, and document findings. Monitor ABG values, and observe for manifestations of hypoxemia, hypercapnia, and acid-base imbalance.

Activity Intolerance. Depleted energy reserves, due to not eating during periods of dyspnea, and impairment of oxygen and carbon dioxide transport leave little oxygen to meet metabolic demands. An appropriate nursing diagnosis is *Activity Intolerance related to decreased oxygen levels for metabolic demands.*

Outcomes. The client will have improved activity tolerance, as evidenced by an ability to perform activities of daily living and a progressive increase in physical activity without excessive dyspnea and fatigue.

Interventions. Assess the client's baseline activity level and response to activity. Note how well the client tolerates activity by assessing for changes in respiratory and pulse rate, marked dyspnea, fatigue, pallor or cyanosis, and dysrhythmias. Schedule activity after treatments or medications. Use oxygen as needed. Gradually increase activity on the basis of tolerance. Balance activity with adequate rest periods.

Teach the client to avoid conditions that increase oxygen demand, such as smoking, temperature extremes, weight gain, and stress. Pursed-lip and diaphragmatic breathing, as well as techniques to lower energy use, should be reinforced. Activities that are tiring should be interspersed with rest.

Provide psychological support and a quiet environment to reduce anxiety and promote rest. Regulate nursing care and visitors as warranted by the client's condition.

Pneumonia is a very common reason for hospital admission. Many institutions provide care using Care Maps. (See the Case Management feature on pneumonia.)

EVALUATION

The level the client will probably attain is monitored every 2 to 3 days. Pneumonia should resolve quickly once the client is receiving antibiotics, provided there are no immune disorders. Older clients may require additional time to fully recover.

PREVENTION

Prevention is the best defense against the spread of pneumonia. When caring for hospitalized clients, (1) wash hands frequently, (2) use gloves appropriately, (3) encourage fluid intake, (4) turn clients every 2 hours, and (5) control clients' pain so they may breathe deeply and cough adequately. Encourage clients to use their incentive spirometer frequently. For clients who have difficulty swallowing or have nasogastric tubes, raise the head of the bed 45 degrees to decrease the risk of aspiration.

Self-Care

Clients with pneumonia who are ambulatory but have an ongoing health problem may require hospitalization. For clients with intact defense mechanisms and good general health, recuperation can often take place at home with rest and supportive treatment; the term "walking pneumonia" is sometimes used to describe this situation.

Chest physiotherapy may be performed for a pre-

CASE MANAGEMENT

Pneumonia

Community-acquired pneumonia may be treated on an outpatient basis, but this is also a very common inpatient diagnosis. Hospitalization should be considered for (1) clients over 65 years of age (2) clients with other risk factors (underlying chronic obstructive lung disease, heart failure, cardiorespiratory disease), (3) immunocompromised clients, or (4) clients with diabetes or cancer, since infection can pose a serious threat. Many facilities have developed clinical pathways for pneumonia.

Critical issues for case management are as follows:

- Obtaining culture specimens promptly before administration of antibiotics
- Administering the first dose of appropriate antibiotic as soon as possible
- Conversion from intravenous (IV) antibiotics to oral administration on day 2 or 3 (depending on decreased white blood cell count, afebrile status, and ability to take fluids).

Assess

- Has there been outpatient treatment with antibiotics that would void culture results?
- Does your baseline assessment give clues to atypical pneumonia or another condition causing concern (atrial fibrillation, pulmonary embolus)?
- Is this client at risk for aspiration, or are there other conditions that may require special monitoring (e.g., blood glucose level, arterial blood gas values)?
- Is the pneumonia bilateral?
- Has the client been admitted often for pneumonia or related problems?
- Does the client smoke, use oxygen, or receive respiratory therapy at home?

Advocate

Clients, especially older adults, may present in a weakened, debilitated state. Cognitive impairments may be worsened by the lack of oxygen, sometimes resulting in labeling of a client as "confused."

Monitor cognitive functioning as the pneumonia diminishes, and remember that a different environment and sensory impairments can also affect the client's behavior.

Encourage movement and exercise between rest periods to prevent worsening of the pneumonia. Administer antibiotics at prescribed intervals, watching for side effects, especially allergic reaction or gastrointestinal problems. Provide liquids, and monitor any swallowing difficulty. Monitor fluid balance (IV and oral fluids) closely, especially if the client is at risk for heart failure. Frequent, small meals may be better tolerated when breathing is difficult.

Talk with clients about how they are managing at home. What caregiver support is available? Will financial needs prevent the client from obtaining needed medications?

Prevent Readmission

- Teach clients about their condition, and encourage completion of an oral antibiotics course at home.
- Emphasize that antibiotics must never be "saved" or shared with other family members.
- Check the status of influenza and pneumonia immunizations; administer as appropriate.
- Teach avoidance of crowded areas as well as hand-washing and secretion disposal.
- Wean the client from oxygen as soon as feasible, and test saturation levels during rest and activity.
- Validate that the client knows how to use any equipment or devices (nebulizer, oxygen, metered dose inhaler) and that the client is familiar with cleaning and safety measures.
- Consider appropriate referrals for home care, pulmonary rehabilitation, and smoking cessation.
- Ensure that the client knows when to follow up with his or her physician any clinical manifestations that require immediate intervention.

Cheryl Noetscher, RN, MS, *Director of Case Management, Crouse Hospital and Community–General Hospital, Syracuse, New York*

scribed period. The client is monitored in a clinic setting until the chest x-ray clears and clinical manifestations abate. Encourage the client to plan for influenza immunization each winter. People who live with the client are also monitored for the onset of pneumonia.

LUNG ABSCESS

Lung abscess is a collection of pus within lung tissue. In its early stages, the abscess resembles a localized pneumonia. If a lung abscess remains unidentified and untreated, tissue necrosis may occur. Lung abscesses are becoming more rare as a result of improved treatment of pneumonia and effective preventive care of clients at high risk for aspiration. Today, abscesses are most often a result of anaerobic bacteria.

Single lung abscesses usually occur distal to a bronchial obstruction. They nearly always create putrid (foul) material. The bronchial obstruction may be due to:

- Aspirated foreign material (e.g., vomitus, mucus, teeth, blood, food, or tissue from upper airway surgery)
- Benign or malignant tumors

Multiple lung abscesses can follow pneumonia caused by necrotizing bacteria (such as *Staphylococcus aureus*, which creates necrotic lung tissue). Bacteria may also arise from septic emboli from infected foci, such as septic phlebitis. Immunosuppressed clients and clients who may aspirate foreign material are at high risk for lung abscesses.

Early assessment findings in a client with a lung abscess are the same as those in a client with bronchopneumonia (i.e., chills, fever, pleuritic pain, cough with abundant sputum). The body attempts to wall off the abscess with fibrous tissue. If the attempt is unsuccessful, the abscess ruptures into a bronchus, causing a cough that produces copious amounts of sputum. The sputum is purulent, foul-smelling, and foul-tasting. After bronchial rupture, hemoptysis often occurs. Chest auscultation reveals decreased breath sounds and dullness to percussion over the affected area. Crackles may be present when the abscess drains.

The diagnosis is commonly confirmed by chest radiography or computed tomography (CT) scan. Sputum cultures assist with identification of the organism.

Outcome Management

Antibiotics are prescribed on the basis of culture results. Although bronchoscopy was once believed to be essential in managing lung abscesses, it is now reserved for clients whose disease fails to improve or who may have malignancy. Surgery is seldom needed because of the success of antibiotic therapy.

Caring for a client with a lung abscess is similar to caring for a client experiencing pneumonia (e.g., promoting hydration, teaching effective cough techniques, and administering postural drainage). Lung abscesses produce copious volumes of sputum. Nursing intervention focuses on removing sputum from the lungs through postural drainage and expectoration. Note the color, quantity, quality, and smell of the expectorated material, including the presence of blood. Use gloves when handling articles contaminated with sputum.

GUIDE TO CLINICAL PATHWAY

Pneumonia

Treatment of the client with pneumonia begins immediately. The care map delineates care beginning 2 hours after admission because immediate treatment has been shown to reduce morbidity. The entire hospital stay is projected as 4 days.

The critical element in early care is to initiate antibiotics. Broad-spectrum intravenous antibiotics are prescribed and must be started within 2 hours of admission, after the drawing of blood for culture analysis, even if no sputum culture specimen has been collected. Then more specific antibiotics are prescribed according to the type of organism being eradicated. Once antibiotics are started, it is expected that the client's dyspnea will improve and that needs for oxygen to maintain oxygen saturation greater than 92% will decrease. Within the first 24 hours, the client is helped to sit in a chair or to walk three times a day. During periods of activity, assess for oxygen desaturation. Use the portable pulse oximetry instrument to continuously monitor oxygen saturation in response to activity.

On day 2 or 3, antibiotics are changed to oral routes if the client has improved clinically, is taking oral foods and fluids, and is afebrile. It is important to instruct the client to complete the entire course of antibiotics after discharge.

The CareMap shown is an excerpt of one that covers emergency department to 24 hours.

Helen Andrews, BSN, RN, *Care Manager, Alegent Health Bergan Mercy Medical Center, Omaha, Nebraska,* and **Linda R. Haddick, MSN, RN,** *Clinical Nurse Specialist, Alegent Health Home Care & Hospice, Omaha, Nebraska*

The sputum may have a foul taste. Provide frequent opportunities for the client to use mouthwash, brush the teeth, and floss. Because long-term antibiotic administration is usually necessary, observe oral mucous membranes for indications of *Candida albicans* overgrowth (i.e., white, cheesy patches). Encourage long-term dental care. Oral nystatin (which the client swishes around the mouth and swallows) may be ordered.

Antibiotic therapy for a lung abscess may be needed for 8 weeks or longer. Clients with lung abscesses must understand the importance of compliance with the medication schedule. The entire course of antibiotics must be taken. Teaching about medications should cover (1) the reasons for taking them, (2) specific directions, such as time of day, frequency, and when to take in relation to food, (3) potential side effects, and (4) what to do if side effects occur. Reassessment after the antibiotics course is completed (e.g., with culture of sputum or chest films) is essential to evaluate the effectiveness of treatment.

PULMONARY TUBERCULOSIS

Tuberculosis (TB) is one of the two most prominent mycobacterial diseases known to humankind. Currently, TB

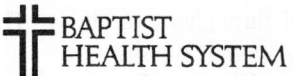

PNEUMONIA CAREMAP
ER 0-2 HRS. AND ER 2-24 HRS.

(Addressograph)

	ER 0-2 HOURS Date: ______	INITIAL Met	INITIAL Not Met	ER 2-24 HOURS Date: ______	INITIAL Met	INITIAL Not Met
General Safety:	Bed rails up x 2, airway precautions, call bell within reach, bed in low position.			Bed rails up x 2, airway precautions, call bell within reach, bed in low position.		
Activity	Up ad lib	___	___	Up ad lib in chair or ambulating at least TID.		
				Goal: Activity Plan established.	___	___
Dietary: Consult Date/Time Completed ___	Diet type ______			Diet type ______		
	Goal: Tolerates > 50% diet.	___	___	**Goal:** Tolerates > 50% diet. 1500-2000cc fluid intake / 24 hr.	___	___
Respiratory: Consult Date/Time Completed ___	SaO2 ______ On (RA) O2 per protocol.			O2 per protocol. Instruct in use of MDI with spacer if indicated.		
	Goal: O2 Sat. > or = 92% Reduced or no respiratory distress.	___	___	**Goal:** O2 Sat. > or = 92%	___	___
Rehab: Consult Date/Time Completed ___						
Discharge Planning: Consult Date/Time Completed ___	Anticipated disposition TCF ___ NH ___ HOME ___ REHAB ___ OTHER ___			Assess discharge needs Refer to Case Management if indicated		
	Goal: Discharge needs identifed	___	___	**Goal:** Discharge needs identified.	___	___
Nursing: Consult Date/Time Completed ___	Elevate head of bed. IV fluids ___ at ___ ml/hr or IV saline lock. **Initial dose of IV ABX within 2 hours.** **DO NOT hold ABX's awaiting collection of sputum specimen.** Instruct in appropriate method of sputum specimen collection. Notify MD if temp > 101.5 if respiration are > 30, SBP < 100.			I&O q 8 hr (D/C when IV fluids stopped D/C IV fluids if tolerating adequate po fluid intake. Elevate head of bed. IV fluids ___ at ___ ml/hr or IV saline lock. If on Vancomycin or Aminoglycoside refer to protocol. Notify MD of temp >101.5, if resp. > 30, SBP < 100. Instruct to cough/deep breathe q 2 hrs. while awake. Encourage increased oral fluid intake. Provide/review patient/family caremap		
	Goal: Initial ABX administered within 2 hrs of arrival. Able to clear upper airway. Able to collect sputum specimen. Sputum specimen acceptable.	___	___	**Goal:** Able to clear upper airway.	___	___
Tests:	CBC, with differential S7, EKG CXR, PA Lateral view, if not already done Blood cultures from 2 sites (prior to 1st dose of ABX) Sputum C&S and gram stain per protocoll					
	Goal: Blood cultures obtained prior to ABX.	___	___			
Other:	Avoid oral antacids if receiving po Quinolones (Consider H2 Blockers).			Pharmacist to review results of gram stain. Avoid oral antacids if receiving PO Quinolones (Consider H2 blocker)		

PNEUMONIA CAREMAP G-99-5043-2 PG REV. 5/4/99

kills more people than any other infectious disease in the world.[4] Before the development of anti-TB drugs in the late 1940s, TB was the leading cause of all deaths in the United States. Drug therapy, along with improvements in public health and general living standards, resulted in a marked decline in incidence over the next three decades. However, between 1985 and 1992, the number of reported TB cases increased by 20%. This increase was attributed to the emergence of the human immunodeficiency virus (HIV) epidemic, recent influxes of immigrants from developing Third World countries, and the deterioration of the nation's health care infrastructure. As a result of renewed efforts at prevention and detection, the number of TB cases is currently declining below the 1985 rate.[42]

There are two prevalent public health concerns in the

United States related to TB. First is the rise in cases of TB due to infection by multidrug-resistant organisms (MDR-TB), which are extremely difficult to treat. It is believed that resistance develops because people either stop taking their medication once they begin to feel well or are noncompliant with treatment as a result of other health problems, such as substance abuse.

The second public health concern is that clients with HIV infection are particularly susceptible to TB because *Mycobacterium tuberculosis*, the organism causing TB, is an extremely *opportunistic* pathogen. In some HIV-seropositive populations, the TB infection rate is 1000-fold higher than the annual rate in the United States. Clients with HIV are at greater risk for acquiring a new infection with rapid progression to active disease or for experiencing reinfection from dormant lesions.

Etiology and Risk Factors

TB is a communicable disease caused by *M. tuberculosis*, an aerobic, acid-fast bacillus (AFB). Tuberculosis is an airborne infection. In nearly all instances, tuberculosis infection is acquired by inhalation of a particle small enough (1 to 5 mm in diameter) to reach the alveolus. Droplets are emitted during coughing, talking, laughing, sneezing, or singing. Infected droplet nuclei may then be inhaled by a susceptible person (host). Before pulmonary infection can occur, the inhaled organisms must resist the lung's defense mechanisms and actually penetrate lung tissue.

Brief exposure to TB does not usually cause infection. People most commonly infected are those who have repeated close contact with an infected person whose disease is not yet diagnosed. Such people include anyone who has repeated contacts with medically underserved clients, low-income populations, foreign-born people, or residents of long-term care facilities or institutional settings. Other high-risk populations are intravenous drug users, homeless people, and people who are occupationally exposed to active TB (health care workers).

In countries that do not have public health programs and those in which TB commonly occurs in cattle, humans may experience bovine TB after drinking raw milk from infected cattle. This form of TB can be prevented by pasteurizing milk and maintaining tuberculin skin-testing programs for cattle.

Pathophysiology

Primary (First) Infection

The first time a client is infected with TB, the disease is said to be a *primary infection*. Primary TB infections are usually located in the apices of the lungs or near the pleurae of the lower lobes. Although a primary infection may be only microscopic (and hence may not appear on x-ray), the following sequence of events is typically observed.

A small area of bronchopneumonia develops in the lung tissue. Many of the infecting tubercle bacilli are phagocytosed (ingested) by wandering macrophages. However, before the development of hypersensitivity and immunity, many of the bacilli may survive within these blood cells and may be carried into regional bronchopulmonary (hilar) lymph nodes via the lymphatic system. The bacilli may even spread throughout the body. Thus, the infection, although small, spreads rapidly.

The primary infection site may or may not undergo a process of necrotic degeneration (*caseation*), which produces cavities filled with a cheese-like mass of tubercle bacilli, dead white blood cells (WBCs), and necrotic lung tissue. In time, this material liquifies, may drain into the tracheobronchial tree, and may be coughed up. The air-filled cavities remain and may be detected on an x-ray.

Most primary tubercles heal over a period of months by forming scars and then calcified lesions, also known as Ghon tubercles. These lesions may contain living bacilli that can be reactivated, even after many years, and cause secondary infection.

Primary TB infections cause the body to develop an allergic reaction to tubercle bacilli or their proteins. This cell-mediated immune response appears in the form of sensitized T cells and is detectable as a positive reaction to a tuberculin skin test. The development of this tuberculin sensitivity occurs in all body cells 2 to 6 weeks after the primary infection. It is maintained as long as living bacilli remain in the body. This acquired immunity usually inhibits further growth of the bacilli and the development of active infection.

The reason active TB disease develops in some clients (instead of being controlled by the acquired immune response and thereby remaining dormant) is poorly understood. However, factors that seem to play a role in the progression from a dormant TB infection to active disease are (1) advanced age, (2) HIV infection, (3) immunosuppression, (4) prolonged corticosteroid therapy, (5) malabsorption syndromes, (6) low body weight (10% or more below ideal weight), (7) substance abuse, (8) presence of other diseases (e.g., diabetes mellitus, end-stage renal disease, or malignancy), and (9) genetic predisposition.

Secondary Infection

In addition to progressive primary disease, reinfection may also lead to a clinical form of active TB, or secondary infection. Primary sites of infection containing TB bacilli may remain latent for years and then may be reactivated if the client's resistance is lowered. Because reinfection is possible and because dormant lesions may be reactivated, it is extremely important for clients who have had a TB infection to be reassessed periodically for new evidence of active disease.

Clinical Manifestations

The detection and diagnosis of TB are achieved through subjective assessment findings and objective test results. The diagnosis can be difficult because TB mimics many other diseases and may occur concurrently with other pulmonary diseases. Nurses and other health care providers should maintain a high index of suspicion for TB in high-risk clients.

The history includes assessing the probability of recent or past exposure to TB as well as the client's occupation, other usual activities, and travel to or residence in countries with a high incidence of TB. A history of exposure to TB is certainly important, but most clients are unaware of exposure. It is advisable to determine whether the client has been previously tested for TB and to obtain the results of that testing.

Figure 62–2 shows the logical progression of the diagnosis and management of TB. Typical findings in pulmonary TB are (1) nonproductive or productive cough, (2) fatigue, (3) anorexia (loss of appetite) and weight loss, (4) low-grade fever, (5) chills and sweats (often at night), (6) dyspnea, (7) hemoptysis, (8) chest pain that may be pleuritic or dull, and (9) chest tightness. Crackles may be present on auscultation.

Primary TB infections may remain unrecognized because they are relatively asymptomatic. Calcified lesions on chest x-ray and a positive skin test reaction are frequently the only indications that a primary TB infection has occurred. Most clients harbor tubercle bacilli for life and never experience active disease because their body defenses are adequate to arrest primary infection. The tubercles heal through fibrosis and calcification. However, infected people face a 10% risk that the primary infection will progress to active disease sometime in their lives. In this situation, the primary complex sites progress and worsen, possibly causing cavitation and the spread of active infection, and the client becomes clinically ill.

Diagnostic Findings

TUBERCULIN SKIN TESTING

Tuberculin skin testing, typically the Mantoux test, is performed on a routine basis in high-risk groups when active TB is suspected. Mantoux testing uses purified protein derivative (PPD) tuberculin to identify TB infection. A small amount of the derivative is administered intradermally to form a wheal in the lower left forearm. The wheal must be examined ("read") in 48 to 72 hours by a trained professional. The presence of induration, not erythema, indicates a positive test result as follows[19]:

- More than 5 mm of induration is considered a positive result for clients with known or suspected HIV infection, intravenous drug users, people in close contact with a known case of TB, and the client with a chest x-ray suggestive of previous TB.
- More than 10 mm of induration is considered positive for clients in all other high-risk groups.
- 15 mm or more of induration is considered positive for clients in low-risk groups.

False-positive reactions to tuberculin skin testing can occur in clients who have other mycobacterial infections or who have received the bacille Calmette-Guérin (BCG) vaccination. False-negative reactions are also possible, especially in people who are immunosuppressed or anergic (impaired ability to react to antigens). For these clients, and for anyone who has a positive skin test reaction, the AFB sputum smear examination and chest x-ray are used to identify active disease. It is critical to initiate respiratory isolation of such clients until AFB sputum results are known.

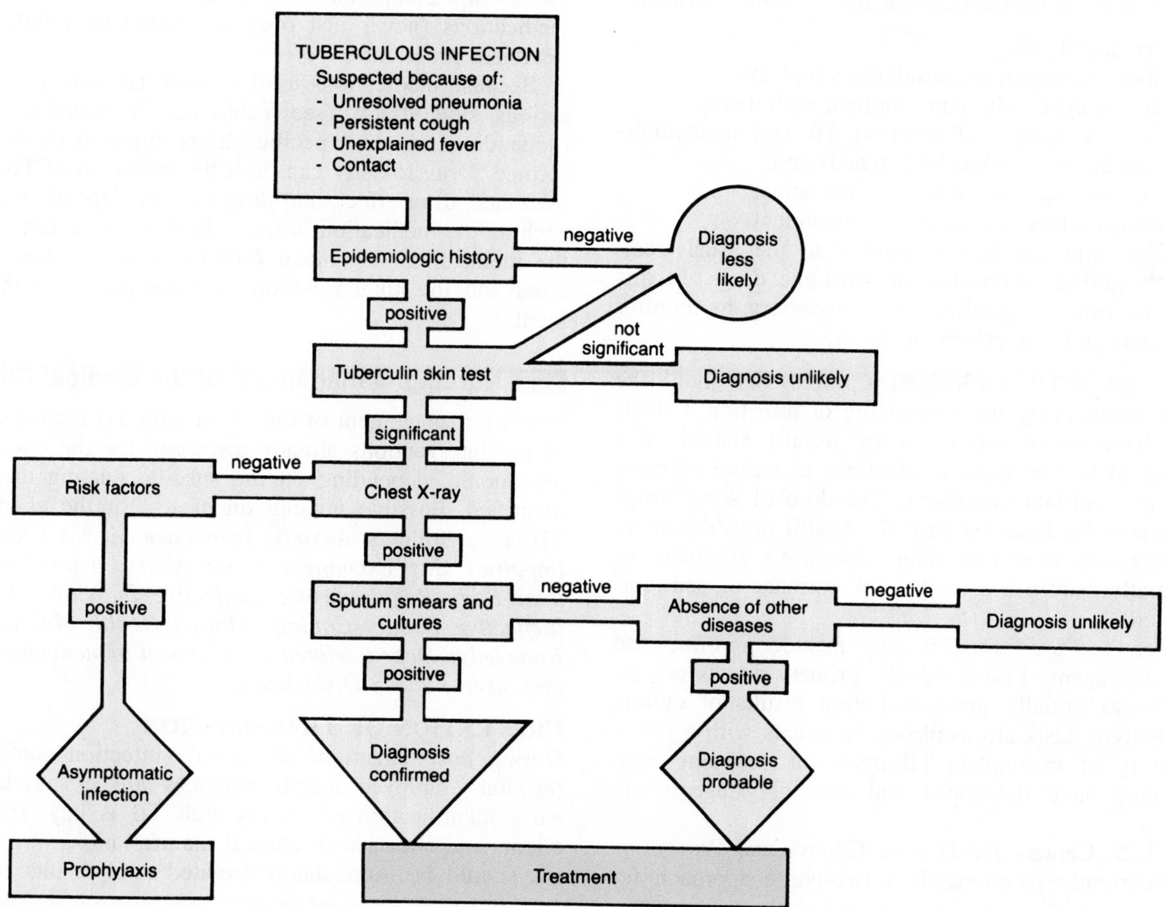

FIGURE 62–2 Algorithm for diagnosis and management of tuberculosis: a logical progression. (Courtesy of the American Lung Association, The Christmas Seal People.)

The term *tuberculin converter* refers to a client who does not show radiologic or bacteriologic evidence of pulmonary TB but whose tuberculin skin test "converts" from a known negative reaction to a known positive reaction. Keep in mind that the absence of a positive (reactive) tuberculin test result does not always mean that TB is absent.

ACID-FAST BACILLUS SMEAR AND CULTURE

A more definitive diagnosis of TB is made from the AFB smear and culture. Three different sputum specimens should be collected on three consecutive mornings. Sputum AFB smears are not extremely sensitive, but the positive result of a sputum AFB smear confirms active disease. A more reliable indicator is a positive culture for *M. tuberculosis*, which does confirm active TB; however, final culture results may not be available for 2 to 12 weeks. Although newer detection tests can generate faster results and show clinical promise, the prevalence of MDR-TB still mandates the use of traditional culture methods for diagnosis.

Outcome Management

Medical Management

Most people with newly diagnosed active TB are not hospitalized. If pulmonary TB is diagnosed in the hospitalized client, the client may be kept in the hospital until therapeutic drug levels are established. Some clients with active TB may be hospitalized for the following reasons:

- They are acutely ill.
- Their living situation is considered a high risk.
- They are thought to be noncompliant with therapy.
- They have a history of previous TB and noncompliance, and the disease has been reactivated.
- Concomitant diseases are present and acute.
- Improvement does not occur after treatment.
- The organisms are highly resistant to the usual treatment, requiring second-line or third-line drugs. In this situation, brief hospitalization is necessary to monitor the effects and side effects of the drugs.

Treatment of TB is a long-term process that should be initiated immediately upon suspicion of infection. Clients with a diagnosis of active TB are usually started on a minimum of two or three medications to ensure elimination of the resistant organisms. The dose of some drugs may initially be large because the bacilli are difficult to kill. Treatment continues long enough to eliminate or substantially reduce the number of dormant or semidormant bacilli.

Medications used for TB may include *first-line* and *second-line* agents (Table 62–2). Primary agents are almost always initially prescribed until results of culture and sensitivity tests are available. In clients with a previous history of incomplete TB treatment, resistant organisms may have developed and secondary agents are used.

The U.S. Centers for Disease Control and Prevention (CDC) currently recommends a two-phase approach for treatment, consisting of (1) an *intensive* phase using two or three drugs, aimed at destroying large numbers of rapidly multiplying organisms and (2) a *maintenance* phase, usually using two drugs, directed at eliminating most remaining bacilli.

The recommended basic treatment regimen for previously untreated clients is 2 months of daily doses of isoniazid and rifampin, plus one or two other drugs, depending on type of organism. This treatment is followed with 4 months of isoniazid and rifampin. Ethambutol or streptomycin may also be used initially until culture and sensitivity test results are obtained and the correct medications are identified. The length of time a client remains infectious varies. Sputum cultures and clinical responses (absence of fever and dyspnea, reduction in cough) are used to evaluate the effectiveness of the therapy.

If compliance with daily dosing is a problem, some TB protocols call for administration of medications two or three times a week rather than daily. Additionally, clients may be assigned to receive *directly observed therapy* (DOT). Such a program is administered in a clinic or physician's office to ensure that clients ingest each dose of medication. In some cities, a noncompliant client may be confined to a hospital or other institution for treatment, according to that city's law. Completion of treatment is critical because incomplete treatment leads to reactivation of TB and the development of drug-resistant strains of TB.

If the medication regimen does not seem effective (e.g., worsening manifestations, continued presence of AFB in sputum, increasing infiltrates or cavity formation on x-ray), the treatment program needs reevaluation, and the client's compliance should be assessed. At least two medications (never just one) are added to a failing TB treatment program.

Because medications used to treat TB have potentially serious side effects (see Table 62–2), baseline studies (depending on the specific drugs prescribed) are performed. Drug toxicity can limit the treatment of TB. Drug tolerance, drug effect, and drug toxicity depend on factors such as the medication dosage, the time since last dosage, the medication's chemical formula, and the client's age, renal and intestinal function, and compliance with treatment.

Nursing Management of the Medical Client

Nursing management of the client with TB includes many of the interventions already discussed for the client with pneumonia, depending on the specific nursing diagnoses identified. Possible nursing diagnoses for the client with TB are as follows: *Anxiety; Ineffective Airway Clearance; Impaired Gas Exchange; Pain; Altered Nutrition: Less than Body Requirements; Ineffective Individual Coping; Ineffective Family Coping; Altered Health Maintenance; Knowledge Deficit related to treatment or noncompliance;* and *Sleep Pattern Disturbance.*

PREVENTION OF TRANSMISSION

During hospitalization, appropriate infection control and hospital employee health practices are essential. First, early identification of clients with TB is key. High-risk clients and clients with clinical manifestations of pneumonia should be immediately isolated until results of AFB smears and cultures are obtained.

Private respiratory isolation rooms should be available. These rooms should be maintained at negative pressure

TABLE 62–2 NURSING IMPLICATIONS FOR MEDICATIONS USED TO TREAT TUBERCULOSIS

Medication and Dosage	Actions	Methods to Evaluate Therapeutic Outcomes	Methods to Evaluate Adverse Outcomes	Nursing Considerations
FIRST-LINE AGENTS				
Isoniazid (INH) 5 mg/kg/day up to 300 mg PO	Unknown; may cause inhibition of myocolic acid synthesis, resulting in disruption of the bacterial cell wall	Decrease of symptoms (cough, night sweats, fever) Fewer bacilli on sputum smear	Monitor hepatic enzymes during the first 3 months of treatment and in clients who are older than 35 years or are alcohol abusers Perform initial eye examination and repeat if visual problems occur	Can cause fatigue, weakness, anorexia, malaise Must be taken on an empty stomach When administered with phenytoin, may lead to phenytoin toxicity
Rifampin (Rifadin) 10 mg/kg/day up to 600 mg PO	Inhibits bacterial RNA synthesis	Decrease of symptoms (cough, night sweats, fever) Fewer bacilli on sputum smear	Use of alcohol or INH increases risk of hepatotoxicity Periodic monitoring of hepatic enzymes required	Should be taken on empty stomach; however, may be taken with meals if severe GI symptoms occur Reduces levels of many drugs; methadone, theophylline, oral contraceptives, oral antidiabetics, oral anticoagulants, protease inhibitors, non-nucleoside reverse transcriptase inhibitors
Rifapentine (Priftin) 600 mg twice weekly PO	Bactericidal activity against intracellular and extracellular *Mycobacterium tuberculosis*	Decrease of symptoms (cough, night sweats, fever) Fewer bacilli on sputum smear	Increases the metabolism of indinavir sulfate (Crixivan), protease inhibitor used in clients with AIDS Monitor hepatic and serum uric acid levels monthly	May turn body secretions red-orange Must be taken with food, as nausea, vomiting, and GI upset are possible Reduces effects of warfarin, phenytoin, sildenafil, oral antiarrhythmics, oral contraceptives, oral antidiabetic agents
SECOND-LINE AGENTS				
Capreomycin or kanamycin 15–30 mg/kg up to 1 g IM	Polypeptide antibiotic	Decrease of symptoms (cough, night sweats, fever) Fewer bacilli on sputum smear	Observe for ototoxicity by obtaining baseline audiology parameters and nephrotoxicity by obtaining baseline renal function measurements Monitor both periodically	Tell client to report dizziness and hearing loss Encourage adequate hydration
Ethionamide (Trecator-SC) 15–20 mg/kg up to 1 g PO	Inhibits peptide synthesis	Decrease of symptoms (cough, night sweats, fever) Fewer bacilli on sputum smear	Observe for hepatotoxicity by obtaining baseline liver function measurements Transient increase in results may occur	Inform client of potential for distorted sense of smell and metallic taste Instruct client to report signs of hypothyroidism

AIDS, acquired immunodeficiency syndrome; GI, gastrointestinal; IM, intramuscularly; PO, by mouth; RNA, ribonucleic acid.

relative to the hallway; negative pressure keeps room air from flowing out into the hallway when the door is opened, thereby avoiding the spread of infectious particles outside the room. Negative-pressure ventilation sends room air directly to the outside, with at least six air exchanges per hour. Additional equipment, such as ultraviolet lamps (proven to kill mycobacteria) and high-efficiency particulate air (HEPA) filters, may also be used.

Personal protective equipment, called *particulate respirators*, is required for all health care workers entering a TB isolation room. When fitted properly, these respirators filter droplet nuclei; the fit of a particulate respirator should be reassessed if there is a change in the wearer's facial shape.

Monitoring health care workers' TB status is essential. Skin testing should be performed yearly in all health care workers who may be exposed to TB. Semi-annual testing should be completed in high-risk areas or where high rates of TB skin test conversion are occurring.

When a client is determined to have TB, public health officials (often nurses) talk with the client and develop a contact list. Everyone with whom the client has had contact is then assessed with a tuberculin skin test and chest x-ray to check for TB infection.

Preventive Therapy

Between 10 and 15 million people in the United States have dormant or asymptomatic TB. Chemoprophylaxis may help many of them avoid active TB and may also prevent initial infection in people recently exposed. Isoniazid preventive therapy (IPT) consists of 300 mg of the drug daily for 6 to 12 months. IPT stops the growth of the bacilli, thus preventing active pulmonary or extrapulmonary TB. IPT is recommended for clients who:

- Are newly infected (have converted tuberculin skin test results but no other indication of active disease)
- Live or closely associate with others who have active TB
- Have significant tuberculin skin test reactions and abnormal chest x-ray findings compatible with those of inactive TB
- Have positive tuberculin skin tests and conditions (e.g., steroid therapy, diabetes mellitus, acquired immunodeficiency syndrome [AIDS]) that place them at increased risk for TB
- Are younger than 35 years of age and have significant tuberculin skin test reactions, even though they may have a normal chest x-ray and no other risk factors

Self-Care

TB treatment is a long process. Nurses in clinics and public health facilities are often responsible for follow-up assessment and monitoring, including (1) determining medication compliance, (2) understanding the pharmacologic actions of medications, (3) monitoring unwanted side effects, (4) collecting follow-up sputum specimens, (5) obtaining serial chest x-rays, and (6) observing for reversal or worsening of initial assessment findings, all of which are part of the ongoing follow-up. It is essential that clients with TB, and their significant others, receive the information summarized in the Client Education Guide for Tuberculosis. Providing complete information and ongoing support helps clients understand the long-term recovery process. The more information clients have and the more personal control they feel they have, the more likely they are to comply with treatment.

Extrapulmonary Tuberculosis

Extrapulmonary tuberculosis (XPTB) is TB that occurs anywhere outside the lungs. Pulmonary TB is the most common form of the disease, but after initial invasion, tubercle bacilli can spread throughout the body via the blood and lymph. *M. tuberculosis* thrives in oxygen-rich areas. Highly aerobic sites, such as the renal cortex, bone growth plates, and meninges, are where XPTB most commonly grows. It may also occur in the genitourinary tract, lymph nodes, pleurae, pericardium, abdomen, and endocrine glands.

Widespread dissemination throughout the body *(miliary tuberculosis)* involves the lungs and many other organs. It is more common in clients who are HIV-seropositive or are 50 years or older. Miliary TB may develop from delayed or late dissemination after immune system compromise in older people who were infected with TB many years earlier.

Despite the severity of the disease, XPTB is often difficult to detect. Assessment findings are frequently nondistinct. Weight loss, fatigue, malaise, fever, and night sweats may or may not be present. The only physical finding that is specific for disseminated TB is a granuloma in the choroid of the retina. Clinical manifestations may precede changes in the chest x-ray.

CLIENT EDUCATION GUIDE

Tuberculosis

- Tuberculosis (TB) is infectious, but it may be cured or arrested if you take your medication as prescribed.
- TB is transmitted by droplet infection and is not carried on articles such as clothing, books, or eating utensils. You do not need to dispose of any possessions.
- Cover your nose and mouth when coughing, laughing, or sneezing.
- Wash your hands very carefully after any contact with body substances, masks, or soiled tissues. Sputum is highly contaminated. Cough into paper tissues, and dispose of them properly.
- Wear a mask in appropriate situations as advised. Make sure the mask is tight-fitting, and change it frequently.
- Activities are usually not restricted for more than 2 to 4 weeks after medication is begun, and you should not be isolated from others as long as you are compliant with the medication therapy.
- Treatment may be needed for a long time. Take your medication exactly as prescribed, and report all side effects to your physician. Do not stop the medication for any reason without the physician's supervision. Keep an adequate supply of medication available at all times to avoid running out. Compliance with treatment is essential.
- Because TB drugs can cause serious side effects, periodic blood work will be required.

Outcome Management

The diagnosis and treatment of XPTB proceed similarly to those of pulmonary TB. However, the treatment period may be longer, and more medications may be used. Treatment depends on the extent, severity, course, and complications of the disease.

NONTUBERCULOUS MYCOBACTERIAL INFECTION

Pathophysiology

Nontuberculous mycobacteria (NTM), also known as MOTT (mycobacteria other than tubercle [bacilli]), are responsible for growing numbers of mycobacterial infections. Although NTM infection is still relatively uncommon, the following changes in disease patterns have appeared: (1) more cases, (2) wider geographical distribution, and (3) new groups of vulnerable hosts, most notably, clients with HIV infection.

NTM are widely distributed in nature (i.e., in food, standing fresh water, salt water, animal bedding, soil, animals, and birds), and most clients acquire their infections from environmental sources rather than from other diseased clients. Infection is common in the southeastern part of the United States and more prevalent in rural areas.

Etiology

The most commonly occurring NTM diseases are caused by *Mycobacterium avium* complex, *Mycobacterium kansasii*, and *Mycobacterium fortuitum*. The primary site of NTM disease is the lungs, although extrapulmonary sites (e.g., liver, spleen, lymph nodes, skin, joints) may occur. Disseminated disease with multiple organ involvement is also possible, most commonly in immunosuppressed clients.

Clinical Manifestations

Pulmonary NTM disease is very similar to TB, although the clinical manifestations may be less severe. Clinical manifestations of the disease include (1) fever, (2) anorexia, (3) night sweats, (4) diarrhea, (5) abdominal pain, and (6) weight loss. Clients with pre-existing bronchopulmonary disease (e.g., bronchiectasis, chronic obstructive pulmonary disease [COPD], or healed pulmonary TB) are at highest risk of pulmonary involvement.

Diagnosis of NTM disease is often difficult because of the widespread distribution of the organisms in the environment. Definitive diagnosis of disease is possible only if NTM are isolated from specimens collected from normally sterile sites (e.g., blood, cerebrospinal fluid, bone marrow, lymph nodes) or through biopsy. However, NTM disease is strongly suspected when (1) a client presents with a clinical syndrome that is compatible with NTM, (2) no other pathogens can be identified, and (3) repeated sputum cultures reveal large numbers of NTM.

Outcome Management

The same medications used to treat TB are prescribed for NTM disease. However, NTM are considerably more resistant to drugs than *M. tuberculosis*. Consequently, combined drug regimens and longer treatment periods are necessary. Treatment typically consists of three to six different medications and lasts for a minimum of 18 to 24 months, continuing until there are no AFB in the sputum specimens collected consecutively for a period of 1 year. As a result, adherence to medical therapy is critical. Clients are often instructed that chemotherapy will be continued for life.[14]

Unsuccessful treatment may result in further lung damage and general debilitation. Regular, daily medication is essential. The more clients understand about the condition and its management, the more likely they will be to complete the full course of medication.

Other aspects of the nursing management of NTM disease are the same as for pulmonary TB (see preceding discussion). Because these diseases are not believed to be transmitted from person to person, however, isolation and measures to control infection, other than good hygiene, are not necessary.

FUNGAL PULMONARY INFECTIONS

Most fungi that are pathogenic to humans limit their activities to the skin. However, the spores of some fungi become airborne and can be inhaled into the respiratory tract, causing pulmonary diseases that, in their chronic forms, produce granulomatous conditions similar to TB. The most common of these are coccidioidomycosis and histoplasmosis. Each has a specific geographical distribution and occurs in people living or traveling in the regions where these fungi are found. Person-to-person transmission is virtually unknown. Opportunistic fungal infections occur in clients with impaired immunity including those who require long-term high dose immunosuppressant therapy, have hematologic malignancies, or have undiagnosed HIV. In fact, histoplasmosis is often a sentinel infection, the first hint that a client is HIV infected.[16]

Coccidioidomycosis is found in the Western Hemisphere, primarily in the San Joaquin Valley of California, Utah, Nevada, New Mexico, Arizona, western Texas, and northern Mexico. The disease is most likely to develop in people engaging in desert recreational activities or working in construction or other occupations that involve digging (e.g., archaeology). The disease is mild and self-limiting in 60% of those affected. Such clients either are asymptomatic or have only mild upper respiratory assessment findings. The remaining 40% experience a syndrome similar to influenza, with cough, fever, pleuritic chest pain, myalgias, and arthralgias. *Erythema multiforme*, a flat, red rash that erupts with dark red papules, occurs in some people.

Etiology

The causative organism of *histoplasmosis*, the fungus *Histoplasma capsulatum*, is endemic to the central and eastern portions of North America, most notably the Ohio River, Missouri River, and Mississippi River valleys. It is also found in South and Central America, India, and Cyprus. This fungus lives in moist soil of appropriate chemical composition, in mushroom cellars, on the floors of chicken houses and bat caves, and in bird droppings, especially those from starlings and blackbirds.

Clinical Manifestations

As with coccidioidomycosis, *H. capsulatum* infections are usually asymptomatic or mild. Clinical manifestations include fever, fatigue, cough, dyspnea, and weight loss of 1 to 2 months in duration.

The diagnosis of fungal pulmonary diseases is usually based on history and clinical assessment findings. Skin testing is also used for coccidioidomycosis and can indicate exposure but not active infection. Chest x-rays may show hilar adenopathy (lymph gland enlargement), small areas of infiltrates, or manifestations of pneumonia. Sometimes, cavities and calcified nodules may form, usually remaining in the lungs as permanent indicators of previous infection.

A few clients may demonstrate disseminated or chronic forms of pulmonary fungal disease. When disseminated disease occurs, central nervous system, liver, spleen, gastrointestinal tract, or musculoskeletal involvement may be present. Chronic disease may result in progressive changes similar to those seen with TB. Emphysema-like pulmonary structural changes may also occur.

Outcome Management

Mild, primary forms of fungal pulmonary disease usually do not require treatment. Progressive, disseminated, or chronic forms are usually treated with intravenous amphotericin B until the client is asymptomatic for 7 to 10 days. This fungicidal antibiotic is quite toxic, and acute reactions (e.g., chills, fever, vomiting, headache, decreased renal function) may occur during its infusion. Antiemetics, antihistamines, antipyretics, or hydrocortisone may be prescribed as premedications. In order to reduce the common problem of thrombophlebitis at the intravenous site, a small amount of heparin may be added to the infusion. Ketoconazole, a less toxic oral medication, may also be used. If the disorder is not responsive to drug therapy, surgical removal of affected areas (e.g., lung cavities) may be necessary.

Nursing management in relation to fungal pulmonary infection consists of (1) providing preventive education to minimize exposure of clients to infectious fungi (i.e., learning to avoid high-risk situations and to recognize early indications of infection) and (2) appropriate support and education for infected clients and their significant others, along with symptomatic management of the disease. Education involves teaching about not only the disease and intervention measures but also reportable indications of complications.

In addition to the pathogenic fungi, common fungal spores may cause serious, potentially fatal pulmonary disease in immunocompromised people. These fungi include *Aspergillus, Blastomyces dermatitidis, Candida,* and *Cryptococcus neoformans.* These infections are also treated with amphotericin B.

CYSTIC FIBROSIS

Cystic fibrosis is a congenital restrictive lung disorder in which the secretions of the exocrine (mucus-producing) glands are abnormal. This disorder affects the sweat glands, respiratory system, digestive tract (particularly the pancreas), and reproductive tract. Cystic fibrosis is the most common inherited genetic disease in the Caucasian population, affecting approximately 1 in 2000 newborns in the United States.

Previously, this condition was considered a "pediatric problem" because it was fatal in childhood. However, advances in early diagnosis and treatment, including antibiotics, chest physiotherapy, and nutrition programs, have extended the median life expectancy into the late 20s or early 30s, with maximum survival documented as high as the seventh decade of life.[37]

Pathophysiology

The mucus-producing glands of the pancreas and lungs hypertrophy and produce excessive secretions that are thick mucoproteins. Tenacious mucus results from failure of the chloride channels to function. Decreased flow of ions and water results in viscid mucus that causes obstruction of the airway. The thick mucus also decreases action of the cilia, leading to stasis of mucus and a medium for infection.

The thick mucus plugs the glands and ducts of the pancreatic acini, intestinal glands, intrahepatic bile ducts, and the gallbladder, causing dilation and fibrosis. These changes result in decreased production of pancreatic enzymes needed for digestion of carbohydrates, fats, and proteins.

Sweat glands, salivary glands, and lacrimal glands are also affected, leading to high concentrations of sodium and chloride in these secretions.

Clinical Manifestations

Pulmonary involvement is the most common and severe manifestation of cystic fibrosis. More than 90% of clients with cystic fibrosis die of severe pulmonary disease. The disease process causes tracheobronchial secretions to become thick and viscous, leading to (1) interference with normal ciliary action, (2) plugging of airways, and (3) creation of a reservoir for bacterial growth and infection. Bronchiectasis may also develop, compounding the infection risk.

Outcome Management

The goals of therapy for cystic fibrosis are to ensure a reasonable quality of life for as long as possible and to prevent or slow the decline in pulmonary functioning. They are achieved by removing secretions, improving aeration, and administering antibiotic agents. Effective clearing of tracheobronchial secretions is promoted by (1) ensuring adequate hydration, (2) administering prescribed mucolytic aerosols, and (3) teaching and supervising effective coughing techniques, use of positive expiratory pressure devices, postural drainage, and chest vibration and percussion. Auscultate the chest before and after therapy, taking note of the quality of lung sounds and the effectiveness of therapy.

Ensure adequate aeration by following the techniques for maintaining clear airways, administering oxygen if hypoxemia is present, maintaining correct body position to facilitate breathing (i.e., sitting up), and performing exercise to improve pulmonary function. Assess the client for manifestations of hypercapnia and other indications of respiratory failure.

Antibiotic therapy has played an important role in extending the life expectancy of clients with cystic fibrosis. Oral antibiotics are often given prophylactically on a routine basis. Intravenous antibiotics are essential during acute infections. Inhaled antibiotics are also being used with more regularity. The choice of antibiotic should be determined by results of sputum culture and sensitivity testing. Infections are most commonly caused by *Pseudomonas aeruginosa,* followed by *S. aureus*. Sputum should be assessed for color, quality, and quantity. All respiratory equipment should be thoroughly cleaned on a routine basis to prevent reinfection from contaminated equipment.

Persistent pulmonary infection with *Pseudomonas* organisms is common in the end stages of cystic fibrosis. Continuous treatment with large doses of intravenous antibiotics is usually indicated. Moderate to severe hemoptysis can occur if the infection causes erosion of pulmonary blood vessels. Blood replacement and temporary cessation of postural drainage may be required.

New treatments for cystic fibrosis have shown moderate success and are still being studied for long-term effects, including:

- Use of synthetically produced DNase, an enzyme that breaks down the deoxyribonucleic acid (DNA) released from neutrophils and causes the "stickiness" of mucus
- Administration of anti-inflammatory drugs (corticosteroids and nonsteroidal anti-inflammatory drugs [NSAIDs]) to decrease the inflammatory response in the respiratory tract epithelium
- Augmentation of the immune defense with supplemental gamma-globulin
- Use of drugs that alter ion movement and thin secretions

Gene therapy is also being evaluated. Gene transfer is possible, but positive results are transient in duration.[37]

Treatment of end-stage disease is primarily concerned with the management of severe complications. Obstruction of the airways leads to a state of hyperinflation. In time, restrictive lung disease is superimposed on the obstructive disease. Pneumothorax (air in the chest cavity) develops in 20% of all adult clients, requiring lung reinflation with chest tubes.

Over time, pulmonary obstruction leads to chronic hypoxemia, hypercapnia, and acidosis. Pulmonary hypertension and, eventually, cor pulmonale may result. Treatment consists of digitalis, diuretics, and oxygen therapy. Clients with severely reduced lung function (forced expiratory volume in 1 second [FEV_1] less than 30% of predicted) whose disease no longer responds to maximal therapy and who are experiencing a decline in quality of life may be candidates for bilateral lung transplantation.

Attention to psychosocial concerns is a nursing priority throughout the course of the disease. In the adult client with cystic fibrosis, psychosocial concerns center on three major areas:

- Disease management (e.g., treatment compliance, sleep disturbance, hemoptysis, nutrition, and hospitalizations)
- Growth and development (e.g., daily activities, work, and sex and reproduction)
- Family relations (e.g., substance abuse, depression, anxiety, and marital problems)

Nursing intervention involves helping clients cope with these problem areas as well as providing emotional support to both clients and their families.

INTERSTITIAL LUNG DISEASE

Interstitial lung diseases (ILDs) comprise a group of diffuse, inflammatory lower respiratory tract disorders. The term *interstitial* is used to indicate that the interstitium of the alveolar walls is thickened and usually fibrotic. The alveolar walls thicken as a result of the accumulation of inflammatory cells. The thickened alveolus becomes nonfunctional.

Etiology

The cause of ILD is not clearly defined. It most commonly develops from idiopathic pulmonary fibrosis, sarcoidosis, and collagen-vascular disorders. ILD can also result from the inhalation of inorganic dust, such as crystalline silica, asbestos, and coal dust, or of organic dust from organisms encountered in farming, use of air conditioning, and animal husbandry. Other possible causes are radiation damage and infectious agents.

Clinical Manifestations

Manifestations of ILD are insidious and nonspecific, such as fatigue, dyspnea, and nonproductive cough. Because the clinical manifestations are nonspecific, ILD may remain undiagnosed for years. The client's history plays a major part in diagnosis because it is important to determine the agents to which the client has been exposed. Clients report progressive dyspnea and often have dyspnea at rest. Physical examination may reveal reduced chest expansion, reflected as a decrease in total lung capacity (TLC). Inspiratory and expiratory crackles are frequently heard. The crackles have a characteristic sound, like the sound of hook-and-loop tape (Velcro) being pulled apart. Clubbing of the finger tips may be present.

Diagnostic assessment includes gallium ventilation-perfusion scans. These scans usually reveal impaired perfusion in the lower lobes and multiple areas of impaired ventilation. The ventilation-perfusion mismatch results in hypoxemia and carbon dioxide retention. Bronchoscopy and biopsy may also be used to confirm ILD.

Outcome Management

Management of a client with ILD is based on the level of respiratory impairment. Inflammation is controlled with corticosteroids. Explain to the client that corticosteroids reduce further impairment but previously injured alveolar-capillary units are permanently damaged. Clients often show subjective improvement while taking steroids, dosage of which can eventually be tapered and stopped. If the offending agent is known, the initial treatment is to remove the client from exposure to the agent. As the disorder progresses, clients are usually treated with inhaled corticosteroids and bronchodilators to help mobilize secretions and oxygen during periods of exercise.

Nursing management is the same as that for clients with restrictive lung disorders.

SARCOIDOSIS

Sarcoidosis is an inflammatory condition that affects many body systems. The disease is characterized by the formation of widespread granulomatous lesions. In addition to lung involvement, which occurs in more than 90% of cases, clients may present with clinical manifestations involving the peripheral lymphatic system, skin, liver, eyes, spleen, bones, salivary glands, joints, nervous system, and heart.

The onset of sarcoidosis is generally between ages 20 and 40 years. The disorder is approximately 14 times more common in African Americans than in Caucasians. Although the male-to-female ratio is about even in the non–African American population, African American women have sarcoidosis twice as frequently as African American men.

Etiology

The cause of sarcoidosis remains unknown, but the disease itself is becoming more fully understood. It is suggested that a triggering agent, which may be genetic, infectious, immunologic, or toxic, stimulates enhanced cell-mediated immune processes at the site of involvement. A series of interactions between T lymphocytes and monocytes-macrophages leads to the formation of *noncaseating* (i.e., having no cheesy necrotic degeneration) granulomas, which are characteristic of the disease. Granuloma formation may regress with therapy or as a result of the disorder's natural course but may also progress to fibrosis and restrictive lung disease. In chronic cases, approximately 10% of clients die of the disease.

Clinical Manifestations

Of clients with sarcoidosis, 30% to 60% are asymptomatic, and the diagnosis is confirmed by chest x-ray.[23] Clients who have pulmonary manifestations usually present with a dry cough and shortness of breath. Chest pain, hemoptysis, or pneumothorax may also be present. Systemic manifestations include fatigue, weakness, malaise, weight loss, and fever. A definitive diagnosis of sarcoidosis is made from tissue biopsy. When lung involvement is suspected, bronchoscopy, bronchoalveolar lavage, mediastinoscopy, or open lung biopsy may be performed.

Outcome Management

Medical management is primarily determined by the extent to which the client's life is disturbed by the manifestations experienced. If the client with sarcoidosis is asymptomatic, management involves ongoing assessment for further disease progression. Obtaining chest x-rays at 6-month intervals is often indicated. When manifestations are present, medical treatment usually consists of systemic corticosteroids to suppress the immune process and often leads to dramatic improvement.

Nursing intervention in clients with sarcoidosis is the same as that in clients with other restrictive lung diseases and hypoxemia. Assess for drug side effects, especially adverse responses to corticosteroids (such as weight gain, change in mood, development of diabetes mellitus). Also assess for signs of improvement, such as increased exercise tolerance, disappearance of initial assessment findings, improved pulmonary function studies, and better oxygenation. If assessment findings worsen, document them, and notify the physician.

NEOPLASTIC LUNG DISORDERS

MALIGNANT LUNG TUMORS

Lung cancer is malignancy in the epithelium of the respiratory tract. At least a dozen different cell types of tumors are included in the classification of lung cancer. The four major types of lung cancer are

- Small cell carcinoma (oat cell carcinoma)
- Squamous cell carcinoma (epidermoid)
- Adenocarcinoma
- Large cell carcinoma

There is no current effective screening test for lung cancer, and the range of treatment options is limited, resulting in frequent poor prognoses. Lung cancer is the leading cause of cancer deaths both in the United States and worldwide. The term *lung cancer* excludes other disorders, such as sarcoma, lymphoma, blastoma, and mesothelioma.

Etiology and Risk Factors

Cigarette smoking is by far the most important risk factor for lung cancer. Ninety per cent of clients who experience lung cancer are, or have been, smokers. Cigarette smoke contains several organ-specific carcinogens. Other carcinogens are inhaled toxins, such as asbestos, arsenic, and pollutants. Genetic predisposition to the development of lung cancer also plays a role in the etiology, as does age, with lung cancer rarely occurring in people younger than 40 years. Finally, TB and low-level radiation are risks for lung cancer.

Pathophysiology

Lung cancers are divided into two major categories: (1) small cell lung cancers (SCLCs) and (2) non–small cell lung cancers (NSCLCs), which include squamous cell carcinoma, adenocarcinoma, and large cell carcinoma. The characteristics of each of these types are described in Table 62–3. In general, survival rates are best for NSCLC, especially with treatment in the early stages. Despite growing knowledge and improving technology, however, overall survival of lung cancer remains low, especially for clients with small cell carcinomas.

Tumor cells grow and invade surrounding lung tissue. The cancerous lung tissue cannot exchange oxygen and carbon dioxide. Airways are invaded, obstructing the flow of air.

TABLE 62–3 OVERVIEW OF MALIGNANT PULMONARY NEOPLASMS

Cell Type	Approximate Incidence	Specific Characteristics	Growth Rate
Epidermoid (squamous cell)	30%–35%	Arises from bronchial epithelium As growth occurs, cavitation may develop in lung distal to tumor; Pancoast's tumor arises in apex and upper lung zones Secondary infections distal to obstructive tumor in bronchioles frequently occur	Slow growth with metastasis not common If metastasis occurs, usually to lymph, adrenals, and liver
Adenocarcinoma	35%–40%	Majority arises from bronchial mucous gland Often subpleural; rarely cavitates; often arises in previously scarred lung tissue Incidence strongly linked to cigarette smoking Increasing incidence in women Bronchioloalveolar cell carcinoma is a subtype	Slow growth Can metastasize throughout lung or to other organs of the body
Large cell	15%–20%	More often peripheral mass, either single or multiple masses Cavitation common May be located centrally, midlung, or peripherally Rare hilar involvement Often grows to large tumor mass before diagnosis	Slow Metastasis may occur to kidney, liver, and adrenals
Small cell (oat cell)	20%–25%	65%–75% manifest as hilar or central mass May compress bronchi Involvement of diaphragm through paralysis of phrenic nerve and hoarseness through paralysis of recurrent laryngeal nerve Pleural and pericardial effusions and tamponade often seen Does not form cavities	Rapid growth Metastasis to mediastinum and to thoracic and extrathoracic structures occurs early

Clinical Manifestations

The warning signals of lung cancer are presented in Box 62–2. In many instances, lung cancer may mimic other pulmonary conditions. Extrapulmonary manifestations may occur before pulmonary manifestations. Specific clinical assessment findings vary according to tumor type, location, and extent as well as pre-existing pulmonary health.

Centrally located pulmonary tumors usually obstruct air flow, producing clinical manifestations such as coughing, wheezing, stridor, and dyspnea. As obstruction increases, bronchopulmonary infection often occurs distal to the obstruction. Chest, shoulder, arm, and back pain may develop as the tumor invades the perivascular nerves. Squamous and small cell tumors often cause hemoptysis. Small cell tumors may also extend into the pericardium, causing pericardial effusion and, possibly, tamponade. Cardiac dysrhythmias are also likely.

Diagnostic Findings

Central pulmonary tumors are easiest to locate and identify with fiberoptic bronchoscopy and sputum cytologic study. During bronchoscopy, bronchial washings or

BOX 62–2 Warning Signals of Lung Cancer

- Any change in respiratory patterns
- Persistent cough
- Sputum streaked with blood
- Frank hemoptysis
- Rust-colored or purulent sputum
- Unexplained weight loss
- Chest, shoulder, back, or arm pain
- Recurring episodes of pleural effusion, pneumonia, or bronchitis
- Unexplained dyspnea

brushings are performed to obtain tumor cells for cytologic and pathologic study. Positive tissue diagnosis is possible 90% of the time.

Peripheral pulmonary tumors often do not produce early assessment findings. In time, pleural pain develops that increases on inspiration, is sharp and severe, and is usually localized. Pleural effusion (see later) also occurs and, along with the pain, limits lung expansion. Only 30% of peripheral lung tumors are successfully categorized by bronchoscopic and cytologic examination.

Pancoast's tumor occurs in the apices of the lungs in both squamous cell and adenocarcinomatous cancers. The tumor is asymptomatic until it extends into surrounding structures. Clinical manifestations are caused by compression of the brachial plexus in the distribution from the eighth cervical nerve to the first two thoracic nerves. This results in arm and shoulder pain on the affected side along with atrophy of the arm and hand muscles. With continuing tumor growth, the ribs over the tumor (usually the first and second ribs) may be invaded, resulting in bone pain. Later, involvement of the cervical sympathetic nerve ganglia may lead to Horner's syndrome. This syndrome consists of miosis (contraction of the pupil), partial ptosis (drooping upper eyelid), and anhidrosis (absence of sweating) on the affected side of the face.

Numerous diagnostic tests may be used to determine the presence and extent of lung cancer. Sputum cytologic study and chest x-ray are most commonly used. CT scans are used to provide detailed anatomic assessment. Magnetic resonance imaging (MRI) can provide high-quality images of the lung and mediastinum to assess for tumor invasion. New imaging techniques use monoclonal antibodies that have an affinity for cancer cells. The antibodies are tagged with technetium and injected into the client. They concentrate in the area of tumor and can be detected by single photon emission computed tomographic (SPECT) images.

Percutaneous transthoracic needle biopsy, mediastinoscopy, or direct surgical biopsy may be required to confirm the diagnosis of certain lung cancers. Radionuclide scans may be used to detect metastasis to the bone, liver, or brain (see Chapter 11).

The tumor-node-metastasis (TNM) classification scheme is used for lung cancer staging (Boxes 62–3 and 62–4; Fig. 62–3). Staging is performed to provide a guideline for the selection of appropriate therapies and the estimation of prognosis. Staging information is valuable in helping clients and their families make treatment decisions and set appropriate short-term and long-term goals.

BOX 62–3 Tumor-Node-Metastasis (TNM) Descriptors for Pulmonary Malignancy

Primary Tumor (T)

Tx

A tumor proven by presence of malignant cells in bronchopulmonary secretions, but not visualized on x-ray or during bronchoscopy, or any tumor that cannot be assessed as in a re-treatment staging

T0

No evidence of primary tumor

Tis

Carcinoma in situ

T1

A tumor that is 3 cm or less in greatest dimension, surrounded by lung or visceral pleura and without evidence of invasion proximal to a lobar bronchus at bronchoscopy

T2

A tumor more than 3 cm in greatest dimension or a tumor of any size that either invades the visceral pleura or has associated atelectasis or obstructive pneumonitis extending to the hilar region; at bronchoscopy, the proximal extent of demonstrable tumor must be within a lobar bronchus or at least 2 cm distal to the carina; any associated atelectasis or obstructive pneumonitis must involve less than an entire lung

T3

A tumor of any size with direct extension into the chest wall (including superior sulcus tumors), the diaphragm, or the mediastinal pleura or pericardium without involving the heart, great vessels, trachea, esophagus, or vertebral body; or a tumor in the main bronchus within 2 cm of the carina without involving the carina

T4

A tumor of any size with invasion of the mediastinum or involving the heart, great vessels, trachea, esophagus, vertebral body, or carina in the presence of malignant pleural effusion

Lymph Nodes (N)

N0

No demonstrable metastases to regional lymph nodes

N1

Metastasis to lymph nodes in the peribronchial or the ipsilateral hilar region or both, including direct extension

N2

Metastasis to ipsilateral mediastinal lymph nodes and subcarinal lymph nodes

N3

Metastasis to contralateral mediastinal, contralateral hilar, ipsilateral or contralateral scalene, or supraclavicular lymph nodes

Distant Metastasis (M)

M0

No (known) distant metastasis

M1

Distant metastasis present; specify site(s)

Modified from the American Joint Committee on Cancer. In Mountain, C. F. (1997). Revisions in the International System for Staging Lung Cancer. *Chest, 111*(6), 1710.

BOX 62–4 Pulmonary Malignancy Staging by Tumor-Node-Metastasis

Stage	TNM Subset
0	Carcinoma in situ
IA	T1N0M0
IB	T2N0M0
IIA	T1N1M0
IIB	T2N1M0 T3N0M0
IIIA	T3N1M0 T1N2M0 T2N2M0 T3N2M0
IIIB	T4N0M0 T4N1M0 T4N2M0 T1N3M0 T2N3M0 T3N3M0 T4N3M0
IV	Any T, any N, and M1

Modified from the American Joint Committee on Cancer. In Mountain, C. F. (1997). Revisions in the International System for Staging Lung Cancer. *Chest, 111*(6), 1710.

METASTASIS

If tumors spread, by either direct extension or metastasis, further clinical manifestations may result. Direct extension to the recurrent laryngeal nerve produces hoarseness. Compression of the esophagus may cause dysphagia. Invasion or compression of the superior vena cava produces superior vena cava syndrome, a potentially life-threatening emergency. Obstruction of venous blood flow leads to clinical manifestations, including (1) shortness of breath, (2) facial, arm, and trunk swelling, (3) distended neck veins, (4) chest pain, and (5) venous stasis. Immediate, palliative surgical treatment may be necessary.

Regional lymph node involvement may produce manifestations due to impaired lymph drainage. Involvement of the mediastinal lymph nodes may result in vocal cord paralysis, dysphagia, diaphragmatic paralysis on the affected side (due to phrenic nerve compression), vena cava compression, and malignant pleural effusion (see later). Usually, when mediastinal lymph nodes are involved, surgical excision of the pulmonary tumor is no longer possible.

Outcome Management

Medical Management

EARLY IDENTIFICATION

Early detection is the key to improving survival rates for clients with lung cancer. When premalignant changes begin, dysplastic cells are identifiable with fiberoptic bronchoscopy and sputum cytologic studies. At this stage, lesions are potentially curable. However, a tumor must be at least 1 cm in diameter before it is detectable on a chest x-ray. Unfortunately, invasion and metastasis have usually already occurred once the tumor reaches this size.

Management of the client with lung cancer depends on tumor type and stage as well as the client's underlying health status. Following diagnosis, primary treatment modalities are surgery, radiation therapy, and chemotherapy.

RADIATION THERAPY

Radiation therapy (radiotherapy) may be used as a potentially curative treatment in clients with locally advanced disease (1) for whom surgery poses an unacceptably high risk, (2) who have technically inoperable tumors, or (3) who refuse thoracotomy. Radiation therapy may also be used in combination with surgery or chemotherapy to improve treatment outcomes.

Radiotherapy is administered over a period of 5 to 6 weeks, either consecutively or in split courses. Doses are limited by the presence of other structures in the treatment area and by normal tissue tolerance. Irreversible fibrotic changes and other pulmonary side effects may

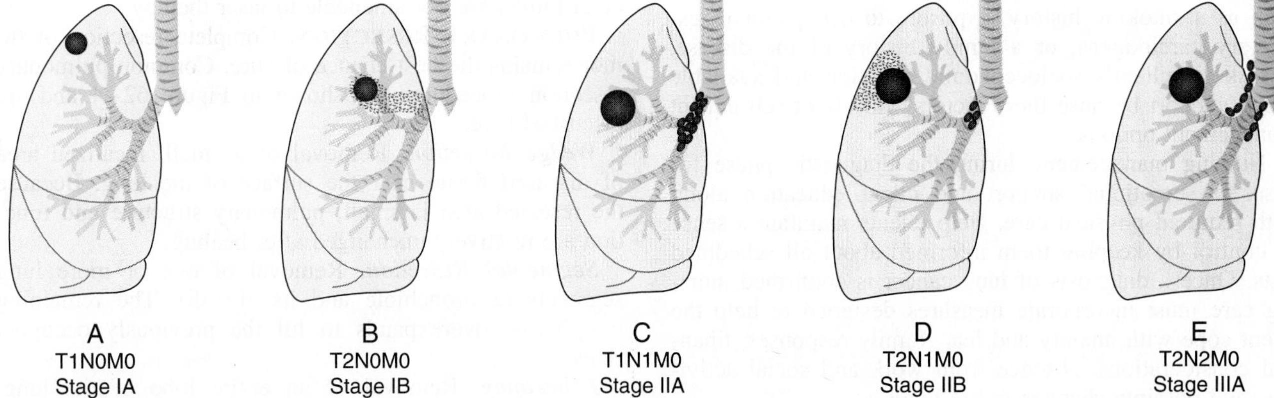

FIGURE 62–3 Example of various stages of lung cancer by the tumor-node-metastasis (TNM) classification system. *A* and *B*, Stage IA and IB disease includes tumors classified as T1 and T2, respectively, with no node involvement or distant metastasis. *C* and *D*, Stage IIA and IIB disease includes tumors classified as T1 and T2, respectively, with metastasis only to the peribronchial or ipsilateral hilar nodes. *E*, Stage IIIA disease includes tumors classified as T2 with metastasis to ipsilateral mediastinal or subcarinal nodes without distant metastasis.

occur. To delineate precisely the area to be irradiated, CT scanning is often performed before treatment begins. This method also minimizes tissue damage to surrounding areas.

Radiotherapy may also be used for palliation of manifestations such as pain, shortness of breath, hemoptysis, and obstruction or compression of bronchi, blood vessels, or esophagus. Irradiation of metastases to the brain and bone may reduce the distressing manifestations associated with these sequelae as well.

CHEMOTHERAPY

The response of lung cancer to chemotherapy depends on the tumor's cell type. SCLC responds well to chemotherapeutic agents because of its rapid growth rate. Results of clinical trials have demonstrated that long-term survival in clients with SCLC can be improved with intensive combination chemotherapy. As a result, chemotherapy is the cornerstone of management of SCLC.

The effectiveness of chemotherapy in the treatment of NSCLC remains controversial. This modality is commonly used in clients treated with surgery or radiation who experience recurrent disease or distant metastasis. However, large-scale studies have failed to demonstrate significantly improved long-term survival rates for such clients. As a result, the decision to use chemotherapy is usually made on an individual basis, depending on the client's previous history, current condition, and acceptance of the risks and side effects involved.

Nursing Management of the Medical Client

DIAGNOSTIC PHASE

The client who is undergoing diagnostic tests for lung cancer faces an uncertain future. If the diagnosis is confirmed, the client can anticipate a variety of physical difficulties, potentially extensive medical treatment, and many emotional changes. The nursing assessment plays a critical role in developing a plan of care that will provide needed support.

The nursing history should include an exploration of the client's chief complaints, particularly cough (productive or nonproductive), dyspnea, pain, and recurrent infection. Ask the client about the presence of risk factors, such as a smoking history, exposure to occupational respiratory carcinogens, or a family history of the disease. Assess the client's socioeconomic situation and available social support because these factors will affect subsequent management options.

Nursing management during the diagnostic phase focuses on emotional support and client education along with required physical care. Help clients maintain a sense of control by keeping them informed about all scheduled tests. Once a diagnosis of lung cancer is confirmed, nursing care must incorporate measures designed to help the client cope with anxiety and fear, family responses, financial considerations, absence from work and social activities, and possible changes in life goals.

TREATMENT PHASE

Nursing care of the client receiving radiation and chemotherapy is detailed in Chapters 18 and 19.

Surgical Management

Surgical intervention is the treatment of choice in early-stage NSCLC. Cure is possible if the disease is still localized to the thoracic cavity and no distant metastases are present. However, only 20% to 25% of clients with NSCLC meet these criteria at the time of diagnosis. For patients who successfully undergo surgical resection, the 5-year survival rate is approximately 35% to 40%.[33]

The role of surgical resection in the treatment of SCLC is limited. Surgery may be effective for clients with the early stages of SCLC, as a component of combined modality therapy. For clients with more advanced disease, surgery causes unnecessary risk and stress, with no valid benefits.

The primary aim of surgical resection is to remove the tumor completely while preserving as much of the normal surrounding lung tissue as possible. The extent of the operation depends on the location and size of the pulmonary tumor and the severity of the underlying pathologic process. Clients with pre-existing pulmonary disease may not be able to tolerate extensive removal of lung tissue.

PREOPERATIVE MANAGEMENT

Extensive pulmonary function testing may be performed before surgery to determine the client's ability to tolerate the proposed surgical intervention. Clients with impaired pulmonary function may be treated with antibiotics, bronchodilating medications, intermittent positive-pressure breathing procedures, and supervised breathing exercises to improve respiratory efficiency. Clients are encouraged to refrain from smoking during the preoperative period because smoking will increase pulmonary secretions and diminish blood oxygen saturation.

SURGICAL PROCEDURES

LASER SURGERY. One surgical treatment modality is laser therapy. Currently, laser therapy is used as a palliative measure for relief of endobronchial obstructions that are not resectable. Laser procedures do not produce systemic or cumulative toxic effects and are well tolerated. Laser therapy may be given in an outpatient setting. However, in order for the laser to be used, the tumor mass must be accessible by bronchoscopy. Therefore, tumors pressing on bronchial tissue from outside the bronchial lumen are not amenable to laser therapy.

PULMONARY RESECTION. Complete resection of tumor remains the best chance of cure. Common pulmonary resection procedures are shown in Figure 62–4 and are discussed here.

Wedge Resection. Removal of a small, localized area of diseased tissue near the surface of the lung. Because the resected area is small, pulmonary structure and function are relatively unchanged after healing.

Segmental Resection. Removal of one or more lung segments (a bronchiole and its alveoli). The remaining lung tissue overexpands to fill the previously occupied space.

Lobectomy. Removal of an entire lobe of the lung. Postoperatively, the remaining lung overexpands to fill the open portion of the thoracic space.

Pneumonectomy. Removal of an entire lung. Once the lung is removed, the involved side of the thoracic cavity

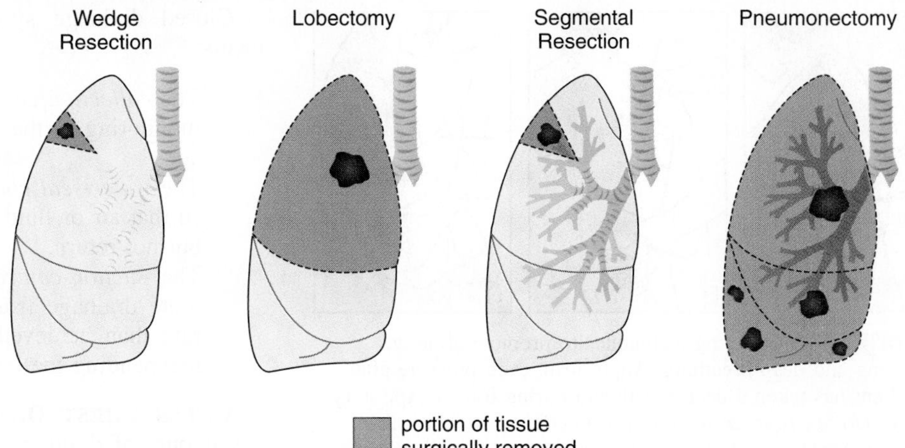

FIGURE 62–4 Pulmonary resections.

is an empty space. In order to reduce the size of the cavity, the surgeon severs the phrenic nerve on the affected side to paralyze the diaphragm in an elevated position. A thoracoplasty, which is the removal of several ribs or portions of ribs to further reduce the thoracic space, may also be performed.

Closed-chest drainage is usually not used after pneumonectomy. The serous fluid that accumulates in the empty thoracic cavity eventually consolidates. The consolidation prevents shifts of the mediastinum, heart, and remaining lung.

CHEST TUBES. Chest surgery causes a pneumothorax on the operated side. During thoracotomy, the parietal pleura is incised, and the pleural space is entered. Atmospheric air rushes into the pleural space. This changes the normally negative pressure in that pleural space to a positive pressure. As a result, the lung recoils to its unexpanded size and remains collapsed. Chest trauma, such as rib fractures, leads to pneumothorax in the same manner. Chest tubes are usually inserted in an operating room during chest surgery. However, in some emergencies, a chest tube may be inserted in a treatment room or at the bedside.

Two catheters are usually placed in the chest following resectional surgery (except pneumonectomy). One catheter (the upper, or anterior, tube) is placed anteriorly through the second intercostal space to permit the escape of air rising in the pleural space. The other catheter (the lower, or posterior, tube) is placed posteriorly through the eighth or ninth intercostal space in the midaxillary line to drain off serosanguineous (consisting of serum and blood) fluid accumulating in the lower portion of the pleural space. The lower tube may have a larger diameter than the upper tube, to enhance fluid drainage. Chest tubes are brought out of the chest wall through stab wounds or through the incisional line. The catheters are secured to the client's skin with sutures.

The two chest tubes may be joined to each other with a plastic Y-junction (and then attached to one closed-chest drainage system). However, it is preferable to leave them separate and to attach them to separate drainage systems. This arrangement makes it possible to monitor air and fluid drainage from each tube and, later, to remove a nondraining tube without disrupting the rest of the system. Flexible drainage tubing connects the chest tube to the drainage collection apparatus. Usually, chest tubes are connected to a closed-chest drainage apparatus before the client leaves the operating room.

Nursing Management of the Surgical Client

PREOPERATIVE ASSESSMENT

Preoperative preparation of the client with lung cancer who is to undergo surgery is the same as for any surgical client but with greater emphasis on assessment and preparation of the respiratory system (see Chapter 15 for discussion of preoperative nursing care).

PREOPERATIVE CARE

Nursing interventions during the preoperative period are aimed primarily at reducing the client's anxiety level. Anxiety results from fear of cancer and its prognosis as well as from fear of the surgical procedure and insufficient knowledge of surgical routines and postoperative self-care activities. The client and family are taught about the following issues:

The anticipated surgical procedure: Assess the client's (and family's) understanding, and give further information as needed.

The early postoperative period: Talk specifically about what will be happening to the client and how he or she can participate in recovery activities. Specific explanations should be given about the presence of chest tubes (except with pneumonectomy) and drainage tubes, intubation and mechanical ventilation, oxygen therapy, and available pain relief measures.

Postoperative exercises: They include (1) respiratory exercises, such as the use of incentive spirometry to maintain effective pulmonary function, (2) splinting techniques to promote effective coughing and deep-breathing (Fig. 62–5), and (3) leg exercises to prevent thrombophlebitis. All of these exercises should be demonstrated preoperatively, and opportunity given for practice and return demonstration.

POSTOPERATIVE ASSESSMENT

During the immediate postoperative period, thorough assessment is essential. Make observations as often as the client's condition warrants. Frequency of observations is determined by the following factors:

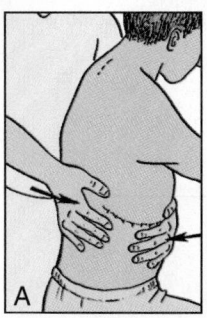

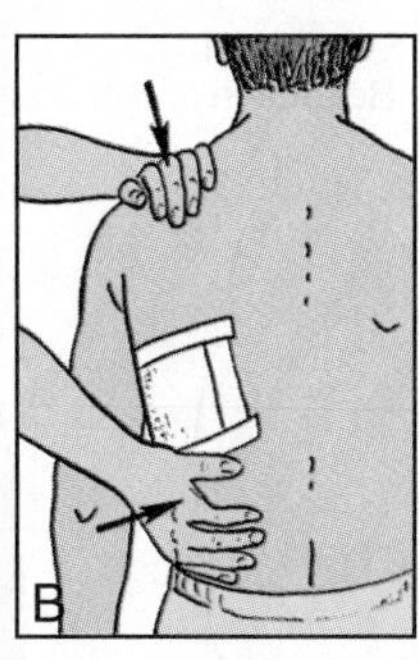

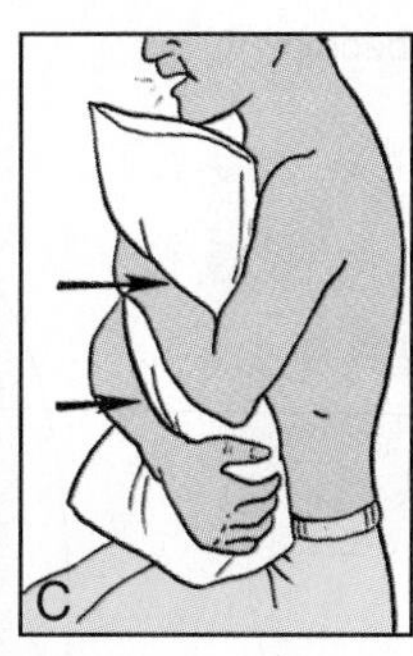

FIGURE 62–5 Splinting techniques to promote effective coughing and deep-breathing. Apply firm, even pressure after the client has taken a deep breath and during forced expiratory cough. Do not squeeze the chest or interfere with chest inspiratory expansion. *A*, Place one hand around the client's back and the other around the incisional area. *B*, Support the area below the incision with one hand while exerting downward pressure on the shoulder on the affected side with the other. *C*, Have the person hug a pillow during forced expiratory cough.

- Amount of anesthesia received and the client's reaction to it
- Amount of intraoperative blood loss
- The client's preoperative condition (e.g., presence of pre-existing medical conditions, such as diabetes and heart disorders)
- The client's response to pain
- Facility protocols

POSTOPERATIVE CARE

Nursing interventions are based on careful assessment and appropriate nursing diagnoses. General postoperative nursing measures are applicable (see Chapter 15). Nursing management specific to thoracic surgery is discussed in the Care Plan.

MAINTAIN CLOSED-CHEST DRAINAGE. Clients have closed-chest drainage after all forms of chest surgery (except pneumonectomy) and some forms of chest trauma.

In closed-chest drainage, the chest drainage system is airtight, or closed, to prevent the effects of atmospheric pressure. Historically, closed-chest drainage was performed with the use of a glass bottle water-seal apparatus (one-, two-, or three-bottle setup) with or without controlled mechanical suction. Most health care facilities have replaced glass bottle water-seal drainage systems with disposable single units, such as the Pleur-evac, Atrium, or Aqua-Seal (Fig. 62–6). However, a knowledge of the basic principles of closed-chest drainage will aid in understanding any specific system.

Closed-chest drainage after thoracotomy or chest trauma is used to:

- Promote evacuation of air and serosanguineous fluid from the pleural space and prevent their reflux
- Help reexpand the remaining lung tissue by reestablishing normal negative pressure in the pleural space
- Prevent mediastinal shift and pneumothorax by equalizing pressures on the two sides of the thoracic cavity

Closed drainage systems have three main compartments:

1. The *collection chamber* collects drainage and allows monitoring of the volume, rate, and nature of drainage.
2. The *water-seal chamber* is used as a one-way valve so that air or fluids can drain from the client's chest but not return.
3. The *suction-control chamber* uses suction to promote drainage from the pleural space (at a greater rate than achieved by gravity alone) and assist in reexpanding the lung.

ASSESS CHEST DRAINAGE. Measure *and* document the amount of drainage coming from the pleural space in the collection chamber. This record helps determine the amount of blood loss and the flow rate of drainage from the pleural space. Disposable plastic systems are manufactured with a marked write-on surface on which to record the amount of drainage. Drainage rates and amounts are used in planning blood replacement therapy and assessing the client's status. As much as 500 to 1000 ml of drainage may occur in the first 24 hours after chest surgery. Between 100 and 300 ml of drainage may accumulate during the first 2 hours; after this time, the drainage should lessen. Excessive drainage or a sudden large increase may require further surgery to determine its cause.

Normally, chest drainage is grossly bloody immediately following surgery, but it should not continue to be so for more than several hours. Assess blood loss by monitoring the rising fluid level in the collection chamber. Suspect hemorrhage if the blood pressure drops and the pulse rate becomes rapid. Check fluid in the drainage collection chamber. If the fluid level has not risen, check the tubes for patency. Notify the surgeon if (1) the drainage remains frankly bloody for longer than the first few postoperative hours, (2) bleeding recurs after it has slowed, or (3) there are any other manifestations of hemorrhage.

ASSESS WATER-SEAL FUNCTION. A water seal provides a one-way valve between atmospheric pressure and subatmospheric (negative) intrapleural pressure. It allows air and fluid to leave the intrapleural space but prevents the back-flow of atmospheric air into the chest.

On expiration, air and fluid in the pleural space travel through the drainage tubing. The air bubbles up through the water seal and enters atmospheric air. On inspiration, the water seal prevents atmospheric air from being sucked back into the pleural space (which would collapse the lung). The fluid in the water-seal compartment is not drawn into the chest cavity because the negative pressures generated during inspiration in the intrapleural space are not high enough to pull the fluid through the drainage tubing. However, fluctuation of the fluid occurs during respiration; this fluctuation is known as "tidaling" (tidal movement) or vacillation.

A closed-chest drainage system must be airtight between the pleural space and the water-seal compartment. Any air leak allows the entry of atmospheric air into the pleural space during inspiration, creating a positive pres-

Text continued on page 1736

THE CLIENT UNDERGOING THORACIC SURGERY

Collaborative Problem. Potential complications of thoracic surgery: pulmonary edema; respiratory insufficiency; tension pneumothorax and mediastinal shift; subcutaneous emphysema; pulmonary embolus; cardiac dysrhythmias; hemorrhage, hemothorax, and hypovolemic shock; and thrombophlebitis.

Outcomes. The nurse will monitor for respiratory, cardiac, and vascular complications.

Interventions	Rationales
1. Monitor for manifestations of respiratory failure: a. Increased respiratory rate b. Dyspnea c. Use of accessory muscles or retractions d. Cyanosis e. Decreased pulse oximetry f. Decreased PaO_2 levels and increased $PaCO_2$ levels g. Restlessness h. Increase in adventitious breath sounds	1. Postoperatively, respiratory insufficiency may result from an altered level of consciousness due to anesthesia and pain medications, incomplete lung reinflation, decreased respiratory effort due to chest pain, and inadequate airway clearance.
2. Monitor for manifestations of tension pneumothorax: a. Severe dyspnea b. Tachypnea and tachycardia c. Extreme restlessness and agitation d. Progressive cyanosis e. Laryngeal and tracheal deviation to unaffected side f. Laterally or medial PMI shift	2. Postoperative tension pneumothorax can result from air leaking through pleural incision lines if closed chest drainage fails to function properly.
3. Observe for subcutaneous emphysema around incision and in the chest and neck: a. Assess progression by periodically marking the chest with a skin-marking pencil at the outer periphery of emphysematous tissue. If neck involvement occurs, measure neck circumference at least every 2 to 4 hours.	3. Subcutaneous emphysema may result from air leakage at pulmonary incision site. a. Rapid progression (i.e., an increase of more than a hand's width in 1 hour) may indicate leakage through the bronchial stump.
b. Keep emergency tracheostomy tray at bedside	b. Severe subcutaneous emphysema in the neck may compress the trachea and may require tracheostomy.
4. Monitor for manifestations of pulmonary embolus: a. Chest pain b. Dyspnea and tachypnea c. Fever d. Hemoptysis e. Indications of right-sided heart failure	4. Pulmonary embolism is a serious potential complication after chest surgery and a significant cause of postoperative hypoxemia.
5. Monitor for signs of acute pulmonary edema: a. Dyspnea b. Crackles c. Persistent cough d. Frothy sputum e. Cyanosis f. Decreased pulse oximetry reading	5. Circulatory overload may result from the reduced size of the pulmonary vascular bed due to surgical removal of pulmonary tissue and delayed reexpansion of the affected lung. Additionally, hypoxia increases capillary permeability, causing fluid to enter pulmonary tissue.
6. Monitor intravenous flow rates. Consult physician if fluid amounts (maintenance plus intermittent medications [e.g., antibiotics]) exceed 125 ml/hr.	6. After chest surgery, intravenous fluids should not exceed 125 ml/hr because of possible circulatory overload.
7. Assess cardiac monitor for the development of cardiac dysrhythmias, particularly atrial fibrillation, atrial flutter, and paroxysmal atrial tachycardia.	7. Cardiac dysrhythmias are fairly common after chest surgery. Rhythm disturbances result from a combination of factors, including increased vagal tone, hypoxia, mediastinal shift, and abnormal blood pH.
8. Assess dressing and incisional area every 4 hours for evidence of bleeding (increase to every 1 to 2 hours if bleeding develops). Assess drainage in closed chest drainage system for signs of bleeding.	8. Blood loss may be great with major thoracic surgery because blood vessels in the thorax are of large diameter and the incision is often large and produces considerable capillary oozing.
9. Monitor for signs of hypovolemic shock: a. Increased pulse b. Decreased blood pressure c. Restlessness and decreased level of consciousness d. Decreased urine output (<30 ml/hr) e. Cool, pale, clammy skin f. Increased respirations	9. The body compensates for lost blood volume by increasing blood flow (through increased heart rate) to vital organs and decreasing peripheral circulation.
10. Monitor for thrombophlebitis: a. Unilateral leg edema b. Calf tenderness, redness, unusual warmth	10. Anesthesia and immobility reduce vasomotor tone, leading to decreased venous return and peripheral pooling of blood.

Care Plan continued on following page

11. Encourage client to perform leg exercises. Discourage placing pillows under knees, crossing the legs, or prolonged sitting. Apply elastic hose or pneumatic compression stockings, if ordered.

11. These measures prevent venous stasis, thus reducing the risk of thrombophlebitis.

Evaluation. The nurse monitors for the development of these complications. Most occur early after surgery, except for pulmonary embolus.

Nursing Diagnosis. Ineffective Airway Clearance related to increased secretions and to decreased coughing effectiveness due to pain.

Outcomes. The client will demonstrate effective airway clearance, as evidenced by clear breath sounds, effective coughing, and adequate air exchange in the lungs.

Interventions	Rationales
1. Once the vital signs are stable, place the client in semi-Fowler position.	1. The upright position enhances lung expansion and facilitates ventilation with minimal effort.
2. Help the client cough and deep-breathe at least every 1 or 2 hours during the first 24 to 48 postoperative hours.	2. Increasing the volume of air in lungs promotes expulsion of secretions.
3. Instruct the client to take a deep breath slowly and to hold it for 3–5 seconds, then exhale; to take a second breath and then, while exhaling, to cough forcefully twice.	3. Coughing helps move tracheobronchial secretions out of the lung. Deep-breathing dilates the airways, stimulates surfactant production, and expands lung tissue.
4. When possible, schedule coughing and deep-breathing sessions at times when pain medication is maximally effective.	4. The less postoperative pain a client experiences, the more effective are coughing and deep-breathing.
5. Assess breath sounds before and after coughing. Provide support and reassurance:	5. This will help in evaluation of coughing effectiveness.
a. Explain that breathing exercises will not damage the lungs or the suture line.	a. Client's fear of "splitting open" the incision may hamper coughing efforts.
b. Manually splint the incision area during coughing and deep-breathing.	b. Physical support of the incision is both comforting and reassuring.
c. Offer sips of warm water.	c. Warm water can aid relaxation and produce more effective coughing.
d. Maintain adequate level of hydration and adequate humidity of inspired air.	d. Fluids and moisture help thin secretions, making them easier to expectorate.
e. Monitor results of chest x-rays.	e. Frequent chest films help detect atelectasis and infection.
f. Evaluate the need for suctioning.	f. If coughing is ineffective, suctioning may be required to remove pulmonary secretions. Suctioning should be performed cautiously so that disruption of pulmonary suture lines is avoided.

Evaluation. Outcomes on effective airway clearance will require days to achieve.

Nursing Diagnosis. Pain related to surgical procedure.

Outcomes. The client will be more comfortable, as evidenced by verbalizing that discomfort is reduced, using less narcotic medication, and moving in bed with less pain.

Interventions	Rationales
1. Assess pain intensity using a self-report measurement tool.	1. Use of a consistent, valid tool promotes communication and evaluation of pain intervention effectiveness.
2. Administer pain medication as ordered.	2. Use of narcotics is a common method of postoperative pain control. Narcotics bind to opiate receptors, decreasing sensations of pain.
3. Observe for side effects of medication used.	3. Side effects are monitored.
4. Offer and instruct clients to ask for pain medication before pain becomes severe.	4. A preventive approach to pain control provides a more consistent level of relief and reduces client anxiety.
5. Assess medication effectiveness and avoid overmedication.	5. Adequate pain relief must be obtained. However, overmedication can depress respirations and the cough reflex.
6. Use nonpharmacologic pain relief measures concurrently.	6. Proper positioning, relaxation techniques, and like measures can augment effects of medications.

Evaluation. Pain will be most acute for 48 to 72 hours postoperatively, requiring narcotics for pain control. Expect pain to subside after that time, and offer less potent narcotics or analgesics.

Nursing Diagnosis. Impaired Physical Mobility related to pain, muscle dissection, restricted positioning, and chest tubes.

Outcomes. The client will maintain physical mobility in the arm and shoulder, as evidenced by regaining of preoperative arm and shoulder function.

Interventions

1. Position client as indicated by phase of recovery and surgical procedure:
   a. Nonoperative side–lying position may be used until consciousness is regained.
   b. Semi-Fowler position (head of bed elevated 30 to 45 degrees) is recommended once vital signs are stable.
   c. Avoid positioning client on operative side if a wedge resection or segmentectomy has been performed.
   d. Avoid complete lateral positioning after pneumonectomy.
2. Gently turn the client every 1 to 2 hours, unless contraindicated.
3. Avoid traction on chest tubes while changing client position. Check for kinking or compression of tubing.
4. Encourage regular ambulation, once client's condition is stable. Maintain supplemental oxygen, if ordered.
5. Begin passive ROM exercises of the arm and shoulder on the affected side 4 hours after recovery from anesthesia. Exercises should be performed two times every 4 to 6 hours through the first 24 postoperative hours, with progression to 10 to 20 times every 2 hours.
6. Active ROM exercises are begun once the client's condition permits.
7. Encourage client to use the arm on the affected side in daily activities (e.g., eating, reaching, grooming). Keep bedside stand on the operative side to encourage reaching. Teach the importance of continued use of the arm after discharge.
8. Carefully assess client's response to activity and exercise. Observe for signs of dyspnea and fatigue.
9. Allow adequate rest periods between activities.

Rationales

1. Repositioning maximizes long expansion and drainage of secretions, promotes ventilation and oxygenation, and enhances comfort.
   a. This position prevents aspiration.
   b. The upright position enhances lung expansion and facilitates chest tube drainage.
   c. Lying on the operative side hinders expansion of remaining lung tissue and may accentuate perfusion of poorly ventilated tissue, thus further impeding normal gas exchange.
   d. Because the mediastinum is no longer held in place on both sides by lung tissue, extreme turning may cause mediastinal shift and compression of the remaining lung.
2. Frequent turning promotes mobilization and drainage of air and fluid from the pleural space. Turning also improves circulation, promotes lung aeration, and enhances comfort.
3. Traction may dislodge the chest tubes. Kinking or compression inhibits drainage and reestablishment of negative intrapleural pressure.
4. Early ambulation improves ventilation, circulation, and morale. Oxygen therapy is used to avoid hypoxia.
5. ROM exercises help prevent adhesion formation in the operative area, which can lead to dysfunction syndrome (i.e., "frozen shoulder").
6. Active ROM exercises prevent adhesions of the incised muscle layers.
7. Regular use of the affected arm and shoulder reduces the possibility of contractures.
8. It may take time for the client's activity tolerance to increase, because the body must adjust to reduced respiratory capacity after resectional surgery.
9. Adequate rest will enable the client to cooperate more fully with activities.

Evaluation. Expect the client to be able to turn independently after 24 hours. Improvement in ROM will require a few days, until pain subsides and the chest tube is removed.

Nursing Diagnosis. Risk for Ineffective Individual Coping related to temporary dependence and loss of full respiratory function.

Outcomes. The client will use adaptive coping mechanisms, as evidenced by verbalizing feelings related to emotional state and taking appropriate actions to regain self-care capabilities.

Interventions

1. Provide opportunity for client to express feelings.
2. Encourage use of positive coping strategies that have been successful in the past.
3. Allow client to have as much control over daily activities and decision-making as is possible.
4. Support and praise all independent activities that promote recovery.

Rationales

1. Loss of normal body function and self-care capabilities can lead to feelings of powerlessness, anger, and grief. Open expression of these feelings can help client begin coping.
2. The use of effective coping actions can decrease feelings of hopelessness and helplessness.
3. Active involvement in the plan of care gives the client a sense of control and promotes return to independence.
4. Emotional support and encouragement help motivate client to continue progress toward independence.

Evaluation. The use of effective coping mechanisms depends on prior coping strategies. This outcome may be met quickly if the client is able to cope with a diagnosis of cancer and has hope for recovery and a support system. On the contrary, coping in the face of a dreaded diagnosis, fear of pain, little hope for recovery, and limited support systems will tax coping mechanisms.

Nursing Diagnosis. Altered Health Maintenance related to self-care after discharge.

Outcomes. Client will be able to maintain health, as evidenced by stating or demonstrating discharge plans.

Interventions	Rationales
1. Provide thorough instruction and preparation for hospital discharge:	1. Thorough understanding promotes compliance and enhances self-care capabilities.
a. Proper wound care	a. Wound care will vary according to condition of incision and client.
b. Continuation of exercise program	b. Continued exercise increases activity tolerance and prevents complications.
c. Precautions regarding activity and environmental irritants	c. Heavy lifting should be avoided. Return to work will depend on client's condition and type of job. However, it is usually possible to return to work within 4 to 6 weeks. Environmental irritants can cause severe coughing episodes.
d. Clinical manifestations to be reported to health care professional	d. Evidence of infection, deteriorating respiratory status, or other complications should be reported promptly.
e. Importance of regular follow-up care	e. The client should be monitored closely for signs of surgical complications, recurrence of malignancy, and metastasis.
f. Community agencies that can provide resources, as needed	f. Community resources can facilitate home management.

Evaluation. Client and family must demonstrate understanding of discharge teaching.

$Paco_2$, partial pressure of arterial carbon dioxide; Pao_2, partial pressure of arterial oxygen; PMI, point of maximal impulse; ROM, range of motion.

sure that collapses the lung. All connections within the drainage system must be tight and secure. However, the water-seal chamber itself *must* have an air vent to provide an escape route for air passing through the water seal from the pleural space.

Observe the Water Seal. Fluid in the water-seal compartment should rise with inspiration and fall with expiration (tidaling). When tidaling is occurring, the drainage tubes are patent and the apparatus is functioning properly. Tidaling stops when the lung has reexpanded or if the chest drainage tubes are kinked or obstructed. If tidaling does not occur:

1. Check to make sure the tubing is not kinked or compressed.
2. Change the client's position.
3. Have the client deep-breathe and cough.
4. *If indicated*, milk the tube (see later). If these measures do not restore tidaling, notify the surgeon. (*Note*: Tidaling may not occur or may be minimal in systems using suction.)

Observe for Bubbling in the Water-Seal Compartment. Bubbling in the water-seal compartment is caused by air passing out of the pleural space into the fluid in the chamber. *Intermittent* bubbling is normal and indicates that the system is accomplishing one of its purposes, that is, removing air from the pleural space.

Continuous bubbling during both inspiration and expiration, however, indicates that air is leaking into the drainage system or pleural cavity. Because air entering the system also enters the pleural space, this situation must be corrected:

1. Locate the source of the air leak, and repair it if you can. Begin by inspecting the chest wall where the catheters are inserted.
2. If a chest catheter is loose or has been partially removed, gently squeeze the skin up around the catheter or apply sterile petrolatum gauze around the insertion site. Determine whether this measure stops the continuous bubbling in the chamber.
3. If the air leak continues, check the tubing, inch by inch, and all the connections. A break in the tubing or a loose connection may be found that can be sealed with tape.
4. If the leak still cannot be located, it may be necessary to replace the drainage system.

Rapid bubbling in the absence of an air leak indicates considerable loss of air, as from an incision or tear in the pulmonary pleura. When this occurs, notify the physician *immediately* so that appropriate measures can be taken to prevent collapse of the lung or mediastinal shift, such as (1) application of suction, (2) increase in the amount of suction, or (3) thoracotomy.

When caring for a client with water-seal drainage, find out whether this particular client's water-seal chamber should be bubbling. Having this knowledge facilitates accurate assessment of the drainage pattern (e.g., if intermittent bubbling changes to constant bubbling or if an apparatus that has not been bubbling begins to bubble).

SUCTION. Suction at 10 to 20 cm H_2O may be applied to a chest drainage system if gravity drainage is not adequate or if a client's cough and respirations are too weak to force air and fluid out of the pleural space through the chest catheters. Additionally, suction may be applied to closed-chest drainage (1) if air is leaking into the pleural space faster than it can be removed by a water-seal apparatus or (2) to speed up the removal of air from the pleural space. Suction is regulated by the height of the water column in the suction chamber. The more fluid in the chamber, the more suction (subatmos-

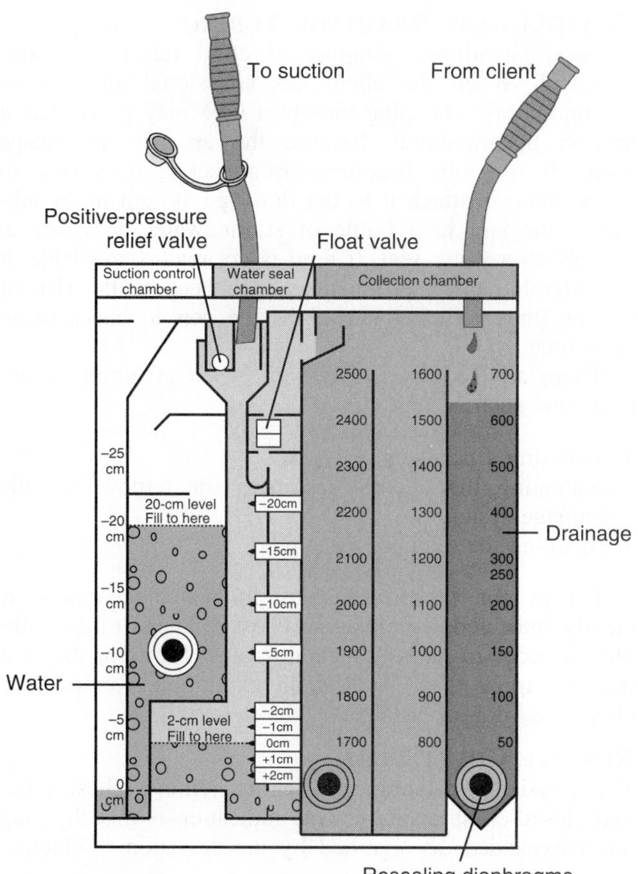

FIGURE 62–6 A commonly used disposable chest drainage system combines the three bottles into a single device. (Courtesy of Deknatel, Fall River, MA.)

pheric pressure) is created. Most clients who require a chest tube postoperatively also need suction for 24 to 72 hours.

If there were no water in the chamber, atmospheric air would go straight from the air vent into the suction source as fast as the suction was applied. Passage of the air through water slows it, and the suction force is controlled. Increasing the source of suction only causes more air to travel through the air vent. The suction applied to the client remains stable. An occluded atmospheric air vent is dangerous because it causes the suction to be applied directly to the pleural cavity. A suction force greater than 50 cm H_2O may cause lung damage.

Assess Suction Apparatus Function. Because most suction regulators can create potentially damaging amounts of suction, the amount of suction in the system must be controlled. Proper functioning of a wet suction control compartment is indicated by continuous bubbling in the suction control chamber. Vigorous bubbling does not increase the amount of suction; rather, it causes the water in the bottle to evaporate more rapidly.

Absence of bubbling in a suction control chamber means that the system is not functioning properly and that the correct level of suction is not being maintained. Possible reasons for malfunction of a mechanical suction apparatus include (1) large amounts of air leaking into the pleural space or into the drainage apparatus and (2) mechanical problems in the regulator (suction power source). The most serious problem is air leaking into the pleural space.

If bubbling in the suction control chamber stops, check for air leaks by briefly clamping the chest drainage tube close to the client's body and observing the chamber.

If bubbling begins in the suction control chamber, there is nothing wrong with either the drainage apparatus or the regulator. The problem is therefore an air leak into the pleural space around the chest tubes. If the air leak cannot be sealed off (e.g., with petrolatum gauze), notify the surgeon immediately.

If bubbling does not begin in the suction control chamber when the chest catheter is clamped, the problem is in the drainage connections or the regulator. Check the system carefully, looking for loose connections and for air leaks around compartment tops and in the tubing (e.g., split tubing). Make sure that the tubing is not kinked, is correctly positioned, and has no dependent loops. If the suction power source appears to be causing the problem, obtain another suction canister and regulator.

Because the chest catheter remains clamped during this inspection, observe the client closely for indications of tension pneumothorax (e.g., dyspnea, tachycardia, hypotension, trachea shift). As soon as the problem is corrected, the fluid in the suction control chamber will begin to bubble. Immediately remove the clamps on the chest catheter.

Some newer drainage systems feature dry suction, which uses a spring or dial mechanism in place of a water column to control the suction level. The advantages include ease in setup, no noise, and provision of higher, more precise levels of suction. However, because you cannot directly visualize the suction level via bubbling with such a system, it is important to assess the suction indicator frequently.

Promote Chest Drainage

Closed-chest drainage systems must always be placed lower (preferably 2 to 3 feet) than the client's chest. Drainage by gravity is thus maintained, and fluid is not forced back into the pleural space. Chest drainage systems must be placed upright on the floor or hung from the foot of the bed.

If the drainage apparatus is on the floor, be careful not to lower a high-low bed or side rails onto it. If a client with closed-chest drainage is to be moved, always keep the chest drainage system below the level of the client's chest.

If the apparatus is placed above the level of the client's chest, even for a moment, fluid from the drainage chamber is siphoned back into the pleural cavity. If absolutely necessary, chest tubes may be double-clamped very briefly during momentary movement of the apparatus above the level of the person's chest (e.g., when moving drainage apparatus from one side of the bed to the other if the tubing is not long enough to allow movement around an end of the bed).

Follow positioning orders carefully. If a client can be positioned on the side that has chest tubes, be sure the client is not lying on (compressing or kinking) the catheters or tubing. This may impair drainage, cause retrograde pressure (forcing drainage back into the pleural cavity), and increase the client's discomfort. Coil the drainage tubing (connecting the chest tube to the drainage apparatus) on the client's mattress so that it falls straight to the drainage apparatus, with no dependent loops. Dependent loops of tubing that contain fluid obstruct fluid flow and create back-pressure, thus impairing air or fluid drainage.

Drainage tubing should be neither too short nor too long. Excessive tubing length causes tangling and kinking. However, make sure the tubing is long enough to allow the person to turn and sit up without pulling on the chest tubes. Each time the client is turned or moved, check the chest tubes to make sure they are not being pulled or displaced. Check the drainage tubing to be certain it is properly positioned.

Tube patency is unlikely to be a problem when chest tubes are evacuating only air or when fluid or blood is draining well by gravity. However, if fragments of a blood clot or lung tissue are visible in the tube, use of chest tube clearance techniques *may* be indicated. Traditionally, nurses have manipulated chest tubes by *milking* or *stripping* (Fig. 62–7).

- To strip a chest tube, gently compress it, and slide one hand down the tubing, away from the client's chest and toward the drainage system. Stabilize the tubing with the other hand so that the tube will not be pulled on or displaced during stripping.
- To milk a chest tube, compress the tube intermittently using a twisting or squeezing motion.

Theoretically, these techniques dislodge clot material from the tube lumen and propel it toward the drainage collection chamber. However, studies have demonstrated no difference in tube patency with or without such manipulation. Additionally, stripping a chest tube can cause complications because it creates excessive negative intrapleural pressure (>100 cm H_2O). Therefore, these techniques should be used with extreme caution, if at all.

Encourage Activity

Encourage a client with closed-chest drainage to cough and deep-breathe frequently. In addition to clearing the bronchi of secretions, these activities promote lung expansion and the expulsion of air and fluid from the pleural space by increasing intrapulmonary and intrapleural pressures.

A client with a chest drainage system can sit up in bed, get in and out of bed, and ambulate without clamping of the chest tubes as long as the apparatus stays upright. Do not exert traction (pull) on the tubing. Various arrangements are used to hold a chest drainage system below waist level during ambulation. The device may be placed in a wheelchair in front of the client. Many disposable units have handles to allow for carrying. If the client's condition warrants, removal of suction during ambulation may be ordered, allowing gravity drainage.

Clamp Chest Drainage Tubing

In most situations, clamping of chest tubes is contraindicated. When the client has a residual air leak or pneumothorax, clamping the chest tube may precipitate a tension pneumothorax because the air has no escape route. If the tube becomes disconnected, it is best to immediately reattach it to the drainage system or to submerge the end in a bottle of sterile water or saline to reestablish a water seal. If fluid is not readily available, it is preferable to leave the tube open because the risk of tension pneumothorax outweighs the consequences of an open tube.

There are occasions, however, when clamping is appropriate, such as:

- Assessing a persistent air leak
- Evaluating the client's readiness for removal of the drainage system
- Changing the drainage system

Except for those occasions in which clamping is clearly indicated, *never* clamp chest drainage tubes without an order to do so. If clamps must be used, the best time to apply them is after an expiration. Remove the clamps as soon as possible.

Remove Chest Tubes

The physician determines when to remove chest tubes and closed-chest drainage. One indication is that the lung has reexpanded, as signified by the cessation of fluctua-

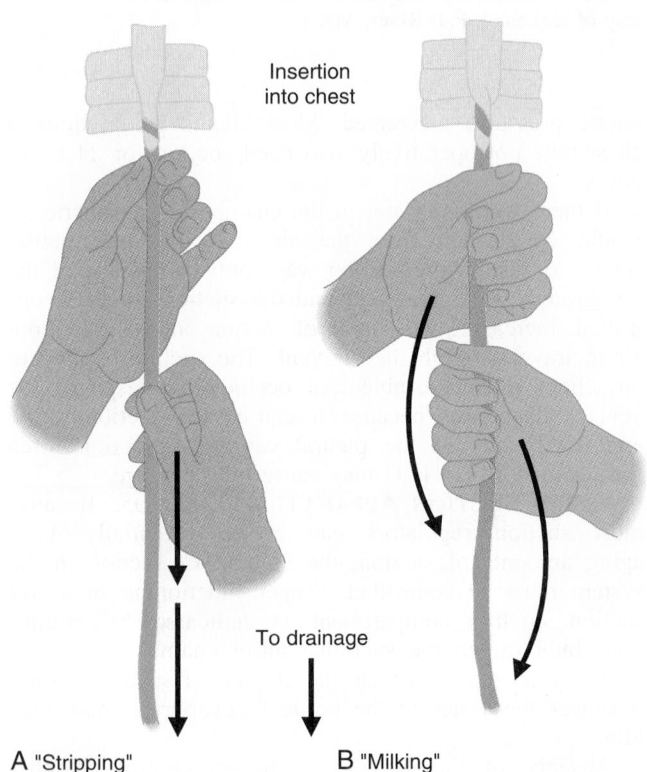

FIGURE 62–7 Stripping *(A)* and milking *(B)* of chest tubes are performed carefully to remove blood clots, but these procedures are not performed routinely.

tion in the water-seal chamber (if suction is not applied). Chest auscultation, chest percussion, and chest x-ray studies confirm lung reexpansion.

Usually, a lung is fully reexpanded after 2 or 3 postoperative days of chest drainage. Chest tubes are generally left in place and connected to drainage systems for an additional 24 hours after all air and significant fluid drainage have stopped. The tubes may be temporarily clamped to see how the client will tolerate their removal. Chest tubes may not be removed if the chest is draining more than 50 to 70 ml of fluid daily. The sooner the chest tubes can be removed, the better. Their presence often contributes to postoperative pain and inactivity. The longer the tubes are in place, the greater the risk of infection. Chest tubes used for treatment of empyema (see later) may be in place longer than tubes placed after chest surgery.

Removal of chest tubes can be moderately painful. The prescribed premedication for pain relief should be administered approximately 30 minutes before the procedure. Assemble equipment as necessary, such as sterile scissors or a suture set to cut sutures securing the tubes, sterile petrolatum gauze, 4×4-inch gauze to cover the wound, and tape.

If chest tubes are accidentally removed, cover the insertion site with sterile petrolatum gauze and notify the surgeon. Observe the client for respiratory distress because tension pneumothorax may develop. If it does, remove the petrolatum gauze to allow air to escape.

BENIGN LUNG TUMORS

Benign pulmonary neoplasms account for fewer than 10% of all primary pulmonary tumors. The term *benign* may be misleading because although they are not directly harmful to the body, some benign tumors may still have serious physiologic effects. Mechanical interference with lung function (e.g., obstruction of a major bronchus) may occur, depending on the tumor's location. In addition, some such tumors may become malignant over time.

The most common benign lung tumor is the hamartoma, which usually arises in peripheral lung parenchyma. This tumor is more common in older men. Other benign tumor types are fibroma, hemangioma, lipoma, and papilloma.

Benign lung tumors are often difficult to diagnose because clients may be asymptomatic. Unless there is preexisting lung disease or major airway obstruction, pulmonary function study results and ABG values are usually within normal limits. The tumor may be first detected on chest x-ray. Confirmatory diagnosis usually requires bronchoscopy or, more commonly, thoracotomy.

Until the diagnosis is confirmed, most clients are quite anxious and fearful of the possibility of cancer. Emotional support is an important adjunct to the physical preparation required for diagnostic procedures.

Surgical intervention is the treatment of choice for all benign neoplasms. Tumor removal promptly alleviates any respiratory manifestations that may have resulted from pressure on lung structures. Postoperative management is the same as that after surgical treatment of malignant lung disease.

OCCUPATIONAL LUNG DISEASES

Etiology and Classification

Lung diseases are among the most common occupational health problems. They are caused by the inhalation of various chemicals, dusts, and other particulate matter that are present in certain settings. Not all clients exposed to occupational inhalants experience lung disease. Harmful effects depend on:

1. Nature of the exposure.
2. Duration and intensity of the exposure.
3. Particle size and water solubility of the inhalant; the larger the particle, the lower the probability of its reaching the lower respiratory tract. Highly water-soluble inhalants tend to dissolve and react in the upper respiratory tract; poorly soluble substances may travel as far as the alveoli.
4. The client's smoking history.
5. Presence or absence of underlying pulmonary disease.

The most commonly encountered occupational lung diseases are described in Table 62–4.

Acute respiratory irritation results from the inhalation of chemicals such as ammonia, chlorine, and nitrogen oxides in the form of gases, aerosols, or particulate matter. If such irritants reach the lower airways, alveolar damage and pulmonary edema can result. Although the effects of acute irritants are usually short-lived, some may cause chronic alveolar damage or airway obstruction.

Occupational asthma is defined as variable air flow obstruction caused by a specific agent in the workplace. It is estimated that between 5% and 20% of all adult asthma cases can be attributed to workplace exposure.[36] By far the greatest number of occupational agents causing asthma are those with known or suspected allergenic properties, such as plant and animal proteins (e.g., wheat flour, cotton, flax, and grain mites). In most cases, the asthma resolves after exposure is terminated. However, hyperactivity of the airways may persist for years.

Hypersensitivity pneumonitis, or allergic alveolitis, is most commonly due to the inhalation of organic antigens of fungal, bacterial, or animal origin. The nature of the exposure and the client's immunologic reactivity determine the pulmonary response. Nonatopic people (i.e., those with no history of allergies) demonstrate a pulmonary response to organic dusts more often than atopic people, although atopic people, too, may exhibit pulmonary reactions.

Pneumoconioses, or the "dust diseases," result from inhalation of minerals, notably silica, coal dust, or asbestos. These diseases are most commonly seen in miners, construction workers, sandblasters, potters, and foundry and quarry workers. Pneumoconioses usually develop gradually over a period of years, eventually leading to diffuse pulmonary fibrosis that diminishes lung capacity and produces restrictive lung disease. Early clinical manifestations are cough and dyspnea on exertion. Chest pain, productive cough, and dyspnea at rest develop as the condition progresses.

TABLE 62–4 CHARACTERISTICS OF OCCUPATIONAL LUNG DISEASE

Disease	Onset of Symptoms	Diagnosis	Treatment	Clinical Course
Acute respiratory irritation	Immediate—within minutes of exposure Pulmonary edema may be delayed for hours	Consistent history Physical findings of respiratory tract irritation	Avoidance of exposure Respiratory support as needed	Resolves in hours to days Pulmonary edema may last days to weeks
Occupational asthma	Immediate—within minutes of exposure Can be delayed up to 6 hours	PFTs demonstrate reduced rates of FEV_1 to FVC Chest x-ray usually normal	Avoidance of exposure Asthma medication Steroids	Resolves within hours Permanent loss of physiologic lung function may occur
Hypersensitivity pneumonitis	Within a few hours of exposure	Chest x-ray findings range from normal to fine or diffuse infiltrates PFTs demonstrate a reduction in vital capacity	Avoidance of exposure Steroids	Symptoms typically lessen in 48 hours Chest x-ray and PFT findings may last for weeks to months or may be permanent
Pneumoconiosis	Requires long-term exposure First manifestation often cough progressing to dyspnea	Restrictive pattern on PFTs Chest x-ray with asbestosis shows interstitial markings in lower lobes and with silicosis shows opacities in upper lobes	Avoidance of exposure Cessation of smoking	Gradual worsening with fatigue, loss of appetite, chest pain, respiratory failure, and death

FEV_1, forced expiratory volume in 1 second; FVC, forced vital capacity; PFTs, pulmonary function tests.

Outcome Management

Early detection is one way to prevent progression of occupational lung disease. The respiratory history should consist of a (1) complete occupational history and questions about the actual job performed rather than title or job description, (2) past as well as current occupations, and (3) exposure to organic and inorganic substances in each job. The physical examination should include assessment of respiratory pattern and effort, presence of cough, lung sounds, and other manifestations indicating potential lung disease. Some employers support ongoing assessment programs (e.g., routine pulmonary function studies or chest x-rays) for workers at risk for occupational lung disorders.

Exposure precautions are essential for avoiding permanent pulmonary disability. Safety measures include adequate ventilation, the wearing of masks, and care in the handling of garments worn in dusty environments.

Nursing intervention for clients experiencing occupational lung diseases is similar to that for clients with other restrictive lung disorders (see following discussion). Supportive measures can help clients adjust their lifestyles to their conditions.

If occupational lung disease is significant, the client may qualify for a disability allowance. Refer clients to community resources, such as federal or state departments of labor, if they have questions about their eligibility for such allowances.

RESTRICTIVE LUNG DISORDERS

Restrictive lung disorders constitute a major category of pulmonary problems. The category includes any disorder that limits lung expansion and produces a pattern of abnormal function on pulmonary function tests characterized by a decrease in TLC.

Etiology

There are many causes of restrictive lung diseases. They may result from conditions affecting lung tissues or extrapulmonary causes. Extrapulmonary causes include neurologic and neuromuscular disorders and disorders affecting the thoracic cage, pleura, and movement of the diaphragm. Obesity may also lead to restrictive lung disorders. Box 62–5 lists restrictive lung disorders.

Clinical Manifestations and Diagnostic Findings

Manifestations vary according to the cause of the restrictive disorder. For example, kyphosis, scoliosis, and kyphoscoliosis result in changes in the thoracic cage (Fig. 62–8). Generally, clients with restrictive lung disease exhibit a rapid, shallow respiratory pattern. Chronic hyperventilation occurs in an effort to overcome the effects of reduced lung volume and compliance. Shortness of breath is experienced, at first only with exertion, but later at rest. ABG measurements reveal alveolar hyperventilation (i.e.,

BOX 62–5 Restrictive Lung Diseases

Restrictive lung diseases are disorders affecting lung volumes and compliance of either chest wall or lung tissue. Their causes are classified as intrapulmonary or extrapulmonary.

Intrapulmonary

Pulmonary fibrosis
Sarcoidosis and other interstitial lung diseases
Pneumonia
Atelectasis
Pneumoconioses
Surgical lung resection
Neoplastic disease

Extrapulmonary

Head or spinal cord injury
Amyotrophic lateral sclerosis
Myasthenia gravis
Muscular dystrophy
Congenital chest wall deformity
Acquired chest wall changes (e.g., kyphosis or scoliosis)
Abdominal distention restricting diaphragmatic movement
Sleep disorders
Poliomyelitis
Pleural effusion
Pleurisy
Excessive obesity

reduced partial pressure of arterial carbon dioxide [Pa_{CO_2}]) during the initial and intermediate phases of the disease process. As the disease progresses, respiratory muscle fatigue may occur, leading to inadequate alveolar ventilation and carbon dioxide retention. Hypoxemia is a common finding, especially in the later stages of restrictive lung disease.

Pulmonary function tests demonstrate impairment of the lungs' bellows action. Commonly, the ratio of FEV_1 to forced vital capacity (FVC), or FEV_1/FVC ratio, is normal or increased (i.e., 75% or more of expected values). The FEV_1/FVC ratio by itself is not an absolute indicator of restrictive lung disorders. Reduced TLC is the primary indicator of the disease. TLC is less than 80% of expected values in clients with restrictive lung disease.

Often a specific diagnosis of restrictive lung disease is made only after extensive testing, including chest x-ray, biopsy, immunologic testing, and tests to differentiate neurologic dysfunction, such as electromyography and cerebrospinal fluid analysis.

Outcome Management

Management is based on the severity of impairment and the ability to reverse the condition. Clients with spinal deformities may be helped by corrective spinal surgery. Likewise, obese clients breathe better after weight loss. Selected clients may benefit from the use of transtracheal oxygen administration or nighttime mechanical ventilation with a mask or cuirass respirator (a device that covers the chest and moves the chest wall out and back through changes in pressure), especially clients who have postpoliomyelitis syndrome.

The primary goals of nursing management of the client with restrictive lung disease are (1) promotion of adequate oxygenation, (2) maintenance of a patent airway, and (3) achievement of the highest possible functional level. Interventions to attain these goals are similar to those used in the treatment of COPD (see Chapter 61). ABG analysis is important for monitoring oxygen needs, acid-base balance, and the effects of physical activity. Pa_{CO_2} values should be monitored because rising carbon dioxide level is an indicator of impending respiratory failure.

Most restrictive lung disorders are not reversible. End-stage disease is characterized by the development of pulmonary hypertension, cor pulmonale, severe hypoxemia, and eventual respiratory failure. Efforts should be made to maintain the client's functional status and quality of life at as high a level as possible.

LUNG TRANSPLANTATION

Lung transplantation is appropriate for clients who have end-stage lung disease that is unresponsive to medical therapy and who are experiencing progressive deterioration in health status. This procedure involves replacement of one or both of the diseased lungs with a lungs from a cadaver donor. Live donor lobar transplantation has also been performed. The success of lung transplantation has improved significantly since the early 1980s and has become a widely accepted treatment for certain pulmonary diseases, such as COPD, cystic fibrosis, pulmonary fibrosis, and pulmonary hypertension.

Preoperative Care

Preoperative assessment consists of both medical and psychosocial evaluation. Once the severity of lung disease is established, the client's physical health is assessed to determine candidacy for transplantation. A battery of tests is performed to rule out active infection and to evaluate cardiac, hepatic, hematopoietic, and renal functions. Psychosocial evaluation focuses on assessing the client's his-

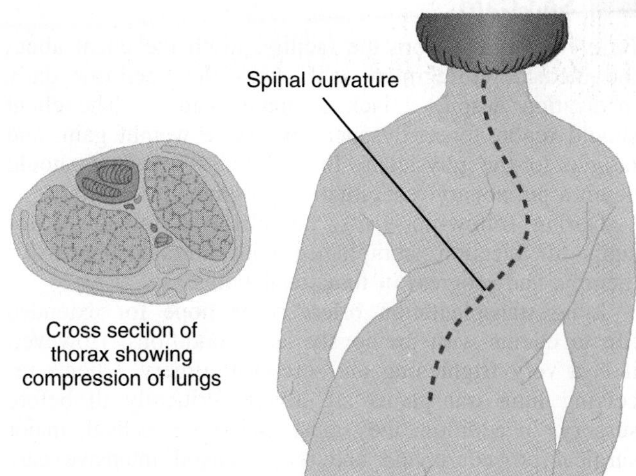

FIGURE 62–8 Thoracic scoliosis. Note the S shape of the spine. These thoracic deformities alter the chest cage space. Lung tissue may be compressed, producing altered lung function (restrictive lung disease).

tory of compliance with medical therapy and medical recommendations as well as his or her ability to cope with stress.[40]

POSTOPERATIVE CARE

Postoperatively, the client is observed for excessive bleeding. Monitor vital signs, hemodynamic pressures, electrocardiogram (ECG), ABG values, transcutaneous oxygen level analysis, and chest tube drainage. Pulmonary edema may develop in the denervated transplanted lung. Therefore, the client may be started on mechanical ventilation with positive end-expiratory pressure (PEEP) for 24 to 48 hours.

Chest x-rays are obtained at least daily. Fluids are restricted, lung sounds are auscultated, and the severity of peripheral edema is monitored. Pain control is extremely important to allow deep-breathing and coughing in addition to chest physiotherapy. Many clients benefit from epidural analgesia. Following extubation, maintain good pain control, and help the client cough, deep-breathe, and use incentive spirometry to expand the lung.

The client who has received a lung is at high risk for infection and transplant rejection. Isolation is used to decrease inadvertent exposure to pathogens. Laboratory values are monitored, especially the WBC and absolute neutrophil counts. Monitor the client for clinical manifestations of infection, such as (1) changes in vital signs (especially fever), (2) local infections at intravenous access sites and incision lines, and (3) changes in respiratory status (excessive secretions, tachypnea, dyspnea, fatigue). Rejection of the transplanted lung may manifest as dyspnea, development of infiltrates on chest x-ray, need for ventilatory support, and fatigue.

Following the initial procedure, the client may experience alterations in self-concept related to changes in (1) appearance, from the side effects of medications such as steroids and immunosuppressants, (2) lifestyle, or (3) work ability and role performance. Be sensitive to these issues, and encourage the client and family to discuss their feelings and explore options.

Self-Care

Before discharge from the facility, teach the client about the medication regimen, and stress the need for daily medication despite a lack of manifestations. The client should report fever, dyspnea, excessive weight gain, and fatigue to the physician. In addition, the client should begin a pulmonary rehabilitation program.

During follow-up visits, the client is monitored for signs of rejection, compliance with immunosuppressive therapy, and progress in functional status.

Lung transplantation offers some hope for extended life to clients with previously fatal conditions. However, it is a very frightening and stressful surgery. Clients receiving lung transplants are always critically ill before surgery. In addition, they must undergo a radical, major surgical procedure and endure prolonged intensive care and isolation procedures. People with transplants also must adapt to an altered self-concept. The client and significant others need constant emotional support for achievement of a successful outcome.

DISORDERS OF THE PLEURA AND PLEURAL SPACE

PLEURAL PAIN

Pleural pain is a common pulmonary manifestation associated with a variety of disorders. It arises from the parietal pleura, which is richly supplied with sensory nerve endings. Pleuritic pain indicates the presence of pleural inflammation (*pleurisy*) due to pneumonia, pulmonary infarction, pleural effusion (see later), or pneumothorax, among others. It is often accompanied by a pleural friction rub that is discovered during chest auscultation.

Pleuritic chest pain often develops abruptly and is usually severe enough that the client seeks medical attention. It commonly occurs on only one side of the chest, usually in the lower lateral portions of the chest wall, and is aggravated by deep-breathing or coughing. Often the client can point directly to the exact location of the pain. However, pleural pain may also be referred to the neck, shoulder, or abdomen. Because other types of chest pain (e.g., cardiac pain, chest wall pain) may be misinterpreted as pleuritic pain, careful assessment is necessary.

Pleuritic pain may restrict normal respiratory efforts, leading to problems with gas exchange and airway clearance. If pain-relieving measures, including administration of prescribed analgesics, do not relieve the pain, the physician may perform an intercostal nerve block (see Chapter 23).

PLEURAL EFFUSION

Pleural effusion is an accumulation of fluid in the pleural space. Pleural fluid normally seeps continually into the pleural space from the capillaries lining the parietal pleura and is reabsorbed by the visceral pleural capillaries and lymphatic system. Any condition that interferes with either secretion or drainage of this fluid leads to pleural effusion.

Causes of pleural effusion can be grouped into four major categories. They are conditions that:

- Increase systemic hydrostatic pressure (e.g., heart failure)
- Reduce capillary oncotic pressure (e.g., liver or renal failure)
- Increase capillary permeability (e.g., infections or trauma)
- Impair lymphatic function (e.g., lymphatic obstruction due to tumor)

Clinical manifestations depend on the amount of fluid present and the severity of lung compression. If the effusion is small (i.e., 250 ml), its presence may be discovered only on a chest x-ray. With large effusions, lung expansion may be restricted, and the client may experience dyspnea, primarily on exertion, and a dry, nonproductive cough caused by bronchial irritation or mediastinal shift. Tactile fremitus may be decreased or absent, and percussion notes may be dull or flat.

PRIMARY PLEURAL EFFUSION

Thoracentesis (see Chapter 59) is used to remove excess pleural fluid. The removed fluid is analyzed to determine whether it is transudate or exudate. *Transudates* are substances that have passed through a membrane or tissue surface. They occur primarily in conditions in which there is protein loss and low protein content (e.g., hypoalbuminemia, cirrhosis, nephrosis) or increased hydrostatic pressure (e.g., heart failure). *Exudates* are substances that have escaped from blood vessels. They contain an accumulation of cells, have a high specific gravity and a high lactate dehydrogenase (LDH) level, and occur in response to malignancies, infections, or inflammatory processes. Exudates occur when there is an increase in capillary permeability.

Differentiating between transudates and exudates helps establish a specific diagnosis. Diagnosis may also require analysis of the fluid for white and red blood cells, malignant cells, bacteria, glucose content, pH, and LDH. Large pleural effusions, whether transudates or exudates, should be drained if they are causing severe respiratory manifestations.

Pleural fluid may be (1) hemorrhagic, or bloody (e.g., if tumor is present or after trauma or pulmonary embolus with infarction), (2) chylous, or thick and white (e.g., after lymphatic obstruction or trauma to the thoracic duct), or (3) rich in cholesterol (e.g., chronic, recurrent effusions due to tuberculosis or rheumatoid arthritis).

If there is a high WBC count and the pleural fluid is purulent, the effusion is called an *empyema*. An empyema of any volume requires drainage and treatment of the infection.

If the pus is not drained, it may become thick and almost solidified or loculated (containing cavities), a condition called *fibrothorax*. Fibrothorax may significantly restrict lung expansion and may require surgical intervention. The procedure, known as *decortication*, involves removal of the restrictive mass of fibrin and inflammatory cells. Decortication is usually not performed until the fibrothorax is relatively solid, so it can be easily removed.

After the procedure, closed-chest drainage with suction is used to reexpand the lung rapidly and fill the pleural space. If the fibrous material has restricted the lung for some time, the lung may not reexpand effectively and further intervention (usually thoracoplasty) may be needed.

■ RECURRENT PLEURAL EFFUSION

In some cases, pleural effusions may recur despite repeated thoracenteses (e.g., malignancy-induced effusions), with resultant compromise of lung function or persistent pleural pain. Treatment of recurrent effusions is accomplished through obliteration of the pleural space. Methods of obliterating the pleural space are as follows:

Pleurectomy (pleural stripping): Surgical stripping of the parietal pleura away from the visceral pleura, which produces an intense inflammatory reaction that promotes adhesion formation between the two layers during healing.

Pleurodesis: Instillation of a sclerosing substance (e.g., unbuffered tetracycline, nitrogen mustard, talc) into the pleural space via a chest tube to create an inflammatory response that causes the pleura to adhere and sclerose to each other.

Because pleural space obliteration creates permanent changes, the client's existing and predicted postprocedure respiratory status must be carefully evaluated. If a large area is involved, significant alterations in ventilatory mechanics (e.g., deep-breathing, coughing) may occur, leading to compromised respiratory function.

After the procedure, closely monitor lung function, including respiratory rate and ventilation pattern. Document alleviation or persistence of pleural pain and watch for indications of a return of the pleural effusion. Pulmonary function studies (see Chapter 59) and ABG measurements should also be performed.

BRONCHOPLEURAL FISTULA

A bronchopleural fistula is a communication between the pleural space and a bronchus. It may occur when an undrained empyema erodes into a bronchus or when the pleural space does not heal spontaneously after removal of a chest tube. A bronchopleural fistula raises the risk of pleural infection and may compromise ventilation and oxygenation.

The management of a client with a bronchopleural fistula is often complex. Bronchopleural fistulae may be slow to heal. The client may be discharged home with a chest tube still in place and connected to a collection system. Teach the client and family how to care for the chest tube and collection system and to recognize both manifestations of irritation at the chest puncture site and changes in chest drainage (e.g., blood) that require the physician to be notified.

METASTATIC PLEURAL TUMORS

Primary tumors in the lungs and other organs often metastasize to the pleura. The primary tumor is usually in a lung but may occur in the breast, ovaries, liver, kidneys, uterus, testicles, or larynx or may result from leukemia or lymphoma. Metastatic pleural disease frequently causes pleural effusions.

Assessment findings in malignant pleural effusion are the same as those in pleural effusion from other causes. Diagnosis of pleural effusion is by chest x-ray examination. The source of the effusion is determined from cytologic examination of pleural fluid obtained by thoracentesis.

Intervention is the same as for any pleural effusion, along with treatment of the primary malignancy.

DISORDERS OF THE DIAPHRAGM

SUBDIAPHRAGMATIC ABSCESS

A subdiaphragmatic abscess may develop as a result of (1) gastrointestinal perforation, (2) surgery of the upper gastrointestinal system, liver, or biliary tract, (3) abdominal trauma, or (4) other intra-abdominal surgery. A subdiaphragmatic abscess produces abdominal and thoracic clinical manifestations that potentially compromise respiratory status.

Thoracic assessment findings consist of pleuritic pain

or pain referred to the shoulder on the affected side. Dyspnea and poor or no diaphragmatic movement are common. Abdominal assessment findings include flank pain or tenderness and a palpable abdominal mass in the region of the abscess. Generalized assessment findings are fever, anorexia, weight loss, and vomiting.

The diagnosis of a subdiaphragmatic abscess is confirmed by chest x-ray. The diaphragm is generally elevated on the affected side. Fluoroscopic studies of diaphragmatic movement reveal limitation or absence of diaphragmatic movement on the affected side. Pleural effusion also commonly occurs. Thoracentesis and analysis of the pleural fluid reveal an exudate. Subdiaphragmatic abscesses may erode and perforate the diaphragm.

Intervention for subdiaphragmatic abscess comprises antibiotic administration, drainage of the abscess, and supportive measures to maintain ventilation and respiratory status. An untreated subdiaphragmatic abscess is nearly always fatal. With treatment, the mortality rate is still high but drops to approximately 25%.

DIAPHRAGMATIC PARALYSIS

Many conditions may affect diaphragm function and result in paralysis, either unilateral or bilateral. The unilateral type of paralysis is more common than the bilateral type.

Etiology

Causes of unilateral diaphragmatic paralysis are as follows:

- Severing of the phrenic nerve during surgery
- Bronchogenic or metastatic tumors
- Neurologic disorders, such as poliomyelitis, encephalitis, herpes zoster, and diphtheria
- Accidental or birth trauma
- Mechanical obstruction (e.g., from aortic aneurysm)
- Infectious processes, such as tuberculosis, pneumonia, pleuritic disorders, and subdiaphragmatic abscess
- Other disorders (e.g., pulmonary infarction, congenital abnormalities)

Causes of bilateral diaphragmatic paralysis include:

- Many neuromuscular disorders, such as amyotrophic lateral sclerosis, muscular dystrophy, and Guillain-Barré syndrome
- Alcohol and lead neuropathies
- Closed-chest trauma
- Anatomic defects, such as congenital absence of the phrenic nerve, traumatic diaphragmatic rupture, and spinal injuries

Clinical Manifestations

Although the diaphragm is the primary muscle of respiration, its role can be assumed in part by the accessory and abdominal muscles. As a result, diaphragmatic paralysis is often difficult to detect.

The diagnosis of unilateral diaphragmatic paralysis is confirmed by fluoroscopy. During the fluoroscopic procedure, the client is asked to "sniff." If paralysis is present, the nonparalyzed side of the diaphragm descends during inspiration (the sniff), and the paralyzed side paradoxically rises. Clients with unilateral diaphragmatic paralysis usually experience dyspnea when lying on the affected side. Dyspnea on exertion is not usual unless there is underlying lung disease. Both TLC and vital capacity (VC) are reduced by about 20%. There is also less ventilation to the affected side, and mild hypoxemia occurs because of shifts of ventilation and blood flow. Pre-existing lung disease combined with unilateral diaphragmatic paralysis may be disabling, depending on the extent of the lung disease.

The effects of bilateral diaphragmatic paralysis are potentially much more severe than those of unilateral paralysis. However, the problem is often subtle and overlooked, especially if the client has a neuromuscular disorder.

Fatigue, disturbed sleep, and morning headache are frequently the only manifestations. A classic manifestation of bilateral paralysis of the diaphragm is increased dyspnea when the client is lying flat on the back (supine). Paradoxical inward abdominal movement during inspiration in the supine position and active use of the accessory muscles of inspiration also occur. The pulmonary effects of bilateral paralysis are pronounced when the client is supine. Functional residual capacity (FRC) is also decreased, as is lung compliance. In the side-lying position, ventilation is preferentially distributed to the uppermost lung tissue and away from blood flow, leading to a significant mismatch of ventilation and perfusion. Severe hypoxemia results. Reduced tidal volume leads to retention of carbon dioxide and respiratory acidosis. Respiratory muscle function decreases during rest and sleep, further compromising respiratory status.

Outcome Management

Little can be done to treat diaphragmatic paralysis. Management is aimed at supporting ventilatory function as needed. If the phrenic nerve is intact, a phrenic nerve pacer may be surgically inserted. However, this measure is possible only if the phrenic nerve can be stimulated (its status is tested first during a fluoroscopic procedure). Use of a phrenic nerve pacer is useful primarily for clients with spinal cord injuries.

Assess the client for subjective indications of hypoxemia or hypercapnia. Monitor ventilatory mechanics (e.g., inspiratory effort, spontaneous VC) and ABGs, observing for trends that indicate deterioration.

Nursing management focuses on maintenance of a patent airway and detection of deteriorating gas exchange. Because inspiration is impaired, the client may need assistance to cough and deep-breathe effectively. Position the client on the unaffected side in the semi-sitting or sitting position. Suction as necessary. Increase hydration to liquify secretions. Administer oxygen as prescribed. If respiratory function declines significantly, the physician and client (or possibly significant others) must decide whether a permanent tracheostomy should be placed and whether mechanical ventilation or other assistance devices (e.g., rocking bed, cuirass respirator) should be used.

CONCLUSIONS

Clients with lung disorders are a challenge to the nurse providing care. In addition to common nursing diagnoses centering on *Impaired Gas Exchange* and *Ineffective Airway Clearance,* the client is often anxious because of the feelings of dyspnea and air hunger. Management of lung disorders consists of methods to open the airway (bronchodilators), clear infection (antibiotics), and improve oxygenation (position, coughing and deep-breathing, oxygen).

THINKING CRITICALLY

1. Your client, who has undergone thoracotomy, has a pleural chest tube connected to water-seal drainage. While your client is being positioned for a bedside chest x-ray, the drainage tubing is inadvertently disconnected from the chest drainage apparatus. What actions should you take?

Factors to Consider. What happens to the normally negative pressure in the pleural space when it is exposed to room air? Is this a dangerous problem?

2. A client with exertional dyspnea is admitted to the unit with a diagnosis of pleural effusion. He has difficulty breathing during the transfer from the cart to bed. You are asked to prepare the client for a thoracentesis. How would you prioritize care? What preparations are necessary for a thoracentesis?

Factors to Consider. What is the purpose of a thoracentesis? How are complications avoided? What clients are at risk for pleural effusion?

BIBLIOGRAPHY

1. Bates, D. V., et al. (1992). Prevention of occupational lung disease. *Chest, 102*(3), 257S.
2. Blumenthal, N. P., Miller, W. T., & Kotloff, R. M. (1997). Radiographic pulmonary infiltrates. *AACN Clinical Issues, 8*(3), 411.
3. Bongard, F. S., Stamos, M. J., & Passaro E. (Eds.). (1997). *Surgery: A clinical approach.* New York: Churchill Livingstone.
4. Boutotte, J. M. (1999). Keeping TB in check. *Nursing 99, 29*(3), 34.
5. Breeding, D. C. (1998). Controlling silica exposures. *Occupational Health and Safety, 67*(10), 178.
6. Brewer, T. F., Heymann, S. J., & Ettling, M. (1998). An effectiveness and cost analysis of presumptive treatment for *Mycobacterium tuberculosis. American Journal of Infection Control, 26*(3), 232.
7. Brogdon, C. F. (1998). Women and cancer. *Journal of Intravenous Nursing, 21*(6), 344.
8. Calianno, C. (1996). Nosocomial pneumonia: Repelling a deadly invader. *Nursing 96, 26*(5), 34.
9. Carpenito, L. J. (2000). *Nursing diagnosis: Application to clinical practice* (8th ed.). Philadelphia: J. B. Lippincott.
10. Clarkson, E. F. (1999). Tuberculosis: An overview. *Journal of Intravenous Nursing, 22*(4), 216.
11. Colice, G. L., & Rubins, J. B. (1999). Practical management of pleural effusions. *Postgraduate Medicine, 105*(7), 67.
12. Corris. P. A. (1997). Prophylaxis post-transplant. *Clinics in Chest Medicine, 18*(2), 311.
13. Donohoe-Dennison, R. (1997). Nurse's guide to common postoperative complications. *Nursing 97, 27*(11), 56.
14. French, A. L., Benator, D. A., & Gordin, F. M. (1997). Nontuberculous mycobacterial infections. *Medical Clinics of North America, 81*(2), 361.
15. Gonzalez-Rothi, R. J. (1997). Resurgent TB: Stopping the spread. *Patient Care, 31*(9), 97.
16. Graybill, J. R., Kaufmann, C. A., & Patel, R. (1999). Treatment of systemic fungal infections. *Patient Care, 33*(19), 50.
17. Hiley, G. J. (1998). Managing the patient with a chest drain: A review. *Nursing Standard, 12*(32), 35.
18. Kemp, C. (1999). Metastatic spread and common symptoms. Part four: Lung cancer, malignant melanoma, multiple myeloma. *American Journal of Hospice and Palliative Care, 16*(3), 545.
19. King, A. B. (1999). Accurately interpreting ppd skin test results. *Nurse Practitioner, 24*(5), 144.
20. King, M. A., & Tomasic, D. M. (1999). Treating TB today. *RN, 99, 62*(6), 26.
21. Konstan, M. W. (1998). Therapies aimed at airway inflammation in cystic fibrosis. *Clinics in Chest Medicine, 19*(3), 505.
22. Long, C. O., Ismeurt, R., & Wilson, L. W. (1995). The elderly and pneumonia: Prevention and management. *Home Healthcare Nurse, 13*(5), 43.
23. Lynch, J. P., Kazerooni, E. A., & Gay, S. E. (1997). Pulmonary sarcoidosis. *Clinics in Chest Medicine, 18*(4), 755.
24. Mandel, J. H., & Baker, B. A. (1989). Recognizing occupational lung disease. *Hospital Practice, 24*(1), 21.
25. Marelich, G. P., & Cross, C. E. (1996). Cystic fibrosis in adults. *Western Journal of Medicine, 164*(4), 321.
26. Markowitz, N., et al. (1997). Incidence of tuberculosis in the united states among HIV-infected persons. *Annals of Internal Medicine, 126*(2), 123.
27. Marshall, B. C., & Samuelson, W. M. (1998). Basic therapies in cystic fibrosis: Does standard therapy work? *Clinics in Chest Medicine, 19*(3), 457.
28. Maurer, J. R., et al. (1998). International guidelines for the selection of lung transplant candidates. *Heart and Lung, 27*(4), 223.
29. Mays, M., & Leiner, S. (1997). Pharmacologic management of common lower respiratory tract disorders in women. *Journal of Nurse-Midwifery, 42*(3), 163.
30. Mountain, C. F. (1997). Revisions in the International System for Staging Lung Cancer. *Chest, 111*(6), 1710.
31. O'Hanlon-Nichols, T. (1996). Commonly asked questions about chest tubes. *American Journal of Nursing, 96*(5), 60.
32. Patterson, G. A. (1997). Indications for unilateral, bilateral, heart-lung, and lobar transplant procedures. *Clinics in Chest Medicine, 18*(2), 225.
33. Quinn, S. (1999). Lung cancer: The role of the nurse in treatment and prevention. *Nursing Standard, 13*(41), 49.
34. Rakel, R. E. (Ed.). (1998). *Conn's current therapy 1998.* Philadelphia: W. B. Saunders.
35. Ramsey, B. W. (1996). Management of pulmonary disease in patients with cystic fibrosis. *New England Journal of Medicine, 335*(13), 179.
36. Redlich, C. A., & Anwar, M. S. (1998). Occupational asthma: Keys to diagnosis and management. *Journal of Respiratory Diseases, 19*(6), 508.
37. Rosenstein, B. J., & Zeitlin, P. L. (1998). Cystic fibrosis. *Lancet, 351*(9098), 277.
38. Ruppert, S. D., Kernicki, J. G., & Dolan, J. T. (1996). *Critical care nursing* (2nd ed.). Philadelphia: F. A. Davis.
39. Sheffield, E. A. (1997). Pathology of sarcoidosis. *Clinics in Chest Medicine, 18*(4), 741.
40. Smith, C. M. (1997). Patient selection, evaluation, and preoperative management for lung transplant candidates. *Clinics in Chest Medicine, 18*(2), 183.
41. Smith, E. L. (1998). Pulmonary metastasis. *Seminars in Oncology Nursing, 14(3), 178.*
42. Sotir, M. J., et al. (1999). Tuberculosis in the inner city: Impact of a continuing epidemic in the 1990s. *Clinical Infectious Diseases, 29*(5), 1138.
43. Stalam, M., & Kaye, D. (2000). Antibiotic agents in the elderly. *Infectious Disease Clinics of North America, 14*(2), 357.
44. Stenton, C. (1998). Managing allergic alveolitis. *The Practitioner, 242*(1584), 200.
45. Vaz, A., et al. (1998). Coccidioidomycosis: An update. *Hospital Practice, 33*(9), 113.
46. Von Nessen, S. (1995). Exercise for patients with cystic fibrosis. *Perspectives in Respiratory Nursing, 6*(2), 5.
47. Yagan, M. B. (1997). Hospital-acquired pneumonia and its management. *Critical Care Nursing Quarterly, 20*(3), 36.
48. Yankaskas, J. R., & Knowles, M. R. (1999). *Cystic fibrosis in adults.* Philadelphia: Lippincott–Williams & Wilkins.

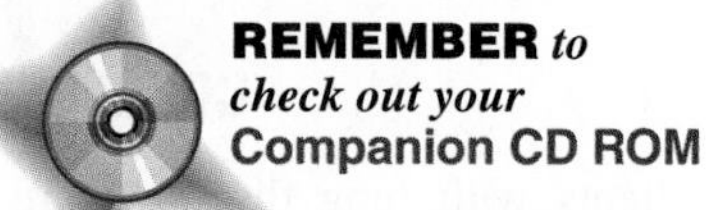

CHAPTER 63 Management of Clients with Acute Pulmonary Disorders

Joyce M. Black

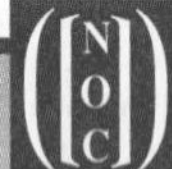

NURSING OUTCOMES CLASSIFICATION (NOC)
for Nursing Diagnoses—Clients with Acute Pulmonary Disorders

Impaired Gas Exchange
Respiratory Status: Gas Exchange
Respiratory Status: Ventilation
Vital Signs Status
Fluid Volume Excess
Electrolyte and Acid-Base Balance
Hydration
Respiratory Status: Ventilation
Inability to Sustain Spontaneous Ventilation
Vital Signs Status
Respiratory Status: Gas Exchange
Respiratory Status: Ventilation

Ineffective Airway Clearance
Aspiration Control
Respiratory Status
Respiratory Status: Gas Exchange
Respiratory Status: Ventilation
Anxiety
Anxiety Control
Symptom Control
Risk for Infection
Immune Status
Risk Control
Tissue Integrity: Skin and Mucous Membranes

Altered Nutrition: Less Than Body Requirements
Nutritional Status
Nutritional Status: Food and Fluid Intake
Nutritional Status: Nutrient Intake
Nutritional Status: Biochemical Measures
Impaired Verbal Communication
Communication Ability
Communication: Expressive Ability
Communication: Receptive Ability
Altered Oral Mucous Membrane
Tissue Integrity: Skin and Mucous Membranes

RESPIRATORY FAILURE

Respiratory failure is a broad, nonspecific clinical diagnosis indicating that the respiratory system is unable to supply the oxygen necessary to maintain metabolism or cannot eliminate sufficient carbon dioxide (CO_2). *Acute respiratory failure* is defined as a partial pressure of arterial oxygen ($Pa{O_2}$) of 50 mm Hg or less or a partial pressure of arterial CO_2 ($Pa{CO_2}$) of 50 mm Hg or more. In clients with chronic hypercapnia, $Pa{CO_2}$ elevations of 5 mm Hg or more from their previously stable levels indicate acute respiratory failure superimposed on chronic respiratory failure.

There are two general types of respiratory failure: (1) hypoxemic and (2) ventilatory. Clients with severe arterial hypoxemia who are minimally responsive to supplemental oxygen despite adequate ventilation have acute *hypoxemic* respiratory failure. Hypoxemic respiratory failure may be caused by diffuse problems such as pulmonary edema, near drowning or adult respiratory distress syndrome (ARDS), or localized problems such as pneumonia, bleeding into the chest, or lung tumors.

Ventilatory failure can result from central nervous system (CNS) depression, inadequate neuromuscular ability to sustain breathing, or excessive respiratory system load. Conditions such as acute deterioration of chronic obstructive pulmonary disease (COPD, sometimes called chronic airflow limitation) and status asthmaticus are other causes of ventilatory failure.

Classically, a client in acute respiratory failure has an elevated $Pa{CO_2}$ directly related to alveolar hypoventilation from either (1) decreased minute ventilation with normal dead space ventilation or (2) normal or increased minute ventilation with increased dead space ventilation. In the first category are clients with normal lungs whose respiratory status is impaired by drugs or diseases affecting respiration (e.g., neuromuscular disorders). In the second category are clients with intrinsic lung diseases such as COPD or severe pneumonia. Lung damage in these clients increases the amount of nonfunctional lung tissue, thus increasing dead space (or wasted) ventilation. Even with normal or increased minute ventilation, they cannot "blow off" (exhale) a sufficient amount of CO_2.

The following material addresses both types of respiratory failure, the conditions that commonly lead to the problem, and the usual management options.

HYPOXEMIC RESPIRATORY FAILURE

■ PULMONARY EDEMA

Pulmonary edema is the abnormal accumulation of fluid in the interstitial spaces surrounding the alveoli with advancement of fluid accumulation in the alveolar sacs. Pulmonary edema is classified by its underlying causes: *Cardiogenic* causes include left ventricular failure, mitral valve stenosis, cardiogenic shock, hypertension, and cardiomyopathy. *Noncardiogenic* causes are shown in Box 63–1. Pulmonary edema can also develop after catastrophic injury to the CNS, such as head injury; this form of pulmonary edema is called *neurogenic* pulmonary edema.

Etiology

Recall the processes guiding fluid movement (see Chapter 12). Normally, fluid moves into the interstitial space at the arterial end of the capillary as a result of hydrostatic pressure in the vessel and returns to the venous end of the capillary due to oncotic pressure and increases in interstitial hydrostatic pressure. Fluid in the interstitial spaces of the lungs is not uncommon. It normally escapes from the microcirculation and enters the interstitium, providing nutrients for the cells. The residual fluid is returned via the lymphatic system. Increased volume of fluid in the pulmonary arteries due to obstruction of forward flow is the most common cause of pulmonary edema. Heart failure is the most common example. Lung tumors can obstruct lymphatic flow and can also lead to pulmonary edema.

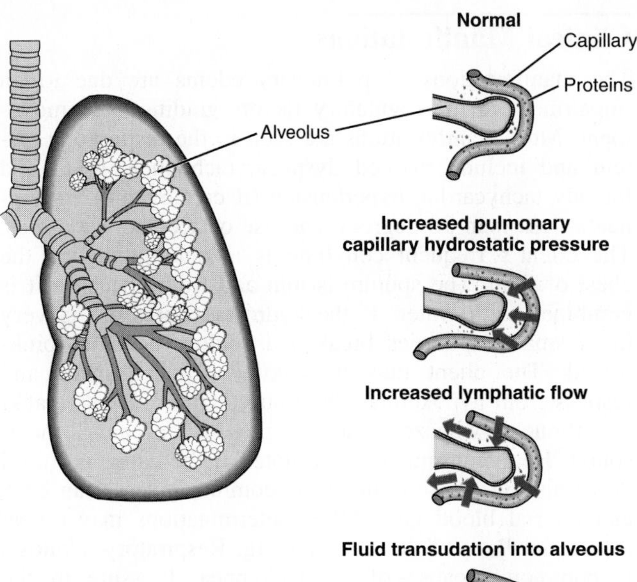

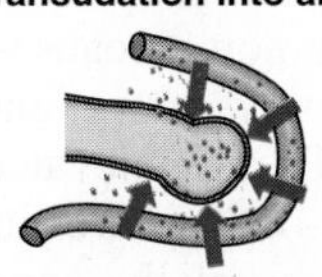

FIGURE 63–1 Progression of pulmonary edema. Pulmonary edema occurs when capillary hydrostatic pressure is increased, promoting movement of fluid into the interstitial space of the alveolar-capillary membrane. Initially, increased lymphatic flow removes the excess fluids but continued leakage eventually overwhelms this mechanism. Gas exchange becomes impaired by the thick membrane. Increasing interstitial fluid pressure ultimately causes leaks into the alveolar sacs, impairing ventilation and gas exchange. (From Hansen, M. [1998]. *Pathophysiology.* Philadelphia: W. B. Saunders.)

BOX 63–1 Causes of Noncardiogenic Pulmonary Edema

- Aspiration of gastric contents, especially if a large amount of HCl is present
- Barotrauma (e.g., with PEEP with mechanical ventilation)
- Drugs (e.g., after administration of narcotics)
- Fluid overload from IV fluids or renal failure
- Hypoalbuminemia (e.g., nephrotic syndrome, hepatic disease, malnutrition)
- Sepsis
- Inhalation of toxic chemicals (e.g., sulfur dioxide, paraquat, phosgene, chlorine, nitrogen oxides)
- High altitudes (>8000 ft)
- Neurogenic stimulus (e.g., increased intracranial pressure, epileptic seizures, head trauma)
- Near-drowning syndrome
- Mechanical ventilation, oxygen toxicity, ARDS
- Malignancies blocking outflow of lymph within the lungs
- Pancreatitis
- Pneumonia
- Smoke inhalation (e.g., trapped in a burning building)
- Unilaterally, after reexpansion of collapsed lung (pneumothorax)

ARDS, adult respiratory distress syndrome; HCl, hydrochloric acid; IV, intravenous; PEEP, positive end-expiratory pressure.

Pathophysiology

Increased hydrostatic pressure in the pulmonary vessels creates an imbalance in the Starling forces, leading to an increase in the fluid filtration into the interstitial spaces of the lung that exceeds the lymphatic capacity to drain the fluid away. Increasing volumes of fluid leak into the alveolar spaces (Fig. 63–1). The lymphatic system drains excess interstitial fluid volume. Additional fluid in the pleura drains into the hilar lymph nodes. If this pathway becomes overwhelmed, however, fluid moves from the interstitium into the alveolar walls. If the alveolar epithelium is damaged, the fluid accumulates in the alveoli. Alveolar edema is a serious late sign in the progression of fluid imbalance.

Hypoxemia develops when the alveolar membrane is thickened by fluid that impairs exchange of oxygen and CO_2. As fluid fills the interstitium and alveolar spaces, lung compliance decreases and oxygen diffusion is impaired. If pulmonary edema has developed because of left ventricular failure, right ventricular failure may occur because the pulmonary artery pressure is elevated. This elevation increases afterload for the right ventricle, resulting in manifestations of right ventricular failure.

Clinical Manifestations

The manifestations of pulmonary edema are due to an impairment in the regulatory factors guiding fluid movement. Most manifestations are seen in the respiratory system and include marked dyspnea, tachypnea, weak and thready tachycardia, hypertension (if cardiogenic), orthopnea at less than 90 degrees, and use of accessory muscles. The client's frequent coughing is an attempt to rid the chest of fluid. The sputum is thin and frothy because it is combined with water. If the hydrostatic pressure is very high, small capillaries break and sputum becomes pink-tinged. The client may be anxious from dyspnea and restless from hypoxemia. Chest auscultation reveals crackles, rhonchi, wheezes, and the presence of an S_3 heart sound. Heart murmur may be noted if the cause is mitral valve disease. Pulse oximetry is commonly less than 85% and arterial blood gas (ABG) determinations may reveal an arterial PaO_2 of 30 to 50 mm Hg. Respiratory alkalosis is common because of the tachypnea. Pressure in the pulmonary artery and pulmonary artery wedge pressure (PAWP) are elevated. The chest x-ray shows areas of "white-out" where fluid has replaced air-filled lung tissue, which normally appears black. Right ventricular failure may also be noted, with manifestations of hepatomegaly, jugular venous distention, and peripheral edema.

Outcome Management

Medical Management

Medical management addresses four areas: (1) correction of hypoxemia, (2) reduction in preload, (3) reduction of afterload, and (4) support of perfusion.

Correcting Hypoxemia

It is imperative to maintain adequate oxygenation, and clients with severe pulmonary edema commonly require oxygen therapy at high FiO_2 levels and may require mechanical ventilation or continuous positive airway pressure (CPAP) if they cannot meet the work of breathing.

Reducing Preload

The client is placed in an upright position. Usually, the client does not lie down because of orthopnea and a feeling of choking when supine. Diuretics are prescribed to promote fluid excretion. Nitrates, such as nitroglycerin, are used for their vasodilative properties. Phlebotomy can be used to remove excessive volumes of blood, although this practice is fairly rare. Older methods of preload reduction included the use of rotating tourniquets; this practice is also rare today. Other management strategies consist of treating the underlying condition.

Reducing Afterload

Afterload is reduced to diminish workload on the left ventricle. Antihypertensive agents, including potent agents such as nitroprusside, are prescribed. Morphine is prescribed to reduce the sympathetic nervous system response and to reduce anxiety from the dyspnea.

Supporting Perfusion

Left ventricular failure is supported by using inotropic medications such as dobutamine. Urine output is monitored closely to determine whether renal perfusion is adequate. An intra-aortic balloon pump (IABP) may be needed (see Chapter 55).

Nursing Management

Assessment

The client with pulmonary edema is assessed quickly upon admission. Anxiety is often marked, and control of dyspnea is imperative. A complete assessment is carried out over the following hours, when the client can breathe more comfortably and answer questions. A baseline weight is recorded, and baseline lung assessment is noted.

Diagnosis, Outcomes, Interventions

Impaired Gas Exchange. The fluid-filled alveoli retard the exchange of gases. Use the nursing diagnosis *Impaired Gas Exchange related to capillary membrane obstruction from fluid* to plan care.

Outcomes. The client will demonstrate improved gas exchange, as evidenced by rising PaO_2 to 55 or 60 mm Hg, oxygen saturation above 90%, normalizing pH, decreasing anxiety and dyspnea, and fewer crackles and rhonchi within 12 hours.

Interventions. Monitor vital signs every 15 minutes initially, until the client is stable, and the electrocardiogram (ECG). Administer oxygen as ordered using a high-flow rebreather bag to maintain oxygenation. Titrate the actual liter flow of oxygen to maintain saturation above 90%. Continuous assessment is needed because the client may not be able to tolerate the work of breathing and may require intubation and mechanical ventilation. Mechanical ventilation and intubation equipment should be nearby. To reduce preload, position the client with the legs in a dependent position. Raising edematous legs increases venous return and will stress the overtaxed left ventricle. Preload is reduced with morphine and nitroglycerin. Morphine can be used to reduce anxiety. Because perfusion to the skin is often compromised, repositioning is important.

Air hunger can lead to panic and feelings of suffocation. Feelings of anxiety in the client can lead to the nurse's empathetic reaction of being out of breath also. Be aware of the "contagiousness" of anxiety and its effect on decision-making. Administer opioids and anxiolytics to control both dyspnea and anxiety. Stay with the client and give breathing using 1 : 1 techniques, such as "Breathe with me, in and out, slowly."[13a]

Fluid Volume Excess. Accumulation of fluid from several causes leads to fluid overload. Use the nursing diagnosis *Fluid Volume Excess related to excess preload.*

Outcomes. The client will demonstrate fluid balance, as evidenced by diuresis (input < ouput), decreased number of crackles and rhonchi, eupnea, weight loss, resolving peripheral edema, and decreased anxiety.

Interventions. Administer furosemide as prescribed to promote diuresis. Place an indwelling catheter to monitor response to diuretics. Monitor urine output, weight, and potassium levels (potassium loss is a side effect of furosemide). Monitor blood pressure to determine whether the client can maintain perfusion without inotropic support. Because oral fluids are restricted, oral care is completed every 2 hours.

TABLE 63–1 RISK FACTORS FOR ACUTE VENTILATORY FAILURE

Imbalances in Load	Imbalances in Neuromuscular Competence
Increased resistance	*Depressed drive*
Bronchospasm	Drug overdose
Airway edema	Brain stem lesions
Retained secretions	Hypothyroidism
Airway obstruction	*Impaired neuromuscular transmission*
Obstructive sleep apnea	Phrenic nerve injury
Elastic recoil in lung	Spinal cord lesion
Alveolar edema	Neuromuscular blocking agents
Infection	Aminoglycosides
Atelectasis	Guillain-Barré syndrome
Elastic recoil in chest wall	Myasthenia gravis
Pleural effusion	Amyotrophic lateral sclerosis
Pneumothorax	Botulism
Rib fractures	*Muscle weakness*
Tumors	Fatigue
Obesity	Electrolyte imbalance
Ascites	Malnutrition
Abdominal distention	Hypoperfusion
Minute ventilation	Hypoxemia
Sepsis	Myopathy

From Schmidt, G., Hall, J., & Wood, L. (1994). Ventilatory failure. In J. Murray & J. Nadel (Eds.), *Textbook of respiratory medicine* (2nd ed.). Philadelphia: W. B. Saunders.

EVALUATION

Expect a fairly rapid response to diuresis and oxygen therapy.

Self-Care

Consider the reasons for development of pulmonary edema when developing a plan for self-care. Clients may need further education on daily weights, dietary choices, and scheduling of medications. Teach the early manifestations of fluid overload so that early intervention is possible.

ACUTE VENTILATORY FAILURE

Ventilatory failure is the inability of the CNS to sustain respiratory drive or inability of the chest wall and muscles to mechanically move air in and out of the lungs.

Etiology and Risk Factors

Two broad categories of problems can lead to acute ventilatory failure: (1) increased load for ventilation and (2) decreased ability or competence of the chest wall and lung to meet oxygen need. The respiratory load placed on the lung to exchange oxygen and CO_2 is impaired by (1) problems of resistance to moving air in and out of the lung, (2) ability of the lung to expand and contract (elastic recoil), and (3) conditions that increase the production of CO_2 or decrease the surface available for exchange of gases. The competence of the nerves and muscles coordinating the movement of the chest can also be impaired by loss of drive to breathe, impaired transmission of signals to the chest and diaphragm, and muscle fatigue. Conditions that can lead to acute ventilatory failure are listed in Table 63–1.

Pathophysiology

Alveolar ventilation is maintained by the CNS acting through nerves and the muscles of respiration to drive breathing. Failure of alveolar ventilation leads to hypercapnia (rising CO_2 levels). When CO_2 levels rise, acidosis develops. Untreated, ventilatory failure leads to death.

In obstructive forms of ventilatory failure, the residual pressure in the chest impairs inhalation and increases the workload of breathing. Functional residual capacity (FRC) is the volume of air remaining in the lung after normal expiration. When end-expiratory alveolar volumes remain above their critical closing point, the alveoli remain open and functioning, allowing oxygen to diffuse into the bloodstream. If alveolar volumes fall below the closing point, the alveoli tend to collapse. When alveoli collapse, no oxygenation of blood flow to the alveoli occurs (Fig. 63–2). The residual volume and FRC are decreased, resulting in a true intrapulmonary shunt (perfusion without oxygenation). Lung compliance is also affected.

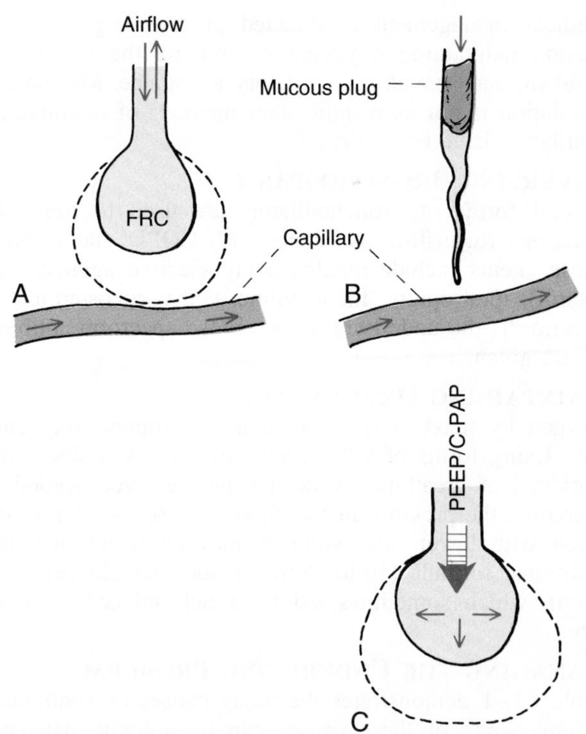

FIGURE 63–2 Effects of positive airway pressure on alveolus. *A,* Normal alveolus. *Dotted line* represents expansion during inspiration. *B,* Collapsed alveolus. Perfusion (continued). *C,* The alveolus is opened by positive pressure. *Dotted line* indicates alveolus during inspiration, and *solid line* indicates end-expiratory alveolar volume. FRC, functional reserve capacity; PEEP, peak end-expiratory pressure; C-PAP, continuous positive airway pressure.

Once alveolar collapse occurs, reinflation necessitates very high opening pressures, the generation of which significantly increases the work of breathing. The hypoxemia resulting from alveolar collapse and the increased oxygen consumption caused by the increased work of breathing may severely compromise the client.

Clinical Manifestations

To avoid frank apnea, recognizing impending ventilatory failure is crucial. Continuous monitoring of high-risk clients indicates changes in respiratory rate, mental status, and patterns of breathing. The client may also verbalize that dyspnea is increasing despite treatment. Altered respiratory patterns can herald impending ventilatory failure. The client's respiratory rate can rise to 50 to 60 breaths per minute, but the breaths are shallow and impaired by spasm of the airway. The rate can also fall to four to six per minute. Clients become confused, less conversant, and less arousable. If the cause is obstruction of the airway, during inspiration the systolic pressure falls as a result of intrathoracic resistance. This change, called *pulsus paradoxus,* is present when systolic blood pressure falls more than 10 mm Hg during inspiration. Pulse oximetry indicates steadily decreasing values, and ABG analysis shows falling PaO_2 and rising $PaCO_2$.

Outcome Management

Medical Management

Medical management is directed at reversing bronchospasm, maintaining oxygenation, treating the underlying problem, and providing ventilatory assistance. Mechanical ventilation is not used until other methods of maintaining ventilation have been tried.

REVERSING BRONCHOSPASM

Several forms of bronchodilators are used to treat obstructions to airflow in clients with COPD and asthma. These agents include inhaled $beta_2$-selective agonists (albuterol), ipratropium, theophylline, and corticosteroids. If infection is the underlying cause, broad-spectrum antibiotics are given.

MAINTAINING OXYGENATION

Oxygen by mask may be adequate to support oxygenation. Using forms of CPAP, such as a mask, reduces the workload of breathing by decreasing the force needed to overcome the pressure in the chest. Outcomes after ventilation with lower tidal volumes may be better than the traditional formula (10 to 15 ml of body weight per kilogram), which sometimes led to stretch-induced lung injury.

MANAGING THE UNDERLYING PROBLEM

Table 63–1 demonstrates the many causes of ventilatory failure. Some of these causes can be quickly managed, such as drug overdose with naloxone, but others require more aggressive treatment. Supportive therapies are used to reverse or control the underlying problem.

MAINTAINING VENTILATION

Mechanical ventilation helps to minimize the work of breathing while effectively promoting gas exchange (oxygenation and ventilation). The client requires an artificial airway (usually by endotracheal tube [ET] intubation initially) and the use of positive-pressure ventilation (PPV). If prolonged intubation is required, the ET tube is replaced with a tracheostomy.

Intubation

The ET tube, a long, slender, hollow tube usually made of polyvinyl chloride, is inserted into the trachea via the mouth or nose. It passes through the vocal cords, and the distal tip is positioned just above the bifurcation of the mainstem of the bronchus (carina). Oral intubation is usually used for short-term airway management. Nasal intubation, a more secure method, is believed to be more comfortable because the tube does not move as much in the airway. However, nasal intubation is not being used in many hospitals because of the risk of sinusitis. The client is supine with all dental bridgework and plates and loose teeth removed because these items can be jarred loose and aspirated during intubation. The client's head is hyperextended, the lower aspect of the neck flexed, and the mouth opened (Fig. 63–3). This position brings the mouth, pharynx, and larynx into a straight line. A laryngoscope is used to hold the airway open, expose the vocal cords, and serve as a guide for the tube into the trachea. ET tubes are inserted only by fully trained health care team members.

Intubation should not cause or exacerbate hypoxia. If the client's neck and mandible are mobile, the procedure usually takes about 30 seconds. Certain pre-existing conditions, such as rheumatoid arthritis of the neck, can make intubation difficult. For clients with expected difficulty of intubation, an oxygen mask can be used to provide oxygen through the mouth. An oxygen saturation monitor may also be used to warn of hypoxemia.

A good practice to remember during difficult intubation is to hold your breath while intubation is attempted. If you must stop to breathe before the client is intubated, the intubation is taking too long. Stop the intubation, reoxygenate the client by mask, and reattempt intubation.

Immediately after ET tube insertion, tube placement is verified by auscultation and chest x-ray to ensure aeration of both sides of the chest. Record in the nurses' notes and on the respiratory flow sheet the point at which the tube meets the lips or nostrils by using the numbers listed on the side of the ET tube. If the tube slips, its correct position can be reestablished quickly.

Secure the ET tube immediately after intubation with adhesive tape, twill tape, or specially designed ET tube holders (Fig. 63–4). Secure a nasotracheal tube in the same way, but place the second of the small strips across the bridge of the nose instead of on the upper lip. Retaping is required only if the tape becomes loose or soiled.

Cuff Inflation

The cuff of an ET tube seals the tube against the tracheal wall to facilitate PPV and protects the respiratory tract from aspiration of foreign material.

The amount of air required to seal an ET tube cuff is reflected by the cuff pressure, which is usually maintained at less than 20 mm Hg. Most ET tubes are designed with soft plastic cuffs for use of high volumes at low pressures. Cuffs are inflated with a volume of air high enough to seal the trachea while exerting the lowest possible pressure on the tracheal wall. Low cuff pressure is neces-

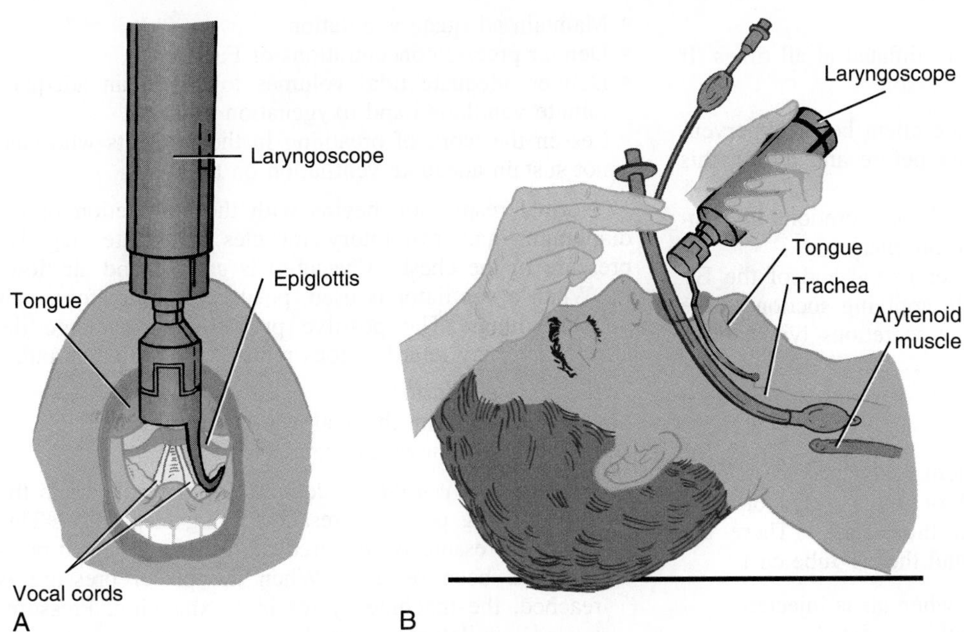

FIGURE 63–3 *A,* A laryngoscope is used to visualize the vocal cords. *B,* The endotracheal tube is inserted with the client's head extended to align the airway.

sary to prevent damage to the tracheal mucosa. Arterial pressures in the tracheal wall are approximately 20 to 25 mm Hg; venous pressures are 18 to 20 mm Hg. Therefore, cuff pressures greater than 18 to 20 mm Hg impair circulation to the tracheal mucosa and necrosis may develop. Assess cuff pressures every 8 hours.

The most common method of cuff inflation (*minimal occlusion volume technique*) aims to provide an adequate seal in the trachea at the lowest possible cuff pressure. Slowly inject air into the cuff while auscultating with a stethoscope placed over the larynx (over the cuff) during a positive-pressure breath. At the point when sounds (from air movement) cease, inflation is stopped, indicating that the cuff is sealed against the tracheal wall.

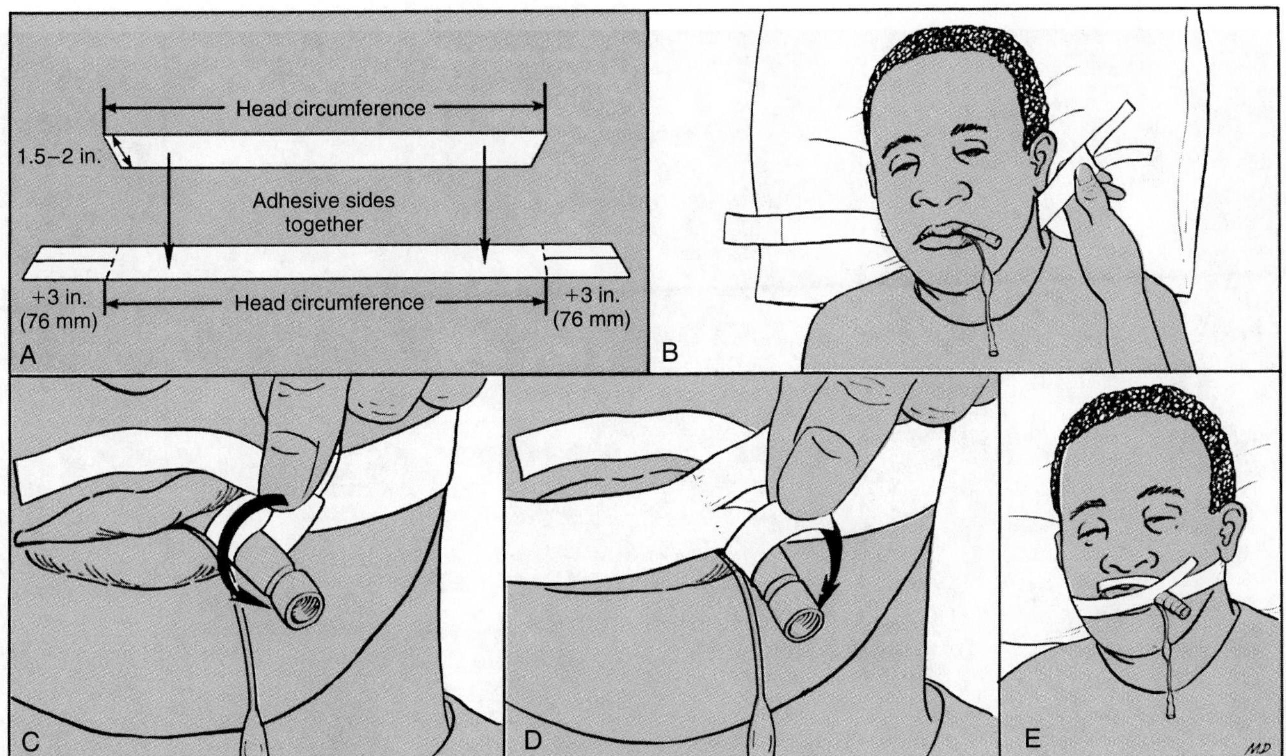

FIGURE 63–4 Securing a cuffed endotracheal tube with tape. *A,* Two strips of tape are torn; one is used to measure head circumference, and the other is 6 inches longer. The tape is placed with the adhesive sides together to form a strip. *B,* Place the strip behind the head and tear one end of the strip in half. *C,* Secure the tube to the upper lip with the untorn end. *D,* Wrap the torn segments around the tube to secure it (*E*).

Cuff Deflation

Generally, ET cuffs should remain inflated at all times. If cuff deflation is required for any reason:

1. Suction the trachea (with the client being hyperventilated and hyperoxygenated before and during this procedure).
2. Clean the area above the cuff of secretions by gently suctioning deep into the oropharynx.
3. Advance the suction catheter to the end of the ET tube. Deflate the cuff while applying suction to the suction catheter so that any secretions lying above the cuff can be removed.
4. Repeat pharyngeal suctioning.

Cuff Leaks

Cuff leaks can be a major problem. They may be caused by a rupture or tear in the cuff or pilot system or by a change in ET tube position in the trachea. There are several signs of a leak in or around the ET tube cuff:

- The pilot balloon is not filling when air is injected.
- The client can talk when the cuff is inflated.
- Air is heard leaking during positive pressure breathing.

If the system is not functional, the ET tube is replaced. Before replacement, increasing tidal volume may help maintain ventilation by compensating for the escaping gas. The client is at high risk for aspiration while the cuff is leaking.

Continuous Mechanical Ventilation

The goals of continuous mechanical ventilation (CMV) are to:

- Maintain adequate ventilation
- Deliver precise concentrations of FiO_2
- Deliver adequate tidal volumes to obtain an adequate minute ventilation and oxygenation
- Lessen the work of breathing in those clients who cannot sustain adequate ventilation on their own.

Normal respiration begins with the contraction of the diaphragm and respiratory muscles to create negative pressure in the chest: A vacuum is created and air flows in. When a ventilator is used, positive pressure forces air into the lungs. The positive pressure can damage the alveoli and may retard venous return and cardiac output.

Types of Ventilators

Several types of mechanical ventilators are available. A control panel is shown in Figure 63–5.

Pressure-cycled ventilators deliver a volume of gas to the airway using positive pressure during inspiration. This positive pressure is delivered until the preselected pressure has been reached. When the preset pressure is reached, the machine cycles into exhalation. Pressure-cycled ventilators are used in only a small portion of clients who require CMV.

Volume-cycled (*volume-controlled* or *volume-limited*) *ventilators* deliver a preset tidal volume of inspired gas. The tidal volume that has been preselected is delivered to the client regardless of the pressure required to deliver this volume. A pressure limit can be set to prevent the occurrence of dangerously high airway pressures.

Time-cycled ventilators terminate when a preset inspiratory time has elapsed. In most of these devices, a pressure limit is also incorporated.

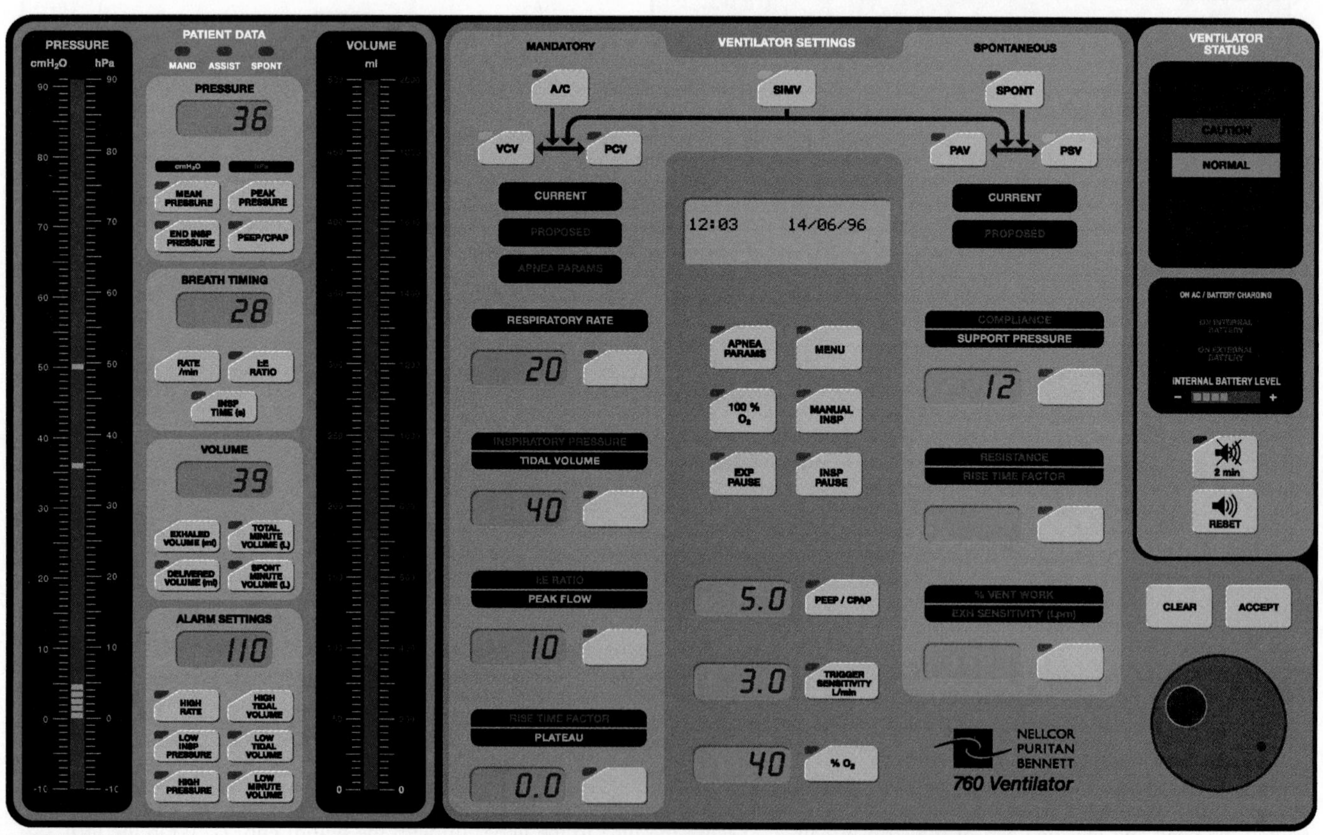

FIGURE 63–5 Nellcor Puritan Bennett 760 Ventilator. (Courtesy of Mallinckrodt, Inc., Nellcor Puritan Bennett Ventilator Division.)

BRIDGE TO CRITICAL CARE

Example of a Ventilator Control Panel

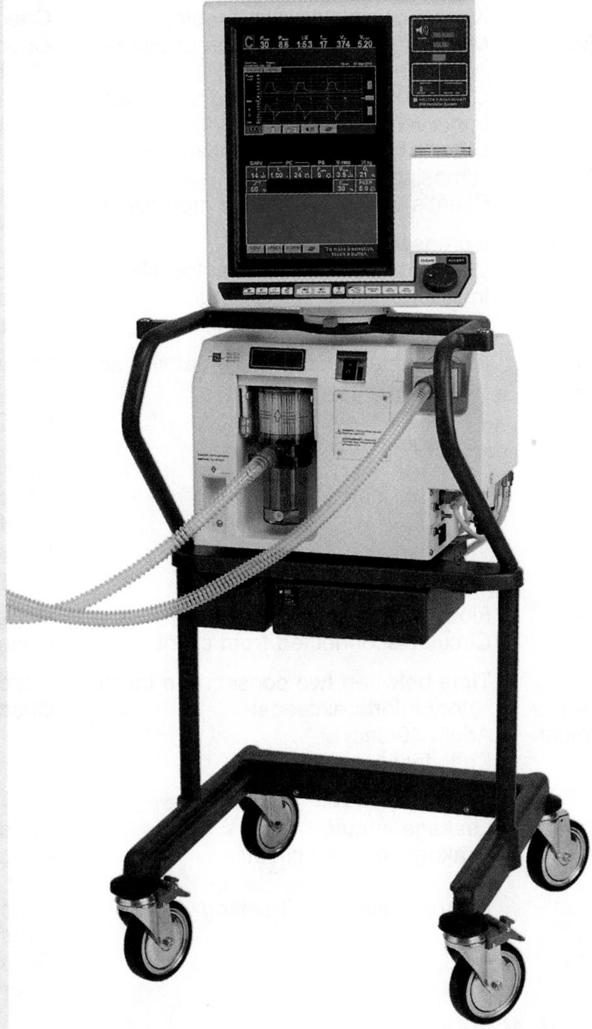

Puritan Bennett 840 Ventilator.

Troubleshooting Alarms

Display Message	Possible Cause	Remedy
HIGH CONTINUOUS PRESSURE	Airway pressure higher than set PEEP plus 15 cm H_2O for more than 15 sec	Check client Check circuit Check ventilator settings and alarm limits
CHECK TUBINGS	Disconnected pressure transducer (expiratory) Blocked pressure transducer (expiratory) Water in expiratory limb of ventilator Wet bacterial filter Clogged bacterial filter	Check ventilator internals on expiratory side Refer to service Replace filter Remove water from tubing and check humidifier settings, i.e., relative humidity Check heater wires in humidifier (if present)
AIRWAY PRESSURE TOO HIGH *Note:* If airway pressure rises 6 cm H_2O above set upper pressure limit, the safety valve opens. Safety valve also opens if system pressure exceeds 120 cm H_2O.	Kinked or blocked client tubing Mucus or secretion plug in endotrachial tube or in airways Client coughing or fighting ventilator Inspiratory flow rate too high Improper alarm setting	Check client Check ventilator settings and alarm limits

Bridge continued on following page

BRIDGE TO CRITICAL CARE *Continued*

Display Message	Possible Cause	Remedy
LIMITED PRESSURE *Note:* Alarm is active only in PRVC and VS modes	Kinked or blocked client tubing Mucus or secretion plug in endotracheal tube or in airways Client coughing or fighting ventilator Improper alarm setting Client's lung/thorax compliance decreasing Client's airway resistance increasing	Check client Check ventilator settings and alarm limits
EXPIRED MINUTE VOLUME TOO HIGH	Increased client activity Ventilator selftriggering (autocycling) Improper alarm limit setting Wet flow transducer	Check client Check trigger sensitivity setting Check alarm limit settings Dry the flow transducer
EXPIRED MINUTE VOLUME TOO LOW	Low spontaneous client breathing activity Leakage in cuff Leakage in client circuit Improper alarm limit setting	Check client Check cuff pressure Check client circuit (perform leakage test if necessary) Check pause time and graphics to verify Consider more ventilatory support for client
EXPIRED MINUTE VOLUME DISPLAY READS 0	Flow transducer faulty Circuit disconnected from client	Replace flow transducer Connect Y-piece to client
APNEA ALARM *Note:* If in VS, ventilator will revert to PRVC. Back-up rate and time must be set.	Time between two consecutive inspiratory efforts exceeds: Adult: 20 sec. Pediatric: 15 sec. Neonate: 10 sec.	Check client Check ventilator settings
PEEP/CPAP AND/OR PLATEAU PRESSURE FAILS TO BE MAINTAINED	Leakage in cuff Leakage in client circuit Improper alarm limit setting	Check cuff pressure Check client circuit (perform leakage test if necessary) Check pause time and graphics to verify Consider more ventilatory support for client

CPAP, continuous positive airway pressure; PEEP, positive end-expiratory pressure; PRVC, pressure-regulated volume control; VS, volume support.

Modified from *Servo Ventilator 300 operating manual 8.0* (1996). Solna, Sweden: Siemens-Elema AB.

Flow-cycled ventilators are triggered to stop when a preset flow rate has been achieved.

Modes of Ventilation

The ventilation mode refers to the way the client receives breaths from the ventilator. There are several conventional modes of CMV (Table 63–2).

Triggering Mechanisms

All breaths given to the client must be initiated or triggered. Triggering mechanisms can be based on (1) time, (2) negative pressure, (3) flow, or (4) volume.

Time-triggered inhalation is used to manage clients who cannot breathe on their own. The ventilator will trigger a breath after a preset time, serving as a back-up in case a client's own breathing rate falls below a preset value.

Negative pressure inhalation is triggered by the initial negative pressure that begins inspiration. As soon as the client initiates a breath, the ventilator is triggered to produce inhalation. The sensitivity of the system is set to reduce the workload of breathing. Pressure fluctuations (e.g., hiccoughs, leaks) can cause premature triggering.

Flow-triggered inhalation occurs when the client can initiate a breath. The ventilator completes the breath by sensing the flow of air into the chest. This system works well in combination with positive end-expiratory pressure (PEEP).

Volume-triggered ventilation occurs when the ventilator completes the breath to maximize inhaled gas volumes.

Alarms

Ventilators have several alarms to assist with their safe use (see Bridge to Critical Care).

Positive End-Expiratory Pressure and Continuous Positive Airway Pressure

PEEP and CPAP are techniques applied during expiration whereby intrathoracic pressures are not allowed to return to ambient atmospheric pressure. The PEEP and CPAP

TABLE 63–2 MODES OF MECHANICAL VENTILATION

Mode	Description
STANDARD MODES	
Continuous mechanical ventilation (CMV)	Ventilator delivers preset tidal volume and respiratory rate. No allowance for spontaneous breaths. Since ventilator is not responsive to client, this can lead to agitation and asynchrony.
Assist/control ventilation (A/C)	Spontaneous inspiratory effort of client triggers ventilator to deliver preset tidal volume. If client does not trigger an assisted breath, ventilator delivers breaths at preset respiratory rate.
Intermittent mandatory ventilation (IMV)	Ventilator delivers preset tidal volume and respiratory rate. Client can take unassisted spontaneous breaths between preset breaths. "Stacking" can occur when voluntary preset breaths occur simultaneously.
Synchronized intermittent mandatory ventilation (SIMV)	Similar to IMV except that preset ventilator breaths are synchronized with client's spontaneous breaths to avoid "stacking" of breaths. Can develop "stacking" of breaths and asynchrony.
Positive end-expiratory pressure (PEEP)	Preset amount of pressure stays in the lungs at the end of exhalation, keeping alveoli open. Used in conjunction with CMV, A/C, IMV, or SIMV
High-frequency ventilation (HFV)	Ventilator delivers breaths at a rate of greater than 60/min and at tidal volumes considerably lower than normal
Inverse ventilation ratio	Inspiration time is lengthened to over half of respiratory cycle. Reduces tendency to collapse alveoli, since they do not empty
Differential lung ventilation	Each lung is ventilated separately; special intubation needed with bifurcated endotracheal tube or two endotracheal tubes
WEANING MODES	
Continuous positive airway pressure (CPAP)	Similar to PEEP, but for the client who is breathing entirely on own (i.e., no ventilator-generated breaths)
Pressure support ventilation (PSV)	Client breathes spontaneously, but ventilator provides a preset level of pressure assistance with each spontaneous breath (inspiration only)
Volume support	Same as pressure support; tidal volume guaranteed
USE OF UNCONVENTIONAL GASES	
Nitric oxide	Relaxes smooth muscle of airway and arterioles. Used in ARDS
Helium	Carries oxygen at a lower density. Used to treat obstruction of large airways
GAS EXCHANGE DEVICES	
Extracorporeal membrane oxygenator (ECMO)	External oxygenation of blood. Blood is removed, oxygenated, and returned to the body without use of heart or lungs
Intravascular oxygenator	An oxygen/carbon dioxide exchange device is implanted in the inferior vena cava

Adapted from Boggs, R. L., & Wooldridge-King, M. (1993). *AACN procedure manual for critical care.* Philadelphia: W. B. Saunders.

are used to apply positive airway pressure that keeps the alveoli open and reduces the amount of shunting, allowing the use of lower levels of FiO_2 (Fig. 63–2*C*). This increased pressure also increases FRC and enhances oxygenation as a result of the enlarged surface area that is available for diffusion. CPAP is applied to a client with spontaneous respiration; PEEP is applied during mechanical ventilation. Positive pressures of 5 to 20 cm H_2O are typically used in adults. Pressures may be adjusted until the level is found that produces the best PaO_2 without producing adverse effects. This level is called "best PEEP."

Risks of PEEP include overdistention of the alveoli, ventilation-perfusion ($\dot{V}/\dot{Q}$) mismatch, subcutaneous emphysema, and decreased cardiac output from increased intrathoracic pressure.

PHYSIOLOGIC CHANGES AFTER MECHANICAL VENTILATION

Many physiologic changes occur when a client is placed on mechanical ventilation. Decreased cardiac output is the most common of these. Normal unassisted respiration begins with subatmospheric pressure. Negative pressure increases during inhalation and decreases during exhalation. Positive pressure applied to the airway has the opposite effect. As positive pressure inflates the lungs, pressure in the thorax builds, decreasing the flow of blood to the vena cava and reducing blood flow to the right atrium of the heart. Exhalation is passive, and pressures return to their normal, resting, subatmospheric level. Positive pressure also briefly affects the left side of the heart by increasing filling and output. This increase is due to the displacement of blood from the pulmonary system into the left ventricle. However, this effect is noted only immediately after institution of PPV.

If PPV is continued for more than a few minutes, blood flow to and from the right ventricle is decreased. This, in turn, decreases the filling of the left ventricle, leading to a lowered cardiac output. The lowered cardiac output is reflected in the hypotension that clients commonly exhibit immediately after receiving mechanical ventilation. It is imperative that blood pressures be monitored closely.

Stretch injury may develop in the alveoli and release inflammatory mediators. The lowest possible tidal volume and PEEP are used.

Other body systems are also affected by PPV. As the diaphragm descends into the abdomen during the inspiratory phase, blood flow to the splanchnic area decreases, sometimes leading to ischemia of the gastric mucosa. Ischemia of the gastric mucosa may be one of the reasons that clients receiving PPV for an extended period have a high incidence of gastrointestinal (GI) bleeding and stress ulcerations. Decreasing blood flow to the splanchnic region also results in decreased blood flow to the kidneys. Decreased blood flow signals the posterior pituitary gland to increase secretion of vasopressin (antidiuretic hormone [ADH]). Elevated vasopressin levels lead to reabsorption of free water in the renal tubular cells, thereby increasing water retention. Lymphatic flow also decreases.

PPV can also cause neurophysiologic changes. When ABG values improve in acute, uncompensated respiratory failure, improved cerebral oxygenation results. A client with compensated *respiratory acidosis* (chronic CO_2 retention) may be adversely affected by positive-pressure breathing owing to "blowing off" (exhalation) of CO_2. Acute alkalosis may occur, producing faintness, dizziness, lightheadedness, and anxiety. If severe alkalosis persists, convulsions, cardiac dysrhythmias, and cerebral edema may occur. Cerebral edema may contribute to intensive care unit (ICU) psychosis.

Oxygen toxicity can develop in clients who receive oxygen at concentrations greater than 70% for as little as 16 to 24 hours. Oxygen free radicals are produced in excess of their normal consumption by antioxidants; oxygen free radicals damage cell membranes, which increases the risk of pulmonary fibrosis. Manifestations of oxygen toxicity include fatigue, lethargy, weakness, restlessness, and nausea and vomiting. Later manifestations include severe dyspnea, coughing, tachycardia, tachypnea, crackles, and cyanosis. Because these manifestations are vague, oxygen concentration is limited to the minimal amount needed to maintain oxygenation.

Nursing Management

The nurse coordinates efforts of the health care team, teaches and supports the client and family, monitors the client's response to ventilation, intervenes to maintain oxygenation and ventilation, and ensures that the client's complex needs are met. See the Care Plan for the Mechanically Ventilated Client.

Neuromuscular Blocking Agents

Sedation is often necessary to maintain ventilation by creating a synchronous respiratory pattern and reduce oxygen demand. In some clients, paralysis with neuromuscular blocking agents is also needed. The most common agents given are vecuronium (Norcuron) and pancuronium (Pavulon). Because neuromuscular blocking agents do not inhibit pain or awareness, they are combined with a sedative or an anxiolytic agent. Pain medication may also be required if the client has pain. If the client is awake, be aware of anxiety or fear related to inability to breathe independently. The story of a nurse on a ventilator is an excellent reminder of a client's perceptions.[13]

Several nursing precautions are needed while these medications are administered. Reorient the client often, and explain all procedures because the client can still hear but cannot move or see. Eye care with lubricating ointment is important.

Long-term use of neuromuscular blocking agents has been associated with prolonged neuromuscular weakness. To avoid these complications, carefully monitor the client's level of paralysis using a peripheral nerve simulator (PNS) (Fig. 63–6). The PNS delivers an electrical stimulus (single, tetanic, or train-of-four) to a nerve. The train of four is the most common stimulus used. The facial, ulnar, posterior tibial, or peroneal nerve can be used; most commonly, the ulnar nerve is used for ongoing evaluation.

Problems with the PNS can give false readings. Poor skin contact, improper electrode placement, or edema of the arm can lead to false-negative readings, suggesting that the client has too high of a blockade. Direct stimulation of the muscle can lead to finger-twitching and may give an erroneous reading. This direct stimulus would provide a false-positive twitch and may lead to administration of more medication than needed. Correlate the PNS response to your clinical observation of the client.

Weaning from a Ventilator

The physician decides when to begin gradually removing, or "weaning," the client from CMV. The modes of the ventilator that depend on the client's initiating a breath can be used as modes for weaning. The decision is usually based on assessments made by nurses and respiratory therapists. The length of time required for successful weaning generally relates to the underlying disease process and to the client's state of health before the ventilator was used. For example, a young client who is recovering from an overdose of drugs can usually be weaned rapidly, but a client with COPD who develops acute respiratory failure and has little or no pulmonary reserve often takes longer and requires much professional patience and skill. Criteria for weaning are shown in Box 63–2.

Techniques for Weaning

Weaning from mechanical ventilation can be accomplished in two ways.

"Rapid" Weaning. The rapid, or T-piece weaning, technique is often used when mechanical ventilation has been instituted only briefly. Start in the morning after the client has had a good night's rest. Place the client in the semi-Fowler position. The ventilator's respiratory rate may be reduced to half the original rate; in some cases, this step may be eliminated. Obtain ABG values in 30 minutes.

Text continued on page 1760

CARE PLAN

THE MECHANICALLY VENTILATED CLIENT

Nursing Diagnosis. Inability to Sustain Spontaneous Ventilation related to imbalance between ventilatory capacity and ventilatory demand

Outcomes. The client will have a normal respiratory rate and pattern, return of arterial blood gases (ABGs) and pulse oximetry to normal, decreased dyspnea, absence of air trapping, and no complications after continuous mechanical ventilation (CMV).

Interventions	Rationales
1. Check ventilator settings, FiO_2, alarms, and connections and endotracheal (ET) tube placement (use cm markings) at beginning of each shift, hourly thereafter, and after any changes.	1. Determine baseline values, and validate that settings are accurate. Ensure that alarms are functional.
2. Assess lung sounds.	2. Lung sounds should be present bilaterally (unless a previous change in lung sounds is known).
3. Check placement of the ET tube, and secure the tube.	3. The visible portion of the ET tube should not change. Check previous records for a mark that is visible (in cm). Securing prevents dislodgment.
4. Use a bite block.	4. A bite block prevents the client from chewing on the tube and ET tube compression.
5. Move the ET tube daily from one side of mouth to the other. Assess for signs of skin or mucous membrane irritation.	5. ET tubes can place pressure on the lips and oral mucosa.
6. Assess for agitation, distress, and "fighting" the ventilator.	6. An incorrect ventilator setup may be providing less air than the client requires.
7. Assess for an obstructed airway. If it is obstructed, manually inflate lungs with a resuscitation bag and 100% oxygen and suction the airway.	7. Airway obstruction with mucus may prevent oxygenation. Providing air to the client is imperative. A common cause of obstruction is retained secretions.
8. Sedate and paralyze the client if ventilator settings and oxygenation are adequate.	8. Sedation and paralysis may be required to prevent mismatch.
9. Medicate the client if pain is indicated.	9. Pain can lead to agitation.
10. Perform passive range-of-motion (ROM) or assisted ROM exercises; transfer the client to a chair when feasible.	10. Immobility leads to decreased respiratory muscle strength.

Evaluation. The timing of goal attainment will vary greatly because of underlying co-morbid conditions. Expect postoperative clients to require CMV for 24 hours or less. Clients with end-stage pulmonary disease may require prolonged ventilatory support.

Nursing Diagnosis. Impaired Gas Exchange and Ineffective Breathing Pattern related to underlying disease process and artificial airway and ventilator system

Outcomes. The client will have improved gas exchange and breathing pattern, ventilation of both lungs, no signs of hypoxemia (O_2 saturation > 92%, respiratory rate < 24/min, no restlessness); ABGs and acid-base balance will return to preintubation level or normal values.

Interventions	Rationales
1. Auscultate lung sounds and respiratory rate and pattern every 1 to 2 hours as needed.	1. Auscultation reveals the amount of fluid and secretion in the lungs; validates that the ET tube is placed correctly so that both lungs can be ventilated; determines ventilatory effectiveness.
2. Provide adequate humidity via the ventilator or nebulizer.	2. This step replaces the function of the upper airway to warm and humidify the inspired air; thins secretions to facilitate their removal.
3. Turn and reposition the client every 2 hours (see Fig. 63–8).	3. Both lungs can be fully ventilated; secretions can be mobilized.
4. Monitor ABG values and pulse oximetry.	4. Degree of oxygenation can be indicated; lack of improvement in ABGs may require a change in interventions.

Evaluation. If the client's underlying problem has been corrected by mechanical ventilation, these outcomes will be met quickly. If the client has a pre-existing pulmonary disease or is acutely ill, it may take several days for attainment of outcomes.

Nursing Diagnosis. Ineffective Airway Clearance related to inability to cough and stimulation of increased secretion formation in the lower tracheobronchial tree from the ET tube.

Outcomes. The client will have improved airway clearance, as evidenced by fewer crackles, fewer rhonchi, and an absence of fever.

Care Plan continued on following page

Interventions	Rationales
1. Assess the need for suctioning: noisy, wet respirations; restlessness; increased pulse and respirations; visible mucus bubbling into the ET tube; rhonchi; and an increase in peak airway pressure.	1. Detecting the need for suctioning early can prevent desaturation.
2. Thoroughly explain the procedure before starting, and provide reassurance to the client throughout.	2. Suctioning can be an uncomfortable and frightening experience.
3. Airway suctioning is performed on an "as-needed" basis, not at regularly scheduled intervals.	3. Suctioning can traumatize the airway and mucosa.
4. Select a catheter of appropriate size. The most common sizes for adults are 12F and 14F.	4. The suction catheter should never exceed half the diameter of an artificial airway or the natural airway it is to enter.
5. Avoid excessive vacuum pressures that may traumatize the airway.	5. The safe range of pressure for adults is 80 to 120 mm Hg.
6. Maintain sterility throughout the procedure. Use closed system for suctioning. Clean gloves can be used for closed suctioning; sterile gloves are needed for open suctioning.	6. Usual cilia clearance and cough are suppressed. Closed systems avoid opening the ET tube and exposing the airway to the environment.
7. Hyperoxygenate before and after each suctioning attempt and after the procedure. Increase the FiO_2 on the ventilator or manually ventilate the client.	7. Providing extra oxygen prevents desaturation from suctioning.

Evaluation. The ability to maintain a clear airway will require several days until the underlying problem (e.g., pneumonia) is stabilized and the client's strength returns.

Nursing Diagnosis. Anxiety related to dependence on CMV for breathing

Outcomes. The client will exhibit decreased anxiety as evidenced by reduction in the level of stress or anxiety and decreased feelings of powerlessness.

Interventions	Rationales
1. Develop a means of communication.	1. Communication allows the client to have needs met.
2. Place a nurse call device within the client's reach.	2. Anxiety is increased when fear of being alone is present.
3. Be available and visible.	3. The client's anxiety is alleviated when not alone.
4. Provide distractions (e.g., television, radio).	4. Anxiety is reduced because the client does not focus on the ventilator and noises.
5. Explain all procedures.	5. The client feels respected and fears are alleviated.
6. Medicate as necessary for anxiety.	6. Antianxiety medications and narcotics may be needed, but use them with caution during weaning because these drugs suppress respiratory drive.
7. Provide privacy.	7. Providing privacy demonstrates respect for the client.
8. Respect the client's rights and opinions.	8. The client feels respected and maintains dignity when included in discussion.
9. Provide a calm environment.	9. A frenzied environment engenders anxiety; if the client becomes anxious, ventilation is more difficult and oxygen needs increase.
10. Explain to the client and family that the client's vocal cords have been bypassed, which prevents talking; encourage them to use other modes of communication.	10. Clients can hear and respond even though they cannot talk.

Evaluation. Expect the client to remain moderately anxious while receiving CMV.

Collaborative Problem. High Risk for Complications of CMV and Positive-Pressure Ventilation (PPV)

Outcomes. The nurse will monitor the client for pulmonary barotrauma, cardiovascular depression, inadvertent extubation, and malposition of the ET tube.

Interventions	Rationales
1. Assess for acute, increasing, or severe dyspnea; agitation; panic; decreased or absent breath sounds; localized hyperresonance; increased breathing effort; tracheal deviation away from the side with abnormal findings; subcutaneous emphysema; and decreasing PaO_2 levels.	1. Barotrauma can lead to pneumothorax or tension pneumothorax.
2. Assess for an acute or gradual fall in blood pressure, tachycardia (early sign), bradycardia (late sign), dysrhythmias, weak peripheral pulses, acute or gradual increase in pulmonary capillary wedge pressure (PCWP), and respiratory "swing" (depression) in arterial or pulmonary artery wave forms during inspiration.	2. Cardiovascular depression can occur after an increase in tidal volume, positive end-expiratory pressure (PEEP), continuous positive airway pressure (CPAP), or with hyperinflation; positive pressure decreases venous return and cardiac output because of an increase in intrathoracic pressure.

Interventions | Rationales (continued)

3. Monitor for signs of inadvertent extubation: vocalization, low-pressure alarm, bilateral decrease in upper lobe airway sounds, gastric distention, clinical manifestations of inadequate ventilation; change in length of portion of ET tube that extends beyond the lip. If inadvertent extubation occurs, notify the physician, because reintubation is necessary; manage ventilation and oxygenation with a self-inflating resuscitation bag.
   - *Rationale:* 3. Inadvertent extubation can be obvious, as when the tube is found in the client's hand; it can also be obscure, as when the tube slips into the hypopharynx or esophagus.
4. Keep an intubation tray readily available.
   - *Rationale:* 4. Intubation supplies may be needed quickly.

Evaluation. Most complications of PPV occur within 48 hours after intubation. Inadvertent extubation can occur at any time.

Nursing Diagnosis. Risk for Infection related to impaired primary defenses in respiratory tract

Outcomes. The client will remain free of infection, as evidenced by clear sputum, no fever, clear lung sounds, no increased difficulty with ventilation (e.g., increased peak inspiratory pressure), white blood cell (WBC) count within normal limits, and respiratory rate less than 24 breaths/min.

Interventions	Rationales
1. Wash your hands thoroughly.	1. Hand-washing reduces spread of infection.
2. Use sterile technique for suctioning.	2. The respiratory tract is considered sterile.
3. Monitor the client for increased breathing effort, localized changes on auscultation, and changes in PaO_2.	3. Infected lung segments transmit sound differently (more solid) and do not permit gas exchange.
4. Provide oral care every 2 hours.	4. The client's mouth becomes dry, and stomatitis may develop from lack of oral secretions.
5. Drain water from ventilator tubing; do not drain water back into the humidifier.	5. Water may become a source of contamination, especially with *Pseudomonas.*
6. Monitor laboratory values, WBC count, and differential.	6. WBC count increases may indicate pulmonary infection.
7. Monitor sputum for changes in color, consistency, amount, and odor.	7. Infection may cause sputum to increase, darken, thicken, and become malodorous.

Evaluation. Infection usually develops after 72 hours of intubation unless the client is immunosuppressed.

Nursing Diagnosis. Altered Nutrition: Less Than Body Requirements related to lack of ability to eat while on a ventilator and to increased metabolic needs

Outcomes. The client will exhibit adequate nutritional intake, as evidenced by (1) stable weight or weight appropriate to height, (2) intake of adequate calorie levels, (3) no signs of catabolism, (4) wound healing, (5) absence of infection, (6) laboratory value within normal limits (prealbumin, total protein, transferrin), and adequate muscle strength to breathe spontaneously.

Interventions	Rationales
1. Provide adequate nutrition (high calorie intake, protein, vitamins, and minerals); provide a nutrition consult, as needed.	1. Intake of about 1200 kcal is adequate to maintain weight; inadequate nutrition decreases diaphragmatic muscle mass, decreases pulmonary function, and increases mechanical ventilation requirements.
2. Begin tube-feeding as soon as it is evident that the client will remain on CMV for a length of time (usually 2–3 days).	2. The client should not be allowed to go into a catabolic state.
3. Avoid excessive carbohydrate loads.	3. Carbohydrate loads may increase carbon dioxide production to the point of producing hypercapnia.
4. Weigh the client daily.	4. Changes in body weight are a reliable indicator of nutritional balance.
5. Monitor intake and output.	5. Fluids are still required, and output should match intake.
6. Assess for complications of tube-feeding: aspiration, diarrhea, constipation.	6. Feed the client while he or she is sitting upright, with the cuff inflated. Check for residual tube feeding every 4 hours (continuous feeding) or before beginning another feeding (intermittent feeding). Diarrhea is often caused by osmotic changes from an excessive concentration of tube feeding or the use of sorbitol-based elixirs; consider reducing the concentration or changing to crushed pills. Constipation is caused by a lack of free water within the feeding; add 100 ml of water every 4 to 6 hours if allowable.
7. If the client cannot tolerate enteral feeding, consider total parenteral feeding (TPN).	7. Clients with decreased gastrointestinal (GI) function may require parenteral nutrition to meet metabolic needs.
8. Monitor bowel sounds.	8. Bowel obstruction and ileus present as changes in bowel sounds.
9. Before tube-feeding or between bolus feedings, obtain pH and guaiac test every 8 hours.	9. A change in pH may indicate an increased risk of gastric stress ulcer. A positive guaiac test indicates bleeding.

Care Plan continued on following page

Evaluation. Malnutrition is preventable. Expect the client's weight to stabilize (unless there is fluid imbalance).

Nursing Diagnosis. Impaired Verbal Communication related to mute state when the ET tube is in place

Outcomes. The client will be able to communicate with health care providers in order to have basic needs met.

Interventions	Rationales
1. Help the client develop a means of communication. Keep a pencil and paper pad or a picture board readily available.	1. With an ET tube passing through the vocal cords, the client cannot cough effectively or speak.
2. Be patient and willing to spend time communicating.	2. Prevents feelings of frustration, and reduces anxiety.

Evaluation. Depending on preexisting problems (language), disease-related problems (confusion), or treatment-related problems (restraints) affecting communication, the timing to develop effective communication may be long or short.

Nursing Diagnosis. Altered Oral Mucous Membranes related to nothing by mouth (NPO) status

Outcomes. The client's gums and mouth will remain moist and ulcer-free.

Interventions	Rationales
1. Provide oral hygiene every 2 hours.	1. Oral mucous membranes dry in 2 hours.
2. Moisten the mouth with solutions that do not contain alcohol or lemon.	2. Alcohol and lemon solutions dry mucous membranes.
3. Moisten lips with lubricant.	3. Lubricants prevent drying, cracking, and excoriation.
4. Brush the client's teeth twice daily.	4. Dental caries are prevented by saliva.
5. Suction oral secretions from mouth.	5. Secretions pool in the oropharynx because of the inflated tracheal cuff.
6. Assess for pressure areas at the corner of the mouth from the ET tube.	6. ET tube repositioning may be required.

Evaluation. Oral mucous membranes can be restored to pink and moist within 24 hours. Oral care, however, is an ongoing need.

If these values are at or near baseline level, place the client on a T-piece at the same FiO_2. Obtain ABG values in 30 minutes. If the ABGs are again at or near baseline level and the respiratory rate is below 25 to 30 breaths/min, extubate. Apply a face tent for high humidity.

Some nurse researchers are questioning the practice of beginning a weaning program in the morning. You may see changes in practice in the next few years based on the correlation of circadian rhythms with ideal time frames for weaning.

"GRADUAL" (SLOW) WEANING. This technique is used after prolonged mechanical ventilation or if a neuromuscular disorder is present. The first step is to ascertain whether spontaneous breathing is present. Once spontaneous breathing has been established, slowly reduce the amount of ventilatory support. Continue to reduce ventilatory support until the client can accept full responsibility for his or her own ventilatory requirements. This process may be accomplished through increasingly longer periods of time on a T-piece (followed by periods of CMV support) or by decreasing the rate of intermittent mandatory ventilation (IMV) or synchronized IMV (SIMV) breaths. This technique may take weeks or even months. Patience is crucial.

Difficulties in Weaning

A first weaning attempt may not be successful for several reasons:

- Decreased muscular strength caused by protein-carbohydrate malnutrition or certain disease processes or caused by incoordination of respiratory muscles from disuse after prolonged CMV
- Increased work of breathing due to increased airway resistance, abdominal distention, a small-diameter artificial airway, upper airway obstruction, or unresolved acute lung diseases
- Increased ventilation requirements
- Difficulty managing secretions
- Psychological factors, such as fear

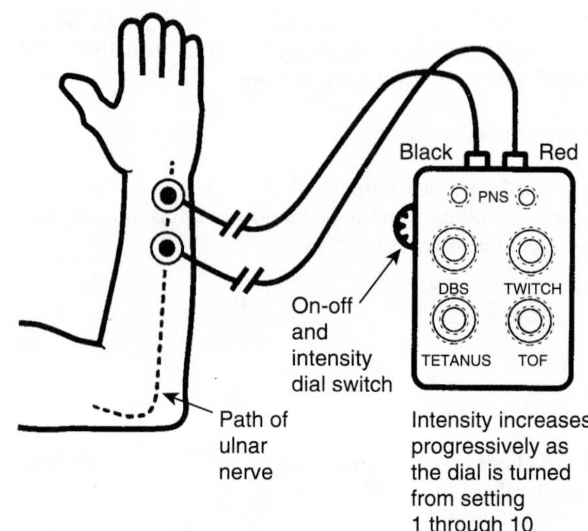

FIGURE 63–6 Peripheral nerve function is assessed with a nerve stimulator. (From Thelan, L. A., et al. [1998]. *Critical care nursing: Diagnosis and management* [3rd ed.]. St. Louis: Mosby–Year Book.)

BOX 63–2 Criteria for a Weaning Trial

Respiratory Criteria

Minute ventilation $\leq$ 15/L min
Respiratory rate $\leq$ 38 breaths/min
Tidal volume $\geq$ 325 ml
Maximum inspiratory pressure ≤ -15 cm H_2O
$FiO_2 \leq 50\%$

Other Criteria

Improvement, correction, or stabilization of the active disease process
Nutritional and fluid status sufficient to maintain the increased metabolic needs and demands of spontaneous respiration
Adequate physical strength and mental alertness
Afebrile status (any infections controlled)
Stable cardiovascular, renal, and cerebral status
Optimal levels of arterial blood gases, electrolytes, hemoglobin, and other laboratory tests

If the first attempt at weaning is not successful, determine the reasons and try to eliminate them in subsequent attempts. Clients who require prolonged ventilatory support and extended periods of weaning often do best in a setting that promotes rehabilitation concepts. These clients can usually be transferred to subacute or extended care facilities.

Extubation

Once the client has been weaned successfully and has demonstrated adequate ventilatory effort and an acceptable level of consciousness to sustain spontaneous respiration, the ET tube may be removed. ET tubes are removed on physician's orders and only by health care team members qualified to reintubate if necessary. The occurrence of laryngospasm and tracheal edema after extubation may occlude the airway, requiring reintubation.

The ET tube is suctioned, the cuff deflated, and the tube removed. Immediately after extubation, the client is usually given oxygen. Assess the client for signs of respiratory distress and hypoxemia, as evidenced by restlessness, irritability, tachycardia, tachypnea, and decreased PaO_2 or increased $PaCO_2$. If these signs are noted, notify the physician and prepare for reintubation.

Some clients are restless and extubate themselves. Because the cuff is not deflated, the tracheal wall can be damaged and bleeding can ensue. In most cases, the client requires reintubation, which must be done swiftly to prevent hypoxemia and to avoid needing to insert the ET tube through swollen tissues. Sometimes, however, the client can be monitored and not reintubated, especially if the time for extubation was approaching.

Dysfunctional Ventilatory Weaning Response

Some clients cannot adjust to lowered levels of mechanical ventilation, and the process of weaning them from the ventilator is delayed. The nursing diagnosis *Dysfunctional Ventilatory Weaning Response related to respiratory muscle fatigue or anxiety* may be used. Manifestations of respiratory muscle fatigue include a respiratory rate more than 30 breaths/min, increased $PaCO_2$, abnormal patterns of breathing, hemodynamic changes such as dysrhythmias, diaphoresis, anxiety, and dyspnea.

An unsuccessful attempt to wean the client may have taken place, resulting in reventilation. When the client can not sustain ventilation independently, the ventilator is set at full ventilation; the client has no spontaneous breaths and, therefore, can rest.

Once the client has rested, attempts at weaning should begin again. Some clients can never be weaned from mechanical ventilation. Those clients can be managed in less acute care units or at home for many years.

Home Care of Ventilater-Dependent Clients

Some clients become stable and can be discharged from acute care and return home. The Bridge to Home Health Care feature provides ways to assist the ventilator-dependent client.

ADULT RESPIRATORY DISTRESS SYNDROME

ARDS is a sudden, progressive form of respiratory failure characterized by severe dyspnea, hypoxemia, and diffuse bilateral infiltrates. It follows acute and massive lung injury that results from a variety of clinical states, often occurring in previously healthy persons. The syndrome was first described in 1967 and has been alternatively referred to by several terms, including shock lung, wet lung, Da Nang lung (from the Vietnam War era), posttraumatic lung, congestive atelectasis, capillary leak syndrome, and adult hyaline membrane disease. Tremendous advances in the treatment of this condition have occurred over the last two decades.

Etiology and Risk Factors

ARDS develops as a result of ischemia during shock, oxygen toxicity, inhalation of noxious fumes or fluids (e.g, gastric acid), or inflammation from pneumonia or sepsis that traumatizes the alveolar capillary membrane. The insult may be directly to lung tissue or indirect, occurring in other body areas. Conditions leading to ARDS are listed in Box 63–3. Early recognition and treatment of these conditions may reduce the risk of ARDS.

Pathophysiology

The hallmark of ARDS is increased permeability of the alveolar membrane, with resultant movement of fluid into the interstitial and alveolar spaces. This leads to the development of noncardiogenic pulmonary edema, which decreases lung compliance and impairs oxygen transport.

Four phases of ARDS have been described:

Phase 1 consists of damage to the capillary endothelium with adhesion of neutrophils and initiation of protease enzymes. Inflammatory responses accompany the pulmonary parenchymal damage, leading to the release of toxic mediators, the activation of complement, the mobilization of macrophages, and the release of vasoactive substances from mast cells.

Phase 2 is further damage to the basement membrane, interstitial space, and alveolar epithelium. Fibrin, blood, fluid, and protein exude into the interstitial

BRIDGE TO HOME HEALTH CARE

Living with a Ventilator

It is essential that the ventilator-dependent child or adult client, family members, and informal caregivers have good communication with the home health nurse, the physician, and community resources. As soon as you obtain physician's orders and establish a plan of care, call the durable medical equipment (DME) supplier to review all of the equipment that will be required in the home setting. You may want to plan a shared visit with the DME supplier to evaluate and coordinate all of the client's equipment needs.

Next, check with the local electric company to ensure that your client will be placed on a list of people to receive priority attention and whose power service will be restored immediately in the event of an electrical failure. The client should have a portable battery-operated ventilator in the home in case of a power failure.

Plan to spend several hours with the family and informal caregivers during your initial home visit. Instruct them about the equipment, ventilator alarms, suctioning devices, dressing changes, and other care requirements. Be certain that they give satisfactory return demonstrations to you. The equipment may be very intimidating to the family. Write as much information as possible; provide the telephone numbers of the home health agency, the equipment supplier, the physician, other pertinent agencies, and yourself to use in case of emergency.

Write instructions about the use of the equipment in terms that the caregivers and family understand. Using large print, use a large piece of paper to make it easy to read and easy to find. It is not unusual to have families or caregivers forget most of the information you have presented after you leave. Remember, the client is probably happy to be back in the home environment, but the family may be very anxious and frightened. Address the availability of respite care or other community resources to provide the family with periods of rest and relaxation.

Equipment noise may be a nuisance. Suggest a radio, television, or cassette player with earphones. If clients can communicate through writing, make sure they have a computer, small chalkboard, or dry erase board. The family and client may want to hire a tutor to teach sign language, but most people learn to read lips.

Keep the room light and open; a bed by a window offers extrasensory stimuli. Caution the family to avoid irritants or pollutants (smoke, animal fur or dander, bird feathers, heavy dust).

Your creativity and imagination can help provide a safe and secure home setting when a ventilator is needed.

Terri Sellin Brown, RN, BSN, *School Nurse, Omaha Public Schools, Omaha, Nebraska*

spaces around the alveoli and increase the distance across the capillary membrane.

Phase 3 occurs when the source of injury persists and more mediators of inflammation are released.

Phase 4 is the irreversible deposition of fibrin into the lung, further decreasing compliance and oxygenation.

Throughout the process, the type II alveolar cells, which produce pulmonary surfactant, are also damaged, which leads to atelectasis and further impairment in lung distensibility and gas exchange. The end result is a significant $\dot{V}/\dot{Q}$ imbalance and profound arterial hypoxemia (see Understanding ARDS and Its Treatment).

Clinical Manifestations

The initial insult of ARDS is followed by a period of apparently normal lung function that may last from 1 to 96 hours. Then hypoxemia rapidly develops and progresses along with decreasing lung compliance and development of diffuse lung infiltrates.

The earliest clinical manifestation of ARDS is usually an increased respiratory rate. Breathing becomes increasingly labored; the client may exhibit air hunger, retractions, and cyanosis. Chest auscultation may or may not reveal the presence of adventitious sounds. If present, abnormal sounds may range from fine inspiratory crackles to widespread coarse crackles. ABG analysis reveals increasing hypoxemia ($Pa_{O_2} < 60$ mm Hg) that does not respond to increased fraction of inspired oxygen levels ($Fi_{O_2} < 40\%$) and compensatory hypocapnia. In the early stages, respiratory alkalosis is present because of hyperventilation. Later, metabolic acidosis develops from increased work of breathing and hypoxemia. The chest x-ray usually demonstrates diffuse, bilateral, and rapidly progressing interstitial or alveolar infiltrates (Fig. 63–7). Bronchial washing and biopsy may be used to determine whether infection is present.

Outcome Management

The keys to successful management of ARDS are early detection and initiation of treatment. The goals of medical management are (1) respiratory support, (2) maintenance of hemodynamic stability, (3) treatment of the underlying cause, when possible, and (4) prevention of complications.

Medical Management

Support Respiration and Ventilation

ET intubation, mechanical ventilation, and PEEP are usually required to maintain adequate blood oxygen levels. Smaller tidal volumes may be used to reduce the risk of lung injury. Other alternative modes of ventilation (e.g., extracorporeal membrane oxygenation [ECMO], intravascular oxygenation) may be employed in some situations. Inverse ratio ventilation (IRV) is one method of increasing mean airway pressure without creating further peak pressures in the alveolus from PEEP. IRV increases the inspiratory portion of each breath to more than half the respiratory cycle.

Nitric oxide (NO) is now being used more often in the treatment of ARDS. NO prevents calcium influx into cells and thereby causes vasodilation. Inhaled NO dilates the capillary bed of the lungs, which in turn reduces the

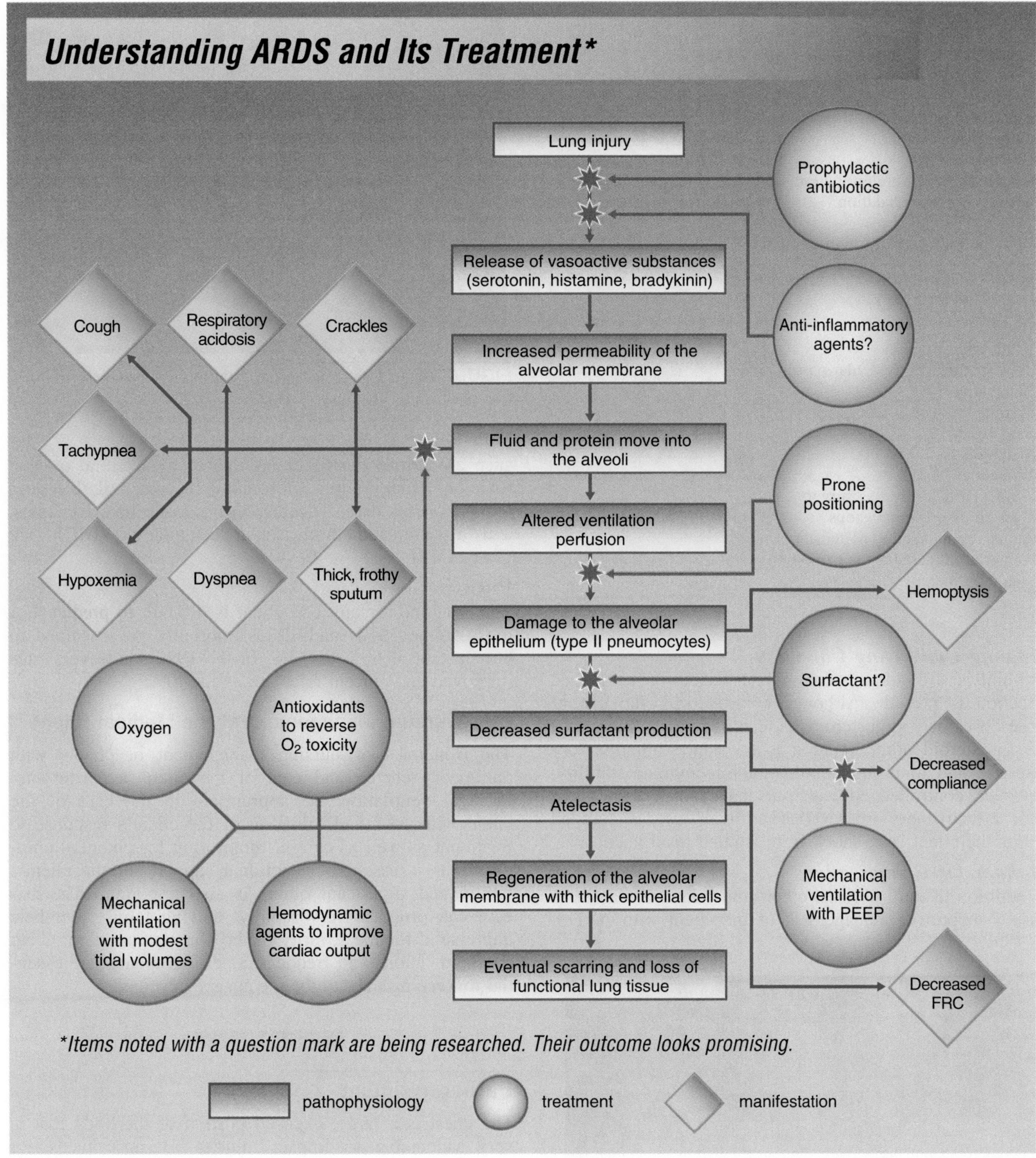

pressure in the pulmonary arteries without lowering systemic blood pressure.

Scavengers of oxygen free radicals are being used. Alpha$_1$-antitrypsin has also been effective in reducing the degradative effect of the proteases. Pharmacologic efforts to inhibit the substances released by the endotoxins, neutrophils, and macrophages are also being explored.[42] To date, no effective method of administering surfactant has been developed.

The prone position has been used to improve oxygenation by changing the distribution of perfusion, sometimes by 50%.[12] Side effects include hypotension, desaturation, and dysrhythmias, although these appear to be short term. The prone position is shown in Figure 63–8.

Maintain Hemodynamic Stability

Hemodynamic monitoring is used to observe the effect of fluids and degree of pulmonary edema. The use of pharmacologic agents in the treatment of ARDS varies according to the client's underlying disease process. Inotropic agents (e.g., dobutamine) may be indicated to improve cardiac output and to increase systemic blood pressure. Fluids are restricted, and diuresis is produced.

BOX 63–3 Risk Factors for Adult Respiratory Distress Syndrome

Direct Pulmonary Trauma

Viral, bacterial, or fungal pneumonias
Lung contusion
Fat embolus
Aspiration (e.g., foreign material, drowning, vomitus)
Massive smoke inhalation
Inhaled toxins
Prolonged exposure to high concentrations of oxygen

Indirect Pulmonary Trauma

Sepsis
Shock
Multisystem trauma
Disseminated intravascular coagulation
Pancreatitis
Uremia
Drug overdose
Anaphylaxis
Idiopathic
Prolonged heart bypass surgery
Massive blood transfusions
Pregnancy-induced hypertension
Increased intracranial pressure
Radiation therapy

Treating Underlying Condition

Antibiotics are administered if suspected or confirmed infection is present. Although controversial, the use of large doses of corticosteroids is also common. The rationale for steroid administration is to reduce inflammatory response and to promote pulmonary membrane stability; however, controlled clinical trials have not demonstrated their effectiveness in ARDS, and their use is avoided unless the client is in shock from adrenal insufficiency.

Monitor for Complications

In addition to lung fibrosis, other complications may arise during supportive management of the client with ARDS, such as cardiac dysrhythmias due to hypoxemia, oxygen toxicity, renal failure, thrombocytopenia, GI bleeding secondary to stress ulcers, sepsis from invasive lines, and disseminated intravascular coagulation (DIC) (see Chapter 75).

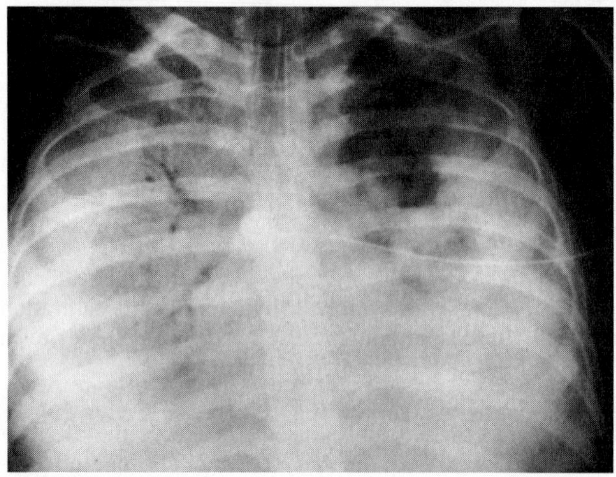

FIGURE 63–7 Adult respiratory distress syndrome (ARDS). This chest x-ray study shows massive consolidation from pulmonary edema following multisystem trauma. (From Fraser, R. G., et al. [1990]. *Diagnosis of diseases of the chest* [3rd ed., p. 493]. Philadelphia: W. B. Saunders.)

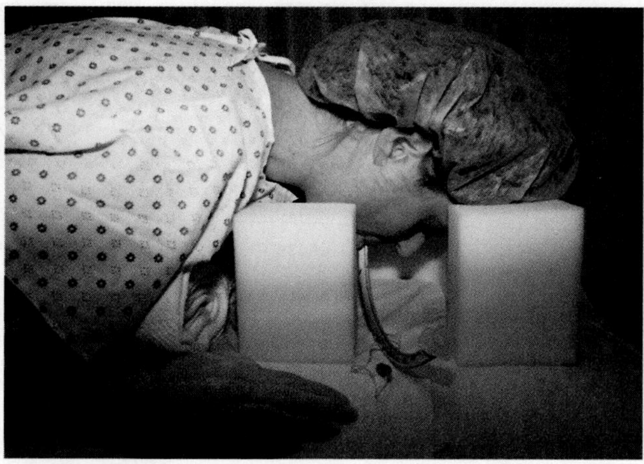

FIGURE 63–8 Use of the prone position to improve ventilation-perfusion. (Courtesy of H.E.A.D. Prone, Inc.)

PROGNOSIS

The outcome for any one client is difficult to predict. For most of the 1970s and 1980s, mortality rates seemed to be constant at 60% to 70%. In the 1990s, however, rates improved and current rates are about 40%.[13]

Nursing Management of the Medical Client

The principles of nursing management of clients with pulmonary edema and care of the client requiring mechanical ventilation are appropriate in the care of the client with ARDS. Evaluation of the client's response to treatment as well as careful monitoring for potential complications is essential. Emotional support for the client's family and significant others is also important. The disease can progress very rapidly, leaving family members unprepared for the severity of the client's condition. Clear communications and frequent condition updates are essential to keeping the family adequately informed.

CHEST TRAUMA

Pathophysiology

The chest is a large, exposed portion of the body that is very vulnerable to impact injuries. Because the chest houses the heart, lungs, and great vessels, chest trauma frequently produces life-threatening disruptions. Injury to the thoracic cage and its contents can restrict the heart's ability to pump blood or the lungs' ability to exchange air and oxygenate blood. Major dangers associated with chest injuries are internal bleeding and punctured organs.

Chest injuries can range from relatively minor bumps and scrapes to severe crushing or penetrating trauma. Chest injuries may be *penetrating* or *nonpenetrating (blunt)*. Penetrating chest injuries may cause an open chest wound, permitting atmospheric air into the pleural space and disrupting the normal ventilation mechanism.

Penetrating chest injuries may seriously damage the lungs, heart, and other thoracic structures.

Blunt injuries are most commonly deceleration injuries associated with motor vehicle crashes. Blunt chest trauma may also result from falls or blows to the chest.

Initial assessment is directed toward identifying and treating immediate life-threatening conditions. Any client with chest trauma should be considered to have a serious injury until it is proved otherwise. Airway patency, adequacy of breathing, and circulatory sufficiency (i.e., presence of shock), or ABCs, are always of primary concern.

Once initial emergencies have been addressed, assess the client more thoroughly (Box 63–4). A medical history helps identify any pre-existing conditions that may further complicate the injury. A thorough physical examination should be performed, with care being taken not to focus only on obvious injuries. Information about the accident (obtained from the injured client or witnesses) assists in the diagnosis of regional as well as anatomic injuries. A chest film and ECG are obtained for detection of possible pulmonary or cardiac impairment.

Outcome Management

Ventilation-perfusion imbalances may result from atelectasis, hemopneumothorax, flail chest, aspiration, or pulmonary contusion. Oxygen or mechanical ventilation may be required. General respiratory status (e.g., rate and depth of respirations, chest movement, spontaneous vital volumes) and ABG values should be monitored closely. Deterioration may indicate previously undetected injury or late-developing complications.

Therapeutic measures such as thoracentesis, chest tube insertion, bronchoscopic aspiration, and thoracotomy (see Chapters 59 and 62) may be indicated. Maintain effective functioning of any equipment used (e.g., chest drainage system). Help the client and significant others understand these procedures and the rationale for their use. Clients with chest injuries may experience significant hypovolemia. Fluid replacement is with blood and blood products, if indicated, or with crystalloid IV solutions (e.g., lactated Ringer's solution, normal saline).

Monitor continually for clinical manifestations of shock. Shock often results from hypovolemia, but in the chest-injured client it may also be caused by cardiac tamponade, cardiac contusion, flail chest, or tension pneumothorax. Central vascular pressure readings (central venous pressure [CVP] or pulmonary artery pressure [PAP]) require careful interpretation. Once the cause of shock is determined, rapid treatment is crucial (see Chapter 81).

Excessive blood loss may further compromise oxygenation. Assess external bleeding carefully, and estimate blood loss. Internal bleeding may result from injuries to the thoracic or abdominal viscera, torn muscles, or fractures. Considerable bleeding (2 L or more) into the pleural space may occur. This is usually detected quickly. Bleeding into areas such as the chest wall (e.g., from torn intercostal muscles) is more difficult to assess. A liter of blood can accumulate between the chest wall muscles without producing much swelling.

A chest-injured person may require large quantities of blood replacement. Until the results of typing and cross-matching are available, the client is given O-negative blood. The volume of blood replacement is determined through assessment of clinical findings, hemodynamic measurements, and laboratory results (e.g., hemoglobin and hematocrit). When possible, surgery is delayed until blood volume is restored.

Pain associated with chest injuries may cause the client to breathe rapidly and shallowly, which leads to atelectasis and pooling of tracheobronchial secretions. Analgesics minimize pain, permit periods of rest and relaxation, and allow the client to cough and to take deeper breaths. Narcotics are most effective if given via the IV route. Intercostal nerve blocks or epidural analgesia may be used in clients with underlying health problems. Splinting the chest may also be helpful.

BOX 63–4 Chest Trauma: Assessment and Interventions

1. Assess "ABCs":
   a. Maintain *a*irway, *b*reathing, and *c*irculation.
   b. Ensure adequate air movement.
2. Obtain a quick history:
   a. What happened?
   b. What was the mechanism of injury?
   c. How long ago did it happen?
   d. Where is the pain? Does it radiate?
   e. Is there anything that makes the pain better or worse?
   f. What does the pain feel like?
   g. How severe is the pain on a scale of 1 to 10?
   h. Is there a significant medical history?
3. Perform a quick (1-minute) assessment for:
   a. Shortness of breath and cyanosis
   b. Vital signs
   c. Skin color and temperature
   d. Wound size and location
   e. Paradoxical chest movement
   f. Distended neck veins
   g. Tracheal deviation
   h. Respiratory stridor
   i. Bilateral breath sounds
   j. Use of accessory muscles
   k. Estimated tidal volume
   l. Subcutaneous emphysema
   m. Sucking chest wounds
   n. Heart sounds
   o. Dysrhythmias
4. Quickly intervene:
   a. Administer oxygen.
   b. Cover any open chest wound.
   c. Control flail segment.
   d. Prepare to insert a chest tube.
   e. Initiate a large-bore intravenous line.

PNEUMOTHORAX

Pathophysiology

Pneumothorax is the presence of air in the pleural space that prohibits complete lung expansion. Air may escape into the pleural space from a puncture or tear in an internal respiratory structure (e.g., bronchus, bronchioles, alveoli). This form of pneumothorax is called *closed (spontaneous) pneumothorax* (Fig. 63–9A). Fractured ribs commonly lead to closed pneumothorax. Air may enter the pleural space directly through a hole in the chest wall (*open pneumothorax*) or diaphragm.

Clinical Manifestations

Clinical manifestations of *moderate* pneumothorax include tachypnea; dyspnea; sudden sharp pain on the affected side with chest movement, breathing, or coughing; asymmetrical chest expansion; diminished or absent breath sounds on the affected side; hyperresonance (tympany) to percussion on the affected side; restlessness; anxiety; and tachycardia.

Clinical manifestations of *severe* pneumothorax include all the preceding and distended neck veins; point of maximal impulse (PMI) of heart beat, or PMI shift; subcutaneous emphysema; decreased tactile and vocal fremitus; tracheal deviation toward the unaffected side; and progressive cyanosis.

Chest x-ray may reveal a slight tracheal shift away from the affected side and retraction of the lung back

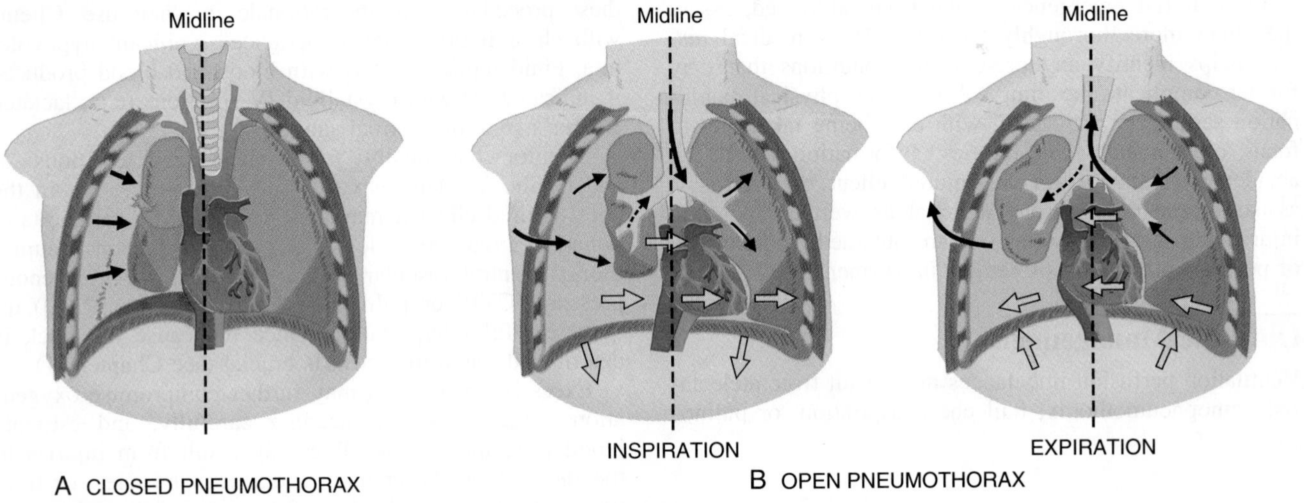

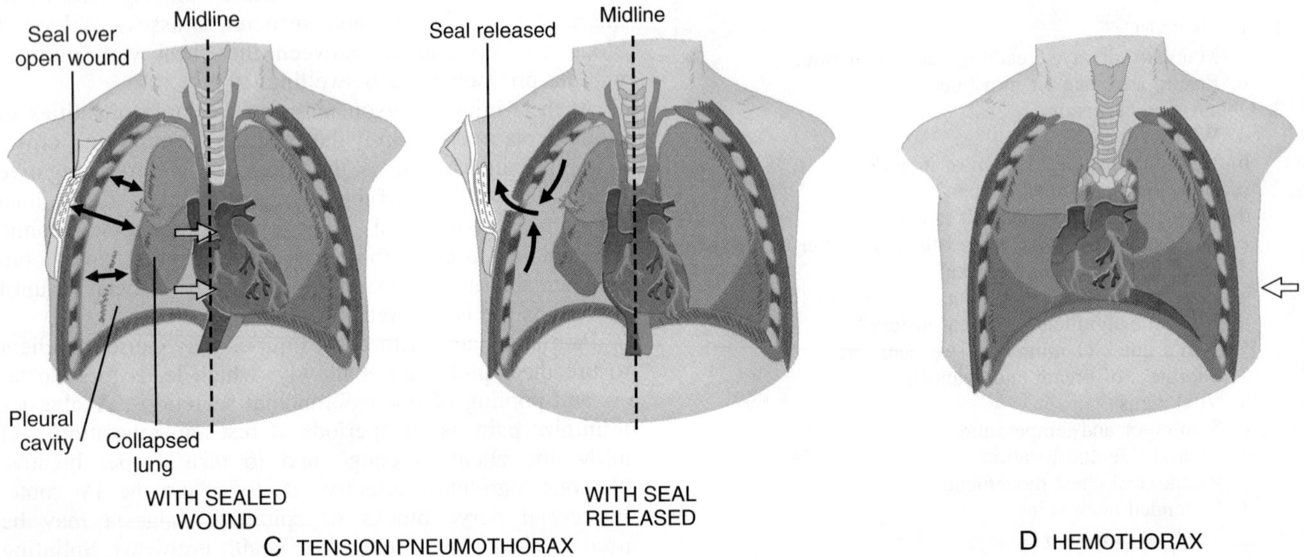

FIGURE 63–9 Pneumothorax.

A, Closed pneumothorax. The lung collapses as air gathers in the pleural space.

B, Open pneumothorax (sucking chest wound). *Solid and dashed arrows* indicate air movement; *open arrows* indicate structural movement. A chest wall wound connects the pleural space with atmospheric air. During inspiration, atmospheric air is sucked into the pleural space through the chest wall wound. Positive pressure in the pleural space collapses the lung on the affected side and pushes the mediastinal contents toward the unaffected side. This reduces the volume of air in the unaffected side considerably. During expiration, air escapes through the chest wall wound, lessening positive pressure in the affected side and allowing the mediastinal contents to swing back toward the affected side. Movement of mediastinal structures from side to side is called mediastinal flutter.

C, Tension pneumothorax. *Left,* If an open pneumothorax is covered (e.g., with a dressing), it forms a seal, resulting in tension pneumothorax with a mediastinal shift. A tear in lung structure continues to allow air into the pleural space. As positive pressure builds in the pleural space, the affected lung collapses, and the mediastinal contents shift to the unaffected side. *Right,* Tension pneumothorax is corrected by removing the seal (e.g., dressing), allowing air trapped in the pleural space to escape.

D, Massive hemothorax (*arrow*) below the left lung, causing collapse of lung tissue.

from the parietal pleura. (In pneumothorax, the collection of air is between the visceral and parietal pleura.) On chest x-ray, pneumothorax is expressed as a percentage. For example, a client may have a complete 100% to a partial 10% pneumothorax. The use of percentages allows for evaluation of progress on subsequent x-rays. If pneumothorax is suspected (but respiratory distress is too severe to permit x-ray confirmation), the physician may insert an 18-gauge needle (emergency thoracentesis) into the second or third intercostal space in the midclavicular line. Aspiration demonstrates whether free air is present in the pleural space.

Outcome Management

Most physicians prefer to insert a chest tube immediately into the pleural space via the fourth intercostal space at the midaxillary or anterior axillary line. The chest catheter is connected to closed chest drainage (see Chapter 62). The catheter permits the continuous escape of air and blood from the pleural space, thus helping the lung expand by reestablishing subatmospheric (negative) pressure in the pleural space (necessary for normal ventilation). Sometimes thoracotomy is done to explore the chest surgically and to repair the site of origin of the pneumothorax or hemothorax.

■ OPEN PNEUMOTHORAX AND MEDIASTINAL FLUTTER

Pathophysiology

An open pneumothorax occurs with sucking chest wounds. With this type of wound, a traumatic opening in the chest wall is large enough for air to move freely in and out of the chest cavity during ventilation (Fig. 63–9*B*). This abnormal movement of air through the chest wound produces a slurping or sucking noise that is audible in a quiet environment.

Etiology

Open sucking chest wounds may result from accidental injuries or surgical trauma. For example, if a chest drainage catheter is accidentally pulled out of a chest, the remaining puncture incision in the chest wall may become a sucking wound.

Outcome Management

When an open sucking chest wound is detected, emergency intervention includes immediately covering the wound securely with anything available. An airtight covering usually prevents tension pneumothorax and preserves ventilation of the opposite lung. Do not waste time looking for a sterile gauze petrolatum dressing (the ideal covering for such a wound) if it is not immediately available. Cover the wound with whatever is at hand (e.g., a towel) right away until someone can bring a sterile petrolatum dressing. When possible, fix the temporary dressing firmly in place with several strips of wide tape.

If the client is conscious and cooperative, ask him or her to take a very deep breath and to try to blow it out while keeping the mouth and nose closed. This pushing effort against a closed glottis helps push air out through the chest wound and reexpand the lung. When the client does this, apply the dressing before the client inhales again.

Stay with the chest-injured client after a dressing has been applied to a sucking wound. Carefully assess for indications of tension pneumothorax and *mediastinal shift* (contents of mediastinum are pushed to the unaffected side of the chest). These complications may develop if the air leak is in the lung or a bronchus; such a situation allows air to escape into the pleural space. In such instances, closing the chest wall wound with an airtight dressing prevents the outflow of escaping air. Thus, an open pneumothorax has been accidentally converted into a tension pneumothorax. If tension pneumothorax appears to be developing after the wound is sealed, immediately unplug the seal to allow the air to escape. Closed chest drainage is necessary to (1) remove the air from the pleural space and (2) allow the lung to reexpand if it is collapsed.

In addition to experiencing dyspnea and collapse of the lung on the affected side, the client with an open pneumothorax may experience *mediastinal flutter.* This complication results from air rushing in and out of the thoracic cavity on the affected side. With inspiration, the mediastinal structures (heart, trachea, esophagus) and collapsed lung are pushed toward the unaffected side. With expiration, these structures then move back toward the affected side. Fluttering, back-and-forth movements of these vital mediastinal structures produce severe cardiopulmonary embarrassment, which is fatal if not treated promptly.

Chest tubes are inserted on the affected side away from the open wound. Surgical closure of the wound may follow. Supplemental high-flow oxygen should be administered.

■ TENSION PNEUMOTHORAX AND MEDIASTINAL SHIFT

Although it is dangerous to have air moving in and out of the pleural space with each respiration (open pneumothorax), the client is at even greater risk when air moves only into the pleural space and cannot move back out (tension pneumothorax). Tension pneumothorax (Fig. 63–9*C*) is a true emergency. Air enters the pleural space with each inspiration, becomes trapped there, and is not expelled during expiration (i.e., one-way valve effect). Pressure builds in the chest as the accumulation of air in the pleural space increases. Tension pneumothorax most commonly occurs with blunt traumatic injuries and is frequently associated with flail chest injuries.

If untreated, tension pneumothorax collapses the lung on the affected side as intrapleural pressure or tension increases, causing a mediastinal shift (mediastinal contents—heart, trachea, esophagus, great vessels—pushed or "shifted" toward the chest's unaffected side). Mediastinal shift may cause (1) compression of the lung in the direction of the shift (i.e., the lung opposite the pneumothorax) and (2) compression, traction, torsion, or kinking of the great vessels; thus, blood return to the heart is dangerously impaired. The latter situation causes a subsequent decrease in cardiac output and blood pressure. Tension pneumothorax produces serious circulatory and pulmonary impairment that can be rapidly fatal. This is a high-priority emergency requiring prompt assessment and intervention.

Clinical Manifestations

Clinical manifestations of tension pneumothorax include (1) marked, severe dyspnea; (2) tachypnea; (3) subcutaneous emphysema in the neck and upper chest; (4) progressive cyanosis; (5) acute chest pain on the affected side; (6) hyperresonance (tympany) to percussion on the affected side; (7) tachycardia; (8) asymmetrical chest wall movement; (9) diminished or absent breath sounds on the affected side; and (10) extreme restlessness and agitation. Other manifestations include (1) neck vein distention; (2) laryngeal and tracheal deviation or shift to the unaffected side; (3) a feeling of tightness or pressure within the chest; (4) a PMI shift laterally or medially; (5) severe hypotension leading to shock; and (6) muffled heart sounds.

A suspected mediastinal shift may be confirmed by x-ray study. Laryngeal and tracheal deviation toward the unaffected side can be detected by gentle palpation and with x-ray study. ABG analysis demonstrates hypoxia and respiratory alkalosis. When mediastinal shift is severe and not immediately corrected, respiratory acidosis may ensue.

Outcome Management

The immediate intervention is to convert *tension* pneumothorax into *open* pneumothorax (a less serious disorder). Large-bore chest tubes (36 to 40 Fr.) are inserted on the affected side at the fifth intercostal space anterior to the midaxillary line. Once tubes are inserted, suction drainage should be established. If a delay is anticipated, a 14- to 18-gauge needle is inserted into the pleural space of the affected side at the level of the second intercostal space at the midclavicular line. Prompt thoracentesis to remove air may be life-saving. As trapped air rushes from a tension pneumothorax, the tension is relieved, the lung should reexpand, and if mediastinal shift is present, it corrects itself. Supplemental oxygen is administered.

HEMOTHORAX

Hemothorax may be present in clients with chest injuries. A small amount of blood (< 300 ml) in the pleural space may cause no clinical manifestations and may require no intervention (blood is reabsorbed spontaneously). Severe hemothorax (1400 to 2500 ml) may be life-threatening because of resultant hypovolemia and tension (Fig. 63–9*D*). Massive hemothorax is associated with 50% to 75% mortality.

Clinical manifestations include respiratory distress, shock, and mediastinal shift. There is dullness to percussion on the affected side.

A chest film confirms a diagnosis of hemothorax. If the client is in severe distress, the physician may aspirate blood from the pleural space by inserting a 16-gauge needle into the fifth or sixth intercostal space at the midaxillary line. To drain intrathoracic accumulations of blood, the physician inserts a large-caliber (36F or larger) chest catheter, which is then connected to a drainage system. An initial drainage of 500 to 1000 ml is considered moderate, and additional treatment may not be required. An initial drainage of 1500 ml or more or continued large amounts of drainage (200 ml/hr) warrants immediate exploratory thoracotomy. Fluid replacement with O-negative blood or autotransfusion of blood should be used.

Surgical repair of active bleeding may be needed.

CHEST FRACTURES

■ FLAIL CHEST

Severe chest injuries that compress the rib cage often produce a "crushed" chest in which the ribs are pushed in on lung tissue. By definition, a flail chest consists of fractures of two or more adjacent ribs on the same side and, possibly, the sternum, with each bone fractured into two or more segments (Fig. 63–10). The flail segment most commonly involves the lateral side of the chest. It is common for a fractured rib end to tear the pleura and lung surface (thereby producing *hemopneumothorax*) and for a crushed chest to have a flail segment. Pulmonary edema, pneumonitis, and atelectasis often develop rapidly when the chest is crushed because fluids tend to increase and collect at the injured site.

The "flail" segment no longer has bony or cartilaginous connections with the rest of the rib cage. Lacking attachment to the thoracic skeleton, the flail section "floats," moving independently of the chest wall during ventilation. This abnormality disrupts the normal bellows action of the thorax by causing *paradoxical motion,* during which the flail portion of the chest and its underlying lung tissue are (1) "sucked in" with inspiration (instead of expanding outward as normal) and (2) "blown out" with expiration, instead of collapsing normally inward. This alteration in normal chest wall mechanics diminishes the client's ability to achieve an adequate tidal volume and to produce an adequate cough. Hypoventilation and hypoxia may result, leading to respiratory failure. Furthermore, mediastinal structures tend to swing back and forth (mediastinal flutter) with significant paradoxical motion. These swings may seriously affect circulatory dynamics, producing elevated venous pressure, impaired filling of the right side of the heart, and decreased arterial pressure.

In addition, pulmonary contusion occurs, resulting in an accumulation of fluid in the affected alveoli, which leads to intrapulmonary shunting and further hypoxia. The full effects of pulmonary contusion may not be manifested until the height of the body's inflammatory response in 24 to 48 hours.

The client with a flail chest commonly experiences emotional and physical distress while trying to breathe in spite of excruciating pain. The client is typically cyanotic and severely dyspneic. Respirations are usually rapid, shallow, and grunting. Paradoxical movement of the chest wall is usually obvious. Hypercapnia and hypoxia worsen as the effort necessary to breathe further depletes the already diminished oxygen supply. Frequent assessment of ABGs is needed to monitor respiratory effectiveness and to detect acidosis. Various factors produce metabolic and respiratory acidosis in chest-injured clients.

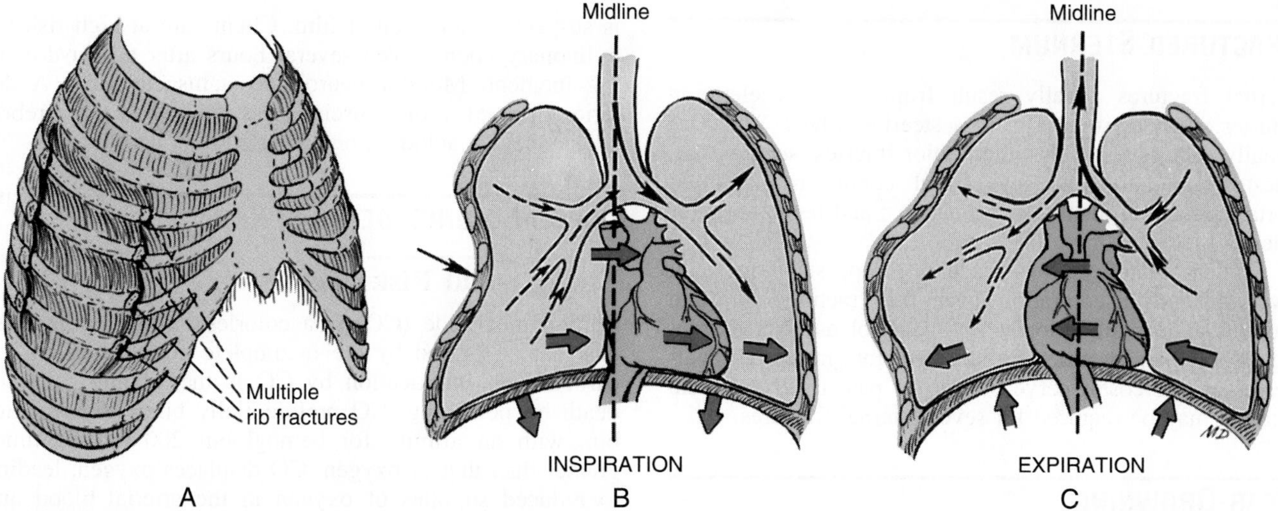

FIGURE 63–10 Flail chest. *Solid and dashed arrows* indicate air movement; *open arrows* indicate structural movement. *A,* A flail chest consists of fractured rib segments that are unattached (free-floating) to the rest of the chest wall. *B,* On inspiration, the flail segment of ribs is sucked inward. The affected lung and mediastinal structures shift to the unaffected side. This compromises the amount of inspired air in the unaffected lung. *C,* On expiration, the flail segment of ribs bellows outward. The affected lung and mediastinal structures shift to the affected side. Some air within the lungs is shunted back and forth between the lungs instead of passing through the upper airway.

Outcome Management

Treatment is usually with intubation and mechanical ventilation, which can accomplish the following:

- Restore adequate ventilation, thus reducing hypoxia and hypercapnia.
- Decrease paradoxical motion by using positive pressure to stabilize the chest wall internally.
- Relieve pain by decreasing movement of the fractured ribs.
- Provide an avenue for removal of secretions.

Internal stabilization with continuous ventilation may require 21 days or more. Muscle relaxants or musculoskeletal paralyzing agents may be administered to reduce the risk of separation of the healing costochondral junctions.

FRACTURED RIBS

Etiology

Rib fractures are common chest injuries, particularly in older adults. Such fractures are usually associated with a blunt injury, such as a fall, a blow to the chest, coughing or sneezing or (more frequently) the impact of the chest against a steering wheel during rapid deceleration. The fifth through the ninth ribs are most commonly affected.

Clinical Manifestations

Clinical manifestations include (1) localized pain and tenderness over the fracture area on inspiration and palpation, (2) shallow respirations, (3) the client's tendency to hold the chest protectively or to breathe shallowly in order to minimize chest movements, (4) bruising or surface markings (sometimes present) at the site of injury, (5) protruding bone splinters if the fracture is compound, and (6) a clicking sensation during inspiration when costochondral separation or dislocation is present.

Fractured ribs predispose to atelectasis and pneumonia because the pain causes shallow breathing and prevents effective coughing. Thus, secretions accumulate, which obstruct the bronchi and become a site of infection. Shallow breathing also reduces lung compliance.

Bone splinters from fractured ribs may cause pneumothorax or hemothorax by puncturing the lung and pleura. Chest films are carefully reviewed for 24 to 48 hours after injury for indications of these complications. Bright-red sputum may be coughed up if the lung has been penetrated. Assess the client for signs of pneumothorax or hemothorax, and report such findings promptly.

Outcome Management

Fractured ribs are generally treated conservatively with rest, local heat, and analgesics. Strapping the ribs is no longer recommended because it restricts deep breathing and can increase the incidence of atelectasis and pneumonia. The pain from fractured ribs usually lasts 5 to 7 days. Complete healing occurs in approximately 6 to 8 weeks.

If pain is severe enough to impair ventilation significantly, a local anesthetic solution may be injected at the fracture site itself. Intercostal nerve blocks may also be used. A client with an underlying chest or heart disease (e.g., COPD, heart failure) may benefit particularly from this type of pain management. A chest film should be taken after this procedure to ensure that pneumothorax has not occurred. Adequate pain control and splinting of the chest during coughing and deep breathing help the client with rib fractures to carry out these painful but vital activities more comfortably. Hospitalization may be required, especially in the elderly, whose vital capacity may be significantly compromised.

Fractured Sternum

Sternal fractures usually result from blunt deceleration injuries, such as impact from a steering wheel. They are usually accompanied by other major injuries, such as flail chest; pulmonary and myocardial contusions; ruptured aorta, trachea, bronchus, or esophagus; and hemothorax or pneumothorax.

Clinical manifestations include sharp, stabbing pain; swelling and discoloration over the fracture site; and crepitus. The main priority is to control associated injuries. A client with a nondisplaced fracture may need analgesics or intercostal nerve blocks for pain relief. Surgical fixation may be required for severe sternal fractures.

Near-Drowning

Clients who initially survive suffocation after submersion in a water or fluid medium are said to have experienced a near-drowning or *immersion syndrome.* Freshwater drowning (i.e., in a swimming pool) is more common than saltwater drowning. Alcohol or drug ingestion, overestimation of swimming skills, hypothermia, hyperventilation, and hypoglycemia are risk factors.

Both freshwater and saltwater wash out alveolar surfactant. Freshwater also changes the surface tension of surfactant. The loss of surfactant leads to alveolar collapse, intrapulmonary shunting, and hypoxemia. Poor perfusion and hypoxemia result in acidosis and eventual pulmonary edema. Near-drowning also compromises the respiratory system and leads to hypoxia, hypercapnia, cardiac arrest, and severe alterations in fluid-electrolyte balance. Bronchospasm, from aspirating water into the lungs, causes most drowning deaths. Cerebral edema from metabolic derangement is a major cause of death.

Outcome Management

Begin assessment and interventions with the ABCs. Obtain a history of the submersion. Include the length of submersion, temperature of the water, any associated injuries, and type of water. Note any respiratory efforts and adventitious sounds. Open the airway while maintaining spinal immobility. Assess the level of consciousness. Look for signs of hypoxia, such as confusion, irritability, lethargy, or unconsciousness. Obtain a complete set of vital signs. Additional injuries may be present, including associated trauma, spinal cord injury from diving, air embolism from scuba diving, and seizures.

For respiratory insufficiency, intubate and ventilate with 100% oxygen and 5 to 10 cm of PEEP to prevent the alveoli from collapsing. If the client is breathing, provide respiratory support with a non-rebreather mask.

Remove the client's wet clothing, and wrap the client in a warm blanket. Core rewarming may be indicated if the client is hypothermic. Rewarm the client slowly to avoid a rapid influx of metabolites (lactic acid) that may be trapped in the cold extremities.

Once the vital functions are stabilized, correct any acid-base or electrolyte abnormalities. Diagnostic studies include ABG analysis, complete blood count, electrolytes, appropriate toxicology studies if alcohol or drug ingestion is suspected, and a chest film. Clients are at high risk for pulmonary edema even several hours after a near-drowning incident. Monitor neurologic status carefully. A deteriorating level of consciousness may indicate cerebral edema, severe acidosis, or increased hypoxia.

Carbon Monoxide Poisoning

Etiology and Risk Factors

Carbon monoxide (CO) is a colorless, odorless, tasteless gas that is formed by the incomplete combustion of any carbon fuel. Intoxication by CO is the leading cause of death by poisoning. CO preferentially binds to hemoglobin, with an affinity for hemoglobin 200 to 230 times greater than that of oxygen. CO displaces oxygen, leading to reduced supplies of oxygen in the arterial blood and development of tissue hypoxia.

Generally, the client gives a history of exposure to CO after being found in an enclosed space in the presence of gases or fire. Faulty furnaces are also associated with CO poisoning. If CO poisoning is due to smoke inhalation, hoarseness, stridor, burns, or soot on the mouth or nose is present. Sputum may be black because of inhalation of soot. In a small number of clients, the skin will appear "cherry red" from high levels of oxygen in arterial blood.

Clinical Manifestations

Clinical manifestations are vague until levels of CO bound to hemoglobin (carboxyhemoglobin, or COHb) are around 40%. Manifestations include headache, vertigo, dizziness, nausea, and dyspnea on exertion when levels are below 20%. Above 20%, the client may have impaired concentration, clumsiness, and throbbing headache. Only when levels exceed 30% are manifestations more evident: irritability, visual changes, impaired thought, and vomiting. At 40% vital signs change and eventually coma ensues when levels are over 50%. The diagnosis is confirmed by measurement of carboxyhemoglobin levels in the blood.

Outcome Management

CO poisoning is treated by inhalation of 100% oxygen to shorten the half-life of CO to around an hour. Hyperbaric oxygen may be required to reduce the half-life of CO to minutes by forcing it off of the hemoglobin molecule. Reasons for CO poisoning must be explored and interventions directed at correcting those problems begun before hospital discharge. If the client's home furnace is faulty, it must be repaired. If the CO poisoning was a suicide attempt, crisis counselors should be used. Long-term neurologic and psychiatric consequences may develop, and the clients should be observed and followed up by their usual health care provider.

CONCLUSIONS

Two forms of respiratory failure exist: hypoxemic and ventilatory. Hypoxemic failure includes problems that lead to failure to transport oxygen and CO_2 across the capillary. Ventilatory failure includes disorders that impair neurologic triggers to breath and neuromuscular movement with respiration. Mechanical ventilation is a common method of treatment for both problems. Chest trauma involves life-threatening problems that demand prompt recognition and treatment.

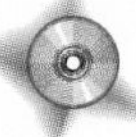

THINKING CRITICALLY

1. **You are caring for a client who is receiving mechanical ventilation. You have just suctioned the client's airway and begin to leave the room when the high-pressure alarm sounds. What should you do?**

Factors to Consider. What changes in the client can trigger the high-pressure alarm? What changes in the ventilator can cause high pressure?

2. **You are going to position the client prone to improve ventilation and perfusion. What considerations should be made before, during, and after the prone position is used?**

Factors to Consider. How can the tubes be moved safely with the client? What complications might occur in a prone position? What procedures cannot be done while the client is prone?

BIBLIOGRAPHY

1. Burns, S. M., et al. (1995). Weaning from long-term mechanical ventilation. *American Journal of Critical Care, 4,* 4.
2. Butler, K. (1995). Psychological care of the ventilated patient. *Journal of Clinical Nursing, 4,* 398.
3. Carroll, P. (1995). A med/surg nurse's guide to mechanical ventilation. *RN, 58*(2), 26.
4. Connelly, B., et. al. (2000). A pilot study exploring mood state and dyspnea in mechanically ventilated patients. *Heart and Lung, 29*(3), 173–179.
5. Jones, C. (1998). Inhaled nitric oxide: Are the safety issues being addressed? *International Critical Care Nursing, 14*(6), 271–275.
6. Kacmarek, R. (1999). Ventilator-associated lung injury. *International Anesthesiology Clinics, 37*(3), 47–64.
7. Klein, D. (1999). Prone positioning in patients with acute respiratory distress syndrome: The Vollman Prone Positioner. *Critical Care Nurse, 19*(4), 66–71.
8. Kosmos, C. (1995). Multype trauma. In S. Kitt (Ed.), *Emergency nursing.* Philadelphia: W. B. Saunders.
9. Lenart, S., & Garrity, J. (2000). Eye care for patients receiving neuromuscular blocking agents or propofol during mechanical ventilation. *American Journal of Critical Care, 9*(3), 188–191.
10. Rice, R. (1995). Home mechanical ventilator management. *Home Healthcare Nurse, 13,* 73.
11. Ruppert, S. D., Kernicki, J. G., & Dolan, J. T. (1996). *Critical Care Nursing* (2nd ed.). Philadelphia: F. A. Davis.
12. Schuster, D., & Kollef, M. (1998). Acute respiratory distress syndrome. In D. Dantzker & S. Scharf (Eds.), *Cardiopulmonary critical care* (3rd ed., pp 415–433). Philadelphia: W. B. Saunders.
13. Spencer, K. (1998). Near breathing: Nurse on a vent. *Plastic Surgical Nursing, 18*(3), 139–140.
13a. Tarizan, A. J. (2000). Caring for dying patients who have air hunger. *Journal of Nursing Scholarship, 32*(2), 137–143.
14. The acute respiratory distress syndrome network. (2000). Ventilation with lower tidal volumes as compared to traditional tidal volumes for acute lung injury and the acute respiratory distress syndrome. *New England Journal of Medicine, 342*(18), 1301–1308.
15. Valta, P., et al. (1999). Acute respiratory distress syndrome: Frequency, clinical course and cost of care. *Critical Care Medicine, 27*(11), 2367–2374.
16. Voggenreiter, G., et al. (1999). Intermittent prone positioning in the treatment of severe and moderate posttraumatic lung injury. *Critical Care Medicine, 27*(11), 2375–2382.
17. Woodruff, D. (1999). How to ward off complication of mechanical ventilation. *Nursing99, 29*(11), 35–39.
18. Wright, J., Doyle, P., & Yoshihara, G. (1996). Mechanical ventilation: Current uses and advances. In J. Clochesy, et al. (Eds.), *Critical care nursing.* Philadelphia: W. B. Saunders.

BRIDGE TO EVIDENCE-BASED PRACTICE

Arterial Oxygen Saturation Monitoring by Pulse Oximetry

QUESTIONS

How accurately do measures of oxygenation using pulse oximetry agree with measures by standard arterial blood gas (ABG) analysis?

What factors affect the accuracy of pulse oximetry?

CITATION

Jensen, L. A., Onyskiw, J. E., & Prasad, N. G. N. (1998). Meta-analysis of arterial oxygen saturation monitoring by pulse oximetry in adults. *Heart and Lung, 27,* 387–408.

STUDIES

Published studies of pulse oximetry in adult clients were located by searching four health science indexes. Because this review used a statistical technique called *meta-analysis* to summarize and compare findings, only studies that supplied the necessary statistics were included. Seventy-four studies published between 1976 and 1994 met the inclusion criteria; approximately 30% were published in the early 1990s.

Many studies compared the percentage of oxygen saturation of hemoglobin (SaO_2) using pulse oximetry with that obtained at the same time using standard ABG analysis (an approach called *repeated measures design*). A variety of participants were represented in the studies, including healthy volunteers, hospitalized clients, cardiac surgical clients, and critically ill clients. Forty-one models of pulse oximeters from 25 manufacturers were studied.

Summary of Findings

Accuracy

The percentage of SaO_2 in arterial blood is widely used as a clinically significant index of oxygenation, and ABG analysis has been the "gold standard" for measuring it. However, the disadvantages of ABG analysis include:

- The need to perform multiple arterial punctures
- The intermittent nature of the information it provides
- Delay between time of sampling and availability of results
- Cost

Pulse oximetry using a finger or ear probe and an oximeter unit is noninvasive, provides immediate and continuous measures, and is relatively inexpensive. Clearly, if pulse oximetry can be established as accurate and precise, it should be widely used.

Pulse oximeters are most accurate when the SaO_2 is in the range of 70% to 100%; in this range, most models were found to be accurate within 2% of the standard ABG analysis value. Overall, few pulse oximeters performed well at an SaO_2 level below 70%.

In 39 studies that provided the essential data for the statistical analysis, the oximetry value and the ABG value had a weighted, average correlation coefficient of .895. (The value is weighted because it has taken into account the number of subjects in each study.) A correlation coefficient (r) of 1.0 would indicate perfect correlation between the values from the two methods. In the studies conducted during the 1990s, the weighted mean correlation coefficient was .899. The highest correlation was in healthy adult volunteers and the lowest in critically ill patients ($r = .760$).

Four studies compared pulse oximetry accuracy with ear and finger probes. Finger probes were found to have a statistically higher correlation with ABG SaO_2 (weighted $r = .967$) than ear probes (weighted $r = .938$).

Factors Affecting Pulse Oximetry Accuracy

Most difficulties in using pulse oximeters produce a blank screen or an error message, indicating problems; however, some circumstances may result in false readings. As mentioned, pulse oximetry readings become less accurate when clients are extremely hypoxic (SaO_2 level <70%).[2, 9, 11, 13, 17] Readings are also inaccurate when abnormalities of the hemoglobin's oxygen-carrying ability (as in carbon monoxide poisoning)[5, 14, 16] or severe anemia is present.[17]

In the three studies on which data were available, the accuracy of pulse oximetry decreased when the blood pressure was low; the weighted average r between pulse oximetry values and ABG values was .582. In one study, the oximeter alarm sounded for systolic blood pressure below 100 mm Hg and accuracy was decreased.[6] In contrast, another study using a different manufacturer's model obtained reliable data when mean arterial pressure was less than 60 mm Hg.[11]

Five studies examined the effect of hypothermia on pulse oximetry. The weighted r from the three studies with the necessary statistics was .665, indicating a relatively low level of accuracy when the client is hypothermic. However, findings are quite variable. In one study, the oximeter did not work properly[17]; in another study the oximeter overestimated the SaO_2[7]; and in another study, high correlations existed whether or not the client was hypothermic.[12]

Whether skin pigmentation affects the accuracy of pulse oximetry is even more uncertain. In the one study in which essential data were provided, the weighted r was .800. In a study that involved testing of two manufacturers' models, there was greater inaccuracy in the subset of African Americans than in the total sample.[3] In clients with high serum bilirubin levels, there was a low correlation between pulse oximetry and ABG—the SaO_2 value was underestimated by the oximeter.[4]

Limitations/Reservations. This soundly conducted statistical analysis of findings from many studies details the extent to which SaO_2 values determined by pulse oximetry correspond with ABG values under a variety of clinical conditions. The report provides much information about the accuracy of specific models of pulse oximeters.

Research-Based Practice

Most pulse oximeters are adequately accurate under various clinical circumstances, but in some clinical situations they may not produce accurate readings. Be aware that pulse oximetry may not record accurate SaO_2 values if the client has any of the following conditions.*

* The direction of error for each of these conditions is provided in the review report.

Arterial Oxygen Saturation Monitoring by Pulse Oximetry *Continued*

- Severe hypoxia (e.g., respiratory arrest)
- Severe anemia
- Sepsis
- Shock
- Hypotension, severe hypertension
- Hypothermia
- Cardiac arrest
- Poor peripheral blood flow (e.g., hypovolemia, peripheral edema, cardiogenic shock)
- Carbon monoxide poisoning (e.g., smoke inhalation, inhalation of fumes from a heating system or motor vehicle)
- High bilirubin levels (liver dysfunction)
- Dark skin pigmentation
- Diseases in which the hemoglobin's oxygen-carrying ability is abnormal
- After receiving intravenous methylene blue dye for a diagnostic procedure

When these conditions exist, pulse oximetry should not be used or it should be used only as a trend detector and the true value of the patient's SaO_2 determined by ABG analysis.

Unfortunately, one or several of these conditions may be present in most critically ill clients. Nevertheless, pulse oximetry is valuable in early detection of a decrease in SaO_2 by providing opportunity to notice deviations from baseline status. The evidence favors the use of finger probes rather than ear probes.

The authors of this meta-analysis caution that pulse oximetry does not present a complete picture of how well body tissues are being oxygenated. Information is not provided about the adequacy of the hemoglobin level, cardiac output, delivery of oxygen to the tissues, or oxygen consumption. Also, carbon dioxide levels and acid-base balance can be obtained only by ABG analysis.

Cited References

1. Barker, S. J., et al. (1993). The effect of sensor malpositioning on pulse oximeter accuracy during hypoxemia. *Anesthesiology, 79,* 248–254.
2. Brodsky, J. B., et al. (1985). Pulse oximetry during one-lung ventilation. *Anesthesiology, 63,* 212–214.
3. Cecil, W. T., et al. (1988). A clinical evaluation of the accuracy of the Nellcor N-100 and the Ohmeda 3700 pulse oximeters. *Journal of Clinical Monitoring, 4,* 31–36.
4. Chaudhary, B. A., & Burki, N. K. (1978). Ear oximetry in clinical practice. *American Review of Respiratory Disease, 117,* 173–175.
5. Douglas, N. J., et al. (1979). Accuracy, sensitivity to carboxyhemoglobin, and speed of response of the Hewlett-Packard 47201A ear oximeter. *American Review of Respiratory Disease, 119,* 311–313.
6. Fahey, P. J., et al. (1983). Clinical evaluation of a new ear oximeter (Abstract). *American Review of Respiratory Disease, 127*(4part2), 129.
7. Gabrielczyk, M. R., & Buist, R. J. (1988). Pulse oximetry and postoperative hypothermia: An evaluation of the Nellcor N-100 in a cardiac surgical intensive care unit. *Anaesthesia, 43,* 402–404.
8. Huffman, L. M. (1989). Pulse oximetry: Accuracy and clinical performance in different practice settings. *Journal of American Association of Nurse Anesthetists, 57,* 475–476.
9. Kagle, D. M., et al. (1987). Evaluation of the Ohmeda 3700 pulse oximeter: Steady state and transient response characteristics. *Anesthesiology, 66,* 376–380.
10. Kissinger, D. P., Hamilton, I. N., & Rozycki, G. S. (1991). The current practice of pulse oximetry and capnometry/capnography in the prehospital setting. *Emergency Care Quarterly, 7,* 44–50.
11. Mihm, F. G., & Halperin, B. D. (1985). Noninvasive detection of profound arterial desaturation using a pulse oximetry device. *Anesthesiology, 62,* 85–87.
12. Peters, K., et al. (1990). Increasing clinical use of pulse oximetry. *Dimensions of Critical Care Nursing, 9,* 107–111.
13. Severinghaus, J. W., Naifeh, K. H., & Koh, S. O. (1989). Errors in 14 pulse oximeters during profound hypoxia. *Journal of Clinical Monitoring, 5,* 72–81.
14. Shippy, M. B., et al. (1984). A clinical evaluation of the BTI BIOX II ear oximeter. *Respiratory Care, 29,* 730–735.
15. Strohl, K. P., et al. (1986). Comparison of three transmittance oximeters. *Medical Instrumentation, 20,* 143–149.
16. Tashiro, C., et al. (1988). Effects of carboxyhemoglobin on pulse oximetry in humans. *Journal of Anesthesia, 2,* 36–40.
17. Tremper, K. K., et al. (1985). Accuracy of pulse oximetry in the critically ill adult: Effect of temperature and hemodynamics (Abstract). *Anesthesiology, 63,* A175.
18. Webb, R. K., Ralston, A. C., & Runciman, W. B. (1991). Potential errors in pulse oximetry: II: Effects of changes in saturation and signal quality. *Anaesthesia, 46,* 207–212.

Sarah Jo Brown, PhD, RN, *Principal and Consultant, Practice-Research Integrations, Norwich, Vermont*

Respiratory Care of Older Adults After Cardiac Surgery

QUESTION

What nursing interventions prevent and decrease the incidence of adverse respiratory-related outcomes in older adults after cardiac surgery?

CITATION

Bezanson, J. (1997). Respiratory care of older adults after cardiac surgery. *Journal of Cardiovascular Nursing, 12,* 71–83.

STUDIES

Although many studies were cited in this review of research-based interventions, the method of identifying the studies cited was not described. Studies from nursing, medical, and interdisciplinary research were included.

A conceptual framework of ventilatory support was used to group the variables that influence respiratory outcomes. The major grouping concepts are (1) pre-episode patient characteristics, (2) processes of patient management, and (3) respiratory-related clinical outcomes. Pre-episode characteristics are depicted as having direct influences on clinical outcomes as well as having indirect influences through their effect on processes of client management. Processes of client management directly influence clinical outcomes.

Summary of Findings

Pre-episode Characteristics of Older Adults (p. 73)

Many respiratory system alterations involving the chest wall and lungs occur as a consequence of aging. Among these changes are diminished respiratory muscle strength,[38] decreased elasticity and recoil of the alveoli,[22, 23, 36] increased chest wall stiffness,[22, 36] and reduced ventilatory responsiveness to hypoxia and hypercapnia.[17] Collectively, these alterations contribute to a decrease in respiratory reserve, which is clinically manifested by reduced coughing efficiency and reduced arterial oxygenation. A study of age and gender differences in clients requiring mechanical ventilation found that men older than 70 years of age had a statistically significant increased incidence of respiratory insufficiency compared with younger men (<70 years). Differences in incidence of respiratory insufficiency were not statistically significant between older and younger women or between older men and women (p. 74).[14]

The presence of disease in adults undergoing cardiac surgery has been associated with development of postoperative pulmonary complications and prolonged mechanical ventilation; these co-morbidities include impaired left ventricular function, angina (pain), diabetes mellitus, and heart failure.[12, 30] Other risk factors include an emergent operation, very low weight, chronic obstructive pulmonary disease (COPD), previous stroke, smoking, and left coronary artery disease.[12] Interestingly, receiving intravenous (IV) antibiotics prior to mechanical ventilation has been associated with ventilator-associated pneumonia.[15] In a study examining the association between psychosocial characteristics and duration of mechanical ventilation,[13] depression, anxiety, and hostility were not associated with either earlier or later extubation. However, a higher positive effect was associated with earlier extubation.

Processes of Patient Management (p. 75)

Anticipated physiologic responses after cardiac surgery include lung injury related to having the heart-lung bypass machine,[25] atelectasis,[6, 19] and increased oxygen consumption related to hypermetabolism.[35] These physiologic responses together with the age-related alterations may contribute to pulmonary complications and prolonged duration of mechanical ventilation in older adults (p. 75). Additionally, decreased level of consciousness following administration of anesthesia and narcotics increases the risk of aspiration and hinders productive coughing effort (p. 75).

Older adults also may have increased vulnerability for aspiration when lying supine, and avoidance of that position may reduce the risk of aspiration.[34] In a study of clients in an intensive care unit (ICU), being over 60 years of age and being supine during the first 24 hours of mechanical ventilation were independently related with development of ventilator-associated pneumonia.[15] Several studies have demonstrated the benefits of right lateral positioning on arterial oxygenation[1, 2]; however, a decrease in pulmonary complications did not occur in a sample of postoperative cardiac surgical clients.[7]

Research findings show that hyperoxygenation prior to endotracheal suctioning with a closed suction system promotes arterial oxygenation.[10] This result is best accomplished using the mechanism of the ventilator rather than the manual resuscitation bag.[24] However, in postoperative cardiac surgery clients hyperinflation of the lungs during hyperoxygenation prior to endotracheal suctioning appears to increase the arterial pressure, which can cause problems in clients with postoperative hypertension.[31, 32] The optimal frequency of endotracheal suctioning remains controversial.[27]

The author of a review of the literature on normal saline instillation before suctioning concluded that this practice may decrease oxygen saturation values[26]; the article was published in 1995. Since then, several studies have demonstrated that saline instillation prior to endotracheal suction adversely affects oxygenation during and after suctioning.[40, 41] The study of 35 clients after coronary artery bypass grafting showed that the group receiving 5 ml of normal saline at the start of suctioning took 3.78 minutes longer to return to baseline mixed venous oxygenation saturation values compared with those not receiving saline.[41]

Predictors of readiness for weaning from mechanical ventilation have been studied in critically ill clients. One study of postoperative cardiac surgery patients identified vital capacity, arterial pH, and mean arterial blood pressure as interdependent predictors of weaning readiness.[9] However, different factors and strategies should probably be used for older adults.[16] Early extubation, defined as less than 8 hours of mechanical ventilation, has been successful in cardiac surgery clients,[4, 8] but its appropriateness in older adults is not certain. In one study, it was considered appropriate in people older than 70 years of age in the absence of co-morbidities and impaired left ventricular functioning (ejection fraction <45%).[8]

The presence of an endotracheal tube after cardiac surgery is stressful to clients,[29] and makes communication with them diffi-

Respiratory Care of Older Adults After Cardiac Surgery *Continued*

cult. Two studies have examined the effects of preoperative arrangements for postoperative communication.[5, 33] In one of the studies,[33] introducing the use of a communication board preoperatively resulted in increased patient satisfaction with communication after discharge from the ICU.

A few studies have examined the role of psychosocial support in promoting comfort and early discontinuation of mechanical ventilation. In a study of men (average age 58 years), a high frequency of spousal visitation was contributory to reduced length of stays in the cardiac surgical ICU.[18] When surgical ICU clients were interviewed 3 days after surgery, closeness and affirming behaviors of visiting family members were often remembered and a majority reported that family visitation provided feelings of comfort and relaxation.[28]

Although effective pain management clearly affects client comfort and ventilation, studies have found inconsistent assessment, administration, and documentation practices in postoperative cardiac surgery clients.[20, 21, 37] In a study of 80 patients, women received smaller doses of IV morphine than men, and older adults were less likely than younger adults to receive prescriptions of acetaminophen with oxycodone.[20] When pain management was documented using a standardized pain flowsheet, clients experienced reduced pain intensity.[37]

Limitations/Reservations. Although this review used research findings as the basis for its recommendations, it is not clear whether *all* studies regarding each recommendation were considered when a recommendation was made. This area of practice is changing rapidly; as a result, much research has been conducted on the various issues related to respiratory care of the postoperative cardiac surgical client since this review was published.

Research-Based Practice

Preoperative assessment of physiologic status, chronic conditions, and pychosocial characteristics helps identify older patients at risk for prolonged ventilatory assistance and pulmonary complications. A cardiac severity scoring system has been developed to assess these risks but has not been validated among older adults.[12] Preoperative assessment can also help identify those clients who are candidates for early extubation. Special arrangements for systematic assessment and client teaching need to be made when clients are admitted on the day of surgery.

Teaching clients slow deep-breathing maneuvers preoperatively can help to improve oxygenation postoperatively. Establishing a simple method for communicating before surgery is important for some people. A picture or word board depicting a few common problems may be useful. Clients also benefit emotionally, and perhaps physiologically, from being allowed frequent, short visits of one or two people who are close to them while they are in the ICU.

The four processes of care that affect respiratory outcomes are (1) suctioning practices, (2) positioning practices, (3) assessing weaning readiness, and (4) pain management. Hyperoxygenation using the mechanical ventilator mechanism prior to endotracheal suctioning has proven benefit. However, the use of normal saline instillation prior to endotracheal suctioning is discouraged, as it has not shown benefit and may adversely affect oxygenation. Elevation of the head of the bed, especially early after intubation, and right lateral positioning, reduce the risk of pneumonia.

Early extubation can be considered for older adults who do not have other conditions precluding it. Algorithms and perioperative clinical pathways have been developed to guide all members of the cardiac surgery team through the processes of care that must be optimized and the decision points involved in providing a safe and timely early extubation. Finally, well-planned pain assessment and management approaches and standardized documentation can improve clients' pain experiences and probably improve their respiratory outcomes.

Cited References

1. Banasik, J. L., et al. (1987). Effect of position on arterial oxygenation in postoperative coronary revascularization patients. *Heart and Lung, 16,* 652–657.
2. Banasik, J. L., & Emerson, R. J. (1996). Effect of lateral position on arterial and venous blood gases in postoperative cardiac surgery patients. *American Journal of Critical Care, 5,* 121–126.
3. Bostick, J., & Wendelgass, S. T. (1987). Normal saline instillation as part of the suctioning procedure: Effects on PaO_2 and amount of secretions. *Heart and Lung, 16,* 532–537.
4. Cheng, DCH. (1995). Pro: Early extubation after cardiac surgery decreases intensive care unit stay and cost. *Journal of Cardiothoracic Vascular Anesthesia, 9,* 460–464.
5. Cronin, L., & Carrizosa, A. (1984). The computer as a communication device for ventilator and tracheostomy patients in the intensive care unit. *Critical Care Nurse, 4,* 72–76.
6. Gamsu, G., et al. (1976). Postoperative impairment of mucous transport in the lung. *American Review of Respiratory Diseases, 114,* 673–679.
7. Gavigan, M., Kline-O'Sullivant, C., & Klumpp-Lybrand, B. (1990). The effect of regular turning on CABG patients. *Critical Care Nursing Quarterly, 12,* 69–76.
8. Gross, S. B. (1995). Early extubation: Preliminary experience in the cardiothoracic patient population. *American Journal of Critical Care, 4,* 262–266.
9. Hanneman, S. K. G. (1994). Multidimensional predictors of success or failure with early weaning from mechanical ventilation after cardiac surgery. *Nursing Research, 43,* 4–10.
10. Harshbarger, S. A., Hoffman, L. A., Zullo, T. G., & Pinsky, M. R. (1992). Effects of a closed tracheal suction system on ventilatory and cardiovascular parameters. *American Journal of Critical Care, 3,* 57–61.
11. Higgins, T. L., et al. (1991). Risk factors for respiratory complications after cardiac surgery (Abstract). *Anesthesia, 75,* A258.
12. Higgins, T. L., et al. (1992). Stratification of morbidity and mortality outcome by preoperative risk factors in coronary artery bypass patients. *Journal of the American Medical Association, 267,* 2344–2348.
13. Ingersoll, G. L., & Grippi, M. A. (1991). Preoperative pulmonary status and postoperative extubation outcome of patients undergoing elective cardiac surgery. *Heart and Lung, 20,* 137–143.
14. King, K. B., et al. (1992). Coronary artery bypass graft surgery in older women and men. *American Journal of Critical Care, 1,* 28–35.
15. Kollef, M. H. (1993). Ventilator-associated pneumonia. *Journal of the American Medical Association, 270,* 1965–1970.
16. Krieger, B. P., et al. (1989). Evaluation of conventional criteria for predicting successful weaning from mechanical ventilatory support in elderly patients. *Critical Care Medicine, 17,* 858–861.
17. Kronenberg, R. S., & Drage, C. W. (1973). Attenuation of the ventilatory and heart rate responses to hypoxia and hypercapnia with aging in normal men. *Journal of Clinical Investigation, 52,* 1812–1819.
18. Kulik, J. A., & Mahler, H. I. M. (1989). Social support and recovery from surgery. *Health Psychology, 8,* 221–238.

Bridge continues on following page

Respiratory Care of Older Adults After Cardiac Surgery *Continued*

19. Matthay, M. A., & Wiener-Kronish, J. P. (1989). Respiratory management after cardiac surgery. *Respiratory Management of Cardiac Surgery, 95,* 424–434.
20. Maxam-Moore, V. A., Wilkie, D. J., & Woods, S. L. (1994). Analgesics for cardiac surgery patients in critical care: Describing current practice. *American Journal of Critical Care, 3,* 31–39.
21. Meehan, D. A., et al. (1995). Analgesic administration, pain intensity, and patient satisfaction in cardiac surgical patients. *American Journal of Critical Care, 4,* 435–442.
22. Mittman, C., et al. (1965). Relationship between chest wall and pulmonary compliance with age. *Journal of Applied Physiology, 20,* 1211–1216.
23. Pierce, J. A., & Ebert, R. V. (1965). Fibrous network of the lung and its changes with age. *Thorax, 20,* 469–476.
24. Preusser, B. A., et al. (1988). Effects of two methods of preoxygenation on mean arterial pressure, cardiac output, peak airway pressure, and post suctioning hypoxemia. *Heart and Lung, 17,* 290–299.
25. Ratliff, N. B., et al. (1973). Pulmonary injury secondary to extracorporeal circulation. *Journal of Thoracic and Cardiovascular Surgery, 65,* 425–432.
26. Raymond, S. J. (1995). Normal saline instillation before suctioning: Helpful or harmful? A review of the literature. *American Journal of Critical Care, 4,* 267–271.
27. Simmons, C. L. (1997). How frequently should endotracheal suctioning be undertaken? *American Journal of Critical Care, 6,* 4–6.
28. Simpson, T. (1991). The family as a source of support for the critically ill adult. *AACN Clinical Issues, 2,* 229–235.
29. Soehren, P. (1995). Stressors perceived by cardiac surgical patients in the intensive care unit. *American Journal of Critical Care, 4,* 71–76.
30. Spivak, S. D., et al. (1996). Preoperative prediction of postoperative respiratory outcome. *Chest, 109,* 1222–1230.
31. Stone, K. S., et al. (1989). Effects of lung hyperinflation on mean arterial pressure and post suctioning hypoxemia, *Heart and Lung, 18,* 377–385.
32. Stone, K. S., et al. (1988). Effect of lung hyperinflation on cardiopulmonary hemodynamics and post suctioning hypoxemia (Abstract). *Heart and Lung, 17,* 309.
33. Stovsky, B., Rudy, E., & Dragonette, P. (1988). Comparison of two types of communication methods used after cardiac surgery with patients with endotracheal tubes. *Heart and Lung, 17,* 281–289.
34. Torres, A., et al. (1992). Pulmonary aspiration of gastric contents in patients receiving mechanical ventilation: The effect of body position. *Annals of Internal Medicine, 116,* 540–543.
35. Tulla, H., et al. (1991). Hypermetabolism after coronary artery bypass. *Journal of Thoracic and Cardiovascular Surgery, 101,* 598–600.
36. Turner, J. M., Mead, J., & Wohl, M. E. (1968). Elasticity of human lungs in relation to age. *Journal of Applied Physiology, 25,* 644–671.
37. Voigt, L., Paice, J. A., & Pouliot, J. (1995). Standardized pain flowsheet: Impact on patient-reported pain experiences after cardiovascular surgery. *American Journal of Critical Care, 4,* 308–313.
38. Wahba, W. M. (1983). Influence of aging on lung function: Clinical significance of changes from age twenty. *Anesthesia and Analgesia, 62,* 764–776.
39. Zuckerman, M., Lubin, B., & Rinck, C. M. (1983). Construction of new scales for the multiple affect adjective check list. *Journal of Behavioral Assessment, 5,* 119–129.

Added References

40. Ackerman, M. H., & Mick, D. J. (1998). Instillation of normal saline before suctioning in patients with pulmonary infections: A prospective randomized controlled trial. *American Journal of Critical Care, 7,* 261–266.
41. Kinloch, D. (1999). Instillation of normal saline during endotracheal suctioning: Effects on mixed venous oxygen saturation. *American Journal of Critical Care, 8,* 231–240.

Sarah Jo Brown, PhD, RN, *Principal and Consultant, Practice-Research Integrations, Norwich, Vermont*

UNIT 14

Sensory Disorders

Anatomy and Physiology Review

The Eyes and Ears

Robert G. Carroll

OVERVIEW

The visual, auditory, and olfactory systems are "distance" senses, bringing information about our environment to our perception. Each system detects the intensity and quality of stimuli, encodes and processes this information, and transmits it to the cerebral cortex. Together these senses provide much of the available information about our environment. This review covers vision and hearing, smell is described in Unit 6.

The *visual apparatus* is specialized to detect light. Light passes through the cornea, aqueous humor, lens, and vitreous humor before striking the retina. The visual receptors —rods and cones—encode data about the intensity and wavelength of light. This information is processed and transmitted through nerve cells of the retina, the optic nerve, and the thalamus before arriving at the visual cortex. The information is constructed in the primary and associated visual cortex into a conscious perception.

The *auditory apparatus* is specialized to detect sound. Sound waves pass through the pinna to the ear drum (tympanic membrane), through the bones of the middle ear, and then to the receptors in the cochlea. The auditory hair cells are arranged on the organ of Corti (the end organ for hearing) and are coded to detect the intensity and frequency of sound. This information passes through the auditory nerve through the lateral lemniscus and, finally, to the auditory cortex. Within the primary and secondary auditory cortex, auditory discrimination occurs.

VISUAL SYSTEM

STRUCTURE OF THE VISUAL SYSTEM

■ EXTERNAL STRUCTURES

The visual system is a complex group of structures that includes the eyeballs, muscles, nerves, fat, and bones. The *ocular adnexa* (Fig. U14–1*A*) are the acessory structures of the eye (muscles, fat, and bone) that support and protect it. The bony orbit (eye socket) surrounds and protects most of the eye so that only a small portion is visible. The orbit is formed from portions of the frontal, lacrimal, ethmoid, maxillary, zygomatous, sphenoid, and palatine bones. These bones are thin and fragile and break easily when pressure is applied to the eye (as in a fistfight). In addition to bone, the orbit also contains fat, various connective tissues, blood vessels, and nerves.

The *eyeball* is moved by six ocular muscles, which are attached to the surface of the globe (Fig. U14–2) and which move the eye through six cardinal gazes. The four rectus muscles (the medial, lateral, superior, and inferior) move the eyes horizontally and vertically. The two oblique muscles (superior and inferior) rotate the eye in circular movements to allow vision at all angles.

The upper and lower *eyelids* are elastic folds of skin that close to protect the anterior eyeball. When the eyelids close, they distribute tear film, which prevents evaporation and drying of the surface epithelium. The elliptic space between the two open lids is the *palpebral fissure.* The corners of the fissure are called the *canthi.* The medial, or inner, canthus is next to the nose; the lateral, or outer, canthus is the outside corner. Oil-secreting *meibomian glands* are embedded in both upper and lower lids (Fig. U14–1*B*).

The *lacrimal gland,* in the upper lid over the outer canthus, produces tears that reach the eyeball through secretory ducts. Tiny openings *(puncti)* in both the upper and lower lids at the inner canthus direct tears to the lacrimal sac. The *nasolacrimal duct* directs the flow of tears into the nose. The tear film is composed of lipids secreted by the meibomian glands and dissolved salts, glucose, urea, protein, and lysozyme secreted by the lacrimal glands. The tear film lubricates, cleans, and protects the ocular surface. Mucus, secreted by goblet cells located in the lids, assists these processes.

■ INNER EYE

The *conjunctiva* is a thin transparent layer of mucous membrane that lines the eyelids and covers the eyeball (Fig. U14–1*C*). The *cornea* is a transparent avascular structure with a brilliant, shiny surface. It is convex in shape, about 0.5 mm thick, and acts as a powerful lens to bend and direct (refract) rays of light to the retina. The cornea is composed of five layers. It derives oxygen from the atmosphere. A rich network of nerve fibers in the outer layer (epithelium) produces a sensation of pain whenever the fibers are exposed or stimulated.

The *sclera* is the fibrous protective coating of the eye. It is white, dense, and continuous with the cornea. In children, the sclera is thin and appears bluish because of the underlying pigmented structures. In old age, it may become yellowish from degeneration.

The *uveal tract,* the middle vascular layer of the eye that furnishes the blood supply to the retina, consists of three structures:

1. The *iris* is a thin, pigmented diaphragm with a central aperture, the pupil. Iris color is determined by the degree of pigmentation in the stromal melanocytes. The interaction of the two iris muscles (sphincter and dilator) determines pupil diameter. Expansion and contraction of the iris regulate the amount of light entering the eye.
2. The *ciliary body* produces and secretes *aqueous humor,* a clear alkaline fluid composed mainly of water, which occupies the space between the iris and the cornea (the anterior chamber of the eye). The ciliary body is in direct continuity with the iris and

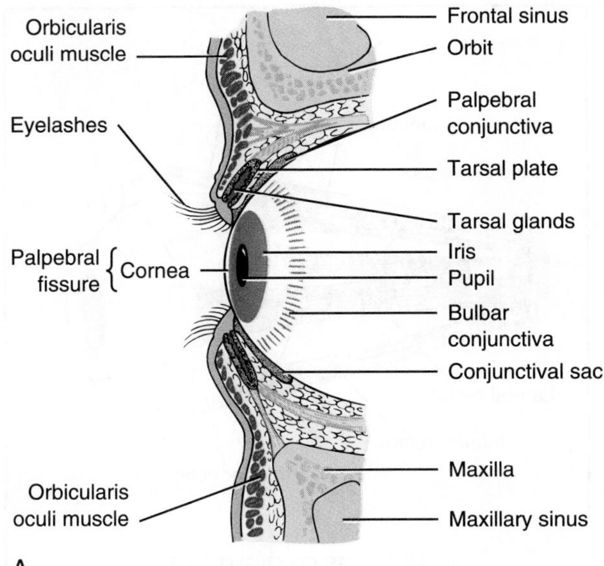

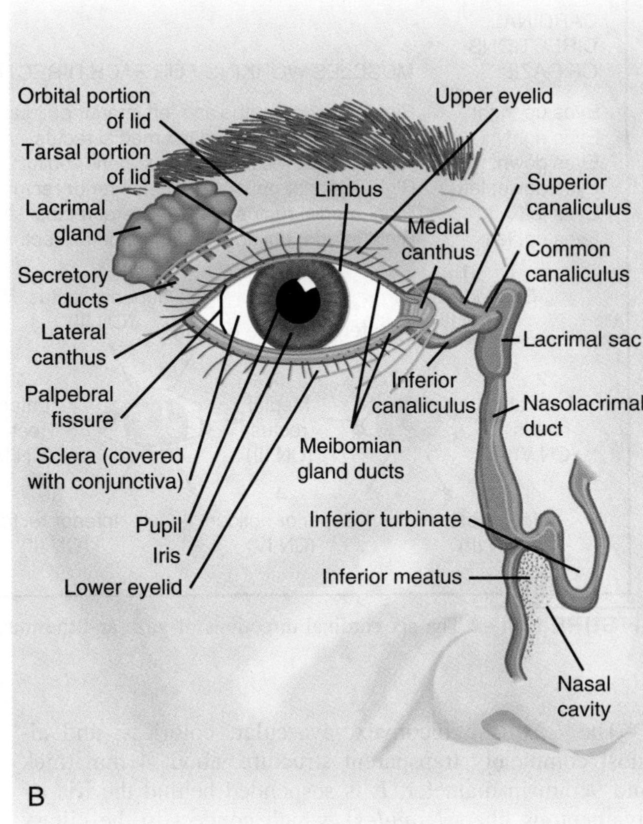

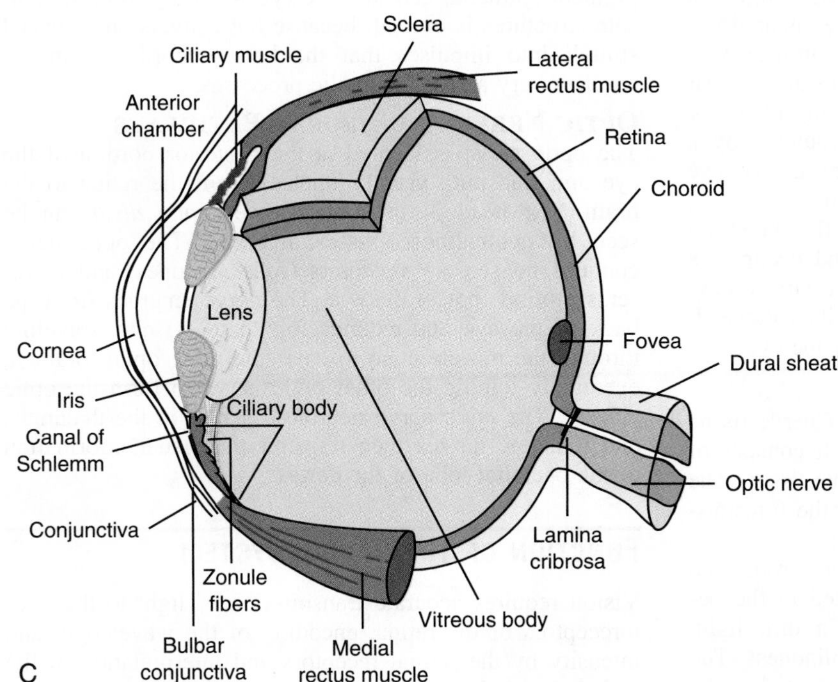

FIGURE U14–1 Surface anatomy of the eye. *A,* Ocular adnexa. *B,* Frontal view of the lacrimal drainage system. *C,* Horizontal section of the eye.

is circular, surrounding the lens. Aqueous humor circulates from the posterior chamber through the pupil into the anterior chamber. The flow continues into the anterior chamber angle and is filtered out through the trabecular meshwork into Schlemm's canal. From there, the aqueous humor is channeled into a capillary network and into episcleral veins. Normal intraocular pressure is maintained as long as there is a balance between the aqueous production and the aqueous humor outflow.

3. The *choroid* is the posterior segment of the uveal tract between the retina and the sclera. It is composed of three layers of vessels and is attached to both the ciliary body and the optic nerve.

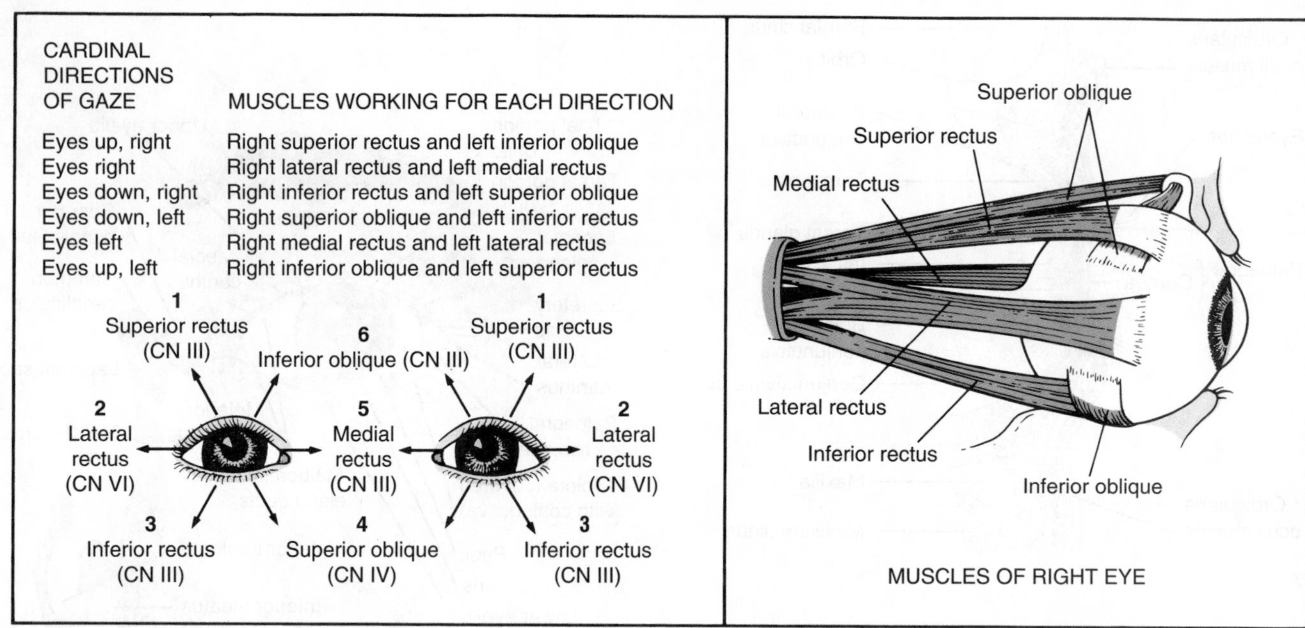

FIGURE U14–2 The six cardinal directions of gaze and the muscles responsible for each.

The *lens* is a biconvex, avascular, colorless, and almost completely transparent structure, about 4 mm thick and 9 mm in diameter. It is suspended behind the iris by ligamentous fibers *(zonules),* which connect to the ciliary body. The sole purpose of the lens is to focus light on the retina. The physiologic interplay of the zonular fibers and elasticity of the lens allows for focusing on nearby or distant objects. The change of focus from distant to near is called *accommodation.* There are no pain fibers or blood vessels in the lens. The lens is surrounded by a transparent envelope (the capsule). The lens of the eye consists of about 65% water and 35% protein.

The *vitreous body* is a clear, avascular, jelly-like structure. Vitreous fluid is thick and viscous, and occupies a space called the *vitreous chamber.* It fills the largest cavity of the eye, accounting for two thirds of its volume. It helps maintain the shape and transparency of the eye.

RETINA

The retina is a thin, semitransparent layer of nerve tissue that forms the innermost lining of the eye. It consists of 10 distinct layers of highly organized, delicate tissue. The retina contains all the sensory receptors for the transmission of light and is actually part of the brain.

There are two types of retinal receptors: rods and cones. About 125 million *rods* are distributed in the periphery of the retina; they function best in dim light. Damage to these structures results in night blindness. The *cones,* numbering about 6 million and concentrated in the center of the retina, provide resolution of small visual angles, resulting in perception of fine details. They are also responsible for color vision.

The center of the retina *(macula)* is an area about 5 mm in diameter. In an ophthalmoscopic examination, it appears as a yellowish spot with a depressed center, the *fovea.* An area 1.5 mm in diameter where only cones are present, the fovea is the point of finest vision. Damage to the fovea can severely reduce central vision.

The retina is composed of many fine layers of neural tissue attached to a single layer of pigmented epithelial cells. The photoreceptor cells in the retina are nourished by the capillaries of the choroid layer just beneath the pigment epithelial cell layer. Oxygen supply to these delicate structures is crucial, because the conversion of visual stimuli into impulses that the brain records as images requires very active metabolic processes.

OPTIC NERVE AND NEURAL PATHWAYS

The optic nerve is located at the posterior portion of the eye and transmits visual impulses from the retina to the brain. The head of the optic nerve *(optic disc)* can be seen by ophthalmoscopic examination. The optic nerve contains no sensory receptors (rods or cones) and represents a blind spot in the eye. The nerve emerges from the back of the eye and extends for 25 to 30 mm, traveling through the muscle cone to enter the bony optic foramen, eventually joining the other optic nerve to form the optic chiasm. The optic nerve neurons synapse in the thalamus, and thalamic nerves then transmit the visual information to the occipital lobe of the cortex.

FUNCTION OF THE VISUAL SYSTEM

Vision requires accurate transmission of light to the photoreceptors of the retina, encoding of the wavelength and intensity by the retinal receptors and interpretation of the coded signals by the visual cortex.

■ TRANSMISSION OF LIGHT

Light passes through the cornea, aqueous humor, lens, and vitreous humor before striking the retina. Blood vessels are opaque, and the cornea, lens, and fovea are sparsely vascularized, which enhances light transmission. The cornea and lens refract light, allowing it to converge to a focal point on the fovea of the retina. Refraction at the lens is regulated by contraction of the ciliary muscles.

Near vision is accomplished by contraction of the ciliary muscles, which increases curvature of the lens and brings near objects into focus on the retina. *Far vision* is accomplished by relaxing the ciliary muscles and flattening the lens. With age, lens elasticity decreases, reducing the ability to accommodate for near vision. Visual abnormalities are corrected by placing an appropriate refractor (eye glasses or contact lens) in the light pathway.

■ VISUAL RECEPTORS OF THE RETINA; CONES AND RODS

Three types of cones are sensitive to specific wavelengths of light, with peak sensitivities in the red, green, and blue wavelengths. Density of the cone receptors is highest in the fovea (the area of highest visual acuity). Bright light causes contraction of the iris, limiting the light entering the eye and focusing the light on the fovea. Exposure to light bleaches retinal photopigments, reducing the receptor responsiveness to subsequent exposure (light adaptation). However, prolonged exposure to dark allows the receptors to recover; cones recover completely in about 5 minutes.

Rods are sensitive to light in the green and yellow wavelengths and impart night *(scotopic)* vision. Rods are distributed throughout the retina, but few rods are in the fovea. In the dark, the iris dilates, admitting light to large portions of the retina. Consequently, night vision is enhanced by looking just to the side of the object of interest. After light exposure, rods recover slowly, taking about 20 minutes to return to peak sensitivity (dark adaptation). Because the rod photopigments are not sensitive to red light, exposure to red light does not interfere with dark adaptation.

■ IMAGE PROCESSING AND THE VISUAL CORTEX

Interneurons in the retina process the receptor output and transmit information via the optic nerve to the thalamus. The thalamus processes information about the wavelength and intensity of the light and relays the information to the visual cortex. Visual space in the cortex is completely crossed; objects appearing on the left side of the body are represented on the right visual cortex and vice versa (Fig. U14–3). The two eyes work as though they were one, focusing on the same point in space and fusing their images so that a single mental impression is obtained. The ability of the eyes to fuse two images into a single image is called *binocular vision,* accounting for one aspect of depth perception.

EFFECTS OF AGING ON VISION

STRUCTURAL CHANGES

Several age-related changes occur in the structures of the eye and surrounding tissue. Eyebrows and eyelashes turn

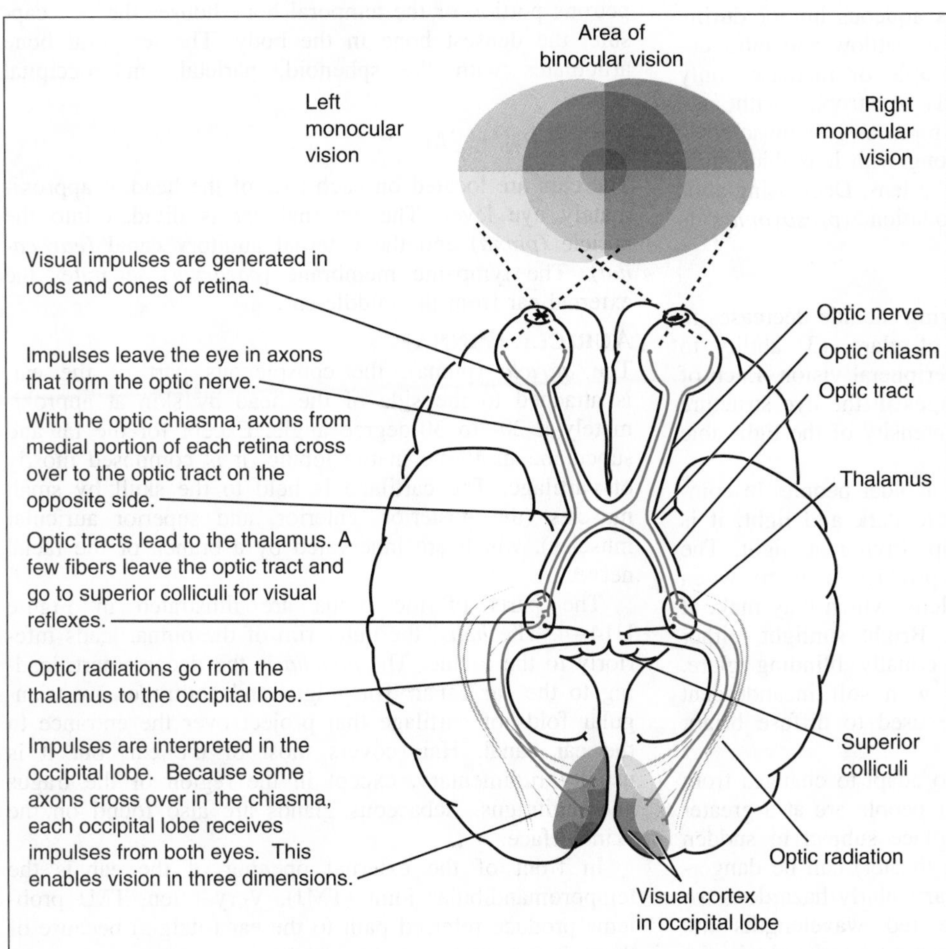

Area of binocular vision
Left monocular vision
Right monocular vision
Visual impulses are generated in rods and cones of retina.
Impulses leave the eye in axons that form the optic nerve.
With the optic chiasma, axons from medial portion of each retina cross over to the optic tract on the opposite side.
Optic tracts lead to the thalamus. A few fibers leave the optic tract and go to superior colliculi for visual reflexes.
Optic radiations go from the thalamus to the occipital lobe.
Impulses are interpreted in the occipital lobe. Because some axons cross over in the chiasma, each occipital lobe receives impulses from both eyes. This enables vision in three dimensions.
Optic nerve
Optic chiasm
Optic tract
Thalamus
Superior colliculi
Optic radiation
Visual cortex in occipital lobe

FIGURE U14–3 Visual pathways from the retina to the occipital lobe. The pathway is partially crossed, so that objects in the visual space of one side are interpreted in the contralateral visual cortex.

gray, and skin around the eyelids becomes wrinkled and loose because of loss of muscle tone and elasticity. Loss of orbital fat causes the eyes to sink deeper into the orbit and sometimes limits the upward gaze. Tear secretions may also diminish, resulting in the condition of dry eyes.

The most frequent and significant age-related change in the eye is the formation of a *cataract.* With age, the thickness and density of the lens increase and the lens becomes progressively yellowed and opaque. Throughout the life span, the lens continues to grow by forming new fiber cells. Although the rate of growth gradually diminishes, the accumulation of cells over time contributes to lens density. Loss of transparency also results from molecular deterioration from absorption of ultraviolet radiation. The yellow material is associated with the development of abnormal fluorescent substances in the aging lens. Although the cloudiness of the lens that occurs with aging decreases visual acuity, it does provide a natural protection for the retina against ultraviolet light. The lens accommodation diminishes because of ciliary muscle atrophy.

The cells of the inner layer of the cornea (endothelium) decrease in number with age. Because this layer does not reproduce lost cells, the ability of this layer to heal after injury or surgery may be compromised. The corneal reflex also may be diminished or absent. Another phenomenon characteristic of aging is the *arcus senilis,* a grayish yellow ring found on the periphery of the cornea surrounding the iris. This ring is thought to be the result of the accumulation of lipids.

The ciliary body produces less aqueous humor during the aging process, but there is less outflow and intraocular pressure remains relatively stable or increases only slightly. The ciliary muscle tends to atrophy with age, and sometimes connective tissue replaces lost muscle tissue. The loss in muscle action along with lens thickening decreases the focusing ability of the lens. Decreasing ability to focus at near accommodation *(presbyopia)* is common.

Visual Changes

The major visual changes with aging include decreases in (1) visual acuity, (2) tolerance of glare, (3) ability to adapt to dark and light, and (4) peripheral vision. Each of these decreases is related to changes in the eye structure and each affects the quality and intensity of the light able to reach the retina.

Glare is a particular problem for older people. In combination with difficulty adjusting to dark and light, it is often the reason older adults stop driving at night. The lights from oncoming vehicles produce a glare when passing through both cornea and lens, which may make it very difficult to discern objects. Bright sunlight, either indoors or outdoors, causes an equally blinding glare. Indoor rooms should be lighted with soft incandescent lights, and sheer curtains can be used to diffuse bright sunlight.

Because the eye takes longer to adapt to changes from dark to light and vice versa, older people are at a greater risk for falls and injuries. Any place subject to sudden changes in lighting (e.g., inside a theater) can be dangerous. Getting up at night can be particularly hazardous for older adults. However, because red wavelengths are longer and are perceived by the cones, a red light in the bathroom at night allows enough vision to function without interfering with dark vision.

Peripheral vision decreases with age and may interfere with social interactions and physical activities. Older adults suffering from loss of peripheral vision may not notice someone sitting next to them. They may also have difficulty finding objects out of their range of vision.

The iris loses pigment with age, and older people may thus appear to have grayish or light blue eyes. The pupil becomes gradually smaller with age. A decrease in pupil size results in a smaller amount of light reaching the retina, meaning that the light must pass through the densest, most opaque area of the lens.

In the posterior chamber, the vitreous body begins to liquefy and collapse. Small pieces of debris from separation and shrinkage of the vitreous body may become visible as "floaters." Although floaters may not obstruct vision, they are an annoyance. Vitreal shrinkage may result in retinal detachment. Additionally, the retina may degenerate as a result of local ischemia and loss of neural function.

AUDITORY SYSTEM

Structure of the Auditory System

The ear is housed in the *temporal bone* of the skull. The temporal bones are two of the eight cranial bones that form part of the base and lateral wall of the skull. The petrous portion of the temporal bone houses the otic capsule, the densest bone in the body. The temporal bone articulates with the sphenoid, parietal, and occipital bones.

■ EXTERNAL EAR

The ears are located on each side of the head at approximately eye level. The external ear is divided into the auricle *(pinna)* and the external auditory canal *(ear canal).* The tympanic membrane *(eardrum)* separates the external ear from the middle ear.

Auricle (Pinna)

The *auricle* (pinna), the conspicuous part of the ear, is attached to the side of the head by skin at approximately a 20- to 30-degree angle. Except for the fat and subcutaneous tissue in the lobule, it is composed mostly of cartilage. The cartilage is held to the skull by small muscles (the posterior, anterior, and superior auricular muscles), which are innervated by a branch of the facial nerve.

The parts of the pinna are illustrated in Figure U14–4. The *helix,* the outer rim of the pinna, leads inferiorly to the lobule. The *concha* is the deepest part, leading to the ear canal. The tragus and antitragus are triangular folds of cartilage that project over the entrance to the ear canal. Hair covers most of the ear, but it is usually rudimentary, except in the region of the tragus and antitragus. Sebaceous glands are also found on the skin surface.

In front of the external opening of the ear is the temporomandibular joint (TMJ). Very often, TMJ problems produce referred pain to the ear (otalgia) because of their shared sensory nerve supply.

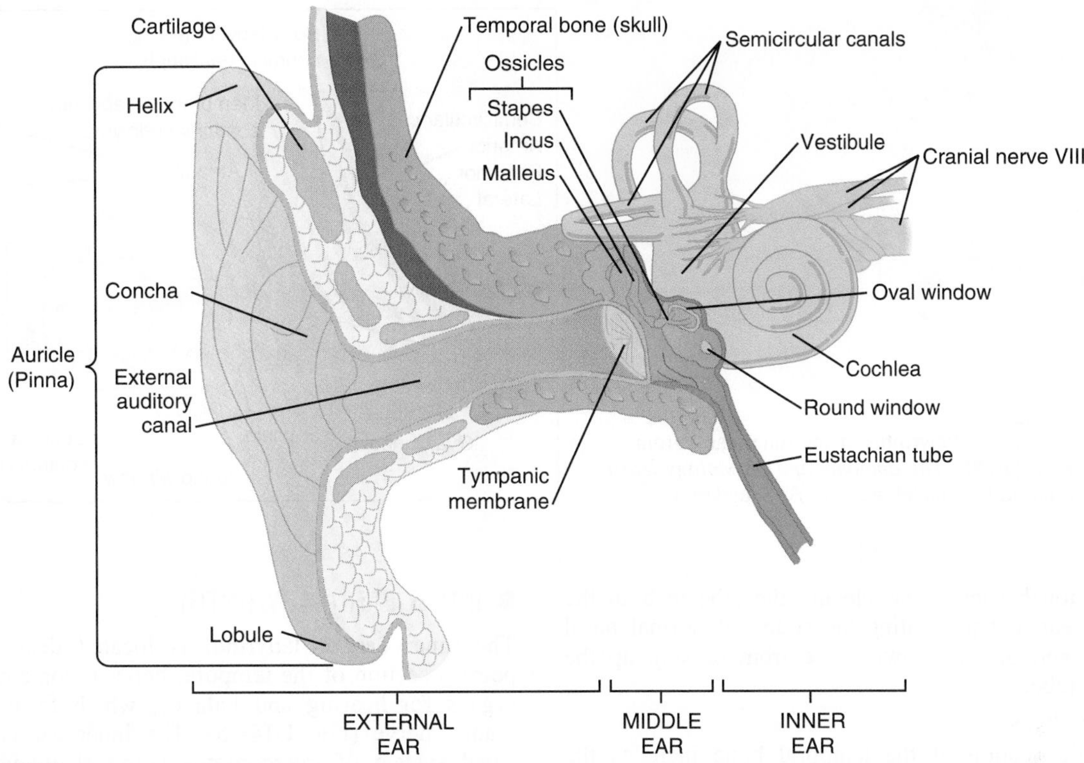

FIGURE U14–4 Anatomy of the ear.

External Auditory Canal (Ear Canal)

The ear canal extends from the concha of the pinna to the tympanic membrane (see Fig. U14–4). This slightly S-shaped canal is approximately 2.5 cm (1 inch) in length and follows an inward, forward, and downward path. The skeleton of cartilage in the outer third is continuous with the cartilage of the pinna. The inner two thirds is a bony canal entering the skull. The lumen of the ear canal is irregularly shaped and is narrowest where the transition from cartilage to bone occurs. The skin covering the cartilage portion is thick, containing sebaceous and ceruminous glands and hair follicles. The sebaceous and ceruminous glands secrete a golden to black substance called *cerumen* (wax). The skin covering the bony portion is very thin.

Tympanic Membrane

The tympanic membrane (eardrum) is an oval disc (~1 cm in diameter); it covers the end of the auditory canal and separates the canal from the middle ear (Fig. U14–4). The eardrum is a thin, translucent, pearly gray membrane obliquely directed downward and inward, so that the posterior part is more accessible than the anterior part. The eardrum consists of three tissue layers:

- An outer epithelial layer continuous with the skin of the ear canal
- A fibrous supporting middle layer
- An inner mucosal layer continuous with the mucosal lining of the middle ear cavity

■ MIDDLE EAR

The middle ear consists of the middle ear cleft and contents: ossicles, oval and round windows, eustachian tube, and facial nerve (see Fig. U14–4). The middle ear lies between the ear canal and the *labyrinth* (inner ear). The middle ear cavity has a mucosal lining.

Ossicles

The middle ear contains the three smallest bones *(ossicles)* of the body, named according to their appearance. The outermost and largest ossicle is the *malleus* (hammer), which is firmly attached to the tympanic membrane. The innermost and smallest ossicle is the *stapes* (stirrup); its footplate occupies the oval window, in direct contact with the perilymph of the inner ear. The *incus* (anvil) lies between the other two and is shaped like a tooth with two roots (see Fig. U14–4).

Windows

The middle ear contains two windows, whose names reflect their shape. The *round window* is an opening in the inner ear from which sound vibrations exit. The *oval window* is an opening in the inner ear into which sound vibrations enter. The oval window is not a true window because the footplate of the stapes bone covers it.

Eustachian Tube

The eustachian tube is a narrow channel approximately 35 mm (1½ inches) long and only 1 mm wide at its narrowest end. This tube connects the middle ear to the nasopharynx (see Fig. U14–4). The structure consists mostly of fibrous tissue, cartilage, and bone; it extends downward, forward, and inward from each middle ear. The eustachian tube is lined with a mucous membrane that is continuous with the lining of the middle ear at one end and with the nasopharynx at the other end. A small section of this tube, originating in the middle ear, remains permanently open. Otherwise, the walls of the tube lightly

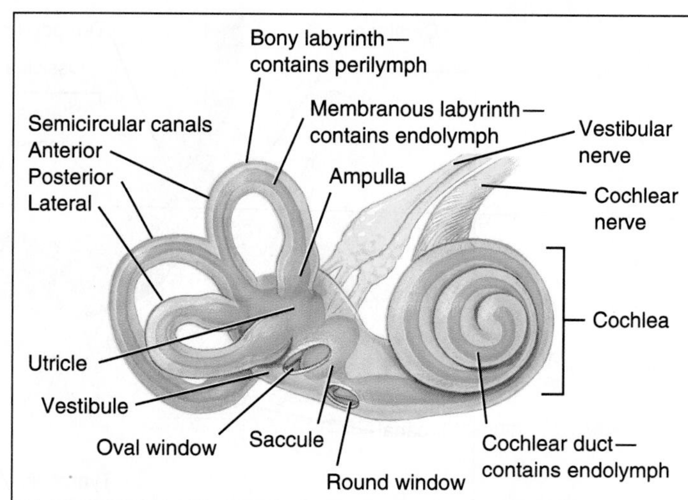

FIGURE U14–5 The labyrinths of the inner ear. (From Applegate, E. J. [2000]. *The anatomy and physiology learning system* [2nd ed.]. Philadelphia: W. B. Saunders.)

oppose or touch each other, closing the tube to both the throat and ear and preventing the sound of normal nasal respiration and of one's own voice from passing up the eustachian tube.

Mastoid Bone

The mastoid section of the temporal bone includes the cone-shaped *mastoid process;* the *mastoid antrum,* a large cavity posteriorly continuous with the middle ear; and the *mastoid air cells,* which extend from the antrum and fill the temporal bone with air pockets.

The mastoid bone is a bony protuberance behind the lower portion of the pinna. The mastoid cavity is close to several important cranial structures: the dura of the temporal lobe, the cerebellar dura, the sigmoid sinus, and the jugular bulb. The middle ear is also bounded by the internal carotid artery. Therefore, infection of the middle ear and mastoid cavities can also involve these structures.

■ INNER EAR (LABYRINTH)

The inner ear or labyrinth is located deep within the petrous section of the temporal bone; it contains the sense organs for hearing and balance, which form the eighth cranial nerve (Fig. U14–5). The inner ear is a complicated system of intercommunicating chambers and connecting tubes composed of two structures:

1. The *bony labyrinth* is the rigid capsule (otic capsule) that surrounds and protects the delicate membranous labyrinth. The *vestibule* connects the cochlea (for hearing) to the three semicircular canals (for balance). The *cochlea,* which looks like a snail shell with 2½ turns, is approximately 7 mm in diameter at the widest part and is structurally divided into three compartments (Fig. U14–6). The upper compartment *(scala vestibuli)* leads from the oval window to the apex of the cochlear spiral. The

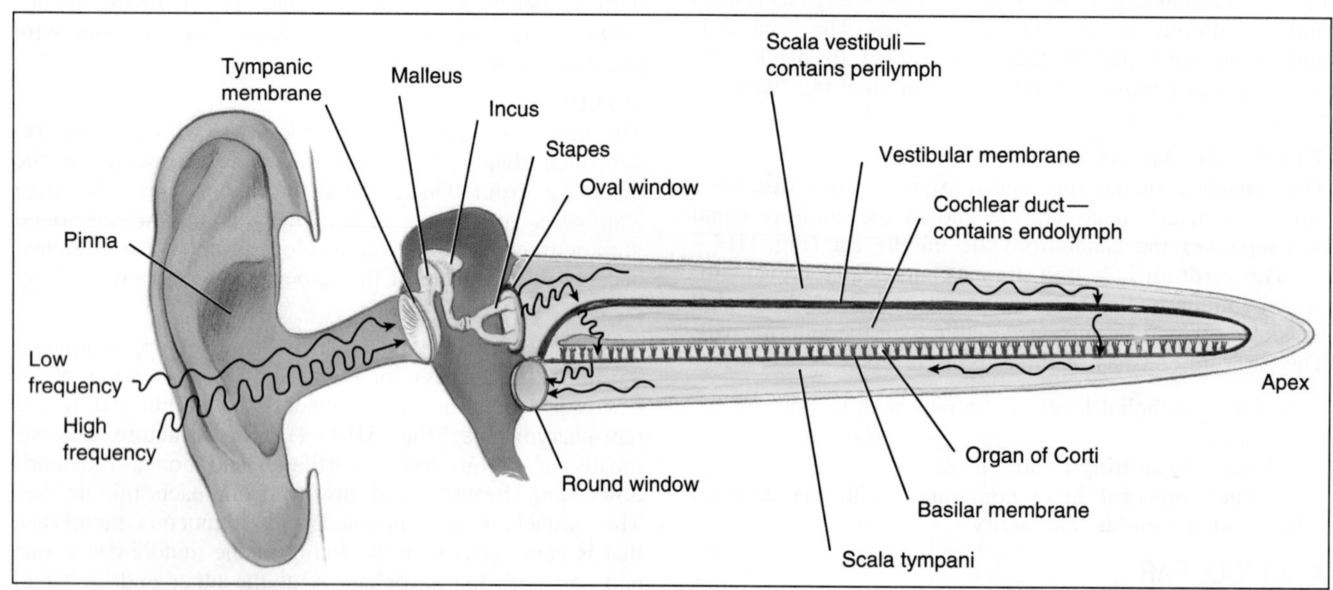

FIGURE U14–6 The uncoiled cochlea, showing the pathway of pressure waves. (From Applegate, E. J. [2000]. *The anatomy and physiology learning system* [2nd ed.]. Philadelphia: W. B. Saunders.)

lower compartment *(scala tympani)* leads from the apex of the cochlear spiral to the round window. The *scala media,* which contains the organ of Corti, lies between the scala vestibuli and scala tympani.

2. The *membranous labyrinth,* lying within but not completely filling the bony labyrinth, is bathed in a fluid called *perilymph,* which communicates with the cerebrospinal fluid (CSF) via the cochlear duct. The membranous labyrinth consists of the utricle, the saccule, the semicircular canals, the cochlear duct, and the *organ of Corti* (the end organ for hearing). The membranous labyrinth contains a different fluid *(endolymph).* This fluid also protects the end organ because it acts as a cushion against abrupt movements of the head.

The three *semicircular canals* are at right angles to each other and are named the anterior (superior), the posterior, and the lateral (horizontal) canal. The horizontal canal lies closest to the middle ear. This arrangement allows detection of movement in all three dimensions.

FUNCTION OF THE AUDITORY SYSTEM

■ EXTERNAL EAR

The ears are a pair of complex sensory organs for both hearing and balance. Their location on either side of the head produces binaural hearing, allows the detection of sound direction, and aids in maintaining equilibrium. The temporal bone provides protection for the organs of hearing and balance. It houses (1) the external and internal auditory canals; (2) the mastoid air cells, which provide an air reservoir for the middle ear; (3) the blood vessels; (4) the facial, vestibular, and auditory nerves; (5) the labyrinth; and (6) the cochlea.

SOUND WAVE CONDUCTION

The head, pinna, and ear canal act as an integrated system to transmit sound vibrations to the eardrum. The external ear actually amplifies certain frequencies. Sound is transmitted from the external ear through the middle ear (which amplifies the sound) to the inner ear (see Fig. U14–6). The funnel shape of the pinna collects and directs sound to the eardrum.

The tympanic membrane, a common membrane between the external ear canal and the middle ear space, protects the middle ear and conducts sound vibrations from the external ear to the ossicles. The sound pressure applied to the stapes (the smallest ossicle) in the oval window is 22 times greater than the sound pressure exerted on the eardrum. The pressure of the sound vibrations is increased as a result of transmission from a larger area to a smaller area, and the lever effect of the ossicular chain. The sound energy, after transformation, is carried by neural elements to the brain for decoding and, thus, hearing.

WAX PRODUCTION

Cerumen (wax) protects the ear. Wax is to the ear what tears are to the eyes. The sticky consistency of the wax and the fine hairs of the ear canal help clean the ear canal of foreign matter and protect it from water damage. Impacted cerumen can cause hearing losses in clients of all ages. At times, wax must be mechanically removed.

■ MIDDLE EAR

SOUND WAVE CONDUCTION

The ossicles transmit sound vibrations mechanically (see Fig. U14–6). The ossicles are held in place by joints, muscles, and ligaments, which also offer some protection from loud sounds. The light weight and the configuration of the ossicles provide an efficient means of transmitting sound vibrations from the air molecules of the external ear to the fluid molecules of the inner ear. Fluids offer more resistance than air and need more force to transmit movement. The ossicular chain produces and magnifies this force in order to move the inner ear fluids.

VENTILATION AND PRESSURE REGULATION

The eustachian tube provides an air passage from the nasopharynx to the middle ear to equalize pressure on both sides of the eardrum. This tube regulates ventilation and pressure, both of which are necessary for normal hearing. During yawning, swallowing, and sneezing, the eustachian tube is opened by the *tensor veli palatini* muscle. The natural opening and closing of the eustachian tube also allows drainage of exudate from the middle ear mucosa. The tube can be forcibly opened by increasing nasopharyngeal pressure. This act (the Valsalva maneuver) is accomplished by attempting to blow air through the nose while holding the nose closed.

The cavity of the mastoid bone and the interconnected arrangement of the air-filled spaces aid the middle ear in adjusting to changes in pressure. The mastoid system acts as a buffer for the middle ear. The system of cavities and air cells also lightens the skull.

■ INNER EAR

HEARING

Sound waves are transmitted by the ossicles to the delicate membrane of the oval window (see Fig. U14–6). These vibrations move the perilymph in the scala vestibuli. The perilymph of the scala vestibuli is continuous with that of the scala tympani at the extreme tip of the "snail shell," called the *helicotrema.* The sound energy vibrations enter through the oval window and exit through the round window.

Vibrations in the perilymph of the scala vestibuli are transmitted through the vestibular membrane *(Reissner's membrane)* to the endolymph that fills the cochlear duct. The cochlear duct is located between the scala vestibuli and the scala tympani. The *organ of Corti,* which is bathed in the endolymph, lies on the basilar membrane in a spiral strip from the basal turn near the round window to the apex at the helicotrema. This organ transforms mechanical sound vibrations into neural activity and separates sound into different frequencies. The electrochemical impulse travels via the acoustic nerve to the brain stem. Auditory nerve input from both ears joins at the lateral lemniscus, reducing the possibility of unilateral deafness from CNS damage. The auditory nerves ascend to the cortex by a variety of pathways, reaching both the primary and secondary auditory regions of the temporal cortex of the brain. Efferent innervation via the acoustic nerve (eighth cranial nerve) reaches the cochlea and vestibule via the internal auditory canal, which also carries the facial nerve (seventh cranial nerve).

Sound is filtered by the ear components. Human auditory sensitivity ranges from 15 to 20,000 Hz. The auditory canal diminishes the passage of sounds with frequencies above 3500 Hz, the higher end of the human voice frequency. The middle ear diminishes passage of sounds with frequencies below 1000 Hz, the lower end of human voice frequency. The muscles of the middle ear decrease sound transmission by uncoupling the ossicles. For example, contraction of the tensor tympani allows reflex adaptation to a noisy environment. Contraction of the stapedius decreases sound transmission while speaking.

BALANCE

The *utricle* and *saccule* are vestibular receptors that position the head as it relates to the pull of gravity. The *semicircular canals* are arranged to sense rotational movements, such as movements or changes in position. Each of the semicircular canals connects with the utricle. Where the canals connect with the utricle is an enlarged portion *(ampulla).* The ampulla contains a cluster of hair cells *(crista),* concerned with dynamic balance. For example, when head position is changed, movement of the endolymph stimulates the hair cells, initiating increased impulses that travel over the vestibular division of the acoustic nerve to the brain. Balance functions in the vestibular system, along with visual cues and musculoskeletal cues, combine to maintain balance. Hearing and balance are partially maintained with the loss of function of one ear.

EFFECTS OF AGING ON HEARING

Many physiologic changes lead to changes in hearing in older people. The hairs become coarser during the aging process; thus, retention of wax is more of a problem. *Presbycusis,* a gradual sensorineural loss caused by nerve degeneration in the inner ear or auditory nerve, is a type of hearing loss that occurs with aging, even in people living in a quiet environment. Loss of auditory neurons in the organ of Corti and cochlear hair cell degeneration create an inability to hear high-frequency sounds. There may also be degeneration of the cochlear conductive membrane and decreased blood supply to the cochlea, leading to inability to hear at all (but especially higher) frequencies. Finally, a loss of cortical auditory neurons leads to diminished hearing and speech comprehension.

CONCLUSIONS

Vision and hearing are two senses that allow distance perception of the environment. Because we rely on these senses for communication with those around us, alterations in either sense can have a profound social and emotional impact. Some reductions in the ability to see or to hear are a normal part of age-related changes.

BIBLIOGRAPHY

1. Applegate, E. J. (2000). *The anatomy and physiology learning system* (2nd ed.). Philadelphia: W. B. Saunders.
2. Guyton, A. C., & Hall, J. (1996). *Textbook of medical physiology* (9th ed.). Philadelphia: W. B. Saunders.
3. Kandel, E. R., Schwartz, J. H., & Jessell, T. M. (1999). *Principles of neural science* (4th ed.). Norwalk, CT: Appleton & Lange.
4. McPhee, S. J., et al. (1999). *Pathophysiology of disease.* New York, McGraw-Hill.
5. Nolte, J. (1999). *The human brain* (4th ed.). St. Louis: Mosby.
6. Silverthorn, D. (1998). *Human physiology.* Upper Saddle River, NJ: Prentice Hall.

CHAPTER 64

Assessment of the Eyes and Ears

Linda A. Vader
Helene J. Krouse

ASSESSMENT OF THE EYE

One of the most important considerations in an ocular assessment is that many ophthalmic disorders are asymptomatic. The four most common preventable causes of permanent vision loss in developed nations are (1) *amblyopia* (reduced visual acuity that is uncorrectable with glasses in the absence of anatomic defects in the eye or visual pathways), (2) diabetic retinopathy, (3) age-related maculopathy, and (4) glaucoma. Routine eye examinations are therefore imperative.

The eye is a unique organ because its external anatomy may be easily assessed. Even the internal eye is visible through the cornea, where blood vessels and central nervous system (CNS) tissue (the retina and optic nerve) may be visualized without the use of x-rays or invasive procedures. The effects of many systemic problems, such as infections, cancer, and vascular and autoimmune disorders, can be detected with an internal eye examination. Clients may voice misconceptions about vision and the eyes (Box 64–1). If you encounter such misconceptions while conducting a physical examination, be prepared to address them.

HISTORY

An ophthalmic history includes (1) demographic data, (2) exploration of current manifestations, (3) past health history, (4) family health history, (5) psychosocial history and lifestyle, and (6) review of systems.

■ BIOGRAPHICAL AND DEMOGRAPHIC DATA

Demographic data relevant to ocular assessment include age and sex. The incidence of cataracts, dry eye, retinal detachment, glaucoma, entropion (eyes turning inward), and ectropion (eyes turning outward) increases with age. Hereditary color vision deficits are more common in men than in women.

■ CURRENT HEALTH

Ocular manifestations may be divided into three basic categories: (1) vision, (2) appearance, and (3) sensations of pain and discomfort.

Chief Complaint

The most common chief complaint is a change or loss of vision, but the complaint may also be less specific, such as headache or eyestrain. Commonly, the client is unable to verbalize a specific complaint. The chief complaint may be as vague as "something is wrong with my eyes."

Symptom Analysis

Whenever possible, characterize clinical manifestations according to rapidity of onset, location, duration, and characteristics (such as frequency and severity). The circumstances surrounding onset as well as the client's response to treatment are important. Record current eye and systemic medications being used and all other current and past ocular disorders.

ABNORMAL VISION

Visual changes or loss of vision may be caused by abnormalities in the eye or anywhere along the visual pathway. Considerations include (1) a refractive (focusing) error; (2) interference from lid *ptosis* (drooping eyelid); (3) clouding or interference in the cornea, lens, aqueous or vitreous space; and (4) malfunction of the retina, optic nerve, or intracranial visual pathway.

Glare or halos may result from uncorrected refractive error, scratches on glasses, dilated pupils, corneal edema, or cataract. Flashing or flickering lights may indicate retinal traction or migraine. Floating spots may represent normal vitreous body strands or the pathologic presence of blood, pigment, or inflammatory cells in the vitreous body. *Diplopia* (double vision) may occur in one eye or both and may be caused by refractive correction, muscle imbalance, or neurologic disorders.

ABNORMAL APPEARANCE

The most common abnormal appearance is a *red eye.* Causes include minor irritation, vascular congestion, subconjunctival hemorrhage, inflammatory disorders, infection, allergy, and trauma (Box 64–2). Other external changes in appearance include growths or lesions, edema, and abnormal position.

BOX 64–1 Common Misconceptions About Vision and the Eyes

The following statements are often passed along as "advice." They are all false.

1. Reading in the dark is harmful to the eyes.
2. Children will outgrow crossed eyes.
3. A cataract is a film growing over the surface of the eye.
4. Cataracts must "ripen" before they are removed.
5. The surgeon takes out the eye to operate on it.
6. A person with failing eyesight should avoid reading to save the eyes.
7. Children must be cautioned not to sit too close to the television.
8. Wearing someone else's glasses may damage your eyes.
9. Misuse of the eyes in childhood results in the need for glasses later in life.
10. Cataracts can be removed by a laser.
11. Emotional stress increases intraocular pressure.

ABNORMAL SENSATION

Eye pain is often poorly localized. Nonspecific complaints include eyestrain, pulling, pressure, fullness, or generalized headache. The pain may be periocular, ocular, or retrobulbar (behind the globe). Foreign-body sensation produces a sharp superficial pain that can be relieved by topical anesthesia. Deeper internal aching may indicate glaucoma, inflammation, muscle spasm, or infection. Reflex spasm of the ciliary muscle and iris sphincter that occurs with inflammation may produce brow ache and *photophobia* (sensitivity to light) or a constricted pupil (*miosis*). Itching is usually a sign of an allergic response. Dryness, burning, grittiness, and mild foreign-body sensation can occur with dry eyes or mild corneal irritation.

Tearing may be due to irritation or an abnormality of the lacrimal system. Increased ocular secretions usually indicate viral or bacterial infections and may also be present in allergic and noninfectious irritations.

■ PAST HEALTH HISTORY

The past health history focuses on systemic disorders commonly associated with ocular manifestations, such as diabetes mellitus, arthritis, hypertension, and thyroid disease.

Childhood and Infectious Diseases

Diseases occurring in childhood with possible ocular sequelae include diabetes mellitus, retinoblastoma, thyroid disorders, rheumatoid arthritis, exposure to sexually transmitted diseases (STDs) such as syphilis and acquired immunodeficiency syndrome (AIDS), and muscular dystrophy. Inquire about vaccinations, particularly for measles (rubella).

Major Illnesses and Hospitalizations

In addition to the just-mentioned systemic diseases, ask about hypertension, multiple sclerosis, myasthenia gravis, and adult onset of thyroid disorders, rheumatoid arthritis, and diabetes mellitus. Ocular diseases and structural problems include refractive errors (and corrective lenses used), strabismus, amblyopia, cataracts, glaucoma, and retinal detachment. If the client wears eyeglasses or contact lenses, ask when the last eye examination took place and when the prescription was last changed. Has the client has been hospitalized or undergone surgery related to the eyes or brain? Is there a history of head trauma or eye trauma related to motor vehicle accidents, sports injury, or other unintentional events?

Medications

Many medications affect the eyes. Prescription drugs include insulin, corticosteroids, oral hypoglycemics, and thyroid replacement hormones. Ask whether the client uses eye drops, and note the name, dose, and frequency taken. Specifically ask about use of over-the-counter eye drops such as natural tears. Over-the-counter preparations that may dry the eyes include antihistamines and decongestants.

Inquire about the use of herbal remedies, dietary supplements such as vitamins, and the consumption of specific foods. Some clients may consume large doses of vitamins A and C and certain foods, believing that these substances will prevent the development of vision problems such as cataracts and macular degeneration.

BOX 64–2 Red Eye

Nurses often encounter a client whose chief complaint is a "red eye." The condition causing the eye to be red (engorgement of the conjunctival vessels) may be a subconjunctival hemorrhage that requires no treatment, or it may be a sign of a serious eye disorder requiring immediate attention. Disorders involving red eye include:

Conjunctivitis—Bacterial, viral, allergic, and irritative
Herpes simplex keratitis—inflammation of the cornea
Scleritis—inflammation of the sclera
Angle-closure glaucoma—sudden occlusion of the anterior chamber angle by iris tissue
Adnexal disease—stye, dacryocystitis, blepharitis, lid lesions (carcinoma), thyroid disease, and vascular lesions
Subconjunctival hemorrhage—accumulation of blood in the potential space between the conjunctiva and the sclera
Pterygium—abnormal growth of tissue that progresses over the cornea
Keratoconjunctivitis sicca—inflammation associated with lacrimal deficiency
Abrasions and foreign bodies—hyperemic response
Abnormal lid function—Bell's palsy, thyroid ophthalmopathy, or lesions that cause ocular exposure

To evaluate a red eye:

1. Check the client's visual acuity with a Snellen chart.
2. Inspect for a pattern of redness.
3. Observe for the presence of discharge.
4. Using a penlight or slit lamp, observe for corneal opacities.
5. Using fluorescein stain, observe corneal defects.
6. Examine the anterior chamber for depth, blood cells, or pus.
7. Examine the pupils for irregularity.
8. Check intraocular pressure.
9. Observe for the pressure of proptosis or a lid disorder.

Allergies

Note allergies to medications and other substances. Has the client ever had an allergic reaction to eye drops or other medications that have affected the eyes? Allergic manifestations include eye redness, tearing, and itching. Determine past allergic reactions not only to medications but also to inhalants (dust, chemicals, or pollens) and contactants (cosmetics or pollens).

■ FAMILY HEALTH HISTORY

Because many ocular disorders tend to be familial, ask specifically about strabismus, glaucoma, *myopia* (nearsightedness), and *hyperopia* (farsightedness). Other common familial disorders include migraine, retinoblastoma, macular degeneration, retinitis pigmentosa, sickle cell anemia, keratoconus, and diabetes mellitus. Lack of a family health history does not necessarily rule out the possibility of a genetic disorder. Some clients do not know the ocular history of family members, and some may be embarrassed or hesitant to share the information.

■ PSYCHOSOCIAL HISTORY

Psychosocial history and lifestyle data significant to the ocular health history include occupational hazards, leisure activities and hobbies, and health management behaviors. A driving history can reveal a vision problem. Ask about the nature of the client's work and hobbies. Is the client exposed to irritating fumes, smoke, or airborne particles? Are safety goggles worn in situations in which eye injury may occur from fragments of metal or sand? Is there insufficient lighting, leading to eyestrain or harsh, glaring light? Leisure and sports activities associated with increased incidence of eye injury include baseball, racquetball, and contact sports; football is associated with a potential for head trauma. Participation in active outdoor activities, such as gardening, hiking, and cross-country skiing, increases the risk of foreign-body injury, abrasion, or penetrating injury. Does the client wear sunglasses or other protective eye gear when outdoors?

Explore health management behaviors related to the eyes. If the client has a systemic disease that affects the eyes, ask whether the client practices self-care measures. For example, does the diabetic client aggressively manage the disease by attempting to regulate blood glucose levels with diet and medication? If the client wears contact lenses, are the lenses cleaned and stored as recommended? Is the client capable of safely taking care of the lenses?

Visual ability is one of several capabilities necessary for a person to operate a motor vehicle. Use tact when assessing a client who may have impaired vision. Clients may not answer truthfully if they feel that driving privileges will be lost.

Briefly review the client's driving history for information that can indicate a vision deficit. Ask if driving at night is difficult because of the need to adjust to the glare from oncoming headlights. Does the client have trouble seeing the dashboard instrument panel at night because of dim lighting? Are traffic or street signs difficult to read while driving? Is the client able to drive in conditions of reduced visibility, such as in rain or fog? Do other vehicles, pedestrians, bicyclists, or objects appear unexpectedly in the peripheral vision while the client is looking straight ahead? Has the client had a motor vehicle accident or "close call" within the past year?

The social stigma of blindness underlies the anxiety that clients experience with actual or potential vision loss. Total loss of vision isolates a person within a different reality. Although most clients are successfully rehabilitated, some losses are permanent. Some people, for a variety of reasons, remain socially isolated. The image of a blind person who is pitied and must accept the charity of others is disturbing.

Not all work environments can be adapted for someone who is visually impaired. Clients with actual or potential vision loss may be faced with barriers in their vocations that force an unwanted change. Age may be a major factor in the client's ability to meet this challenge. Self-esteem is closely related to one's roles in a particular lifestyle. Loss of control in personal, family, and work situations can be devastating. The issue of dependence versus independence may also be a factor in the client's ability to cope with the stressors of vision loss.

■ REVIEW OF SYSTEMS

The review of systems (ROS) relevant to the eyes includes asking about manifestations such as headaches and problems with sinusitis. Determine whether manifestations occur in association with pain or discomfort, visual changes, swelling, redness, or drainage from the eye. Ask about the time of day and the season of year during which manifestations occur as well as about sensitivity to light. Detailed questions are presented in Box 9–2.

PHYSICAL EXAMINATION

Your role and scope of practice in ophthalmic assessment and examination vary according to state nurse practice acts, institutions, and employer guidelines. Regardless of the level of responsibility in any practice situation, you must be knowledgeable about ophthalmic clinical manifestations and diagnoses as they relate to the holistic approach to client care.

Examination of the eyes includes assessment of external structures, using inspection and palpation, extraocular movements (EOMs), visual acuity, and visual fields (peripheral vision). If you have advanced clinical assessment skills, you may perform tonometry and examine the internal eye structures with an ophthalmoscope. For an example of an assessment recording, see Physical Assessment Findings in the Healthy Adult: The Eye.

Observe the client's body structure and features for obvious deformities and apparent age. For example, the hand deformities or abnormal gait of a client with arthritis may be a clue to the diagnosis of an associated eye disorder of keratoconjunctivitis sicca (*dry eye syndrome*) in a client who reports itching and burning eyes.

■ EXTERNAL EYE

External eye structures include the eyebrows, eyelashes, eyelids, the lacrimal apparatus, anterior portion of the eyeballs, conjunctivae, sclerae, corneas, anterior chambers, pupils, and irises. Inspect and palpate these structures while the client sits at eye level.

PHYSICAL ASSESSMENT FINDINGS IN THE HEALTHY ADULT

The Eye

Inspection

Visual acuity 20/20. Eyebrows full, mobile. Eyelashes curve out and away from eyelids. Ptosis absent. Eyelids without lesions or inflammation. Eyes moist. Palpebral conjunctivae pink; bulbar conjunctivae clear. Scleral color even, without redness. Corneal light reflection symmetrical. PERRLA, directly and consensually. Cornea smooth; lens and anterior chamber clear. Irises evenly colored. EOMs full, without nystagmus. Conjugate movement. No strabismus. Visual fields full to confrontation.

Palpation

Eyeballs firm. Orbits without edema. No regurgitation from puncta. Tenderness absent over lacrimal apparatus.

Funduscopic Examination

Red reflexes visualized. AV ratio approximately 2:3. Vessels without tortuosity, narrowing, pulsation, or nicking. Disc margins clear, no cupping, cup-to-disc ratio 1:3. No evidence of retinal hemorrhage, patches, spots.

AV, artery-to-vein; EOM, extraocular movement; PERRLA, pupils equal, round, reactive to light and accommodation.

Eye Position

Assess eye position for symmetry and alignment. Sunken or protruding eyes, such as protrusion of one eye or both eyes (*exophthalmos*) are an abnormal finding.

Eyebrows

Inspect the eyebrows for symmetry, hair distribution, skin conditions, and movement. The eyebrows normally move up and down smoothly under control of the facial nerves. Hair loss of the lateral aspects occurs with aging. The skin may be dry and flaking (i.e., dandruff), which is abnormal.

Eyelids and Eyelashes

Examine the eyelids and eyelashes for placement and symmetry. When open, the upper lids rest at the top of the irises and the lower lids at the bottom so that the sclerae are not visible above or below the irises. Sagging of the upper lids that covers part of the pupil (ptosis) is abnormal. Ptosis may occur with aging but also results from edema, third cranial nerve disorders, and neuromuscular disorders. Check for effective closure by asking the client to close the eyes. Eyelids that turn inward *(entropion)* or outward *(ectropion)* can result in corneal irritation. Lid eversion and inversion are often related to aging tissues but may result from facial nerve paresis, scarring, or allergies. Elevate the eyebrows to inspect the upper lids for lesions. Inspect the lower lids by asking the client to open the eyes. Examine the skin of the eyelids and orbit by palpating for texture, firmness, mobility, and integrity of the underlying tissues.

Blink Response

Blinking is an involuntary reflex that occurs bilaterally up to 20 times a minute. Rapid, infrequent, or asymmetrical blinking is abnormal.

Eyeballs

Palpate the eyeballs for symmetry and firmness. Instruct the client to close the eyes and look down. Place the tip of the index fingers on the upper eyelids, over the sclerae, and palpate gently. Normally, the eyeballs feel firm and symmetrical, not asymmetrical, hard, or soft. If you have advanced clinical skills, you may perform tonometry to measure ocular pressure (see Internal Eye Examination).

Lacrimal Apparatus

Examine the lacrimal apparatus by retracting the upper lid and having the client look down so that part of the lacrimal gland may be visualized. Observe this area for swelling or tenderness. The eye surface should be moist, without excess tearing. Inspect the area between the lower lid and the nose, which should be free of edema. Gently palpate the area over the lower orbit rim near the inner canthus (over the lacrimal sac). There should be no regurgitation of fluid from the sac or puncta.

Conjunctivae and Sclerae

Inspect the conjunctivae and sclerae for color changes, texture, vascularity, lesions, thickness, secretions, and foreign bodies. The bulbar conjunctivae are colorless and transparent, allowing the sclerae to be seen. Small blood vessels may be visible. In white people, the sclerae are white; in people with dark skin, they may appear light yellow. Wear gloves to inspect the palpebral conjunctivae, and wash your hands both before and after this portion of the examination.

Retract the lower eyelids to expose the conjunctivae without applying pressure to the eyeballs. You (or the client) should gently push the lower lids down against the bony orbit while the client looks up. Healthy conjunctivae are pink to light red; paleness or a bright red color is abnormal. If the lower palpebral conjunctivae are normal, the upper palpebral conjunctivae usually are not inspected. If examination is necessary, evert the upper eyelids by gently grasping the eyelashes of the upper lid and pulling down while the client looks down. Place a cotton-tipped applicator just above the lid margin, and turn the upper lid inside out over the applicator. After the inspection, return the eyelid to its normal position by gently pulling the eyelashes forward while the client looks up.

Corneal Reflex

The corneal reflex test is performed to assess the function of the fifth (trigeminal) cranial nerve. Instruct the client to keep the eyes open and look straight ahead. Bring a sterile cotton wisp from behind the client and touch it lightly to the cornea. Blinking and tearing indicate that the nerves are intact. Use a separate wisp for each eye. An alternative method is to use a syringe or the bulb from an otoscope to gently puff air across the cornea, eliciting the blink-and-tear response. A client wearing contact lenses may not respond to the same degree as someone who does not wear them because of insensitivity to the stimulus.

Cornea

Inspect the cornea from an oblique angle while shining a penlight on the corneal surface. The irises are easily visible. In older adults, a thin, grayish white ring around the edge of the cornea (*arcus senilis*) may be seen. Abnormalities include surface irregularity and cloudiness (opacity).

Anterior Chamber

Using the same oblique angle and penlight, inspect the anterior chamber while observing the cornea. The chambers should appear clear and transparent with no cloudiness or shadows cast upon the irises. The depth of the chamber between the cornea and iris normally is about 3 mm. Shallower or deeper chambers are abnormal; refer the client to an ophthalmologist.

Iris and Pupil

Inspect the iris and pupil. The iris should light up with oblique lighting from the penlight and should have a consistent color. Bulging or uneven coloring is abnormal. When light shines into the eyes, the iris constricts as the optic nerves are stimulated, causing the pupil to become smaller. Dim lighting causes the pupil to dilate. Inspect the pupils for size, equality, shape, and ability to react to light and accommodation. Pupils are normally black, round, with smooth borders, and the same size. The actual size depends on the level of lighting, effect of medications that alter iris contractility, changes in intracranial pressure, or lesions impinging on the optic nerve.

Dim the light to test pupil reactions to light and accommodation. Instruct the client to look straight ahead. To test direct response to light, bring the penlight in from the side to shine directly over the center of the pupil. The illuminated pupil should constrict briskly and evenly. Repeat this maneuver on the other eye. Both eyes should react to the same degree. Test consensual response by observing one pupil while the penlight is shone on the opposite pupil. Both pupils should constrict to the same degree, although the consensual response is slightly slower.

Test accommodation by holding the penlight 4 to 6 inches (10 to 15 cm) away from the client's nose. Instruct the client to look first at the penlight, then at the distant wall straight ahead, and then back at the penlight. While the client gazes from near to far and back again, observe the pupils' response to changes in distance. The pupils should dilate when the client looks at the far point and should constrict when the client looks at the near object. Then move the penlight toward the bridge of the client's nose, observing the pupils for convergence and constriction.

Results of the pupil assessment that are normal are recorded as PERRLA (*p*upils *e*qual, *r*ound, and *r*eactive to *l*ight, and *a*ccommodation). Abnormal results include light intolerance *(photophobia),* irregular or unequal pupils, or pupils that do not react to light or accommodation. Pupil abnormalities may be caused by neurologic disease, intraocular inflammation, iris adhesions, systemic or ocular medication side effects, or surgical alteration, or they may be benign variations of normal findings.

Ocular Motility

Evaluation of ocular motility provides information about the extraocular muscles; the orbit; the oculomotor, trochlear, and abducent nerves; their brain stem connections; and the cerebral cortex. Ask the client to track a target with both eyes as it is moved in each of the six cardinal directions of gaze (see Fig. 64–1). Note the speed, smoothness, range, and symmetry of movements and observe for unsteadiness of fixation (*nystagmus*).

The eyes normally move in parallel to each other, smoothly and in unison. Test the function of the oculomotor, trochlear, and abducent nerves by asking the client to look straight ahead while you stand directly in front. Hold a penlight approximately 12 inches (30 cm) from the client's eyes. Instruct the client to keep the head still and to follow the penlight's movements with the eyes only. Move the penlight slowly and smoothly through the six cardinal positions of gaze, being careful not to go beyond the client's field of vision. Move the penlight in an orderly manner from the center outward along each of the six directions; pause briefly to observe for nystagmus, then return to the center. Nystagmus is an involuntary rapid, oscillating movement of the eyeball and is considered an abnormal finding except for slight nystagmus in the extreme lateral gazes (e.g., end-point nystagmus). If the eyes do not move in parallel or if the upper eyelid covers more than a tiny portion of the iris, note the conditions as abnormal findings.

Corneal Light Reflex Test

The corneal light reflex test (Hirschberg's test) determines eye alignment. Shine a penlight at the bridge of the client's nose from a distance of 12 to 15 inches (30 to 38 cm) while the client stares straight ahead. Observe where the light reflects from both corneas; the reflection should be symmetrical. Asymmetrical reflection is abnormal and may indicate *strabismus,* a disorder in which the eye axes cannot be directed to the same object. A constant deviation of ocular alignment is termed *tropia.* Deviation toward the nose is called *esoptropia,* a deviation away from the nose is called *exotropia,* and a vertical (up or down) deviation is called *hypertropia.* Latent deviations are seen only when one eye is covered and are called *phorias* (e.g., *esophoria* and *exophoria*).

Cover-Uncover Test

This test assesses eye muscle function and alignment for tropia and phoria. Ask the client to stare straight ahead at a fixed point approximately 20 inches (51 cm) away. Cover one of the client's eyes with an opaque card while you observe the uncovered eye for lateral or medial movement as it focuses on the fixed point. There should be no movement. Remove the eye cover, and observe that

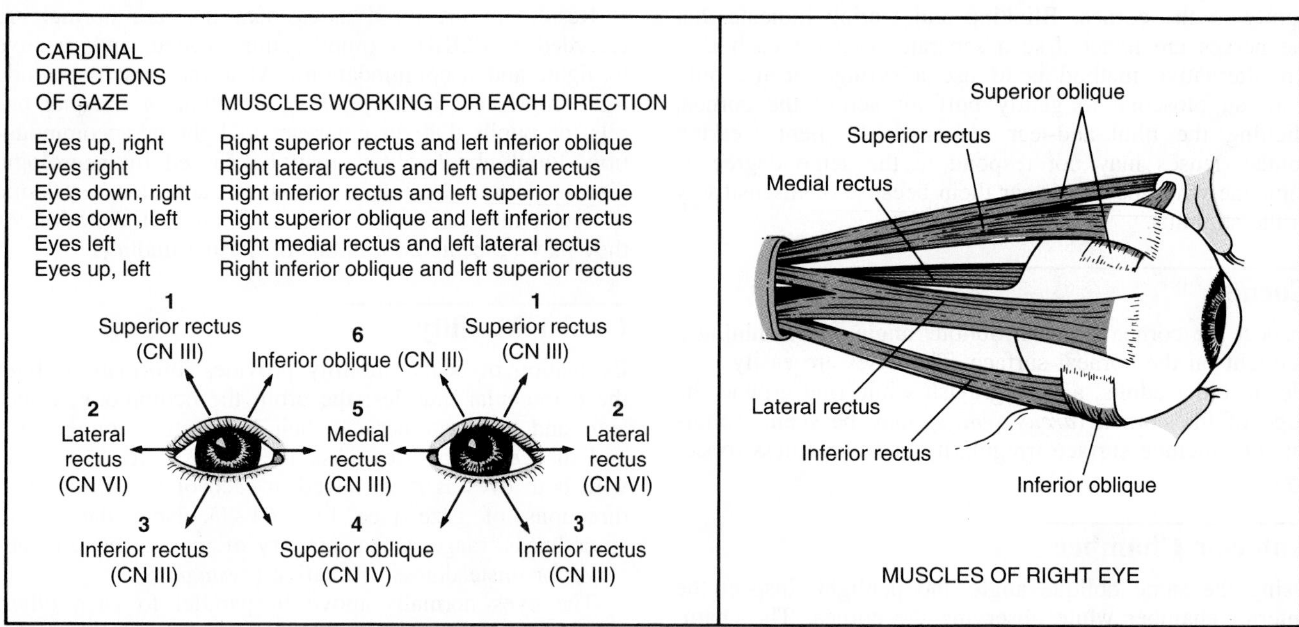

FIGURE 64–1 The six cardinal directions of gaze and the muscles responsible for each: (1) right, (2) left, (3) up and right, (4) up and left, (5) down and right, and (6) down and left. CN, cranial nerve.

eye for movement as it focuses on the fixed point; again, there should be no movement. Repeat the maneuvers for the opposite eye. The test may need to be repeated several times to confirm abnormal findings of strabismus.

Vision

VISUAL ACUITY

Testing visual acuity is the standard and routine method used to determine the clarity of the ocular media (cornea, lens, and vitreous) and the function of the visual pathway from the retina to the brain. Although abnormal acuity implies an uncorrected refractive error or pathologic process, normal acuity does not exclude disease of the visual system. Visual acuity is assessed in one eye at a time, then in both eyes together, with the client comfortably seated. Begin with the right eye while covering the left eye with an occluder or opaque card. Test visual acuity with and without corrective lenses. Visual acuity is traditionally measured with the Snellen chart (Fig. 64–2*A*) at a distance of 20 feet; at this distance, rays of light from an object are practically parallel and little effort of accommodation is required. In rooms that are shorter than 20 feet, mirrors or projection may be used to achieve the required distance. Charts may also be reduced proportionately to compensate for distance. Adaptations may be needed for the client who is illiterate or who does not speak English; variations of the Snellen chart are available for these clients. The numbers and symbols can be used in lieu of letters. There must be adequate lighting for the client to see.

Begin by asking the client to read the smallest line of symbols or letters that is seen. Credit the client for the smallest line of print that is read with more than 50% accuracy. Record the results according to the standardized numbers printed next to the lines on the chart. The sizes of the symbols are identified according to the distances at which they are normally visible. For example, the largest symbols can be read 200 feet away by people with unimpaired vision. The results of visual acuity testing are expressed as a fraction. The numerator denotes the distance the client is from the chart letters, and the denominator denotes the distance from the chart at which a client with normal vision can see the chart letters. Examples of results are as follows:

- Vision that is 20/20 is normal; that is, the client is able to read at 20 feet what a person with normal vision can read at 20 feet.
- A client with a visual acuity of 20/60 can read at a distance of 20 feet only what a client with normal vision can read at 60 feet.
- The client with *myopia* (nearsightedness) has results of 20/30 or greater, signifying that the client can read at 20 feet only what a person with normal vision can read at 30 feet (or greater).
- *Hyperopia* (farsightedness) results are 20/15 or less; that is, the client can read at 20 feet what a person with normal vision can read at 15 feet (or less).
- A result of 20/15 indicates better-than-average visual acuity.
- *Legal blindness* is defined as 20/200 or less with corrected vision (glasses or contact lenses) or less than 20 degrees of visual field in the better eye.

When the client cannot distinguish the largest letter on the chart, ask the client to read the number of fingers held up in front of him or her at a distance of 3 feet (CF = count fingers). If the client cannot distinguish fingers, ask whether the client perceives hand movements (HM = hand motion). Finally, determine whether the client can perceive light (LP = light perception). NLP indicates no light perception.

Test near vision with a card or newsprint held 12 to 14 inches (30 to 36 cm) from the client's eyes (Fig. 64–

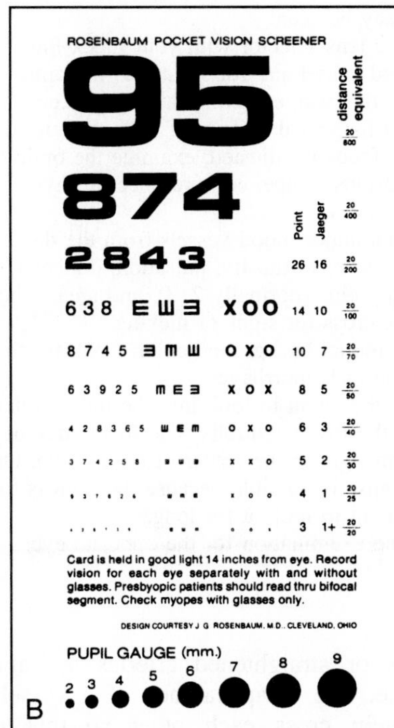

FIGURE 64–2 *A*, Snellen's chart, for assessment of visual acuity. *B*, A Rosenbaum pocket vision screener. The charts are not pictured to scale with respect to one another. (*B*, Courtesy of SMP Division, Cooper Laboratories [P.R.], Inc., San German, Puerto Rico.)

2*B*). Corrective lenses are worn if needed. The client with normal vision can read the material at that distance. Complaints of blurring or attempts by the client to move the card either closer or farther away signal abnormal near vision.

If the client becomes familiar with the letters through repeated examination, have the client read the letters backward. If the client can read most of the letters in a particular line but misses one or two, document the visual acuity as 20/40–2.

VISUAL FIELDS

Visual field testing is used to evaluate peripheral vision. It may be accomplished by the *confrontational method* (Fig. 64–3) or with a computerized instrument. The confrontational method assumes that the examiner has normal peripheral vision.

The client sits facing you approximately 2 feet (60 cm) away. The client's eyes and yours should be at the same level. Both you and the client cover the eyes directly opposite to one another with an opaque cover (e.g., your right eye and the client's left eye) and stare at each other's uncovered eye. Hold a small object, such as a penlight, in your free hand, holding it equidistant between yourself and the client, just out of view at the periphery of the visual field. Starting with the superior field, slowly bring the penlight down between the client and yourself until the client states that he or she can see it. (You should be able to see the penlight at the same time.)

Repeat this maneuver at 45-degree angles, progressing through the superior, temporal, inferior, and nasal fields until all are tested. You may need to position the penlight slightly behind the client to adequately test the temporal fields. Repeat the test for the other eye. Normal visual fields extend approximately 50 degrees superiorly, 90 degrees laterally, 70 degrees inferiorly, and 60 degrees medially. Gross visual field defects can be detected and, if found, refer the client for further examination.

A variety of manual and computerized visual field testing equipment may be used to permit more accurate, reproducible detection and quantification of *scotoma* (an area of decreased visual function). CNS disorders, such as a brain lesion or syphilis, and ocular disorders, such as glaucoma or retinal detachment, can alter visual fields.

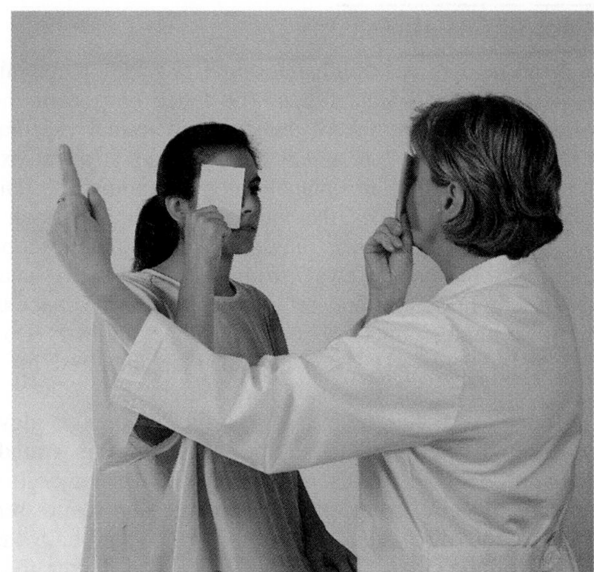

FIGURE 64–3 Confrontational method of assessment of visual fields. (From Jarvis, C. [1996]. *Physical examination and health assessment* [2nd ed.]. Philadelphia: W. B. Saunders.)

Special Testing of Vision

COLOR VISION

Color vision problems are genetic and acquired in both men and women. Men are more often affected with inherited losses in color vision (7%), and women are affected to a lesser degree (0.5%). Nutritional problems, optic nerve disorders, and problems with the fovea centralis can also alter color perception.

Color vision testing is not always part of a routine eye examination. It is used most often in screening people seeking a license to operate a motor vehicle or for employment in which color discrimination is important. A common test involves the use of color plates on which numbers are outlined in primary colors and surrounded by "confusion" colors. The person with color vision problems is unable to recognize the figure. One such test consists of 84 chips of color that are matched in terms of increasing hues.

Central Area Blindness Assessment

The Amsler grid is a 20-cm square that is divided into 5-mm squares with a dot in the center. The grid is used to detect and follow the development of central area blindness (scotoma), such as occurs in macular degeneration. The client wears glasses, closes one eye, and holds the grid 12 inches from the face (the usual reading distance). The client fixes vision on the central dot and describes any areas of distortion or absences in the grid.

■ INTERNAL EYE

Internal eye structures are visible only with illumination such as that provided by an ophthalmoscope. This instrument is used to inspect the structures posterior to the iris, including the lens and fundus (which includes the retina, retinal vessels, choroid, optic disc, macula, and fovea). Using the ophthalmoscope requires considerable skill and practice.

Direct Ophthalmoscopy

The hand-held direct ophthalmoscope provides a magnified (×15) image of the fundus (posterior portion of the eye) and a detailed view of the disc and retinal vascular bed. Ophthalmoscopy is a part of a general physical examination as well as an ophthalmologic examination. Dilating the eye enhances the view, although a darkened room may cause adequate dilation. The ophthalmoscope is held 1 to 2 inches away from the client's eye and, through a light source and reflective mirrors, the macula, optic disc, and retinal vessels can be examined (Box 64–3 and Fig. 64–4). The view may be impaired by a cloudy cornea or the presence of a cataract.

Normally, the red reflex is a bright red-orange glow seen through the pupil. The optic disc appears round, with well-defined margins (except in the nasal margin), and a creamy pink color. The physiologic cup (depressed center of the disc) should be no larger than half the diameter of the optic disc. Retinal veins are darker than arteries and radiate from the disc. Veins are slightly thicker than arteries and should be free of pulsation. Tortuous vessels or straightened arteries are abnormal, as is nicking (i.e., the disappearance of a vessel where an artery and vein cross each other so that one vessel looks discontinuous). The retinal background is pink in whites, and dark and heavily pigmented in people with a dark complexion. Choroidal vessels may appear as linear orange streaks. A normal retina is shown in Figure 64–4.

The fundus is the only site in the body where the vascular bed may be observed directly. Thus, funduscopic examination yields information about many systemic diseases. Abnormal findings include an altered arteriovenous ratio, narrowed arteries, widened veins, pinched-off vessels, abnormal arterial light reflex, excessive tortuosity, numerous arteriovenous nickings, exudates, white patches, and focal hemorrhage.

BOX 64–3 Guidelines for Using an Ophthalmoscope

1. Assemble the ophthalmoscope by attaching the head to the handle.
2. Darken the room.
3. Turn on the ophthalmoscope light by depressing the rheostat button and turning the rheostat to the brightest light.
4. Turn the aperture selector to a large round circle of light.
5. Turn the lens selector dial to zero.
6. Instruct the client to stare straight ahead and to focus on a distant object.
7. Leave both of your eyes open during the examination. Learn to suppress visual stimulation from the eye that is not looking through the viewing aperture.
8. Hold the ophthalmoscope while steadying the client's head with your free hand.
9. Approach the client from the side at approximately a 45-degree angle and a distance of 15 inches. Direct the light into the client's pupil.
10. Move slowly closer to the client's eye, keeping the light directed on the pupil. If the client blinks, hold your position steady until the client's eye opens again. At approximately 15 inches, visualize the red reflex, then the anterior chamber. Moving closer, look at the lens. Finally, when very close (1 to 2 inches), vessels of the fundus may be seen.
11. Adjust the lens selector with your index finger to focus on a blood vessel and follow it into the optic disc.
12. Focus on the disc, adjusting the lens selector as needed to correct for visual deficits of both you and the client. Once the focus is adjusted, examine the optic disc (for color, margins, shape, and presence of physiologic cup; see Fig. 64–6).
13. Follow the major blood vessels from the disc and look for evidence of tortuosity, pulsation, diameter, ratio of arteries to veins (normally 2:3), and areas where arteries and veins cross for signs of nicking.
14. Note the retinal background color. Look for the presence of exudate or hemorrhage.
15. Last, ask the client to look into the light so that you can examine the fovea centralis. The fovea may be seen as a tiny bright light in the center of the macula. Only a very brief glimpse is possible because the light is too bright for the client to look at for long.
16. Repeat the examination for the opposite eye.

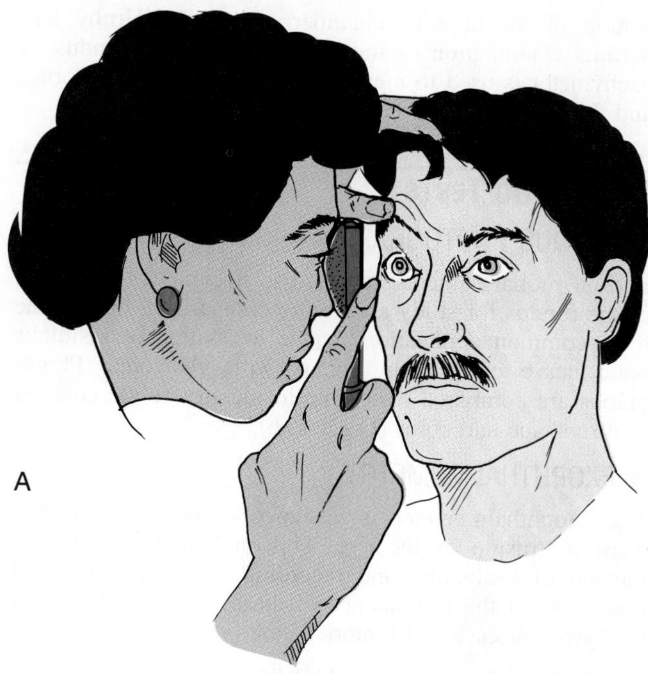

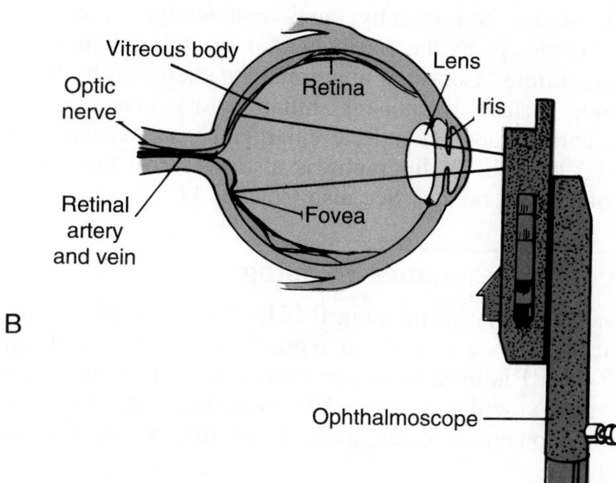

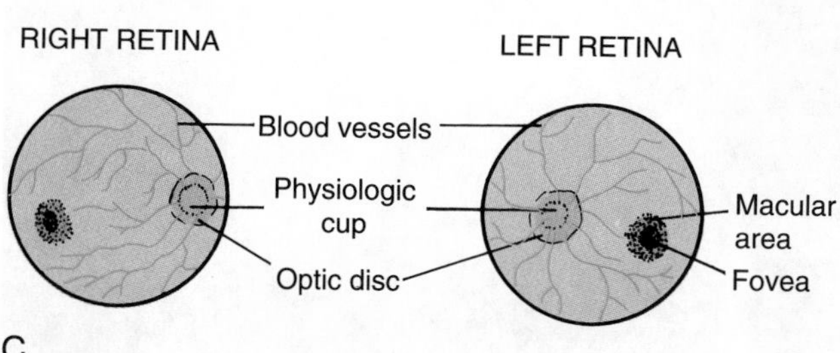

FIGURE 64–4 *A,* The examiner uses the right hand to hold the ophthalmoscope to the right eye to examine the client's right eye. The examiner uses the left hand and left eye when examining the client's left eye. Note the positioning of the examiner's free hand, which is placed to steady the client's head and to slightly retract the eyebrow. *B,* The examiner sees what appears in the angle of light through the viewing aperture. *C,* The actual area of retina visualized depends on the dilation of the pupil. Note the structures that may be examined.

Indirect Ophthalmoscopy

Indirect ophthalmoscopy provides a stereoscopic picture over a large area of the retina. The light source comes from a head-mounted light. The examiner holds a convex lens in front of the client's eye and, through a viewing device attached to the headband, sees an inverted reversed image. The indirect ophthalmoscope provides for binocular visual inspection with depth perception and permits a wider field of view compared with the direct method.

Tonometry

Tonometry is a method of measuring intraocular fluid pressure with the use of calibrated instruments that indent or flatten the corneal apex. The eye can be thought of as an enclosed compartment through which there is a constant circulation of *aqueous humor,* which maintains the shape of the eye with a relatively uniform pressure within the globe. As the pressure increases, the eye becomes firmer and a greater force is required to cause the same amount of indentation. Pressures between 8 and 21 mm Hg are considered within the normal range.

The two most common types of tonometers are the hand-held tonometer and applanation tonometer (Fig. 64–5). The portable hand-held instrument may be used in an office, clinic, emergency department, or operating room or at the bedside. It measures the amount of tension on the cornea. First the cornea is anesthetized with a topical anesthetic eye drop. While the client sits and looks straight forward, the tonopen is held perpendicular to the cornea and tapped several times directly on the

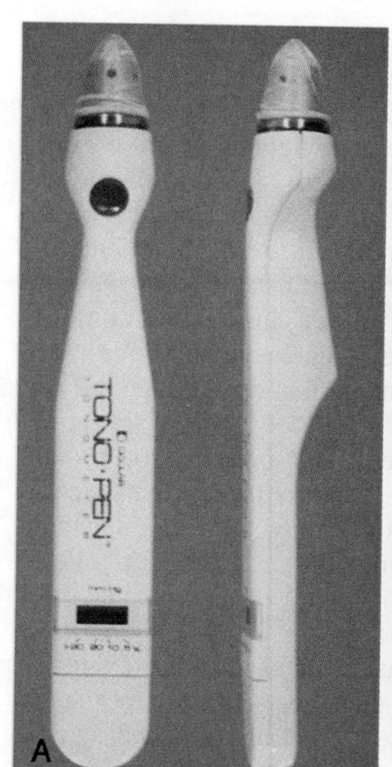

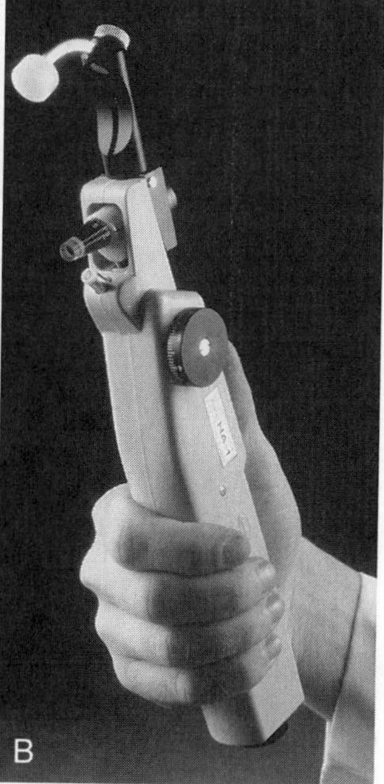

FIGURE 64–5 *A, Left and right,* Tonometer, seen from two viewpoints (Courtesy of Ophthalmic Photography at the University of Michigan W. K. Kellogg Eye Center, Ann Arbor.) *B,* Hand-held applanation tonometer. (Courtesy of Kowa Optimed, Torrance, CA.)

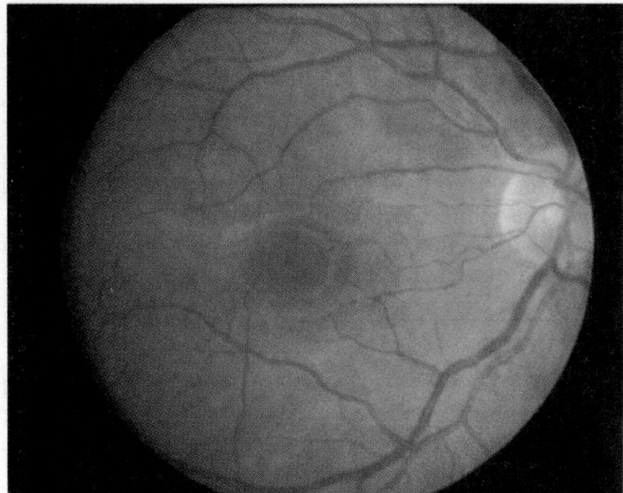

FIGURE 64–6 A normal fundus. (Courtesy of Ophthalmic Photography at the University of Michigan W. K. Kellogg Eye Center, Ann Arbor.)

cornea. A computer chip in the instrument averages the readings and notes the standard deviation.

An applanation tonometer, which may either be handheld or attached to a slit-lamp microscope, measures the amount of force required to flatten the corneal apex by a standard amount. Anesthetic eye drops are also used beforehand.

Intraocular pressure is noted in the client record with a large T. The top number indicates the pressure in the right eye and the bottom number, the left eye.

Slit-Lamp Examination

The slit-lamp microscope is used to illuminate and examine the anterior segment of the eye under magnification. A linear slit beam of incandescent light is projected onto the globe, illuminating an optical cross-section of the anterior chamber. The angle of illumination, length, width, and intensity of the light may be adjusted. The client sits, and the head is stabilized by an adjustable chin rest and forehead strap. Details of the lid margins, lashes, conjunctiva, tear film, cornea, iris, lens, and aqueous humor can be studied. At the highest magnification setting, the abnormal presence of red or white blood cells in the aqueous humor may be visualized. The presence of protein (flare), called an *anterior chamber reaction,* that accompanies intraocular inflammation may also be detected. Normal aqueous humor is optically clear, without cells or flare. The presence of cells and flare is documented as 1 to 4+.

Fluorescein dye is often used in a slit-lamp examination to highlight corneal irregularities. Sterile paper strips containing fluorescein dye are wetted and touched against the inner surface of the lower lid, instilling the yellow dye into the tear film and onto the corneal surface. A blue filter is attached to the light beam, causing the dye to fluoresce. The dye highlights defects in the cornea.

In addition to the applanation tonometer, several other devices may be attached to the slit lamp to expand the scope of the examination. A gonioscope provides visualization of the anterior chamber angle. The Hruby lens permits examination of the vitreous body and fundus. A pachymeter is used to measure the thickness of the cornea and the anterior chamber.

DIAGNOSTIC TESTS

■ FUNDUS PHOTOGRAPHY

Special retinal cameras are used to document fine details of the fundus for study and future comparison. One of the most common applications is the evaluation of insidious optic nerve changes in clients with glaucoma. Photographs are compared over time to identify subtle changes in disc shape and color (Fig. 64–6).

■ EXOPHTHALMOMETRY

The exophthalmometer is designed to measure the forward protrusion of the eye. This instrument provides a method of evaluating and recording the progression and regression of the prominence of the eye in disorders such as thyroid disease and tumors of the orbit.

■ OPHTHALMIC RADIOGRAPHY

X-ray study, tomography, and computed tomography (CT) are useful in the evaluation of orbital and intracranial conditions. Common abnormalities evaluated by these methods include neoplasms, inflammatory masses, fractures, and extraocular muscle enlargement associated with Graves' disease. Radiography is also useful in the detection of foreign bodies. See also Chapter 11.

Magnetic Resonance Imaging

Magnetic resonance imaging (MRI) allows obtaining multidimensional views without repositioning the client (Fig. 64–7). MRI is used to image edema, areas of demyelination, and vascular lesions. However, the availability of MRI equipment is often limited and the examination is lengthy.

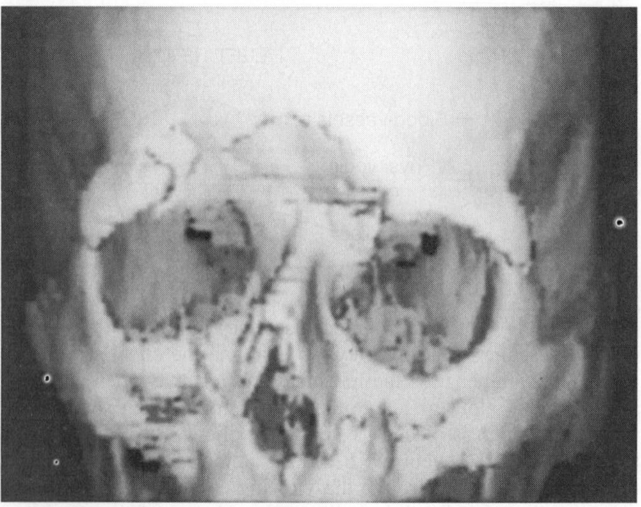

FIGURE 64–7 A magnetic resonance imaging (MRI) scan showing massive facial fractures. Note the three-dimensional appearance obtained with MRI.

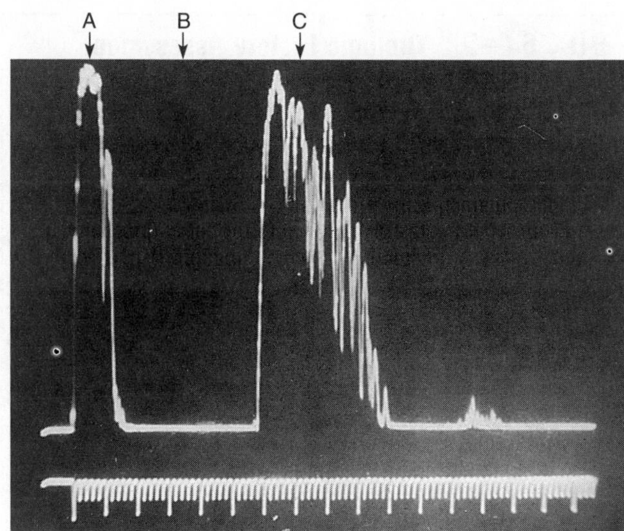

FIGURE 64–8 A normal A-scan ultrasound study of the eye. The sound beam is aimed in a straight line, and echoes are displayed as spikes. The amplitude depends on the density of the reflecting tissue and perpendicularity of the probe. *A,* Cornea and lens. *B,* Clear vitreous. *C,* Retina and choroid.

Ultrasonography

Ultrasonography uses high-frequency sound waves transmitted through a probe placed directly on the eyeball. As the sound waves bounce back off the various tissue components, they are collected by a receiver and amplified on an oscilloscope screen. Sound waves derived from the most distal structures arrive last, having traveled the farthest (Fig. 64–8). A-scan ultrasonography is used to measure axial length, the distance from the cornea to the retina, to determine the refractive power of an intraocular lens in cataract surgery. B-scan ultrasonography may be used to evaluate the characteristics of a lesion, as well as its size and growth over time, or the presence of a foreign body.

■ OPHTHALMODYNAMOMETRY

Ophthalmodynamometry is a test that consists of exerting pressure on the sclera with a spring plunger while the central retinal vessels emerging from the disc through an ophthalmoscope are observed. This instrument gives an approximate measurement of the relative pressures in the central retinal arteries and indirectly assesses carotid arterial flow on either side. Ophthalmodynamometry is indicated in the neurologic evaluation of clients who complain of "blacking out" of vision in one eye (*amaurosis*), spells of weakness on one side of the body, or other manifestations of cerebral ischemia. A difference of more than 20% in the diastolic pressures between the two eyes suggests insufficiency of the carotid arterial system on the side with the lower pressure.

■ ELECTRORETINOGRAPHY

An electrical potential exists between the cornea and retina of the eye. Because the retina is neurologic tissue, the retina exhibits certain electrical responses when stimulated by light. Electroretinography (ERG) measures the change in electrical potential of the eye caused by a diffuse flash of light. For this test, electrodes incorporated into a contact lens are placed directly on the anesthetized eye. Because eye movements disrupt the values of the test, the client must be able to fixate on a target while keeping the eyes still. Normal ERG findings signify functional integrity of the retina. Retinal diseases that may be evaluated with ERG include retinitis pigmentosa (progressive degeneration of photoreceptor cells), massive ischemia, disseminated infection, or toxic effects from drugs or chemicals.

■ VISUAL EVOKED RESPONSE

Visual evoked response (VER) is similar to ERG, in that it also measures the electrical potential resulting from a visual stimulus. The entire visual pathway from the retina to the cortex may be evaluated through the placement of electrodes on the scalp. Reduced speed of neuronal conduction, as with demyelination in optic neuritis, results in an abnormal response. Retinal or optic nerve disease may be diagnosed by stimulation of each eye separately.

■ FLUORESCEIN ANGIOGRAPHY

Fundus photography is enhanced by the use of fluorescein dye whose molecules emit green light when stimulated by blue light. The client sits in front of a retina camera after the pupils are dilated. A small amount of fluorescein dye is injected into an antecubital vein. The dye circulates throughout the body before eventual excretion by the kidneys. As the dye passes through the retinal and choroidal circulation, it can be visualized and photographed because of its ability to fluoresce (Fig. 64–9). A rapid sequence of pictures captures the initial rapid perfusion of the retinal and choroidal vessels. Later photos may demonstrate the gradual leakage of dye from abnormal vessels. Changes in blood flow, ischemia, and hemorrhage may be detected. Because it can so precisely delineate areas of

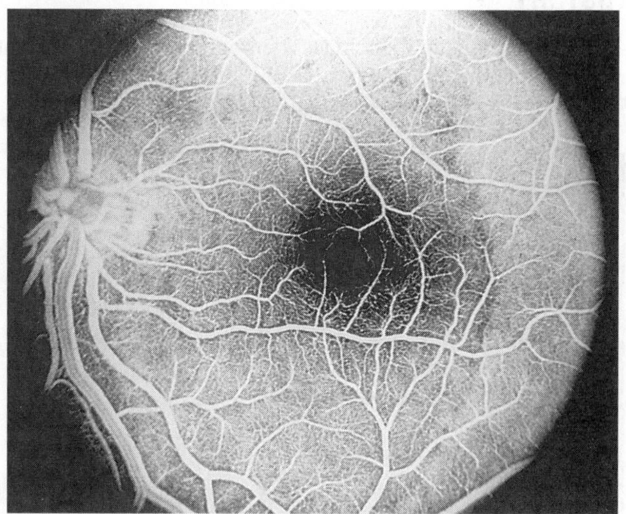

FIGURE 64–9 A normal fluorescein angiogram. The normal pattern of fluorescein angiography can be divided into three phases: (1) The *filling phase* (pictured) takes 8 to 20 seconds. (2) The *recirculation phase* starts 0.5 second after the filling phase and lasts 3 to 5 minutes. (3) The *late phase* lasts 30 to 60 minutes. Photographs are taken before injection, at half-second intervals for 20 seconds, then at intervals of 5 minutes.

abnormality, it is an essential guide for planning laser treatment of retinal vascular disease.

You may administer the intravenous (IV) fluorescein dye injection under an ophthalmologist's direction. First assess the client's general health status and identify any allergies. Allergic reactions to other dye injections, such as for an IV pyelogram [IVP] or cholangiogram, should be considered before the fluorescein injection. Diphenhydramine may be prescribed prophylactically. Although anaphylactic shock is a rare occurrence, emergency equipment should be located nearby. Occasionally, a client's vasovagal response to the dye may include vertigo, nausea, and momentary loss of consciousness. Obtain a consent for the procedure. Explain that during the injection the client may experience a warm sensation. The client will also hear the mechanics of the camera taking rapid-sequence photographs and experience bright flashes of light.

After the examination, encourage the client to increase intake of fluids because the dye is excreted through the kidneys. During the next 24 hours, the urine will be yellowish, and light-complexioned clients may experience a temporary yellow tint to the skin that will fade within a few hours as the dye is excreted. Because the pupils are dilated before the examination, it may be necessary to wear dark glasses for several hours until the pupils can constrict again in the presence of light.

ASSESSMENT OF THE EAR

The otologic history can be an important assessment tool and should be obtained before audiometric testing. Certain behavioral cues can indicate hearing impairment (Box 64–4). Collect significant data by conducting a thorough interview. Include the specific items in the otologic history (Box 64–5).

HISTORY

An otologic history includes demographic data, current clinical manifestations, past health history, family health

BOX 64–4 Clues Suggesting Hearing Impairment

Any adult who exhibits one or more of the following traits may be experiencing hearing impairment:

- Is irritable, hostile, hypersensitive in intercliental relations
- Has difficulty hearing upper frequency consonants (Sl, Sh)
- Complains about people mumbling
- Turns up volume on television
- Asks for frequent repetition and answers questions inappropriately
- Loses sense of humor, becomes grim
- Leans forward to hear better or turns head to preferred side
- Shuns large-group and small-group audience situations
- Shuns areas with increased background noise
- Might appear aloof and "stuck up"
- Complains of ringing in the ears
- Has an unusually soft or loud voice

BOX 64–5 Otologic History Assessment Guide

Current Problem

What changes are you having in your hearing?
Do you have any of the following manifestations?

Distortion of hearing	Yes No
Differences in the pitch of sound	Yes No
Noise in your ear	Yes No
Fullness or pressure in your ear	Yes No
Pain in your ear	Yes No
Drainage from your ear	Yes No
Have you ever had a hearing examination?	Yes No

If yes, why?
What were the results?

Use of Hearing Aids

Are you wearing hearing aids now?	Yes No
Are your hearing aids effective?	Yes No
How old are your hearing aids?	L ___ yr R ___ yr

Associated Problems

Do you have any of the following manifestations?

Head noise or ringing	Yes No
Feeling dizzy or unsteady	Yes No
Blurred vision	Yes No
Double vision	Yes No
Numbness in the hands or feet	Yes No
Weakness in the arms or legs	Yes No
Tingling around the mouth or face	Yes No
Loss of consciousness or blackouts	Yes No
Fainting	Yes No
Convulsions or seizures	Yes No

Risk Factors

Have you ever worked around loud noises?	Yes No
How long? ________ yr	
Do you still work around loud noise?	Yes No
Do you wear ear protection?	Yes No

Past Health History

Did you have hearing problems as a child?	Yes No
Did you have frequent ear infections as a child?	Yes No
Did you ever have a perforation in your eardrum?	Yes No
Did you ever get hit in the ear?	Yes No
Have you had ear surgery?	Yes No

If yes,

	Date	Operation	Surgeon
Right ear	____	____	____
Left ear	____	____	____

Do you have any food or medication allergies?
Please list and describe your reaction.

Family History

Do you have family members who were hard of hearing before 50 years old?
If yes, explain.

Have any members of your family ever had ear surgery?
If yes, explain.

history, psychosocial history, and review of systems. Ear problems often result from childhood illnesses or abnormalities associated with adjacent structures. The history interview is essential for determining current problems related to the ear.

■ BIOGRAPHICAL AND DEMOGRAPHIC DATA

Demographic data relevant to otologic assessment include the client's age. Hearing impairment may occur as a consequence of the aging process (Table 64–1).

■ CURRENT HEALTH

Chief Complaint

The most common chief complaints include the following:

- Hearing loss
- Pain
- Tinnitus
- Ear drainage
- Loss of balance
- Vertigo
- Dizziness

The client may also complain of associated nausea or vomiting. Complete a symptom analysis to determine onset, duration, frequency, and precipitating and relieving factors. Explore the client's past health history to determine the chronicity of the problem and the probable cause (see Box 64–5).

Symptom Analysis

Hearing loss may occur suddenly or gradually and can accompany the normal aging processes. The loss may be conductive, sensorineural, or related to a CNS disorder. The client may report inability to hear certain words or sounds or that sounds are muffled.

Pain may be perceived as a feeling of fullness in the ear. It may be intensified by movement and relieved by holding the head still or by applying heat. Ear pain may occur as a result of related problems of the nose, sinuses, oral cavity, or pharynx.

Ear drainage can be bloody (sanguineous), clear (serous), mixed (serosanguineous), or contain pus (purulent). Drainage may also be accompanied by an odor.

Tinnitus (ringing in the ears) may be reported as high-pitched or low-pitched, roaring, humming, hissing, or loud and persistent. Tinnitus may occur more commonly at certain times of the day and may involve one or both ears.

Loss of balance may be accompanied by vertigo or dizziness. *Vertigo* is a sensation of motion while the person is not moving. A client may feel that either he or she or the room is moving. *Dizziness* is a sensation of unsteadiness and a feeling of movement within the head or lightheadedness.

TABLE 64–1 CHANGES IN AUDITORY ACUITY CAUSED BY AGING

Anatomic Changes	Physiologic Changes
Degeneration of basilar conductive membrane of cochlea	Decreased ability to hear at all frequencies but greater at higher frequencies
Degeneration of cochlear hair cells	Decreased ability to hear high-frequency sounds
Decreased vascularity of cochlea	Loss of hearing equal at all frequencies
Loss of auditory neurons in spiral ganglia of organ of Corti	Loss of ability to hear high-frequency sounds
Loss of cortical auditory neurons	Diminished hearing and speech comprehension

■ PAST HEALTH HISTORY

Childhood and Infectious Diseases

Common childhood diseases involving the ears include the following:

- Acute middle ear infections (otitis media)
- Eardrum perforations resulting from otitis media
- Complications of ear infections such as chronic otitis media, frequent upper respiratory tract infection, and acute and chronic sinus infections

Infectious diseases with ear sequelae include mumps, measles, and meningitis. Specifically inquire whether the client has been immunized for mumps, measles, and *Haemophilus influenzae* type b (Hib). In utero exposure to maternal influenza or rubella may result in congenital hearing loss in the child. Premature birth is also associated with hearing problems.

Major Illnesses and Hospitalizations

Inquire about a history of upper respiratory tract infections. Has the client had a tonsillectomy or adenoidectomy? Does the history include ear surgery? Has the client had trauma to the head or ear, such as a severe blow or sustained loud noise exposure or concussion from sudden changes in air pressure (such as may occur in an explosion)? Does the history include chronic eardrum perforation?

Medications

Certain medications can damage the vestibulocochlear nerve (eighth cranial nerve), with resultant hearing loss, tinnitus, or disturbances in equilibrium. Aspirin is a common cause of tinnitus. Other drugs include aminoglycosides, analgesics, salicylates, quinine, chemotherapeutic agents, and antiprotozoal agents (Box 64–6). Obtain a complete medication history for prescription and over-the-counter drugs and herbal remedies.

Review the use of herbal remedies. Ginger (*Zingiber officinale*) is known for its anti-nausea effect and may be used for the relief of motion sickness. Ginkgo biloba (*Ginkgo biloba*) has been used for tinnitus and vertigo.

Allergies

In addition to asking about allergies to medications and other substances, inquire about allergies resulting in nasal

BOX 64–6 Selected Ototoxic* Drugs

Aminoglycoside Antibiotics

Streptomycin
Neomycin
Gentamicin
Tobramycin
Amikacin
Kanamycin
Minocycline
Netilmicin

Other Antibiotics

Vancomycin
Viomycin
Polymyxin B
Polymyxin E
Erythromycin
Capreomycin
Chloramphenicol

Other Drugs

Chemotherapeutic agents (bleomycin, cisplatin, nitrogen mustard)
Salicylates
Quinine drugs
Quinidine
Chloroquine

Diuretics

Furosemide
Ethacrynic acid
Acetazolamide
Bumetanide
Mannitol

Chemicals

Metals (lead, mercury, gold, arsenic)
Alcohol
Aniline dyes
Caffeine
Carbon monoxide
Nicotine
Potassium bromate
Povidone-iodine

* Substances toxic to the ear.

stuffiness and congestion. Close proximity of the eustachian tubes to the nasal mucosa may also result in edema, which obstructs the flow of air between the middle ear and nose so that air pressure cannot be equalized.

FAMILY HEALTH HISTORY

Ask about a history of hearing loss or ear surgery among family members. Determine the age at onset for hearing loss or changes in hearing acuity.

PSYCHOSOCIAL HISTORY

Psychosocial and lifestyle factors that influence the incidence of hearing impairment include occupational hazards, environmental exposure, and leisure activities and hobbies. Ask about exposure to loud noises (Table 64–2), including type, frequency, and duration. Is protective ear gear worn? Sound intensity is measured in units known as *decibels*. Ordinary speech level measures about 50 decibels (dB); heavy traffic is about 70 dB; at above 80 dB, noise becomes uncomfortable to the human ear. Exposure to levels greater than 85 to 90 dB for months or years causes cochlear damage.

Does the client swim, especially in water that may be contaminated? Has the client had problems with "swimmer's ear"? Does the client use earplugs to prevent water from entering the ear canal? Contaminated water can provoke an external ear infection and, if the tympanic membrane is perforated, may lead to infection in the middle ear.

Explore the client's ear hygiene habits. Does the client put objects into the ear, such as pencils, hairpins, or cotton-tipped applicators? Inserting objects such as these can traumatize the ear canal and damage or perforate the tympanic membrane.

REVIEW OF SYSTEMS

The review of systems related to the ear includes asking about problems with the nose, sinuses, mouth, pharynx, and throat. Has the client experienced head trauma, loss of balance, dizziness, or vertigo. Detailed questions for the review of systems are found in Box 9–2.

PHYSICAL EXAMINATION

Physical examination of the ear includes assessment of hearing acuity, balance, and equilibrium. Because the external ear is completely visible, it is easy to identify anatomic landmarks and to assess abnormalities. The eardrum reveals important information regarding the middle ear. However, because much of the middle ear and inner ear is inaccessible to direct examination, you must make inferences indirectly by testing auditory and vestibular function. See Physical Assessment Findings in the Healthy Adult: The Ear.

INSPECTION AND PALPATION

External Ear

Gross examination of both ears should precede individual examination of either ear. Use inspection and palpation to assess the external ear. Note size, configuration, and angle of attachment to the head. Observe the configuration of the pinna for gross deformity. Note whether the ears protrude and the degree of protrusion, the color of the skin of the ears, and whether additional skin tags are present. The skin of the ear should be smooth and without breaks or inflammation, especially in the crevice behind the ear. Note any lumps, skin lesions, or cysts, and record approximate size and location.

Perform palpation and manipulation of the pinna to detect tenderness, nodules, or *tophi* (small, hard nodules in the helix that are deposits of uric acid crystals characteristic of gout). During palpation, move the pinna, feel the mastoid area, and press on the tragus, noting any pain or discomfort, which may indicate inflammation or infection.

TABLE 64–2 DECIBEL (dB) RATINGS AND HAZARDOUS TIME EXPOSURE OF COMMON NOISES

Typical Level* (dB)	Example	Dangerous Time Exposure
0	Lowest sound audible to human ear	
30	Quiet library, soft whisper	
40	Quiet office, living room, bedroom away from traffic	
50	Light traffic at a distance, refrigerator, gentle breeze	
60	Air conditioner at 20 ft, conversation, sewing machine	
70	Busy traffic, noisy restaurant (constant exposure)	Critical level begins
80	Subway, heavy city traffic, alarm clock at 2 ft, factory noise	More than 8 hr
90	Truck traffic, noisy home appliances, shop tools, lawnmower	Less than 8 hr
100	Chain saw, boiler shop, pneumatic drill	2 hr
120	Rock concert in front of speakers, sandblasting, thunderclap	Immediate danger
140	Gunshot blast, jet plane	Any length of exposure time is dangerous
180	Rocket launching pad	Hearing loss is inevitable

* Sound levels refer to intensity experienced at typical working distances. Intensity drops 6 dB with every doubling of distance from noise source. (Courtesy of American Academy of Otolaryngology–Head and Neck Surgery, Washington, DC.)

Ear Canal

Direct Observation

Inspection of the ear canal is carried out by direct observation, otoscopy, or microscopic examination. For direct observation, ask the adult to tip his or her head slightly to the opposite side while you pull the pinna up, back, and out. Use a penlight to inspect the ear canal for any abnormalities such as extreme narrowing, excessive wax, redness, scaliness, swelling, drainage, cysts, or foreign objects. None of these signs should be present. Visualization of the eardrum with this method would be unlikely.

Otoscopy

The eardrum is located at the end of the only skin-lined canal in the body. Proper visualization requires illumination and magnification for accurate assessment. An otoscope is portable, and otoscopic examination is the most common method used. An otoscope is a device (Fig. 64–10) consisting of a handle, a light source, a magnifying lens, and an attachment for visualizing the ear canal and eardrum. A pneumatic device attached to the otoscope is used for injecting air into the ear canal to test the mobility and integrity of the eardrum.

Specula for the otoscope come in various sizes. Since

PHYSICAL ASSESSMENT FINDINGS IN THE HEALTHY ADULT

The Ear

Inspection

Auricles symmetrical, superior portion level with outer canthus of eye. Outer canals clear. Preauricular and postauricular areas without swelling, masses, or lesions. AC > BC, bilaterally. No lateralization. Whisper heard at 3 feet.

Palpation

Tenderness over tragus and mastoid absent. No masses.

Otoscopic Examination

Soft cerumen present in canals. No discharge. TMs intact, gray. Cone of light at 4:00 in right ear and at 7:00 in left ear. Landmarks visualized. No retraction or bulging. TM freely movable with pneumatic pressure.

AC, air conduction; BC, bone conduction; TM, tympanic membrane.

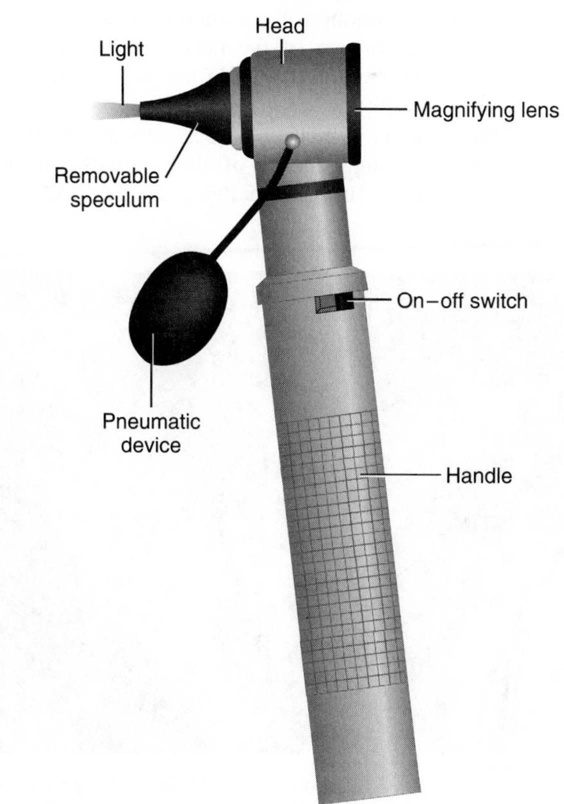

FIGURE 64–10 An otoscope.

the diameter of the meatus and the length of the ear canal vary, select the speculum with the largest diameter that fits comfortably into the ear canal. Check the light source for brightness. If the light appears yellowish or dim (like a flashlight with weak batteries), recharge or replace the batteries.

Hold the otoscope with the dominant hand, positioning it so that your hand rests against the client's head (Fig. 64–11). If the client moves suddenly, the otoscope will also move, thereby reducing the likelihood of damaging the external canal during examination. With your nondominant hand, pull the pinna up, back, and out (in the adult), thus straightening the ear canal. While this is done, gently tilt the client's head away from you and insert the speculum slowly and carefully into the ear canal. Bring your eye close to the magnifying lens to visualize the ear canal and eardrum. When a pneumatic bulb is present, advance the otoscope far enough to make a secure seal.

Observe the ear canal while the speculum is entering and leaving. Move the otoscope in a circular fashion to visualize the entire ear canal. Note abnormalities such as extreme narrowing of the ear canal, nodules, redness, scaliness, swelling, drainage, cysts, foreign objects, and excessive wax. Visualization of the eardrum is impaired by most of these abnormalities. Sometimes the ear canal must be cleaned of wax, dead skin, and other debris. Wax and debris can be removed with a cerumen spoon (wax curet), suction aspirator, or irrigation.

Cerumen should not interfere with the examination when the amount is small. Cerumen is normally present in the external ear and varies in color from light yellow to black. Cerumen that is impacted in the ear canal is a common cause of hearing loss, especially in the elderly. Therefore, assess the amount of cerumen present.

Distinguishing landmarks of the normal eardrum (Fig. 64–12) are (1) the annulus, the fibrous border that attaches the eardrum to the temporal bone; (2) the short process of the malleus, which protrudes into the eardrum superiorly; (3) the long process of the malleus (manubrium); (4) the umbo of the malleus, at the point of maximal concavity and attaches to the center of the eardrum; (5) the pars flaccida, a small triangular area above the short process of the malleus; and (6) the pars tensa, the remaining and largest portion of the eardrum.

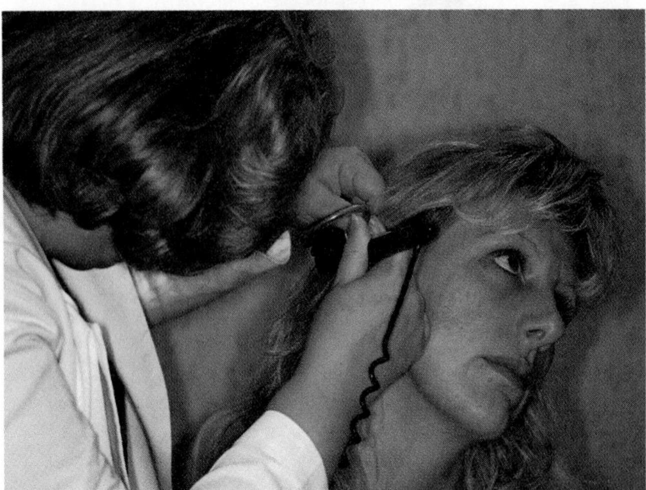

FIGURE 64–11 Use of the otoscope. Hold the otoscope handle between the thumb and fingers. Pull the pinna backward and upward in the adult to straighten the auditory canal.

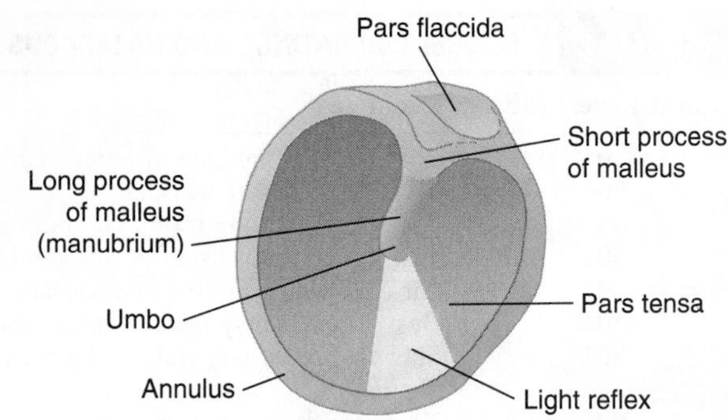

FIGURE 64–12 Normal right eardrum (tympanic membrane).

The normal eardrum is slightly conical, translucent, shiny and smooth, and pearly gray in color. The position of the drumhead is oblique with respect to the ear canal. In the presence of disease, not only does the color of the eardrum change; other abnormalities are also manifested, such as retraction, bulging, or perforation of the eardrum and a white plaque (*tympanosclerosis*) on the eardrum.

Carefully inspect the entire eardrum, including the border (annulus), rotating the otoscope as needed. A cone of light reflex should be present on the eardrum in the lower anterior quadrant. The umbo and the long and short process of the malleus should be easily visible through the eardrum.

Test the mobility of the eardrum by using the pneumatic device of the otoscope to inject a small puff of air into the ear canal. Observe the eardrum for normal movement. An adequate seal is important to perform this maneuver accurately.

TESTS FOR AUDITORY ACUITY

Assessment of the middle and inner ear for hearing is accomplished by sophisticated methods of indirect testing (e.g., audiometry and vestibular testing). However, a gross assessment of hearing can be made simply through conversation, by evaluating the logical sequence of replies and the appropriateness of the responses. Gross assessments can be made at the bedside or in the office.

Test each ear separately to estimate hearing ability. Begin by occluding one of the client's ears with a finger. Then, while standing a foot away, whisper two-syllable numbers softly toward the unoccluded ear and ask the client to repeat the numbers. Increase the intensity of your voice from a soft, medium, or loud whisper to a soft, medium, or loud voice. If you suspect that the client is lip-reading, turn the client's face to one side. Ask the client whether hearing is better in one ear than in the other ear. If auditory acuity between the two ears is different, test the ear that hears better first. Next, produce noise in the better-hearing ear by rapidly but gently moving the finger in the client's ear canal while the other ear is tested.

Although the ticking of a watch tick can also be used to test hearing, it produces a higher-pitched sound, which is less relevant to functional hearing compared with the voice test.

The tuning fork also provides a general estimate of hearing loss. A frequency of 512 Hz is recommended. The two major tuning fork tests date from the 19th century and are named after their originators: Weber and Rinne.

Weber Test

The Weber test is used to assess conduction of sound through bone. Set the tuning fork into vibration by striking the tines on your hand. Place the rounded tip of the handle on the center of the client's forehead or nasal bone (Fig. 64–13*A*). Placement on the teeth (even false teeth) is a reliable option. Does the client hear the tone in the center of the head, the right ear, or the left ear? Normally, the sound is heard equally in both ears by bone conduction. If there is a sensorineural (nerve) hearing loss in one ear, the sound is heard in the unaffected ear. With a conductive (air conduction) hearing loss, the sound is heard better in the affected ear.

Rinne Test

The Rinne test compares air conduction to bone conduction and helps to differentiate conductive from sensorineural hearing loss. Shift the vibrating tuning fork between two positions: first against the mastoid bone for bone conduction (Fig. 64–13*B*) and then 2 inches from the opening of the ear canal for air conduction (Fig. 64–13*C*). Move the tuning fork when the client no longer hears the sound by bone conduction, and ask the client to indicate whether the tone is louder in front of or behind the ear. Ask the client to state when the tone is no longer heard by air conduction.

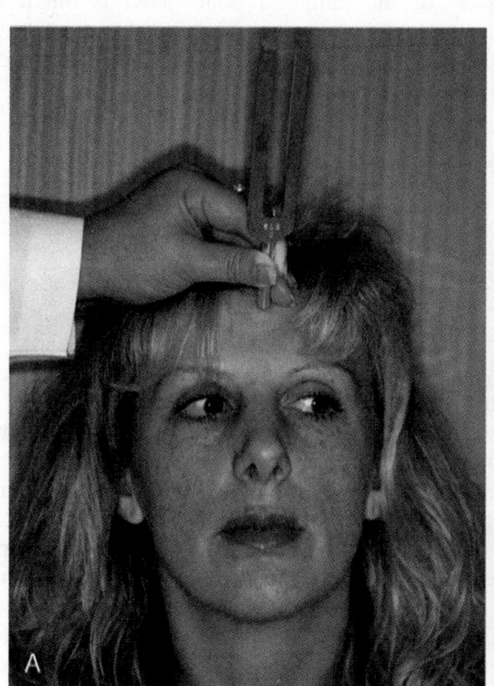

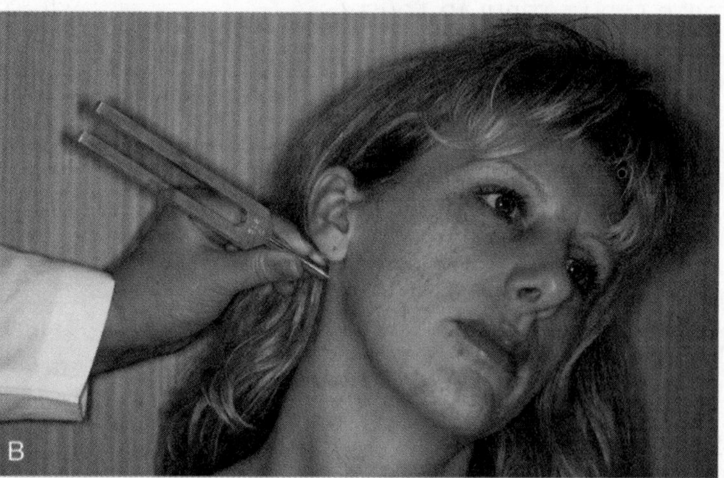

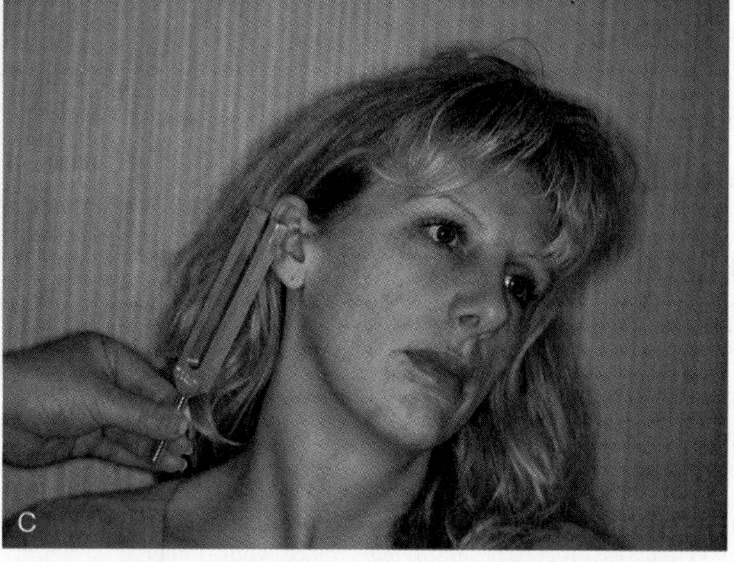

FIGURE 64–13 Weber and Rinne tests for hearing impairment. The Weber test is used to detect lateralization of hearing; the Rinne test distinguishes conductive hearing loss from sensorineural hearing loss. The two tests should be performed consecutively. *A,* For the Weber test, use a vibrating tuning fork, placed on the client's head to produce a centrally located stimulus. The client should hear the sound equally in both ears. The tone is louder in an ear with unilateral conductive loss and quieter in an ear with unilateral sensorineural loss. *B,* Perform the Rinne test to characterize the unilateral hearing loss as either conductive or sensorineural. Hold a vibrating tuning fork on the mastoid bone. *C,* When the client no longer hears the sound, place the tuning fork about 2 inches from the external ear. When the tone is louder through air than through bone, the Rinne test finding is positive, which indicates either normal hearing or a sensorineural hearing loss. A negative Rinne test finding, or louder bone conduction than air conduction, indicates a conductive loss.

Normally, sound is heard twice as long or as loud by air conduction than it is by bone conduction. Results are as follows:

- In *normal* hearing, air conduction is greater than bone conduction (a positive Rinne test finding).
- With a *conductive* hearing loss, bone conduction sounds louder or longer than air conduction sounds (a negative Rinne test finding).
- With a *sensorineural* hearing loss, the client hears better by air conduction (a positive Rinne test finding).

Conductive hearing loss results when the pathways of normal sound conduction are blocked. Because vibrations against the mastoid bone can bypass the obstruction, bone conduction lasts longer or sounds louder than air conduction. In *sensorineural* hearing loss, the acoustic nerve is less able to perceive vibrations from either bone or air; therefore, normal patterns are reported by the client.

■ TESTS FOR VESTIBULAR ACUITY

Romberg Test

Assess the inner ear for balance by performing a Romberg test. The client stands with feet together, arms by the sides, and eyes closed. Note the ability to maintain an upright posture with only a minimal amount of sway. Stand close to the client to offer balance support if needed. If the client loses balance, this is a positive Romberg sign, suggesting a vestibular ear problem or cerebellar ataxia.

A *tandem* Romberg test should also be performed. Instruct the client to walk forward and backward, heel-to-toe. A peripheral vestibular lesion may cause marked swaying or falling. A client without pathologic vestibular change can usually maintain balance, depending on age.

A *past-pointing test* can also indicate a labyrinthine disorder. While the client is seated, facing you with eyes open, hold out your index finger at the client's shoulder level. Instruct the client to touch your finger with the right index finger. Ask the client to lower the arm, close the eyes, and touch your finger again. Repeat the procedure, testing the client's left index finger. Observe and record the presence or absence, as well as the degree and direction, of past-pointing. A labyrinthine disorder can lead to past-pointing when the eyes are closed. Cerebral lesions are indicated when past-pointing occurs whether the eyes are open or closed.

Test for Nystagmus

Nystagmus is involuntary, rhythmic oscillation of the eyes associated with vestibular dysfunction. Nystagmus occurs normally when a client watches a rapidly moving object or looks beyond 30 degrees laterally (*end-point nystagmus*). To assess for *gaze nystagmus,* place your finger directly in front of the client at eye level. Ask the client to follow (track) the finger without moving the head. Starting at the midline, slowly move your finger toward the client's right ear and then the left ear, but not more than 30 degrees laterally, superiorly, or inferiorly. Observe the client's eyes for any jerking movements. For example, if the eyes jerk quickly to the left, and drift slowly back to the right, the client has left spontaneous (*horizontal*) nystagmus. Nystagmus is named for the direction of the fast phase. Nystagmus can be horizontal, vertical, or rotary.

DIAGNOSTIC TESTS

■ TESTS FOR AURAL STRUCTURE

The temporal bone and its structures are easily examined by radiography (x-ray study). The oldest, but not necessarily most useful, study is x-ray examination of the mastoid bone. More recent radiographic techniques have largely been replaced by imaging studies (see Chapter 11).

Computed Tomography

CT without contrast medium is the most commonly ordered CT scan for imaging of the temporal bone. Contrast is not generally needed because most bony structures are well seen. Contrast may be used to delineate vascular or soft tissue structures.

Magnetic Resonance Imaging

MRI reveals membranous organs as well as nerves and blood vessels of the temporal bone. MRI is the test of choice for tumors of the temporal bone. Contrast can be used for enhancement. For certain diagnostic assessments, both MRI and CT scans are obtained.

Arteriography

Arteriography is used to assess vascular abnormalities in the temporal bone.

■ TESTS FOR AUDITORY FUNCTION

Audiometric Tests

Audiology may be broadly called the science of hearing. Audiometric tests are performed to measure hearing and comprehension. A hearing test is performed in a soundproof booth by an audiologist. An audiometer is an electronic instrument used to test hearing by producing sounds of varying pure-tone frequencies between 250–8000 Hz and loudness. The unit of measure of hearing, the decibel (dB), is a logarithmic function of sound intensity. The average normal adult has a hearing threshold of 0 to 20 dB hearing loss. The greater the threshold level, the poorer the hearing sensivity. The client is asked to signal the audiologist by raising a hand or pressing a button when a tone is heard; the responses are plotted on a graph called an *audiogram* (Fig. 64–14). Earphones are used for the audiogram.

Normal hearing is a range established nationally by testing the hearing levels of people of all ages. A client with normal hearing ability has 80% or more hearing, depending on age.

Some audiometric tests are performed by computer-assisted instruments. The objective of these special tests is to reveal whether a disorder is in the cochlea, acoustic nerve, or brain stem.

AUDIOGRAPHY

The components of hearing are tested through assessment of air conduction, bone conduction, and speech. Air con-

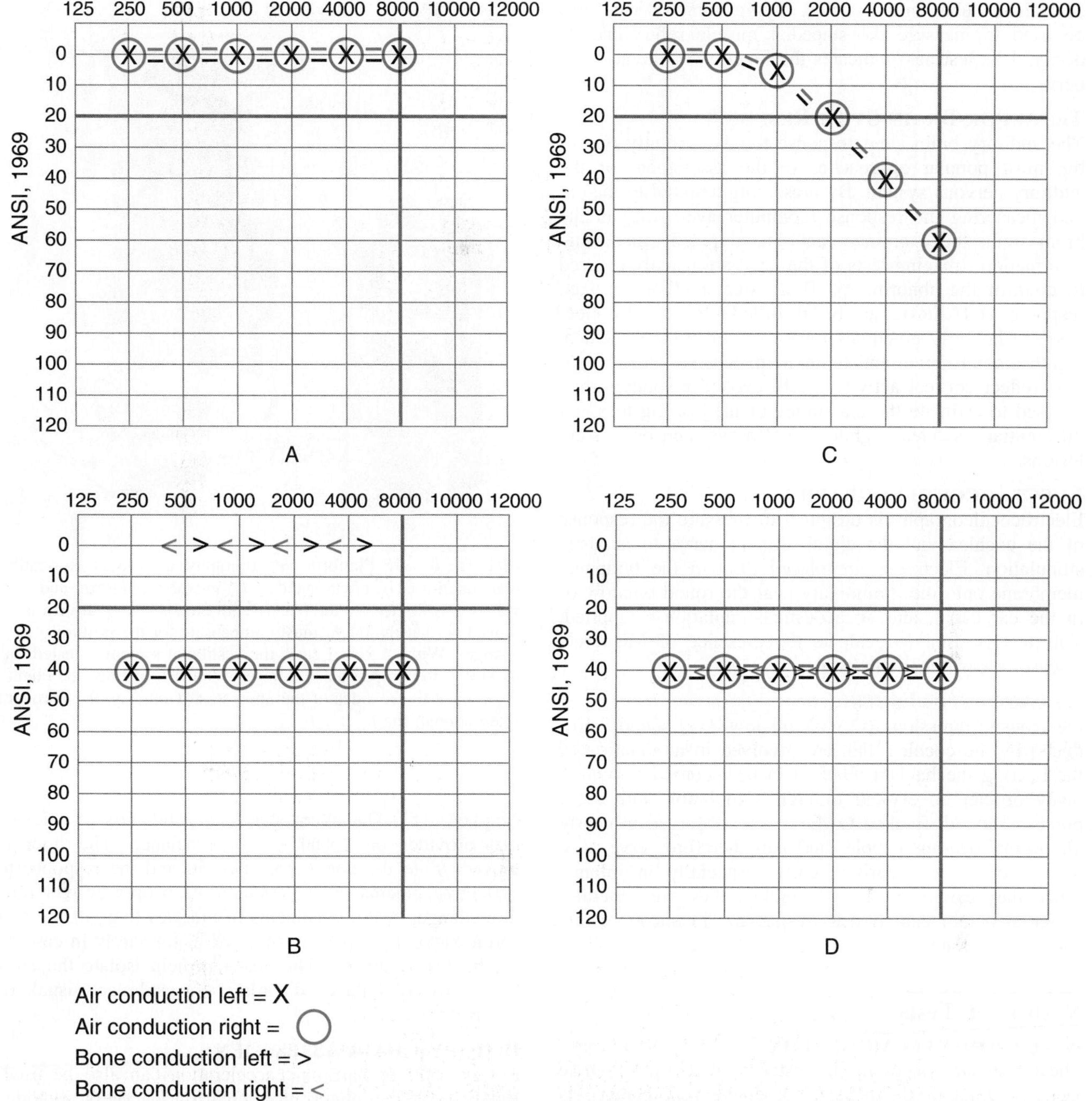

FIGURE 64–14 Audiograms showing types of hearing. *A,* Normal hearing. *B,* Conductive hearing loss. *C,* High-frequency hearing loss. *D,* Sensorineural hearing loss. (Courtesy of Arnold G. Schuring, M.D.)

duction is assessed by presenting tones through the earphones. When the examiner varies the loudness and frequency of tones, a hearing level is established. Bone conduction is assessed by presenting tones through a bone conduction oscillator placed behind the ear on the mastoid bone. The bone conduction level is the level at which the cochlea can hear, bypassing the middle ear structures, and is referred to as the *nerve hearing level.* A difference between air and bone conduction signifies a conductive hearing loss. When air and bone conduction are the same, either normal hearing or a *sensorineural* (nerve) hearing loss exists. Speech evaluation includes (1) *speech reception threshold* (the level of speech hearing), which serves as a check on the reliability of the air conduction test, and *speech discrimination* (the ability to understand the spoken word).

TYMPANOMETRY

A popular test used for differentiating problems in the middle ear is tympanometry, or impedance audiometry. This test measures compliance (mobility) and impedance (opposition to movement) of the tympanic membrane and ossicles of the middle ear. The examiner applies positive, normal, and negative air pressure into the external meatus and measures the resultant sound energy flow, which is traced on a graph called a *tympanogram.* Abnormalities on the tympanogram reveal dysfunction of the middle ear, eustachian tube, and ossicles. Tympanometry can also be used to measure the stapedial muscle reflex and its decay. This test also indicates the function of the acoustic nerve.

Tests for Brain Stem Response

The auditory brain stem response test is currently one of the most popular approaches to the assessment of the auditory nervous system. By presenting a sound to the ear and measuring the response (computer averaging) in the brain stem, the examiner can obtain specific diagnostic information. Imaging tests of the head are usually ordered to confirm the abnormality. Brain stem auditory evoked responses (BAERs) can be recorded from scalp electrodes. The early potentials reflect activity in the cochlea, eighth cranial nerve, and brain stem. Later evoked potentials reflect cortical activity. Early evoked responses may be used to estimate the magnitude of the hearing loss and differentiate cochlea, eighth cranial nerve, and brain stem lesions.

Electrocochleography

Electrocochleography is designed to measure the response of the cochlea and the eighth cranial nerve to acoustic stimulation. Electrodes are placed through the tympanic membrane onto the promontary near the round window or in the ear canal, and an acoustic stimulation is applied. This test is used to evaluate the presence of Ménière's disease or perilymphatic fistula.

Otoacoustic Emissions

Otoacoustic emissions (OAEs) are low-level sounds, produced by the cochlea, that are involved in modulation of the hearing mechanism. OAEs can be recorded spontaneously or can be evoked through stimulation with short bursts of sound. Evoked OAEs can be observed in nearly all normal-hearing people, and can therefore serve as a useful screen for hearing acuity, especially in infants. Since they can be measured quickly, they are generally easier to obtain than BAERs, especially in uncooperative and crying infants.

Vestibular Tests

Electronystagmography

The vestibular system can be tested by electrophysiologic means. Although the physical assessment of balance is important, the most common objective measurement of balance is accomplished by electronystagmography (ENG). The ENG instrument was developed to measure nystagmus (involuntary, rapid eye movement) in response to stimulation of the vestibular system. This stimulation includes testing the client at rest in different positions for both the eyes and the head, and with different temperatures of air or water in the ear canals, thus stimulating the semicircular canals. The different test results give a recording (electronystagmogram) that reflects the status of each labyrinth and can indicate CNS system disorders.

Platform Posturography

Platform posturography, performed while the client is standing, is another balance test that helps to identify, quantify, and localize the source of balance disorders (Fig. 64–15). The client stands in a tall box-like device that provides no visual cues for balance. The floor is moved while the client stands on it, and the response to correcting balance is recorded. Most people correct posture changes with adjustments in muscles (e.g., of the feet and ankles). The client is strapped in for safety in case he or she loses balance. This test can help isolate the etiologic basis of balance disorders as vestibular, visual, or proprioceptive.

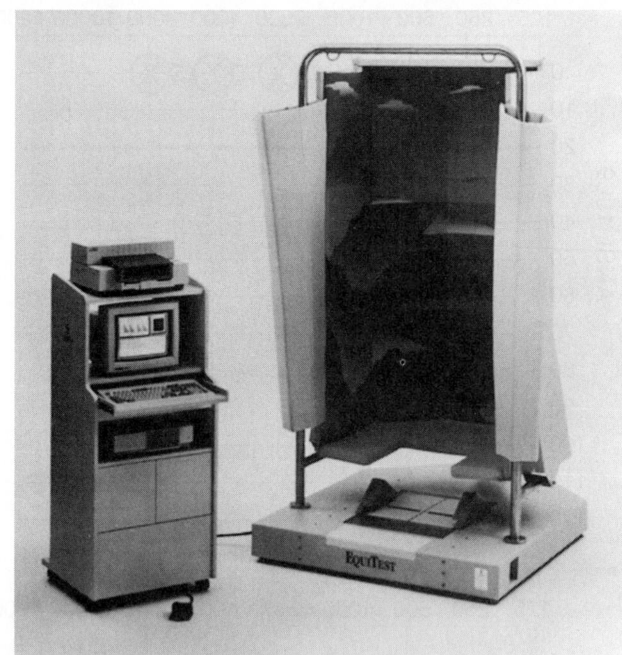

FIGURE 64–15 Platform posturography, used to assess vestibular function. The client stands on a movable platform, and vision is restricted by the panels with clouds. The platform is moved so that the client must compensate for the postural changes. Without visual cues, the vestibular system is tested for its ability to compensate. Because of the risk of falls, the client is strapped to the sides of the apparatus. (Courtesy of Neurocom International, Inc.)

Rotary Chair Assessment

Rotary chair or harmonic acceleration can also be used. Rotation of the client in a chair in darkness provides information about vestibular dysfunction and the level of central compensation.

■ LABORATORY TESTS

Blood Tests

Blood tests that are diagnostic for systemic abnormalities are only secondarily significant for ear disease. For example, an elevated white blood cell (WBC) count suggests an infection but is not diagnostic of ear disease. In the presence of clinical signs of ear infection, and in the absence of other signs of infection, however, an elevated WBC count does suggest acute ear infection. Other blood tests are useful for diagnosis of autoimmune diseases and other systemic illnesses that can affect hearing and balance.

Cultures

Drainage samples from the ear canal are sometimes obtained for culture to identify an infecting organism. This is rarely necessary in choosing an antibiotic for acute infections. When long-term drainage is present, such as in chronic otitis media, cultures are more helpful because multiple pathogenic organisms can be present.

Tests for the Presence of Cerebrospinal Fluid

When clear drainage is found in the ear, a dilemma is presented. Is this cerebrospinal fluid (CSF) or serous drainage? A fistula from the inner ear to the middle ear can drain CSF. This pathway can also lead to meningitis by retrograde contamination. Therefore, an analysis of clear fluid drainage from the ear or nose is often helpful in the diagnosis.

Tissue Specimens

Biopsy specimens of abnormal tissue from the ear canal or from other tissue harvested during surgery are necessary to rule out a malignancy and to identify unusual problems. In an infected ear, abnormal tissue is readily identified with visual assessment. If the surgeon is in doubt about the findings, a tissue sample is taken for pathologic examination.

CONCLUSIONS

Understanding the complexity of ocular structures and the physiology of vision is essential to providing comprehensive nursing care for clients with ocular disorders. Ophthalmic Registered Nurses perform the roles of educator, technician, counselor, and coordinator in the diagnostic setting.

Hearing and balance are vital to a person's safety and independence. Understanding the physiology of hearing and balance is essential to providing comprehensive nursing care for clients with ear disorders.

BIBLIOGRAPHY

1. Eagle, R. (1999). *Eye pathology: An atlas and basic text.* Philadelphia: W. B. Saunders.
2. Goldblum, K. (Ed.). (1997). *Ophthalmic nursing core curriculum.* Dubuque, IA: Kendall.
3. Jarvis, C. (2000). *Physical examination and health assessment* (3rd ed.). Philadelphia: W. B. Saunders.
4. Kanski, J. (1999). *Clinical ophthalmology* (4th ed.). Oxford: Butterworth Heinemann.
5. Sigler, B., & Schuring, L. T. (1993). *Ear, nose and throat disorders.* St. Louis: Mosby–Year Book.
6. Silverman, C. A. (1998). Audiologic assessment and amplification. *Primary Care, 25* (3), 545–581.
7. Thompson, J. M., & Wilson, S. F. (1996). *Health assessment for nursing practice.* St. Louis: Mosby–Year Book.
8. Vaughan, D, Asbury, T., & Riordan-Eva, P. (1995). *General ophthalmology* (14th ed.). Norwalk, CT: Appleton & Lange.

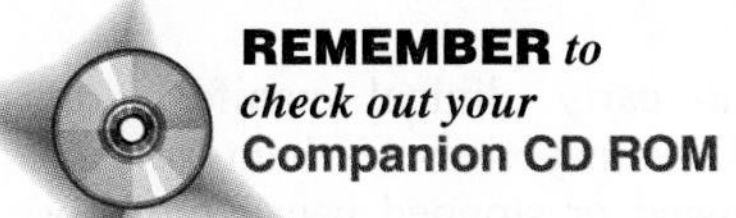

CHAPTER 65

Management of Clients with Visual Disorders

Linda A. Vader

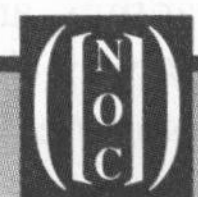

NURSING OUTCOMES CLASSIFICATION (NOC) for Nursing Diagnoses—Clients with Visual Disorders

Anticipatory Grieving
Coping
Grief Resolution
Psychosocial Adjustment: Life Change
Ineffective Management of Therapeutic Regimen
Compliance Behavior
Knowledge: Treatment Regimen
Participation: Health Care Regimen
Treatment Behavior: Illness or Injury
Knowledge Deficit
Knowledge Deficit: Treatment Procedure
Knowledge Deficit: Regimen
Sensory/Perceptual Alterations (Visual)
Anxiety Control
Body Image
Vision Compensation Behavior

The role that vision plays in our lives is difficult to define because it is so deeply personal and intimate. It is the connection between the mind and the body and the rest of the world. The visual pathway is a multidimensional system with many structures and processes subject to trauma or disorders. When there is a failure of any part along the visual pathway, the result is loss of vision.

Loss of vision is closely associated with the loss of independence. Even simple tasks become difficult to perform without assistance. Seeing what food is being served at the table, selecting clothes for color and design, avoiding objects while walking, and reading books, magazines, or personal mail are no longer possible. The visually impaired person must adapt to this loss in order to maintain control in the daily affairs of life.

The nursing diagnosis *Sensory/Perceptual Alterations* is commonly identified for clients with visual problems or impairment. Nursing interventions focus on providing a safe environment and education for self-care. The most important assessment you can make, however, should address your client's grieving process. Visual impairment is more than a physiologic deficit. It is a loss that has physical, emotional, and spiritual effects on the person afflicted. Even minor changes in vision can provoke feelings of anger and frustration in people who must rely on clear and sharp vision in their work (e.g., airline pilots, artists, photographers, architects). Permanent and profound loss of vision can result in morbid grieving, in which an individual is unable to cope with or adapt to life changes.

Surveys have shown that most people are more afraid of going blind than dying of cancer. Although we have made some improvements in the way our society views and provides for people who are physically challenged, blind people are frequently regarded with pity. Loss of vision is a threat to a person's independence, self-esteem, and self-control.

GLAUCOMA

Glaucoma comprises a group of ocular disorders characterized by increased intraocular pressure, optic nerve atrophy, and visual field loss. It is estimated that more than 80,000 people in the United States are blind as a result of glaucoma. The incidence of glaucoma is about 1.5%, and in blacks between ages 45 and 65 years, the prevalence is at least five times that of whites in the same age group. In most cases, blindness can be prevented if treatment is begun early.

Classification

Many terms are used to describe the various types of glaucoma:

Primary and *secondary glaucoma* refer to whether the cause is the disease alone or another condition.

Acute and *chronic* refer to the onset and duration of the disorder.

Open (wide) and *closed* (narrow) describe the width of the angle between the cornea and the iris (Fig. 65–1*A*). Anatomically narrow anterior chamber angles predispose people to an acute onset of *angle-closure glaucoma.*

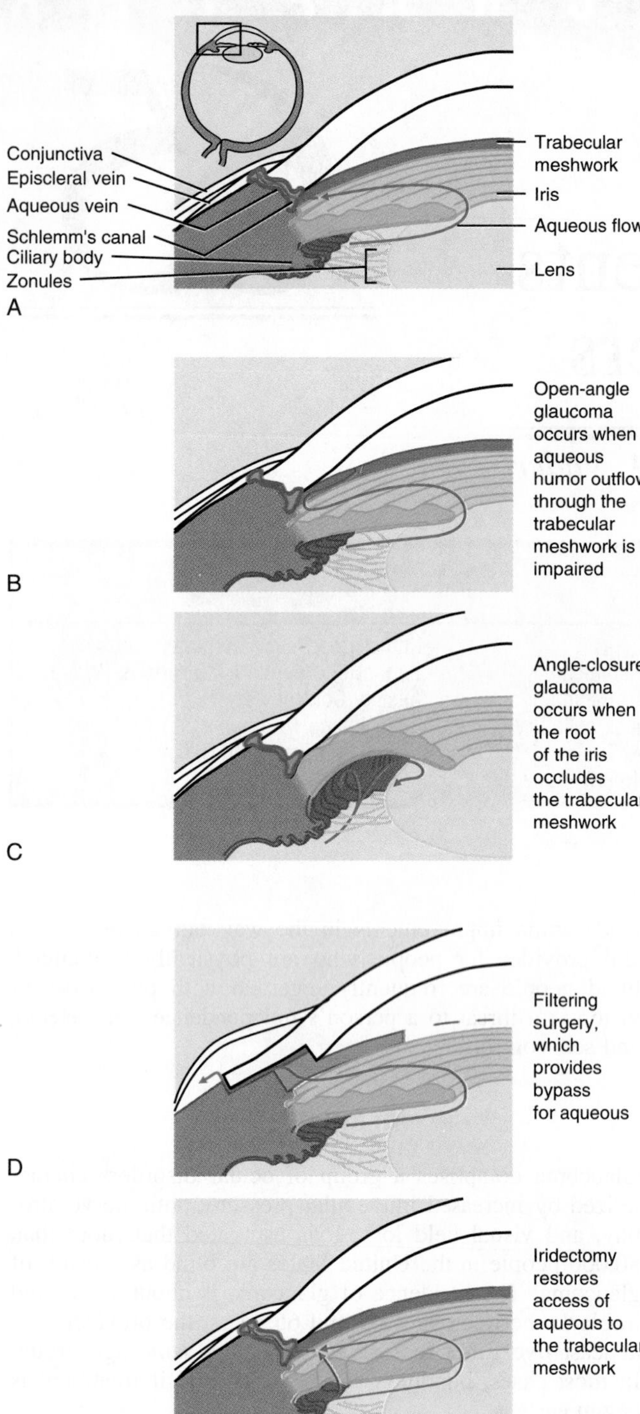
Conjunctiva
Episcleral vein
Aqueous vein
Schlemm's canal
Ciliary body
Zonules
A
Trabecular meshwork
Iris
Aqueous flow
Lens
Open-angle glaucoma occurs when aqueous humor outflow through the trabecular meshwork is impaired
B
Angle-closure glaucoma occurs when the root of the iris occludes the trabecular meshwork
C
Filtering surgery, which provides bypass for aqueous
D
Iridectomy restores access of aqueous to the trabecular meshwork
E

FIGURE 65–1 *A,* Normal flow of aqueous humor. *B,* Open-angle glaucoma occurs when aqueous humor outflow is impaired by the trabecular meshwork. *C,* Angle-closure glaucoma occurs when the root of the iris occludes the trabecular meshwork. Filtering surgery (*D*) and iridectomy (*E*) restore flow of aqueous humor through the trabecular meshwork.

Primary Open-Angle Glaucoma

Primary open-angle glaucoma, the most common form, is a multifactorial disorder that is often genetically determined, bilateral, insidious in onset, and slow to progress. This type of glaucoma is often referred to as the "thief in the night" because no early clinical manifestations are present to alert the client that vision is being lost. Aqueous humor flow is slowed or stopped because of obstruction by the trabecular meshwork (Fig. 65–1*B*).

Angle-Closure Glaucoma

An acute attack of angle-closure glaucoma can develop only in an eye in which the anterior chamber angle is anatomically narrow. The attack occurs because of a sudden blockage of the anterior angle by the base of the iris (Fig. 65–1*C*).

Other Forms of Glaucoma

Low-tension glaucoma resembles primary open-angle glaucoma. The angle is normal, the optic nerves are cupped, and the visual fields show characteristic glaucomatous effects (peripheral vision deficits). These changes, however, develop in the presence of statistically normal intraocular pressures. Although the pressure readings are in the normal range, treatment is indicated to lower the pressure even further to avoid progressive optic nerve damage and visual field loss.

Secondary glaucoma is a result of increased intraocular pressure that has developed for other problems, such as postoperative edema. Edematous tissue may inhibit the outflow of aqueous humor through the trabecular meshwork. Delayed healing of corneal wound edges may result in epithelial cell growth into the anterior chamber.

Congenital glaucoma is rare, the result of developmental abnormalities in anterior chamber angle structures, the cornea, and the iris.

Etiology and Risk Factors

Approximately 90% of primary glaucoma occurs in people with open angles. Because there are no early warning clinical manifestations, it is imperative that regular ophthalmic examinations include tonometry and assessment of the optic nerve head (disc). The most common cause of chronic open-angle glaucoma is degenerative change in the trabecular meshwork, resulting in decreased outflow of aqueous humor. Hypertension, cardiovascular disease, diabetes, and obesity are associated with the development of glaucoma. Increased intraocular pressure also results from inflammation of filtering structures in uveitis. Encroachment by a rapidly growing tumor and chronic use of topical corticosteroids may also produce manifestations of open-angle glaucoma. The cause of *low-tension glaucoma* is not known.

Secondary glaucoma may occur as a result of trauma. Lens displacement, hemorrhage into the anterior chamber, lacerations, and contusions can disrupt the flow pattern of aqueous humor. Smoking, ingestion of caffeine or large amounts of fluids, alcohol, illicit drugs, corticosteroids, altered hormone levels, posture, and eye movements may cause varying transient increases in intraocular pressure.

Congenital glaucoma is caused by an arrest of development of the anterior chamber angle structures at about the 7th month of fetal life.

Pathophysiology

Intraocular pressure is determined by the rate of aqueous humor production in the ciliary body and the resistance to outflow of aqueous humor from the eye. Intraocular pressure varies with diurnal cycles (the highest pressure is usually on awakening) and body position (increased when lying down). Normal variations do not usually exceed 2 to 3 mm Hg. Intraocular pressure and blood pressure are independent of each other, but variations in systemic blood pressure may be associated with corresponding variations in intraocular pressure. Increased intraocular pressure may result from hyperproduction of aqueous humor or obstruction of outflow. As aqueous fluid builds up in the eye, the increased pressure inhibits blood supply to the optic nerve and the retina. These delicate tissues become ischemic and gradually lose function.

Clinical Manifestations

Clinical manifestations of glaucoma include increased intraocular pressure, cupping or indentation of the optic nerve head (disc), and visual field defects. As intraocular pressure increases, the head of the optic nerve is pressed inward. Visual field defects are the result of the loss of blood supply to areas in the retina. The individual response to intraocular pressure varies; some clients sustain damage from relatively low pressures, whereas others sustain no damage from high pressure. The degree of increased pressure that causes ocular damage is not the same in every eye, and some clients may tolerate a pressure for long periods that would rapidly blind another.

In clients with *acute angle-closure glaucoma,* the aqueous flow is obstructed and intraocular pressure becomes markedly elevated, causing severe pain and blurred vision or vision loss. Some clients see rainbow halos around lights, and some experience nausea and vomiting.

Depending on the primary factor, *secondary glaucoma* may be acute or chronic. The ocular manifestations, however, are the same as in angle-closure glaucoma.

An ophthalmoscopic examination shows atrophy (pale color) and cupping (indentation) of the optic nerve head. The visual field examination is used to determine the extent of peripheral vision loss (see visual fields earlier). In *chronic open-angle glaucoma,* a small crescent-shaped *scotoma* (blind spot) appears early in the disease. In *acute angle-closure glaucoma,* the fields demonstrate larger areas of significant loss of vision.

In clients with *angle-closure glaucoma,* a slit-lamp examination may demonstrate an erythematous conjunctiva and corneal cloudiness. The anterior chamber aqueous humor may also appear turbid (hazy), and the pupil may be nonreactive. Slit-lamp examination is used in *open-angle glaucoma* to look for secondary causes and associated findings. Intraocular pressure is measured at the slit lamp with the applanation tonometer. Increased intraocular pressure (>23 mm Hg) indicates the need for further evaluation. Gonioscopy is performed to determine the depth of the anterior chamber angle and to examine the entire circumference of the angle for any abnormal changes in the filtering meshwork.

Outcome Management

The goal of management is to facilitate the outflow of aqueous humor through remaining channels and to maintain intraocular pressure within a range that prevents further damage to the optic nerve. If intraocular pressure is very high, it must be reduced to retain vision. If vision is lost, the goals are to restore independence for the client.

Medical Management

REDUCE INTRAOCULAR PRESSURE (PROMOTE AQUEOUS FLOW)

Several medications are used to promote aqueous flow in *narrow-angle glaucoma:* (1) topical miotics, which act by constricting the pupil, (2) topical epinephrine, which increases outflow, (3) topical beta-blockers or alpha-adrenergics, which suppress the secretion of aqueous humor, and (4) oral carbonic anhydrase inhibitors, which also reduce the production of aqueous humor. Figure 65–2 shows the sites of action for various drugs.

Also shown in the figure are sites of action for drugs used to treat *open-angle glaucoma.* Mydriatic agents dilate the pupil by inhibiting the parasympathetic nervous system and blocking acetylcholine. Cycloplegic agents paralyze the ciliary muscle and the dilator muscle of the iris, causing both pupillary dilation and paralysis of accommodation. These dilating agents are contraindicated in narrow-angle glaucoma, because further dilation of the pupil restricts outflow of aqueous humor.

REDUCE INTRAOCULAR PRESSURE

In emergent situations in which intraocular pressure must be brought under control, an oral osmotic agent may be administered in the form of glycerin (Osmoglyn). The agent is supplied in a variety of strengths, and the percentage of the solution ordered is closely checked against what is supplied. The diuretic action of glycerin lowers intraocular pressure. Diabetic clients often receive a synthetic glycerin such as isosorbide (Ismotic) to reduce the effect on blood glucose levels. The average dose for an adult is 1.5 g/kg oral solution of 100 g/220 ml (45%), which may be repeated several times until the intraocular

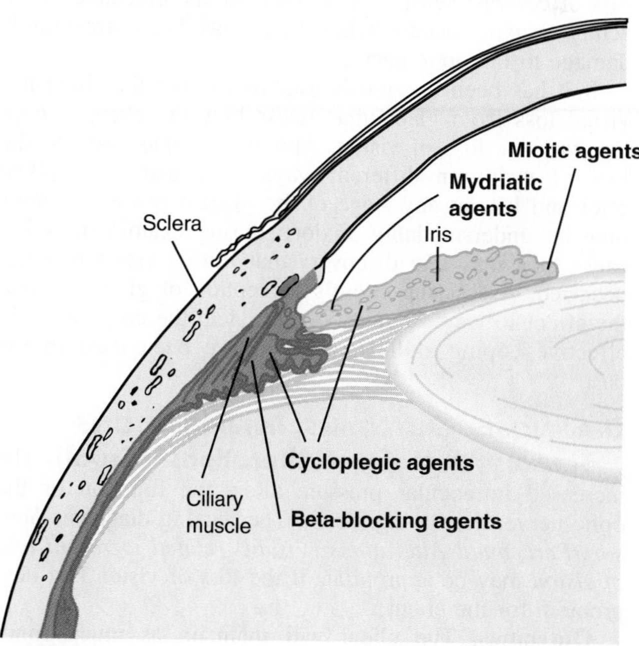

FIGURE 65–2 Sites of action of mydriatic, beta-blocking, cycloplegic, and miotic agents.

pressure is reduced to a tolerable level. If the glycerin is not already flavored, the extreme sweetness and viscosity may be made more palatable by mixing it with equal parts of a tart juice such as lemon. Serving the solution over cracked ice also makes it more palatable. After 3 hours, encourage the intake of water and other liquids to prevent mild to moderate dehydration and make sure the client can get to the bathroom during the diuretic phase.

Intravenous (IV) mannitol, a potent osmotic diuretic, may be used to arrest extremely high intraocular pressure. It should be used only for management of a glaucoma crisis under close nursing and medical supervision. Carefully evaluate the client's cardiovascular and renal status before treatment is begun. Document baseline vital signs before treatment and frequently during the infusion. Because mannitol tends to crystallize, the bottle may need to be warmed before it is administered. Do not use the vial while crystals are present. An in-line micropore filter should also be used to prevent infusion of any crystal particles.

Nursing Management of the Medical Client

ASSESSMENT

Nursing assessment includes establishing demographic data of age and race because open-angle glaucoma occurs most often in clients over 40 years of age and in blacks. Determine whether there is a family history of glaucoma or other eye problems and whether the client has had ocular surgery, infections, or trauma. An accurate list of current medications is imperative because over-the-counter medications (such as antihistamines) may dilate the pupil, increasing the risk for angle-closure glaucoma. Always note a history of allergic reactions, particularly to medications or dyes.

Ask the client to describe any changes in vision. Although the manifestations of primary open-angle glaucoma are insidious, the client may describe blind spots in the periphery or an overall decreased visual acuity with loss of contrast sensitivity. Decreased uncorrectable visual acuity usually occurs when there has been irreversible damage to the optic nerve.

If it has been previously established that the client has visual loss from glaucoma, assess how the client is coping with the loss of vision. Although people adapt to the loss of vision in different ways, they usually manifest grief and loss at any stage of the disease process. Clients may be understandably anxious during examinations because they may fear discovery that further vision loss has occurred. Assess the client's perception of glaucoma and the effect it has on quality of life. Help the client identify effective coping skills that may have been used in the past.

DIAGNOSIS, OUTCOMES, INTERVENTIONS

Sensory/Perceptual Alterations (Visual). The increased intraocular pressure alters the function of the optic nerve, decreasing vision. The nursing diagnosis *Sensory/Perceptual Alterations (Visual) related to recent loss of vision* may be appropriate if the loss of vision is a new problem for the client.

Outcomes. The client will maintain as much functional vision as possible, report no further loss of vision, adapt to any visual loss, be able to perform activities of daily living (ADL), and recognize clinical manifestations of complications.

Interventions. Reassure the client that although some vision has been lost and cannot be restored, further loss may be prevented by adhering to the treatment plan.

Anticipatory Grieving. Vision lost to glaucoma is irreparable. Even with the most aggressive medical and surgical management, vision loss may progress. A typical nursing diagnosis would therefore be *Anticipatory Grieving related to loss of vision.* Significant loss of vision represents the need for compromise and adaptation for both client and family.

Outcomes. The client will express grief, describe the meaning of the loss, and share the grief with significant others.

Interventions. Assess the causative and contributing factors that may delay the work of grieving and promote family cohesiveness. The social stigma of blindness underlies the anxiety that clients experience with actual or potential loss of vision. Total loss of vision isolates a person within a different reality. Although most clients are successfully rehabilitated, some losses are permanent. Also, some people, for a variety of reasons, remain socially isolated. The image of a blind person who is pitied and must accept the charity of others is disturbing.

Use therapeutic communication to express empathy as the client relates expected and actual losses that are due to loss of vision. People with actual or potential loss of vision may be faced with barriers in their vocations that force an unwanted change. Not all jobs and work environments are adaptable for a person who is visually impaired. Age may be a major factor in the person's ability to meet this challenge.

Self-esteem is closely related to the roles of people in their particular lifestyle. Loss of control in personal, family, and work situations can be devastating. The issue of dependence versus independence may also be a factor in the person's ability to cope with the stressors of vision loss.

Risk for Ineffective Management of Therapeutic Regimen (Individuals). The regimen for eye drops and oral medications to control glaucoma ranges from simple to complex. This diagnosis should be stated as *Risk for Ineffective Management of Therapeutic Regimen (Individuals) related to complex medication schedule.*

Outcomes. The client will describe the disease process and the regimen for disease control, and will relate how the medication routine will be incorporated into ADL.

Interventions. The client may need to instill as many as three or four different eye drops from one to six times a day. Constricting eye drops are usually prescribed four times a day, and beta-blockers are usually prescribed every 12 hours; however, the eye drops may be needed every 4 to 6 hours. The schedule is designed to provide the best possible control of intraocular pressure around the clock.

Medications are an integral part of the treatment and care of a client with glaucoma, and nursing interventions must thus be directed at the client's ability to understand and comply with prescribed therapy.

First, determine the client's current level of knowledge. Provide necessary information about glaucoma and its treatment in understandable terms. Diagrams may be helpful to the client and significant others. Because treatment for glaucoma is often complex, involving both oral and topical ophthalmic medications, review a written plan of care in large print with the client and family. To maximize compliance, ensure that the plan of care fits into the client's lifestyle.

The administration of eye drops is a critical component of self-care for the client with glaucoma. After instructing the client and family on the technique of instillation, validate the client's or family's ability to properly instill eye drops by asking for a demonstration. Be sure to include discussion of medications and their side effects. Table 65–1 lists additional guidelines for teaching the client about eye drops.

EVALUATION

Independent self-care is the area for evaluation in the medically managed client. Evaluate the client's ability for self-care (a short-term outcome) and compliance with the medical regimen (a long-term outcome).

Modifications for Elderly Clients

Older clients with arthritic or shaking hands have difficulty instilling their own eye drops. Instruct the client to lie down on a bed or sofa. Tilting the head back can lead to loss of balance. The eye drop regimen for glaucoma requires accurate timing. Older clients may need visual reminders, such as a check-off list, and may also need to use a timer or an alarm clock to help them remember.

TABLE 65–1 TEACHING THE CLIENT ABOUT EYE DROPS FOR GLAUCOMA

Medication	Teaching Aspects
Pilocarpine HCl	Usually given three to four times a day A miotic, causing pupillary constriction to open Schlemm's canal Space out administration, beginning on awakening and ending at bedtime. May cause blurred vision after instillation Brow ache has been reported Consider use of thin gel strips (a timed-release form) to improve compliance
Timolol maleate and other beta-blockers (e.g., levobunolol)	Usually given every 12 hours Decreases production of aqueous humor Space out administration Contraindicated in clients with asthma and chronic obstructive pulmonary disease Assess for bradycardia before administration
Carbonic anhydrase inhibitors (e.g., acetazolamide)	Inhibits production of aqueous humor Available as tablets and in sustained-release capsules Side effects include anorexia and tingling in the hands and feet

Surgical Management

When maximal medical therapy fails to halt the progression of visual field loss and optic nerve damage, surgical intervention is recommended. Many procedures are used to improve aqueous humor outflow; however, no operation has been uniformly successful.

LASER TRABECULOPLASTY. The use of the laser to create an opening in the trabecular meshwork is often indicated before filtering surgery is considered. The laser produces scars in the trabecular meshwork, causing tightening of meshwork fibers. The tightened fibers allow increased outflow of aqueous humor. Intraocular pressure is reduced through improved outflow in about 80% of cases. The effect of the laser treatment decreases with time, and the procedure may need to be repeated. Medical treatment is usually continued.

TRABECULECTOMY. Trabeculectomy is the creation of an opening through which the aqueous fluid escapes. A half-thickness scleral flap is loosely sutured over the created opening through which the fluid escapes, again resulting in subconjunctival absorption of aqueous humor (Fig. 65–1*C*).

FILTERING PROCEDURES. Operations such as trephination, thermal sclerostomy, and sclerectomy create an outflow channel from the anterior chamber into the subconjunctival space (Fig. 65–1*D*). Aqueous humor is absorbed through the conjunctival vessels. In about 25% of cases, the opening closes because of scar tissue formation and reoperation is necessary. Such filtering procedures are less successful in young and black clients, who tend to have an increased ability to produce thicker scar tissue. Topical corticosteroids are used postoperatively because their anti-inflammatory action inhibits proliferation of fibroblasts at the surgical site.

IRIDECTOMY. Iridectomy is the creation of a new route for the flow of aqueous humor to the trabecular meshwork. The laser is used to create the new opening in the iris (Fig. 65–1*E*).

OTHER TECHNIQUES. 5-Fluorouracil (5-FU), mitomycin, and other antimetabolites are sometimes injected subconjunctivally because they also inhibit fibroblast proliferation and thereby reduce postoperative scarring. Ocular implantation devices (e.g., Molteno implant, Baerveldt seton) are sometimes used to control the flow of aqueous humor in clients with complicated types of glaucoma. A device is sutured to the outer surface of the eyeball on the sclera between the ocular muscles. A tiny probe is inserted under the scleral flap directly into the anterior chamber that directs the flow of aqueous humor more posteriorly than in the more common filtering procedures.

CYCLODESTRUCTIVE PROCEDURES. When other surgical procedures have failed, cyclocryotherapy (application of a freezing tip) or cyclophotocoagulation may be used to damage the ciliary body and decrease production of aqueous humor.

Nursing Management of the Surgical Client

PREOPERATIVE CARE

Preoperative nursing care includes preparing the client for a surgical procedure that may be performed in either an outpatient or inpatient setting (see Chapter 15).

Laser therapy is most commonly performed in a clinic or office, including use of a topical anesthetic. Explain both the expected outcome of the procedure and the "popping" sounds and flashing lights that the client will experience. Explain that there will be a waiting period (usually 1 to 2 hours) after the procedure to evaluate a possible rise in intraocular pressure. Because of the instability of the intraocular pressure, the client should arrange for a friend or family member to accompany him or her and to provide transportation.

POSTOPERATIVE CARE

When the client returns from the operating room, the eye is covered with a patch and a metal or plastic shield for protection. Instruct the client not to lie on the operative side to avoid pressure on the surgical site. When the effects of perioperative sedation have diminished, the client may walk about and eat as desired.

Frequent monitoring of intraocular pressure is necessary because the surgical site is microscopic. Assess the client for unrelieved pain, nausea, and decreased vision. When healing is delayed, the anterior chamber may not re-form. Intraocular pressure readings may be 2 to 5 mm Hg, or the anterior chamber may even be flat. If the anterior chamber does not re-form, another surgical procedure may be required. The wound also may seal tightly, causing intraocular pressure to rise above normal levels; such a case also warrants reoperation.

Self-Care

The postoperative plan must include client education and evaluation of the home environment and available care. Because the level of independence varies with each client, use information supplied by the client and family or friends to assess how much support may be needed. Although many clients with glaucoma undergo repeated surgical procedures, carefully review the information each time. Client and family education includes the following steps:

1. Manifestations of infection (redness, swelling, drainage, blurred vision, pain).
2. Manifestations of increased intraocular pressure (unrelieved pain, nausea, decrease in vision).
3. The rationale for eye protection (shield or eyeglasses at all times) to protect from light and trauma.
4. Medications and eye drop instillation technique.
5. Scheduled return visit date and time.
6. Treatment of the surgical site:
   a. Carefully clean the area around the eye with warm tap water and a clean washcloth.
   b. Do not rub or apply pressure over the closed eye, which may damage healing tissue.

CATARACTS

A *cataract* is an opacity of the lens. Although cataract formation is usually associated with aging, there are several other causes. Some degree of cataract formation is to be expected in most people over 70 years of age. More than a million cataract operations are now being performed annually in the United States. A person with a normal life span is likely to undergo a cataract operation more than any other major surgical procedure.

The most common cataract is the *age-related* or *senile* type. Worldwide, cataract is the primary cause of reduced vision and blindness. Senile cataracts usually begin around the age of 50 years and consist of cortical, nuclear, or posterior subcapsular opacities, which may coexist in various combinations. In *cortical* cataracts, spokelike opacifications are found in the periphery of the lens. They progress slowly, infrequently involve the visual axis, and often do not cause severe loss of vision. Nuclear sclerotic cataracts are a result of a progressive yellowing and hardening of the central lens (nucleus). Most people over age 70 years have some degree of nuclear sclerosis. Posterior subcapsular opacities occur centrally on the posterior lens capsule and cause visual loss early in their development because they lie directly on the visual axis.

Etiology and Risk Factors

The cumulative exposure to ultraviolet light over a person's life span is the single most important risk factor in cataract development. People who live at high altitudes or who work in bright sunlight, such as commercial fishermen, appear to experience cataract formation earlier in life. Glass blowers and welders without eye protection are also at higher risk.

Cataracts may develop as a result of many other systemic, ocular, and congenital disorders.

Systemic disorders include diabetes, tetany, myotonic dystrophy, neurodermatitis, galactosemia, Lowe's syndrome, Werner's syndrome, and Down syndrome.

Intraocular disorders include iridocyclitis, retinitis, retinal detachment, and onchocerciasis.

Infections (German measles, mumps, hepatitis, poliomyelitis, chickenpox, infectious mononucleosis) during the first trimester of pregnancy may cause *congenital* cataracts.

Blunt trauma, lacerations, foreign bodies, radiation, exposure to infrared light, and chronic use of corticosteroids may also result in cataracts.

Pathophysiology

Cataract formation is characterized chemically by a reduction in oxygen uptake and an initial increase in water content followed by dehydration of the lens. Sodium and calcium contents are increased; potassium, ascorbic acid, and protein contents are decreased. The protein in the lens undergoes numerous age-related changes, including yellowing from formation of fluorescent compounds and molecular changes. These changes, along with the photoabsorption of ultraviolet radiation throughout life, suggest that cataracts may be caused by a photochemical process.

Cataracts progress through the following clinical stages of development:

Immature cataracts are not completely opaque, and some light is transmitted through them, allowing useful vision.

Mature cataracts are completely opaque. The former term for this stage was *ripe*. Vision is significantly reduced.

Intumescent cataracts are those in which the lens absorbs water and increases in size. The lens may be mature or immature. The increase in size may result in glaucoma.

Hypermature cataracts are those in which the lens proteins break down into short-chain polypeptides that leak out through the lens capsule. The pieces of protein are engulfed by macrophages, which may obstruct the trabecular meshwork, causing phacolytic glaucoma.

Clinical Manifestations

Clients experience blurred vision, sometimes monocular diplopia (double vision), photophobia (light sensitivity), and glare because the opacity of the lens obstructs the reception of light and images by the retina. Clients usually see better in low light when the pupil is dilated, which allows for vision around a central opacity. There is no complaint of pain. A cloudy lens can be observed (Fig. 65–3).

A cataract should be suspected when the red reflex seen with the direct ophthalmoscope is distorted or absent. Although cataracts can usually be easily identified with the direct ophthalmoscope, an accurate determination of the type and extent of the lens change requires a slit-lamp examination.

Outcome Management

Surgical Management

There is no known treatment other than surgery that prevents or reduces cataract formation. The goal of cataract surgery is to remove the opacified lens. Since the 1980s, cataract surgery has improved dramatically as a result of the operating microscope, new instrumentation, improved suture material, smaller incisions, and refinement of the intraocular lens implant. The lens is surgically removed by an intracapsular or extracapsular procedure (Fig. 65–4).

Intracapsular cataract extraction (ICCE) consists of removing the lens, including the lens capsule. *Extracapsular* cataract extraction (ECCE) consists of removing the lens and the anterior portion of the lens capsule. The posterior lens capsule is left intact. Although ICCE is highly successful and still performed, ECCE is by far the most common procedure in the United States. The primary reason for performing ECCE is to allow insertion of a posterior chamber intraocular lens inside the remaining capsule, which results in fewer postoperative complications.

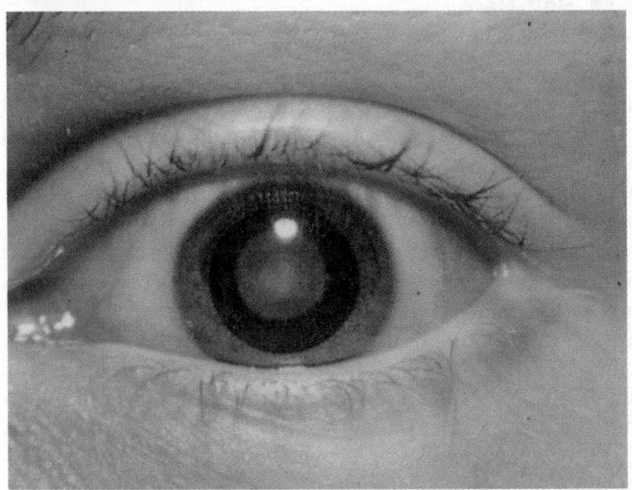

FIGURE 65–3 The cloudy appearance of a lens affected by cataract. (Courtesy of Ophthalmic Photography at the University of Michigan W. K. Kellogg Eye Center, Ann Arbor.)

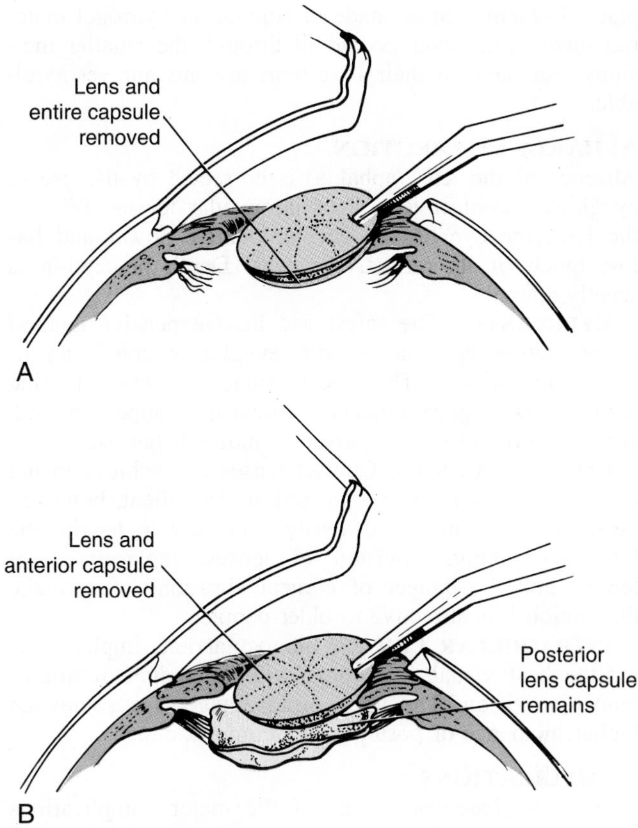

FIGURE 65–4 Surgical approaches to lens removal for cataracts. *A,* Intracapsular cataract extraction. *B,* Extracapsular cataract extraction.

Phacoemulsification is an extracapsular technique that uses ultrasound vibrations to break up the lens material. Pieces of the anterior lens capsule and the lens are removed by suction through the phacoemulsifier tip. With this "small incision" technique, a much smaller incision in the eye is necessary. Only one to three sutures are needed, and in some cases none at all is required. Wound healing in small-incision surgery occurs at the same rate as in larger-incision techniques.

Cataract surgery is often performed while the client is under IV conscious sedation. An IV injection of methohexital sodium (Brevital) or thiopental (Pentothal) induces a few minutes of light anesthesia while the retrobulbar injection of local anesthetic solution is given. Cataract surgery is also successfully performed with a topical anesthetic.

Intraocular Lens Implantation

After extraction of the cataract, a new lens is inserted in the posterior chamber, or the client is left without a lens. Although there are many styles of intraocular lenses, they all consist of two basic parts: (1) a clear spherical optic lens usually made of polymethyl methacrylate (Plexiglas) and (2) footplates or haptic lenses to hold the lens in place. Foldable lenses made of silicone or hydrogel material have been developed to fit through the smaller incisions, but data on their long-term use are not yet available.

APHAKIA CORRECTION

Absence of the lens (aphakia) is corrected by the use of eyeglasses, contact lenses, or intraocular lenses. Without the lens, the eye has no accommodative power and has lost much of its refractive power. Depth perception is greatly altered.

EYEGLASSES. The safest and least expensive method of correcting aphakia is with eyeglasses consisting of very thick lenses. The disadvantage, however, is that thick lenses magnify objects. Vertical lines appear curved, and it is difficult for the person to judge distances.

CONTACT LENSES. Contact lenses can achieve visual correction with much less distortion. The client, however, must have the manual dexterity necessary to handle the lenses. Cleaning, insertion of lenses, replacement of lenses, and the danger of corneal abrasions often make this option less attractive to older people.

INTRAOCULAR LENSES. Intraocular lens implants offer the best visual correction, with immediate return of binocular vision. The main disadvantage is a somewhat higher incidence of postoperative complications.

COMPLICATIONS

Secondary glaucoma is one of the major complications that may occur after cataract extraction. As a result of postoperative edema in the ocular tissues, a certain rise in intraocular pressure is anticipated and expected. This elevation most often resolves within 24 to 72 hours. If prolonged intraocular pressure persists, medical therapy may be necessary.

Postoperative infection, bleeding, macular edema, and wound leaks are also possible. The incidence of retinal detachment is higher in the first 12 months after cataract surgery.

Following ECCE, the posterior capsule may become opacified, which is called an *after-cataract* or *secondary membrane.* Subcapsular lens epithelial cells may regenerate lens fibers, which can obstruct vision. This postoperative complication occurs fairly frequently and used to require a second operation to remove the opacified tissue. The neodymium:yttrium-aluminum-garnet (Nd:YAG) laser is being used to create an opening in the capsule through pulses of laser energy that cause tiny "explosions" in the target tissue. Complications of this technique include a transient rise in intraocular pressure and possible damage to the intraocular lens.

Nursing Management of the Surgical Client

ASSESSMENT

During the history and physical examination, ask the client about any predisposing factors (trauma, systemic diseases, medications such as corticosteroids, and other ocular problems). Visual acuity (both distant and near) in each eye is documented. Ask the client to describe visual disturbances. The client's visual acuity may be relatively close to normal ranges, yet the client may experience difficulty in performing ADL. The client's individual perception of the quality of vision is an important factor in determining the need for surgery.

DIAGNOSIS, OUTCOMES, INTERVENTIONS

Sensory/Perceptual Alterations (Visual). Removal of the clouded lens reduces glare and cloudy vision. Improvement in visual acuity is related to the type of correction. Intraocular lens implantation provides the best visual correction. Contact lenses provide a good correction, and eyeglasses provide functional correction. None of these corrections provide the same visual acuity as the natural lens of the eye. Although vision may be greatly improved, there may still be varying degrees of change in depth perception. Write the nursing diagnosis as *Sensory/Perceptual Alterations (Visual) related to lens extraction and replacement.*

Outcomes. The client will gain improved vision and will adapt to changes in visual correction.

Interventions. Adaptation is the key issue in caring for the client having cataract surgery. Nursing interventions are based on assisting the client to gain or maintain as much independence as possible. Evaluate the client's lifestyle, abilities, and home environment. A 55-year-old client who is an architect and otherwise healthy may have an early cataract removed because it interferes with his work in areas where bright light is used. A 75-year-old diabetic client who is retired and mainly watches television has entirely different needs.

Unless there are other ocular complications or health factors, cataract surgery is performed on an outpatient basis. When clients are admitted to the hospital or surgical facility, determine their current level of knowledge and understanding of the perioperative events. Preoperative eye drops may include a dilating agent such as tropicamide (Mydriacyl) to facilitate the surgery. A cycloplegic cyclopentolate (Cyclogyl) may also be administered to paralyze the ciliary muscles.

EVALUATION

Adaptation to restored normal vision is usually rapid. Adaptation to limited vision requires more time based on individual variations.

Self-Care

After cataract surgery, clients are expected to return for a follow-up visit the next morning and again at 1 week and at 1 month. Postoperative care includes observation of the ocular dressing, if present, and assessment of the client's ability to perform ADL at the preoperative level. Nausea and vomiting are no longer an expected outcome of the surgical procedure but, if present, should be reported immediately. Prolonged vomiting may result in increased intraocular pressure and wound dehiscence. The eye patch is usually removed the next morning but may be removed after a few hours if the client has limited vision in the other eye. Instruct the client to wear a metal or plastic shield to protect the eye from accidental injury and not to rub the eye. Glasses may be worn during the day. The Client Education Guide provides instructions to be followed after cataract removal.

Restrictions on postoperative activity vary according to the practice of the ophthalmologist. Generally, the client

CLIENT EDUCATION GUIDE

Care After Cataract Removal

Leave the eye patch in place.
For 24 hours, limit your activity to sitting in a chair, resting in bed, and walking to the bathroom.
Do not rub your eye.
You can wear your glasses.
Do not lift more than 5 pounds (the weight of a gallon of milk).
Do not strain (or bear down).
Do not sleep on the side of your body that was operated on.
Take your eye drops.
Take acetaminophen (e.g., Tylenol) as needed for pain or itching.
DO NOT take aspirin or drugs containing aspirin.
Report any pain that is unrelieved, redness around the eye, nausea, or vomiting.
Wear eye shield to protect your eye.

should avoid heavy lifting (>5 pounds) or straining in the early postoperative period.

Eye care for the client after cataract surgery is the same as that for glaucoma clients (see Glaucoma). Postoperative eye medications may include antibiotics, corticosteroids, or both. Assess the client's or family's ability to instill eye drops appropriately. Review the rationale and schedule for the medications with the client and family. Postoperative discomfort should be minimal to moderate and is usually relieved by acetaminophen. Clients commonly experience an itching sensation after cataract surgery. Instruct the client to report any pain that is unrelieved. Review the clinical manifestations of infection and increased intraocular pressure with the client and family.

Depending on the client's age, ability, and availability of assistance, make a referral for home health care if indicated. Adjustment to changes in vision also varies with the individual client.

RETINAL DISORDERS

RETINAL DETACHMENT

Rhegmatogenous retinal detachment (secondary to a tear in the retina) is characterized by a retinal hole, liquid in the vitreous body with access to the hole, and subsequent fluid accumulation between the retina and the retinal pigment epithelium. The liquid seeps through the hole and separates the retina from its blood supply. Without intervention, the detachment continues to spread and the detached retina loses the ability to function. It may become increasingly detached over a period of hours to years.

Etiology and Risk Factors

Retinal detachment occurs mainly in the adult eye. The overall incidence is 1 in 15,000 people per year, but the risk of detachment increases after age 40 and most often occurs between the ages of 50 and 70.

Predisposing factors to retinal detachment include aging, cataract extraction, degeneration of the retina, trauma, severe myopia, previous retinal detachment in the other eye, and a family history of retinal detachment. Retinal holes and tears usually occur from spontaneous vitreous traction, but there may be abnormal adhesions between the retina and vitreous body secondary to diabetic retinopathy, injury, or other ocular disorders. Atrophy of the vitreous body may also result in a retinal tear.

Pathophysiology

If the retina is separated from its choroidal blood supply, it will die. The retinal tissues are at a high risk for avascular necrosis because they are delicate structures and have a high metabolic rate.

Clinical Manifestations

Characteristic clinical manifestations of retinal detachment are described by clients as a shadow or curtain falling across the field of vision. Shadows or black areas in the field of vision are the result of separation of visual receptors from the neural pathway (Fig. 65–5). No pain is associated with a detached retina. The onset is usually sudden and may be accompanied by a burst of black spots or floaters indicating that bleeding has occurred as a result of the detachment. The person may also see flashes of light caused by separation of the retina.

Examination with a direct and indirect ophthalmoscope reveals the portion of the retina involved and the extent of the detachment (Fig. 65–6). A scleral depressor also may be used externally on the lid or conjunctiva to assist in rotating the eyeball and to indent the retina for increased viewing ability. Areas of detachment appear bluish gray, as opposed to the normal red-pink color. Retinal tears are most often horseshoe-shaped but may be round.

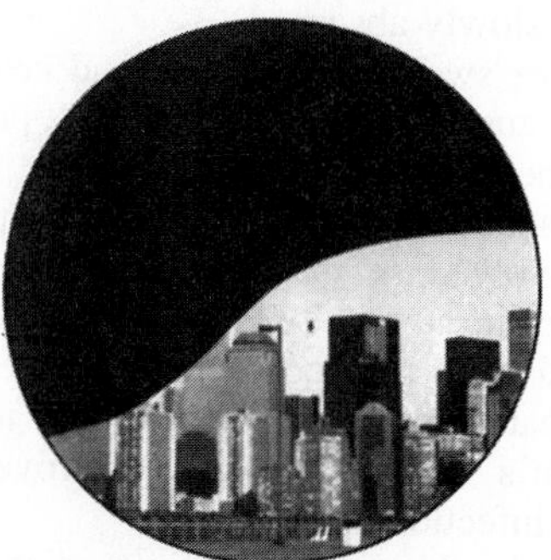

Detached Retina

FIGURE 65–5 Vision of a client with retinal detachment. (Courtesy of National Industries of the Blind, Wayne, NJ.)

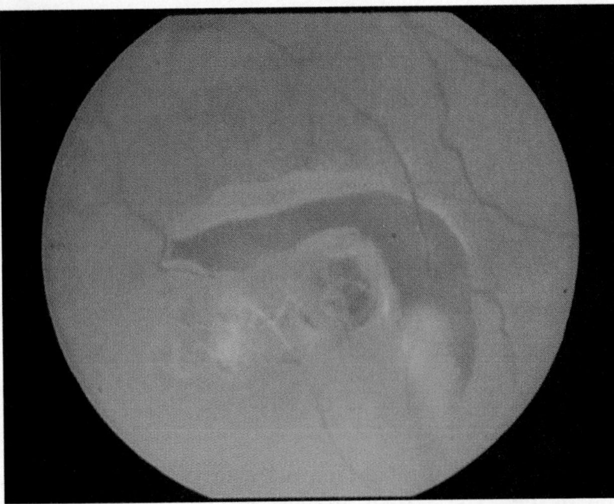

FIGURE 65–6 Bluish-gray appearance of areas of retinal detachment. (Courtesy of Ophthalmic Photography at the University of Michigan W. K. Kellogg Eye Center, Ann Arbor.)

Surgical Management

There is no known medical treatment for a detached retina. The goal of surgical repair of retinal detachment is to place the retina back in contact with the choroid and to seal the accompanying holes and breaks. Often *cryopexy* (use of a freezing probe) or laser photocoagulation is used to seal the hole if it has not progressed to detachment. Both methods create inflammation around the area, which scars and seals the hole. If not treated promptly, a retinal detachment may progress to involve the macula, which greatly compromises visual acuity. A retinal detachment requires urgent intervention.

The surgical procedure to place the retina back in contact with the choroid is called *scleral buckling* (Fig. 65–7). The sclera is actually depressed from the outside by rubber-like silicone (Silastic) sponges or bands that are sutured in place permanently. In addition to the buckling procedure, an intraocular injection of air or sulfahexafluoride (SF6) gas bubble, or both, may be used to apply pressure on the retina from the inside of the eye. This holds the retina in place by gravitational force during the healing phase. Postoperative positioning of the client maximizes the tamponade effect of the air or gas bubble. The bubble is slowly absorbed.

Postoperative swelling of tissues and cells in the anterior chamber caused by the inflammatory process or compromise of the venous drainage system may result in increased intraocular pressure. Because of the fragility of the tissues involved in the repair, re-detachment of the retina may occur at any time. At times, the retina has been separated from its blood supply long enough so that, even when reattached, it no longer has useful function and the client's vision does not improve significantly. Postoperative infection is also a risk.

The client should not expect immediate return of vision. Postoperative inflammation and the dilating drops interfere with vision. As healing takes place over weeks and months, vision may improve gradually.

Nursing Management of the Preoperative Client

ASSESSMENT

When the history has been obtained and the physical examination is being performed, assess the client's visual changes in both eyes. Visual field loss occurs in the opposite quadrant of the actual detachment. For example, a tear in the temporal region, which is affected more frequently, creates a visual defect in the nasal area. The pupil must be widely dilated for a retinal examination. Tell clients that they will experience an extremely bright light and will be asked to change their gaze frequently to facilitate the examination.

DIAGNOSIS, OUTCOMES, INTERVENTION

Sensory/Perceptual Alterations (Visual). The extent of loss of vision is related to the portion of the retina involved. Giant retinal tears involving the entire retina may result in temporary blindness, whereas peripheral tears may not interfere with central vision at all.

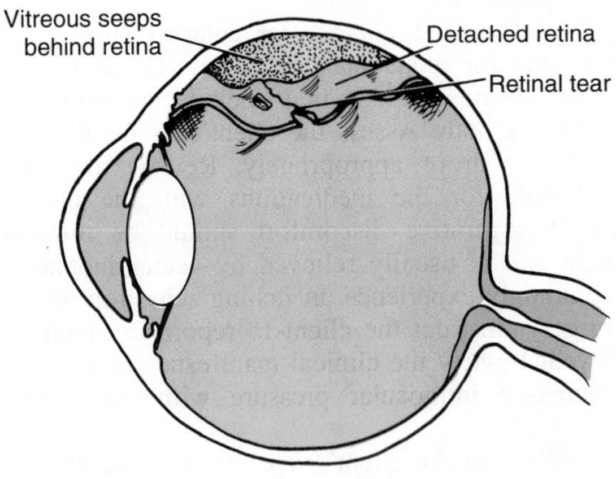

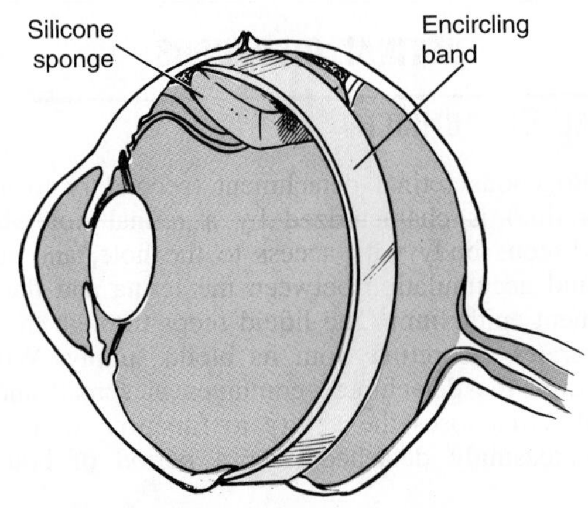

FIGURE 65–7 Scleral buckling to repair a detached retina. A silicone sponge implant is placed over the tear and held in place with an encircling band. When the buckle is tightened, the implant indents the sclera, holding the choroid and retina together.

Healing involves delicate neurologic tissue, and visual improvement may be gradual over several months. Write the nursing diagnosis as *Sensory/Perceptual Alterations (Visual) related to decreased retinal function.*

Outcomes. The client will maintain as much functional vision as possible, as evidenced by reporting no further loss of vision; adapting to any visual loss; and demonstrating an ability to perform ADL, to instill eye medications, and to recognize clinical manifestations of complications.

Interventions. The focus of the care plan is to help the client cope with the fears and reality of loss of vision and adapt to changes in vision. The client must be aware of the clinical manifestations of further loss of vision. See the Bridge to Home Health Care feature for suggestions on how to assist clients.

Knowledge Deficit. Assess the client's current level of knowledge and understanding of the implications of retinal detachment and the expectations for the surgical procedure The most common nursing diagnosis used before surgery is *Knowledge Deficit related to impending surgery, unknown outcomes, and expectations.*

Outcomes. The client will express understanding of the planned operation, expected outcomes for restoration of vision, and role in his or her own care after surgery.

Interventions. Provide preoperative teaching. Preoperative nursing care involves preparing the client for outpatient surgery or an overnight stay in the hospital. Because retinal detachment repair may take several hours, general anesthesia is used commonly. The pupil must be widely dilated before the operation, and the client may be given a sedative.

EVALUATION

Determine whether the client has adapted to imposed changes in vision. You may need to find help at home for independent living until sight returns or the client adapts to changes in vision.

Nursing Management of the Postoperative Client

Observe the eye patch for any drainage. Blood loss in retinal detachment surgery is minimal, and only serous drainage is expected on the postoperative dressing. Assess level of pain and presence of nausea.

Activity restrictions may be necessary if an air or gas bubble has been injected. The client needs to be positioned so that the bubble can apply maximal pressure on the retina by the force of gravity. This position, usually head down and to one side, is maintained for several days. Provide suggestions for comfort and support with the positioning (pillows under stomach, elbows, or ankles).

Posterior segment surgery, such as scleral buckling procedures, causes considerably more discomfort than anterior segment procedures do. Ocular muscles are separated, and the globe is manipulated to reach the posterior portions of the eyeball. Narcotics may be needed during the first 24 hours after surgery. Nausea and vomiting may also require management.

BRIDGE TO HOME HEALTH CARE

Coping with Failing Vision

Providing a safe home environment for the client with failing vision is essential. Promoting an autonomous lifestyle is desirable. Assessing the client's ability to remain safely at home is an important responsibility of home health care nurses.

Basic emergency procedures can be implemented by the use of nationwide services such as Lifeline. This service provides a portable electronic device usually worn around the client's neck or wrist. By simply pushing the button, immediate contact is made with emergency personnel. The toll-free phone number is 1-800-852-5433.

Local telephone companies can provide special adaptive equipment for 9-1-1 access. Telephones that can be programmed and have lighted or large numbers are available in most retail stores.

Home safety precautions can be simple. Burns can be prevented by color-coding water faucets. Use red for hot water and blue for cold water. Marking the "Off" dials on stoves and microwave ovens with colored tape or paint reduces the chance of injury.

Adequate lighting is essential. During the day, natural light is preferable. Open drapes or shades to provide ample light. Replace light bulbs with the highest wattage recommended.

Removal of hazards, such as throw rugs, clutter, and unnecessary furniture, can promote unrestricted ambulation. Handrails can be installed in hallways, in bathrooms, and on steps to prevent falls. Equipment such as canes, walkers, raised toilet seats, and bathtub rails promote safety. These items are available at medical supply stores.

Many commercial products are now marketed that can be of great assistance in the home. Pill organizers are clearly marked boxes with the day of the week and the times pills are to be taken. These can be filled by family members for a week at a time. Electronic lamp timers and voice-activated switches will allow the client to function more independently.

Access to a television and a radio is important. Large-print newspapers and reading materials help keep the client in touch with current events. The local library and the American Association for the Blind can provide assistance in obtaining needed items.

Creativity and planning can allow the client to remain at home in a safe environment for as long as possible.

Bernadette Mruz, RN, *Clinical Manager, Visiting Nurse Association of Omaha, Omaha, Nebraska*

IV acetazolamide (Diamox) may be used to reduce increased intraocular pressure. The intraocular pressure is monitored closely during the first 24 hours. Encourage the client to resume a regular diet and fluids as tolerated. The eye patch and shield are removed the next morning. Redness and swelling of the lids and conjunctiva should be expected from the surgical manipulation. After several days, the swelling and ecchymosis of the lids subside, but the conjunctiva may remain red or pink for a few weeks.

Postoperative eye medications generally include an antibiotic-steroid combination eye drop to prevent infection and reduce inflammation. Cycloplegic agents are prescribed to dilate the pupil and relax the ciliary muscles, which decreases discomfort and helps prevent the formation of iris adhesions to the corneal endothelium (synechiae). Either warm or cold compresses may be applied for comfort several times a day.

Self-Care

Because retinal detachment surgery is often performed on an urgent basis, the client rarely has an opportunity to plan for the surgery. Evaluate the home environment, and assist the client and family in preparing for any necessary support. Although the eye patch is usually removed early in the postoperative period, clients commonly have decreased functional vision in the eye.

Instruct the client to clean the eye with warm tap water using a clean washcloth. Warm compresses may be continued at home. Either an eye shield or glasses should be worn during the day, and the shield should be worn during naps and at night. Advise the client to avoid vigorous activities and heavy lifting during the immediate postoperative period. If an air or gas bubble has been injected, it may take several weeks to be totally absorbed. Clients are advised to avoid air travel during this time because the gas and air expand at high altitudes.

DIABETIC RETINOPATHY

Diabetic retinopathy is a progressive disorder of the retina characterized by microscopic damage to the retinal vessels, resulting in occlusion of the vessels. As a result of inadequate blood supply, sections of the retina deteriorate and vision is permanently lost.

Etiology and Risk Factors

Diabetic retinopathy is one of the leading causes of blindness worldwide. All diabetic people are at risk for retinopathy, although there appears to be a strong correlation between incidence and severity of retinopathy and duration of the disease and blood glucose control. Approximately 30% to 40% of the diabetic population has some degree of retinopathy. Clients who have had diabetes for 15 to 20 years have an 80% to 90% risk for development of retinopathy.

Pathophysiology

There are two types of diabetic retinopathy: (1) background *(nonproliferative)* and (2) *proliferative.* In background retinopathy, early pathologic changes demonstrate the hyperpermeability and weakening of the retinal vessels. The capillaries develop tiny dot-like outpouchings (microaneurysms), and the retinal veins become dilated and tortuous. Multiple hemorrhages occur from these defective vessels. Retinal edema is caused by leaking capillaries, and after the serous fluid is absorbed, a yellowish precipitate ("hard exudate") remains. Hemorrhages, exudates, and ischemia contribute to impaired vision, particularly if these occur on or around the macula. Progressive retinal ischemia stimulates the growth of new but ineffective blood vessels. These new and fragile blood vessels proliferate and grow into the vitreous body. These vessels leak, hemorrhage, and undergo fibrous changes that may form bands that pull on the retina, causing detachment. This process is called *proliferative retinopathy* (Fig. 65–8). With increasing ischemia, microinfarcts of the nerve fiber layer, called "cotton-wool spots," appear.

Clinical Manifestations

Clients experience a wide range of visual disturbances and fluctuations. Retinal vessel hemorrhage into the vitreous space obstructs vision with black spots or floaters or may result in complete loss of vision. Areas of retinal ischemia become blind spots. Macular edema causes decreased central vision.

Outcome Management

To reduce the occurrence of hemorrhage and retinal detachment in progressive retinopathy, the argon laser is used to photocoagulate the blood vessels. Hundreds and even thousands of microscopic photocoagulation applications (burns) are systematically placed around the peripheral retina, avoiding the central area that includes the macula and the optic disc. When a hemorrhage does not clear spontaneously over time, a vitrectomy (removal of a portion of the vitreous humor) may be performed. A vitrectomy may also be needed to release the traction of membranes on the retina.

Nursing interventions for the client with diabetic retinopathy are focused on assessment and management of diabetes. Elevations in blood glucose levels cause a temporary decrease in visual acuity. Because retinopathy is generally progressive, the client will need to cope with increasing visual deficits. Community referrals for rehabilitation and aids for low vision often provide useful assistance. Visiting nurses often prepare insulin injections for the upcoming week, because clients cannot see well enough to do this accurately.

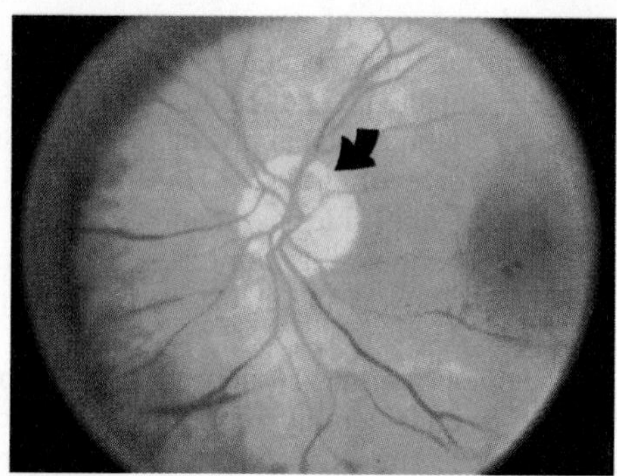

FIGURE 65–8 Proliferative diabetic retinopathy. Neovascularization covers one fourth to one third of the optic disc (*arrow*). (Standard photograph No. 10A of the Modified Airlee House Classification of Diabetic Retinopathy. Courtesy of the Early Treatment Diabetic Retinopathy Study Research Group.)

RETINITIS PIGMENTOSA

Retinitis pigmentosa is a genetic disorder that initially destroys the rods of the eye. Because the rods perceive black and white vision, the earliest manifestation is noticed during childhood as night blindness. Over the next several years, manifestations progress until a total loss of peripheral vision occurs. In time, central vision is also lost. No treatment is available to slow or stop this disorder. Genetic counseling is advised.

Retinal infections in clients with acquired immunodeficiency syndrome (AIDS) are discussed at the end of this chapter.

AGE-RELATED MACULAR DEGENERATION

Previously known as *senile macular degeneration,* age-related macular degeneration is an atrophic degenerative process that affects the macula and surrounding tissues, resulting in central visual deficits. Age-related macular degeneration is found to some degree in most adults over age 65 years. It is one of the most common causes of visual loss in older people. The exact cause is unknown, but the incidence increases with each decade in people over 50 years of age. It may be hereditary.

Age-related macular degeneration falls into two groups: (1) nonexudative *(dry)* and (2) exudative *(wet).* Both types are usually bilateral and progressive.

DRY MACULAR DEGENERATION

Nonexudative age-related macular degeneration is characterized by atrophy and degeneration of the outer retina and underlying structures. Yellowish round spots *(drusen)* may be seen on the retina and macula with an ophthalmoscope. Drusen are deposits of amorphous material from the pigment epithelial cells of the retina. Over time, these spots increase, enlarge, and may calcify.

WET MACULAR DEGENERATION

At the exudative stage of age-related macular degeneration, Bruch's membrane, which lies just beneath the pigment epithelial cell layer of the retina, becomes compromised. This results in serous fluid leaks from the choroid, with accompanying proliferation of choroidal blood vessels. A dome-shaped retinal pigment epithelium may be seen when examining the fundus. These leaks produce a visual effect called *metamorphopsia,* which is the blurred, wavy distortion of vision. The client may also notice a blurred scotoma or decreased central visual acuity (Fig. 65–9). Fundus photography and angiography may be performed on a regular basis to document and evaluate changes.

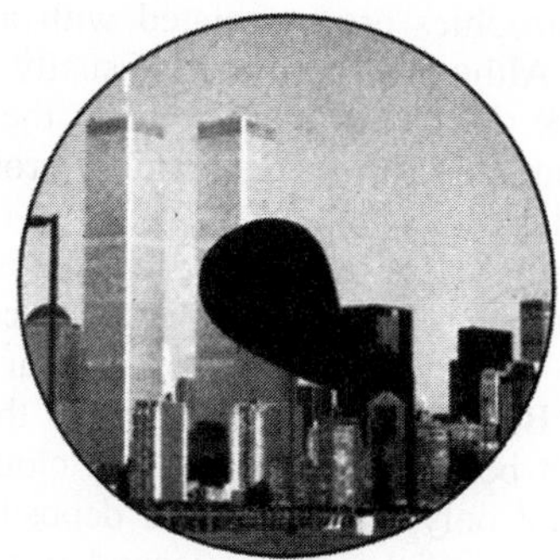

Macular Degeneration

FIGURE 65–9 Vision of a client with macular degeneration. (Courtesy of National Industries for the Blind, Wayne, NJ.)

Outcome Management

There is no known means of medical treatment or prevention of age-related macular degeneration. Further damage from exudative macular degeneration sometimes may be arrested by the use of argon photocoagulation, even though laser damage to the retina in this area results in a blind spot. When the fovea is involved, central vision is lost and the only helpful measures are low-vision aids.

The client with age-related macular degeneration is threatened with the loss of central vision (see Bridge to Home Health Care). To evaluate changes in vision, teach the client to use the Amsler chart at home. You may assist the client to maximize remaining vision with low-vision aids and community referral to a low-vision specialist and low-vision support groups.

RETINAL ARTERY OCCLUSION

Occlusion of the retinal artery or vein can cause loss of vision. The most common causes of occlusion are emboli from atherosclerosis, valvular heart disease, and increases in blood viscosity. The retinal artery can also be occluded from embolized plaque in the carotid artery or from spasm. Retinal artery occlusion causes a sudden, unilateral, painless loss of vision. The severity of the visual loss ranges from total loss, when the central artery is occluded, to a loss of a visual field, when a branch of the artery is blocked. Retinal vein occlusion is due to systemic vascular disorders, venous stasis, hypertension, or increased blood viscosity.

Outcome Management

Retinal artery occlusion is an emergency. Management includes intermittent massage of the eyeball by a physician to move an embolus from the central artery into a branch and increased oxygenation (95% oxygen for 10 minutes). Surgery can include anterior chamber paracentesis to reduce intraocular pressure and to move the embolus. Anticoagulants are used in the early phases of occlusion.

CORNEAL DISORDERS

CORNEAL DYSTROPHIES

Corneal dystrophies comprise a group of hereditary and acquired disorders of unknown cause, characterized by deposits in the layers of the cornea and alteration of the corneal structure. Specific corneal dystrophies characteristically appear at different ages. They may be stationary or slowly progressive throughout life. The most common form, Fuchs' dystrophy, usually begins in a person's 20s or 30s, affects more women than men, and is slowly progressive.

Corneal dystrophies are associated with all five layers of the cornea. Although the disease usually originates in the inner layers (Descemet's membrane, the stroma, and Bowman's membrane), the degeneration, erosion, and deposits affect all layers.

Fuchs' dystrophy is characterized by deposits in Descemet's membrane that look like warts. Descemet's membrane becomes thickened, and defects appear in the endothelial layer. Because the integrity of the cornea is compromised, it becomes edematous and cloudy. Vision is compromised not only by the corneal deposits but also by the altered structure of the cornea secondary to the edema.

The cornea is evaluated by slit-lamp examination. Fluorescein staining is used to enhance visualization of surface corneal defects. Corneal scrapings may be taken with a sterile spatula for further staining and microscopic evaluation. Specular micrography (see Diagnostic Tests in Chapter 64) may be used to evaluate the corneal endothelium.

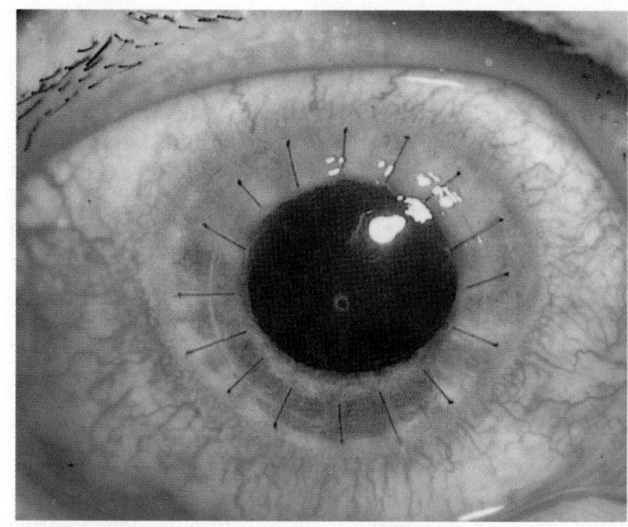

FIGURE 65–11 Clinical appearance of the eye after keratoplasty. (Courtesy of Ophthalmic Photography at the University of Michigan W. K. Kellogg Eye Center, Ann Arbor.)

Surgical Management

Corneal Transplantation

The goal of corneal transplantation *(keratoplasty)* is to improve the clarity of vision. This operation may be indicated for serious corneal conditions, including corneal dystrophy. *Penetrating* keratoplasty denotes full-thickness corneal replacement; *lamellar* keratoplasty denotes a partial-thickness procedure.

Because there is a direct relationship between age and health of the endothelial layer of the cornea, young donor tissue is preferred. Donor eyes are obtained from cadavers, must be enucleated soon after death because of rapid endothelial cell death, and must be stored in a preserving solution. Storage, handling, and coordination of donor tissue with surgeons are provide by a network of state eye bank associations around the country.

Corneal transplantation surgery is usually performed with the client under local anesthesia (Fig. 65–10). The surgeon prepares a donor cornea first by using a trephine to cut a corneal button with a radius of usually 7.0 to 8.5 mm. The recipient cornea is prepared in the same manner; however, it is usually cut 0.5 mm smaller so that there is an overlap by the donor cornea, which is then sutured into place. Figure 65–11 shows the eye after keratoplasty.

Graft rejection or failure may occur at any time after transplantation. It can result from unsuitable storage of donor tissue, dystrophy of the donor's endothelium, surgical trauma, or immunologic rejection. Wound leakage, bleeding into the anterior chamber, glaucoma, cataract, and infection are other complications that may occur. At the first sign of graft rejection, when the cornea becomes cloudy and edematous and when there is an anterior chamber reaction (presence of white blood cells or protein) (Fig. 65–12), topical steroids are prescribed in fre-

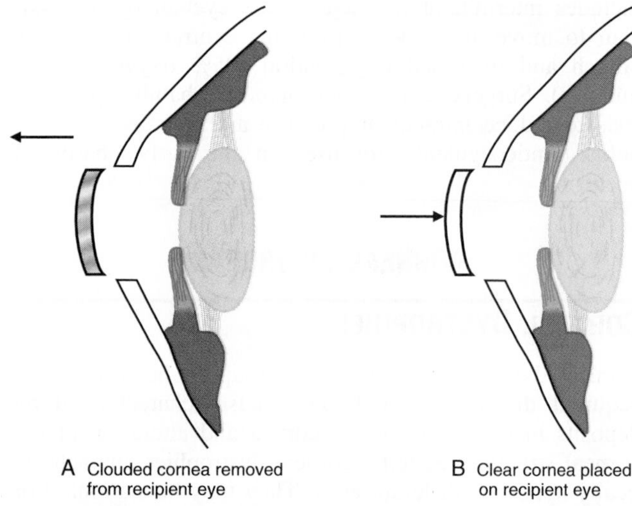
A Clouded cornea removed from recipient eye
B Clear cornea placed on recipient eye

FIGURE 65–10 Steps for corneal transplantation (penetrating keratoplasty). *A,* The diseased cornea is removed with a trephine. *B,* The donor cornea is placed on the eye and stitched in place with extremely fine suture material.

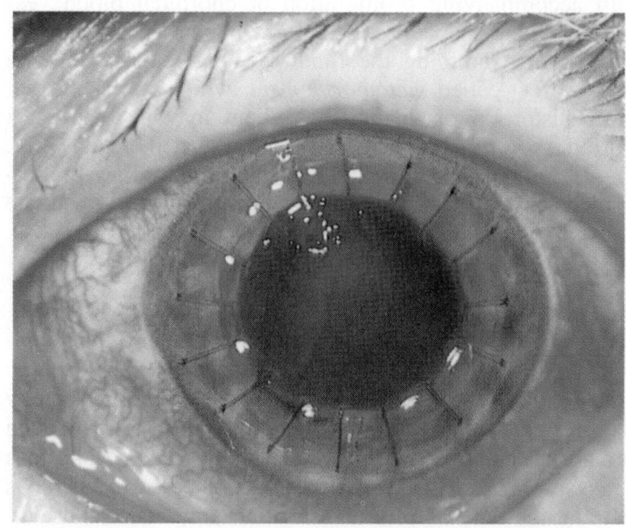

FIGURE 65–12 Acute graft rejection. (Courtesy of Ophthalmic Photography at the University of Michigan W. K. Kellogg Eye Center, Ann Arbor.)

quent doses to control the inflammatory response and to reverse the rejection reaction. In severe cases, a second transplantation may be necessary.

Nursing Management of the Postoperative Client

Corneal transplant surgery is usually performed as outpatient surgery. Postoperatively, the client returns from the operating room with an eye patch and protective shield in place. Observe the patch for signs of drainage. There is no blood loss associated with this procedure. The client should experience only mild to moderate discomfort, which should be relieved by acetaminophen. Unrelieved pain may indicate a rise in intraocular pressure and should be reported to the surgeon. Because the eye patch is to be in place until the following morning, assess the client's ability for self-care and advise the client and family about the hazards of monocular vision (see postoperative care for retinal detachment).

The eye is examined the next morning with the slit lamp. Depending on the extent of preoperative visual limitations, most clients experience improved vision immediately. Instruct clients, however, not to raise their expectations for full vision too high. Vision continues to improve gradually because the healing process may take up to a year or more. Glasses or contact lenses are usually needed to obtain the best result. Many months may be required for restoration of vision, and revisions in the care plan may be needed.

Self-Care

Postoperative eye drops usually include an antibiotic and a corticosteroid. Topical corticosteroid therapy may be needed indefinitely. Discharge instructions include the rationale for the medications and proper instillation technique. It is important for the client to wear eye protection in the form of regular glasses, sunglasses, or a protective shield to prevent injury to the eye. Advise the client never to rub the eye. The area around the eye may be cleaned with warm tap water using a clean washcloth.

Teach the client and family to recognize the clinical manifestations of graft rejection. A mnemonic tool may be useful in teaching the client to remember the signs of graft rejection (RSVP):

R, redness
S, swelling
V, decreased vision
P, pain

Teach the client and family to recognize the signs of increased intraocular pressure and infection.

Advise the client to evaluate vision in the eye each day. A picture on the wall or some object in a well-lighted room should be selected as a point of reference. If a change in vision from the day before is noted, the client should reevaluate his or her vision in a few hours. If no improvement is noted or if vision is worse, the client should notify the physician. Because graft rejection may occur at any time (even years) after the surgery, advise the client to make the vision check a routine part of ADL for the rest of his or her life.

CORNEAL INFECTION: KERATITIS

The corneal epithelium is normally an effective barrier against microorganisms. Once it is compromised from disease or trauma, the underlying stromal layer becomes an excellent culture medium for a variety of organisms. Dry eyes or ineffective eyelid closure predisposes the eye to keratitis. Clients who have a systemic collagen disorder, such as rheumatoid arthritis, are particularly susceptible to corneal infections and ulceration.

The client's eyes tear more than usual because the cornea produces tears to reduce the irritation. Sensitivity to light is due to the irritated nerve endings in the cornea, and blurred vision results from the inability of the cornea to provide the proper refractive surface. Clients with a corneal defect from an infection experience a great deal of discomfort, which is worsened by eyelid movement. The eye appears infected and indurated. Fluorescein staining of the cornea outlines the affected area, which can be viewed through the slit lamp or with a hand-held flashlight.

Corneal infections may develop into ulcerations that severely compromise the integrity of the eye (Fig. 65–13). Sources of infection include bacteria (e.g., *Staphylococcus aureus, Pseudomonas aeruginosa, Streptococcus pneumoniae*), fungi *(Candida, Aspergillus)*, viruses (adenovirus, herpes simplex, herpes zoster), and protozoa *(Acanthamoeba)*. Clinical findings under slit-lamp examination are specific to particular organisms. Hypopyon (a layer of white cells in the anterior chamber) may accompany corneal ulceration.

Outcome Management

The goal of treatment is to eradicate the infection, prevent further injury to the cornea, and promote comfort and healing.

Medical Management

Topical antibiotic, antifungal, and antiviral therapy is prescribed, with the frequency of instillation based on the

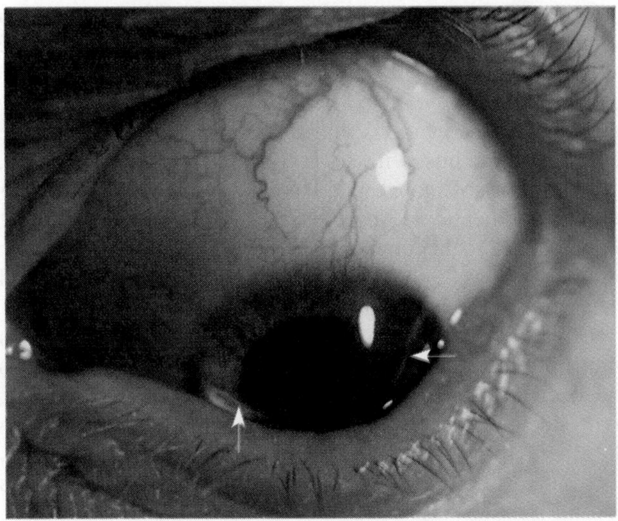

FIGURE 65–13 A corneal ulcer (*arrows*). (Courtesy of Ophthalmic Photography at the University of Michigan W. K. Kellogg Eye Center, Ann Arbor.)

severity of the infection to prevent progression to perforation and to promote healing. Maximal therapy includes the alternating instillation of two broad-spectrum eye drops every 15 minutes around the clock. As the infection begins to respond to the medication, frequency of administration is gradually decreased. Systemic IV medication may be prescribed as well.

To aid the healing process, surgical intervention may be necessary. *Tarsorrhaphy* (suturing the eyelid closed) promotes healing by decreasing eyelid blinking and by decreasing evaporation of the corneal tear film. For corneal perforation, a conjunctival flap may be performed to cover the defect. Tissue adhesive, a kind of "superglue," may also be used to seal the perforation. A soft contact lens may be used as a bandage to maintain the seal. Large perforations may require either lamellar (partial-thickness) or penetrating (full-thickness) keratoplasty.

When medical and surgical interventions fail, *enucleation* (removal of the entire eyeball) may be necessary (see nursing care of ocular melanoma). In some cases, *evisceration* (removal of orbital contents only) may be indicated. The scleral shell is left intact along with the ocular muscles, which allows for improved ocular prosthetic fit and function.

Nursing Management

Although the early stages of corneal infection are often managed at home, the client may need to be hospitalized for the management of a severe corneal ulcer. If the client and family have been instilling frequent eye drops at home, the client may be fatigued from lack of sleep as well as anxious about possible loss of vision. Assess the client's level of discomfort and methods of coping with the stress of pain and lack of sleep. Often at this stage, the client is not coping well at all. When eye drops are given every 15 minutes around the clock, the schedule is a challenge not only for the client but for you as well. Hand-washing is particularly important in this situation and is carried out even if gloves are worn to instill the drops. The threat of losing eyesight compels many clients to watch the clock for fear that you will forget to administer the eye drops. You can build the client's trust and reduce anxiety by scrupulous adherence to the time schedule.

The client's eye may need to be cleaned frequently because the medications and excessive tears will become dried and the lids will stick together. Warm tap water, applied with soft gauze pads, is used. The combination of tearing, medications, and cleaning may cause the skin of older clients to become excoriated. Antibiotic ophthalmic ointment may be applied to the lower lid margin and cheek to reduce irritation.

Effective sleep and rest are nearly impossible, with interruptions every 15 minutes. The client rarely reaches the deeper stages of sleep, and most experience restless, light sleep in stages 1 and 2. In addition to the eye pain the client may already be experiencing, some eye drops, such as fortified bacitracin, may cause stinging that lasts several minutes.

You can institute several measures to comfort the client. Outline a daily routine of care, based as much as possible on the client's normal routine at home. Because there are many interruptions to the client's personal time and space, identify at least two periods of time during the day when the client may rest or nap, with the only interruption being the nurse who comes in to administer the eye drops. Post a sign on the door to the client's room for privacy during these rest times. You and the client may also agree that you will not open topics of conversation during this time but will quietly instill the eye drops. Adopt this same routine during the client's normal nighttime. Some clients are actually able to sleep during instillation of eye drops at night; however, establish this routine with the client in advance. Older clients, who are accustomed to more stage 2 sleep than younger clients, are able to rest more effectively. Because younger clients tend to become confused and irritable more often, speak to the client before touching him or her. Oral analgesics are given at regular intervals, and mild sleeping medications may be helpful at bedtime.

Clients usually become adapted to this regimen of interruptions after the first 48 hours. As the cornea begins to show improvement, the eye drops may be reduced in frequency to every 30 minutes and then to every hour. Most clients do not notice a great deal of difference in the every-30-minute routine, but when the routine is reduced to every hour, they begin to sleep more heavily as the body attempts to compensate for lost sleep. At the end of an hour, the client may complain to you that it has seemed like only a few minutes since the last interruption. Intense dreaming may also be experienced during this time.

Self-Care

At discharge from the facility, the client should be able to demonstrate how to properly instill eye drops. The client will also understand the importance of complying with the medication regimen. Instruct the client and family about the clinical manifestations of increasing infections. The eye may continue to be cleaned with warm tap water at home. Assess the home environment if the client's vision is greatly reduced. Referrals for rehabilitation also may be necessary.

UVEAL TRACT DISORDERS: UVEITIS

Uveitis is an inflammation of the uveal tract that can affect one or more parts (iris, ciliary body, choroid). Uveitis commonly occurs in its acute form from a hypersensitivity reaction or in its chronic form following microbial infection. Clients complain of pain, blurred vision, and photophobia. There is marked redness of the eye, and the pupil is usually constricted. Cells (white blood cells) and flare (protein), called an "anterior chamber reaction," are seen in the anterior chamber fluid with the slit lamp.

The primary cause of discomfort in clients with uveitis is ciliary body muscle spasm. A cycloplegic medication such as atropine effectively relieves the spasm, and the dilation of the pupil prevents the inflamed iris from adhering to the lens and the corneal endothelium from forming synechiae. Topical steroid drops are prescribed to reduce the inflammation.

MALIGNANT OCULAR TUMORS

OCULAR MELANOMA

Although fewer than 1% of the people in the United States are affected by malignant ocular tumors, treatment of these tumors can be a challenge for both client and nurse. Choroidal melanomas are often detected during a routine ocular examination because there is no pain associated with the development of the tumor. By the time the tumor has grown large enough to obstruct vision, there may be involvement of the macula and metastasis.

Outcome Management

The goal of treatment is to care for the malignancy while preserving the eye.

Medical Management

When ocular melanoma is discovered early, radiation therapy alone may be the treatment of choice. Radiation therapy to the eye is accomplished through insertion of a tiny plate or plaque about the size of a dime that holds tiny seeds of radioactive iodine 125. The plaque is sutured to the sclera directly over the site of the tumor. It is left in place for several days, depending on the required dose, and then removed. Both insertion and removal are performed in the operating room.

During treatment, a lead shield is placed over the eye. Radiation exposure to the nurse who cares for the client is minimal—a small fraction of a chest x-ray study. Despite this extremely low exposure, the routine restrictions for hospital personnel and visitors are implemented for the sake of consistency. Hospitalization for treatment with radioactive iodine is required, depending on regulations.

During the client's hospitalization for this treatment, provide support and encouragement for the client. The plaque is only mildly to moderately uncomfortable, and discomfort should be relieved with acetaminophen. The difficult challenge for clients is confinement to their room with limitations on visitors at a time when support is essential. Eye medications include a cycloplegic agent and an antibiotic-steroid eye drop.

Surgical Management

ENUCLEATION

The goal of surgical removal is to preserve life by removing the tumor. Removal of the entire eyeball (enucleation) has been the traditional method of treatment and may be combined with radiation treatments. Exenteration (removal of the eyeball and surrounding tissues and bone) may also be necessary. The goal for clients following enucleation is adaptation to monocular vision and return to their former level of independence.

Enucleation surgery is usually performed with the client under general anesthesia, but IV conscious sedation may also be used. The ocular muscles are dissected from the eyeball, which is removed by severing the optic nerve and vessels at the back. An acrylic sphere covered by donor scleral tissue is usually placed within the capsule of tissue that formerly held the eyeball. Scleral tissue encourages fibrovascular ingrowth, which prevents migration and extrusion of the implant. A soft plastic scleral shell is placed in the visible outer portion of the socket as a support until a permanent prosthesis can be made. A newer type of implant, hydroxyapatite, which is made of the same inorganic material present in human bone, is now being used.

Several weeks later, a central hole is drilled into the sphere and covering tissues. A peg (which later fits into a depression on the posterior surface of the artificial eye) is then inserted into the hole. The movement of the implant by the muscle cone is transferred directly to the prosthesis. With the artificial eye being primarily supported by the peg instead of the lids and socket tissues, there are fewer cosmetic and structural complications.

Nursing Management

The client undergoing enucleation for a malignant tumor is stressed not only by the threat of cancer but also by disfigurement of the face. Assess the client's response, home, and family for support mechanisms. Nursing interventions are focused on assisting the client to grieve for the lost body part and lost vision and to identify coping mechanisms that will facilitate rehabilitation.

PREOPERATIVE CARE

Assist the client in preparing for the surgical procedure. Most often, the client is made aware of the tumor at a routine office visit. Surgery is usually scheduled within a few days. Recognizing that the client is most appropriately in a state of shock and denial, carefully explain the perioperative events. Although it is possible to have an enucleation as an outpatient procedure, the client may stay overnight in the hospital.

POSTOPERATIVE CARE

Provide routine postoperative care. The client returns from the operating room with a pressure dressing over the eye. Assess the dressing for bleeding using standard postoperative routines. Clients are understandably anxious about the removal of the dressing the next morning. Prepare the client by explaining how the eye and conformer will appear. The socket and lids will be swollen, and the white plastic conformer is visible. Determine the client's or family's ability to care for the wound postoperatively.

Some clients fear that their appearance will frighten others, especially children. In this case, an eye patch may be worn during the 4 to 6 weeks before the prosthesis is fitted but should not be worn continuously. Eventually, the eye prosthesis can be worn and looks pleasingly normal (Fig. 65–14). Refer to a fundamentals of nursing textbook for insertion and removal of the prosthesis.

The area around the lids may be cleaned with warm tap water with a clean washcloth. Soap and water should be kept away from the socket. If the plastic conformer accidentally comes out, it should be washed and replaced. Antibiotic ophthalmic ointment is usually ordered to be instilled in the socket once or twice a day.

Self-Care

Adjustment to monocular vision is a challenge the client begins to face immediately. Depth perception is altered, and the client needs to exercise caution in walking,

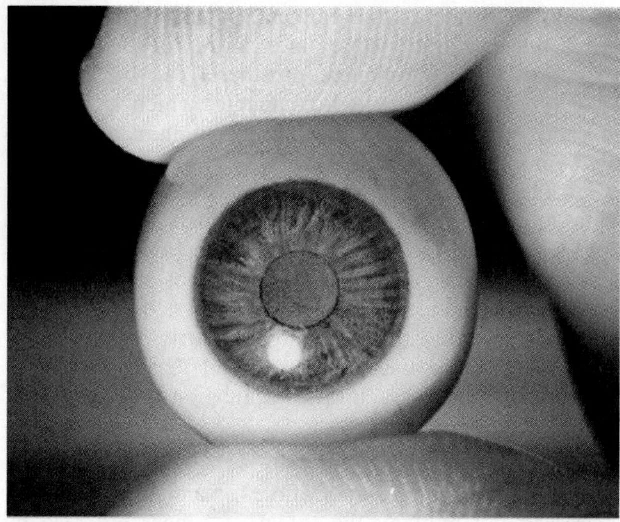

FIGURE 65–14 An ocular prosthesis. (Courtesy of Ophthalmic Photography at the University of Michigan W. K. Kellogg Eye Center, Ann Arbor.)

crossing streets, and driving. Advise the client to practice ADLs until visual and body adjustments are made.

Emphasize the need for extra precaution with the remaining eye. Eye protection should be worn when engaging in any activity that might even remotely result in an injury. Many clients are advised to wear glasses even if no correction is needed.

RETINOBLASTOMA

Retinoblastoma is a highly malignant intraocular tumor. The tumor occurs in two forms: sporadic (60%) and inherited (40%). The neoplasm arises from mutations in the primitive neuroectodermal tissue of the retina. It is a relatively rare form of cancer, occurring most often in children.

Clinical manifestations are difficult to detect early because they are not obvious. In children, parents usually notice a whitish appearance of the pupil *(cat's eye reflex)* and strabismus. Decreased vision, *proptosis* (protruding eye), and pain are late signs. Retinoblastomas grow rapidly along the optic nerve and invade the brain.

Treatment of mild or moderate forms of retinoblastoma includes radiation, photocoagulation, and cryotherapy to save vision. Eyes with extensive retinal destruction or glaucoma are enucleated (see later). Adults who have survived retinoblastoma are at increased risk for other malignancies, especially osteogenic sarcoma.

EYELID TUMORS

Basal cell and squamous cell carcinomas of the lids are the most common malignant tumors of the eyelids. These tumors appear more frequently in people with fair complexions who have had chronic exposure to the sun. Malignant lid tumors are most often (90% to 95%) of the basal cell type and frequently appear on the lower lid as nodules that gradually enlarge, becoming scaly and ulcerated. Benign tumors of the lids are very common and often increase in frequency as people age. Melanocytic nevi (moles) and verrucae (warts) commonly appear on the lids and lid margins. Xanthelasma appears as yellow, wrinkled patches, which are actually lipid deposits under the skin of the eyelids. These benign lesions may be removed for cosmetic reasons.

Malignant tumors may be removed and treated by various methods, such as electrodesiccation, cryotherapy, and surgery. When the tumor is large, reconstruction may be required.

EYELID, LACRIMAL, AND CONJUNCTIVAL DISORDERS

DRY EYE SYNDROME

Dry eye syndrome is a condition in which tear production is inadequate. It most commonly occurs in women between 50 and 60 years of age. Three primary causes are lacrimal gland malfunction, mucin deficiency, and mechanical abnormalities that prevent the spread of tears across the surface of the eye. The lacrimal gland can be genetically malformed or malformed because of injury or infection. Tear production is also decreased in Sjögren's syndrome, an autoimmune disorder that commonly accompanies rheumatoid arthritis. Facial nerve (seventh cranial nerve) palsy disrupts tear production. Conjunctivitis and mumps can obstruct the gland. Some medications, such as antihistamines, atropine, and beta-adrenergic blocking agents, decrease tear production.

Mucin, a substance produced by the goblet cells in the eyelid, maintains an even layer of tears across the surface of the eye. The absence of mucin allows the tear film to break up, leaving "dry spots" on the cornea. Mucin deficiency is seen in clients with vitamin A deficiency and those taking medications such as antihistamines and beta-adrenergic blocking agents.

Mechanical abnormalities include problems with eyelid structure, eyeball extrusion, and misuse of contact lenses.

Manifestations include burning, itching eyes and a sensation of "something" in the eye. The term *keratoconjunctivitis sicca* is used to describe the problem.

Management includes determining the degree of injury to the cornea. Artificial tears (eye drops and lubricants) can be used. In addition, some clients benefit from using airtight goggles at night to prevent tear evaporation. Postmenopausal women have found some relief from estrogen replacement. Surgery can be used to open the lacrimal duct or to repair lid problems.

Other eyelid, lacrimal, and conjunctival disorders are discussed in Table 65–2.

REFRACTIVE DISORDERS

Light is bent (refracted) as it passes through the cornea and lens of the eye. Refractive errors exist when light rays are not focused appropriately on the retina of the eye.

Three basic abnormalities of refraction occur in the eye: (1) myopia, (2) hyperopia, and (3) astigmatism. Optical correction is important to distinguish between visual loss caused by disease and visual loss caused by refractive error. *Refractometry* is the measurement of refractive error and should not be confused with *refraction,* the

TABLE 65–2 EYELID, LACRIMAL, AND CONJUNCTIVAL DISORDERS

Disorder	Definition	Appearance	Management
Dacryocystitis	Inflammation of lacrimal gland		Antibiotics, daily massage of the lacrimal system
Hordeolum (stye)	Infection of glands of eyelids	Redness and swelling of a localized area of the eyelid	Warm compresses and antibiotics; may need to be incised and drained
Chalazion	Chronic granuloma of meibomian gland	Painless, localized swelling of the lid margin	If cosmetically distracting, may be surgically removed
Blepharitis	Chronic, bilateral inflammation of eyelids	Itching and burning of the eyes, eyes appear red, scales noted on the lashes	Wash eyelids with baby shampoo, water, and cotton-tipped applicators; antibiotic ointments may be prescribed
Conjunctivitis	Inflammation of conjunctiva from various microorganisms	Redness, tearing, and exudation of eyelid; may progress to eyelid drooping, abnormal tissue growth	Antibiotic eye drops
Entropion	Turning in eyelid margin	Inversion of lower eyelid; dry and irritated eyes	Surgical resection
Ptosis	Drooping of eyelid from several causes	Irritation of eye caused by drying, loss of tears	Artificial tears; surgical correction needed; sometimes glasses used to life redundant skin
Lagophthalmos	Inadequate closure of eyelids	Irritation of eye caused by drying	Artificial tears, eye shields at night; surgical correction
Absence of blinking	Lack of blinking seen with Parkinson's disease and hyperthyroidism	Blinking less than 20 times a minute	Artificial tears; eye shields at night

method used to determine which lens or lenses (if any) will most benefit the client.

MYOPIA

Myopia, or *nearsightedness,* is a condition in which the light rays come into focus in front of the retina (Fig. 65–15*A*). In this case, the refractive power of the eye is too strong and a concave, or minus, lens is used to focus light rays on the eye. In most cases, myopia is caused by an eyeball that is longer than normal, which may be a familial trait. Transient myopia may occur with the administration of a variety of medications (sulfonamides, acetazolamide, salicylates, and steroids) and has been associated with other disorders, such as influenza, typhoid fever, severe dehydration, and large intakes of antacids (for stomach ulcers).

Correction is accomplished with eyeglasses or contact lenses.

HYPEROPIA

The hyperopic, or *farsighted,* eye is deficient in its ability to focus light rays. The focal point falls behind the eye, and, consequently, the image that falls on the retina is blurred (see Fig. 65–15*B*). Vision may be brought into focus by placing a convex, or plus, lens in front of the eye. The lens supplies the magnifying power that the eye is lacking. Hyperopia may be caused by an eyeball that is shorter than normal or a cornea that has less curvature than normal. Because children have a greater ability to

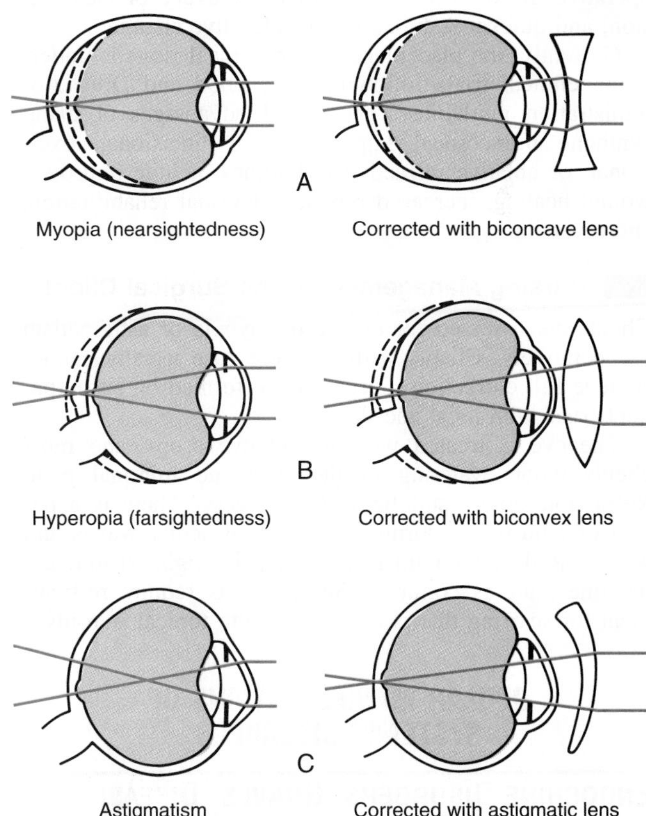

FIGURE 65–15 *A–C,* Common refractive disorders and their correction. *Dashed lines* in *A* and *B* indicate normal eye contour.

accommodate, they are less often affected than adults. Demands for close work and reading usually bring on manifestations of headache or eyestrain.

Correction is based on a person's age and individual needs and complaints.

ASTIGMATISM

Astigmatism is a refractive condition in which rays of light are not bent equally by the cornea in all directions, so that a point of focus is not attained (see Fig. 65–15*C*). In most instances, astigmatism is caused because the curvature of the cornea is not perfectly spherical. This is the cause of poor vision for both distant and near objects.

Astigmatism is corrected with cylindrical lenses.

Surgical Management

Several techniques and methods of surgical correction for myopia and hyperopia were developed in the 1990s. Short-wavelength, high-energy ultraviolet radiation lasers are being used to reshape the corneal surface. In photorefractive keratectomy (PRK) for myopia, the central cornea is flattened with the excimer laser. The same laser may be used to reshape the cornea by steepening the central curvature to correct hyperopia.

Laser in situ keratomileusis (LASIK) is a procedure in which an extremely thin layer of the cornea is peeled back for the laser reshaping on the middle layer of the cornea and then put back in place. Although the LASIK procedure is more difficult to perform, there is less postoperative discomfort, a more rapid recovery of clear vision, and quicker stabilization of refractive change.

Currently, the placement of intracorneal rings is undergoing clinical trials following U.S. Food and Drug Administration guidelines. Theoretical advantages of using synthetic intracorneal implants versus incisional, excisional, or ablative refractive techniques include improved wound healing, increased rapidity of visual rehabilitation, and reversibility.

Nursing Management of the Surgical Client

Clients are assessed for degree of myopia or astigmatism preoperatively. Clients with a severe case usually cannot achieve full correction. Surgery is performed on an outpatient basis with local anesthesia.

The eye is treated with steroid eye drops, and most clients report watering of the eyes and minimal pain. Refraction slowly stabilizes after surgery. There is a period of adjustment during which visual acuity waxes and wanes. Reduced contrast sensitivity in night vision and daytime glare is common. Some clients require re-treatment for scarring that is unresponsive to topical steroids.

OCULAR MANIFESTATIONS OF SYSTEMIC DISORDERS

ENDOCRINE DISORDERS: GRAVES' DISEASE

Graves' disease may exist with or without any clinical evidence of thyroid dysfunction. Ocular manifestations include retraction of both upper and lower lids, resulting in a staring or frightened expression (Stellwag's sign), and lid lag (Graefe's sign), the retarded lowering of the upper lid when looking down (Fig. 65–16). When the gaze is changed from down to up, the globe then lags behind the upper lid. Other signs are infrequent blinking, marked fine tremor with lid closure, and jerky movements on lid opening.

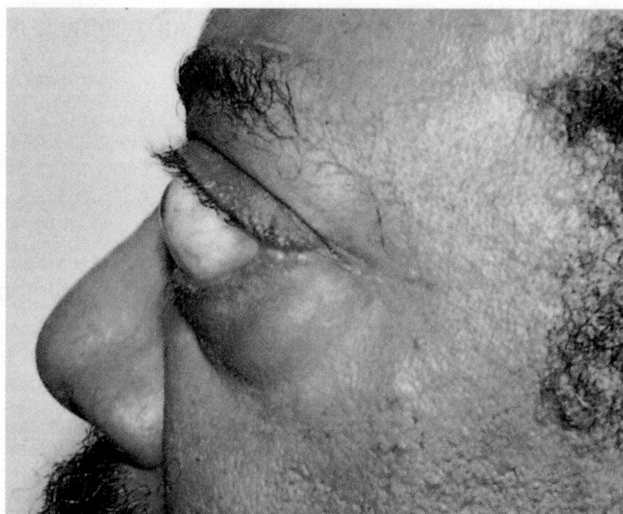

FIGURE 65–16 Graves' exophthalmos. (Courtesy of Ophthalmic Photography at the University of Michigan W. K. Kellogg Eye Center, Ann Arbor.)

The globes enlarge because of the increased size of extraocular muscles, edema of tissues, and excess orbital fat. The eye develops proptosis (forward protrusion of the eyeballs), which is called exophthalmos. Subsequent degeneration of muscle tissue leads to fibrosis, which restricts muscle movement, resulting in double vision.

Outcome Management

As a primary measure, adequate control of thyroid abnormalities is essential. Diuretics as well as steroid therapy and radiotherapy may be indicated.

Surgical interventions include corrective lid surgery and tarsorrhaphy for lid retraction to protect the cornea. Decompression of the orbit, which usually involves removal of the inferior and medial walls of the orbit, may be necessary to accommodate proliferative orbital fat and enlarged ocular muscles. Ocular muscle surgery may also be indicated.

The extent of the surgical procedure is likely to determine whether the client undergoing an orbital decompression requires a hospital stay. If the surgery is extensive, suction drains may be placed at the operative sites. Drainage is usually serosanguineous. It is important that the client sleep with the head elevated to reduce postoperative swelling.

Advise the client to expect redness, swelling, and ecchymoses around the eyes and lids. In the immediate postoperative period, check the client's visual acuity with a near vision card every hour to monitor the possibility of pressure on the optic nerve (see Thinking Critically). Caution the client to modify normal activities for the first 2 weeks after surgery.

Rheumatoid and Connective Tissue Disorders

Sjögren's syndrome includes keratoconjunctivitis sicca, a common condition in which tear secretion is reduced, in association with a systemic disorder such as rheumatoid arthritis, psoriatic arthritis, connective tissue disorders, sarcoidosis, or Crohn's disease. Manifestations include ocular irritation and foreign-body sensation. Frequent instillation of lubricating eye drops or ointment is effective in most cases.

Several ocular problems may be associated with systemic lupus erythematosus (SLE), a connective tissue disorder. The eyelids may be involved, with the discoid lesions characteristic of the disease. Punctate epithelial keratopathy and secondary Sjögren's syndrome may also occur. Retinopathy of SLE produces cotton-wool spots and increased retinal vessel fragility, as in diabetes. Optic neuropathy can also occur.

Neurologic Disorders

Approximately 90% of clients with myasthenia gravis have ocular involvement. In most cases, it is the presenting manifestation. *Ptosis* (drooping of the eyelid) is bilateral but may be asymmetrical. Diplopia is frequently in the vertical plane. Nystagmus is also present. Ocular myopathy and cranial nerve palsy may develop later, as may *ophthalmoplegia* (paralysis of all extraocular muscles). Medical treatment is supportive and includes systemic steroids.

There is also a close association between optic neuritis and multiple sclerosis. Approximately three fourths of women and one third of men with optic neuritis have multiple sclerosis at 15-year follow-up. Typically, an attack of optic neuritis starts with acute onset of loss of vision in one eye, with periocular discomfort made worse by movement of the eye. Visual impairment is progressive over 2 weeks and usually resolves after 4 to 6 weeks. Recovery may take longer and may be incomplete. Medical treatment consists of oral, IV, and retrobulbar steroids.

Circulatory Disorders

The primary response of retinal arterioles to hypertension is a narrowing. In clients with chronic hypertension, the blood-retina barrier is disrupted in small areas, resulting in increased vascular permeability. Funduscopic examination reveals vasoconstriction, leakage, and arteriosclerosis. Hypertensive retinopathy is graded for severity on a scale of 1 to 4, with 4 the most severe. Systemic hypertension is also associated with an increased risk of retinal vein occlusion. There is no known treatment for retinal vein occlusion.

Immunologic Disorders

Ocular complications affect approximately 75% of clients with acquired immunodeficiency syndrome (AIDS). In many cases, it is the presenting ocular manifestations that may lead to diagnosis of human immunodeficiency virus (HIV) infection. Cytomegalovirus (CMV) *retinitis* is the most common opportunistic ocular infection. This sight-threatening condition occurs in 30% of clients with AIDS. It is often asymptomatic until it is well established, when the client begins to notice visual field loss, "floaters," or other vague vision problems. A unilateral lesion with the appearance of a cotton-wool spot often develops with white irregular borders associated with hemorrhages. Small lesions may be seen beyond the edges. The retina in the center of the lesion becomes thin and tears easily. Loss of vision is involved and central vision is greatly diminished.

Clients with CMV retinitis require IV therapy, usually through placement of a long-term indwelling catheter. Ganciclovir or foscarnet sodium is administered over several weeks in the hospital or through home care. Because progression is rapid, early treatment is essential and may prevent involvement of the other eye. Careful monitoring of side effects and response to the medication is imperative.

Other infectious ocular conditions that may occur in people with HIV disease are bacterial corneal ulcers (syphilis, staphylococcosis), fungal corneal ulcers (candidiasis, cryptococcosis, histoplasmosis, sporotrichosis), and protozoan (toxoplasmosis, pneumocystosis) and viral infections (herpes simplex).

Noninfectious ocular manifestations in people with HIV infection include HIV retinopathy and neoplastic processes such as Kaposi's sarcoma and non-Hodgkin's lymphoma, which appear around the ocular adnexa. AIDS retinopathy is seen in more than 50% of clients with HIV infection. Direct ophthalmoscopy reveals the presence of cotton-wool spots, retinal hemorrhages, and other microvascular anomalies. The lesions of AIDS retinopathy are indistinguishable from the retinopathy of diabetes or hypertension. They usually occur in the superficial retina and resolve over a period of a few weeks, whereas CMV retinitis lesions will expand. Kaposi's sarcoma and non-Hodgkin's lymphoma present around the eyelids and orbit with diplopia, ptosis, conjunctival edema, or hemorrhage. Diagnosis is confirmed with imaging, needle biopsy, and systemic work-up. Treatment of Kaposi's sarcoma is usually conservative and may include radiotherapy.

Evaluation of extraocular muscle function is important because lymphoma may increase intracranial pressure, which may lead to cranial nerve palsies and altered eye position. Surgical correction of extraocular muscle positioning may be necessary for resolving diplopia or for cosmetic reasons.

Lyme Disease

Lyme disease *(Borrelia burgdorferi),* transmitted by the bite of a tick, consists of three stages. The initial stage involves a lesion and erythema around the bite, accompanied by regional lymphadenopathy, malaise, fever, headache, myalgia, arthralgia, and frequently conjunctivitis. Several weeks to months later, the second phase is associated with neurologic and cardiac problems. Along with these problems, there may be cranial nerve palsies, uveitis, optic neuropathy, keratitis, choroiditis, and exudative retinal detachments. Rheumatologic complications may develop in the third stage, which may occur over several years. Tetracycline and penicillin are effective in treating the initial infection and in preventing late complications.

CONCLUSIONS

To provide comprehensive nursing care for clients, it is essential to understand the complexity of ocular structures and the physiology of vision. The specialty practice of ophthalmic nursing is devoted to caring for clients with eye disorders. Ophthalmic Registered Nurses perform the roles of caregiver, advocate, educator, counselor, technician, coordinator, and researcher. Ophthalmic nursing care not only is directed at those biologic systems that are affected by an actual or potential deficit but also is an integration of how actual or potential visual deficits affect the individual as an entire being.

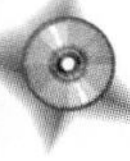

THINKING CRITICALLY

1. **Your client is a 72-year-old retired carpenter who has undergone outpatient cataract surgery. He and his wife live an hour away from the surgery center, where they received instructions to call the emergency number if any unusual pain or nausea. They have an appointment to return for a follow-up evaluation the next morning. After supper, the client's wife calls to report that her husband has a headache. She says that her husband also has an upset stomach, but she thinks he feels queasy because he ate some spicy food. The client does not want his wife to drive him back at night and thinks she should not have bothered to call because they have an appointment in the morning. How would you proceed? What further assessment data are needed? What are the likely complications following cataract surgery, and what are their clinical manifestations?**

Factors to Consider. Might the headache and upset stomach be related to the cataract surgery, or are they likely to be unrelated?

2. **Your client, a 55-year-old woman with Graves' ophthalmopathy, has undergone surgery in the late afternoon today for a right orbital decompression. An incisional drain is in place at the right temple with a bulb attached for suction. The surgeon has ordered postoperative vision checks with a near vision card every hour throughout the night. The surgery lasted more than 3 hours; general anesthesia was used, and the client is still sedated. Her right eye is extremely swollen; she is unable to open it to read the vision card. She winces and cries when her operative eye is touched, and she is so sleepy that she cannot respond by reading the vision card. What should you do to carry out the surgeon's postoperative orders?**

Factors to Consider. Are such severe eye pain and swelling normal postoperative findings? How would you assess the eye? How would you rouse the client to perform these crucial eye assessments?

BIBLIOGRAPHY

1. Allen, P., & Shepherd, J. (1998). The ophthalmic registered nurse's responsibility to the adult patient with low vision. *Insight, 23*(2), 53.
2. Benson, W., & Lanier, J. (1998). Current diagnosis and treatment of corneal ulcers. *Current Opinion in Ophthalmology, 9*(4), 45.
3. Burris, T. (1998). Intrastomal corneal ring technology: Results and indications. *Current Opinion in Ophthalmology, 9*(4), 9.
4. D'Ambrosio, F. (1999). Assessing disability in the patient with cataracts. *Current Opinion in Ophthalmology, 10*(1), 42.
5. Dolphin, K. (1998). Complications of postenucleation/evisceration implants. *Current Opinion in Ophthalmology, 9*(5), 75.
6. Eagle, R. (1999). *Eye pathology: An atlas and basic text.* Philadelphia: W. B. Saunders.
7. Emery, J. (1999). Capsular opacification after cataract surgery. *Current Opinion in Ophthalmology, 10*(1), 42.
8. Fishbaugh, J. (1995). Look who's driving now? Visual standards for driver's licensing in the United States. *Insight, 20*(4), 11–20
9. Gills, J., Loyd, T., & Cherchio, M. (1995). Anesthesia, preoperative, and postoperative medications. *Current Opinion in Ophthalmology, 6,* 31–35.
10. Gimbel, H., & Levy, S. (1998). Indications, results, and complications of LASIK. *Current Opinion in Ophthalmology, 9*(4), 3.
11. Goldblum, K. (Ed.). (1997). *Ophthalmic nursing core curriculum.* Dubuque, IA: Kendall Publishing.
12. Gramer, E., & Tausch, M. (1995). The risk profile of the glaucomatous patient. *Current Opinion in Ophthalmology, 6,* 78–88.
13. Grehn, F. (1995). The value of trabeculotomy in glaucoma surgery. *Current Opinion in Ophthalmology, 6,* 52–60.
14. Harding, J. (1995). Epidemiology, pathophysiology, and world blindness. *Current Opinion in Ophthalmology, 6,* 27–30.
15. Haller, J. (1998). Retinal detachment. *Focal Points, 16*(5), 1–14.
16. Kanski, J. (1999). *Clinical ophthalmology* (4th ed.). Oxford: Butterworth Heinemann.
17. L'Esperance, F. (1998). Choosing the appropriate photorefractive keratoplasty patient. *Focal Points, 16*(9), 1–14.
18. Miller, N., & Newman, N. (1999). *Clinical neuro-ophthalmology: The essentials* (5th ed.). Baltimore: Williams & Wilkins.
19. O'Brart, D. (1999). The status of hyperopic LASIK. *Current Opinion in Ophthalmology, 10*(4), 247.
20. O'Day, B. (1999). Employment barriers for people with visual impairments. *Journal of Visual Impairment and Blindness, 93*(10), 627–642.
21. Pieramici, D., & Bressler, S. (1998). Age-related macular degeneration and risk factors for the development of choroidal neovascularization in the fellow eye. *Current Opinion in Ophthalmology,* 38.
22. Recchia, F., Conolly, B., & Benson, W. (1998). Ocular manifestations of diabetes. *Current Opinion of Ophthalmology, 9*(6), 64.
23. Rowen, S. (1999). Preoperative and postoperative medications used for cataract surgery. *Current Opinion in Ophthalmology, 10*(1), 29.
24. Schubert, H. (1998). Ocular manifestations of systemic hypertension. *Current Opinion in Ophthalmology, 9*(6), 93.
25. Shields, J., & Shields, C. (1999). *Atlas of eyelid and conjunctival tumors.* Philadelphia: Lippincott–Williams & Wilkins.
26. Smith, S. (1999). Non-proliferative diabetic retinopathy and macular edema. *Insight, 24*(2), 59–64.
27. Sperber, L., & Dodick, J. (1995). Laser therapy in cataract surgery. *Current Opinion in Ophthalmology, 6,* 22–26.
28. Stewart, W. (1995). The effect of lifestyle on the relative risk to develop open-angle glaucoma. *Current Opinion in Ophthalmology, 6,* 3–9.
29. Stewart, W. (1999). Perspectives in the medical treatment of glaucoma. *Current Opinion in Ophthalmology, 10*(2), 99.
30. Trobe, J. (1993). *The physician's guide to eye care.* San Francisco: American Academy of Ophthalmology.
31. Vader, L. (1996). The significance of cultural values in vision loss. *ABNF Journal, 1*(3), 69–71.
32. Vader, L. (2000). Ophthalmic nursing. In N. Burden (Ed.), *Ambulatory surgery nursing.* Philadelphia: W. B. Saunders.
33. Vaughan, D., Asbury, T., & Riordan-Eva, P. (1995). *General ophthalmology* (14th ed.). Norwalk, CT: Appleton & Lange.
34. Wason, B., & McMillan, J. (1998). *Macular degeneration.* Berkeley, CA: Hunter House Publishers.
35. Whitaker, R., & Whitaker, V. (1999). Glaucoma: What the ophthalmic nurse should know. *Insight, 24*(3), 86.

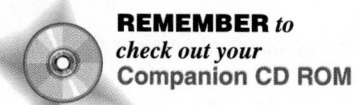

CHAPTER 66

Management of Clients with Hearing and Balance Disorders

Helene J. Krouse

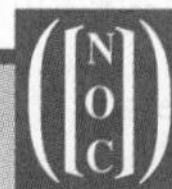

NURSING OUTCOMES CLASSIFICATION (NOC)
for Nursing Diagnoses—Clients with Hearing and Balance Disorders

Nausea
Comfort Level
Hydration
Nutritional Status: Food and Fluid Intake
Symptom Severity

Impaired Adjustment
Acceptance: Health Status
Psychosocial Adjustment: Life Change
Self Esteem

Impaired Social Interaction
Communication Ability
Social Interaction Skills

Impaired Verbal Communication
Communication Ability
Communication: Expressive Ability
Communication: Receptive Ability

Ineffective Denial
Psychosocial Adjustment: Life Change

Ineffective Individual Coping
Caregiver Stressors
Coping
Quality of Life
Role Performance

Risk for Injury
Risk Control: Hearing Impairment
Safety Behavior: Fall Prevention

Risk for Loneliness
Family Coping
Loneliness
Social Involvement

Social Isolation
Social Interaction Skills
Well-being

Hearing Impairment

Hearing impairment ranges from minor difficulty in understanding words or hearing certain sounds to total deafness. Hearing impairment is the nation's primary disability: one in 15 Americans is affected. By the year 2050, approximately one in five clients in the United States will be 55 years or older; of these estimated 58 million people, 26 million are expected to have hearing impairment. Of the 10 million people in the United States with a hearing loss who are now 65 years or older, more than 90% have a sensorineural hearing loss. Because of fear, misinformation, lack of information, and vanity, many clients do not admit that they have a hearing problem. Up to 80% of all hearing impairments are caused by hearing nerve disorders, for which no cure is currently available. Hearing impairments diminish the quality of life for a third of adults between 65 and 75 years of age.

Etiology and Risk Factors

Many factors influence the type and amount of hearing loss. Hearing loss is not an actual disorder but is a clinical manifestation of many possible problems. Both common and uncommon causes of hearing impairment are examined in this chapter. Hearing loss can be classified into three main areas:

- Conductive hearing loss (i.e., otosclerosis, trauma)
- Sensorineural hearing loss (i.e., presbycusis, noise-induced, and sudden hearing loss)
- Mixed hearing loss

Conductive hearing loss results from interference of sound transmission through the external ear and middle ear. It may be caused by (1) anything that blocks the external ear, such as wax, infection, or a foreign body, (2) thickening, retraction, scarring, or perforation of the tympanic membrane, or (3) any pathophysiologic changes in the middle ear that affect or freeze one or more of the ossicles.

Sensorineural hearing loss is caused by impairment of the function of the inner ear, the eighth cranial nerve, or the brain. Causes are congenital and hereditary factors, noise injury, aging and degenerative processes, Ménière's disease, and ototoxicity. Systemic disorders, such as autoimmune disease, syphilis, certain collagen disorders, and diabetes, may cause sensorineural hearing losses. Most recently, cigarette smoking and exposure to environmental tobacco smoke have been associated with age-related hearing loss.

In a *mixed hearing loss*, both conductive and sensorineural hearing components are present simultaneously. A client with a perforated eardrum and presbycusis has both conductive and sensorineural hearing losses.

CONDUCTIVE HEARING LOSS

Ear Obstructions

Obstruction of the ear is most commonly caused by impacted cerumen. Although the ear canal is self-cleaning, cerumen may become impacted from a disorder or from improper cleaning. The elderly are more susceptible to cerumen impaction because hair in the ear becomes coarser with age and traps the wax. Some people produce more cerumen in the ear canal and require a regular routine for eliminating excessive buildup of wax in the ear canal. Insertion of cotton-tipped swabs into the ear canal can create further impaction of ear wax or can even traumatize the ear canal or perforate the eardrum.

Ear obstruction can also be caused by a wide array of foreign bodies that fit into the ear canal and impede conduction of sound waves. The most common foreign bodies found in the adult ear are pieces of cotton and insects. Foreign bodies commonly seen in children consist of small toys, beads, insects, and food, such as kernels of corn. Teach clients to avoid inserting hard instruments into the ear and to avoid obstructing the ear canal with objects.

Infection

Many infections can lead to hearing loss. An infection of the inner ear, called *labyrinthitis,* can be either viral or bacterial in origin. Viral labyrinthitis can be associated with recent respiratory tract infections, measles, mumps, or rubella. Bacterial labyrinthitis, which is rare, is associated with otitis media or meningitis. Otitis media is a common disorder of the middle ear. Repeated infections or allergic inflammation can lead to fluid accumulation behind the eardrum, causing dampening of the sound being conducted to the inner ear. In addition, drainage, perforation, or scarring of the tympanic membrane can result in a conductive hearing loss. Otitis media and other infectious ear processes are discussed later in the chapter, under the heading Otalgia.

Otosclerosis

Otosclerosis, or hardening of the inner ear, is a genetic disorder in which repeated resorption and redeposition of abnormal bone gradually leads to fixation of the footplate of the stapes in the oval window (Fig. 66–1*A*). The immobility of the footplate prevents transmission of sound vibration into the inner ear, leading to conductive hearing loss. This disorder occurs twice as often in women and is ten times more prevalent in whites. The disorder is autosomally dominant with variable penetrance and, therefore, can be transmitted to offspring if only one parent has the disorder.

Tympanosclerosis

Tympanosclerosis is the result of repeated infection and trauma to the tympanic membrane. It consists of a deposit of collagen and calcium within the middle ear that can harden around the ossicles, causing a conductive hearing loss. Tympanosclerotic deposits can also be found mounded in the middle ear or as plaque on the tympanic membrane.

Trauma to the Tympanic Membrane

The tympanic membrane can be damaged by trauma. Increased pressure from a hand slap, falling in water, sports injuries, cleaning the ear with a sharp instrument, and industrial accidents involving welding sparks can rupture the thin membrane. Trauma to the tympanic membrane from a blast or blunt injury can involve the middle ear, causing a fracture or dislocation of the ossicles and tearing of the tympanic membrane. Also, the facial nerve is vulnerable to trauma. A basilar skull fracture involves the temporal bone and, depending on the fracture site, causes ossicular damage as well as facial nerve paralysis and sensorineural hearing loss. Care of clients with facial fracture is discussed in Chapter 49. When the tympanic membrane is perforated, infection is a concern.

SENSORINEURAL HEARING LOSS

Presbycusis

Presbycusis is a progressive hearing loss found predominantly in the elderly. This degenerative process involves changes in the labyrinthine structures over time. The client initially experiences a decrease in high-frequency sound. At times, *tinnitus,* or the perception of noise in the ear, accompanies this decline in hearing.

Sudden Hearing Loss

Sudden (idiopathic) hearing loss (SHL) is a fairly common condition in which the client loses hearing in an ear

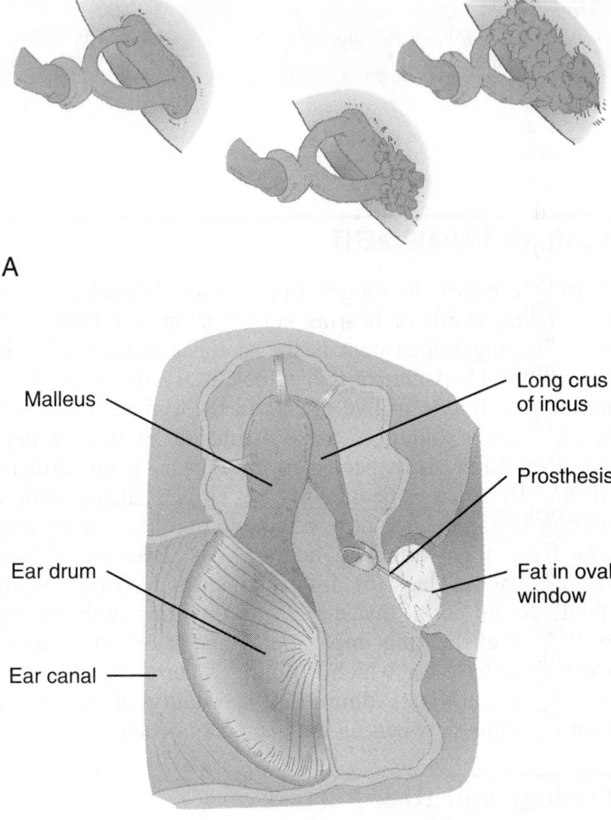

FIGURE 66–1 *A*, Stapedial otosclerosis. The immovable footplate prevents sound transmission. *B*, Stapedectomy.

within minutes or hours. This condition is almost exclusively unilateral. Although the exact cause of sudden sensorineural hearing loss has not been determined, postmortem examinations of temporal bones suggest that the disease involves a viral infection of the inner ear. Prompt early intervention with oral corticosteroids has been shown to at least partially restore the lost hearing in many patients with sudden hearing loss. In the United States alone, approximately 4000 new cases of sudden hearing loss are reported annually.

Sensorineural hearing loss of abrupt onset can sometimes occur from discrete causes. Some of these specific causes are (1) rapid infectious processes, such as meningitis or mumps, (2) ototoxic agents, (3) trauma, (4) metabolic disturbances, and (5) immunologic disorders. In most cases of SHL, however, no specific cause is found.

Congenital Hearing Loss

Congenital episodes of sensorineural hearing loss are not uncommon. These losses can be severe and present at the time of birth or can develop during childhood or early adulthood and gradually worsen with time. Congenital hearing loss often results in total deafness. It can occur either in a genetic pattern within families or spontaneously. Both autosomal recessive and autosomal dominant methods of transmission have been documented. In milder cases of congenital hearing loss, the individual may not be aware of a loss until hearing is screened for work or school. In families with a history of congenital hearing loss, infant screening is essential to allow early detection of the problem and rehabilitation of congenitally deaf infants.

Noise-Induced Hearing Loss

Noise-induced hearing loss is a specific type of sensorineural hearing loss that most often occurs over time from repeated acoustic trauma from loud noise. The major causes are industrial noise, use of firearms, and listening to loud music. Traumatic injury associated with a sudden loud noise, such as a blast, can also result in noise-induced hearing loss.

Benign and Malignant Tumors

Both benign and malignant tumors of the temporal bone can involve the inner ear and lead to sensorineural hearing loss. The most common benign tumor is an acoustic neuroma or schwannoma of the eighth cranial nerve. The tumor usually develops in the internal auditory canal, the bony channel through which the vestibular nerve passes as it leaves the inner ear. The tumor presses on the nerve, which then sends false signals to the brain. If the vestibular portion of the nerve is compressed, the client is unable to interpret stimuli about position and movement. If the cochlear branch is compressed, the client experiences tinnitus. The first clinical manifestation is often partial or complete sensorineural hearing loss followed by tinnitus. The client may also report dizziness.

Other tumors in the cerebellopontine angle likewise involve the seventh and eighth cranial nerves as they enter the internal acoustic meatus. Malignant tumors invade the entire inner ear, usually spreading from the middle ear and mastoid system.

Meniéré's Disease

Ménière's disease is a disorder that affects both vestibular and auditory function. It is caused by excess endolymph (clear intracellular fluid in the membranous labyrinth of the inner ear) in the vestibular and semicircular canals. Hearing loss is fluctuant, and usually subtle and reversible in the early stages. Later, the hearing loss becomes permanent. Although Ménière's disease is associated with sensorineural hearing loss, the most prominent clinical manifestation is vertigo (feeling that the surroundings or one's own body is revolving). Therefore, it is fully discussed in the section Balance Disorders.

Central Auditory Dysfunction

Central auditory dysfunction is a phenomenon whereby the central nervous system (CNS) cannot interpret normal auditory signals. Central auditory dysfunction, also known as central deafness, is a rare form of sensorineural hearing loss. Diseases that alter the CNS, such as cerebrovascular accidents and tumors, can cause central deafness.

MIXED HEARING LOSS

Some causes of hearing impairment can result in both sensorineural and conductive hearing losses. These types of losses are referred to as *mixed hearing loss.* Clients with mixed hearing loss present with clinical manifestations associated with both sensorineural and conductive hearing losses.

Prevention and Screening

A major nursing responsibility is the identification of hearing impairment in clients in both hospital and community settings. The different types of hearing loss are listed in Box 66–1. Identification of clients at risk for hearing loss and adequate protection of the ears are important to maintain normal function. The American

BOX 66–1 Types of Hearing Loss

Air conduction hearing loss: Loss of hearing through the external and middle ear.
Bone conduction hearing loss: Loss of hearing through the inner ear.
Central hearing loss: Loss of hearing from damage to the brain's auditory pathways or auditory center.
Conductive hearing loss: Loss of hearing in which air conduction is worse than bone conduction and involves the external and middle ear.
Fluctuating hearing loss: A sensorineural hearing loss that varies with time.
Functional hearing loss: Loss of hearing for which no organic lesion can be found.
Mixed hearing loss: Both sensorineural and conductive hearing loss.
Neural hearing loss: A sensorineural hearing loss originating in the eighth cranial nerve or brain stem.
Sensorineural hearing loss: Loss of hearing involving the cochlea and hearing nerve; bone and air conduction equal but diminished.
Sensory hearing loss: A sensorineural hearing loss in the cochlea and involving the hair cells and nerve endings.
Sudden hearing loss: A sensorineural hearing loss with a sudden onset.

Conductive hearing loss results from interference with conduction in the external and middle ear; sensorineural hearing loss in the inner ear; and mixed hearing loss in all three areas.

Speech-Language-Hearing Association (ASHA) has recommended specific guidelines for annual hearing screenings for children 3 to 10 years old who are at risk for hearing impairment.

Primary prevention is aimed at minimizing the risks from trauma, noise exposure, use of ototoxic drugs, and infectious diseases, such as meningitis, mumps, and measles. To reduce the risk of head trauma, young clients should be instructed to wear protective headgear or helmets when participating in sports. People should avoid insertion of hard instruments or objects into the ear canal to prevent obstruction, trauma, or perforation. Individuals in occupations with high noise exposure should be instructed to wear earplugs and to avoid prolonged exposure. Exposure to noise levels in excess of 80 decibels (dB) throughout an 8-hour day is considered excessive and should be avoided. In addition, teenagers need to be aware that listening to extremely loud music in enclosed spaces, such as cars, can contribute to hearing loss.

Secondary prevention involves early detection of hearing impairment through screening and referral of any ear problems. Hearing screenings are important to detect hearing impairment in children that can be related to congenital, infectious, or allergic processes. Hearing tests and ear examinations should be performed in clients 65 years and older and in people experiencing hearing difficulties. When administering drugs with ototoxic side effects, monitor clients for vertigo, lessened hearing acuity, and tinnitus. If any of these manifestations occurs, the client or nurse must stop the ototoxic medication and promptly notify the physician.

Tertiary prevention focuses on maintenance of optimal function through hearing rehabilitation programs, proper use and care of hearing aids, and implementation of coping and communication strategies.

Pathophysiology

Conductive hearing loss is the result of interference of sound transmission into and through the external ear and middle ear. The inner ear is not affected in a pure conductive loss; therefore, sound transmission from the inner ear to the brain is normal. Normal movement of sound vibrations through the ear canal, tympanic membrane, or ossicles is impeded because of the nature of the disease process involved in the conductive loss. Sound is perceived as faint or distant, but it remains relatively clear. Most conductive hearing losses are correctable by medical or surgical treatment.

Sensorineural hearing loss, however, results from disease or trauma to the organ of Corti or auditory nerve pathways of the inner ear leading to the brain stem. Normal reception and transmission of sound waves is disrupted. Sound is distorted and faint. Sensorineural hearing losses are usually permanent and are generally not correctable by medical or surgical treatment.

Clinical Manifestations

Most hearing loss is gradual and goes unnoticed by the client until several incidents of communication problems have occurred. Significant others and co-workers are usually aware of the client's hearing problem long before the client realizes or admits to the problem. However, a small loss of hearing goes unnoticed and does not cause manifestations. Health care providers should be alert for the following manifestations of hearing loss in a client:

- Failure to respond to oral communication
- Inappropriate response to oral communication
- Excessively loud speech
- Abnormal awareness of sounds
- Strained facial expressions
- Tilting of head when listening
- Constant need for clarification of conversation
- Faulty speech articulation
- Listening to radio and television at increased volume

The hearing impaired, or "hard-of-hearing" client may repeat the information, even incorrectly, or may ask for clarification. Clients with a hearing loss can also experience distorted or abnormal sounds. Sometimes a sound is heard at different pitches for each ear; this is called *diplacusis*. A sound may cause a rapid increase in loudness; this is called *recruitment*. These abnormal sounds can cause discomfort.

The onset of a conductive hearing loss can be sudden or progressive. In cases of fluid in the middle ear, hearing loss is often bilateral but is usually restored with medical or surgical treatment. In other conductive processes, such as otosclerosis, clinical manifestations consist of slow progressive hearing loss with changes noted even in adolescence. Hearing loss is usually bilateral but may be asymmetrical. Other manifestations are mild tinnitus, recurrent vertigo, and postural imbalance. It is common for the client to speak in a very soft voice.

If damage to the tympanic membrane is suspected, such as perforation, examination of the client may reveal a conductive hearing loss and serous drainage in the ear canal. The hearing loss found with a total perforation of the eardrum is approximately 35 dB (one third of the hearing range). With small perforations, no loss may be present. If a perforation is present, damage to the ossicles should be suspected. Diagnostic findings of conductive hearing loss include greater bone conduction than air conduction on Rinne's test. If hearing loss is greater in one ear, Weber's test shows lateralization to the more affected ear. Pure tone audiometry confirms hearing loss. *Speech discrimination* (understanding of words) is usually maintained.

Noise-induced hearing loss is characterized by a greater loss in the higher frequencies. Sudden or fluctuating hearing losses are recognized as separate disorders from routine sensorineural hearing loss. Although fluctuating losses usually suggest syphilis or Ménière's disease, sudden sensorineural hearing losses are believed to be viral in origin. Recognition of these patterns is important because medical treatment of such disorders can result in significant improvements in hearing.

A characteristic of a severe hearing loss is the loss of discrimination. To some clients, a hearing loss feels like a blockage or fullness in the ear or an inability to distinguish the direction of sounds.

Tinnitus accompanies most sensorineural hearing losses and is very annoying. Tinnitus literally means "ringing" but can actually sound like roaring, the chirping of crickets, or, occasionally, music. Tinnitus is not a disease but a very distressing manifestation, and it is sometimes a warning sign of hearing loss or other, more serious problems. Ear noise that cannot be heard by an observer is classified as *subjective tinnitus*, which is the most common kind. Any ear noise that can be heard by someone other than the client is called *objective tinnitus*. In some clients, the tinnitus becomes the problem, and the underlying cause may be forgotten.

The major nursing responsibility in a client with tinnitus is to perform a thorough history and assessment of the onset, frequency, constancy, and level of intensity of the tinnitus. Unilateral tinnitus merits a complete neuro-otologic evaluation with the goal of ruling out the possibility of a tumor, most likely an acoustic neuroma. The nurse must keep in mind that tinnitus is a manifestation of an underlying pathologic process that warrants further referral.

Table 66–1 presents clinical manifestations of conductive and sensorineural hearing losses. Diagnostic measures include (1) testing for hearing of pure tones on audiometry, (2) speech reception and discrimination, (3) tympanometry, and, (4) sometimes, brain stem auditory evoked responses. Tones are presented using earphones (air conduction) and vibrators (bone conduction). The minimal level at which the client can hear is determined. The *speech reception threshold* is the lowest intensity at which the client can correctly repeat 50% of the words presented. The speech discrimination test is a measure of the client's ability to understand speech when it is presented at a volume that is easily heard.

Outcome Management

Medical Management

The goals for medical management of the client with hearing impairment are (1) to restore hearing loss, (2) to assist hearing, (3) to manage tinnitus, and (4) to implement aural rehabilitation.

Restore Hearing Loss

Hearing loss that results from blockage or fullness in the ear associated with an infectious process may be restored to normal with administration of antibiotics for bacterial infections or acyclovir and oral corticosteroids for herpesvirus infections. In the case of sudden hearing loss, prompt administration of oral corticosteroids is used in an attempt to lessen the progressive hearing loss or to reverse a sudden loss. If ototoxicity is suspected, the administration of all ototoxic medications is discontinued. Most sensorineural hearing loss cannot be reversed with medical or surgical intervention. Conductive hearing loss, in contrast, is often amenable to surgical correction.

Assist Hearing

Unfortunately, most hearing losses are permanent, and hearing cannot be restored. The use of hearing aids and assistive listening devices can greatly improve the client's ability to communicate and interact with others.

Hearing aids amplify sound in a controlled manner. They are used by both *hearing-impaired* clients (those with slight or moderate hearing loss) and *deaf* clients (those with severe or profound hearing loss). Hearing aids make sound louder but do not improve the quality of sound. Therefore, clients with decreased discrimination benefit less from a hearing aid. The hearing aid amplifies all background noises, such as hospital machinery, background conversation in restaurants, footsteps, and department store noises, as well as speech. These noises may mask conversation or confuse the hearing-impaired client, especially one who is elderly.

A client should undergo a trial period before purchasing a hearing aid to see whether he or she can adapt to its use. In fact, in most states, such a trial period is mandatory. Bilateral (binaural) aids may be desirable.

Several types of hearing aids are available, and they vary according to size and location. Hearing aids can be worn in the following locations:

- In the ear
- In the ear canal
- Behind the ear (postauricular)
- In eyeglasses
- In the middle of the chest (body-worn aid)

Regardless of type, the hearing aid consists of four parts:

1. Microphone to receive sound waves from the air and change sounds into electrical signals.
2. Amplifier to increase the strength of electrical signals.
3. Receiver (loudspeaker) to change the electrical signals into sound waves.
4. Battery to provide the electrical energy needed to operate the hearing aid.

On all types of hearing aids but the body-worn type, all four components are housed in one small case. The louder sounds are then directed into the ear through a custom-molded earpiece (Fig. 66–2).

The evolution in hearing aid design has led to smaller and more effective aids. Small hearing aids are available

TABLE 66–1 CLINICAL MANIFESTATIONS OF CONDUCTIVE AND SENSORINEURAL HEARING LOSSES

	Conductive Hearing Loss	Sensorineural Hearing Loss
Voice quality	Soft voice	Loud voice
Effect of environmental noise on hearing	Hearing improved	Hearing made worse
Speech discrimination	Good	Poor
Ability to hear on telephone	Good	Poor
Lateralization on Weber's test	To diseased ear	To normal ear
Result of Rinne's test	Negative, AC<BC	Positive, AC>BC

AC, air conduction; BC, bone conduction.

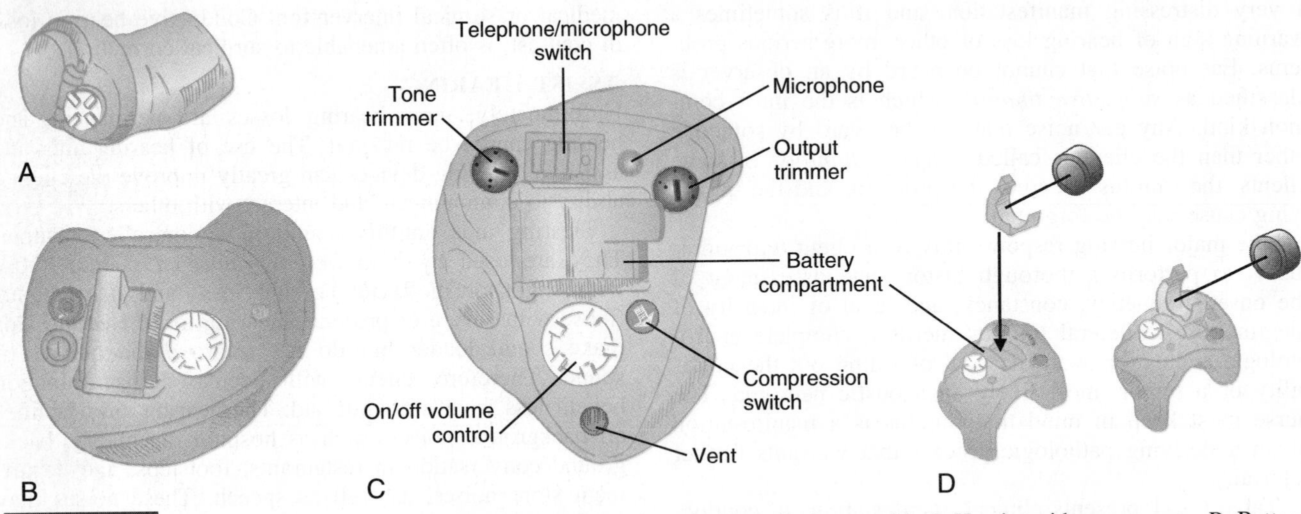

FIGURE 66–2 Types of hearing aids and components. *A*, In-the-canal aid. *B*, In-the-ear aid. *C*, Hearing aid components. *D*, Battery compartment. (Courtesy of Arnold G. Schuring, M.D.)

that fit into the ear canal. The latest advancement in hearing aids is digital processing. Another advancement is directional microphones, which enhance the voice of a speaker in front of the client and suppress background noise. Programmable hearing aids allow the selection of various amplification patterns by the user, and may have some added benefit for clients. Hearing aid technology will continue to advance.

Assistive listening devices help the hearing-impaired client hear the television or radio as well as use the telephone. Stationary devices called teletypewriters and a portable instrument called a Telecommunication Device for the Deaf (TDD) are used for telephone communication by the profoundly deaf. A flashing light signals the presence of a dial tone, a busy signal, or a ring. When another teletypewriter or TDD is reached, messages are typed and displayed on a screen or printed. Other devices, such as flashing lights that alert a deaf person to a ringing doorbell, alarm clock, or smoke alarm, are available. Hearing dogs are trained to be sensitive to certain noises, such as the telephone, doorbells, and crying children. On hearing the sound, a hearing dog moves back and forth between the client and the sound to alert the client.

Manage Tinnitus

Tinnitus can be a very distressing disorder associated with the sensorineural hearing loss. Many approaches have been tried to alleviate this problem, including biofeedback, electrostimulation, hypnosis, medication, hearing aids, and tinnitus maskers. They have all met with minimal success. Tinnitus maskers appear quite similar to hearing aids except that they generate noise. The tinnitus masker is of benefit only while it is being used. However, every approach for the relief from tinnitus is only moderately successful, at best. Clients should be counseled to avoid unproven treatments for tinnitus. The nurse and family must be alert to manifestations of depression if the tinnitus is chronic. The quality of the spouse's support of the client with tinnitus has been shown to be strongly correlated with role function. In addition, the nurse should be alert to spousal interaction and should facilitate problem-solving as needed.

Implement Aural Rehabilitation

Aural rehabilitation may improve communication if (1) hearing loss is irreversible or is not amenable to surgical intervention or (2) the client elects not to have surgery. The purpose of aural rehabilitation is to maximize the hearing-impaired client's communication skills.

Hearing is one of our primary modes of communication. Rehabilitation is directed toward teaching the client to more effectively use the other senses, those of vision, touch, and vibration, and to maximize the use of any remaining hearing ability. The outcome of rehabilitation is affected by all demographic variables and the severity of impairment. As with other forms of rehabilitation, success depends partly on the client's level of motivation.

Speech reading, the current term used for lip reading, is an important means of communication. Speech reading is the process of understanding vocal communication by the integration of lip movements with facial expressions, gestures, environmental clues, and conversation contexts. Speech reading is difficult without auditory cues, for several reasons. Many movements for speech are rapid, many sounds are similar (*b, m, p*), and the production of certain sounds in any language is not visible. The hearing-impaired client must guess at a high percentage of words. Knowledge of this fact alone helps the nurse be more understanding of the client who is using this communication approach.

Because of reduced auditory feedback (the inability of hearing-impaired clients to monitor their own speech), the clearness, pitch quality, or rate of the client's speech may deteriorate. These changes may alter the efficiency of communication and reduce the intelligibility of speech. The goal of speech training is to conserve, develop, or prevent deterioration of speech skills.

Last, but still important, is sign language. Sign language allows communication by hand signals that represent different letters of the alphabet, words, and phrases.

Nursing Management of the Medical Client

ASSESSMENT

The client's ability to communicate may be informally assessed during the history. The nurse should assess the client's ability to follow conversation. During the interview, the nurse should look for answers to the following questions:

1. Does the client admit to having a hearing loss and difficulty communicating or blame other people for not speaking clearly?
2. In what settings does the client have more problems with hearing or communicating?
3. Are family members, co-workers, and friends aware of the hearing problem? Are they supportive of the client, making communication easier and including him or her in conversation? Do others feel frustrated or angry when the client cannot hear correctly or does not respond? Does the client feel left out? Embarrassed?
4. Does the client try to understand spoken words? Or does he or she withdraw or refuse to participate, letting others do the talking?
5. Does the client wear a hearing aid? Does it appear to work?

Occasionally, laboratory, radiologic, and vestibular examinations are used for assessment. In an otology office, the nurse may have the responsibility of performing the history, otologic examination, and screening audiometry. The history is often the most important part of the clinical assessment, as previously described (see questionnaire in Chapter 64). The extent of assessment of the sensorineural hearing loss depends on the setting and the nurse's educational preparation and experience. Nurses should be able to inspect the outer ear and grossly assess auditory acuity.

Visualization of the ear canal and tympanic membrane is accomplished with the otoscope. Cerumen in the canal or on the eardrum can interfere with the examination and may need to be removed. The blind removal of ear wax with an ear syringe should be performed only if the ear is free of other abnormalities, such as an infection or perforation of the eardrum.

Impacted accumulations of ear wax may be softened and loosened for removal by alternating instillations of glycerin and hydrogen peroxide eardrops. The eardrops are warmed to body temperature and used daily as directed for 1 to 2 weeks. The ear is then irrigated gently with warm water for removal of the softened wax or cleaned under magnification with a cerumen spoon. Wax on the tympanic membrane should be removed by a otolaryngologist or an advanced-practice nurse in otaryngology. However, the removal of cerumen can lead to irritation from mildly caustic commercial products.

DIAGNOSIS, OUTCOMES, INTERVENTIONS

Impaired Verbal Communication. Clients who have lost their ability to hear are best managed with the nursing diagnosis *Impaired Verbal Communication related to effects of hearing loss.*

Outcomes. The client will develop effective methods to communicate needs and will be included in conversation.

Interventions. When normal conversation is impossible, writing may be used successfully by clients who have good comprehension of English (or their primary language). Writing may cause frustration when the client's primary language is American Sign Language because it is grammatically different from standard English. Visual aids, such as pictures, diagrams, and models, may also improve the nurse's ability to explain medical terminology or procedures. An expert interpreter should be used when other attempts to communicate have failed or when speed and accuracy are critical. The National Registry of Interpreters for the Deaf (NRID) has local chapters and offers certification for qualified individuals. Box 66–2 lists common nursing interventions to improve communication with hearing-impaired clients. They can apply to all clients, regardless of the type or severity of hearing loss.

Many hearing-impaired clients live in the community. Nurses may see these clients for their hearing problems or for many other problems. The Bridge to Home Health Care addresses approaches to home care of hearing-impaired clients.

BOX 66–2 Common Nursing Interventions for Hearing-Impaired Clients

- Get the client's attention by raising your arm or hand.
- Stand with a light on your face; this helps the client to speech-read.
- Talk directly to the client while facing him or her.
- Speak clearly, but do not overaccentuate words.
- Speak in a normal tone; do not shout. Shouting overuses normal speaking movements so may cause distortion, and may be too loud for the client with sensorineural damage. If the client has conductive loss only, it is sometimes helpful to make the voice louder without shouting.
- If the client does not seem to understand what is said, express it differently. Some words are difficult to "see" in speech reading, such as "white" and "red."
- Move closer to the client and toward the better-hearing ear.
- Write out proper names or any statement that you are not sure was understood.
- Do not smile, chew gum, or cover the mouth when talking.
- Remember that a client's inattention may indicate tiredness or lack of understanding.
- Use phrases to convey meaning rather than one-word answers. State the major topic of the discussion first, and then give details.
- Do not show annoyance by careless facial expressions. Clients who are hard of hearing depend more on visual clues for understanding.
- Encourage the use of a hearing aid if it is available; allow the client to adjust it before speaking.
- In a group, repeat important statements, and avoid making asides to others in the group.
- Avoid the use of the intercommunication system, because this may distort sound and cause poor communication.
- Do not avoid conversation with a client who has hearing loss. It has been said that to live in a silent world is much more devastating than to live in darkness, and clients with hearing loss appear to have more emotional difficulties than do those who are blind.

BRIDGE TO HOME HEALTH CARE

Living with a Severe Hearing Loss

People are often reluctant to admit that they have a hearing impairment. This reluctance results in difficulty with verbal communication, inability to follow instructions, and social isolation. To maximize communication, reduce background noise (turn off the television or radio), face the person, and speak clearly without shouting. Sometimes, the only way to communicate is by writing. Develop written materials for repeated use. Include introduction materials (e.g., your name, your agency's name, the purpose of your visit), reportable problems, and treatment regimens.

In many cases, hearing loss is due to accumulation of cerumen. Use an otoscope to visualize the ear canal. If cerumen is present, a physician may need to remove it. If you are responsible for removing the cerumen, contact the physician to discuss a prescription for an ear irrigation solution, instill the solution, and evaluate the amount and color of drainage.

When people experience a hearing loss, they need a medical evaluation and a hearing aid evaluation. Many older adults are reluctant to wear a hearing aid for various reasons. It is a visual sign of an impairment, it is expensive, and it necessitates leaving home for evaluation, fitting, and follow-up appointments. If a client's reluctance is due to cosmetic reasons, show pictures of hearing aids and discuss individuals who wear hearing aids, such as former President George Bush.

If cost is a problem, consider a referral to a social worker to identify local resources. Currently, Medicare pays for the cost of a hearing evaluation and little for the hearing aid; Medicaid usually pays for the hearing aid. Consider other financial resources, such as the American Association of Retired Persons and local hearing aid vendors. When leaving home is a problem, check whether a vendor will make a home visit. If this is not a possible, suggest that the client use a head-set amplifier that can be purchased from a local electronics store.

Teaching is an important nursing intervention related to hearing impairment. It involves cleaning the devices and changing the batteries. Also, evaluate the client's ability to use the telephone and answer the door. Local telephone companies can equip the telephone with an adjustable volume control, hearing aid adapters, loud ringing signals, and a Telecommunication Device for the Deaf (TDD). A TDD allows the hearing-impaired individual to communicate by typing information into a specially designed device. To receive information, the receiver must have a specific TDD telephone number. Teach the client with a TDD about TDD telephone numbers for an emergency response, and provide information about the home health agency and community resources.

It is important to involve informal caregivers, significant others, and family members in the management of a hearing impairment. Teach these people to maximize communication with a variety of techniques and adaptive equipment.

Gail F. Wilkerson, RN, MSN, CS, *Disease Management Specialist, Heart Failure, Group Health Plan, St. Louis, Missouri*

Ineffective Individual Coping. The individual with a loss of hearing goes through the same stages of grieving as others experiencing a loss. Rehabilitation cannot begin until some acceptance of the hearing loss has taken place, leading to the nursing diagnosis *Ineffective Individual Coping related to recent loss of hearing.*

Outcomes. The client will discuss or will demonstrate problem-solving–based coping strategies, as evidenced by the following:

1. Taking the initiative to inform others of the hearing impairment and requesting that they assist with communication by using techniques that promote comprehension.
2. Not experiencing feelings of embarrassment, frustration, or withdrawal.
3. Not blaming others for failure to communicate effectively.
4. Avoiding situations and environments, such as noisy areas, that impair hearing.

Interventions. Work with the client and family on methods to enhance communication and thereby enhance coping. Encourage the client to role-play how he or she might tell people about the hearing impairment and indicate what techniques should be used to help hearing. Self-help groups, such as Self-Help for Hard of Hearing People (SHHH), located in Bethesda, Md., can assist with resources, information, and support for clients and their families.

Impaired Social Interaction. Clients with hearing losses can experience fears of inadequacy, feelings of inferiority, depression, and varying degrees of stress and isolation. The nursing diagnosis *Impaired Social Interaction related to perceived inability to interact with others secondary to hearing loss* can be used to guide interventions.

Outcomes. The client will exhibit a willingness to be involved in social situations, as evidenced by (1) attempting to become a part of social events, (2) conversing with others, (3) indicating lessened feelings of inadequacy, and (4) responding appropriately to questions asked (not fabricating answers to cover hearing loss).

Interventions. The ASHA urges that all clients with hearing impairments *not* be grouped into one category. Each client is unique and has an individual hearing problem. The nurse functions as a role model in accepting the client as an individual and demonstrating effective communication techniques.

Work with the client to enhance coping, encourage continued social involvement, and advocate the use of various organizations to their fullest extent. Many agencies and associations exist for the hearing-impaired client. Services are offered by audiology clinics and sponsored by universities, hospitals, community programs, state or local departments of health, the Department of Veterans Affairs (VA), and national organizations.

Knowledge Deficit. Clients with new hearing aids need information about their care and proper use. Therefore, *Knowledge Deficit related to lack of previous exposure to a hearing aid* is an important nursing diagnosis.

Outcomes. The client will have greater knowledge about the hearing aid, as evidenced by proper use and care of the aid.

Interventions. The hearing aid user should know how to care for the aid (Box 66–3) and what to do if the device does not work. Gain a basic knowledge of the hearing aid to help with insertion for clients who are ill. Encourage the client to use the hearing aid and to store it safely when not using it. Turn the device off before removal to prevent squealing feedback. The maintenance of a hearing aid is becoming less of a problem today. Usually, the aid is returned to the dealer for factory repair while the client uses a "loaner" hearing aid. Unlicensed assistive personnel often care for clients with hearing aids. Delegation of care of the hearing aid and the hearing-impaired client is shown in the Management and Delegation feature.

Cost has been cited as a major factor in the non-use of hearing aids. Clients needing financial assistance should be referred to the state department of vocational rehabilitation, the local Lions Club, and, in some states, Medicaid.

EVALUATION

A client with a new hearing loss or disorder needs frequent evaluation to determine the severity of hearing loss, coping strategies, and ability to adequately communicate. Because many forms of hearing loss are permanent or progressive, long-term evaluation should also be performed to be certain the client is adapting positively. Also determine whether the client has questions about the equipment used for hearing rehabilitation and the need for further education.

BOX 66–3 Care of a Hearing Aid

- Turn the hearing aid off when it is not in use.
- Open the battery compartment at night to avoid accidental drainage of battery power.
- Keep an extra battery available at all times.
- Wash the ear mold frequently (daily if necessary) with mild soap and warm water, and use a pipe cleaner to cleanse the cannula.
- Dry the ear mold completely before reconnecting it to the hearing aid.
- Do not wear the hearing aid when you have an ear infection.

What to Do if the Hearing Aid Fails to Work

- Check the on-off switch.
- Inspect the ear mold for cleanliness.
- Examine the battery for correct insertion.
- Examine the cord plug for correct insertion.
- Examine the cord for breaks.
- Replace the battery, cord, or both, if necessary. The life of batteries varies according to the amount of use and power requirements of the aid. Batteries last 2 to 14 days.
- Check the position of the ear mold in the ear. If the hearing aid "whistles," the ear mold is probably not inserted properly into the ear canal, or you need to have a new ear mold made.

MANAGEMENT AND DELEGATION

Hearing Aids

Caring for hearing aids and helping clients with maintenance of these devices may be delegated to unlicensed assistive personnel. Clients with new hearing aids need individualized teaching provided by you, the Registered Nurse. You are to evaluate the client's understanding of the instruction. Before delegating hearing aid care, consider the following issues:

- The client's learning needs. Are these new hearing aids? Does the client have a new hearing loss disorder? If so, you should instruct the client to care for these devices and provide consistent teaching.
- The competency level of the unlicensed assistive personnel who will potentially perform hearing aid care. Unlicensed assistive personnel may not provide the initial instruction but may reinforce the instructions that you have provided.

Instruct unlicensed assistive personnel caring for the client with hearing aids to:

- Encourage the use of hearing aids and independent care by clients without cognitive impairment.
- Provide safe storage of the hearing aids when not in use (in the client's personal case or another small storage device). If the client is hospitalized, ensure that the case is labeled with the client's name and location.
- Turn the device off when it is not in use. If the aid is to be off for a prolonged duration (such as during the night or sleeping hours), open the battery compartment to avoid additional drainage of battery power.
- Cleanse the ear mold with mild soap and water each day or as needed.
- Completely dry the ear mold prior to reconnecting it to the hearing aid.
- Help the client insert the ear mold into the ear. If the hearing aid makes a whistling noise, the device is not inserted properly into the ear. At this point, it may be necessary for you to further assess placement in the ear canal.
- Allow the client to adjust the volume prior to speaking.
- Speak clearly in a normal tone to the client. Do not shout.
- Turn off the device before removing it to prevent squealing "feedback."

Findings that are immediately reportable to you are (1) difficulty with placement in the ear, (2) redness or drainage in the ear, (3) mechanical failure of the device, and (4) other issues of concern to the client.

Kimberly Elgin, BSN, RN, *Clinician III, Clinical Manager, Surgical Services, University of Virginia Health System, Charlottesville, Virginia*

Surgical Management

Surgery is usually not warranted for sensorineural hearing loss. However, because mixed, conductive, and sensorineural hearing loss exists, surgery may be performed (1) to restore the conductive hearing loss, (2) to remove tumor, and (3) to assist hearing in profoundly deaf people.

Restore Conductive Hearing

The most common cause of conductive hearing loss is serous otitis media (see later). Although most commonly seen in children, this disorder can occur at any age. In cases of serous otitis media and persistent conductive hearing loss that do not resolve after 2 to 3 months of medical management, an incision into the tympanic membrane and an evacuation of fluid can be performed with the client under local or general anesthesia. This procedure, known as *myringotomy*, will restore hearing. It is discussed later in this chapter.

Another type of conductive hearing loss that can be treated medically or corrected surgically results from otosclerosis. Because speech discrimination is usually unimpaired, simple amplification of sound is quite effective. People who are at high risk of otosclerosis or who are not candidates for surgery can be given medications in an attempt to reduce the severity of the bony fusion. Sodium fluoride has been given to replace the hydroxyl ion in bone and decrease resorption. In addition, calcium gluconate and vitamin D have been used to retard bone resorption. If hearing is stable, these minerals and vitamins are given for only 2 years. The clinical efficacy of these medications remains unsubstantiated.

Stapedectomy. Surgical intervention for otosclerosis has been very successful. *Stapedectomy* is a surgical procedure whereby the damaged stapes is removed and replaced with a stainless steel, polytetrafluoroethylene (Teflon), or plastic prosthesis (Fig. 66–1*B*). The oval window is grafted with absorbable gelatin sponge (Gelfoam) or tissue grafts. Stapedectomy was once a common middle ear procedure. However, the pool of clients with otosclerosis is dwindling, and today, stapedectomy is performed less and less often.

The client must be free of otitis externa and otitis media before surgery. To reduce the risk of bleeding, the client should use no aspirin or products with aspirin for 1 week before surgery. Preoperative and postoperative audiograms and tympanograms are performed to test hearing acuity levels.

After surgery, the client is often instructed to lie on the nonoperative ear with the head of the bed elevated. This position helps reduce edema and prevent dislodgment of the prosthesis. Antibiotics are prescribed. The packing in the ear canal should not be disturbed. Upon discharge from the hospital, the client is told to report the acute onset of vertigo. To reduce the risk of development of a perilymph fistula (rupture of the oval window, which permits leakage of perilymph fluid), the client should avoid excessive exercise, straining, and activities that may lead to head trauma. If the client needs to blow the nose, it should be done gently, one nostril at a time. The client should sneeze with the mouth open. No airplane travel is allowed for a month.

Hearing aids may still be required after stapedectomy, and the client's hearing will need to be reevaluated. Complications of the operation include granuloma formation and perilymph fistula. Either complication may result in profound deafness and persistent vertigo. Hearing loss may also develop after surgery from middle ear adhesions or shifting of the prosthesis.

Tumor Excision

Surgery is usually recommended for treatment of acoustic neuroma. Current microsurgical techniques often allow preservation of hearing and usually enable resection of the tumor without injury to the facial nerve. In older clients, especially those with total deafness in the affected ear, a more conservative, nonsurgical approach is sometimes taken, because acoustic neuroma is benign and very slow growing.

Assist Hearing in Profound Deafness

Use of implantable hearing devices (IHDs) may be appropriate in various clients. There are three types of implantable hearing devices: cochlear implants, temporal bone stimulators, and middle ear implants.

Cochlear Implants. Cochlear implants provide auditory sensation to clients with severe to profound sensorineural hearing loss who cannot benefit from a hearing aid (Fig. 66–3). Preoperative vestibular testing is highly recommended for all clients in whom a cochlear implant is being considered.

The cochlear implant contains a small computer that changes the spoken word to electrical impulses. The impulses are transmitted across the skin to an implanted coil that carries the impulse to the hearing nerve endings in the cochlea by means of an electrode introduced through the round window. The most effective cochlear implants use multiple-frequency channels. In multichannel cochlear implants, up to 22 electrodes are inserted along the cochlear partition. The surgery for insertion of a cochlear implant is similar to mastoid surgery. The success of a cochlear implant varies widely, ranging from minimal improvement in auditory awareness to the ability to understand speech on the telephone.

Temporal Bone Stimulators (Bone Hearing Devices). In some cases of hearing loss, sound can be transmitted by applying a stimulation directly to the temporal bone, thereby transmitting sound through the skull to the inner ear. For clients with a conductive hearing loss, a device is available in which the receiver is implanted under the skin into the skull. The external device transmits the sound through the skin. This device is worn above the ear rather than in the ear canal. Because some conductive hearing losses cannot be surgically repaired, the temporal bone stimulator may provide an alternative rehabilitative method to conventional hearing aids. It is not widely used at the present time.

Middle Ear Implants (Semi-Implantable Device). A variety of implantable devices are being evaluated for sound amplification. However, many challenges have to be met before a workable device is available. This method of hearing aid technology is still in the research stage.

Otalgia

Otalgia is defined as pain in the ear, or earache. Otalgia can be primary in origin (i.e., coming from a disorder in

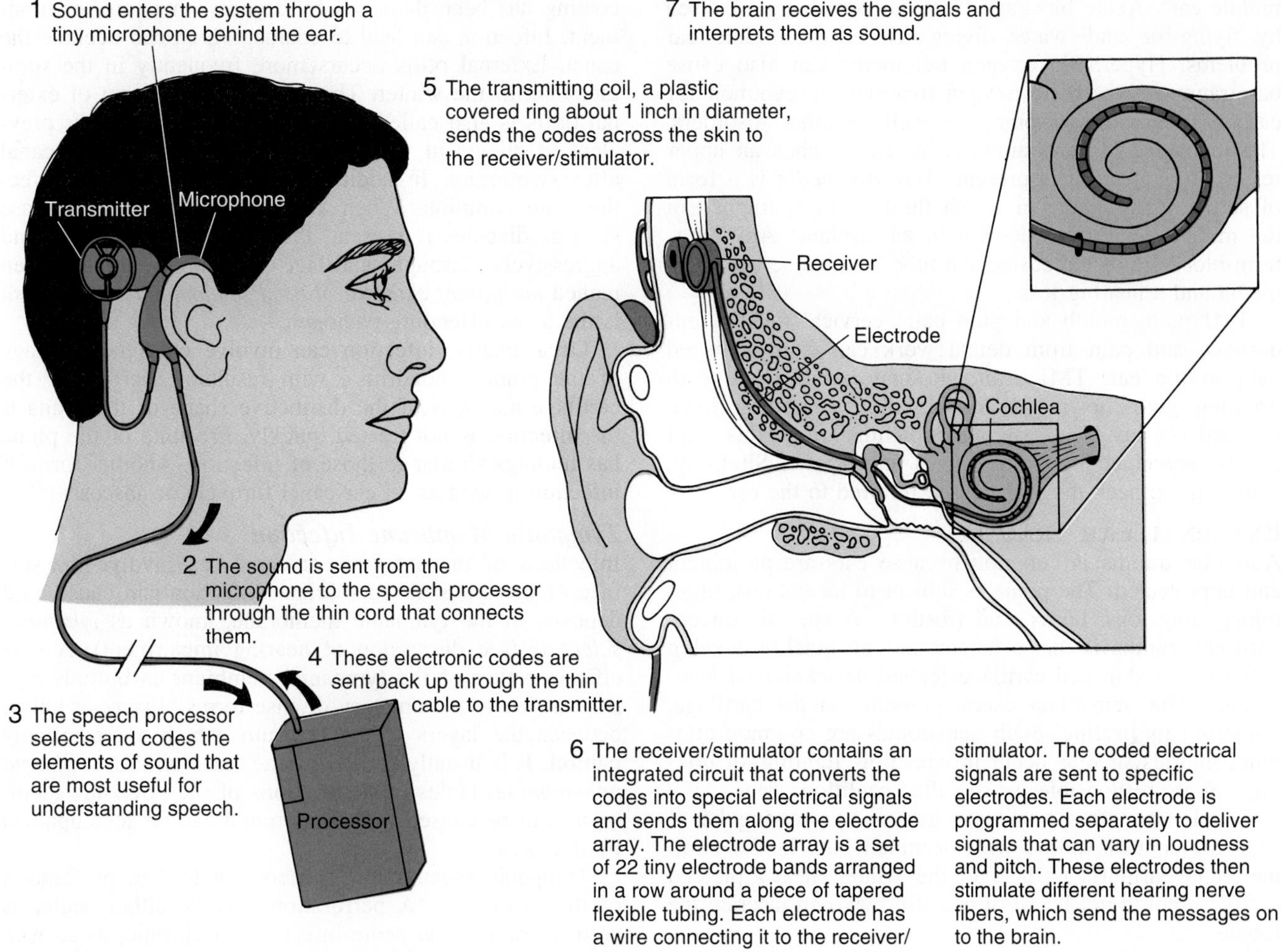

1 Sound enters the system through a tiny microphone behind the ear.
7 The brain receives the signals and interprets them as sound.
5 The transmitting coil, a plastic covered ring about 1 inch in diameter, sends the codes across the skin to the receiver/stimulator.
Transmitter
Microphone
Receiver
Electrode
Cochlea
2 The sound is sent from the microphone to the speech processor through the thin cord that connects them.
4 These electronic codes are sent back up through the thin cable to the transmitter.
3 The speech processor selects and codes the elements of sound that are most useful for understanding speech.
Processor
6 The receiver/stimulator contains an integrated circuit that converts the codes into special electrical signals and sends them along the electrode array. The electrode array is a set of 22 tiny electrode bands arranged in a row around a piece of tapered flexible tubing. Each electrode has a wire connecting it to the receiver/stimulator. The coded electrical signals are sent to specific electrodes. Each electrode is programmed separately to deliver signals that can vary in loudness and pitch. These electrodes then stimulate different hearing nerve fibers, which send the messages on to the brain.

FIGURE 66–3 Cochlear implant to restore hearing.

the ear) infectious, or referred (i.e., coming from a disorder outside the ear). Otalgia from ear pain can be the result of infection in the external or middle ear or of trauma to the ear and head. Referred otalgia can be caused by disorders in the temporomandibular joint (TMJ), cranial nerves, face, scalp, pharynx, tonsils, thyroid, trachea, teeth, or cervical muscles.

Etiology and Risk Factors

Otalgia can be related to infectious processes in the external and middle ear. Bacterial contaminants can enter the ear through insertion of unclean articles, such as fingers or toys. Insertion of any sharp objects into the ear canal can traumatize the skin and provide an open medium for infection. Instillation of contaminated solutions into the ear or swimming in polluted water raises the risk for development of ear infection and inflammation. Clients with recent upper respiratory infections, eustachian tube dysfunction, and allergies are also at increased risk for ear infections.

Infectious and neoplastic processes of the pharynx can also cause referred otalgia. It is not uncommon for patients with acute tonsillitis to complain of significant ear pain, even though the ears may be normal on examination. Otalgia following tonsillectomy is universal and is not a manifestation of infection. In clients with unilateral otalgia and a history of smoking, consideration must be given to a neoplastic process of the lateral pharynx, especially if there are concurrent manifestations, such as hoarseness or dysphagia. Examination of the lower pharynx by means of a fiberoptic endoscope is necessary in the smoker with persistent hoarseness, and referral to an otolaryngologist is indicated.

Trauma to the head, temporal bone, and ear can also result in ear pain. Engaging in contact sports without protective headgear can result in severe trauma to the head, injuring the hearing apparatus. A blow to the ear by an object such as a ball or hand can cause local or diffuse pain in the area. Noise trauma from a blast or loud noise may create a ringing sensation that is perceived as painful and uncomfortable. Nerve damage may be accompanied by an intolerance to even soft sounds, resulting in severe pain. Exposure to extremely hot or cold temperatures can lead to burns or severe frostbite, respectively, of the external ear.

Blockage of the eustachian tube and otalgia can be the result of enlarged adenoid tissue and tonsils in children, middle ear infections often associated with upper respiratory infections, and *barotrauma* (pressure injury to the middle ear). Acute blockage from altitude changes caused by flying or underwater diving will cause middle ear problems. Hyperbaric oxygen treatments can also cause barotrauma. Hyperbaric oxygen treatment is common for carbon monoxide poisoning as well as other disorders. The incidence of barotrauma is increased when an upper respiratory infection is present. *Aerotitis media* is a form of serous otitis media in which fluid or air is trapped in the middle ear during descent in an airplane. Any long-term blockage of the eustachian tube leads to serous otitis media and a hearing loss.

TMJ pain, mouth and gum pain, cervical muscle tenderness, and pain from dental work can cause referred pain to the ear. TMJ arthralgia may result from teeth grinding, gum chewing, excessive talking, or biting down on hard objects. The resultant inflammation to this joint can be perceived by the client as an earache. Similarly, stress on the neck muscles can be referred to the ear.

External Ear Trauma

Auricular trauma is common because ears are prominent and unprotected. The pinna is subject to lacerations, blunt injury, abrasions, burns, and frostbite. A special concern with ear trauma is that a hematoma can quickly develop between the skin and cartilage (called *perichondrial hematoma*). The hematoma exerts pressure on the cartilage, impairing its healing. Such hematomas are common after blunt injuries such as occur in wrestling, fighting, or boxing and are responsible for so-called cauliflower ear.

People can often avoid ear trauma by wearing headgear for contact sports, wide-brimmed hats in the summer, and earmuffs or hats in the winter; heavy pierced earrings should not be worn because they can lacerate the lobule.

Foreign Bodies

Surprisingly, a wide array of foreign bodies fit into the ear canal. The most common foreign body found in the adult ear is either a piece of cotton or, most annoying, an insect.

Ear pain from obstruction usually results from the buildup of matter in the ear canal, which leads to pressure and pain. Clients may also report decreased hearing, a sense of fullness, a throbbing sensation, and itching. The onset, duration, frequency, and intensity of manifestations should be noted.

Eustachian Tube Disorders

Because the eustachian tube connects the middle ear to the nasopharynx, pharyngeal disorders also cause eustachian tube dysfunction and, thus, secondary middle ear problems. For example, a common disorder is blockage of the eustachian tube by enlarged adenoid tissue in children. In adults, swelling of the mucosa in the eustachian tube during an upper respiratory infection can lead to serous otitis media (see later). For persistent unilateral blocked eustachian tube, a malignant tumor must be ruled out as the cause.

Ear Infections

Otitis Externa

The most common problems found in the external ear are infections, primarily bacterial or fungal. The most frequent infection, called *external otitis,* involves the external ear canal. Infection begins when the protective waxy coating has been damaged by dryness, moisture, or treatment. Infection can lead to edema, which can occlude the canal. External otitis occurs more frequently in the summer than in the winter. The most common form of external otitis is also called *swimmer's ear,* because it is prevalent in clients in whom water remains in the ear canal after swimming. In addition, opportunistic fungal infections are common. When a debilitating systemic disease such as diabetes is present, the external otitis can spread aggressively through cartilage and bone and is then named *malignant external otitis*; *Pseudomonas aeruginosa* is the usual offending pathogen.

Occasionally, infection can involve only the cartilage of the pinna (chondritis), with resultant necrosis of the cartilage and loss of the distinctive shape of the pinna if the infection is not treated quickly. Frostbite of the pinna has findings similar to those of infection. Another form of infection is seen as an ear canal furuncle or abscess.

Tympanic Membrane Infection

Infections of the external ear canal can involve the surface of the tympanic membrane. Infection can cause hard deposits in the tympanic membrane, known as *tympanosclerosis* (see discussion of hearing impairment). A specific infection of the tympanic membrane is bullous myringitis. This inflammatory disease forms blisters or bullae between the layers of the eardrum, which are extremely painful. It is usually caused by the bacterium *Mycoplasma pneumoniae.* Holes or perforations of the tympanic membrane can be caused by infection and can be accompanied by drainage.

Tympanic membrane disorders can lead to perforation of the membrane. A perforation may be either acute, as seen in trauma and acute infection, or chronic, as seen in repeated infection. An acute perforation has a better chance of healing spontaneously than does a chronic perforation.

Otitis Media

Otitis media is the most prevalent disorder of the middle ear. It is most common in children, but it does occur in adults. When an infection is sudden in onset and short in duration, the diagnosis is acute suppurative otitis media. When the infection is repeated, usually causing drainage and perforation, the problem is chronic otitis media. Chronic otitis media is often due to gram-negative organisms, such as *Pseudomonas, Staphylococcus,* and *Klebsiella.* Anaerobes such as *Bacteroides* have also been identified in culture analysis of specimens from the ear. Infection can cause swelling of the mucosa throughout the middle ear and eustachian tube. At times, *serous otitis media* is found in conjunction with upper respiratory infections or allergies.

Chronic otitis media can lead to tympanic membrane retraction, adhesive otitis media, or necrosis of the tympanic membrane (perforations) or of the ossicles. Both problems create a conductive hearing loss. Necrosis of the bone covering of the facial nerve may cause facial paralysis. Because of the anatomy of the temporal bone, middle ear infection can also lead to brain abscesses that are life-threatening if not treated properly. Cholesteatoma, another complication, is discussed later.

Subsequent to infectious otitis media or allergic disease, fluid may form in the middle ear, known as serous otitis media. This fluid is formed when a vacuum develops in the middle ear, caused by a blocked eustachian tube. When the swelling subsides, the fluid may be too thick to drain. Tympanometry is a useful diagnostic assessment to distinguish a normal ear from one with a middle ear effusion.

Mastoiditis

The mastoid system is a series of air cells contained within the temporal bone that communicate with the middle ear. Before the discovery of antibiotics, a mastoid infection was a life-threatening event. Now, acute mastoiditis is very rare, although chronic mastoiditis does sometimes occur. With repeated middle ear infections, the mastoid cavity becomes a significant part of the problem, increasing the amount of drainage. A chronic infection also leads to the development of cholesteatoma (see later).

Drainage from the mastoid cavity via the ear canal is the most likely sign to appear. The drainage courses through the middle ear and out the tympanic membrane through a perforation. Tenderness over the mastoid cavity behind the ear points to an infection but usually is caused by an acute exacerbation of chronic mastoiditis rather than an acute mastoiditis. The protrusion of the pinna as a result of swelling over the mastoid may be part of this process.

Cholesteatoma

Cholesteatoma is a cyst in the middle ear or mastoid system that is lined with squamous epithelium and filled with keratin debris. Often, infection is present in the mass of the cholesteatoma. Although cholesterol granules can be present in the specimen, yielding the term cholesteatoma, they are not the primary pathologic process.

Cholesteatoma most often results from chronic otitis media or marginal perforation of the tympanic membrane. Clients have conductive hearing loss and foul-smelling discharge from the ears. Although it is a benign growth, the cholesteatoma causes erosion of the surrounding structures, leading to other problems, such as brain abscesses, vertigo, and facial paralysis. Fortunately, these complications are uncommon.

OTHER MASSES

Benign masses of the external ear canal are usually cysts that arise from a sebaceous gland or, more rarely, from the cerumen glands. Cysts can also be congenital in nature. Bony protrusions seen in the bony portion of the ear canal are called *exostoses*. The skin covering an exostosis is normal. If the skin is red, the mass is usually an abscess. Infectious polyps found in the ear canal arise from either the tympanic membrane or, more commonly, the middle ear, through a hole in the tympanic membrane.

Malignant tumors are also found in the external ear. The cutaneous carcinomas are most often basal cell carcinoma on the pinna and squamous cell carcinoma in the ear canal. If not treated, the carcinomas can invade underlying structures; squamous cell carcinoma may spread throughout the temporal bone. Rare tumors of the cerumen glands are of the adenoma cell type. Masses of the external ear are diagnosed through physical examination and biopsy to rule out malignancy. Surgical excision may be required.

Both benign and malignant tumors can involve the tympanic membrane, but they seldom arise from it. However, an infectious glandular polyp can be isolated to the tympanic membrane. Tumors in the middle ear can be seen through or may protrude through the tympanic membrane.

The most common benign growth in the middle ear is an infectious polyp. A facial nerve neuroma is found along the course of the facial nerve. Malignant tumors involving the middle ear can be primary or secondary.

The same tumors that arise in the middle ear can be found in the mastoid cavity. Because the mastoid cavity is connected to other air cells throughout the temporal bone and is close to the brain, malignant tumors at this location carry a poor prognosis.

Pathophysiology

Otalgia related to a problem in the ear is usually the result of an inflammatory process that can be caused by trauma or infection. Inflammation causes chemical mediators to be released into the tissue and the chemotaxis of leukocytes to the damaged area, resulting in tissue edema, pain, heat, and redness. This inflammatory process results in swelling of tissue that impinges on nerve endings and surrounding areas, causing the otalgia. Masses such as tumors grow and press on nearby tissue and nerves, causing pain. Sometimes, the infection or mass erodes into tissue and bone as in cholesteatoma and causes further inflammation and pain.

Otalgia can also be caused by referred pain to the ear. In conditions such as TMJ or cervical adenopathy, the pain does not originate in the ear. However, the neuronal pain pathways for these processes cross over and are perceived in the ear. Although the perception of pain in the ear is real, the cause of the pain is not related to a pathologic process in that area.

Clinical Manifestations

In the case of head trauma and damage to the tympanic membrane, clients often report an episode of brief but intense otalgia. Blunt injury to the auricle can result in a blue or reddish purple, tense swelling over the pinna. Perichondrial hematomas can develop and, left untreated, form a hypertrophic scar known as a cauliflower ear, which is an occupational hazard for boxers. However, if the tympanic membrane is ruptured from barotrauma or otitis media, the client often notes a sudden *relief of pressure and pain.* Pain is not usually elicited on palpation of the external ear; this phenomenon usually provides a differential diagnosis between problems of the external ear and middle ear. Disorders involving the tympanic membrane are painful, perhaps the most painful of all middle ear disorders. Hearing loss may be noted but is often reversible.

Ear pain from obstruction usually results from the buildup of matter in the ear canal, which leads to pressure and pain. Clients may also report decreased hearing, a sense of fullness, a throbbing sensation, and itching. The onset, duration, frequency, and intensity of manifestations should be noted.

Pain in the external ear is the most common clinical

manifestation of infection. Pain ranges from mild to severe and is generally unilateral. Pain is more intense when the ear canal is swollen. Painful sites are tender because of the close proximity of bone (a hard surface) when the ear is palpated. A clue to early external otitis is tenderness when the pinna is gently pulled on, in contrast to otitis media, in which touching the ear does not cause pain. A forerunner of pain in external otitis is itching in the ear canal. Inflammation (redness) is easily identified with an otoscope. At different stages of infection, drainage will be found from the ear canal. In early infectious disorders, the drainage may be clear rather than discolored by pus.

Manifestations of otitis media include ear pain and an immobile tympanic membrane. Because the tympanic membrane is a semitransparent membrane, what lies beneath it is visible. It can also become discolored or displaced. Therefore, both fluid and infection can be seen in the middle ear. The tympanic membrane may be dull or red instead of the normal pearly gray. The eardrum may be normal, perforated, infected, retracted, or bulging, according to the disease process involved.

In addition, the client may report bubbling, crackling, or popping sensations in the ear, especially during swallowing. There is a sense of fullness in the ear and conductive hearing loss that fluctuates.

Suppurative otitis media is invasion of the middle ear by virulent organisms and formation of pus, often accompanied by purulent *otorrhea* (drainage). Clinical manifestations include intense ear pain, fever, mild to moderate conductive hearing loss, thickened and bulging tympanic membrane, and occasional dizziness.

Outcome Management

Medical Management

The goals of medical management are to (1) promote healing, (2) alleviate pain, and (3) restore normal function of the ears.

PROMOTE HEALING

EAR IRRIGATION. The ear is commonly irrigated to cleanse the external auditory canal or to remove impacted wax, debris, or foreign bodies in order to promote healing. Irrigation is not used in clients with a history or clinical suspicion of perforated eardrum. Ear irrigation is performed as follows.

Warm the irrigating solution (usually water) to body temperature, and place it in the irrigating syringe. Protect the client's clothes with a plastic drape, and place a kidney-shaped basin below the ear to catch the irrigating solution. Have the client sit with the ear to be irrigated toward you and the head tilted toward the other ear. In the adult, pull the external ear upward and backward (or in children pull external ear directly back) and direct the tip of the syringe along the upper wall of the ear canal (Fig. 66–4). The canal should not be completely obstructed by the syringe to allow the back-flow of solution.

Sometimes the client is instructed to use a medicinal ear irrigation solution. The most common solution for ear irrigation is boric acid and alcohol, which is obtained by prescription. This solution cleanses the ear of debris and infection and provides a drying agent. A 2- or 3-oz ear

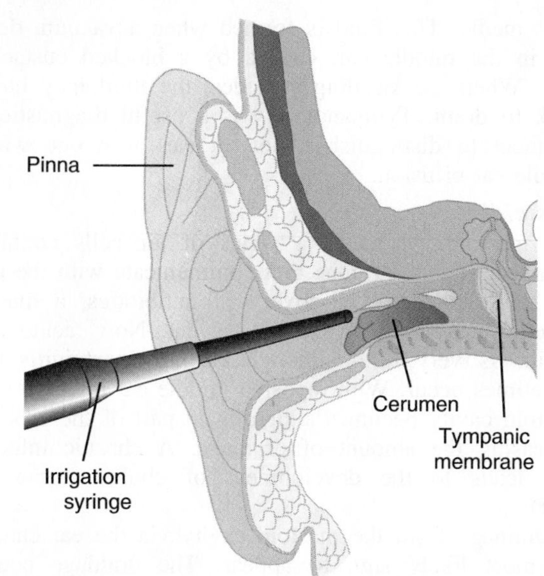

FIGURE 66–4 Ear irrigation. The tip of the syringe is directed along the upper wall of the ear canal.

syringe is needed for irrigation. A family member performs the irrigation for the client. Usually, the ear irrigation is followed by the use of eardrops.

When charting the ear irrigation, include the type of irrigation solution used and the nature of returned solution, regarding amount, texture, color of cerumen, and type of debris. In addition, instruct the client to report pain, vertigo, or nausea during the procedure.

ANTIBIOTICS. Local and systemic antibiotics are the cornerstone of preventing and managing infectious processes. However, the first rule of treating infection is meticulous cleaning of the site so that the local antibiotic can reach the infected area. Suction, irrigation, or manual removal of matter with a cotton-tipped swab can be used. Regular application of antibiotic-steroid eardrops for a week is required.

If the ear canal is swollen shut, a wick must be inserted to allow the drops to penetrate the canal. Eardrops are placed directly on the wick. Commercially prepared wicks or single pieces of ¼-inch gauze can be used. The wick serves not only as a bandage but also as an excellent vehicle to medicate the ear canal. The wick is gently inserted into the ear canal by means of forceps while the external ear is gently pulled upward and backward. The wick is usually slightly less than 1 inch in length (Fig. 66–5). The client should lie on the unaffected side for 3 to 5 minutes to allow gravity to promote movement of the medication into the ear canal. If the infection is generalized or severe, systemic antibiotics are used. An infection that involves cartilage has to be treated aggressively and quickly with systemic antibiotics to avoid complications.

With any form of otitis media, appropriate antibiotic therapy may be necessary. If drainage is present, a specimen may be collected for culture analysis and sensitivity testing. However, most episodes of acute otitis media do not produce drainage, and the specific bacterial cause need not be identified. Otitis media is generally a very easily managed disease, but if it is not treated properly, it

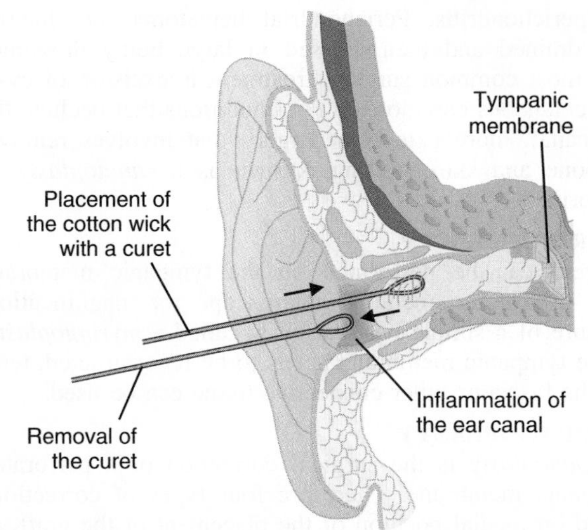

FIGURE 66–5 Administration of antibiotics for otitis externa. A curet with a cotton wick around it is placed into the ear canal. The wick is gently placed into the canal, and an antibiotic or treatment solution is added to the wick.

can lead to sinusitis, meningitis, and brain abscess because of the proximity of the ear to other tissues.

Suppurative otitis media is managed with systemic antibiotics, topical antibiotic drops, and analgesics. If otitis media becomes chronic, myringotomy may be required to ventilate the middle ear and equalize pressure between the middle ear and external ear. Because infection starts in the middle ear, the problems in the mastoid cavity are avoided by early use of antibiotics with otitis media.

ALLEVIATE PAIN

Because external otitis is one of the most painful disorders of the ear, appropriate analgesics are required. Pain persists for 24 to 48 hours after treatment is initiated. Once the swelling and drainage are reduced by treatment, in about 48 hours, the pain subsides.

RESTORE NORMAL FUNCTION AND REMOVE FOREIGN BODIES

Removal of foreign bodies from the ear canal can be quite difficult. The external auditory canal is an exquisitely sensitive, elliptical, cylinder-like structure. In adults, it is about 24 mm long and has two anatomic points of narrowing. Objects caught behind these narrow points create the greatest problems for removal. If perforation of the tympanic membrane is deemed unlikely and the object is not tightly wedged, you can irrigate the external canal with warm water. Direct the stream of water superiorly and anteriorly into the ear canal and around the object (see Fig. 66–4). Water pressure builds up and forces the object outward. It often takes about 200 to 300 ml of water to remove an object. Do not irrigate vegetable foreign proteins, such as beans, because they would swell and become even more difficult to remove.

For removal of a live insect, the ear canal is filled with mineral oil, lidocaine, or an ether-soaked cotton ball, *not water,* to kill or stupefy the insect. Water would cause the insect to swell and become more difficult to remove.

The least traumatic method of removing a foreign body is with the aid of an operating microscope. The nurse should not spend a long time attempting to remove an object from the ear without asking for help. After removing the object, inspect the tympanic membrane and ear canal for manifestations of trauma. If trauma is noted, the client should be treated for external otitis and seen again in 4 to 5 days.

Nursing Management of the Medical Client

ASSESSMENT

When obtaining the history of the pain, ask the client about what events have triggered the ear pain, paying special attention to a recent history of:

- Upper respiratory tract infection
- Travel by airplane
- Exposure to very loud noises
- Trauma to the head
- Stressors that lead to teeth grinding or dental work

The nurse first observes the external ear for redness, swelling, lumps, scaling, crusting, or drainage, either serous or purulent. During assessment of the external ear, manipulation of the ear is important. If the client complains of pain when any part of the ear is palpated, an abscess, a lesion, or some kind of inflammatory process of the ear canal is suspected. If an otoscopic examination is performed, care must be taken not to cause the client unnecessary pain. An abscess may be close to the opening of the canal, where the pressure of the speculum may cause greater pain.

During physical examination, determine the presence of pain with swallowing, neck rotation, palpation of the face and head (over the sinuses), palpation of the mastoid process, and manipulation of the pinna. Assess the TMJ by inserting your index fingers into the external auditory canals and applying pressure anteriorly while the client opens and closes the mouth. TMJ syndrome may cause pain, clicking, or crepitation of the joint during movement.

DIAGNOSIS, OUTCOMES, INTERVENTIONS

Altered Protection. Because of tissue damage from trauma, foreign body, or pathogen, the nursing diagnosis *Altered Protection related to tissue destruction* may be appropriate in the client with otalgia.

Outcomes. The client will not develop an infectious process or will experience resolution of infection without complications.

Interventions. Monitor for clinical manifestations of infection, and administer antibiotics as prescribed. Other medications, such as antihistamines, decongestants, and steroid nasal sprays, may be ordered to reduce inflammation that can damage tissue. Teach the client to complete the entire prescription of the antibiotic even though manifestations may have cleared (see the Client Education Guide).

During an infectious process, instruct the client to avoid getting water in the ear while bathing or showering by using earplugs or placing cotton balls coated with petroleum jelly in the ear canal.

Eardrops may also be prescribed for bacterial or fungal infections, which are often seen in otitis externa. Various irrigations of the mastoid system and middle ear are used for chronic infections along with antibiotic eardrops or

CLIENT EDUCATION GUIDE

Infection of the Tympanic Membrane, Middle Ear, or Mastoid Cavity

To prevent further infections:

- Take medications for allergic or upper respiratory infections.
- Avoid water in the ear (such as while showering, shampooing the hair, or swimming) with a tympanic perforation. Use an earplug.
- Irrigate your ear with an ear syringe. Tip your head so that the solution runs into your ear.
- During treatment for infection, avoid getting water in the ear. If the possibility exists, place two pieces of cotton in the ear, the first piece dry and the second piece saturated with petroleum jelly.
- Seek medical attention for manifestations of decreased hearing, pain in the ear, or drainage from the ear.

powders. In chronic otitis media with discharge, both broad-spectrum oral antibiotics and topical antibiotic drops are used.

Pain. Otalgia may be caused by a process in the ear or may be referred from a source outside the ear, resulting in the nursing diagnosis *Pain related to inflammation in the external or middle ear or from referred pain in the head and neck area.*

Outcomes. The client will be able to relieve pain and achieve an acceptable comfort level.

Interventions. Otalgia is managed by treating the primary problem. Comfort can be promoted by using anesthetic ear solutions or systemic analgesics. After the physician has prescribed the analgesic therapy, instruct the client as to the amount, frequency, and duration. Other measures are application of heat by warm compress, a soft diet, a quiet environment, and positioning of the client with the affected ear down.

The client with TMJ syndrome should avoid chewing and hyperextension of the jaw (e.g., for dental examination and care). He or she should also try to stop grinding the teeth. A specially fitted mouth guard to be worn while sleeping can be helpful in preventing teeth grinding at night.

In the case of eustachian tube dysfunction or barotrauma, teach the client how to facilitate opening of the eustachian tube. Chewing gum, sucking hard candy and swallowing often, yawning, and blowing air out against closed nostrils (Valsalva maneuver) help open the tube.

EVALUATION

The positive outcome for the client with otalgia depends on (1) the thoroughness of the instructions provided by the nurse and (2) the client's compliance with the prescribed treatment regimen. Ongoing assessment of the client to achieve resolution of infectious and inflammatory processes contributing to the otalgia are key to effective management.

Surgical Management

The surgical treatment of infections involves incision and drainage in the acute phase for abscesses and, at times, for perichondritis. Perichondrial hematomas are incised and drained and then dressed in large bulky dressings. The most common surgical treatment is excision of cysts and cutaneous carcinomas. For conditions that occlude the ear canal, more extensive surgery that involves removal of bone and skin grafting, known as a *canaloplasty,* is performed.

MYRINGOPLASTY

Surgery can be performed on the tympanic membrane with use of an operating microscope for magnification. Closure of a simple perforation is called a *myringoplasty.* If the tympanic membrane needs to be reconstructed, temporalis fascia or other connective tissue can be used.

TYMPANOPLASTY

Tympanoplasty is the surgical correction of a perforated tympanic membrane. There are four types of corrections based on medial position of the placement of the graft, as follows:

Type I: Graft rests on malleus
Type II: Graft rests on incus
Type III: Graft attaches to head of stapes
Type IV: Graft attaches to footplate of stapes

When the eustachian tube is stable, postoperative hearing results worsen as one proceeds from type I to type IV tympanoplasty. Under favorable conditions, type I tympanoplasty should result in normal or near-normal restoration of conductive hearing loss, whereas type IV should result in approximately a 30-db air-bone gap. In tympanoplasty, a graft is placed to restore the damaged tympanic membrane. The location of the graft depends on the original defect. Sometimes tympanostomy (ventilation) tubes are inserted.

OSSICULOPLASTY

The surgical procedure of ossicular reconstruction is called *ossiculoplasty.* Various methods of repositioning these tiny ear bones are now in use. In addition, various synthetic prostheses have been used to reconnect the ossicles to carry sound. In an attempt to prevent extrusion of the prostheses, tissue is combined with the prostheses to rebuild the ossicles. This semibiologic method is used in different forms by most otologic surgeons (Fig. 66–6).

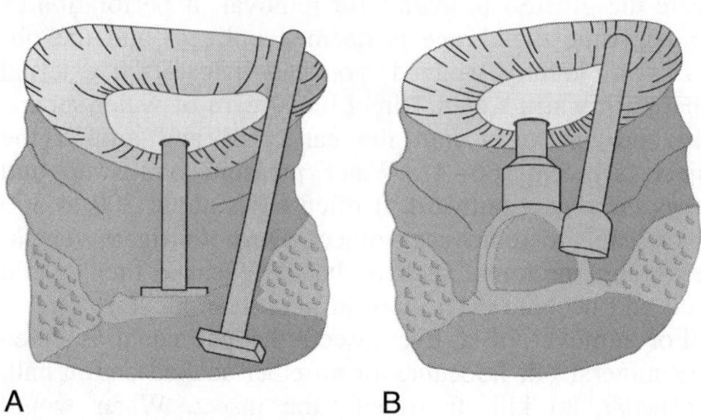

FIGURE 66–6 Middle ear prostheses used for reconstruction. *A*, Ossicle columella prosthesis (total ossicular replacement). *B*, Ossicle cup prosthesis (partial ossicular replacement). (Courtesy of Arnold G. Shuring, M.D.)

Laser surgery can be performed in chronic ear disease for a cholesteatoma associated with the stapes.

Myringotomy

An incision into the tympanic membrane through which fluid is removed by suction is called *myringotomy*. To keep the incision open and to prevent a recurrence of fluid, various types of transtympanic tubes can be inserted into the incision. These tubes extrude by themselves in 3 to 12 months and rarely have to be removed. More permanent tubes (T tubes) with larger flanges may be used for clients who require repeated myringotomies.

Mastoidectomy

Radical mastoidectomy removes the contents of the mastoid bone for control of infection and cholesteatoma. However, because the radical mastoidectomy sacrificed hearing, a modified radical mastoidectomy was developed to save the remaining middle ear structures. With the advent of antibiotics, simple mastoidectomy became possible, which maintained a normal-appearing ear canal. Because radical and modified mastoidectomies exteriorize the mastoid cavity to the external ear canal, they are known as *open* or *canal wall–down mastoidectomies*. *Closed* or *canal wall–up mastoidectomies* are simple mastoidectomies with modifications that are performed in conjunction with tympanoplasty and ossiculoplasty to retain or regain hearing. Today, even the open mastoidectomy is performed with various tympanoplasties.

Nursing Management of the Surgical Client

Preoperative Care

The scope of nursing activities for the client undergoing surgery for otalgia can be as broad as a preoperative assessment performed in an office or clinic or as limited as an assessment performed in the holding area of the surgical suite. Before surgery, an audiogram and tympanogram are obtained to assess preoperative hearing acuity. The client's level of knowledge about the procedure, expectations, and mental readiness for surgery are evaluated along with the physiologic status.

The client undergoing ear surgery should be told what to expect during the procedure, because local anesthesia with sedation is often used. Instructions should be given about the duration of the procedure, the estimated length of hospital stay, and immediate postoperative instructions. Very often, fear of the unknown can be decreased by an understanding of the events that will occur.

Postoperative Care

Pain is not usually a major problem, but mild analgesia may be required. Vertigo or lightheadedness may occur when the client ambulates for the first time. Clients should be supervised when ambulating on the day of surgery to protect them from falling. Some clients who are quite vertiginous exhibit nystagmus (see Chapter 64) from stimulation of the inner ear. The vertigo usually passes very quickly and seldom requires medication.

The ear rarely bleeds after surgery. A small amount of serosanguineous drainage on a cotton ball is expected. After most ear procedures, only a cotton ball is needed in the ear, although a dressing over the ear may be necessary after tympanomastoidectomy. The Client Education Guide lists precautions that the client should be aware of after ear surgery.

Immediate postoperative instructions may include the following:

1. Positioning should be specified, such as the client lying with operated ear up for several hours after surgery.
2. If necessary, the client should blow the nose gently one side at a time.
3. The client should sneeze or cough with the mouth open.
4. Participation in water sports or activities is prohibited.

Normal occurrences in the initial period after ear surgery may include the following:

- Decreased hearing in operated ear from surgical packing (people may sound like they are talking in a barrel)
- Noises in the ear, such as cracking or popping
- Minor earache and discomfort in cheek and jaw
- Ear swelling

Balance Disorders

As already described, *vertigo* is the perception that either oneself or one's surroundings are moving. The person with vertigo usually remains seated or supine to prevent falling. Vertigo is often described as "dizziness." However, dizziness, which can involve feelings of disorientation in space or lightheadedness, is different. Vertigo results from imbalance of neural signals from the vestibular system in the ears. The imbalance of signals is interpreted by the brain as constant motion in space.

Disorders of balance and coordination result from problems of the vestibular system and "righting" reflexes. Balance can also be affected by problems outside the

CLIENT EDUCATION GUIDE

Precautions After Ear Surgery

To prevent injury and promote healing:

- Continue to blow your nose gently one side at a time and to sneeze or cough with your mouth open for 1 week after surgery.
- Avoid physical activity for 1 week and exercises or sports for 3 weeks after surgery.
- Return to work as recommended, usually 3 to 7 days after surgery (3 weeks if work is strenuous).
- Avoid heavy lifting, especially after stapedectomy.
- Change the cotton ball in your ear daily as prescribed.
- Keep your ear dry for 4 to 6 weeks after surgery.
- Do not shampoo for 1 week after surgery.
- Protect your ear when necessary with two pieces of cotton (outer piece saturated with petroleum jelly).
- Avoid airplane flights for the first week after surgery. For sensation of ear pressure, hold your nose, close your mouth, and swallow to equalize pressure.
- Wear noise defenders in loud environments.
- Report any drainage other than a slight amount of bleeding to the physician.

vestibular system. Very few problems are more private than those involving one's sense of balance. Balance problems may be debilitating and may also cause embarrassing gait problems, which can jeopardize safety. More than 90 million Americans aged 17 years or older have experienced vertigo or a balance problem. Vertigo is second only to chronic pain as the most common symptom reported in America today.

Etiology and Risk Factors

Although vertigo and dizziness are not synonymous, they both relate to a sense of balance and equilibrium. Dizziness, vertigo, and syncope (fainting) are all manifestations of one of the following types of problems:

- Peripheral vestibular disorders (i.e., labyrinthine or inner ear)
- Central disorders (i.e., medullary, cerebellar, or cortical)
- Systemic disorders (i.e., cardiovascular or metabolic)

Peripheral vestibular disorders involve a disorder in the labyrinth or internal ear. Central disorders result from a problem in the brain or nerves, such as a tumor of the eighth cranial nerve (acoustic neuroma) or stroke. Systemic disorders begin in a nerve or organ outside the cranium (e.g., orthostatic hypotension, hypoglycemia). Examples of common causes of vertigo and dizziness, grouped by etiology, are presented in Box 66–4.

Little can be done to reduce the risk of balance disorders. Clients should be treated early for manifestations of ear problems. Clients at high risk for falling as a result of vertigo should stand up slowly to prevent injury and should keep a light on at all times to enable visual cues to lessen the disequilibrium. Finally, situations that lead to vertigo should be avoided. Motion sickness occurs normally if the provocative stimulus is present. Humans are not evolutionarily adapted to special environmental situations, such as deep-sea diving, high-speed flying, and space travel. Vertigo or dizziness may occur in these environments.

BOX 66–4 Disorders Associated with Vertigo and Dizziness

Peripheral Labyrinthine (Inner Ear) Disorders

Benign paroxysmal positional vertigo (BPPV)
Labyrinthitis
Ménière's disease
Cholesteatoma

Central Nervous System Disorders

Cerebellar lesions
Temporal lobe lesions
Tumors of cranial nerve VIII (e.g., acoustic neuroma)
Stroke

Systemic Disorders

Diabetes
Postural hypotension
Arthritis
Hypoglycemia
Multiple sclerosis
Parkinson's disease
Allergies

PERIPHERAL VESTIBULAR DISORDERS

Benign Paroxysmal Positional Vertigo

Benign paroxysmal positional vertigo (BPPV) is a common cause of vertigo. It tends to follow head injury and viral infections of the inner ear. BPPV is due to *cupulolithiasis,* the presence of calcium crystals in the semicircular canals. These crystals are normally deposited on small hair-like structures in the ear called otoliths, and they slow responses to head movement. When they are dislodged, head movement creates a hypersensitive response. BPPV is provoked when the head is placed in certain positions, usually hyperextended and to one side. Clinical manifestations usually consist of brief attacks of rotational vertigo, a rapid head tilt to the affected ear, and a lag time of 3 to 6 seconds between change of position and vertigo with nystagmus. It is usually self-limited and resolves spontaneously over weeks to months.

Labyrinthitis (Vestibular Neuronitis)

Labyrinthitis is infection or inflammation of the cochlear or vestibular portion of the inner ear or both. Causes are not fully understood, but the syndrome tends to occur in spring and early summer and to be preceded by an upper respiratory infection. A virus has therefore been implicated but has never been isolated. Three classic manifestations are reported: vertigo, nausea, and vomiting. There are no hearing changes. Vertigo is usually sudden in onset; it peaks in 24 to 48 hours and then gradually subsides over 1 to 2 weeks. Supportive treatment is usually given during the wait for the underlying problems to clear.

Ménière's Disease

As mentioned previously, Ménière's disease is caused by excess endolymph in the vestibular and semicircular canals. Normal vestibular activity depends on stability of fluid pressure. Ménière's disease causes hearing changes and vertigo. It is discussed under balance disorders because the vertigo is often the most troublesome manifestation in the early stages.

Ménière's disease is an episodic illness that waxes and wanes, often remaining quiescent for many years and then reappearing. A cluster of manifestations develops, consisting of (1) paroxysmal whirling vertigo, (2) fluctuating hearing loss, (3) tinnitus, and (4) aural fullness. Only one or two manifestations may be present initially. Vertigo is characterized by remission and relapses without apparent cause, although the manifestations become less severe in time. The initial attacks consist of approximately 30 minutes of intense vertigo, which commonly provokes nausea and vomiting. Remaining stationary reduces vertigo.

A sensorineural hearing loss (see hearing impairment) that may be reversible in the early stages is a serious consequence of Ménière's disease. Control of episodes of the disease is usually possible, although a cure is not yet available. Clients are treated with low-sodium diets, diuretics, and balance exercises. Surgery, which is another option, is discussed later.

Central Disorders of Balance

Dizziness may be a manifestation of a transient ischemic attack (TIA) ("small stroke"). A temporary loss of blood flow to the brain leads to several manifestations, depending on the brain area that is not being perfused. Clients can experience momentary losses of consciousness, transient numbness, tingling, weakness, and changes in speech. TIAs should be reported and treated aggressively to prevent true ischemic changes.

Systemic Disorders Leading to Vertigo

Physiologic Vertigo

Physiologic vertigo is involved in common disorders such as motion sickness. In these conditions, vertigo is minimal or absent, but autonomic manifestations are present. Motion sickness leads to perspiration, nausea, vomiting, increased salivation, yawning, and malaise. Physiologic vertigo can usually be suppressed by supplying sensory cues that come from other stimuli. For example, motion sickness from reading in a car can be reduced by looking out the window at the moving environment.

Presbystasis

A disorder that is recognized more and more is presbystasis, or disequilibrium of aging. Because of the generalized degenerative changes that occur in aging, balance and stability are affected. In addition to the labyrinth, balance also depends on the visual system and the proprioceptive changes in the muscles. Because all three systems are involved in aging, the elderly have difficulty with stability, which results in falls and subsequent trauma.

Orthostatic Hypotension

Orthostatic hypotension is a sudden drop in blood pressure and dizziness upon sitting or standing. The manifestations noted are lightheadedness and faintness, not vertigo, which is due to inadequate cerebral blood flow. The elderly are at high risk of orthostatic hypotension because of atherosclerosis and the use of medications that lead to diuresis or hypotension (e.g., furosemide, calcium-channel blockers). Orthostasis is diagnosed through assessment of positional blood pressure changes. Clients should be taught to change position slowly, and medications may require adjustment if blood pressure is too low.

Pathophysiology

The body maintains balance and equilibrium by responding to an intricate network of information. The ability to maintain balance depends on the intactness of four systems:

- Vestibular system (the labyrinth or inner ear)
- Visual system (the eyes)
- Proprioceptive system (the somatosensory nerves of joints and muscles)
- Cerebellar system (the coordinator)

The sensations transmitted from the ears, the eyes, and the somatosensory nerves are integrated in the brain stem and cerebellum and perceived in the cerebral cortex. Gradual interference of vestibular input causes compensatory changes that allow the brain to adjust slowly. Quick changes demand more adjustments than can be made. Infections can destroy the nerve and alter transmission of messages. Overproduction of endolymph can slow transmission of messages and lead to the perception that the body is in constant motion. Head trauma can shake free calcium carbonate crystals on the utricular macule and alter endolymph movement.

Clinical Manifestations

Vertigo is the most common clinical manifestation in a client with a balance problem. The clinical manifestations of balance disorders vary widely depending on (1) the cause, (2) the location (one or both ears), (3) the client's age at onset, (4) the extent of the loss of vestibular function, and (5) the rapidity with which damage occurs. Disease in the external ear, middle ear, and inner ear usually leads to vertigo that is sudden, transient, and accompanied by vagal manifestations (e.g., nausea, vomiting, sweating, and pallor). The vertigo that is associated with cerebrovascular lesions does not follow a pattern; however, tinnitus and hearing loss are usually not present.

An important differentiation is whether the vertigo is associated with hearing loss. The close anatomic relationship between the balance and hearing systems sometimes causes the sensation of vertigo in conjunction with a hearing loss. However, in most instances, vertigo is present without a hearing loss. It is also important to distinguish between vertigo from vestibular problems and other forms of vertigo. Table 66–2 differentiates the two forms of vertigo.

Dizziness is described by clients in such varied terms that it is almost impossible to define. Not all the terms listed here suggest true vertigo. The nurse should record

TABLE 66–2 VESTIBULAR AND NONVESTIBULAR VERTIGO

	Vestibular	Nonvestibular
Common descriptions	Spinning (environment moves), on a merry-go-round	Lightheadedness, feeling of being dissociated from body, swimming, giddiness, spinning inside (environment stationary)
Clinical manifestations	Drunkenness, tilting, motion sickness, off-balance	
Course of illness	Episodic	Constant
Precipitating factors	Head movement, position change	Stress, hyperventilation, cardiac dysrhythmia, orthostatic hypotension
Associated manifestations	Nausea, vomiting, tinnitus, hearing loss, impaired vision, unsteadiness	Perspiration, pallor, paresthesias, palpitations, syncope, difficulty concentrating, tension headache; anxiety

the terms or description the client uses to help find the actual cause. Clinical manifestations include, but are not limited to:

- Staggering
- Giddiness
- Lightheadedness
- Disorientation
- Visual blurring
- Veering in one direction while walking
- Unsteadiness
- Reeling
- Faintness
- Wooziness
- Shakiness
- Instability
- Wobbliness
- Bewilderment
- Confusion
- Being dazed
- Clumsiness
- Sense of floating
- Sense of falling
- Weakness
- Vague feeling of uncertainty

Even after the vertigo has abated, anxiety tends to persist. Clients are very worried about having another "attack."

For the client with vertigo, the differential diagnosis may be accomplished by means of a thorough medical assessment, including audiometry, vestibular tests, imaging evaluation, and, sometimes, laboratory studies. Clients who have had vertigo may become quite anxious when they think about experiencing it again. Because vertigo is only a clinical manifestation, the diagnosis and treatment of the underlying disease are important. Unlike with vision or hearing problems, no single organ is responsible for balance problems. Therefore, the diagnosis, treatment, and rehabilitation of the client with a balance problem can be difficult as well as frustrating.

Outcome Management

Medical Management

Two main treatment goals guide the medical management of the client with vertigo. They are (1) suppression of the CNS and the vestibular system and (2) vestibular rehabilitation.

Suppress the Central Nervous System and Vestibular System

Treatment of acute vertigo involves several medicines, which are called antivertigo agents. These medicines tend to suppress the balance system or the CNS, allowing recovery over time. They should be used judiciously in clients with BPPV because they slow recovery of function. Other medicines used for specific disorders are antibiotics, steroids, diuretics, tranquilizers, and vitamins.

Promote Vestibular Rehabilitation

Vestibular rehabilitation is a recognized form of control for vertigo. Because the balance system can compensate, head and total body exercises are performed by the client to hasten compensation. Usually, physical therapists are involved in structuring this treatment. Vestibular rehabilitation uses all three organ systems that provide balance.

The exercises included in vestibular rehabilitation are performed as follows:

1. While lying in bed, slowly then quickly turn the eyes up, down, and from side to side, and the head forward, backward, and from side to side.
2. Perform the same exercises while sitting; in addition, bend forward and pick up objects from the ground.
3. While standing, perform the previously mentioned exercises; in addition, change from sitting to standing position with the eyes open and then closed, and turn around in between (i.e., change direction as well as position with eyes open and closed).
4. While moving about, walk up and down steps with the eyes open and then closed, or play games involving stooping and stretching, such as basketball.

It is believed that when vertigo is induced by these exercises, a tolerance for it is acquired. Clients should perform these exercises from the time of the acute attack and continue until they are free of manifestations for two consecutive days. Driving a car safely needs to be addressed with clients who have vertigo.

A specific intervention strategy that is currently being utilized involves a series of manipulative interventions known as the *Epley maneuvers*. These maneuvers, which are used specifically for BPPV, are designed to facilitate return of dislodged otoliths to their more normal position within the labyrinth. The Epley maneuvers are essentially a more direct, rapid method to restore normal function and are of variable efficacy.

Nursing Management of the Medical Client

Assessment

Nursing assessment of the client with a balance problem should consist of the following areas:

1. A client interview to obtain a health history and specific information about the onset and characteristics of the balance problem and associated hearing problems. Attempt to distinguish the type of vertigo reported, and note aggravating conditions (e.g., head movement).
2. An interview with a family member to determine the effects of the client's balance problem on others.
3. Assessment of the effect of the vertigo on the client's performance of the activities of daily living.

The importance of the history and interview cannot be overemphasized. An adequate description of vertigo should include information about the onset, exacerbating and alleviating factors, associated clinical manifestations, and predisposing factors in the medical history, as previously described. All clients bring some degree of anxiety regarding this illness to the examina-

BOX 66–5 Assessment Guide for Clients with Balance Disorders

A. When you are dizzy, do you experience any of the following sensations? Please read the entire list first. Then circle the numbers of those sensations that describe what you experience most accurately.
   1. Lightheadedness
   2. Tendency to lose balance or to fall
   3. Objects spinning or turning around you
   4. Sensation that you are turning
   5. Headache
   6. Nausea or vomiting
   7. Pressure in the head

B. Please fill in the blank spaces.
   1. When did the dizziness first occur? ______
   2. Is your vertigo constant? ______
   3. Does it come in attacks? ______
   4. How often do attacks occur? ______
   5. How long are the attacks? ______
   6. Does vertigo occur only in certain positions? ______
      When upright? ______
      When lying flat? ______
      Turning to the right? ______
      Turning to the left? ______
   7. Have you ever stumbled or fallen because of vertigo? ______
   8. Do you know of anything that will stop the vertigo or make it better? ______
      Make your vertigo worse? ______
      Bring on an attack? ______
   9. Did you ever injure your head? ______
   10. Do you take any medications regularly (e.g., tranquilizers; oral contraceptives; barbiturates; a course of antibiotics, such as streptomycin, neomycin)? ______
   11. Do you use tobacco in any form? ______
       Alcohol? ______
   12. Have you worked for long in a noisy environment? ______
   13. Do you suffer easily from motion sickness? ______

tion. Balance problems can have devastating effects on a client's behavior. The disruption of the client's routine, the severity of the "attacks," and the fear of the unknown can make the client agitated, anxious, or depressed. The nurse must be aware of these feelings and must demonstrate self-confidence, patience, courtesy, and gentleness.

A structured questionnaire such as the one shown in Box 66–5 should be completed by the client. These questions can also be used to facilitate the interview. However, the interview should be guided by client cues. A gross assessment of the client's balance can be made by watching the client's gait. Evidence of instability may be noted if the client touches the wall or walks with a wide-based, waddling gait.

The same inspection, palpation, and otoscopic examination should be performed for the client with a balance problem as was performed for the client with hearing loss (see earlier discussion). The client must be questioned for the loss of hearing and tinnitus, which can accompany a balance problem.

DIAGNOSIS, OUTCOMES, INTERVENTIONS

Nursing care of the client with vertigo is detailed in the Care Plan.

Surgical Management

Approximately 5% or less of all clients with vertigo undergo surgical intervention.

ENDOLYMPHATIC SAC SURGERY

The endolymphatic sac procedures include decompression and various forms of shunts to the CNS or mastoid cavity. The intent of these procedures is to lessen the fluid pressure within the labyrinth and control the vertigo of Ménière's disease. Forty-four studies have been conducted over the past decade to determine the efficacy of endolymphatic sac procedures. A collective review of the results of 1800 cases of various surgical approaches to the endolymphatic sac found that 22% of clients had improved hearing, 53% had no change in hearing acuity, and 25% had worsened hearing as determined by the established guidelines. Refinement of surgical approaches and outcomes research on these techniques continues to be important.

LABYRINTHECTOMY

Labyrinthectomy is a form of surgery designed to destroy the labyrinth and eliminate its abnormal input. It is performed through the oval or round window (membranous limits of cochlear and inner ear). This is a destructive procedure that removes the membranous labyrinth, either subtotally through the oval window or totally through the mastoid bone. Any remaining hearing is sacrificed.

In a nonsurgical approach to labyrinthectomy, an ototoxic drug can be injected through the tympanic membrane into the middle ear in order to destroy the hair cells of the vestibular system. This procedure is carried out over a series of visits and is designed to decrease the abnormal vestibular signal in the affected ear. A secondary and sometimes unavoidable effect is concurrent cochlear toxicity. Clients are treated until their vestibular manifestations improve significantly, with the goal of preserving as much hearing as possible.

VESTIBULAR NERVE RESECTION

Vestibular nerve resection is a highly effective procedure performed to alleviate vertigo. Vestibular nerve resection can be performed through the labyrinth (sacrificing hearing) or around the labyrinth (saving hearing). The retrolabyrinthine surgical approach is the most common form of surgical control for vertigo today. This method preserves the inner ear structures and approaches the vestibular nerve from behind the semicircular canal. Alleviation of the client's vertigo is usually immediate. Because of the compensation by all of the other structures related to maintaining balance, a client can function with only one labyrinth.

C A R E   P L A N

THE CLIENT WITH VERTIGO

Nursing Diagnosis. Risk for Injury related to tendency to lose balance.

Outcomes. The client will reduce the risk of injury by moving slowly, remaining immobile when dizzy, and using aids for ambulation if gait and balance are unstable.

Interventions	Rationales
1. While the client is at bed rest:	1. Basis for intervention:
a. Encourage the client to move in bed slowly.	a. Slow movement allows the vestibular system time to regain balance and integrate messages.
b. Minimize the client's head movement during acute attacks.	b. Eye and head movements often aggravate vertigo.
c. Darken the room.	c. Darkness may help reduce acute vertigo.
d. Avoid startling the client to reduce reflexic head movement.	d. The risk of vertigo caused by sudden movement is reduced.
e. Help the client with hygiene as needed while encouraging independence.	e. Assistance protects the client from slipping. Complete care may be needed.
f. Keep the side rails up and the bed in low position when the client is in bed. Place call light, phone, and personal articles within the client's reach.	f. Side rails remind the client to call for help. A low bed position limits distance to the floor in case of falls from bed. Placing articles within reach decreases the client's risk of falling when reaching for articles.
g. Help with ambulation as needed.	g. Reduces risk of falls.

Evaluation. Expect this outcome to be met over several days. Look for small improvements, and encourage the client.

Nursing Diagnosis. Risk for Impaired Adjustment related to a required change in lifestyle secondary to unpredictability of vertigo.

Outcomes. The client will adjust to or modify his or her lifestyle to decrease disability and exert maximal control and independence within limits imposed by vertigo and balance disorder.

Interventions	Rationales
1. Encourage the client to identify personal strengths and roles that can still be fulfilled.	1. Encouragement fosters positive self-esteem.
2. Encourage the client to talk about feelings, personal perception of danger, and perception of his or her own coping skills and limitations.	2. Allows nurse to provide individualized support.
3. Encourage the client to make decisions and assume responsibility for self-care.	3. Personal responsibility helps the client to maintain a sense of control.
4. Provide information about vertigo and how to prepare for attacks.	4. Education promotes a problem-solving approach to managing the disorder.
5. Encourage the client to perform balance exercises.	5. Balance exercises reduce the severity of attacks by training the central nervous system to adjust to changes in position.
6. Include the client's family and significant others in discussions.	6. Family involvement promotes awareness and, hopefully fosters support.

Evaluation. Achievement of this outcome rests almost entirely on the client's willingness to modify a previous lifestyle and his or her ability to overcome limits that can be felt from vertigo.

Nursing Diagnosis. Impaired Verbal Communication related to decreased hearing and tinnitus.

Outcomes. The client will report satisfaction with ability to communicate.

Interventions	Rationales
1. Assess the client's hearing acuity and audiogram results.	1. Assessment results provide factual information on the severity of hearing loss.
2. Speak distinctly and enunciate words without shouting.	2. Clear speech facilitates hearing and comprehension.
3. Use picture boards or write to communicate.	3. These are alternate methods of communication.
4. Assess the client for hearing aid candidacy, and make needed referrals.	4. Hearing aids augment sound.

continued

Evaluation. This outcome may require several days to achieve. Hearing loss is reversible in early stages but may become permanent if prolonged.

Nursing Diagnosis. Risk for Fluid Volume Deficit related to decreased oral intake and loss of fluids through emesis.

Outcomes. The client will maintain adequate fluid volume, as evidenced by normal blood pressure, normal pulse rate, quick skin turgor, moist oral mucous membranes, and adequate urine output.

Interventions	Rationales
1. Assess the client's pulse, respiration, and blood pressure every 4 hours (if stable).	1. Hypotension and tachycardia are indicators of dehydration.
2. Assess the client's skin turgor, oral mucous membranes, oral intake, and urine output every 8 hours (if stable).	2. Decreased skin turgor, dry mucous membranes, and oliguria are indicators of dehydration.
3. Compare intake with output, and consider intravenous fluids if the output is greater than intake for several hours.	3. Intake should equal output over 24 hours. Urine output should be 20–30ml/hr. Intravenous fluids are another access for fluids.
4. Encourage the client to drink fluids.	4. Lost fluids should be replaced.
5. Teach the client to avoid caffeinated beverages.	5. Caffeine is a vestibular stimulant.
6. Administer antiemetics as ordered, and observe for side effects of medications given.	6. Antiemetics reduce the risk of emesis and allow for increased oral intake.
7. Encourage the client to try resting on the unaffected ear.	7. Gravity facilitates drainage from the affected ear.

Evaluation. If the client's nausea can be controlled, fluid balance should be achievable within 24 to 48 hours.

Nursing Diagnosis. Powerlessness related to feelings of loss of control secondary to unpredictability of vertigo.

Outcomes. The client will verbalize ways to maintain control and respond to vertigo.

Interventions	Rationales
1. Assess the client's cognitive appraisal of illness.	1. Cognitive appraisal of the illness provides information about the client's perception of the illness and how much control the client feels he or she has over vertigo.
2. Assess the client's previous coping strategies.	2. The client will use previous coping strategies during this new stress.
3. Help the client develop coping strategies based on past coping skills and situational support available to the client.	3. Reuse effective past coping strategies. Situation support can help bridge the client's return to society.
4. Stress the importance of maintaining or resuming normal activities or developing diversionary activities.	4. Reduces the risk that client will become disabled by vertigo. Activity also reduces depression.
5. Provide needed information about vertigo: a. Information about prescribed medications b. Manifestations requiring medical attention (e.g., a sudden loss of hearing, a change in the current level of hearing, visual disturbances, weakness or numbness in the extremities, seizures, loss of consciousness, or progressive worsening of vertigo)	5. Encourages the use of problem-solving and coping.
6. Refer the client to support groups in the community.	6. The client may benefit from interaction with others and may learn effective methods to cope with the disorder.

Evaluation. Feelings of powerlessness may require weeks to months to resolve, especially if vertigo is chronic.

CONCLUSIONS

Nurses caring for clients with hearing and balance problems need to focus on safety and on promoting independence. Many hearing-impaired clients live a normal life with hearing augmentation and aural rehabilitation. Clients who have diminished hearing or balance disorders are at increased risk for injury because of lack of awareness of the risks or from losing balance. Infections of the ears remain common, but excellent antibiotics have reduced the incidence of chronic problems caused by infections. Tumors of the ear are rare, but when they occur, they are quite destructive.

THINKING CRITICALLY

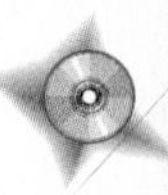

1. A middle-aged man comes to the health clinic with ear pain and difficulty hearing. He had some serous drainage 1 day ago but does not recall any recent infection (throat or ear). The problem has persisted intermittently over the past 6 months and is getting progressively more painful and occurring more frequently. If surgery were deemed necessary for this client, how would you prepare him? What discharge teaching might need to be completed for this client after ear surgery?

Factors to Consider. What preoperative assessments are needed? How should equal pressures be maintained on the tympanic membrane? What normal occurrences might the client expect in the initial period following surgery?

2. **An elderly woman reveals a 10-year history of ear infection. She is experiencing sensorineural hearing loss associated with presbycusis, which affects older people. During her clinic appointment, she tells the nurse that her right ear is painful and is keeping her awake at night. She explains that she can hear most sounds, although sounds on the right side seem to be coming through a filter. She has been using her eardrops as directed but has stopped taking her oral antibiotic because she felt better 2 days ago. She requests information about daily medication or a surgical procedure that might alleviate the problem. How should you respond to this client's request? How do age-related changes contribute to her problem?**

Factors to Consider. What is the assessment focus for this client? What is the prognosis for the client with presbycusis? What type of teaching does the client require?

BIBLIOGRAPHY

1. Balkany, T., Hodges, A. V., & Luntz, M. (1996). Update on cochlear implantation. *Otolaryngologic Clinics of North America, 29*(2), 277–289.
2. Clendaniel, R. A., & Tucci, D. L. (1997). Vestibular rehabilitation strategies in Ménière's disease. *Otolaryngologic Clinics of North America, 30*(6), 1145–1158.
3. Cruickshanks, K. J., et al. (1998). Cigarette smoking and hearing loss: The epidemiology of hearing loss study. *Journal of the American Medical Association, 279*, 1715–1719.
4. Cummings, C. W., et al. (1998). *Otolaryngology-head and neck surgery* (3rd ed.). St. Louis: Mosby–Year Book.
5. Fairbanks, D. N. F. (1999). *Antimicrobial therapy in otolaryngology–head and neck surgery* (9th ed.). Alexandria, VA: American Academy of Otolaryngology–Head and Neck Surgery.
6. Gershman, K., & Nielsen, C. (1995). Prevention and screening in the nursing home. *Clinics in Primary Care, 22*(4), 731–753.
7. Girardi, M., & Konrad, H. R. (1998). Vestibular rehabilitation therapy for the patient with dizziness and balance disorders. *ORL–Head and Neck Nursing, 16*(4), 13–21.
8. Glasscock, M. E., & Stambaugh, G. E. (1990). *Surgery of the ear.* Philadelphia: W. B. Saunders.
9. Grant, I. L. & Welling, D. B. (1997). The treatment of hearing loss in Ménière's disease. *Otolaryngologic Clinics of North America, 30*(6), 1123–1144.
10. Hughes, G. B., et al. (1996). Sudden sensorineural hearing loss. *Otolaryngologic Clinics of North America, 29*(3), 393–405.
11. Jamieson, D. G., Brennan, R. L., & Cornelisse, L. E. (1995). Evaluation of speech enhancement strategy with normal-hearing and hearing-impaired listeners. *Ear and Hearing, 16*(3), 274–286.
12. Jerger, J., et al. (1995). Hearing impairment in older adults: New concepts. *Journal of the American Geriatric Society, 43*(8), 928–935.
13. Karver, S. B. (1998). Otitis media. *Primary Care, 25*(3), 619–632.
14. La Rosa, S. (1998). Primary care management of otitis externa. *The Nurse Practitioner, 23*(6), 125–128, 131–133.
15. Linstrom, C. J. (1998). Cochlear implantation: Practical information for the generalist. *Primary Care, 25*(3), 583–612.
16. Maniglia, A. J. (1996). State of the art on the development of the implantable hearing device for partial hearing loss. *Otolaryngologic Clinics of North America, 29*(2), 225–243.
17. Monsell, E. M., & Harley, R. E. (1996). Eustachian tube dysfunction. *Otolaryngologic Clinics of North America, 29*(3), 466–444.
18. Nobel, W., Ter-Horst, K., & Byrne, D. (1995). Disabilities and handicaps associated with impaired auditory localization. *Journal of the American Academy of Audiology, 6*(2), 129–140.
19. Pollock, K. J. (1995). Ménière's disease: A review of the problem. *ORL–Head and Neck Nursing, 13*(2), 10–13.
20. Seidman, M. D., & Jacobson, G. P. (1996). Update on tinnitus. *Otolaryngologic Clinics of North America, 29*(3), 455–465.
21. Sigler, B., & Schuring, L. T. (1993). *Ear, nose and throat disorders.* St. Louis: Mosby–Year Book.
22. Silverman, C. A. (1998). Audiologic assessment and amplification. *Primary Care, 25*(3), 545–581.
23. Slattery, W. H., & Fayad, J. N. (1997). Medical treatment of Ménière's disease. *Otolaryngologic Clinics of North America, 30*(6), 1027–1066.
24. Society of Otorhinolaryngology–Head and Neck Nurses. (1994). *Guidelines for otorhinolaryngology head and neck nursing practice.* New Smyrna Beach, FL: Author.
25. Telian, S. A., & Shepard, N. T. (1996). Update on vestibular rehabilitation therapy. *Otolaryngologic Clinics of North America, 29*(2), 359–661.
26. Weber, P. C., & Adkins, W. Y., Jr. (1997). The differential diagnosis of Ménière's disease. *Otolaryngologic Clinics of North America, 30*(6), 977–986.

UNIT 15

Cognitive and Perceptual Disorders

Anatomy and Physiology Review
The Neurologic System

Joyce M. Black

The nervous system is the body's most organized and complex structural and functional system. It profoundly affects both psychological and physiologic function. This unit discusses the importance of the nervous system to human function and the major consequences of neurologic disorders.

CENTRAL NERVOUS SYSTEM

The brain and spinal cord are known collectively as the *central nervous system* (CNS). The CNS is divided into three major functional divisions:

1. Higher-level brain or cerebral cortex
2. Lower brain level (basal ganglia, thalamus, hypothalamus, midbrain, pons, medulla, cerebellum)
3. Spinal cord

These structures are protected by a rigid bony encasement, three layers of membranes, a fluid cushion, and a blood-brain or blood–spinal cord barrier.

BRAIN

The brain is the largest and most complex part of the nervous system. It is composed of more than 100 billion neurons and associated fibers. The brain tissues have a gelatin-like consistency. This semi-solid organ weighs about 1400 g (~3 pounds) in the adult.

■ CEREBRUM

The cerebrum is divided by a deep groove (longitudinal fissure) into two sections called *cerebral hemispheres.* A transverse fissure separates the cerebrum from the cerebellum. The outermost layer of the cerebrum, the *cerebral cortex,* is only 2 to 5 mm thick. Directly beneath the cerebral cortex are varying thicknesses of association tracts above the commisural tracts, known as the *corpus callosum* (Fig. U15–1).

The cerebral cortex is composed of gray matter (predominantly nerve cell bodies and dendrites) formed into raised convolutions, or gyri. Approximately 75% of the neuronal cell bodies in the brain are found in the cortex. The shallow grooves between the gyri *(sulci)* divide the cerebral cortex into five lobes: frontal, parietal, occipital, temporal, and central (insula) (Fig. U15–2).

The term *neocortex* is often used to refer to the cerebral cortex. The neocortex includes all of the cerebral cortex except the olfactory portions and the hippocampal regions.

Both the left cortex and the right cortex interpret sensory data, store memories, learn, and form concepts. However, each hemisphere dominates the other in many functions. In most people, for example, the *left* cortex has dominance for systematic analysis, language and speech, mathematics, abstraction, and reasoning. The *right* cortex has dominance for assimilation of sensory experiences, such as visual-spatial information, and activities such as dancing, gymnastics, music, and art appreciation.

In the frontal lobes, the precentral gyrus (motor cortex) controls voluntary motor activity. Most of these fibers cross to the opposite side of the brain at the medulla and descend via the spinal cord as the lateral corticospinal tracts. The area anterior to the precentral gyrus (the premotor area) is also associated with voluntary motor activities. *Broca's area,* lying anterior to the primary motor cortex and superior to the lateral sulcus, coordinates the complex muscular activity of the mouth, tongue, and larynx, which makes expressive (motor) speech possible. Damage to this area leaves the client unable to speak clearly, a disorder called *Broca's aphasia.*

The *prefrontal areas* control (1) attention over time (concentration); (2) motivation, (3) ability to formulate or select goals; (4) ability to plan; (5) ability to initiate, maintain, or terminate actions; (6) ability to self-monitor, and (7) ability to use feedback (called "executive functions"). These same areas are thought to contribute to reasoning, problem-solving activities, and emotional stability by inhibiting the limbic areas of the cerebrum (see later).

Each *parietal lobe,* located posterior to the central sulcus of Rolando, contains a primary somatic (tactile) receptive area and the somatic (tactile) association areas. The post-central gyrus and the posterior portion of the paracentral lobule are the primary receptive (interpretation) areas for tactile sensations (e.g., temperature, touch, pressure). The association areas occupy the remainder of the parietal lobe. Concept formation and abstraction are carried out by the parietal association areas. The right parietal areas are also dominant for spatial orientation and awareness of size and shapes (stereognosis) and body position (proprioception). The left parietal areas assist with right-left orientation and mathematics.

Each *occipital lobe* contains a primary visual receptive (interpretation) area and visual association areas. The primary visual cortex is on either side of the calcarine sulcus. The other areas of the occipital cortices are visual association areas. Visual memories are stored in these areas, which contribute to our ability to visually recognize and understand our environment.

Each *temporal lobe* is located under (caudal to) the lateral sulcus. The temporal lobe contains a primary auditory receptive area and secondary auditory association areas. Spoken language memories are stored in the left temporal auditory association areas. All other sound memories that are not language (e.g., music, various animal sounds, other noises) are stored in the right temporal lobe auditory areas. Damage to these areas would leave us unable to understand spoken or written language or

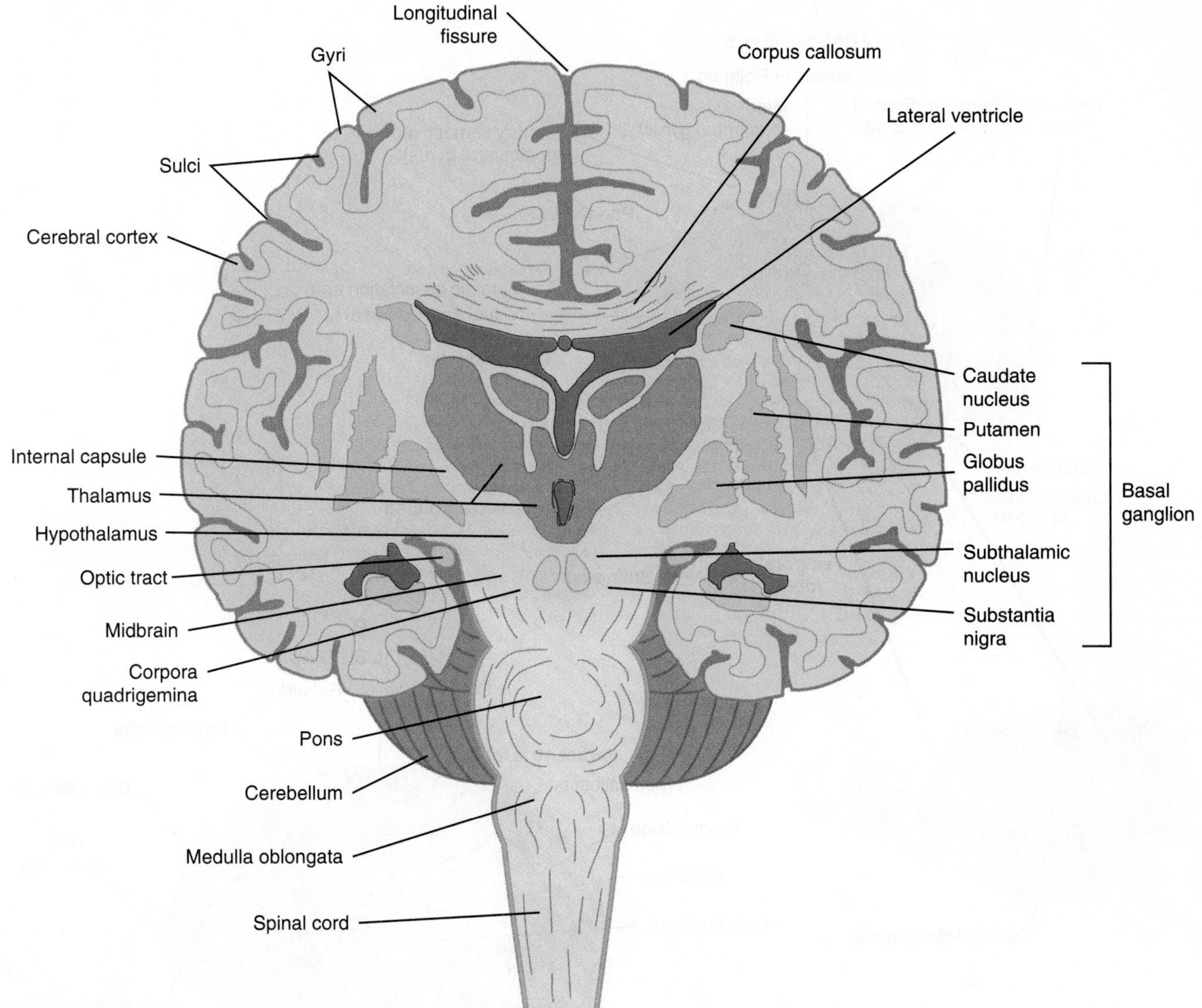

FIGURE U15–1 Structures of the brain (coronal section).

to recognize music or other environmental sounds. Cells that facilitate understanding language reside in Wernicke's area.

The *central (insula) lobe* is located deep within the lateral sulcus and is surrounded by the frontal, parietal, and temporal lobes. Nerve fibers for taste pass through the parietal lobe to the insular lobe. Many association fibers leading to other parts of the cerebral cortex pass through this lobe.

■ HIPPOCAMPUS

The hippocampus, a part of the medial section of the temporal lobe, plays an essential role in the process of *memory,* a very complex phenomenon. Three levels of memory have been identified:

1. *Short-term (recent) memory* is lost after seconds or minutes.
2. *Intermediate memory* lasts days to weeks and eventually is lost.
3. *Long-term (remote) memory* is stored and lasts a lifetime.

Theories about the physiologic basis of memory suggest that reverberating neuronal messages cause short-term memory and that actual neuronal structural changes lead to long-term memory. The hippocampus assists in the conversion of short-term memory into intermediate and long-term memory in the thalamus. The association fibers of the frontal, parietal, temporal, and occipital lobes as well as the diencephalon is important in long-term memory.[2]

■ BASAL GANGLIA

The basal ganglia consist of several structures of subcortical gray matter buried deep in the cerebral hemispheres. These structures include the caudate nucleus, putamen, globus pallidus, substantia nigra, and subthalamic nucleus. The basal ganglia serve as processing stations linking the cerebral cortex to thalamic nuclei. Almost all the motor and sensory fibers connecting the cerebral cortex and the spinal cord travel through the white matter pathways near the caudate nucleus and putamen ganglia. These pathways are known as the *in-*

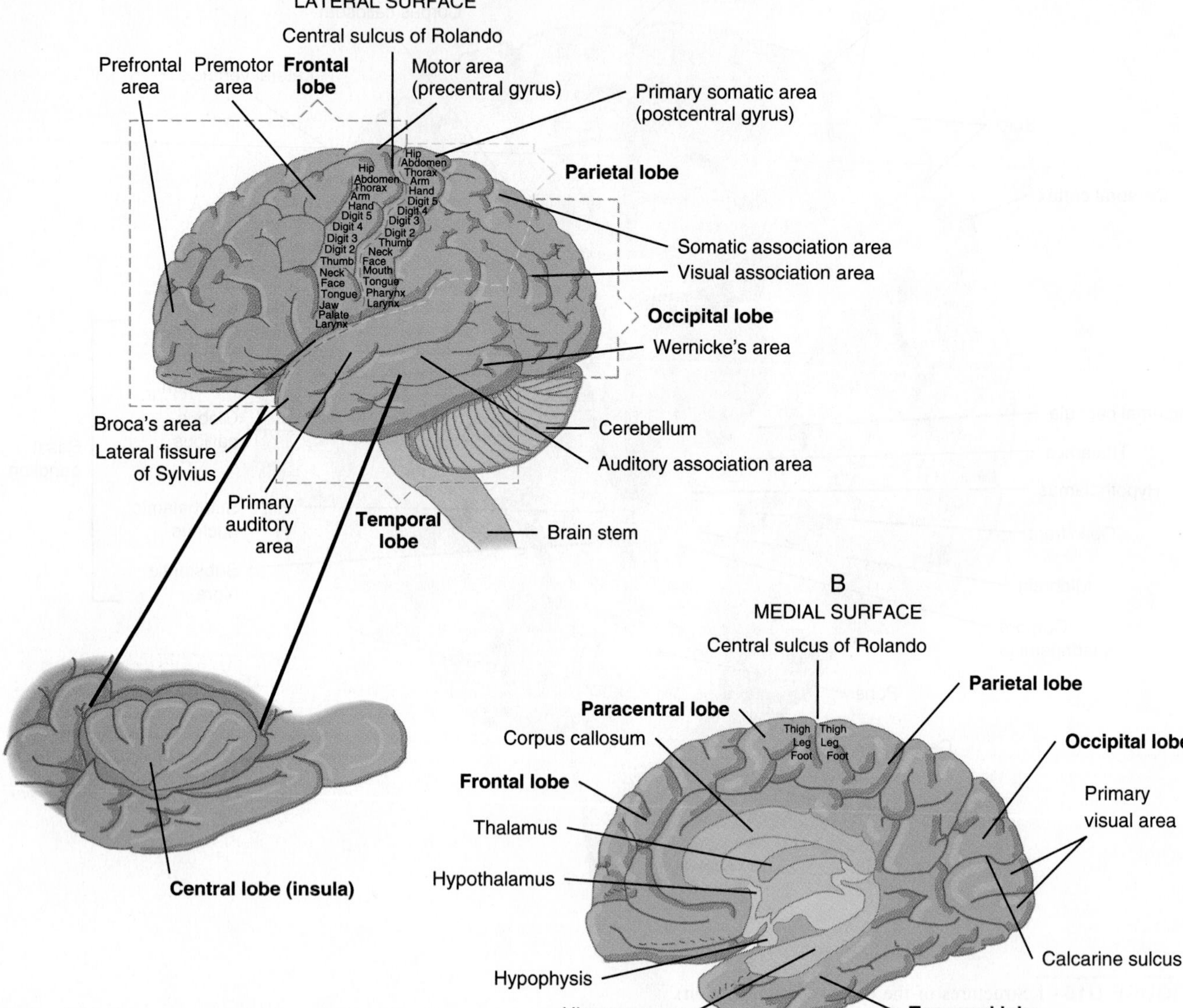

FIGURE U15–2 The lateral *(A)* and medial *(B)* surfaces of the cerebral cortex. The central lobe is the fifth lobe.

ternal capsule. The basal ganglia, along with the corticospinal tract, is important in controlling complex motor activity.

■ DIENCEPHALON

The diencephalon is composed of the thalamus and the hypothalamus. The *thalamus* lies between the cerebral hemispheres and superior to the brain stem. Its gray matter surrounds the lateral edges of the third ventricle. The *hypothalamus* forms the floor of the third ventricle. Other important structures found in and near the diencephalon include (1) the optic tracts and optic chiasm, (2) the pituitary gland on the floor of the diencephalon, and (3) the pineal gland on the roof of the diencephalon.

The thalamus channels all ascending (sensory) information, except smell, to the appropriate cortical cells. The hypothalamus regulates autonomic nervous system (ANS) functions such as heart rate, blood pressure, water and electrolyte balance, stomach and intestinal motility, glandular activity, body temperature, hunger, body weight, and sleep-wakefulness. It also serves as the master over the pituitary gland by releasing factors that stimulate or inhibit pituitary gland output.

■ LIMBIC SYSTEM

The limbic system is made up of many nuclei, including parts of the medial portion of the frontal and temporal lobes (hippocampus), thalamus, hypothalamus, and the basal ganglia. It is considered the center for feelings and control of emotional expression (fear, anger, pleasure, sorrow). The limbic system (the temporal lobe component) also receives nerve fibers from the olfactory bulbs and thus plays an essential role in the interpretation of smells.

■ BRAIN STEM

The brain stem is composed of the midbrain, pons, and medulla oblongata (Table U15–1). These structures are

TABLE U15–1 **BRAIN STEM STRUCTURES AND THEIR FUNCTIONS**

Structures	Functions
MIDBRAIN	
Corpora quadrigemina	
Superior colliculi	Visual reflexes
Inferior colliculi	Auditory reflexes
Cerebral aqueduct	
Origin of CN III and IV	
Ascending sensory pathways	
Reticular formation	
Red nuclei	Motor pathways to spinal cord, cerebellum
Paired crura cerebri	Afferent/efferent cerebellar pathways
Substantia nigra	Part of basal ganglia
Descending motor pathways	
PONS	
Fourth ventricle	
Nuclei of inferior colliculus	Auditory processing
Nuclei of CN V, VI, VII	
Locus ceruleus	Secretes norepinephrine
Raphe nuclei	Secretes serotonin
Ascending sensory pathways	
Medial lemniscus, auditory pathway	Proprioceptive pathways
Descending motor pathways	
Medial longitudinal fasciculi	Efferent pathway to spinal cord
Pyramids (corticospinal, corticobulbar, corticopontine)	Voluntary motor
Reticular formation	
Respiratory centers	
Pontine nuclei; pontocerebellar fibers	
MEDULLA OBLONGATA	
Fourth ventricle	
Central canal	
Raphe nuclei	Secretes serotonin
Ascending sensory pathways	
Medial lemniscal pathways	Proprioceptive pathways
Spinothalamic tracts	Pain pathways
Trigeminothalamic tracts	Tactile, temperature
Lateral lemnisci	Auditory pathways
Nuclei of CN VIII, IX, X, XI, XII	
Olive and vestibular-cerebellar systems	
Reflex centers: respiratory, vasomotor, cardiac, coughing, swallowing, sneezing, vomiting	
Reticular formation	
Descending motor pathways (pyramids)	Voluntary motor

CN, cranial nerve.

continuous segments of the diencephalon nuclei. They are composed of ascending pathways, the reticular formation, cranial nerves and their nuclei, and descending autonomic and motor pathways.

RETICULAR FORMATION

The reticular formation is composed of a complex network of gray matter (nuclei), ascending reticular pathways, and descending reticular pathways. Its nuclei extend from the superior part of the spinal cord to the diencephalon and communicate with the basal ganglia, cerebrum, and cerebellum.

The reticular formation assists in regulation of skeletal motor movement and spinal reflexes. It also filters incoming sensory information to the cerebral cortex. Approximately 99% of sensory information is disregarded as unessential. One component of the reticular formation, the reticular activating system, controls the sleep-wake cycle (see Chapter 22) and consciousness.

CEREBELLUM

The cerebellum is composed of gray and white matter. The cortex of the cerebellum is a thin layer of gray matter arranged in parallel long and deep gyri, called *folia,* and separated by cerebellar sulci (Fig. U15–3). Deep fissures divide the cerebellum into three lobes, but the functional division of the cerebellum consists of a right and left hemisphere separated by a narrow band of white matter called the *vermis.* An extension of dura mater, the falx cerebelli, partially separates the hemispheres.

The cerebellum integrates sensory information related to position of body parts, coordinates skeletal muscle movement, and regulates muscle tension, which is necessary for balance and posture. Three pairs of nerve tracts (cerebellar peduncles) provide the communication pathways. The inferior peduncles are sensory (afferent) pathways from the spinal cord and medulla, which carry information related to the position of body parts to the cerebellum. The middle peduncles carry information from the cerebral cortex to effector cells that control voluntary (purposeful) motor activities. The cerebellum also receives sensory input from the receptors in the muscles, tendons, joints, eyes, and inner ear. After this information is integrated and analyzed, the cerebellum sends impulses via the superior peduncles (efferent pathways) to the brain stem and spinal cord and then to the appropriate body parts (effectors) to make connections.

Most of the tracts in the cerebellum travel through various nuclei without crossing. Therefore, the right cerebellar hemisphere predominantly affects the right (ipsilateral) side of the body and vice versa.

SPINAL CORD

The spinal cord, that portion of the CNS surrounded and protected by the vertebral column, is continuous with the medulla and lies within the upper two thirds of the vertebral canal (the cavity within the vertebral column). The lower spinal cord terminates caudally in a cone-shaped structure known as the *conus medullaris* at the level of the first (L1) and second (L2) lumbar vertebrae. The spinal cord is subdivided into four areas: (1) cervical cord, (2) thoracic cord, (3) lumbar area, and (4) sacral cord (conus medullaris) (Fig. U15–4).

Within the spinal cord, butterfly-shaped gray matter (mostly unmyelinated) is surrounded by mostly myelinated white matter. The white matter consists of *ascend-*

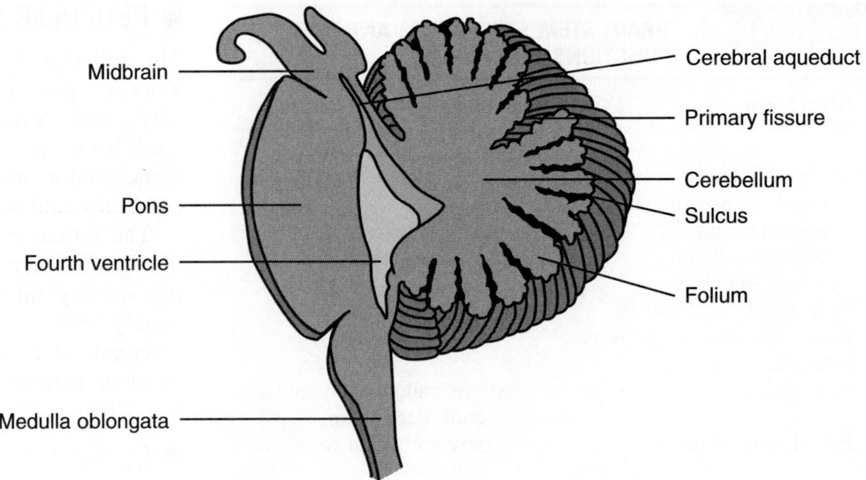

FIGURE U15–3 Sagittal view of the brain stem, fourth ventricle, and cerebellum.

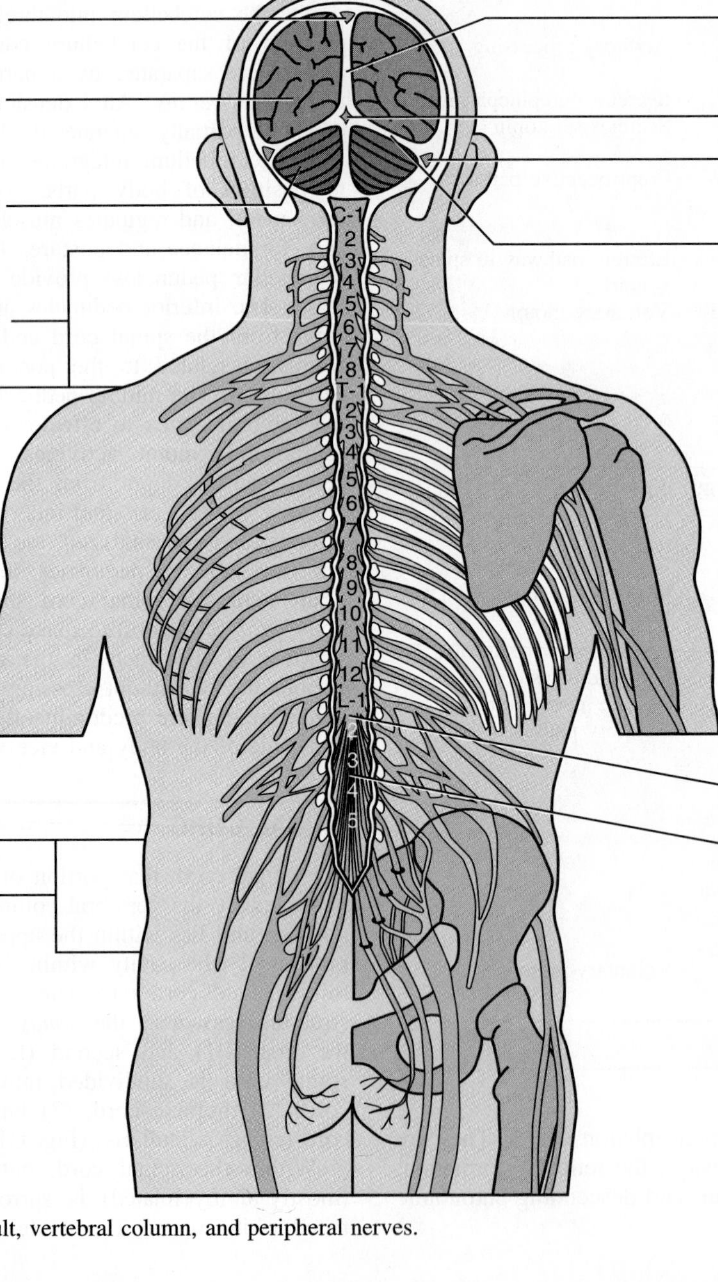

FIGURE U15–4 Cranial vault, vertebral column, and peripheral nerves.

ing tracts and *descending tracts* that conduct nerve impulses between the brain and the cells outside the CNS. The cell bodies in the gray matter are grouped into clusters of nuclei and laminae (a defined group or column of cells). The tracts in the white matter are arranged into three paired columns: posterior, lateral, and anterior (Fig. U15–5, *inset*).

■ ASCENDING AND DESCENDING PATHWAYS

The *ascending (sensory) pathways* in the spinal cord eventually terminate in the cerebral and cerebellar cortex. Motor impulses from the brain, which travel through the *descending pathways,* terminate in the muscles and glands. For example, a spinothalamic tract, which is a sensory tract, begins in the spinal cord and ends in the parietal lobe. The corticospinal tract is a descending tract that originates in the frontal lobe of the cerebral cortex, travels through the spinal cord, and terminates in the muscle cells. These motor neurons, which originate in the frontal lobe and continue through the corticospinal tract, are also referred to as *upper motor neurons. Lower motor neurons* are cells that begin in the anterior horn of the spinal cord and pass into the spinal nerves.

Table U15–2 summarizes the specific functions of the major brain and spinal cord tracts.

Many of the tracts communicating with the cerebral cortex cross (decussate), but not all cross at the same place. The term *contralateral* refers to tracts that cross at the medulla and ascend or descend to the opposite side of the body; *ipsilateral* (same-sided) tracts do not cross. For example, sensory tracts (including the anterior spinothalamic, posterior, and anterior spinocerebellar tracts) cross in the medulla as they ascend to the cerebral cortex. Therefore, the sensory neurons in the cerebral cortex interpret sensory stimuli from the contralateral side of the body.

The lateral corticospinal spinal tract (the pyramidal tract) crosses at the medulla as it descends from the frontal lobe of the cerebral cortex to the spinal cord. The posterior spinocerebellar tracts are ipsilateral tracts and thus coordinate muscular function on the same side of the body. The crossing of the lateral spinothalamic tract is unique.

PROTECTIVE AND NUTRITIONAL STRUCTURES

■ CRANIUM AND VERTEBRAL COLUMN

Eight bones that fuse early in childhood compose the cranium. The fused junctions are called *sutures.* The cranium encloses the brain structures and serves as a source of protection.

The floor, or basilar plate, of the cranial vault has three depressions, called *fossae.* The frontal lobes lie in the anterior fossa. The temporal lobes and the base of the diencephalon lie in the middle fossa. The cerebellum rests in the posterior fossa.

The vertebral column, a flexible series of vertebrae, surrounds and protects the spinal cord. The vertebral column consists of seven cervical vertebrae, 12 thoracic vertebrae, five lumbar vertebrae, five sacral vertebrae fused into a sacrum, and four coccygeal vertebrae fused into a coccyx. Ligaments hold the vertebrae together, and discs between the vertebrae prevent the bones from rubbing together.

■ MENINGES

The meninges, three membranes enveloping the brain and spinal cord, are predominantly for protection (Fig.

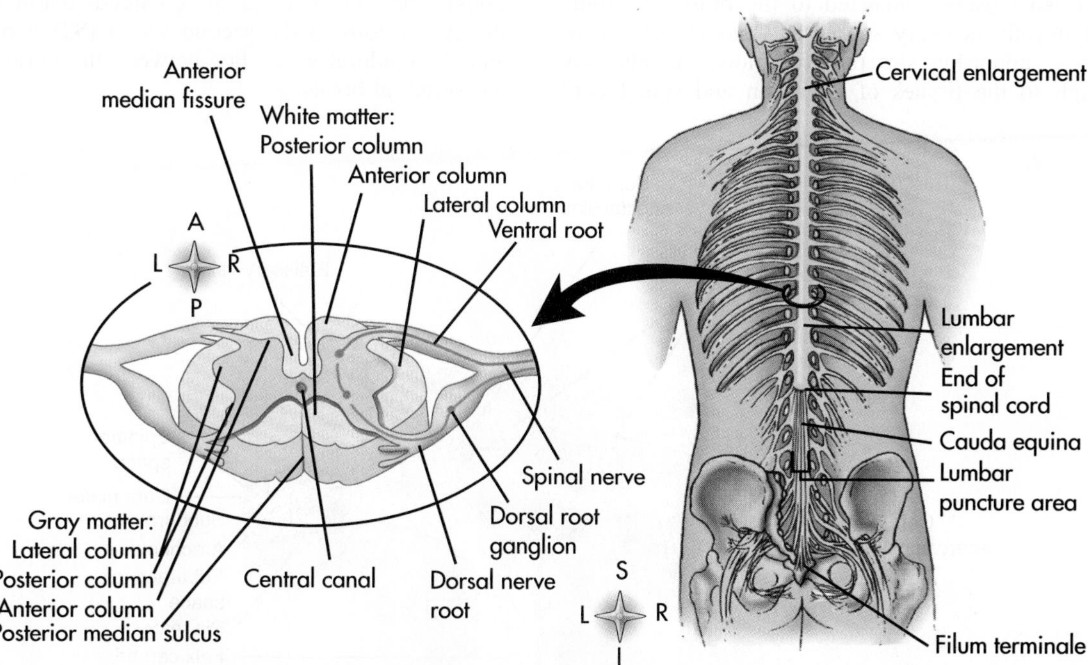

FIGURE U15–5 The spinal cord ends at L-2. *Inset,* Transverse section *(left)* of the spinal cord. (From Thibodeau, G., & Patton, K. [1999]. *Anatomy and physiology* [4th ed., p. 381]. St. Louis: Mosby.)

TABLE U15–2 MAJOR NERVE TRACTS OF THE SPINAL CORD

Tract	Location	Function
ASCENDING TRACTS		
Fasciculus gracilis	Posterior column	Touch, pressure, body movement, position
Fasciculus cuneatus	Posterior column	
Spinothalamic		
Lateral	Lateral column	Pain, temperature
Anterior	Anterior column	Light (crude) touch
Spinocerebellar		
Posterior	Lateral column	Coordination of muscle movements
Anterior	Lateral column	
DESCENDING TRACTS		
Corticospinal		
Lateral	Lateral column	Voluntary motor
Ventral	Anterior column	Voluntary motor
Reticulospinal		
Lateral	Lateral column	Autonomic nervous system fibers, muscle tone, sweat glands
Anterior	Anterior column	
Medial	Anterior column	
Rubrospinal	Lateral column	Coordination of muscle movements

U15–6). Each layer, the pia mater, arachnoid, and dura mater, is a separate membrane.

The *pia mater* is a vascular layer of connective tissue and is so closely connected to the brain and spinal cord that it follows every sulcus and fissure. This layer serves as a supporting structure for blood vessels passing through to the tissues of the brain and spinal cord. The pia mater and astrocytes together form the membrane part of the blood-brain barrier (see Blood-Brain Barrier).

The *arachnoid,* a thin layer of connective tissue, extends from the top of each gyrus to the top of the adjacent gyrus; it does not extend into the sulci and fissures. The space between this layer and the pia mater is known as the *subarachnoid space.* Cerebrospinal fluid (CSF) flows through this space.

The cranial *dura mater* is a tough, nonstretchable vascular membrane with two layers. The *outer* dura mater is actually the membrane (periosteum) of the cranial bones. The *inner* dura mater forms the plates that separate the two cerebral hemispheres (falx cerebri), the cerebrum and the brain stem and cerebellum (tentorium cerebelli), and the cerebellar hemispheres (faly cerebelli). The tentorium cerebelli is a landmark term that is often used by clinicians to separate parts of the brain; it is often referred to as "tentorium." *Supratentorial* refers to the cerebrum and all the structures superior to the tentorium cerebelli; *infratentorial* refers to structures inferior to the tentorium cerebelli—the brain stem and the cerebellum.

Brain spaces that often fill with blood after head trauma include the potential space (the *subdural space*) between the inner dura mater and the arachnoid and the *epidural space* between the dura mater and the periosteum.

The meninges anchor the spinal cord. The pia mater, which closely surrounds the spinal cord, continues from the tip of the conus as a thread-like structure (the *filum terminale*) to the end of the vertebral column, where it is anchored into the ligament on the posterior side of the coccyx. The denticulate ligaments extend laterally from the pia mater to the dura mater to suspend the spinal cord from the dura mater.

Two common spaces that are commonly accessed by physicians are the subarachnoid space (for diagnostic studies) and the epidural space (for delivery of medications). The subarachnoid space extends below the level of the spinal cord to the second sacral (S2) vertebral level, and the epidural space lies between the dural sheath and the vertebral bones.

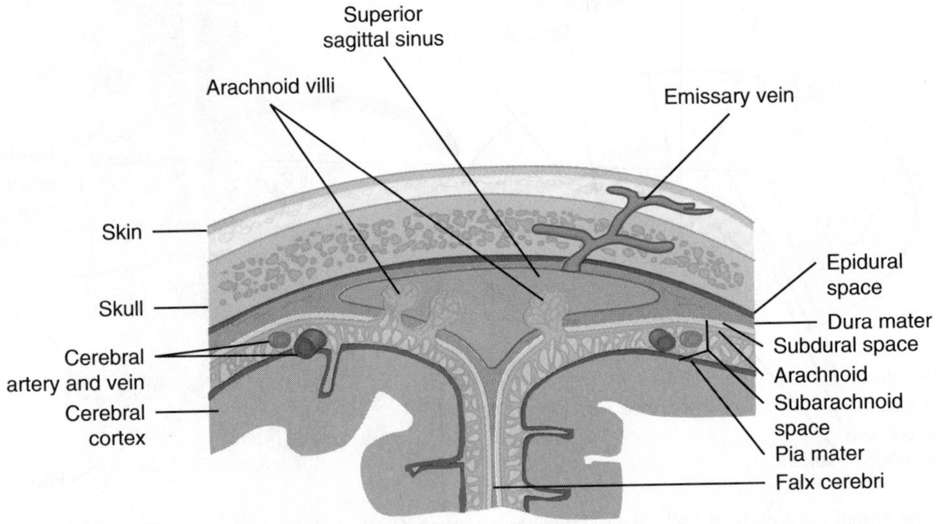

FIGURE U15–6 The meninges (coronal section through the superior sagittal sinus).

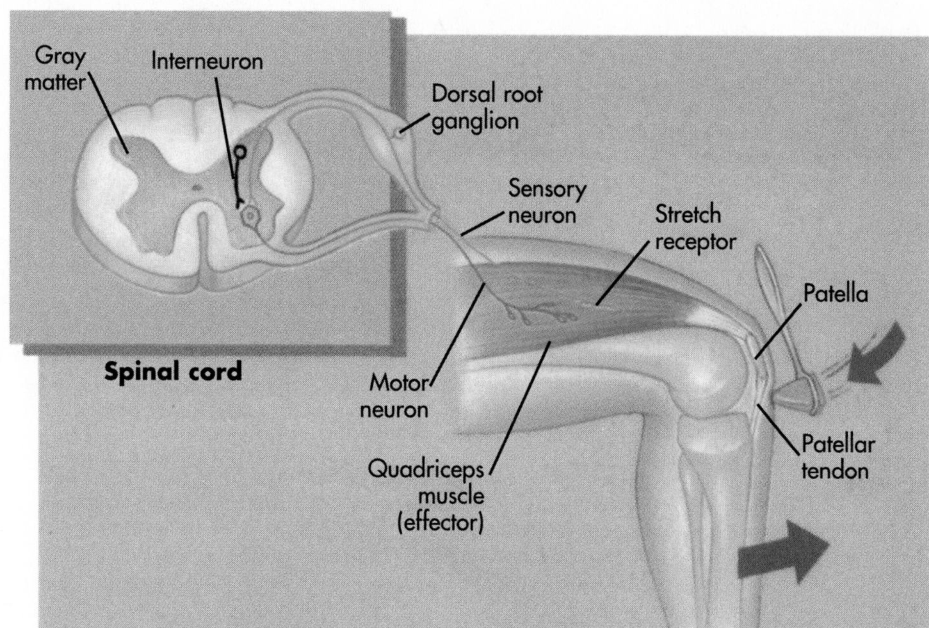

FIGURE U15–7 Patellar reflex and neural pathway involved in the reflex response. (From Thibodeau, G., & Patton, K. [1999]. *Anatomy and physiology* [4th ed., p. 428]. St. Louis: Mosby.)

■ REFLEX MECHANISMS

Our unconscious automatic responses to internal and external stimuli, known as *reflex responses,* provide many homeostatic functions. Although the spinal cord is often thought of as the reflex center, it is not the only site for reflex regulation. Many of the complex reflexes controlling heart rate, breathing, blood pressure, swallowing, sneezing, coughing, and vomiting are found in the brain stem.

Some intrinsic reflex circuits in the spinal cord create patterns of movement (flexion and extension) that are the basis for posture and forward progression. Other reflex circuits are the bases for spinal cord reflexes, which include the myotatic (deep tendon, stretch) reflex, the flexor withdrawal reflex, the crossed extension reflex, and the extensor thrust reflex. Visceral-somatic reflexes can also excite or inhibit the motor neurons, producing changes in muscle tone and even movement.

Neuromuscular spindles monitor muscle stretch. As a muscle stretches, increased firing of spindles leads to contraction of the same muscle, commonly seen as the *knee-jerk reflex.* The Golgi tendon organs are sensory nerve endings that protect against excessive contraction.

Simple reflexes require only two or three neurons; for example, the knee-jerk reflex requires only a sensory and a motor neuron. The *withdrawal reflex* helps prevent or decrease tissue injury when a body part touches a potentially harmful object. The harmful stimuli are sent via the sensory neuron to the interneuron in the spinal cord for interpretation and the response message is sent via the motor neuron, resulting in the withdrawal response (Fig. U15–7).

■ CEREBROSPINAL FLUID AND THE VENTRICULAR SYSTEM

CSF is a clear, colorless fluid. Approximately 100 to 160 ml of CSF circulates through the ventricles and within the subarachnoid space. When a person is lying in a horizontal position, the average CSF pressure is 100 to 180 mm Hg.

About two thirds of the CSF is made in the choroid plexus of the four ventricles, primarily in the lateral ventricles. Small amounts are produced by ependymal, arachnoid, and other brain cells. The choroid plexus is a network of blood vessels within the pia mater that is in direct contact with the lining of the ventricles. The choroid plexuses together produce approximately 500 ml of CSF per day. If CSF were allowed to accumulate, it would exert enough pressure to damage the brain. Normally, however, it is absorbed into the blood at the same rate at which it is formed.

The ventricular system is a series of cavities within the brain. CSF flows from each of the lateral ventricles via the foramen of Monro into the third ventricle (Fig. U15–8). The third ventricle is midline just beneath the fornix. CSF drains from the third ventricle through the aqueduct of Sylvius into the fourth ventricle. The fourth ventricle is located in the brain stem just anterior to the cerebellum. From the fourth ventricle, CSF passes via one of three foramina (two foramina of Luschka and one foramen of Magendie) into a large subarachnoid space that lies behind the medulla and below the cerebellum, called the *cisterna magna.* The cisterna magna is continuous with the subarachnoid space, which surrounds the brain and spinal cord.

Eventually, the CSF circulates upward into the region of the superior sagittal sinus where it is absorbed across the arachnoid villi. The arachnoid granulations are extensive tufts of pia-arachnoid that along with the inner dura extend into the superior sagittal sinus and permit one-way flow of CSF into the sinus.

■ BLOOD-BRAIN BARRIER

Three brain barriers (blood-brain, blood–CSF, and brain-CSF) primarily regulate and maintain an optimal and stable chemical environment for neurons. Brain barriers are either physical barriers or physiologic processes (transport systems) that slow movement of certain substances from one CNS compartment to another by regulating ion movement between the compartments. Physical barriers include tight junctions of the endothelial cells lining the capillaries, pores of the capillaries of the choroid plexuses, the

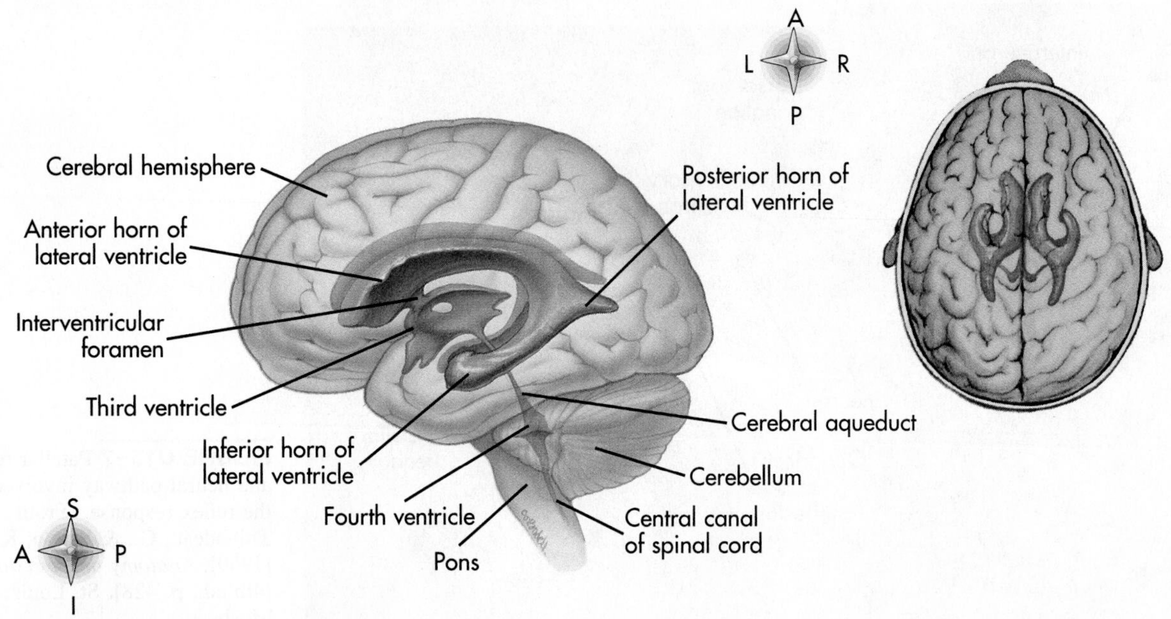

FIGURE U15–8 The ventricles of the brain produce and circulate cerebrospinal fluid. (From Thibodeau, G., & Patton, K. [1999]. *Anatomy and physiology* [4th ed., p. 378]. St. Louis: Mosby.)

basement membrane (ependymal cells) next to the choroid plexuses, and the pial-glial membrane.

An intact blood-brain barrier may prevent some drugs from crossing into the brain, a fact that must be considered when medications are prescribed for nervous system disorders. Certain events, including dilutional hyponatremia, acute hypertension, high doses of some anesthetics, vasodilation, and hypercarbia, can increase the permeability of the blood-brain barrier.

Blood Supply

The brain requires one third of the cardiac output and uses 20% of the body's oxygen. Glucose is catabolized or burned for its energy. Gray matter has higher metabolic needs than white matter. The brain receives 750 to 900 ml of blood flow per minute. Blood flow is regulated by levels of carbon dioxide. When carbon dioxide levels rise, a negative feedback mechanism causes vasodilation.

The vertebral arteries and the internal carotid arteries (Fig. U15–9) provide the arterial supply to the brain.

ARTERIAL SUPPLY

The *vertebral arteries* branch from the subclavian arteries, travel through the transverse foramina in the cervical vertebrae, and enter the cranial vault through the foramen magnum. The vertebral arteries are located on the anterolateral surface of the medulla. At the junction of the medulla and pons, the vertebral arteries join to form the basilar artery. The basilar artery bifurcates at the midbrain level to form two posterior cerebral arteries. The vertebral artery system supplies the brain stem, the cerebellum, the lower portion of the diencephalon, and the medial and inferior regions of the temporal and occipital lobes.

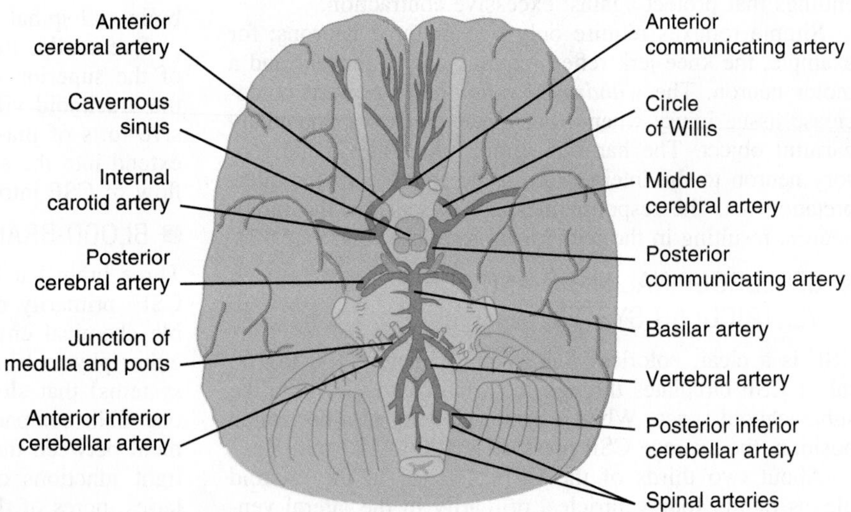

FIGURE U15–9 Inferior view of the cerebral circulation.

The *internal carotid arteries* branch from the common carotid arteries and enter through the carotid canals at the base of the skull. The internal carotid arteries bifurcate into the anterior and middle cerebral arteries. Near this bifurcation, the circle of Willis (a ring of blood vessels at the base of the brain) is formed by the posterior cerebral arteries, posterior communicating arteries, internal carotid arteries, anterior cerebral arteries, and anterior communicating branches. The internal carotid arteries supply the upper diencephalon, basal ganglia, lateral temporal and occipital lobes, and parietal and frontal lobes. The middle cerebral arteries supply large portions of the frontal, parietal, temporal, occipital, and insular lobes and the basal ganglia, internal capsule, and thalamus. The anterior cerebral arteries supply the medial portions of the frontal and parietal lobes and the upper basal ganglia and internal capsule (see Fig. U15–9).

The spinal cord derives its arterial blood supply from small spinal arteries that branch off larger arteries, including the vertebral, ascending cervical, deep cervical, intercostal, lumbar, and sacral arteries. These arteries and their branches form the three main arteries of the spinal cord, the anterior spinal artery and a pair of posterior spinal arteries, which extend the length of the cord.

■ VENOUS SUPPLY

Most of the venous blood from the head returns to the heart through the internal jugular veins, the external jugular veins, and the vertebral veins.

Venous distribution is similar to arterial distribution of the spinal cord. The venous system drains into the venous sinuses located between the dura mater and the periosteum of the vertebral column.

CELLS OF THE NERVOUS SYSTEM

■ STRUCTURE

Nervous tissue consists mainly of *neuroglia* and *neurons* (as well as vascular and some connective tissues). Neurons are responsible for communication, and neurological cells provide support for the activity of neurons. The brain and spinal cord constitute the CNS.

■ NEUROGLIA

Glial cells, collectively called neuroglia, provide structure and support for neurons. They are plentiful, with a ratio of glial cells to neurons high as 50:1! They also control ion concentrations within the extracellular space and contribute to the transport of nutrients, gases, and waste products between neurons and the vascular system and the CSF. Clinically, these cells are responsible for the development of many intracranial tumors. Four types of neuroglial cells exist (Fig. U15–10).

In addition to these functions, each type of glial cell has specific functions.

Astrocytes supply nutrients to the neurons. They have specialized contacts with blood vessels in the pial-glial

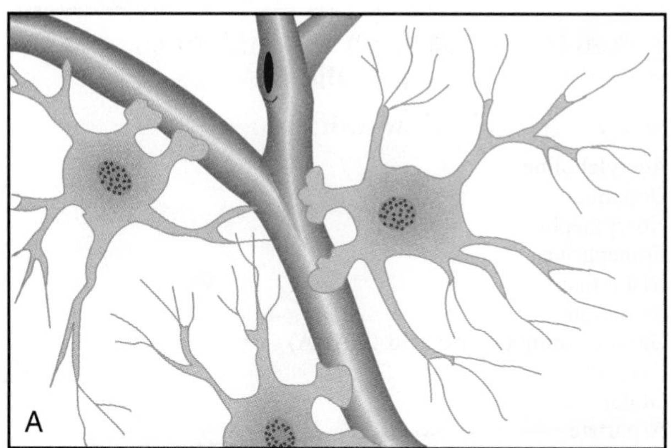

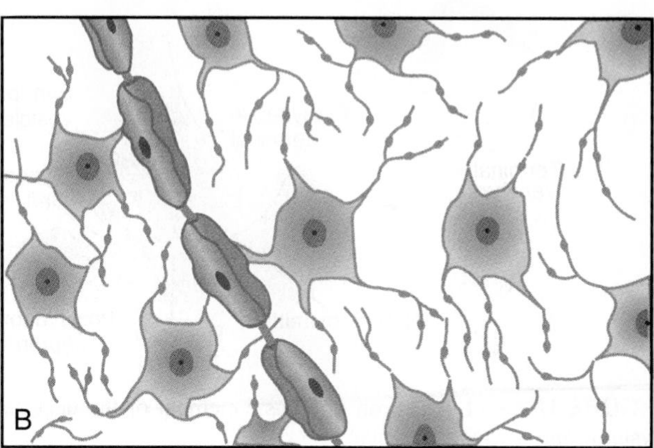

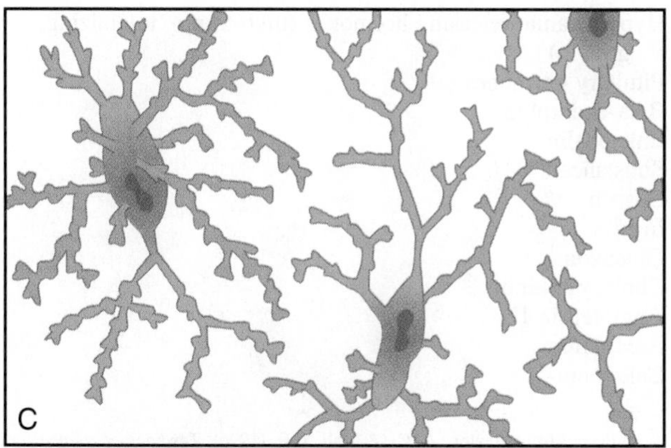

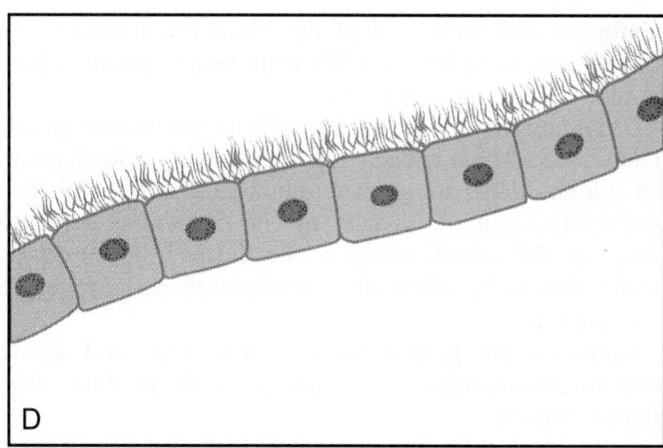

FIGURE U15–10 Neuroglial cells. *A*, Astrocytes along the capillary. *B*, Oligodendrocytes along the nerves. *C*, Microglia (phagocytes). *D*, Ependymal cells form a sheet that lines fluid cavities in the brain.

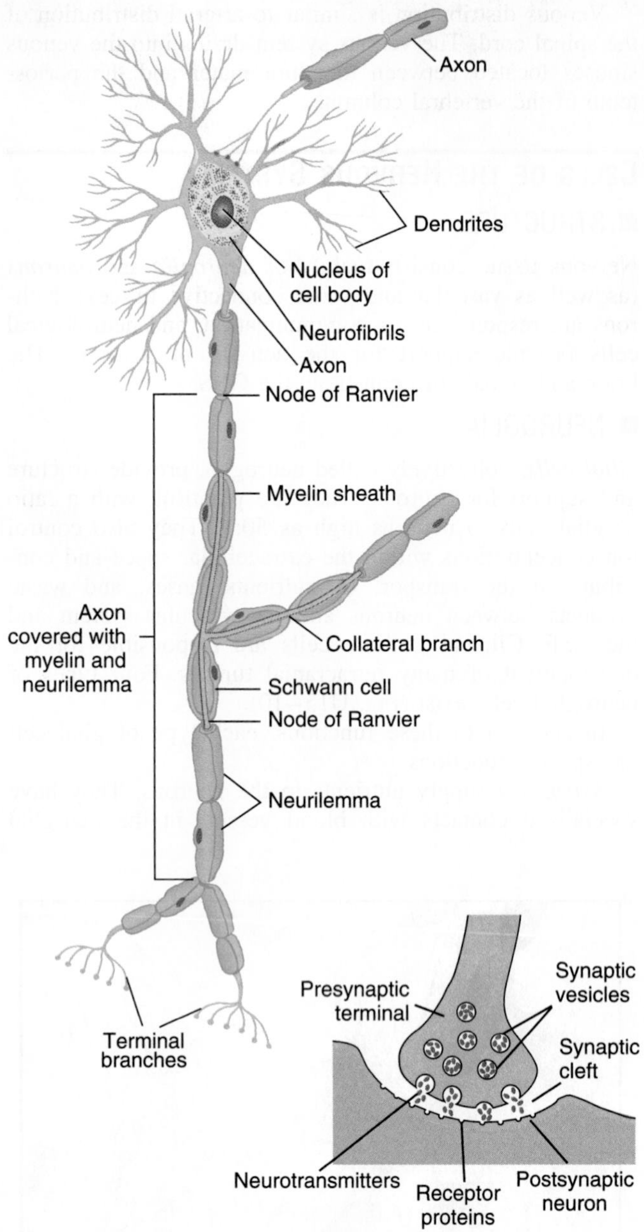

FIGURE U15–11 A neuron (the basic element of the nervous system) and a chemical synapse.

membrane and form part of the blood-brain barrier. Astrocytes appear to be the CNS cells that respond to brain trauma by forming scar tissue.

Oligodendrocytes are comparable to the Schwann cells in the PNS. These cells wrap themselves around axons, and the spiraled part of their membrane is referred to as *myelin.* The outermost part of the Schwann cells also make up the *neurilemma,* a sheath that surrounds the myelin sheath. Neurilemma is essential to nerve regeneration (see later).

Microglia are phagocytic scavenger cells and are related to macrophages. They phagocytose products from injured neurons.

Ependymal cells line the ventricles, choroid plexuses, and the central canal that extends through the spinal cord. They create a one-cell-layered membrane that allows regulated diffusion of substances between the interstitial fluid and the CSF.

■ NEURONS

A neuronal cell body *(soma)* is like other cells, in that it contains most of the organelles seen in other cells. Unique structures in the neuron include *neurofibrils,* which are networks of thread-like structures supporting other structures. *Nissl bodies* are dark-staining sections of rough endoplasmic reticulum and are unique to the neuron.

Tree-like *dendrites* carry messages to the neuronal cell body; *axons* carry messages away from the cell body (Fig. U15–11).

Three types of neurons exist:

1. *Unipolar* neurons have only one nerve fiber leaving the cell body, but they branch to form a dendrite and axon. Unipolar neurons often send general sensory signals.
2. *Multipolar* neurons send motor signals.
3. *Bipolar* neurons are often utilized in the pathways of special sensory systems (eyes, nose, and ears).

Synapses, very important in nerve function, are small spaces between neurons and their muscular or glandular target organs. As a message travels down the neuron, it reaches a synapse that it must cross in order to "jump" to

BOX U15–1 Common Neurotransmitters and Neuropeptides

Small-Molecule Transmitters

Acetylcholine
Dopamine
Norepinephrine
Epinephrine
Histamine
Serotonin
Gamma-aminobutyric acid (GABA)
Glycine
Glutamate
Aspartate
Nitric oxide

Neuropeptides

Hypothalamic-releasing hormones (thyrotropin, luteinizing, growth)
Pituitary hormones
Beta-endorphin
Enkephalin
Substance P
Gastrin
Insulin
Glucagon
Cholecystokinin
Angiotensin II
Bradykinin
Calcitonin

Adapted from Guyton, A. C., & Hall, J. E. (1996). *Textbook of medical science* (9th ed., pp. 572–573). Philadelphia: W. B. Saunders.

the next neuron. There are two types of synapses; *chemical* synapses dominate. In an *electrical synapse,* the electrical nerve impulses of two cells cross directly through a very small separation (called *gap junctions* or a *nexus*) from the presynaptic to the postsynaptic cell; this type of synapse is found in smooth and cardiac muscle cells.

Chemical substances called *neurotransmitters* are discharged into the space *(cleft)* between two neurons and propel the message onto the next neuron. Transmitters are manufactured in the cell body, and transported anterograde to the terminals *(knobs),* stored, and secreted from the vesicles in the first neuron *(presynaptic neuron)* into the synaptic cleft (see Fig. U15–11). The neurotransmitter excites, inhibits, or modifies signals to the second neuron (postsynaptic neuron) by interacting with the receptors on its membrane. More than 100 neurotransmitters have been identified. Box U15–1 lists the more common transmitters.

IMPULSE CONDUCTION

■ RESTING POTENTIAL

A neuron not conducting a nerve impulse is said to be "resting." Although it is resting, it remains charged and potentially ready to fire. The potential to fire is produced by a difference in electrical charge between the interstitial fluid outside the neuron and the intracellular fluid within (Fig. U15–12). The inside of the nerve cell is electrically negative, the interstitial fluid electrically positive. A resulting membrane potential, measured in millivolts (mV) results from this difference in electrical potential between the two compartments. The *resting membrane potential* (RMP) of neurons is between −45 and −75 mV. The RMP in a neuron is −70 mV; in cardiac and skeletal cells it is −90 mV.

The cell is *depolarized* when an influx of sodium makes the membrane potential more positive (i.e., rising to zero). In most cells, this is due to an electrical stimulus transmitted by an adjacent cell.

As the membrane potential rises during depolarization, it reaches a specified level *(threshold).* When threshold is reached, the excited cell is committed to full action potential because the cell follows an all-or-none phenomenon.

Repolarization is the restoration of the membrane polarity, and sodium and potassium are returned to their usual places via the sodium-potassium pump.

After an action potential is generated, no segment of the nerve fiber can conduct another action potential for a brief period of time (<1 ms). This interval is called the *absolute refractory period.* Sodium and potassium are returning to their original locations during this period, and sodium cannot enter the nerve cell. During the next period, called the *relative refractory period,* only a stimulus stronger than ordinary can produce an action potential. On average, a return to a resting potential takes approximately 10 to 30 ms.

■ NERVE IMPULSES

Because neurons are arranged in chain-like pathways, impulses must travel from one cell to another quickly. In nerve cells, the impulse begins at the axon. When the action potential reaches the presynaptic knob at the dendrite, the membrane's permeability to calcium increases, allowing increased calcium influx. Calcium promotes fusing of the vesicles with the membrane and release of the neurotransmitters inside. Some neurotransmitters are transported back into the vesicles *(reuptake).* Others are decomposed by an enzyme process. For example, acetylcholinesterase decomposes acetylcholine at the postsynaptic membrane.

■ MYELIN

Myelin surrounds most large nerve fibers and is separated by nodes of Ranvier. Action potentials are generated only at the nodes and thus they skip between them rather than depolarize the entire membrane. This jumping characteristic is known as "saltatory conduction." Conduction using this process is very rapid. Neurons with their axons covered by myelin are called *myelinated nerve fibers;* neurons with little or no myelin are called *unmyelinated nerve fibers.* Myelinated fibers in the CNS compose the *white matter* in the brain and spinal cord. *Gray matter* consists of cell bodies which are unmyelinated. The speed of the nerve impulse conduction is also related to the

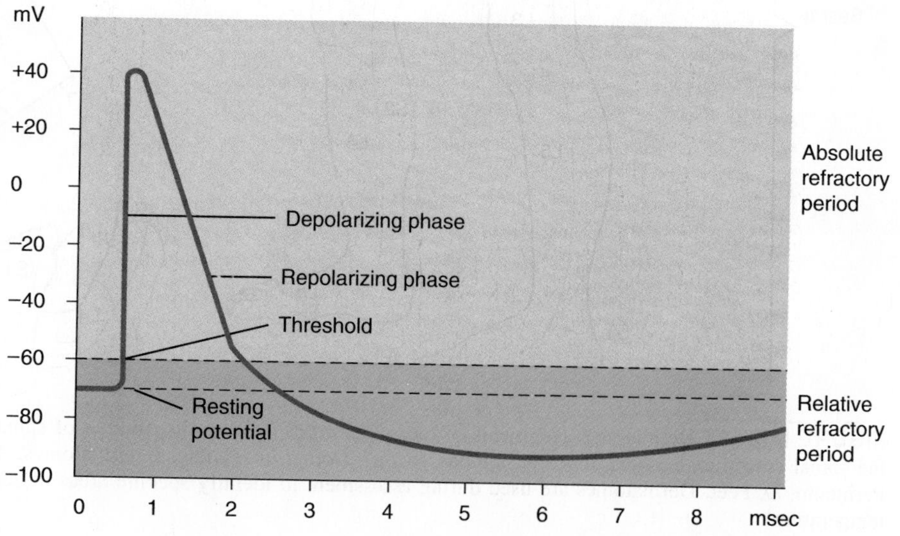

FIGURE U15–12 Generation of nerve impulses. The resting membrane potential is shown at −70 mV.

diameter of the fiber; the greater the diameter, the faster the impulse.

■ RECEPTORS

Receptors are biologic transducers, using the stimulus of one form of energy—mechanical, electrical, chemical, thermal or light—to initiate the "electrical" energy of the nerve impulse. Although sensory receptors may be stimulated by more than one form of energy, each receptor is especially sensitive to a particular form of energy.

Receptors exhibit a phenomenon known as *adaptation,* a decreased receptor sensitivity in response to steady continuous stimuli. Slow-adapting receptors can maintain the lower rate of discharge for minutes to even hours. Fast-adapting receptor bursts of impulses terminate less than 1 second after initiation of the stimulus. The mechanism of adaptation is not known.

Receptors respond more effectively to change than to continuous stimulation. This characteristic of nerve "fatigue" is protective.

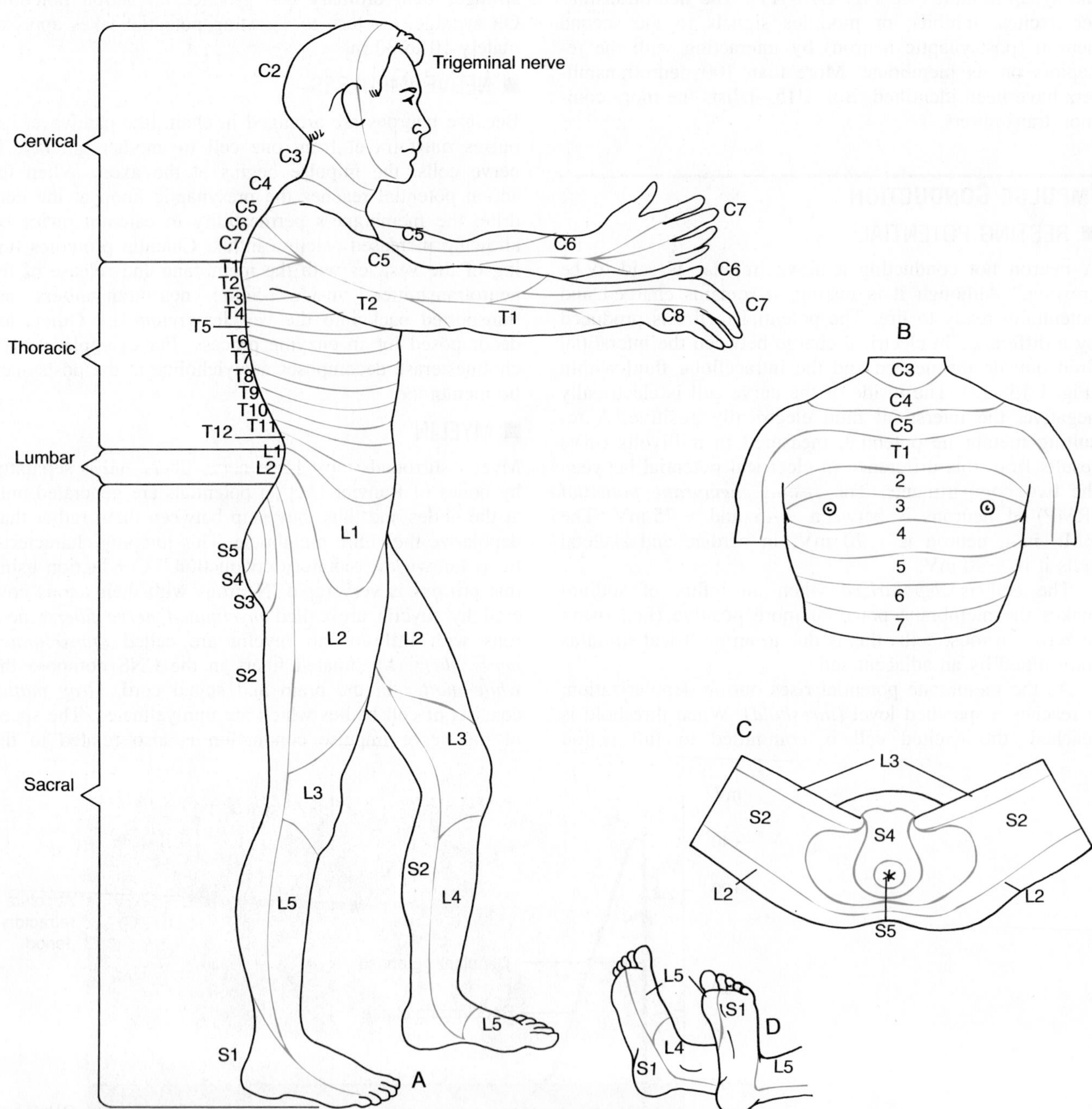

FIGURE U15–13 Dermatomes (segments of the spinal cord) indicate distribution of spinal nerves. *Solid lines* divide the regions of the spinal cord (i.e., cervical, thoracic, lumbar, sacral). *Dotted lines* indicate dermatomes. *A*, Torso and limbs. *B*, Anterior chest. *C*, Perineum. *D*, Feet. Dermatomes are used during assessment to identify specific areas of sensory impairment (e.g., touch, pain, temperature).

PERIPHERAL NERVOUS SYSTEM

The PNS includes all neurons other than those in the brain and spinal cord. It consists of pathways of nerve fibers between the CNS and all outlying structures in the body. Included in the PNS are 12 pairs of cranial nerves and 31 pairs of spinal nerves.

Nerves that conduct impulses to the brain and spinal cord are called *sensory (afferent) neurons.* Nerves that conduct impulses away from the brain and spinal cord are called *motor (efferent) neurons.* Most nerves are mixed, having both sensory and motor components.

SPINAL NERVES

The spinal nerves develop from a series of nerve rootlets that collect laterally as spinal roots. Each spinal nerve consists of a *dorsal (sensory) root* and a *ventral (motor) root* which unite to form a spinal nerve. The dorsal root emerges from the posterolateral cord. The ventral root emerges from the anterolateral spinal cord. There are 31 pairs of spinal nerves: eight pairs of cervical nerves, 12 pairs of thoracic nerves, five pairs of lumbar nerves, five pairs of sacral nerves, and usually one pair of coccygeal nerves (see Fig. U15–4). The specific area of sensory reception for each dorsal root is called a *sensory dermatome* (Fig. U15–13).

The peripheral nerves that are formed into plexuses have specific names. There are three major plexuses:

1. The *cervical plexus* supplies the muscles and skin of the neck and branches to form the phrenic nerve, which innervates the diaphragm.
2. The *brachial plexus* supplies the muscles and skin of the shoulder, axilla, arm, forearm, and hand. It branches to form the ulnar, median, and radial nerves.
3. The *lumbosacral plexus* supplies sensory and motor impulses to the muscles and skin of the perineum, gluteal region, thighs, legs, and feet. Its many branches include the pudendal, gluteal, femoral, sciatic, tibial, and common fibular nerves.

CRANIAL NERVES

Twelve pairs of cranial nerves arise from the brain. Most of the cranial nerves are composed of both motor and sensory neurons, although a few cranial nerves carry only sensory impulses (Fig. U15–14). Except for the olfactory and optic nerves, whose nuclei lie just below the cere-

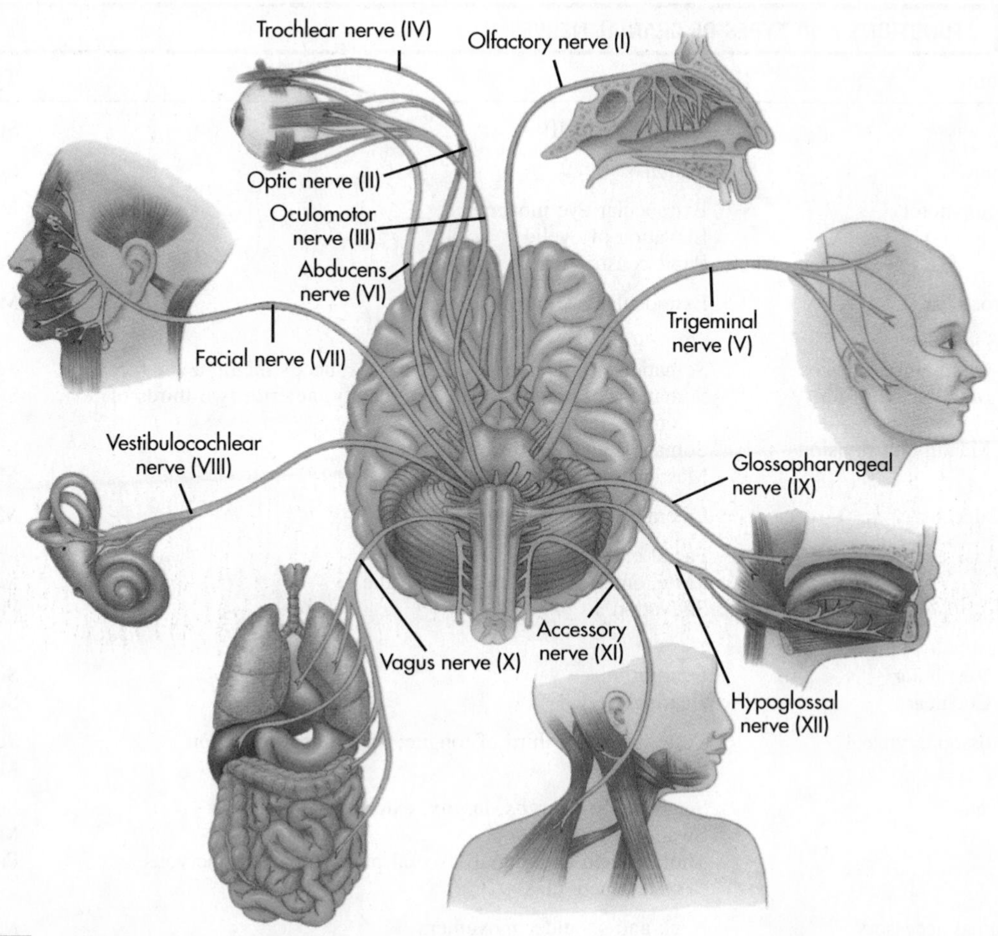

FIGURE U15–14 Ventral surface of the brain showing the attachment of the cranial nerves. (From Thibodeau, G., & Patton, K. [1999]. *Anatomy and physiology* [4th ed., p. 420]. St. Louis: Mosby.)

brum, all the other cranial nerve nuclei lie within the brain stem. Table U15–3 presents the 12 pairs of cranial nerves.

AUTONOMIC NERVOUS SYSTEM

The autonomic nervous system (ANS) is the part of the PNS that coordinates involuntary activities, such as visceral functions, smooth and cardiac muscle changes, and glandular responses. Although it can function independently, its primary control is from the brain and spinal cord. The ANS has two divisions: the *sympathetic* and *parasympathetic nervous systems.* The efferent ANS fibers travel within some cranial and spinal nerves. These two systems are highly integrated and interact with each other to maintain a stable internal environment.

Unlike the *somatic* neurons, which usually are single neurons linking the CNS to a muscle or gland, the ANS has a *two-neuron chain* prior to the effector organ. The terminal of the first neuron is located in the CNS and synapses with nerve fibers whose cell bodies are within an autonomic ganglion. The axon of the second neuron (postganglionic fiber) carries impulses to the target viscera. An exception is the adrenal medulla, which is innervated directly by preganglionic fibers. The medulla is actually composed of postganglionic neurons that secrete adrenaline into the bloodstream during an "adrenaline rush."

The *sympathetic nervous system* coordinates activities used to handle stress and is geared for action as a whole for short periods of time. The preganglionic neurons of the sympathetic nervous system emerge from the spinal cord via the motor (ventral) roots of the thoracic and upper two lumbar spinal nerves (T1-L2) (see Fig. U15–14). Preganglionic axons are short; postganglionic axons are long.

The *parasympathetic nervous system* is associated with conservation and restoration of energy stores and is geared to act locally and discretely for a longer duration. The preganglionic fibers emerge from the brain stem via the cranial nerves and from the spinal cord via the sacral spinal nerves at S2-4. These preganglionic fibers have long axons that synapse with the postganglionic neurons in ganglia close to or located within the organs to be innervated. Each postganglionic neuron has a relatively short axon. Most organ systems, but not all, have both parasympathetic and sympathetic innervation. Approximately 75% of the parasympathetic fibers are in the vagus nerve.

Table U15–4 lists the effects of both the sympa-

TABLE U15–3 FUNCTIONS AND TYPES OF CRANIAL NERVES

	Name	Function	Type
I	Olfactory	Olfaction (smell)	Sensory
II	Optic	Vision	Sensory
III	Oculomotor	Extraocular eye movement Elevation of eyelid Pupil constriction	Motor Parasympathetic
IV	Trochlear	Extraocular eye movement	Motor
V	Trigeminal		
	Ophthalmic division	Somatic sensations of cornea, nasal mucous membranes, face	Sensory
	Maxillary division	Somatic sensations of face, oral cavity, anterior two thirds of tongue, teeth	Sensory
	Mandibular division	Somatic sensation of lower face Mastication (chewing)	Sensory Motor
VI	Abducens	Lateral eye movement	Motor
VII	Facial	Facial expression Taste, anterior two thirds of tongue Salivation	Motor Sensory Parasympathetic
VIII	Vestibulocochlear		
	Vestibular	Equilibrium	Sensory
	Cochlear	Hearing	Sensory
IX	Glossopharyngeal	Taste, posterior third of tongue; pharyngeal sensation Swallowing	Sensory Motor
X	Vagus	Sensation in pharynx, larynx, external ear Swallowing Thoracic and abdominal visceral parasympathetic nervous system activities	Sensory Motor Parasympathetic
XI	Spinal accessory	Neck and shoulder movement	Motor
XII	Hypoglossal	Tongue movement	Motor

TABLE U15–4 EFFECTS OF THE SYMPATHETIC AND PARASYMPATHETIC NERVOUS SYSTEMS ON ORGANS

Organ	Effect of Sympathetic Stimulation	Effect of Parasympathetic Stimulation
Eye		
Pupil	Dilation (alpha)*	Constriction
Ciliary muscle	Slight relaxation (far vision)	Constriction (near vision)
Glands	Vasoconstriction and slight secretion	Stimulation of copious secretion (containing many enzymes for enzyme-secreting glands)
Nasal		
Lacrimal		
Parotid		
Submandibular		
Gastric		
Pancreatic		
Sweat glands	Copious sweating (cholinergic)	Sweating on palms of hands
Apocrine glands	Thick, odoriferous secretion	None
Heart		
Muscle	Increased rate ($beta_1$) Increased force of contraction ($beta_1$)	Slowed rate Decreased force of contraction (especially of atria)
Coronaries	Dilated ($beta_2$); constricted (alpha)	Dilation
Lungs		
Bronchi	Dilation ($beta_2$)	Constriction
Blood vessels	Mild constriction	? Dilation
Gut		
Lumen	Decreased peristalsis and tone ($beta_2$)	Increased peristalsis and tone
Sphincter	Increased tone (alpha)	Relaxation (most times)
Liver	Gluconeogenesis, glycogenolysis ($beta_2$)	Slight glycogen synthesis
Gallbladder and bile ducts	Relaxation	Contraction
Kidney	Decreased output and renin secretion	None
Bladder		
Detrusor	Relaxation (slight) ($beta_2$)	Contraction
Trigone	Contraction (alpha)	Relaxation
Penis	Ejaculation	Erection
Systemic arterioles		
Abdominal viscera	Constriction (alpha)	None
Muscle	Constriction (alpha) Dilation ($beta_2$) Dilation (cholinergic)	None
Skin	Constriction	None
Blood		
Coagulation	Increase	None
Glucose	Increase	None
Lipids	Increase	None
Basal metabolism	Increase up to 100%	None
Adrenal medullary secretion	Increase	None
Mental activity	Increase	None
Piloerector muscles	Contraction (alpha)	None
Skeletal muscle	Increased glycogenolysis ($beta_2$) Increased strength	None
Fat cells	Lipolysis ($beta_1$)	None

*Sympathetic nervous system composed of alpha, $beta_1$, and $beta_2$ receptors.
Adapted from Guyton, A. C., & Hall, J. E. (1996). *Textbook of medical science* (9th ed., pp. 774–775). Philadelphia: W. B. Saunders.

thetic and parasympathetic nervous systems on different organs. These functions and responses are related to the type of neurotransmitter released. The preganglionic fibers of the sympathetic and parasympathetic nerves and the postganglionic fibers of the parasympathetic nerves release acetycholine. The postganglionic fibers of the sympathetic nerves release norepinephrine. Fibers secreting acetylcholine are called *cholinergic fibers;*

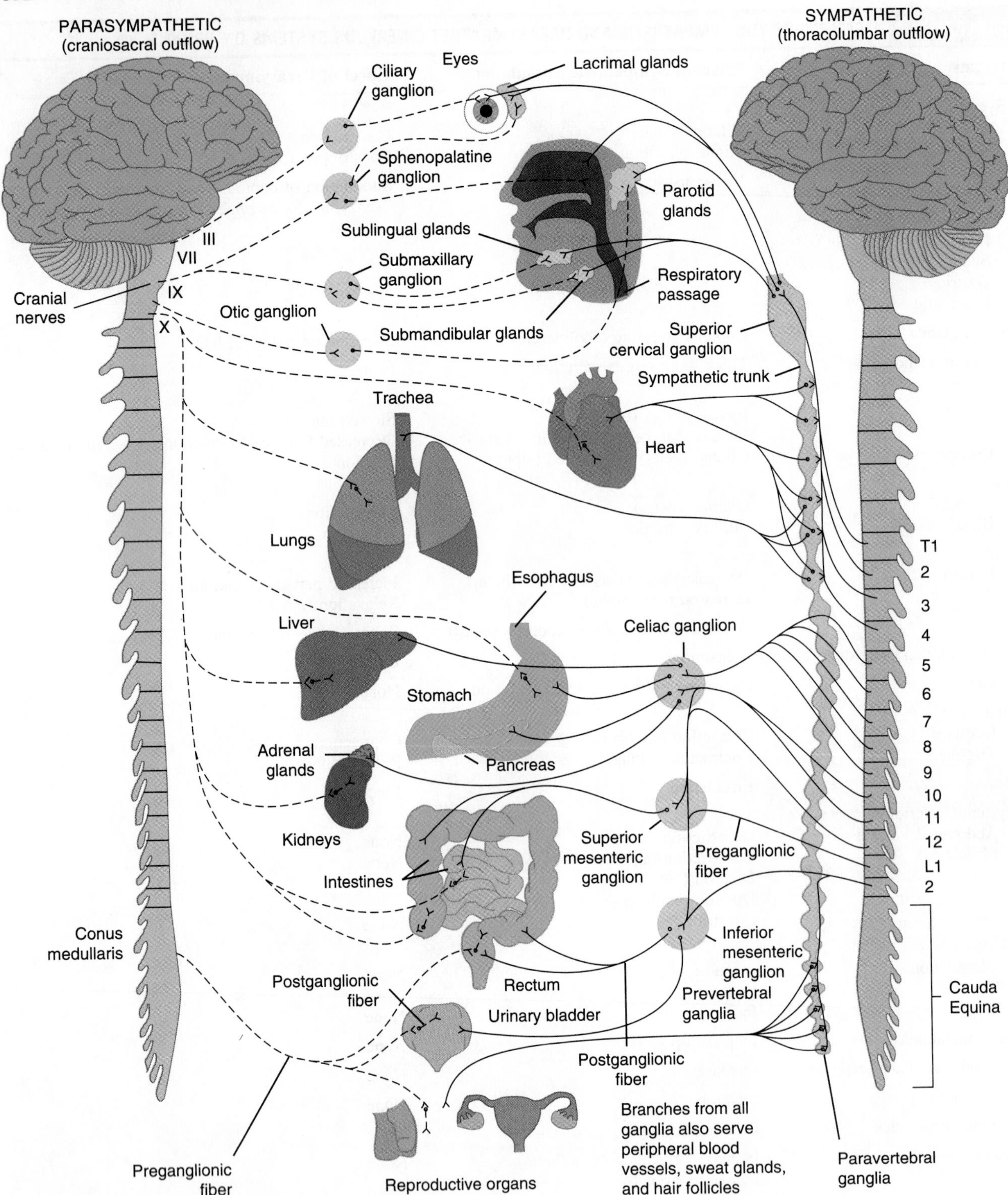

FIGURE U15–15 Autonomic nervous system.

fibers secreting norepinephrine are called *adrenergic fibers.*

The complexity of the sympathetic and parasympathetic response also depends on the type of receptor that combines with the neurotransmitter. The sympathetic nervous system has four types of receptors: alpha$_1$, alpha$_2$, beta$_1$, and beta$_2$. The parasympathetic nervous system has muscarinic and nicotinic receptors.

EFFECTS OF INJURY ON THE NERVOUS SYSTEM

■ REGENERATION

For many years, it was thought that nerve cell bodies were not able to regenerate; however, it appears that CNS cortical neurons do attempt to regenerate. PNS regeneration can occur if only the axon in the PNS is injured. Initially, there is breakdown of the myelin sheath and axon. The axon swells and fragments while the myelin sheath disintegrates distal to the injury. The cell body takes up water. Macrophages phagocytose the breakdown products. Neurilemma cells migrate into the emerging space (Fig. U15–16).

The injured axon tip forms a new plasma membrane. A few days after injury, sprouts emerge from the tip. Peripheral nerve sprouts enter the distal stump and often come in contact with a neurilemma cord, which serves as a guide. The regenerating axon grows along the cord at a rate of 4 mm/day. Later, the neurilemma cells encapsulate the regenerating nerve fibers. With time, the axon and myelin sheath both thicken. Axons within the CNS sprout and form growing tips but appear unable to sustain the metabolic responses necessary for extensive regeneration. It is believed that the axon tip is not able to penetrate the glial scar formed at the injury site, such as after spinal cord injury.

An uninjured axon may sprout a collateral branch at a node of Ranvier that may enter into an adjacent denervated neurilemma cord. Collateral nerve regeneration occurs in both the PNS and the CNS, for example, after peripheral nerve trauma or inflammation of a peripheral nerve, as in Bell's palsy.

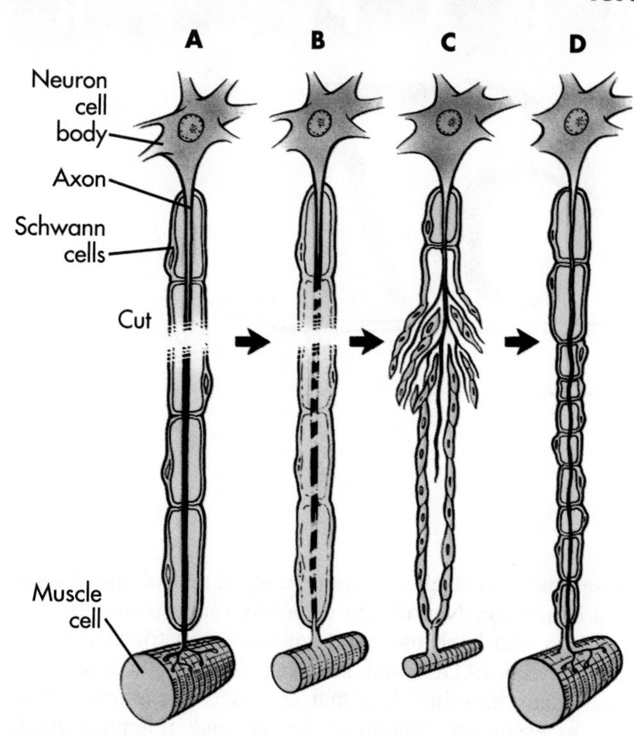

FIGURE U15–16 Regeneration of peripheral nerve tissue. *A*, An injury results in a cut nerve. *B*, Immediately after the injury, the distal portion of the axon degenerates, as does its myelin sheath. *C*, The remaining neurilemma cells tunnel from the point of injury to the effector. New Schwann cells grow within this tunnel, maintaining a path for regrowth of the axon. Meanwhile, several growing fibers reach the tunnel. *D*, The neuron's attachment is reestablished. (From Thibodeau, G., & Patton, K. [1999]. *Anatomy and physiology* [4th ed., p. 353]. St. Louis: Mosby.)

Effects of Aging on the Nervous System

Neurons undergo senescence. Intracellular, cellular, and biochemical changes occur. Lipofuscin accumulates in the cell. Neurofibrillary tangles and senile plaques develop. After we reach 30 years of age, neurons decrease in number and neuroglial cells increase in size and number. The number of dendrites decreases, but the intrinsic dendritic changes are quite variable in hippocampal areas of the brain on postmortem examination in the normal aging population. Variations in dendrite length, stability, and growth have been attributed to compensatory response to death of dendrites.

Aging has little effect on sensory and primary memory but causes a decrease in working memory, including longer retrieval times for short-term memory, categorization, and episodic memory. Dendritic changes are quite pronounced in pathologic conditions such as Alzheimer's disease (see Chapter 72). The axons also change in normal aging; their diameters thin, and the receptors decrease in number.

CONCLUSIONS

The nervous system has three major divisions:

1. The CNS regulates higher-level process, such as thought and vital functions.
2. The PNS provides pathways to the CNS.
3. The ANS coordinates involuntary activities such as digestion.

The neuron is the structural and functional unit of the nervous system. The typical neuron is composed of a cell body, one axon, and several dendrites. The impulses along the nerve are carried through the action of several electrolytes. Neurotransmitters carry the impulse from neuron to neuron.

BIBLIOGRAPHY

1. Guyton, A. C., & Hall, J. E. (1996). *Textbook of medical science* (9th ed.). Philadelphia: W. B. Saunders.
2. Hanson, M. (1998). *Pathophysiology.* Philadelphia: W. B. Saunders.
3. Lewis, B. (1992). *AANA Journal* Course: Update for nurse anesthetists: Blood-brain barrier function alteration during anesthesia. *Journal of the American Association of Nurse Anesthetists, 60*(6), 573–577.
4. Sur, M., & Cowey, A. (1995). Cerebral cortex: Function and development. *Neuron, 15,* 497–505.
5. Tower, D. B. (1992). A century of neuronal and neuroglial interactions, and their pathological implications: An overview. In A. C. H. Yu, et al. (Eds.), *Progress in brain research* (Vol. 94, pp. 3–17). New York: Elsevier Science.

CHAPTER

67

Assessment of the Neurologic System

Mary Vorder Bruegge

Assessment of a client experiencing a neurologic disorder is a challenge. Neurologic disorders range from simple to complex and have profound consequences for activities of daily living (ADL) and survival. Neurologic assessment establishes baseline data that are used to compare ongoing assessments, diagnose actual and potential health problems, manage client care, and evaluate the outcome. Because of the complexity of the nervous system, neurologic assessment is both multifaceted and lengthy. The three main components of a neurologic assessment are

- A comprehensive history
- A neurologic physical examination
- General and specific neurodiagnostic studies

Assessment is both anatomic and functional. Continuous observations of the client are made and compared with baseline data. Astute observations are essential because many neurologic changes occur subtly. Nurses collect data on the client's ability to function physically (e.g., self-care deficit) and mentally (e.g., confusion and altered problem solving). Finally, because many neurologic disorders are serious, the nurse provides skillful, crisis-oriented support for the client and significant others.

This chapter presents basic neurologic assessment procedures. Additional assessment techniques for specific neurologic disorders are discussed throughout Unit 15. Novice practitioners may follow the assessment sequence described in this chapter to avoid missing parts of a complex examination. Advanced clinicians may develop a preferred sequence based on experience. The sequence suggested in Table 67–1 integrates cranial nerve and reflex testing into motor and sensory examinations.

HISTORY

The history consists of biographical data, the chief complaint and symptom analysis, past health history, family health history, psychosocial history, and review of systems.

■ BIOGRAPHICAL AND DEMOGRAPHIC DATA

Biographical data comprise demographic, administrative, and insurance information. Often included are (1) a personal profile or brief description of the client, (2) the source of the history (e.g., client or a significant other), and (3) the client's mental status (indicating the reliability of the data). Neurologic problems often affect mental status, sometimes making it difficult to obtain an accurate history directly from the client.

■ CURRENT HEALTH

Chief Complaint

Obtain a detailed description of the events that have led the client to seek care. Avoid suggesting manifestations to the client, and use open-ended questions.

Symptom Analysis

Determine the onset and sequence of manifestations and their progress. Describe neurologic disease processes accurately to facilitate the diagnostic process. Ask the client to describe manifestations using his or her own words. Use a symptom analysis to elicit manifestation characteristics and their progression (see Chapter 9).

The health history guides the physical examination. For example, a complaint of dizziness cues a focus on examination of the eyes, ears (vestibular nerve), and cerebellar function instead of motor and sensory functions. Detailed neurologic examination is indicated when the client reports behavioral changes, altered level of consciousness (LOC), growth and development problems, pain, changes in motor or sensory function, infection, or trauma. Assess for neurologic problems that may be related to other problems, such as alcohol and recreational drug use, metabolic imbalances, and metastatic lesions.

■ PAST HEALTH HISTORY

Childhood and Infectious Diseases and Immunizations

Collect data regarding common childhood diseases and immunizations. Diseases associated with neurologic sequelae include rubella, rubeola, cytomegalovirus infection, herpes simplex, influenza, and meningitis. Ask whether the client has completed the recommended immunization schedule. Public health resources provide schedules for

Text continued on page 1879

TABLE 67–1 NEUROLOGIC ASSESSMENT GUIDELINES

Functional Category	Specific Category	Area of Nervous System Involved	Assessment Technique	Examples of Disorders
1. Consciousness (awareness of self and environment)	Arousal response to verbal, tactile, and visual stimuli	Reticular activating system (mesencephalon, diencephalon) Both hemispheres	Is client alert? What is attention span? Is there normal response to visual and auditory stimuli? Reaction to loud noises, shaking, deep pressure over eye orbits or sternum? Are vital signs, pupils, and reflexes normal?	Elevation: insomnia, agitation, mania, delirium Depression: somnolence, lethargy, semicoma, coma
2. Mentation	Thinking	Cerebral hemispheres plus specific regional functions	Is client oriented (time, place, person)?	Disorientation
	Insight, judgment, planning	Frontal lobe, with association fibers to other areas of cerebrum	Does client recognize implication of illness? Are goals congruent with abilities? How would client respond to given situation (e.g., house on fire)?	Lack of judgment, inattention to grooming, appearance, and personal habits
	Fund of information	Basic biologic intellect (frontal lobe) integrated into other areas	Calculation ability, knowledge of current events consistent with educational level. Who is U.S. president?	Impairment—functioning not congruent with level of education
	Memory	Temporal lobe and association to most other areas of cortex		
	Recent	Hippocampus	What did client eat for breakfast? What happened yesterday?	Organic brain disease
	Past	Frontal lobe	Recall past events during taking of history	Lapses of memory for past events may coincide with past CNS problems (e.g., trauma, infection, psychic trauma)
	Feeling (affect) (congruence of response to stimulus)	Limbic system (usually involves both hemispheres)	Compare observed with expected reactions. Are emotions labile? Appropriate?	Blunted affect: hysteria, schizophrenia, bilateral frontal lobe lesions
	Perceptual distortions (illusions, hallucinations)	General and specific cortical areas in hallucinations	Observations for behavior indicating perceptual problems. Ask client	Irritative lesions of cortex may → hallucinations (occipital cortex → visual, postcentral gyrus → somatic sensation, uncus → smell)
3. Language and speech	Dysarthria (defects in articulation, enunciation), and rhythm in speech	Impairment of muscles of tongue, palate, pharynx, or lips (may be due to ↓ impulses or incoordination) Brain stem, cerebellum, or extraneural causes; CN V, VII, IX, X, XII	Have client repeat a difficult phrase (e.g., "Susie sells seashells by the seashore")	Slurring, slowness, indistinctness, nasality, break in normal speech rhythm (i.e., speech of intoxication); amyotrophic lateral sclerosis; pseudobulbar palsy; myasthenia gravis

Table continued on following page

TABLE 67–1 NEUROLOGIC ASSESSMENT GUIDELINES *Continued*

Functional Category	Specific Category	Area of Nervous System Involved	Assessment Technique	Examples of Disorders
	Dysphonia (abnormal production of sounds from larynx)	Many extraneural causes Recurrent laryngeal nerve problems (part of vagus); CN X	Is client hoarse? Whispered voice is intact Use indirect laryngoscopy findings	Compression of recurrent laryngeal nerve by bronchogenic carcinoma of left mainstem bronchus Left atrial hypertrophy
		Medulla (area of nucleus of CN X)		Brain stem tumors, occlusion of posterior inferior cerebellar or vertebral artery
	Aphasia (inability to use and understand written and spoken words)	Fluent (receptive) left temporal and parietal lobes (Wernicke's area)	Observe vocal expression, written expression, comprehension of spoken and written language, and gesture communication	Cerebrovascular disease of middle cerebral artery Trauma, tumor, abscess, etc., in left temporal and parietal lobe areas
		Nonfluent (expressive) Broca's area (lateral) inferior portion of frontal lobe of dominant side		Damage to Broca's area or association fibers (stroke, tumor, etc.)
		Global (combined)		
	Agnosia (inability to recognize objects or symbols by means of senses)	Primarily in parietal temporal and occipital areas	Sense organs intact? Can the client recognize objects by sight, touch, hearing, etc.?	Cerebrovascular disease
4. Motor function	Expression (facial)	CN VII	Symmetry of smile, frown, raising of eyebrows	Central facial weakness (upper motor neuron dysfunction); weakness of lower half of face Causes: cerebral vascular accident, corticobulbar tract Peripheral facial weakness (lower motor dysfunction); weakness of entire half of face Causes: Bell's palsy, brain stem tumor, fracture of temporal bone
	Eating (chewing, swallowing)	CN V, VII, IX, X, XII	Strength of masticator muscles, gag reflexes, ability to swallow	Tetanus, peripheral spasm of muscle; amyotrophic lateral sclerosis, medullary tumor; pseudobulbar palsy may be associated with dysarthria
	Eye movements	CN III, IV, VI	Extraocular movement, pupil size, reactivity, pupils react equally to accommodation, diplopia, nystagmus	Cerebral peduncle pressure → CN III dysfunction, cavernous sinus thrombus → CN III, IV, VI problem Muscular problems (e.g., myasthenia gravis, hyperthyroid) Horner's syndrome (ptosis, constricted pupil), anisocoria

TABLE 67–1 **NEUROLOGIC ASSESSMENT GUIDELINES** *Continued*

Functional Category	Specific Category	Area of Nervous System Involved	Assessment Technique	Examples of Disorders
	Moving	Motor precentral gyrus (pyramidal) and cerebellar systems, basal ganglia, CN XI, spinal cord, upper motor neuron, (brain → spinal cord via corticospinal tract)	Gait, heel-to-toe walking, presence or absence of involuntary movements, coordination, muscle tone, mass, strength, Romberg's test, ability to shrug shoulders and to rise from chair	*Upper motor neuron:* Brain and cord-sparing anterior horn cell Tone ↑ ↑ (spastic) Bulk ↓ due to atrophy of disuse Reflexes ↑ ↑ due to loss of central inhibition No fasciculations Frequent clonus
		Lower motor neuron (motor cells of cranial and spinal nerves and anterior horn cells → peripheral muscles)		*Lower motor neuron:* Segment anterior horn cell peripheral nerve Tone ↓ ↓ (flaccid) Bulk ↓ due to tone loss Reflexes ↓ or absent due to loss of anterior horn cell Fasciculations No clonus
		Involves cerebellum		*Cerebellar problem →* loss of coordination and balance
5. Sensory function	Seeing	CN II: optic, occipital lobe	Acuity, visual fields, funduscopy	Field test: loss in retina or optic nerve → loss in eye involved, optic chiasm → bitemporal hemianopsia Optic tract → homonymous hemianopsia, parietal lobe → quadrant problems (inferior), temporal lobe → superior quadrant problems ↑ Intracranial pressure → papilledema (raised disc → hemorrhage)
	Smelling	CN I: temporal lobe (uncus)	Ability to detect familiar odors	Usually ↓ smell due to extraneural causes (e.g., upper respiratory infection, allergy, smoking), olfactory groove; meningioma, olfactory hallucinations

Table continued on following page

TABLE 67–1 NEUROLOGIC ASSESSMENT GUIDELINES *Continued*

Functional Category	Specific Category	Area of Nervous System Involved	Assessment Technique	Examples of Disorders
	Hearing	CN VIII: cochlear division, temporal lobe	Acuity of hearing, presence or absence of unusual sounds, Weber's and Rinne tests	May have conductive (nerve OK) or neural hearing loss; Ménière's syndrome (tinnitus, hearing loss, vertigo, and nystagmus), basilar skull fracture → otorrhea Brain stem vascular dysfunction or tumors → ↓ hearing
	Taste	CN VII, IX: insula lobe	Ability to differentiate sweet, salt, sour, and bitter	Brain stem or insula lesions → ↓ taste; extraneural causes, smoking, poor oral hygiene
	Feeling (sensory)	Peripheral nerves → Dermatomes → Spinal cord → Tracts (leading to) Pain-temperature–tactile, anterolateral system, proprioception, stereognosis, dorsal roots → thalamus leading to somasthetic area (postcentral gyrus, parietal lobe)	Pain: pinprick Touch: cotton touched to skin Proprioception: check where digit is in space Vibration: place vibrating tuning fork on bony prominence Temperature: test tubes of cold and warm water laid against skin; person identifies whether hot or cold	Polyneuropathy (e.g., diabetes, anemia) Spinal cord lesions → dermatome alterations Upper pons → thalamus, contralateral loss Thalamus → contralateral loss + paresthesia Thalamus → cortex → cortical sensory loss
6. Bowel and bladder function	Bowel function	Afferent Spinal nerve S3–5 External sphincter (voluntary control) Internal sphincter Spinal nerve S3–5 Autonomic nervous system Cerebral cortex	Check for fecal impaction or incontinence Check muscle tone	Fecal incontinence with lesions S3–5 Anal anesthesia—conus medullaris and tabes dorsalis May be extraneural causes Loss of inhibitory control (e.g., stroke)
	Bladder function	Autonomic nervous system Afferent Spinal nerve T9–L2, S2–4 Pudendal nerve Efferent Spinal nerve T11–L2 External sphincter (voluntary) Spinal nerve S2–4 Cerebral cortex	Feels when bladder is full, complete emptying. Does client have urgency, frequency?	Urinary incontinence Flaccid bladder Spastic bladder Loss of inhibitory control (e.g., stroke) May be extraneural causes

C, cervical; CN, cranial nerve; CNS, central nervous system; L, lumbar; S, sacral; T, thoracic.
↑, increase; ↑ ↑, significantly increased; ↓, decreased; ↓ ↓, significantly decreased; →, may affect or lead to.

childhood immunizations as well as recommendations for travelers to foreign countries.

Major Illnesses and Hospitalizations

A number of major illnesses are associated with neurologic changes, such as diabetes mellitus, pernicious anemia, cancer, infections, and hypertension. Advanced liver disease and renal disease result in metabolic disturbances, fluid and electrolyte imbalances, and acid-base changes that affect mental function. Inquire about hospitalization, injury, or surgery for neurologic system problems, such as head trauma, seizures, stroke, and crushing tissue injury. Has the client undergone a neurologic diagnostic study, such as electroencephalography (EEG), electromyography (EMG), or computed tomography (CT)? Results of such diagnostic studies provide valuable data for future comparison.

Medications

The medication history covers all medicines that the client is taking or has taken, both prescription and over-the-counter, including herbal preparations. Specifically, ask about aspirin, anticonvulsants, stimulants and depressants, sedatives, anticoagulants, narcotics, tranquilizers, and antihypertensive medications. Many preparations for allergies and colds contain ingredients that cause drowsiness. Inquire about the current or past use of recreational drugs, the type of drug, and the duration of use.

Common herbal preparations used for neurologic problems are as follows:

- CNS stimulants: betel nut (*Areca catechu*); ephedra (*Ephedra sinica, E. vulgaris, E. nevadensis*), also known as Ma huang, and illegal in some areas; nutmeg (*Myristica fragrans*).
- Sedatives/hypnotics: chamomile (*Matricaria recutita, Chamaemelum nobile*); gotu kola (*Centella asiatica*); hops (*Humulus lupulus*); kava kava (*Piper mythysticum*); St. John's wort (*Hypericum perforatum*); valerian (*Valeriana officinalis*).
- Antidepressives: *Ginkgo biloba*; sage (*Salvia officinalis*); St. John's wort. Sage can be used as an aid for dizziness, as can *G. biloba*. *G. biloba* has also been indicated for treating tinnitus, short-term memory loss, and headache.
- Analgesics: cayenne (*Capsicum*), taken internally for headache and toothache or applied externally for neuralgia; feverfew (*Tanacetum parthenium*), used in the treatment and prophylaxis of migraine headaches; white willow (*Salix purpurea, S. fragilis, S. daphnoides*), used as an analgesic and antipyretic.
- Antihypertensive or anti-stroke effects: garlic (*Allium sativum*); *G. biloba*; onion (*Allium cepa*); reishi mushroom (*Ganoderma lucidum*).

Growth and Development

The growth and development history may help determine whether neurologic dysfunction was present at an early age. The perinatal history may contain data about in utero exposure to viruses (rubella), maternal consumption of alcohol, tobacco, or other drugs, and radiation. Ask whether the client's mother carried to full term during her pregnancy. Premature birth increases the risk of neurologic damage from inadequate oxygenation and intracranial bleeding if ventilator support was used. A difficult or prolonged labor and delivery can result in hypoxia or use of forceps for delivery, with consequent central and peripheral neurologic damage.

At what age did the client accomplish major developmental tasks, such as walking and talking? Was the client able to participate in games, sports, and other childhood activities with peers? Did the client have any problems with coordination, balance, or agility?

■ FAMILY HEALTH HISTORY

Ask about a family history of neurologic disorders to determine the presence of genetic risk factors. Inquire about epilepsy, Huntington's disease, amyotrophic lateral sclerosis, muscular dystrophy, hypertension, stroke, mental retardation, and psychiatric disorders.

■ PSYCHOSOCIAL HISTORY

An understanding of personal psychosocial factors (e.g., educational background, level of performance, and personality changes) enhances assessment. Inquire about changes that have occurred in daily routines. Ask about changes in sleep patterns, exercise routines, hobbies and recreation, occupation, perceived stressors, and sexual interest and performance. Is there risk of exposure to neurotoxic fumes or chemicals, such as pesticides, paints, or bonding agents (glue), or does the client spend time in an inadequately ventilated living area or workspace?

■ REVIEW OF SYSTEMS

Neurologic disorders often subtly affect the ability to function in an integrated fashion. Ask the client to describe any neurologic manifestations, such as behavior changes, mood swings, loss of consciousness, seizures, headaches, dizziness, vertigo, memory deficits, speech or motor function problems (e.g., unstable balance or posture, gait changes, tics, tremors), and sensory function problems (e.g., vision changes, pain, paresthesia or tingling, paralysis). Significant neurologic assessment data include those given in Box 67–1. Detailed questions for the review of systems can be found in Chapter 9, Box 9–2.

The client who has a neurologic problem may be unaware of its presence. Attempt to supplement and corroborate the history and review of systems by speaking with a family member or significant other who knows the client well. Ask specifically about mental or physical changes that have been noticed.

PHYSICAL EXAMINATION

The physical examination is intended to detect abnormalities in neurologic functioning. Variations in client age, physical condition, and LOC determine how detailed an examination can be. A comprehensive neurologic examination is described here. Adapt the examination to the client's level of neurologic function. Box 67–2 is a guide for adapting the assessment in various situations. A suggested sequence for the physical examination is as follows:

BOX 67–1 Manifestations Related to Neurologic Assessment

Eye
Visual loss
Diplopia
Ptosis
Proptosis

Ear, Nose, and Throat
Infections
Hearing loss
Tinnitus
Dizziness
Vertigo
Voice change
Dysphagia
Changes in taste or smell
Experiences of unusual smells

Cardiovascular
Syncope
Palpitations
Hypotension
Hypertension
Vertigo
Transient ischemic attacks
Stroke

Neurologic
Weakness
Numbness
Paresthesias
Headache
Pain
Altered thinking
Speech difficulty
Vomiting
Vertigo
Ataxia
Fainting
Seizures
Any loss of consciousness
Distortions of reality
Use of consciousness-altering drugs
Disorientation
Altered sleep patterns
Changes in ability to speak, read, or understand language
Changes in memory of recent or remote events
Changes in ability to concentrate

Skin
Hair and nail changes

Musculoskeletal
Tremor
Weakness
Altered coordination
Staggering
Difficulty climbing stairs

1. Vital signs.
2. Mental status (including language and communication).
3. Head, neck, and back.
4. Cranial nerves (including pupils).
5. Motor system.
6. Sensory function.
7. Reflexes.
8. Autonomic nervous system.

Neurologic findings are summarized in the accompanying feature called Physical Assessment Findings in the Healthy Adult: Neurologic System.

■ VITAL SIGNS

Although cortical changes occur first (e.g., LOC), vital signs are assessed first because neurologic disorders can cause life-threatening changes in vital signs. Clients who have cervical spinal cord injuries exhibit a classic triad of hypotension, bradycardia, and hypothermia related to the loss of sympathetic nervous system function. Inadequate perfusion of vital organs may result from hypotension if the blood pressure is not sustained.

Changes in vital signs can also accompany the late stages of increased intracranial pressure (ICP). The body attempts to provide an adequate supply of oxygen and glucose to the brain by increasing the blood flow to the brain to compensate for the elevated ICP. *Cushing's response* consists of elevated systolic blood pressure, widened pulse pressure, and bradycardia. Respiratory rate and rhythm can be altered by increased ICP on the brain stem.

■ MENTAL STATUS

Document general data about the client's mental status (e.g., LOC, orientation, memory, mood and affect, intellectual performance, judgment and insight, and language and communication). The mental status examination is discussed in Chapter 9.

Level of Consciousness

The *LOC* is the most sensitive indicator of changes in neurologic status. Consciousness is maintained by the cerebral hemispheres and reticular activating system. Test LOC by using stimuli to determine arousal. Stimuli include verbal, visual, tactile, and noxious agents, such as painful pressure.

When assessing LOC, begin by observing spontaneous behavior before using stimuli; then provide stimuli, and make observations regarding the response. Start with a visual cue, such as walking in front of the client or waving hello. If a response is not elicited, provide verbal stimulation. Use touch and painful (noxious) stimuli only if the client does not respond to the milder forms of stimulation.

If a painful stimulus is needed to elicit a response, it should be a central stimulus, such as sternal pressure, supraorbital ridge pressure, or sternocleidomastoid muscle pinch. Although nail bed pressure may be used, it is a

BOX 67–2 The Initial Neurologic Examination in the Clinical Setting

The sequence in which the neurologic examination is performed and the amount of time devoted to each step are dictated by the client's situation. For example, assessment of the head-injured client in the emergency department requires evaluation of vital signs, pupil reactivity, level of consciousness, and motor response. These clients may not be stable or cooperative enough to allow completion of the cranial nerve and sensory response assessment. Spinal cord–injured clients, however, are usually coherent and able to participate in the sensory examination. The sensory assessment information is essential for documenting changes in the status of spinal cord–injured clients.

As clients become more stable and cooperative, the examination can be performed in more depth and with less frequency. Remember that neurologically impaired clients frequently experience fluctuations in status. Alter the assessment schedule and technique to detect and report these fluctuations.

Following are suggested modifications in the screening neurologic examination that may be made on the basis of the client's initial presentation:

- *Initial examination for diagnosis and triage*:
  - Client history based on chief complaint
  - Physical examination including vital signs
  - Level of consciousness
  - Pupillary response
  - Brain stem function (corneal reflex)
  - Motor and sensory functions in all four extremities
- *If the client is conscious and stable*:
  - Complete baseline neurologic examination
  - Focused examinations at prescribed levels
- *If the client is conscious and unstable*:
  - Quick baseline physical assessment
  - Frequent focused examinations until client is stable
  - Vital signs
  - Level of consciousness
  - Pupillary response
  - Brain stem function
  - Motor and sensory functions in extremities
  - Spinal cord function
- *If the patient is unconscious but stable*:
  - Vital signs
  - Level of consciousness and ability to arouse
  - Cranial nerve function
  - Motor and sensory functions
  - Pathologic reflexes
- *If the patient is unconscious and unstable*:
  - Vital signs
  - Level of consciousness
  - Cranial nerve function
  - Motor and sensory functions relative to the ability to test for them
  - Pathologic reflexes
  - Frequent focused examinations on ongoing basis (hourly or more often)
- *If spinal cord involvement is suspected:*
  - Motor functions in detail with testing of specific muscle groups
  - Sensory function
  - Reflexes
  - Bowel and bladder functions
  - Vital signs

peripheral stimulation and may elicit a spinal reflex response rather than a central, or brain, response. Noxious stimuli are also discussed in Chapter 68.

Document the location and type of stimuli applied along with the client's response so that the results can be accurately compared with those of future examinations. Terms such as "alert," "lethargic," "stuporous," "semicomatose," and "comatose" are vague. Avoid these terms unless your agency has explicit definitions for them to maintain consistency.

The *Glasgow Coma Scale* is an assessment tool designed to note trends in a client's response to stimuli (see Chapter 73). The original Glasgow Coma Scale was developed for use with head-injured clients. Many variations of this scale now exist for use with other client populations.

Orientation

Establish *orientation* to time, place, person, and event (or situation); for instance, ask What is your name? What year is this? What kind of place is this? Where are you? What brought you to the hospital today?

Memory

Identify gross deficits in long-term and short-term memory with simple tests. Test *long-term memory* when the client relates the past health history. (Of course, another source must be able to validate the data.) Test *short-term memory* by (1) stating three words for the client to remember (e.g., red, Broadway, three), (2) asking the client to say the words immediately, and (3) then asking the client to repeat them after a few minutes.

Mood and Affect

Assess mood by asking the client to describe how he or she feels. Assess affect (1) by the way the client appears (e.g., euphoric, depressed) and (2) from the reports of significant others. Is the client's affect appropriate to the situation?

Intellectual Performance

Intellectual performance consists of the fund of knowledge and calculation ability. Ask the client to identify com-

PHYSICAL ASSESSMENT FINDINGS IN THE HEALTHY ADULT

Neurologic System

Inspection

Mental Status. Oriented to person, place, time, and situation. No difficulty recalling recent and past events. Serial 7s deferred. Mood and affect congruent; cooperative, and pleasant. Thought process clear and logical. Demonstrates effective problem solving. Speech articulate, clear, and fluent.

Head, Neck, and Back. Normocephalic without obvious lesions. Maintains head position. Spine in straight alignment with normal cervical, thoracic, and lumbar curves. Neck and back have full range of motion.

Cranial Nerves.

CN I. Discerns smell of coffee, cinnamon, alcohol.

CN II. Visual acuity per Snellen's chart is OU = 20/20. Visual fields full to confrontation. Optic disc margins sharp, no cupping; cup-to-disc ratio is 1:3. Retina: Arteriovenous ratio is 2:3, without nicking. Fovea visualized.

CN III, CN IV, CN VI. PERRLA, direct and consensual. Accommodation present. EOMs intact without nystagmus or strabismus. Cover-uncover test negative. Corneal light reflections symmetrical.

CN V. Opens and closes mouth; chews, clenches teeth, and moves jaw side to side voluntarily. Sensation intact to forehead, cheeks, and chin. Corneal reflexes present.

CN VII. Face movements symmetrical with smiling, frowning, eyebrow raising, lip pursing, and cheek puffing. Discerns sweet, salty, sour, and bitter tastes (also CN IX).

CN VIII. Gross hearing intact. Whisper heard at 3 ft. Air conduction greater than bone conduction bilaterally.

CN IX and CN X. Tongue and uvula midline. Uvula and soft palate rise in midline with phonation. Gag reflex present bilaterally. Swallows, coughs, and speaks without difficulty.

CN XI. Performs shoulder shrugs. Turns head against resistance. Maintains head position against resistance.

CN XII. Tongue protrudes midline without deviation; pushes side to side with equal strength.

Motor Function. Muscle groups symmetrical. Gross and fine motor coordination intact. Moves all extremities through range of motion. Romberg's test negative. Pronator drift absent. Gait smooth, steady. Maintains balance walking on toes and heels. Rapid alternating movements and point-to-point maneuvers performed without difficulty.

Sensory Function. Sensation to light touch, pain, and vibration intact distally and over trunk, neck, and face. Position sense of fingers and toes intact. Stereognosis and graphism present bilaterally. Two-point discrimination: 2 mm on index fingers. Discerns two-point simultaneous stimulation.

Palpation

Head, Neck, and Back. Skull without lesions or tenderness; smooth and firm. Neck and paravertebral muscles firm, relaxed, and nontender. No pain or tenderness over spinous processes.

Motor Function. Muscle groups firm and elastic; strength rated as 5/5.

Percussion

Reflexes. Deep tendon reflexes rated 2+ (on a scale of 0–4+) in triceps, biceps, wrists, knees, and ankles. Plantar reflexes present. Abdominal reflexes present in all four quadrants.

Auscultation

Vascular Flow. Absence of bruit over carotid arteries bilaterally.

monly known people, places, events, and the like. Assess calculation ability by asking the client to count by 7s (*serial 7s*) or 3s. If the client is unable to perform reversed serial 7s, have the client perform simple addition or subtraction (e.g., 3 + 4 = ?, 13 − 5 = ?).

Judgment and Insight

Judgment and insight include reasoning, abstract thinking, problem solving, and the client's perception of the situation. Assess reasoning, abstract thinking, and problem-solving for indications of major problems with thought content (see Chapter 9).

Listen to how the client answers questions. Are the answers logical? Do they relate to the question? Can the client concentrate and remain focused, or is the client easily distracted? Assess abstract thinking by asking the client to explain a proverb such as "A rolling stone gathers no moss." Evaluate reasoning and problem-solving by describing a situation and asking the client to give a solution. For example, "What would you do if you lost your house keys?" Assess insight and perception by asking the client to give an opinion about what might be the cause of the chief complaint.

Language and Communication

Language and communication assessment tests the ability to express and comprehend one's environment. Grossly evaluate *expression* and *comprehension* during the initial interview. Does the client initiate speech? Is speech fluent and appropriate?

Assess speech quality. Is speech clear and intelligible, or garbled because of facial droop or poor dentition? Note the content of speech (orientation, intellect, logic). Assess speech for articulation problems (usually motor disorders) or comprehension or expression problems (aphasic disorders).

Does the client follow verbal commands? Evaluate the client's ability to communicate and understand verbally, in writing, mathematically, and nonverbally.

COMPREHENSION AND EXPRESSION. Comprehension and expression are then assessed in more depth. Test the *ability to comprehend spoken language* by asking the client to follow basic commands ("Show me your right thumb," "Stick out your tongue"). To determine comprehension of written language, ask the client to read several words or sentences and explain them. Write a simple command ("Stick out your tongue"), and have the client read and then perform the command.

Evaluate *expression* as the client responds to questions that require more than a nod or a *yes* or *no* answer. Evaluate speech for flow, choice of words, and completion of phrases or sentences. If the client is expressively aphasic), test comprehension by asking *yes* or *no* questions or by having the client follow simple verbal commands. Assess written expression by having the client write answers to simple questions on paper (e.g., "Write your name and address").

INTEGRATED SENSORY FUNCTIONS. *Integrated sensory functions* involving language are often tested with this portion of the neurologic examination. Have the client perform simple addition or subtraction without writing. Ask the client to orally identify common objects, such as a pen, a key, and a watch. These skills require integration of cortical functioning (calculation) and visual recognition with expressive speech.

■ HEAD, NECK, AND BACK

Examine the head, neck, and spine using inspection, palpation, percussion, and auscultation. Tumors, vascular disorders, traumatic disorders, and problems involving the vertebrae and surrounding muscles may be detected through examination.

Inspection

Inspect the head for size, shape, contour, and symmetry. Note any ecchymosis (bruising) around the eyes or behind the ears. Anterior basilar skull fractures often result in "raccoon eyes," with periorbital ecchymosis and, occasionally, drainage of cerebrospinal fluid (CSF) from the nares. Middle fossa basilar skull fractures often result in ecchymosis over the mastoid process behind the ears (Battle's sign) and drainage of blood, CSF, or both from the ears.

Palpation

Palpate the skull lightly for nodules or masses and to supplement inspection findings. Wear gloves if there are open or draining areas. The skull normally feels smooth and firm. Areas of bogginess or depressions are abnormal. Palpation of neck muscles may identify masses or tender areas. Ask the client to flex the neck with the chin touching the chest; look for nuchal (back of the neck) rigidity, which is a sign of meningeal irritation.

Inspect and palpate spine alignment. Note any deviation from the normal curvatures. Palpate the paravertebral muscles for masses, tenderness, and spasm (also see Chapter 25).

Percussion

Gentle percussion over the spinous processes may produce pain or tenderness, which are abnormal findings.

Auscultation

Auscultation of major neck and other vessels may reveal bruits or other abnormal sounds suggesting an abnormality. Use the bell of the stethoscope to auscultate the carotid arteries. Bruits result from turbulent flow, usually a sign of atherosclerotic disease.

■ CRANIAL NERVES

The cranial nerves are referred to by specific name or Roman numeral. Cranial nerve (CN) examination is important for two reasons. First, CN III through CN XII arise in the brain stem. Testing their function provides information about the brain stem and related pathways. Second, three reflexes involving cranial nerves are called *protective reflexes* (corneal, gag, and cough reflexes). The presence or absence of protective reflexes indicates the ability to protect the eye surfaces and airway. This is especially important in unconscious patients.

Normal cranial nerve reflexes require an appropriately received stimulus (input) that produces an appropriate response (output). During testing of cranial nerves, the absence of a normal response may indicate (1) failure to receive stimuli (input failure), (2) failure to respond appropriately (output failure), or (3) a combination of input and output failure. Determining which problems exist is often a challenge. For example, vision is a function of CN II, and pupillary light response is a function of both CN II and CN III (Fig. 67–1; see Table 67–1). The structure and function of the cranial nerves are discussed in the Anatomy and Physiology review for Unit 15.

Olfactory Nerve (CN I): Smell

The function of CN I is purely sensory. Ask the client to smell and then identify an aromatic, nonirritating odor (e.g., coffee, isopropyl alcohol, toothpaste) with each nostril separately and with the eyes closed. Test with several different odors. If the client can perceive any one smell, consider the nerve functional.

Although inability to smell *(anosmia)* may develop in older people, problems such as basal skull fracture or olfactory groove tumor also may be responsible. Other possible causes of anosmia are cribriform plate fracture, an olfactory bulb or a tract tumor, and previous sinus disorders or surgery.

Optic Nerve (CN II): Vision

CN II has a purely sensory function. Assessment of the optic nerve involves the following steps:

1. Inspecting the globe for foreign bodies, cataracts, inflammation, or other obvious abnormalities. Details of eye assessment are given in Chapter 64.
2. Testing *visual acuity*. Have the client read a newspaper, a sign (from a distance), or a Snellen's chart. Eyeglasses should be worn during the test if the

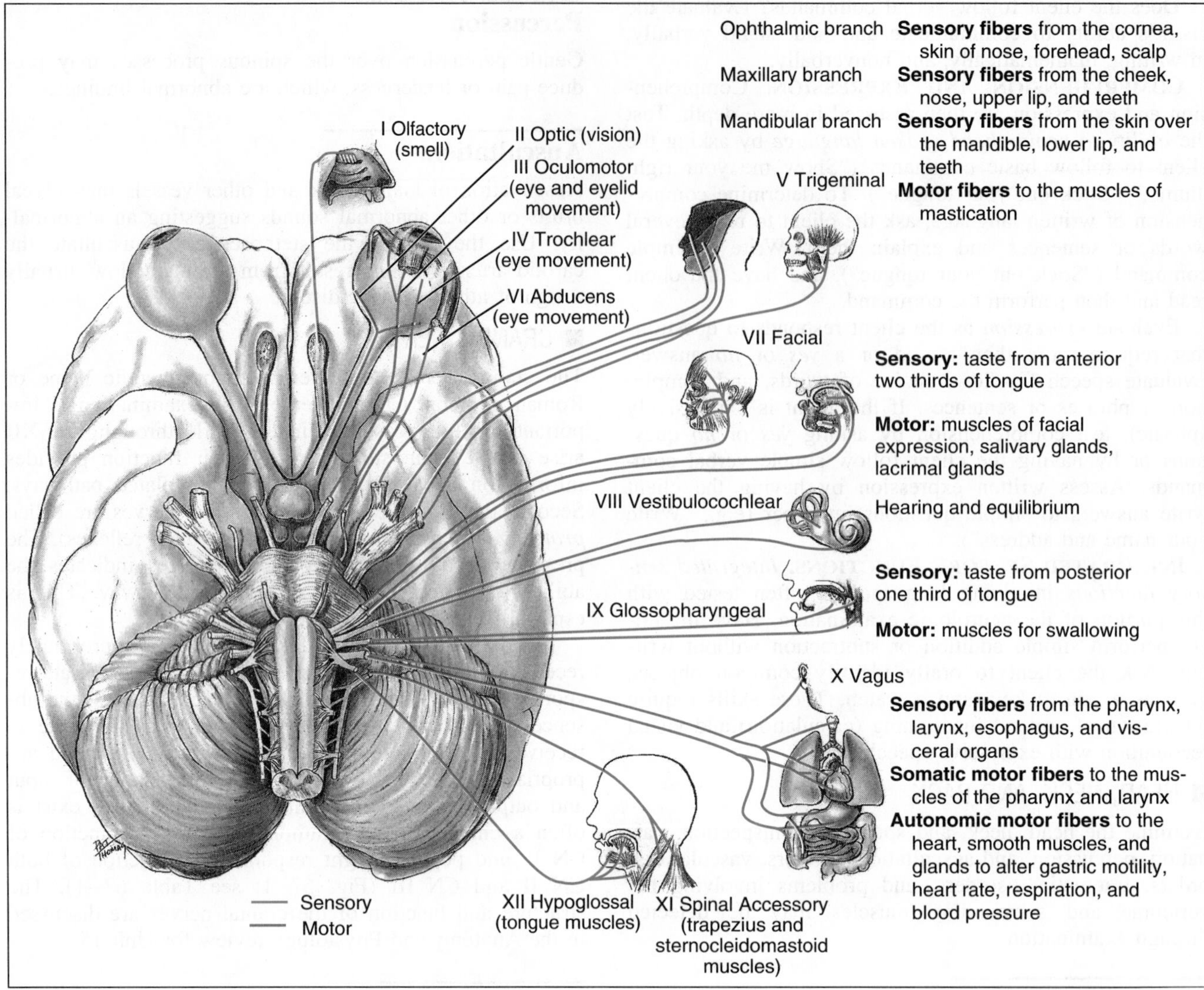

FIGURE 67–1 Distribution of the cranial nerves. Study this figure along with Table 67–1.

client usually wears them. Refraction errors are not significant in neurologic assessment.

3. Testing *visual fields* to determine whether vision is absent in one or more directions or in a portion of the visual field, such as half of the visual field, the middle portion, or both sides. Such losses may indicate various problems and may correlate with the area of the brain involved.
4. Examining the eye fundus with an ophthalmoscope. Gross inspection of the eyes and examination of the fundus can provide information about neurologic disease. Possible causes of abnormal findings include trauma to orbit or eyeball; fracture of optic foramen; diabetic retinopathy; laceration or blood clot in the brain's temporal, parietal, or occipital lobes; and increased ICP (e.g., papilledema).

Oculomotor (CN III), Trochlear (CN IV), and Abducens (CN VI) Nerves: Eyes and Eye Movement

CN III, CN IV, and CN VI have only motor components. CN III controls pupil constriction and elevation of the upper lid. Pupils should be equal in size and round. In approximately 20% of the population, *anisocoria* (unequal pupils) is a normal finding. Older clients who have undergone cataract surgery with lens implants may have irregular, nonreactive pupils. This finding does not indicate neurologic damage. Note pupil size before shining a light into the client's eyes. Document each pupil's size and shape.

Approach the pupil from the temporal side while the client looks straight ahead. Test each pupil for both direct and consensual responses (pupillary constriction) to a light. A *direct response* occurs in the eye being tested. A *consensual response* occurs in the other eye. A direct response indicates an intact connection in the midbrain between CN II and the ipsilateral CN III. An intact consensual response indicates a connection between CN II and the contralateral CN III via a connection in the midbrain.

Test *accommodation* (eyes able to focus on both near and far objects) by having the client look across the room (away from the light source) and then at your fingers held about 6 inches from the client's nose. Normally, the lens shape changes and the pupils constrict. The notation

PERRLA (*p*upils *e*qual, *r*ound, *r*eactive to *l*ight and *ac*commodation) indicates that these functions are normal. When testing *pupillary light reflex* only (not accommodation), the abbreviation *PERL* (*p*upils *e*qual, *r*eactive to *l*ight) is used.

CN III lies over the edge of the uncal portion of the temporal lobe. Increased ICP or edema causes that area of the brain to shift, and CN III is stretched. This disruption of the CN III pathway causes either a sluggish response or absence of response to light. This response can be unilateral or bilateral, depending on the site and severity of edema. *Hippus*, the rhythmic constriction and dilation of a pupil, is caused by early compromise of CN III with increased ICP; it is not seen in all clients. Destruction of part of CN III can cause *ptosis* (drooping of the eyelid). Disorders or pressure on a specific side of CN III can cause the ipsilateral pupil to dilate, the eyelid to droop, and the eye to deviate outward.

CN III, CN IV, and CN VI coordinate to control eye movements in all six cardinal directions of gaze (see Chapter 64). Test the function of these nerves by having the client hold the head still and follow your finger or another object as it is moved in all directions of gaze. *Conjugate gaze* allows for the eyes to move in a coordinated effort for binocular vision (two images "merged" into one). *Disconjugate gaze* often occurs due to weakness of one or more extraocular muscles. *Diplopia* (double vision) occurs with disconjugate gaze because the two images are not "merged." If a client has diplopia but no muscle weakness can be demonstrated, shine a light so it reflects on both eyes. The area of reflection is normally symmetrical, meaning that the client has a conjugate gaze. In disconjugate gaze, the light's reflection is asymmetrical (i.e., not the same in both eyes).

If *extraocular movements* are intact, document as "EOMs intact." Also observe for *nystagmus* (involuntary eye movements), seen as fine, rhythmic eye movements that can be vertical or horizontal. Possible causes of abnormal findings include (1) pressure on CN III, CN IV, or CN VI at the brain stem due to fracture of the orbit; (2) increased ICP; and (3) tumor at or trauma to the base of the brain. An inability to look down or to walk down steps because of a visual disturbance might be related to CN IV dysfunction. Inability of an eye to move laterally outward is associated with compression of or damage to CN VI.

Trigeminal Nerve (CN V)

CN V has a motor division and a sensory division. The motor division innervates the muscles of mastication. Test CN V function by asking the client to clamp the jaws shut, open the mouth against resistance, open the mouth widely, move the jaw from side to side, and make chewing movements. A normal CN V allows all these activities. Document any asymmetry in the temporal muscles.

The sensory division mediates all sensations for the entire face, scalp, cornea, and nasal and oral cavities. With the client's eyes closed, test sensations such as pain (e.g., pinprick), touch (e.g., wisp of cotton), and temperature (e.g., hot and cold test tubes of water) on both sides of the face from the top of the head (vertex) to the chin.

Test the *corneal reflexes* by gently touching the cornea with a sterile wisp of cotton or gently stroking the eyelash. (Omit this test during the screening examination.) The normal response is brisk eyelid blinking. The corneal reflex involves CN V and CN VII. CN V is the afferent (sensory) arc, and CN VII controls closure of the eye (motor). Possible causes of abnormal findings include a tumor at or trauma to the base of the brain, a fracture of the orbit, and trigeminal neuralgia.

Facial Nerve (CN VII)

CN VII has both a motor division and a sensory division. The motor division innervates muscles controlling facial expression. Observe the face for symmetry and the ability to use facial muscles. Ask the client to smile, frown, raise the forehead and eyebrows, tightly close the eyes and resist attempts to open them, whistle, show the teeth, and puff out the cheeks. Test the anterior part of the tongue for taste by asking the client to close the eyes and protrude (stick out) the tongue. Then place a taste substance on one side of the anterior tongue. Have the client keep the tongue protruded while identifying the taste. Ask the client to rinse the mouth or drink a small amount of water before testing the other side. Test taste on each side with sweet, salty, acidic or sour (e.g., vinegar or lemon), and bitter (e.g., coffee) substances.

Common abnormalities noted with CN VII dysfunction include (1) loss of the nasolabial fold, (2) inability to close the eye and blink reflexively, (3) facial asymmetry, (4) drooling, (5) difficulty swallowing secretions, (6) loss of tearing, and (7) loss of taste on the anterior two thirds of the tongue. Possible causes of abnormal findings are Bell's palsy, temporal bone fracture, and peripheral laceration or contusion of the parotid region.

The lower half of the facial muscles, especially around the mouth, also receive innervation from the voluntary motor area of the frontal lobes. Deficits of lower facial muscles can be related to a lesion in the contralateral frontal lobe (i.e., client who has had a stroke and has a flattened nasolabial fold and facial droop on the opposite side retains the ability to close the eyelid on the same side of the face). Deficits on the lower half of the face only are called *central deficits* because the lesion is in the CNS. A deficit involving both the upper face and lower face is called a *peripheral deficit* because the lesion involves CN VII, which is a peripheral nerve.

Vestibulocochlear or Acoustic Nerve (CN VIII)

CN VIII is a sensory nerve with two divisions: cochlear and vestibular. The cochlear nerve permits hearing. Test *auditory acuity* by having the client listen to and report on a whispered voice, rustling fingers, or a tuning fork at various distances from the ear. Test *bone and air conduction* with a tuning fork. Audiometry may be used for a precise assessment.

The vestibular nerve helps maintain equilibrium by coordinating the muscles of the eye, neck, trunk, and extremities. *Equilibrium tests* include Romberg's and caloric tests (oculovestibular reflex) and electronystagmography. (Hearing and equilibrium assessment is described in Chapter 64.) Possible causes of abnormal findings include Ménière's syndrome and acoustic neuroma.

Glossopharyngeal (CN IX) and Vagus (CN X) Nerves

CN IX and CN X have both motor and sensory components. Because of overlapping innervation of the pharynx, assess these nerves together. Ask the client to open the mouth widely and say "Ah." Observe the position and movement of the uvula and palate. The palate should rise symmetrically, and the uvula should at the midline. Test the *gag reflex* by gently touching each side of the pharynx with a tongue depressor, which normally elicits a brisk response. Use a small amount of water to assess the ability to swallow. Test the posterior third of the tongue for taste, as with CN VII (perform when testing CN VII). Dysfunction of CN IX includes loss of taste and sensation of the glossopharyngeal nerve.

To test the function of CN X, ask the client to cough and to speak. Damage to CN X causes an ineffective cough and a weak, hoarse voice. To differentiate areas of weakness, ask the client to vocalize different sounds: "kuh-kuh" (soft palate), "mi-mi" (lips), "la-la" (tongue). Possible causes of abnormal findings include brain stem trauma or tumors, neck trauma, and stroke.

Spinal Accessory Nerve (CN XI)

CN XI has only a motor component. It innervates the sternocleidomastoid muscle and the upper portion of the trapezius muscle. Ask the client to (1) elevate the shoulders (with and without resistance), (2) turn (not tilt) the head to one side and then the other, (3) resist attempts to pull the chin back toward the midline, and (4) push the head forward against resistance. Disorders may produce drooping of a shoulder, muscle atrophy, weak shoulder shrug, or weak turn of the head. Possible causes of abnormal findings include neck trauma, radical neck surgery, and torticollis.

Hypoglossal Nerve (CN XII)

CN XII has only a motor component. This nerve innervates the tongue. Ask the client to open the mouth widely, stick out the tongue, and rapidly move the tongue from side to side and in and out. Document any deviation from midline. Assess strength by having the client push the tongue against the inside of the cheek while applying external pressure. Possible causes of abnormal findings include neck trauma associated with major blood vessel damage.

■ MOTOR SYSTEM

Assessing the motor system thoroughly involves numerous procedures. The following discussion focuses on the screening examinations and common abnormalities.

Muscle Size

Inspect all major muscle groups bilaterally for symmetry, hypertrophy, and atrophy.

Muscle Strength

Assess the power in major muscle groups against resistance (see Chapter 25). Assess and rate muscle strength on a 5-point scale in all four extremities, comparing one side with the other, as follows:

5/5 = Normal full strength. Muscle is able to move actively through the full range of motion against the effects of gravity and applied resistance.
4/5 = Muscle is able to move actively through the full range of motion against the effect of gravity with weakness to applied resistance.
3/5 = Muscle is able to move actively against the effect of gravity alone.
2/5 = Muscle is able to move across a surface but cannot overcome gravity.
1/5 = Muscle contraction is palpable and visible; trace or flicker movement occurs.
0/5 = Muscle contraction or movement is undetectable.

Next, test for subtle weakness in upper and lower extremities. For upper extremities, have the client hold the arms straight out in front with the palms up ("like holding a tray"). Ask the client to close the eyes and to maintain the position. A *pronator drift* is said to be present if one arm pronates and falls lower than the other. For the lower extremities, have the client walk on the heels, then on the toes. This tests dorsiflexion, plantiflexion, and balance.

Assessment of specific muscle groups evaluates deficits in certain areas, such as spinal cord disorders. Disorders of muscle strength may be exhibited as weakness on one side of the body, in both lower extremities, or in both upper and lower extremities.

If asymmetry is detected, ask the client or family whether it is long-standing or recent. Consider the client's age and physical condition when interpreting the results of muscle strength testing. One would not expect the same strength from a physically fit young client as from an elderly or debilitated client. If abnormalities are found in muscle power, more detailed assessment may be conducted with procedures such as EMG (see later in this chapter).

Muscle Tone

Assess muscle tone while moving each extremity through its range of passive motion. When tone is decreased *(hypotonicity),* the muscles are soft, flabby, or flaccid; when tone is increased *(hypertonicity),* the muscles are resistant to movement, rigid, or spastic. Note the presence of abnormal flexion or extension posture.

Muscle Coordination

Muscle coordination assessment consists of testing rapid alternating movements, point-to-point maneuvers, and maintenance of truncal balance and head position. Test *rapid alternating movements* by asking the client to touch (approximate) each finger to the thumb quickly in succession. Alternatively, ask the client to pat the thighs first with the palms, then with the back of the hands, and to repeat the patting quickly.

For *point-to-point testing*, hold up an index finger approximately 18 inches from the client. Ask the client to first touch his or her nose with a finger, then touch your index finger, and then touch the nose again. Repeat this several times while you move your index finger to different locations. Perform the test for the client's right and left hands. Test lower extremity coordination by asking the client to place the heel of the foot below the other knee and then to slide the heel down the shin toward the great toe. Repeat for the other leg.

Assess *truncal balance* with the client sitting. Can the client remain upright without support? Gently push the client to a leaning position. Can the client return to an upright position? Note *head position* by observing the ability to move the head while following your movements.

Disorders related to coordination indicate cerebellar or posterior column lesions. The defining characteristics of cerebellar dysfunction are (1) ataxia, (2) intention tremor (tremor upon nearing the object), (3) nystagmus, (4) ocular dysmetria (inability to gaze on an object), and (5) dysdiadochokinesia (arresting one motor impulse and substituting an opposite one).

Gait and Station

Assess gait and station by having the client stand still, walk, and walk in tandem (i.e., one foot in front of the other in a straight line). Walking involves the functions of motor power, sensation, and coordination. The ability to stand quietly with the feet together requires coordination and intact *proprioception* (sense of body position). If the client has difficulty standing, assess further to determine whether the client is weak or unsteady. If the client is weak, you need to protect the client from falling. Box 67–3 includes terms used to describe gait disorders.

Movement

Examine the muscles for fine and gross abnormal movements. Examples of fine movements are *fasciculations* (involuntary ripples or twitches that occur while the client is relaxed), which may indicate lower motor neuron disease. Examples of more grossly abnormal movements, often representing extrapyramidal disease, are described in Box 67–4.

Move all joints through a full range of passive motion. Abnormal findings include pain, contractures, and muscle resistance.

Test for *apraxia* (inability to carry out a learned movement on command in the absence of weakness or paralysis). Ask the client to perform a common activity, such as tying shoes or combing hair. Apraxia is present if a client can follow other commands (indicating intact comprehension), has the motor strength to move the extremity involved, but cannot carry out the command.

BOX 67–4 Abnormal Movements Associated with Extrapyramidal Disease

Akinesia: reduced body movement in the absence of weakness or paralysis; habitual movements (e.g., swinging arms) limited or absent
Athetosis: gross, writhing, worm-like movements of body, face, or extremities
Ballismus: a form of chorea; involuntary dramatic movements of arms and legs (*hemiballismus* involves only one side)
Bradykinesia: slow movement
Chorea: discrete, jerky, purposeless movements in distal extremities and face
Dystonia: prolonged twisting movements
Myoclonus: sudden muscle contractions of varying intensity that may involve a small part of one extremity or the entire body; may violently fling a client to the floor
Tic: involuntary movement of groups of muscles in stereotypic patterns; may be physical or psychogenic in origin; pathologic causes of tics include Tourette's syndrome and tic douloureux
Tremors: involuntary trembling or quivering; may vary in direction, amplitude, rhythmicity, parts involved, speed, and timing in relation to rest or activity; types include parkinsonian, familial, and senile

BOX 67–3 Terms Associated with Gait Disorders

Ataxic: staggering and unsteady
Double step: alternate steps differing in length or rate
Dystonic: irregular and nondirective
Dystrophic or broad-based: legs far apart; weight shifting from side to side (waddling)
Equine: high steps
Festinating: walking on toes at an accelerating pace
Helicopod: feet (or foot) making a half-circle with each step
Hemiplegic: paralyzed on one side; paralyzed limb swings outward; foot drags; arm on affected side does not swing freely
Parkinsonian: short, accelerating steps; shuffling; forward-leaning posture; head, hips, and knees flexed; difficulty starting and stopping
Scissors: legs crossed while walking with short, slow steps
Spastic: stiff, short steps; toes catch and drag; legs held together; hips and knees flexed
Steppage: foot and toes lifted high; heel comes down heavily
Tabetic: high steps; foot slaps down

Motor Testing of Unconscious Patients

In this chapter, the term "patient" is used to describe the client who is unconscious and who cannot be an active participant in care. The family is considered the client in these situations.

An unresponsive patient can be tested only for response to painful stimuli (e.g., reflex withdrawal of limbs, wincing, grimacing). Although a pain stimulus is used, the response is usually recorded as a motor system response. These responses are often incorporated into the motor scale of the Glasgow Coma Scale.

Use deep pain to elicit a sensory response when an unconscious patient is unresponsive to superficial stimuli. Use minimal stimulation to assess cerebral response to pain with techniques such as rubbing the sternum, applying pressure to the orbital rim, or squeezing the sternocleidomastoid muscle. Nail bed pressure may be used; however, the stimulus is a peripheral source of pain and may produce a spinal segment reflex response even in the absence of cerebral function. Document the site and type of stimulus used so that the examination can be adequately reproduced at a later time. Note the patient's response to the noxious stimuli. Following are the most common responses to painful stimuli:

- *Localization:* Patient reaches for the source of the stimulus and attempts to push the examiner away.
- *Flexion withdrawal:* Patient moves without purpose and may exhibit minimal movement, grimacing, or wincing.
- *Abnormal flexion (decorticate posturing):* Patient flexes, adducts, and internally rotates the wrists and arms to the chest and rigidly extends the legs. This posture indicates damage in the corticospinal tracts near the cerebral hemispheres that has left the rubrospinal tract intact.
- *Abnormal extension (decerebrate posturing):* Patient extends and pronates the arms while rigidly extending the legs. This posture indicates damage in the upper brain stem.
- *No response:* There is no visible reaction to painful stimuli.

SENSORY FUNCTION

The sensory function examination incorporates assessment of responses to superficial and mechanical sensations as well as cortical discrimination. Sensory assessment involves testing for touch, pain, vibration, position (proprioception), and discrimination. Assessment of hearing, vision, smell, and taste is also sensory assessment. Sensory assessment may identify dermatomes as having normal, absent, reduced, exaggerated, or delayed sensation. Dermatomes are discussed in the Anatomy and Physiology review for Unit 15.

A complete sensory examination is possible only on a conscious client because the client's cooperation is required. Always test sensation with the client's eyes closed. Help the client relax.

Conduct sensory assessment systematically. Test a particular area of the body, then test the corresponding area on the other side. Begin testing a selection of dermatomes that represent cervical, thoracic, lumbar, and sacral segments of the spinal cord. If you note a sensory loss, you can perform a more detailed testing of surrounding dermatomes. Document asymmetrical findings (those varying from one side to the other). If the client has a sensory loss, document the area of loss and where normal sensation begins. Sensation assessment may be documented on a body chart of dermatomes.

Superficial Sensation

Test superficial sensations by stimulating the skin in symmetrical areas on each side of the body according to dermatome distribution. Test *superficial pain* by alternating the sharp and dull ends of a broken cotton applicator. The wooden broken end is pointed enough for testing sharp sensation, yet dull enough not to break the skin. The cotton swab end serves as the dull stimulus. Use a new swab for each client to eliminate concern about cross-contamination from one client to another.

TOUCH AND PAIN

Ask the client to close the eyes. Explain that the client will feel a sharp or a dull stimulus. Demonstrate how sharp and dull feel. Touch the client with the dull end of the swab. Then apply a painful stimulus with the pointed end. Move from the fingers to the shoulders. Alternate the two stimuli inconsistently (so that the client cannot predict which is being used), and ask the client to distinguish sharp from dull. Then test from the toes to the thighs. Finally, test the anterior and posterior trunk and the buttocks.

Keep the dermatomal pattern in mind while testing. Where there is a loss of the sense of pain, test for awareness of temperature. Otherwise, it is not necessary to test for temperature because pain and temperature sensations travel on related pathways.

OTHER MODALITIES

Other modalities for testing superficial sensation in the conscious client include using a cotton wisp to assess *light touch.* Follow the same guidelines as for testing superficial pain sensation, stimulating symmetrical areas of the dermatomes.

Temperature sensation is not assessed routinely. Perform the test only when pain and light touch responses are abnormal. Use two test tubes, one filled with warm water and one with cold water. Check first to ensure that the warm water is not too hot. Assess each major dermatome symmetrically. Alternatively, use the side of the tuning fork, which is usually cold, to test for awareness of temperature.

Mechanical Sensation

Mechanical sensations are assessed with vibration and proprioception.

VIBRATION

Use a tuning fork to test for vibration. Place the end of a vibrating tuning fork on a distal bony prominence, such as a finger or great toe joint. Ask the client to indicate when the vibration is felt and when it is no longer felt. Once the client indicates that the sensation has stopped, test your own joint to see whether you can feel vibration. You serve as the control. If the client reports that the sensation has stopped but you can still sense a clear vibration, the client has reduced vibratory sense. If the client does not feel vibration at all, move the tuning fork proximally to test the wrist, elbow, or ankle.

PROPRIOCEPTION

Test proprioception by holding the side of the client's fingertips, then the great toes, between thumb and index finger. As each of the client's fingers and toes are gently flexed and extended, ask the client to state when movement is felt and in what direction. If impairment is detected, test more proximal joints.

Discrimination

Cortical discrimination depends on the ability to integrate and interpret sensory stimuli in the parietal lobe. Included are tests for stereognosis, graphism, extinction phenomenon, and simultaneous two-point stimulation.

To test *stereognosis* (i.e., discernment of the form and configuration of objects felt, or three-dimensional discrimination), place three small, familiar objects, such as a coin, a key, and a paper clip, one at a time in the client's hands. Ask the client to identify each with the eyes closed.

To test *graphism* (recognition of the form and configuration of written symbols), trace different separate letters and numbers on the client's palm with the blunt end of a pen. Ask the client to identify each with the eyes closed. Orient the figures so that they are right-side-up for the client.

To test for the *extinction phenomenon* (simultaneous stimulation), prick the client's skin at the same point on the two sides of the body at the same time. Ask the client to state whether one or two pricks are felt.

To perform *two-point stimulation* (two-point discrimination), simultaneously prick the skin with two pins at varying distances apart to identify the smallest distance at which the client can perceive two pricks. Normal distances at which two-point discrimination is lost are: upper arms, 75 mm; thighs, 75 mm; back, 40 to 70 mm; chest, 40 mm; forearms, 40 mm; palms, 8 to 12 mm; toes, 3 to 8 mm; fingertips, 2.8 mm; and tongue, 1 mm.

Abnormalities of sensation include:

- *Dysesthesias:* well-localized irritating sensations, such as warmth, cold, itching, tickling, crawling, prickling, and tingling
- *Paresthesias:* distortions of sensory stimuli (e.g., light touch may be experienced as burning or painful sensation)
- *Anesthesia:* absence of the sense of touch
- *Hypoesthesia:* reduced sense of touch
- *Hyperesthesia:* pathologic (abnormal) overperception of touch
- *Analgesia:* absence of the sense of pain
- *Hypalgesia:* reduced sense of pain
- *Hyperalgesia:* increased sense of pain
- *Agraphesthesia:* inability to identify symbols traced on the palm when the eyes are closed
- *Astereognosis:* loss of sense of three-dimensional discrimination

Figure 67–2 summarizes patterns of sensory loss. Sensory changes are part of the normal aging process. Careful assessment of such changes is the basis of nursing intervention for elderly clients. Table 67–1 contains guidelines for assessment.

■ REFLEX ACTIVITY

Reflex testing evaluates the integrity of specific sensory and motor pathways. Reflex arcs consist of:

- Receptor (sensory) organ
- Afferent (sensory) nerve
- Connection in the central nervous system (brain or spinal cord)
- Efferent (motor) nerve
- Effector (motor) organ

Reflex activity assessment, always a part of neurologic assessment, provides information about the nature, location, and progression of neurologic disorders.

Normal Reflexes

Two types of reflexes are normally present: (1) superficial, or cutaneous, reflexes and (2) deep tendon, or muscle-stretch, reflexes (Table 67–2).

SUPERFICIAL (CUTANEOUS) REFLEXES

Superficial (cutaneous) reflexes are elicited by stimulation of the skin or mucous membranes. The stimulus is produced by stroking a sensory zone with an object that will not cause damage. Superficial reflexes (i.e., abdominal, plantar, corneal, pharyngeal [gag], cremasteric, and anal) are absent in pyramidal tract disorders. For example, they are absent on the affected side after a cerebrovascular accident (stroke).

ABDOMINAL REFLEX. Lightly stroking the skin on an abdominal quadrant normally contracts the abdominal muscle, moving the umbilicus toward the stimulated side.

PLANTAR REFLEX. Scratching the foot's outer aspect of the plantar surface (outer sole) from the heel toward the toes normally contracts or flexes the toes in clients older than 2 years of age.

CORNEAL REFLEX. Gently touching the cornea with a wisp of cotton causes reflex blinking. For example, to test the left eye, have the client look up and to the right, and bring the cotton wisp in from the side so the client cannot see your hand; then very gently touch the outer edge of the cornea.

In an unconscious patient, you can test the corneal reflex by holding the eyelids open and placing a drop of sterile saline on the cornea. This technique prevents inadvertent corneal abrasions.

PHARYNGEAL (GAG) REFLEX. Gentle stimulation with a tongue blade at the back of the throat and pharynx normally produces gagging. The corneal and pharyngeal reflexes are usually assessed with the cranial nerves, discussed earlier.

CREMASTERIC REFLEX. Stroking the inner thigh of a man normally elevates the ipsilateral testicle.

ANAL REFLEX. Stimulate the perianal skin or gently insert a gloved finger into the rectum. Normal response is contraction of the rectal sphincter.

DEEP TENDON (MUSCLE-STRETCH) REFLEXES

Deep tendon reflexes are also called muscle-stretch, or myotactic, reflexes because reflex muscle contraction normally results from rapid stretching of the muscle. This is produced by sharply striking a muscle tendon's point of insertion with a sudden, brief blow of a reflex hammer (Fig. 67–3 and Box 67–5).

Reflexes commonly assessed include the Achilles tendon, patella, biceps, and triceps as follows:

- An *ankle jerk* (plantiflexion of the foot) is produced by tapping the Achilles tendon.
- A *knee jerk, quadriceps jerk,* or *patellar reflex* (leg extension) is produced by tapping the quadriceps femoris tendon just below the patella.
- A *biceps jerk* (forearm flexion) is produced by tapping the biceps brachii tendon.
- A *triceps jerk* (forearm extension) is produced by tapping the triceps brachii tendon at the elbow.

OTHER NORMAL REFLEXES

Some normal reflexes involve structures other than skeletal muscles. For example, reflex mechanisms help maintain respiration and keep blood pressure within normal limits. Reflex salivation may follow the taste (or smell) of food. Flashing a light in an eye causes the pupils of both eyes to constrict (*light reflex* or *pupillary reflex*; see also the discussion of cranial nerve assessment).

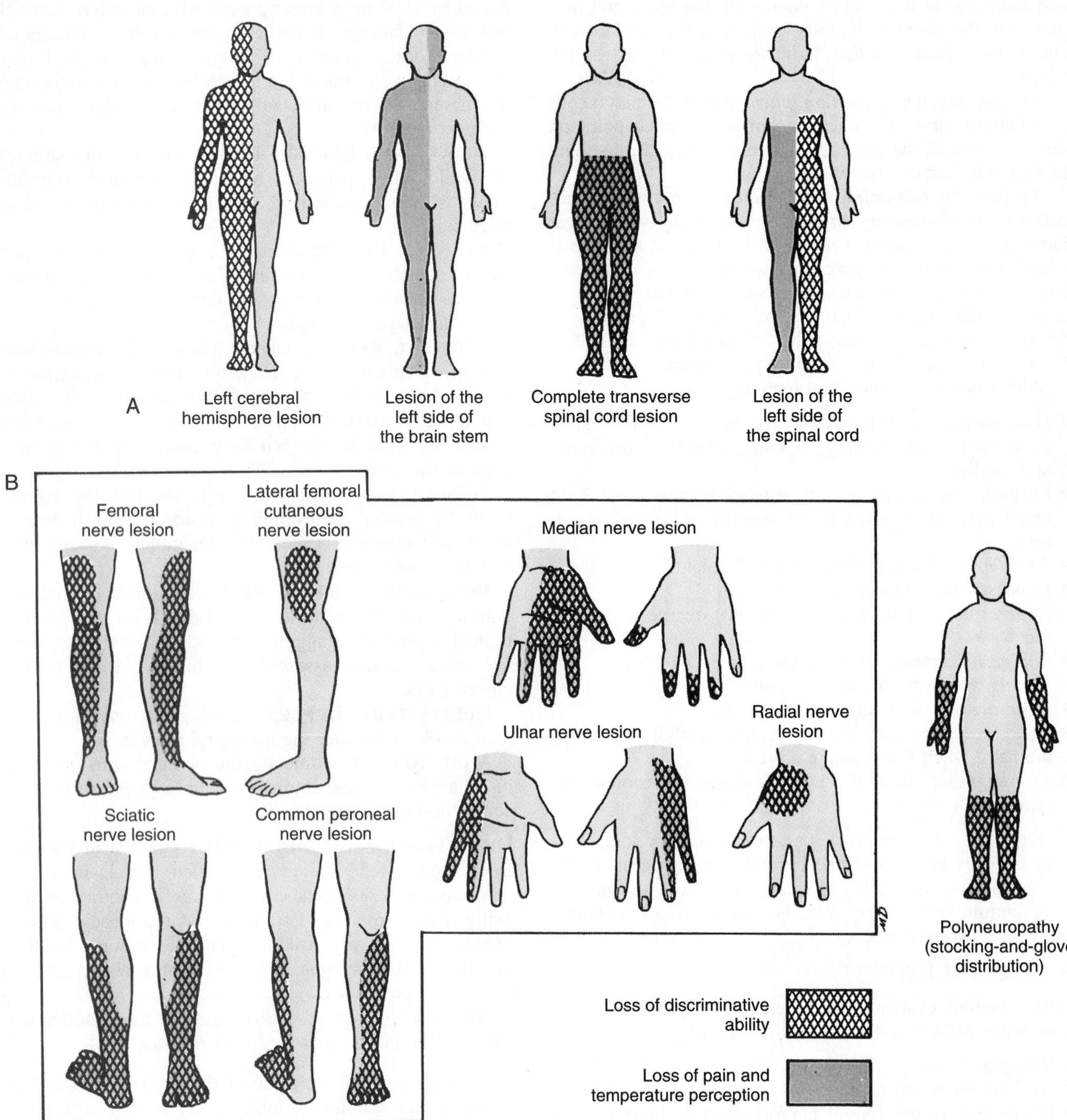

FIGURE 67–2 Patterns of sensory loss with brain and spinal cord disorders *(A)* and peripheral nerve lesions *(B)*.

Abnormal Reflexes

Pathologic reflexes indicate neurologic disorders, often related to the spinal cord or higher centers. These responses include Babinski's, jaw, palm-chin (palmomental), clonus, snout, rooting, sucking, glabella, grasp, and chewing reflexes.

BABINSKI'S REFLEX. Test Babinski's reflex by gently scraping the sole of the foot with a blunt object. To elicit the reflex, start the stimulus at the midpoint of the heel, and move upward and laterally along the outer border of the sole to the ball of the foot. Continue the stimulus across the ball of the foot (without touching the toes) toward the medial side and off the foot. Alternatively, start the stimulus at the midlateral sole and carry it down toward the heel. A normal response is plantiflexion of the toes. An abnormal response (presence of Babinski's reflex) is dorsiflexion of the great toe and, often, fanning of the other toes (Fig. 67–4). In extreme circumstances, a Babinski reflex may be accompanied by dorsiflexion of

TABLE 67–2 **IMPORTANT REFLEXES**

Reflex	Assessment Technique	Expected Response	Pathway Involved
TENDON REFLEXES			
Biceps reflex	A blow on the examiner's thumb placed over the biceps tendon	Flexion of elbow	C5-6
Brachioradialis reflex (supinator)	Styloid process of radius is tapped while forearm is in semiflexion and semipronation	Flexion of elbow, fingers, and hand with supination of forearm	C5-6
Triceps reflex	Strike on triceps tendon just above the olecranon	Extension of elbow	C6-8 (C7 primarily)
Patellar reflex (knee jerk)	Tap on patellar tendon	Leg extends	L2-4
Achilles reflex (ankle jerk)	Tap on Achilles tendon	Plantar flexion of foot	S1-2
SUPERFICIAL REFLEXES			
Corneal reflex	Light touch at the corneoscleral junction	Closure of eyelids	CN V, VII
Palatal and pharyngeal reflexes	Light touch to soft palate and pharynx	Elevation of palate; gagging	CN IX, X
Abdominal reflexes	Stroke skin of upper, middle, and lower abdomen toward umbilicus	Contraction of abdominal wall toward stimulus	Upper: T7-9 Middle: T9-11 Lower: T11-12
Cremasteric reflex	Stroke medial surface of upper thigh	Elevation of ipsilateral scrotum and testicle	T12-L2
Anal reflex	Stroke perianal region	Contraction of external anal sphincter	S3-5
Plantar reflex (normal)	Stroke sole of foot	Flexion of toes	L4-S2
Plantar reflex (pathologic; Babinski's sign)	Stroke sole of foot	Dorsiflexion of great toe and fanning of other toes	L4-S2

C, cervical; CN, cranial nerve; L, lumbar; S, sacral; T, thoracic.
Adapted from Mitchell, P. A., et al. (1988). *AANN's neuroscience nursing: Phenomena and practice.* Norwalk, CT: Appleton & Lange.

the foot at the ankle and flexion at the knee and hip (called triple flexion).

When exaggerated deep reflexes are present, superficial reflexes are usually diminished or absent and pathologic reflexes (e.g., Babinski's reflex) are observed.

JAW REFLEX. The jaw reflex is also called mandibular reflex or "jaw jerk." Have the client relax the mouth, leaving it open slightly. Then tap gently on the lower jaw below the mouth. The jaw normally contracts and closes the mouth as a result of downward tapping. This reflex is absent in most clients but may be present in clients who have lesions in the corticobulbar tract above the mid-pons.

PALM-CHIN (PALMOMENTAL) REFLEX. The palm-chin reflex is produced by vigorous, rapid irritation on the mound of the palm at the thumb's base with a blunt instrument, which causes the chin muscles to pull up on the same side.

CLONUS. Clonus consists of rapidly alternating joint flexions and extensions resulting from continuous rhythmic contractions of a stretched muscle. This is not like a normal stretch reflex, which typically produces one reflex action. With clonus, the action continues. Support the leg at the knee, and help the client relax the leg. Rapidly flex the foot, and hold it in a flexed position. The flexion stretches the calf muscles and causes repeated "beats" of clonus if this reflex is present.

SNOUT REFLEX. A brisk midline tap above or below the mouth results in pursing of the lips. This reflex is normal in infants but is abnormal in adults.

ROOTING REFLEX. Stroking the side of the face causes the mouth to open and the head to turn to the stimulated side. This reflex is normal in infants but is abnormal in adults.

SUCKING REFLEX. Touching the lips with a blunt object results in movement of the tongue, lips, and jaws. This reflex is normal in infants but is abnormal in adults.

GLABELLA REFLEX. Tapping the forehead between the eyebrows results in sustained closure of the eyelids.

GRASP REFLEX. Placing an object in the palm of the hand causes the fingers to curl around it.

CHEWING REFLEX. A tongue blade placed between the teeth results in the tight closing of the jaws.

Grading Reflex Activity

Figure 67–5 shows the grading and documentation of superficial reflexes. Although 1+ or 3+ responses are not

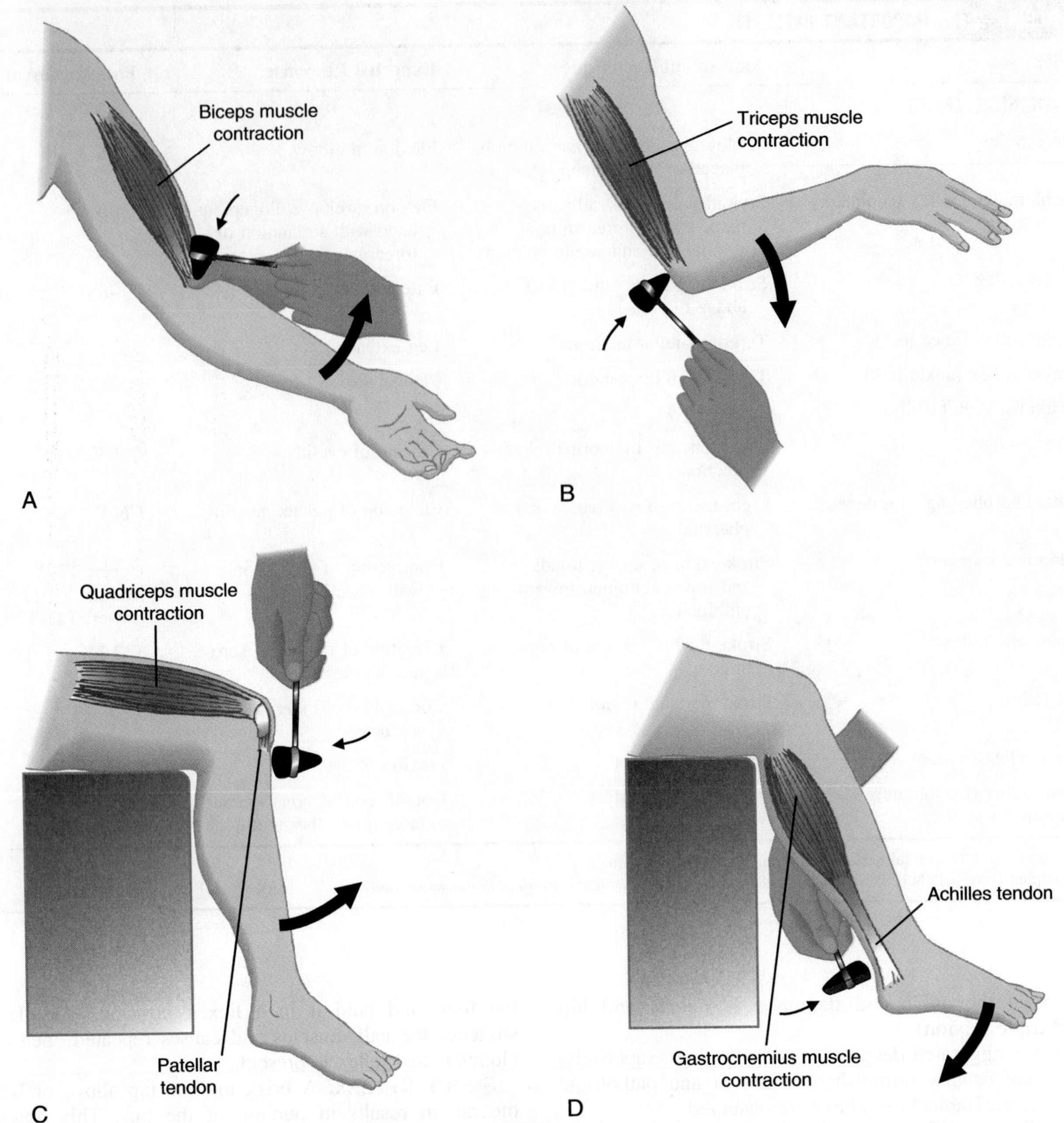

FIGURE 67–3 Deep tendon (muscle-stretch) reflexes. *A*, Biceps jerk (C5–6). *B*, Triceps jerk (C7–8). *C*, Patellar reflexes (L2–4). *D*, Ankle jerk (S1–2).

considered normal, they may not be significant findings. Asymmetrical responses are more significant. Abnormal reflexes may be present in both neurologic and metabolic disorders. Table 67–2 summarizes important reflexes.

■ AUTONOMIC NERVOUS SYSTEM

The autonomic nervous system cannot be examined directly. The system consists of sympathetic and parasympathetic innervation of many body organs. The functioning of the system is evaluated by a full body systems assessment. Clinical manifestations of autonomic nervous system disorders occur in many body systems. Unit 15 focuses on neurologic disorders (e.g., heatstroke, autonomic dysreflexia). Disorders of other portions of the autonomic system are discussed in the cardiac, urinary, digestive, reproductive, and endocrine chapters of this book.

Examples of activity under autonomic nervous system influence are:

- Increased or decreased heart rate
- Peripheral vasoconstriction or vasodilation
- Bronchoconstriction or bronchodilation
- Increased or decreased peristalsis
- Constriction or dilation of the pupil

Review any medications the client is taking. Many medications have side effects involving the parasympathetic or sympathetic nervous system.

BOX 67–5 Guidelines for Assessment of Deep Tendon Reflexes

Use the following guidelines when assessing deep tendon reflexes:

1. Test deep tendon reflexes with the client either sitting or supine.
2. Support the joint where the tendon is being tested so that the attached muscle is relaxed.
3. Use the pointed end of a triangular reflex hammer to strike over small areas while you place your thumb over the biceps tendon. Use the flat end of the hammer to strike over larger areas, such as the Achilles tendon.
4. Hold the reflex hammer loosely between thumb and fingers so it can swing in an arc.
5. Swing the reflex hammer using only wrist motion, not the arm or elbow.
6. Tap the tendon briskly.
7. Note the speed, force, and amplitude of reflex responses.
8. Compare reflex responses on the two sides of the body.
9. Grade reflexes on a 0 to 4+ scale. Consider the strength of the reflex in relation to the bulk of the muscle mass.

Repeat testing of reflexes graded 0 or 1+ by using the technique of reinforcement (see next phase). Note in the record that *reinforcement* was used. Reinforcement is a maneuver used to enhance deep tendon reflex responses when they are graded 0 or 1+. Reinforcement maneuvers for various deep tendon reflexes are as follows:

1. Ask the client to perform isometric contraction of other muscles, which may increase the generalized reflex response.
2. For the upper extremities, have the client either clench the teeth together or contract the quadriceps muscles (i.e., push the thighs against the table).
3. For the lower extremities, have the client lock the fingers together and try to pull them apart at the same time you test the tendon.

■ FUNCTIONAL ASSESSMENT

A client who has a neurologic disorder may experience problems that disrupt basic function either permanently or temporarily. Ability to cope effectively with ADL (ability to meet basic needs) is often altered. For example, a client may have problems seeing, hearing, breathing, walking, talking, or eating. Remember, a client with a neurologic disorder may be frustrated just trying to do the things most people take for granted.

Functional assessment can be incorporated into the neurologic examination as well as into the daily care of the client. During the examination, note any deficits the client experiences and how the client manages them. Ask the client or family what changes have been made in daily routines to accommodate deficits. Document not only the deficit but also the functional response. Examples include:

- *Motor strength of right arm 4/5:* The client reports independence in ADL but notices difficulty in carrying books or groceries with the right arm.
- *Diplopia:* The client uses an eye patch, alternating the side covered every few hours to reduce the headache and nausea caused by diplopia.

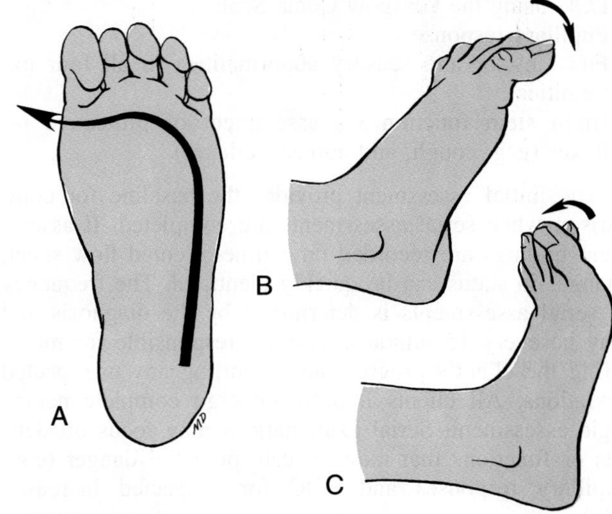

FIGURE 67–4 Babinski's reflex. *A*, Test maneuver: Using a blunt point, scratch the sole of foot as shown. *B*, Normal response (absence of Babinski's response) is plantiflexion of the toes. *C*, Abnormal response (presence of Babinski's response) is dorsiflexion of the big toe and often a fanning of the other toes.

- *Right gaze preference:* The client overcomes gaze preference and moves the eyes past the midline to the left when asked. The client turns the head to the left to see visitors enter a room.

■ CLINICAL APPLICATIONS

Initial assessment for diagnosis and triage of the client with a possible neurologic deficit consists of a history, a *brief* physical examination, and a neurologic examination. The *initial* neurologic examination usually includes assessments of the following (see Box 67–2):

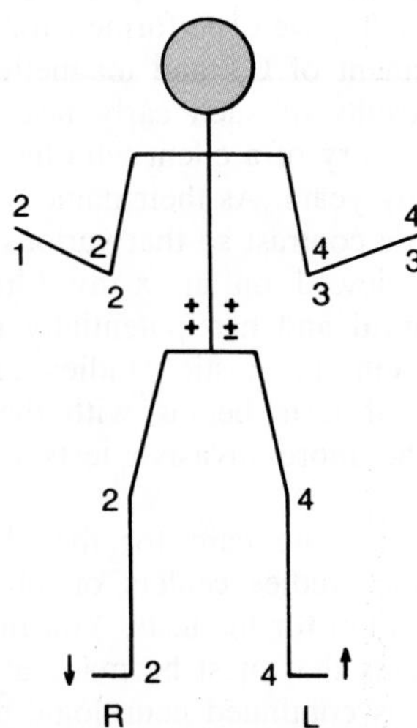

FIGURE 67–5 Documentation of muscle-stretch and superficial reflexes in left hemiparesis. Muscle-stretch reflex grades: 0, absent; 1, diminished; 2, normal; 3, brisker than normal; 4, hyperactive (clonus). Superficial reflex grades: 0, absent, ±, equivocal or barely present; +, normally active.

- LOC using the Glasgow Coma Scale
- Pupillary response
- Focal motor and sensory abnormalities in all four extremities
- Brain stem function via assessment of protective reflexes (gag, cough, and corneal reflexes)

The initial assessment provides the baseline for comparison when serial assessments are completed. If assessment findings are recorded on a time-oriented flow sheet, changes in status can be quickly identified. The frequency of serial assessments is determined by the diagnosis and may be every 15 minutes. You are responsible for monitoring the client's progress and reporting any unexpected deviations. All clients initially undergo complete neurologic assessment. Serial examinations may focus on deficits or functions that may indicate potential danger (e.g., pupillary responses and LOC for suspected increased ICP).

Thorough assessment and reporting of changes in a client serve a major role in determining the plan of care. Often the client's current condition (e.g., a decreased level of responsiveness and a change in pupillary reaction) is compared with initial data.

Because nurses are with clients consistently, it is the nurse's responsibility to develop sound assessment skills and to recognize trends in the client's condition that warrant further care. In no other area of practice are subtle changes as important to detect and act on than in the care of the client with a neurologic disorder.

DIAGNOSTIC TESTS

The complexity of the CNS combined with the relative inaccessibility of the brain requires study by indirect techniques. Early techniques, such as lumbar puncture, plain x-ray study, EEG, and pneumoencephalography, have provided the foundation for new techniques that allow more detailed examination of the brain structure, blood supply, and metabolism.

Air contrast studies, such as pneumoencephalography and ventriculography, were performed for assessment before the development of CT and magnetic resonance imaging (MRI). Results of such early tests may be found recorded in the history of a client who has had neurologic disorders for many years. As their name implied, the tests used air to provide contrast so that various portions of the brain could be viewed on an x-ray film. Air contrast studies were painful and had potentially serious side effects. Today's neurodiagnostic studies are much safer. This description of tests begins with the least invasive and moves to the more invasive tests of structure and then of function.

The focus of nursing care for the client who is to undergo diagnostic studies centers on physical and psychological preparation for the tests. You must plan for the specific assessments that must be made after the study is completed, such as continued neurologic assessment. Determine which components of the neurologic examination you will use in serial assessments before and after the test. These findings will be compared with results of the baseline neurologic examination. Before a diagnostic study, educate the client and family about the purpose of the study, the preparation needed, and the client's role during the test.

After the diagnostic procedures have been performed, assess the client for possible side effects and neurologic changes, and help the client understand the results of the studies, as needed. More information on diagnostic testing can be found in Chapter 11.

■ NONINVASIVE TESTS OF STRUCTURE

Skull and Spinal X-ray Studies

Skull x-ray studies reveal the size and shape of the skull bones, suture separation in infants, fractures or bony defects, erosion, calcification, sella turcica erosion, and pineal gland shift (>12 years of age). Spinal x-ray studies show fractures, dislocation, compressions, curvature, erosion, narrowed spinal cord, and degenerative processes.

The nurse may accompany clients who are confused, combative, or ventilator dependent to the radiology department to assist with client positioning and cooperation during the examination. If a spinal fracture is suspected, the neck is immobilized before the client is moved for the x-ray films. A lateral view of the cervical spine is taken first because the x-ray study can usually be conducted with minimal movement to determine whether fractures have occurred. Multiple views of the cervical spine are needed to rule out fracture. Until the results are known, maintain preprocedure precautions, such as spinal immobilization.

Computed Tomography

PROCEDURE

The primary purpose of CT scanning is to detect intracranial bleeding, space-occupying lesions, cerebral edema, and shifts of brain structures. Infarctions, hydrocephalus, and cerebral atrophy can also be identified. Advances in technology have expanded the uses of CT. Spiral CT utilizes injection of contrast material followed by rapid image sequencing to study movement of the contrast material through the cerebral blood vessels. Xenon CT uses inhaled xenon gas, which is absorbed into the blood stream, to enhance views that depict regional cerebral blood flow.

Aneurysms and arteriovenous malformations (AVMs) are best detected by angiography. The basilar cisterns and posterior fossa are not as well visualized on CT scans because these areas reveal high-density contrast between bone and air-filled sinuses (Fig. 67–6).

CT scans can be used for stereotactic procedures. Before the scan, a frame is applied to the client's head with pins inserted into the skull. The scan is performed with the frame in place. The computer marks reference measurements on the scan to guide the location of treatment.

PREPROCEDURE CARE

Answer any questions the client and family have about the CT scan. Explain that fasting usually is not required for CT of the head. If you think that the client might become nauseated, adjust the intake of food and fluids accordingly. For example, some clients prefer a light meal to reduce nausea, with others preferring an empty stomach before the test.

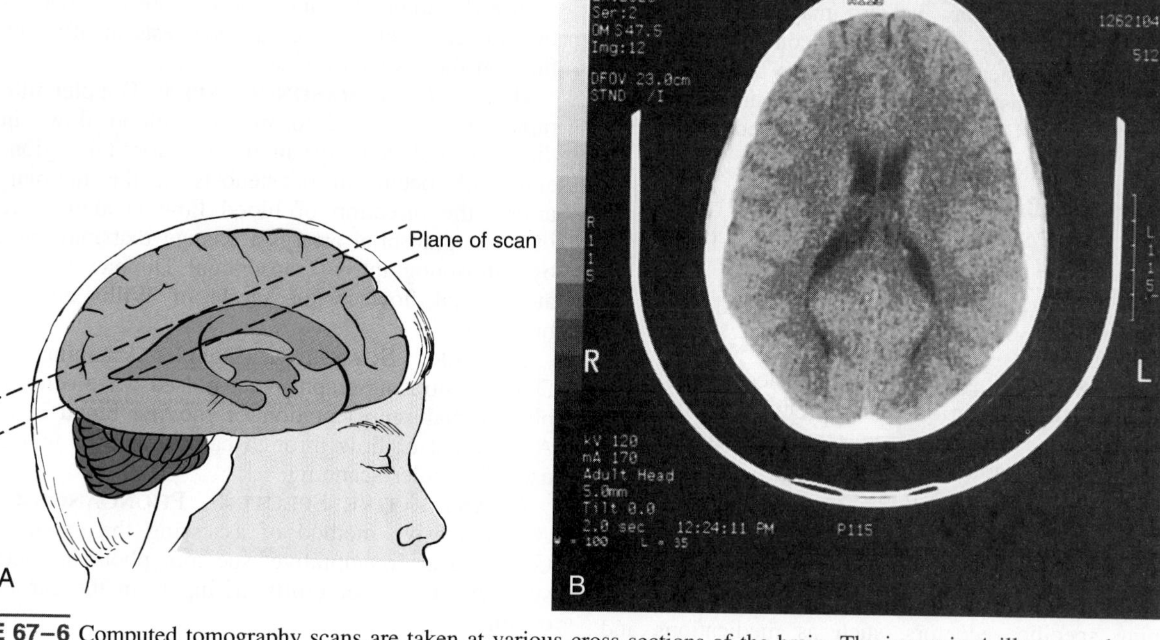

FIGURE 67–6 Computed tomography scans are taken at various cross-sections of the brain. The image in *A* illustrates the cross-section used for the scan shown in *B*.

Explain that a contrast agent may be used. Because some agents are iodine-based, ask whether the client has allergies to iodine or contrast material (see Chapter 11). If the client does not have an intravenous (IV) infusion, such an infusion will be established before the study begins. Before the test in which contrast material is to be used, check that informed consent has been obtained.

Postprocedure Care

After the test, assess the client for reactions to contrast media and check other specific observations, such as presence of hematoma at the injection site and manifestations of IV infiltration of contrast material or fluids. Report infiltration of contrast medium to the radiologist. The client can resume normal activities unless other diagnostic tests are planned.

If a stereotactic frame was used during CT, it is to be left in place until the stereotactic procedure is completed. The frame may be a source of anxiety, and light sedation may be ordered to help keep the client relaxed.

Serial neurologic examinations are necessary after any testing to evaluate the potential effects on the client's neurologic function from contrast media, transportation to a new environment, or sedation. Assess the client before and after the CT scan.

Magnetic Resonance Imaging

Procedure

MRI provides more anatomically detailed pictures than are available with CT (Fig. 67–7). MRI has several advantages over CT. MRI can detect disorders in white matter pathways caused by loss of myelin, as in multiple sclerosis, better than CT. MRI can evaluate cerebral infarction within hours of the event; CT would not demonstrate the stroke for several days. Contrast material can be used with MRI to delineate blood flow through cerebral blood vessels in more detail than is possible with CT.

Preprocedure Care

Teach the client and family about the purpose of the test, what the client will hear and feel during the examination, and the client's role during the test. Before the test, the client should remove all metal-containing objects. IV fluid pumps must be removed immediately before the test. Spe-

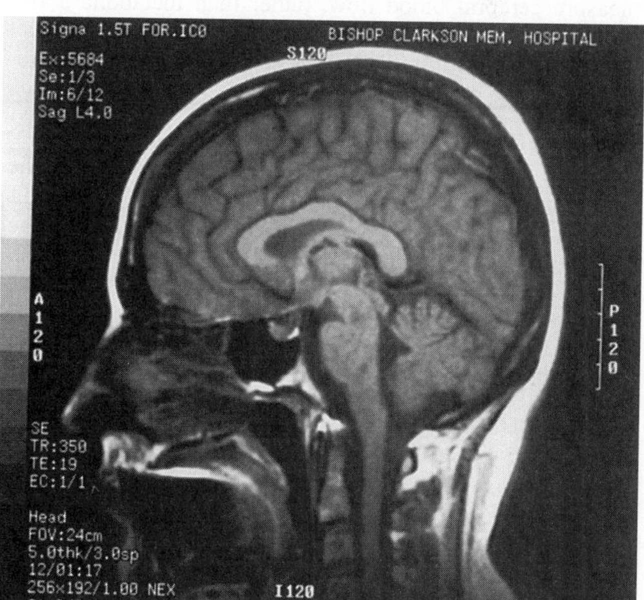

FIGURE 67–7 A normal magnetic resonance image. This sagittal section shows the cerebrum, ventricles, cerebellum, and medulla.

cial MRI-compatible monitoring devices, such as pulse oximeters and ECG leads, can be left in place.

Usually, the client may eat and may take prescribed medications before the examination. If contrast material is to be used, ask whether the client tends to become nauseated easily and adjust the intake of food and fluids accordingly. Chapter 11 details the MRI procedure and client care.

POSTPROCEDURE CARE

After the test, the client can resume previous activities.

Positron Emission Tomography

PROCEDURE

Positron emission tomography (PET) enables visualization of physiologic function in body areas. Often, the function of diseased tissue is different from that of normal tissues. PET has three primary uses:

- Determining the amount of blood flow to specific body tissues
- Revealing how adequately tissues use blood or nutrients, such as oxygen
- Mapping specific receptors, such as medications and neurotransmitters

PET can be used to measure cerebral blood flow, cerebral glucose metabolism, and oxygen extraction. PET is used in the diagnosis of stroke, brain tumors, and epilepsy, and to chart the progress of Alzheimer's disease, Parkinson's disease, head injury, schizophrenia, and manic-depressive illness.

A major disadvantage of PET is its high cost. The procedure requires its own positron to manufacture high-energy radioactive tracers; a PET system can cost $5 million initially. As a result, a modification of the procedure, called single-photon emission computed tomography (SPECT), has been developed. SPECT uses less precise but more stable and more readily available isotopes to measure cerebral blood flow, rather than metabolic activity as measured with PET. SPECT appears to be an effective diagnostic tool. A PET scan is shown in Chapter 11, Figure 11–6.

PREPROCEDURE CARE

Educate the client and family about the purpose of the test, what the client will hear and feel during the examination, and the client's role during the test. In contrast to CT and MRI equipment, the PET scanner is absolutely quiet. Clients must fast for 4 hours before the scan. If the client is diabetic, it is preferred that the blood glucose level be below 150 g/dl. Clients who are agitated may require sedation before the scan.

POSTPROCEDURE CARE

After the test, the client can resume usual activities.

Tests for Vascular Abnormalities

The noninvasive tests described here are useful in assessing cerebrovascular disorders.

OPHTHALMODYNAMOMETRY. Ophthalmodynamometry is used to compare the retinal artery pressures in the eyes. It may help in the diagnosis of extracranial vascular disease. While the retina is observed through an ophthalmoscope, pressure (or suction) is applied to the eyeball with a dynamometer and readings are obtained. A reduction in retinal artery pressure suggests insufficient carotid flow on the ipsilateral side.

DOPPLER ULTRASONOGRAPHY. Doppler ultrasonography may be used to measure blood flow (including direction and velocity) in the supraorbital region. In clients with occlusion or stenosis of the internal carotid artery, the direction of blood flow is altered (reversed) in the supraorbital artery, a change that may be detected by ultrasonography. Transcranial Doppler studies evaluate arterial flow in the circle of Willis and its major branches.

DOPPLER SCANNING. Doppler scanning combines Doppler ultrasonography with pulsed wave echocardiography. Visual representation of moving blood is obtained. Assessment of flow through carotid arteries is a common use of Doppler scanning.

QUANTITATIVE SPECTRAL PHONOANGIOGRAPHY. A noninvasive method of assessing the extent of carotid stenosis, quantitative spectral phonoangiography is spectral analysis of bruits arising from the carotid bifurcation.

■ INVASIVE TESTS OF STRUCTURE

Lumbar Puncture

PROCEDURE

In a client undergoing a lumbar puncture (LP), also known as a *spinal tap*, a needle is inserted into the subarachnoid space in the lumbar region of the spine below the level of the spinal cord. CSF can be withdrawn from or substances can be injected into this space.

LP is performed for assessment and therapeutic purposes. LP enables assessment of CSF pressure and collection of CSF for evaluation. When meningitis or subarachnoid hemorrhage is suspected, the CSF is examined for white blood cells and blood. A *myelogram* is a x-ray study in which contrast material is injected into the subarachnoid space after CSF is removed in order to examine the spinal canal. Therapeutically, LP is used to administer spinal medications and anesthetics.

Even though LP is generally a safe procedure, it is associated with potential hazards. The procedure can be uncomfortable. The client feels pressure in the lower back and may experience pain if a nerve root is touched with the needle during insertion. The potential complications of LP are CSF leakage, infection, intervertebral disc damage, and brain herniation.

A space-occupying lesion within the cranium, such as a tumor or bleeding, increases ICP. Therefore, LP is not performed in clients with papilledema (a sign of increased ICP), suspected intracranial lesions, increased ICP, or infection of the skin at the puncture site. CT scans are used in these clients to rule out masses before an LP is performed. If an LP were performed in a client with increased ICP, there would be a rapid decrease in CSF pressure around the spinal cord. This change in pressure might allow the structures within the brain to drop (herniate) into the spinal canal. The process of herniation creates pressure on the vital centers in the medulla (cardiac and respiratory centers) and may cause sudden death.

Preprocedure Care

Educate the client and the family about the purpose of LP, what the client will feel, and the client's role during the examination. Obtain an informed consent. If possible, the client should empty the bladder and bowels before the procedure. The client lies on one side with the legs pulled onto the abdomen and the head tucked into the chest in order to open the spaces between the vertebrae. The client must lie still during the test. Sedation may be ordered before the procedure.

Assemble the necessary equipment in the client's room. Lumbar puncture trays containing all the needed equipment are available. In addition, have laboratory request forms available and a marking pencil to label the samples of spinal fluid.

Intraprocedure Care

LP to remove a sample of CSF is described here; however, the same general principles apply to any LP procedure.

1. Position the client on the side (lateral recumbency) with the back close to the edge of the bed. Place a pillow under the flank so that the spinous processes are horizontal. Use additional pillows between the knees and under the head to keep the spine horizontal.
2. Ask the client to draw the knees up to the abdomen and the chin onto the chest (Fig. 67–8). Help the client maintain this curved position to separate and increase space between the vertebrae so that the needle can be inserted more easily.
3. Stand in front of the client, and place one hand behind the client's knees and the other around the neck. Keep the client's upper shoulder from falling forward, thus preventing rotation of the spine. (An alternative position is to have the client sitting up with the head and chest bent toward the knees.)
4. After a local anesthetic is given, the physician places a small needle into the space between the vertebrae in the lower back. In adults, the needle is inserted about level with the top of the iliac crests (hip bones) or at the next lower vertebral level (usually between the third and fourth or fourth and fifth lumbar vertebrae). In adults, the spinal cord normally ends at the lower border of the first lumbar vertebra. Thus, the puncture site is low enough to avoid spinal cord injury.
5. The needle bevel is usually held parallel to the longitudinal fibers of the dura. This position limits the size of the dural tear and reduces the risk of CSF leak.
6. Local pain may occur as the needle passes the dura mater. Ask the client to mention additional discomfort, which may indicate misplacement of the needle.

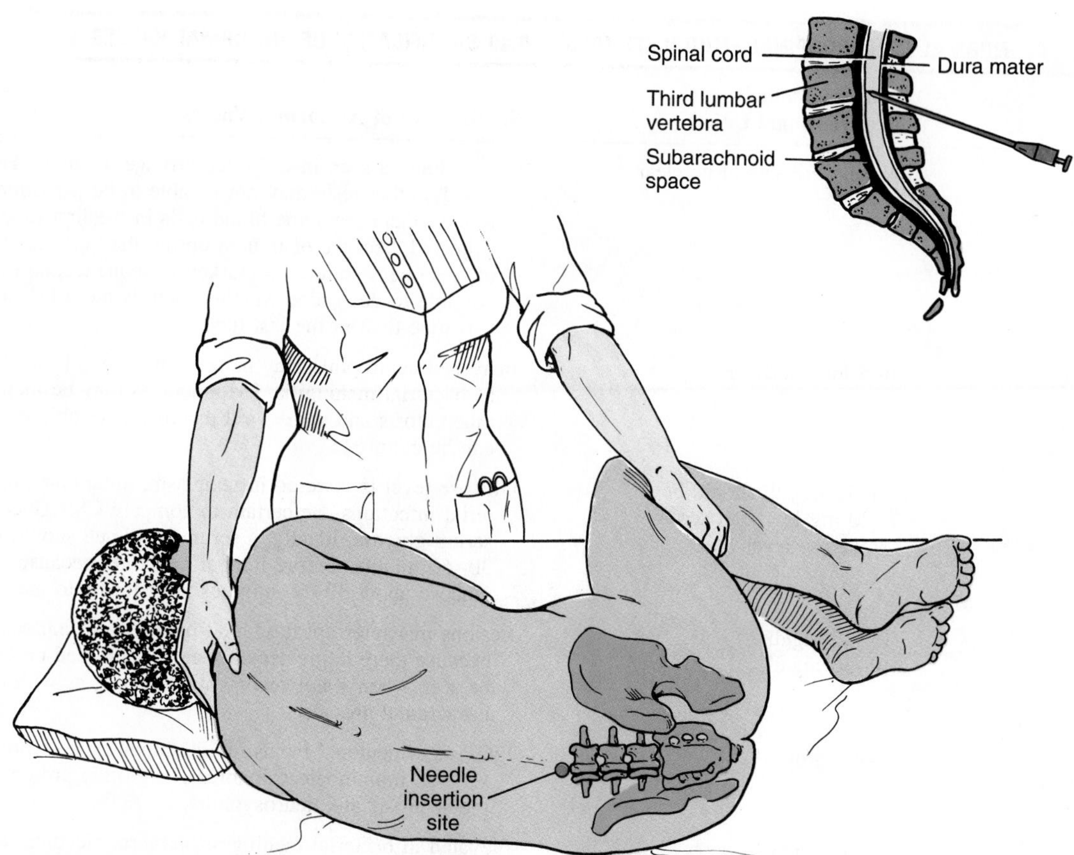

FIGURE 67–8 Lumbar puncture. Position the client laterally, with the knees drawn up to the abdomen and the chin brought down to the chest. This position increases the spaces between the vertebrae. The sterile lumbar puncture needle is inserted as shown, between the third and fourth (or fourth and fifth) vertebrae and enters the subarachnoid space.

7. When the needle has entered the subarachnoid space, the physician removes the stylus and attaches a stopcock and manometer to measure CSF pressure. The first stabilized CSF pressure is the opening pressure. Normal opening CSF pressure with the client in a horizontal position is 6 to 13 mm Hg (80 to 180 mm H_2O). Pressures exceeding 15 mm Hg (200 mm H_2O) are abnormal. Normally, CSF pressure oscillates (fluctuates) in the manometer, readily responding to coughing, straining, and changes in the person's breathing. If there is a blockage in the spinal canal, the CSF pressure may not oscillate.
8. CSF specimens are collected in a series of small sterile test tubes, numbered in sequence of collection (e.g., No. 1, No. 2). Two to 3 ml of CSF is collected in each tube; 8 to 10 ml may be removed.
9. The needle is withdrawn, and the physician places a dry sterile dressing over the puncture site.

In adults, CSF is assessed for cells, chloride, glucose, protein, and lactate dehydrogenase (LDH) as well as pressure. Table 67–3 lists common abnormalities of CSF. In the analysis of CSF, the first vial obtained is not assessed for blood because it may contain blood from the puncture.

POSTPROCEDURE CARE

Record vital signs after the LP. Sometimes, lying flat for several hours is prescribed. The client can eat and drink as before the test. Drinking extra fluids will help restore CSF volume. If the CSF pressure measurement indicated a high ICP, assess the client for decreasing LOC, which would indicate rising ICP.

Post-LP headache (spinal puncture headache, spinal headache) is typically throbbing, bifrontal, and suboccipital, developing a few hours to several days after an LP. The headache is probably due to continuing CSF leakage through the opening in the dura made by the needle. As a result of the leak, the CSF circulating around the cranium is depleted. The fluid loss allows abnormal movement of the brain in the skull. When the brain moves, tension is placed on the meninges and venous sinuses, causing pain. The headache is usually relieved when the client lies down and is made worse with sitting up or with a sudden jolt of the head. Such headaches usually disappear within 24 hours but may last for several days.

To reduce the risk of post-LP headache, have the client remain in bed after the examination. Although physician's orders may differ, an average time in bed is 3 hours. Encourage fluids to replace the CSF withdrawn during the test. Once a headache begins, treatment may be bed rest in a dark, quiet room and the administration of analgesics and fluids.

If the headache continues, an epidural blood patch may be required. Blood is withdrawn from the client's vein and injected into the epidural space, usually at the LP site. The blood acts as a fibrin patch to seal the hole in

TABLE 67–3 NORMAL CEREBROSPINAL FLUID (CSF) VALUES AND SIGNIFICANCE OF ABNORMAL VALUES

Substance	Normal Value (Conventional Units)	Significance of Abnormal Values
Blood	None; CSF should be clear	Gross blood is seen in CNS hemorrhage. If the CSF is grossly bloody, other tests may not be able to be performed. Rarely, there are some blood cells in the first tube of CSF collected, because of trauma during the tap. The collection of specimens should be marked in sequence, so that it is possible to determine whether there is more blood in the first tube than in the last tube.
Cells	0–5 mononuclear	Increased neutrophils may be seen in bacterial infections such as bacterial meningitis. Lymphocytes may be increased in tuberculosis and some viral disorders. Aerobic pathogens can be cultured.
Glucose	50–75 mg/dl, should be 20 mg less than serum glucose level	Glucose level is lowered in neoplasm, inflammation, and bacterial infections. Be certain to compare CSF glucose with serum glucose. Ideally, a serum specimen should be drawn 30–60 minutes before lumbar puncture, because it takes glucose about 30–60 minutes to diffuse into the CSF.
Protein Albumin	15–45 mg/dl 10–30 mg/dl	Lesions that interrupt the blood-brain barrier increase proteins because there is greater diffusion. Decreased proteins can be seen when water reabsorption occurs, as with elevated intracranial pressure.
IgG Oligoclonal bands	1–4 mg/dl Absent	IgG and oligoclonal bands (an abnormal type of protein band seen on immunoelectrophoresis) are often present in multiple sclerosis and neurosyphilis.
Pressure	70–180 mm H_2O	Elevated in bacterial meningitis, cerebral bleeding, and tumors. Decreased in conditions that obstruct CSF flow, such as tumors of the spinal canal.

CNS, central nervous system; CSF, cerebrospinal fluid; IgG, immunoglobulin G.

the dura and prevent further CSF leakage. Blood patches cannot be performed in a client who has bleeding tendencies or infection at the puncture site.

Myelography

Myelography is an x-ray examination of the spinal cord and vertebral canal following introduction of contrast material into the spinal subarachnoid space (Fig. 67–9). It is used to study the spinal canal and subarachnoid space. This study is a valuable assessment tool when the spinal cord is thought to be compressed (e.g., by a herniated intervertebral disc or an encroaching tumor). Myelography is used to identify spinal cord disorders, such as intramedullary tumors, AVMs, and syringomyelia.

In the radiology department, an LP is performed, a small amount of CSF is withdrawn, and contrast material is injected. With the needle in place, the client is turned onto the abdomen and secured to the table. While the radiologist observes with fluoroscopy, the table is slowly tilted. Tilting causes the column of contrast material to move up or down within the subarachnoid space, permitting visualization of the desired areas. Standard films are taken. If the contrast material used is water-soluble, it is not removed from the spinal column. In some cases, the myelogram is followed by a CT scan of the spine to evaluate the contrast-enhanced structures.

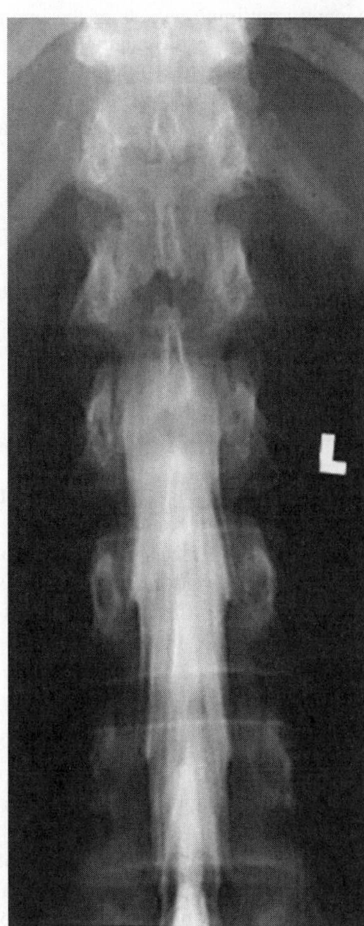

FIGURE 67–9 A myelogram of the lumbar spine shows contrast dye flowing throughout the subarachnoid space without obstruction.

Preparation for a myelogram requires hydration for at least 12 hours before the procedure. After the myelogram, the client remains flat in bed if oil-based contrast material was used; the head of the bed is elevated 15 to 30 degrees if water-based contrast material was used. Usually, the client remains in bed 6 to 8 hours and then resumes normal activity. Encourage the client to drink extra fluids. Assess neurologic status frequently.

Back pain (ranging from mild discomfort to severe pain) in the area of the needle insertion may develop and may last a few days. Also, the client may experience a stiff neck and headache for a few days, particularly if the contrast medium was allowed to rise to high cervical levels. The discomfort is usually relieved by having the client lie flat and by administration of fluids and analgesics (see LP discussion).

Cisternal Puncture

Cisternal puncture involves puncture of the cisterna magna (a small reservoir of CSF between the cerebellum and medulla). This procedure is performed either to drain CSF or to obtain a specimen if there is a block in the spinal subarachnoid space or if LP is contraindicated. CT and MRI have largely replaced this procedure.

A short-beveled needle is inserted below the occipital bone, between the first cervical lamina and the rim of the foramen magnum. Fluoroscopy is used to guide exact placement of the needle. If the client has a lesion on the spinal cord, the upper edge of the lesion can be determined by contrast material injected via the cisternal puncture. If there is any concern about the client's ability to cooperate and hold still, sedation or general anesthesia may be used. Positioning the client and subsequent assessments and interventions are essentially the same as those for LP.

Cerebral Angiography

A *cerebral angiogram* consists of injection of contrast material into an artery to visualize intracranial circulation (Fig. 67–10). Angiography is the procedure used most often to visualize aneurysms, AVMs, major vessel displacement, vascular occlusion, and thrombi. Cerebral angiography is not only invasive; it is also a procedure in which small errors can result in permanent disability or death. Meticulous attention must be given to the client before, during, and after angiography.

PROCEDURE

A catheter is inserted into the femoral artery and guided with a fluoroscope into the carotid or vertebral arteries. This approach has replaced previous approaches in which the carotid, vertebral, or brachial vessel was punctured directly. A femoral artery puncture is less traumatic, and local complications, such as infection and bleeding at the puncture site, occur away from the neck. Once the vessels are reached, the contrast agent is injected and a series of x-ray films is taken from lateral, anteroposterior, and oblique approaches. Sequential views show the movement of the contrast material in the vessels.

After the catheter is removed, a sterile dressing is placed over the puncture site and firm pressure is applied to the site for 10 minutes to prevent hematoma formation.

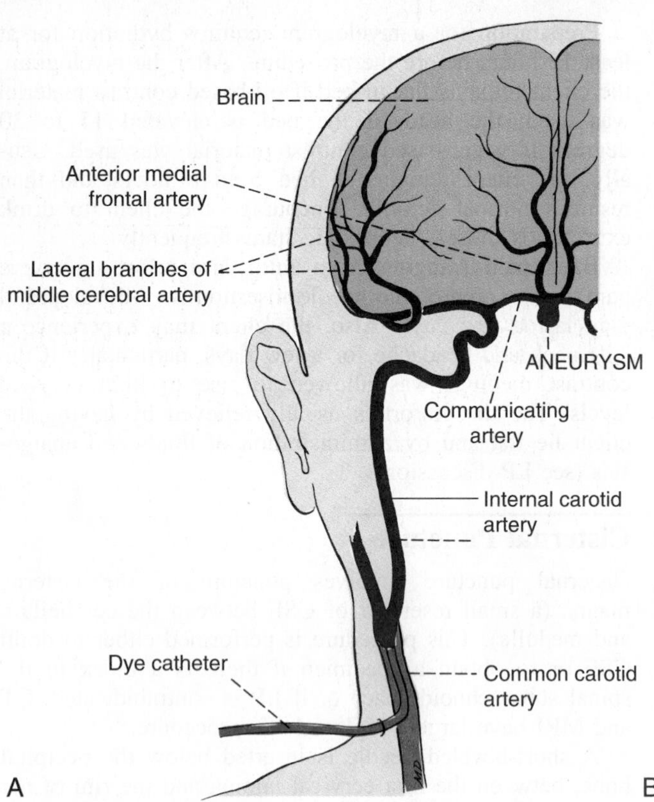

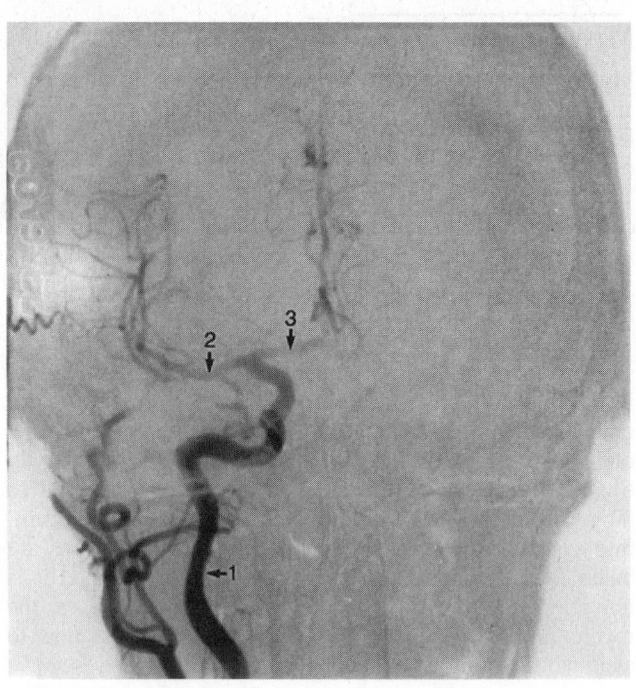

FIGURE 67–10 Cerebral angiography allows x-ray visualization of the brain's vascular system when a contrast dye is injected arterially. *A*, Insertion of dye through a catheter in the common carotid artery, subsequently outlining vessels of the brain. *B*, An angiogram using the subtraction technique. 1, Internal carotid artery. 2, Middle cerebral artery. 3, Middle meningeal artery.

Sandbags and a pressure dressing may be used to provide firm pressure after the first 10 minutes. The injection site may be tender.

INTERVENTIONAL ANGIOGRAPHY. A polymer glue or small balloons are used to occlude feeding vessels in tumors or AVMs. Blocking the feeding vessels reduces the size and vascularity of the tumor or AVM, thus diminishing the need for, and the complications of, its surgical removal. Interventional angiography also enables balloon angioplasty to be performed in order to expand atherosclerotically narrowed cerebral vessels.

DIGITAL VENOUS ANGIOGRAPHY. Computerized digital video subtraction systems allow visualization of vascular structures. Much less contrast medium is required compared with that needed for cerebral angiography. A central venous line is necessary to inject the contrast medium. Raw data are stored in digital form and can be retrieved at any time. Images with the best vascular visualization are selected and subjected to electronic manipulation to improve image detail.

Indications for digital venous angiography include:

- Assessment for transient ischemic attacks
- Serial follow-up evaluations for known carotid stenoses
- Assessment of intracranial tumors
- Postoperative assessment of aneurysms
- Follow-up evaluations after extracranial-intracranial bypass procedures
- Assessment of dural venous sinuses

Three to four venous injections of contrast material are usually required for a complete diagnostic craniocerebral study. The only potential complication is a reaction to the contrast material.

PREPROCEDURE CARE

Educate the client and family about the purpose of the test, what the client will experience, and the client's role during the procedure. Before the test, the client may not take anything by mouth for 4 to 6 hours but should be kept well hydrated. IV fluids may be prescribed. Document the neurologic status of the client to serve as a baseline measure after the examination. The client should remove any metal items from the head, such as barrettes and earrings. Report allergies to iodine.

During the test, the client is given an injection of local anesthetic before placement of the catheter. The client may have a warm flushed feeling when the contrast material is injected. The client is continually assessed for neurologic deterioration while the angiogram is being performed.

POSTPROCEDURE CARE

After the test, assess for complications, which are rare. They include (1) local and systemic allergic reactions to the contrast medium, (2) spasm or occlusion of the vessel by a clot, (3) hemorrhage, and (4) obstructive clot formation above a femoral injection site. Assess for reactions to the contrast material. Spasm or occlusion of the target vessels causes symptoms similar to those of a stroke (see Chapter 70.) Clot formation at the injection site also causes ischemic reactions in the affected area. These adverse reactions are usually reversible and rarely cause permanent damage.

Complications vary according to their cause. For example, indications of centrally located reactions include changes in LOC, aphasia, hemiplegia (paralysis of one side of the body), hemiparesis (muscular weakness or partial paralysis of one side of the body), convulsive seizures, and increased focal symptoms. A hematoma in the neck may cause difficulty in breathing or swallowing. If the hematoma is large, it may compress the trachea and esophagus, requiring emergency tracheostomy. Nausea, vomiting, extremity numbness or weakness, speech disturbances, profuse sweating, and alterations in LOC may indicate a delayed reaction to the contrast material.

After angiography, position the client safely and comfortably and maintain the prescribed bed rest. Clients undergoing diagnostic angiograms may need to stay in bed only 4 hours. If interventional treatment was performed, the client may have to remain in bed longer.

Check the injection site frequently for bleeding and hematoma formation. Keep the affected extremity (arm or leg) or neck straight to prevent vessel kinking and clot formation. Assess vital signs (every 15 minutes for 1 hour, then every 30 minutes for 1 hour, then every hour for 4 hours), pulses distal to the puncture site, color and temperature of the extremity, and the ability to move the distal extremity. The client can usually resume a regular diet.

Cerebral Perfusion Studies

When brain death is suspected, cerebral perfusion can be assessed. The patient is injected with technetium 99m (^{99m}Tc), a radioisotope. The ability of ^{99m}Tc to perfuse from blood vessels into brain tissue is assessed with a scanner. In patients who are clinically brain-dead, there is no uptake of the substance by the cerebrum or cerebellum. The radioisotope is injected, and the scanner can be brought to the bedside to evaluate perfusion. Although brain death can be determined by clinical examination, the perfusion study is used when the clinical findings are clouded by the previous use of long-acting sedative medications.

NONINVASIVE TESTS OF FUNCTION

Electroencephalogram

An electroencephalogram is a measurement of the electrical activity of the superficial layers of the cerebral cortex. It records the electrical potentials from neuron activity within the brain in the form of wave patterns. The intensity and pattern of electrical activity are influenced by the reticular activating system. The wave characteristics depend on the extent of cortical activity. Waveform patterns can be affected by (1) structural lesions, such as tumors, subdural hematomas, and areas of infarction, (2) infections, (3) degenerative processes, and (4) metabolic disorders.

Several distinct wave patterns are found in recordings of clients without brain disorders. Wave patterns are called delta, theta, alpha, or beta, depending on their appearance (amplitude and frequency). EEG waves are shown in Figure 67–11. EEG wave patterns change with aging and disease; for example, beta activity increases with age.

PROCEDURE

Electrodes are attached to the client's scalp (Fig. 67–12). The waveforms are amplified and recorded on a moving paper strip, much as for an electrocardiogram. The recordings are interpreted according to the characteristics, frequency, and amplitude of brain waves.

If the patient is comatose or is unable to be moved, a bedside study can be performed. For routine diagnostic examination, the client is taken to an EEG laboratory, a more controlled environment. The scalp is cleaned, and

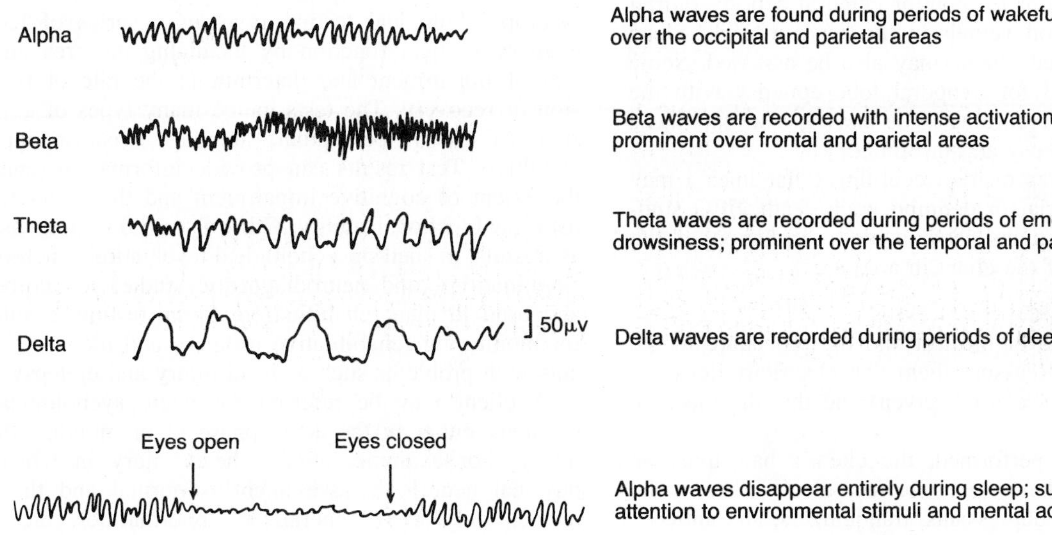
Alpha
Alpha waves are found during periods of wakefulness; prominent over the occipital and parietal areas
Beta
Beta waves are recorded with intense activation of the CNS; prominent over frontal and parietal areas
Theta
Theta waves are recorded during periods of emotional stress or drowsiness; prominent over the temporal and parietal areas
Delta
50μv
Delta waves are recorded during periods of deep sleep
Eyes open
Eyes closed
Alpha waves disappear entirely during sleep; sudden alerting; attention to environmental stimuli and mental activity
1 sec

FIGURE 67–11 Electroencephalographic waves. (Modified from Guyton, A. C., & Hall, J. [Eds.]. [1996]. *Textbook of medical physiology* [9th ed.]. Philadelphia: W. B. Saunders.)

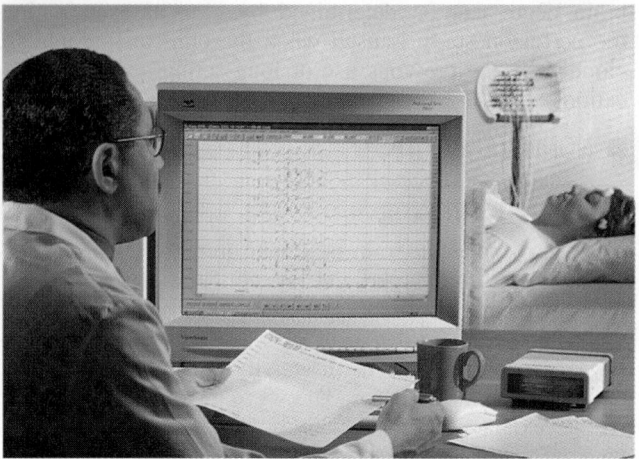

FIGURE 67–12 Client undergoing an electroencephalogram.

electrodes are applied to the scalp and ear lobe (for reference) with special conductive gel. Leads can also be placed in the nasopharynx to assess waveforms from the temporal lobe.

The first portion of the test is performed with the client as relaxed as possible to obtain a baseline recording. Further readings are taken while the client is hyperventilating, sleeping, or viewing flickering lights. Hyperventilation alters acid-base balance (respiratory alkalosis) and decreases cerebral blood flow. Flickering lights may trigger seizures. Sleep may evoke abnormal EEG patterns not present while the client is awake. The client may be kept awake the night preceding the test or may be sedated to induce sleep.

The electroencephalogram is used to assess seizure disorders. The results are diffusely abnormal in various metabolic disturbances, toxic conditions (e.g., drug overdose), coma, organic brain syndrome, and infections such as meningitis and encephalitis. The device may be used in the operating room to monitor cerebral activity during surgery on the blood vessels in the head or neck. Sleep patterns in depressed clients may also be assessed. Some clients are assessed for temporal lobe epilepsy with the use of a 24-hour recording. The device also facilitates diagnosis of narcolepsy and insomnia.

Absence of waves on the recording ("flat lines") may be one of the criteria for defining brain death. EEG studies of comatose patients show a high correlation of flat EEGs with death of the client in a coma.

Preprocedure Care

Explain the purpose of the test and the procedure to the client and family. Reassure them that electricity does not enter the brain (shock is not given) and that the machine cannot read minds.

Before EEG is performed, the client's hair must be shampooed. Stimulants (e.g., coffee, alcohol, tea, cola, and cigarettes), antidepressants, tranquilizers, and anticonvulsants should be avoided for 24 to 48 hours before the test. Sometimes sleep is withheld. If the client will be asked to sleep for a portion of the test, sleep should be minimized the night before the test. The client will be asked to relax during the test because anxiety can block alpha rhythms and produce artifacts from increased muscle tone in the head and neck. Send adequate supplies (i.e., IV fluids or oxygen) to the laboratory with the client.

If EEG is being performed to evaluate the possibility of brain death, artifacts must be kept to a minimum. Electrode manipulation, electrical interference, respirator cycling, and someone walking in the room can cause artifacts. Follow agency guidelines when EEG is performed at the bedside.

Postprocedure Care

After EEG, the client can resume previous activity, medications, and diet. If seizure activity is possible, follow precautions to avoid seizures. The hair can be washed, and acetone may be used to remove the electrode paste or gel from the scalp and hair.

Evoked Potential Studies

Evoked potential (EP) studies are a form of EEG in which brain waves are monitored as various stimuli are given. The test is used to assess the function of the cerebral hemispheres and the brain stem. A variety of types of stimuli are used, such as auditory, somatosensory, and visual. Typical stimuli are flashing lights, buzzing tones, and peripheral nerve stimulation. EP studies can be used to assess blindness, deafness, and brain stem injury. Specific brain signals can be accentuated and others filtered out, allowing assessment of brain waves from other areas.

EP studies are carried out in the same fashion as EEG studies. EP studies can detect abnormalities even if the client is sedated or paralyzed with neuromuscular blocking agents. Some clinicians believe that EP studies are more reliable than clinical assessments in predicting neurologic recovery in comatose, head-injured patients. Nursing interventions are the same as for the client undergoing an EEG study except in the explanation of the variations between the tests.

Neuropsychological Testing

Neuropsychological testing involves a series of tests to evaluate cortical function by localizing the area and extent of impairment and determining the rate of progression or recovery. The tests gauge many types of abilities, such as motor, perceptual, language, visuospatial, and cognitive. Test results can provide information regarding the extent of cognitive impairment and the effect it may have on functional ability. Clinical manifestations as well as results of neuropsychological evaluations, neurologic examinations, and neurodiagnostic studies are correlated and used to plan rehabilitation. Serial testing is valuable for monitoring rehabilitative progress and recovery in clients with problems such as head injury and epilepsy.

A client may be referred for neuropsychological assessment either in the acute phase of or months after an injury. For example, after a head injury in which the physical neurologic assessment is normal and the EEG reveals only mild generalized abnormalities, the client may complain of being unable to work because of persistent headaches. Test results may be used to make recommendations about treatment, including educational and vocational rehabilitation.

Neuropsychological tests measure deficits in coping skills by assessing the skills directly. They may be helpful when deficits in adaptive abilities are suspected. An individual test may be performed in the case of a disorder with only one specific manifestation, or a complete series of tests with extended evaluation may require several hours or days of testing. The client's level of performance is compared with scores representing normal performance levels. General measures of intelligence (e.g., Wechsler Adult Intelligence Scale) as well as tests of emotional and personal adjustment (e.g., the Minnesota Multiphasic Personality Inventory) are used.

Testing may be nonspecific in implicating the presence of brain damage or very narrow in scope with sensitivity for certain areas of the brain. Results may indicate that something is wrong but may be unable to identify the specific problem.

Memory loss is common after head injury and in neurologic disorders. Skills such as reading, which have been stored in the brain over the years, may be retained, in contrast to new learning or short-term memory, which may be impaired. An impaired memory may interfere with the effectiveness of client teaching and the client's ability to learn. A brain-injured client with damage to the limbic system, especially the hippocampus, amygdala, or areas of the temporal and prefrontal lobes, is a candidate for neuropsychological testing to determine memory loss.

Testing can identify problems in cognitive, psychomotor, and affective domains. Left hemisphere lesions impair factual information functions, like problem-solving, decision-making, and judgment. Client and family teaching must be modified to address these deficits.

Both the right and left hemispheres are involved with psychomotor learning. The right hemisphere controls visuospatial abilities, and the left controls verbal instructions and sequencing of activities. Repetition and time are needed for the individual to perform activities automatically. Memory loss that is identified from damage to the right or left hemisphere and is causing affective learning deficits can be improved with role modeling and one-to-one and group therapy. Documentation of client behavior and functional abilities assists the neuropsychologist in following the client's progress and recovery.

■ INVASIVE TESTS OF FUNCTION

Caloric Testing

The oculovestibular reflex, or *caloric test,* provides information about the function of the vestibular portion of CN VIII and pathways in the pons and midbrain. It aids in the differential diagnosis of brain stem lesions (see also Chapter 68).

The test is performed only in an unconscious patient to determine the presence of brain stem function. Check that the ear canal is patent and that the tympanic membrane is intact. Ice-cold water is introduced into the auditory canal. If brain stem function is intact, the eyes move in a conjugate fashion slowly toward the irrigated side and then quickly move back to midline. With brain stem death, this nystagmus pattern does not occur. Oculovestibular tests are contraindicated for patients with perforated eardrums or with acute labyrinthine disease. As with pupil signs, abnormalities in eye movements help to localize the area of a disorder. They also help differentiate between structural and metabolic causes of coma.

Peripheral Nerve Studies

ELECTROMYOGRAPHY. EMG is used to measure and document electrical currents produced by skeletal muscles, called *muscle action potentials.* Small needle electrodes are inserted into muscles. The electrical potentials of each muscle are amplified, transmitted to an oscilloscope, and displayed on a screen. The recording can be made audible and documented on paper (Fig. 67–13).

EMG provides objective diagnostic information for various neuromuscular disorders. EMG can differentiate between primary muscle disease and disease secondary to denervation. It helps identify specific primary muscle diseases. The results may indicate a transmission defect at the neuromuscular junction, such as myasthenia gravis. The procedure can be used to help differentiate diseases of the anterior horn cells from those primarily of peripheral nerves. Peripheral nerve degeneration and regeneration can be monitored with EMG before clinical manifestations appear.

NERVE CONDUCTION VELOCITY STUDY. A nerve conduction velocity study, often performed in conjunction with EMG, is used to evaluate the excitability and conduction velocities of motor and sensory nerves. It is helpful in identifying peripheral nerve disorders. A stimulating electrode and a recording electrode are placed to test specific nerves (usually on a limb). The time required for the passage of a nerve impulse from the point of stimulation to the point of recording is measured precisely. Conduction velocity is calculated. Both motor and sensory modalities are altered in peripheral nervous system disorders (e.g., carpal tunnel syndrome), whereas only motor

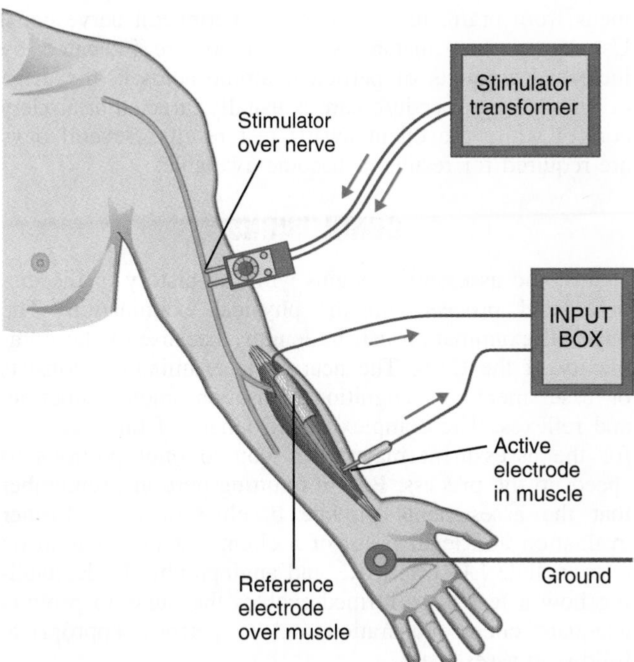

FIGURE 67–13 Electromyography measures and documents electrical currents produced by skeletal muscles. A stimulator is placed over the peripheral nerve being tested. A small pin is inserted into the muscle being assessed for nerve innervation, and a ground wire is placed on the client's skin.

fibers are affected in chronic disease of the anterior horn cell or motor nerve roots.

Explain the procedure. The client should avoid all stimulants, depressants, and sedatives for 24 hours before the test. There may be discomfort when the electrodes are inserted. If many muscles are tested, there may be residual discomfort. There may be a mild electrical shock during the procedure. The client lies flat and may be asked to move various muscles at specific times during the test. Clients with neuritis may have residual pain after testing. Mild analgesic medications may be needed.

Muscle Biopsy

Muscle biopsy is used in the diagnosis of neuropathies and myopathies. It is useful in distinguishing neurogenic from myopathic processes. However, muscle histologic findings are nonspecific for any neurogenic atrophy. An EMG is helpful in locating those muscle areas that are most abnormal. It is important that areas that have been traumatized by needle electrodes be avoided when tissue is taken for biopsy. Care of the biopsy site is needed.

Cellular Assessment

Chromosome analysis assists diagnosis of some abnormal neurologic conditions and provides the basis for genetic counseling in families with evidence of congenital neurologic malformations. Chromosomes can be prepared for microscopic examination from tissue culture of cells obtained from peripheral blood, bone marrow, or skin.

Mental retardation and convulsive seizures may result from neurologic dysfunction associated with inborn errors of metabolism. Diagnosis of carbohydrate and lipid metabolism disorders may require measurements of specific enzyme concentrations in blood cells or in biopsy specimens from brain, muscle, liver, or peripheral nerve cells. Usually, protein metabolism disorders are indicated by increased amounts of particular amino acids in the urine or blood. Postprocedure care is usually directed at anxiety control while the client awaits test results. Several days are required for results to become available.

CONCLUSIONS

Neurologic assessment begins with the history of the disorder and proceeds to the physical examination. The physical examination can be lengthy because of the complexity of the CNS. The neurologic examination consists of assessments of cognition, sensation, motor function, and reflexes. The complexity and length of time required for the assessment may tempt you to omit portions to speed up the process. Before omitting portions, remember that the assessments provide baseline data for further evaluation and legal proof of a client's status. Diagnostic tests include LP, CT, MRI, and angiography. Understanding how a test is performed enables the nurse to provide adequate client preparation and to perform appropriate follow-up assessments.

BIBLIOGRAPHY

1. ———. (1996). Adult screening for cognitive and functional impairment. *Nurse Practitioner, 21*(4), 112–115.
2. The American Association for Neuroscience Nurses. (1996). *Core curriculum for neuroscience nursing*. Chicago: Author.
3. Baker, D. (1993). Assessment and management of impairments in swallowing. *Nursing Clinics of North America, 28*(4), 793–805.
4. Barker, E. (1994). *Neuroscience nursing*. St. Louis: Mosby–Year Book.
5. Barker, E., & Moore, K. (1992). Neurological assessment. *RN, 55*(4), 28–35.
6. Bell, T. A., et al. (1992). Transcranial Doppler: Correlation of blood velocity measurement with clinical status in subarachnoid hemorrhage. *Journal of Neuroscience Nursing, 24*(4), 215–219.
7. Biller, J. (1997). *Practical neurology*. Philadelphia: Lippincott-Raven.
8. Bondy, K. (1994). Assessing cognitive function: A guide to neuropsychological testing. *Rehabilitation Nursing, 19*(1), 24–30.
9. Brocklehurst, R., Tallis, J., & Fillit, H. (1992). *Textbook of geriatric medicine and gerontology* (4th ed.). New York: Churchill Livingstone.
10. Buzea, C. E. (1995). Understanding computerized EEG monitoring in the ICU. *Journal of Neuroscience Nursing, 27*(5), 292–297.
11. Cason, C. L., & Sample, J. C. (1995). Preparatory information for myelogram. *Journal of Neuroscience Nursing, 27*(3), 182–187.
12. Chernecky, C., & Berger, B. (1997). *Laboratory tests and diagnostic procedures* (2nd ed.). Philadelphia: W. B. Saunders.
13. DiDonato, O., & Schaffer, V. (1994). The importance of outcome data in brain injury. *Rehabilitation Nursing, 19*(4), 219–228.
14. Gilman, S. (1992). Advances in neurology: Part 2. *New England Journal of Medicine, 326*(25), 1671–1676.
15. Gilman, S. (1998). Imaging the brain: Part I. *New England Journal of Medicine, 338*(12), 812–820.
16. Gilman, S. (1998). Imaging the brain: Part II. *New England Journal of Medicine, 338*(13), 889–896.
17. Gilroy, J. (1990). *Basic neurology* (2nd ed.). New York: Pergamon Press.
18. Guyton, A., & Hall, J. (1996). *Textbook of medical physiology* (9th ed.). Philadelphia: W. B. Saunders.
19. Hickey, J. V. (1997). *Clinical practice of neurological and neuroscience nursing*. Philadelphia: Lippincott-Raven.
20. Hudak, C. M., & Gallo, B. M. (1997). Quick review of neurodiagnostic testing. *American Journal of Nursing, 97*(7), 16CC–16FF.
21. Jarvis, C. (2000). *Physical examination and health assessment* (3rd ed.). Philadelphia: W. B. Saunders.
22. Lauren, N., et al. (1989). Cerebral perfusion imaging with technetium-99m HM-PAO in brain death and severe central nervous system injury. *Journal of Nuclear Medicine, 30*(10), 1627–1635.
23. Lederman, R. (1996). Lumbar puncture: Essential steps to a safe and valid procedure. *Geriatrics, 51*(6), 51–58.
24. Lewis, A. M. (1999). Neurologic emergency! *Nursing, 29*(10), 54–56.
25. Lower, J. (1992). Rapid neuroassessment. *American Journal of Nursing, 92*(6), 38–48.
26. Lucke, K. T., Kerr, M. E., & Chovanes, G. (1995). Continuous bedside cerebral blood flow monitoring. *Journal of Neuroscience Nursing, 27*(3), 164–173.
27. McDonagh, A. (1991). Getting your patient ready for a nuclear medicine scan. *Nursing 91, 21*(2), 53–57.
28. McGruder, J., et al. (1988). Headache after lumbar puncture: Review of the epidural blood patch. *Southern Medical Journal, 81*(10), 1249–1252.
29. Monti, E., Kerr, M., & Bender, C. (1995). Monitoring neuromuscular function. *Journal of Neuroscience Nursing, 27*(4), 252–256.
30. O'Hanlon-Nichols, T. (1999). Neurologic assessment. *American Journal of Nursing, 99*(6), 44–50.
31. Pressman, E., Zeidman, S., & Summers, L. (1995). Primary care for women: Comprehensive assessment of the neurological system. *Journal of Nurse-Midwifery, 40*(2), 163–71.
32. Reid, R., et al. (1989). Clinical use of technetium-99m HM-PAO for determination of brain death. *Journal of Nuclear Medicine, 30*(10), 1621–1626.
33. Shier, D., et al. (1996). *Hole's human anatomy and physiology* (7th ed.). Dubuque, IA: Wm. C. Brown.
34. Solomon, E. P. (1992). *An introduction to human anatomy and physiology* (2nd ed.). Philadelphia: W. B. Saunders.
35. Sur, M., & Cowey, A. (1995). Cerebral cortex: Functional development. *Neuron, 15,* 497–505.
36. Swartz, M. H. (1997). *Textbook of physical diagnosis* (3rd ed.). Philadelphia: W. B. Saunders.

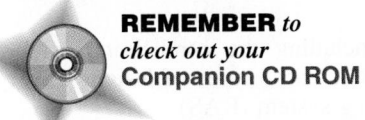

CHAPTER 68

Management of Comatose or Confused Clients

Chris Stewart Amidei

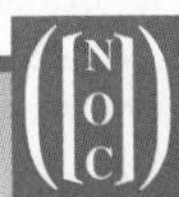

NURSING OUTCOMES CLASSIFICATION (NOC) for Nursing Diagnoses—Comatose or Confused Clients

Altered Family Processes
Family Coping
Family Normalization
Family Participation in Professional Care
Grief Resolution
Social Support
Altered Nutrition: Less Than Body Requirements
Nutritional Status: Nutrient Intake
Nutritional Status: Biochemical Measures
Nutritional Status: Body Mass
Altered Oral Mucous Membranes
Oral Health
Tissue Integrity: Skin and Mucous Membranes
Altered Thought Processes
Cognitive Orientation
Distorted Thought Control
Communication Ability
Bowel Incontinence
Bowel Elimination
Bowel Continence
Caregiver Role Strain
Caregiver Emotional Health
Caregiver Lifestyle Disruption
Caregiver Performance: Direct Care
Caregiver Physical Health
Caregiver Stressors
Caregiver Home Care Readiness
Caregiver Patient Relationship
Knowledge: Health Resources
Social Support
Risk for Aspiration
Neurologic Status
Respiratory Status: Gas Exchange
Respiratory Status: Ventilation
Risk for Disuse Syndrome (Contractures)
Immobility Consequences: Physiologic
Joint Movement: Passive
Mobility Level
Muscle Function
Risk for Fluid Volume Deficit
Electrolyte and Acid-Base Balance
Hydration
Nutritional Status: Food and Fluid Intake
Thermoregulation
Urinary Elimination
Risk for Impaired Skin Integrity
Immobility Consequences: Physiologic
Tissue Integrity: Skin and Mucous Membranes
Tissue Perfusion: Peripheral
Risk for Injury
Neurologic Status
Risk Control
Safety Status: Falls
Safety Status: Physical Injury
Risk for Suffocation
Aspiration Control
Neurological Status: Consciousness
Respiratory Status: Gas Exchange
Sleep Pattern Disturbance
Rest
Sleep

Perhaps more than any other clients we encounter, clients who are comatose or confused need to be cared for in a holistic manner. All aspects of physiologic and psychological function need to be addressed. Even if clients cannot interact with the environment, the nurse must care for them in a respectful and dignified manner. It is important for family members to see that their loved ones are spoken to and cared for in a professional and caring way.

The brain serves many functions in the body. In contrast to other body systems that monitor and regulate a group of functions, such as the gastrointestinal (GI) tract regulating digestion, the nervous system monitors and regulates all other body systems. Some of these functions are self-protective, including the ability to think, be awake, respond appropriately to the environment, and move about. Other functions are automatic, such as the regulation of body temperature and protective reflex responses. When these protective functions are lost, the clinical manifestations reflect the complexity of the nervous system.

The term *patient* is used in this chapter to describe the client who is comatose. It is assumed that such a client cannot be an active participant in care and that the *family* serves as the *client* in these circumstances.

DISORDERS OF CONSCIOUSNESS

Consciousness is a state of being that has two important aspects: (1) wakefulness and (2) awareness of self, environment, and time. *Awareness of self* means that the client can identify himself or herself. *Awareness of environment* indicates that the client can identify his or her present location and reason for being there. *Awareness of time* indicates that a client knows the date, month, and year and can identify common current facts, such as the name of the President of the United States.

Unconsciousness can be brief, lasting for a few seconds to an hour or so, or sustained, lasting for a few hours or longer. To produce unconsciousness, a disorder must (1) disrupt the ascending reticular activating system, which extends the length of the brain stem and up into the thalamus, (2) significantly disrupt the function of both cerebral hemispheres, or (3) metabolically depress overall brain function, as in a drug overdose.

Coma is a state of sustained unconsciousness in which the patient (1) does not respond to verbal stimuli, (2) may have varying responses to painful stimuli, (3) does not move voluntarily, (4) may have altered respiratory patterns, (5) may have altered pupillary responses to light, and (6) does not blink. In general, the longer the coma lasts, the more likely that it is irreversible and due to a permanent disorder in the brain structure. Duration of coma is also associated with mortality and outcome; the longer the coma, the higher the mortality rates, and the poorer the neurologic outcome.[4]

Etiology and Risk Factors

Two kinds of disorders produce sustained coma (Fig. 68–1):

1. Structural lesions in the brain that place pressure on the brain stem or the structures within the posterior cranial fossa, including the cerebellum, midbrain, pons, and medulla. These types of lesions affect the reticular activating system (RAS).
2. Metabolic disorders and diffuse lesions, which impair wakefulness and awareness by reducing the supply of oxygen and glucose, which are necessary energy substrates, or by allowing waste products to accumulate in the brain.

Structural causes of coma include brain tumors, head trauma, and cerebral hemorrhage. The brain can be a site for tumors to metastasize from many organs, such as breast and lung, or tumors may arise from the brain itself. Automobile and motorcycle accidents, physical assaults, gunshot wounds, and falls are common causes of head injury. The impact of the initial injury causes damage. A cascade of events also occurs in response to the initial injury, characterized by edema and ischemia. Clients with head injury (see Chapter 73) may also have sustained injury to the chest or airway, which increases the risk of hypoxia. Cerebral hemorrhage can occur as a consequence of hypertension or from rupture of a vascular anomaly. Hemorrhage causes coma by placing pressure on brain tissue.

There are many metabolic causes of coma. The term *metabolic* is used to describe any problem that alters brain metabolism. Most metabolic comas originate in organ systems outside the brain. *Hypoxia* is a common cause of metabolic coma. Blood loss, high altitudes, or carbon monoxide poisoning may deprive the brain of oxygen. *Ischemia,* inadequate tissue levels of oxygen, may occur with cardiac disorders in which cardiac output is decreased, such as cardiac arrest or even

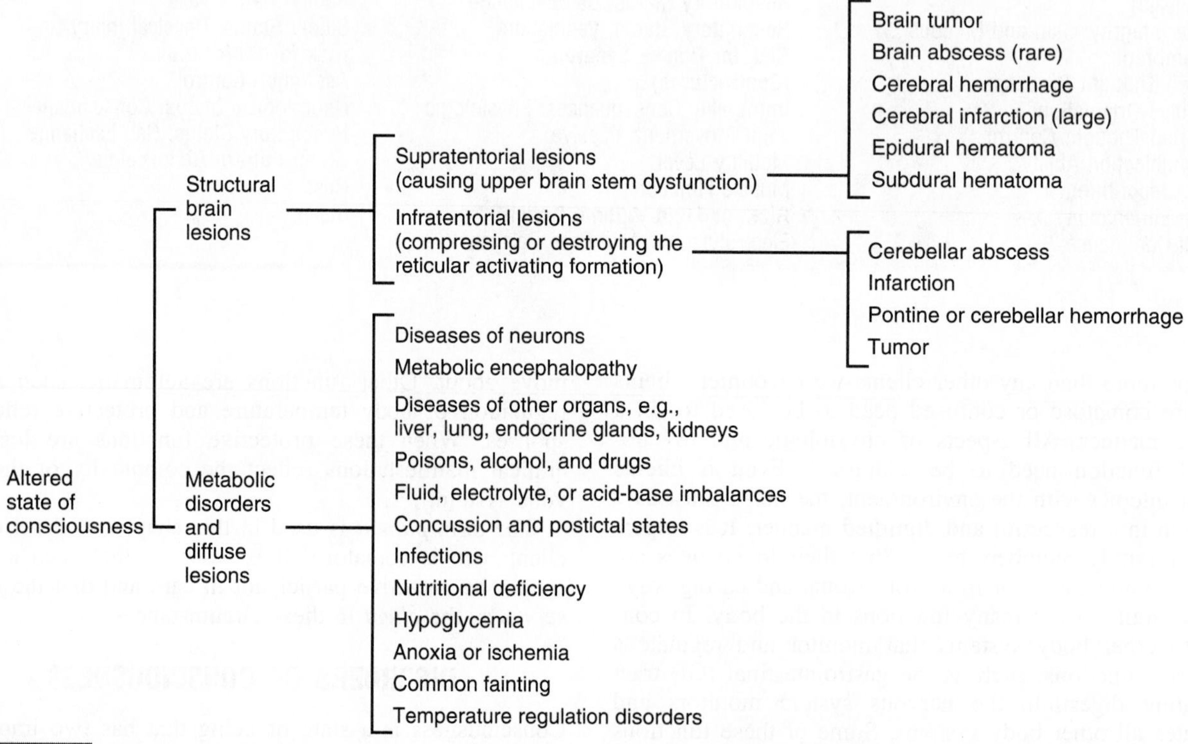

FIGURE 68–1 Some causes of altered states of consciousness. *Supratentorial* lesions are located *above* the dura roofing in the cerebellum, which separates the cerebellum from the cerebrum. *Infratentorial* lesions lie *beneath* the dura roofing in the cerebellum.

fainting. Disorders of the liver, lungs, and kidney may produce coma through the accumulation of metabolic waste products. Many other factors affect brain metabolism, including toxins, hypoglycemia, fever, infections such as encephalitis, and fluid, electrolyte, or acid-base imbalances.

Pathophysiology

Consciousness is a complex function controlled by the RAS and its integrated components. The RAS begins in the medulla as the reticular formation (RF) (Fig. 68–2). The reticular formation connects to the RAS, which is located in the midbrain, which then connects to the hypothalamus and thalamus. Integrated pathways connect to the cortex via the thalamus and to the limbic system via the hypothalamus. Feedback systems also connect at the brain stem level. The reticular formation produces wakefulness, whereas the RAS and higher connections are responsible for awareness of self and the environment. Diffuse cortical connections allow maximum integration of all conscious-related activities.

Disorders that affect any part of the RAS can produce coma. To produce coma, a disorder must affect both cerebral hemispheres or the brain stem itself. Disorders affect these areas in one of three ways:

1. Direct compression or destruction of structures responsible for consciousness. A tumor or hemorrhage in the brain stem or swelling in the cerebral hemispheres can cause coma in this manner.
2. Decrease in availability of oxygen or glucose, both of which are needed for cerebral metabolism. Hypoxia and ischemia are the most common causes; without oxygen and glucose, the brain cannot form the chemicals necessary to carry out its functions.
3. Toxic effects of substances on structures of the RAS. Toxic wastes from liver or kidney disease, bacterial invasion from meningitis, and metabolites from drug overdose are examples of such substances.

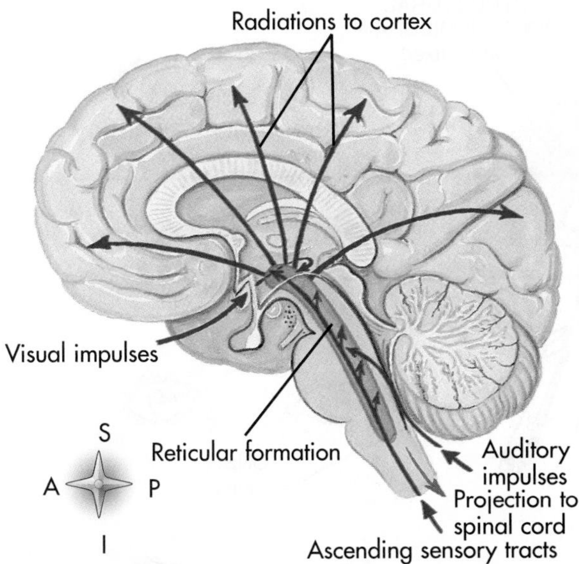

FIGURE 68–2 The reticular activating system (RAS) consists of centers in the brain stem reticular formation along with fibers conducting to the centers from below and fibers conducting from the centers to widespread areas of the cerebral cortex. A functioning RAS is essential for consciousness. (From Thibodeau, G., & Patton, K. [1999]. *Anatomy and physiology* [4th ed., p. 395]. St. Louis: Mosby.)

TABLE 68–1 DIFFERENTIAL MANIFESTATIONS OF STRUCTURALLY INDUCED AND METABOLIC COMA

Mechanism	Manifestations
Supratentorial mass lesions compressing or displacing the diencephalon or brain stem	Initiating sign is usually focal cerebral dysfunction Signs of dysfunction progress cephalocaudad Neurologic signs at any given time point to one anatomic area (e.g., frontal lobes, thalamus) Motor signs are often asymmetrical
Infratentorial mass of destruction causing coma	History of sudden onset of coma Localizing brain stem signs precede or accompany onset of coma and always include oculovestibular abnormality Cranial nerve palsies "Bizarre" respiratory patterns that appear at coma onset
Metabolic coma	Confusion and stupor commonly precede motor signs Motor signs usually are symmetrical Pupillary reactions usually are preserved Asterixis, myoclonus, tremor, and seizures are common Acid-base imbalance with hyperventilation or hypoventilation is common

The causes may overlap. The exact location of involvement as well as the extent of the problem and the time frame of its occurrence determine the depth of coma.

Clinical Manifestations

Masses located in the supratentorial area (above the dura roofing the cerebellum) of the brain cause a fairly predictable set of clinical manifestations (Table 68–1). Supratentorial lesions can involve the entire cortical or subcortical level of the brain tissue, as with ischemia. The disorder may also be located in one hemisphere, as with tumor. These masses first produce manifestations such as headache, localized sensorimotor deficits, aphasia, visual loss, and seizures. The manifestations are related to the specific area of the brain affected.

For example, if the client has a mass in the frontal lobe, early clinical manifestations may consist of headaches, memory deficits, or partial seizures. *Partial seizures* are seizures occurring in one area of the body, such as the hand. As the mass expands, manifestations worsen because the mass places pressure on nearby areas. This pressure may cause a unilateral sensorimotor deficit (e.g., client cannot raise the right leg or has numbness in the right leg), aphasia, or a deficit in the visual field (blind in one half of the visual field). The client usually has intact pupillary and oculocephalic reflexes (see later). If the mass is not detected or cannot be treated and so progresses, coma eventually develops. Coma indicates that the mass has grown and now compresses structures deep in the brain stem.

Disorders of the infratentorial area (located beneath the dura roofing the cerebellum) cause the client to suddenly lose consciousness either (1) by directly affecting the RAS or its pathways or (2) by invading the brain stem or reducing its blood supply. Infratentorial lesions may produce unusual respiratory patterns (Fig. 68–3). The medulla houses the center for rhythmic breathing. This center's function is lost as consciousness decreases, and the lower brain stem begins to regulate breathing by responding to changes primarily in the carbon dioxide levels as well as in acid-base balance and oxygen levels. The result is a very irregular breathing depth and pattern. The mass or edema in the brain commonly compresses the cranial nerves, and various cranial nerve palsies can be seen, in particular, abnormal eye movements and loss of pupillary reactivity to light. Specific patterns of pupil size and reactivity to light occur when pressure is exerted at various levels (see Fig. 68–3).

Coma caused by a metabolic disorder more often is manifested as the presence of bilateral or symmetrical findings, because the disorder affects the entire brain rather than just one section. The patient usually demonstrates confusion and stupor before any physical signs are noticed. Physical signs of coma due to a metabolic disorder include tremor, asterixis (flapping tremors of the hands), myoclonus (a single, sudden jerking movement), and seizures. Pupillary response is usually normal unless the condition is related to drug overdose. Depending on the underlying cause, acid-base imbalances may be noted. For example, metabolic acidosis would be present in a patient with diabetic coma.

Level of consciousness is the single most important indicator of neurologic function. In the comatose patient, this indicator is lost and other indicators of neurologic function must be evaluated. Information about motor response, pupil size and reactivity to light, presence or absence of oculocephalic and oculovestibular responses, and breathing pattern can localize the level of involvement and determine the depth of coma. For discussion on these indicators, see Chapter 73.

Some patients in coma awaken slowly and begin to respond normally. They often require physical, occupational, and speech therapy in order to return to maximal levels of function. Irreversible coma is caused by damage to any area of the brain that destroys the patient's ability to respond to the environment. The brain stem and cerebellum remain intact, however, so that vital functions, such as heart, lung, and gastrointestinal functions, continue. Patients can remain in irreversible coma for years. Significant ethical and legal debates have arisen regarding the maintenance of nutritional intake for such a patient, particularly when a patient's family questions the rationale for artificial feeding.

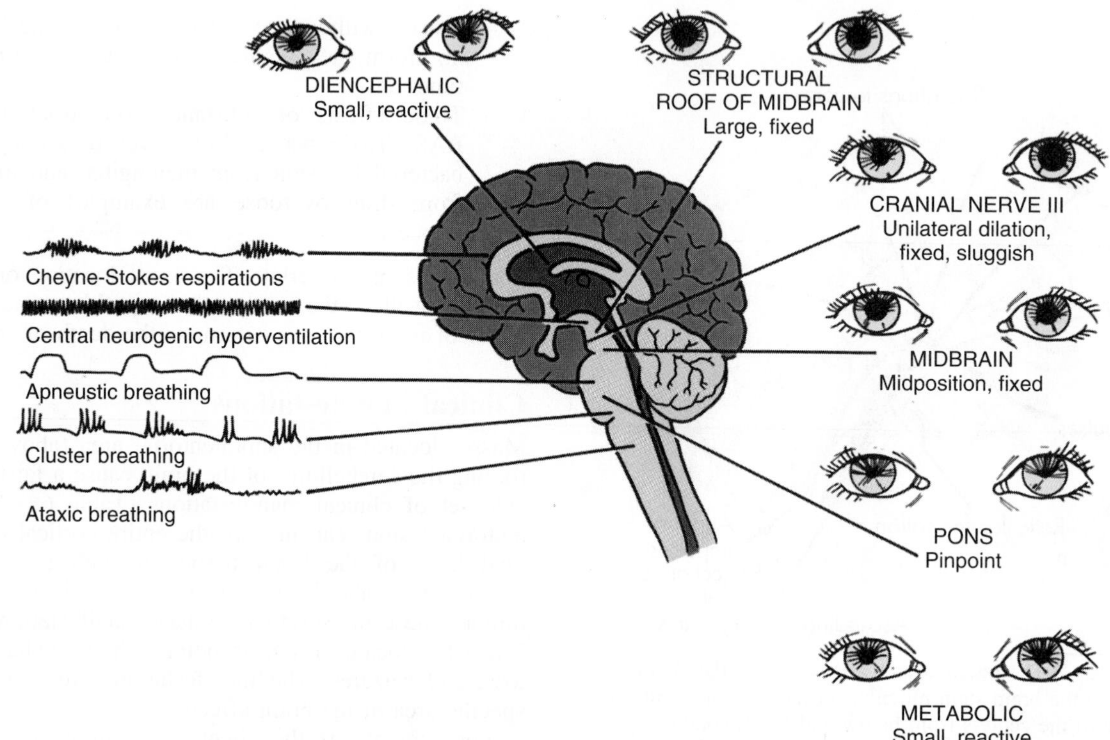

FIGURE 68–3 Respiratory patterns and appearances of the pupil associated with lesions of various neurologic structures. Cheyne-Stokes respiration may occur because of altered cerebral perfusion deep within the cerebral hemisphere or from within the diencephalon.

Diagnostic Findings

The neurologic examination is supplemented by diagnostic testing. Tests identify structural or physiologic abnormalities that affect brain function.

Computed Tomography and Magnetic Resonance Imaging. A computed tomography (CT) or magnetic resonance imaging (MRI) scan usually provides data that indicate whether the cause of the coma is structural. In coma, a CT scan is usually performed first because it is quicker. Tumors or areas of bleeding are evident on the scan. Sometimes the patient requires emergency surgery to remove the mass or drain the fluid and thereby relieve pressure. In metabolic coma, the structures may appear unremarkable, or edema or diffuse nonspecific changes may be seen.

Lumbar Puncture. A lumbar puncture can be performed when it is known, from data provided by the CT or MRI scans, that the patient does not have an expanding intracranial mass. Obtaining this information prior to lumbar puncture avoids the risk of herniation due to sudden changes in cerebrospinal fluid (CSF) pressures (low in the spinal column and high in the ventricles). A lumbar puncture can assist in the diagnosis of infection or bleeding as a cause of coma. CSF may be cloudy or bloody when the patient has an infection or bleeding into the ventricles or the subarachnoid space.

Electroencephalography. Electroencephalography (EEG) can be used to determine whether the patient is comatose because of continuous seizures. EEG results are abnormal in many patients with structural and metabolic coma and do not serve as a clear diagnostic tool. A portion of the general population may have abnormal EEG results as well.

Laboratory Tests. Liver and kidney function as well as glucose level may be evaluated through blood tests. A urine or blood toxicology screen may be useful in distinguishing drug-induced coma. Blood oxygenation tests may be used to evaluate for hypoxia. Other laboratory tests may be ordered specific to the patient's situation. Chapter 67 covers specific neurologic diagnostic tests.

Tests for Abnormal Reflexes

Oculocephalic Reflex Response. The *doll's eye reflex* is movement of the eyes in the direction opposite to that in which the head is moved; for example, doll's eye reflex is considered present if the eyes move to the right when the head is rotated to the left, and vice versa (Fig. 68–4). This test can be performed only in unconscious patients, because conscious patients have voluntary control over eye movements. The presence of the doll's eye reflex indicates that brain stem function is preserved. The reflex is absent or impaired in patients with brain stem problems. The doll's eye test should never be performed in comatose patients with suspected or known cervical spine injury because the head movement required may produce permanent spinal cord damage.

Patients in metabolic coma, except for that caused by barbiturate or phenytoin (Dilantin) poisoning, retain ocular reflexes. The brain stem in a comatose patient may be functioning even in the absence of the doll's eye reflex. Other agents and disorders can block the eye's response. Neuromuscular drugs, such as succinylcholine, and Ménière's disease, which destroys the labyrinth in the ear, cause absence of the oculocephalic response. In the patient without Ménière's disease or evidence of neuromuscular drugs, however, absence of the oculocephalogyric response supports the diagnosis of brain death.[4, 6]

Oculovestibular Reflex Response. If oculocephalic responses are absent, an oculovestibular (caloric) test can be performed to test cranial nerves III, IV, VI, and VIII (see Chapter 67). A normal response to instillation of iced water into one ear canal is seen as smooth movement of both eyes with nystagmus toward the irrigated ear (see Fig. 68–4*C*). Instillation of warm water results in eye movement away from the irrigated ear. *Nystagmus* is the involuntary oscillation of the eyeballs; it may be horizontal, vertical, oblique, rotary, or mixed, with various rates of movement.

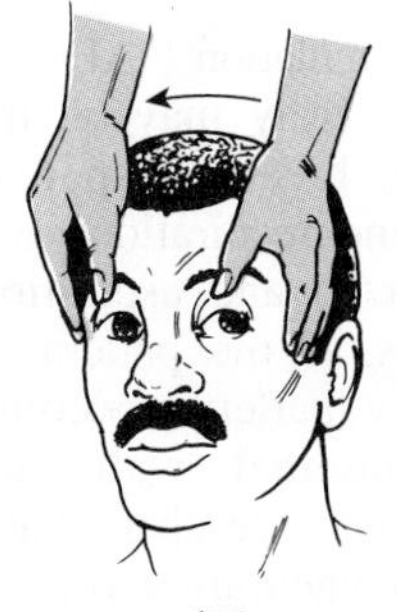
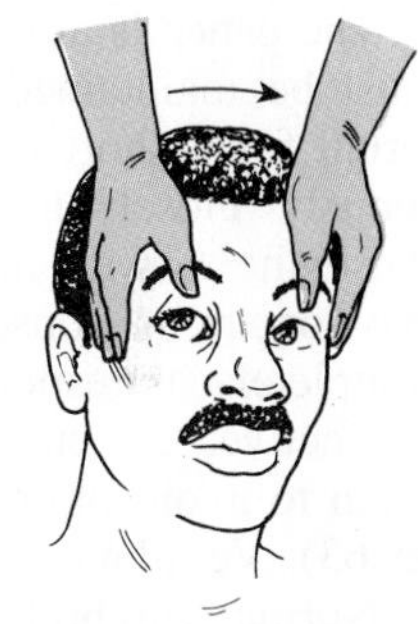

A. NORMAL REACTION:
Eyes move in direction opposite to head movement when head is turned

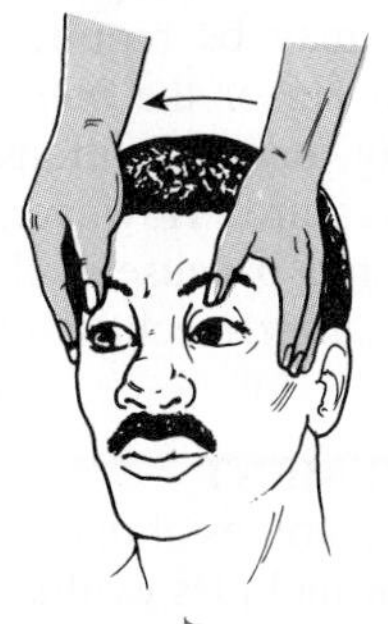
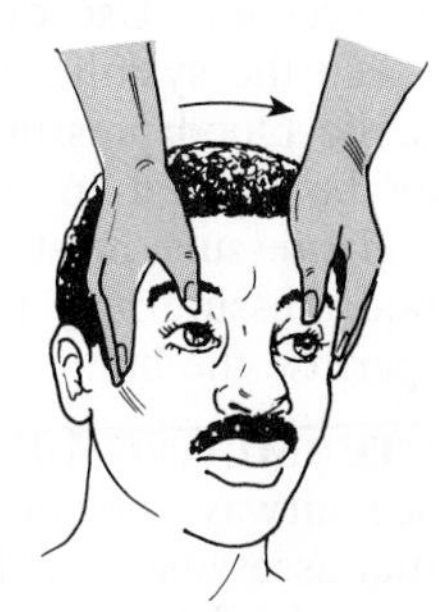

B. ABNORMAL REACTION:
Eyes remain in fixed position in skull when head is turned

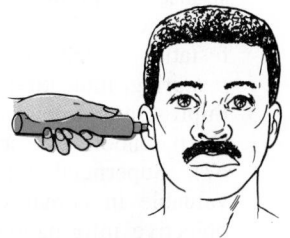

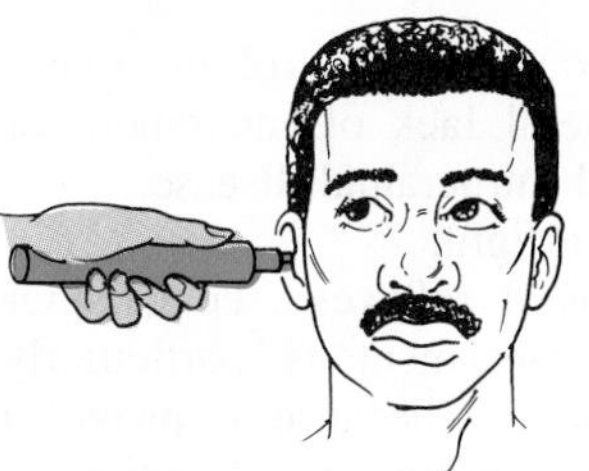

C. NORMAL CALORIC:
Eyes deviate to side of ice water application

D. ABNORMAL CALORIC:
Eyes do not deviate

FIGURE 68–4 *A* and *B,* Normal and abnormal doll's eye reflexes (oculocephalic response). *C* and *D,* Normal and abnormal caloric test results (oculovestibular response).

Failure to produce eye movement and nystagmus with the instillation of warm or cold water into the ear canal indicates an altered brain stem, with a few exceptions. The use of ototoxic drugs, barbiturates, sedatives, phenytoin, or tricyclic antidepressants or the presence of Ménière's disease may produce a false-negative caloric test result. In a patient without these conditions, the absence of an oculovestibular reflex supports the diagnosis of brain death.

A caloric test is contraindicated in a patient with a ruptured tympanic membrane (eardrum) or otorrhea (ear discharge). This test is usually performed only in comatose patients because awake patients may vomit in response to the stimulation of CN VIII.

Outcome Management

The goals of medical management are to preserve brain function and to prevent additional brain injury. The primary focus is on maintaining the supply of oxygen and glucose to the brain.

The patient's airway, breathing, and circulation ("ABCs") must be maintained. A nasal or oral airway may be inserted for a short time. If the patient is breathing spontaneously, closely monitor the airway and respirations because the airway may become obstructed and aspiration may occur as consciousness decreases. If the patient is completely unresponsive or respiratory patterns become ineffective, an endotracheal tube is inserted, with care taken to avoid injury to the cervical spine (see also Chapter 63). Ventilation and supplemental oxygen are given.

Normal cerebral perfusion is promoted through monitoring of blood pressure and maintenance of the systolic pressure between 100 and 160 mm Hg. Blood pressures lower or higher than these levels may alter cerebral perfusion pressure. Use of vasoactive agents may be required to keep the systolic pressure at 100 mm Hg or the *mean* systolic blood pressure above 80 mm Hg, or medications may be needed to lower the blood pressure. However, blood pressure must be cautiously lowered because high blood pressure may represent a compensatory mechanism to perfuse the brain.

DETERMINING LEVEL OF INVOLVEMENT

Once airway, breathing, and circulation are established, initial assessment of the comatose patient includes evaluation of the following factors:[11]

1. Level of consciousness, through observation of response to stimuli.
2. Presence or absence of localizing neurologic manifestations, such as unilateral lack of movement or posturing, indicating focal intracranial disease.
3. Pupil size and reactivity to light.
4. Deep tendon and superficial reflexes (see Chapter 67). Superficial reflex assessment is particularly valuable in comatose patients because it provides objective information about brain stem function in the absence of consciousness. Assess the corneal reflex carefully to avoid corneal abrasion.
5. Response to noxious stimuli. First, loud verbal stimuli and then shaking are performed to produce a response. If none is noted, the examiner applies a painful stimulus, such as pressure to the sternum, nail beds, or supraorbital notch. Care must be taken not to damage skin underlying the areas where pressure is applied. Other aspects of sensory assessment are not possible or are unreliable in comatose patients.
6. Evidence of trauma. Trauma may be the result of coma rather than the cause of it (e.g., a tongue bite may result from a seizure). Examine the ears for ruptured eardrums and otorrhea.
7. Determination of serum oxygenation, blood alcohol, blood urea nitrogen, ammonia, and glucose levels if manifestations suggest a metabolic disorder.
8. History from significant others (or observers of what has happened), if possible.

REVERSING COMMON CAUSES OF COMA

Immediate interventions for the patient in a coma include treatment of common causes of coma while assessment of neurologic status and diagnostic testing continue. For example, after a blood specimen is drawn for testing, intravenous (IV) glucose is given to reverse potential insulin reactions. Many comatose patients are malnourished and subject to Wernicke's encephalopathy related to alcohol abuse. These patients are commonly given thiamine, especially if they are given glucose.

If the patient is having repetitive seizures, coma and brain damage can follow. The patient is given IV diazepam or lorazepam to stop the seizures. If the patient is not intubated, closely monitor the airway because of the respiratory depressant effects of these medications.

Many metabolic causes of coma lead to acid-base, fluid, and electrolyte imbalances. The patient's acid-base balance should be restored quickly. Fluid imbalances should be restored slowly to prevent rebound fluid shifts into the brain (see Chapter 12). Isotonic saline is usually given if the patient is dehydrated, and fluids are withheld if the patient is fluid-overloaded. If cerebral edema is present, osmotic diuretics may be used to promote shifting of extracellular brain fluid back into the plasma. Other medications, such as steroids, barbiturate therapy, and neuromuscular blocking agents, decrease intracranial pressure (ICP) through more indirect means. (Electrolyte imbalances are covered in Chapter 13.)

If infection is suspected, specimens for culture are obtained from the blood, nose, throat, and wounds (if present). Once such specimens have been collected, antibiotics are given if infection is suspected. Body temperature should be normalized as much as possible by means of antipyretics, air circulation, and cooling mattresses. Care must be taken to ensure that the patient does not shiver, because shivering increases ICP.

Coma from drug overdose may be reversed by specific antidotes if the ingested drug can be identified. Often, however, the specific drug ingested is not known. A blood specimen should be collected for a toxicity screen. Narcotic overdose may be reversed with naloxone. Because the duration of action of naloxone is 2 to 3 hours shorter than that of most narcotics, naloxone may need to be readministered. Seizures resulting from cocaine overdose can be treated with diazepam. Patients with cocaine overdose often have cardiac dysrhythmias and irregular respirations. Gastric lavage may be used to remove ingested agents, followed by instillation of activated charcoal.

Structural causes of coma may require surgery to decompress the cranial vault. Burr holes may be created to drain a subdural hematoma. A craniotomy may be performed to remove a tumor or intracerebral hematoma. A ventricular catheter or shunt may be placed to relieve hydrocephalus.

To stimulate your thought process, see Thinking Critically at the end of this chapter for the description of a scenario involving a client with coma from a hypertensive hemorrhage.

PREVENTING COMPLICATIONS

If the coma is prolonged, initiate enteral feeding to promote nutrition and prevent muscle wasting. Parenteral nutrition may be used if paralytic ileus is present. Take care to avoid hyperglycemia, which can exacerbate brain injury in the presence of ischemia. However, brain cells have a high glucose need compared with other cells; supplying the cell need without causing brain damage requires a delicate balance.

Prevent the complications of immobility, such as pneumonia and pressure ulcers, with frequent turning or the use of an oscillating bed. Continue to reposition the patient to relieve skin pressure unless the bed provides more than 40 degrees of rotation. The eyes may need to be taped closed to avoid corneal abrasion. Suctioning may be needed to keep the airway clear and prevent pneumonia. Passive range-of-motion exercises keep joints mobile and minimize muscle wasting. Position the extremities in correct alignment to prevent contractures. Use sequential compression stockings to prevent deep venous thrombosis (DVT); low-dose heparin may also be ordered. All of these complications are continually assessed for and are treated promptly if they occur.

OUTCOMES

In the past, little information was available on which to base a prediction about the outcome for a patient in coma. Most of the time, a "wait-and-see" approach was taken. Today, the family and the health care team should have some idea of the probable eventual outcome for the patient. It is discouraging and inappropriate to vigorously treat a patient who has no chance of recovery, but it is even more inappropriate to deny treatment to a patient with a reasonable chance of recovery.

Coma after head injury has a statistically better outcome than coma associated with medical illness.[9] About 50% of patients in coma from head injury die, many instantly. Immediate treatment may somewhat improve the outcome for those who reach the hospital. Recovery in traumatic cases is closely linked to age; the younger the patient, the better the recovery. Severely abnormal neuro-ophthalmologic signs reflecting brain stem dysfunction imply a poor prognosis; approximately 90% of patients with such signs either die or remain in near-vegetative states.[4]

The absence of pupillary, corneal, or oculovestibular responses during the early stages of coma is highly predictive of mortality or significant morbidity (e.g., persistent vegetative state). The recovery of these responses and a return to purposeful movement correlate with a better prognosis. Patients who lapse into coma as a result of metabolic disorders have an extremely poor prognosis if the coma lasts more than 1 week.

Coma stimulation, application of planned meaningful, multimodality sensory stimulation, has been suggested as a measure to enhance outcome from coma. Clinical validity of coma stimulation has not been clearly established. The type of stimulation, timing of application, and outcomes measures used vary among studies, making it difficult to determine whether coma stimulation is of benefit.[5] Nonetheless, the nurse is encouraged to interact with comatose patients through all their sensory systems.

Nursing Management of the Medical Client

ASSESSMENT

Frequent, systematic, and objective nursing assessment of the comatose patient, including neurologic status, is essential. Serial observations are important for comparison and to facilitate prompt reporting of even subtle changes in status. Even if assessment findings seem insignificant for long periods, documentation provides an objective pattern and an important baseline for future observations. Assessment of consciousness is most effective when the assessments are performed by a consistent nurse. The neurologic assessment is performed as often as every 15 minutes during the first few hours of coma. Depending on the patient's condition, assessments may need to be continued hourly for several days.

The Critical Monitoring feature lists the neurologic manifestations of a person who is unconscious. Presenting manifestations are ordered according to the degree of seriousness. Remembering these subtle changes in assessment helps in early identification of a patient's improvement or worsening. A decrease in the patient's Glasgow Coma Scale (GCS) score also indicates worsening. The GCS is the most common neurologic assessment tool used in clinical practice (see Chapter 73).

Although neurologic assessment is the priority evaluation, the entire body of a comatose patient must be periodically observed because the patient is unable to offer any specific complaints. Complications either of the initial condition causing coma or of immobility can arise at any time during the course of care. If surgery has been performed, postoperative assessments must be performed as well.

DIAGNOSIS, OUTCOMES, INTERVENTIONS

This section describes interventions appropriate for all comatose patients regardless of the cause of the coma. Interventions specific to particular etiologic factors are described elsewhere (e.g., hepatic coma in Chapter 47, and uremic coma in Chapter 34).

Comatose patients are completely dependent on others because their protective reflexes are impaired. Nursing intervention provides the safety normally afforded by protective reflexes. Coma is often life-threatening and requires aggressive medical intervention. Physicians are concerned with establishing a medical diagnosis and prescribing appropriate treatment; nurses are responsible for meeting basic human needs and preventing the complications associated with coma. Nurses are also responsible for assessing and intervening to reduce ICP.

Altered cerebral tissue perfusion is one of the highest risks for a patient with an altered level of consciousness. This outcome is often seen as a direct consequence of

CRITICAL MONITORING

Manifestations of Changes in Neurologic Status

"Change" is the key word. Notify the physician whenever there is a change in the client's neurologic status. The following manifestations are listed in the order that indicates a *worsening* in the client's condition. Remember, a client may display a "transient" deterioration in neurologic responses that does not warrant calling a physician. For example, after you have just performed suctioning of the client's airway or have turned the client, you would anticipate a possible change in neurologic status. If you hyperoxygenate the client and ensure proper positioning for venous return from the jugular veins and airway maintenance, however, any signs of increased deficit should last only a few seconds or no more than 4 or 5 minutes. Signs of increased deficit that last longer than this increase the risk for irreversible brain injury.

Normal

Alert, oriented to person, place, time
Responds appropriately to verbal commands
Eyes open spontaneously with any stimulus, unless in a deep sleep

Abnormal; Changes Due to Altered Perfusion of the Cerebral Cortex

Altered level of consciousness
Altered perception of time, then place, and lastly person
Motor deficits (e.g., hemiparesis, hemiplegia)
Speech deficits (e.g., expressive or receptive speech or both)
Memory deficits (e.g., recent, intermediate, remote)
Hyperreflexia
Babinski's sign
Seizures
Decorticate rigidity
Emotional lability
Altered sensory interpretation
Cheyne-Stokes respiration
Headache, nausea, vomiting, papilledema

Abnormal; Changes Due to Altered Perfusion Just Inferior to the Cortex

Pupillary changes: asymmetry of size, shape, or time-responsiveness
Loss of reaction to direct light
Visual field changes (e.g., homonymous hemianopsia; see Chapter 69)

Abnormal; Changes Due to Altered Perfusion of the Diencephalon

Altered temperature; first high fevers, then hypothermia
Cheyne-Stokes respiration

Abnormal; Changes Due to Altered Perfusion of the Posterior Pituitary Gland

Diabetes insipidus (decreased antidiuretic hormone)

Abnormal; Changes Due to Altered Perfusion of the Midbrain

Dysfunction of CN III (loss of reaction to indirect or consensual light, dysconjugate eye movement)
Dysfunction of CN IV (dysconjugate eye movement)
Central neurogenic hyperventilation

Abnormal; Changes Due to Altered Perfusion of the Upper Pons

Dysfunction of CN V (altered sensory function to cornea, nasal membranes, face, oral cavity, tongue, teeth, or altered mastication)
Dysfunction of CN VI (altered lateral eye movement)
Dysfunction of CN VII (altered facial expression, taste, and salivation)
Central neurogenic hyperventilation
Abnormal extension posture
Pinpoint pupils

Abnormal; Changes Due to Altered Perfusion of the Lower Pons

Apneustic breathing
Flaccidity

Abnormal; Changes Due to Altered Perfusion of the Medulla

Dysfunction of CN VIII (altered equilibrium and hearing)
Dysfunction of CN IX (altered taste, pharyngeal sensations, and cough and swallowing)
Dysfunction of CN X (altered sensations in pharynx, larynx, external ear, and altered cough and swallowing; altered parasympathetic nervous system functions in thoracic and abdominal viscera)
Dysfunction of CN XI (altered neck and shoulder movement)
Dysfunction of CN XII (altered tongue movement)
Projectile vomiting
Cushing's triad (increased systolic blood pressure, wide pulse pressure, bradycardia)
Ataxic (Biot's respiration)

CN, cranial nerve.

increasing ICP. Nursing management of this problem is described in Chapter 73.

Risk for Suffocation. Clients who are unconscious cannot swallow because of loss or suppression of the gag or coughing reflex and thus are at risk for suffocation. Airway obstruction is the most common source of harm to patients with decreased consciousness. Write the diagnosis as *Risk for Suffocation related to loss of gag reflex.*

Outcomes. The client will exhibit no signs of accidental suffocation or airway obstruction as evidenced by (1) clear lung sounds, (2) equal lung expansion, and (3) absence of stridor, cyanosis, and pallor.

Interventions. For initial airway management, an oral airway can be inserted in an unconscious patient. Endotracheal intubation, with the use of a ventilator, may be required to maintain airway patency or improve ventilation.

For extended airway management, a tracheostomy may be required to (1) allow long-term continuous mechanical ventilation, (2) facilitate removal of tracheobronchial secretions, and (3) separate the upper and lower airways (see Chapter 60).

Risk for Aspiration. The lack of effective airway clearance and gag reflex puts the comatose patient at very high risk for aspiration. Write the diagnosis as *Risk for Aspiration related to lack of effective airway clearance and loss of gag reflex.*

Outcomes. The patient will exhibit no signs of aspiration, as evidenced by (1) clear lung sounds, (2) no stridor, (3) absence of fever, (4) minimal amounts of clear mucus upon suctioning, and (5) clear lungs as demonstrated by chest x-ray.

Interventions. Monitor results of arterial blood gas (ABG) analysis and pulse oximetry to determine the level of oxygenation provided by ventilators or oxygen. Assess breath sounds every 1 to 2 hours in acutely ill patients. Keep suctioning equipment available.

Perform tracheobronchial suctioning as needed, not routinely, to prevent or decrease the accumulation of secretions from immobility, the lack of a cough and sigh reflex, or pneumonia. Not suctioning a person who cannot expectorate his or her own secretions can cause hypoxia and result in neurologic damage. Suctioning should be gentle, and the catheter should not remain in the airway for longer than 10 seconds. While suctioning, observe the cardiac monitor for dysrhythmias (e.g., premature ventricular contractions) secondary to hypoxia. Hyperoxygenating the patient before, during, and after suctioning decreases the risk of dysrhythmias. Hyperoxygenation and limiting the suctioning time to 10 seconds also minimizes increased ICP associated with suctioning. Never suction the nasal passages in the patient with a basilar skull fracture because the suction catheter can enter the cranial cavity.

A comatose patient may lack pharyngeal reflexes and be unable to swallow. Pneumonia secondary to aspiration is a common cause of death in unconscious patients. To reduce the risk of aspiration, never give a comatose patient fluids to swallow. Secretions also accumulate in the posterior pharynx and may be aspirated. If the patient is intubated, make sure the cuff is inflated. Suction the upper trachea and posterior pharynx as often as necessary to remove secretions. After tracheal suctioning, the same suction catheter can be used for oral or pharyngeal suctioning, but not vice versa. Also, turn the patient from side to side every 2 hours to facilitate drainage of secretions and prevent pneumonia.

While performing mouth care, place a comatose patient in a lateral position to prevent aspiration. If facial paralysis is present, keep the affected side uppermost. Keep the patient's mouth open by placing an oral airway or bite block between the teeth. Pay close attention to the roof of the mouth in patients who breathe through the mouth for long periods. Crusts of dried sputum may form, break off, and be aspirated. Use of artificial moisturizers may help prevent crust formation; however, frequent oral care is the best prevention.

As consciousness returns and the client begins to respond to verbal stimuli and has a gag reflex, test the client's ability to suck and to swallow liquids. Before the test, position the client in high Fowler's position, and have suction equipment nearby in case it is needed. Use a thick juice, nectar, or ice chips rather than water; liquid of a thick consistency is easier to swallow. Place about 1 teaspoon of liquid into the back of the mouth. Observe for swallowing. Suction as needed to prevent aspiration. If a client cannot suck through a straw or drink from a glass because of facial paralysis, place fluids into the unaffected side of the mouth with an aseptic (Asepto) syringe. Watch for difficulty in swallowing. Suction as needed.

If there is any question about a client's ability to swallow, a formal swallowing evaluation should be performed by a speech therapist. Clients who cannot swallow for long periods may require placement of a gastrostomy tube. Many rehabilitation and extended-care facilities require the use of gastrostomy tubes rather than nasogastric (NG) tubes because there is less risk of aspiration with gastrostomy tube-feedings.

Clients with impaired swallowing require special instruction. Swallowing can be stimulated by having the client lean the head forward and, after taking fluid, quickly tip the head backward. Stroking the anterior neck may also promote swallowing.

Once a client can safely swallow, begin oral nutrition with small liquid feedings, progressing to a soft diet. Discontinue tube-feedings only when the client can take adequate nutrition orally. Many clients are fed orally during the daytime and tube-fed at night to maintain adequate nutrition.

When changing from tube-feeding to oral feeding, turn off the tube-feeding several hours before the meal. This will stimulate the appetite. When a client begins to eat independently, be reassuring and encouraging. Remind the client to eat slowly and to swallow after each bite. Position the client sitting up as tolerated.

Altered Oral Mucous Membranes. Several factors can lead to altered oral mucous membranes. The comatose patient usually has an NPO (nothing by mouth) order, is unable to swallow, and breathes through the mouth. A possible nursing diagnosis might be *Altered Oral Mucous Membranes related to mouth breathing.*

Outcomes. The patient will maintain intact oral mucous membranes, as evidenced by oral and nasal mucous membranes that are pink, moist, and without lesions, crusts, or bloody drainage.

Interventions. Using a flashlight and tongue depressor, inspect the patient's mouth every 8 hours. Keep the patient's lips coated with a water-soluble lubricant to prevent encrustation, drying, and cracking. Carefully inspect a paralyzed cheek for crusts or other conditions requiring intervention. Provide oral hygiene to prevent excessive drying of oral mucous membranes and complications such as parotitis, aspiration, and respiratory tract infections.

At least twice a day, brush the patient's teeth with a small toothbrush, and rinse the mouth. Clean the oral mucous membranes (especially the roof of the mouth), tongue, and gums with sponge toothbrushes. Avoid using agents containing lemon or alcohol, because they dry the membranes. While performing mouth care in an unconscious patient, suction excess secretions to prevent aspiration. Toothbrushes with suction attachments are now available in many health care agencies.

Nasal passages may become occluded because an unconscious patient is unable to sniff, blow, sneeze, or otherwise clear the nose. To clear the nasal passages of mucus and crust formations, gently swab the nose with an applicator moistened with water or normal saline. Then apply a thin coat of water-soluble lubricant with a cotton-tipped applicator.

Do *not* clean the nasal passages or ears of a patient with a basilar skull fracture. If bleeding occurs from the ears or nose, or if CSF (a watery discharge) appears to be draining from these areas, notify the physician.

Risk for Impaired Skin Integrity. Normal reflexes reduce the risk of skin ischemia by signaling conscious (even sleeping) persons to shift their body weight. Comatose patients have lost these protective reflexes and are completely immobile. Sometimes patients are agitated and can shear the skin with frequent nonpurposeful movements; this diagnosis also applies to these patients. Write the diagnosis as *Risk for Impaired Skin Integrity related to immobility.*

Outcomes. The patient will have intact skin, as evidenced by no reddened areas over bony prominences and no areas or signs of skin irritation or dryness.

Interventions. Provide nursing intervention for all self-care needs, including bathing and care of the hair, skin, and nails. Patients often scratch themselves as the depth of unconsciousness lessens; therefore, keep the nails trimmed. Patients who are comatose for long periods may be lifted occasionally into a bathtub half-filled with warm water. It may be helpful to apply solutions high in fatty acids (e.g., Castile soap, baby oil, or cold cream) daily and to bathe the patient weekly to prevent loss of cutaneous oils as well as skin irritation and dryness.

Perineal care should be performed at least every 8 hours and after every episode of incontinence. If perineal care is not effective for a woman with vaginal discharge or odor, consult the physician about the use of cleansing douches.

When the patient cannot respond to local tissue hypoxia from being in one position for an extended time, the risk of pressure ulcers increases. Patients should be repositioned at least every 2 hours. If repositioning is impossible because of the patient's medical condition, place the patient on a special mattress or bed (Fig. 68–5). However, the use of a special bed does not eliminate the need to pad bony prominences and assess the skin every 4 hours. In addition, meet the nutritional needs of the patient to reduce the risk of pressure ulcers.

Risk for Contractures. Normal movement and stretch are needed to prevent tightening of one group of muscles. When muscle groups are not used during periods of immobility, contractures of joints can develop. Footdrop is of special concern. Write the diagnosis as *Risk for Contractures related to disuse.*

Outcomes. The patient will maintain full range of motion in any joint, as evidenced by an absence of contractures. Another outcome could be that the client will have a reduced risk of contractures, as evidenced by (1) a

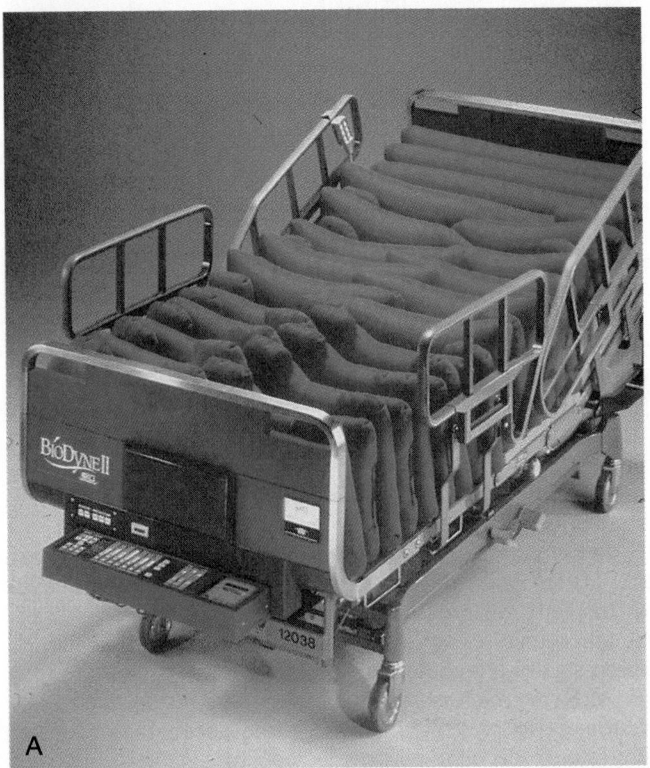

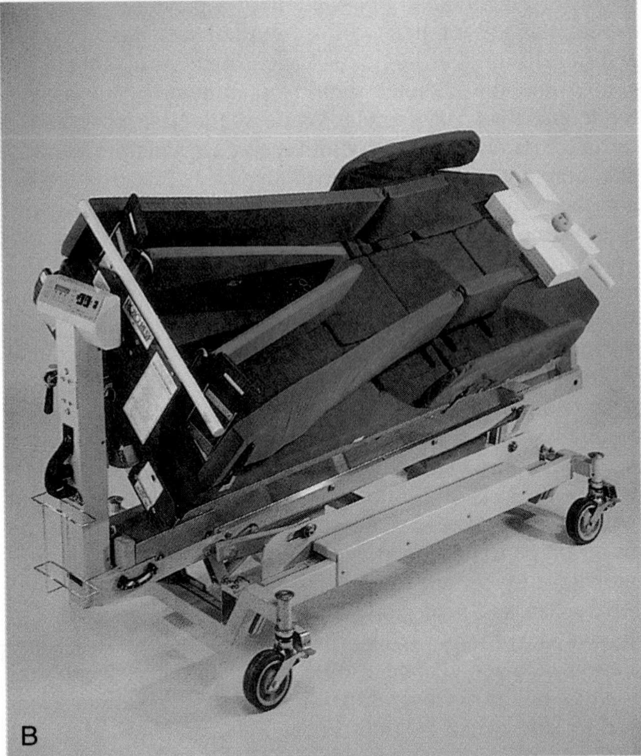

FIGURE 68–5 *A,* BioDyne, an oscillating air support surface. *B,* Roto Rest, an oscillating bed. Both devices are used to treat hypoxemia and to reduce the incidence of nosocomial pneumonia. Roto Rest is also used for clients with spinal cord injury and skeletal traction. (Courtesy of Kinetic Concepts, Inc., San Antonio, TX.)

normal range of motion, (2) an absence of flexed arms and legs, and (3) no manifestations of footdrop.

Interventions. Prevent contractures by maintaining the patient's extremities in functional positions with proper support. Hand and forearm splints prevent flexion contracture of the fingers and wrists. Orthotic devices or high-top athletic shoes are used to support the feet. Remove the support devices every 4 hours to perform skin care and passive exercises. Assess the heel closely.

Altered Nutrition: Less Than Body Requirements. Comatose patients cannot eat and yet have normal or even increased metabolic needs, so they can quickly become malnourished. Write the diagnosis as *Altered Nutrition: Less Than Body Requirements related to inability to eat and swallow.*

Outcomes. The patient will demonstrate the following signs of adequate nutrition: (1) stable weight, (2) adequate calories for age, height, and weight, (3) intake equaling output, (4) healing of incisions and wounds within 12 to 14 days, and (5) hemoglobin, blood urea nitrogen, total lymphocyte count, total protein, and serum albumin values within normal limits for age and sex.

Interventions. IV fluids are begun on admission for comatose patients. Initially the IV site provides access to the circulatory system for the administration of medications. Because fluid intake is restricted and only limited amounts of glucose and few electrolytes are given by the IV route, an IV infusion cannot be considered nutritional support. Consider that a 1-L solution of 5% dextrose provides only 200 kilocalories!

Just because a patient is comatose, never assume that hunger is not present and that caloric needs are reduced. In fact, the opposite is true; such a patient's caloric needs are usually increased. Nutritional and fluid needs of comatose patients are usually met through enteral feedings because of the risk of aspiration with the oral route. If the patient does not have paralytic ileus or delayed gastric emptying and if bowel sounds are audible, start enteral feedings (see Management and Delegation feature on enteral nutrition).

The nutritional requirements of a patient in coma are complex; a complete nutritional assessment with comparison of height and weight charts, laboratory tests, and clinical examination is essential. There is a marked increase in metabolic needs. Malnutrition increases the morbidity and mortality of neurologically ill patients. Diarrhea and delayed gastric emptying may result from malabsorption. Healing cannot take place in the presence of a negative nitrogen state. Immunodeficiency, with increased risk of infection, sepsis, stress ulcers, weight loss, skeletal muscle protein wasting, and lung tissue catabolism leading to diaphragmatic weakness with respiratory reduction, results from prolonged calorie and protein deprivation. Starvation can lead to death.

Nursing responsibilities in tube-feeding of comatose patients are critical because these patients cannot communicate and may have lost protective cough and gag reflexes. The possible complications from enteral feeding, and their prevention, are described here:

1. Vomiting and aspiration if the stomach is overfilled or the head of the patient is below the level of the stomach, such as during chest physiotherapy. When tube-feeding a patient, elevate the head of the bed at least 30 degrees to minimize possible aspiration.
2. Tube dislocation into trachea or lungs, causing aspiration. Some facilities use blue food coloring to tint the formula; then, if suctioned secretions are blue, aspiration is suspected. Comatose patients are often

MANAGEMENT AND DELEGATION

Preparing Enteral Nutrition

Enteral nutrition may be delivered via oral, nasal, gastrostomy, or jejunostomy tubes. Gastrostomy or jejunostomy tubes are most commonly used because they pose a lower risk of aspiration. The delivery of enteral nutrition, including the verification of tube placement, is your responsibility. You may choose to delegate the reconstitution or preparation of enteral feedings to assistive personnel. Before delegating the preparation of tube feeding or refilling the nutrition reservoir bag, consider the following:

- Your abdominal assessment does not reveal abdominal distention, pain, discomfort, or complaints of nausea. Your examination includes verification of tube placement, and the residual volume is less than 50% of the previous hour's intake. The presence of any of these findings would prompt you to delay the tube feeding and notify the physician of your examination findings.
- You have checked the physician's order for the type and rate of tube feeding to be delivered.
- Instruct assistive personnel in the proper dilution and handling of enteral feeding. (*Hint:* When mixing powdered enteral feedings, always place the powder in the mixing container before the water; this will ensure that the powder dissolves fully.)
- Instruct assistive personnel to place a 4-hour supply of feeding in the reservoir bag and to store the remaining mixture in a refrigerator for future use. Label the storage container with the client's name, date on which mixture was prepared, and description of mixture.
- Although assistive personnel may prime the pump, you must set the pump and ensure that the flow rate matches the ordered flow rate.
- You are responsible for performing any irrigation of the tube.
- You may delegate care of gastrostomy and jejunostomy tube site to assistive personnel.
- You are responsible for monitoring fluid and nutritional balance via input and output and changes in weight.

Describe findings that are immediately reportable to you for assistive personnel. They include any difficulty in preparing the enteral feeding and client complaints of fullness, nausea, or vomiting.

Verify the competence of assistive personnel in performing these tasks during orientation and annually thereafter.

Donna W. Markey, MSN, RN, ACNP-CS, *Clinician IV, Surgical Services, University of Virginia Health System, Charlottesville, Virginia*

restless. Tape the tube securely to prevent dislodgment. Aspiration may occur if a feeding tube is pulled out during a feeding session or whenever it is unclamped. During feeding sessions, cloth wristlets or wrist restraints may be needed.

Verify NG tube placement by aspirating for gastric contents. Some agency policies and some manufacturers of small-bore tubes require checking tube placement by listening with a stethoscope for "whooshing" while instilling air through the tube. Never tube-feed a patient in the supine position unless all other positions are impossible. Leave the head of the bed elevated 30 degrees for at least 30 minutes after bolus feedings.

3. Ulcerated or crusted nares due to local pressure from the feeding tube.
4. Tracheoesophageal fistula, that is, breakdown of the anterior esophageal wall from prolonged contact between the NG tube and a tracheostomy tube. This complication is manifested by gastric contents in tracheal secretions. Notify the physician immediately.
5. Trauma to the gastric mucosa if the tube's distal end hardens, as may happen over time.
6. Delayed gastric emptying. Check residual volumes every 4 hours. If the residual volume is more than 100 ml, delay the feeding for 1 hour, then reassess. Assess bowel sounds, and check for gastric distention; if this complication persists after several hours, notify the physician. If there is a high suspicion that the patient has a bowel obstruction, do not return the gastric residue to the stomach.
7. Fluid volume deficit if hypertonic tube-feedings are given. To prevent this problem, ensure that the patient receives approximately 1 ml of fluid for every kilocalorie of feeding. Depending on the agency's policy, this intervention may require consultation with the dietitian or the physician.
8. Constipation or diarrhea, which may develop from the osmolarity of the feeding, the use of liquid medications with a sorbitol base, or a too rapid infusion.
9. Sacral pressure ulcers from continued positioning in the semi-Fowler position. Turn the patient 30 degrees lateral (to the side) with the head of the bed elevated to reduce pressure on the sacrum.

Risk for Fluid Volume Deficit. The comatose patient cannot drink fluids or respond to normal thirst mechanisms. Such a patient is therefore at *Risk for Fluid Volume Deficit.* Recall that hypertonic tube-feedings also increase this risk.

Outcomes. The patient will demonstrate these indications of fluid balance: (1) intake and output being equal for 24, 48, and 72 hours, (2) stable body weight, (3) no signs of excessive perspiration, diarrhea, or vomiting, (4) serum glucose, hematocrit, and blood urea nitrogen, creatinine, sodium, potassium, and chloride values within normal limits, and (5) moist oral mucous membranes with absence of tongue furrows.

Interventions. Important aspects in maintaining fluid and electrolyte balance in unconscious patients are (1) accurate documentation of intake and output, (2) daily weighing with comparison of trends, and (3) assessment and documentation of conditions that may increase fluid volume deficit (e.g., diaphoresis, polyuria, diarrhea, vomiting, hypertonic tube-feedings).

Before fluid and electrolyte intervention is planned for a comatose patient, carefully assess the fluid-electrolyte status. The coma itself may have a fluid or electrolyte cause. Blood tests such as blood glucose, hematocrit, blood urea nitrogen, or creatinine, serum sodium, potassium, chloride, and carbon dioxide measurements help determine fluid and electrolyte status (see Chapters 12 and 13). Dehydration and water intoxication (true hyponatremia) are common causes of electrolyte imbalance associated with coma.

Always avoid overhydration in a patient receiving IV fluids because of the risk of cerebral edema. Diuretics may be prescribed to correct fluid overload and reduce edema. Monitor the response to these medications. When evaluating the response to any diuretic, empty the indwelling catheter before administering the diuretic. Evaluation of the response should consider the diuretic given, the dose, and the patient's renal status.

Risk for Injury. It may not be apparent that the comatose patient is at *Risk for Injury* because he or she does not move. If the coma starts to lighten, however, the patient can move and, without protection, could fall or be injured. In addition, use caution when moving the patient, who cannot voice pain. Although the loss of the corneal blink reflex, which increases the risk of corneal abrasions, is also a type of injury, it is addressed as a collaborative problem. Nursing interventions for a loss of the corneal blink reflex are discussed in Chapter 73.

Outcomes. The patient will not sustain injury, as evidenced by an absence of abrasions or bruises and experiencing no falls from bed.

Interventions. Keep the side rails up on the bed and the bed in the lowest position whenever the patient is not receiving direct care or is unattended. Observe seizure precautions for anyone who has a history of seizure or is at risk of seizure. Protect the patient from injury during seizures or periods of agitation (e.g., use padded side rails, keep the patient's nails short and filed). It is of utmost importance to protect the patient's head. Give the prescribed seizure medication on time to maintain a high seizure threshold. If a dose of the medication is missed for any reason (e.g., vomiting), notify the physician. Antiepileptic medication should not be withheld without a physician order.

Give adequate support to the limbs and head when moving or turning an unconscious patient. Limbs without tone may dislocate if they are allowed to fall unsupported. Always turn an unconscious patient toward you or someone else to prevent falls. Protect an unconscious patient from external sources of heat (e.g., heating pads).

Do not restrain the patient unless it is absolutely necessary because restraint is likely to worsen confused and combative behavior. If restraints are used, they must be released at least every 2 hours for range-of-motion exercises and skin checks. Do not leave unstable patients unattended. Attempt to manage the patient's behaviors without restraints first. "Sitters," hospital volunteers, or family members or friends may be able to provide attendant services. Avoid oversedation because it may alter respirations, which increases ICP and masks changes in a patient's level of consciousness.

Fecal Incontinence. Once a paralytic ileus is corrected, the patient will produce feces. Most patients are incontinent because voluntary control is required for the function of the external anal sphincter. Write the diagnosis as *Fecal Incontinence related to inability to respond to normal cues about evacuation;* also consider *High Risk for Impaired Skin Integrity related to fecal incontinence.*

Outcomes. The patient will have reduced fecal incontinence, as evidenced by (1) a bowel movement every 2 to 3 days and (2) no signs of fecal impaction.

Interventions. Plan interventions to (1) control bowel movements, (2) maintain the patient's normal elimination schedule, and (3) prevent fecal impaction or constipation. As soon as the patient is able, begin a program of bowel retraining. Maintain a regular schedule, administering stool softeners and suppositories, and performing digital removal of stool at approximately the same times each day. Examine the abdomen frequently for distention. Constipation and fecal impaction may occur. Small, frequent liquid stools may indicate impaction. If diarrhea or constipation persists, assess for possible causes, such as medications, enteral feedings, and intestinal bacterial infections.

Caution: Consult with the physician prior to performing digital removal of stool in a patient with an altered level of consciousness. This intervention has been known to induce seizures and may increase ICP. Rectal application of an anesthetic jelly prior to the stimulus decreases this risk.

Altered Family Processes. Having a family member in a coma is a significant stressor for the family. A possible diagnosis is *Altered Family Processes related to uncertain future or impending death of a family member.* Individualize the etiology portion of the diagnosis to fit the specific patient and family.

Outcomes. Family members will exhibit positive coping behaviors, as evidenced by (1) showing an ability to solve problems, (2) meeting the needs of other family members, and (3) asking questions about the patient that indicate understanding of previous teaching.

Interventions. The significant others of a comatose patient are often very stressed. It is difficult for the family when they cannot communicate with the patient. The uncertainty of not knowing whether the patient will recover is a major stressor. Include family members in the patient's care to the extent that they can and want to be involved. Family members need information and realistic hope.

It is important for the family to see the patient receiving high-quality, professional, and caring nursing care. For example, talk to the patient as if he or she can understand. Initially, this behavior will seem awkward, but in time, it will feel appropriate. Tell the patient that he or she will be turned to the side, bathed, and so on, before performing the task. Depending on the depth of the coma, the patient's sense of hearing may still be intact. Therefore, speak to the patient as if he or she can hear, and tell the family to do the same. Comatose patients have awakened and reported that they remember hearing specific voices.

The family is often in a state of shock, needing someone to recognize their needs and help them through this difficult situation. They may experience various conflicting feelings, such as guilt and anger. The Client Education Guide suggests ways for the patient's family members to cope with these feelings.

Allow significant others to stay with the patient when and where possible. At times, family members may become zealous about attending and may stay at the patient's bedside continuously. Encourage family members to care for themselves also by eating regular meals and obtaining adequate sleep. Have them consider using external support systems (e.g., neighbors and church groups). Tell them that they will be telephoned if any significant changes occur in their loved one's status, and ask them to leave a phone number where they can be reached. Encourage family members to phone if they have questions or concerns.

Social workers may be contacted to provide additional support. Some hospitals, especially tertiary care centers, have "family homes," where family members who must travel a long distance to the hospital may stay to be close to the hospital and the patient.

EVALUATION

The patient may remain comatose for a few hours or even months. Some comatose patients (e.g., patients with diabetic coma) awaken and make a complete recovery while in the hospital. Therefore, some expected outcomes have brief time frames (e.g., airway obstruction), whereas others are prolonged, requiring frequent reevaluation (e.g.,

CLIENT EDUCATION GUIDE

When a Loved One Is in an Altered State of Consciousness

Family Instructions

Seeing a loved one in this state causes a roller coaster of feelings (e.g., denial, anger, depression, guilt, bargaining). There is no "correct" order for these feelings; they may recur even after one thinks they have been worked through. These and other feelings are normal. It is important to "give yourself permission" to feel, so that you can work through the grieving process.

Talk to and touch your loved one. Research supports the positive benefit of talking to and touching the person.

Become involved in the care of your loved one, including decisions about how he or she will be cared for.

Learn about the devices and equipment used to monitor and treat your loved one.

Stay informed of your loved one's condition. Ask a nurse to repeat or explain information provided by the physician and to clarify any medical jargon that you do not understand.

If the physician has indicated that there is no chance for your loved one's recovery, refocus your energies into hoping for a peaceful death. Consider organ donation; this has helped other families with their healing.

Join a support group, whether your loved one is expected to die or to stay at this level of altered consciousness for an indeterminate time. Through reaching out, you may be able to find strength and meaning in this tragedy.

family coping). Your evaluation may identify a need for revision of the care plan.

Modifications for Elderly Clients

The older patient in a coma requires the same quality of care as patients in other age groups. However, the older patient is at higher risk for all complications of immobility, especially pressure ulcers and pneumonia. Urinary retention is common in elderly men because of prostatic enlargement. Finally, fully assess the patient for the common disorders of aging (e.g., diabetes) that might be the cause of the coma.

Self-Care

The site to which a patient with coma is discharged from an acute care setting depends totally on (1) the condition of the patient, (2) the cause of the coma, and (3) the level of family support available. If the patient is recovering from coma, plan for placement in a rehabilitation center. Patients remaining in coma but showing slow recovery may be placed in an extended-care facility until they can participate in rehabilitation.[3, 12] Coma stimulation programs, although not readily available, provide an alternative for the patient who is slow to recover.[3–5]

If the patient is in a coma and is not expected to awaken but may live for a time with nutritional support, placement in a skilled nursing center is common.[4] In these centers, supportive care is given. Family members usually specify how aggressively they wish the patient to be treated in the event of a deterioration in status. Your role in discharge of the comatose patient centers on communication with the receiving nurses and the family. If the patient is ventilator-dependent or combative, special consideration is required for transport to the new facility. Provide a complete plan of care.

CONFUSIONAL STATES

Confusion is a mental state marked by alterations in thought and attention deficit, followed by problems in comprehension. It is accompanied by a loss of short-term memory and, often, irritability alternating with drowsiness. Confusion is a common clinical manifestation in many neurologic and metabolic disorders.

Sundowning is defined as agitation, confusion, and restlessness that occurs after the sun sets.[12] However, diurnal variations may be responsible for these changes as well.[1]

Confusion has been shown to increase both morbidity and length of hospital stay. This relationship has major implications in terms of cost containment, especially because people older than 85 years are the fastest-growing age group in the United States.

Etiology and Risk Factors

There are many causes of confusion. Common causes of acute confusion are alcohol withdrawal and drug ingestion. Confusion can also follow fever, heart failure, head injury, and use of anesthetics. Other causes of confusion are hypoxia, hypoglycemia, severe fluid and electrolyte disorders, sepsis, liver or renal failure, poisons, and drug overdose.

Delirium and dementia are classifications of types of confusion. Three features are common to all types of *delirium:*

- A disturbance of consciousness with a reduced ability to focus, sustain, or shift attention
- A change in cognition (memory, language, disorientation) or development of a perceptual disturbance that is not better accounted for by a pre-existing, established, or evolving dementia
- A change that develops over a short time (hours to days) and may fluctuate during the course of the day

Several classifications of delirium have each of the three common features but specific causes. They are (1) delirium related to a general medical condition, (2) delirium due to substance intoxication (prescribed drugs, over-the-counter medications, or street drugs), (3) delirium due to substance withdrawal, (4) delirium with multiple causes, and (5) delirium "not otherwise specified."[7, 10]

Dementia is the chronic form of confusion. As with delirium, there are common features in the many types of dementia. They are as follows:

- The development of multiple memory impairments
- One or more of the following cognitive disturbances: *aphasia* (problems with expressing speech or understanding sounds), *apraxia* (inability to convert a thought to action), *agnosia,* (inability to recognize objects), impaired executive functioning
- Significant impairment and decline in social or occupational functioning
- A gradual onset and continuing cognitive decline

The classifications of dementia include the four common features with variable causes and characteristics. There are many subtypes of dementia of the Alzheimer's type. Essentially, all other causes, such as central nervous system (CNS) disorders, systemic conditions, substance-induced conditions, depression, and schizophrenia, must be ruled out. The other types of dementia are (1) vascular dementia (multi-infarct), (2) dementia secondary to other general medical conditions, (3) substance-induced persisting dementia, (4) dementia with multiple causes, and (5) dementia "not otherwise specified."[6, 9]

An in-depth discussion of the care related to specific types of delirium and dementia, as well as the memory changes that occur in clients with amnesic disorders and other cognitive disorders not meeting the criteria for any of the preceding classifications, is beyond the scope of this book. The reader should refer to a psychiatric textbook for this information. This discussion focuses on the general care of a client with confusion. However, because dementia of the Alzheimer's type is a growing problem, Chapter 72 details the pathologic processes and care related to this type of degenerative disease.

Risk factors leading to confusion vary with the specific etiologic factors. In general, the proper management of various diseases, such as diabetes mellitus, would reduce the incidence of confusion. Disorders such as Alzheimer's disease have no known prevention at this time, although new drugs may slow disease progression. Avoid the use of any medications that contribute to confusion in people who are at risk for confusion.

Pathophysiology

Three mechanisms account for the development of *acute confusion:* (1) damage to the brain with swelling or loss of oxygen, blood, or both (functional disorder), (2) impairment of the action of the nervous system by chemicals or other substances (metabolic disorder), and (3) the rebound overactivity of a previously depressed center in the brain. Chemicals that cross the blood-brain barrier, such as alcohol, impair the metabolism of neuronal cells. When the drug action wears off or the drug is withdrawn from the client, the lower centers in the brain are overactive. This overactivity accounts for the development of acute confusion, combativeness, and other abnormal behaviors.

Chronic confusional states are due to disorders that cause brain tissue destruction, biochemical imbalances, or compression of the brain. For example, people with Alzheimer's disease lack acetylcholine, a neurotransmitter that is necessary for short-term memory. Other disorders causing chronic confusion may be inherited; may be secondary to a transmissible agent, as with Creutzfeldt-Jakob disease; or may follow diseases such as encephalitis.

Clinical Manifestations

The earliest sign of a brain disorder is a *disorder of attention.* The client may report the loss of concentration or may appear preoccupied. At the same time, restlessness, emotional lability, insomnia or drowsiness, and vivid nightmares may begin. Clients may appear anxious and may fear that they are "going crazy." As the disorder progresses, stupor and coma develop. Behaviors seen in the client are reflective not of personality but of the cause of the disorder. For example, barbiturate or alcohol abuse and withdrawal and liver disorders cause agitated delirium. In contrast, anoxia and kidney and lung disorders are associated with a quieter response. Disorders that develop rapidly are more likely to cause an agitated response than those that develop slowly.

Fluctuations in cognition (the ability to think and reason) are common in clients with metabolic brain disorders. Clients may be totally irrational one moment and lucid the next. Some of the fluctuations are caused by the environment. Delirious clients become more disoriented at night, in unfamiliar surroundings, when they hear unfamiliar noises or see unfamiliar people, or when restraints are used. The lack of a window in the room has caused many clients to become disoriented.

Loss of memory for recent events is a hallmark of metabolic brain disorders. The client commonly has difficulty with both immediate recall and abstract thought. Clients who are delirious quickly lose orientation to time. Normal people can readily recall six or seven digits forward and five or six backward and identify the commonalities between an orange and an apple or a tree and a bush; delirious clients cannot do these things. However, the client's general intelligence level can affect the behaviors observed. If possible, the client's level of education should be known before the assessment.

Perceptual errors (e.g., mistaking the nurse for a daughter) as well as hallucinations, illusions, and delusions are common accompaniments of delirium.

Hallucinations are sensations occurring in the absence of external stimuli. A client may hear, see, feel, smell, or taste something that is not present. The client may or may not realize that the experience is "not real." Unfortunately, the most common hallucinations involve rodents and unfriendly animals (e.g., snakes, spiders). These visions are very frightening.

Illusions differ from hallucinations, in that illusions are the misinterpretation of something actually in the environment. For example, if a client sees a shadow on the drape and mistakes it for a real person, the client is experiencing an illusion.

Delusions are thoughts or beliefs that have no basis in fact. For example, a client may think that he or she has been robbed or poisoned, when there is no basis for this belief.

There are no specific diagnostic tests for confusion. The client may undergo CT or MRI scanning to determine whether there is a structural cause for the confusion, such as a tumor or stroke. In addition, a series of laboratory studies may be performed to look for a metabolic cause. Common studies include a complete blood count, electrolyte measurements, determination of vitamin B_{12} and folate levels, thyroid and liver function studies, drug toxicity screening tests, and an EEG. A lumbar puncture may be performed for the analysis of CSF.

Outcome Management

Medical Management

In all care settings, the medical management of the confused client begins by determining the cause of the confusion and correcting it, if possible.[7] When no specific cause is found, the medical management focuses on controlling manifestations. Sometimes medications can be given to calm agitation. Nutritional needs also must be monitored.

Nursing Management of the Medical Client

ASSESSMENT

A thorough history is required for assessment of the confused client. The history should include the onset of the confusion, past medical illnesses, work and occupational history, and past injuries. Disorders such as diabetes or liver failure may be out of control and responsible for the confusion. The client may have been exposed to heavy metals or toxic wastes at work. Record past injuries, especially head injury. Depending on the level of confusion, the client may not be able to answer each question, and you may need to rely on the family or others who have been with the client. Review medications, including over-the-counter drugs and nutritional supplements.

Specific questions about the client's ability to handle routine financial transactions or home safety with tasks such as cooking, dressing, and driving will help determine whether the client can be safely returned home or is in need of an alternative arrangement. At times, the family may report a change in personality, such as apathy, social isolation, disinterest in current events, and irritability. Record these observations because they may be clinical manifestations of Alzheimer's disease or frontal lobe lesions.

The confused client requires ongoing assessment with the Mini-Mental State Examination (see Chapter 67). This examination is much more sensitive than other tools for serial evaluations of confused clients.[13] Analyze the data collected to determine whether the confusion is improving, worsening, or unchanged.

The confused client is often combative and argumentative. Observe for factors in the client's environment that may affect confusion. Assess whether the client is able to refrain from self-injury or injury to others. If not bedridden, the client may wander about and become lost or injured if harmful items are not secured (e.g., knives).

Confusion can occur in clients of any age or culture and from variable causes. The nurse's role as a client advocate supersedes personal bias related to any of these variables.

DIAGNOSIS, OUTCOMES, INTERVENTIONS

This section describes interventions appropriate to the confused client, regardless of the cause, with an emphasis on the issue of safety.

Altered Thought Processes. Use the nursing diagnosis *Altered Thought Processes related to failure in memory and lack of self-protective behavior to address needs for safety.*

Outcomes. The client will have improved thought processes, as evidenced by (1) higher scores on the Mini-Mental State Examination and (2) decreased frequency of hallucinations, illusions, and delusions.

Interventions. The confused client will benefit from consistency in the environment and care routine. Keep objects, such as the tray table and bedside chair, in the same place. If possible, the same staff member should care for the client. Give the client short explanations as events occur, such as "You need an x-ray" and "Please sit in the wheelchair." Saying to a confused client, "In 2 hours, an x-ray tech will be coming to take you for a CT scan," is useless, because such a client will neither understand nor remember it. Response time may be slowed in confusion; allow the client time to respond.

Reorient the client as often as necessary, but use caution about the specific communication used. Clients with chronic untreatable confusion do not benefit from reorientation and may become more agitated when you attempt to reorient them. For example, in one study in which a 92-year-old client was told repeatedly that her mother or father could not possibly be alive, the client reacted each time as if it was the first time she had been told and grieved deeply.[13] For these selected clients, avoid re-orienting, and "go along" with the confusion. Of course, when the client is at risk of injury, safety precautions are foremost. Clocks and calendars in the room also help with reorientation. The use of familiar objects is helpful when a client's remote memory is intact. For example, the use of a quilt from home on the bed may help the confused client recognize the bed as his or her own.

Promote reduction of unfamiliar noise because it adds to confusion. The client's room should be quiet and softly lighted without producing shadows.

Consistency in care of a client with confusion requires communication among caregivers. This communication occurs not only through the oral reporting method but also in the care plan and documentation records.

Risk for Injury. Confusion greatly increases risk of harm. The client cannot interpret, or may not be able to respond to, environmental stimuli that precede danger. Write the nursing diagnosis as *Risk for Injury related to the unpredictable behavior and inability to interpret environmental stimuli.*

Outcomes. The client will not sustain injury and will not injure others.

Interventions. The client must be protected from self-injury. The client should be in a room near the nursing station so that assessments can be performed every 30 to 60 minutes. In addition, the bed should be in the low position. Structure the client's environment to minimize injury; remove any extraneous equipment.

The routine use of physical restraints (e.g., side rails, cloth restraints) or chemical restraints (e.g., medication) is discouraged.[8] The use of side rails and restraints does not guarantee that clients will not fall and often either makes them more agitated or leads to more severe injury when they do fall. Alternatives to restraints include the use of sitters for ongoing observation and placement of the patient in an area permitting constant observation, such as the nursing station. If all other alternatives have been unsuccessful and restraints are used, make frequent assessments and record the data. Cloth restraints must be removed every 2 hours to assess the skin beneath them and perform range-of-motion exercises. Chemical restraint (e.g., tranquilizers) can result in greater confusion and tremors (extrapyramidal symptoms).

The client with brain alteration is not in control of his or her behavior. Behaviors may be unpredictable, irrational, or impulsive, or the client may be frightened and suspicious. Never "punish" a confused client for inappropriate behavior or remarks. Instead, remember that these personality changes are a result of brain lesions, and adjust the care plan accordingly. If a client is agitated, provide reassurance and a calm environment. Redirect or distract the client. Monitoring systems may be used for clients who wander.

Confused elderly clients are at increased risk for falls. A formal fall risk assessment should be completed. Some institutions have programs for clients who are at risk for falling or who have fallen. These programs include frequent assessments, routine toileting, bed and wandering monitors, and environmental changes (mattress on the floor, use of a lap buddy). Trying to ambulate to the bathroom is a common time for falls, and toileting should be offered routinely (every 2 hours).

Sleep Pattern Disturbance. A common problem seen in confused clients consists of daytime napping and nighttime hallucinations. This problem is stated as *Sleep Pattern Disturbance related to alterations in usual sleep habits.*

Outcomes. The client will have improved sleep patterns, as evidenced by (1) sleeping 4 to 6 hours continuously at night and (2) not sleeping as often during the day.

Interventions. Plan nighttime interventions to allow 4 to 6 hours of uninterrupted sleep. Recall that a sleep cycle requires 1½ to 2 hours, and the loss of REM (rapid eye movement) sleep can increase confusion. When you enter the room at night, assess the client for REM. If REM is present, the client should be allowed to complete the REM portion of the sleep cycle. You should return later to care for the client.

Keep the client active during the day so that there is

some fatigue by nighttime. Daytime sleeping is a difficult pattern to break, and the client may have to be kept awake for this pattern to be reversed. Bedtime routines should be developed. Avoid the use of caffeinated beverages and alcohol, which may prevent sleep. For the elderly client, the normal changes in sleep with aging need to be considered, such as the greater use of short naps and less sleep during the night. Sleeping medications are seldom given to the confused client because they often alter sleep cycles and rob the client of REM sleep. See Chapter 21 for further information about sleep disorders.

Risk for Caregiver Role Strain. The unfamiliar behavior of the confused client or the stress of providing continual care for the client at home may increase stress in the family and alter their ability to cope. This diagnosis is stated as *Risk for Caregiver Role Strain related to long-term, stressful, and complex care required by family member.*

Outcomes. The client's family members will maintain their own physical and psychological health, as evidenced by (1) improved use of support systems, (2) obtaining of adequate equipment to provide care, (3) limited use of addictive drugs for coping, (4) interaction with friends and extended family (as desired), and (5) appropriate analysis of the client's condition.

Interventions. Teach the family to monitor for the effects of confusion. When confusion is a new problem for the client, the family will be distressed by the behavior. Explain to the family that the client is not able to control behavior or speech at this time. Assess whether the client becomes calm or agitated when the family is present, and advise visitations accordingly. If possible, the need for and use of restraints should be explained to the family before they see a client in restraints. The family may become very upset when they see their loved one "tied" to a bed. Advance explanations can avert some of this reaction. There have been instances in which a client suffered an injury because the family did not understand the purpose for the restraints and untied them.

See Management and Delegation: Physical Restraints.

MANAGEMENT AND DELEGATION

Physical Restraints

The use of physical restraints to protect a client from self-harm or injury, or to manage a client at risk for disruption of medical therapies, is a decision made collaboratively between you and the physician and may include consultation with other members of the interdisciplinary team. The serious decision to use physical restraints is made after your comprehensive assessment and evaluation of previous interventions and alternatives.

A clear goal is the use of the least restrictive device for the shortest interval possible. Regulatory agencies consider the use of restraints to be a high-risk intervention. Death and injury have been associated with restraint use in hospital environments. Your clinical site should provide you with clear guidelines regarding the use of restraints and the role of unlicensed assistive personnel in caring for restrained clients.

Before delegating care of the client in physical restraints, consider the following:

- Have the client and family been informed and educated regarding the need for restraints to protect the client? Your education of the client and family should include standards of care and discussion of what factors lead to discontinuation of restraints.
- Have you assessed the client to determine the most appropriate type of restraint? The restraint must be the right size. Follow the manufacturer's recommendations for sizing. Never use anything other than a manufactured device that has been approved by the Food and Drug Administration.
- Have you obtained a physician's order for the use of restraints? In addition to the initiation order for restraints, there should be ongoing discussion of the need to continue restraint use with the interdisciplinary team and physician order updates every 24 hours.

Your assessment of the client's safety and comfort needs must occur at regular intervals as defined by your institution. You are accountable for assessing and documenting the client's condition, the client's response to restraints, and the safety and comfort interventions provided.

Consider the following points when delegating components of care to assistive personnel:

- Be very clear about the type of restraint being used. In addition to applying restraints according to the manufacturer's instructions, restraints are to be secured only to the bed frame or chair with slip knots.
- Explain that restraints are never used as a punishment.
- Clients with altered mental status experiencing unmet elimination needs may become agitated. Instruct assistive personnel to offer assistance with elimination at regular intervals.
- Provide specific expectations and a time schedule for observation of the client.
- Instruct on how to remove restraints one at a time in agitated clients.
- How to respond to clients who ask for the restraints to "be cut-off" by re-explaining the need for them.

You may delegate these components of care to assistive personnel:

- Assistance with activities of daily living, such as bathing, grooming, and feeding
- Active or passive range of motion
- Turning and repositioning the client. They should be instructed to re-secure restraints after position changes.

Describe for the assistive personnel the findings that are immediately reportable to you. Such findings may include skin redness or irritation noted at points of contact with the restraint device, changes in color or movement of areas distal to the restraint, the client's unplanned removal of a restraint, disruption of a medical therapy, and the client's complaints of discomfort or distress. Verify the competency of assistive personnel in caring for restrained patients during orientation and in an ongoing manner thereafter.

Kathleen Rea, BSN, RN, *Clinician III, Clinical Manager, Surgical Services, University of Virginia Health System, Charlottesville, Virginia*

Choosing the placement site for a confused client being discharged from the hospital varies with the cause of confusion. If the confusion is acute and full recovery is expected, the patient may be able to go home under the care of family members. If the confusion is chronic, the patient needs either care or supervision at home or placement in an extended-care facility. Some communities offer adult day care and respite services that give family members relief from the constant care of the confused person. See Chapter 72 for care of the client with Alzheimer's disease at home.

Advise the family to have legal counsel determine the client's competence and the need for guardianship or durable power of attorney. The family may also need to grieve the loss of the client's previous functional role, personality, companionship, and so on. Assess for evidence of violence in the caregiver and the client. Caregiver violence is possible, especially if the client was violent toward the caregiver in the past.

Help the caregiver find respite care and personal time to meet his or her own needs and to learn stress management techniques. Female caregivers are especially vulnerable to social isolation.

EVALUATION

Most of the time, confusion will require many months to abate. The diagnosis of a chronic, progressive condition such as Alzheimer's disease or dementia of the Alzheimer type may require an entire change in care plan prioritization. These conditions are discussed in Chapter 72.

Modifications for Elderly Clients

It is common, but incorrect, to believe that elderly people naturally undergo a marked deterioration in mental function. In general, elderly people have difficulty recalling new information but their remote memory is intact. In addition, depression occurs in 20% to 30% of the elderly. Depression may follow the loss of friends, spouse, health, and independence and may lead to manifestations such as memory loss and confusion.

Older adults are particularly at risk for confusion during hospitalization.[10] They are dealing not only with the stress of being ill but also with the stress of an unfamiliar environment. Elderly clients may rely heavily on familiar landmarks and routines to help them maintain an independent lifestyle. These cues are often lost in the hospital or extended-care setting. A large percentage of the population in hospital and extended-care settings are elderly, who typically have other conditions that contribute to confusion. Confusion is best managed by using a team approach and teaching unlicensed personnel to (1) introduce themselves at the beginning of a work shift, (2) use the same time for the client's sleep, naps, and meals, (3) routinely place the client on the toilet or commode, (4) talk to the client about the past, (5) gently redirect lost or wandering clients, and (6) encourage self-care (eating, dressing, and so on).

CONCLUSIONS

Clients who are confused or comatose are vulnerable to many complications, including injury, aspiration, malnutrition, and skin breakdown. Nurses provide a lifeline for these clients, giving protection and promoting normal body functions. The families of these clients require therapeutic management because they face many difficult decisions.

THINKING CRITICALLY

1. A 48-year-old man is brought to the emergency department by ambulance. His wife states that he had been shaving in the bathroom when she heard a thud. She found him unresponsive on the floor. How do you intervene?

Factors to Consider. What was the client's neurologic baseline when he was received in the emergency department? What other clinical manifestations did the client display? Were there any physical signs of injury to his head or other parts of his body? Does he have any other significant medical history or allergies?

2. You are caring for a 72-year-old woman who recently underwent repair of a hip fracture. Her husband indicates that she had recently been confused, which led to her falling and fracturing her hip. How do you intervene?

Factors to Consider. What do you include in your assessment? What kinds of interventions do you need to consider? How do you involve her family?

BIBLIOGRAPHY

1. Davis, A. E., & White, J. J. (1995). Innovative sensory input for the comatose brain-injured patient. *Critical Care Nursing Clinics of North America, 7*(2):351–361.
2. Foreman, M. D., et al. (1999). Standard of practice protocol: Acute confusion/delirium. *Geriatric Nursing 20*(3), 147–152.
3. Giacino, J. T., et al. (1997). Development of practice guidelines for assessment and management of the vegetative and minimally conscious states. *Journal of Head Trauma Rehabilitation, 12*(4), 36–51.
4. Hamel, M. B., et al. (1995). Identification of comatose patients at high risk for death or severe disability. *Journal of the American Medical Association, 273*(23), 1842–1848.
5. Helwick, L. D. (1994). Stimulation programs for coma patients. *Critical Care Nurse, 8*, 47–51.
6. Hickey, J. V. (1997). Management of the unconscious patient. In *The clinical practice of neurological and neurosurgical nursing* (4th ed.). Philadelphia: J. B. Lippincott. 275–294.
7. Mentes, J., et al. (1999). Acute confusion indicators: Risk factors and prevalence using MDS data. *Research in Nursing and Health, 22*(2), 95–105.
8. Rogers, P. D., & Bocchino, N. L. (1999). Restraint-free care: Is it possible? *American Journal of Nursing, 99*(10), 26–34.
9. Rosenwasser, R. H., & Schneck, M. J. (1996). Initial evaluation and management of acute coma. *Hospital Medicine, 32*(12), 39–44.
10. Shedd, P. P., Kobokovich, L. J., & Slattery, M. J. (1995). Confused patients in the acute care setting: Prevalence, intervention, and outcomes. *Journal of Gerontological Nursing, 21*(4), 5–12.
11. Stewart-Amidei, C. (1991). Assessing the comatose patient in the intensive care unit. *AACN Clinical Issues in Critical Care Nursing, 2*(4), 613–622.
12. Talbot, L. R., & Joanette, Y. (1998). Postcomatose unawareness in a brain-injured populaton. *Journal of Neuroscience Nursing, 30*(2), 129–134.
13. Wallace, M. (1994). The sundown syndrome. *Geriatric Nursing, 15*(3), 164–166.

REMEMBER *to check out your* Companion CD ROM

CHAPTER 69

Management of Clients with Cerebral Disorders

Melanie Minton

NURSING OUTCOMES CLASSIFICATION (NOC)
for Nursing Diagnoses—Clients with Cerebral Disorders

Altered Health Maintenance
Knowledge: Health Behaviors
Knowledge: Treatment Regimen
Treatment Behavior: Illness
Altered Thought Processes
Cognitive Ability
Cognitive Orientation
Decision-Making
Altered Tissue Perfusion: Cerebral
Cognitive Ability
Neurologic Status
Neurologic Status: Central Motor Control
Neurologic Status: Consciousness
Tissue Perfusion: Cerebral
Anticipatory Grieving
Aggression Control
Coping
Family Coping
Grief Resolution
Psychosocial Adjustment: Life Change
Anxiety
Aggression Control
Anxiety Control
Coping
Decreased Adaptive Capacity: Intracranial
Electrolyte and Acid-Base Balance
Fluid Balance
Neurologic Status: Autonomic
Neurologic Status: Cranial Sensory/Motor Function
Neurologic Status: Spinal Sensory/Motor Function
Ineffective Individual Coping
Aggression Control
Coping
Decision-Making
Impulse Control
Role Performance
Risk of Injury
Safety Status: Falls Occurrence
Safety Status: Physical Injury
Symptom Control
Risk for Spiritual Distress
Anxiety Control
Coping
Grief Resolution
Hope
Quality of Life
Spiritual Well-Being

SEIZURE DISORDERS

In this chapter, an important distinction is made between seizures and epilepsy. A *seizure* is a sudden, abnormal electrical discharge from the brain that results in changes in sensation, behavior, movements, perception, or consciousness. A seizure may occur in isolation or with some acute problem within the central nervous system (CNS), such as a low blood glucose level, drug or alcohol withdrawal, or traumatic brain injury. *Epilepsy* is a chronic disorder of recurrent seizures. An isolated, single seizure does not constitute epilepsy.[20, 24, 46, 48]

EPILEPSY

Epilepsy is derived from the Greek *epilepsia,* meaning "seizure." In early times, epilepsy was viewed as being of divine origin and was called the "sacred disease" because someone with epilepsy was thought to be "seized" or struck down by the gods. An epileptic syndrome is composed of paroxysmal neurologic dysfunction causing recurrent episodes of one or more of the following manifestations: loss of consciousness, convulsive movements or other motor activity, sensory phenomena, and behavioral abnormalities. About 2.3 million Americans are known to have seizures or epilepsy. About 181,000 new cases of seizures and epilepsy are documented annually.[20, 24, 45, 47]

The last two decades have brought significant advances in the understanding, diagnosis, and treatment of epilepsy. Despite improvements in electroencephalographic monitoring, neuroimaging, and surgery, however, a cure has not been found.

Etiology and Risk Factors

Epilepsy can be caused by any process that disrupts the stability of the neuronal cell membrane. A variety of conditions are associated with an extremely high likelihood of onset of a chronic seizure disorder. One of the best examples of such conditions is severe, penetrating head trauma, which is associated with up to a 50% risk of the development of epilepsy. This association suggests that the injury results in a long-lasting pathologic change in the CNS that transforms a presumably normal neural network into one that is abnormally hyperexcitable.

The identified mechanism responsible for such malfunction is unknown. Possible theories include neuronal structural impairment, abnormalities involving the sodium-potassium pump, and changes in various neurochemicals.[20, 48] Hypersensitive neurons can be found throughout the brain and spinal cord. The neuronal cell membrane appears to be more permeable and more sensitive to various offending factors. An epileptogenic focus may develop at the location of increased cell membrane permeability. The epileptogenic focus may be limited to a specific area or encompass the entire cortical surface.

Seizures are classified as *genetic, acquired,* or *idiopathic.*[39] What is not well understood is how these three factors may cause the seizure threshold to be lowered, thereby increasing the possibility of seizures. For example, with idiopathic seizures, what is the offending agent? Is it structural, neurochemical, or a combination of several factors?

Idiopathic epilepsy most often begins before the age of 20 years and rarely begins after age 30. Seizures beginning in newborns and infants are often caused by congenital brain defects, birth injuries, or metabolic problems such as anoxia, hypoglycemia, or hypocalcemia. Although the underlying cause may be perinatal, seizures may not begin for many years, often with onset during puberty. Other than in children under age 5 years, the highest incidence of new-onset epilepsy is in people older than 65. The increased risk in this age group is attributed to the increase in conditions that cause neurologic changes in this group. These include cerebrovascular disease, tumor, delirium, Alzheimer's disease, infection, accumulated trauma, and chronic alcoholism, as well as the aging process itself.[20, 24, 26, 46, 48]

When the cause of seizures is known, the disorder is called *secondary epilepsy.* After age 20, generalized seizures usually have an identifiable cause. These causes include traumatic brain injury, brain tumor, and infection. Approximately two thirds of cases of epilepsy are idiopathic; the remainder are from secondary causes.

Pathophysiology

When the integrity of the neuronal cell membrane is altered, the cell begins firing with increased frequency and amplitude.[20, 46, 48] When the intensity of the discharges reaches a threshold, the neuronal firing spreads to adjacent normal neurons. Discharges in the brain stem cause muscle contraction and possibly loss of consciousness. The excitation of the cells can spread to the spinal cord.

Normally, excitatory messages from a single hypersensitive neuron in the cerebral cortex are modulated by deeper structures (e.g., thalamus and brain stem) (Fig. 69–1). In epilepsy, these bursts of electrical activity from the cortex are not controlled or modulated. These discharges block normal inhibition and perpetuate a feedback loop. Eventually, inhibitory neurons in the cortex, anterior thalamus, and basal ganglia slow the neuronal firing. This inhibition interrupts the seizure and produces an intermittent contraction-relaxation phase. Once the epileptogenic neurons are exhausted and inhibitory processes build, the seizure stops. These later events depress CNS action and impair consciousness. This period of impaired consciousness after a seizure, called a *postictal state,* may be manifested as sleep, confusion, or fatigue.

Seizure activity increases the need for adenosine triphosphate (ATP) and also cerebral oxygen consumption. Supplies of oxygen and glucose are rapidly consumed. To meet these demands, the cerebral blood flow increases by during a seizure. If the seizure is ongoing (as in status epilepticus), severe hypoxia and lactic acidosis occur and may result in brain tissue destruction.[20, 34, 45]

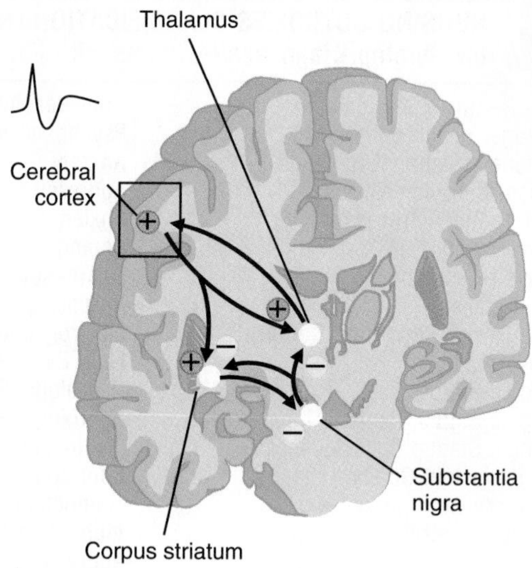

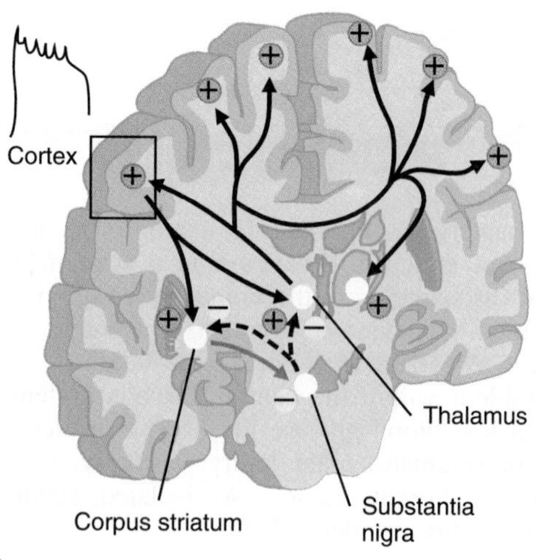

FIGURE 69–1 *A,* Normally, excitatory messages from the cerebral cortex are modulated by deeper structures. *B,* In clients with epilepsy, bursts of activity from the cortex are not modulated and these bursts spread. (From Devinsky, O. [1994]. Seizure disorders. *Clinical Symposia, 46*(1), 1–54. Adapted from an original illustration in *Clinical Symposia,* illustrated by John Craig, M.D., copyright by Ciba-Geigy Corporation.)

Clinical Manifestations

Epilepsy has been classified according to the age at onset, cause, area of origin, abnormalities on the electroencephalogram (EEG), and clinical type of seizure. The International Classification of Epileptic Seizures, used here, is based on the clinical seizure type and on EEG findings during seizures (the ictal period) and between seizures (the interictal period). According to this classification of epilepsy, the neurologic abnormality may be limited to a specific part or focus of the brain—hence the term "partial seizures"—may involve the entire cortical surface, to produce a generalized seizure. Using these two major categories, epileptologists can classify the major forms of epilepsy.[41]

Partial (Focal, Local) Seizures with No Loss of Consciousness

Partial seizures are the most common type of epilepsy. The first clinical and electroencephalographic changes indicate initial activation of neurons in one part of the cerebral hemisphere. They are further classified according to whether or not consciousness is impaired. There are four types of simple partial seizures that do not impair consciousness. These include seizures with motor signs, those with somatosensory or "special senses" signs, those with autonomic manifestations, and psychic manifestations.[41]

Motor Signs. Partial seizures with motor signs arise from a focus in the region of the brain's motor cortex. The resulting motor activity (seizure) occurs in the part of the body innervated by motor neurons originating in the affected region of the cortex. Because the hand and fingers have the largest cortical representation, many focal motor seizures begin with convulsive movement in an upper extremity. Involuntary movements may spread centrally and involve the entire limb, and even the same side of the face and lower extremity. This progression or spread is known as the jacksonian march. The client also may exhibit changes in posture or spoken utterances.[41]

Somatosensory or "Special Senses" Manifestations. If the epileptogenic focus is in the parietal region, the client experiences sensory phenomena such as numbness and tingling in the affected area. If the focus is in the occipital region, the client may experience bright, flashing lights in the field of vision opposite the side of the focus. Likewise, the client can have changes in speech or taste. Involvement of the posterior temporal area of the dominant hemisphere (usually the left) causes difficulty with speaking, or aphasia.[41]

Autonomic Manifestations. Stimulation of the autonomic system produces epigastric sensations, pallor, sweating, flushing, piloerection (goose flesh), pupillary dilation, tachycardia, and tachypnea.[41]

Psychic Manifestations. Seizures arising in the anterior temporal lobe can begin with psychic manifestations. These seizures frequently begin with an aura, a subjective sensation that helps localize the focus. An aura may be a strange smell, noise, or sensation preceding a seizure, or a sense of "rising" or "welling up" in the epigastric region. Visual distortions and feelings such as déjà vu are common.[41]

Complex Partial Seizures

There are two types of complex partial seizures: complex partial seizures with automatisms and partial seizures evolving into generalized seizures.

Complex Partial Seizures with Automatisms. The most characteristic features of a complex partial seizure are the accompanying *automatisms.* These automatic behaviors include purposeless repetitive activities such as lip-smacking, chewing, patting a part of the body, or picking at clothes while in a dreamy state. Inappropriate or antisocial behavior may also automatically occur during the seizure. This unusual behavior may cause the client to be viewed as psychotic or otherwise mentally disturbed. However, some abnormalities are very subtle and may not be detected by an untrained observer.

Temporal lobe seizures usually last 2 to 3 minutes but may last up to 15 minutes. The client is usually unaware of any activity during the seizure and may be confused or drowsy postictally. Attempts to restrain the client during a seizure may induce combative and uncooperative behavior.[41]

Partial Seizures Evolving to Secondary Generalized Seizures. These seizures start from a particular focus, and then the electrical discharges spread throughout the brain. Clinically, the client first shows focal signs; for example, one side of the face moves, and then the whole body becomes involved. Consciousness is lost if the discharges spread throughout the brain.[41]

Generalized Seizures

Generalized seizures lead to a loss of consciousness. They can be convulsive or nonconvulsive. Generalized seizures begin with manifestations involving both hemispheres. Consciousness may be impaired, which may be the first clinical manifestation. About one third of seizures are generalized. Types of generalized seizures are absence, myoclonic, clonic, tonic, tonic-clonic, and atonic.[41]

Absence Seizures. Absence seizures occur in childhood and early adolescence. "Grand mal" or partial seizures may develop at any time in patients who have had absence seizures.[41]

Myoclonic Seizures. Myoclonic seizures involve sudden uncontrollable jerking movements of either a single muscle group or multiple groups, sometimes causing the client to fall. The client loses consciousness for a moment and then is confused postictally. These seizures often occur in the morning, and clients often report that they spill their coffee with their fall.[41]

Clonic Seizures. The clinical manifestations of clonic seizures include rhythmic muscular contraction and relaxation lasting several minutes. Distinct phases of clonic seizures are not easily observed.[41]

Tonic Seizures. Tonic seizures include an abrupt increase in muscular tone and muscular contraction. In addition, with tonic seizures there is a loss of consciousness and the presence of autonomic signs. Tonic seizures may last from 30 seconds to several minutes.[41]

Tonic-Clonic Seizures. Formerly known as "grand mal" seizures, tonic-clonic seizures are the type of seizures most closely associated with epilepsy. Actually, however, this type of generalized seizure comprises only 10% of all seizures. A tonic-clonic seizure typically proceeds as follows:

1. Aura may or may not be present.
2. Sudden loss of consciousness may occur.
3. In the tonic phase, the entire body becomes rigid (Fig. 69–2*A*). If standing or sitting, the client falls stiffly to the floor. A cry may be uttered. Respirations are interrupted temporarily, and the client may become cyanotic. The jaw is fixed and the hands are clenched. The eyes may be opened wide; the pupils are dilated and fixed. The tonic phase lasts 30 to 60 seconds. At the end of this phase the client breathes deeply.
4. The clonic phase begins next, with rhythmic, jerky contraction and relaxation of all body muscles, especially those of the extremities (Fig. 69–2*B*). The client is usually incontinent and may bite the lips, tongue, or inside of the mouth. Excessive saliva is blown from the mouth, which creates frothing at the lips.
5. An entire tonic-clonic seizure may last from 2 to 5 minutes, after which the client enters the postictal phase, during which he or she relaxes and remains totally unresponsive for a time. The client may rouse briefly and then go into a postictal sleep lasting 30 minutes to several hours. This sleep may be followed by general fatigue, depression, confusion, or headache, all of which gradually resolve. The client has complete amnesia for the seizure episode and may feel nauseated, stiff, and sore. Bruising may occur as the result of falls. Petechial hemorrhages may develop on the face and chest due to the vasovagal responses. Falling during the seizure may cause other injury.

Tonic-clonic seizures vary in frequency from many times daily to once or twice a year. Tonic-only and clonic-only seizures may also occur.[20, 41, 45]

ATONIC SEIZURES. Atonic seizures are associated with a total loss of muscle tone. They may be mild, with the client briefly nodding the head, or the client may fall to the floor. Consciousness is impaired only briefly.[41]

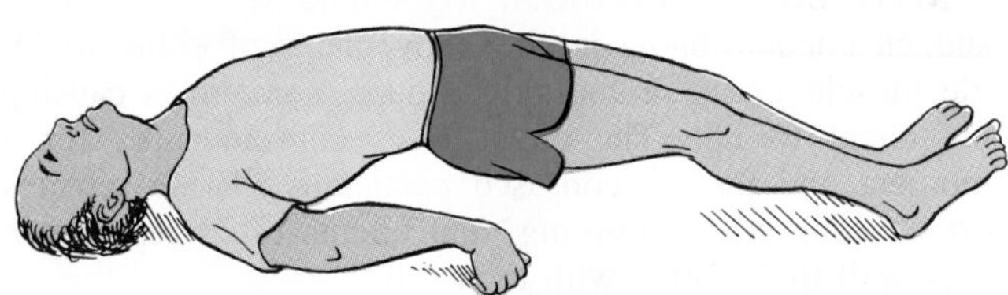

A Tonic phase

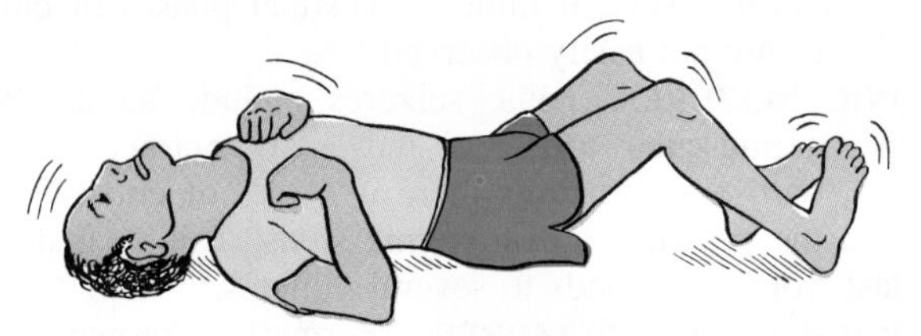

B Clonic phase

FIGURE 69–2 *A*, The tonic phase of a seizure is marked by loss of consciousness, falling, crying, and generalized stiffness. There may be incontinence. *B*, During the clonic phase, there is jerking of the limbs and salivary frothing.

DIAGNOSTIC TESTS

The major diagnostic tool for assessment of clients suspected of having epilepsy is the EEG (see Chapter 68). This test assists in (1) locating the focus of abnormal electrical discharges, if present; (2) establishing a diagnosis of epilepsy; and (3) identifying the specific type of seizures. The EEG records only the electrical activity of the cerebral cortex. With this limitation, a normal EEG tracing does not always exclude a diagnosis of epilepsy, and EEG abnormalities do not always confirm the diagnosis. During a seizure, EEG abnormalities involve all parts of the cortex. Between seizures, clients with epilepsy may show EEG abnormalities not characteristic of seizure disorders. An ambulatory EEG study can be used to clarify suspected seizures that are occurring frequently. The monitor used is similar to a Holter monitor. Long-term video EEG monitoring may also be used to rule out pseudoseizures.

Occasionally, diagnostic tests such as skull radiography, computed tomography (CT), and magnetic resonance imaging (MRI) are used to rule out brain lesions that can trigger seizures. Positron emission tomography (PET) and single photon emission computed tomography (SPECT) may be helpful to measure cerebral blood flow in clients undergoing surgery for epilepsy. As important as the EEG and other diagnostic studies are, a complete seizure profile and history must be established. The seizure profile includes a baseline neurologic examination and description of the seizure activity, as well as laboratory studies.[20, 47]

Outcome Management

Medical Management

The goals of management of clients with seizures and epilepsy are to prevent injury during seizures, to eliminate factors that precipitate seizures, to diagnose and treat the cause of the seizure, and to control seizures to allow a desired lifestyle.

PREVENTION OF INJURY DURING A SEIZURE

During a seizure, the major goals are to maintain the airway, to prevent injury to the client, to observe the seizure activity, and to administer appropriate anticonvulsant medications. Today, "seizure precautions" as identified in a hospital setting refers to the availability of an oral airway and suction equipment. In the home or the community, turning the person to his or her side displaces the tongue and usually results in an open airway once the tonic phase has ceased. Any tight clothing around the person's neck is loosened.

The person experiencing a seizure usually requires protection from the environment. For example, objects should be moved out of the way so that he or she does not strike the head or extremities. Put a pillow or folded blanket under the affected person's head, but do not flex the neck sharply or close the airway.

Observers' descriptions of a seizure can be very helpful in making a diagnosis, especially if the descriptions include details such as the sequence in which phenomena occurred. Instruct the family and unlicensed assistive personnel to make the following observations:

- How long did the seizure last?
- Where in the body did the seizure begin and how did it progress?
- Did the client's eyes and/or head deviate?
- Were the respirations labored or frothy?
- Was the client incontinent?
- Did the client lose consciousness?
- What were the types of movements and what body parts moved?
- Eliminating factors that precipitate seizures

For decades the main antiepileptic drugs (AEDs) were phenytoin (Dilantin), phenobarbital, carbamazepine (Tegretol), and valproate sodium (Depakote). Since the 1990s, other AEDs have been approved and show promising effectiveness. Currently available antiepileptic drugs appear to act primarily by blocking the initiation or spread of seizures.

Phenytoin, carbamazepine, valproic acid, and lamotrigine inhibit sodium-dependent action potentials, blocking the burst and firing neurons in a seizure focus. Phenytoin also appears to suppress seizure spread through inhibition of specific voltage-gated calcium channels.

Benzodiazepines and barbiturates augment inhibition by distinct interactions with gamma-aminobutyric acid (GABA) receptors (see Anatomy and Physiology review). Valproic acid elevates the concentration of GABA in the brain, perhaps through interaction with enzymes involved in the synthesis (glutamic acid decarboxylase) and catabolism (GABA transaminase) of GABA. Gabapentin, which is a structural analog of GABA, appears to increase GABA levels by enhancing GABA synthesis and release and may also cause a decrease in glutamate synthesis. The two most effective drugs for absence seizures, ethosuximide and valproic acid, probably acts by reducing calcium conduction in thalamic neurons.

In contrast to the relatively large number of antiepileptic drugs that can attenuate seizure activity, there are no drugs known to prevent the formation of a seizure focus after CNS injury in humans. The eventual development of such "antiepileptogenic" drugs will provide an important means of preventing the emergence of epilepsy after injuries such as head trauma, stroke, and CNS infection.

The use of AEDs is not without adverse effects. Although myriad adverse effects can occur, for the most part they can be grouped into three categories; idiosyncratic, dose-related, and allergic reactions. It is the responsibility of the nurse, as well as of other health care team members, to instruct the client about the action, dosing, and possible side effects of the various AEDs.

Medical intervention focuses on prescribing AEDs to arrest or prevent seizures. Table 69–1 lists and describes the most common anticonvulsants. Developing a program of correctly prescribed anticonvulsants requires weeks of medication adjustment by trial and error. The desired outcome pharmacologic management is monotherapy (use of

TABLE 69–1 MEDICATIONS USED TO TREAT EPILEPSY

Proposed Mechanism/ Drug	Action	Therapeutic Outcome	Adverse Outcomes	Dosing
Phenytoin	Stabilizes the neuronal membrane	Reduces partial and generalized tonic-clonic seizures	Unsteady gait, slurred speech, confusion, nausea, hypothermia, coma	Narrow window of therapeutic effectiveness; requires frequent monitoring of blood levels to prevent overdosage Associated with many drug-drug interactions Can be given IV for seizures; however, can suppress respirations and heart rate
Phenobarbital	Prolongs postsynaptic potential; prolongs chloride channel opening and GABA activity	Reduces partial and generalized tonic-clonic seizures	Hypotension, cardiac dysrhythmias, dizziness, lethargy, CNS excitement	Parenteral solutions are highly alkaline; dilute and monitor closely Controlled substance Long half-life; use cautiously in clients with impaired renal or hepatic function Abrupt withdrawal may precipitate seizures in clients with epilepsy
Ethosuximide (Zarotin)	Reduces calcium conductance in thalamus	Drug of choice for simple absence seizures	Ataxia, drowsiness, sedation, behavioral changes	Use cautiously in clients with hepatic disease

CNS, central nervous system; GABA, gamma-aminobutyric acid.

one anticonvulsant medication).[20, 46] Large doses of a single anticonvulsant are often more helpful than smaller doses of several drugs.

Ideally, initial treatment begins with a single drug (primary anticonvulsant) until either seizure control is attained or unacceptable side effects appear. If side effects become intolerable before seizures are controlled, another drug is added. Combining medications does carry the potential risk of drug-drug interactions, which decrease effectiveness.

Nursing Management of the Medical Client

The management of epilepsy does not usually involve hospitalization. However, a client may initially be hospitalized for assessment, diagnosis, and education immediately after a first seizure (i.e., in a person with previously undiagnosed epilepsy). Hospitalization may also be required if seizures become uncontrolled or if status epilepticus develops. Nurses have a role in assessing for altered health maintenance related to knowledge deficit or other barriers, anticipating risk of injury, and providing support for clients and their families who experience life changes related to seizure disorders.

ASSESSMENT

Assessment of clients not actively experiencing seizures includes the following:

- History, including prenatal, birth, and developmental history; family history; age at seizure onset; history of all illnesses and trauma; previous brain surgery or stroke; complete description of seizures, including precipitating factors; and presence of an aura
- Medication use and postictal symptoms
- Psychosocial assessment, including mental status examination
- Complete physical examination, focusing on neurologic signs (usually, physical findings between seizures are normal)

DIAGNOSIS, OUTCOMES, INTERVENTIONS

Altered Health Maintenance. This nursing diagnosis is appropriate for clients who are having difficulty adjusting their life to their epileptic condition. Knowledge deficit of the significance of managing the AED regimen is a common problem. State the diagnosis as *Altered Health Maintenance related to chronic disorder (epilepsy) management.*

Outcomes. The client will have improved health maintenance related to knowledge deficit, as evidenced by maintaining routine dosing, consulting a physician whenever there is a problem, and wearing a medical alert identification tag or bracelet.

Intervention. Provide the client with verbal information and written reinforcement about (1) how anticonvulsants prevent seizures, (2) the importance of taking prescribed medication regularly, and (3) care during seizures. Consult with the client to plan ways to make taking medication part of daily activities (e.g., keeping medication by the toothbrush). Also, help the client to identify factors that precipitate seizures and ways of avoiding these factors. Such factors include increased stress, lack of sleep, emotional upset, and alcohol use. See the Client Education Guide on Epilepsy for other important teaching information.

EVALUATION

The short-term outcomes for the client who is experiencing a seizure are usually met within hours. An example is that the seizure stops and the client returns to the previous level of functioning. Nursing care of clients with confirmed epilepsy should focus on the long-term outcomes with self-care.

Modifications for Elderly Clients

With the increasing frequency of epilepsy in the elderly population, nurses need to be more aware of the changes in pharmacokinetics in this age group. Concurrent disease, foods, and drug-drug interactions affect absorption of anticonvulsant medication. A decrease in albumin, as is commonly seen in the older adult, can increase the free plasma level of these drugs. Decreased metabolism can increase the half-life of these drugs, and decreased elimination can result in higher plasma levels.

Enteral feedings inhibit the absorption of phenytoin (Dilantin). Therefore, the feeding should be turned off 2 hours before and after administration of phenytoin, or the dose should be altered on the basis of plasma levels. Altered vitamin D metabolism with phenytoin increases the risk of osteoporosis. Carbamazepine (Tegretol) carries an increased risk of slowed cardiac conduction and heart failure; hyponatremia secondary to increased secretion of antidiuretic hormone, especially if the client is on a low-sodium diet; and altered cholesterol metabolism in the elderly population. Valproate (Depakene) carries an increased risk of causing hyperammonemia in older clients, leading to hepatic dysfunction, decrease in platelets, and toxicity related to its longer half-life in this population.[20, 24, 46–48]

Surgical Management

For approximately 75% of clients with seizures, medical management with AEDs and follow-up evaluation suf-

> **CLIENT EDUCATION GUIDE**
>
> **Epilepsy**
>
> **Client Instructions**
>
> - Take prescribed dosages of medications to maintain your blood levels.
> - Consult your physician if you are unable to take medication because of illness.
> - Observe for side effects of anticonvulsant drugs. Do not stop taking medications because of annoying side effects; this is very dangerous. Consult your physician first.
> - Notify the physician if seizure activity is not being controlled. Provide specific descriptions of the seizure activity.
> - Do not take any over-the-counter medications without consulting with your physician.
> - Obtain a medical alert identification card (or bracelet or tag) with the name of the drug, dosage, and frequency, and your physician's name and phone number. Carry this identification with you at all times.

fices. The remaining 25% continue to have seizures. For about 5% of people with epilepsy, surgery is recommended to control the disease.

The safest and most effective surgical treatment is cortical resection of the anterior temporal lobe for complex partial seizures.[10, 13] Criteria for resection include (1) failure of the medical approach and (2) localization and identification of a focus of abnormal discharge that is easily accessible surgically and is located in the "dispensable" areas of the cerebral cortex. Dispensable areas are those for which there is a duplicative area in the cortex.

Thorough assessment is necessary before surgery. This is usually done in three phases:

Phase 1 involves using video EEG to locate the epileptogenic focus. This stage can also include SPECT and PET studies.[41] Intelligence quotient (IQ) testing and psychological assessments are usually performed.[45, 63]

Phase 2 is used when surface EEG electrodes are not sensitive enough to locate the seizure focus exactly. Depth electrodes are placed in the temporal and frontal lobes of the brain or in the subdural space. These techniques allow detailed maps of the brain for surgery.[17]

Phase 3 involves cerebral angiography with *Wada's test* to determine hemispheric dominance and location of the speech center. The functional supremacy of one cerebral hemisphere is crucial to language function.

Wada's test is a method of determining which side of the brain is dominant for speech production. An injection of amobarbital sodium (Amytal Sodium) is introduced into the left internal carotid artery. If the left hemisphere is dominant, speech is arrested for 1 or 2 minutes, followed by misnaming and misreading for 8 to 9 minutes altogether. After 30 minutes, the process is repeated in the right internal carotid artery. The physician looks for changes in sensation, abstract thought, and coordination.

Postprocedural care is the same as for cerebral angiography (see Chapter 68).[49]

CORTICAL RESECTION/CORPUS CALLOSOTOMY. Corpus callosal resection is considered palliative surgery designed to make the seizures more tolerable. It involves the excision of one section of cortex to reduce the spread of epileptic discharges (Fig. 69–3*A*). One complication, called *disconnection syndrome,* results when the pathways responsible for communication from one hemisphere to another are severed. Clinical manifestations range from motor apraxias and mutism to minimal losses detected only on neuropsychological testing. Staged resections are now performed to reduce the risk of disconnection syndrome.[44, 62]

TEMPORAL LOBECTOMY. This form of curative surgery for epilepsy is performed to remove the area in which the seizures begin without causing neurologic or cognitive deficits (Fig. 69–3*B*). If the dominant hemisphere is removed, the client experiences some language defects for a few weeks. Visual defects from loss of visual projection fibers are compensated for quickly.[44, 62]

HEMISPHERECTOMY. Removal of most of the cortex of one hemisphere is done in children with intractable seizures to control those that are injurious, not to stop all seizures (Fig. 69–3*C*).[44, 62]

VAGAL NERVE STIMULATOR IMPLANTATION. The implantation of a vagal nerve stimulator (VNS) offers clients another treatment modality. Although the underlying mechanism is not fully understood, the VNS is believed to provide a stimulus that desynchronizes the abnormal uncontrolled electrical discharge of the brain activity during a seizure. One study has reported that the benefit from VNS increases over time. For example, 40%

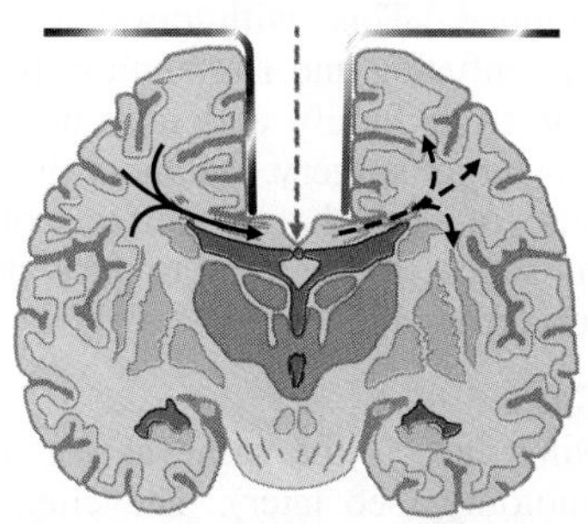

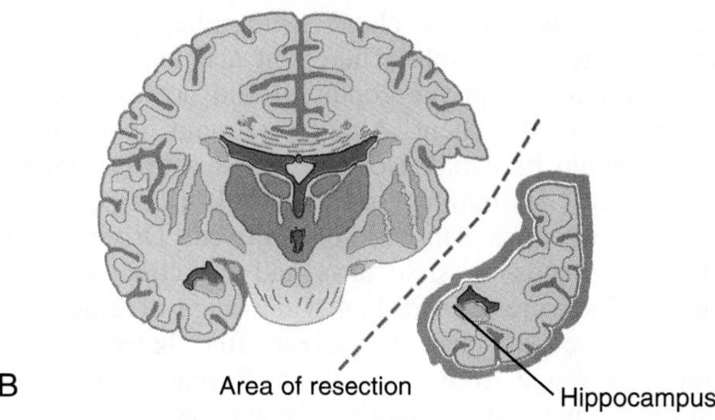

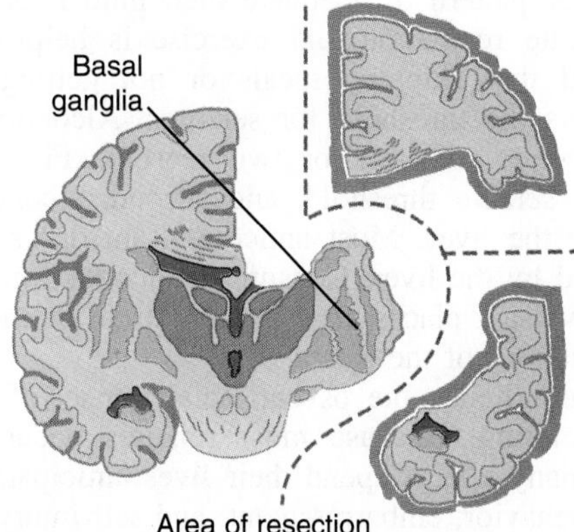

FIGURE 69–3 Surgery for epilepsy can consist of corpus callosotomy *(A),* temporal lobectomy *(B),* or hemispherectomy *(C).* (From Devinsky, O. [1994]. Seizure disorders. *Clinical Symposia, 46*(1), 1–54. Adapted from an original illustration in *Clinical Symposia,* illustrated by John Craig, M.D., copyright by Ciba-Geigy Corporation.)

to 45% of clients continue to experience a decrease in the frequency of seizures at 18 months after implantation of the VNS.[36, 45, 52, 59]

Nursing Management of the Surgical Client

PREOPERATIVE CARE

The role of the nurse during the evaluation phase before surgery is to provide support and education. Clients who have epilepsy have been trying to control their seizures for most of their lives. Now, as part of the preoperative assessment, the health care team needs to observe the client during seizure activity. Therefore, AEDs are tapered and discontinued. This withdrawal of effective medication is often confusing and frightening. In addition, some clients are far from family and may be rethinking their decision to undergo surgery. Memory impairments are common because of both the side effects of medications and postictal states. Be certain to provide written material and reinforce education often.[26, 33, 45]

POSTOPERATIVE CARE

Postoperative nursing care is the same as for any client undergoing a craniotomy (see later). The client is often placed in an intensive care unit (ICU) to facilitate frequent assessment. Anticonvulsant medications are resumed immediately after surgery as well as after leaving the hospital.[33, 43]

Self-Care

It is important for the client with epilepsy to live as normal a life as possible. The client and family members must learn to accept the condition and not exaggerate it or overprotect the client. Although certain dangerous activities should be avoided or performed with special safeguards (e.g,. swimming or horseback riding), a wide range of activities can still be enjoyed. Driving motor vehicles depends on state laws and the client's medical control of seizures. There is a wide range of time during which the client must be seizure-free before driving. Times can range from 3 months to 2 years. This restriction on driving can be emotionally and economically devastating for clients of all ages and socioeconomic backgrounds.

A regular pattern of adequate diet, fluid intake, sleep, and moderate recreation and exercise is helpful. Many clients find that skipping meals or not getting enough sleep lowers the threshold for seizures. Alcoholic beverages are contraindicated for two reasons. First, alcohol lowers the seizure threshold, and second, alcohol is detoxified by the liver. Most anticonvulsant drugs are also metabolized by the liver. Consuming alcohol while taking an anticonvulsant places an increased strain on the metabolizing functions of the liver.

For some clients, the psychosocial impact of epilepsy is overwhelming. Because most seizures occur without warning, many clients spend their lives anticipating inappropriate behavior, embarrassment, and self-injury. Clients with epilepsy often have a poor self-image, feelings of inferiority, self-consciousness, guilt, anger, depression, and other emotional problems. Education and support groups can help clients deal with the emotional impact of epilepsy.

The client and family members should be taught that epilepsy is a chronic disorder that requires long-term management. Even though the client may have been seizure-free for some time, it is important to take medication as prescribed. Phenytoin, a common anticonvulsant, leads to excessive gingival (gum tissue) growth. Brushing two to three times daily helps retard gingival growth. Some clients have excess gingival tissue excised every 6 to 12 months. Medications may also cause diplopia, ataxia, sedation, and bone marrow depression. Most anticonvulsant drugs require periodic monitoring of serum drug levels, liver function, and complete blood counts. Clients with epilepsy should always wear or carry identification stating that they have epilepsy and providing the name and telephone number of their physician.

If the client is able to recognize that certain activities trigger the seizure, the activities can be avoided, or the client can be desensitized in some cases. For example, flickering lights can trigger seizures. Fluorescent lights and flickering shadows from trees on the road while driving during the late afternoon are common precipitants of seizures. If the client experiences an aura, precautions should be taken immediately to prevent self-injury from the impending seizure—for example, lying down on the ground or floor or, if driving a vehicle, pulling over to the side of the road and lying on the seat. Instruct clients to carry a large pillow in the vehicle or to use the arms to protect the head.

Some clients with epilepsy cannot find employment if they admit to having seizures. However, falsifying job applications can result in dismissal from employment. These factors contribute to a higher incidence of depression among clients with epilepsy. Nurses can educate the public regarding epilepsy and help to dissipate prejudices. When discussing the long-term impact of epilepsy with the client, be empathetic but realistic. It is hoped the client can accept the lifestyle limitations of the disorder and not be overwhelmed by them.[5]

The client's family needs to know what to do in the event of a seizure. The affected person should be protected from self-injury. Clothing should be loosened, the head protected from impact, and sharp objects in the environment removed. The person should not be forcibly restrained during a seizure but protected from self-injury. Hard objects or fingers should not be inserted into the mouth. People experiencing a seizure do not swallow the tongue—a common misconception. However, the tongue can occlude the airway, and positioning the head is important to protect the airway. After the head is protected from injury, the person should be placed in a side-lying position to displace the tongue and allow oral secretions to drain from the airway. Someone should stay with the person until full consciousness has returned. An ambulance should be called if the seizure lasts for longer than 10 minutes, if another seizure occurs before consciousness returns, if there is respiratory difficulty on evidence of injury, or if the person is pregnant.

Various organizations are working at public education, introduction of appropriate legislation, and assisting people with epilepsy. In the United States, these include the Epilepsy Foundation of America and Epilepsy Services. Similar organizations exist in other countries.

SEIZURES

Not all seizures are epilepsy. Not only do clients differ in their susceptibility to experiencing a seizure; there are also variations in seizure thresholds. For example, seizures may be induced by high fevers in children who are otherwise normal and who never develop other neurologic problems, including epilepsy.

The cause of seizures varies widely in adults. Brain tumors are the most common cause. Seizures are often the first manifestation of an intracranial mass. Traumatic brain injury is another common cause of seizures in young adults. With severe closed head injuries, seizures occur in a small percentage of clients. However, with open head injuries in which the skull and dura are penetrated, the incidence of seizures rises markedly.

Cerebrovascular disease is the most common cause of seizures in clients over age 50. These seizures usually accompany a stroke. In other vascular lesions, such as arteriovenous malformations (AVMs), seizures may be the first manifestation.

CNS infections frequently produce seizures, either in the acute phase of infection or chronically thereafter. Seizures can be a sequela of viral infections, brain abscesses, and meningitis. Postinfectious encephalitis can cause persistent seizures.

Toxic substances that interfere with brain metabolism or with the supply of oxygen or glucose to the brain can cause seizures. Alcohol is one of the most frequently ingested toxins and can cause seizures either during ingestion or during withdrawal. Chronic substance abuse, especially of barbiturates, can lead to seizures when the drug is withdrawn (see Chapter 24).

Simulated convulsive episodes may occur in clients with psychiatric disorders. These are called "pseudoseizures." One key to differentiating between pseudoseizures and actual seizures is to look for stereotypical movements and a paroxysmal nature of the episodes. Clients with recurrent seizures exhibit the same stereotypic movements with each seizure. Clients exhibiting pseudoseizure make different movements with each seizure.[33, 47]

Management of the client who is experiencing a single seizure focuses on protecting the client during the seizure and then identifying and correcting the underlying problem. Care of clients during a seizure is as discussed earlier.

Controversy exists over the best pharmacologic approach to seizure management. Many authorities recommend a single antiepileptic drug therapy approach, which decreases the risk of drug interactions and adverse effects, makes monitoring easier, and increases client compliance.

STATUS EPILEPTICUS

Etiology

Status epilepticus, a medical emergency, is a state in which a client has continuous seizures or seizures in rapid succession, without regaining consciousness, lasting at least 30 minutes. The most common cause of status epilepticus is the sudden withdrawal of anticonvulsant medication. During a seizure, the brain's metabolic needs increase dramatically. If these heightened requirements continue without opportunity for the body to recover, the supply of glucose and oxygen to the brain becomes inadequate, and permanent brain damage may occur.

Outcome Management

The major goals in managing a client with status epilepticus are to establish and protect the airway, to control the seizure, and to monitor for cessation or other outcomes.

The airway is maintained and aspiration prevented by placing the client in a side-lying position, suctioning the airway, and providing oxygen. Recall that oxygen offers nothing to a client who is apneic; therefore, intubation may be necessary to ventilate and oxygenate the client.

Anticonvulsant medications are given to terminate seizures and to prevent exhaustion. Intravenous (IV) infusion is begun immediately and maintained during treatment. Status epilepticus is treated with diazepam in doses of 5 to 10 mg (0.2 mg/kg) given every 10 to 20 minutes, for a total dose of up to 30 mg in an 8-hour period. Lorazepam (0.1 mg/kg) can also be given in 4-mg doses given over 2 to 5 minutes, repeated every 10 to 15 minutes to a maximum of 8 mg (0.2 mg/kg). In addition, phenytoin can be given to a total dose of 15 to 18 mg/kg by slow IV push (no more than 50 mg/min). Assess the client for bradycardia and heart block while phenytoin is given. If this agent is not effective, diazepam or lorazepam can be used. Because all of these medications can depress respiration, emergency ventilation equipment should be readily available.

If diazepam or lorazepam is not effective, pentobarbital can be used to bring on a barbiturate coma and suppress brain activity. Inducing coma is used only after the anticonvulsant treatments have been tried and have not been unsuccessful. The client in barbiturate coma is ventilator-dependent and requires nursing care in an ICU.

A last resort involves the use of general anesthesia. If a general anesthetic agent or a neuromuscular blocking agent such as vecuronium bromide (Norcuron) is required, the client requires mechanical ventilation, continuous EEG monitoring, and hemodynamic monitoring.

The client's neurologic status is assessed frequently. Even when the status epilepticus has been controlled, the client may be unresponsive for a period of time. Absence of signs of seizure does not mean the seizure has stopped. The manifestations may not be evident. Semiconscious clients thought to be in a postictal state have been found to be still experiencing seizure. After the seizures have been controlled, maintenance anticonvulsants are prescribed.

Clients experiencing status epilepticus are especially difficult for significant others to watch. They need support and assessment. Always explain to family members the treatment being given.[20, 24, 33, 45–47]

BRAIN TUMORS

Brain tumors are identified as primary or secondary lesions. Tumors arising from the brain or its supporting structures are called *primary* brain tumors; those metastasizing from other areas in the body are *secondary* tumors. Brain tumors may also be referred to as *intra-axial* or *extra-axial.* Intra-axial tumors are those originating from the glial cells (cells supporting the neurons) and arise from within the cerebrum, cerebellum, or the brain stem. Extra-axial tumors have their origin in the skull, meninges, cranial nerves, or pituitary gland.

The Central Brain Tumor Registry for the United States (CBTRUS) estimates that the overall incidence for primary brain and CNS tumors is 11.5 cases per 100,000 person-years. This registry estimates that 35,000 new primary brain tumors are diagnosed yearly. The incidence of brain tumors appears to be increasing but may reflect improved and earlier diagnosis.[2, 12, 50, 51]

Etiology

A clear etiologic factor has not been established for any of the primary brain tumors. Although the type of cell that gives rise to the tumor can often be identified, the mechanism causing the cells to act abnormally remains unknown. Most primary brain tumors do not metastasize out of the brain to other areas. Neuroscience researchers are searching for the answers. Familial tendencies, immunosuppression, and environmental factors are being considered.[2, 12, 14, 50, 51]

Pathophysiology

Space-Occupying Lesions

Brain tumors are described as "space-occupying lesions." This phrase explains that the tumor displaces normal tissue or occupies normal tissue spaces. When normal brain tissue is compressed, normal brain tissue cannot function and may become necrotic.

Increased Intracranial Pressure

Not only are the tumors space-occupying lesions; they often produce considerable cerebral edema. The skull is a rigid, box-like structure, containing little room for expansion of any of the intracranial contents. Brain tumors cause progressively increased intracranial pressure (ICP) which leads to displacement of brain structures with herniation of the brain (see Chapter 72).

Intracranial Tumors

Intracranial tumors may arise from neurons (neuromas) or from the support cells, the neuroglial cells (gliomas). Brain tumors can be encapsulated, nonencapsulated, and/or invasive. Much confusion exists with regard to the pathologic and histologic nomenclature. Historically, staging or grading scales identified tumors as grade I (benign) through grade IV or V (malignant). A more recent, three-tiered system from the World Health Organization (WHO) labels tumors according to the maturity of the tumor cells—for example, "mature cells, benign," or "immature cells, malignant"[32, 44, 62] (see Box 69–1).

Glial Tumors. Gliomas are tumors of the neuroglia (supporting brain tissue). Astrocytomas are the most common type of glial cell tumor and can be found throughout the brain and/or spinal cord. These tumors occur in adults and children. Depending upon the exact location, clinical manifestations may result in increased ICP or focal compression.[44, 62]

Oligodendrogliomas. Oligodendroglial cells are found in the CNS and produce myelin. Oligodendrogliomas are tumors of the white matter of the brain. They tend to develop in the cortex of the frontal and parietal lobes. This tumor is fairly slow-growing and calcifies, which makes it recognizable on x-ray studies. The calcification may contribute to the development of seizures as a presenting clinical manifestation. Oligodendrogliomas peak in clients between the ages of 30 and 50 years. Clinical manifestations in addition to seizures are headache, personality changes, and papilledema.[44, 62]

Ependymomas. The ependymal cells line the ventricles and form the inner lining of the spinal cord. Ependymomas may be found anywhere within the CNS; however, there is an increased incidence in the fourth ventricle and intramedullary (within the spinal cord tissue). This tumor affects all age groups. Manifestations are caused by ventricular obstruction and include headache, vomiting, diplopia, dizziness, ataxia, vision changes, and motor and sensory abnormalities.[44, 62]

Pituitary Tumors. Pituitary tumors are usually slow-growing tumors that involve only the anterior lobe of the pituitary gland or extend into the floor of the third ventricle. Most of these are benign, small, and encapsulated. Manifestations can be related to hypofunctioning of the gland and include visual field defects, irregular or absent menstrual cycles, infertility, decreased libido, impotence, decreased body hair, and decreased production of pituitary-stimulating hormones; this decrease results in decreased thyroid and adrenal function. Hypersecretion can also occur and is related to the hormones that are in excess. Combinations of hyposecretion and hypersecretion can also be seen. Manifestations of pituitary tumors are often overlooked for months because they are so diverse. Clients are usually diagnosed by testing blood for the presence of pituitary-stimulating hormones.[44, 62]

Tumors of Supporting Structures. These tumors include meningiomas and acoustic neuromas.

Meningiomas. Meningiomas are common benign tumors that may involve all meningeal layers; however,

BOX 69–1 Schema for Classifying Brain Tumors*

Astrocytoma	Increased number of astrocytes; mature astrocytes; normally developed astrocytes
Anaplastic astrocytoma	Increased number of less mature astrocytes; possibility of mitotic figures (mitotic figures represent increased cellular division and malignant changes)
Glioblastoma multiforme	Increased number of astrocyte cells; immature astrocytes; presence of mitotic figures; hemorrhage, necrosis, swelling, and obscure tumor margins

* This schema of astrocytoma, anaplastic tumor, and glioblastoma multiforme is also used for the astrocytoma, ependymoma, and oligodendroglioma.

these tumors are believed to originate in the arachnoid cells (Fig. 69–4). Most meningiomas are benign, but some tumors may become malignant.[13] Meningiomas may be found in the brain or spinal cord. They are slow-growing and occur at any age, most commonly at midlife and in women. Manifestations depend on location of the tumor and can be quite diverse. Outcomes are related to the site of the tumor. Recurrence is a concern.[33, 44, 62]

Acoustic Neuromas. Acoustic neuromas are tumors of the Schwann cells of the eighth cranial nerve, the acoustic nerve. Manifestations are tinnitus, dizziness, and unilateral hearing loss. If the tumor is allowed to grow, it can displace the other cranial nerves—especially cranial nerves IV to X—and the brain stem. An excellent outcome can be expected with surgical resection and preservation of the remaining cranial nerves. However, most clients experience at least temporary tinnitus, balance problems, and facial weakness after surgery.[23, 44, 62]

METASTATIC BRAIN TUMORS. Metastatic brain tumors are those with primary sites outside of the brain. Cancers of the lung, breast, and kidney and malignant melanoma are the major sources of metastatic brain cancers. The tumor location may also be within the brain or on the arachnoid. The common locations of brain tumors are shown in Figure 69–4.

Clinical Manifestations

General clinical manifestations are caused by changes in cerebral function resulting from edema and increased ICP. The classic triad of clinical manifestations is headache, nausea, and vomiting. Papilledema, which for diagnostic purposes is often substituted for one component of the triad, is not a manifestation; however, it is a hallmark of increased ICP.

MENTAL STATUS CHANGES

As in any neurologic or neurosurgical disorder, a change in the level of consciousness (LOC) or sensorium is often

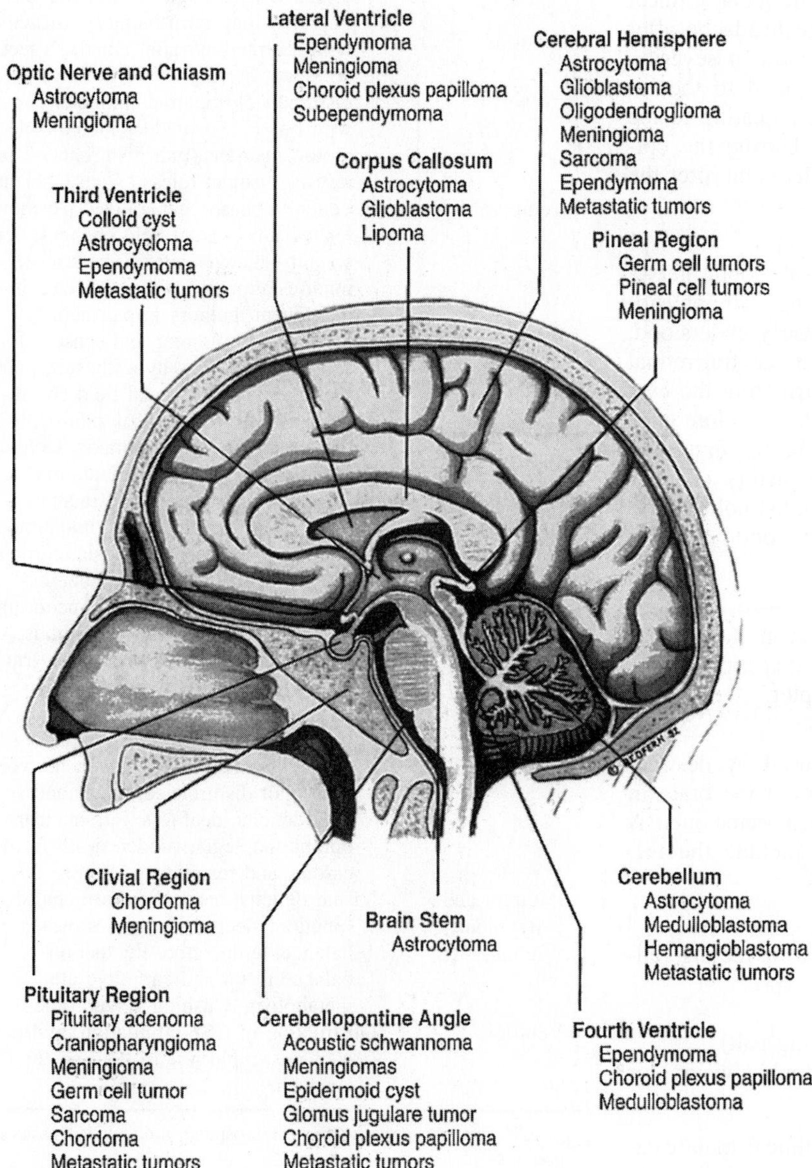

FIGURE 69–4 Common intracranial tumors and their usual locations. (From Murphy, G. P., Lawrence, W., & Lenhard, R. E. [1995]. American Cancer Society *Textbook of clinical oncology* [2nd ed., p. 381]. Atlanta: American Cancer Society.)

noted. Mental and emotional status changes such as lethargy and drowsiness, confusion, disorientation, and personality changes may be found.

Headaches

Headaches may be localized or generalized and are most severe in the frontal or occipital region. They are usually intermittent, are of increasing duration, and may be intensified by a change in posture or straining. Recurrent, severe headaches in a client who was previously free of headaches, or recurrent headaches in the morning, increasing in frequency and severity, may indicate an intracranial tumor and indicate the need for further assessment.

Nausea and Vomiting

Classically, the clinical manifestations of nausea and vomiting are believed to occur because of pressure on the medulla, where the vomiting center is found. The occurrence of these manifestations may be related to generalized swelling, cerebral edema, increasing headache, and/or stimulation of the chemoemetic trigger zone (CETZ). The CETZ has numerous neural connections from areas within the cerebral hemispheres that transmit or synapse with the vomiting center in the medulla. In a frequent clinical scenario, the client complains of a severe headache after lying flat in bed. As the headache increases in severity, the client may also experience nausea related to the involvement of the CETZ. With increasing signaling to the vomiting center, the client then vomits. During the episode of emesis the client may hyperventilate and after the episode may note that the headache is less severe.

Papilledema

Compression of the second cranial nerve, the optic nerve, may result in papilledema. The underlying pathophysiologic mechanism of papilledema is not clearly understood. The cause may be increased pressure in the central retinal vein as a result of obstructed venous return from the eye. Papilledema, also known as "choked disc," is common in clients with intracranial tumors and may be the first sign. Early papilledema does not cause visual acuity changes and can be detected only through an ophthalmologic examination. Prolonged papilledema causes optic atrophy and severely diminished visual acuity.

Seizures

Seizures, focal or generalized, are common in clients with intracranial tumors, especially cerebral hemisphere tumors. See previous discussion in this chapter.

Localized Manifestations

Localized clinical manifestations are caused by destruction, irritation, or compression of the part of the brain in or near the tumor. Blood supply to the affected area is also impaired. Localized manifestations include the following:

- Focal weaknesses (e.g., hemiparesis)
- Sensory disturbances, including absence of feeling (anesthesia) or abnormal sensation (paresthesia)
- Language disturbances
- Coordination disturbances (e.g., staggering gait)
- Visual disturbance such as diplopia (double vision) or visual field deficit (monopia)

As with other cranial disorders, the clinical manifestations associated with a brain tumor correlate with the area of the brain involved. Table 69–2 lists specific clinical manifestations based on tumor location. As an intracranial tumor enlarges, it shifts intracranial structures, which may lead to herniation.

Despite the availability of extremely sensitive and sophisticated equipment, brain tumor diagnosis is often delayed because of difficulty recognizing early manifestations. No two adults with the diagnosis of brain tumor present with the same clinical manifestations. Older clients, especially, fail to report such problems during regular examinations because they forget or think that the manifestations are "just part of growing old."

TABLE 69–2 CLINICAL MANIFESTATIONS OF BRAIN TUMORS BY LOCATION

Location	Clinical Manifestations
Frontal lobe	Disturbed mental state, apathy, inappropriate behavior, dementia, depression, emotional lability, inattentiveness, inability to concentrate, indifference, loss of self-restraint and social behavior, impaired long-term memory, difficulty with abstraction, quiet but flat affect, dominant hemisphere expressive speech disturbance, impaired sphincter control with bowel and bladder incontinence, motor disorders, gait disturbances, paralysis, "frontal release signs," seizures
Temporal lobe	Receptive aphasia, generalized psychomotor seizures, visual field changes, personality changes, ataxia, headache, manifestations of increased ICP, tinnitus, recent memory impairment
Parietal lobe	Sensory deficits, motor and sensory focal seizures, agnosias, hypesthesias, paresthesias, dyslexia, visual field cut, diminished appreciation of side opposite the tumor, headache, apraxia, tactile inattention, right/left disorientation
Occipital lobe	Headache, manifestations of increased ICP, visual impairment (homonymous hemianopsia), visual agnosia, cortical blindness, hallucinations, seizures
Cerebellar	Unsteady gait, falling, ataxia, incoordination, tremors, head tilt, nystagmus, CSF obstruction/hydrocephalus, truncal ataxia if vermis is tumor site
Brain stem	Vertigo, dizziness, vomiting, CN III–XII palsies/dysfunction, nystagmus, decreased corneal reflex, headache, vomiting, gait disturbance, motor and sensory deficits, deafness, intranuclear ophthalmoplegia, sudden death from cardiac and respiratory failure
Pituitary and hypothalamus	Visual deficits, headache, hormonal dysfunction, sleep disturbances, water imbalance, temperature fluctuations, imbalance in fat and carbohydrate metabolism, Cushing's syndrome
Ventricle	Obstruction of CSF circulation, hydrocephalus, rapid rise in ICP, postural headache

CN, cranial nerve; CSF, cerebrospinal fluid; ICP, intracranial pressure.

Diagnostic Findings

If an intracranial tumor is suspected, noninvasive studies such as CT, MRI, and x-ray examination are performed (Fig. 69–5). Other disorders may be ruled out with EEG, radionuclide scans, angiogram, or a lumbar puncture. A stereotactic biopsy may confirm the diagnosis of a brain tumor and help in planning chemotherapy and radiation therapy. Three-dimensional thresholding techniques help visualize the tumor's location in the brain and can assist with plans for resection. PET scans can also be used to study the biochemical and physiologic effects of the tumor.

Outcome Management

Medical Management

For the adult client with a brain tumor, there are many options for treatment. Regardless of which treatment modality is selected, there are several goals. First and foremost, the initial goal is to remove and/or reduce as much of the tumor burden as possible. Additional goals include managing increased ICP, controlling and/or preventing of seizures, and monitoring for motor or sensory deficits and cranial nerve deficits.

Intervention depends on the type and location of the intracranial tumor and the client's medical condition. Management is always interdisciplinary, with several members forming a clinical team to support the client through care.

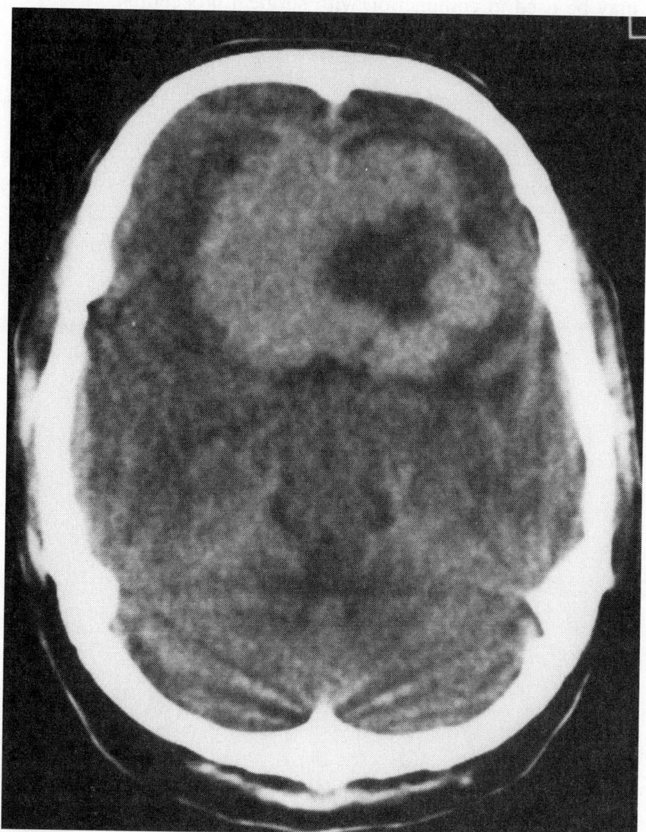

FIGURE 69–5 Magnetic resonance image revealing a midline frontal meningioma.

Surgical intervention may range from biopsy to total removal of the brain tumor. The primary goal of surgery, whether biopsy or resection, is to arrive at the histologic/pathologic diagnosis. Surgical resection decreases the tumor bulk or burden, making other treatments and adjunctive therapeutic treatments more effective. With only a few exceptions, all clients with brain tumors require surgical intervention.

Surgical Management

CRANIOTOMY

The term *craniotomy* means to surgically create an opening into the skull. A craniectomy (removal of a portion of the cranium) may be performed for decompression. Regardless of the type of tumor and the extent of tumor removed, today the neurosurgeon has many methods to remove tumor (see Table 69–3).

Intraoperatively the client may be positioned in various ways to facilitate exposure and visualization. Such positions and/or head-supporting frames have the potential to cause skin pressure on the head, edema of the face, and muscle soreness, especially in the neck. Preoperatively and/or postoperatively, a ventriculostomy—in which a catheter is inserted through a burr hole into the ventricle—may be needed to drain cerebrospinal fluid (CSF) or blood. Drains may be used if a large area of dead space remains after the removal of the tumor.

TRANSSPHENOIDAL HYPOPHYSECTOMY

Transsphenoidal hypophysectomy may be used for clients with pituitary tumors, if the tumor is small and housed within the sella turcica (bony structure housing the pituitary gland). The initial incision for this procedure is made horizontally at the junction of the inner aspect of the upper lip and gingiva, extending bilaterally to the canine teeth. From this incision a surgical area is created beneath the nasal cartilage, extending superiorly through and up to the floor of the sella turcica. At this location, the area of the floor of the sella turcica is accessed, and the tumor is removed (Fig. 69–6). Fat and/or muscle grafts, using tissue from the abdomen or upper thigh, are implanted at the surgical site to assist in healing, of the hypophysectomy operative wound. Nasal packing may or may not be used.

After any brain surgery the client is closely assessed for injury to and edema of the brain. Specific complications from intracranial surgery depend on the area of surgery and the procedure being performed. Examples include increased ICP, motor or sensory deficits and cranial deficits, seizures, CSF leak, wound infection, and CNS infections. If there is loss of significant functions, these problems can be psychosocially and physically devastating. Some postoperative complications gradually resolve, but others are permanent.

General postoperative complications after intracranial surgery do not differ from those after other forms of surgery. Complications may occur as the result of anesthesia, narcotics, or immobility. Ecchymosis and periorbital edema may be present after intracranial surgery but are transient. These changes affecting the appearance of the eyes and the face overall can be very frightening to the client as well as to the family members.

TABLE 69-3 SURGICAL OPTIONS FOR BRAIN TUMOR DIAGNOSIS AND EXCISION

Procedure	Description
Cortical mapping	Intraoperative cortical EEG recording and monitoring, facilitating areas for greater resection without loss of eloquent motor and/or sensory functions
Stereotactic surgery	Localization of a specific target within a three-dimensional space: with the client stabilized in a head frame, the tumor is imaged using either CT or MRI; data from the scans are analyzed by a computer and a trajectory location is identified; stereotactic procedures may be used for biopsy or craniotomy
Frameless stereotactic localization systems	External devices are placed preoperatively and the client's body is scanned using CT or MRI; scanning data are transferred to the operating room, allowing determination of the boundaries of the lesion by means of a surgical "wand"
Brain-mapping technique	Utilizes viewing wand to precisely identify location of specific anatomical functions—i.e., motor, sensory, and/or speech; methods developed include localizing tumors not only with ultrasound techniques but with various wandlike structures
Intraoperative ultrasonography	Utilizes a hand-held device to differentiate tumors with a cystic component; ultrasound techniques allow identification of tumor margins
Laser surgery	Destroys tumor tissue without causing adjacent edema or damage
Neuro-endoscopic techniques	For treatment of third and/or lateral ventricle lesions; this approach provides access to lesions in areas otherwise difficult to locate
Intraoperative imaging techniques	Real-time CT or MRI imaging in the operating room is evolving and holds great promise; such imaging affords safer and better resections as a result of improved visualization
Ultrasonic aspirator	Suction-like device used in removing solid tumors
Direct cortical stimulation	Electrical current is directed to a specific area in the brain, causing a visible movement of the corresponding body part
Somatosensory evoked potentials (SSEPs)	Measurement of electrical response of specific areas (e.g., visual, auditory, brain stem); after the function of such critical areas has been determined, these areas can be avoided during surgical manipulation
Embolization	Decreases blood supply to the tumor; may be used in conjunction with surgical procedures
Photodynamic therapy	Combination of a sensitizing agent and laser surgery; goal is for the "sensitizing" agent to make the tumor more visible or "fluorescent" when the laser is used
Polymer wafer implants	Chemotherapeutic wafers are placed in the tumor bed; currently, carmustine is available, and other agents are being tested

CT, computed tomography; EEG, electroencephalography; MRI, magnetic resonance imaging.

Nursing Management of the Surgical Client

PREOPERATIVE CARE

Today more than at any other time, the role of the nurse caring for the client with the diagnosis of a brain tumor is diverse. The nurse in the neurosurgeon's office begins preoperative teaching. The nurse is usually the first person the client sees when being admitted for diagnostic procedures. During the perioperative and the postoperative periods, the nurse prepares the client for various transitions in the continuum of care.

Preoperative assessment includes the routine assessment data (see Chapter 15). In addition, obtain a detailed history and physical examination to provide a baseline for comparison of neurologic data. Obtain and record data on the following:

- Vital signs; LOC, orientation to person, place and time; ability to follow instructions; pupil equality, size, reactivity, accommodation, and reaction to light; extraocular eye movements; and cranial nerve function
- Limb strength and movement—note limited or exaggerated movements, pronator drift, hand grip, dorsiflex-

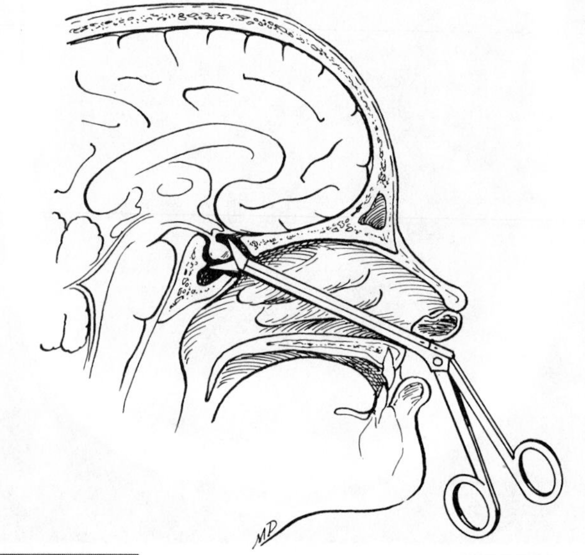

FIGURE 69-6 Transsphenoidal hypophysectomy for the excision of pituitary tumors.

ion/plantiflexion, any paresis or paralysis, or sensory abnormalities
- Manifestations of increased ICP, such as changes in Glasgow Coma Scale score, difficulties in problem-solving, limited memory, changes in pupil response, or loss of limb strength or movement

Preoperative interventions are similar to those for the care of other clients before surgery (see Chapter 15). In addition, the client undergoing a craniotomy requires hair removal at the surgical site. If the operation is for treatment of cancer, the client and family members may have considerable anxiety over the potential outcome. Offer explanations and clarification as needed. Be certain not to offer empty promises about recovery.

POSTOPERATIVE CARE

The postoperative care of the client after craniotomy is shown in the accompanying Care Plan. See also the information on care of clients with increased ICP in Chapter 74.

Postoperative care after pituitary surgery using a transsphenoidal approach includes prohibition of the use of straws for drinking any fluid, to prevent trauma to oral/gingival incision site. Frequent oral hygiene is provided, and a cool vaporizer mist may be used to keep oral mucous membranes moist. The nasal drip pad ("moustache" dressing pad) is assessed frequently for bloody and/or clear fluid (CSF). The donor site and dressings are also assessed, and dressings are changed as needed.

A fairly common effect of pituitary surgery is the development of transient diabetes insipidus (DI) as a result of decreased secretion of antidiuretic hormone (ADH). The main clinical manifestations of DI are polyuria (large urine volumes) and polydipsia (increased thirst). Clients with DI produce large volumes (2 to 15 L/day) of dilute urine with a specific gravity of 1.005 or less. These clients require laboratory assessment of serum and urine levels of sodium and osmolality. Aside from the inconvenience of polyuria, the client often suffers no serious side effects from DI unless deprived of oral or IV fluids. When this happens, circulatory collapse (hypovolemic shock) and hypertonic encephalopathy occur as a result of fluid shifts in the brain. Usual treatment is with IV vasopressin (Pitressin) or inhalation desmopressin (DDAVP). Long-acting forms of these agents can be used for the treatment of chronic DI.

Medical Management

Surgical excision is completed initially to reduce the bulk of the brain tumor, or to excise it completely, in most clients. After surgery when an exact histological diagnosis has been obtained, the client is given adjuvant therapy including radiation therapy and chemotherapy. A complete discussion of these modes of cancer treatment can be found in Chapters 18 and 19; this material is also applicable to the care of clients with brain cancer.

RADIATION THERAPY

Conventional radiotherapy utilizes two different machines to deliver the radiation: the linear accelerator and the cobalt machine. Both of these machine are used in treating brain tumors. With conventional radiotherapy, the standard dose for primary brain tumors is approximately 6000 Gy given four to five times a week for a 4- to 6-week period. For clients with metastatic tumors, a standard dose of radiation is approximately 3000 Gy. The exact dose depends on tumor characteristics, volume of tissue to be irradiated, and the goals of radiation therapy. Radiation treatments are usually given over shorter periods of time to allow for protection of normal surrounding tissues. The cancer cells in CNS tumors tend to be more slowly dividing; therefore, the tumor response often takes longer. This concept is important for clients to understand, as they may be disappointed when they do not see effects during or immediately following irradiation.

As in many areas of medicine, new methods of treatment and improved delivery devices are helping clients daily. This is also the case with radiation therapy. Newer methods of delivery and more sophisticated machines are available. Table 69–4 offers examples of advances made in the area of radiotherapy for clients with brain tumors.[2] Additional forms of radiation therapy, although not considered conventional and, more important, not readily available are heavy particle radiation therapy, fast neutron radiotherapy, photodynamic therapy, and boron neutron capture therapy.[2] In spite of its wide use, radiation therapy is not without consequences. Effects may be acute, early, delayed, or late delayed; see Chapter 19.

CHEMOTHERAPY

In addition to surgery and radiotherapy, chemotherapy is used in the management of brain tumors. As part of a multimodality approach, chemotherapy may be given before, during, or after other therapies. The goal of chemotherapy is to match the appropriate agent with the appropriate cell cycle phase and then attack the rapidly dividing cells. However, there are several challenges in the use of chemotherapy in the treatment of brain tumors: the blood-brain barrier blocks transportation, there are few data to guide specific dose schedules, and the mitotic cycle of brain tumor cells is very long. Today, there does not appear to be one chemotherapy agent that can overcome all of the challenges.

The nitrosoureas are the most frequently used and effective chemotherapy agent for brain tumors. Examples of these drugs are carmustine (BCNU) and lomustine (CCNU). For the client with a brain tumor, the chemotherapy regimen may involve oral medication; IV solutions; intra-arterial routes; or intraventricular, intra-tumor, or epidural administration; or the use of other implanted devices, such as the Ommaya reservoir[8] (see Chapter 19, Fig. 19–3).

Some progress has been made in delivery of chemotherapy across the blood-brain barrier. Of recent interest is the use of substances to open up the blood-brain barrier. In opening or unlocking the blood-brain barrier, certain agents may enter and directly bind with the CSF and/or have a direct effect on the tumor. The osmotic diuretic mannitol may be used to disrupt the blood-brain barrier, allowing for greater drug concentration. There are also newer chemotherapeutic agents that cross the blood-brain barrier.[2, 5, 16, 18] As with the treatment of any cancer invading the body and especially the brain, the hope lies in future research. Biologic response modifiers and modula-

THE CLIENT WHO HAS UNDERGONE CRANIOTOMY

Nursing Diagnosis. Risk for Altered Tissue Perfusion: Cerebral related to edema or bleeding after craniotomy.

Outcomes. The client will have intracranial pressure (ICP) less than 15 mm Hg, mean arterial pressure (MAP) greater than 70 mm Hg, cerebral perfusion pressure (CPP) greater than 50 mm Hg, neurologic assessments and vital signs at baseline values or improved, no clinical manifestations of increased ICP and/or herniation, and body temperature less than 38.5° C.

Interventions	Rationales
1. Assess neurologic status and vital signs frequently and compare with baseline values.	1. A change in level of consciousness is the first sign of increasing intracranial pressure (ICP).
2. Elevated head of bed to 30 degrees.	2. Elevation facilitates venous drainage and reduces edema.
3. Maintain head and neck in neutral alignment.	3. This facilitates venous drainage and reduces edema.
4. Change position slowly.	4. Rapid changes in position increase cerebral blood flow and pressure.
5. Avoid a Valsalva maneuver.	5. Straining during coughing, movement in bed, or moving bowels increases ICP.
6. Monitor intake and output frequently.	6. Excess fluids can promote edema; dehydration can decrease cerebral arterial flow.
7. Monitor pulse oximetry and arterial blood gases.	7. The cerebrum is sensitive to lack of oxygen, and damage can occur within minutes after onset of hypoxia.
8. Suction airway as needed.	8. Routine suctioning not advised because it stimulates cough and increases ICP; however, sputum plugs cause retention of carbon dioxide and need to be removed because carbon dioxide increases cerebral blood flow and pressure.

Evaluation. Depending on the etiology of edema or amount of bleeding, it may require hours to days to control ICP.

Nursing Diagnosis. Ineffective Individual Coping related to fear of changes in body image, role performance, or life expectancy.

Outcomes. The client will have improved individual coping, as evidenced by statements indicating feelings of self-worth, behaviors demonstrating self-worth, and less use of dependent behaviors.

Interventions	Rationales
1. Encourage family members/significant others to assist in meeting need for close contact.	1. Family members may also fear that they will injure the client.
2. Anticipate needs.	2. Anxiety increases feelings of loneliness.
3. Offer praise and encouragement during ongoing assessment of client's readiness to move toward more competent coping.	3. Positive reinforcement helps to guide future steps toward independence.
4. Reduce environmental stress by minimizing interruptions and stimuli.	4. Noise and frequent interruptions may decrease needed sleep and alter ability to cope.
5. Provide opportunities for expression and ventilation of feelings.	5. Problem-solving coping styles are initiated by talking about feelings and issues.
6. Utilize consistent personnel.	6. A therapeutic relationship is easier to maintain than to build.
7. Establish trust relationship; follow through on promises.	7. Feelings of fear and anxiety are reduced.

Evaluation. Coping skills will wax and wane over time. Expect periods of coping and periods of failure to cope with changes in prognosis.

Nursing Diagnosis. Anxiety related to uncertain future and prognosis.

Outcomes. The client will have decreased anxiety and express fears and concerns openly.

Interventions	Rationales
1. Repeat information; provide information in different forms; encourage the client and/or significant other to write down questions and/or concerns.	1. Depending on the type of tumor, the location of the tumor, and/or motor or sensory deficits, the client may be faced with the loss of specific functions and the possibility of having a malignancy. Appropriate interventions may help the client better understand the prescribed plan of care.
2. Encourage open communication between the client, significant others, and members of the health care team.	2. Having a diagnosis of brain cancer may immobilize all of the normal coping mechanisms of the client and significant others.
3. Involve the client's clergy or hospital chaplain if desired.	3. Spiritual support is crucial at times of serious illness for the client, family members, and significant others. The client need not be "religious" to gain support from clergy.

Evaluation. Anxiety should be controllable in a short time. However, changes in response to therapy or other outcomes will increase anxiety.

Nursing Diagnosis. Risk for Altered Thought Processes related to neurologic changes from edema or surgical excision of sections of brain or tumor.

Outcomes. The client will make decisions and process information at expected levels, express and identify anger, exercise control over own behavior, and make appropriate choices, and/or cease hostile behavior.

Interventions	Rationales
1. Allow client to verbalize concerns, and channel these concerns to the appropriate person.	1. Problem-solving coping begins with verbalization of concerns.
2. Offer reasonable choices to client.	2. Feelings of control can be reestablished by offering choices to client. All options must be safe and implementable for the client.
3. Assist client to recognize alternatives and the implications of choices.	3. This measure helps client with problem-solving abilities.
4. Report client's status to client, and allow for opportunity to make decisions about treatment or no treatment.	4. Do not keep facts from the client. The client has the right to know his or her diagnosis and to be a part of decisions about care.
5. Inform family about physiologic reasons for behavior, and teach them how to respond to client.	5. The family needs to be informed about any abnormal behavior and how best to respond to it.
6. Use a consistent approach to inappropriate behavior; establish contracts if needed.	6. Consistent approaches help the client relearn acceptable ways of personal expression.
7. Maintain nonjudgmental behavior.	7. The nurse realizes that the client's outbursts are not personal attacks but due to the disease or feelings of loss of control.

Evaluation. Expect restoration of thought and behavior control to take weeks or months. Long-term coping by the family is important.

Nursing Diagnosis. Anticipatory Grief related to potential loss of function, previous abilities, or life from brain cancer or surgery.

Outcomes. The client will have resolution of grief or progression through stages of grief, as evidenced by expression of feelings, maintaining hope, identifying problems with changes in body function, seeking help with anticipated problems, or developing realistic plans for the future.

Interventions	Rationales
1. Acknowledge reality, but do not force its acceptance.	1. Denial is a powerful defense mechanism; clients will examine reality when they are ready.
2. Establish regular time to spend with client, family members, and/or significant others for the exclusive purpose of discussing feelings and concerns.	2. Discussions about feelings can be difficult; giving the client time to plan and prepare facilitates the discussion.
3. If denial is beneficial, respond by listening with and reflecting statements by client.	3. It is important to understand that not all clients reach acceptance of their disease; some remain in complete denial.
4. Accept emotions and assist client, family members, and/or significant others to clarify them.	4. This measure reinforces the ideas that emotional response is normal and that family members should be accepting of the client at all stages of grief.
5. Assess perceptions about realistic goals and the future.	5. Inaccurate perceptions about the future can prevent or stall planning.
6. Have the client list those activities he or she wants to perform/resume.	6. Plans for the future can be uplifting.

Evaluation. Expect each client and family to cope differently with grief over losses or impending death. Clients may go through the "typical" stages in order or go back and forth between them.

tion of the immune system are two of the keys that scientists hope may hold the answers.

The care of the client with a brain tumor is a challenging task for all involved. The client should not feel abandoned or uninformed during any portion of the care or treatment. To assist the client, family members, significant others, and the health care team, the American Cancer Society as well as the American Brain Tumor Association provides valuable information.

HEMORRHAGIC CEREBROVASCULAR DISORDERS

There are two types of hemorrhagic cerebrovascular disorders (CVDs): (1) intracerebral hemorrhage (ICH) (see Chapter 70) and (2) subarachnoid hemorrhage (SAH). The following section discusses SAH resulting from bleeding due to intracranial aneurysms and AVMs.

TABLE 69–4 RADIATION THERAPY MODALITIES FOR TREATMENT OF BRAIN TUMORS

Procedure	Description
Interstitial radiation Also called brachytherapy, tumor implants, tumor seeding, and/or radioactive pellets	Temporary or permanent placement of radioactive substances in the tumor bed Advantages include minimal effects to the surrounding tissue Generally not advised in large tumors because of secondary swelling and edema Disadvantages: implantation does require a surgical procedure; because of the radioactive substances, the client must be protected and isolated to prevent exposure to family members and health care personnel
Stereotactic radiosurgery, stereotactic radiotherapy	Allows for a high dose of radiation beams to be directed precisely to a small brain tumor in a single session If multiple sessions are required, technique is called stereotactic radiotherapy Gamma knife, linear accelerator, or cyclotron is used to deliver the radiation Best used on small, round, well-defined tumors The Peacock technique incorporates stereotaxis, radiosurgery, and computers to deliver radiation exactly to the tumor, skipping over vital areas that may be embedded in the tumor such as nerves or blood vessels
Hyperthermia	Application of heat into the tumor; electrodes with small catheters/antennae are placed through burr holes in the skull into the tumor bed; using computer-assisted stereotactic methods, the heat is delivered into the tumor Several features of brain tumors make tumor cells more susceptible to the increased temperature: poor blood supply, hypoxic areas, and increased acidity; these factors alone allow the increased temperature to kill the tumor cells Nerve cells in the brain can tolerate temperatures up to 40° C before cellular death occurs Hyperthermia uses heat from radiofrequency or microwave sources
Radiation sensitizing therapy	Use of various pharmacologic agents as "sensitizers" to make the tumor more responsive to radiation therapy and other therapies
Intraoperative radiation	Direct irradiation of the tumor while exposed in surgery; bypasses normal tissues
Conformal radiation	High or higher dose of external radiation "conformed" to match tumor's shape; the goal is to deliver a uniform amount of radiation to the entire tumor
Radioactive monoclonal antibodies	Antibodies that are cloned or mated to kill tumor cells

SUBARACHNOID HEMORRHAGE

SAH is the occurrence of bleeding into the subarachnoid space. SAH most often develops from traumatic brain injury (TBI) (see Chapter 73), intracranial aneurysms, and AVMs. Other potential causes of SAH include brain tumors (see earlier discussion), blood dyscrasias, and anticoagulant therapy.

Etiology

An SAH can occur when any of the aforementioned conditions weakens the artery, causing either a leaking or rupturing of the artery. Trauma is the leading cause of SAH, and intracranial aneurysms are the second leading cause of SAH. The majority of intracranial aneurysms are congenital or developmental.

ANEURYSMS

An intracranial aneurysm is from a weakness in the tunica media, the middle layer of the blood vessel. The most common type of intracranial aneurysm is the saccular or berry aneurysm. These congenital aneurysms are present from birth and begin to weaken over time. The muscular walls of the artery weaken and lead to formation of a sac-like or berry-like structure.

Conditions that hasten the development of this type of aneurysm are hypertension, atherosclerosis, the aging process, and stress.[44, 62] Greater than 25% of all clients with intracranial aneurysms present with multiple intracranial aneurysms. Statistically, SAH is more common in females than in males.[44, 62]

Intracranial aneurysms are found more often in the anterior cerebral circulation (internal carotid artery and its branches—the anterior cerebral artery [ACA], the middle cerebral artery [MCA], and the posterior cerebral artery [PCA])—than in the posterior cerebral circulation, including the vertebral and basilar arteries. Intracranial aneurysms are found in locations where normal anatomic weaknesses occur—that is, in bifurcations and trifurcations.

Pathophysiology

Saccular aneurysms occur at the bifurcations of the large arteries at the base of the brain and rupture into the subarachnoid space in the basal cisterns. Approximately 85% of aneurysms occur in the anterior circulation, mostly in the circle of Willis. The common sites include the junction of the anterior communicating artery with the ACA, the junction of the PCA with the internal carotid artery, and the bifurcation of the MCA. The top of the basilar artery, the junction of the basilar artery and the superior cerebellar artery or the anterior inferior cerebellar artery, and the junction of the vertebral artery and the posterior inferior cerebellar artery comprise most of the remainder (see Fig. 69–7).

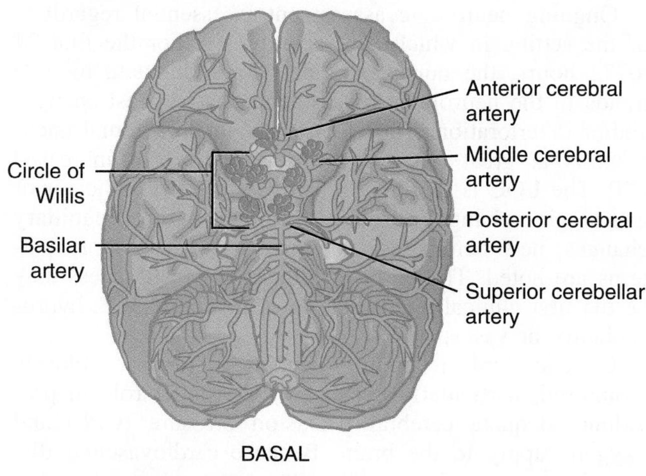

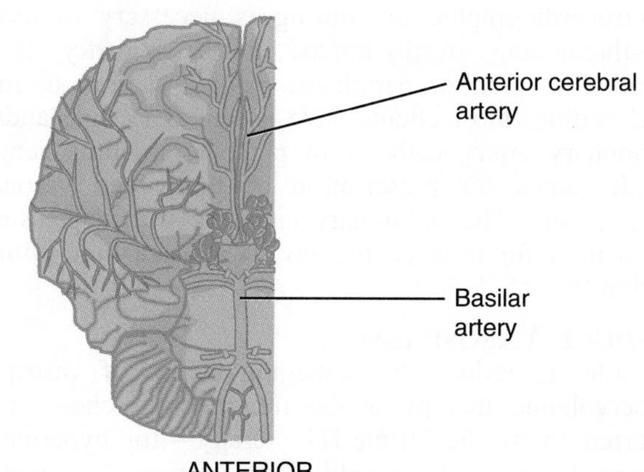

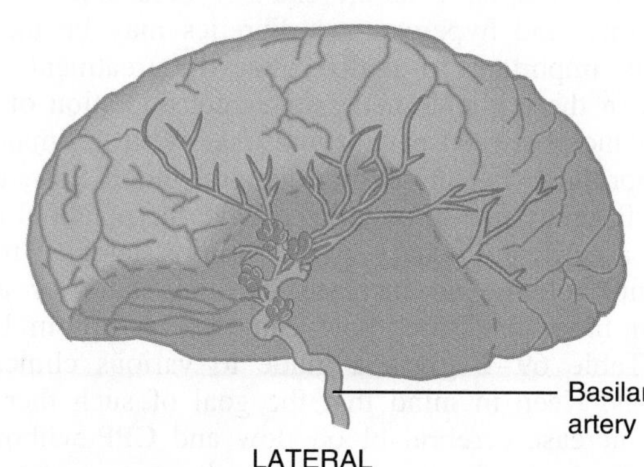

FIGURE 69–7 Common locations of cerebral aneurysms.

As an aneurysm develops, it often forms a neck with a dome. The arterial internal elastic lamina disappears at the base of the neck. The media thins, and connective tissue replaces smooth muscle cells. At the site of rupture (most often the dome), the wall thins, and the tear that allows bleeding is often no more than 0.5 mm long. It is not possible to predict which aneurysms are likely to rupture, but limited data suggest that most ruptured aneurysms are large, averaging 7 mm in diameter.

Vasospasm is defined as the constriction or narrowing of the cerebral vessels. Narrowing of the arteries at the base of the brain regularly occurs after SAH. This vasospasm causes ischemia and infarction. Vasospasm is a very serious consequence and is the major cause of delayed morbidity or death. Although the precise mechanism of delayed vasospasm is uncertain, it seems related to direct effects of clotted blood and its breakdown products on the artery. In general, the more blood there is surrounding the arteries, the more likely that there will be symptomatic vasospasm.

Clinical Manifestations

Aneurysms are found during incidental assessment, such as a work-up for headache, or may be detected because of a mass effect, when the accumulated blood pushes on other structures. Occasionally, mild premonitory manifestations are present, such as mild headache, confusion, fainting, or vertigo. However, the onset of the hemorrhage is usually sudden. The client experiences a sudden, severe headache, often accompanied by vomiting, often describing the headache as "the worst headache I have ever had."

The client may lose consciousness immediately or may become confused and lethargic and gradually become comatose within hours, or may remain conscious and coherent. Generalized seizures may occur. Manifestations of meningeal irritation (e.g., nuchal rigidity, photophobia, back pain) are often present, caused by blood in the subarachnoid space. Depending on the location and size of the aneurysm and the SAH, focal clinical manifestations may be noted (e.g., motor or sensory deficits, speech and cranial nerve deficits). Retinal hemorrhages may be present. Various grading scales have been developed. Table 69–5 presents criteria for the Hunt-Hess scale and the Fisher scale.

Manifestations of vasospasm vary according to the specific arterial territories involved. However, collateral

TABLE 69–5 GRADING SCALES FOR SUBARACHNOID HEMORRHAGE

HUNT-HESS CLINICAL GRADING SCALE FOR CLIENTS WITH ANEURYSMAL SAH

Grade	Clinical Criteria
I	Alert, minimal headache
II	Alert, moderate to severe headache (cranial nerve palsy allowed)
III	Lethargic or confused or mild focal deficit
IV	Stuporous, moderate to severe hemiparesis, possibly early decerebrate rigidity
V	Deep coma, decerebrate rigidity, moribund appearance

FISHER SCALE FOR CT GRADING OF CLIENTS WITH SUSPECTED ANEURYSMAL SAH

Grade	CT Criteria
1	No SAH on CT scan
2	Thin SAH (<1 mm)
3	Thick SAH (>1 mm)
4	Intracerebral or intraventricular hemorrhage, with no or thin SAH (<1 mm)

CT, computed tomography; SAH, subarachnoid hemorrhage.

blood flow may prevent the appearance of some expected manifestations. Spasm of the MCA typically causes contralateral hemiparesis and dysphasia (dominant hemisphere). Proximal ACA vasospasm causes abulia (faulty problem-solving) and incontinence, whereas severe vasospasm of the PCA causes hemianopia. Severe spasm of the basilar or vertebral arteries occasionally produces focal brain stem ischemia. All of these focal neurologic manifestations may develop over a few days, fluctuate, or present abruptly.

Manifestations of ischemia appear 4 to 14 days after the hemorrhage, most frequently at about 7 days. The severity and distribution of vasospasm determine whether infarction occurs subsequently.

Diagnosis of SAH is usually based on history and physical examination. The hallmark of aneurysmal rupture is presence of blood in the CSF. In about 80% of affected clients, enough blood is present to be visualized on a non-contrast CT scan obtained within 72 hours. A small hemorrhage may not be seen on CT scan. If the scan neither establishes the diagnosis of SAH nor demonstrates a mass lesion or obstructive hydrocephalus, a lumbar puncture is performed to establish the presence of subarachnoid blood. Lumbar puncture is contraindicated when pressure is high in the cerebrum.

CT scan may identify blood in the subarachnoid space, intracerebral clots, and large clots surrounding an aneurysm. However, cerebral angiography is the definitive diagnostic test. A four-vessel study provides adequate visualization of the carotid and vertebrobasilar circulation. An angiogram usually provides information about the aneurysm location and type, vessels supplying the aneurysm, presence of an intracerebral blood clot, and presence of cerebral vasospasm.[44, 62] Depending on the client's condition, angiography may be performed immediately or when the client's condition stabilizes. (See Chapter 11 regarding angiography.)

Outcome Management

Medical Management

The client with an SAH resulting from an intracranial aneurysm presents a challenge to all members of the interdisciplinary health care team. Until the 1980s it was not unusual to place a client on bedrest, imposing severe physical and environmental limitations (complete bedrest for 10 to 14 days, dimming lights, feeding the client, keeping the room quiet, and minimizing visitors). This management approach was believed to lessen the effects of the SAH, allowing for better visualization during surgery and decreasing swelling and cerebral edema. Many innovations have developed over the intervening years to cause a paradigm shift not only in the treatment interventions but also in the medical and nursing management.[44, 62] Today, treatment is often instituted within 24 hours of onset of the headache, and the client typically makes a full recovery.

The goals for the management of a client with SAH include maintaining cerebral perfusion pressure, controlled ICP, minimizing effects of vasospasm, managing hydrocephalus, managing cardiac dysrhythmias, and preventing bleeding (or rebleeding).

Ongoing neurologic assessment is essential regardless of the setting in which care is provided. For the first 24 to 72 hours, the nurse examines the serial data to note trends in the neurologic assessments that suggest changes and/or deterioration. The client with an intracranial aneurysm is at great risk for the development of increased ICP. The LOC is the most sensitive and early indicator of neurologic change, usually evident before pupillary changes, new hemiparesis, or changes in respiratory patterns are noted. The onset of lethargy or restlessness may be the first clinical manifestation of increased ICP, hydrocephalus, or vasospasm.

Cardiac and respiratory function is also closely monitored, particularly because of the direct role in providing adequate cerebral perfusion pressure (CPP) and oxygen supply to the brain. Because cardiovascular disease is common in people with aneurysms, continuous electrocardiographic monitoring is necessary to identify life-threatening dysrhythmias. Pulse oximetry is imperative to monitor peripheral oxygen saturation. In the ICU setting, most clients have a central IV line and/or a pulmonary artery catheter in place to monitor hemodynamic status for prescription of fluids and vasoactive medications. The pulmonary capillary wedge pressure is often used for targeted therapy to manage fluid administration.[11, 21, 44, 54, 55, 63]

Reduce Vasospasm

In order to reduce the damaging effects of vasospasm, hypervolemic therapy is the treatment of choice (often referred to as the "triple-H" therapy—for hypertension, hypervolemia, and hemodilution). Various therapies are utilized. For example, calcium channel blockers, vasopressor agents, and hyperosmotic diuretics may be indicated. It is important to realize that the treatment of vasospasm in these clients necessitates consideration of a delicate balance between benefit and risk. With the major goal of improving and increasing cerebral blood flow, as well as CPP, many measures utilized have the potential to precipitate a cardiopulmonary crisis. Simply stated, if the client cannot tolerate an increase in fluid status or an increase in blood pressure, how can the vasospasm be relieved? Table 69–6 gives a guide to various clinical interventions. Keep in mind that the goal of such therapies is to increase cerebral blood flow and CPP without producing cerebral infarction or cardiopulmonary compromise.[11, 54, 60]

Maintain Cerebral Perfusion Pressure

Medical and nursing management focuses on maintaining blood pressure to facilitate CPP. The blood pressure must be maintained to keep the systemic pressure at a level high enough to provide adequate CPP, yet not so high to cause rebleeding. Various medications and or infusions are used to maintain the blood pressure approximately 10% above the patient's normal pressure. In addition to medications supporting the blood pressure, blood products, and albumin are used when indicated. When the blood pressure exceeds the acceptable range, antihypertensive and diuretic agents are used to decrease the blood pressure slowly. Any sudden decrease in blood pressure will have a dramatic effect on the cerebral blood flow, as well as on the CPP, and may increase the risk of cerebral infarction.[60]

TABLE 69–6 EXAMPLE TREATMENT PROTOCOL FOR VASOSPASM

Intervention	Rationale
1. Continuous observation and assessment of neurologic status.	Alterations provide information concerning increasing vasospasm.
2. Maintain patent airway with Po_2 values greater than 85 mm Hg and Pco_2 between 25 and 30 mm Hg.	Prevent cerebral hypoxia; hypercapnia increases cerebral blood flow.
3. Hemodynamic monitoring used with assessment parameters to be determined. For example, check PA pressures q 1 to 2 hr, PCWP q 2 to 4 hr, and cardiac outputs q 8 hr.	Desired wedge pressures 14–16 mm Hg. Hemodynamic readings give indications of effects of "triple-H" therapy (see text) not only on cardiopulmonary system but on intracranial vessels as well.
4. If PCWP <10 mm Hg, notify physician; may order fluid challenge. If PCWP >20 mm Hg, notify physician; may order diuretic.	Desired state of fluid balance to maintain an increase in cerebral blood flow.
5. Maintain infusion rate at 100–150 ml/hr to 225–250 ml/hr; albumin or plasma if needed; IV mannitol 1–2 ampules q 4–6 hr.	Maintain perfusion via "triple-H" therapy. Mannitol produces some vasodilation, which can increase cerebral blood flow.
6. Packed RBCs or whole blood if hematocrit less than 30%.	For volume replacement if hemodilution becomes excessive in client.
7. Dopamine 400 mg in 250 D_5W to maintain systolic BP and/or MAP between specified values.	Increases cardiac output and increases cerebral blood flow.
8. Nimodipine (Nimotop) 60 mg q 4 hr for at least 3 wk.	Calcium channel blocker; promotes relaxation of blood vessels, decreasing vasospasm.
9. Morphine as required.	Sedative effect; allows for continuous monitoring.
10. Accurate I&O q 1 hr.	Fluid balance is crucial to maintaining CPP.

BP, blood pressure; CPP, cerebral perfusion pressure; D_5W, 5% dextrose in water; I&O, (fluid) input and output; MAP, mean arterial pressure; PA, pulmonary artery; Pco_2, partial pressure of carbon dioxide; PCWP, pulmonary capillary wedge pressure; Po_2, partial pressure of oxygen; RBCs, red blood cells.

Surgical Management

To successfully treat the aneurysm requires either a surgical procedure or endovascular intervention. If surgery is the chosen treatment, many different procedures may be used; however, the one most commonly used is clipping of the intracranial aneurysm. Aneurysms not anatomically suited to clipping can be wrapped in a surgical gauze material and/or coated with an acrylic material.[44, 60, 62]

Endovascular Therapy and Embolization

An embolization procedure involves clotting of the aneurysm by means of platinum coils, wires, or embolic substances. An interventional radiologist performs the procedure in an angiography suite. An cerebral angiogram is first performed to facilitate advancing a catheter to the selected vessel(s) in the brain. Once the neck of the aneurysm is visualized, a small platinum wire is guided carefully into the aneurysm. Each coil is advanced until it curls into a ball shape inside the aneurysm, not allowing arterial blood to flow into the aneurysmal sac. As each coil is fitted into the sac, a small current of electricity is deployed that breaks the solder and leaves the coils in the aneurysm. When the aneurysm becomes embolized, thrombosing begins. To complete the procedure, an angiogram is performed.

After embolization, the client is admitted to the ICU. The client may receive heparin for 12 to 24 hours after the procedure. The catheter sheath (from the angiogram site) remains in the femoral/groin area with a saline infusion to maintain patency of the artery. Care of the femoral/groin site includes assessing the puncture site for bleeding and hematoma formation, as well as frequent checking of peripheral pulses of the legs. The client is instructed to remain flat in bed and to avoid bending the leg at the groin. Nursing measures to maintain comfort are provided as indicated. Ongoing and frequent assessment of neurologic status is required.

Complications. Minimal complications result from the embolization procedure. If the aneurysm has not bled, there is a risk of bleeding at the time of embolization. Other problems may be related to the cerebral angiogram (see Chapter 67). Regardless of the treatment utilized, one factor of importance not only in selection of the treatment protocol but also in the clinical course is whether or not the aneurysm has ruptured or bled.[37, 54, 57, 60] If the SAH aneurysm ruptures, the client experiences a hemorrhagic stroke (see Chapter 70).

Aneurysm Clipping

Surgical obliteration of the aneurysm with a metal clip eliminates the risk of rebleeding. A craniotomy incision is used, and the aneurysm is isolated. A metal clip is placed over the neck of the aneurysm. The timing of surgery is based on the clinical status and the grade of the aneurysm. Clients with grade I or II aneurysms are operated on within 3 days of the SAH event. Clients with lesions of grades III to V undergo clipping later on, between 10 and 14 days. Surgery is delayed while vasospasm is present. Operating on vessels in spasm increases mortality and morbidity. For clients with high-grade aneurysms, the risk of rebleeding is less than that for morbidity and mortality of early surgery. Unfortunately, medical instability, delay in transfer from one hospital to another, or client or family reluctance to consent to surgery may also delay prompt intervention.

Postoperatively, the client's neurologic status is carefully monitored. The usual postoperative care is given, including cardiac monitoring. As with any neurologic disorder, the physician must be promptly notified about any neurologic changes.

ARTERIOVENOUS MALFORMATIONS

Etiology and Pathophysiology

AVMs are vascular lesions composed of a tangled array of arteries and veins. AVMs have abnormal communication between artery and vein, wherein the blood is shunted directly from artery to vein, skipping the capillary bed. One major artery (a common example is the MCA) and an adjacent vein form the origin of the AVM, called the *nidus* of the malformation. Going to and from the nidus are multiple feeding vessels. Most AVMs are congenital, resulting from failure of capillary formation in utero. Some AVMs have been associated with traumatic brain injuries, wherein the blood is shunted around a hematoma.[45, 61, 63] AVMs range in size from small to those encompassing an entire hemisphere.

AVMs may be found in the brain or spinal cord. Intracranially, the majority of AVMs are found in the cerebral hemispheres. In the spinal cord, AVMs predominantly occur on the posterior aspect of the cord. Depending on the size of the malformation, the number of feeders, and the magnitude of circulatory steal, the AVM can bleed or undergo thrombosis, resulting in transient to permanent spinal cord damage.

Clinical Manifestations

The onset of clinical manifestations may be seen at any age; however, increased incidence is noted in clients under 40 years of age. Manifestations are related to the anatomy of the malformation and the vessels involved and occur as the result of the vessels' weakening and shunting of blood in the tortuous mass. Manifestations may also be due to increasing size of the AVM. As the AVM expands, the anomalous vessels dilate and require more blood. The process of acquiring more blood flow is referred to as circulatory "steal." In this phenomenon, blood is diverted (stolen) from normal areas to maintain flow through the anomalous vessels. Consequently, localized hypoperfusion and hypoxia occur in the tissue adjacent to the AVM.

When the AVM bleeds, the client may present with any of the following: complaints of headache, seizures, SAH, or infracerebral hemorrhage. Once an AVM has bled, there is a 25% chance of rebleeding.

Outcome Management

The management of AVMs is similar to that of intracranial aneurysm. Nursing goals are comparable to those for aneurysm management, with limitation of activity, seizure control, and blood pressure management. The goals of AVM treatment are complete and permanent obliteration of the lesion. This goal may be accomplished with surgery, endovascular embolizations, or radiosurgery. The client's condition and the characteristics of the AVM determine the course of treatment. For example, in a client who has had a large SAH, vasospasm may develop. In this case, treatment is delayed until the vasospasm is decreased or resolved. With an improvement in the clinical status of the client, a treatment plan can then be developed.[44, 60, 62]

Clients commonly require a combination of treatments. Surgical resection may be the preferred treatment. Depending upon the size and location of the aneurysm, the client may undergo serial embolizations, and surgery is the final form of treatment. For the serial embolizations, a thrombosing agent, histoacryl glue may be used. The goal of the embolization is to place the glue as close to the nidus of the AVM as possible.

Another treatment option for cerebral AVMs is radiosurgery. This approach may constitute the main treatment or may be used in combination with other therapies. Radiosurgery consists of direction of a focused beam of radiation toward the nidus of the AVM. The dose delivered is determined by the size of the AVM. The use of radiotherapy is recommended with small AVMs.

For example, research is ongoing with "liquid coils" (coils that take the shape within the vascular lesion) and new coatings on currently used coils. The future holds the answers to the treatment and management of hemorrhagic cerebral disorders.[44, 60, 62]

INFECTIONS

BACTERIAL MENINGITIS

Bacterial meningitis is characterized by inflammation of all the meninges; however, the organisms predominantly involve the arachnoid and subarachnoid spaces. The infection spreads throughout the subarachnoid space via the CSF around the brain and spinal cord and usually involves the ventricles.

Etiology

Almost any bacteria entering the body can cause meningitis. The most common are meningococci (*Neisseria meningitidis*), pneumococci (*Streptococcus pneumoniae*), and *Haemophilus influenzae.* These organisms are often present in the nasopharynx. It is not known how they enter the bloodstream and the subarachnoid space. *S. pneumoniae* and *N. meningitidis* are found most often in adults. Factors predisposing to bacterial meningitis include traumatic brain injury, systemic infection, postsurgical infection, meningeal infection, anatomic defects, and other systemic illnesses. Toxins such as intrathecal drugs or tumor cytokines may directly trigger meningeal irritation.

Pathophysiology

The route of entry into the intact CNS is uncertain. Invasion may occur through the choroid plexus (across the blood-brain barrier) or within monocytes as a component of normal cellular movement. Little change occurs in brain structure in the early stages of meningitis. Later in bacterial meningitis, inflammation leads to formation of exudate. The arachnoid and pia tissues become thickened, and adhesions form, especially in areas where there normally is an increased amount of CSF. The arteries supplying the subarachnoid space, may be engorged with blood, leading to rupture or thrombosis of these vessels.

Clinical Manifestations

The classic manifestations of meningitis are nuchal rigidity (rigidity of the neck), Brudzinski's sign and Kernig's sign, and photophobia. To assess for *Kernig's sign,* begin with the client recumbent and the thigh flexed at a right angle to the abdomen, and with the knee flexed at a 90-degree angle to the thigh. Then extend the client's lower leg. In meningeal irritation, extending the leg upward causes pain, spasm of the hamstring muscles, and resistance to further leg extension at the knee (Fig. 69–8*A*). To assess for *Brudzinski's sign,* with the client supine lift the head rapidly up from the bed. If meningeal irritation is present, forward neck flexion produces flexion of both thighs at the hips and flexure movements of the ankles and knees (Fig. 69–8*B*).

Other general manifestations related to infection are also present, such as fever, tachycardia, headache, prostration, chills, fever, nausea, and vomiting. The client may be irritable at first but, as the infection progresses, appears acutely ill and confused, stuporous, or semicomatose. Seizures may occur. A petechial or hemorrhagic rash may develop. CSF is cloudy. Gram stain of the CSF reveals organisms in 70% to 80% of cases.[39] When the organism cannot be identified, bacterial antigens can be determined. *Haemophilus influenzae* is frequently detected with this technique. Clients with bacterial pneumomeningitis demonstrate the following:

- Moderately elevated CSF pressures
- Elevated CSF protein (normal, 15 to 45 mg/dl)
- Decreased CSF glucose (normal 60 to 80 mg/dl, or two-thirds of the serum glucose value)
- Elevated white blood cell count, usually increased (100 to 10,000/cm^3), with predominantly polymorphonuclear leukocytes

Outcome Management

Bacterial meningitis constitutes a medical emergency. If untreated, it can be fatal within hours to days. Medical diagnosis is made by assessment of clinical manifestations and is confirmed by isolating the causative organism from the CSF. The use of antibiotics has reduced the mortality rate for all types of bacterial meningitis. Prognosis varies according to the causative organism. The mortality rate is less than 5%.[40] Deaths most often occur in newborn infants and in older adults. Complications are rare but may include septic shock, vasomotor collapse, seizures, and increased ICP due to hydrocephalus, brain swelling, and fluid overload. Residual neurologic deficits are rare in adults.[31]

Intervention depends on the causative microorganism and the source of the infection. Empiric therapy in bacterial meningitis includes cephalosporins, rifampin, and vancomycin. The empirical use of penicillin or ampicillin in the treatment of CNS infections is avoided because of the beta-lactamase–producing *H. influenzae* and *N. meningitidis.* It is believed that the cephalosporins are more potent against the beta-lactamase organisms. Chloramphenicol and trimethoprim-sulfamethoxazole are recommended for clients allergic to penicillin. Once the organism is known, antibiotics with greater sensitivity may be used. High doses of the appropriate antibiotic are usually prescribed for at least 10 days. If the primary focus of infection is located in the frontal area, such as the parasinuses, or if cranial osteomyelitis is present, surgery may be indicated after the acute phases of meningitis have subsided.

A unique problem in treating CNS infection is that an intact blood-brain barrier prevents complete penetration of the antibiotic. However, inflammation inhibits the blood-brain barrier, so for a short time, antibiotics penetrate the CNS. Antibiotics are given intravenously; the blood-brain barrier recovers as inflammation subsides, and high doses are required in order to reach the CSF.

Adequate fluid and electrolyte balance must be maintained. Frequent assessment of the neurologic status is indicated to detect early signs of increasing ICP and seizures. Anticonvulsants may be prescribed for seizure prevention.

Outbreaks of meningitis can be a major health problem in the community, especially when they occur in schools. Refer to your facility's isolation protocols.

BACTERIAL TOXINS

Toxins produced by several pathogenic bacteria have a special affinity for the nervous system. They cause conditions such as tetanus, diphtheria, and botulism. Tetanus, a preventable disease, is caused by the anaerobic spore-forming rod *Clostridium tetani.* Tetanus may be found in

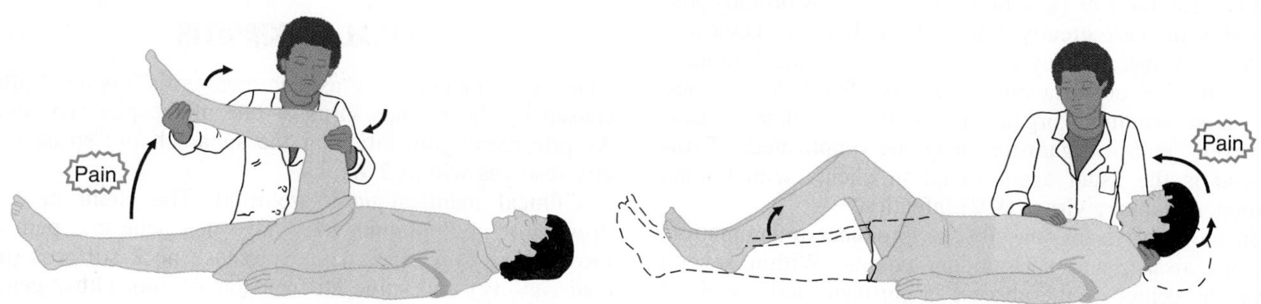

FIGURE 69–8 Assessment of meningeal irritation. *A,* Kernig's sign. *B,* Brudzinski's sign.

people with some form of trauma and no history of tetanus immunization. Bacteria enter the CNS from a wound in which the spores were introduced and produced a toxin. The toxin enters the blood stream from the wound and travels to the central and peripheral nervous systems. It is important to note that with wounds that are closer to the head, the neurotoxin causes tetanus more quickly.

Clinical Manifestations

Clinical manifestations may be limited to painful muscular spasms and contractions in the affected extremity. However, generalized tetanus is more common, with painful, involuntary muscular contractions involving the neck and facial muscles, especially cheek muscles, the jaw becomes locked closed (trismus), resulting in a grotesque grinning expression (risus sardonicus). The involuntary muscular contractions may further involve the pharyngeal and respiratory muscles, neck, trunk, and limbs. The affected muscles become rigid, with occurrence of painful paroxysms of tonic contractions in response to even the slightest external stimuli. The client may also exhibit seizures as a result of airway problems and/or hypoxia.

Outcome Management

Interventions for the acute care of the client with tetanus include the respiratory support with possible mechanical ventilation, use of neuromuscular blocking agents, surgery to debride any associated wounds, a single dose of tetanus immune globulin (Hyper-Tet), a 10-day course of penicillin G (tetracycline, erythromycin, and chloramphenicol are alternative agents), enteral feedings, and prophylactic anticoagulation to prevent thrombus. The overall mortality rate for tetanus is 25% to 50%, even in modern facilities with extensive resources. Tetanus is best prevented by immunization and regular booster doses of the toxoid.

BRAIN ABSCESS

A brain abscess is a collection of either encapsulated or free pus within brain tissue arising from a primary focus elsewhere (e.g., ear, mastoid sinuses, nasal sinuses, heart, distal bones, lungs, or primary bacteremia). The frontal lobe is the most common site of a brain abscess. They vary in size. A large abscess may involve most of one cerebral hemisphere. Other abscesses are microscopic. Brain abscesses are relatively rare and when they occur, it is most common in persons under age 30. Morbidity and mortality increase greatly with multiple brain abscesses.

A brain abscess may occur after penetrating traumatic brain injuries or intracranial surgery. Staphylococci are the most common organisms in trauma-related cases; however, many organisms may be implicated. *Toxoplasma* is the usual agent found in clients with human immunodeficiency virus (HIV) infection.

In its early stages, the abscess produces inflammation, necrotic tissue, and surrounding edema. Within several days, the center of the abscess is purulent, and a wall of granulation tissue forms, encapsulating the abscess. Infection may spread through thin places in the wall of the capsule, resulting in development of additional abscesses.

Clinical Manifestations

Clinical manifestations of a brain abscess are essentially the same as those seen with any space-occupying brain lesion. Headache and lethargy are the most common manifestations. Manifestations of infection (e.g., fever, chills) are present about half the time. The client may experience drowsiness, confusion, and a depressed mental status as a result of the cerebral edema, increasing ICP, and the intracranial effects of the brain abscess. Transient focal neurologic disorders (e.g., weakness on one side, loss of speech) occur when the abscess is located in a specific area such as the motor or speech area. Early manifestations may subside, and then within a few days or weeks, indications of increasing ICP may develop (e.g., recurrent headaches, changes in LOC focal or generalized seizures).

Medical diagnosis of brain abscess is made by CT and MRI.

Outcome Management

Pyogenic brain abscess may be treated with antibiotic therapy alone or antibiotics combined with surgical aspiration or excision. Needle aspiration may be performed stereotactically (guided by CT imaging) with the use of local anesthesia. Corticosteroids may also be given to reduce cerebral edema. Penicillin is the antibiotic of choice for this type of infection. When antibiotics are used to treat the abscess, follow-up CT scans are used to monitor progress.[6, 31]

VIRAL INFECTIONS

Neurologic viral infections are usually associated with systemic viral infections and can be devastating. Viruses may enter the body via the respiratory system, mouth, or genitalia or from an insect or animal bite. The organism invades the CNS via the cerebral capillaries and choroid plexus or along peripheral nerves. Viruses multiply in the body and cause viremia (blood infected with viruses). Some viruses appear to have an affinity for specific cell types within the CNS.

There is no adequate treatment for most CNS viral infections. Immunizations are available for a few viral conditions (e.g., poliomyelitis, rabies). However, they are not available for most viral encephalitides. At present, mass immunization is practical only for acute anterior poliomyelitis. The best control of other viral disorders is to identify and eliminate vectors responsible for their transmission.[29, 31]

VIRAL MENINGITIS

Acute viral meningitis ("aseptic meningitis") is most often caused by the mumps virus or one of the picornaviruses. Aseptic meningitis infecting the subarachnoid space usually resolves within 2 weeks.

Clinical manifestations are mild. The client may be drowsy or photophobic, may have headache and pain on moving the eyes, and may experience neck stiffness (nuchal rigidity) and spine stiffness on flexion. Other generalized manifestations include weakness, rash, and painful extremities. Fever and signs of meningeal irritation may be present. Physical examination reveals the presence of nuchal rigidity and Brudzinski's and Kernig's signs. Acute and convalescent serologic testing and appropriate viral cultures may identify the specific virus.

Interventions for clients with aseptic meningitis are related to symptom management. Keep the client at bed rest during the acute phase. Plan interventions to relieve headache, control fever, and increase comfort. If seizures occur, anticonvulsants are prescribed.[29, 31]

VIRAL ENCEPHALITIS

Encephalitis is an inflammation of the brain parenchyma from viral invasion. The two most common viral infections are arthropod-borne virus (arbovirus) encephalitis and herpes simplex type 1 virus encephalitis. Also, the viruses that cause viral meningitis may cause severe viral encephalitis.

The course of the illness is unpredictable. Of the clients who recover, a significant percentage have some disability, including mental deterioration, personality changes, and hemiparesis. Residual disability is even higher with eastern equine encephalitis.

Viral encephalitis begins like any acute febrile illness with headache, fever, malaise, and sore throat. Later the client experiences alterations in level of consciousness and sensorium (confusion progressing to disorientation and lethargy progressing to coma). In addition, motor or sensory deficits, seizures, hyperirritability, cranial nerve involvement, and increased ICP may be present.

ARBOVIRUS ENCEPHALITIS

Arbovirus encephalitis is caused by arboviruses that multiply in a blood-sucking vector (e.g., mosquito, tick) and are transmitted to humans by the insect's bite. The incidence of diseases caused by arboviruses is characteristically seasonal and geographic. Become familiar with those in your area. In the United States, they occur in late summer and early fall. The most common types of encephalitides are the St. Louis and eastern and western equine forms of encephalitis.

The infection sites are usually microscopic and scattered throughout the cerebral gray and white matter except in eastern equine encephalitis, in which major parts of a lobe or hemisphere may be destroyed. Two thirds of people who acquire eastern equine encephalitis either die or develop severe residual disabilities including mental retardation, seizures, blindness, deafness, speech disorders, and hemiplegia.

Clinical manifestations with all arbovirus encephalitides are similar. The onset is gradual in adults and older children, with headache, nausea, vomiting, listlessness, and fever. After a few days, seizures, nuchal rigidity, stupor, and coma develop. Photophobia, hemiparesis, and asymmetrical reflexes may be present. Fever and neurologic manifestations subside within 2 weeks if the client does not develop irreversible CNS changes or die.[29, 31]

HERPES SIMPLEX VIRUS ENCEPHALITIS

Herpes simplex virus encephalitis occurs at any time of year and throughout the world. It affects particularly middle-aged people.

The gradually evolving initial clinical manifestations are similar to those of other acute encephalitides. However, this virus has an affinity for the inferomedial portions of the frontal and temporal lobes. The client soon becomes acutely ill with headache, fever, vomiting, and, often, seizures. If the infection is not aggressively treated, temporal lobe swelling leads to transtentorial herniation, coma, and brain death.

A biopsy may be done in an attempt to identify the herpes virus. Although biopsy is definitive for the disease, there are risks. MRI is an effective and safe diagnostic tool.

Intervention for herpes simplex encephalitis is a 10-day course of IV acyclovir, an antiviral agent. To be effective, it must be given early in the course of the disease. Despite treatment, the course of the disease may be unrelenting. The prognosis is grave but not hopeless, however, there is significant mortality with this infection. Of people who survive, many are left with severe neurologic and mental disabilities such as global dementia, seizures, and aphasia.

Nursing intervention is a challenge. An acutely ill client is often restless and combative and exhibits bizarre behavior. Extensive rehabilitation is often needed. The client needs careful protection from injury, and the family requires supportive care. If residual behavior changes and mental deterioration develop, assist the family to adjust to changes in the client. Refer the family to agency or community support groups.[29, 31]

FUNGAL INFECTIONS

Fungi may cause meningitis, meningoencephalitis, intracranial thrombophlebitis, or brain abscess. CNS fungal infections are rare. When they do occur, these infections are usually complications of another condition. Conditions that increase the risk of fungal infections include those that interfere with the body's normal flora or suppress the immune response, such as acquired immunodeficiency syndrome (AIDS), leukemia, organ transplantation, diabetes, and collagen-vascular disease.

Cryptococcosis is the most frequent CNS fungal infection. The cryptococcus, a common soil fungus, can cause granulomatous meningitis. Small granulomas and cysts are found within the cortex, and large granulomas and cystic nodules are found deep within the brain. This organism is an opportunist, and the incidence of cryptococcosis has risen since the onset of the AIDS epidemic. Clinical manifestations vary, and diagnosis is confirmed by finding *Cryptococcus neoformans* in the CSF. If untreated, this infection is fatal within a few weeks.

Mucormycosis, a malignant infection of cerebral vessels, is a rare complication of diabetic acidosis. It begins in the nose and paranasal sinuses and spreads to the brain. It may be associated with fungal meningitis.

CNS fungal infections produce clinical manifestations similar to those of bacterial infections. The main intervention for these infections is administration of IV amphotericin B, flucytosine, or fluconazole. With this treatment, recovery is almost certain, except for clients with advanced infection or other, overwhelming, fatal diseases. Cryptococcal meningitis in clients with AIDS is highly refractory and is associated with a 50% to 60% relapse rate.

PARASITIC INFESTATIONS

In South America and Mexico, the parasite most commonly affecting the CNS is *Cysticercus.* The tapeworm, in larval form, causes a systemic infestation. Raw or undercooked pork may contain tapeworms, which are passed into the gastrointestinal tract, where they grow. The worm enters the bloodstream and establishes a cyst, commonly within the muscles and brain tissue. The cyst, which may be 3 to 15 mm in diameter, contains the larvae of the tapeworm. These larvae die approximately 18 months after infestation. Calcification of the cyst and inflammation follow. Clients may have more than one cyst.

CT or MRI studies identify the cysts. Cysticercosis titers may be identified in the blood and CSF; however, surgical biopsy is often performed to confirm the diagnosis.

The drug praziquantel is used to treat cysticercosis. The mechanism of action is to eliminate the tapeworm from the gastrointestinal system. If pharmacologic treatment is ineffective, surgical excision of the cyst may be recommended.[29, 31]

TOXOPLASMOSIS

The most common opportunistic infection of the CNS in clients who have AIDS is toxoplasmosis. It is usually manifested as single or multiple brain abscesses. Initial clinical manifestations are headache, confusion, lethargy, and low-grade fever. More than 65% of clients develop such focal signs as weakness, ataxia, speech disturbances, apraxia, seizures, and sensory disturbances.[34]

Treatment consists of administration of pyrimethamine (Daraprim), sulfadiazine or clindamycin (Cleocin), and leucovorin (folinic acid or Wellcovorin). If a therapeutic response is seen, the client is kept on maintenance dosages.

HEADACHE

Headache, the most common of pains, may occur either in the absence of organic disease or as a manifestation of serious disease. Most headaches are transient and of only moderate or slight severity. However, a few types are chronic, intense, and recurrent over a period of months or years. Headache is a manifestation of an underlying disorder, rather than a disease itself. The cause of headache must be identified so that appropriate treatment can be given.

Clients often self-treat headaches with over-the-counter medications. Most headaches do not indicate serious disease. However, encourage clients with persistent or recurrent headaches to seek neurologic assessment. Serious disorders that typically produce headache include intracranial tumors and hemorrhage, CNS infections, acute systemic infections, TBI, cerebral hypoxia, severe hypertension, and acute or chronic diseases of the eye, ear, nose, or throat.

Assessment of headaches includes detailed history, psychosocial assessment, and physical examination. Neurologic assessment is particularly important. Possible neurologic diagnostic tests include skull x-ray studies, CT, EEG, and lumbar puncture with CSF examination.

History should determine (1) location of the pain, intensity, and paths of radiation; (2) character of the headache (e.g., sharp, dull, throbbing); (3) mode of headache onset, duration, and frequency; (4) methods used to treat the headache; (5) presence of localized tenderness; (6) associated phenomena or precipitating factors; and (7) familial incidence.

Classification and Etiology

TENSION HEADACHE

Tension headaches result from muscle contraction (Fig. 69–9*A*). This type of headache is described as a tight bandlike discomfort that is unrelenting, with few headache-free intervals. The pain typically builds slowly, fluctuates in severity, and may persist more or less continuously for many days. Triggers include fatigue and stress. The diagnosis of tension headache is confirmed when the headaches occur more often than 15 days a month. Clients may report that the head feels as if it is in a vise or that the posterior neck muscles are tight. In some patients, anxiety or depression coexists with tension headache.

CLUSTER HEADACHES

Cluster headaches are sometimes classified as a form of migraine (Fig. 69–9*B*). These headaches have a cyclical pattern of one to three short-lived attacks of periorbital pain lasting from 4 to 8 weeks, with an increased incidence in spring and fall. These headaches also have quiescent periods lasting months to years. Cluster headaches occur more often in men.

The headache lasts between 15 minutes and 3 hours. It may occur one to four times each day and may awaken the client from sleep. The pain is described as deep, boring, intense pain of such severity that the client has difficulty remaining still. The client may also develop Horner's syndrome with constricted pupils, injected conjunctiva, unilateral lacrimation, and rhinorrhea during the headaches. Cluster headaches are triggered by consumption of alcohol.

Propranolol and amitriptyline are largely ineffective. Lithium is beneficial for cluster headache and ineffective in migraine. The most satisfactory treatment is the administration of drugs to prevent cluster attacks until the bout is over. Effective prophylactic drugs are prednisone, lithium, methysergide, ergotamine, and verapamil. Lithium appears to be particularly useful for the chronic form of the disorder. A 10-day course of prednisone, followed by a rapid taper, may interrupt the pain bout for many clients.

For the attacks themselves, oxygen inhalation (9 L/min via a loose mask) is the most effective modality; inhalation of 100% oxygen for 15 minutes is often necessary. The self-administration of intranasal lidocaine, either 4% topical or 2% viscous, to the most caudal aspect of the inferior nasal turbinate can produce a ganglionic block that is usually remarkably effective in terminating an attack.

MIGRAINE HEADACHES

Migraine headache is often considered to be a "vascular" headache, vasospasm and ischemia of intracranial vessels being the cause of the pain (Fig. 69–9*C*). These head-

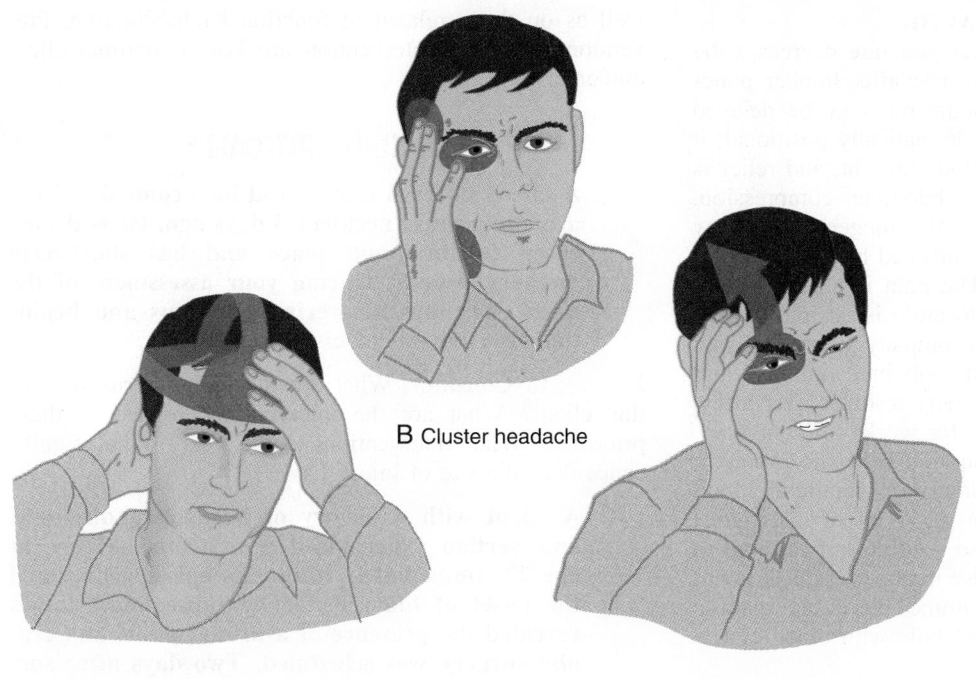

FIGURE 69–9 Types of headaches. The red areas show the regions of greatest pain. *A,* Muscle contraction headache. *B,* Cluster headache. *C,* Migraine headache.

aches usually begin in puberty and are more common in women, often associated with hormonal changes following the menstrual cycle. About 66% of cases of migraine are familial.

Migraine headaches last between 4 and 72 hours, with headache-free intervals between attacks. The headache is most often unilateral, but pain may occur on alternate sides with different attacks. Pain is described as throbbing and pulsatile. Photophobia, phonophobia, anorexia, nausea, vomiting, and focal neurologic signs are often present. Some clients have a visual aura that precedes the headache by 10 to 60 minutes (usually 20 minutes). The client sees a jagged edge of light in the visual fields. Other premonitory manifestations occur 12 to 24 hours before an attack and may include euphoria, fatigue, yawning, and craving for sweets. Migraine headache can be triggered by relief of intense stress, missing meals, or tyramine-rich foods. See the accompanying Client Education Guide.

Typically, the client finds pain relief in a quiet, dark environment. When aspirin and acetaminophen alone fail, the addition of butalbital, caffeine, ibuprofen (600 to 800 mg), and naproxen (375 to 750 mg) is often useful. Isometheptene compound, 1 to 2 capsules, is effective for mild to moderate "common migraine." When these measures fail, more aggressive therapy should be considered. Drug absorption is impaired during migrainous attacks because of reduced gastrointestinal motility. Delayed absorption occurs in the absence of nausea and is related to the severity of the attack and not its duration. Therefore, when oral agents fail to cure, alternative therapies, including rectal ergotamine, subcutaneous sumatriptan, parenteral dihydroergotamine, and IV chlorpromazine and prochlorperazine, should be tried.

Today a number of drugs are available with the capacity to stabilize migraine. They must be taken daily. The decision of whether to use this approach depends on the frequency of attacks and on how well acute treatment is working. The occurrence of at least two or three attacks per month may be an indication for this approach. There is usually a lag of 2 weeks before an effect is seen. The major drugs are propranolol, amitriptyline, valproate, verapamil, phenelzine, and methysergide.

CLIENT EDUCATION GUIDE

Migraine Headache

Client Instructions

- Many things can trigger a migraine headache. Find out what things trigger your headaches and avoid those triggers. If this is not possible, consult your physician about adjusting the dosage of your medication.
- If menstruation and ovulation are triggers, consult your physician for adjustments to your medication dosage.
- Alcohol temporarily increases the diameter of your blood vessels (a process called vasodilation), which may trigger migraines.
- Some foods, such as chocolate, cheese, citrus fruits, coffee, pork, and dairy products, contain substances that may trigger migraines.
- Low food intake may lead to a low blood glucose (sugar) level (hypoglycemia), which can trigger migraines. Eat small, frequent meals to decrease this risk.
- Stress management is essential. Adjust your lifestyle to reduce fatigue and exposure to bright sunlight, heat, or humidity. Get enough sleep. If you are having trouble managing the stresses in your life, seek expert guidance.

Lumbar Puncture Headache

Loss of CSF volume with lumbar puncture decreases the brain's supportive cushion. Headache after lumbar puncture usually begins within 48 hours but may be delayed for up to 12 days. Head pain is dramatically positional; it begins when the client sits or stands upright, and relief is obtained upon reclining or with abdominal compression. The longer the client is upright, the longer the latency before head pain subsides. It is worsened by head shaking and jugular vein compression. The pain is usually a dull ache but may be throbbing; its location is occipitofrontal. Nausea and stiff neck often accompany headache, and occasionally blurred vision, photophobia, tinnitus, and vertigo are reported. The pain usually resolves over a few days but may on occasion persist for weeks to months.

Treatment with IV caffeine sodium benzoate promptly terminates headache in most clients. An epidural blood patch accomplished by injection of 15 ml of autologous whole blood rarely fails for those who do not respond to caffeine. The mechanism for these treatment effects is not certain. The blood patch has an immediate effect, making it unlikely that sealing off a dural hole with blood clot is its mechanism of action.

Postconcussion Headache and Syndrome

After seemingly trivial head injuries and particularly after rear-end motor vehicle collisions, many clients report varying combinations of headache, dizziness, vertigo, and impaired memory. Anxiety, irritability, and difficulty with concentration are other hallmarks of *postconcussion syndrome.* Manifestations may remit after several weeks or persist for months and even years after the injury.

Postconcussion headaches may occur whether or not a client was rendered unconscious by head trauma. Typically, findings on neurologic examination are normal, with the exception of the behavioral abnormalities. Chronic subdural hematoma may on occasion mimic this disorder. Although the cause of postconcussive headache disorder is not known, it should not in general be viewed as a primary psychological disturbance. It often persists long after the settlement of pending lawsuits.

Treatment is symptomatic support. Repeated encouragement that the syndrome eventually remits is important.

Other Causes of Headache

Head pain may also develop from disorders of the eyes, ears, teeth, and paranasal structures. Headaches may result from errors of refraction, glaucoma (with increased intraocular pressure), inflammation, and ocular muscle disturbances (see Chapter 65). Pain associated with sinus infection is usually caused by irritation and inflammation of sinus openings. Sinus walls are less sensitive. The pain of a sinus headache may be relieved or eliminated by decongestants and analgesics. Sometimes antibiotics are needed. Surgery to drain the sinuses may also be required (see Chapter 60).

CONCLUSIONS

Because of the complexity of brain disorders and the emotional reactions of the client and family members to these problems, neurologic nursing is one of the most challenging areas of nursing practice. Common nursing problems center on cerebral perfusion and cognition as well as on those related to functional rehabilitation. Prevention and early intervention are key to optimal client outcome.

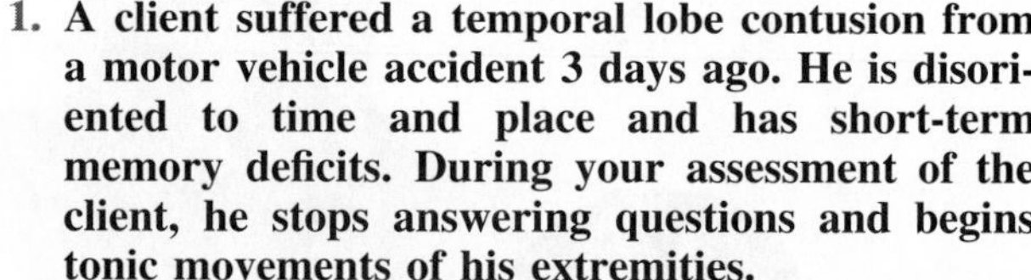

THINKING CRITICALLY

1. **A client suffered a temporal lobe contusion from a motor vehicle accident 3 days ago. He is disoriented to time and place and has short-term memory deficits. During your assessment of the client, he stops answering questions and begins tonic movements of his extremities.**

Factors to Consider. What are the highest priorities for this client? What are the interventions related to these priorities? What interventions come next? What significance does the site of injury have?

2. **A client with a history of headaches, dizziness, and vertigo experienced a first-time seizure at age 27. Immediately after this episode, he noted the onset of blurred vision. Subsequent studies revealed the presence of a brain tumor, and cranial surgery was scheduled. Two days after surgery, the client is transferred to the regular unit. What are your responsibilities regarding monitoring for an increase in intracranial pressure? What are the general interventions for the client after craniotomy?**

Factors to Consider. What is the major complication following intracranial surgery? How do the general interventions prevent complications associated with this type of surgery?

3. **A client is seen in the emergency department at 9 AM on Monday morning. His chief complaint is a severe headache. He states: "I am having the worst headache of my life. The pain awakened me around 5 AM and has gotten worse and worse." On examination the patient is found to have a score of 15 on the Glasgow Coma Scale, complains of nausea, and has a stiff neck. The left-hand grip is slightly weaker than the right-hand grip, and there is a slight pronator drift of the left arm. In addition, there is flattening of the left nasolabial fold. A computed tomography scan of the brain reveals moderate hemorrhage on the right side with increased blood present in the right sylvian fissure. What tests would you expect to be ordered? What complications are important to assess for in this client?**

Factors to Consider. What problem is probably in progress? Is the client a surgical candidate, either at present or later on?

4. **You are caring for a client who had a malignant brain tumor resected 72 hours ago. During previous assessments, she was alert and oriented; her pupils were equal, round, reactive to light, and accommodative (PERRLA), her eyes opened spontaneously; and she was moving all four extremities equally and on command. Her Glasgow Coma Scale (GCS) score was 15. Now, however, she is slow to respond, although still oriented to**

person, place, and time. Her right pupil is equal in size to the left but exhibits a sluggish reaction to direct light. Her left pupil responds normally. She still responds to verbal commands appropriately, has equal motor strength, and opens her eyes spontaneously. Thus, her score on the GCS is still 15. You decide to notify the physician. Why?

Factors to Consider. How sensitive is the Glasgow Coma Scale? What abnormality may be indicated by the decreased response time and the change in pupil reaction?

BIBLIOGRAPHY

1. American Association of Neuroscience Nursing. (1978). Core Curriculum for Neurosurgical Nurses. Chicago.
2. American Brain Tumor Association. (2000). A Primer of Brain Tumors (7th ed.). Chicago.
3. American Council for Headache Education. (1996). Available: *http://www.achnet.org/whatcause.html,* 1–9.
4. Anderson, S. I., et al. (1999). Mood disorders in patients after treatment for primary intracranial tumors. *British Journal of Neurosurgery, 13*(5), 480–485.
5. Barad, M. B. (1999). Functional assessment for transitions in patient acuity. In *Nursing Clinics of North America, 34*(3), 607–620.
6. Bauman, C. K. (1997). Multiple bilateral cerebral abscesses with hemorrhage. *Journal of Neuroscience Nursing, 29*(1), 4–14.
7. Bauman, G. S., et al. (1998). Bihemispheric malignant glioma: One size does not fit all. *Journal of Neuro-oncology, 28,* 83–89.
8. Berweiler, U., et al. (1998). Reservoir systems for intraventricular chemotherapy. *Journal of Neuro-Oncology, 38,* 141–143.
9. Billings, C. V. (1980). Emotional first aid. *American Journal of Nursing, 80*(11), 2006–2009.
10. Breslau, N., et al. (2000). Headache and major depression. *Neurology, 54*(2), 308–313.
11. Brisman, M. H., & Bederson, J. B. (1997). Surgical management of subarachnoid hemorrhage. *New Horizons, 5*(4), 376–386.
12. (2000). *CA: A Cancer Journal for Clinicans, 50*(1), 12–13.
13. Coke, C. B., et al. (1998). Atypical and malignant meningiomas: An outcome report of 17 cases. *Journal of Neuro-oncology, 39,* 65–70.
14. Davis, F., & Preston-Martin, S. (1998). The epidemiology of brain tumors. In D. Bigner, et al. (Eds.), *Russell and Rubinstein's pathology of tumors of the nervous system* (6th ed.). London: Edward Arnold.
15. Davis, M., & Lucatorto, M. (1994). Mannitol revisited. *Journal of Neuroscience Nursing, 26*(3), 170–174.
16. Dawson, H., & Segal, M. B. (1996). *Physiology of the CSF and blood-brain barriers.* New York: CRC Press.
17. Dewar, S., et al. (1996). Intracranial electrode monitoring for seizure location: Indications, methods and the prevention of complications. *Journal of Neuroscience Nursing, 28*(5), 280–292.
18. Doolittle, N., et al. (1998). Blood-brain barrier disruption for the treatment of malignant brain tumors: The national program. *Journal of Neuroscience Nursing, 30*(2), 81–90.
19. Engle, G. (1964). Grief and grieving. *American Journal of Nursing, 64*(9), 93–98.
20. Engle, J., & Pedley, T. A. (Eds.). (1998). *Epilepsy—a comprehensive textbook* (Vols. I, II, and III). Philadelphia: Lippincott-Raven.
21. Faylor, C. R. (1999). Using transcranial Doppler to augment the neurological examination after aneurysmal subarachnoid hemorrhage. *Journal of Neuroscience Nursing, 31*(5), 285–293.
22. Fisher, C. M., et al. (1980). Relation of cerebrovasospasm to subarachnoid hemorrhage visualized by computerized tomographic scanning. *Neurosurgery, 6*(1), 1–9.
23. Gormely, W. B., et al. (1997). Acoustic neuromas: Results of current surgical management. *Neurosurgery, 41*(1), 50–60.
24. Gumnit, R. (1997). *Living well with epilepsy* (2nd ed.). Minneapolis: Demos Vermande.
25. Gurney, J., et al. (1999). The contribution of nonmalignant tumors to CNS tumor incidence rates among children in the United States. *Cancer Causes and Control, 10*(2), 101–105.
26. Hickey, J. V. (1997). *The clinical practice of neurological and neurosurgical nursing.* Philadelphia: Lippincott-Raven.
27. Huether, S. E., & McCance, K. L. (1996). *Understanding pathophysiology.* St. Louis: Mosby–Year Book.
28. Hunt, W. E., & Hess, R. M. (1968). Surgical risks as related to time of intervention in the repair of intracranial aneurysms. *Journal of Neurosurgery, 28,* 14–20.
29. Johnson, R. T. (1996). Emerging viral infections. *Archives of Neurology, 53,* 18–22.
30. Kajs-Wylie, M. (1999). Antihypertensive therapy for the neurological patient: A nursing challenge. *Journal of Neuroscience Nursing, 31*(3), 142–151.
31. King, D. (1999). Central nervous system infection. *Nursing Clinics of North America, 34*(3), 761–771.
32. Kleihues, P., et al. (1993). The new WHO classification of brain tumors. *Brain Pathology, 3,* 225–268.
33. Long, L., & Reeves, A. (1997). The practical aspects of epilepsy: Critical components of comprehensive patient care. *Journal of Neuroscience Nursing, 29*(4), 249–254.
34. McCarthy, B., et al. (1998). Factors associated with survival in patients with meningioma. *Journal of Neurosurgery, 88,* 831–839.
35. Moloney, M. F., et al. (2000). Caring for the woman with migraine headaches. *Nurse Practitioner,* 2000 Feb.; *25*(2), 17–41.
36. Morris, G. L., et al. (1999). Long-term treatment with vagus nerve stimulation in patients with refractory epilepsy. *Neurology, 53*(7), 1731–1735.
37. Morrison, S. R. (1997). Guglielmi detachable coils: An alternative therapy for surgically high-risk aneurysms. *Journal of Neuroscience Nursing, 29*(4), 232–237.
38. Noebels, J. (1998). Genetics and epilepsy. In Ozuna, J., et al. (Eds.), *Clinical nursing practice in epilepsy* (Vol. 2, pp. 4–7). Secaucus: Churchill Communications.
39. *Radiation therapy and you: A guide to self-help during treatment.* Bethesda, MD: National Institutes of Health, National Cancer Institute. NIH Publ. No. 97–2227, Revised October 1993; reprinted January 1997.
40. Raskin, N. H. (1996). Approach to the patient with migraine. *Hospital Practice, 31*(2), 93–106.
41. Santillli, N., & Sierzant, T. (1987). Advances in the treatment of epilepsy. *Journal of Neuroscience Nursing, 19,*143–144.
42. Sargent, J., et al. (1995). Oral sumatriptan is effective and well tolerated for the acute treatment of migraine. *Neurology, 45*(suppl. 7), S10–S14.
43. Schiller, Y., et al. (2000). Discontinuation of antiepileptic drugs after successful epilepsy surgery. *Neurology, 54*(2), 346–349.
44. Schmidek, H. H., & Sweet, W. H. (1995). *Operative neurosurgical techniques* (3rd ed., Vols. I and II). Philadelphia: W. B. Saunders.
45. Shafer, P. O. (1999). Epilepsy and seizures—advances in seizure assessment, treatment and self-management. *Nursing Clinics of North America, 34*(3), 743–759.
46. Shafer, P. O. (1999). New therapies in the management of acute or cluster seizures and seizure emergencies. *Journal of Neuroscience Nursing, 31*(4), 224–230.
47. Shah, S. M., & Kelly, K. M. (1999). *Emergency, neurology—principles and practices.* Cambridge: Cambridge University Press.
48. Spencer, D. C., et al. (2000). The role of intracarotid amobarbital procedure in evaluation of patients for epilepsy. *Surgery, 42*(3), 302–325.
49. Surawiez, T. S., et al. (1998) Brain tumor survival: Results from the National Cancer Data Base. *Journal of Neuro-Oncology, 40,* 151–160.
50. Surawiez, T. S., et al. (1999). Results from the Central Brain Tumor Registry of the United States, 1990–1994. *Neuro-oncology* [On-line]. Available: Doc No. 98–13.
51. Surveillance, Epidemiology, and End Results (SEER). (1998). Cancer statistics review, 1973–1995 U.S. populations. Bethesda, MD: National Cancer Institute.
52. Snively, C., et al. (1998). Vagal nerve stimulator as a treatment for intractable epilepsy. *Journal of Neuroscience Nursing, 30*(5), 286–289.
53. Solomon, G. (1997). Update on therapeutics of headache—diagnosis and treatment of headache in the primary care setting. Available: *http://www.sgim.org/meetings/am20/ws/headache.html,* 1–13.
54. Tamargo, R. J., et al. (1997). Aneurysmal subarachnoid hemorrhage: prognostic features and outcomes. *New Horizons, 5*(4), 364–374.

55. Vale, F. L., et al. (1997). The relationship of subarachnoid hemorrhage and the need for postoperative shunting. *Journal of Neurosurgery, 86,* 462–466.
56. Vannemreddy, P. S. S. V., et al. (2000). Glioblastoma multiforme in a case of acquired immunodeficiency syndrome: Investigating a possible oncogenic influence of human immunodeficiency virus on glial cells. *Journal of Neurosurgery, 92,* 161–164.
57. Vinuela, F., et al. (1997) Guglielmi detachable coil embolization of acute intracranial aneurysm: Perioperative anatomical and clinical outcome in 403 patients. *Journal of Neurosurgery, 86,* 475–482.
58. Vitners, H. V. (1998). *Diagnostic neuropathology.* New York: Marcel Dekker.
59. Vonck, K., et al. (1999). Long-term results of vagus nerve stimulation in refractory epilepsy. *Seizure, 8,* 328–334.
60. Walters, K. (2000). Personal communication.
61. Walters, P. 1990). Chemo: A nurse's guide to action, administration, and side effects. *RN, 53*(2), 52–67.
62. Youmans, J. R. (Ed). (1996). *Neurological surgery: A comprehensive reference guide to the diagnosis and management of neurosurgical problems.* Philadelphia: W. B. Saunders.
63. Yundt, K. D., et al.(1996). Hospital resource utilization in the treatment of cerebral aneurysms. *Journal of Neurosurgery, 85,* 403–409.

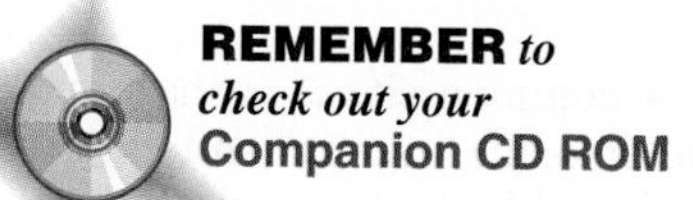

CHAPTER 70

Management of Clients with Stroke

Catherine A. Kernich

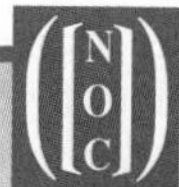

NURSING OUTCOMES CLASSIFICATION (NOC)
for Nursing Diagnoses—Clients with Stroke

Altered Cerebral Tissue Perfusion
Neurologic Status: Consciousness
Tissue Perfusion: Cerebral
Altered Tissue Perfusion
Risk for Aspiration
Neurologic Status
Swallowing Status
Impaired Physical Mobility
Ambulation: Walking
Ambulation: Wheelchair
Body Positioning: Self-Initiated
Joint Movement: Active
Mobility Level
Transfer Performance
Hyperthermia
Thermoregulation
Risk for Impaired Skin Integrity
Immobility Consequences: Physiologic
Tissue Integrity: Skin and Mucous Membranes
Self-Care Deficit
Self-Care: Activities of Daily Living
Self-Care: Eating
Self-Care: Dressing
Self-Care: Bathing
Self-Care: Hygiene
Risk for Injury
Neurologic Status
Safety Behavior: Fall Prevention
Safety Behavior: Home Physical Environment
Safety Status: Falls Occurrence
Safety Status: Physical Injury
Altered Nutrition: Less Than Body Requirements
Nutritional Status: Food and Fluid Intake
Nutritional Status: Biochemical Measures
Nutritional Status: Body Mass
Impaired Verbal Communication
Communication: Expressive Ability
Communication: Receptive Ability
Muscle Function
Altered Thought Processes
Cognitive Ability
Cognitive Orientation
Information Processing
Memory
Visual Sensory/Perceptual Alteration
Vision Compensation Behavior
Risk Control: Visual Impairment
Unilateral Neglect
Self-Care: Activities of Daily Living
Ineffective Individual Coping
Coping
Role Performance
Social Support
Caregiver-Patient Relationship

STROKE—SCOPE OF THE PROBLEM

Stroke is a term used to describe neurologic changes caused by an interruption in the blood supply to a part of the brain. The two major types of stroke are *ischemic* and *hemorrhagic*. Ischemic stroke is caused by a thrombotic or embolic blockage of blood flow to the brain. Bleeding into the brain tissue or the subarachnoid space causes a hemorrhagic stroke. Ischemic strokes account for approximately 83% of all strokes. The remaining 17% of strokes are hemorrhagic.

Cerebrovascular disorders are the third leading cause of death in the United States and account for approximately 150,000 mortalities annually. An estimated 550,000 people experience a stroke each year.[42] When second strokes are considered in the estimates, the incidence increases to 700,000 per year in the United States alone.[6] Stroke is both the leading cause of adult disability and the primary diagnosis for long-term care.[14] There are 3 million stroke survivors living with varying degrees of disability in the United States. Along with a high mortality rate, strokes produce significant morbidity in people who survive them. Of the stroke survivors, 31% require assistance with self-care, 20% require assistance with ambulation, 71% have some impairment in vocational ability up to 7 years following the stroke, and 16% are institutionalized.[31]

The advent of thrombolytic therapy for the treatment of acute ischemic stroke has revolutionized the care of the client following a stroke. Before 1995, health care professionals could offer only supportive measures and rehabilitation to stroke survivors.[12] New therapies can now prevent or limit the extent of brain tissue damage caused by acute ischemic stroke. Thrombolytic therapy must be administered as soon as possible after the onset of the stroke; a treatment window of 3 hours from the onset of manifestations has been established. To convey this sense of urgency regarding the evaluation and treatment of stroke, health care professionals now refer to stroke as brain attack. Public education is focused on prevention, recognition of manifestations, and early treatment of brain attack.[42, 49]

Etiology and Risk Factors

ISCHEMIA

Ischemia occurs when the blood supply to a part of the brain is interrupted or totally occluded. Ultimate survival of ischemic brain tissue depends on the length of time it is deprived plus the degree of altered brain metabolism. Ischemia is commonly due to thrombosis or embolism (Fig. 70–1). Thrombotic strokes are more common than embolic strokes.

Strokes can also be "large vessel" and "small vessel." Large vessel strokes are caused by blockage of a major cerebral artery, such as the internal carotid, anterior cerebral, middle cerebral, posterior cerebral, vertebral, and basilar arteries. Small vessel strokes affect smaller vessels that branch off the larger vessels to penetrate deep into the brain.

Thrombosis

A thrombus starts with damage to the endothelial lining of the vessel. Atherosclerosis is the primary culprit. Atherosclerosis causes fatty material to deposit and form plaques on vessel walls. These plaques continue to enlarge and cause stenosis of the artery. Stenosis alters the usual smooth flow of blood through the artery. Blood swirls around the irregular surface of the plaques, causing platelets to adhere to the plaque. Eventually, the vessel lumen becomes obstructed. Rarely, occlusion is due to inflammation of the arteries, called *arteritis* or *vasculitis*.

A thrombus may develop anywhere along a carotid artery or its branches. A common site is at the bifurcation of the common carotid into the internal and external carotid arteries. Thrombotic stroke is the most common type of stroke in people with diabetes.

Lacunar strokes are small vessel strokes. The endothelium of smaller vessels is primarily affected by hypertension, which causes a thickening of the vessel wall and stenosis. Lacunar infarctions are also common in people with diabetes mellitus.

Embolism

The occlusion of a cerebral artery by an embolus causes an embolic stroke. An embolus forms outside the brain, detaches, and travels through the cerebral circulation until it lodges in and occludes a cerebral artery. A common embolus is plaque. A thrombus can detach from the internal carotid artery at the site of an ulcerated plaque and travel into the cerebral circulation. Chronic atrial fibrillation is associated with a high incidence of embolic stroke. Blood pools in the poorly emptying atria. Tiny clots form in the left atrium and move through the heart and into the cerebral circulation. Mechanical prosthetic heart valves have a rougher surface than the normal endocardium and can cause an increased risk of clots. Both bacterial and nonbacterial endocarditis can be sources of emboli. Other sources of emboli include tumor, fat, bacteria, and air. Any cerebrovascular territory may be affected. The incidence of cerebral embolism increases with age.

HEMORRHAGE

Intracerebral hemorrhage results from rupture of a cerebral vessel, which causes bleeding into brain tissue. Intracerebral hemorrhage is most often secondary to hypertension and is most common after age 50 years. These hemorrhages usually produce extensive residual functional

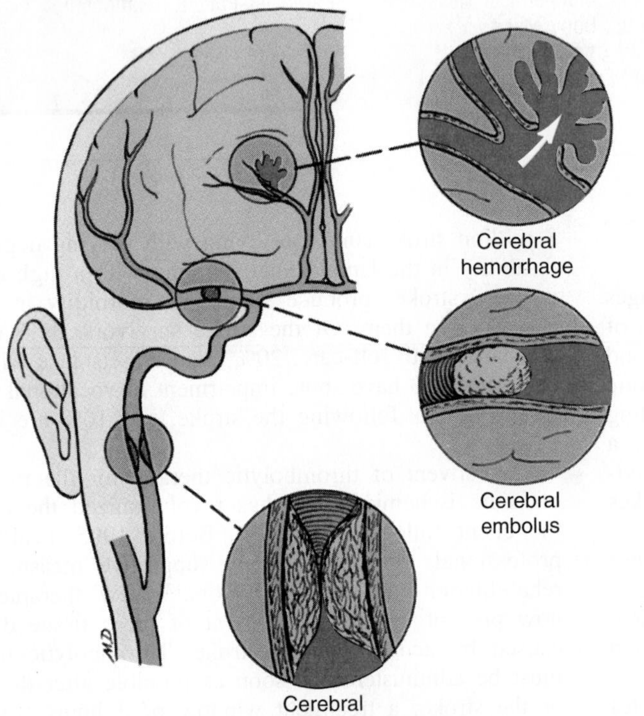

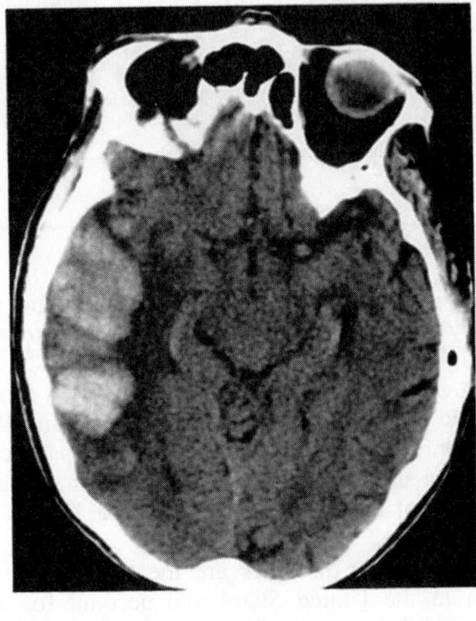

FIGURE 70–1 *A*, Events causing stroke. *B*, Magnetic resonance image showing a hemorrhagic stroke in the left cerebrum.

loss and have the slowest recovery of all types of stroke. The overall mortality of intracerebral hemorrhage varies between 25% and 60%.[22] The volume of the hemorrhage is the single most important predictor of client outcome.[20, 22] Bleeding may also occur from rupture of an aneurysm or a vascular malformation. The effects of these hemorrhages depend on the site and the extent of the bleeding.

OTHER CAUSES

Cerebral arterial spasm, caused by irritation, reduces blood flow to the area of the brain supplied by the constricted vessel. Spasm of short duration does not necessarily cause permanent brain damage.

Hypercoagulable states, including protein C and protein S deficiencies and disorders of the clotting cascade, can cause thrombosis and ischemic stroke. Compression of cerebral vessels may result from a tumor, large blood clot, swollen brain tissue, brain abscess, or other disorders. These causes are fairly rare.

RISK FACTORS

There has been a gradual decline in the incidence of stroke and stroke mortalities in many industrialized countries in recent years. This is due to stroke prevention through the increased recognition and treatment of risk factors. Modifiable risk factors can be reduced or eliminated through lifestyle changes. Hypertension is the most important modifiable risk factor for both ischemic and hemorrhagic stroke. Adequate blood pressure control is associated with a 38% reduction in stroke incidence.[4]

Cardiovascular disease and atrial fibrillation are also associated with an increased risk of stroke. Diabetes mellitus increases the risk of stroke and morbidity and mortality after stroke. The mechanism is related to macrovascular changes in people with diabetes mellitus. Prior stroke, carotid stenosis, and a history of transient ischemic attacks (TIAs) are considered modifiable risk factors for stroke. Reduction in the risk factors for initial stroke may prevent stroke recurrence.[41] Early recognition and treatment of carotid stenosis and treatment of TIAs with antiplatelet agents reduce the risk of stroke.

Other modifiable risk factors for stroke include hyperlipidemia, cigarette smoking, excessive alcohol consumption, cocaine use, and obesity. Stroke is uncommon in women of childbearing age. However, high-dose estrogen oral contraceptives combined with hypertension, cigarette smoking, migraine headaches, and increasing age increase the risk of stroke in women.[17] Conversely, hormone replacement therapy in postmenopausal women may decrease their risk of stroke.

Client education is aimed at stroke prevention. *Primary* prevention of stroke includes:

- Maintaining an ideal body weight
- Maintaining safe cholesterol levels
- Smoking cessation
- Using low-dose estrogen contraceptives only in the absence of other risk factors
- Reducing alcohol consumption
- Eliminating illicit drug use

Secondary prevention includes:

- Adequate blood pressure control
- Care of diabetes mellitus
- Treatment of cardiovascular disease, TIA, and atrial fibrillation

Nonmodifiable risk factors cannot be prevented or treated. Advancing age is one of the most significant risk factors for stroke. The incidence of stroke in men is slightly higher than that in women. Stroke is more prevalent in African Americans than in whites or Hispanics.[25] This is probably related to the increased incidence of hypertension and diabetes mellitus in this group.[6] Family history of stroke increases one's risk for stroke.

Pathophysiology

The brain is very sensitive to a loss of blood supply. Unlike other body tissues, such as muscle, the brain cannot resort to anaerobic metabolism in the absence of oxygen and glucose. The brain is perfused at the expense of other less vital organs to preserve cerebral metabolism. Hypoxia can cause cerebral ischemia. Short-term ischemia leads to temporary neurologic deficits or a TIA. If blood flow is not restored, brain tissue sustains irreversible damage or infarction within minutes. The extent of infarction depends on the location and size of the occluded artery and the adequacy of collateral circulation to the area it supplies.

Ischemia quickly alters cerebral metabolism. Cell death and permanent changes can occur within 3 to 10 minutes. The client's baseline oxygen level and ability to compensate determine how quickly irreversible changes occur. Blood flow can be altered by localized perfusion problems, such as stroke, or generalized perfusion problems, such as hypotension or cardiac arrest. Cerebral perfusion pressure must fall to two thirds of normal (a mean arterial pressure of 50 mm Hg or below) before the brain does not receive adequate blood flow. These numbers assume a normal baseline of blood flow. A client who has lost compensatory autoregulation experiences manifestations of neurologic deficit sooner.

Decreased cerebral perfusion is usually caused by occlusion of a cerebral artery or intracerebral hemorrhage. Occlusion produces ischemia in the brain tissue supplied by the affected artery and edema in the surrounding tissue. Cells in the center of the stroke area, or the core, die almost immediately following stroke onset. This is referred to as *primary neuronal injury.* A zone of hypoperfusion also exists around the infarcted core. This zone is called the *penumbra.*[19] The size of this zone depends on the amount of collateral circulation present. Collateral circulation describes the vessels that augment the major circulatory vessels of the brain. Differences in the size and number of collateral vessels help explain variations in the severity of manifestations experienced by clients with strokes in the same anatomic area.

A cascade of biochemical processes occurs within minutes of cerebral ischemia. Neurotoxins including oxygen free radicals, nitric oxide, and glutamate are released. Local acidosis develops. Membrane depolarization occurs. This results in an influx of calcium and sodium. Cytotoxic edema and cell death are a result. This is secondary neuronal injury. Penumbral neurons are highly susceptible to the effects of the ischemic cascade. The area of edema after ischemia may lead to temporary neurologic deficits.

Edema may subside in a few hours or sometimes in several days, and the client may regain some function.

Most intracerebral hemorrhages are caused by the rupture of arteriosclerotic and hypertensive vessels. Most intracerebral hemorrhages are very large. Therefore, it is not surprising that hemorrhage into the brain causes the most fatalities of all strokes. Aneurysms are weakened outpouchings in a vessel wall. Although cerebral aneurysms are usually small (2 to 6 mm in diameter), they can rupture. An estimated 6% of all strokes are caused by aneurysm rupture. A stroke secondary to bleeding often produces spasm of cerebral vessels and cerebral ischemia because the blood outside of the vessels acts as an irritant to the tissues.

Clinical Manifestations

General findings of stroke unrelated to specific vessel sites include headache, vomiting, seizures, changes in mental status, fever, and changes on the electrocardiogram (ECG). ECG changes include T-wave changes, shortened PR interval, prolonged QT interval, premature ventricular contractions, sinus bradycardia, and ventricular and supraventricular tachycardias.[7]

EARLY WARNINGS

Manifestations of impending ischemic stroke include transient hemiparesis, loss of speech, and hemisensory loss. Manifestations of a thrombotic stroke develop over minutes to hours to days. The slow onset is related to the increasing size of the thrombus, with partial and then complete occlusion of the affected vessel. In contrast, manifestations of embolic strokes occur suddenly and without warning.

Hemorrhagic stroke occurs rapidly, with manifestations developing over minutes to hours. Common manifestations include severe occipital or nuchal headaches, vertigo or syncope, paresthesias, transient paralysis, epistaxis, and retinal hemorrhages.

Manifestations of deficit must persist longer than 24 hours to be diagnostic of stroke. TIAs are focal neurologic deficits lasting less than 24 hours.

SPECIFIC DEFICITS AFTER STROKE

Stroke manifestations can be correlated with the cause (Table 70–1) and with the area of the brain in which perfusion is impaired (Table 70–2). The middle cerebral artery is the most common site of ischemic stroke. The client's deficit also varies according to whether the dominant or the nondominant side of the brain is affected. The degree of deficit can also vary from little impairment to serious functional loss.

Hemiparesis and Hemiplegia

Hemiparesis (weakness) or hemiplegia (paralysis) of one side of the body may occur after a stroke. These deficits are usually caused by a stroke in the anterior or middle cerebral artery, leading to an infarction in the motor strip of the frontal cortex. Complete hemiplegia involves half of the face and tongue as well as the arm and leg of the ipsilateral side of the body. Infarction in the right side of the brain causes left-sided hemiplegia, and vice versa, because nerve fibers cross over in the pyramidal tract as they pass from the brain to the spinal cord. Strokes causing hemiparesis or hemiplegia usually affect other cortical areas in addition to the motor strip. As a result, hemiparesis and hemiplegia are often accompanied by other manifestations of stroke, including hemisensory loss, hemianopia, apraxia, agnosia, and aphasia. Muscles of the thorax and abdomen are usually not affected because they are innervated from both cerebral hemispheres.

When voluntary muscle control is lost, strong flexor muscles overbalance the extensors. This imbalance can cause serious contractures. For example, a hemiplegic client's affected arm tends to rotate internally and to adduct, because adductor muscles are stronger than abductors. The elbow, wrist, and fingers also tend to flex. The affected leg tends to rotate externally at the hip joint, flex at the knee, and plantar flex and supinate at the ankle joint (Fig. 70–2).

Aphasia

Aphasia is a deficit in the ability to communicate. Aphasia may involve any or all aspects of communication, including speaking, reading, writing, and understanding spoken language. The primary language center is usually located in the left cerebral hemisphere and is affected by stroke in the left middle cerebral artery. There are several different types of aphasia. The most common are described here.

Wernicke's (sensory or *receptive) aphasia* affects speech comprehension as a result of an infarction in the temporal lobe of the brain. *Broca's (expressive* or *motor) aphasia* affects speech production as a result of an infarction in the frontal lobe of the brain. Branches of the

TABLE 70–1 CLINICAL MANIFESTATIONS OF THE VARIOUS CAUSES OF CEREBROVASCULAR ACCIDENT

Cause	Clinical Manifestations
Thrombosis	Tends to develop during sleep or within 1 hour of arising Ischemia is produced gradually; therefore, the clinical manifestations develop more slowly than those caused by hemorrhage or emboli Relative preservation of consciousness Hypertension
Embolism	No discernible time pattern, unrelated to activity Clinical manifestations occur rapidly, within 10–30 seconds, and often without warning May have rapid improvement Relative preservation of consciousness Normotension
Hemorrhage	Typically occurs during active, waking hours Severe headache and nuchal rigidity occur (if client is able to report manifestations) Rapid onset of complete hemiplegia, occurs over minutes to 1 hour Usually results in extensive, permanent loss of function with slower, less complete recovery Rapid progression into coma

TABLE 70–2 CLINICAL MANIFESTATIONS OF CEREBROVASCULAR ACCIDENTS ASSOCIATED WITH AREA OF BRAIN AFFECTED

Location	Middle Cerebral Artery	Anterior Cerebral Artery	Posterior Cerebral Artery	Internal Carotid Artery	Vertebrobasilar System	Anteroinferior Cerebellar (Lateral Pontine)	Posteroinferior Cerebellar
Motor changes	Contralateral hemiparesis or hemiplegia, face and arm deficits greater than leg	Contralateral hemiparesis, foot and leg deficits greater than arm, footdrop, gait disturbances	Mild contralateral hemiparesis (with thalamic or subthalamic involvement) Intention tremor	Contralateral hemiparesis with facial asymmetry	Alternating motor weaknesses Ataxic gait, dysmetria (uncoordinated actions)	Ipsilateral ataxia Facial paralysis	Ataxia Paralysis of larynx and soft palate
Sensory changes	Contralateral hemisensory alterations Neglect of involved extremities	Contralateral hemisensory alterations	Diffuse sensory loss (thalamic)	Contralateral sensory alterations	Contralateral hemisensory impairments	Ipsilateral loss of sensation in face, sensation changes on trunk and limbs	Ipsilateral loss of sensation in face, contralateral on body
Visual or ocular changes	Homonymous hemianopia Inability to turn eyes toward affected side	Deviation of eyes toward affected side	Pupillary dysfunction (brain stem) Loss of conjugate gaze, nystagmus Loss of depth perception Cortical blindness Homonymous hemianopia	Homonymous hemianopia Ipsilateral periods of blindness (amaurosis fugax)	Double vision Homonymous hemianopia Nystagmus, conjugate gaze paralysis	Nystagmus	Nystagmus
Speech changes	Dyslexia, dysgraphia, aphasia	Expressive aphasia	Perseveration Dyslexia	Aphasia if dominant hemisphere is involved	Dysarthria		Dysarthria
Mental changes	Memory deficits	Confusion, amnesia Flat affect, apathy Shortened attention span Loss of mental acuity	Memory deficits		Memory loss Disorientation		
Other changes	Vomiting may occur	Apraxia (inability to carry out purposeful movements in nonaffected areas) Incontinence	Visual hallucinations	Mild Horner's syndrome Carotid bruits	Drop attacks Tinnitus, hearing loss Vertigo Dysphagia Coma or locked-in syndrome	Horner's syndrome Tinnitus, hearing loss	Horner's syndrome Hiccups and coughing Vertigo Nausea, vomiting

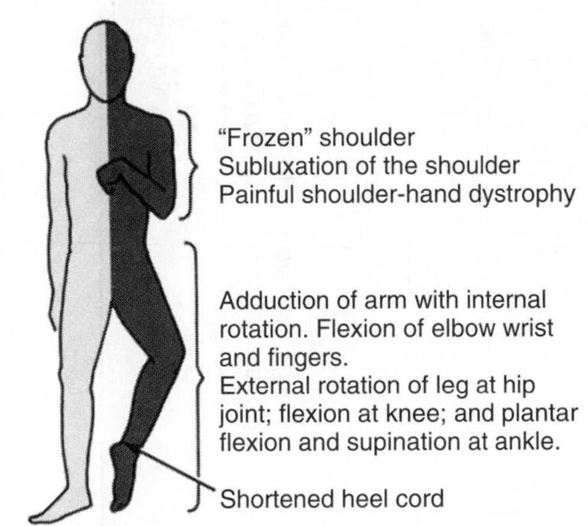

FIGURE 70–2 Hemiplegic contractures. The elbow is bent, the wrist is flexed, and the fingers are curled into palmar flexion; the knee is bent and the heel cord is shortened.

middle cerebral artery supply both areas. *Global aphasia* affects both speech comprehension and speech production.

Other methods of classifying aphasia are by fluency or by the degree of difficulty in articulation. Clients with fluent aphasia (Wernicke's) have speech that is well articulated and grammatically correct but lacks content. Clients with nonfluent aphasia (Broca's) have varying degrees of difficulty in producing speech, and what words are spoken are uttered slowly, with great effort and poor articulation. Clients with global aphasia typically repeat the same sounds they hear and have poor comprehension.

Sensory or fluent aphasias involve loss of the ability to comprehend written, printed, or spoken words. A client with acoustic aphasia can hear the sounds of speech, but the parts of the brain that give meaning to these sounds are damaged. Clients have difficulty understanding what is being said. They hear sound but cannot make sense of it, because they cannot understand the symbolic communication associated with the sound. Visual aphasia is similar. Affected clients cannot read words but can see them. They cannot understand the symbolic content of printed or written symbols.

Motor or nonfluent aphasias include aphasias in which the ability to write, make signs, or speak is lost. For example, with motor aphasia, words may be recalled but the client cannot combine speech sounds into words and syllables. Pure motor or pure sensory aphasias are rare. Most aphasias are mixed, affecting both expressive and receptive elements.

Most aphasias are partial rather than complete. The severity of aphasia varies with the area involved and the extent of cerebral damage. Severe damage may deprive the client of any meaningful relationship with the environment and family. Global aphasia can be so extensive that neither expressive nor receptive language abilities are retained. Early determination of the client's yes-no reliability facilitates communication. Verbal skills are often the best. Reading and writing are usually more impaired. The use of gestures can aid in communication.

Aphasia is frequently associated with hemiplegia involving the dominant hemisphere. The speech center for a right-handed client is usually located in the left cerebral hemisphere; the speech center for a left-handed client may be in the brain's right or left side. Thus, a right-handed client with right-sided hemiplegia usually has aphasia because the speech center is in the damaged left hemisphere. Most people have left-sided speech dominance.

Dysarthria

Dysarthria is imperfect articulation that causes difficulty in speaking. It is important to differentiate between dysarthria and aphasia. With dysarthria, the client understands language but has difficulty pronouncing words and may slur them, enunciating poorly. No disturbance is evident in grammar or in sentence construction. A dysarthric client can understand verbal speech and can read and write (unless the dominant hand is paralyzed, absent, or injured).

Dysarthria is caused by cranial nerve dysfunction from a stroke in the vertebrobasilar artery or its branches. It may result from weakness or paralysis of the muscles of the lips, tongue, and larynx or from a loss of sensation. In addition to speaking problems, clients with dysarthria often have difficulty chewing and swallowing because of poor muscle control.

Dysphagia

Swallowing is a complex process requiring the function of several cranial nerves. The mouth must open (cranial nerve V), the lips must close (cranial nerve VII), and the tongue must move (cranial nerve XII). The mouth must sense the quantity and quality of the food bolus (cranial nerves V and VII) and must send messages to the swallowing center (cranial nerves V and IX). During swallowing, the tongue moves the food bolus toward the oropharynx. The pharynx elevates and the glottis closes. Contraction of the pharyngeal muscles transports food from the pharynx to the esophagus. Peristalsis moves food to the stomach. A stroke in the territory of the vertebrobasilar system causes dysphagia.

Apraxia

Apraxia is a condition affecting complex motor integration and therefore can result from a stroke in several areas in the brain. In apraxia, the client cannot carry out a skilled act such as dressing in the absence of paralysis. A client with apraxia may be able to conceive or conceptualize the content of messages to send to muscles. However, the motor patterns or schema necessary to convey the impulse message cannot be reconstructed. Thus, accurate "instructions" do not reach the limb from the brain, and the desired action or movement does not happen. Apraxia ranges from relatively simple to highly complex disorders. For example, a client may have less difficulty writing than speaking or vice versa.

Visual Changes

Vision is a complex process controlled by several areas in the brain. Parietal and temporal lobe strokes may interrupt visual fibers of the optic tract en route to the occipital cortex and impair visual acuity. Depth perception and visual perception of horizontal and vertical planes may also be impaired. In clients with hemiplegia, this causes motor performance problems in gait and posture (Fig. 70–3). Clients may or may not be aware of a perceptual difficulty, but it may cause them to be accident-prone and

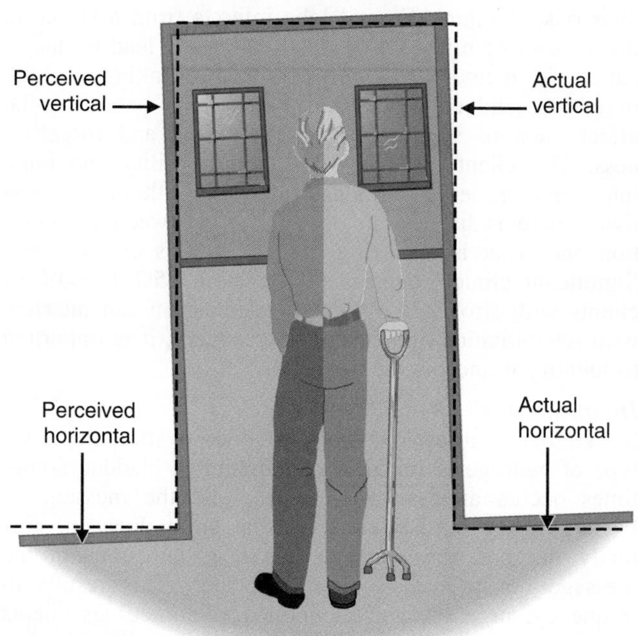

FIGURE 70–3 Perceptual disturbances in hemiplegia. Such disturbances can be both unpleasant and unsafe.

their behavior to appear bizarre. Visual disorders may interfere with a client's ability to relearn motor skills. Infarcts affecting the function of cranial nerves III, IV, and VI may produce cranial nerve palsies and result in diplopia.

HOMONYMOUS HEMIANOPIA. Homonymous hemianopia (Fig. 70–4) is a visual loss in the same half of the visual field of each eye, so the client has only half of normal vision. For example, the client may see clearly on one side of the midline but see nothing on the other side. Clients with homonymous hemianopia cannot see past the midline without turning the head toward that side.

HORNER'S SYNDROME. Horner's syndrome is the paralysis of sympathetic nerves to the eye, causing sinking of the eyeball, ptosis of the upper eyelid, slight elevation of the lower lid, constriction of the pupil, and lack of tearing in the eye.

Agnosia

Agnosia is a disturbance in the ability to recognize familiar objects through the senses. The most common types are visual and auditory. Agnosia may result from an occlusion of the middle or posterior cerebral arteries supplying the temporal or occipital lobes.

A client with visual agnosia sees objects but is unable to recognize or attach meaning to them. Disorientation occurs because of an inability to recognize environmental cues, familiar faces, or symbols. Such a client may examine objects curiously but be unable to determine their function. This can cause considerable self-care deficit when common, necessary objects, such as silverware, clothing, or toilet articles, are unfamiliar. Visual agnosia greatly increases the risk for injury because the client cannot recognize danger or symbols that warn of danger. Extensive visual agnosia can produce such extreme be-

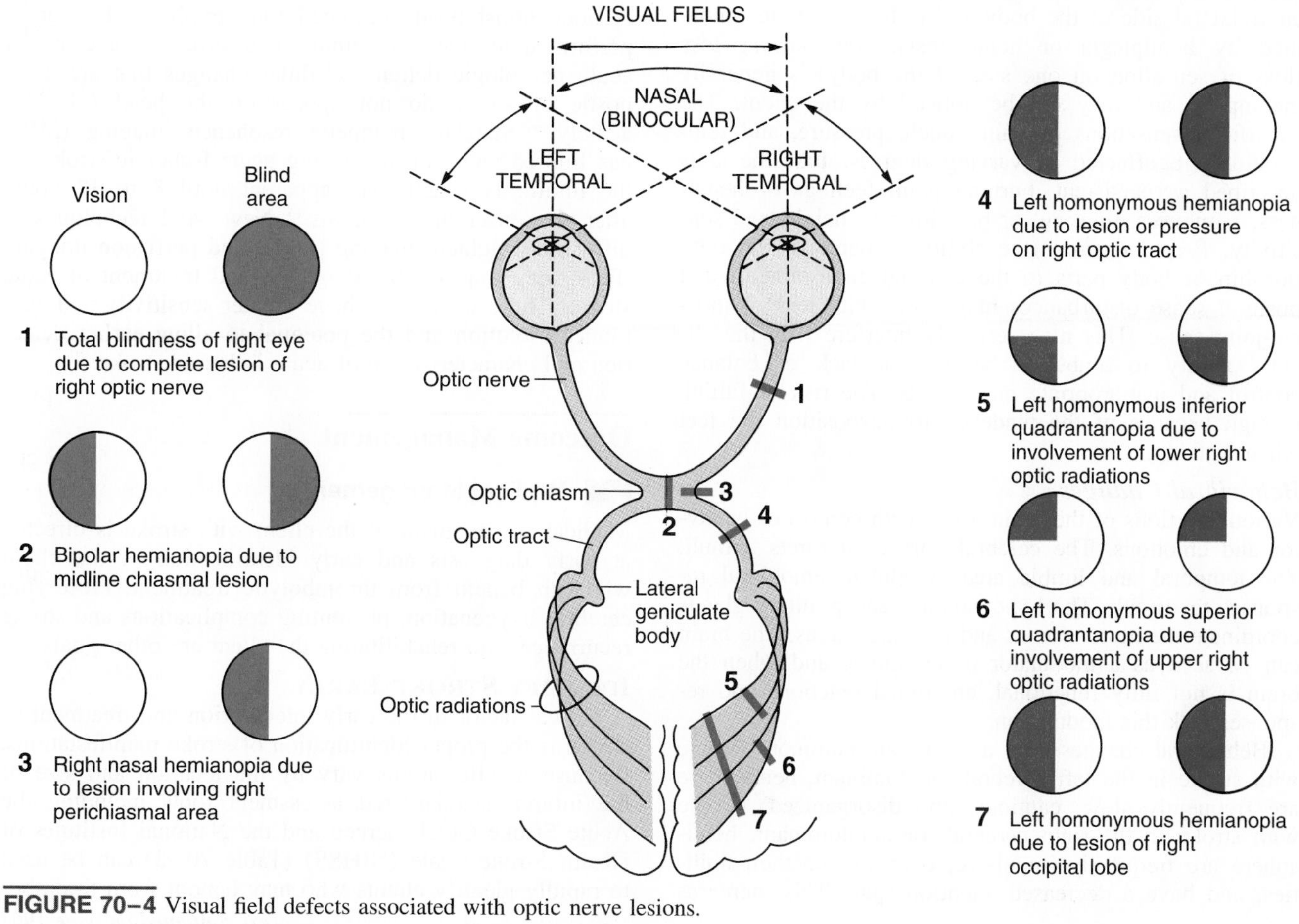

VISUAL FIELDS
NASAL (BINOCULAR)
LEFT TEMPORAL
RIGHT TEMPORAL
Vision
Blind area
Optic nerve
Optic chiasm
Optic tract
Lateral geniculate body
Optic radiations

1 Total blindness of right eye due to complete lesion of right optic nerve

2 Bipolar hemianopia due to midline chiasmal lesion

3 Right nasal hemianopia due to lesion involving right perichiasmal area

4 Left homonymous hemianopia due to lesion or pressure on right optic tract

5 Left homonymous inferior quadrantanopia due to involvement of lower right optic radiations

6 Left homonymous superior quadrantanopia due to involvement of upper right optic radiations

7 Left homonymous hemianopia due to lesion of right occipital lobe

FIGURE 70–4 Visual field defects associated with optic nerve lesions.

havioral effects that the client's condition may be inaccurately diagnosed as diffuse dementia.

A client with auditory agnosia cannot attach meaning to sounds in the absence of hearing loss or decreased level of consciousness. Some degree of aphasia is almost always present. Often, these people are initially considered hysterical or psychotic.

Unilateral Neglect

Unilateral neglect is the inability of a person to respond to stimulus on the contralateral side of a cerebral infarction. Clients with injury to the temporoparietal lobe, inferior parietal lobe, lateral frontal lobe, cingulate gyrus, thalamus, and striatum as a result of a middle cerebral artery occlusion most commonly develop neglect. Because of the dominance of the right hemisphere in directing attention, neglect is most commonly seen in clients with right hemisphere damage.

Clinical manifestations of unilateral neglect include failure to (1) attend to one side of the body, (2) report or respond to stimuli on one side of the body, (3) use one extremity, and (4) orient the head and eyes to one side. Unilateral neglect may be accompanied by inaccurate beliefs about the position of a limb in space or its existence or ownership. For example, a man with unilateral neglect may not believe that his arm is part of his body, he may be unaware of his arm's position, or he may deny that a limb is paralyzed when it is.

Sensory Deficits

Several types of sensory changes can result from a stroke in the sensory strip of the parietal lobe supplied by the anterior or middle cerebral artery. The deficit is on the contralateral side of the body and is frequently accompanied by hemiplegia or hemiparesis. *Hemisensory* loss (loss of sensation on one side of the body) is generally incomplete and may not be noticed by the client. The superficial sensations of pain, touch, pressure, and temperature are affected in varying degrees. Paresthesia is described as persistent, burning pain; feelings of heaviness, numbness, tingling, or prickling; or heightened sensitivity. *Proprioception* (the ability to perceive the relationship of body parts to the external environment) and postural sense disturbances may occur with loss of muscle-joint sense. This may seriously interfere with the client's ability to ambulate because of lack of balance control and inappropriate movements. The risk of falling is high because of the tendency to misposition the feet when walking.

Behavioral Changes

Various portions of the brain assist with control of behavior and emotions. The cerebral cortex interprets stimuli. The temporal and limbic areas modulate emotional responses to stimuli. The hypothalamus and pituitary glands coordinate the motor cortex and language areas. The brain can be seen as a modulator of emotions, and when the brain is not fully functional, emotional reactions and responses lack this modulation.

Behavioral changes after a stroke are common. People with stroke in the left cerebral, or dominant, hemisphere are frequently slow, cautious, and disorganized. People with stroke in the right cerebral, or nondominant, hemisphere are frequently impulsive, overestimate their abilities, and have a decreased attention span. This increases their risk of injury. Frontal lobe infarcts from a stroke in the anterior or middle cerebral arteries may lead to disturbances in memory, judgment, abstract thinking, insight, inhibition, and emotion.[49] The client may exhibit a flat affect, lack of spontaneity, distractibility, and forgetfulness. The client may have emotional lability and burst into tears or, less commonly, laughter without provocation. There is little or no relationship between the emotion and what is occurring in the person's environment. Significant clinical depression occurs in 25% to 60% of clients with strokes.[18, 23] Because depression can interfere with rehabilitation and functional recovery, it is important to identify it and initiate treatment.[35]

Incontinence

Stroke may cause bowel and bladder dysfunction. One type of neurogenic bladder, an uninhibited bladder, sometimes occurs after stroke. Nerves send the message of bladder filling to the brain, but the brain does not correctly interpret the message and does not transmit the message not to urinate to the bladder. This results in frequency, urgency, and incontinence. Sometimes clients with a type of neurogenic bowel seem fixated on having a bowel movement. Other causes of incontinence may be memory lapses, inattention, emotional factors, inability to communicate, impaired physical mobility, and infection. The duration and severity of the dysfunction depend on the extent and location of the infarct.[9]

DIAGNOSTIC FINDINGS

With the advent of thrombolytic therapy in the treatment of acute ischemic stroke, accurate brain imaging plays an important role in the diagnosis and treatment of stroke.[15] A noncontrast head computed tomography (CT) scan is performed to rule out hemorrhagic stroke as a cause of acute neurologic deficits. Cellular changes that are diagnostic of stroke do not appear on the head CT scan acutely.[39] Standard magnetic resonance imaging (MRI) has limited value in diagnosing acute ischemic stroke, as the infarct is usually not apparent until 8 to 12 hours after the onset of symptoms.[15] New MRI techniques—diffusion-weighted imaging (DWI) and perfusion imaging (PI)—may improve the diagnosis and treatment of acute stroke. These techniques have greater sensitivity and anatomic resolution and the potential to allow earlier detection and characterization of acute ischemic stroke.[37]

Outcome Management

Medical Management

Medical management of the client with stroke is directed at early diagnosis and early identification of the client who can benefit from thrombolytic treatment. Preserving cerebral oxygenation, preventing complications and stroke recurrence, and rehabilitating the client are other goals.

IDENTIFY STROKE EARLY

A critical factor in the early intervention and treatment of stroke is the proper identification of stroke manifestations. Because manifestations vary by the location and size of the infarct, standardized assessment tools including the Acute Stroke Quick Screen and the National Institutes of Health Stroke Scale (NIHSS) (Table 70–3) can be used to rapidly identify clients who may benefit from thrombo-

Text continued on page 1963

TABLE 70–3 NATIONAL INSTITUTES OF HEALTH (NIH) STROKE SCALE

Administer stroke scale items in the order listed. Scores should reflect what the patient does, not what the clinician thinks the patient can do. Except where indicated, the patient should not be coached (i.e., repeated requests to patient to make a special effort).

Instruction	Scale Definition
1a. Level of Consciousness The investigator must choose a response, even if a full evaluation is prevented by such obstacles as an endotracheal tube, language barrier, or orotracheal trauma or bandages. A **3** is scored only if the patient makes no movement (other than reflexive posturing) in response to noxious stimulation.	0 = Alert, keenly responsive 1 = Not alert, but arousable by minor stimulation to obey, answer, or respond 2 = Not alert, requires repeated stimulation or painful stimulation to make movements (not stereotyped) 3 = Responds only with reflex motor or autonomic effects, or totally unresponsive, flaccid, areflexic
1b. LOC Questions The patient is asked the month and his or her age. The answer must be correct—there is no partial credit for being close. Aphasic and stuporous patients who do not comprehend the questions will score **2**. Patients unable to speak because of endotracheal intubation, orotracheal trauma, severe dysarthria from any cause, language barrier, or any other problem not secondary to aphasia are given a **1**. It is important that only the initial answer be graded and that the examiner not "help" the patient with verbal or nonverbal cues.	0 = Answers both questions correctly 1 = Answers one question correctly 2 = Answers neither question correctly
1c. LOC Commands The patient is asked to open and close the eyes and then to grip and release the nonparetic hand. Substitute another one-step command if the hands cannot be used. Credit is given if an unequivocal attempt is made but not completed due to weakness. If patients do not respond to command, the task should be demonstrated to them (pantomime) and score the result (i.e., follows none, one, or two commands). Patients with trauma, amputation, or other physical impediments should be given suitable one-step commands. Only the first attempt is scored.	0 = Performs both tasks correctly 1 = Performs one task correctly 2 = Performs neither task correctly
2. Best Gaze Only horizontal eye movements will be tested. Voluntary or reflexive (oculocephalic) eye movements will be scored, but caloric testing is not done. If the patient has a conjugate deviation of the eyes that can be overcome by voluntary or reflexive activity, the score will be **1**. If a patient has an isolated peripheral nerve paresis (CN III, IV, or VI), score a **1**. Gaze is testable in all aphasic patients. Patients with ocular trauma, bandages, pre-existing blindness, or other disorder of visual acuity or fields should be tested with reflexive movements, and a choice made by the investigator. Establishing eye contact and then moving about the patient from side to side will occasionally clarify the presence of a gaze palsy.	0 = Normal 1 = Partial gaze palsy; this score is given when gaze is abnormal in one or both eyes, but where forced deviation or total gaze paresis is not present 2 = Forced deviation or total gaze paresis not overcome by the oculocephalic maneuver
3. Visual Visual fields (upper and lower quadrants) are tested by confrontation, using finger counting or visual threat as appropriate. Patient must be encouraged, but if he or she looks at the side of the moving fingers appropriately, this can be scored as normal. If there is unilateral blindness or enucleation, visual fields in the remaining eye are scored. Score **1** only if a clear-cut asymmetry, including quadrantanopia, is found. If patient is blind from any cause, score **3**. Double simultaneous stimulation is performed at this point. If there is extinction, patient receives a **1** and the results are used to answer question 11.	0 = No visual loss 1 = Partial hemianopia 2 = Complete hemianopia 3 = Bilateral hemianopia (blind including cortical blindness)

Table continued on following page

TABLE 70–3 NATIONAL INSTITUTES OF HEALTH (NIH) STROKE SCALE *Continued*

Instruction	Scale Definition
4. Facial Palsy Ask or use pantomime to encourage the patient to show teeth or smile and close eyes. Score symmetry of grimace in response to noxious stimuli in the poorly responsive or noncomprehending patient. If facial trauma or bandages, orotracheal tube, tape, or other physical barrier obscures the face, these should be removed to the extent possible.	0 = Normal symmetrical movement 1 = Minor paralysis (flattened nasolabial fold, asymmetry on smiling) 2 = Partial paralysis (total or near total paralysis of lower face) 3 = Complete paralysis (absence of facial movement in the upper and lower face)
5 and 6. Motor Arm and Leg The limb is placed in the appropriate position: extend the arms 90 degrees (if sitting) or 45 degrees (if supine) and the leg 30 degrees (always tested supine). Drift is scored if the arm falls before 10 seconds or the leg before 5 seconds. The aphasic patient is encouraged using urgency in the voice and pantomime but not noxious stimulation. Each limb is tested in turn, beginning with the nonparetic arm. Only in the case of amputation or joint fusion at the shoulder or hip may the score be **9**, and the examiner must clearly write the explanation for scoring as a **9**.	0 = No drift; limb holds 90 degrees (or 45 degrees) for full 10 seconds 1 = Drift; limb holds 90 degrees (or 45 degrees) but drifts down before full 10 seconds; does not hit bed or other support 2 = Some effort against gravity; limb cannot get to or maintain (if cued) 90 degrees (or 45 degrees), drifts down to bed but has some effort against gravity 3 = No effort against gravity; limb falls 4 = No movement 9 = Amputation, joint fusion; explain: 5a = Left arm 5b = Right arm
	0 = No drift; leg holds 30 degrees for full 5 seconds 1 = Drift; leg falls by the end of the 5-second period but does not hit bed 2 = Some effort against gravity; leg falls to bed by 5 seconds but has some effort against gravity 3 = No effort against gravity; leg falls to bed immediately 4 = No movement 9 = Amputation, joint fusion; explain: 6a = Left leg 6b = Right leg
7. Limb Ataxia This item is aimed at finding evidence of a unilateral cerebellar lesion. Test with eyes open. In case of visual defect, ensure testing is done in intact visual field. The finger-nose-finger and heel-shin tests are performed on both sides, and ataxia is scored only if present out of proportion to weakness. Ataxia is absent in the patient who cannot understand or is hemiplegic. Only in the case of amputation or joint fusion may the item be scored **9**, and the examiner must clearly write the explanation for not scoring. In case of blindness, test by touching nose from extended arm position.	0 = Absent 1 = Present in one limb 2 = Present in two limbs If present, is ataxia in Right arm: 1 = Yes 2 = No 9 = Amputation or joint fusion; explain: Left arm: 1 = Yes 2 = No 9 = Amputation or joint fusion; explain: Right leg: 1 = Yes 2 = No 9 = Amputation or joint fusion; explain: Left leg: 1 = Yes 2 = No 9 = Amputation or joint fusion; explain:
8. Sensory Sensation or grimace to pinprick when tested or withdrawal from noxious stimulus in the obtunded or aphasic patient. Only sensory loss attributed to stroke is scored as abnormal, and the examiner should test as many body areas (arms [not hands], legs, trunk, face) as needed to accurately check for hemisensory loss. A score of **2**, "severe or total," should only be given when a severe or total loss of sensation can be clearly demonstrated. Stuporous and aphasic patients will therefore probably score **1** or **0**. The patient with brain stem stroke who has bilateral loss of sensation is scored **2**. If the patient does not respond and is quadriplegic, score **2**. Patients in coma (question 1a = 3) are arbitrarily given a **2** on this item.	0 = Normal; no sensory loss 1 = Mild to moderate sensory loss; patient feels pinprick is less sharp or is dull on the affected side, or there is a loss of superficial pain with pinprick but patient is aware he or she is being touched 2 = Severe to total sensory loss; patient is not aware of being touched

TABLE 70–3 NATIONAL INSTITUTES OF HEALTH (NIH) STROKE SCALE *Continued*

Instruction	Scale Definition
9. Best Language A great deal of information about comprehension will be obtained during the preceding sections of the examination. The patient is asked to describe what is happening in the attached picture, to name the items on the attached naming sheet, and to read from the attached list of sentences. Comprehension is judged from responses here as well as to all of the commands in the preceding general neurologic examination. If visual loss interferes with the tests, ask the patient to identify objects placed in the hand, repeat, and produce speech. The intubated patient should be asked to write a sentence. The patient in coma (question 1a = 3) will arbitrarily score **3** on this item. The examiner must choose a score in the patient with stupor or limited cooperation, but a score of **3** should be used only if the patient is mute and follows no one-step commands.	0 = No aphasia; normal 1 = Mild to moderate aphasia; some obvious loss of fluency or facility of comprehension, without significant limitation on ideas expressed or form of expression. Reduction of speech and/or comprehension, however, makes conversation about provided material difficult or impossible. For example, in conversation about provided materials examiner can identify picture or naming card from patient's response. 2 = Severe aphasia; all communication is through fragmentary expression; great need for inference, questioning, and guessing by the listener. Range of information that can be exchanged is limited; listener carries burden of communication. Examiner cannot identify materials provided from patient response. 3 = Mute, global aphasia; no usable speech or auditory comprehension
10. Dysarthria If the patient is thought to be normal, an adequate sample of speech must be obtained by asking patient to read or repeat words from the attached list. If the patient has severe aphasia, the clarity of articulation of spontaneous speech can be rated. Only if the patient is intubated or has other physical barriers to producing speech may the item be scored **9**, and the examiner must clearly write an explanation for not scoring. Do not tell the patient why he or she is being tested.	0 = Normal 1 = Mild to moderate; patient slurs at least some words and, at worst, can be understood with some difficulty 2 = Severe; patient's speech is so slurred as to be unintelligible in the absence of or out of proportion to any dysphasia, or is mute/anarthric 9 = Intubated or other physical barrier; explain:
11. Extinction and Inattention (formerly Neglect) Sufficient information to identify neglect may be obtained during the prior testing. If the patient has severe visual loss preventing visual double simultaneous stimulation, and the cutaneous stimuli are normal, the score is normal. If the patient has aphasia but does appear to attend to both sides, the score is normal. The presence of visual spatial neglect or anosognosia may also be taken as evidence of neglect. Because neglect is scored only if present, the item is never untestable.	0 = No abnormality 1 = Visual, tactile, auditory, spatial, or personal inattention or extinction to bilateral simultaneous stimulation in one of the sensory modalities 2 = Profound hemi-inattention or hemi-inattention to more than one modality; does not recognize own hand or orients to only one side of space
Additional item, not part of the NIH Stroke Scale score.	
12. Distal Motor Function The patient's hand is held up at the forearm by the examiner, and patient is asked to extend his or her fingers as much as possible. If the patient cannot or does not extend the fingers, the examiner places the fingers in full extension and observes for any flexion movement for 5 seconds. The patient's first attempts only are scored. Repetition of the instructions or of the testing is prohibited.	0 = Normal (no flexion after 5 seconds) 1 = At least some extension after 5 seconds but not fully extended; any movement of the fingers that is not a command is not scored 2 = No voluntary extension after 5 seconds; movement of the fingers at another time is not scored a. Left arm b. Right arm

CN, cranial nerve; LOC, level of consciousness.
Modified from National Institutes of Health, Bethesda, MD.

lytic therapy.[39, 46] The assessment must be complete and accurate to provide a baseline for ongoing assessments.

The initial assessment of the client who is thought to have had a stroke includes level of consciousness, pupillary response to light, visual fields, movement of extremities, speech, sensation, reflexes, ataxia, and vital signs. These data are often recorded and scored on the Glasgow Coma Scale (GCS). In addition, if intracranial pressure monitors are in place, baseline pressure values and waveforms should be noted.

A complete history of the presenting problem as well as past medical and social history provides data about the cause of the stroke. This information also guides stroke treatment. The time of onset of manifestations must be determined, as thrombolytic therapy must be administered within 3 hours of the onset of manifestations. A history of hypertension or cardiac valve disorders is commonly associated with stroke.

MAINTAIN CEREBRAL OXYGENATION

Emergency care of the client with stroke includes maintaining a patent airway. The client should be turned on the affected side if he or she is unconscious, to promote drainage of saliva from the airway. The collar of the shirt should be loosened to facilitate venous return. The head should be elevated, but the neck should not be flexed. The person should be kept quiet, and emergency help should be contacted.

Once the client is in the emergency department (ED), a patent airway is maintained and oxygen is supplied. If the client demonstrates poor ventilatory effort, intubation and mechanical ventilation may be required to prevent hypoxia and increased cerebral ischemia. An ECG is performed to assess for cardiac disorders, such as atrial fibrillation, that increase the risk for embolic stroke. Blood pressure is also evaluated, and hypertension may be reduced with vasodilators. Caution is exercised when treating blood pressure, as lowering the blood pressure too far may lower cerebral perfusion pressure and increase cerebral ischemia.[19, 39] Laboratory tests for hematology, chemistry, and coagulation are obtained to rule out stroke-mimicking conditions and to detect bleeding disorders that would increase the risk of bleeding during thrombolytic therapy.

RESTORE CEREBRAL BLOOD FLOW

The client is evaluated as a candidate for thrombolytic therapy once an intracerebral hemorrhage is ruled out. The goal of thrombolytic therapy is recanalization of the occluded vessel and reperfusion of ischemic brain tissue.[13, 26] Thrombolytic agents are exogenous plasminogen activators, which dissolve the thrombus or embolus blocking the cerebral blood flow.[27] Clients who receive recombinant tissue plasminogen activator (rt-PA) within 3 hours of the onset of stroke are 30% more likely to have minimal or no disability from acute ischemic stroke without an increase in mortality.[31, 38]

There are several contraindications to thrombolytic therapy:

- More than 3 hours from onset
- Intracranial hemorrhage on CT scan
- Rapidly improving stroke manifestations or TIA
- Recent stroke, intracranial surgery, or head trauma
- Uncontrolled hypertension
- Conditions that may increase the risk for systemic bleeding, such as active internal bleeding within 21 days, a major surgery within 14 days, or current use of oral anticoagulants, are also contraindications for thrombolytic therapy.

Treatment should begin immediately after the client is deemed to be a candidate for rt-PA. The dose of rt-PA for acute ischemic stroke is 0.9 mg/kg administered intravenously over 1 hour. Ten per cent of the total dose is given as a bolus over 1 minute prior to the initiation of the intravenous dose.[32, 38, 39] The pharmacologic half-life of rt-PA is approximately 5 to 7 minutes. After thrombolytic therapy, the client is sent to the intensive care unit (ICU) for careful monitoring of blood pressure, neurologic status, and bleeding.

The risk-benefit ratio for the use of thrombolytic therapy must be considered in certain client populations. The choice of whether to pursue aggressive treatment focuses on several factors, such as the client's age, his or her preference (if known), the presence and severity of other disorders, the size of the infarction, how much time has elapsed since the infarction, and the rehabilitation potential. The risk of intracerebral hemorrhage after rt-PA is greater in clients with early signs of a major infarct on CT scan.[47, 50] People with severe neurologic deficits at presentation (NIHSS > 22) are at increased risk for intracerebral hemorrhage and poor outcome.[39, 50]

At present, the treatment for most clients with large areas of infarction or large intracerebral hemorrhage is supportive care. It is hoped that future research can improve the treatment outcomes for these clients.

PREVENT COMPLICATIONS

Bleeding

Following the administration of rt-PA, the client is monitored for potential complications of rt-PA, which may include intracranial hemorrhage and systemic bleeding.[1] In the initial studies of rt-PA in acute ischemic stroke, symptomatic intracranial hemorrhage occurred in 6.4% of clients within the first 36 hours after treatment.[31] Intracranial hemorrhage carries a mortality rate of greater than 50%.[26] All fatal intracranial hemorrhages occurred within the first 24 hours of treatment.[1] The expanding clot of an intracranial hemorrhage destroys brain tissue. The pressure of the clot also disrupts blood flow and causes additional ischemia. Increased intracranial pressure (ICP) results from the space-occupying clot and surrounding edema of ischemic tissue. This can lead to midline shift of intracranial contents, possible brain stem herniation, and death. To decrease the risk of intracranial or systemic bleeding, anticoagulants and antiplatelet medications are not recommended until 24 hours after administration of rt-PA.[5]

Stringent blood pressure management is the single most important measure to prevent intracranial hemorrhage after thrombolysis.[1] Frequent vital signs and neurologic checks are necessary to prevent hypertension and detect signs of intracranial hemorrhage. Hypertension frequently accompanies acute ischemic stroke. Therefore, blood pressure is usually not treated unless it increases to 185 mm Hg systolic or 105 mm Hg diastolic.[1] In addition, the mean arterial pressure should be lowered no more than 10% and in gradual increments.[43] This is less likely to lead to hypoperfusion and worsening cerebral ischemia.

An intracranial hemorrhage should be suspected if the client has new complaints of headache, nausea and vomiting, or sudden change in level of consciousness. An intracranial hemorrhage should be assumed with any acute worsening of neurologic function until it can be ruled out by CT scan. If the rt-PA is still infusing, the infusion should be stopped. A complete blood count, coagulation studies, and type and cross are done. If a head CT scan reveals intracranial hemorrhage, fresh frozen plasma with fibrinogen or cryoprecipitate is administered to correct coagulopathies.

Systemic bleeding may also occur as a complication of rt-PA. Clinical manifestations include change in level of consciousness (LOC), tachycardia, hypotension, and cool, clammy, and pale skin. Thrombolytic therapy may be stopped depending on the site and severity of the bleeding.[19]

Cerebral Edema

Increased ICP is a potential complication of large ischemic strokes.[29] Increased ICP is also a potential complication of intracerebral hemorrhage, either primary or secondary to thrombolytic therapy. Manifestations of increased ICP include change in LOC, reflex hypertension, and worsening neurologic status. Invasive monitoring of ICP is done for those clients with decreased LOC who are at high risk for increased ICP. All clients are placed on bed rest with the head of the bed elevated to 30 degrees to decrease ICP and to facilitate venous drainage. Ideally, the degree of head elevation is based on the response of the client's ICP for those clients on ICP monitoring.[30, 44]

External *ventriculostomy* drainage is sometimes used to reduce pressure from cerebrospinal fluid (CSF) accumulation. A burr hole is placed through the skull, and a catheter is passed into the lateral ventricle to allow for controlled drainage of CSF. Blood pressure is closely monitored. The goal is to maintain blood pressure low enough to prevent another stroke or hemorrhage without decreasing cerebral perfusion. The client may require continuous mechanical ventilation and hyperventilation to decrease ICP. Mannitol, an osmotic diuretic, helps in lowering increased ICP. Surgical evacuation of the intracerebral hematoma may be performed. Increasing ICP, central herniation, and brain stem hemorrhage lead to death from depression of the vital centers in the medulla, that is, brain stem failure.

Stroke Recurrence

The incidence of stroke recurrence in the first 4 weeks after acute ischemic stroke ranges from 0.6% to 2.2% per week.[48] The risks of anticoagulation include intracranial hemorrhage, systemic bleeding, and death. Therefore, the general use of heparin in all clients with acute ischemic stroke is no longer recommended. Heparin is indicated to prevent stroke recurrence in clients at risk for cardiogenic emboli. Initially, unfractionated heparin is administered intravenously, and then warfarin is administered orally. Intravenous (IV) heparin is delivered with an infusion pump for accurate and safe delivery. Monitoring of clotting times is important to detect overanticoagulation, which increases the risk of bleeding. Activated partial thromboplastin time (aPTT) should be at 1.5 to 2.5 times control for anticoagulation to be effective.

After a therapeutic anticoagulant level has been achieved with heparin therapy, warfarin is begun. Because warfarin has a long half-life, the physician initiates the warfarin therapy while the client is still receiving IV heparin. Once the client has a therapeutic response to warfarin, in about 24 to 48 hours, the physician discontinues the heparin and continues the warfarin therapy. The therapeutic International Normalized Ratio (INR) for prophylaxis against cardiogenic embolization is 2.0 to 3.0.[43] Clients receiving anticoagulation therapy should be assessed for bruising, hematuria, blood in feces, bleeding from mucous membranes, and new-onset or worsening headaches.

The long-term risk for stroke recurrence is 4% to 14% per year.[1] Antiplatelet agents, including aspirin, ticlopidine, and clopidogrel, decrease the risk for secondary stroke by 20% to 25%.[7, 40] Antiplatelet agents inhibit platelet function to decrease the risk of thrombus formation. The selection of the specific antiplatelet agent is individualized according to the client's medical history.

Aspiration

Clients with stroke are at high risk for aspiration pneumonia, which is the direct cause of death in 6% of strokes.[3] Aspiration is most common in the early period and is related to loss of pharyngeal sensation, loss of oropharyngeal motor control, and decreased LOC. Oral food and fluids are generally withheld for 24 to 48 hours. If the client cannot eat or drink after 48 hours, alternate feeding routes are used, such as tube-feeding or hyperalimentation. When the swallowing mechanism has returned, the client can be fed orally. Progressive feeding programs for dysphagia are based on the degree of swallowing ability.

Other Potential Complications

Other complications of stroke depend primarily on the location of the lesion or infarcted tissue. If the brain stem is affected, blood pressure fluctuations, altered respiratory patterns, and cardiac dysrhythmias are all possible. Physical injury related to the client's inability to realize his or her limitations can occur. Complications of immobility can also occur.

Coma can follow strokes of various causes. The blood supply to the brain stem or reticular activating system, which controls consciousness, may have been directly occluded. Similarly, the deep structures of the thalamus that relay information to the cerebral cortex may be involved. Vascular occlusion of the internal carotid artery or one of its major branches may also decrease LOC. Sometimes the cerebral edema that follows stroke may produce midline shifts, resulting in coma.

Hyperthermia is treated immediately with antipyretics. Temperature elevations lead to increased cerebral metabolic needs, which in turn cause cerebral edema and increased risk for cerebral ischemia. In addition, a hypothermia blanket or ice packs may be required to reduce body temperature. Causing the client to shiver should be avoided, however, because shivering increases oxygen consumption and ICP. If seizures develop, phenytoin (Dilantin) or phenobarbital may be used.

Strokes caused by occlusive disease (e.g., thrombus, embolus) rarely cause sudden death. When stroke is fatal, death may occur within 3 to 12 hours, but it more often occurs between 1 and 14 days after the original episode. Typically, with any type of fatal stroke, a rise in temperature, heart rate, and respiratory rate occurs along with deepening coma several hours or days before death. These are a result of damage to the vasomotor and heat-regulating centers. See the Case Study.

Rehabilitation After Stroke

From the onset of stroke, interventions are aimed at maximizing the client's physical and cognitive recovery.[16] Early premobilization efforts are aimed at preventing the complications of neurologic deficit and immobility. After the first few days of the acute event, cerebral edema has usually subsided and the residual deficits of stroke can be identified. Clients with stroke and their families face diffi-

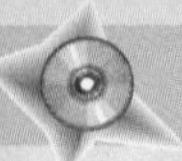

Meningioma, Fractured Hip, and Possible Cerebrovascular Accident

Mrs. Olsen is a 72-year-old white woman who resides at Shady Oaks Care Center. She fell today and could not get up again because of the pain. An x-ray obtained at the nursing home showed a proximal femoral fracture near the right hip joint. She has been transferred to your hospital for a preoperative medical evaluation in preparation for possible surgical repair of her right hip fracture later today.

Mrs. Olsen has a history of a meningioma, which has been resected three times. Two days ago, the client had an episode of apparent dysfunction of the left upper and lower extremities associated with a period of hypertension and agitation, all of which resolved within 24 hours. Mrs. Olsen also has a history of deep vein thrombosis (DVT) following one of her surgical procedures, but is not receiving long-term anticoagulation therapy. What ramifications will this have for her current treatment?

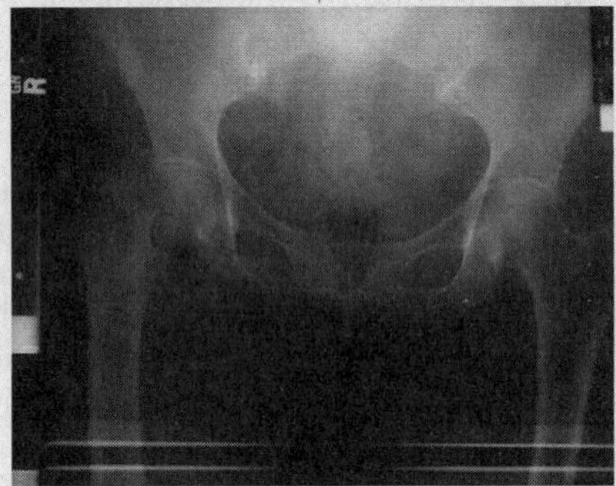

■ Radiograph of Mrs. Olsen's fracture of the proximal femur, near the right hip joint.

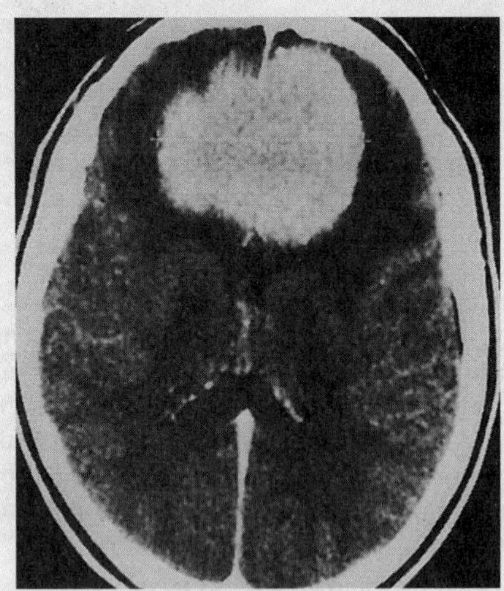

■ This contrast CT scan shows Mrs. Olsen's meningioma before resection.

Nursing Admission Assessment

Mrs. Olsen has lived at Shady Oaks since her last craniotomy, after which she developed seizures and was given a regimen of phenytoin. The daughter states that her mother has had several falls during the past several days and seems imbalanced at times when she changes position.

Mrs. Olsen is a World War II immigrant from Denmark, where her siblings continue to live. Since her last craniotomy, she has been lapsing into intervals during which she uses her native language and believes that her daughter is her sister Ingrid. Consider the implications of this in your preoperative preparations. Mrs. Olsen denies discomfort at this time.

Mrs. Olsen taught high school mathematics until the time of her first craniotomy 10 years ago. Her husband died of a myocardial infarction last year.

Selected Admission Laboratory Values	
RBC	3.76 million/mm^3
Hb	11.7 g/dl
Hct	34%
WBC	10,200/mm^3
Sodium	141 mEq/L
Potassium	4.3 mEq/L
Chloride	101 mEq/L
CO_2	22 mEq/L
Glucose	157 mg/dl
ABO/Rh type	O^+
Phenytoin level	7.6 μg/ml

Nursing Physical Examination

Height: 5′6″
Weight: 135 lb (61.4 kg)
Vital signs: BP = 170/90; TPR = 99.6, 102, 22
LOC: Awake, alert, slightly confused; daughter states that she is asking in Danish where she is and what happened
EENT: PERRLA, evidence of cranial surgical scars on right frontal region, slight left facial droop, hand grasps equal
Cardiac: Regular rate and rhythm without gallop or murmur
Pulmonary: Clear bilaterally
Abdominal: Soft, nontender, active bowel sounds
Genitourinary: Foley catheter inserted in ER draining clear yellow urine
Peripheral pulses: 3/4 without edema, some shortening of right lower extremity

Initial Treatment Plan

Meds: Phenytoin (Dilantin) 200 mg PO or IV bid
IV: D_5LR TKO
Diet: NPO
Activity: Bed rest with mattress overlay and trapeze

Additional assessments: Vital signs, neurologic checks, and neurovascular assessments checks q 4 h
Treatments: Ice to right hip continuously
Diagnostic tests: CT scan of head

Mrs. Olsen's CT scan revealed no further progression of her meningioma. She successfully underwent surgery for endoprosthetic replacement of the right proximal femur. Postoperatively, the surgeon orders:

- Advance diet as tolerated
- Soft wrist and Posey restraints as needed to protect self
- Physical therapy to initiate progressive ambulation with weight-bearing as tolerated
- Incentive spirometer while awake
- Medical therapy: cefazolin (Ancef) 1 g IV q 8 h × 4, Lovenox 30 mg SC q 12 h, docusate sodium (Colace) 100 mg PO daily, meperidine (Demerol) 75 mg with hydroxyzine (Vistaril) 25 mg IM q 3 h prn; and Vicodin 500 mg q 4 h prn.

Mrs. Olsen pulls out her Foley catheter 36 hours postoperatively. The urine had become cloudy and odorous. Recordings of the time and amount of voiding and trimethoprim-sulfamethoxazole (Bactrim) 1 tablet PO bid are ordered. Consider the factors that precipitated the need for this drug.

Mrs. Olsen continues to speak primarily in Danish. Because she is incontinent, she requires disposable undergarments. She also refuses to eat, and the nurse is unable to determine why. The IV infusion was discontinued after Mrs. Olsen pulled it out during her bath. Attempts at ambulation have been unsuccessful because of communication difficulties. A Danish interpreter is not available, and although Mrs. Olsen's daughter speaks Danish, she has had to return to her job and family responsibilities. The physician is planning to release Mrs. Olsen to Shady Oaks tomorrow.

Discharge Criteria

Average LOS (insurance certification): 8.5 days with transfer to skilled care on day 5.
Complete transfer form.
Initiate social services referral to coordinate transfer.

Questions to Be Considered

1. Mrs. Olsen becomes increasingly agitated while in restraints. What alternative measures might the nurse consider to protect Mrs. Olsen? Discuss the ethical implications surrounding physical and chemical restraints.
2. Consider the implications that Mrs. Olsen's neurologic problems—the meningioma, seizures, and a possible CVA—may have had in relationship to her fall. What other factors may have contributed to the fall? What actions should the nurse take to protect her from future injury?
3. Based on her admission assessment data, calculate Mrs. Olsen's score on the Glasgow Coma Scale. What influence does Mrs. Olsen's use of the Danish language have on your calculation? How is her situation different from someone who is not bilingual?
4. How has Mrs. Olsen's recovery been compromised because of her lack of mobilization? Identify potential complications that may occur as a result of immobility. How may they be prevented? Discuss methods of communication you might use to facilitate Mrs. Olsen's recovery and rehabilitation.
5. Discuss the effects that Mrs. Olsen's refusal to eat will have on the processes of wound healing and immunity.
6. Review the nursing implications and related patient education for administration of phenytoin and trimethoprim-sulfamethoxazole.
7. Compare and contrast brain tumors in terms of treatment and prognosis.

---

bid, twice daily; CO_2, carbon dioxide; CT, computed tomography; CVA, cerebrovascular accident; D_5LR, 5% dextrose in lactated Ringer's solution; ER, emergency room; EENT, ears, eyes, nose, throat; Hb, hemoglobin; Hct, hematocrit; μg, micrograms; IV, intravenous; LOC, level of consciousness; LOS, length of stay; NPO, nothing by mouth; PERRLA, pupils equal, round, reactive to light and accommodation; PO, orally; prn, as needed; RBC, red blood cell; SC, subcutaneous; TKO, to keep open; TPR, temperature, pulse, respirations; WBC, white blood cell count.

cult adjustments as the acute stages pass and residual disabilities become obvious.

Previously it had been thought that damage to the central nervous system (CNS) was irreversible. Now it has been shown that even in adults with significant brain injury, relearning can take place. It is extremely important that relearning take place as soon as possible after the injury. Early rehabilitation makes this relearning possible. Clients recover most of their function during the first 3 to 6 months after stroke but may continue to demonstrate modest improvement for 6 to 12 months after stroke.[23]

An interdisciplinary rehabilitation team is necessary to assist and support clients and their families during this time. Assessing the functional abilities of the client and setting realistic goals are part of this approach. To optimize recovery, all clinicians should use the Clinical Practice Guidelines developed by the Agency for Health Care Policy and Research (AHCPR) on post-stroke rehabilitation to guide care of a client suffering from a stroke.[35, 36]

Because stroke is a common health care problem, many facilities have developed clinical pathways to guide care. (See CareMap and Guide to Clinical Pathway.)

The recommended plan of care includes using interdisciplinary services to:

- Document the client's condition and course fully, including deficits, status of other diseases, complications, changes in status, and functional status before stroke
- Begin physical activity as soon as the client's medical condition is stable; use caution with early mobilization in clients with progressing neurologic deficit, subarachnoid or intracerebral hemorrhage, severe orthostatic hypotension, acute myocardial infarction, or acute deep vein thrombosis
- Assist in managing general health functions throughout all stages of treatment, such as managing dysphagia, nutrition, hydration, bladder and bowel function, sleep and rest, co-morbid conditions, and acute illnesses

- Prevent complications, including deep vein thrombosis and pulmonary embolism, aspiration, skin breakdown, urinary tract infections, falls, spasticity and contractures, shoulder injury, and seizures
- Prevent recurrent strokes through control of modifiable risk factors, oral anticoagulation, antiplatelet therapy, or surgical intervention
- Assess throughout acute and rehabilitation stages
- Use reliable standardized instruments for evaluation
- Evaluate for formal rehabilitation during acute stage
- Choose individual or interdisciplinary program based on the client's and family's needs; success of the program requires full support and active participation of the client and family; families must be involved at the outset
- Choose the local rehabilitation program that best meets the client's and family's needs

INTERDISCIPLINARY MANAGEMENT

Several other disciplines join to facilitate recovery of the client following a stroke. It is the coordinated effort of the entire team that best serves the client and family.

GUIDE TO CLINICAL PATHWAY

Stroke

The care of a client with a stroke revolves around quick diagnosis and treatment. Some strokes, if detected early, can be treated with fibrinolytic medications. This care map guides the care of a client with a completed stroke. The expected length of stay is 5 days to diagnose and treat the stroke and to begin rehabilitation of the client and family.

By the second day of hospitalization, the client will have undergone computed tomography, carotid Doppler imaging, and echocardiography. On day 2, a key aspect of recovery is to initiate rehabilitation by the physical, occupational, and speech-language therapists. These therapists continue to treat the client following hospital discharge.

Because the stroke can still be evolving at day 2, neurologic status must be accurately assessed; review the techniques for this assessment. Assessment of changes in cognition is the key indicator of changes in intracranial pressure. Continue to teach the client not to get up without assistance. Monitor the client for aspiration, seizures, and bleeding from anticoagulant therapy. Expect to monitor prothrombin time, partial thromboplastin time, and the International Normalized Ratio to regulate the amount of anticoagulation needed. The amount of heparin infused may vary throughout the day.

Monitor blood pressure carefully; elevations in blood pressure can injure the brain and increase the risk of bleeding. Follow precautions closely to maintain blood pressure in desired range.

The CareMap is reprinted with permission from Baptist Health System.

The CareMap shown is an excerpt of one that covers emergency department admission through day 5.

Helen Andrews, BSN, RN, *Care Manager, Alegent Health Bergan Mercy Medical Center, Omaha, Nebraska,* and **Linda R. Haddick, MSN, RN,** *Clinical Nurse Specialist, Alegent Health Home Care & Hospice, Omaha, Nebraska*

Physical Therapy

Physical therapists work with the client to build strength and preserve range of motion (ROM) and tone in noninvolved muscles. Physical therapy also builds ROM and tone and retrains muscles affected by the stroke. The client also works on balance and proprioception skills. This may enable the client, with continued improvement, to sit on the edge of the bed and to eventually ambulate. Exercise and bed mobility skills are taught at the client's bedside, as are wheelchair mobility and transfers. Clients who would benefit from the use of an orthosis are identified and instructed on how to apply and remove it. A hemiplegic client is usually able to ambulate using a quad cane following gait training.

Occupational Therapy

Occupational therapists work with the client to relearn activities of daily living (ADL) and to use assistive devices that promote independence. For example, a client with hemiplegia may be able to dress if the clothing can be closed with self-fastening tape (Velcro) fasteners rather than buttons.

Many clients experience severe pain in the affected shoulder and hand after a stroke. This pain can be so severe that it results in lack of balance and loss of ROM, which further restricts mobility and self-care. Overstretching from turns and transfers can aggravate the problem. Some clients have experienced partial dislocation or subluxation of the shoulder both from having the shoulder pulled on and from the weight of the arm pulling it. Chronic subluxation results in shoulder-hand syndrome, characterized by a painful or frozen shoulder and hand edema. Occupational therapists assist in treating this problem and in instructing the client and caregivers in proper transfer and positioning techniques to prevent further injury.

Speech Therapy

Speech pathologists work with the client to foster the maximum amount of speech recovery possible through relearning, accentuation of speech sounds, or use of alternative communication devices. The speech pathologist also assesses the client's swallowing mechanism and makes recommendations for initiation and progression of foods and fluids to decrease the risk of aspiration.

Case Management

Case managers are often assigned to clients following stroke. Their role is to facilitate all care providers and to advocate for the client and family. (See Case Management feature.)

Nursing Management of the Medical Client

ASSESSMENT

Ongoing assessments of all body systems are needed. The use of a standardized neurologic assessment tool such as the GCS assists the nurse in documenting changes in the client's status and in monitoring progress. In addition to the neurologic assessment, the client's heart sounds, heart rate and rhythm, respiratory rate and rhythm, temperature, levels of nutrition, ability to swallow, bladder and bowel elimination, communication, and sexuality need to be assessed. The client's and family's psychosocial and learning needs should be assessed daily.

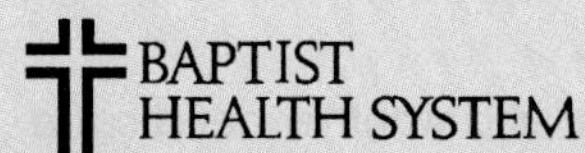

CVA/TIA CAREMAP
DAY 2 AND DAY 3

	DAY 2 Date: ______	INITIAL Met	Not Met	DAY 3 Date: ______	INITIAL Met	Not Met
General Safety:	Bed rails up, call light within reach, fall precautions, seizure precautions, bleeding precautions, airway precautions.			Bed rails up, call light within reach, fall precautions, seizure precautions, bleeding precautions, airway precautions.		
Activity	Note PT/OT/ST treatment recommendations &/or activity as tolerated.			Progress as tolerated.		
	Goal: Tolerates activity progression.	____	____	**Goal:** Performs ADL's as independently as possible with adaptive equipment.	____	____
Dietary: Consult Date/Time Completed ____	Diet as tolerated. If not tolerating diet, consider calorie counts.			Diet as tolerated. If not tolerating diet, consider calorie counts. Instruct re: food/drug interaction if applicable.		
	Goal: Tolerates > 50% diet.	____	____	**Goal:** Tolerates > 50% diet. Food/Drug Interaction Education Initiated.	____ ____	____ ____
Respiratory: Consult Date/Time Completed ____	Wean O2 if indicated.			Wean O2 as indicated		
	Goal: SaO2 ≥ 92% on RA &/or with supplemental O2.	____	____	**Goal:** SaO2 ≥ 92% on RA or with supplemental O2.	____	____
Rehab: Consult Date/Time Completed ____	Continue PT/OT/ST as ordered.			Continue PT/OT/ST as ordered.		
	Goal: Tolerates activities/Rehab	____	____	**Goal:** Tolerates activities/Rehab progression.	____	____
Discharge Planning: Consult Date/Time Completed ____	Continue to assess discharge disposition Rehab to recommend appropriate disposition/ needs @ D/C.			Continue to assess discharge disposition. Rehab to recommend appropriate disposition/ needs @ D/C. Assess home equipment needs if planned discharged to home. Identify community resources needed.		
	Goal: Discharge plan initiated.	____	____	**Goal:** Refer to TCF/Rehab (Easy St)/NH/ Home Health as ordered.	____	____
Nursing: Consult Date/Time Completed ____	VS & neuro checks q 4 h, I & O q 8 h. Notify MD if: Change in neuro status Systolic BP≥220 &/or DBP≥110 HR ≥ 150 or ≤ 50 RR ≥ 30 Temp ≥ 101 IV fluids - NS (Avoid D5W). DVT prophylaxis: Sequential hose for non-ambulating patients. Following swallowing guidelines as indicated. Elevate weak/flaccid upper extremity on pillow. Refer to CVA/TIA Patient Info. Handbook and CVA Patient/Family Caremap.			VS & neuro checks q 8 h, I & O q 8 h. Notify MD if: Change in neuro status Systolic BP≥220 &/or DBP≥110 HR ≥ 150 or ≤ 50 RR ≥ 30 Temp ≥ 101 IV fluids - NS (Avoid D5W). DVT prophylaxis: Sequential hose for non-ambulating patients. Swallowing guidelines as indicated. Elevate weak/flaccid upper extremity on pillow. Refer to CVA/TIA Patient Info. Handbook and CVA Patient/Family Caremap.		
	Goals: Neuro status stable with no deterioration. No evidence of aspiration, swallowing management continues. Vital signs within parameters. Pt./Family education continued.	____ ____ ____ ____	____ ____ ____ ____	**Goals:** Neuro status stable with no deterioration. No evidence of aspiration, swallowing management continued. Vital signs within parameters. Pt./Family education continued.	____ ____ ____ ____	____ ____ ____ ____
Tests:	PT monitoring if on heparin protocol. PT/INR if on Coumadin.			PT monitoring if on heparin protocol. PT/INR if on Coumadin.		
Other:	BP/Anticoagulation/DVT prophylaxis option (see orders). Avoid Nifedipine (Procardia).			BP/Anticoagulation/DVT prophylaxis option (see orders). Avoid Nifedipine (Procardia).		

CVA/TIA CAREMAP G-99-5013A-3PG REV. 11/8/99

DIAGNOSIS, OUTCOMES, INTERVENTIONS

Altered Cerebral Tissue Perfusion. Perfusion of the cerebrum is critical for survival and long-term outcome. Therefore, it should be the first priority in care of clients with acute stroke. Decreased cerebral blood flow may be secondary to thrombus, embolus, hemorrhage, edema, or spasm. Ongoing assessment and intervention are required beyond the critical stage. Data that indicate that the risk for altered perfusion has become an actual problem are shown in Box 70–1.

Outcomes. The client will have improved cerebral tissue perfusion, as evidenced by ICP less than 15 mm Hg, cerebral perfusion pressure (CPP) greater than 65 mm Hg, no type A waves (when using intracranial monitors), no

CASE MANAGEMENT

Stroke

Because of the prevalence of cardiovascular disease in the United States, stroke (brain attack) is one of the most common conditions seen in acute care. It can also be a high-cost diagnosis-related group (DRG) and can result in a prolonged length of stay. Many hospitals have developed clinical pathways in an attempt to decrease the variability of treatment, to decrease the length of stay, and to control cost. These measures result in positive outcomes for clients, because transfer to rehabilitation occurs earlier, allowing clients to start recovery sooner.

Assess

- Has the client had an ischemic or hemorrhagic stroke?
- What manifestations is the client experiencing?
- Has the client had previous transient ischemic attacks or strokes?
- Is this a life-threatening situation, with the client in critical care, or is the stroke completed, allowing therapy to begin?
- In the case of hemorrhagic stroke, is surgery anticipated?
- What other conditions are present that might make it more difficult to treat the stroke (hypertension, diabetes, atrial fibrillation, polycythemia)?

Assess the client's ability to swallow immediately; take measures to prevent aspiration. In the case of continued swallowing difficulty, assess the need for a feeding tube.

Assess deficits and determine how they will affect the client's care plan (e.g., hemiparesis, hemiplegia, aphasia, visual changes, incontinence). Although it may be difficult, begin exercises and physical therapy evaluation and treatments as soon as possible. Assess the need for referral to other professionals such as social workers or speech therapists.

Advocate

Stroke is an unexpected event causing many life decisions and changes for the client and family. Depending on the severity of the stroke and whether deficits are transitory or permanent, family members may be called on to determine treatment or resuscitation decisions.

Try to determine whether the client has advance directives or has named a health care proxy. Because many clients and family members will be older, they may be overwhelmed and need assistance from pastoral care or social work staff. Depending on the need for rehabilitation or long-term placement, financial assessments or applications for assistance may be necessary.

Be aware of the emotional stress on the client and family as they deal with the impact of change, possibly from a fully independent state to one requiring a great deal of assistance. Carefully explain diagnostic tests and treatments such as computed tomography (CT) scans, magnetic resonance imaging (MRI), Doppler studies, and anticoagulant therapy.

Prevent Readmission

If the stroke has been minor and the client can return home, assess the need for ongoing nursing care and physical or speech therapy. Focus on returning the client to optimal functioning.

Ensure that manifestations of stroke are recognized and that the client understands the urgency of care. Work with the client to reduce risk factors such as hypertension, hypercholesterolemia, obesity, and smoking. Ensure that medication regimens are understood, especially anticoagulant therapy and follow-up blood work. Families must know about and be prepared to deal with depression or emotional lability, which may occur.

Many clients need short-term rehabilitation before returning home. Entrance into a rehabilitation program is advisable as soon as the client is stable and can tolerate the program requirements. Intensive speech, physical, and occupational therapy can assist the client to regain function and to develop living skills despite deficits.

Cheryl Noetscher, RN, MS, *Director of Case Management, Crouse Hospital and Community–General Hospital, Syracuse, New York*

reports of headache, no decreases in LOC, and stable or improving GCS score.

Interventions. Serial assessments of these data may be required as often as every 15 minutes for unstable clients to every 2 to 4 hours for stable clients. Analyze data for trends, and if the client is deteriorating neurologically, notify the physician. Manifestations of progressive deterioration include decreasing LOC, changes in motor or sensory function, pupillary changes, respiratory difficulty, and development of visual or perceptual defects or aphasia.

Maintain the client's blood pressure, within the range prescribed by the physician, to maintain perfusion without promoting cerebral edema. Maintain normothermia to reduce cerebral glucose and oxygen consumption. Cluster nursing interventions to reduce unneeded movement and stimulation. Elevate the head of the bed 30 degrees to reduce cerebral edema. Maintain the client's head in neutral position to improve venous drainage.

BOX 70–1 Manifestations Indicating an Actual Change in Cerebral Perfusion

- Intracranial pressure greater than 15 mm Hg sustained for 15 to 30 seconds or longer
- Cerebral perfusion pressure less than 70 mm Hg
- Decrease in Glasgow Coma Scale score of two or more points from baseline
- Decreasing levels of consciousness
- Mean arterial pressure of less than 80 mm Hg or systolic blood pressure less than 100 mm Hg
- Bradycardia
- Altered pattern of breathing
- Loss of response to painful stimuli
- Change in pupil size or response to light
- Headache
- Vomiting
- Abnormal flexion or extension posturing

Administer medications to improve cerebral tissue perfusion as prescribed. The drugs prescribed to decrease risk for further thrombus formation include anticoagulants or antiplatelet agents. Nimodipine, a calcium-channel blocker, is used to treat vasospasm secondary to subarachnoid hemorrhage.[11]

Delirium and restlessness should be controlled, with sedatives if necessary. Be certain, however, that restlessness is not the result of treatable causes, such as hypoxia, full bladder, bowel impaction, or pain. Restraints should be avoided, because they often increase agitation and intracerebral pressure.

Straining at stool or with excessive coughing, vomiting, lifting, or use of the arms to change position should be avoided, because the Valsalva maneuver increases intracerebral pressure. Mild laxatives and stool softeners are often prescribed.

Altered Tissue Perfusion. Because of the increased risk for systemic bleeding secondary to the use of thrombolytic therapy or anticoagulation, altered tissue perfusion is an important nursing diagnosis. Write the nursing diagnosis as *Altered Tissue Perfusion related to prolonged bleeding times secondary to use of thrombolytic agents or anticoagulation.*

Outcomes. Hemorrhage will be prevented, as evidenced by the absence of bleeding and by normal vital signs.

Interventions. For the client who is receiving thrombolytic therapy, certain interventions can prevent systemic bleeding. These include no arterial punctures or insertions of nasogastric tubes for 24 hours after the infusion; monitor all puncture sites and body fluids for signs of bleeding for 24 hours; and maintain bed rest for 24 hours after completion of the infusion. Gingival bleeding and oozing from intravenous sites were associated with intracranial hemorrhage.[1] Pressure may be applied to any compressible bleeding sites.

For the client who is receiving anticoagulation, monitor the aPPT and INR and adjust the client's dosage based on the physician's orders. Report any signs of bleeding to the physician immediately.

Risk of Aspiration. An increased risk for aspiration is listed here because of its importance in maintaining airway and oxygenation. Not all clients are at risk for aspiration after stroke, and their risk depends on the time since injury and area of infarction. When considering this diagnosis, use the following causes of aspiration to guide your problem-solving: impaired swallowing, depressed cough and gag reflexes, and decreased LOC.

Outcomes. The client will remain free of clinical manifestations of aspiration, as evidenced by easily managing saliva, no choking or coughing while eating, no fever, and no crackles or rhonchi.

Interventions. Assess the client for clinical manifestations of aspiration, such as fever, dyspnea, crackles and rhonchi, confusion, and decreased PaO_2 in arterial blood gases. Use caution in feeding the client, either orally or enterally. If the client is receiving enteral feedings, add food coloring to the tube-feeding to assist with identifying aspiration via suctioned aspirate. Monitor chest x-ray results, and report findings of pulmonary infiltrate.

Impaired Physical Mobility. Almost all clients have some degree of immobility after a stroke. In the early phases of stroke recovery, the client may be completely immobile and need assistance just to turn over in bed. Later in recovery, mobility may only be hampered in one extremity. Various causes can be used to individualize this diagnosis. These include (1) loss of muscle tone secondary to flaccid paralysis or spasticity and (2) reluctance to move associated with fear of self-injury or prolonged disuse.

Outcomes. The client will achieve maximal physical mobility within the limitations imposed by the stroke, as evidenced by more normal movement of the affected extremity, improved muscle strength, and effective use of adaptive devices.

Interventions. Assess the client's degree of muscle strength to use as a baseline value and for determining and evaluating outcomes. A comprehensive assessment by a physical therapist helps to determine appropriate activity levels.

Encourage Bed Exercises. Encouraging clients with hemiplegia to exercise while they are at bed rest not only prepares them for later activities but also offers hope and a sense of optimism about recovery. A hemiplegic client can learn to move the weak leg by sliding the unaffected leg under it to lift and move the weak leg. The client can also use the unaffected arm to move the affected arm and hand. Keep in mind that clients may have difficulty crossing the midline.

Frequent gluteal and quadriceps muscle setting exercises during the day help prepare the client for later ambulation. Begin with five repetitions, and increase gradually to 20 repetitions each time. Instruct the client as follows:

1. *Gluteal setting:* "Pinch" or contract the buttocks together and count to five. Then relax and count to five. Repeat.
2. *Quadriceps setting:* Contract the quadriceps muscles, on the anterior portion of the thigh, while raising the heel and trying to squash a rolled towel placed under the popliteal fossa against the mattress. While keeping the muscle contracted, count to five. Then relax and count to five. Repeat. Perform on both legs if possible. Start quadriceps setting exercise as soon as the client is conscious. The quadriceps muscle is the most important in giving knee joint stability in walking.

Help the Client Sit Up. Help the client out of bed as soon as the client's condition is medically stable. Remember, however, that hemiplegia can severely affect balance. Assistance is needed to provide security and safety. Raise the head of the bed slowly to reduce orthostatic hypotension.

When the client first sits up, support the affected side, especially the back and the head. Gradually, the client learns to sit alone with the head of the bed elevated and then to sit on the edge of the bed with the feet on a firm surface. Help the client maintain balance by extending the affected arm and placing the palm flat on the bed. Be patient and encouraging as the client regains balance. When the client is sitting in a chair, support the weak side with pillows.

Eventually, the client learns to raise the weak leg with the unaffected leg and to swing both legs laterally over the side of the bed onto the floor. It is safest to have the client pivot on the unaffected leg. Therefore, position the chair at a right angle to the unaffected side.

Teach the Client How to Use a Wheelchair. A hemiplegic client needs to learn safe transfers from the bed to the chair, commode, or wheelchair. The Client Education Guide shows one method. The client with hemiplegia can propel a wheelchair with the unaffected arm and leg; one-arm-drive wheelchairs also are available. Once the client is in a wheelchair, his or her level of independence increases greatly. Deficits in spatial relations, decreased awareness, and unilateral neglect can result in problems such as falling and running into doors. Clients must not be allowed to perform wheelchair self-transfers until they have demonstrated competence.

Promote Walking. A tilt table may be used in physical therapy to help the client assume a standing position if difficulty with balance is a problem. The client can begin standing as soon as the quadriceps muscles on the unaffected side have normal strength. Have the client seated on the edge of the bed. Encourage the client to rise, using the muscle power of the unaffected leg. The client may tend to swing around toward the affected side. Gradually, the client learns to take increasing amounts of weight onto the weaker side.

Despite weakness in the affected limb, a hemiplegic

CLIENT EDUCATION GUIDE

Transfer from Bed to Wheelchair by a Hemiplegic Client

Lock the wheelchair for safety, and keep it beside the bed on your unaffected side.

Use your unaffected arm and leg (*A* and *B*) to move your affected arm and leg.

As your legs drop over the edge of the bed, swing your torso up to a sitting position (*C*).

Push yourself up to a standing position (*D*) by using your unaffected arm and leg.

Reach across the wheelchair (*E*) to grasp the far arm of the chair, and turn to seat yourself.

Shading on the right side of the client indicates the affected side.

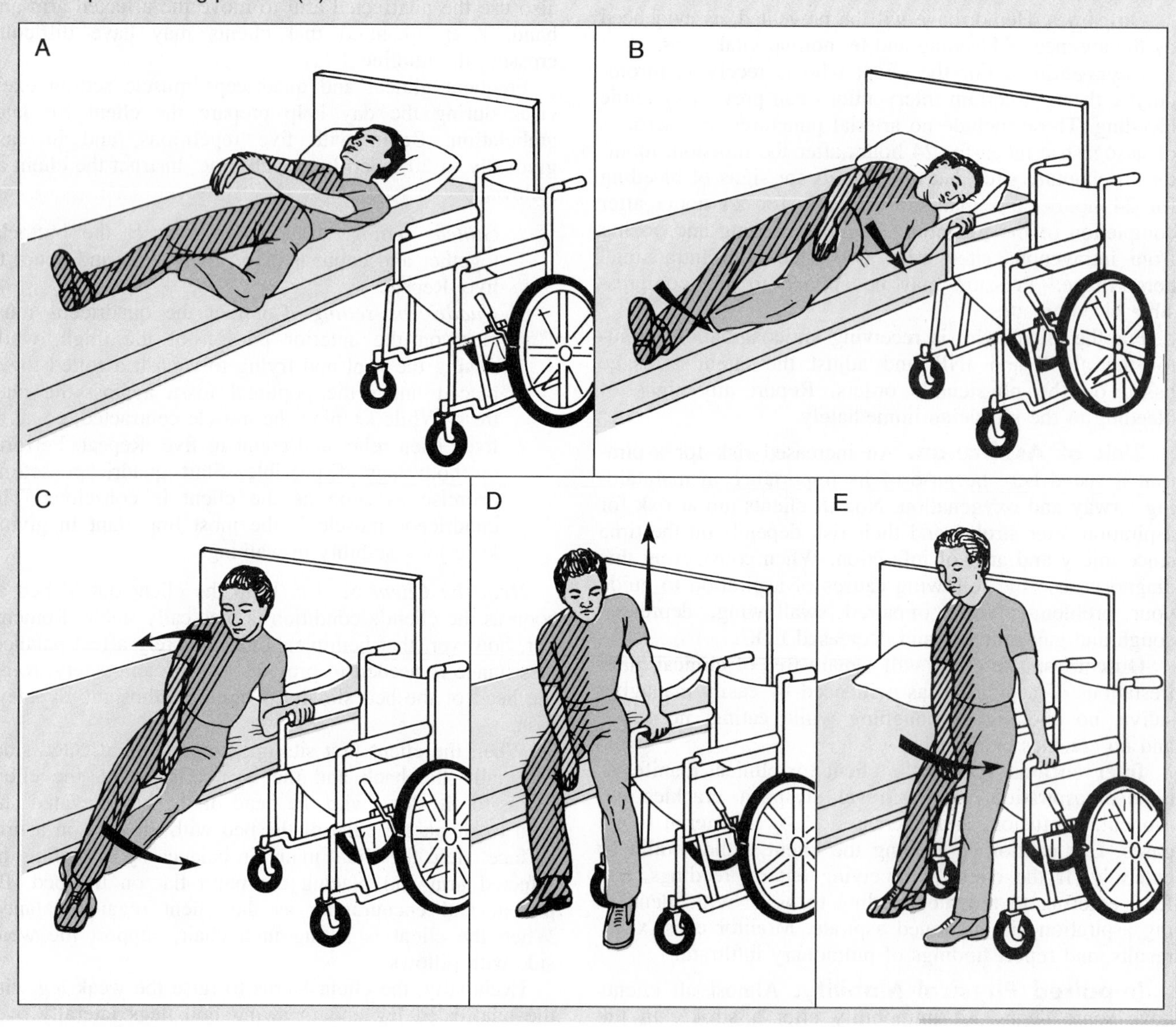

client often develops an extensor reflex, which facilitates standing. Position yourself on the weaker side when helping the client to stand. To avoid pulling on the affected arm and increasing the risk for shoulder injury, provide support with ambulation by using a gait belt. A quad cane should be used on the unaffected side to allow walking with a three-point gait.

Most hemiplegic clients can be taught to walk. Remind them to keep the body weight forward over the feet. Practice is important for learning to walk correctly. Incorrect habits, once developed, may be difficult to overcome later. Supervise clients carefully until they can safely walk alone without fear of falling. When walking, the client should not show circumduction or toe scraping or stoop forward. Heel-toe walking with a reciprocal gait pattern is the goal of ambulation.

Teach Bracing. If bracing is used, teach the client and family how to apply and remove the brace, to observe skin for breakdown, to give proper skin care, and to care for the brace itself.

Hyperthermia. Bleeding or edema of the hypothalamus can lead to ischemia of the thermoregulatory center of the brain.

Outcomes. The client will experience decreasing temperature or will have normal temperature.

Interventions. Treat fever with antipyretics. A hypothermia blanket may be used to bring down a high temperature quickly. When hypothermia blankets are used, assess the skin frequently for pressure points and cold injury. Shivering must be avoided because the muscle activity increases body temperature. Keeping the feet warm with blankets may decrease shivering. Phenothiazines may be used to help stabilize neuronal membranes if fever is related to damaged brain structures.

Risk for Impaired Skin Integrity. The loss of protective sensation and decreased ability to move increases the risk for injury to the skin. In addition, skin damage may develop from friction and shearing or increased skin fragility from inadequate nutritional status or edema.

Outcomes. The client's skin will remain intact, as evidenced by an absence of stage I pressure ulcer development and an absence of manifestations of redness from friction or shearing.

Interventions. Assess the skin every 2 hours. Change the position of a client with hemiplegia or decreased LOC every 2 hours. Develop a written turning schedule for other health care providers and family members to follow. When positioning the client on the affected side, make sure that body weight does not harm affected limbs. Support the affected arm and leg when turning and positioning a hemiplegic client. Complete shoulder and hip dislocation can occur if the flaccid extremity is not supported properly. Place a pillow between the client's legs to provide support. The client may be able to tolerate lying only for 30 minutes on the affected side because of the impaired circulation or pain.

Risk for Contracture. One of the normal activities of the brain is to inhibit spastic muscle contraction. Early in stroke recovery, flaccidity is usually present because of a loss of cerebral connections for afferent sensory and efferent motor nerves. During recovery, affected muscles may be spastic because the injured brain cannot inhibit spastic muscle contraction. Therefore, the diagnosis *Risk for Contracture* is due to flaccid paralysis or spasticity.

Outcomes. The client will have absence of contractures, joint ankylosis, and muscle shortening, as evidenced by maintaining normal ROM.

Interventions. Assess the client's ROM in both the involved and noninvolved joints. These findings can be used as a baseline and as an expected outcome.

Perform passive ROM exercises two times daily after the first 24 hours following a stroke unless otherwise prescribed. Motor impulses usually begin to return between 2 and 14 days after a stroke. The affected part (initially flaccid) becomes spastic as the spinal cord motor systems establish their autonomy and the potential for contractures increases. Passive ROM exercises are more difficult to perform once affected muscles begin to tighten.

Do not force extremities beyond the point of initiating pain or continuous spasm. Always support the joint you are exercising, and move the extremity smoothly, without jerking movements. Frequent passive ROM exercises (1) prevent joint immobility, tendon contractures, and muscle atrophy; (2) stimulate circulation; and (3) help reestablish neuromuscular pathways. By performing these exercises before dressing and undressing the client, you may facilitate self-care.

Teach the client to use the unaffected hand to lift the weak arm and to put it through ROM exercises. Exercise each finger separately. While the client is in bed, teach him or her (1) to exercise the affected arm by grasping it at the wrist with the unaffected hand and raising it above the head and (2) to stretch and rub the fingers of the affected hand several times each day. Active ROM to the unaffected extremities assists in maintaining or increasing muscle strength.

Once some voluntary movement returns, encourage the client with assisted movements. As motor strength increases, resisted movements may strengthen weakened muscles and help restore muscle bulk. Shoulder slings are not recommended because they may increase the risk of contractures.

Several interventions are used to reduce the risk for joint contracture:

1. Allow the client to sit upright for short periods only; sitting can contribute to hip and knee flexion deformities.
2. When the client is on one side, do not flex the hip acutely.
3. Do not place a pillow under the affected knee when the client is supine; this encourages flexion deformity and impedes circulation.
4. If the client's knees tend to hyperextend, place a folded towel under the knee for short periods while the client is lying supine.

If the client can tolerate the prone position, place the client in this position for 15 to 30 minutes several times a day, with a small pillow placed under the pelvis (from the umbilicus to the upper third of the thigh) to hyperextend the hip joints.

Prevent foot drop, heel cord shortening, and plantiflexion by (1) avoiding pressure on the feet, (2) performing frequent passive ROM exercises, and (3) having the client sit in a chair as soon as possible with the feet flat on the floor. While the client is in bed, keep the foot flexed at 90 degrees by using high-top tennis shoes or orthotics.

A trochanter roll, extending from the crest of the ilium to midthigh, prevents external hip rotation by wedging under the projection of the greater trochanter and stopping the femur from rolling. Trochanter rolls increase the risk of skin impairment; assess the skin beneath the roll often.

When the client is in bed, prevent adduction of the affected shoulder by placing a pillow in the axilla, between the upper arm and the chest wall, to keep the arm abducted about 60 degrees. Keep the arm slightly flexed in a neutral position. Place the forearm on another pillow with the elbow above the shoulder and the wrist above the elbow. This position stretches the shoulder's internal rotators. Elevating the arm also helps prevent edema and resultant fibrosis.

Place the affected hand in a position of function (i.e., slightly supinated with fingers slightly flexed and the thumb in opposition). Frequent passive ROM exercises are important. The use of splints to prevent flexion contractures is more effective if the splints are designed individually by occupational therapists and scheduled for on-and-off periods to allow for skin assessment and ROM. Squeezing a rubber ball is not recommended because it promotes flexion when extension is desired.

The weight of an immobile arm may cause pain and movement limitation (frozen shoulder) or subluxation of the shoulder joint. Prevent these by supporting a completely flaccid arm with a pillow when the client is in bed or seated in a chair.

Self-Care Deficit. Self-care deficits may range from not being able to reach with a weak arm to full dependence on others. This diagnosis is applicable if an achievable outcome can be obtained. Clients with complete paralysis and cognitive deficits may not be able to perform self-care. Other diagnoses may be more applicable, such as *Impaired Physical Mobility* and *Impaired Skin Integrity.* Several diagnoses can be used to describe *Self-Care Deficit,* including *Impaired Physical Mobility, Visual Sensory/Perceptual Alterations, Unilateral Neglect,* or *Altered Thought Processes.*

Outcomes. The client will perform as many ADL as possible within limitations, as evidenced by use of adaptive devices and techniques.

Interventions. Initially, a client who has had a stroke may need considerable help with all self-care activities, including washing, eating, and grooming. Encourage clients to perform as many self-care activities as possible and to use the affected arm to avoid the tendency to do everything with the unaffected arm. This activity helps preserve independent self-care, prevents complications of immobility, and enhances self-esteem.

Remember, stroke clients are easily frustrated and may need a lot of encouragement. Self-care activities provide an excellent opportunity for family teaching. Family members find it very difficult to watch a loved one struggle with a task, and they often perform the task for the client. Explain how it benefits the client to be as independent as possible.

In clients with diplopia, an eye patch over one eye removes the second image and promotes better vision. Alternating the patch daily helps to maintain the function and strength of the extraocular muscles in both eyes. Provide mouth care at least three or four times a day, giving special attention to the affected side of the tongue and mouth. Focus rehabilitation plans on self-care deficits and ADL.

Risk for Injury. The *Risk for Injury* and trauma continues throughout recovery from stroke. It may also extend into the home environment, where clients attempt to perform former activities, such as cooking or driving. Factors that increase the risk for injury include decreased LOC, weakness, flaccidity, spasticity, impulsive behavior, altered thought processes, and motor, visual, and spatial-perceptual impairments.

Outcomes. The client will remain free from injury, as evidenced by an absence of abrasions, burns, or falls. The client will also seek needed help to perform tasks that are beyond his or her capabilities.

Interventions. Keep the side rails of the bed raised for clients with recent hemiplegia to protect them from rolling out of bed. As recovery proceeds, the client may pull against side rails when sitting up or turning. Once the client can get out of bed unassisted, half side rails may be more useful. Full side rails hinder ambulation.

A client with impaired sensation is especially prone to injury. Frequent skin inspections for manifestations of injury are essential. Visual disturbances may also increase a hemiplegic client's potential for injury. Weakness on one side makes clients susceptible to falls. Remind clients to walk slowly, rest adequately between intervals of walking, use effective lighting, and look where they are going. Be especially alert during toileting. Make sure that support staff and family members know not to leave these clients alone in the bathroom.

Altered Nutrition. Use the nursing diagnosis *Altered Nutrition: Less Than Body Requirements* if your client has an inability to swallow secondary to stroke. Support the diagnosis with data on intake and output, ability to swallow, caloric intake and weight change over the past 3 days, hemoglobin, hematocrit, albumin, prealbumin, and lymphocyte count over the past 3 days.

Outcomes. The client will demonstrate signs of adequate nutrition, as evidenced by (1) maintenance of stable weight; (2) consumption of adequate calories for age, height, and weight; (3) intake equaling output; (4) hemoglobin and hematocrit levels within normal limits for age and sex; (5) lymphocyte count, prealbumin, and albumin levels within normal limits; and (6) healing of incisions and wounds within 12 to 14 days, as applicable.

Interventions. Carefully assess the client's diet to ensure adequate nutrition. Assess total intake. Feeding clients with partial paralysis of the tongue, mouth, and throat requires patience and care for prevention of choking and aspiration. Clients often fear choking and are embarrassed and frustrated by eating difficulties. Consequently, they may avoid eating and may not obtain adequate nutrition. Give supplemental meals as necessary. If the client cannot swallow at all, tube-feeding may be used. With help and encouragement, hemiplegic clients can usually learn to feed themselves. Many helpful orthotic devices are available through consultation with an occupational therapist. These might include utensils with built-up handles or scoop plates. Make mealtimes pleasant and unhurried. Serve food attractively and at an appropriate temperature.

Feeding can be very frustrating for a dysphagic client, especially if the caregiver is not familiar with the client's specific disabilities. Support personnel and family members need to be taught basic feeding techniques. These people also need to be informed of each client's individual needs and limitations. To facilitate feeding, assess the following and intervene as necessary. The speech pathologist can recommend additional feeding techniques based on the client's specific deficits and needs.

Promote Head Control. If the client has limited or no voluntary head control, placing a hand on the forehead may help. The caregiver approaches the client from the midline rather than from the side so that the client does not have to turn the head to be fed. Remind the client not to throw the head back to propel food, because this can lead to aspiration. The head should be midline and flexed slightly forward.

Assist in Positioning. Have the client in an upright position, as close to 90 degrees as possible, either in bed or in a chair. Support the client's head to counteract hyperextension.

Promote Mouth Opening. If the client does not open the mouth, lightly touch both lips with the tip of a spoon. If this does not work, apply light pressure with a finger to the chin just below the lower lip. Ask the client to open at the same time. Stroking the muscle under the chin (digastric muscle), without crossing the midline, also stimulates mouth opening.

Stimulate Mouth Closing. If a client does not close the lips, swallowing is more difficult. Stimulate lip closure by stroking the lips with a finger or ice or by applying gentle pressure just above the upper lip with your thumb or forefinger.

Help the Client with Swallowing. A dysphagic client must concentrate on swallowing. A quiet environment, free from distractions, is helpful. Feed the client slowly and offer small amounts. Begin feeding the client with foods that require no chewing and are easy to swallow (Table 70–4). Gradually progress to foods that require more chewing and swallowing effort as tolerated. Alternate liquids with solids whenever possible to prevent food from being left in the mouth. Avoid nonthickened liquids. Place food in the unaffected side of the mouth. Encourage the client to chew each bite thoroughly. After clients have swallowed, teach them to check for food on the paralyzed side by turning the head to the unaffected side and sweeping the mouth with the tongue.

Impaired Verbal Communication. The inability to speak is very frustrating for clients. Early recognition of this problem decreases some of the frustration in meeting everyday needs. Loss of verbal communication is

TABLE 70–4 PROGRESSIVE FEEDING PROGRAM FOR CLIENTS WITH DYSPHAGIA

	Stage I	Stage II	Stage III	Stage IV
Description	Severe swallowing difficulty	Chewing and swallowing difficulty with various textures	Less difficulty swallowing, beginning to control foods better in mouth, able to tolerate various food textures and consistencies	Able to swallow most foods very well
Meats	Puréed meat with gravy, baby food, egg yolks	Junior baby food meats with gravy; scrambled, soft, or poached eggs; cottage cheese	Ground meat with gravy, soft meats (tuna) in casseroles, macaroni and cheese, fish without bones, chopped meats	Soft diet
Starch	Mashed potatoes with gravy	Muffins (no seeds), pancakes, French toast, cooked cereal (thick)	Toast (no seeds), rice, soft baked potato	Soft foods
Vegetables	Puréed	Junior vegetables	Peas, squash, cooked carrots; avoid stringy foods (celery, spinach)	Soft foods
Fruits	Puréed	Cooked fruit, ripe banana, soft canned fruit	Grapefruit and orange sections; peeled ripe peaches, pears, and nectarines	Soft foods
Dessert	Custard, pudding	Cakes (no seeds, nuts)	Pies, cakes, sherbet, ice cream	Soft foods
Liquids	None	None	Thick liquids, nectars, strained cream soups, eggnog, liquid caloric supplements, milk shakes	May be able to have thickened liquids

usually caused by ischemia of the dominant cerebral hemisphere, leading to loss of the function of muscles that produce speech.

Outcomes. The client will be able to effectively communicate, the client's needs will be understood and met, and the client will indicate understanding of the communication of others.

Interventions. Communication involves the dual processes of sending and receiving language. Although either can be affected, the expressive deficit is usually greater than the receptive deficit after initial recovery. Clients may understand more than they can respond to.

Most aphasic clients regain some speech through spontaneous recovery or speech therapy. Speech therapy should be started early. Occasionally, residual brain function is not adequate for an aphasic client to relearn the complicated processes of communication. A picture board may be helpful.

Assessment of dysarthria usually includes examination of the peripheral muscles of speech, tests for specific speech skills, and assessment of the client's functional ability based on the clarity of speech in conversation. Speech therapy is beneficial for many dysarthric clients.

Reinforce the lessons that a speech therapist has initiated. Remember, the client may have a short attention span. Use every encounter to encourage and support communication, yet be careful not to cause frustration and fatigue. In general, when working with an aphasic client, speak at a slower rate and give the client time to respond. Listen and watch carefully when an aphasic client attempts to communicate. Try hard to understand. This reduces the client's frustration. Anticipate an aphasic client's needs, to reduce feelings of communication helplessness.

When a client *cannot identify objects by name,* give the client practice in receiving word images. For example, point to an object and clearly state its name. Then ask the client to repeat the word.

When a client *cannot understand spoken words or has receptive difficulty,* repeat simple directions until they are understood. Do not shout. The client can hear. Speak slowly and clearly. Talk without pressing for a response. Use nonverbal methods of communication to reinforce your words. Stand within 6 feet, and face the client directly. Gradually shift topics of conversation, and tell the client when you are going to change the topic.

When a client has *difficulty with verbal expression,* give the client practice in repeating words after you. Begin with simple words and then progress to simple sentences.

Help the family to communicate with the aphasic client. Act as a role model for such communication by being calm, patient, and gentle. Explain how damaging it can be to the client's self-image if others appear embarrassed or amused by the client's attempts to communicate. Likewise, the family should not do all of the speaking for the client.

Always try to put aphasic clients at ease. Reduce the feelings of panic that may occur when they first realize that they cannot communicate as before. The fact that others understand the problem is helpful. Offer calm reassurance. Demonstrate use of the call light and allow the client to practice. Use gestures and one-step commands.

Risk for Corneal Abrasion. Following stroke, clients may lose their ability to blink. Without a blink reflex, the cornea will dry and become abraded. The collaborative problem is *Risk for Corneal Abrasion.*

Outcomes. Monitor the client for risk factors for the development of corneal abrasion, including absence of eye closure or blinking and lack of eye moisture.

Interventions. Protect the eye with an eye patch if no blinking is noted. Instill prescribed artificial tears or consult the physician for a prescription if none exists.

Altered Thought Processes. Sometimes it is difficult to make a diagnosis of *Altered Thought Processes* unless you spend some time with the client. Asking simple or common questions may get fixed, yet correct, answers. Often, after spending a morning with a client, you may note difficulty with thought processing that was not evident on first assessment. Changes in behavior may be caused by alterations in body image, sensation, vision, mobility, and perception. Cerebral edema may also increase confusion.

Outcomes. The client will have reduced confusion, as evidenced by recall of information, improved Mini-Mental State examination scores, decreased agitation, cooperation with interventions, and appropriate responses to questions about recent and past events.

Interventions. Try to prevent disorientation by reorienting the client as LOC improves. Continually reorient a confused client. Glasses and hearing aids assist the client in maintaining awareness of the environment and thus improve thought processes. Activity such as sitting up in a chair for meals or at scheduled times throughout the day also improves LOC and orientation. Position a calendar and a clock where the client can see them. Stroke contributes to altered behavioral patterns, including confusion, memory loss, and emotional lability. To decrease agitation, explain all nursing activities before initiating them. Avoid sensory overload.

Visual Sensory/Perceptual Alterations. Ischemia of visual pathways can lead to altered vision. The client may not notice you when you approach from one side or may not eat food from one side of the food tray. A thorough assessment of visual fields is usually needed for this diagnosis.

Outcomes. The client will successfully compensate for altered visual perceptions, as evidenced by safely performing ADL and safely compensating for visual deficit through scanning or other techniques.

Interventions. Approach the client from the side that is not visually impaired. Position the call light and telephone on that side. If possible, position the bed so that the client's side that is not visually impaired is toward the center of the room. Teach clients to position the head to increase the visual field. Warn hemiplegic clients to be very careful when crossing streets because they may not see traffic approaching from the affected side. An eye patch over one eye in clients with diplopia removes the second image and assists vision.

A client with perceptual deficits benefits from simplicity. A busy or noisy environment is difficult to interpret and may increase confusion. Reduce complexity and the need for decision-making. For example:

1. Obtain clothing that is simply designed and easy to put on.
2. Give brief, simple directions.
3. Prepare food trays with a minimum number of utensils, dishes, and foods.

Unilateral Neglect. *Unilateral Neglect* is a pattern of lack of awareness of one side of the body. The client behaves as if that part is simply not there. He or she does not look for the paralyzed limb when moving about. It is caused by damage to portions of the nondominant cerebral hemisphere. Unilateral neglect creates increased risk of injury. It is possible to relearn to look for and to move the limb.

Outcomes. The client will be able to compensate for unilateral neglect, as evidenced by being free from injury and demonstrating an increased awareness of the neglected body side.

Interventions. Initially, adapt the environment to the deficit by focusing on the client's unaffected side. Greet the client as you enter the room, especially if the entrance is toward the neglected side. Keep personal care items and a bedside chair and commode on the unaffected side. Set up the client's food tray toward the unaffected side. Position the client's extremities in correct alignment. Gradually begin to focus the client's attention to the affected side. Move the personal items, bedside chair, and commode to the affected side. Assist the client from the affected side. Have the client groom the affected side first. Cue the client to scan the entire environment and remind the client to keep track of the affected extremities.

Ineffective Individual Coping. Coping strategies are quite varied among people. Any major illness or change in the body challenges a client's or family's coping skills. This process is particularly true after a stroke because of the physiologic changes and frustrations associated with the resulting deficits. The term *coping* refers to the use of all forms of coping strategies: emotional, cognitive, support systems, and risk appraisal.

Outcomes. The client will develop effective coping strategies, as evidenced by appropriate lifestyle modifications, use of the assistance of others, and appropriate social interactions.

Interventions. After a stroke, the client may experience grief over lost mobility, inability to communicate, alterations in sensation and vision, and loss of roles within society. Stroke clients express feelings of profound suffering related to the sudden, devastating changes that accompany stroke.[2, 34] Be understanding and kind. Supportive statements are often helpful, such as "I am sure it's hard for you not to be able to dress alone." The client needs to feel listened to and cared about.

Loss of independence is of particular concern for the stroke client.[45] Care for clients in a way that encourages their independence. Arrange the environment and anticipate needs to reduce frustration. Praise all successes, however small. Break a long-term goal into several short-term goals so the client can experience successes along the way. For example, a long-term goal may be to walk independently, but short-term goals such as sitting on the side of the bed and ambulating with a quad cane will allow the client to have successes and the long-term goal will seem more attainable. Inappropriate behavior may occur. When necessary, point out the behavior in a matter-of-fact manner and ask them to stop. Significant others often need help to understand that these behaviors may be caused by damage to the inhibitory centers in the brain or they may be a part of the normal grief response. Provide support by helping the client and family to understand this.

Aphasic clients often express their emotional state by irritability and "moodiness." These frustrated clients are often anxious, bewildered, and depressed. Emotional lability may also be present. Accept such behavior in a matter-of-fact but kind manner, without embarrassment. Help families by encouraging short visits by one or two people. If children are allowed to visit, ensure that they are adequately supervised.

Psychosocial Nursing Diagnoses. Various psychosocial nursing diagnoses may be appropriate for clients experiencing stroke, depending on the client and the circumstances. These include *Altered Family Processes* (see Chapter 9), *Diversional Activity Deficit, Anxiety, Fear, Powerlessness, Self-Esteem Disturbance,* and *Social Isolation.* Shift in spousal roles often occurs. The ways in which a couple copes will determine how satisfying their lives are after a stroke.[45] Include significant others in the plan of care. Let them help care for the client if they wish. Provide them with the information they need to understand the client's condition. Many clients with strokes are in ICUs during the acute phase. The complexity of equipment and activity within an ICU may be frightening to the client and to significant others. Explain carefully what is happening, and provide opportunities for questions and discussion. Give frequent reassurance and support.

EVALUATION

Evaluate the degree of outcome attainment on an ongoing basis. After a stroke, some outcomes, such as cerebral perfusion, are achieved early; others, such as self-care deficit, may require long-term rehabilitation. Monitor progress toward outcomes, working with both the client and the family.

Surgical Management

Several criteria are used to identify candidates for rapid evacuation of the hematoma in hemorrhagic stroke. The clients most likely to benefit from surgery are those who are younger than 70 years of age, can open their eyes and follow commands, have elevated ICP (>30 mm Hg), or are rapidly deteriorating neurologically. Clients who have large blood clots removed often can recover a substantial portion of speech. Surgery is usually not performed in clients with bleeding in deep cerebral structures such as the basal ganglia or thalamus.

Most therapies are aimed at reducing increased ICP.[22] Surgery is also performed on some intracranial aneurysms and on the carotid arteries to reduce the risk for stroke.

Modifications for Elderly Clients

Because stroke affects older people more than others, the nursing care discussed here does not have to be significantly altered for older clients. Older people often have multiple medical problems that must be monitored and treated simultaneously.

Self-Care

Clients who have experienced a stroke often are transferred to a rehabilitation unit after they are medically stable. The client is evaluated for rehabilitation potential, and plans are made for ongoing therapy. The plan of care established during acute care can continue. The major nursing diagnoses and collaborative problems include *Impaired Physical Mobility, Self-Care Deficit, Impaired Verbal Communication, Risk for Contracture, Altered Nutrition: Less Than Body Requirements,* and *Ineffective Individual Coping.*

Three adjuncts to discharge from rehabilitation settings to home are:

- Self-medication
- Use of therapeutic passes
- Rehabilitation home visits

Self-medication means that clients can manage their own medications. Goals are to help the client learn about the medications, including dosage, action, and side effects. Provide a supervised trial to evaluate the client's knowledge and compliance and to enable clients to develop increased responsibility for their own care. A clear and accurate medication chart is helpful.

Therapeutic passes allow the client to return to home or family for short stays. They facilitate discharge planning and improve the transition into the community. Passes help the stroke survivor adjust to the home environment and to practice self-care activities at home and help the family adjust to living with the stroke survivor and to any alterations in physical, cognitive, and emotional functioning. Clients and family members can practice problem-solving and can perform some physical care skills needed after discharge from the facility. Much effort goes into planning for the passes and preparing the client and family. Passes are usually for 8 hours at first and then are increased to a weekend. When the client returns to the facility, the client and family discuss any difficulties they had during the pass interval. Team members intervene with information, retraining, or procurement of needed supplies.

For the *rehabilitation home visit,* team members, including the nurse, social worker, and physical and occupational therapists, visit the client's home. The purpose is to evaluate the accessibility of the home and the safety of the home environment based on the client's level of functioning, specifically, the client's ability (1) to get in and out of the house; (2) to perform specific tasks in each room; (3) to transfer onto and off of the toilet, bed, and chair; and (4) to move about from room to room. The client's ability to safely use the telephone and various appliances is also evaluated. On the basis of findings from the visit, the team recommends home modifications, further teaching, or adaptive equipment.

The family needs a clear understanding of the client's residual deficits. If spatial or perceptual deficits or unilateral neglect is present, emphasize the need for assistance with daily activities and the need for adherence to safety precautions to prevent injury. Writing lists of tasks or activities may help clients with impaired memory. Reinforce measures to improve mobility and the ability to perform ADL. The client should have a plan for exercises. Of equal importance, the family and client need to have realistic expectations about the client's abilities, so they can encourage independence when and where the client is able.

Provide written documentation of any anticoagulant schedule as well as a list of warning signs of bleeding. Reinforce the need for caution when the client is using sharp instruments and tools. If appropriate, contact sports must be curtailed while the client is receiving anticoagulants. The INR is closely monitored, and medications are adjusted as needed. The client should be taught to carry Medic-Alert identification.

Provide information about community resources that can assist the client and family with home management and adjustments to residual deficits. These resources include Meals-on-Wheels, the American Heart Association, stroke support groups, social services, local service groups to assist with the purchase of equipment, and individual and family counselors.

At times, the stroke client may not be able to tolerate the intensive therapy of a rehabilitation setting, and placement in an extended care facility may be necessary. This is usually very stressful for the client and family, particularly an older spouse. In some cases, care by nurses and allied health professionals in the home may prevent placement in an extended care facility. If both partners are older or in poor health, placement in an extended care facility may be the only option. This can create feelings of guilt and abandonment. Emotional support must be provided to both the client and family members. Education in how to choose a facility and how to monitor care can be helpful.

TRANSIENT ISCHEMIC ATTACKS

Transient ischemic attacks (TIAs) are sudden, brief episodes of neurologic dysfunction caused by temporary, focal cerebral ischemia. Recovery is complete. By definition, a TIA lasts less than 24 hours, and most TIAs last only 5 to 20 minutes. TIAs lasting greater than 1 hour are often caused by small infarcts.[4] TIAs often serve as warning signs of an impending stroke. In fact, one third of people with untreated TIAs experience a stroke within 5 years.[4]

Etiology and Risk Factors

During a TIA, a transient decrease in blood supply to a focal area of the cerebrum or brain stem occurs. Many factors can cause this ischemia. Thromboembolism from ulcerated plaque on the carotid arteries is the most common cause of TIAs, accounting for 80% of cases. Thromboemboli may originate in the vertebrobasilar system. Other sources of emboli include blood clots forming on diseased or prosthetic heart valves, atrial fibrillation, or breakdown of plaque.

Pathophysiology

The pathophysiology of a TIA is similar to that of a stroke. The major differences are the short duration of ischemia and the lack of permanent deficits.

Clinical Manifestations

Manifestations of TIAs vary, depending on which area of the brain is affected. Common manifestations of a TIA in the carotid artery circulation include a rapid onset of weakness or numbness in an arm or leg, aphasia, and visual field cuts. Manifestations of a TIA in the vertebrobasilar circulation include two or more of the following: vertigo, diplopia, dysphagia, dysarthria, and ataxia.

TIAs are often recurrent; however, some clients have only one or two episodes before having a complete stroke. TIAs may occur for 2 to 6 years before cerebral infarction, or clusters of TIAs may first appear only a few hours or days before a cerebral infarction. Between episodes, neurologic assessment findings are normal.

The diagnosis of TIA is confirmed by the client's reported clinical manifestations. The causes of the TIA and potential risk for stroke are diagnosed by the following examinations:

1. Auscultation for a carotid bruit.
2. CT to rule out stroke or other causes of neurologic deficit.
3. Doppler, computed tomographic angiography (CTA), or magnetic resonance angiography (MRA) studies of the carotid arteries.
4. Cerebral angiogram.
5. ECG to assess for atrial fibrillation.
6. Transthoracic or transesophageal echocardiography (TTE and TEE, respectively) to rule out mural thrombosis and valvular disorders.

The results of the noninvasive carotid artery studies, which include the Doppler, CTA, and MRA, determine whether the more invasive cerebral angiogram is performed. The TTE is often performed before the TEE as it is less invasive; however, the TEE may better visualize prosthetic valves and the left atrium.

Conditions that mimic a TIA include intracranial hemorrhage, seizures, hypoglycemia, migraine, and inner ear disorders.

Outcome Management

Medical Management

Preventing the progression of a TIA to a stroke is the goal of medical management. Every effort is made to determine the cause of the TIAs. Another important medical intervention is to identify and decrease the client's modifiable risk factors for stroke.[7] Antihypertensives or antiplatelet drugs may be prescribed. Warfarin may be administered for emboli of cardiac origin.

Teach the client and family about the manifestations of stroke, risk factors for stroke, and emergency care if a stroke occurs at home. If the client is hospitalized, assess neurologic status frequently for progressive ischemia.

Clients experiencing TIAs are often afraid that they are having a stroke. They need emotional support and education during this stressful time. The diagnostic work-up as well as the manifestations themselves can produce anxiety. Thorough, simple explanations of upcoming events can help. Stress the importance of completing the work-up. Baseline neurologic status must be recorded for postoperative comparison.

Surgical Management

Clients who are considered for surgery are those who have a low risk for postoperative morbidity and mortality and one of the following: (1) asymptomatic carotid artery disease with greater than 60% stenosis or (2) symptomatic carotid artery disease with greater than 70% stenosis.[21, 28] In these clients, the incidence of stroke with surgical management is significantly reduced compared with those with medical management. Clients considered at increased risk for postoperative morbidity and mortality include those with coronary artery disease, pulmonary disease, and moderate to severe stroke on the ipsilateral side.[21, 28] Surgery is usually performed only on stenotic arteries, not on those that are totally occluded. A client may require bilateral endarterectomy. The interval between surgeries is determined by the client's tolerance of the procedure and the likelihood of symptom progression from the remaining stenotic vessel.

Most surgeons perform cerebral angiography before carotid artery surgery to accurately quantitate the degree of carotid stenosis.[21] The risk for stroke or death from cerebral angiography is 1%.[21] Vast improvements in technology of noninvasive carotid artery studies allow surgeons to use the data to guide the planning for surgery.[28] Preoperative aspirin is often administered to decrease the formation of embolism at the carotid suture line. If the client is receiving heparin, it is usually stopped on arrival to the operating room.

CAROTID ENDARTERECTOMY

Carotid endarterectomy is useful in preventing stroke. Carotid endarterectomy is the opening of the carotid artery to remove obstructing and embolizing plaque (Fig. 70–5). After coronary artery bypass, it is the second most common vascular surgical procedure. An incision is made on the anterior border of the sternocleidomastoid muscle. The vessel is clamped, and the plaque or atheroma is removed. There is a potential for decreased cerebral perfusion during the operation because the artery must be clamped during the procedure. Some surgeons use intraoperative electroencephalogram (EEG) and transcranial Doppler monitoring to detect decreased cerebral perfusion while the carotid artery is clamped. In addition, some surgeons shunt blood from below the targeted carotid artery incision to above it to provide a temporary blood supply to the brain. The client is admitted to the ICU for monitoring of neurologic and vital signs and is usually discharged the following day.

PROGNOSIS. Follow-up Doppler studies are performed at 3 months postoperatively to assess for artery patency and again at 6 months to 1 year to detect restenosis on the operated side and disease on the nonoperated side. Restenosis occurs in approximately 5% of clients after carotid endarterectomy.[21]

COMPLICATIONS. Neurologic complications of carotid endarterectomy include:

- Embolization during surgery, causing cerebral vessel occlusion and ischemia
- Thrombosis of the artery at the endarterectomy site, causing cerebral ischemia
- Inadequate cerebral perfusion from intolerance of the temporary artery clamping during surgery

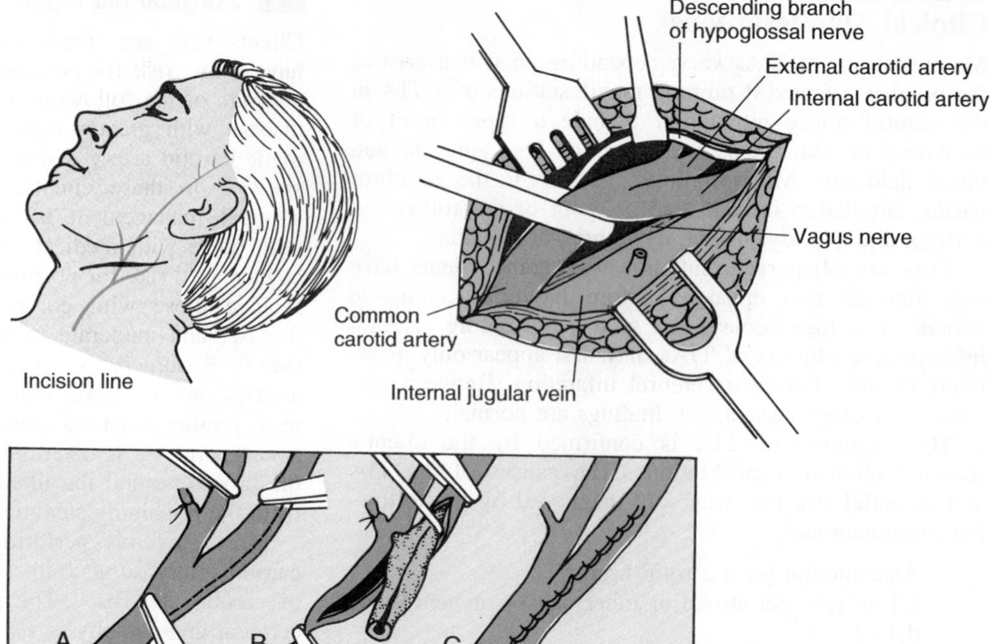

FIGURE 70–5 Carotid endarterectomy. *A*, The common carotid artery is clamped, and an incision is made along the carotid bifurcation. *B*, Plaque is removed. Sometimes portions of the artery are also removed and reconstructed with vein grafts or polyester, such as Dacron. *C*, The artery is sutured closed, and the clamps are removed.

OTHER TECHNIQUES

Recent advances in microcatheter and microballoon technology have lead to the investigational use of interventional neurovascular procedures to treat and prevent cerebrovascular disorders.[10] Results of studies in the use of carotid angioplasty and stenting have been promising. The less invasive procedures would treat severe carotid stenosis in a less invasive way than traditional surgery.[8]

Cerebral angioplasty is similar to coronary angioplasty. A balloon catheter is threaded through the arterial system via the femoral artery to the area of carotid stenosis. A small balloon is inflated to dilate the lesion. A stent catheter can also be used to further open the area of stenosis. The Food and Drug Administration (FDA) views both of these procedures to be experimental. The complications and complication rate are comparable to those of carotid endarterectomy.

Nursing Management of the Surgical Client

Postoperative care after carotid endarterectomy includes neurologic assessments every 1 to 2 hours. Immediately report indications of deterioration of neurologic status. In addition, several cranial nerves are in close proximity to the operative site. The function of the following cranial nerves is assessed: facial (VII), vagus (X), spinal accessory (XI), and hypoglossal (XII). Cranial nerve dysfunction is usually temporary but may last for months. The most common cranial nerve damage causes vocal cord paralysis, difficulty managing saliva, or tongue deviation.

Keep the client's head aligned in a straight position to help maintain airway patency and to minimize stress on the operative site. Antiplatelet agents are often administered. The client can lie supine or on the side, as long as the neck is not flexed.

Elevate the head of the bed when vital signs are stable. Local applications of cold to the operative site may be prescribed.

Frequently assess the client's breathing pattern, pulse, and blood pressure. Maintain the client's blood pressure within 20 mm Hg of the preoperative normal values. Hypertension or hypotension may lead to hemorrhage, ischemia, or occlusion of the anastomosis. Labile blood pressure is a common problem after surgery. Baroreceptors located in the lining of the carotid sinus are one of the primary mechanisms of maintaining normotension. Manipulation of the baroreceptors during surgery causes a short-term disruption in blood pressure regulation.

Observe the operative site. Airway obstruction can occur from excessive swelling of the neck or hematoma formation. Bleeding and hemorrhage are a concern because anticoagulation from intraoperative heparin is not yet reversed. Risk factor modification is essential to the long-term success of the surgery and the general health of the client.[24]

Client and Public Education

The general public has limited knowledge of the manifestations of stroke. In one study, only slightly more than half of the respondents could name at least one stroke manifestation.[33] In addition, only 68% could name a risk factor for stroke.[33] A public education campaign is under way to promote awareness of the manifestations of a stroke. In this campaign, stroke is referred to as "brain attack" to indicate the need for emergency care with the same intensity as a heart attack. Prompt recognition allows for early treatment of a stroke, which may lessen residual deficits and decrease disability. Recognition and modification of risk factors for stroke is the most important prevention available.

CONCLUSIONS

Stroke is being managed today as a treatable problem if it is recognized early. However, because of the limited knowledge of the public about early warning signs, many clients still suffer the consequences of stroke. Treatment of the client with stroke is aimed at maximizing function and preventing disability.

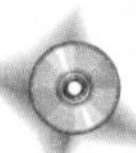

THINKING CRITICALLY

1. A 70-year-old man had a left-sided stroke 2 days ago. While obtaining his assessment, you note that his blood pressure is elevated at 200 mm Hg systolic; his usual systolic blood pressure is 140 to 160 mm Hg. He is receiving oxygen at 5 L, but his oxygen saturation has dropped from 95% to 88% in the last hour. The client was oriented to person, place, and time an hour ago but has become increasingly restless and slightly confused. The confusion has led him to pull out a nasogastric tube that had been placed for nutritional maintenance. What other neurologic assessments should you do? What is the first priority? Is the suddenness of this change significant?

Factors to Consider. How has the client's assessment changed from baseline values? Is there any relationship between the increased blood pressure and the hypoxia? Is the removal of the nasogastric tube an immediate problem?

BIBLIOGRAPHY

1. Barch, C., et al., and the NINDS rt-PA Stroke Study Group. (1997). Nursing management of acute complications following rt-PA in acute ischemic stroke. *Journal of Neuroscience Nursing, 29*(6), 367–372.
2. Berquist, W. H., McLean, R., & Kobylinski, B. A. (1994). *Stroke survivors.* San Francisco: Jossey-Bass Publishers.
3. Bernardine, G. L., & Mayer, S. A. (1999). Cardiac and pulmonary complications of cerebrovascular disease. *The Neurologist 5*(1), 24–32.
4. Biller, J., & Love, B. B. (2000). Ischemic cerebrovascular disease. In W. G. Bradley (Ed.), *Neurology in clinical practice: Principles of diagnosis and management* (3rd ed.). Boston: Butterworth-Heinemann.
5. Braimah, J., et al., and the NINDS rt-PA Stroke Study Group. (1997). Nursing care of acute stroke patients after receiving rt-PA therapy. *Journal of Neuroscience Nursing, 29*(6), 373–383.
6. Broderick, J., et al. (1998). The Greater Cincinnati/Northern Kentucky stroke study: Preliminary first-ever and total incidence rates of stroke among blacks. *Stroke, 29*(2), 415–421.
7. Caplan, L. R. (1998). 10 most commonly asked questions about stroke. *The Neurologist, 4*(4), 227–231.
8. Cates, C. (2000). 10 most commonly asked questions about carotid angioplasty and stenting. *The Neurologist, 6*(1), 58–62.
9. Chan, H. (1997). Bladder management in acute care of stroke patients: A quality improvement project. *Journal of Neuroscience Nursing, 29*(3), 187–190.
10. Clark, W. M., Barnwell, S. L., & Nesbit, G. M. (1997). Potential role of interventional neurovascular therapy for cerebrovascular disease. *The Neurologist, 3*(2), 95–103.
11. Counsell, C., et al. (1995). Nimodipine: A drug therapy for treatment of vasospasm. *Journal of Neuroscience Nursing, 27*(1), 53–55.
12. Daley, S., et al., and the NINDS rt-PA Stroke Study Group. (1997). Education to improve stroke awareness and emergent response. *Journal of Neuroscience Nursing, 29*(6), 393–398.
13. Deibert, E., & Diringer, M. N. (1999). The intensive care management of acute ischemic stroke. *The Neurologist, 5*(6), 313–325.
14. Donnarumma, R., et al., and the NINDS rt-PA Stroke Study Group. (1997). Overview: Hyperacute rt-PA stroke treatment. *Journal of Neuroscience Nursing, 29*(6), 351–355.
15. Fisher, M., & Albers, G. W. (1999). Applications of diffusion-perfusion magnetic resonance imaging in acute ischemic stroke. *Neurology, 52,* 1750–1756.
16. Gelber, D. A., & Callahan, G. D. (1999). Neurorehabilitation. *The Neurologist, 5*(5), 271–278.
17. Hershey, L. (1999). 10 most commonly asked questions about stroke in women. *The Neurologist, 5*(3), 166–168.
18. Hinkle, J. L. (1998). Biological and behavioral correlates of stroke and depression. *Journal of Neuroscience Nursing, 30*(1), 25–31.
19. Hock, N. (1998). Neuroprotective and thrombolytic agents: Advances in stroke treatment. *Journal of Neuroscience Nursing, 30*(3), 175–184.
20. Jeffrey, S. (1998). Managing the "dynamic process" of hemorrhagic stroke. *Neurology Reviews,* 28–29.
21. Johnson, C. J., & Jones, C. E. (1997). Carotid artery surgery. *The Neurologist, 3*(3), 146–154.
22. Kase, C. S. (2000). Intracerebral hemorrhage. In W. G. Bradley (Ed.), *Neurology in clinical practice: Principles of diagnosis and management* (3rd ed.). Boston: Butterworth-Heinemann.
23. Kelly-Hayes, M., & Paige, C. (1995). Assessment and psychologic factors in stroke rehabilitation. *Neurology, 45*(suppl. 1), S29–S32.
24. Leonard, A. (1996). Carotid endarterectomy: A nursing perspective. *Journal of Neuroscience Nursing, 28*(2), 99.
25. Liskay, A. M. (1999). Stroke: Are you at risk? *The Neurologist, 5*(1), 53–54.
26. Lyden, P. D., et al. (1997). Intravenous thrombolysis for acute stroke. *Neurology, 49,* 14–29.
27. Macabasco, A. C., & Hickman, J. L. (1995). Thrombolytic therapy for brain attack. *Journal of Neuroscience Nursing, 27*(3), 138–149.
28. Macdonald, R. L. (1996). Controversies in the management of carotid stenosis. *Journal of Neuroscience Nursing, 28*(2), 93–98.
29. Manno, E. M., et al. (1999). The effects of mannitol on cerebral edema after large hemispheric cerebral infarct. *Neurology, 52,* 583–587.
30. Mayer, S. A., & Dennis, L. J. (1998). Management of increased intracranial pressure. *The Neurologist, 4*(1), 2–12.
31. Mayo, N. E., et al. (2000). There's no place like home: An evaluation of early supported discharge for stroke. *Stroke, 31*(5), 1016–1023.
32. National Institute of Neurological Disorders and Stroke rt-PA Stroke Study Group. (1995). Tissue plasminogen activator for acute ischemic stroke. *New England Journal of Medicine, 333*(24), 1581–1587.
33. Pancioli, A., et al. (1998). Public perception of stroke warning signs and knowledge of potential risk factors. *Journal of the American Medical Association, 279*(16), 1288–1292.
34. Pilkington, F. B. (1999). A qualitative study of life after stroke. *Journal of Neuroscience Nursing, 31*(6), 336–347.
35. Post-stroke Rehabilitation Guideline Panel. (1995). *Post-stroke rehabilitation: Assessment, referral and patient management. Quick reference guide for clinicians. No. 16.* Rockville, MD: U.S. Department of Health and Human Services, Agency for Health Care Policy and Research Pub. No. 95-0663.
36. Post-stroke Rehabilitation Guideline Panel. (1995). Post-stroke rehabilitation: Clinical practice guidelines. *American Family Physician, 52*(2), 461–470.
37. Prichard, J. W., & Grossman, R. I. (1999). New reasons for early use of MRI in stroke. *Neurology, 52,* 1733–1736.
38. Quality Standards Subcommittee of the American Academy of Neurology. (1996). Practice advisory: Thrombolytic therapy for acute ischemic stroke. Summary statement. *Neurology, 47,* 835–839.
39. Rapp, K., et al., and the NINDS rt-PA Stroke Study Group. (1997). Code stroke: Rapid transport, triage and treatment using rt-PA therapy. *Journal of Neuroscience Nursing, 29*(6), 361–366.
40. Raps, E. C., & Galetta, S. L. (1995). Stroke prevention therapies and management of patient subgroups. *Neurology, 45*(suppl. 1), S19–S24.
41. Sacco, R. L. (1995). Risk factors and outcomes for ischemic stroke. *Neurology,* 45(2 suppl. 1):S10–S14.
42. Selman, W. R., Tarr, R., & Landis, D. M. D. (1997). Brain attack: Emergency treatment of ischemic stroke. *American Family Physician, 55*(8), 2655–2662.
43. Shepard, T. J., & Fox, S. W. (1996). Assessment and management of hypertension in the acute ischemic stroke patient. *Journal of Neuroscience Nursing, 28*(1), 5–12.

44. Simmons, B. J. (1997). Management of intracranial hemodynamics in the adult: A research analysis of head positioning and recommendations for clinical practice and further research. *Journal of Neuroscience Nursing, 29*(1), 44–49.
45. Smith, G. R., & Mahoney, C. (1995). Coping and marital equilibrium after stroke. *Journal of Neuroscience Nursing, 27*(2), 83–89.
46. Spilker, J., et al., and the NINDS rt-PA Stroke Study Group. (1997). Using the NIH Stroke Scale to assess stroke patients. *Journal of Neuroscience Nursing, 29*(6), 384–392.
47. Suarez, J. L., et al. (1999). Predictors of clinical improvement, angiographic recanalization, and intracranial hemorrhage after intra-arterial thrombolysis for acute ischemic stroke. *Stroke, 30,* 2094–2100.
48. Swanson, R. A. (1999). Intravenous heparin for acute stroke: What can we learn from the megatrials? *Neurology, 52,* 1746–1750.
49. Testani-Dufour, L., & Marano Morrison, C. A. (1997). Brain attack: Correlative anatomy. *Journal of Neuroscience Nursing, 29*(4), 213–222.
50. Toni, D., et al. (1996). Hemorrhagic transformation of brain infarct: Predictability in the first 5 hours from stroke onset and influence on clinical outcome. *Neurology, 46,* 341–345.

REMEMBER *to check out your* **Companion CD ROM**

CHAPTER 71

Management of Clients with Peripheral Nervous System Disorders

Anne Marie Johnson Fredrichs

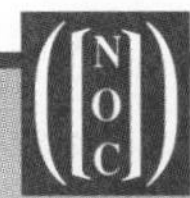

NURSING OUTCOME CLASSIFICATION (NOC) for Nursing Diagnoses—Clients with Peripheral Nerve Disorders

Activity Intolerance
Ambulation: Walking
Activity Tolerance
Pain: Disruptive Effects
Altered Role Performance
Role Performance
Psychosocial Adjustment: Life Change
Altered Tissue Perfusion: Peripheral
Sensory Function: Cutaneous
Tissue Perfusion: Peripheral

Altered Urinary Elimination
Urinary Continence
Urinary Elimination
Anxiety
Psychosocial Adjustment: Life Change
Symptom Control
Body Image Disturbance
Acceptance: Health Status
Self-Esteem

Chronic Pain
Body Image
Hope
Role Performance
Self-Esteem
Social Interaction Skills
Impaired Physical Mobility
Mobility Level
Pain Level
Pain
Comfort Level
Pain Level

This chapter examines disorders of the peripheral nerves and cranial nerves. The autonomic disorders are discussed in Chapter 72. Disorders of the spinal cord, apart from spinal cord injury, also are presented. Spinal cord injury is discussed in Chapter 73.

LOWER BACK PAIN

The spine is a mechanical organ that has been described as a crane with the ability to support weight, maintain balance, and counter numerous daily strains during normal work and recreational activities. Although it has tremendous ability to withstand most mechanical stresses, it can be stressed beyond its limits. Forces that exceed the capacity of the tissues to stretch can lead to injury and pain. Low back pain is the second most common reason for visits to a physician. The treatment of low back costs $70 to $100 billion yearly.

Etiology

The origin of back pain is not well known and has never been fully described. Many groups have given up trying to describe the cause of lower back pain and instead have listed several *red flag* conditions that are associated with the problem. Three groups of problems lead to back pain:

1. *Biomechanical* origins include compression of the discs, herniation of the disc, torsion injury, or vibration. These problems are seen when clients have occupations that require strenuous or repetitive lifting in a stooped position or occupations that require operating vibrating machinery.
2. *Destructive* origins include infection, tumors, and rheumatoid disorders.
3. *Degenerative* problems include osteoporosis and spinal stenosis.

Vertebrae can also be affected by osteoporosis. Osteoporotic vertebrae can collapse and lead to compression of the nerve roots. The spinal canal can narrow and compress the nerves; this problem is called *spinal stenosis.* It usually occurs in older people. Severity can range from entrapment of one nerve root to compression of the entire cord.

Other disorders include those that have no clear physiologic cause, yet lead to loss of income and pain. There is a growing body of data that show strong psychological influences on the response of clients to lower back pain. The primary determining factors for disability from low back pain appear to be based on whether the client is depressed, unhappy in a work setting, or involved in litigation. These psychosocial issues do not mean the pain is not real. The manner in which the brain processes pain may be implicated. The psychosocial aspects may suppress the serotoninergic pathways and limit the secretion of endorphins.

Back Strain

Back strain is an acute injury leading to lower back pain. Back strain occurs when the client flexes the back without bending the knees or makes rotating movements, creating significant stress on the intervertebral disc and muscles of the lower back.

Disc Herniation

An intervertebral disc is a pad that rests between the centers of two adjacent vertebrae. Discs provide cushions for spinal movement. The intervertebral disc is composed of three parts:

1. *Cartilaginous plates* act as the superior and inferior limits of the disc. These plates are composed of hyaline cartilage and cover the top and bottom of the vertebrae.
2. The *annulus fibrosus* is a ring of tissue that gives size and shape to the disc and holds the nucleus pulposus in place.
3. The *nucleus pulposus* is a semigelatinous material that forms the center of the disc and provides the cushioning effect.

Strenuous activity or degeneration of the disc or vertebrae can allow the disc to move from its normal location. Displacement of intervertebral disc material may be referred to as *prolapse, herniation, rupture,* or *extrusion.* Ruptured intervertebral discs may occur at any level of the spine. Lumbar discs are more likely to rupture than cervical discs because of the force of gravity; continual movement in this region; and improper movements of the spine, as with lifting or turning. As in spinal cord injury, thoracic disc disorders are the least common.

More than half of people with clinical manifestations of a herniated disc give a history of a previous back injury. Heavy physical labor, strenuous exercise, and weak abdominal and back muscles increase the risk of herniated disc. Repeated stress progressively weakens the disc, resulting in bulging and herniation.

Lordosis

Lordosis is an excessive backward concavity in the lumbar spine. It is commonly associated with sagging shoulders, medial rotation of the legs, and an exaggerated pelvic angle. Excessive lordosis may result in swayback and kyphosis. Back pain is common.

Spondylolisthesis

Spondylolisthesis is the forward slipping of one vertebra. It commonly occurs at L4–L5, where the upper vertebra slips forward out of alignment. Spondylolisthesis is graded from 1 to 4. Grades 1 and 2 are managed conservatively; for grades 3 and 4, surgery with fusion is usually required for stabilization (Fig. 71–1).

Spondylolysis

Spondylolysis is a structural defect in the lamina or neural arch of the spine. The vertebral arch slips forward. The lumbar spine is most commonly involved.

Spinal Stenosis

Spinal stenosis (Fig. 71–2) is due to ligamentous infolding and hypertrophy of the bone. It produces pressure on the entire spinal cord. If compression remains untreated, weakness or paralysis of the innervated muscle groups may result.

Pathophysiology

The pathophysiology of lower back pain is a source of fascination, frustration, and often confusion by clinicians and scientists who attempt to treat and study clients with this problem. The spine is the only organ that consists of bones, joints, ligaments, fatty tissue, multiple layers of muscles, peripheral nerves, sensory ganglia, autonomic ganglia, and the spinal cord. These structures, in turn, are fed by an intricate system of arteries and veins. The movement of the spine is complex and injury to the spine and other structures leads to unique patterns of pain.

Compressive loads have different effects on the intervertebral disc, body of the vertebrae, facets, and spinal ligaments. Under compressive loads, the annular fibers of the discs are stretched. The vertebrae are also compressed and may fracture at the end-plates. Spinal ligaments tend to buckle easily, and the facet joints offer little resistance to compression.

The result is that the disc can herniate. When the disc only bulges, the annulus remains intact. With herniation, the annulus usually is torn, allowing extrusion of the nucleus pulposus (see Fig. 71–2). Compression of spinal nerve roots may result from herniation of the disc. The discs that separate and pad the vertebrae are innervated with fine nerve endings. When a lumbar disc impinges on the sciatic nerve, the condition with its resulting pain is called *sciatica.* Sciatica is a severe, usually activity-dependent, intermittent pain in the leg that occurs along the course of the sciatic nerve and its branches.

Clinical Manifestations

Rupture or herniation of a lumbar disc leads to lower back pain that radiates down the sciatic nerve into the posterior thigh as a result of compression of the spinal nerve roots. Typically, the pain of sciatica begins in the

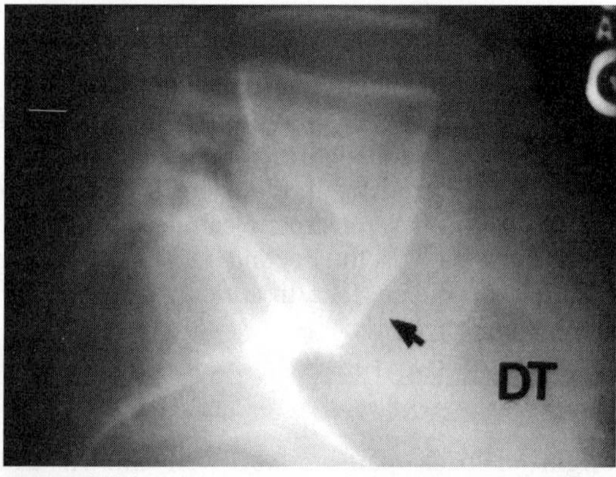

FIGURE 71–1 Preoperative radiograph of spondylolisthesis. Note the slippage of the vertebrae. (Courtesy of James Manz, M.D., Mayo Clinic, Eau Claire, WI.)

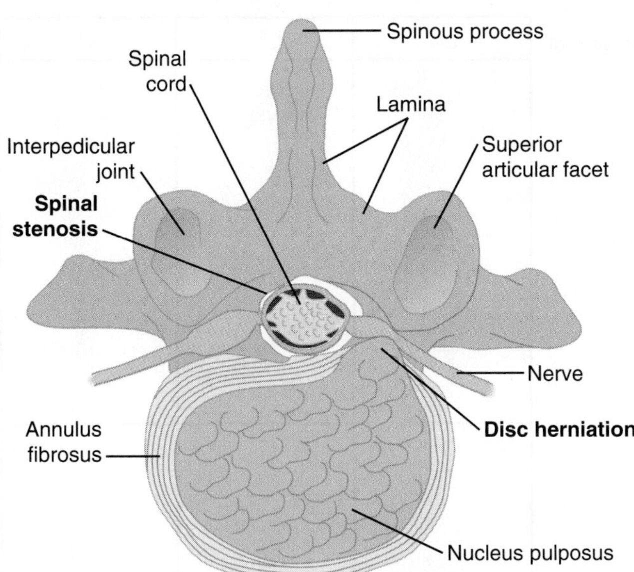

FIGURE 71–2 The usual causes of low back pain are disc herniation and spinal stenosis.

buttocks and extends down the back of the thigh and leg to the ankle. Disc herniation can also lead to groin pain. The client also has muscle spasms and hyperesthesia (numbness and tingling) in the area of distribution of affected nerve roots. The pain is exacerbated by straining (coughing, sneezing, defecation, bending, lifting, and straight-leg raising) or prolonged sitting and is relieved by side-lying with the knees flexed. Any movement of the lower extremities that stretches the nerve causes pain and involuntary resistance. Straight-leg raising on the affected side is limited. Complete extension of the leg is not possible when the thigh is flexed on the abdomen (Lasègue sign). There may be depression of deep tendon reflexes.

Manifestations of spinal stenosis usually begin slowly and are due to pressure placed on nerve roots as they exit the vertebrae. The most common manifestations are aching pain with standing and walking, paresthesias, and heaviness in the legs that progresses as the client walks. There is rapid improvement in manifestations with trunk flexion, stooping, or sitting. The manifestations of spinal stenosis must be differentiated from claudication.

Diagnostic Findings

X-ray studies may show spinal degenerative changes (at any level) that may indicate disc problems but usually do not show a ruptured disc. Osteophytes and narrowed disc interspaces are degenerative changes visible on radiographs. Other spinal disorders (e.g., spinal tumors, vertebral fracture, rheumatoid arthritis, and osteoarthritis) can lead to the same manifestations.

Magnetic resonance imaging (MRI) may show spinal stenosis (narrowing of the spinal canal), extrusion of disc material into the spinal canal, and impingement of a spinal nerve root (Fig. 71–3).

Myelography may show narrowing of the disc space and impingement of a spinal nerve root. This modality can identify the level of herniation and may be used to rule out other spinal diseases. It is typically performed if MRI is not conclusive.

A computed tomography (CT) scan usually is done after myelography. This sequence allows better imaging with only one administration of contrast material. CT scanning may show spinal stenosis or other changes associated with degenerative disc disease. CT scans are more useful at the thoracic or lumbar level than the cervical level.

Discography is the injection of a water-soluble imaging material into the nucleus pulposus. It is used to determine internal changes in the disc. During the injection, information is recorded about the amount of dye accepted and the pressure needed to inject the material. Clients can have allergic responses to the contrast agent and develop disc space infections from the injection. Electromyography of the peripheral nerves also may be used to localize the site of the ruptured disc. Paraspinal mapping and somatosensory evoked potentials may be used for diagnosis.

Outcome Management

Medical Management

Goals of medical care include reducing pain and spasms, improving mobility, and repairing any structural problems in the spine or discs.

Initial assessment of the client with lower back pain is designed to help pinpoint the cause. The client's medical history is obtained to help determine whether a serious underlying condition is responsible for the pain, such as a fracture, tumor, or infection. The client's psychological and socioeconomic history is obtained because such prob-

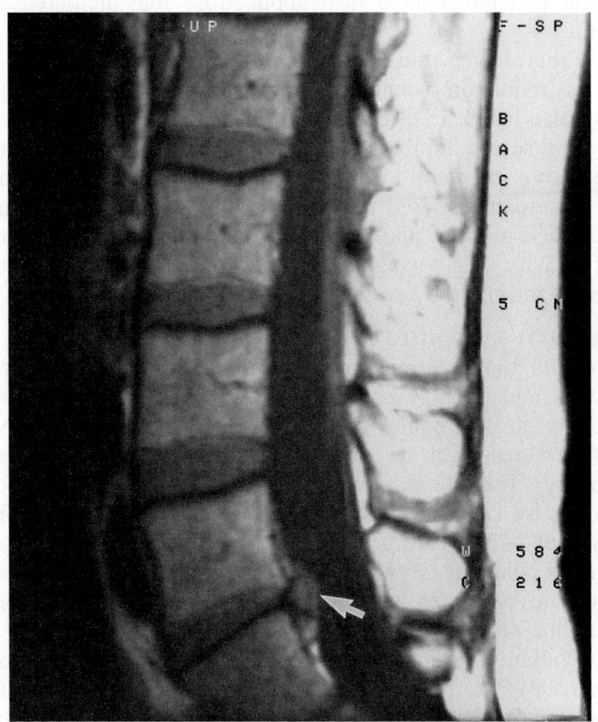

FIGURE 71–3 Magnetic resonance image of the lumbar spine shows herniation of the disc between L5 and S1.

lems can complicate assessment and management. The client also is asked to rate the pain. Physical examination is used to determine whether lumbar nerve roots are involved by testing for reflexes, muscle strength, and the presence of neurologic deficits (Fig. 71–4).

Control Pain and Spasms

Initial care of acute lower back pain is directed at managing the client's pain and directing activities. Pain usually is managed with nonsteroidal anti-inflammatory drugs (NSAIDs) or COX-2 inhibitors, muscle relaxants, and, at times, narcotics. Ice may be used to reduce pain with acute disc herniation for the first 48 hours. After that time, heat usually is a better analgesic. A semi-sitting position (in a recliner chair) usually is comfortable and promotes forward lumbar spine flexion and reduces back strain. Other positions of comfort include (1) the supine position with pillows under the legs and (2) the lateral position, in which the client lies on the unaffected side with a thin pillow between the knees with the painful leg flexed to reduce tension on the sciatic nerve. Lying in a prone position and sleeping with thick pillows under the head should be avoided. Physical therapists may be able to relieve pain and spasm with stretching exercises and ultrasonic heat treatments. Work space or equipment modifications may also be necessary.

If the client has nonspecific lower back pain, manipulation may be used by a physical therapist or chiropractor. *Spinal manipulation* is the use of the hands on the spine to stretch, mobilize, or manipulate the spine and paravertebral tissues. It usually is performed for clients with manifestations that last more than 1 month. The Agent for Health Care Policy and Research (AHCPR)[1] review panel found no evidence that spinal traction with weights was effective in reducing lower back pain. Although unproven, deep ultrasonic heat treatment and moist local heat applications may help reduce pain.

Progressive muscle relaxation exercises and other stress reduction techniques can be helpful. Muscle stretching also has been effective for fascial pain.

For severe lumbar disc problems with leg pain, conservative intervention involves 2 to 4 days of bed rest on a firm mattress. Bed rest relieves back pain by relieving the back muscles and vertebrae of the stresses. The forces of gravity (e.g., weight of the head with cervical problems) and motion can increase back pain during activity.

Improve Mobility

Activity modifications are prescribed to reduce back irritation and to prevent debilitation from inactivity. Most clients do not require bed rest; in fact, more than 4 days of bed rest can be debilitating and actually slow recovery. The client is taught to minimize the stress of lifting by keeping objects close to the body and to avoid twisting when lifting. Sitting may worsen leg pain, and clients who sit at work should change positions often. Aerobic activities should be prescribed to help avoid debilitation.

Walking, stationary bicycling, and back strengthening exercises can be performed. Exercise may begin within the first 2 weeks after injury, and each activity should be performed for 20 to 30 minutes, two or three times a week, for best aerobic conditioning.

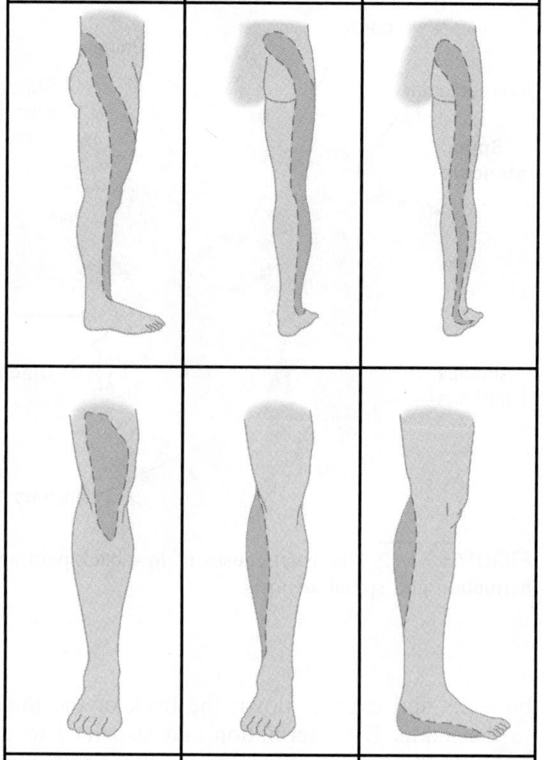

Nerve root	L4	L5	S1
Pain			
Numbness			
Motor weakness	Extension of quadriceps	Dorsiflexion of great toe and foot	Plantar flexion of great toe and foot
Screening Exam	Squat and rise	Heel walking	Walking on toes
Reflexes	Knee jerk diminished	None reliable	Ankle jerk diminished

FIGURE 71–4 Assessment of lumbar nerve root compromise includes testing for motor weakness and reflexes and eliciting pain (screening examination). (Redrawn from Agency for Health Care Policy and Research. [1994]. *Acute low back problems in adults: Assessment and treatment. Quick reference guide for clinicians,* No. 14. Rockville, MD: Author.)

Work activities need to be individualized for each client based on job requirements. See the Client Education Guide on lower back care.

A back brace or corset may be prescribed for a client with a ruptured lumbar disc. Back supports usually are not recommended once clinical manifestations are relieved, however, because restricted back motion progressively weakens muscles and causes further degeneration of spinal structures. Exercise to strengthen the back and abdominal muscles helps prevent further problems if the exercises are done daily throughout life.

Nursing Care of the Medical Client

Nursing care focuses on assisting the client to adjust his or her lifestyle to reduce the risk of further back injuries. Many clients are frustrated with the lack of cure of their back pain. Clients have become accustomed to having a well-defined cause of a problem and a well-researched approach for management. Many clients with lower back pain have pain for years without relief. This level of chronic pain can lead to depression and personality or relationship difficulties. Nurses remain sensitive to the exasperation felt by the clients as well as the health care team.

Nurses are actively involved in teaching the client safe methods to lift and bend, how to lie down and how to rise from bed to avoid twisting, and how to take NSAIDs correctly to reduce the risk of gastric ulceration. If the client requires narcotics for pain, instruct the client to eat high-fiber foods to reduce constipation and not to operate machinery or drive. The Client Education Guide on lower back care can be used to teach clients.

Surgical Management

Surgery is indicated in clients with spinal disc problems when (1) sciatica is severe and disabling, (2) manifestations of sciatica persist without improvement or worsen, and (3) physiologic evidence of specific nerve root dysfunction is present. Surgery also is used to stabilize spinal fractures and to correct scoliosis and kyphoscoliosis. Some surgeons use other criteria.

CHEMONUCLEOLYSIS

Chymopapain is a proteolytic enzyme isolated from papaya latex that is used as a meat tenderizer. Injected into the disc, chymopapain digests the protein in the disc and shrinks it. It is contraindicated in people with multiple allergies and in people allergic to papaya. Immediate and delayed (after 15 days) allergic responses have been reported. Its use has been abandoned by most practitioners.

PERCUTANEOUS DISCECTOMY

Herniated disc material can be excised with a trocar to remove the center of the disc. The laser also is used to destroy the damaged disc.

MICRODISCECTOMY

Microdiscectomy is the use of microsurgical instruments to remove the herniated fragment of disc. Use of this technique results in less trauma to the surgical site compared with standard surgery, and more tissue integrity is preserved. Advantages of microsurgery include (1) minimal nerve root retraction, (2) preservation of an intact joint capsule (no bone is removed), (3) improved hemostasis, and (4) minimal stripping of the muscle and fascia from the spine.

DECOMPRESSIVE LAMINECTOMY

The term *laminectomy* is confusing and is used loosely. The term *laminectomy* means complete removal of the bone between the spinous process and the facet; this seldom is necessary. The more correct term for what is done is a *laminotomy*, or the creation of a hole in the lamina.

Decompressive laminectomy is surgical removal of the posterior arch of a vertebra, exposing the spinal cord (Fig. 71–5). This procedure gives access to the spinal canal for (1) removing a spinal cord tumor, (2) removing portions of the facets, or (3) decompressing bone infringement on the spinal cord. Sometimes foraminotomy is performed to enlarge the intervertebral foramen if it is narrowed and osteophytic processes (overgrowth of bone) entrap the nerve root and impinge on neural structures.

SPINAL FUSION/ARTHRODESIS

Spinal fusion is the placement of bone grafts (bone chips) between vertebrae (Fig. 71–6). The new bone that grows fuses the two vertebrae and immobilizes them to reduce the pain. Usually no more than five vertebrae are fused; fusing more than five vertebrae causes considerable loss of movement in the spine. The bone graft may be obtained from a bone bank or the anterior-superior iliac crest. During healing, the graft gradually grows onto the vertebrae and forms a bone union. This bone union causes permanent stiffness in the area. The stiffness is hardly noticed in the lumbar area after a while but is noticeable in the cervical area. The client cannot be guaranteed that back pain will be relieved permanently or that further surgery will not be required.

SPINAL FUSION WITH INSTRUMENTATION

Metal rods may be used to straighten and fuse the spine in disorders such as scoliosis or multiple vertebral fractures. Other devices also can be used to provide additional support while the bones heal in a fused manner (Fig. 71–7).

COMPLICATIONS

General potential complications after spinal disc surgery at any level include infection and inflammation, injury to nerve roots, dural tears, cauda equina syndrome, and hematoma. Non-union of the surgical area also is a risk and

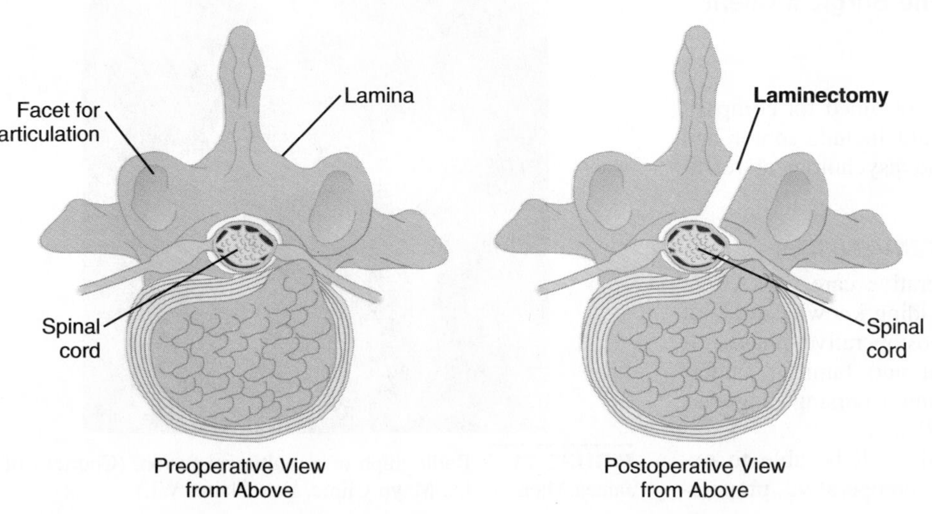

FIGURE 71–5 Laminectomy for the interlaminal removal of a herniated disc.

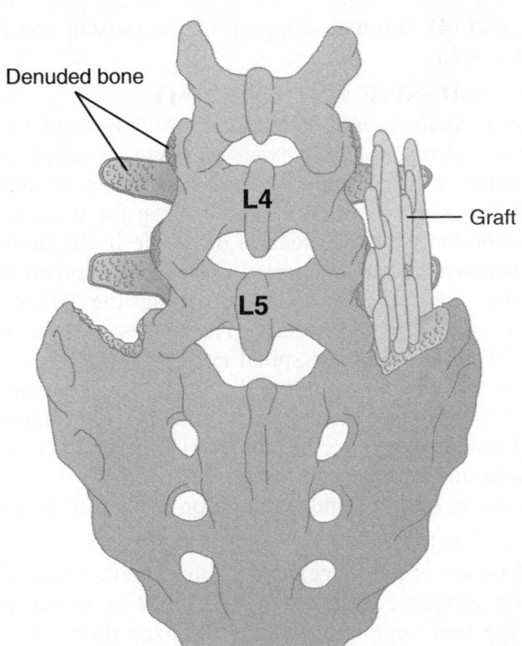

FIGURE 71–6 Lumbar interbody spinal fusion. Bone grafts are taken from the iliac crest and inserted between the vertebrae. The bed of raw bone is shown on the left, and the graft material is shown in place on the right.

is associated with smoking. Some surgeons assess serum nicotine levels prior to surgery to reduce the risk of non-union and validate statements of smoking cessation.

PROGNOSIS

The AHCPR reviewed outcomes of surgery for lower back problems.[1] In general, lumbar discectomy often relieved manifestations of pain faster than continued medical management in people with severe and disabling leg pain. In other people with no leg pain, however, there appeared to be little difference in outcome between discectomy and conservative care. Most clients who had chymopapain injections required eventual discectomy for permanent pain relief. More study is needed to determine who is best served by the various techniques; client preference also plays a big role in the technique chosen.

Nursing Management of the Surgical Client

PREOPERATIVE CARE

ASSESSMENT

A baseline neurologic assessment is obtained for comparison after surgery. Assessment should include motor and sensory function of extremities and psychological readiness for surgery.

DIAGNOSIS, OUTCOMES, INTERVENTION

Knowledge Deficit. Perioperative care of a client having spinal surgery includes providing knowledge about the preoperative, operative, and postoperative phases. It also includes evaluating the client and family's understanding of the experience. A common nursing diagnosis in this circumstance is *Knowledge Deficit.*

Outcomes. The client and family will be able to explain the surgical procedure, the preoperative preparations, and the postoperative precautions and needs. The client will demonstrate safe mobility, including logrolling and transfer to and from the bed.

Interventions. Include the family in preoperative education. Explain to the client that frequent turning follows surgery and that correct turning protects the back and helps the recovery process. Explain the logrolling method of turning, the necessity for limitations on activity to prevent damage (flexion, extension, or twisting) to the surgical site, and the importance of not straining. Advise the client to ask for help rather than stretch to reach for objects. Stool softeners are given daily while the client is in the hospital to minimize straining with bowel movements. Clients with a recent injury may not be permitted to ambulate before surgery. For these clients, explain and demonstrate.

Encourage clients who smoke to stop smoking. Smoking increases cardiovascular complications and increases the risk of poor wound healing and non-union if a fusion is performed.

If a fusion is to be done, clients need to be evaluated for autologous blood donations. Two to 3 units should be donated, the last one at least 1 week before the surgery. Elderly clients may require more time for blood donation. A fusion also necessitates informing the client of the bone graft site and the additional pain associated with the autograft bone donor site.

The client may also need changes in the home setting. These changes should be considered before surgery and include location of bathroom, devices needed for ambulation, ability to use the shower, and toilet seat risers.

Fear and Anxiety. Many people fear postoperative problems such as paralysis and chronic pain. *Fear and Anxiety* is a common nursing diagnosis in this situation.

Outcomes. The client will express a low level of fear or anxiety related to the upcoming surgery and will use positive coping strategies to decrease fear or anxiety.

Interventions. Encourage the client and family to express their concerns and fears about the spinal surgery. Concerns and fears should be allayed whenever possible. For example, clients need to be aware that some edema is

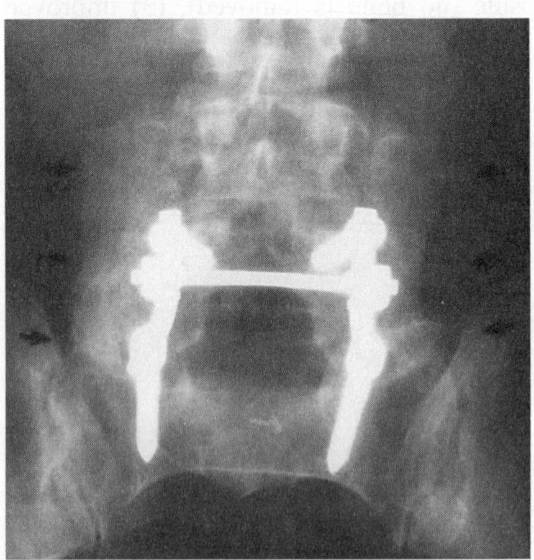

FIGURE 71–7 Radiograph of a multilevel fusion. (Courtesy of James Manz, M.D., Mayo Clinic, Eau Claire, WI.)

expected at the surgical site, and some of the preoperative deficit may still exist after surgery but should improve as the edema lessens.

EVALUATION

Preoperative education should allay some of the concerns of the client and family. Do not expect all anxiety to be relieved; in fact, some new areas of concern may arise. If questions come up about the operation, ask the surgeon to answer them. Do not attempt to provide information outside of your area of expertise.

POSTOPERATIVE CARE

ASSESSMENT

After spinal surgery, assessment is similar to that performed for other surgical clients. A head-to-toe assessment is done. Dressings and drains are checked. Evaluate the level of pain and the response to analgesia. Assess neurologic function by asking the client to move his or her legs and feet and comparing the results with those of the baseline evaluation.

Question the client about the presence of numbness or tingling and changes in sensation or pain. These paresthesias are a consequence of the edema from the surgery but should improve. If progressive weakness or paralysis of the lower extremities, loss of sphincter control, anal numbness, or urinary retention (called the *cauda equina syndrome*) occur, notify the physician immediately. Emergency surgical decompression may be required.

Clients who have had fusions are on bed rest longer and are at higher risk for deep venous thrombosis. Compression devices may be used to improve venous return. Observe for and report any manifestations of deep venous thrombosis: positive Homans' sign, redness or swelling in the leg, or sudden chest pain or dyspnea. Assess the wound for bulging or clear drainage, which may indicate cerebrospinal fluid leakage. If the client has had an anterior approach, usual care for abdominal surgery is required (e.g., assessment of ileus).

Disc problems often create fears and concerns related to pain, treatments, sexual activity, possible length of illness, and possible lifestyle changes. Provide psychosocial support to the client and family. Impaired mobility and altered urinary or bowel elimination also are common problems experienced after disc surgery. Considerations about employment and finances should be referred to a social worker.

DIAGNOSIS, OUTCOMES, INTERVENTIONS

Pain. Pain secondary to incisional trauma and edema is an expected response after spinal surgery. Write this common postoperative nursing diagnosis as *Pain related to tissue trauma secondary to back (and/or abdominal) incision.*

Outcomes. The client will express comfort, such as level 3 on a scale of 0 to 10.

Interventions. Although acute incisional pain is present, often the pain in an extremity is significantly less after herniated disc surgery. Many surgeons inject long-acting local anesthetics into disc spaces during surgery. This injection gives the client immediate relief from pain and promotes a positive attitude toward the outcome of surgery. Often the pain recurs on the second postoperative day. This recurrence is due to the increase in swelling and the fact that the local anesthetic is wearing off.

Acute postoperative pain can be managed by using a basal dose of a narcotic with an intravenous (IV) pump in combination with a patient-controlled analgesia (PCA) dose for pain peaks (breakthrough pain) not controlled by the continuous dose. Another method of providing basal (continuous) pain medication is by intravenous drip or epidural catheter. If the client is on as-needed (prn) pain management, teach the client to keep pain levels tolerable by asking for narcotics before the pain is too great. Ice may be applied to the incision using an abdominal wrap that holds sheets of ice along the lumbar area and reduces the risk of ice burns.

Impaired Physical Mobility. Clients who have spinal surgery have varying degrees of mobility limitations. The diagnosis can be written as *Impaired Physical Mobility related to pain, leg weakness, prolonged immobility, or fear of pain and spasms.* Choose the etiologic mechanism that best fits your client.

Outcomes. The client will resume a maximal level of progressive activity, starting with logrolling on the day of surgery, progressing to independent movement from the bed to a standing position, followed by independent ambulation before discharge.

Interventions. Encourage the client to move the legs and feet while on bed rest to promote venous return. Alternating compression stockings may be used to promote venous return. Keep the bed linens loose at the foot of the bed to promote movement. If the client requires assistance to turn or when turning to place a bedpan, turn the client in the logrolling manner. A fracture bedpan is used to reduce back arching and strain.

When the client is being transferred to bed postoperatively, at least four people should assist. Transfer devices, such as a sliding board, may be used with adequate help. Transfer the client gently and smoothly, with the spine supported and properly aligned at all times.

Immediately after lumbar discectomy, the client typically is not turned for an hour or so but remains flat to aid hemostasis. Begin side-to-side logrolling, and repeat every 2 hours. If a dural tear was repaired, the surgeon may order the client to remain flat longer to minimize the risk of cerebrospinal fluid leak or a tear in the dural sutures. While clients are immobile and supine, elevate the heels from the bed.

After lumbar fusion, the bed generally is kept flat. The client logrolls from side to side, usually beginning about 4 hours after surgery, then every 2 to 4 hours thereafter. Twisting the client's spine or twisting at the hips must be avoided. Ensure safety during turning to prevent straining of the spine or rolling off the bed. It is beneficial to have extra help in turning a client the first few times after spinal surgery. Spinal bone grafts are delicate and heal slowly. Eventually, turning is permitted without help, while keeping the spine rigid.

It is common for the client to have spasms and pain with turning, and pain medication should be administered before moving. If the client is receiving medication by PCA administer the medication about 10 minutes before moving the client. The advanced dose provides pain control without the immediate nausea and flushing that many clients develop. Once the client is turned, tilt the client back onto pillows to reduce pressure on the iliac crest. Back strain may then be reduced by (1) keeping the client's spine straight, (2) flexing the upper leg and placing a pillow between the legs, and (3) placing a pillow to support the upper arm and prevent the upper shoulder from sagging. If the iliac crest has been used as a donor site, the client may not be able to turn onto that side because of pain. Abdominal incisions should be splinted to reduce pain.

Follow the surgeon's orders on how high the head of the bed can be elevated. Use a pressure-reduction mattress to reduce the risk of pressure ulcers if the client had spinal surgery for fracture stabilization or will be in bed for a long time. Use of a trapeze over the bed is contraindicated because it promotes twisting. The call light and PCA control are placed so that the client can touch them without straining. Once the client is allowed to reach for things, objects should be placed conveniently.

If a client is supine after spinal surgery (e.g., is using a bedpan), the lower back muscles may be relaxed somewhat if pillows are placed under the entire length of the legs. This placement may also prevent thrombophlebitis in the femoral vessels. Do not flex the client's knees by placing anything under the popliteal space; this is hazardous because it increases the risk of deep venous thrombosis. A sign is placed on the bed describing the prescribed position for the bed. Instruct the client clearly about contraindicated activities and positions.

To assist the client into a chair, keep the bed flat, and teach the client to roll onto the side (Fig. 71–8). Then push the torso from the bed with the arms to rise from the bed. This technique has often been used by clients with long-standing back pain and may be familiar to the client. If the client has had long-standing back pain before surgery, review the client's technique for rising from the bed. Usually the client is assisted to a chair the morning after surgery. Be sure to follow the physician's activity prescriptions.

After spinal surgery, a brace or corset may be required temporarily to support the spine. Clients who have lumbar or thoracic spinal fusions may wear a fiberglass brace. Initially, back braces or corsets may be worn all the time, whether the client is in or out of bed. As the client's muscles strengthen, the use of braces or corsets usually is decreased. Casts may be used for a while after any thoracic spinal surgery for clients with unstable thoracic spines (e.g., thoracic spinal cord trauma).

Altered Urinary Elimination. After spinal surgery, urinary retention may occur. Most commonly, it occurs because of pain and spasms when resting supine and as a side effect of narcotics. Retention also occurs when the cauda equina is affected. Write the nursing diagnosis as *Risk for Altered Urinary Elimination related to pain and spasms with movement, inability to void in a supine position, and side effects from narcotics.*

Outcomes. The client will resume normal bladder emptying by the time he or she is ambulating.

Interventions. Assess for bladder distention and pain 8 hours after surgery. If the client's bladder is distended and painful on palpation, noninvasive measures should be tried first. The client is commonly catheterized with an in-and-out catheter (straight catheterization) twice, after which an indwelling catheter is placed. It may be used for the first few days until the client is ambulating and using less pain medication. When the catheter is removed, generally clients can urinate when sitting or standing rather than lying supine. If the bladder is full or cannot be emptied completely, the physician may order straight catheterization to check for residual urine.

Risk for Paralytic Ileus. The most common bowel problem after laminectomy and spinal fusion is

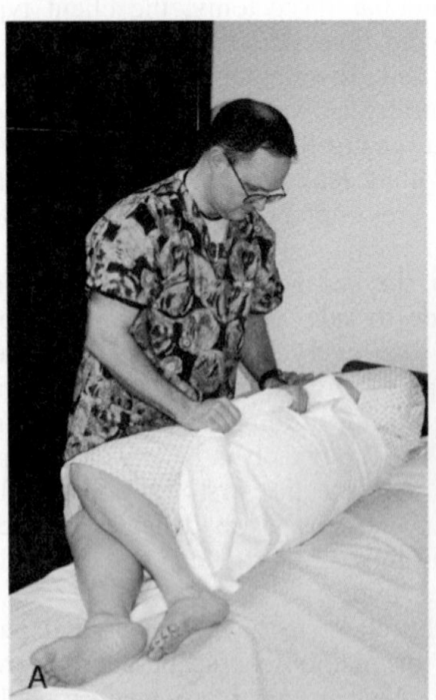

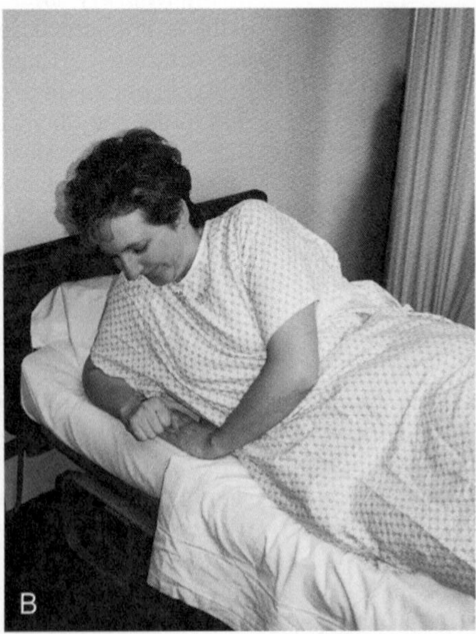

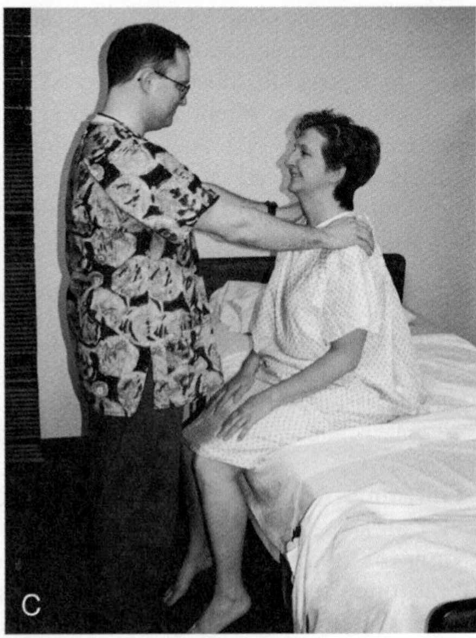

FIGURE 71–8 Helping the client stand after lumbar fusion. *A,* Logroll the client to the edge of the bed using a turning sheet if needed. Leave the bed in that position. *B,* The client pushes off the bed with the hand and the other elbow to sit up without twisting. The client drops her legs off the side of the bed at the same time. *C,* With the client seated on the edge of the bed, the nurse assesses for orthostatic hypotension. The client stands from the bed without flexing the back.

paralytic ileus. This loss of bowel sounds and abdominal distention is due to lack of peristalsis from a sudden loss of parasympathetic function innervating the bowels and manipulation of the intestines in anterior approaches to spinal surgery.

Outcomes. The nurse can expect return of normal bowel function, including normal bowel sound patterns, and evacuation without straining, by the time the client is ambulating. This problem is expressed as a collaborative situation; therefore, the outcome is written in terms of the nurse's actions. The nurse's actions cannot independently alter the outcome, as occurs with nursing diagnoses.

Interventions. Assessment findings with paralytic ileus include nausea, vomiting, a hard abdomen, and absence of bowel sounds. The client is assessed every 4 hours postoperatively for bowel distention.

If the client has paralytic ileus or if ileus is expected to develop as a result of extensive manipulation during surgery, a nasogastric tube connected to low intermittent suction is inserted and the client takes no fluid or food by mouth (NPO status). When a client's gag reflex and bowel sounds have returned and the client passes gas or has a bowel movement, a clear liquid diet is prescribed and the client progresses to a regular diet.

Bowel dysfunction may occur for several days postoperatively. Inactivity often causes problems with bowel elimination. Bowel movements are documented. Fluids are forced as ordered; a regular time for bowel movements and bowel care is encouraged; fiber is provided in the diet (when allowed), and prescribed medications and enemas (e.g., stool softeners, mild bulk laxatives, or a suppository) are administered. Instruct the client not to strain for a bowel movement because this increases pain and cerebrospinal fluid pressure. Often, clients find it difficult or impossible to defecate when lying flat. A bowel movement may not occur until sitting up is possible.

Evaluation. Expect pain to be controlled with mild to moderate narcotic analgesics, bowel and bladder function to be intact, the client to be able to walk steadily for several yards, and the client to be able to eat before discharge.

Self-Care

Approximately 80% of the population experience lower back pain at some point in their lives. About 10% of clients who seek medical attention for back pain have herniated discs. Because of the frequency of herniated disc problems, health promotion is an essential activity for health care providers. The Client Education Guide provides suggestions for lower back care.

CERVICAL DISC DISORDERS

Discs may become entrapped in the cervical spine. The process is similar to that with herniated lumbar discs.

CLIENT EDUCATION GUIDE

Lower Back Care

- Get out of bed by rolling onto one side near the edge of the mattress. Push up to a straight position by pushing off the bed with your arms, while keeping your spine straight, and swing your legs over the edge. Avoid twisting while getting up.
- Do not sleep while partially reclined or sitting in a chair. Sleep on a bed with a firm (not hard) mattress.
- Avoid riding in or driving a car for a long distance or time. Sit erect without slouching.
- Avoid low couches and chairs, and use your leg muscles when rising from a chair; a recliner chair is usually comfortable.
- When you must stand for a long time, bend one knee to reduce stress on your lower back by elevating one foot on a stool.
- Maintain a body weight that is close to ideal.
- Exercise and walk or swim to strengthen your back and abdominal muscles. Wear low-heeled shoes.
- Eat a diet high in fiber and fluids to soften bowel movements and reduce strain. When adding fiber to your diet, add it slowly over days.
- Use proper body mechanics when lifting. Get adequate help if the object is heavy. Use the muscles of your legs, not your back, by bending at the knees to get close to the object being lifted. Never turn and lift at the same time.

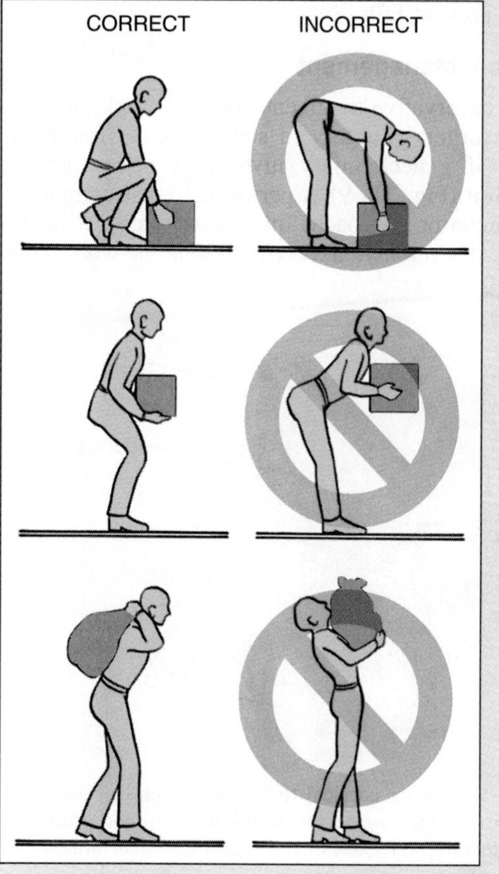

Manifestations include arm pain, neck pain and spasms, and loss of function (grip strength) and changes in sensation in the hands.

Outcome Management

Medical Management

Initial treatment is with NSAIDs, muscle stretching, and teaching proper body mechanics. Opinions differ concerning the advisability of performing head and neck range-of-motion exercises in the presence of significant cervical disease. Tell the client to avoid activities that increase cervical disc pain. To prevent neck extension when in bed, only one flat pillow (to prevent neck flexion) is recommended. The neck should not be hyperextended. Intermittent traction may be applied for cervical disc herniation (5 to 8 pound weight) to relieve pain. The head of the bed may be elevated slightly with cervical traction. Otherwise, it is best kept flat when cervical pain is present. A review of posture at work is important for clients who work at computer terminals. Keyboards, screens, and written materials should be kept at a height that reduces strain on the neck and shoulders.

A soft cervical collar may be prescribed for mild to moderate cervical disc problems to keep the head slightly flexed. After fracture of a cervical vertebra, cervical disc rupture, or whiplash injury, the client may wear a neck brace (fitted so that the chin rests on a cup and the neck is kept hyperextended), a hard collar (which extends up under the chin and prevents flexion of the neck), or a soft collar. Neck braces tend to limit vision; people wearing them cannot look down at their feet. Safety awareness is important to prevent falls.

Surgical Management

Sometimes conservative treatment does not work, and clients require surgery. Surgery to stabilize bone fragments is necessary if a neck injury involves a bone fracture. Cervical fusion (Fig. 71–9) is performed most commonly through an anterior approach. Immediately after a posterior cervical discectomy, a cervical collar is worn (Fig. 71–10). A hard cervical collar usually is prescribed after fusion. Complications after posterior cervical surgery include soft tissue hematoma, air embolism, and subcutaneous wound dehiscence. Complications after anterior cervical surgeries include laryngeal nerve damage and injury to neck structures, such as the carotid arteries, trachea, esophagus, and soft tissue.

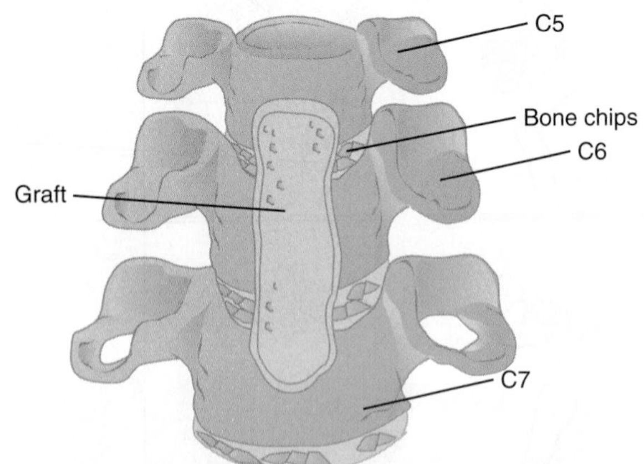

FIGURE 71–9 Anterior cervical fusion. A trough has been cut into the anterior cervical spine for insertion of an iliac graft as a splint. The intervertebral spaces have been filled with bone chips.

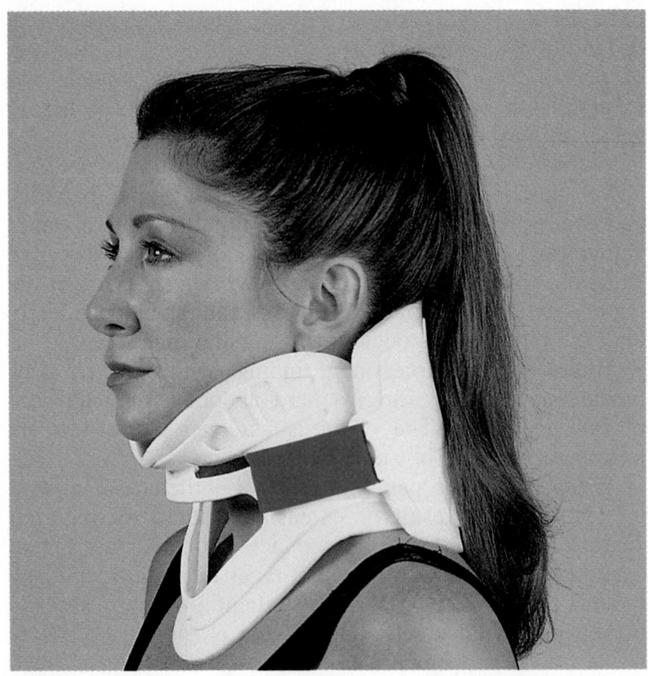

FIGURE 71–10 A cervical collar with a chin piece. This orthosis provides additional support for the head and some restriction of cervical spine motion. (Courtesy of Zimmer, Inc., Dover, OH.)

After microdiscectomy, the client may have the head of the bed elevated to whatever position is comfortable. After cervical spine fusion, the surgeon indicates the degree of head elevation for comfort and to reduce edema. Make sure the spine is in anatomic alignment. The client's head may be elevated, and a folded small towel, bath blanket, or small pillow is placed under the head to maintain spinal alignment while the client lies supine or on the side.

Assess and document the client's neurologic status frequently. The development or worsening of a neurologic deficit must be reported promptly to the surgeon. During the first 24 hours after an anterior cervical discectomy, assess the client's ability to breathe, check the operative site for excessive swelling, and look for shifting of the trachea and changes in the client's voice. Laryngeal nerve damage during surgery may cause permanent vocal impairment, such as hoarseness. If a spinal fusion was performed with the anterior cervical discectomy, the surgeon is notified if radicular pain recurs suddenly. This pain could mean that the bone graft has moved out of place and surgery needs to be repeated. Assess the client for indications of postoperative improvement, such as absence of paresthesias.

After surgery on the cervical spine, watch for indications of respiratory paralysis resulting from cord edema. Emergency tracheostomy equipment is kept at hand.

Tell the client that it is not unusual for preoperative manifestations to persist for a few days secondary to edema at the operative site, although these manifestations are usually less uncomfortable. Difficulty swallowing and throat discomfort are usually present for several days and usually are due to local irritation from the endotracheal tube. A soft diet, throat lozenges, a viscous lidocaine (Xylocaine) solution, humidified air, minimal talking, and other comfort measures lessen the discomfort.

A wound drain may be present and is usually removed by the surgeon on the second postoperative day, after drainage has decreased. Bladder and bowel management are the same as for clients after lumbar surgery. Cervical surgery may affect the parasympathetic chain, causing urinary retention.

Self-Care

With shorter postoperative hospital stays, most clients are discharged before suture or staple removal. Instruction for care of the incision includes keeping the sutures or staples clean and dry and noting any increased redness or drainage from the wound. Clients need clear instructions on walking, lifting, driving, and returning to work. Most clients can resume activity 6 weeks after surgery. Specific physician instructions need to be followed.

Prolonged sitting or standing in one position strains the healing back. Contraindicated activities vary. Instruct the client to ask the surgeon when it will be safe to perform activities that could damage the back (e.g., climbing stairs, lifting a weight heavier than 5 pounds, prolonged travel, sexual activity, sports, exercise, and driving a car). Clients must not smoke. Smoking reduces blood supply to the tissues and delays healing. The Client Education Guide lists other suggestions for home care after a cervical laminectomy or fusion.

CLIENT EDUCATION GUIDE

Home Care After Cervical Laminectomy or Fusion

- Keep the incision clear and dry. Change dressings when damp or soiled.
- Report redness, swelling, odor, or pain in the incision.
- Wear the collar at all times for 6 weeks or until your physician gives you permission to stop.
- You may wash under the collar with mild soap. Dry the skin well.
- If the collar is hard and needs cleaning, you should lie flat, remove the front of the collar, and wash the front first, using the back of the collar for neck support. Then replace the front of the collar and turn onto a pillow for support. Open one side of the collar and wash the back of your neck, then repeat on the other side.
- If the collar itches, a small silk scarf between the neck and the collar may provide some comfort.
- If a soft collar is prescribed, stockinettes made of soft fiber that fit over the collar can be purchased. Purchase two stockinettes so that when one is soiled, it can be removed, laundered, and replaced when dry.
- Riding in a car is permissible, but driving is not allowed until your physician has given you permission.

POST-POLIO SYNDROME

Poliomyelitis is an acute form of paralysis characterized by destruction of motor cells in the spinal cord and brain stem. The disease has been controlled since the 1950s, when mass immunization was used. Post-polio syndrome can develop in polio survivors 30 years after the original disease, however.

Post-polio syndrome is a new onset of progressive weakness, fatigue, decreased temperature tolerance, emotional distress, dysphagia, pain in the joints and muscles, and respiratory problems. The onset is insidious, and weakness occasionally extends to muscles that were not involved during the initial illness. The prognosis generally is good; progression to further weakness is usually slow, with plateau periods of 1 to 10 years. The syndrome is thought to be due to progressive dysfunction and loss of motor neurons that compensated for the neurons lost during the original infection and not to persistent or reactivated poliovirus infection.

The fatigue from post-polio syndrome is treated with pyridostigmine (Mestinon). Side effects of increased muscle twitching, nausea, diarrhea and frequency are common. The weakness is treated with strengthening exercises, steroids to reduce inflammation, and electrical stimulation. Other manifestations also are treated symptomatically.

Post-polio syndrome can be discouraging for clients who have successfully adapted to their disease and disability. Respiratory distress may bring back memories of the initial disease and treatment in an iron lung (an early form of a respirator in which the client's entire body was cocooned in a metal tube). Further restrictions are difficult to accept. Emotional support is vital. Teach the client to balance rest and activity.

SYRINGOMYELIA

Syringomyelia is often associated with the Arnold-Chiari malformation (an abnormal protrusion of the medulla into the spinal canal) or spina bifida. Syringomyelia consists of abnormal cavities filled with dense, glue-like tissue in the spinal cord substance, especially the cervical cord. Scar tissue surrounds the cysts. Syringomyelia is characterized by (1) muscular weakness and wasting; (2) sensory defects; and (3) indications of injury to the long tracts of the spinal cord, such as hyperreflexia.

These disturbances may begin at any age but most often occur between ages 30 and 40. Syringomyelia often occurs with other developmental defects. Kyphosis (abnormal increased convexity in curvature of the thoracic spine when viewed from the side), scoliosis (lateral deviation in the normally straight vertical line of the spine), and clubfoot often occur with syringomyelia.

Early manifestations of cervical syringomyelia often include:

- Atrophy, weakness, and fibrillations of the small muscles of the hands
- Loss of pain sensation in the fingers or forearms
- Weakness and atrophy of the shoulder girdle muscles
- Horner's syndrome, characterized by upper eyelid ptosis, pupil constriction, anhidrosis (absence of sweating), and flushing of the affected side of the face

- Nystagmus
- Vasomotor and trophic disturbances of the upper extremities

Although there is segmental loss or impairment of pain and temperature sensation, sensation for light touch remains. Segments of sensory loss may be separated by zones of normal sensation. Spasticity, ataxia, or paralysis of the lower extremities may occur as well as disturbed bladder control if the lumbosacral region of the spinal cord is involved. Cranial nerve involvement may produce additional problems, such as impairment of facial pain and temperature sensation, loss of the corneal reflex (necessitating protection of the eye), dysphagia, dysarthria, laryngeal stridor (possibly necessitating tracheostomy), nystagmus, and atrophy and fibrillation of the tongue muscles.

Syringomyelia may progress rapidly at first, then become quiescent for many years. Some people live 40 years after onset. Others become incapacitated (from paralysis or sensory defects) or die within a few years.

Treatment includes relieving increased pressure on the cord from the fluid content of the cavities within the spinal canal. The fluid buildup can be removed and cerebrospinal fluid outflow restored by direct surgical drainage or by shunt placement.

SPINAL TUMORS

Spinal tumors are similar in nature and origin to intracranial tumors but occur much less often. They are most common in young or middle-aged adults and most commonly involve the thoracic region. Spinal tumors may occur outside of the spinal cord, such as in the meninges, nerve roots, or vertebrae (extramedullary), or within the substance of the spinal cord (intramedullary). Neurofibromas and meningiomas are the most common spinal cord tumors. Both are benign and operable and may not produce permanent damage if removed early.

Clinical Manifestations

Clinical manifestations of spinal tumors vary according to their location. Extramedullary tumors cause manifestations by compressing the spinal cord or some of its nerve roots or by occluding blood vessels supplying the cord. Early characteristics of spinal cord compression include pain, sensory loss, muscle weakness, and muscle wasting. Progressive cord compression is manifested by spastic weakness below the level of the lesion, decreased sensation, and increased reflexes. Severe cord compression at the cervical level destroys cord function and produces quadriplegia; compression at the thoracic or lumbar level results in paraplegia.

Intramedullary tumors produce more variable clinical manifestations. High cervical cord involvement causes spastic quadriplegia and sensory changes. Tumors in descending areas of the spinal cord produce motor and sensory changes appropriate to functions at that level.

Medical diagnosis is made after a complete general neurologic examination. Diagnostic testing includes a spinal radiograph, CT scan, MRI, and a myelogram, individually or serially.

Outcome Management

Intervention for spinal tumors usually is surgery, radiation therapy, or both. Immediate surgery is indicated if compression of the cord or nerve roots is evident. Often, surgery results in marked improvement or complete restoration of function, especially if the tumor is benign and encapsulated (e.g., meningioma or lipoma). Functional improvement is less common if cord necrosis has developed, however. Complete surgical removal of an intramedullary tumor is rare. Partial resection followed by radiation may improve the client's condition. Usually, the course of the condition is gradually progressive.

VASCULAR SPINAL CORD LESIONS

As with stroke, spinal cord vascular lesions may be caused by rupture, thrombosis, or embolism. Trauma is the usual cause of hemorrhage into the spinal cord. Thrombosis of the spinal vessels usually is secondary to meningitis or to compression of the vessels by tumors, granulomas, or abscesses in the epidural space.

MYELOMALACIA

Myelomalacia is softening or infarction of the spinal cord from spinal artery occlusion. Prognosis is poor. There is little or no return of normal function to the involved areas. Myelomalacia is suspected when indications of transverse myelitis develop suddenly.

Assessment findings in myelomalacia depend on the level of the lesion in the cord. There is always motor paralysis and dissociated sensory loss below the level of the lesion, accompanied by paralysis of bladder and bowel sphincters. Paralysis usually is bilateral but rarely complete. Initially the limbs are flaccid, and no deep tendon or superficial reflexes are elicited, as in spinal shock. After several weeks, spasticity, hyperreflexia, and clonus develop.

Intervention focuses on maintaining body functions, preventing complications of immobility, and providing pain relief. The client usually begins intensive rehabilitation 12 to 14 hours after onset of manifestations.

HEMATOMYELIA

Hematomyelia is hemorrhage into the substance of the spinal cord. It almost always follows trauma but may be caused by vascular malformation or a bleeding disorder.

Clinical manifestations usually develop suddenly, immediately after spinal injury, and depend on the size of the hemorrhage. After trauma, it is important to differentiate between hematomyelia and a vertebral fracture-dislocation. Immediate surgery to relieve cord compression is indicated if fracture-dislocation is evident on radiograph. Spinal angiography, spinal CT scans, and MRI enable visualization of vascular lesions. Some of these lesions are treated by ligating their feeding vessels, others by excising the entire malformation.

Management is the same as for myelomalacia. If surgery is needed, postoperative care is similar to that given to clients with other forms of spinal surgery.

NEUROSYPHILIS

Neurosyphilis is a chronic or late stage of syphilis involving infection of the brain, spinal cord, or both. The oculomotor nerves may be affected, leading to an inability of the pupil to react to light, called an *Argyll Robertson pupil.* The posterior columns and nerve roots of the spinal cord may be affected, which is called *tabes dorsalis.*

Clinical Manifestations

Because these are sensory nerves, the most common manifestation is pain. The pain can occur almost anywhere in the body, although abdominal pain is most common. The pain is severe enough to be confused with gastric ulcers and gallbladder disease. In addition to pain, areas of paresthesias may be noted. A common finding in tabes dorsalis is the loss of position sense in the feet and legs. As a result, clients walk with a slapping step. They are at increased risk for falls when walking in the dark because they must rely on visual cues for placement of their feet with each step. Because the gait is abnormal, bone alignment with walking is altered. Eventually the foot is abnormally shaped (called *Charcot's joint*). This alteration in foot structure can lead to foot ulcerations because the client bears the body weight on abnormal areas. The brain also can be involved in later stages of syphilis. A general deterioration of mental status can develop.

Outcome Management

With improved case finding and the use of penicillin to treat syphilis in its early stages, the management of syphilis is improving. With development of resistant strains of organisms and a rise in the incidence of sexually transmitted diseases, however, problems may recur in the future.

DISORDERS OF THE CRANIAL NERVES

Cranial nerves can be affected in many ways by various nervous system disorders. For example, they may be affected secondarily by compression resulting from increased intracranial pressure, or they may be damaged directly as a result of head injuries. Only the two most common disorders specific to the cranial nerves, not those associated with other disorders, are discussed here. Other cranial nerve disorders exist. Regeneration of the cranial nerves can occur except for the first (olfactory) or second (optic) cranial nerve because these nerves are actually part of the central nervous system.

TRIGEMINAL NEURALGIA

Chronic irritation of the fifth cranial nerve results in trigeminal neuralgia. Approximately 15,000 cases are diagnosed each year in the United States. Although most commonly occurring in people 50 to 70 years old, trigeminal neuralgia can occur in adults of any age. Approximately 60% of clients are women. The trigeminal nerve has three divisions: ophthalmic, maxillary, and mandibular (Fig. 71–11). Trigeminal neuralgia may occur in any one or more of these divisions.

Etiology

Causes of trigeminal neuralgia can be *intrinsic* or *extrinsic* lesions within the nerve itself, such as gross abnormalities of the axon or myelin, as may occur with multiple sclerosis. Extrinsic lesions are outside the trigeminal root and include mechanical compression by tumors, vascular anomalies, dental abscesses, or jaw malformation.

Clinical Manifestations

Trigeminal neuralgia is characterized by intermittent episodes of intense pain of sudden onset. The pain rarely is relieved by analgesics. Tactile stimulation, such as touch and facial hygiene, and talking may trigger an attack. Trigeminal neuralgia is more prevalent in the maxillary and mandibular distributions and on the right side of the face. Bilateral trigeminal neuralgia is rare but does occur. The pain from trigeminal neuralgia can become so intense that the client ponders suicide.

None of the current diagnostic studies identify trigeminal neuralgia. A CT scan, MRI, and angiography can identify a causative lesion. The diagnosis is made on the basis of an in-depth history, with attention paid to triggering stimuli and the nature and site of the pain.

A careful history is obtained from the client regarding stimuli that trigger an attack. This information is used to plan care so as to minimize triggering events. The client's dental hygiene and nutritional intake are evaluated. These clients often do not eat enough to meet their daily nutritional needs and neglect their teeth because of the pain.

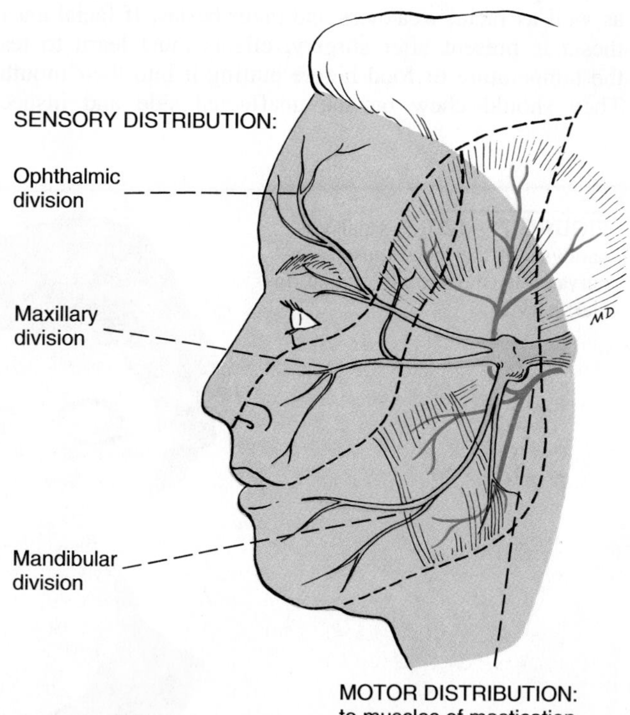

Figure 71–11 Distribution of the trigeminal nerve. Trigeminal neuralgia develops along the course of this nerve.

Outcome Management

Anticonvulsant agents such as carbamazepine (Tegretol) are often prescribed as the initial treatment of trigeminal neuralgia. These drugs may dampen the reactivity of the neurons within the trigeminal nerve. For some clients, these medications are all the treatment that is needed. Liver impairment may result from administration of carbamazepine and phenytoin. Liver enzymes must be monitored before and during therapy. If the client cannot tolerate the dose needed for pain control, phenytoin can be used. These medications should be used cautiously in clients with a history of alcohol abuse. Baclofen (Lioresal) is an antispasmodic that may be used alone or in conjunction with anticonvulsants. Narcotics are not particularly effective in relieving trigeminal neuralgia pain.

Help clients use and improve any pain control strategies they have developed. Clients with trigeminal neuralgia need emotional support to help them deal with pain that has often been present for a long time.

Surgery includes nerve blocks with alcohol and glycerol; peripheral neurectomy; and percutaneous radiofrequency wave forms, which create lesions that alter pain transmission. The relief obtained with these procedures is not always permanent. Complications include development of facial paresthesias and muscular weakness. These procedures, being less invasive, often are tolerated better by elderly or debilitated clients.

More invasive techniques involve major surgical procedures. Microvascular decompression involves removing the vessel from the posterior trigeminal root. A rhizotomy is the actual resection of the root of the nerve. With these procedures, craniotomy is required to allow access to the nerve.

Complications include those of any surgical procedure as well as facial weakness and paresthesias. If facial anesthesia is present after surgery, clients must learn to test the temperature of food before putting it into their mouth. They should chew on the unaffected side and inspect mucous membranes for irritation. Assess for aspiration and advance the diet slowly. Teach clients to use a water jet device instead of a toothbrush for dental hygiene, and advise them to visit the dentist as soon as possible after surgery.

If the corneal reflex has been impaired, the client needs to be taught eye care. During the acute postoperative period, apply eye drops and a protective shield. The client assumes these tasks with supervision, then independently.

BELL'S PALSY

Pathophysiology and Etiology

Bell's palsy affects the motor aspects of the facial nerve, the seventh cranial nerve (Fig. 71–12). Bell's palsy is the most common type of peripheral facial paralysis. It affects women and men in all age groups. It is most common between ages 20 and 40 years.

Bell's palsy results in a unilateral paralysis of the facial muscles of expression. There is no evidence of a pathologic cause. Facial paralysis may be central or peripheral in origin. Central facial palsy is an upper motor neuron paralysis or paresis. Sometimes it produces dissociation of motor function. In this situation, the client cannot voluntarily show his or her teeth on the paralyzed side but can show them with emotional stimulation, such as that causing smiles or laughter. This phenomenon is called *voluntary emotional dissociation.*

Clinical Manifestations

Typical assessment findings on the affected side include (1) upward movement of the eyeball on closing the eye (Bell's phenomenon), (2) drooping of the mouth, (3) flattening of the nasolabial fold, (4) widening of the palpebral fissure, and (5) a slight lag in closing the eye. Eating may be difficult.

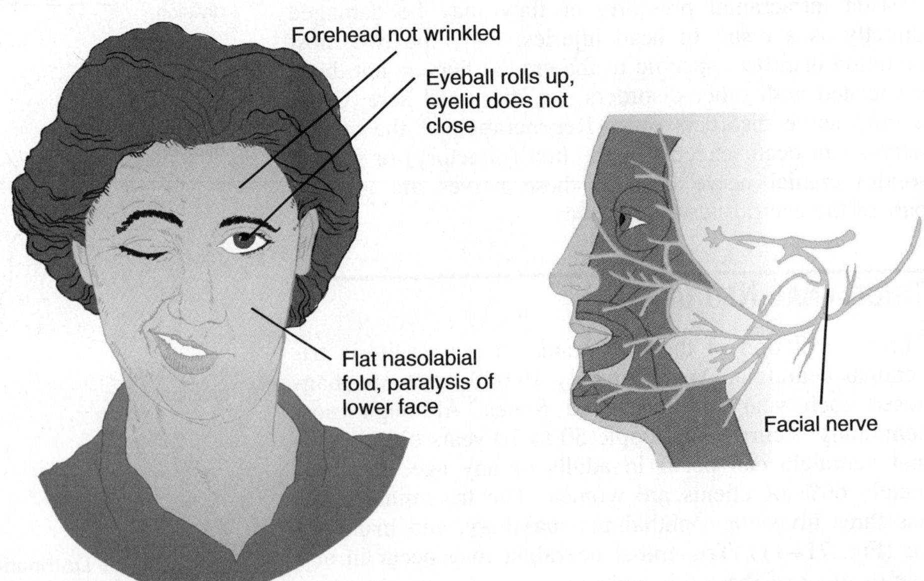

FIGURE 71–12 Bell's palsy is paralysis of the facial muscles innervated by the seventh cranial (facial) nerve.

Outcome Management

There is no known cure for Bell's palsy. Palliative measures include:

- Analgesics if discomfort occurs from herpetic lesions
- Corticosteroids to decrease nerve tissue edema
- Physiotherapy, moist heat, gentle massage, and stimulation of the facial nerve with faradic current
- Corneal protection with an artificial tears solution, sunglasses, an eye patch at night, and periodic gentle closure of the eye

Clients experiencing Bell's palsy often think they have had a stroke. Reassure the client that this is not the case. Most clients recover from Bell's palsy within a few weeks without residual manifestations. If permanent complete facial paralysis occurs, surgery may be necessary. Anastomosis of the peripheral end of the facial nerve with the spinal accessory or hypoglossal nerve may allow closure of the eye during sleep and restores tone to the facial musculature.

UPPER MOTOR NEURON LESIONS

Because the lower motor neurons (LMNs) send instructions for the muscles to contract, it follows that certain pathways in the central nervous system influence the activity of the LMNs that facilitates and inhibits muscle contractions. Several known pathways that arise from the higher brain centers influence the activity of the LMNs. These pathways constitute the upper motor neurons (UMNs). The UMNs originate in the motor strip of the cerebral cortex and in multiple brain stem nuclei. From the cortex, these axons pass through the internal capsule; most of them cross over in the medulla and descend in the spinal cord through the corticospinal tracts. A few do not cross in the brain but cross later in the spinal cord.

The corticospinal tracts are responsible primarily for precise, fine, voluntary motor movements. They also assist in modulating muscle tone and reflexes to some degree. Any lesion that destroys the UMNs results in contralateral paralysis, such as is seen with cerebrovascular accident (stroke). Initially the involved area is flaccid and hyporeflexic. The flaccidity gradually recedes, and the reflex arc becomes hyperactive because of the lack of inhibition by the UMNs. Muscle tone is hypertonic, and the extremity becomes spastic. Despite the spasms, the muscle becomes atrophied from disuse. The atrophy seen with UMN lesions occurs later than that seen with LMN problems. The Babinski reflex is present.

LOWER MOTOR NEURON LESIONS

LMNs consist of the anterior horn cells located in the anterior gray matter of the spinal cord. They also are located in the motor cranial nuclei of the brain stem. Each anterior horn cell has a long axon that leaves the cord by the anterior spinal root and extends out the peripheral nerve, eventually synapsing at the motor endplate of a neuromuscular junction. These structures form a motor unit that controls skeletal muscle activity, both voluntary and reflex activity. They are the last cells to carry information from the nervous system out to the muscles.

LMN lesions often are associated with spinal cord injury or tumors and surgery on the aorta, which alters blood flow to the spinal cord. When a lesion develops in the LMNs, flaccid muscle weakness or paralysis, loss of reflexes, loss of muscle tone, and atrophy of the involved muscles develop. The degree to which these clinical manifestations develop depends on the extent of the lesion. Each anterior horn cell innervates several separate muscle fibers, and because several anterior horn cells exist at each spinal level, a lesion confined to one spinal segment may not damage all of the anterior horn cells innervating an entire muscle. This type of lesion would cause muscle weakness rather than paralysis.

Paralysis occurs when a lesion involves the column or anterior horn cells in several spinal segments. If all the peripheral motor nerves are involved, the entire muscle becomes flaccid. The muscles atrophy early because of lack of innervation.

DISORDERS OF THE PERIPHERAL NERVES

Peripheral nerves can be injured in many ways—from bone fractures, stretching of the nerves, infections, vascular or metabolic disturbances, constriction by fascial bands, pressure from tumors, trauma associated with perforating wounds, injection of drugs, and exposure to chemicals or toxins. *Neuropathy* is nerve damage from any cause. *Mononeuropathy* is injury to a single nerve as a result of localized injury. *Polyneuropathy* is diffuse damage to many nerves as a result of toxic agents or metabolic disturbances. The peripheral nerves subjected most commonly to external pressure are the median, radial, ulnar, sciatic, common peroneal, tibial, and long thoracic nerves. The common peroneal nerve (a terminal branch of the sciatic) is injured more frequently than any other nerve. Because of its course and distribution, the sciatic nerve is exposed to internal and external trauma and inflammation more than any other nerve. The median nerve most often is injured by constriction from fascial bands. The axillary nerve may be injured as the result of an allergic reaction to serum injections or secondary to improper crutch walking. The sciatic nerve may be injured directly during medication injections. It may also be secondarily injured from diffusion of injected solutions. Any peripheral nerve can be injured by bone fractures or perforating wounds.

Assessment findings with nerve damage depend on the type of nerve injured and the extent of damage. Damaged motor nerves cause clinical manifestations, such as flaccid paralysis, muscle wasting, and reflex loss in the muscle innervated by the injured nerve. Damaged mixed nerves or sensory nerves cause vasomotor and trophic disturbances after partial or complete interruption of the nerve. After partial injury or incomplete division of a nerve, the person may experience stabbing pains, paresthesias (pins-and-needles sensation), and occasionally the burning pains of causalgia. Damaged sensory nerves cause loss of sensation in the nerves' area of anatomic distribution.

PERIPHERAL NEUROPATHIES

■ CUMULATIVE TRAUMA DISORDERS

Cumulative trauma disorders (CTDs) include a group of overuse syndromes that predominantly affect the wrist and hand. They are also often called *repetitive strain injuries* because some repetitive work activities seem to cause or exacerbate manifestations. There are several forms, and some are listed in Table 71–1. The client often describes fatigue, with aching and tiredness during the activity. Rest generally relieves manifestations in this first clinical stage. Later the client reports manifestations that persist into the next day. Finally the client complains of chronic aching, fatigue, and weakness despite rest. In attempts to minimize the incidence and effects of cumulative trauma disorders, health specialists in business and industry have modified work tasks, work stations, tools or equipment, and the work environment (see Table 71–1).

■ CARPAL TUNNEL SYNDROME

Carpal tunnel syndrome (CTS) is an entrapment neuropathy that occurs when the median nerve is compressed as it passes through the wrist along a pathway to the hand. The tunnel, called the *carpal tunnel,* is bordered by the flexor retinaculum, a band of fibrous tissue that prevents the wrist tendons from bowing when the wrist is flexed. Compression causes sensory and motor changes in the thumb, index finger, middle finger, and radial aspect of the ring finger. CTS also leads to atrophy of the radial half of the thenar eminence.

Etiology

CTS may develop spontaneously without a known cause or may result from disease or injury. The most commonly reported cause of CTS is repetitive motion of the wrist, with the wrist in constant flexion. A higher incidence of CTS is reported among homemakers, factory workers, bricklayers, cashiers, musicians, secretaries, and computer operators. Pregnancy, hypothyroidism, gout, and rheumatoid arthritis are other conditions associated with CTS.

Clinical Manifestations

Initially the client may be awakened at night by pain and paresthesia. Although these initial manifestations are temporary and relieved by shaking the hand, later stages may be accompanied by motor loss (e.g., progressive weakness, inability to perform fine motor activities), burning or numbness in the thumb, index finger, or middle finger, and daytime pain.

Assessment of the client begins with a thorough history, including occupational tasks. Diagnostic assessment for CTS includes assessing for Tinel's and Phalen's signs (Fig. 71–13*A* and *B*). Tinel's sign is the development of tingling in the hands and fingers when the wrist is tapped. Phalen's test is assessing for the development of numbness and tingling after forceful flexion of the wrists for 20 to 30 seconds (see Fig. 71–13*B*).

Finally the wrist compression test is done. The test involves manual application of 30 seconds of pressure over the flexor retinaculum (Fig. 71–13*C*). If paresthesias develop after compression, the result is positive. The wrist compression test is 87% accurate in the diagnosis of CTS. Electromyography procedure also may be used in differential diagnosis to rule out other possible causes.

Outcome Management

Initially, the wrist is splinted in a neutral position to prevent mechanical irritation of the nerve. Injection of steroids into the flexor tendons is done less frequently now because of reported problems with scarring, median nerve damage, and infection. In addition to rest, pyridoxine HCl (vitamin B_6) has been helpful. For some clients, pain can be relieved by gently squeezing the distal metacarpal heads together with the affected hand, palm up; in some instances, stretch of digits III and IV also is required. This maneuver also may help in the clinical diagnosis of CTS.

Surgery is indicated with (1) severe manifestations of long duration, (2) muscle atrophy, or (3) progressive sensory loss in the fingers and hand. Regional anesthesia is used for carpal tunnel release (decompression of the median nerve by transecting the transverse carpal ligament). Carpal tunnel release can be performed by opening the wrist or through an endoscope. The transverse ligament is divided to relieve pressure.

After surgery, blood flow is assessed hourly by checking the color, capillary refill, and warmth of the finger tips. When the anesthetic has worn off, assess the fingers for sensation.

Initially, postoperative care centers on wrist immobilization using bulky dressings and a wrist splint. The arm is elevated on pillows to reduce edema. Encourage the client to try to move the fingers, even though they are splinted. After the dressings are removed, progressive exercises, including flexion, extension, and gripping, are begun. The client often returns to the same type of work, so that recovery of strength and flexibility are imperative. Work site analysis should also be completed to avoid reinjury.

The client and family are the care providers beyond the immediate postoperative period. Because this surgery usually is performed on an outpatient basis, provide detailed instructions on home care. The Client Education Guide lists suggestions for home care after carpal tunnel release.

■ ULNAR NERVE SYNDROME

Lying within a bony groove at the elbow, the ulnar nerve is susceptible to compression from direct trauma to the elbow (e.g., hitting the funny bone) or from changes within the groove that gradually squeeze the nerve. Repeated mild trauma (e.g., habitual leaning of the elbows on a hard surface such as experienced by truck drivers) can injure the ulnar nerve. Sensory changes occur in the ulnar aspect of the hand and wrist. The usual treatment for ulnar nerve compression at the elbow is surgical transplantation of the ulnar nerve.

■ TARSAL TUNNEL SYNDROME

Tarsal tunnel syndrome is the counterpart of CTS in the lower extremity. In this syndrome, the posterior tibial nerve is trapped beneath the flexor retinaculum and deep fascia along the foot's medial border.

TABLE 71–1 REPETITIVE MOTION INJURIES

Condition	Manifestations	People/Occupations at Risk	Usual Treatment
NECK			
Tension neck syndrome	Stiff, aching neck; headache	Typists, keypunch operators, cashiers, and others who must maintain a restricted posture	Prevention is key: (1) pause frequently when typing or keying to stretch about 30 sec every 30 min; (2) place screen directly in front of typist, avoid twisting; (3) place material to be typed at eye level if possible; avoid having materials to be typed consistently on one side of typist; conservative*
Cervical syndrome	Pain on flexion or extension of the neck with radiation down the arm	Common in people who assume awkward positions for a long time, such as painters, dentists	Conservative,* cervical collar, surgery
SHOULDER			
Thoracic outlet syndrome	Numbness, pain, ischemia, and weakened pulse in upper extremity with hyperextension of the shoulder	Overhead assembly workers, automobile repair mechanics, letter carriers	Conservative,* transcutaneous nerve stimulation, surgery
Supraspinatus tendinitis	Pain on elevating arm above 70 degrees at the shoulder	People who must maintain abduction with elbow extended—painters, construction workers	Conservative,* physical therapy, steroid injections
Bicipital tendinitis	Pain over the bicipital tendon in bicipital groove	Window washers, construction workers, shipping clerks	Conservative,* physical therapy, steroid injections
ELBOW, HAND, AND WRIST			
Lateral or medial epicondylitis (tennis elbow)	Local pain and pain on resisted hand motion	Repeated and forceful rotation of the forearm with the wrist bent; can be seen in bowlers, tennis players, and pitchers	Conservative,* steroid injections, surgery
de Quervain's tenosynovitis (inflammation of the extensor pollicus brevis tendons)	Gradual onset of pain, and sometimes swelling of the radial styloid; popping sensation on extension of the thumb	Middle-aged women and those subject to repetitive stress of the thumb	Conservative,* steroid injections, surgery
Carpal tunnel syndrome	Pain and paresthesias on percussion over the median nerve at the wrist (Tinel's sign) or with flexed wrists pressed together (positive Phalen's maneuver); night pain after 3–4 hr of sleep, morning stiffness, daytime numbness	Repetitive forced hand movements, keypunch operators, cashiers, typists, people with degenerative joint disease	Prevention is key: (1) while typing pause frequently at least 30 sec every 30 min; (2) adjust keyboard so the elbows are at 90 degree angle and wrists are straight; (3) do not rest wrists on a hard surface or restpad; wrists should "float" above keyboard; (4) use a light touch when striking the keys; conservative,* steroid injections, surgery
Ulnar nerve entrapment	Pain and paresthesias on percussion of the ulnar nerve over the epicondyle (Tinel's sign); local swelling and tissue hypertrophy around elbow	Rheumatoid arthritis clients, occupational stress on elbow	Conservative,* surgery

*Conservative treatment consists of restriction of the harmful motion, splinting (if appropriate and only for short periods of time or at night), application of ice or heat, mild analgesics and nonsteroidal anti-inflammatory drugs, and gentle stretching exercises.

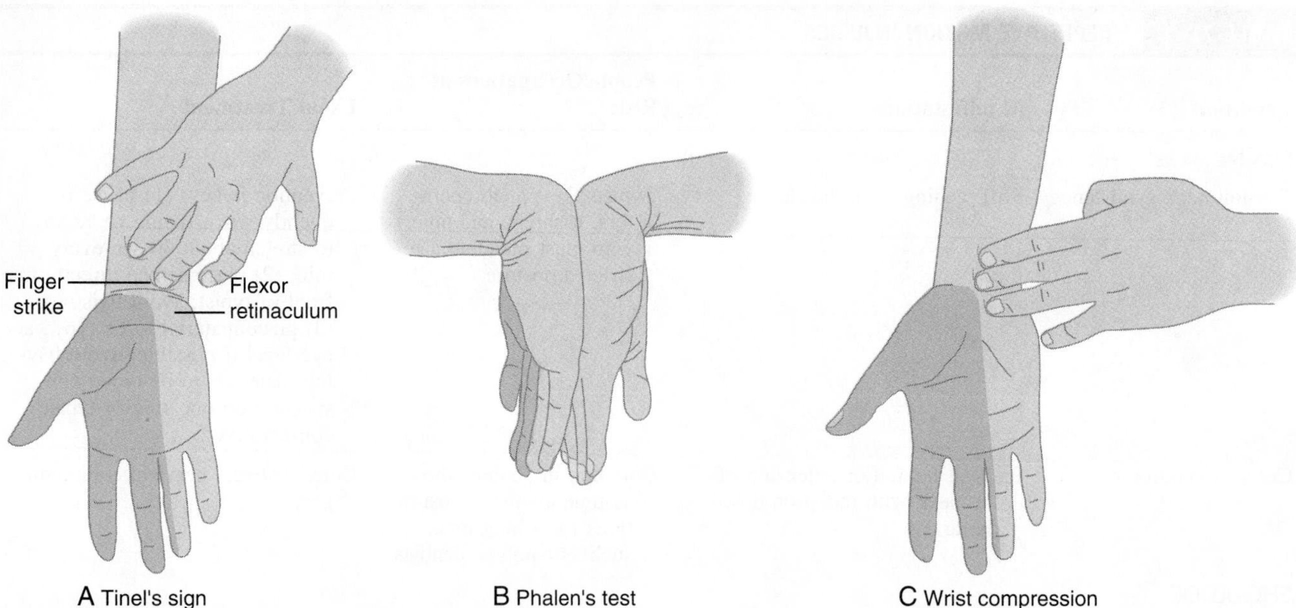

FIGURE 71–13 Clinical examination of carpal tunnel syndrome includes tests for Tinel's sign (*A*), Phalen's sign (*B*), and wrist compression (*C*). Each of these maneuvers elicits numbness and pain in the thumb, the index and middle fingers, and the radial aspect of the ring finger if carpal tunnel syndrome is present.

DUPUYTREN'S CONTRACTURE

Dupuytren's contracture, a permanent flexor contracture of the fourth and fifth fingers, is inherited as an autosomal dominant trait. It is common in people of Northern European descent and is more common in alcoholics and diabetics.

In severe forms of contracture, a longitudinal fibrous cord forms, which extends from the fingers to the palm and pulls the fingers into a locked position. Milder forms are characterized by less contracture and fewer nodules in the palmar fascia.

Ten years or more may pass before surgery is necessary. The decision to operate is usually made when the client can no longer lay the hand outstretched on a table.

CLIENT EDUCATION GUIDE

Home Care After Carpal Tunnel Release

- Check the circulation in your hand; notify the physician if you notice: increased swelling that results in the hand or fingers becoming pale, tingly, or cold; rings too tight to remove; or if any of these manifestations are present even without swelling.
- Keep the affected wrist elevated as much as possible, using the splint to immobilize the wrist area.
- Flex and extend your fingers hourly during waking hours.
- Observe for signs of infection: odorous dressing, fever, or increased pain at the incisional site.
- Use analgesia as directed for pain relief.
- Restrict lifting for 2 months.
- Wear a splint for 7 to 14 days after surgery or until the sutures are removed.
- Avoid getting the incision site wet until after the sutures are removed.

The operation consists of excision of part of the palmar fascia. After surgery, the hand is dressed in a large compression dressing. Range-of-motion movements are encouraged. Frequent assessments of capillary refill and finger color are needed. Splints may be used at night to promote extension. Many months of physical therapy may be needed, and full function may not be achievable.

GANGLION

The most common soft tissue mass found in the hand or wrist is a ganglion, a firm cystic lesion that often is located deep in the tissues. Trauma or degenerative changes in the fibrous joint capsule are thought to contribute to development of a ganglion. Depending on its location, the ganglion can compress the median nerve, leading to CTS. The benign cyst, which consists of clear mucinous fluid enclosed in a fibrous capsule, is found most often on the dorsum of the wrist.

To relieve pain or numbness, the ganglion may be aspirated or the cyst surgically excised. The area may then be injected with a corticosteroid before a pressure dressing and splint are applied. NSAIDs are commonly used for pain or discomfort. Wrist ganglions may recur in 30% of affected clients.[16]

PERIPHERAL NERVE INJURIES

Nerves can be injured in common household accidents (cut on glass) or in severe motor vehicle accidents. Assessment includes full examination of the hand, a discussion of the client's occupation, and documentation of the dominant hand.

Conservative management may include splinting, ice, elevation of the limb, or administration of NSAIDs and analgesic agents, or a combination of these. If a peripheral nerve is traumatically severed, the ends should be surgically anastomosed to enable healing. The nearer the site of injury occurs to the central nervous system, the less chance of regeneration. When nerves are damaged only slightly, mild edema occurs at the injury site. This edema may cause temporary manifestations of motor and/or sensory loss that recede in a few days or possibly weeks.

Postoperative care of clients having nerve repair or grafting includes elevation of the extremity. Elevation is critical to reducing edema and improving venous return. The procedure usually is performed with local anesthesia; therefore, assessment of neurovascular status is not conclusive until the anesthesia has worn off. Color, warmth, movement, sensation, capillary refill, and strength are assessed. Some of these assessments can be hampered by dressings, but as many as possible should be performed.

Monitor the finger tips for blood flow with Doppler laser or standard Doppler ultrasonography and temperature probes. The temperature of the hand is usually less than the core temperature, and the surgeon indicates acceptable ranges of temperature. Physical therapy begins within a few days to promote movement after severe injuries.

If the injury is severe, the client may have recurring dreams about the accident and the injury. These dreams are generally normal post-traumatic responses, but if they are bothersome to the client, a psychiatric consultant may be helpful.

PERIPHERAL NERVE TUMORS

Although solitary tumors (generally neurofibromas) may develop on any peripheral nerve, multiple tumors occur most often and are part of a syndrome known as *neurofibromatosis (von Recklinghausen's disease).* This hereditary disorder is characterized by multiple tumors of the spinal and cranial nerves along with involvement of many other systems. The disease usually is not life-threatening, and lesions are excised only when they interfere with normal activity. Intracranial and intraspinal tumors usually are removed.

Surgery for peripheral nerve tumors is generally performed on an outpatient basis. In the recovery room, the dressings are checked for drainage; circulation, motion, and sensation in the extremity are assessed. Clients are encouraged to perform range-of-motion exercises. Clients and family members are taught the manifestations of circulatory compromise and infection, medication management, and care of the dressing and incision.

CONCLUSIONS

Physical and psychological impairments vary with the degree of damage as well as the client's response and ability to cope with body changes. The coping response is not always related to the degree of physiologic damage. A client can have facial paralysis or trigeminal neuralgia and be more compromised psychologically than a client with spinal cord injury who has strong coping skills. It is imperative that nurses comprehend the severity of the client's dysfunction as it relates to quality of life as well as the impact it has on family dynamics.

THINKING CRITICALLY

1. The client, a 34-year-old woman, had undergone a lumbar laminectomy done earlier today. A previous assessment showed that movement and sensation of both lower extremities were intact. During the current postoperative assessment, she stated that her right toes felt numb, and the dorsiflexion and plantiflexion of the right foot are a little weaker than earlier. She has requested an analgesic because she is starting to get a headache. What are the priorities for her care? What assessments and interventions might be used?

Factors to Consider. What assessment methods can be used to determine the extent of vascular insufficiency? What type of neurologic checks should be done?

BIBLIOGRAPHY

1. Agency for Health Care Policy and Research (AHCPR). (1994). *Acute low back problems in adults: Assessment and treatment.* No. 95-0642. Rockville, MD: U.S. Department of Health and Human Services: Public Health Service, AHCPR.
2. Atroshi, I., et al. (1999). Symptoms, disability, and quality of life in patients with carpal tunnel syndrome. *Journal of Hand Surgery, 24*(2), 398–404.
3. Burge, P., et al. (1997). Smoking, alcohol and the risk of Dupuytren's contracture. *Journal of Bone and Joint Surgery (Br), 79*(2), 206–210.
4. Chen, T. Y. (2000). The clinical presentation of uppermost cervical disc protrusion. *Spine, 25*(4), 439–442.
5. Freidman, R. A. (2000). The surgical management of Bell's palsy: A review. *American Journal of Otolaryngology, 21*(1), 139–144.
6. Geary, S. (1996). Nursing management of cranial nerve dysfunction. *Journal of Neuroscience, Nursing, 27*(2), 102–108.
7. Halderman, S. (1999). Low back pain: Current physiological concepts. *Neurological Clinics, 17*(1), 1–16.
8. Hall, H. (1999). Surgery: Indications and options. *Neurological Clinics, 17*(1), 113–130.
9. Kloen, P. (1999). New insights in the development of Dupuytren's contracture: A review. *British Journal of Plastic Surgery, 52*(8), 629–635.
10. Kuric, J. (1995). Spinal cord tumors. *Critical Care Nursing Clinics of North America, 7*(1), 151–157.
11. Laine, D. E. (1999). Low back pain and carpal tunnel syndrome: Two troublesome presentations in the workplace. *Advances in Nurse Practitioners, 7*(6) 49–50, 74.
12. LeCompte, C. M. (1997). Post polio syndrome: An update for the primary health care provider. *The Nurse Practitioner, 22*(6), 133–154.
13. Maksud, D. (1993). Psychological adjustments to hand injuries: Nursing management. *Plastic Surgical Nursing, 13*(4), 72–76.
14. Manente, G., et al. (1999). A relief maneuver in carpal tunnel syndrome. *Muscle and Nerve, 22*(11), 1587–1589.
15. Massy-Westropp, N., Grimmer, K., & Bain, G. (2000). A systematic review of the clinical diagnostic tests for carpal tunnel syndrome. *Journal of Hand Surgery, 25*(1), 120–127.
16. McConaghy, D. J. (1994). Trigeminal neuralgia: A personal review and nursing implications. *Journal of Neuroscience Nursing, 26*(2), 85–89.
17. Neatherlin, J. S., & Brillhart, B. (1996). Body image in preoperative and postoperative lumbar laminectomy patients. *Journal of Neuroscience Nursing, 27*(1), 43–46.
18. Postacchini, F. (1999). Management of herniation of the lumbar disc. *Journal of Bone and Joint Surgery (Br), 81*(4), 567–574.
19. Swenson, R. (1999). Differential diagnosis: A reasonable clinical approach. *Neurological Clinics, 17*(1), 43–64.
20. Thorsteinsson, G. (1997). Management of post-polio syndrome. *Mayo Clinic Proceedings, 72,* 627–638.

CHAPTER 72

REMEMBER *to check out your* **Companion CD ROM**

Management of Clients with Degenerative Neurologic Disorders

Amy Perrin Ross

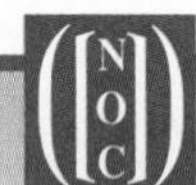

NURSING OUTCOMES CLASSIFICATION (NOC)
for Nursing Diagnoses—Clients with Degenerative Neurologic Disorders

Activity Intolerance
Activity Tolerance
Energy Conservation
Self-Care: Activities of Daily Living (ADL)
Altered Thought Processes
Cognitive Ability
Cognitive Orientation
Information Processing
Memory
Altered Urinary Elimination
Urinary Continence
Urinary Elimination
Caregiver Role Strain
Caregiver Emotional Health
Caregiver Performance: Direct Care
Caregiver Performance: Indirect Care
Caregiver Physical Health
Caregiver Stressors
Caregiver Well-Being
Depression Control
Knowledge: Health Resources
Constipation
Bowel Elimination
Hydration
Impaired Physical Mobility
Body Positioning: Self-Initiated
Joint Movement: Active
Mobility Level
Impaired Verbal Communication
Communication Ability
Communication: Expressive Ability
Communication: Receptive Ability
Cognitive Orientation
Distorted Thought Control
Knowledge Deficit
Knowledge: Disease Process
Knowledge: Health Resources
Knowledge: Medication
Risk for Injury
Neurological Status
Risk Detection
Safety Behavior: Fall Prevention
Safety Behavior: Home Physical Environment
Safety Status: Falls Occurrence
Risk for Self Care Deficit
Self-Care: Activities of Daily Living (ADL)
Mobility Level
Self Care Deficit
Self-Care: Activities of Daily Living
Urge Incontinence
Tissue Integrity: Skin and Mucous Membranes
Urinary Continence
Urinary Elimination
Self-Esteem Disturbance
Self-Esteem
Body Image
Social Support

Degenerative neurologic disorders pose a great challenge to the client, the family, and the caregiver, whether it is the nurse, a family member, or a significant other. By their very nature, these disorders cause progressive decline in neurologic function. Some progress relatively quickly (over months to 1 or 2 years) whereas others progress more gradually, sometimes over decades. Common nursing diagnoses for clients with these disorders are *Altered Thought Processes, Memory Deficit, Visual-Perceptual Alteration, Impaired Physical Mobility, Incontinence, Self-Care Deficit,* and *Impaired Individual and Family Coping.* A major goal of intervention is to help the client achieve an optimal level of functioning in light of chronic neurologic deficits.

The diagnosis of degenerative neurologic disease is most often made in an outpatient setting. However, hospital admission may be necessary when acute relapses or life-threatening events occur. Many clients return to their homes and have regular follow-up in outpatient clinics; however, some may require rehabilitation, in either inpatient or outpatient settings, for newly acquired deficits. Other clients may require transfer to long-term care facilities because of significant decline in ability to provide self-care. Still other clients may not survive their acute illness.

ALZHEIMER'S DISEASE

Alzheimer's disease (AD) is the most common form of dementia among people 65 years of age and older. Dementia is intellectual deterioration severe enough to interfere with occupational or social performance. It involves progressive decline in two or more areas of cognition, usually memory and language, calculation, visuospatial perception, constructional praxis, judgment, abstraction, or personality. AD constitutes at least half of all dementias (see Chapter 68 for a general discussion of dementia).

AD affects about 4 million Americans. Slightly more than half of these people receive care at home, and the remainder receive institutional nursing care. The prevalence of AD doubles every 5 years after the age of 65. In fact, some estimates indicate that nearly half of all people over age 85 years have AD.

Etiology and Risk Factors

The cause of AD has not been found, although several risk factors have been identified. As can be seen by the statistics listed earlier, increasing age is a risk factor. Genetic factors can influence AD. At least five chromosomes (1, 12, 14, 19, 21) are involved in some forms of familial AD. Four genetic loci have also been identified as contributing to AD, including the amyloid precursor gene, the presenillin 1 gene, the presenillin 2 gene, and the apolipoprotein E gene. However, these loci do not account for all of the genetic risk. Further, the lack of 100% concordance in studies of identical twins implies that environmental, metabolic, and other factors also may play a role.

Nearly all people with Down's syndrome develop dementia and the pathologic features of AD. Current research is investigating the role of vascular disease and the onset of the clinical manifestations of AD. Female sex, head trauma, lack of education, and myocardial infarction have been linked to AD, but these associations are weak.[6] Some have postulated that aluminum intoxication, disordered immune function, and viral infection may be etiologic, but these factors have not been proven. A role for genetic testing is yet to be defined.

Although the major risk factors for AD (age, family history) cannot be controlled, efforts to reduce the incidence of head trauma and cardiovascular disease may help reduce the incidence of AD and other types of dementia.

Pathophysiology

Alois Alzheimer first described presenile dementia in 1907. He used a new staining technique of human brain tissue to demonstrate the pathologic changes. The changes he noted are now termed *neurofibrillary tangles* and *neuritic (amloid) plaques* (Fig. 72–1). The neuritic plaque is a cluster of degenerating nerve terminals, both dendritic and axonal, that contain amyloid protein. During metabolism, the amyloid precursor protein becomes embedded in the membrane of the neuron. Its effect on the neuron is being studied. These plaques develop first in neocortex and the hippocampus areas of the brain used for memory and other cognitive functions. Neurofibrillary tangles are abnormal neurons in which the cytoplasm is filled with bundles of abnormal protein called *paired helical filaments.* The term "association" is used to describe all the intellectual activities of the cerebral cortex. These functions include learning and reasoning, memory storage and recall, language abilities, and even consciousness.

Gross brain changes evident in clients with AD include thickening of the leptomeninges, shrunken gyri, widened sulci, enlarged ventricles, hippocampal shrinkage, and generalized atrophy.

In addition to structural changes, neurotransmitter changes are evident in the brain of clients with AD. A decline in cholinergic neurons in the basal nucleus leads to loss of choline acetyltransferase in the neocortex and hippocampus. Also affected are neuronal systems that project to the neocortex: the noradrenergic locus ceruleus and the serotonergic dorsal raphe nucleus in the brain stem. These two areas also contain neurofibrillary tangles. Involved neurons in the neocortex include those using corticotropin-releasing factor, somatostatin, and glutamate. Some of the changes are also due to oxidation.

Clinical Manifestations

Clinically, AD is characterized by a relentless impairment of decision-making that generally begins insidiously and can progress for a decade or so. The onset of AD typically occurs in late middle age (age 65 years and older), although some familial cases occur in a person's 40s and 50s.

First Stage

The sequence of loss of higher cognitive functions is a helpful clue in establishing the clinical diagnosis. The clinical progression of manifestations is usually divided into three stages (Box 72–1).

Memory disturbance is usually the first feature of the disease. Family members or co-workers often notice the

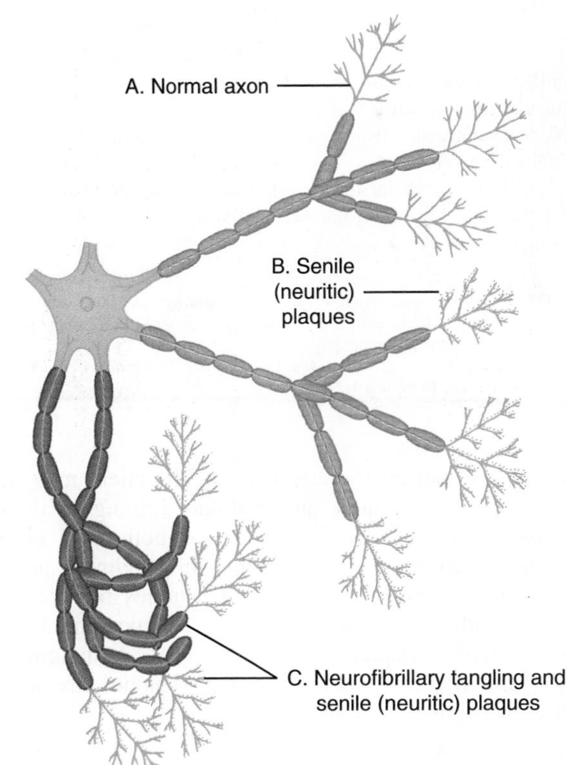

FIGURE 72–1 Neurofibrillary tangles. In clients with Alzheimer's disease and some other neurologic disorders, these tangles replace the normal neuronal cytoplasm. The tangles are often seen with senile plaques and appear throughout the cortex, hippocampus, and amygdala. The number of plaques and tangles correlates roughly with the severity of the dementia. *A,* Normal axon. *B,* Senile plaques on ends of axon. *C,* Neurofibrillary tangles and senile plaques replacing normal axon.

BOX 72-1 Common Clinical Manifestations in Each Stage of Dementia of the Alzheimer's Type

Stage I (duration of disease 1–3 years)

Memory—new learning defective, remote recall mildly impaired
Visuospatial skills—topographic disorientation, poor complex constructions
Language—poor wordlist generation, anomia
Personality—indifference, occasional irritability
Psychiatric features—depression or delusions in some
Motor system—normal
EEG—normal
CT/MRI—normal
PET/SPECT—bilateral posterior parietal hypometabolism/hyperperfusion

Stage II (duration of disease 2–10 years)

Memory—recent and remote recall more severely impaired
Visuospatial skills—poor constructions, spatial disorientation
Language—fluent aphasia
Calculation—acalculia
Praxis—ideomotor apraxia
Personality—indifference or irritability
Psychiatric features—delusions in some
Motor system—restlessness, pacing
EEG—slowing of background rhythm
CT/MRI—normal or ventricular dilation and sulcal enlargement
PET/SPECT—bilateral parietal and frontal hypometabolism/hypoperfusion

Stage III (duration of disease 8–12 years)

Intellectual functions—severely deteriorated
Motor—limb rigidity and flexion posture
Sphincter control—urinary and fecal incontinence
EEG—diffusely slow
CT/MRI—ventricular dilation and sulcal enlargement
PET/SPECT—bilateral parietal and frontal hypometabolism/hypoperfusion

EEG, electroencephalogram; CT, computed tomography; MRI, magnetic resonance imaging; PET, positron emission tomography; SPECT, single photon emission computed tomography.

From Cummings, J. L., & Benson, D. F. (1992). *Dementia: A clinical approach.* Boston: Butterworth-Heinemann.

memory loss before the client does. The client may demonstrate poor judgment and problem-solving skills and become careless in work habits and household chores. The client may do well in familiar surroundings and may be able to follow well-established routines but lacks the ability to adapt to new challenges. The person may become irritable, suspicious, or indifferent. Agitation, apathy, dysphoria, and aberrant motor behavior are associated with cognitive impairments.

SECOND STAGE

In the second stage of illness, the client may demonstrate *language disturbance,* characterized by impaired word-finding and circumlocution (talking around a subject rather than about it directly). Later, spontaneous speech becomes increasingly empty, and paraphasias (words used in the wrong context) are used. Clients may repeat words and phrases just spoken by themselves (*palilalia*) or by others (*echolalia*). Motor disturbance (*apraxia*) is characterized by difficulty in using everyday objects such as a toothbrush, comb, razor, and utensils. Apraxia combined with forgetfulness can create serious safety problems. The person may leave a stove burner on in the kitchen or forget to extinguish a cigarette. Indifference worsens, and restlessness with frequent pacing appears. *Hyperorality* (the desire to take everything into the mouth to suck, chew, or taste) may develop. Swallowing may become difficult.

Depression and irritability may worsen, and delusions and psychosis may appear. The person fears personal harm, theft of property, or infidelity of the spouse. Clients may see bugs crawling on the bed or throughout the house. Wandering at night is common. Occasional incontinence may occur.

THIRD STAGE

In the final stage, virtually all *mental* and *speech abilities* are lost. Voluntary movement is minimal, and the limbs become rigid with flexor posturing. Urinary and fecal incontinence are frequent. The person has lost all ability for self-care.

Diagnostic Findings

Because there is no definitive test for AD, the diagnosis is made by exclusion of known causes of dementia (e.g., toxic or metabolic alterations, drug side effects, cerebrovascular disease, neoplasm, and infection). The diagnosis is confirmed with (1) the presence of dementia involving two or more areas of cognition, (2) insidious onset, steady progression, and (3) loss of normal alertness.[14] When these criteria are applied, nine of 10 people given this diagnosis have AD confirmed at autopsy. Postmortem examination of the brain is the only way an AD diagnosis can be confirmed. The brain is viewed under the microscope for the presence of neuritic plaques and neurofibrillary tangles.

Diagnostic assessments such as electroencephalogram (EEG), computed tomography (CT), and magnetic resonance imaging (MRI) are frequently used in the diagnosis of AD. Position emission tomography (PET) has also been used. In general, these studies rule out other causes of dementia, such as seizures and cerebral bleeding, but do not identify AD. EEG changes may not appear until the later stages. CT and MRI usually reveal atrophy that is greater than what would be considered normal for age.

Finally, laboratory studies are performed to rule out metabolic and drug-related causes of dementia. These studies include urinalysis, complete blood count (CBC), erythrocyte sedimentation rate (ESR), electrolytes, blood urea nitrogen (BUN) and creatinine values, thyroid and liver function tests, calcium, serum B_{12} levels, syphilis serology, and human immunodeficiency virus (HIV) testing.

Outcome Management

There is no cure for AD. Results of studies in which acetylcholine (ACh) precursors (choline, lecithin, and deanol) and anticholinesterase agents (physostigmine and tetrahydroaminoacridine) are used to enhance memory and cognitive function have been disappointing. Tacrine (Cognex) inhibits breakdown of acetylcholinesterase in the brain, allowing more ACh to be available for nerve impulse transmission. Because of potential liver toxicity, liver function test results must be checked weekly for 18 weeks. Donepezil (Aricept), another cholinesterase inhibitor, is a reversible, selective anticholinesterase that produces minimal peripheral side effects. Donepezil is given only once a day, which is helpful for people in the early stages who are responsible for managing their own medications. Rivastigmine, a relatively selective pseudo-irreversible inhibitor of acetylcholinesterase, which is used in Europe, recently received an approval letter from the Food and Drug Administration (FDA). In an effort to combat the effect of oxygen free radicals, alpha-tocopherol (vitamin E) and selegiline have been studied. Both agents have been reported to delay the development of the later stages of AD[36] and show some improvement in levels of independent and behavioral manifestations. An extract of Ginkgo biloba may improve cognitive function for 6 to 12 months.[20] Propentofylline has been effective in the management of AD.

Most pharmacologic therapy is primarily aimed at treating behavioral problems, although behavioral and environmental manipulations are often more effective. Low-dose antipsychotic agents such as haloperidol (Haldol) can be effective for agitation and confusion. The lowest effective dose should be used and should be given just before bedtime. Sometimes twice-a-day dosing is required. Adverse side effects such as akathisia (motor restlessness), parkinsonian symptoms, tardive dyskinesia, orthostatic hypotension, anticholinergic symptoms (urinary retention and confusion), and sedation should be monitored. Antidepressants (e.g., nortriptyline and desipramine) that carry few anticholinergic side effects, fluoxetine, and trazodone are helpful for depression (Table 72–1).

Nursing Management of the Medical Client

ASSESSMENT

When AD is suspected, a complete history should be taken to assess for other causes of dementia. Data should be obtained from the client, family, and co-workers (if possible). Secondary sources are used because the client is often unaware of a problem with thought processing and minimizes it. Ask specific questions about difficulties with activities of daily living (ADL), increasing forgetfulness, and changes in personality. Assess past medical history for previous head injury or surgery, recent falls, headache, and a family history of AD. A Mini-Mental State examination may provide objective data for ongoing evaluation of the client (see Chapter 67).

AD has a profound impact on psychosocial behaviors. Ask about the client's reactions to changes in routine or in the environment. It is not uncommon for a client with AD to become very agitated over small changes, and apathy, social isolation, and irritability may be noted. As the brain continues to atrophy and the limbic system becomes dysfunctional, the client may become paranoid, use abusive language, and become suspicious of others.

AD has a profound impact on the family. Assess the family for strengths and weaknesses, their ability to provide care for the client, and their financial concerns. In large centers, the assessment of the client and family is performed through a team approach. The Client Education Guide provides instructions and resources for caregivers of people with AD.

DIAGNOSIS, OUTCOMES, INTERVENTION

Impaired Verbal Communication. Use the nursing diagnosis *Impaired Verbal Communication related to neuronal degeneration* to describe the client with AD.

Outcomes. The client's needs will be communicated effectively, as evidenced by making his or her needs

TABLE 72–1 PHARMACOLOGIC TREATMENT OF BEHAVIORAL PROBLEMS IN DEMENTIA OF THE ALZHEIMER'S TYPE

Problem	Treatment Options
Suspiciousness, paranoia, sundowning	Behavioral Environmental Correct sensory impairment Low-dose antipsychotics Loxapine (5–25 mg/day) Causes fewer EPS More sedative Low-potency antipsychotic Risperidone (1–4 mg/day) Observe for EPS Haloperidol (0.25–1.0 mg/day)
Anxiety	Treat underlying physical problems (pain, dyspnea, urinary urgency, sensory impairment) If acute, offer reassurance If related to confusion, use antipsychotics If diffuse or chronic, use short-acting benzodiazepine (e.g., oxazepam) Avoid non-benzodiazepine sedative-hypnotics, especially barbiturates Role of buspirone unclear
Acute catastrophic reactions	Lorazepam 1–4 mg IM Haloperidol 2–5 mg IM
Insomnia	Environmental, behavioral If associated confusion, use low-dose antipsychotics If associated depression, use: Nortriptyline Doxepin If associated restlessness with antipsychotic treatments: Lorazepam Observe for disinhibition or increased confusion Ambien
Angry or violent outbursts	Very difficult to control Behavior log is key to determine relationship to stimuli such as: Pain from arthritis or other chronic illness Urinary problems Constipation Low-dose antipsychotic Risperidone, loxapine, clozapine Carbamazepine Lithium

EPS, extrapyramidal symptoms such as restlessness, drooling, stiffness, shuffling, cogwheel rigidity (like Parkinson's disease); IM, intramuscularly.

CLIENT EDUCATION GUIDE

Caring for Family Members with Alzheimer's Disease

Client Instructions

Be sure that you have verbal and written information about the disease, the results of diagnostic testing (including the results of neuropsychological testing), legal and financial resources, and social support resources such as support groups.

Meet regularly with your health care providers to discuss the demands of caring for people with Alzheimer's, strategies for reducing stress, and resources for support.

Contact the local branches of national and regional Alzheimer's groups. A good place to start for information is the National Alzheimer's Association, 919 Michigan Ave., Suite 1000, Chicago, IL 60661. Call 1-800-272-3900.

Many caregivers have also found it helpful to read various publications.

known and interacting meaningfully with others. This outcome is often possible only in the early stages. In later stages, a more appropriate outcome might be expressed as the client's needs are interpreted appropriately.

Interventions. In the initial stage of AD, the client's receptive and expressive language skills are relatively intact. You must be prepared to adapt to the communication level of the client. If the client speaks only single words or short phrases, you should do likewise. It is best to speak slowly and simply, with a firm volume and low pitch. The tone of voice should always be calm and reassuring and project control of the situation. However, when language becomes impaired in the second stage of the illness, be prepared to apply new techniques for communicating with the client.

Nonverbal behavior can provide you with clues. Clients with AD often avert their eyes, look down, back away, and increase hand gesturing when they do not understand. If they are frustrated, angry, or hostile, they may increase motor activity by pacing, rattling doorknobs, waving their arms or shaking their fists, frowning, raising their voice volume and pitch, or tightening their facial muscles. These behaviors should signal staff to increase their alertness, search for the cause of the distress, and prepare to intervene.

Interventions can include the following:

- Decreasing environmental stimuli
- Approaching the client calmly and with assurance
- Taking care not to place any demands on the client
- Gently distracting the client
- Making sure that all verbal and nonverbal communication cues are concordant
- Using multiple sensory modalities (visual, auditory, and tactile) to send the message but not all forms at the same time

The client's memory loss can be an advantage in distracting him or her from the stressful situation. If removed from the situation and provided with a calm, nonthreatening environment, clients may forget why they are upset. Elicit listening behavior by reaching out and touching, holding a hand, putting an arm around the waist, or in some way maintaining physical contact with the client. Dementia sufferers can perceive nonverbal behavior of others and can become agitated or upset if they sense negative nonverbal behavior from them.

The identification of pain or discomfort in clients with advanced AD is also difficult. Behavioral indicators of discomfort include noisy breathing, negative vocalization (constant muttering, making sounds with a negative quality), a sad or frightened facial expression, frowning, tense body language, and fidgeting.

Altered Thought Processes. Neuronal degeneration also affects thought processing. State this diagnosis as *Altered Thought Processes related to neuronal degeneration.*

Outcomes. The client will have appropriate thought processing, as evidenced by retention of information to maximal capacity, maintaining orientation to maximal capacity, and sharing meaningful life experiences.

Intervention. Because memory deficit occurs in all stages of AD, you must continually apply interventions to enhance memory. Reorient the client as necessary by placing a calendar and clock in obvious places. Because the client's long-term memory is retained longer than short-term memory, allow clients to reminisce. Become aware of a client's past experiences so that they can be shared meaningfully. Repetition is useful for ensuring maximal retention of information by the client.

Risk for Injury. Altered thought processes lead to impaired judgment and forgetfulness. These changes increase risk for injury. State this common diagnosis as *Risk for Injury related to impaired judgment, forgetfulness, and motor impairments* (specify).

Outcomes. The client's physical and environmental safety will be maintained, as evidenced by the absence of physical injury and the existence of a safe living environment.

Interventions. Impaired judgment, forgetfulness, and motor impairment can make any environment unsafe for the client with AD. In the home, electrical devices, toxic substances, loose rugs, hot tap water, inadequate lighting, and unlocked doors can be sources of injury. Teach family members how to eliminate these safety hazards. In the inpatient setting, ensure that clients cannot leave the premises without being noticed, that they wear an identification badge in case they become lost, and that doors and windows are secured. Dangerous objects should be kept out of reach, and potentially dangerous activities, such as cooking, should be supervised. The client's driving skill should be evaluated at regular intervals. See Bridge to Home Health Care on safety solutions.

Self-Care Deficit. State the diagnosis of self-care problems as *Self-Care Deficit related to loss of memory and motor impairments.*

Outcomes. Clients will maintain self-care ability, as evidenced by completing the tasks they are capable of performing and receiving assistance with ADL they are incapable of performing.

Interventions. Encourage the client with AD to do as much as possible, as long as it is safe and appropriate. Carefully balance helping the client with maintaining his or her autonomy; this can boost the client's confidence

BRIDGE TO HOME HEALTH CARE

Safety Solutions for People with Alzheimer's Disease

To live with damaged thinking and judgment is to live at risk. People with Alzheimer's disease cannot take responsibility for their own safety. They are unable to evaluate the potential consequences of their actions and they forget quickly. Verbal reminders and written notes have little value, but there are many other ways to promote safety.

Older people love to live surrounded by their treasures. Although a neat home is always safer than a cluttered one, anticipate that only small changes can be made. Suggest moving knickknacks so that the edges of surfaces can be used for balance. Retain the existing furniture arrangements, but consider removing or altering furniture with sharp corners, rocking chairs that tip easily, coffee tables, and fragile antiques. Block off unsafe areas by placing a sturdy chair in front of them. Eliminate hazards such as trailing wires, extension cords, or telephone cords. Caution caregivers to watch for paper or wooden objects that are tossed into gas fireplaces.

Most accidents happen in the kitchen and the bathroom. Therefore, it is important to thoroughly assess how the person with Alzheimer's disease uses those areas. Disable stoves by removing knobs, installing a special switch behind the stove, removing a fuse, or turning the stove off at the breaker. Because people may retain over-learned food preparation skills, they may be able to safely use sharp utensils and hot surfaces but do need to be supervised. Encourage them to participate in meal preparation by doing single steps of a task, such as tearing lettuce for a salad or putting plates on the table.

Remove rugs and runners that tend to slide, especially those in the bathroom. Install grab bars to help prevent falls during transfers into or out of the tub or shower. Bars should be attached to structural supports rather than drywall or plaster. Consider using a raised toilet seat if rising is difficult and a bedside commode at night if urgency is a problem. Bath benches with non-skid feet are best, and hand-held showers minimize the need for the person to move about. Lower the temperature on the water heater to 120° F so that the water cannot become hot enough to scald anyone. If hot pipes are exposed, cover them with insulation.

While walking is good exercise and can reduce stress, wandering can become a safety issue. If the environment is secured with a fence, camouflaged doors, or locks, people with dementia may move freely within a relatively safe area, reducing the stress of caregivers who are afraid to let them out of sight. It is important to balance freedom, safety, and client rights. If wandering away from home is a potential hazard, the Alzheimer's Association has an excellent program called "Safe Return." More information about this low-cost program is available by calling 1-800-272-3900.

Tammi G. Hardiman, RN, BSN, *Nurse Consultant, Community Services Quality Assurance, Department of Social and Health Services, State of Washington, Arlington, Washington*

and self-respect, which can be very fragile during the early and middle stages of the disease. Give the client plenty of time to complete a task. Constantly encouraging, urging, and reminding the client in a step-by-step approach are necessary.

Urge Incontinence. AD clients develop urge incontinence as cortical neurons degenerate and no longer provide inhibition of the micturition and defecation responses. State this diagnosis as *Urge Incontinence related to neuronal degeneration and forgetfulness.*

Outcomes. The client will have optimal continence of bladder and bowel, as evidenced by having clean, dry clothing and bedding as much as possible; having intact skin; and voiding appropriately in the bathroom.

Interventions. Anticipation of elimination needs and scheduled voiding and defecation times can help in the initial stages. The client may show nonverbal signs of needing to void or defecate, like restlessness, grasping the genital area, or picking at clothing. Sometimes the client forgets where the bathroom is located. Having clear, bright signs indicating where the bathroom is and frequently taking the client there may help control incontinence. Fluid intake after the dinner meal can be restricted to help maintain continence during the night.

Try to arrange a bowel program to coincide with the client's usual pattern. In the later stages of AD, clients may need to wear incontinence pads during the day and external urinary drainage devices at night. Indwelling catheters should be avoided because of the risk of infection and injury.

Caregiver Role Strain. Family members and especially caregivers (usually a spouse or adult child) of clients with AD face a great deal of emotional and physical burden. State this diagnosis as *Caregiver Role Strain related to grieving the loss of a family member to AD, change in social role, and intense demands for time commitment and provision of care.*

Outcomes. The family will demonstrate decreased role strain, as evidenced by voicing their emotional concerns, seeking appropriate assistance, and providing adequate care for the client.

Interventions. Family members grieve the loss of the person they used to know. Each decline in cognitive function becomes another source of grief. Two stages of grief in the family have been described.

The process of grief begins during the caregiving stage and continues after the client's death. Normal family routines are lost, and the relationship between the family member and the dementia sufferer changes. Factors that have the most profound effect on the emotional well-being of caregivers include incontinence, overdemanding behavior, and the need for constant supervision.

Wives tend to experience a higher degree of emotional burden as caregivers than husbands do. Paradoxically, the closer the emotional bond between caregiver and dementia sufferer, the less the strain for the caregiver. Conversely, a low past level of intimacy is associated with an increased level of both perceived strain and depression in the spouse caregiver. Caregivers are most likely to be depressed if they feel a loss of control over their spouse's behavior, if they feel unable to cope with the impact of caregiving, and if they perceive the situation to be stable and to affect everything.

Studies have not determined that formal support of the caregiver (home visits by special practitioners, chore workers, and day care workers) relieves the caregiver's burden more than informal support (family member visits and support groups). The Alzheimer's Disease and Related Disorders Association has local chapters that offer support groups in many major cities in the United States (Phone: 1-800-272-3900).

Interview family members to determine their understanding of the diagnosis and prognosis of AD and to allow them to discuss their concerns about caring for the client.

- Do they know about community resources?
- Do they have someone to call when they can no longer cope with caregiving?

The home environment should be evaluated for safety before the client is sent home from the hospital.

- Is the home on a busy street?
- Can doors be secured so that the client cannot get out without supervision?
- Are potentially dangerous appliances out of reach?

A variety of options are available to caregivers. Chore service workers can help with household chores and relieve the caregiver of these duties. Other paid help can provide in-home respite care by observing the dementia sufferer while the caregiver tends to business outside the home, seeks social interaction, or meets recreational needs.

Adult day care provides time away from home for the dementia sufferer. Day care usually offers a lunchtime meal as well as several hours of scheduled activities that are tailored to the client's abilities. These activities may include games, crafts, music, and exercise.

Respite care involves admission to an extended care facility for a few days to a few weeks to allow the caregiver time to recover from the demands of providing 24-hour care (See the Bridge to Home Health Care on respite for caregivers).

BRIDGE TO HOME HEALTH CARE

Respite Care for Caregivers of People with Alzheimer's Disease

When providing home care for people with Alzheimer's disease, be alert to how well the caregivers themselves are managing their own health. If *their* health fails as a result of the stress of caregiving, the person with Alzheimer's may need to be placed in a nursing home much sooner than expected.

You can help caregivers find physical and emotional respite by following these suggestions:

- Encourage caregivers to be realistic about what needs they can meet for their loved ones and what needs they cannot meet.
- Suggest that caregivers make a list of all the tasks they perform for the person with Alzheimer's. Next to each task, have them write down who else could do the job. (Caregivers may find that they are performing some tasks that their loved ones could still do for themselves.) This exercise will help caregivers identify tasks that they could delegate to someone else.
- Help caregivers identify friends and neighbors who can offer them support, take the caregiver out for dinner, or stay with the person with Alzheimer's while the caregiver gets some precious time alone. Often, friends of caregivers are more supportive than family members, because friends can maintain more objectivity.
- Know the community resources that provide in-home day care for people with Alzheimer's.
- Encourage caregivers to share their knowledge and experience with newly assigned health care staff to foster a team approach in care. Caregivers often fear that "no one will care for my loved one like I do." They are right.
- Know the community centers that provide day care outside the home. Find out about the qualifications of the staff, cost of services, eligibility criteria, availability of financial assistance, daily activities at the centers, and environment of the centers. Having firsthand knowledge of the centers will help you guide families as they make choices.
- Encourage caregivers to try a day care community center for at least 2 to 3 weeks, knowing that it is normal when their loved one does not like the new experience at first. Sometimes caregivers are more likely to accept assistance if they know they are "just having a trial period for a few weeks."
- Encourage caregivers to make use of support groups offered by the local chapter of the Alzheimer's Disease and Related Disorders Association.
- Validate the caregiver's feelings of anger, guilt, exhaustion, and frustration. Let caregivers know that you understand how bad things can get at home, even though people with Alzheimer's may appear alert and pleasant when company visits.
- Caregivers may complain about "going crazy" as they watch their loved ones perform tedious, repetitive tasks. For example, when they pick up fallen leaves one leaf at a time rather than raking up the leaves. Help caregivers analyze activities in terms of safety. Does the activity harm the person with Alzheimer's? If not, caregivers can reframe their perceptions of the activity and accept it as harmless.
- Know the assisted living facilities that offer extended care for caregivers who want to go away for trips. Use these times to help the caregiver begin planning for long-term care in an assisted living facility or nursing home. Caregivers may consider long-term care when the person with Alzheimer's begins to wander at night, stops eating, becomes incontinent, or becomes belligerent or violent with the caregiver.
- Laugh with caregivers. Help them realize that finding humor in the absurdities of life can make it possible to deal with a situation that might otherwise be unbearable.

Cyndy Hunt Luzinski, RN MS, *Community Nurse Case Manager, Poudre Valley Health System, Fort Collins, Colorado*

Nursing home care is usually the final and most difficult and trying option for a caregiver. This decision creates guilt, self-doubt, and anxiety; however, it may be the only option when the caregiver suffers burnout and becomes unable to provide adequate care. Table 72–2 lists nursing guidelines for meeting family needs.

When the person with AD reaches the terminal stage of illness, questions about end-of-life treatments arise.

- Should a feeding tube be used to provide nourishment?
- Should antibiotics be used to treat pneumonias or other infections?
- Should cardiopulmonary resuscitation be used?

Ideally, decisions about these questions are raised and discussed with the client and family members before the person loses the capacity to make decisions.

Two forms of *advance directives* (means of expressing one's wishes about life-sustaining treatment after losing the mental capacity to make informed decisions) are available. One is the *living will,* a written document signed by the individual (while he or she is still mentally capable of making informed decisions) in the presence of a witness. The living will lists conditions under which the person wishes life-sustaining treatments to be withheld or withdrawn. The other advance directive is a *durable power of attorney for health care.* This is a legal document in which the person (while still mentally capable) assigns someone to act on his or her behalf in matters of health care decisions if the person loses decisional capacity (e.g., becomes demented).

EVALUATION

Continually evaluate the degree of expected outcome attainment. You should expect progress toward outcomes to be slow. If the client is transferred to a new center (e.g., hospital), some regression can be expected. Family evaluation should be completed on regular intervals.

CREUTZFELDT-JAKOB DISEASE

Etiology

Creutzfeldt-Jakob disease (CJD) is a subacute CNS disorder that produces progressive dementia, myoclonus, and distinctive EEG changes. CJD is a unique disease that can apparently arise from two separate mechanisms, genetic and infectious. People with the genetic form have a mutated gene. The infectious form does not develop from a known virus or other pathogen; therefore, words like *virion, slow virus,* and *prion* are sometimes used to describe the etiologic agent. Several reports document human-to-human spread of CJD from cornea transplants, dural allografts, human pituitary growth hormone injections, and reuse of stereotactic EEG electrodes that had been previously implanted in a person with CJD. Apparently, a group of infected cadavers were used for growth hormone replacement. Incubation periods have ranged from 4 to 21 years, which indicates the enormous difficulty of tracing the infection. Additional cases may still appear in people who received the hormone before its discontinuation in 1985. In 1996, CJD was associated with ingestion of infected beef. This led to the popular term "mad cow disease."

The incidence of CJD peaks in the age group 40 to 70 years. It affects both sexes equally. A higher incidence has been noted in Libyan-born Jewish people and in some groups from Chile and the former Czechoslovakia.

Clinical Manifestations

Manifestations include vague psychiatric or behavior changes suggesting a personality change. About one third of clients report weight loss, anorexia, insomnia, malaise, and dizziness for a period of weeks to months. In the early stages, there is progressive memory loss, visual impairment, and dysphagia. Within a few weeks or months, a relentlessly progressive dementia develops and marked deterioration is noted from week to week. Myoclonus (twitching) is usually present. Deterioration is rapid, with 90% of clients dying within 1 year.

A definitive diagnosis attempts to differentiate CJD from AD. AD has a more protracted course and no myoclonus or EEG changes. Lithium toxicity can mimic the manifestations, but they clear within about 2 weeks after discontinuation of the drug. Brain biopsy during hospitalization or on autopsy is the usual method of establishing a definitive diagnosis.

Outcome Management

No effective treatment is available, and CJD appears to be uniformly fatal. Nursing care is directed at supportive care, preventing skin breakdown, furnishing nutrition, and providing emotional support to the client and family. Families require much support, care, and concern as they try to cope with the sudden onset of this debilitating disease and with managing the day-to-day care of the client.

Although CJD can be transmitted, the risk to health care workers and others having contact with the client is no more than that to the general population. Isolation of clients is not indicated, but personnel should wear gloves when handling tissues, blood, and spinal fluid. Accidental skin contact with possibly infected material should be followed by washing in 10 normal sodium hydroxide or a solution of 5% household chlorine bleach. The agent can be inactivated on surfaces by using a 10% bleach solution for 1 hour. Surgical and pathologic instruments should be steam-autoclaved for 1 hour at 132° C. No organs, tissue, or tissue products from clients with CJD or any other ill-defined neurologic disorders should be used for transplantation or replacement therapy.

HUNTINGTON'S DISEASE

Huntington's disease (HD), also known as *Huntington's chorea,* is a genetically transmitted degenerative neurologic disease. It is characterized by abnormal movements (chorea), intellectual decline, and emotional disturbance. Clinical manifestations usually begin in the 30s and 40s, although occasionally they begin in young adulthood or even in children. Women and men are equally affected. The disease is relentlessly progressive, leading to disabil-

TABLE 72–2 NURSING GUIDELINES FOR MEETING THE NEEDS OF THE FAMILY OF THE CLIENT WITH DEMENTIA OF THE ALZHEIMER'S TYPE

Goals	Selected Interventions
PHYSICAL	
Monitor chronic health problems or physical limitations of family caregiver	Obtain health history of family caregiver to identify past and new health problems
Identify development of new health problems	Support family in following through with routine health examinations
	Refer family members to physician when health problems are observed
	Assess family's understanding of medical management of own health problems
	Teach family members to preserve own health in order to continue caring for patient with Alzheimer's disease
Identify cues for stress	Emphasize family's need for adequate nutrition, hydration, exercise, and rest
Examine somatic health problems	Help family members to be alert to signs of caregiver stress
PSYCHOSOCIAL	
Assist family in coping positively with stress	Instruct family to get respite regularly for rest and relaxation
	Teach stress management techniques (i.e., relaxation, supportive relationships, goal setting, time management, diversion)
Identify destructive methods of coping (i.e., alcohol, drugs, tobacco, overeating or undereating, physical abuse of patient)	Refer family to physician, therapist when stress remains unmanageable even with social or psychological resources
Assess family dynamics	Refer signs of physical abuse to adult protective services
Assist family members in dealing with role change and conflict	Recognize the family's role, discuss capacity to provide care, and give reinforcement for care provided
	Counsel family in dealing with role conflicts, unmet expectations, or interpersonal conflicts
	Teach family the need to maintain roles and social activities outside caregiving experience
	Administer burden interview
	Reinforce family's attempt to cope
	Acknowledge family fears of being unable to continue with caregiving
If need for support identified, direct family members to sources	Refer family to a support group to share with others in similar situations
	Refer family to nearest office on aging or Alzheimer's Disease and Related Disorders Association, Inc. (ADRDA) to identify benefits in community available to Alzheimer's disease clients
Identify family's mixed emotions (i.e., depression, anger, resentment, pity, embarrassment, guilt)	Listen to family and facilitate sharing of emotions and feelings in supportive, empathic environment
Identify alternative plans for care if family members or social support systems become unable to provide care or are ineffective	Counsel and support family if patient placed in care of others (i.e., day care, respite service, home care, nursing home); allay feelings of guilt
	Facilitate family meeting to identify time for socialization
Identify financial limitations	Encourage family to be specific about financial limitations
	Offer family referrals (legal, financial, or social service) for information on eligibility for private, county, state, or federal financial support for home services, and advise and counsel regarding power of attorney or guardianship, trust or estate planning
Assess family's ability to make funeral plans	Help family anticipate and cope with grief process
	Assist family in making prefuneral arrangements
	Address family's fear regarding the possible role of heredity in development of Alzheimer's disease and assist in making decision regarding autopsy

TABLE 72–2 NURSING GUIDELINES FOR MEETING THE NEEDS OF THE FAMILY OF THE CLIENT WITH DEMENTIA OF THE ALZHEIMER'S TYPE *Continued*

Goals	Selected Interventions
ENVIRONMENTAL	
Identify compatibility of environment with family and client	Conduct a family meeting to discuss relationship of family, patient, and environment
Assess learning needs regarding client care tasks	Teach management of concurrent physical health problems of the client with Alzheimer's disease Include family in development of patient care plan Teach family to encourage the client to continue daily habits to extent possible Complete behavior problems checklist Anticipate likely problems and teach how to manage them Teach environmental modification (consistent, simple, calm routines) to maximize family endurance and enhance safety Teach family to relate to patient with creative connectedness (touch, humor, flexibility, reminiscence, music, planned activities)
Assess family need and desire for information about Alzheimer's disease and how it affects the client's behavior	Assist family in understanding symptoms related to memory loss, nature of the illness, symptoms, stages of disease progression, and behavior manifestations Provide written material to reinforce education and understanding (i.e., *The 36-Hour Day, Coping and Caring: Living with Alzheimer's Disease;* literature from local, state, or national ADRDA chapters) Supply ADRDA 24-hour hotline number: 1-800-621-0379

Adapted from Stevenson, J. P. (1990). Family stress to home care of Alzheimer's disease patients and implications for support. *Journal of Neuroscience Nursing, 22*(3), 185.

ity and death within 15 to 20 years. Death usually results from respiratory complications caused by aspiration.

The disease is autosomal dominant; offspring of an affected person have a 50% chance of inheriting the disease. Because HD does not skip generations, offspring who have not inherited the disease will not pass it on to their offspring. The abnormal gene has been isolated on chromosome 4.

Pathophysiology

The pathologic changes of HD involve degeneration of the striatum (caudate and putamen) in the basal ganglia. Other subtle changes occur in the cortex and cerebellum, namely, loss of neurons and an increased number of glial cells (gliosis). The degeneration of the caudate nucleus leads to a reduction in several neurotransmitters, including gamma-aminobutyric acid, ACh, substance P, and metenkephalin, and their synthetic enzymes. This change leaves relatively higher concentrations of the other neurotransmitters, dopamine and norepinephrine. The relative excess of dopamine in HD, a disorder of excessive movement, can be contrasted to the lack of dopamine in Parkinson's disease (PD), a disorder of lack of movement.

Clinical Manifestations

Emotional disturbances and mental deterioration may precede the abnormal movements. The person may become negative, suspicious, and irritable. This condition may progress to depression and psychosis. Temper outbursts and sexual promiscuity may also occur. Severe mood swings are common. Cognitive decline progresses, and eventually the person becomes demented, incontinent, and completely unable to care for himself or herself.

The abnormal movements in HD are subtle at first. The person may appear restless or fidgety. The person may be aware of these movements and try to mask them by making them seem to be parts of intentional movements, such as head scratching or leg crossing. As the disease progresses, the rapid, jerky choreiform movements become more pronounced and involve all muscles. The person is constantly in motion. Stress, emotional situations, and attempts to perform voluntary movement can aggravate the abnormal movements. During sleep, the movements diminish or disappear.

The diagnosis of HD is made on the basis of clinical manifestations and family history, because there is no specific diagnostic test for the disease itself. CT or MRI imaging of the brain may show atrophy of the head of the caudate, but this factor alone is not diagnostic of HD.

Outcome Management

There is no known treatment to cure or alter the course of HD. Haloperidol, a dopamine blocker, can control the abnormal movements and some behavioral manifestations.

Diazepam can be used to lower anxiety, aiding in control of movements. Antidepressants can help depression.

LATE-STAGE DYSPHAGIA

One of the most common and dangerous problems in the middle to late stages is dysphagia. Several interventions should be tried. Medications need to be evaluated for their anticholinergic and sedative effects, which may impair swallowing. Mealtimes should be free of stress and clutter and have an unhurried atmosphere. Use of adaptive eating utensils can encourage and extend independence in eating. The diet should include foods that are easy to swallow and form a bolus in the mouth (e.g., canned peaches, chopped meat in gravy and mashed potatoes, custards). Many clients with HD require high caloric intake because of excessive movements and should try eating frequent, small meals containing high-calorie foods. Clients should sit upright when eating. While swallowing, they should keep the chin down toward the chest. They can be trained to hold their breath before swallowing and cough after each mouthful is swallowed to clear the throat of any residual food.

Nursing Management

If the client continues to have difficulty eating and loses weight despite dietary and environmental modifications, a feeding tube may become necessary. However, artificial feeding methods often frighten families, and they pose ethical dilemmas about prolonging life. Nurses can help clients and their families make these difficult decisions by clarifying the issues and providing information on the types, risks, benefits, and long-term effects of artificial feeding methods.

Poor control of oral and respiratory muscles can make communication difficult. The nurse can assist the family to develop signals such as raising a hand or keeping the eyes open or closed for yes and no responses. If physical signals are not an option, cards with printed words may be helpful. Keep communication simple and unstrained. Repeat words that are understood to let the client know that communication has been successful.

Excessive movements and falls may cause physical injury and can restrict independence. Pads on wheelchairs and beds, shin guards, and walking belts can prevent injury. Aids for ambulation (e.g., walking behind a wheelchair) can extend independence. Clothing should be light and simple to don and doff.

HD has a major impact on the family, not only because of the burden of caregiving but also because of the risk to offspring of inheriting the disease. Many ethical dilemmas surrounding the issue of privacy can surface in cases of HD. Whether test results are positive or negative, the results are of interest to the spouse, other family members, employers, and insurers. However, principles of confidentiality forbid disclosure of medical information to anyone unless the client consents. Be sensitive to the client's desire for confidentiality but use this opportunity to teach the client about the effect the disease may have on other family members. Because a blood test is now available to check for the presence of the abnormal gene, family members face difficult choices about whether to find out if they have the Huntington gene.

MULTIPLE SCLEROSIS

Multiple sclerosis (MS) is a chronic demyelinating disease that affects the myelin sheath of neurons in the CNS. The myelin sheath is essential for normal conduction of nerve impulses. Patches of myelin deteriorate at irregular intervals along the nerve axon, causing slowing of nerve conduction. Axonal destruction also occurs in MS.

The onset of MS usually occurs between ages 20 and 40, and it affects women twice as often as men. Whites are affected more often than Hispanics, blacks, or Asians. The disease is most prevalent in the colder climates of North America and Europe. If someone is born in an area of high risk for MS and moves to an area of low risk after age 15, the person carries the risk of the area of origin.

Etiology and Risk Factors

The exact cause of MS is unknown. Most theories suggest that MS is an immunogenetic-viral disease, that is, an immune-mediated demyelination triggered by a viral infection. A genetic susceptibility apparently alters the body's immune response to viral infection. Multiple genes are probably involved. However, the only consistently identified disease locus is on the HLA gene complex on chromosome 6.

A variety of precipitating factors can precede the onset or an exacerbation of MS, such as infection, physical injury, emotional stress, pregnancy, and fatigue. Most pregnancy-related exacerbations occur 3 months post partum and may relate more to the stress of labor and fatigue during the puerperium than to the pregnancy itself.

Pathophysiology

Myelin is a highly conductive fatty material that surrounds the axon and speeds conduction of nerve impulses along the axon. In MS, *plaques* form along the myelin sheath, causing inflammation, edema, and eventually scarring and destruction (Fig. 72–2). Plaques are characterized by primary demyelination and death of oligodendrocytes in the center of the lesion. Initially, perivascular inflammatory cells (autoreactive T cells) invade the myelin-covered axons in the CNS. This is followed by extensive gliosis or scarring by astrocytes and aberrant attempts at remyelination, with oligodendrocytes proliferating at the edges of the plaque. When edema and inflammation subside, some remyelination occurs but is often incomplete.

Although plaques may occur anywhere in the white matter of the CNS, the areas most commonly involved are the optic nerves, cerebrum, and cervical spinal cord.

Clinical Manifestations

The wide variety of manifestations possible with MS and the unpredictable nature of the disease pose many challenges to the client and family. The course of illness varies from person to person. Four clinical patterns have been identified (Fig. 72–3). The most common initial pattern is *relapsing-remitting* MS. Clients experience manifestations that eventually remit with little or no progression of disability.

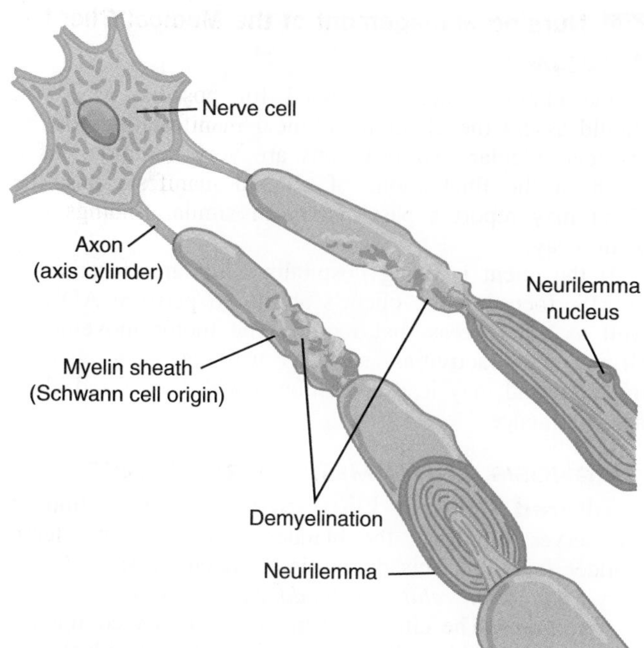

FIGURE 72–2 Changes in the nerve sheath, as seen in multiple sclerosis. Myelin is made by the oligodendrocyte and coats peripheral nerves, facilitating nervous impulse. In clients with multiple sclerosis, the myelin degenerates in patches, causing nerve transmission to become erratic.

The random distribution of MS plaques leads to several clinical manifestations:

- Weakness or tingling sensations (paresthesias) of one or more extremities caused by involvement of the cerebrum or spinal cord
- Vision loss from optic neuritis
- Incoordination that is due to cerebellar involvement
- Bowel and bladder dysfunction as a result of spinal cord involvement

Bladder dysfunction can take several forms, depending on which neural pathways are affected. Dysfunction may involve hesitancy, frequency, loss of sensation, incontinence, and retention. There may be increased or decreased detrusor, bladder neck, or external sphincter tone, or a combination of these problems. The ultimate bladder dysfunction, however, is usually hyperreflexia in association with sphincter dyssynergia (sphincter contraction during detrusor contraction).[3] Proper diagnosis of the type of bladder dysfunction requires a thorough history, laboratory assessment of kidney function, and identification of possible infection. If bladder emptying is defective, further investigation with urography, cystoscopy, and urodynamic studies should be performed.

Constipation is commonly experienced by clients with MS. Dysfunction can result from one or more of the following factors: spinal cord lesion, immobility, dehydration, medications, and nutritional deficiencies. Stool incontinence, although more rare, is also possible. Sexual dysfunction can also occur as a result of lesions in the ascending or descending autonomic and sensory fibers in the spinal cord.

Fatigue is a common manifestation of MS and usually one of the most disabling. Spasticity can reduce energy, inhibit motor control, and interfere with self-care, sexuality, vocational responsibilities, and recreation.

Because MS strikes young adults during their years of establishing a family and an occupation, the impact of the disease can be devastating. Depression often occurs in clients, but it is not clear whether depression is a reaction to disability or a function of the disease itself. Others may experience euphoria, emotional instability, or apathy.

Because there is no definitive test for MS, clinicians rely on a detailed history, clinical findings, and a variety of diagnostic tests. The history often reveals several episodes of neurologic dysfunction, separated by time and by different locations in the CNS. Current research looking at clients who experience only one manifestation such as optic neuritis is changing the way clinicians diagnose MS.

Diagnostic tests include:

- CSF evaluation for the presence of oligoclonal banding
- Evoked potentials of the optic pathways and auditory system to assess the presence of slowed nerve conduction
- MRI of the brain and spinal cord to determine the presence of MS plaques

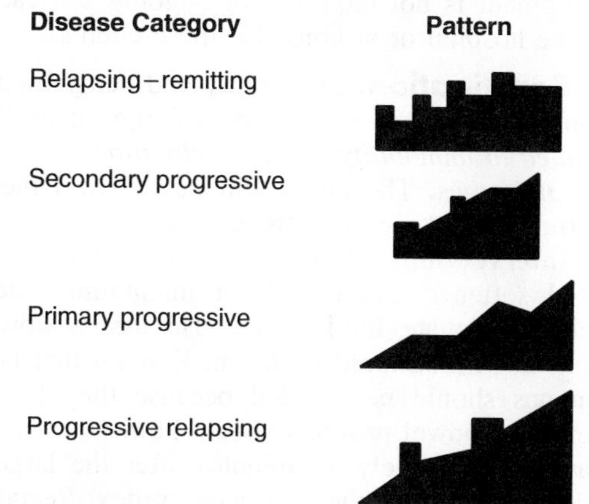

Disease Category
Pattern
Definition
Relapsing–remitting
Episodes of acute worsening with recovery and a stable course between relapses
Secondary progressive
Gradual neurologic deterioration with or without superimposed acute relapses in a client who previously had relapsing–remitting multiple sclerosis
Primary progressive
Gradual, nearly continuous neurologic deterioration from the onset of manifestations
Progressive relapsing
Gradual neurologic deterioration from the onset of manifestations but with subsequent superimposed relapses

FIGURE 72–3 Clinical patterns of multiple sclerosis. (Modified from Lublin, F. D., & Reingold, S. C. [1996]. Defining the clinical course of multiple sclerosis: Results of an international survey. *Neurology, 46,* 907–911.)

Outcome Management

Treatment generally falls into one of three categories: (1) treatment of acute relapses, (2) treatment aimed at disease management, and (3) symptomatic treatment.

Treating Acute Relapses

Treatment of acute relapses usually involves the use of intravenous (IV) or oral corticosteroids, which have both anti-inflammatory and immunosuppressive properties. They are often used to enhance recovery from an exacerbation. Methylprednisolone is standard therapy for acute exacerbations sometimes followed by an oral prednisone taper. Azathioprine (Imuran) and cyclophosphamide (Cytoxan), other immunosuppressive agents, may be used for more severe exacerbations or progressive MS.

Treating Exacerbations

Interferon β_{1b} (Betaseron) is used for ambulatory clients with relapsing-remitting MS. Interferon β_{1b} is a genetically engineered complex protein with both antiviral and immunoregulatory properties that can reduce the number of MS exacerbations. The drug is injected subcutaneously every other day. Interferon β_{1a} (Avonex) is also available for the treatment of relapsing forms of MS. In addition to reducing the number and severity of relapses, interferon β_{1a} provides a delay in disability in placebo-controlled studies.

The third disease-modifying agent avaliable for use in the United States is glatiramer acetate (Copaxone), a synthetic polypeptide approved for use in relapsing-remitting MS. It is not an interferon but is believed to work by mimicking myelin basic protein and interrupting the inflammatory cascade to prevent damage to myelin.

Side effects of the interferons include fever, fatigue, and flu-like manifestations. Clients on interferon β_{1a} have also reported increased depression and injection site reactions. Copaxone does not produce the interferon-type side effects of fever and flu-like manifestations, but rare episodes of face flushing, chest tightness, and shortness of breath lasting less than 15 minutes have been reported. Numerous other therapeutic agents are undergoing clinical trials.

Symptomatic Treatment

Several strategies are available for symptomatic management in MS. Pharmacologic interventions can be used for bladder dysfunction (oxybutynin, propantheline); constipation (psyllium hydromucilloid, bisacodyl pills or suppositories); fatigue (amantadine, modafinil); spasticity (baclofen, diazepam, dantrolene); tremor (propranolol, phenobarbital, clonazepam); and dysesthesias and trigeminal neuralgia (carbamazepine, phenytoin, amitriptyline).

Transcutaneous electrical nerve stimulation (TENS) is also helpful for dysesthesias. Areas of numbness should be inspected regularly to prevent injury and development of pressure ulcers. Skin should be kept dry and free of urine and feces. A seat cushion that distributes pressure should be used for wheelchair-bound clients with insensate buttock skin. Blindness or severely impaired vision may occur. In this case, refer the client to Services for the Blind for rehabilitation. Cognitive and perceptual impairment necessitates psychometric and functional testing for accurate assessment and rehabilitation services.

Nursing Management of the Medical Client

Assessment

If the client is being assessed for possible MS, you should assess the client for clinical manifestations of the disorder. Ocular manifestations are very common. As a result of the fluctuations of clinical manifestations, the client may report a past history of similar findings that went away.

If the client is being hospitalized for an exacerbation of MS, focus on the client's ability to perform ADL as well as other areas that require fine motor movements. Gross motor activities, such as walking, may also be impaired and may lead to problems with bowel and bladder continence.

Diagnosis, Outcomes, Interventions

Altered Urinary Elimination. Demyelination of the nerves supplying the bladder may result in altered bladder function. This diagnosis is stated as *Altered Urinary Elimination related to bladder dysfunction.*

Outcomes. The client will maintain urinary continence and normal bladder filling, as evidenced by residual volumes of less than 100 ml, application of appropriate bladder elimination procedures, and verbalization of personal satisfaction with urinary elimination status.

Interventions. The following interventions are for neurogenic bladder, the most common type of bladder dysfunction in MS.

Fluid intake should be maintained at 2000 ml/24 hours, ideally, 400 to 500 ml with each meal and 200 ml at midmorning, midafternoon, and late afternoon. Avoiding fluid intake after the evening meal reduces the need for emptying the bladder during the night.

Voiding should be attempted every 3 hours during waking hours. If voiding is not successful, a catheter should be inserted into the bladder and then removed once emptying is complete. This is called *intermittent catheterization.* If the volume of catheterized urine exceeds 500 ml, catheterization may need to be scheduled more frequently.

Instruct the client on how to do self-catheterization if he or she is capable. A clean red rubber catheter can be reused for up to 1 week, as long as it is washed thoroughly with soap and water and placed in a clean, tightly sealed plastic bag after every catheterization. Sterile equipment is not required for ongoing self-catheterization in the hospital or at home for these clients.

Constipation. Immobility and demyelination lead to constipation. State this common diagnosis as *Constipation related to immobility and demyelination.*

Outcomes. The client will have bowel movements of normal consistency and frequency.

Interventions. A high-fiber diet, bulk formers, and stool softeners are useful for maintaining stool consistency. Adequate fluid intake also assists bowel elimination; 2000 ml should be taken. Explain that laxatives and enemas should be avoided because they lead to dependence. A bowel program should be performed every other day, approximately 45 minutes after the largest meal, to take advantage of the gastrocolic reflex. Rectal evacuation may be augmented by the use of glycerin or bisacodyl suppositories or digital stimulation.

Activity Intolerance. State this common diagnosis as *Activity Intolerance related to fatigue and muscle weakness.*

Outcomes. The client will demonstrate improved activity tolerance, as evidenced by (1) maintaining a balance between work, rest, and exercise and recreation; (2) performing ADL without excessive fatigue; (3) using energy-saving devices and techniques; (4) avoiding elevations in environmental and body temperatures; and (5) consuming a diet adequate in calories and protein for body size, frame, and age.

Intervention. Because fatigue can be precipitated by warm temperatures, the environment should be kept cool. If air conditioning is unavailable, cool baths and ice packs may help lower body temperature.

Assist the client to plan activities at his or her peak energy level, which is usually in the morning. This schedule promotes optimal synchrony between circadian rhythms and the client's physical demands. The client should plan for periods of rest throughout the day. Collaboration with the physical and occupational therapist can reveal methods to reduce energy consumption with repeated tasks and apply adaptive devices for ambulation and toileting. The drugs amantadine (Symmetrel) and modafinil (Provigil) may alleviate fatigue in some clients.

Impaired Physical Mobility. Several problems lead to difficulties with mobility. State this diagnosis as *Impaired Physical Mobility related to weakness, contractures, spasticity, and ataxia.*

Outcomes. The client will achieve optimal physical mobility, as evidenced by improved or maintained range of motion in all joints, optimal control of spasticity, and effective use of adaptive aids.

Interventions. Although some clients are bothered by painful muscle spasms, others may rely on spasticity to stabilize weak limbs during transfers and ambulation. Spastic muscles must be stretched at least twice daily through their full range of motion. The drug baclofen (Lioresal) provides synaptic inhibition of spinal reflexes, which can reduce spasticity, although it may increase weakness and fatigue in some clients. Diazepam (Valium), tizanidine (Zanaflex), and dantrolene (Dantrium) are other antispasmotic drugs. Surgical intervention or nerve blocks may be necessary if contractures develop. Monitor the effect of medications on spasticity, promote activity to decrease spasms, and utilize spasms for muscle strength when transferring.

Advise that strengthening exercises for muscle weakness (paresis) must be done with caution because they can exacerbate paresis by causing muscle fatigue. However, selective strengthening of nonaffected or less affected muscles can enhance physical function and well-being. Range-of-motion exercises should be performed at least twice daily. Active movement is preferable to passive movement. Correct body alignment should be maintained to reduce the risk of contractures. Splints may help maintain position and provide support for weak hands and ankles. Ataxia and tremor of the extremities can be lessened by the use of small weights applied to the distal extremities or the use of weighted utensils. Weakness and fatigue can worsen ataxia. Ambulation aids such as a cane or a walker may be necessary.

Risk for Self-Care Deficit. Clients with MS may experience a decline in self-care abilities. State this diagnosis as *Risk for Self-Care Deficit related to muscle weakness.*

Outcomes. The client will reduce the risk for self-care deficits by using ADL aids.

Interventions. Clients may require aids, such as wheelchairs or canes, to perform ADL and ambulate. The performance of ADL may be enhanced if counters and tabletops are adjusted to a comfortable working height. Work in combination with the physical therapist, occupational therapist, social worker, and home health nurse to identify, purchase, and teach the client how to use ADL aids.

Knowledge Deficit. The client with a new diagnosis of MS often lacks knowledge about MS, its unpredictable course, and the role of stress in MS. State this diagnosis as *Knowledge Deficit related to new diagnosis of MS.*

Outcomes. The client will have more knowledge about MS, as evidenced by stating facts about the course of MS and the role of stress in MS.

Interventions. The client with MS needs to have a clear understanding of the unpredictability of this disorder. The client may be free of manifestations for many weeks to months, even years, and then experience them. If the client can identify stressors that exacerbate the clinical manifestations, sometimes these stressors can be avoided. The National Multiple Sclerosis Society can be an excellent resource for education and support. For clients on one of the three disease-modifying agents, each company has a support program to offer education, financial information, and support for people with MS and their families.

Self-Esteem Disturbance. Because of the age of the client, loss of independence and fear of disability can be devastating. Psychosocial diagnosis is important in providing holistic care. State this diagnosis as *Self Esteem Disturbance related to loss of independence and fear of disability.*

Outcomes. The client will achieve improved self-esteem, as evidenced by verbalizing awareness that personal goals and body image will need to be adjusted, willingness to maintain appropriate independence, and positive thoughts and statements about self.

Intervention. Regardless of the cause of disturbance in self-esteem, carefully assess the individual and family history for the presence and type of depressive episodes and the clinical manifestations. Identify previous treatment for depression, including psychotherapy and drug therapy. By assessing the client's problem-solving strategies, you can identify coping behavior strengths and defense mechanisms such as denial, avoidance, or intellectualization that the client may use to mask depression.

Evaluate the client's social support system, which contributes to a sense of well-being. Grieving the loss of function in MS can lead to a reactive depression and require provision of support group therapy for both the client and family. Some clients may not benefit from this kind of therapy, however, because they may see people whose condition is much worse than their own and may fear developing that level of disability. On-line computer services for MS clients can provide a means of social support.

EVALUATION

The degree of expected outcome attainment should be evaluated on an ongoing basis. Most outcomes are long-term and may require weeks to months to attain.

GUILLAIN-BARRÉ SYNDROME

Etiology

Guillain-Barré syndrome (GBS) is an inflammatory disease of unknown origin that involves degeneration of the myelin sheath of peripheral nerves. GBS is seen worldwide and affects people of all ages and races. Since the virtual elimination of poliomyelitis, GBS has become the most common cause of acute generalized paralysis, with an annual incidence of 0.75 to 2.0/100,000 population. In one half to two thirds of cases, an upper respiratory or gastrointestinal infection precedes the onset of the syndrome by 1 to 4 weeks.

Although many organisms have been suspected, including *Cytomegalovirus* and Epstein-Barr virus, *Campylobacter jejuni* is the organism most often implicated. This gram-negative rod is found in poultry, pets, raw milk, and contaminated water. *C. jejuni* targets the myelin sheath. Macrophages penetrate the basal lamina surrounding the axon, displace the Schwann cell from the myelin sheath, and phagocytose the myelin lamellae. An association between HIV and GBS has also been reported, and clients with GBS should be tested for HIV.

Clinical Manifestations

A characteristic feature is ascending weakness, usually beginning in the lower extremities and spreading, sometimes rapidly, to the trunk, upper extremities, and even the face. The weakness evolves over hours to days, with maximal deficit by 4 weeks in 90% of cases. Deep tendon reflexes are lost. Paresthesias (tingling sensation) in the limbs may occur early in the course of the illness.

This *initial phase* is usually followed by a *plateau phase* during which the disease no longer seems to progress but the client does not recover functions initially lost. Deep, aching muscle pain in the shoulder girdle and thighs is common. The two most dangerous features of the disease are respiratory muscle weakness and autonomic neuropathy involving both the sympathetic and parasympathetic systems. The latter feature can involve orthostatic hypotension, hypertension, pupillary disturbances, sweating dysfunction, cardiac dysrhythmias, paralytic ileus, and urinary retention.

The third phase of the disease is the *recovery phase.* Improvement and recovery occur with remyelination. However, if nerve axons are damaged, some residual deficits may remain. Remyelination occurs in a descending pattern; the functions lost last are thus the first to be regained. Recovery is usually maximal at 6 months, although severe cases may take up to 2 years for maximal recovery. Fortunately, 85% to 90% of clients with GBS recover completely.

Diagnosis of GBS is based on history and physical examination, cerebrospinal fluid (CSF) examination, and electrophysiologic studies. The CSF contains increased protein, with few or no white blood cells. Nerve conduction velocity is slowed, although it may be normal in the early stage of the illness. Conduction block, a diminution in amplitude or an absence of elicited muscle action potentials from stimulation of a peripheral nerve, also occurs.

Outcome Management

The focus of therapy is supportive care. Monitor respiratory or cardiovascular status carefully: vital signs, serial measurement of vital capacity, peripheral oxygen saturation, and electrocardiography. When vital capacity falls to 15 ml/kg of body weight, intubation and artificial ventilation are usually necessary. Early treatment with plasmapheresis may accelerate recovery, although the exact mechanism for this effect is not known (hypotheses include the removal of circulating antibodies or other humoral myelinotoxic or immunopathogenic factors). Intravenous immunoglobulin G (IVIG) therapy may prove to be the treatment of choice because it can be administered easily and can be given with other drugs simultaneously (plasmapheresis removes co-medication jointly with adverse disease factors).

During the first several days after hospital admission, it is crucial to assess the client's respiratory, swallowing, and autonomic function (see the Critical Monitoring feature). Assess the following at least every 4 hours: vital signs, forced vital capacity, swallowing, strength in the extremities, and intake and output balance. If ascending

CRITICAL MONITORING

Respiratory Distress with Guillain-Barré Syndrome

Monitor the client for:

- Complaints of headache
- Myoclonic jerks
- Drowsiness
- Confusion
- Restlessness
- Reduced cough
- Decreased ability to move pulmonary secretions

Assess pulmonary function studies for:

- Decreased forced vital capacity (<15 ml/kg)
- Decreased tidal volume (<3–4 ml/kg)
- Decreased maximum inspiratory pressure (<10–20 cm H_2O)
- Decreased maximum expiratory pressure (<40 cm H_2O)

Assess arterial blood gases for:

- Decreased PAO_2 (<80 mm Hg on 50% FIO_2 with normal PCO_2)
- Alveolar-arterial gradient > 300 on 50% FIO_2
- $PaCO_2$ > 50 mm Hg
- Vd/Vt > 0.6

FIO_2, fraction of inspired oxygen; $PaCO_2$, partial pressure of arterial carbon dioxide; PAO_2, partial pressure of arterial oxygen; Vd/Vt, ratio of dead space volume to tidal volume.

weakness is noted, increase the frequency of assessment to every 2 hours or even more often. Cardiac monitoring and supplemental oxygen are often needed. Common complications include bladder infection, deep vein thrombosis, pulmonary emboli, pneumonia, and syndrome of inappropriate antidiuretic hormone (SIADH).

Interventions to control infection and prevent complications of immobility are vital. Proper body alignment should be maintained to prevent deformities and injury to paralyzed limbs. Once the client's condition is stabilized, rehabilitative interventions can be implemented.

Assist the client in coping with the progressive nature of GBS. During the early stages, clients are frightened because their paralysis can ascend rapidly. They are often admitted to an acute care agency with progressive weakness and within days are completely paralyzed. Clients fear they will never recover. Help clients in verbalizing their fears, and offer support and encouragement that although the disorder is progressive, most clients gain full recovery. Encouragement is not hollow, however. The client is not taught to expect immediate resolution but is assisted to realize the usual time frames for recovery.

PARKINSON'S DISEASE

Classification

PD is an idiopathic syndrome characterized by disability from tremor and rigidity. Various other forms of parkinsonism cause similar clinical manifestations but have known causes. They include:

- *Postencephalitic* parkinsonism, which occurred after the large epidemic of encephalitis in 1919
- *Drug-induced* parkinsonism, occurring after long-term use of phenothiazines
- *Toxin-induced* parkinsonism, sometimes resulting from carbon monoxide, mercury, or manganese exposure
- Exposure to agricultural herbicides and pesticides (being studied)
- Trauma injury to the midbrain

PD is the most common form of parkinsonism. PD involves degeneration of dopamine-producing cells in the substantia nigra, which leads to degeneration of dopaminergic neurons in the basal ganglia. Once cell loss in the substantia nigra reaches 80%, manifestations appear. The cause of nigral cell degeneration is not known. The net result of the loss of dopaminergic neurons is an imbalance of dopamine in relation to ACh in the basal ganglia, which leads to the clinical characteristics of PD.

Clinical Manifestations

PD most often develops in people in their 60s, although it can strike much younger people as well. It occurs worldwide. About 1% of people over age 50 have PD. The disease has six cardinal features: (1) tremor at rest; (2) rigidity; (3) bradykinesia (slow movement); (4) flexed posture of the neck, trunk, and limbs; (5) loss of postural reflexes; and (6) freezing movement.

Early in the disease, the client may notice a slight slowing in the ability to perform ADL (*bradykinesia*). A general feeling of stiffness (rigidity) may be noticed, along with mild diffuse muscular pain. *Tremor* is a common early sign that usually occurs in one of the upper limbs. It occurs at rest and involves a coarse "pill-rolling" movement of the thumb against the fingers that can vary in intensity and distribution. Voluntary movement stops or reduces the tremor in some people; however, others may have tremor during voluntary movement (intention tremor) as well.

Bradykinesia makes voluntary movements difficult to execute. When manifestations are severe, total lack of movement (*akinesia*) may occur and the client is literally frozen in one spot. Bradykinesia also affects gait. Initially, there may be a slight stiffness of one leg while walking, and the ipsilateral arm may be held flexed at the elbow and abducted at the shoulder. The person may catch or drag one foot. Later, when both sides of the body are involved, the typical shuffling gait with short steps may develop. There is lack of associated swinging of the arms while walking. In advanced PD, the client stands with head, shoulders, and spine flexed forward, giving the appearance of a stooped posture (Fig. 72–4).

The face of someone with advanced PD appears stiff, mask-like, and without expression. The speech is low in volume, monotonous in tone, and slow. Words are poorly articulated (dysarthria). Saliva may flow involuntarily from the mouth because of the lack of spontaneous swallowing.

PD does not usually affect intellectual ability; however, a dementia similar to that of AD develops in 15% to 20% of clients with PD. Mood disturbance can occur, and emotional stress may intensify clinical manifestations.

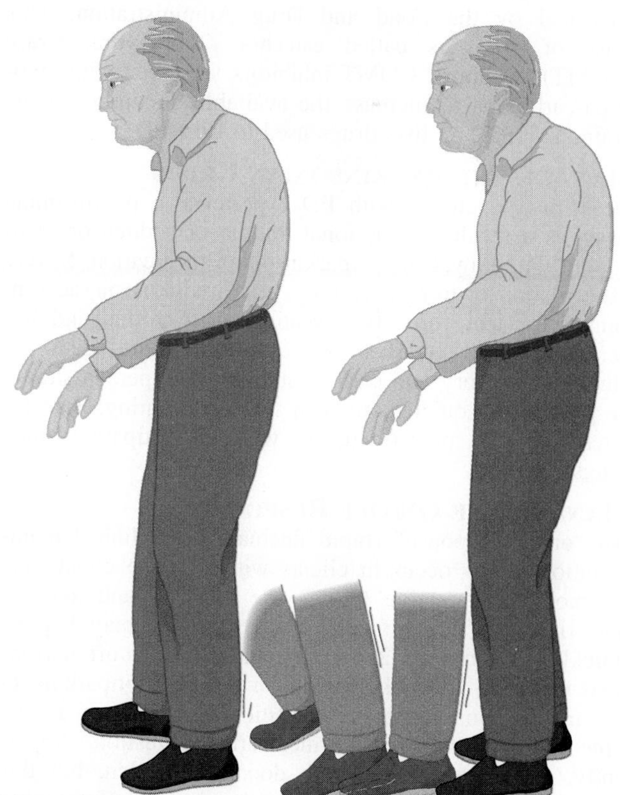

FIGURE 72–4 Gait changes seen in Parkinson's disease. Some of the clinical manifestations of Parkinson's disease are stooped posture, bradykinesia, and a festinant gait.

The course of the disease is slowly progressive. The person becomes more rigid and more disabled, eventually requiring full assistance with ADL.

Outcome Management

The manifestations of PD can be relieved by various medications, particularly levodopa and anticholinergic drugs. The purpose of levodopa is to provide dopamine to the basal ganglia. The purpose of anticholinergic drugs is to block release of acetylcholine, thereby creating a better balance between acetylcholine and dopamine. The most common levodopa drug is carbidopa-levodopa (Sinemet). Levodopa is a synthetic metabolic precursor of dopamine. Dopamine itself cannot be used because it cannot cross the blood-brain barrier. Carbidopa must be given with levodopa because it prevents peripheral metabolism of levodopa, allowing levodopa to reach the brain.

The benefit of the drug seems to decline with prolonged use. The therapy is more effective in treating bradykinesia and rigidity than tremor. The dosage of levodopa is gradually increased until the optimal therapeutic response is achieved. This process may take several months. When the daily dose of levodopa approaches the desired level, the client often has involuntary dyskinesias (jerky, writhing movements), especially of the face, mouth, and tongue. Some clients prefer this stage to being severely bradykinetic, because at least they can be mobile and perform voluntary movements more easily.

In 1998, a new class of drug treatment for PD was approved by the Food and Drug Administration. This class of drugs is called catechol *O*-methyltransferase (COMT) inhibitors. COMT inhibitors are given with levodopa-carbidopa to increase the available dopamine in the brain. Table 72–3 lists drugs used to treat PD.

Manage the Parkinsonian Crisis

Occasionally, clients with PD experience a parkinsonian crisis as a result of emotional trauma or sudden or inadvertent withdrawal of antiparkinsonian medication. Severe exacerbation of tremor, rigidity, and bradykinesia, accompanied by acute anxiety, sweating, tachycardia, and hyperpnea, occur. Intervention for parkinsonian crisis includes respiratory and cardiac support. The person should be placed in a quiet room with subdued lighting. Barbiturates may be prescribed, as well as antiparkinsonian drugs.

Manage the On/Off Response

An "on/off response" (rapid fluctuation of clinical manifestations) may occur in clients with PD; the client may be mobile and active ("on") one moment and akinetic and rigid ("off") the next. This transition may happen quickly, within 1 to 2 minutes. Initially, the off periods tend to occur 3 to 4 hours after a dose of antiparkinsonian medication. Later, the transition may happen at any time and be unrelated to medication ingestion. Apparently, off periods are due to dopamine deficit, but this factor is not clear. A person experiencing on/off response may be temporarily helped by shortening the interval between medication doses or by gradually increasing the total dosage.

Medications such as ropinirole may be given in addition to other PD medications to help smooth out the fluctuations.

Nursing Management of the Medical Client

Nursing care of the PD client includes health assessment, medication instruction and monitoring, liaison with other members of the health care team, and client and family education. Case managers are often used to guide transitions from one facility to the next (see Case Management: The Older Adult).

Advise the client to maintain fluid intake of 2L/24 hours and to increase intake of dietary fiber. Stool softeners and mild laxatives can be used. A regular time for bowel movements should be established, usually a half-hour after the morning or evening meal.

Teach the client various techniques to enhance voluntary movement. Clients often need to try different strategies on their own to find what helps most. Some clients grasp coins in their pocket to reduce embarrassing hand tremor. Others grip the arms of a chair. Mental thoughts, such as walking over imaginary lines, can aid ambulation. One client finds that tossing small scraps of paper in front of him aids his walking; another finds that rocking back and forth helps initiate movement. Encourage daily range of motion exercises to avoid rigidity and contractures. Remind the client to maintain good posture and to avoid flexion of the neck and shoulders. The client should sleep on a firm mattress. When resting, the client should avoid using a pillow to prevent flexion of the spine. Periodically lying prone also helps.

Because self-care activities are performed more slowly by the client with PD, extra time should be allowed for completion of tasks such as dressing, bathing, and eating. Warming trays can keep food hot. Recommend rest periods during meals to avoid aspiration.

As PD progresses, clients become rigid and unresponsive to verbal stimuli. During these stages, continue to treat clients with dignity, speaking to the clients rather than ignoring them.

Teach the client about home safety. Loose carpeting should be removed. Grab bars should be placed in the bathroom. An elevated toilet seat should be installed. Clients with severe tremor should avoid carrying hot liquids. Walking aids such as a cane or walker can provide added stability (see the Client Education Guide).

The client and family need emotional support. Support groups are available in most major cities. Refer the client and family to the American Parkinson Disease Association.

Surgical Management

Surgical interventions are used for PD. Intractable tremor may be ameliorated by thalamotomy or pallidotomy. Autologous transplantation of adrenal medullary tissue into the brains of PD clients, in the hope that these cells will produce dopamine, has yielded disappointing results. Fetal tissue transplantation has produced better results, although no cases resulted in complete reversal of parkinsonian symptoms.[2] Transplantation of genetically engineered cell lines or vector-mediated gene transfection might ultimately prove to be the most effective strategy for the surgical treatment of PD.[2]

TABLE 72–3 PHARMACOLOGIC MANAGEMENT OF PARKINSON'S DISEASE

Drug Classification and Example	Action	Indications	Common Side Effects	Nursing Implications
ANTICHOLINERGICS				
Trihexyphenidyl (Artane) Benztropine (Cogentin) Procyclidine (Kemadrin) Ethopropazine (Parsidol)	Inhibit action of endogenous acetylcholine and muscarine agonists to block the excitatory effect of the cholinergic system	Tremor, rigidity, drooling	Dry mouth, constipation, blurred vision, confusion, hallucinations	Usually contraindicated in clients with acute-angle glaucoma and tachycardia; monitor pulse and blood pressure during periods of dosage adjustment; administer with meals; do not withdraw medication suddenly
ANTIHISTAMINES				
Diphenhydramine (Benadryl)	Mild anticholinergic	Tremor, rigidity, insomnia	Dry mouth, lethargy, confusion	Use with caution in clients with seizures, hypertension, hyperthyroidism, heart and renal disease, and diabetes; administer with meals or antacids
DOPAMINERGICS				
Amantadine (Symmetrel)	Cause release of dopamine in central nervous system	Rigidity, bradykinesia	Dizziness, ataxia, insomnia, leg edema	Monitor client for postural hypotension, do not administer at bedtime
Carbidopa-levadopa (Sinemet)		Tremor, rigidity, bradykinesia	Orthostatic hypotension, nausea, hallucinations, dystonia, dyskinesias	Monitor blood pressure; use elastic stockings to increase venous return; monitor client for urinary retention
DOPAMINE AGONISTS				
Bromocriptine (Parlodel)	Activate dopamine receptors in the central nervous system	Fluctuation of manifestations, dyskinesia, dystonia	Hallucinations, mental fogginess, orthostatic hypotension, confusion	Monitor blood pressure and mental status
Pergolide (Permax)			Orthostatic hypotension, nausea, insomnia	Monitor blood pressure; do not administer at bedtime
COMT INHIBITORS				
Tolcapone	Enhance effect of dopamine	Adjuvant treatment	Diarrhea, elevated liver enzymes	Monitor liver enzymes
Encapone	Enhance effect of dopamine	Adjuvant treatment	Nausea, headache	Monitor for levodopa side effects
MAO INHIBITORS				
Selegiline (Deprenyl)*	Inhibit monoamine oxidase B, an enzyme that converts chemical byproducts in the brain into neurotoxins that prevent substantia nigra cell death	Adjuvant treatment	Nausea, dizziness, confusion, hallucinations, dry mouth	Monitor for levodopa side effects, as selegiline may increase effect of levodopa

*One study showed that levodopa in combination with selegiline provided no clinical benefit over levodopa alone in treating early, mild Parkinson's disease. Moreover, mortality was significantly higher when these two drugs were used together. (See Lees, A. J. [1995]. *British Journal of Medicine, 311,* 1602–1607.[23])

COMT, catechol-*O*-methyltransferase; MAO, monoamine oxidase.

CASE MANAGEMENT

The Older Adult

As technology and medication advances have increased the human life span, nurses will frequently be challenged to care for older adult clients experiencing an exacerbation of a chronic condition (such as chronic obstructive pulmonary disease) or who have an acute medical-surgical problem (such as a myocardial infarction) accompanied by multiple co-morbidities (e.g., hypertension, diabetes). You can assist these clients by using case management principles.

Assess

Avoid stereotyping as you perform your assessment, remembering that a client's cognitive changes may result from unfamiliarity with the environment or acute illness, such as an infection or electrolyte imbalance.

- Why has this client entered the health care system (Lack of caregiver or support services? Change in care needs or medications? Sensory changes? Pain management? Recent loss or depression? Poor nutrition or lack of education? Not understanding the care regimen?)
- Is there evidence of physical or psychological abuse or neglect?
- Are there environmental or safety barriers at home?
- Are there financial or insurance concerns, or does this older client need help to apply for assistance?
- Is there a pattern of frequent readmissions?

Work with the case manager, social worker and other team members to resolve these issues before discharge.

Advocate

Consider assignment to a primary nurse.

Allow extra time to explain procedures and treatments; help older adult clients participate in planning care and decision-making rather than deferring to family members. Even cognitively impaired clients can make some choices.

Decisions about advance directives and limitation of treatment may not always coincide with what you believe should be done, but respect such judgments when the client is informed and capable of making decisions. Encourage clients to select health proxies and make wishes known.

Clinical pathway time frames may need to be modified because of age and co-morbidities. Complete documentation of progress toward expected outcomes can ensure reimbursement and appropriate length of stay.

Prevent Readmission

Maintaining or improving baseline nutrition, hydration, mobility and ambulation are paramount to success after hospital discharge. Complicated medication regimens necessitate that you provide a good explanation as well as a written schedule for the client to follow. Changes in lifestyle or place of residence may be necessary and unexpected.

Observe the client's ability to perform the treatments needed; obtain equipment, nursing services, and prescriptions.

Teach preventive measures, such as flu shots and when to call the physician. If possible, follow up by phone after discharge to see that the care plan is being followed and to answer questions.

Cheryl Noetscher, RN, MS, *Director of Case Management, Crouse Hospital and Community–General Hospital, Syracuse, New York*

MYASTHENIA GRAVIS

Etiology

Myasthenia gravis (MG) is an autoimmune disease that presents as muscular weakness and fatigue that worsens with exercise and improves with rest. The manifestations result from a loss of ACh receptors in the postsynaptic neurons of the neuromuscular junction. The cause of MG is unknown, but 80% of people with the generalized form of the disease have elevated titers of antibodies to the ACh receptor in their serum. MG may appear at any age, although there are two peaks of onset. In early-onset MG, at age 20 to 30 years, women are more often affected than men. In late-onset MG, after age 50, men are more often affected. The overall incidence of MG is 0.4 per 100,000 and the prevalence is 0.5 to 5.0 per 100,000.

Clinical Manifestations

The primary feature of MG is increasing weakness with sustained muscle contraction. For instance, if the person is asked to hold the arms up, the power of muscle contraction diminishes and the arms gradually drift downward. After a period of rest, the muscles regain their strength. Muscle weakness is greatest after exertion or at the end of the day.

Ocular manifestations are most common, with *ptosis* (drooping of the upper eyelid) or *diplopia* (double vision) occurring in many clients. Ptosis is due to weakness of the levator palpebrae muscles of the eye. If not present at the time of examination, ptosis can be elicited by prolonged upward gaze, which creates fatigue of the muscle.

Diplopia is a result of weakness or fatigue of the extraocular muscles. Other manifestations are weakness of the orbicularis oculi muscles (which help close the eye), the facial muscles, the muscles of chewing and swallowing, and the limbs. Weakness of the facial and levator palpebrae muscles produces an expressionless face, with droopy eyelids, smoothed features, and a tendency for the mouth to hang open.

An attempt to smile often turns into a snarl because of the weakness. A person may hold a hand under the jaw to keep it closed. Dysphagia and a nasal quality to speech occur when the muscles of chewing and swallowing are involved. In severe cases, respiratory muscle weakness may occur, which may necessitate intubation and mechanical ventilation (see myasthenic crisis).

The course of MG varies, and there may be remissions and exacerbations. Clinical manifestations may progress quickly or slowly and may fluctuate from day to day. The severity of the disease varies greatly from person to person.

Diagnostic Findings

The diagnosis of MG is based on the clinical presentation and can be confirmed by testing the client's response to anticholinesterase drugs. These drugs inhibit cholinesterase, an enzyme that breaks down ACh in the neuromuscular junction, thereby allowing more ACh to bind to the remaining ACh receptors. Edrophonium (Tensilon) is a short-acting drug that is given intravenously *(Tensilon test)*. A test dose of 2 mg (for adults) is injected first. If no untoward reaction occurs (such as increased weakness, change in heart rate or rhythm, nausea, or abdominal cramps), the remaining 8 mg is injected. The client is then observed for objective signs of improvement in muscle strength. The effect is transitory, wearing off after 3 to 5 minutes. Another drug, neostigmine methylsulfate (Prostigmin), may be used because of its longer duration of effect on muscle strength (1 to 2 hours), which allows better analysis of its effect.

When either drug is used, IV atropine sulfate should be available to inject as an antidote. This medication counteracts any severe cholinergic reactions (cardiac dysrhythmias or abdominal cramping). Electromyography (EMG) helps confirm the diagnosis. Repetitive stimulation of the nerve with recording from the involved muscle shows a characteristic decrementing response of the muscle action potential.

Outcome Management

There is no cure for MG. Pharmacologic intervention consists of two groups of medications: (1) short-acting anticholinesterase compounds and (2) corticosteroids. The most effective anticholinesterase drugs are pyridostigmine (Mestinon) and neostigmine (Prostigmin). Dosages are highly individualized, based on physiologic response to the medication. The goal is to achieve the maximum benefit (muscle strength and endurance) with the fewest

CLIENT EDUCATION GUIDE

Parkinson's Disease

Client Instructions

Make sure that you understand how to take your medications, the importance of following the correct diet, and what side effects you can expect from your medications.

To avoid rigidity and the development of contractures:

- Exercise and stretch regularly.
- Perform the exercises recommended in your self-help booklets.
- Exercise first thing in the morning, when your energy levels are highest.
- Exercise in bed if getting to the floor is difficult.
- Get out of a chair by bending over slowly so that your head is over your toes; avoid soft, deep chairs.

If your health care provider has told you that you have bradykinesia (slow movements):

- Rock back and forth to get going.
- Imagine that you are stepping over an imaginary line when you walk.
- Throw small objects (e.g., small scraps of paper) in front of you to practice fine motor movements.
- Count to yourself while walking.
- Visualize your intended movement.

If you have a tremor:

- Hold change in your pocket or squeeze a small rubber ball.
- Use both hands to accomplish tasks.
- Lie face down on the floor and relax your entire body.
- Sleep on the side that has the tremor.

If you have trouble getting dressed:

- Dress and undress in front of a mirror.
- Use adaptive devices such as long-handled shoehorns and button fasteners.
- Buy clothes with self-fasteners (e.g., Velcro) and slide-locking buckles.

To ensure safety:

- Wear good, sturdy shoes.
- Use a cane or walker.
- Concentrate on standing upright.
- Consciously pick up your feet to take steps.
- Remove all throw rugs, electrical cords, and clutter from the floor.
- Make sure that you have adequate lighting.
- Arrange essential items so that they are within easy reach.
- Use a bath chair and a handheld shower nozzle.
- Have grab bars installed in the bathroom.
- Have a raised toilet seat installed

To ensure good communication:

- Pause between every few words.
- Exaggerate the pronunciation of words.
- Finish saying the final consonant of a word before starting to say the next word.
- Express ideas in short, concise phrases.
- Plan what to say.
- Face the listener.

To ensure adequate swallowing and prevent aspiration:

- Think through the steps of swallowing:
  - Keep your lips closed.
  - Keep your teeth together.
  - Put food on your tongue.
  - Lift your tongue up and back.
  - Swallow.
- Eat slowly, taking small bites.
- Chew hard and move food around with your tongue.
- Finish one bite before taking another.

To keep saliva from building up in your mouth:

- Make a conscious effort to swallow saliva often.
- Keep your head in an upright position so saliva will collect in the back of your throat and stimulate automatic swallowing.
- Swallow excess saliva before attempting to speak.

side effects (excessive salivation, sweating, nausea, diarrhea, abdominal cramps, or tachycardia). Corticosteroids (usually prednisone) are directed toward reducing the levels of serum ACh receptor antibodies. Corticosteroids may temporarily worsen symptoms; however, this is followed by gradual improvement in muscle strength.

After a peak of improvement is reached and maintained for several weeks, the dosage of both prednisone and anticholinesterase medication may be gradually decreased. A low maintenance dose of alternate-day prednisone may be effective for many months or years. Precautions with any steroid therapy are important, including potassium supplements if indicated and liberal use of antacids.

Potential complications of steroid use are cataracts, hypertension, diabetes, fluid retention, delayed wound healing, insomnia, and osteoporosis. Other treatments include azathioprine (Imuran) and cyclosporine (Sandimmune), which reduce the level of circulating ACh receptor antibodies, and plasmapheresis and IVIG.

PLASMAPHERESIS

Plasmapheresis is an adjunctive therapy for clients with refractory MG. It is a process by which plasma is separated from formed elements of blood. The plasma is discarded and the packed red blood cells are joined with albumin, normal saline, and electrolytes and returned to the client. The purpose is to remove plasma proteins containing antibodies that are believed to cause MG. Plasmapheresis may produce transient improvement in clients who have actual or pending respiratory failure.

Usually, three to five treatments given once daily over 5 to 7 days are required. Potential complications include myasthenic or cholinergic crisis and, rarely, hypovolemia. Muscle strength should be assessed before and after the procedure, with particular attention paid to vital capacity, swallowing ability, diplopia, and ptosis, to evaluate the effectiveness of the treatment.

COMPLICATIONS

Two major complications of MG may occur: *myasthenic crisis* and *cholinergic crisis* (Box 72–2).

MYASTHENIC CRISIS. Clients with moderate or severe generalized MG, especially those who have difficulty swallowing or breathing, may experience a sudden worsening of their condition. This is usually precipitated by an intercurrent infection or sudden withdrawal of anticholinesterase drugs, but it may occur spontaneously. If an increase in the dosage of the anticholinesterase drug does not improve the weakness, endotracheal intubation and mechanical ventilation may be required. In many instances, drug responsiveness returns in 24 to 48 hours, and weaning from the respirator can proceed.

CHOLINERGIC CRISIS. Cholinergic crisis occurs as a result of overmedication. The muscarinic effect of a toxic level of anticholinesterase medication causes abdominal cramps, diarrhea, and excessive pulmonary secretions. The nicotinic effect paradoxically worsens weakness and can cause bronchial spasm. If respiratory status is compromised, the client may need intubation and mechanical ventilation.

Nursing Management of the Medical Client

Clients with MG are usually managed in an outpatient setting. When clients are hospitalized for diagnosis or during a crisis, the following nursing management procedure may be pertinent.

Because MG may involve the muscles of respiration, the client may experience dyspnea and ineffective cough and swallow mechanisms. This may lead to aspiration and pneumonia. Encourage deep breathing and coughing. Have suction equipment available at the bedside; instruct the client on how to use it. Instruct the client to sit upright when eating, to swallow only when the chin is tipped downward toward the chest, and never to speak while food is in the mouth. Oxygen and, in severe cases, mechanical ventilation may be required.

In MG, weakness is usually greatest following exertion and at the end of the day. Activities should be carefully planned to include rest periods so that energy is conserved and the muscles have a chance to regain their strength. Rearrangement of the home environment may help prevent unnecessary energy expenditure. Vocational retraining may be indicated for those who can no longer meet the physical demands of their jobs. Clients with severe disease or an acute exacerbation will be totally dependent on nursing care for ADL. This level of care requires that complications of immobility be avoided.

BOX 72–2 Myasthenic and Cholinergic Crises in Clients with Myasthenia Gravis

Myasthenic Crisis Is Caused by Undermedication

Clinical Manifestations

Sudden marked rise in blood pressure due to hypoxia
Increased heart rate
Severe respiratory distress and cyanosis
Absent cough and swallow reflex
Increased secretions, increased diaphoresis, and increased lacrimation
Restlessness, dysarthria
Bowel and bladder incontinence

Intervention

Increased doses of cholinergic drugs as long as the client responds positively to edrophonium treatment
Possible mechanical ventilation if respiratory muscle paralysis is acute

Cholinergic Crisis Is Caused by Depolarization Block Resulting from Excessive Medications

Clinical Manifestations

Weakness with difficulty swallowing, chewing, speaking, and breathing
Apprehension, nausea, and vomiting
Abdominal cramps and diarrhea
Increased secretions and saliva
Sweating, lacrimation, fasciculations, and blurred vision

Intervention

Discontinue all cholinergic drugs until cholinergic effects decrease
Provide adequate ventilatory support
1 mg intravenous atropine may be necessary to counteract severe cholinergic reactions

Provide the client and family with information about MG and its treatment (see end of chapter). They should be aware of adverse reactions of both anticholinesterase drugs and steroids. Explain how to recognize myasthenic and cholinergic crises and how to have a plan to seek medical intervention, if necessary.

Surgical Management

Thymectomy can be used for treatment. The thymus gland, located in the superior mediastinum, is important during fetal growth for development of the immune system. It is usually atrophied and nonfunctioning in adulthood. The effect of thymectomy is not fully understood. It may alter some immunologic control mechanism that affects the production of antibodies to the ACh receptor, or it may eliminate a trigger to antibody production. Thymectomy is indicated for clients with thymoma, selected clients with generalized MG without thymoma, and selected clients with disabling ocular MG.[14] The procedure is recommended early in the course of the disease. Nursing management is similar to care following thoracic surgery.

EATON-LAMBERT (MYASTHENIC) SYNDROME

Eaton-Lambert syndrome (also called *myasthenic syndrome*) is a myasthenia-like condition in which weakness is noted in the limbs. It is characterized by defective release of ACh possibly caused by autoantibodies (IgG). Eaton-Lambert syndrome is found almost exclusively in people with oat cell carcinoma of the lung and has been noted less often in people with cancers of the prostate, stomach, rectum, and breast.

The onset is insidious, and clinical manifestations are progressive. In comparison with MG, diplopia is less common and there is proximal weakness of the legs, arms, and pelvic girdle. There is reduced muscle action potential when muscle is stimulated, but repetitive stimulation augments muscle action. Weakness tends to develop with exertion, although some clients have a temporary increase in power when muscles are repeatedly stimulated. Autonomic dysfunction is common, presenting as dry mouth, impotence, and peripheral paresthesias.

Treatment is directed at the primary cancer. Guanidine HCl may improve manifestations by increasing ACh release. Plasmapheresis and immunotherapy have also been used. Calcium-channel blockers can worsen the transmission defect. Because MG can precede the development of cancer by many years, clients with Eaton-Lambert syndrome should be assessed yearly for the development of cancer.

AMYOTROPHIC LATERAL SCLEROSIS

Amyotrophic lateral sclerosis (ALS) is the most common of the motor neuron diseases. It is an age-dependent, fatal paralytic disorder also known as *Charcot's disease* and *Lou Gehrig's disease.* Onset is usually in middle age. Men are affected more often than women. The overall incidence of ALS is 0.4 to 1.8 per 100,000, and the prevalence is 4 to 6 per 100,000.

Clinical Manifestations

ALS involves degeneration of both the anterior horn cells and the corticospinal tracts. Consequently, both upper and lower motor neuron clinical manifestations are seen. Lower motor neuron clinical manifestations include weakness, atrophy, cramps, and fasciculations (irregular twitchings of muscle fibers or bundles). Upper motor neuron signs include spasticity and hyperreflexia. Involvement of the corticobulbar tracts causes dysphagia (difficulty swallowing) and dysarthria (slurred speech). The sensory system is not involved, and cognition is not affected. The client remains alert and mentally intact throughout the course of the disease.

The course of the disease is relentlessly progressive. Death usually results from pneumonia caused by respiratory compromise within 2 to 5 years.

Weakness typically begins in the upper extremities and progressively involves the upper arms and shoulders and then the muscles of the neck and throat. The trunk and lower extremities are usually not affected until late in the disease. When the intercostal muscles and diaphragm become involved, respirations are shallow and coughing is ineffective. Cognition, as well as bowel and bladder sphincters, remains intact, even when the client is totally debilitated. In some cases, weakness begins in the brain stem, causing problems with speech and swallowing. This is called *bulbar ALS.*

Diagnosis of ALS is made by the clinical presentation and EMG. EMG criteria for the diagnosis of ALS include the presence of widespread anterior horn cell dysfunction with fibrillations, positive waves, fasciculations, and chronic neurogenic motor unit potential changes in multiple nerve root distribution in at least three limbs and the paraspinal muscles in the presence of normal sensory responses.

Outcome Management

Supportive therapy was the only intervention for ALS until riluzole (Rilutek) was approved in 1996. Its mechanism of action is unknown, but it is thought to have a neuroprotective effect. The drug extends the life of ALS clients by a few months. Clients with ALS are usually admitted to health care facilities only twice in their illness, first for diagnosis and later in the final stage of debilitation.

Supportive nursing care is an important aspect of managing the ALS client. In the outpatient arena, the nurse can provide ongoing assessment of daily living needs and make suggestions for modifications in activity level, clothing, and diet. Often, just allowing the client or family to talk about problems reduces anxiety and helps them find solutions to problems.[19] Interventions should be aimed at conserving energy. Activities should be spaced during the day. Muscle stress, strenuous activity, and extremes of hot and cold should be avoided. Leg braces, canes, and walkers can prolong independence in ambulation. Hand braces, special utensils, and adaptive devices such as buttonhooks can help with dressing and self-feeding. Pressure ulcers are not usually a problem because the sensory system remains intact and the client can feel when pressure on a body part is too great.

In the acute care setting, gather information from the client and family about communication needs and which positions are best for respiration, handling secretions, eating, and turning routines.

Encourage fluid intake regularly, when the client is not fatigued. Proper positioning is imperative. Providing a cup with a spout may prevent liquid from running out of the corners of the mouth. Give liquids by using a large syringe with short tubing on the tip. The tube is placed on the anterior portion of the tongue, and gentle force is used to deliver small amounts of liquid.

Encourage small, frequent, high-nutrient feedings. Tell the client to sit upright, with the head slightly flexed forward while eating. Papase tablets placed under the tongue 10 minutes before meals can make thick saliva less sticky. Plenty of time should be allowed for eating, and the client should not attempt to speak while food is in the mouth. Have suction equipment available during meals to reduce the risk of aspiration of food and secretions that become lodged in the mouth and pharynx. The head may need to be stabilized with a soft cervical collar. Consult the dietitian for special diet recommendations.

Although speech remains intelligible, the client can be trained to slow the rate of speech and exaggerate articulation. As manifestations progress, the client may need to repeat words or have an interpreter (usually the spouse). At this stage, it is important to eliminate extraneous noise, face the client when he or she is talking, and maintain eye contact. When the client's speech contains only one-word phrases or is no longer possible, writing can be an effective means of communicating and should be encouraged. When writing is no longer possible, a speech pathologist can provide communication devices such as alphabet boards and portable memo writers.[9]

If the client is a smoker, encourage him or her to stop. Exposure to people with respiratory infections should be avoided. Remind the client to use good posture. Pulmonary function tests should be performed regularly to assess ventilatory status. Clients generally experience respiratory fatigue when vital capacity is less than 1.5 L. Some clients can be taught to use their abdominal muscles to enhance respirations when the intercostal muscles and diaphragm become weak. A sign of pending respiratory insufficiency is shortness of breath while eating.

Encourage the client and family to talk about the losses they are experiencing and the feelings associated with them. Family members should be encouraged to take time for rest and activities away from the client. Refer the client and family to an ALS support group.

Eventually, clients face the difficult choice of deciding whether they will accept artificial ventilation. Encourage them to discuss this with family and friends and to seek input from ALS support groups. Encourage clients to complete advance directives to indicate whether they desire life-sustaining treatments such as cardiopulmonary resuscitation, but this should be reassessed at regular intervals. Clients may change their minds on the basis of their experience with their illness, changes in their subjective appreciation of their quality of life, or changes in their evaluation of the benefits and burdens of life-sustaining measures as they come to terms with the imminence of death.[21]

CONCLUSIONS

Degenerative neurologic disorders have many causes, including viruses, autoimmune responses, and heredity. Some have no known cause. In general, they are relentlessly progressive, slowly taking away both physical and mental ability. Nurses should focus care on the management of clinical manifestations and prevention of complications. Family support throughout the process of care is essential.

THINKING CRITICALLY

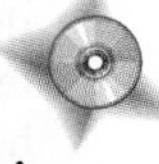

1. A 52-year-old man with multiple sclerosis is wheelchair-bound and has a neurogenic bladder. He complains of a sudden onset of generalized weakness, fever, and chills and is admitted to the hospital. What priorities should be set for his care?

Factors to Consider. What do generalized weakness, fever, and chills suggest in *any* client? If your client has not been following good bladder management, how can you intervene?

2. A 70-year-old man with Parkinson's disease is admitted to the hospital after experiencing severe nightmares and periods of confusion. During lucid periods, he is very disturbed by these manifestations. At other times, he believes that his wife is participating in a conspiracy to harm him. What assessments and interventions should you consider?

Factors to Consider. Are hallucinations and paranoia typical manifestations of Parkinson's disease? Might the client's manifestations be related to treatment or to some cause other than Parkinson's disease?

3. A 41-year-old woman with myasthenia gravis is taking pyridostigmine and prednisone. She is complaining of increased fatigue and weakness and has difficulty breathing. What concerns should you have?

Factors to Consider. Might the client's difficult breathing be related to her fatigue and weakness? Could these manifestations be related to myasthenia gravis or its treatment?

BIBLIOGRAPHY

1. Acorn, S., & Andersen, S. (1990). Depression in multiple sclerosis: Critique of the research literature. *Journal of Neuroscience Nursing, 22*(4), 209–214.
2. Ahlskog, J. E. (1993). Cerebral transplantation for Parkinson's disease: Current progress and future prospects. *Mayo Clinic Proceedings, 68,* 578–591.
3. Andrews, K. L., & Husmann, D. A. (1997). Bladder dysfunction and management in multiple sclerosis. *Mayo Clinic Proceedings, 72,* 1176–1183.
4. Bansil, S., Cook, S. D., & Rohowsky-Kochan, C. (1995). Multiple sclerosis: Immune mechanisms and update on current therapies. *Annals of Neurology 37*(suppl. 1), S87–101.
5. Brown, P. (1997). The risk of bovine spongiform encephalopathy ('mad cow disease') to human health. *Journal of the American Medical Association, 278*(12), 1008–1011.

6. Coleman, L. M., Fowler, L. L., & Williams, M. E. (1995). Use of unproven therapies by people with Alzheimer's disease. *Journal of the American Geriatrics Society, 43,* 747–750.
7. Corey-Bloom, J., et al. (1995). Diagnosis and evaluation of dementia. *Neurology, 45,* 211–218.
8. Corey-Bloom, J., Galaski, D., & Thal, L. J. (1994). Clinical features and natural history of Alzheimer's disease. In D.B. Calne (Ed.), *Neurodegenerative diseases* (pp. 631–645). Philadelphia: W. B. Saunders.
9. Cummings, J. L., & Benson, D. F. (1992). *Dementia, a clinical approach.* Boston: Butterworth-Heinemann.
10. Franco, D. A., & Bashir, R. M. (1996, December). Current concepts in Guillain-Barré syndrome. *Nebraska Medical Journal,* 406–411.
11. Hillel, A. D., & Miller, R. (1989). Bulbar amyotrophic lateral sclerosis: Patterns of progression and clinical management. *Head and Neck, 11*(1), 51–59.
12. Hogancamp, W. E., Rodriguez, M., & Weinshenker, B. G. (1997). The epidemiology of multiple sclerosis. *Mayo Clinic Proceedings, 72,* 871–878.
13. Hunt, V. P., & Walker, F. O. (1989). Dysphagia in Huntington's disease. *Journal of Neuroscience Nursing, 21*(2), 92–95.
14. Hurley, A. C., et al. (1992). Assessment of discomfort in advanced Alzheimer patients. *Research in Nursing and Health, 15*(5), 369–378.
15. Jones, P. S., & Martinson, I. M. (1992). The experience of bereavement in care givers of family members with Alzheimer's disease. *Image—The Journal of Nursing Scholarship, 24*(3), 172–176.
16. Kernich, A., & Kaminski, H. J. (1995). Myasthenia gravis: Pathophysiology, diagnosis, and collaborative care. *Journal of Neuroscience Nursing, 27,* 207–215.
17. Khoury, S. J., & Weiner, H. L. (1998). Multiple sclerosis: What have we learned from magnetic resonance imaging studies? *Archives of Internal Medicine, 158,* 565–573.
18. Lang, A. E., & Lozano, A.M. (1998). Parkinson's disease. *New England Journal of Medicine 339*(16), 1130–1143.
19. Lanska, D. J. (1990). Indications for thymectomy in myasthenia gravis. *Neurology, 40*(12), 1828–1829.
20. Le Bars, P. L., et al. (1997). A placebo-controlled, double-blind, randomized trial of an extract of ginkgo biloba for dementia. *Journal of the American Medical Association, 278*(16), 1327–1332.
21. Lees, A. J. (1995). Comparison of therapeutic effects and mortality data of levodopa and levodopa combined with selegiline in patients with early, mild Parkinson's disease. *British Journal of Medicine, 311,* 1602–1607.
22. Lucchinetti, C. F., & Rodriguez, M. (1997). The controversy surrounding pathogenesis of the multiple sclerosis lesion. *Mayo Clinic Proceedings, 72,* 665–678.
23. Mayeux, R., & Chun, M. (1995). Dementias. In L. P. Rowland (Ed.), *Merritt's textbook of neurology* (9th ed.). Baltimore: Williams & Wilkins.
24. Mayo Foundation for Medical Education and Research. (1996, October). Alzheimer's disease: Living with a 'long goodbye.' *Mayo Clinic Health Letter* (suppl.), 1–8.
25. McKhann, G., et al. (1984). Clinical diagnosis of Alzheimer's disease: Report of the NINCDS-ADRDA Work Group under the auspices of Department of Health and Human Services Task Force on Alzheimer's Disease. *Neurology, 34*(7), 939–944.
26. Mega, M., et al. (1996). The spectrum of behavioral changes in Alzheimer's disease. *Neurology, 46*(1), 130–135.
27. Mezey, M., et al. (1996). Life-sustaining treatment decisions by spouses of patients with Alzheimer's disease. *Journal of the American Geriatrics Society, 44*(2), 144–150.
28. Mocsny, N. (1991). Precautions to prevent the spread of Creutzfeldt-Jakob disease. *Journal of Neuroscience Nursing, 23*(2), 116–119.
29. Nowotny, M. L. (1998). My journey with amyotrophic lateral sclerosis. *Journal of Neuroscience Nursing, 30*(1), 68–70.
30. Pericak-Vance, M. A., et al. (1997). Complete genomic screen in late-onset familial Alzheimer disease: Evidence for a new locus on chromosome 12. *Journal of the American Medical Association, 278*(15), 1237–1241.
31. Post, S. G., et al. (1997). The clinical introduction of genetic testing for Alzheimer disease: An ethical perspective. *Journal of the American Medical Association, 277*(10), 832–836.
32. Robinson, B. E. (1997). Guideline for initial evaluation of the patient with memory loss. *Geriatrics, 52*(12), 30–39.
33. Rodriguez, M. (1997). Multiple sclerosis: Insights into molecular pathogenesis and therapy. *Mayo Clinic Proceedings, 72,* 663–664.
34. Ropper, A. H. (1992). The Guillain-Barré syndrome. *New England Journal of Medicine, 326*(17), 1130–1136.
35. Rudick, R. A., et al. (1997). Management of multiple sclerosis. *New England Journal of Medicine, 337*(22), 1604–1611.
36. Sano, M., et al. (1997). A controlled trial of selegiline, alphatocopherol, or both as treatment for Alzheimer's disease. *New England Journal of Medicine, 336*(17), 1216–1222.
37. Silverstein, M. D., et al. (1991). Amyotrophic lateral sclerosis and life-sustaining therapy: Patients' desires for information, participation in decision making, and life-sustaining therapy. *Mayo Clinic Proceedings, 66*(9), 906–913.
38. Tienari, P. J. (1994). Multiple sclerosis: Multiple etiologies, multiple genes? *Annals of Medicine, 26,* 259–269.
39. van der Meche, F. G. A. (1994). The Guillain-Barré syndrome: Plasma exchange or immunoglobulin intravenously? *Journal of Neurology, Neurosurgery, and Psychiatry, 57*(suppl.), 33–34.
40. Vrabec, N. J. (1997). Literature review of social support and caregiver burden, 1980 to 1995. *Image—The Journal of Nursing Scholarship, 29*(4), 383–388.

CHAPTER

73

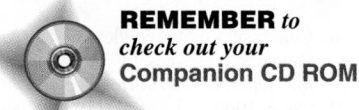

Management of Clients with Neurologic Trauma

Norma D. McNair

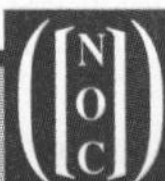

NURSING OUTCOMES CLASSIFICATION (NOC)
for Nursing Diagnoses—Clients with Neurologic Trauma

Altered Family Processes
Family Coping
Family Functioning
Psychosocial Adjustment: Life Change
Role Performance
Altered Health Maintenance
Health Belief: Perceived Resources
Knowledge: Health Resources
Risk Detection
Social Support
Altered Nutrition: Less Than Body Requirements
Nutritional Status: Food and Fluid Intake
Altered Oral Mucous Membrane
Oral Health
Tissue Integrity: Skin and Mucous Membrane
Altered Thought Processes
Cognitive Ability
Cognitive Orientation
Information Processing
Neurologic Status: Consciousness
Altered Tissue Perfusion: Cerebral
Cognitive Ability
Neurologic Status: Consciousness
Tissue Perfusion: Cerebral
Anticipatory Grieving
Grief Resolution
Psychosocial Adjustment: Life Change
Chronic Pain
Comfort Level
Depression Control
Pain: Disruptive Effects
Pain: Psychological Response
Constipation
Bowel Elimination
Hydration
Impaired Gas Exchange
Respiratory Status: Ventilation
Vital Signs Status
Impaired Physical Mobility
Ambulation: Wheelchair
Sensory Function: Proprioception
Transfer Performance
Impaired Skin Integrity
Tissue Integrity: Skin and Mucous Membranes
Inability to Sustain Spontaneous Ventilation
Neurologic Status: Central Motor Control
Vital Signs Status
Ineffective Airway Clearance
Aspiration Control
Respiratory Status: Airway Patency
Respiratory Status: Ventilation
Ineffective Family Coping: Compromised
Family Coping
Family Normalization
Ineffective Individual Coping
Coping
Information Processing
Role Performance
Social Support
Ineffective Thermoregulation
Thermoregulation
Post-Trauma Syndrome
Coping
Fear Control
Risk for Aspiration
Cognitive Ability
Immobility Consequences: Physiologic
Neurologic Status
Respiratory Status: Ventilation
Risk for Impaired Skin Integrity
Immobility Consequences: Physiologic
Tissue Integrity: Skin and Mucous Membranes
Risk for Injury
Neurologic Status
Risk Control
Sexual Dysfunction
Sexual Functioning
Role Performance
Total Incontinence
Neurological Status
Tissue Integrity: Skin and Mucous Membranes
Urinary Continence

The complexity of the central nervous system (CNS) allows the human organism to evaluate information about the outside world. Failure of the brain or the spinal cord to accurately process information prevents the affected person from accurately performing tasks and may impair interactions with others as well as self-appraisal.

Admission of a client with CNS trauma to the emergency department requires rapid mobilization of a trauma team. The team provides initial assessment and resuscitation of the trauma victim and performs triage to the appropriate radiologic studies and surgical service. Ultimately, the management of a client with a head injury, spinal cord injury, or combination of neurologic injuries is directed by the neurosurgical service. This chapter examines the needs of clients with CNS trauma, including head and spinal cord injuries.

INCREASED INTRACRANIAL PRESSURE

Intracranial pressure (ICP) is the pressure exerted in the cranium by its contents: the brain, blood, and cerebrospinal fluid (CSF) (Fig. 73–1). ICP is measured with a

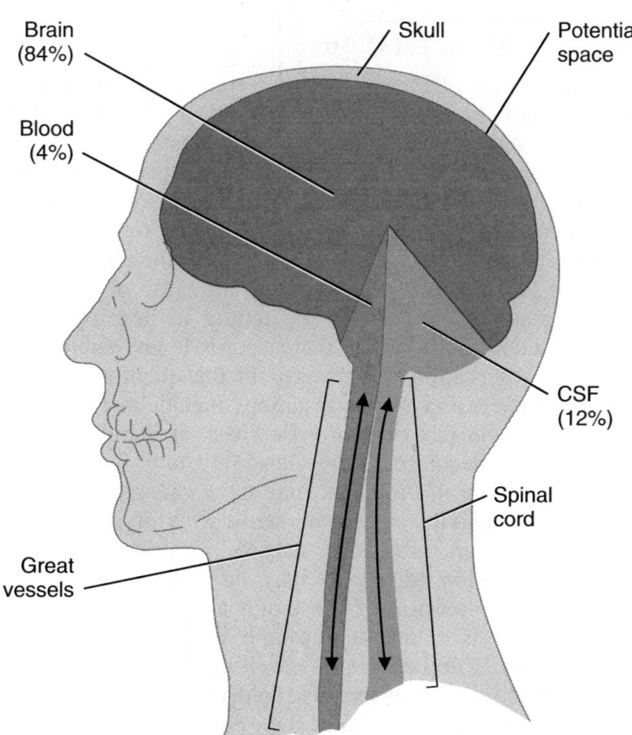

FIGURE 73–1 Components of the intracranial vault.

monitor in either the ventricle, the brain parenchyma, or the subarachnoid space. The normal ICP is 5 to 15 mm Hg. Pressures over 20 mm Hg are considered to represent *increased ICP,* which seriously impairs cerebral perfusion. Recognition of increased ICP is one of the most important assessments made by nurses caring for clients with neurologic disorders.

Cerebral perfusion pressure (CPP) is the amount of blood flow from the systemic circulation that is required to provide adequate oxygen and glucose for brain metabolism. *Mean arterial pressure* (MAP) represents the average pressure during the cardiac cycle. It is calculated by adding the systolic pressure to twice the diastolic pressure and dividing by 3. (Diastole is twice as long as systole.) The formula for calculating cerebral perfusion pressure is as follows:

$$CPP = MAP - ICP$$

When MAP and ICP are equal, there is no CPP and brain perfusion ceases. Therefore, it is crucial to keep ICP and MAP controlled.

Etiology and Risk Factors

Increased ICP is most often associated with a space-occupying lesion, a cerebral infarction, an obstruction to the outflow of CSF, an abscess, an ingested or accumulated toxin, impaired blood flow to or from the brain, vasodilation from increased carbon dioxide ($PaCO_2$) or decreased partial pressure of oxygen (PaO_2), systemic hypertension, or increased intrathoracic pressure. Risk factors include head injury, brain tumors, cerebral bleeding, hydrocephalus, and edema from surgery or injury.

Pathophysiology

The skull is a hard, bony vault filled with brain tissue, blood, and CSF. A balance between these three components maintains the pressure within the cranium. The modified Munro-Kellie hypothesis, a theory for understanding ICP, states that because the bony skull cannot expand, when one of the three components expands, the other two must compensate by decreasing in volume in order for the total brain volume and pressure to remain constant.

As an intracranial mass enlarges, initial compensation occurs through *displacement of CSF* into the spinal canal. The ability of the brain to adapt to increasing pressure without increasing ICP is called *compliance.* The movement of CSF out of the cranium is the first and major compensatory mechanism, but it can accommodate increasing intracranial volume only to a point. When the compliance of the brain is exceeded, the ICP rises, clinical manifestations develop, and other compensatory efforts to reduce pressure begin.

The second form of compensation is *reduction of blood volume* in the brain. When blood flow is reduced by 40%, cerebral tissue becomes acidotic. When 60% of blood flow is lost, the electroencephalogram (EEG) begins to change. This stage of compensation alters cerebral metabolism, eventually leading to brain tissue hypoxia and areas of brain tissue ischemia.

The last stage of compensation and the most lethal is *displacement of brain tissue* across the tentorium, under the falx cerebri, or through the foramen magnum into the spinal canal. This process is called *herniation* and often results in death from brain stem compression. The brain is supported within various intracranial compartments (Fig. 73–2). The supratentorial compartment contains all of the brain tissue from the top of the midbrain upward. This section is divided into right and left chambers by the tough, inelastic fibers of the falx cerebri. The supratentorial compartment is separated from the infratentorial compartment (containing the brain stem and cerebellum) by the tentorium cerebelli. The brain is capable of some movement within these compartments. Pressure increases in one compartment affect surrounding areas of lower pressure.

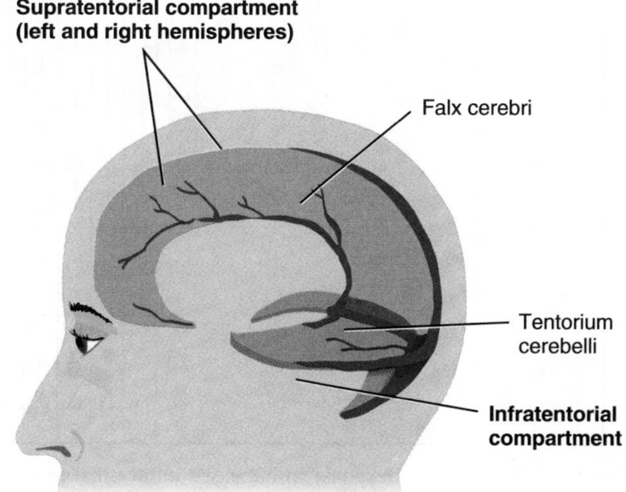

FIGURE 73–2 The intracranial compartments.

With regard to ICP maintenance, *autoregulation* is the occurrence of compensatory changes in the diameter of the intracranial blood vessels designed to maintain a constant blood flow during changes in cerebral perfusion pressure. Autoregulation is lost with increasing ICP. Small increases in brain volume can then cause dramatic increases in ICP, with a longer time required to return to baseline level. When ICP approaches systemic blood pressure, cerebral perfusion decreases and the brain suffers severe hypoxia and acidosis.

CEREBRAL EDEMA

The terms *cerebral edema, brain swelling,* and *increased ICP* are sometimes used interchangeably, but they are not the same. Cerebral edema and brain swelling are causes of increased ICP. An increase in brain bulk caused by an increase in cerebral blood volume is called *brain swelling. Brain edema,* in contrast, is an increase in the fluid content surrounding the tissues of the brain, such as in the extracellular spaces or the white matter, or within the cells themselves. The distinction between these two conditions is important because the interventions differ.

After head injury, edema develops as a result of a disruption of the blood-brain barrier. This type of edema is similar to other forms of edema, such as that seen in a sprained ankle. The fluid contains electrolytes, proteins, and blood. Edema reaches its maximum within 48 to 72 hours after brain surgery or injury. The fluid returns to the systemic circulation via the CSF or the venous system. This form of edema is usually treated with osmotic diuretics.

Brain swelling is also caused by increased blood volume resulting from dilated cerebral blood vessels. Brain swelling appears to be the major mechanism responsible for increasing ICP and for decreasing the size of the ventricles when compensation occurs. This form of swelling may be treated with therapeutic hyperventilation using mechanical ventilation to cause vasoconstriction.

Clinical Manifestations

Manifestations of increased ICP are caused by traction on the cerebral blood vessels from swelling tissues and by pressure on the pain-sensitive dura mater and various structures within the brain and eye. The pathologic process of increased ICP actually comprises several entities that occur at the same time. No single set of clinical manifestations occurs in all clients. Indications of increased ICP relate to the location and cause of the raised pressure and to the speed and extent of its development.

The manifestations of increased ICP are subtle, and diligent observation for changes in the client's condition is necessary. Clinical manifestations include *any* alteration in level of consciousness (restlessness, irritability, confusion), and a decrease in the Glasgow Coma Scale (GCS) score. In addition, the client may have changes in speech, pupillary reactivity, motor or sensory ability, or cardiac rate and rhythm. Headache, nausea, vomiting, or blurred or double vision (diplopia) may be reported. The optic nerve is an extension of the brain, and increased tension in the skull is transmitted to the optic nerve to cause papilledema. Papilledema is swelling and hyperemia of the optic disc and can be observed only through an ophthalmoscope. Early detection (i.e., before clinical manifestations develop) by means of periodic ophthalmologic examination and ICP monitoring in the critical care unit can greatly improve a client's outcome.

Cushing's triad—increased systolic blood pressure with widened pulse pressure and bradycardia—is a late response and indicates severe increased ICP with failure of autoregulation. Respiratory patterns progress from Cheyne-Stokes respiration to central neurogenic hyperventilation to apneustic breathing and ataxic breathing as ICP increases (see Chapter 68). Hyperthermia is typically present when the hypothalamus is first affected by the increase in pressure, followed by hypothermia as ICP increases (Fig. 73–3).

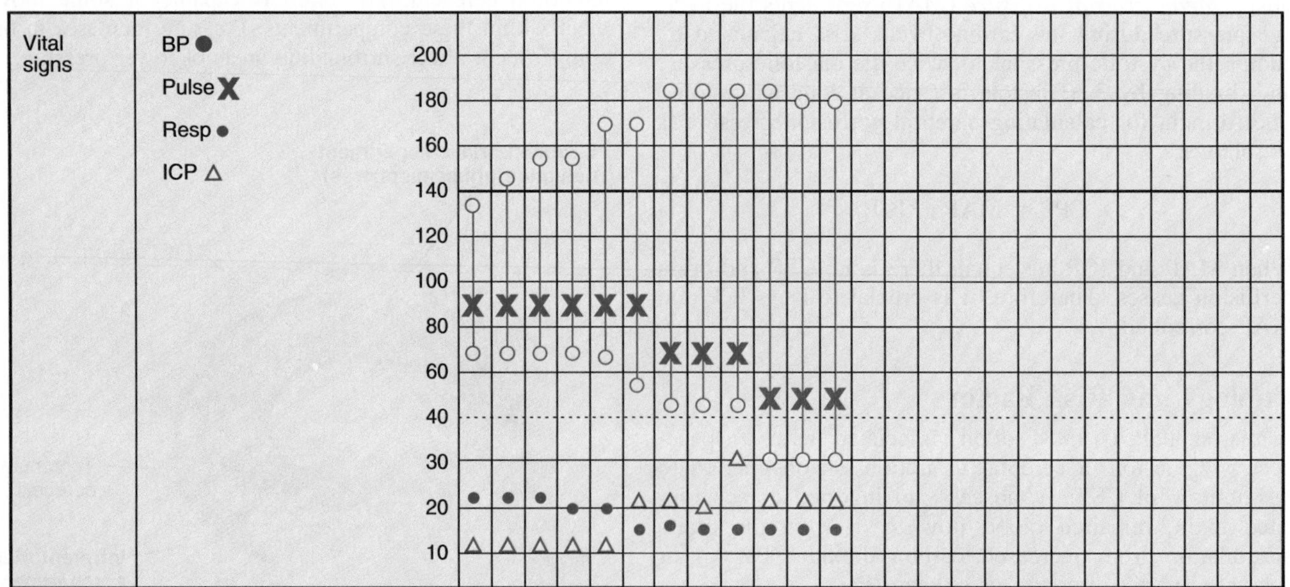

FIGURE 73–3 A late response to increased intracranial pressure is Cushing's triad (also called Cushing's response): bradycardia, systolic hypertension, and a wide pulse pressure, which result from pressure on the medulla. These manifestations can occur with intracranial hypertension or herniation. Alterations in the respiratory pattern also accompany Cushing's triad.

Common diagnostic studies that are performed to determine the source of increased ICP include skull radiography, computed tomography (CT) scanning, and magnetic resonance imaging (MRI). A lumbar puncture is not usually performed because of the risk of causing herniation of the brain stem when the pressure of the CSF in the spinal cord is lower than in the cranium. In addition, the CSF pressure at the lumbar level is not always an accurate reflection of the intracranial CSF pressure.

HERNIATION SYNDROMES

Herniation syndromes have been classified into five types (Fig. 73–4). These conditions occur late in the course of increased ICP and represent the body's last attempt to restore normal brain volume and pressure through displacement of blood, brain tissue, or CSF.

Herniation, regardless of the type, always constitutes an emergency. *Notify the physician immediately of any manifestations that indicate a worsening of the client's condition due to increasing ICP.*

SUPRATENTORIAL HERNIATION SYNDROMES

TRANSCALVARIAL HERNIATION. Transcalvarial herniation occurs with open head injuries when brain tissue is extruded through an unstable skull fracture. Clinical manifestations vary greatly depending on the location and extent of the open skull fracture.

CENTRAL TRANSTENTORIAL HERNIATION. Central transtentorial herniation is the end result of the downward displacement of the diencephalon through the tentorial notch. It is caused by injuries or masses located in the cerebral cortex or on the outward perimeter of the cerebrum.[73] An early indication of central transtentorial herniation is a rapid change in the level of consciousness. As the pressure increases, changes in respiratory patterns are seen: first, Cheyne-Stokes respirations and then central neurogenic hyperventilation; later, apneustic breathing and also ataxic breathing (Biot's respiration); and, finally, apnea (see Chapter 68). Pupils become small but at first remain reactive, with progression to a dilated and fixed state. Pathologic reflexes begin with Babinski's sign (see Chapter 67) and then progress from abnormal flexion to abnormal extensor posturing. Doll's eye reflex and a positive response to caloric testing are noted when brain stem function is still intact but are absent if the brain stem dies (see Chapter 68). The Critical Monitoring feature in Chapter 68 lists the specific areas of brain involvement that are correlated with pathologic manifestation.

LATERAL TRANSTENTORIAL HERNIATION. Lateral transtentorial herniation occurs from displacement by masses in or along the temporal lobe. It is also called *uncal herniation,* because as the temporal lobe is compressed, the uncus (the anteromedial portion of the hippocampus) and/or the hippocampal gyrus shift from the middle fossa through the tentorial notch into the posterior fossa.[73] As the herniation progresses, the pupils first become sluggish in response to light and then become unresponsive; lack of response is seen first in the ipsilateral pupil and then in the contralateral pupil, secondary to third cranial nerve compression at the midbrain level. Other progressive clinical manifestations include a decreasing level of consciousness (stupor to coma), Cheyne-Stokes respirations followed by central neurogenic hyperventilation, and abnormal flexor posturing that progresses to abnormal extensor posturing.

CINGULATE HERNIATION. Cingulate herniation occurs when the frontal lobes of the cerebrum are compressed, resulting in compression of the cingulate gyrus (an arch-shaped convolution situated just above the corpus callosum) under the falx cerebri.[73] Manifestations are related to cerebral artery compression resulting in ischemia and congestion, edema, and increasing ICP.

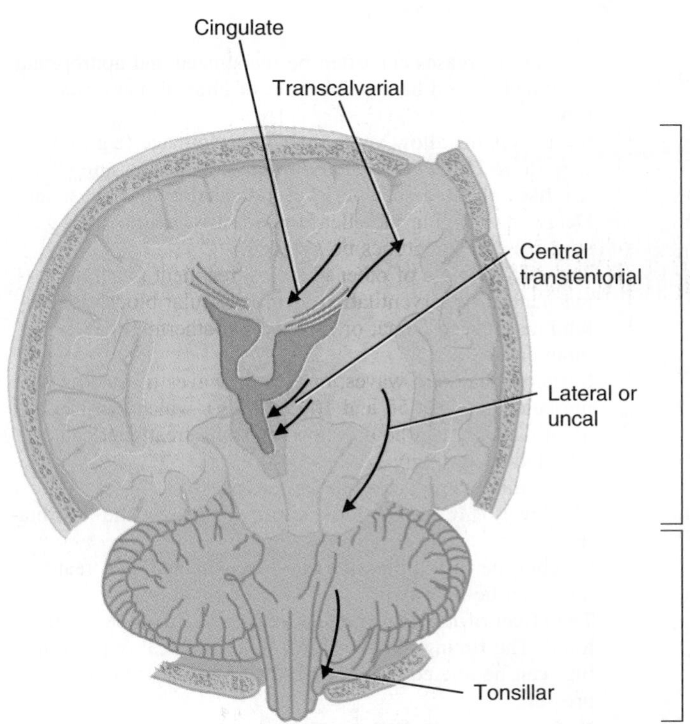

FIGURE 73–4 Types of intracranial herniation. In *transcalvarial* herniation, edematous brain tissue is extruded through the skull. In *central* transtentorial herniation, the lesion is located centrally or superiorly in the cranium, and compression of central and midbrain structures may result. In *lateral,* or *uncal,* herniation the lesion is located laterally within the cranium and can cause pressure on the midbrain. *Cingulate* herniation occurs between the two frontal lobes; the brain is pressed under the falx cerebri. In *tonsillar* herniation, the cerebellar tonsils are driven between the posterior arch of the atlas and the medulla and may be compressed.

INFRATENTORIAL (TONSILLAR) HERNIATION SYNDROME

Tonsillar herniation, also known as *cerebellar herniation,* occurs when the cerebellar tonsil shifts through the foramen magnum, compressing the medulla and upper portion of the spinal cord. Increasing pressure in the posterior fossa, often secondary to cerebellar bleeding, is the usual underlying problem. Manifestations often progress rapidly and include erratic changes in blood pressure, pulse rate, and breathing; decreased level of consciousness; an arched, stiff neck; and quadriparesis.

Outcome Management

The goals of medical management are to decrease ICP, to maintain optimal neurologic function, and to ready the client for rehabilitation.

DECREASE INTRACRANIAL PRESSURE

Emergency care of the client at high risk for development of increased ICP focuses on maintaining the airway, improving breathing, and promoting circulation. Immediate interventions may include intubation followed by hyperventilation, osmotic diuretics, and elevation of the head to promote venous drainage.

HYPERVENTILATION. Carbon dioxide causes cerebral blood vessels to dilate. By increasing the ventilator settings to cause hyperventilation, a hypocarbic (low carbon dioxide) blood level is created. A partial pressure of CO_2 ($Paco_2$) level between 30 and 35 mm Hg results in vasoconstriction of the cerebral blood vessels, leading to decreased blood flow and thus decreased ICP. It is also important to maintain oxygenation. The swollen or bruised brain has an increased need for oxygen and glucose because of an increased metabolic rate. The Pao_2 must be kept between 90 and 100 mm Hg.

MANNITOL. Mannitol, a hyperosmotic agent, is the preferred agent for treating increased ICP because it does not cross an intact blood-brain barrier and has fewer rebound effects.[15] It is given in doses of 0.25 g to 1.0 g/kg intravenously. Hyperosmotic agents increase intravascular pressure by drawing fluid from the interstitial spaces and from the brain cells. If the blood-brain barrier is damaged, the medication enters the brain and increases swelling. Renal function, electrolytes, and serum osmolality need to be monitored when the client is receiving mannitol. Diuresis is expected, and the client may become dehydrated with the excessive use of mannitol. Dehydration is manifested by increased serum sodium and osmolality values.

CEREBRAL PERFUSION. Vasoactive medication, given either to raise or lower blood pressure, may be required to maintain CPP at a normal level. CPP is a result of the relationship between blood pressure and ICP. If the physician has not left orders to treat blood pressure changes, notification must occur if the blood pressure range is below 100 or above 150 mm Hg systolic. Often, physician orders specify titration of medication to maintain the CPP at greater than 70 mm Hg.

PREVENTION OF COMPLICATIONS. Antibiotics may be prescribed, especially with an open head injury, the placement of an ICP monitor, or an infection in another body system. Infections increase metabolism and thus also raise ICP.

Anti-seizure medication (e.g., phenytoin, phenobarbital, diazepam) may be given prophylactically to reduce the risk of seizures. Seizures significantly increase metabolic requirements and cerebral blood flow and volume and thus increase ICP. Chapter 69 describes the care of the client with seizures.

Intravenous (IV) fluids are given by IV pump to help monitor the amount of fluids given. The client is maintained in an euvolemic state. Hypertonic IV solutions are avoided because of the risk of promoting cerebral edema.

Temperature reduction decreases metabolism and cerebral blood flow and thus ICP. Antipyretics may be used, but a hypothermic blanket is more commonly the intervention of choice. Muscle relaxants are given to prevent shivering.

MONITOR INTRACRANIAL PRESSURE

Continuous ICP monitoring is used for clients experiencing conditions associated with potentially elevated ICP (e.g., head trauma, preoperative and postoperative aneurysms, tumors, posterior fossa lesions). Use of ICP monitors has several benefits (Box 73–1). However, ICP monitoring devices never replace serial clinical observations of the client's condition.

Several methods of ICP monitoring are available. The most common types measure CSF pressure in the ventricles, brain parenchyma, or subarachnoid space. Intraventricular catheters, parenchymal catheters, and subarachnoid bolts give more accurate results than the epidural catheters, but their use carries a higher incidence of infection. The intraventricular catheter is the most accurate type of intracranial monitor, and it can be used to drain CSF, but it has the highest risk of infection. The screw (bolt) is placed into the subarachnoid space, which allows pressure readings but not removal of fluid. The third

BOX 73–1 Benefits of Intracranial Pressure Monitoring

- Pressure increases can often be recognized and appropriate treatment started before the onset of clinical manifestations.
- Some systems allow ventricular fluid drainage (e.g., three-way stopcock device) when the intracranial pressure (ICP) has risen above a specific level indicated by the physician.
- Delays in bringing the client to definitive treatment (e.g., surgery) can sometimes be avoided.
- The effectiveness of other types of treatment (such as mechanical hyperventilation, neuromuscular blockade, barbiturate-induced coma, or induced hypothermia) can be monitored.
- Sustained pressure waves, or plateau waves (occurring at pressures between 50 and 100 mm Hg), which can cause brain damage, can be detected early and treatment can be adjusted accordingly.
- Intracranial compliance can be measured.
- The level of ICP elevation can provide prognostic information.
- Cerebral perfusion pressure can be calculated and treatment can be adjusted.
- The effect of nursing interventions on ICP can be monitored. The timing of procedures that raise ICP (e.g., turning) can be altered to coincide with periods of "lower" pressure.

common type is an intraparenchymal monitor. It measures pressure in brain tissue. All of the monitoring devices carry a risk of infection owing to their invasive nature. Most surgeons prescribe antibiotics, limit the length of time for which the ICP monitor remains in place, and monitor CSF samples on a regular basis. The accompanying Bridge to Critical Care describes the nurse's role in caring for clients with these devices.

Monitoring ICP also allows the measurement of intracranial compliance. Introducing a known volume of fluid into the ventricle and measuring its effect on ICP tests compliance. Detecting a change in the critical relationship between volume and pressure allows early treatment before the onset of clinical manifestations or sustained elevated ICP. Measurements of cerebral perfusion pressure (CPP) can be made with ICP monitors. Ideally, CPP should be maintained at greater than 70 mm Hg.

PREVENT COMPLICATIONS

Intracranial Hypertension

Intracranial hypertension is defined as an ICP of 20 to 25 mm Hg and can lead to a fatal herniation of the brain. When the herniation occurs at the level of the medulla, death is imminent. Mannitol administration, hyperventilation, sedation, and CSF drainage constitute the usual steps in management of intracranial hypertension.

BARBITURATES. Some clients require large doses of barbiturates to treat uncontrolled ICP. Barbiturate therapy requires sophisticated monitoring and special training, but its use has been associated with increased survival outcomes. The client is intubated and placed on ventilatory support, and a pulmonary artery catheter is inserted.

Pentobarbital, 5 to 10 mg/kg by slow IV injection over 60 minutes, is given in a loading dose, followed by a maintenance dose of 1 mg/kg per hour until the ICP is under control or until the EEG shows a burst suppression pattern 6 to 10 seconds' duration. Pentobarbital may cause a decrease in the blood pressure, so the MAP should not be allowed to fall below 80 mm Hg.

Monitor serum drug levels daily; the dose should be reduced if serum levels exceed 5 mg/dl or if the burst suppression pattern on the EEG lasts longer than 10 seconds. Monitor temperature because barbiturates reduce metabolism, thereby cooling the body. If the temperature falls below 36° C, active warming is indicated.

Continue pupillary assessment. Even when a client is in a coma, the pupils dilate if the brain stem becomes compressed. Notify the physician of this change. Barbiturate therapy eliminates the client's normal protective functions. The client is completely dependent on nursing care for all basic needs (see Chapter 68). Wean clients slowly from barbiturate therapy to prevent rebound intracranial hypertension.

NEUROMUSCULAR BLOCKING AGENTS. Nondepolarizing neuromuscular blocking agents are sometimes used to induce skeletal muscle relaxation and to promote synchronous breathing during mechanical ventilation. Decreasing muscle activity may be necessary to control ICP. Nurses use a peripheral nerve stimulator to monitor for adequacy of drug dosage as well as for the risk of overdose (see Chapter 63). Pentobarbital and neuromuscular blocking agents usually are not given concomitantly. If the client is receiving a neuromuscular blocking agent, sedation and analgesia must be given, as the neuromuscular blocking agents do not provide it.

Other Complications

Other complications of increased ICP include Cushing's stress ulcer (which results from decreased mucosal blood flow and hypersecretion of acid from overstimulation of the vagal nuclei), neurogenic pulmonary edema, diabetes insipidus, and syndrome of inappropriate secretion of antidiuretic hormone (SIADH). These complications are described in Table 73–1.

Nursing Management Assessment

ASSESSMENT

GLASGOW COMA SCALE. The Glasgow Coma Scale (GCS) is the most commonly used neurologic assessment tool in clinical care (Box 73–2). This scale provides objective measurement of three essential components of the neurologic examination: spontaneity of eye opening, best verbal response, and best motor response. The total of the three scores can range from 3 to 15. The client who is unresponsive to painful stimuli, does not open the eyes, and has complete muscular flaccidity has a score of 3. The client who is oriented, opens the eyes spontaneously, and follows commands scores 15. A score of 8 or less indicates coma. Because the scoring of the GCS is based on the client's ability to respond and to communicate, the following criteria may render the GCS invalid:

- The client is intubated and cannot speak.
- Eyes are swollen closed.
- The client is unable to communicate in English.
- The client has a hearing loss.
- The client is blind.
- The client is aphasic.
- The client is paralyzed or hemiplegic.

The first GCS score recorded for the client becomes the baseline score. Subsequent scores allow assessment of trends or changes in neurologic status. The GCS also can be used to recognize disorders as well as to predict outcomes. The use of consistent criteria for client assessment is more important than the specific tool used. Specific behaviors dictating a given score should be indicated. If variations occur in scoring criteria, the value of the scale is lost, and serious changes in the client's condition can be overlooked or treated unnecessarily (Fig. 73–5). More detailed neurologic assessments are conducted to identify specific trends in responses.

LEVEL OF CONSCIOUSNESS. The first change in a client who presents with altered cerebral tissue perfusion is a change in the level of consciousness (LOC). When decreased LOC is noted, serial and detailed assessments are required until the client has achieved maximum recovery. To eliminate the subjectivity associated with use of terms such as "lethargy," "obtundation," "semi-coma," or "coma," the GCS both objectifies the client's LOC and assists in identifying very subtle changes.

PUPIL RESPONSE. A pupil check includes assessing pupil appearance and physiologic response. The affected pupil is usually on the same (ipsilateral) side as the brain lesion, whereas the motor and sensory deficits are usually on the opposite (contralateral) side. Be careful not to mistake a prosthetic eye for a fixed pupil.

BRIDGE TO CRITICAL CARE

Intracranial Pressure Monitoring

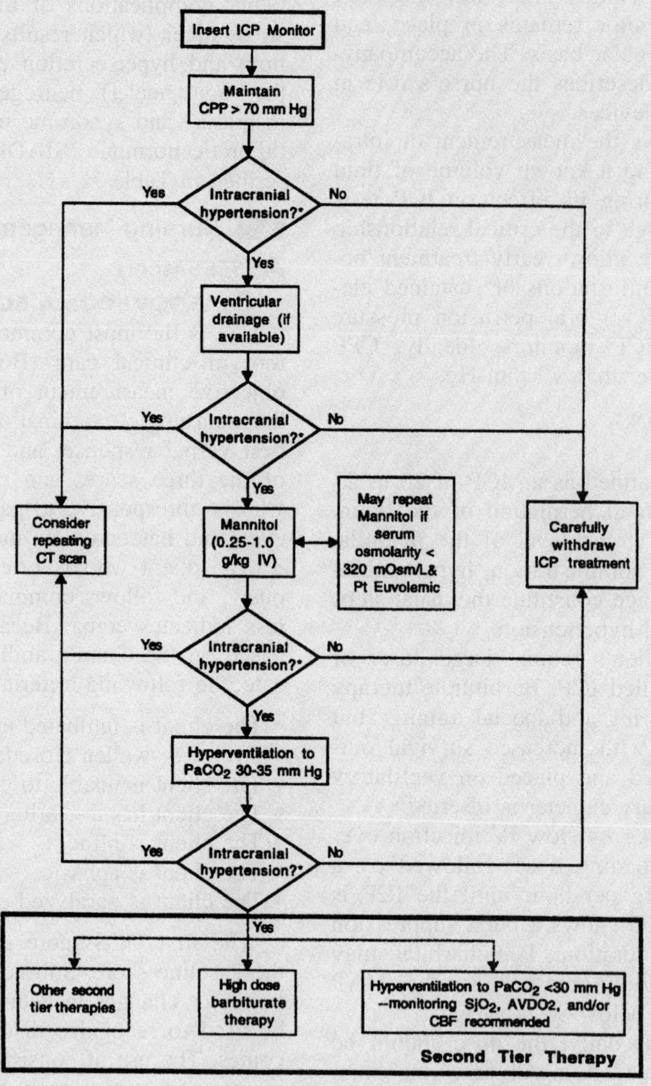

Intracranial Pressure Waveforms

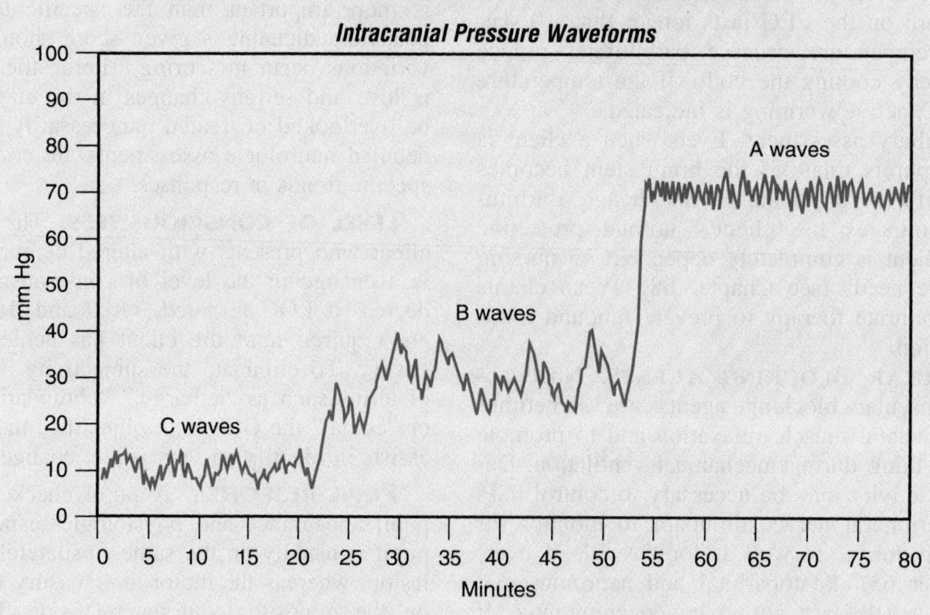

BRIDGE TO CRITICAL CARE *Continued*

The shape of the waves is influenced by cardiac pulsations and respirations as well as by intracranial pressure (ICP).

- *C waves* occur four to eight times per minute and reflect fluctuations in arterial pressure. C waves are not considered significant.
- *B waves* occur at intervals of 30 seconds to 2 minutes and represent increases in ICP to 50 mm Hg. They may be precursors to A waves.
- *A waves* are most pronounced when the amount of cranial contents is increased. Also called *plateau waves,* A waves represent recurrent ICP elevations to 100 mm Hg. An A wave may be caused by coughing or straining but, if recurrent or sustained, may indicate a reduced ability of the brain to compensate. The client may also show other manifestations of increasing ICP.

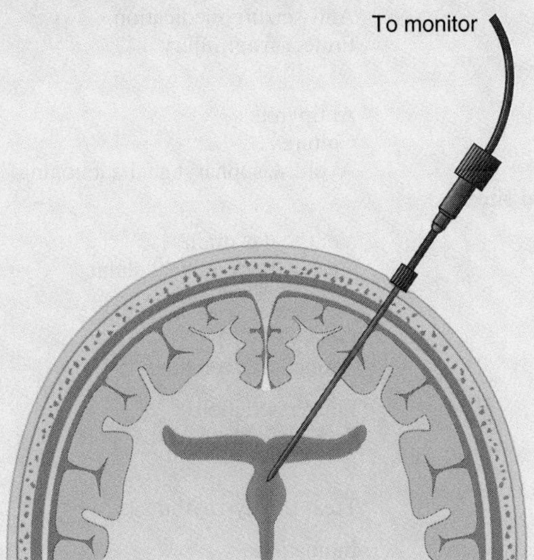

Ventricular catheter (ventriculostomy)

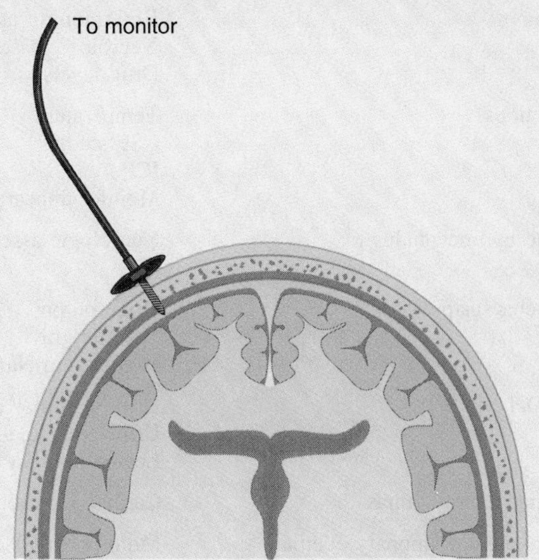

Subarachnoid screw (bolt)

General Interventions for Monitoring Intracranial Pressure

- Ensure that the tubing is long enough to allow the client to be moved in bed but that it is no longer than 14 feet. Use of tubing longer than 14 feet may cause inaccurate readings.
- Be careful to prevent kinks in the tubing.
- Place the catheter at the preset level of the transducer to take a reading.
- Use sterile technique when setting up the device.
- Monitor for manifestations of infection.
- Notify the physician if the readings show damping (lessening of amplitude) of the waves. The catheter may need to be flushed by the physician.
- If inaccurate readings occur, check for:
  - Leaks in the system
  - Differences in the height of the transducer and the device
  - Kinks in the tubing
  - Client activity or behavior involving performance of the Valsalva maneuver
  - Obstruction in the system

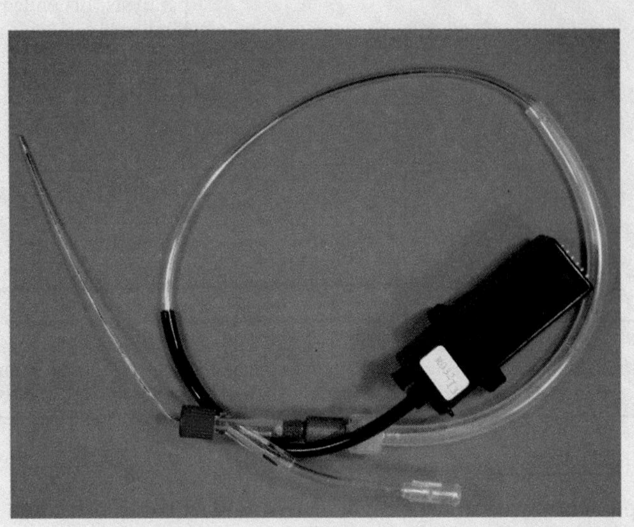

Pupil Equality. Document pupil equality, noting the relative size of each pupil.

Pupil Size. Estimate the size of each pupil in millimeters (mm) before and after light stimulation. A penlight provides more accurate data than obtainable with a flashlight owing to the smaller size of the light and the ability to focus the beam directly at the pupil.

Pupil Position. Note whether the pupil is positioned in the midline or deviated from midline.

Pupil Reaction to Light. Bring the penlight from the lateral aspect of the client's head toward the eye. Observe for constriction in that eye as well as in the opposite eye. Then test the opposite eye in the same way. The detection of subtle change may require four ap-

TABLE 73–1 COMPLICATIONS OF HEAD INJURY

Condition	Assessment	Treatment
Cerebral edema	ICP monitor Neurologic assessment	CSF drainage Diuresis Sedation
Stress ulcers	NPO status Monitor nasogastric drainage output for blood	Histamine blockers
Seizures	EEG monitoring Neurologic assessment Drug levels	Anti-seizure medication Protect from injury
Infections	Temperature CSF studies ICP Monitor appearance of affected site(s)	Antipyretics Cultures Avoid nasopharyngeal suctioning
Acute hydrocephalus	Neurologic assessment	Ventricular drain Ventriculoperitoneal shunt
Diabetes insipidus	Urine output >200 ml/hr Specific gravity <1.005 High serum Na^+ level	Free water replacement DDAVP Maintain euvolemia
SIADH	Urine output <30 ml/hr Urine specific gravity >1.020 Low serum Na^+ level	Fluid restriction Sodium replacement
Cardiac dysrhythmias	Cardiac monitoring	Treat the dysrhythmia
Neurogenic pulmonary edema	Monitor ABGs, SpO_2, pulmonary secretions	Intubation Mechanical ventilation Treatment similar to that for ARDS (see Chapter 63)
Subarachnoid hemorrhage/aneurysms	Monitor for exopthalmos, cranial nerve paralysis, distended orbital and periorbital veins Monitor CSF for blood	Notify physician of changes in neurologic examination or of other signs of subarachnoid hemorrhage
Altered behavior	Monitor orientation and memory	Reorient client Educate family regarding behavior
Post-trauma response	Monitor for headache, poor concentration, dizziness, irritability, sensitivity to noise, restlessness, depression, easy fatigability, anxiety, impaired memory	Educate client and family about possible sequelae of head injury Request physician visit if symptoms persist Encourage cognitive rehabilitation if symptoms persist

ABG, arterial blood gas; ARDS, adult respiratory distress syndrome; CSF, cerebrospinal fluid; DDAVP, 1-deamino(8-D-arginine) vasopressin; EEG, electroencephalogram; ICP, intracranial pressure; Na^+, sodium ion; NPO, nothing by mouth; SIADH, syndrome of inappropriate secretion of antidiuretic hormone; SpO_2, oxygen saturation (as measured by pulse oximetry).

proaches with the penlight. Brisk and equal constriction of the pupils to direct and indirect light is a normal response. Sluggish or unequal direct or indirect (consensual) response is abnormal. Anisocoria, or unequal pupils, occurs normally in about 17% of the population, with one pupil being about 1 mm larger. It is important to ascertain information about pupil inequality from the client or family members so that an unnecessary procedure is not performed.

Pupil Shape. Normally, pupils are round. Describe abnormal shapes with a drawing. Pupils may be oddly shaped owing to previous eye surgery. A pupil that looks oval may be early evidence of increasing ICP.

Pupil Accommodation. Normally, the size of the pupil and the lens (which is not visible to the naked eye) accommodate (adjust) to varying focal lengths. Having the client focus on a distant object and then quickly focus on a close object tests accommodation. Pupils should become smaller as the object is brought nearer the eye and should dilate when the object is moved away from the eye. Accommodation is often not tested in the acute care setting owing to the inability of the client to cooperate.

The acronym PERRLA is often used in practice and indicates that the *p*upils are *e*qual, *r*ound, and *r*eactive to *l*ight and *a*ccommodation. Notify the physician immediately if any change occurs in the pupillary response.

BOX 73–2 Assessment of Clients Using the Glasgow Coma Scale

The Glasgow Coma Scale (GCS) is a numeric expression of cognition, behavior, and neurologic function. It is the most commonly used scale and was designed to measure level of consciousness and severity of injury through eye opening, verbal responsiveness, and motor response. The total of the three scores ranges from 3 to 15, with 3 the most severe and 15 normal. Assessments of abstract thought and problem-solving should be combined with the GCS to give a more complete picture of neurologic status.

Documentation should contain specific descriptive terms. For example, instead of just indicating that the client is "stuporous," record the evidence of stupor that you observe: "no response to verbal commands, responded only to tracheal suctioning with abnormal flexor posturing." Words such as "lethargic," "stuporous," or "comatose" are open to individual interpretation, and a clear description of behavior is less likely to be misunderstood.

Scale Components

Eye Opening

Observe eye opening without speaking to the client. Does the client open the eyes and look around? If the eyes are closed, call the client's name. If no response is noted, raise your voice. If there is still no response, use a mildly painful stimulus, given in the central part of the body, such as squeezing the trapezius muscle or rubbing the sternum.

Avoid supraorbital pressure, as it can cause damage to the eyes. Pinching of the body can cause severe bruising and is unnecessary in a neurologic examination.

Motor Response

Asking the client to follow specific commands such as "Raise your right arm" or "Wiggle your toes" assesses motor responses. Do not ask the client to squeeze your hand because grasp is a reflexive response that can occur with head injury. If agency protocol lists grasp as a neurologic assessment component, ask the client to "let go" after grasping, to measure cognitive ability to control movement.

In a client who is unable to follow commands, observe the response to a painful stimulus. Responses may include (1) localizing (trying to remove the stimulus), (2) withdrawing, and (3) posturing. In addition, a response may not be elicited and the client may remain motionless.

Compare the right and left sides and the upper and lower extremities. Record the best response while also recording any abnormality that indicates decreased movement in a particular extremity.

Motor Activity

Motor activity assessment is the measure of strength of voluntary movement of the arms and legs. If a client cannot cooperate with testing, paralysis may be difficult to detect. Observe the client carefully. If a client is restless, paralysis may become obvious because the paralyzed part does not move as other body parts move. Additional information may be obtained by:

1. Comparing the tone of one side of the body with that of the other.
2. Lifting the arms or legs on both sides, releasing them, and watching them drop to the bed.
3. Observing the position of the limbs at rest.

If a client can cooperate, assessing "drift" may demonstrate subtle tone and strength alterations. For this assessment, have the client hold both arms up in front of the body with palms upward and eyes closed. Muscles are weak if one arm "drifts" (gradually moves) downward or if the hand pronates (turns over). This maneuver is often referred to as the *pronator drift test.*

Posturing

Review posturing in Chapter 68. As the client's intracranial pressure increases at the cortical level, abnormal flexor posturing occurs. As pressure reaches the pons level, abnormal extensor posturing occurs. When the pressure reaches further to the medullary level, flaccidity is noted, or response is totally lacking—the gravest of all signs.

Verbal Response

Verbal responses assess the client's orientation to self, environment, and time. Ask appropriate questions such as the following: "What is your name? Where are you? What is the month, year, season, nearest holiday?" Avoid asking questions about the date or day of the week.

Being hospitalized can alter accuracy of that response even in a person with normal cognitive function. Structure the conversation to elicit information that can be verified by family members, such as home address or employer's name. In many cases, a slight degree of confusion is not noticeable until some time is spent with the client. An apparently oriented client may ask the same question a few minutes after it was originally asked and answered, or the client may have "learned" the answers to common questions such as "What is your name?" and "What hospital are you in?" Therefore, it is helpful to reassess the client regularly to check memory or to challenge cognitive integrity with various questions. In addition, observing the course of a normal conversation may give evidence of confusion or disorientation.

Scoring

After obtaining the data for all three parts of the GCS, total the points for each part and compare the score obtained with the client's baseline score. If a decrease in the score of even 1 point occurs, complete a detailed neurologic assessment, including pupillary responses, and notify the physician.

EYE MOVEMENT. Document eye movement changes. Observe the position of the eyes when assessing the pupils. The eyes should move together. If dysconjugate (not together) movement is noted, the physician should be notified.

VITAL SIGNS. Initially, vital signs should be assessed every 15 minutes until they are stable. Body temperature should be monitored every 2 hours. If hypothermia or hyperthermia occurs, continuous temperature monitoring should be used. Trends in vital signs and respiratory patterns should be analyzed. As ICP increases and herniation occurs at the level of the medulla, Cushing's response occurs (see Fig. 73–3).

Vital sign changes are *late* changes. See the following discussion of altered cerebral tissue perfusion for care of a client with increasing ICP. Once the vital signs begin to

MISSION HOSPITAL
REGIONAL MEDICAL CENTER

ADULT NEURO FLOW SHEET

TIME

GLASGOW COMA SCALE		Eyes Open	
		Best Motor	
		Best Verbal	
		TOTAL	
VOLUNTARY MOTOR	Right	upper extremity	
		lower extremity	
	Left	upper extremity	
		lower extremity	
CRANIAL NERVES	PUPILS Right	Size	
		Reaction	
	PUPILS Left	Size	
		Reaction	
	EOMS	Conjugate	
		Dysconjugate	
		Tracking Right	
		Left	
		Blink Reflex	
		Gag Reflex	
		Facial Symmetry	

TIME

KEY

MOTOR
5+ Normal Power
4+ Weakness
3+ Anti-gravity
2+ Not anti-gravity
1+ Trace
0 No movement

Pupil Size
B = Brisk
S = Sluggish
A = Absent

2mm 3mm 4mm 5mm

6mm 7mm 8mm

✓ = Present
O = Absent
S = Symmetrical
A = Asymmetrical

Date

Speech Patterns: ______

Comments: ______

GLASGOW COMA SCALE		
Eyes Open	4	Spontaneously
	3	To verbal command
	2	To Pain
	1	No Response
Best Motor Response	6	Obeys Commands
	5	Localize Pain
	4	Flexion to pain withdraw
	3	Flexion Decorticate
	2	Extension to pain (decerebrate)
	1	No Response to pain
Best Verbal Response	5	Oriented
	4	Confused
	3	Inappropriate words
	2	Incomprehensible sounds
	1	No Response

Unit ______

R.N. Signature ______ Shift: ______

R.N. Signature ______ Shift: ______

R.N. Signature ______ Shift: ______

ADDRESSOGRAPH

#408 10/89 Adult Neuro Flow Sheet

A

FIGURE 73–5 *A*, A neurologic observation chart. (Courtesy of Mission Hospital Regional Medical Center, Mission Viejo, CA.)

NEUROLOGIC FLOW SHEET

1. Glasgow Coma Scale (GCS). Three areas are assessed: Best eye opening, Best motor response, and Best verbal response. Assign the appropriate numerical score for each category (1st box—best eye, 2nd box—best motor, and 3rd box—best verbal). Place the total score in the fourth box (total score 3-15).

2. Voluntary Motor is evaluated by assessing each extremity on both the right and left side. Note **symmetry vs. asymmetry.** In the cooperative patient, voluntary motor strength is assessed by asking the patient to close their eyes and hold their arms straight ahead with palms up for about 30 seconds. The leg strength is evaluated by asking the patient to push downward against the examiner's hands.

Scoring: Normal power (5+) is the score given if the patient's arms stay in the same position and/or if the legs have equal strong power.

Weakness (4+) is the score given if one of the pt.'s arm drifts downward (hands may pronate) or if the leg strength is diminished. Some resistance to force is noted.

Anti-gravity (3+) is the score given if the patient is able to move an extremity above the plane of gravity (ie flexing & extending a hand up/down against gravity).

Not anti-gravity (2+) is the score given to a patient who can move the extremity back and forth on the bed but not against the forces of gravity.

Trace movement (1+) is the score given to a patient who can move an extremity slightly.

No movement (0) is the score given if a patient cannot move the extremity.

3. **Cranial Nerve Exam:**

Pupillary response: Each pupil is assessed individually. Note the size of the pupil prior to shining the light into the eye. Place your hand at the bridge of the nose to block light to the opposite eye. Using the penlight, shine the light from outside the right eye to midpoint across the eye to assess the direct light reflex. Note the pupillary constriction (Brisk, sluggish, or non-reactive) in the right eye. Also, observe for constriction in the left pupil (consensual light reflex). Repeat the above steps for the left eye observing the direct light reflex in the left eye and the consensual reflex in the right eye. Document the pupil size (prior to light in the eye) and the reaction on the flow sheet.

Extra-ocular movements (EOMS's) are tested on patients who are awake enough to follow instructions. Ask the patient to follow your fingers with his eyes without moving the head. Move your fingers in a figure H and observe both eyes as they move across/up/down. **Conjugate eye movements** occur when both eyes move in parallel motion. **Dysconjugate eye movements** occur when the eyes do not move in a lateral direction together (one eye may move laterally while the other is fixed or moves in another direction). **Tracking** occurs when the patient is consciously following someone's or something's movement around the room. Place a check for present or a 0 for absent.

The Blink reflex is elicited by lightly stroking the patient's eyelashes. When the eyelids are closed, the eyelids will flutter slightly if the reflex is present. In the conscious alert patient, observe for blinking. Place a check for present or a 0 for absent.

The Gag reflex is evaluated by asking the alert, cooperative patient to cough or swallow. If the patient is unable to do so or is unconscious, take a long cotton tipped swab and stroke the back of the patient's throat. Note if the reflex is present (place a check) or absent (place a 0).

Muscles of the face: Note the muscle symmetry of the facial muscles. Note the ability of the eyelids to open spontaneously and equally. Ask the patient to close their eyes as tightly as possible. Note asymmetry. Ask the patient to smile—note the corners of the mouth to identify symmetrical patterns. Ask the patient to frown/wrinkle his forehead—note the symmetry of the muscles. Place a S for symmetrical and an A for asymmetrical.

Speech patterns: Note if speech is clear, slurred, rambling, or aphasic.

Comments: Utilize this section to elaborate on any abnormal findings or document other pertinent data.

Sign your name and document shift worked. Complete the date/unit and addressograph. The neurological flow sheet is for a 24 hour period. Each day at 7 am, obtain a new flow sheet. Document your findings in the appropriate time box.

B

FIGURE 73–5 *Continued B*, Neurologic flow sheet.

deteriorate, many other changes have already occurred, such as a decrease in LOC. Ongoing monitoring for such changes is imperative; do not wait for vital signs to change, as the delay may prove fatal for the client. Any changes in neurologic status may be very significant and must be reported to the physician, no matter how minor they may seem.

DIAGNOSIS, OUTCOMES, INTERVENTIONS

Altered Cerebral Tissue Perfusion. If your patient is in a coma because of increased ICP, use this diagnosis to reflect the risk to cerebral tissue perfusion. Write the diagnosis as *Altered Cerebral Tissue Perfusion related to increased ICP.* The term *patient* is used to refer to a person in a coma. The *client* in this case is the patient's family, who serves as his or her advocate.

Outcomes. The patient will maintain normal cerebral perfusion, as evidenced by (1) stable or improving levels of consciousness; (2) stable or improving GCS score; (3) ICP of 15 mm Hg or less; (4) no restlessness, irritability, or headache; and (5) no pupillary changes, no seizures, no widening pulse pressure, no respiratory irregularity, and no hypertension or bradycardia.

Interventions. Administer the medications ordered to reduce cerebral edema (e.g., osmotic diuretics) and to decrease the risk of seizure (e.g., anticonvulsants), and monitor the patient's response to these medications. If the patient's baseline manifestations of increased ICP are not improving, if the patient's status deteriorates, or if seizures develop, notify the physician. Also, consult the physician for medication to promote bowel evacuation without straining, as straining increases ICP. Disimpaction is not advised because of the vasovagal response that occurs.

Position the Patient. Place the patient supine with the head elevated 30 degrees unless contraindicated (e.g., with some spinal injuries, some aneurysms). Keep the patient's head in a neutral position to facilitate venous drainage from the brain. Avoid extreme rotation and flexion of the neck because these positions compress the jugular veins and increase ICP. Also avoid extreme hip flexion because this position increases intra-abdominal and intrathoracic pressure, which increases ICP.[75] As coma lightens, the patient may become disoriented and combative, making it difficult to maintain proper positioning. If restraints must be used, remember that they often increase agitation, which increases ICP.

Maintain a Patent Airway. Patients need to maintain a patent airway even in the presence of increased ICP. Suctioning assists in preventing buildup of secretions and CO_2 and a resultant elevation of ICP. Adequately oxygenate intubated patients before initiating suctioning, between suctioning efforts, and after suctioning. Try to limit suctioning to three passes, and limit each pass to 10 seconds. Recall that nasal drainage may indicate a dural tear; therefore, suctioning of the nares is contraindicated because of the risk of meningitis.

Balance Fluid Levels. In the past, only small amounts of fluids were administered to clients with head injury, in an effort to decrease cerebral edema. Current data indicate that fluid restriction may actually reduce blood volume and decrease cerebral circulation. The lack of volume causes the blood to be thick and sluggish and may also decrease the mobilization of nutrition and toxins into and out of the circulation. Evidently, patients should be maintained in a euvolemic state rather than a fluid-restricted state. Fluid restriction may be appropriate for certain conditions (such as SIADH) but otherwise is contraindicated. Strict intake and output measurement is still necessary to assess fluid balance.

Control Body Temperature. Hyperthermia increases ICP because of the increased metabolic demand. Therefore, notify the physician immediately if hyperthermia occurs. If a patient's ICP is being managed with a hypothermia blanket, notify the physician if the patient's response is not within the prescribed parameters. Observe for shivering because this phenomenon also increases metabolism and ICP. Assess for skin breakdown if cooling blankets are used for extended periods, and especially in patients who are thin.

Monitor Intracranial Pressure. The ICP reading should be less than 15 mm Hg, the MAP reading 80 mm Hg or above, and the CPP reading above 70 mm Hg.

Plateau waves (A waves) are noted when ICP goes above 50 mm Hg and can be sustained for longer than 5 minutes. Whenever these sustained pressures are present, assess for contributing factors and intervene appropriately. For example, neck flexion, excessive hip flexion, airway secretions, excess water in the ventilator tubing, taping the endotracheal tube tightly over the jugular veins, and discussing the patient's condition at the bedside all have been known to increase ICP. Spacing and planning of nonessential nursing interventions (e.g., turning the patient) for when the patient's ICP is not elevated help to prevent plateau waves. Plateau waves may not be obvious on the ICP monitor screen; a printout generated at a slow rate may be required for accurate observation of these waves. Whenever ICP is over 20 mm Hg, interventions to decrease ICP should begin.

Assessing the ICP monitor site for infection and leakage, using sterile technique for dressing and drainage bag changes, and maintaining a closed system are helpful in preventing infection or in promoting early intervention if infection occurs. If CSF drainage is required, most systems have a stopcock for attaching the tubing and drainage bag that maintains the closed system, decreasing the likelihood of infection. The system is opened only to change the drainage bag. The drainage bag is changed with strict sterile technique.

EVALUATION

Evaluate the client's response to treatment as often as every 15 minutes, progressing to hourly, then every 2 to 4 hours, and every 8 hours as the client improves. Once the physician has determined that the client's clinical condition has been optimized, the frequency and extent of evaluation can diminish even further. In the immediate and acute stages, anticipate ongoing modification in the care plan to help the client reach maximum recovery.

Surgical Management

Various surgical techniques are used to treat increased ICP. Optimally, the cause of increased ICP is located and removed. Other techniques include surgical placement of a ventriculoperitoneal shunt to allow drainage if CSF circulation is blocked (Fig. 73–6) and decompressive sur-

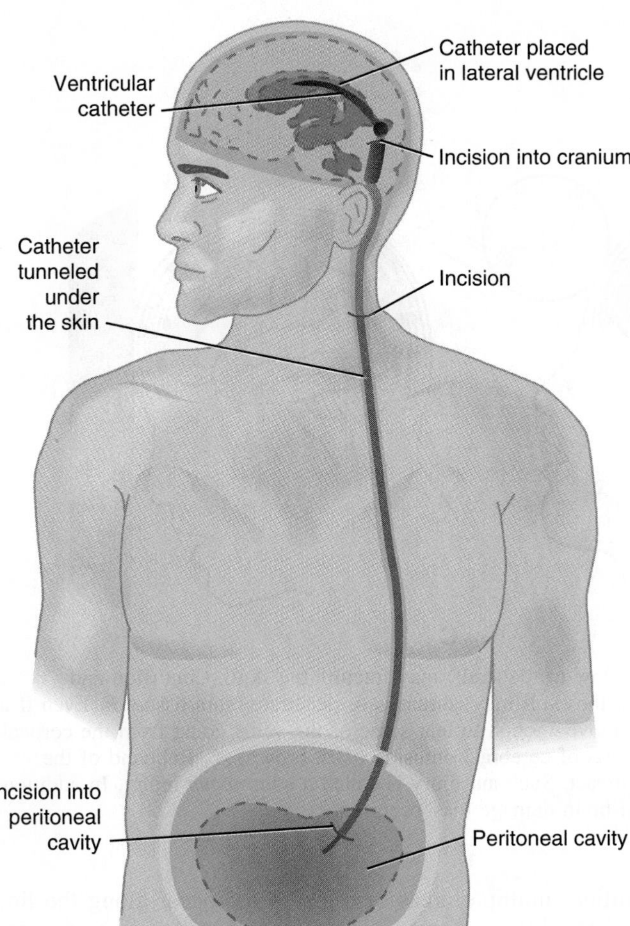

FIGURE 73–6 Ventriculoperitoneal shunt placed for chronic hydrocephalus.

gery. The latter is done by removing some brain tissue (e.g., part of the temporal lobe) to give the remaining structures room to expand. If compliance is low during surgery, the bone flap removed to gain access to the brain is not replaced, or the dura may not be closed. Subsequent surgery is then required to repair the defect. Postoperative care is the same as that required after craniotomy (see Chapter 69).

TRAUMATIC BRAIN INJURY

Traumatic brain injury is an insult to the brain capable of producing physical, intellectual, emotional, social, and vocational changes. In the United States, a head injury is experienced approximately every 15 seconds. Head injuries occur in about 7 million Americans every year. Among these head-injured people, more than 500,000 are hospitalized, 100,000 experience chronic disability, and approximately 2000 are left in a persistent vegetative state.[40]

Head injuries are fatal in more than 30% of cases before the injured person arrives at the hospital owing to the seriousness of the injury. An additional 20% of people die later because of secondary brain injury.[30] Secondary brain events include ischemia from hypoxia and hypotension, secondary hemorrhage, and cerebral edema.

Clients with traumatic head injuries often have other major injuries, including injury to the facial structures, lungs, heart, cervical spine, abdomen, and bones. Facial fractures and lung injuries may contribute to respiratory insufficiency. Airway obstruction and decreased ability to breathe (e.g., from pulmonary contusion, flail chest, pneumothorax) contribute to respiratory insufficiency and poor oxygenation of the brain and other tissues. Ischemia of brain tissue may result.

Hemorrhagic shock in clients with multiple trauma is rarely caused by head injury alone. Frequently, shock is due to ruptured abdominal organs or musculoskeletal injuries (e.g., fractured femur and pelvis). Circulation may be further compromised by cardiac contusion and associated dysrhythmias.

Etiology and Risk Factors

Of clients admitted to the emergency room, 50% have evidence of ingestion of alcohol or other substances of abuse. Most are males younger than 30 years of age. Peak occurrence is during evenings, nights, and weekends. Motor vehicle accidents are the leading cause of head injuries. Other causes are assaults, falls, and sports-related injuries.

A major risk factor for head injury is alcohol consumption. Alcohol slows reflexes and alters cognitive processes and perception. These physiologic changes increase the chances of being involved in an accident or altercation. A second risk factor is driving without seat belts.

MECHANISMS OF INJURY

Head injuries are caused by a sudden force to the head (Fig. 73–7). The results are complex. Three mechanisms contribute to head trauma:

An *acceleration* injury occurs when the immobile head is struck by a moving object (Fig. 73–7*A*).

Deformation refers to injuries in which the force results in deformation and disruption of the integrity of the impacted body part, as in a skull fracture (Fig. 73–7*B*).

If the head is moving and hits an immobile object, a *deceleration* injury occurs (Fig. 73–7*C*). An example is an automobile accident in which the head hits the steering wheel.

In an *acceleration-deceleration* injury, a moving object hits the immobile head and the head then hits an immobile object. Acceleration-deceleration injuries are also associated with *rotation injury,* in which the brain is twisted within the skull.

Blunt Trauma

Blunt trauma occurs when the head strikes an immobile object. Acceleration and deceleration injuries often result from blunt trauma. These are complex injuries involving several cranial structures, including brain parenchyma and vessels. Because the brain is able to move within the skull, movement of the brain can result in injuries at different locations. The brain is partially tethered (at its base) and is also suspended in CSF. Therefore, a blow to the skull can cause the hemispheres to twist on the fixed brain stem.

As the brain moves, it scrapes over the skull's irregular inner prominences, which bruise and lacerate brain

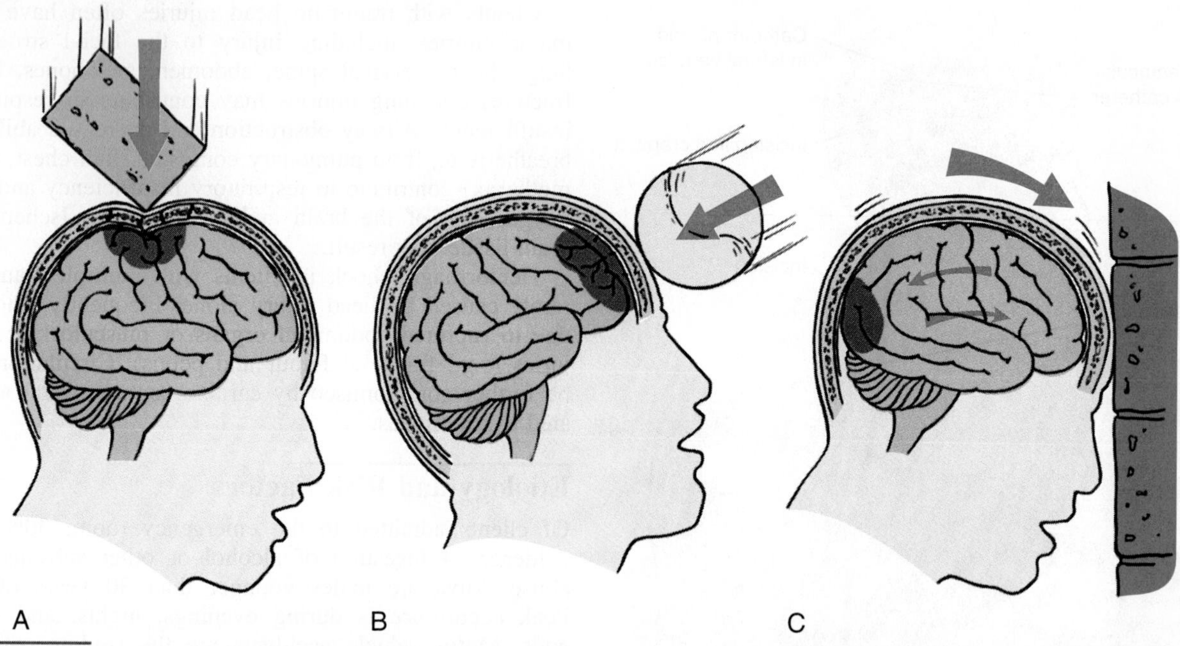

FIGURE 73–7 Some mechanisms of head injury. *A,* Direct injury (a blow to the skull) may fracture the skull. Contusion and laceration of the brain may result from fractures. Depressed portions of the skull may compress or penetrate brain tissue. *B,* Even if a blow to the skull does not result in fracture, it may cause the brain to move enough to tear some of the veins going from the cortical surface to the dura. Subdural hematoma may then develop. Note the areas of cerebral contusion (dark brown). *C,* Rebound of the cranial contents may result in an area of injury opposite the point of impact. Such an injury is called a *contrecoup* injury. In addition to the direct damage sustained in the three injuries depicted, additional brain damage may occur.

tissue. Disruption of the brain's small surface blood vessels may occur. Changes in capillary integrity lead to fluid shifts and petechial hemorrhages. Cranial nerves, nerve tracts, larger blood vessels, and other structures may be stretched, twisted, or rotated, and their functions disrupted.

Penetrating Trauma

Penetrating injuries include those made by foreign bodies (e.g., knives or bullets) or those made by bone fragments from a skull fracture. The damage caused by a penetrating injury often relates to the velocity with which a penetrating object pierces the skull and brain. Bone fragments from a skull fracture may cause local brain injury by lacerating brain tissue and damaging other structures (e.g., nerves, blood vessels). If a major blood vessel is severed or ruptured, a large clot (hematoma) may form, with resultant damage to adjacent or remote structures (e.g., brain compression as in a herniation syndrome). Thus, a hematoma can itself cause extensive brain tissue damage.

High-velocity objects (e.g., bullets) produce shock waves in the skull and brain. The shock waves may significantly damage brain structures beyond those in the object's path. Frequently, penetrating wounds create an open communication between the external environment and the cranial cavity. Thus, infection is a possible complication.

Coup-Contrecoup Injuries

A *coup* (French for "blow") injury occurs immediately at the point of impact. Because of movement within the skull, the same blow may cause injury on the opposite side of the brain, that is, a contrecoup injury (see Fig. 73–7*C*). *Contrecoup* is French for "counterblow." In addition, multiple areas of injury often occur along the line of the blow's force. Tissue around major injured areas often swells, which increases damage to the brain (Fig. 73–8).

PRIMARY INJURIES

Primary injury results directly from the impact itself. It is contrasted with secondary injury, which is caused by hypoxia, hypercapnia, hypotension, and intracranial hypertension. The secondary problems occur hours to days after the initial impact.

Scalp Injuries

Scalp injuries can cause lacerations, hematomas, and contusions or abrasions to the skin. These injuries may be unsightly and bleed profusely. Clients with minor scalp injuries not accompanied by damage to other areas do not require hospitalization. The care of these injuries is discussed in Chapter 82.

Skull Fractures

Skull fractures are often caused by a force sufficient to fracture the skull and cause brain injury. The fractures themselves do not signal that brain injury is also present. However, skull fractures often cause serious brain damage. Depressed skull fractures injure the brain by bruising it (resulting in a contusion) or by driving bone fragments into it (causing lacerations). The site of a fracture and the extent of brain injury may not correlate.

The three types of skull fractures are as follows:

- *Linear skull fractures* appear as thin lines radiographically and do not require treatment; they are important only if there is significant underlying brain damage.
- *Depressed skull fractures* may be palpated and are seen radiographically.

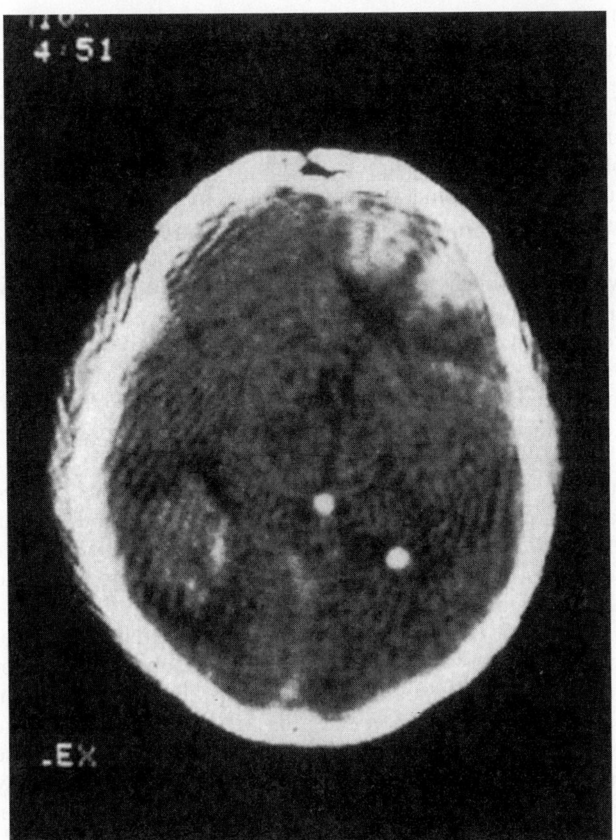

FIGURE 73–8 A magnetic resonance imaging scan showing coup-contrecoup injury after head injury.

- *Basilar skull fractures* occur in bones over the base of the frontal and temporal lobes. These are not observable on plain radiographs but may be manifested as ecchymosis around the eyes or behind the ears.

Brain Injuries

A single classification of brain injuries does not exist. However, the terms *open, closed, contusion,* and *concussion* are often applied to brain injuries. Open head injuries are those that penetrate the skull. Closed injuries are from blunt trauma.

CONCUSSIONS. A concussion is head trauma that may result in loss of consciousness for 5 minutes or less and retrograde amnesia. There is no break in the skull or dura, and no visible damage on a CT or MRI scan.

CONTUSIONS. Contusions are associated with more extensive damage than that from concussions. With contusions, the brain itself is damaged, often with multiple areas of petechial and punctate hemorrhage and bruised areas in brain tissue. Diffuse axonal injury resulting in anatomic disruption of the white matter may result from serious contusions. Microscopic nerve fiber lesions also occur. Abnormalities may be located primarily in one area of the brain, but other areas may also be injured. This is particularly true of brain stem contusions, which are a very serious type of lesion.

DIFFUSE AXONAL INJURY. Diffuse axonal injury is the most severe form of head injury because there is no focal lesion to remove. The injury involves the tissue of the entire brain and occurs at the microscopic level. Diffuse axonal injury is classified as mild, moderate, or severe. With mild diffuse axonal injury, loss of consciousness lasting 6 to 24 hours is characteristic, and there may be short-term disability associated with it. With moderate diffuse axonal injury, coma lasting less than 24 hours is the predominant clinical feature, with incomplete recovery on awakening. Severe diffuse axonal injury involves primary injury to the brain stem. The patient may present with abnormal posturing and in coma, but there is no evidence of cerebral edema or increased ICP. Diffuse axonal injury begins with immediate loss of consciousness, prolonged coma, abnormal flexion or extension posturing, hypertension, and fever.

Focal Injuries

EPIDURAL HEMATOMA. An epidural hematoma, also called an *extradural hematoma,* forms between the skull and the dura mater (see Fig. 73–9). It occurs in about 10% of severe head injuries and is usually associated with a skull fracture. An epidural hematoma occurs from injury to the extracerebral blood vessels, most often the middle meningeal artery. Bleeding is almost always continuous, and a large clot forms, which separates the dura from the skull.

Manifestations are usually acute in onset because the bleeding is often arterial. With an epidural hematoma, the following sequence of events may occur:

1. The client is unconscious immediately after head trauma.
2. The client awakens and is quite lucid.

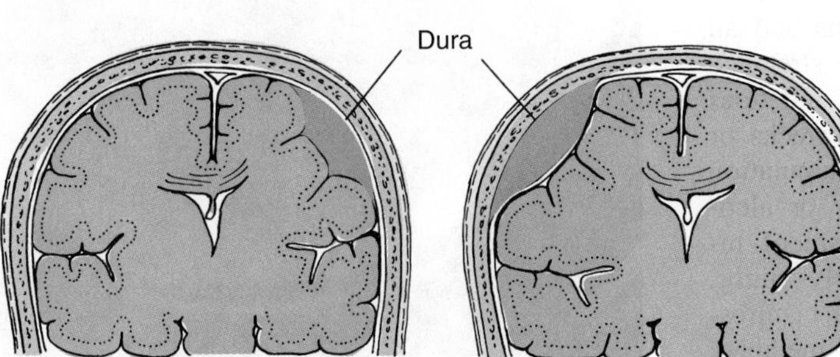

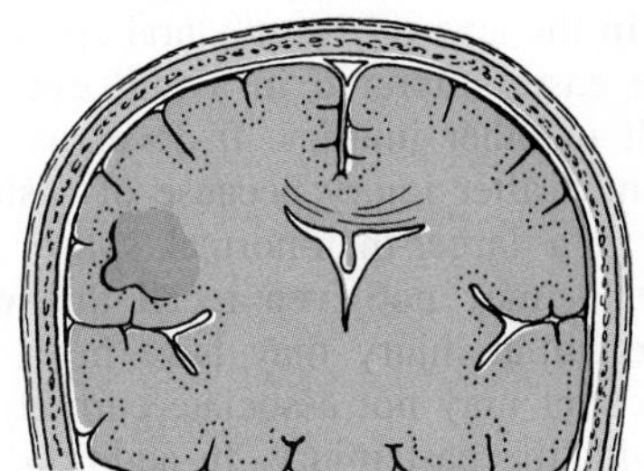

FIGURE 73–9 Formation of a hematoma after head injury.

3. LOC occurs and pupil dilation response rapidly deteriorates, with onset of eye movement paralysis, on the same side as that of the hematoma.
4. The client lapses into a coma.

Although these manifestations are often described as "classic" for an epidural hematoma, few clients present with such classic manifestations, and astute assessment is necessary to prevent death.

Skull radiography and CT scanning confirm the diagnosis. Rapid diagnosis and prompt intervention are essential with an epidural hematoma. Careful, ongoing assessment of neurologic status is also necessary.

SUBDURAL HEMATOMA. Subdural hematoma is a collection of blood in the subdural space (i.e., between the dura mater and arachnoid mater). The tearing of the bridging veins over the brain causes most subdural hematomas.

Subdural hematomas may be classified as acute, subacute, or chronic, depending on how rapidly clinical manifestations develop. Another classification recognizes only acute and chronic, combining the acute and subacute categories.

Acute and Subacute Subdural Hematoma. Acute subdural hematoma usually results from brain or blood vessel laceration. Acute subdural hematomas are a serious complication requiring prompt treatment, because they compress and distort an already damaged, edematous brain. Acute subdural hematoma is symptomatic within 24 to 48 hours of injury. Acute subdural hematoma is seen in approximately 24% of clients with severe head injuries.

Clinical manifestations of acute subdural hematoma are similar to those of acute epidural hematoma. The onset and development of the clinical manifestations may be somewhat slower because the bleeding is more often venous, rather than arterial. Symptom recognition may be difficult because subdural hematoma is often associated with moderate or severe brain injury. A patient developing an acute subdural hematoma may remain unconscious after injury or may have a variable LOC (depending on the extent of injury). A conscious client usually has a headache. The client may become irritable and confused and lapse into a coma or show a fluctuating LOC. Manifestations of increasing ICP appear. Subtle changes in LOC and development of lateralizing changes (i.e., on one side) such as hemiparesis, pupillary dilation, or extraocular eye movement paralysis may be the only findings.

Chronic Subdural Hematoma. Chronic subdural hematoma is most common in older and alcoholic clients (Fig. 73–10). These clients experience atrophy of the brain, which results in stretching of the bridging veins and an increase in the size of the subdural space. These stretched veins are easily ruptured in a fall, even if the fall does not result in other injuries. It develops several weeks or even months after injury because of a slow accumulation of fluid in a larger-than-normal space. Elderly or alcoholic clients may not even recall the mechanism of injury. The initial injury may have been relatively minor, and the client may not associate current clinical manifestations with the past injury. In addition, family members may not recognize the subtle neurologic changes or may not give credence to them because of the client's age.

Gradually, the enlarging blood clot creates pressure on the brain. There is an interval during which the client appears to be recovering or seems completely recovered. Later, manifestations of neurologic deterioration develop. The client may become drowsy, inattentive, and incoherent and display personality changes. Headaches are another prominent symptom. These indications of chronic subdural hematoma may be overlooked until focal or lateralizing signs appear (e.g., hemiparesis, pupil signs). Changes in LOC continue, and LOC may fluctuate widely. Clinical assessment with subdural hematoma is similar to that with epidural hematomas. Surgical intervention usually consists of placing several burr holes or performing a craniotomy to remove the hematoma. Treatment results depend on the client's condition before surgery and the degree of primary brain tissue damage.

A client who has undergone evacuation of a chronic subdural hematoma usually has a drain placed in the cavity to prevent reaccumulation of the fluid and blood. These clients are typically kept flat during the immediate postoperative period. This allows the brain to reexpand to fill the cranial cavity.

INTRACEREBRAL HEMATOMA. Intracerebral hematomas occur less often than epidural or subdural hematomas. They are caused by bleeding directly into brain tissue and may occur at the area of injury, some distance away, or deep within the brain. These hematomas cause problems with increased ICP. Surgical resection may cause as much damage as the clot itself and is usually not

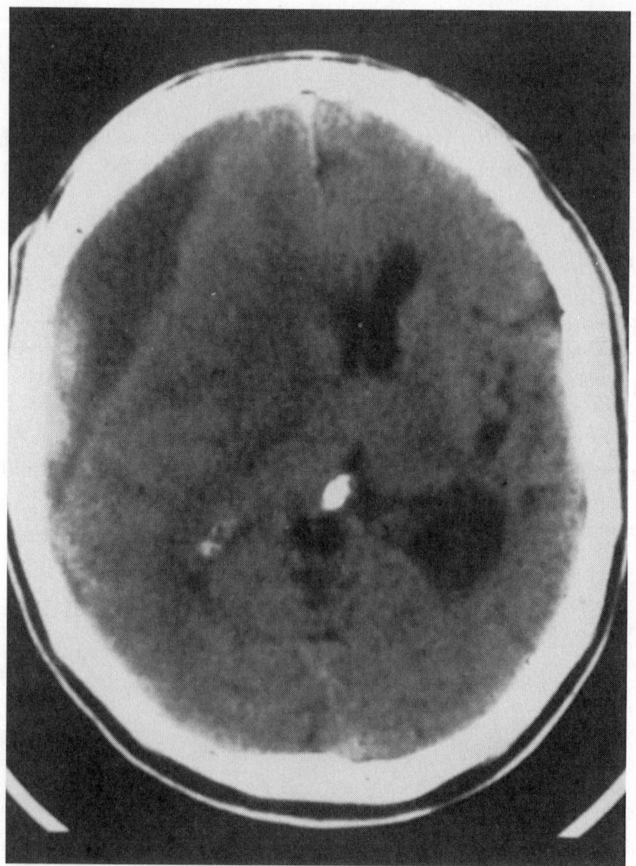

FIGURE 73–10 Magnetic resonance image of a chronic subdural hematoma with an area of acute bleeding, causing a severe midline shift.

performed unless the clot is easily accessible. Clinical manifestations are similar to those that occur with epidural or subdural hematomas, although hemiplegia is more common than hemiparesis. Many assessment findings relate to the lesion's mass effect. Various other clinical manifestations may also be present, depending on the location of the intracerebral hematoma. A diagnosis is established as with other types of hematomas. One form of hematoma, called *delayed traumatic intracerebral hematoma,* occurs after a few days. It is most common in persons with disseminated intravascular coagulation, hypertension, a history of alcohol abuse, or hypoxia. It carries a poor prognosis.

Pathophysiology

A concussion usually causes injury to the brain that is reversible. Some biochemical and ultrastructural damage, such as depletion in mitochondrial adenosine triphosphate and changes in vascular permeability, also can occur.[82]

Major head injuries cause direct damage to the parenchyma of the brain. Kinetic energy is transmitted to the brain, and bruising analogous to that seen in soft tissue injuries results. A blow to the surface of the brain leads to rapid brain tissue displacement and disruption of blood vessels, leading to bleeding, tissue injury, and edema.

Clients with diffuse axonal damage have microscopic injury to the axons in the cerebrum, the corpus callosum, and the brain stem. Widespread white matter injury, white matter degeneration, neuronal dysfunction, and global cerebral edema are characteristic features.

Studies have noted a significantly increased mortality rate in the client who experiences hypotension especially early in the post-injury time frame. When autoregulation is disrupted, as in head injury, cerebral hypoperfusion leads to brain tissue ischemia. Hypoxia has a lesser effect on mortality so long as cerebral perfusion is adequate, because the brain can extract extra oxygen for short periods of time. The combination of arterial hypotension and hypoxemia is significant in the progression of secondary injury. Other causes of secondary brain injury include increased ICP, respiratory problems, electrolyte imbalance, and infection.

Reperfusion injury occurs when ischemia is reversed and blood flow is reestablished; it also leads to secondary injury. Reperfusion injury is probably caused by oxygen free radicals, which are normal byproducts of aerobic metabolism that usually break down into oxygen and water. In cell injury, breakdown of these radicals is impaired so that they accumulate, causing destruction of nucleic acids, proteins, carbohydrates, and lipids and, eventually, cell membranes in the brain tissue. Currently, research is targeted at developing neuroprotective agents that prevent delayed injury progression.[30]

Clinical Manifestations

Skull Fractures

Other than a history of skull fracture, clients may not have clear manifestations of the injury. Therefore, they need careful ongoing assessment. They may develop other clinical signs, including the following:

- CSF or other fluid draining from the ear or nose
- Evidence of various cranial nerve injuries
- Blood behind the tympanic membrane
- Periorbital ecchymoses (bruises around the eyes)
- Later, a bruise over the mastoid process (Battle's sign)

Indications of cranial nerve and inner ear damage may be noted at the time of the initial injury or may not appear until later. They include the following:

- Vision changes from optic nerve damage
- Hearing loss from auditory nerve damage
- Loss of the sense of smell from olfactory nerve damage
- Squint or fixed, dilated pupil and loss of some eye movements from oculomotor nerve damage
- Facial paresis or paralysis (unilateral) from facial nerve damage
- Vertigo caused by damage from otoliths in the inner ear
- Nystagmus from damage to the vestibular system

Basilar skull fractures, depressed fractures, and other open (compound) fractures allow communication between the external environment and the brain. Infection is therefore a possible complication. See Chapter 69 for a discussion of brain abscess and meningitis. Increasing ICP with basilar skull fractures can be difficult to assess because the pressure is not exerted on the motor strip of the frontal lobes, which means that there will be no weakness in the contralateral extremities. Assess for subtle changes in vital signs, especially heart rate and rhythm and breathing patterns.

Concussions

After concussion, observers report a loss of consciousness for 5 minutes or less. Retrograde amnesia, post-traumatic amnesia, or both may be present. The duration of amnesia may directly correlate with the severity of the concussion. The client usually presents with headache and dizziness and may complain of nausea and vomiting. There is no break in the skull or dura, and no visible damage is seen on CT or MRI scans.

Contusions

The clinical manifestations of contusions are varied, partly because any area of the brain can suffer contusion. Contusions are often associated with other serious injuries, including cervical fractures. Secondary effects (e.g., brain swelling and edema) accompany serious contusions. Increased ICP and herniation syndromes may result. Contusions may be divided into cerebral contusions and brain stem contusions.

Cerebral Contusions. Manifestations of cerebral contusions vary, depending on which areas of the cerebral hemispheres are damaged. An agitated, confused head-injured client who remains alert may have a temporal lobe contusion. Hemiparesis in an alert head-injured client may indicate a frontal contusion. An aphasic head-injured client may have a frontotemporal contusion. Other findings indicate contusions in other areas. Although these findings correlate with cerebral contusion, they do not rule out other abnormalities, such as a developing mass lesion. Adverse changes in the client's condition require immediate medical attention. If treated early, these complications may be reversible.

Brain Stem Contusions. Brain stem contusions render a client immediately unresponsive or partially comatose, because of significant brain stem disruption. Typically, an altered LOC continues for at least several hours and usually days or weeks. The client may regain partial consciousness within hours or remain in a coma.

Damage to the reticular activating system may render the client permanently comatose. Other neurologic abnormalities are present and are usually symmetrical (i.e., evenly distributed on both sides of the body). Some may be lateralized (asymmetrical, or on one side of the body only), indicating development of a secondary event, such as a hematoma.

In addition to the altered LOC that is always present with brain stem contusion, respiratory, pupillary, eye movement, and motor abnormalities may occur.

- Respirations may be normal, periodic, very rapid, or ataxic.
- Pupils are usually small, equal, and reactive. Damage to the upper brain stem (third cranial nerve) may cause pupillary abnormalities.
- Loss of normal eye movements may occur because pathways controlling eye movements traverse the midbrain and pons.
- The client may respond to light or noxious stimuli by purposeful movements, such as pushing the stimulus away, or the client may have no response to stimuli (i.e, may be in a flaccid state). In the presence of profound alteration in LOC, flexion and extension posturing may be elicited with or without noxious stimuli (see Chapter 68).

Brain stem contusions do not usually injure the brain stem alone. Localized swelling or direct injury to the hypothalamus may produce autonomic nervous system effects. The client may have a high temperature and a rapid pulse and respirations and may perspire profusely. These effects may wax and wane but, if sustained, can lead to serious complications.

These clinical manifestations often vary from one observation to another, whereas findings with a developing hematoma are more consistent. Careful documentation of assessment findings to identify patterns or trends in the client's condition is important.

Diagnostic assessments such as CT or MRI scanning may reveal fractures and areas of bleeding or brain shift (see Fig. 73–10). Lumbar puncture can also be used to assess for bleeding within the subarachnoid space, provided that any possibility of increased ICP has been ruled out. Currently, CT scans can identify blood in the subarachnoid space, and lumbar punctures are rarely done for this purpose.

Outcome Management

Major goals in the care of severely head-injured clients are as follows:

- Prompt recognition and treatment of hypoxia and acid-base disorders that can contribute to cerebral edema
- Control of increasing ICP resulting from factors such as cerebral edema or expanding hematoma
- Stabilization of other conditions

Medical Management

The medical management of severely head-injured clients focuses on supporting all organ systems while recovery from the injuries takes place. This involves (1) ventilatory support, (2) management of fluid balance and elimination, and (3) management of nutrition and gastrointestinal function. Head trauma affects all systems of the body, and managing its effects requires a holistic perspective. Clinical manifestations may be the result of the initial head injury or may arise from a complicating process.

Initial Management. The initial management of clients with head injury is the same as for any other injured client: airway, breathing, and circulation. There is a high association of cervical fracture with head injury; therefore, the client must be immobilized at the scene of the injury. Lateral cervical spine x-ray films are obtained before the client's head is moved, or the immobilization devices are removed for these studies. The client with head injury is protected from possible complications of cord injury by immobilizing the head and neck immediately, using a cervical collar or sandbags until a collar can be obtained.

If intubation is necessary, a jaw thrust maneuver must be used. A baseline assessment of the client's motor and sensory function is obtained at the scene of the accident. Interventions include lowering the ICP with hyperventilation by mechanical ventilation or by manually ventilating the client with a bag-valve-mask device.

An IV line is placed and fluids are given to stabilize the blood pressure. Head injury alone does not cause major loss of blood. If substantial blood loss is suspected, look for other injuries (e.g., fractures, abdominal injury, severe scalp laceration).

A complete history including the mechanism of injury is important. These data allow the physician to determine the probable extent of injury and allow the emergency department personnel to prepare for the client's arrival. Open head wounds should be covered and pressure applied to control bleeding unless there appears to be an underlying depressed or compound skull fracture.

Do not attempt to remove foreign objects or any penetrating objects from the wound. Uncomplicated scalp wounds (that do not lie over depressed or compound skull fractures) are anesthetized with a local anesthetic agent, cleansed, and sutured. In the emergency department, primary and secondary surveys of the client's injuries are performed. Resuscitation continues with fluid administration.

Laboratory studies are performed, as are necessary radiologic studies. If any identified injuries require emergency surgery, the client is taken directly to the operating room (OR) before admission to the intensive care unit (ICU). Once the client is stabilized enough for transfer to the ICU, the neurosurgical and trauma teams and the nursing staff maintain ongoing care.

Ongoing Management. Ongoing care to reduce ICP is the focus of critical care. Osmotic diuretics, hyperventilation, and adequate oxygenation continue. The cerebral metabolic rate is reduced with sedatives, paralytic agents, antipyretics, barbiturates, and hypothermia. Morphine is a frequently used narcotic for the head-injured client. It reduces pain and can be given intravenously. Respiratory depression is controlled in the client who is intubated and ventilated. Paralytic agents may be used to promote adequate ventilation and should be administered in conjunction with a sedative and an analgesic, because paralytic agents have no sedative or analgesic effect.

PROGNOSIS. Not many clients die instantly from head injury. However, many head-injured clients die within the first few minutes after injury from shock or impaired respiration. Early death may also result from brain stem damage. According to the results of several studies, coma duration is the best predictor of damage severity because it correlates highly with probability of death, intellectual deficit, and social skill impairment. These studies classified a *mild* head injury as loss of consciousness for 20 minutes or less, a *moderate* head injury as 21 to 59 minutes of unconsciousness, and *severe* head injury as coma for 1 hour or more.[12]

Nursing Management

A description of the mechanism of injury is helpful in understanding the nature of a head injury. Whenever there are witnesses to the accident, information obtained can be valuable in determining the extent of the injury. Information about the client's activity and LOC before and after the injury is also helpful. Also important is whether the client was conscious at all or unconscious after injury.

As soon as possible after head injury, assess and document the client's vital signs and neurologic status. This initial assessment and the data obtained from witnesses at the accident scene establish a baseline for later observations. Carefully document all assessment findings. Assessment data collection is described earlier in this chapter.

The physician should be promptly notified of any findings that indicate the possible development of complications. It is particularly difficult to assess the condition of a head-injured client who has ingested large amounts of alcohol or other drugs before injury, because the effects of these substances may obscure significant clinical abnormalities.

DIAGNOSIS, OUTCOMES, INTERVENTIONS

Many nursing and collaborative problems are present in the client with a head injury, such as risk for *Ineffective Airway Clearance, Altered Tissue Perfusion,* seizures, paralysis, infection, diabetes insipidus, and *Post-trauma Syndrome.* Other problems that a client with a head injury may experience include the following:

- Risk for Contractures
- Impaired Skin Integrity
- Altered Oral Mucous Membranes
- Altered Nutrition
- Altered Fluid Volume
- Risk for Injury
- Risk for Increased ICP
- Altered Thought Processes
- Altered Family Processes

Nursing diagnoses for these problems are discussed in Chapters 68 and 69. Investigation of the underlying cause of these problems and the interventions for them must be individualized according to the client's needs.

Risk for Ineffective Airway Clearance. The client with traumatic brain injury may have an altered state of consciousness and may not be able to expectorate secretions. The client is also at increased risk for aspiration.

Outcomes. The client will have effective airway clearance. The upper airway should be free of secretions. Respirations should be of a regular rate (16 to 22 respirations per minute), rhythm, and depth. Breath sounds should be clear in both lungs, and the chest should have symmetrical movement. The trachea should be in a midline position, and there should be no dyspnea or accessory muscle use. Aspiration should be prevented. The PaO_2 should be maintained greater than 90 mm Hg and $PaCO_2$ between 30 and 35 mm Hg initially. The chest film should be clear.

Interventions. Nursing actions aimed at maintaining adequate airway clearance include clearing the mouth and oral pharynx of foreign bodies (e.g., broken teeth) and suctioning the oropharynx and trachea every 1 or 2 hours and as needed. Avoid suctioning the nasopharynx until after a basilar fracture or meningeal tear is ruled out. A semiprone, lateral position may facilitate drainage of secretions and prevent aspiration but is contraindicated with increased ICP or a cervical fracture. Humidified oxygen, endotracheal intubation, mechanical ventilation, or a tracheostomy may be required to maintain the client's PaO_2 and $PaCO_2$ within set parameters.

Altered Cerebral Tissue Perfusion. In clients who suffer from traumatic brain injuries, another appropriate nursing diagnosis is *Risk for Altered Cerebral Tissue Perfusion secondary to hypotension, hypertension, intracranial hemorrhage, hematoma, or other injuries.*

Outcomes. The client will have adequate cerebral tissue perfusion. The client will have a stable or improving LOC with a stable GCS score and an ICP of less than 15 mm Hg. Temperature will be maintained at less than 38.5° C. The client's blood pressure will be maintained within established parameters. Urinary output will be at a minimum of 30 ml per hour and not greater than 200 ml per hour. Laboratory values will remain within normal limits.

Interventions. Although anticipatory, prudent monitoring is key to early detection of altered cerebral tissue perfusion; nursing interventions can actually prevent, delay, or minimize altered cerebral perfusion. These interventions are discussed earlier in this chapter. Briefly, they include maintaining all physiologic parameters within normal limits, positioning the client for optimal venous return, and monitoring extracerebral systems for complications. Communicating a client's neurologic status accurately and completely through verbal reporting and documentation is essential to early identification of change and early intervention. ICP monitoring may be required (see earlier).

Surgical Management

Conditions that may require surgery include subdural and epidural hematomas, depressed skull fractures, and penetrating foreign bodies. An epidural clot may be surgically evacuated through burr holes (Fig. 73–11) or a craniotomy. During surgery, the wound may be drained and bleeding vessels ligated. After surgery, nursing care is the same as for any client recovering from a craniotomy. Simple skull depressions are treated electively by surgically elevating the depressed bone tissue, removing fragments, and repairing lacerated dura. Compound depressed skull fractures are immediately treated surgically. The scalp, skull, and devitalized brain are debrided, and the

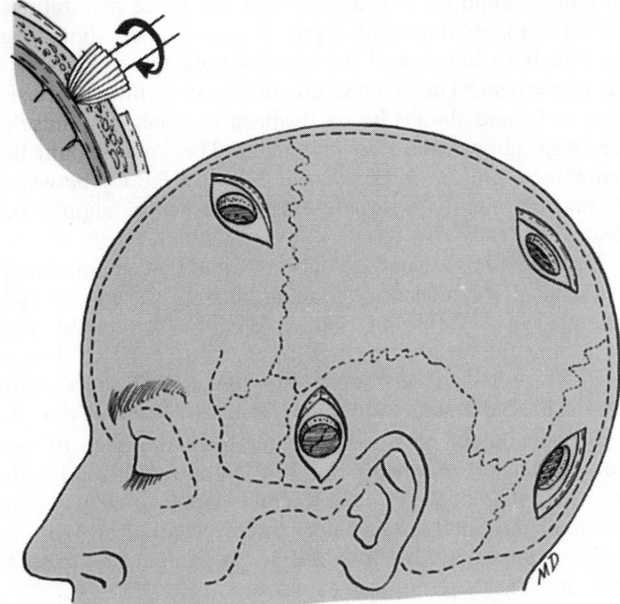

FIGURE 73–11 Placement of burr holes in the skull.

wound is cleaned thoroughly. Unless all foreign material is removed, a brain abscess or seizures may develop. Debridement of a penetrating wound or depressed skull fracture frequently leaves a cranial defect that is cosmetically unsightly. The defect may be surgically corrected by cranioplasty at a later time.

ICP is reduced as much as possible before surgery. Baseline neurologic data are documented. Informed consent needs to be obtained from the family if the patient is unconscious or confused. After surgery, provide nursing care for the client following the guidelines for craniotomy (see Chapter 69).

Self-Care

Clients with possible head injury or mild head injury were previously hospitalized for observation for a minimum of 6 hours (ideally for 48 hours) because of the risk of extradural hemorrhage. If the client is sent home, give clear instructions to help the client's caregiver assess for complications (see the accompanying Client Education Guide).

Rehabilitation

Most clients hospitalized for more than 48 hours because of a head injury ultimately require some rehabilitation. Clients with mild head injury may be overlooked in the population of people who need follow-up care. Mild head injuries can cause headache, memory difficulties, difficulty performing simple tasks, and irritability. These clinical manifestations may persist for a month or longer.

Rehabilitation may take place in an inpatient or outpatient setting, depending on the client's condition. Rehabilitation may include physical, occupational, speech, and cognitive therapy and is essential in returning the client to maximal function. Nurses play a major role in the rehabilitation of the head-injured client and in the education of significant others.

More severely injured clients may be sent to rehabilitation facilities with feeding tubes or tracheostomy tubes in place. Clients and families need assistance in choosing a new health care facility that can deliver the level of care needed. If recovery is unlikely, the client may need to be transferred to an extended-care facility. Because many head-injured clients are young, previously healthy people, placement in a nursing home may be a very difficult reality for family members to accept. Teaching and support can greatly improve coping. Involvement of disciplines such as social services, pastoral care, or discharge planning can increase the family members' understanding of the next phase of care.

The rehabilitation of clients with brain injuries is challenging. In some cases, community reintegration is unsuccessful. Studies have reported improvement in the client's ability to lead a productive life with the use of interdisciplinary techniques that include rehabilitation in cognition, compensatory techniques, social skills, emotional adjustment, leisure skills, physical fitness, and health maintenance. Most clients require 6 months in a rehabilitation program.[52]

Modifications for Elderly Clients

Although most head injuries do not occur in the elderly population, diagnosis is often more difficult in older adults because of an atypical presentation. These clients also experience more complications. An older client may be less able to tolerate respiratory problems or cardiac dysrhythmias. The presence of chronic diseases such as chronic obstructive pulmonary disease or heart failure can make managing ventilation and fluid balance more difficult. If any type of mental impairment was present before the injury, recovery to full independence is less likely. Poor stamina and medical complications may impede rehabilitation.

SPINAL CORD INJURY

Injury to the spinal cord can range in severity from mild flexion-extension "whiplash" injuries to complete transection of the cord with permanent quadriplegia. Trauma to

CLIENT EDUCATION GUIDE

Monitoring Family Members After Head Injury

Family Instructions

- Observe your family member for 24 hours.
- Take him or her to the hospital immediately if you notice any of the following:
  - Increased drowsiness or confusion
  - Inability to be awakened
  - Vomiting
  - Convulsions
  - Bleeding or drainage from the nose or ears
  - Weakness in either arm or leg
  - Loss of feeling in either arm or either leg
  - Blurring of vision
  - Slurring of speech
  - Enlargement or shrinkage of one pupil

the cord can occur at any level but most commonly occurs in the cervical and lower thoracic–upper lumbar vertebrae. This finding is due in part to the support given by the ribs to the thoracic spine and the flexibility of the cervical and lumbar spinal segments.

Although this discussion focuses on nursing management of *acute* spinal cord injury (SCI), it should be remembered that there are approximately 200,000 spinal cord–injured people living in the United States.

Etiology and Risk Factors

Trauma is the most common cause of SCI. Each year about 10,000 people sustain such injury. Most are males between the ages of 16 and 30 years. Nine per cent of injuries occur in people over the age of 60. Traumatic spinal cord injuries are most often caused by automobile or motorcycle accidents, gunshot or knife wounds, falls, and sports mishaps. Over half of all SCIs involve the cervical spine, and the rest occur in the thoracic, lumbar, and sacral spinal segments.

The feeling of immortality often experienced by adolescents and young adults contributes strongly to their risk of SCI. Young people may believe they can engage in dangerous behavior without being injured. The use of alcohol and illicit drugs can reinforce this belief in immortality. A young person who has experienced the devastation of SCI may best deliver the message of primary prevention. In several nationwide programs, head-injured and spinal cord–injured people are available to speak at school-sponsored educational programs.

Nontraumatic disorders may also result in SCI. These problems include the following:

- Cervical spondylosis with myelopathy (spinal canal narrowing with progressive injury to the cord and roots)
- Myelitis (infective or noninfective)
- Osteoporosis, causing vertebral compression fractures
- Syringomyelia (central cavitation of the cord)
- Tumors, both infiltrative and compressive
- Vascular diseases, usually infarction or hemorrhage

Whatever the cause, SCI produces distinctive and debilitating damage. Nowhere else in the body can a local insult produce such devastation in proportion to the extent of tissue involved.

FLEXION-ROTATION, DISLOCATION, AND FRACTURE-DISLOCATION INJURIES

By far the most common spinal cord injuries are flexion injuries. When a person strikes the head against the steering wheel or windshield, the spine is forced into acute hyperflexion (Fig. 73–12). Rupture of the posterior ligaments results in forward dislocation of the vertebrae. Blood vessels may be damaged, leading to ischemia of the spinal cord. The cervical spine, usually at the C5–6 level, is most commonly affected by a flexion injury. In the thoracic-lumbar spine, this type of injury is most frequently seen at the T12–L1 level.

HYPEREXTENSION INJURIES

Hyperextension injuries result after a fall in which the chin hits an object and the head is thrown back (see Fig. 73–12). The anterior ligament is ruptured, with fracture of the posterior elements of the vertebral body. Hyperextension of the spinal cord against the ligamentum flavum can lead to dorsal column contusion and posterior dislocation of the vertebrae. Complete transection of the cord can follow a hyperextension injury, although transection of the cord is rare. Clients who present with complete lesions of the spinal cord do not necessarily have transection of the cord. Complete lesions of the cord result in loss of all voluntary movement and sensation below the lesion and loss of reflex function in isolated segments of the cord.

COMPRESSION INJURIES

Compression injuries are often caused by falls or jumps in which the person lands directly on the head, sacrum, or feet (see Fig. 73–12). The force of impact fractures the vertebrae, and the fragments compress the cord. Disc and bone fragments may be propelled into the spinal cord upon impact. The lumbar and the lower thoracic vertebrae are the most commonly injured regions after a compression impact when the person lands on the feet. If the person lands on the head (as in diving into shallow water), the injury is to the cervical spine. About 50% of these injuries result in incomplete lesions. Incomplete lesions occur when some of the spinal tracts remain intact.

UNIQUE CERVICAL INJURIES

Three types of fractures are unique to the cervical spine (Fig. 73–13):

1. *Fractures of the odontoid process* (the odontoid process is the superior projection of the bone on C2) may be intact, with no detectable movement, or may be displaced, with movement and entrapment of the spinal cord.
2. A *hangman's fracture* is a bilateral fracture through the pedicles of C2, separating the posterior elements from the body of the vertebra.
3. The *Jefferson fracture* involves bursting of the ring of C1. The spinal canal usually widens.

These injuries are usually associated with other spinal injuries. Clients with these cervical fractures either die of the injury immediately or are stable and may walk into the emergency department reporting only neck pain.

Pathophysiology

SCIs most often occur as a result of injury to the vertebrae. The most common sites of injury are at the C1–2, C4–6, and T11–L2 vertebrae. These segments of the spine are the most mobile and therefore most easily injured.

The cord is injured as the result of acceleration, deceleration, or another force (e.g., impact) applied to the spine. The forces injure the spinal cord by compressing, pulling, or tearing the tissues. Microscopic bleeding occurs immediately after injury, primarily in the gray matter of the cord. Within the first hour, edema develops and often spreads along segments of the spinal cord. Arachidonic acid and its metabolites (prostaglandins, thromboxanes, and leukotrienes) cause edema. Cord edema peaks within 2 to 3 days and subsides within the first 7 days after injury. Although the site of the initial injury has the most edema and bleeding, some edema and bleeding extend at least for two cord segments on either side of the

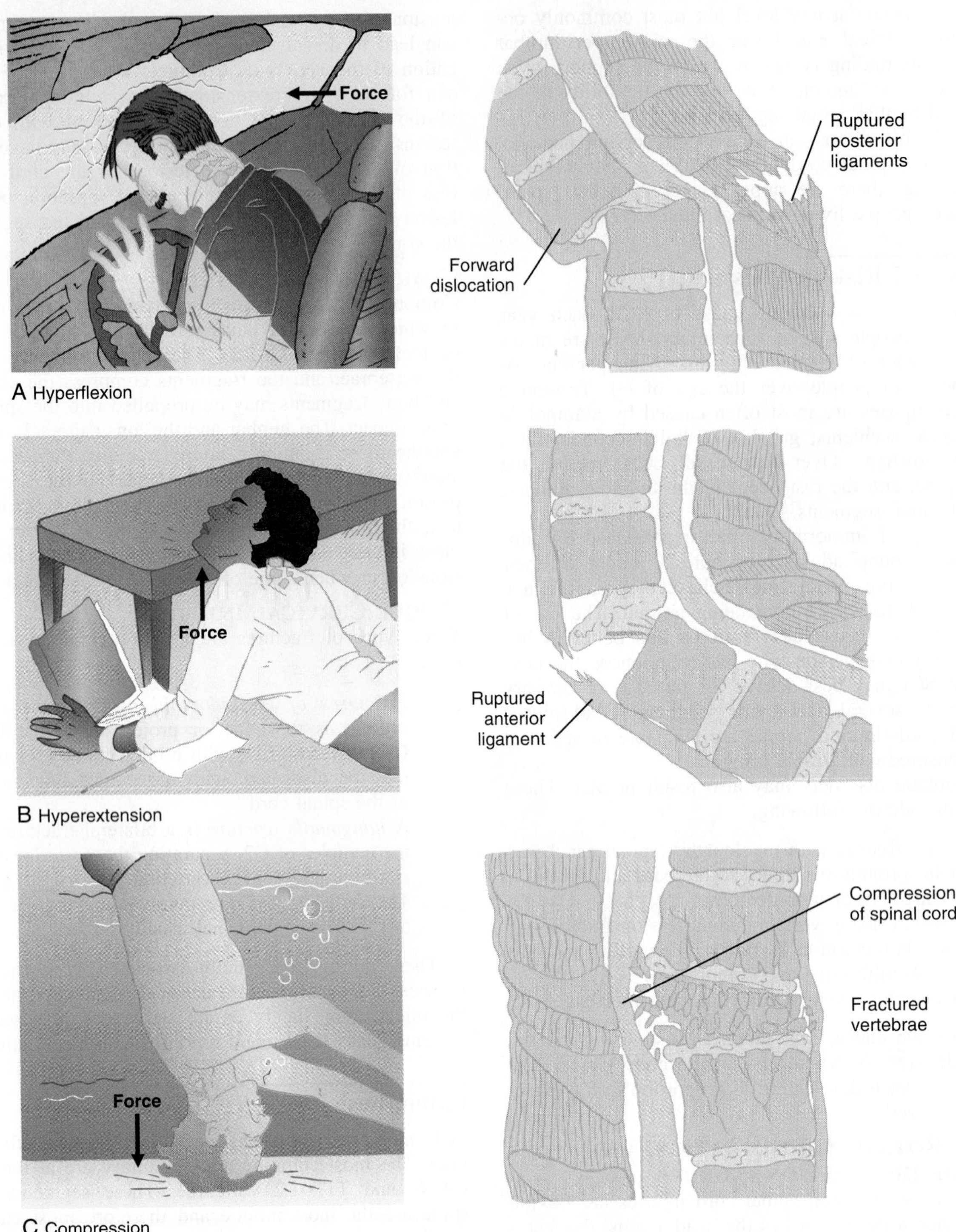

FIGURE 73–12 Patterns of cervical spine injury. *A,* Flexion injury of the cervical spine ruptures the posterior ligaments. *B,* Hyperextension injury of the cervical spine ruptures the anterior ligaments. *C,* Compression fractures crush the vertebrae and force bony fragments into the spinal canal.

injury. The edema of the cord leads to temporary loss of sensation and function. Spinal cord tissue injury is related to the initial insult, biochemical changes, and hemodynamic instability. Therefore, immediately after injury, it is not easy to determine the ultimate degree of permanent impairment.

Further changes include fragmentation of the axonal covering and loss of myelin. Phagocytic cells can injure surviving axons as they scavenge cellular debris. Chemotactic and inflammatory mediators further extend tissue necrosis. Macrophages engulf the spinal cord tissue and may cause a central cavity (called post-traumatic syringomyelia) to develop as early as 9 days after injury.

In addition, the oligodendroglial cells that support the cord are lost. Injury to the cord leads to rapid loss of axonal conduction from ion changes, such as very rapid

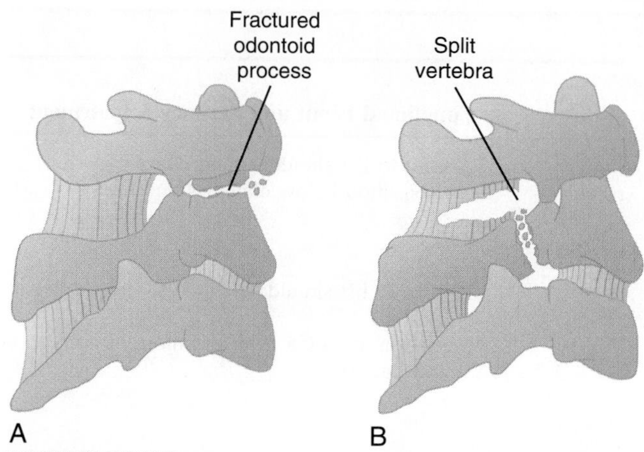

FIGURE 73–13 Fractures of the cervical spine. *A,* Odontoid fractures are fractures of the superior projection of C2 that normally projects into C1. Stabilization is required for healing. *B,* Hangman's fractures are of the pedicle of C2. The vertebra is split in half. These fractures are usually treated with a halo brace. A third type of cervical spine fracture called Jefferson's fracture is described in the text.

increases in extracellular potassium and influx of calcium into the cell. Finally, free radicals are produced. Free radicals are normally found in the body but are quickly controlled by antioxidant enzyme systems. When the antioxidant systems are overwhelmed, the free radicals damage tissues.

The physiologic response to SCI extends beyond changes within the spinal cord. For example, the sympathetic nervous system stress response results in reduced perfusion of the gastrointestinal tract and reduced production of gastric mucus to protect the lining. Ulceration and bleeding may develop.

Spasticity is the increased tone or contraction of muscles, producing stiff movements. Various CNS injuries or diseases such as SCI, cerebrovascular accidents, and cerebral palsy may result in spasticity. After SCI, the brain can no longer influence reflex movements through the spinal cord. Eventually, the lower part of the cord, using spinal reflexes, begins to work automatically. Spinal reflex activities include the flexor withdrawal reflex and reflex emptying of the bladder and bowel. These primitive spinal mechanisms, normally kept inactive by higher centers, are "released" when the normal inhibitions of the higher centers are destroyed. As recovery progresses, flexor responses are interspersed with extensor spasms. These movements ultimately develop into predominantly extensor activity. The client's limbs spasm into extension with movement. Spasticity may remain indefinitely or may gradually decrease over time.

Clinical Manifestations

Level of Injury

The initial clinical manifestations of acute SCI depend on the level and extent of injury to the cord. Below the level of injury or lesion, the following functions are lost:

- Voluntary movement
- Sensation of pain, temperature, pressure, and proprioception (ability to know where the body is in space)
- Bowel and bladder function
- Spinal and autonomic reflexes

The level of injury may be described in terms of (1) skeletal injury and (2) neurologic level of injury. Skeletal injury refers to the vertebral damage demonstrated by x-ray study. The criterion of the American Spinal Injury Association (ASIA) is useful in describing the level of spinal cord involvement: *The neurologic level of injury is the lowest segment of the spinal cord with bilateral intact sensory and motor function.* Assess sensory function according to dermatomes to identify the areas of skin with normal sensation. Motor function is measured by testing myotomes to identify muscles with active movement and full range of motion (ROM) against gravity. The ASIA Impairment Scale is:

- Normal with sensory and motor function preserved
- Incomplete with the majority of motor function preserved
- Incomplete with nonfunctional motor function preserved
- Incomplete with only sensation preserved
- Complete with loss of sensation and motor function

Injury to the cervical cord produces quadriplegia. Injuries above the C4 level may be fatal because of loss of innervation to the diaphragm and intercostal muscles. Without immediate rescue breathing after the accident, the injured person will die of respiratory failure. Today, with the general public's knowledge of cardiopulmonary resuscitation, many people survive this injury to the cervical spine. Injuries to the remainder of the cervical spine create specific patterns of motor loss (Table 73–2). Note that a person with a C7 injury is able to lift the shoulders, elbows, and wrists and has some hand function, but below C7 there remains no motor function or sensation.

Injuries to the thoracic or lumbar spinal segment produce paraplegia. People with such injuries have function in their upper extremities and can be mobile in a wheelchair or with crutches and braces. People with L5 injury can extend the great toe and dorsiflex the ankle. They have no sensation in the perianal area, calf, heel, or small toe.

Changes in Reflexes

Reflexes, which normally cross the spinal cord and return to the stimulated limb, are absent in early SCI because of spinal cord edema. Blood pressure and temperature in denervated (without nervous function or innervation) areas fall markedly and respond poorly to reflex stimuli.

After cord edema subsides, some body functions may return by reflex (e.g., control of the urinary bladder), but they lack integration with other visceral activities. Visceral activities may be initiated by atypical stimuli. For example, scratching the skin may cause vasodilation, sweating, and urination. Nervous system lesions may produce a type of defective urinary bladder function known as *cord bladder.* For example, stimulation of the skin on the lower abdomen or thighs may cause reflex urination. This form of cord bladder is called an *automatic bladder.* Such stimulation may also cause reflex ejaculation and priapism (persistent abnormal penile erection without sexual desire) in paralyzed men.

TABLE 73–2 SPINAL CORD INJURY AND IMPAIRMENT

Level of Injury	Functional Limit and Sensory Impairment
C5	Ability to lift shoulders and elbows (partial) No sensation below clavicles
C6	Ability to lift shoulders, elbows, and wrists (partial) Sensation as in C5 level but more in arms and thumbs
C7	Ability to lift shoulders, elbows, wrists, and hands (partial) Sensation as in C6 level with more in arms and middle fingers
C8	Ability to lift shoulders, elbows, wrists, and hands (partial) Sensation as in C7 level with more in arms and little fingers
T4	Ability to use arms and hands normally No sensation below nipple line
T6	Ability to use intercostal muscles No sensation below sixth intercostal space
L2	Ability to use abdominal muscles and flex hips No sensation below midanterior thigh level or in perianal area

Muscle Spasms

Intense and painful muscular spasms of the lower extremities occur following a traumatic complete transverse spinal cord lesion. In assisting the client and the family members to understand these movements, it should be explained that these muscle spasms are involuntary and do not mean that voluntary movement is returning. This information, although disappointing, is essential.

Muscle spasms range in intensity from mild muscular twitching to vigorous mass reflexogenic states. Extreme, involuntary muscle spasms can actually throw a client out of bed or wheelchair. Bed side rails are kept up and restraining straps are comfortably secured over the client lying on a stretcher. Muscle spasms, often aggravated by cold weather, prolonged periods of sitting, or emotionally upsetting events, may become intolerable. Reflex spasms may be triggered by extrinsic or visceral stimuli, such as a distended bladder.

Emotion (e.g., anxiety, crying, anger, laughing) or cutaneous stimulation (e.g., tickling, stroking, pinching) may initiate spastic movements. By learning to recognize events that trigger such reflex spasms, the client may use these potentially annoying movements to achieve functional activities such as urination.

Autonomic Dysreflexia

Autonomic dysreflexia, also known as autonomic hyperreflexia, is a life-threatening syndrome. It is a cluster of clinical manifestations that results when multiple spinal cord autonomic responses discharge simultaneously. This syndrome, observed in as many as 85% of clients with cord injury above the T6 level, can occur anytime after spinal shock has resolved. Dysreflexia often resolves 3 years after injury, but it may recur. The manifestations of autonomic dysreflexia result from an exaggerated sympathetic response to a noxious stimulus below the level of the cord lesion. Common stimuli are bladder and bowel distention but may also be pressure ulcers, spasms, pain, pressure on the penis, excessive rectal stimulation, bladder stones, ingrown toenails, abdominal abnormalities, or uterine contractions.

Exaggerated sympathetic responses cause the blood vessels below the level of injury to constrict. As a result, the client develops hypertension (with pressures possibly as high as 300 mm Hg), a pounding headache, flushing above the level of the lesion, nasal stuffiness, diaphoresis, piloerection ("gooseflesh"), dilated pupils with blurred vision, bradycardia (30 to 40 beats per minute [BPM]), restlessness, and nausea. The manifestations are a result of compensatory efforts to overcome the severe hypertension. Initially, baroreceptors sense the hypertensive stimuli and stimulate the parasympathetic nervous system, which results in vasodilation above the level of cord injury (headache, flushing) and bradycardia. The problem is that the visceral and peripheral vessels do not dilate because the efferent impulses cannot pass through the damaged cord. Thus, the overall effect is one of extreme hypertension. Seizures and cerebral hemorrhage occur in approximately 10% to 15% of cases. See the later discussion on Risk for Autonomic Dysreflexia for interventions.

Clinical Syndromes Causing Partial Paralysis

Five spinal cord syndromes cause partial paralysis (Fig. 73–14): central cord syndrome, anterior cord syndrome, Brown-Séquard syndrome, conus medullaris syndrome, and cauda equina syndrome. Each has distinctive neurologic features.

Central Cord Syndrome. Central cord syndrome (most common with hyperextension-hyperflexion injuries) produces more weakness in the upper extremities than in the lower. This type of injury occurs most often in the older adult who has a pre-existing spinal stenosis. This injury may also occur in a person who lands on the head such as when diving into shallow water and hitting the bottom. The common mechanism of injury is a fall forward. The weakness is caused by edema and hemorrhage in the central area of the cord, which is predominantly occupied by nerve tracts to the hands and arms.

Anterior Cord Syndrome. A lesion in the anterior spinal cord causes anterior cord syndrome, with complete motor function loss and decreased pain sensation. Deep pressure, position sense, and two-point discrimination sensations remain intact. Often the anterior spinal artery is affected, causing an infarction of spinal cord tissue. Cervical cord concussion may produce various degrees of motor and sensory deficit, which completely resolve within hours. Occasionally, cervical cord trauma produces only root injuries, which may paralyze isolated muscles or muscle groups in the arms and shoulders. These deficits are usually permanent.

Brown-Séquard Syndrome. Brown-Séquard syndrome is caused by lateral hemisection of the cord (i.e., when half the cord is cut or otherwise damaged), as a bullet wound or knife wound. This injury results in ipsilateral motor paralysis, loss of vibratory and position sense, and contralateral loss of pain and temperature sensation.

Conus Medullaris Syndrome. Conus medullaris syndrome follows damage to the lumbar nerve roots and the conus medullaris in the spinal cord. The client usually has bowel and bladder areflexia and flaccid lower extremities. The bulbospongiosis penile (erection) and micturition reflexes may be preserved when damage is limited to the upper sacral segments of the spinal cord.

Cauda Equina Syndrome. Injury to the lumbosacral nerve roots below the conus medullaris results in the cauda equina syndrome. The client experiences areflexia of the bowel, bladder, and lower extremities.

Spinal Shock

The immediate response to cord transection is called *spinal shock.* The client with SCI experiences complete loss of skeletal muscle function, bowel and bladder tone, sexual function, and autonomic reflexes. Loss of venous return and hypotension also occur. The hypothalamus cannot control temperature by vasoconstriction and increased metabolism; therefore, the client's body assumes the environmental temperature. Spinal shock is most severe in clients with higher levels of SCI. Clients with thoracic or lumbar injuries are often unaffected owing to the sparing of the sympathetic nervous system with these levels of injury.

Spinal shock may last for 1 to 6 weeks. Indications that spinal shock is resolving include return of reflexes, development of hyperreflexia rather than flaccidity, and return of reflex emptying of the bladder. The earliest reflexes recovered are the flexor reflexes evoked by noxious cutaneous stimulation. The return of the bulbospongiosus reflex in male patients is also an early indicator of recovery from spinal shock. Babinski's reflex (dorsiflexion of the great toe with fanning of the other toes when the sole of the foot is stroked) is an early-returning reflex.

Diagnostic Findings

Initially, full spinal x-ray films are obtained. If a high-level cervical lesion is suspected, films of the odontoid bone viewed through the open mouth may be required. CT scans may be obtained after the client has achieved hemodynamic and ventilatory stabilization. These studies provide more information regarding the nature of fractures and the status of the spinal cord. They are also useful when a fracture is not seen on x-ray films but neurologic deficit is present. MRI may also be used to locate the level of the lesion. Although controversial, myelography may be used if SCI is suspected and the degree of deficit is increasing. Somatosensory evoked potentials (SSEPs) are used to establish the extent of injury and are often performed within 48 hours of admission.

Outcome Management

Both the initial (especially during the first hour after injury) and long-term interventions provided for a client who has sustained an SCI significantly influence the following:

- The extent of the injury and associated deficits
- How well the person survives the acute phase of injury
- The success of recovery and rehabilitation

People with SCI can lead productive and, in many cases, independent lives. As with head injury, information

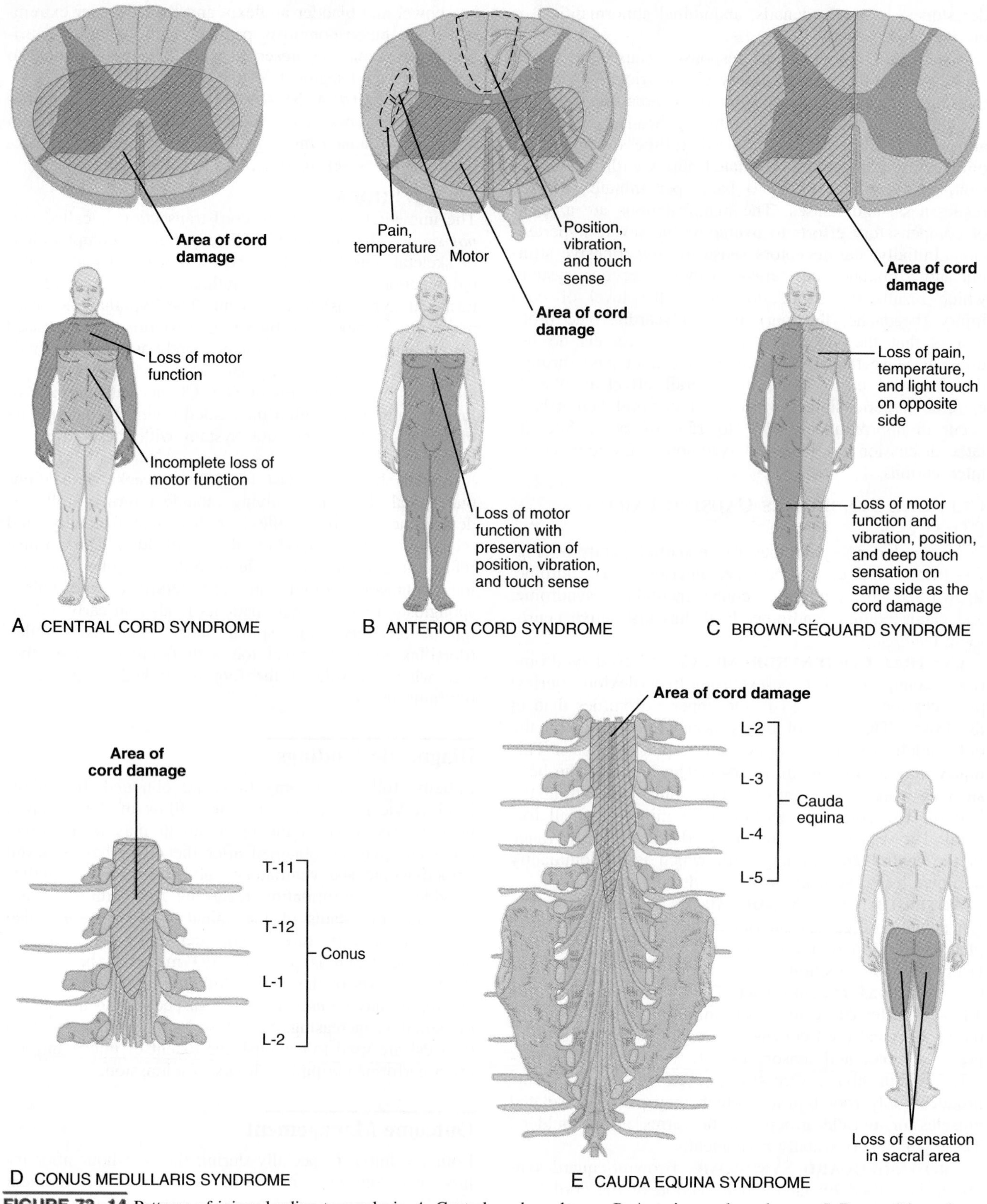

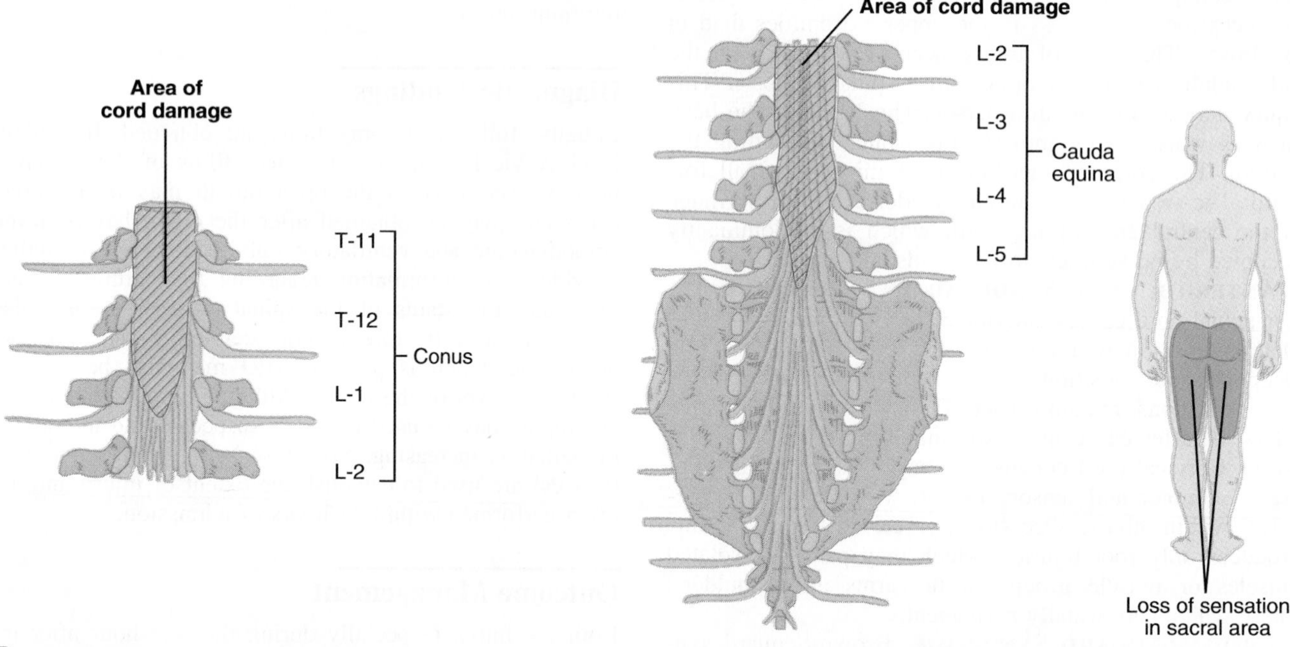

FIGURE 73–14 Patterns of injury leading to paralysis. *A,* Central cord syndrome. *B,* Anterior cord syndrome. *C,* Brown-Séquard syndrome. *D,* Conus medullaris syndrome. *E,* Cauda equina syndrome.

obtained from witnesses to the accident can assist in diagnosis and treatment. Information from witnesses or the client should include mechanism of injury, presence and duration of loss of consciousness, and impairment of motor function. It is also important to diagnose SCI correctly. Delays in diagnosis can be attributed to alcohol intoxication, concomitant head injury, or other multiple injuries.

Initial Care

At the scene of the accident, the injured person should be moved only when there are adequate numbers of people to accomplish this with immobilization of the spine. The neck should be stabilized in a neutral position without flexion or extension until a fixed immobilizing device can be applied. Cervical traction should not be applied. Without x-ray films to guide movements, the spinal cord can be injured. The simplest method of immobilizing the spine is to place the affected person on a spine board and to secure the spine with a hard collar around the neck and self-fastening ties across the torso and legs. Transparent stiff collars have become popular because they allow visualization of the carotid arteries and trachea. Excellent on-the-scene care has increased the number of persons who are neurologically intact despite vertebral column fractures.[28] Accurate reporting of the person's baseline deficits is essential to help the physician plan the aggressiveness of treatment interventions.

Spinal trauma is often associated with other injuries such as head injury, chest trauma, extremity fractures, and abdominal injury. Anyone who has sustained multiple trauma should be handled as if spinal injuries were present until assessment proves otherwise. In handling a client suspected of having a cervical spine injury, the spine is kept in neutral alignment and flexion is prevented.

If turning is required, a *logrolling* maneuver is used. The client is placed in a supine position on a firm surface. The head is supported in alignment with the body and is immobilized with a firm, padded cervical collar. Some physicians use halter traction immediately to keep the cervical spine aligned and prevent movement. Clothing is cut off rather than removed. The client is transported on a flat, firm stretcher with the neck immobilized. SCI-trained personnel should remain with the client while x-ray studies are taken to ensure that the cervical spine is not moved.

Cervical spine injury may produce respiratory distress. When difficulty breathing is noted, immediate action is taken to maintain a patent airway and to provide adequate oxygenation. It is important that the client's neck not be hyperextended during intubation; therefore, the jaw thrust technique is used. Suctioning is performed as necessary to maintain a patent airway. Mechanically assisted ventilation is required when definite loss or impairment of respiratory muscle function occurs. Respiratory parameters can be used to guide a decision to mechanically ventilate the client. Serial decreases in vital capacity along with an increase in partial pressure of arterial carbon dioxide ($PaCO_2$) constitute a good predictor of impending pulmonary failure. A vital capacity of less than 15 ml/kg is cause for serious concern.

In the emergency department, a client who has sustained a severe cervical injury should be placed immediately in skeletal traction to immobilize the cervical spine and reduce the fracture and dislocation. Gardner-Wells tongs are inserted through the outer table of the skull (Fig. 73–15). Traction is applied to the tongs via rope, pulleys, and weights. Traction weight is begun with 10 to 20 pounds (4.5 to 9.1 kg) and is gradually increased to accomplish bone reduction. When proper alignment is obtained and verified by x-ray examination, the traction weight may be lessened to maintain the reduction. Traction is not used to stabilize and immobilize thoracic or lumbar spinal fractures or fracture-dislocations because there is no effective way to provide it. Therefore, the spine is kept in alignment, and logrolling is used as needed, until surgical stabilization can be performed.

A cross-table lateral x-ray film of the cervical spine is obtained before transport of the injured person. Lateral and anteroposterior x-ray studies are not usually sufficient. To visualize lower cervical fractures, it is necessary to either apply downward traction to the arms or have the arms in the swimmer's position during x-ray examination.

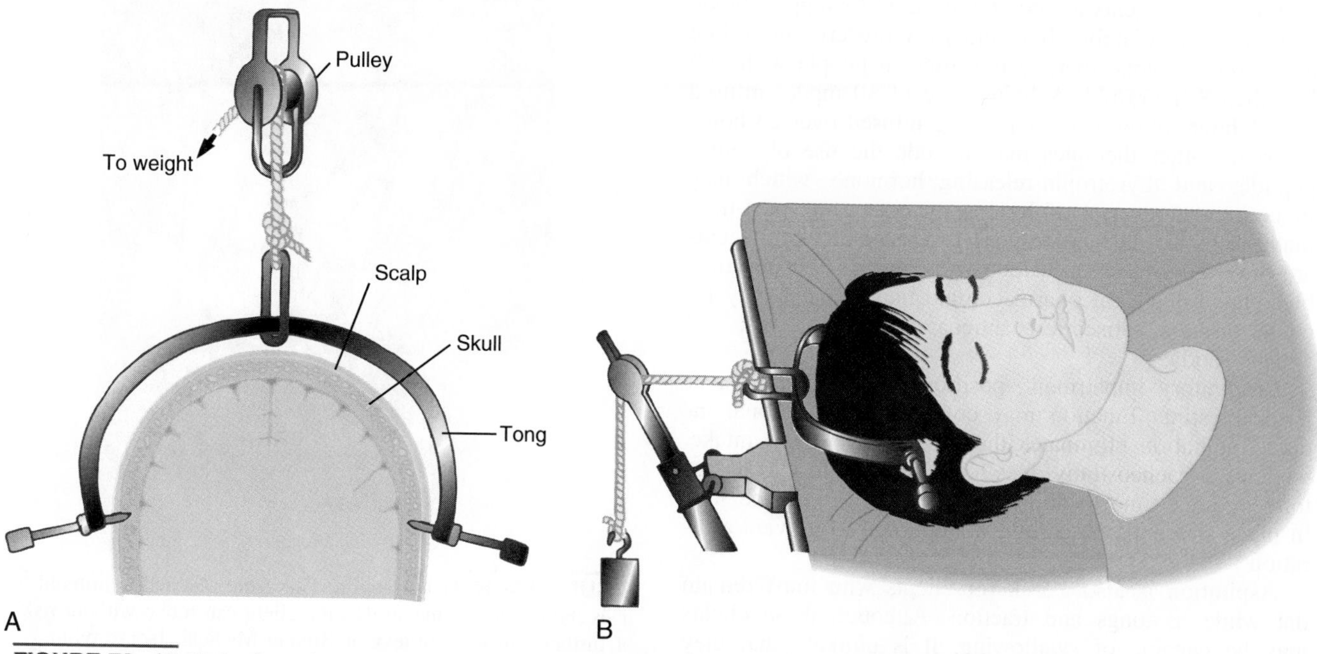

FIGURE 73–15 Skeletal traction for cervical injuries. *A,* Crutchfield tongs. *B,* Gardner-Wells tongs.

If a high-level cervical lesion is suspected, a view of the odontoid bone through the open mouth may be required. A brief but thorough neurologic examination is made to assess the extent of injury and to establish a baseline of function and involvement for later comparison.

Common emergency interventions include insertion of an IV line and infusion of normal saline, insertion of an indwelling catheter, administration of high-dose steroids, administration of vasoactive medications to maintain systolic blood pressure, insertion of a nasogastric tube, and provision of oxygen if oxygen saturation is low.

Once orthopedic and medical stabilization of the fracture has been achieved, the client is transferred to an ICU or to an SCI center. It is important that the client be appropriately immobilized before transport.

Medical Management

Once the client's spine and emergency medical conditions have been stabilized, a complete neurologic assessment is performed. Several associated injuries are commonly seen with SCI. These include orthopedic injury to the spine, head injury, chest injury, abdominal injury, and genitourinary injury. Some of these injuries may not be immediately evident in the emergency department, and ongoing assessments are made until the problem is ruled out.

The client is monitored for spinal shock and the effects of hypotension, bradycardia, and decreased cardiac output. Respiratory compromise may occur if the client develops diaphragmatic fatigue; mechanical ventilation may be needed. Arterial blood gases are monitored closely. The client may be transferred to a kinetic treatment bed to reduce the risk of pressure ulcer development, improve pulmonary function, and minimize complications of immobility. These beds are shown in Chapter 68, Figure 68–5.

Potential complications include atelectasis, pneumonia, bradycardia, hypotension, deep vein thrombosis, gastrointestinal bleeding, pressure ulcers, joint contractures, and psychological dysfunction such as denial and depression.

Vasoactive agents are commonly used to support blood pressure immediately after injury. Short-term high-dose methylprednisolone therapy is started in people with SCI less than 8 hours old. A bolus dose of 30 mg/kg infused over 1 hour followed by 5.4 mg/kg infused over 23 hours is usual. Other therapies may include the use of neuropeptides and thyrotropin-releasing hormone, which may induce some reversal of lesions by decreasing post-traumatic ischemia. Histamine-2 (H_2) receptor-blocking agents are often given to reduce the risk of gastric and intestinal bleeding. Long-term pharmacologic management may include urinary antiseptics, anticoagulants, laxatives, and antispasmodics.

Respiratory impairment, position, emotional status, or gastrointestinal function may compromise nutritional intake. Intubation eliminates the possibility of oral intake, whereas a tracheostomy does not. Clients with a tracheostomy require time to adjust to swallowing with the tube in place and must be carefully monitored to prevent aspiration.

Aspiration is also a risk for clients who must remain flat while in tongs and traction. Although these clients may be capable of swallowing, it is unlikely that they will be able to safely consume enough food to meet their metabolic needs. Clients wearing a halo jacket (Fig. 73–16) often experience difficulty eating because the halo jacket immobilizes the head. They should be encouraged to take small bites, eat slowly, and concentrate on swallowing.

Depression is a common reaction to SCI and may be associated with inhibition of the appetite. Choosing when and what to eat may be one of the few areas of control left to the person with SCI. As much free choice of dietary intake as is feasible should be encouraged.

Any of these conditions can severely limit a spinal injury client's oral intake at a time when a high-calorie, high-protein diet is needed. Enteral feeding or total parenteral hyperalimentation is often prescribed until oral intake is sufficient to meet the body's needs.

Initial Nursing Management of the Client with Spinal Cord Injury

ASSESSMENT

A holistic assessment approach is essential in planning for nursing care of clients with SCI. Every system of the body is affected with these injuries. A complete baseline assessment is obtained initially. The results of subsequent assessments are then compared with the baseline results. Specific components in the assessment of the client with an SCI depend on the client's phase of treatment. Therefore, assessment is addressed within the following sections.

Careful monitoring of hemodynamic parameters is essential. Heart rate, blood pressure, temperature, respirations, fluid balance, and peripheral oxygen saturation (as determined by pulse oximetry) should be monitored continuously.

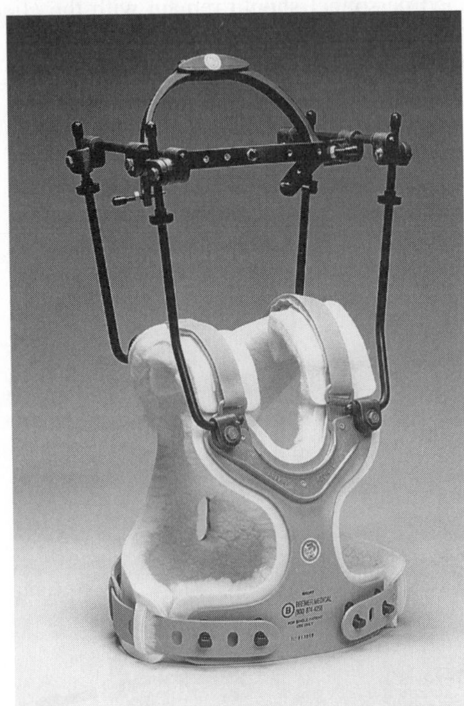

FIGURE 73–16 Halo traction. This form of traction immobilizes the cervical spine so that the client can move without risk of further injury. (Courtesy of Bremer Medical, Jacksonville, FL.)

If the client is conscious, ask whether there is any pain. Determining whether the client can feel a touch or a pinprick in the feet, legs, trunk, hands, and arms tests sensation. Levels of sensation are documented according to dermatomes. To assess motor function, ask the client to wiggle toes, move ankles, flex knees, and move hands and arms. The location, symmetry, and strength of muscle movement are documented (Table 73–3). The major reflexes—that is, the Achilles, patellar, biceps, and triceps tendon reflexes—are briefly tested. Assessment for intact sensation in areas such as the perineum is also necessary. If the patient is unresponsive, assessment is more limited. Assess respiratory status by observing for spontaneous movement and thorax expansion. Sensation and movement of extremities are assessed by watching the client for a few moments or by applying a painful stimulus (nail bed pressure) and observing for withdrawal.

Usually the client is awake and may be concerned about obtaining pain relief, the chances of survival, and the safety of any other people in the accident. Once these issues are addressed, the client may begin to appraise the severity of his or her own injury.

Rehabilitation begins when the client is admitted to the acute health care facility. During the acute stage, nursing and medical attention is appropriately focused on immediate needs. However, it is also imperative to remember that the client probably will have severe residual disabilities and must make major lifestyle changes. Care provided in the acute period can significantly affect the client's later life. Prevention of complications such as infection, pressure sores, and contractures facilitates rehabilitation and reduces suffering, disability, and expense. Challenges in care of clients with SCI is presented in the Case Study.

DIAGNOSIS, OUTCOMES, INTERVENTIONS

Risk for Hypotension. Clients suffering from SCI are at risk for the development of hypotension. The collaborative problem of *Risk for Hypotension* is related to vasodilation and the inability to vasoconstrict, rather than to volume depletion.

Outcomes. Expected outcomes for collaborative problems address actions of the nurse, rather than client outcomes. The problem is within the physician's domain; therefore, nurses monitor for it.

The nurse will monitor for hypotension. The client will have no manifestations of pulmonary fluid overload. The client's systolic blood pressure will remain greater than 90 mm Hg. The heart rate will be maintained at more than 60 BPM.

Interventions. Hypotension associated with spinal shock is initially treated with IV fluid. It is important to remember that fluid depletion is not the cause of hypotension; rather, lack of reflexes is the cause. Therefore, fluid resuscitation should be carefully monitored to avoid fluid overload, which can lead to pulmonary edema. Vasopressor agents are often given in the acute phase of SCI to maintain blood pressure.

TABLE 73–3 MOTOR ASSESSMENT AFTER SPINAL CORD INJURY

Spinal Nerve(s)	Assessment Technique
C4–5	Shoulders are shrugged against downward pressure of examiner's hands
C5–6	Arm is pulled up from resting position against resistance
C7	From the flexed position, arm is straightened out against resistance
C7	Index finger is held firmly to thumb against resistance to pull it away
C8	Hand grasp strength is evaluated
L2–4	Leg is lifted from the bed against resistance
L2–4	From flexed position, knee is extended against resistance
L5–S1	Knee is flexed against resistance
L5	Foot is pulled up toward nose against resistance
S1	Foot is pushed down (as in stepping on automobile gas pedal) against resistance

Inability to Sustain Spontaneous Ventilation, Ineffective Airway Clearance, Impaired Gas Exchange. Cervical-level SCI carries a high risk of respiratory compromise. Any or all three of these nursing diagnoses may be appropriate.

Outcomes. The client will show no signs of respiratory compromise, as evidenced by clear lung sounds; PaO_2, PCO_2, pH, and oxygen saturation values within normal limits; unlabored respirations; and normal vital capacity.

Interventions. Chest physical therapy can help mobilize secretions and prevent pneumonia, as can suctioning and assisted coughing. When spinal cord edema has temporarily impaired respiratory function, mechanical ventilation is used to support respiration. Intubation and ventilation can be frightening to a person who has been able to breathe independently. Provide reassurance that mechanical ventilation will probably not be permanent. Clients may also be placed on a kinetic bed in order to maximize pulmonary function. Sedation is administered as needed after intubation.

For extended airway management, a tracheostomy may be required to allow for long-term controlled ventilation, to facilitate the removal of tracheobronchial secretions, and to seal off the esophagus from the trachea for the prevention of aspiration. An abdominal binder is often used to provide abdominal support, to facilitate diaphragmatic breathing, and to increase venous return.

Risk for Aspiration. Clients with a tracheostomy or ineffective airway clearance or in whom the gag reflex is absent are at higher risk for aspiration. Aspiration is a common cause of morbidity in spinal cord–injured clients.

Outcomes. The client will exhibit no signs of aspiration, as evidenced by clear lung sounds; absence of stridor and fever; minimal amounts of clear mucus upon suctioning; and PaO_2, $PaCO_2$, pH, and oxygen saturation values within normal limits.

Interventions. Suctioning equipment should be kept available and breath sounds assessed every 1 or 2 hours in acutely ill clients. The results of arterial blood gas analysis and pulse oximetry are monitored to determine the degree of oxygenation provided with mechanical ven-

Spinal Cord Injury

Ben Brown is a 21-year-old college junior who was admitted to the intensive care unit (ICU) via the emergency department for evaluation and treatment of a spinal cord injury (SCI) sustained in a diving accident. Consider the type of fracture most typical from this kind of accident. He is accompanied by his fiancée and his parents.

Admission Orders

Admit to ICU
Routine vital signs
Neurologic checks every hour for 24 hours
Bed rest; may logroll side to side
Maintain position of hard cervical collar
NPO status
Foley catheter with dependent drainage
IV Decadron 10 mg now and 4 mg every 4 hours
No sedation
CT scan of head and neck without contrast agent

Skeletal tongs are applied at the bedside, and cervical traction is instituted.

Nursing Admission Assessment

Ben is awake, alert, and cooperative. He has no known allergies. He states that he is an engineering major in college and is planning to be married this spring. His fiancée is an elementary education major. During the assessment, Ben makes several jokes and does not talk about or ask about his lack of sensation or movement below the nipple line. Consider the level of spinal injury that would be reflected by these manifestations.

Nursing Physical Assessment

Height: 6′2″ Weight: 170 lb (77.3 kg)
Vital signs: BP 150/90 TPR 97.6 90 22
LOC: Alert and oriented ×3
EENT: PERRLA
Cardiac: Sinus rhythm without ectopic beats, S_1 and S_2 readily audible without rubs or murmur
Pulmonary: Lung sounds clear bilaterally, diminished from the mid-lung fields to the bases
Abdominal: Abdomen is flat with active bowel sounds in all four quadrants
Genitourinary: Foley catheter in place and draining clear straw-colored urine
Peripheral pulses: 2/2, without edema noted

The CT scan reveals a compression fracture at C6 with multiple bone fragments in the spinal canal. There is no evidence of transection of the spinal cord. Consider the alternatives available to Ben for treatment of this type of injury. Ben continues to display lack of sensation and movement below the nipple line. Yesterday, Ben pushed his lunch tray on the floor and threw a flower vase at the wall. Ben's fiancée left the room in tears and stated: "The wedding is off." Consider the stage of grieving in which these manifestations might occur.

Ben is fitted for a halo brace and is scheduled to be transferred to a regional rehabilitation facility at the end of the week: "Oh, great—I'm being turfed to the freak ward." Consider the possible responses to this remark that Ben's nurse could make.

Discharge and Post-treatment Considerations

Average length of stay: 4.6 days in acute care facility followed by rehabilitation stay dictated by client's rehabilitation potential
Client transfer sheet: include most current assessment, medical treatment plan and previous laboratory work, and radiology reports
Community referrals: SCI support group, social services referral for home care or assisted living arrangements after discharge

Questions to Be Considered

1. This morning Ben complained of an excruciating headache, and BP was 210/110. Identify the etiologic factors that might cause these manifestations and the nursing interventions.
2. Compare and contrast the sensory and motor deficits expected for various levels of SCI. Include C1–2, C4–6, T4–6, L1–5, and S1–5 in your discussion. Identify the rehabilitation potential and priority nursing actions for each of these categories.
3. Identify the teaching on sexual function that is necessary for clients with SCI. When should this teaching begin?
4. Identify the key nursing actions for clients in skeletal traction for cervical injuries. Compare these nursing actions with those given after treatment for these injuries.
5. Consider the risks and benefits of halo traction versus spinal fusion for the treatment of cervical injuries.
6. Compare and contrast the nursing roles and priorities of the acute or critical care nurse and the rehabilitation nurse in caring for clients with SCI.
7. Compare and contrast the traumatic and nontraumatic disorders that may result in SCI. Consider how the source of the injury may influence nursing care.

BP, blood pressure; CT, computed tomography; EENT, eye-ear-nose-throat; IV, intravenous; LOC, level of consciousness; LOS, length of stay; NPO, nothing by mouth; PERRLA, pupils equal, round, and reactive to light and accommodation; TPR, temperature, pulse, respirations.

tilation or supplemental oxygen administration. Tracheobronchial suctioning is performed frequently to prevent or reduce the accumulation of secretions from immobility, lack of a cough reflex, or pneumonia. Monitor the electrocardiogram for dysrhythmias (e.g., premature ventricular contractions) due to hypoxia during suctioning.

Ineffective Thermoregulation. Thermoregulation may be altered because of loss of hypothalamic control of the sympathetic nervous system in clients with SCI above the T6 level.

Outcome. The client will maintain normothermic status.

Interventions. Rectal or core temperature is monitored every 4 hours during the first 72 hours after injury. Skin surfaces are palpated for areas of warmth, coolness, and moisture. Control the environmental temperature by using bed linens as needed to warm the client, eliminating drafts in the room, and using hypothermia blankets cautiously.

EVALUATION

The problems identified in the early period of SCI care should resolve within 72 hours, especially if there are no other serious injuries or medical problems. If the client remains in an ICU for a prolonged time, implement other aspects of SCI care as discussed later on.

Surgical Management

Surgical intervention for progressive neurologic deficit is indicated for any of the following:

- Compound fractures and penetrating wounds of the spine
- Presence of bone fragments in the spinal canal
- Syndrome of acute anterior spinal cord trauma[37]

Some neurosurgeons and orthopedic surgeons recommend decompressive laminectomy for complete SCIs. In this type of surgery, the laminae of the vertebrae are removed to minimize pressure on the spinal cord. Others believe that laminectomy should not be used routinely to treat SCI. Similarly, some surgeons recommend stabilization by surgical fusion within the first few days after trauma, whereas others do not. Insertion of metal plates and screws or the use of bone grafts or a combination of these accomplishes fusion.

Cervical fractures can also be allowed to heal with stabilization of bone fragments achieved by immobilization in a brace or halo jacket (see Fig. 73–16). The halo jacket has a ring that is fixed to the skull with pins. This ring is then attached to the jacket by rods. This system provides the traction required to maintain cervical alignment. A halo jacket allows early mobilization and rehabilitation. The wrench that comes with the brace should always be taped to the front of the jacket, to allow quick removal in case of emergency. Never grasp the rods to help reposition the client. If the client has some mobility remaining, always assist during the client's first attempt at any activity. The halo jacket changes the client's center of gravity, making falls a constant risk. Perform pin site care around the pin insertion sites daily. Refer to your agency's policy manual for guidelines.

Burst fractures of the thoracic and lumbar spinal segments can be treated with body casts, Harrington rods, or other devices for spine stabilization. Spine stabilization devices are commonly inserted through a posterior incision (Fig. 73–17). After the operation, perform the usual postoperative assessments, including an assessment of the neurovascular status of the legs. Chest tubes and nasogastric tubes are inserted during surgery. The client is logrolled to facilitate maintenance of respiration and skin perfusion. Pain is managed with continuous-infusion or injected narcotics. The client usually is fitted for a body brace, and mobilization begins on the fourth day.

Complications of surgery include infection and poor wound healing, as well as those related to anesthesia. Both infection and impaired wound healing are more likely to occur in a malnourished client.

Spinal Cord Injury Rehabilitation

In 1970, the United States Rehabilitation Service Administration adopted a model system for rehabilitation of spinal cord–injured people. The key to the system is the use of multidisciplinary teams of physicians, nurses, and allied health care providers (physical therapists, occupational therapists, speech and language pathologists) to reduce morbidity, maximize functional recovery, and promote independence.

ESTABLISH FUNCTIONAL GOALS

Prediction of functional ability after SCI can generally be guided by the degree of residual muscle function (Table 73–4). Clients with all levels of injury and of all ages benefit from rehabilitation. The client and family are involved in all phases. The client delegates needed skills to another caregiver so that care can be provided at home. The skills learned in a rehabilitation setting must be adapted to the home environment and community setting before hospital discharge. This process can be accomplished by use of therapeutic weekend passes and partici-

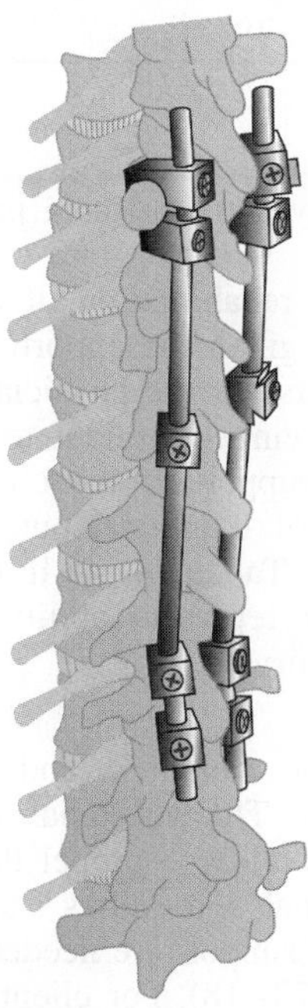

FIGURE 73–17 Fractures of the spine are often stabilized with internal fixation devices.

TABLE 73–4 **FUNCTIONAL GOALS IN REHABILITATION AFTER SPINAL CORD INJURY**

Spinal Cord Level	Muscle Function	Functional Goals
C1–2	No phrenic nerve function	Respirations managed with phrenic pacemaker
C3–4	Neck control; scapular elevators; diaphragm function may be weak or absent	Manipulate electric wheelchair with breath control, chin control, or voice activation
C5	Fair to good shoulder control; functional deltoids/biceps; elbow flexion	Dress upper trunk; turn self in bed with or without arm slings Propel wheelchair with hand splints or after tenodesis Assist in getting into and out of bed May learn to write or type
C6	Good shoulder control; wrist extension; supinators	Dress upper trunk; sometimes dress lower trunk Propel wheelchair with hand rim projections Self-feeding with hand splints Transfer from wheelchair to bed with or without minimal assistance (e.g., sliding board) Assist in getting to and from bedside commode; self-catheterization
C7	Possibly weak shoulder depression; weak elbow extension; some hand function; triceps	Independent in transfer to bed, car, and toilet Total dressing independence Propel wheelchair with standard hand rims Self-feeding with no assistive devices
T1–4	Good to normal upper extremity muscle function; intrinsic muscles of the hand; no trunk control	Independent in transfer to bed, car, and toilet Total dressing independence Propel wheelchair with standard hand rims Self-feeding with no assistive devices Transfer from wheelchair to floor and return Propel wheelchair up and down curb Transfer from wheelchair to tub and return
T5–L2	Partial to good trunk stability	Total wheelchair independence Limited ambulation with bilateral long leg braces and crutches (injury at T12 or below)
L3–4	All trunk-pelvic stabilizers intact; hip flexors, adductors, quadriceps	Ambulation with short leg braces with or without crutches, depending on level of injury
L5–S3	Hip extensors, abductors; knee flexors; ankle control	No equipment needed if plantiflexion is strong enough for push-off at end of stance

pation in community activities as a part of the rehabilitation process.

In all phases of rehabilitation, it is imperative that a motivated client be given the opportunity to perform any skill, even if the nurse or the physician can accomplish it more quickly. Allowing the client to attempt a complex skill demonstrates support of the client's self-care abilities. A description of functional outcomes for rehabilitation is provided in Table 73–4. It is intended to be a guide and may not represent ability in all clients with various levels of injury.

Promote Mobility

Wheelchairs provide mobility, and having the proper wheelchair is crucial. The wheelchair design must provide the client with the ability to propel the chair and prevent development of spinal deformities and pressure ulcers. A high back and head support are needed for clients without arm function (Fig. 73–18). For clients who can use their arms, the back of the wheelchair should be at the level of the scapula and the wheelchair should be lower than normal to facilitate transfers. Cushions help reduce pressure and the risk of pressure ulcers. However, cushions do not prevent pressure ulcers, and weight shifts are still needed every 10 to 15 minutes of time spent in the wheelchair. Physical therapists work with the client to teach how to transfer from bed to a wheelchair, from a wheelchair into and out of a car, and from the wheelchair onto a toilet.

Current emphasis is on strengthening muscles rather than using braces. However, back braces may be prescribed after lumbar spinal injury or for intervertebral disc problems. More frequently, a thoracolumbosacral orthosis is used. This device is a custom-made plastic brace with front and back pieces that attach together with self-fastening straps. This brace provides stability for the healing spine. The nurse is responsible for supervising the unlicensed professional whenever he or she is assisting with positioning transfers for a client with a spinal abnormality.

Reduce Spasticity

Spasticity often interferes with positioning and functional activities. Spasticity does serve to maintain muscle bulk

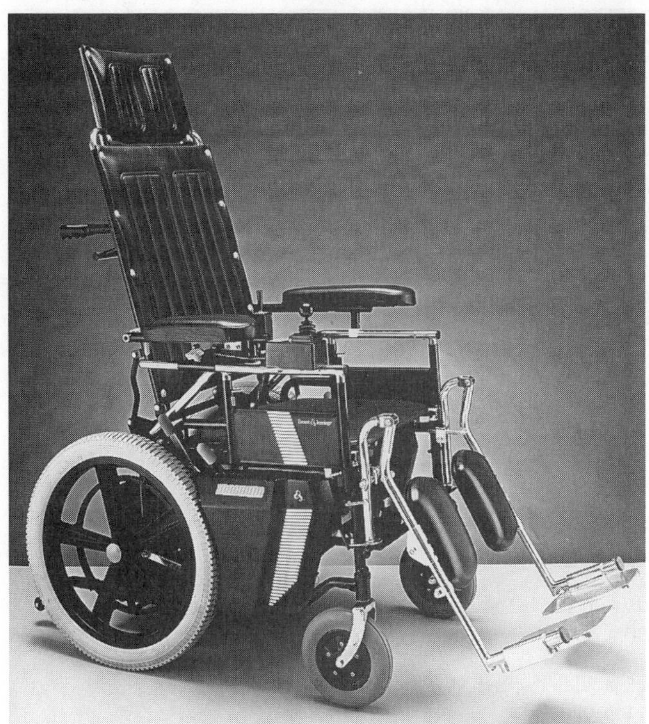

FIGURE 73–18 A wheelchair with power hand controls for clients with C1–3 cervical spine injury. A respirator can be attached to the wheelchair. (Courtesy of Everett and Jennings, St. Louis, MO.)

and venous return and can aid in transfers. Treatment includes range-of-motion (ROM) exercises and antispasmotic medications such as baclofen, dantrolene sodium, and clonidine. Medications for the treatment of spasms are given only when the spasms cause discomfort or safety concerns.

Improve Bladder and Bowel Control

The term *neurogenic bladder* is used to describe bladder control changes that occur with both upper and lower motor neuron disorders. Upper motor neuron disorders produce a spastic or reflex bladder. Lower motor neuron disorders produce a flaccid bladder. There are many ways to manage the bladder, and treatment options must be tailored to fit the client's preferences and lifestyle as well as his or her functional abilities.

Most clients with arm function are taught to empty their bladder using the Credé maneuver over the bladder to relax the sphincter and express urine (see Bladder Retraining in the nursing management section later on). To ensure complete emptying, this method is often combined with other techniques such as catheterization and use of external catheters. Intermittent catheterization reduces the risk of infection and bladder stone formation caused by indwelling catheters. Clients with injuries at the C6 level and lower can perform self-catheterization, although the technique requires adequate hand function and the ability to manage lower extremity clothing. External catheters are used for men who void between catheterizations or for those who leak urine during bladder spasms.

Suprapubic catheters seem to offer the advantages of less infection and urethral injury over indwelling catheters. Indwelling catheters are not ideal from a medical standpoint but are preferred by many clients because of the ease of management. Complications include infection, bladder stones, urethral damage, and a reported increased incidence of bladder cancer. A neurogenic bladder may also be managed pharmacologically with medications such as bethanechol (Urecholine) to stimulate bladder contraction. Urine-acidifying agents may also be prescribed to reduce the risk of infection.

A neurogenic bowel is similar to a neurogenic bladder in that the client cannot control defecation. The goal is to develop a bowel elimination method that is convenient, effective, and least expensive for the client. Sufficient fluid and fiber intake is essential. When fiber is added to or increased in the diet, it must be done slowly to avoid cramping and diarrhea. Stool softeners and bulk laxatives may also be used.

Bowel movements of clients with upper motor neuron damage are generally regulated with suppositories or digital stimulation every day, or every other day to reduce the risk of autonomic dysreflexia. A lower motor neuron neurogenic bowel is more difficult to regulate, and often the client requires manual removal of impacted material.

Prevent Pressure Ulcers

Anesthetic skin is associated with any increased frequency of pressure ulcers. During the acute care period, the risk of pressure ulcer development is related to the level of injury, completeness of the injury, and duration of immobilization. Guidelines based on many studies recommend that clients be turned or have their weight shifted at least every 2 hours. The Agency for Health Care Policy and Research (AHCPR) guidelines for prevention of skin injury include completing a daily systematic skin inspection, using proper positioning techniques (to minimize shearing and friction effects), maintaining adequate nutritional support, minimizing environmental exposure (i.e., excessive moisture or dryness), and avoiding massage over bony prominences. Prevention of pressure ulcers should include use of pressure-relieving devices (such as cushions or specialty bed). Wheelchair-bound clients are taught to relieve pressure every 15 minutes.

Reduce Respiratory Dysfunction

Respiratory dysfunction is a significant cause of morbidity and mortality after SCI. The diaphragm may be the only functional muscle active in respiration because the intercostal and abdominal muscles are often paralyzed. Vital capacity and inspiratory reserve volume are markedly diminished. The client should be taught to use incentive spirometry and diaphragmatic breathing to enhance vital capacity. Glossopharyngeal breathing uses the tongue and muscles of the pharynx to force air into the lungs. This technique enhances vital capacity and promotes chest expansion.

Promote Expression of Sexuality

Sexual function in spinal cord–injured men depends on the location of the lesion (Table 73–5). Reflex erection is possible in some clients with upper motor neuron lesions and also with some lower motor neuron lesions. Ejaculation is possible with lower motor neuron lesions and if the lesion is more caudal. Unfortunately, the fertility rate is about 5%, but it is hoped that this rate will improve

TABLE 73–5 SEXUAL FUNCTION IN CLIENTS WITH SPINAL CORD INJURY

Sexuality	Reproductive Functioning	Special Considerations for Contraceptive Methods
FEMALES		
Lesions at C1–3: Reflex lubrication is probable; erogenous areas may develop above injury; libido is intact **Lesions at C4–6:** Psychogenic lubrication is unlikely; nongenital orgasm may be experienced **Lesions at C7:** Able to use hands for holding and caressing **Lesions at T12–L5:** Psychogenic stimulation of the clitoris, lubrication, labial swelling, and skin flush are possible but unlikely	Menstruation and fertility unaffected Pregnancy is not affected Incidence of bladder infection during pregnancy increases Risk of autonomic hyperreflexia during labor and delivery increases	Birth control pills are contraindicated when circulatory problems are present Thrombophlebitis and other problems could go undetected owing to lack of sensation in extremities Intrauterine devices may be contraindicated because of pelvic inflammatory disease Client must be able to assess for vaginal bleeding
MALES		
Lesions at C1–3: Reflex erection is caused by genital stimulation psychogenic erection is not possible; erogenous zones above injury site may develop; libido is intact **Lesions at C4–6:** Reflex erection is possible; nongenital orgasm may be experienced; no ejaculation; oral sex is possible; libido is intact **Lesions at C7:** Holding and caressing with hands is possible **Lesions at T12–L6:** Psychogenic stimulation and erection are possible; no reflex erection **Lesions at S2–4:** Reflex erection is possible; ejaculation is possible but may be retrograde	Semen can be obtained from the bladder of clients who have retrograde ejaculation For clients who cannot ejaculate, semen can be obtained through glandular vibratory stimulation In general, semen quality is impaired, with poor motility the most common abnormality Some clients are candidates for penile prosthesis	Client or partner may apply condom

with advances in technology. It is becoming a common practice for semen to be collected and frozen for later in vivo fertilization. Sexual dysfunction is approached from two avenues: psychological counseling and education about technological advances in the facilitation of sexual activity. Erection can be restored with external aids, an implantable penile prosthesis, or medications.

Female clients retain fertility after SCI. Problems with sexual function generally relate to positioning and the lack of vaginal lubrication. These problems can usually be addressed through client education.

Control Pain

Long-term pain occurs in almost all spinal cord–injured clients with intact sensation. Dysesthetic pain, which is distal to the site of injury, is extremely disabling. It is similar to the phantom pain experienced after amputation. It is described as cutting, burning, piercing, radiating, or tightening. The usual treatment is with non-narcotic analgesics and transcutaneous nerve stimulators. A prn (as-needed) approach to pain management is not recommended for chronic pain. However, routine analgesics may need to be supplemented with other pain-relieving medications given prn during a client's pain peaks.

Reduce Abnormal Bone Growth

Heterotopic ossification is the formation of bone in abnormal locations, occurring most often around the hips and knees after SCI. The client may develop swelling in the joint or loss of ROM. Heterotopic ossification is diagnosed by x-ray study or bone scan. Treatment includes the use of etidronate disodium (Didronel) and ROM exercises of the affected joints. Sometimes the bone is removed surgically.

Promote Psychological Adjustment

Psychological counseling is ongoing. Commonly, spinal cord–injured clients participate in peer group counseling sessions in which experiences and solutions are shared to help newly injured clients to cope better with their losses. Vocational rehabilitation may help clients reach their maximum rehabilitation potential.

Ongoing Nursing Management of the Client with Spinal Cord Injury

ASSESSMENT

The client usually is transferred from the ICU after becoming hemodynamically stable. Clients with high cervical injuries may remain on ventilators. The care of the ventilator-dependent client is discussed in Chapter 63. Some of the nursing diagnoses that applied in the critical care unit may still apply after transfer. The client remains at risk for skin impairment and may still have difficulty swallowing, with attendant risk for aspiration. A baseline assessment should be completed upon transfer.

DIAGNOSIS, OUTCOMES, INTERVENTIONS

Impaired Physical Mobility. SCI causing permanent impaired physical mobility produces problems with ambulation and potential complications arising from immobility. The relevant diagnosis is *Impaired Physical Mobility related to inability to move upper and/or lower extremities secondary to paralysis.*

Outcomes. The client will have maximal physical mobility, as evidenced by absence of tendon contractures, joint ankylosis, and muscle shortening and will demonstrate effective use of adaptive devices.

Interventions. Throughout the acute and rehabilitative phases of nursing care, make every effort to maximize functional abilities and independence by encouraging the client to perform independently any activities of daily living (ADL) for which capability remains.

Provide Positioning and Adaptive Equipment. Improper positioning of the client in the bed or chair and lack of joint movements (e.g., related to spasticity or immobility) lead to tendon contractures, joint ankylosis, and muscle shortening. Interventions to prevent such problems include the following:

- Frequent position changes
- Proper positioning of joints
- Use of splints and removable casts
- Intermittent turning to a prone position
- Positioning of upper extremities away from the body
- Draping of bed linen over frames to keep pressure off the feet
- Keeping knee joints flexed 15 degrees when the client is supine
- Use of active and passive conditioning exercises (see Risk for Contractures later on)

Wristdrop and footdrop are inevitable sequelae in paralyzed extremities unless specific preventive measures are used. Footdrop may be prevented by keeping the client's feet firmly supported in dorsiflexion at right angles to the hips to counteract the force of gravity on weakened muscles. Many devices are available to prevent footdrop. Skin must be frequently assessed to prevent associated skin breakdown. Support a paralyzed arm in a sling when the client is out of bed and in a cock-up splint when the client is in bed. Usually, the hand end of the splint is elevated 2 inches to support the wrist, and the fingers are maintained in a position of function. Posterior molded casts may be used instead of splints to support a paralyzed wrist while the client is in bed. For some clients, pillows and a hand roll are adequate.

Assist with Transfers and Ambulation. Rehabilitative programs often require strength and endurance. To prepare a client for ambulation, the unaffected parts of the body must be strengthened and suitable exercises started early. Tolerance for activity gradually increases. Take care not to fatigue the client. Periods of planned rest and recreation are important.

Physical therapy is essential for all clients with SCI. Paraplegic clients need to learn various transfers in order to become self-sufficient. One transfer method is illustrated in Figure 73–19. Learning to sit up precedes learning to transfer. Many paralyzed clients become mobile by using a wheelchair. Many types of wheelchairs are available, and selection needs to be made carefully, according to individual needs.

The brace or corset should be applied before the client is assisted to get out of bed. A thin, knitted undershirt is worn under the brace or corset to protect the skin and to keep the appliance clean. To apply the brace or corset, turn the client to one side, place the appliance against the back, and then roll the client back into it. The brace or corset is secured while the client lies supine. As recovery and rehabilitation progress, many clients learn to apply their own brace or corset while in bed. Others continue to need help. The degree of arm and hand function determines the client's ability to apply a brace.

Weight-bearing begins as early as possible after SCI. Weight-bearing stimulates osteoblastic activity and thus decreases demineralization of bone *(osteoporosis)* that develops with prolonged immobilization. Use of a standing board or tilt table assists the person to gradually tolerate a standing position. Having the client assume a standing position periodically each day also helps prevent contrac-

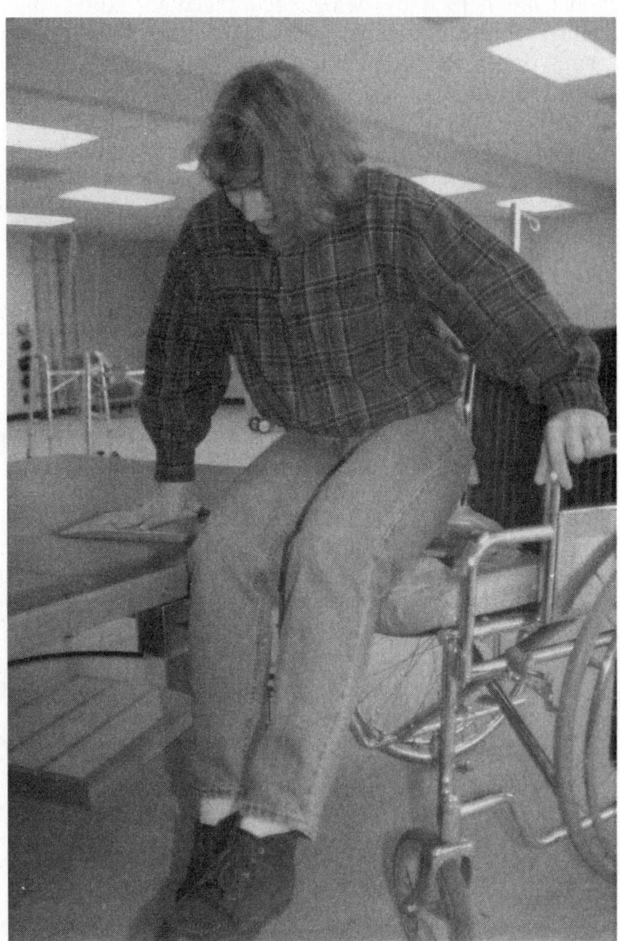

FIGURE 73–19 Bed-to-wheelchair lateral transfer using a sliding board.

tures (e.g., hip contractures resulting from long periods of sitting).

Take care in helping clients to stand or sit in a chair for the first time. Because of the effects of loss of muscular activity on the peripheral venous system, these clients are prone to orthostatic hypotension. Always check blood pressure before and after transfers. Syncope during a wheelchair transfer may be avoided in the quadriplegic client by use of an abdominal binder, thigh-high support hose, and slowly elevating the head of the bed to 90 degrees. Using a recliner or a wheelchair with an adjustable back will help achieve gradual elevations.

Clients easily lose balance when wearing braces, particularly the halo brace, and must be very careful to avoid falling. The accompanying Client Education Guide describes the use of a halo vest. A brace feels surprisingly heavy at first, especially if the client is weak. For safety, shoes, rather than slippers or just stockings or socks, should be worn during ambulation. Shoes should tie or have self-fastening straps for firm support and have a low heel. High-top athletic shoes give added support. Slick soles, high or narrow heels, and stockinged feet are hazardous. Wearing shoes also helps prevent footdrop when the client lies down.

The fit, comfort, and appearance of braces, corsets, and shoes are important to the client. Try to accommodate the preferences of clients who want to be as stylish as possible as well as benefit from therapeutic garments. Disabled clients are helped by being encouraged to express their feelings concerning their self-image and by having their desires taken into consideration when being fitted for therapeutic garments. Some garments can be painful when first worn. The pain worsens if the garments do not fit properly. The client's skin should be inspected frequently, especially at first, because pressure sores can develop very quickly.

Ineffective Airway Clearance. Airway clearance may be impaired because of paralysis of the abdominal and intercostal muscles. The relevant nursing diagnosis is *Ineffective Airway Clearance related to inability to cough.*

Outcomes. The client will participate in "quad-assisted" coughing, remain afebrile, and have normal blood gas or pulse oximetry values and clear sputum.

Interventions. Use the "quad-assisted" cough maneuver to promote airway clearance. As for the Heimlich maneuver, place a fist or heel of the hand between the umbilicus and the xiphoid process. Press inward and upward during the client's cough. Other interventions, such as turning, hydration, and chest physical therapy, may also be used.

Risk for Contractures. Active ROM is severely limited or nonexistent in the upper extremities and nonexistent in the lower extremities in a client with cervical cord damage; it is also nonexistent in the lower extremities in a client with thoracic or lumbar cord damage. This deficit increases the risk for contractures. The nursing diagnosis is *Risk for Contractures related to inability to move purposefully.*

Outcomes. Monitor the client for changes in ROM in all joints. The client will have no change in ROM compared with the level before injury.

Interventions. Passive exercises prevent contractures and painful reflex dystrophies of the hand and shoulder.

CLIENT EDUCATION GUIDE

Use of a Halo Vest

- The vest or the halo ring bolts are to be adjusted only by the neurosurgeon or by someone designated to do so. If the bolts become loose, tell your physician.
- Use fleece or foam inserts to relieve discomfort at pressure points.
- Keep the vest lining dry. If the fleece gets wet, dry it with a hair dryer (on a cool setting); do not allow the fleece to become matted.
- Clean the pins at least once a day; cleaning agents include soap and water applied using cotton-tipped swabs, alcohol swabs, or shampoo soap if hair is being washed. Crusts can be removed using hydrogen peroxide or alcohol. Ointments and antiseptics are not recommended for routine care. Use a separate sterile swab for each pin site.
- Report redness, swelling, drainage, open areas around the pin (tracking), pain, tenderness, or a clicking noise from the pin site. Retightening is usually necessary during the first 24 to 48 hours for the first week.
- Recheck the pins every 2 to 3 weeks.
- Wash the skin under the vest. Use a bath towel wrung out in hot water (alcohol is permitted) and pull it back and forth. Do not use soap, lotion, or powder because it cannot be removed adequately. Assess daily for skin breakdown under the vest using a flashlight. Showering is prohibited. A sponge bath or tub bath with minimal water to prevent the vest liner from getting wet may be permitted. When the hair is shampooed, the shoulders and neck of the vest must be protected with plastic. Do not use any products other than shampoo on your hair (no dyes, tints, sprays, or conditioners).
- When getting out of bed, roll onto your side and push on the mattress with your arm; sitting straight up puts too much stress on the front pins. *Never use the metal frame for turning or lifting!*
- A rolled towel or pillowcase between the back of your neck and the bed or next to your cheek when lying on your side and raising the head of the bed will increase sleeping comfort.
- Adapt your clothing to fit over the halo, or select clothing with button, self-fastening, or zipper closures. The vest will be needed for about 3 months, followed by a hard collar.
- Eat food products high in protein and calcium to promote bone healing.
- Have the correct size of wrench with you in case of an emergency. The anterior portion of the vest including the anterior bolts can then be loosened as necessary; the posterior portion of the vest should remain in place to provide stability for the spine during cardiopulmonary resuscitation.

Adapted from Reid, B., & Marr, J. (1990). *Health professional's guide to caring for the client with a halo vest* (pp. 1–12). Jacksonville, FL: Bremer Medical.

Such exercises may be prescribed as soon as 48 to 72 hours after injury. Active exercises, massage, and electrical stimulation may also be prescribed. Begin shoulder and arm exercises early. Strength in these areas and in the chest and back is essential for effective self-transfers and ambulation when the lower spine is stable enough to permit mobilization.

Self-Care Deficit. The client who has suffered an SCI is often unable to perform many self-care activities.

Outcomes. The client will independently perform as many ADL tasks as possible. If unable to independently perform an activity, the client will be able to direct a caregiver's performance. These goals will be evaluated by observing successful performance of ADL by the client or under the client's direction.

Interventions. Self-care deficit can lead to a feeling of powerlessness. Assisting the client to maximize independence can lessen this feeling. The client is assisted with muscle-strengthening exercises and the use of adaptive devices. Clients with high cervical injuries are able to perform very few activities independently. Allow them adequate time to accomplish whatever tasks they can. If help with ADL is needed, adapt nursing care to the client's routine. In collaborating to maintain intact oral mucous membranes, a schedule is established for brushing teeth at least twice daily and cleaning the tongue, roof of the mouth, and gums with agents not containing lemon or alcohol.

Risk for Altered Nutrition: Less Than Body Requirements. After traumatic injury there is increased metabolic demand because of the response to stress and the body's requirements for healing. The relevant nursing diagnosis is written *Risk for Altered Nutrition: Less Than Body Requirements related to increased metabolic demand and inability to access nutrients.* Anorexia related to depression may be another etiologic factor.

Outcomes. The client will not experience excessive weight loss (more than 10 lb) during hospitalization.

Interventions. The client should be weighed on admission to obtain a baseline measurement. Nutrient supplementation should begin by 72 hours after injury if the client is not eating. Enteral feeding can be used if the client has bowel sounds. If the client still has paralytic ileus, hyperalimentation is commonly used. Weigh the client at least once a week to monitor progress.

Total Incontinence. Observe the client carefully for indications of faulty bladder control and infection, including incontinence, retention, urgency, dribbling, frequency, enuresis, and precipitate micturition. Document such observations and inform the physician. The relevant nursing diagnosis is written *Total Incontinence related to paralysis.*

Outcomes. The client will have improved bladder control, as evidenced by no infection and emptying of the bladder every 4 to 6 hours.

Interventions. Nursing intervention is planned to prevent urinary tract infection, to preserve existing bladder capacity and muscle tone, and to establish and maintain a routine pattern of elimination requiring minimal artificial assistance.

Urinary bladder atony (absence of tone) may last several weeks or months after SCI. In clients with upper motor neuron lesions, when spinal shock subsides and the reflexes return, as evidenced by an increase in rectal tone, a reflex contraction will empty the bladder. During the period of atony, a retention catheter may be inserted to prevent bladder distention and keep the client dry and comfortable. Bladder overdistention causes stretching and fissure formation—a predisposing factor for infection—and may result in bladder rupture. When sensory pathways are damaged, the client does not feel the discomfort of bladder distention. However, prolonged catheter use also predisposes to infection. Therefore, catheterization every 6 hours is preferred over a retention catheter.

Urinary complications may be avoided by periodically examining the client for bladder distention, accurately documenting fluid intake and output, using aseptic technique when handling urinary catheters, and observing for signs of bladder infection. Encourage the client to drink water to keep the urine diluted, which lessens the possibility of infection. Urine acidifiers may be prescribed.

Urinary complications occur because of incomplete emptying of the bladder, necessitating catheterization. Catheterization may predispose the client to infection and vesicoureteral reflux, which may lead to kidney complications. Renal calculi, pyelonephritis, and hydronephrosis are major causes of considerable disability and even death in paralyzed clients.

To prevent development of renal calculi, encourage the client to drink about 3000 ml of fluid per day, unless contraindicated by other medical conditions. This is sufficient to maintain a minimal urinary output of 2000 ml per day. Drinking this much fluid may increase incontinence but is necessary to prevent renal calculi.

Bowel Incontinence or Constipation. Bowel dysfunction is a common but manageable problem in a client with SCI. This common nursing diagnosis is written as *Constipation related to paralysis.*

Outcomes. The client will have reduced risk of bowel incontinence or constipation, as evidenced by a bowel movement every 1 to 2 days, no signs of fecal impaction, no incontinence, and no signs of hyperreflexia.

Interventions. Nursing intervention is planned to prevent constipation, distention, and impaction; to detect and treat these conditions if they occur; and to reestablish habitual, controlled bowel movements by conditioned reflex activity. Paralytic ileus is common after SCI. By frequently assessing bowel sounds and documenting the passage of stool, return of peristalsis can be determined, and the client can resume oral intake. The client is observed carefully for indications of constipation, diarrhea, or tenesmus (straining at stool). If the bowel becomes impacted, a cleansing enema may be prescribed to initially empty the lower bowel. However, enemas should be avoided for long-term bowel management. A paraplegic or quadriplegic client cannot retain an enema solution, nor can the degree of intestinal distention be felt. Therefore, enemas must be administered carefully to avoid overdistending the intestine with excessive fluid; 500 ml or less is usually given.

The client's intake of fluid and food and elimination patterns are documented. The routine daily pattern of bowel elimination is established, with the client using suppositories and other means of stimulating evacuation until reflex evacuation occurs.

A daily fluid intake of 3000 ml per day is important for proper bowel function as well as bladder function. Also, the diet must be high in bulk and roughage such as bran, whole grains, fresh and dried fruits, and leafy green and raw vegetables. A stool softener such as docusate sodium (Colace) may be taken daily, but laxatives should be carefully administered. Bulk-forming medications (e.g., psyllium hydrophilic mucilloid [Metamucil]) are very effective for spinal cord–injured clients so long as adequate hydration is maintained.

Risk for Impaired Skin Integrity. Clients with SCI are at higher risk of impairment of skin integrity because of immobility and loss of protective functions.

Outcomes. The client will have intact skin, as evidenced by no reddened areas over bony prominences and no areas or signs of skin irritation or dryness.

Interventions. The spinal cord–injured client cannot respond to the sensory cues to local tissue hypoxia resulting from being in one position for an extended period of time. Impaired skin sensation occurring with quadriplegia and paraplegia predisposes the client to the development of pressure ulcers and other injuries. Spinal cord–injured clients should be placed on pressure-reducing beds or mattresses. However, the use of these special beds does not eliminate the need to assess the skin every 2 to 4 hours and does not eliminate the risk of pressure ulcers. In addition, the client's nutritional needs must be met to reduce the risk of pressure ulcers.

A client with spinal fractures may be placed on a Roto-Rest bed. A Roto-Rest bed is currently popular for management of clients with SCI or other disorders requiring prolonged immobilization (see Chapter 68, Fig. 68–5). It is equipped with supportive packs and straps that keep the body in neutral alignment while it continuously oscillates from side to side. If rotation is greater than 35 degrees, the continuous motion helps prevent skin breakdown, reduce urinary stasis, and promote lung aeration. Unfortunately, the constant movement may also stimulate peristalsis, resulting in severe diarrhea. Some clients also experience disorientation from the constant movement and have reported fear of falling. Staff members should remain with the client initially to provide emotional support and reassurance. Also, it is important to pull window curtains at night, as a client in a Roto-Rest bed who can see himself or herself "floating" in the window reflection can become disoriented or frightened.

Chronic Pain. Clients with SCI may experience pain at the level of the injury and radiating along spinal nerves originating in the area. Phantom pain may also be experienced. The onset of pain is usually later than for muscle spasms. Some paraplegic and quadriplegic clients experience both pain and spasm. Pain most often occurs in the lower extremities.

Outcomes. The client will experience adequate pain relief, as evidenced by verbalization of improvement in comfort, ability to rest without interruption by pain, and ability to participate in therapies without hindrance by pain.

Interventions. Analgesics such as aspirin and nonsteroidal anti-inflammatory drugs (NSAIDs) may be prescribed. Narcotics are seldom used after the initial injury and are contraindicated in clients with high cervical-level injuries because of the risk of respiratory depression.

Clients with thoracic pulmonary injuries tend to breathe more shallowly to avoid pain. Inadequate depth of respirations can lead to complications. Give prescribed pain medication and encourage deep-breathing and coughing to aerate the lungs and remove secretions from the respiratory tract.

Antispasmodics, NSAIDs, and non-narcotic analgesics are prescribed for pain associated with spasticity. Surgery (e.g., neurectomy, chordotomy) is sometimes required for pain relief.

Risk for Autonomic Dysreflexia. Autonomic dysreflexia/hyperreflexia is a serious complication of SCI when injury is above the T6 level. This collaborative problem is documented as *Risk for Autonomic Dysreflexia related to spinal cord injury.*

Outcomes. The nurse will monitor for clinical manifestations of autonomic dysreflexia and respond to them quickly.

Interventions. Assess the client for sudden onset of severe hypertension, severe throbbing headache, profuse diaphoresis, flushing of the skin above the level of the lesion, nasal stuffiness, pilomotor spasm, blurred vision, nausea, and bradycardia. (See the Critical Monitoring feature.)

Educate the client about early warning signs and symptoms of autonomic dysreflexia and the importance of calling for a nurse immediately should any occur. Adaptive call lights are available to facilitate calling for assistance. If autonomic dysreflexia does occur, institute the following measures:

1. Elevate the head of the bed to a sitting position immediately.
2. Check blood pressure.
3. Check for possible sources of irritation (e.g., kinked or clogged catheter or distended bladder or lower bowel).
4. Remove the stimulus if it can be done quickly. Once the source of irritation is removed, manifestations of autonomic dysreflexia usually subside.
5. If blood pressure remains elevated, antihypertensive medication (nitrates, hydralazine, guanethidine, or diazoxide) may be administered according to pre-

CRITICAL MONITORING

Features of Autonomic Dysreflexia

- Severe hypertension (up to 300 mm Hg)
- Pounding headache
- Flushing (above the level of the lesion)
- Piloerection
- Diaphoresis
- Dilated pupils, blurred vision
- Nasal stuffiness
- Bradycardia (pulse < 60 BPM)
- Restlessness
- Nausea

scription or procedural policy (intravenously, intranasally, or sublingually).
6. If there is no order or policy or if these measures do not correct the problem, notify the physician.

Once manifestations have subsided, observe the client's vital signs and neurologic status closely for 3 to 4 hours. If an antihypertensive medication has been given, the client may become hypotensive after the stimulus is removed. Autonomic dysreflexia may recur if the stimulus is not completely removed. If the identified source is bladder distention, use caution when emptying the bladder. Remove 500 ml every 5 to 15 minutes. If the identified source of irritation is bowel distention, be very careful when removing the impacted material from the bowel. An anesthetic lubricant is used, and another nurse must monitor the client's blood pressure every few minutes. The stimulation of trying to remove the impacted material can increase the severity of the autonomic response. When a quadriplegic client complains of a headache, *do not automatically give analgesics without first checking the blood pressure.*

Risk for Injury. In clients with SCI, another appropriate nursing diagnosis is *Risk for Injury related to abnormal reflexes, spasms, and corneal drying.* Corneal abrasions may result unless proper interventions are instituted.

Outcomes. The client will sustain no injuries due to spasms, as evidenced by no abrasions or bruising. Corneal abrasions will not occur.

Interventions. Injections should be avoided whenever possible. Medications should be given orally or IV if needed. When injections are unavoidable, give above the level of the cord lesion whenever possible. Absorption may be compromised in denervated areas of the body with impaired capillary and precapillary circulation. Moisten the cornea with natural tears every 4 hours for a client with altered blinking reflexes.

Clients can also be injured from involuntary spasms. Avoid unnecessary stimulation of areas that elicit reflex spinal automatisms. When such reactions do occur, an unembarrassed, accepting response helps relieve the client's anxiety and embarrassment. Gentle, slow hyperextension of a limb in spasm can often override the trigger points and interrupt the spasm. Abnormal spinal reflexes make people respond to stimuli in ways that may be puzzling to them and others unless the origin of such responses is explained. For example, stimulation of the limbs (perhaps toe flexion while the person's foot is being dried) may cause mass flexion of the upper and lower extremities. Mass flexion reactions may be accompanied by massive contractions of the abdominal wall, evacuation of the urinary bladder and bowel, and automatic response such as sweating, flushing, penile erection, or pilomotor reactions below the level of the lesion.

Risk for Thrombophlebitis. Muscular activity is a major factor in venous circulation. A paralyzed client experiences slowed venous return and pooling of blood in dependent limbs. These phenomena constitute the basis for the diagnosis *Risk for Thrombophlebitis.*

Outcomes. Monitor for thrombophlebitis, as evidenced by unilateral leg edema, erythema, and warmth.

Interventions. In the acute phase of SCI, antiembolism stockings, sequential compression devices, and subcutaneous heparin may be used prophylactically.

Education is vital to preventing vascular complications and minimizing their impact. Teach the client the importance of all preventive activities. During assessment of the legs for signs of clot formation (i.e., redness and unilateral swelling and warmth), explain the components of assessment, and emphasize the importance of incorporating this activity into daily routines. Measuring calf diameter on both legs daily to detect any changes is a more objective way of assessing swelling. Clients also learn not to cross their legs while sitting in a wheelchair.

Ineffective Individual Coping. When the reality of the injury and the permanence of deficit are understood, coping skills may need to be taught. The nursing diagnosis can be written as *Ineffective Individual Coping related to paralysis.*

Outcomes. The client will use adaptive coping strategies and resources appropriately.

Interventions. Clients need to find appropriate methods for coping with new approaches to performing ADL and managing bodily functions. The learning needs of spinal cord–injured clients and their family members are complex and ongoing. In the acute phase, education about spinal anatomy and physiology is needed. This teaching begins in the acute phase of hospitalization and should be incorporated into all aspects of care. Successful learning in this stage affects the client's entire life.

Anticipatory Grieving. Clients with SCI experience many changes (e.g., functional ability, role definition, body image, and financial security). Grief is a normal response to these losses. Write the diagnosis as *Anticipatory Grieving related to multiple losses.*

Outcomes. The client will progress through the grieving process and develop adaptive coping strategies, as evidenced by verbalizing his or her feelings about the injury and the future, participating in community activities, and expressing positive thoughts about the future.

Intervention. Adjusting to paralysis is difficult physically and psychosocially for the client and family. Family members may experience the same reactions as those experienced by the disabled client, and may need the same kind of help. Sudden paralysis in a previously healthy, active person can be devastating. Typically, the sudden lifestyle changes brought about by serious SCI produce a grief reaction. The reaction may involve initial shock and denial, leading to depression and anger. Crying and talking about the injury may be helpful. Social services or pastoral care may also be of assistance during this time of grief.

It takes time to adjust to disability and to develop ways of coping. Psychological adjustment occurs when the client can function appropriately in the real world.

A client may use psychological defense mechanisms in adjusting to paralysis. When caring for such a client, assess the possible reasons for observed behavior. Hostility, depression, anger, or withdrawal may be upsetting to staff and family. These emotions and behaviors represent coping mechanisms and should not be taken personally.

Paralysis may cause complex changes in self-concept and body image. In the acute phase, immobilization can contribute to sensory deprivation and its consequences (e.g., hallucinations). Providing visual, auditory, and tactile stimulation as desired by the client may minimize the experience of deprivation.

Paralyzed clients are often helped initially by being with others who are experiencing similar problems. Clients should be allowed to wear their own clothing as soon as possible and encouraged to be out of bed and out of the hospital room. Planned social activities may reduce feelings of social isolation and may help clients regain self-confidence. Peer counseling, in which newly disabled clients are provided with opportunities to talk with others who have adjusted to similar disabilities, may be helpful.

A sense of security is particularly important for a newly paralyzed client adjusting to enforced dependency. A paralyzed client should always have a means of summoning help, yet needs to learn that it is safe to be alone at times. Blow lights, minimal-pressure call lights, pads, and voice-activated call lights are now available in many settings.

Gradually, the client develops trust in his or her abilities and resources and relinquishes some reliance on others. These feelings and attitudes develop slowly as the client experiences genuinely trustworthy relationships.

To avoid unnecessary frustrations, try to keep the client's environment comfortable, with necessary items conveniently placed. It is difficult and depressing for the client to have to ask for help repeatedly. Although recent advances have been made in the rehabilitation prognosis of paraplegic and quadriplegic clients, it is important to be realistic as well as optimistic. Nurses need to understand the tremendous lifestyle changes disabled clients must make. Some people can be rehabilitated to a level of near-independence: walking (perhaps with braces or other appliances), driving a car, and coping with full-time employment outside the home. Quadriplegic clients usually rely on a wheelchair and other devices and appliances.

Most paralyzed clients can become productive and happy. One well-known SCI victim, the actor Christopher Reeve, has been serving as a positive role model regarding *abilities* that remain after SCI. Even if some clients are unable to be "productive," all disabled clients have a right to a satisfying, happy life. Although many paralyzed clients achieve complete rehabilitation, others lead lives that are difficult, frustrating, and psychophysiologically complex. At times, severe mental depression develops. Depression is assessed, and professional counseling is offered as indicated. Unfortunately, ideations of suicide are frequent.

Ineffective Family Coping: Compromised. A family is a unit. A trauma as devastating as SCI to one of the members of the family unit affects the entire family. The relevant nursing diagnosis can be written *Ineffective Family Coping: Compromised related to multiple changes in the family roles.*

Outcomes. The client and family members will identify areas of significant or potential loss and changes in family roles, work together to overcome obstacles, seek appropriate support services, and be able to restore a supportive family structure.

Interventions. The injury affects not only physical functioning but also the psychological, vocational, educational, and social aspects of life. An organized team approach is vital to helping the injured client and family cope with lifestyle changes. Nurses are often the first health care professionals to assess client and family coping. An open, empathetic manner can allow the people involved to express their grief and uncertainty and to ask questions. Educate the family about the normal grief response. Also carefully probe into persistent denial of grief or lack of progression through grieving. Encouraging as much optimism as possible while remaining truthful and realistic may help SCI survivors to face the future.

Assess the previous roles of the client and other family members and how they have handled stressful situations or losses. Identify the family's sources of strength. Assess patterns of interaction between family members; their spiritual, social, and economic status, their lifestyle, and cultural or ethnic influences should also be noted. These variables often influence how the family responds to grief. Sometimes the nurse can play a valuable role simply by giving family members permission to have a day off from visiting.

Ineffective Management of Therapeutic Regimen (Individual). Clients with SCI have bladder function changes. Bladder emptying has to be learned using a different approach, and bowel retraining is often necessary. A common nursing diagnosis in this circumstance is *Ineffective Management of Therapeutic Regimen (Individual).*

Outcomes. The client will be able to manage his or her bowel and bladder or instruct others how to do so.

Interventions. One of the most common stimuli for autonomic dysreflexia, a life-threatening complication in people with SCI, is bladder distention. Therefore, intervention leading to bladder management is crucial.

Promote Bladder Retraining. When the initial indwelling catheter is removed, a program of intermittent catheterization is commonly prescribed to empty the bladder regularly every 4 to 6 hours for several weeks. During this time, the client is taught methods of emptying the bladder without catheterization. Such methods promote urination by increasing intra-abdominal pressure on the bladder. For some clients with SCI, urinary flow can be initiated by using the Credé maneuver, the Valsalva maneuver, or the rectal stretch.

The *Credé maneuver* involves placing the fist or fingers directly over the bladder and pressing down toward the pubic bone with a kneading motion. This motion is continued until the bladder is empty.

The *Valsalva maneuver* involves inhaling deeply, holding the breath, and bearing down as hard as possible, as if for a bowel movement.

The *rectal stretch* involves inserting a lubricated, gloved finger into the rectum. When the anal sphincter is relaxed, the client maintains the relaxation by gently pulling on the sphincter. This relaxes the perineal floor. The Valsalva maneuver is performed at the same time.

Urination may also be prompted by reflex stimulation. The following stimuli may be successful: tapping the suprapubic area; stroking the glans penis, thigh, or vulva; tugging pubic hairs; or flexing the toes. The client or caregiver may apply the stimulation. As training continues, less stimulation is needed to initiate urination.

Catheterization may be required at home. Teach the client and caregiver clean, rather than sterile, technique. This technique has the same infection rate as for sterile insertion methods used for home catheterization. Suprapubic catheters may be inserted for long-term bladder management.

Occasionally, a surgical procedure such as sphincterotomy may be necessary. The bladder then empties continuously. An external, condom-type catheter connected to a closed drainage bag may be used to collect urine in men. External appliances for females are not consistently effective.

Teach Bowel Retraining. Bowel retraining is possible for most paraplegic and quadriplegic clients. It involves developing controlled bowel movements by conditioned reflex activity. Begin bowel retraining as soon as feasible. Ensure privacy during the daily bowel routine, and if possible, have the client sitting upright. When possible, include appropriate family members in the bowel retraining program, as they may be involved in this aspect of long-term management. Always assess the family members' willingness to participate in such care. If the sexual partner is also responsible for hygiene and personal care, problems in role separation and intimacy may result. These issues should be openly discussed between partners.

With an effective bowel program, a client has a bowel movement once a day or every other day and is not incontinent at other times. Attaining continence may influence a paralyzed client's vocational future and positively affect ability to have satisfying social relationships. It can also give the client the confidence to cope with other problems.

Sexual Dysfunction. Spinal cord–injured clients are often concerned about sexuality and their ability to achieve sexual fulfillment. They often worry about such concerns long before they express them to others. Nurses are often asked about sexuality issues before other professionals are approached, perhaps because nurses provide intimate care. Such care can promote a high degree of trust.

Outcomes. The client will develop personally satisfying and socially acceptable means of expressing sexuality, as evidenced by interacting appropriately in social situations, verbalizing the effects of the injury on sexual function, discussing sexual issues with a health care team member, verbalizing methods of sexual expression, and verbalizing understanding of contraceptive implications.

Interventions. Some clients discuss their own sexual potential directly. Others refer to it subtly or appear crude in the way they introduce the topic, such as making inappropriate sexual comments or gestures. Such behaviors are attempts to acknowledge sexuality. Try to look beyond the behavior to the underlying emotional concerns. Acknowledge the client's concerns and offer to open a discussion, by saying, for example, "You seem concerned about your sexuality, James. This is a common concern that others with spinal cord injury have had. Sometimes talking about it helps. If you like, we can talk about how this has affected you, and when you are ready, I can share with you interventions that have helped others who have had similar problems."

To be helpful, nurses need to be able to talk about sexuality without embarrassment. They also need accurate information about "normal" sexuality and how physiologic changes that occur because of the injury affect sexual function.

The client can be referred to another person or an agency if appropriate. Referral should not be made too hastily, however. If a client talks with a nurse about this subject, it is probably because the client feels most comfortable speaking with that nurse at that time. Allow the client to lead the conversation, which may be difficult. Professionals must be aware that they do not always know what a client needs and wants and should listen carefully to the client's voiced concerns.

Generally, a physiologic sexual response requires an intact nervous system. For example, psychogenic erection requires an intact spinal cord with preservation of S2–4 nerve roots and spinal reflexes; ejaculation is a function of skeletal muscle controlled by the somatic center in the pudendal nerve originating in the S2–4 roots; and orgasm involves contraction of both smooth and skeletal muscle. It should be remembered, however, that there is more involved in sexual expression than physiologic response.

To some extent, sexual function can be predicted by the level of the spinal cord lesion (see Table 73–5). For example, psychogenic erection is often difficult or impossible after SCI. However, although physical limitations certainly exist, every person is different. Many men do have reflex erections after SCI. Many disabled people enjoy "paraorgasm" (phantom orgasm) by developing alternative erogenous zones. The genitals are not the only body areas in which sexual stimulation is possible, and intercourse is not the only means of sexual expression.

Some people find it disappointing, perhaps devastating, that they can no longer function sexually as they did before the injury. However, they can be helped to learn new ways of giving and receiving sexual pleasure. Sex and relationship counseling is sometimes helpful. Some form of sexual expression is possible for anyone, regardless of disability. Before making specific suggestions for alternative expressions of sexuality, discussion with the client should occur to identify past sexual behavior and cultural taboos. Some clients may find some methods of giving and receiving sexual pleasure unacceptable. Lack of a sexual partner may be a deterrent but should not preclude discussion of sexuality. Society as a whole is becoming progressively more open about sexuality.

Increasingly, the parenting potential of disabled people is receiving societal attention. Physical assessment is needed to determine a client's ability to reproduce. Male infertility is a frequent complication of SCI because of testicular atrophy, decreased sperm formation, and infrequent ejaculation. Most men are unable to ejaculate after SCI. Women usually remain fertile and can conceive and deliver a child. Adoption is a viable option, and conception by artificial insemination is possible.

Disabled people may have contraception concerns. Little is known about the effects of various kinds of contraceptives on disabled people. Oral contraceptives may be contraindicated. Paralyzed women often have slowed circulation, increasing the potential circulatory complications of oral contraceptives. To use an intrauterine device, a woman must have feeling in her pelvis to be able to recognize early manifestations of pelvic inflammatory disease. Many paralyzed women do not have such sensation. Barrier devices, such as a diaphragm, a condom, or foam, may be used if at least one partner has enough manual dexterity to insert the diaphragm or foam or put on the condom.

Risk for Injury. Sensory loss poses serious problems for paralyzed clients because they cannot feel the pain or pressure that normally warns of tissue damage.

Outcomes. The client will be free of injury, as evidenced by absence of abrasions, reddened areas, ulcerations, or burns.

Interventions. Spinal cord–injured clients should not wear tight, restrictive clothing or ill-fitting shoes or braces. They need to develop the habit of preventive thinking to avoid potential danger. Dangerous situations include getting too close to heaters, radiators, and fireplaces and using heating pads or hot-water bottles. Burns can be a serious problem because impaired circulation delays healing. External heat should not be applied if there is a loss of sensation, and the bath water should not be too hot.

Regular foot and nail care is required to prevent overgrown nails from rubbing or cutting the skin and to prevent ingrown nails. Instruct the client not to cut corns or calluses; cutting too deep is easy to do and may lead to a foot infection. Cocoa butter or oils without alcohol may be used to soften calluses and reduce cracking.

Altered Health Maintenance. SCI results in many alterations in physiologic functioning that place the client at risk for maintaining normal health status. A possible nursing diagnosis is *Altered Health Maintenance.*

Outcomes. The client and family members will be able to meet the client's needs, as evidenced by intact skin, bowel and bladder continence, ability to transfer into and out of a wheelchair, absence of infection, maintenance of appropriate weight, and satisfaction with personal relationships.

Interventions. Teaching should be conducted in short sessions, using easily understood terms. For example, teach the caregiver the importance of providing good skin care on the hands and skinfolds to prevent *Candida* overgrowth. Complex tasks should be taught in steps, with return demonstrations provided by the client or caregiver.

Most spinal cord–injured people are transferred from an acute care hospital to a rehabilitation facility. After functional capabilities have been maximized, the person is then discharged from the rehabilitation facility. The accompanying Bridge to Home Health Care feature provides suggestions for helping caregivers support the client with SCI who lives at home.

EVALUATION

Spinal cord–injured clients are hospitalized for a long time. Therefore, certain functions important to expected outcomes need to be evaluated frequently, such as respiratory and cardiac function. Other expected outcomes will not be achieved for months, such as independence in ADL. The plan of care must reflect these individual needs of the client.

Modifications for Elderly Clients

For older adults with SCI, the most important modification of the nursing care plan is increased vigilance. Older people are more prone to the complications of immobility. A person with heart failure may have difficulty breathing when lying flat. Before initiation of halo traction in this age group, some neurosurgeons perform a temporary prophylactic tracheostomy, because the older client has difficulty swallowing oral secretions and eating. Older people are also more susceptible to sensory deprivation. The nurse must make sure the client has his or her eyeglasses and hearing aid. If a window or clock is not within range of vision, the client should be reoriented as needed. Discharge plans for elderly clients may be complicated if the caregiver is also elderly. The spouse of an older spinal cord–injured person may not have the physical strength to provide the needed care. Learning to provide home care may also be problematic.

Self-Care

Paraplegic clients can usually live independently. Most quadriplegic clients need assistance with daily activities. Depending on the amount of assistance needed and the specific situation, this care may be provided by family members or by a part-time or full-time paid attendant. By using a wheelchair, clients may become completely independent in ADL, with minimal help of social services personnel, a home health aide, or family members. Many clients drive and hold outside jobs.

Ventilator-dependent people who cannot obtain in-home care and others who do not have the personal or financial resources for in-home care may have no option except institutional living. The problem of limited government resources for all clients requiring rehabilitative care remains an important ethical issue in nursing. Group living situations, especially for young adults, are becoming more available, however.

CONCLUSIONS

Disorders of the spinal cord and peripheral nervous system range from life-threatening SCIs to temporary peripheral nerve compressions. The physical and psychological impairments vary with the degree of damage as well as the client's response to and ability to cope with the body changes. The coping response is not always related to the degree of physiologic damage. A client who has facial paralysis or trigeminal neuralgia can be more compromised psychologically than a client with SCI who has developed strong coping skills. It is imperative that nurses comprehend the severity of the client's dysfunction as it relates to quality of life, as well as the impact it has on family dynamics.

Management of the client with SCI is complex and multidisciplinary. Successful rehabilitation provides the client with the opportunity to be productive in society in spite of severe neurologic deficit.

THINKING CRITICALLY

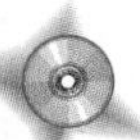

1. **A 23-year-old man was admitted from the emergency department (ED) after a car accident in**

which he sustained a concussion and thoracic injuries with thoracic spinal cord involvement. The client's baseline data included loss of consciousness for 15 minutes, headache, nausea, and inability to move or feel any sensation from his thorax down. One hour after this man arrived in the intensive care unit (ICU), additional assessment changes included inability to move fingers and hands and to flex or extend the arms. Shoulder movement was still intact. He was fully conscious and his vital signs were stable. What critical interventions initiated in the ED need to be continued in the ICU? What do these changes in data indicate? What nursing interventions are appropriate both initially and as precautions?

Factors to Consider. What are the implications when a high thoracic injury occurs? What changes indicate ascending cord dysfunction?

2. **A 22-year-old man was admitted 4 hours after sustaining a C6 spinal cord compression injury. No neurologic deficits were found, but his blood alcohol level was very high on admission. Initially, he kept falling asleep after you completed your assessments. Gardner-Wells tongs with 10 pounds of traction were placed. Now that the client is more awake, he has begun thrashing his arms and attempting to roll over in bed. What are the priorities for his care? What nursing interventions should be used?**

Factors to Consider. What is the purpose of the Gardner-Wells tongs? How would edema and microscopic bleeding compromise recovery in this client?

3. **The client, a 34-year-old woman, had a lumbar laminectomy done earlier in the day. An earlier assessment showed that movement and sensation of both lower extremities were intact. During the current postoperative assessment she states that her right toes feel numb, and the dorsiflexion and plantiflexion of the right foot are a little weaker than earlier. She has requested an analgesic because she is starting to get a headache. What are the priorities for her care? What assessments and interventions might be used?**

Factors to Consider. What assessment methods can be used to determine the extent of vascular insufficiency? What type of neurologic checks should be done?

BIBLIOGRAPHY

1. American Association of Neuroscience Nurses. (1997). *Clinical guideline series: Intracranial pressure monitoring.* Chicago: Author.
2. American Spinal Injury Association (ASIA). (1992). *Standards for neurological and functional classification of spinal cord injury.* Chicago: Author.
3. Bauman, W. A., & Spungen, A. M. (2000). Metabolic changes in persons after spinal cord injury. *Physical Medicine and Rehabilitation Clinics of North America, 11*(1), 109–140.
4. Bell, G. B. (1999). Spinal cord injury, pressure ulcers, support surfaces. *Ostomy and Wound Management, 45*(6), 48–50, 52–53.
5. Brain Trauma Foundation. (1995). *Guidelines for the management of severe head injury.* Chicago: Author.
6. Bryce, T. N., & Ragnarsson, K. T. (2000). Pain after spinal cord injury. *Physical Medicine and Rehabilitation Clinics of North America, 11*(1), 157–168.
7. Buckley, D. A., & Guanci, M. M. (1999). Spinal cord trauma. *Nursing Clinics of North America, 34*(3), 661–687.
8. Cantella, D. (1999). Sports-related spinal cord injuries. *Critical Care Nursing Quarterly, 22*(2), 14–19.
9. Chen, D., & Nussbaum, S. B. (2000). The gastrointestinal system and bowel management following spinal cord injury. *Physical Medicine and Rehabilitation Clinics of North America, 11*(1), 45–56, viii.
10. Clear, D., & Chadwick, D. W. (2000). Seizures provoked by blows to the head. *Epilepsia, 41*(2), 243–244.
11. Cruz, J. (1996). Adverse effects of pentobarbital on cerebral venous oxygenation of comatose patients with acute traumatic brain swelling: Relationship to outcome. *Journal of Neurosurgery, 85,* 758–761.
12. Cruz, J., et al. (1998). Severe acute brain trauma. In J. Cruz (Ed.), *Neurological and neurosurgical emergencies* (pp. 405–436). Philadelphia: W. B. Saunders.
13. Davis, B., & Handy, C. (1996). Cellulitis: An unreported complication of long-term SCI patients. *SCI Nursing, 13*(2), 35–38.
14. Dennis, G. C., et al. (2000). Somatosensory evoked potentials, neurologic examination and MRI for assessment of spinal cord decompression. *Life Science, 66*(5), 389–397.
15. Dubendorf, P. (1999). Spinal cord injury pathophysiology. *Critical Care Nursing Quarterly, 22*(2), 31–35.
16. Fortune, J. B., et al. (1995). Effect of hyperventilation, mannitol and ventriculostomy drainage on cerebral blood flow after head injury. *Journal of Trauma, 39,* 1091–1097.
17. Fowler, S. B., et al. (1995). Pharmacological interventions for agitation in head-injured patients in the acute care setting. *Journal of Neuroscience Nursing, 27*(2), 119–123.
18. Geary, S. (1996). Nursing management of cranial nerve dysfunction. *Journal of Neuroscience Nursing, 27*(2), 102–108.
19. Germon, K. (1994). Intracranial pressure monitoring in the 1990s. *Critical Care Nursing Quarterly, 17*(1), 21–32.
20. Goldstein, B. (2000). Musculoskeletal conditions after spinal cord injury. *Physical Medicine and Rehabilitation Clinics of North America, 11*(1), 91–108, viii–ix.
21. Gregory, R. J. (1995). Understanding and coping with neurological impairment. *Rehabilitation Nursing, 20*(2), 74–78.
22. Guerra, W. K. W., Piek, J, & Gaab, M. R. (1999). Decompressive craniectomy to treat intracranial hypertension in head injured patients. *Intensive and Critical Care Medicine, 25*(11), 1327–1329.
23. Gupta, A. K., & Bullock, M. R. (1998). Monitoring the injured brain in intensive care: present and future. Hospital Medicine 59(9), 704–713.
24. Hanson, C. W. (1998). Acute respiratory failure in neuroemergencies. In J. Cruz (Ed.), *Neurological and neurosurgical emergencies* (pp. 21–38). Philadelphia: W. B. Saunders.
25. Hickey, J. V. (1997). Craniocerebral injuries. In J. V. Hickey (Ed.), *The clinical practice of neurological and neurosurgical nursing* (4th ed., pp. 385–417). Philadelphia: J. B. Lippincott.
26. Hickey, J. V. (1997). Intracranial pressure: Theory and management of increased intracranial pressure. In J. V. Hickey (Ed.), *The clinical practice of neurological and neurosurgical nursing* (4th ed., pp. 295–328). Philadelphia: J. B. Lippincott.
27. Hickey, J. V. (1997). Vertebral and spinal cord injuries. In J. V. Hickey (Ed.), *The clinical practice of neurological and neurosurgical nursing* (4th ed., pp. 419–465). Philadelphia: J. B. Lippincott.
28. Hilton, G. (1994). Secondary brain injury and the role of neuroprotective agents. *Journal of Neuroscience Nursing, 26*(4), 251–255.
29. Jacobs, D. G., & Westerbrand, A. (1998). Antibiotic prophylaxis for intracranial pressure monitors. *Journal of the National Medical Association, 90*(7), 417–423.
30. Kavchak-Keyes, M. A. (2000). Autonomic hyperreflexia. *Rehabilitation Nursing, 25*(1), 31–35.
31. Kelly, D. F. (1995). Alcohol and head injury: An issue revisited. *Journal of Neurotrauma, 12,* 883–890.
32. Kirshblum, S. (1999). Treatment alternatives for spinal cord injury related spasticity. *Journal of Spinal Cord Medicine, 22*(3), 199–217.
33. Kirshblum, S. C., & O'Connor, K. C. (2000). Levels of spinal cord injury and predictors for neurologic recovery. *Physical Medicine and Rehabilitation Clinics of North America, 11*(1), 1–27, vii.

34. Lanig, I. S., & Peterson, W. P. (2000). The respiratory system in spinal cord injury. *Physical Medicine and Rehabilitation Clinics of North America, 11*(1), 29–43, vii.
35. Linsenmeyer, T. A. (2000). Sexual function and infertility following spinal cord injury. *Physical Medicine and Rehabilitation Clinics of North America, 11*(1), 141–156, ix.
36. Little, J. W., et al. (2000). Neurologic recovery and neurologic decline after spinal cord injury. *Physical Medicine and Rehabilitation Clinics of North America, 11*(1), 73–89.
37. Lovasik, D. (1999). The older patient with a spinal cord injury. *Critical Care Nursing Quarterly, 22*(2), 20–30.
38. Marcotte, P. J., Shaver, E. G., & Weil, R. J. (1998). Acute spinal disorders. In J. Cruz (Ed.), *Neurological and neurosurgical emergencies* (pp. 363–403). Philadelphia: W. B. Saunders.
39. Marion, D. W., & Speigel, T. P. (2000). Changes in the management of severe traumatic brain injury: 1991–1997. *Critical Care Medicine, 28*(1): 16–8.
40. McNair, N. D. (1996). Intracranial pressure monitoring. In J. M. Clouchesy, et al. (Eds.), *Critical Care Nursing* (2nd ed., pp. 289–307). Philadelphia: W. B. Saunders.
41. McNair, N. D. (1999). Traumatic brain injury. *Nursing Clinics of North America, 34*(3), 637–659.
42. Mitcho, K., & Yanko, J. R. (1999). Acute care management of spinal cord injuries. *Critical Care Nursing Quarterly, 22*(2), 60–79.
43. Nayduch, D., Lee, A., & Butler, D. (1994). High-dose methylprednisolone after acute spinal cord injury. *Critical Care Nurse, 14*(4), 69–78.
44. Neatherlin, J. S., & Brillhart, B. (1996). Body image in preoperative and postoperative lumbar laminectomy patients. *Journal of Neuroscience Nursing, 27*(1), 43–46.
45. Neatherlin, J. S. (1999). Foundation for practice: Neuroassessment for neuroscience nurses. *Nursing Clinics of North America, 34*(3), 573–592.
46. Peterson, P. L., et al. (1998). Initial evaluation and management of neuroemergencies. In J. Cruz (Ed.), *Neurological and neurosurgical emergencies* (pp. 1–20). Philadelphia: W. B. Saunders.
47. Quint, D. J. (2000). Indications for emergent MRI of the central nervous system. *Journal of the American Medical Association, 283*(7), 853–855.
48. Ramson, K. P., et al. (1998). Neuroemergency nursing. In J. Cruz (Ed.), *Neurological and neurosurgical emergencies* (pp. 467–501). Philadelphia: W. B. Saunders.
49. Richmond, T., Metcalf, J., & Daly, M. (1995). Requirements for nursing care services and associated costs in acute spinal cord injury. *Journal of Neuroscience Nursing, 27*(1), 47–52.
50. Rosner, M. J., Rosner, S. D., & Johnson, A. H. (1995). Cerebral perfusion pressure: Management protocol and clinical results. *Journal of Neurosurgery, 83,* 949–1062.
51. Rovlias, A., & Kotson, S. (2000). The influence of hyperglycemia on neurologic outcome in patients with severe head injury. *Neurosurgery, 46*(2), 335–342.
52. Sandel, M. E., et al. (1998). Neurorehabilitation. In J. Cruz (Ed.), *Neurological and neurosurgical emergencies* (pp. 503–546). Philadelphia: W. B. Saunders.
53. Segatore, M. (1999). Corticosteroids and traumatic brain injury: Status at the end of the decade of the brain. *Journal of Neuroscience Nursing, 31*(4), 239–250.
54. Seidl, E. C. (1999). Promising pharmacological agents in the management of acute spinal cord injury. *Critical Care Nursing Quarterly, 22*(2), 44–50.
55. Shaddinger, D. E. (1996). An acute spinal cord injury: My family's perspective. *Journal of Neuroscience Nursing, 27*(4), 236–239.
56. Shpritz, D. W. (1999). Neurodiagnostic studies. *Nursing Clinics of North America, 34*(3), 593–606.
57. Stewart-Amidei, C. (1998). Neurologic monitoring in the ICU. *Critical Care Nursing Quarterly, 21*(3), 47–60.
58. Thurman, D. J., et al. (1999). Traumatic brain injury in the United States: A public health perspective. *Journal of Head Trauma Rehabilitation, 14*(6), 602–615.
59. Veltman, R. H., et al. (1993). Cognitive screening in mild brain injury. *Journal of Neuroscience Nursing, 25*(6), 367–372.
60. Winemuller, M. K., et al. (1999). Prevention of venous thromboembolism in patients with spinal cord injury: Effects of sequential pneumatic compression and heparin. *Journal of Spinal Cord Medicine, 23*(3), 182–191.
61. Yundt, K. D., & Diringer, M. N. (1997). The use of hyperventilation and its impact on cerebral ischemia in the treatment of traumatic brain injury. *Critical Care Clinics, 13*(1), 163–184.
62. Zasler, N. D. (1994). Mild traumatic brain injury and post-concussive disorders: Neuromedical and medicolegal caveats. *Network, 5*(3), 3–5.

UNIT 16

Protective Disorders

Anatomy and Physiology Review

The Hematopoietic System

Joyce M. Black

Enemies of many kinds and in great numbers assault the body during a lifetime. Injury can lead to bleeding, and wounds are common. The body is also threatened by hordes of microorganisms. The body defends itself against attack by viruses, bacteria, and other parasites by using two sets of separate but interrelated functions: (1) *resistance* (called by some innate immunity) and (2) *immunity*. Both of these systems must be present and operating properly in order to block establishment of infectious agents, to minimize damage caused by disease in progress, and to expel, destroy, or isolate infectious agents that gain access to inner tissues.

Through time, the old and new defenses merged together to form a sort of three-layered approach providing both *surveillance* ("inside" threats) and *defense* ("outside" threats) functions. The importance of these mechanisms to our health and well-being becomes apparent when the defenses of a healthy body are compromised by infection or suppressed by medication or chemotherapy. Parts of the defense system in a healthy body may function inappropriately to reject organ and tissue transplants and may produce autoimmune disease or hypersensitivity states that cause pathologic changes and sometimes death.

RESISTANCE: A FORM OF NONSPECIFIC DEFENSE

The first line of defense in the body is the aspect of resistance that stops a threatening agent or condition. Defenses provide a form of resistance against disease by combatting anything not recognized as *self.* Resistance components are usually the first to encounter infectious agents or parasites. Many of these functions operate independently of the immune system but, as shown later, some of the components and features participate in or amplify acquired immune responses.

SURFACE DEFENSES

Intact skin and mucous membranes are sufficient to provide barriers that prevent penetration to underlying tissues by many pathogens. Lysozyme in tears and bile in the gut inhibit gram-positive bacteria; hydrochloric acid in the stomach is lethal to all pathogens; and fatty acids help protect the skin from infectious agents. Surface-clearing mechanisms (such as washing of oral surfaces by saliva, tear-washing, urine-flushing, the mucociliary escalator in the trachea), mucoperistaltic propulsion in the small intestine, and the cough reflex prevent attachment of invading organisms. Autochthonous (natural) flora interfere with colonization of pathogens by both *niche* (function) and *habitat* (location) *competition.*

The *reticuloendothelia system* (RES) includes mononuclear phagocytic cells (macrophages). Fixed (attached) macrophages in the sinusoids of the liver, spleen, and bone marrow monitor the circulating blood and remove all foreign particulates and any moribund self cells. Resident mobile macrophages in lymph nodes remove foreign particulate matter. Macrophages in the alveolar spaces are the most active of the RES cells and help remove inspired particulates that reach the lower recesses of the lung.

ORGANS OF THE IMMUNE AND HEMATOLOGIC SYSTEMS

The organs of the immune and hematologic systems are shown in Figure U16–1. There are both peripheral and central organs.

■ PERIPHERAL LYMPHOID TISSUE

Peripheral lymphoid tissues are sites for antigen processing and presentation and for T-cell and B-cell activation. These are the only locales for the production of the molecules and cells that serve as effector units of the immune response.

LYMPH NODES

Lymph nodes are mostly small organs (many are less than 5 mm in diameter) that are present throughout the body interconnected by means of lymph vessels. Their structure is fairly complex and provides both RES and immune functions. The lymph node receives fluid, particulates, and solutes that are taken up by lymphatic capillaries from distal tissue sites. Resident macrophages within the node monitor the lymph fluid passing through for the presence of foreign particulates and remove them by phagocytic action. Antigenic substances, either particulates or solutes, are taken up by the macrophages or dendritic cells serving as antigen-presenting cells (APCs). Immunocompetent cells in the lymph node can give rise to either a humoral immune response or a cell-mediated immune response. The masses of cells called lymph or medullary cords also exist as a site of secondary humoral immune responses.

Lymph nodes are found in large numbers in the thoracic and abdominal cavities. Those lying close to the body surface are called *superficial nodes.* Cervical nodes lie alongside the neck, axillary nodes in the armpit, and inguinal nodes in the crease between the upper thigh and the trunk. When inflamed, these nodes become swollen and may be palpated, serving as diagnostic signs.

LYMPH NODULES

The structure of the lymph nodules is much less organized than that of the lymph nodes. The nodules occur in the mucosal epithelium lining the respiratory, gastrointestinal (GI), and urogenital tracts. Antigenic materials are translocated across a dome epithelium through a special

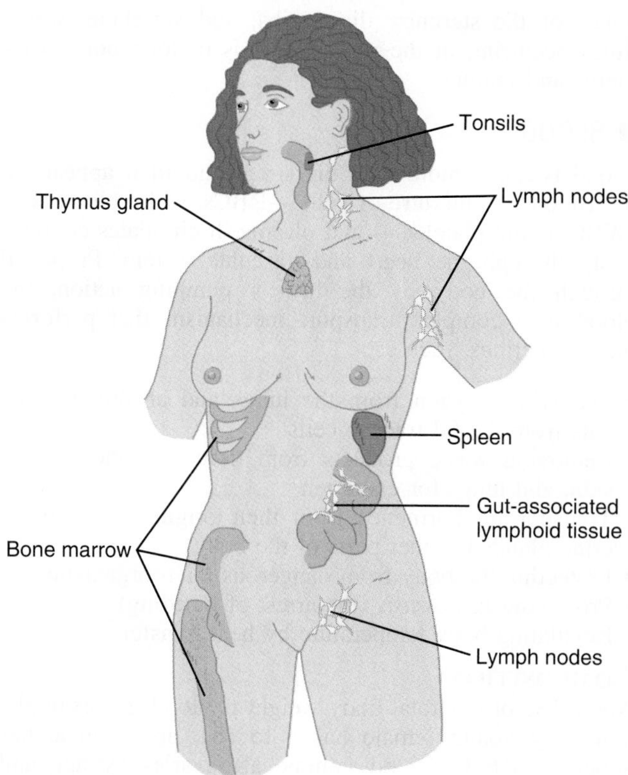

FIGURE U16–1 Organs of the immune system. The bone marrow, spleen, lymph nodes, tonsils, and gut-associated lymphoid tissue (GALT) function in both specific and nonspecific immunity, whereas the thymus functions primarily in specific immunity.

cell (M cell). The translocated material is deposited directly into the nodule structure where it is taken up by APCs. Immunocompetent B cells in lymph nodules produce either immunoglobulin E (IgE) or IgA. These two classes of immunoglobulins provide for the development either of allergy of the immediate hypersensitivity type (atopy) or of a mucosal immune response.

■ CENTRAL LYMPHOID ORGANS

SPLEEN

The spleen is the largest lymphoid organ in the body. Its defensive functions include the blood-clearing process via fixed macrophages in sinusoids as well as serving as a major site of humoral immune responses to blood-borne antigens. The splenic pulp is divided into red zones and white zones. The white zones are accumulations of lymphocytes and APCs. Loss of the spleen or diminished function due to injury or infection greatly increases the risk of infection with extracellular bacteria.

Other functions of the spleen include (1) assisting in recycling iron by capturing hemoglobin released from destroyed red blood cells (RBCs) and (2) performing pitting (removal of particles from RBCs without destroying the cell itself).

THYMUS

The thymus is a lymphoepithelial organ located in the mediastinum, the thoracic cavity between the lungs and above the heart. The thymus reaches peak development during childhood. After puberty, it begins to atrophy but remnants persist into old age. The thymus is an endocrine organ that secretes hormones that contribute to the maintenance and function of peripheral T-cell populations. The interior of the early thymus is filled with thymocytes from the bone marrow and from a high rate of cell replication within the organ.

A fundamental paradigm in immunology is the rearrangement of germ line genes during differentiation of lymphocytes in the central lymphoid tissues, leading to the production of molecules for the recognition of antigen. In both cell types, the antigen recognition unit is inserted into the membrane with the antigen-reactive ends extending out into the extracellular environment. The T cell uses the T-cell antigen receptor, and the B cell has a tetrapeptide monomer called *surface immunoglobulin* (SIg). The individual cells each have a unique receptor capable of reacting only with a single antigenic determinant (Fig. U16–2). Each specifically reacting cell is called a *clonotype*; when properly stimulated by antigen, the clonotype produces effector units (either antibody molecules or specially reactive cells) and a memory cell clone, both of which have the identical specificity of the original clonotype.

The positive and negative selection processes acting on cells in the thymus make it possible for the mechanism to discriminate between *self* and *non-self* in immune function. This distinction is accomplished by making antigen recognition absolutely dependent on the variable but individually unique composition of the transcription products of gene loci located in the major histocompatibility region of the genome.

Class I major histocompatibility complex (MHC) molecules are found on nearly all nucleated cells in the body and represent a major antigenic distinction between individuals of a given species with different genotypes. This

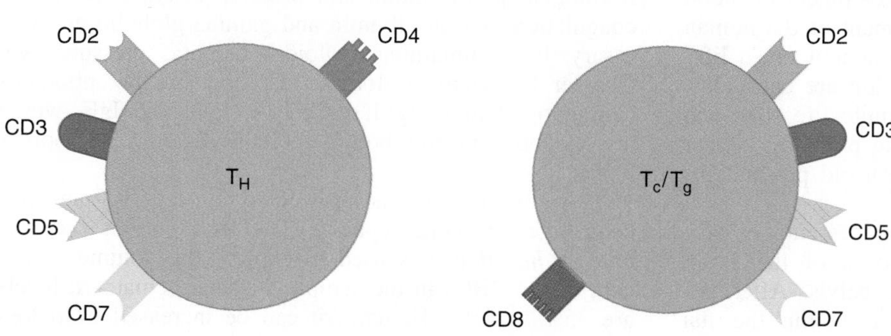

FIGURE U16–2 T cells can be distinguished by distinctive molecules located on their cell surfaces. They are called cluster designations (CDs). All mature T cells carry markers known as T2 (or CD2), T3 (or CD3), T5 (or CD5), and T7 (or CD7). T helper (T_H) cells carry a T4 (CD4) marker, and suppressor and cytotoxic T (T_c/T_g) cells carry a T8 (CD8) marker.

molecule is necessary for antigen recognition by T cells with CD8 surface markers. Class II MHC molecules are found on some APCs, on all B cells, and on antigen-activated T cells. This molecule is necessary for antigen recognition by T cells with CD4 surface markers. MHC antigens in humans were intitially discovered on leukocyte membranes and are thus called *human leukocyte antigens* (HLAs). It is this recognition system that forms the basis for the rejection of foreign or transplanted tissue. The cells in the recipient's immune system recognize the surface HLA proteins of the donor's tissue as being nonself.

BONE MARROW

Bone marrow constitutes one of the largest organs in the body, with an aggregate weight in adults of about 3000 g (comparable in mass to the liver). Based on visual appearance, the marrow mass was originally described as being either red or yellow. *Red marrow* consists of a mass of supporting cells surrounding aggregates of hematopoietic cells and interspaced with sinusoidal capillaries.

Yellow marrow has a large number of adipose cells, which accounts for its characteristic light color. This portion, or compartment, of the marrow is generally not active in hematopoiesis in a normal healthy person. However, following severe blood loss or the development of a sustained state of hypoxia, the yellow marrow can be converted into a red marrow state and production of blood cells initiated.

Function of Bone Marrow

Bone marrow provides for the following:

- Maintenance of a self-renewing pluripotent stem cell population from which all blood cells are derived
- An environment for the differentiation and maturation of blood cells
- A storage site for large numbers of neutrophils and erythrocytes
- Transformation of undifferentiated lymphocytes into mature B cells
- A site of antibody production in a secondary immune response to thymic-dependent antigens administered intravenously

Sinusoids bearing fixed macrophages serve an RES function in blood clearing. This is a defensive action based on the phagocytic activity of the macrophages attached to the luminal side of the marrow sinuses. These phagocytes, part of the RES or mononuclear phagocytic system, monitor the blood for the presence of foreign particulate matter, remove it, and destroy it.

FORMATION OF BLOOD CELLS. *Hematopoiesis*, the important process of formation and development of blood cells, begins very early in the development of the human embryo and must persist unabated throughout one's lifetime. The demands made on this function are enormous. Cells in the peripheral blood have a finite life span and must be continuously renewed at a rate probably greater than 10 billion cells/day. For a 100-year-old person, this would amount to more than 10^{14} cells.

During childhood, all blood cells are essentially produced in marrow sites of the flat bones of the skull, clavicle, sternum, ribs, vertebrae, and pelvis. After puberty, hematopoiesis becomes localized within the flat bones of the sternum, ilium, ribs, and vertebrae, sometimes occurring in the proximal ends of long bones (humerus and femur).

■ BLOOD

Blood is much more than the simple liquid it appears to be. Blood is a mixutre of cells—RBCs, white blood cells (WBCs), and platelets—and plasma. It circulates continuously through the heart and vascular system. Propelled through the body by the heart's pumping action, the blood is a complex transport mechanism that performs many functions, such as:

- Supplying oxygen from the lungs and absorbed nutrients from the GI tract to cells
- Removing waste products from tissues to the kidney, skin, and lungs for excretion
- Transporting hormones from their origin in the endocrine glands to other parts of the body
- Protecting the body from dangerous microorganisms
- Promoting *hemostasis* (the arrest of bleeding)
- Regulating body temperature by heat transfer

COMPOSITION

About 8% of our total body weight is blood; for example, a healthy young female has 4 to 5 L and a male has about 5 to 6 L. Blood volume also varies by age and body composition. There is an inverse relationship between blood volume and kilograms of body weight. The less body fat, the more blood per kilogram of body weight is present.

Arterial blood is bright red because of the oxygen bound to hemoglobin and oxygen within RBCs. Venous blood is dark red because of its lower oxygen content. Blood is three to four times more viscous (thick) than water. Specific gravity is 1.048 to 1.066. Blood is slightly alkaline, with a pH of 7.35 to 7.45 (neutral pH is 7.0).

PLASMA

Plasma, the liquid portion of the blood, is one of the three major blood fluids (along with interstitial and intracellular fluids). Plasma makes up about 55% of the blood, and solid suspended particles (blood cells and platelets) compose the other 45%. The major function of plasma is to maintain the blood volume within the vascular compartment.

A straw-colored, watery substance, plasma is composed of 92% water, 7% proteins, and less than 1% nutrients, metabolic wastes, respiratory gases, enzymes, hormones, clotting factors, and inorganic salts. The proteins include serum albumin (alpha-globulin, and alpha$_2$-globulin, beta-globulin, and gamma-globulin) as well as fibrinogen, prothrombin, and proteins essential for blood coagulation. Serum albumin and gamma globulin are necessary for maintaining colloidal osmotic pressure (see Chapter 12). Gamma globulin also contains the antibodies (immunoglobulins) IgM, IgG, IgA, IgD, and IgE, which are essential in the body's defense against microorganisms.

If a tube of blood is allowed to stand or is spun in a centrifuge, the cells separate. The term *packed cell volume* or *hematocrit* is used to express the volume or per cent of the RBCs in the sample. Normal hematocrit levels are 35% to 45%. Hematocrit can be increased from loss of plasma (e.g., dehydration) or increased production of RBCs (polycythemia). Low hematocrit levels are seen in overyhydration and low numbers of RBCs (Fig. U16–3). The WBCs and platelets make up less than 1% of the blood volume. These cells form a buffy coat or white layer and are seen at the interface of the RBCs and plasma.

Hematopoiesis

Stem cells are poorly characterized, undifferentiated cells that exist within the red marrow. These totipotent, or pluripotent, stem cells are self-replicating and maintain a small population throughout the lifetime of the individual. Following stimulation by one or more signal molecules called *poietins,* the stem cells can undergo differentiation into erythrocytes (RBCs), megakaryocytes, and leukocytes. The steps of hematopiesis and the divisions of each cell, once it takes a committed path, are shown in Figure U16–4.

Control of Hematopoiesis

Much of the mechanism of hematopoietic regulation that stimulates the initial differentiation of stem cells and controls the early differentiation of the expanding cell lines is either not known or is poorly characterized. The so-called *hematopoietic inductive environment* is provided mainly by growth factors. These growth factors (*cytokines*) control cell growth, proliferation, and differentiation. Growth factors are usually identified by using acronyms that are a legacy from original studies of colony-forming cells. The suffix "-CSF" (colony-stimulating factor) describes the growth factor that stimulates or regulates the development of the corresponding cell type identified by the prefix "CFU-." For example, G-CSF is the growth factor for CFU-G (colony-forming unit–granulocytic series), and M-CSF is the growth factor regulating the development of monocytes (CFU-M). Other growth factors, interleukins (ILs), are given numbers to distinguish between different molecules; IL-1 is derived from macrophages, IL-3 from activated T cells, and so forth.

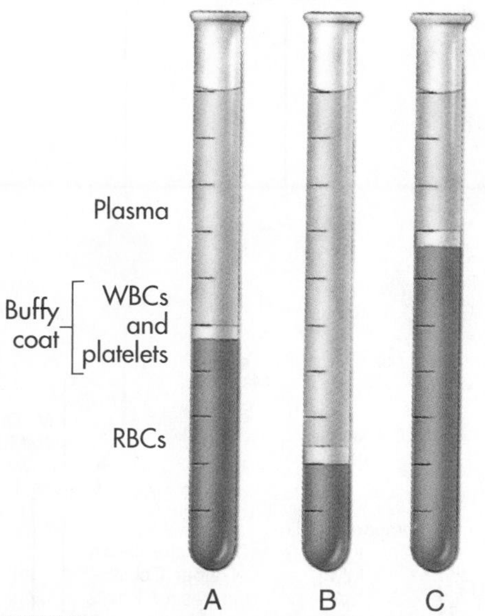

FIGURE U16–3 Tubes showing hematocrit levels of normal blood, anemia, and polycythemia. Note the buffy coat located between the packed red blood cells (RBCs) and the plasma. *A,* A normal percentage of RBCs. *B,* Anemia (a low percentage of RBCs). *C,* Polycythemia (a high percentage of RBCs). WBCs, white blood cells. (From Thibodeau, G., & Patton, K. [1999]. *Anatomy and physiology* [4th ed., p. 529]. St. Louis: Mosby.)

Red Blood Cells

RBCs (erythrocytes) carry oxygen or hemoglobin to the cells and carbon dioxide back to the lungs. RBCs also assist with acid-base balance. They contain carbonic anhydrase, an enzyme that joins carbon dioxide to water to form carbonic acid. The acid dissociates to form bicarbonate and hydrogen ions, which diffuse out of the RBC.

The mature RBC has no nucleus and is only 7.5 μm in diameter. Each RBC has a depression on the flat surface which provides a thin center and thicker edges. The RBC's unique structure supplies a very large surface area relative to its volume and allows the cell to change shape passively as it is transported through capillaries that are smaller than 7.5 μm. The average RBC count is 5,500,000 cells/mm^3 of blood.

Packed within each RBC are about 200 to 300 million molecules of hemoglobin. Each hemoglobin molecule is composed of four protein chains (globin). The globin is bound to a heme group that contains one iron atom. In healthy men, 100 ml of blood contains 14 to 16 g of hemoglobin. Women have slightly less, about 12 to 14 g. When hemoglobin levels fall to less than 10 g, anemia exists.

Erythrocyte Production

The production of erythrocytes is termed *erythropoiesis.* Everyday RBCs are produced at a very rapid rate. Normally, every minute of the day, more than 100 million RBCs are formed to replace an equal number of destroyed cells. The rate of RBC production increases when oxygen levels decrease, during pregnancy and under the influence of erythropoietin. Healthy bone marrow has the capacity to increase its production of erythrocytes six to eight times over the normal rate and is thus able to keep pace with increased destruction or loss of RBCs. This response mechanism can maintain a remarkably constant number of erythrocytes within each of us.

Erythrocytes are produced in the red bone marrow. Required for this process are (1) precursor cells, (2) a proper microenvironment, and (3) adequate supplies of iron, vitamin B_{12}, folic acid, protein, pyridoxine, and traces of copper. If any of these factors is missing, the resultant erythrocytes will be fragile, misshapen, abnormally large or small, deficient in hemoglobin, or too few in number. Erythrocytes arise from nucleated cells called *hematopoietic stem cells. Stem cells* can maintain a constant population of newly differentiating cells. Differentiation takes about 7 days and involves about six stages (Fig. U16–5).

Immature erythrocytes leave the bone marrow via veins in the marrow and enter the general circulation as reticulocytes. After their release from the marrow sites, the reticulocytes travel to the spleen, where they undergo conditioning and evolve into mature erythrocytes before being released into the general circulation.

The life span of RBCs is about 105 to 120 days. As erythrocytes age, they become increasingly fragile and eventually rupture. The released hemoglobin and the empty membranes ("ghost cells") are taken up by macro-

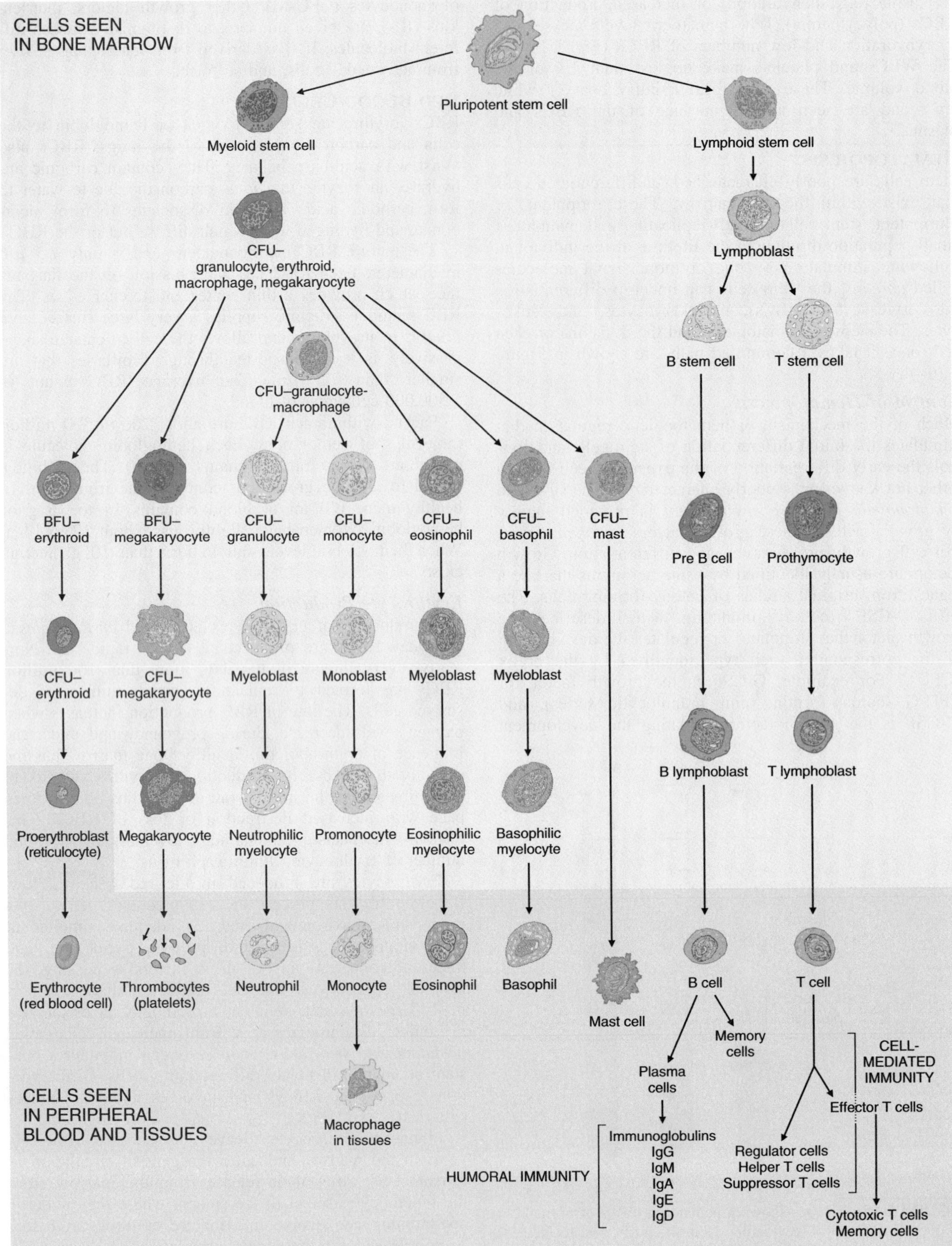

FIGURE U16–4 Hematopoietic cascade. The pluripotent stem cell is the origin of all cells. Once a pathway is chosen, the cell is committed to the final cell type.

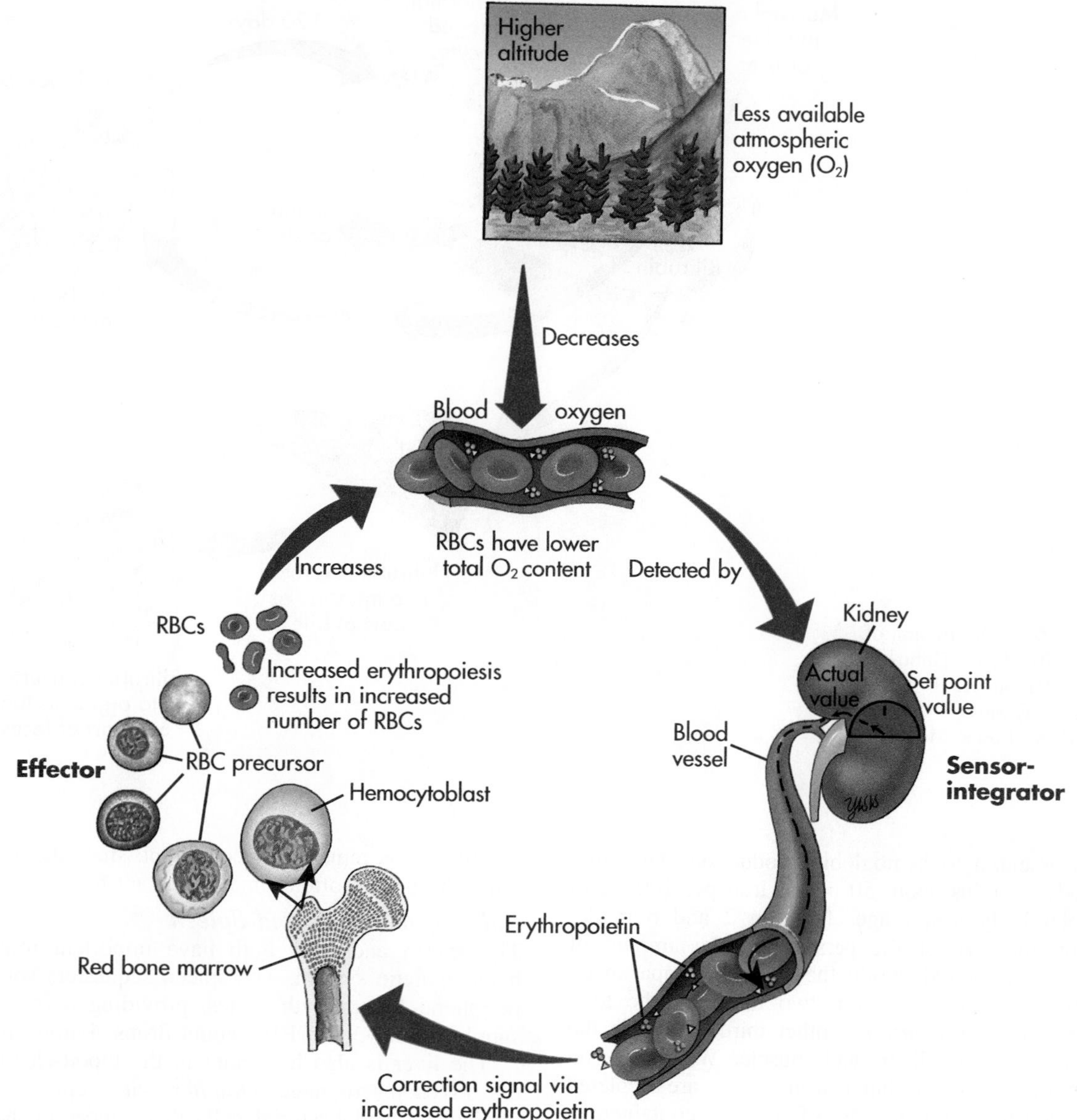

FIGURE U16–5 Erythropoiesis. In response to decreased blood oxygen, the kidneys release erythropoietin, which stimulates erythrocyte production in the red bone marrow. (From Thibodeau, G., & Patton, K. [1999]. *Anatomy and physiology* [4th ed., p. 533]. St. Louis: Mosby.)

phages within the liver, spleen, lymph nodes, and bone marrow. The hemoglobin is broken down into heme (iron and porphyrin) and globin (polypeptide chain) fractions. The iron of the heme fraction is returned to the liver, spleen, and bone marrow to be reused in making hemoglobin. The liver converts the porphyrin of the heme fraction into bilirubin, an orange pigment, and secretes it into the bile to be excreted from the body in the feces and urine (Fig. U16–6). During periods of increased RBC destruction (e.g., in hemolytic anemia), excessive amounts of bilirubin are formed and may accumulate in the body's tissues.

Nutritional Influences on Red Blood Cell Production

Vitamin B_{12} is essential for normal RBC maturation and nervous system functions. Because it is not synthesized in the body, vitamin B_{12} must be a component of the daily diet. Animal products such as meat and dairy products are the only sources of this vitamin. In this context, vitamin B_{12} is called *extrinsic factor* (meaning outside the body). When released from food during gastric digestion, vitamin B_{12} binds with an autogenous glycoprotein called *intrinsic factor* (inside the body) present in the duodenum, and the complex is transported to the distal ileum, where specific receptors in the mucosa bind vitamin B_{12} for absorption into the blood.

Folic acid, a B-group vitamin, is necessary for RBC formation and maturation; unlike vitamin B_{12}, however folic acid does not play a role in nervous system function. The molecule is synthesized by many plants and bacteria. Major dietary sources of folic acid are vegetables and fruits. Cooking destroys some forms of folic acid.

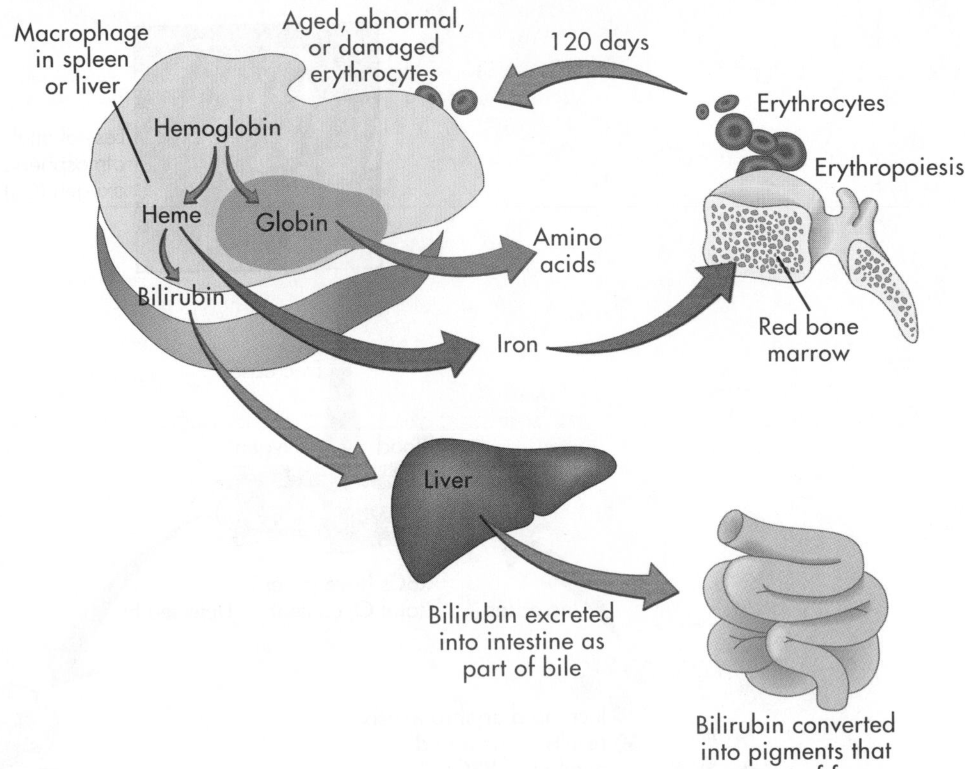

FIGURE U16–6 Destruction of red blood cells. (From Thibodeau, G., & Patton, K. [1999]. *Anatomy and physiology* [4th ed., p. 534]. St. Louis: Mosby.)

Iron is essential to hemoglobin production. The adult human body contains about 50 mg of iron per 100 ml of blood. Total body iron ranges between 2 and 6 g, depending on the size of the person and the amount of hemoglobin sequestered within the cellular compartment. Hemoglobin accounts for about two thirds of the total iron (called *essential iron*). The other third resides in the bone marrow, spleen, liver, and muscle. When an iron deficiency develops, the latter iron stores are depleted first, followed by a gradual loss of the iron contained in hemoglobin.

Megakaryocytes and Platelets

Platelets *(thrombocytes)* have two essential roles in hemostasis: (1) occlusion of small openings in blood vessels (a hemostatic function) and (2) provision of chemical components in the molecular cascade leading to coagulation (a thromboplastic function).

Individual platelets are produced by a fragmentation process from giant multinucleated cells in the red bone marrow called *megakaryoctes* (see Fig. U16–4). The earliest percursor in this transformation sequence, a megakaryoblast, is large (~30 mm in diameter), has a basophilic cytoplasm, and, when mature, contains multiple nuclear equivalents. The time required for the formation of human platelets is about 5 days. Cytoplasmic extensions from megakaryoblasts are extruded into sinusoids, and platelets are formed by fragmentation at the terminal ends of the filaments. Normal human marrow may have up to 6 million megakaryocytes per kilogram of body weight, with each megakaryocyte being able to give rise to a thousand or more individual platelets. Platelet production in a normal person appears to be under tight control and is remarkably consistent, since the numbers in a healthy person often remain constant for years.

Roles of the Liver and Spleen

The spleen and liver both have important roles in the hematopoietic system. The spleen sequesters some of the peripheral blood erythrocytes, providing a ready reserve supply whenever the RBC count drops significantly.

The liver is also important in the blood-clearing process. Fixed macrophages *(Kupffer cells)* remove inanimate particulates and bacterial cells that appear in the peripheral blood. The roles of the liver in hematopoiesis are mostly indirect and consist of:

- Production of small quantities of erythropoietin
- Synthesis of plasma proteins and clotting factors
- Decomposition of hemoglobin into bilirubin
- Storage of iron in the form of *ferritin*

Hemostasis

Normal hemostasis is a process that repairs vascular breaks to reduce blood loss from blood vessels while maintaining the flow of blood through the vascular system. The three components of the hemostatic mechanism are (1) the blood vessels, (2) the platelets (or thrombocytes), and (3) coagulation factors. These components accomplish hemostatis in three stages (Fig. U16–7):

1. The vascular phase, in which *vasoconstriction* of the vessels occurs.
2. Formation of a platelet plug.
3. Coagulation or formation of a fibrin clot. Once the fibrin clot has served its purpose, it is balanced by *fibrinolysis* (clot dissolution), thus preventing thrombosis.

Whenever bleeding results from injury or disease, the blood vessels that supply the damaged site constrict. Vasoconstriction slows the flow of blood to the injured area, decreasing blood loss. Vasoconstriction results from muscular tissue and reflex nervous system reactions. *Serotonin,* a potent local vasoconstrictor, is secreted by cells in the small intestine and promotes blood vessel constriction on injury.

Adequate numbers of cells (150,000 to 400,000/mm^3) are required in the peripheral blood for hemostasis. When platelets come into contact with an alteration of the endothelial cell lining of a blood vessel, they become sticky and adhere to one another, thus sealing the surface of the vessel lining. Platelets also release intracellular storage granules, which include substances that can stimulate circulating platelets and cause them to acquire new adhesive properties. These platelet constituents can activate additional platelets that aggregate to form a *thrombus.*

Platelets control hemostasis unless large blood vessels have been damaged. If bleeding is severe, coagulation factors must join with platelets to form a permanent clot. The coagulation system consists of a series of interactions that result in the formation of a fibrin clot. The system consists of clotting proteins (except factor IV), that is, factors that circulate in the plasma (except factor III, which is released from damaged cells) in an inactive state.

The formation of a fibrin clot can result from activation of one of two pathways: *intrinsic* or *extrinsic.* Various factors are needed by these two pathways for completion of a final common pathway that results in a fibrin clot.

The *extrinsic pathway* is initiated when tissue injury occurs outside the vessels, such as a burn. Damaged tissues release factor III (tissue thromboplastin), which initiates the clotting cascade to form activated factor X, which leads to the final common pathway of clot formation.

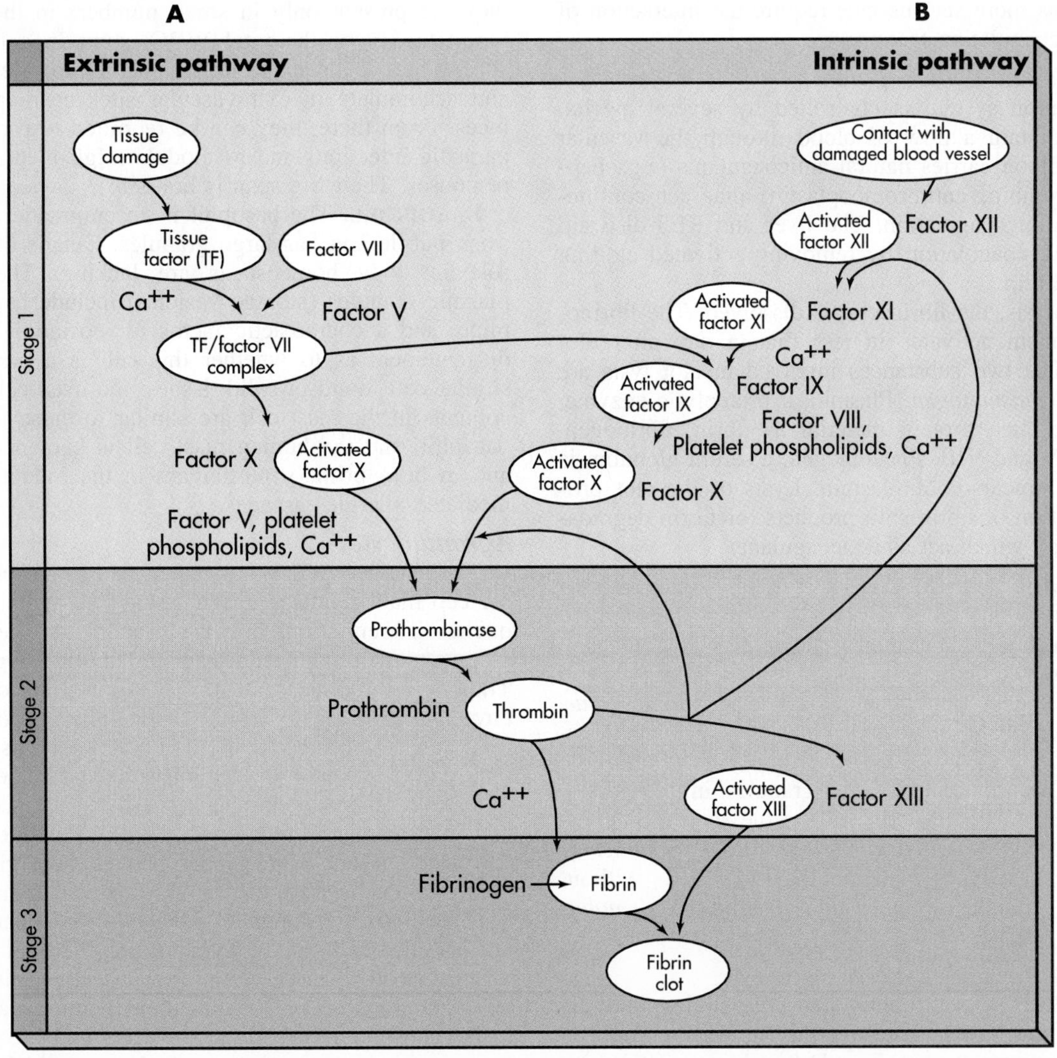

FIGURE U16–7 Clot formation. *A,* Extrinsic clotting pathway. *Stage I:* Damaged tissue releases tissue factor (TF), which with factor VII and calcium ions activates factor X. Activated factor X, factor V, phospholipids, and calcium ions form prothrombinase. *Stage 2:* Prothrombin is converted to thrombin by prothrombinase. *Stage 3:* Fibrinogen is converted to fibrin by thrombin. Fibrin forms a clot. *B,* Intrinsic clotting pathway. *Stage 1:* Damaged vessels cause activation of factor XII. Activated factor XII activates factor XI, which activates factor IX. Factor IX, along with factor VIII and platelet phospholipids, activates factor X. Activated factor X, factor V, phospholipids, and calcium ions form prothrombinase. *Stages 2* and *3* take the same course as in the extrinsic clotting pathway. (From Thibodeau, G., & Patton, K. [1999]. *Anatomy and physiology* [4th ed., p. 543]. St. Louis: Mosby.)

The *intrinsic pathway* involves the blood itself (i.e., antigen-antibody reactions and endotoxins) or damage to the blood vessels. All factors for the intrinsic system are present in the plasma. This pathway is initiated when factor XII is exposed to a foreign surface, which initiates a cascade of enzymatic reactions to activate factor X, leading to the common pathway.

Activated factor X is responsible for the conversion of prothrombin to thrombin and of soluble fibrinogen to an insoluble fibrin clot. The protein fibrin forms dense interlacing threads that entrap erythrocytes and platelets. The platelets then release a contractile protein, which causes shrinkage and retraction of the clot into a firm, insoluble fibrin mass. The process of retraction squeezes out the clear yellow serum. Serum differs from plasma, in that it does not contain clotting factors.

In some cases, formation of a fibrin clot is unnecessary because hemostasis occurs at an early stage. Temporary clots are sometimes insufficient. For example, bleeding from a small pinprick can normally be ended by a platelet plug, whereas more serious cuts require the interaction of the various coagulation factors.

Fibrinolysis and Anticoagulants

The coagulation system is controlled by several mechanisms to maintain a flow of blood through the vascular space. The blood carries natural anticoagulants (e.g., heparin, antithrombin, antithromboplastin) that act continuously to inhibit coagulation. The liver and RES also aid in controlling coagulation by removing activated clotting factors and fibrin.

In fibrinolysis, the fibrin clot is dissolved. The fibrinolytic mechanism activates in less than a day after clot formation. The two substances involved in clot lysis are *plasmin* and *plasminogen.* Plasmin, a proteolytic enzyme, can dissolve such protein material as fibrin, fibrinogen, and factors V and VIII. Plasminogen, a serum globulin, is the inactive precursor of plasmin. Lysis of the clot produces formation of fibrin split products (or fibrin degradation products), which act as anticoagulants.

White Blood Cells (Leukocytes)

There are five types of WBCs, or *leukocytes,* classified according to the presence or absence of granules and the staining characteristics of their cytoplasm. As a group, the leukocytes appear brightly colored when stained. *Granulocytes* are derived from a myeloid stem cell that differentiates (see Fig. U16–4). Granulocytes include three types of WBCs that have large granules in their cytoplasm. Their names are derived from the staining properties: (1) *neutrophils,* (2) *eosinophils,* and (3) *basophils.*

There are two types of agranulocytes (WBCs without cytoplasmic granules): (1) *monocytes* and (2) *lymphocytes.*

Granulocytes

Neutrophils. Neutrophils stain very light pink-purple with netural dyes. The granules in their cytoplasm make them appear "coarse," and they have nuclei with many lobes. Because of the appearance of their nuclei, they are also called polymorphonuclear leukocytes ("polys").

The neutrophil is the primary cell to respond during an acute inflammatory response (see Fig. U16–4). About 90% of mature neutrophils remain in the bone marrow, a storage arrangement that enables the body to quickly release large numbers of these cells when inflammation occurs in perimeter tissues. The remaining 10% of neutrophils in the peripheral blood are subdivided, about half and half, into a circulating cell group and a cell group that adheres to endothelial linings in small blood vessels.

Thus, a complete blood count (CBC) for a healthy person accounts for only about 5% of the total number of mature neutrophils actually present in the body at that time. The increases seen in peripheral WBC counts during episodes of inflammation are the result of large numbers of neutrophils being released from the bone marrow reserve. If the inflamed state is prolonged, the supply of mature cells with lobed nuclei will be exhausted, and immature neutrophils with a banded nucleus will appear in the circulating blood (shift to the left). The neutrophil's life span is hours to 3 days.

Eosinophils. Eosinophils contain numerous large granules that stain orange. Under normal circumstances, mature eosinophils do not remain long in the marrow; they are present only in small numbers in the peripheral blood (<3% of the total WBC count in a healthy person). These cells exit the peripheral blood compartment and accumulate in extravascular sites near epthelial surfaces. From there, they can be recruited to protect against parasitic infections and to modulate IgE-mediated allergic responses. Their life span is hours to 3 days.

Basophils. The basophil is an enigmatic cell type. It sains purple and has large granules. Details of its normal role in body homeostasis are lacking. The intracytoplasmic granules (storage vesicles) include heparin, histamine, and a chemotactic factor for eosinophils. There is disagreement as to whether this cell is a precursor to a similar cell found in solid tissues: the mast cell. Vesicular contents in the mast cell are similar to those found in the basophil, and the human mast cell is known to bind IgE and to be a primary participant in the induction of IgE-mediated allergic cascades.

Agranulocytes

Monocytes. The monocyte is derived from a precursor cell that is indistinguishable from a myelobast. Subsequent differentiation, however, leads to a cell structure that is markedly different from that of the granulocyte. The monocyte released from the bone marrow into the circulation is a hypoactive phagocytic cell. After becoming attached to sinusoidal endothelium in the spleen, bone marrow, and liver, or after emigrating from the blood into lung, connective, lymphoid tissue, this cell becomes transformed into a *macrophage* with full phagocytic function.

In earlier times some macrophages were given special names when they were discovered: alveolar macrophages (dust cells) in the lungs, histiocytes in connective tissues, and Kupffer cells in the liver. In the 1920s, it was recognized that all of these cells formed a large, dispersed cell population whose major functional feature was phagocytosis. These cells constitute the RES and are responsible for removing all foreign particulate material that enters the body.

The macrophage is attracted secondarily to acute inflamed sites and is the characteristic cell in chronic and in many secretory T cell–orchestrated inflammatory lesions. Some macrophages also have immune functions by serving as antigen-processing cells and APCs.

LYMPHOCYTES. In their mature form, lymphocytes are assigned to one of three groups according to the presence of characteristic surface markers and cell function (see Fig. U16–2): (1) Some lymphocytes are programmed in the thymus to become *T cells;* (2) others are programmed in the bone marrow become *B cells;* and (3) some lymphocytes, not identifiable as either T or B cells, are *null cells.*

B cells function in antibody-mediated immune responses helping to defend the body against invasive types of bacteria, bacterial toxins, and some viruses.

T cells are the basis of cell-mediated immune functions that defend against facultative and obligate intracellular pathogens, fungi, and viruses.

Null lymphocytes, sometimes called *natural killer cells,* defend against some viral infections and are able to destroy some tumor cells.

The Natural Killer Cell System. Natural killer (NK) cells are a poorly understood group of lymphoid cells that make up about 5% to 10% of the circulating lymphoctes. They are involved in killing some tumor cells and some virally infected cells. Their cytotoxicity can be enhanced by exposure to cytokines, which convert a naive NK cell into a lymphokine-activated cell. After binding to a target cell, the NK cell secretes special protein molecules called *perforins* into the intercellular space. The perforins cause holes to form in the target cell membrane in a manner analogous to the membrane attack complex (MAC) of complement. Interestingly, people who have normal T-cell and B-cell populations but who are deficient in NK cells experience repetitive life-threatening infections by viruses such as varicella and cytomegalovirus.

Inflammation

Inflammation is a complex response to sublethal injury to a tissue, having both local and systemic consequences. The process can be initiated by products released from damaged cells, by components from microbial cells, and by the interaction of effector units and antigen. Within the injured tissue site, the first indication is a transient constriction followed by a sustained dilation of small blood vessels. Swelling at the site is caused by the escape of plasma (with its solutes: complement, fibrinogen, immunoglobulins). At about the same time that the vessels are responding, WBCs begin to stick to the vascular endothelium, a process called *margination.* Neutrophils are the first to escape from the vessels *(diapedesis)* and, in response to a chemotactic gradient, accumulate at the site of injury.

After a few hours, monocytes from the local circulation and macrophages present in local connective tissues begin to infiltrate the site of injury and soon replace the neutrophils as the dominant cell type. In a limited type of injury, the healing and resolution begin shortly afterward (see Chapter 16). Some cytokines produced by stimulated macrophages act locally to stimulate vascular changes and to activate fibroblasts and other cells. The same or other cytokines are distributed systemically and help to initiate the *acute phase response.* This systemic response accompanies a strong local inflammatory response. Many aspects of the acute phase response are initiated by the action of cytokines produced by stimulated macrophages. These stimulatory molecules include IL-1, tumor necrosis factor (TNF), and IL-6. The systemic responses of the host include (1) elevation of serum cortisol; (2) induction of fever; (3) leukocytosis; (4) the de novo appearance of C-reactive protein, an opsonizing protein that aids in phagocytosis; (5) increased production of complement components; and (6) increased production of siderophores (iron-binding proteins).

IMMUNITY

We can become immunized by *direct* (active) or *indirect* (passive) means as follows:

1. *Active* immunity; we produce effector units following stimulation by an antigen.
2. *Natural* immunity is produced by disease and environmentally acquired allergies.
3. *Artifical* immunity is produced via vaccinations and allergies from therapeutic drugs.
4. *Passive* immunity; we receive effector units produced by an animal, another human, or by gene-engineering procedures.

Natural immunity is produced via colostrum (topological protection in humans) and across the placenta (systemic protection in humans). Artificial immunity is produced through pooled gamma (immune)-globulin, RH_0(D) immune globulin (RhoGAM), and genetically engineered human antibody.

ACQUIRED IMMUNITY

Four types (or compartments) of active immunity are identified based on the type and body location of the effector units:

1. *Humoral immunity.* The effector units are immunoglobulins (IgM, IgG, and IgA) present in the peripheral blood.
2. *Mucosal immunity.* The effector unit is an immunoglobulin (secretory IgA) present in mucous secretions of the respiratory tract, GI tract, and urogenital tract.
3. *Cell-mediated immunity.* The effector units are cytotoxic T cells that circulate in peripheral blood and are present in peripheral lymphoid tissues.
4. *Atopic hypersensitivity (type I hypersensitivity).* The effector unit is IgE, which is attached to surface receptors on mast cells found in connective tissues and subsurface tissues of the respiratory and GI tract.

THE PRIMARY IMMUNE RESPONSE AND THE IMMUNE CASCADE

A primary immune response arguably occurs only once (Fig. U16–8). The quality and quantity of the primary immune response depend on many factors, some of which are host-related whereas others depend on the composition of the antigen and how it is presented to the recipient. The primary immune response can be divided into three stages (the immune cascade).

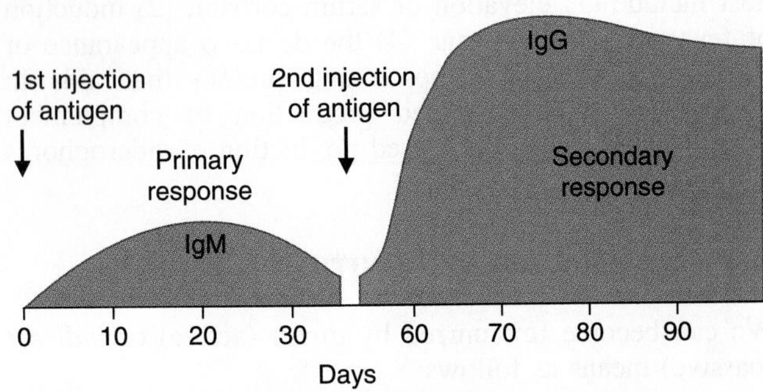

FIGURE U16–8 Primary and secondary antibody response. The second exposure of an antigen to the host causes a more rapid, stronger, and longer-acting response than the first exposure, owing to the presence of memory cells. Immunoglobin M (IgM) is most often produced in the primary response, whereas IgG is more likely to be produced predominantly in the secondary response.

PHASE I: AFFERENT PHASE

Application or Exposure to the Antigen

Topical (skin) exposure is successful only with certain materials called *proantigens.* Examples of these substances include plant secretions (poison oak, poison ivy), salts of nickel and chromium, and formaldehyde. Mucosal exposure, through epithelia in the respiratory, GI, or urogenital tract, is triggered by foods (strawberries, peanuts), drugs (aspirin), pollens, or house dust. Parenteral (subcutaneous, intradermal, intravenous) exposure is via vaccines, allergens for testing, and so forth.

Transport of Antigen

Lymph nodules lie immediately under modified mucosal epithelium (bearing M cells in the gut). No transport of antigen is required. Antigen deposited into solid tissues gains access to draining lymphatics and is then carried to the nearest regional lymph node. Antigen introduced intravenously localizes in the white pulp of the spleen. Proantigens applied to the skin are absorbed and, in conjunction with Langerhans cells in the subepithelial tissues, are coupled with an autogenous protein. The resultant complex is transported to a regional lymph node.

Arrival of Antigen

Arrival of antigen in peripheral lymphoid tissue is followed by its uptake by APCs.

Any exogenous molecule or any cell that does not have the self-markers of the recipient can serve as an antigen. Antigens may be natural, artificial, or synthetic.

Natural antigens include unmodified bacteria, fungi, viruses, parasites, foreign tissue cells, and large individual molecules such as proteins.

Artificial antigens are natural antigens that have been altered, usually to produce a vaccine: killed or attenuated bacteria, inactivated viruses, and toxoids.

Synthetic antigens are not found in nature but are produced in the laboratory (e.g., molecules genetically engineered to improve current or proposed immunization protocols).

The reactive sites of antigens are called determinant sites (or *epitopes*) and consist of three to five monosaccharide or amino acid residues that act together as a unit. The determinant sites are complementary to the reactive sites of the T cell antigen receptor (on T cells) and the serum immune globulin (SIg) (on B cells). Each natural antigen has many different epitopes, each of which is capable of stimulating a specific B-cell or T-cell clonotype (Fig. U16–9).

PHASE 2: CENTRAL PHASE

In phase 2, the central phase, antigen is taken up by or becomes affiliated with processing and presenting cells. Protein antigens are processed intracellularly by the APCs into peptide fragments, and the fragments, in association with the major histocompatibility molecules. They are placed on the surface of the APCs for presentation to T cells or to B cells that react to antigen in solute form, or they are adsorbed to the surfaces of follicular dendritic cells. T and B lymphocytes become activated and produce effector units and memory clonotypes.

PHASE 3: EFFERENT PHASE

Effector units and memory clonotypes are exported to all body sites. If residual antigen remains in the tissues, effector units may combine with it, causing manifestations until the antigen is neutralized or removed. Residual antigen is most often seen with obligate or facultative intracellular parasites or pathogens. This condition is not likely to occur with an extracellular pathogen.

The Secondary Immune Response

The secondary immune response occurs when a person who has been previously immunized with an antigen is rechallenged later with the same substance. This second (and any subsequent) response is characterized by several features that distinguish it from the primary immune response. Effector units are generally produced in greater quantity for a longer period of time, and antibody molecules may exhibit a higher affinity for antigen (see Fig. U16–8).

ANTIGEN PROCESSING AND PRESENTATION

T-cell recognition of antigen is limited to peptide fragments presented by an APC in conjunction with an MHC molecule. The recognition process is assisted by CD4 or CD8 molecules on the T cell surface. Class I MHC mole-

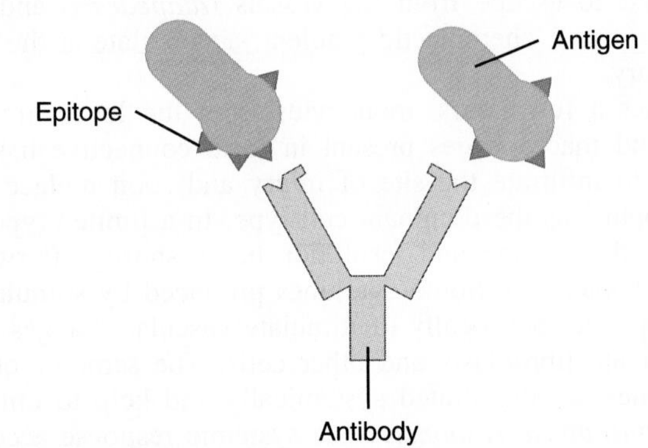

FIGURE U16–9 Epitopes protrude from the surface of an antigen and combine with the appropriate receptor of an antibody, much as a key fits into a lock.

cules are used to present peptides to CD8 cells, and class II molecules present peptides to CD4 cells. This recognition process is said to be self-MHC–restricted; that is, the APC and the T cell both must have the same MHC molecules (each must recognize the other as self). The cells that can function as APCs in peripheral lymphoid tissue sites are B cells, dendritic cells, and some macrophages. Other locations include endothelial cells in peripheral vasculature (in humans) and Langerhans cells in the skin.

■ B CELLS AND THE ANTIBODY RESPONSE

B cells recognize antigen in one of two forms:

1. When free, unprocessed antigen, characteristically carbohydrate is encountered, the response is limited; only IgM is produced, and there are no memory B clonotypes developed.
2. When proteins or protein conjugates are used as antigens, the APCs must first process the molecules to produce peptide fragments, which are combined with MHC molecules and then presented to T helper cells (Fig. U16–10).

The activated T cells secrete cytokines, which assist the B cell in responding to its own set of determinant sites present on the protein antigen. The cytokines stimulate growth and maturation in B cells, induce isotype switching, and make possible the development of memory clonotypes in both T and B cell lines.

After being activated by antigen and stimulated by cytokines, the B cell is transformed morphologically and physiologically into a distinct cell type: the *plasma cell.* Plasma cells are highly differentiated and specialized cells that are capable of producing large quantities of secreted immunoglobulin.

■ IMMUNOGLOBULINS

Antibodies, or immunoglobulins, are a family of glycoprotein molecules that are present in the body as solutes in body fluids (plasma and mucous secretions) and attached to a group of cells in solid tissues. Once attached, they inactivate and bind to antigens to facilitate phagocytosis and initiate inflammation by activating the complement cascade (Fig. U16–11). The terminal amino acid residues react with receptors on the surface of macrophages, neutrophils, B cells, and mast cells. There are five types (Table U16–1).

IGG. IgG is available to react with any antigen that gains access to the circulating blood, either by opsonizing it for accelerated uptake by RES cells or by activating complement via the classic pathway. When inflammation occurs in extravascular tissues, IgG is carried out of the vascular compartment to the septic site. IgG is the immunoglobulin that crosses the placenta and protects the newborn during the first few months of life. There are four sublcasses of IgG based on variation in amino acid composition in the heavy chain.

IGA. IgA is the predominant immunoglobulin in saliva, tears, colostrum, breast milk, and intestinal and bronchial secretions. The secretory (or mucosal) form of IgA serves to prevent the adherence of microorganisms to mucosal epithelium and thus supplements resistance mechanisms

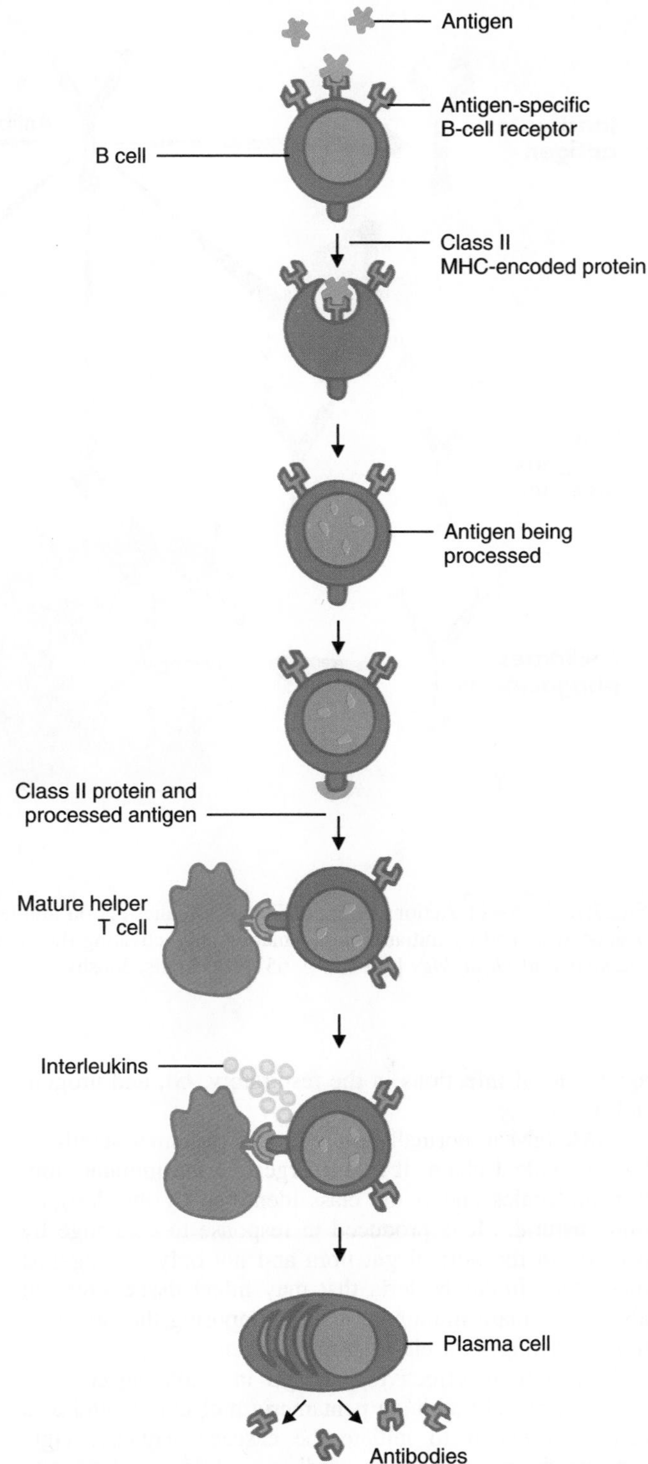

FIGURE U16–10 Activation of B cells to make antibody. The B cell uses its receptor to bind matching antigen, which it engulfs and processes. The B cell then presents a piece of antigen, bound to class II protein, on its surface. The complex binds to the mature T helper cell, which releases interleukins that transform the B cell into an antibody-secreting plasma cell. (Redrawn from Schindler, L. W. [1991]. *Understanding the immune system.* Washington, DC: National Institutes of Health.)

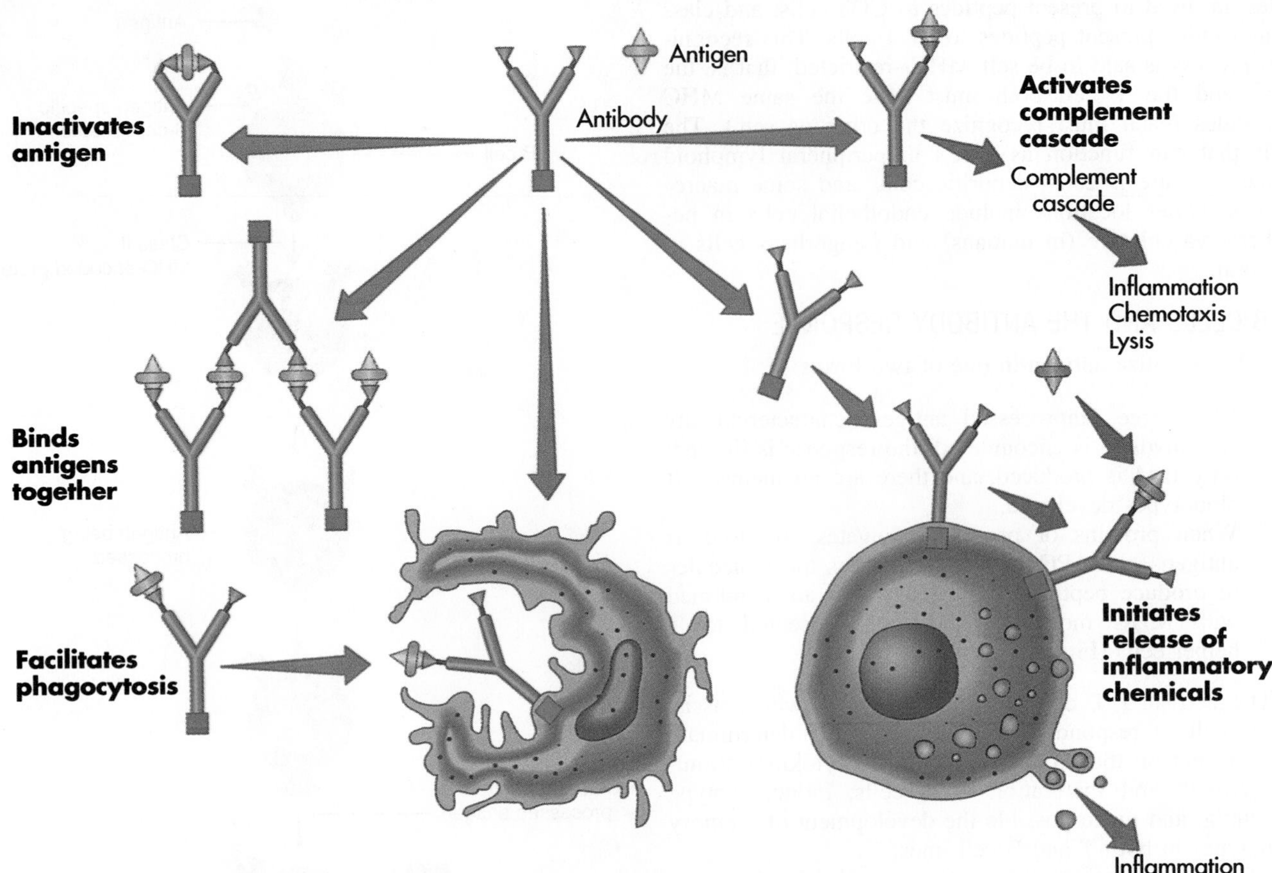

FIGURE U16–11 Actions of antibodies. Antibodies act on antigens by inactivating and binding them together to faciliate phagocytosis and by initiating inflammation and activating the complement cascade. (From Thibodeau, G., & Patton, K. [1999]. *Anatomy and physiology* [4th ed., p. 652]. St. Louis: Mosby.)

against local infections in the respiratory, GI, and urogenital tracts.

IGM. IgM is normally present as a pentamer stabilized by a peptide J chain. It is the largest of the immunoglobulin molecules and is the class identified by the designation "natural." It is produced in response to challenge by bacteria in the normal gut flora and not only acts against these and similar bacteria that may infect tissue sites but also is the main immunoglobulin composing the isoagglutinins reacting with blood group antigens.

IgM is more effective than IgG in activating complement, since only a single pentameric molecule bound to a cell is sufficient to initiate the cascade sequence (IgG requires the presence of two adjacent molecules bound to the cell surface). IgM is the early antibody seen in response to a thymic-dependent antigen and is the sole antibody produced against a thymic-independent antigen.

IGE. In most people, IgE is normally present only in trace amounts within the blood. Exceptions are people who have active atopic allergies or who are infected with parasitic worms. In humans, IgE is normally bound to a surface receptor on mast cells, where, following antigen binding, it triggers the release of chemical mediators such as histamine, which helps initiate the cascade of events leading to the expression of atopic allergy.

IGD. IgD contributes fewer than 1% of the total circu-

TABLE U16–1 CLASSES AND CHARACTERISTICS OF IMMUNOGLOBULINS (Ig)

Class	% of Total	Characteristics
IgG	75	Present in circulation and tissue spaces Opsonizes antigen Activates complement Transferred transplacentally The first Ig synthesized in secondary immune response
IgA	15	Present in the circulation and seromucous secretions Prevents adherence of microorganisms to mucosal surface
IgM	10	Present primarily in the circulation Powerful agglutinating antibody The first Ig of the primary immune response Activates complement
IgE	<1.0	Mediates hypersensitivity reactions Binds to mast cells and triggers mediator release
IgD	<1.0	Lymphocyte differentiation Full function unknown

lating immunoglobulins. The physiologic function of IgD is unknown. It is present in large numbers on the cell membrane of naive B lymphocytes, and its only role is thought to be for antigen recognition.

Monoclonal Antibodies

Monoclonal antibodies are immunoglobulins that can be synthesized by fusing a normal plasma cell (for antibody) with a myeloma cell (for longevity). The products of such a hybrid cell are immunoglobulins with an identical specificity. Current technology enables large quantities of immunoglobulins with almost any specificity to be produced at reasonable cost. Because they have a single specificity, they are widely used in research and for diagnostic and therapeutic regimens. Some of the applications include leukocyte identification, parasite and pathogen identification, quantitative estimation of peptide hormones, antitumor therapy, immunosuppression, and fertility control.

Complement and Amplification of Antibody Function

Complement refers to a group of proteins existing as solutes in plasma. When activated, the various components react in a cascade fashion. Complement activated by antibodies form holes in a bacterium's plasma membrane. Sodium and water diffuse into the cells and cause them to swell and burst (Fig. U16–12). Plasma complement can be activated by either of two methods: (1) a classic pathway requiring the participation of antibody and (2) an alternative pathway that is independent of antibody.

The alternative pathway is the older from an evolutionary standpoint and is a major contributor to defense against pathogens. Surface molecules of many bacterial species can initiate the complement cascade, leading to the destruction of the bacterial cell either indirectly by opsonization or by direct cell lysis.

Activation of complement by the classic pathway must be preceded by the interaction of antigen with antibody (either IgG or IgM). The advantage of this pathway is that complement can be recruited to assist in the removal of any solute or of any cell against which antibody can be produced.

T Lymphocytes and Cell-Mediated Immunity

Cell-mediated immunity (CMI) includes immune responses in which antibodies are not involved. CMI is vital in protecting the body against infection by viruses, slow-growing bacteria, and fungal infections. It also has a major role in immunosurveillance, reacting to abnormal clones of self cells, some of which are malignant. Such altered self cells can be destroyed in early stages by cytotoxic T cells or by NK cells, preventing them from becoming established tumors. Other CMI functions include primary rejection of allografts and development of delayed hypersensitivity reactions such as contact derma-

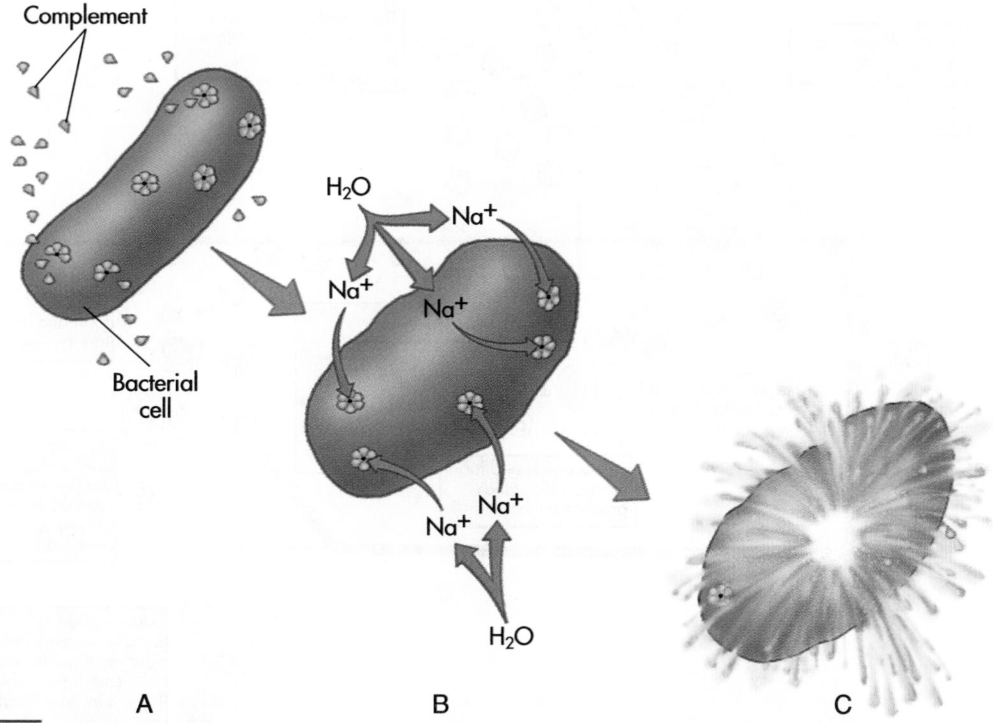

FIGURE U16–12 Complement fixation. *A*, Complement molecules activated by antibodies form doughnut-shaped complexes in a bacterium's plasma membrane. *B*, Holes in the complement complex allow sodium (Na^+) and then water (H_2O) to diffuse into the bacterium. *C*, After enough water has entered, the swollen bacterium bursts. (From Thibodeau, G., & Patton, K. [1999]. *Anatomy and physiology* [4th ed., p. 653]. St. Louis: Mosby.)

titis (poison oak) and hypersensitivity to products of the tubercle bacillus. Many, if not all, of the biologic actions of T lymphocytes are mediated through the secretion of factors called lymphokines (cytokines). Although humoral and cell-mediated responses are often discussed separately, these two arms of the immune system work together (Fig. U16–13), sometimes inseparably, and failure or malfunction in one part of the system frequently alter the effectiveness of the other.

The T lymphocytes that play a predominant role in CMI belong to a variety of T cell subsets. Some have a regulatory function and are designated as *T helper cells* or *T suppressor cells;* others act as effector cells. Cytokines from antigen-activated T helper cells assist B cells to mature and produce antibody and also modulate the maturation and function of cytotoxic T cells (see Fig. U16–13). The importance of T helper cell function is reflected by the severe consequences seen when it is suppressed by physical or chemical means or depleted during infection with human immunodeficiency virus (HIV); the T helper cell is a primary target of HIV. The decline of T helper cells in infected people is almost inevitably followed by recurrent episodes of opportunistic infections and the development of malignancy in people with acquired immunodeficiency syndrome (AIDS).

The homeostatic reduction or suppression of B and T cell responses to antigen is no longer considered to be restricted to a single suppressor cell population (once thought to be a subset of T cells bearing the CD8 marker). It is now hypothesized that this type of negative regulation may be a function of essentially all T cells. Whether a given cell will act to produce a positive immune response (produce effector units) or will mediate a negative response (tolerance) may be a function of the mechanism by which an individual T cell is activated by antigen.

The cytotoxic T lymphocyte reacts individually with target cells to establish a contact boundary that is required for target cell destruction. The intimate contact between the target cell and the cytotoxic T lymphocyte is mediated by an antigen-specific process and allows the cytotoxic T lymphocyte to release lytic molecules (*porins*)

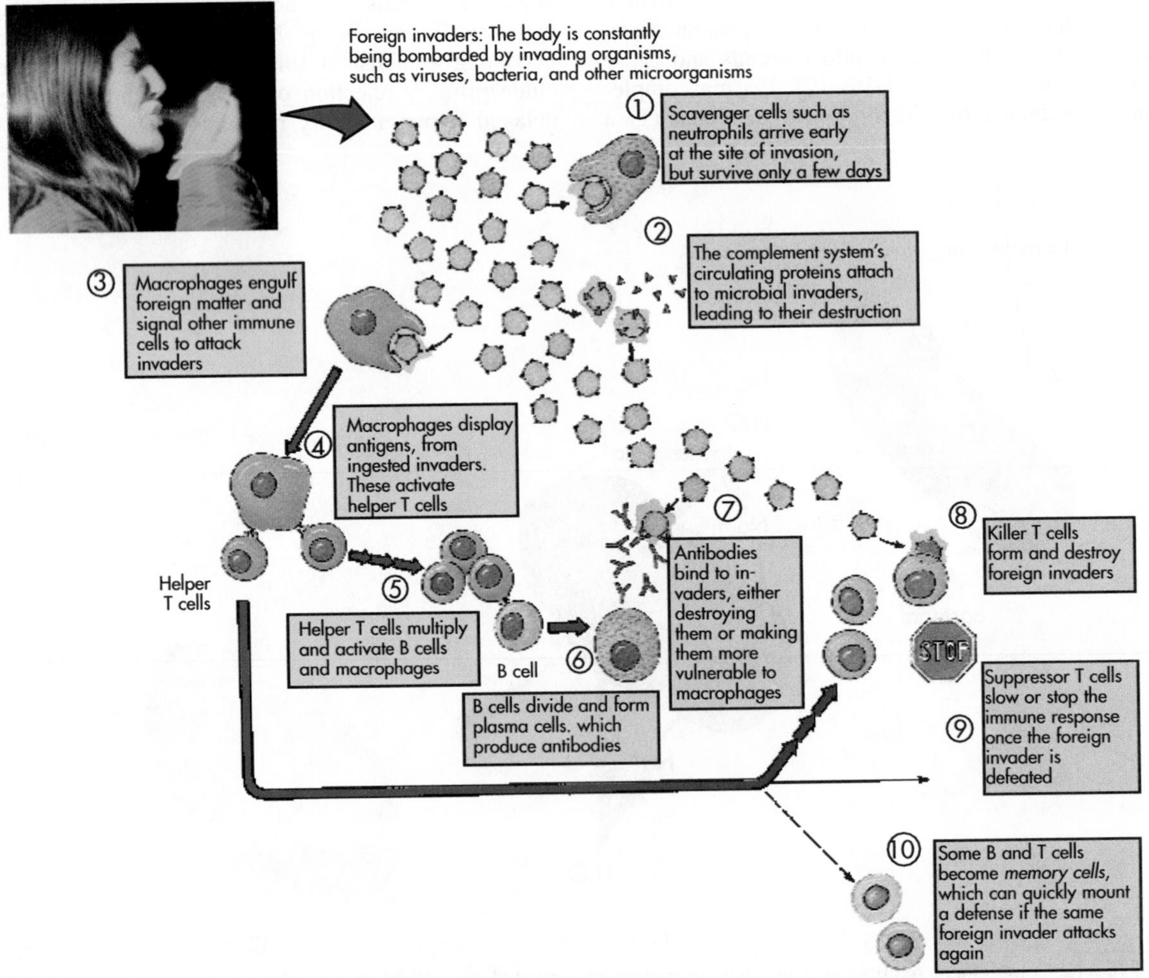

FIGURE U16–13 The protective systems include both arms of defense. Sneezing decreases exposure to the virus. Humoral immunity is shown in steps 1 and 2, cell-mediated immunity in steps 3 and 10. (From Thibodeau, G., & Patton, K. [1999]. *Anatomy and physiology* [4th ed., p. 657]. St. Louis: Mosby.)

directly into the membrane of the target cell. Cytokines produced and released by the cytotoxic T lymphocyte during the cell contact phase enhance the action of porins. The cytotoxic T lymphocyte function is to kill viral-infected host cells, malignant cells, and cells in allograft transplants.

CYTOKINES

The *cytokine* is a general term for cell-derived factors that mediate interactions between cells. Cytokines produced by lymphocytes are called *lymphokines;* those produced by monocyte-macrophage cells are called *monokines.* Some of these factors are called interleukins, indicating service as regulatory signals between various leukocytes (Table U16–2).

Cytokines are a diverse group of proteins with four areas of function:

1. Enhancement of mononuclear phagocytes.
2. Regulation of lymphocyte growth, differentiation, maturation, and secretory activities.
3. Inflammation.
4. Systemic effects such as fever induction and induction of hemopoietic activity in the bone marrow.

One of the best known cytokines is *IL-1,* originally described in the early 1960s. Produced by macrophages, it plays a role in induction of fever, acts as a coactivator of T cells, assists in activation of B cells and NK cells, and initiates the acute phase response.

TABLE U16–2 MAJOR CYTOKINES

Cytokine	Principal Effects
Interleukin-1 (IL-1)	Lymphocyte activation Macrophage and neutrophil stimulation Stimulation of acute phase proteins Fever and sleep Pituitary hormone regulation
Interleukin-2 (IL-2)	Enhances T cell growth and function
Interleukin-3 (IL-3)	Stimulates differentiation of hematopoietic cells (colony-stimulating factor)
Interleukin-4 (IL-4)	B cell growth factor
Interleukin-5 (IL-5)	B cell growth and differentiation
Interleukin-6 (IL-6)	B cell growth and differentiation Stimulates the acute phase response
Colony-stimulating factor	Stimulates division and differentiation of bone marrow stem cells
Interferon	Antiviral factor
Tumor necrosis factor	Activates macrophages, granulocytes, and cytotoxic cells Cachexia Mediates septic shock Increases leukocyte adhesion Enhances antigen presentation

IL-2 is also well known from its first identification as a T-cell growth factor. The growth-enhancing function was crucial in the original studies of some of the retroviruses. Current research efforts are directed toward finding an application for IL-2 for treatment of malignant conditions.

IL-3 and *IL-4* are necessary for inducing antigen-stimulated B cells to undergo isotype switching to change from synthesis and secretion of IgM to IgG (or IgA or IgE). IL-3 also stimulates bone marrow stem cells to differentiate into monocytic and granulocytic precursors.

Interferons (IFNs) are another group of molecules that serve as intercellular messengers. There are three major types:

1. IFN-α, produced by many cells.
2. INF-β, produced by fibroblasts.
3. IFN-γ, produced by T lymphocytes.

All interferons have antiviral activity and have a down-regulating effect on proliferation of both normal and malignant cells.

Tumor necrosis factor acts as a growth factor for fibroblasts and has a necrotizing effect on tumor cells. TNF participates in inducing the acute phase response, and is apparently one of the major factors in inducing endotoxic shock (sometimes seen in infections with gram-negative bacteria). This cytokine is thought to be a major cause of infection-related cachexia.

BLOOD GROUPS AND BLOOD TYPING

Human RBCs display antigens that are either glycoproteins or glycolipids on the surface of the membrane. Together the various blood group systems contribute more than 400 characterized antigens. Antigens are inherited from the parents. Fewer than a dozen of these blood group antigens attract frequent clinical notice, and of these only the ABO and rhesus (Rh) systems are major determinants of compatibility testing.

■ THE ABO BLOOD GROUP SYSTEM

The ABO blood type is inherited as an autosomal trait. The four major blood types of clinical importance in this genetic system are A, B, AB, and O. Blood is typed according to the antigens found on the RBC and the antibodies found in the serum.

For the antibodies to be formed, usually there must be exposure to foreign or homologous RBC antigens through pregnancy or transfusion. The major exceptions are the A and B antigens, for which there are structurally similar proteins in the environment, resulting in antibody formation against the missing A or B or AB antigen by the age of 3 months.

The two major antigens within the blood group system are antigens A and B. We may have one (type A or type B), both (type AB), or neither (type O) antigen on our RBCs. There also are two major antibodies found in the serum: anti-A and anti-B. A client with type A blood would have anti-B antibodies; a client with type B blood, anti-A antibodies; a client with type O blood, anti-A and anti-B antibodies; and a client with type AB blood, neither antibody (Table U16–3).

TABLE U16-3 THE ABO BLOOD GROUP SYSTEM

Blood Type	Agglutinogens on RBCs	Agglutinins in Plasma	Frequency in United States
A	A	Anti-B	41%
B	B	Anti-A	10%
AB	A and B	None	4%
O	None	Anti-A and anti-B	45%

RBCs, red blood cells.

■ THE Rh SYSTEM

The Rh blood groups are nearly equal in clinical importance to the ABO groups. Although Rh serology involves more than 20 different antigens, the D antigen has the most clinical significance because of the high risk of formation of an anti-D in an Rh-negative recipient. The term *Rh-positive* means that the client has the D antigen; the *Rh-negative* client has no D antigen.

The most striking difference between the ABO and Rh systems is that in the ABO system, there is spontaneous development of antibodies directed against A and B antigens not present on the RBC. In the Rh system, antibody formation is never spontaneous. Instead, a client must first be exposed to the Rh antigen, for example, through a blood transfusion or pregnancy. Thus, clients with Rh-negative blood, transfused for the first time with Rh-positive blood, do not experience a reaction because their blood does not yet contain anti-Rh antibodies (anti-D). About 50% of people, however, develop sensitivity and form antibodies against the D antigen as a result of exposure to it from transfusion or pregnancy. Should a sensitized client receive a second transfusion or have a second pregnancy with exposure to the D antigen, some degree of RBC destruction will occur. However, it is usually possible to prevent sensitization from occurring the first time by administering a single dose of anti-Rh antibodies in the form of Rh_0(D) immune globulin (RhoGAM) immediately following exposure to the D antigen.

THE HLA SYSTEM

HLAs are also called *histocompatibility antigens* because the antigens (glycoproteins) are found on the surface of most cells in the body except RBCs (including circulating and tissue cells). The HLA system is a series of closely linked genes located on the short arm of chromosome 6. The major function of the HLA antigen is regulation of the immune response, distinguishing self from non-self. This plays a major role in the rejection of transplanted tissues when donor and recipient HLA antigens do not match. There also is an association between HLA antigens and some diseases. For example, in ankylosing spondylitis, the association with HLA factor is so strong that HLA typing can be used diagnostically.

CONCLUSIONS

The immune system is extremely complex. It has evolved through the years to become a pervasive and highly structured group of complex functions that defend the body against pathogens and parasites from the outside and are able to detect and attack altered self cells that pose threats to organismal homeostasis.

BIBLIOGRAPHY

1. Ader, R., & Cohen, N. (1993). Psychoneuroimmunology: Conditioning and stress. *Annual Review of Psychology, 44,* 53.
2. Arai, K., et al. (1990). Cytokines: Coordinators of immunity and inflammatory responses. *Annual Review of Biochemistry, 59,* 783.
3. Hedrick, S. M. (1992). Dawn of the hunt for nonclassical MHC function. *Cell, 70,* 177.
4. Knight, S. C., & Stagg, A. J. (1993). Antigen-presenting cell types. *Current Opinion in Immunology, 5,* 374.
5. Lanzavecchia, A. (1993). Identifying strategies for immune intervention. *Science, 260,* 937.
6. Ogawa, M. (1993). Review: Differentiation and proliferation of hematopoietic stem cells. *Blood, 81,* 2844–2854.
7. Spivak, J., et al. (1996). Cell cycle–specific behavior of erythropoietin. *Experimental Hematology, 24*(2), 141–150.
8. Springer, T. A. (1990). Adhesion receptors in the immune system. *Nature, 346,* 425.
9. Tomlinson, S. (1993). Complement defense mechanisms. *Current Opinion in Immunology, 5,* 83.
10. Virella, G. Patrick, C. C., & Goust, J. M. (1993). Diagnostic evaluation of lymphocyte functions of cell-mediated immunity. *Immunology Series, 58,* 291.
11. von Boehmer, H., & Kisielow, P. (1991). How the immune system learns about self. *Scientific American, 265*(4), 74.
12. Williams, W. J., et al. (1995). *Hematology* (5th ed.). New York: McGraw-Hill.
13. Young, J. D. E., & Cohn, Z. A. (1988). How killer T cells kill. *Scientific American, 258*(1), 38.

CHAPTER 74

Assessment of the Hematopoietic System

Mary A. Allen

HISTORY

The nature of the presenting problem determines the focus of the health history for the hematopoietic system. Clients may present with manifestations suggesting a hematologic or an immunologic problem.

■ BIOGRAPHICAL AND DEMOGRAPHIC DATA

When assessing the hematopoietic system, note the client's age, sex, race, ethnicity, and family health history. The immune response is diminished in both very young and older people. Some hematologic and immunologic disorders occur more frequently at certain ages, in women or men, and in those of a particular race or ethnic background. In addition, the normal values of some hematologic tests have age-specific and sex-specific norms. For example, hemoglobin and hematocrit levels are lower in women, particularly during the menstrual years, than in men. Hemoglobin values in blacks are approximately 0.5 g/dl lower than in whites.

Collect family health history data because several hematologic and immunologic disorders are inherited. Note occupations, housing, and hobbies to identify possible exposure to chemicals, radiation, and allergens. Inquire about residence and work locations to determine environmental triggers of allergic responses.

■ CURRENT HEALTH

Chief Complaint

Disorders of the hematopoietic system often affect all organs and tissues of the body, resulting in widespread pathophysiologic manifestations. Manifestations may be vague and nonspecific, such as fatigue, malaise, fever, anorexia, weight loss, and chronic diarrhea. In general, anemias often manifest with fatigue, paleness, and weakness; bleeding disorders with bruising, petechiae, epistaxis, and bleeding gums; and immunodeficiencies with recurrent infections, fever, and chronic diarrhea. Allergic manifestations range from mild to severe and can be systemic or organ-specific such as integumentary, respiratory, gastrointestinal, or cardiovascular reactions. Conduct a symptom analysis (see Chapter 9). The Review of Systems outlines the body systems, their common hematopoietic findings, and the possible pathophysiologic bases.

All material in this chapter is in the public domain, with the exception of any borrowed figures or tables.

Symptom Analysis

TIMING. Ask the client when the manifestations began and whether the onset was abrupt or gradual. Manifestations of anemias and immunodeficiencies can develop over time. Bleeding disorders may be present since childhood or may have a recent onset. Some allergic manifestations begin in childhood, whereas others develop later in life. Ask which allergens trigger a response and whether allergies are seasonal in appearance. Determine how long the allergic manifestations last and whether they are relieved or persist once the allergen is removed.

QUALITY AND QUANTITY. How long do bleeding episodes last and how severe are they? Does blood ooze from a site or does sudden, massive bleeding occur? (Sudden bleeding is less common than prolonged, slow hemorrhage.) How often do bleeding episodes occur and how long do they last? What does the client do to stop them? Ask about injury or physical trauma resulting in a break in the skin's integrity. Does the client report associated manifestations, such as lymph node swelling, edema, fever, pain, tenderness, pruritus, redness, or drainage?

Note allergic manifestations such as rhinitis, sneezing, nasal stuffiness, postnasal drip, sore throat, voice changes, hoarseness, wheezing, persistent cough, dyspnea, malaise, fatigue, tearing, or altered hearing acuity. Manifestations vary, depending on the nature of the allergen and individual sensitivity patterns. A symptom analysis for each reported manifestation assists in identifying the allergen.

SEVERITY AND LOCATION. Fatigue is the most common manifestation of anemia. Is more rest than usual needed? Is endurance affected? Ask the client to compare how activities and activity tolerance have changed over time (e.g., in the past month compared to a year ago).

Attempt to quantify the severity of bleeding tendency. Does the client bruise easily? Has bleeding into the joints occurred? For menstruating women, ask whether the number and saturation of sanitary products used during a recent cycle has increased from the usual pattern.

Do allergic manifestations present as simple skin rashes, nasal stuffiness, and cough, or are they more severe such as wheezing and respiratory distress? Do different allergens trigger different responses? Has the client ever experienced an anaphylactic reaction?

Precipitating Factors. Hepatic, splenic, or renal diseases may manifest as hematologic or hemorrhagic problems. Anticoagulant medications can precipitate bleeding episodes. Bone marrow suppression can lead to anemia, leukopenia, and thrombocytopenia. Causative agents include antineoplastic drugs, some antibiotics, and radiation. Other hematologic effects from certain drugs include hemolysis and disruption of platelet aggregation.

Has the client recently been exposed to infectious agents? Does the client take corticosteroids or other immunosuppressive drugs, thus increasing the risk of infection? Systemic and local infections can result from broken skin integrity, ingrown nails, or puncture wounds. Altered lymph vessel structure (from surgical disruption, trauma, neoplasm, or scarring from radiation) can lead to edema, particularly in an extremity.

The major types of allergic triggers include (1) inhalants (pollens, molds, spores, dust mites, trees, grasses, animal dander), (2) contact agents (dyes in clothing, fibers, cosmetics, metals in jewelry, plant oils and secretions, topical drugs, numerous chemicals), (3) ingested agents (foods, food additives, drugs), (4) injectable agents (drugs, vaccines, insect venom).

Aggravating and Relieving Factors. Medications containing salicylates, including many over-the-counter (OTC) drugs, can aggravate bleeding tendencies (see later). Is the client's edema aggravated by dependent positioning or tight, restrictive clothing? Does elevation of the affected body part reduce or relieve swelling? Are elastic support garments worn to reduce or prevent edema?

What relieves allergic manifestations (antihistamines, antipruritic agents)? What does the client use for relief from a rash? Is an inhaled medication needed for respiratory manifestations?

PAST HEALTH HISTORY

Assess for hematologic disorders by asking whether there is a history of anemia; concurrent disorders, such as renal, liver, or autoimmune disease; cancer; or organ transplantation.

Assess for bleeding disorders. Ask whether the disorder may be related to genetic factors, exposure to toxins, or liver disease. Cirrhosis, hepatitis, and other liver diseases can result in reduced production of clotting factors as well as reduced clearance of factors that inhibit clotting or promote fibrinolysis.

When assessing the client with a bleeding disorder, ask the following: How long has there been a bleeding problem? Was it present in childhood, or has it appeared recently? Do any family members have a history of bleeding disorders? Is the bleeding linked to any specific event or procedure? For example, does severe bleeding occur with menses or following minor trauma, a tooth extraction, minor surgery (including circumcision), shaving, or participation in contact sports? Does the client have frequent nosebleeds (epistaxis)? Is there a history of bleeding into the joints or cavities? Does the client bruise easily or report petechiae? How severe are bleeding episodes, and how long do they last? Is bleeding slow and prolonged or sudden and massive?

Immunodeficiencies may be present at birth or may develop later in life and may be iatrogenic (i.e., a result of treatment with cytotoxic agents, corticosteroids or other immunosuppressants, or radiation). Immunodeficiencies may also result from protein-deficiency malnutrition, protein-losing enteropathy, nephrotic syndrome, or hypercatabolic states (major trauma, severe thermal injury) Immunodeficiencies may be related to loss of anatomic integrity from instrumentation (catheters), impaired dermatologic barrier function (burns, psoriasis, atopic dermatitis), mucosal inflammation (atopic diseases, irritants such as cigarette smoke), or mucociliary elevator dysfunction (cystic fibrosis or the immotile cilia syndrome).

Ask the client about indications of a possible immunodeficiency: poor or delayed wound healing; chronic diarrhea; unusually frequent bacterial infections; unusually severe viral infections; development of an infection with an unusual microorganism (fungus or protozoa); exposure to human immunodeficiency virus (HIV) through sexual activity, injection drug use, transfusion of blood or blood products, or other source; or family history of recurrent infection.

When assessing lymphatic problems, inquire about trauma or other injury, especially to an extremity. Has the client had a recent infection or neoplasm? Edema may be related to altered anatomy or disorders affecting the vascular system, such as heart failure, deep vein thrombosis, or renal disease.

Ask whether allergic manifestations have been present since childhood. Can the client identify triggers? Is there a seasonal pattern associated with the manifestations? Has hospitalization or emergency treatment been necessary for a severe allergic reaction? Was desensitization therapy (allergy shots) undertaken, and was it effective?

Childhood and Infectious Diseases

Did the client experience an unusually severe course of measles, mumps, or other infectious diseases of childhood? Were there severe reactions to vaccinations, especially immunizations with live virus vaccines such as measles and mumps? Are vaccinations current? (See Chapter 9.)

Major Illnesses and Hospitalizations

Ask about major illnesses and hospitalizations. Has the client received a blood or blood product transfusion, and for what reason? Have there been retroperitoneal, intracranial, or paratracheal hemorrhages? Were there problems or reactions to the blood or blood products? Does the client know his or her blood type, including Rh factor? This information is important for the pregnant client who is Rh-negative (see Chapter 37).

Has the client recently donated blood or blood components? Donating whole blood, erythrocytes, leukocytes, platelets, or plasma may affect laboratory values for days or weeks.

Ask the client about the occurrence of any major illnesses, including (1) cancer, (2) lymphoproliferative diseases (lymphoma, leukemia, multiple myeloma), (3) infection (HIV-1, HIV-2, rubella, cytomegalovirus, influenza, varicella zoster), (4) systemic inflammatory diseases (rheumatoid arthritis, systemic lupus erythematosus, sarcoidosis, vasculitis), (5) diabetes mellitus, (6) renal or liver disease, and (7) sickle cell disease.

Is there a history of diseases involving the terminal ileum, Crohn's disease, tropical sprue, ulcers, or severe atrophic gastritis? Ask the client to describe the disorder and its treatment.

Operations

Surgical procedures can influence the development of hematologic disorders or immunodeficiency. For example, cardiac valve replacement may cause erythrocyte hemolysis and subsequent anemia. Anemia may also occur following partial or total gastrectomy or removal of the terminal portion of the ileum because of the consequent reduction in absorption of vitamin B_{12}. Surgical removal of duodenal tissue can decrease iron absorption and thus produce iron deficiency anemia. Splenectomy increases the risk of overwhelming infections with encapsulated bacteria such as *Streptococcus pneumoniae*. Surgical instrumentation and loss of anatomic integrity increase the risk of infection.

Medications

Note the client's past and current use of both prescription and over-the-counter drugs as well as herbal or complementary remedies. Many medications can prolong bleeding, cause hemolysis of red blood cells, or through selective or general bone marrow suppression, produce anemia, thrombocytopenia, or leukopenia. Medications can also inhibit folic acid absorption from the intestine, leading to folic acid deficiency and anemia.

Inquire whether the client takes medications that can cause hemolysis: (1) antihypoglycemic (antidiabetic) agents, such as chlorpropamide, glyburide, and tolbutamide; (2) cardiovascular medications, such as mefenamic acid, methyldopa, and procainamide; and (3) antibiotics, including sulfonamides and penicillins.

Ask about current or recent anticoagulant therapy or antithrombolytic treatment. The anticoagulants heparin and warfarin prolong bleeding, and heparin may also cause immune-mediated thrombocytopenia. The thrombolytic agents streptokinase, tissue plasminogen activator (t-PA), and urokinase also prolong bleeding.

A wide range of medications can affect platelet function or cause thrombocytopenia. Ask about over-the-counter medications containing aspirin or other nonsteroidal anti-inflammatory drugs (NSAIDs) that can interfere with platelet aggregation and prolong bleeding.

Has the client taken corticosteroids, antineoplastic agents (cyclophosphamide, chlorambucil, cisplatin, etoposide), other immunosuppressants (gold salts, NSAIDs), or therapies (irradiation) for the treatment of cancer or autoimmune diseases? These agents may suppress bone marrow production of blood cells or the immune response. Effects may continue long after the medications have been stopped. Treatment with cytotoxic agents or high doses of corticosteroids can mask fever and other manifestations until an infection is serious and widespread.

Has the client received other medications for which myelosuppression is an adverse effect? These include chloramphenicol, cephalosporins, penicillin, tetracycline, sulfonamides, d-penicillamine, amphotericin B, antimalarials, captopril, phenothiazines, or antithyroid drugs.

Determine whether the client has received intravenous immune globulin (IGIV) or intramuscular immune globulin (IMIG) to treat an immunoglobulin deficiency or other condition.

Herbal preparations to ask the client about include comfrey (*Symphylum officinale*), echinacea (*Echinacea angustifolia, E. pallida, E. purpura*), evening primrose (*Oenothera biennis*), ginseng (*Panax ginseng, P. quinquefolius, Eleutherococcus senticosus*), goldenseal (*Hydrastis canadensis*), licorice (*Glycyrrhiza glabra, G. uralensis*), maitake (*Grifola frondosa*), St. John's wort (*Hypericum perforatum*), and stinging nettle (*Urtica dioica*). Topical comfrey acts as an anti-inflammatory on wounds. Herbs used to boost the immune system include echinacea, evening primrose, ginseng, goldenseal, and maitake. St. John's wort has antiviral actions. Licorice is used to reduce inflammation, fight viruses and bacteria, and reduce asthma and allergy manifestations. Stinging nettle is used as a hay fever remedy. Products associated with anticancer properties include vitamins E and C, beta-carotene, selenium, garlic (*Allium sativum*), and green tea. Folic acid (vitamin B_6) and cobalamin (vitamin B_{12}) are necessary to prevent pernicious anemia.

Allergies

If there is a history of transfusions with blood or blood products, ask about complications. Reactions to blood products include fever, chills, back or flank pain, wheezing, headache, vomiting, urticaria (hives), and shock.

Ask the client about past episodes of allergic reactions. Is there a seasonal pattern to the episodes? What manifestations developed? What treatment was given, and was it effective? Inquire about food and drug allergies or sensitivities. Has the client ever had an anaphylactic reaction or been hospitalized for an allergic reaction? Has the client had desensitization treatment with allergy injections. If so, was it effective?

Has the client undergone procedures requiring administration of radiopaque contrast medium, or is this likely in the future? Clients with a history of allergies or asthma may be at higher risk of a reaction to these media and may be candidates for low-ionic-contrast media or pretreatment with medications to reduce the risk of serious reaction. Previously, clients often were asked about allergies to shellfish or iodine before administration of radiopaque contrast media because it was thought that iodine-based cross-reactions could occur. However, seafood allergies are immunoglobin E (IgE)–mediated reactions to the muscle protein tropomyosin that is present in shellfish and mollusks and do not involve reactions to iodine. Conversely, most reactions to radiopaque contrast media do not appear to be IgE-mediated and are unrelated to allergies to tropomyosin or iodine.

■ FAMILY HEALTH HISTORY

Explore the family history for (1) anemia; (2) thrombocytopenia; (3) bleeding disorders, such as hemophilia or von

Willebrand's disease; (4) congenital blood disorders, such as sickle cell anemia; (5) jaundice; (6) infections that are unusually frequent, unusually severe, or caused by an unusual organism; (7) delayed healing; (8) cancer; or (9) autoimmune disease. A family history of neonatal jaundice or early cholecystectomy (gallbladder removal) may indicate a genetic hematologic disorder.

Ask the client to identify allergies and sensitivities in family members, particularly atopic reactions. Hay fever tends to occur among family members.

■ PSYCHOSOCIAL HISTORY

Hematopoietic disorders can result in physiologic changes that affect the client's psychosocial status and ability to perform activities of daily living (ADL). Assess for work-related problems, sexual dysfunction, and fatigue that may interfere with role performance. Encourage the client to discuss current levels of stress and whether they seem to relate to the appearance of allergic manifestations. How does the client react to allergic manifestations? For example, some people break out in hives when under emotional stress. Their appearance triggers more emotional distress and can lead to further outbreaks. A cycle may develop that is difficult to interrupt.

Occupation

Ask about occupational exposure to agents that might predispose the client to the development of hematopoietic disorders: radiation, aromatic hydrocarbons (kerosene, gasoline), benzene (used in manufacture of pharmaceuticals, rubber, leather, and explosives), inorganic arsenics, trinitrotoluene, insecticides, weed killers, lead, and phenylbutazone. Exposure to toxic chemicals and ionizing radiation may occur in several industries (chemicals, plastics, ceramics, steel, metal refinery); in the manufacturing of rubber tires, shoes, incandescent lamps, vacuum tubes, glue, and varnish; in nuclear reactors, uranium mines, research laboratories, hospital radiology, or sterile supplies; and in farming and horticulture.

Does the client have sufficient energy to perform normal activities and occupational tasks? Do fatigue, dyspnea, or other manifestations interfere with a productive lifestyle? Has the client missed time from work or school, resulting in financial loss or other economic concerns, such as health or life insurance eligibility?

Exposure to allergens at work may trigger reactions. Ask about the heating and cooling systems if airborne allergens are suspected.

Geographical Location and Environment

Geographical location may be associated with exposure to possible health hazards. Living at altitudes above 10,000 feet may result in increased hemoglobin levels and other physiologic adaptations. Immunologic disorders may be more prevalent in certain geographical areas. High levels of air pollution can increase the incidence of allergy-related respiratory problems. Ask about home and work environments. Are pets, house plants, or fresh-cut flowers present? What type of vegetation is in the immediate vicinity?

Nutrition

The hematopoietic system depends on the adequate intake of protein, calories, vitamins (A, B_{12}, folic acid), minerals, and trace elements such as iron and zinc. Inadequate intake of any of these substances can lead to anemia or immunodeficiency. Assess for conditions that increase nutritional needs, such as pregnancy, lactation, and hypercatabolic states that occur with thermal injuries. When assessing anemia, obtain a dietary history focusing on the intake of foods such as meat, fish, eggs, dairy products, whole grains, dark green vegetables, legumes, and nuts. Strict vegetarians who do not eat foods of animal origin may be at higher risk for a deficiency anemia, especially related to inadequate intake of vitamin B_{12} (see Chapter 28).

Does the client have allergies to foods or food additives? Do these allergies limit the intake of specific nutrients as previously identified? A food diary is useful to help identify food-related allergic reactions. See Chapter 28 for further discussion.

Habits

Assess the client's current and past use of tobacco (including exposure to second-hand smoke that can aggravate allergies), alcohol, and illicit drugs. Excessive use of alcohol in particular often results in poor nutrition, folic acid deficiency, and decreased immunity as well as acute or chronic loss of blood from gastritis and esophageal varices. Many substances, most notably alcohol, damage the structure and function of liver cells, decreasing the production of clotting factors and reducing the clearance of factors that promote clot dissolution; the result is a bleeding tendency.

■ REVIEW OF SYSTEMS

General manifestations of hematopoietic disorders include fatigue, malaise, weakness, and fever. Specific manifestations can vary if the disorder is related to anemia, bleeding, or immunodeficiency. Allergic manifestations can be general or specific.

Anemia is characterized by pallor, weakness, and lightheadedness; severe anemia manifests with chronic severe fatigue, exertional dyspnea, headache, or vertigo. Clients with bleeding disorders manifest petechiae, purpura, and ecchymoses (bruises); spontaneous bleeding from the nose, gingiva, vagina, and rectum; oozing of blood from cuts and venipuncture sites; jaundice; conjunctival or retinal hemorrhage; hemoptysis, hematemesis, hematuria, and back and flank pain.

Clients with hemophilia and other congenital coagulation disorders have a history of lifelong bleeding tendencies, such as (1) excessive or prolonged bleeding after circumcision or dental extraction; (2) repeated episodes of spontaneous bleeding into joints (hemarthrosis), and (3) life-threatening hemorrhages (retroperitoneal, intracranial, paratracheal).

Clients with immunodeficiencies have a history of recurrent infections, especially of mucous membranes (e.g., oral cavity, anorectal area, genitourinary tract, respiratory tract); poor wound healing; diarrhea; and manifestations of systemic activation of the inflammatory response (fever, malaise, fatigue, anorexia, unexplained weight loss, headache, and irritability). Clients with allergies may have rhinitis, sinusitis, urticaria, and pruritus.

Skin

Integumentary manifestations may be pallor (anemia); pruritus and ruddy skin (polycythemia vera); jaundice (bile pigment accumulation from hemolytic anemia), dry skin, dry hair, brittle nails, and spoon-shaped concave nails with longitudinal ridges (iron deficiency anemia); petechiae, especially of the lower legs and hard palate (thrombocytopenia), purpura, and ecchymoses (thrombocytopenia and bleeding disorders); delayed wound healing, lymphadenopathy, and severe acne or acne scars (immunodeficiency); and rashes, urticaria, pruritus, dryness, and scaling (allergies).

Assess for local inflammation (redness, heat, swelling, pain). Clients with severe neutropenia or immunosuppression may be unable to mount the inflammatory response of fever, redness, and pus formation.

Eyes

Ocular manifestations include visual disturbances (anemia, polycythemia), blindness (retinal hemorrhage related to thrombocytopenia or bleeding disorder), scleral jaundice (hemolytic anemia) and conjunctivitis, tearing, eye rubbing, styes, and dark circles or "allergic shiners," or "raccoon eyes" (allergies).

Ears

Aural manifestations are vertigo or tinnitus (severe anemia). Bleeding disorders may manifest as blood in the external auditory canal or as a bluish tympanic membrane, suggesting blood in the middle ear. Immunodeficiencies can manifest as chronic otitis media, mastoiditis, and hearing impairment related to chronic infections (eardrum rupture, scarring, perforated tympanic membrane) or treatment with ototoxic drugs.

Nose

Nasal manifestations include epistaxis (thrombocytopenia and bleeding disorders); crusting around nares, sinopulmonary drainage, and indications of chronic sinusitis (immunodeficiency); and sneezing, sniffling, rhinitis, nasal polyps, nasal voice quality, a crease across the bridge of the nose from chronic rubbing, and stuffiness (allergies).

Mouth

Oral manifestations include a smooth, glossy, bright red, and sore tongue (pernicious anemia, iron deficiency anemia); gingival bleeding (thrombocytopenia, bleeding disorders); and oral ulcers (aphthous, herpetic), candidiasis, gingivitis, periodontitis, dental caries, and tooth loss (immunodeficiencies). The tonsils may be absent without a history of tonsillectomy, or they may be enlarged, inflamed, or pustular. Lip and tongue swelling, frequent throat clearing from postnasal drip, sore throat, itching of the palate, throat, or neck, and hoarseness can occur (allergies).

Lungs

Respiratory manifestations include dyspnea and orthopnea (anemia, sickle cell crisis), wheezing, frequent cough, ineffective cough, and respiratory arrest (allergies).

Cardiovascular System

Cardiovascular manifestations include tachycardia, palpitations (compensatory mechanism to increase cardiac output secondary to anemia), murmurs, particularly systolic (increased volume and velocity of blood through valves related to anemia), and angina (decreased oxygen supply to the heart related to rapid-onset anemia).

Gastrointestinal Tract

The gastrointestinal system may be affected by dysphagia (mucous membrane atrophy related to iron deficiency anemia), abdominal pain (sickle cell disease, retroperitoneal bleeding, acute hemolysis), hepatomegaly, splenomegaly (hemolytic anemia resulting in increased need for removal of erythrocytes), hematemesis and melena (thrombocytopenia and bleeding disorders), vomiting, cramping, and diarrhea (allergies).

Genitourinary Tract

Urinary manifestations include hematuria (hemolysis and bleeding disorders). Reproductive manifestations are amenorrhea and menorrhagia (iron deficiency and bleeding disorders) and decreased fertility (severe anemia).

Musculoskeletal System

Musculoskeletal manifestations are back pain (hemolysis), sternal tenderness and excruciating bone pain (sickle cell crises), and joint pain (hemarthroses or bleeding into joints, often related to hemophilia).

Nervous System

Neurologic manifestations are headache and confusion (anemia, polycythemia); brain hemorrhage (thrombocytopenia or a bleeding disorder); and peripheral neuropathy, paresthesias, and loss of balance (pernicious anemia). The client may experience mental depression (hematopoietic disorders that cause fatigue, discomfort, and acute and chronic problems related to a disease process) or coping difficulties related to a diagnosis of life-threatening illness.

PHYSICAL EXAMINATION

The physical examination of the hematopoietic system can entail both a complete head-to-toe examination and examinations of specific systems, depending on the nature of the client's problem. For example, anemia or fever can cause tachycardia and systolic ejection murmur; immunodeficiency manifested by repeated episodes of pulmonary infections may result in adventitious breath sounds. (See Chapters 54 and 59 for discussions of cardiac and respiratory assessment, respectively.) The Physical Assessment Findings in the Healthy Adult feature outlines expected findings.

The portions of the lymphatic system accessible for a physical examination are the superficial lymph nodes, liver, and spleen (see Chapter 42). Note the presence of a surgical splenectomy scar. Assess the superficial lymph nodes using inspection and palpation. Supplement the findings from the history and physical examination with results from laboratory tests and specific diagnostic studies.

Inspection

Inspect surfaces overlying the lymph nodes for masses, scars, swelling, and redness. Note extremity swelling or edema. Look for symmetry and compare with the contralateral side.

Palpation

Use a methodical approach to examine the lymph nodes; do not overlook single nodes or chains of nodes. Palpate nodes for location, size, shape, consistency, symmetry, discreteness, mobility, tenderness, temperature, overlying edema, or red streaks. Avoid excessive pressure to discern small, yet palpable nodes. Chapter 10 describes the palpation technique.

Lymph nodes are generally nonpalpable. However, small (≤1 cm in diameter), single, round, soft, mobile, nontender nodes are common, particularly in the head, neck, and inguinal areas, and are usually not significant. Nodes that are inflamed, tender, large (>1 cm in diameter), hard, matted together, or fixed to underlying structures are abnormal. Describe their characteristics thoroughly. If you see a mass, palpate the area and compare with the contralateral side. The supraclavicular area is a frequent site of metastatic disease; investigate palpable nodes in this site.

PHYSICAL ASSESSMENT FINDINGS IN THE HEALTHY ADULT

Hematopoietic System

Inspection

Alert and oriented; febrile. Skin color even, without pallor, flushing, jaundice, bruises, or petechiae. Lumps or masses absent, no draining lesions. Sclerae white. Lingual papillae visible; oral lesions absent. Eupneic. Joints not swollen; full range of motion

Palpation

Lumps, masses absent. Lymph nodes, liver, and spleen nonpalpable and nontender. Joints nontender. Several round, small (<0.5 cm), discrete, soft, mobile nodes palpable in submandibular area

Auscultation

Heart sounds regular, without murmurs or palpitations

The nodes of the head and neck and the clavicular and epitrochlear areas are most easily palpated while the client is sitting. Palpate inguinal and popliteal nodes when the client is lying down. Axillary nodes may be palpated with the client sitting or lying. Specific guidelines for palpating the lymph nodes are presented in Table 74–1. Palpation techniques are shown in Chapter 10, Figure 10–3.

DIAGNOSTIC TESTS

Diagnosis of hematologic, bleeding, or immunologic disorders depends primarily on laboratory analysis. There is no particular preprocedure or postprocedure care associated with the simple blood tests that are involved in most hematopoietic assessments.

Although dozens of specific tests are used to diagnose individual disorders, all cases generally call for (1) a complete blood count (CBC) to determine the number of leukocytes, erythrocytes, and platelets; (2) a white blood cell (WBC) differential count to indicate the relative percentages of the different leukocytes; (3) coagulation studies such as prothrombin time (PT), partial thromboplastin time (PTT), and bleeding time; and (4) a peripheral blood smear for red blood cell morphology to differentiate various anemias and blood dyscrasias.

The diagnosis of deficiency anemias may require measuring serum levels of iron, total iron-binding capacity (TIBC), transferrin saturation, ferritin, folic acid, and vitamin B_{12} (Table 74–2). Bone marrow aspiration and biopsy are performed to determine both the cellularity of the bone marrow and the morphology of the cells present. The diagnosis of particular hematologic disorders requires specialized blood tests, such as the Schilling test, hemoglobin electrophoresis, and measurement of levels of specific clotting factors. These specialized tests are discussed in Chapter 75.

■ HEMATOLOGIC TESTS

Complete Blood Count

The CBC includes the red blood cell (RBC) count, hemoglobin, hematocrit, RBC indices, WBC count with or without differential, and platelet count. Table 74–3 presents reference values for the CBC. Table 74–4 reviews the effects of diseases, disorders, and conditions on the CBC and the RBC indices.

RED BLOOD CELL COUNT. The RBC count measures the number of RBCs per cubic millimeter (mm^3) of blood. This value is useful in verifying findings from other hematopoietic tests for diagnosis of anemia and polycythemia. Normal values vary with age and sex.

HEMOGLOBIN LEVEL. A hemoglobin determination is used to evaluate the hemoglobin content (and thus the iron status and oxygen-carrying capacity) of erythrocytes by measuring the number of grams of hemoglobin per deciliter (100 ml) of blood. This measurement helps to indicate anemias and polycythemia. Normal hemoglobin levels vary with age and sex.

HEMATOCRIT LEVEL. Often used in place of the RBC count, the hematocrit is a measure of the volume of RBCs in whole blood expressed as a percentage. This test is useful in the diagnosis of anemia, polycythemia, and

TABLE 74–1 SEQUENCE AND PALPATION TECHNIQUE FOR LYMPH NODES

Nodes	Location	Palpation Technique
Occipital	Posterior at base of skull and lateral to cervical spine	Flex the client's neck forward slightly to relax the trapezius. Palpate right and left node centers simultaneously.
Posterior auricular (mastoid)	Behind auricle of ear, over outer surface of mastoid process	Palpate over both mastoid processes simultaneously.
Preauricular (anterior auricular)	In front of tragus of ear	Palpate right and left sides simultaneously, anterior to the tragus and posterior to the temporomandibular joint.
Retropharyngeal (tonsillar)	Near angle of jaw at jaw margin	Flex the client's neck slightly in the midline. Palpate behind both jaw angles simultaneously.
Submandibular (submaxillary)	Along medial border of mandible, between angle of jaw and chin	Palpate along the medial borders of the mandible from the angle of the jaw toward the chin. Palpate right and left node centers simultaneously.
Submental	At the midline, posterior to tip of mandible under chin	Palpate with one hand under the client's chin just behind the tip of the mandible. Steady the client's head with the free hand if necessary.
Anterior superficial cervical chain	Along and over (anterior to) sternocleidomastoid, in anterior triangle	Flex the client's neck forward to relax the sternocleidomastoid. Palpate one side at a time. Palpate slowly against the sternocleidomastoid, progressing from the clavicle toward the jaw.
Posterior superficial cervical chain	Along anterior edge of trapezius, in posterior triangle	Flex the client's neck to relax the trapezius muscles. Palpate slowly against the trapezius muscles, progressing from the mastoid processes toward the clavicles.
Deep cervical chain	Under sternocleidomastoid	Flex the client's neck laterally toward the side being examined to relax the muscles and soft tissue. Palpate one side at a time. Hook the thumb (on one side) and fingers (on the other side) around the sternocleidomastoid muscle to feel deep to the muscle. Progress from the jaw toward the sternum.
	Along anterior edge of sternocleidomastoid, in anterior triangle	With the client's neck still flexed laterally, palpate along the anterior edge of the sternocleidomastoid from the sternum to the jaw angle. Repeat on the opposite side of the neck.
Supraclavicular (scalene)	Above clavicle, in angle formed by clavicle and sternocleidomastoid	Flex the client's neck sharply with one hand and encourage the client to relax the shoulders so that clavicles drop. Palpate one side at a time with fingers over the client's right clavicle lateral to the sternocleidomastoid. Ask the client to inhale deeply while pressing in and behind the clavicle. Repeat using the right hand to palpate the client's left node centers.
Infraclavicular	Below the clavicle, in midclavicular area	Palpate the right and left sides simultaneously, pushing in and up, under the clavicles.
Axillary (anterior pectoral, midaxillary, and posterior subscapular)	In the axilla (performed during breast examination)	Palpate one side at a time, anteriorly, centrally, and posteriorly. If the client is sitting, support the client's right forearm with your right hand and use the finger tips of your left hand to palpate, starting low in the anterior axilla, advancing higher to the central nodes, then to the posterior nodes. If nodes are palpable, try to slide fingers beneath to evaluate. Repeat on the other side (see Chapter 37).
Epitrochlear (cubital)	Medial surface of upper arm in groove between the biceps and triceps muscles (included in breast examination)	Flex the client's elbow about 90 degrees, support the elbow with one hand and palpate with the other. Feel for nodes in the fossa, about 3 cm proximal to the medial epicondyle of the humerus (see Chapter 37).
Inguinal	Superior (horizontal) chain, just below inguinal ligament Inferior (vertical) chain: close to upper portion of great saphenous vein	Have the client lie supine with knee slightly flexed. Palpate one side at a time, rolling fingers along the inguinal ligament.
Popliteal	In popliteal fossae on lateral aspect of the knee	Have the client lie supine with the knee slightly flexed. Palpate one side at a time.

abnormal hydration states. The hematocrit value is roughly three times the hemoglobin concentration. Normal values vary with age and sex.

Red Blood Cell Indices. RBC indices are measures of erythrocyte size and hemoglobin content. These values derive from the RBC count and hemoglobin level. Table 74–5 describes the three RBC indices: mean corpuscular volume, mean corpuscular hemoglobin, and mean corpuscular hemoglobin concentration. The indices are helpful in assessing the various anemias.

TABLE 74–2 LABORATORY TESTS USED IN THE DIAGNOSIS OF ANEMIA

Test	Normal Value
Iron	50–150 μg/dl
Total iron-binding capacity (TIBC)	250–350 μg/dl
Transferrin	250–430 mg/dl
Transferrin saturation	20%–55%
Ferritin	Men: 15–200 μg/ml Women: 11–200 μg/ml
Folate	7–20 μg/ml
Vitamin B_{12}	200–800 pg/ml
Schilling test (vitamin B_{12} absorption)	8.5%–28% excretion in 24–48 hr

dl, deciliter; ml, milliliter; μg, microgram; pg, picogram.

PLATELET COUNT. The platelet count measures the number of platelets (thrombocytes) per cubic millimeter of blood. Platelets have a key role in blood clotting. The count is valuable in assessing the severity of thrombocytopenia (abnormally low platelet count), which can result in spontaneous bleeding, as well as thrombocytosis (abnormally high platelet count).

WHITE BLOOD CELL COUNT. The WBC count measures the number of WBCs in a cubic millimeter (mm^3) of blood. It is used to detect infection or inflammation and to monitor a client's response to or adverse effects of chemotherapy or radiation therapy.

WHITE BLOOD CELL DIFFERENTIAL. The WBC differential determines the proportion of each of the five types of WBCs in a sample of 100 WBCs. To determine the actual (absolute) count of a specific WBC type, multiply the total WBC count by the cell percentage reported in the differential. The differential helps in evaluating the body's capacity to resist and overcome infections, in detecting and classifying leukemias and other disorders, and in detecting allergies and helminthic infections.

Peripheral Blood Smear

A peripheral blood smear is obtained to determine variations and abnormalities in erythrocytes, leukocytes, and platelets. Cells of normal size and shape are termed *normocytes;* cells of normal color are *normochromic.* Abnormalities of erythrocyte size, shape, and color usually indicate some form of anemia (Table 74–6).

Reticulocyte Count

A reflection of RBC production, the reticulocyte count measures the responsiveness of the bone marrow to a diminished number of circulating erythrocytes. Specifically, this test measures the number of reticulocytes released from the bone marrow into the blood. An increased reticulocyte count indicates increased erythrocyte production, probably because of excessive RBC destruction (hemolytic anemia) or loss (hemorrhage). A decrease in the reticulocyte count may indicate bone marrow failure or pernicious anemia. The reticulocyte count is also used to evaluate the effectiveness of treatment of pernicious anemia and bone marrow failure.

Antiglobulin Tests

The *direct* antiglobulin test (Coombs' test) is used to (1) detect certain antigen-antibody reactions between serum antibodies and RBC antigens, (2) differentiate between various forms of hemolytic anemia, (3) determine unusual blood types, and (4) identify hemolytic disease in newborns. This test examines erythrocytes for the presence of antibodies (agglutinins) that damage erythrocytes without causing clumping or hemolysis. It is used to crossmatch blood for blood transfusions, test umbilical cord blood for erythroblastosis fetalis, and diagnose acquired hemolytic anemia.

The *indirect* antiglobulin test identifies antibodies to erythrocyte antigens in the serum of clients who have a greater than normal chance of developing transfusion reactions. Both the direct and the indirect tests are agglutination procedures that use a suspension of RBCs.

Coagulation Screening Tests

Laboratory studies are the most crucial for pinpointing the type and cause of bleeding disorders (Table 74–7). Initially, four basic laboratory tests are performed to discern whether the bleeding problem is related to a platelet, coagulation, or vascular defect: (1) platelet count, (2) PT, (3) PTT, and (4) bleeding time. Most bleeding disorders are diagnosed by the PT and PTT.

TABLE 74–3 NORMAL VALUES FOR COMPLETE BLOOD COUNTS IN ADULTS

Measure	Value*
ERYTHROCYTES	
RBC count (number of cells/mm^3 of blood)	Women: 4.2–5.4 million/mm^3 Men: 4.7–6.1 million/mm^3
Hemoglobin (oxygen-carrying pigment of RBC)	Women: 12–16.0 g/dl Men: 13.5–18.0 g/dl
Hematocrit (% volume of RBCs in whole blood)	Women: 37%–47% (pregnancy >33%) Men: 42%–52%
Reticulocytes	0.5%–2% of total erythrocytes
LEUKOCYTES	
WBC count (number of cells/mm^3 of blood)	4000–9000/mm^3
WBC differential	
Granulocytes	
Neutrophils	55%–70%
Eosinophils	1%–4%
Basophils	0.5%–1.0%
Agranulocytes	
Lymphocytes	20%–40%
Monocytes	2%–8%
PLATELETS	
Platelet (thrombocyte) count (number of cells/mm^3 of blood)	150,000–450,000/mm^3

*Normal values may differ significantly among laboratories. g/dl, grams per deciliter; mm^3, cubic millimeter; RBC, red blood cell; WBC, white blood cell

TABLE 74–4 DISEASES, DISORDERS, AND CONDITIONS AFFECTING THE COMPLETE BLOOD COUNT (CBC), AND RED BLOOD CELL (RBC) INDICES

CBC, RBC Index	Increased by	Decreased by
RBC count	Polycythemia vera, cardiac and pulmonary disorders characterized by cyanosis, dehydration, acute poisoning	Anemia, fluid overload, recent hemorrhage, leukemia
Reticulocyte count	Hemolytic anemia, hemorrhage, following effective treatment for pernicious anemia	Bone marrow failure, pernicious anemia
Hemoglobin	Hemoconcentration from polycythemia or dehydration	Hemodilution (fluid overload), anemia, recent hemorrhage
Hematocrit	Hemoconcentration from loss of fluid, dehydration, polycythemia	Hemodilution, anemia, acute massive blood loss
Mean corpuscular volume	Pernicious anemia, macrocytic anemia, folic acid or vitamin B_{12} deficiency anemias	Microcytic anemia, iron deficiency anemia, hypochromic anemia, thalassemia, lead poisoning
Mean corpuscular hemoglobin	Macrocytic anemia	Microcytic anemia
Mean corpuscular hemoglobin concentration	Spherocytosis	Microcytic anemia, hypochromic anemia, thalassemia, iron deficiency anemia
WBC count	Infection, leukemia, tissue necrosis	Bone marrow depression
Neutrophils	Inflammatory disease or response, tissue necrosis (burns, myocardial infarction), granulocytic leukemia and other malignancies, acute stress response, bacterial infection	Bone marrow depression, viral diseases, drugs (chemotherapy, some antibiotics, psychotropics)
Eosinophils	Allergic reactions, parasitic infections, skin diseases, neoplasms, pernicious anemia	Stress response, Cushing's syndrome
Basophils	Leukemia, some hemolytic anemias, polycythemia vera	Corticosteroids, allergic reactions, acute infections (*Note:* decline is unlikely to be detected because normal count is 0%–2%)
Lymphocytes	Infectious mononucleosis, chronic bacterial infections, tuberculosis, pertussis, lymphocytic leukemia	AIDS, corticosteroids, immunosuppressive drugs
Monocytes	Infections (tuberculosis, malaria, Rocky Mountain spotted fever), collagen-vascular diseases, monocytic leukemia	Drug therapy, prednisone
Platelet count	Malignancies, polycythemia vera, splenectomy (rebound thrombocytosis)	Idiopathic thrombocytopenia purpura, aplastic anemia, hemolytic disorders, chemotherapeutic drugs or radiation, hypersplenism or splenomegaly, infiltrative bone marrow disease, disseminated intravascular coagulation, viral infections, AIDS

RBC, red blood cell; WBC, white blood cell; AIDS, acquired immunodeficiency syndrome.

TABLE 74–5 RED BLOOD CELL INDICES

Mean Corpuscular Volume (MCV)	Mean Corpuscular Hemoglobin (MCH)	Mean Corpuscular Hemoglobin Concentration (MCHC)
Measures average size or volume of individual RBC; differentiates anemias into microcytic, normocytic, and macrocytic	Measures hemoglobin content within one RBC of average size	Measures average hemoglobin concentration within 100 ml (1 dl) of packed RBCs
Formula: $\frac{Hct}{RBC}$	Formula: $\frac{Hb}{RBC}$	Formula: $\frac{Hb}{Hct}$
Normal value: 80–95 μm	Normal value: 27–31 pg	Normal value: 32–36 g/dl of packed RBCs
MCV <80 μm means abnormally small (i.e., *microcytic*) RBCs MCV >94 μm means abnormally large (i.e., *macrocytic*) RBCs	MCH <27 pg indicates hemoglobin deficiency, hypochromic RBCs MCH >32 pg indicates macrocytic cells with abnormally large volume of hemoglobin MCH >35.5 suggests spherocytosis	MCHC <32 g/dl indicates hemoglobin deficiency MCHC remains normal when MCH >32 g/dl because cells are oversized (i.e., fewer cells can be packed together within 1 dl)

Hb, hemoglobin; Hct, hematocrit; RBC, red blood cell; μm, micrometer; pg, picogram; g/dl, grams per deciliter.

TABLE 74–6 ABNORMALITIES OF THE ERYTHROCYTE

Abnormality	Characteristics of Abnormal Cell	Conditions Characterized by Abnormality
Anisocytes	Vary from normal in size	Any of the anemias
Poikilocytes	Abnormally shaped (e.g., tear- or club-shaped)	Any of the anemias; most bizarre shapes seen in the severe anemias
Microcytes	Abnormally small (<6 mm)	Microcytic anemias (e.g., iron deficiency anemia, thalassemia major)
Macrocytes	Abnormally large (>9 mm)	Macrocytic anemias (e.g., pernicious anemia, folic acid deficiency anemia)
Hypochromic cells	Pale appearance because of abnormally low hemoglobin content	Any of the anemias
Spherocytes	Relatively small and round rather than biconcave	Hereditary spherocytosis, warm antibody-induced immunohemolytic disease
Schistocytes	Fragmented, with bizarre shapes (e.g., triangles, spirals)	Hemolytic anemia, thrombotic thrombocytopenic purpura
Sickle cells	Crescent- or sickle-shaped from presence of abnormal hemoglobin (Hb S)	Sickle cell anemia
Target cells	Thin, with small amount of hemoglobin in center	Hemoglobin C diseases, thalassemia major, sickle cell anemia
Metarubricytes	Nucleated	Severe anemia

Because the normal and therapeutic ranges for PT vary according to the type of reagent used in the assay, the PT is standardized by conversion to the International Normalized Ratio (INR). For most clinical conditions that necessitate anticoagulation, the recommended INR is 2 to 3.5. Clients with mechanical prosthetic valves or recurrent systemic embolism need higher INR levels. PT may be performed with a finger stick sample at the point of care via a portable laser photodetector.

Additional coagulation screening tests are (1) the D-dimer, which confirms diagnosis of disseminated intravascular coagulation (DIC), (2) the fibrinogen level, which is low in DIC, and (3) fibrin degradation products (FDP) which are elevated in DIC.

Bone Marrow Aspiration and Biopsy

Bone marrow aspiration and biopsy are used to assess and identify most blood dyscrasias (e.g., aplastic anemia, leukemias, pernicious anemia, thrombocytopenia). Examination of the bone marrow reveals the number, size, and shape of the RBCs, WBCs, and platelet precursors. Hematologists examine marrow cells for various maturational abnormalities. Bone marrow aspiration and biopsy may be performed by a physician or a specially trained nurse. The practitioner may elect to perform the biopsy first and the aspiration second. Bone marrow samples are most commonly taken from the posterior iliac crests. An alternative site for specimens is the sternum.

Preprocedure Care

Prepare the client for the test. Explain the purpose of the procedure and what to expect. Advise the client that there will be pain during the procedure. Verify that the client has signed an informed consent form. Provide sedation as prescribed. Some protocols use conscious sedation or anesthesia (see Chapter 15).

Procedure

Help the client assume the lateral decubitus position, with the side from where the biopsy will be taken uppermost. Clean the client's skin with an antiseptic solution such as povidone-iodine. A local anesthetic is administered to numb the skin and subcutaneous tissue to the level of the periosteum. Applying ice to the contralateral side reduces pain.

Bone Marrow Aspiration. The skin is incised with a scalpel. The bone marrow aspiration needle containing an obturator is inserted through the incision to the bone cortex and into the marrow space. Once the needle is in place, the obturator is removed. A syringe is then attached to the needle, and about 1 ml of marrow is withdrawn. Because the marrow space itself cannot be anesthetized, removal of the marrow usually produces moderate to severe pain of short duration. The pain usually stops as soon as suction on the marrow space is stopped. The marrow is ejected onto labeled slides. The needle is withdrawn. Specimens should be sent to the laboratory immediately.

Bone Marrow Biopsy. The bone marrow biopsy needle is advanced through the soft tissue to the periosteum of the biopsy site. The obturator is removed, and the biopsy needle is advanced into the cortex. After the cortex is penetrated, the biopsy needle is advanced another 2 to 3 cm through the bony trabeculae. The needle is rotated several times in a circular back-and-forth motion to cut the core sample and then is withdrawn. A small probe is used to remove the core sample from the end of the biopsy needle, and the sample is placed in formalin. Specimens are labeled and sent to the laboratory immediately.

Postprocedure Care

After the procedure, apply pressure until bleeding stops. Most clients require only a small bandage over the site because bleeding is usually minimal. However, many clients who require bone marrow aspiration are thrombocytopenic and may need a longer period of pressure to stop bleeding. A pressure dressing and sandbag may be applied in these cases. Instruct the family to observe the site frequently on the day of the procedure and for several

TABLE 74–7 LABORATORY TESTS USED IN THE DIAGNOSIS OF HEMORRHAGIC DISORDERS

Name of Test	Purpose	Normal Values	Interpretation of Findings
Platelet count	Measures number of circulating platelets in venous or arterial blood	150,000–450,000/mm^3	Low count results in prolonged bleeding time and impaired clot retraction; diagnostic of thrombocytopenia
Prothrombin time (PT)	Determines activity and interaction of factors V, VII, and X, prothrombin, and fibrinogen; determines dosages of oral anticoagulant drugs	11–15 sec (one-stage) INR: 2–3.5	Prolonged PT is seen in clients receiving anticoagulant therapy; with low levels or deficiencies of fibrinogen, clotting factors II, V, VII, and X; impaired prothrombin activity; in the presence of circulating anticoagulants as seen in SLE
Partial thromboplastin time (PTT, aPTT)	Complex method for testing the normalcy of intrinsic coagulation process; employed to identify deficiencies of coagulation factors, prothrombin, and fibrinogen; used to monitor heparin therapy	25–38 sec	Prolongation of time indicates coagulation disorder that is related to deficiency of a coagulation factor; not diagnostic for platelet disorders
Thrombin time	Measures functional fibrinogen available, as shown by the time needed to form fibrin clot after thrombin is added	10–15 sec	Prolonged time indicates DIC or hypofibrinogenemia; presence in blood of excess heparin or other anticoagulants
Thromboplastin generation test (TGT)	Measures generation of thromboplastin; if result abnormal, second stage is done to identify missing coagulation factor	<12 sec (100%)	Abnormal values found in hemophilia
Fibrinogen level	Measures level of fibrinogen	200–400 mg/dl	Abnormally low values may indicate DIC, liver disease, congenital or acquired afibrinogenemia
Fibrin split products (FSPs), fibrin degradation products (FDPs) test	Measures products that result from breakdown of fibrin	Less than 10 μg/ml	Abnormally high levels are seen in DIC; helpful in monitoring fibrinolytic therapy
D-dimer	Measures a specific product resulting from breakdown of fibrin	Less than 0.5 μg/ml	Abnormallly high levels confirm the diagnosis of DIC; screen for abruptio placentae (placental abruption)
Activated clotting time	Crude measure of coagulation process in venous blood; used to control heparin therapy; commonly used during cardiovascular surgery and in the ICU	7–120 sec (depends on type of activator used)	Prolonged time occurs in severe coagulation problems and therapeutic administration of heparin
Bleeding time	Measures ability to stop bleeding after a small puncture wound	3–8 min in adults (varies with test method)	Prolonged bleeding time occurs in vascular maladies and after aspirin ingestion
Capillary fragility test (tourniquet test, Rumpel-Leede test)	Crude test of vascular resistance and platelet number and function; a BP cuff is placed on the arm and inflated to a pressure midway between systolic and diastolic BP for 5 min; petechiae in area are counted	No petechiae	Petechiae (five or more) are seen in thrombocytopenia and vascular purpura
Clot retraction	Indicates function and number of platelets; measures time needed for contraction of an undisturbed clot	50%–100% in 24 hr	Clot retraction is retarded in thrombocytopenia; clot is small and soft in thrombasthenia (functional disturbance of platelets)

BP, blood pressure; DIC, disseminated intravascular coagulation; ICU, intensive care unit; INR, International Normalized Ratio; mg/dl, milligrams per deciliter; μg, microgram; SLE, systemic lupus erythematosis.

TABLE 74–8 LYMPHOCYTE IMMUNOPHENOTYPING

Cell	Total Lymphocyte Count (%)	Absolute Count	Decreased	Increased
CD3 (mature T cells)	56%–77%	860–1880/mm³	AIDS, chronic lymphocytic leukemia, SCID, immunosuppressive therapy	Acute lymphocytic leukemia, infectious mononucleosis, multiple myleoma
CD19 (total B cells)	7%–17%	140–370/mm³	Acute lymphocytic leukemia, SCID	Chronic lymphocytic leukemia, multiple myeloma, SLE
CD4 (T helper cells)	32%–54%	530–1190/mm³	AIDS	—
CD8 (T killer/suppressor cells)	24%–37%	430–1060/mm³	AIDS	—

mm³, cubic millimeter; AIDS, acquired immunodeficiency syndrome; SLE, systemic lupus erythematosus; SCID, severe combined immunodeficiency disease.

days thereafter for clients with an increased risk for bleeding. Clients may experience some discomfort or pain and may require a mild analgesic.

■ IMMUNOLOGIC STATUS TESTS

Most immunodeficiencies can be identified through three blood tests requiring no preprocedure or postprocedure care: (1) WBC and differential, (2) immunoglobulin levels, and (3) total serum complement. Additional immunodeficiencies can be determined through more complex tests, including lymphocyte immunophenotyping, measures of immunoglobulin subclasses, complement assays, and the presence of specific antibodies (after immunizations or exposure to antigens as with communicable diseases).

Lymphocyte Immunophenotyping

Lymphocyte subpopulation analysis by flow cytometry measures total numbers and percentages of B lymphocytes, T lymphocytes, and T lymphocyte subsets (CD4, CD8) in a peripheral blood sample. Table 74–8 lists normal levels of T and B lymphocytes and conditions in which abnormal levels of T and B cells occur.

Advanced lymphocyte assays (not detailed here) include

- Mixed lymphocyte culture reaction with the client as stimulator and the client as responder
- Lymphoproliferation assays using chemicals such as phytohemagglutinin (PHA) or concanavalin A (ConA) to stimulate T cells and pokeweed mitogen to stimulate B cells
- Tests of natural killer cell activity
- Tests for deficiencies of adenosine deaminase and purine nucleoside phosphorylase

Immunoglobulin Isotypes

The immunoglobulin isotype examination measures the serum level of the various immunoglobulins: IgG, IgA, IgM, IgD, and IgE (Table 74–9). Subclasses of IgG may also be measured (IgG1, IgG2, IgG3, IgG4).

Complement Assays

Immunodeficiencies or disorders that are related to a lack of normal levels of complement components may be detected by the level of the total serum complement (CH50) or may require measuring levels of specific complement components such as C3 and C4. In rare cases, functional complement assays are required to diagnose complement disorders. Table 74–10 provides normal complement levels.

Radiography

Congenital absence of thymic tissue (diagnostic of certain immunodeficiencies) or tumor of the thymus gland (associated with myasthenia gravis) can be detected by a chest radiograph (see Chapter 11).

Other radiographic procedures may be performed to assist the diagnosis of allergy-related disorders. X-ray films and computed tomography (CT) may be ordered to assess the integrity of the sinuses (see Chapter 11).

Lymphangiography allows visualization of the lymphatic system to assess malignancy, metastases, or obstruction. Following local anesthesia administration, blue dye is injected into the dorsa of the feet and is taken up

TABLE 74–9 IMMUNOGLOBULIN (Ig) ISOTOPES

Immunoglobulin	Normal Range (mg/dl)
IgG	550–1990
IgG1	280–1020
IgG2	60–790
IgG3	14–240
IgG4	11–330
IgM	45–145
IgA	70–310
IgE	0.01–0.04
IgD	0–8

mg/dl, milligrams per deciliter.

TABLE 74-10 COMPLEMENT ASSAYS

Test	Normal Range
Total serum complement (CH50)	75–160 U/ml
C3	55–177 mg/dl
C4	15–50 mg/dl

mg/dl, milligrams per deciliter; U/ml, units per millilter.

by the lymphatics. When a lymphatic channel is located, a surgical incision into the channel allows insertion of a catheter. An oil-based dye is injected, and its progress through the lymphatic system is monitored with x-rays taken over 1 to 2 days.

Postprocedure care and complications are similar to those for angiography (see Chapter 11). Explain that the dye colors the urine blue until it is completely excreted. The dorsa may also remain blue for months.

Skin Tests

Skin tests confirm sensitivity to a specific allergen. A known antigen is placed on or directly beneath the skin to detect the presence of antibodies. Antigens are applied by one of three methods:

1. *Patch tests* (see Chapter 48).
2. *Scratch tests* (also known as *tine tests* or *prick tests*). Antigens are applied to superficial scratches that cut the outer layer of skin. The skin is then covered with gauze.
3. Intradermal allergy tests involve injecting a small amount (usually 0.1 ml) into the intradermal layer of the skin. Intradermal testing is the most accurate method but carries a higher risk of severe allergic reaction.

Take a thorough client history of allergies, and explain the purpose of the test and the procedure. Verify the specific antigens prescribed by the physician for testing, and ensure the availability of emergency resuscitation equipment in the event of an anaphylactic reaction.

Nurses often administer skin tests and interpret test results. Observe the client for the following. An immediate, positive reaction can appear within 10 to 20 minutes after antigen application, marked by erythema and wheal formation. Positive reactions indicate an antibody (B cell) response to a previous exposure to the antigen; they also suggest that the client is allergic to the substance causing the reaction. Negative reactions may be inconclusive, indicating the need for further assessment. Negative results may indicate that (1) antibodies have not formed to the specific antigen, (2) the antigen was deposited too deeply into the skin (subcutaneously rather than intradermally), or (3) the client is immunosuppressed as a result of disease or therapy (chemotherapy, corticosteroids, radiation therapy, or long-acting antihistamines that can mute an allergic response).

Problems following skin testing range from minor itching and discomfort at the injection site (common) to anaphylaxis (rare). Relieve itching and minor discomfort with the application of cool compresses and topical corticosteroids. If ulceration of the injection site occurs, keep the area clean and dry. Anaphylaxis is potentially lethal. Clients who have known anaphylactic reactions to specific antigens should never be tested for allergy to that substance. Anaphylaxis is treated with the administration of oxygen and subcutaneous epinephrine and by establishing intravenous access for administration of corticosteroids, antihistamines, and other medications, such as bronchodilators.

DELAYED-TYPE HYPERSENSITIVITY SKIN TESTING. T-cell responsiveness may be evaluated by DTH skin testing. Antigens to which people have been immunized (mumps, tetanus) or to which they commonly have been exposed (*Candida albicans*) are injected intradermally into the ventral forearm. After 24 to 72 hours, people with normal T-cell immunity exhibit an area of hard, reddened swelling (*induration*) at the injection site. The localized thickening and redness indicate accumulation of sensitized T lymphocytes at the site of antigen administration. Absence of induration may indicate *anergy* (a state of immunologic hyporesponsiveness) and an inability to react to common antigens. Anergy is associated with congenital T-cell immunodeficiency, malnutrition, cancer, HIV infection, immunosuppressant therapy, and, in the elderly, aging of the immune system.

DTH antigens are most accurately administered by separate intradermal injections of mumps antigen, *C. albicans* antigen, and tetanus toxoid fluid (1:5 dilution). Other antigens such as streptokinase, streptodornase, or trichophytin may be used but may be less reliable in assessment of T-cell immunity.

A commercial kit (CMI Multitest, Merieux, France) permits the simultaneous administration of several DTH antigens as well as a positive and a negative control. However, the kit may be less reliable for tuberculosis screening because it contains *old tuberculin* rather than *purified protein derivative* (PPD). For consistency, it is best if the same person administers and reads the skin test.

PROCEDURE

Use a 1-ml syringe with a 1/2-inch 26 to 27 gauge needle to administer the antigen. Select a site on the ventral surface of the forearm, avoiding veins or bruises. Clean the skin with alcohol, and allow it to dry. Stretch the skin taut. Inject 0.1 ml of the antigen intradermally, producing a wheal 6 to 10 mm in diameter. Circle the area with a marking pen. If more than one antigen is administered, administer each antigen 5 cm apart. Document the site of administration of each antigen using a schematic drawing.

POSTPROCEDURE CARE

After 48 to 72 hours, palpate the site for induration. Use a flexible ruler to measure the area of induration; redness alone is not significant. Induration of 5 mm or more with erythema indicates a positive response to the antigen and probable intact cell-mediated immunity. Record the results.

Food Allergy Testing

Food allergies are evaluated by skin testing or by either a *challenge diet* or *elimination diet.* In the challenge diet, the suspected food is eaten by the client in increasingly larger amounts until a reaction occurs. Reactions range from erythema, itching, and rash to vomiting or diarrhea. Manifestations such as fatigue, depression, or restlessness are not conclusive. In the elimination diet, foods are eliminated from the diet, one by one, until manifestations are relieved. Reactions may indicate an allergy to food additives or the food itself.

CONCLUSIONS

The hematopoietic system is extremely complex. Understanding the structure, function, and assessment of the hematopoietic system will help you care for clients with any of the wide variety of disorders that affect this highly complex system.

BIBLIOGRAPHY

1. Anderson, K. N. (Ed.). (1998). *Mosby's medical, nursing, and allied health dictionary.* St. Louis: Mosby–Year Book.
2. Bates, B. (1995). *A guide to physical examination and history taking* (6th ed.) Philadelphia: J. B. Lippincott.
3. Bennett, J. C., & Plum, F. (Eds.). (1996). *Cecil textbook of medicine* (20th ed.). Philadelphia: W. B. Saunders.
4. Chernecky, C. C., & Berger, B. J. (Eds.). (1997). *Laboratory tests and diagnostic procedures* (2nd ed.). Philadelphia: W. B. Saunders.
5. Coakley, F. V., & Panicek, D. M. (1997). Iodine allergy: An oyster without a pearl? *American Journal of Roentgenology, 169*(4), 951–952.
6. Conn, H. F., Clohency, R. J., & Conn, R. B. (Eds.). (1997). *Current diagnosis.* Philadelphia: W. B. Saunders.
7. Corbett, J. (1996). *Laboratory tests and diagnostic procedures with nursing diagnoses* (4th ed.). Stamford, CT: Appleton & Lange.
8. Freeman, T. M. (1998). Anaphylaxis: Diagnosis and treatment. *Primary Care, 25*(4), 809–817.
9. Gibbar-Clements, T., Shirrell, D., & Free, C. (1997). PT and APTT: Seeing beyond the numbers. *Nursing, 27*(7), 49–51.
10. Goyette, R. E. (1997). *Hematology: A comprehensive guide to the diagnosis and treatment of blood disorders.* Los Angeles: Practice Management Information Corporation (PMIC).
11. Gruchalla, R. S. (1998). Drug allergies. *Primary Care, 25*(4), 791–807.
12. Guyton, A. C., & Hall, J. E. (1996). *Textbook of medical physiology* (9th ed.). Philadelphia: W. B. Saunders.
13. Hash, R. B. (1999). Intravascular radiographic contrast media: Issues for family physicians. *Journal of American Family Practice, 12*(1), 32–42.
14. Henry, J. B. (Ed.). (1996). *Clinical diagnosis and management by laboratory methods* (19th ed.). Philadelphia: W. B. Saunders.
15. Jarvis, C. (2000). *Physical examination and health assessment* (3rd ed.). Philadelphia: W. B. Saunders.
16. Kee, J. L. (1995). *Laboratory and diagnostic tests with nursing implications* (4th ed.). Norwalk, CT: Appleton & Lange.
17. Kurt J., et al. (Eds.). (1998). *Harrison's principles of internal medicine* (13th ed.). New York: McGraw-Hill.
18. Mandell, G. L., Douglas, R. G., & Bennett, J. E. (1995). *Principles and practice of infectious diseases* (4th ed.). New York: Churchill Livingstone.
19. Metcalfe, D. D. (1998). Food allergy. *Primary Care, 25*(4), 819–829.
20. Pagana, K. D., & Pagana, T. J. (1997). *Mosby's diagnostic and laboratory reference* (3rd ed.). St. Louis: Mosby–Year Book.
21. Seidel, H. M., et al. (1995). *Mosby's guide to physical examination* (3rd ed.). St. Louis: Mosby–Year Book.
22. Stellato, C., & Adkinson, N. F. (1998). Pathophysiology of contrast media anaphylactoid reactions: New perspectives on an old problem. *Allergy, 53*(12), 1111–1113.
23. Stevens, M. L. (1997). *Fundamentals of clinical hematology.* Philadelphia: W. B. Saunders.
24. Tierney, L. M., McPhee, S. J., & Papadakis, M. A. (Eds.). (1998). *Current medical diagnosis and treatment 1998* (36th ed.). Stamford, CT: Appleton & Lange.
25. Treseler, K. M. (1995). *Clinical laboratory and diagnostic tests: Significance and nursing implications* (3rd ed.). Stamford, CT: Appleton & Lange.
26. Watson, J., & Jaffee, M. S. (1995). *Nurse's manual of laboratory and diagnostic tests* (2nd ed.). Philadelphia: F. A. Davis.

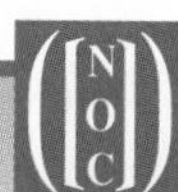
REMEMBER *to check out your* **Companion CD ROM**

CHAPTER 75

Management of Clients with Hematologic Disorders

Linda Yoder

NURSING OUTCOMES CLASSIFICATION (NOC) for Nursing Diagnoses—Clients with Hematologic Disorders

Activity Intolerance
Activity Tolerance
Circulation Status
Endurance
Pain: Disruptive Effects
Altered Protection
Coagulation Status
Infection Status
Altered Perfusion
Tissue Perfusion: Skin and Mucous Membranes
Tissue Perfusion: Peripheral
Fatigue
Activity Tolerance
Comfort Level
Energy Conservation
Rest
Quality of Life
Knowledge Deficit
Knowledge: Disease Process
Knowledge: Energy Conservation
Pain
Comfort Level
Pain Control
Pain: Disruptive Effects
Pain Level
Symptom Control
Symptom Severity

This chapter discusses disorders affecting red blood cells (erythrocytes), the spleen, platelets, and clotting factors. Priorities of nursing care center around lack of oxygenated blood flow and risk of hemorrhage. Leukemia and lymphoma are discussed in Chapter 78.

DISORDERS AFFECTING RED BLOOD CELLS

THE ANEMIAS

Anemia is a reduction in red blood cells (RBCs), which in turn decreases the oxygen-carrying capacity of the blood. Not a disease in itself, anemia reflects an abnormality in RBC number, structure, or function. The prevalence of anemia increases with age; an estimated 20% of older adults are anemic. However, anemia cannot be assumed to be caused simply by aging without the exclusion of reversible causes. The elderly client should be fully assessed for an underlying cause of anemia.

Etiology

Major causes of anemia are deficiencies and abnormalities of RBC production or excessive blood loss or destruction of RBCs.

Hematopoiesis is reviewed in the Anatomy and Physiology review preceding this unit. RBCs are produced in bone marrow. The requirements for RBC production, called *erythropoiesis,* include precursor cells (*reticulocytes*), adequate supplies of iron, vitamin B_{12}, folic acid, protein, pyridoxine, and traces of copper. If any of these factors is missing, the RBCs will be fragile, misshapen, of abnormal size, lacking hemoglobin, or too few in number.

Anemia may be due to acute or chronic blood loss. Increased destruction of RBCs can result from extrinsic sources, physical causes such as prosthetic heart valves, or thrombotic thrombocytopenic purpura. It also can result from antibodies, as in transfusion mismatch; from infectious agents and toxins; or from other causes, such as hypersplenism or osmotic and physical injury to the cell seen in sickle cell disease.

Classification

Anemias are classified according to the size of the RBC. Normal RBCs are shown in Figure 75–1*A*. *Normocytic anemia* is anemia with normal RBC size and shape. This form of anemia is commonly due to blood loss, chronic disease, and bone marrow suppression with chemotherapy. *Microcytic anemia* is defined as anemia with small RBCs and low levels of hemoglobin in each RBC. Common causes of microcytic anemia include iron deficiency due to protein malnutrition and occult gastrointestinal (GI) bleeding with gastritis or colon cancer. *Macrocytic anemia* is characterized by large RBCs. Common causes include vitamin B_{12} and folic acid deficiency. Anemias can also be due to defective hemoglobin in which case, the condition is called *sickle cell anemia* (Fig. 75–1*B*).

Pathophysiology

Transport of oxygen is impaired with anemia. Hemoglobin is lacking or the number of RBCs is too low to carry adequate oxygen to tissues, and hypoxia develops.

Clinical Manifestations

Manifestations accompanying anemia differ, depending on the severity and speed of blood loss, the chronicity of the anemia, the age of the person, and the presence of other disorders. Tissue hypoxia is the underlying cause of all manifestations accompanying anemia. Other manifestations listed below are due to the underlying problem.

Clients often appear pale, particularly of palm lines, nail beds, conjunctivae, and circumoral area. Because of tissue hypoxia, clients are fatigued. There may be shortness of breath, dyspnea on exertion, or palpitations. Hypotension is common, especially if the client has lost blood. If the client has GI bleeding, tarry stools may be present. If heart failure develops, orthopnea, angina, tachycardia, dependent edema, bruits, and tachypnea may occur.

Clients with mild anemia (hemoglobin of 10–12 g/dl) are usually asymptomatic. If manifestations do occur, they typically follow strenuous exertion. Clients with moderate anemia may suffer from dyspnea, palpitations, diaphoresis with exertion, and chronic fatigue. Some clients with severe anemia, such as those with chronic renal failure, may be asymptomatic because their anemia develops gradually.

The RBC count, hemoglobin level, and hematocrit confirm the presence of anemia. A bone marrow specimen may be required to confirm the type of anemia. A peripheral blood smear (RBC indices) is needed to determine the size of the RBC.

Outcome Management

Medical Management

The goals of care for clients with anemia include (1) alleviating or controlling the causes, (2) relieving the manifestations, and (3) preventing complications. Management of the anemias ranges from specific treatments to symptomatic care. Treatment also varies in intensity and duration because some anemias resolve after blood transfusion, others resolve within a few weeks or months, and still other forms require lifelong intervention.

ALLEVIATE AND CONTROL THE CAUSES

Four common forms of anemia along with specific interventions are discussed next.

RELIEVE MANIFESTATIONS

Oxygen Therapy

Oxygen therapy may be prescribed for clients with severe anemia because their blood has a reduced capacity for oxygen. Oxygen helps prevent tissue hypoxia and lessens the workload of the heart as it struggles to compensate for the lower hemoglobin levels.

Erythropoietin

Subcutaneous injections of erythropoietin can be given to treat anemias of chronic disease. For this drug to be effective, the client must have bone marrow capable of producing RBCs and sufficient nutrients to produce RBCs.

Iron Replacement

Iron can be given to augment oral intake. Oral forms of iron are usually given for mild forms of anemia. The medications of choice are ferrous sulfate (Feosol), 0.325 g orally three times a day with meals; ferrous gluconate (Fergon), 0.3 g orally twice a day; and intramuscular (IM) iron dextran (Imferon), 100 to 250 mg. Clients usu-

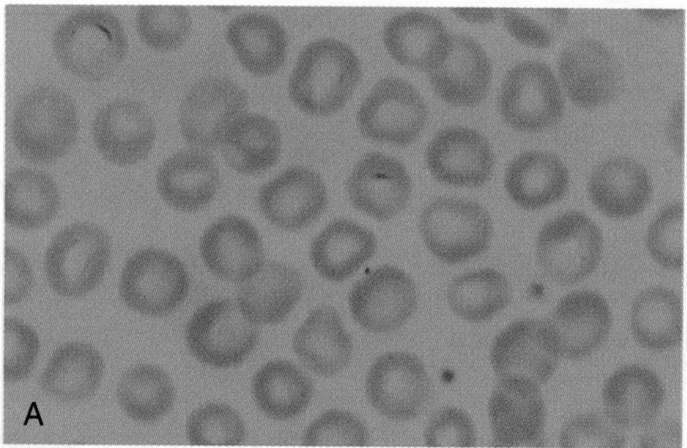

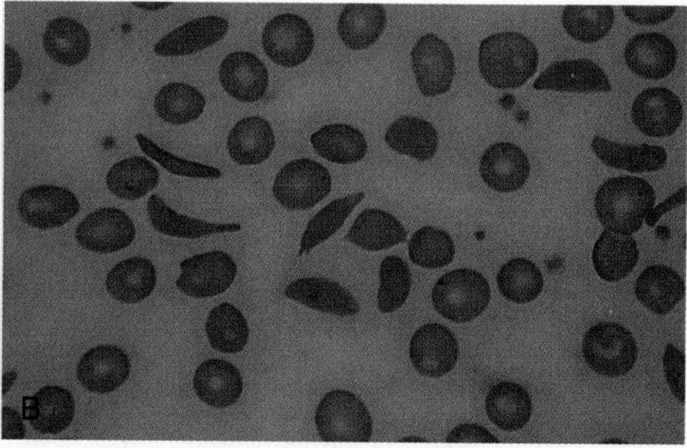

FIGURE 75–1 *A*, Normal red blood cells. *B*, Sickle cell anemia. (Magnification ×875.) Note the elongated and sickle-shaped cells. (From Rodak, B. [1995]. *Diagnostic hematology* [pp. 83, 257]. Philadelphia: W. B. Saunders.)

ally receive iron supplements for at least 6 months for repletion of the body stores. Parenteral iron therapy is administered to clients who (1) have an intolerance to oral iron preparations, (2) habitually forget to take their medications, or (3) continue to suffer blood losses. Iron dextran is the parenteral drug of choice. The client typically feels more energetic and has an increased appetite within 48 hours. Peak reticulocytosis occurs at about day 10. RBC indices and hemoglobin content gradually return to normal. Because of the high risk of allergic reaction, if iron is to be given intravenously, the physician usually administers the first dose.

Blood Transfusions

Blood transfusions are valuable in treating anemia resulting from acute blood loss and also may benefit clients with severe chronic anemia (hemoglobin < 6 g/dl) who have responded poorly to other forms of therapy. Packed RBCs may be given to clients who have lost blood in surgery or due to trauma. The Joint Commission on Accreditation of Healthcare Organizations (JCAHO) requires that all blood transfusions be evaluated to confirm that clear medical indications for the transfusion exist and that the client responds as expected. The physician's order for transfusion should specify blood component, volume, and rate of infusion. Table 75–1 describes blood components.

Blood is administered after informed consent is obtained. Consent includes an explanation of medical indications for homologous transfusion and its benefits, risks, and alternatives. Documentation of informed consent may consist of a form in the medical record stating that this information was presented in a manner understandable to the client (e.g., "Risks of and alternatives to blood transfusion were explained, and the client consented"). If the client is clinically unable to consent to transfusion, a reasonable effort should be made to secure consent from a family member. If no family member is available or time does not allow, place a note to this effect in the chart. Assess the client's understanding of the transfusion, and accurately respond to questions and concerns.

Two alternatives to homologous (random) blood transfusion should be considered: *autologous* and *directed* (designated) donation. Clients who do not have leukemia or bacteremia should be offered the option of donating their own blood before a scheduled surgical procedure when there is a reasonable expectation that blood will be required. Although the risk-benefit ratio should be evaluated, experience to date indicates that even clients with heart disease and other high-risk conditions tolerate donating blood well. The elimination of disease transmission, alloimmunization, and other potential transfusion complications makes this a reasonable option for many surgical clients.

Autologous donations can be made every 3 days if the donor's hemoglobin remains at or above 11 g/dl. For the blood to be maintained in a liquid state, donations should begin within 5 weeks of the transfusion date. RBCs can be stored frozen for 10 years, but the expense involved and time required for final preparation limit this practice to those who have extremely rare blood types. Donations should cease at least 3 days before the date of transfusion.

Another commonly used method of autologous blood collection is intraoperative, postoperative, or post-traumatic blood salvage. Blood is suctioned from body cavities, joint spaces, and other closed operative or trauma sites. Tissue debris and other sterile contaminants may necessitate special processing such as washing. Salvaged blood must be reinfused within 6 hours of collection.

A second option is for transfusion recipients to designate their own donors. Directed donations have not decreased the risk of contracting human immunodeficiency virus (HIV) infection. In fact, directed donors appear to have a higher incidence of hepatitis. This is probably due to the fact that a large percentage of directed donors are giving blood for the first time, and first-time donors commonly test positive for hepatitis surrogate markers. Despite this evidence, clients frequently feel more comfortable identifying their donors. Discuss all of these options with the client in sufficient time to permit donation and blood testing.

PRETRANSFUSION TESTING. The client's major concern is likely to be the safety of the transfusion, specifically the risk of contracting acquired immunodeficiency syndrome (AIDS). Provide accurate information for the client, and begin efforts to ensure a safe and effective transfusion before the blood or component is collected. For many decades, prospective donors have been asked two categories of questions: (1) those intended to protect the donor from possible risks of donation, and (2) those intended to protect the recipient from risks of transfusion.

To reduce the risk of HIV transmission to blood recipients, there has been a marked increase in the second group of questions. In addition, donors are required to read information about behaviors known to increase the risk of HIV infection; in most collection centers, they are questioned directly about their involvement in such activities.

Finally, a method must be made available for donors to indicate anonymously that their unit is or is not safe for transfusion. In addition to obtaining a thorough donor history, many diagnostic tests for serologic and infectious disease are routinely performed on the donor's blood.

When a need for blood is identified, several tests are done to confirm that the client's blood is compatible with that of the donor. First, the recipient's ABO and Rh type are identified. To determine the presence of antibody other than anti-A or anti-B, an antibody screen is performed. This test (the "indirect antiglobulin test") is done by adding the recipient's serum to donor RBCs known to have a certain set of minor blood group antigens. Coombs' serum (antihuman globulin) is added to facilitate visibility of cellular agglutination, an indicator of antigen-antibody complex formation. The results are viewed macroscopically and microscopically. More than 400 minor RBC antigens have been identified in RBCs, each of which can stimulate the production of an antibody. However, only the few (~30) that are of sufficiently potent antigenicity to be clinically significant are included in the routine antibody screen.

It is not uncommon for chronically transfused clients to develop multiple antibodies. Identifying the antibodies and obtaining blood from donors who do not possess the antigens can significantly complicate the testing procedure and lengthen the time required for blood preparation.

Blood products containing RBCs may be further tested for compatibility to crossmatch testing. For this procedure, donor RBCs are combined with the recipient's se-

TABLE 75–1 BLOOD COMPONENTS

Whole Blood	Red Blood Cells	Platelet Concentrates	Fresh Frozen Plasma	Cryoprecipitate	Granulocyte Concentrates	Plasma Derivatives	Coagulation Factor Concentrates
COMPOSITION							
RBC, plasma, plasma proteins (globulins, antibodies), 63 ml of anticoagulant-preservative	RBC with CPDA-1 solution (anticoagulant-preservative only), final hematocrit no higher than 80% (80% RBC, 20% plasma) RBC with 100 ml additive solution, final hematocrit about 55%–60%	Single-unit platelets contain a minimum of 5.5×10^{10} (1 unit) platelets in 50–70 ml of plasma obtained by separating platelet-rich plasma from 1 unit of fresh whole blood; 6–10 units may be pooled for 1 transfusion Single-donor platelets contain a minimum of 3.0×10^{11} platelets (6 units) obtained from single donor by use of automated cell separator during apheresis; recipient exposed to fewer donors, which decreases complications	91% water, 7% protein (globulin, antibodies, clotting factors), and 2% carbohydrates Freezing within 8 hr of collection preserves all clotting factors	Each unit contains about 80–120 units of factor VIII (antihemophilic factor) that represents 50% of antihemophilic factor originally present in unit, vWF, 250 mg of fibrinogen, and 20%–30% of factor XIII present in a unit of whole blood, suspended in 10–20 ml of plasma	Unit obtained by granulocytaphresis contains a minimum of 1.0×10^{10} granulocytes, variable amounts of lymphocytes (usually <10%), 30–50 ml of RBC and 100–400 ml of plasma, and 6–10 units of platelets; the platelets can be separated from the unit if the granulocyte recipient is not thrombocytopenic	*Albumin:* 96% albumin, 4% globulin and other proteins extracted from plasma; available as a 5% solution, oncotically equivalent to plasma, and also a concentrated 25% solution *Plasma protein fraction:* 83% albumin and 17% globulins extracted from plasma; less pure than albumin and has higher degree of contamination with other plasma proteins; in 5% solution only	*Factor VIII:* Lyophilized concentrate containing large quantities of factor VIII; prepared from large pools of donor plasma, but heat treatment during fractionation process significantly reduces risk of transmitting viral disease *Factor IX:* Lyophilized concentrate containing large quantities of factor IX; also contains factors II, VII, and X; product prepared from large pools of donor plasma, but heat treatment during fractionation process significantly reduces risk of transmitting viral disease
VOLUME							
500 ml/unit	250–350 ml/unit 350–400 ml/unit	50–70 ml/unit 200–400 ml/unit	200–250 ml	5–10 ml/unit	200–400 ml with platelets 100–200 ml without platelets	Albumin: 250 and 500 ml (5%); 50 and 100 ml (25%)	Multiple-dose vial

ABO/Rh COMPATIBILITY							
The ABO type of the donor should be identical with the recipient's Rh− blood can be given to an Rh− or Rh+ recipient	A can match with A or O; B can match with B or O; O can match only with O; AB can match with A, B, or O Rh− blood can be given to either Rh+ or Rh− recipient	Whereas platelets have no ABO or Rh antigens, they are suspended in 200–400 ml of plasma containing donor antibodies and a small number of RBC ABO and Rh compatibility is recommended	A can match with A or AB; B can match with B or AB; AB can match only with AB; O can match with A, B, AB, or O Rh− and Rh+ blood can be given to either Rh+ or Rh− recipient	Cryoprecipitate contains no RBC and a small volume of plasma ABO crossmatching not needed, and plasma compatibility preferred but not required	Granulocytes contain a significant number of RBC and plasma; therefore, ABO of donor should be identical with recipient's Rh− components may be transfused to an Rh+ recipient	Antibodies destroyed during processing; therefore, compatibility not a factor	Antibodies destroyed during processing, so compatibility not a factor
SPECIAL CONSIDERATIONS							
Whole blood transfusion is rarely indicated Treatment with specific blood components is usually recommended	RBC may be viscous, thus 0.9% saline may be added to achieve optimal flow rates For some clients, a leukocyte depletion filter may be used to prevent complications	Because platelet concentrates contain few RBC, crossmatch testing is not required Plasma ABO and Rh compatibility is recommended, especially when the total volume of the transfusion exceeds 150–200 ml Only filters specially designed for platelet transfusion should be used	Plasma carries same risk of disease transmission as does whole blood If only volume expansion is required, products of choice are crystalloid or colloid solutions, such as saline or albumin Plasma contains no RBC, and Rh compatibility and crossmatching are not required ABO compatibility must be confirmed before administration	Single units of cryoprecipitate may be pooled into 1 container by the blood collection center If individual bags are issued, 0.9% saline may need to be added to rinse residual cryoprecipitate from bags and tubing	Granulocytes have short survival (<24 hr); infuse as soon as possible Granulocyte concentrates contain a significant number of RBC; pretransfusion testing recommended Increased incidence of febrile, nonhemolytic reactions with granulocyte transfusions; infuse slowly, observe client closely; premedication with an antihistamine, acetaminophen, steroids advised Do *not* administer amphotericin B within 4 hr of granulocyte transfusion to avoid pulmonary insufficiency	PPF and albumin cannot transmit hepatitis or HIV infection; the pasteurization process used to prepare the products destroys such viruses Hypotension has been associated with rapid infusion of PPF; 25% albumin can cause a significantly increased blood pressure because of its ability to draw fluid into the intravascular space	Factor VIII and factor IX assays should be performed at appropriate intervals to assess response Factor VIII concentration lacks vWF and should not be used in treatment of von Willebrand's disease

Table continued on following page

TABLE 75–1 BLOOD COMPONENTS *Continued*

Whole Blood	Red Blood Cells	Platelet Concentrates	Fresh Frozen Plasma	Cryoprecipitate	Granulocyte Concentrates	Plasma Derivatives	Coagulation Factor Concentrates
OUTCOMES							
Prevention or resolution of hypovolemic shock and anemia In a nonbleeding adult, 1 unit of whole blood should increase hematocrit by 3% and hemoglobin by 1 g/dl	Resolution of manifestations of anemia In a nonbleeding adult, 1 unit of RBC should increase hematocrit by 3% and hemoglobin by 1 g/dl	Prevention or resolution of bleeding due to thrombocytopenia or platelet dysfunction 1 unit should raise peripheral platelet count 5000–10,000/mm^3 if underlying cause is resolved or controlled Efficacy of platelet transfusion can be determined by obtaining platelet counts at 1 hr and 18–24 hr after infusion	Treatment effectiveness is assessed by monitoring coagulation function, specifically, PT and PTT, or by specific factor assays	Correction of factor VIII, vWF, factor XIII, and fibrinogen deficiency; cessation of bleeding in uremic clients Laboratory values required to assess effectiveness of treatment	Improvement in or resolution of infection No increase in peripheral WBC count usually seen after granulocyte transfusion in adults, although increase may be seen in children An improvement in clinical condition because of resolving infection is the only measure of treatment effectiveness	The client will acquire and maintain adequate blood pressure and volume support	The client will develop hemostasis because of increased levels of factor VIII and factor IX activity

CPDA-1, citrate-phosphate-dextrose-adenine; FFP, fresh-frozen plasma; HIV, human immunodeficiency virus; IV, intravenous; PPF, plasma protein fraction; PT, prothrombin time; PTT, partial thromboplastin time; RBC, red blood cells; vWF, von Willebrand's factor; WBC, white blood cells.

rum and Coombs' serum. After an inoculation period, the results are viewed microscopically. If no RBC agglutination has occurred, the crossmatch is compatible. Crossmatching adds very little to the safety of transfusion (0.01% to 0.1%) if a negative antibody screen is initially obtained. In these situations, the Coombs' phase can be eliminated to shorten the procedure and reduce cost.

Routine serologic testing requires a 10-ml clotted sample and a 7-ml citrated sample. Approximately 1 hour is required for testing in routine situations. In the event of a medical emergency, O-negative RBCs and AB plasma can be safely administered to most clients without serologic testing.

Failure to correctly label the samples used for blood bank testing may lead to fatal errors. Several precautionary measures should be taken to reduce this risk. Label the sample at the bedside after asking the client to state his or her name and comparing it with the name on the identification bracelet. If the client cannot state his or her name, identity should be confirmed by a family member or other person familiar with the client whenever possible. The date and initials of the phlebotomist must be written on the sample label. Many institutions have adopted a secondary identification system. Several commercial systems are available; each is designed to ensure that the sample used for crossmatch has been drawn from the client who receives the transfusion.

Delayed Transfusion Complications. Complications can occur days to years after a transfusion. Fever, mild jaundice, and decreased hematocrit may indicate a delayed hemolytic reaction. Hemolysis of RBCs may occur 3 days to several months after the transfusion if an antibody was undetected during crossmatch testing and RBCs containing that antigen were transfused. Usually no medical treatment is required.

Iron overload may occur in clients receiving more than 100 units of blood over a period of time, such as clients with aplastic anemia. The normal iron level of 2 to 3 g usually remains constant because iron is metabolized at a fixed rate. Each unit of RBCs contains an additional 200 mg of iron. In clients who receive more than 100 units of RBCs, excess iron stores in major organs often develop. Complications of iron overload include cardiac myopathies (pericarditis, arrhythmias, heart failure), thyroid insufficiency, endocrine and pancreas malfunction (glucose intolerance), liver fibrosis, profound anemia, and skin discoloration. Cardiomyopathies related to iron overload are a frequent cause of death in the chronically transfused client. Deferoxamine, which chelates and removes accumulated iron via the kidneys, may be administered intravenously or subcutaneously to prevent this potentially fatal complication.

Post-transfusion graft-versus-host disease (GVHD) can occur if donor lymphocytes engraft and divide in the marrow spaces of an immunocompromised recipient. Manifestations are fever, rash, diarrhea, and hepatitis. This frequently fatal complication can be prevented by irradiation of all cellular components before administration to high-risk clients.

Many diseases can be transmitted through blood transfusion. The most common is hepatitis C. Although manifestations are milder than those seen with hepatitis B, chronic liver disease and cirrhosis may develop. Hepatitis B should be considered if the recipient experiences anorexia, malaise, nausea, vomiting, dark urine, and jaundice within 4 to 6 weeks of transfusion. Elevated alanine aminotransferase (ALT) and aspartate aminotransferase (AST) levels are frequently seen, indicating liver damage that may be permanent. Hepatitis B and C are treated symptomatically. With advances in donor testing and screening in the United States, the risk of hepatitis has decreased to about 3%.

On rare occasions, HIV-1 is transmitted from an infected donor to a blood recipient. The client may be asymptomatic for several years or may have flu-like manifestations in 2 to 4 weeks. Whereas more than 25,000 cases of transfusion-associated AIDS were reported before routine donor testing in 1985, the incidence has decreased to 1 in 100,000 to 150,000 as a result of careful donor screening and testing.

Nursing Management

Assessment

The general nursing care of clients with anemia includes adequate assessment by the nurse to help identify the cause of the anemia and client education. You can help in diagnosis by taking a complete health history focusing on the elements outlined in Chapter 74. Client teaching is extremely important in treating the anemias because most of the care takes place in an outpatient clinic or the client's home. Help the client and family become knowledgeable about self-care in both preventing and treating anemia.

Diagnosis, Outcomes, Interventions

Activity Intolerance. Write the diagnosis as *Activity Intolerance related to decreased blood supply or low hemoglobin levels, as evidenced by fatigue, dyspnea, pallor, and tachycardia.*

Outcomes. The client will tolerate activity, as evidenced by walking increasing distances, or sitting up without fatigue, dyspnea, pallor, or tachycardia.

Interventions. A unit of packed RBCs may be administered to improve overall blood volume or increase hematocrit (see blood transfusion earlier).

Obtain Venous Access. The gauge of the needle used for transfusion varies with the product being infused. When packed RBCs weighing less than 300 g are infused, a 20-gauge or larger needle is needed to achieve maximal flow rate. If a smaller-gauge needle must be used, the RBCs can be diluted with 0.9% saline. To prevent hemolysis, add no solution other than normal saline to blood components.

Components containing a significant volume of plasma or other diluent can be safely infused at a rapid rate through smaller-gauge needles or catheters. A central venous catheter is an acceptable access option for blood transfusion. However, a large volume of refrigerated blood infused rapidly into the ventricle of the heart may cause cardiac dysrhythmias. Warming the blood can reduce the risk of this complication.

Another issue of concern is the use of multilumen catheters, which may allow blood to mix with incompatible solutions and medications as they exit the catheter tips. Experience indicates that the circulation achieved through a blood vessel suitable for central line placement results in rapid mixing of fluids. As a result, no harmful effects have been reported.

Request Blood Release. Blood bank regulations state that refrigerated components may not be returned to inventory if they have been warmed to more than 10° C (50° F). To meet this requirement, most transfusion medicine services consider 30 minutes to be the maximal allowable time out of monitored storage. To avoid wasting a scarce commodity, certain procedures should be performed before blood is requested.

An IV catheter appropriate for transfusing the requested component should be functional, flushed with normal saline, and maintained at a keep-vein-open (KVO) rate. Vital signs should then be taken and recorded. Fever may be a reason for delaying the transfusion. In addition to masking a possible manifestation of an acute transfusion reaction, fever can also compromise the efficacy of platelet transfusions.

Premedication also may be required if the client has a history of adverse reactions. In many cases, febrile reactions can be prevented by administering acetaminophen. A history of allergic reactions may warrant prophylactic administration of antihistamines (e.g., diphenhydramine HCl). To ensure effectiveness, administer oral medication 30 minutes before the transfusion is started. IV medication may be given immediately before the transfusion is initiated.

Blood should be released from the blood bank only to adequately trained personnel. The name and identification number of the recipient must be provided and a permanent record of this information maintained in the blood bank. So that delivery to the wrong client is avoided, blood should be transported to only one client at a time.

Confirm Blood Acceptability. The most crucial phase of transfusion is confirming product compatibility and verifying the client's identity. Before going to the client's bedside, verify ABO and Rh compatibility, usually by comparing the bag label with the medical record and forms issued from the blood bank. Also check the bag label to ensure that the correct component has been issued and for date of expiration. Components expire at midnight of the day marked on the bag unless otherwise specified.

Inspect the unit for leaks, abnormal color, clots, excessive air, and bubbles. Check carefully for important labels (such as "autologous," "directed") or instructions (such as "use leukocyte-depleting filter"). Cellular components (whole blood, RBCs, and platelets) for an immunosuppressed client should be clearly marked *irradiated.* Clients with Hodgkin's or non-Hodgkin's lymphoma, acute leukemia, or congenital immunodeficiency disorders and bone marrow transplant recipients may develop posttransfusion GVHD if lymphocytes contaminating cellular components engraft and divide. Transfusions from first-degree family members may also cause fatal GVHD. A small dose of radiation delivered to the component before release from the blood bank renders the lymphocytes incapable of mitotic action.

At the bedside, compare the name and number on the identification bracelet with the tag on the blood bag. If applicable, check the secondary identification system. The American Association of Blood Banks recommends that two qualified people perform this critical step.

Infuse Blood. Most blood products should be infused through administration sets designed specifically for this use. The set usually contains a 170-mm filter designed to trap fibrin clots and other debris that accumulates during blood storage. Most standard filters can filter 4 units of blood.

Tubing is available in two basic configurations: straight or Y-type. The use of Y-type tubing simplifies the process of adding normal saline to RBCs and provides ready access to a saline flush if the transfusion must be interrupted. Straight tubing usually has a medication injection site a few inches from the needle. If an adverse reaction develops, a keep-vein-open saline drip initiated at this site maintains patency of the IV line but avoids exposure to the 30 to 50 ml of blood remaining in the tubing and filter. Change the administration set every 4 to 6 hours, or according to institution policy, to reduce the risk of septicemia.

Several types of infusion devices are available to regulate and monitor the flow of IV solutions. There are basically two types:

- Infusion controllers, which regulate flow by gravity
- Infusion pumps, which deliver solutions under pressure

Infusion controllers may be used with all blood products if they are designed to function with opaque solutions. However, the negative pressure exerted by the peristaltic or syringe-like cassette action of infusion pumps may cause RBC hemolysis. If the transfusion product contains a significant number of RBCs, consult the manufacturer before a pump designed for crystalloid and colloid solutions is used.

If manual pressure cuffs are used to increase RBC flow rate, the pressure should not exceed 300 mm Hg. Do not use standard sphygmomanometers for this purpose because they do not exert uniform pressure against all parts of the bag.

Blood warmers may be used to prevent hypothermia, which can be induced by rapid infusion of large volumes of refrigerated blood. Neonatal exchange transfusion, plasma exchange, surgery, and trauma are all clinical situations that may require the use of a blood warmer. Other clients of concern are those with cold agglutinin disease. These clients have antibodies that react at temperatures under 37° C (98.6° F). Systemic circulatory cooling can cause intravascular agglutination. This condition may be detected during serologic testing. Once this client has been identified, the transfusion service may recommend the use of a blood warmer for all transfusions.

Two types of devices are approved by blood bank regulatory agencies for warming blood. For dry heating, a bag is placed between two aluminum heating plates or a disposable cuff-style bag is wrapped around a cylindrical aluminum heating element. A second type uses warm water to increase the temperature of the blood. Water baths containing water warmed to 37° C (98.6° F) may be used only if they have been specifically designed for warming blood. The blood bag should never be fully immersed in water.

Monitor During the Transfusion. The first 10 to 15 minutes of any transfusion are the most critical. If a major ABO incompatibility exists or a severe allergic reaction such as anaphylaxis occurs, it is usually evident within the first 50 ml of the transfusion. Therefore, it is recommended that the transfusion begin slowly and that the client be closely monitored. If no evidence of a reaction is noted within the first 15 minutes, flow can be increased to the prescribed rate.

Before leaving the client unattended, instruct the client to report anything unusual immediately. Take and record vital signs before the transfusion begins, after the first 15 minutes, and every hour until 1 hour after the transfusion has been discontinued. Check vital signs immediately if the client displays any untoward manifestations.

The recommended rate of infusion varies with the blood component being transfused. Components such as platelets, plasma, and cryoprecipitate may be infused rapidly, but take care to avoid circulatory overload, especially with geriatric clients and clients with cardiac disease. For avoiding the risk of septicemia, infusions should not exceed 4 hours. If the client's size or medical condition does not allow infusion within 4 hours, the unit may be split into smaller aliquots in the blood bank.

Regulatory agencies require complete documentation of the transfusion, including identification of personnel starting and ending the transfusion, unique product number, and outcome (e.g., "no reaction noted"). If an adverse reaction does occur, document the manifestations, actions taken, and future recommendations in the client's medical record.

Watch for Transfusion Reaction. Exposure to foreign blood elements may mediate immunologic and nonimmunologic reactions affecting all major body systems. Consider any unusual manifestation occurring during or immediately after a transfusion a potential reaction. Monitor unconscious patients closely because manifestations of a reaction may be inhibited in the unconscious state. The acute reactions most frequently seen are described in Table 75–2.

Whereas treatment may vary depending on the manifestations, follow certain standard procedures when a reaction is suspected. In all cases, stop the transfusion and keep the intravenous line open with normal saline. Treat life-threatening manifestations such as respiratory or circulatory failure immediately. Contact the client's physician and the blood bank. According to institutional policy, obtain appropriate laboratory samples. Samples used to evaluate a reaction include blood and urine. Free hemoglobin found in either indicates that RBCs have hemolyzed, the most serious serologic finding.

To avoid clouding the diagnostic picture by venous trauma, obtain blood samples from a large peripheral vein using at least a 19-gauge needle. The blood sample is also used to repeat ABO and Rh typing, antibody screening, and direct antiglobulin testing. A discrepancy in results between initial and repeat testing may indicate that incompatible blood was transfused. When future transfusions are required, special processing (e.g., washing) may then be performed in the blood bank to reduce the risks of another adverse reaction.

Altered Tissue Perfusion. The lack of circulating blood volume can create tissue hypoxia. State this diagnosis as *Altered Tissue Perfusion related to loss of blood volume.*

Outcomes. The client will have adequate tissue perfusion, as evidenced by normotension, warm extremities, heart rate between 60 and 100 beats/min, ability to perform activities of daily living or walk without dyspnea or tachycardia.

Interventions. Monitor vital signs and peripheral pulses, peripheral skin temperature, and activity tolerance. Clients should receive adequate food and fluids to assist with blood volume and provide protein for hemoglobin manufacturing. Keep the client warm, adding blankets to the feet for additional comfort.

Altered Nutrition: Less Than Body Requirements. Write the nursing diagnosis as *Altered Nutrition: Less than Body Requirements related to disease, treatment, or lack of knowledge of adequate nutrition.*

Outcomes. The client will have nutritional deficiencies corrected and optimal nutrition will be achieved, as evidenced by blood test results reaching normal range, improved tolerance for activity, and anemia resolved.

Interventions. Teach the basics of good nutrition; encourage a diet high in protein, iron, and vitamins with frequent small meals. Encourage foods cooked in iron pots and ingestion of foods such as liver (the richest source), oysters, lean meats, kidney beans, whole wheat bread, kale, spinach, egg yolks, turnip tops, beet greens, carrots, apricots, and raisins. Document the client's weight. Encourage good oral hygiene.

Risk for Ineffective Management of Therapeutic Regimen (Individuals). This nursing diagnosis is related to the client's self-care ability and the ability to take iron preparations.

Outcomes. The client will verbalize correct dosage of, route of, and indications for iron preparations, as evidenced by correct administration of iron medications and an absence of complications.

Interventions. Inform the client that iron salts are gastric irritants and should always be taken after meals. Liquid iron preparations should be well diluted and taken through a straw (undiluted liquid iron stains teeth). Constipation, commonly seen during iron therapy, can be avoided by a high-fiber diet and use of stool softeners or laxatives as required. Avoid consumption of coffee and tea with iron; absorption is hampered by the tannates. To administer parenteral iron medications, use Z track methods (see Fundamentals textbooks for a review).

EVALUATION

Resolution of anemia requires time. When packed RBCs are used, anemia will be corrected immediately. When oral iron preparations are used, it takes weeks for anemia to resolve and the client will thus need assessments at intervals to monitor the progress of therapy.

Modifications for Elderly Clients

Older clients are at risk for iron deficiency anemia because of poor nutritional intake and a decreased absorption of iron in the intestine. These clients also require complete assessment for diagnosis of the cause of the anemia. They often experience chronic blood loss from a variety of diseases that also may cause anemia, and differential diagnosis is thus required.

TABLE 75–2 ACUTE TRANSFUSION REACTIONS

Reaction	Cause	Clinical Manifestations	Management	Prevention
IMMUNOGENIC				
Allergic Incidence: 1%	Sensitivity to foreign proteins in plasma	Urticaria, flushing, itching (no fever)	Administer antihistamines as directed If manifestations mild and transient, transfusion may resume	Treat prophylactically with antihistamines
Febrile, nonhemolytic Incidence: 0.5%–1.0%	Sensitization to donor white blood cells, platelets, or plasma proteins	Sudden chills and fever (rise in temperature > 1° C [1.8° F]), headache, flushing, anxiety, muscle pain	Give antipyretics as prescribed; avoid aspirin in thrombocytopenic clients	Consider leukocyte-poor blood products (filtered, washed, or frozen) if fever occurs more than once
Acute hemolytic Incidence: 1:25,000 Fatal: 2:1 × 10^6	Infusion of ABO-incompatible red blood cells	Chills, fever, low back pain, flushing, tachycardia, tachypnea, hemoglobinuria, hemoglobinemia, hypotension, vascular collapse, bleeding, acute renal failure, shock, cardiac arrest, death	Treat shock Maintain blood pressure Give diuretics as prescribed to maintain urine flow Insert indwelling catheter or measure hourly output Dialysis may be needed	Meticulously verify recipient from sample collection to transfusion
Anaphylactic Incidence: 1:150,000	Infusion of IgA proteins to IgA-deficient recipient who has developed anti-IgA antibodies	Anxiety, urticaria, wheezing progressing to cyanosis, shock, and possible cardiac arrest	Initiate CPR if indicated Have epinephrine ready for injection (0.4 ml of a 1:1000 solution SC)	Give blood components from IgA-deficient donors or remove *all* plasma by washing
NONIMMUNOGENIC				
Circulatory overload Estimated Incidence: 1:10,000 (not usually reported to blood bank)	Infusion of blood at a rate too rapid for size, cardiac status, or clinical condition of recipient	Cough, dyspnea, pulmonary congestion (rales), headache, hypertension, tachycardia, distended neck veins	Place client in upright position with feet in dependent position Administer diuretics, oxygen, and morphine as prescribed Phlebotomy may be required	Adjust transfusion volume and flow rate on basis of client size and clinical status If slow transfusion will exceed 4 hr, request that unit be aliquoted into smaller volumes
Septicemia Incidence: very rare	Transfusion of component contaminated with microorganism	Rapid onset of chills, high fever, vomiting, diarrhea, marked hypotension, and shock	Treat manifestations and administer antibiotics, IV fluids, vasopressors, and steroids as directed Obtain culture of client and blood containers	Collect, process, store, and transfuse blood according to industry standards Infuse within 4 hr of starting time

CPR, cardiopulmonary resuscitation; IG, immunoglobulin; IV, intravenous; SC, subcutaneously.

IRON DEFICIENCY ANEMIA

Etiology and Risk Factors

Iron deficiency anemia is associated with either inadequate absorption or excessive loss of iron; it is a chronic, microcytic, hypochromic anemia (see Fig. 75–1*B*). Iron deficiency anemia is caused by an inadequate supply of iron needed to synthesize hemoglobin. Iron is essential to the oxygen-carrying function of heme; without it, the marrow produces RBCs that are deficient in hemoglobin concentration.

The major risk factors for iron deficiency anemia are (1) chronic blood loss, (2) insufficient intake of iron, (3) impaired absorption of iron, and (4) excessive demands for RBC production. An average diet supplies the body with about 12 to 15 mg/day of iron, of which only 5% to 10% (0.6 to 1.5 mg) is absorbed. The amount of iron normally absorbed daily is sufficient for meeting the needs of women past childbearing age and healthy men, but it does not meet the greater needs of menstruating and pregnant women, adolescents, children, and infants. These five groups must have a higher daily intake of iron. Economic constraints, poor dentition, and lack of interest in food preparation commonly lead to iron deficiency in older people. Fortunately, the GI tract can increase its absorption of iron from 10% daily to about 20% to 30% daily. In this way, the body often compensates for diminishing iron stores due to inadequate iron intake or excessive iron loss.

Iron is stored in the form of ferritin, an iron-phosphorus-protein complex that contains about 23% iron. It is formed in the intestinal mucosa when ferric iron joins with the protein apoferritin. Ferritin is stored in the tissues, primarily in the reticuloendothelial cells of the liver, spleen, and bone marrow.

Normal iron excretion is less than 1 mg/day. Iron is excreted in urine, sweat, bile, and feces and from the skin in desquamated cells. The average woman loses another 15 mg monthly during menses. Menstruation is the most common cause of iron deficiency in women. GI tract bleeding is a common etiologic factor in men; it may result from peptic ulcers, hiatal hernia, gastritis, cancer, hemorrhoids, diverticula, ulcerative colitis, or salicylate poisoning. It may also be associated with gastritis from the use of aspirin, steroids, or nonsteroidal anti-inflammatory drugs (NSAIDs). Bleeding from the GI tract is usually chronic and occult (too small to be seen). A chronic blood loss of as little as 2 to 4 ml/day can result in iron deficiency anemia, because every 2 ml of blood contains 1 mg of iron. The body can compensate for such losses to some degree by excreting less than 0.5 mg of iron daily rather than the normal 1 mg.

Alteration in the mucosa of the duodenum and proximal jejunum (as in chronic diarrhea, malabsorption syndromes such as celiac disease, and gastrectomy) affects iron absorption, predisposing to iron deficiency states. Tannates (in tea and coffee), carbonates, the chelating agent ethylenediaminetetraacetic acid (EDTA), and the medicinal antacid magnesium trisilicate all hinder nonheme iron absorption.

Clinical Manifestations

In mild cases of iron deficiency anemia, the client is asymptomatic; in more severe cases, assessment reveals the general manifestations of anemia, including:

- Peripheral blood smears revealing microcytic and pale (hypochromic) RBCs
- A hemoglobin level decreased to as low as 6 to 9 g/dl
- Moderately reduced total RBC count, rarely dropping below 3 million cells/mm^3
- Reduced mean corpuscular volume, mean corpuscular hemoglobin, and mean corpuscular hemoglobin concentration
- Serum iron level (normally 50 to 150 mg/dl) decreased to 10 mg/dl
- Total iron-binding capacity elevated to 350 to 500 mg/dl (normal is 250 to 350 mg/dl)
- Complete absence of hemosiderin (an insoluble form of storage iron) from bone marrow
- Immunoradiometric serum ferritin level below normal

Outcome Management

Management of iron deficiency anemia focuses on (1) diagnosis of and correction of the underlying cause and (2) treatment through diet and supplemental iron preparations. Once the diagnosis of iron deficiency anemia is confirmed, studies are conducted to find the cause. Radiographic studies (GI tract series), stool examination for occult blood, esophagoscopy, gastroscopy, and sigmoidoscopy are commonly done to identify the site of blood loss.

Supplemental iron is administered to increase iron available in the blood. Oral and injectable forms of iron are available (see earlier).

MEGALOBLASTIC ANEMIA

Anemias caused by deficiencies of vitamin B_{12} and folic acid are called megaloblastic anemias because they are characterized by the appearance of megaloblasts (large, primitive RBCs) in blood and bone marrow. Other common features are:

- Leukopenia, a decreased number of white blood cells (WBCs)
- Thrombocytopenia, a decreased number of platelets
- Oral, GI, and neurologic manifestations
- A favorable response to injections of either vitamin B_{12} or folic acid

PERNICIOUS ANEMIA

Etiology and Risk Factors

Pernicious anemia is a type of macrocytic anemia caused by failure of absorption of vitamin B_{12} (cobalamin). It is the most prevalent form of vitamin B_{12} deficiency in the United States and Canada. Cobalamin is released from its protein-bound state by an acidic gastric environment. Lack of gastric acid may lead to pernicious anemia, however; the most common cause is lack of intrinsic factor, a glucoprotein produced by parietal cells of the gastric lining. Vitamin B_{12} is absorbed in the terminal ileum; if that portion of the bowel is surgically resected, absorption cannot occur. The cause of pernicious anemia may also be from an autoimmune response. Ninety per cent of people with pernicious anemia have autoantibodies that react specifically against parietal gastric cells, and 60% have anti-intrinsic factor antibody.

Without vitamin B_{12}, deoxyribonucleic acid (DNA) synthesis and cell replication are impaired. RBC precursors do not divide normally, and large, poorly functioning RBCs are created. Erythropoiesis (from impaired folic acid from the lack of vitamin B_{12}) and production of myelin on nerves (from vitamin B_{12} directly) are greatly affected.

Clinical Manifestations

The major manifestations of pernicious anemia are low hemoglobin, hematocrit, and RBC levels. The diagnosis is based on the presence of anemia, GI manifestations, and neurologic disorders; laboratory blood and bone marrow tests; absence of gastric hydrochloric acid (HCl) and a favorable response to a vitamin B_{12} "therapeutic trial." The Schilling test measures the absorption of orally administered radioactive vitamin B_{12} (tagged with cobalt 60) before and after parenteral administration of intrinsic factor. This procedure detects lack of intrinsic factor and is the definitive test for pernicious anemia.

Gastric secretion analysis to check for the presence of free HCl is another important test; most clients with pernicious anemia have low-volume gastric secretions with a high pH and free hydrochloric acid. Furthermore, these findings do not change, even after the administration of histamine, which normally stimulates gastric secretion.

Outcome Management

VITAMIN B_{12}

Clients with pernicious anemia need both immediate treatment and lifelong therapy with maintenance vitamin B_{12}. During the acute phase of illness, the client may be given vitamin B_{12} injections. The response to the injections is usually quick and dramatic, often occurring within 24 to 48 hours. Within 72 hours, reticulocytes begin to increase; by the end of the first week, the total RBC count rises significantly. Cardiovascular involvement usually lessens with improved erythropoiesis. Peripheral nerve function may improve with treatment.

IRON SUPPLEMENTS

Additionally, the client may need oral iron supplementation if the hemoglobin level fails to rise in proportion to an increased RBC count. As stated earlier, iron deficiency may be an etiologic factor in pernicious anemia and must be corrected if it is present. Iron deficiency anemia can also develop during treatment of pernicious anemia. Injections of vitamin B_{12} may cause a rapid regeneration of RBC that depletes iron. As a result, the hemoglobin level remains low, although the total RBC count rises. Once the acute stage of the illness is past, the client with pernicious anemia must undertake a lifelong program of maintenance therapy. Monthly injections of vitamin B_{12} are needed to avoid relapse. The nurse plays a vital role in educating clients with this disorder on the importance of continuous care.

Encourage the client to eat a diet high in folic acid and iron to supplement the medication used to treat the anemia. If the cause involves altered absorption of vitamin B_{12}, nutritional supplements are useless. If the disease is related to decreased intake of the vitamin, a diet high in vitamin B_{12} is encouraged.

FOLIC ACID

Folic acid is sometimes given with vitamin B_{12} to clients with a history of poor nutrition. Folic acid can be dangerous, however, because it may intensify neurologic problems, and large doses of folate may obscure a vitamin B_{12} deficiency. Therefore, a therapeutic trial of folate should never be given before pernicious anemia is ruled out.

DIGESTANTS

Digestants to enhance the metabolism of vitamins, such as HCl diluted in water and given with meals, are often used during the first few weeks of vitamin B_{12} therapy.

ANEMIA CAUSED BY FOLIC ACID DEFICIENCY

Etiology and Risk Factors

Anemia associated with folic acid deficiency is very common. There are many causes, most of which are the same as those of vitamin B_{12} deficiency. Usually, folic acid deficiency results from a diet lacking in such foods as green leafy vegetables, liver, citrus fruits, and yeast. Clients with chronic alcoholism, because of their typically inadequate diets, are particularly at risk. High levels of alcohol in the blood also partially block the response of the bone marrow to folic acid, which thereby interferes with erythropoiesis.

Folic acid deficiency, like vitamin B_{12} deficiency, can develop with malabsorption syndromes (e.g., sprue, celiac disease, steatorrhea). Certain medications can also impede folic acid absorption and utilization. For example, a serious anemia may develop under the following conditions:

- Long-term use of anticonvulsant medications (e.g., primidone, phenytoin, phenobarbital)
- Administration of antimetabolites (e.g., folic acid antagonists, purine, pyrimidine analogs) to clients with cancer and leukemia
- Use of certain oral contraceptives

Finally, folic acid deficiency may occur with increased demands for folate, such as during the growth spurts of infancy and adolescence.

Folic acid, like vitamin B_{12}, is necessary for DNA synthesis; unlike pernicious anemia, however, folic acid deficiency does not cause neurologic manifestations. Anemia due to folic acid deficiency has a slow and insidious onset. The client, often thin and emaciated, usually appears quite ill. The client's malnourished and debilitated state frequently leads to other deficiencies, for example, of iron, protein, minerals, and other vitamins. Some clients may also have an electrolyte imbalance and neurologic manifestations may develop as a result of thiamine, calcium, or magnesium deficiency (commonly linked with alcoholism). Cirrhosis of the liver and bleeding varices further complicate anemia for the alcohclic client.

The megaloblastic anemia caused by folic acid deficiency is the same as that seen in pernicious anemia. The diagnosis is confirmed by blood smear and bone marrow examinations. With folic acid deficiency, the serum folate level is less than 4 ng/ml (normal, 7 to 20 ng/ml): the Schilling test finding is normal; HCl is probably present in the gastric juice; neurologic manifestations are absent; and the client responds favorably to a therapeutic trial of 50 to 100 mg folic acid administered intramuscularly daily for 10 days.

Outcome Management

For correction of anemia caused by folate deficiency, the client receives oral doses of folic acid 0.1 to 5.0 mg/day until the blood profile improves or until the cause of intestinal malabsorption is corrected. Clients with malabsorption syndromes may need parenteral folic acid initially, followed by maintenance therapy with oral doses. Folic acid is administered intramuscularly in the form of folinic acid (leucovorin calcium injection). Additionally, vitamin C is sometimes prescribed because it increases the role of folic acid in promoting erythropoiesis.

APLASTIC ANEMIAS

Aplastic anemia is caused by bone marrow that is severely hypoplastic (underdeveloped), that is, devoid of erythroid, myeloid, and megakaryocytic cell lines. Hypoplastic bone marrow results in anemia, leukopenia, and thrombocytopenia. When all three cellular elements are suppressed, the condition is known as *pancytopenia.* Aplastic anemia affects people of all ages, and men and women are equally susceptible. The incidence of aplastic anemia is about 4 per million population. *Congenital* aplastic anemia (*Fanconi's anemia*) usually occurs in childhood.

Etiology and Risk Factors

Acquired aplastic anemia may result from either an autoimmune mechanism or a direct injury by *myelotoxins.* Three groups of myelotoxins are:

1. Agents that always cause marrow damage when received in sufficiently large doses, such as radiant energy (x-rays, radium, and radioactive isotopes of gold or phosphorus), benzene and its derivatives, alkylating agents, and antimetabolites used to treat malignant tumors. Radiation causes the bone marrow to stop producing blood cells by inhibiting mitosis, or cell division, and antimetabolites used in cancer therapy block the synthesis of purines or nucleic acids.
2. Agents that occasionally cause marrow failure, such as chloramphenicol (Chloromycetin, the drug most commonly linked with aplastic anemia), sulfonamides, quinacrine, phenylbutazone, the anticonvulsants phenytoin and mephenytoin, and gold compounds.
3. Agents that have been linked with aplastic anemia in only a few cases, such as streptomycin, tripelennamine, DDT, meprobamate, hair and aniline dyes, and carbon tetrachloride.

The onset of aplastic anemia may be insidious or rapid. In idiopathic or hereditary cases, the onset is usually gradual. When bone marrow failure results from a myelotoxin, however, the onset may be explosive, with quickly developing manifestations. If the condition does not reverse itself when the offending agent is removed, it can be fatal.

Clinical Manifestations

Manifestations of pancytopenia are particularly severe. The RBC count and leukocyte and platelet counts all decline. The three conditions then develop: (1) normocytic anemia, (2) neutropenia, and (3) thrombocytopenia. The RBC count is usually below 1 million/mm^3, with a low reticulocyte count. The client reports progressive fatigue, lassitude, and dyspnea. The leukocyte count may be less than 1000/mm^3 (normal range, 5000 to 10,000/mm^3). The client, therefore, suffers from an increased susceptibility to infection, because without leukocytes the body cannot adequately battle bacteria and other invading organisms. If the absolute neutrophil count drops below 500/mm^3, a fulminating bacterial infection may develop, often from the client's own normal flora. The platelet count may fall below 30,000 to 15,000/mm^3 (normal range, 150,000 to 450,000/mm^3, which usually causes bleeding into the skin and mucous membranes. The client is also at risk for retinal hemorrhage and intracranial hemorrhage. If the platelet count is severely reduced, the client may hemorrhage spontaneously.

The diagnosis of aplastic anemia and pancytopenia is based on the differential blood count, the client's manifestations, history of exposure to a myelotoxin, and bone marrow examination.

Outcome Management

The client with pancytopenia is often critically ill. Prompt medical attention and skillful nursing care are necessary. The first step in halting the process of aplastic anemia is immediate withdrawal of the offending agent or drug.

Monitor any client undergoing radiotherapy or receiving a medication that is a suspected myelotoxin for marrow failure by frequent complete blood counts (CBCs). A significant drop in the RBC, leukocyte, or platelet count signals the need to stop the drug. Usually, stopping a suspected agent is followed by a rise in the CBC. Unfortunately, marrow failure due to chloramphenicol may progress despite discontinuation of the drug. If aplastic anemia develops from a suspected myelotoxic agent, blood transfusions are the mainstay of therapy until bone marrow activity signals recovery. Because the marrow of the aplastic client is severely depressed, cellular blood components should be irradiated before transfusion to inactivate lymphocytes and to prevent transfusion-associated GVHD (see Chapter 78). If the marrow does not recover and long-term RBC support is required, iron overload often results. Before iron chelating therapy became available, this complication was a leading cause of death.

Bone marrow transplantation is now the treatment of choice in aplastic anemia when (1) an autoimmune phenomenon is suspected or (2) the bone marrow fails to regenerate after discontinuation of myelotoxic agents. Currently, transplantation can take place only if the client has a human leukocyte antigen (HLA)–matched donor. Comparing the results of clients treated by bone marrow transplantation with conventional therapy of steroids and androgens reveals a 2-year survival rate of 60% to 80% with bone marrow transplantation versus 25% for those treated conventionally.

HEMOLYTIC ANEMIA

Hemolytic anemias are due to a shortening of the RBC life span, abnormal destruction of RBCs by macrophages or a hyperactive spleen, or failure of the bone marrow to replace destroyed RBCs.

The client with hemolytic anemia suffers from all the general manifestations of anemia discussed earlier (lassitude, fatigue, etc.). Renal failure may be a complication of severe hemolysis. It is caused by excretion of an increased load of RBC degradation products.

Laboratory findings indicative of hemolytic anemia usually include normocytic anemia, reticulocytosis due to increased efforts of the bone marrow to compensate for excessive erythrocyte destruction, increased RBC fragility, shortened erythrocyte life span, hyperbilirubinemia, increased fecal and urinary urobilinogen, and (in cases of massive intravascular hemolysis) hemoglobinemia.

Treatment includes removal of the offending agent. Adequate fluids are given to flush the kidneys. In addition, sodium bicarbonate or sodium lactate are administered to alkalize the urine, which decreases the likelihood of precipitation in the renal tubules. Splenectomy may be required.

SICKLE CELL ANEMIA AND SICKLE CELL TRAIT

Sickle cell anemia is an inherited disorder of hemoglobin synthesis resulting in tissue hypoxia and obstruction of blood vessels. It primarily affects the world's black population (Fig. 75–2). Worldwide, sickle cell anemia is the most common form of anemia. Sickle cell trait is a milder form of the disorder. The trait is prevalent in Africa, possibly because the abnormal hemoglobin is more resistant to the parasite that causes malaria, which is endemic in some areas.

Etiology and Risk Factors

The genetic defect results in substitution of the amino acid valine for glutamine on one of the globin chains of the hemoglobin molecule. This sickle cell hemoglobin (Hb S) is less soluble than the normal adult hemoglobin (Hb A). Hb S also assumes a sickle or crescent shape when deoxygenated. As shown in Figure 75–2, whether a client will have sickle cell anemia, sickle cell trait, or neither depends on the genes for hemoglobin inherited from each parent.

Pathophysiology

Sickle cell anemia is named for the appearance of the RBC when blood oxygen decreases. The cell assumes a sickle, or crescent, shape (Fig. 75–1*D*). Once the RBC sickles, it becomes rigid, and the blood becomes more viscous and may obstruct capillary blood flow, causing further hypoxia and, consequently, more sickling. Thus, a vicious circle ensues. The organs most vulnerable to infarction and necrosis are the brain and kidneys, because of their constant demand for oxygen, and the bone marrow and spleen, because of their normally sluggish circulation.

The mechanisms that precipitate the various forms of sickling crises remain unclear. However, two major factors are definitely linked with the sickling of cells: (1) hypoxia, due to low oxygen tension, and (2) an increased blood viscosity, due to an increased concentration of sickled cells. Exposure to low oxygen tensions (e.g., at high

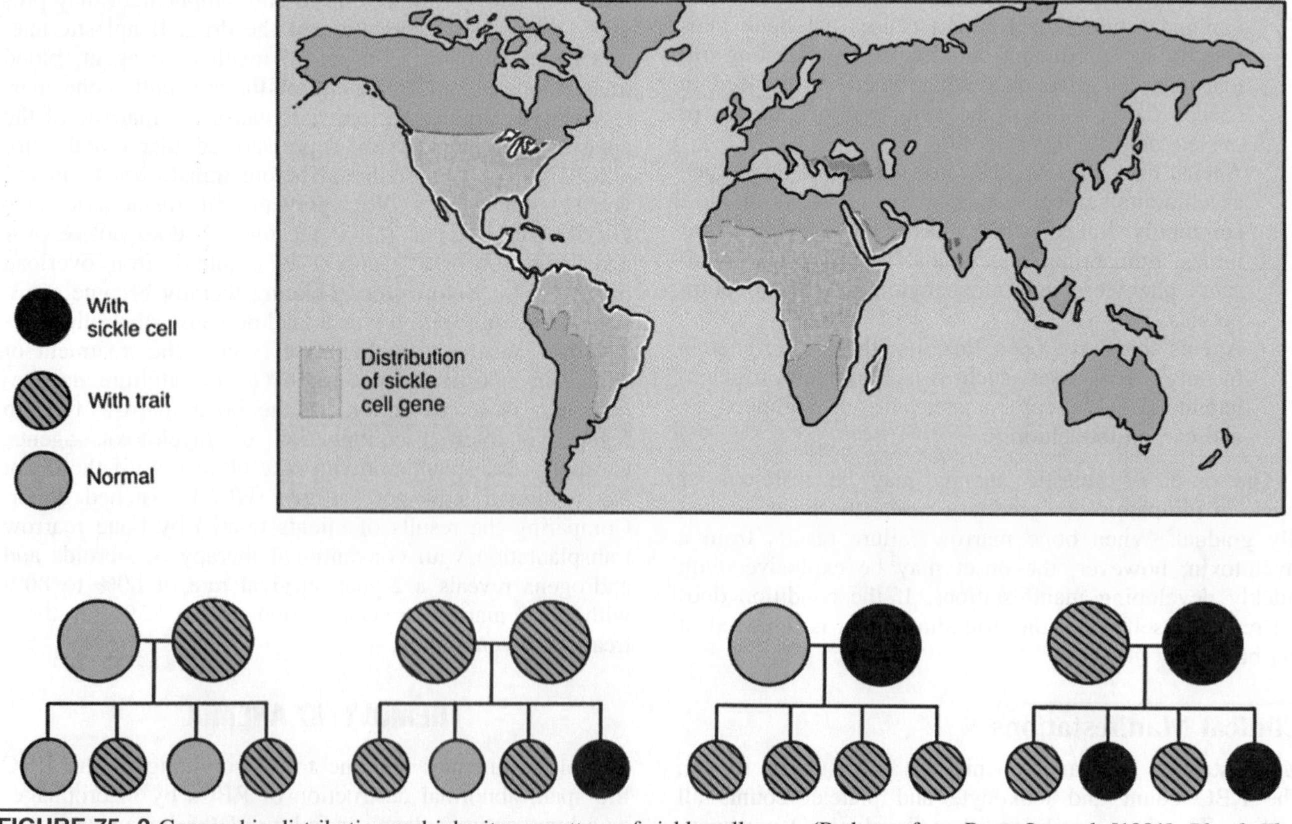

FIGURE 75–2 Geographic distribution and inheritance pattern of sickle cell gene. (Redrawn from Page, J., et al. [1981]. *Blood: The river of life.* Washington, DC: Torstar Books.)

altitudes, flying in nonpressurized planes, exercising strenuously, or undergoing anesthesia without receiving adequate oxygenation) results in hypoxia. Although both Hb S and Hb A have the same solubility when oxygenated, deoxygenation of the blood drastically affects Hb S.

Sickle cell crisis is an acute exacerbation of the disorder due to respiratory infections or other stressors that reduce blood oxygen levels. Five causes have been described:

1. Vaso-occlusive or pain crisis: Pain originating from an area of vascular occlusion. This type shows no change on hematologic examination.
2. Aplastic crisis: in bone marrow hypoplasia with decreased hemoglobin and RBCs; pain may be present.
3. Hemolytic crisis: RBC destruction and fever.
4. Sequestration crisis: a result of sudden and massive trapping of RBCs by visceral organs, such as the spleen.
5. Mixed crisis: manifestations of more than one type.

Clinical Manifestations

Sickle cell anemia is usually manifested after a child is 6 months old, when fetal hemoglobin is no longer present. Occasionally, clinical manifestations do not appear until adulthood. Young children who have the disease do not grow properly because of anemia. Weakness and fatigue are also present. Developmental delays in sexual maturity and retarded growth may be seen.

Sluggish circulation leads to edema of the hands and feet. Jaundice or pallor may be present. Infarctions in the spleen are so common that, after childhood, the spleen of most sickle cell anemia clients is small and scarred. Leg ulcers are found in about 75% of older children and adults with the disease. Other manifestations include necrosis of the head of the femur, possibly leading to osteomyelitis and necrotic bone marrow with development of infection, joint pain, renal medullary ischemia resulting in diminished capacity to concentrate urine, priapism, pulmonary infarctions, myocardial infarctions, and cerebrovascular accidents. Hyperactivity of the bone marrow leads to spindly legs, a short trunk, and a tower-shaped skull.

Sickle cell crisis is characterized by:

- Cardiac systolic murmurs, dysrhythmias, heart enlargement
- Dyspnea, chest pain, cyanosis
- Sensorimotor manifestations of increased intracranial pressure due to cerebral hemorrhaging
- Renal manifestations of uremia, such as decreased urinary output and edema

Diagnostic Findings

Hemolytic anemia develops from the destruction of sickle cells; hemoglobin values usually lie in a range of 12 to 18 g/dl, depending on age and sex. An elevated bilirubin level from the released hemoglobin may result in gallstone formation (cholelithiasis). Four laboratory procedures demonstrate the presence of Hb S in either homozygous or heterozygous carriers:

- Stained blood smear
- Sickle cell slide preparation
- Sickle-turbidity tube test
- Hemoglobin electrophoresis

Stained Blood Smear

A stained blood smear is examined for the presence of sickle cells.

Sickle Cell Slide Preparation

A blood specimen is observed for the sickling phenomenon after deoxygenation of the blood. This test is accurate but time-consuming.

Sickle-Turbidity Tube Test

The sickle-turbidity tube test is an excellent mass screening test to detect Hb S. After a finger prick, blood is mixed with Sickledex solution in a test tube. Five minutes later, the specimen is observed for cloudiness, which indicates the presence of Hb S. Solutions mixed with normal hemoglobin remain clear. Although the test demonstrates Hb S, it does not differentiate sickle cell disease from the trait.

Hemoglobin Electrophoresis

Hemoglobin electrophoresis differentiates sickle cell anemia from sickle cell trait. By means of an applied electric field, the various types of hemoglobin within a blood specimen are separated. If a blood specimen contains both Hb S and Hb A, the client is heterozygous—has sickle cell trait. If Hb S is 75% to 100% of the total and the rest Hb F or Hb A_2, the client is homozygous—has sickle cell anemia.

Many African Americans are unaware that they carry the sickle cell trait and that they can transmit this trait to their offspring. Consequently, researchers are perfecting mass screening tests for the detection of Hb S among the black population. Clients having only the sickle cell trait may never be detected unless they are exposed to extremely low oxygen tension (e.g., mountain climbing, flying in a nonpressurized plane), extremely hard work or exercise, or pregnancy. When exposed to extreme stressors, the client with the trait may experience manifestations of sickle cell disease.

Outcome Management

Medical Management

Treatment of sickle cell anemia consists chiefly of supportive care (e.g., rest, oxygen, IV administration of fluids and electrolytes to ensure adequate hydration, sedation, and analgesics).

In some cases, the slow administration of packed RBCs or partial exchange transfusion helps relieve severe anemic manifestations. During episodes of increased risk (e.g., surgery, pregnancy), some clients benefit from *hypertransfusion* (or transfusions until more than 50% of the circulating RBCs are of donor origin).

Anticoagulants, steroids, and cobalt treatments have all been used without success to reverse the sickling process. Clients with sickle cell disease have an increased need for folic acid and, therefore, usually receive a daily oral supplement to prevent increased anemia from folate deficiency. Prophylactic penicillin may also be ordered. Hydroxyurea and erythropoietin are being used in clinical trials in an attempt to increase fetal hemoglobin in clients with a diagnosis of sickle cell disease.

Nursing Management

ASSESSMENT

Assess the client for the pattern of data that may indicate sickle cell crisis. Assess for the ability of the family and client to cope with the disorder and understanding of the disease and the triggers of crisis.

DIAGNOSIS, OUTCOMES, INTERVENTIONS

Pain. Because of the joint swelling secondary to sickling crisis, one nursing diagnosis is *Pain related to joint swelling.*

Outcomes. The client will experience diminished pain, relieved, as evidenced by verbalization of pain relief and reliance on less opiates for control of pain.

Intervention. Assess for pain every 2 to 4 hours, and administer analgesics as needed according to orders; monitor for effectiveness of analgesia. Apply heat to joints as ordered. Provide rest periods. Administer fluids to prevent dehydration and recurrence of pain crisis. Increase oral fluid intake, and monitor intake and output.

Knowledge Deficit. Another nursing diagnosis is *Knowledge Deficit related to disease, treatment, and prevention of crises.*

Outcomes. The client will understand the disease, treatment, and prevention of crises, as evidenced by the client's statements and the absence of crises.

Interventions. When educating clients about sickle cell anemia or sickle cell trait, remember to:

1. Explain the nature of the disease, and give the client a chance to express feelings and ask questions.
2. Encourage African American parents to have themselves and their children tested for the presence of Hb S.
3. Advise the client to have routine medical examinations that include an RBC count.
4. Encourage young adults who carry Hb S to ask their physician for genetic counseling before marrying or having children.
5. Alert young women with sickle cell anemia that pregnancy carries a very high risk for them.
6. Explain that pulmonary or renal complications, or both, may develop.
7. Explain how to prevent crises, such as (a) avoiding high altitudes and flying in nonpressurized planes (because oxygen tension is lowered under these conditions) and (b) taking caution against becoming dehydrated and to call a physician if vomiting, diarrhea, high fever, or any other cause of water loss develops.

EVALUATION

An appropriate outcome for the client with sickle cell disease is that the disease will remain in remission as long as possible. It is impossible to prevent every crisis; however, with education and an effort by the client, the number of attacks can be reduced.

POLYCYTHEMIA VERA

Polycythemia vera, the excessive bone marrow production of erythrocytes, leukocytes, and platelets, is caused by excessive activation of pluripotent stem cells. The inordinate mass production of these three cell lines results in (1) an increase in blood viscosity; (2) an increase in the total blood volume, which may be twice or even three times greater than normal; and (3) severe blood congestion of all tissues and organs. Because of these problems, the client suffers many manifestations, including an increased risk of clot formation.

Clinical Manifestations

In its early stages, polycythemia usually remains asymptomatic (an increased hematocrit level may be an incidental finding). However, hypervolemia and hyperviscosity may lead to dizziness, headache, tinnitus, visual disturbances, and other manifestations, depending on the body system affected. The client may also have a ruddy complexion (plethora) and dusky, red mucosa; cardiovascular hypertension (with dizziness, headache, and a sense of fullness in the head) and heart failure (shortness of breath, orthopnea); increased clotting leading to cerebrovascular accident, myocardial infarction, or peripheral gangrene; and bleeding (hemorrhage in capillaries, venules, and arterioles), which causes rupture of vessels; GI peptic ulcers, enlargement of liver and spleen; and skeletal gout (painful swollen joints, usually the big toe) characterized by an increased uric acid level.

Diagnostic findings include (1) an RBC count as high as 8 to 12 million/mm^3; (2) hemoglobin level of 18 to 25 g/dl; (3) hematocrit greater than 54% in men and 49% in women; (4) platelet count usually increased; (5) normal arterial blood gases (ABG) values; (6) hyperplastic bone marrow; and (7) a serum uric acid level three to four times normal.

Outcome Management

The goals of care in polycythemia vera are twofold: reduction of (1) blood volume and viscosity and (2) bone marrow activity. These decreases are accomplished through phlebotomy, administration of myelosuppressive agents, and radiation therapy. Emergency phlebotomy can be used to remove 500 to 2000 ml of blood until the hematocrit reaches 45%. Subsequent phlebotomies should be carried out as frequently (monthly) as necessary to maintain the hematocrit at about 45%. As iron deficiency supervenes, RBC production will be retarded, so that clients managed by phlebotomy alone may require as few as two or three phlebotomies a year.

Myelosuppressive agents can be used to retard the bone marrow. Radioactive phosphorus sometimes produces remissions that last from 6 months to 2 years. Other drugs include chlorambucil, busulfan, and hydroxyurea. Radiation therapy may be used to reduce the production of RBCs in the marrow.

DISORDERS AFFECTING WHITE BLOOD CELLS

White blood cells (WBCs), also called *leukocytes,* are divided into two groups:

- *Granulocytes* (polymorphonuclear leukocytes)
- *Agranulocytes* (mononuclear cells)

Granulocytes, in turn, are divided into three groups: (1) neutrophils, (2) basophils, and (3) eosinophils. The names denote affinity for the dyes used in staining. Agranulocytes include lymphocytes (B and T) and monocytes.

Plasmacytes (plasma cells) are derived from B lymphocytes. Plasmacytes are formed within the bone marrow and lymph nodes and are active in producing immunoglobulins (antibodies). Leukemia and lymphoma are discussed in Chapter 78.

AGRANULOCYTOSIS

Agranulocytosis (granulocytopenia, malignant neutropenia) is an acute, potentially fatal blood dyscrasia characterized by profound *neutropenia* (a reduced number of circulating neutrophils). Because neutrophils make up roughly 93% of all granulocytes, the terms *neutropenia* and *agranulocytosis* are often used interchangeably. Agranulocytosis is a fairly rare condition. For unknown reasons, females are much more susceptible to this condition than males, although even among females, agranulocytosis is relatively rare.

Etiology and Risk Factors

Agranulocytosis results either from the failure of neutrophil production to keep pace with destruction of the cells or from increased destruction of neutrophils, which removes them from circulation. Chemotherapy, radiation, and aplastic anemia all reduce or stop neutrophil production through interference with granulopoiesis. The most common cause of agranulocytosis is drug toxicity or hypersensitivity. Two groups of agents are capable of suppressing granulocyte production:

1. Agents that always produce neutropenia when given in sufficiently large doses over time, such as many cancer chemotherapeutic agents, ionizing radiation, and benzene.
2. Agents that produce neutropenia only in clients particularly sensitive to the drug, such as tranquilizers (chlorpromazine), antithyroid agents (propylthiouracil), anticonvulsants (phenytoin), antibiotics (chloramphenicol), and phenylbutazone.

Agranulocytosis can occur in clients with anemias related to diminished erythropoiesis (e.g., aplastic and megaloblastic anemias). It may also accompany certain diseases (e.g., tuberculosis, typhoid fever, malaria, uremia).

Accelerated destruction of neutrophils can result from infection, autoimmune disease, and idiosyncratic reactions to many drugs. The destruction may be so rapid that production cannot keep up with it. If agranulocytosis is not reversed when the cause is removed, the client will require an allogeneic bone marrow transplant for survival.

Pathophysiology

Failure to produce adequate numbers of white blood cells prevents normal surveillance and phagocytosis; infection from the neutropenia is a common sequela. Neutrophils constitute a swift and powerful defense against invading microorganisms. Consequently, decreases in their number result in a greater susceptibility to bacterial invasion, especially when the client's absolute neutrophil count (ANC) drops below $500/mm^3$.

Clinical Manifestations

The manifestations of agranulocytosis are a result of the neutropenia. Typically, the onset of this acute disease is rapid. For the first 2 or 3 days, severe fatigue and weakness occur, next followed by a sore throat, ulcerations of the pharyngeal and buccal mucosa, dysphagia, high fever, weak and rapid pulse, and severe chills. Without prompt antibiotic treatment, the disorder usually causes death within a week. The mucous membranes of the throat and mouth are particularly vulnerable.

The diagnosis of agranulocytosis rests on the following:

- Leukopenia, evidenced by WBC counts of 500 to $3000/mm^3$ with extreme reduction in polymorphonuclear cells (0 to 2%)
- Bone marrow examination revealing an absence of granulocytes, a maturational arrest of young developing cells, or an increased number of myeloid precursors (signifying peripheral granulocyte destruction)
- Cultures of urine, blood, and ulcerative lesions in the throat and mouth that are positive for bacteria, usually gram-positive cocci
- A history of exposure to an offending agent as well as all the aforementioned findings (with many clients medicating themselves with potentially dangerous drugs; all drugs taken within the past 6 to 12 months need to be investigated)

Outcome Management

Treatment of clients with agranulocytosis involves eliminating potentially toxic agents that may be responsible for marrow suppression. Agranulocytosis caused by toxic substances is usually reversed within 2 to 3 weeks after their elimination.

Surveillance cultures of blood, throat, sputum, urine, and stool should be taken at frequent intervals to monitor the status of infections. Combinations of broad-spectrum antibiotics are usually administered until the offending organism is identified. Untreated infectious processes in this situation carry a mortality rate of 80%.

Treatment of agranulocytosis includes various *colony-stimulating factors,* such as granulocyte colony-stimulating factor (G-CSF), granulocyte macrophage colony-stimulating factor (GM-CSF), and erythropoietin (EPO). These are given after the offending agent has been eliminated.

MULTIPLE MYELOMA

Multiple myeloma is a B-cell neoplastic condition characterized by abnormal malignant proliferation of plasma cells secreting a monoclonal paraprotein, accumulation of mature plasma cells in the bone marrow, and complications throughout the body as a result of dissemination of the disease (e.g., lytic bone lesions and osteoporosis, hematopoietic suppression, hypercalcemia, proteinuria, and renal failure). Risk factors include an increased incidence in some families, ionizing radiation, and occupational chemical exposures.

Pathophysiology

Multiple myeloma is characterized by an abnormal proliferation of plasma cells. With this overproduction of plasma cells, bone destruction also occurs. In addition to bone destruction, multiple myeloma is characterized by disruption of RBC, leukocyte, and platelet production, which results from plasma cells crowding the bone marrow. Impaired production of these cell forms causes anemia, increased vulnerability to infection and bleeding tendencies, respectively.

Clinical Manifestations

Once manifestations appear, they typically involve the skeletal system, particularly the pelvis, spine, and ribs. Some clients have backache or bone pain that worsens with movement. Others suffer sudden pathologic fractures accompanied by severe pain. In time, skeletal destruction increases and the client may develop sternum and rib cage deformities. Diffuse osteoporosis usually appears, accompanied by a negative calcium balance. The skull shows multiple osteolytic lesions. Loss of calcium and phosphorus from damaged bones eventually leads to the development of renal stones, particularly in immobilized clients.

Diagnostic Findings

Diagnosis of multiple myeloma rests on radiographic studies, bone marrow biopsy, and blood and urine examination. Radiographic studies reveal diffuse lesions in the bone, widespread demineralization, and osteoporosis. The bone marrow contains large numbers of immature plasma cells. Normally, plasma cells constitute 5% of the bone marrow cell population. Because of the abnormal number of plasma cells producing immunoglobulins, peripheral blood samples sent for plasma electrophoresis reveal a large amount of abnormal immunoglobulins. Another diagnostic manifestation of multiple myeloma is the appearance of Bence-Jones protein in the urine, consisting of monoclonal immunoglobulin light chains.

Outcome Management

Management is aimed at early recognition and treatment of complications of the disease. Clients with hypercalcemia often become anorectic, nauseated, drowsy, confused, and disoriented and may require hospitalization. Not all clients with multiple myeloma should be treated. Manifestations, physical findings, and laboratory data must be considered. In some cases, treatment might be withheld and the client re-evaluated in 2 to 3 months. If overt manifestations are present, chemotherapy is the preferred initial treatment. Palliative radiation should be limited to clients with disabling pain from a well-defined location that has not been responsive to chemotherapy. Autologous or allogeneic bone marrow transplantation is also an option.

Suppress the Bone Marrow

There is some controversy over the most effective chemotherapy regimen. Therapy with melphalan and prednisone or a combination of alkylating agents can be effective. Prednisone and melphalan given orally for a period of 4 to 7 days and repeated at 4- to 6-week intervals produces positive results in 50% to 60% of clients. Leukocyte and platelet counts are monitored regularly and doses adjusted until modest cytopenia occurs. Combination chemotherapy, commonly melphalan, cyclophosphamide, carmustine (BCNU), vincristine (Oncovin), and prednisone, has shown a 70% to 75% response rate. This therapy may continue for 1 to 2 years, but relapse almost always occurs when chemotherapy is discontinued. Interferon-alfa appears to be beneficial in prolonging the duration of remission.

Reduce Serum Calcium Levels

In the past, corticosteroids such as high-dose dexamethasone, mithramycin, furosemide, and IV hydration were commonly prescribed for hypercalcemia; however, newer agents now exist. Etidronate disodium (Didronel) or gallium nitrate (Ganite) and IV hydration are effective. The newest and most effective agent is pamidronate sodium (Aredia).

Administer fluids in adequate amounts to maintain an output of 1.5 to 2.0 L/day. Clients with multiple myeloma usually require about 3 L of fluid per day. The client needs sufficient fluid not only to dilute the calcium overload but also to prevent protein from precipitating in the renal tubules, even after effective treatment with chemotherapy. Administer medications to increase calcium excretion and to decrease calcium loss from bone, such as furosemide (Lasix), steroids, and plicamycin, etidronate, gallium, or pamidronate.

If the client is able, encourage activity that places stress on the long bones to increase calcium resorption. Antiemetics may be required for relief of nausea and vomiting. Small, frequent feedings may be better tolerated, and stool softeners may be routinely required. Closely monitor intake, output, and blood studies to determine effectiveness of treatment. Weigh the client daily so that any significant loss can be noted and corrected.

Closely monitor the client's mental status. If disorientation or confusion occurs, remove sharp objects and other potentially hazardous items from the environment. The side rails should be raised, and light restraints may be required.

Teach significant others the manifestations of hypercalcemia and to report them immediately to the physician. Instruct family members or significant others on how to institute safety measures to prevent falls and injuries. The client may need some assistive devices at home, such as a toilet riser and handhold bars in the bathroom. Measure the client's calcium level at regular intervals for assessment of the development of hypercalcemia.

INFECTIOUS MONONUCLEOSIS

Pathophysiology and Etiology

Infectious mononucleosis, also known as glandular disease or the "kissing disease," is a self-limiting condition characterized by painful enlargement of the lymph nodes, lymphocytosis, sore throat, and fever. Primarily a disease of the young, it usually strikes children between the ages of 3 and 5 years and young adults between the ages of 15 and 25 years. The greatest incidence occurs among college students, medical students, and nurses. Although this disease usually occurs sporadically, epidemic forms may sweep through colleges and children's homes.

The cause of infectious mononucleosis is Epstein-Barr virus (EBV), a herpesvirus. Although the mode of transmission remains unknown, the disease may be transmitted through the oropharyngeal route during close contact, as with kissing.

Clinical Manifestations

The onset of infectious mononucleosis follows an incubation period of 2 to 6 weeks. Before frank clinical manifestations present, the person may experience fatigue, headaches, malaise, and myalgias. Subsequently, assessment reveals temperatures up to 39° C (102.2° F), pharyngitis, and lymphadenopathy that is more pronounced in the cervical regions. In 10% to 15% of those affected, a maculopapular rash develops, closely resembling the rash of rubella. Splenic enlargement causes left upper quadrant pain. Nervous system involvement may lead to severe headache. In rare cases, liver involvement may develop into a hepatitis-like syndrome.

When infectious mononucleosis is severe, two complications may develop: (1) splenic rupture resulting from the infiltration of the spleen by massive numbers of lymphocytes and (2) streptococcal pharyngitis (Vincent's angina) secondary to bacterial invasion of the throat.

The diagnosis of infectious mononucleosis is based on three criteria: (1) physical assessment, (2) laboratory tests, and (3) the Paul-Bunnel test.

The WBC count usually ranges from 12,000 to 20,000/mm^3, of which 50% are lymphocytes and monocytes and 10% to 20% are large, atypical lymphocytes. The *mono spot test* is also performed with a throat swab. It detects anti-EBV antibodies and is positive in 50% of cases within the first week and 90% of cases in the fourth week.

Outcome Management

No specific intervention either mitigates or shortens the disease process. Because infectious mononucleosis must simply run its course, treatments are directed at control of manifestations. Bed rest is recommended until fever is resolved. Acetaminophen, cool sponge baths, and a large fluid intake help control fever. Warm saline throat irrigation may relieve the sore throat. Aspirin is avoided because of the risk of Reye's syndrome. Contact sports must be avoided to reduce the risk of splenic rupture.

Although complications sometimes develop, the prognosis for clients with infectious mononucleosis is generally excellent. The febrile phase of this disorder typically lasts 2 to 4 weeks. During the long convalescence, the client slowly regains strength and energy.

SPLENIC RUPTURE AND HYPERSPLENISM

Etiology

The most frequent indication for splenectomy is rupture of the spleen complicated by severe hemorrhage. Causes of splenic rupture include:

- Trauma (e.g., automobile accidents, bullet or knife wounds, severe blows to the spleen).
- Accidental tearing of the splenic capsule during surgery on neighboring organs
- Disease of the spleen that causes softening or damage (e.g., infectious mononucleosis and malaria)

In hypersplenism, a second important indication for splenectomy, the spleen destroys, in excessive numbers, one of the blood cell types (i.e., erythrocytes, leukocytes, or platelets). Primary hypersplenism occurs in idiopathic thrombocytopenic purpura and congenital spherocytosis. Some etiologic factors associated with secondary hypersplenism include lymphomas (including Hodgkin's disease), leukemia, polycythemia vera, acute infections (including infectious mononucleosis), chronic infections, malaria, syphilis, hemoglobinopathy, and cirrhosis of the liver.

Clinical Manifestations

Manifestations of hypersplenism include moderate to massive splenomegaly, anemia, leukopenia, or thrombocytopenia, and a compensatory increase in the production of the affected cell line by the bone marrow. Overactivity of the spleen develops either as a primary condition of unknown origin or as a condition secondary to another disease.

Laboratory indications for splenectomy include granulocytopenia of less than 500/mm^3 and thrombocytopenia of less than 20,000/mm^3.

Outcome Management

Primary hypersplenism can be alleviated by splenectomy. Splenectomy is palliative only for clients with secondary hypersplenism because the surgery has little or no effect on the course of the primary illness. When the diagnosis is confirmed, it is important to teach the client to prevent complications associated with the specific cytopenia.

The spleen has an important role in the phagocytosis of circulating opsonized organisms. After splenectomy, young children are at high risk for fulminant infections due to *Streptococcus pneumoniae, Haemophilus influenzae, Neisseria meningitidis,* and other encapsulated organisms. Continuous prophylactic antibiotics may be advisable during the early years or indefinitely. Adults are also at increased risk for infection, especially during the first 3 years after surgery. The splenectomized client should be advised to seek medical treatment at the earliest manifestations of infection.

The unique functions performed by the spleen are eventually taken over by other organs. However, the loss of the spleen due to cessation of function or splenectomy does require the client to be monitored for potentially serious complications. The nursing care of the client undergoing splenectomy is generally the same as that discussed in Chapter 15 for any client undergoing surgery.

DISORDERS OF PLATELETS AND CLOTTING FACTORS

Disorders of hemostasis affecting platelets and clotting factors include (1) hemorrhagic disorders, (2) purpura, and (3) coagulation disorders.

HEMORRHAGIC DISORDERS

Normal clot formation and lysis depend on (1) intact blood vessels, (2) an adequate number of functioning platelets, (3) sufficient amounts of the 12 clotting factors, and (4) a well-controlled fibrinolytic system. Consequently, the four basic problems underlying hemorrhagic (bleeding) disorders are as follows:

- Weak, damaged vessels that rupture easily or spontaneously
- Platelet deficiency (*thrombocytopenia*) due to hypoproliferation, excessive pooling of platelets in the spleen, or excessive platelet destruction
- Deficiency or total lack of one of the clotting factors
- Excessive or insufficient fibrinolysis

Disorders of hemostasis fall into two major categories: *purpura* and *coagulation* (Box 75–1).

The diagnosis of a hemorrhagic disorder depends on a complete health and family history, physical examination, and laboratory tests for platelet and clotting defects. The history usually offers numerous clues to the type of bleeding problem and its cause.

If the history indicates a bleeding disorder, examine the client for overt manifestations of bleeding. Petechiae (tiny hemorrhagic spots caused by intradermal or submucosal bleeding) are usually present in vascular and thrombocytopenic purpuras. The presence of *ecchymoses* (large, blotchy, subcutaneous hemorrhagic areas), *hematomas* (subdermal hemorrhage), and *hemarthrosis* (blood within the joints) points to *hemophilia.* However, ecchymoses may develop in any hemorrhagic disorder. Clients who hemorrhage severely from several areas during childbirth or a major surgical procedure may have a fibrinogen deficiency. In addition to any evidence of bleeding, search for manifestations of hepatic cirrhosis (e.g., hepatomegaly, jaundice) and splenomegaly. Laboratory studies provide the most crucial evidence for pinpointing the type and cause of a bleeding disorder.

Clients with hemorrhagic disorders need to understand (1) why they are at risk for bleeding, (2) the manifestations of bleeding, and (3) preventive measures to avoid bleeding. Those who can be managed by home health care should be referred to appropriate health care agencies. Clients with bleeding disorders should carry an identification card at all times that indicates their diagnosis, name of physician or health care agency, and blood type. Assess each client before even minor invasive procedures, such as dental extractions, to rule out a history of bleeding disorders.

BOX 75–1 Classification of Disorders of Hemostasis

Purpura

Vascular defect purpura
- Familial hemorrhagic telangiectasia
- Anaphylactoid purpura (allergic purpura)
- Toxic purpura

Platelet disorder purpura
- Idiopathic thrombocytopenic purpura
- Secondary thrombocytopenias

Coagulation Disorders

Hemophilia
Hypoprothrombinemia
Disseminated intravascular coagulation (DIC)

IDIOPATHIC THROMBOCYTOPENIC PURPURA

Idiopathic thrombocytopenic purpura (ITP) is an autoimmune bleeding disorder characterized by the development of autoantibodies to one's own platelets, the binding of autoantibodies to antigens, and the destruction of platelets in the spleen and, to a lesser extent, in the liver. Normally, platelets survive 8 to 10 days within the circulation; in ITP, however, platelet survival is as brief as 1 to 3 days or less. In most cases, ITP takes a course of remissions and exacerbations that, in untreated cases, may continue for years.

Clinical Manifestations

Clinical manifestations include petechiae, ecchymosis, epistaxis, bleeding from the gums, and easy bruising. Women may have extremely heavy menses or bleeding between periods.

Diagnostic findings that confirm the presence of ITP include:

- A platelet count below 100,000/mm^3
- Prolonged bleeding time with normal coagulation time (all coagulation factors are present and normal)
- Increased capillary fragility, as demonstrated by the tourniquet test
- Positive platelet antibody screening
- Bone marrow aspirate containing normal or increased numbers of megakaryocytes

Complications of ITP include (1) cerebral hemorrhage, which proves fatal in 1% to 5% of clients with ITP; (2) severe hemorrhages from the nose, GI tract, and urinary system; (3) bleeding into the diaphragm, which can result in pulmonary complications; and (4) nerve pain, extremity anesthesia, or paralysis resulting from the pressure of hematomas on nerves or brain tissues.

Outcome Management

The treatment of choice for clients with ITP is steroids to inhibit the macrophage ingestion of the antibody-coated platelets. Plasmapheresis is sometimes used as short-term therapy until the steroid therapy takes effect. If the client is actively bleeding or requires surgery, IV gamma globulin can be used to increase the platelet count.

If the client does not have a sustained remission, splenectomy may be needed (see earlier). In 60% to 80% of cases, removal of the spleen results in complete and permanent remission. The effectiveness of splenectomy is believed to be related to the removal of the site of premature destruction of the antibody-sensitized platelets.

Danazol (Danocrine) has been used with success in some clients. Immunosuppressive therapy used in refractory cases includes vincristine, vinblastine (Velban), azathioprine (Imuran), and cyclophosphamide.

Nursing care of clients at high risk for bleeding is discussed in Chapter 78.

COAGULATION DISORDERS

The coagulation disorders stem from a defect in the clotting mechanisms. One or more of the clotting factors is depleted or absent. The important coagulation disorders discussed here are (1) hypoprothrombinemia, (2) disseminated intravascular coagulation (DIC), and (3) the hemophilias.

HYPOPROTHROMBINEMIA

Pathophysiology

Hypoprothrombinemia refers to a deficiency in the amount of circulating prothrombin. Prothrombin is a protein produced in the liver and normally found in the blood. For prothrombin synthesis to take place, vitamin K (a fat-soluble vitamin) must be present in the liver to act as a catalyst. Hypoprothrombinemia develops from a vitamin K deficiency or liver disorder or from an overdose of aspirin, coumarin, or coumarin-derivative anticoagulant (such as warfarin), which antagonizes the action of vitamin K.

The fat-soluble vitamin K is largely synthesized by bacteria in the small intestine, a classic example of symbiosis. The bacteria do more than their share, since we excrete large amounts of the vitamin. There is no standard dietary daily allowance. Because vitamin K is fat-soluble, it depends on the presence of bile for absorption. Once absorbed, vitamin K catalyzes prothrombin synthesis within the liver cells. Vitamin K deficiency is seen in newborns, who arrive with a limited supply and a largely sterile digestive tract, and in clients with GI tract disorders that interfere with the absorption of vitamin K, such as (1) malabsorption syndrome and jaundice due to bile duct obstruction; (2) liver damage so extensive that liver cells cannot produce bile or synthesize prothrombin; and (3) prolonged sulfonamide or antibiotic administration that sterilizes the bowel, thereby halting vitamin K manufactured by GI tract bacteria.

Dicumarol is an effective anticoagulant, interfering with vitamin K in prothrombin synthesis. In excessive doses, prothrombin time is prolonged. If the prothrombin time is too long, the danger of bleeding or spontaneous hemorrhage increases.

Clinical Manifestations

The major manifestations of hypoprothrombinemia are ecchymosis after minimal trauma, epistaxis, postoperative hemorrhage from the incision, hematuria, gastrointestinal tract bleeding, and prolonged bleeding from a venipuncture. The outstanding laboratory finding is a prolonged prothrombin time.

Outcome Management

Treatment of hypoprothrombinemia aims at the underlying cause. For example, vitamin K deficiency resulting from malabsorption is corrected through intramuscular or IV administration of vitamin K, such as phytonadione (AquaMEPHYTON) or menadione (Synkayvite). If overdosage with a coumarin anticoagulant is the underlying problem, anticoagulant therapy is stopped. To normalize the prothrombin time, phytonadione is administered orally for minor bleeding problems or intravenously for hemorrhage. Finally, if prothrombin deficiency results from liver disease, concentrates of prothrombin or of prothrombin and factors VII, IX, and X may be transfused.

DISSEMINATED INTRAVASCULAR COAGULATION

DIC is a complex and important coagulation disorder characterized by two apparently conflicting manifestations: (1) diffuse fibrin deposition within arterioles and capillaries, with resultant widespread clotting, and (2) hemorrhage from the kidneys, brain, adrenal glands, heart, and other organs occurs following activation of clotting factors and fibrinolytic enzymes throughout arterioles and capillaries. DIC is often called a "consumptive coagulopathy" because of the depletion of platelets.

Etiology and Risk Factors

The causes of DIC are many, and there is considerable overlap among the syndromes that precede its occurrence. Sepsis is the leading cause; up to 73% of clients with sepsis develop DIC. Four categories of causative factors are:

- Introduction of tissue coagulation factors into the circulation
- Damage to vascular endothelium
- Stagnant blood flow
- Infection

Box 75–2 lists conditions that may precipitate DIC.

Pathophysiology

Two pathways can initiate DIC. An extrinsic pathway of massive tissue damage due to burns or trauma or an intrinsic pathway due to damage to the endothelium release thromboplastic substances that result in activation of

BOX 75–2 Conditions That May Precipitate Disseminated Intravascular Coagulation

Shock
Cirrhosis
Purpura fulminans
Glomerulonephritis
Acute fulminant hepatitis
Acute bacterial and viral infections

Conditions that may cause the release of platelet factor III:

- Fat emboli
- Snakebites

Hemolytic processes caused by:

- Infection
- Transfusion reactions
- Immunologic disorders

Tissue damage caused by:

- Trauma
- Heat stroke
- Extensive burns
- Transplant rejections
- Surgery—particularly if extracorporeal circulation was used

Conditions that may cause the release of thromboplastin from tissues:

- Neoplastic growths
  - Acute leukemias
  - Prostatic cancer
  - Bronchogenic cancer
  - Giant cavernous hemangioma
- Obstetric conditions
  - Abruptio placentae (placental abruption)
  - Retained dead fetus
  - Amniotic fluid embolism

thrombin, which in turn activates fibrinogen and results in deposition of fibrin throughout the microcirculation. The formation of fibrin results from increased generation of thrombin, suppression of anticoagulation mechanisms, and delayed removal of fibrin due to impaired fibrinolysis (see Understanding DIC and Its Treatment).

Platelet aggregation or adhesiveness is increased; this enables fibrin clots and microthrombi to form in the brain, kidneys, heart, and other organs, causing micro-infarcts and tissue necrosis. RBCs become trapped in the fibrin strands and are destroyed (hemolysis). The resultant sluggish circulation of blood reduces the flow of nutrients and oxygen to the cells. Platelets, prothrombin, and other clotting factors are consumed in the process, which compromises coagulation and predisposes to bleeding.

Excessive clotting activates the fibrinolytic mechanism, which causes the production of fibrin degradation products. Fibrin degradation products act to inhibit platelet clotting functions, which causes further bleeding. Ultimately, with lysis of clots and depletion of clotting factors, the blood loses its ability to clot.

Clinical Manifestations

The onset of DIC is usually acute and develops within days to hours after an initial assault to the body system, such as shock. Subacute DIC may not be apparent initially but may become fulminant as the clinical course progresses. Chronic cases of DIC characteristically develop in clients with cancer or in women carrying a dead fetus.

Manifestations may be mild or extremely severe. They include purpura, petechiae, and ecchymoses on the skin, mucous membranes, heart lining, and lungs; prolonged bleeding from venipuncture; severe, uncontrolled hemorrhage during surgery or childbirth; oliguria and acute renal failure; and convulsions and coma. Ischemia of the peripheral tissue leads to coolness and mottling of the extremities.

The prognosis for clients with DIC varies. The condition may be self-limiting. On the other hand, hemorrhage, organ damage (especially acute respiratory distress syndrome), or even death may occur within a few days or even a few hours if associated with gram-negative sepsis. In severe cases, the mortality rate reaches 80%.

Diagnostic Findings

Diagnostic findings in severe cases of DIC indicate that the hemostatic mechanism has failed totally. A prolonged prothrombin time and activated partial thromboplastin time, very low (and falling) platelet count (<100,000/mm^3), low plasma levels of coagulation inhibitors, and prolonged clotting times are common findings. Table 75–3 lists the laboratory tests used in the diagnosis of DIC.

Outcome Management

Medical Management

The treatment of DIC is currently under investigation as researchers attempt to validate the most suitable means of managing this syndrome. To treat DIC successfully, clinicians must (1) correct the basic problem (such as infection, delivery of a fetus, surgery, or irradiation for cancer), (2) reverse the pathologic clotting, (3) control bleeding and shock, (4) detect occult bleeding, (5) measure blood loss, (6) administer blood products and medication as prescribed, and (7) observe for and report transfusion reactions and medication side effects.

Manifestations of thrombosis are treated with IV heparin, which interrupts the clotting cascade by blocking thrombi. The use of heparin is controversial and is reserved for clients with thrombosis seen as acute renal failure to skin ischemia. Low doses are given, such as 300 to 500 units per hour by continuous infusion. Antithrombin III, a natural inhibitor of coagulation, such as the drug desirudin, might be more effective than heparin and is being studied. Washed packed RBCs are administered to replace blood volume lost through hemorrhage without administering anticoagulant substances.

Cryoprecipitate is given for depletion of factors V and VIII. Administration of antithrombin III (in fresh frozen

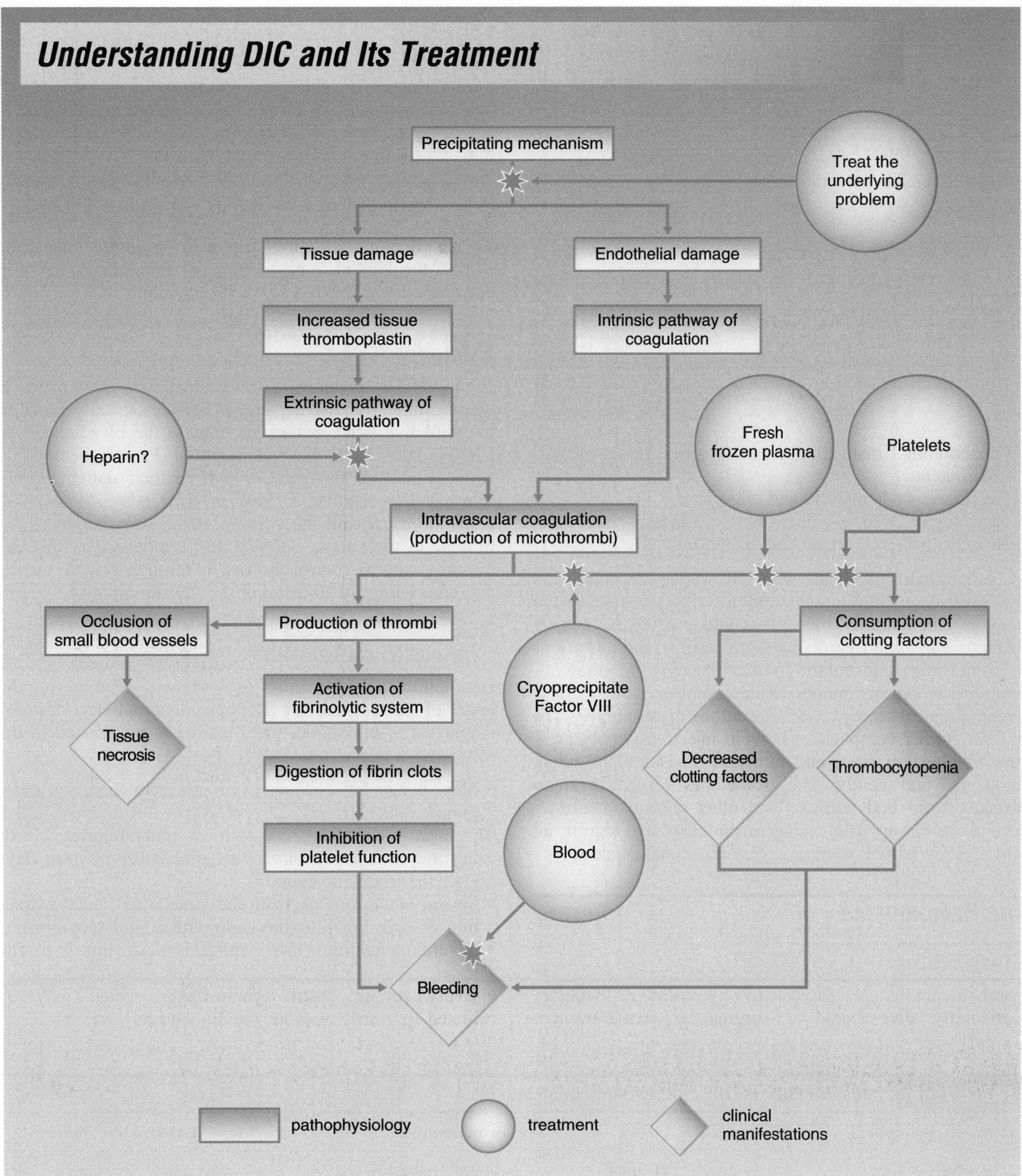

plasma) shortens the course of the disorder and reduces the complications of DIC. When bleeding cannot be controlled with heparin, aminocaproic acid (Amicar) is given. Cardiac, renal, and electrolyte studies should be followed closely during its use.

Several new agents to control bleeding and reverse laboratory manifestations of DIC are being studied. The protease inhibitors gabexate and aprotinin (Trasylol) have been used with some success. These drugs are still considered investigational.

Nursing Management

Assess all body systems for the effects of DIC, including:

- Integumentary bleeding or oozing of blood from venipuncture sites or mucosal surfaces and wounds, pallor, petechiae, ecchymoses, and hematomas
- Respiratory tachypnea, hemoptysis, orthopnea, and basilar rales
- Cardiovascular tachycardia and hypotension

TABLE 75-3 LABORATORY TESTS USED IN DIAGNOSIS OF DISSEMINATED INTRAVASCULAR COAGULATION

Test	Results
Prothrombin time	Prolonged
Partial thromboplastin time	Usually prolonged
Thrombin time	Usually prolonged
Fibrinogen level	Usually depressed
Platelet count	Usually depressed
Fibrin degradation products	Elevated
Protamine sulfate test	Strongly positive
Factor assays II, V, VII	Reduced

- GI abdominal distention, guaiac-positive stools or gastric contents
- Genitourinary hematuria and oliguria
- Neurologic vision changes, dizziness, headache, changes in mental status, and irritability

Nursing care of clients with DIC varies, depending on the severity of the process. Generally, the goal is to monitor and quantify blood loss and provide supportive therapy with blood components to resolve manifestations of hemorrhage and control further bleeding. Monitor appropriate laboratory values to determine treatment effectiveness and observe for manifestations of thrombosis. To prevent further complications, avoid injections, apply pressure to bleeding sites, and turn and reposition the client frequently and gently. DIC sometimes results in overt bleeding from body orifices and other clinical manifestations that are very frightening to the client and significant others. They will all require intense emotional support.

THE HEMOPHILIAS

Classification

The hemophilias are characterized by prolonged bleeding, particularly after accidental, surgical, or dental trauma. There are three major types of hemophilia: (1) hemophilia A (*classic* hemophilia), (2) hemophilia B (*Christmas disease*), and (3) von Willebrand's disease.

Hemophilia A, the most common of the congenital coagulation disorders, is due to a deficiency in the procoagulant protein factor VIII. The major characteristics of the hemophilias are compared in Table 75-4. Because classic hemophilia makes up 80% of all hemophilias, the discussion of manifestations and treatment refers only to this type.

The hemophilias are relatively common disorders. Within the United States alone, an estimated 25,000 clients are afflicted with a form of hemophilia.

Etiology

Hemophilia is genetically transmitted in a sex-linked (X chromosome) recessive pattern. Females usually transmit the defective gene, but males express the bleeding disorder. Females rarely have hemophilia. Female hemophilia carriers transmit the gene to half of their daughters and transmit the disorder to half of their sons. Males with hemophilia transmit the gene to all of their daughters but to none of their sons. Because this is a hereditary disease, the only way to control the risk is through genetic testing and counseling for decreasing the transmission.

Clinical Manifestations

Hemophilia may be mild or severe, depending on the level of factor VIII or IX coagulant activity. Usually diagnosed in childhood, this disorder is manifested in the following ways:

- Slow persistent bleeding from cuts, scratches, and other minor traumas
- Delayed hemorrhage that follows minor injuries; bleeding may not start from a site until hours or even days after the traumatic event
- Severe hemorrhaging from the gums after dental extraction or even brushing the teeth with a hard toothbrush
- Severe, sometimes fatal, epistaxis after injury to the nose
- Overwhelming gastric hemorrhage, which may be linked to gastric disorders such as ulcers

TABLE 75-4 COMPARISON OF THE THREE FORMS OF HEMOPHILIA

Form of Hemophilia	Etiology	Transmission	Major Laboratory Findings
Hemophilia A (classic hemophilia)	Inherited factor VIII (antihemophilic globulin) deficiency	Transmitted as sex-linked *recessive* trait; transmitted by females; occurs in males and, rarely, homozygous females	Coagulation time prolonged but bleeding time normal; factor VIII missing from plasma
Hemophilia B (Christmas disease)	Inherited factor IX (plasma thromboplastin component) deficiency	Transmitted as sex-linked *recessive* trait; transmitted by females; occurs in males and, rarely, homozygous females	Laboratory findings and symptoms same as in hemophilia A; factor IX missing
von Willebrand's disease	Inherited factor VIII deficiency and defective platelet dysfunction	Transmitted as autosomal *dominant* trait to both sexes; occurs in both males and females	Both coagulation time and bleeding time prolonged; low factor VIII levels; platelet adhesiveness decreased

- Recurrent hematoma formation in the deep subcutaneous tissue, in the intramuscular tissues, and around the peripheral nerves

If nerves are compressed by hematomas, the client suffers severe pain, anesthesia of the innervated part, nerve damage, and paralysis. In addition, muscular atrophy sometimes results.

Finally, recurrent *hemarthrosis* (bleeding into the joints) is common in untreated cases and may result in serious joint deformity and permanent crippling. Hemarthrosis affects the knees, ankles, elbows, wrists, fingers, hips, and shoulders, in that order. All of this bleeding can be controlled with the administration of the missing factor (VIII or IX).

Platelet function, platelet count, bleeding time, and prothrombin time are normal. The activated partial thromboplastin time (a pTT) is prolonged. Quantitative assays for factor VIII determine the severity of the disease.

Outcome Management

The goals of care for clients with hemophilia are as follows:

- Stop topical bleeding as quickly as possible
- Raise the level of antihemophilic factor (AHF) in the plasma, thereby temporarily supplying the missing factor causing hemorrhage;
- Prevent complications leading to and caused by bleeding

Immediate transfusion of factor VIII or IX concentrate is the primary treatment. Although plasma and cryoprecipitate contain factor VIII, concentrates have a known AHF content and carry less risk of blood volume overload. As a result of the volume of blood products required, hepatitis and HIV infection represent the major infectious risks, but improved purification techniques now used routinely in the preparation of concentrated factors have virtually eliminated this threat. Because the procoagulant activity of AHF disappears rapidly, clients need transfusions every 12 hours until bleeding stops.

Transfusion of packed RBCs or WBCs are used only to replace blood volume when there has been severe loss. Prophylactic transfusion of factor VIII to a level of 50% above normal is recommended in cases of minor injury, surgery, and dental extractions.

One major complication is linked to repeated transfusions and AHF therapy. About 5% of persons with hemophilia become sensitized to AHF and develop autoimmune anti-AHF antibodies. In clients with low titers of factor VIII antibodies, major and life-threatening hemorrhages are treated with massive doses of factor VIII from animal sources (bovine and porcine), inactivated prothrombin complex concentrates (Konyne 80, Proplex T), or activated prothrombin complex concentrates (Feiba VH Immuno, Autoplex T). Clinicians are using various experimental treatments such as immunosuppressive therapy to combat this problem. Topical bleeding can usually be temporarily controlled by applying pressure to the injured site, packing the area with a fibrin foam, and applying topical hemostatics such as thrombin.

Hemarthrosis may be controlled if the client receives AHF in the early stages of bleeding. Joint immobilization and local chilling (such as packing ice around the joint) may bring relief. If pain is severe, it may be necessary to aspirate blood from the joint. Once bleeding stops and swelling subsides, the client should perform active range-of-motion exercises without weight-bearing to prevent further complications, such as deformity and muscle atrophy.

The prognosis for clients with hemophilia has greatly improved since the discovery of AHF. Before this, 50% of people with hemophilia died before they reached their 5th year; today, death rarely occurs after minor trauma. Home infusion of AHF ensures that treatment is instituted at the first manifestation of bleeding, with complications thus prevented. Clinicians have developed training programs with strict guidelines. When these guidelines are carefully followed, clients with hemophilia lose less time from work or school and need fewer visits to the emergency department. Fatalities mainly follow the development of autoimmune antibodies (anti-AHF) and retroperitoneal bleeding after internal hemorrhage.

Analgesics and corticosteroids often reduce joint pain and swelling. In mild hemophilia, the use of IV desmopressin may eliminate the need for AHF. Desmopressin acts by causing an increase in plasma factor VIII activity.

Although most clients with hemophilia are successfully maintained with home health care, they may be seen in the hospital during acute bleeding episodes or for nonrelated treatments. If even a minor invasive procedure is planned, it is crucial to assess the factor VIII level and administer a sufficient quantity of factor concentrate before the procedure. During routine medical examinations, these clients should be assessed for frequency of bleeding episodes and effectiveness of home therapy. Examine joints for manifestations of bleeding and related atrophy.

During client teaching, review routine situations that increase the client's risk of bleeding, such as contact sports, minor invasive procedures, falls, and cuts. Teach the client to recognize early manifestations and why it is critical to intervene with treatment immediately. Discuss situations that require medical consultation. Provide teaching about bleeding precautions for prevention of injury or trauma that may precipitate a bleeding episode. Effective and prompt administration of factors to reduce the incidence of bleeding episodes and resultant complications, such as joint atrophy, is a priority. The client will need to learn IV infusion administration techniques to control the bleeding.

CONCLUSIONS

Hematologic diseases are complex disorders that require the nurse to understand the hematopoietic system. The nurse is often involved in the administration of blood and blood products for treatment of these various disorders. Many of the blood disorders are life-threatening; others are easily controlled with proper nutrition or regular medication.

Because blood and blood product transfusions are widely used in the treatment of hematologic disorders, it is vital that you understand this procedure, the implications of these procedures, and the proper techniques of administration so the client will receive safe and effective care.

THINKING CRITICALLY

1. **A 62-year-old client underwent a gastric resection for peptic ulcer disease 3 months ago at a hospital in another state. She comes to the nursing clinic complaining of shortness of breath and fatigue with minimal physical exertion. She currently takes ranitidine (Zantac). What assessments should you make now?**

Factors to Consider. What is the significance of the history of gastric resection? How might this contribute to the client's lethargy? What might be causing the shortness of breath and fatigue? What laboratory results would be appropriate to evaluate? What teaching should you consider with this client?

2. **A 40-year-old client has recently been told that she has multiple myeloma. She has been admitted to the oncology inpatient unit for initial evaluation and treatment. On her 4th day after admission, she becomes confused and difficult to arouse. Bowel sounds are diminished, and she begins to vomit. What priority assessment should you make now?**

Factors to Consider. What might predispose the client to this change in her level of consciousness? What additional assessments would you need to make? What interventions should you anticipate at this time?

BIBLIOGRAPHY

1. Bataille, R., & Harousseau, J. (1997). Multiple myeloma. *New England Journal of Medicine, 336*(23), 1657–1664.
2. Boyland, L., & Gleeson, C. (1999). Clinical management: The management of anemia. *European Journal of Palliative Care, 6*(5), 145–148.
3. Bunn, H. F. (1997). The pathogenesis and treatment of sickle cell disease. *New England Journal of Medicine, 337*(11), 762–769.
4. Cella, D., & Bron, D. (1999). The effect of epoetin alfa on quality of life in anemia cancer patients. *Cancer Practice, 7*(4), 177–182.
5. Charache, S., and Investigators of the Multicenter Study of Hydroxyurea in Sickle Cell Anemia. (1995). Effect of hydroxyurea on the frequency of painful crises in sickle cell anemia. *New England Journal of Medicine, 332*(20), 1317–1322.
6. George, J., et al. (1998). Drug-induced thrombocytopenia: A systemic review of published case reports. *Annals of Internal Medicine, 129*(11), 886–890.
7. Gobel, B. H. (1999). Disseminated intravascular coagulation. *Seminars in Oncology Nursing, 15*(3), 174–182.
8. Goldberg, M., Murphy, S., & Wallach, H. (1998, September 30). Myeloproliferative disorders. *Patient Care,* 37–57.
9. Hawkins, R. (1999). Disseminated intravascular coagulation. *Clinical Journal of Oncology Nursing, 3*(3), 127, 131.
10. Johns, A. (1998). Overview of bone marrow and stem cell transplantation. *Journal of Intravenous Nursing, 21*(6), 356–360.
11. Lee, E. J., Phoenix, D., Brown, W., & Jackson, B. (1997). A comparison study of children with sickle cell disease and their non-disease siblings on hopelessness, depression and perceived competence. *Journal of Advanced Nursing, 25,* 79–86.
12. Levi, M., & Cate, H. T. (1999). Disseminated intravascular coagulation. *New England Journal of Medicine, 341*(8), 586–592.
13. McBrien, N. (1997). Thrombotic thrombocytopenic purpura. *American Journal of Nursing, 97*(2), 28–29.
14. Paquette, R. L., et al. (1995). Long-term outcome of aplastic anemia in adults treated with antithymocyte globulin: Comparison with bone marrow transplantation. *Blood, 85*(1), 283–290.
15. Richer, S. (1997). A practical guide for differentiating between iron deficiency anemia and anemia of chronic disease in children and adult. *The Nurse Practitioner, 22*(4), 82–103.
16. Schilling, R. F., & Williams, W. J. (1995). Vitamin B_{12} deficiency: Underdiagnosed, overtreated? *Hospital Practice (Office Edition), 30*(7), 47–52; discussion 52, 54.
17. Stephan, F., et al. (1999). Thrombocytopenia in a surgical ICU. *Chest, 115*(5), 1363–1370.
18. Vichinsky, E. P., and The Preoperative Transfusion in Sickle Cell Disease Study Group. (1995). A comparison of conservative and aggressive transfusion regimens in the perioperative management of sickle cell disease. *New England Journal of Medicine, 333*(4), 206–213.
19. Worrall, L. M., Thompkins, C. A., & Rust, D. M. (1999). Recognizing and managing anemia. *Clinical Journal of Oncology Nursing, 3*(4), 153–160, 180–182.
20. Young, N. S., & Maciejewski, J. (1997). The pathophysiology of acquired aplastic anemia. *New England Journal of Medicine, 336*(19), 1365–1372.

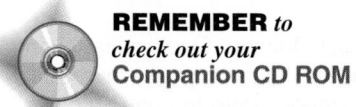

CHAPTER 76

Management of Clients with Immune Disorders

Linda Ludy Scott

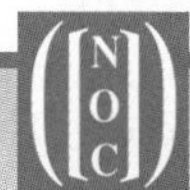

NURSING OUTCOMES CLASSIFICATIONS (NOC) for Nursing Diagnoses—Clients with Immune Disorders

Altered Health Maintenance
Health Belief: Perceived Resources
Health-Promoting Behavior
Health-Seeking Behavior
Knowledge: Health Behaviors
Knowledge: Health Promotion
Knowledge: Health Resources
Knowledge: Treatment Regimen
Participation: Health Care Decisions
Psychosocial Adjustment: Life Change
Risk Detection
Self-Direction of Care
Social Support
Treatment Behavior: Illness or Injury

Latex Allergy Response
Immune Hypersensitivity Control
Symptom Severity
Tissue Integrity: Skin and Mucous Membranes

Risk for Latex Allergy Response
Immune Hypersensitivity Control
Knowledge: Health Behaviors
Risk Control
Risk Detection
Tissue Integrity: Skin and Mucous Membranes

The immune system constitutes the body's defense system against invading foreign substances. A functioning immune system must protect the body from potential pathogens. An immune system that is malfunctioning predisposes an individual to the development of a wide variety of diseases, ranging from severe infection to autoimmune disease, and the resultant tissue injury. The Unit 16 review describes the normally functioning immune system; this chapter looks at alterations in the immune system and how these changes affect the human organism.

HYPERSENSITIVITY DISORDERS

As health care providers, nurses deal with allergic conditions far more often than might be suspected. Allergic rhinitis, asthma, and dermatitis are just a few examples of these immunologic diseases.

The tendency to develop allergies involving immunoglobulin E (IgE) antibody formation is known as *atopy.* The terms *atopic, allergic,* and *hypersensitive* are frequently used interchangeably. *Allergy* (or, more appropriately, hypersensitivity) describes the increased immune response to the presence of an allergen, also known as an *antigen.* Between 10% and 20% of the population has allergies. We cannot exactly predict who will have allergies; however, there is a higher incidence of allergies among children of allergic parents.

People must progress through a two-step process to become allergic. Step 1 starts with *sensitization.* Sensitization occurs when an individual develops IgE antibodies against a substance that is inhaled, ingested, or injected. Newly formed IgE antibodies stick to basophils and mast cells, found in the skin's mucosal surfaces and the respiratory and gastrointestinal (GI) tracts. Hypersensitivity can be claimed only after IgE antibodies against a certain foreign substance have formed and are bound to the surface of tissue mast cells and circulating basophils.

Hypersensitivity does not produce any of the manifestations typically associated with allergic disease. It is not until step 2, *reexposure to the allergen,* that allergic manifestations such as sneezing, asthma, and anaphylaxis occur. Even though the cellular events for all immediate allergic reactions tend to be similar, there are differences in the clinical sequelae that occur, based on the state of the individual's host defenses, the nature of the allergen, the concentration of the allergen, the route by which the allergen enters, the amount of allergen exposure received, and which organ is affected.

Etiology and Risk Factors

HOST DEFENSES. Some people are more susceptible to hypersensitivity than others for reasons that are unclear. Specific IgE formation can be influenced by vital infections, especially those caused by cytomegalovirus (CMV) and mononucleosis. Factors such as air pollution, sex, age, and exposure to second-hand smoke may all influence manifestations of allergies.

Nature of the Allergen. Allergens are proteins capable of inducing IgE antibody, thus triggering an allergic response. Molecules that combine with proteins to produce antibodies are called *haptens.* Haptens, along with other environmental allergens, are carried on vectors that may become airborne (e.g., pollen, dust particles, animal dander). Contact with these allergens causes sensitization and atopy and evokes the acute manifestations of allergy. Some haptens (e.g., penicillin) are highly antigenic.

Concentration of the Allergen. Higher concentrations usually result in hypersensitivity responses of greater intensity. Lower concentrations of the allergen may then cause severe manifestations when reexposure occurs.

Route of Entrance into the Body. Routes by which allergens enter the body include inhalation, injection, ingestion, and direct contact. Most allergens are inhaled.

Exposure to the Allergen. Sensitization to allergens is necessary in order for hypersensitivity to occur. A few factors that influence the likelihood of development of allergy are a person's age at the time of exposure (exposure early in life), the type of allergen (house dust mite, cockroach, various medications, and pollen), the allergen load (lower levels are capable of inducing specific IgE production), and the month of a person's birth (a greater affinity for allergies is seen in those born in the spring and fall).

Pathophysiology

The key intermediate in allergic disease is the IgE antibody. The production of IgE in response to an allergen renders an individual allergic. There are two general categories of hypersensitivity reactions: (1) *immediate* (humoral or antigen-antibody) and (2) *delayed* (cell-mediated).

Immediate Reaction. The immediate (antigen-antibody) reaction occurs within minutes after exposure to the allergen. The resultant IgE production mediates the immediate response by activating mast cells and basophils, causing them to degranulate and release mediators such as histamine.

The mediators, whether preformed or newly formed after activation, are able to increase vascular permeability, dilate vessels, cause bronchospasm, contract smooth muscle, and ignite other inflammatory cells. Table 76–1 describes chemical mediators of the allergic reaction, their action, and the associated manifestations.

Manifestations of mediator release vary, depending on the organ where the mediators' receptors are found. For example, histamine is a preformed mast cell mediator that has receptors in various organs, including skin, oral and nasal mucosa, lungs, and the smooth muscle in the GI tract. Once histamine binds to its receptor, it can cause many reactions. Vasodilation causes edema; smooth muscle contraction results in dangerous airway narrowing; and glandular stimulation leads to increased mucus secretion in the nose, lungs, and GI tract.

Newly formed mediators, including lipid mediators and cytokines, are made after the mast cell has been activated and have similar actions to those of histamine, but their effects tend to last much longer. Once released into the blood and after binding to their receptors, these mediators cause more bronchial smooth muscle contraction, vasodilation in the skin, nasal congestion, and edema.

Delayed Reaction. The delayed (cell-mediated or late-phase) reaction is seen when there is a prolonged response to the initial allergen. T cells govern the delayed inflammatory response that occurs approximately 2 to 8 hours after mast cells have been activated by the initial allergen exposure.

Hypersensitivity reactions are divided into four main types (Table 76–2):

- I, Immediate or anaphylactic
- II, Cytolytic or cytotoxic
- III, Immune complex
- IV, Cell-mediated or delayed

Type I (Anaphylactic) Hypersensitivity

The anaphylactic response (described previously) is a rapidly occurring reaction mediated by IgE antibodies. The allergen binds to IgE antibodies, which are attracted to the surface of mast cells and basophils, causing release of mediators (see Table 76–1). Examples of type I hypersensitivity reactions include anaphylaxis, allergic rhinitis, asthma, and acute allergic drug reactions.

Type II (Cytolytic or Cytotoxic) Hypersensitivity

Cytolytic or cytotoxic reactions are complement-dependent and thus involve IgG or IgM antibodies. The antigen-antibody binding results in activation of the complement system and destroys the cell upon which the antigen is bound, usually a circulating blood cell, thus causing tissue injury. Examples of tissue injury caused by type II hypersensitivity include hemolytic anemia, Rh hemolytic disease in the newborn, autoimmune hyperthyroidism, myasthenia gravis, and blood transfusion reactions.

During a blood transfusion, blood group incompatibility causes cell lysis, which results in a transfusion reaction. The antigen responsible for initiating the reaction is a part of the donor red blood cell membrane. Manifestations of a transfusion reaction result from intravascular hemolysis of red blood cells. They include headache and back pain (flank), chest pain similar to angina, nausea and vomiting, tachycardia and hypotension, hematuria, and urticaria.

Transfusions of more than 100 ml of incompatible blood can result in severe, permanent renal damage, circulatory shock, and death. Therefore, if manifestations develop, stop the transfusion at once, maintain an open intravenous (IV) line, check the client's vital signs, and notify the physician immediately. For detailed nursing interventions related to transfusion reactions, see Chapter 75.

Type III (Immune Complex) Hypersensitivity

Immune complex reactions result when antigens bind to antibodies leading to tissue injury. The molecular size of the antigen-antibody complexes is an important feature in eliciting immune complex reactions. Larger complexes are rapidly cleared by phagocytic cells. The smaller complexes formed in antigen excess persist longer in the circulation because they are not as easily captured by

TABLE 76–1 CHEMICAL MEDIATORS OF THE ALLERGIC REACTION

Mediator	Action	Manifestations
Histamine	Dilates blood vessels and increases vascular permeability	Erythema, tissue swelling, and shock
	Constricts smooth muscles in the bronchial airways	Shortness of breath and wheezing
	Stimulates nerve endings	Itching and painful skin
	Increases mucus production in the airways and GI tract	Congestion, gastric reflux, and heartburn
Platelet-activating factor	Dilates the blood vessels and constricts the bronchial airways	Same as for histamine
	Aids in the secretion and aggregation of platelets	Same as for histamine
Eosinophil chemotactic factor of anaphylaxis (ECF-A)	Increases eosinophil migration	Inflamed airways
Neutrophil chemotactic factor	Increases neutrophil migration	Inflamed airways
Heparin	Anticoagulation	Increased bleeding and bruising
Bradykinin	Slows smooth muscle contraction	Mucous plugging
	Increases vascular permeability	Swelling
	Increases mucus production	Congestion
LIPID MEDIATORS OR SRS-A		
Leukotrienes	Increase vascular permeability Increase smooth muscle contraction	Same as for histamine
Prostaglandin D	Constricts bronchial airways	Wheezing, shortness of breath, and cough
	Vasodilation	Flushing and swelling
Cytokines (IL-4, IL-5, TNF-α)	Allow cells to influence the activity and development of other unrelated cells Aid in eosinophil production Increase vascular permeability	Inflammation, edema, and fibrosis

GI, gastrointestinal; IL, interleukin; SRS, slow-reacting substance of anaphylaxis; TNF, tumor necrosis factor.

phagocytic cells in the spleen and liver. Inflammation results and leads to acute or chronic disease of the organ system in which the immune complexes were deposited.

Immune complex–mediated inflammation is produced by IgG or IgM antibodies, antigen, and complement. The mediators of inflammatory injury include the complement cleavage peptides, which can activate mast cells, neutrophils, monocytes, and other cells. Release of lysosomal

TABLE 76–2 TYPES OF HYPERSENSITIVITY REACTIONS

	Type	Causative Component	Pathologic Process	Reaction
I	Immediate/anaphylactic	IgE	Mast cell degranulation ↓ Histamine and leukotriene release	Anaphylaxis Atopic diseases Skin reactions
II	Cytolytic/cytotoxic	IgG IgM Complement	Complement fixation ↓ Cell lysis	ABO incompatibility Drug-induced hemolytic anemia
III	Immune complex	Antigen-antibody complexes	Deposition in vessels and tissue walls ↓ Inflammation	Arthus reaction Serum sickness Systemic lupus erythematosus Acute glomerulonephritis
IV	Cell-mediated/delayed	Sensitized T cells	Lymphokine release	Tuberculosis Contact dermatitis Transplant rejection

Ig, immunoglobulin.

granules from white blood cells and macrophages causes further tissue injury.

The antigen may be tissue-fixed or released locally, as in Goodpasture's syndrome, in which circulating antibodies react with autologous antigens in the glomerular basement membranes of the kidneys, causing inflammation of the glomerulus.

Antigen-antibody complexes are formed in the bloodstream and get trapped in capillaries or deposited in vessel walls, causing urticaria, arthritis, arteritis, or glomerulonephritis.

Alternatively, antigen-antibody complexes may form in the joint space, with resultant synovitis, as in rheumatoid arthritis.

The Arthus reaction is a localized area of tissue necrosis that results from immune complex hypersensitivity.

The antigen may also be circulating, as in serum sickness. Serum sickness develops 6 to 14 days after injection with a foreign serum. Deposition of complexes on vessel walls causes complement activation, with resultant edema, fever, inflammation of blood vessels and joints, and urticaria. Classic serum sickness is rare, because large doses of heterologous sera (e.g., horse antisera to human lymphocytes) are seldom used.

However, a serum sickness–like reaction may occur after administration of such medications as penicillin, sulfonamides, streptomycin, thiouracils, and hydantoin compounds. Rather than being dominated by cutaneous vasculitis, these reactions more often manifest with fever, arthralgias, lymphadenopathy, and urticaria. The illness is usually benign and self-limiting. It resolves after the offending medication is discontinued.

Nursing care of the client with serum sickness depends on the severity of the reaction. For a mild reaction, care includes control of fever and pain with aspirin and antihistamines. For a severe reaction, care may require steroids.

Serum sickness can be prevented by avoiding allergen exposure. Obtain an allergy history and information about any previous reactions to drugs or vaccines. Document findings in the client's chart, care plan, and medication record so that the risk of subsequent exposure will be minimized.

TYPE IV (CELL-MEDIATED, LATE-PHASE OR DELAYED) HYPERSENSITIVITY

In cell-mediated hypersensitivity, sensitized T cells respond to antigens by releasing lymphokines, some of which direct phagocytic cell activity. This reaction occurs 24 to 72 hours after exposure to an allergen. Delayed hypersensitivity is induced by chronic infection (e.g., tuberculosis) or by contact sensitivities, as in contact dermatitis.

Type IV reactions occur after the intradermal injection of tuberculosis antigen or purified protein derivative (PPD). If the client has been sensitized to tuberculosis, sensitized T cells react with the antigen at the injection site. The reaction leads to edema and fibrin deposits, which result in the induration characteristic of a positive tuberculosis reaction.

Graft-versus-host disease (GVHD) and transplant rejection are also type IV reactions. In GVHD, immunocompetent donor bone marrow cells (the graft) react against various antigens in the bone marrow recipient (the host). Various clinical manifestations result, including skin, GI, and hepatic lesions. Transplant rejection and GVHD are discussed in Chapter 80.

Contact dermatitis is another type IV reaction that occurs after sensitization to an allergen, commonly a cosmetic, adhesive, topical medication, drug additive (such as lanolin added to lotions), or plant toxin (such as poison ivy). With the first exposure, no reaction occurs but antigens are formed. On subsequent exposures, hypersensitivity reactions are triggered, which lead to itching, erythema, and vesicular lesions.

Clinical Manifestations

During an allergic response, mast cell activation and the release of chemical mediators result in increased vascular permeability, edema, dilation of blood vessels, smooth muscle contraction, bronchospasm, and increased mucus secretion in the nose, lungs, and GI tract.

The diagnosis of an allergic disease is based on the client's history, manifestations experienced during or after allergen exposure, and the results from commonly used allergy tests. Common allergy tests include (1) skin testing; (2) radioallergosorbent test (RAST), which is used for measuring IgE levels to certain allergens in vitro; (3) pulmonary function tests (PFTs) to diagnose asthma; and (4) blood assays for IgE levels.

SKIN TESTING. The health care practitioner introduces a small quantity of allergen into the skin by quickly pricking, scratching, or puncturing it or by using intradermal injection. A wheal and flare reaction usually occurs soon after the allergen is introduced into the skin if the client is allergic. Skin testing is generally considered safe, but it always carries a risk of causing a systemic reaction such as anaphylaxis.

Intradermal testing or injecting the known allergen directly below the skin is the most accurate skin test but is linked to a higher incidence of severe allergic reactions. Therefore, it should be used with extreme caution and under close supervision. A patch test can be used to evaluate contact allergies; the allergen is applied directly to the skin and then covered with a gauze dressing.

Nurses often administer skin tests and interpret test results. An *immediate* reaction (i.e., appearing within 10 to 20 minutes after the injection), marked by erythema and wheal formation greater than 3 mm of the positive control (usually histamine), denotes a positive reaction. *Positive* reactions indicate antibody response to previous exposure to this antigen and suggest the person is allergic to the particular substance that causes the reaction. *Negative* reactions may be inconclusive, requiring further assessment. Negative results may indicate the following: (1) antibodies have not formed to this antigen, (2) the antigen was deposited too deeply into the skin (e.g., subcutaneously), (3) the client is immunosuppressed from disease or therapies (e.g., steroids, chemotherapy, radiation therapy), or (4) the client has taken antihistamines within the past 72 hours.

Problems that arise from skin testing range from minor itching to anaphylaxis. Itching and discomfort at the injection site are common and can be relieved by the application of cool compresses, topical steroid or antihistamine creams, and oral antihistamines such as diphenhydramine (Benadryl). Ulceration of the injection site is best treated by keeping the area clean and dry. Anaphylactic shock is a rare but potentially lethal complication of skin testing. A client with a history of an anaphylactic reaction to a substance should never undergo skin testing for an allergy to that substance. This is especially true of allergens such as penicillin, which can produce lethal anaphylaxis in susceptible clients.

Radioallergosorbent Test. RAST uses the principle of immunoabsorption and reveals elevated levels of allergen-specific IgE associated with atopy. The allergen of interest is first bound to some solid surface, usually a paper disc. The client's blood is then incubated with the disc. If the client has antibodies specific to the allergen being tested, they bind to that allergen. The unbound antibodies are washed away, and the level of antigen-specific IgE can be measured. This test is somewhat less sensitive than skin testing and is more time-consuming and costly.

Pulmonary Function Test. PFTs are done to confirm the diagnosis or to evaluate the respiratory status in asthmatic disease, to assess the severity of lung obstruction, and to guide the medical treatment of asthma. The principal abnormality associated with asthma is reversible airway obstruction, reflected by a reduction in the forced expiratory volume measured in 1 second (FEV_1). Reversibility is noted if an increase of more than 10% in the FEV_1 is noted after giving a bronchodilator such as albuterol (Ventolin).

Blood Assays. Immunometric blood assays measure the total amount of IgE normally present in the circulation. Most studies have shown that blood concentrations of IgE are increased in the presence of allergic disease. However, a normal or even decreased level may occur in IgE-mediated sensitivities. Elevated serum eosinophil levels also may suggest hypersensitivities.

Outcome Management

Medical Management

Allergies are among the most common disorders seen in the medical community. The client often requires a combination of treatments, ranging from avoidance of known allergens to environmental control and immunotherapy.

Identify Allergen

It is imperative to obtain a detailed history, perform a thorough assessment and examination, and ensure that appropriate diagnostic tests are performed. The clinician must know the times of the year during which manifestations occur in order to determine a correct diagnosis on the basis of the offending allergen. If year-round manifestations are present, find out whether they are worse at any time.

Avoid Allergen

Avoidance of the allergen is often the easiest, cheapest, and safest way of dealing with allergies. However, identification of the specific allergen is sometimes difficult, especially if the client refuses, cannot afford, or cannot locate allergen-testing services. Even if the allergen can be identified, complete avoidance may not be possible, as with pollens and food additives.

Control Environment

Environmental control sometimes helps eliminate airborne allergens. Figure 76–1 illustrates ways to desensitize a room. These environmental controls, combined with air filters that remove small particles from the air, can help eliminate many allergens.

Administer Medications

Atopic clients benefit greatly from selected prescriptions and over-the-counter medications. Usually, clients self-administer these agents, although in some settings the nurse or a family member administers them.

Antihistamines. Antihistamines are the major group of prescription and over-the-counter drugs used to alleviate allergic manifestations. These medications relieve sneezing, rhinitis, itching, and other manifestations of allergic rhinitis. They bind to the H_1 receptor. Traditional antihistamines such as diphenhydramine (Benadryl) pass the blood-brain barrier and can produce significant drowsiness. Because newer agents (cetirizine [Zyrtec], fexofenadine [Allegra], and loratadine [Claritin]) do not cross the blood-brain barrier (or do so poorly), they do not cause the drowsiness that limits the use of older medications.

Decongestants. Decongestants (oral sympathomimetics) help relieve nasal congestion by stimulating the alpha-adrenergic receptors that control the capillary sphincters at the entrance to the venous plexuses of the turbinates. Decongestants act primarily on turbinate swelling and are more effective and rapid in onset when used topically rather than orally. However, because the prolonged use of topical nasal sprays can cause rhinitis medicamentosa (recurrence of congestion), it is advisable to limit their use to no more than 1 week. These drugs can be combined with antihistamines to treat the multiple manifestations of allergy.

Steroids. Corticosteroids, anti-inflammatory agents, and immunosuppressants can be used to treat allergic manifestations. Corticosteroids are the most effective drug for the treatment of rhinitis. Oral steroids are in general more effective and rapid in onset than topical forms, but their systemic effects can produce a myriad of complications. Topical steroid creams can be used to treat dermatitis. Beclomethasone dipropionate (Beconase), triamcinolone (Nasacort), flunisolide (Nasarel), budesonide (Rhinocort), and fluticasone (Flonase) are nasal sprays useful in treating allergic rhinitis, and they evoke few systemic side effects.

Aerosols. Cromolyn sodium is a topical or aerosol medication used to treat allergic rhinitis (Nasalcrom) and asthma (Intal). Its mechanism of action is not completely understood, but it helps prevent the release of chemical mediators (e.g., histamine and leukotrienes) from mast cells during both immediate and late-phase reactions. Cromolyn sodium should be administered before allergen exposure. It should be started a week before allergy season to be most effective in the treatment of seasonal allergic rhinitis. It must be used on a regular basis and, unfortunately, dosing is required three to four times a day.

Inhaled steroids are fundamental to the treatment of asthma. New inhaled steroids with a greater topical potency ratio and fewer systemic effects allow greater control in asthma management. Fluticasone (Flovent), triamcinolone (Azmacort), and beclomethasone (Vanceril) are examples of inhaled steroids.

Anticholinergics. Anticholinergics are used primarily to treat allergic rhinitis and rhinorrhea caused by

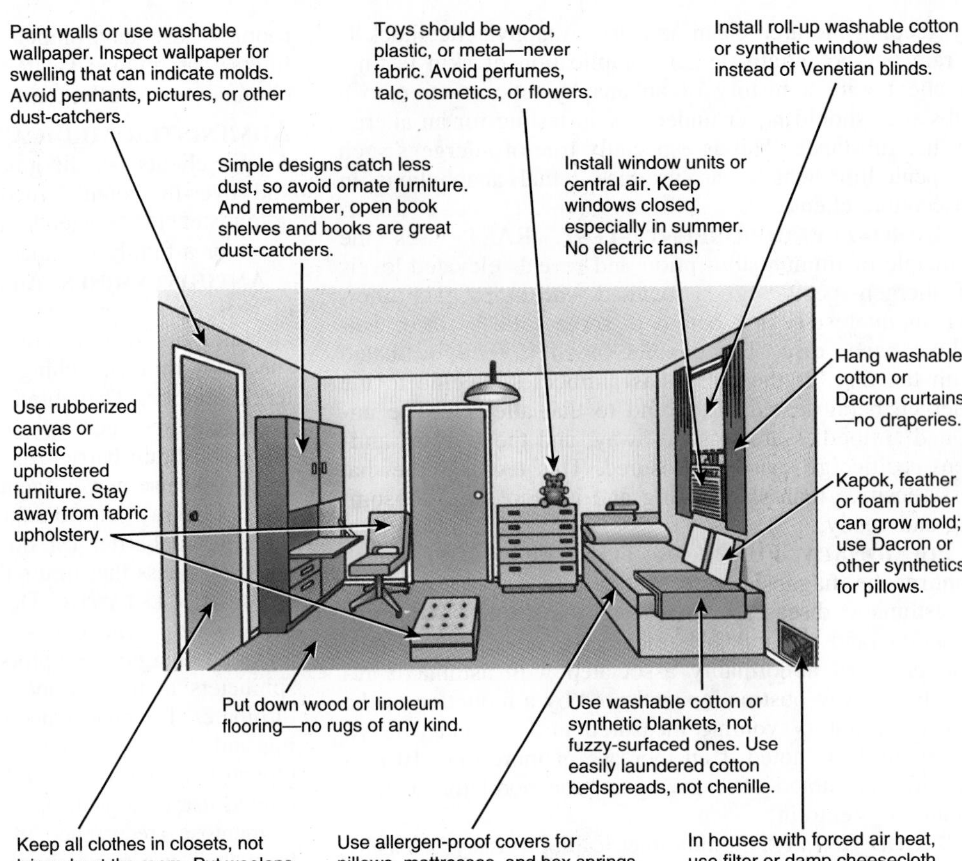
Paint walls or use washable wallpaper. Inspect wallpaper for swelling that can indicate molds. Avoid pennants, pictures, or other dust-catchers.
Toys should be wood, plastic, or metal—never fabric. Avoid perfumes, talc, cosmetics, or flowers.
Install roll-up washable cotton or synthetic window shades instead of Venetian blinds.
Simple designs catch less dust, so avoid ornate furniture. And remember, open book shelves and books are great dust-catchers.
Install window units or central air. Keep windows closed, especially in summer. No electric fans!
Hang washable cotton or Dacron curtains —no draperies.
Use rubberized canvas or plastic upholstered furniture. Stay away from fabric upholstery.
Kapok, feather or foam rubber can grow mold; use Dacron or other synthetics for pillows.
Put down wood or linoleum flooring—no rugs of any kind.
Use washable cotton or synthetic blankets, not fuzzy-surfaced ones. Use easily laundered cotton bedspreads, not chenille.
Keep all clothes in closets, not lying about the room. Put woolens in zipper bags—avoid mothballs, insect sprays, tar paper, or camphor.
Use allergen-proof covers for pillows, mattresses, and box springs. Since zipper leaks act as jets, spraying dust, tape over zippers. Don't store anything under the bed.
In houses with forced air heat, use filter or damp cheesecloth over inlet to reduce dust circulation. Change every two weeks. Keep bed away from vent.

FIGURE 76–1 Controlling the environment of a room. Dacron is a trade name for polyester. (Courtesy of A. H. Robins Company, Richmond, VA.)

the common cold. Ipratropium (Atrovent) was a major advance in the therapeutic regimen for asthma. It does not cross the blood-brain barrier and is relatively free of side effects. Anticholinergics are also available in oral forms in combination with antihistamines and decongestant preparations (Dura-Vent DA, Extendryl SR).

BRONCHODILATORS. Beta$_2$ agonists are commonly used to control bronchospasm in asthma. Albuterol (Ventolin) and other short-acting bronchodilators have proved to be well tolerated. The drawback of the older bronchodilators is their short duration of action (only 4 to 6 hours), which limits their use for manifestations experienced at night. This problem has been addressed with the new generation of long-acting beta$_2$ agonists such as salmeterol (Serevent).

ANTILEUKOTRIENES. Antileukotrienes are used to treat manifestations of asthma and anaphylaxis. They block the synthesis or action of leukotriene mediators, which are known to contribute to airway edema, smooth muscle contraction, and the process of inflammation. These drugs include zafirlukast (Accolate) and zileuton (Zyflo).

PROMOTE DESENSITIZATION

Immunotherapy ("desensitization therapy") is designed for the treatment of type I, IgE-mediated hypersensitivity reactions. Precise doses of allergens are injected at intervals over a prolonged period. The doses are increased gradually over time. Immunotherapy increases IgG antibody levels and may increase suppressor T-cell function. Specific IgG interferes with IgE binding to allergens and thus mitigates the hypersensitivity response. Immunotherapy is widely used in the treatment of allergic rhinitis (hay fever), for which its greatest success has been achieved. It also is used for Hymenoptera sensitivity (bee, yellow jacket, wasp, and hornet stings) with reportable success. There is some controversy regarding the efficacy of this treatment in the management of asthma.

Nurses often administer these injections and assess and treat side effects. Clients are asked to wait at least 30 to 40 minutes after receiving the injections so that immediate reactions can be treated. Side effects are similar to those seen in skin testing.

Nursing Management of the Medical Client

ASSESSMENT

As a nurse, you play a crucial role in obtaining a detailed medical history of the client and ensuring that appropriate diagnostic tests are performed. The most important part of evaluating the allergic client is the history. The history should elicit all of the client's current manifestations. It is important for clinicians to know whether the manifestations are always present or what times of the year they worsen.

Indoor allergens are causing increasing amounts of distress. House dust mites and cockroach and animal allergens are problematic and are present year-round in many homes. Assess whether animals are present in the home and, if so, how many. Is the house filled with plants that may harbor mold spores? Is the client exposed to moist rooms such as a basement that is constantly damp?

Environmental factors such as smoke may exacerbate manifestations. Where these manifestations present is very important to ascertain. Many occupations involve exposure to certain allergens such as smoke, latex, chemicals, and animals. Manifestations may be reported as worse during the workweek versus the weekend. Inquiries such as these help to narrow down possible causes of manifestations.

DIAGNOSIS, OUTCOMES, INTERVENTIONS

Altered Health Maintenance. The key nursing diagnosis for the client with hypersensitivity disorders is *Altered Health Maintenance related to lack of knowledge of disease process, treatment regimen and risk control methods.*

Outcomes. The client will follow a mutually agreed on health maintenance plan that includes stated understanding of disease process, treatment regimen, and control of risk factors.

Interventions

Provide Teaching. Although clients usually self-administer medications, as described under the medical management section, you are responsible for instructing clients and significant others about these medications. The client needs to learn what the medication is, why it is being prescribed, how to take it, when to take it, and what the possible side effects might be. In addition, the client needs to know what to do during an anaphylactic reaction (see Anaphylaxis).

If an inhaler is prescribed, the client must be taught how to use it correctly (see Chapter 61). A spacer (an attachment added to the inhaler that holds the medication in the additional chamber or space until the client inhales) may be recommended to help the client obtain the maximal effect. Some clients are taught to perform desensitization injections themselves. In this case, teach clients the proper injection technique and the signs of any untoward reactions to the medications.

Clients may need to carry medications for anaphylaxis with them at all times. In such instances, clients should also wear a medical-alert bracelet. Other nursing interventions are described in the following sections under specific disorders.

EVALUATION

It is expected that the client will obtain relief from allergic manifestations when the treatment regimen is followed. The client will be able to avoid or control risk factors for allergic manifestations. Ideally, the client will be able to avoid anaphylactic events and obtain treatment before serious problems develop.

ALLERGIC DISORDERS

FOOD ALLERGY

Adverse food reactions can be classified in one of two ways: (1) *food allergies,* which occur by a specific IgE-mediated response to the offending food, such as food-induced anaphylaxis from peanuts, and (2) *food intolerances,* which do not result from an IgE-mediated response but which cause manifestations such as diarrhea and vomiting. The prevalence of food intolerances is much higher than that of food allergies.

A thorough history is the most important factor in the diagnosis of food allergy or intolerance. Food allergies can be determined through skin testing. Food diaries (a record of events, including dietary intake for subsequent episodes) are used to provide insight for the correct diagnosis. The standard of diagnosis in food allergy is the double-blind, placebo-controlled food challenge. The suspected food is eliminated from the diet for 10 to 14 days. Antihistamines are not to be taken for at least 24 hours before the challenge, and a fasting state should be maintained for 12 to 18 hours before testing. The challenge starts with the introduction of a very low dose of the suspected food, and the dose is gradually increased every 20 to 30 minutes until a reaction is noted or the amount of food present in a normal feeding is reached. *Elimination diets* are also used and consist of removing one food at a time until the adverse manifestations are relieved.

Measuring serum blood tryptase levels can also prove helpful, because elevations in tryptase occur and are detectable in the blood for up to 2 hours after a severe systemic reaction. However, negative results do not rule out a positive reaction.

See Bridge to Home Health Care: Immunosuppression and Health.

ATOPIC DERMATITIS

Atopic dermatitis occurs in about 10% of the population. Clients typically have a history of or complaints about itchy skin, in addition to a history of rashes in the area of skin creases. Other common complaints are of generally dry skin initially experienced in children younger than 2 years of age, accompanied by manifestations of asthma, hay fever, or dermatitis. Lesions of atopic dermatitis are red and pruritic, contain exudates, and are maculopapular in younger clients, becoming drier and thicker as clients age. The lesions are typically found on the cheeks, scalp, and forehead; in later years, they may occur on the trunk and extremities.

Medical Management

Treatment is aimed at controlling and reducing the manifestations because there is no true cure. Antihistamines are used with good results to help alleviate the itch-scratch cycle that is common to atopic dermatitis. The mainstay of therapy is topical corticosteroids, which control the inflammation in the skin lesions. Gels penetrate more effectively but are drying. Ointments should be used in more severe cases, because they promote hydration; however, some clients do not care for them, because they are oily and become messy in the heat. Creams and lotions are the least penetrating but are preferred by most clients. They are absorbed quickly and promote comfort. Antibiotics may be needed to treat superficial skin infections caused by intense pruritus and scratching.

BRIDGE TO HOME HEALTH CARE

Managing Immunosuppression and Nutrition

The client who is immune-compromised faces numerous challenges related to nutrition, one of the most fundamental human needs. Anorexia, fatigue, weakness, nausea, and vomiting make it difficult to maintain or improve weight and nutritional status. Sometimes as a result of treatments and medications, immune-suppressed clients experience painful mouth sores and an altered sense of taste. Foods that they previously enjoyed no longer "taste right," and the act of eating holds little pleasure.

Conserving energy and enhancing adequate caloric intake are the ways to maintain nutritional status. Clients who have willing family members or friends should let them assist with meal preparation and clean-up. They should eat frequent, small amounts of high-calorie, nutritious foods that are flavorful and easy to prepare, ingest, and digest. Some clients do not like common supplements like canned shakes because of their thick texture. Adding ice to these drinks can make them more palatable and does not alter the calorie content. Homemade shakes can be made using yogurt, ice cream, or whole milk and adding fruit or concentrated fruit juice. Shakes can be prepared in advance and frozen for later use.

Mouth ulcers can be "painted" with a 4:1 mixture of aluminum/magnesium hydroxide (e.g., Maalox) and lidocaine (Xylocaine) to make eating more pleasant. Clients need to avoid constipation because it is likely to affect their appetite adversely. A daily routine of dried prunes or apricots, stool softeners, and gentle abdominal massage can help immensely.

Maximize your client's dietary success by encouraging full use of the senses. For example, caregivers can bake bread or cookies so that the aroma will stimulate appetite. Ask your client to visualize warm bread with melting butter, jam, or peanut butter. Encourage your client to eat meals with healthy family members and friends. Even snacking together can help maintain social interaction and minimize the isolation that many immune-suppressed individuals experience. Isolation breeds depression. Depression can have dire effects on appetite.

Clients who have poorly functioning immune systems need to evaluate the safety of their food choices and preparation. It is essential that all food handlers wash their hands carefully. Thoroughly clean fresh food; avoid other food that may harbor bacteria. Clients may want to avoid dining away from home, because they risk exposure to infection amid large groups of people. Food prepared for restaurants, vendors, picnics, or other social functions may harbor bacteria such as *Escherichia coli* or *Salmonella*. Even people with healthy immune systems can become seriously ill from these organisms; for people with immunosuppression, they can be deadly.

Some clients need total parental nutrition (TPN) in order to achieve adequate caloric intake. Although TPN may be necessary for survival, it provides nutrition in a rather unnatural way. Allow clients to have some degree of control by incorporating the therapy into their usual nighttime routines. Early risers should "hook-up" early in the evening so they can enjoy the morning time, when they usually have the most energy. "Night-owls" may want to use the opposite schedule. Clients whose gastrointestinal systems still function should continue to take some food by mouth. This helps to preserve the ability to taste and swallow and to maintain fundamental social and cultural connections.

Jeannine Mueller Harmon, RN, CS, MSN, FNP, *Family Nurse Practitioner, Metropolitan State University, St. Paul, Minnesota*

Nursing Management of the Medical Client

Teach clients the importance of environmental control. A key strategy is to minimize allergen exposure and physical stimuli that provoke pruritus. Explain that the client can reduce itching by avoiding severe changes in temperature, wearing loose cotton clothing, using gentle detergents, and rinsing clothing completely. Advise them to avoid chemical irritants, emotional stress, aeroallergens such as dust and animal dander, and dietary allergens. Teach the client general skin care measures, such as how to:

1. Maintain good skin hydration by bathing in lukewarm water
2. Use gentle soaps (e.g., Basis, Dove)
3. Apply a lubricant like Alpha Keri, petroleum jelly, Eucerin, or Aquaphor to the skin immediately after bathing
4. Avoid scratching
5. Keep fingernails trimmed to avoid infection

URTICARIA

Urticaria (or hives) is a cutaneous reaction associated with several different causes. It occurs in as many as 25% of all people at some point in time. Hives that are present daily or intermittently over a period of less than 6 weeks are termed *acute* urticaria. Hives present for more than 6 weeks are referred to as *chronic* urticaria.

Lesions of urticaria tend to be papules or plaques that fade within 24 hours. They do not leave areas of hyperpigmentation. Hives are round or oval and range in size from a few millimeters to several centimeters.

Mast cells and their mediators may play a key role in urticaria, causing intense pruritus and vascular changes. A lesional skin biopsy to identify which types of inflammatory cells are present in the lesion is useful in structuring treatment. Some known provoking stimuli of urticaria are medications, foreign substances, foods and food additives, infections, insect bites and stings, contact irritants, inhalants, heat, cold, light, and pressure.

Medical Management

Although management focuses on identifying and eliminating any known causative factors, in approximately 80% of chronic cases no cause of urticaria is found. All clients with urticaria should be cautioned about aspirin and nonsteroidal anti-inflammatory drugs (NSAIDs), which may exacerbate existing hives. Opiates or narcotics should be used cautiously as well, because they are typically mast cell degranulators.

Antihistamines are the mainstay of therapy for urticaria. Nonsedating antihistamines are recommended during the day; more sedating antihistamines may be preferred at night. Doxepin (Sinequan), a tricyclic antidepressant, is sometimes used for treatment because of its actions on both H_1 and H_2 receptors. Corticosteroids should not be used except for short-term therapy.

Nursing Management of the Medical Client

Urticaria tends to evoke anxiety and frustration in both clients and clinicians. The most effective treatment is to eliminate any triggers. Help the client identify factors that may be suspect, and suggest elimination diets and challenges if foods or food additives are thought to provoke manifestations. Encourage clients to avoid initiating physical factors, such as pressure from tight clothing, heat, vibration, sunlight, and rubbing of the skin. Good skin hydration is mandatory; counsel the client to avoid harsh soaps and irritants and to apply moisturizing lotions after bathing while the skin is still damp.

ANAPHYLAXIS, INSECT STING ALLERGY, AND LATEX ALLERGY

The most common causes of anaphylaxis are drugs, foods, latex exposure, and insect bites and stings. Common food offenders in adults are peanuts, tree nuts, and shellfish (Table 76–3). Insect stings cause many deaths in the United States every year. The incidence of anaphylaxis related to latex exposure, especially in health care workers, has dramatically increased since the 1990s with the increased use of latex gloves.

Anaphylactic events commonly present with hives and angioedema and often with dyspnea, wheezing, syncope, hypotension, nausea, vomiting, diarrhea, abdominal pain, flushing, headache, rhinitis, substernal pain, and itching. Cardiovascular collapse, shock, and respiratory obstruction, which can occur immediately and without other manifestations, are the primary cause of death from anaphylaxis. Although manifestations usually begin 5 to 30 minutes after the offending trigger has been encountered, there can be a delay of an hour or more. The more rapid the onset, the more severe the episode.

The incidence of anaphylaxis related to insect stings ranges from 0.3% to 3% in the general population. The sting insects are members of the order Hymenoptera. People may be allergic to one or all of the stinging insects, but the sting of the yellow jacket is the most common cause of allergy. Common reactions to an insect sting include pain, swelling, and redness that may be localized or extend over a large area. The swelling usually peaks in 24 to 48 hours and may last for 7 to 10 days. There are no factors that identify those at potential risk for anaphylaxis from an insect sting other than a prior history. Those who have had severe anaphylaxis have an 80% chance of another reaction.

Health care workers are at particular risk for latex allergy. Workers with allergies to latex also have a high incidence of reactions to certain foods, such as chestnuts, bananas, kiwi, and papaya. Manifestations range from simple dermatitis to generalized itching, urticaria, sneezing, coughing, wheezing, hypotension, and shock on exposure. The diagnosis of type I hypersensitivity to latex is confirmed by in vivo skin testing with raw latex extracts or in vitro blood assays that measure specific IgE responses to latex.

TABLE 76–3 COMMON AGENTS CAUSING ANAPHYLAXIS

DRUGS	
Penicillins (most common)	Vancomycin
Cephalosporins	Amphotericin B
Tetracyclines	Polymyxin
Streptomycin	Bacitracin
Kanamycin	Aspirin, other anti-inflammatory agents
Neomycin	Colchicine
Heparin	Tranquilizers
Protamine	
FOODS	
Peanuts	Milk
Seafood	Citrus fruits
Eggs	Strawberries
Nuts	Legumes
INSECT VENOMS	
Hymenoptera (honeybees, wasps, yellow jackets, hornets, fire ants)	
BIOLOGICALS	
Heterologous antisera (especially equine)	
Enzymes	
Hormones	
Vaccines (especially egg-cultured types)	
BLOOD PRODUCTS	
Plasma	
Cryoprecipitate	
Whole blood	
Gamma globulin	
ALLERGEN EXTRACTS	
Skin-testing agents	
Desensitization	
DIAGNOSTIC AGENTS	
Sulfobromophthalein	
Iodinated contrast media	

Medical Management

Anaphylaxis is treated by (1) subcutaneous epinephrine injection, (2) removing or discontinuing the causative agent, (3) administering emergency oxygen, (4) maintaining an open airway, (5) placing the client in the Trendelenburg position, and (6) giving supportive IV fluids, such as 0.9% normal saline or lactated Ringer's solution as necessary.

Nursing Management of the Medical Client

Nursing Diagnoses. *Risk for Latex Allergy and Latex Allergy Response* are more specific nursing diagnoses for latex allergy reactions. Most of the interventions for these diagnoses have been described under the nursing diagnosis *Altered Health Maintenance.* In addition, the incidence and severity of anaphylactic reactions are decreased by both general and specific measures. Take a thorough history for drug, food, insect, pollen and animal allergies from every client. Counsel all clients with a history of anaphylaxis or anaphylactic-like reactions to carry epinephrine with them at all times in the form of Epi-Pen or Ana-Kit for self-injection. Recommend that they carry a medical-alert bracelet or necklace and an identification card in their wallet or purse and that they register with the proper authorities.

ALLERGIC RHINITIS

Manifestations of allergic rhinitis are persistent and show seasonal variation. Nasal manifestations are often accompanied by eye irritation, which causes pruritus, erythema, and excessive tearing. Numerous allergens may cause these manifestations, such as tree pollens (most common in the spring), grasses (summer), ragweed (fall), or dust mites and animal dander (year-round).

When the nasal mucosa is exposed to an allergen, a series of events is set in motion. Allergen exposure increases the production of IgE, which binds to the receptors on mast cells and basophils and eventually causes a release of mediators. The mediator release leads to increased swelling and blockage of the nose, watery discharge, sneezing, and nasal itching.

Medical Management

Nasal glucocorticoid sprays are used with good results for the treatment of allergic rhinitis. The newer, nonsedating antihistamines are beneficial in maintaining control over allergic rhinitis and are a crucial component of therapy.

Nursing Management of the Medical Client

Educating the client is the most important component of therapy. Teach clients to avoid allergens and to use air filters and air conditioning. Emphasize that compliance with medication is essential. Explain the reasoning behind daily medication use as well as how to adjust the medication to control minor flare-ups and to prevent progression of the disease.

ASTHMA

Because the diagnosis and treatment of asthma account for a substantial number of outpatient visits in allergy clinics, a heightened awareness and thorough understanding of the disease are warranted. See Chapter 61 for a thorough discussion of asthma management.

CONCLUSIONS

The immune system is a complex, interrelated system that affects the whole body. As a nurse, you must understand immune responses in order to provide clients with complete and individualized care. Because the care of these clients requires multifaceted interventions, you must be able to develop and implement complex care plans to meet their needs.

THINKING CRITICALLY

1. **L. S. is a 41-year-old woman admitted for surgery. After surgery, she was to receive prophylactic IV cephalosporin but received a dose of penicillin by mistake. She has a known allergy to penicillin. With a history of allergy to penicillin, what type of hypersensitivity reaction is L. S. most likely to experience? Using the concepts of hypersensitivity, explain this process.**

Factors to Consider. What reactions might the nurse expect? What should be the nurse's first actions? What medications might the nurse expect the physician to prescribe to treat this reaction? How can such a reaction be prevented from occurring in the future?

2. **A. W. is a 21-year-old college student admitted with an asthmatic attack that has not responded to his usual treatments. He is admitted for a course of IV medications and respiratory treatments. When you enter the room to start the IV line, his wheezing is audible. He is also anxious and gasping for air. What actions should you implement? What problems might you experience when you start the IV line?**

Factors to Consider. After the acute phase is over, what might the nurse assess to determine the cause of the asthma attack and why the typical interventions were unsuccessful? What additional teaching might be required?

3. **R. H. is a newly graduated Registered Nurse on an oncology unit. She has been wearing gloves more than ever during the past 2 weeks following orientation. A rash develops on her hands, and she complains of itching all over her body. What type of allergic reaction might be occurring? What actions to assess the allergy should be taken?**

Factors to Consider. Can R. H. expect to continue in her new job? Does the organization have a responsibility to keep her employed?

BIBLIOGRAPHY

1. Aaronson, D. (1998). Side effects of rhinitis medications. *Journal of Clinical Immunology, 101*(2), S379–S383.
2. Blaylock, B. (1995). Latex allergies: Overview, prevention and implications for nursing care. *Ostomy Wound Management, 41*(5), 10–15.
3. Boguniewicz, M. (1997). Advances in the understanding and treatment of atopic dermatitis. *Current Opinion in Pediatrics, 9,* 577–581.
4. Burks, A., et al. (1998). Atopic dermatitis and food hypersensitivity reactions. *Journal of Pediatrics, 132*(1), 132–136.
5. Costa, J., Weller, P., & Galli, S. (1997). The cells of the allergic response. *Journal of the American Medical Association, 278*(22), 1815–1822.
6. DeShazo, R. (1997). Future trends in allergy and immunology. *Journal of the American Medical Association, 278*(22), 2024–2025.

7. Donohoe, M. (1997). Allergic diseases. *Lippincott's Primary Care Practice, 1*(2), 117–128.
8. Gift, A. G., & Pugh, L. C. (1993). Dyspnea and fatigue. *Nursing Clinics of North America, 28*(2), 373–384.
9. Glaspoli, I. (1997). Stinging insect allergies: Assessing and managing. *Australian Family Physician, 26*(12), 1395–1401.
10. Kaplan, A. (1997). Treatment of chronic urticaria. *Western Journal of Medicine, 167*(5), 348.
11. Kim, K., Safadi, G., & Sheikh, K. (1997). Diagnostic evaluation of type I latex allergy. *Annals of Allergy, Asthma and Immunology, 80,* 66–76.
12. Kumar, A., Busse, W. (1996). Clinical aspects of anti-inflammatory therapy in asthma. *Current Opinion in Pulmonary Medicine, 2*(1), 40–47.
13. Leff, A. (1998). Pharmacologic management of asthma. *Journal of Clinical Immunology, 101,* S397–S399.
14. Lemanske, R. (1998). A review of the current guidelines for allergic rhinitis and asthma. *Journal of Clinical Immunology, 101,* S392–S396.
15. Lemanske, R., & Busse, W. (1997). Asthma. *Journal of the American Medical Association, 278(22),* 1855–1873.
16. Lundeberg, M., et al. (1997). Diagnosis of latex allergy. *Allergy, 52,* 1042–1043.
17. Naclerio, R., & Solomon, W. (1997). Rhinitis and inhalant allergens. *JAMA, 278*(22), 1842–1848.
18. Negro, J., et al. (1997). Leukotrienes and their antagonists in allergic disorders. *Allergy Immunopathology, 25*(2), 104–112.
19. Nettina, S. (1997). Patient with recurrent episodes of hives: Answers and discussion of allergic disorders case study. *Lippincott's Primary Care Practice, 1,* 351–354.
20. Nilsson, G., Metcalfe, D. (1996). Contemporary issues in mast cell biology. *Allergy and Asthma Proceedings, 17*(2), 59–63.
21. Rachelefsky, G. (1998). Pharmacologic management of allergic rhinitis. *Journal of Clinical Immunology, 101,* S367–S369.
22. Rumsaeng, V., & Metcalf, D. (1998). Asthma and food allergy. *Nutrition Reviews, 56*(1), S153–S160.
23. Sabroe, R., & Greaves, M. (1997). Food allergy. *Journal of the American Medical Association, 278*(22), 1888–1894.
24. Schoenwetter, W. (1996). Safe allergen immunotherapy: The correct allergen, the appropriate client, the adequate dose. *Postgraduate Medicine, 100*(2), 123–126, 131–135.
25. Slavin, R. (1998). Complications of allergic rhinitis: Implications for sinusitis and asthma. *Journal of Allergy and Clinical Immunology, 101,* S357–S360.
26. Storms, W. (1998). A comprehensive diagnostic approach to upper airway disease. *Journal of Allergy and Clinical Immunology, 101,* S361–S363.
27. Volcheck, G., & Li, J. (1997). Subspecialty clinics: Allergic diseases. Exercise-induced urticaria and anaphylaxis. *Mayo Clinic Proceedings, 72,* 140–147.
28. Weber, R. (1997). Immunotherapy with allergens. *Journal of the American Medical Association, 278*(22), 1881–1887.
29. Wheeler, A., & Drachenberg, K. (1997). New routes and formulations for allergen-specific immunotherapy. *Allergy, 52*(6), 602–612.
30. Workman, M. L. (1995). Essential concepts of inflammation and immunity. *Critical Care Nursing Clinics of North America, 7*(4), 601–615.

CHAPTER

77

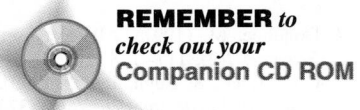

Management of Clients with Autoimmune Disease

Joyce M. Black

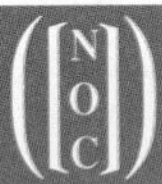

NURSING OUTCOMES CLASSIFICATION (NOC)
for Nursing Diagnoses—Clients with Autoimmune Disease

Activity Intolerance
Self-Care: Activities of Daily Living
Endurance
Altered Health Maintenance
Health Promoting Behavior
Knowledge: Health Promotion
Knowledge: Treatment Regimen
Participation: Health Care Decisions
Social Support
Altered Role Performance
Coping
Depression Control
Psychosocial Adjustment: Life Change
Role Performance

Altered Tissue Perfusion: Peripheral
Tissue Perfusion: Peripheral
Sensory Function: Cutaneous
Chronic Pain
Comfort Level
Depression Control
Pain Control
Pain: Psychological Response
Fatigue
Activity Tolerance
Endurance
Energy Conservation
Sleep
Quality of Life

Impaired Social Interaction
Role Performance
Social Involvement
Impaired Physical Mobility
Ambulation: Walking
Mobility
Self-Care: Activities of Daily Living

Imagine trying to wear an antique suit of armor 24 hours a day. Consider how it would limit your movements. Think about how painful it would be if some of the joint hinges were rusty. Walking or even moving would cause you to feel tired and worn out. For many people living with rheumatoid arthritis or one of the other connective tissue disorders referred to as "rheumatic disorders," life is like living in a painful suit of armor.

More than 100 different connective tissue disorders, or collagen disorders, have been identified,[11] and one in every seven persons, more than 37 million people, have evidence of some form of arthritis. The term *rheuma,* meaning "flux," was used in the first century. Early physicians believed that these diseases originated in the brain as viscous fluid, "a bad humor," which flowed down into the body and attacked joints. We use a more common term, *arthritis,* which means inflammation of a joint.

Connective tissue, the most abundant tissue in the body, is found as loose connective tissue, dense connective tissue, elastic connective tissue, hematopoietic tissue, and strong connective tissue (Box 77–1). The primary functions of connective tissue are to bind cells, organs, and tissues together; to provide warmth; and to permit ease of mechanical movement. Collagen and elastin are the major components of connective tissue. The underlying problem in connective tissue disorders is alteration or disruption of the protein component in the collagen.

The most common disorders are osteoarthritis, osteoporosis, gout, rheumatoid arthritis, systemic lupus erythematosus (SLE), scleroderma, and ankylosing spondylitis. Less common disorders include rheumatic syndromes associated with infectious agents, metabolic and endocrine diseases associated with rheumatic states, connective tissue neoplasms, extra-articular disorders, and miscellaneous disorders associated with joint symptoms. Disorders with an autoimmune cause are discussed in this chapter. Other orthopedic disorders are discussed in Chapter 26. Although the conditions have different clinical patterns, pain and impaired mobility are common problems with these disorders. Many connective tissue diseases are autoimmune disorders without a known cause or cure. Most of these disorders are chronic and follow a course of progressive deterioration. Before the specific disorders can be discussed, an understanding of autoimmunity is important.

This chapter includes material written for the fifth edition by Cleda L. Meyer.

BOX 77–1 Types of Connective Tissue

Loose connective tissue
- Areolar
- Adipose
- Reticular

Dense connective tissue
- Tendons
- Fascia
- Dermis
- Submucosa of gastrointestinal tract
- Fibrous joint capsules

Elastic connective tissue
- Walls of the aorta
- Part of the trachea and bronchi
- Vocal cords
- Some ligaments

Hematopoietic tissue

Strong supportive tissue
- Cartilage
- Bone
- Ligaments

AUTOIMMUNITY

Connective tissue disorders are caused by problems with the immune system. The immune system provides antibodies that recognize and destroy antigens. Antigens can include bacteria, fungi, parasites, viruses, our own damaged tissues, or foreign bodies (e.g., wood splinters). Antibodies can recognize "self" and "non-self" markers. All cells with a nucleus have protein markers on their cell membranes, known as *major histocompatibility complexes* (MHCs). Foreign cells also have cell markers, called *antigenic determinants* or *epitopes.* Properly functioning antibodies recognize both types of markers and either attack them or leave them alone, as appropriate.

Crucial to the process of immunity is the ability to recognize normal tissue and *not* invade or destroy it. When the immune system loses its ability to distinguish normal from abnormal tissue, normal tissue is destroyed. This process is called *autoimmunity;* the disorder arising therefrom is called *autoimmune disease.* There is now compelling evidence that a growing number of disorders are due to autoimmune responses.

Autoimmune disorders form a spectrum; for example:

At one end of the spectrum are conditions in which autoantibodies are directed at a single organ or tissue, resulting in local tissue damage. A classic example is Hashimoto's thyroiditis, in which autoantibodies have absolute specificity for the thyroid tissues (see Chapter 43).

At the other end of the spectrum is SLE (discussed later). In SLE, autoantibodies react with virtually every cell. The result is widespread lesions throughout the body.

In the middle of the spectrum falls Goodpasture's syndrome, in which autoantibodies destroy the basement membrane of the lungs and kidneys, leading to disease in these organs (see Chapter 35).

THEORIES ON AUTOIMMUNITY

Although it would be appealing to explain all autoimmune disorders by a single mechanism, there are a number of ways in which normal tolerance of self is bypassed. More than one defect might be present in a disorders and the defects may vary from one disorder to the next. Furthermore, the development of autoimmune disorders is through the interaction of immunologic, genetic, and environmental components. Not everyone with the same genetic susceptibility will have an autoimmune disorder. Therefore, other factors, such as the environment, probably play a role. Here we can only scratch the surface of a rapidly evolving area of health care.

Normal T helper cell tolerance is crucial to the prevention of autoimmunity. Developing T cells that can recognize normal tissues are usually deleted in the peripheral T cell pools and therefore never reach the tissues. In an autoimmune disorder, this tolerance is bypassed.

Several theories have been proposed to explain the etiology of autoimmune diseases. Genetic predisposition seems to be an important factor. Human leukocyte antigen (HLA) genes are frequently associated with autoimmune disorders. Certain genes appear to increase the risk substantially. The HLA-B27 phenotype is present in 95% of clients with ankylosing spondylitis. However, not everyone with HLA-B27 develops ankylosing spondylitis because of differences in the way the antigen is presented to the immune system.

Modification of the Molecule

If a potentially damaging molecule, called an autoantigenic determinant, is attached to a new carrier, part of the new complex may be recognized as foreign. This process can happen with drugs or microorganisms. Some drugs, like the antihypertensive agent methyldopa, alter the surface of the red blood cell (RBC). This change makes the damaged RBC look foreign and it is attacked (Fig. 77–1*A*).

Release of Sequestered Antigens

The release theory proposes that the self-antigens are isolated from the immune system within an organ during the neonatal period. When the organ is damaged later in life, these antigens are exposed to the immune system, which does not recognize them as self and therefore destroys the damaged cells. Bacteria, viruses, and parasites can degrade collagen and gamma-globulin. There are specific autoantibodies developed for gamma-globulin called *rheumatoid factors* (RFs), which are described later (Fig. 77–1*B*).

Molecular Mimicry

Several infectious agents cross-react with human tissues because of similarities between the molecular segments or epitopes of the foreign antigens and the person's own cells. Rheumatic heart disease sometimes follows streptococcal infection because an antibody to the streptococcal M protein cross-reacts with the M protein in the sarcolemma of the cardiac muscle. Once the infectious agent provokes tissue damage, the process continues because tissue injury releases more self-antigens (Fig. 77–1*C*).

Interaction of T Cells and B Cells

One of the tolerance mechanisms is inactivation of T lymphocytes when fully competent B lymphocytes are present. This normal process is called *clonal anergy.* Sev-

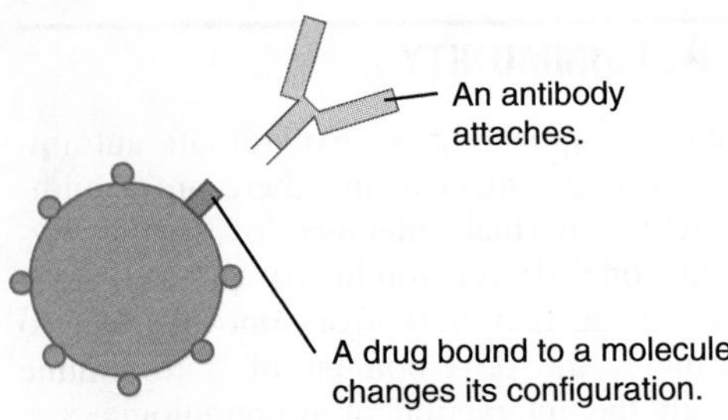
An antibody attaches.
A drug bound to a molecule changes its configuration.
A Modification of the molecule

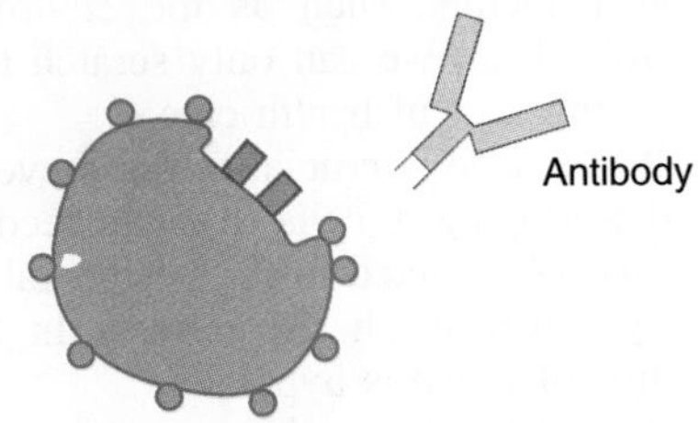
Antibody
B Release of sequestered antigens

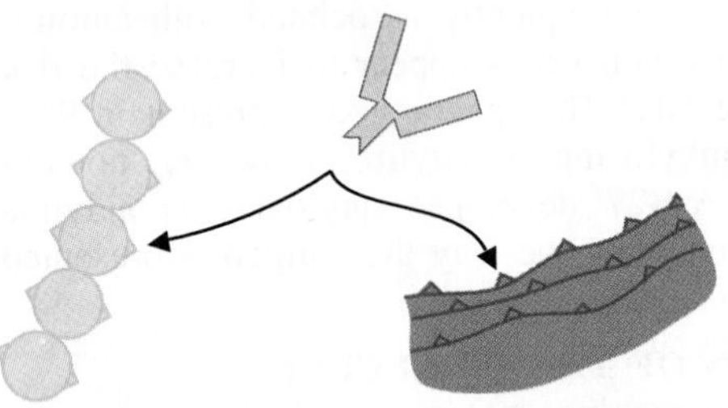
Streptococcus viridans bacteria are attacked.
A sarcolemma with a similar configuration is also attacked.
C Molecular mimicry

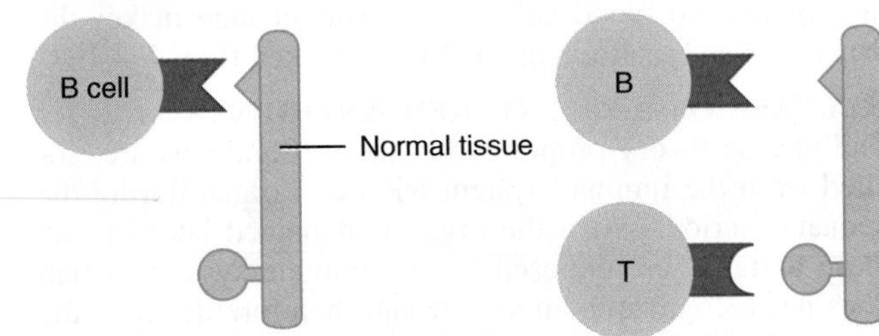
B cell
Normal tissue
B
T
Normal state: A B cell is not stimulated without a T cell.
When a T cell is stimulated, a B cell is also triggered.
D Interaction of B cells and T cells

FIGURE 77–1 Theories of autoimmunity. *A,* Molecule modification. *B,* Release of antigens. *C,* Molecular mimicry. *D,* B- and T-cell interaction.

eral microorganisms are capable of producing polyclonal (antigen-nonspecific) B cells. Failure of this process leads to the production of nonspecific B lymphocytes. *Epstein-Barr virus* (EBV) is often cited as a cause of autoimmune disorders (Fig. 77–1*D*).

Any loss of T suppressor cell function contributes to autoimmunity. Conversely, excessive T cell help may drive B cells to extremely high levels of autoantibody production. Enhanced T helper cell function is seen in people with SLE.

RHEUMATOID ARTHRITIS

Rheumatoid arthritis (RA) is an autoimmune connective tissue disease that most commonly causes inflammation of the joints and joint deformity. RA affects about 1% of the worldwide population,[11] and more than 3 million people in the United States have RA. The incidence is two to three times higher in women until age 65 years, when men are affected equally. Clinical manifestations are most likely to occur in women during the menopausal years (ages 48–52). A 35-year review of research studies showed that median life expectancy for people with RA was shortened by 7 to 10 years in men and 3 to 7 years in women.[27]

Etiology and Risk Factors

A combination of factors, rather than a single cause, appears to be responsible for the onset of RA. RA occurs in genetically predisposed people, and is probably triggered by an unknown infectious agent. Some evidence shows an association of EBV, parvovirus, and other viruses[11] with RA. Seventy per cent of people with RA have the HLA-D4 and HLA-DR1 genes, a fact that supports a possible genetic predisposition. An initial self-limited infection may trigger an autoimmune attack against synovial membranes.

Pathophysiology

The initial infection induces inflammation of the synovial membranes (synovitis). T lymphocytes migrate into the inflamed area, activating monocyte-macrophage and B lymphocytes. In most clients, the antibodies produced during this activation are autoantibodies in the immunoglobulin M (IgM) class. The altered antibodies (*rheumatoid factors* [RFs]) form immune complexes with IgG that are deposited in the synovial membranes, where they stimulate local inflammation. See Understanding Rheumatoid Arthritis and Its Treatment.

Joint deformity in RA occurs from repeated episodes of inflammation. The damage to the joint occurs in four distinct phases (Fig. 77–2):

1. The mechanism of the first phase, *initiation,* is not understood. Some changes in the synovial lining are present.
2. During the *immune response* phase, large numbers of infiltrating lymphocytes (T cells, most of them CD4 cells) and RFs are present in the synovial fluid. These antibodies trigger the release of complement, which attracts leukocytes and macrophages to the area. RFs also stimulate the release of prostaglandins, which attract more leukocytes to the synovial fluid. Cytokines normally stimulate remodeling and rebuilding of cartilage; however, in RA this process is disrupted and cartilage is destroyed.
3. As the disease process continues during the *inflammatory* phase, the resultant swelling damages tiny blood vessels in the synovial membrane, which contains the synovial fluid. In response to this damage, the body releases arachidonic acid and lysosomal enzymes. Oxygen radicals are also present.

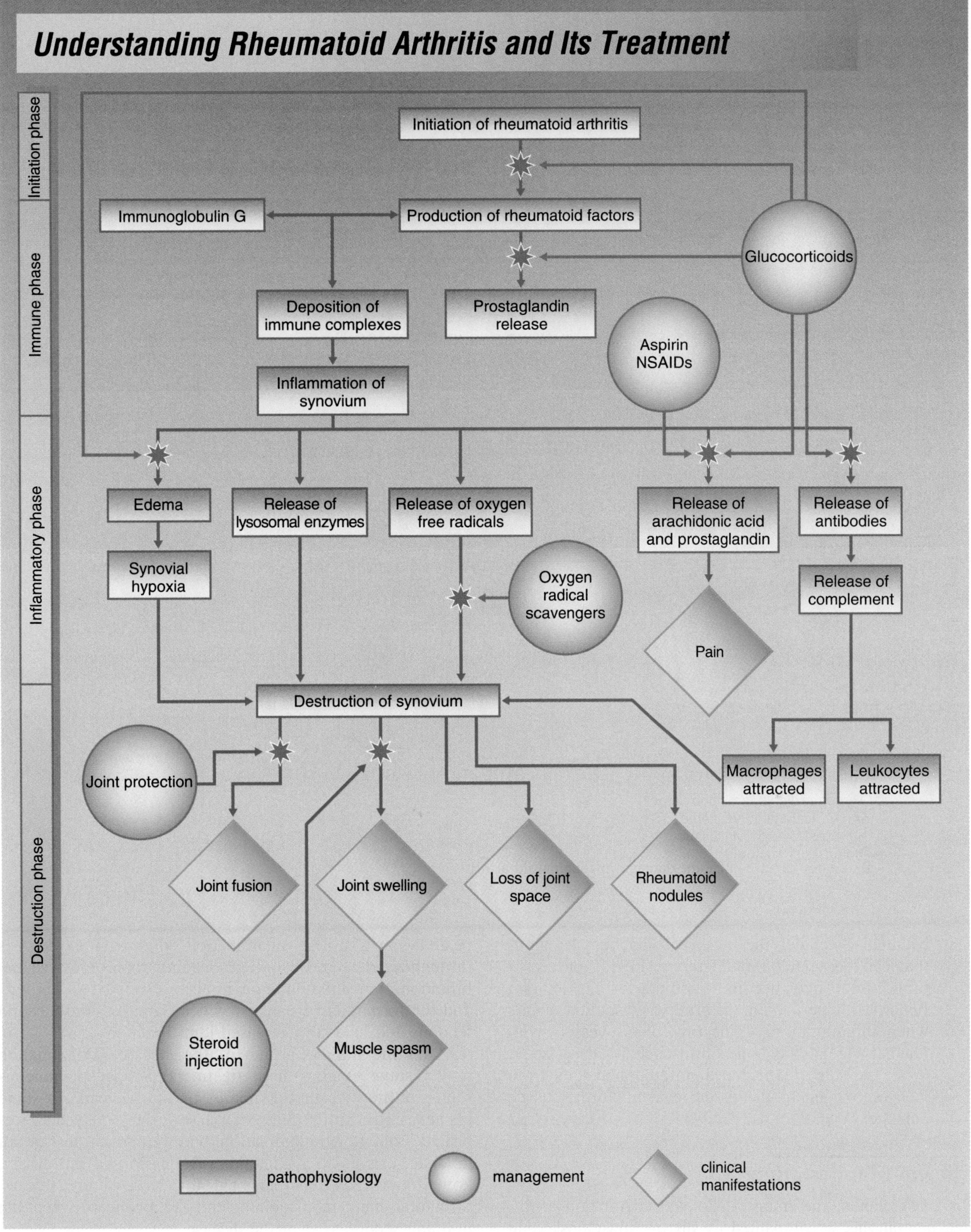

These substances create fissures in the surface of the synovium. They intensify the inflammation, eventually causing cells to enlarge and change into hyperactive stromal cells that thicken the membrane.

4. The *destruction* phase occurs over time. If the inflammatory process is not arrested, a thickened fibrous scar tissue (pannus) is formed. Pannus adheres to the articular surface of the cartilage and

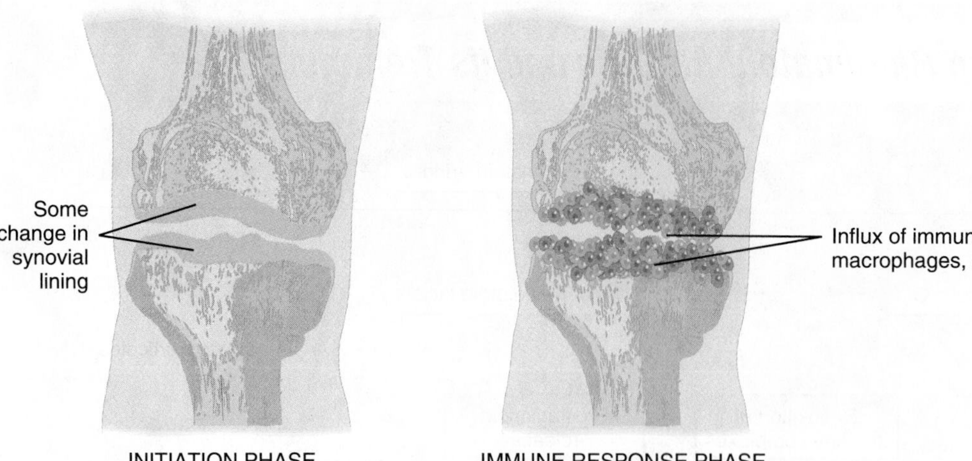

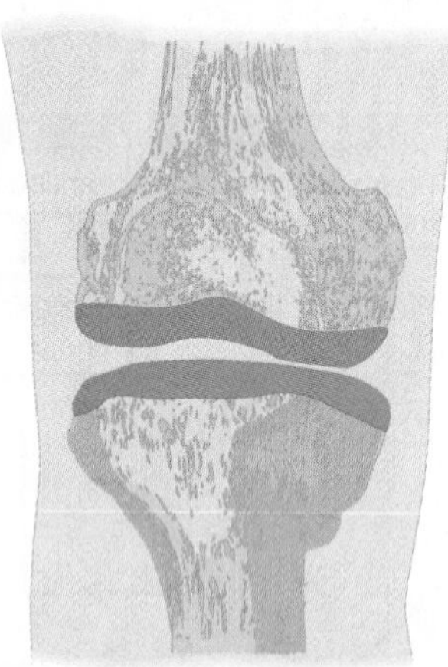

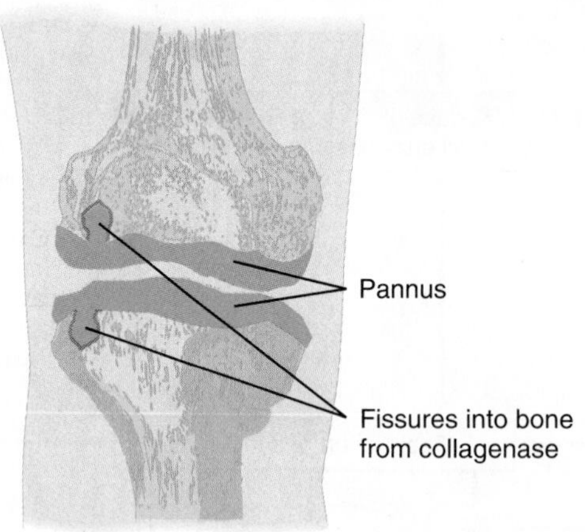

FIGURE 77–2 The four phases of joint damage in rheumatoid arthritis.

eventually invades the bone, causing bony erosions that can be seen on radiographs. In this phase, fibrous tissue may become calcified, leading to joint fusion with permanent deformity. Vasculitis occurs when inflammation of the tiny blood vessels with platelets, leukocytes, and fibrin occludes the vessels. When vessels are occluded, infarction results from lack of oxygen to the tissue, causing further tissue damage.

Clinical Manifestations

For most clients, the manifestations of RA begin as increasing fatigue, accompanied by diffuse musculoskeletal pain, low-grade fever, anorexia, and weight loss. Stiffness occurs after inactivity, such as sleep or prolonged sitting. In fact, the duration of morning stiffness is one measure of the severity of RA.

With the passage of time, the manifestations become more sustained. The more common course includes repeated periods of inflammation of varying degrees throughout the course of RA, leading to progressive debilitation. The inflammation is accompanied by synovitis and the formation of pannus, which damages muscles and tendons and leads to decreased joint function.

After the initial flare-up of the disease, inflammation may resolve even without treatment, and a spontaneous remission may occur for months or 1 to 2 years. In some instances, this remission may last up to 25 years. Repeated bouts of inflammation and remission lead to a gradual loss of joint function. Remission is not likely, however, if RA has persisted for more than 2 years. Structural damage of joints tends to occur between the first and second year of the disease.

Since RA is a systemic disease, clinical manifestations may occur in various parts of the body; however, the joints are generally affected first. Joints tend to be affected symmetrically. For example, if one wrist is affected, the other is likely to be affected also. The wrist, proximal interphalangeal (PIP), and metacarpophalangeal

(MCP) joints are usually involved first. Joint swelling is more apparent in the morning after an accumulation of fluid during the night.

Clinical manifestations of RA are divided into (1) *articular,* or within the joint (e.g., synovitis, hand deformity, muscle spasm and weakness, rheumatoid nodules) and (2) *extra-articular,* or outside the joint (e.g., Sjögren's syndrome, vasculitis, pulmonary fibrosis, pericarditis, nerve compression, Felty's syndrome).

Synovial fluid is a protective cushion that permits free joint articulation. Inflammation inside the synovial capsule, spreading into synovial fluid, results in swelling, warmth, pain, and increased pressure on surrounding tissue. The inflammatory process of synovitis causes the tendons and ligaments to become shortened and less flexible, leading to deformity. The wrist, PIP, and MCP joints are most commonly involved. The result of this involvement is three types of hand deformity (Fig. 77–3):

1. *Ulnar drift* occurs when synovitis stretches and damages the tendons. Eventually, the tendons become shortened and fixed. An imbalance of damaged extensor tendons and intact flexor tendons causes the *subluxation* (drift) of the MCP joint.
2. *Boutonnière deformity* results from flexion of the PIP joint and hyperextension of the distal interphalangeal (DIP) joint extensor tendon, causing it to shift.
3. *Swan-neck deformity* is due to flexion contracture of the MCP joint, hyperextension of the PIP, and flexion of the DIP. Muscle spasm occurs in RA when the muscles are stretched over inflamed joints. The abnormal position of enlarged bone ends and inflamed muscles leads to further deformity. Pain and swelling cause the client to avoid using the joint or to move the joint guardedly, further weakening the muscles.

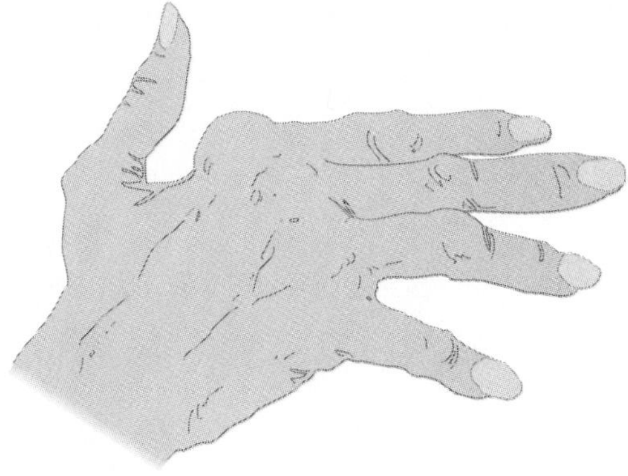
Ulnar drift

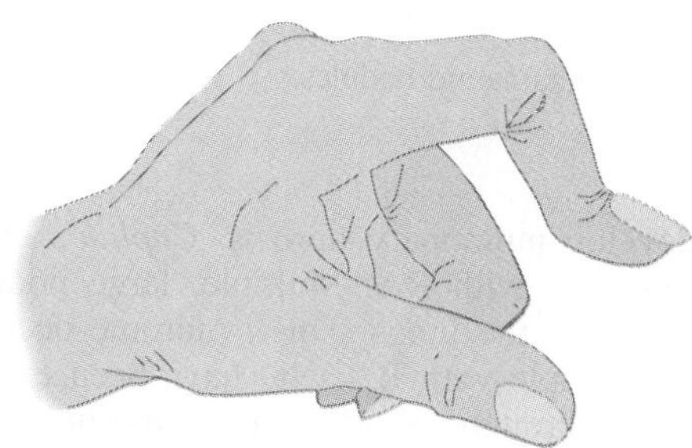
Boutonnière deformity

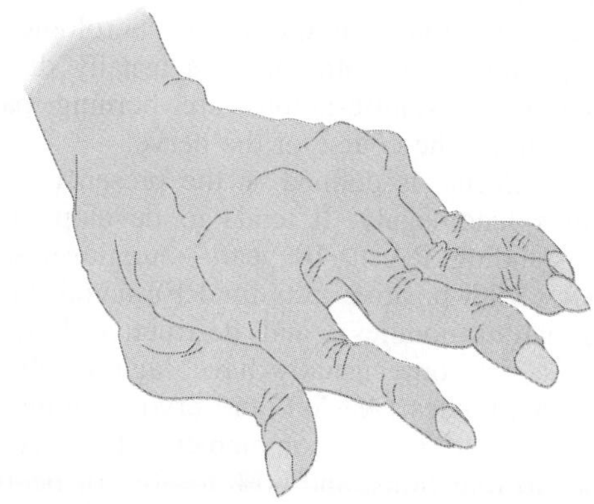
Swan-neck deformity

FIGURE 77–3 Three types of hand deformity characteristic of clients with rheumatoid arthritis.

Rheumatoid nodules are composed of granulation tissue surrounding a central core of fibrous debris. These firm, nontender nodules are usually in subcutaneous tissue, although they have been found in visceral organs, including the lungs and the heart. They tend to develop during exacerbations of the disease. The most common sites are the wrist, carpal, knee, and elbow joints, and MCP and PIP joints of the fingers (Fig. 77–4). Rheumatoid nodules behind the knee may be tender, and this tenderness may be mistaken for a positive Homans' sign.

Extra-articular manifestations of RA may occur at any time in the course of the disorder and may, at times, overshadow the articular manifestations. These systemic manifestations must be treated quickly because they are major predictors of morbidity and even mortality.

Ocular problems are commonly associated with connective tissue disorders. Many of the problems are potentially blinding. The most common ocular problem seen in RA is *Sjögren's syndrome,* (see later). These people usually have scleritis and episcleritis. Episcleritis produces redness in the eye and some discomfort but no pain, and there is seldom a discharge. It rarely, if ever, causes loss of vision. Episcleritis is a benign self-limiting problem that seldom requires treatment. In contrast, scleritis can lead to blindness and severe ocular pain. Untreated, the problem can lead to ulcers of the cornea and glaucoma.

Vasculitis is actually a group of disorders, including polyarteritis nodosa, systemic necrotizing vasculitis, and allergic granulomatous angiitis. All of these disorders result in necrotizing inflammation of the blood vessels. Circulating immune complexes are deposited in the blood vessels, causing inflammation and damage to large and small vessels. The result is end-stage organ damage. The specific manifestations vary, depending on the organs affected.

Pulmonary fibrosis, a common problem in clients with RA, is caused in part by smoking. Up to 28% of persons

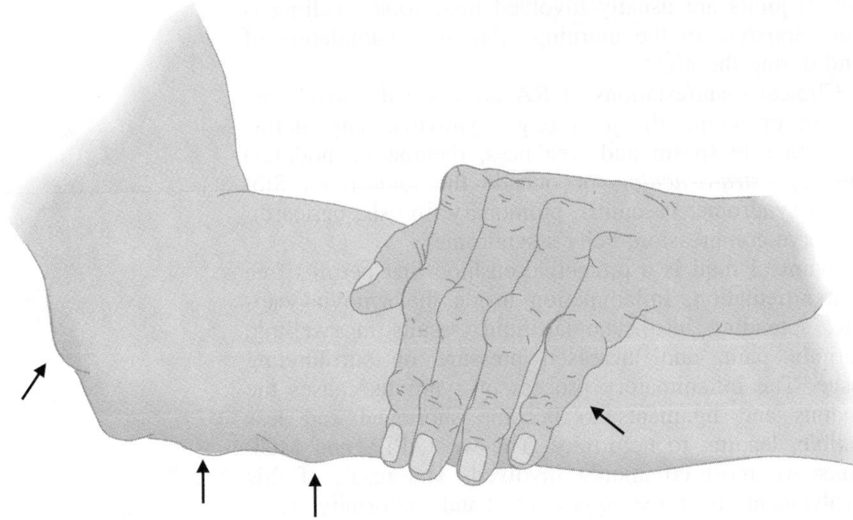

FIGURE 77–4 Rheumatoid nodules.

with RA develop pulmonary fibrosis. *Caplan's syndrome* is pneumoconiosis with RA. Multiple, large nodules are present throughout the lungs. This syndrome occurs most commonly in people with RA who have been exposed to silica, usually through occupational exposure, such as granite workers.

Pericarditis is the most common cardiac disorder in people with RA (~50%). Mitral and aortic valve disease have been noted.

Nerve compression in RA leads to neurologic impairment. Peripheral nerve entrapment is usually due to extensive synovitis. Manifestations are burning pain and paresthesias along the course of the nerve.

Felty's syndrome is defined as the presence of leukopenia with splenomegaly. It tends to develop in people with long-standing RA (>10 years' duration), seropositive RA (RA with positive tests for RF), nodular RA (RA with rheumatoid nodules), and destructive RA. People with Felty's syndrome usually have high levels of RF, antinuclear antibodies (ANAs), and cryoglobulins and diminished levels of serum complement. The neutropenia predisposes to infections, and 60% to 90% of people with Felty's syndrome develop pneumonia or joint infections. Felty's syndrome is usually managed with disease-modifying antirheumatic drugs for RA, such as gold salts or methotrexate.

Clients presenting with manifestations suggestive of RA actually have RA only if the following criteria are met:

- Morning stiffness lasting at least 1 hour
- Swelling of three or more joints
- Swelling of the wrist, PIP, or MCP joints
- Symmetrical joint swelling
- Rheumatoid nodules
- Positive results on tests for RF
- Changes on hand radiographs typical of RA, specifically erosions or bony decalcification

The first four criteria must be present for at least 6 weeks. A definite diagnosis requires that four of these seven features be present at the same time.

Diagnostic Findings

Additional manifestations are visible only on x-ray studies, which are of value in diagnosis and in the evaluation of treatment. High-resolution films, as used in mammography, aid in the early detection of bony erosions. Radiographs are also helpful for identifying narrowing of the joint spaces and loss of cartilage (Fig. 77–5). These ero-

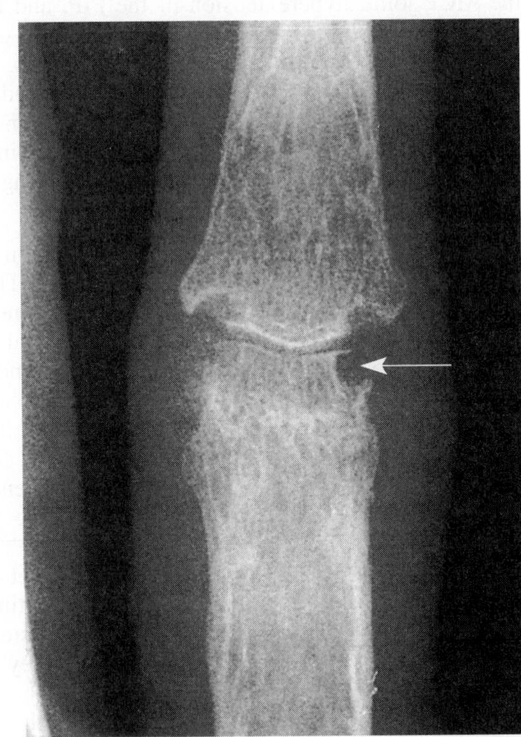

FIGURE 77–5 X-ray of an interphalangeal joint affected by rheumatoid arthritis. Pocket erosion is shown with the arrow. Pocket erosions can spread into trabecular bone and weaken the bone surface. There is also joint space narrowing and soft tissue swelling. (From Resnick, D., Berthiaume, M. J., & Sartoris, D. [1993]: Imaging. In W. N. Kelley, et al. [Eds.], *Textbook of rheumatology* [4th ed., p. 600]. Philadelphia: W. B. Saunders.)

sions may first be detected at the edges of the bone that have direct contact with the inflamed synovium. The formation of pannus and osteoporotic changes may also be detected on x-ray film.

Laboratory tests for the presence of RF aid in definitive diagnosis; however, elevations in RF levels take a while to appear. Within the first 3 months after the onset of clinical manifestations, test results for RF are positive in only 25% of people with RA; after 1 year, however, RF is found in 80% of people with RA. Nevertheless, RF is not specific for RA and may be found in 3% of the population without any clinical manifestations of RA.

Other laboratory findings in RA include an accelerated erythrocyte sedimentation rate (ESR), elevated serum globulins, and a positive test for C-reactive protein. A secondary finding is normochromic, normocytic anemia, which is often found in chronic disease. Synovial fluid may be aspirated for examination. Abnormal findings in the synovial fluid of clients with RA include reduced viscosity and white blood cell (WBC) counts as high as 50,000/mm^3.

Outcome Management

Medical Management

The goals for clients with RA are to relieve pain, reduce inflammation, protect articular surfaces, maintain function, and control systemic involvement. The management of RA uses a balanced program of pharmacologic therapy with nonsteroidal anti-inflammatory drugs (NSAIDs), education, physical therapy, occupational therapy, and psychosocial therapy. With this balanced program, many clients with RA are able to maintain function and continue active, productive lifestyles. If these measures are unsuccessful, pharmacologic therapy with disease-modifying antirheumatic drugs may be used. Corticosteroid therapy, surgery, and therapy with experimental drugs are reserved for RA resistant to less aggressive approaches.

For most clients with RA, diagnosis and treatment occur in a community setting. Part of the initial and ongoing assessment of people with RA involves determining their degree of functional impairment. The American College of Rheumatology identifies four categories for rating functional ability in people with arthritis:

1 = normal function
2 = adequate function for normal activities
3 = limited function for activities of daily living (ADL)
4 = inability to function independently

Relieve Pain and Inflammation

Medical management of RA involves four general approaches (Table 71–1):

1. Aspirin and other NSAIDs as well as simple analgesics are used to control the local inflammatory process. Anti-inflammatory medications impair the natural action of the mediators of inflammation (arachidonic acid, prostaglandins, and oxygen radicals). These drugs work on the end process of inflammation, and the client's response to these drugs is usually quick and easily noticed. However, because these drugs do not reverse the initial arthritic processes in RA, bone edges remain rough and weakened, and inflammation returns once the effects of the drugs subside.
2. Although low-dose oral glucocorticoids have been widely used to suppress inflammation, they may also retard the development and progression of bone erosions.
3. A variety of agents classified as disease-modifying or slow-acting antirheumatic drugs appear to decrease elevated levels of acute-phase reactants in treated clients and are thought to modify the destructive capacity of the disease. Other agents, the immunosuppressive and cytotoxic drugs, ameliorate the disease process in some clients.
4. Intra-articular glucocorticoids can provide transient relief when systemic medical therapy has failed to resolve inflammation.

A "last-resort" approach that can be entertained involves the use of investigational therapies, including combinations of disease-modifying antirheumatic drugs (DMARDs) and other experimental agents. Substituting *omega-3 fatty acids,* such as eicosapentaenoic acid found in certain fish oils, for dietary omega-6 essential fatty acids, found in meat, has provided symptomatic improvement in clients with RA. Some nontraditional approaches also have been claimed to be effective (e.g., diet, plant and animal extracts, vaccines, hormones, topical preparations). Many of these are costly, and none has been shown to be effective. However, belief in their efficacy ensures their continued use by some clients.

Whole-body rest can decrease joint inflammation in RA, and many clients with RA find that an afternoon nap reduces fatigue and helps them cope with the rest of the day. In addition, rest of specific joints with splints protects the joints and facilitates healing. However, the use of rest requires a fine balance; once inflammation subsides, the client should begin activity again to preserve as much joint function as possible. Of interest is that when people with RA have strokes, the joints affected by RA lose their inflammation. Clearly, activity and strain exacerbate the inflammation.

Protect Articular Surfaces

Joint protection and alleviation of discomfort are important aspects of the management of RA. Joint protection techniques and techniques for carrying out tasks without pain are typically taught by an occupational therapist and reinforced by nurses. Table 77–2 lists the principles of joint protection and strategies for lessening discomfort.

Maintain Function

Range of Motion Exercises. Safe and effective exercises strengthen weakened muscles and improve function. Exercises may be carried out in group activities or independently. Daily range-of-motion (ROM) exercises are an important component of this program and do relieve pain. Isometric exercises help maintain muscle function, even when the client wears splints. Physical therapists also measure clients for orthoses, splints, and assistive devices that may be necessary in advanced disease. A correct fit of such devices is important to preserve a functional joint and maintain skin integrity. Physi-

TABLE 77–1 MEDICATIONS USED IN THE TREATMENT OF RHEUMATOID ARTHRITIS

Class	Example	Action	Therapeutic Outcomes	Adverse Outcomes	Dosing
Anti-inflammatory	Aspirin (Ecotrin)	Inhibits synthesis of prostaglandin	Reduction in pain and inflammation	Increased bleeding tendencies, gastric ulceration	Take with food, milk, or antacid; toxic levels cause tinnitus; observe for dark stools (occult bleeding)
Nonsteroidal anti-inflammatory drugs (NSAIDs)	Ibuprofen (Motrin, Advil)	Inhibits prostaglandin synthesis by blocking precursor enzymes	Reduction in joint pain and inflammation	GI upset, gastritis, GI bleeding Dizziness Decreased platelet aggregation	Do not crush enteric-coated forms Take with food or milk
Nonsteroidal anti-inflammatory agents (COX-2)	Celecoxib (Celebrex)	Inhibits COX-2 enzymes	Decrease in joint pain, tenderness, and swelling	GI upset No effect on platelet aggregation	Take with food or milk
Glucocorticoids	Prednisone	Decreases inflammation by suppressing the migration of WBCs and the immune response	Marked reduction in pain and inflammation	Delayed wound healing, insomnia, increased appetite Addison's crises if withdrawn suddenly or during periods of intense stress	Take with food or milk Taper dose slowly
Disease-modifying antirheumatic drugs (DMARDs)	Methotrexate	Immunosuppressive	Inhibits DNA synthesis	Bone marrow suppression, nausea and vomiting	Take on an empty stomach Monitor CBC, differential, and platelet counts

CBC, complete blood count; COX, cyclooxygenase; DNA, deoxyribonucleic acid; GI, gastrointestinal; WBC, white blood cell.

cal therapists also help clients learn the correct methods of using walkers and wheelchairs when the lower extremities are severely impaired by RA.

OCCUPATIONAL THERAPY. Occupational therapists teach clients ways to avoid placing strain on weak joints. For example, to protect joints during ADL, they may instruct clients to use both hands to carry items or may teach clients with weak grips how to use jar openers, levers attached to doorknobs, and other adaptive devices. Occupational therapists can also recommend workplace modifications and modifications in clothing to assist in dressing. For example, they might advise wearing clothing with self-fastening fabric (e.g., Velcro) closures rather than zippers. Occupational therapy promotes independence and enhances self-esteem.

CONTROL SYSTEMIC INVOLVEMENT

Anti-inflammatory medications are used to control systemic involvement. Most clients' manifestations can be managed with aspirin, cyclooxygenase (COX-2) inhibitors, and NSAIDs. Sometimes anti-inflammatory treatments call for corticosteroids, slow-acting antirheumatic drugs, and some experimental medications (see Table 77–1).

ASPIRIN. Aspirin (acetylsalicylic acid) is a prostaglandin inhibitor used to decrease inflammation. Aspirin has historically been one of the first drugs used to treat RA. However, it is used less often today because the high doses required in RA leave the client susceptible to troublesome side effects, such as gastrointestinal (GI) irritation and bleeding, impaired platelet function, and ototoxicity. To achieve anti-inflammatory effects, the therapeutic dose of aspirin is 2.4 to 3.6 g/day. At these high doses, aspirin is frequently toxic. In addition, to sustain therapeutic blood levels, aspirin must be taken four times a day, and such frequent dosing often leads to problems with compliance with the medication regimen. As with the other NSAIDs, clients should be instructed to take aspirin with food and watch for clinical manifestations of GI bleeding, easy bruising, and tinnitus. Few clients tolerate the doses needed to achieve therapeutic benefit.

CYCLOOXYGENASE 2 INHIBITORS. Celecoxib is an anti-inflammatory agent that inhibits COX-2 enzymes while allowing normal activity of COX-1 enzymes. Celecoxib has been shown to be effective at all doses studied in providing pain relief and anti-inflammatory relief while reducing the GI side effects more than naproxen, an anti-inflammatory agent that inhibits both COX-1 and COX-2 enzymes.

OTHER NSAIDS. NSAIDs are used extensively to decrease inflammation and provide pain relief in clients with RA. Many NSAIDs are available over the counter at low doses. The most common NSAIDs are ibuprofen (Motrin, Advil), naproxen (Naprosyn), tolmetin (Tolectin), sulindac (Clinoril), piroxicam (Feldene), diclofenac (Voltaren), and ketoprofen (Orudis). The therapeutic effect of these drugs is to inhibit prostaglandin synthesis, thus decreasing the pain and swelling that accompany the inflammatory response. Unfortunately, because NSAIDs suppress prostaglandin production, they also decrease production of gastric mucus and intestinal bicarbonate. These unwanted changes in the GI mucosa greatly increase the risk of bleeding and ulceration. These drugs are therefore usually taken with food, and a histamine receptor antagonist such as ranitidine (Zantac) is usually prescribed concurrently to reduce secretion of stomach acids.

NSAIDs also decrease platelet adherence ("stickiness") and therefore increase the risk of bleeding. Clients therefore need to be taught to watch for bruising and clinical manifestations of GI bleeding. When about to undergo surgery or dental work, clients should also inform the surgeon or dentist of their current medications.

Most NSAIDs permit simpler dosing schedules and have fewer side effects than aspirin. Nevertheless, clients need to be taught the importance of using the prescribed dosage and the need for continued medical monitoring during therapy.

GLUCOCORTICOIDS. Glucocorticoids, such as prednisone and cortisone, have both anti-inflammatory and immunosuppressive effects; however, they do not directly modify RA. Long-term use of these drugs is accompanied by serious side effects, such as adrenal suppression, osteoporosis, paper-thin skin, delayed healing, and cataracts. The health care provider, therefore, usually tries to control manifestations with other medications first. The lowest possible dose to establish control of pain and inflammation is used. The dose is reduced as soon as possible to keep the client on the smallest dose that keeps the symptoms under control. The dosage must be increased during periods of major physiologic stress, such as illness or surgery, because the suppressed adrenal glands cannot respond with the usual cortisol boost during stress. Careful monitoring of the client taking glucocorticoids is essential because of the serious complications that result from their long-term use.

When inflammation and tenderness are localized to particular joints, intra-articular injections of corticosteroids may be helpful. Reduced pain and improved function may last for weeks or months after these injections. Corticosteroid injections have been useful in delaying surgery for carpal tunnel syndrome, and they can decrease the need for larger oral doses of corticosteroids. Intra-articular injection of corticosteroids is a sterile procedure requiring careful skin preparation. The physician first aspirates excess fluid, then injects the corticosteroids. The client should keep the needle insertion area clean, dry, and covered with a sterile dressing for the first 24 hours after the procedure.

TABLE 77–2 PRINCIPLES OF JOINT PROTECTION AND STRATEGIES FOR LESSENING DISCOMFORT

Principles of Joint Protection	Strategies for Lessening Discomfort
Respect pain (fear of pain can lead to inactivity; ignoring pain can lead to joint damage)	Carry out activities and exercise only to the point of fatigue or discomfort Reduce the time spent in doing painful activities Avoid doing activities (other than gentle ROM) when joints are inflamed
Balance work and rest	Rest 5–10 min periodically when doing tasks that take more time Get sufficient sleep Take a 30-min rest during the afternoon
Reduce effort by joints	Slide objects rather than lift them Store items at convenient heights Avoid stooping, bending, or overreaching Sit to work whenever possible
Avoid positions of stress on joints	Avoid tight pinch or grip: use built-up handles and holders for objects such as toothbrushes and pens Avoid turning fingers toward the little finger: turn fingers toward the thumb Avoid wrist flexion and rotation during stirring (e.g., use spoon like a dagger) Use two hands to lift or carry objects Always consider adaptive devices (jar opener, reachers, built-up keys)
Use larger, stronger joints	Lift with palm and forearm instead of fingers Use a backpack, waist pack, or shoulder bag instead of a handbag
Use joints in most stable positions	Avoid or minimize excessive stretch of joint ligaments (e.g., rise from chair symmetrically and avoid leaning to either side) Maintain good posture
Avoid remaining in one position	Change position (or stretch) every 20 min Balance sitting tasks with those that require moving around
Avoid activities that cannot be stopped	Break activities into defined parts

ROM, range of motion.
From Maher, A., Salmond, S., & Pellino, T. (Eds.). (1994). *Orthopedic nursing.* Philadelphia: W. B. Saunders.

SLOW-ACTING ANTIRHEUMATIC DRUGS. Slow-acting antirheumatic drugs (SAARDs), also called disease-modifying antirheumatic drugs (DMARDs), are gaining acceptance for primary therapy. These medications—gold salts, antimalarials, immunosuppressive agents, and *d*-penicillamine—seem to slow progression of RA by blocking the immunologic aspects of inflammation. However, like other drugs used in the treatment of RA, they do not correct the underlying cause of the disease. Previously used for clients who did not respond adequately to symptomatic therapy, these drugs are being used more aggressively to arrest clinical manifestations and thus decrease joint destruction. They may be used alone or in combination with NSAIDs. Because DMARDs are generally slow-acting, they must be taken for several months before an effective response becomes noticeable. Some of these agents are also used in cancer treatment. Because the doses in RA are much lower than those used in cancer treatment, the side effects are therefore decreased, but careful monitoring for toxicity is still important.

EXPERIMENTAL DRUGS. Experimental drugs are also used in the treatment of RA. Such drugs include biologic response modifiers, immunomodifiers, antioxidants, and inhibitors of cartilage metabolism. Of course, when these drugs are used, clients are monitored closely so that therapy can be adjusted to avoid or decrease side effects.

The stress of living with a chronic disease such as RA, with pain and loss of independent function, can lead to depression. Altered body image, sexual problems, and decreased ability to work outside the home also contribute to depressed mood. Depressed clients report more pain and fatigue and decreased activity, with further loss of independence and function.

Outcomes

Living with a progressive, painful, chronic debilitating condition like RA presents many problems. Current therapeutic regimens enable many people to preserve function and lead productive lives with less pain. The psychosocial problems associated with this disease present additional challenges. The median life expectancy of persons with RA is shortened by 3 to 7 years. The increased mortality rate seems to be limited to clients with more severe articular disease and can be attributed largely to infection and GI bleeding. Drug therapy also may play a role in the increased mortality rate seen in these individuals. Factors correlated with early death include disability, disease duration or severity, glucocorticoid use, age at onset, and low socioeconomic or educational status.

Nursing Management of the Medical Client

The primary nursing goal in the management of a client with RA is to promote the healthiest possible life for the client. The nurse's role is to assess, educate, coordinate treatments, facilitate adaptations in the home, reevaluate periodically, and serve as client advocate. Providing information to help the client deal with chronic pain, comply with treatment, and cope with a chronic disease are some of the challenges faced in managing clients with RA. The nurse provides information and encourages the client's self-management by allowing choices about when to exercise, which adaptive equipment to use, and what other self-care techniques to employ. Clients with RA appreciate caring and empathy by the nurses.

See the Bridge to Home Health Care feature on independent living.

ASSESSMENT

Nursing assessment begins by identifying the client's concerns and needs. The history should include information about the duration of clinical manifestations and ways the client has been managing those manifestations, particularly pain. It is important to identify other conditions that the client may have. The client's current understanding of RA and the coping strategies used for dealing with pain and fatigue are important. Determine the methods that the client is now using to obtain pain relief (and the amount of pain that the client considers tolerable). Find out what methods the client is using for joint protection.

Evaluate the amount of swelling and pain in each joint, and the number of affected joints (to obtain a "joint count"). Recall that disease severity is based on the joint count, laboratory findings, and radiographic changes. In addition, physiologic measures of function such as a timed walk, measures of grip strength, and results of self-report instruments that evaluate flexion and extension enable further evaluation of functional impairment and the impact of the disease on the client's life. Assess for current clinical manifestations in the client's eyes, heart, lungs, and peripheral nerves. It is important to note new manifestations and marked changes in previous clinical manifestations.

RA can be a crippling disorder. After 10 to 15 years with the disorder, less than one half of clients can still perform their own ADL. These physical limitations can greatly alter the client's usual role in the family, ability to work gainfully, ability to participate in family events, and ability to be an active sexual partner. Extreme fatigue and pain usually lead to early bedtimes and a reluctance to socialize. In addition, physical changes in the body can lead to lowered self-esteem. Western society values beauty and youth. Clients may find it psychologically difficult to be seen in public and deal with stares brought on by a hand deformity and other changes. As the client grieves the loss of a healthy, youthful body, thoughts of suicide can occur. Be sensitive to these issues and bring them into the discussion if the client or family hints at suicidal thoughts. Despite these changes, however, RA does not have to be a crippling disorder; with good medical and nursing care, many clients can maintain a healthy, productive, active lifestyle.

In caring for clients with RA, the nurse also acts as a liaison to obtain orders and arrange appointments with physical therapists, occupational therapists, and other providers. In rural settings, where these "extra" services are limited, you may need to provide supplemental information that these specialists would otherwise provide, and you may need to use printed resources to help clients.

DIAGNOSIS, OUTCOMES, INTERVENTION

Chronic Pain. The primary diagnosis of clients with RA is *Chronic Pain related to inflammation and swelling from pressure on surrounding tissues, joint deformity, and joint destruction.* The amount of pain that these clients

BRIDGE TO HOME HEALTH CARE

Increasing Independent Living with Rheumatoid Arthritis

Because the development of rheumatoid arthritis is often insidious, it is important to identify clients who are having difficulty managing in their homes and provide health education and home modification information before their problems become significant. Pain, fatigue, and joint deformities often limit clients' ability to perform normal reach and grasp patterns, and, therefore, limit their ability to perform daily tasks. Examples of such tasks are turning knobs, obtaining items from the refrigerator and cupboard shelves, getting dressed, writing, and using the phone. Mobility may be impaired to the extent that it is difficult to get on and off chairs or the toilet, and to stand long enough to prepare a meal or take a shower.

Clients commonly feel as if they cannot control pain and fatigue because of the dramatic fluctuations they experience. Clients may react by insisting that they perform tasks even during acute inflammatory stages, a decision that may increase joint stress, pain, and deformity. In contrast, other clients may stop performing some activities of daily living (ADL) and may become reliant on others. This latter decision may decrease their overall daily activity level, leading to weakness and dependence. All of these clients need accurate information.

Clients who have rheumatoid arthritis often experience joint pain with activity. For example, pain can occur when they attempt to lift a milk carton. Clients may experience pain long after a task is performed, as when they sustain the pinch needed to use an eating utensil. They need to identify situations that increase their pain so that they and their health care providers can problem-solve and determine the best use of adaptive methods and devices. Without this understanding, clients may become reluctant to use various beneficial approaches. For example, to decrease joint pain, clients should consider using devices such as large-handled eating utensils and using a small pitcher of milk instead of a heavy milk carton.

The disease process and daily, repetitive joint strain can lead to joint stress and deformity. When clients struggle each day to get out of a low recliner chair or obtain heavy dishes from a shelf above shoulder height, they may create further deformity and pain. Use health education to help clients understand this relationship and become more receptive to beneficial changes, such as higher chairs or rearranging the kitchen.

It is critical that clients maintain consistent range of motion and strength activities as well as ADL while using the correct joint protection and energy-conservation methods. Before clients use the assistance of housekeepers and home health aides, or lift-up chairs and other equipment, the potential benefits and disadvantages must be carefully calculated. When introduced at the appropriate times, such assistance may allow clients to remain in their own homes. If assistance is introduced before occupational and physical therapists have completed evaluations, it may lead to further dependence and deterioration.

Health education should incorporate the client's goals and lifestyle. Clients need information about the link between their disease and ADL and how they can positively influence this link. To be successful, clients need to use adaptive methods and devices correctly and balance their rest and activity in addition to taking medications. The home health care team is responsible for providing clients with tools and options that will promote independence and productivity at present and in the future. In this way, clients can make choices about their lifestyles and maintain maximum independence within their homes.

Linda J. Svatora, OTR/L, MBA, *Occupational therapist, Visiting Nurse Association of Omaha, Omaha, Nebraska*

experience permeates all aspects of their life. Recall the earlier analogy of living in a rusty armored suit.

Outcomes. The client's pain will be controlled at a level that permits the client to perform ADL.

Interventions. Chronic pain must be managed to allow the client to perform daily activities and function normally, to increase mobility, and to reduce fatigue. Teach the client the purpose and expected action of prescribed analgesics. You can use a handout to describe which side effects the client should report. Other pain relief interventions may include the use of heat or cold, exercise, and massage. Paraffin baths have been used for arthritis of the hands; however, the greatest benefit from this intervention occurs when the client exercises immediately after the treatment. Cold therapy is applied by cold packs, ice massage, immersion, or vapocoolant sprays. Although heat or cold may reduce pain, they may not be effective in decreasing inflammation. Transcutaneous electrical nerve stimulation (TENS) units have been used to reduce pain and local joint inflammation if only one or two joints are involved. Caution should be used when applying topical creams, rubs, or sprays (see the Client Education Guide).

Relaxation techniques, such as guided imagery, help some people cope with pain. Classes to teach coping techniques have been effective in decreasing pain and anxiety. When correctly performed, massage may also help relieve muscular aches and pain; however, it is important to massage only the surrounding muscles. *Never massage acutely inflamed joints;* doing so may aggravate inflammation.

Many clients with RA are perceived as demanding and manipulative. This misconception has stemmed from clients' attempts to control what little of their world they can. Chronic pain and fatigue often push coping skills to the limit. With what little energy is left, these clients attempt to control other parts of their lives. Approach these clients with compassion and appreciation for their problems. Many of their idiosyncrasies, such as statements like "Don't put the covers over my toes," are attempts to reduce pain. There is no such thing as a rheumatoid personality.

Impaired Physical Mobility. Another common nursing diagnosis is *Impaired Physical Mobility related to pain, stiffness, and joint deformity.* Using the armored suit analogy, you can see how movement of any kind is hampered when most or all of the articular joints are inflamed.

Outcomes. The client will maintain mobility at the highest possible level to carry out desired activities.

CLIENT EDUCATION GUIDE

Using Topical Pain Relievers

Topical pain relievers work in several ways, depending on their ingredients. Some, which contain salicylates, the substance found in aspirin, may penetrate through the skin to the joint and reduce pain. Other pain relievers contain ingredients such as menthol or camphor that irritate the skin and distract attention from the actual pain. Still others contain capsaicin, a substance found in hot peppers, which reduces the pain signal to the brain.

Regardless of the mechanism of action of the pain reliever, the Arthritis Foundation recommends that topical pain relievers be only one part of a comprehensive treatment program that includes medication, exercise, rest, joint protection, and, in severe cases, surgery.

Convey these additional instructions to the client as follows:

- Read and follow the directions of the package.
- Wash your hands after every application.
- Keep topical pain relievers away from your eyes, mucous membranes, cuts, or irritated skin.
- If you are allergic to aspirin or are taking an anticoagulant ("blood thinner"), talk with your physician before using any rubs, creams, or sprays that contain salicylates.
- Keep all topical pain relievers out of the reach of children.

Interventions. Encourage the client to stay active. In cooperation with a physical therapist or trained exercise physiologist, help the client to develop an exercise program to preserve ROM while protecting joints. Maintaining function and mobility are necessary for the client to manage self-care activities.

Exercise can decrease morning stiffness, pain, and fatigue and enhance the client's self-esteem. Participating in group exercise programs, such as community water exercise programs (Fig. 77–6), provides social support and strengthens coping. Seek programs led by arthritis-certified instructors who monitor movement for adequate joint protection. Each session should include a warm-up period, full ROM exercises, endurance exercises, muscle-strengthening exercises, and cool-down exercises. Clients may use analgesics prior to exercise to permit increased freedom of movement. If a joint becomes painful during the exercise and the pain persists for 2 hours or more after the exercise, the activity should be modified.

Fatigue. Fatigue is a complex physiologic process involving the muscles, heart, lungs, and immune system. Clients with RA often experience fatigue, in part because of their chronic inflammatory process, pain, and depression. The diagnosis you may be working with is *Fatigue related to chronic inflammation, pain, or depression.*

Outcomes. The client will develop methods to balance rest and activity and will express satisfaction with his or her current level of activity and energy.

Interventions. Help the client to explore reasonable options for gaining enough sleep and finding time during the day to rest or nap. This may require changes in job performance or work relationships (if others need to do the client's work while he or she rests). Be sensitive to these concerns, and ask if your suggestions are reasonable in the client's personal setting. Practitioners can find it easy to say "be sure to rest now" without determining the feasibility of this protocol. For example, if the client is a young mother, she may need to send her young children to a neighbor for an hour or two each afternoon or nap while the children nap.

Altered Role Performance, Body Image Disturbance, Self-Esteem Disturbance. Several psychosocial nursing diagnoses may apply to the client with RA. Choose the one that best fits the client. All of these diagnoses may be related to chronic pain, the need for others to perform previous roles, feelings of helplessness,

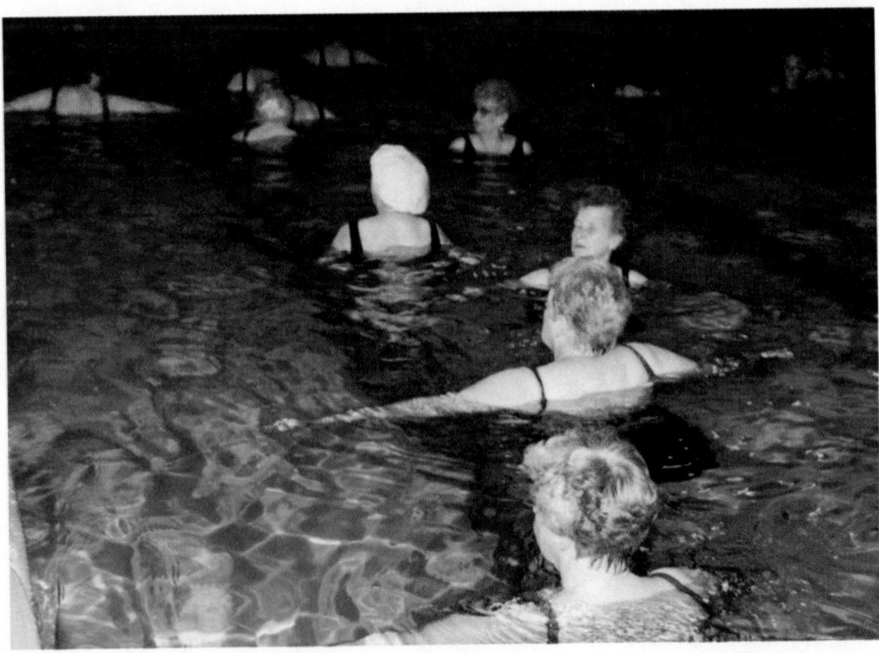

FIGURE 77–6 A community water exercise program. Many clients with rheumatoid arthritis find that water exercise helps to control pain and disability and improves exercise tolerance. The people in this class demonstrate the importance of keeping the shoulders submerged to allow the buoyancy of the water to protect their joints.

and feelings of embarrassment. We next present several avenues of care; select those that apply best to the particular client.

Outcomes. Although the actual outcomes statement depends on the client's particular diagnosis, most outcomes focus on the client's being able to express improved satisfaction with the problem. The problems identified by the three psychosocial diagnoses are usually very closely related, and improvement in one area can lead to improvement in others.

Interventions. The disease itself alters appearance, and in the client given corticosteroids several side effects from these medications can lead to alterations in self-esteem. Corticosteroids cause abnormal deposition of fat in the face (giving the client a "moon face" appearance) and shoulders (causing a "buffalo hump"); other side effects include acne, paper-thin skin that bruises easily, striae, and weight gain. Because of these and other side effects, the prescriber must always consider the risk-benefit ratio when initiating corticosteroid therapy. Also, the client may question the use of corticosteroids because the physical changes caused by them can be humiliating, even though the medications slow the inflammation. Most of these changes are permanent, and the client needs time to work through a new body image. Changes in body image take months to accept. Be sensitive to negative self-talk by the client, and express acceptance of the client's appearance; suggest clothing options to minimize visible changes.

The client and family will need time to plan for and accept the changes in the client's ability to perform previous tasks. Initially, it may seem easy to fill the role of two people in the home, and clients and their families may seem wary of efforts to encourage them to think about this change over the years that follow. Clients may also think initially that they will be able to go back to work full-time and that joint inflammation is only temporary. Be sensitive to this type of denial, and work with the client and family "where they are." Gradually, as the disease progresses, clients and families may need additional help as they try to come to terms with the long-term implications of the disease.

Risk of Ineffective Management of Therapeutic Regimen (Individuals). A final nursing diagnosis for the medically managed client with RA is *Risk for Ineffective Management of Therapeutic Regimen related to complex medications, schedules, high risk of side effects from medications, health maintenance, and self-care.* The management of any chronic disorder is complex, and the management of RA is no exception. Clients often have to take several types of medications with many undesirable side effects. They must plan for exercise and rest, and cope with daily pain and stiffness.

Outcomes. The client will make informed decisions about the management of the disease that will lead to a satisfactory quality of life despite the disease.

Interventions. Education focuses on coping skills, alternative methods of managing pain, joint protection, exercise, and adaptations for retaining functional independence. Inadequate knowledge may contribute to noncompliance with treatment regimens. Also, because of the pattern of remissions and exacerbations characteristic of RA, people tend to become discouraged with their prescribed treatments. Likewise, the medications used in the treatment of RA may provide only moderate pain relief, and many are slow-acting. Clients with RA therefore are susceptible to "quack" cures and unproven remedies (Box 77–2).

Unproven arthritis remedies are treatments that in scientific studies have not been shown to work and to be safe. Proven treatments for arthritis must show in repeated, controlled scientific tests that they work by meeting one or more of the following goals:

- Pain reduction
- Reduction of inflammation
- Safe joint mobility
- Avoidance of stress damage to joints

Proven treatments also must show how safe they are. The benefits of a treatment in controlling arthritis should be greater than the risk of unwanted or harmful effects. Some unproven remedies are harmless, others are harmful, and still others have health effects that are unknown. Even if an unproven remedy is in itself harmless, it can still have a detrimental effect if it causes a person to stop or slow down proven treatments to control arthritis. Nevertheless, despite the many problems that people with RA face daily, many of these people courageously overcome these problems to maintain active, productive lives. There are news groups on America On-Line for arthritis that clients or health care providers can access and World Wide Web browsers can go to *http://www.arthritis.org.*

EVALUATION

The process of RA is slow to improve. It takes several weeks to months for the expected outcomes for most of these diagnoses to be met. When joints are already severely damaged and pain is uncontrollable, joint replacement becomes an option. These and other surgical therapies are discussed under Surgical Management.

Modifications for Elderly Clients

Older adults can slowly succumb to the pain and immobility associated with the disease, becoming complacent and sedentary. Some of these people with RA virtually *never* leave home for fear of pain and embarrassment about being slow to walk and move. Help these clients to find ways of improving mobility by having them work among other clients of their own age and abilities. In addition, elderly clients are often being treated for several other problems, such as lung or heart disease, each with its own treatment regimen. The proper integration of all of these medications and other treatments is important.

Surgical Management

Surgical procedures may be helpful for clients with arthritis. Surgery may be used to relieve pain, improve function, and correct deformities. Previously, surgery was considered only late in the course of arthritis, often after severe joint destruction or deformity had developed. Now, however, early surgery is used to prevent deformities during the early phases or active stages of the disease.

TENDON TRANSFER AND OSTEOTOMY

Tendon transfers can prevent progressive deformity caused by muscle spasm. During these procedures, nod-

BOX 77–2 Unproven Remedies for Arthritis

Harmless

Copper bracelets
Mineral springs
Uranium mines
Vibrators
Vinegar and honey

Harmful

Dimethyl sulfoxide (DMSO)
Large doses of vitamins
Drugs with hidden ingredients such as corticosteroids
Snake venom

Unknown

Biofeedback
Diets
Fish oil
Lasers
Yucca

The Arthritis Foundation estimates that most people with arthritis have tried an unproven arthritis remedy at some point.
One in 10 people who have tried unproven arthritis remedies report harmful side effects, according to a Health and Human Services survey.
An estimated $1 billion is spent yearly on unproven arthritis remedies.
Any unproven remedy, no matter how harmless, can become harmful if it stops or delays someone from seeking a prescribed treatment program from a physician.

How To Determine Whether a Remedy Is Unproven

It may be difficult to spot an unproven remedy at first glance. The only source of information about a remedy may be what is given out by its promoters. People with arthritis should be cautious if the proposed remedy falls into one or more of the following categories:

- *Works for all types of arthritis:* There are more than 100 types of arthritis and treatments vary for each kind.
- *Uses case histories and testimonials:* Claims of individuals helped by a treatment need to be backed up by repeated studies on large numbers of people.
- *Cites only one study:* A single study may obtain results that other studies cannot repeat. A number of scientists must repeat the same study and get similar results for a treatment to be considered proven. A single study may, however, suggest a treatment that may have promise and should be studied further.
- *Cites a study without a control group:* Use of a control group helps show that results are due to the new treatment, not to another factor.
- *Does not list contents:* Some advertisements for a miracle drug for arthritis feature just aspirin at a high price. Other treatments contain corticosteroids and other powerful drugs. These drugs may cause severe side effects and should not be taken without a doctor's supervision.
- *Has no warnings about side effects:* There should be warnings on the label or instructions stating who should not use the treatment.
- *Claims to be based on a secret formula:* Scientists share their discoveries so that other experts in arthritis can review and question their findings.

Courtesy of the Arthritis Foundation, Atlanta.

ules or benign bony tumors (*exostoses*) may be surgically removed and flexion contractures surgically relieved. *Osteotomies* (excising or cutting through bone) may improve the function of deformed joints or limbs. For example, a femoral head osteotomy may give symptomatic relief by changing the position of the head of the femur when it is being subjected to the stress of impact against the acetabulum. Postoperative care varies, depending on the joint treated. In general, joints operated on are immobilized for a short time and then remobilized with physical therapy.

SYNOVECTOMY

Synovectomy (surgical removal of synovia, as in the elbows, wrists, fingers, or knees) may be used in clients with RA to help maintain joint function. With RA, joint destruction begins in the synovial tissue and then proceeds to involve bone, cartilage, and other structures. Early synovectomy helps prevent recurrent inflammation. Short-term immobilization is needed after surgery.

ARTHRODESIS

Arthrodesis is an operation to produce bony fusion of a joint. Most commonly, arthrodesis is used for clients with bone loss after joint infection, with tumors, with musculoskeletal trauma, and with paralysis. Arthrodesis can also help certain clients with RA or degenerative arthritis to regain some mobility. The surgeon usually uses metal screws and plates to fuse the joint. Although arthrodesis immobilizes the joint, the procedure eliminates much of the pain of the arthritic process and improves the client's functional mobility. The ankle is the joint most commonly treated with arthrodesis, usually to relieve post-traumatic arthritis, although the hip and knee can also be fused.

Despite its limited benefits, arthrodesis also has its drawbacks. It often results in stiffness in adjacent joints and increases the energy required for ambulation. It is possible, at times, to convert some fused joints to arthroplasties later in life. Bone grafts can also be used to stabilize the joint when desired union fails to occur after arthrodesis or when the use of screws or other devices is inadvisable. After surgery, the limb is casted. Nursing care is the same as for clients with casts (see Chapter 27).

JOINT REPLACEMENT

Joint replacement (*arthroplasty*) is the surgical replacement of natural diseased joints or joint components with

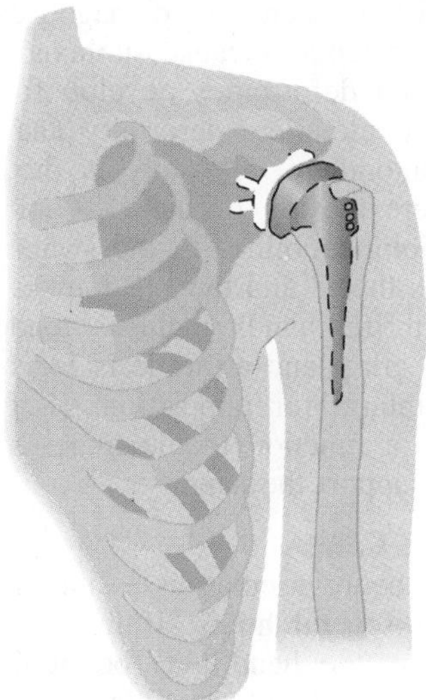

FIGURE 77–7 Total shoulder arthroplasty.

artificial joints or joint components. The operation restores motion to a joint and function to the muscles, ligaments, and other soft tissue structures that control a joint. The concept of joint replacement surgery is actually several hundred years old, but the modern ideas of joint replacement began in the 1960s, with the development of replacement components for the hip joint made of stainless steel and polyethylene (a lightweight plastic). Soon after, replacement joints were designed for the knee, shoulder, elbow, and fingers.

Today, joint prostheses are still a combination of a metal surface articulating with a polyethylene surface. The metal surfaces are made of strong, lightweight alloys such as cobalt-chromium and titanium-aluminum-vanadium. Both surfaces of an arthritic joint are replaced. If only one surface is replaced, the prosthesis would rub against the remaining tissue and not relieve pain or improve function. Arthritic joints can be replaced. Arthroplasty of the shoulder, elbow, and fingers is discussed next; hip and knee replacement is described in Chapter 26 following discussion of osteoarthritis.

Shoulder Arthroplasty

Disorders of the shoulder that require arthroplasty are much less common than those problems in weight-bearing joints. Although the shoulder is classified as a ball-and-socket joint, it permits more mobility than any other joint in the body. The large head of the humerus articulates against, not inside, the small glenoid cavity. This freedom of movement comes at the expense of stability. No inherent stability exists in the shoulder joint. The shoulder relies on soft tissue and ligaments for stability, particularly the rotator cuff muscle-tendon unit.

Four muscles and their tendons compose the rotator cuff, which allows the normal shoulder to move through three planes: flexion and extension, abduction and adduction, and internal rotation and external rotation.

Shoulder pain can have several causes; it is thus important to determine the true cause of the problem before treatment begins. Common manifestations of glenohumeral disorders include difficulty in flexion and extension and increased pain with attempted movement. An increase in joint stiffness may occur after sleeping. Local injections of steroids and physical therapy can usually delay surgery.

Shoulder arthroplasty is the replacement of the humeral head and glenoid articulating surface with a metal and polyethylene prosthesis (Fig. 77–7). The primary indication for total shoulder replacement is pain caused by incongruity of the glenoid and humeral head. Improvement in function and ROM is a secondary objective of the operation. Usual problems that are treated with total shoulder arthroplasty are RA, osteoarthritis, fractures, and dislocations. There are no specific age limitations, but the client must be well motivated and be a reasonable surgical risk. In many clients with RA, the rotator cuff is thin and diseased. This is a disadvantage for full recovery of shoulder function.

Contraindications include infection and inability to comply with rehabilitation, such as clients with physiologic (e.g., neuropathy) or psychological problems. Complications include brachial nerve palsy, prosthetic loosening, joint dislocation or subluxation, and impingement syndrome.

POSTOPERATIVE CARE

Nursing assessment includes neurovascular examination of the operative arm at least every 4 hours (see the Critical Monitoring feature). A possible complication is development of impingement syndrome because of the proximity of the brachial plexus. Hemovac drainage should be less than 100 ml during the first 12 hours. Elevate the head of the bed 30 degrees to reduce swelling and improve comfort. Aggressive pain management is needed; the shoulder arthroplasty usually causes more pain during the first 24 hours than the other joint replacements.

Patient-controlled analgesia (PCA) works well when supplemented with non-narcotic anti-inflammatory agents

CRITICAL MONITORING

Postoperative Brachial Plexus Compromise

- To assess median nerve status, have the client grasp your hand. Note the strength of the first and second fingers. A weak grip may indicate compromise of the median nerve.
- To assess radial nerve status, note the movement of the client's thumb toward the palm, and back to neutral. Problems with this motion may indicate compromise of the radial nerve.
- To assess ulnar nerve status, have the client spread all the fingers wide and resist pressure. Weakness against pressure may indicate compromise of the ulnar nerve.
- To assess cutaneous nerve status, assess for flexion of the biceps by having the client raise the forearm. Poor biceps flexion may indicate compromise of the cutaneous nerve.
- To assess axillary nerve status, have the client push the elbow outward against pressure. Hold the arm still while you palpate the deltoid for contraction. Weak contraction may indicate compromise of the axillary nerve.

(e.g., ketorolac tromethamine [Toradol]). Ice is applied to the shoulder. It may be difficult for the client to find a comfortable position to lie in; position the shoulder for comfort without forcing it into motion. Place the client's personal items within easy reach of the nonoperative arm.

After surgery, the client's arm is placed in a sling or Velpeau bandage. Clients with rotator cuff repair wear a light brace to prevent abduction and external rotation. A shoulder continuous passive motion (CPM) device can be used for all three planes of motion. Initially, the shoulder is placed in forward flexion and external rotation. Shoulder rehabilitation begins quickly after surgery and continues for about 6 weeks. For no other joint is rehabilitation as important as for the shoulder. The shoulder is placed through progressive external and internal ROM, hyperextension, and finally exercises with resistance once the rotator cuff has healed (~6 weeks). Usually, the client can be taught how to use the nonoperative arm to move the operative arm through ROM.

Elbow Arthroplasty

Early forms of elbow arthroplasty were metal-to-metal hinges, replacing the hinge structure of the elbow joint. Few of these prostheses are used today because they loosen after 2 to 3 years. Later, hinge joints were made that contained metal and polyethylene. This metal and plastic joint allows for some medial to lateral and rotational movements. A nonhinged elbow joint contains a metal and polyethylene component.

Indications for elbow arthroplasty are pain, mechanical instability, and bilateral elbow arthrodesis (fusion of the elbow). It is also possible to correct pain in the elbow by resecting the olecranon; this is called a *resection arthroplasty*. Severe RA is the most common indication for total elbow arthroplasty. After surgery, the arm is dressed in compressive dressings or splinted, and wound drains are placed.

POSTOPERATIVE CARE

Postoperative care includes elevating the arm above the shoulder for 4 to 5 days. Assess the client every 4 hours for ulnar nerve entrapment. Check the client's hand strength; especially assess the thumb and index finger's ability to pinch and ability to adduct the fourth and fifth fingers. The ulnar nerve lies close to the posteromedial surface of the elbow. This nerve is called the "funny bone" because of the uncomfortable sensation in the arm and fingers when it is hit.

Assess for radial and ulnar pulses and capillary refill. Some institutions use pulse oximetry to continuously assess tissue perfusion. Pain is managed with PCA narcotics. Elbow flexion and extension are allowed as tolerated. Personal items should be placed within easy reach of the nonoperative arm.

An occupational therapist should guide the client on how to modify ADL. Clients should not lift more than 5 pounds or begin triceps and biceps strengthening exercises for 3 months. The client will never be able to lift heavy items or play sports with the operative arm.

Hand Arthroplasty

Various hand deformities develop from the synovitis of RA (see Fig. 77–4). Synovitis stretches the central portion of the extensor tendon, causing it to shift. Eventually, the tendons become shortened and fixed. *Ulnar drift* occurs when the imbalance of damaged extensor tendons and intact flexor tendons cause subluxation of the MCP joint. Other hand deformities develop from synovitis of the PIP joint: boutonnière deformity and swan-neck deformity. A boutonnière deformity is flexion of the PIP joint and hyperextension of the DIP joint. There is no loss of MCP joint mobility. In the swan-neck deformity, the DIP joint is flexed and the PIP joint is hyperextended. Surgery of arthritic hands includes tendon transfers to improve pinch grasp and arthrodesis for strength and position of the thumb for opposition. Hinge implants are placed to restore function to the fingers. Fluff dressings are applied to support the hand.

POSTOPERATIVE CARE

After surgery, neurovascular assessments are performed every hour for several hours. If the client has regional block anesthesia, the hand may be numb. The hand is elevated off the bed to prevent ulnar pressure. The hand is usually placed in a stockinette and suspended from the bed. An opening is made to assess the fingers. Encourage the client to exercise the fingers 10 times every hour, attempting full extension and flexion. Finger exercises reduce edema and pain. Place the client's personal items within easy reach of the nonoperative arm. If the opposite hand is equally deformed from RA, the client is quite helpless and will require assistance with most components of ADL.

Encourage the client to use the nonoperative arm as much as possible. Some clients may express great concern about being dependent. Promote independence, and praise actions that foster self-care.

Rehabilitation is a long process. Most clients are fitted with outrigger splints with rubber bands that allow exercise with resistance after 1 week. Therapy continues for several weeks to assist the client to regain strength and control.

Modifications for Elderly Clients

Older clients may have adapted to RA very well but often find any further dependency needed after surgery difficult to handle. They tend to be slower in their recovery from total joint replacement. They may require prolonged hospitalization in an extended care facility or subacute care setting until they regain adequate mobility to function independently or with some assistance and safety.

SYSTEMIC LUPUS ERYTHEMATOSUS

SLE is a chronic, inflammatory, autoimmune disorder characterized by a wide array of clinical manifestations in vascular and connective tissue. *Lupus* is the Latin word for wolf, referring to a belief in the 1800s that the rash associated with this disease was caused by a wolf bite. Although this red butterfly rash is distinctive in some clients, it is absent in others.

There are two types of lupus erythematosus (LE): systemic and discoid. There is also a reversible form of lupus that is caused by reactions to various medications. SLE is the most severe form of the disorder; however, if well controlled, it can also be mild. Discoid LE is a mild form of the disorder that involves only the skin. The face, neck, and upper chest are usually affected.

SLE is relatively rare, occurring in 1 in 2000 persons. It most commonly develops in younger women between

BOX 77–3 Medications Associated with Lupus-Like Syndrome

Definite

Hydralazine
Procainamide

Possible

Chlorpromazine
Ethosuximide
Hydantoin
Isoniazid
Methyldopa
d-Penicillamine
Oral contraceptives
Practolol
Quinidine

ages 15 and 40 years. It is also more common in African Americans, followed by Asians and then whites. It is almost 10 times more common in women than in men. This suggests a hormonal influence.[13]

Etiology and Risk Factors

The cause of SLE is unknown. Certain factors, such as genetic predisposition, infection, environmental irritants, physical and emotional stress, and exposure to ultraviolet B radiation, have been implicated. It is suggested that the genetic predisposition for the disease is present in some clients and a virus or some other agent triggers it, resulting in disease occurrence. This theory is as yet unsupported. SLE also has a familial tendency; when a twin has the disease, the incidence is 25% to 50% greater in the other twin than in the general population.

Several medications have been implicated in the development of a reversible form of lupus-like syndrome (Box 77–3). These drugs bind to and alter deoxyribonucleic acid (DNA), possibly enhancing the response. There may also be a correlation between the client's ability to metabolize the medication and a predisposition to SLE.

Pathophysiology

People with SLE produce several autoantibodies. The primary autoantibodies produced are directed at the cell nuclei and are called antinuclear antibodies (ANAs). SLE produces autoantibodies against double-stranded (ds) DNA, and the presence of these antibodies in the serum is considered typical of SLE. Normally, the T suppressor cells prevent autoantibody formation. In SLE, a defect in the T suppressor cell prevents this protective process. Natural killer (NK) cell function is also suppressed; NK cells cannot kill abnormal cells as readily. There are inherited defects in complement factors and cell surface receptors that normally assist with clearing immune complexes.

ANAs do not cause much of cellular destruction alone, primarily because ANAs do not come in contact with intact cell nuclei. When cells die, the nuclei are released and then bind to the ANAs. The immune complex that is formed triggers the inflammatory response, which is the primary cause of tissue damage. In addition, the immune complex is large and is often deposited in tissues. Deposition of this complex causes even more tissue damage by initiating the complement cascade and further increasing inflammation. A common site of deposition is the basement membrane of the kidney, which leads to glomerulonephritis. The complexes can also cause vasculitis, or inflammation of the vessels, resulting in a decrease of oxygen in organs and tissues. The immune complexes can also be deposited in the heart and brain.

Clinical Manifestations

SLE is not a single specific disorder, and therefore manifestations can vary greatly among people. About 90% of clients have polyarthritis and polyarthralgias. Pain is most common in the small joints of the hands, feet, wrists, and knees. Clients also have nonspecific manifestations, such as weight loss, fever, malaise, and lethargy. Many of the manifestations of SLE are due to the deposition of immune complexes in the tissues. The course of SLE also has exacerbations or flares and controlled periods (remissions).

ACUTE FORMS

Manifestations of acute SLE may include fever, musculoskeletal aches and pains, butterfly rash on the face, pleural effusion, basilar pneumonia, generalized lymphadenopathy, pericarditis, tachycardia, hepatosplenomegaly, nephritis, delirium, convulsions, psychosis, and coma.

CHRONIC FORMS

Manifestations of chronic SLE depend on the organs involved but may include fever, malaise, weight loss, cutaneous discoid LE lesions, erythematosus of exposed skin, generalized lymphadenopathy, severe hemolytic anemia, thrombocytopenic purpura, hypersplenism, pericarditis, pleural effusion, tachycardia, peripheral vascular syndromes (e.g., Raynaud's phenomenon, gangrene) (Fig. 77–8), ulcerative mucous membrane lesions, abdominal pains, nausea, vomiting, anorexia, bloody stools, hepatic dysfunction, hepatomegaly, focal glomerulitis progressing

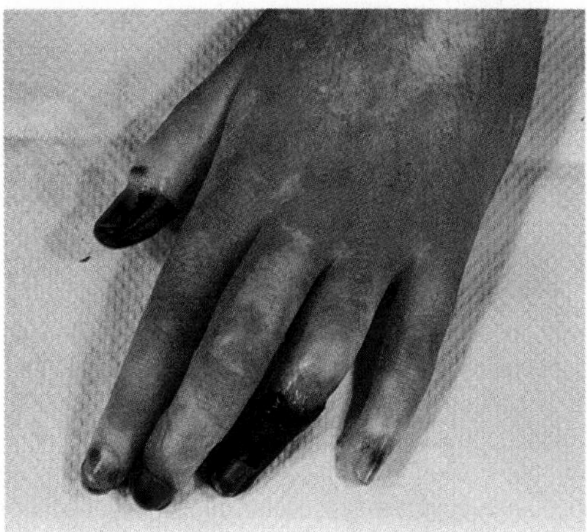

FIGURE 77–8 Vasospasm that occurs with advanced systemic lupus erythematosus can lead to gangrene of the fingers.

to glomerulonephritis, myalgia, arthralgia, neuritis, hemiplegia, psychosis, convulsions, and coma.

Diagnostic Findings

Diagnostic findings include the presence of LE cells (autoantibodies) in the serum, and the severity of SLE usually correlates with the degree of LE cell formation. Clients with SLE also have decreased complement levels; immune antibodies to DNA anti-samarium in the serum; increased gamma-globulin fraction due to increased antibody production; decreased levels of RBCs, WBCs, and platelets; and an elevated ESR.

At some point, abnormalities in the kidneys can be noted on an intravenous pyelogram; a barium enema might reveal colonic ulceration; a magnetic resonance imaging study might reveal central nervous system (CNS) involvement; and an electrocardiogram or echocardiogram might show cardiac changes.

Outcome Management

Medical Management

The goals of care for the client with SLE focus on (1) maintenance of skin integrity, (2) promotion of a healthy lifestyle and reduction of stress, (3) maintenance of proper nutrition, (4) promotion of comfort, (5) increase in the client's independence, and (6) maintenance of emotional well-being. The client is examined every 3 months with a complete blood count, determination of creatinine and cholesterol levels, urinalysis, and sometimes serum C3, C4, and anti-ds DNA.

Management of SLE is based on the organ systems involved. For example, if the client has cardiac involvement with either pericarditis or pleural effusion, intravenous pulse methylprednisolone may be used for 3 days, followed by oral prednisone. Cutaneous manifestations are managed with antimalarial agents. Most treatments are with medications; an algorithm has been developed to guide care (Fig. 77–9). Plasmapheresis may also be used to remove circulating autoantibodies and immune complexes from the blood before organ and tissue damage occur. The efficacy of this treatment has not been determined.

Clients with SLE require more than medications for proper management. Advise the client of lifestyle changes needed to reduce the risk of coronary artery disease, including management of hypertension, smoking cessation, and prevention of obesity and hyperlipidemia. Hypertension is aggressively managed with medications because it commonly leads to renal failure and death. Advise the client to reduce salt, fat, and cholesterol intake.

People in the United States have been called sun worshipers because they strive for a "healthy tan." Of course, tanning is dangerous to everyone, but the client with SLE must consider the sun an enemy. Photosensitivity is common; in many clients with SLE a rash develops after sun exposure as a result of stimulation of inflammatory processes.

All SLE clients receiving corticosteroids or immunosuppressants should receive the pneumococcal pneumonia vaccine and yearly influenza vaccine. Teach clients to report any signs of infection quickly. If possible, sulfa antibiotics should be avoided because of their tendency to cause allergy and flares of SLE. Ongoing dental care is important to avoid a potential source of systemic infection. Yearly ophthalmologic examinations are also important to monitor for side effects of antimalarial therapy and to detect and treat cataracts secondary to long-term corticosteroid use.

Renal disease, such as nephritis leading to renal failure, is a common outcome. Again, high-dose corticosteroids are given initially. If the creatinine level rises above 3 mg/dl, dialysis is considered.

Strides have been made in treating life-threatening SLE with allogeneic stem cell transplantation. This procedure may offer hope to clients with acute forms of SLE who have had a poor response to 3 or more months of high-dose corticosteroids and immunosuppressive agents.

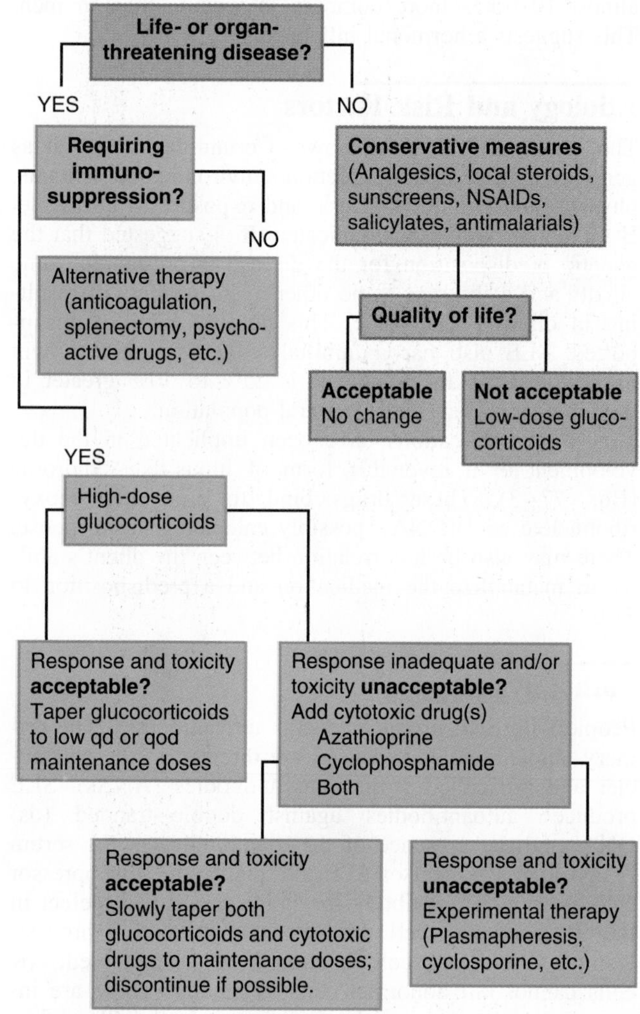

FIGURE 77–9 An algorithm for the management of clients with systemic lupus erythematosus. NSAIDs, nonsteroidal anti-inflammatory drugs. (From Hahn, B. H. [1993]. Management of systemic lupus erythematosus. In W. N. Kelley, et al. [Eds.], *Textbook of rheumatology* [4th ed.]. Philadelphia: W. B. Saunders.)

Nursing Management of the Medical Client

Nursing intervention for clients with SLE depends on how the client responds to the condition and on the severity and specific types of clinical manifestations. In a newly diagnosed client, you can expect knowledge deficits with respect to the diagnosis itself, prescribed drug therapies, and the prognosis. Explain how to relieve anxiety and avoid misunderstandings. This is particularly important in terms of the prescribed medications. Advise the client and significant others of the actions, side effects, and potential interactions of prescribed medications, especially corticosteroids.

During follow-up visits, review changes in all body systems. A physical examination is needed, with attention given to skin, muscles, and joints. CNS involvement is common, and a complete psychosocial assessment is important to detect changes in cognition and emotional stability.

During exacerbations, provide physiologic support to prevent skin breakdown, maintain nutritional and metabolic status, and minimize the risk of opportunistic infection. Also, provide emotional support to the client facing a chronic, potentially fatal disease. Clients may experience grief reaction following diagnosis, with exacerbations, or both. Allow for verbalization of these feelings. In such situations, be supportive and understanding; when necessary, refer the client or family members for counseling.

Outcomes

In general, the clinical pattern and prognosis of SLE are variable. The illness may develop rapidly with an acute fulminant course. More commonly, it develops insidiously and becomes chronic, with remissions and exacerbations. The course of the disorder is more severe when onset occurs at a young age. The survival rate has improved dramatically in recent years, although the disease is still potentially fatal. More than 95% of clients are alive 5 years after diagnosis. Improvements in treatments mean that clients can now live for many years.

The leading cause of death in clients with SLE is renal failure. There is some degree of kidney involvement causing progressive changes within the glomeruli in most clients with SLE. With progression of SLE nephritis, the glomeruli become increasingly abnormal and accumulate immune complex deposits. Once 75% of the glomeruli have been affected, the client shows manifestations of renal failure. The heart is the other major organ involved in SLE. The immune complexes are deposited in the coronary vessels, myocardium, and pericardium. CNS involvement, usually leading to cerebral infarction, can also occur.

PROGRESSIVE SYSTEMIC SCLEROSIS (SCLERODERMA)

Progressive systemic sclerosis (PSS) is a disorder caused by excessive collagen deposition, microvascular injury, and changes in humoral and cellular immunity. PSS is commonly known as *scleroderma,* although the skin is not the only organ system affected by the progressive sclerosis. Actually, this is a connective tissue disease characterized by fibrosis and degenerative changes of the skin, synovium, digital arteries, and parenchyma and small arteries of the internal organs.

Etiology

The exact etiologic mechanisms of PSS are not fully understood. Excess deposition of collagen is the characteristic feature of PSS, but the cause of excess collagen production is not known. However, the collagen that is produced is normal in other aspects. Vascular changes include fibrosis of the endothelium of small arterioles. Endothelial damage and cell death activate platelets and cause more inflammation. The activated platelets also lead to vasoconstriction and increased capillary permeability and recruit other inflammatory cells (e.g., fibroblasts) into the area. Alterations in humoral immunity are seen in the development of antibodies to type IV collagen found in the basement membranes of tissues. People with PSS have hypergammaglobulinemia, with the greatest increase in immunoglobulin G (IgG). Cellular immunity is also altered. In PSS, T lymphocytes accumulate in involved tissues; therefore, circulating T lymphocytes may be slightly decreased.

Clinical Manifestations

Scleroderma is classified into two categories: localized and generalized.

Localized scleroderma is the less severe form and affects primarily the skin. It may involve muscles and bones but does not affect the internal organs. Localized scleroderma is further divided into *morphea* and *linear* forms. Morphea is the development of skin lesions that are hard, oval, and white with a purple ring around them. Morphea often improves in time. Linear scleroderma is seen as a skin lesion that looks like a thick line of skin. It often begins in childhood and develops on the arms, legs, or forehead. The lesion can extend into the muscle and bone beneath it and alter growth.

Generalized scleroderma (true PSS) involves the skin and many other internal organs such as the kidneys, lungs, joints, muscles, cardiovascular system, and digestive system. Generalized PSS can also be further divided into *limited subcutaneous* and *diffuse subcutaneous* forms, often called CREST:

*C*alcinosis is the development of small white calcium deposits beneath the skin. The lumps may break open and drain a chalky fluid.

*R*aynaud's syndrome, common in most clients with PSS, consists of spasms of the arteries and arterioles. Spasms can occur spontaneously but most often are brought on by exposure to cold or emotional stress.

*E*sophageal motility is decreased from excessive deposits of collagen and muscle atrophy.

*S*clerodactyly is scleroderma of the fingers and toes.

*T*elangiectasia is permanent dilation of the capillaries, arterioles, and venules.

Limited subcutaneous scleroderma usually has a slow onset and may take 10 to 20 years before manifestations appear. Manifestations are usually one of the CREST forms. Prognosis is favorable. Diffuse subcutaneous scleroderma affects the entire body and most of the manifestations of CREST appear.

Progressively fatal PSS is associated with a generalized skin thickening and invasion into internal organs. Common clinical manifestations include subcutaneous edema, fever, and malaise. The skin becomes thickened and hide-like and loses normal skinfolds (Fig. 77–10). Ulcerations around the fingertips and subcutaneous calcification occur. Polyarthritis and polyarthralgias are also present. Dysphagia due to esophageal dysfunction, from abnormalities in motility, and later from fibrosis, occurs in about 90% of clients. Fibrosis and atrophy of the GI tract cause hypermotility and malabsorption. Diffuse pulmonary fibrosis and pulmonary vascular disease are reflected by low oxygen-diffusing capacity and decreased lung compliance. Hypertensive uremic syndrome, resulting from obstruction in small renal vessels, is serious. RF may be present in a small number of clients. Mild anemia is often present. An elevated ESR and hypergammaglobulinemia are also common. PSS typically progresses slowly. When death occurs, it is usually from infection or renal or cardiac failure.

Outcome Management

Treatment of PSS is supportive and symptomatic. The primary goal of medical treatment is to trigger a remission of the disease. Steroids and immunosuppressants are used to treat the disease, often in high doses.

Nursing interventions are directed at control of clinical manifestations. One of the major areas of concern is skin care to prevent breakdown and ulceration. The skin should be carefully inspected daily so any injury or breakdown is noted and treatment begun immediately. Teach the client to use gentle soaps and nonalcohol astringent lotions to maintain skin integrity.

Helping the client control acute pain, which is sometimes associated with Raynaud's phenomenon, polyarthralgia, and polyarthritis, is another important nursing function. The client must learn to avoid activities that might trigger pain. This includes actions such as joint protection behaviors, avoiding extreme cold, wearing gloves when hands are exposed to cold (even when removing food from the freezer), eliminating smoking, and resting the painful part when pain is acute.

If the client is experiencing esophageal dysfunction, modification of the diet may be necessary. Clients usually tolerate small, frequent, bland feedings better than three regular meals a day. The client also should learn to sit up for at least 1 hour after meals to promote digestion and food motility. Histamine receptor antagonists and antacids may be prescribed to decrease the acidity some clients feel.

The client will need continued follow-up care and monitoring. As with SLE, the client also needs psychosocial support to cope with this chronic debilitating disease. Encourage the client to continue to receive psychological support as needed after hospitalization.

ANKYLOSING SPONDYLITIS

Ankylosing spondylitis (AS), or *Marie-Strumpell disease,* is a chronic, progressive inflammation of the spine and sacroiliac joints. It affects 1% of the population, mostly males. The exact cause of AS is not known, but transmission is genetic. The joints of the sacroiliac begin to inflame and then ossify (fuse) as the joints and disc spaces are replaced by bone. The process moves up the spinal column until the spine is stiff and rigid, and then the disorder extends into the hips, knees, and shoulders.

AS begins insidiously in adolescence or young adulthood, usually with morning backache and stiffness in the lumbar area. The pain and stiffness subside with movement but return with inactivity. Other manifestations include iritis, arthritis or arthralgia, weight loss, and malaise. In advanced stages of AS, the client is rigid and stooped forward (Fig. 77–11). The spine is rigid and looks like bamboo shoots on radiographs. Laboratory tests reveal increased HLA-B27. ESR and RF are usually negative.

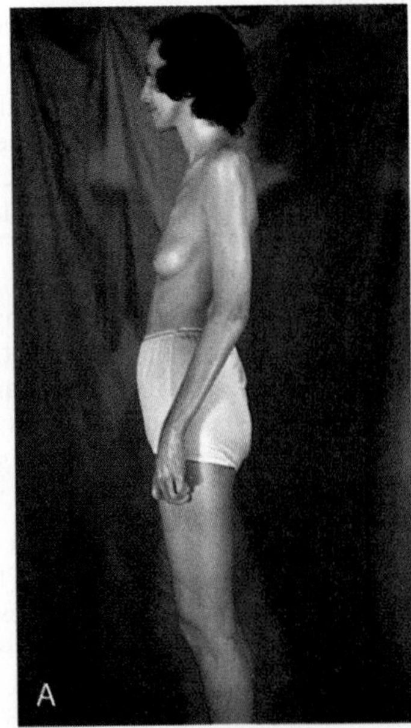

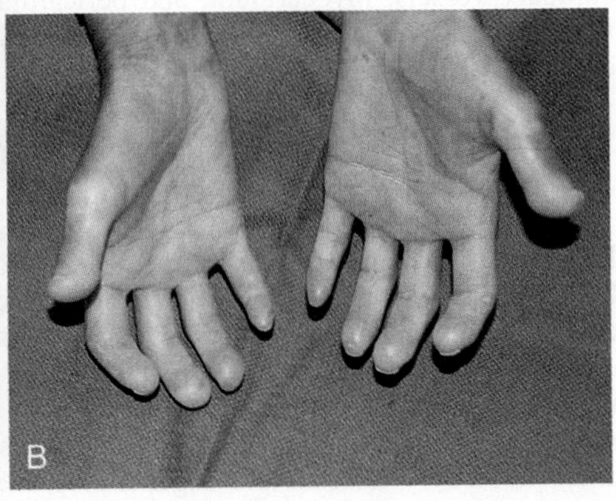

FIGURE 77–10 *A,* Long-term scleroderma. *B,* Appearance of the hands in a client with scleroderma.

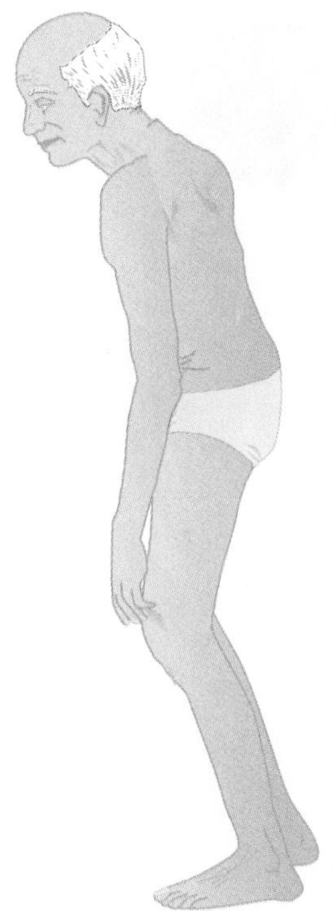

FIGURE 77–11 Posture of a client with advanced ankylosing spondylitis.

Outcome Management

There is no management to prevent or slow the progress of AS. Since stiffening of the spine is inevitable, the goals of management are to relieve pain, maintain optimal posture, and prevent respiratory involvement from minimal chest movements. Pain is usually treated with NSAIDs and heat. Instruct the client to try to maintain an erect posture and to rest frequently throughout the day. Splints and back braces are helpful for support.

Surgical management may include osteotomy for marked deformities of the hip or spine. Occasionally hip or knee arthroplasty is used.

SJÖGREN'S SYNDROME

Sjögren's syndrome, a chronic inflammatory disorder of the eyes, can be a primary problem or secondary to RA. It involves a decrease in lacrimation and salivation caused by obstruction of the secretory ducts by immune complexes. People with Sjögren's syndrome exhibit dry eyes (keratoconjunctivitis sicca) and a dry mouth (xerostomia).

Common manifestations include swelling of the lacrimal ducts and parotid glands and fatigue. This disorder affects mainly women, who experience an additional manifestation of vaginal dryness. Almost half of people with Sjögren's syndrome also exhibit another connective tissue disorder, especially RA.

Diagnostic tests reveal hypergammaglobulinemia and the presence of RF, ANAs, and anti-extractable nuclear antigen. Autoantibodies against salivary duct antigens are also found. If the client also has RA, the treatment is directed at the underlying arthritis. Artificial tears are helpful for keeping the eyes moist and preventing corneal abrasions. Artificial saliva can be used for the xerostomia. If the syndrome is left untreated, the client can develop visual problems, oral ulcerations, dental caries, and dysphagia.

Clients with Sjögren's syndrome have difficulty when going to surgery. Placing these clients on NPO (nothing by mouth) status can cause great oral discomfort because saliva secretion is decreased. Artificial saliva should be used. In addition, these clients are at risk for corneal abrasion because of the low humidity in the surgery suite. Ocular lubricants should be used preoperatively.

FIBROMYALGIA SYNDROME

Not all people complaining of musculoskeletal pain have arthritis. Fibromyalgia syndrome is an increasingly recognized chronic musculoskeletal pain disorder of unknown cause. It occurs in about 2% of the general population, predominately in girls and young women. Active research is being conducted to find the cause; some data indicate that there may be alterations in several hormones (e.g., adrenocorticotropic hormone, growth hormone) and the hypothalamus-pituitary-adrenal axis.

Clinical Manifestations

Clinical manifestations include fatigue, morning stiffness, non-refreshing sleep due to lack of stage 4 sleep, and postexertional muscle pain. About one third of clients have associated problems such as irritable bowel syndrome, tension headaches, premenstrual syndrome, numbness and tingling, and Raynaud's phenomenon. Fatigue is the most common clinical manifestation, and the most common cause of the fatigue is chronic depression. The physical examination is often unremarkable unless attention is paid to the tender points (Fig. 77–12).

Palpate these points with moderate pressure with the pulp of your thumb or forefinger. Intersperse examination of tender points with examination of nontender points to avoid anticipation reactions if every point is associated with pain.

Outcome Management

Management includes L-tryptophan to increase sleep, tricyclic antidepressants to inhibit serotonin uptake, benzodiazepines for the treatment of anxiety associated with depression, and corticosteroids and NSAIDs for pain control. Low-intensity exercise is also important and helps to decrease pain. Biofeedback, acupuncture, and hypnotherapy have also been used to help manage nonmuscular problems such as functional diarrhea, tension headache, and fatigue. The efficacy of these treatments is yet to be fully ascertained.

Many clients with fibromyalgia perceive themselves to be significantly disabled and have a reduced quality of life that rivals conditions such as RA and terminal emphysema. Clients with fibromyalgia have difficulty coping with "daily hassles" and this, in turn, increases the psychological stress. Cognitive behavioral therapy is often effective in providing these clients a sense of control over their lives.

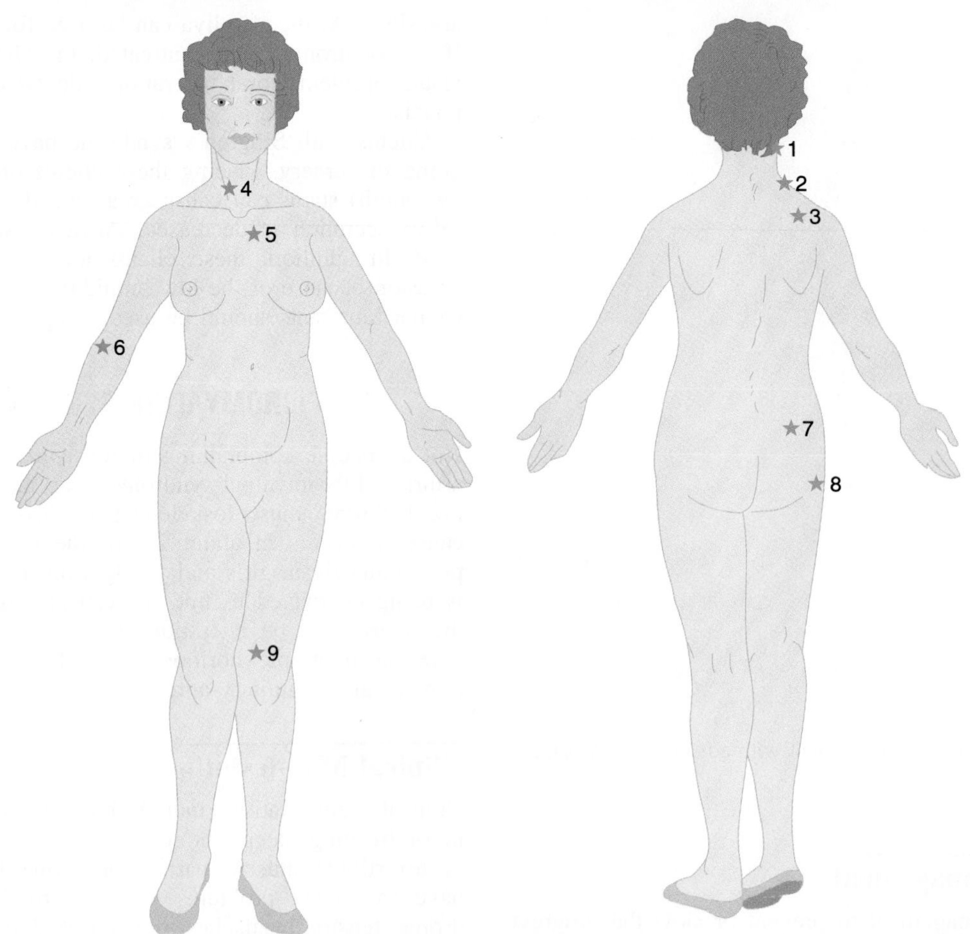

FIGURE 77–12 The nine paired tender points recommended by the 1990 American College of Rheumatology Criteria Committee for establishing a diagnosis of fibromyalgia. 1, Insertion of the nuchal muscles into the occiput. 2, Upper border of the trapezius—midportion. 3, Muscle attachments to the upper medial border of the scapula. 4, Anterior aspects of C5 and C7 intertransverse spaces. 5, Second rib space—about 3 cm lateral to the sternal border. 6, Muscle attachments to the lateral epicondyle—about 2 cm below the bony prominence. 7, Upper outer quadrant of the gluteal muscles. 8, Muscle attachments just posterior to the greater trochanter. 9, Medial fat pad of the knee proximal to the joint line. Eleven or more tender points in conjunction with a history of widespread pain are characteristic of the fibromyalgia syndrome. (From Bennett, R. [1993]: The fibromyalgia syndrome. In W. N. Kelley, et al. [Eds.], *Textbook of rheumatology* [4th ed., p. 472]. Philadelphia: W. B. Saunders.)

POLYMYOSITIS AND DERMATOMYOSITIS

Polymyositis is an acute or chronic inflammatory disorder of the striated muscles causing symmetrical weakness. When there is a rash associated with polymyositis, the condition is referred to as *dermatomyositis.* As with other connective tissue diseases, polymyositis and dermatomyositis are characterized by periods of remission and exacerbation and are chronically progressive. This disorder is twice as common in women as in men and occurs equally among all races. People between ages 30 and 60 are most at risk. Polymyositis may be associated with a malignancy.

Clinical manifestations of the disease, besides the symmetrical muscle weakness and rash, include polyarthralgia, polyarthritis, and Raynaud's phenomenon. Clients with dermatomyositis have characteristic heliotrope B (lilac) rash and periorbital edema. The muscle weakness can lead to problems with speaking and swallowing. Diagnostic tests reveal positive ANAs and focal deposition of complement, IgG, and IgM in vessels of the involved muscles.

These disorders are treated with high-dose corticosteroids and immunosuppressants. Nursing care is mainly supportive. Monitor the client's ability to swallow so that aspiration does not occur.

VASCULITIS

Vasculitis comprises a group of disorders leading to inflammation and necrosis of blood vessel walls. Soluble immune complexes are deposited in blood vessel walls in areas where capillaries have increased permeability. After deposition, the immune system is activated and the complex is destroyed along with the blood vessel wall. These disorders include polyarteritis nodosa, systemic necrotizing vasculitis, and allergic granulomatous angiitis. Inflammation and damage to large and small vessels result in end-stage organ damage.

Specific manifestations vary, depending on the organs affected. Steroids are the treatment of choice for these disorders.

REITER'S SYNDROME

Reiter's syndrome is a triad of arthritis, urethritis, and conjunctivitis. The syndrome is triggered by genitourinary or gastrointestinal infections, especially *Chlamydia.* Other manifestations may include prostatitis, penile or vaginal lesions, and urethral discharge. Achilles tendon and plantar fascia inflammation also occur. HLA-B27 is present in most clients and indicates an immunologic aspect.

The syndrome is treated with steroid therapy and aggressive physical therapy. NSAIDs may be used to treat the joint pain. Antibiotics are not used, since no organism can be obtained for culture.

The major nursing concerns are with pain and stiffness. Most problems are similar to those seen in clients with RA.

POLYMYALGIA RHEUMATICA AND CRANIAL ARTERITIS

Polymyalgia rheumatica is a clinical syndrome occurring more commonly in women than in men. It is a disease of aging, rarely occurring before age 60 years. It is characterized by pain and stiffness in the neck, shoulder, back, and pelvic girdle, especially in the morning. Headaches or painful areas on the head may be present. The client also may have a low-grade fever or temporal arteritis. Laboratory findings include an elevated ESR, mild anemia, and possible elevation of immunoglobulins. Steroids usually produce symptomatic relief within days.

Giant cell arteritis, also known as temporal or cranial arteritis, is also a disease of older people. The client often has manifestations of polymyalgia rheumatica for months, then suddenly experiences the severe headaches associated with temporal arteritis. The onset of this disorder is usually sudden, with severe pain often appearing in the temporal area. The pain also may be felt in the occipital area, face, jaw, or side of the neck. It is usually associated with hyperesthesia, which makes any touch exquisitely painful. The client may experience visual changes, including sudden onset of blindness in one or both eyes.

It is very important to diagnose and treat this disorder before blindness occurs. Because older women are often affected, their complaints of decreased vision and headaches are sometimes ignored as normal aging. Treatment is with corticosteroids, which are highly effective in controlling this disorder.

MIXED CONNECTIVE TISSUE DISEASE

Mixed connective tissue disease is a combination of several connective tissue diseases. Clients have manifestations that are not typical of any one disorder. This diagnosis is applied to about 10% of clients with connective tissue disease. Frequent combinations are SLE and PSS and RA. Mixed connective tissue diseases are managed according to their manifestations. Often clients are managed as if they had SLE. The term mixed connective tissue disease is used less frequently today.

LYME DISEASE

Lyme disease is one form of rheumatic joint disease with a known cause. It is included as a connective tissue disorder because the skin, joints, nervous system, and heart are involved. This complex multisystem disease is caused by the tick-borne spirochete *Borrelia burgdorferi.* Clinical manifestations found from 3 to 32 days after the bite may include a red flat rash that clears in the center, severe headache, stiff neck, fever, chills, myalgias, joint pain, severe malaise, and fatigue.

The disease can be treated with a course of antibiotic therapy. Doxycycline is the most common antibiotic used. Neurologic abnormalities may occur if treatment is ineffective. Intra-articular steroids and NSAIDs may be used to relieve joint inflammation and pain. Long-term effects include fatigue and arthralgia for many years after the initial infection.

SECONDARY ARTHRITIS

WHIPPLE'S DISEASE

Whipple's disease is a secondary arthritis associated with a GI disorder. The disease was first described in the early 1900s as a condition characterized by arthralgias, diarrhea, abdominal pain, and weight loss. Other manifestations include fever, lymphadenopathy, and increased skin pigmentation. The disease can affect almost every organ system in the body. Whipple's disease occurs most commonly in middle-aged white men. Although an organism was described as the cause, it was not isolated until 1992.

Treatment of Whipple's disease consists of broad-spectrum antimicrobial agents.

OTHER DISORDERS CAUSING ARTHRITIS

Other conditions that may produce arthritis-type symptoms include Crohn's disease, ulcerative colitis, tuberculosis, hyperthyroidism, hyperparathyroidism, sickle cell anemia crisis, and psoriasis. Treatment of the primary condition usually leads to a decrease in the severity of the arthritis.

CONCLUSIONS

Autoimmune disorders most often lead to problems of the joints, such as rheumatoid arthritis, and problems with other connective tissues, such as scleroderma. These chronic problems and resulting pain and deformity quickly test the resources of the client. Client education for self-care is critical. Most of these problems have no cure, so the nurse considers the effects of chronic pain, multiple treatments, and progressive deformity on self-concept, role performance, and family systems.

THINKING CRITICALLY

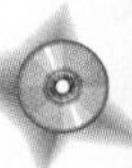

1. **You are working in an outpatient clinic and receive a call from a 66-year-old woman who is**

experiencing a flare-up of rheumatoid arthritis. She was seen 2 days ago in the clinic and given a high dose of prednisone. Now, she reports epigastric abdominal pain. A symptom analysis reveals the following: her pain has a burning quality, is worse between meals, is relieved by food, and is aggravated by coffee. She has taken some over-the-counter ibuprofen for the pain but states, "It didn't help." What other information do you need to collect? What interventions would you advise?

Factors to Consider. Consider the side effects of corticosteroids and NSAIDs.

2. **A 55-year-old woman with a history of joint pain is scheduled for a total hip replacement. She has experienced increasing pain while walking and hopes to be able to walk pain-free so she can resume her job as a waitress. What nursing assessments are pertinent to this type of condition and proposed surgery? How realistic is the client's desire to return to work as a waitress?**

Factors to Consider. How will assessments help in the prevention of postoperative complications? Are clients able to return to an improved level of functioning following joint replacement surgery?

BIBLIOGRAPHY

1. Albert, L. J., & Inman, R. D. (1999). Molecular mimicry and autoimmunity. *New England Journal of Medicine, 341*(27), 2068–2074.
2. Awerbach, M. (1995). Different concepts of chronic musculoskeletal pain. *Annals of Rheumatic Disease, 54*(5), 331–332.
3. Belza, B. L., et al. (1993). Correlates of fatigue in older adults with rheumatoid arthritis. *Nursing Research, 42,* 93–99.
4. Bertsch, C. (1995). CREST syndrome: A variant of systemic sclerosis. *Orthopaedic Nursing, 14*(2), 53–60.
5. Bonafede, R. D., Downey, D. C., & Bennet, R. M. (1995). An association of fibromyalgia with primary Sjögren's syndrome. *Journal of Rheumatology, 22*(1), 133–136.
6. Carson, D. A., & Tan, E. M. (1995). Apoptosis in rheumatic disease. *Bulletin on the Rheumatic Diseases, 44*(1), 1–3.
7. Dav, P. C., & Callahan, J. P. (1994). Immune modulation during treatment of systemic sclerosis with plasmapheresis and immunosuppressive drugs. *Clinical Immunology and Immunopathology, 76*(2), 159–165.
8. Dildy, S. (1996). Suffering in people with rheumatoid arthritis. *Applied Nursing Research, 9*(4), 177–183.
9. Goldenberg, D. (1995). Fatigue in rheumatic disease. *Bulletin on the Rheumatic Diseases, 44*(1), 4–7.
10. Halverson, P. B. (1995). Extraarticular manifestations of rheumatoid arthritis. *Orthopaedic Nursing, 14*(4), 47–50.
11. Harris, E. (1993). Etiology and pathogenesis of rheumatoid arthritis. In W. N. Kelley, et al. (Eds.), *Textbook of rheumatology.* Philadelphia: W. B. Saunders.
12. Johnson, R. L. (1993). Total shoulder arthroplasty. *Orthopaedic Nursing, 12*(1), 14–22.
13. Kuper, B., & Failla, S. (2000). Systemic lupus erythematosus: A multisystem autoimmune disease. *Nursing Clinics of North America, 35*(1), 253–266.
14. Legerton, C. W. (1995). Systemic sclerosis: Clinical management of its major complications. *Rheumatic Disease Clinics of North America, 21*(11), 203–216.
15. Meyer, C. L., & Hawley, D. J. (1994). Characteristics of participants in water exercise programs compared to patients seen in a rheumatic disease clinic. *Arthritis Care and Research, 7*(2), 85–89.
16. Mikanowicz, C., & Leslie, M. (2000). Polymyalgia rheumatica and temporal arteritis: A case presentation. *Nursing Clinics of North America, 35*(1), 245–252.
17. Minor, M. A., & Brown, J. D. (1993). Exercise maintenance of persons with arthritis after participation in a class experience. *Health Education Quarterly, 20*(1), 83–95.
18. Morrow, A. K., Parker, J. C., & Russell, J. L. (1994). Clinical implications of depression in rheumatoid arthritis. *Arthritis Care and Research, 7*(2), 58–63.
19. Neuberger, G. B., et al. (1993). Promoting self-care in clients with arthritis. *Arthritis Care and Research, 6*(3), 141–148.
20. Osial, T. A., Jr., Cash, J. M., & Eisenbeis, C. H., Jr. (1993). Arthritis-associated syndromes. *Primary Care, 20,* 857–879.
21. Parker, J. C., et al. (1992). Psychological factors, immunologic activation, and disease activity in rheumatoid arthritis. *Arthritis Care and Research, 5*(1), 196–201.
22. Rankin, J. A. (1995). Pathophysiology of the rheumatoid joint. *Orthopaedic Nursing, 14*(4), 39–46.
23. Riott, I. M. (1994). Autoimmune disease. In *Essential immunology* (8th ed., pp. 412–418). Cambridge, MA: Blackwell Scientific Publications.
24. Seltzer, E., et al. (2000). Long term outcome of persons with Lyme disease. *Journal of the American Medical Association, 283*(5), 609–616.
25. Sisk, T. D., & Wright, P. E. (1992). Arthroplasty of shoulder and elbow. In A. H. Crenshaw (Ed.), *Campbell's operative orthopaedics* (pp. 627–673). St. Louis: Mosby–Year Book.
26. Vale, D. (2000). Recognition and management of Sjogren's syndrome: Strategies for the advanced practice nurse. *Nursing Clinics of North America, 35*(1), 267–278.
27. Wolfe, F., et al. (1994). The mortality of rheumatoid arthritis. *Arthritis and Rheumatism, 37,* 481–494.
28. Workman, M. L. (2000). Immune mechanisms in rheumatic disease. *Nursing Clinics of North America, 35*(1), 175–188.

REMEMBER *to check out your* **Companion CD ROM**

CHAPTER 78

Management of the Client with Leukemia and Lymphoma

Linda Yoder

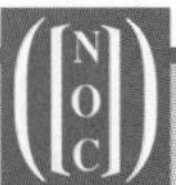

NURSING OUTCOMES CLASSIFICATION (NOC) for Nursing Diagnoses—Clients with Leukemia and Lymphoma

Altered Nutrition: Less Than Body Requirements
Nutritional Status
Nutritional Status: Food and Fluids
Nutritional Status: Nutrient Intake
Sensory Function: Taste and Smell

Altered Oral Mucous Membranes
Immune Status
Infection Status
Oral Health
Self-Care: Oral Hygiene
Pain Level
Swallowing Status
Tissue Integrity: Skin and Mucous Membranes

Altered Protection
Coagulation Status
Coping
Immune Status
Infection Status
Nutritional Status

Altered Role Performance
Coping
Depression Level
Family Functioning
Psychosocial Adjustment: Life Change

Anticipatory Grieving
Coping
Family Coping
Grief Resolution
Sleep

Body Image
Acceptance: Health Status
Body Image
Self-Esteem

Death Anxiety
Dignified Dying
Fear Control
Depression Level

Diarrhea
Bowel Elimination
Electrolyte/Acid-Base Balance
Fluid Balance
Hydration
Symptom Severity

Dysfunctional Grieving
Coping
Family Coping
Grief Resolution
Role Performance

Energy Field Disturbance
Spiritual Well-Being
Well-Being

Fatigue
Activity Tolerance
Endurance
Energy Conservation
Nutritional Status: Energy
Psychomotor Energy

Hopelessness
Depression Control
Depression Level
Hope
Quality of Life
Sleep

Impaired Skin Integrity
Tissue Integrity: Skin and Mucous Membranes

Ineffective Denial
Acceptance: Health Status
Anxiety Control
Fear Control

Nausea
Comfort Level
Hydration
Nutritional Status: Food and Fluid Intake
Symptom Severity

Pain
Comfort Level
Pain Control
Pain Level
Symptom Control
Well-Being

Risk for Ineffective Management of Therapeutic Regimen
Knowledge Therapeutic Regimen

Risk for Infection
Immune Status
Nutritional Status

Sexual Dysfunction
Acceptance
Sexual Functioning

Spiritual Distress
Anxiety Control
Coping
Dignified Dying
Hope
Quality of Life
Spiritual Well-Being
Well-Being

Cancers of the hematopoietic system are disorders resulting from the proliferation of malignant cells that originate in the bone marrow, thymus, and lymphatic tissue. Blood cells that originate in bone marrow are called *hematopoietic cells;* cells that originate in the lymph are called *lymphoid cells.* Leukemia is cancer of the bone marrow, and lymphoma is cancer of the lymphoid tissue.

LEUKEMIA

Leukemia is a malignant disease of the blood-forming organs. Leukemia accounts for 8% of all human cancers and is the most common malignancy in children and young adults. Half of all leukemias are classified as acute, with rapid onset and progression of disease resulting in 100% mortality within days to months without appropriate therapy. The remaining leukemias, classified as chronic, have a more indolent course. In children, 80% of leukemias are lymphocytic, with 20% nonlymphocytic. In adults, the percentages are reversed, with 80% being nonlymphocytic.

Etiology and Risk Factors

Although the cause of leukemia is unknown, several risk factors are associated with leukemia, including (1) genetic factors, (2) exposure to ionizing radiation and chemicals, (3) congenital abnormalities (i.e., Down's syndrome), and (4) presence of primary immunodeficiency, and infection with the human T-cell leukemia virus type 1 (HTLV-1). Genetic factors increase the risk of leukemia. A high incidence of acute leukemias and *chronic lymphocytic leukemia* (CLL) is reported in certain families. Hereditary abnormalities associated with an increased incidence of leukemia are Down's syndrome, Fanconi's aplastic anemia, Bloom's syndrome, ataxia telangiectasia, trisomy 13 (Patau's syndrome), Wiskott-Aldrich syndrome, and congenital X-linked agammaglobulinemia. Identical twins, fraternal twins, and siblings of children with leukemia are also at increased risk. In *chronic myelogenous leukemia* (CML), more than 90% of clients have the Philadelphia chromosome, an abnormal chromosome (see Chronic Leukemia).

Overexposure to ionizing radiation is a major risk factor for development of leukemia, with the disease developing years after the initial exposure. Alkylating agents used to treat other cancers, especially in combination with radiation therapy, increase a person's risk of leukemia. Workers exposed to chemical agents, such as benzene, an aromatic hydrocarbon, are at a much higher risk.

Causal risk factors acting together with a genetic predisposition can alter nuclear deoxyribonucleic acid (DNA). The leukemic cell is then unable to mature and respond to normal regulatory mechanisms. Abnormal chromosomes are reported in 40% to 50% of clients with acute leukemia, and certain chromosomes are repeatedly more involved than others. It appears that a mutation in a single cell gives rise to some leukemias.

Pathophysiology

In normal bone marrow, efficient regulation ensures that cell proliferation and maturation are adequate to meet a person's needs. Pluripotent stem cells commit to differentiate along the myeloid or lymphoid pathway in the presence of growth factors. In leukemia, control is missing or abnormal. Leukemia is an uncontrolled proliferation of leukocytes. This lack of control causes normal bone marrow to be replaced by immature and undifferentiated leukocytes or *blast cells* (Fig. 78–1). Abnormal, immature leukocytes then circulate in the blood and infiltrate the blood-forming organs (liver, spleen, lymph nodes) and other sites throughout the body.

The French-American-British (FAB) Cooperative Group developed a classification system that is universally accepted. Under this system, acute leukemias are classified on the basis of morphologic characteristics and histochemical staining of blast cells, which indicates the percentage of immature cells in the bone marrow (Table 78–1).

Acute Leukemia

For the leukemic process to be termed *acute,* at least 50% of the marrow cells must be immature. *Acute lymphoblastic leukemia* (ALL) is most common in children (median age, 11 years). *Acute nonlymphocytic leukemia* (ANLL) is more common in adults (median age, 67 years). Leukemias are considered clonal disorders, in that a single cell undergoes transformation, and leukemic cells then proliferate. An interesting paradox is that leukemic cells apparently divide more slowly and take longer to synthesize DNA than other blood precursors do. Acute leukemia is not caused by rapid cellular proliferation but instead is caused by the blocking of blood cell precursors. Leukemic cells accumulate relentlessly in most affected individuals, and they compete with normal cellular proliferation. Acute leukemia has also been termed an *accumulation disorder* as well as a *proliferation disorder.*

The development of leukemia occurs in the most primitive blood precursors, pluripotent stem cells, which give rise to all other blood cells (see in the Hematologic A & P review for Unit 16). The leukemia blasts, or precursor cells, literally "crowd out" the marrow and cause cellular proliferation of the other cell lines to cease. Normal granulocytic, monocytic, lymphocytic, erythrocytic, and megakaryocytic stem cells cease to function, causing pancytopenia (a reduction in all cellular components of the blood). Transformation also may occur specifically in the granulocyte-monocyte series and not in the erythrocyte series.

Chronic Leukemia

Chronic leukemia is classified as CML or CLL. CML originates in the pluripotent stem cell. Initially, the marrow is hypercellular with most cells normal. Typically, the peripheral blood smear reveals leukocytosis and thrombocytosis with an increased production of granulocytes. In 90% of cases, examination of the bone marrow cells during metaphase shows a translocation called the *Philadelphia chromosome.* After a relatively slow course for a median period of 4 years, the client with CML invariably enters a *blast crisis* that resembles acute leukemia.

Blast crisis results in the death of more than 70% of clients with CML. During this phase, increasing numbers of blasts (immature myeloid precursor cells, especially myeloblasts, the most primitive granulocyte precursors) proliferate in the blood and bone marrow. In blast crisis, the blasts and promyelocytes (another myeloid cell precursor type) exceed 20% in the blood and 30% in the marrow. Increased fibrotic tissue in the marrow is another manifestation of blast crisis. Leukopenia, thrombocytopenia, and anemia also are evident. Without treatment, death usually occurs within 6 months of onset.

CLL is characterized by the proliferation of early B lymphocytes and is an indolent leukemia most often seen

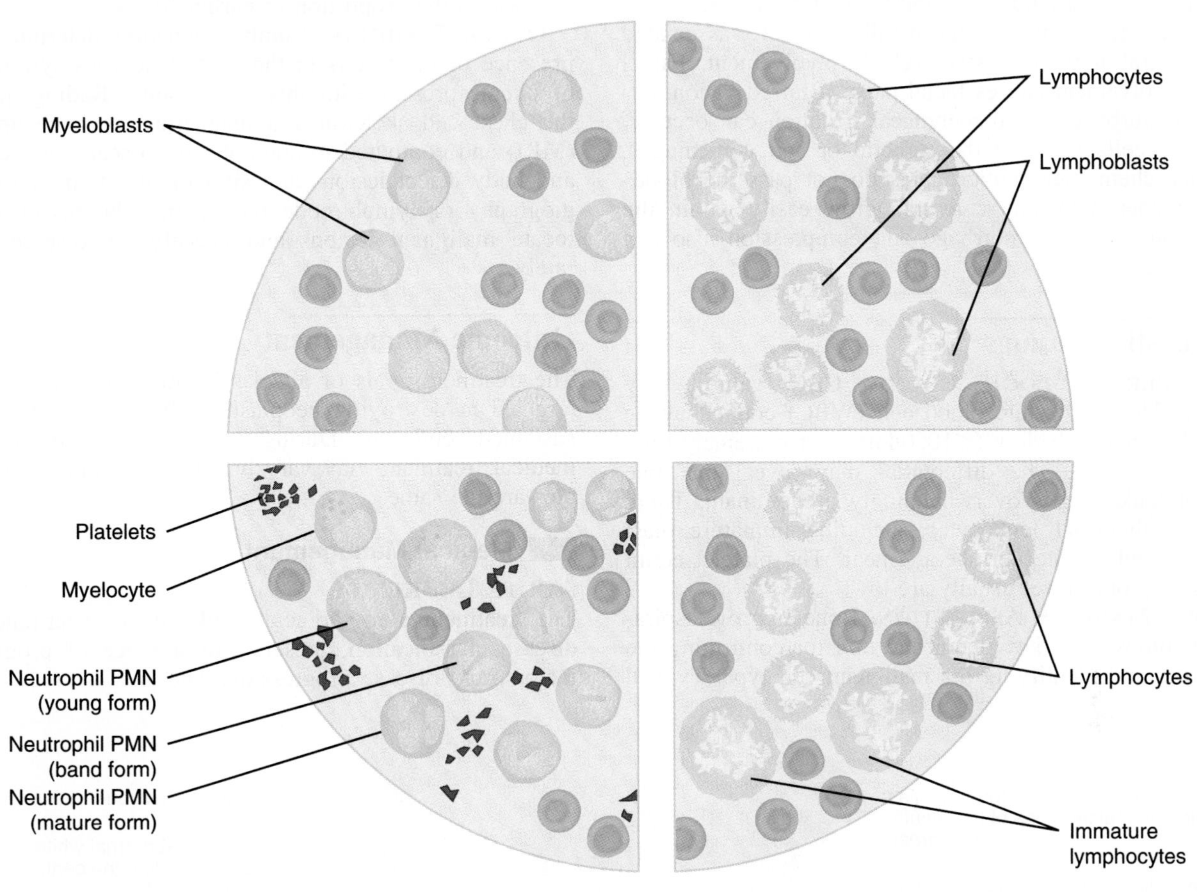

FIGURE 78–1 Comparison of types of leukemia.

in men older than 50 years of age. It is usually discovered when the complete blood count (CBC) is performed as part of a routine physical examination. A peripheral blood smear reveals increased numbers of mature and slightly immature lymphocytes. As the disease progresses, lymphocytes infiltrate the lymph nodes, liver, spleen, and ultimately the bone marrow. A staging system is based on the extent of lymphocyte infiltration. Progression of the disease may take 15 years.

Clinical Manifestations

The manifestations of all types of leukemia are similar. The clinical history usually reveals anemia, thrombocytopenia, and leukopenia.

Clinical manifestations of bone marrow depression include fatigue caused by anemia, bleeding resulting from thrombocytopenia (reduced numbers of circulating platelets), fever caused by infection, anorexia, headaches, and papilledema. Bleeding can occur in the skin, gums, mucous membranes, and gastrointestinal (GI) and genitourinary tracts. Bleeding also is the underlying cause of petechiae and ecchymosis (discoloration visible through the skin).

Anorexia is associated with weight loss, diminished sensitivity to sour and sweet tastes, wasting away of muscle, and difficulty swallowing. Liver, spleen, and lymph node enlargement are more common in ALL than in

TABLE 78–1 FRENCH-AMERICAN-BRITISH (FAB) CLASSIFICATION OF ACUTE LEUKEMIA

Acute lymphocytic leukemia
- L1 Common childhood leukemia
- L2 Adult acute lymphocytic leukemia
- L3 Rare subtype, blasts resembling those in Burkitt's lymphoma

Acute myeloblastic leukemia

Granulocytic
- M1 Myeloblastic leukemia without maturation
- M2 Myeloblastic leukemia with maturation
- M3 Hypergranular promyelocytic leukemia

Monocytic
- M4 Myelomonocytic leukemia
- M5 Monocytic

Erythroid
- M6 Erythroleukemia

ANLL. Splenomegaly and hepatomegaly usually occur together. The leukemic client commonly experiences abdominal pain and tenderness and breast tenderness.

Headache, vomiting, and papilledema are associated with central nervous system (CNS) involvement. Facial nerve involvement causes facial palsy. Blurred vision, auditory disturbances, and meningeal irritation can occur if leukemic cells infiltrate the cerebral or spinal meninges. Because chemotherapeutic agents do not pass the blood-brain barrier, leukemia cells can grow easily within the CNS. Intracranial hemorrhage and compression also can occur (Fig. 78–2).

Diagnostic Findings

COMPLETE BLOOD COUNT. CBC values vary greatly. The total white blood cell (WBC) count may be normal, abnormally low (<1000/mm³), or extremely high (>200,000/mm³). The differential may reveal that one type of leukocyte is overwhelmingly predominant. There may be abnormal leukocytes, including immature blast forms, noted on the peripheral smear. The platelet count and hemoglobin level usually are low.

BONE MARROW ASPIRATION. Bone marrow aspiration or biopsy is a key diagnostic tool for confirming the diagnosis and identifying the malignant cell type. Typical findings in the bone marrow aspirate and biopsy are an overall increase in the number of marrow cells with an increase in the proportion of earlier forms.

OTHER FINDINGS. Lumbar puncture determines the presence of blast cells in the central nervous system; 5% of clients present with this abnormality. Radiography of the chest and skeleton and magnetic resonance imaging (MRI) and computed tomography (CT) scans of the head and body detect lesions and sites of infection. Lymphangiography or lymph node biopsy may be performed to locate malignant lesions and classify the disease accurately.

Outcome Management

The treatment goals of all classifications of leukemia are targeted at destroying neoplastic cells and maintaining a sustained remission. During each phase of therapy, the medical treatment may vary but the basic nursing principles are the same.

Medical Management

ACUTE LEUKEMIA

The treatment plan for acute leukemia is determined by disease classification, presence or absence of prognostic factors, and disease progression. The goal of treatment is

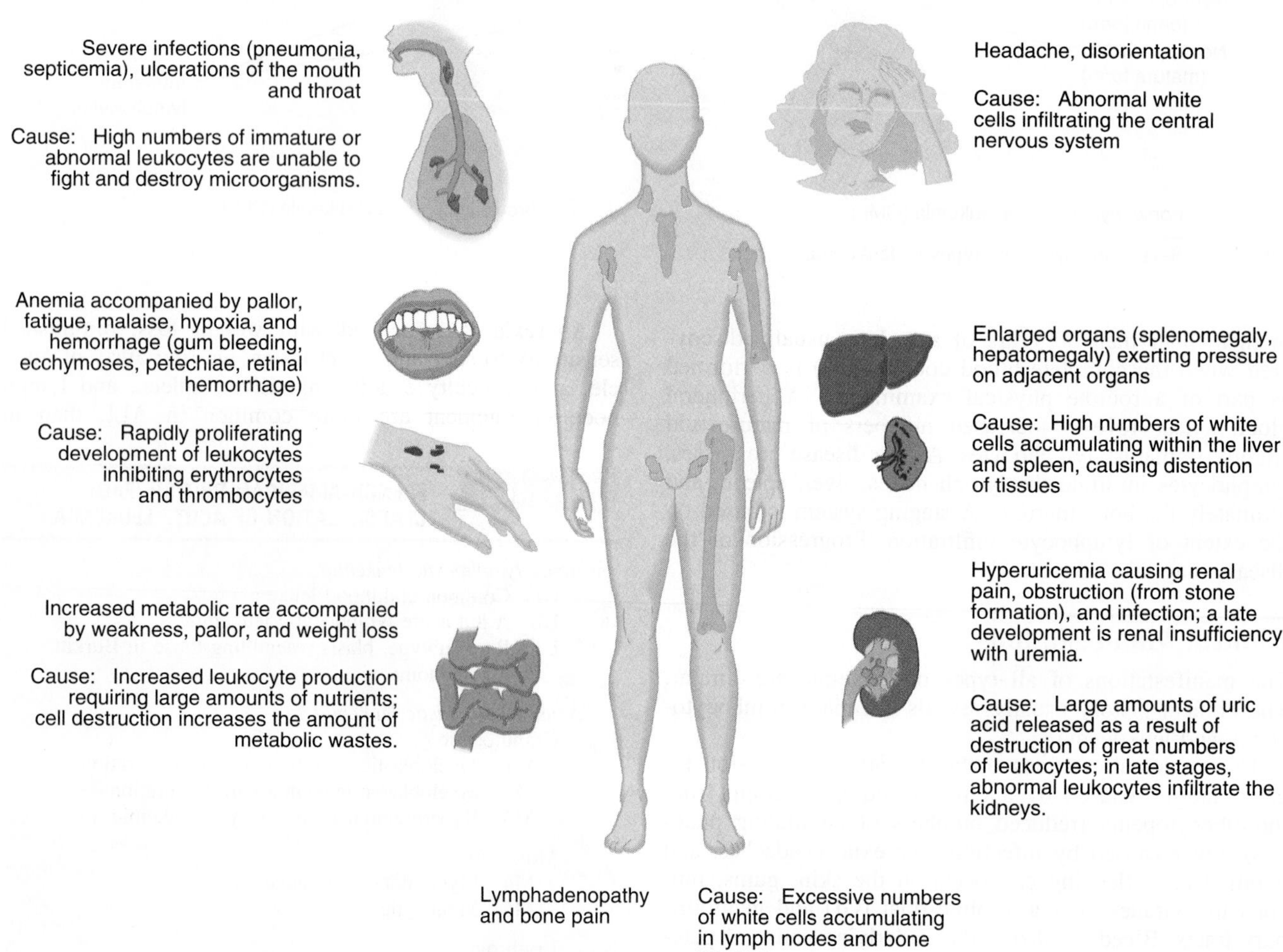

FIGURE 78–2 Clinical manifestations and pathophysiologic bases of leukemia.

complete remission with restoration of normal bone marrow function; this means a level of blast cells in the marrow less than 5%. Approximately 60% to 80% of adults with ALL achieve complete remission, with 35% to 45% surviving 2 years. The cure rate remains low without bone marrow transplantation, however. Of adults with ANLL, 60% to 70% achieve complete remission, with about 25% surviving 5 years or more.

Destruction of Neoplastic Cells

CHEMOTHERAPY. Chemotherapy is given to destroy the malignant cells of the bone marrow. The treatment protocol for acute leukemia involves three phases:

1. *Induction phase.* The client receives an intensive course of chemotherapy designed to induce complete remission. The usual criteria for complete remission are blast cells less than 5% of the bone marrow cells and normal peripheral blood counts. Both conditions must be sustained for at least 1 month. Once remission is achieved, the consolidation phase begins.
2. *Consolidation phase.* Modified courses of intensive chemotherapy are given to eradicate any remaining disease. Usually, a higher dose of one or more chemotherapeutic agents is administered.
3. *Maintenance phase.* Small doses of different combinations of chemotherapeutic agents are given every 3 to 4 weeks. This phase may continue for a year or more and is structured to allow the client to live as normal a life as possible. This phase is used more commonly with ALL.

TUMOR LYSIS SYNDROME. A potentially fatal complication resulting from the treatment of acute leukemia, tumor lysis syndrome is a group of metabolic complications associated with the rapid destruction of a large number of WBCs. If the WBC count is high when chemotherapy is initiated, rapid cell lysis can lead to: (1) increased serum uric acid, phosphate, and potassium levels and (2) decreased serum calcium levels. Manifestations include confusion, weakness, numbness, bradycardia, electrocardiographic (ECG) changes, and dysrhythmias (hyperkalemia); numbness, tingling, muscle cramps, seizures, tetany, and ECG changes (hypocalcemia); and uric acid crystalluria, renal obstruction, and acute renal failure (hyperuricemia). Acute tumor lysis syndrome can be prevented by increasing intravenous (IV) hydration, alkalizing the urine, and administering allopurinol (Zyloprim).

REPLACING CELLS AND CONTROLLING INFECTION. Current treatment modalities for acute leukemia destroy normal and aberrant cells. Therapy is aimed at preventing and resolving the complications of acquired and induced pancytopenia—anemia, bleeding, and infection. Transfusions of red blood cells (RBCs) and platelets may be required until the marrow produces mature cells. If the client requires IV infusions of RBCs and amphotericin B, an antifungal agent, they should be separated by at least 1 hour so that adverse (e.g., allergic) reactions, can be detected.

RADIATION THERAPY. Radiation therapy may be administered as an adjunct to chemotherapy when leukemic cells infiltrate the CNS, skin, rectum, and testes or when a large mediastinal mass is noted upon diagnosis (as may occur in ALL).

CHRONIC MYELOGENOUS LEUKEMIA

The goal of therapy in the chronic phase of CML is to control leukocytosis and thrombocytosis. When unwanted cells accumulate, apheresis is a method of blood collection in which blood is withdrawn. The unwanted component is separated, and the remainder of the blood is returned to the client. *Apheresis* is usually performed with use of automated blood cell separators designed to selectively remove the desired blood element. *Leukapheresis* may be performed to lower an extremely high peripheral leukocyte count quickly and to prevent acute tumor lysis syndrome, but results are temporary (Fig. 78–3). Likewise, for thrombocytosis of 2 million/mm^3, *thrombocytapheresis* may be necessary. If painful splenomegaly develops, irradiating or removing the spleen relieves this manifestation.

The most widely used medications are interferon alfa and hydroxyurea, which are given orally and intravenously. Clients with a blast crisis (Fig. 78–4) require intensive chemotherapy with the same agents as used in acute leukemia. These drugs can destroy leukemic blast cells, transform them into normal granulocytes, or prevent leukemic cells from inhibiting formation of normal granulocytes. Unfortunately, drugs are usually ineffective in achieving long-term remission.

CHRONIC LYMPHOCYTIC LEUKEMIA

The goal of therapy in CLL is palliation or symptom control. Local radiation to the spleen may be given as a palliative treatment to reduce complications. Two complications seen during the later stages are hemolytic anemia resulting from autoimmune disorder, and hypogammaglobulinemia, which further increases susceptibility to infection. Antibiotics, transfusions of RBCs, and injections of gamma-globulin concentrates may be required for these clients. Leukapheresis is performed when the WBCs are great enough to cause vascular thrombosis or embolism, especially in clients who are unresponsive to chemotherapy.

Chemotherapy

Chlorambucil (Leukeran) or cyclophosphamide (Cytoxan) may be given orally to reduce manifestations of CML. Chemotherapy generally is given for 2 weeks of every month. When anemia (stage III) and thrombocytopenia (stage IV) develop, daily oral prednisone is given as an adjunct to the alkylating agents. Prednisone has a marked lymphocytolytic effect and may stimulate the production of RBCs and platelets. Fludarabine is a new chemotherapeutic agent that appears effective in treating CLL.

Nursing Management of the Medical Client

ASSESSMENT

Obtain a thorough health history to aid in diagnosis and treatment. The initial history and physical examination provide baseline data to facilitate assessment of complications of ablative chemotherapy and radiation therapy. Be sure to obtain a thorough health history from the client and family members. The severity and longevity of the manifestations of leukemia are important facts to obtain and document.

Ask the client about risk factors and causative factors. Age is important to note because the incidence of leukemia increases with age. The client's occupation and hob-

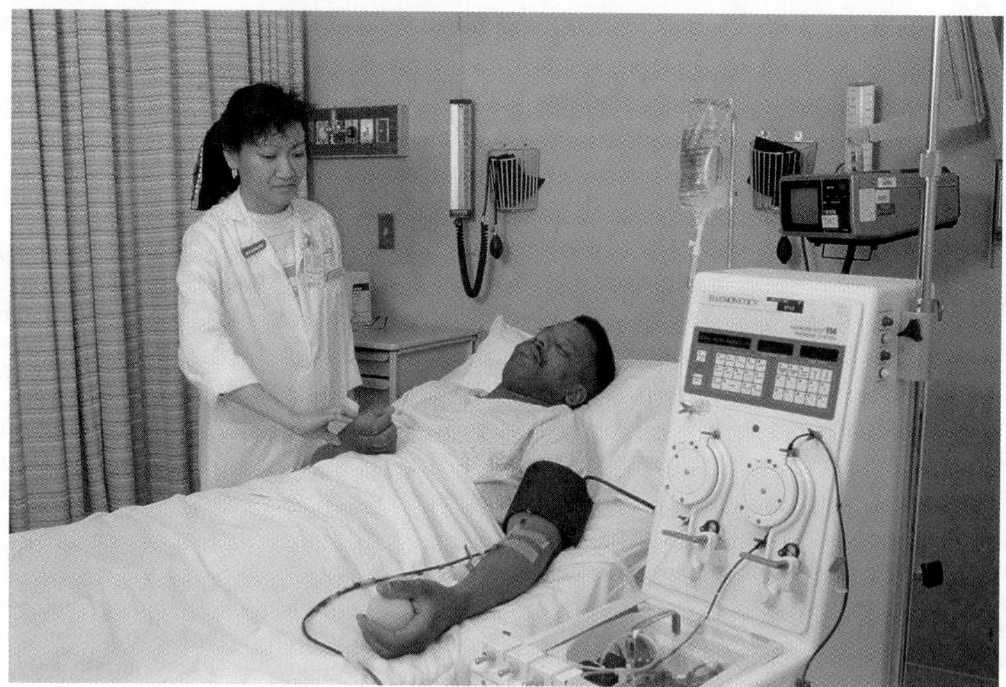

FIGURE 78–3 The white blood cell (WBC) level can be temporarily lowered by leukapheresis. Several automated blood cell separators effectively remove large numbers of WBCs and return red blood cells and plasma to the client. The Haemonetics V50 cell separator is commonly used to perform this procedure.

bies may also give hints about environmental exposures. Previous illnesses and medical history may indicate risk factors.

Because leukemia increases the risk of infection resulting from loss of WBC function, ask about the frequency and severity of infections, such as colds, pneumonia, bronchitis, and unexplained fever, during the past 6 months. Leukemia reduces the production of RBCs. The client may report activity intolerance, headache resulting from cerebral hypoxia, increased sleepiness, decreased attention span, anorexia, and weight loss.

The loss of platelet function increases the risk of bleeding. The client may report a tendency to bleed or bruise easily (e.g., nosebleeds), inability to stop bleeding from small nicks, bleeding in saliva with toothbrushing, increased menstrual flow, or blood in stool or urine.

Physical examination findings may include the manifestations shown in Figure 78–2. A complete head-to-toe assessment is performed. Clients with leukemia or blast crisis may have tachycardia, hypotension, tachypnea, murmurs or bruits, and increased capillary fill time resulting from low RBC counts. Skin and mucous membranes may

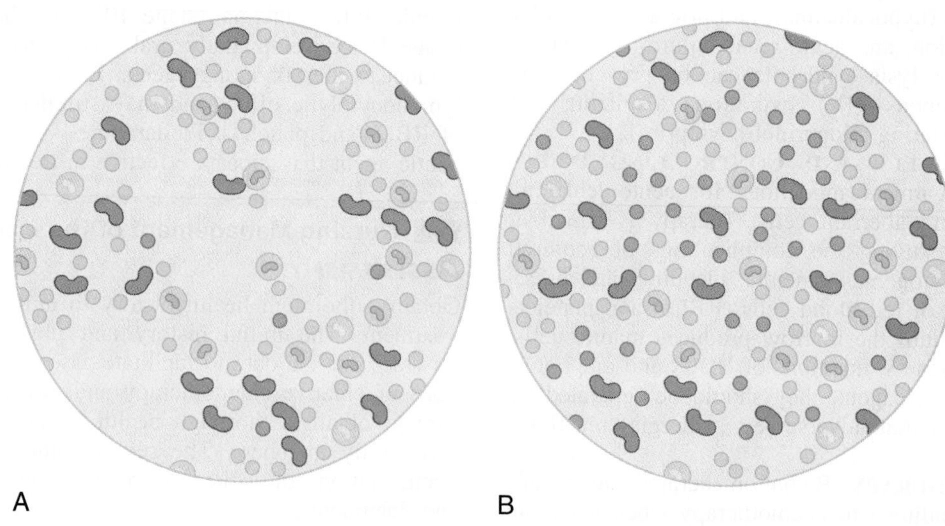

FIGURE 78–4 *A,* Microscopic view of a normal bone marrow specimen showing a normal distribution of blood cell types and fatty spaces. Blast cells appear as round, dark gray circles. *B,* During blast crisis, the number of blast cells increases and fatty spaces shrink.

show evidence of bruising and bleeding. Petechiae (small raised red spots) may be present. Lymph node enlargement may be present. If the leukemic cells have infiltrated the spleen or liver, abdominal tenderness may be noted. If the leukemic cells have infiltrated the brain, the client may be confused, have seizures, or become comatose.

The therapeutic relationship initiated during assessment is used to support the psychosocial needs of clients and their families. Leukemia is a life-threatening illness, and working with the client and family as a team is beneficial. Educating the client is an ongoing process to increase understanding of the disease and may help in obtaining compliance with treatment.

The nursing role during the acute phases of leukemia is extremely challenging because the client has many physical and psychosocial needs. Modern therapies offer hope for remission and possibly cure for some clients, but leukemia is still a diagnosis equated with pain, expensive long-term therapy, and potential death.

DIAGNOSIS, OUTCOMES, INTERVENTIONS

Risk for Sepsis. The diagnosis is written as *Risk for Sepsis related to neutropenia or leukocytosis secondary to leukemia or treatment.*

Outcomes. Infection will be prevented or will be discovered early and treated effectively, as evidenced by a neutrophil count greater than 1000/mm³, an absence of fever, and no respiratory difficulty.

Interventions. Institute required hand-washing for everyone coming in contact with the client. The client's risk for infection is estimated by calculating the absolute neutrophil count (ANC) (Box 78–1). The client should be in protective isolation if the ANC count is below 500/mm³. Visitors with possible communicable diseases should be screened for the presence of infection, and visitors or staff with colds or respiratory infections should not be allowed near the client. Avoid all live plants, flowers, and stuffed animals in the client's room.

The client should be on a low-bacteria diet that excludes raw fruits and vegetables. Assist the client with a daily bath using antimicrobial soap. Encourage the client to perform meticulous oral hygiene several times a day. Female clients should not douche and should avoid the use of tampons. Daily stool softeners are ordered to reduce the risk of anal fissures. Avoid insertion of rectal suppositories and rectal thermometers. Oral, axillary, or tympanic temperature should be taken every 4 hours and the physician notified if a temperature is higher than 38° C (100.5° to 101° F) or lower than 36° C (97° to 97.5° F). Fever may be the only manifestation in a neutropenic client. Assess the cause of fever before initiation of therapy by obtaining specimens of blood, sputum, urine, central line sites, and other potential sources of infection for culture.

Administer antibiotics as ordered. Therapy usually consists of multiple IV broad-spectrum antibiotics administered on alternating schedules. Administer analgesics as ordered for relief of discomfort, avoiding aspirin if the client is thrombocytopenic. Aspirin or aspirin-containing products also should be avoided because they may mask fever.

Invasive procedures should be avoided if possible. Provide meticulous skin decontamination before venipunctures. Maintain sterile occlusion of central venous catheters and perform routine dressing care according to institutional policy. Change IV tubing according to agency policy.

Monitor the client closely for manifestations of fungal or viral infections (i.e., increased respirations, rales, dyspnea, changed oral mucosa). Monitor the respiratory rate and auscultate breath sounds regularly. Viral and fungal pneumonia are common causes of death in the neutropenic client.

Risk for Hemorrhage. The client eventually becomes thrombocytopenic because of the progression of the disease or because of chemotherapy treatment, leading to the nursing diagnosis of *Risk for Hemorrhage related to thrombocytopenia secondary to either leukemia or treatment.*

Outcomes. Bleeding as a result of injuries, such as falls, punctures, cuts, or other environmental hazards, will be prevented or will be diagnosed and treated successfully, as evidenced by absence of bleeding and a platelet count greater than 20,000/mm³.

Interventions. Institute bleeding precautions, as follows:

- Provide soft toothbrushes or nonimpregnated cotton swabs or sponges for oral hygiene; avoid flossing, hard toothbrushes, and commercial mouthwashes.

BOX 78–1 Determining the Absolute Neutrophil Count

A leading complication in oncology clients is infection, and to recognize this risk, the absolute neutrophil count (ANC) is calculated daily. The ANC (or granulocyte count) provides a numeric estimate of the client's immune status, risk for bacterial infection, and need for reverse isolation. For example, the client with leukemia may have a high white blood cell (WBC) count or a normal count. On calculating the ANC, however, you may find that the client is at high risk for infection. For example, if a client had a WBC count of 9000 mm³, composed of 10% segmented neutrophils (segs), 60% blast cells, and 30% other WBCs, this client would have an increased risk of infection because the functional neutrophils are only 900.

Three numbers are required:

- Banded neutrophil count
- Segmented neutrophil count
- Total WBC

Obtain these numbers from the complete blood cell count and differential. The total WBC count is composed of five types of cells; the results from the laboratory show the total count and the percentage of each WBC type. For example, on the differential counts, the value next to monocytes represents the percentage of monocytes among the total number of WBCs.

Then use the following formula to calculate the ANC:

$$(\% \text{ band} + \% \text{ segs}) \times \text{total WBC count} = \text{ANC}$$

Example:

$$(2\% \text{ bands} + 55\% \text{ segs}) \times 1600 = 912$$

When the ANC is less than 1000, the client is at risk for bacterial infection.

When the ANC count is less than 500, the client is at high risk for bacterial infection.

- Instruct the client to avoid blowing or picking the nose, straining at bowel movements, douching or using tampons, or using nonelectric razors. Men and women should use only electric razors to shave with during the neutropenic phase.
- Do not give any injections, intramuscularly or subcutaneously, and do not insert rectal suppositories.
- Do not give medications containing aspirin, and instruct the client to avoid aspirin-containing medications.
- Avoid urinary catheters whenever possible. If a catheter must be inserted, use the smallest size possible, lubricate it well, and insert it gently.
- Avoid mucosal trauma during suctioning. Remove all potential hazards and sharp objects from the environment.
- Use a pressure-reducing mattress, and turn the client frequently to prevent pressure sores. Use bed cradles to protect extremities.
- Avoid overinflation of the blood pressure cuff, and rotate the cuff to different sites. Avoid prolonged use of tourniquets.
- Use only paper tape, and avoid strong adhesives that may cause skin adhesions.

Teach the client and significant others or family members to institute bleeding precautions during periods of thrombocytopenia. Monitor the client at least every 4 hours for manifestations of bleeding, such as ecchymosis, petechiae, epistaxis, gingival bleeding, hematuria, occult blood in stools, enlarged abdominal girth, disorientation, confusion, and changes in level of consciousness. All urine, stools, and emesis should be tested for blood. Take and record vital signs routinely, noting manifestations of altered tissue perfusion related to anemia (increased respirations and pulse, decreased blood pressure).

Check the platelet count, hemoglobin level, and hematocrit daily. Report a hemoglobin level of less than 10 g/dl and a platelet count of less than 20,000/mm^3. Administer packed RBCs and platelets as ordered. Keep a current blood sample in the laboratory for crossmatching if needed in an emergency.

Fatigue. Fatigue is a common complaint by clients. It may be cumulative, a gradually worsening response to treatments for cancer, low hematocrit, low hemoglobin, altered blood glucose levels, decreased oxygen saturation levels, abnormal electrolyte levels, or unintentional weight loss. Fatigue is the greatest about 2 to 3 days after IV chemotherapy. The nursing diagnosis is written *Fatigue related to side effects of treatments, low hemoglobin levels, pain, lack of sleep, or other causes* as made evident by the client. A scale to rate fatigue numerically is used, such as the Piper Fatigue Scale (see Chapter 22).

Outcomes. The client will report less fatigue, plan adequate rest periods, and be able to do an increasing amount of usual activities with decreasing assistance from others.

Interventions. Assess the physical, psychological, and treatment-related causes of fatigue. Encourage exercise to maintain strength. Ask a physical therapist to assist with bed and strengthening exercises. An occupational therapist may be able to offer suggestions or devices to conserve energy. If the client has thrombocytopenia or fever or has just received chemotherapy (past 24 hours), exercise is not encouraged to avoid injury. If possible, administer cisplatin and interferon at night to reduce the fatigue. Advocate for adequate pain relief, minimizing interruptions and reducing visitors when rest is needed. Outpatient chemotherapy is best scheduled on Fridays for clients who continue to work allowing them to rest over the weekend.

Altered Nutrition. The client usually experiences decreased appetite and decreased nutritional intake as a result of the effects of radiation therapy and chemotherapy on the GI tract. Write the diagnosis as *Altered Nutrition: Less Than Body Requirements related to anorexia, pain or fatigue.*

Outcomes. The client will maintain adequate nutrition, maintain body weight, as evidenced by stable weight, adequate caloric intake, and maintenance of fluid and electrolyte balance.

Interventions. Administer antiemetics, as ordered, around the clock to prevent nausea and vomiting. Premedicate the client with sufficient antiemetics before meals to encourage food and fluid intake. Administer local and IV analgesics, as ordered, to relieve pain caused by mucositis.

Discuss daily dietary requirements with the client and provide high-carbohydrate meals and oral supplements. Allow the client to make food selections. Cold foods, shakes, and sandwiches are tolerated better than hot or spicy foods. Small, frequent feedings may be tolerated better than three large meals a day. Monitor weight daily. If the client cannot tolerate food for an extended period, begin total parenteral nutrition (TPN), as ordered, and monitor intake. The client's own digestive system should be used as long as possible, with TPN used as a last resort. Use antidiarrheal agents as needed to treat diarrhea. Coordinate and plan rest periods and activities of daily living in increments as needed to minimize fatigue.

Body Image Disturbance. Most clients experience body image disturbance. The nursing diagnosis is written as *Body Image Disturbance due to alopecia, weight loss, and fatigue.*

Outcomes. The client will be able to demonstrate and discuss understanding of the disease condition and the temporary nature of changes in body image and energy.

Interventions. Inform the client before treatment of the potential for hair loss over the entire body. Encourage the use of scarves, hats, or wigs as desired. Explain the temporary nature of alopecia, although the hair may have a different color or texture when it returns.

Encourage the client to balance rest with exercise and activities to maintain muscle tone without developing severe fatigue. Discuss daily dietary requirements with the client, and provide high-carbohydrate meals and oral supplements in an attempt to help clients maintain their body weight and an appearance that is acceptable to them.

Risk for Reproductive or Sexual Dysfunction. Many clients experience reproductive or sexual dysfunction. The nursing diagnosis is written *Reproductive and/or Sexual Dysfunction related to the effects of chemotherapy or radiation therapy on reproductive organs.*

Outcomes. The client will be able to discuss the potential for sterility and decreased libido that may result from therapy.

Interventions. Describe the normal cellular destruction that might lead to temporary or permanent destruction of reproductive function in the client. Inform the client that sexual libido may be altered during and after the acute phase of the illness because of fatigue or other side effects of therapy. Provide the client with emotional support and references to support groups. Provide manuals for alternative sexual positioning and techniques. In appropriate cases, inform the client of reproductive alternatives, such as sperm banking and artificial insemination.

Risk for Ineffective Management of Therapeutic Regimen (Individuals) and Risk for Ineffective Management of Therapeutic Regimen: Families. Because hospital lengths of stay have become shorter and many oncology clients receive their care in outpatient settings, there is *Risk for Ineffective Management of Therapeutic Regimen (Individuals) and Risk for Ineffective Management of Therapeutic Regimen: Families* related to the chronic nature of the disease process and the risk for complications.

Outcomes. The client and family will manage the therapeutic regimen, as evidenced by effective medication administration, an absence of infections, no hemorrhage, and the client's ability to remain independent at home.

Interventions. After the induction phase of therapy is completed successfully, the client frequently returns home to recover and await subsequent courses of therapy that may be given on an outpatient basis, if no serious complications arise. It is common for clients to return home with anemia and thrombocytopenia. They also may suffer from the residual effects of chemotherapy or radiation therapy, such as loss of appetite, nausea, and mucositis. Some clients find it difficult to leave the security of the hospital setting because of significantly altered body image, fatigue, and fear.

Teach the client and significant others how to recognize manifestations of complications as well as appropriate actions to take. Inform them of measures to ensure safety and to reduce risks of bleeding and infection. Provide phone numbers of nursing personnel they can call with questions and for suggestions for interventions. The client and family should be referred to an oncology clinical nurse specialist or case manager as soon as possible after diagnosis. These nurses often assist the client and family concerning the disease process, the planned treatment, and strategies for successful transition from the hospital to home and outpatient care.

EVALUATION

The desired outcome for the client with leukemia is that the disease will become a chronic condition that the client and family can cope with in a positive manner. If acute leukemia does not respond to therapy, the client's life expectancy is short.

Surgical Management

BONE MARROW TRANSPLANTATION

To achieve cure with acute leukemia, BMT is the current recommended treatment. Allogeneic BMT presents a treatment option for clients younger than 60 years of age who have a suitable HLA-matched donor. Transplantation performed during the first remission has a higher success rate than transplantation performed during repeated remissions or in the blast phase of chronic leukemia. BMT is discussed later in this chapter.

Modifications for Elderly Clients

Older clients are at greater risk for chronic leukemia. The treatment of chronic leukemia in older clients is less vigorous. BMT is an option in the elderly if they are otherwise fit and if their organ systems can endure the stress of the procedure. Some older adults with excellent physical and psychological functioning have done quite well with BMT.

LYMPHOMAS

Primary tumors originating from the lymphatic system were identified in 1932. Lymphoma is the most common tumor of the lymphoid system, with about 55,000 new cases diagnosed annually. Lymphomas are tumors of primary lymphoid tissue (thymus and bone marrow) or secondary tissue (lymph nodes, spleen, tonsils, and intestinal lymphoid tissue). Most lymphomas are neoplasms of secondary lymphoid tissue and involve mostly lymph nodes, the spleen, or both. Malignant lymphoid cells sometimes are found in circulating blood, indicating bone marrow involvement. The major subdivisions of malignant lymphomas are *Hodgkin's lymphoma* (*Hodgkin's disease* [HD]) and *non-Hodgkin's lymphoma* (NHL). Bone marrow involvement occurs more often in non-Hodgkin's lymphoma than in HD.

HODGKIN'S DISEASE

In 1832, Hodgkin described a disease characterized by relentless enlargement of lymph nodes beginning in the neck and spreading throughout the body. He also reported that biopsy tissue showed a distinctive large cell, called a *Reed and Sternberg cell,* for the scientists who named it. Today the disease is called *Hodgkin's disease* and is known to be cancer of the lymph, or a lymphoma. Incidence rates differ with respect to age, gender, geographic locations, and socioeconomic class. Approximately 7500 new cases of HD are diagnosed annually. The male-to-female ratio is 1.4:1.

In economically advantaged countries, the incidence of HD is bimodal, with the first peak occurring in the mid-20s and the second peak occurring after age 50. In economically underdeveloped countries, the overall incidence of HD is lower than in developed countries but the incidence of HD before age 15 is higher, with only a modest increase into young adulthood. The incidence in people older than age 60 is declining, probably because of improved diagnostic techniques that classify NHL more correctly.

Etiology

The exact cause of HD is unknown, although indirect evidence indicates a viral cause. The Epstein-Barr virus (EBV) is believed to be a causative agent. EBV-associated lymphomas are well documented in clients who have received organ transplants or who have an immunodeficiency disease. A two-fold to three-fold increase of HD is seen among clients who have a history of mononucleosis, a disease caused by EBV. Researchers have shown that 30% to 50% of HD specimens contained EBV genome fragments in the diagnostic Reed-Sternberg cells.

Some studies indicate a genetic predisposition for HD. The disease occurs more frequently in Jews and among first-degree relatives. Siblings were shown to have a two-fold to five-fold increased risk, and same-sex siblings have a nine-fold increased risk. An increased risk was found among parent-child pairs but not among spouses, suggesting a genetic rather than infectious cause. Research continues in an attempt to identify the genetic role in the development of HD.

Pathophysiology

Cancerous transformation occurs from a particular site in the lymph node. With continuing growth, the entire node becomes replaced, with zones of necrosis obscuring the normal nodular pattern. The mechanism of growth and spread of Hodgkin's disease remains unknown. Some have suggested that the disease progresses by extension to adjacent structures. It also may disseminate by the lymphatics because lymphoreticular cells inhabit all tissues of the body except the CNS. Hematologic spread also may occur, possibly by means of direct infiltration of blood vessels.

Clinical Manifestations

Clients often are asymptomatic and may present with painless lymphadenopathy. Enlarged lymph nodes most commonly are found in the supraclavicular, cervical, and mediastinal regions (Fig. 78–5). Local manifestations produced by lymphadenopathy usually are caused by pressure or obstruction. Involvement of the extremities can be manifested by pain, nerve irritation, and obliteration of the pulse. Clients may experience a nonproductive cough, with the chest radiograph revealing a mediastinal mass, which is present in 50% of clients.

Pericardial involvement can occur by direct invasion from mediastinal lymph nodes. This involvement can cause pericardial friction rub, pericardial effusion, and engorgement of neck veins. Other manifestations arise when enlarged lymph nodes obstruct or compress an adjacent structure (e.g., edema of the face, neck, and right arm secondary to superior vena cava compression or renal failure secondary to urethral obstruction).

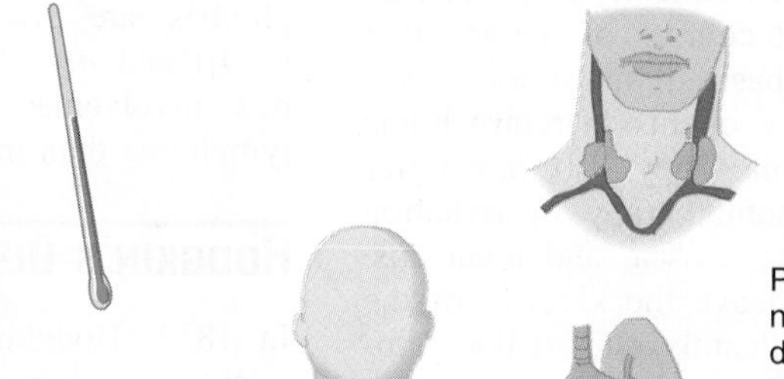

Severe pruritus is an early sign.
Cause: Unknown
Irregular fever usually present; temperature is elevated for a few days, then drops to normal or subnormal for several days; continuous high fever may indicate impending death.
Cause: Apparently related to neoplastic involvement of internal nodes or viscera
Jaundice
Cause: Obstruction of the bile ducts as a result of liver damage causes bilirubin to accumulate in the blood and discolor the skin.
Hepatosplenomegaly
Cause: Dissemination of the disorder from the lymph nodes to other organs
Renal failure
Cause: Ureteral obstruction by enlarged lymph nodes
Progressive anemia accompanied by fatigue, malaise, anorexia
Cause: Erythrocyte life span is shortened; erythropoiesis is unable to keep pace with erythrocyte destruction.
Edema and cyanosis of the face and neck
Cause: Enlarged lymph nodes place pressure on veins, obstructing drainage of this area.
Pulmonary symptoms including nonproductive cough, stridor, dyspnea, chest pain, cyanosis, and pleural effusion
Cause: Mediastinal lymph node enlargement, involvement of the lung parenchyma, and invasion of the pleura
Alcohol-induced pain in the bones, in involved lymph nodes, or around the mediastinum occurs immediately after drinking alcohol and lasts for 30 to 60 minutes.
Cause: Unknown
Bone pain, vertebral compression
Cause: Dissemination of disease from the lymph nodes to the bones
Paraplegia
Cause: Compression of the spinal cord resulting from extradural involvement
Nerve pain
Cause: Compression of the nerve roots of the brachial, lumbar, or sacral plexuses

FIGURE 78–5 Clinical manifestations and pathophysiologic bases of Hodgkin's disease.

If the tumor infiltrates the spine and presses on the spinal cord, manifestations of spinal cord compression can develop. Manifestations range from early back pain with motor weakness and sensory loss to loss of motor function, urinary retention, constipation, and other manifestations of compression of the cord late in the disease.

Associated clinical manifestations of unexplained weight loss of more than 10% of body weight in 6 months, frequent drenching night sweats, and fever above 38° C also may be present. Pruritus is a systemic manifestation that can be significant if it is recurrent. These additional manifestations are known as *B* symptoms for staging purposes; they occur in greater frequency in older clients and are negatively related to the prognosis.

The diagnosis is confirmed by lymph node and bone marrow biopsy. A chest radiograph to evaluate complaints of persistent cough or dyspnea may identify mediastinal involvement. The extent of disease is determined by CT scans of the thoracic, abdominal, and pelvic areas as well as gallium scans of mediastinal or hilar lymph nodes and lymphangiography of the lower extremities. If the extent of the disease cannot be determined by these diagnostic tests and confirmation of abdominal disease is necessary for determining treatment choice, a staging laparotomy may be performed.

STAGING

HD is divided into categories, or stages, according to the microscopic appearance of the involved lymph nodes, the extent and severity of the disorder, and the prognosis. Accurate staging of HD is important for determining treatment options. Table 78–2 shows the Cotswold Staging Classification, which modified the Ann Arbor classification system, primarily to incorporate the newer diagnostic tests and the evidence that bulky disease is an important prognostic indicator.

Outcome Management

Since the advent of combination chemotherapy, adult HD has become one of the most curable malignancies, resulting in a long-term survival rate of about 70%. The goal of therapy for clients with stage I and II disease is to achieve long-term disease-free survival with minimal acute and long-term complications that affect quality of life. Treatment consists of radiation therapy alone or combined with chemotherapy.

ERADICATION OF TUMOR CELLS

Radiation treatment for HD involves three locations: the mantle, the para-aortic region, and the pelvis (Fig. 78–6). The mantle field encompasses the submandibular, cervical, infraclavicular, axillary, mediastinal, subcarinal, and hilar lymph nodes. In clinical stage I and II disease, combined chemotherapy and radiation therapy are recommended for clients with unfavorable prognostic indicators. Most cancer centers classify B symptoms (fever, night sweats, and unexplained weight loss), high erythrocyte sedimentation rate (ESR), or large mediastinal adenopathy as poor prognostic factors. Some centers include large numbers of site involvement and older age as poor prognostic indicators.

Chemotherapy has become the primary treatment strategy, with or without radiation therapy, in stage I and II disease with poor prognostic indicators and in clients with advanced HD. There are numerous chemotherapy regimens for HD. For years, MOPP (mechlorethamine, vincristine [oncovin], procarbazine, prednisone) was the gold standard of therapy; however, ABVD (doxorubicin [Adriamycin], bleomycin, vinblastine, dacarbazine) has emerged as the best alternative to MOPP. The primary advantages of ABVD are its ease of delivery in full doses, fewer side effects, and less risk of subsequent development of leukemia. With proper treatment, the 20-year disease-free survival rate of HD is 70% to 80% and the overall survival rate, with salvage chemotherapy for clients who relapse, is 80% to 95%.

Research has shown that clients with advanced stage disease (II and IV) may achieve better treatment results with MOPP plus ABVD than with MOPP alone. Other studies showed that ABVD alone can achieve results similar to MOPP plus ABVD. Many physicians recommend ABVD alone given for as many cycles as required to achieve a complete remission, plus two consolidation cycles (usually six cycles total). The use of radiation therapy in advanced disease is individualized to the client, especially those with local-regional disease problems.

Clients who relapse after definitive HD therapy generally require some type of systemic therapy, which depends on the type of initial therapy used. Therapies range from chemotherapy and wide-field radiation to high-dose chemotherapy with autologous or allogeneic stem cell

TABLE 78–2 COTSWOLD STAGING CLASSIFICATION FOR HODGKIN'S DISEASE

Stage I	Involvement of a single lymph node region or a lymphoid structure (e.g., spleen, thymus, Waldeyer's ring)
Stage II	Involvement of two or more lymph node regions on the same side of the diaphragm (i.e., the mediastinum is a single site, hilar lymph nodes are lateralized). The number of anatomic sites should be indicated by a subscript (e.g., II_2)
Stage III	Involvement of lymph node regions or structures on both sides of the diaphragm: III_1: With or without involvement of splenic, hilar, celiac, or portal nodes III_2: With involvement of para-aortic, iliac, or mesenteric nodes.
Stage IV	Involvement of extranodal site(s) beyond that designated E.
DESIGNATION APPLICABLE TO ANY DISEASE STAGE	
A	No manifestations
B	Fever, drenching sweats, weight loss (B symptoms)
X	Bulky disease: >⅓ the width of the mediastinum <10 cm maximal dimension of nodal mass
E	Involvement of a single extranodal site, contiguous or proximal to a known nodal site.
CS	Clinical stage
PS	Pathologic stage

Data from Bennett, J. C., et al. (1996). *Cecil textbook of medicine* (20th ed.). Philadelphia: W. B. Saunders.

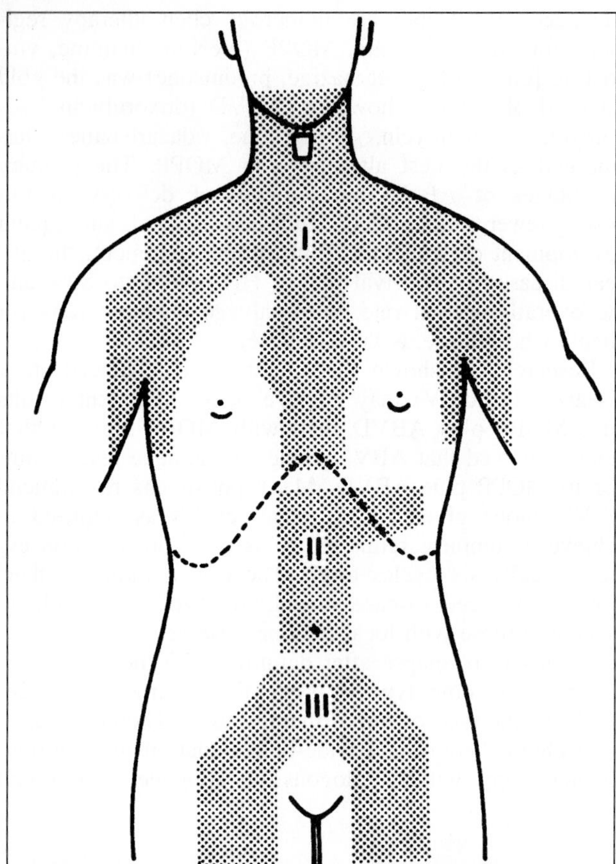

FIGURE 78–6 Radiation fields in therapy for Hodgkin's disease. *Shaded areas* represent the three treatment fields. The *mantle field* is the uppermost field (I). Lungs and vocal cords are protected by lead blocks; the heart and thyroid gland are within the field. The *para-aortic field,* or middle field (II), extends from the diaphragm to just above the bifurcation of the aorta. When the spleen has not been removed, this field is extended to include the entire spleen and splenic hilum. The *pelvic* or *inverted Y field* is the lowest field (III). It encompasses the pelvic and inguinal nodes and includes a large area of bone marrow. (From Murphy G. P., Lawrence, W., & Lenhard, R. E. [1995]. *American Cancer Society textbook of clinical oncology.* [2nd ed.]. Atlanta: American Cancer Society.)

transplant. Of clients with stages I to II HD, 20% to 30% relapse within 5 years after radiation therapy. In these cases, the use of combination chemotherapy produces a 57% to 62% disease-free survival at 10 years. At the National Cancer Institute, a 93% second complete remission rate was seen in clients with initial remissions longer than 12 months after chemotherapy. The positive results of several studies investigating the use of stem cell transplant have provided the basis for recommending bone marrow and stem cell transplantation for all HD clients who relapsed or did not respond to any primary chemotherapy, regardless of the length of the initial remission.

Complications

The complications related to HD are numerous because they are a result of the disease itself, radiation therapy, chemotherapy, or a combination of several of these factors (Table 78–3).

Nursing Management of the Medical Client

Obtain a thorough health history from the client and family members. The severity and longevity of the manifestations of lymphoma are important facts to obtain and document. Nurses play an essential role in symptom management associated with therapy. Because of the side effects of chemotherapy, clients may ask for a reduction of the dosage or may want to stop therapy completely. Provide clients with information regarding the effect of reducing or stopping therapy on long-term survival.

Explain to clients that they may have an impaired antibody response to vaccination. Clients who are projected to undergo chemotherapy are given *Haemophilus influenzae* type B, meningococcal, and pneumococcal vaccines before initiating therapy. Nurses are key to ensuring that these vaccines are provided at the appropriate time.

NON-HODGKIN'S LYMPHOMA

NHL comprises a group of malignancies with a common origin in the lymphoid cells. They are heterogeneous in cellular origin, morphologic appearance, and clinical behavior. The American Cancer Society estimates approximately 55,000 new cases of NHL annually and 25,000 related deaths in the United States.

NHL is seven times more common than HD. Between 1973 and 1991, there was a 73% increase in the incidence of NHL. Part of this increase was attributed to

TABLE 78–3 COMPLICATIONS OF HODGKIN'S DISEASE

Problem	Cause
Thyroid dysfunction Thymic hyperplasia	Underlying disease, therapy, or both
Hypothyroidism Thyroid cancer	Direct or indirect radiation exposure
Sexual dysfunction Male impotence Male and female infertility Female dyspareunia	Underlying disease, therapy, or both
Herpes zoster or varicella	Underlying disease, therapy, or both
Pulmonary dysfunction Pneumonitis (acute, chronic, or both)	Direct or indirect radiation exposure, bleomycin, nitrosoureas, radiation recall
Cardiac dysfunction Cardiomyopathy	Mediastinal radiation therapy, pericarditis (acute), doxorubicin, radiation recall
Pericarditis (chronic)	Mediastinal radiation therapy
Dental caries	Salivary changes related to radiation therapy
Myelodysplastic syndrome	Therapy, especially if age >40 yr or lymphocytic leukemia
Non-Hodgkin's lymphoma	Therapy
Solid tumors	Direct or indirect radiation exposure

acquired immunodeficiency syndrome (AIDS). NHL is about 60 times more common in people with AIDS than in the general population of the United States. NHL is the sixth most common cause of cancer-related deaths in the United States. Men are affected more often than women, and the incidence is higher in whites than other races. Survival outcomes are better for women than men and for people younger than 65 years of age. NHL can occur in any age group, but an increase in incidence occurs in the 50s and 60s. Because the average age at diagnosis is in the 50s, the number of years of life lost to these malignancies ranks NHL fourth in economic impact among cancers in the United States.

Etiology

No hereditary, ethnic, or dietary risk factors have been associated with NHL. An increased risk is associated with immunodeficiency states, autoimmune disorders, and infectious physical and chemical agents. As with HD, a viral or bacterial cause has been implicated (EBV, HTLV-1, human herpesvirus 8, *Helicobacter pylori*). A greater than expected incidence of NHL is reported in people with ataxia-telangiectasia, Wiskott-Aldrich syndrome, and Chédiak-Higashi syndrome.

Classifications

Terminology describing NHL is complex, inconsistent, and ambiguous, and there are several classifications. Rappaport's widely used classification, developed in 1956, distinguishes two major histopathologic patterns: nodular and diffuse (Table 78–4). These two patterns in NHL illustrate two different pathologic states. The nodular (and diffuse, well-differentiated lymphocytic) pattern involves nodal and extranodal sites. The diffuse pattern does not show the cell aggregates that are evident in the nodular pattern.

Based on expanding knowledge of the lymphatic system physiology, six distinct classification systems emerged worldwide in the 1970s. To standardize terminology, the Revised European-American Lymphoma (REAL) classification system was proposed in 1994. This classification includes all lymphoma types and the extra-nodal lymphomas not included in the other classification systems.

TABLE 78–4 RAPPAPORT STAGING CLASSIFICATION

Grade	Characteristics
Low grade	Diffuse, lymphocytic, well differentiated Nodular, lymphocytic, poorly differentiated Nodular, mixed, lymphocytic and histiocytic
Intermediate grade	Nodular, histiocytic Diffuse, lymphocytic Diffuse, mixed, lymphocytic and histiocytic
High grade	Diffuse, histiocytic Diffuse, lymphoblastic Diffuse, undifferentiated

Pathophysiology

In clients with NHL, an abnormal proliferation of neoplastic lymphocytes occurs. The cells remain fixed at one phase of development and continue to proliferate. Both T and B lymphocytes mature in the lymph nodes. Clinical manifestations are due to mechanical obstruction of the enlarged lymph nodes. Lymphocytic infiltration of the abdomen or oropharynx also can occur.

Clinical Manifestations

Clients with NHL present with localized or generalized lymphadenopathy. The cervical, axillary, inguinal, and femoral chains are the most frequent sites of lymph node enlargement. The swelling is generally painless, and the nodes have enlarged and transformed over months or years. Extranodal sites of involvement are the nasopharynx, GI tract, bone, thyroid, testes, and soft tissue. Some clients have retroperitoneal and abdominal masses with abdominal fullness, back pain, ascites (fluid in the peritoneal cavity), and leg swelling.

Several sites of involvement in NHL are not common in HD, such as Waldeyer's ring (lymphoid tissue that encircles the tonsils), the stomach, the small and large bowel, mesenteric lymph nodes, the thyroid, the skin, the pancreas, the kidneys, and the CNS. With diffuse NHL, clinical manifestations are variable and generally involve more systemic findings. Clients also may experience systemic *B* symptoms, including night sweats, fever, and weight loss. Approximately one third of clients have hepatomegaly or splenomegaly.

Certain other clinical conditions mimic the malignant lymphomas, including tuberculosis, syphilis, systemic lupus erythematosus, lung cancer, and bone cancer. A thorough diagnostic evaluation is required.

Diagnostic Findings

Blood work includes a CBC, ESR, and peripheral smear to rule out other causes of lymphadenopathy, such as mononucleosis. Blood cultures and other serologic studies for viral and autoimmune diseases provide important differential information. Elevated lactate dehydrogenase (LDH) levels may be seen in advanced NHL.

A lymph node biopsy is an important diagnostic tool. Indications for biopsy are

- Adenopathy for longer than 3 weeks, which progresses in size or spreads to other areas
- *B* symptoms that cannot be attributed to other causes
- Abnormal blood test results indicative of lymphoma
- Radiographs that suggest possible extranodal involvement

Because of the aggressive nature of AIDS-related NHL, any symptomatic client at increased risk or known to be positive for human immunodeficiency virus (HIV) should have a biopsy to rule out high-grade lymphoma.

Just as in HD, once the diagnosis of NHL is made, disease staging should take place. Noninvasive imaging techniques, such as CT and MRI, are useful tools in the initial staging of NHL. Renal and liver function tests are performed to determine the presence of extranodal involvement. Bilateral bone marrow biopsies are important because metastasis to the bone marrow is common, especially in low-grade disease.

Outcome Management

Many classification systems are used to differentiate NHL according to histologic type and cytologic characteristics. Treatment varies based on the histology and stage of the tumor. The treatment of a low-grade lymphoma is different from that for high-grade disease. Low-grade tumors tend to progress slowly and often are asymptomatic for long periods; the natural course of the disease may fluctuate considerably over 5 to 10 years with or without treatment. Low-grade cells eventually transform into a more aggressive disease process, however, and quickly cause the death of the client. Because of this process, indolent NHL is believed to be incurable, and many controversies exist concerning treatment standards, especially in clients who have disseminated disease.

The progression of intermediate-grade and high-grade lymphomas is similar to that of other cancers. Because of their higher growth fraction, however, these tumors tend to be more sensitive to chemotherapy and radiation therapy; there is a higher response rate when these tumors are treated. Combination chemotherapy is used to produce tumor shrinkage and remission. Cyclophosphamide and doxorubicin are active against lymphoma. Various combination drug regimens that include these two drugs are used in the treatment of NHL. Controversy regarding first-line standard of care therapy still exists. Studies comparing various treatment protocols affirmed the practice of using CHOP (cyclophosphamide, hydroxydaunorubicin [doxorubicin], vincristine [oncovin], prednisone) as first-line therapy in many academic and community settings.

For clients with low-grade NHL in stage I to II, radiation therapy alone may be curative, although there are reports of recurrence past 10 years. Depending on whether the disease is supradiaphragmatic or subdiaphragmatic, single-mode therapy includes mantle and inverted *Y* field irradiation (see Fig. 78–6). Management of stage III to IV low-grade lymphoma with any therapy is controversial. In clients who are asymptomatic, a watch-and-wait approach may be used. In some studies comparing clients treated with aggressive initial chemotherapy versus those using watchful waiting, the disease-free survival at 4 years was striking (51% in the treatment group versus 12% in the observed clients). There was no difference in the overall survival of the groups, however. Such findings contribute to the ongoing confusion as to the best initial treatment of such clients.

Clients with stage III to IV intermediate-grade lymphoma require combination chemotherapy as an immediate intervention. Clients who are older than 60 years of age and have elevated LDH levels, poor performance status, and stage III to IV intermediate disease are at higher risk and should be offered aggressive regimens that provide higher-dose intensities.

The diagnosis of a high-grade NHL warrants immediate and aggressive treatment. Clients may present with rapidly growing disease that has the potential to double in bulk in days or hours. Treatment includes dose-intense chemotherapy, with or without radiation therapy, and prophylactic CNS therapy. It is necessary to provide prophylaxis for the CNS because the blood-brain barrier prevents chemotherapy from getting into CNS spaces. Without such treatment, lymphoma cells may look for "sanctuary" in the CNS (CNS metastasis). High-grade NHL clients also are excellent candidates for bone marrow or stem cell transplantation because the tumors respond dramatically to high-dose chemotherapy, which is part of the preparative regimen of transplant.

Many clients (30% to 60%) with NHL do not achieve a complete remission and require salvage therapy to control the disease; however, none of the salvage therapies offer the client more than a small likelihood of surviving another 24 months after treatment. Biologic response modifiers (BRMs) and monoclonal antibodies (rituximab) have been used with varied success.

Nursing Management of the Medical Client

ASSESSMENT

Although the appearance of an enlarged lymph node in the absence of infection may cause worry, 56% of healthy adults may experience cervical adenopathy. Any enlargement of lymph nodes warrants further evaluation.

The work-up for NHL begins with a thorough history and physical examination. On examination, lymph nodes involved in infectious processes may be tender or painful, whereas lymphomatous nodes tend to be firm and "rubbery" and are found in generalized patterns. Carcinomatous nodes often are hard and sometimes matted to one another or fixed to underlying structures in contiguous or regional patterns. Other hallmarks of lymphoma, such as systemic *B* symptoms (fever, night sweats, unexplained weight loss), are seen in 20% to 30% of clients, but these manifestations also may be seen in other disease states, such as certain infections and connective tissue diseases.

The heterogeneous nature of NHL challenges nurses to meet a variety of physical and psychosocial needs for both clients and their families. The client and family members are confronted with managing a demanding diagnosis and treatment and the effects of the disease on daily routines. Health care professionals often assume that clients with supportive families manage well, but family members do share the strain of the illness, are deeply affected (psychologically, financially, and perhaps physically), and need ongoing support. It is crucial that nurses adapt their plans of care for these clients along the disease trajectory which can wax and wane for many years.

DIAGNOSIS, OUTCOMES, INTERVENTIONS

The nursing diagnosis, outcomes, and interventions for HD and NHL are the same as those for the client with leukemia.

Nursing Diagnoses. These clients are *At Risk for Sepsis, At Risk of Bleeding* (as a result of thrombocytopenia secondary to treatment), *At Risk for Sexual/Reproductive Dysfunction,* prone to *Altered Nutrition,* and *At Risk for Ineffective Management of Therapeutic Regimen* (Individuals and Families).

Outcomes. The desired outcome for the client with lymphoma is that the disease will become a chronic condition that the client and family can cope with in a positive manner. If the disease becomes terminal, the outcome should include a death with dignity, in which comfort measures and psychological support are emphasized.

Interventions. Interventions for these problems were discussed previously for leukemic clients.

EVALUATION

Physiologic problems may resolve quickly with medication. Psychological diagnosis will require prolonged intervention.

BONE MARROW TRANSPLANTATION

Since the 1970s, BMT has progressed from a treatment of last resort to a viable therapeutic modality for a variety of hematologic, malignant, and nonmalignant disorders. Peripheral stem cell transplantation and autologous transplants have further revolutionized the field. The status of the disease to be treated by BMT is an important determinant of the outcome for the client. When BMT is performed in clients with acute leukemia in full relapse, the disease-free survival rates approximate 15%, whereas BMT mortality falls dramatically in clients with chemotherapy-induced remission.

INDICATIONS

Bone marrow transplant may be considered as a treatment for clients with the following:

- Aplastic anemia
- Malignant disorders, specifically myelodysplastic syndromes, leukemia (certain types of acute leukemic, chronic leukemic, and preleukemic states), lymphoma, multiple myeloma, neuroblastoma, and selected solid tumors (breast cancer, ovarian cancer, testicular cancer, poor-risk germ cell tumors)
- Nonmalignant hematologic disorders, such as Fanconi's anemia, thalassemia, and sickle cell anemia
- Immunodeficiency disorders, such as severe combined immunodeficiency disease and Wiskott-Aldrich syndrome

BONE MARROW HARVESTING

Sources of Bone Marrow

There are three types of bone marrow donors: (1) allogeneic, (2) syngeneic, and (3) autologous.

ALLOGENEIC BONE MARROW. Allogeneic bone marrow is obtained from a relative or unrelated donor having a close HLA type. This was the most common type of marrow transplant but it carried the highest rate of morbidity and mortality because of complications of incompatibility such as graft-versus-host disease (GVHD). The rate of allogeneic transplants has dropped with the drop in the birth rate and the increased use of autologous and peripheral stem cell transplants.

SYNGENEIC BONE MARROW. Syngeneic marrow is donated by an identical twin. Although syngeneic marrow is a perfect HLA match, which eliminates the risks of marrow rejection, the incidence of leukemic relapse is higher than when an allogeneic donor is used because GVHD is considered to have an antileukemic effect.

AUTOLOGOUS BONE MARROW. Autologous marrow is removed from the intended recipient during the remission phase to allow another course of ablative therapy to be given if a relapse occurs. Although autologous marrow eliminates the risk of adverse immunologic responses, such as GVHD and graft rejection, relapse after autologous BMT is a frequent occurrence. This relapse may be due to contamination of the harvested bone marrow by malignant cells or to failure of pretransplant chemotherapy to eradicate completely the tumor cells from the body. The role of techniques used to purge residual tumor cells from marrow (chemotherapy, monoclonal antibodies) remains uncertain because of the absence of controlled trials.

Histocompatibility Testing for Allogeneic and Syngeneic Transplantation

Immunologic recognition of the differences in HLA antigens is the first step in host transplant rejection. The HLA system antigens are a complex set of protein structures found on the surface membrane of all human nucleated cells, solid tissues, and circulating blood cells except red blood cells. This genetically inherited mixture of antigens is considered representative of the tissue type of each person.

Siblings have a 1 in 4 chance of having identical sets of HLA antigens. This situation would provide the optimally matched allogeneic bone marrow donor. Because of the complexity of the HLA system, nonrelated clients have less than a 1 in 5000 chance of having identical HLA types. The establishment of the National Bone Marrow Donor Program (NMDP) in 1986 has given hope to many clients who do not have a compatible relative donor. As of June 2000, approximately 1 million donors are listed in the NMDP's registry, with about 25,000 new volunteer donors added to the registry every month. This has increased the use of unrelated donors for allogeneic transplants.

ALLOGENEIC DONOR PREPARATION

An extensive work-up is performed for ensuring compatibility and the mental and physical well-being of the prospective donor. This evaluation includes histocompatibility testing, medical history, physical examination, chest film, ECG, laboratory evaluation (complete blood count, chemistry profile, viral testing, rapid plasma reagin test [syphilis], ABO and Rh blood typing, coagulation studies), and psychological testing (may include psychiatric consultation).

Before marrow harvest, an informed consent, including potential donor complications (pain, fever, hematoma), must be obtained. In rare instances, the donor may experience serious adverse effects from general anesthesia. Because of the potential for significant blood loss during the harvesting process, syngeneic and allogeneic donors are required to donate autologous blood for reinfusion before the procedure.

Newborns currently are being used as potential donors through the use of their cord blood, which is rich in stem cells. Some parents are being encouraged to freeze their newborn's cord blood for future use, especially if there is a history of cancer in the family.

Marrow Collection

When collecting marrow, the client or donor is given general or spinal anesthesia in the operating room. The marrow is obtained in 2- to 5-ml aliquots from the marrow spaces of the posterior and, occasionally, anterior iliac crest and sternum. Numerous skin punctures may be required; the aspiration needle is redirected to various marrow spaces without being withdrawn. A total of 400 to 800 ml of marrow usually is obtained. The blood is placed in heparinized tissue culture media and filtered for removal of fat and bone particles. Marrow can be infused immediately or frozen in a solution containing dimethyl sulfoxide (DMSO), which preserves stem cells in the frozen state.

Peripheral Stem Cell Collection

Peripheral stem (progenitor) cells are harvested by apheresis or leukapheresis, a process that removes blood through a large-bore catheter and runs it through a machine that removes the stem cells before returning the blood to the client. Because stem cell concentration is much lower in peripheral blood compared with bone marrow, a process to increase the concentration in the peripheral blood must be initiated first. To increase the number of circulating stem cells, a stimulus, such as a colony-stimulating factor (CSF), interleukins (ILs), fusion molecules (made from a combination of a CSF and IL-3), or some chemotherapeutic agents, may be given to the donor before the stem cell harvest. As mentioned earlier, the umbilical cord of newborns also is rich in stem cells.

Once the stem cells are harvested, they are preserved in the same manner as bone marrow. The engraftment of stem cells occurs at approximately the same rate as or slightly faster than with marrow transplantation.

Allogeneic Transplant

Recipient Preparation

The physical and psychological evaluation of the recipient is similar to that of the donor. Additional testing may be required to stage existing disease accurately. The recipient must undergo a preparative regimen before transplantation. Such a regimen serves three purposes:

1. Malignant cells are destroyed.
2. The immune system is inactivated, which reduces the risk of GVHD in allogeneic transplant clients.
3. The marrow cavities are emptied to provide space for implantation of the transfused stem cells.

Common protocols combine total body irradiation and high doses of a single chemotherapeutic agent (cyclophosphamide is one of the most common agents used) or fractionated/high doses of multiple agents. A multilumen central venous catheter is inserted to provide suitable access for marrow infusion as well as for antibiotics, blood products, hyperalimentation, and frequent blood sampling.

Bone Marrow Infusion

The infusion of the marrow is commonly anticlimactic after the client has undergone the rigorous preparatory chemotherapy and radiation therapy (often referred to as the *conditioning regimen*). The marrow usually is administered immediately after the conditioning regimen is complete. Marrow is administered from a large blood infusion bag by a multilumen catheter, using an infusion pump, or small volumes may be prefiltered and given by IV push by a physician.

The BMT client remains pancytopenic until the transplanted stem cells make their way to the medullary cavities, where subsequent growth and reconstitution of the marrow are confirmed. Indications of successful engraftment are an increase in platelets and RBCs in the peripheral blood count. This change may occur 14 days after marrow infusion. Each day that recovery is delayed places the client at added risk. Graft rejection is evident if the bone marrow fails to produce peripheral blood cells after several weeks.

Nursing Management

Nursing management of BMT clients follows the plan of care for any completely immunosuppressed client. Clients receiving allogeneic transplants must be observed closely for manifestations of GVHD. Potential immediate adverse reactions are allergic (urticaria, chills, fever), volume overload, and pulmonary complications secondary to fat emboli. Renal damage may occur from too many erythrocytes. The period immediately after transplant is crucial. Multisystem failure related to ablative therapy is common, as are immune reactions caused by the transplanted cells.

GRAFT-VERSUS-HOST DISEASE

The most common and potentially disastrous complication of allogeneic BMT is GVHD, which may occur 7 to 30 days after infusion of viable lymphocytes. The donor T lymphocytes form an immunologic reaction against the host cells. The clients at highest risk for development of GVHD are those who have had allogeneic BMT. Of those clients, risk is greatest when the donor mismatched two to three antigens and when the client is older than age 30 years. There remains a moderate risk (35% to 50% incidence) in clients who have HLA-identical donors.

Acute Graft-Versus-Host Disease

Acute GVHD is staged according to the organ system affected (Table 78–5). It usually affects the gut, skin, lungs, or liver. *Stage I* GVHD occurs in many allogeneic transplant clients. Skin manifestations may resolve without treatment. Systemic complications may be treated with immunosuppressive drug therapy.

Therapy for GVHD includes high doses of methylprednisolone, antithymocyte globulin, antilymphocyte globulin, cyclosporine, and anti–T cell immunotoxins. These also leave the client immunosuppressed and vulnerable to infection. The prognosis and treatment depend on the severity of the syndrome. Acute GVHD that does not respond to treatment greatly increases the morbidity and mortality of BMT.

Nursing management of clients with stage I GVHD is shown in the Care Plan.

TABLE 78–5 STAGES OF ACUTE GRAFT-VERSUS-HOST DISEASE

Stage	Skin Manifestations	Liver Manifestations	Gastrointestinal Manifestations
1	Maculopapular rash >25% body surface area	Bilirubin 2–3 mg/dl	Diarrhea 500–1000 ml/day
2	Maculopapular rash 25%–50% body surface area	Bilirubin 3–6 mg/dl	Diarrhea 1000–1500 ml/day
3	Generalized erythroderma	Bilirubin 6–15 mg/dl	Diarrhea >1500 ml/day
4	Desquamation and bullae	Bilirubin >15 mg/dl	Abdominal pain or ileus

C A R E P L A N

■ THE CLIENT WITH STAGE I GRAFT-VERSUS-HOST DISEASE

Nursing Diagnosis: Risk for Injury related to graft-versus-host disease

Outcome: Client exhibits resolution of early graft-versus-host disease (GVHD) as evidenced by healing of skin, return of liver functions to normal, resolution of diarrhea and abdominal cramping, normal serum electrolytes, and control of pain.

Interventions	Rationales
1. Assess client's or significant other's knowledge of GVHD.	1. The client or significant other also can monitor for clinical manifestations and by reporting them early enhance treatment.
2. Teach client or significant other about the early manifestations of GVHD and to report them: a. Erythematosus rash on palms, soles, ears and trunk b. Anorexia, abdominal cramping, diarrhea, nausea, vomiting	2. Client is ambulatory and may not recognize the need to report these data to the nurse.
3. Determine baseline status or skin condition, liver function (alkaline phosphatase, bilirubin), and gastrointestinal function before donor marrow infusion.	3. Baseline data guide assessments of further data.
4. Assess for manifestations of GVHD at day 25 post-transplant.	4. The median onset time of GVHD is 25 days after bone marrow transplant.
5. Administer prescribed preventive agents.	5. Medications such as methotrexate and cyclosporine are used to suppress response.
6. Monitor magnesium levels daily.	6. Cyclosporine can induce seizures in hypomagnesemic clients.
7. Monitor renal function daily.	7. Bilirubin levels rise in GVHD.
8. Irradiate all blood products before infusing.	8. Irradiation prevents the infusion of immunocompetent T lymphocytes.
9. Bathe daily in warm saline or warm Hibiclens solution diluted to 1:8 with sterile water. Pat skin dry.	9. Skin care is important to reduce the risk of infection and avoid injury to the skin.
10. Apply prescribed lotions to the moist skin after bathing.	10. Keeping the skin moist reduces the risk of cracks, which increase the risk of infection.
11. Monitor characteristics of stools. If diarrhea develops, keep the client on NPO (nothing by mouth). Administer antidiarrheal agents, and test all stools for blood.	11. Diarrhea is a manifestation of GVHD. Blood loss through stool may require transfusion for replacement.
12. Monitor intake and output strictly, and record daily weights.	12. GVHD can lead to dehydration. Clients receiving chemotherapeutic agents need ample fluids during administration to prevent renal damage.

CHRONIC GRAFT-VERSUS-HOST DISEASE

Chronic GVHD, a long-term form of the disease with less acute manifestations, may occur even if the client has not experienced acute GVHD. Chronic GVHD appears approximately 100 days after transplantation; it may affect the liver, GI system, oral mucosa, and lungs as well as the skin. Chronic GVHD resembles autoimmune collagen-vascular disorders, such as systemic lupus erythematosus. It is characterized by scleroderma-like skin fibrosis and Sjögren's syndrome, in which the mucosa and lacrimal ducts are abnormally dry.

Diagnosis of chronic GVHD is confirmed by skin and oral mucosal biopsy. Although severe GVHD usually is fatal, researchers believe that a complete absence of this immune reaction increases the risk of leukemic relapse. This situation may be due to a beneficial graft-versus-leukemic reaction that mild GVHD stimulates. In allogeneic BMT recipients with GVHD stages II through IV, the relapse rate is 2.5 times lower than in syngeneic recipients or allogeneic recipients without GVHD.

CONCLUSIONS

Leukemia and lymphoma are complex diseases affecting physiologic and psychological aspects of the client and the family. Nursing care focuses on protecting the client from infection resulting from loss of WBC function, protection from hemorrhage resulting from loss of platelet function, and protection from hypoxia resulting from loss of RBC function.

THINKING CRITICALLY

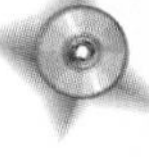

1. A 68-year-old woman is admitted with acute nonlymphocytic leukemia (ANLL). She is receiving chemotherapy. Her white blood cell count is 1000; 3% are banded neutrophils, and 54% are segmented neutrophils. What, if any, precautions are needed?

Factors to Consider. How is her risk of sepsis determined? Why does body temperature serve as one marker of infection? What precautions are followed?

2. A 34-year-old man with acute myelogenous leukemia comes to the outpatient oncology facility for his second round of chemotherapy. Three days later, the client calls the clinic nurse and is complaining of bleeding gums. What is the priority problem you should address? What instructions should the clinic nurse give the client at this time?

Factors to Consider. What pathologic process underlies the client's manifestations? Are there laboratory results you would want to check? What other precautions should you institute on the basis of the client's other manifestations and the laboratory data? What other data are significant to collect at this time?

BIBLIOGRAPHY

1. Bean, C. A. (1997). Acute lymphocytic leukemia: Nursing care, psychosocial issues, and discharge education. *Oncology Nursing Forum, 24*(6), 961–962.
2. Bilodeau, B. A., & Fessele, K. L. (1998). Non-Hodgkin's lymphoma. *Seminars in Oncology Nursing, 14*(4), 273–283.
3. Buchsel, P. C., Leum, E. W., & Randolph, S. R. (1996). Delayed complications of bone marrow transplantation: An update. *Oncology Nursing Forum, 23*(8),1267–1291.
4. Coleman, S. (1995). Bone marrow transplantation: Issues for critical care nurses: An overview of the oral complications of adult patients with malignant hematological conditions who have undergone radiotherapy or chemotherapy. *Journal of Advanced Nursing (England), 22*(6), 1085–1091.
5. Courtens, A. M., & Abu-Saad, H. H. (1998). Nursing diagnoses in patients with leukemia. *Nursing Diagnosis, 9*(2), 49–61.
6. De Meyer, E. S., Fletcher, M. A., & Buchsel, P. C. (1997). Management of dermatologic complications of chronic graft versus host disease: A case study. *Clinical Journal of Oncology Nursing, 1*(4), 95–104.
7. Ezzone, S. A. (1999). Tumor lysis syndrome. *Seminars in Oncology Nursing, 15*(3), 202–208.
8. Fernsler, J., & Fanuele, J. S. (1998). Lymphomas: Long-term sequelae and survivorship issues. *Seminars in Oncology Nursing, 14*(4), 321–328.
9. Hays, K., & McCartney, S. (1998). Nursing care of the patient with chronic lymphocytic leukemia. *Seminars in Oncology, 25*(1), 75–79.
10. Hogan, D. K., & Rosenthal, L. D. (1998). Oncologic emergencies in the patient with lymphoma. *Seminars in Oncology Nursing, 14*(4), 312–320.
11. Hurley, C. (1997). Ambulatory care after bone marrow or peripheral blood stem cell transplantation. *Clinical Journal of Oncology Nursing, 1*(1), 19–21.
12. Johns, A. (1998). Overview of bone marrow and stem cell transplantation. *Journal of Intravenous Nursing, 21*(6), 356–360.
13. Kosits, C., & Callaghan, M. (2000). Rituximab: A new monoclonal antibody therapy for non-Hodgkin's lymphoma. *Oncology Nursing Forum, 27*(1), 51–59.
14. McGuire, D. B., et al. (1998). Acute oral pain and mucositis in bone marrow transplant and leukemia patients: Data from a pilot study. *Cancer Nursing, 21*(6), 385–393.
15. Roach, M. (1998). Nurses manage recombinant interleukin-2 side effects in elderly patients with leukemia. *Oncology Nursing Forum, 25*(1), 29–30.
16. Sheely, L. C. (1996). Sleep disturbances in hospitalized patients with cancer. *Oncology Nursing Forum, 23*(1), 109–111.
17. Shelton, B. K., Baker, L., & Stecker, S. (1996). Critical care of the patient with hematologic malignancy. *AACN Clinical Issues 7*(1), 65–78.
18. Skalla, K. (1996). The interferons. *Seminars in Oncology Nursing, 12*(2), 97–105.
19. Stolar, K. (1999). A graft versus host disease prevention and management tool: A mechanism for improving continuity of care. *Oncology Nursing Forum, 26*(6), 977–978.
20. Vogelsang, G. B. (2000). Advances in the treatment of graft-versus-host disease. *Leukemia (England), 14*(3), 509–510.
21. Wagner, N. D., & Quinones, V. W. (1998). Allogeneic peripheral blood stem cell transplantation: Clinical overview and nursing implications. *Oncology Nursing Forum, 25*(6), 1049–1055.
22. Warmkessel, J. H. (1997). Caring for patients with non-Hodgkin's lymphoma. *Nursing, 27*(6), 48–49.
23. Yeager, K. A., et al. (2000). Implementation of an oral care standard for leukemia and transplantation patients. *Cancer Nursing, 23*(1), 40–47.

UNIT

17

Multisystem Disorders

REMEMBER *to check out your* Companion CD ROM

CHAPTER 79

Management of Clients with Acquired Immunodeficiency Syndrome

Peter J. Ungvarski

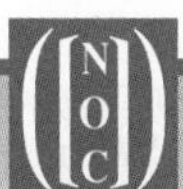

NURSING OUTCOMES CLASSIFICATION (NOC) for Nursing Diagnoses—Clients with HIV/AIDS

Altered Nutrition: Less Than Body Requirements
Nutritional Status
Nutritional Status: Food and Fluid Intake
Nutritional Status: Nutrient Intake
Effective Management of Therapeutic Regimen: Individual
Adherence Behavior
Compliance Behavior
Family Participation in Professional Care
Knowledge: Treatment Regimen
Participation: Health Care Decisions
Risk Control
Symptom Control
Fatigue
Activity Intolerance
Endurance
Energy Conservation
Nutritional Status: Energy
Psychomotor Energy
Hyperthermia
Immune Status
Thermoregulation
Pain
Comfort Level
Pain Control
Pain: Disruptive Effects
Pain Level

The human immunodeficiency virus (HIV) infects people worldwide and results in the destruction of the body's host defenses and immune system. By 1999, HIV infected more than 47 million people throughout the world, with an estimated 6 million people newly infected each year. HIV kills more people than any other infectious disease and ranks fourth among the leading causes of death worldwide.

For many years, because of our lack of understanding and effective treatment, HIV was considered a rapidly progressing fatal disease. Today, HIV infection is viewed more optimistically as a chronic disease that can be controlled with appropriate health care. However, the cost of such health care (~$12,000 yearly per person) limits its accessibility to developed, industrialized nations such as the United States. Because many parts of the world, such as Africa and Asia, lack adequate economic resources to treat this disease, HIV infection continues to be a rapidly progressing fatal illness in these areas.

From both a medical and nursing perspective, clinical management parallels the HIV illness trajectory. Once infected with HIV, a person who receives appropriate treatment can live for many years and continue to function without major problems. In the latter stages of disease, for a variety of reasons to be discussed, the illness progresses, wearing out the immune system. The person is then given the diagnosis acquired immunodeficiency syndrome (AIDS).

Because of this dual clinical picture, the material presented in this chapter is divided into (1) caring for the person with HIV disease and (2) caring for the person with AIDS. Remember, that advances and breakthroughs occur rapidly in this area of health care; you must seek additional information to stay up to date.

Etiology and Risk Factors

ETIOLOGY

The etiologic agent associated with AIDS was first isolated by French scientists in 1983 and named the *lymphadenopathy-associated virus.* One year later, an American scientist claimed the discovery of the etiologic agent and named it the *human T-cell lymphotropic virus type III.* Although both scientists actually identified the same virus, much confusion took place. In 1986, the International Society on the Taxonomy of Viruses renamed the virus, calling it the human immunodeficiency virus. In that same year, much to everyone's surprise, a second and distinctly different strain of the virus was discovered in Africa. Therefore, since 1986, the scientific names to distinguish between the two viruses are HIV-1 and HIV-2.

This was a major—and alarming—discovery because it was the first clue that HIV could change its appearance, or mutate, very rapidly. The capability of HIV to mutate rapidly is often referred to as *genetic promiscuity,* and it has become the hallmark of this virus, creating a monumental challenge for scientists and researchers alike. HIV-1 is distributed worldwide, but it is most prevalent in Europe and the United States. HIV-2 predominates in west African nations but has been isolated in other parts of the world. By 1999, approximately 79 cases of HIV-2 had been identified in the United States; most of the infected people had been born in Africa. Most worldwide infections are HIV-1.

By 1996, scientists discovered that HIV-1 had also mutated several times. It has two major subtypes, or *clades,* designated (1) HIV-1 major (group M) viruses and (2) HIV-1 outlier (group O) viruses.

HIV-1 Group M

Group M viruses have been assigned to 10 genetic subtypes, designated HIV-1, group M, subtype A, B, C, D, E, F, G, H, I, and J, according to the phylogenetic analysis of their genes. The distribution of subtypes varies worldwide. For example, whereas subtype B predominates in North America and Europe, subtypes A, B, C, and E have been identified in India. There is concern that subtypes other than B will invade the United States, because American service personnel assigned to overseas duty who have become infected with HIV-1 have been found to be infected with subtypes A, D, and E.

It is important to mention these complexities to illustrate the rapidly changing nature of HIV. The virus poses a considerable challenge to researchers investigating new drugs to treat the disease or developing vaccines because their work is usually limited to one specific subtype of HIV-1. Indeed, vaccine trials have demonstrated that a vaccine for one subtype may not work for other subtypes.

HIV-1 Group O

The designation O was deliberate, because this mutation was an outlier and differed from the others, in that it cannot be detected with the routine HIV antibody tests used in the United States. Group O was primarily identified in west and central Africa, with a few isolated cases found through special tests in France and the United States. The Centers for Disease Control and Prevention (CDC) is working with the manufacturers of HIV-1 antibody test kits to ensure that testing methods are reconfigured to detect HIV-1 group O as well as group M.

RISK FACTORS

Modes of transmission have remained constant throughout the course of the HIV pandemic. The virus is spread through certain sexual practices, through exposure to blood, and through perinatal transmission. The patterns in the spread of HIV changed considerably during the first 19 years of the epidemic in the United States. Comparing the 1980s with the 1990s, significant increases have been noted in intravenous (IV) drug users, women, and heterosexuals. Although most Americans infected with HIV continue to be men who have sex with men, the overall number has decreased considerably. This decline, however, has been limited to white men; the number of new HIV infections among racial and ethnic minority men who have sex with men continues to increase, as outlined in the Diversity in Health Care feature. In young adults (ages 19 to 29 years), the number of new infections has been increasing, especially in the South and Midwest. HIV infection and AIDS are the second leading causes of death among adults ages 25 to 44 years.

Perhaps the most overlooked population in the HIV epidemic is adults over age 50 years. By 1999, about 11% of the nation's total number of reported AIDS cases were in this age group. People over age 50 years may not be tested promptly for HIV because they and their health care providers may not perceive them to be at risk for this disease. Women over age 50 years are acquiring HIV infection primarily through heterosexual contact. Although the largest numbers of AIDS and HIV cases have been reported in large cities, such as New York and San Francisco, there has been a shift of newly diagnosed infections to small cities and rural areas, especially in the South and Midwest.

The principal mode of transmission of HIV throughout the world has been through sexual exposure. With the exception of Australia, Europe, and the United States, most HIV transmission has been through heterosexual activities. One important lesson that health care professionals have learned from the HIV epidemic is that sexual *practices,* not sexual *preferences,* place people at risk for sexually transmitted diseases (STDs). Homosexual men who do not engage in unprotected anus-penile sex or expose themselves to another person's body fluids are no more at risk for acquiring HIV infection than anyone else; similarly, heterosexual or homosexual couples in long-term, monogamous relationships are at low risk. The problem of unsafe sexual encounters outside of these relationships does, however, pose a risk.

Sexual practices that are *completely safe* include (1) autosexual activities (such as masturbation), (2) mutually monogamous relationships between noninfected partners, and (3) abstinence. *Very safe* sexual practices include non-insertive activity. Insertive practices with a condom are considered *probably safe* as long as the condom does not break and no contact with body fluids occurs. Everything else is considered risky. Other cofactors, such as engaging in sexual activities while under the influence of drugs or alcohol, having multiple sex partners, and the presence of sores in the genital area, increase the risk of acquiring HIV. Although the number of reported cases is small, oral sexual practices, whether performed on a man or a woman, have been implicated as a possible transmission activity.

Transmission by exposure to blood is a very broad category that encompasses numerous possible routes. The most obvious are through the administration of blood or blood products, transplantation of donated tissue or organs, and implantation of semen contaminated with HIV. Prevention of HIV infection by any of these means is possible by donor exclusion (excluding persons from high-risk groups), routine serologic testing of donated tissues or fluids for HIV antibodies, and heat inactivation of

DIVERSITY IN HEALTH CARE

HIV and AIDS in Minority Populations

Culture is an important variable in understanding the transmission and prevention of the human immunodeficiency virus (HIV) and acquired immunodeficiency syndrome (AIDS) because of the disproportionate occurrence of the disease in minority populations. AIDS affects many aspects of life that have cultural meanings, such as reproduction, birth, death, the roles of women, and sexuality.[2] Health care workers are challenged to understand the complex factors that account for the disproportionate occurrence of HIV and AIDS in minorities. Understanding these factors is the first step in finding interventions to prevent the further escalation of the HIV/AIDS epidemic. Clearly, health care workers must become "culturally competent" if they are to work effectively with their various patient groups in preventing and treating HIV disease.

The Problem

Minorities are disproportionately affected by HIV and AIDS. This is clearly represented by the HIV and AIDS statistics in the United States.[1] Cumulative case reports for people with AIDS through 1998 indicate that 58.6% were black or Hispanic. Specifically, by the end of 1997, the number of African-Americans living with AIDS *increased* from 32.7% of people with AIDS in 1992 to 39.2% in 1997. For Hispanics, the same category of figures *increased* from 17% in 1992 to 19.4% in 1997. For whites, the figures *decreased* from 1992 to 1997. In 1992, the number of whites with AIDS was 49%; this figure declined to 40% in 1997.[6]

The elimination of HIV and AIDS through preventing their spread is, at present, the only viable goal. Culture is an important variable in understanding HIV and AIDS because it is apparent in values, attitudes, and behaviors associated with everyday life. Consequently, health care workers must become *culturally competent*[4]; that is, they must:

- Develop an awareness of one's own sensations and beliefs
- Demonstrate knowledge and understanding of the client's culture
- Accept and respect cultural differences
- Adapt care to be congruent with the client's culture

Cultural competence facilitates assessments and interventions with culturally diverse populations. It includes the recognition that the Western biomedical explanation of HIV and AIDS is viewed as limited by ethnic minorities. One can only speculate how this variable influences the finding that people reported with AIDS increasingly represent those whose diagnosis was too late for them to benefit from treatment, people who did not seek care or did not have access to care, or people for whom treatment failed.[6] Consequently, health care workers should become familiar with alternative lay beliefs and explanations regarding AIDS and appropriate intervention.

An example is provided by the research of Suarez and colleagues.[5] Building on the fact that Hispanics residing in the United States are disproportionately affected by HIV infection and AIDS, these researchers investigated the beliefs and practices of Hispanics who were receiving medical care for their HIV infection. More than three quarters of the study population reported that they engaged in folk, religious, and other alternative healing practices.

Interventions

HIV infection and AIDS have provided an opportunity to focus on prevention and to understand how disease interacts with the complexities of culture. HIV prevention and treatment programs ideally are based on the following goals[2]:

- To use and enhance cultural beliefs, values, and roles as core elements of the intervention process
- To use traditional gender roles as well as the role of the family in health education and care as a starting point
- To enhance beneficial beliefs and practices that relate to HIV disease
- To clarify misperceptions that feed fear and stigma
- To modify harmful beliefs or negative attitudes and practices within the context of positive ethnocultural and community values

There is promising evidence that culturally sensitive theory-based interventions can be successful in reducing the HIV risk-associated sexual behavior of adolescents. For example, Jemmott and associates[3] noted that African American adolescents are at a high risk for contracting HIV and AIDS but that little is known about what interventions to reduce risk are most effective. Their research was designed to evaluate the effects of abstinence and safer sex HIV risk-reduction interventions on the sexual risk behaviors of inner-city African American adolescents. The study interventions were based on cognitive-behavioral theories. The interventions were designed to be educational, entertaining, and culturally sensitive. For example, each intervention incorporated the theme "Be Proud, Be Responsible" for yourself and your community. The interventions involved group discussions, videos, games, brainstorming, experiential exercises, and skill-building activities. The results suggest that both abstinence and safer sex interventions can reduce HIV sexual risk behaviors, but safer sex interventions may be especially effective with sexually experienced adolescents and may have longer-lasting effects.[3]

The elimination of HIV and AIDS through prevention is a viable goal. HIV and AIDS have provided an opportunity to focus on prevention and understand how disease interacts with the complexities of culture. If we continue to ignore the complexities of HIV and AIDS, it will not be long before the next great global epidemic demonstrates that ignorance and prejudice are the greatest human risks.[1]

For further information on HIV/AIDS and minority populations, the following selected resources may be consulted:

African American AIDS Policy and Training Institute
3418 Huxley Street
Los Angeles, CA 90027
Tel: 323-663-4194
Fax: 323-666-8846
e-mail: *info@aaainstitute.org*
Web site: *http://www.aaainstitute.org*

AIDS Education Services for Minorities
http://www.accessatlanta.com/community/groups/aesm

American Red Cross African American AIDS Program
http://www.redcross.org/hss/HIVAIDS/afam/index.html

CDC National Prevention Information Network
http://www.cdcnpin.org

Chart continued on following page

DIVERSITY IN HEALTH CARE *Continued*

Centers for Disease Control and Prevention
Divisions of HIV/AIDS Prevention
http://www.cdc.gov/nchstp/hiv_aids

Community HIV/AIDS Technical Assistance Network (CHATAN)
National Coalition of Hispanic Health and Human Services Organizations (COSSMHO)
1501 Sixteenth Street, NW
Washington, DC 20036
Tel: 202-387-5000
Fax: 202-797-4353
e-mail: *info@cossmho.org*
Web site: *http://www.cossmho.org/hiv.html*

Gay and Lesbian Latino AIDS Education Initiative (GALAEI)
1233 Locust Street
Philadelphia, PA 19107
Tel: 215-985-3382
Fax: 215-985-3388
Web site: *http://www.critpath.org/galaei*

Hispanic AIDS Awareness Program (Programa de Informacion Sobre el SIDA)
2350 Coral Way, Suite 301
Miami, FL 33145
Tel: 305-860-0780
Fax: 305-860-0580
e-mail: *HAAP@emservices.com*
Web site: *http://www.emservices.com/haap*

Minority AIDS Project
5149 Jefferson Boulevard
Los Angeles, CA 90016-3836
Tel: 213-936-4949
Fax: 213-936-4973
e-mail: *Paul519@aol.com*
Web site: *http//www.geocities.com/Hollywood/9930/map.html*

National Minority AIDS Council
1931 13th Street, N.W.
Washington, DC 20009
Tel: 202-483-6622; 800-559-4145
Fax: 202-483-1135
e-mail: *info@nmac.org*
Web site: *http://www.nmac.org*

"Race/Ethnicity and HIV/AIDS," in *The Body: An AIDS and HIV Information Resource*
Web sites: *http://thebody.com/whatis/race.html*
http://thebody.com/bbs/forums.html

U.S. Department of Health and Human Services, Office of Minority Health Resource Center:
"Minority HIV/AIDS Initiative"
Tel: 1-800-444-6472
e-mail: *info@omhrc.gov*
Web site: *http://www.omhrc.gov/omh/aids/aidshome.htm*

University of California, San Francisco:
"HIV InSite: Gateway to AIDS Knowledge"
Web site: *http://HIVInSite.ucsf.edu*

References

1. Bradley-Springer, L. (1999). The complex realities of primary prevention for HIV infection in a "just do it" world. *Nursing Clinics of North America, 34*(1), 49–70.
2. Flaskerud, J. (1999). Culture and ethnicity. In P. Ungvarski, & J. Flaskerud (Eds.), *HIV/AIDS: A guide to primary care management.* Philadelphia: W. B. Saunders.
3. Jemmott, J., Jemmott, L., & Fong, G. (1998). Abstinence and safer sex: HIV risk-reduction interventions for African American adolescents. *Journal of the American Medical Association, 279*(19), 1529–1536.
4. Paulanka, B., & Purnell, L. (1998). *Transcultural health care: A culturally competent approach.* Philadelphia: F. A. Davis.
5. Suarez, M., Raffaelli M., & O'Leary, O. (1996). Use of folk healing practices by HIV-infected Hispanics living in the United States. *AIDS Care, 8*(6), 683–690.
6. U.S. Department of Health and Human Services, Public Health Service, Centers for Disease Control and Prevention. (1998). *HIV/AIDS Surveillance Report,* 10(2).

Joyce Larson-Presswalla, PhD, RN, *President, "Culture Counts," Marketing Coordinator, James A. Haley Veterans Hospital, Tampa, Florida*

certain blood products, such as factor VIII concentrate. Other means of preventing HIV infection related to blood products are autologous (self-donated) blood programs and limiting the administration of any blood product to situations in which it is absolutely necessary.

Use of injected drugs accounts for the largest number of HIV infections through exposure to contaminated blood. The only *absolutely safe* injection drug use behavior is not to inject. *Very safe* practice with injected drugs is to use sterilized injection paraphernalia and never share needles and syringes. A *probably safe* practice is to clean injection paraphernalia with full-strength bleach before injecting, although disposable needles and syringes are difficult to clean. Anything else is considered risky. Other cofactors that increase the chances of acquiring HIV by drug injection include the seroprevalence of HIV in the geographical location of the drug user, the social setting of injection drug use (e.g., "shooting galleries," where injection paraphernalia is shared), and the frequency of injection.

Needle exchange programs provide sterile injection equipment, latex condoms, counseling, and access to social and health programs, including drug detoxification treatment. Numerous studies have shown that needle exchange programs decrease the spread of HIV and hepatitis B and C and do not increase or promote injection drug use. Despite the proven success of this approach to disease prevention, state and federal legislators have been reluctant to appropriate funds to support this model of care. In the United States, because of existing attitudes about IV drug use, needle exchange programs may operate as legal, illegal but tolerated, or illegal or underground programs. In Europe, where the approach to preventing disease has received more favorable support, governments providing national health care services for their citizens have found that needle exchange programs not only have reduced the incidence of disease but also have significantly reduced health care spending for diseases associated with IV drug injection.

Occupational exposure to blood is a potential problem not only for health care workers but also for members of other occupations, such as police and corrections officers. The state of Connecticut legalized the sale of sterile needles and syringes in certain drugstores and found that they not only reduced the incidence of needle sharing in IV drug users but also resulted in a significant decrease in the number of occupationally acquired needle-stick injuries in police officers.

The problem of HIV transmission to health care workers by clients is an ongoing concern of workers, employers, and public health officials. In the United States, by January 1999, the cumulative total number of health care workers with documented, occupationally acquired HIV or AIDS was 54. The number with possible (less clear evidence) transmission was 134. Although most health care workers occupationally infected with HIV acquired the virus after percutaneous exposure, other modes of transmission included mucocutaneous exposure and direct exposure to HIV in the laboratory setting. The actual average risk to a health care worker for exposure to HIV is extremely low (0.3% after a needle-stick or sharp instrument injury and 0.09% after a mucous membrane exposure). The risk, when an exposure occurs, is increased in situations in which a deep injury occurs, when there is visible blood on the device causing the injury, when the device involved was previously placed in a client's artery or vein, and when AIDS was diagnosed in the source client who died within 60 days after the health care worker's exposure (presumably because concentrations of HIV in the blood are very high at this time).

Accidental needle-stick exposure poses the greatest hazard to health care workers. As a health care worker, you should learn and follow Standard Precautions when handling blood and body fluids and when performing procedures that could expose you to blood and body fluids. When any incident reflects potential exposure to blood-borne pathogens, seek medical treatment immediately. The U.S. Public Health Service has issued guidelines for evaluating and treating exposures to HIV. In the case of high-risk exposures, they recommend that combination antiretroviral therapy be given for at least 4 weeks for post-exposure prophylaxis.

In the United States, only one case of HIV transmission from a health care worker to clients has been documented. It was reported in 1990 and involved a Florida dentist. Six clients reportedly became infected with HIV after receiving dental care. The circumstances of this case implied inadequate disinfection and sterilization of instruments in the dental office. Since this incident, retrospective (look-back) studies of possible HIV transmission from infected health care workers to clients have not identified any other cases in the United States. In 1999, one additional case of HIV transmission from a health care worker to a client was reported in France. An HIV-positive physician who was injured during orthopedic surgery transmitted HIV to the client. The surgeon acquired HIV in 1983 when he sustained an injury while operating on an HIV-infected client.

Perinatal HIV exposure can occur during pregnancy, during vaginal delivery, and post partum through breast-feeding. Of all babies born to HIV-infected women worldwide, about 23% are infected. The risk of transmission from mother to child (*vertical transmission*) increases if viral activity is high and the CD4+ titer is low, which is usually the case in later stages of HIV disease, when the diagnosis is AIDS. Clinical trials were conducted to see whether giving pregnant women antiretroviral therapy for HIV could reduce the risk by controlling HIV activity and raising the CD4+ cell count; administration of zidovudine reduced the rate of vertical HIV infection from 23% to 8%. The CDC has published guidelines for the use of zidovudine and other antiretroviral therapies for pregnant women and their newborn infants. Although no increase in birth defects has been noted in babies born to mothers who took zidovudine during pregnancy, one newer antiretroviral agent (efavirenz) caused birth defects in animal trials and should be avoided during pregnancy.

The only absolute method of preventing perinatal exposure is to avoid pregnancy. All health care workers should discuss HIV infection as part of routine prenatal care with all clients, because many mothers may be unaware that they are infected with HIV. Infected women who carry to term should be advised against breast-feeding, as this has been implicated as a mode of HIV transmission.

Primary prevention of HIV infection for exposed individuals is an emerging concept being applied not only to health care workers but also to the treatment of other accidental exposures. Post-exposure prophylaxis is being used as a health maintenance strategy by some clinicians for people who:

- Have unprotected anal or vaginal intercourse
- Have receptive oral intercourse with ejaculation
- Share needles with an infected partner
- Have a single-event exposure, such as a rape
- Intend to stop high-risk behaviors

Considerable controversy surrounds the use of post-exposure prophylaxis except in cases of rape, and the ethical aspects of providing such treatment continue to be discussed.

Since 1987, about 15 experimental HIV vaccines have been tested on more than 2000 healthy people. Vaccines are being developed to prevent HIV infection (preventive vaccine) and to treat people infected with HIV (therapeutic vaccine). To date, vaccine development has focused on recombinant vaccines structured from HIV envelope glycoproteins gp120 and gp160. Trials have begun with about 5000 volunteers to determine the effectiveness of these vaccines. One major drawback to soliciting volunteers for these trials is the possibility that they will have a false-positive result for HIV after receiving the vaccine because their bodies have developed antibodies to the virus. This may pose a problem for these people when HIV testing is required, such as when they are seeking employment or applying for insurance.

Pathophysiology

HIV-1 is a member of the lentivirus subfamily of human retroviruses. Diseases caused by lentiviruses are characterized by an insidious onset with progressive involvement of the central nervous system (CNS) and may result in disorders of the immune system. HIV-1 is one of five viruses in the lentivirus family (Fig. 79–1). The others are HIV-2 and human T-lymphotropic virus (HTLV) types I, II, and IV.

A retrovirus belongs to the family Retroviridae and

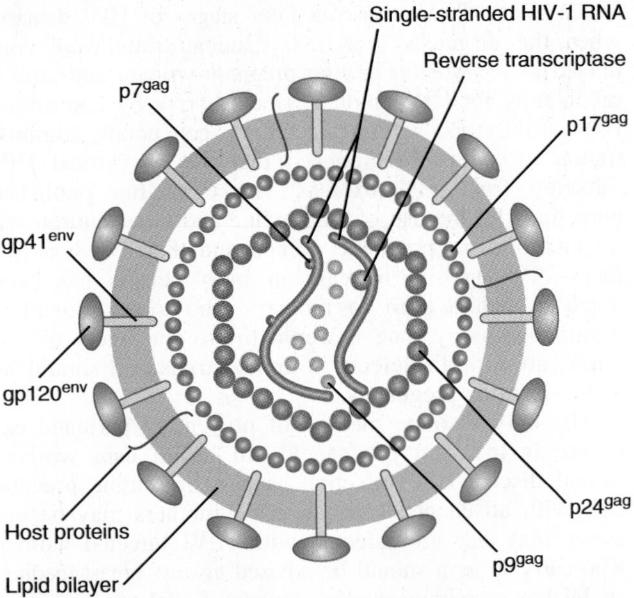

FIGURE 79–1 Schematic diagram of the human immunodeficiency virus-1 (HIV-1) virion. RNA, ribonucleic acid. Redrawn from Sande, M., & Volberding, P. [1997]. *The medical management of AIDS* [5th ed.]. Philadelphia: W. B. Saunders, p. 18.)

possesses ribonucleic acid (RNA)-dependent deoxyribonucleic acid (DNA) polymerase (reverse transcriptase). HIV infects T helper cells (T4 lymphocytes), macrophages, and B cells. HIV does not directly affect the central nervous system or peripheral neurons, astrocytes, or oligodendrocytes. HIV infection in the central nervous system is indirectly caused by neurotoxins produced by infected macrophages or chemical substances produced by the dysregulation of cytokines and chemokines.

T helper cells are infected more readily than are other cells. The depletion of T helper cells occurs in the following steps:

1. Once inside the host, HIV attaches to the target cell membrane by way of its receptor molecule, $CD4^+$.
2. The virus is uncoated, and the RNA enters the cell.
3. The enzyme known as reverse transcriptase is released, and viral RNA is transcribed into DNA.
4. This newly created DNA moves into the nucleus and the DNA of the cell.
5. A provirus is created when the viral DNA integrates itself into the cellular DNA or genome of the cell.
6. Once the provirus is in place, its genetic material is no longer pure cell but part virus.
7. The cell may function abnormally.
8. The host cell dies, and viral budding occurs (Fig. 79–2). The new virus proceeds to infect other cells.

The main target for HIV is the T4 helper cell; however, the "glue" to which HIV is attracted is the $CD4^+$ molecule, which acts as the receptor for HIV on the T4 helper cell. Even though the $CD4^+$ molecule is also found on other cells, such as macrophages and monocytes, clinicians usually refer to T4 helper cells as $CD4^+$ cells. Therefore, in articles, research papers, or laboratory reports about HIV the labels *T4, T4 helper, CF4⁺* and *CD4⁺ T helper cell* are used synonymously. Other substances known as *chemokines* act as messengers to facilitate entry of HIV into cells. Examples of such chemokines are cysteine-cysteine receptor 3 (CCR3) and CCR5. In 1996, scientists discovered that certain people have a genetic defect in the CCR5 gene and, despite repeated exposure to HIV, never become infected.

The $CD4^+$ T helper cells are the regulating cells in the immune system. They interact with monocytes, macrophages, cytotoxic T cells, natural killer cells, and B cells. In the analogy of an orchestra and a conductor, the T cells are the "conductor" of the immune system, directing all of the activity ("music") produced by the other immune cells ("orchestra"). Therefore, it is apparent that the loss of the $CD4^+$ T helper cells results in chaos. The body loses its basic ability to maintain a consistent state of health. With significant losses of these regulatory cells, the HIV-infected person become highly susceptible to acquired infection and pathogens that have previously caused disease may reactivate and also cause infection. A prime example is the varicella zoster virus, which may have caused chickenpox in an HIV-infected person as a child and may reactivate as shingles when the $CD4^+$ T-cell count drops to low levels.

The average laboratory range for the $CD4^+$ T-cell count is 500 to 1600 mm^3. A gradual physiologic decline occurs in these cells over the life of an individual. In fact, $CD4^+$ T-cell counts in newborns are almost double those of an adult. In the adult, $CD4^+$ cell counts below $200/mm^3$ are considered dangerously low and infection is

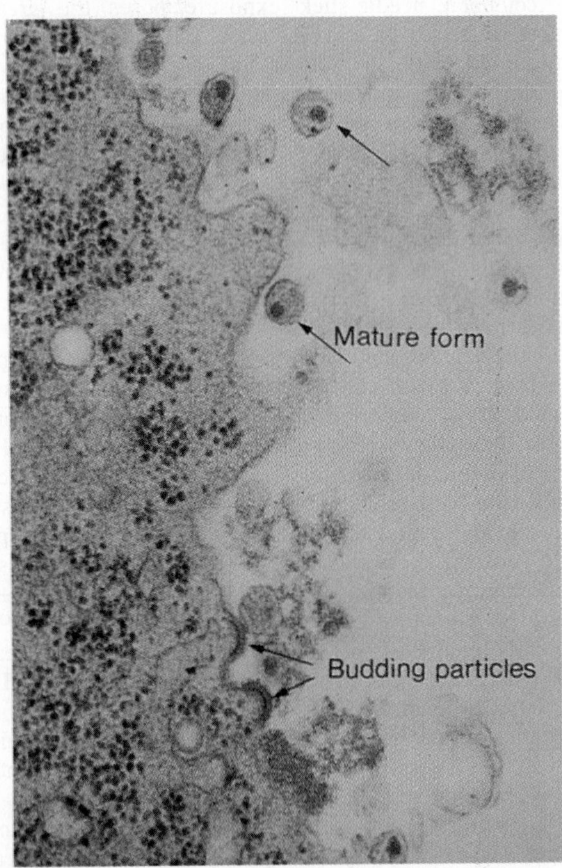

FIGURE 79–2 Human immunodeficiency virus. Electron micrograph of the virus budding from a T lymphocyte. (From Friedman-Kien, A., & Cockerell, C. [1996]. *Color atlas of AIDS* [2nd ed.]. Philadelphia: W. B. Saunders, p. 11.)

likely to develop. Other laboratory changes that indicate immune dysfunction include:

- An overall decline in the total numbers of white blood cells
- Decreases in both the total number and percentage of lymphocytes
- Significant changes in the $CD4^+/CD8^+$ ratio
- Decreased $CD4^+$ T-cell test findings
- Absent or decreased skin test reactivity *(anergy)*
- Increased immunoglobulin levels

The cause of all this damage to the immune system is the extensive amount of HIV activity that takes place in the body of an infected person from the time of infection. HIV replicates at a very rapid rate. In fact, it may produce 10 million new *virions* (viral particles) daily. Although a person with HIV may be asymptomatic and $CD4^+$ cell counts may be within the normal range, insidious destruction of the immune system is taking place. Antiretroviral drugs play a key role in interrupting the HIV disease process by inhibiting the ability of the virus to replicate, thus reducing the amount of circulating virus in the body and halting its destructive activity. Once this happens, the immune system begins to heal and restore itself, as noted by rising $CD4^+$ cell counts.

There are numerous challenges to sustaining the beneficial effects of antiretroviral therapy. The biggest problem is the ability of HIV to mutate and to become resistant to antiretroviral drugs. When this happens, the infected person is said to have drug failure manifested by a rise in viral load and a decline in $CD4^+$ cell counts. The combination of drugs must then be changed. Because two to three drugs are usually ordered at one time and fewer than 15 drugs have been approved to treat HIV infection, the number of combinations that can be prescribed is limited. Additionally, although the drugs can contain the disease in plasma, the virus can hide in many other cells in the body. Finally, because most antiretroviral agents do not cross the blood-brain barrier in the CNS, treatment of CNS problems caused by HIV infection can be very difficult.

The course of HIV illness often varies from person to person. Several cofactors may accelerate the immunodeficiency, including malnutrition, continued use of injected drugs and recreational substances, allergic conditions, genetics, age, pregnancy, gender, and presence of infections. In some instances, research has clearly implicated some of these cofactors as contributing to a more rapid decline in $CD4^+$ cell levels; for others, the evidence is less clear. Factors that have been linked to increased mortality and morbidity include lower socioeconomic status, lack of access to adequate care, receiving care in a hospital with limited AIDS experience, and being treated by a physician with little experience in AIDS care.

Overall, comparing the 1980s with the 1990s, survival among clients with AIDS has doubled. Most authors attribute increases in survival to the introduction of drugs to prevent opportunistic infections when the $CD4^+$ count falls below 200 mm^3 and to the use of antiretroviral agents to treat HIV disease.

To illustrate further the differences observed in HIV-infected people, scientists have reported that about 5% of them are perfectly healthy after many years and show no signs of disease progression. These *long-term non-progressors:*

- Have had documented evidence of HIV infection for more than 10 years
- Are asymptomatic
- Have normal, stable immune profiles
- Have never required any treatment for HIV disease

Long-term non-progressors appear to produce vigorous amounts of serum antibodies that keep HIV activity at extremely low levels, thus preventing immune system damage. Do not confuse a long-term non-progressor with a *long-term survivor,* defined as someone who has lived for more than 8 years after an AIDS diagnosis, who shows all clinical and laboratory manifestations of disease, and who continuously requires treatment.

Although the principal target of HIV is the immune system, considerable damage occurs to other parts of the body as a direct result of HIV in body tissues. A few examples of clinical conditions that can be directly attributed to HIV include cranial and peripheral neuropathies, uveitis, cardiomyopathy, pneumonitis, malabsorption in the small intestine, nephritis, cervicitis, arthritis, psoriasis, gonad dysfunction, and adrenalitis. Additionally, damage to the hematologic system, which is due in part to impaired blood cell production, commonly results in anemia, granulocytopenia, and thrombocytopenia throughout the course of disease.

In addition to managing HIV disease, clinicians are challenged with addressing those illnesses that existed before the person acquired HIV infection. These not only require continuing treatment and attention but also may complicate the course of illness. Frequently encountered pre-existing and co-morbid conditions seen in HIV-infected clients include, but are not limited to, alcoholism, drug dependence, liver disease, kidney disease, psychiatric illness, and a history of STDs. As therapy improves and people with HIV disease live longer, they will also require treatment for such illnesses as cancer, coronary artery disease, chronic obstructive lung disease, hypertension, and diabetes, all of which may occur in the aging population not infected with HIV.

Clinical Manifestations

As knowledge has evolved regarding the HIV disease process, the CDC has developed and revised numerous classification systems (Box 79–1). The most recent classification system for HIV disease in adults and adolescents is based on two monitoring parameters used to follow a client: (1) laboratory data ($CD4^+$ cell counts) and (2) clinical presentation (the person's clinical manifestations of diseases). The period in which a person becomes infected is referred to as *primary infection.* If HIV is detected in a client at the time of initial infection, the client is considered to be in category A.

Primary infection is the initial period after a person has acquired HIV, usually through a high-risk behavior (e.g., certain sexual practices or IV drug use). The length of time that primary infection lasts varies from several weeks to a few months. During primary infection, 50% to 70% of people become sick. Many clinicians are unaware of this fact and tend to think that primary infection is

BOX 79–1 Human Immunodeficiency Virus (HIV) Classification System for Adolescents and Adults

The Centers for Disease Control and Prevention (CDC) classification system for HIV-infected adolescents and adults emphasizes the importance of $CD4^+$ lymphocyte testing in clinical management. The classification system is divided into laboratory and clinical categories as follows.

	Clinical Categories		
Laboratory Categories ($CD4^+$ Cell Categories)	**A Asymptomatic, Acute (Primary) HIV or PGL**	**B Symptomatic, Not A or C Conditions**	**C AIDS-Indicator Conditions**
$\geq$500 mm^3	A1	B1	C1
200–499 mm^3	A2	B2	C2
<200 mm^3 AIDS-indicator T-cell count	A3	B3	C3

Shaded areas in the chart are *AIDS-defining* categories. *Laboratory* categories are based on the most recent $CD4^+$ cell count. *Clinical* categories describe the clinical status of the client and the presence or absence of certain diseases.

Category A

One or more of the following conditions occurring in an adolescent or adult with documented HIV infection. Conditions listed in categories B and C must not have occurred.

- Asymptomatic HIV infection
- PGL
- Acute (primary) HIV infection with accompanying illness or history of acute HIV infection

Category B

Symptomatic conditions occurring in an HIV-infected adolescent or adult that are not included among conditions listed in clinical category C and that meet at least one of the following criteria:

- The conditions are attributed to HIV infection or indicate a defect in cell-mediated immunity
- The conditions are considered by physicians to have a clinical course or management that is complicated by HIV infection

Examples of conditions in clinical category B include, but are not limited to, the following:

- Bacterial endocarditis, meningitis, pneumonia, or sepsis
- Candidiasis, vulvovaginal; persistent for more than 1 month, or poorly responsive to therapy
- Candidiasis, oropharyngeal (thrush)
- Cervical dysplasia, severe; or carcinoma
- Constitutional manifestations, such as fever (38.5° C) or diarrhea lasting more than 1 month
- Hairy leukoplakia, oral
- Herpes zoster (shingles), involving at least two distinct episodes or more than one dermatome
- Idiopathic thrombocytopenic purpura
- Listeriosis
- Nocardiosis
- Pelvic inflammatory disease
- Peripheral neuropathy

Category C

Any condition listed in the 1987 surveillance case definition of acquired immunodeficiency syndrome (AIDS) and affecting an adolescent or an adult. The conditions in clinical category C are strongly associated with severe immunodeficiency, occur frequently in HIV-infected clients, and cause serious morbidity or mortality. According to the classification system, HIV-infected clients would be classified on the basis of both the lowest accurate (not necessarily the most recent) $CD4^+$ lymphocyte determination *and* the most severe clinical condition diagnosed, regardless of the client's current clinical condition. Specific diseases that are considered AIDS-defining diagnostic categories include:

- Candidiasis of bronchi, trachea, or lungs
- Candidiasis, esophageal
- Cervical cancer, invasive
- $CD4^+$ T lymphocyte cell count < 200 mm^3 ($<14\%$)
- Coccidioidomycosis, disseminated or extrapulmonary
- Cryptococcosis, extrapulmonary
- Cryptosporidiosis, chronic intestinal (more than 1 month duration)
- Cytomegalovirus disease (other than liver, spleen, or nodes)
- Cytomegalovirus retinitis (with loss of vision)
- Encephalopathy, HIV-related
- Herpes simplex: chronic ulcer or ulcers (>1 month duration), bronchitis, pneumonitis, or esophagitis
- Histoplasmosis, disseminated or extrapulmonary
- Isosporiasis, chronic intestinal (>1 month duration)
- Kaposi's sarcoma
- Lymphoma, Burkitt's (or equivalent term)
- Lymphoma, immunoblastic (or equivalent term)
- Lymphoma, primary, of brain
- *Mycobacterium avium* complex or *M. kansasii,* disseminated or extrapulmonary
- *Mycobacterium tuberculosis,* any site (pulmonary or extrapulmonary)
- *Mycobacterium,* other species or unidentified species, disseminated or extrapulmonary
- *Pneumocystis carinii* pneumonia
- Pneumonia, recurrent
- Progressive multifocal leukoencephalopathy
- Salmonella septicemia, recurrent
- Toxoplasmosis of brain
- Wasting syndrome due to HIV

PGL, persistent generalized lymphadenopathy.
Adapted from Centers for Disease Control and Prevention. (1992). 1993 revised classification system for HIV infection and expanded surveillance case definition for AIDS among adolescents and adults. *Morbidity and Mortality Weekly Report, 41*(RR-17), 1–19.

silent. In addition to constitutional manifestations (fever, fatigue, lymphadenopathy, nausea, vomiting), the infected person may experience headache; truncal (torso and arms) rash; ulcers of the mouth, genitals, or both; thrush; pharyngitis; diarrhea; hepatomegaly; myalgia; arthralgia; anemia; thrombocytopenia; and leukopenia. In some people, the manifestations are mild and comparable to those of mononucleosis. Other people have severe manifestations and may need hospitalization.

During primary infection, a sudden and intense burst of HIV activity results in a high viral load and a dramatic drop in the $CD4^+$ cell count. In fact, the $CD4^+$ cell count may drop at the time of primary infection to below 100 mm^3, with the concomitant development of an AIDS-defining illness. This is also the period in which most newly infected people develop antibodies to HIV, which can then be detected through enzyme immunoassay testing. There is a "window" period for *seroconversion* (the time it takes for a newly infected person to develop antibodies to HIV that can be detected in a laboratory specimen). On average, antibodies can be detected in 4 to 12 weeks.

Unfortunately, in most instances the diagnosis is not confirmed at the time of primary infection, either because the person does not seek medical care or because the clinician does not take an adequate history that raises the suspicion of HIV infection. This is quite a serious situation, because preliminary studies have shown that starting antiretroviral therapy at the time of initial infection may prevent damage to the immune system and to other body systems. Table 79–1 lists the parts of the health history needed to detect a client's HIV exposure risk.

Except in certain instances, as when seeking a federal job or when testing infant umbilical cord blood, the decision to seek an enzyme immunoassay test for HIV antibodies is left up to the individual. Testing also involves pretest and post-test counseling. Laws governing the reporting of HIV antibody test results vary from state to state, and testing may be performed either anonymously or confidentially. If the enzyme immunoassay result is positive, a second test, the Western blot, is performed to confirm a positive HIV status.

If testing is performed too early in the initial infection period, a false-negative result may occur. A few cases of outliers also did not test positive for up to 3 years after becoming infected. False-positive results are extremely rare but may occur in clients with autoimmune disorders, such as lupus erythematosus, or in clients who have taken part in HIV vaccine studies.

Other methods for detecting HIV infection include home test kits, salivary tests, and urine tests. The marketability, cost, and popularity have limited the use of home test kits thus far. Saliva test results are as accurate as serologic testing, but the urine test is slightly less accurate.

In general, test results are reported as (1) positive, (2) negative, or (3) indeterminate. A *positive* result means that the person is HIV-infected, but it does not predict the future course of disease. A *negative* result means that HIV antibodies were not detected. Indeterminate results usually mean that the enzyme immunoassay test was positive but the Western blot test did not confirm those findings. Repeated testing on indeterminate results often shows an HIV-negative antibody test. Repeated testing later is commonly recommended as a means of validating initial test results.

The period following primary infection is one in which the person usually remains asymptomatic for many years. Therefore, clients with HIV disease are commonly categorized in group A for extended periods. Although the clients have no obvious major manifestations they may start to notice recurrent infections of the sinuses or respiratory tract or may feel increasing fatigue. Although no significant disease is apparent, viral destruction takes place throughout the body. A major portion of this destructive activity occurs in lymph tissue and results in a slowly declining $CD4^+$ cell count. The damage to lymphatic structures also has a negative effect on the quality of $CD4^+$ cells that are continuously produced within the body. After a while, although the numbers may be adequate, $CD4^+$ cells lose their ability to contain the destructive nature of HIV.

Since the beginning of the HIV epidemic, the focus of clinical monitoring has been on evaluating the quantity of $CD4^+$ cells. In essence, $CD4^+$ cell counts are an indirect measurement of the clinical course of HIV disease, showing the end result of HIV activity. In 1996, *viral load testing* became available to directly measure how much viral activity was occurring in a person with the disease. Viral load tests measure the amount of HIV RNA in plasma, quantify HIV activity, determine prognosis, indicate the need for treatment, evaluate the biologic response to treatment, and detect treatment failure. $CD4^+$ cell counts should not be a substitute for viral load testing, because the correlation between the two results is weak. High viral loads may not always correlate with clinical manifestations and a low $CD4^+$ cell count, and vice versa. Viral load results may be reported in copies per milliliter (e.g., 10,000 copies/ml). The actual numbers may be reported as follows:

- Decimal numbers, as in 10,000 copies
- Exponents, as in 10^4, where the exponent 4 indicates the number of zeros after the 1
- A logarithm, in this case 4, which indicates 10^4 or 10,000

Thus, a report that sets viral activity at 5 logs would be interpreted as 10^5 or 100,000 copies/ml.

As the disease progresses, manifestations such as thrush or vulvovaginal candidiasis usually appear, which are distinct manifestations of an underlying immunodeficiency. This development is what commonly causes people to seek HIV antibody testing. Those who have symptomatic illness are then classified into group B (see Box 79–1). Eventually, a client with HIV infection develops one or more AIDS-defining diseases and is finally classified into group C. Once again, this may be the first time that HIV infection is discovered.

Outcome Management for HIV Infection

Medical Management of the Client with HIV Infection

The outcomes for medical and nursing management of the client infected with HIV are to maintain the person's

TABLE 79–1 ACTUAL OR POTENTIAL RISKS FOR EXPOSURE TO HUMAN IMMUNODEFICIENCY VIRUS (HIV): THE HEALTH HISTORY

SOCIAL HISTORY	
Sexual activities	Sex with men, women, or both Preferred sexual activities Absolutely safe behavior: abstinence or mutually monogamous with a noninfected partner Very safe behavior: noninsertive sexual practices Probably safe behavior: insertive sexual practices using condoms and spermicide Risky behavior: everything else Use of condoms (both male and female), including application, removal, use of lubricants, and difference in condom efficacy Engaging in sex with multiple partners Use of mood-affecting drugs before or during sexual activities Whether HIV infection has been diagnosed in anyone with whom the client has had sexual relations
Needle exposure	Use of drugs via intravenous route Sharing of needles, syringes, and other drug paraphernalia Other needle-exposure activities, such as tattoos, acupuncture, treatment by unskilled individuals or "folk doctors," or sharing prescribed drugs between friends Whether HIV disease has been diagnosed in anyone with whom client has shared needles
Occupational history	Current employment status Client's occupation and responsibilities in relation to risk potential for HIV exposure Whether client experienced any exposures Type of health care follow-up the client has pursued since exposure Client's knowledge of signs and symptoms of seroconversion and need for follow-up
Travel	Within the past 10 years Sexual activities when traveling in areas with many AIDS cases, such as New York, California, New Jersey, Texas, Florida, Haiti, or Zaire Treatment for illnesses or accidents while traveling Immigration history and potential exposures in country of origin
FAMILY HISTORY	
Medical and mental health problems	Substance use in the home or by other family members Tuberculosis HIV infection Other pertinent data
DRUG HISTORY	
Use of mood-altering drugs	Alcohol, marijuana, cocaine, crack, LSD, Quaaludes (methaqualone), amphetamines, barbiturates, tranquilizers, amyl or butyl nitrite ("poppers"), heroin, "crystal meth," or "ecstasy" Route of administration: oral, inhalation (including sniffing, snorting, and smoking), intravenous, or subcutaneous ("skin-popping") Any current or previous treatment for substance abuse
MEDICAL HISTORY	
HIV testing	Whether testing has ever been recommended Where testing was done Test results Whether client has documentation of test and results
Major diseases	Hemophilia Treatment with clotting replacements, such as factor VIII Other pertinent disorders
Transfusion	Whether client was donor or recipient
Sexually transmitted diseases	Syphilis, gonorrhea, amebiasis, herpes simplex (oral or genital), *Giardia lamblia* enteritis, *Chlamydia,* condylomata, trichomoniasis, or pelvic inflammatory disease Other pertinent disorders

AIDS, acquired immunodeficiency syndrome; LSD, lysergic acid diethylamide.

health, initiate and maintain an effective antiretroviral regimen, and prevent infectious complications. This requires health care follow-up at specified intervals and an understanding that, to achieve these outcomes, the client has to make lifestyle changes.

Maintain Health

Initiating a plan of care for any client infected with HIV requires a detailed laboratory and clinical assessment not only for the initial evaluation but also on an ongoing basis. Initial and follow-up laboratory testing provides invaluable information on disease progression, serves as a guide for treatment decisions, and determines the efficacy of treatment prescribed. A complete blood count is needed to identify anemia, thrombocytopenia, leukopenia, and developing infections. Multichannel chemistry panels and urinalysis reveal renal, liver, metabolic, or nutritional disease. Both tests are repeated at 6- to 12-month intervals to detect any abnormalities resulting from disease progression or prescribed drugs. These results are also needed to modify dosages of antiretroviral drugs for clients with impaired kidney or liver function.

An annual tuberculin skin test detects mycobacterial disease, and a chest x-ray identifies pulmonary problems. For women, a pregnancy test and Papanicolaou (Pap) smear are usually performed. Pap smears are performed twice during the first year after a diagnosis of HIV infection and then at least annually. Screening for venereal diseases includes testing for syphilis, gonorrhea, and *Chlamydia.* These are repeated annually if the client is sexually active. Hepatitis A and B antibody testing is performed to identify acute or prior infection and to determine the need for immunization. Although no vaccine is yet available, hepatitis C antibody testing may also be performed because there is a high incidence of hepatitis C in people infected with HIV.

Testing for pathogens known to cause opportunistic infections in people infected with HIV includes serologic tests intended to detect previous exposure to toxoplasmosis, histoplasmosis, cryptococcosis, and cytomegalovirus. For seronegative clients, repeated testing may reveal a primary exposure. For seropositive clients, rising titers of antibodies to these pathogens indicate the need for prophylactic therapy.

Finally, $CD4^+$ cell counts, ratios, and percentages are performed to determine the degree of immunodeficiency, and viral load testing is ordered to calculate the amount of viral activity. Viral load test result interpretations are as follows:

- $<$ 10,000 copies/ml: poses a low risk for AIDS
- 10,000 to 100,000 copies/ml: doubles risk for AIDS
- $>$ 100,000 copies/ml: poses a high risk for AIDS

The initial test, without any treatment, may reveal viral loads of 80,000 to 1 million copies/ml or even higher. These same tests are repeated at intervals determined by the presence or absence of manifestations or disease in the client through the course of illness. Because several viral load tests have been approved for use, clinicians are advised to use the same viral load test when performing serial measurements to control variations in test results. Diseases such as influenza, herpes, or pneumonia, as well as testing immediately after the influenza vaccine is administered, can cause a temporary rise in test results. Therefore, testing should be deferred in any of these situations.

Initiate and Maintain Antiretroviral Therapy

The decision to treat HIV disease should involve both the primary care provider and the client. Many clients, because of personal experience or preference, may refuse recommended antiretroviral therapy. Clinicians should, in a noncoercive manner, provide as much objective information as possible so that the person with HIV can make an informed choice about taking these drugs. Because of the accumulating data indicating increased survival in people who receive antiretroviral therapy, most clinicians would recommend starting an antiretroviral combination therapy regimen.

Current guidelines recommend that therapy begin when the viral load is 5000 to 10,000 copies/ml and when the client has evidence of clinical or immunologic deterioration ($CD4^+$ cell count <500 mm^3) or when the viral load is more than 20,000 copies/ml, regardless of clinical manifestations. Many clinicians also recommend that antiretroviral therapy be started close to primary HIV infection or as soon as HIV infection is identified. They reason that less damage is done to the immune system the sooner therapy is started.

Three classes of antiretroviral agents have been approved in the United States:

- Nucleoside reverse transcriptase inhibitors (NRTIs)
- Protease inhibitors (PIs)
- Non-nucleoside reverse transcriptase inhibitors (NNRTIs)

NRTIs block HIV replication by protecting noninfected cells. PIs render HIV particles noninfectious in cells already infected with HIV. NNRTIs work in a manner similar to that of nucleoside analogs. Table 79–2 presents the three classes of antiretrovirals. The goals of therapy are to inhibit the replication of HIV, reduce the viral load to undetectable levels, and stabilize the disease.

The first NRTI, approved in March 1987, was zidovudine (Retrovir, AZT). The original dosage was 1,200 mg/day taken at specified intervals. The most profound side effect was myelosuppression, resulting in anemia and leukopenia, which often required repeated transfusions. Many people currently infected with HIV remember the difficult experience of a friend or loved one and consequently may be reluctant to try antiretroviral therapy. By 1990, research demonstrated that 600 mg/day of zidovudine (half the original dose) was sufficient to achieve the desired effects. Other NRTIs include didanosine (Videx, ddI, approved in 1991), zalcitabine (Hivid, ddC, approved in 1992), stavudine (Zerit, d4T, approved in 1994), lamivudine (Epivir, 3TC, approved in 1995), a combination of lamivudine and zidovudine (Combivir, approved in 1997), and abacavir (Ziagen, approved in 1998).

Eager anticipation preceded the approval of PIs, a new class of drugs, because large numbers of clients developed resistance to NRTIs. PIs include saquinavir (Invirase or Fortovase, approved in 1995), indinavir (Crixivan, approved in 1996), ritonavir (Norvir, approved in 1996), nelfinavir (Viracept, approved in 1997), and amprenavir (Agenerase, approved in 1999). The newest class of

TABLE 79–2 ANTIRETROVIRAL THERAPY FOR HUMAN IMMUNODEFICIENCY VIRUS (HIV) INFECTION

Drug	Adverse Outcomes	Adult Dosing	Nursing Implications
NUCLEOSIDE REVERSE TRANSCRIPTASE INHIBITORS			
Abacavir (Ziagen)	Fatigue, changes in liver function tests, headache, abdominal pain, constipation, diarrhea, nausea, vomiting, insomnia, skin rash, and dizziness	300 mg PO bid	During the first 4 weeks of therapy, client should stop treatment immediately if flu-like manifestations develop and keep getting worse (fever, rash, malaise, nausea, vomiting, diarrhea) Once a hypersensitivity reaction is noted the drug should not be restarted (rechallenged) May be taken with or without food
Didanosine (Videx, ddI)	Pancreatitis (abdominal pain, nausea, vomiting), peripheral neuropathy (tingling, burning, numbness, or pain in the finger tips or feet), anxiety, headache, irritability, inability to sleep, restlessness, dry mouth, nervousness, and rash	>60 kg—*tablets:* 200 mg PO q 12 h; *powder:* 250 mg PO q 12 h <60 kg—*tablets:* 125 mg PO q 12 h; *powder:* 167 mg PO q 12 h	Give on an empty stomach 30 minutes before or 2 hours after a meal Tablets can be chewed, crushed, or dispersed in water (when dispersed, use within 1 hour); powder should be mixed only in drinking water Pediatric powder is mixed into solution by pharmacist and is stable for 30 days if refrigerated Must be separated by 1 hour from other drugs
Lamivudine (Epivir, 3TC)	Peripheral neuropathy (tingling, burning, numbness, or pain in the hands, arms, feet, or legs), pancreatitis (nausea, vomiting, severe abdominal or stomach pain), unusually tired or weak, fever, chills or sore throat, skin rash, headache, nausea, malaise, diarrhea, cough, insomnia, dizziness, muscle pain, joint pain, abdominal cramps, and dyspepsia	>50 kg—150 mg PO bid <50 kg—2 mg/kg PO bid	Give in combination with other antiretrovirals, never as monotherapy May take without regard to food Store at room temperature Tell client to avoid alcohol Report persistent severe abdominal pain, nausea, vomiting, and numbness or tingling
Lamivudine/zidovudine (Combivir)	Headache, malaise, fever, chills, nausea, vomiting, diarrhea, anorexia, abdominal pain and cramps, neuropathy, insomnia, dizziness, nasal manifestations, musculoskeletal pain, rash, neutropenia, and anemia	1 tablet (contains 150 mg of lamivudine and 300 mg of zidovudine) PO bid	May be taken with or without food
Stavudine (Zerit, d4T)	Numbness, tingling, or pain in the hands or feet, headache, diarrhea, chills and fever, nausea, vomiting, muscle pain, loss of strength or energy, insomnia, anxiety, joint pain, back pain, loss of appetite, nervousness, and dizziness	>60 kg—40 mg PO q 12 h <60 kg—30 mg PO q 12 h	Compounded with lactose; lactose intolerant clients can take LactAid (lactase enzyme) tablets before taking stavudine May take without regard to food Tell client to avoid alcohol Report tingling, burning, pain, or numbness of hands or feet
Zalcitabine (Hivid, ddC)	Numbness, tingling, burning, and pain in lower extremities, abdominal pain, nausea, vomiting, rash, gastrointestinal intolerance, fever, sore throat, headache, fatigue, nausea, pruritus, muscle pain, difficulty swallowing, and arthralgia	0.75 mg PO q 8 h	Store tablets at room temperature Best taken on an empty stomach Swallow tablets whole with plenty of water

Zidovudine (Retrovir, AZT)	Fatigue, muscle pain, headache, nausea, vomiting, insomnia, anemia (pale skin, unusually tired or weak), neutropenia (fever, chills, sore throat), confusion, mental changes, seizures, and bluish-brown bands on fingernails	As prophylaxis for vertical transmission of HIV: **maternal use after first timester**—200 mg PO tid or 300 mg PO bid; **during delivery**—2 mg/kg IV loading dose over 30–60 minutes followed by continuous infusion of 1 mg/kg/hour until the cord is clamped As treatment: 200 mg PO tid or 300 mg PO bid	Store capsules and syrup at room temperature Protect from light May take without regard to food Take with food to decrease nausea, but avoid high-fat meal because it impairs absorption Infusion should be given over at least 60 minutes Give in combination with other antiretrovirals except during pregnancy, when it can be given as monotherapy
PROTEASE INHIBITORS			
Amprenavir (Agenerase)	Nausea, vomiting, rash, diarrhea, flatulence, fatigue, headache, and perioral paresthesia	1200 mg PO bid	During the first few weeks of therapy, observe for skin reactions; Stevens-Johnson syndrome has been reported
Indinavir (Crixivan)	Kidney stones (blood in urine, sharp back pain), nausea, diarrhea, vomiting, abdominal pain, headache, insomnia, altered taste, dizziness, generalized weakness, and asymptomatic hyperbilirubinemia May increase triglycerides May cause hyperglycemia May cause fat redistribution in the body	800 mg PO q 8 h	Give in combination with other antiretrovirals, never as monotherapy Store at room temperature Take on an empty stomach or with a light meal (high-fat, high-protein meals decrease blood levels by 77%) Give at least 1 hour apart if given with didanosine Must drink at least 1.5 liters of water daily Compounded with lactose; lactose intolerant clients can take LactAid tablets before taking indinavir Extremely moisture sensitive; keep in original container with desiccants; do not pre-pour into medication box; do not keep in bathroom Blood glucose should be monitored
Nelfinavir (Viracept)	Diarrhea, flatulence, nausea, abdominal pain, generalized weakness, and rash May increase triglycerides May cause hyperglycemia May cause fat redistribution in the body	750 mg PO tid or 1250 mg PO bid	Give in combination with other antiretrovirals, never as monotherapy Loperamide will control diarrhea Oral powder may be mixed with a small amount of water, milk, dietary supplement, chocolate milk, or pudding Do not mix with acidic foods, such as apple sauce, apple juice, or orange juice, because doing so produces a bitter taste Once mixed, consume entire contents within 6 hours Take with food for optimal absorption Blood glucose should be monitored

Table continued on following page

TABLE 79–2 ANTIRETROVIRAL THERAPY FOR HUMAN IMMUNODEFICIENCY VIRUS (HIV) INFECTION *Continued*

Drug	Adverse Outcomes	Adult Dosing	Nursing Implications
Ritonavir (Norvir)	Nausea, vomiting, diarrhea, loss of appetite, abdominal pain, taste alterations, headache, dizziness, sleepiness, tingling sensation or numbness around the lips, hands, or feet, fatigue, weakness May increase liver enzymes and triglycerides May cause hyperglycemia May cause fat redistribution in the body	Initially, 300 mg PO q 12 h, increasing by 100 mg PO q 12 h to a maximum of 600 mg PO q 12 h	Store capsules and solution in refrigerator and protect from light Refrigeration of solution not necessary if used within 30 days, but store below 77° F Take with food (increases blood levels) Taste of oral solution may be improved by mixing with plain or chocolate milk, pudding, or ice cream within 1 hour of dosing; by dulling the taste buds through chewing on ice, Popsicles (frozen dessert), or spoonfuls of partially frozen orange or grape juice; by eating peanut butter before administration to coat the mouth; or by chewing gum or hard candies after taking the dose Tobacco decreases blood levels Blood glucose should be monitored Alcohol intake can worsen manifestations (ritonavir oral solution contains alcohol)
Saquinavir (Invirase, Fortovase)	Nausea, diarrhea, ulcers in mouth, abdominal discomfort, abdominal pain, burning or prickling sensation, skin rash, weakness, and headache May increase triglycerides May cause hyperglycemia May cause fat redistribution in the body	Invirase, 600 mg PO tid; Fortovase, 1200 mg PO tid	Compounded with lactose; lactose intolerant clients can take LactAid tablets before taking saquinavir Take with a full meal; high-fat meal increases blood levels Photosensitivity can occur; use sunscreen or protective clothing Blood glucose should be monitored
NON-NUCLEOSIDE REVERSE TRANSCRIPTASE INHIBITORS			
Delavirdine (Rescriptor)	Diffuse, itchy, maculopapular rash, nausea, arthralgia, insomnia, changes in dreams, headache, diarrhea, fatigue, and increased liver enzymes	Initially, 200 mg PO tid for 14 days, then 400 mg PO tid	May take without regard to food
Efavirenz (Sustiva)	52% of clients in clinical trials experienced central nervous system and psychiatric manifestations, including dizziness, nightmares, confusion, insomnia, somnolence, cognitive impairment, amnesia, agitation, depersonalization, hallucinations, and euphoria; other side effects include nausea, vomiting, diarrhea, rash, and fatigue	600 mg PO once daily at bedtime	Do not give to pregnant women; birth defects occurred in animal studies Most side effects disappear after 2–4 weeks of therapy
Nevirapine (Viramune)	Rash, fever, nausea, headache, abnormal liver function tests, stomatitis (sores or ulcers in mouth), numbness, muscle pain, hepatitis (yellow skin, diarrhea, nausea, headache)	Initially 200 mg daily PO for 14 days, then 200 mg PO bid or 400 mg PO once daily	May take without regard to food

Note: Except for zidovudine, which may be prescribed as monotherapy for pregnant women, all of the antiretrovirals are prescribed in combinations of three or more at once.
bid, twice a day; h, hour; IV, intravenous; PO, by mouth; q, every; tid, three times a day.

drugs, the NNRTIs, includes nevirapine (Viramune, approved in 1996), delavirdine (Rescriptor, approved in 1997), and efavirenz (Sustiva, approved in 1998).

Perhaps the greatest challenge in treating HIV infection has been the genetic promiscuity of this virus. As stated earlier, HIV mutates rapidly. In the presence of an antiretroviral drug, it can develop resistance to the drug and continue to grow in the presence of the drug. Three types of drug resistance are of concern:

- *Genotype resistance,* in which the virus mutates
- *Phenotype resistance,* in which the virus shows a decrease in sensitivity to the drug
- *Cross-resistance,* in which the virus, having developed resistance to one drug, becomes resistant to other drugs in that class

Monotherapy (prescription of one antiretroviral agent at a time) is more likely to result in drug resistance than combination therapy. *Subtherapeutic* levels of a drug also lead to drug resistance. Subtherapeutic levels can occur when the client does not take the prescribed dosage, does not take doses at specified intervals, or both, and can also occur when other prescribed drugs interact with the antiretroviral drug and cause lower blood levels.

In an attempt to prevent drug resistance, clinicians order combination therapy, believing that combinations of drugs "confuse" the virus, thus interfering with its ability to develop resistance. Unfortunately, preliminary data show that even in combinations of three drugs at once, resistance develops to one or more of the agents being taken. Combination therapy includes two or more drugs given simultaneously from the NRTI group either exclusively or in combination with a PI or an NNRTI. The goal is to find combinations that are the least toxic and that produce the largest and most long-lasting viral response (lowest viral load) and the best immune response (highest $CD4^+$ cell counts).

Evaluation of the efficacy of antiretroviral therapy is based on the client's clinical manifestations and on laboratory tests of viral load and $CD4^+$ cell counts. The most reliable objective determinant is viral load testing, which is performed 3 to 4 weeks after initiating or changing therapy. If the decrease in viral load is not at least three times the original laboratory reports, or decreased by at least 0.5 log, the therapy is usually changed. Repeated testing to make sure that the drugs are working is usually performed at 3- to 4-month intervals.

Drug failure, in which the ordered combination is no longer effective, can occur after trying several standard combinations or antiretrovirals. The challenge to the clinician at that point is to try combinations of four to six drugs in an effort to suppress HIV activity once again. This approach to therapeutic intervention is commonly called *salvage therapy.* In many instances, salvage therapy fails because the HIV-infected person has developed drug resistance to most of the available drugs.

Studies are also being conducted to identify other chemotherapeutic strategies to control HIV infection. Scientists are looking at the use of HIV vaccines as a therapeutic strategy to stimulate host responses and control viral replication. Research continues to investigate the development of *immunomodulators,* drugs designed to modulate or reconstitute the immune system. Drugs being studied include tumor necrosis factor alpha (TNF-α), interleukin-2 (IL-2), IV immune globulin, and interferon alfa. IL-2 used in adults and IV immune globulin used in children have shown some promising effects.

PREVENT INFECTION

By 1986, surveillance data indicated that in more than 80% of people with HIV disease, *Pneumocystis carinii* pneumonia occurred at least once before death. Studies eventually showed that morbidity and mortality could be significantly reduced by giving a drug prophylactically for *P. carinii* pneumonia. Since 1989, the U.S. Public Health Service has recommended that all HIV-infected clients with a $CD4^+$ cell count below 200 mm^3 receive prophylaxis for *P. carinii* pneumonia. Drugs include trimethoprim-sulfamethoxazole (TMP-SMX); dapsone; dapsone, pyrimethamine, and leucovorin; aerosolized pentamidine; or atovaquone. Alternatives include intermittent parenteral pentamidine, pyrimethamine-sulfadoxine, clindamycin plus primaquine, atovaquone, and IV trimetrexate. TMP-SMX and dapsone also provide protection against toxoplasmosis.

Although surveillance data alone do not reflect the true incidence of infection with *Mycobacterium avium-intracellulare* complex, postmortem examinations revealed that more than 60% of HIV-infected people had an active infection. Since 1993, the U.S. Public Health Service has recommended that all HIV-infected clients with a $CD4^+$ cell count below 50 mm^3 receive prophylaxis for *M. avium-intracellulare* complex. Recommended drugs include clarithromycin, azithromycin, and rifabutin. However, these drugs may interact with antiretrovirals.

All HIV-infected clients with a positive result to a tuberculin skin test that have no evidence of active tuberculosis should receive 9 months of preventive therapy with isoniazid. Pyridoxine should be added to reduce the potential for peripheral neuropathy. An alternative regimen is rifabutin and pyrazinamide for 2 months. However, these drugs may interact with antiretrovirals.

Other recommended prophylactic measures include prevention of respiratory infections using pneumococcal vaccine and influenza vaccine and prevention of traveler's diarrhea, when traveling to countries where diarrhea is common, using antimicrobials such as ciprofloxacin. Finally, prophylactic medication may be ordered to prevent cytomegalovirus infection, recurrent candidiasis, cryptococcosis, or histoplasmosis.

Nursing Management of the Client with HIV Infection

ASSESSMENT

To help a client with health maintenance behaviors, do not restrict your nursing assessment to the client's immediate clinical status. Instead, focus on potential problems that may be encountered during the illness trajectory. For example, federal legislation passed in 1996 barred states from providing Medicaid to illegal immigrants to the United States. It is of no value to tell people that they need regular health care follow-up if they have no insurance and no money to pay for it. Social work intervention is needed to find an alternative source of health care services, such as the federally funded AIDS Drug Assistance Program, which provides more than just drugs. If the client lives alone and has no one willing to assist, he or she may need to be placed in an institution when the illness progresses. As a coordinator of care, you should have information readily available to identify problems and plan ahead.

Before performing any teaching, evaluate the client's existing level of knowledge about HIV infection. Some clients may know very little. Others may be very knowledgeable and may have even suspected they were infected but avoided being tested. Try to assess exactly what the client does or does not know about transmission and health-promoting behaviors before you make any assumptions.

The psychological burden of HIV disease can be overwhelming. Crisis points at which you can anticipate anxiety, fear, or depression include the following:

- Time of the initial HIV-positive diagnosis
- Time of the initial AIDS diagnosis
- Changes in treatment
- Development of new manifestations
- Recurrence of problems or relapse
- Terminal illness

Psychological conflicts that clients commonly experience include fear of transmitting HIV to others, constant worry about developing an infection, guilt about a previous lifestyle, and changes in personal relationships. Social stressors may include disclosure of one's HIV status, stigma conferred by that status, insecurity about employment and insurance, and loneliness and social isolation.

DIAGNOSIS, OUTCOMES, INTERVENTIONS

Effective Management of Therapeutic Regimen: Individual. The primary nursing diagnosis encountered with newly diagnosed HIV infection is *Effective Management of Therapeutic Regimen: Individual, related to behaviors that will improve the level of health and prevent complications.* Although some clients may know about HIV disease, it is unlikely that they know all that can be done to improve their health.

Outcomes. The client will know about HIV disease, how to prevent transmission, how to manage the disease, and how to prevent complications.

Interventions

Provide Education. Health teaching should be ongoing and repeated at frequent intervals. An HIV-infected person can adopt several behaviors that not only improve immune function but also increase a sense of well-being. The content outline for teaching health maintenance includes stress management, exercise, safe sex practices, procreation and HIV infection, nutrition (with emphasis on a high-protein, high-calorie, low-fat diet), food and water safety, skin care, hair care, routine mouth care, proper hand-washing, environmental cleaning and safety, pet care, limiting alcohol consumption, use of injected drugs, travel safety and avoiding exposure to infectious pathogens, importance of health care follow-up, and understanding and interpreting viral load tests and $CD4^+$ cell counts.

Carefully explain viral load test results to your clients because many people misunderstand the results. When successful therapy begins, the viral load drops from very high levels, such as 750,000 copies/ml, down to what are called "undetectable" levels. However, most laboratory personnel can detect HIV copies down to only 400 copies/ml. Because anything lower cannot be measured, the laboratory report reads "undetectable levels." Although this is great news and indicates the success of the prescribed regimen, it does not mean that the person no longer has HIV infection. Some clients with HIV infection leave their primary care provider thinking that they are disease free and no longer at risk of spreading HIV. This must be clarified whenever you report laboratory results to a client; emphasize that the client must still practice safer sex, avoid sharing needles, and so on.

Encourage clients to tell their health care providers about any self-prescribed therapies they may be taking, because they may have a positive or negative influence on the outcomes of care. Keep track of over-the-counter medications because they may interact with prescribed therapies. Some clients may also obtain drugs through buyers' clubs or underground pharmacies. This may not only be detrimental to the effectiveness of prescribed treatments but may also have an adverse effect on observations made during a drug trial.

Some clients may opt to try alternative or complementary treatments, including (1) spiritual or psychological interventions (e.g., guided imagery, meditation, faith healing); (2) nutritional alternatives (e.g., a Macrobiotic diet; (3) drug and biologic therapies, (e.g., homeopathy, oxygen, ozone therapy); and (4) physical forces (e.g., acupuncture, acupressure, massage therapy). In most cases, these choices can have a positive effect on the person's emotional well-being but may also have a negative effect. For example, a Macrobiotic diet can lead to vitamin and mineral deficiencies as well as weight loss. Herbal remedies may cause nausea, vomiting, diarrhea, or CNS depression. Despite these effects, some clients may continue to use these methods.

Initiate and Maintain Antiretroviral Therapy. One of the most important aspects of providing nursing care to the HIV-infected client is helping with the antiretroviral regimen. Studies suggest that clients with chronic diseases such as hypertension and diabetes take their prescribed drugs about 50% of the time. In contrast, to sustain the durability and efficacy of antiretroviral therapy, clients must maintain about a 90% compliance rate. This places high expectations on both the HIV-infected client and the physicians and nurses. Because therapy is now recommended early in the course of HIV infection, within weeks after the initial infection, you should discuss the potential benefits and risks of antiretroviral therapy. Potential benefits include:

- Control of HIV replication and mutation, with reduction in viral load
- Prevention of destruction of the immune system and loss of $CD4^+$ T helper cells
- Delayed progression to AIDS-defining illnesses
- Decreased risk for development of HIV resistance to drugs
- Decreased risk drug toxicity (drugs are started when the client is healthier)
- Increased survival with HIV disease (the most important benefit)

Potential risks include:

- Reduced quality of life from adverse drug effects and the inconvenience of a complex regimen
- Earlier development of drug resistance
- A limited number of drugs available to respond to drug resistance
- Unknown long-term toxicity of antiretroviral therapy
- Unknown duration of the effectiveness of current antiretroviral therapies

The decision of whether to take antiretrovirals is ultimately up to the client. The regimens ordered are commonly complex and require the client to take large numbers of pills daily, often at exactly spaced intervals, such as every 8 hours rather than simply three times a day. Didanosine must be taken on an empty stomach and separated by time from all other medications. Saquinavir must be taken with a high-fat meal. Indinavir must be taken with a low-fat meal. Liquid preparations often taste horrible, and the client must try various strategies to mask the taste. All of the drugs have side effects to which the person must learn to adjust and control. They also interact with numerous other drugs. These drug-drug interactions are usually not life-threatening, but they may interfere with antiretroviral blood levels, causing subtherapeutic effects, drug resistance, and drug failure. Instruct all clients taking antiretrovirals as follows:

- Take the drug at specified intervals.
- Do not skip a dose.
- Do not increase or decrease the number of pills you take.
- Follow meal and fluid requirements.
- If side effects occur, tell your physician or nurse. If side effects are significant, ask your primary care provider for information or medication to help manage them.
- Store all drugs as instructed.
- If you do not want to take the drugs, tell your primary care provider.
- If you take the drugs only periodically, it would be better not to take them at all. Discuss this with your physician or nurse.
- Remember, the treatment plan is yours. If you do not agree with it, discuss it with your physician or nurse.

Because of the concern over the development of drug resistance and drug failure, several studies have been started on methods to help people infected with HIV adhere to their drug regimens. Several strategies have proved very helpful, especially when used together:

1. Write out the client's drug and meal schedule, explaining when to eat and when to take which drugs (Table 79–3).
2. Provide the client with an electronic reminder. Research suggests that the main reason why people with HIV miss a drug dose is because they "forget." An alarm set to go off at the next dosing time can keep the client from forgetting.
3. Provide a large pill box with removable sleeves so that the client can conveniently carry the day's supply of drugs.

This combination of interventions can be used for any client with a chronic condition who must take medications daily.

Other strategies that enhance drug adherence behaviors include (1) ongoing supervision (telephone follow-up or home visits), (2) providing the client with written information about drugs and how to take them, and (3) interactive teaching sessions in which the client provides return demonstrations. Primary care providers also need to incorporate cultural and religious beliefs when addressing drug adherence behaviors. Meal planning because of fat content requirements or dietary restrictions or preferences, as well as the need to abstain from food and water on certain days because of religious practices, may be necessary.

Prevent Infection. Nursing strategies to prevent infection include health teaching and helping the client take

TABLE 79–3 SAMPLE MEDICATION AND MEAL SCHEDULE

Time	Comments	Medicine to Take	Box Label to Use
7 AM	Eat *breakfast* and drink a full glass (8 oz) of fluid	Zerit, Epivir, LactAid, Fortovase, Norvir, multivitamin, Biaxin, Bactrim, sulfadiazine, pyrimethamine, leucovorin	AM
12 noon	Eat *lunch,* and drink a full glass (8 oz) of fluid	Sulfadiazine	Noon
7 PM	Eat *supper,* and drink a full glass (8 oz) of fluid	Zerit, Epivir, LactAid, Fortovase, Norvir, Biaxin, sulfadiazine	PM
10 PM	Eat a snack, and drink a full glass (8 oz) of fluid	Sulfadiazine	Bed
During the night	If you get up during the night, drink a full glass (8 oz) of fluid		

Note: Take Fortovase and Norvir with food. These drugs are not absorbed well if taken on an empty stomach.

drugs properly to prevent opportunistic infections. Health teaching focuses on safer sex practices not only to prevent HIV transmission but also to keep from acquiring STDs. Practicing food and water safety can prevent such diseases as salmonellosis, cryptosporidiosis, and toxoplasmosis. Maintaining skin and mucous membrane integrity with good skin and mouth hygiene can reduce the incidence of candidiasis.

EVALUATION

Evaluation includes the client's understanding of teaching that has been provided and the choices that each person may make. If a client chooses not to adopt a recommended behavior, it does not mean that the client is noncompliant. People with HIV who smoke may find that their stress level rises too high when they try to quit, even when using a nicotine patch or gum. Such clients may choose to continue to smoke. Health care providers can have a difficult time evaluating the outcomes of teaching and weighing them against the client's free choice. Remember, the ultimate decision about following a health care provider's advice belongs to the client. The client's decisions do not reflect failure on the part of the health care professional.

Evaluation of a client's ability to adhere to a prescribed drug regimen includes both subjective and objective techniques. *Subjective* evaluation is by self-report; clients and their care partner describe the client's ability to take all prescribed medications. *Objective* analysis of the success of the plan of care is by laboratory evaluation of CD4+ cell counts and viral load. Avoid "pill counting" as a way to evaluate whether a client is taking drugs as prescribed. This should be performed only if the client wants this intervention and participates. Pill counts have been used for many years by nurses as a sort of policing activity when they find a client is not following a drug regimen properly. Today, pill counts are considered by many nurse experts to be a waste of time because clients often simply discard leftover pills if they know that a nurse will be performing a pill count.

A totally different situation exists when minimal learning takes place because of cognitive impairment. It is well documented that problems with thinking or memory may exist and go unidentified if they are not obvious. This is more likely to occur in clients with less than a 12th grade education and in clients over age 50. In such a situation, a care partner should be designated, who receives all information when it is provided to the client. Whenever the care partner cannot make a clinic or office visit, provide telephone teaching and document that you accomplished this.

Outcome Management for AIDS

As both the quantity and quality of CD4+ cells diminish, "AIDS-indicator" diseases occur. The categories of AIDS-defining illnesses include opportunistic infections, cancers, and other conditions specific to HIV disease. The four main types of opportunistic infections are (1) bacterial, (2) fungal, (3) protozoal, and (4) viral. Bacterial infections are the easiest to treat, and viruses are the most difficult. Neoplasms associated with AIDS include Kaposi's sarcoma, non-Hodgkin's lymphoma, and invasive cervical cancer. Two other conditions that are unique to AIDS are (1) HIV encephalopathy and (2) HIV wasting syndrome. Since the introduction of combination antiretroviral therapy in 1996, the onset of AIDS-defining illness has been delayed and treating these diseases has become easier.

Medical Management of the AIDS Client

PREVENT AND TREAT OPPORTUNISTIC INFECTIONS

Most of the pathogens responsible for opportunistic infections are ubiquitous; that is, they are all around us. *P. carinii* is in the air we breathe. The reason most people do not become sick from this organism is that their immune systems are intact. Once the regulators of the immune system (CD4+ cells) are destroyed by HIV, however, infection occurs. Most opportunistic infections result from secondary reactivation of previously acquired pathogens rather than from a new or primary infection. For example, most people are infected with *P. carinii* in the early preschool years, when it causes respiratory manifestations and is probably dismissed as a common cold. The child's intact immune system brings the infection under control. However, the organism remains dormant in the person's body. The potential then exists that if an immunodeficiency occurs, the organism can reactivate, causing disease again. This concept applies to any person with an immunodeficiency, regardless of the cause. To illustrate further, clients with cancer who receive chemotherapy and become immunodeficient may also develop infection from *P. carinii.*

Single opportunistic infections are rare, and clients may have multiple infections. Many of the opportunistic infections that occur in people with HIV are not curable. Because the immune system no longer has the strength to contain the infection, it becomes chronic and requires lifetime suppressive therapy. Helping the client comply with the antibiotic regimen to keep opportunistic infections under control is an essential part of the care planning process. Because the client must take antibiotics for extended periods, drug resistance may develop, and both physicians and nurses must constantly observe the client for recurrence of manifestations that may indicate the infection is reactivating and the drugs no longer work.

Bacterial Infections

***MYCOBACTERIUM TUBERCULOSIS* INFECTION.** Co-infection with *M. tuberculosis* (TB) and HIV is common, especially in large metropolitan areas. Because the bacterium is airborne, the presence of an immunodeficiency makes the person with HIV very susceptible to TB. All HIV-infected people should be tested annually to detect new or active infection. Nosocomial spread of TB among clients hospitalized and placed on AIDS units has been a problem. Manifestations of active infection are categorized as constitutional, pulmonary, or extrapulmonary. Constitutional manifestations include fever, chills, weight loss, night sweats, lymphadenopathy, and fatigue. Pulmonary manifestations may include cough, dyspnea, chest pain, and hemoptysis. Extrapulmonary presentation may involve lymph nodes, bones, joints, liver, spleen, central nervous system, skin, gastrointestinal tract, mass lesions, urine, and blood.

The recommended therapy includes a combination of drugs that may include isoniazid, rifampin, pyrazinamide, and either ethambutol or streptomycin. Drug selection is based on culture and sensitivity reports and potential drug-drug interactions with antiretrovirals already being taken.

Multi-drug–resistant TB was identified as an emerging problem in the United States around 1987. By 1990, significant numbers of cases were identified, especially among people with HIV infection. Studies attributed the development of multi-drug–resistant TB to physicians prescribing insufficient numbers of drugs to treat new cases of TB and once again the development of TB strains resistant to the most widely prescribed agents, isoniazid and rifampin. Based on drug sensitivity reports, second-line therapy for multi-drug–resistant TB includes ciprofloxacin, ofloxacin, kanamycin, amikacin, capreomycin, ethionamide, cycloserine, aminosalicylic acid, or clofazimine as single drug or combination therapy.

In institutional settings, clients are placed in respiratory isolation until sputum tests reveal that they are no longer infectious. In many cases of multi-drug–resistant TB, despite therapy, sputum results indicate the presence of organisms; it is not uncommon to have clients remain in respiratory isolation until discharge. TB is a reportable communicable disease, and health care professionals are required to report new cases to local health authorities.

Follow-up care focuses on management of clinical manifestations. Monitoring drug compliance is essential to ensure effective treatment and to prevent recurrent active disease. In cities where multi-drug–resistant TB has become a significant problem, local health departments have established monitoring programs (known as *directly observed therapy*), in which health care workers travel to client locations and watch them take their medications. Psychological stressors for the client include coping with the stigma of both HIV and TB.

***MYCOBACTERIUM AVIUM* COMPLEX.** *M. avium* complex is also sometimes called *M. avium-intracellulare.* The organism exists in soil, water, animals, eggs, and unpasteurized dairy products. Not all members of the *Mycobacterium* family of bacteria are communicable. *M. avium* complex is referred to as an atypical, noncommunicable mycobacterial disease. Because most people with HIV develop active disease and the risk of infection increases with $CD4^+$ cell counts below 50 mm^3, prophylaxis to prevent infection is recommended. Additionally, *M. avium* complex infection is much easier to prevent than to treat.

The clinical presentation of *M. avium* complex infection includes fever, night sweats, fatigue, anorexia, weight loss, abdominal pain, and diarrhea. Because the disease is difficult to treat and side effects of the medications are numerous, the decision whether to treat *M. avium* complex infection depends on the severity of manifestations and the presence of renal or hepatic disease. Two to six drugs may be used at one time, including some combination of azithromycin, clarithromycin, clofazimine, ethambutol, ciprofloxacin, rifabutin, and amikacin.

Follow-up care focuses on managing clinical manifestations because they may persist despite drug therapy. It is important to evaluate the client's ability to comply with the prescribed therapy because some clients may decrease the dosage of prescribed pills on their own to minimize side effects. Both clients and their care providers need to be taught that this is not a communicable disease.

SALMONELLOSIS. *Salmonella* infection can be prevented by teaching the client about food and water safety and proper food handling. Infection occurs after ingestion of contaminated food, including (1) beef, pork, poultry, and eggs; (2) drinking contaminated water; (3) ingesting contaminated drugs or diagnostic agents; (4) directly handling contaminated feces; or (5) sexual activity involving oral-anal contact. Food handlers may be asymptomatic carriers, and pets, especially turtles, may be a source of exposure. Presenting clinical manifestations include fever, night sweats, fatigue, anorexia, weight loss, abdominal pain, and diarrhea. Treatment includes ampicillin, chloramphenicol, trimethoprim-sulfamethoxazole, ciprofloxacin, or norfloxacin. Follow-up care focuses on management of manifestations, including preventing and managing skin breakdown in the perianal region.

BACTERIAL PNEUMONIA. Recurrent bacterial pneumonia is common among IV drug users. Predisposing factors include needle sharing, environmental exposure, heavy alcohol use, smoking, and inadequate nutrition. Pathogens most often associated with bacterial pneumonia, seen in people infected with HIV, are *Streptococcus pneumoniae* and *Haemophilus influenzae.* The risk of bacterial pneumonia increases when the $CD4^+$ cell count is below 200 mm^3. Antibiotic treatment is based on culture and sensitivity reports. Follow-up care includes focusing on behavioral changes that decrease the possibility of recurrence (such as smoking cessation, adequate nutrition, and using clean needles to inject drugs).

Pneumococcal vaccination should be given at 5-year intervals. Prophylactic therapy prescribed to prevent *P. carinii* pneumonia or *M. avium* complex may provide some protection against recurrent bacterial pneumonia.

Fungal Infections

CANDIDIASIS. *Candida albicans* not only is ubiquitous (in soil and food, on fomites) but also is a commensal organism normally found on the skin and in the mouth, vagina, and large intestine. Most infections are *endogenous;* that is, the person's own organism is the source of the infection. *Nosocomial* spread in hospitals and nursing homes can also occur. Human-to-human transmission can occur from mother to infant during vaginal delivery and between sexual partners. Clinical presentation is related to the site of infection: dysphagia with esophagitis, oral lesions with thrush, cutaneous lesions with intertrigo, vulvovaginal irritation and discharge with vaginitis, and constitutional symptoms with disseminated disease. Treatment is also site-dependent:

- For *oral/esophageal candidiasis,* clotrimazole troches, nystatin suspension, ketoconazole, fluconazole, and amphotericin B oral suspension (for esophagitis only)
- For *intertrigo* and *vaginitis,* clotrimazole, miconazole, ketoconazole, fluconazole, imidazole, and itraconazole (for nail infection)
- For *disseminated disease,* amphotericin B, with or without flucytosine

Follow-up care includes teaching routine skin and mouth care. Encourage the client to eat 8 ounces of yogurt made from live cultures (*Lactobacillus acidophi-*

lus) to help control recurrent infection with *Candida*. For recurrent, frequent episodes or after a severe episode, prophylactic therapy with fluconazole, ketoconazole, or itraconazole may be ordered.

CRYPTOCOCCOSIS. *Cryptococcus neoformans* is ubiquitous and found in pigeon droppings, nesting places, soil, fruit, and unpasteurized fruit juices. The organism is aerosolized and inhaled. As an AIDS-indicator disease, it causes lung and brain infection. HIV-infected smokers are more prone to development of cryptococcosis. Clinical manifestations primarily involve the CNS but can also include the lungs, skin, and mouth.

CNS manifestations include low-grade fever, fatigue, headaches, nausea, vomiting, and altered mental status. Pulmonary manifestations include cough, dyspnea, and pleuritic chest pain. Cutaneous and oral manifestations include painless lesions that may mimic Kaposi's sarcoma or molluscum contagiosum. Treatment includes amphotericin B, with or without flucytosine, fluconazole, or itraconazole. Maintenance lifetime suppressive therapy is required with fluconazole, itraconazole, or amphotericin B, and follow-up care focuses on assisting with medication compliance and monitoring for recurrence of symptoms that indicate resistance to maintenance drug therapy.

HISTOPLASMOSIS. *Histoplasma capsulatum,* a fungus endemic to certain regions of the United States, is most prevalent in the middle, central, and south central states and Puerto Rico. Therefore, people with HIV disease and living in these areas are susceptible to the disease. When diagnosed in other parts of the country (e.g., New York, California), the disease usually appears in a client who either grew up in or traveled to the endemic regions. Manifestations include fever; weight loss; enlarged lymph nodes, liver, and spleen; abdominal pain; oral and skin lesions; anemia; leukopenia; and thrombocytopenia.

Treatment includes amphotericin B, itraconazole, or fluconazole. Maintenance lifetime suppressive therapy (itraconazole or amphotericin B) is required. Follow-up care focuses on helping with drug compliance and monitoring for recurrence of manifestations that indicate resistance to maintenance drug therapy.

COCCIDIOIDOMYCOSIS. *Coccidioides immitis* is a fungus endemic to the southwestern United States. It was originally discovered in the San Joaquin Valley in southern California and is also referred to as *valley fever.* As an AIDS-defining diagnosis, it is commonly seen in people infected with HIV residing in Arizona, California, Nevada, New Mexico, Texas, and Utah. When diagnosed in other parts of the United States, the disease usually appears in a client who either grew up in or traveled to the endemic regions. Clinical presentation includes fever, dyspnea, fatigue, weight loss, and cough.

Treatment includes amphotericin B, ketoconazole, itraconazole, or fluconazole. Maintenance lifetime suppressive therapy is required using fluconazole, itraconazole, or amphotericin B. Follow-up care focuses on helping with drug compliance and monitoring for recurrence of manifestations that indicate resistance to maintenance drug therapy.

Protozoal Infections

PNEUMOCYSTOSIS. *P. carinii* is a ubiquitous organism that is airborne and can be found in the lungs of humans and animals. Most healthy people have had a primary infection by 4 years of age. Although most of the literature suggests that *P. carinii* infection in people with HIV is a secondary appearance of a previously acquired pathogen (reactivation), more recent information has revealed that some clients have different strains of the organism, which may indicate that reinfection is possible through airborne transmission.

Clinical presentation can be elusive, and about 7% of clients with the infection are asymptomatic. With *P. carinii* pneumonia, coughing is a frequent first manifestation. The pneumonia begins with a nonproductive cough and progresses to a productive cough. Eventually, the client has fever and dyspnea on exertion and then dyspnea at rest. Extrapulmonary *P. carinii* infection can occur in the eyes, ears, lymph nodes, heart, spleen, liver, and pleural space and on the skin.

Clients who are receiving prophylaxis for *P. carinii* pneumonia sometimes also go on to have infection because of poor drug compliance, unusual or erratic pharmacokinetics, or development of drug resistance. Treatment may be with trimethoprim-sulfamethoxazole, pentamidine, atovaquone, trimethoprim-dapsone, clindamycin-primaquine, or trimetrexate. Maintenance lifetime suppressive therapy is required with trimethoprim-sulfamethoxazole, pentamidine aerosol, atovaquone, dapsone, or clindamycin-primaquine. Follow-up care focuses on helping with drug compliance and monitoring for recurrence of manifestations that indicate resistance to maintenance drug therapy.

TOXOPLASMOSIS. *Toxoplasma gondii* is ubiquitous in nature and is acquired through ingestion of contaminated meat (lamb and pork), vegetables, eggs, and unpasteurized dairy products. The only documented human-to-human transmission noted is from mother to fetus, if the mother acquires primary infection during pregnancy. Toxoplasmosis can also be acquired through direct handling of contaminated cat feces. However, fewer than 1% of domestic cats are infected with *T. gondii.* A veterinarian can perform a simple blood test to determine whether a cat is infected. Studies of cat owners infected with HIV have not shown any increased risk for the development of toxoplasmosis. The potential for the development of toxoplasmosis increases when the $CD4^+$ cell count is below 100 mm^3. If trimethoprim-sulfamethoxazole or dapsone is prescribed for *P. carinii* pneumonia prophylaxis, the drug would provide prophylaxis against toxoplasmosis as well.

Clinical manifestations of CNS infection include headache, impaired cognition, hemiparesis, aphasia, ataxia, vision loss, cranial nerve palsies, motor problems, and seizures. Infection can also involve the heart, lungs, skin, stomach, abdomen, and testes. Treatment includes pyrimethamine plus sulfadiazine, dexamethasone, phenytoin, leucovorin, clindamycin plus pyrimethamine, clarithromycin, or azithromycin. Maintenance lifetime suppressive therapy calls for pyrimethamine plus sulfadiazine plus leucovorin or clindamycin plus pyrimethamine plus leucovorin. Follow-up care focuses on helping with drug compliance and monitoring for recurrence of manifestations that indicate resistance to maintenance drug therapy.

CRYPTOSPORIDIOSIS. *Cryptosporidium* is found in mammals, birds, reptiles, and fish. The primary mode of transmission in people infected with HIV is through the ingestion of contaminated food or water. Water-borne transmission can occur when drinking supplies become contaminated, including municipal water supplies, because chlorine does not destroy the organism. Boiling water for 1 minute destroys this organism.

Cryptosporidial disease can also be acquired from contaminated swimming pools, from handling infected animals, and through anal-oral sexual contact with an infected person. When cryptosporidiosis occurs in immunocompetent people, the disease is self-limiting. In an immunodeficient person with HIV, the disease is chronic and causes malabsorption, dehydration, and malnutrition. It can lead to death. Clinical presentation includes profuse diarrhea, steatorrhea (1 to 25 L/day), flatulence, abdominal cramping and pain, anorexia, nausea, vomiting, profound weight loss, fever, fatigue, myalgia, and electrolyte imbalance.

There is no effective treatment for cryptosporidiosis. Drugs that may be tried include paromomycin, letrazuril, azithromycin, clarithromycin, nitazoxanide, and symptomatic therapy to decrease peristalsis and control pain. Spontaneous remission has occurred once combination antiretroviral therapy was started, presumably because the immune system restores itself and controls the disease. Special attention is also needed to manage skin breakdown in the perianal region. Clients with cryptosporidiosis are vulnerable to depression and social isolation.

ISOSPORIASIS. *Isospora belli* is a parasite that is transmitted through contact with infected animals or humans or contaminated water. The disease is often seen in immigrants from Mexico, Haiti, and Central America. Clinical manifestations of the disease include diarrhea, anorexia, nausea, vomiting, weight loss, abdominal pain, and fever. Drug therapy includes trimethoprim-sulfamethoxazole or pyrimethamine plus leucovorin. Treatment is usually successful, and lifetime suppressive therapy is not usually required.

Viral Infections

CYTOMEGALOVIRUS DISEASE. Cytomegalovirus (CMV) is ubiquitous in humans throughout the world. Almost everyone eventually becomes infected with CMV, which is transmitted through direct contact with infected secretions, including saliva, cervical fluid, urine, semen, breast milk, feces, and blood. In people infected with HIV, CMV infection can be asymptomatic or can cause chorioretinitis, pneumonitis, encephalitis, adrenalitis, colitis, esophagitis, hepatitis, or cholangitis.

Drugs used to treat CMV infection systemically include ganciclovir, foscarnet, and cidofovir. Treatment also may involve intraocular ganciclovir implants or intravitreal injection of ganciclovir, foscarnet, or cidofovir. Maintenance lifetime suppressive therapy is required using any of these drugs. Follow-up care focuses on helping with drug compliance and monitoring for recurrence of manifestations that indicate resistance to maintenance drug therapy.

HERPES SIMPLEX. Herpes simplex virus (HSV) is ubiquitous and is spread by direct contact with infected secretions. HSV-1 is present in oral secretions, and HSV-2 is present in genital secretions. Transmission also takes place with "symptom-free excretors" (people previously infected with HSV and with no apparent lesions). Clinical presentation includes painful vesicular lesions that coalesce and rupture. Lesions usually occur in the oral, genital, or perianal region. HSV can also cause encephalitis, esophagitis, bronchitis, keratitis, pericarditis, and hand infection.

Treatment includes acyclovir, foscarnet, or famciclovir. Topical acyclovir also relieves pain and itching associated with skin lesions. Follow-up care focuses on monitoring the client for recurrent disease. Chronic disease requires lifetime suppressive therapy with acyclovir.

PROGRESSIVE MULTIFOCAL LEUKOENCEPHALOPATHY. Progressive multifocal leukoencephalopathy is caused by the JC virus (initials of the first client in whom it was discovered). The JC virus is ubiquitous in nature and appears to infect most middle-aged people. Active disease in people infected with HIV results in limb weakness, ataxia, cognitive impairment, vision loss, speech impairment, and headache. In the latter stages of illness, it progresses to dementia, blindness, paralysis, and death.

There is no effective therapy, but drugs that may be used include acyclovir, foscarnet, adenine arabinoside, cytosine arabinoside, and interferon alfa. There have been reports of spontaneous remission of this disease once combination antiretroviral therapy is started, presumably because the immune system restores itself and controls the disease. Follow-up care focuses on palliative therapy, safety measures, and preventing complications from immobility.

TREAT NEOPLASMS

Kaposi's Sarcoma

Four types of Kaposi's sarcoma may be encountered in clinical practice:

- Classic Kaposi's sarcoma, which tends to occur in older men who are black, of Mediterranean descent, or from certain Jewish populations
- African Kaposi's sarcoma, seen in Africa
- Transplant Kaposi's sarcoma, seen in people who receive organ transplants
- HIV-related Kaposi's sarcoma, which differs from the others in that it runs a fulminant course, is disseminated throughout the body, and results in shorter survival

HIV-related Kaposi's sarcoma is the only form associated with HIV disease. It has been diagnosed predominantly in men who have sex with men and is thought to be associated with a sexually transmitted pathogen that then predisposes the person to development. A new type of herpesvirus, named human herpesvirus type 8 (HHV-8), is suspected. Kaposi's sarcoma differs from most AIDS-defining diseases, in that it is unrelated to low $CD4^+$ cell counts and can occur early in HIV infection.

Clinical presentation typically starts with an initial "patch" that is flat and pink, looks like a bruise, and is symmetrical on both sides of the body. Later, it turns into dark violet or black plaques (see Fig. 49–19). Clinical presentation of the lesions can include the mouth, skin, mucous membranes, head, neck, torso, limbs (soles of feet), genitals, lung, brain, intestines, testes, liver, spleen, pancreas, adrenal gland, and lymph nodes. They can be painful.

Treatment depends on the extent of tumors (tumor burden), $CD4^+$ cell count, associated manifestations and diseases, and the client's functional ability. Local therapy includes radiation, localized chemotherapy, and cryotherapy. Systemic therapy includes vincristine, vinblastine, etoposide, doxorubicin, daunorubicin, bleomycin, and interferon alfa, with or without an HIV-specific antiretroviral agent. Experimental therapies under investigation include possible treatment of the underlying viral cause of Kaposi's sarcoma with foscarnet or ganciclovir. Initially, several therapies may be tried, which may be effective in suppressing the course of Kaposi's sarcoma; eventually, however, the clinical decline in the client's condition makes continued treatment impossible.

Non-Hodgkin's Lymphoma

Non-Hodgkin's lymphoma tends to occur late in the course of HIV disease and is related to low CD4+ cell counts. The primary sites of occurrence are the brain, gastrointestinal tract, bone marrow, and liver. The initial clinical presentation may be nonspecific and include fever, night sweats, and weight loss, all of which are associated with *M. avium* complex infection, TB, and CMV infection.

Treatment includes methotrexate, bleomycin, doxorubicin, cyclophosphamide, vincristine, and dexamethasone. Despite aggressive treatment, the prognosis is poor except in clients on combination antiretroviral therapy, who tend to survive longer.

Invasive Cervical Cancer

Cervical intraepithelial neoplasia (CIN), the precursor to cervical cancer, occurs at a high rate in women infected with HIV, progresses more rapidly, is less responsive to therapy, and is related to low CD4+ cell counts. In early stages of disease, the client is asymptomatic. Cervical dysplasia is usually detected by Pap smear. Early clinical manifestations include postcoital bleeding, metrorrhagia, and a blood-tinged vaginal discharge. Manifestations of more extensive disease include back, pelvic, and leg pain; weight loss; vaginal bleeding; anemia; lymphadenopathy; and edema of the legs.

Treatment of CIN can include conization, laser therapy, cryosurgery, electrocautery, or hysterectomy. For invasive cancer, treatment may involve surgery, radiation, and chemotherapy with cisplatin, vincristine, bleomycin, or mitomycin. Follow-up care focuses on recurrent disease and control of manifestations and metastasis.

Treat Conditions Specific to AIDS

AIDS Dementia

HIV encephalopathy, also referred to as *AIDS dementia complex,* appears to affect the very young and older HIV-infected clients and clients with anemia and weight loss. In addition, HIV-infected people with less than a 12th grade education may be more likely to show clinical manifestations. Manifestations include cognitive dysfunction, motor problems, and behavioral changes. Cognitive manifestations include an inability to concentrate, decreased memory, impaired judgment, and slowed thinking. Motor impairment may be manifested as leg weakness, ataxia, and clumsiness. Behavioral changes can range from apathy, reduced spontaneity, and social withdrawal to irritability, hyperactivity, anxiety, mania, and delirium.

The staging system for AIDS dementia complex is as follows:

- Stage 0: normal
- Stage 0.5: minimal
- Stage 1: mild
- Stage 2: moderate
- Stage 3: severe
- Stage 4: end stage

Some studies have shown a favorable response to combination antiretroviral therapy. Delirium with agitation can be treated with haloperidol, lorazepam, or molindone. Follow-up monitoring focuses on detecting the progression of AIDS dementia complex and on evaluating the client's ability to safely maintain independent living and comply with prescribed therapies.

HIV Wasting Syndrome

Weight loss occurs at some point in more than 90% of people with HIV-infected infection. *HIV wasting* is defined as profound involuntary weight loss (>10% of total body baseline weight) and either chronic diarrhea or chronic weakness and fever. The primary causes of HIV wasting syndrome are reduced food intake, malabsorption of nutrients, and altered metabolism of nutrients. The clinical evaluation of a client with HIV wasting syndrome includes an attempt to determine the cause. For example, if the origin is a gastrointestinal (GI) infection (e.g., salmonellosis), treating the underlying infection usually alleviates the progressive weight loss. In men with HIV infection, low testosterone levels lead to weight loss, a trend that can be reversed with testosterone replacement.

Once wasting has begun, treatment usually results in only partial recovery. The goal of drug therapy is to stimulate appetite, produce weight gain, and increase lean muscle mass. Weight gain that results in increased body fat is of little benefit. Drugs used to treat HIV wasting syndrome include oxandrolone, thalidomide, megestrol acetate, and dronabinol. The latter two drugs usually result in weight gain that is primarily fat. The drug used most successfully to treat wasting is human growth hormone. Follow-up therapy includes constant assessment for factors that may interfere with the plan of care (cognitive impairment, severe fatigue, or a lack of resources to buy or prepare food).

Nursing Management of the AIDS Client

In advanced HIV disease, the goal of nursing care is to diagnose and treat human responses to actual or potential health problems related to the development of clinical manifestations and the diagnosis of AIDS. All efforts are directed at controlling manifestations. Actual or potential problems seen in people with AIDS include fever, fatigue, weight loss, nausea, diarrhea, dry and painful mouth, dry skin, skin lesions, pain, dyspnea, cough, impaired cognition, impaired vision, insomnia, and sexual dysfunction. Common nursing diagnoses that have been identified through nursing research associated with the diagnosis of AIDS are presented in Box 79–2. Four problems that affect most AIDS clients are described here. Also see the HIV Case Study and Bridge to Home Care Health.

Assessment

Assessment of clinical manifestations should include both subjective and objective data. All clinical manifestations should be quantified. The easiest way to measure the severity of a clinical manifestation is by asking the client to rate it on a scale from 0 to 10, with 0 being no

Human Immunodeficiency Virus (HIV)

Edith Jones is a white woman, age 50 years, who presents to an outpatient clinic with complaints of fever, fatigue, "swollen glands," and a sore throat. She is an elementary school teacher and states that she believes she has been exposed to some virus in her classroom. She is concerned because the manifestations have not resolved as quickly as they usually do when she catches a "classroom bug."

Nursing Assessment

Mrs. Jones is alert and cooperative. She says that she has had these manifestations for the past 2 weeks. She has a 17-year-old daughter. Mrs. Jones relates that her husband was killed in a car accident 5 years ago and that she has recently begun dating again. She fears that the stresses of a new relationship and raising a teenager are catching up with her. She states, "Dating has changed so much since before I was married. Maybe I'm just too old to start dating again." Consider the factors that place Mrs. Jones at risk for contracting HIV.

Nursing Physical Assessment

Height: 5′6″
Weight: 140 lb (63.6 kg)
Vital signs: blood pressure, 120/80; TPR, 99.0, 90, 20
LOC: alert and cooperative
EENT: mouth and pharynx are reddened, submaxillary and tonsillar lymph nodes are readily palpable
Cardiac: heart tones are regular, S_1 and S_2 are readily audible with no murmurs or rubs noted
Pulmonary: lung sounds are clear bilaterally
Abdominal: abdomen is flat with hyperactive bowel tones
Genitourinary: deferred
Peripheral pulses: 2/2, without edema

A complete blood count (CBC) is ordered.

CBC Results	
RBC	4.0 μl
Hb	12.0 g/dl
Hct	36%
WBC	2500 μl
Neutrophils	80%
Basophils	2%
Lymphocytes	14%
Monocytes	4%
Platelets	100 × 10^9/L

Consider the pathophysiologic factors that might cause the alterations noted in these results. A more detailed dating history obtained from Mrs. Jones reveals that she has had sexual intercourse with three different men during the past 12 months and did not use condoms. When questioned further, she insists that these men told her that she was the only woman they were dating and that she did not realize she needed to get a more detailed sexual history from them. She is reluctant to contact these men now because she is no longer seeing any of them.

An enzyme immunoassay and a $CD4^+$ cell count are ordered. Mrs. Jones is instructed to call the clinic in 5 days to obtain her results. Her enzyme immunoassay is positive for antibodies to HIV, and her $CD4^+$ cell count is 75/mm^3. Mrs. Jones is instructed to return to the clinic for follow-up tests and treatment. A Western blot, HIV RNA viral load test, and purified protein derivative (PPD) skin test by Mantoux method are performed. The Western blot confirms the diagnosis of HIV, and the initial HIV RNA viral load is 11,000 copies/ml. Mrs. Jones' PPD result is negative.

Mrs. Jones remains reluctant to talk about her prior sexual activities, but she does agree to contact her three recent sexual partners and tell them about her diagnosis. She is more concerned about what to tell her daughter and her parents. "I certainly haven't set a very good example for my daughter. I wonder if I'll live long enough to see her married," she states.

Her primary care provider explains that she could consider initiating antiretroviral therapy because her viral load is above 10,000 copies/ml and her $CD4^+$ cell count is low. However, considering the fact that variations may occur with these test results, the primary care provider schedules her for a second HIV RNA viral load and $CD4^+$ count. In the meantime, teaching is begun regarding the basics of HIV infection and prevention of transmission.

More tests reveal an HIV RNA viral load of 13,500 copies/ml and a $CD4^+$ count of 64 mm^3. After discussing treatment options with her primary care provider, Mrs. Jones agrees to start antiretroviral therapy.

Initial Antiretroviral	Therapy Orders
Combivir	1 tablet orally twice a day
Sustiva	600 mg orally at bedtime

Consider other teaching and referrals that should be made at this time.

Mrs. Jones returns to the clinic in 3 weeks for follow-up laboratory work. Her HIV RNA viral load is now reported as being undetectable, and her $CD4^+$ is now 90/mm^3. Mrs. Jones exclaims "Maybe I don't really have AIDS after all." Consider appropriate responses that could be made to this remark. Mrs. Jones is instructed to continue the same drug regimen and to return to the clinic on a regular basis for follow-up.

Case Study continued on following page

Discharge and Post-treatment Considerations

Average length of stay: outpatient only
Complete client instruction (including diet, medications, safe sexual practices, infection prevention, support groups, and follow-up appointments)
Community referral: HIV support group

Questions to Be Considered

1. Compare and contrast the practical and ethical considerations of treatment options for clients with and without health insurance coverage. Identify alternate sources of funding for clients without private health insurance.
2. Identify the precautions that Mrs. Jones should take to protect herself from secondary infections and to protect others from becoming infected with HIV. Considering her $CD4^+$ count, should she receive any prophylactic therapy to prevent an opportunistic infection?
3. Discuss the medication teaching necessary for the various antiretroviral drugs. What implications do these drugs have for nursing practice?
4. Identify the assessment and laboratory findings that would indicate Mrs. Jones had progressed to acquired immunodeficiency syndrome (AIDS).
5. Compare and contrast the nursing care required for the HIV client versus the AIDS client.
6. Discuss safe sexual practice and how this information might be most effectively conveyed to the various at-risk populations. Include age, race, marital status, socioeconomic, and geographical factors in your discussion.
7. Compare and contrast the assessment data that would indicate a client with HIV is coping positively with the illness. Identify measures to promote effective coping.

EENT, eyes, ears, nose, throat; Hb, hemoglobin; Hct, hematocrit; μl, microliters; LOC, level of consciousness; RBC, red blood cell count; RNA, ribonucleic acid; TPR, temperature, pulse, respirations; WBC, white blood cell count.

problem at all and 10 being the worst possible. This method works very well for most manifestations, such as fatigue and pain. Fever assessment can be made easy if the client is willing to keep a fever diary (writing down his temperature whenever he takes it). For clients who have no scale at home, you will have to rely on their self-report about how they look and how their clothes fit to detect trends in weight.

Pain is a subjective experience. The single most reliable indicator of the existence and intensity of acute pain and any related discomfort or distress is the client's self-report. Neither behavior nor vital signs can substitute for

BRIDGE TO HOME HEALTH CARE

Living with HIV/AIDS

People who have a diagnosis of HIV or AIDS face a very different future today than even 5 years ago because of recently developed medications and treatments. They have new and complex challenges because they are living longer. If you provide care in community settings such as homes or clinics, expect to work as a team member with clients, other health care providers, clients' partners, significant others, children, extended family members, and the community to deal with the challenges and help provide the highest quality care possible. Become familiar with community resources that are available to clients and their families. Transportation to health care facilities, the location of the pharmacy and grocery store, availability of volunteers and respite programs, financial assistance, and career counseling or job retraining are examples of needed resources.

Because the client's immune system is compromised, it is important to teach the client and caregivers how to prevent infections and use standard precautions. Instruct about proper food handling, water and sanitation, linens, and dressings. Find out about the health status of others in the home, especially those who have or are at high risk for acute or chronic health problems. Such information will help you develop a successful plan of care.

Become comfortable discussing sexual issues and family planning or contraception with clients. If you are not able to do this, refer your clients to someone who is knowledgeable and who can deal with these issues in a confidential manner.

The spiritual and emotional health needs of people who live with HIV and AIDS must be addressed. The stress of living with a serious illness can take its toll on the clients and those near to them. Encourage the client and others to express their feelings and listen to them; you may hear many significant and difficult issues. Allow clients and family members to deal with the issues, and help them achieve resolution and closure. Consider a referral to a mental health expert, a spiritual counselor, or a social worker when appropriate.

Be alert for signs of family violence, spouse abuse, or child abuse. Stress, cognitive impairment, loss of work, expenses, and difficulties related to illegal drug use and sales can contribute to these problems. Know related regulations, and contact proper authorities when needed.

Clients who have HIV and AIDS usually need to take many medications to be administered on a specific schedule. Determine whether clients can manage their medications themselves or need assistance and whether they have adequate knowledge about the medications. Make sure the medication schedule is reasonable and encourages compliance. Assess for drug allergies and for potential drug interactions that can occur when various physicians prescribe many drugs.

Considering your own safety is essential when you provide community-focused services to any clients. If you are visiting areas with high crime rates or known drug use, talk to your clients and their families and ask for their assistance. It may be safer to schedule your visits in the mornings. You may need to be accompanied by a volunteer or agency escort who is familiar with the area and neighborhood. Always try to blend into the neighborhood, be alert for signs of trouble, and leave immediately if you sense trouble.

Pamela J. Nelson, RN, MS, *Assistant Professor of Nursing, Bethel College, St. Paul, Minnesota*

BOX 79–2 Common Nursing Diagnoses for Clients with Human Immunodeficiency Virus and Acquired Immunodeficiency Syndrome

Altered Oral Mucous Membrane
Altered Thought Processes
Altered Nutrition: Less Than Body Requirements
Altered Health Maintenance
Altered Protection
Anxiety
Bathing/Hygiene Self-Care Deficit
Body Image Disturbance
Diarrhea
Death Anxiety
Dressing/Grooming Self-Care Deficit
Fatigue
Fluid Volume Deficit
Hyperthermia
Impaired Physical Mobility
Impaired Skin Integrity
Impaired Tissue Integrity
Ineffective Management of Therapeutic Regimen
Ineffective Breathing Pattern
Knowledge Deficit
Nausea
Pain
Powerlessness
Risk for Altered Body Temperature
Risk for Caregiver Role Strain
Risk for Ineffective Individual Coping
Risk for Injury
Sensory/Perceptual Alterations
Sleep Pattern Disturbance
Toileting Self-Care Deficit

that self-report. A client may be in excruciating pain even while smiling or laughing to cope with it. Trying to figure out whether a client has pain when the client is actually reporting pain is a waste of time.

DIAGNOSIS, OUTCOMES, INTERVENTIONS

Hyperthermia. An important nursing diagnosis for a client with AIDS is *Hyperthermia related to chronic HIV infection, secondary opportunistic infection, malignancy, autoimmune disorders, diarrhea, dehydration, allergic response to medications, or infection at IV sites, catheters, drains, and incisions.*

Outcomes. After discussing the finding of assessment and the nursing diagnosis, select interventions in concert with the client, care partner, or both to control fever and replace fluid loss.

Interventions. Because of the underlying immunodeficiency and impaired inflammatory response, clinical manifestations of infection, including fever, may be greatly muted. Nonpharmacologic interventions include keeping the client in a warm room to avert shivering and applying a sheet and a loosely woven blanket. Avoid fanning the bed covers, exposing skin, or rapidly removing clothing that might cause chilling.

Avoid counterproductive treatments, such as tepid water sponge bathing, which causes defensive vasoconstriction and has not been shown to be an effective coolant in fever. Indeed, sponge baths can cause shivering and can be distressing. Avoid alcohol sponging as well, which also causes vasoconstriction, shivering, and toxic fumes. The alcohol also can be absorbed cutaneously, causing hypoglycemia.

Increase caloric and fluid intake by providing a plan for six feedings distributed over 24 hours and high-protein, high-calorie nutritional supplements, especially if the client has anorexia. Provide 2 to 2.5 L of fluid to drink daily.

Maintain comfort and safety by providing dry clothes and bed linens made out of cotton rather than synthetics. Use emollient creams for dry skin. Monitor mental status frequently, especially when the client has a fever. Evaluate the client's need for assistance with all activities of daily living. Teach the client how to manage chronic recurrent night fever and night sweats by:

- Taking the antipyretic agent of choice before going to sleep
- Having a change of bedclothes nearby in case a change is necessary
- Keeping a plastic cover on the pillow
- Placing a towel over the pillow in case of profuse diaphoresis
- Keeping liquids at the bedside to drink

Pharmacologic treatment can include aspirin, nonsteroidal anti-inflammatory drugs (NSAIDs), or acetaminophen. Follow-up should include comparing patterns of use of these agents with laboratory evaluation of hepatic and hematologic abnormalities, as well as interactions with other agents.

Fatigue. Another common nursing diagnosis is *Fatigue related to chronic HIV infection, anemia, secondary opportunistic infection, malnutrition, dehydration, prolonged immobility, and psychological and situational factors.*

Outcomes. After discussing and validating the findings of assessment and nursing diagnosis, select interventions in concert with the client, care partner, or both to increase self-awareness of fatigue, associated clinical manifestations, environmental factors affecting fatigue, and activity tolerance. Identify interventions to highlight the importance of resting when needed and accepting assistance when needed. Develop a plan for a lifestyle that keeps the client independent, socially active, and involved in activities of daily living.

Interventions. Promote self-care and self-awareness by having the client keep a daily fatigue diary for at least 1 week to identify sources of fatigue and appropriate interventions, as well as patterns of peak fitness. Advise the client to avoid coffee, tobacco, and alcohol, any of which may increase fatigue in some people. Promote adequate sleep by increasing the amount of sleep each day. Reduce the amount of sleep-cycle interruptions by preparing for sleep and keeping needed items at the bedside (e.g., ice water, a urinal, and a towel to absorb perspiration).

Promote rest and activity by developing a written 24-hour schedule of daily activities that alternates short activities with rest periods. Identify activity priorities, such as eating breakfast and then resting before bathing in the morning, as opposed to the reverse. Evaluate the client's needs and point out ways to conserve energy, such as sitting down while dressing, shaving, or preparing food; sitting on a shower chair while bathing; or using disposable items for eating so that no cleanup is needed. Help the client write up a plan for rest and activities that progresses from daily to weekly. Encourage the client to always plan activities ahead of time.

Prepare an exercise schedule (immobilization may lead to decreased endurance and increased fatigue) and plan exercises at peak energy times (after a rest period). Follow the exercises with rest. Aerobic exercise, which increases endurance, can reduce fatigue. Additional natural techniques that may be of benefit include progressive muscle relaxation, acupressure, massage, reflexology, imagery and visualization, autogenic relaxation, reframing and positive affirmations, therapeutic touch, and social support and support groups

Altered Nutrition: Less Than Body Requirements. A frequently encountered nursing diagnosis is *Altered Nutrition: Less Than Body Requirements related to increased nutrient requirements, decreased food intake secondary to side effects of medications and infection such as an anorexia, nausea, vomiting, altered taste, or impaired swallowing or chewing, diarrhea, fatigue, depression, or impaired cognition.*

Outcomes. After discussing and validating the findings of assessment and the nursing diagnosis, select interventions in concert with the client, care partner, or both to increase food intake, preserve lean body mass, and provide adequate levels of all nutrients.

Interventions

Minimize Anorexia. Minimize factors contributing to anorexia. For *hyperosmia* (an increased sense of smell), avoid cooking odors by keeping windows open and the home well aerated. Encourage meals that include cold foods. For *hyposmia* (a decreased sense of smell), use spices such as basil, oregano, rosemary, thyme, cloves, mint, cinnamon, or lemon juice to enhance smell. For alterations in sense of taste (especially related to distaste for red meat), marinate meat in a commercial marinade, wine, or vinegar before cooking it, and use substitutes for red meat, such as eggs, peanut butter, tofu, cheeses, poultry, and fish.

Prevent Weight Loss. Weight loss can be a significant problem for clients who live alone or who have fatigue or depression. Interventions include:

- Eating small meals frequently throughout the day
- Eating high-calorie snacks or commercially prepared supplements (liquids or bars)
- Indulging in favorite foods
- Consuming more nutrient-dense foods and beverages rather than filling up on low-calorie items
- Drinking liquids 30 minutes before eating instead of with meals
- Preparing meals (such as soups or casseroles) ahead of time so they can be divided into individual servings and frozen until ready to use
- Keeping easy-to-prepare foods on hand, such as frozen dinners, canned foods, and eggs
- Encouraging the client to dine with friends or family
- Getting family members and friends involved in meal preparation; the pleasant atmosphere they can provide may stimulate the client's appetite

Many communities have home food delivery service for people with AIDS as well.

Improve Food Intake. Minimize factors related to difficulty in chewing, dysphagia (difficulty in swallowing), or odynophagia (painful swallowing) by advising clients to avoid rough foods, such as (1) raw fruits and vegetables; spicy, acidic, or salty foods; (2) alcohol or tobacco; (3) excessively hot or cold foods; and (4) sticky foods, such as peanut butter; and (5) slippery foods, such as gelatin, bologna, and elbow macaroni. Encourage the client to:

- Eat foods at room temperature
- Choose mild foods and drinks, such as apple juice rather than orange juice
- Eat dry grain foods (such as breads, crackers, and cookies) after softening them in milk, tea, or another mild beverage
- Eat nonabrasive foods that are easy to swallow, such as ice cream, pudding, well-cooked eggs, noodle dishes, baked fish, and soft cheese
- Eat Popsicles (frozen dessert) to numb pain
- Use a straw when drinking
- Tilt the head forward or back to make swallowing easier

Increase the Availability of Food. Minimize factors related to the client's inability to obtain food by evaluating his or her financial resources and the need for referral for Medicaid, food stamps, or other services. Evaluate the client's home and ability to prepare and obtain food. Look for such problems as an absence of cooking facilities and the need for alternative housing arrangements. Explore community resources that provide free meals.

Teach Nutritional Requirements. If the client has no metabolic condition that requires a special diet, the prescribed diet for people with HIV disease should include high-protein, high-calorie, low-fat foods. Help the client plan a 24-hour menu, and review the essential elements of a low-microbe diet and food safety and preparation. Nutritional teaching should, as much as possible, follow the client's usual pattern of food intake rather than expect the client to follow a totally new, unfamiliar prescription for meal planning.

Pain. A common nursing diagnosis is *Pain related to arthralgia, myalgia, or neuropathy associated with HIV disease, mass lesions associated with opportunistic infection(s) or cancer, side effects of medications, co-morbid disease such as diabetic neuropathy, or interventions such as surgery.*

Outcomes. After discussing and validating the findings of assessment, select interventions in concert with the client, care partner, or both to reduce the incidence and severity of pain, communicate effectively about pain experiences, and enhance comfort and satisfaction.

Interventions

Provide Comfort Measures. Non-drug interventions include identifying activities of daily living that seem to increase the intensity and severity of pain. Provide additional comfort measures, such as using a pressure-relieving mattress, positioning and supporting limbs comfortably when in bed or a chair, and using a "pull sheet" to move clients or help them change positions. For institutionalized clients, encourage family members or significant others to bring in familiar objects, such as pillows and blankets, favorite photographs, religious articles, personal clothing, cologne, make-up, face powder, and other cosmetics.

Provide Physical Therapy. Physical therapy can be very helpful in managing pain. The physical therapist can provide:

- Exercise to maintain or increase physical activity levels and endurance
- Ultrasound and physical treatments, such as application of heat or cold, to reduce musculoskeletal pain
- Therapeutic massage
- Instruction and supervision in using a transcutaneous electrical nerve stimulation (TENS) device, commonly called a *TENS unit*

Administer Pain Medications. Pharmacologic treatments usually include *non-opioid analgesics,* such as aspirin and acetaminophen for mild pain, (2) *weak opioids,* such as codeine and oxycodone for moderate pain, and (3) *strong opioids,* such as morphine for severe pain. For neuropathic pain (such as HIV-associated polyneuropathy, acute and postherpetic neuralgia, and nucleoside toxicity with didanosine, zalcitabine, and stavudine), adjuvants such as ibuprofen may be used as well as amitriptyline, desipramine, nortriptyline, doxepin, carbamazepine, divalproex, phenytoin, gabapentin, or mexiletine.

Primary care providers should anticipate several changes in prescriptions for analgesics when starting the client with a pain control regimen. A major error in initial pain management occurs when a clinician prescribes a 2-week supply of an analgesic, assumes that the prescription works, and has no further contact until the client returns 2 weeks later for follow-up. On the contrary, during the initial phase of pain control, the clinician should have daily contact with the client, even if by telephone, and should anticipate schedule changes. Dosage frequency should be adjusted to prevent pain from recurring once the duration of analgesic action is determined. Similarly, it is a waste of money to prescribe large amounts of an analgesic, such as a 30-day supply, knowing that the orders will change. Orders for opioid analgesics should include "rescue" doses for breakthrough pain when regularly scheduled doses are insufficient.

Orders for analgesics as needed (prn) result in delays in administration and intervals of inadequate pain control. Tell clients and their care partners that the client may sleep for extended periods and may appear very drowsy during the first few days of a pain control regimen. Although this may result in part from the initial effects of the drug, it probably also reflects exhaustion and the need for rest as a result of sleep deprivation caused by pain. This situation usually reverses itself within a few days after a scheduled pain management regimen is begun.

Clients may refuse an analgesic if they are not in pain or may forgo it when they are asleep. Explain that this decision may lower blood analgesia levels and cause a resurgence of pain and failure of the pain control plan. Although the anti-inflammatory effects of aspirin are highly effective as an analgesic adjuvant, because aspirin inhibits platelet function, it may be contraindicated if the client has a low platelet count.

Helpful guidelines for managing pain in the injecting drug user include (1) having a single practitioner prescribe medications, (2) refusing to refill lost prescriptions, (3) carefully rationing narcotic prescriptions, and (4) limiting rescue doses of narcotic analgesics on a monthly basis. Clients who are in recovery for narcotic addiction and are being treated with methadone maintenance still experience pain and in most instances require higher and more frequent doses of analgesia than a narcotic-naive client would. Some antiretroviral drugs, such as nevirapine and ritonavir, interfere with the half-life of methadone and may decrease its blood levels. The client will experience mild withdrawal symptoms. Increasing the daily dose of methadone usually resolves the problem.

Because diarrhea is common in clients with HIV disease, especially when protease inhibitors are prescribed, the constipating effects of analgesics may actually be beneficial. Evaluate each client's response to therapy instead of automatically using stool softeners when initiating the pain control plan.

Encourage Complementary Therapies. Complementary therapies that may be used include cognitive-behavioral interventions, such as education and instruction in pain control, relaxation exercises, imagery, music distraction, biofeedback, and therapeutic touch.

EVALUATION

It is expected that the client, care partner, or both will be able to (1) identify appropriate measures to take for a fever, (2) initiate and maintain adequate hydration and nutrition, and (3) demonstrate the ability to take and record the client's temperature accurately. Although infection-related fever can be controlled with appropriate antibiotic therapy, this problem can be expected to recur throughout the illness.

It is expected that the client, care partner, or both will be able to (1) identify causative factors that increase fatigue, (2) plan a schedule of paced activity for a 24-hour period, (3) demonstrate the ability to participate in a program of exercise, and (4) verbalize a decrease in the client's fatigue for a 24-hour period. Fatigue is a manifestation that can be expected to recur throughout HIV disease, especially because it is a side effect of some antiretroviral medications, such as zidovudine and ritonavir.

It is expected that the client will maintain or increase weight. It is expected that the client, care partner, or both will (1) identify factors related to anorexia, difficulty in chewing, dysphagia, or odynophagia; (2) identify sufficient resources to obtain and prepare food or make use of social work interventions employed to obtain food stamps or public assistance; (3) identify ways to increase protein and calorie intake; (4) identify key concepts in planning a low-microbial diet; and (5) select a balanced 24-hour menu. The client's weight will fluctuate during the course of HIV disease related to the development of new disease processes and the side effects of prescribed medications.

It is expected that the client, care partner, or both will (1) identify aggravating factors or precipitating factors related to the pain experienced, (2) identify measures to control pain, and (3) verbalize a decrease in the amount and type of pain experienced over 24 hours. Pain may be either chronic or acute, depending on the cause. In most instances, it can be managed effectively, as with any client with another diagnosis.

CONCLUSIONS

HIV continues to be a major threat to human health worldwide. At one time or another, you will care for a person with HIV infection or AIDS. To provide adequate care for a person with HIV infection, you must understand the illness trajectory and the therapeutic interventions needed to maintain health. Always seek expert guidance when starting to care for a client with HIV infection or AIDS. The nature of care is very complex, and the client's clinical needs are numerous.

THINKING CRITICALLY

1. **A 30-year-old woman presents with fever, fatigue, lymphadenopathy, thrush, diarrhea, and pain in her muscles and joints. She has a rash on her torso and arms. What questions would you ask to determine her possible exposure to HIV? How will the client be evaluated and treated?**

Factors to Consider. What tests confirm the diagnosis of AIDS? How is the $CD4^+$ cell count used? What is the purpose of the viral load test? What treatment may be used?

2. **You are working in a homeless shelter and are scheduled to present a 20-minute program on AIDS prevention. A small class of four men and three women have gathered. They are all known to you, and you suspect that one couple may be infected with HIV. What should you plan to teach?**

Factors to Consider. What main areas of HIV education should be addressed? What is an effective method of communicating this information?

3. **Your HIV-infected female client leaves the physician's office and comes over to you and says, "I don't have HIV anymore. The doctor just told me that my viral load was undetectable." How would you respond?**

Factors to Consider. What does an undetectable viral load test result mean? What would you tell this client about safer sex practices and becoming pregnant?

4. **Your 40-year-old male client with AIDS and *P. carinii* pneumonia is about to be discharged from the hospital. His $CD4^+$** cell count is 35. He asks you what he should do now. What teaching would you provide?

Factors to Consider. When does a person with HIV infection get an AIDS diagnosis? Does this client need any medication for his pneumonia? Given the fact that the $CD4^+$ cell count is 35, does he need any medication to prevent any other opportunistic infections?

BIBLIOGRAPHY

1. American Dietetic Association. (1994). Position of the American Dietetic Association and the Canadian Dietetic Association: Nutrition intervention in the care of persons with human immunodeficiency virus infection. *Journal of the American Dietetic Association, 94,* 1042–1045.
2. Anastasi, J. K., & Sun Lee, V. (1994). HIV wasting: How to stop the cycle. *American Journal of Nursing, 94,* 18–24.
3. Bartlett, J. (1997). *Medical management of HIV infection.* Available: *http://www.hopkins-aids.edu.*
4. Breitbart, W., & McDonald, M. V. (1996). Pharmacologic pain management in HIV/AIDS. *Journal of the International Association of Physicians in AIDS Care, 2*(7), 17–26.
5. Centers for Disease Control. (1992). 1993 Revised classification system for HIV infection and expanded surveillance case definition for AIDS among adolescents and adults. *Morbidity and Mortality Weekly Report, 41* (RR-17), 1–19.
6. Centers for Disease Control and Prevention. (1998). *HIV/AIDS Surveillance Report, 10*(2), 1–39.
7. Centers for Disease Control and Prevention. (1999). *1999 USPHS/IDSA guidelines for the prevention of opportunistic infections in persons infected with human immunodeficiency virus.* Atlanta: Author.
8. Centers for Disease Control and Prevention. (1999). *Guidelines for the use of antiretroviral agents in HIV-infected adults and adolescents.* Atlanta: Author.
9. Dolin, R., Masur, H., & Saag, M. (Eds.). (1999). *AIDS therapy.* New York: Churchill Livingstone.
10. Ferris, F. D., et al. (1995). *A comprehensive guide for the care of persons with HIV disease: Module 4 palliative care.* Toronto, Canada: Mount Sinai Hospital and Casey House Hospice.
11. Friedman-Kien, A., & Cockerell, C. (1996). *Color atlas of AIDS* (2nd ed.). Philadelphia: W. B. Saunders.
12. Gorbach, S., Bartlett, J., & Blacklow, N. (1998). *Infectious diseases* (2nd ed.). Philadelphia: W. B. Saunders.
13. Hinkle, K. (1991). A literature review: HIV seropositivity in the elderly. *Journal of Gerontological Nursing, 7*(10), 12–17.
14. Jewitt, J. F., & Hecht, F. M. (1993). Preventive health care for adults with HIV infection. *Journal of the American Medical Association, 269*(9), 1144–1153.
15. Katsufrakis, P. (Ed.). (1997). HIV/AIDS management in office practice. *Primary Care Clinics in Office Practice. 24*(3), 469–690.
16. Lipsky, J. J. (1996). Antiretroviral drugs for AIDS. *Lancet, 348,* 800–803.
17. Mellors, J. W., et al. (1996). Prognosis in HIV-1 infection predicted by the quantity of virus in plasma. *Science, 272*(5265), 1167–1170.
18. National Institute of Allergy and Infectious Diseases. (1997). HIV persists and can replicate despite prolonged combination therapy. *NIAD News.*
19. Rosenberg, E., & Cotton, D. (1997). Primary HIV infection and the acute retroviral syndrome: The urgent need for recognition. *AIDS Clinical Care, 9*(3), 19, 23–25.
20. Sande, M., & Volberding, P. (1997). *The medical management of AIDS* (5th ed.). Philadelphia: W. B. Saunders.
21. Sherman, D. (Ed.). (1999). HIV/AIDS update. *Nursing Clinics of North America, 34*(1), 1–256.
22. Ungvarski, P. J. (1995). Meeting the challenge of AIDS. *Imprint, 42*(4), 51–54.
23. Ungvarski, P. J. (1996). Waging war on HIV wasting. *RN, 59*(2), 26–32.
24. Ungvarski, P. J. (1996). Challenges for the urban home care provider: The New York experience. *Nursing Clinics of North America, 31*(1), 81–95.
25. Ungvarski, P. J. (1997). Update on HIV infection. *American Journal of Nursing, 97*(1), 4–52.
26. Ungvarski, P. J. (1997). Adherence to prescribed HIV-1 protease inhibitors in the home setting. *Journal of the Association of Nurses in AIDS Care, 8*(Suppl.), 37–45.
27. Ungvarski, P. J., & Flaskerud, J. H. (Eds.). (1999). *HIV/AIDS: A guide to primary care management* (4th ed.). Philadelphia: W. B. Saunders.
28. Zeller, J. M., Swanson, B., & Cohen, F. L. (1993). Suggestions for clinical nursing research: Symptom management in AIDS patients. *Journal of the Association of Nurses in AIDS Care, 4*(3), 13–17.

CHAPTER 80

Management of Clients Requiring Transplantation

Connie White-Williams

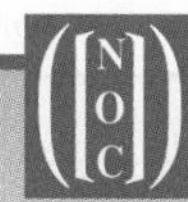

NURSING OUTCOMES CLASSIFICATION (NOC)
for Nursing Diagnoses—Clients Requiring Transplantation

Altered Nutrition: More Than Body Requirements
Nutritional Status: Food and Fluid Intake
Nutritional Status: Nutrient Intake
Weight Control
Altered Protection/Risk for Infection
Immune Status
Knowledge: Infection Control
Risk Control
Treatment Behavior: Illness or Injury
Tissue Integrity: Skin/Mucous Membrane
Wound Healing: Primary Intention
Wound Healing: Secondary Intention

Effective Management of Therapeutic Regimen: Individual
Adherence Behavior
Compliance Behavior
Family Participation in Professional Care
Knowledge: Treatment Regimen
Participation: Health Care Decisions
Risk Control
Symptom Control
Pain
Comfort Level
Pain Control
Pain: Disruptive Effects
Pain Level

Risk for Ineffective Individual Coping
Coping
Decision Making
Impulse Control
Information Processing
Role Performance
Social Support
Risk for Injury
Knowledge: Personal Safety
Risk Control
Risk Detection
Safety Behavior: Personal
Symptom Control

The field of organ transplantation has evolved from the early beginnings of experimental kidney transplantation to the current practice of multiple organ transplantation. The advances made have been due largely to the increased knowledge in the areas of immunology and organ preservation, recipient and donor selection, and management of postoperative complications.

Organ transplantation is needed when an organ is irreversibly diseased or injured, leading to end-stage organ failure. Transplantation offers people with end-stage organ failure a chance to live longer and to overcome conditions that were once considered hopeless. Thus, nurses have an increasing opportunity to care for clients with end-stage disease who are awaiting transplantation or who have undergone organ transplantation. In addition, nurses may also play a vital role in identification of potential donors and their management during the donor maintenance period.

Historical Perspective

Transplantation had its beginnings in the 17th century with blood transfusions; however, the era of modern transplantation originated with a tooth replacement by John Hunter in the 18th century.[19] In 1912, Alexis Carrel developed the techniques for surgical suturing and vascular anastomosis that opened the pathway to solid organ transplantation.[25] Much of the work during the succeeding years focused on immunology, the importance of ABO and Rh blood group compatibility, and, later, the development of histocompatibility testing, all of which are crucial to organ transplantation today.[26, 33] In 1943, Medawar[39] described the immune response of acute rejection, and by 1970 the relationship between donor and recipient histocompatibility in the role of acute rejection was recognized.[56]

Although many attempts at kidney transplantation were

made in the early 1900s, it was not until 1954 that Merrell and Murray performed the first successful kidney transplantation, between identical twin brothers.[19] Experimental heart transplantation took place in the early 1900s. Hardy transplanted a chimpanzee heart (xenograft) into a 68-year-old man in 1964. In 1967, Barnard performed the first human-to-human heart transplant.[5, 19] The first lung transplantation was performed by Hardy in 1963.[11] Experimental liver transplantation began in the 1950s. The first human liver transplantation was performed in 1963 by Starzl.[53] Figure 80–1 presents a summary of the number of transplantation procedures reported by the United Network of Organ Sharing (UNOS).[61]

With current success and survival statistics, these procedures are no longer deemed experimental. Organ transplantation is clearly an option for clients with end-stage organ disease. Much of the success is due to the availability of new immunosuppressive therapies, advances in organ preservation, improved surgical techniques, and the recognition of risk factors that affect survival after transplantation. Because transplant recipients now live longer, however, numerous social, economic, ethical, and quality of life (QOL) issues have arisen.

Related Issues

■ COST

Average costs for the surgical procedure plus 5-year post-transplantation expenses are approximately $172,000 for kidney transplantation, $317,000 for heart transplantation, $312,000 for lung transplantation, and $394,000 for liver transplantation.[60] The Social Security Act was amended in 1972 to cover the cost of dialysis and transplantation for end-stage renal disease. Although coverage by private insurance companies, health maintenance organizations, (HMOs), preferred provider organizations (PPOs), and Medicare/Medicaid has increased, the high

Number of U.S. Transplants: 1988 to December 31, 1998 by Organ and Donor Type*

ORGAN	DONOR TYPE	YEAR OF TRANSPLANT PROCEDURE										
		1988	1989	1990	1991	1992	1993	1994	1995	1996	1997	1998
KIDNEY*	CADAVER	7231	7087	7782	7733	7696	8171	8384	8602	8571	8613	8938
	LIVING	1812	1903	2094	2393	2536	2850	3008	3347	3605	3797	4017
	TOTAL	9043	8990	9876	10126	10232	11021	11392	11949	12176	12410	12955
LIVER	CADAVER	1713	2199	2677	2931	3031	3404	3592	3879	4013	4101	4384
	LIVING	0	2	14	22	33	36	60	46	53	69	66
	TOTAL	1713	2201	2691	2953	3064	3440	3652	3925	4066	1470	4450
PANCREAS*	CADAVER	244	413	526	529	554	772	840	1018	1013	1056	1216
	LIVING	5	4	2	1	3	2	2	7	11	6	2
	TOTAL	249	417	528	530	557	774	842	1025	1024	1062	1218
HEART	CADAVER	1670	1696	2095	2122	2170	2295	2338	2361	2342	2294	2340
	LIVING†	7	9	12	4	1	2	3	0	1	0	0
	TOTAL	1677	1705	2107	2126	2171	2297	2341	2361	2343	2294	2340
LUNG	CADAVER	33	93	202	401	535	660	708	849	790	912	829
	LIVING	0	0	1	4	0	7	15	23	20	18	20
	TOTAL	33	93	203	405	535	667	723	872	810	930	849
HEART-LUNG	CADAVER	74	67	52	51	48	60	70	69	39	61	45
	LIVING	0	0	0	0	0	0	0	0	0	0	0
	TOTAL	74	67	52	51	48	60	70	69	39	61	45
INTESTINE‡	CADAVER			5	12	22	34	23	44	43	65	68
	LIVING			0	0	0	0	0	1	2	2	1
	TOTAL			5	12	22	34	23	45	45	67	69
TOTAL*	CADAVER	10965	11555	13339	13779	14056	15396	15955	16822	16811	17102	17820
	LIVING	1824	1918	2123	2424	2573	2897	3088	3424	3692	3892	4106
	TOTAL	12789	13473	15462	16203	16629	18293	19043	20246	20503	20994	21926

* In this table, Simultaneous Kidney-Pancreas transplants are counted *twice*, both in Kidney Transplants and in Pancreas Transplants. The number of Simultaneous Kidney-Pancreas transplants performed in each year were: 1988–170, 1989–334, 1990–459, 1991–452, 1992–493, 1993–661, 1994–748, 1995–918, 1996–859, 1997–853, 1998–965.

† Living heart donors donate their healthy heart when they become heart-lung recipients. This is called a domino transplant.

‡ Data on Intestine transplants were not collected prior to April 1994. At that time, information was collected retrospectively for transplantations performed January 1990–March 1994.

Note: Double kidney, double lung, and heart-lung transplants are counted as one transplant. All other multiorgan transplants are being included in the total for each individual organ transplanted.

Based on UNOS Scientific Registry data as of April 19, 1999. Data subject to change based on future data submission or correction.

FIGURE 80–1 Number of transplant procedures in the United States, 1988–1998. (Modified from United Network of Organ Sharing [UNOS], Richmond, VA.)

cost remains a factor for clients who wish to undergo transplantation. In 1996, Medicare extended the coverage of immunosuppressive medications to 3 years after transplantation, which was a positive step toward helping clients financially.

■ SHORTAGE OF ORGAN DONORS

The shortage of organ donors is the most significant limitation to transplantation. There are simply not enough organs for the thousands of clients waiting for transplantation. As of the year 1999, the number of clients with end-stage disease waiting for an organ were as follows: 41,135 for a kidney; 4203 for a heart; 3195 for a lung; 12,618 for a liver; and 444 for a pancreas.[61] Required request/referral and presumed consent programs are being implemented to increase organ donation. Also, the transplantation community is investigating methods to increase donor organ supply. For example, redefining brain death to include cerebral death and anencephaly, use of xenotransplantation (transplanting organs from one species to another), and expanding the donor criteria to include older donors and living extrarenal donors (as in lobar transplantation of lung or liver) all are methods to increase donor organ supply.

■ ETHICAL CONSIDERATIONS

Many moral and ethical issues surround transplantation. Religious and cultural customs and beliefs related to death and organ donation and transplantation create challenges for health care professionals (Table 80–1). As ways to increase the organ donor pool are explored, additional ethical dilemmas may be encountered. The future trends for transplantation include more living-related donation and new experimentation such as cell transplantation. As nurses, it is important to be knowledgeable about these issues and communicate and discuss dilemmas with peers and professionals.

DEFINITION OF DEATH. There continues to be debate on the issue of death and how it is defined. The Uniform Determination of Death Act states that "an individual is considered dead if sustaining either (1) irreversible cessation of circulatory and respiratory function or (2) irreversible cessation of all functions of the entire brain, including the brain stem."[55] Different criteria are recognized for children and infants. In clients in chronic vegetative states or in anencephalic infants, brain stem function is intact but body and mental functions are not. Should death be redefined to include these people as donors? In transplantation, there will always be the dilemma of too few organs available in the face of the need to respect the life of people in a vegetative state who may be potential donors.

BUYING AND SELLING OF ORGANS. The National Organ Transplant Act of 1984 prohibits the sale of human organs and tissues. In addition, the Uniform Anatomical Gift Act of 1968 prohibits the sale or purchase of body parts or organs.[55] The conflict arises with respect to property rights. Supporters of organ sales believe that people own their bodies and have the right to do what they wish with their bodies—including the sale of their organs. The legal sale of blood plasma and sperm, which are body fluids, fuels the debate. The sale of organs in the United States is unlawful. A change in the law would alter the existing practice of free, altruistic donation.

PRISONERS AS DONORS OR RECIPIENTS. A number of concerns arise in exploring solutions to the organ donor shortage. Once again, payment for organs enters the picture. Should prisoners be allowed to donate a kidney or bone marrow for a reduced sentence? This practice would not comply with current altruistic donation. In the same context, should a convicted criminal be allowed to be a transplant recipient? Some authorities believe that being a convicted criminal should not be an exclusion criterion, whereas others argue that it should be an exclusion criterion because of the prisoner's limited life expectancy outside prison.

NON–HEART-BEATING DONORS. Other potential organ donors are people who have experienced a respiratory or circulatory death. The hearts of these potential donors have stopped beating at the time of organ recovery. Ethical issues arise with the brain death definition and when death occurs after asystole.

XENOTRANSPLANTATION. Xenotransplantation, the transplantation of organs, tissues, or cells from one species to another (e.g., transplantation of a baboon heart into a human body), has been proposed as one answer to the organ donor shortage. Many medical and ethical issues become considerations with this concept. Medical issues include organ rejection, new modes of infection transmission, and incompatible immune system responses. Ethical considerations include informed consent, the use of animals as donors, potential benefits versus risks, and public health issues.

OUTCOME MANAGEMENT

■ CLIENTS WITH END-STAGE ORGAN DISEASE

REFERRAL AND RECIPIENT SELECTION

A primary responsibility of the transplantation team is to transplant organs into clients who have the best chance for a long-term successful outcome. It is expected that the transplant recipient will experience an improvement in functional status, maintain long-term graft function, and enjoy improved QOL. This result is accomplished by the selection of an appropriate candidate. The transplantation evaluation is a complex, multidisciplinary process that is usually initiated after a referral by the primary physician. The evaluation begins with an initial assessment of medical records and an examination of the client by the transplantation team. On the basis of findings from the client's history and physical examination, the transplantation team determines whether the client should undergo further evaluation for transplantation. A depiction of the referral and evaluation process can be seen in Figure 80–2.

The goals of the evaluation process are to determine:

- The medical necessity for transplantation
- The surgical feasibility of the procedure
- Risk factors and the proper timing of transplantation
- Psychosocial suitability
- Immunologic status

The evaluation can be performed on either an inpatient or outpatient basis and usually takes 3 to 5 days. During this period, extensive testing is completed, client education is provided, and the client and family members meet the members of the transplantation team. Tests and proce-

TABLE 80–1 RELIGIOUS AND CULTURAL CUSTOMS AND BELIEFS RELATED TO DEATH AND ORGAN DONATION/TRANSPLANTATION

Religious or Cultural Group	Death	Organ Donation/Transplantation
Religious Groups		
Adventist	Dead are asleep until return of Jesus Christ	Individual and family may receive or donate organs
Baha'i	No official rituals	Both permitted
Baptist	Desire clergy present	Both approved if donor not endangered
Buddhist	"Last rite" chanting may be practiced at bedside	Matter of individual conscience
Church of Christ	No official rituals	No official position
Church of God	"Home-going ritual"	No conflict
Church of Jesus Christ of Latter Day Saints (Mormons)	Proper to bury dead in ground; cremation is discouraged	Personal choice; reflection encouraged
Eastern Orthodox Church	"Last rites"; cremation discouraged	No conflict; both are permitted
Episcopalian	"Last rites" not mandatory; desirable—Litany at the Time of Death read	No conflict if donor is not violated
Friends (Quakers)	Do not believe in life after this life	Both are permitted
Grace Brethren	No "last rites"; burial or cremation permitted	No conflict; they encourage both
Greek Orthodox	"Last rites"	Organ transplantation has always been acceptable
Hindu	Certain prescribed rites followed by priest; bodies cremated	No conflict
Islamic (Muslim, Moslem)	Patient must confess sins and beg forgiveness before death; family present	Organ donation provided that donors consent in advance in writing; not stored in organ banks
Jehovah's Witness	No official "last rites"	Do not encourage organ donation; a matter for the individual conscience; all organs drained of blood before transplantation
Judaism	Relatives and close friends remain with the deceased; no cremation	Donation or transplantation of organs requires rabbinical consultation
Lutheran	"Last rites" are optional	Both are acceptable and encouraged
Mennonite	No formal prescribed action	No conflict; both acceptable
Methodist, United	Believe in divine punishment after death; good rewarded, evil punished	Encourages both
Pentecostal (Assembly of God, Foursquare Church)	No official "last rites"	No official position
Presbyterian	Read scripture and pray	Encourage and endorse organ donation
Roman Catholic	"Last rites"	Transplantation and organ donation permissible
Russian Orthodox	Do not believe in autopsies, embalming, or cremation	Donation/transplantation of kidneys, eyes and tissues permitted; heart donation/transplantation not allowed
Cultural Groups		
African American	Funeral attendance symbolizes respect; "sticking together"; cultural rituals and quick "pulling together" by the family facilitates this process	No conflict with organ donation/transplantation
American Indian	Burial practices vary among tribal groups	Information not available
Black Muslim	Carefully prescribed procedure for washing and shrouding and funeral rites	Will accept a transplant if needed to live

TABLE 80–1 RELIGIOUS AND CULTURAL CUSTOMS AND BELIEFS RELATED TO DEATH AND ORGAN DONATION/TRANSPLANTATION *Continued*

Religious or Cultural Group	Death	Organ Donation/Transplantation
Chinese American	Chinese have an aversion to death and to anything concerning it; funeral rituals crucial to the well-being of descendants	Information not available
Hispanics (Puerto Rican, Mexican, Latino)	Spirit of the dying person needs reassurance from the living; a wake held 1 day prior to funeral; use of funeral home popular; "luto" (or mourning) is marked by wearing black and subdued behavior	No conflicts; whole family participates in the decision
Japanese American	Among Buddhists death is considered a passage; rituals: body of a dead loved one is prepared by close family member and given a bath of warm water, purification rites before the body is wrapped in a white kimono	Organ donation a matter of individual conscience
Southeast Asian Americans (Vietnamese, Cambodian, Laotian, Hmong)	Oldest male makes decisions; death of an infant is deeply mourned; expressions of grief vary	Information not available
West Indian (Haitian, Jamaican, Dominican Republican)	Death arrangements are usually made by the male kinsman of the deceased; death caused by angry voodoo spirits can give rise to conflicting feelings of guilt and anger	Permitted according to the specific religious beliefs of the individual

Data from McQuay, J. E. (1994). Cross-cultural customs and beliefs related to health crises, death, and organ donation/transplantation: A guide to assist health care professionals understand different responses and provide cross-cultural assistance. *Critical Care Nursing Clinics of North America, 7*(3), 581–594, an appendix adapted from Turner, J. W. (1987). Appendix: Attitudes and requirements of various religious groups. In DeGroot, K. D., & Damato, M. B. *Critical care skills* (pp. 389–395). Norwalk, CT: Appleton & Lange.

dures performed during the evaluation are listed in Table 80–2. These tests provide the transplantation team with information regarding the status of all organ systems, infections, coexisting medical conditions, organ-matching, and the psychosocial issues that may affect the client and family. Psychosocial factors include neurocognitive status, coping skills, compliance history, availability of support systems, financial status, and extent of resources (Table 80–3). An example of an evaluation summary sheet to be completed for transplantation candidates is depicted in Figure 80–3.

The details of the evaluation process may vary between transplantation centers and with the organs being evaluated. It is important for you to understand the evaluation process and to know the indications for and contraindications to transplantation. In addition, preoperative education is an important responsibility of the nurse. The goal of education of the potential organ recipient is to provide the client and family with factual information regarding the waiting time for an organ, the surgical procedure, and the post-transplant regimens, including diet, exercise, medication, routine follow-up, complications and return to "normal" life expectations (return to work). Many centers provide this education using several teaching skills such as one-to-one teaching, group classes and/or written information. The client uses this information to make an informed decision to undergo transplantation.

If contraindications are found during the transplantation evaluation (Box 80–1), the transplantation team reviews treatment options with the client and family. If no contraindications are found, the client can then be listed on the national waiting list according to criteria established by UNOS, a nationwide system dedicated to the equitable sharing and distribution of donor organs.

LISTING FOR TRANSPLANTATION AND WAITING FOR A DONOR ORGAN

The criteria for listing a client for transplantation are governed by UNOS and vary according to the organ to be transplanted. These criteria include urgency, blood type, and recipient weight and height.

Stable clients wait at home or near the transplantation center. Many clients choose local housing such as an apartment. A few centers provide hospital-owned housing dedicated to use by pre- and post-transplantation clients and their families. Cellular telephones or beeper systems must be available to allow the transplantation team to contact the client at any time. Usually, a client who lives at a distance from the transplantation center requiring more than 2 hours' travel time must relocate or arrange air transportation to arrive at the center within an acceptable time.

Unstable clients wait in the hospital, often in an intensive care unit. Some clients, particularly those awaiting heart transplantation, may live outside the hospital with continuous inotropic support. Intermittent hospitalization

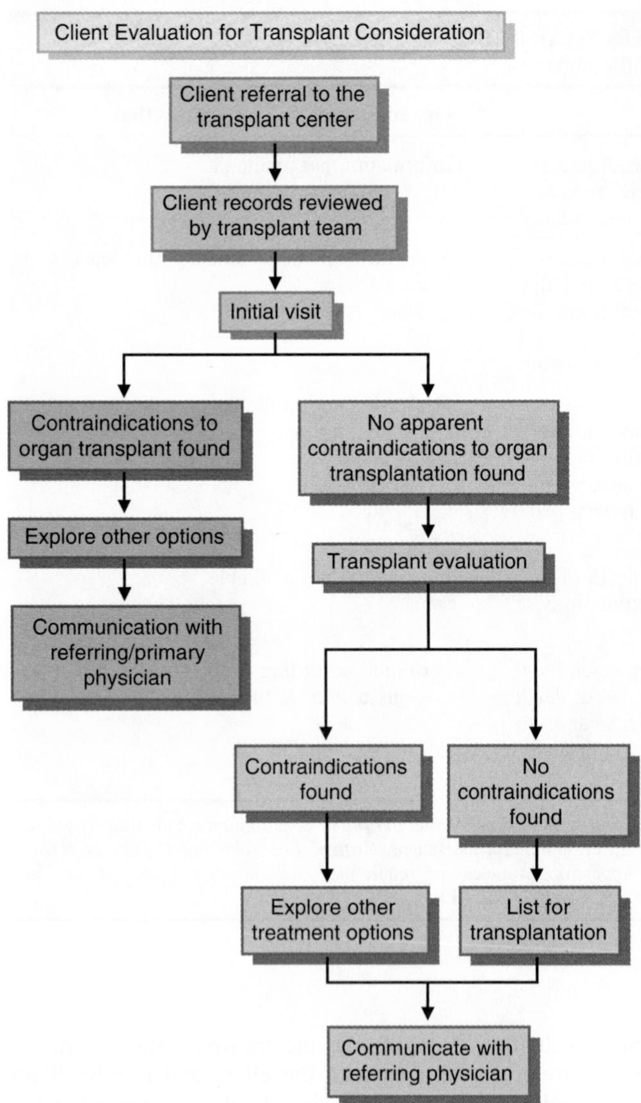

FIGURE 80–2 Client evaluation for transplantation.

may be needed throughout the waiting period. In heart transplantation candidates who become hemodynamically unstable, the use of an intra-aortic balloon pump or a ventricular-assist device may be necessary. Clients waiting for renal transplantation may be receiving dialysis, and those waiting for lung transplantation may require ventilator assistance. In liver transplantation candidates, mechanical assistance devices are not used during the wait for the transplant. Cardiac or pulmonary rehabilitation before transplantation is beneficial to optimize the client's strength and aerobic capacity.

Waiting for transplantation is perhaps the most stressful time for clients and families as they cope with terminal illness, altered lifestyles, financial strain, and impending surgery. Both the client and family members may experience feelings of anxiety, depression, and helplessness.[23, 46] An often forgotten but important component of transplantation nursing is the care of clients with end-stage organ disease who are waiting for transplantation. The transplantation nurse may care for clients while they wait in the hospital for a donor organ, in the clinic setting, or in the home. This wait may be days, months or even years, and it is natural for the nurse to develop strong personal and professional relationships with these clients.

Along with the intense nursing that is involved in keeping the client alive during the waiting period, emotional stress may develop in nurses caring for these clients. It is important for nurses to have periodic meetings to discuss their feelings and difficult cases and to develop plans of care for the clients. More than 80,000 people in the United States die from end-stage renal disease, while 30,000 receive dialysis each year.[2, 4] Approximately 1.1 million Americans were expected to experience a new or recurrent heart failure by year 2000.[1] Cirrhosis is the fourth leading cause of death, accounting for 25,000 deaths yearly.[3, 22] It is important for transplantation nurses to understand that while there may be many happy moments when an organ becomes available for the clients, there will also be tragedies when death occurs before an organ is located. Working with transplantation clients can be both emotionally draining and frustrating during the waiting period for organ availability. Nurses can strive to provide excellent care for the client but have little control over the availability of organs. It is important that emotional support be provided not only for health care staff members and their families but also for transplantation clients and their families. Many centers have established support groups vital to the emotional well-being of the people involved.

During the waiting time, the nurse, as part of the transplantation team, and the client with end-stage organ disease begin to establish a trusting relationship, participate in the client's education, and work together to grasp the realities of life after transplantation. Many clients and their families unrealistically expect that transplantation will cure all life's problems. The problems of end-stage organ disease may be resolved, but new problems associated with transplantation, including medication side effects, rejection, infections, and financial limitations, are frequently encountered. Help the client understand the post-transplantation regimen, and explain what to expect once the client is discharged from the hospital.

ORGAN DONATION AND RECOVERY

The gifts of organ and tissue by donation are a vital part of transplantation. Without the gracious decision of the donor or donor family to give the "gift of life" by donation, there would be no post-transplantation miracles.

If the potential donor is a living relative, careful physical and psychosocial assessment is necessary. Potential donors must be psychologically evaluated as to their real desire to donate an organ, usually a kidney, and the ability to make a lifelong adjustment to having one kidney. To avoid conflict of interest, evaluation of the donor is commonly done by a team different from that caring for the recipient. Discussions with the donor should be held in strict confidence; if the potential donor decides not to donate, the medical team frequently cites a physical contraindication, in order to allow continued acceptance of that person by the other family members.

Several legislative initiatives have advanced issues of donation and transplantation. In 1968, the Uniform Anatomical Gift Act, aimed at increasing volunteer organ donation, became law. Included in this law were the specifications for notifying legal next of kin of donation wishes, uniform donor cards, and designation of donation

TABLE 80–2 EVALUATION FOR ORGAN TRANSPLANTATION

GENERAL

Complete medical history and physical examination
Psychiatric and social evaluation
Laboratory studies
- Electrolyte and metabolic profile
- Liver function tests
- Hematologic profile
- Fasting cholesterol/lipid profile
- Arterial blood gas analysis
- Urinalysis, urine specific gravity determination
- Creatinine clearance determination
- ABO blood typing
- Antibody screen
- Human leukocyte antigen (HLA) tissue typing
- Lymphocyte cytotoxicity screen (assay for preformed reactive antibodies)

Virologic and microbiologic profile testing for the following:
- Cytomegalovirus (CMV)
- Toxoplasmosis
- Human immunodeficiency virus (HIV)
- Hepatitis B surface antigen (HBsAg)
- Hepatitis C antibody
- Epstein-Barr virus (EBV)
- Syphilis: Veneral Disease Research Laboratory (VDRL) assay
- Tuberculosis: Purified protein derivative (PPD) testing with controls

KIDNEY

Laboratory studies
Glomerular filtration rate determination
Radiographic and radionuclide scanning studies
- Renal ultrasound examination
- Kidney-urethra-bladder radiographic series
- Renal radionuclide scanning
- Renal angiography
- Magnetic resonance imaging
- Renal biopsy
- Cystourethrography

HEART

Radiographic and radionuclide scanning studies
- Posteroanterior (PA) and lateral chest radiographs
- Sinus and panoramic films
- Resting radionuclide angiography
- Pulmonary function tests
- Ventilation-perfusion lung scan
- Nuclear magnetic resonance imaging when indicated
- CT studies when indicated
- Resting and exercise gas exchange studies

Cardiac catheterization
Two-dimensional echocardiography
Electrocardiography

LIVER

Laboratory studies: additional blood work for diagnosis of specific liver disease may be indicated
Radiographic and radionuclide scanning studies
- Ultrasound examination of liver and biliary tree
- CT scan of head
- CT scan of abdomen with liver volumes
- Endoscopic retrograde cholangiopancreatography
- Percutaneous transhepatic cholangiogram
- Pulmonary and cardiac evaluation

LUNG

Radiographic and radionuclide scanning studies
- CT scan of chest
- Ventilation-perfusion scan
- Pulmonary function tests
- Cardiac evaluation

CT, computed tomography.

preference on the driver's license. The National Transplant Act of 1984 addressed medical, legal, ethical, and social issues of donation such as requiring national scientific registries for assessment by the federal government and declaring it illegal to buy and sell human organs.[55]

TABLE 80–3 CONSIDERATIONS IN THE PSYCHOSOCIAL EVALUATION FOR TRANSPLANTATION

Demographics	**Health maintenance**
Age	Oxygen requirements
Marital status	Dialysis
Support systems	Compliance with medication regimen
	Compliance with clinical appointments
Financial	**Transportation**
Insurance	Ability to get to clinic or hospital
Savings	Travel time to transplantation center
Social habits	**Home environment**
Smoking	Telephone
Drinking	Running water
Illicit drugs	Trailer/home (e.g., financial? steps? cleanliness?)
Coping skills	Heating and air conditioning

Also, the Organ Procurement and Transplant Network (OPTN) was established to create a national client registry and to coordinate organ allocation and distribution. UNOS is under contract from the U.S. Department of Health and Human Services to operate OPTN.[43]

The Omnibus Budget Reconciliation Act (OBRA) of 1986 requires hospitals to have written policies and procedures for identification and referral of potential donors. Under the 1987 Organ Donation Request Act, consideration of the donor's religious beliefs is mandated, and guidelines are set forth to guide the health care team's approach to next of kin for donor consent, attainment of consent, and notification of the organ procurement organization (OPO).

OBRA also requires transplantation centers and OPOs to be members of OPTN. OPOs are nonprofit organ recovery services in the United States that constitute an integral link in the identification, acceptance, and management of the potential organ donor. In addition to the coordination of organ recovery, transplant procurement coordinators within the OPO provide professional and public education, assist hospitals during donor evaluation, and offer family counseling. Other responsibilities of the procurement coordinators are assisting in donor manage-

PRINT IN BLACK INK CONFIDENTIAL

ORGAN EVALUATION SUMMARY SHEET

Name: (Last, First, Middle) | Sex

Date of Birth (M/D/Y) | Age | Race (UNOS def) | Hospital Number

SS Number | Phone: Home | Phone: Work

Stamp Patient Keyplate Here

Address | Occupation | Number living children: | Admit Date:

❑ Spouse, or… ❑ Companion (check one) Name | Years Married/Together | Discharge Date:

Travel Distance from UAB (miles) | Travel Time by Auto to UAB (miles) | Spouse/Companion Occupation | Number Pregnancies: | UAB MD:

Referring MD:

Referring MD Address:

Med Hx (check all that apply) ❑ Gout: Dt:____ Last:____ ❑ Hypertension: Dt:____ ❑ Pancreatitis: Dt:______ ❑ Hepatitis: Dt:________ ❑ Diverticulitis: DtDx:______ ❑ Prior Transfusions: #____ ❑ CVA: Dt Last:________ ❑ TIA: Dt Last:________ ❑ Carotid Bruit: ❑ L ❑ R ❑ CEA: ❑ L yr__ ❑ R yr__ ❑ Diabetes; Insl: ❑ Y ❑ N ❑ Peripheral Embolus: yr____ ❑ Pul. Emb: mo/yr______ ❑ Nephrolithiasis: Yr.Last____ ❑ Asthma/COPD/Emphysema ❑ Peripheral Vas Disease ❑ Renal Insufficiency ❑ Perm Pacemaker: mo/yr 1st___ mo/yr last___ ❑ Peptic Ulcer: Dt:____ ❑ G.I. Bleed:

Cardiac History:
Primary Cardiac Diagnosis, check one (reason for tx):
❑ Ischemic ❑ Idiopathic ❑ Myocarditis
❑ Congenital (& congen valvular) ❑ Post partum
❑ Acquired valvular (not isch) ❑ Alcoholic
❑ Other: ________________
Comments: ________________
❑ Chronic anticoagulation (Coumadin), yr started:____

❑ Angina History: Class at present____(I–IV)
❑ CHF History. Onset:___/___; Class now:___
❑ Congenital Heart Disease Surgery: #:______
❑ Valvular Heart Disease Surgery: #:______
TypeSurg: ________________ yr:____
TypeSurg: ________________ yr:____
TypeSurg: ________________ yr:____
TypeSurg: ________________ yr:____

❑ CABG: #:______ year(s):________
❑ V. Tach:(❑ Stable ❑ Arrest) ❑ V. Fib
❑ EP Study: ❑ + inducible: (❑ VT ❑ VF) Dt:____
❑ A Fib/A Flutr: (❑ Parox. ❑ Chronic) Dt:______
❑ Cardiac Arrest? Date(s):________
❑ **ICD** Placed: Date:___/____ Location:______
*Manufacturer:________ Model:______
❑ LV thrombus (documented)

Other Medical Problems (specify):

Non-cardiac Surgical History (specify, with dates):

Allergies/Intolerences (specify, with sign/symptom):

Habits | Tobacco: | Alcohol: | Drug:

Social: | Insurance: | Covers Transplant? | Psychiatric:

Neuropsychology: Grade 1–5, 1=poor, 5=excellent | Neurophology: | Psychiatric: | Compliance: | Support: | Knowledge: | Planning: | Coping:

Comments:

Dental Evaluation:

Significant Physical Exam | Height: | Weight: | HEENT:

Lungs: | Cardiovascular:

Abdomen: | Extremities:

Neuro: | Rectal: | **Hemacult x 3:**

D/C Meds: | RN:

Laboratory Tests

Chemistry Date:	Na	K	Cl	Mag	HCO3	Glucose	BUN	Creat	Uric Acid	Calcium	Phospho	T Bili	Ind Bili	Dir Bili
	Alk Phos	LDH	GOT	GGT	CPK		T Choles	Triglycer	HDL	CAD Risk	Alk Phos	Creatinine Clearance: = ______ *ml/mr* ___*mg*(T.Vol)/14.4/___*mg/dl*(SerCreat)		
Hematology Date:	Hct	Hg	WBC	Segs	Bands	Eosino	Lymphs	Other	PT	INR	PTT	Platelets	TProt	Albu

Allotype Data Date:	PRA, flow	PRA, Specificity:	AB Screen	HLA	A	A	B	B	Bw	Bw	Cw	Cw
	ABO Blood Type & Rh	Coomb's Test			DR	DR	DR	DR	DQ	DQ	DPw	DPw

Infectious Dis. Screening Date:	General	HIV:	IFA Toxo:	RPR:	Hepatitis	HBs Ag	HBs Ab	HB core Ab	TB	24 hr	48 hr	72 hr
		CMV:	Herpes:	EBV:		HepA IgM	HepA IGG	Hep C Ab	PPD			
									Controls			

CHF Eval Date:	Free T4	T4	T3RIA	TSH	Sed Rate	RA Latex	Ferritin	Serum Iron	TIBC

Other Tests | UA: Date: | If Female: HCG | If Male: Prostate Spec. Ag

Electrocardiogram Date: | If Female: Mammograms: Date:

Chest X-Ray Date: | Sinus X-Rays Date:

24 Hour Holter: Date: | Abdominal Ultrasound:: Date:

Echocardiogram: Description: ________________ Echo: LV EF: ______%
Date: (__________): LVd_____mm MR:_____ TR:_____ AI:_____ PI:_____ Est. PA systolic pressure:________mmHg RV EF: ______%

VQ Lung Scan Date: | Radionuclide Ventriculogram (MUGA) Date: | MUGA LV EF = %

Pulmonary Function Testing Date: Interpretation: | FVC (value/%) | FEV1 (value/%) | FEF 25%–75% (value/%) | MaxVC (value/%) | DLCO (value/%)

ABGs on | Ph | PO2 | PCO2 | Saturation | COHb

Rest/Exercise Gas Exchange Data Date: | Total Exercise Time | Anaerobic Threshold | VO2 Max (peak)

Cardiac Cath Data

Coronary Angiograms
Date:
Location:

Date	H.R.	AoSyst	AoDiast	RAm	PAs	PAd	PAm	PCWP	C.O.	C.I.	PVR	SVR	IV Meds & dose/NTG During Cath

Other Tests:

Final Disposition: ❑ Listed for Tx: date__________ Status @ listing:______ ❑ Not listed due to:

❑ If checked, explanted heart should be sent to pathology as diagnosis not confirmed prior to transplant

FIGURE 80–3 Transplantation evaluation summary sheet. (Courtesy of University of Alabama–Birmingham Heart and Lung Program.)

BOX 80–1 General Contraindications to Organ Transplantation

- Presence of active systemic infection (bacteremia, fungemia, viremia)
- Malignant disease (except skin cancer and some primary tumors of the diseased organ)
- Active peptic ulcer disease
- Active abuse of alcohol or other substances
- Severe damage to organ system(s) other than that to be transplanted (such as severe cardiovascular dysfunction in the potential liver transplant recipient)
- Severe psychiatric disease
- Demonstration of past or current inability to comply with a prescribed medical regimen
- Lack of a functional social support system
- Lack of sufficient financial resources to pay for surgery, hospitalization, medication, and follow-up care

ment, arranging transportation to and from the donor hospital, and assisting surgical personnel in the operating room. The procurement coordinator provides information to the clinical transplantation coordinator and the transplantation surgeon throughout the recovery process.

OPOs are either hospital-based or independent. They must meet criteria mandated by the Health Care Finance Administration (HCFA), which includes (1) arranging for appropriate tissue typing, (2) demonstrating a working relationship with 75% of hospitals within the OPO area, (3) discussing accounting procedures, (4) providing a method of transport of donated organs, (5) submitting center-specific data, (6) cooperating with local tissue banks, and (7) having a governing board of directors.

ROLE OF THE NURSE IN ORGAN DONATION

The nurse plays an important role in organ donation and recovery with early identification of potential donors, referral to the OPO, and assisting in the medical management of the organ donor.[16] The nurse may act as a liaison with donor families or may be involved in the clinical management of the donor. This nursing role can be a very emotional experience. A nurse involved in this process must acknowledge the personal loss incurred when faced with the brain death of a donor client. The nurse then begins to focus on managing that client's vital systems until donation is completed.

The nurse's identification of a potential organ donor is a vital link to transplantation. To be a donor, a person must meet certain criteria, including sustaining an injury resulting in brain death. According to the Uniform Determination of Death Act, "An individual is dead if he has sustained either irreversible cessation of circulatory and respiratory functions or irreversible cessation of all functions of the brain, including the brain stem, as determined in accordance with accepted medical standards."[55]

The nurse may be the first to recognize the manifestations of brain death, including lack of responsiveness; absence of cough, gag, or corneal reflexes; and lack of response to painful stimuli. These findings should be reported to the physician. Refer all clients who meet brain death criteria to the local OPO. It is most often a nurse who notifies the OPO of the potential donor. Notification should occur when brain death is imminent, to allow the procurement coordinator to become familiar with the potential donor's case. Figure 80–4 depicts the organ donor referral and triage procedure.

The first step in the donation process is awareness of potential organ donors. Organ donors are people who have suffered an injury leading to brain death. The most common causes of injury are head trauma, cerebrovascular accidents (CVAs), subarachnoid hemorrhage, and primary brain tumors. Once a potential donor is identified, the organ procurement agency should be notified. The next steps are documentation of brain death and family consent of donation.

Next, medical management of the potential donor begins. The goal of donor management is to maintain optimal conditions ensuring functional and infection-free organs for transplantation. This goal is accomplished by the diligent management of hydration and tissue perfusion, oxygenation, infection control, diuresis, and temperature regulation. Common problems encountered in management of the potential donor are hypotension, shock, electrolyte imbalances, disseminated intravascular coagulation (DIC), and loss of thermoregulation. The ideal organ donor is a person who unfortunately has suffered a fatal injury resulting in brain death who was otherwise healthy

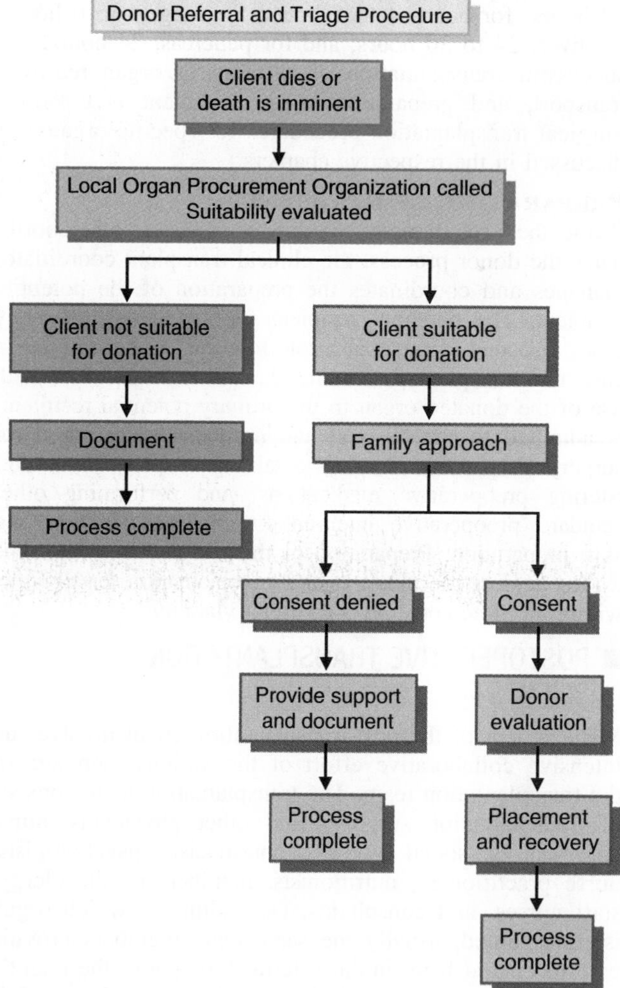

FIGURE 80–4 Organ recovery process.

and infection-free. Criteria for organ donation are listed in Table 80–4.

Initiation of the organ donor process should proceed according to hospital policy. Organ recovery occurs in the operating room only after (1) identifying a potential donor, (2) notifying an OPO, (3) diagnosing brain death, (4) obtaining family consent, and (5) managing the donor until organ removal is complete.

ORGAN RECOVERY

Multiple organ procurement, or recovery of more than one type of organ from a single donor, is standard practice. As many as four separate surgical teams may be present in the operating room, each focusing on recovery of one organ. Usually, a separate surgical team prepares the recipient for the new organ. After a midline incision is made, dissection of organs occurs. Once cross-clamping of the aorta is done and cardioplegia is begun, the heart is removed. Then lungs, liver, and finally kidneys are procured.

The organs are preserved in a cold storage solution selected by the transplantation center. Examples of such solutions are University of Wisconsin solution (UW solution), Euro-Collins solution, Belzer's solution, and other, institution-specific solutions. Organs are preserved in a sterile storage solution, packed in ice, and transported to the recipient in a cooler.

Viability times for donated organs vary. Standard periods after organ recovery are as follows: for kidney, 48 to 72 hours; for heart, 4 to 5 hours; for lung, 4 to 6 hours; for liver, 24 to 30 hours; and for pancreas, 24 hours. For successful transplantation, the timing of organ removal, transport, and preparation of the recipient is essential. Surgical transplantation procedures for specific organs are discussed in the respective chapters.

PREPARATION OF RECIPIENT

While the procurement coordinator manages and coordinates the donor process, the clinical transplant coordinator manages and coordinates the preparation of the potential recipient. The potential recipient (or recipients—in many cases a second client is also told to come to the hospital in case the transplantation team encounters a problem with use of the donated organ in the primary potential recipient) is admitted to the hospital and immediately prepared for surgery. Preparation involves obtaining blood work, administering preoperative medications, and performing other standard preoperative interventions such as shaving and skin preparation. Preparation of the recipient may become a race against the clock as the transplantation team works within the time constraints of organ viability.

POSTOPERATIVE TRANSPLANTATION CLIENTS

Management of the post-transplantation client involves an intensive collaborative effort of the various members of the transplantation team. The transplantation team consists of transplantation surgeons and other physicians, nurse coordinators, social workers, pharmacists, psychologists, nurse practitioners, nutritionists, members of the clergy, staff nurses, and consultants. Depending on which organ is transplanted, usually the same team members provide care to clients from initial referral throughout the client's lifetime. In many cases, kidney or liver transplant recipients return to their referring physicians for long-term

TABLE 80–4 CONDITIONS OF PARTICIPATION FOR ORGAN DONATION

CONDITIONS OF PARTICIPATION

The Department of Health and Human Services (HHS), in an attempt to optimize donor potential and abate the critical shortage of organs for transplantation, issued the Hospital Conditions of Participation (COP) for Medicare and Medicaid on June 22, 1998. This rule took effect on August 21, 1998, and requires all U.S. hospitals to adopt a "routine notification" policy or mandates that hospitals have and implement written protocols to ensure that the organ procurement organization (OPO) is notified of all deaths. According to the COP, the hospital must, "in a timely fashion," notify the OPO of individuals who die or whose death is imminent," thus eliminating the need for hospital staff to identify a potential donor.* All patients who die should be considered a potential organ and/or tissue donor.

Routine notification ensures that an individual who is most familiar with the current criteria on donation, specifically the OPO, evaluates every individual who dies to determine suitability for donation. If the policy were consistently followed, routine notification would make it virtually impossible for the hospital not to refer all potential organ donors. Thus, routine notification places the decision-making and determination of medical suitability for a person to be a donor in the hands of the procurement and transplant community, not in the hands of hospital staff.

This rule is designed not to exclude hospital professionals from the process but, rather, to ensure that the procurement professionals are included.

Five stipulations are contained in the COP:

- A hospital must have an agreement with an OPO and must contact the OPO in a timely manner about all individuals who die or whose death is imminent. The OPO will then determine medical suitability for donation.
- Every hospital must have an agreement with a designated eye and tissue bank to cooperate in the recovery of eyes and tissues.
- Every hospital must ensure that the family of every potential donor is offered the option to donate organs and/or tissues or not to donate.
- Every hospital must work in collaboration with the OPO and tissue or eye bank in educating their staff, participating in death records to identify potential donors and maintain potential donors during the donor management period while necessary testing and the placement of organs and tissues take place.
- Every hospital must provide organ-transplant–related data, as requested by the national Organ Procurement and Transplantation Network and the U.S. Scientific Registry of Transplant Recipients and the OPOs.†

* Final Rule: *Federal Register,* Vol. 63, No. 119, June 22, 1998. 42 CFR Part 482.4.5. Department of Health and Human Services: Health Care Financing Administration. Medicare and Medicaid Programs; Hospital Conditions of Participation; Identification of Potential Organ, Tissue and Eye Donors and Transplant Hospitals, Provision of Transplant Related Data.

† From Chabalewski, F. L. et al. *Donation and transplantation: Into the new millennium.* Available: *www.medscape.com,* October 5, 2000.

Source: United Network for Organ Sharing.

care. Nursing care should be designed to recognize life-threatening clinical problems, to prevent complications, and to promote the client's return to normal activities with improved QOL.

Basic Immunology Related to Transplantation

To effectively care for the transplant client, you must understand basic immunology concepts related to transplantation (see Chapters 74 and 76). The immune response elicits mechanisms that direct the body to recognize transplanted organs as foreign (non-self). Although this immune response is normal, it is the goal of immunosuppressive agents to alter this immune response in transplanted clients.

The innate or nonspecific immune responses consist of natural mechanisms for the protection of the client against foreign antigens. These natural defenses are present at birth, lack memory, and do not need prior exposure for antigens to develop. Innate immunity mechanisms include physical barriers, chemical barriers, and leukocyte reactions, all of which play a role in the body's immune response.

Acquired or specific immunity involves mechanisms elicited by the lymphoid system. Lymphoid cells include plasma cells and lymphocytes. Lymphocytes constitute 30% of the white blood cells (WBCs) and are responsible for the recognition of antigens. These lymphocyte defense mechanisms recognize foreign antigens and can elicit rejection of transplanted organs. Two types of lymphocytes can elicit a response: B lymphocytes, which mediate a humoral immune response through the production of antibodies, and T lymphocytes, which are derived from maturing stems cells in the thymus and act to defend the body by interaction with an antigen with a sensitized T lymphocyte.[8, 48] There are regulator (T helper and T suppressor) and effector (cytoxic and memory) T lymphocytes.

In humans, the genetic factor used to determine specific antigen recognition is called the major histocompatibility complex (MHC). The MHC is the human leukocyte antigen (HLA) gene complex, located on chromosome 6. Antigens of the HLA complex are divided into two classes: class I comprises HLA types, A, B, and C; class II consists of HLA types DR, DQ, and DP. Histocompatibility testing is used to minimize specific immune responses to the transplanted organ. The type of histocompatibility testing varies according to the organ transplanted and with time limitations. Before transplantation, the potential recipient undergoes ABO typing, Rh typing, and HLA tissue typing. An assay for preformed reactive antibodies (PRAs) determines the presence of preformed antibodies to HLA antigens. Results range from zero to 100%. If a potential recipient is found to have antibodies against specific HLA antigens, a donor organ with those antigens is not suitable for transplantation.

Several types of cross-matching procedures can be performed to identify the presence of antibodies in the potential recipient to antigens located on the lymphocytes of the potential donor. A positive result on cross-matching means that antibodies are present, and transplantation is usually inadvisable because of the associated higher risk of rejection. A negative result on cross-matching means that no antibodies are present, with a reduced risk of rejection.

Immunosuppression

The goal of immunosuppressive therapy involves the delicate balance of adequately suppressing the immune response to prevent organ rejection without developing complications from the therapy itself. This intricate balance of the immunosuppressive medication regimen is individualized for each client. The transplantation team aims to keep the dose of each drug within the therapeutic range. Management of the immunosuppressive regimen is crucial to long-term outcomes in post-transplantation clients; for example, excessive immunosuppression may lead to increased risk of infection, liver or kidney insufficiency, joint necrosis, cataracts, or malignancies, whereas inadequate immunosuppression may lead to rejection of the transplanted organ. Although in many cases long-term graft acceptance can be maintained with less drug as time goes by, most clients require immunosuppression for life to prevent rejection of the transplanted organ.

Immunosuppressive agents are utilized in the post-transplantation population in three categories of use: induction, maintenance, and anti-rejection. Specific agents and dosages vary according to category of use. Protocols are dependent on the type of organ(s) transplanted, transplantation center–specific practices, and the client's history and current health status. See Table 80–5 for nursing implications for the major immunosuppressive agents.[6, 21, 50, 51, 62] Most transplantation centers use multiple-drug regimens containing agents that act on various functions of the immune system and also minimize side effects. Many new immunosuppressant medications are currently being developed and tested in the United States and Europe.

Complications

Rejection

Transplantation of allografts (organs transplanted between genetically different individuals in the same species) elicits an immune response in which the antigens in tissue of the transplanted organ are recognized as foreign; hence, a series of events occur, resulting in rejection of the organ. Rejection is classified into three types: (1) hyperacute, (2) acute, and (3) chronic (Fig. 80–5).

Hyperacute Rejection. Hyperacute rejection can occur within minutes to hours of implantation of the organ. It is caused by the presence of antibodies. Usually, a destructive humoral or B-cell reaction to antigens on the vascular endothelium results in organ necrosis. Most hyperacute rejection episodes can be prevented by previous PRA assay, histocompatibility testing, and cross-matching. If hyperacute rejection occurs, treatment options are limited. Clients who have received kidney or kidney-pancreas transplants may need to return to dialysis. Clients who have received other organ transplants may receive plasmapheresis, which is a procedure utilized to remove circulating antibodies from the blood. If this measure fails, re-transplantation is indicated.

Acute Rejection. Acute rejection usually occurs in the first 3 months after transplantation; however, it can occur at any time, particularly if the immunosuppression regimen is altered or if an infection develops. Acute rejection can be either a purely cellular immune response mediated by T cells or an antibody-mediated response, or a combination of the two.[31] Diagnosis is based on clinical

TABLE 80–5 NURSING IMPLICATIONS FOR IMMUNOSUPPRESSIVE AGENTS USED IN TRANSPLANTATION

Agent	Action(s)	Indication	Potential Effects	Dosing Considerations
Cyclosporine (Neoral, Sandimmune)	Inhibits production of T lymphocytes Suppresses activity of T lymphocytes Inhibits IL-2 production	Prevention and treatment of organ rejection	Hypertension Renal dysfunction Tremor Hirsutism Gum hyperplasia	Gelatin capsules Oral solution IV solution Brand-name and generic preparation available Monitor trough levels and drug interactions
Tacrolimus (FK506)	Prevents synthesis of IL-2	Prevention and treatment of organ rejection	Tremor Diabetes Renal dysfunction Hypertension Nausea	Capsules Pediatric suspension IV solution Monitor trough levels and drug interactions
Corticosteroids—anti-inflammatory agents				
Methylprednisolone (Solu-Medrol)	Inhibits IL-1 Inhibits production of T lymphocytes	Adjunctive immunosuppressive agent for prevention and treatment of organ rejection	Diabetes Cataracts Obesity Muscle weakness GI bleeding Cushingoid state Osteoporosis	Tablets IV solution Give with anti-ulcer medications for high doses
Immunosuppressive antimetabolites				
Azathioprine (Imuran)	Interferes with DNA and RNA synthesis Inhibits proliferation of T and B lymphocytes	Prevention of organ rejection	Leukopenia Anemia Hepatoxicity Nausea Neoplasia	Tablets IV solution Allopurinol potentiates action
Mycophenolate mofetil (CellCept)	Selectively inhibits de novo purine synthesis of activated T and B lymphocytes	Prevention of organ rejection	Diarrhea Leukopenia Vomiting Sepsis	Capsules Tablets IV solution
Monoclonal Antibodies				
Muromonab-CD3 (Orthoclone OKT3)	Blocks function of CD3 molecule and inhibits T lymphocyte function	Treatment of organ rejection	Flu-like syndrome Anaphylactic response	IV solution; give via filter Chest film, vital signs should be monitored
Daclizumab (Zenapax), basiliximab (Simulect)	IL-2 antagonist that inhibits activation of lymphocytes	Prevention of organ rejection	Fever Fatigue GI distress	IV solution
Polyclonal Antibodies				
Antithymocyte globulin (ATG) Antilymphocyte globulin (ALG)	Depletes number of circulating T lymphocytes	Treatment of organ rejection	Fever Chills Leukopenia Thrombocytopenia Fatigue	IV solution; give via filter

GI, gastrointestinal; IL, interleukin.

manifestations, laboratory data, or results of tests such as organ biopsy. Clinical manifestations of rejection are listed in Box 80–2.

Treatment usually consists of high-dose steroids; if recurrent episodes occur, muromonab-CD3 (Orthoclone OKT3) may be administered.

CHRONIC REJECTION. Chronic rejection evolves gradually, usually after the first 3 months after transplantation. It may be the result of frequent episodes of acute rejection, increased ischemic time, or cytomegalovirus (CMV) infection. Chronic rejection results in progressive loss of graft function. The transplanted organ develops a persistent, perivascular inflammation associated with focal myocyte necrosis. Chronic rejection is treated in similar fashion to test for acute rejection; however, re-transplantation may be required as a result of the progressive deterioration of organ function.

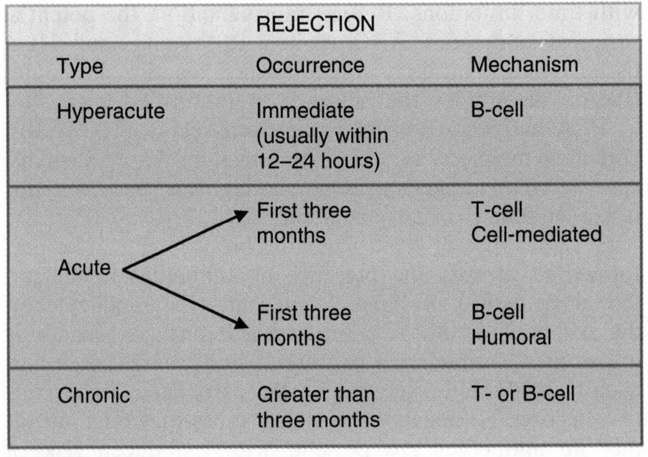

REJECTION
Type
Occurrence
Mechanism
Hyperacute
Immediate (usually within 12–24 hours)
B-cell
Acute
First three months
T-cell Cell-mediated
First three months
B-cell Humoral
Chronic
Greater than three months
T- or B-cell

FIGURE 80–5 Transplant rejection.

BOX 80–2 Clinical Manifestations of Graft Rejection

- Fever
- Graft tenderness
- Fatigue
- Heart: shortness of breath, irregular heart beat
- Lung: shortness of breath
- Abnormal laboratory test results
  - Kidney: ↑ serum creatinine, blood urea nitrogen levels
  - Liver: ↑ total bilirubin, liver enzyme levels
  - Pancreas: ↑ urine amylase

Infection

Infection is the leading cause of morbidity and mortality after transplantation. Many factors contribute to the potential risk of infection, including the client's age, nutritional status, medical condition before transplantation, infection history and exposure, and the immunosuppressive regimen. Infections seen in transplant recipients are usually the result of immunosuppression or altered immune defenses.[15, 47] During the first month after transplantation, nosocomial infections are common; then, between 1 and 6 months, opportunistic infections such as *Pneumocystis carinii* pneumonia, candidiasis, and CMV infection occur.[40, 57] The lungs are the most common site for infection, followed by blood, urine, and the gastrointestinal tract. Common infections seen in transplant recipients are listed in Table 80–6. Infection is the most common indication for hospital readmission after transplantation.[30]

Malignancy

The development of post-transplantation malignancies caused by the immunodeficient state is well documented.[45] Types of malignancies seen in the post-transplantation population include basal cell and squamous cell carcinomas of the skin and lip, seen most commonly, followed by the lymphoproliferative disorders and cancers of the vulva, perineum, and lungs.[45] Reduction in the level of immunosuppression, surgical resection, chemotherapy, and radiation therapy are treatment options.

All clients should be screened for development of cancer after transplantation. Routine gynecologic examinations, including mammography and cervical smear in women; annual prostate-specific antigen (PSA) testing in men; and regular physical examination of neck and groin lymph nodes should be performed to detect any problems. Report any unusual lesions to the transplantation team. In addition, monitor clients who are seronegative for Epstein-Barr virus for conversion to seropositivity, which may place them at higher risk for lymphoproliferative disease after transplantation.[65] Clients need to be educated to use sun screen products with a sun protection factor (SPF) of 15 or greater and to wear protective clothing to help prevent skin malignancies.

■ CLIENTS RECEIVING A SPECIFIC ORGAN TRANSPLANT

RENAL TRANSPLANTATION

The potential renal transplant recipient has end-stage renal disease, most commonly the result of hypertension, diabetic nephropathy, or a hereditary or congenital disorder.[49] In most cases the renal transplant candidate is anemic and fatigued and has been maintained on chronic hemodialysis (see Chapter 36). Contraindications to renal transplantation include seropositivity for the human immunodeficiency virus (HIV), active infection, severe coronary artery disease with left ventricular dysfunction, malignancy, severe peripheral vascular disease, severe carotid artery disease, and chronic active hepatitis.

Unlike the heart, lung, liver, or pancreas transplantation candidate, the kidney transplantation candidate has several potential donors: living related, living non-related, and cadaver. Eighty-five per cent of all renal transplants are from cadaveric donors.

Extensive histocompatibility testing is completed for renal transplantation, because evidence now indicates that six antigen matches are necessary for long-term graft survival. Six-antigen-matching means that six antigens recognized on recipient HLA tissue typing match six antigens found on donor HLA tissue typing. A negative

TABLE 80–6 COMMON INFECTIONS AFTER TRANSPLANTATION

Infecting Organism	Site(s) Affected	Therapeutic Agent of Choice
Bacteria		
Gram-negative bacilli		Ticarcillin-clavulanate (Timentin)
Klebsiella	Lung	
Pseudomonas	Blood	Gentamicin
Escherichia coli	CNS	
Legionella	Lung	
Enterobacter		
Gram-positive cocci		Vancomycin
Enterococci		
Staphylococci		
Streptococci		
Viruses		
Cytomegalovirus	Lung Blood GI tract	Ganciclovir
Varicella-zoster virus	Skin Blood	Acyclovir
Protozoa		
Toxoplasma gondii	Transplanted organ Lung Liver	Pyrimethamine Sulfadiazine Folinic acid
Pneumocystis	Lung	Trimethoprim-sulfamethoxazole
Fungi		
Aspergillus	Lung CNS	Amphotericin B
Candida	Oral mucosa	Nystatin Fluconazole Amphotericin B

CNS, central nervous system; GI, gastrointestinal.

result on cross-matching is required for transplantation to occur.

Nursing Care. Nursing care of the renal transplant recipient is focused on the recognition and prevention of complications. Ongoing assessment of renal function—by determination of blood urea nitrogen (BUN), serum creatinine, glomerular filtration rate (GFR), fluid intake and output, weight, and serum electrolytes—is routine in these clients. If indicated, a renal scan or ultrasound study may be used to detect complications. Renal biopsy may be performed to make a definitive diagnosis, as rejection, acute tubular necrosis (ATN), and obstructive complications have similar manifestations.

Goals are to maintain hydration, promote diuresis, avoid fluid overload, and prevent infection. Complications after renal transplantation include fluid and electrolyte imbalances, ATN, obstructive or vascular complications, rejection, and infection. Clinical manifestations of potential complications in the renal transplantation client are decreased urine output, graft tenderness or pain, rising serum creatinine level, fever, and weight gain.

Pancreas and Pancreas-Kidney Transplantation

Pancreas transplantation is indicated for the client with type 1 diabetes mellitus to restore normal glucose metabolism.[54] Pancreas-kidney transplantation is performed in the diabetic client with end-stage renal disease (see Chapter 45).[20, 59] Contraindications are the same as in renal transplantation.

Nursing Care. Nursing care includes monitoring for fluid and electrolyte imbalances, especially BUN, serum creatinine, bicarbonate, and CO_2. Urine amylase is also monitored to assess pancreatic function. Clinical manifestations of graft thrombosis are a sudden rise in serum glucose, severe graft pain, and increased serum creatinine with combined kidney-pancreas transplantation.

Heart Transplantation

Potential candidates for heart transplantation are usually New York Heart Association class III or IV and younger than 65 years of age and have a life expectancy of less than 12 months. The most common diseases treated by heart transplantation are coronary artery disease and cardiomyopathy.[12] Contraindications to heart transplantation include malignancy; active infection; autoimmune disorders; irreversible kidney, lung, or liver disease; and severely elevated pulmonary vascular resistance. Relative contraindications, which vary between transplantation centers, are peptic ulcer disease, CVA, peripheral vascular disease, diabetes mellitus, and obesity.[42]

When listed for transplantation, candidates are evaluated periodically, usually every 4 to 6 weeks, to monitor their overall condition. Stable clients wait at home or near the hospital, and clients who are hemodynamically unstable wait at the hospital. Clients who become critically ill may need continuous inotropic infusions or ventricular-assist devices.

Cardiac Transplantation Physiology Alterations

Unique to the cardiac transplant recipient is cardiac transplant denervation. Denervation occurs after orthotopic transplantation, in which the vagus nerve is severed. The resultant lack of vagal nerve stimulation results in (1) a higher resting heart rate, (2) a gradual increase in heart rate with exercise and delayed return to baseline, (3) absence of angina, and (4) enhanced response to certain drugs (e.g., adrenaline, adenosine) and decreased response to other drugs (e.g., atropine, digoxin).[7] Finally, two P waves may be detected on the electrocardiogram resulting from the presence of both donor and recipient heart sinoatrial (SA) nodes. It is important to note that only the donor heart SA node regulates the electrical conduction of the heart.

Nursing Care. The nursing assessment is a vital component in the care of the cardiac transplant recipient. The physical assessment should include auscultation of heart and breath sounds and assessment of pedal pulses and of the jugular vein for distention. Ongoing assessment of renal and liver function and monitoring of immunosuppressant drug levels and the complete blood count (CBC) are important in the overall care of the client. Complications seen after heart transplantation include organ dysfunction, rejection, infection, coronary vasculopathy, and malignancy.[10, 13, 38] Chest radiography is used to monitor possible lung infection, whereas echocardiography and endomyocardial biopsy are utilized to detect rejection. Clinical manifestations of rejection include fever, shortness of breath, fatigue, presence of S_3 or S_4 heart sound, decreased blood pressure, decreased ejection fraction, and jugular vein distention.

Liver Transplantation

Indications for liver transplantation include chronic irreversible liver disease due to a number of underlying disorders. In adults, the most common indications are cirrhosis secondary to chronic hepatitis, cryptogenic cirrhosis, primary biliary cirrhosis, and primary sclerosing cholangitis (see Chapter 47).[9, 41] Contraindications to liver transplantation are center-specific and may include portal vein thrombosis, active alcoholism, active infection, malignancy outside the hepatobiliary system, and advanced cardiopulmonary disease. The client evaluation takes into account technical feasibility and optimal timing of surgery in addition to the usual physical and psychosocial indications.

Nursing Care. The postoperative care of the liver transplant client is complex. Nursing care focuses on monitoring graft function, managing fluid and electrolyte imbalances, preventing problems with other organ systems, and assessing for signs of rejection or infection. Clinical manifestations of rejection include fever, elevation of liver enzymes, and change in color, amount, and consistency of bile drainage through the T tube.

Diagnosis of rejection is confirmed by liver biopsy. In addition, a sudden increase in the International Normalized Ratio (INR) (a system for reporting prothrombin values), serum bilirubin, or liver enzymes may indicate a complication such as hepatic artery thrombosis or biliary obstruction. If neurologic status is affected, serum ammonia levels may be monitored. Finally, as in all organ transplantation procedures, renal function, immunosuppressant drug levels, and white blood cell (WBC) count should be closely monitored.

Lung Transplantation

The lung transplantation candidate has end-stage pulmonary disease; is generally younger than 65 years of age for single-lung transplantation, 60 years for two-lung transplantation, or 55 years for heart-lung transplantation; and is able to participate in pulmonary rehabilitation (i.e., is not wheelchair-dependent).[32, 58] The decision on whether to perform a single-lung or double-lung procedure varies among transplantation centers but is based on the likelihood of achieving the best outcome and most improvement in QOL.

Contraindications to lung transplantation are active malignancy, positive results on hepatitis B antigen assay, hepatitis C, autoimmune disorders, and dysfunction of organ(s) other than the lungs. Risk factors that affect eligibility include symptomatic osteoporosis, the need for steroid therapy in doses greater than 20 mg/day, severe musculoskeletal disease, impaired nutritional status (malnutrition or obesity), the need for mechanical ventilation, and colonization with fungi or atypical mycobacteria.[37]

Lung Transplantation Physiology Alterations. Removal of native lung and lung replacement entail denervation of the transplanted lung. Denervation interferes with autonomic nervous system communication, resulting in dysfunctional ciliary movement, loss of cough reflex, and changes in mucus production, which lead to ineffective clearance of airway secretions. Health maintenance interventions to maintain patent airways are chest vibropercussion, postural drainage, and use of an incentive spirometer.

Nursing Care. The postoperative care of the lung transplant recipient is gratifying. It is a pleasure to watch a pre-transplantation oxygen-dependent client gasping for breath become an active person requiring no oxygen after transplantation. Immunosuppressant drug levels, electrolyte determinations, liver function tests, CBC, chest radiography, and pulmonary function tests are important monitoring tests in this population.

Complications include surgical side effects, graft dysfunction, rejection, infection, and bronchiolitis obliterans, or obliterating bronchiolitis (OB). OB is the greatest limiting factor to long-term survival after lung transplantation. OB is progressive in nature, resulting in severe shortness of breath, and must be treated aggressively. Usual medical management may include administration of intravenous steroids, cytolytic therapy (with OKT3), administration of thymoglobulin, photopheresis, and retransplantation. Goals in nursing management are to prevent and recognize complications and to promote return to a functional lifestyle.

Self-Care

Before discharge from the hospital, pertinent information is discussed with the client and family members. Postoperative education after transplantation can be quite challenging, because many clients are discharged between 1 and 2 weeks after surgery. Many institutions provide client education booklets. Information discussed with the client and family is presented in Box 80–3.

Of special importance are knowledge of the clinical manifestations of rejection and infection and indications for contacting the transplantation team. A schedule of return appointments is usually given at discharge. Most clients reside close to the transplantation center for 2 to 8 weeks before going home. This proximity allows for frequent medical visits, ongoing education, and familiariza-

BOX 80–3 Client and Family Education After Transplantation

- Members of transplantation team
- When to call the transplant coordinator
- Immunosuppression
  - Administration of medications
  - Side effects of medications
- Rejection
  - Definition, manifestations, diagnosis, treatment
- Infection
  - Definition, manifestations, diagnosis, treatment
- Routine care
  - Temperature
  - Weight
  - Skin care
  - Incision care
  - Fluid intake and output
  - Pedal pulses
  - Incentive spirometry
  - Clinic schedule
- Diet after transplantation
- Activities after transplantation
  - Precautions
  - Exercise
  - Physical therapy
- Self-care
  - Blood pressure
  - Blood glucose levels
  - Medical identification bracelet and card
  - Sun exposure
  - Sexual activity
  - Sending specimens for laboratory monitoring tests
  - Vacations
  - Over-the-counter medicines to be avoided
  - Driving
  - Birth control
- Psychosocial issues
  - Physical appearance
  - Family participation and support
  - Writing to the donor family
  - Cost of transplantation
- Health maintenance
  - Dental care
  - Ophthalmologic examinations
  - Gynecologic examinations
  - Yearly evaluations of transplant

tion of the client with the postoperative regimen. It also allows the client to become more independent and resume self-care responsibilities. Often it is the nurse who is best able to monitor compliance with the medical regimen and to identify difficulty coping with the post-transplantation regimen. Once the client returns home, it may be necessary for a home health nurse to provide wound care, perform intravenous infusions, or perform other nursing care measures. Findings on home visits are communicated to the transplantation coordinator.[44] Box 80–4 lists nursing diagnoses related to care of the post-transplantation client.

Meticulous follow-up evaluation (assessing for manifestations of rejection, infection, or other complications) is essential to the long-term well-being of the post-transplantation client. Long-term care of the transplant recipient requires communication between the client and transplantation team. Each client should be assessed for infection, rejection, malignancy, organ dysfunction, and adverse signs of immunosuppression such as diabetes, hypertension, abnormalities on liver function testing, and gastrointestinal distress.

Psychosocial issues that should be investigated are financial status, family dynamics, and return to work. The social worker at the transplantation center can assist the client with insurance questions, medication assistance programs, and ways of dealing with the financial stresses of transplantation.

Health maintenance areas to evaluate are screening by mammography and Papanicolaou (Pap) smears in women, colon cancer screening, and immunizations such as with the influenza vaccine and pneumococcal vaccine (Pneumovax). Routine dental and ophthalmologic examinations should be scheduled. Communication with the referring physician or the primary health care provider is also important. Constant relaying of information including laboratory findings, clinic visit results, and follow-up plans should occur between the transplantation center and the client's primary health care provider.

QUALITY OF LIFE AFTER TRANSPLANTATION

Examining quality of life (QOL) before and after transplantation is becoming a common practice in all areas of organ transplantation. Not only the traditional factors of survival and morbidity but also how the client functions, copes, and lives after the transplantation operation are now perceived as important. The diabetic client who is no longer insulin-dependent or the client who had end-stage renal disease who no longer requires dialysis has experienced a major change in lifestyle. Although there are challenges related to immunosuppressive therapy, most clients who undergo successful transplantation report improved QOL. Research studies may evaluate QOL at a specific period either before or after transplantation.[17, 23] Differences in the effects of drug treatment, device intervention, or medical therapy on QOL may be examined also.[29]

Hathaway reported improved QOL in renal transplant recipients regardless of race or gender of the client.[27] Hathaway also completed a longitudinal study of 91 kidney transplant recipients who underwent QOL testing before transplantation and at 6 and 12 months after transplantation. The Sickness Impact Profile, the Adult Self-Image Scale, and the Personal Resource Questionnaire were used for this study. Variables that predicted post-transplantation QOL were employment status, the number of transplantation-related hospitalizations, and available social support.[28] White-Williams and colleagues found that males reported better QOL than that described by females both before heart transplantation and at 6 months after transplantation.[63]

Grady and colleagues reported on compliance at 1 year and at 2 years after heart transplantation in 120 recipients. Compliance was measured with the Heart Transplant Compliance Instrument developed for this study. The heart transplant recipients had no difficulty following medication regimens but did have difficulty with diet, exercise, and taking their vital signs.[24]

De Geest and associates also examined compliance with taking medications in heart transplant recipients. They found that compliance with immunosuppressive medication was high; however, clients who were considered "moderate noncompliers" had a higher incidence of late acute rejection episodes. The findings in this study suggest that client compliance plays a pivotal role in long-term outcome after transplantation.[14]

Limbos and colleagues studied QOL in women before and after lung transplantation. Overall QOL improved after transplantation; however, the women reported impairments with sexuality and body satisfaction.[34] Manzetti reported that a health maintenance program of education and exercise improved QOL in clients awaiting lung transplantation.[36] Similarly, LoBiondo-Wood and colleagues reported improved QOL over time in 41-post–liver transplantation clients.[35] Long-term studies of QOL should enable nurses to understand and appreciate the impact of chronic illnesses and transplantation on clients and families.

BOX 80–4 Nursing Diagnoses for the Post-Transplantation Client

- *Altered Nutrition: Risk for More Than Body Requirements* related to side effects of immunosuppressant agents/*Risk for Less Than Body Requirements* related to increased caloric needs after transplantation
- *Altered Protection and Risk for Infection* related to immunosuppression required after organ transplantation
- *Effective Management of Therapeutic Regimen* related to post-transplantation regimen
- *Pain* related to transplantation surgery
- *Risk for Ineffective Individual Coping* after transplantation related to increased stress, anxiety, fear, and lifestyle changes
- *Risk for Injury:* rejection of transplanted organ related to impaired immunocompetence; malignancy/diabetes/hypertension related to immunosuppression

CONCLUSIONS

Nursing care of the transplantation client is both challenging and extremely rewarding. With thorough understanding of the end-stage disease process and its manifestations, the organ donation and recovery process, and postoperative management, the nurse has the unique ability to work as a member of the interdisciplinary team caring for this group of clients. The nurse may serve as primary care provider, client advocate, and liaison with other team members. To maximize QOL, caring for the client and family must focus on both the physical and psychosocial aspects of transplantation, including not only medical treatments but also nursing interventions that address the client's specific QOL issues. If psychosocial issues are not fully explored, the client is likely to experience poorer satisfaction with the post-transplantation outcome. Meticulous medical care, long-term follow-up, and addressing physical and psychosocial QOL issues all are important components of management to improve both survival and QOL in the population of clients who have undergone organ transplantation.

THINKING CRITICALLY

1. A client has been receiving dialysis for several years awaiting kidney transplantation. She is notified that a kidney donor has been found and that she should proceed to the hospital. What teaching will be completed before she goes to surgery? What psychosocial care should be offered?

Factors to Consider. What teaching and support will the family require? What are the ramifications if the donor kidney is found to be an unsuitable match for the client?

2. A client has recently undergone heart transplantation and is to be discharged from the hospital in 2 days. What client education should be completed? What education should be completed for the family?

Factors to Consider. What living arrangements are required for the client after discharge? What are the long-term concerns related to financial factors, QOL issues, and long-term immunosuppressive therapy?

3. At a pre-transplantation support group, a client makes the following statement: "I think I may need to buy my new organ." How should the nurse react to this statement? What ethical issues are raised by this statement?

Factors to Consider. What other ethical considerations regarding organ donation should the transplantation nurse be aware of?

BIBLIOGRPHY

1. American Heart Association. Available: *http://www. americanheart.org.*
2. American Kidney Foundation. Available: *http://www.kidney.org.*
3. American Liver Foundation. Available: *http://www.liverfoundation.org.*
4. Baily, M. A. (1988). Economic issues in organ substitution technology. In D. Mathieu (Ed.), *Organ substitution technology: Ethical, legal and public policy issues.* Boulder, CO: Westview.
5. Barnard, C. N. (1967). A human cardiac transplant. *South African Medical Journal, 41,* 1271–1274.
6. Beniaminovitz, S., et al. (1999). Use of daclizumab decreases the frequency of early allograft rejection: De novo heart transplant recipients. *Journal of Heart and Lung Transplantation, 18,* 47.
7. Britow, M. R. (1990). The surgically denervated transplanted human heart. *Circulation, 82,* 658–660.
8. Campbell, P., & Halloran, P. F. (1996). Antibody-mediated rejection. In K. Solz, L. Racusen, & M. Billingham (Eds.), *Solid organ transplant rejection.* New York: Marcel Dekker.
9. Coleman, J., Mendoza, M., & Bindon-Peiler, P. (1991). Liver disease that leads to transplantation. *Critical Care Nurse, 13,* 41–50.
10. Constanzo-Nordin, M., et al. (1992). Cardiac allograft vasculopathy: Relationship with acute cellular rejection and histocompatibility. *Journal of Heart and Lung Transplantation 11,* S90.
11. Cooper, J. D. (1995). Historical perspective lung transplantation. In G. Patterson & L. Couraud (Eds.), *Lung transplantation.* New York: Elsevier.
12. Costanzo, M., et al. (1995). Selection and treatment of candidates for heart transplantation. *Circulation, 92,* 3593–3612.
13. Costanzo, M., et. al., & The Cardiac Transplant Research Database Group. (1996). Heart transplant coronary artery disease detected by angiography: A multi-institutional study. *Journal of Heart and Lung Transplantation, 15,* S39.
14. De Geest, S., et al. (1998). Late acute rejection and subclinical noncompliance with cyclosporine therapy in heart transplant recipients. *Journal of Heart and Lung Transplantation, 17,* 854–863.
15. Dummer, J. (1990). Infection complications of transplantation. In M. Thompson & A. Brest (Eds.), *Cardiac transplantation* (pp. 163–178). Philadelphia: F. A. Davis.
16. Ehrle, R., Shafer, T., & Nelson, K. (1999). Referral, request, and consent for organ donation: Best practice—a blueprint for success. *Critical Care Nurse, 19*(2), 21–33.
17. Evans R. W., et al. (1985). The quality of life of clients with end stage renal disease. *New England Journal of Medicine, 312,* 553–559.
18. Fishman, J., & Rubin, R. (1998). Medical progress: Infection in organ transplant recipients. *New England Journal of Medicine, 338,* 1741–1751.
19. Flye, M. (Ed.). (1989). History of transplantation. In *Principles of organ transplantation.* Philadelphia: W. B. Saunders.
20. Freise, C, et al. (1999). Simultaneous pancreas-kidney transplantation: An overview of indications, complications and outcomes. *Western Journal of Medicine, 170,* 11–18.
21. Gaber, A., et al. (1998). Results of the double-blind randomized, multicenter phase II clinical trial of Thymoglobulin versus Atgam in the treatment of acute graft rejection episodes after renal transplantation. *Transplantation, 66,* 29–37.
22. Galamobos, J. (1979). *Cirrhosis.* (*Major problems in internal medicine* series [Vol. 17]). Philadelphia: W. B. Saunders.
23. Grady, K., Jalowiec, A., & White-Williams, C. (1995). Predictors of quality of life in patients with advanced heart failure awaiting transplantation. *Journal of Heart and Lung Transplantation, 14,* 2–10.
24. Grady, K., et al. (1998). Patient compliance at one year and two years after heart transplantation. *Journal of Heart and Lung Transplantation, 17,* 383–394.
25. Guthrie, C. (Ed.). (1912). Applications of blood vessel surgery. In *Blood vessel surgery.* New York: Longmans, Green.
26. Hansen, T., Carreno, B., & Sachs, D. (1993). The major histocompatibility complex. In W. Paul (Ed.), *Fundamental immunology* (3rd ed., pp. 577–628). New York: Raven Press.
27. Hathaway, D., et al. (1996). Racial and gender differences in quality of life prior to and following kidney transplantation. *Proceedings of the Tenth Annual Southern Nursing Research Society Conference.*
28. Hathaway, D., et al. (1998). Post kidney transplantation quality of life prediction models. *Clinical Transplantation, 12,* 168–174.
29. Hilbrands, L., Hoitsma, A., & Koene, R. (1995). The effect of immunosuppressive drugs on quality of life after renal transplantation. *Transplantation, 59,* 1263–1270.
30. Hosendpud, J., et al.(1998). *The Registry of the International Society for Heart and Lung Transplantation: 15th Official Report—1998, 17,* 656–668.
31. Hruban, R. H., Baldwin, W. M., & Sanfilippo, F. (1996). Immunopathology of rejection. In K. Solz, L. Racusen, & M. Billingham (Eds.), *Solid organ transplantation rejection.* New York: Marcel Dekker.
32. Kaiser, L., & Cooper, J. D. (1992). The current status of lung transplantation. *Advances in Surgery, 25,* 259–307.
33. Landsteiner, K. (1928). Cell antigens and individual specificity. *Journal of Immunology, 15,* 589–600.

34. Limbos, M., Chan, C., & Kesten, S. (1997). Quality of life in female lung transplant candidates and recipients. *Chest, 112,* 1165–1174.
35. LoBiondo-Wood, G., et al. (1997). Impact of liver transplantation on quality of life: A longitudinal perspective. *Applied Nursing Research, 10*(1), 27–32.
36. Manzetti, J., et al. (1994). Exercise, education and quality of life in lung transplant candidates. *Journal of Heart and Lung Transplantation, 13,* 297–305.
37. Maurer, J., et al. (1998). International guidelines for the selection of lung transplant candidates. *Journal of Heart and Lung Transplantation, 17,* 703–709.
38. McGiffin, D., et al. (1995). Cardiac transplant coronary artery disease: A multivariable analysis of disease development and morbid events. *Journal of Thoracic and Cardiovascular Surgery, 108*(6), 1081–1089.
39. Medawar, P. B. (1945). A second study of the behavior and fate of skin homografts in rabbits: A report to the War Wounds Committee of the Medical Research Council. *Journal of Anatomy, 69,* 157–176.
40. Miller, L., et al. (1994). Infection after heart transplantation: A multiinstitutional study. *Journal of Heart and Lung Transplantation, 13,* 353.
41. National Digestive Disease Advisory Board. (1990). Conference on Liver Transplantation, Arlington, VA.
42. O'Connell, J., et al. (1992). Cardiac transplantation: Recipient selection, donor procurement, and medical follow-up: A statement for health professionals from the Committee on Cardiac Transplantation of the Council on Clinical Cardiology, American Heart Association. *Circulation, 86,* 1061–1079.
43. Office of Organ Transplantation. (1987). *The status of organ donation and coordination serves: Report to Congress for fiscal year 1987.* Washington, DC: U.S. Department of Health and Human Services.
44. Olesen, M., Leum, E., & Randolph, S. (1999). *Heart failure, transplantation and the role of the home care.* Resources.
45. Penn, I. (1991). Cancer in the immunosuppressed organ recipient. *Transplantation Proceedings, 23,* 1771–1772.
46. Reither, A. M. (1990). Psychiatric aspects of transplantation. In S. L. Smith (Ed.), *Tissue and organ transplantation: Implications for professional nursing practice.* St. Louis: Mosby-Year Book.
47. Rubin, R. (1988). Infection in the renal and liver transplant client. In R. Rubin & L. Young (Ed.), *Clinical approach to infection in the compromised host* (2nd ed., pp. 557–621). New York: Plenum Press.
48. Sabatine, M., & Auchincluss, H. (1996). Cell-mediated rejection. In K. Solz, L. Racusen, & M. Billingham (Eds.), *Solid organ transplant rejection.* New York: Marcel Dekker.
49. Shapiro, R., & Simmons, R. L. (1992). Renal transplantation. In T. Starzl, et al. (Eds.), *Atlas of organ transplantation.* New York: Gower.
50. Shumway, S. J., & Frist, W. H. (1995). Immunosuppressants. In S. J. Shumway & N. E. Shumway (Eds.), *Thoracic transplantation.* Cambridge: Blackwell Science.
51. Simulect. Novartis Product Insert. East Hanover, NJ.
52. Spector, N., Connolly, M., & Garrity, E. (1996). Lung transplant rejection: Obliterative bronchiolitis. *American Journal of Critical Care, 5,* 366–372.
53. Starzl, T. E., et al. (1963). Homotransplantation of the liver in humans. *Surgery, Gynecology and Obstetrics, 117,* 659–676.
54. Sutherland, D. E. R., Gruessner, R. W. G., & Gores, P. F. (1994). Pancreas and islet transplantation: An update. *Transplantation Reviews, 8*(4), 185–206.
55. Task Force on Organ Transplantation. (1986). *Organ transplantation: Issues and recommendations.* (HRP-0906976.) Rockville, MD: Health Resources and Services Administration.
56. Terasaki, P. I., Marchioro, P. L., & Starzl, T. E. (1965). *Histocompatibility testing.* Washington, DC: National Academy of Sciences.
57. Tolkoff-Rubin, N. E., & Rubin, R. H. (1992). Infection in organ transplant recipients. In S. Gorback, J. Bartlett, & N. Blacklon (Eds.), *Infectious diseases.* Philadelphia: W. B. Saunders.
58. Trulock, E. (1993). Recipient selection. *Chest Surgery Clinics of North America, 3*(1), 1–18.
59. Trusler, L. A. (1991). Simultaneous kidney-pancreas transplantation. *ANNA Journal, 18*(5), 487–491.
60. United Network of Organ Sharing (UNOS). (1997). *Annual report of the U.S. Scientific Registry for Transplant Recipients and Organ Procurement and Transplantation Network—Transplant data.* Richmond, VA: Author.
61. United Network of Organ Sharing (UNOS) OPTN and Scientific Registry Data, April 19, 1999.
62. White-Williams, C. (1993). Immunosuppressive therapy after cardiac transplantation. *Critical Care Nurse Quarterly, 16*(2), 1–10.
63. White-Williams, C., Jalowic, A., & Grady, K. (1997). Gender differences in quality of life outcomes before and 6 months after heart transplantation. *Journal of Heart and Lung Transplantation, 16,* 100.
64. Williams, T. (1995). Rejection in lung transplantation. In G. Paterson (Ed.), *Lung transplantation.* New York: Elsevier.
65. Zangwill, S., et al. (1998). Incidence and outcome of primary Epstein-Barr virus infection and lymphoproliferative disease in pediatric heart transplant recipients. *Journal of Heart and Lung Transplantation, 17,* 116–120.

REMEMBER *to check out your* **Companion CD ROM**

CHAPTER 81

Management of Clients with Shock and Multisystem Disorders

Louise Nelson LaFramboise

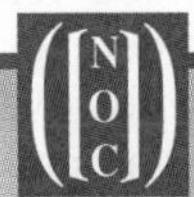

NURSING OUTCOMES CLASSIFICATION (NOC) for Nursing Diagnoses—Clients in Shock

Altered Tissue Perfusion: Cerebral, Cardiopulmonary, Renal, Gastrointestinal, Peripheral
Bowel Elimination
Cognitive Ability
Electrolyte and Acid-Base Balance
Fluid Balance
Hydration
Neurologic Status
Neurologic Status: Consciousness
Neurologic Status: Central Motor Control
Pain Level
Sensory Function: Cutaneous
Swallowing Status
Tissue Perfusion: Cerebral
Tissue Perfusion: Pulmonary
Tissue Perfusion: Cardiac
Tissue Perfusion: Abdominal Organ
Tissue Perfusion: Peripheral
Tissue Integrity: Skin and Mucous Membrane
Urinary Elimination
Vital Signs Status

SHOCK

Shock is a complex clinical syndrome that may occur at any time and in any place. It is a life-threatening condition often requiring team action by many health care providers, including nurses, physicians, laboratory technicians, pharmacists, and respiratory therapists. Shock causes thousands of deaths and unknown numbers of permanent injuries each year. The economic impact of shock is staggering, with health care costs for treatment of shock in the billions of dollars each year. Because shock is potentially lethal, debilitating, and costly, it is essential that nurses identify clients at risk for shock, recognize the early assessment findings indicating shock, and initiate appropriate interventions before shock ensues.

Shock is defined as failure of the circulatory system to maintain adequate perfusion of vital organs. Disorders leading to inadequate tissue perfusion result in decreased oxygenation at the cellular level. Inadequate oxygenation results in anaerobic cellular metabolism and accumulated waste products in cells. If this condition is untreated, cell and organ death occur.

Shock is commonly divided into three major classifications:

- Hypovolemic
- Cardiogenic
- Distributive

Hypovolemic shock is due to inadequate circulating blood volume resulting from hemorrhage with actual blood loss, burns with a loss of plasma proteins and fluid shifts, or dehydration with a loss of fluid volume. It is the most common type of shock and develops when the intravascular volume decreases to the point where compensatory mechanisms are unable to maintain organ and tissue perfusion.

Cardiogenic shock is due to inadequate pumping action of the heart because of primary cardiac muscle dysfunction or mechanical obstruction of blood flow caused by myocardial infarction (MI), valvular insufficiency caused by disease or trauma, cardiac dysrhythmias, or an obstructive condition, such as pericardial tamponade or pulmonary embolus. Cardiogenic shock occurs in 10% to 15% of all clients following MI and carries an associated mortality rate of up to 80%. Cardiogenic shock after an MI usually occurs when 40% or more of the myocardium has been damaged.

Sometimes the term *obstructive shock* is used to include conditions that lead to a sudden obstruction of blood flow (i.e., cardiac tamponade, tension pneumothorax, pulmonary embolism). Obstructive causes are discussed within the topic of cardiogenic shock because the ability of the heart to pump effectively is the primary problem.

Distributive shock (also called *vasogenic shock*) is due

to changes in blood vessel tone that increase the size of the vascular space without an increase in the circulating blood volume. The result is a relative hypovolemia (total fluid volume remains the same but is redistributed). Distributive shock is further divided into three types:

- *Anaphylactic shock,* a severe hypersensitivity reaction resulting in massive systemic vasodilation
- *Neurogenic shock,* or interference with nervous system control of the blood vessels, such as with spinal cord injury (especially cervical spine injury), spinal anesthesia, or severe vasovagal reactions caused by pain or psychic trauma
- *Septic shock,* caused by a release of vasoactive substances

Some amount of neurogenic shock is seen with all spinal cord injuries. More dramatic cases of neurogenic shock are seen with cervical spine injuries. The duration of neurogenic shock is usually 1 to 6 weeks, provided there has been no irreparable cord injury. The incidence of septic and anaphylactic shock is variable. Clients who are at risk for either type of shock should be monitored closely.

Etiology and Risk Factors

All causes of shock focus on some component of blood distribution throughout the body. There can be an insufficient quantity of blood (hypovolemic shock), an incompetent pump (cardiogenic shock), or an ineffective delivery of blood (distributive shock).

Hypovolemic Shock

The primary event precipitating hypovolemic shock is a large reduction in the circulating blood volume so that the body's metabolic needs cannot be met. Hypovolemic shock may be due to a loss of plasma or blood. Conditions that may cause a reduction in the circulating volume include hemorrhage, burns, and dehydration.

Health promotion activities to prevent hypovolemic shock include client education to avoid injuries that would put someone at risk for hypovolemic shock (see Client Education Guide later). Health maintenance activities are the use of oxygen and maintenance of fluid and electrolyte balance. To restore health, monitor the client with telemetry and hemodynamic monitoring, and give vasoactive medications and blood and fluid replacements as ordered.

Hemorrhage

Hemorrhage is the loss of blood. Clinical manifestations may begin to appear with a blood volume deficit of 15% to 25%, or about 500 to 1500 ml in an adult with a normal circulating volume. Shock fully develops if a previously healthy client loses about one third of the normal circulating blood volume of 5 L.

The loss of smaller amounts of blood may cause shock in clients less able to compensate rapidly (e.g., older people with decreased vascular tone and impaired cardiac function). The extent to which shock develops after blood loss also depends on the length of time over which the blood loss occurs. Clients experiencing slow blood loss over a period of days or weeks tolerate their blood loss better than clients whose blood loss occurs rapidly over minutes or hours. Hypovolemic shock following trauma is typically the result of hemorrhage. The classes of hemorrhage and the associated assessment findings are listed in Table 81–1.

Burns

Hypovolemic shock produced by burns occurs most often in people with large partial-thickness or full-thickness burns. It is caused primarily by a shift of plasma from the vascular space into the interstitial space. In addition to these fluid losses or shifts, the client may have cardiac dysfunction that is due to the presence of *myocardial depressant factor* (MDF), a polypeptide (see later). MDF affects the contractility of cardiac muscle by depressing myocardial muscle function. The result is impaired cardiac output, even in the presence of a normal circulating volume. Shock related to burns is discussed in Chapter 50.

TABLE 81–1 ASSESSMENT FINDINGS AND CLASSIFICATIONS OF ACUTE HEMORRHAGE*

Assessment Finding	Class I	Class II	Class III	Class IV
Blood loss (%)	<15	15–30	30–40	>40
Blood loss (ml)	<750	750–1500	1500–2000	>2000
Pulse rate/min	<100	>100	>120	>140
Respiratory rate/min	Normal (14–20)	20–30	30–40	>35
Blood pressure	Normal	Normal	Decreased	Decreased
Pulse pressure	Normal or increased	Decreased	Decreased	Decreased
Central nervous system/ mental status	Slightly anxious	Mildly anxious	Anxious, confused	Confused, lethargic
Urinary output (ml/hr)	>30	20–30	5–15	Negligible
Intravenous fluid replacement	Crystalloid at 3 ml/1 ml of blood loss	Crystalloid at 3 ml/1 ml of blood loss	Crystalloid plus blood at 3 ml/1 ml of blood loss	Crystalloid plus blood at 3 ml/1 ml of blood loss

*Assumes a normal 70-kg man.

Data from American College of Surgeons Committee on Trauma. (1997). *Advanced trauma life support student manual* (p. 98). Chicago: Author.

Other causes of hypovolemic shock that may produce fluid shifts similar to those in burns include nephrotic syndrome, severe crush injuries, starvation, surgery, and conditions causing plasma fluids to accumulate in the abdominal cavity (e.g., cirrhosis of the liver, pancreatitis, and bowel obstruction).

Dehydration

Shock may also occur from either reduced oral fluid intake or significant fluid losses (e.g., rigorous exercise causing fluid loss from sweating and insensible fluid loss through the respiratory tract and hot environments). Loss of fluid, leading to dehydration-induced hypovolemic shock, may occur in people with excessive urine output or prolonged vomiting or diarrhea. Clients with chronic illnesses, especially older people, may be at increased risk because of impaired recognition of thirst or an inability to obtain fluids, inadequate maintenance of chronic conditions (i.e., increased blood glucose levels with diabetes), or inadequate monitoring of therapeutic regimens (i.e., diuretic-induced dehydration). With prolonged fluid deficit, all compartments—intravascular, interstitial, and intracellular—are depleted.

Cardiogenic Shock

Cardiogenic shock results primarily from an inability of heart muscle to function adequately or mechanical obstructions of blood flow to or from the heart. As with other causes of shock, the lack of blood flow decreases tissue and organ perfusion.

Myocardial Infarction

Impaired heart muscle action is most often caused by MI (see Chapter 58). The area of dead or dying tissue that occurs with infarction impairs contractility of the myocardium, and the cardiac output decreases. Impaired myocardial contractility may also occur with blunt cardiac trauma, cardiomyopathy, and heart failure.

Prevention of cardiogenic shock related to MI begins with health promotion activities directed at client education for decreasing the risk factors associated with coronary artery disease (e.g., increasing exercise and modifying dietary intake). Supportive oxygenation and administration of inotropic agents and vasodilators are health maintenance activities. An intra-aortic balloon pump (IABP) may be needed for health restoration.

Clients in cardiogenic shock may also develop some degree of hypovolemic shock. This is most often due to the therapeutic use of diuretics or to edema in the extremities or other dependent areas (caused by inadequate cardiac pumping activity and venous congestion).

Obstructive Conditions

Several types of mechanical obstructions to blood flow may cause cardiogenic shock:

1. *Large pulmonary embolism.* An *embolus* is usually the result of a blood clot that breaks loose in a person with deep vein thrombosis (DVT). This embolus travels through the venous system to the right side of the heart and into the pulmonary artery. The size of the embolus determines at what point it lodges in the pulmonary artery. A large embolus can inhibit perfusion of a major portion of the lung field, resulting in an increased workload for the right ventricle.
2. *Pericardial tamponade* is an accumulation of blood or fluid in the pericardial space that compresses the myocardium and interferes with the myocardium's ability to expand.
3. A *tension pneumothorax* is a significant amount of air in the pleural space compressing the heart and great vessels, thus interfering with venous return to the heart.

Other Causes of Cardiogenic Shock

Additional causes of cardiogenic shock include (1) cardiac valvular insufficiency from trauma or disease, (2) myocardial aneurysms (usually due to previous MI or congenital abnormalities), (3) rupture of a valvular papillary muscle, (4) ventricle rupture, (5) aortic stenosis, (6) mitral regurgitation, and (7) cardiac dysrhythmias.

Clients with hypovolemic shock are also at risk for cardiogenic shock. The myocardium normally receives its blood supply during diastole. When the heart rate increases to compensate for the decreased volume and to increase cardiac output, diastole is shortened, leading to insufficient time for the coronary arteries to fill with blood. Because these arteries supply blood to the myocardium, the myocardial oxygen supply is impaired. The increased heart rate also increases the myocardium's need for oxygen, predisposing the myocardium to injury because of the decreased blood flow and resultant decreased oxygen supply. In addition, the decreased venous return associated with hypovolemia results in decreased coronary artery perfusion and inadequate oxygenation of the myocardium.

Finally, shock results in the release of MDF and lactic acid, which depresses myocardial function.

DISTRIBUTIVE (VASOGENIC) SHOCK

Distributive shock results from inadequate vascular tone. Blood volume remains normal, but the size of the vascular space increases dramatically because of massive vasodilation. The result is maldistribution of the blood because of decreased blood pressure (BP) and lack of blood returning to the heart, which is why it is often referred to as "relative" hypovolemia. The volume of blood remains constant, but the blood has pooled because of increased capacity of the vascular system.

After extensive vasodilation, the BP, return of venous blood to the heart, and cardiac output are decreased. As with other forms of shock, tissue anoxia and cell destruction result. The massive vasodilation present with distributive shock has several major causes.

Acute Allergic Reaction (Anaphylactic Shock)

Anaphylactic shock occurs as a result of an acute allergic reaction from exposure to a substance to which the client has been sensitized. Common sensitizing agents are penicillin, penicillin derivatives, bee stings, chocolate, strawberries, peanuts, snake venom, iodine-based contrast for x-rays, foods, and nonsteroidal anti-inflammatory drugs (NSAIDs).

Reexposure to the foreign substance results in the offending antigen binding to previously made immunoglobulins (i.e., IgE) located on the mast cell. This binding causes the release of several chemical mediators from the cell, such as histamine, platelet-activating factor, leukotrienes, and prostaglandins (see Chapter 76). Manifestations include massive vasodilation, urticaria (hives), laryngeal edema, and bronchial constriction. Without prompt treatment, a person with anaphylactic shock will die of cardiovascular collapse and respiratory failure.

To help prevent the onset of anaphylactic shock, teach clients to avoid precipitators and to use an epinephrine injection (e.g., Epi-Pen). Encouraging clients to wear medical alert bracelets and to seek allergy desensitization also decreases their potential for anaphylactic shock.

Spinal Cord Injury (Neurogenic Shock)

With injury to the cervical spine, the autonomic nervous system is affected. Below the level of injury, there is blocking of sympathetic nervous stimulation and the parasympathetic system goes unopposed. This unopposed stimulation causes vasodilation, decreased venous return, decreased cardiac output, and decreased tissue perfusion. Teaching clients safety measures may help prevent spinal cord injury and neurogenic shock.

Health maintenance actions are to protect the client's spine, maintain the client's airway and breathing, provide circulatory support, and provide for thermoregulation. Health restoration involves rehabilitation when the client is stable.

Infection (Septic Shock)

Sepsis is the systemic response to infection. The process begins with the growth of various microorganisms at the site of infection. Organisms may invade the bloodstream directly (leading to positive blood cultures) or may remain in one area. The organisms release various substances into the bloodstream. These substances include structural parts of the organism, such as endotoxins and elements synthesized by them called *exotoxins.* Once these substances are released into the body, they activate the complement cascade. A complex shock picture occurs (see later). Septic shock is lethal, with a mortality rate of up to 50%.

Encouraging clients to treat infections immediately and completely may help reduce the incidence of septic shock. Older and immunocompromised clients should be monitored closely for infection, and treatment should begin immediately when infection is diagnosed. Shock is a serious development. Identify high-risk clients, and implement measures to prevent shock whenever possible.

Pathophysiology

Remember, adequate circulating volume is dependent on three interrelated components of the cardiovascular system: (1) the heart, (2) vascular tone, and (3) blood volume. A minor impairment in one component is compensated for by the other two. Prolonged or severe impairments lead to shock. Some of the problems with decreased organ and tissue perfusion in shock are due to failure of the normal mechanisms.

Blood flows throughout the body because of its driving pressure as it leaves the left ventricle (LV). Nowhere else in the cardiovascular system is blood under as high a pressure as it is in the LV. About 100 ml of blood (called *stroke volume*) leaves the LV at systolic BP about 80 times a minute. Because the metabolic demands are continuous rather than intermittent, blood is delivered into muscular walled arterioles, where it can be stored and released more consistently into the capillaries. From here, blood flows slowly through the capillaries that have greatest demand. (For example, when you run, more blood flows to your legs and lungs and less flows to your gastrointestinal (GI) tract. After you eat, the opposite is true.)

The microcirculation has the potential capacity to hold a great volume of blood. Nonetheless, the capillaries normally are relatively ischemic, containing only about 5% of the body's volume of blood. Typically, blood flow through the capillary bed is influenced by the varying needs of the cells located near the vessel. The capillaries open on demand of the cells adjacent to them. The size of the body's larger blood vessels is regulated by the autonomic nervous system, but this is not true for the microcirculation. Arteriole and capillary sphincters are separate mechanisms governed by different controls.

The microcirculation is relatively autonomous as a functional entity. Its patterns of behavior (in both normal and abnormal situations) are highly independent of the vasomotor influences affecting the systemic circulation lying next to it. The systemic circulatory bed and the microcirculatory bed apparently do not have sensing devices that would allow a unified, coordinated response throughout the entire circulation. Thus, events occurring within one bed do not influence events in the other. The relative autonomy of the microcirculation and the lack of coordination between it and the systemic circulation are important in determining the course of events in shock.

In the capillaries, nutrients in the blood are delivered to interstitial spaces to be picked up by the cells and wastes are transported to the capillary. The microcirculation is governed locally by vasoactive substances released into the area by the actions of various types of cells. This local regulation is a sensitive mechanism that can adjust blood flow from moment to moment according to tissue needs. The capillaries eventually join and meet veins that deliver blood to the heart. Veins have no muscle and are very low-pressure systems in which blood returns to the heart by using one-way valves. Veins can also store very large amounts of blood.

Two major receptors sense blood flow and volume and help the body make needed adjustments. The *arterial baroreceptor,* located in the aortic arch, senses how full the system is. If pressure in the muscular arterioles is low because of increased demand, the baroreceptor stimulates the sympathetic nervous system. This stimulation results in increased cardiac output, by increasing rate and stroke volume, and through increased muscle tension on the arteriole walls (*systemic* or *peripheral vascular resistance*). If BP was low to begin with, there is insufficient pressure for perfusion at the capillary end.

On the right side of the heart is the *atrial baroreceptor,* which measures the fluid volume returning to the heart. It also stimulates the sympathetic nervous system and constricts vessels storing blood in areas that are not considered vital to survival. The heart and brain are the organs considered most vital to survival. All other areas are considered less essential to survival.

Chemoreceptors are also located in the aortic arch and carotid bodies. These receptors sense decreased pH and increased partial pressure of arterial carbon dioxide ($PaCO_2$). When tissues do not receive adequate blood, they maintain their metabolism using an anaerobic pathway. A product of this pathway is lactic acid. When there is inadequate perfusion, carbon dioxide (CO_2) accumulates in the tissues. If breathing is also impaired, CO_2 is not exhaled. When these changes are sensed by chemoreceptors, respiratory rate and depth increase and cardiac output increases to correct the imbalance.

A juxtaglomerular receptor in the kidney measures blood flow to the kidney. When blood volume falls, the cells in the receptor release renin. Renin begins a cascade of response (angiotensin I, angiotensin II) that eventually produces potent peripheral vasoconstriction. In addition, antidiuretic hormone (ADH) is released when osmoreceptors in the hypothalamus are triggered. Osmoreceptors sense the osmolality, that is, how "concentrated" the blood is. When osmolality is increased, ADH release prevents diuresis, increases water returned to the body from the kidney and thus increases total blood volume.

All of these receptors and hormones maintain volume and thus arterial pressure. When the circulatory system is functioning properly, mean arterial pressure (MAP) is maintained at normal levels (70 to 105 mm Hg):

$$MAP = \frac{(\text{systolic} + [2 \times \text{diastolic}])}{3}$$

MAP is the average effective pressure that drives blood through the systemic organs. If MAP is not maintained at normal or near-normal levels, tissues are inadequately perfused.

If one of the three components of circulation fails, other parts of the system initiate compensatory mechanisms. For example, vasoconstriction and increased cardiac output may be used to compensate for decreased volume. As long as two of these factors can maintain a satisfactory compensatory action, adequate blood circulation can be maintained even though the third factor is not functioning normally. If compensatory mechanisms fail or if more than one of the three factors necessary for adequate circulation malfunction, circulatory failure results and shock develops.

STAGES OF SHOCK

Early Compensation Stage

During the initial or compensated stage of shock, cardiac output is slightly decreased because of loss of actual or relative blood volume. During this stage, the body's compensatory mechanisms can maintain BP within a normal to low-normal range and can maintain tissue perfusion to the vital organs. During the compensatory phase, the systemic circulation and microcirculation work together. Both undergo a major readjustment in which their activities are coordinated to preserve the entire system. Figure 81–1 illustrates these readjustments.

Decompensation Stage

If shock and the compensatory vasoconstriction persist, the body begins to decompensate and the systemic circulation and microcirculation no longer work in unison. As vasoconstriction continues, the supply of oxygenated blood to the tissues is reduced. This results in anaerobic metabolism and lactic acidosis. Acidosis and the increasing $PaCO_2$ cause the microcirculation to dilate. This dilation causes decreased venous return and decreased circulation of reoxygenated blood.

Lactic acidosis also causes increased capillary permeability and relaxation of the capillary sphincters. Relaxation of the sphincters allows increased blood in the capillaries and increased capillary pressure. This increased pressure along with the increased capillary permeability allows fluid to move out of the vascular space and back into the tissues. In doing so, the microcirculation has reversed its pattern and is trying to secure for itself (and the tissue it supplies) more of the limited supply of available blood. Thus, the blood supply is progressively retained in the capillary bed and blood pools in the microcirculation. Because the cells demand greater perfusion time, many or most of the capillaries remain open at any one time, increasing the vascular space in the microcirculation.

Increased vascular capacity, decreased blood volume, or decreased heart action reduces the MAP. In turn, the pressure gradient for the venous return of blood decreases. This also contributes to venous pooling of blood, decreased venous return to the heart, and decreased cardiac output.

Because there are no feedback systems within the body to change this pattern, the cycle of events becomes progressively more severe. Eventually, the circulation is totally disrupted. Once the vascular space enlarges (because of vasodilation of the microcirculation), even a normal blood volume cannot fill all these small vessels and the larger ones as well. The result is a low central venous pressure (CVP), except in cardiogenic shock, and inadequate venous return to the right side of the heart, with a further decrease in cardiac output.

This resultant decrease in circulating volume and capillary flow does not allow adequate perfusion and oxygenation of the vital organs. With the prolonged decrease in capillary blood flow, the tissues become hypoxic. This cycle of events is illustrated in Figure 81–2.

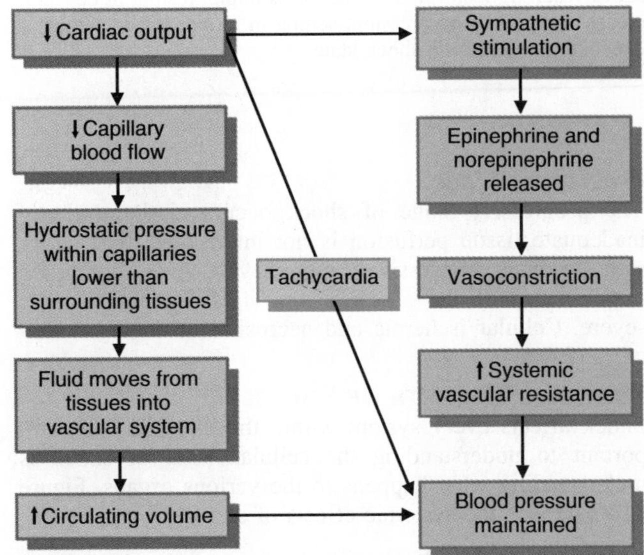

FIGURE 81–1 Compensated stage of shock. Regardless of the cause, a decreased cardiac output is generally the stimulus that precipitates the body's response to compensate for the hypovolemia (relative or actual) to maintain blood pressure.

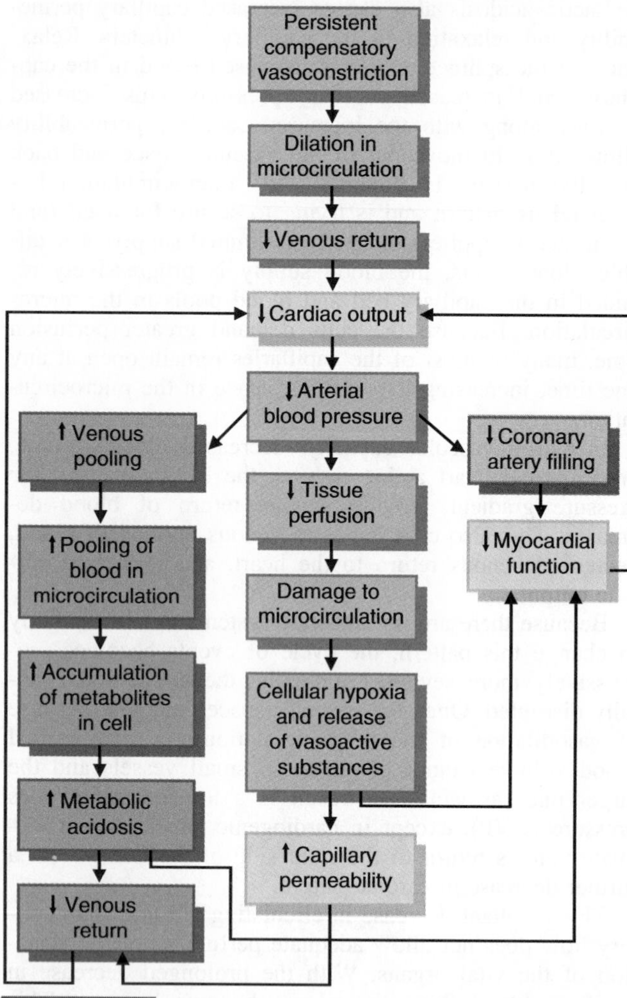

FIGURE 81–2 Vicious cycle of events occurring in shock. The shock syndrome can be initiated anywhere in the cycle, depending on the precipitating cause (e.g., impaired myocardial function due to myocardial infarction, blood loss due to trauma, or the release of vasoactive toxins due to sepsis). Hypovolemic shock resulting from blood loss, for example, results in decreased arterial blood pressure, setting in motion a cascade of events that worsen the shock state.

Progressive Stage

The progressive stage of shock occurs if the cycle of inadequate tissue perfusion is not interrupted. The shock state becomes progressively more severe, even though the initial cause of the shock is not itself becoming more severe. Cellular ischemia and necrosis lead to organ failure and death.

SYSTEMIC EFFECTS OF SHOCK

Shock affects every system within the body. Equally important to understanding the cellular level of shock is understanding what happens to the various organs. Figure 81–3 depicts the systemic effects of shock.

Respiratory System

Getting oxygen in (*ventilation*) and delivering oxygenated blood to the tissues (*perfusion*) are crucial for survival. Shock produces prolonged circulatory insufficiency. This leads to variable and inadequate perfusion of certain organs and tissues, particularly at the microcirculation level. Such circulatory deprivation results in tissue hypoxia and anoxia. Hypoxia and anoxia can be tolerated for a short time. As the time lengthens, the chances of recovery diminish. A lack of oxygen appears to initiate the progressive stage of shock. The greater the difference between the amount of oxygen available and the amount needed, the more rapidly progressive shock develops. If sufficient oxygen is available to the cells to meet the body's needs, progressive shock is less likely to occur.

Despite many advances in shock prevention, early recognition, and management, respiratory failure continues to be a major cause of death in shock. The magnitude of this problem surfaced during the Vietnam War when soldiers sustaining massive injuries and profound blood loss were successfully resuscitated only to die several days later of acute respiratory distress syndrome (ARDS) (see Chapter 63). Although ARDS remains the greatest contributing factor to respiratory failure, other causes of respiratory failure during shock include aspiration and loss of neurologic control of breathing.

ACID-BASE BALANCE. To function properly, cells depend on adequate circulation to receive nutrients, electrolytes, and oxygen and to remove waste products. Oxygen and nutrients are essential to life because they make possible chemical transformations resulting in the synthesis of adenosine triphosphate (ATP). ATP is the ultimate source of energy for life processes.

When oxygen is not present, ATP is produced through a different set of reactions called *anaerobic metabolism.* Although production of ATP in this manner is a useful emergency measure, it is inefficient compared with the normal process of *aerobic (oxidative) metabolism.* Anaerobic metabolism produces anaerobic metabolites, such as lactic acid (which causes intracellular acidity with consequent cellular damage) and substrates of the adenylic acid system (which depress the heart) (Fig. 81–4).

In response to the chemoreceptors sensing decreased pH, the rate and depth of respirations are increased to "blow off" (exhale) CO_2 in an attempt to compensate for the metabolic acidosis. This results in respiratory alkalosis. However, the cellular hypoxia is caused not by inadequate ventilation but by inadequate tissue perfusion. Therefore, the increased respiratory effort does little to correct the problem.

Because lactic acid is not exhaled, it accumulates in tissue fluids, which thus become increasingly acidic. Eventually, metabolic acidosis is produced. During metabolic acidosis, blood pH and bicarbonate levels fall. Pyruvate, lactate, phosphate, and sulfate levels rise. Unless circulation is restored, the acidotic reaction resulting from metabolic acidosis ultimately kills the cells. The buildup of lactic acid causes such a severe local acidosis that cellular enzymes are inactivated. As a result, the cells soon die.

Respiratory alkalosis or *respiratory acidosis* (induced by pulmonary ventilatory or diffusion changes) may be superimposed on the metabolic acidosis. As perfusion and oxygen delivery to the tissues decrease, cellular energy production decreases. To compensate, cells increase anaerobic metabolism, which results in the buildup of lactic acid in the cell. As the pH of the cells decreases, lysosomes within the cell explode, releasing powerful, de-

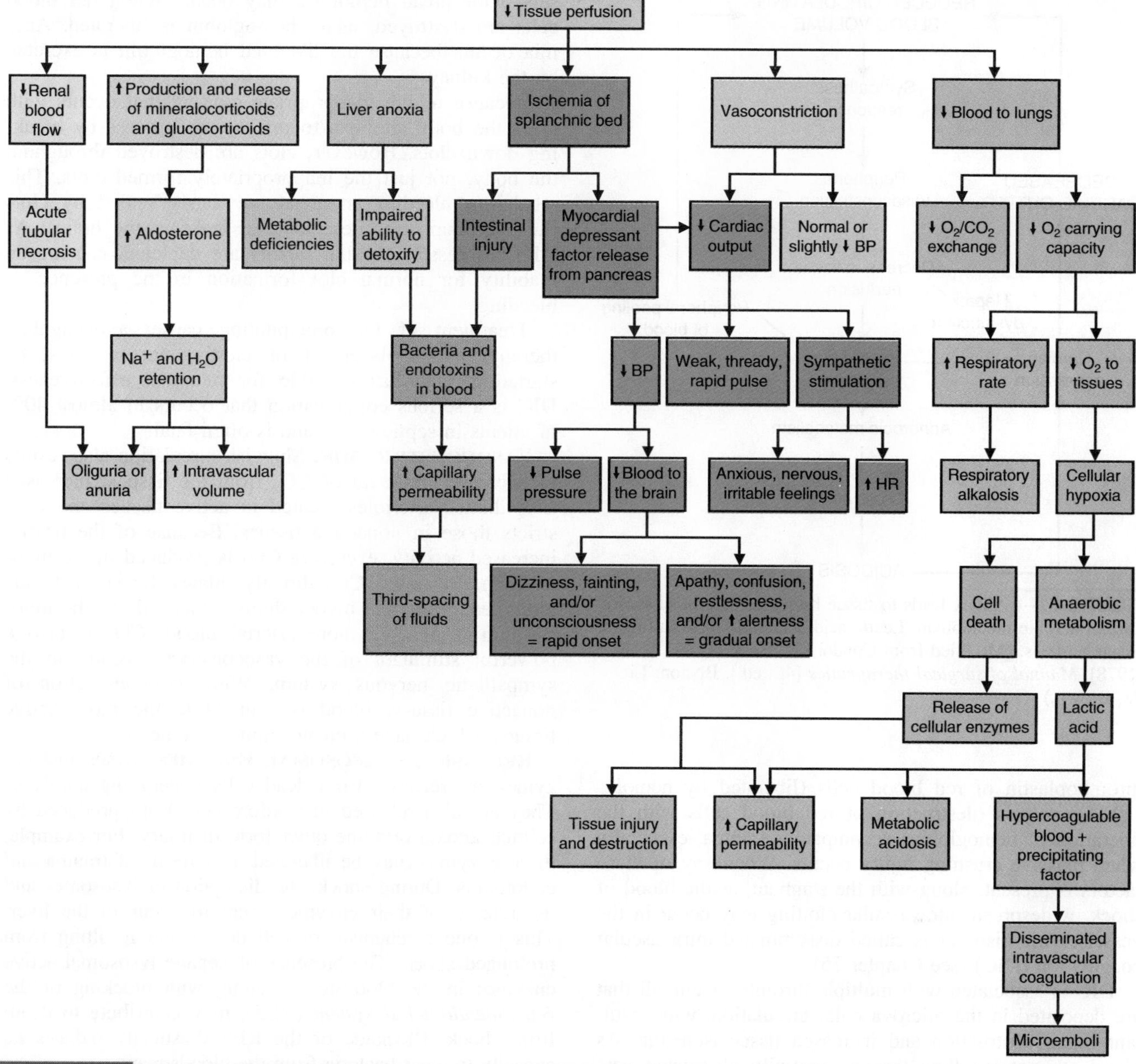

FIGURE 81–3 Systemic effects of shock.

structive enzymes. These enzymes destroy the cellular membrane and digest the cell contents. Once this process begins, the cellular changes are irreversible. The final result is cellular death (Fig. 81–5).

Cardiovascular System

MYOCARDIAL DETERIORATION. As shock progresses, the heart deteriorates. Cardiac deterioration is one of the major causes of death in shock. Although the exact cause of myocardial depression is unclear, much attention has been directed at MDF. MDF, a polypeptide with vasoactive properties, is released in response to ischemia of the GI tract. It causes a significant reduction in cardiac output, even in the presence of a normal circulating volume of blood. Another factor contributing to cardiac deterioration may be myocardial zonal lesions, which appear in the myocardium after ischemia or infarction. Cells in these areas do not fully repolarize and thus interfere with the usual efficient electrical conduction in the heart, which results in impaired contraction and possibly cardiac failure.

Cardiac depression is often compensated for by the large cardiac reserve of a normal person. Because of this reserve, the heart can deteriorate to less than one third (sometimes less than one fifth) of its normal pumping strength without measurable evidence of cardiac failure.

DISSEMINATED INTRAVASCULAR COAGULATION. During shock, tissue hypoxia results from the sluggish movement of blood in the capillaries. Anaerobic metabolism begins, increasing the production of lactic acid. The slow-moving acidic blood is hypercoagulable; however, it does not coagulate unless a clot-initiating factor is present. Such factors include bacterial endotoxins and

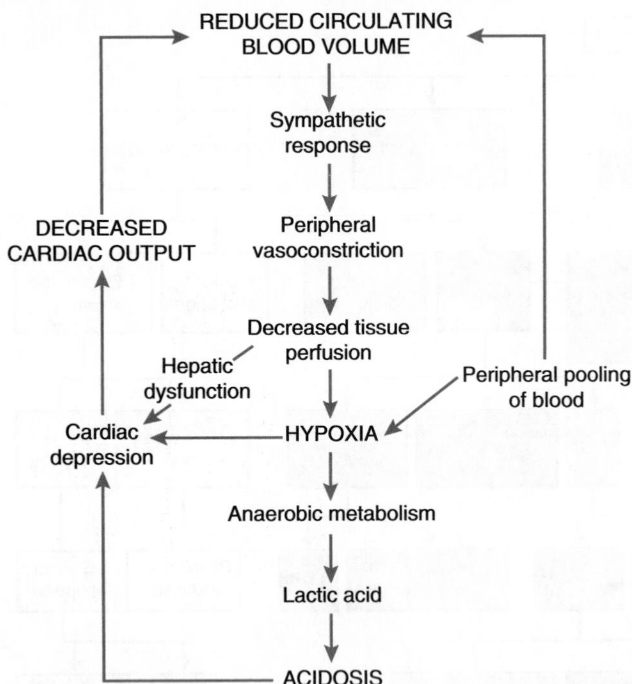

FIGURE 81–4 Shock leads to tissue hypoxia, with blockage of normal aerobic metabolism. Lactic acid accumulates, resulting in tissue acidosis. (Modified from Condon, R. E., & Nyhus, L. M. [1978]. *Manual of surgical therapeutics* [4th ed.]. Boston: Little, Brown.)

thromboplastin of red blood cells (liberated by hemolysis). Hemolysis (destruction of red blood cells with the liberation of hemoglobin) accompanies trauma, especially when massive crushing injury occurs. When any of these factors is present, along with the stagnant, acidic blood of shock, widespread intravascular clotting may occur in the vessels. This disorder is called disseminated intravascular coagulation (DIC) (see Chapter 75).

DIC is associated with multiple thrombi or emboli that are deposited in the microvascular circulation, with resultant organ obstruction and increased tissue ischemia. As blood attempts to flow through partially obstructed vessels, widespread hemolysis may occur. When red blood cells are destroyed, again hemoglobin is liberated. Anemia occurs because the liberated hemoglobin is excreted by the kidneys.

Because of the inappropriate clotting that occurs with DIC, the body attempts to reverse the process by breaking down clots. However, clots are destroyed throughout the body, not just the inappropriately formed clots. This results in bleeding in areas previously sealed by clots (i.e., venipuncture sites, vascular leaks in the brain). As DIC progresses, clotting factors are depleted, causing an inability for normal clot formation in the presence of bleeding.

Treatment of the precipitating cause, anticoagulant therapy, and replacement of clotting factors must be started as soon as possible for maximal effectiveness. DIC is a serious complication that occurs in almost 40% of clients in septic shock and is often fatal.

VASOCONSTRICTION. Sluggish circulation also results in decreased removal of CO_2 from the tissues. Increased CO_2 dilates arterioles located in active tissues and constricts those in nonactive tissues. Because of the heart's increased activity, excessive CO_2 is produced in the myocardium. Increased CO_2 directly dilates the coronary arteries leading to the myocardium, which allows the myocardium to receive more arterial blood. CO_2 is also a powerful stimulant of the vasoconstrictor center in the sympathetic nervous system. With vasoconstriction of nonactive tissues, blood is shunted to the more active tissues, which have a greater immediate need.

RELEASE OF LYSOSOMAL ENZYMES. Lysosomal enzymes are released from dead cells undergoing autolysis. They are also released just before cell death produced by cellular anoxia or some other form of injury. For example, these enzymes may be liberated as a result of trauma and endotoxins. During shock, the disruption of lysosomes and the release of their enzymes seem to occur in the liver. This is one mechanism of cell destruction resulting from prolonged shock. The presence of hepatic lysosomal active enzymes in the bloodstream, along with blocking of the *reticuloendothelial system* (RES), may contribute to death from shock. Blockade of the RES drastically reduces its capacity to clear bacteria from the bloodstream.

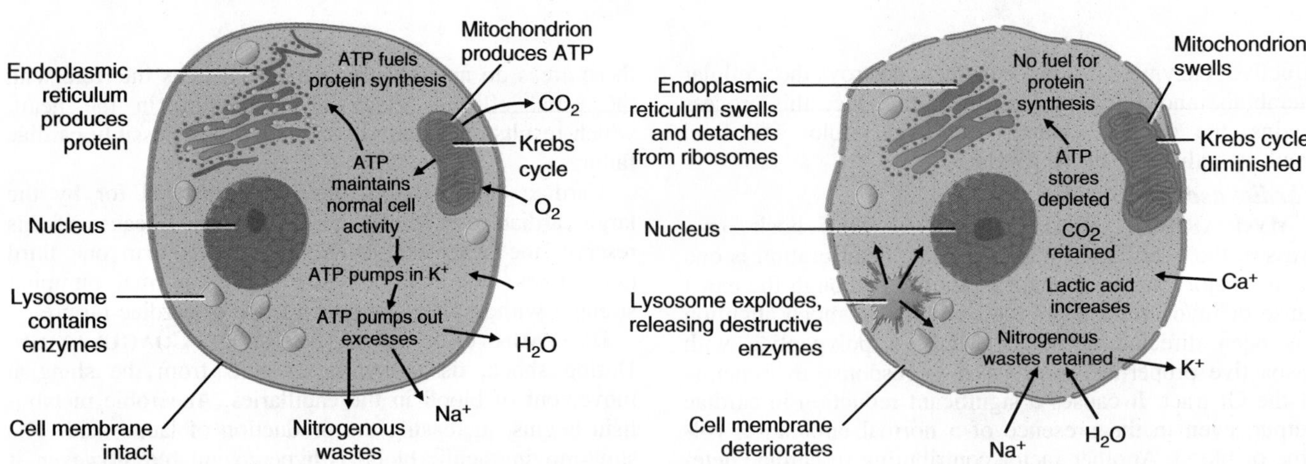

FIGURE 81–5 *Left,* Normal cell. *Right,* Alterations in cell function during late shock. ATP, adenosine triphosphate; Ca^+, calcium; CO_2, carbon dioxide; H_2O, water; Na^+, sodium; O_2, oxygen.

Lysosomal enzymes become most active in an acid pH range. Thus, as long as normal acid-base balance is maintained within the body, these enzymes are repressed within normal cells. During shock, however, the accompanying metabolic acidosis accelerates the activation of these enzymes in hypoxic tissues. The activation of lysosomal hydrolases within the cells and their release into the circulation markedly exacerbate the tissue injury that occurs during shock. The release of active lysosomal proteases and other enzymes from damaged tissue into the bloodstream and their action on extracellular and intracellular structures probably contribute to the progression of injury from cell to cell.

Vasoactive Substances. Vasoactive substances are highly variable in promoting vasoconstriction or vasodilation in a person experiencing shock. The influence they exert may be altered by factors such as pH, the specific tissue (e.g., heart, lung), the presence of drugs or other substances, serum electrolyte levels, and the sensitivity of the end organ.

Catecholamines. Catecholamines, such as epinephrine and norepinephrine, are present early in shock and are related to the fight-or-flight response. Their general effects are to increase blood flow to the brain, heart, and striated (skeletal) muscle and to decrease blood flow to the skin, kidneys, and splanchnic bed. Although the initial effect of vasoconstriction in the skin, kidneys, and splanchnic bed (GI tract) serves to increase the intravascular volume, sustained vasoconstriction contributes to stagnant hypoxia and cellular death.

Histamine. Histamine causes vasodilation, increased capillary permeability, bronchoconstriction, coronary vasodilation, and cutaneous reactions (flares, wheals). The effects of histamine are especially obvious in anaphylactic and septic shock.

Vasoactive Polypeptides. Among the more important vasoactive polypeptides that appear to play significant roles in shock are:

1. *Bradykinin.* A kinin peptide, bradykinin is known to produce vasodilation, increased capillary permeability, smooth muscle relaxation, pain, and infiltration of an area with leukocytes. Kinins appear to be most active in late shock. They may be a factor in the development of pulmonary insufficiency associated with shock.
2. *Angiotensin.* Angiotensin results from the action of renal renin on angiotensinogen. This potent substance causes vasoconstriction and increased vascular resistance. Although similar to norepinephrine in effect, angiotensin may produce fewer negative effects. Its role in sodium and water retention (through the stimulation of aldosterone secretion) is discussed under the adrenal response.
3. *MDF.* MDF is a vasoactive polypeptide that contributes to cardiac failure in clients in shock by depressing cardiac muscle contraction.

Neuroendocrine System

GENERAL ADAPTATION SYSTEM (GAS) RESPONSE. Neuroendocrine responses during shock are defensive reactions that occur during the body's stage of resistance in the general adaptation syndrome (GAS). Recall that the length of the stage of resistance varies among people and is determined by a body's ability to compensate for its deficiencies. Hence, one person may be able to combat shock longer than another. For example, a previously healthy person may have a longer stage of resistance against shock compared with a client who is debilitated before shock develops.

ADRENAL RESPONSE. Some basic features of the neuroendocrine responses include (1) the release of epinephrine and norepinephrine from the adrenal medulla (which results in increased respiratory and heart rates, increased BP, increased blood flow to organs, decreased blood flow to peripheral tissues) and (2) the release of mineralocorticoids (which control fluid and electrolyte balance) and glucocorticoids (which affect energy and tissue resistance) from the adrenal cortex.

Increased production of adrenocortical mineralocorticoid hormones occurs. The main mineralocorticoids—aldosterone and desoxycorticosterone—help to increase intravascular fluid volume by stimulating the kidneys to retain sodium and hence water. The renal tubular conservation of sodium occurs with any type of fluid loss or blood volume depletion. Aldosterone is essential to conservation of sodium. Because water is retained in the body along with sodium, urine excretion is diminished during shock. This fluid is retained in the bloodstream in an effort to increase blood volume. Increasing the volume of blood in this way is aimed at increasing venous return, cardiac output, and BP.

PITUITARY RESPONSE. Of major importance in regulating water and sodium balance are aldosterone and ADH, also called *vasopressin.* ADH is produced by the posterior pituitary gland. The blood's osmolality (osmotic concentration) increases with dehydration. This stimulates osmoreceptors in the hypothalamus to release ADH from the posterior pituitary gland. Via the blood, the ADH is carried to the kidneys. There it causes the body to retain water.

Various components of the sympathoadrenal (sympathetic part of the autonomic nervous system and adrenal medulla) response to a major stressor are shown in Figure 81–6.

Metabolic Response. Generally, the hormonal response to stress rapidly provides fuel for the body's various tissues, organs, and systems. These fuels (e.g., amino acids, fatty acids, and glucose) are produced by the breakdown of food. These substances are then chemically converted into energy, resulting in the formation of ATP. ATP is the main source of energy produced and used inside the body's cells.

The glucocorticoids, particularly hydrocortisone, mobilize energy stores. During the initial phase of shock, the body's small stores of available carbohydrate are rapidly depleted. It then becomes necessary to mobilize protein and fat stores to meet the body's energy requirements. Protein catabolism and negative nitrogen balance occur as part of the metabolic response, because of gluconeogenesis (resulting from glucocorticoid action) and starvation.

NEUROLOGIC RESPONSE. With shock, cerebral blood flow and cerebral metabolism may become insufficient to maintain normal mental functioning and level of consciousness. Brain cells are highly sensitive to a shortage of oxygen and glucose and to fluid imbalances. When the brain becomes hypoxic, the cerebral vessels dilate to re-

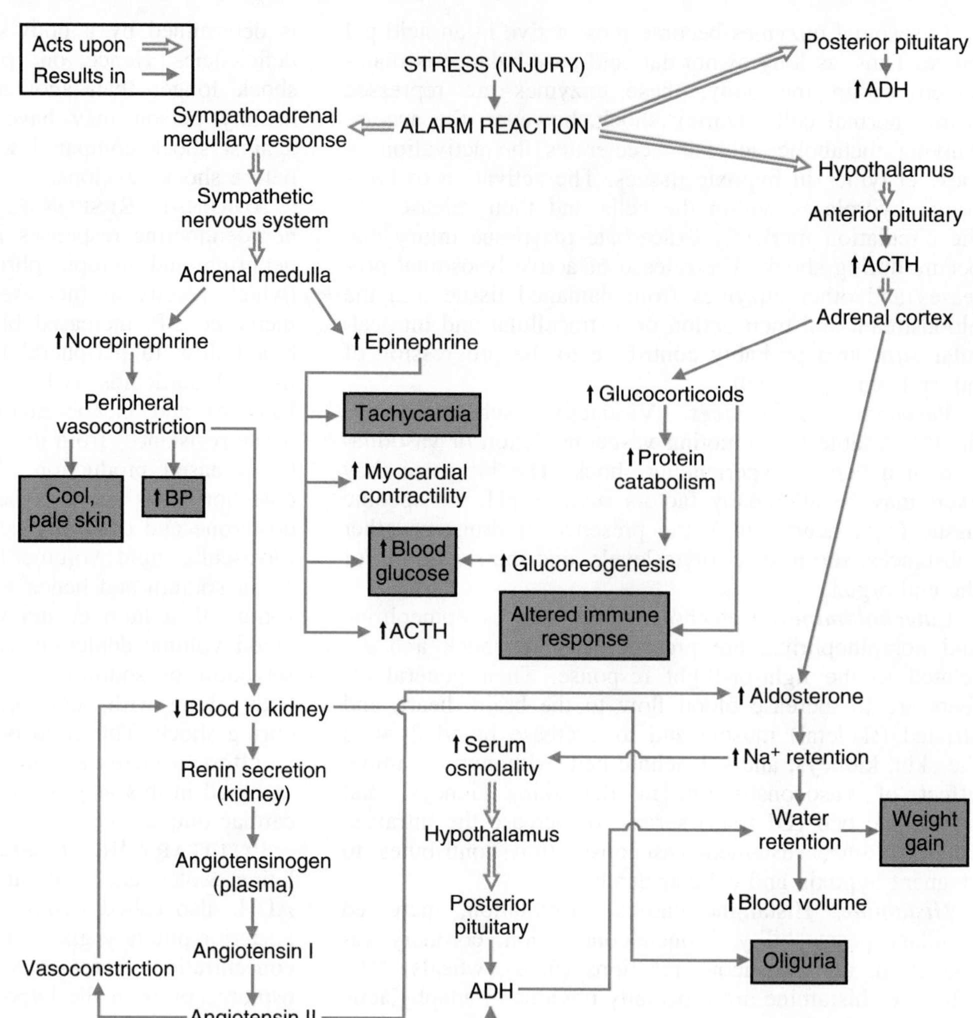

FIGURE 81–6 Components of the neuroendocrine response to a major stressor. Readily observed clinical signs as well as laboratory values are indicated by the boxes. ACTH, adrenocorticotropic hormone; ADH, antidiuretic hormone; BP, blood pressure.

store blood flow. Likewise, blood is diverted to the brain from the other, less vital organs.

Immune System

All forms of shock severely depress macrophages, which are located in both the blood and tissues. The capacity of macrophages to remove bacteria and the constantly formed endotoxins from the bloodstream is greatly reduced. Alterations in the blood itself are partially due to tissue hypoxia and impairment of monitoring activities of the macrophage. The stasis, sludging, tendency for venular thrombosis, impaired capillary permeability, and subnormal vascular reactivity that occur during shock can all be traced to macrophage dysfunction.

The impaired ability of macrophages to ward off toxic agents is critical. Reduced blood flow through the intestines during shock extensively impairs the integrity of intestinal tissue. This results in the movement of normal GI flora across the impaired intestinal tissue into the bloodstream, leading to a possible bacteremic state. The person in a state of shock is more susceptible than normal to bacterial products, particularly bacterial endotoxins, because of alterations in macrophage function.

Gastrointestinal System

Under sympathetic stimulation, vagal stimulation to the GI tract slows or stops, resulting in ileus with an absence of peristalsis. A lack of nutrient blood supply to the intestines increases the risk of tissue necrosis and sepsis.

GI changes appear to have a more important role in the progression of shock than previously thought. The submucosa of the intestine becomes ischemic early in shock. If ischemia is prolonged, actual tissue necrosis of intestinal mucosa occurs. The intestinal arterioles and venules seem highly susceptible to the extensive vasoconstriction that occurs during shock. The massive amount of tissue destruction within the intestines that results from vasoconstriction and tissue anoxia is sufficient to cause death even if bacteria are not present. Bacteria and their toxins contribute to shock by escaping into the systemic circulation following destruction of the intestinal mucosa barrier.

Shock causes serious changes in the functions of the liver, the major organ of detoxification. The liver also suffers from this impaired circulation and appears to be a source of toxic materials. Normally, the liver protectively traps and disposes of toxic materials (released from the bowel contents) that are products of bacterial enzyme actions. During shock, the anoxic liver develops metabolic deficiencies, has an impaired ability to detoxify, and may release vasoactive substances. In addition, enhanced bacterial invasion of the liver from the intestine apparently occurs.

Finally, during shock, pooling of blood occurs in the viscera. Pooling of blood in the liver and portal bed may result from masses of agglutinated (clotted) blood plugging numerous small hepatic vessels, sinusoids, and intrahepatic radicles of the portal vein and hepatic artery.

Renal System

The rate of urinary production reflects visceral blood flow and body fluid balance. Thus, urinary output indicates the status of circulation through the vital organs. Adequate urinary output indicates adequate circulation even if the arterial blood pressure is below normal.

ALTERED CAPILLARY BLOOD PRESSURE AND GLOMERULAR FILTRATION. Glomerular filtration within the kidneys depends on the pressure at which the blood is circulating through the glomerular capillaries. Usually, the average capillary pressure of blood is much higher in the glomeruli than in other capillaries. Interestingly, under usual circumstances, the kidneys can maintain this heightened capillary pressure in the glomeruli in spite of changes in systemic BP. Afferent arterioles supplying the glomeruli dilate as the BP falls and constrict as it rises. However, eventually this adaptive mechanism cannot protect the kidneys against damage from a falling systemic BP.

During shock, when blood volume and BP decline steadily, glomerular filtration is progressively reduced, which leads to an inability of the kidneys to excrete sodium and water. To compensate, the body excretes some sodium and water through the sweat glands. Damaged kidneys also lose their crucial ability to regulate electrolyte and acid-base balance.

Inadequate perfusion of renal capillaries is believed to be the cause of early renal failure in shock. The afferent and efferent arterioles constrict, shunting blood away from the glomeruli. Later, if shock persists, actual renal shutdown occurs from focal tubular necrosis. Unfortunately, vasoconstriction in the kidneys may continue for a prolonged period of time after the systemic BP is restored to normal levels.

RENAL ISCHEMIA. During shock, the kidneys may experience renal ischemia. Because the kidneys have a high rate of metabolism, they are highly susceptible to injury of the tubule cells when the blood supply is deficient. When injury to the kidneys is extensive and renal failure ensues, acute tubular necrosis (ATN) occurs. With appropriate intervention, including careful fluid administration, the kidneys can heal. Normal kidney function usually returns after 10 to 14 days.

Clinical Manifestations

SYSTEMIC MANIFESTATIONS OF SHOCK

Because shock affects every system within the body, there are numerous clinical manifestations. The body is made up of many cells, which may function or malfunction at different stages of metabolic impairment. Subjective complaints are usually nonspecific and may not be particularly helpful to the clinician attempting to diagnose shock and treat the client. The client may report feeling sick, weak, cold, hot, nauseated, dizzy, confused, frightened, thirsty, or short of breath. Observable and measurable manifestations (Fig. 81–7) are often conflicting. BP, cardiac output, and urinary output are usually (but not always) decreased. Respiratory rate is usually increased. Variable indicators of shock include alterations in heart rate, core body temperature, skin temperature, systemic vascular resistance, and skin color. Dyspnea, altered sensorium, and diaphoresis may be present. The manifestations discussed in the sections that follow are usually present in people with shock of any type.

Respiratory System

Rapid, shallow respirations (tachypnea) typically occur during shock because of decreased tissue perfusion. The

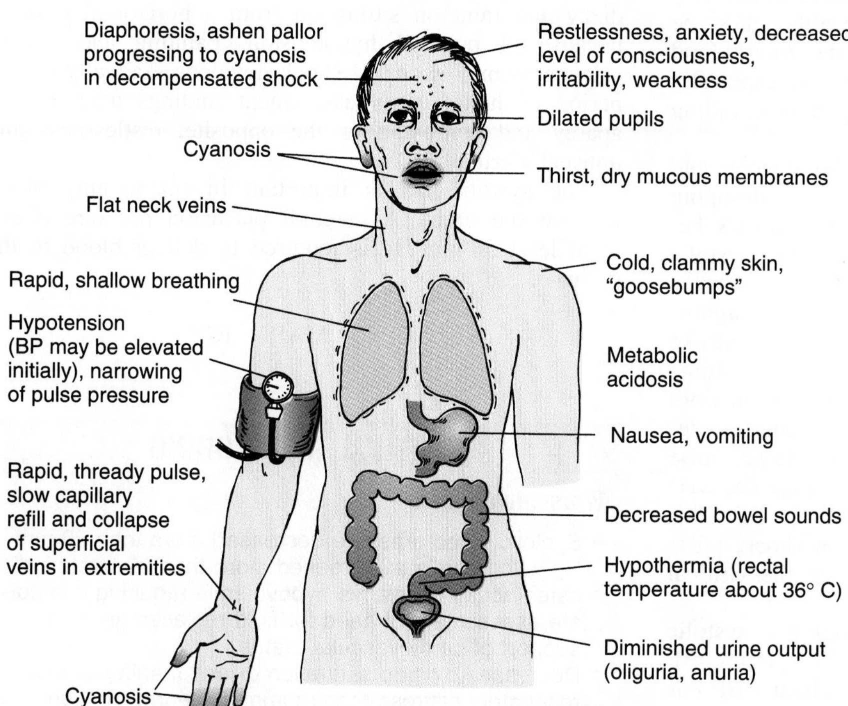

FIGURE 81–7 Clinical manifestations of the client with hypovolemic shock.

respiratory rate increases as the blood's oxygen-carrying capacity decreases. These changes may signal the development of hypoxemia and respiratory alkalosis.

Cardiovascular System

TACHYCARDIA. During shock, the pulse rate usually increases as a result of increased sympathetic stimulation. Tachycardia (rapid heartbeat) occurs in an attempt to maintain adequate cardiac output when the blood's circulating volume is declining. With increased rate, the pulse becomes typically weak and thready. At the onset of shock, the pulse rate does not relate as directly to the severity of shock as does BP. This is because in the early stage of shock, worry, excitement, and fear may influence the heart rate out of proportion to the underlying conditions. However, when emotional factors are no longer significant, serial observations of the pulse rate over a period of time are highly useful to assess the client's condition and the direction of the shock state and to evaluate the effectiveness of intervention.

Older clients (with and without various degrees of heart block) and clients taking beta-blockers are exceptions to this event. Their heart rates may show little change despite the presence of conditions causing circulatory failure (e.g., hemorrhage). The pulse rate may become extremely slow in the terminal stages of shock and is usually slow in neurogenic shock.

HYPOTENSION. The systolic BP indicates the integrity of the heart, arteries, and arterioles. The diastolic BP indicates the resistance (*systemic vascular resistance* [SVR] or *vasoconstriction*) of blood vessels. For example, an increasing diastolic BP indicates increasing systemic blood vessel resistance. Conversely, a declining diastolic BP indicates decreasing SVR. When the diastolic BP falls significantly, vasoconstriction is being lost as a compensatory mechanism. When vasoconstriction is replaced by marked vasodilation, there is no resistance to blood flow and an adequate BP is difficult to maintain.

Usually, the BP begins to fall when total blood volume is decreased by about 15% to 20%; although some people may lose as much as 25% of the total blood volume without having a fall in BP. This is especially true in young adults; therefore, in young adults, falling BP is a *very* late manifestation of shock.

Typically, as shock progresses, both the systolic and diastolic BPs drop, with the systolic pressure dropping more than the diastolic. The pulse pressure narrows because it is equal to the difference between the systolic and diastolic BPs.

During shock, pulse pressure is actually more significant than BP because it tends to parallel cardiac stroke volume. The pulse pressure is affected by stroke volume (amount of blood ejected by the LV during contraction) and by peripheral resistance. If stroke volume is decreased from a decreased circulating blood volume, pulse pressure decreases. In shock, pulse pressure may decrease even in the presence of an acceptable systolic BP. This may provide a clue to worsening shock. In shock, pulse pressure is often less than 20 mm Hg. See the Critical Monitoring feature.

To maintain coronary circulation, a minimal systolic BP of 60 to 70 mm Hg is necessary. In interpreting BP readings, it is important to know what the client's BP has been. A systolic BP of 100 mm Hg or less is significant for clients whose systolic BP usually ranges from 110 to 140 mm Hg. When a client is supine, a decline in BP may be a late finding. Hypotension by itself is not shock. Healthy clients often have BP readings lower than textbook normal values.

Additional problems need to be considered in assessment of BP that make BP an unreliable criterion for assessing the presence and severity of shock. In the early, compensated stages of shock, BP changes are generally unreliable because the arterial pressure may actually be normal or slightly elevated even though shock is present. In fact, blood volume deficits of 1 L or more may occur even though arterial and venous pressures are normal or elevated. When severe vasoconstriction is present, BP may be normal even though the circulation is actually highly inadequate. Conversely, the blood flow may be adequate even though BP is decreased (e.g., because of mechanisms such as vasodilation).

Valuable information about the level of arterial pressure in clients with vasoconstriction can be gained by assessing the strength of the femoral pulses. Doppler study may also be appropriate to obtain an accurate peripheral BP. With displaced or depleted blood volume, it is important to consider adequate venous filling. Hypovolemia, whether actual or relative, causes superficial veins to flatten. This change may hamper attempts to insert intravenous (IV) catheters for fluid replacement.

NEUROENDOCRINE SYSTEM. Early in shock, hyperactivity of the sympathetic nervous system with increased secretion of epinephrine usually causes the client to feel anxious, nervous, and irritable. Anxiety and worry are seen in the client's facial expressions.

Assessment findings associated with lack of blood to the brain are determined by the suddenness with which the shock develops and by its severity. With sudden, severe shock, the body may not have time to initiate its compensatory adjustment mechanisms. Consequently, the brain is deprived of its blood supply. The client may feel dizzy and faint on sitting up from a horizontal position because of postural hypotension. Fainting and unconsciousness may occur. If shock develops gradually over a period of hours, early assessment findings may include apathy and confusion or the opposite, restlessness and unusual alertness.

The systolic BP is important in maintaining blood flow to the brain. A cerebral perfusion pressure (CPP) of at least 50 mm Hg is required to deliver blood to the brain

$$CPP = MAP - ICP$$

CRITICAL MONITORING

Worsening Shock

- Systolic blood pressure decreased more than 20 mm Hg with heart rate increased more than 20 beats indicates actual or relative hypovolemia requiring immediate assessment of need for fluid replacement and support of cardiovascular status.
- Decreased oxygen saturation or any manifestations of respiratory distress require immediate intervention.

where ICP is intracranial pressure. Usually, a decrease in systolic BP is accompanied by a reduced flow of blood to the brain. The brain's vessels, like those of the heart, however, are not constricted by the vasoconstrictor center in the medulla oblongata. Thus, blood from the peripheral vessels can be shifted to the brain as an emergency compensatory measure.

A client's level of consciousness decreases as circulation to brain tissue becomes increasingly impaired. Confusion, agitation, and restlessness may occur. In trauma situations, restlessness can be mistaken for pain. If narcotics are given, the client's situation may be worsened or it may be difficult to detect worsening hypoxia. Drowsiness and stupor are more likely in shock related to severe infection than in shock caused by trauma and hemorrhage. As compensatory mechanisms fail, apathy may ensue. Ultimately, a comatose condition may be reached.

Renal System

A fall in urinary volume, often the earliest manifestation of developing shock, may occur even while arterial BP and pulse remain stable. Although urinary output is one of the most sensitive indices in shock, any form of shock that develops very rapidly shows other manifestations before decreased urinary output is noticed.

Urinary output should be kept above 0.5 ml/kg/hr. If the hourly output diminishes significantly, treatment must be instituted to prevent renal failure. Urinary flow of less than 20 ml/hour can cause ATN from inadequate renal circulation.

Clinical Manifestations of Specific Types of Shock

Hypovolemic Shock

Initially, urine osmolality and specific gravity increase because of sodium and water reabsorption, which attempts to support circulating volume. As altered tissue perfusion and the hypovolemic shock progress, urine osmolality and specific gravity decrease because of the kidneys' inability to reabsorb sodium and water.

Sympathetic nervous system stimulation of the skin leads to marked diaphoresis. Clients sweat profusely, which increases insensible fluid loss, leading to further hypovolemia and temperature instability. Sympathetic stimulation also results in increased pulse and respirations and decreased tissue perfusion to the skin, causing the skin to feel cool and clammy and to appear pale.

Cyanosis may indicate either decreased tissue perfusion or decreased oxygenation or both. Cyanosis is a late manifestation of decreased oxygenation.

Cardiogenic Shock

Because of the impaired muscle action or mechanical obstruction that caused the cardiogenic shock, blood is inadequately pumped through the heart. This results in a back-up of blood. When the shock is due to right-sided heart failure, this back-up is evidenced as jugular venous distention and increased CVP. (See Chapters 55 and 62 for discussions of cardiac tamponade and tension pneumothorax.) When the shock is due to left-sided failure, blood backs up into the pulmonary circulation, resulting in pulmonary edema, crackles in the lungs, and increased pulmonary capillary wedge pressure (PCWP). As in hypovolemic shock, there is stimulation of the sympathetic nervous system because of decreased cardiac output and decreased BP and all of its resultant clinical manifestations.

Distributive Shock

Anaphylactic Shock. Initially, the client may complain of a vague feeling of uneasiness or a feeling of impending doom. The massive vasodilation that occurs with anaphylaxis may cause complaints of headache as well. This may be followed by severe anxiety, dizziness, disorientation, and loss of consciousness.

Respiratory involvement may be apparent through a variety of manifestations. The initial complaint may be a feeling as though there were a lump in the throat. This is due to laryngeal edema and is followed by hoarseness, coughing, dyspnea, and stridor. Diffuse wheezes and a prolonged expiratory phase are heard on auscultation. If a pulse oximeter is in use, there may be a rapid decline in oxygen saturation.

Additional complaints may include pruritus and urticaria. Direct observation may also demonstrate edema of the eyelids, lips, or tongue (angioedema).

Neurogenic Shock. In neurogenic shock, abnormal distribution of fluid volume occurs from interruption or loss of innervation. Exceptions to the usual clinical manifestations are bradycardia and hypotension (which cannot be corrected because of loss of the ability of vasoconstriction). Below the level of injury, skin temperature takes on the same temperature as the room (poikilothermia). Skin is dry to the touch because of an inability to sweat.

Septic Shock. In the early stages of septic shock, the body experiences massive vasodilation. Warm, dry, flushed skin is apparent during this hyperdynamic stage of septic shock. The compensatory increase in cardiac output and resultant increased perfusion of the skin give this stage the name "warm shock." During later stages, when compensatory mechanisms fail, the release of MDF and decreased venous return result in decreased perfusion and "cold shock," or the hypodynamic stage. At this point, the skin becomes pale, cold, clammy, and mottled. Body temperature drops to subnormal levels. Auscultation of the lungs reveals crackles and wheezes, which develop secondary to pulmonary congestion as ARDS ensues. In addition to the clinical manifestations seen with shock in general, changes in the level of consciousness may include drowsiness and stupor progressing to coma.

Diagnostic Assessment

Diagnostic assessments of clients in shock should include oxygenation, organ perfusion, and fluid balance. Assessment of respiratory status can be accomplished to some degree by noninvasive procedures such as spirometry, pulse oximeter, or arterial blood gases (ABGs).

ABG analysis may also be done to determine whether the metabolic acidosis that occurs with shock is being effectively combated by hyperventilation. A low $Paco_2$, along with low pH and bicarbonate levels (metabolic acidosis), indicates that hyperventilation is trying to compensate. However, a rising $Paco_2$ in the presence of a persistently low pH indicates that respiratory assistance is needed. It is also important to monitor Pao_2 levels to determine whether the client is being adequately oxygenated. (See Critical Monitoring and Chapter 63 for discussions of respiratory interventions.)

CVP measurement is one of the first invasive assessments made in the presence of shock to estimate fluid loss. A pulmonary artery or Swan-Ganz catheter may also be inserted to assist with assessments of fluid status, cardiac function, and tissue oxygen consumption.

Other noninvasive assessment and monitoring tools are the cardiac monitor and the 12-lead electrocardiogram (ECG). Laboratory studies include a complete blood count, blood chemistry, and blood and body fluid cultures for certain clients.

Outcome Management

Treatment should generally be instituted for shock whenever at least two of the following three conditions occur: systolic BP of 80 mm Hg or less, pulse pressure of 20 mm Hg or less, and pulse rate of 120 or more. Pulse pressure is calculated by subtracting diastolic BP from systolic BP and normally is between 30 and 50 mm Hg.

The therapeutic management of shock has changed markedly over recent years. Lowering the head, raising the feet, and administering potent vasoconstrictor drugs were once the foundation of treatment for a client in shock. Now, emphasis is placed on maintaining adequate circulating volume, positions that do not interfere with pulmonary ventilation, and the use of medications having both vasoconstrictor and vasodilator effects.

Medical Management

Correct the Causative Factor

Assessment and an accurate differential medical diagnosis, which establish the specific cause of the shock state, form the basis for treatment. The differential medical diagnosis is usually readily made unless the shock is in an advanced stage, in which several specific forms of shock may exist at the same time. Some forms of shock more easily recognized are hypovolemic shock that is due to extensive burns or trauma and cardiogenic shock with severe chest pain and acute MI. Septic shock is probably the most difficult shock state to diagnose because of its insidious onset and complex manifestations.

Improve Oxygenation

Maintaining the client's airway is vital to the treatment of shock. In all types of shock, supplemental oxygen is administered to protect against hypoxemia. Oxygen can be delivered via a nasal cannula, a mask, a high-flow non-rebreathing mask, an endotracheal tube, or a tracheostomy tube.

Endotracheal intubation, or tracheostomy, may be performed to rest an exhausted client during severe or prolonged shock and to correct respiratory failure. By increasing the rate of pulmonary ventilation (through spontaneous or mechanical hyperventilation), it is possible to compensate for minor degrees of metabolic acidosis. This increased "blowing off" of carbon with hyperventilation begins to compensate for acid-base imbalance. Positive end-expiratory pressure (PEEP) may be added when the client is being mechanically ventilated. This assists in preventing atelectasis and may provide a higher PaO_2 for the client at a lower oxygen concentration setting. The goal of therapy is to maintain a PaO_2 greater than 50 mm Hg and an SaO_2 greater than 90% to avoid anaerobic metabolism. If the chest is congested, chest physical therapy, including vibration, percussion, and postural drainage, may be required.

Sometimes the interventions discussed cannot establish optimal tissue oxygenation. In these instances, hyperbaric oxygenation (HBO) or extracorporeal membrane oxygenation may be used. HBO involves the administration of 100% oxygen under 2 to 3 atm of pressure. This raises tissue oxygen tension to normal or above-normal levels. HBO requires the use of special chambers, which usually are available only in highly specialized institutions.

Extracorporeal membrane oxygenation is most commonly used in adults as a temporary intervention for refractory ARDS. Arterial and venous catheters are inserted, and some of the client's blood is diverted through them into a machine that artificially oxygenates the blood. This is a relatively expensive form of therapy and is usually done only in large medical centers.

Restore and Maintain Adequate Perfusion

The primary aim in treating shock is to maintain an adequate circulating blood volume. Unless this is accomplished early, subsequent therapeutic measures are of no avail, and death can be anticipated. In addition, other treatment adjuncts are necessary, which are discussed in the sections that follow. The adjuncts facilitate the distribution of blood to the body and enhance perfusion and oxygenation of the tissues with the circulating blood.

Administer Vasoactive Medications

Table 81–2 lists vasoactive medications commonly used to treat shock.

Vasoconstrictors. Vasoconstrictors elevate the systemic BP by constricting peripheral arterioles. Vasoconstrictor agents may be used briefly in shock if compensatory vasoconstriction is unable to maintain blood flow to vital organs. They may also be used to correct hypotension secondary to vasoconstrictor nerve paralysis, as in spinal anesthesia or conditions associated with massive vasodilation. However, vasoconstrictors should not

TABLE 81–2 VASOACTIVE MEDICATIONS USED IN SHOCK MANAGEMENT

Medication	Action
High-dosage dopamine (Intropin); norepinephrine (Levophed); phenylephrine (Neo-Synephrine)	Systemic vasoconstriction, especially in the gastrointestinal tract, skin, and kidney
Amrinone (Inocor); epinephrine (Adrenalin); dobutamine (Dobutrex); isoproterenol (Isuprel)	Increased heart rate, increased contractility
Amrinone; dobutamine; epinephrine; isoproterenol; nitroprusside (Nipride)	Vasodilation of blood vessels in heart and skeletal muscle
Low-dosage dopamine	Vasodilation of renal and mesenteric blood vessels
Amrinone; nitroglycerin (Tridil); nitroprusside	Relaxation of vascular smooth muscle

be used exclusively but should be given concomitantly with IV fluids in an attempt to restore adequate circulation and perfusion.

Perfusion of vital organs with blood is impossible when systolic BP is below 50 mm Hg. Usually, the goal of using vasoconstrictors is to achieve and maintain a mean BP of 70 to 80 mm Hg, which is sufficient to perfuse tissues. Generally, attempts to increase the BP beyond this level are not advisable because vasoconstrictors increase the heart's oxygen demand and may cause fatal dysrhythmias. Vasoconstrictors are used with extreme caution in cardiogenic shock. Other major adverse effects of vasoconstrictors include decreased renal and splanchnic blood flow, excessive or sudden rise in arterial BP (which may precipitate heart failure), pulmonary edema or LV decompensation, and gangrene of the fingers and toes from prolonged vasoconstriction.

Although the use of vasoconstrictors during shock is being critically evaluated, they do favorably increase blood flow to the brain and heart in severely hypotensive clients. Reduced tissue perfusion when systolic pressures are below 60 to 70 mm Hg may precipitate MI or a cerebrovascular accident.

VASODILATORS. Agents that induce vasodilation or inhibit vasoconstriction may promote recovery from shock in which intensive vasoconstriction is contributing to the problem. These include adrenergic blocking agents, ganglionic blocking agents, and direct-acting peripheral vasodilators.

Adrenergic blockade prevents harmful effects of prolonged vasoconstriction such as increased pressure in capillaries, promoting fluid loss from the vascular to the interstitial compartment, and altered blood flow, especially in the splanchnic area. Prolonged vasoconstriction also impairs cellular nutrition and allows accumulation of waste products. Adrenergic blockade prevents these changes in circulation and may also induce opposite beneficial changes.

Vasodilators may be helpful during shock when vasoconstriction is severe and persists even though fluids have been infused in what should be adequate amounts for fluid replacement. Vasodilators may be administered to try to inhibit vasoconstriction of peripheral blood vessels (the result of norepinephrine from sympathetic stimulation) so that blood can be redistributed to enhance tissue perfusion and increase vascular volume.

When shock is caused by hypovolemia, rapid and adequate fluid replacement is essential before vasodilators are used. Vasodilators are dangerous because they lower arterial blood pressure if they are given while circulating blood volume is deficient. When the circulating blood volume is inadequate, the body depends on vasoconstriction to try to maintain arterial pressure. However, when the vascular space is full and cardiac venous return is adequate, vasodilation should open arterioles in the lungs and elsewhere. This lets blood circulate, increasing cardiac output and capillary perfusion without lowering systemic BP. In fact, a vasodilator may produce a dramatic, sustained rise in the systemic arterial pressure.

Keep clients who are receiving vasodilators lying relatively flat. Elevation of the head can produce dangerous orthostatic hypotension. Older clients may have sclerotic blood vessels and may not tolerate the hypotension that may accompany administration of vasodilators. In this situation, a cardiotonic drug (such as dobutamine) may be given with the vasodilator to increase cardiac output.

Vasoconstrictor medications are sometimes given in combination with vasodilator medications. This may be done to offset the profound effects that may occur with some vasoconstrictors and to provide the benefits both types of drugs have to offer.

Characteristically, impaired tissue perfusion is correctable during early shock. However, it may be fatal if treatment is not received or is inadequate. In the later stages of shock, impaired tissue perfusion becomes "irreversible," leading to death in spite of treatment. However, treatment for "irreversible" shock is never abandoned while the client remains alive. Before a client's shock state is viewed as probably irreversible, restoration of circulating volume and identification and treatment of occult bleeding, any factors interfering with cardiopulmonary function, and overwhelming infection must be attempted.

During shock intervention, all of the basic pathophysiologic changes associated with the development of shock must be corrected. Some problems that must often be treated are the vascular problem of vasoconstriction, with the diminished tissue perfusion it causes; the intravascular problem of coagulation and sludging of blood cells; and the extravascular problem of extravasation of fluid into the extravascular space.

Assist Circulation

Mechanical devices that assist circulation or decrease the heart's workload may be used as temporary measures in managing clients in shock. Examples of these include the military or medical antishock trousers (MAST), IABP, and external counterpulsation device. (See Chapter 56 for more information.)

MAST GARMENT. MAST, also called pneumatic antishock garment (Fig. 81–8), encases the lower part of the body in a one-piece, three-chambered (one abdominal and two leg chambers) suit from the lower costal margin to the ankles. The external pressure provided by the MAST garment causes increased vascular resistance and reduces the diameter of blood vessels in the abdomen and legs. This results in impedance of blood flow and may decrease leakage into the tissues, resulting in increased perfusion of vital organs. Cardiac output and arterial BP increase.

MAST garments are most often used in trauma situations occurring outside the hospital setting for management of massive blood loss with no obtainable BP, fluid loss other than hemorrhage, and cardiac arrest caused by severe fluid or blood loss. They also help further reduce bleeding in areas being compressed, immobilize fractures of the femur and pelvis, and facilitate insertion of the IV line by increasing upper extremity cardiac output and vein filling. The use of MAST garments continues to be controversial because the decreased perfusion in the lower extremities leads to acidosis in the compressed tissues. MAST garments may be contraindicated in cardiogenic shock.

INTRA-AORTIC BALLOON PUMP. An IABP is used primarily in clients with cardiogenic shock and after open heart surgery. The heart's ability to adequately pump blood is augmented by a balloon-tipped catheter placed in

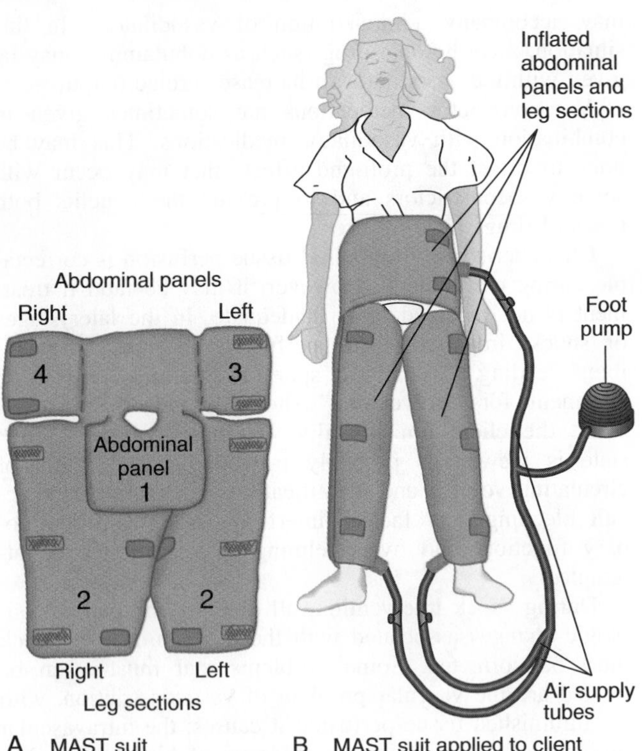

FIGURE 81–8 MAST suit, or pneumatic antishock garment. *A,* The suit is composed of two leg compartments and an abdominal compartment. *B,* MAST suit in place. Abdominal and leg compartments are attached to air tubes and a foot pump for inflation. MAST, *M*ilitary *A*nti*s*hock *T*rousers.

the descending thoracic aorta. The catheter is attached to a unit that inflates during diastole and deflates just before systole. This counterpulsation displaces blood back into the aorta and improves coronary artery circulation. In cardiogenic shock, use of the IABP reduces preload, allowing the heart to more efficiently empty, thereby increasing cardiac output. Details of the IABP are found in the Bridge to Critical Care feature on IABP in Chapter 56.

External Counterpulsation Device. This device uses the same general principles as an IABP but is applied externally to the legs. The legs are encased in air- or water-filled tubular bags connected to a pumping unit. Pressure is applied to the legs during diastole and is released in systole.

Modified Trendelenburg Position. A client in shock is usually placed in a modified Trendelenburg position with the lower extremities elevated 30 to 45 degrees, the knees straight, the trunk horizontal or very slightly raised, and the neck comfortably positioned with the head level with the chest or slightly higher (Fig. 81–9). This position promotes increased venous return from the lower extremities without compressing the abdominal organs against the diaphragm.

Elevating the legs mobilizes blood that has pooled in the lower extremities. As a result of gravity, the additional circulating blood increases venous return to the heart, thus improving cardiac output. The position is of temporary value in moderate hypovolemia. However, it does not help in severe hypovolemia, because the extremities have very little blood in them in such a state. Generally, the modified shock position is not used with cardiogenic shock, when there is already circulatory overload.

The traditional Trendelenburg position (head down, with legs elevated at least 30 degrees above the head) was once the classic shock position but is no longer used for shock management because it compresses the abdominal contents against the diaphragm, interfering with pulmonary excursion, and promotes congestion of blood in the brain, possibly contributing to cerebral edema.

Replace Fluid Volume

The mainstay of hypovolemic shock therapy is expansion of circulating blood volume by IV administration of blood or other appropriate fluids. Fluid replacement should be administered through large-bore peripheral lines, central venous lines, or both.

Various fluids are given to correct specific problems, such as electrolyte or protein deficiencies or other defects of the blood, including acidosis and hyponatremia. However, in treating hypovolemic shock, the immediate results of therapy seem to depend less on the type of fluid administered for fluid replacement than on the amount of fluid administered. Generally, enough fluid is given to exceed the normal blood volume. In part, this "extra" fluid is required because the vascular space is expanded as a result of dilation of the microcirculation. Additional fluid is also administered to replace intracellular fluid that was mobilized into the circulation as an early response to the hypovolemia.

In replacing fluids, enough volume must be administered to fill the capillaries and run through into the veins. Such fluid replacement maintains CVP and provides an adequate venous return to the heart. This promotes additional cardiac output. In addition, adequate fluid replacement decreases the blood catecholamine level and thus produces a vasodilation that promotes capillary flow. Adequate flow of fluids in the capillaries in turn perfuses tissues and prevents sludging and coagulation of blood within the vessels. Carefully monitor IV fluid replacement therapy to prevent circulatory overload. Hypervolemia can be lethal; thus aggressive fluid replacement should be tapered off when urinary output is at least 60 ml/hour, BP is greater than 100 mm Hg, or the heart rate is 60 to 100 beats per minute.

IV fluids used in shock management may include warmed crystalloids or balanced salt solutions, colloids,

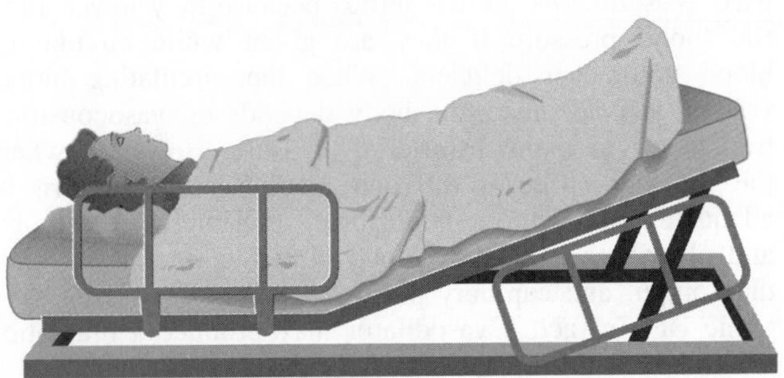

FIGURE 81–9 Positioning of the person in shock. This position is a modification of Trendelenburg's position and includes elevating the legs, leaving the trunk flat, and elevating the head and shoulders slightly.

and blood. Dextrose and water should not be used to resuscitate a client; once the dextrose is metabolized, only hypotonic water remains, which leads to greater fluid shifts.

CRYSTALLOID OR BALANCED SALT SOLUTIONS. During hypovolemic shock, the loss of circulating blood volume is also associated with redistribution of extravascular fluid. A sizable amount of fluid (about 4 L in moderately severe shock) leaves the interstitial space. This is in addition to fluid lost from the circulating volume. Thus, fluid replacement therapy must replace both blood lost from the circulation and fluid lost from the interstitial space. About two thirds of the crystalloid solution administered moves out of the vascular space into the tissues. To assist with fluid administration, a three-to-one rule has been developed. For a client's estimated blood loss, three times as much crystalloid solution must be administered for adequate volume resuscitation. Crystalloid solutions that may be administered include normal saline, Ringer's lactate, or half-normal saline.

Electrolyte solutions such as Ringer's lactate help expand extracellular volume, reduce viscosity, and prevent sludging. In a client with impaired liver function, a solution containing lactate could further compound the problem of lactic acidosis because lactate is converted to bicarbonate by the liver. If the liver is functioning normally, lactate does not accumulate. Because the liver is not an organ of primary perfusion during times of stress for the body, other solutions should be considered before Ringer's lactate.

Abnormalities of electrolyte and acid-base balance are corrected with the specific substance needed rather than with a solution that administers multiple electrolytes and acid-base components. Therapy is gauged by serial ABG and electrolyte determinations.

COLLOID SOLUTIONS. Colloid solutions contain proteins normally too large to exit at the capillary; thus they remain in the vascular compartment and increase osmotic pressure of the capillaries. This increased osmotic pressure helps retain fluid in the vascular compartment and maintain circulating volume. These solutions may be used in conjunction with crystalloid solutions in treating hypovolemic shock in an attempt to maintain an adequate circulating volume. The most commonly used colloid solutions include plasma and its components, plasma substitutes (e.g., dextran), oxygen-carrying solutions other than blood (e.g., perfluorochemicals), and hetastarch. (See discussions of blood and blood transfusions, Chapter 75.) Colloid solutions are often not used in initial fluid resuscitation after major burn injury. The capillary leakage is large enough that even the proteins escape.

Plasma is sometimes used in treating clients with low serum protein levels in an effort to control fluid escape from the vascular system. Fresh frozen plasma (FFP) is the form commonly used to improve serum protein levels. FFP may be administered after massive transfusions to restore some clotting factors deficient in "banked" blood. Because FFP requires 15 to 30 minutes to thaw, it is not used in initial fluid resuscitation with shock.

Albumin may also be used to achieve adequate osmotic pressure. Occasionally, it is administered when sufficient amounts of other fluids fail to restore an adequate circulating volume. Use of albumin is controversial because it may move into the pulmonary interstitial space, drawing water along with it. Thus, albumin may contribute to the development of ARDS.

Dextran may be used in both high- and low-molecular-weight forms. By initiating therapy with low-molecular-weight dextran and then progressing to high-molecular-weight forms, the incidence of hypersensitivity reactions to dextran can be lowered. The advantage in using dextran is that it contains large molecules that should effectively and rapidly expand the intravascular volume. Dextran can interfere with blood type and crossmatch procedures and with clotting factors. It should therefore be used only after type and crossmatch have been done and until blood is available for transfusion.

Although the administration of crystalloids, albumin, and blood has been the standard treatment of hypovolemic shock for many years, several new substances have been introduced for shock management. Perfluorochemicals such as Fluosol are non-blood, oxygen-carrying solutions that remain in the circulation for about 12 to 24 hours. Major limitations associated with the use of perfluorochemicals relate to limited immediate availability (the product must be stored frozen), administration of 80% to 100% O_2 for the solution to be effective, and accumulation of the chemicals in the body. Advantages include the high solubility of perfluorochemicals, making them readily available to the tissues, and their acceptability to clients whose religious beliefs prohibit the use of blood products. Perfluorochemicals have been researched since the 1970s and are still considered experimental at this time. Hetastarch is a glycogen-like synthetic colloid that has been used to treat hypovolemic shock and also may provide alternatives to blood administration.

BLOOD. When hemorrhage is the primary cause of shock, the rapid administration of large volumes of packed cells or whole blood may be necessary. Type-specific, crossmatched blood is the most desirable form of blood replacement. However, if the client is hemorrhaging, it may be necessary to administer type-specific, uncrossmatched blood: O-negative blood or O-positive, low–antibody titer blood. Women should receive Rh-negative blood.

When shock resulting from hemorrhage is treated, crystalloid is usually given as an initial emergency treatment to sustain blood pressure. Later, the acute anemia resulting from hemorrhage must be corrected by administration of packed cells for the prevention of hypoxemia.

During fluid replacement, a normal red blood cell mass should be maintained. Fluids given in excess of normal volume should be fluids other than blood so that they can be easily removed from the circulation by the kidneys once the shock is corrected. If the normal red blood cell mass is exceeded, it is difficult for the body to get rid of the excess red blood cells after the vascular volume contracts to normal (after adequate perfusion of tissues with blood is achieved). Because dangers also are involved in blood transfusions, blood should not be used if another fluid can satisfactorily maintain an adequate oxygen-carrying capacity and can sufficiently increase blood volume. Clients can become so dilute that there are relatively few blood cells as the result of up to 8 to 12 L of fluid being administered in only a few hours.

Provide Autotransfusion

Autotransfusion involves collecting and retransfusing blood into the same client. Autotransfusion is used in the prevention or treatment of existing hypovolemic shock caused by hemorrhage. It is common in the treatment of chest injuries.

Evaluate Fluid Replacement

Often, fluid replacement is the only treatment required for shock. However, it is difficult to evaluate whether fluid replacement is adequate. Internal losses of circulating fluid volume, including whole blood, into areas of traumatized tissue, infection, and so forth are difficult to estimate. If a vasoconstrictor drug has been administered or if prolonged vasoconstriction occurs, an additional considerable loss of circulating volume may also occur because of vasoconstriction. Large volumes of IV fluid may be administered either until systemic BP, urinary volume, and lactate levels become relatively normal or until central venous or pulmonary artery pressures, or both, become elevated.

Infusion of blood or other fluids usually continues only as long as the CVP is low, that is, below 4 cm H_2O or 2 mm Hg. When the CVP is higher than normal (e.g., above 15 cm H_2O or 11 mm Hg), benefit cannot be expected from the continued infusion of fluids or blood beyond maintenance amounts. When the CVP is low and the lungs are clear, with no indications of congestive heart failure, fluids are administered to improve the return of blood to the heart. However, some clients have a normal or low CVP in spite of faulty LV function. They readily develop congestive failure or pulmonary edema. Thus, a low or normal CVP does not always mean that fluid administration is advisable.

IV fluid administration should be stopped before extremely high elevations of pulmonary artery pressure occur if there is an adequate systemic response. An adequate volume of circulating fluid causes an ample venous return to the right side of the heart and increases the right-sided output. Pulmonary artery hypertension may develop if continued pulmonary obstruction is present because of coagulation in the microcirculation or vasoconstriction. This appears as increased pulmonary artery pressure. In the presence of right-sided heart failure, this increased pressure may back up through the right side of the heart, causing an abnormal elevation in CVP. Vasodilators may help open this partially blocked pulmonary microcirculation.

PREVENT COMPLICATIONS

Prevent Renal Impairment

Impaired kidney function and ATN may result from inadequate renal tissue perfusion, as discussed earlier. In an attempt to prevent acute renal damage, the urinary output is monitored with an indwelling catheter, and diuretics (e.g., furosemide) may be given. Correcting metabolic acidosis (see Chapter 14) and using other measures to increase blood volume and improve cardiac output also benefit the kidney as well as other tissues. If tubular necrosis is present, peritoneal dialysis or hemodialysis may be needed until regeneration of functioning renal tubular epithelium occurs. (See also Chapter 36.)

During shock, urinary output should be measured and compared with normal urinary production. The normal rate of urinary excretion from the kidneys is 1 ml/minute or 60 ml/hour. A client who becomes acutely hypovolemic or is experiencing a redistribution of circulating volume cannot maintain an hourly output of 40 to 60 ml of urine. Decreased urinary output (oliguria) typically occurs in shock. Often during shock, the urinary output may stop completely (anuria). When this occurs, the client is said to be in renal shutdown or renal failure.

Oliguria does not contraindicate the administration of large volumes of fluid in the treatment of shock. In fact, restoring renal capillary perfusion along with that of other vital capillaries restores urine volume production as long as tubular necrosis is not already present. Fluid administration may prevent ATN in the kidneys.

A large amount of tissue damage (e.g., crush injuries) may cause a release of myoglobin from muscle tissue. Because the myoglobin molecule is large, a type of mechanical renal failure may result from attempts to excrete large amounts of myoglobin. Fluid administration is again important to decrease damage to the tubules.

Prevent Gastrointestinal Bleeding

An early physiologic response to shock is a decrease in splanchnic circulation. This reduces the blood supply to the stomach and bowel, causing inadequate gastrointestinal tissue perfusion and delayed gastric emptying; thus, vomiting with aspiration of gastric contents into the lung may occur. For this reason and for diagnostic purposes, nasogastric (NG) suction is often used during treatment of shock. A double-lumen, 16 Fr. NG tube is usually used in adults.

Assess gastric aspirate periodically for blood. Guaiac solution or Hemoccult tablets and reagent can be used to check for blood; litmus paper checks the pH to determine the acidity of the stomach. Promptly report new findings of blood or increases in the amount of blood. Histamine blockers and proton pump inhibitors are used to reduce gastric acid in the stomach. Antacids may also be instilled through the tube when the pH is acidic.

When shock is caused by gastrointestinal bleeding, other NG tubes may be used. If the suspected cause of bleeding is a gastric ulcer, a 36 Fr. Ewald tube may be used. This tube's many large holes facilitate saline lavage and removal of blood clots. If esophageal varices are suspected or present, a Sengstaken-Blakemore tube is often used. This triple-lumen tube exerts pressure on the lower portion of the esophagus and the upper portion of the stomach, where varices are most prominent. Pressure is created by esophageal and gastric balloons inflated with air. Gentle traction is applied to keep the balloons in proper position (see Chapter 47).

The medical management of shock has been discussed in general. Tables 81–3, 81–4, and 81–5 give some of the specific interventions for hypovolemic, cardiogenic, and distributive shock, respectively.

PROVIDE PHARMACOLOGIC MANAGEMENT

Antibiotics

Antibiotics are essential when shock is due to infection. If septic shock is suspected, a blood specimen for culture and sensitivity is taken at once, and broad-spectrum antibiotics are started even though the specific infectious organism has not yet been identified. When the blood sample is drawn, samples of urine, sputum, and fluid from

TABLE 81–3 SUMMARY OF THE MANAGEMENT OF HYPOVOLEMIC SHOCK

Etiology	Clinical Situation	Intervention*
Blood loss	Massive trauma Gastrointestinal bleeding Ruptured aortic aneurysm Surgery Erosion of vessel from lesion, tubes, or other devices DIC	Stop external bleeding with direct pressure, pressure dressing, tourniquet (as last resort) Reduce intra-abdominal or retroperitoneal bleeding by applying MAST garment or prepare for emergency surgery Administer lactated Ringer's solution or normal saline Transfuse with fresh whole blood, packed cells, fresh frozen plasma, platelets, or other clotting factors, if significant improvement does not occur with crystalloid administration Use non-blood plasma expanders (albumin, hetastarch, dextran) until blood is available Conduct autotransfusion if appropriate
Plasma loss	Burns Accumulation of intra-abdominal fluid Malnutrition Severe dermatitis DIC	Administer low-dose cardiotonics (dopamine, dobutamine) Administer lactated Ringer's solution or normal saline Administer albumin, fresh frozen plasma, hetastarch, or dextran if cardiac output is still low
Crystalloid loss	Dehydration (e.g., diabetic ketoacidosis, heat exhaustion) Protracted vomiting, diarrhea Nasogastric suction	Administer isotonic or hypotonic saline with electrolytes as needed to maintain normal circulating volume and electrolyte balance

*Assumes that airway management and cardiac monitoring are ongoing.
DIC, disseminated intravascular coagulation; MAST, *m*ilitary or *m*edical *a*ntishock *t*rousers.

TABLE 81–4 SUMMARY OF THE MANAGEMENT OF CARDIOGENIC SHOCK

Etiology	Clinical Situation	Intervention*
Mycocardial disease or injury	Acute myocardial infarction Myocardial contusion Cardiomyopathies	Fluid-challenge with up to 300 ml of normal saline solution or Ringer's lactate to rule out hypovolemia, unless heart failure or pulmonary edema is present Insert CVP or pulmonary artery catheter; monitor cardiac output, pulmonary artery pressure, and PCWP; administer IV fluids to maintain left ventricular filling pressure of 15–20 mm Hg Administer inotropics (e.g., dopamine or dobutamine) Vasodilators (e.g., sodium nitroprusside, nitroglycerin, calcium-channel blockers, morphine) Diuretics (e.g., mannitol or furosemide) Cardiotonics (e.g., digitalis) Beta-blockers (propranolol) Glucocorticosteroids† Intra-aortic balloon pump or external counterpulsation device if unresponsive to other therapies
Valvular disease or injury	Ruptured aortic cusp Ruptured papillary muscle Ball thrombus	Same as above: if rapid response does not occur, prepare for prompt cardiac surgery
External pressure on the heart interferes with heart filling or emptying	Pericardial tamponade due to trauma, aneurysm, cardiac surgery, pericarditis Massive pulmonary embolus Tension pneumothorax Ascites Hemoperitoneum Mechanical ventilation	Relieve tamponade with ECG-assisted pericardiocentesis; repair surgically if it recurs Thrombolytic (streptokinase) or anticoagulant (heparin) therapy; surgery for removal of clot Relieve air accumulation with needle thoracostomy or chest tube insertion Relieve fluid accumulation with paracentesis Reduce inspiratory pressure
Cardiac dysrhythmias	Tachydysrhythmias Bradydysrhythmias Pulseless electrical activity	Treat dysrhythmias; be prepared to initiate CPR, cardiac pacing

*Assumes that airway management and cardiac monitoring are ongoing.
†Controversial.
CPR, cardiopulmonary resuscitation; CVP, central venous pressure; ECG, electrocardiogram; IV, intravenous; PCWP, pulmonary capillary wedge pressure.

TABLE 81–5 SUMMARY OF THE MANAGEMENT OF DISTRIBUTIVE SHOCK

Etiology	Clinical Situation	Intervention*
Anaphylactic shock	Allergy to food, medicines, dyes, insect bites, stings, or latex	Prepare for surgical management of the airway Decrease further absorption of antigen (e.g., stop IV fluid, place tourniquet between injection or sting site and heart if feasible) Epinephrine (1:100) 2 inhalations every 3 hours, *or* Epinephrine (1:1000) 0.2–0.5 ml every 5–15 min given subcutaneously, *or* Epinephrine (1:10,000) 0.5–1.0 ml every 5–15 min given at a rate of 1 mg/min IV fluid resuscitation with isotonic solution Diphenhydramine HCl or H_1-receptor antagonist IV Theophylline IV drip for bronchospasm Steroids IV Vasopressors (e.g., norepinephrine, metaraminol bitartrate, high-dosage dopamine) Gastric lavage for ingested antigen Ice pack to injection or sting site Meat tenderizer paste to sting site
Septic shock	Often gram-negative septicemia but also caused by other organisms in debilitated, immunodeficient, or chronically ill clients	Identify origin of sepsis; culture all suspected sources Vigorous IV fluid resuscitation with normal saline Empirical antibiotic therapy: until sensitivities are reported If suspected organism is gram-positive, vancomycin is used; if suspected organism is gram-negative, give expanded-spectrum penicillin or a cephalosporin and aminoglycoside Administer cardiotonic agents (e.g., dopamine or dobutamine, norepinephrine, isoproterenol, digitalis, calcium) Naloxone (narcotic antagonist) Prostaglandins Monoclonal antibodies Temperature control (both hypothermia and hyperthermia are noted) Heparin, clotting factors, blood products if DIC develops
Neurogenic (spinal) shock	Spinal anesthesia Spinal cord injury	Normal saline to restore volume Treat bradycardia with atropine Vasopressors (e.g., norepinephrine, metaraminol bitartrate, high-dosage dopamine, and phenylephrine) may be given Place client in modified Trendelenburg's position
Vasovagal reaction	Severe pain Severe emotional stress	Place client in a head-down or recumbent position Give atropine if bradycardia and profound hypotension; eliminate pain

*Assumes airway management and cardiac monitoring are ongoing.
DIC, disseminated intravascular coagulation; IV, intravenous.

draining wounds, sinuses, and so forth are also taken for culture. The antibiotic selected depends on the cause of the infection and should not be initiated until after all cultures have been taken. However, once cultures have been obtained, treatment with empirical broad-spectrum antibiotics should be initiated. Cephalosporins, gentamicin, and aminoglycosides may be used in combination until specific culture and sensitivity information is available. Antibiotics may also be administered along with appropriate surgical management to clients with open or potentially contaminated wounds who are experiencing hypovolemic shock.

Monoclonal Technology

Multiple therapies that specifically target the mediators of septic shock are currently being researched. Monoclonal antiendotoxin (e.g., HA-1A and E5) neutralizes the endotoxin or toxicity of the offending pathogen or the immune response itself. Interleukin-1 receptor agonists, anti-tumor necrosing factor antibodies, and platelet activating factor inhibitors are also in research trials for their effectiveness in reducing the morbidity and mortality from septic shock. Research results to date on these three therapies are mixed, but researchers continue to search for the solution in preventing the significant negative outcomes of septic shock.

Heparin

The anticoagulant effect of heparin may help prevent complications or treat DIC. The dosage is usually adjusted according to clotting studies. Heparin is also used because of the prolonged immobility often associated with shock. Immobility predisposes clients to venous thrombosis and pulmonary emboli. The treatment of DIC may include heparin administration to minimize consumption of clotting factors. Heparin also may be appropriate for clients with ARDS if the primary cause of the respiratory insufficiency is suspected to be DIC or massive microembolism.

Steroids

Steroids have several effects that may assist the client in neurogenic shock after spinal cord injury. They are given to reduce edema in the cord and have been shown to improve recovery. They assist in treatment by stabilizing lysosomal membrane and preventing intracellular release of enzymes. Complications from high-dose steroid therapy include acute gastrointestinal bleeding, aggravation of diabetes, and immunosuppression. Steroids used to be given to treat septic shock, but mortality was not reduced and the practice was abandoned.

Naloxone

Naloxone (Narcan), an opiate antagonist, is commonly used to treat narcotic and synthetic narcotic overdosages. During stress, opiate-like substances known as enkephalins and endorphins are released from the brain. Although the mechanisms of action are not clear, endorphins may play a role in capillary bed vasodilation found in all forms of shock. Studies indicate that when naloxone is administered to animals not in shock, no significant cardiovascular effects are noted. However, when administered during shock, naloxone reverses the hypotension and decreases cardiac contractility. It is believed that naloxone blocks the effects of endorphins and enkephalins.

Epinephrine

Epinephrine is the drug of choice for emergency treatment of allergic reactions (anaphylaxis). Epinephrine inhibits histamine release and antagonizes its effects on end organs, resulting in reversal of the bronchial constriction, increased capillary permeability, and vasodilation, which occur with acute anaphylactic reactions. The overall effect is improved respiratory status and cardiovascular stability.

Diphenhydramine

Anaphylaxis can also be treated with antihistamines, like diphenhydramine (Benadryl). This medication acts primarily to relieve clinical manifestations associated with anaphylaxis rather than to stop the release of histamine. Therefore, epinephrine is always administered first in treating anaphylaxis.

Histamine H_2-Receptor Antagonists

Histamine H_2-receptor antagonists, which inhibit gastric acid secretion, may be administered intravenously to a client experiencing shock to prevent stress ulcers. They may be prescribed in combination with oral antacids. Stress ulcers are often lethal complications of severe illness or injury produced by continuous shunting of blood from the gastrointestinal tract from extended sympathetic nervous system stimulation.

Narcotics

The need for pain relief may be obvious in clients experiencing different types of shock. However, the use of narcotics for pain management may, unfortunately, be dangerous. Narcotics interfere with vasoconstriction, and vasoconstriction may be the mechanism by which the client's BP is maintained. Morphine sulfate, however, causes pooling of blood in the extremities and contributes to a decrease in anxiety. These effects may prove useful for the client in cardiogenic shock.

Cardiotonic Medications

Medications that improve myocardial contraction are basic in treating those forms of shock that decrease cardiac output (e.g., hypovolemic shock and cardiogenic shock):

- Digitalis is often used if there is evidence of cardiac failure. By strengthening and slowing the heart beat, digitalis supports a weakened heart and may reduce the heart rate to a more normal level.
- Lidocaine, bretylium, quinidine, and procainamide may treat dysrhythmias that tend to reduce cardiac efficiency. However, these medications reduce myocardial contractility.
- Atropine may treat bradycardia, which predisposes clients to cardiogenic shock.

Calcium

Calcium is needed for normal functioning of the nervous and cardiovascular systems and for blood clotting. The value and dosages of calcium in treating shock are not clear. However, calcium may be administered if impaired cardiac function is evident. Calcium may precipitate toxic effects in a person who has received digitalis. It is given only with extreme caution to such a person. Monitor for evidence of digitalis toxicity (e.g., bradyarrhythmias or tachyarrhythmias, ST-segment depression).

Calcium chloride should be given intravenously only. Calcium gluconate may be given intramuscularly but is very irritating to tissues. Although calcium chloride and calcium gluconate are both available as 10% solutions, they are not identical in concentration. Do not substitute one for the other. Indications of hypocalcemia may be subtle. Careful assessment is essential. (See discussions of calcium in Chapter 13.)

Nursing Management of the Medical Client

Nursing outcomes are similar to medical outcomes in that the overall goals of care are to correct the causative factor if possible, improve oxygenation, restore and maintain adequate tissue perfusion, and prevent complications. However, a majority of the interventions provided for clients in shock require a physician's order and are not independent nursing actions. The nurse's major responsibilities in shock include assessment of the client's condition and timely and accurate performance of dependent interventions.

ASSESSMENT

Because a client's condition can change rapidly in shock, frequent nursing assessment is essential. Documentation of the progress and response to interventions needs to be concise, yet convey the client's status minute by minute.

Initiate a flow sheet containing all pertinent data in an easily read format. This flow sheet must accompany the assessments are essential in treating shock. Blood chemistries, blood gases, oxygen saturations, and electrolytes need to be determined frequently and reported promptly so therapy can be adjusted to the client's rapidly changing physiologic status.

The first step in assessing a person in shock is a general overview, giving attention to airway, breathing, and circulation (ABC). Once the airway is patent, air exchange is adequate, a pulse is present, and the cervical spine is immobilized (if it is a trauma situation), perform a rapid, cursory initial head-to-toe physical assessment. The initial assessment goal is to identify major problems and gross abnormalities. Give further detailed attention to specific injuries or problems after shock is stabilized.

IMPROVE OXYGENATION. Several assessments should be performed to determine that no airway or breathing problems exist. To determine airway patency, assess for the presence of noisy respirations and check for obstructions. Listen to lung sounds to determine adequate air movement. Assess the respiratory rate and effort to evaluate the adequacy of breathing. Evaluate chest wall expansion and assess for chest wall bulges or defects. Monitor for tracheal deviation, which could indicate tension pneumothorax.

When caring for clients experiencing shock, carefully differentiate nursing diagnoses concerning pain and impaired gas exchange. Restlessness is an assessment finding common to both and can thus be easily misinterpreted. Too often, clients who are restless, especially trauma victims, are given narcotics because their behavior is incorrectly interpreted as resulting from pain. However, the restlessness frequently is actually due to hypoxia, and narcotics worsen the problem. The decision to administer narcotics is often a nursing decision. It is important to assess the need for these medications carefully. Attention to positioning, splinting of injured areas, breathing techniques, and comfort measures may provide safer and more effective pain relief than narcotics. (Pain is discussed in detail in Chapter 23.)

RESTORE AND MAINTAIN ADEQUATE PERFUSION. To complete the critical assessment of ABCs, circulation must be evaluated. Assess the client's pulse, blood pressure, skin color, temperature, heart sounds, peripheral pulses, state of hydration, and skin perfusion (e.g., capillary refill time <3 seconds). Check the condition of the mucous membranes, sclera, and conjunctivae; the presence of pallor or cyanosis; and fullness of the neck veins (jugular venous distention, which may suggest right heart failure and cardiogenic shock).

It is imperative that the adequacy of blood volume be determined prior to administration of narcotics to a client suffering from acute, multiple trauma. Narcotic administration causes vasodilation, which results in severe hypotension or shock. If a narcotic is administered intramuscularly to a client in shock, it also may not be completely absorbed because of the vasoconstriction that is present. Because the client experiences little or no pain relief, then a second injection may be given. Once fluid resuscitation is complete and the circulating volume is restored, the client may absorb both doses of the narcotic. No one in shock should be given intramuscular medications.

When narcotics are appropriate for a client in shock, they are most effective if administered intravenously in small doses. When caring for trauma victims, especially those with massive injury, remember that the extent of the injury does not necessarily coincide with the amount of pain being experienced. Careful assessment is necessary once narcotic administration seems safe (in terms of the client's hemodynamic status). Assess the client's blood pressure more closely after IV administration of narcotics to watch for hypotension.

Even though a person in shock may feel cold and may be hypothermic, do not apply heat to the skin. Heat application dilates peripheral blood vessels and draws blood away from the vital organs (where it is life-sustaining) into the vessels of the skin. This interferes with the body's initial compensatory mechanism of peripheral vasoconstriction. Heat also increases the body's metabolism. In turn, this increases the need for oxygen and puts an added strain on the heart.

This does not mean that the person is kept in a cold environment. The environment is kept warm because it is important that the person not become chilled. Chilling and shivering require energy expenditure needed to maintain vital functions. Chilling also contributes to sludging of blood in the microcirculation. Hypothermia slows the heart, increases the likelihood of ventricular fibrillation, and inhibits the body's reparative processes.

After potentially life-threatening problems are treated, take complete vital signs, with BP taken in both arms to rule out other causes of hypovolemic shock (i.e., thoracic dissection, aneurysm). It is important to take postural vital signs if applicable and if it is safe to do so. Do not take postural vital signs if the client has multiple traumatic injuries; if there is evidence of vertebral, pelvic, or femoral fracture; or if hypotension already exists. Clients with postural hypotension should not be sent to the x-ray department for upright films until they are adequately volume-resuscitated. If x-rays must be taken, clients require constant attendance by a nurse who monitors vital signs, administers IV fluids if necessary, and provides guidance to x-ray department personnel regarding movement, positioning, and timing of studies.

Measurement of postural vital signs is taken when there is a history or presence of significant blood loss, unexplained tachycardia, a history of fluid loss (e.g., diarrhea, vomiting, diuretic therapy, or third-space loss), unexplained syncope, blunt chest or abdominal trauma, or abdominal pain.

Alternative Methods of Blood Pressure Monitoring. Often when a client is in shock, it is difficult to hear the BP with a standard stethoscope. Two commonly used techniques to obtain BP measurements are palpation of the radial or brachial pulse during deflation of the BP cuff and use of a Doppler instrument. When palpation is used, the first palpable pulse noted during deflation of the cuff is the systolic BP. Document the BP as such (e.g., 90/palp). A Doppler amplifies arterial and venous pulsations by ultrasonography. Various Doppler probes are available and are used instead of a stethoscope to measure BP. Systolic BP is easily heard by placing the probe over the brachial artery after applying transmission gel. The diastolic BP is not obtainable when the Doppler is used.

For clarity and accuracy, document the method by which BP readings are taken (in addition to the readings themselves) and whether palpation or a Doppler monitor is used. This is important because these readings may be higher or lower than those obtained in the standard way with a cuff and stethoscope. Likewise, document whether readings are obtained by automatic BP machines even though readings from these machines may not differ from those taken in the standard way.

Direct measurement of arterial BP by use of an arterial line often is done during shock. Discussion of arterial lines is found in Chapter 55.

Temperature Monitoring. An accurate core temperature measurement is important in assessing a client in shock. Sometimes an indwelling flexible rectal probe connected to a continuous display monitor is more accurate and less traumatic than intermittent rectal temperature measurements with a standard thermometer. Core temperature can also be measured with a thermometer inserted by the manufacturer into an indwelling urinary catheter. Tympanic temperatures are commonly used in critical care settings and provide core temperature measurements. Core temperature can also be obtained if the client has a thermodilution (Swan-Ganz) catheter in place.

Oral temperature measurement is neither accurate nor safe. During shock, the buccal mucosa is poorly perfused, and the client should be receiving oxygen by mask or nasal prongs. (Because clients in shock are hypoxemic, the procedure of removing the oxygen long enough to obtain an oral temperature is not routinely recommended.)

Cardiac Monitoring. For assessment and evaluation purposes, the electrical activity of the heart needs to be continuously monitored in all clients in shock, regardless of age. Nurses caring for clients experiencing shock need to be able to initiate cardiac monitoring, recognize cardiac dysrhythmias, and initiate treatment for any potentially lethal dysrhythmias that occur (see Chapter 57).

During the initial resuscitation period, it may be more appropriate to place the ECG monitor electrodes on the client's shoulders rather than on the chest. This placement does not interfere with chest film findings. It also allows better access to the chest for thoracic procedures such as insertion of chest tubes, pericardiocentesis, and CVP line placement. Once the client is stabilized, the electrodes may be moved to the chest.

Hemodynamic Monitoring. Measurement of CVP is one hemodynamic technique that may be used in initial shock management, especially with hypovolemic shock. However, because CVP only provides information regarding preload, peripheral intra-arterial lines or a pulmonary artery catheter is inserted as soon as possible. Blood volume needs to be expanded as the vascular space enlarges, and CVP measurements are used to determine the amount of fluid needed to fill the enlarging vascular space. The rate of fluid replacement is adjusted to maintain the desired CVP. It is serious if the CVP continues to fall in spite of fluid replacement. This means that the rate and volume of fluid replacement are not sufficient to meet the client's physiologic needs.

Peripheral arterial catheters are commonly used in shock to measure arterial BP and MAP and to obtain blood samples for chemical and blood gas analysis. These catheters are usually placed in the radial artery but may also be placed in the femoral or brachial arteries. Pulmonary artery and PCWP measurements are monitored to assess left-sided heart function and to guide fluid administration. These pressures are measured through a Swan-Ganz catheter. The PCWP corresponds to the LV end-diastolic pressure. This is the pressure in the LV just before contraction. A rise in this pressure in a client with cardiogenic shock may indicate left-sided heart failure. A low value in a client with hypovolemic shock may indicate that volume replacement is needed. In a client with septic shock, lower values would be expected during the warm phase and higher values during the cold phase.

Depending on the type of Swan-Ganz catheter used, additional measurements may be obtained. Some catheters have a fiberoptic tip that allows measurement of oxygen saturation of hemoglobin in the venous blood (Svo_2). Svo_2 is measured in the pulmonary artery, just before the blood's reoxygenation in the lungs. This reading gives an average of the tissue's uptake or use of oxygen in the body. The normal range for Svo_2 is 60% to 80%. When the Svo_2 falls below 60%, it may indicate either decreased arterial oxygenation or increased tissue oxygen demand. If the Svo_2 is greater than 80%, the indication, in relation to shock, is that the oxygen is unable either to reach the tissues or to be extracted by the tissues.

Most Swan-Ganz catheters also have a thermistor bead just proximal to the balloon. This may be used to determine cardiac output by a thermodilution technique. A fourth lumen opens at the level of the right atrium, and CVP measurements (preload) can be obtained through this lumen.

Monitoring Cardiac Output. Cardiac output, measured in liters per minute, is the amount of blood pumped by the LV into the aorta each minute. During shock, cardiac output may be decreased because of myocardial damage resulting from an MI or, in hypovolemic shock, from inadequate volume replacement.

Because of the widespread use of Swan-Ganz catheters and the ease of performing measurements, cardiac output monitoring is used in managing all types of shock. These measurements assess overall cardiac function and the function of the LV. Factors that may alter cardiac output include heart rate, SVR, age, body size, exercise, and (in persons with cardiac problems) decreased filling or emptying of the LV.

Cardiac index is the cardiac output divided by the body surface area. Cardiac output as a separate reading does not take into account the amount of tissue that needs to be perfused. By figuring body size into the calculation, a more accurate assessment is obtained.

SVR can be determined by using the cardiac output and the MAP. SVR measures afterload and provides information regarding vasoconstriction or vasodilation. Decreased SVR indicates systemic vasodilation and may indicate the need for administration of vasoconstrictors. Increased SVR indicates systemic vasoconstriction and the potential need for vasodilators. Arterial BP and cardiac function should always be taken into consideration before administering vasoconstrictors or vasodilators.

PREVENT COMPLICATIONS. Although it is important to begin assessments and interventions with the ABCs, additional assessments are necessary to evaluate the client's overall condition and prevent complications. Additional assessments important in preventing complications include evaluation of:

- Level of consciousness and orientation ×3 (i.e., person, place, time)
- Ability to move extremities
- Sensation in all extremities
- Hand grasps
- Response to verbal and painful stimuli
- Pupil size and reaction to light
- Presence of abnormal posturing; presence, location, intensity, and duration of pain and what relieves the pain
- Bowel sounds
- Abdominal distention or rigidity
- Circumference of abdomen or extremities
- Presence of lacerations, contusions, ecchymoses, petechiae, and purpura (also check for bruising over flank area)
- Bone deformities
- Presence of medical alert tags or bracelets

RENAL IMPAIRMENT. An indwelling urinary catheter is a simple means of monitoring a client during shock. Continuously measuring urinary flow provides important information about peripheral blood flow and kidney function. Because the amount of urine excreted during shock is often very small, it is important to have an accurate, calibrated urine collector. In some settings, the catheter may be attached to a urimeter collector or to a more complex electric urimeter.

Urinary volume changes can be highly important as an index of the success or failure of therapy. Minimal (<0.5 ml/kg/hr) or absent urinary output indicates treatment is not successful. Increasing urinary output is a favorable sign. Assess the client's urinary output routinely and record it at least every hour.

DIAGNOSIS, OUTCOMES, INTERVENTIONS

Altered Tissue Perfusion. The nursing diagnosis *Altered Peripheral Tissue Perfusion* can be used to describe the reduced tissue perfusion and inadequate effective circulating intravascular blood volume. This diagnosis does not describe the oxygen-carrying capacity of the blood, but rather the volume of circulating blood and its ability to reach the tissues. The diagnosis can be written *Altered Peripheral Tissue Perfusion related to actual or relative (specify type) hypovolemia secondary to shock (specify type).* Other potential nursing diagnoses for the client in shock are listed in Box 81–1.

Outcomes. Nursing care of the client with shock is complex. Specific nursing and medical interventions vary according to individual needs and the setting in which care is delivered (e.g., emergency department versus intensive care unit). However, four major outcomes of care are desired:

1. Adequate blood flow (tissue perfusion) and cellular oxygenation are achieved to maintain the integrity of the tissue or organ.
2. The metabolic needs of the tissue or organ are reduced or maintained.
3. The client and family will cope effectively during the acute stage of shock.
4. The client and significant others will understand the cause of the problem and will modify their lifestyle to minimize or eliminate the causative factor.

Interventions. In caring for clients with altered tissue perfusion, your responsibilities are as follows:

- Provide continuous assessment of the client. Cardiovascular and respiratory changes can occur rapidly, and interventions must be adjusted promptly. Document observations clearly and concisely.
- Help decrease tissue oxygen demand. Because shock states can double the body's O_2 consumption, promote factors that decrease tissue oxygen need. Interventions aimed at decreasing total body work, pain, anxiety, and temperature will decrease tissue oxygen demand.
- Help the client (and family) to feel physically and emotionally comfortable.
- Facilitate expression of concerns and questions by the client and family. For example, try to reduce the client's fears and anxieties about what is happening and about the equipment being used.
- Keep equipment and supplies (e.g., suction, emergency drugs) available and in working order.

BOX 81–1 Potential Nursing Diagnoses for the Client in Shock

Activity Intolerance
Altered Family Processes
Altered Nutrition: Less than Body Requirements
Altered Role Performance
Altered Thought Processes
Altered Tissue Perfusion: Cerebral, Cardiopulmonary, Renal, Gastrointestinal, Peripheral
Anticipatory Grieving
Anxiety
Body Image Disturbance
Constipation
Decreased Cardiac Output
Fear
Fluid Volume Deficit
Impaired Gas Exchange
Impaired Physical Mobility
Impaired or Risk for Impaired Skin Integrity
Impaired Verbal Communication
Ineffective Airway Clearance
Ineffective Breathing Pattern
Ineffective Family Coping: Compromised
Pain
Personal Identity Disturbance
Self-Esteem Disturbance
Self-Care Deficit: Feeding, Bathing/Hygiene, Dressing/Grooming, Toileting
Sensory/Perceptual Alterations: Visual, Auditory, Kinesthetic, Gustatory, Tactile
Sleep Pattern Disturbance
Spiritual Distress

- Implement appropriate, planned nursing interventions to prevent complications that can develop from enforced immobilization.
- Provide adequate pain relief, because pain intensifies shock. Base this intervention on careful assessment.
- Provide care to the family.

A client in shock is extremely ill and may die. In addition, the stress of the situation is compounded by emergency medical treatment, with all the people, equipment, and movement this entails. During shock management, nurses have to attend to numerous delegated medical care activities. However, there must be sufficient nursing resources to provide psychosocial care (e.g., reassurance, emotional support) to the client and family. All of these people involved may be frightened, anxious, confused, and very dependent.

Keep the client's family informed of what is happening. They need information on which to base decisions. Because of the family's anxiety, the nurse may need to calmly repeat information several times. See the Client Education Guide for information to be conveyed. Remember that the client and significant others may be experiencing "psychological shock." They often need (and greatly appreciate) opportunities to discuss with care providers their important concerns.

Do not keep loved ones away from the client unnecessarily. Because of limited space, there may be times when they have to wait in another room for a period of time. However, they should not be kept away long and should be given a reasonable explanation of why it is necessary to leave their loved one.

A client experiencing shock requires emotional support. When caught up in the sudden drama of an emergency or critical care, health professionals sometimes forget that the experience and setting are often new and very frightening for the client. Unfortunately, "dehumanization" of the client may occasionally occur during the rush of emergency treatment. Whether a client appears to be conscious or not, always explain what is happening. Keep the atmosphere as quiet and orderly as possible. Eliminate unnecessary chatter. Commonly, recovered clients remember hearing what was said and were aware of what happened to them even though they appeared to be unconscious.

Among a nurse's greatest responsibilities are providing support, comfort, and advocacy to clients receiving care and to their significant others. In nursing clients who are critically ill and experiencing shock, this is very important.

CLIENT EDUCATION GUIDE

Shock

- It is difficult to prevent the occurrence of shock because the causes are often unpredictable. If your family member is in shock, obtain precise, consistent information about his or her current status and prognosis.
- Learn about the monitoring equipment in use.
- Learn how to communicate with the client who is intubated or unconscious.
- Learn how to demonstrate love and caring to someone surrounded by equipment.
- Participate in your family member's care during the hospital stay; this increases your ability to provide care at home.
- Learn how to prevent recurrence if the cause was avoidable.

EVALUATION

It is expected that the client will achieve adequate tissue perfusion and make a full recovery without complications from the type of shock being experienced, be transferred to a medical unit, and eventually be dismissed to home. Recovery from the cause of the shock may be delayed because of the complications created from the shock episode (e.g., wound healing).

Surgical Management

Although surgical interventions that can help in shock states are limited, they may be very useful in trauma situations. In hypovolemic shock caused by trauma, surgery can be performed in an attempt to control sources of bleeding. Once bleeding has been controlled, interventions aimed at restoring adequate fluid volume are more effective.

Self-Care

Shock must be fully resolved before a client is transferred or discharged (unless the client is being transported for the treatment of shock). Clients who survive shock find that recovery from the precipitating problem is delayed. They may also experience some feelings of confusion, depression, or grief when they realize that they lived through a very critical illness.

MULTIPLE ORGAN DYSFUNCTION SYNDROME

Single organ failure (e.g., heart failure, renal failure) has long been recognized as a cause of mortality and morbidity in critically ill clients. In trauma centers in the late 1960s, a new form of organ failure was recognized, that of sequential failure of the lungs, liver, and kidneys usually followed by death. By the 1970s, the syndrome of sequential organ failure was well described. Today, this problem is named *multiple organ dysfunction syndrome* (MODS), *multiple organ system failure,* or *multiorgan system failure* and is considered to be present when two or more organs fail. More recently, the precursor to MODS has been labeled as *systemic inflammatory response syndrome* (SIRS).

Etiology and Risk Factors

There are several causes of MODS, including dead tissue, injured tissue, infection, perfusion deficits, and persistent sources of inflammation such as pancreatitis or pneumonitis. Acute lung injury is usually present in some form. People known to be at high risk for developing MODS include those with impaired immune responses such as the elderly, clients with chronic illnesses, clients with malnutrition, and clients with cancer. In addition, clients with prolonged or exaggerated inflammatory responses are at risk, including victims of severe trauma and clients with sepsis.

Prevention is a primary direction of current therapy. Source control is a major emphasis. Whenever possible, the potential source of sepsis or inflammation is excised or removed (e.g., full-thickness burn wound). Unfortunately, the source cannot be removed in many cases, such as pneumonia, pancreatitis, soft tissue injury, and hematoma. When the source cannot be removed, empirical antimicrobial agents are used to reduce risk.

It would be helpful to clinicians to be able to predict which clients are at the highest risk, but accurate prediction remains elusive. The most predictive variables appear to be the ratio of arterial oxygen tension (PaO_2) to the fraction of inspired oxygen (FiO_2) on day 1; the plasma lactate on day 2; the serum bilirubin on day 6; and the serum creatinine of day 12 postinjury. When nurses note these predictors, increased surveillance should begin.

Pathophysiology

In the healthy person, the normal integrated inflammatory immune response (IIR) functions to protect tissue from microbial invasion and rid the body of cellular debris and foreign material. The IIR is a continual process of responses until the insult slows and the client's condition stabilizes. The IIR stops once it is no longer needed. SIRS is a case of unchecked inflammatory responses. MODS is the end result of the prolonged response.

Most inciting events start with a local injury from trauma, infection, or lack of perfusion. Bacteria introduced into the wound or allowed to grow in necrotic tissues because of a decreased immune response activate the systemic inflammatory responses. Bacteria release toxins that activate systemic mediators of inflammation. Activation of the systemic response is an effort to "recruit help" to battle the invasion of microorganisms.

Once the inflammatory response becomes systemic, it is controlled by chemical mediators of inflammation. Mediators include bradykinin, complement, histamine, interleukin-1, prekallikrein, prostaglandins, and tumor necrosis factor. These powerful mediators of inflammation induce a systemic response. Endothelial cells are a common target for some mediators. The endothelium is destroyed, and blood flow is reduced to the tissues. Endothelial damage is produced by endotoxins from bacteria, tumor necrosis factor, interleukin-1, platelet activating factors, and many others. When this inflammatory response is unchecked, it produces damage to organs and tissues by altering perfusion, disturbing oxygen supply or demand, or changing metabolic dysfunctions. Metabolism increases under the direction of mediators such as cortisol and the catecholamines.

Many organs "respond" to MODS. The lungs are usually the first to malfunction, because of the large surface area of pulmonary epithelium combined with the presence of bacterial contamination from systemic blood return. The GI tract is the second system to malfunction, and it propagates conditions for further deterioration of other organs. Once the GI tract is malfunctioning, bacteria quickly relocate from tract to other organs. Additionally, the hypermetabolic state increases gastric acid production, increasing the risk of ulceration and bleeding. The most serious metabolic problem is hypermetabolism. The hypermetabolic state is continued by cell-to-cell communication and the sympathetic nervous system responding in its usual "fight-or-flight" response.

Classification

There are two types of MODS. *Primary* MODS results directly from "a well-defined insult in which organ dysfunction occurs early and is directly attributed to the insult itself."[1] The direct insult initially causes a localized inflammatory response that may or may not progress to SIRS. An example of primary MODS is a primary pulmonary injury, such as aspiration. Only a small percentage of clients develop primary MODS.

Secondary MODS is a consequence of widespread systemic inflammation, which develops after a variety of insults, and results in dysfunction of organs not involved in the initial insult.[1] The client enters a hypermetabolic state that lasts for 14 to 21 days. During this time, the body engages in autocatabolism that causes profound changes in the body's metabolic processes. Unless the process can be stopped, the outcome for the client is death. Secondary MODS occurs with conditions such as septic shock and ARDS.

Clinical Manifestations

There is usually a precipitating event to MODS, including aspiration, ruptured aneurysm, or septic shock, which is associated with resultant hypotension. The client is resuscitated; the cause is treated; and the client appears to do well for a few days. The following possible sequence of events often develops.

The client experiences SIRS before MODS develops. Within a few days, there is an insidious onset of a low-grade fever, tachycardia, increased numbers of banded and segmented neutrophils on the differential count (called a left shift), and dyspnea with the appearance of diffuse patchy infiltrates on the chest x-ray. The client often has some deterioration in mental status, with reasonably normal renal and hepatic laboratory results. Dyspnea progresses, and intubation and mechanical ventilation are required. Some evidence of consumptive coagulopathy (DIC) is usually present. The client is usually stable hemodynamically and has relative polyuria, an increased cardiac index (>4.5 L/min), and systemic vascular resistance of under 600 dynes cm^{-5}. Clients often have increased serum glucose levels in the absence of diabetes. Some physicians use the criteria presented in Table 81–6 to make the diagnosis of MODS.

Between 7 and 10 days, the bilirubin level rises and continues to rise, followed by an increase in serum creatinine. Blood glucose and lactate levels continue to rise because of the hypermetabolic state. Other progressive changes include excretion of urinary nitrogen and protein combined with decreased levels of serum albumin, prealbumin, and retinol binding protein. Bacteremia with enteric organisms is also common. In addition, infections from *Candida* and viruses such as herpes and cytomegalovirus are common. Surgical wounds display delayed healing, and pressure ulcers may develop. During this time, the client needs increasing amounts of fluids and inotropic medications to keep blood volume and cardiac

TABLE 81–6 MODIFIED APACHE II CRITERIA FOR DIAGNOSIS OF MULTIPLE ORGAN DYSFUNCTION SYNDROME

CARDIOVASCULAR FAILURE (PRESENCE OF ONE OR MORE OF THE FOLLOWING)

Heart rate <54 beats/min
Mean arterial pressure ≤49 mm Hg (systolic pressure ≤60 mm Hg)
Occurrence of ventricular tachycardia or ventricular fibrillation
Serum pH ≤7.24 with a $PaCO_2$ of ≤40 mm Hg

RESPIRATORY FAILURE (PRESENCE OF ONE OR MORE OF THE FOLLOWING)

Respiratory rate ≤5 breaths/min or ≥49 breaths/min
$PaCO_2$ ≥50 mm Hg
Alveolar-arterial oxygen difference ≥350 mm Hg (calculate as follows, at sea level: (713 × % oxygen in inspired gas) − $PaCO_2$ − PaO_2)
Dependent on ventilator or CPAP on the second day

RENAL FAILURE (PRESENCE OF ONE OR MORE OF THE FOLLOWING)

Urine output ≤479 ml/24 hr or ≤159 ml/8 hr
Serum BUN ≥100 mg/dl (35.7 mmol/L)
Serum creatinine ≥3.5 mg/dl (309 μmol/L)

HEMATOLOGIC FAILURE (PRESENCE OF ONE OR MORE OF THE FOLLOWING)

WBC count ≤1000/μl (1 × 10^9/L)
Platelets ≤20,000/μl (20 × 10^9/L)
Hematocrit ≤20%

NEUROLOGIC FAILURE

Glasgow Coma Scale score ≤6 (in absence of sedation)

HEPATIC FAILURE (PRESENCE OF BOTH OF THE FOLLOWING)

Serum bilirubin ≥6 mg%
Prothrombin time ≥4 sec over control in the absence of systemic anticoagulation

CPAP, continuous positive airway pressure; BUN, blood urea nitrogen; WBC, white blood cell.

From Knaus, W. A., & Wagner, D. P. (1989). Multiple systems organ failure: Epidemiology and prognosis. *Critical Care Clinics, 5*(2), 221.

preload near normal and to replace fluids lost through polyuria.

Between day 14 and day 21, the client is unstable and appears close to death. The client may lose consciousness. Renal failure worsens to the point of considering dialysis. Edema may be present because of low serum protein levels. Mixed venous oxygen levels may rise because of problems with tissue uptake of oxygen caused by mitochrondial dysfunction. Lactic acidosis worsens, liver enzymes continue to rise, and coagulation disorders become impossible to correct.

Prognosis

If the process of MODS is not reversed by day 21, it is usually evident that the client will die. Death usually occurs between days 21 and 28 after the injury or precipitating event. Not all clients with MODS die; however, MODS remains the leading cause of death in the intensive care unit (ICU), with mortality rates from 50% to 90% despite the development of better antibiotics, better resuscitation, and more sophisticated means of organ support. For those clients who survive, the average duration of ICU stay is about 21 days. The rehabilitation, which is directed at recovery of muscle mass and neuromuscular function, lasts about 10 months.

Outcome Management

Medical Management

RESTRAIN THE ACTIVATORS

Manifestations of potential infection must be quickly treated to restrain the activators of MODS. If the agent is known, antibiotics to which the organism is sensitive should be administered. If the organism is not known, broad-spectrum antibiotics are given. Antibiotics are sometimes directed at the probable organism (an empirical treatment). Early aggressive management of sources of infection should be carried out. For example, the client may need to have a large infected wound incised and drained or necrotic tissue excised. Extreme caution must be taken to avoid infecting the client. These clients have many invasive monitors and may have open wounds. Unfortunately, clients in critical care units exist in a paradox. The ICU is the only environment with sophisticated equipment and health care professionals to provide safe care, yet it is an environment where the risk of infection is higher. In addition, there is a high prevalence of multiresistant organisms, such as vancomycin-resistant *enterococci* (VRE) and methicillin-resistant *Staphylococcus aureus* (MRSA).

Because the lungs are often the first organs to fail, they require special attention. Aggressive pulmonary care is needed in all clients who are at risk of MODS. Interventions may be as simple as coughing and deep breathing to ambulation. The client's oxygen saturation should be monitored.

Because malnutrition develops from the hypermetabolism and the GI tract often seeds other areas with bacteria, some clinicians require the client to be fed enterally. They believe that feeding enhances perfusion and decreases the bacterial load and the effects of endotoxins. Nutrient intake is usually 30 to 35 kcal/kg/day of carbohydrates. Fats are restricted to 0.5 to 1 g/kg/day. Proteins are given to the client via modified amino acids. Some practitioners administer protein until a rise in plasma transferrin or prealbumin is noted. Increases in these values indicate hepatic protein synthesis rather than a breakdown of body stores. Decontamination of the GI tract and pharynx has been found to decrease infection but has shown no effect on the death rate from MODS.

CONTROL THE MEDIATORS

Controlling the mediators of inflammation is directed at (1) general levels of care and (2) specific treatments targeted at the problem cells. Maintenance of a positive nitrogen balance via nutrition, promotion of sleep and rest, and management of pain are important general care areas. Specific treatments include monoclonal antibodies to control mediators such as interleukin-1, endotoxins, and tumor necrosis factors. These therapies are shown in Table 81–7. Outcomes from research in these treatments are conflicting, and it appears that there is no "magic bullet" to cure the problem. Development of more specific monoclonal antibodies is ongoing.

Protect the Affected Organs

Care is directed toward maintaining the function of organs that fail with MODS. The client is intubated and mechanically ventilated in order to maintain adequate oxygenation. Oxygen is given to the client until blood levels of lactate decrease toward normal. Elevated serum lactate levels indicate the use of anaerobic metabolism. Nurses must recognize that certain clinical problems further increase the need for oxygen. Problems such as fever, seizures, and shivering increase oxygen demands. These problems should be controlled with medications or environmental changes (e.g., warming).

Fluids and inotropic drugs are used to support hemodynamic parameters. The client often becomes more unstable and needs continuous monitoring. Nutritional support is also critical to reduce the catabolism that accompanies hypermetabolism. Dialysis is often used to reduce azotemia from renal failure.

Nursing Management of the Medical Client

Care of the client with MODS is multifaceted, balancing the needs of one system against the needs of another while trying to maintain optimal functioning of each system. Nursing diagnoses appropriate for the client with MODS are determined by the system involved and the clinical manifestations identified.

The number of independent nursing interventions for the client with MODS is very limited. The overall goal for nursing is effective client and family coping. This complex disorder taxes the client and family. Nurses must remain sensitive to the needs of the family. Caring for the family of critically ill clients is a challenge in that understanding, predicting, and intervening with families in crisis is less exact than the calculation of oxygen needs. There are no easy formulas to use to provide hope, courage, coping, and caring. Nurses must remain alert to the needs of the family as well as the client during this stressful time.

TABLE 81–7 SUMMARY OF POTENTIALLY USEFUL THERAPIES FOR MULTIPLE ORGAN DYSFUNCTION SYNDROME

Rationale	Therapy
Treatment of infection	Monoclonal antibodies Passive antibody protection Gut decontamination regimens
Support of gut function	Mucosal trophic agents: e.g., glutamine, bombesin, ketone bodies Early enteral feeding Regulation of gut microbial flora
Improved resuscitation	Hypertonic saline In-line sensors Tissue-specific sensors Noninvasive monitoring
Endothelial cell protection	PAF inhibitors WBC adherence inhibition Antioxidant therapy Eicosanoid modulation
Modulation of macrophage function	n3 polyunsaturated fatty acids Signal transduction modulation
Stimulation of lymphocyte function	Arginine w3 polyunsaturated fatty acids

PAF, platelet activating factor; WBC, white blood cell.
From Lekander, B. J., & Cerra, F. B. (1990). The syndrome of multiple organ failure. *Critical Care Clinics of North America* 2(2), 338.

CONCLUSIONS

This chapter has discussed shock under three major classifications: hypovolemic, cardiogenic, and distributive. The pathophysiology, clinical manifestations, and medical and nursing management have been presented. Shock is a critical condition with a high mortality rate. Early diagnosis and intervention are necessary for the best possible outcomes. Multiple organ dysfunction syndrome is a syndrome of multiple organs progressively failing because of prolonged inflammatory responses.

THINKING CRITICALLY

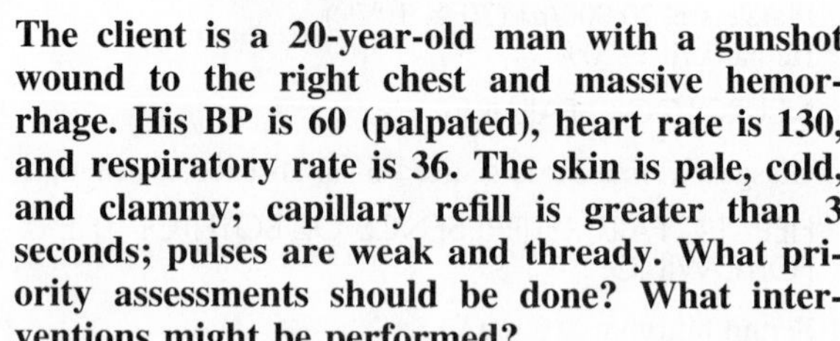

1. **The client is a 20-year-old man with a gunshot wound to the right chest and massive hemorrhage. His BP is 60 (palpated), heart rate is 130, and respiratory rate is 36. The skin is pale, cold, and clammy; capillary refill is greater than 3 seconds; pulses are weak and thready. What priority assessments should be done? What interventions might be performed?**

Factors to Consider. What do his vital signs tell you? What injuries might have occurred with a major chest trauma? How can his need for fluid and blood replacement best be met?

2. **A 69-year-old man was brought to the emergency department by a rescue squad. He had undergone a colon resection 2 weeks ago. His wife said that he was having increased difficulty breathing and he could feel his heart beating in his chest. He also has seemed "slower" to her. He is not moving as fast as usual and gets very dizzy when he stands up. He almost passed out, which is why she called the rescue squad. What priority assessments should be done? What interventions might be performed?**

Factors to Consider. What might be happening that could lead to all of the problems with breathing, dizziness, and confusion? What risk might be present as a result of the surgery?

3. **A 65-year-old man in the coronary care unit had an acute myocardial infarction (MI) 3 days ago. The monitor alarms and assessments reveal that his BP is 76/50; respiratory rate is 20. His pulse**

is rapid (128) and thready. His skin is cool and diaphoretic, with a slight ashen color; the capillary refill is greater than 3 seconds. The client is restless and confused. What priority assessments should be done? What interventions might be performed?

Factors to Consider. What form of shock can quickly develop in a client after an MI? Does he need fluid resuscitation to increase his blood pressure? Why or why not? What medications are commonly used to support a heart in distress? Are special forms of monitoring needed while these medications are used?

BIBLIOGRAPHY

1. American College of Chest Physicians/Society of Critical Care Medicine Consensus Conference Committee. (1992). Definitions for sepsis and organ failure and guidelines for the use of innovative therapies in sepsis. *Critical Care Medicine, 20*(6), 864–874.
2. Astiz, M. E., & Rackow, E. C. (1998). Septic shock. *The Lancet, 351,* 1501–1505.
3. Biro, G. P., et al. (1995). Oxyradical generation after resuscitation of hemorrhagic shock with blood or stroma-free hemoglobin solution. *Artificial Cells, Blood Substitutes, and Immobilization Biotechnology, 23*(6), 631–645.
4. Bone, R. C., et al. (1995). A second large controlled clinical study of E5, a monoclonal antibody to endotoxin: Results of a prospective, multicenter, randomized, controlled trial. *Critical Care Medicine, 23*(6), 994–1005.
5. Bone, R. C., Sprung, C. L., & Sibbald, W. J. (1992). Definitions for sepsis and organ failure. *Critical Care Medicine, 20*(6), 724–726.
6. Brass, N. J. (1994). Predisposition to multiple organ dysfunction. *Critical Care Nursing Quarterly, 16*(4), 1–7.
7. Bunn, H. F. (1995). The role of hemoglobin based blood substitutes in transfusion medicine. *Transfusion Clinique et Biologique, 2*(6), 433–439.
8. Campbell, J. (1997). Anaphylaxis. *Professional Nurse, 12*(6), 429–432.
9. Cashin, S. (1996). Is there a role for prehospital intramuscular adrenaline in anaphylaxis? *Australian Journal of Emergency Care, 3*(1), 11–15.
10. Crowley, S. R. (1996). The pathogenesis of shock. *Heart and Lung, 25*(2), 124–134.
11. DeJong, M. J. (1997). Clinical snapshot: Cardiogenic shock. *American Journal of Nursing, 97*(6), 40–41.
12. Evangelisto, M. (1997). Latex allergy: The downside of standard precautions. *Today's Surgical Nurse, 19*(5), 28–33.
13. Fehlings, M. G., & Louw, D. (1996). Initial stabilization and medical management of acute spinal cord injury. *American Family Physician, 54*(1), 155–162.
14. Fisher, D., & Sawin, K. (1998). Pearls for practice: Latex allergy in the primary care setting. *Journal of the American Academy of Nurse Practitioners, 10*(5), 203–208.
15. Graham, P., & Brass, N. J. (1994). Multiple organ dysfunction: Pathophysiology and therapeutic modalities. *Critical Care Nursing Quarterly, 16*(4), 8–15.
16. Green, T. (1997). Systems and diseases. The immune system. Part I. Anaphylaxis. *Nursing Times, 93*(42), 60–63.
17. Kavanagh, R. J., Radhakrishnan, D., & Park, G. R. (1995). *Care of the Critically Ill, 11*(3), 114–119.
18. Kellum J. A., & Decker, J. M. (1996). The immune system: Relation to sepsis and multiple organ failure. *AACN Clinical Issues: Advanced Practice in Acute and Critical Care, 7*(3), 339–350, 459–460.
19. Kimmings, A. N., Gouma, D. J., & van Deventer, S. J. H. (1994). Endotoxin in the pathogenesis of gram-negative sepsis. *Care of the Critically Ill, 10*(4), 170–173.
20. Levins, T. T., & Brown, K. K. (1995). Hemodynamic puzzle: Critical interventions in septic shock. *American Journal of Nursing, 95*(1), 20–21.
21. Livingston, D. H., Mosenthal, A. C., & Deitch, E. A. (1995). Sepsis and multiple organ dysfunction syndrome: A clinical-mechanistic overview. *New Horizons, 3*(2), 257–266.
22. Maier, R. V., & Bulger, E. M. (1996). Endothelial changes after shock and injury. *New Horizons, 4*(2), 211–223.
23. McCloskey, R. V., et al. (1994). Treatment of septic shock with human monoclonal antibody HA-1A. *Annals of Internal Medicine, 121*(1), 1–5.
24. McMahon, K. (1995). Multiple organ failure: The final complication of critical illness. *Critical Care Nurse, 15*(6), 23–30.
25. Monchik, K. O. (1998). Prehospital management of acute pulmonary edema with accompanying cardiogenic shock. *Emergency Medical Services, 27*(8), 35–36, 39–41, 56.
26. O'Donnell, L. (1996). Complications of MI: Beyond the acute stage. *American Journal of Nursing, 96*(9), 25–30.
27. O'Neal, P. V. (1994). How to spot early signs of cardiogenic shock. *American Journal of Nursing, 94*(5), 36–41.
28. Nose, Y. (1998). Oxygen-carrying macromolecules: Therapeutic agents for the treatment of hypoxia. *Artificial Organs, 22*(7), 618–622.
29. Ostrow, C. L., Hupp, E., & Topjian, D. (1994). The effect of Trendelenburg and modified Trendelenburg positions on cardiac output, blood pressure, and oxygenation: A preliminary study. *American Journal of Critical Care, 3*(5), 382–386.
30. Shoemaker, W. C., et al. (1996). Resuscitation from severe hemorrhage. *Critical Care Medicine, 24* (suppl. 2), S12–S23.
31. Smail, N., et al. (1995). Role of systemic inflammatory response syndrome and infection in the occurrence of early multiple organ dysfunction syndrome following severe trauma. *Intensive Care Medicine, 21*(10), 813–816.
32. Stapczynski, J. S. (1999, June). *Septic shock* [On-line]. Available: *www.emedicine.com/emerg/topic533.htm.*
33. Talan, D. A. (1997). Sepsis and septic shock. *Emergency Medicine Clinics of North America, 29*(3), 54–56, 61, 65–68.
34. Wardle, E. N. (1997). New research findings in septic shock/endotoxaemia. *Care of the Critically Ill, 13*(6), 222–224, 226.
35. Wiessner, W. H., Casey, L. C., & Zbilut, J. P. (1995). Treatment of sepsis and septic shock: A review. *Heart and Lung, 24*(5), 380–392.
36. Williams, J. G., Bernstein, S., & Prager, M. (1998). Effect of melatonin on activated macrophage TNF, IL-6, and reactive oxygen intermediates. *Shock, 9*(6), 406–411.
37. Young, J. S., Fernandez, M., & Meredith, J. W. (1997). The effect of oxygen delivery-directed resuscitation on splanchnic and hepatic oxygen transport after hemorrhagic shock. *Journal of Surgical Research, 71*(1), 87–92.

REMEMBER *to check out your* **Companion CD ROM**

CHAPTER 82

Management of Clients in the Emergency Department

Judy Selfridge-Thomas

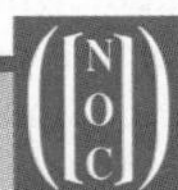

NURSING OUTCOMES CLASSIFICATION (NOC) for Nursing Diagnoses—Clients in the Emergency Department

Acute Confusion
Cognitive Ability
Distorted Thought Control
Information Processing
Memory
Neurologic Status: Consciousness
Sleep
Decreased Cardiac Output
Cardiac Pump Effectiveness
Circulation Status
Tissue Perfusion: Abdominal Organs
Tissue Perfusion: Peripheral
Vital Signs Status
Fluid Volume Excess
Electrolyte and Acid-Base Balance
Fluid Balance
Hydration
Fluid Volume Deficit
Electrolyte and Acid-Base Balance
Fluid Balance
Hydration
Nutritional Status: Food and Fluid Intake
Hypothermia
Thermoregulation
Impaired Gas Exchange
Electrolyte and Acid-Base Balance
Respiratory Status: Gas Exchange
Respiratory Status: Ventilation
Tissue Perfusion: Pulmonary
Vital Signs Status
Impaired Physical Mobility
Ambulation: Walking
Ambulation: Wheelchair
Body Positioning: Self-Initiated
Joint Movement: Active
Mobility Level
Sensory Function: Proprioception
Transfer Performance
Impaired Skin Integrity
Tissue Integrity: Skin and Mucous Membranes
Wound Healing: Primary Intention
Wound Healing: Secondary Intention
Ineffective Airway Clearance
Aspiration Control
Respiratory Status: Airway Patency
Respiratory Status: Gas Exchange
Respiratory Status: Ventilation
Ineffective Breathing Patterns
Respiratory Status: Airway Patency
Respiratory Status: Ventilation
Vital Signs Status
Ineffective Individual Coping
Aggression Control
Coping
Decision Making
Impulse Control
Information Processing
Role Performance
Social Support
Pain
Comfort Level
Pain Control
Pain: Disruptive Effects
Pain Level
Risk for Infection
Dialysis Access Integrity
Immobility Consequences: Physiologic
Immune Status
Immunization Behavior
Knowledge: Infection Control
Nutritional Status
Risk Control
Risk Control: Sexually Transmitted Diseases (STDs)
Risk Detection
Tissue Integrity: Skin and Mucous Membranes
Treatment Behavior: Illness or Injury
Wound Healing: Primary Intention
Wound Healing: Secondary Intention
Risk for Poisoning
Knowledge: Medicine
Medication Response
Risk Control
Risk Control: Drug Use
Risk Detection
Safety Behavior: Home Physical Environment
Self-Care: Nonparenteral Education
Self-Care: Parenteral Medication
Suicide: Self-Restraint
Sensory Perceptual Alterations
Anxiety Control
Body Image
Cognitive Ability
Cognitive Orientation
Distorted Thought Process
Energy Conservation
Hearing Compensation Behavior
Vision Compensation Behavior

During the mid-1960s, the need for the specialization of emergency services throughout the United States was identified as a national priority in order to reduce the associated morbidity and mortality resulting from catastrophic illness or injury. Since then, the specialties of emergency medicine, emergency nursing, and prehospital care services have grown. In the United States, more than 100 million clients use emergency departments (EDs) for health care services each year.[41] The scope of these services ranges from treatment of acute conditions that threaten the loss of life, limb, or vision to management of non-urgent, chronic conditions.

EMERGENCY MEDICAL SERVICES

The Emergency Medical Services (EMS) system encompasses all aspects of emergency care. Federal, state, and county EMS systems are designed to complement each other. The systems are responsible for establishing, regulating, and monitoring the components involved in the provision of emergency care. These components include such entities as 911 telephone access systems, Emergency Medical Technician (EMT) and paramedical personnel scopes of practice, ground and air ambulance services, dispatch communication between points of incident and responding personnel, and telecommunications between paramedical personnel and specialty-designated EDs known as *base station hospitals.* EMS systems are also instrumental in the coordination of activities for management of disaster situations.

Two goals of the EMS system are (1) to provide emergency care to a client as quickly as possible and (2) to assure that the "right client arrives at the right hospital in the least amount of time." Consequently, EMS systems are involved with specialty-designated hospital departments and EDs such as local or state trauma centers, burn centers, and pediatric care centers.

EMERGENCY NURSING

Emergency nursing was officially recognized as a specialty in 1970. The national association representing these nurses is the Emergency Nurses Association (ENA). Its current membership comprises more than 25,000 nurses who have chosen this area of professional nursing.

According to the ENA, the definition of emergency nursing involves

> . . . the assessment, diagnosis, and treatment of perceived, actual or potential, sudden or urgent, physical or psychosocial problems that are primarily episodic or acute. These may require minimal care or life-support measures, education of patient and significant others, appropriate referral and knowledge of legal implications.[13]

In addition to provision of direct client care, other multifaceted roles exist within emergency nursing. The emergency nurse may be involved in the initial triaging of clients according to illness severity, may perform as a mobile intensive care nurse (MICN) by directing prehospital care personnel via telecommunication, and frequently may provide client care in the prehospital environment. Community clinics utilize ED nurses, and many emergency nurses have become active in injury prevention programs at both national and local levels. Advanced practice roles such as clinical nurse specialists and nurse practitioners are used in many EDs throughout the United States. Nurses in these advanced practice roles often have a master's degree–level of education or higher in addition to specialty certification.

Nurses employed in an ED must be prepared to provide care to clients of all age groups who may have any possible illness or injury. It is often cited that emergency nurses must have an understanding of almost all disease processes specific to any age group. Unfortunately, ED nursing is not usually addressed in depth in generic nursing programs. The education of ED nurses frequently occurs through hospital orientation programs, post-employment internship courses, and continuing education programs. ED nurses can obtain national specialty certification through an examination process. A certified ED nurse can use the credential of Certified Emergency Nurse (CEN).

LEGAL ISSUES

Nurses deal with a variety of legal issues in whatever specialty area they practice. The ED is no exception; however, certain issues are of paramount importance in this setting.

FEDERAL LEGISLATION

Past federal legislation has mandated that any client who presents to an ED seeking treatment must be rendered aid regardless of financial ability to pay for services. Since the mid-1980s, additional specific legislation was enacted requiring ED personnel to stabilize any client considered medically unstable before transfer to another health care facility—the Consolidated Omnibus Budget Reconciliation Act (COBRA) of 1986 and the Omnibus Budget Reconciliation Act (OBRA) of 1990.[2] This stabilization must occur regardless of the client's financial ability to pay for services. ED personnel who transfer clients to another institution without first providing this initial stabilization can incur substantial fines and penalties, as can the hospital administration.

Clients with various illnesses seek health care services in the ED, even with the proliferation of managed health care plans and gatekeeping policies.[41] Financial reimbursement for rendered services has been denied to EDs from managed health care plans after retrospective determinations that the client's problem did not constitute a true emergency. Again, legislation has been enacted (Emergency Medical Treatment and Active Labor Act [EMTALA] legislation of 1988, 1989, 1990, and 1994)[2] requiring that a medical screening examination be performed on all ED clients before solicitation of information about ability to pay. This medical screening examination must be inclusive enough to determine whether the client requires emergency medical treatment or is in active labor. Violations of this legislation can again result in fines and penalties. Every congressional year, new legislation is proposed in an attempt to provide appropriate emergency medical treatment to the public while continuing to acknowledge cost-containment issues.

CONSENT TO TREAT

Most adult clients who receive treatment in the ED give voluntary consent to the standard and usual treatment performed in this setting. In some instances, however, a client is deemed unable to give consent for treatment. This inability may be due to the critical nature of the client's illness or injury or to other conditions, such as an altered level of consciousness. In these instances, emergency care may be rendered to the client under the implied emergency doctrine.[1] This doctrine assumes that the client would consent to treatment to prevent death or disability if the client were so able.

Children under the age of legal majority must have the consent of their parent or legal guardian for medical care to be rendered. Exceptions include (1) emancipated minors; (2) minors seeking treatment for communicable diseases, including sexually transmitted diseases, injuries from abuse, and alcohol or drug rehabilitation; and (3) minor-aged females requiring treatment for pregnancy or pregnancy-related concerns. Some states also allow the adult caregiver with whom the child resides to give treatment authorization even though that caregiver may not be the parent.

The issue of informed consent in the ED is the same as in any other health care setting. Adult clients must be informed about the necessity of required treatments, expected outcomes, and potential complications. Clients must also be mentally competent and understand the information being explained. As in any other setting, a mentally competent adult client always maintains the right to refuse treatment or withdraw previously given consent.

RESTRAINTS

Restraining a client while he or she is in the ED may at times become necessary. The need for restraint usually arises because the client is becoming agitated or possibly violent. Hard leather or chemical restraints are used if the client is in danger of injuring self or others. If restraints are required, departmental guidelines for their use must be followed.[1] A physician's order for applying restraints along with the client's behavior mandating the use of restraints must be documented. The client must be periodically reevaluated both for the continued need for restraints and for integrity of distal circulation, motor movement, and sensory level of the restrained extremities. The findings must be documented. Offering water to the client and providing opportunities to urinate or relieve other body needs are required, as is documentation of this nursing care. No client may be kept in restraints against his or her will unless the client's behavior indicates the existence of safety issues.[1]

Clients in the ED who have psychological conditions that render them a danger to themselves or to others, or who are unable to provide food or shelter for themselves, can be held on a legal psychiatric restraining order. This order mandates that such clients be placed in a locked psychiatric facility for their protection for a maximum of 72 hours. Within that 72-hour period, the client must be evaluated by a psychiatrist to determine whether the legal order needs to be extended or whether the client can be released back into society.

MANDATORY REPORTING

Every state has mandatory reporting regulations that affect emergency nurses. Incidents and conditions may need to be reported to federal, state, or local authorities or to the Department of Public Health, Department of Motor Vehicles, coroner's offices, or animal control agencies. The types of incidents requiring reporting are suspected child, sexual, domestic, and elder abuse; assaults; motor vehicle crashes; communicable diseases such as hepatitis, sexually transmitted diseases, chicken pox, measles, mumps, meningitis, tuberculosis, and food poisoning; seizure activity; death; and animal bites. Every ED has written policies regarding these mandatory reports.

EVIDENCE COLLECTION AND PRESERVATION

Recognition of unusual circumstances surrounding a client's injury or death is an important aspect of ED nursing because of the associated legal implications. Not only must the legal authorities be notified; in many instances, the ED nurse may be required to collect and preserve evidence taken from the client. This evidence can include bullets, weapons, clothing, and body fluid specimens.

All collected evidence must be identified by the client's name, hospital identification number, date and time of evidence collection, type of evidence and source (e.g., venipuncture, hematoma, aspiration vomitus, swab), and the initials and/or signature of the person collecting the evidence. Once the evidence has been collected, its preservation and the maintenance of the "chain of custody" is extremely important. Tables 82–1 to 82–3 relate to evidence collection.

VIOLENCE

Violence directed against ED personnel has become an issue of concern during the past decade.[24, 35] The environment inherent in the ED, the emotional circumstances often surrounding the illness or injury that affect both clients and family members, and the increasingly violent

TABLE 82–1 EVIDENCE COLLECTION IN THE EMERGENCY DEPARTMENT

Evidence	Collection/Container
Glass fragments, bullets, broken fingernails, paint chips, loose hair follicles, fibers, or trace evidence such as soil	Place each item in a paper envelope or specimen container.
Head or pubic hair samples	Collected samples from combings and cuttings are each placed in a paper envelope.
Blood (from both venipuncture and possible hematoma evacuation), urine, gastric washings, or vomitus	A 20- to 30-ml sample placed in a sealed container.
Swabs from wounds, membranes, or orifices	Air-dry before placing in a collection container or paper envelope.

From Selfridge-Thomas, J. (1995). *Manual of emergency nursing* (p. 382). Philadelphia: W. B. Saunders.

TABLE 82–2 TIPS FOR PRESERVING EVIDENCE IN THE EMERGENCY DEPARTMENT

1. Minimally handle the body of a deceased person.
2. Place paper bags on the hands and feet and possibly over the head of a deceased person to protect trace evidence or residue.
3. Place wet clothing in individual paper bags. Do not use plastic bags, as wet clothes can "sweat," thereby destroying evidence.
4. Photograph inflicted wounds or injury before cleansing or repair.
5. Do not insert invasive tubes through pre-existing wounds or holes (e.g., do not place chest tubes through chest wounds or intravenous catheters through needle track marks).
6. Do not cut clothing through evidence holes such as stab wounds or bullet wounds.
7. Collect the client's personal items such as written notes, drugs or medications, and items from clothing pockets.
8. Do not allow family members, significant others, or friends to be alone with the client.

From Selfridge-Thomas, J. (1995). *Manual of emergency nursing* (p. 382). Philadelphia: W. B. Saunders.

trends in the United States all play a role in this unfortunate phenomenon. Administrative changes have been made in some EDs to enhance both public and health care worker safety. These measures have included the installation of items such as metal detectors, "panic buttons," bullet-proof glass, and lock-down doors at public entrances; increasing the visibility of security guards; utilizing patrol guard dogs; and instituting visitor control policies.[35]

Education of ED personnel in violence prevention is also of paramount importance. The following areas are crucial to address:

- Recognizing potentially violent clients and situations
- Identifying verbally and physically abusive signs from clients, family members, or friends
- Understanding the importance of instinct or "gut reactions"
- Using simple communication strategies to defuse potentially problematic situations
- Requiring clients to completely undress before physical examination
- Minimizing the presence of "potential weapons" in client care areas such as scalpels, needles, excess tubing attached to oxygen flow meters, scissors, stethoscopes worn around the neck, and personal jewelry
- Restraining clients, when necessary, using a team approach
- Avoiding becoming a hostage in a volatile situation

Once a violent situation has erupted, the protection of ED personnel and others in the department is of utmost concern. Any means necessary to ensure their safety must be undertaken.

TABLE 82–3 MAINTAINING "CHAIN OF CUSTODY" OF EVIDENCE IN THE EMERGENCY DEPARTMENT

1. Label all collected evidence with client information data.
2. Document all collected evidence with the date and time and the initials of the person collecting evidence.
3. Document all transfers of evidence from one person to another and include the reason for transfer of evidence.
4. Obtain signatures of the person releasing evidence and of the person receiving evidence.
5. *Never* leave collected evidence unattended.

From Selfridge-Thomas, J. (1995). *Manual of emergency nursing* (p. 383). Philadelphia: W. B. Saunders.

ETHICAL ISSUES

The ethical issues confronting ED nurses usually concern end-of-life concerns. Initial resuscitation and stabilization of clients in critical condition constitutes universal standard practice in the ED. At times, however, the desired outcome of client survivability is not achievable.

UNEXPECTED DEATH

When death occurs in the ED setting, it is usually sudden and unexpected, even if the client has had a prolonged illness. The unexpected nature of the death, or impending death, can present ethical dilemmas for both the survivors and the ED personnel. One such issue deals with the length to which resuscitation is performed. This is usually a physician's decision; however, family members may at times have input. Allowing family members or significant others to be present during client resuscitation is becoming more common. This practice is not necessarily disruptive to the resuscitation process, and it can be of comfort to the survivors and the involved ED personnel.[4, 23]

When death does occur, the ED nurse and the ED physician have important roles in informing the family:

- Inform the family of the client's death, and refer to the deceased client by name.
- Provide the family with an explanation of the course of events related to the death; use simple explanations.
- Offer the family an opportunity to view the body if desired. If a child has died, allow the parent to hold the child if they so desire. Providing the parent with a lock of the child's hair may be comforting.
- Help the family to focus on decisions requiring immediate attention such as taking possession of the deceased person's valuables, postmortem examination if desired or required, possible organ or tissue donation, and funeral home selection.
- Inform family members when they can leave the ED setting.
- Provide community agency referral as needed.

ADVANCE DIRECTIVES

In 1991, Congress enacted the Patient Self-Determination Act (PSDA). This act allows a client, or the client's health care proxy, to make determinations related to end-of-life measures.[9] Emergency care personnel are obligated to abide by the client's advance directive decisions, if that information is available and provided in writing. When this written information is not available, ED personnel have a responsibility to stabilize and/or resuscitate any client according to standard treatment guidelines regardless of a family member's expressed wishes.

ORGAN AND TISSUE DONATION

Issues related to potential organ or tissue donation often arise in the ED setting. Once a potential donor is identified, the surviving family members need to be approached. A team approach involving a physician, a nurse, and possibly an organ procurement coordinator is optimal. Utmost dignity and professionalism must be maintained. (Chapter 80 reviews religious and cultural customs and beliefs related to death and organ transplantation.) Remember, whatever decision the family makes regarding organ or tissue donation, that decision must be supported by health care personnel.

COMPONENTS OF EMERGENCY CARE

Even though treatment decisions in the ED may at first appear to occur in a chaotic fashion, there is an inherent order in the timing and choice of interventions performed throughout a client's stay. The organizational flow of events involves client triage (prioritizing), nursing assessment of the client, diagnostic testing, formulation of diagnoses, outcome management, evaluation, disposition, and documentation.

TRIAGE

Whether clients arrive via ambulance or are ambulatory, they are triaged at some point by either an ED physician or an ED nurse. The purpose of this triage process is to expediently determine the severity of a client's problem or condition. The acuity level of the presenting problem is rated according to predetermined categories; the most frequently used ratings are *emergent, urgent,* and *non-urgent.* Table 82–4 provides a definition for each of these categories.

TABLE 82–4 THREE-CATEGORY TRIAGE RATING IN THE EMERGENCY DEPARTMENT

Emergent category: Client must be treated immediately; otherwise, life/limb/vision is threatened.

Urgent category: Client requires treatment, but life/limb/vision is not threatened if care cannot be provided within 1 to 2 hours.

Non-urgent category: Client requires evaluation and possible treatment, but time is not a critical factor.

Once an initial determination is made about the severity of the client's condition, a more in-depth nursing and medical assessment is completed. Appropriate diagnostic testing and specific interventions are performed using a team approach as emergency physicians and nurses work collaboratively to provide appropriate and expeditious management of the client's problem.

NURSING ASSESSMENT

The nursing assessment process for any client entering the ED is divided into the *primary* assessment and the *secondary* assessment (Fig. 82–1).

The purpose of the *primary assessment* is to immediately identify any client problem that poses a threat, immediate or potential, to life, limb, or vision. Information is gathered primarily through objective data. If any abnormalities are found during the primary assessment, immediate interventions such as cardiopulmonary resuscitation (CPR) and Advanced Life Support (ALS) must be instituted to aid in preserving the client's life, limb, or vision. The primary assessment is made using the ABC mnemonic:

A Airway patency
B Breathing effectiveness
C Circulation (both peripheral and organ-specific)

For any client arriving in the ED who has been involved in a major traumatic injury, the primary assessment must also include an evaluation of the cervical spine area for any potential injury.

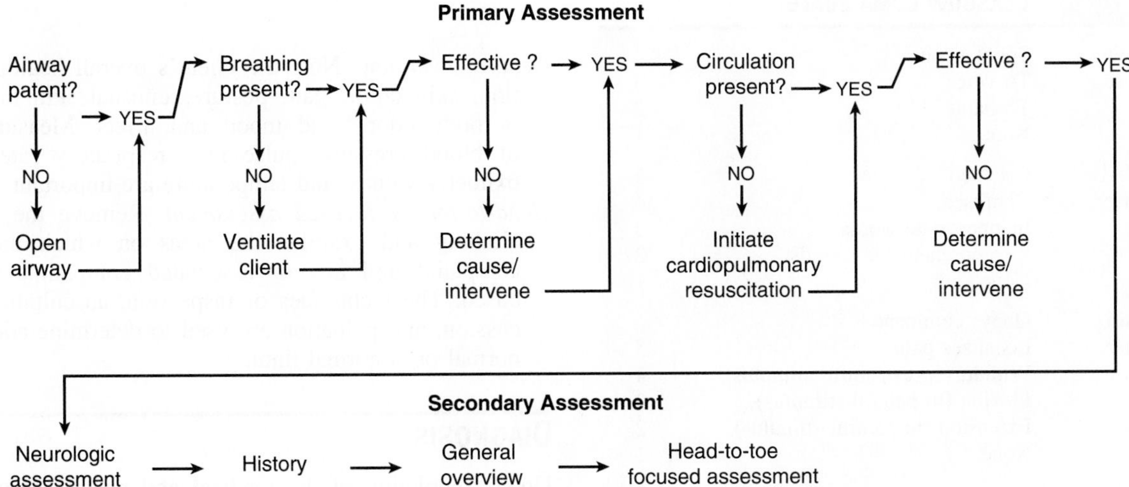

FIGURE 82–1 Primary and secondary assessment process.

Once it is determined that a client's ABC status is satisfactory, the *secondary assessment* is performed to identify any other non–life-threatening problems the client may be experiencing. Both subjective information and objective data are obtained. The secondary assessment includes the following elements.

Neurologic assessment. Determine the client's (1) level of consciousness; (2) orientation to person, place, time, and event; (3) Glasgow Coma Scale (GCS) score (Table 82–5); (4) pupillary size, equality, and reaction to light and accommodation; and (5) motor movement and strength of hand grips and pedal pushes.

History. Elicit the nature of the client's chief complaint, duration of the problem, mechanism of injury from blunt or penetrating forces (Table 82–6), associated manifestations related to the primary problem, past pertinent medical history, current medications and compliance, use of over-the-counter (OTC) medications or herbs, routine use of alcohol or illicit drugs, known medication allergies, and immunization history. Women of childbearing age may need to be questioned about the date of the last normal menstrual period (LNMP), number of pregnancies and outcomes, and age at onset or at end of menstruation.

Pain. The most frequent complaint for which clients seek emergency care is related to pain. Obtaining specific information regarding pain patterns can be extremely helpful. Asking questions according to the PQRST mnemonic often provides useful information:

- *P Provokes:* Are there any specific factors that cause the pain to increase or decrease?
- *Q Quality:* What descriptive terminology identifies the type of pain—dull, sharp, colicky, pressure?
- *R Region/Radiation:* Where is the pain located? Does it move to other areas?
- *S Severity:* Use a rating scale of 1 to 10 to describe pain severity, with 1 indicating no or minimal pain and 10 representing severe pain.
- *T Timing:* How long has the pain been present? Are there cycles related to when the pain is present or absent?

TABLE 82–5 GLASGOW COMA SCALE

Eye-opening response	Spontaneous	4
	To voice	3
	To pain	2
	None	1
Best verbal response	Oriented	5
	Confused	4
	Inappropriate words	3
	Incomprehensible sounds	2
	None	1
Best motor response	Obeys command	6
	Localizes pain	5
	Withdraws (to painful stimulus)	4
	Flexion (to painful stimulus)	3
	Extension (to painful stimulus)	2
	None	1
Total		3–15

TABLE 82–6 HISTORY QUESTIONS RELATED TO INJURY

MOTOR VEHICLE CRASHES

- Were you the driver or passenger?
- Were you wearing a seatbelt or shoulder harness (or both) correctly?
- Did the airbag deploy?
- Did you hit the steering wheel or the dashboard? If so, with what part of your body?
- Did you lose consciousness? If so, for how long?
- How fast was the vehicle going?
- What did the vehicle hit?
- Did the vehicle hit a moving object or a nonmoving object? (Paramedical personnel may provide information describing the condition of the car.)
- Where is your pain?
- How far were you thrown from the car?
- What is the condition of the other passengers?

BLUNT INJURY FROM FALLS

- How far did you fall?
- What precipitated the fall?
- What did you land on?
- Where is your pain?
- Did you lose consciousness?

GUNSHOT WOUNDS

- How long ago did the incident occur?
- How many shots did you hear?
- What type of gun was it?
- From what direction do you think the bullet entered your body?
- How far away was the assailant?
- Where is your pain?

PENETRATING WOUNDS OR STAB WOUNDS

- How long ago did the injury occur?
- How many times were you stabbed?
- How long was the knife or sharp object?
- How far in did the sharp object go?
- From what direction were you stabbed?
- Where is your pain?

From Kitt S., et al. (Eds.). (1995). *Emergency nursing: A physiologic and clinical perspective* (2nd ed.). Philadelphia: W. B. Saunders.

General overview. Note the client's overall health condition, skin color, gait, posture, unusual skin markings or body odors, and mood and affect. Measurements of blood pressure, pulse rate, respiratory rate, pulse oximetry values, and temperature are important.

Head-to-toe or focused assessment. Remove the client's clothing and examine the areas on which the chief complaint and any or associated complaints are focused. The techniques of inspection, auscultation, percussion, and palpation are used to determine additional normal or abnormal findings.

DIAGNOSIS

Upon completion of the medical and nursing assessment process, diagnostic tests (radiographic, cardiology, laboratory, special studies) may be initiated. Once all pertinent information has been collected, a working diagnosis is formulated. The physician provides a medical diagnosis; in addition, the ED nurse may incorporate a variety of nursing diagnoses. These diagnoses provide a framework on which to build a plan of appropriate client care.

OUTCOME MANAGEMENT

Necessary client care interventions may be initiated by the ED nurse, the ED physician, or other health care providers. There is frequent collaboration among all health care providers involved, and interventions are assigned priority according to the severity of the client's condition.

EVALUATION

The desired goal in client care is to achieve positive client outcomes after medical or nursing management. This is an integral component of ED nursing care. If the client's condition does not improve with initial interventions, the plan of care must be reexamined and additional interventions may be required.

CLIENT DISPOSITION

All clients entering the ED are eventually discharged from the ED. They may be transferred to another health-care facility, admitted to the hospital, or released to home or another facility. Most clients are released to home following treatment. Before being discharged from the ED, a client and/or family members must be given both oral and written instructions concerning follow-up care. These instructions should identify the client's diagnosed problem, explain necessary continued treatments, describe potential complications, and specify time frames for rechecks and the name of the physician to whom the client is being referred. These instructions should be presented in both oral and written form in the client's primary language. At times, a hospital or family interpreter may be required to accomplish this outcome.

NURSING DOCUMENTATION

Because ED nurses frequently are responsible for an assigned area, zone, or "pod" within the department and clients enter and exit those areas on a continual basis, nursing documentation is of paramount importance. Include the recording of all assessment findings, diagnostic tests, interventions and management, responses to treatment, achieved outcomes, and client education. Documentation needs to be complete but concise. It provides an ongoing record of the client's condition and responses. The format may be a flow sheet, narrative, or computer-generated format or a combination of these.

EMERGENCY CONDITIONS

INEFFECTIVE AIRWAY CLEARANCE

A compromised or ineffective airway may be due to either complete or partial airway obstruction. Common causes of airway compromise include the presence of a foreign object in the airway, airway edema, airway infection, facial or airway injury, and tongue obstruction.[37, 38]

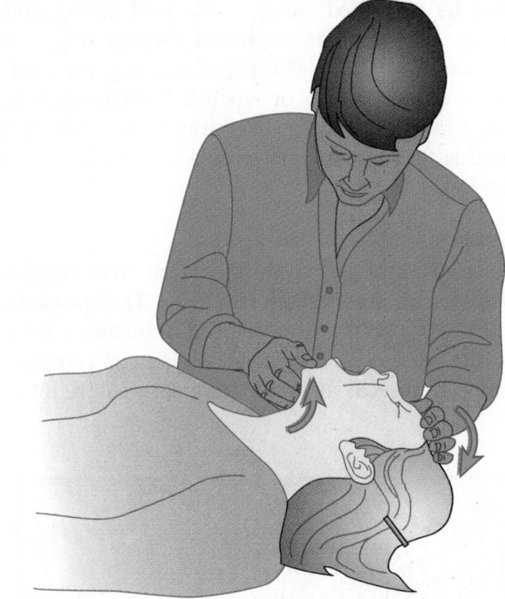

FIGURE 82–2 Chin lift maneuver to open the airway.

Clinical Manifestations

The clinical manifestations of airway compromise include absence of respirations, drooling, stridor, intercostal or substernal retractions, cyanosis, and agitation. A decreased level of consciousness may lead to airway compromise as a result of obstruction of the posterior pharynx by the relaxed tongue.

Outcome Management

REMOVE OBSTRUCTION

If an obstruction is present, the airway should be opened by a chin lift or jaw thrust maneuver (Figs. 82–2 and 82–3). If either of these maneuvers opens the client's airway, patency is maintained via the insertion of a nasopharyngeal tube or oral airway device. If these maneuvers fail to relieve the obstruction, more aggressive interven-

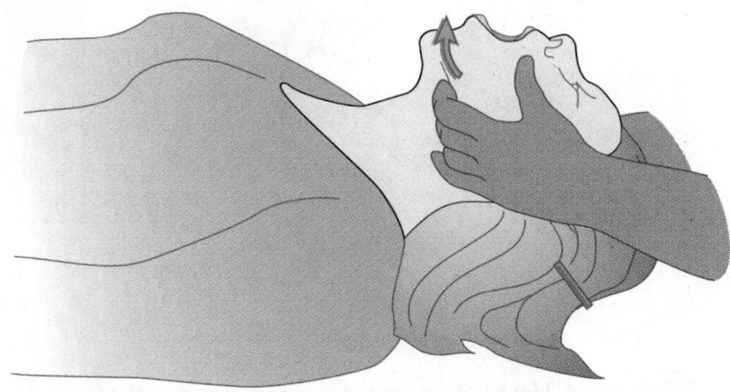

FIGURE 82–3 The jaw thrust maneuver to open the airway is the preferred method for use in clients with head or cervical neck injury.

tions must be instituted, such as (1) performing abdominal or chest thrusts if an aspirated foreign object is the suspected cause (Fig. 82–4), (2) suctioning the oral cavity to remove secretions or visible foreign objects, (3) intubating via the nasal or oral route, and (4) assisting with creating a surgical airway via a cricothyroidotomy (Fig. 82–5).

INTUBATE

In some cases, oral or nasal intubation may require the use of *rapid-sequence induction* (RSI). This procedure is used in awake clients who require intubation either to maintain the airway or as a mechanism to provide adequate ventilation. RSI is most frequently used in clients who have sustained a head or spinal injury and in clients who are rapidly tiring from the effort of maintaining respirations. RSI involves (1) establishing venous access; (2) hyperventilating the client with 100% oxygen; and (3) administering an intravenous (IV) general barbiturate or anesthetic medication such as thiopental 3 to 5 mg/kg, fentanyl (Sublimaze) 3 to 15 μg/kg, ketamine (Ketalar) 1 to 2 mg/kg, etomidate (Amidate) 0.3 mg/kg, or propofol (Diprivan) 2.0 mg/kg, followed immediately by the administration of an IV muscle-paralyzing agent such as succinylcholine (Anectine) 1.5 to 2.0 mg/kg.[12] Once the client loses consciousness and adequate muscle relaxation and paralysis have been obtained, intubation with ventilation using 100% oxygen is implemented.

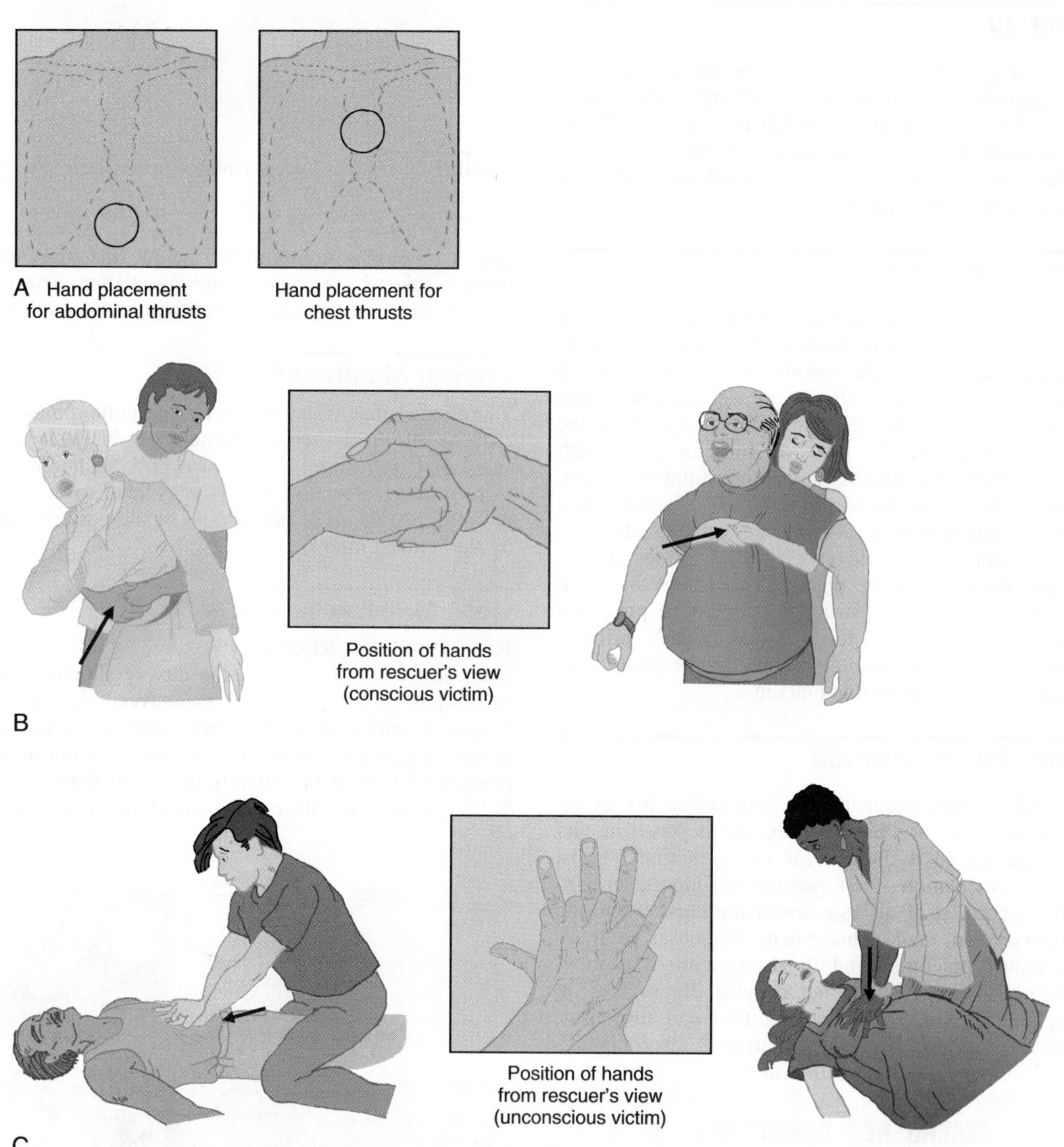

FIGURE 82–4 Heimlich maneuver, used for removal of foreign bodies blocking the upper airway. Vigorous upward chest or abdominal thrusts produce a rush of air that expels the foreign body. The abdominal thrust is the original Heimlich maneuver. The chest thrust is an adaptation that is useful for obese or pregnant victims. Use four quick thrusts in the positions shown. *A,* Hand placement. *B,* Maneuver for conscious victims. *C,* Maneuver for unconscious victims.

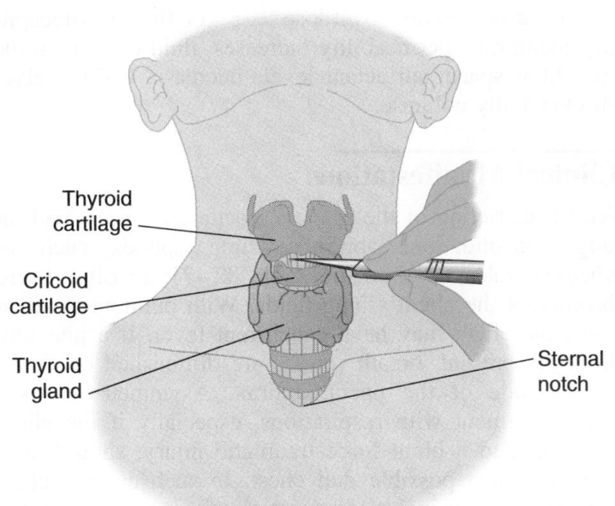

FIGURE 82–5 A cricothyrotomy procedure is performed to create a temporary airway. An opening is made into the trachea and is maintained with a small plastic tube.

VERIFY ENDOTRACHEAL TUBE PLACEMENT

After an oral intubation procedure, the ED nurse is immediately responsible for auscultation of the client's chest during assisted ventilation to confirm the presence of equal bilateral breath sounds. If breath sounds are heard over the epigastric area, the endotracheal tube must be removed, the client hyperventilated, and the procedure reattempted. Breath sounds heard more prominently over the upper right chest indicate that the endotracheal tube has advanced too far into the right main bronchus. The tube needs to be pulled back and breath sounds reassessed. Once the presence of equal and bilateral breath sounds is confirmed, the tube is secured in place, and a chest film is obtained to document correct tube placement.

Securing and maintaining a patent airway constitute the first priority in any ED client. Other treatments directed at the cause of airway compromise will then be instituted. These measures may include administration of IV medications if infection or local edema is present.

IMMOBILIZE THE SPINE

If the client with an actual or potential airway problem has had a traumatic injury, simultaneous stabilization of the client's cervical, thoracic, and lumbar spine must be instituted and maintained to prevent any further possible spinal injury. Stabilization is accomplished utilizing a team approach and involves the following steps: (1) manually stabilizing the client's head and cervical spine; (2) applying a hard cervical collar around the client's nuchal area; (3) placing the client on a long, rigid backboard; (4) securing the client to the backboard; (5) placing immobilization devices, such as rolled towels, at the side of the client's head/neck; and finally (6) placing a strip of adhesive tape across the client's forehead and immobilization devices and then onto the back board (see Fig. 82–6).

INEFFECTIVE BREATHING PATTERNS

Breathing patterns are affected if a client is either hyperventilating or hypoventilating. The normal respiratory rate for an adult is between 12 and 20 breaths/minute; children normally have faster respiratory rates until approximately the age of 10 years.

■ HYPERVENTILATION

Clinical Manifestations

Respiratory rates faster than normal constitute tachypnea and, in many cases, hyperventilation. Common causes for hyperventilation include anxiety reactions, pulmonary infections, and metabolic deviations.[37, 38] With excessive and prolonged hyperventilation, carbon dioxide levels de-

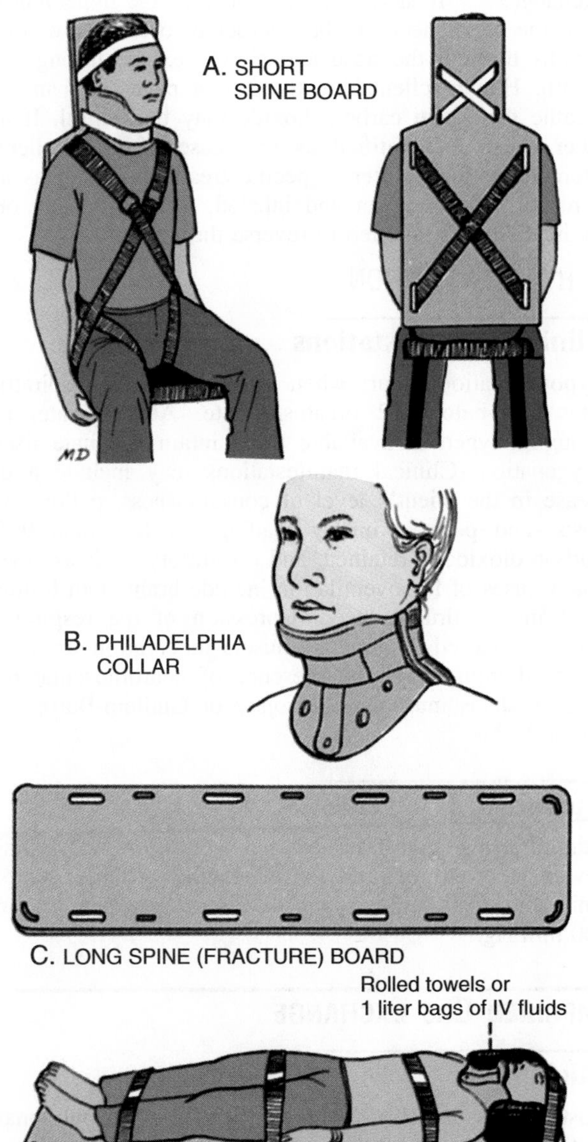

FIGURE 82–6 Spine-immobilizing devices. *A,* The short spine board is applied to a client who is seated (e.g., in an automobile) and is applied along with a cervical collar before extrication of the person from the vehicle. *B,* The Philadelphia collar, a two-piece, hard, molded plastic device, can be applied without manipulating the neck and provides good immobilization of the cervical spine. *C,* The long spine (fracture) board is made of wood and contains cut-out sections along the sides for securing restraining straps and for lifting the injured client.

crease, and respiratory alkalosis can result. The client may report numbness and tingling sensations in the distal extremities or around the lips, along with carpal or pedal spasms. A sensation of chest pain may also be present. Frequently this condition is caused by client anxiety, but it is important to also investigate other possible causes, such as pain, aspirin toxicity, diabetic ketoacidosis, fluid loss, central nervous system (CNS) lesions, and pulmonary embolism.

Outcome Management

The goals of treatment are to return the client's breathing pattern and rate to normal and to restore normal gas exchange.[37, 38] If anxiety is the cause of the hyperventilation, the client needs to be instructed to take slow, deep breaths through the nose and slowly exhale through the mouth. Having clients breathe into a paper bag and rebreathe their own carbon dioxide may be helpful. If another cause is identified as the reason for the client's altered breathing pattern, specific treatments such as administration of oxygen and inhaled, intravenous, or oral medications are initiated to reverse the process.

■ HYPOVENTILATION

Clinical Manifestations

Hypoventilation occurs when an adult client's respiratory rate falls below 12 breaths/minute. At this rate, not enough oxygen is available to maintain adequate tissue oxygenation. Clinical manifestations may include a decrease in the client's level of consciousness, pallor, cyanosis, and pulse oximetry readings of less than 96%. Carbon dioxide is retained, and respiratory acidosis develops. Causes of hypoventilation include brain stem lesions, head injury, drug-induced depression of the respiratory center, impaired respiratory muscle innervation from spinal cord injury, and the presence of neuromuscular diseases such as muscular dystrophy or Guillain-Barré syndrome.[37, 38]

Outcome Management

Administering high-flow oxygen via a bag-valve-mask device is often required to reduce the systemic hypoxemia and to return oxygen levels to between 80 and 100 mm Hg.

IMPAIRED GAS EXCHANGE

Etiology

Obstructions, infections, and injury within the pulmonary system can lead to the development of gas exchange abnormalities. Common causative disorders include asthma, reactive airway disease, chronic obstructive pulmonary disease, pulmonary embolism, bronchitis, pneumonia, tuberculosis, pneumothorax, and chest injuries such as a flail chest.[6, 8, 14, 20, 37, 38]

A less common cause of a gas exchange problem is noncardiac pulmonary edema, which results from acute damage to the alveolocapillary membrane. This damage can occur from inhalation injury, near-drowning, sepsis, trauma, and narcotic overdose.[37, 38] As the alveolocapillary membrane permeability increases, fluid collects in the interstitial space, surfactant levels decrease, and the alveoli eventually collapse.

Clinical Manifestations

With constriction of the bronchi, accumulation of fluid, or lung consolidation, abnormal lung sounds such as wheezes, rales, or rhonchi (Table 82–7) are often heard throughout the client's lung fields. With pulmonary infections, the client may have concurrent fever. If a pneumothorax is present, breath sounds are diminished or absent on the side of the pneumothorax. Asymmetrical chest wall movement with respirations, especially if the client has sustained a blunt force traumatic injury, should raise suspicion of a possible flail chest. In such cases a chest film provides valuable diagnostic information about the cause of the client's problem. A ventilation-perfusion (V/Q) scan can aid in the diagnosis of pulmonary embolism.

Outcome Management

ADMINISTER OXYGEN

Oxygen therapy with a flow rate of between 2 and 10 L/min via nasal cannula or face mask is the priority intervention for clients with an obstructive or infectious cause of ineffective gas exchange.

ADMINISTER MEDICATIONS TO OPEN AIRWAYS

Oxygen administration is frequently followed by administering aerosolized bronchodilator medications such as metaproterenol (Alupent) or albuterol (Ventolin) in order to open constricted upper or lower bronchi.[28] Subcutaneous epinephrine 1 : 1000 may be administered to relax constricted bronchi and to reduce the degree of airway or bronchial edema.[16] Administration of steroid medications, either intravenously or orally, is a frequent therapy.[20] A client with a suspected pulmonary embolus may be given IV thrombolytic medications, such as tissue-type plasminogen activator (t-PA [Activase]), to lyse the offending embolus and also heparin to prevent the formation of new emboli.

MINIMIZE SPREAD OF INFECTION

Infectious diseases that are the cause of impaired gas exchange are treated with IV or oral antibiotic medications. A client thought to have a highly contagious pulmonary disease such as tuberculosis must be isolated

TABLE 82–7 RESPIRATORY SOUNDS ASSOCIATED WITH ILLNESS

Illness	Lung Sounds
Asthma	Wheezes
COPD	Rales, rhonchi, wheezes
Bronchitis	Rhonchi
Pneumonia	Rhonchi, abnormal bronchial sounds
Tuberculosis	Rhonchi, abnormal bronchial sounds
Bronchiolitis	Wheezes

COPD, chronic obstructive pulmonary disease.

from the general ED client population. The use of a high-efficiency particulate air (HEPA) filter mask placed over the nose and mouth is indicated to prevent spreading of aerosol droplets.[29] ED personnel caring for the client may also need to wear this type of mask to decrease exposure risks.

■ TRAUMATIC PNEUMOTHORAX

A pneumothorax can be classified as a simple pneumothorax, open pneumothorax, or tension pneumothorax (Fig. 82–7).[26] In a *simple pneumothorax,* air from the bronchus, bronchioles, or alveoli escapes into the pleural space and diminishes lung expansion capacity. With an *open pneumothorax,* a traumatically created opening in the client's chest wall allows air to move freely into and out of the thoracic cavity during inspiration and exhalation. A tension pneumothorax occurs when air continues to become trapped in the pleural cavity with no mechanism of escape during the exhalation process. This type of pneumothorax is an emergent condition.

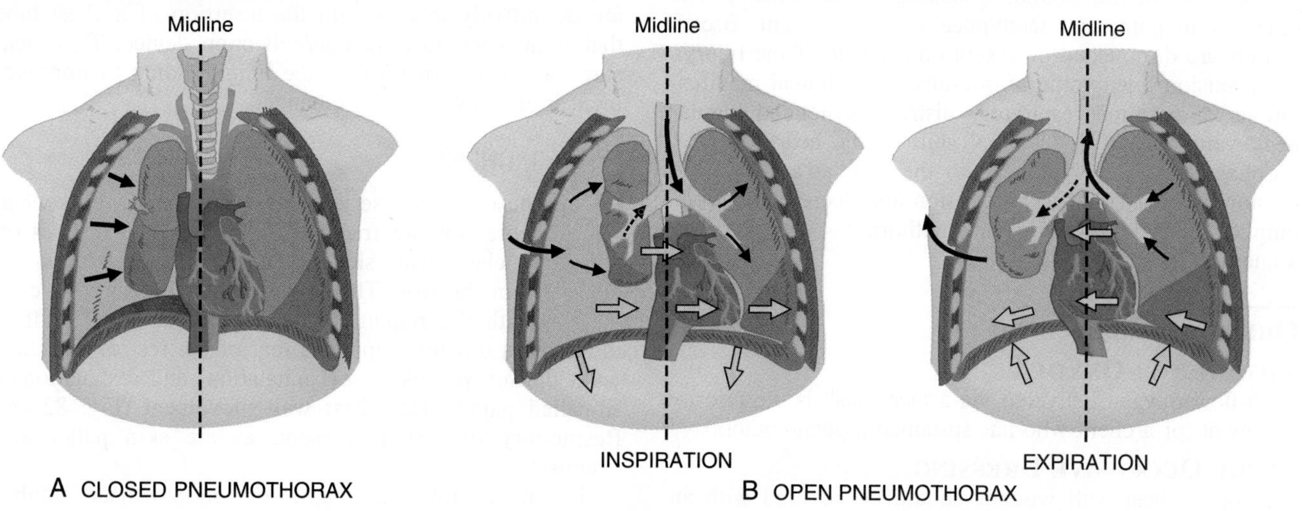

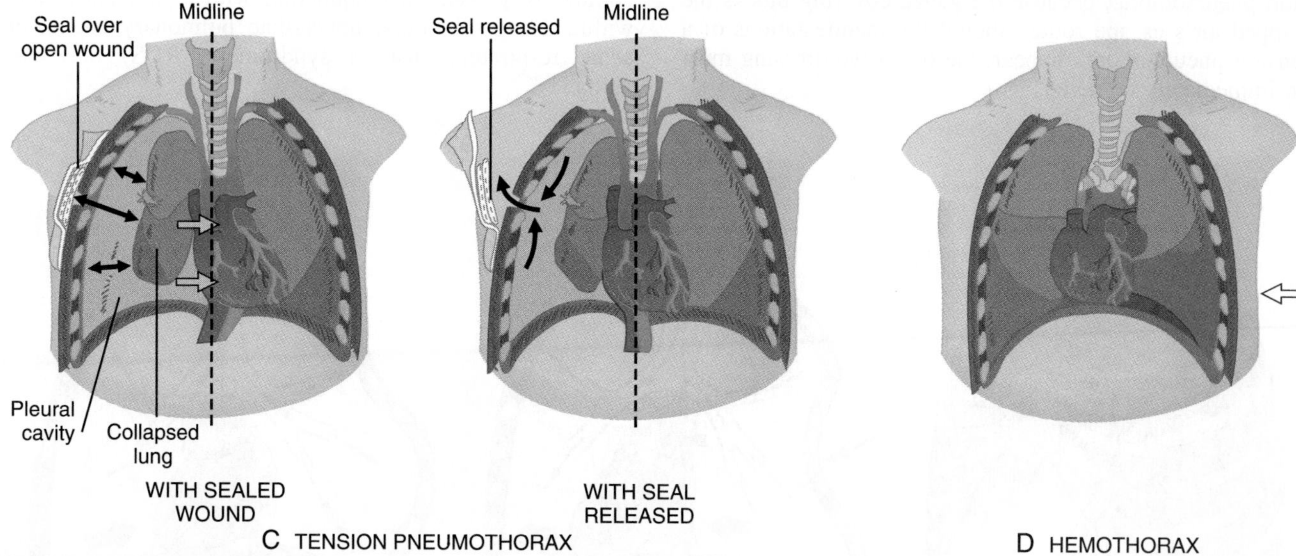

FIGURE 82–7 Pneumothorax.

A, Closed pneumothorax. The lung collapses as air gathers in the pleural space.

B, Open pneumothorax (sucking chest wound). *Solid arrows* indicate air movement; *open arrows,* structural movement. A chest wall wound connects the pleural space with atmospheric air. During inspiration, atmospheric air is sucked into the pleural space through the chest wall wound. Positive pressure in the pleural space collapses the lung on the affected side and pushes the mediastinal contents toward the unaffected side. This reduces the volume of air in the unaffected side considerably. During expiration, air escapes through the chest wall wound, lessening positive pressure in the affected side and allowing the mediastinal contents to swing back toward the affected side. Movement of mediastinal structures from side to side is called mediastinal flutter.

C, Tension pneumothorax. *Left,* If an open pneumothorax is covered (e.g., with a dressing), it forms a seal, and tension pneumothorax with a mediastinal shift develops. A tear in lung structure continues to allow air into the pleural space. As positive pressure builds in the pleural space, the affected lung collapses, and the mediastinal contents shift to the unaffected side. *Right,* Tension pneumothorax is corrected by removing the seal (e.g., dressing), allowing air trapped in the pleural space to escape.

D, Hemothorax. Massive hemothorax (*arrow*) below the left lung causes collapse of lung tissue.

Clinical Manifestations

A simple pneumothorax can occur spontaneously but is frequently associated with penetrating injury forces delivered to the chest or with blunt forces causing a rib fracture. Pain with respirations is present, as is the auscultative finding of unequal breath sounds. Pulse oximetry readings are less than 94%.

An obvious chest wound is present with an open pneumothorax, as this type of pneumothorax is most commonly caused by penetrating injury forces. As air moves into and out of the wound, a sucking sound is heard. The client is in pain, and tachypnea will be present. Breath sounds are diminished or absent on the side of the injury.

A tension pneumothorax produces the clinical manifestations of extreme respiratory distress, distended jugular neck veins, and a mediastinal shift of the heart, trachea, esophagus, and great vessels to the side away from the tension pneumothorax. Hypotension and decreased cardiac output are other findings. Pneumothorax is diagnosed by a chest radiograph.

Outcome Management

Administer Oxygen

High-flow oxygen delivered via a face mask is the priority treatment for a client who has sustained a pneumothorax.

Apply Occlusive Dressing

Any open chest wall wounds should be covered with an occlusive gauze dressing, but this intervention may convert an open pneumothorax into the more dangerous tension pneumothorax because the gauze covering blocks the trapped air's escape route. Should the manifestations of a tension pneumothorax appear, the occlusive dressing must be immediately removed.

Release Trapped Air

If a tension pneumothorax is thought to be the cause of respiratory distress and if it has not been iatrogenically produced by covering an open chest wound, a 14- to 16-gauge catheter needle is immediately inserted into the client's anterior chest wall on the affected side at the second midclavicular intercostal space.[25] This life-saving intervention allows the immediate release of trapped air and decompresses the pleural cavity.

Place Chest Tube

The simple, open, and tension varieties of pneumothorax are definitively treated with the insertion of a chest tube that is attached to a suction/collection device. This measure aids in reexpansion of the lung, leading to improvement in the client's gas exchange.

■ FLAIL CHEST

A flail chest involves serious rib fractures. It occurs when two or more ribs are fractured in two or more places on the same chest wall side or when the sternum is detached from the ribs. The fractured segment has no connection with the remaining rib cage. This segment then moves in a direction opposite that of the rest of the chest wall during processes of inhalation and exhalation—so-called paradoxical chest wall movement (Fig. 82–8). Respiratory distress is present, as are skin pallor and cyanosis.

Treatment involves nasal or endotracheal intubation and mechanical ventilation with positive end-expiratory pressure (PEEP). Pulmonary contusions are commonly present in conjunction with a flail chest, and within 24 to 48 hours, noncardiac pulmonary edema or acute respiratory distress syndrome (ARDS) may develop.[19, 25]

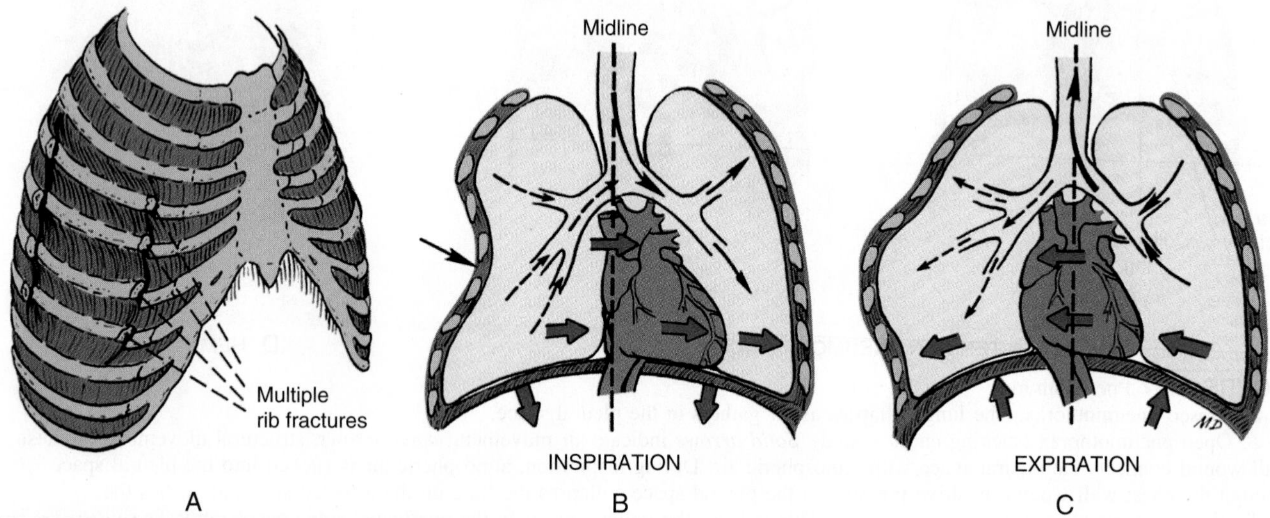

FIGURE 82–8 Flail chest. *Dashed arrows* indicate air movement; *solid arrows,* structural movement. *A,* A flail chest consists of fractured rib segments that are unattached (free-floating) to the rest of the chest wall. *B,* On inspiration, the flail segment of ribs is sucked inward. The affected lung and mediastinal structures shift to the unaffected side. This compromises the amount of inspired air in the unaffected lung. *C,* On expiration, the flail segment of ribs bellows outward. The affected lung and mediastinal structures shift to the affected side. Some air within the lungs is shunted back and forth between the lungs instead of passing through the upper airway.

Fluid Volume Deficit

A decrease in circulating blood volume leads to fluid volume deficit and, subsequently, to decreased tissue perfusion. Therefore, any condition producing a profound volume deficit necessitates immediate intervention. The more common causes of volume loss include shock due to acute hypovolemia, dehydration, and major burn injuries.[37, 38] Clients can lose blood volume through either internal or external active bleeding. The internal bleeding sites usually associated with large volume loss include the posterior nasal passages, aortic vessel injury or dissecting aneurysm, pulmonary vasculature, stomach, liver, spleen, uterus or fallopian tube, and fractures of the pelvis and femur. Illness leading to prolonged vomiting or diarrhea can also produce large fluid losses. "Third-spacing" volume loss or interstitial volume sequestering associated with major burn injury occurs approximately 12 hours after injury (see Chapter 50).

As volume loss occurs, various compensatory mechanisms act to produce vasoconstriction of the vasculature, retain fluid via the renal tubules, and increase cardiac output.[36] These compensatory mechanisms—such as stimulation of the sympathetic nervous system; the release of renin, angiotensin, aldosterone, and antidiuretic hormones; and fluid shifts—continue in an effort to restore tissue perfusion, thus ensuring cell survival. However, these mechanisms are limited in scope, and if the lost volume is not restored, eventually cellular structures incur irreversible damage from the oxygen debt, and death ensues.[36]

Clinical Manifestations

The client often provides a history of recent injury or illness with associated volume loss. Clinical manifestations may include agitation or decreasing level of consciousness, pale and diaphoretic skin, delayed capillary refill time of longer than 2 seconds, tachycardia, tachypnea, decreased urinary output, and hypotension.[36–39] Positive orthostatic vital signs (a decrease in systolic blood pressure by 20 mm Hg and an increase in pulse rate by 20 beats/min associated with the client changing from a lying to an upright position) may be present in clients with a mild to moderate volume loss. If blood has accumulated in the thoracic cavity (hemothorax) or abdominal cavity, percussion over the area elicits a dull sound. A collection of blood under the thoracic diaphragm or in the peritoneal cavity can produce Kehr's sign (referred shoulder pain unrelated to injury) or a rigid, hard abdomen with increased rebound tenderness upon palpation.

Diagnostic testing is directed at locating the source of any internal bleeding. Tests may include radiography, ultrasonography, and computed tomography (CT) scans of the chest, pelvis, extremities, or abdomen. The laboratory tests of blood typing, complete blood count (CBC), hemoglobin concentration and hematocrit, and electrolyte panel are performed on collected blood samples. A urine specimen should be tested for specific gravity and the presence of blood and leukocytes and, in females, for pregnancy. If gastrointestinal bleeding is suspected, a nasogastric tube is passed and the aspirate tested for the presence of blood. Stool is tested for blood.

A diagnostic peritoneal lavage (DPL) procedure is occasionally performed in unstable clients who have sustained abdominal injury. A peritoneal catheter is inserted into the client's peritoneal cavity, and 1 L of normal saline is infused. The fluid is then drained, via gravity, from the peritoneal cavity back into the emptied fluid bag. The fluid is examined for the presence of blood, bile, feces, amylase, and white blood cells to determine whether organs within the peritoneal cavity have been injured (Fig. 82–9).

Diagnostic testing not only helps in identifying the source and severity of volume loss but also aids in determining whether the client requires immediate surgery or hospital admission.

Outcome Management

Treatment is directed at preventing further volume loss and replacing fluid volume.[36–38]

Maintain Blood Flow to Vital Organs

High-flow oxygen is delivered via face mask to provide additional oxygen to tissues. Positioning the client in a supine position with the legs elevated is appropriate.

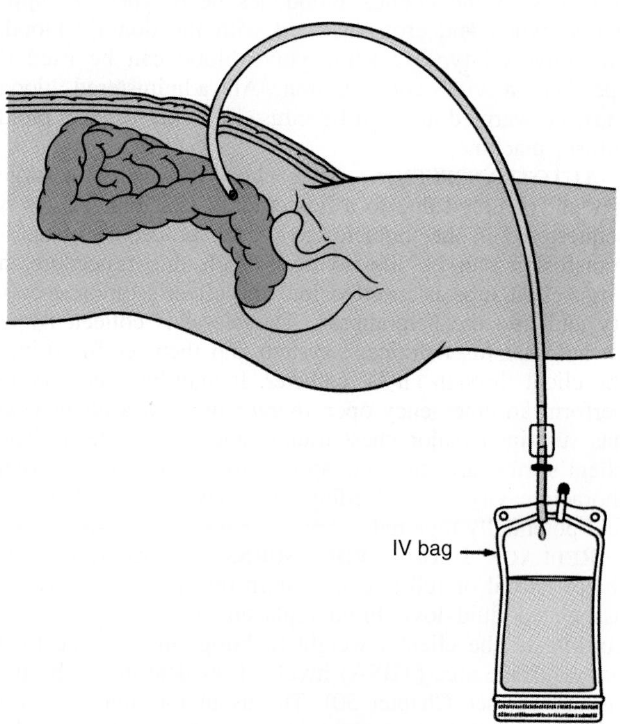

INTERPRETATION OF RESULTS

Positive result	Free-flowing blood on aspiration Grossly bloody lavage return >100,000 RBC/mm3 >500 WBC/mm3 Exit of lavage fluid from urinary or thoracic catheters
Equivocal result	50,000–100,000 RBC/mm3 100–500 WBC/mm3
Negative result	<50,000 RBC/mm3 <100 WBC/mm3

FIGURE 82–9 Diagnostic peritoneal lavage.

STOP OR DECREASE BLEEDING

If external bleeding is present, direct pressure should be applied to control further blood loss. The application of tourniquets and clamping of exposed vessels should be avoided if possible. If the bleeding source is the posterior nasal passages, the client needs to be seated and leaning forward in a high Fowler position. Nasal packing is required.

REPLACE FLUIDS

Venous access must be obtained using a large-bore catheter (14 to 16 gauge). Usually two IV sites are required for fluid replacement. At the time of vein cannulation, blood samples should also be obtained for laboratory testing.

CRYSTALLOIDS. Crystalloid fluids (normal saline, lactated Ringer's solution) are the replacement fluids of choice. They should be warmed and administered at a ratio of 3 : 1 (3 L of solution for every 1 L of volume loss) in an adult.

COLLOIDS. Colloid fluids (e.g., blood, hetastarch, albumin) may also be given fluid resuscitation. These fluids contain proteins and are infused at a 1 : 1 ratio (1 unit of solution for every 1 unit of blood loss). Blood can be administered as whole blood or as packed red blood cells. It is best if the client's blood has been typed or, optimally, typed and cross-matched with the donor's blood, but universal type O Rh-negative blood can be used if speed is a vital consideration. All administered blood must be warmed and can be infused quickly using a rapid infuser machine.

AUTOTRANSFUSION. After chest trauma, if a large amount of blood due to a hemothorax (see Fig. 82–7) is sequestered in the thoracic cavity, the procedure of autotransfusion can be life-saving.[31] With this procedure, a large chest tube is inserted into the client's thoracic cavity and into the hemothorax. The blood is collected into an autotransfuser drainage system and then reinfused into the client through an IV catheter. It may be necessary to perform an emergency open thoracotomy on a client who has sustained major chest trauma and is near death. The client's ribs are cut and spread to expose the internal thoracic cavity. Any bleeding sites may then be identified and potentially repaired.

REPLACE FLUIDS FOR BURNS. Clients who have major partial or full-thickness burn injuries are at risk for associated fluid loss. Fluid replacement is calculated according to the client's weight in kilograms and the total body surface area (TBSA) involved, as determined by the *rule of 9*s (see Chapter 50). The usual formula is 2 to 4 ml of fluid × body weight in kilograms × TBSA. The calculated amount of fluid is used as the total fluid replacement volume required over the 24-hour period from the time of injury. One half of the total fluid amount is infused in the first 8-hour period, one fourth of the fluid amount in the second 8-hour period, and the remaining one fourth amount in the last 8-hour period.

INSTITUTE OTHER MEASURES

Once fluid resuscitation is begun, other interventions can be instituted. A nasogastric tube is passed to prevent vomiting and possible aspiration. In clients with gastrointestinal bleeding, gastric lavage is performed using room-temperature normal saline instilled and aspirated through the nasogastric tube. An indwelling urinary catheter is inserted for the purpose of measuring urinary output. The client with volume loss is prone to the development of mild hypothermia. Keeping the client warm with blankets, warming lights, and infusion of warmed fluids aids in maintaining a normal body temperature. Continual monitoring of cardiac rate and rhythm, blood pressure, pulse oximetry readings, respiratory rate, and temperature is indicated.

FLUID VOLUME EXCESS

Clients who have an excess of fluid volume can concurrently have pulmonary congestion, leading to respiratory distress. Although clients with renal failure experience fluid volume excess, the disorder most commonly associated with fluid overload in the ED is heart failure. Heart failure results in fluid excess because of the inability of the cardiac muscle to function effectively. Ejection fraction decreases, pressure in the left ventricle increases, and eventually pressure increases affect the left atrium and right ventricle and atrium.[30]

Clinical Manifestations

The clinical manifestations of heart failure include agitation or restlessness, tachypnea and increased respiratory effort, respiratory rales, distended jugular neck veins, tachycardia, skin pallor, diaphoresis, ascites, and pitting dependent edema. Pulse oximetry readings are less than 94%, and the client may also cough up excessive, frothy sputum. Cardiac dysrhythmias, such as atrial fibrillation, may be noted with cardiac monitoring.[30]

Because these clients often have a chronic history of heart failure, their daily medication regimen usually includes digoxin, furosemide (Lasix), and potassium. Electrolyte imbalances are common, and serum levels of digoxin must be assessed via laboratory studies. Chest films provide information about the severity of the heart failure.

Outcome Management

IMPROVE OXYGENATION

Treatment is directed at improving the client's ability to breathe. Positioning the client in a high Fowler position facilitates the ability to breathe. Oxygen is administered at a high flow rate via face mask, although this intervention may be difficult for the client to tolerate. If respiratory fatigue develops, the client must be intubated in order to provide adequate ventilation. The use of rapid-sequence induction (RSI) before intubation may be indicated. A newer method of treating respiratory failure associated with heart failure involves the use of a tight-fitting mask placed over the client's nose and mouth and then connected to a mechanical ventilator.[34]

ADMINISTER MEDICATIONS

Establishing venous access for medication administration is necessary. The common medications include nitroglycerin 5 to 10 μg/minute given by IV infusion, furosemide (Lasix) 40 to 100 mg given intravenously, and morphine sulfate 2 to 10 mg given intravenously. If serum digoxin levels are subtherapeutic and the client is not hypokalemic, then digoxin may be administered 0.6 to 1 mg intravenously. Dobutamine, angiotensin-converting enzyme (ACE) inhibitor, and beta-blocker medications may be administered cautiously in some settings to reduce cardiac preload and to produce inotropic effects.[16]

MONITOR RESPONSE TO TREATMENT

Continual monitoring of the client's response to treatment is of paramount importance. Assessment should include level of consciousness, cardiac status, blood pressure, respiratory rate and effort, pulse oximetry, and urinary output.

DECREASED CARDIAC OUTPUT

Any illness or injury that has a direct effect on the heart can produce a decrease in cardiac output. Such disorders include cardiac dysrhythmias, acute myocardial infarction, cardiac injury, cardiac tamponade, and cardiac infection or myopathy.[37, 38]

When cardiac output decreases, tissue perfusion is adversely affected. Cardiac output (CO) is determined by stroke volume (SV) and heart rate (HR):

$$CO = SV \times HR$$

Therefore, a reduction in stroke volume or an alteration in heart rate has a direct effect on cardiac output. Cardiac dysrhythmias and acute myocardial infarction directly affect heart rate. Acute myocardial infarction also reduces stroke volume as a result of the death of cardiac muscle. Cardiac tamponade results in compression of the cardiac muscle by the collection of blood or fluid in the pericardial sac. This effect produces a decrease in stroke volume. Infection and cardiac myopathy also affect the cardiac muscle structures, thereby reducing stroke volume.

Clinical Manifestations

Depending on the cause of the reduced cardiac output, clients may present with differing clinical manifestations. Dysrhythmias are self-evident on cardiac monitoring. The most prominent manifestations include chest pain, skin pallor, diaphoresis, hypotension, nausea, and agitation or a decrease in level of consciousness. External chest wall injury may be evident with cardiac contusions. Cardiac tamponade produces the additional manifestations of distended jugular neck veins and muffled heart sounds. Fever may be present with cardiac infections.

Diagnostic tests include cardiac monitoring, chest radiography or ultrasonography, and laboratory studies. Levels of the cardiac enzymes creatine kinase (CK) and the CK-MB fraction and of the cardiac markers myoglobin and troponin T and troponin I are especially important in diagnosing the occurrences of a myocardial infarction.[17] Treadmill stress testing and dobutamine stress echocardiography (DSE) may also be performed to aid in the evaluation of chest pain.[43]

Outcome Management

IMPROVE CARDIAC OUTPUT

The goal of treatment is to improve cardiac output.[40, 41] High-flow oxygen should be administered via face mask, and venous access should be secured for the administration of medications. Supraventricular tachycardic dysrhythmias are frequently treated with the IV adenosine (Adenocar) 6 mg, whereas bradycardic rhythms may be treated with IV atropine 0.5 to 2 mg or with the insertion of a cardiac pacemaker. Lidocaine 1 mg/kg is administered to clients with premature ventricular contractions provided that they are not associated with a bradycardic rhythm. Clients who have sustained a cardiac contusion from traumatic injury may also develop cardiac dysrhythmias. For further discussion of dysrhythmia treatment, see Chapter 57.

INCREASE CORONARY ARTERY BLOOD FLOW

An acute myocardial infarction is often caused by an embolus or thrombus that occludes a coronary artery. Initially, nitroglycerin, administered sublingually or intravenously, and morphine sulfate are given to reduce pain and to produce vasodilation of the coronary arteries. Treatment may then involve the administration of oral aspirin, thrombolytic IV medications, and IV heparin or the more invasive procedure of percutaneous transluminal coronary angioplasty (PTCA). Beta-blocker therapy is also instituted in clients who do not have concurrent heart failure or cardiogenic shock.[7, 17]

Clients who have received thrombolytic medications must be continuously monitored for the presence of active bleeding. Other monitoring parameters include pain relief, cardiac rate and rhythm, blood pressure, pulse oximetry readings, and respiratory rate.

REMOVE PERICARDIAL FLUID

Blunt or penetrating force injury to the left chest can cause cardiac tamponade. If this injury is suspected or diagnosed, treatment involves pericardiocentesis (Fig. 82–10). A long spinal needle attached to a 60-ml syringe is inserted beneath the xiphoid into the pericardial sac. The accumulated blood is removed, compression of the ventricles is relieved, and cardiac output is restored.

TREAT INFECTIOUS CAUSES

Infections of the heart structures, such as pericarditis or endocarditis, may be treated with pain-relieving medications and/or antibiotics. Pericarditis is frequently caused by a viral organism, whereas endocarditis is of bacterial origin and requires antibiotic therapy.

PAIN

Pain is the most common complaint of clients seeking emergency care. Pain can be caused by almost any entity; therefore, identifying the source of pain is of paramount importance. The sensation of pain may be the only complaint, or pain may be associated with other clinical evidence of illness or injury. Pain is assessed as described earlier in the chapter.

Outcome Management

PROMOTE COMFORT

Pain relief is the goal of treatment and may be provided by administering oral, intramuscular, or IV analgesic or narcotic medications.[42] With isolated orthopedic injuries, such as digit injuries, pain relief may be obtained by injecting affected nerves with anesthetizing medications.

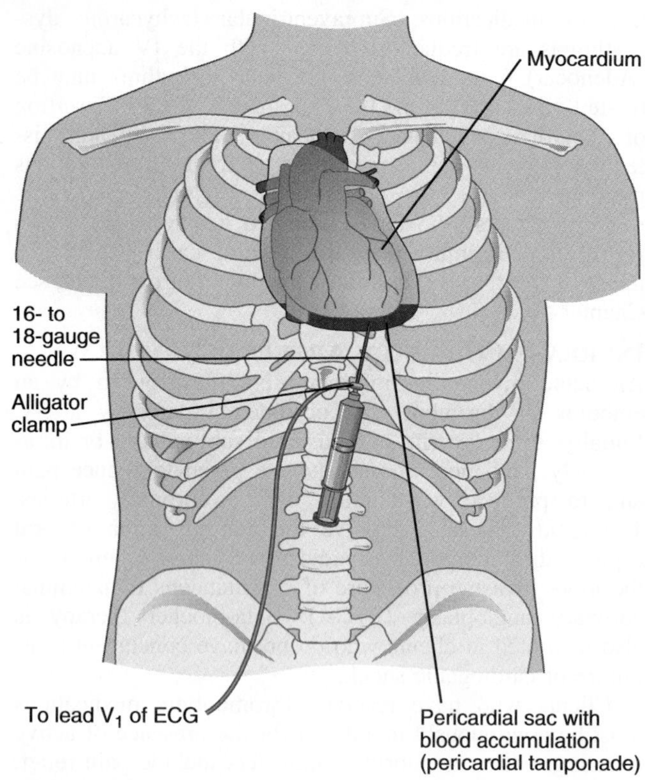

FIGURE 82–10 Pericardiocentesis procedure. (Modified from Kosmos, C. A. [1995]. In Kitt, S., et al. [Eds.], *Emergency nursing: A physiologic and clinical perspective* [2nd ed., p. 66]. Philadelphia: W. B. Saunders.)

Client comfort measures should also be instituted. Measures may include client positioning to ease stress on painful areas, elevating injured extremities, applying ice or cool compresses to injured areas, and attempting to make the room environment comfortable for the client.

Induce Conscious Sedation

Instituting conscious sedation is a routine practice in many EDs. This procedure involves controlled pharmacologic depression of the level of consciousness that nevertheless allows maintenance of the client's reflexes to protect the airway as well as spontaneous ventilation.[40] Conscious sedation is most commonly induced with medications such as midazolam (Versed), ketamine (Ketalar), or fentanyl (Sublimaze).[40] Dose and route of administration vary with the agent used. The most common routes are intramuscular (IM), IV, and nasal. The ED nurse's responsibility is to continually monitor the client for airway patency, oxygen saturation levels, cardiac activity, and response to physical or verbal stimulation until recovery from the anesthesia has occurred. The duration of sedation may be anywhere from 30 to 60 minutes. The only two absolute contraindications to conscious sedation are (1) hemodynamic instability and (2) refusal by a competent client or a parent.

ACUTE CONFUSION

Clients can have an altered level of consciousness from many causes. Underlying disorders such as cerebrovascular accident (CVA), metabolic abnormalities, seizure, intoxication, or injury need to be considered.[37, 38] A helpful guide to use in attempting to determine the cause is the "vowels-TIPS" mnemonic: A, alcohol; E, epilepsy, encephalopathy, endocrine; I, insulin; O, overdose; U, underdose or uremia; T, trauma; I, infection; P, psychogenic; S, stroke or shock.

The normal state of wakefulness and consciousness is controlled by the reticular activating system (RAS) and the brain's cerebral hemispheres. Various factors can produce a decreased state of wakefulness: impairment of the CNS from lesions or hemorrhage; a decreased supply of oxygen, blood, or glucose to cerebral tissues; and exposure to, ingestion of, or withdrawal from substances toxic to cerebral tissue.

Family members or prehospital personnel may be the only sources for obtaining historical information. It is extremely important to determine any known illnesses of the client, current medications, recent injury, known alcohol or drug use, and duration of the client's altered mental state.

Clinical Manifestations

Clinical manifestations vary according to the cause of the client's illness or injury. The Glasgow Coma Scale score is less than 15. Pupil size and equality may be altered. Unequal pupil size and reaction may indicate compression of the third cranial nerve caused by increased intracranial pressure. Small, pinpoint pupils may signify opiate overdose, pontine hemorrhage, cholinesterase poisoning, or recent use of miotic eye drops. Cranial nerve abnormalities and unilateral decreased muscle strength may be present with a recent CVA. Tongue lacerations can indicate recent seizure activity. Pale, cool, clammy skin can occur with shock or hypoglycemia. Fresh needle marks on the skin indicate recent IV drug use. A petechial rash on the skin can be an indication of a lethal bacterial meningitis. Bruising of the face, eyes (raccoon eyes), or mastoid process (Battle's sign) or a bluish hue to the tympanic membrane can indicate recent head injury and an associated basilar skull fracture.[37, 38]

Diagnostic testing involves first obtaining a bedside serum glucose level. Other laboratory studies may be indicated, including serum levels of specific medications, serum and urine toxicology screening tests, CBC, blood cultures, electrolyte panel, arterial blood gas analysis, and urinalysis. Urine specimens should also be tested for the presence of myoglobin, as clients who have been comatose for a prolonged time can develop rhabdomyolysis, resulting from ischemia and damage to large muscle groups. Other diagnostic studies include electrocardiogram (ECG), chest film, and brain CT scan. Occasionally a lumbar puncture may need to be performed.

Outcome Management

Establish and Maintain Airway

The first treatment priority in a client with an altered level of consciousness is establishing and maintaining the airway. If required, oral or nasal airway devices should be inserted, or preparations for intubation should be undertaken. During interventions directed at maintaining airway patency, spinal immobilization should also be considered if there is any suspicion that a traumatic injury may have occurred. High-flow oxygen via a face mask must be administered to provide supplemental oxygen to brain tissue.

Establish Vascular Access for Appropriate Medications

Venous access must be secured for possible IV fluid or medication administration. If a bedside glucose level reading is less than 45 mg/dl, 50% dextrose (D_{50}) is administered intravenously. If the bedside glucose level reading indicates a high level of glucose, therapy should be instituted for treatment of diabetic ketoacidosis or hyperglycemic hyperosmolar nonketotic coma (Chapter 45).

Naloxone (Narcan) 2 to 4 mg intravenously may also be administered. If the cause of the alteration in consciousness is an opiate overdose, naloxone reverses the process.

If a CVA is considered to be the cause of the client's altered level of consciousness, treatment may involve administering an IV thrombolytic medication.[5] The thrombolytic drug can be administered only after the brain CT scan has been obtained and examined by a radiologist to rule out a nonhemorrhage cause of the stroke. Research is currently being conducted on the early administration of brain-protective medications for the treatment of a CVA.[33]

If tonic-clonic seizure activity begins, the client is medicated with diazepam (Valium) 5 to 10 mg intravenously to terminate the seizure. This intervention may need to be followed by IV administration of phenytoin (Dilantin). Phenytoin must be diluted in normal saline solution and infused at a rate of less than 50 mg/minute.

IV antibiotic medications are administered in any client with known or suspected bacterial infection within the brain tissue or cerebrospinal fluid. In clients with bacterial meningitis, this can be a life-saving intervention.

Monitor Intoxicated Clients and Treat Toxicity States

Intoxicated clients with an altered level of consciousness must be monitored in the ED for a minimum of 4 to 6 hours. Treatment involves IV fluid support and nutritional supplementation with thiamine, multivitamins, and occasionally folic acid. If the level of consciousness does not improve within 4 to 6 hours, a brain CT scan should be done. It is not unusual for these clients to have suffered minor head trauma during their intoxicated state, with subsequent development of a subdural hematoma.

Monitor Clients with Head Trauma and Treat the Injuries

Neurologic trauma can result in minor disturbances such as a concussion (Table 82–8). The majority of head-injured clients are released to home without any definitive treatment. Before leaving the ED, the client and or family members must be given instructions on manifestations that indicate worsening of the client's condition.

Other types of neurologic trauma, such as skull fractures, cerebral edema, subdural hematomas, epidural hematomas, and cerebral contusions, may require operative intervention. The client must be closely monitored in the ED for any manifestations of increasing intracranial pressure. Diuretic medications such as mannitol may be administered intravenously to prevent or diminish cerebral edema.[26]

TABLE 82–8 CLASSIFICATION OF CONCUSSION

Grade	Clinical Manifestations
I	No loss of consciousness; transient confusion (lasting a few minutes); rapid return to normal functioning; no amnesia
II	Brief loss of consciousness; mild confusion; some amnesia, usually anterograde
III	Loss of consciousness for less than 6 hours; profound confusion; anterograde and retrograde amnesia
IV	Loss of consciousness for more than 6 hours; confusion; anterograde and retrograde amnesia

Prevent Injury

Safety is an important issue in a client with an altered level of consciousness. The client may need to be positioned on the left side, and frequent oral suctioning may be necessary. If in place, spinal immobilization must be maintained. Bed side rails must be up and locked in position at all times. Clients are monitored for changes in level of consciousness along with cardiac rate and rhythm, blood pressure, pulse oximetry, and respiratory rates.

Sensory Perceptual Alterations

Altered vision is the most common complaint associated with sensory perceptual changes. Such alterations can be caused by infection, inflammation, or trauma.[18, 37, 38]

Clinical Manifestations

The client may be able to provide information related to the visual changes and the circumstances surrounding the onset of the changes. The affected eye should be assessed for discharge from the eye, excessive tearing, redness of the conjunctiva, presence of a ciliary flush (a ring of inflammation surrounding the corneal-scleral junction), obvious foreign objects, presence of a cloudy cornea, extruded globe contents, and obvious ecchymosis, laceration, or trauma to the eye and surrounding structures. A baseline visual acuity test must be performed in any client with a complaint related to the eye.

Changes in vision can be present with non-urgent conditions such as conjunctivitis. This infection of the conjunctival tissue is highly contagious. Foreign objects or chemicals in the eye, corneal abrasions, and deep structure infections or injury are more significant problems, and the client usually presents with a complaint of pain as well as visual changes.

Outcome Management

Anesthetizing ophthalmic drops can be placed in the affected eye to diminish pain and allow for a more thorough examination of the eye. Superficial conjunctival infections are treated with topical ophthalmic antibiotic drops or ointments. Small superficial foreign objects are removed by the ED physician. For exposure to harmful chemicals, the eye must be irrigated with a minimum of 1 L of normal saline. After irrigation, the pH of the eye is checked; if it has not returned to normal (pH 6 to 7), irrigation may need to be continued. If corneal abrasions are present, the client is given oral pain relief medications and topical ophthalmic antibiotic medication. Patching of the affected eye is not recommended.

More serious problems associated with the eye necessitate an immediate consultation with or referral to an ophthalmologist.[11] These problems include complaints of sudden changes in or loss of vision with or without pain, impaled foreign objects, extensive injury, and globe rupture. Any client who receives treatment from the ED physician for an eye problem should be instructed to be rechecked within 24 hours by his or her primary physician or an ophthalmologist.

INFECTION

Clients frequently present to the ED because of an infectious process. The infection may be caused by either viral or bacterial organisms. The source of the infection may be localized, or the infection may have spread to surrounding tissues or be systemic. It also may be contagious.

Clinical Manifestations

The type of clinical manifestations depends upon the organism causing the infection, the extent of the infection, and the location of the infection.[37, 38] Bacterial infections usually produce more obvious and severe manifestations than those seen in viral infections. With bacterial infections, the client may have a fever. Older adults and neonates frequently have subnormal temperatures with an infectious process. The client may have pain at the site of the infection, such as the ear, throat, abdomen, genitourinary tract, or an area of skin. Meningeal infections can also produce headache, vomiting, neck pain, and occasionally petechiae. Pulmonary infections are frequently accompanied by productive cough and sputum. Erythema, edema, lymphadenopathy, and observable discharge or pus may be present with ear, throat, or skin infections. A skin rash may also be the presenting problem.

A systemic infectious process can lead to septic shock, in which endotoxins from bacterial organisms are released into the circulation. The client is acutely ill and may have clinical manifestations of fever, tachycardia, hypotension, and decreased urinary output. In later stages of sepsis, the client may become hypothermic, the skin may have a mottled appearance, and the level of consciousness becomes diminished.[36] These findings are usually associated with a high mortality rate.

A primary decision must be made about whether the infection is considered contagious to other clients in the ED. If the infection is thought to be contagious, the client must be isolated as quickly as possible from other clients. It then becomes important to identify the primary source of the infection. The ears, throat, lungs, skin, and genital and pelvic areas must be assessed for evidence of infection. A chest film is obtained, in addition to possible abdominal and pelvic ultrasound studies. Laboratory studies include a urinalysis, CBC, and culture of discharge and blood specimens. If the source of the infection has not been identified, a lumbar puncture may be required.

Outcome Management

ADMINISTER MEDICATIONS

Treatment involves administering antibiotic medications selected according to the identified or probable source of the infection. These agents may be administered orally, intramuscularly, or intravenously. The antipyretic medications acetaminophen (Tylenol) and ibuprofen can be administered orally to reduce fever. Other treatments to reduce fever involve undressing the client and allowing heat to dissipate into the environment. Cooling the client using tepid bath water is not routinely performed. Abscesses due to skin infections may need to be incised, drained, and packed.

MONITOR AND TREAT SEPSIS

If sepsis is suspected, it is important to also administer high-flow oxygen to the client, infuse IV fluids of normal saline, and insert a nasogastric tube and an indwelling urinary catheter. Additional infused medications, after antibiotic administration, may include dopamine and corticosteroids. The client must be closely monitored for changes in blood pressure, heart rate, respiratory rate, oxygen saturation, cardiac rhythm, urinary output, level of conscious changes, and prolonged bleeding times. These clients are at risk for disseminated intravascular coagulopathy (DIC).

IMPAIRED PHYSICAL MOBILITY

Any injury to the musculoskeletal system can lead to a decrease in the client's mobility.[32] Other causes of impaired mobility are injuries to the vertebral bodies and possibly the spinal cord. Sprains of ligaments, fractures to bones, dislocated joints, muscle strains, and amputated extremities or digits are the majority of problems for which clients seek emergency care related to mobility deficits.

Spinal cord injury can involve edema of the cord, with transitory or minimal deficits; cord edema can be marked; or the cord can actually be severed. With marked edema or cord severance, deficits are usually devastating and permanent. Neurogenic shock can develop with loss of the sympathetic component of the autonomic nervous system. With only the parasympathetic nervous system functioning, massive vasodilation occurs, and tissue perfusion is decreased.

Clinical Manifestations

Clinical manifestations with the majority of musculoskeletal injuries include swelling around the injured area, presence of ecchymosis, obvious deformity of the area, palpable tenderness, and limited movement of the area. Amputations are self-evident, and depending upon whether a complete or partial amputation has occurred, active bleeding may be minimal or profuse. With a complete amputation, active bleeding is minimal as a result of constriction of the severed vessels. It is important that the ED nurse assess the effectiveness of circulation, motor movement, and presence and degree of sensation distal to any musculoskeletal injury.

An injury to the spinal cord produces either or both motor and sensory deficits below the level of injury. If the injury is in the upper thoracic or cervical area, the diaphragm and thoracic intercostal muscles can be affected, leading to respiratory compromise.[22, 37, 38] A client with neurogenic shock has warm and dry skin, hypotension, and bradycardia, with no movement or sensation below the level of injury.

Radiographic films of the injured area are obtained to aid in identifying fractures. Depending upon the extent of the injury, additional laboratory tests or other diagnostic studies may be performed.

Outcome Management

Treat Sprains, Strains, and Fractures

Treatment of extremity sprains and fractures consists of immediately elevating the extremity above the level of the client's heart, applying ice to the area, and immobilizing the extremity with pillows or cardboard splints.[22] Oral, intramuscular, or IV pain medication may also need to be administered. More definitive immobilization of the area with the application of splints, molds, or immobilizers is accomplished before the client leaves the ED. Lower extremity injuries may require the client to use crutches. Detailed crutch-walking instructions must be provided (Table 82–9), and the client should be able to demonstrate adequate use of the crutches to the ED nurse.

Pain-relieving medication is also administered to clients with muscle strains.[21, 27] Once clients achieve relief of pain, they are usually discharged to home with instructions to rest and to apply alternating ice and heat to the injured area for the next 24 hours.[21]

Reduce Dislocations

A joint dislocation requires reduction in the ED. This procedure is performed by the ED physician. Pain-relieving and muscle-relaxant medications may need to be administered before the reduction procedure. Once joint reduction has been achieved, a post-reduction radiographic film must be obtained. After successful reduction, the joint is immobilized with the required orthopedic device.

TABLE 82–9 CRUTCH-WALKING INSTRUCTIONS

1. Measure for correct size of crutches—with client standing, measure from 3.75–5.0 cm below the axillary fold to a point on the floor 10 cm in front of the client and 15 cm lateral to the small toe.
2. With client standing, shoulders and back are straight, elbows flexed at 30 degrees, wrists extended, and hands dorsiflexed. Do not bear weight on axilla.
3. Three-point gait sequence involves movement of the weaker leg with both crutches simultaneously.
4. To go down stairs, place crutches on affected side, place weight on unaffected leg, place crutches on next lower step, and bring unaffected leg down to share the work of lowering the body with the support of the crutches.
5. To walk up stairs, place crutches on affected side a half-step width from the lowest step, place weight on hands, and lift the stronger leg to the step.

From Kitt S., et al. (Eds.). (1995). *Emergency nursing: A physiologic and clinical perspective* (2nd ed.). Philadelphia: W. B. Saunders.

Treat Amputation

The goal in the management of a client who has sustained an amputation is to attempt to salvage the part so that possible replantation can occur.[21, 37, 38] Any profuse bleeding from the stump should be controlled with direct pressure. The use of tourniquets and clamps is discouraged, as these measures can further damage the injured tissue. If the client has sustained significant blood loss, high-flow oxygen is administered, venous access is established, and replacement fluids are given.

The stump is then gently cleansed with normal saline. The amputated part is wrapped in sterile gauze moistened with normal saline. It is then placed in a plastic bag or container, and the plastic bag or container is placed on ice. The amputated part should *never* be placed directly on ice, as freezing of the tissues will result, making replantation impossible. The client is given pain-relieving medications and possible tetanus prophylaxis with tetanus and diphtheria toxoids (Td) 0.5 ml if more than 5 years have elapsed since the last tetanus immunization.

Treat Spinal Cord Injury

Clients with a spinal cord injury must be maintained in complete spinal immobilization. At a minimum, a cross-table lateral cervical spine radiograph is required, and this study may be followed by more extensive spinal films or a CT scan. When a high thoracic or cervical injury is present, the client may become fatigued with the effort of maintaining respirations. The need for nasal intubation and assisted ventilation must be considered. IV fluids are necessary to maintain perfusion. Administration of high-dose IV steroids such as methylprednisolone (Solu-Medrol), 30 mg/kg over 15 minutes and then 5.4 mg/kg by infusion over the following 23 hours, may be considered to reduce cord edema.[23, 40, 41] IV administration of high-dose dopamine to counteract parasympathetic nervous system effects is another treatment consideration. This therapy, however, must be instituted cautiously, as the vasoconstrictive effect may decrease perfusion to the injured cord. A nasogastric tube and indwelling urinary catheter are inserted.

The client must be kept warm with blankets and heating lights as necessary, because often the ability to regulate internal body temperature has been lost. Stabilization of cervical fractures may involve applying Gardner-Wells tongs with traction or a halo traction device. Monitoring of body temperature, cardiac rate and rhythm, blood pressure, respiratory rate and effort, pulse oximetry, urinary output, and changes in sensory and motor movement is vital.

Impaired Skin Integrity

Skin and soft tissue injury is a common problem encountered in the ED. Injury to the skin and surrounding soft tissue can occur from sharp objects, blunt force injury, scraping mechanisms, or bites resulting in lacerations, contusions, abrasions, avulsions, or puncture wounds.[37, 38]

Clinical Manifestations

Once the skin barrier has been interrupted, the potential for infection is increased. Skin flora and other bacteria now have access to the underlying structures. After injury to the skin, natural, or secondary, healing processes occur, resulting in skin closure and scarring. Primary closure, or suturing, of skin wounds also closes the skin and reduces the amount of scarring. Wounds caused by forces in which bacteria were deeply embedded in the tissues, or that are older than approximately 12 hours, are not routinely managed by primary closure. Diagnostic tests may involve radiographic films of the wound area. Such studies are important if there is any suspicion that a foreign object may be embedded in the wound.

Outcome Management

Skin and soft tissue wounds can occur anywhere on the body. Scalp and facial lacerations often bleed profusely because of the high vascularity of these areas. Direct pressure over the wound is usually sufficient to control bleeding.

CLEANSE THE WOUND

Cleansing of wounds is best achieved using high-pressure irrigation and normal saline solution. Directing the stream flow from a 20- to 30-ml syringe directly into the wound adequately cleanses most wounds.[39] A minimum of 100 ml of solution should be used. Shaving an area around a wound to remove hair is controversial. In most instances, shaving is not necessary and absolutely should NEVER be performed on a wound located in a client's eyebrow.

Open wounds often need to be anesthetized before cleansing and most definitely must be anesthetized before primary repair is attempted. A cotton ball can be saturated with a topical solution of tetracaine-adrenaline-cocaine (TAC) or lidocaine-epinephrine-tetracaine (LET) and then applied directly to a face or scalp wound, so long as it is not used near mucous membranes. Other anesthetic agents include lidocaine 1% or 2%, with or without epinephrine, and bupivacaine (Marcaine) 0.25% or 0.5%, with or without epinephrine. Anesthetic agents with epinephrine should never be injected into wounds located on the fingers, toes, ears, nose, or penis because of the vasoconstricting effects of epinephrine. Bupivacaine provides a longer anesthetic effect than that obtained with lidocaine.

CLOSE THE WOUND

Small, superficial wounds may be closed with adhesive paper strips or Dermabond glue. It is important to evert and bring the wound edges close together and then apply the paper strips or glue.[39]

Larger wounds that are gaping, involve injury to deeper structures, and are located in high-tension areas or over joints need to be sutured for optimal healing. The type of suture material required varies depending upon the size and location of the open wound (Table 82–10).

Abrasion injuries are not sutured. Abrasion injuries need to be thoroughly cleansed in order to remove any particles or debris left in the wound. If particles do remain in the wound, a tattooing effect results with the healing process. Human and animal bites are not routinely sutured because of the highly contaminated nature of the wound. The wound is thoroughly irrigated, and prophylactic antibiotic medications are frequently administered. Animal bites should be reported to the local animal control authorities.

TABLE 82–10 SUTURE MATERIAL

Suture Size	Indicated Use: Body Area(s)
2–0, 3–0	Tissue subjected to strong tensile forces (e.g., knees, elbows, over joints)
3–0, 4–0	Epidermal and dermal layers, except for face
5–0, 6–0	Facial area

APPLY A DRESSING

Protective dressings must be applied to wounds before the client leaves the ED. The majority of dressings involve first applying a thin layer of antibacterial ointment or gauze impregnated with petrolatum (Vaseline) or other occlusive substance. Then dry, sterile gauze is applied for padding, followed by a wrap of woven gauze (Kling or Kerlix). Adhesive tape is used to hold the dressing in place.

ADMINISTER TETANUS AND RABIES PROPHYLAXIS

Clients must be questioned about their tetanus immunization status. Table 82–11 presents current recommendations for tetanus prophylaxis. Td 0.5 ml is the preferred agent for active immunization in adults. Should passive immunization be necessary, human tetanus immune globulin (TIG) 250 units is administered. If both preparations must be administered, separate sites for injection should be selected.

Rabies prophylaxis should be considered in clients who have been bitten by dogs, cats, skunks, raccoons, bats, squirrels, or opossums, even though the incidence of rabies is low in the United States.[16] Prophylaxis is especially important if the animal cannot be located and placed under quarantine for an observation period. The

TABLE 82–11 TETANUS PROPHYLAXIS IN WOUND MANAGEMENT

Immunization History (No. of Doses)	Clean Minor Wounds		All Other Wounds	
	*Td**	*TIG†*	*Td*	*TIG*
Uncertain	Yes	No	Yes	Yes
0–2	Yes	No	Yes	Yes
3 or more	No (Yes, if >10 yr since last dose)	No	No (Yes, if >5 yr since last dose)	No

Modified from Centers for Disease Control and Prevention: *MMWR Morbidity and Mortality Weekly Report,* 1989–1990.

* Td, tetanus and diphtheria toxoids: used for persons 7 years of age or older. For children younger than 7 years, diphtheria-pertussis-tetanus (DPT).

† TIG, tetanus immune globulin (Hypertet).

dose of human rabies immune globulin (RIG) for passive immunization is 20 units/kg, with as much as possible injected into and around the wound site and the remainder of the dose injected intramuscularly in the buttocks. For active immunization with human diploid cell vaccine (HDCV), the dose is 1 ml initially and again on days 3, 7, 14, and 28 following the bite incident.

INSTRUCT ON WOUND CARE

Instructions related to the care of the wound are given to the client and/or family member before they leave the ED. These instructions should identify the manifestations of infection and explain care of the wound and timing for a follow-up appointment with the appropriate physician for a recheck of the wound and for another appointment for removal of sutures.

POISONING

ACCIDENTAL AND INTENTIONAL POISONINGS

Poisonings are either accidental or intentional. Accidental poisonings occur more commonly in the pediatric age group, whereas intentional poisonings are more frequent in the adolescent and adult population. Poisoning can also occur from injected venom, such as snake or insect bites.

Obtaining accurate information about the offending substance, amount, and time of ingestion or exposure can be difficult. Details may be available from family or friends. Other important information to obtain is whether the client has vomited since the exposure, whether the client has been depressed or had any previous episodes of intentional poisoning, and any other associated details.

Clinical Manifestations

Assessment must be directed toward the intactness of the client's ABCs (airway, breathing, and circulation). There may be very few outward clinical manifestations that aid in determining the substance that was was ingested, inhaled, or injected.

Diagnostic tests may include electrocardiography and continual cardiac monitoring. Blood and urine specimens need to be obtained for toxicology screening and testing. In many cases the results of these tests are not rapidly available. Chest films may aid in diagnosing possible aspiration. If envenomation is the source of poisoning, bleeding and coagulation studies must be performed.

Outcome Management

MAINTAIN AIRWAY

If the client demonstrates a decrease in level of consciousness, initial interventions include establishing and maintaining a patent airway, possibly with airway adjunct devices. Oxygen should be administered, and venous access should be obtained.

REMOVE OFFENDING SUBSTANCE

Treatment is directed at removing or absorbing the offending substance. If the substance was injected, naloxone 2 to 4 mg may be administered intravenously. If the client's level of consciousness is decreased and the substance was ingested, a large nasogastric (Ewald) tube is passed either nasally or orally and gastric lavage performed. This procedure involves instilling approximately 250–500 ml normal saline solution through the tube and then removing the solution either with a syringe or gravity drainage into a collection bag. This process is repeated until the returned contents are clear. Then liquid-activated charcoal and a cathartic are instilled through the Ewald tube and allowed to remain in the stomach. The charcoal aids in absorbing any other remaining particles of the toxic substance.

Awake and alert clients are given liquid-activated charcoal to drink. Occasionally, the charcoal slurry may cause the client to vomit, and an additional dose of the charcoal may be required. The purpose of activated charcoal is again to quickly absorb the ingested toxic substance to minimize its harmful effects. Syrup of ipecac is not routinely administered[3]; it is not effective in removing the toxic substance, unless the ingestion has occurred within the previous 30 minutes, as its emetic effect prolongs the time until activated charcoal can be administered. Clients who have ingested an alkaline-based substance are not given syrup of ipecac, charcoal, or any substance that can cause emesis.

If a specific toxic substance exposure is known and an antidote is available, the antidote is administered. Table 82–12 provides a list of the more common poisoning substances and antidotes.

TABLE 82–12 POISONINGS AND ANTIDOTES

Toxic Substance	Treatment
Beta-blocker medications	Treat hypotension initially with fluids; if unsuccessful, administer glucagon 100–150 μg/kg IV followed by 2–5 mg/hr by infusion
Calcium channel-blocker medications	Calcium chloride 5–10 ml IV, or calcium gluconate 10–20 ml IV
Carbon monoxide	100% oxygen; possibly use of hyperbaric chamber
Iron	Deferoxamine (Desferal) 80 mg/kg IV or IM and repeated q 8 hr
Isoniazid (INH)	Pyridoxine (vitamin B_6) IV in a dose equivalent to amount ingested (gram for gram); if ingested amount is unknown, administer 5 g IV over 3–5 min, then repeat q 3–5 min until seizures are controlled
Methanol, ethylene glycol	50% ethanol 0.7 g/kg, or 7 ml/kg of 10% ethanol IV; continuous IV infusion of 0.07 to 0.1 g/kg/hr to maintain blood ethanol concentration between 100 and 200 mg/dl
Phenothiazine medications	Diphenhydramine (Benadryl) 0.5–1 mg/kg IV or benztropine (Cogentin) 1–2 mg IM

PROVIDE PSYCHIATRIC EVALUATION AS NEEDED

Any client who is in the ED because of an intentional poisoning must have a psychiatric evaluation before discharge and release from the ED. Many communities have psychiatric evaluation teams (PETs) that provide this service.

■ SNAKE BITE

Snake antivenin is available for clients who have been envenomated by a pit viper (a poisonous snake). The area of the envenomation may be swollen and ecchymotic, and pain may be present at the site. Pit viper venom produces both proteolytic and hemotoxic effects. Massive swelling producing a compartment syndrome may develop, and a coagulation disorder such as DIC may result. The wound area should be gently cleansed. Ice should not be applied to reduce swelling. Antivenin is administered intravenously, but skin or conjunctival testing must be performed before administering the antivenin.[10]

HYPERTHERMIA

Hyperthermic emergencies are usually the result of environmental exposure. The geriatric population is at the greatest risk for developing hyperthermia. The types of hyperthermic problems are heat cramps, heat exhaustion, and heat stroke.[37, 38] Heat stroke is the most severe.

Clinical Manifestations

Muscle spasms of the arms and legs are evident with heat cramps. Often there is a depletion of sodium because the client has been perspiring excessively. Excessive sweating can lead to dehydration and heat exhaustion. The client may complain of headache, dizziness, nausea, and weakness. Mild hypotension can be present, and the skin is frequently cool and clammy to the touch.

Heat stroke is an emergent condition. The client is often comatose. Other clinical manifestations include hypotension, tachycardia, hot and flushed-appearing skin, and a core temperature of greater than 105° F (40.5° C).

Outcome Management

ADMINISTER FLUIDS AND ELECTROLYTES

For the client with mild heat cramps, administering oral fluids with electrolytes and removal from the hot environment are usually the only necessary treatments. Treatment of a client with heat exhaustion also involves removal from the hot environment and administering either oral or IV fluids to correct the problem.

RESOLVE HEAT STROKE

Heat stroke treatment involves establishing and maintaining a patent airway, administering high-flow oxygen, and establishing venous access. IV normal saline is administered to restore fluid volume. Cooling measures must be instituted quickly. These measures include removing all clothing from the client; spraying tepid mist over the client's body and using a fan to increase air flow; placing ice packs on the scalp and neck and in the axillae and groin; and using a cooling blanket. Gastric lavage with cool saline and peritoneal dialysis may be necessary. Cooling measures should continue until the client's body temperature is 101° F (38.4° C).[37, 38] As the temperature decreases, administering chlorpromazine (Thorazine) or diazepam (Valium) may be required to reduce shivering.

A nasogastric tube and indwelling urinary catheter must be inserted. Continual cardiac, pulse oximetry, blood pressure, respiratory rate, and temperature monitoring are performed.

HYPOTHERMIA

Clinical Manifestations

A body temperature of below 94° F (34.4° C) indicates the condition of hypothermia. The development of hypothermia is usually unintentional and involves accidental and prolonged exposure to cold temperatures.

Hypothermia severity can be divided into stages depending upon the client's core temperature. Different clinical manifestations are present with each stage (see Table 82–13).

Outcome Management

REWARM THE CLIENT

After the establishment and maintenance of a patent airway, heated high-flow oxygen administration, and venous access with warmed fluid replacement, treatment is then directed at rewarming the client. Rewarming must be done slowly, as the hypothermic client is especially prone to the development of ventricular fibrillation and cardiovascular collapse if blood is returned too rapidly to a cold heart. Rewarming methods include the following[37, 38]:

1. *Passive warming*
   a. Removing wet clothing
   b. Covering the client with warm blankets
   c. Placing the client in a warm room

TABLE 82–13 STAGES OF HYPOTHERMIA

Stage	Clinical Manifestations
Mild: 93° to 95° F (34.0°–35° C)	Person is conscious and alert but may have lethargy and confusion Shivering Bradycardia or tachycardia
Moderate: 86° to 93° F (30°–34° C)	Decreased level of consciousness or coma Hypoventilation Bradycardia Atrial fibrillation Hypovolemia Cessation of shivering Possible hyperglycemia due to underutilization of glucose
Severe: <86° F (<30° C)	Coma Fixed and dilated pupils Bradycardia Apnea Hypotension Ventricular fibrillation Asystole

2. *Active warming*
   a. Immersing the client in a warm bath (104° F [40° C])
   b. Placing the client on a warming blanket
   c. Placing radiant lamps over the client
3. *Active core warming*
   a. Infusing warmed IV fluids
   b. Providing heated, humidified supplemental oxygen
   c. Performing warm fluid lavage (peritoneal, gastric, bladder, or colonic lavage)
   d. Performing continuous arteriovenous rewarming (CAVR), hemodialysis, or cardiopulmonary bypass

Insertion of a nasogastric tube and indwelling urinary catheter is an additional component of care. Continual cardiac, pulse oximetry, blood pressure, respiratory rate, and temperature monitoring must be instituted.

■ FROSTBITE

Hypothermia to the extremities can lead to frostbite injury. The feet, hands, nose, ears, and cheeks are most commonly affected.[37, 38] Damage to the tissues occurs, and peripheral blood flow is reduced. The area may appear red and swollen or may be pale in color. Formation of blisters containing either clear or purple bloody fluid may be seen. Rewarming of the frostbitten area should begin once the client is removed from the cold environment. The frostbitten part should be immersed in heated water at 105° to 115° F (40.6° to 46.1° C). The frostbitten area needs to be handled gently so that blood-filled blisters remain intact. Loose, sterile, bulky dressings are then applied and changed daily. The rewarming process is painful; therefore, pain-relieving medications must be administered.

INEFFECTIVE INDIVIDUAL COPING

Clients present to the ED not only with medical and traumatically induced problems but with psychological issues as well. Psychological disorders can range from mild anxiety to psychosis to deep depression. It is important that clients with psychological problems be taken as seriously as clients seeking treatment for medical problems.

A brief mental status examination needs to be conducted to assess the client's behavior, speech patterns, mood and affect, thought processes, and judgment and insight. Has the client recently experienced a crisis-producing situation? Is the client experiencing auditory or visual hallucinations? A physical examination must be performed to identify any concurrent medical condition that may be compounding the problem.

It is important to communicate with the client in a calm, nonjudgmental, and accepting manner. Focusing the client on reality and explaining expected behaviors constitute part of the therapeutic communication process. In some cases, involuntary psychiatric hospitalization may be required. Should the client be discharged from the ED, providing outside agency assistance and referral can be helpful.

CONCLUSIONS

Providing care to clients in the ED setting can be challenging and rewarding. An understanding of the principles of emergency care is the cornerstone of the specialty of emergency nursing. The majority of clients present to the ED without a working diagnosis but only a cadre of clinical manifestations. Therefore, assessing each client using an organized approach is paramount for the ED nurse in order to be able to establish care priorities and to institute appropriate interventions. The nursing process from assessment to evaluation is continually utilized. The scope of ED nursing is constantly changing and expanding beyond the hospital walls into the areas of community practice and community education.

THINKING CRITICALLY

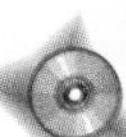

1. A 23-year-old man walks into the emergency department. He tells you that he was in a motor vehicle accident about 4 hours ago. The police were at the scene, but he refused to be transported to the emergency department because he felt fine; he went home. At home, however, the client started to experience worsening shoulder and posterior neck pain. His mother urged him to come to the emergency department. He tells you that he has "numbness" in his fingers and a "tingling" feeling in his right elbow. If you were the triage nurse, what potential problems would you consider that this client might have? Would you classify the client as emergent, urgent, or nonurgent? What measures should you take to ensure the client's safety?

Factors to Consider. What injuries sustained in a motor vehicle accident might account for the client's manifestations?

2. A 35-year-old man was brought in to the emergency department by the city police, who were arresting him for drunk and disorderly conduct. He had been involved in a barroom brawl, during which he acquired several small lacerations about the face and arms from broken glass, a hit to the head, and kicks to his ribs. He is conscious, verbally abusive, and threatening to fight his way out of the emergency department because he wants "to go home and be left alone." He has twice threatened you with bodily harm if you persist in preventing him from leaving. How would you proceed with this case?

Factors to Consider. Whom should you call? Would it be appropriate to sedate this client? What should you do if the client actually harms you physically?

3. A 60-year-old man has arrived at the emergency department with a complaint of headache. He states that he never had headaches until about 2 weeks ago, when he began awakening in the morning with head pain. The headache would go away each day after he had been up and around for a few hours and had taken aspirin. In the last few days, however, neither aspirin nor acetaminophen has helped and the headache has become nearly continuous. His wife states that his speech and balance have been "off" a little. He

wonders whether there can be any connection between his headaches and a recent fall or a recent elevation in blood pressure. Describe how you would proceed with an evaluation of this client. What further information should you elicit from him? What is your assessment priority? What triage classification would be best for this client? What interventions should you anticipate?

Factors to Consider. What diagnostic assessments should you anticipate? What should you include in your physical examination and nursing history?

4. **The client, a 70-year-old man, has been brought to the emergency department by ambulance. His wife states that he has become increasingly confused over the past few months. Within the past few days, he has become worse, is difficult to awaken in the morning, and is "sleepy" all day. This situation progressed until today, when the client's wife could not keep him awake at all; she called an ambulance and had him brought in. The client has a long history of hypertension, coronary artery disease, diabetes mellitus, and depression. Ambulance records show evidence that the client is difficult to arouse, but upon aggressive stimulation he "wakes up" and can follow basic commands. His vital signs are stable, but his pulse is slow and irregular. Blood pressure is now lower than his "norm." His wife has brought his medications with her in a large paper bag. What is your priority assessment? What should you include in your physical assessment? What interventions should you anticipate?**

Factors to Consider. What body systems should you assess? What diagnostic studies should you anticipate?

BIBLIOGRAPHY

1. Andrews, M., Goldberg, K., & Kaplan, H. (1996). *Nurses' legal handbook* (3rd ed.). Springhouse, PA: Springhouse Corporation.
2. Baier, F. E. (1993). Implications of the Consolidated Omnibus Budget Reconciliation "antidumping" legislation for emergency nurses. *Journal of Emergency Nursing, 19*(2), 115–120.
3. Bartscherer, D. J. (1997). Syrup of ipecac: Appropriate use in the emergency Department. *Journal of Emergency Nursing, 23*(3), 251–253.
4. Belanger, M. A., & Reed, S. (1997). A rural community hospital's experience with family-witnessed resuscitation. *Journal of Emergency Nursing, 23*(3), 238–239.
5. Bethel, S. A. (1997). Intravenous thrombolytic therapy for stroke emergencies. *Journal of Emergency Nursing, 23*(4), 344–346.
6. Brucker, J. M. (1998). Respiratory syncytial virus. *ADVANCE for Nurse Practitioners, 6*(2), 61–65.
7. Buhse, M. (1998). Quick thinking needed: Early management of acute myocardial infarction. *ADVANCE for Nurse Practitioners, 6*(8), 29–35.
8. Coakley-Maller, C., & Shea, M. (1997). Respiratory infections in children. *ADVANCE for Nurse Practitioners, 5*(9), 21–27.
9. Cornell, S. (1998). Advance directives: Whose death is it, anyway? *ADVANCE for Nurse Practitioners, 6*(7), 68–70.
10. Deer, P. J. (1997). Elapid envenomation: A medical emergency. *Journal of Emergency Nursing, 23*(6), 574–577.
11. DelGross, C., & Smally A. J. (1997). A 24-year-old male with eye trauma. *Clinical Reviews, 7*(10), 142–144.
12. Dronen, S. C. (1998). Pharmacologic adjuncts to intubation. In J. R. Roberts & J. R. Hedges (Eds.), *Clinical procedures in emergency medicine* (3rd ed.). Philadelphia: W. B. Saunders.
13. Emergency Nurses Association (1999). In J. Dains, et al. (Eds.), *Standards of emergency nursing practice* (4th ed., pp. 59–64). St. Louis: Mosby–Year Book.
14. Frakes, M. A. (1997). Asthma in the emergency department. *Journal of Emergency Nursing, 23*(5), 429–435.
15. Gerchufsky, M. (1996). Collaring a killer: What you need to know about rabies. *ADVANCE for Nurse Practitioners, 4*(9), 49–52
16. Dambro, M. R., & Griffith, J. A. (1996, September). Griffith's 5-minute clinical consult: Congestive heart failure. *Clinical Reviews,* 138–139.
17. Hahn, M. S. (1995). Matters of the heart. *ADVANCE for Nurse Practitioners, 3*(9), 13–17.
18. Hahn, M. S. (1996). Common eye problems in primary care. *ADVANCE for Nurse Practitioners, 4*(3), 27–31.
19. Harrahill, M. (1998). Flail chest: A nursing challenge. *Journal of Emergency Nursing, 24*(3), 288–289.
20. Higgins, B., & Barrow, S. (1998). Asthma in adolescents. *ADVANCE for Nurse Practitioners, 6*(2), 28–37.
21. Jagmin, M. G. (1995). Musculoskeletal emergencies. In S. Kitt, et al. (Eds.), *Emergency nursing: A physiologic and clinical perspective* (2nd ed.). Philadelphia: W. B. Saunders.
22. Jaworski, M. A. (1995). Spinal trauma. In S. Kitt, et al. (Eds.), *Emergency nursing: A physiologic and clinical perspective* (2nd ed.). Philadelphia: W. B. Saunders.
23. Jezierski, M. (1993). Foote Hospital Emergency Department: Shattering a paradigm. *Journal of Emergency Nursing, 19*(3), 266–267.
24. Keep, N., et al. (1992). California Emergency Nurses Association's informal survey of violence in California emergency departments. *Journal of Emergency Nursing, 18*(5), 433–439.
25. Kosmos, C. A. (1995). Multiple trauma. In S. Kitt, et al. (Eds.), *Emergency nursing: A physiologic and clinical perspective* (2nd ed). Philadelphia: W. B. Saunders.
26. Leccese, C. (1997). Reducing the toll of brain injury: New guidelines offer principles for intervention. *ADVANCE for Nurse Practitioners, 5*(6), 57–60.
27. McIntosh, E. (1997). Low back pain in adults. Guidelines for the history and physical exam. *ADVANCE for Nurse Practitioners, 5*(8), 16–25.
28. Maller, C. C. (1995). Adult asthma management: All things considered. *ADVANCE for Nurse Practitioners, 3*(9), 20–26.
29. Mathias, S., & Hodgdon, A. K. (1997). Resurgence of tuberculosis: Implications for emergency nurses. *Journal of Emergency Nursing, 23*(5), 425–428.
30. Miller, S. K. (1997). Congestive heart failure: Clinical assessment and pharmacologic management. *ADVANCE for Nurse Practitioners, 5*(6), 17–27.
31. Murdock, M. A., & Roberson, M. L. (1993). Reported use of autotransfusion systems in initial resuscitation areas by one hundred thirty-six United States hospitals. *Journal of Emergency Nursing, 19*(6), 486–490.
32. O'Hanlon-Nichols, T. (1998). A review of the adult musculoskeletal system. *American Journal of Nursing,* 98(6), 48–52.
33. Richman, E. (1996). Acute stroke interventions: Proactive strategies to preserve brain tissue. *ADVANCE for Nurse Practitioners, 4*(4), 79–97.
34. Reynolds, J. E. (1997). Noninvasive ventilation for acute respiratory failure. *Journal of Emergency Nursing, 23*(6), 608–610.
35. Sarnese, P. M. (1997). Assessing security in the emergency department: An overview. *Journal of Emergency Nursing, 23*(1), 23–26.
36. Selfridge-Thomas, J. (1995). Shock. In S. Kitt, et al. (Eds.), *Emergency nursing: A physiologic and clinical perspective* (2nd ed.). Philadelphia: W. B. Saunders.
37. Selfridge-Thomas, J. (1997). *Emergency nursing: An essential guide for patient care.* Philadelphia: W. B. Saunders.
38. Selfridge-Thomas, J. (1995). *Manual of emergency nursing.* Philadelphia: W. B. Saunders.
39. Walters, G. K. (1996). Managing soft tissue wounds: Caveats for everyday practice. *ADVANCE for Nurse Practitioners, 4*(3), 37–54.
40. Ward, K. R., & Yealy, D. M. (1998). Systemic analgesia and sedation for procedures. In J. R. Roberts & J. R. Hedges (Eds.), *Clinical procedures in emergency medicine* (4th ed.). Philadelphia: W. B. Saunders.
41. Williams, R. M. (1997). Are emergency departments really the most expensive place of all? *Journal of Emergency Nursing, 23*(4), 292–294.
42. Winslow, E. H. (1998). Effective pain management. *American Journal of Nursing, 98*(7), 16HH–16II.
43. Zielinski, S., Pavey, S., & Dunham, S. (1998). Dobutamine stress echocardiogram: Emergency department evaluation of chest pain. *Journal of Emergency Nursing, 24*(3), 240–246.

Fever-Related Interventions

QUESTIONS

When are interventions to control fever most beneficial to a critically ill client?
How is fever most effectively managed in the critically ill?

CITATION

Henker, R. (1999). Evidence-based practice: Fever-related interventions. *American Journal of Critical Care, 8,* 481–487.

STUDIES

Approximately 30 research reports from biologic, critical care, nursing, and medical journals were reviewed and integrated. Four animal studies were included. The method of assembling the studies was not described, and tables summarizing the studies cited were not provided. The author rated the strength of the evidence for each recommendation using the levels of the American Association of Critical-Care Nurses (AACN) Research-Based Practice Protocols.*

Summary of Findings

When Should Fever Be Treated in the Critically Ill? (p. 481)

Physiologic Responses Associated with Fever (p. 482)

Four animal studies demonstrating that fever is a beneficial host defense response were cited. Although fever may be beneficial to survival, in treating humans other factors such as the client's comfort and demands that fever makes on cardiopulmonary physiology must be considered. Fever, possibly in association with bacterial endotoxins, causes increased oxygen consumption, heart rate, serum levels of norepinephrine and epinephrine, and cardiac output.[23, 28] In a clinical study,[2] the heart rate of critically ill patients with temperatures greater than 37.8° C (100° F) was significantly higher than those with temperatures less than that level (average of 111 beats per minute for the first group, 94 for the latter).

Elevated Body Temperature in Clients with Head Injuries (p. 483)

The use of moderate hypothermia for treatment of clients with traumatic brain injury may improve outcomes. Two studies have found that hypothermia decreased intracranial pressure (ICP),[17, 25] and three studies found that clients treated with hypothermia had higher Glasgow Coma Scale scores.[6, 16, 17] Two studies indicated that in patients with head injuries the brain temperature tends to be higher than the core temperature,[9, 24]

Fever in Clients with Sepsis (p. 483)

Studies of the effects of fever in clients with sepsis are difficult to interpret because of the multiple factors that can affect outcomes. However, these clients are an interesting group to study because altered thermoregulation causes some of them to be hypothermic and others to be febrile. In a study of 500 clients with bacteremia or fungemia, the survival rate of 405 in whom fever developed was higher than in the relatively hypothermic clients.[29] In a large clinical trial,[5] the 9% of the septic population with hypothermia had a much worse prognosis than the febrile clients with sepsis. Compared with febrile clients, hypothermic clients had a higher incidence of central nervous system (CNS) dysfunction, shock, clotting abnormalities, inability to recover from shock, and death. The authors concluded that hypothermia associated with sepsis syndrome is related to poor clinical outcomes. In a randomized, double-blind clinical trial of 455 clients, treating sepsis with ibuprofen decreased fever, tachycardia, oxygen consumption, and lactic acidosis but did not reduce the incidence or duration of shock or respiratory distress syndrome, nor did this treatment improve survival.[1]

How Is Fever Most Effectively Treated in the Critically Ill?

Clinical Comparison of Antipyretic Agents and Physical Cooling

Antipyretic agents, tepid sponging, iced cloths, and cooling blankets are often used to reduce fever. Two important issues of concern when these interventions are used are the effect on core body temperature and the associated cardiovascular responses. In a study of 21 clients with neurologic dysfunction, these three methods were compared in terms of time required to return to 100° F and shivering.[19] No difference was found in the time required; however, the small size of each group may have made a difference impossible to detect even if it existed. Clients cooled by acetaminophen and a hypothermia blanket demonstrated significantly more shivering compared with clients cooled by acetaminophen alone or by acetaminophen and sponging. Another small study of 14 patients[10] compared acetaminophen alone (n = 5), acetaminophen and cooling blanket (n = 3), and cooling blanket alone (n = 6); after 3 hours, the mean pulmonary artery temperature of the first group increased 0.2 of a degree, whereas it decreased on average 0.4 and 0.3 of a degree in the other two groups. These were the only studies found by the reviewer comparing treatments of fever in critically ill clients.

Physical Cooling

In a study of the care of critically ill clients, cooling blankets were used to treat fever in clients whose body temperature was above 39.7° C; most were receiving mechanical ventilation or had acute disease of the CNS[21]; 41% of the 94 episodes of fever in this study were treated with cooling blankets. Four

*Recommendation levels of the AACN Research-Based Practice Protocols[4]: level 1, manufacturer's recommendation only; level 2, theory-based, no research data to support the recommendation—expert consensus group recommendation; level 3, laboratory data but not clinical data to support the recommendation; level 4, limited clinical studies to support the recommendation; level 5, clinical studies in more than one or two different populations or situations; and level 6, clinical studies in a variety of populations and situations.

Bridge continued on the following page

Fever-Related Interventions *Continued*

cooling blanket temperatures (7.2° C, 12.8° C, 18.3° C, 23.9° C) were evaluated in a random assignment study of 89 febrile, critically ill clients.[3] The clients were placed between two cooling blankets and were also given acetaminophen. No statistically significant difference was found among the four groups in terms of amount of time required to decrease temperature, but clients were more comfortable at the higher temperatures. Although there was no difference in the average time in which clients started shivering, less shivering occurred with warmer blanket temperatures. These findings were interpreted as meaning that warmer blanket temperatures provide similar rates of cooling, possibly less shivering, and greater comfort to patients. No reports were found evaluating the effectiveness of one versus two blankets or anterior versus posterior placement of cooling blankets.

The effectiveness of cooling with tepid water sponging, ice packs, and exposure of more body surface to room air has received surprisingly little attention. A study comparing acetaminophen, external cooling, and metamizole (an analgesic) in 20 critically ill adults found external cooling with cloths soaked in ice water was the most effective method of decreasing core body temperature; the administration of acetaminophen was the least effective.[22] A chart review study examined the temperature responses of 88 febrile medical-surgical patients to administration of acetaminophen alone and acetaminophen in combination with physical cooling.[7] Temperatures decreased in 82 (92%) of the clients, with an average decrease of 2.4° C. Ice packs were the most commonly used means of physical cooling; of five patients treated with acetaminophen and ice packs, three experienced a decrease in temperature, whereas two experienced a small increase.

In summary, physical cooling is effective but the relative benefits of various methods of physical cooling have not been studied, nor has the extent to which physical cooling interventions other than the cooling blanket induce shivering.

Antipyretic Agents (p. 485)

In one study of critically ill adults[15] a combination of acetaminophen and paralytic agents was found to decrease oxygen consumption, cardiac output, and heart rate. As mentioned earlier, in the critically ill, acetaminophen was less effective than external cooling[10, 22] and less effective than metamizole in decreasing body temperature.[22] The extent to which acetaminophen is absorbed in the gastrointestinal tract of the critically ill may be a factor in its effectiveness, although one study comparing burn patients with heathy volunteers found no difference in drug absorption in the two groups.[20]

Another study of 27 critically ill clients with a variety of problems[26] documented wide variations in drug level 60 minutes after administration. No studies compared oral administration with rectal administration in critically ill persons. Two studies of young children after surgery[13, 18] suggest that absorption of acetaminophen is faster and better via the upper gastric route than via the rectal route.

No studies were found comparing the effects of various antipyretics on fever in critically ill clients. In two studies of febrile children, peak levels of oral acetaminophen were reached in 0.5 to 1.0 hour after administration, whereas peak levels of oral ibuprofen occurred from 1.0 to 1.5 hours.[2, 14] A comparison of oral acetaminophen (650 mg) to three doses of intramuscular ketorolac (15, 30, and 60 mg), a nonsteroidal anti-inflammatory drug, in healthy adult volunteers found that those who received 60 mg of ketorolac had the smallest increase in temperature after injection with an endotoxin; those who received 30 mg of ketorolac had increases similar to those who were given acetaminophen.[27]

"Other Methods of Treating Fever" (p. 486)

Cooling by blowing cold air across the skin surface (convective cooling) has not been studied as extensively as rewarming with warm air. Another approach involving the wrapping of extremities over peripheral skin sensors has been used to decrease shivering. In a randomized study of clients receiving amphotericin B, the responses of 20 subjects whose extremities were wrapped were compared to those of the control group.[11] The duration of shivering episodes in the control group was longer than what was experienced by the extremity-wrapped group.

Limitations/Reservations. Critically ill clients are a widely diverse group and many have multisystem dysfunctions. As a result, separating the effects of fever from those of underlying disease and dysfunction is difficult. CNS dysfunctions and variations in blood flow in particular make evaluation of fever interventions difficult to study. Hence, the body of research is affected by multiple uncontrolled variables.

An important uncontrolled variable is the manner in which the interventions were delivered. Many of the studies did nothing to ensure that the interventions were delivered in a consistent manner or that temperatures were measured in the same way; such lack of control decreases the likelihood of detecting an effect of the interventions on fever.

In addition, many of the studies are small, suggesting that the lack of difference in intervention effectiveness found in some of these studies might be the result of an inadequate sample size, not a true difference in intervention effectiveness. Hence, this body of research lacks findings from high quality studies in which clinicians can have confidence, and many questions remain regarding whether, how, and when to intervene to manage fever.

Research-Based Practice

The benefits of fever as a host defense mechanism and an indicator of disease must always be weighed against the metabolic, cardiovascular, and pulmonary demands (i.e., energy expenditures) imposed by fever. These demands may not be tolerated by older or debilitated persons, infants, and those with coronary heart disease, heart failure, or pulmonary disease. When a person is at risk to not tolerate fever, intervention to reduce temperature is indicated.

If the fever is determined to be of infectious origin, antibiotic treatment of the underlying infection will be started. In fever of a noninfectious or an infectious basis, interventions may need to be instituted to control the fever itself until the underlying disorder can be brought under control. A common form of intervention is to administer antipyretic medication (e.g., aspirin, acetaminophen, paracetamol, metamizole). However, the benefits of these medications alone in critically ill clients are not well supported by the research findings of this review; in several studies, acetaminophen or metamizole when

Fever-Related Interventions *Continued*

used alone either did not reduce temperature or was not as effective as physical cooling.

Some form of physical cooling should be considered as a means of reducing temperature in critically ill clients; options include removing bed linens, tepid water sponging, placement of ice water–cooled cloths on the client, or the use of a circulating cooling blanket. Physical cooling may be most effective when used in combination with an antipyretic medication. However, the high incidence of shivering associated with the use of cooling blankets must be kept in mind. From the findings of one study, cooling blanket temperatures in the range of 23.9° C should be used to avoid shivering and to promote comfort. Wrapping of extremities, using the method suggested by Holtzclaw,[12] may prevent shivering and its associated costs in some cases. Every attempt should be made to prevent shivering, and when it does occur, it should not be allowed to continue because it can drive temperatures higher while imposing metabolic and cardiovascular burdens.

Regarding client outcomes, the evidence regarding reducing the fever of patients with sepsis is inconclusive. There are more advantages associated with reducing fever in clients with head injury.

From the evidence assembled for this review, one can only conclude that there are many gaps in the research base regarding management of fever in the critically ill. The literature does not address all the decisions clinicians make in managing fever. Until more research is available, clinicians must combine the little research-based knowledge that is available with considerable experience-based knowledge and close observation of how individual clients respond to antipyretic medications, physical cooling, or both. Also, nurses and physicians who treat particular critically ill populations on a regular basis may have additional insights regarding what works best.

References

1. Bernard, G. R., et al. (1997). The effects of ibuprofen on the physiology and survival of patients with sepsis. *New England Journal of Medicine, 336,* 912–918.
2. Brown, R. D., et al. (1992). Single-dose pharmacokinetics of ibuprofen and acetaminophen in febrile children. *Journal of Clinical Pharmacology, 32,* 231–241.
3. Caruso, C. C., et al. (1992). Cooling effects and comfort of four cooling blanket temperatures in humans with fever. *Nursing Research, 41,* 68–72.
4. Chulay, M. (1998). Information for contributors. *AACN Research-Based Practice Protocols.* Aliso Viejo, CA: American Association of Critical-Care Nurses.
5. Clemmer, T. P., et al. (1992). The Methylprednisonolone Severe Sepsis Study Group: Hypothemia in the sepsis syndrome and clincial outcome. *Critical Care Medicine, 20,* 1395–1401.
6. Clifton, G. L., et al. (1993). A phase II study of moderate hypothermia in severe brain injury. *Journal of Neurotrauma, 10,* 263–271.
7. Grossman, et al. (1995). Current practices in fever management. *Journal of Medical-Surgical Nursing, 4,* 193–198.
8. Haupt, M. T., & Rackow, E. (1983). Adverse effects of febrile state on cardiac performance. *American Heart Journal, 105,* 763–768.
9. Henker, R. A., Brown, S. D., & Marion, D. W. (1998). Comparison of brain temperature with bladder and rectal temperatures in adults with severe head injury. *Neurosurgery, 42,* 1071–1075.
10. Henker, R., et al. (1997). Core temperature and cardiovascular responses to antipyretics in febrile critically ill adults [Abstract]. *Critical Care Medicine, 25,* A23.
11. Holtzclaw, B. J. (1990). Control of febrile shivering during amphotericin B therapy. *Oncology Nursing Forum, 17,* 521–524.
12. Holtzclaw, B. (1993). The shivering response. *Annual Review of Nursing Research, 11,* 31–55.
13. Hopkins, G. S., Underhill, S., & Booker, P. D. (1990). Pharmacokinetics of paracetamol after cardiac surgery. *Archives of Disease in Childhood, 65,* 971–976.
14. Kelley, M. T., et al. (1992). Pharmacokinetics and pharmacodynamics of ibuprofen isomers and acetaminophen in febrile children. *Clinical Pharmacology and Therapeutics, 52,* 181–189.
15. Manthous, C. A., et al. (1995). Effect of cooling on oxygen consumption in febrile critically ill patients. *American Journal of Respiratory and Critical Care Medicine, 151,* 10–14.
16. Marion, D. W., et al. (1993). The use of moderate therapeutic hypothermia for patients with severe head injuries: A preliminary report. *Journal of Neurosurgery, 79,* 354–362.
17. Marion, D. W., et al. (1997). Treatment of traumatic brain injury with moderate hypothermia. *New England Journal of Medicine, 336,* 540–546.
18. Montgomery, C. J., et al. (1995). Plasma concentrations after high-dose (45 mg*kg^{-1}) rectal acetaminophen in children. *Canadian Journal of Anaesthesia, 42,* 982–986.
19. Morgan, S. P. (1990). A comparison of three methods of managing fever in the neurological patient. *Journal of Neuroscience Nursing, 22,* 19–24.
20. Oliver, Y.-P. H., et al. Evaluation of gastric emptying in severe, burn-injured patients. *Critical Care Medicine, 21,* 527–531.
21. O'Donnell, J., et al. (1997). Use and effectiveness of hypothermia blankets for febrile patients in the intensive care unit. *Clinical Infectious Diseases, 24,* 1208–1213.
22. Poblete, B., et al. (1997). Metabolic effects of IV propacetamol, metamizol, or external cooling in critically ill febrile sedate patients. *British Journal of Anaesthesia, 78,* 123–127.
23. Revhaug, A., et al. (1988). Inhibition of cyclo-oxygenase attenuates the metabolic response to endotoxin in humans. *Archives of Surgery, 123,* 162–170.
24. Rumana, C. S., et al. (1998). Brain temperature exceeds systemic temperature in head-injured patients. *Critical Care Medicine, 26,* 562–567.
25. Shiozaki, T., et al. (1993). Effect of mild hypothermia on uncontrollable intracranial hypertension after severe head injury. *Journal of Neuorsurgery, 79,* 363–368.
26. Tarling, M. M., et al. (1997). A model of gastric emptying using paracetamol absorption in intensive care patients. *Intensive Care Medicine, 23,* 256–260.
27. Vargas, R., et al. (1994). Evaluation of the antipyretic effect of ketorolac, acetaminophen, and placebo in endotoxin-induced fever. *Journal of Clinical Pharmacology, 34,* 848–853.
28. Weinberg, J. R., et al. (1989). Studies on the circulation in normotensive febrile patients. *Quarterly Journal of Experimental Physiology, 74,* 301–310.
29. Weinstein, M. P., et al. (1983). The clinical significance of positive blood cultures: A comprehensive analysis of 500 episodes of bacteremia and fungemia in adults. II: Clinical observations with special reference to factors influencing prognosis. *Reviews of Infectious Diseases, 5,* 54–70.

Sarah Jo Brown, PhD, RN, *Principal and Consultant, Practice-Research Integrations, Norwich, Vermont*

Quality of Life After Organ Transplantation

QUESTIONS

Does quality of life (QOL) improve from the pre-transplantation to the post-transplantation period?
Is QOL in transplant recipients better than QOL in other similarly ill comparison groups?
Is QOL in transplant recipients similar to or better than QOL in healthy people?

CITATION

Dew, M. A., Switzer, G. E., Goycoolea, J. M., Allen, A. A., DiMartini, A., Kormos, R. L., and Griffith, B. P. (1997). Does transplantation produce quality of life benefits? A quantitative analysis. *Transplantation, 64,* 1261–1273.

"Quality of life" was defined as well-being in three areas of well-being: (1) physical functioning, (2) mental/cognitive health, and (3) social functioning. Within each of these functional areas, several variables were analyzed. For example, in physical functioning the following seven variables were analyzed: ambulation, mobility, pain, fatigue, sleep, activities of daily living, and perceived physical status.

STUDIES

Published studies conducted from 1972 through 1996 were located; 218 were included in the analysis. Studies of kidney recipients were most prevalent, followed by studies of heart, liver, and bone marrow recipients. Studies of pancreas/kidney-pancreas and lung/heart-lung recipients were considerably less common. The 218 studies included almost 15,000 recipients and varied widely in sample size and study design. Most studies assessed recipients just once, most often within the year after surgery, but 36% of the studies observed recipients from 1 to 3 years. Only 9% of the studies followed recipients more than 3 years after surgery.

Summary of Findings

Does Quality of Life Improve From Before to After Transplantation? (p. 1267)

Seventy-six studies evaluated clients before and then again after transplantation. In general, QOL improved with the procedure, but variations by area of functioning and by transplant type occurred. Across transplant types, 86% of the studies documented improvement in physical functioning, 67% in social functioning, and 62% in mental/cognitive functioning.

Physical functioning was improved, according to all (100%) studies involving pancreas/kidney-pancreas recipients and all studies involving lung/heart-lung recipients. In contrast, 67% of the studies involving bone marrow recipients found improvement. The proportion of studies finding improvement in the other transplant types fell between these two levels. Within the mental/cognitive area, more than 80% of the studies involving kidney recipients found improvement, whereas only 32% of studies involving pancreas/kidney-pancreas recipients did. For social functioning, all (100%) studies involving lung/heart-lung recipients found improvement; in contrast, only 50% of bone marrow transplant studies found improvement. Thus, despite the considerable variation among the transplant types and across the three functional areas, in most studies recipients experienced improved QOL after transplantation.

Is Quality of Life in Transplant Recipients Better Than Quality of Life in Other Similarly Ill Comparison Groups? (p. 1268)

Eighty-four studies addressed this issue, typically comparing recipients to people with similar conditions who did not receive transplants. The majority of studies (58%) found that physical functioning for transplant recipients was better than that of ill comparison groups. Although some studies examining mental/cognitive and social functioning found advantages for transplant recipient over comparison groups, most *did not* find advantages; instead, the majority of studies noted that mental/cognitive and social functioning in recipients were the same or poorer than in comparison groups.

Studies of lung/heart-lung recipients found the greatest advantage for transplant recipients over similarly ill comparison groups; the group with the least documented improvement, when compared with a similar ill group, were bone marrow recipients. Again, each group of recipients (i.e., by transplant type) varied somewhat across the three areas of functioning.

Is Quality of Life in Transplant Recipients Similar to or Better Than Quality of Life in Healthy Samples? (p. 1270)

Although a few of the 67 studies that addressed this issue found that QOL in recipients was equal to or better than that in healthy people, the majority of the studies noted a poorer quality of life in all three areas of functioning. Heart and lung/heart-lung recipients compared most favorably, whereas no studies of bone marrow recipients or pancreas/kidney-pancreas found QOL in recipients to be at least as good as that in healthy persons.

In summary, although transplantation may not restore QOL to previous levels, the evidence has established clear QOL benefits. The specific nature and degree of benefits depend on the type of transplantation procedure.

Other Issues

Recipients rated their overall QOL as "high." This high rating is somewhat at odds with the more modest improvements in the specific areas of functioning. The researchers who conducted the meta-analysis suggest that this is because transplant clients feel that they have been given the gift of an extended life. This perception probably leads to a redefinition of "normal" life and an increased valuing of life even when their daily lives have difficulties. Importantly, the longitudinal studies found QOL either to be stable or to improve over the first 1 to 7 years after transplantation.

Limitations/Reservations These findings do not mean that every transplant client will realize an improved QOL, although the research evidence regarding the change in QOL from before to after surgery on average is impressive. All studies considered averaged experiences of all those in the sample. For this question, an average result means that most recipients experienced a higher QOL. For others, QOL stayed the same; however, a few recipients may have even experienced a decline in QOL. The authors note that most of the studies in this analysis were conducted in the pre-cyclosporine or pre-FK506 era. These

Quality of Life After Organ Transplantation *Continued*

two medications have been found to improve QOL in some recipients.

Research-Based Practice

Because the benefits in QOL vary from one type of transplantative procedure to another, nurses caring for clients who have undergone a particular type of procedure should look at the findings of this meta-analysis that specifically pertain to that population. Only some of those specific findings have been presented in this synopsis.

The fact that most recipients rated their overall QOL as high, even though they admitted having problems and difficulties in specific areas of functioning, indicates that a person's perception of QOL is a very personal and subjective assessment—"personal" in that QOL depends on personal values and priorities. For example, physical functioning may be most important determinant of QOL for some people because it affects independence and the ability to get out in the world. Other people may not view independence and mobility as this important and may say instead, "I can't do what I use to do, but as long as I can take care of most of my own bodily functions, I'm okay. The important thing is that I have my wits about me and can make my own decisions."

Rating one's QOL is relative because the experience of having a life-threatening illness changes how one thinks about life in general and about one's own life in particular. From the outside, someone's life may look as if it is shaped by medication schedules, treatment procedures, side effects, and limitations; To the person living that life, however, there may be sufficient joys to make it worthwhile, even rich. Health providers often focus on the problems and difficulties, neglecting to take the time to talk with clients about what is going on in their lives that brings meaning, enjoyment, and social connectedness. Nurses must be careful to not make any assumptions about an individual client's QOL, particularly if they do not know the client well.

Nurses must also be aware that when clients rate their overall QOL, they are using some kind of standard. For some people, that standard may be their QOL before they became ill; others may evaluate their QOL as it is in the present; and others still may base their rating on how they think their QOL will be or would have been had they not undergone the transplantation surgery. Still others may look at another person who they think has a life that is more constrained and difficult than their own and may compare their QOL to that person's QOL. Most people have an amazing capacity to adapt to difficult circumstances and to continue to find meaning in life. This analysis of QOL studies speaks to that capacity just as much as it documents the objective benefits of organ transplantation technology.

Nurses working with a particular population of transplant clients acquire insights into the post-transplant issues that clients may encounter. This knowledge can be combined with the findings of this meta-analysis to help clients and families who are considering transplantation to think through the effects a transplant is likely to have on their lives. The information in this meta-analysis regarding the experiences of the recipients of a particular type of transplant can be used as long as the nurse remains aware that these findings are based on the average experience and are not a guarantee of how things will be for any one client.

Sarah Jo Brown, PhD, RN, *Principal and Consultant, Practice-Research Integrations, Norwich, Vermont*

Religious Beliefs and Practices Affecting Health Care

Religious Group	Beliefs and Practices
WESTERN RELIGIONS	
Judaism	
Orthodox and some Conservative Jewish groups	*Care of women:* A woman is considered to be in a ritual state of impurity whenever blood is coming from her uterus, such as during menstrual periods and after the birth of a child. During this time, her husband does not have physical contact with her. When this time is completed, she will bathe herself in a pool called a *mikvah.* Be aware of this practice, and be sensitive to the husband and wife because the husband will not touch his wife. He cannot assist her in moving in the bed; the nurse must do this. An Orthodox Jewish man will not touch any women other than his wife, daughters, and mother. *Dietary rules:* (1) Kosher dietary laws include the following: no mixing of milk and meat at a meal; no consumption of food or any derivative thereof from animals not slaughtered in accordance with Jewish law; use of separate cooking utensils for milk and milk products; if a client requires milk and meat products for a meal, the dairy foods should be served first, followed later by the meat. (2) During Yom Kippur (Day of Atonement), a 24-hour fast is required, but exceptions are made for those who cannot fast because of medical reasons. (3) During Passover, no leavened products are eaten. (4) The client may say benediction of thanksgiving before meals and grace at the end of the meal. Time and a quiet environment should be provided for this. *Sabbath:* Observed from sunset Friday until sunset Saturday. Orthodox law prohibits riding in a car, smoking, turning lights on and off, handling money, and using television and telephone. Nurses need to be aware of these customs when caring for observant Jews at home and in the hospital. Medical or surgical treatments should be postponed if possible. *Death:* Judaism defines death as occurring when respiration and circulation are irreversibly stopped and no movement is apparent. (1) Euthanasia is strictly forbidden by Orthodox Jews, who advocate the strict use of life support measures. (2) Prior to death, Jewish faith indicates that visiting of the person by family and friends is a religious duty. The Torah and Psalms may be read and prayers recited. A witness needs to be present when a person prays for health so that if death occurs, God will protect the family and the spirit will be committed to God. Extraneous talking and conversation about death are not encouraged unless initiated by the client or visitors. In Judaism, the belief is that people should have someone with them when the soul leaves the body; thus, family and/or friends should be allowed to stay with the client. After death, the body should not be left alone until buried, usually within 24 hours. (3) When death occurs, the body should be untouched for 8 to 30 minutes. Medical personnel should not touch or wash the body but should allow only an Orthodox person or the Jewish Burial Society to care for the body. Handling of a corpse on the Sabbath is forbidden to Jewish persons. If need be, the nursing staff may provide routine care of the body, wearing gloves. Water in the room should be emptied, and the family may request that mirrors be covered to symbolize that a death has occurred. (4) Orthodox Jews and some Conservative Jews do not approve of autopsies. If an autopsy must be done, all body parts must remain with the body. (5) For Orthodox Jews, the body must be buried within 24 hours. No flowers are permitted. A fetus must be buried. (6) A 7-day mourning period is required by the immediate family. Family members must stay at home except for Sabbath worship. (7) Organs or other body parts such as amputated limbs must be made available for burial for Orthodox Jews, who believe that all of the body must be returned to earth. *Birth control and abortion:* Artificial methods of birth control are not encouraged. Vasectomy is not allowed. Abortion may be performed only to save the mother's life.

Table continued on following page

Religious Group	Beliefs and Practices
WESTERN RELIGIONS *(Continued)*	
	Organ transplantation: Although it has been assumed that donor organ transplantation is not permitted by Orthodox Jews but is allowed with rabbinic consent, using an organ to save a life is encouraged.* *Shaving:* The beard is regarded as a mark of piety among observant Jews. For the very Orthodox, shaving should not be done with a razor but with scissors or electric razor, because a blade should not contact the skin. *Head covering:* Orthodox men wear skull caps at all times, and women cover their hair after marriage. Some Orthodox women wear wigs as a mark of piety. Conservative Jews cover their heads only during acts of worship and prayer. *Prayer:* Praying directly to God, including a prayer of confession, is required for Orthodox Jews. Provide quiet time for prayer.
Reform Jews	*Care of women:* Reform Jews do not observe the rules against touching. *Dietary rules:* Reform Jews usually do not observe kosher dietary restriction. *Sabbath:* Usual custom is to worship in temples on Friday evenings. No strict rules. *Death:* Reform Jews advocate use of life support without heroic measures. They allow cremation but suggest that ashes be buried in a Jewish cemetery. *Organ transplantation:* Donation or transplantation of organs allowed with permission of a rabbi. *Head covering:* Men usually pray without wearing skull caps.
Christianity Roman Catholic	*Holy Eucharist:* For clients and health care providers who are to receive communion, abstinence from solid food and alcohol is required for 15 minutes (if possible) prior to reception of the consecrated wafer. Medicine, water, and nonalcoholic drinks are permitted at any time. If a client is in danger of death, the fast is waived because the reception of the Eucharist at this time is very important. *Anointing of the sick:* The priest uses oil to anoint the forehead and hands and, if desired, the affected area. The rite may be performed on any who are ill and desire it. Clients receiving the sacrament seek complete healing and strength to endure suffering. Prior to 1963, this sacrament was given only to clients at time of imminent death; be sensitive to the meaning this has for the client. If possible, call a priest before the client is unconscious but you may also call when there is sudden death, because the sacrament may also be given shortly after death. Record on the care plan that this sacrament has been administered. *Dietary habits:* Obligatory fasting is excused during hospitalization. However, if there are no health restrictions, some Catholics may still observe the following guidelines: (1) Anyone 14 years or older must abstain from eating meat on Ash Wednesday and all Fridays during Lent. Some older Catholics may still abstain from meat on all Fridays of the year. (2) In addition to abstinence from meat, persons 21 to 59 years of age must limit themselves to one full meal and two light meals on Ash Wednesday and Good Friday. (3) Eastern Rite Catholics are stricter about fasting and fast more frequently than Western Rite Catholics, and it is important for you to know if a client is Eastern or Western. *Death:* Each Roman Catholic should participate in the anointing of the sick as well as the Eucharist and penance before death. The body should not be shrouded until after these sacraments are performed. All body parts that retain human quality must be appropriately buried or cremated. *Birth control:* Contraception is prohibited except for abstinence or natural family planning. Referral to a priest for questions about this can be of great help. You can teach the techniques of natural family planning if you are familiar with them; otherwise, this should be referred to the physician or to a support group of the church that instructs couples in this method of birth control. Sterilization is prohibited unless there is an overriding medical reason. *Organ donation:* Donation and transplantation of organs are acceptable as long as the donor is not harmed and is not deprived of life. *Religious objects:* Rosary prayers are said using rosary beads. Medals bearing the images of saints, relics, statues, and scapulars are important objects that may be pinned to a hospital gown or pillow or may be at the bedside. Take extreme care not to lose these objects, because they have special meaning to the client.
Eastern Orthodox	*Holy Eucharist:* The priest is notified if the client desires this sacrament. *Anointing of the sick:* The priest conducts this rite in the hospital room.

Religious Group	Beliefs and Practices
WESTERN RELIGIONS *(Continued)*	
	Dietary habits: Fasting from meat and dairy products is required on Wednesday and Friday during Lent and on other holy days. Hospital clients are exempt if fasting is detrimental to health. *Special days:* Christmas is celebrated on January 7 and New Year's Day on January 14. This is important to know when you are caring for a client who is hospitalized on these days. *Death:* Last rites are obligatory. This is handled by an ordained priest who is notified by the nurse while the client is conscious. The Russian Orthodox Church does not encourage autopsy or organ donation. Euthanasia, even for the terminally ill, is discouraged, as is cremation. *Birth control:* Contraception as well as abortion is not permitted.
Protestant	*Holy Communion:* Notify clergy if the client desires.
Assemblies of God (Pentecostal)	*Anointing of the sick:* Members believe in divine healing through prayer and the laying on of hands. Clergy is notified if client or family desires this. *Dietary habits:* Abstinence from alcohol, tobacco, and all illegal drugs is strongly encouraged. *Death:* No special practices. *Other practices:* Faith in God and in the health care providers is encouraged. Members pray for divine intervention in health matters. Encourage and allow time for prayer. Members may speak in "tongues" during prayer.
Baptist (over 27 different groups in the United States)	*Holy Communion:* Clergy should be notified if the client desires. *Dietary habits:* Total abstinence from alcohol is expected. *Death:* No general service is provided, but the clergy does minister through counseling, prayer, and Scripture as requested by the client or family, and the client is encouraged to believe in Jesus Christ as Savior and Lord. *Other practices:* The Bible is held to be the word of God. Either allow quiet time for Scripture reading, or offer to read to the client.
Christian Church (Disciples of Christ)	*Holy Communion:* Open communion is celebrated each Sunday and is a central part of worship services. Notify the clergy if the client desires it, or the clergy may suggest it. *Death:* No special practices. *Other practices:* Church elders as well as clergy may be notified to assist with meeting the client's spiritual needs.
Church of the Brethren	*Holy Communion:* Is usually received within church, but clergy may give it in the hospital when requested. *Anointing of the sick:* Practices for physical healing as well as spiritual uplift are held in high regard by the church. The clergy is notified if the client or family desire. *Death:* The clergy is notified for counsel and prayer.
Church of the Nazarene	*Holy Communion:* Pastor will administer if the client wishes. *Dietary habits:* The use of alcohol and tobacco is forbidden. *Death:* Cremation is permitted, and term stillborn infants are buried. *Other practices:* A belief in divine healing but not to the exclusion of medical treatment. Clients may desire quiet time for prayer.
Episcopal (Anglican)	*Holy Communion:* The priest is notified if the client wishes to receive this sacrament. *Anointing of the sick:* Priest may administer this rite when death is imminent, but it is not considered mandatory. *Dietary habits:* Some clients may abstain from meat on Fridays. Others may fast before receiving the Eucharist, but fasting is not mandatory. *Death:* No special practices. *Other practices:* Confession of sins to a priest is optional; if the client desires this, the clergy should be notified.
Lutheran (18 different branches)	*Holy Communion:* Notify the clergy if the client desires this sacrament. Clergy may also inquire about the client's desire. *Anointing of the sick:* The client may request an anointing and blessing from the minister when the prognosis is poor. *Death:* A service of Commendation of the Dying is used at the client's or family's request.

Table continued on following page

Religious Group	Beliefs and Practices
WESTERN RELIGIONS *(Continued)*	
Mennonite (12 different groups)	*Holy Communion:* Served twice a year, with foot-washing a part of the ceremony. *Dietary habits:* Abstinence from alcohol is urged for all. *Death:* Prayer is important at time of crisis, and contacting a minister is important. *Other practices:* Women may wear head coverings during hospitalization. Anointing with oil is administered in harmony with James 5:14 when requested.
Methodist (over 20 different groups)	*Holy Communion:* Notify the clergy if a client requests it prior to surgery or another health crisis. *Anointing of the sick:* If requested, the clergy will come to pray and sprinkle the client with olive oil. *Death:* Scripture reading and prayer are important at this time. *Other practices:* Donation of one's body or part of the body at death is encouraged.
Presbyterian (10 different groups)	*Holy Communion:* Given when appropriate and convenient, at the hospitalized client's request. *Death:* Notify a local pastor or elder for prayer and Scripture reading if desired by the family or client.
Quaker (Friends)	*Holy Communion:* Because Friends have no creed, there is a diversity of personal beliefs. One belief is that outward sacraments are usually not necessary because there is the ministry of the Spirit inwardly in such areas as baptism and communion. *Death:* Believe that the present life is part of God's kingdom and generally have no ceremony as a rite of passage from this life to the next. Personal beliefs and wishes need to be ascertained, and you can then act on the client's wishes.
Salvation Army	*Holy Communion:* No particular ceremony. *Death:* Notify the local officer in charge of the Army Corps for any soldier (member) who needs assistance. *Other practices:* The Bible is seen as the only rule for one's faith, and the Scriptures should be made available to a client. The Army has many of its own social welfare centers, with hospitals and homes where unwed mothers are cared for and outpatient services provided. No medical or surgical procedures are opposed, except for abortion on demand.
Seventh-day Adventist	*Holy Communion:* Although this sacrament is not required of hospitalized clients, the clergy are notified if the client desires. *Anointing of the sick:* The clergy are contacted for prayer and anointing with oil. *Dietary habits:* Because the body is viewed as the temple of the Holy Spirit, healthy living is essential. Therefore, the use of alcohol, tobacco, coffee, and tea and the promiscuous use of drugs are prohibited. Some are vegetarians, and most avoid pork. *Special days:* The Sabbath is observed on Saturday. *Death:* No special procedures. *Other related practices:* Use of hypnotism is opposed by some. Persons of homosexual or lesbian orientation are ministered to in the hope of correction of these practices, which are believed to be wrong. A Bible should always be available for Scripture reading.
United Church of Christ	*Holy Communion:* Clergy are notified if the client desires to receive this sacrament. *Death:* If the client desires counsel or prayer, notify the clergy.
Other	
Christian Science	*Dietary habits:* Because alcohol and tobacco are considered drugs, they are not used. Coffee and tea are often declined. *Death:* Autopsy is usually declined unless required by law. Donation of organs is unlikely, but is an individual decision. *Other practices:* Adherents do not normally seek medical care, because they approach health care in a different, primarily spiritual, framework. They commonly utilize the services of a surgeon to set a bone but decline drugs and, in general, other medical or surgical procedures. Hypnotism and psychotherapy are also declined. Family planning is left to the family. They seek exemption from vaccinations but obey legal requirements (e.g., report infectious diseases and obey public health quarantines). Nonmedical care facilities are maintained for those needing nursing assistance in the course of a healing. *The Christian Science Journal* lists available Christian Science nurses. When a Christian Science believer is in the hospital, allow and encourage time for prayer and study. Clients may request that a Christian Science practitioner be notified to come.

Religious Group	Beliefs and Practices
WESTERN RELIGIONS *(Continued)*	
Jehovah's Witnesses	*Dietary habits:* Use of alcohol and tobacco is discouraged, because these harm the physical body. *Death:* Autopsy is a private matter to be decided by the persons involved. Burial and cremation are acceptable. *Birth control and abortion:* Use of birth control is a personal decision. Abortion is opposed on the basis of Exodus 21:22–23. *Organ transplantation:* Use of organ transplants is a private decision. If an organ is transplanted, it must be cleansed with a nonblood solution. *Blood transfusions:* Blood transfusions violate God's laws and are therefore not allowed. Clients do respect physicians and will accept alternatives to blood transfusions. These might include use of nonblood plasma expanders, careful surgical techniques to decrease blood loss, use of autologous transfusions, and autotransfusion through use of a heart-lung machine. Nurses should check unconscious patients for medical alert cards that state that the person does not want a transfusion. Since Jehovah's Witnesses are prepared to die rather than break God's law, you need to be sensitive to the spiritual as well as the physical needs of the client.
Church of Jesus Christ of Latter-day Saints	*Holy Communion:* A hospitalized client may desire to have a member of the church priesthood administer this sacrament. *Anointing of the sick:* Mormons commonly are anointed and given a blessing by laying on of hands before going to the hospital and after admission. *Dietary habits:* Abstinence from the use of tobacco; beverages with caffeine such as cola, coffee, and tea; alcohol and other substances considered injurious. Mormons eat meat but encourage the intake of fruits, grains, and herbs. *Death:* Burial of the body is preferred. A church elder should be notified to assist the family. If need be, the elder will assist the funeral director in dressing the body in special clothes and will give other help as needed. *Birth control and abortion:* Abortion is opposed except when the life of the mother is in danger. Only natural means of birth control are recommended. Artificial means can be used when the health of the woman is at stake (including emotional health). *Personal care:* Cleanliness is very important to Mormons. A sacred undergarment may be worn at all times by Mormons and should be removed only in emergency situations. *Other practices:* Allowing quiet time for prayer and the reading of the sacred writings is important. The church maintains a welfare system to assist those in need. Families are of great importance, and visiting should be encouraged.
Unitarian Universalist Association	*Death:* Cremation is often preferred to burial. *Other practices:* Use of birth control is advocated as part of responsible parenting. Strong support for a woman's right to choice regarding abortion is maintained. Unitarian Universalists advocate donation of body parts for research and transplants.
Unification Church	*Baptism:* No baptism. *Special days:* Sunday mornings are used to honor Reverend and Mrs. Moon as the true parents, and members get up at 5:00 AM, bow before a picture of the Moons three times, and vow to do what is needed to help the Reverend accomplish his mission on earth. *Death:* Adherents believe that after death one's place of destiny will depend on his or her spirit's quality of life and goodness while on earth. In the afterlife, one will have the same aspirations and feelings as before, when on earth. Hell is not a concern, because it will not be a place as heaven grows in size. Persons who leave the Unification Church are warned that Satan may try to possess them. *Other practices:* All marriages must be solemnized by Reverend Moon in order to be part of the perfect family and have salvation. The church supplies its faithful members with life's necessities. Members may use occult practices to have spiritual and psychic experiences.
Islam	*Dietary habits:* No pork or alcoholic beverages allowed. All halal (permissible) meat must be blessed and killed in a special way. This is called *zabihah* (correctly slaughtered).

Table continued on following page

Religious Group	Beliefs and Practices
WESTERN RELIGIONS *(Continued)*	
	Death: Prior to death, family members ask to be present so that they can read the Koran and pray with the client. An Imam may come if requested by the client or family but is not required. Clients must face Mecca and confess their sins and beg forgiveness in the presence of their family. If the family is unavailable, any practicing Muslim can provide support to the client. After death, Muslims prefer that the family wash, prepare, and place the body in a position facing Mecca. If necessary, the health care providers may perform these procedures as long as they wear gloves. Burial is performed as soon as possible. Cremation is forbidden. Autopsy is also prohibited except for legal reasons, and then no body part is to be removed. Donation of body parts or organs is not allowed, because according to culturally developed law, persons do not own their bodies. *Abortion and birth control:* Abortion is forbidden, and many conservative Muslims do not encourage the use of contraceptives because this interferes with God's purpose. Others feel that a woman should only have as many children as her husband can afford. Contraception is permitted by Islamic law. *Personal devotions:* At prayer time, washing is required, even by those who are sick. A client on bed rest may require assistance with this task before prayer. Provision of privacy is important during prayer. *Religious objects:* The Koran must not be touched by anyone ritually unclean, and nothing should be placed on top of it. Some Muslims wear *taviz,* a black string on which words of the Koran are attached. These should not be removed and must remain dry. Certain items of jewelry, such as bangles, may have religious significance and should not be removed unnecessarily. *Care of women:* Because women are not allowed to sign consent forms or make a decision regarding family planning, the husband needs to be present. Women are very modest and frequently wear clothes that cover all of the body. During a medical examination, the woman's modesty should be respected as much as possible. Muslim women prefer female physicians. For 40 days after giving birth and also during menstruation, a woman is exempt from prayer because this is a time of cleansing for her.
American Muslim Mission	*Dietary habits:* In addition to refusing pork, many will not eat traditional African American foods, such as corn bread and collard greens. *Death:* The family is contacted before any care of the deceased is performed. There are special procedures for washing and shrouding the body. *Other practices:* Quiet time is necessary to permit prayer. Members are encouraged to use African American physicians for health care. Because these clients do not smoke, their request for a nonsmoking roommate should be honored.
EASTERN RELIGIONS	
Hinduism	*Dietary habits:* Some sects are vegetarian, believing meats and intoxicants to be too stimulating to the senses. *Belief about illness:* Hindus view illnesses as a result of misuse of the body or a consequence of sins committed in a previous life. They do not oppose medical treatment, but they view its effect as transitory. They believe that praying for health is the lowest form of prayer. *Death:* See death as a union with Brahman (God) achieved through prayers, ritual, purity, self-control, detachment, truth, nonviolence, charity, and compassion toward all creatures. Following death, one will be reborn (reincarnated) into a future life based on the behavior in this life. The record of behavior is called *karma.* Eventually, the process of rebirth stops, which is called *moksha.* A priest may be called at the time of death, and may tie a thread around the neck or waist as a blessing. The family washes the body, and it is cremated. *Other practices:* Offer daily worship at a shrine in the home. Daily offering to god, and morning and evening rites. Society is organized into castes, or strata. People are born into a caste, and the caste shapes one's entire life. Hindus practice a discipline of the mind and body, called yoga, to reach God. In the highest state, a meditating yogi does not see, hear, taste, feel, or smell. Beyond good and evil, time and space, he is one with God.

Religious Group	Beliefs and Practices
EASTERN RELIGIONS *(Continued)*	
Buddhism	*Death:* Buddhists believe that salvation depends on one's own right living; they believe in reincarnation. Buddhists can speed the process toward Nirvana, the goal of all humanity's striving, through acts of merit. Meditation, worship, and prayer are some of the acts of merit. Buddhists may drive themselves into more and more ritual or contemplation in the hope that their last moments of consciousness may be filled with thoughts worthy enough to elevate them to a higher existence. Last rites of chanting may be performed at bedside. *Renunciation:* The most important Buddhist feasts. Young boys are taught to despise the world's vanity, and the boy spends a night in a nearby monastery.
Taoism/Confucianism	*General beliefs:* Founded on ethical principles of Confucius. God is not clearly defined as in other religions. Taoism is a mixture of magic and religion. Believers hold that humans and nature are inseparable, and that if heaven is upset, earth does not prosper. This relationship is described as *yin* and *yang,* which are two interplaying forces. When *yin* and *yang* are in balance, good occurs. *Death:* The dead are remembered in all festivals. The fate of the dead in the afterworld depends not only on the life they led but also on being properly honored after death. Otherwise they may become demons. Graves are mounds like those dedicated to the gifts of the soil. Graves and houses must be in harmony with the universe, otherwise evil will befall the occupants.

*The American Scene. (2000). *Hadassah* (suppl, Summer), 4.
Modified from Carson, V. B. (1989). *Spiritual dimensions of nursing practice.* Philadelphia: W. B. Saunders.

A Health History Format That Integrates the Assessment of Functional Health Patterns

Functional Health Pattern	Assessment
Health perception–health management	Quality of usual and current health rated on a scale of 1 to 10 Self-rating of the importance of health on a scale of 1 to 10 Perceived ability to control and manage health Resources used in health management including primary health care provider Self-care measures to maintain or prevent disruption of health status Health habits (e.g., seat belt use, diet, alcohol consumption, tobacco use) Complete description of present health problem (i.e., chief complaint) Expectations for outcome of current health problem Expectations for care givers Previous illnesses or hospitalizations, reaction to these events, and their outcomes Developmental history, including childhood illnesses and immunizations Ability to manage and comply with recommended treatment of health problems Current medications, including over-the-counter and recreational (street) drugs Allergies Environmental factors affecting health (e.g., occupation, home, leisure) Socioeconomic factors affecting health (e.g., financial concerns, health care insurance, living conditions) Knowledge and use of community resources to manage health Family history
Nutritional-metabolic	Recall of usual food and fluid intake for the past 24 hours Comparison of the 24-hour recall diet to typical pattern of diet intake Quality of appetite Dietary restrictions (medical order) Food preferences and dislikes Use of food supplements (e.g., vitamins) Knowledge level of dietary recommendations (e.g., Food Guide Pyramid, recommended dietary allowances, special dietary guidelines) Past alterations in dietary habits (e.g., bulimia nervosa, anorexia nervosa) Usual weight Minimum and maximum weight range Recent weight gain or loss (how much? time span? intentional?) Social significance of food Who shops for food items? Who usually prepares meals? Religious or cultural beliefs affecting diet or meal preparation Ability to swallow and chew Are there any feeding problems?
Elimination	
Bowel	Usual bowel habits, including frequency, time of day, color, consistency, assistive devices used (e.g., laxatives, suppositories, enemas), constipation, diarrhea Change in bowel habits; describe
Bladder	Usual frequency, amount, color of voiding Assistive devices used (e.g., self-catheterization) Problems with frequency, urgency, burning, retention, incontinence, dribbling, dysuria, polyuria, nocturia
Skin	Condition, color, temperature, turgor, lesions, edema, pruritus
Activity-exercise	Description of usual daily activities Weekend schedule, if different from daily Occupation-related activities Leisure activities including hobbies Description of exercise regimen Limitation in ambulation, bathing, dressing, toileting, and feeding Dyspnea with exertion Fatigue

Functional Health Pattern	Assessment
Sleep-rest	Usual sleep habits including bedtime, hours of sleep obtained, wake-up time Problems falling asleep or staying asleep Sleep aids used, including medications, food, beverages, and sexual intercourse Rating of quality of sleep obtained (does client feel rested?) Periods of decreased wakefulness during the day Naps or rest periods
Cognitive-perceptual	Ability to understand Educational level obtained Self-rating of intelligence level Ability to communicate with others Ability to make decisions and the relative ease or difficulty experienced with decision-making Ability to see, hear, feel, taste, smell Compensations made for sensory deficits and their effectiveness Problems with vertigo, heat or cold intolerance Pain (including a symptom analysis) Desire to learn
Self-perception–self-concept	Description of self, including strengths and weaknesses Major concerns Health goals Body image and feelings about self Level of satisfaction with current age Perceived developmental level Emotional status Effect of illness on self-perception Personal factors contributing to illness, recovery, health maintenance
Role relationship	Language, quality of speech and relevancy Ability to express self Family life, including family members and their relationships to client Roles client and family members fill Interpersonal relationships within family Support systems within family, including person client feels closest to Family-related problems including living arrangements, parenting, marital problems, abuse Occupation and job-related role expectations Problems at work Societal relationships beyond family or work Most important person to client Type of neighborhood or community in which client lives Participation in social groups (e.g., church, synagogue, clubs) Perceived contributions to society
Sexuality-reproductive	Level of satisfaction with role as male or female Anticipated changes related to health problem (e.g., fertility, libido, impotence, pregnancy, contraception, menstruation) Sexual activity, including how long client has been sexually active, number of partners, use of contraceptives Known exposure to venereal diseases, including human immunodeficiency virus infection Level of satisfaction with intercourse Problems with intercourse (e.g., premature ejaculation, impotence, pain, bleeding)
Female	Menstrual history including age at menarche, description of typical cycle, last menstrual period, age at menopause, or manifestations of menopause Obstetric history including number of pregnancies, number of births, problems during pregnancy or labor and delivery Practice of breast self-examination, knowledge of technique, compliance Last Pap test and results, frequency of pelvic examinations and Pap tests
Male	Circumcision Age at climacteric and description of manifestations experienced Practice of testicular self-examination, knowledge of technique, compliance Prostate examination, prostate-specific antigen test and results

Table continued on following page

Functional Health Pattern	Assessment
Coping–stress tolerance	Coping strategies used and their effectiveness Personal loss or major changes in past year Comfort and security needs Most stressful event in life and reaction to it Use of stress management techniques and their effectiveness (e.g., eating, sleeping, self-medication, counseling, exercise, biofeedback) Effect of stress on lifestyle and ability to function, including decision-making
Value-belief	Most important value to client Sources of strength and hope Importance of religion, type, and frequency of worship Life goals Values influencing decision-making and ability to resolve moral questions Recent changes in values or beliefs Conflict in values or beliefs with those of significant others Spirituality needs, particularly during time of illness or hospitalization

Laboratory Values of Clinical Importance in Medical-Surgical Nursing

Reference laboratory values can provide guidelines for the clinician to use when assessing clients with a wide variety of problems. The laboratory values given here are for reference only and are not absolute normal values. Remember, there is no sharp dividing line between normal and abnormal. Clients with only slightly elevated values may have apparent disease, whereas those with more elevated values may not. Trends in laboratory values are often much more important than the single value.

When analyzing laboratory values, consider the following questions:

- Is the value an expected abnormal finding? For example, creatinine is normally elevated in clients with renal failure.
- Is the value an unexpected abnormal finding? For example, elevated blood glucose levels in a client without diabetes may signal a disease.
- Is the value an unexpected normal finding? For example, a client with angina and probable myocardial infarction would be expected to have elevated isoenzymes. Normal levels may mean that the client has another cause of chest pain.
- Is the value an expected normal finding? For example, a healthy client should have a normal complete blood count.

Use the analytic technique as a guide to determine when to call the physician. Remember, the laboratory only reports findings; nurses help interpret their significance.

Appendix C summarizes the common laboratory diagnostic studies for use as a quick reference. A complete explanation of the diagnostic study and its meaning is covered in the appropriate section (such as liver function studies in Chapter 47). This Appendix simply provides a convenient way to check the normal values for the most common diagnostic studies. For details concerning the meaning of the value, see the appropriate section in the text.

The following abbreviations are used throughout the laboratory studies:

g = gram
kg = kilogram
mg = milligram (10^{-3})
μg = microgram (10^{-6})
ng = nanogram (10^{-9})
pg = picogram (10^{-12})
L = liter
ml = milliliter
dl = deciliter (100 ml)
fL = femtoliter
mm = millimeter
mm^3 = cubic millimeter
U = unit
mU = milliunit
μU = microunit
mOsm = milliosmole
mol = mole
μmol = micromole
nmol = nanomole
pmol = picomole
fmol = femtomole (10^{-15})
mEq = milliequivalent
μm = micrometer

REFERENCE VALUES IN HEMATOLOGY*

Test		Conventional Units	SI Units
Acid hemolysis test (Ham)		No hemolysis	No hemolysis
Alkaline phosphatase, leukocyte		Total score 14 to 100	Total score 14 to 100
Cell counts			
Erythrocytes			
Males		4.6 to 6.2 million/mm^3	4.6 to 6.2 × 10^{12}/L
Females		4.2 to 5.4 million/mm^3	4.2 to 5.2 × 10^{12}/L
Children (varies with age)		4.5 to 5.1 million/mm^3	4.5 to 5.1 × 10^{12}/L
Leukocytes, total		4500 to 11,000/mm^3	4.5 to 11.0 × 10^9/L
Leukocytes, differential	*Percentage*	***Absolute***	***Absolute***
Myelocytes	0	0/mm^3	0/L
Band neutrophils	3 to 5	150 to 400/mm^3	150 to 400 × 10^6/L
Segmented neutrophils	54 to 62	3000 to 5800/mm^3	3000 to 5800 × 10^6/L
Lymphocytes	25 to 33	1500 to 3000/mm^3	1500 to 3000 × 10^6/L
Monocytes	3 to 7	300 to 500/mm^3	300 to 500 × 10^6/L
Eosinophils	1 to 3	50 to 250/mm^3	50 to 250 × 10^6/L
Basophils	0 to 1	15 to 50/mm^3	15 to 50 × 10^6/L
Platelets		150,000 to 400,000/mm^3	150 to 400 × 10^9/L
Reticulocytes		25,000 to 75,000/mm^3 (0.5% to 1.5% of erythrocytes)	25 to 75 × 10^9/L
Coagulation tests			
Bleeding time (template)		2.75 to 8.0 min	2.75 to 8.0 min
Coagulation time (glass tubes)		5 to 15 min	5 to 15 min
D-Dimer		<0.5 μg/ml	<0.5 mg/L
Factor VIII and other coagulation factors		50% to 150% of normal	0.5 to 1.5 of normal
Fibrin split products (Thrombo-Welco test)		<10 μg/ml	<10 mg/L
Fibrinogen		200 to 400 mg/dl	2.0 to 4.0 g/L
Partial thromboplastin time (PTT)		20 to 35 sec	20 to 35 sec
Prothrombin time (PT)		12.0 to 14.0 sec	12.0 to 14.0 sec
Coombs' test			
Direct		Negative	Negative
Indirect		Negative	Negative
Corpuscular values of erythrocytes			
Mean corpuscular hemoglobin (MCH)		26 to 34 pg/cell	26 to 34 pg/cell
Mean corpuscular volume (MCV)		80 to 96 μm^3	80 to 96 fL
Mean corpuscular hemoglobin concentration (MCHC)		32 to 36 g/dl	320 to 360 g/L
Haptoglobin		20 to 165 mg/dl	0.20 to 1.65 g/L
Hematocrit			
Males		40 to 54 ml/dl	0.40 to 0.54 volume fraction
Females		37 to 47 ml/dl	0.37 to 0.47 volume fraction
Newborns		49 to 54 ml/dl	0.49 to 0.54 volume fraction
Children (varies with age)		35 to 49 ml/dl	0.35 to 0.49 volume fraction
Hemoglobin			
Males		13.0 to 18.0 g/dl	8.1 to 11.2 mmol/L
Females		12.0 to 16.0 g/dl	7.4 to 9.9 mmol/L
Newborns		16.5 to 19.5 g/dl	10.2 to 12.1 mmol/L
Children (varies with age)		11.2 to 16.5 g/dl	7.0 to 10.2 mmol/L
Hemoglobin, fetal		<1.0% of total	<0.01 of total
Hemoglobin A_{1C}		3% to 5% of total	0.03 to 0.05 of total
Hemoglobin A_2		1.5% to 3.0% of total	0.015 to 0.03 of total
Hemoglobin, plasma		0 to 5.0 mg/dl	0 to 3.2 μmol/L
Methemoglobin		30 to 130 mg/dl	19 to 80 μmol/L
Sedimentation rate (ESR)			
Wintrobe			
Males		0 to 5 mm/hr	0 to 5 mm/hr
Females		0 to 15 mm/hr	0 to 15 mm/hr
Westergren			
Males		0 to 15 mm/hr	0 to 15 mm/hr
Females		0 to 20 mm/hr	0 to 20 mm/hr

*For some procedures, reference values may vary, depending on the method used.

Modified from Conn, R. B., Borer, W. Z., & Snyder, J. W. (1997). *Current diagnosis* (9th ed., pp. 1235–1241). Philadelphia: W. B. Saunders; and data from Malarkey, L. M., & McMorrow, M. E. (2000). *Nurses' manual of laboratory tests and diagnostic procedures* (2nd ed.). Philadelphia: W. B. Saunders.

REFERENCE VALUES FOR BLOOD, PLASMA, AND SERUM*

Test	Conventional Units	SI Units
Acetoacetate plus acetone		
Qualitative	Negative	Negative
Quantitative	0.3 to 2.0 mg/dl	3 to 20 mg/L
Acid phosphatase, serum (thymolphthalein monophosphate substrate)	0.11 to 0.60 U/L	0.11 to 0.60 U/L
Adrenocorticotropin, plasma (ACTH)		
8:00 AM	10 to 80 pg/ml	2–18 pmol/L
Alanine aminotransferase, serum (ALT, SGPT)	1 to 45 U/L	1 to 45 U/L
Albumin, serum	3.3 to 5.2 g/dl	33 to 52 g/L
Aldolase, serum	0.0 to 7.0 U/L	0.0 to 7.0 U/L
Aldosterone, plasma		
Standing	5 to 30 ng/dl	140 to 830 pmol/L
Recumbent	3 to 10 ng/dl	80 to 275 pmol/L
Alkaline phosphatase, serum (ALP)		
Adult	35 to 150 U/L	35 to 150 U/L
Adolescent	100 to 500 U/L	100 to 500 U/L
Child	100 to 350 U/L	100 to 350 U/L
Ammonia nitrogen, plasma	10 to 50 μmol/L	10 to 50 μmol/L
Amylase, serum	25 to 125 U/L	25 to 125 U/L
Anion gap, serum, calculated	8 to 16 mEq/L	8 to 16 mmol/L
Ascorbic acid, blood	0.4 to 1.5 mg/dl	23 to 85 μmol/L
Aspartate aminotransferase, serum (AST, SGOT)	1 to 36 U/L	1 to 36 U/L
Base excess, arterial blood, calculated	0 ± 2 mEq/L	0 ± 2 mmol/L
Bicarbonate		
Venous plasma	23 to 29 mEq/L	23 to 29 mmol/L
Arterial blood	21 to 27 mEq/L	21 to 27 mmol/L
Bile acids, serum	0.3 to 3.0 mg/dl	0.8 to 7.6 μmol/L
Bilirubin, serum		
Conjugated	0.1 to 0.4 mg/dl	1.7 to 6.8 μmol/L
Total	0.3 to 1.1 mg/dl	5.1 to 19 μmol/L
Calcium, serum	8.4 to 10.6 mg/dl	2.10 to 2.65 mmol/L
Calcium, ionized, serum	4.25 to 5.25 mg/dl	1.05 to 1.30 mmol/L
Carbon dioxide, total, serum or plasma	24 to 31 mEq/L	24 to 31 mmol/L
Carbon dioxide tension, blood (PCO_2)	35 to 45 mm Hg	35 to 45 mm Hg
β-Carotene serum	60 to 260 μg/dl	1.1 to 8.6 μmol/L
Catecholamines, plasma		
Epinephrine (supine)	<50 pg/ml	<273 pmol/L
Norepinephrine (supine)	110 to 410 pg/ml	650 to 2,423 pmol/L
Ceruloplasmin, serum	23 to 44 mg/dl	230 to 440 mg/L
Chloride, serum or plasma	96 to 106 mEq/L	96 to 106 mmol/L
Cholesterol, serum or EDTA plasma		
Desirable range	<200 mg/dl	<5.20 mmol/L
LDL Cholesterol	60 to 180 mg/dl	1.55 to 4.65 mmol/L
HDL Cholesterol	30 to 80 mg/dl	0.80 to 2.05 mmol/L
Copper	70 to 140 μg/dl	11 to 22 μmol/L
Cortisol, plasma		
8:00 AM	6 to 23 μg/dl	170 to 630 nmol/L
4:00 PM	3 to 15 μg/dl	80 to 410 nmol/L
10:00 PM	<50% of 8 AM value	<0.5 of 8 AM value
Creatine, serum		
Males	0.2 to 0.5 mg/dl	15 to 40 μmol/L
Females	0.3 to 0.9 mg/dl	25 to 70 μmol/L

Table continued on following page

REFERENCE VALUES FOR BLOOD, PLASMA, AND SERUM* *Continued*

Test	Conventional Units	SI Units
Creatine kinase, serum (CK, CPK)		
Males	55 to 170 U/L	55 to 170 U/L
Females	30 to 135 U/L	30 to 135 U/L
Creatine kinase MB isozyme, serum	<5% of total CK activity <5% ng/ml by immunoassay	<5% of total CK activity <5% ng/ml by immunoassay
Creatinine, serum	0.6 to 1.2 mg/dl	50 to 110 μmol/L
Ferritin, serum	20 to 200 ng/ml	20 to 200 μg/L
Fibrinogen, plasma	200 to 400 mg/dl	2.0 to 4.0 g/L
Folate		
Serum	3.0 to 18.0 ng/ml	6.8 to 41.0 nmol/L
Erythrocytes	145 to 540 ng/ml	330 to 1220 nmol/L
Follicle-stimulating hormone, plasma (FSH)		
Males	4 to 25 mU/ml	4 to 25 U/L
Females	4 to 30 mU/ml	4 to 30 U/L
Postmenopausal	40 to 250 mU/ml	40 to 250 U/L
γ-Glutamyltransferase, serum	5 to 40 U/L	5 to 40 U/L
Gastrin, (fasting) serum	0 to 110 pg/ml	0 to 110 ng/L
Glucose (fasting), plasma or serum	70 to 115 mg/dl	3.9 to 6.4 nmol/L
Growth hormone, plasma (HGH)	0 to 6 ng/ml	0 to 6 μg/L
Haptoglobin, serum	26 to 165 mg/dl	0.20 to 1.65 g/L
Immunoglobulins, serum		
IgG	640 to 1350 mg/dl	6.4 to 13.5 g/L
IgA	70 to 310 mg/dl	0.70 to 3.1 g/L
IgM	90 to 350 mg/dl	0.90 to 3.5 g/L
IgD	0.0 to 6.0 mg/dl	0.0 to 60 mg/L
IgE	0.0 to 430 ng/ml	0.0 to 430 μg/L
Insulin (fasting), plasma	5 to 25 μU/ml	36 to 179 pmol/L
Iron, serum	75 to 175 μg/dl	13 to 31 μmol/L
Iron-binding capacity, serum		
Total	250 to 410 μg/dl	45 to 73 μmol/L
Saturation	20% to 55%	0.20 to 0.55
Lactate		
Venous blood	5.0 to 20.0 mg/dl	0.6 to 2.2 mmol/L
Arterial blood	5.0 to 15.0 mg/dl	0.6 to 1.7 mmol/L
Lactate dehydrogenase, serum (LD, LDH)	110 to 220 U/L	110 to 220 U/L
Lipase, serum	10 to 140 U/L	10 to 140 U/L
Lipids, total, serum	400 to 800 mg/dl	4.0 to 8.0 g/L
Luteinizing hormone, serum (LH)		
Males	1 to 9 mU/ml	1 to 9 U/L
Females		
Follicular phase	2 to 10 U/L	2 to 10 U/L
Midcycle peak	15 to 65 U/L	15 to 65 U/L
Luteal phase	1 to 12 U/L	1 to 12 U/L
Postmenopausal	12 to 65 U/L	12 to 65 U/L
Magnesium, serum	1.3 to 2.1 mg/dl	0.65 to 1.05 mmol/L
Osmolality	275 to 295 mOsm/kg H_2O	275 to 295 mOsm/kg H_2O
Oxygen, blood, arterial, room air		
Saturation (SaO_2)	95% to 98%	95% to 98%
Partial pressure (PaO_2)	80 to 100 mm Hg	80 to 100 mm Hg
pH, arterial blood	7.35 to 7.45	7.35 to 7.45
Phenylalanine, serum (Guthrie test)	<2 mg/dl	121 μmol/L
Phosphate, inorganic, serum	3.0 to 4.5 mg/dl	1.0 to 1.5 mmol/L
Potassium, serum	3.5 to 5.0 mEq/L	3.5 to 5.0 mmol/L

REFERENCE VALUES FOR BLOOD, PLASMA, AND SERUM* *Continued*

Test	Conventional Units	SI Units
Prolactin, serum		
Males	1 to 15 ng/ml	1 to 15 μg/L
Females	1 to 20 ng/ml	1 to 20 μg/L
Protein, serum		
Total	6.0 to 8.0 g/dl	60 to 80 g/L
Albumin	3.5 to 5.5 g/dl	35 to 55 g/L
α_1-Globulin	0.2 to 0.4 g/dl	2 to 4 g/L
α_2-Globulin	0.5 to 0.9 g/dl	5 to 9 g/L
β-Globulin	0.6 to 1.1 g/dl	6 to 11 g/L
γ-Globulin	0.7 to 1.7 g/dl	7 to 17 g/L
Pyruvate, blood	0.3 to 0.9 mg/dl	0.03 to 0.10 mmol/L
Sodium, serum or plasma	135 to 145 mEq/L	135 to 145 mmol/L
Testosterone, plasma		
Males	300 to 1200 ng/dl	10.4 to 41.6 nmol/L
Females	20 to 75 ng/dl	0.7 to 2.6 nmol/L
Pregnant	40 to 200 ng/dl	1.4 to 6.9 nmol/L
Thyroglobulin	3 to 42 ng/ml	3 to 42 μg/L
Thyroid-stimulating hormone, serum (TSH)	0.4 to 4.8 μIU/ml	0.4 to 4.8 mIU/L
Thyroxine, free, serum (FT_4)	0.9 to 2.1 ng/dl	12 to 27 pmol/L
Thyroxine, serum (T_4)	4.5 to 12.0 μg/dl	58 to 154 nmol/L
Triglycerides, serum, after 12 hr fast	40 to 150 mg/dl	0.4 to 1.5 g/L
Triiodothyronine, serum (T_3)	70 to 190 ng/dl	1.1 to 2.9 nmol/L
Triiodothyronine uptake, resin (T_3RU)	25% to 38% uptake	0.25 to 0.38 uptake
Urate		
Males	2.5 to 8.0 mg/dl	150 to 480 μmol/L
Females	2.2 to 7.0 mg/dl	130 to 420 μmol/L
Urea, serum or plasma	24 to 49 mg/dl	4.0 to 8.2 nmol/L
Urea nitrogen, serum or plasma	11 to 23 mg/dl	8.0 to 16.4 nmol/L
Viscosity, serum	1.4 to 1.8 × water	1.4 to 1.8 × water
Vitamin A, serum	20 to 80 μg/dl	0.70 to 2.80 μmol/L
Vitamin B_{12}, serum	180 to 900 pg/ml	133 to 664 pmol/L

*For some procedures, reference values may vary, depending on the method used.

Modified from Conn, R. B., Borer, W. Z., & Snyder, J. W. (1997). *Current diagnosis* (9th ed., pp. 1235–1241). Philadelphia: W. B. Saunders; and data from Malarkey, L. M., & McMorrow, M. E. (2000). *Nurses' manual of laboratory tests and diagnostic procedures* (2nd ed.). Philadelphia: W. B. Saunders.

REFERENCE VALUES FOR URINE*

Test	Conventional Units	SI Units
Acetone and acetoacetate, qualitative	Negative	Negative
Albumin		
Qualitative	Negative	Negative
Quantitative	10 to 100 mg/24 hr	0.15 to 1.5 μmol/24 hr
Aldosterone	3 to 20 μg/24 hr	8.3 to 55 nmol/24 hr
δ-Aminolevulinic acid	1.3 to 7.0 mg/24 hr	10 to 53 μmol/24 hr
Amylase	<17 U/hr	<17 U/hr
Amylase/creatinine clearance ratio	0.01 to 0.04	0.01 to 0.04
Bilirubin, qualitative	Negative	Negative
Calcium (usual diet)	<250 mg/24 hr	<6.3 nmol/24 hr
Catecholamines		
Epinephrine	<10 μg/24 hr	<55 nmol/24 hr
Norepinephrine	<100 μg/24 hr	<590 nmol/24 hr
Total free catecholamines	4 to 126 μg/24 hr	24 to 745 nmol/24 hr
Total metanephrines	0.1 to 1.6 mg/24 hr	0.5 to 8.1 μmol/24 hr
Chloride (varies with intake)	110 to 250 mEq/24 hr	110 to 250 nmol/24 hr
Copper	0 to 50 μg/24 hr	0 to 0.80 μmol/24 hr
Cortisol, free	10 to 100 μg/24 hr	27.6 to 276 nmol/24 hr
Creatine		
Males	0 to 40 mg/24 hr	0.0 to 0.30 mmol/24 hr
Females	0 to 80 mg/24 hr	0.0 to 0.60 mmol/24 hr
Creatinine	15 to 25 mg/kg/24 hr	0.13–0.22 mmol/kg/24 hr
Creatinine clearance (corrected to 1.73 m^2 body surface area)		
Males	110 to 150 ml/min/1.73 m^2	110 to 150 ml/min/1.73 m^2
Females	105 to 132 ml/min/1.73 m^2	105 to 132 ml/min/1.73 m^2
Dehydroepiandrosterone		
Males	0.2 to 2.0 mg/24 hr	0.7 to 6.9 μmol/24 hr
Females	0.2 to 1.8 mg/24 hr	0.7 to 6.2 μmol/24 hr
Estrogens, total		
Males	4 to 25 μg/24 hr	14 to 90 nmol/24 hr
Females	5 to 100 μg/24 hr	18 to 360 nmol/24 hr
Glucose (as reducing substance)	<250 mg/24 hr	<250 mg/24 hr
Hemoglobin and myoglobin, qualitative	Negative	Negative
17-Hydroxycorticosteroids		
Males	3 to 9 mg/24 hr	8.3 to 25 μmol/24 hr
Females	2 to 8 mg/24 hr	5.5 to 22 μmol/24 hr
5-Hydroxyindoleacetic acid		
Qualitative	Negative	Negative
Quantitative	2 to 6 mg/24 hr	10 to 31 μmol/24 hr
17-Ketosteroids		
Males	8 to 22 mg/24 hr	28 to 76 μmol/24 hr
Females	6 to 15 mg/24 hr	21 to 52 μmol/24 hr
Magnesium	6.0 to 10 mEq/24 hr	3.0 to 5.0 mmol/24 hr
Metanephrines (see Catecholamines)		
Osmolality	38 to 1,400 mOsm/kg H_2O	38 to 1,400 mOsm/kg H_2O
pH	4.6 to 8.0	4.6 to 8.0
Phenylpyruvic acid, qualitative	Negative	Negative
Phosphate	0.4 to 1.3 g/24 hr	13 to 42 mmol/24 hr
Porphobilinogen		
Qualitative	Negative	Negative
Quantitative	<2.0 mg/24 hr	<9 μmol/24 hr

REFERENCE VALUES FOR URINE* *Continued*

Test	Conventional Units	SI Units
Porphyrins		
Coproporphyrin	50 to 250 μg/24 hr	77 to 380 nmol/24 hr
Uroporphyrin	10 to 30 μg/24 hr	12 to 36 nmol/24 hr
Potassium	25 to 125 mEq/24 hr	25 to 125 mmol/24 hr
Pregnanediol		
Males	0.0 to 1.9 mg/24 hr	0.0 to 6.0 μmol/24 hr
Females		
Proliferative phase	0.0 to 2.6 mg/24 hr	0.0 to 8.0 μmol/24 hr
Luteal phase	2.6 to 10.6 mg/24 hr	8 to 33 μmol/24 hr
Postmenopausal	0.2 to 1.0 mg/24 hr	0.6 to 3.1 μmol/24 hr
Pregnanetriol	<2.5 mg/24 hr	<7.4 μmol/24 hr
Protein		
Qualitative	Negative	Negative
Quantitative	10 to 150 mg/24 hr	10 to 150 mg/24 hr
Protein-creatinine ratio	<0.2	<0.2
Sodium (usual diet)	60 to 260 mEq/24 hr	60 to 260 mmol/24 hr
Specific gravity, random	1.003 to 1.030	1.003 to 1.030
Urate (usual diet)	250 to 750 mg/24 hr	1.5 to 4.4 mmol/24 hr
Urobilinogen	0.5 to 4.0 mg/24 hr	0.6 to 6.8 μmol/24 hr
Vanillylmandelic acid (VMA) (4-hydroxy-3-methoxy-mandelic acid)	1 to 8 mg/24 hr	5 to 40 μmol/24 hr

*For some procedures, reference values may vary, depending on the method used.

Modified from Conn, R. B., Borer, W. Z., & Snyder, J. W. (1997). *Current diagnosis* (9th ed., pp. 1235–1241). Philadelphia: W. B. Saunders; and data from Malarkey, L. M., & McMorrow, M. E. (2000). *Nurses' manual of laboratory tests and diagnostic procedures* (2nd ed.). Philadelphia: W. B. Saunders.

REFERENCE VALUES FOR THERAPEUTIC DRUG MONITORING (Serum)

	Therapeutic Range	Toxic Levels	Proprietary Names
Antibiotics			
Amikacin	25 to 30 μg/ml	Peak > 35 μg/ml Trough > 10 μg/ml	Amikin
Chloramphenicol	10 to 20 μg/ml	>25 μg/ml	Chloromycetin
Gentamicin	5 to 10 μg/ml	Peak > 12 μg/ml Trough > 2 μg/ml	Garamycin
Tobramycin	5 to 10 μg/ml	Peak > 10 μg/ml Trough > 2 μg/ml	Nebcin
Vancomycin	5 to 10 μg/ml	Peak > 40 μg/ml Trough > 10 μg/ml	Vancocin
Anticonvulsants			
Carbamazepine	5 to 12 μg/ml	>15 μg/ml	Tegretol
Ethosuximide	40 to 100 μg/ml	>150 μg/ml	Zarontin
Phenobarbital	15 to 40 μg/ml	Vary widely because of developed tolerance	Luminal
Phenytoin	10 to 20 μg/ml	>20 μg/ml	Dilantin
Primidone	5 to 12 μg/ml	>15 μg/ml	Mysoline
Valproic acid	50 to 100 μg/ml	>100 μg/ml	Depakene
Analgesics			
Acetaminophen	10 to 20 μg/ml	>250 μg/ml	Tylenol Datril
Salicylate	100 to 250 μg/ml	>300 μg/ml	Aspirin Bufferin

Table continued on following page

REFERENCE VALUES FOR THERAPEUTIC DRUG MONITORING (Serum) *Continued*

	Therapeutic Range	Toxic Levels	Proprietary Names
Bronchodilator			
Theophylline (aminophylline)	10 to 20 μg/ml	>20 μg/ml	Theo-Dur
Cardiovascular Drugs			
Amiodarone (specimen must be obtained more than 8 hr after last dose	1 to 2 μg/ml	>2 μg/ml	Cordarone
Digitoxin (specimen must be obtained 12 to 24 hr after last dose)	15 to 25 ng/ml	>35 ng/ml	Crystodigin
Digoxin (specimen must be obtained more than 6 hr after last dose)	0.8 to 2.0 ng/ml	>2.4 ng/ml	Lanoxin
Disopyramide	2 to 5 μg/ml	>7 μg/ml	Norpace
Flecainide	0.2 to 1.0 ng/ml	>1 ng/ml	Tambocor
Lidocaine	1.5 to 5.0 μg/ml	>6 to 8 μg/ml	Xylocaine
Mexiletine	0.7 to 2.0 ng/ml	>2 ng/ml	Mexitil
Procainamide	4 to 10 μg/ml	>12 μg/ml	Pronestyl
(measured as procainamide + *N*-acetyl procainamide)	8 to 30 μg/ml	>30 μg/ml	
Propranolol	50 to 100 ng/ml	Variable	Inderal
Quinidine	2 to 5 μg/ml	>6 μg/ml	Cardioquin Quinaglute Quinidex
Tocainide	4 to 10 ng/ml	>10 ng/ml	Tonocard
Psychopharmacologic Drugs			
Amitriptyline (measured as amitriptyline + nortriptyline)	120 to 150 ng/ml	>500 ng/ml	Elavil Endep Limbitrol Triavil
Bupropion	25 to 100 ng/ml	Not applicable	Wellbutrin
Desipramine (measured as desipramine + imipramine)	150 to 300 ng/ml	>500 ng/ml	Norpramin Pertofrane
Imipramine (measured as imipramine + desipramine)	125 to 250 ng/ml	>400 ng/ml	Janimine Tofranil
Lithium (obtain specimen 12 hr after last dose)	0.6 to 1.5 mEq/L	>1.5 mEq/L	Lithobid
Nortriptyline	50 to 150 ng/ml	500 ng/ml	Aventyl Pamelor

Modified from Conn, R. B., Borer, W. Z., & Snyder, J. W. (1997). *Current diagnosis* (9th ed., pp. 1235–1241). Philadelphia: W. B. Saunders; and data from Malarkey, L. M., & McMorrow, M. E. (2000). *Nurses' manual of laboratory tests and diagnostic procedures* (2nd ed.). Philadelphia: W. B. Saunders.

REFERENCE VALUES IN TOXICOLOGY

	Conventional Units	SI Units
Arsenic, blood	3.5 to 7.2 μg/dl	0.47 to 0.96 μmol/L
Arsenic, urine	<130 μg/24 hr	<1.7 μmol/24 hr
Bromides, serum, inorganic	<100 mg/dl Toxic above 140 to 1000 mg/dl	14 to 100 mmol/L Toxic above 14 to 100 mmol/L
Carboxyhemoglobin, blood Symptoms occur	<5% saturation >15% saturation	<0.05 saturation >0.15 saturation
Ethanol, blood	<0.05 mg/dl <0.005%	<1.0 mmol/L
Marked intoxication	300 to 400 mg/dl 0.3% to 0.4%	65 to 87 mmol/L
Alcoholic stupor	400 to 500 mg/dl 0.4% to 0.5%	87 to 109 mmol/L
Coma	>500 mg/dl >0.5%	>109 mmol/L
Lead, blood	<25 μg/dl	1.2 μmol/L
Lead, urine	<80 μg/24 hr	<0.4 μmol/24 hr
Mercury, urine	<30 μg/24 hr	<150 nmol/24 hr

Modified from Conn, R. B., Borer, W. Z., & Snyder, J. W. (1997). *Current diagnosis* (9th ed., pp. 1235–1241). Philadelphia: W. B. Saunders; and data from Malarkey, L. M., & McMorrow, M. E. (2000). *Nurses' manual of laboratory tests and diagnostic procedures* (2nd ed.). Philadelphia: W. B. Saunders.

REFERENCE VALUES FOR CEREBROSPINAL FLUID

	Conventional Units	SI Units
Cells	<5/mm³ All mononuclear	<5 × 10^6/L All mononuclear
Electrophoresis	Predominantly albumin	Predominantly albumin
Glucose	50 to 75 mg/dl (20 mg/dl less than serum)	2.8 to 4.2 mmol/L (1.1 mmol/L less than serum)
IgG		
Children <14 yr	<8% of total protein	<0.08 of total protein
Adults	<14% of total protein	<0.14 of total protein
IgG index $\frac{\text{CSF/serum IgG ratio}}{\text{CSF/serum albumin ratio}}$	0.3 to 0.6	0.3 to 0.6
Oligoclonal banding on electrophoresis	Absent	Absent
Pressure, opening	70 to 180 mm H_2O	70 to 180 mm H_2O
Protein, total	15 to 45 mg/dl	150 to 450 mg/L

Modified from Conn, R. B., Borer, W. Z., & Snyder, J. W. (1997). *Current diagnosis* (9th ed., pp. 1235–1241). Philadelphia: W. B. Saunders; and data from Malarkey, L. M., & McMorrow, M. E. (2000). *Nurses' manual of laboratory tests and diagnostic procedures* (2nd ed.). Philadelphia: W. B. Saunders.

REFERENCE VALUES FOR SEMEN ANALYSIS

	Conventional Units	SI Units
Volume	2 to 5 ml	2 to 5 ml
Liquefaction	Complete in 15 min	Complete in 15 min
Leukocytes	Occasional or absent	Occasional or absent
Count	60 to 150 million/ml	60 to 150 × 10^6/ml
Motility	>80% motile	>0.80 motile
Morphology	80% to 90% normal forms	0.80 to 0.90 normal forms
Fructose	>150 mg/dl	>8.33 mmol/L

Modified from Conn, R. B., Borer, W. Z., & Snyder, J. W. (1997). *Current diagnosis* (9th ed., pp. 1235–1241). Philadelphia: W. B. Saunders; and data from Malarkey, L. M., & McMorrow, M. E. (2000). *Nurses' manual of laboratory tests and diagnostic procedures* (2nd ed.). Philadelphia: W. B. Saunders.

REFERENCE VALUES FOR TESTS OF GASTROINTESTINAL FUNCTION

Test Name	Conventional Units
Bentiromide	6-hr urinary arylamine excretion > 57% excludes pancreatic insufficiency
β-Carotene, serum	60–250 ng/dl
Fecal fat estimation	
Qualitative	No fat globules seen by high-power microscope
Quantitative	<6 g/24 hr (>95% coefficient of fat absorption)
Gastric acid output	
Basal	
Males	0.0–10.5 mmol/hr
Females	0.0–5.6 mmol/hr
Gastric acid output *(continued)*	
Maximum (after histamine or pentagastrin)	
Males	9.0–48.0 mmol/hr
Females	6.0–31.0 mmol/hr
Ratio: basal/maximum	
Males	0.0–0.31
Females	0.0–0.29
Secretin test, pancreatic fluid	
Volume	>1.8 ml/kg/hr
Bicarbonate	>80 mEq/L
D-Xylose absorption test, urine	>20% of ingested dose excreted in 5 hr

Modified from Conn, R. B., Borer, W. Z., & Snyder, J. W. (1997). *Current diagnosis* (9th ed., pp. 1235–1241). Philadelphia: W. B. Saunders.

Index

Note: Page numbers in *italics* indicate illustrations; those followed by t indicate tables; and those followed by b indicate boxed material.

A

B

C

G

I

J

K

M

N

V

W

X

Y

Z

STANDARD AND TRANSMISSION-BASED PRECAUTIONS

STANDARD PRECAUTIONS FOR THE CARE OF ALL PATIENTS	
Hand-washing	Wash your hands immediately after removing gloves, between client contacts, and after contact with blood, body fluids, secretions, excretions, and contaminated equipment or articles.
Gloves	Wear gloves when touching mucous membranes or nonintact skin, and when touching blood, body fluids, secretions, excretions, and contaminated items.
Mask, eye protection, face shield	Wear a mask, an eye protector, or a face shield during procedures that are likely to generate splashes or sprays of blood, body fluids, secretions, and excretions.
Gown	Wear a gown during procedures that are likely to generate splashes or sprays of blood, body fluids, secretions, and excretions.
Client care equipment	Handle soiled client care equipment in a manner that prevents skin and mucous membrane exposure, contamination of clothing, and transfer of microorganisms to other clients and environments. Reusable equipment must be cleaned and reprocessed appropriately.
Environmental control	Ensure adequate procedures for the routine care, cleaning, and disinfection of client furniture, equipment, and environmental surfaces.
Linen	Handle soiled linen in a manner that prevents skin and mucous membrane exposure, contamination of clothing, and transfer of microorganisms to other clients and environments.
Sharps	Do not recap used needles. Do not bend, break, or manipulate used needles by hand. Place used needles, scalpels, and other sharps in puncture-resistant, labeled sharps containers.
Client resuscitation	Use a mouthpiece, resuscitation bag, or other ventilation device to avoid mouth-to-mouth resuscitation.
Client placement	Use a private room for a client who contaminates the environment or cannot assist in maintaining appropriate hygiene.
ADDITIONAL TRANSMISSION-BASED PRECAUTIONS	
Contact precautions[3]	1. Place client in a private room or with another client who is infected with the same organism. The client should remain in the room unless it is essential to leave. 2. Wear gloves when entering the room, and change them after contact with infective material such as feces or wound drainage. 3. Wash your hands with an antimicrobial agent immediately after removing gloves while still in the client's room. 4. Wear a gown if you anticipate contact with infected material. 5. Do not share client care equipment if possible. If you must share equipment, clean and disinfect it between client contacts. 6. Take additional precautions to prevent the spread of vancomycin-resistant organisms.[2]
Droplet precautions[3]	1. Place client in a private room or with another client who is infected with the same organism. The door to the room may remain open. The client should remain in the room unless it is essential to leave. 2. Wear a mask when working within 3 feet of the client. Have the client wear a mask during transport outside the room.
Airborne precautions[3]	1. Place client in a negative-pressure isolation room with at least six air exchanges per hour. Air from the room must be discharged to the outdoors or through a high-efficiency filter before the air is circulated to the other areas in the hospital. The room door must remain closed. 2. Wear a mask when entering the room. Have the client wear a mask during transport outside the room. All persons entering the room should wear a mask. 3. Follow additional CDC guidelines for preventing the transmission of tuberculosis.[1]

Data from Centers for Disease Control and Prevention (CDC). (1994). Guidelines for preventing the transmission of *Mycobacterium tuberculosis* in health-care facilities. *Morbidity and Mortality Weekly Report, 43*(RR-13), 1–132[1]; Centers for Disease Control and Prevention (CDC). (1995). Recommendations for preventing the spread of vancomycin resistance: Recommendations of the Hospital Infection Control Practices Advisory Committee (HICPAC). *Morbidity and Mortality Weekly Report, 44*(RR-12), 1–13[2]; and Garner J. S., & Hospital Infection Control Practices Advisory Committee. (1996). Guidelines for isolation precautions in hospitals. *Infection Control and Hospital Epidemiology, 17,* 54–80.[3]